Endocrinology and Metabolism

NOTICE

Endocrinology and Metabolism

THIRD EDITION

EDITORS

Philip Felig, M.D.
Attending Physician
Senior Medical Staff
Lenox Hill Hospital
New York, New York

John D. Baxter, M.D.
Professor of Medicine
Chief, Division of Endocrinology
Parnassus and Mount Zion Campuses
Director, Metabolic Research Unit
University of California, San Francisco

Lawrence A. Frohman, M.D.
Edmund F. Foley Professor and Chairman
Department of Medicine
University of Illinois College of Medicine
Physician-in-Chief
University of Illinois Hospital
Chicago, Illinois

McGRAW-HILL, INC.
HEALTH PROFESSIONS DIVISION

New York St. Louis San Francisco Auckland Bogotá Caracas
Lisbon London Madrid Mexico City Milan Montreal New Delhi
San Juan Singapore Sydney Tokyo Toronto

Endocrinology and Metabolism

1234567890 KGPKGP 98765

ISBN 0-07-020448-9

This book was set in Century Schoolbook by
ATLIS Graphics & Design, Inc.
The editors were J. Dereck Jeffers and Mariapaz Ramos Englis;
the production supervisor was Clara Stanley;
text and cover designer was N.S.G. Design;
the index was prepared by Alexandra Nickerson.
Quebecor Printing/Kingsport was printer and binder.

The book is printed on acid-free paper.

Library of Congress Cataloging-in-Publication Data

Endocrinology and metabolism / editors, Philip Felig, John D. Baxter,
Lawrence A. Frohman. — 3d ed.
p. cm.
Includes bibliographical references and index.
ISBN 0-07-020448-9 :
1. Endocrinology. 2. Endocrine glands—Diseases. 3. Metabolism—Disorders. I. Felig, Philip, date. II. Baxter, J. D. (John D.), date. III. Frohman, Lawrence A.
[DNLM: 1. Endocrine Diseases—metabolism. WK 100 E536 1995]
RC648.E464 1995
616.4—dc20
DNLM/DLC
for Library of Congress

To our wives, children,
and
grandchildren

Florence; Clifford, Minna, Noam, and Yair; David and Anna Marie; and Elliot
PF

Lee, Leslie, and Gillian
JDB

Barbara; Michael, Stella, and Evan; Marc, Susan, Alicia, Hannah, and Zoe; Erica, Mitchell, and Aaron; and Rena
LAF

Contents

Contributors xxxi
Preface xxxv

PART I GENERAL ENDOCRINOLOGY

1 **Introduction to the Endocrine System** **3**
John D. Baxter, Lawrence A. Frohman, and Philip Felig

Definitions and Scope of Endocrinology 3
Types of Hormones and Their Synthesis and Release 5
Circulation of Hormones 6
Hormone Metabolism 7
Regulation of Hormone Levels 7
Hormone Uptake and Internalization 8
Mechanisms of Hormone Action 8
Regulation of Hormone Responsiveness 9
Classification of Hormone Action 9
Evolution of the Endocrine System 9
Simple and Complex Regulation 9
Origin of Hormones and Other Regulatory Ligands 10
Origin of Receptors and Other Mediators of Regulatory Ligand Actions 11
Diversification of Families of Hormones 11
Evolution of the Endocrine Glands 11
Integration of the Endocrine System 12
Integrated Action of a Given Class of Hormone 12
Hormone Synergisms: Recruitment of Multiple Hormones for Coordinated Responses 12
Hormone Antagonisms: Fine Tuning of Metabolism 13
Mechanisms for Attenuating or Terminating the Response 13
Actions of Hormones 13
Intermediary Metabolism and Growth 13
Highly Specific Functions 13
Disorders of the Endocrine System 14
Hormone Deficiency Syndromes 14
Hormone Excess Syndromes 16
Multiple Endocrine Syndromes 17
Abnormalities of Endocrine Glands Not Associated with Hormonal Imbalance 18
Clinical Assessment of Endocrine Status 18
History and Physical Examination 18
Laboratory Testing 18
Treatment of Endocrine Diseases 20
Hormone Agonist and Antagonist Therapy 20
References 21

2 **The Clinical Manifestations of Endocrine Disease** 23
Lawrence A. Frohman, Philip Felig, and John D. Baxter
Generalized Symptoms 23
Weakness and Fatigue 24
Weight Loss 24
Weight Gain 24
Body Temperature 25
Skin 25
Nose, Voice, and Tongue 26
Gastrointestinal System 26
Hemopoietic System 27
Cardiovascular System 28
Urinary Tract 28
Sexual Function 29
Bones and Joints 30
Central Nervous System 31
Neuromuscular Abnormalities 31
Ophthalmic Abnormalities 32

3 **Gene Expression and Recombinant DNA in Endocrinology and Metabolism** 35
David G. Gardner and Barry J. Gertz
Genes and Their Expression 35
DNA Structure and Replication 35
Chromatin 37
RNA Structure and Function 38
Gene Expression 39
Regulation of Gene Expression 42
Gene Evolution 44
Mechanisms of Genetic Disease 44
Recombinant DNA Technology 45
Hybridization 46
DNA Sequencing 47
Sources of DNA for Molecular Cloning 48
Polymerase Chain Reaction 51
Transfer of Cloned Genes into Mammalian Cells 52
Transgenic Animals 53
Production of Medically Important Proteins by Recombinant DNA Techniques 55
Products of Recombinant DNA Technology 56
New Drug Delivery Systems 57
Use of DNA in the Diagnosis of Genetic Disease 57
Potential for Human Gene Therapy 58
Impact for Molecular Biology on Medicine 60
References 61

4 **Biosynthesis, Secretion, and Metabolism of Hormones** 69
Gordon N. Gill
Peptide Hormones 69
Biosynthesis of Messenger RNA 69
Biosynthesis of Peptide Hormones 72
Secretion, Transport, and Metabolism of Peptide Hormones 77

Steroid Hormones 78
Cholesterol Substrate for Steroid Hormone Formation 79
The Rate-Controlling Step in Steroid Hormone Synthesis 80
Pathway of Steroid Hormone Biosynthesis 81
Tropic Regulation of Steroid Hormone Synthesis 84
Transport and Metabolism of Steroid Hormones 85
Thyroid Hormone 86
Iodine Metabolism 86
Anatomy of a Distinctive Biosynthetic Pathway 87
Transport and Metabolism 88
References 89

5A Molecular Mechanisms of Hormone Action: Control of Target Cell Function by Peptide and Catecholamine Hormones 91
Kevin J. Catt

General Aspects of Hormone Action 91
Classes of Hormone Action and Domains of Hormonal Control 91
Local Hormonal Regulation: Paracrine and Autocrine Secretion 93
Peptide Hormone Receptors 94
Binding Properties of Peptide Hormone Receptors 95
The Nature of Hormone-Receptor Interactions 96
Hormonal Activation of Receptors 97
Receptor Occupancy and Activation of Target Cell Responses 97
Chemical and Physical Properties of Peptide Hormone Receptors 98
Receptor Structure and Function 99
Ligand-Gated Ion Channels 99
G Protein–Coupled Receptors 102
Growth Factor Receptors 108
Transmembrane Signal Transduction Mechanisms 111
G Proteins and Signal Transduction 111
The GTP-Binding Protein Superfamily 116
Receptor Phosphorylation and Hormone Action 119
Intrinsic Receptor Signaling Domains 120
Protein Tyrosine Phosphatases 121
Hormone Receptors and Target Cell Desensitization 122
Synthesis and Regulation of Peptide Hormone Receptors 124
Biosynthesis and Expression of Plasma Membrane Receptors 124
Receptor Regulation in Endocrine Target Cells 125
Effects of Receptor Regulation on Cell Responses 127
Fate of the Hormone-Receptor Complex 127
Intracellular Mediators of Peptide Hormone Action 130
The Second Messenger Hypothesis 130
Guanylate Cyclase, Cyclic GMP, and cGMP-Dependent Protein Kinase 137
Nitric Oxide: A New Signaling Molecule 138
Calcium and Calcium-Dependent Enzyme Systems 139
Hormone Action and Phospholipid Metabolism 147
Signal Transduction to the Nucleus 157
Cytokine Receptor Signaling 158
Hormonal Regulation of Early Response Genes 159
References 161

5B Molecular Mechanisms of Hormone Action: Regulation of Target Cell Function by the Steroid Hormone Receptor Supergene Family 169
Jan Carlstedt-Duke, Anthony Wright, Martin Göttlicher, Sam Okret, and Jan-Åke Gustafsson

Mechanisms of Action of Steroid Hormones 169
Plasma Binding Steroid Hormones 173
Structures of Steroid Hormone Receptors 173
Steroid Binding 173
Chaperone Proteins 174
Dimerization 175
Phosphorylation 176
Intracellular Localization 176
Steroid Hormone Antagonists 177
Activation by Nonsteroidal Entities 178
Regulation of Steroid Receptor Levels and Responsiveness 178
Mechanism of Gene Regulation by Nuclear Receptors 178
DNA Binding by Nuclear Receptors 178
Mechanism of Transcriptional Transactivation by Nuclear Receptors 180
Synergistic Transactivation by Nuclear Receptors 181
Negative Regulation by Nuclear Receptor Proteins 181
Genetic Defects in Receptor Function 182
Steroid Receptors and Oncogenesis 182
Orphan Receptors: Novel Members of the Steroid Receptor Gene Superfamily 183
Common Characteristics of Orphan Receptors 183
Properties of Specific Orphan Receptors 185
Physiologic Roles of Orphan Receptors 186
Thyroid Hormone Receptors 187
Thyroid Hormones and Their Mechanism of Action 187
Structure of TRs 187
TRs as Dominant Repressors 188
Possible Functional Significance of Multiple TR Forms and Subtypes 188
Heterodimers with TRs and Other Proteins 188
Familial Thyroid Hormone Resistance and TRs 188
Receptors for Retinoic Acid and Its Analogues 189
Biology of Retinoids 189
Retinoic Acid Receptors and Their Possible Functional Significance 189
A Role for RXR in RAR and Other Nuclear Receptor Functions 190
References 191

6 Hormone Assays 201
A. Eugene Pekary and Jerome M. Hershman

Bioassays 201
In Vivo Assays 201
In Vitro Assays 202
Cytochemical Assays 202
Complementarity of in Vivo and in Vitro Assays 203
Nomenclature 203
Types of Immunoassays 203
Labeled Analyte and Reagent Limiting 203
Reagent Excess and Labeled Antibody 204
Free and Total Hormone Measurements 205
Immunoassay Reagents 206
Binding Proteins 206
Labels 208
Separation Systems 209
Liquid-Phase Precipitation 210
Solid-Phase Adsorption 210

Solid-Phase Precipitation *210*
Homogeneous Assay Systems 210
Fluorescence Polarization *210*
Amplitude-Modulated Enzyme Assays *210*
Receptor Assays 211
Chromatographic Assays 211
Chromatography *211*
Detection *211*
Immunoassay Optimization and Validation 212
General Considerations *212*
Detection Limits *212*
Specificity *212*
Interference 213
Sample Matrix Effects *213*
Heterophilic Antibodies *213*
Complement and Rheumatoid Factors *214*
Enzyme Contaminants *214*
Drug Interference *214*
Hemodynamic Effects *214*
Quality Control 214
Future Trends 215
References 215

PART II NEUROENDOCRINOLOGY AND THE PITUITARY

7 Neuroendocrinology **221**
Mark E. Molitch
General Concepts in Neuroendocrinology 221
Overview of the Brain-Hypothalamic-Pituitary-Target Organ Regulation 221
Neuron-Neuron Interactions *221*
Hypophysiotropic Hormones *223*
Feedback Loops *224*
Anatomic Aspect 226
Hypothalamus *226*
Median Eminence and Hypothalamic-Pituitary Portal System *227*
Pituitary *230*
Hypophysiotropic Hormones 231
Thyrotropin Releasing Hormone *232*
Gonadotropin Releasing Hormone *235*
Somatostatin *239*
Corticotropin Releasing Hormone *242*
Growth Hormone Releasing Hormone *245*
Prolactin Inhibiting Factor *247*
Prolactin Releasing Factor *248*
Neurotransmitters 248
Biosynthesis and Metabolism of Bioaminergic Neurotransmitters *248*
Anatomic Pathways of Bioaminergic Neurotransmitters *248*
Neuropharmacology of Bioaminergic Neurotransmitters *250*
Amino Acid Neurotransmitters *251*
Neuropeptides *251*
The Pineal Gland 254
Anatomy *254*
Pineal Hormones and Neurotransmitters *254*
Pineal and Biological Rhythms *256*
CNS Rhythms and Neuroendocrine Function 257
Neuroendocrine Disease 259

7 (Continued)

Disease of the Hypothalamus 259
Effects of Hypothalamic Disease on Pituitary Function 264
Effects of Hypothalamic Disease on Other Neurometabolic Functions 268
Neuroendocrine Alterations in Systemic Disease 271
Other CNS Disorders 274
References 275

---

8 Diseases of the Anterior Pituitary **289**
Lawrence A. Frohman
Pituitary Gland 289
Anatomy 289
Blood and Nerve Supply 289
Embryology 290
Cell Types 291
Anterior Pituitary Hormones 293
Corticotropin-Related Peptides 293
Glycoprotein Hormones 297
Somatomammotropic Hormones 303
Hypopituitarism 313
Etiology 313
Primary Hypopituitarism 313
Secondary Hypopituitarism 316
Clinical Features 317
Differential Diagnosis 319
Diagnostic Procedures 320
Treatment 324
Pituitary Tumors 327
Classification 327
Signs and Symptoms 328
Diagnostic Procedures 330
Differential Diagnosis 336
Therapy 339
Pituitary Tumors Associated with Hormone Hypersecretion 341
Growth Hormone-Secreting Pituitary Tumors: Acromegaly 341
Prolactin-Secreting Tumors: Amenorrhea-Galactorrhea Syndrome 349
ACTH-Secreting Tumors: Cushing's Disease 357
Glycoprotein-Secreting Tumors 363
Details of Hypothalamic-Pituitary Testing 363
ACTH 363
TSH 365
LH and FSH 366
Growth Hormone 366
Prolactin 368
References 369

---

9 Posterior Pituitary **385**
Gary L. Robertson
Posterior Pituitary Hormones 385
Anatomy 385
Chemistry 385
Biosynthesis and Release 386
Regulation of Secretion 387
Distribution and Clearance 395
Biological Action 396
Thirst 398
Maintenance of Salt and Water Balance 399

Pathology 402
Decreased Secretion 402
Pathophysiology 405
Diagnosis 409
Therapy 412
Pathologic Hyperfunction 415
Etiology and Pathophysiology 415
Diagnosis 419
Therapy 420
Tests Used in Diagnosis 421
Hypofunction 421
Hyperfunction 422
General Considerations 423
References 423

PART III THYROID DISEASE

10 The Thyroid: Physiology, Thyrotoxicosis, Hypothyroidism, and the Painful Thyroid 435
Robert D. Utiger
Anatomy and Physiology 435
Clinical Anatomy 435
Chemistry of Thyroid Hormones 436
Thyroid Hormone Biosynthesis 436
Therapy 339
Transport and Cellular Binding of Thyroid Hormones 441
Biochemical Actions of Thyroid Hormones 443
Regulation of Thyroid Hormone Production 445
Evaluation of Thyroid Function 450
Physiologic Variables Affecting Pituitary-Thyroid Function and Tests 455
Alterations in Serum Thyroid Hormone Binding 457
Nonthyroidal Illness 459
Effects of Specific Disorders on Thyroid Function 463
Effects of Various Drugs on Thyroid Function 464
Thyrotoxicosis 465
Pathophysiology of Thyrotoxicosis 466
Causes of Thyrotoxicosis 467
Clinical Manifestations of Thyrotoxicosis 473
Laboratory Diagnosis of Thyrotoxicosis 477
Treatment of Thyrotoxicosis 479
Special Situations 485
Extrathyroidal Manifestations of Graves' Disease 488
Hypothyroidism 492
Pathophysiology of Hypothyroidism 492
Causes of Hypothyroidism 492
Clinical Manifestations of Hypothyroidism 498
Laboratory Diagnosis of Hypothyroidism 503
Treatment of Hypothyroidism 504
Special Situations 506
The Painful Thyroid 507
Subacute Thyroiditis 508
Hemorrhage in a Thyroid Nodule 508
Radiation Thyroiditis 508
Suppurative Thyroiditis 508
References 509

11 The Thyroid: Nodules and Neoplasia **521**
Gerard N. Burrow

Goiter 521
Classification of Goiter and Thyroid Neoplasia 521
Historical Overview 521
Etiology of Goiter 522
Endemic Goiter 524
Sporadic Goiter 526
Nontoxic Goiter 530
Solitary Thyroid Nodules 533
Factors Predisposing to Thyroid Cancer 533
Physical Characteristics 534
Laboratory Diagnosis 534
Management of a Solitary Thyroid Nodule 537
Thyroid Carcinoma 539
Classification 539
Incidence of Thyroid Carcinoma 539
The Effects of Radiation on the Development of Thyroid Carcinoma 540
Natural History of Thyroid Carcinoma 541
Evaluation of Thyroid Carcinoma 543
Therapy for Thyroid Carcinoma 543
Thyroid Lymphoma 545
Subsequent Follow-Up 545
Medullary Carcinoma of the Thyroid 546
References 549

PART IV ADRENAL DISEASE

12 The Adrenal Cortex **555**
Walter L. Miller and J. Blake Tyrrell

Embryology, Anatomy, and History 555
History 555
Embryology and Development 556
Anatomy 557
Steroid Hormone Biosynthesis 559
Chemistry of Steroid Hormones 559
Cholesterol: The Precursor of Steroid Hormones 560
3β-Hydroxysteroid Dehydrogenase/Δ^5-Δ^4 Isomerase 567
P450c17: 17α Hydroxylase/17,20-Lyase 568
P450c21:21-Hydroxylase 569
P450c11: 11β Hydroxylase/18-Hydroxylase/18-Oxidase 570
17-Ketosteroid Reductase/17β-Hydroxysteroid Oxidoreductase 571
Other Steroidogenic Enzymes 571
Steroid Synthesis in the Fetal Adrenal 573
Regulation of Adrenal Steroidogenesis 573
Regulation of Glucocorticoids 573
Regulation of Mineralocorticoids 580
Regulation of Adrenal Androgens 583
Plasma Steroids and Their Disposal 584
Quantities of Steroids Produced 584
Inhibitors of Adrenal Steroid Biosynthesis 585
Physical State of Steroids in Plasma 586
Metabolism of Adrenocortical Steroids 590
Variations in Steroid Metabolism 592
Molecular Mechanisms and Physiologic Actions 593
Definition of a Glucocorticoid 593

Molecular Mechanisms of Glucocorticoid Hormone Action 593
Glucocorticoid Agonists and Antagonists 595
Structure-Activity Relations of Glucocorticoids: Basis for Biological Activity 595
Actions of Glucocorticoids 596
Definition of a Mineralocorticoid 610
Molecular Mechanisms of Mineralocorticoid Action 610
Mineralocorticoid Agonists and Antagonists 611
Physiologic Actions of Mineralocorticoids 612
Actions of Adrenal Androgens and Estrogens 614
Laboratory Evaluation of Adrenocortical Function 614
Plasma Cortisol and Related Steroids 614
Urinary Corticosteroids 617
Cortisol Production Rate 618
Dexamethasone Suppression Tests 618
Tests of Pituitary-Adrenal Reserve 620
Metyrapone Testing 622
CRH Testing 622
Insulin-Induced Hypoglycemia 623
Mineralocorticoids 623
Plasma Androgens 623
Urinary Androgens 624
Clinical Utility 624
Adrenocortical Function in Children 624
Disorders of Steroid Hormone Synthesis 626
Introduction 626
21-Hydroxylase Deficiency 627
3β-Hydroxysteroid Dehydrogenase Deficiency 638
P450c17 (17α-Hydroxylase/17, 20-Lyase) Deficiency 639
P450c11 Deficiency 640
Congenital Lipoid Adrenal Hyperplasia 641
Adrenocortical Insufficiency 642
Primary Adrenocortical Insufficiency (Addison's Disease) 642
Secondary Adrenocortical Insufficiency 651
Diagnosis 652
Treatment 654
Prognosis and Survival 657
Hypoaldosteronism 657
Adrenocortical Hyperfunction 659
Cushing's Syndrome 659
Adrenal Tumors 665
Problems in Diagnosis 668
Hyperaldosteronism 678
References 680

13 Diseases of the Sympathochromaffin System 713
Philip E. Cryer

Sympathochromaffin Physiology 714
Biochemistry of the Catecholamines 714
Physiology of Adrenergic Axon Terminals and Chromaffin Cells 715
Biological Effects of the Catecholamines 720
Integrated Physiology of the Sympathochromaffin System 722
The Biological Roles of Epinephrine and Norepinephrine:Hormones and Neurotransmitters 724
Sympathochromaffin Pathophysiology 726
Pheochromocytoma 726
Generalized Autonomic Failure 732
Hypoglycemia 736

13 (Continued)

The Sympathochromaffin System in Other Endocrine-Metabolic Disorders 738
Other Endocrine Disorders 740
Diagnostic Testing 740
Measurement of Catecholamines and Their Metabolites 740
Indirect Tests of Autonomic Function 743
References 743

---

14 The Endocrinology of Hypertension 749
John D. Baxter, Dorothee Perloff, Willa Hsueh, Edward G. Biglieri

General Features of Hypertension 749
Epidemiology 749
Genetic and Environmental Influences 752
Regulation of Blood Pressure 753
Complications of Hypertension 753
Hormonal Modifiers of Blood Pressure 754
The Renin-Angiotension System 754
Mineralocorticoids 767
Glucocorticoids 770
Corticotropin (ACTH) 771
Estrogens, Progestins, and Androgens 772
Thyroid Hormone 772
Vasopressin 772
Erythropoietin 772
Growth Hormone 773
Calcitonin Gene–Related Peptide 773
Calcium-Regulating Hormones 773
Endothelin 774
Nitric Oxide (Endothelium-Derived Releasing Factor) 774
Endothelium-Derived Hyperpolarizing Factor (EDHF) 776
Atrial Natriuretic Peptides 776
Catecholamines and the Autonomic Nervous System 779
Prostaglandins and Other Eicosanoids 780
Kallikreins and Kirins 780
Ions, Hormones, and Blood Pressure 781
Evaluation of Hypertensive Patient 794
Clinical History 794
Laboratory Tests 795
Renovascular Hypertension 797
Pathology of Renovascular Hypertension 798
Natural History of Renal Artery Lesions 801
Initiating the Evaluation for Renovascular Hypertension 802
Specific Diagnostic Studies for Renovascular Hypertension 803
Therapy for Renovascular Hypertension 808
Primary Aldosteronism 812
Occurrence and Classification 817
Pathophysiology 821
History and Physical Findings 822
Hypertension 822
Diagnostic Procedures 822
Treatment 830

Other Low-Renin Hypertension Syndromes 832
Deoxycorticosterone-Excess Hypertension 832
Syndrome of Apparent Mineralocorticoid Excess 834
Spironolactone-Unresponsive Subgroup (Liddle's Syndrome) 834
Primary or Secondary Glucocorticoid Resistance 835
Cushing's Syndrome 835
References 835

15 Glucocorticoid Therapy 855
J. Blake Tyrrell
Physiologic and Pharmacologic Actions of Glucocorticoids in Relation to Steroid Therapy 855
Therapeutic Influences 855
Adverse Influences 857
Molecular Mechanisms for Glucocorticoid-Mediated Therapeutic Influences 858
Kinetic Considerations 859
Manifestations of Iatrogenic Cushing's Syndrome 859
Comparisons with Spontaneous Cushing's Syndrome 859
Ocular Changes 859
Avascular Necrosis of Bone 860
Osteoporosis 860
Infections 861
Myopathy 861
Atherosclerosis 862
Dose and Time Dependency and Reversibility 862
Diagnosis of Iatrogenic Cushing's Syndrome 862
Determinants of Glucocorticoid Potency 862
Bioavailability 862
Distribution 863
Metabolism and Clearance 863
Concentration at Sites of Action 864
Agonist Activity 865
Overall Estimation of Glucocorticoid Potency 865
Variations in Sensitivity to Glucocorticoids: Glucocorticoid Resistance 865
Glucocorticoid Preparations 866
Steroids with Glucocorticoid Activity Available for Therapy 866
Orally and Parenterally Active Preparations 866
Intraarticular Preparations 866
Topical Preparations 867
Inhaled Corticosteroids 868
ACTH 868
Some General Principles 868
Selection of Patients 868
Need for Empirical Data 869
Short-Term versus Long-Term 869
Testing the Sensitivity 869
Dose-Response Considerations 869
The Use of Adjunctive Therapy 870
Specific Measures to Reduce Side Effects 870
Cognizance of Objective Criteria 870
The Circadian Rhythm 871
Adjusting the Dose 871
Alternate-Day Therapy 871
Special Situations 873
Pregnancy 873
Diabetes 873
Surgery 873
Psychiatry 873

15 **(Continued)**

Peptic Ulcer 873
Pediatrics 874
Kaposi's Sarcoma 874
Withdrawal of Glucocorticoids and Suppression of the Hypothalamic-Pituitary-Adrenal Axis 874
Kinetics and Dosage Required for Suppression 874
Kinetics of Return to Normal Axis Function 875
Steroid Withdrawal Syndromes 877
Evaluation of Axis Function 878
Withdrawal Protocols and Indications for Steroid Coverage 878
References 879

PART V GONADAL DISEASE

16 **The Testis** **885**
Richard J. Santen
Anatomy 885
Central Nervous System and Hypothalamic-Pituitary Axis 885
Testes 886
Physiology 891
Hypothalamic-Pituitary-Leydig Cell Axis 891
Hypothalamic-Pituitary-Germ Cell Axis 907
Interactions between the LH-Leydig Cell and FSH-Germ Cell Axes 910
Prolactin Effects on Male Reproduction 911
Clinical Evaluation of the Hypothalamic-Pituitary-Testicular Axis 911
Assessment of Hormonal Status 911
Biological Effects of Sex Steroids on Target Organs 913
Genetic Tests 913
Structural and Functional Assessment 914
Age-Dependent Physiologic Changes in Testicular Function 916
Prepuberty 916
Puberty 916
Clinical Disorders 917
Introduction 917
Hypogonadotropic Syndromes 917
Hypogonadotropic Hypogonadism 928
Treatment of Hypogonadism 935
Germinal Cell Failure 938
Overview 938
Hypergonadotropic Syndromes 938
Eugonadotropic Germinal Cell Failure 940
Sinopulmonary-Infertility Syndrome 941
Genetic Syndromes 941
Autoimmunity 942
Approach to the Diagnosis of the Infertile Male 942
Disorders Associated with Nonphysiologic Secretion of Gonadotropins 943
Gonadotropin-Producing Tumors 943
Precocious Puberty 943
Cryptorchism 944
Pathophysiology 944
Rationale for Treatment 946
Treatment 947
Gynecomastia 947
Overview 947
Physiologic Forms of Gynecomastia 948

Pathologic Forms of Gynecomastia 948
Evaluation 949
Treatment 950
Impotence 951
Male Contraception 951
Testicular Tumors 952
Androgen-Dependent Neoplasia 952
Secondary Endocrine Treatments 953
Complete Androgen Blockade 954
References 955

---

17 The Ovary: Basic Principles and Concepts
A. Physiology 973
Gregory F. Erickson
Anatomy 973
Morphology 973
Blood Vessels 973
Innervation 975
Histology 975
Ovarian Follicles 975
Preantral Follicles 975
Antral Follicles 979
Ovarian Interstitial Cells 982
Corpora Lutea 985
Biogenesis of Ovarian Hormones 987
Steroids 987
Ovarian Cytodifferentiation: Underlying Control Mechanisms 991
The Granulosa Cell 991
The Interstitial Cells 993
Follicle Development: Control Mechanisms 998
Recruitment 998
Atresia 999
Selection 999
Ovulation 1002
Physiologic Correlates of Ovarian Activity with Aging 1004
The Fetal Period 1004
Premenarche 1004
Menarche 1004
Postmenarche: The Normal Menstrual Cycle 1006
Menopause 1008
The Concept of Ovarian Growth Factors 1009
Conclusion 1009
References 1010

B. Clinical 1016
Robert I. McLachlan, Neil McClure, David L. Healy, and Henry G. Burger
Ovarian Disorders in Teenagers 1016
Primary Amenorrhea 1016
Menarcheal Menorrhagia 1021
Ovarian Disorders in Young Adults 1021
Secondary Amenorrhea 1021
Polycystic Ovary Syndrome 1027
Virilization and Hirsutism 1030
Female Infertility: Diagnosis of Ovulatory Dysfunction 1032
Menorrhagia and Dysmenorrhea 1036
Premenstrual Syndrome 1040

17 (Continued)

Ovarian Disorders in Middle Age 1040
Endocrinology of the Menopause 1040
Climacteric Symptoms 1041
Postmenopausal Problems 1043
Long-Term Hormone Replacement Therapy 1044
Postmenopausal Bleeding 1046
Chemical Contraception and Contragestation 1046
New Progestogens 1047
References 1048

18 Sexual Differentiation 1053
Jeremy S. D. Winter and Robert M. Couch
Normal Sex Determination and Sexual Differentiation 1053
Genetic Sex 1054
Gonadal Sex 1058
Differentiation of the Genital Ducts 1060
Differentiation of the Urogenital Sinus and External Genitalia 1061
Hormonal Sex: Differentiation of the Hypothalamic-Pituitary-Gonadal Axis 1062
Abnormal Sexual Differentiation 1068
Errors of Primary Sex Determination 1068
Errors of Sexual Differentiation 1078
Clinical Approach to Disorders of Sexual Differentiation 1096
The Newborn with Abnormal Genitalia 1096
Virilization during Childhood or Adolescence 1099
Delayed Puberty, Amenorrhea, and Infertility 1099
References 1099

PART VI FUEL METABOLISM

19 The Endocrine Pancreas: Diabetes Mellitus 1107
Philip Felig and Michael Bergman
Physiology of Fuel Metabolism 1108
Carbohydrate Metabolism 1108
Fat Metabolism 1119
Interactions of Fat and Carbohydrate Medium 1123
Amino Acid Metabolism 1125
Insulin 1128
Glucagon 1146
Catecholamines 1150
Glucocorticoids 1150
Growth Hormone 1151
Insulin-Like Growth Factors 1151
Pancreatic Polypeptide 1152
Regulatory and Counterregulatory Hormones 1152
Fuel-Hormone Interactions 1152
Diabetes Mellitus 1156
History 1156
Definition and Classification 1156
Etiology 1159
Prediction and Prevention 1164
Pathogenesis 1165
Pathophysiology 1170
Diagnosis 1174
Prevalence 1179

Pathology 1179
Clinical Manifestations 1181
Pathogenesis of Diabetic Complications 1193
Mortality 1197
Treatment 1197
Hyperglycemic-Ketoacidotic Emergencies 1219
Pregnancy and Diabetes 1225
Lipoatrophic Diabetes 1232
Secondary Diabetes 1233
References 1235

20 Hypoglycemia **1251**
Harry Shamoon
Definition 1251
Signs and Symptoms 1251
Neuroglycopenia 1251
Sympathoadrenal Symptoms 1252
Other Symptoms and Signs 1252
Tests for Evaluation of Hypoglycemia 1253
Plasma Insulin 1253
C Peptide 1253
Proinsulin 1254
Supervised Prolonged Fasting 1254
Oral Glucose Tolerance Test 1254
Other Tests 1255
Classification 1255
Fasting Hypoglycemia 1255
Reactive Hypoglycemias 1264
Induced Hypoglycemias 1265
Diagnostic and Therapeutic Approach to Fasting Hypoglycemia 1266
References 1267

21 Obesity **1271**
John M. Amatruda and Stephen Welle
Definition and Diagnosis of Obesity 1271
Medical Complications of Obesity 1273
Cardiovascular Disease 1247
Metabolic Disorders 1277
Cancer 1279
Endocrine Disorders 1279
Skeletal Disorders 1280
Pulmonary Disorders 1281
Miscellaneous Disorders 1281
Etiology of Obesity 1281
Genetic Factors 1282
Environmental Factors 1283
Energy Expenditure 1283
Food Intake 1286
Endocrine Systems and the Autonomic Nervous System 1289
Summary 1290
Other Causes of Obesity 1290
Treatment of Obesity 1290
Prevention 1290
Exercise 1291
Behavioral Modification 1294

21 (Continued)

Diet 1294
Fad Diets 1299
Drugs 1299
Surgery for Morbid Obesity 1301
Summary 1303
References 1303

22 Disorders of Lipid Metabolism **1315**
D. Roger Illingworth, P. Barton Duell, and William E. Connor
The Plasma Lipoproteins 1315
Lipoprotein Classification 1316
Lipoprotein Composition 1316
The Apoproteins 1318
Lipoprotein Structure 1320
Synthesis and Catabolism of Lipids and Lipoproteins 1320
Lipids 1320
Enzymes and Transfer Proteins Active in Lipoprotein Metabolism 1321
Lipoprotein Metabolism 1322
Atherogenicity of Individual Lipoprotein Particles 1325
The Hyperlipidemias 1326
Classification of Hyperlipidemias 1326
Criteria for the Diagnosis of Hyperlipoproteinemia 1327
Secondary Hyperlipidemias 1330
Hypercholesterolemia 1335
Familial Hypercholesterolemia 1335
Familial Defective Apolipoprotein B-100 1342
Combined Hypercholesterolemia and Hypertriglyceridemia 1343
Hypertriglyceridemia 1348
Disorders of High-Density Lipoproteins 1353
Familial Apolipoprotein A-I and C-III Deficiency 1354
Familial Apo-A-I, C-III, A-IV Deficiency 1355
HDL Deficiency with Planar Xanthomas 1355
Lecithin Cholesterol Acyltransferase Deficiency 1355
Fish Eye Disease 1355
Familial Apo-A-I Variants 1355
Familial Hypoalphalipoproteinemia 1355
Tangier Disease 1355
Familial Hyperalphalipoproteinemia 1357
Other Lipoprotein Disorders 1357
Abetalipoproteinemia 1357
Hypobetalipoproteinemia 1359
Chylomicron/Retention Disease 1359
Familial Lecithin Cholesterol Acyltransferse Deficiency 1359
Sterol Storage Diseases 1360
Atherosclerosis 1360
Xanthomas 1362
Acid Cholesteryl Ester Hydrolase Deficiency 1362
Familial Diseases with Storage of Sterols Other Than Cholesterol 1363
Cerebrotendinous Xanthomatosis 1363
Sitosterolemia and Xanthomatosis 1364
Dietary Treatment of Hyperlipidemia 1366
The Effects of Specific Nutrients on the Plasma Lipids and Lipoproteins 1367
Implementation of the Single-Diet Concept for the Treatment of Hyperlipidemia 1374
A Phased Approach to the Dietary Treatment of Hyperlipidemia 1378

Pharmaceutical Agents for the Treatment of Hyperlipoproteinemia 1380
Bile Acid Sequestrants 1381
Nicotinic Acid 1382
HMG CoA Reductase Inhibitors 1383
Probucol 1385
Clofibrate 1386
Gemfibrozil 1387
Miscellaneous Agents 1387
Future Advances 1388
The Surgical Treatment of Hyperlipoproteinemia 1390
Surgical Procedures in Homozygous Familial Hypercholesterolemia 1390
Treatment of Special Patient Populations 1390
Laboratory Tests in the Diagnosis of Hyperlipidemias 1392
Collection and Handling of the Sample 1392
Lipid Determinations 1392
Lipoprotein Separations 1392
Additional Laboratory Tests 1393
References 1394

PART VII CALCIUM AND BONE METABOLISM

23 Mineral Metabolism 1407
Gordon J. Strewler and Michael Rosenblatt
Cellular and Extracellular Calcium Metabolism 1407
Parathyroid Hormone 1409
Anatomy and Embryology of the Parathyroid Glands 1409
Biosynthesis, Processing, and Secretion of Parathyroid Hormone 1409
Metabolism of Parathyroid Hormone 1414
Assay of Parathyroid Hormone 1415
Biological Effects and Mechanisms of Action of Parathyroid Hormone 1416
Calcitonin 1431
Introduction and Historical Notes 1431
Biological Effects and Mechanism of Action 1432
Biochemistry and Molecular Biology 1433
Calcitonin as a Therapeutic Agent 1434
Vitamin D 1437
Historical Introduction 1437
Biosynthesis and Chemistry 1437
Absorption, Activation, and Transport of Vitamin D 1438
Further Metabolism of $1\alpha,25\text{-}(OH)_2D$ *1443*
Vitamin D Nutrition 1443
Cellular Basis of Vitamin D Action 1444
Actions of Vitamin D in Intestine, Bone, and Kidney 1445
Assay of Vitamin D Metabolites 1448
Hypercalcemia 1449
Introduction 1449
The Defense Against Hypercalcemia 1449
Approach to the Hypercalcemic Patient 1450
Primary Hyperparathyroidism 1452
Malignancy-Associated Hypercalcemia 1467
Other Hypercalcemic Disorders 1474
Hypocalcemia 1477
Classification of Hypocalcemic Disorders 1477
Approach to the Hypocalcemic Patient 1478
Clinical Manifestations of Hypocalcemia 1478
Hypoparathyroidism 1480

23 (Continued)

Pseudohypoparathyroidism 1482
Other Hypocalcemia Disorders 1487
Treatment of Hypocalcemia 1487
Disorders of Phosphate Metabolism 1489
Phosphate Homeostasis 1489
Disorders Causing Hypophosphatemia 1492
Disorders Causing Hyperphosphatemia 1494
Disorders of Magnesium Metabolism 1494
Magnesium Balance 1495
Hypomagnesemia 1495
Hypermagnesemia 1497
Testing 1497
Serum Chemistries 1497
Urinary Determinations 1497
Testing for Pseudohypoparathyroidism 1498
References 1499

24 Metabolic Bone Disease **1517**
Frederick R. Singer
Clinical Evaluation of Metabolic Bone Disease 1517
History and Physical Examination 1517
Clinical Chemistry 1517
Radiology and Nuclear Medicine 1519
Bone Biopsy 1519
Osteomalacia and Rickets 1521
Clinical Presentation 1521
Bone Pathology 1523
Classification and Pathogenesis 1524
Vitamin D Abnormalities 1524
Hypophosphatemia 1526
Miscellaneous 1528
Treatment 1529
Osteoporosis 1530
Clinical Presentation 1530
Bone Pathology 1533
Classification and Pathogenesis 1534
Prevention 1538
Treatment 1540
Osteopetrosis 1541
Renal Osteodystrophy 1542
Clinical Presentation 1542
Bone Pathology 1543
Pathogenesis 1543
Treatment 1544
Hereditary Hyperphosphatasia 1546
Fibrous Dysplasia 1546
Paget's Disease of Bone 1547
Clinical Presentation 1547
Bone Pathology 1550
Pathogenesis 1551
Treatment 1551
References 1554

25 Nephrolithiasis **1565**
Bruce Ettinger and Karl L. Insogna
Introduction 1565
Epidemiology 1565
Classification of Calculi by Clinical Presentation 1565
Classification of Calculi by Crystalline Structure 1565
Quantitating Clinical Stone Events 1566
Theories of Stone Pathogenesis 1566
Physical Chemical Aspects of Stone Formation 1567
Evaluation and Treatment 1568
Cystinuria 1573
History 1573
Genetics 1573
Pathophysiology of Cystinuria 1573
Dependence of Cystine Solubility on Urinary pH 1573
Dependence of Cystine Excretion on Salt Intake 1574
Effect of Cysteine-Complexing Agents 1574
Clinical Findings 1574
Clinical Evaluation 1575
Treatment 1575
Uric Acid Stones 1577
Epidemiology 1577
Purine Metabolism and Uric Acid Excretion 1577
Uric Acid Solubility in Urine 1578
Risk Factors for Uric Acid Stones 1578
Effect of Diet on Urinary pH and Uric Acid Excretion 1578
Gout and Uric Acid Stones 1578
Other Clinical Disorders Associated with Uric Acid Stones 1579
Differentiating Uric Acid from Other Purine-Related Stones 1579
Mechanisms of the Effect of Allopurinol on Uric Acid 1579
Efficacy of Medical Treatment of Uric Acid Lithiasis 1580
Evaluation 1580
Therapy 1580
Calcium Phosphate Stones 1581
Crystalline Forms of Calcium Phosphate 1581
Effect of pH on Solubility of Calcium Phosphate 1581
Renal Tubular Acidosis 1581
Pathophysiology of Stone Disease in Renal Tubular Acidosis 1582
Incomplete Renal Tubular Acidosis 1582
Evaluation 1583
Treatment 1583
Magnesium Ammonium Phosphate Stones 1583
Terminology 1583
History and Epidemiology 1583
Pathophysiology 1584
Bacteriology 1584
Clinical Risk Factors 1584
Serious Morbidity from MAP Stones 1584
Evaluation 1584
Treatment 1584
Calcium Oxalate and Mixed Calcium Stones 1585
Epidemiology 1585
Physical Chemistry 1586
Natural History of Calcium Oxalate Lithiasis 1586
Risk Factors 1587
Evaluation: Calcium Oxalate Stones 1602
Treatment of Calcium Oxalate Nephrolithiasis 1605
Closing Comments 1609
References 1609

PART VIII MISCELLANEOUS DISORDERS

26 Disorders of Growth and Development **1619**
Margaret H. MacGillivray

Biological Stages of Growth 1619
Control of Growth Processes 1619
- *Genetic Factors 1620*
- *Peptide Growth Factors and Hormonal Influences 1620*
- *Insulin-Like Growth Factors 1621*
- *Hormonal Regulation 1626*
- *Nutrition 1633*

Physiology of Skeletal Growth 1633
Developmental Stages 1634
- *Intrauterine Life 1634*
- *Infancy: Birth to 2 Years of Age 1634*
- *Childhood 1635*
- *Adolescence 1635*

Short Stature 1636
- *Clinical Approach to Short Stature 1636*
- *Causes of Short Stature 1640*

Growth Excess 1657
- *Normal Variants 1657*
- *Pathologic Overgrowth 1658*

Appendix: Details of Testing Procedures in Children 1665
- *Pituitary-Hypothalamic Evaluation 1665*
- *Adrenal Function Tests 1667*

References 1668

27 Gastrointestinal Hormones and Carcinoid Syndrome **1675**
Jan Redfern and Thomas M. O'Dorisio

Localization and Distribution of GI Peptides 1675
Biological Actions and Clinical Applications 1677
- *Somatostatin 1677*
- *Gastrin 1681*
- *Cholecystokinin 1682*
- *Secretin 1683*
- *Vasoactive Intestinal Polypeptide 1684*
- *Gastric Inhibitory Polypeptide (Glucose-Dependent Insulinotropic Peptide) 1685*
- *Motilin 1686*
- *Pancreatic Polypeptide Family 1687*
- *Neurotensin 1687*
- *Substance P 1688*

Carcinoid Syndrome 1688
- *Pathology 1689*
- *Symptoms 1690*
- *Pathophysiology 1690*
- *Diagnosis 1691*
- *Differential Diagnosis 1694*
- *Treatment 1694*
- *Prognosis 1695*

References 1695

28 **Multiglandular Endocrine Disorders** **1703**
Leonard J. Deftos, Bayard D. Catherwood, and Henry G. Bone III

Multiple Endocrine Neoplasia Type 1 (MEN 1) 1703
Definition and History 1703
Components of the Syndrome 1703
Clinical Evaluation 1706
Epidemiology 1707
MEN in Other Species 1707
Pathogenesis 1707
Management 1708
Multiple Endocrine Neoplasia Type 2 (MEN 2) 1709
Medullary Thyroid Carcinoma 1709
Pheochromocytoma 1715
Hyperparathyroidism 1716
Multiple Mucosal Neuromas (MMN) 1716
Treatment 1717
Pluriglandular Endocrine Insufficiency Syndromes 1717
Pluriglandular Autoimmunity with Addison's Disease 1718
Thyroid Disease and Diabetes Mellitus without Addison's Disease 1724
Other Disorders 1724
Diagnosis, Complications, and Surveillance 1724
Genetics of Pluriglandular Endocrine Insufficiency Syndromes 1726
Nonautoimmune Pluriglandular Dysfunction 1726
References 1726

29 **Ectopic Hormone Production** **1733**
Glenn D. Braunstein

General Principles 1733
Paraneoplastic Syndromes 1733
Eutopic versus Ectopic Hormone Production 1733
Importance of Ectopic Hormone Production 1735
Criteria for Ectopic Hormone Production 1736
Frequency of Ectopic Hormone Production 1738
Etiology of Ectopic Hormone Production 1741
Therapy 1744
Hormones as Tumor Markers 1745
Specific Syndromes 1747
Hypercalcemia of Malignancy 1747
Ectopic POMC/ACTH Syndrome 1754
Syndrome of Inappropriate Antidiuresis in Cancer 1758
Hypoglycemia Associated with Malignancy 1761
Oncogenic Osteomalacia 1764
Ectopic Growth Hormone and Growth Hormone Releasing Hormone Production 1766
Ectopic Production of Placental Proteins 1768
Paraneoplastic Erythrocytosis 1769
Ectopic Production of Calcitonin 1770
Other Hormones Produced by Tumors 1771
References 1772

30 **Hormone-Responsive Tumors** **1785**
Christopher C. Benz

General Aspects Concerning the Development of Hormone-Responsive Tumors 1787
Steroids as Carcinogens and Tumor Promoters 1787

30 (Continued)

The Role of Oncogenes and Tumor Suppressor Genes in Hormone-Responsive Tumors 1789
Epidemiologic Features of Hormone-Responsive Tumors 1790
Primary Modalities of Endocrine Intervention 1793
Cellular Mechanisms Mediating Hormone Response 1795
Receptor Mechanisms Mediating Hormone Response 1798
Clinical Characteristics of Hormone-Responsive Cancers 1799
Breast Cancer 1799
Endometrial Cancer 1803
Prostate Cancer 1805
References 1807

---

31 Hormones, Aging, and Endocrine Disorders in the Elderly 1813
John E. Morley

Theories of Aging 1816
Hormonal Changes 1817
Growth Hormone and IGF-I 1817
Prolactin 1817
Hypothalamic-Pituitary-Thyroid Axis 1818
Hypothalamic-Pituitary-Adrenal Axis 1818
Sex Hormones 1819
Hormones Associated with Water Metabolism 1821
Frailty, Hormones, and Aging 1822
Growth Hormone 1822
Testosterone 1823
Estrogens 1823
Vitamin D, Type II (Age-Related) Osteopenia, and Hip Fracture 1823
Sexuality and Aging 1825
Males 1825
Females 1827
Diabetes Mellitus 1827
Hyperglycemia of Aging 1827
Should Blood Glucose Be Controlled in Older Individuals? 1827
Special Features in the Management of Older Diabetics 1828
Diet in Older Diabetics 1828
Oral Hypoglycemia Agents 1828
Insulin 1829
Monitoring Treatment 1829
Diabetes in Nursing Home Residents 1829
Summary 1830
Nutritional Disorders 1830
Conclusion 1831
References 1831

---

32 Hormones and Athletic Performance 1837
David C. Cumming

Energy Supply and Physical Work 1837
Evaluating Hormonal Response to Exercise and Training 1837
Effects of Physical Activity and Training on Endocrine Function 1838
Growth Hormone in Exercise 1838
ACTH-Cortisol Axis 1840
Exercise and the ACTH-Cortisol Axis 1840
The Effect of Physical Training 1840
Influence of Circadian and Other Rhythms 1841
Physiologic Significance 1841

Prolactin and Exercise 1841
Effects of Training on Prolactin 1842
Mechanisms 1842
TSH-Thyroid Axis 1842
Acute Responses 1842
Effect of Training 1842
Endogenous Opiates in Exercise and Training 1843
Response to Acute Physical Activity 1843
Effects of Training 1843
Physiologic Significance of the Exercise-Associated Opiate Increase 1844
Opiates, Exercise, and Appetite Suppression in Humans 1845
Summary 1846
Endocrine Regulation of Fluid Balance during Physical Work 1846
Arginine Vasopressin, Exercise, and Training 1846
Aldosterone, Exercise, and Training 1847
Insulin and Glucagon in Exercise 1847
Insulin and Exercise 1847
Glucagon and Exercise 1848
Effects of Training 1848
Catecholamines in Exercise 1848
Epinephrine and Norepinephrine 1848
Control of Catecholamine Release 1849
Effects of Catecholamine Release 1849
Effects of Training 1849
Dopamine Responses to Exercise 1849
Exercise, Training, and the Hypothalamic-Pituitary-Gonadal Axis 1849
Acute Exercise and the HPG Axis in Men 1850
Short-Term Exercise and the HPG Axis 1850
Mechanism of Exercise-Associated Testosterone Increase 1850
The Effects of Prolonged Exercise on the HPG Axis in Men 1851
Effects of Endurance Training on the HPG Axis in Men 1852
Symptomatic Impairment of the HPG Axis in Men 1852
Mechanisms of Long-Term Activity-Associated Suppression of Circulating Testosterone Levels 1853
Exercise and the Reproductive System in Women 1853
Acute Exercise-Associated Changes in Reproductive Hormones 1853
Reproductive Effects of Exercise in Women 1854
The Psychological Stress of Training and Competing 1854
The Physical Stress of Training and/or Competition 1854
Body Composition and Nutrition 1855
Predisposition of Menstrual Irregularity 1856
The Endocrinology of Exercise-Associated Reproductive Dysfunction 1856
Summary 1857
Use of Performance-Enhancing Endocrine Drugs (Doping) in Competitive and Recreational Sports Activity 1857
Mens Sana in Corpore Sano: Ethical Aspects of Doping in Sports 1857
Anabolic Steroids 1858
The Use of Anabolic Steroids by Athletes 1860
Other Ergogenic Aids 1865
Growth Hormone 1865
Erythropoietin 1865
References 1866

Index 1887

Contributors

JOHN M. AMATRUDA, M.D. [21]
Director, Institute for Metabolic Disorders
Miles Research Center
West Haven, Connecticut
Department of Medicine
Endocrine/Metabolism Unit
University of Rochester
Rochester, New York

JOHN D. BAXTER, M.D. [1, 2, 14]
Professor of Medicine
Chief, Division of Endocrinology
Parnassus and Mount Zion Campuses
Metabolic Research Unit
University of California, San Francisco
San Francisco, California

CHRISTOPHER C. BENZ, M.D. [30]
Associate Professor of Medicine
University of California, San Francisco
San Francisco, California

MICHAEL BERGMAN, M.D., F.A.C.P. [19]
Director, Cardiovascular Clinical Research
Schering-Plough Research Institute
Kenilworth, New Jersey
Clinical Professor of Medicine
New York Medical College
Valhalla, New York

EDWARD G. BIGLIERI, M.D. [14]
Professor of Medicine, Emeritus
University of California, San Francisco
San Francisco, California

HENRY G. BONE III, M.D. [28]
Senior Staff Physician
Henry Ford Hospital
Bone and Mineral Division
Detroit, Michigan

GLENN D. BRAUNSTEIN, M.D. [29]
Professor of Medicine
UCLA School of Medicine
Chairman, Department of Medicine
Cedars-Sinai Medical Center
Los Angeles, California

HENRY G. BURGER, M.D. [17B]
Professor and Director
Department of Endocrinology
Prince Henry Institute of Medical Research
Clayton, Victoria, Australia

Note: Numbers in brackets refer to chapters written or co-written by the contributors.

GERARD N. BURROW, M.D. [11]
Dean and Professor of Medicine
Yale University School of Medicine
New Haven, Connecticut

JAN CARLSTEDT-DUKE, M.D. [5B]
Department of Medical Nutrition
Karolinska Institute
Huddinge University Hospital
Novum, Huddinge, Sweden

BAYARD D. CATHERWOOD, M.D. [28]
Professor of Medicine
Associate Professor of Anatomy and Cell Biology
Emory University School of Medicine
Chief, Endocrinology and Metabolism
Atlanta Veterans Affairs Medical Center
Atlanta, Georgia

KEVIN J. CATT, M.D., Ph.D. [5A]
Chief
Endocrinological Reproductive Research Branch
National Institute of Child Health and Human Development
Bethesda, Maryland

WILLIAM E. CONNOR, M.D. [22]
Professor of Medicine
Division of Endocrinology, Diabetes, and Clinical Nutrition
Department of Medicine
Oregon Health Sciences University
Portland, Oregon

ROBERT M. COUCH, M.D. [18]
Assistant Professor
Department of Pediatrics
University of Alberta
Edmonton, Alberta, Canada

PHILIP E. CRYER, M.D. [13]
Professor
Metabolism Division
Washington University School of Medicine

DAVID C. CUMMING, M.B., Ch.B., F.R.C.O.G., F.R.C.S.C. [32]
Professor
Department of Obstetrics and Gynecology and Medicine
Division of Endocrinology
University of Alberta
Edmonton, Alberta, Canada

LEONARD J. DEFTOS, M.D. [28]
Professor of Medicine
Endocrine Section
University of California and the San Diego VA Medical Center
La Jolla, California

P. BARTON DUELL, M.D. [22]
Assistant Professor
Division of Endocrinology, Diabetes, and Clinical Nutrition
Department of Medicine
Oregon Health Sciences University
Portland, Oregon

GREGORY F. ERICKSON, Ph.D. [17A]
Professor
Department of Reproductive Medicine
University of California, San Diego
La Jolla, California

BRUCE ETTINGER, M.D. [25]
Senior Investigator
Division of Research
Kaiser Permanente Medical Care Program
Oakland, California
Clinical Professor of Medicine
University of California, San Francisco
San Francisco, California

PHILIP FELIG, M.D. [1, 2, 19]
Attending Physician
Senior Medical Staff, Lenox Hill Hospital
New York, New York

LAWRENCE A. FROHMAN, M.D. [1, 2, 8]
Edmund F. Foley Professor and Chairman
Department of Medicine
University of Illinois College of Medicine
Physician-in-Chief
University of Illinois Hospital
Chicago, Illinois

DAVID G. GARDNER, M.D. [3]
Professor of Medicine
University of California, San Francisco
San Francisco, California

BARRY J. GERTZ, M.D., Ph.D. [3]
Senior Director, Clinical Pharmacology
Merck, Sharpe, and Dohme Research Laboratories
Rahway, New Jersey

GORDON N. GILL, M.D. [4]
Professor of Medicine
Co-Director, Division of Endocrinology and Metabolism
Associate Chair for Scientific Affairs
Department of Medicine
University of California, San Diego
La Jolla, California

MARTIN GÖTTLICHER, M.D. [5B]
Center for Biotechnology
Karolinska Institute
Huddinge, Sweden

JAN-ÅKE GUSTAFSSON, M.D. [5B]
Chairman
Department of Medical Nutrition
Karolinska Institute
Huddinge University Hospital
Huddinge, Sweden

DAVID L. HEALY, M.D. [17B]
Professor
Monash University
Department of Obstetrics and Gynaecology
Monash Medical Centre
Clayton, Victoria, Australia

JEROME M. HERSHMAN, M.D. [6]
Professor of Medicine, UCLA School of Medicine
Chief, Endocrinology and Metabolism Division
Wadsworth VA Hospital
West Los Angeles Veterans Affairs Medical Center
Los Angeles, California

WILLA HSUEH, M.D. [14]
University of Southern California Medical Center
Los Angeles, California

D. ROGER ILLINGWORTH, M.D. [22]
Department of Medicine
Division of Endocrinology
Oregon Health Sciences University
Portland, Oregon

KARL L. INSOGNA, M.D. [25]
Associate Professor of Medicine
Yale University School of Medicine
Director, Yale Bone Center
New Haven, Connecticut

MARGARET H. MACGILLIVRAY, M.D. [26]
Professor
Department of Pediatrics
State University of New York
School of Medicine at Buffalo
Buffalo, New York

NEIL MCCLURE, M.D. [17B]
Monash University
Department of Obstetrics and Gynaecology
Monash Medical Centre
Clayton, Victoria, Australia

ROBERT I. MCLACHLAN, M.D. [17B]
Prince Henry's Institute of Medical Research
Clayton, Victoria, Australia

WALTER L. MILLER, M.D. [12]
Professor of Medicine
Department of Pediatrics and the Metabolic Research Unit
University of California, San Francisco
San Francisco, California

MARK E. MOLITCH, M.D. [7]
Professor of Medicine
Center for Endocrinology, Metabolism, and Molecular Medicine
Department of Medicine
Northwestern University Medical School
Chicago, Illinois

JOHN E. MORLEY, M.B. B.Ch. [31]
Dammert Professor of Gerontology
Department of Medicine
St. Louis University Medical School and Geriatric Research
Education and Clinical Center
St. Louis Veterans Administration Medical Center
St. Louis, Missouri

THOMAS M. O'DORISIO, M.D. [27]
Professor of Internal Medicine and Physiology
Director, Division of Endocrinology and Metabolism
Department of Internal Medicine
The Ohio State University College of Medicine
Columbus, Ohio

SAM OKRET, M.D. [5B]
Department of Medical Nutrition
Karolinska Institute
Huddinge University Hospital
Huddinge, Sweden

A. EUGENE PEKARY, PH.D. [6]
Supervisory Research Chemist
Endocrinology Research Laboratory
Veterans Administration West Los Angeles Medical Center
Adjunct Professor of Medicine
Department of Medicine
University of California - Los Angeles
Los Angeles, California

DOROTHEE PERLOFF, M.D. [14]
Clinical Professor of Medicine
University of California, San Francisco
San Francisco, California

JAN REDFERN, Ph.D. [27]
Medical Director, Project House, Inc.
University Plaza
Hackensack, New Jersey
Formerly Research Assistant Professor
Department of Internal Medicine
University of Texas Southwestern Medical Center at Dallas
Dallas, Texas

GARY L. ROBERTSON, M.D. [9]
Professor
Department of Medicine
Program Director
General Clinical Research Center
Northwestern University Medical School
Chicago, Illinois

MICHAEL ROSENBLATT, M.D. [23]
Robert H. Ebert Professor of Molecular Medicine
Harvard Medical School
Director, Harvard–MIT Division of Health Sciences and Technology
Chief, Division of Bone and Mineral Metabolism
Beth Israel Hospital
Vice-President, Biology Research and Molecular Biology
Merck, Sharpe, and Dohme Research Laboratories
Boston, Massachusetts

RICHARD J. SANTEN, M.D. [16]
Professor and Chairman
Department of Internal Medicine
Wayne State University
Detroit, Michigan

HARRY SHAMOON, M.D. [20]
Professor of Medicine
Division of Endocrinology and Metabolism
Department of Medicine, Diabetes Research and Training Center
Albert Einstein College of Medicine
Bronx, New York

FREDERICK R. SINGER, M.D. [24]
Medical Director, Osteoporosis/Metabolic Bone Disease Laboratory
Saint John's Hospital and Health Center
Director, Skeletal Biology Laboratory
John Wayne Cancer Institute
Santa Monica, California
Clinical Professor of Medicine
UCLA School of Medicine
Los Angeles, California

GORDON J. STREWLER, M.D. [23]
Professor of Medicine
University of California, San Francisco
Chief, Endocrine Unit
Veterans Affairs Medical Center
San Francisco, California

J. BLAKE TYRRELL, M.D. [12, 15]
Clinical Professor of Medicine
Chief
Parnassus and Mount Zion Campuses
University of California, San Francisco
San Francisco, California

ROBERT D. UTIGER, M.D. [10]
Clinical Professor of Medicine
Harvard Medical School
Deputy Editor
New England Journal of Medicine
Boston, Massachusetts

STEPHEN WELLE, Ph.D. [21]
Associate Professor of Medicine and Physiology
University of Rochester
Rochester, New York

JEREMY S.D. WINTER, M.D., F.R.C.P.C. [18]
Professor
Department of Pediatrics
University of Manitoba
Head, Section of Endocrinology and Metabolism
University of Alberta
Edmonton, Alberta, Canada

ANTHONY WRIGHT, M.D. [5B]
Center for Biotechnology
Karolinska Institute
Huddinge, Sweden

Preface

In the seven years that have elapsed since the publication of the Second Edition of *Endocrinology and Metabolism,* there has been an enormous increase in our knowledge of basic concepts of cellular and molecular biology, genetics, and intracellular signaling mechanisms. As a result, our understanding of the etiology and pathophysiology of endocrine and metabolic disorders and our approach to diagnosis and treatment have been advanced. This increase in our knowledge base has heightened the challenge of providing a textbook that properly balances a discussion of basic principles with the details of diagnosis and management of disease entities.

As in the previous editions, we have attempted to achieve this balance between basic science and clinical management in a manner that is useful for the clinical endocrinologist as well as the research-oriented scholar and trainee in endocrinology. To that end, this edition involves extensive revision or entirely new chapters as well as the addition of chapters dealing with subjects not previously covered (Hormones and Aging; Hormones and Athletic Performance). In addition to blending basic science and clinical management in the chapters dealing with specific disorders, we have retained the format of an introductory series of chapters. These deal with general principles of the organization and molecular and cellular biology of the endocrine system, the clinical presentation of endocrine disease, and the principles of endocrine testing.

We are grateful to our contributors for the enormity and the excellence of their efforts. We acknowledge with special thanks the contribution and support of our colleagues at McGraw-Hill, J. Dereck Jeffers, Editor-in-Chief, and Mariapaz Ramos Englis, Senior Editing Manager.

PART I

General Endocrinology

CHAPTER 1

Introduction to the Endocrine System

John D. Baxter

Lawrence A. Frohman

Philip Felig

DEFINITIONS AND SCOPE OF ENDOCRINOLOGY

The endocrine system, along with the nervous system, has evolved to provide mechanisms for communication between cells and organs. Such systems have been critical for the development and function of multicellular organisms that in higher species such as humans have rather sophisticated control systems. These systems regulate and thus permit growth and development, reproduction, homeostasis, and responses to changes in the environment such as provocative stimuli and stress.

The term *endocrine* refers to the process of the secretion of biologically active substances into the body. This contrasts with the term *exocrine,* which refers to external secretion, generally via anatomically identifiable ducts, such as into the gastrointestinal tract. As the term is ordinarily used, an endocrine gland or cell is one that secretes substances, referred to as *hormones,* that exert regulatory functions, typically in cells other than those in which they are produced. The term *hormone* is derived from a Greek verb meaning "to set in motion." Strictly speaking, then, a hormone is a substance that is secreted by one cell and travels through the circulation, where it exerts actions on other cells (Fig. 1-1).

In order to act, hormones must interact with other loci on or in the target cell. These sites are termed *receptors* (Chap. 5). Thus, a receptor is a locus to which the hormone binds in order to elicit its actions. A receptor has two functions. First, it must be able to distinguish the hormone from all the other chemicals present in the circulation and bind it. Thus, a receptor must be capable of binding the hormone tightly enough and also must not bind extraneous substances. The hormone-binding sites on receptors have evolved to have unique configurations that are complementary to the hormones they bind. In general, these hormone-receptor interactions are noncovalent in nature and are reversible. Second, the receptor must be able to transmit the information gained from the binding to trigger a cellular response. Thus, substances that bind hormones, even tightly, but do not trigger subsequent responses are not receptors; examples include *transport proteins* (discussed below) and the enzymes involved in hormone biosynthesis or metabolism (see Chap. 4).

These simple distinctions serve to define endocrinology, receptors, and hormones in most cases. Thus, for example, insulin (Chap. 19) is secreted from an endocrine gland, the pancreatic islets; travels in the circulation; and associates with insulin receptors present on most tissues, where the hormone-receptor interaction triggers numerous responses involved in regulating the metabolism of carbohydrates and other substances. Parathyroid hormone (PTH) (Chap. 23) is synthesized in and released from the parathyroid glands, travels through the circulation, and binds to several target tissues, where it regulates calcium homeostasis. In addition to these clear examples, there are numerous others in which the distinctions may appear to be fuzzy and imprecise. In most cases these seeming discrepancies are more apparent than real.

A major area of overlap in terms of the function of regulatory molecules involves the nervous system, and an entire discipline—neuroendocrinology—has evolved to address the relation between the nervous and endocrine systems (Fig. 1-1). This is discussed in detail in Chap. 7. Overall, the nervous system has evolved to release regulatory substances from nerve cells or their axons that act across synaptic junctions on adjacent cells. Sometimes these substances, or *neurotransmitters,* travel considerable distances to act, but when they do so, they in general travel along the axons (Fig. 1-1). Acetylcholine, catecholamines, and dopamine are well-known neurotransmitters.

The brain is also an endocrine gland (Chap. 7; Fig. 1-1). It is the major source for some hormones. The hypothalamic releasing hormones or factors include thyrotropin releasing hormone (TRH), corticotropin releasing hormone (CRH), growth hormone

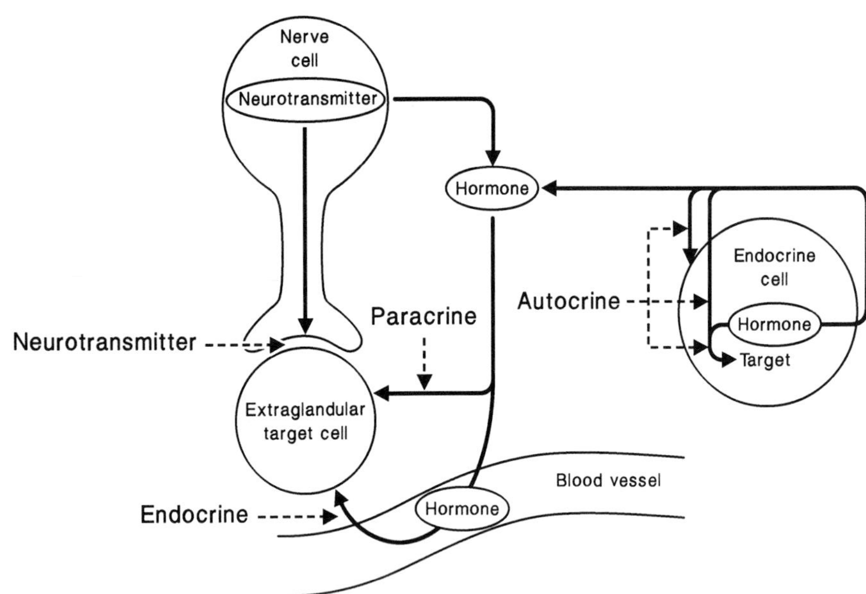

FIGURE 1-1 Distinctions between the endocrine and nervous systems and between the various types of hormone action: hormone (endocrine), autocrine, and paracrine. See the text for details.

releasing hormone (GHRH), gonadotropin releasing hormone (GnRH), somatostatin, and dopamine; all are produced in the hypothalamus, from which they travel through the hypophyseal portal system to stimulate or inhibit the synthesis and release of pituitary hormones. Some of the hormones of the anterior pituitary (Chap. 8) and all those of the posterior pituitary (Chap. 9) are also synthesized in the hypothalamus.

Since both the nervous and endocrine systems gradually came to use various ligands to serve their regulatory functions, it is not surprising that the same or related ligands can be used both as neurotransmitters and as hormones. Thus, both norepinephrine, secreted from nerve endings, and epinephrine, secreted from the adrenal medulla, act through adrenergic receptors (Chap. 13). Dopamine is a well-established neurotransmitter that is also active after it travels through the circulation. The brain produces a number of other hormones (Chap. 7). Prolactin, growth hormone, pro-opiomelanocortin (POMC), renin, and atrial natriuretic factor are examples of these brain hormones, but brain production probably contributes negligibly to the circulating levels of these substances. Therefore, if they exhibit biological activity (something not yet established), they probably play a local role in regulation. If this is true, they may be neurotransmitters. How can these overlaps be resolved in terms of definition? For the most part, the answers are simple. If a given ligand is released into the circulation to act, it is a hormone; if it is released from a nerve terminal to act locally, it is a neurotransmitter. The same substance can be both a neurotransmitter and a hormone.

The nervous and endocrine systems are also related in other ways. Thus, in many cases the function of endocrine tissues is controlled by the autonomic nervous system. Endocrine glands such as the pituitary, pancreatic islets, renal juxtaglomerular cells, and the adrenal gland respond to neural stimulation. Again, while the overlaps are obvious, the definitions can still be simple, and the same cell can function as both an endocrine cell and a nerve cell.

The designation of endocrine tissue has of necessity broadened with recent advances in the understanding of endocrinology: some tissues are specialized specifically as endocrine glands, while other endocrine glands also serve other functions. Examples of the first type include the thyroid, pituitary, parathyroid, and adrenal glands and the pancreatic islets. The central nervous system, by contrast, serves other functions, and the ovaries and testes, in addition to producing hormones, also produce oocytes and sperm, respectively. The atrium of the heart produces atrial natriuretic factor (Chap. 14); the liver, insulin-like growth factor I (IGF-I; also called somatomedin; Chap. 26) and angiotensinogen (the precursor to angiotensin II; Chap. 14); the kidney, erythropoietin[1] and the active form of vitamin D_3 (1,25-OH cholecalciferol; Chap. 23); the gastrointestinal tract, gastrin, somatostatin, cholecystokinin, and others (Chap. 27); and cells of the immune system, numerous hormones such as interleukins, interferons, and tumor necrosis factor.[2,3]

Do hormones need to travel through the circulation to act? No. Locally released hormones can act on cells in the immediate vicinity of their release (Fig.

1-1). Growth factors can be released in tissues such as bone (Chap. 24). Somatostatin is released by the pancreatic delta cells (Chap. 19) and has the potential to suppress insulin release by beta cells and glucagon release by alpha cells (Chap. 19). Prostaglandins and other eicosanoids are in all likelihood released to act on cells in their immediate vicinity. This type of intracellular communication has been termed *paraendocrine* or *paracrine* and thus has been incorporated into the general discipline of endocrinology (Fig. 1-1).

Hormones can also act on the cells that produce them. This type of communication has been termed *autocrine* (Fig. 1-1). Such actions are probably important in cancer cells. Certain oncogenes encode analogues of growth factors or their receptors that enhance the progression of the malignant state.[4–6] Insulin has an inhibitory effect on its own secretion, independent of changes in blood glucose levels (Chap. 19).

Still other examples can be cited in which semantic distinctions become fuzzy and overlaps occur between endocrinology and other disciplines. For instance, renin of renal origin is ordinarily considered a hormone, but rather than acting on other cell types, it functions as an enzyme in the bloodstream to release angiotensin I from its substrate, angiotensinogen (Chap. 14). The regulators of the immune response, such as the interleukins,[2,3] the growth factors (Chap. 26), erythropoietin,[1] and other factors, function as hormones or in paracrine or autocrine regulation but are ordinarily not considered hormones even though they should be.

Since common clinical problems in endocrinology are due either to an excess or to a deficiency of a hormone, it is not surprising that classically, endocrinology was signal-level-oriented, with the dominant consideration being how much or how little of the hormone was present. Over time, the signal-level consideration has been expanded to include reserve. For example, the diagnosis of adrenal insufficiency is based not on a random measurement of plasma cortisol in the unstressed state but on the extent to which cortisol can be released in response to provocative stimuli (Chap. 12). Increasingly, attention has also been focused on the response limb of the endocrine system. In interpreting the significance of a hormone's concentration in the blood, it is equally critical to know how sensitive the target cells are to that hormone. Some syndromes have features of hormone deficiency in the presence of elevated or normal hormone levels that are due to decreased responsiveness to hormones. Pseudohypoparathyroidism (Chap. 23), testicular feminization (Chap. 16), generalized resistance to thyroid hormone (Chap. 10), vitamin D–resistant rickets (Chap. 24), and type II diabetes mellitus (Chap. 19) are examples. Rarely recognized are states with features of hormone excess and normal to low hormone levels. A group of patients with the stigmata of primary aldosteronism and low plasma levels of aldosterone (Chap. 14) may fit this model. In low-renin essential hypertension, there may be an isolated feature of hormone hyperresponsiveness with increased sensitivity of adrenal glomerulosa aldosterone production to angiotensin II (Chap. 14). Normoprolactinemic galactorrhea is believed to result from increased breast sensitivity to prolactin (Chap. 8). The diseases cited above are due predominantly to specific genetic defects. In addition, cellular sensitivity to hormones is extensively regulated by the same (homologous) hormone and by other factors (Chap. 5); the most common feature is negative regulation of responsiveness by the homologous hormone. It is especially important to utilize this information when one is administering hormone therapy for endocrine or other diseases.

TYPES OF HORMONES AND THEIR SYNTHESIS AND RELEASE

A number of types of molecules have evolved to regulate body processes: peptides, lipids, and amino acid analogues all serve as hormones (Fig. 1-2). Sophisticated mechanisms have also evolved to synthesize these hormones. The types of hormones that exist and the mechanisms by which they are synthesized are discussed in detail in Chap. 4 and in the chapters on specific hormonal systems. These hormones and mechanisms of synthesis are discussed here only in outline form to provide perspective.

Peptide hormones vary in size, composition, number of chains, modification of groups, and mechanisms of production. Thus, whereas growth hormone is a single chain of 191 amino acids (Chaps. 8 and 26), TRH is a cyclized tripeptide with modified amino groups (Chaps. 4, 7, and 10). The glycoprotein hormones—thyroid stimulating hormone (TSH), luteinizing hormone (LH), follicle stimulating hormone (FSH), and chorionic gonadotropin (CG)—all have two peptide chains, one of which (α chain) is common to all, while the other (β chain) is unique for each member of the set (Chaps. 4 and 8). Insulin, by contrast, consists of two chains that are derived from a single gene product (preproinsulin) (Chaps. 4 and 19). Many hormones, such as corticotropin (ACTH; 39 amino acids), β-endorphin (29 amino acids), and insulin, are proteolytic products of a larger precursor protein (Chaps. 4, 7, and 8). Some hormones (e.g., FSH) are glycosylated, whereas others (e.g., ACTH in humans) are not (Chap. 4).

The steroid hormones and prostaglandins are derived from the lipids cholesterol and arachidonic acid, respectively (Chap. 4). They are synthesized through a series of reactions that modify their parent compounds.

The amino acid analogues include epinephrine, norepinephrine, dopamine (Chap. 13), and thyroid

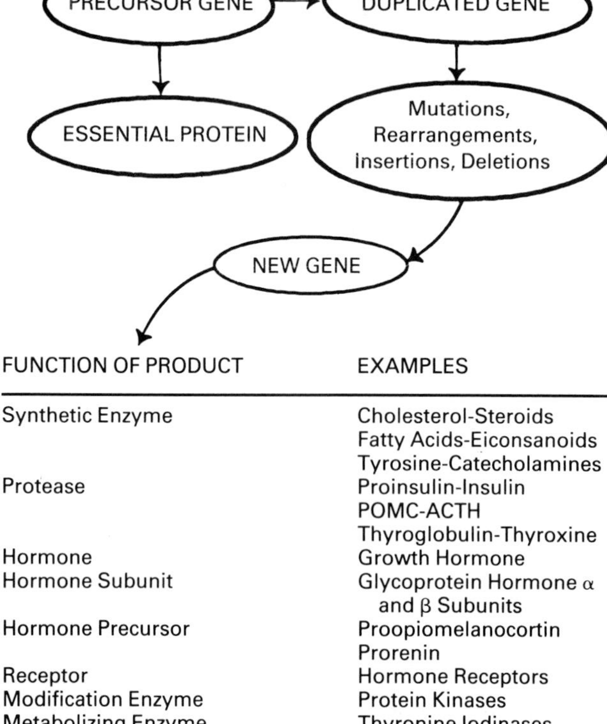

FUNCTION OF PRODUCT	EXAMPLES
Synthetic Enzyme	Cholesterol-Steroids Fatty Acids-Eiconsanoids Tyrosine-Catecholamines
Protease	Proinsulin-Insulin POMC-ACTH Thyroglobulin-Thyroxine
Hormone	Growth Hormone
Hormone Subunit	Glycoprotein Hormone α and β Subunits
Hormone Precursor	Proopiomelanocortin Prorenin
Receptor	Hormone Receptors
Modification Enzyme	Protein Kinases
Metabolizing Enzyme	Thyronine Iodinases

FIGURE 1-2 Evolution of the endocrine system. Genes encoding proteins that perform critical functions were duplicated. These duplicated genes then underwent rearrangements, deletions, mutations, and insertions, leading to derivative genes that perform the biosynthetic and regulatory functions of the endocrine system.

hormones (Chaps. 4 and 10), which are all derived from tyrosine, and 5-hydroxytryptamine, derived from tryptophan.

A variety of control mechanisms regulate hormone synthesis, release, and removal. In general, the fine-tuning of hormone levels involves influences on production and release, with the removal mechanisms showing less variation. There are marked variations in terms of the regulation of production and release. For example, with insulin, the pancreatic beta cells can store several days' supply of the hormones; the stimuli to insulin release (e.g., hyperglycemia) result in an early release that reflects the discharge of stored insulin, followed by a slower release associated with an increase in insulin production (Chap. 19). With steroids, by contrast, there is little storage of the hormone, and the stimuli to release increase the production of new hormone that is released relatively rapidly (Chap. 4).

In general, the endocrine glands secrete the form of the hormone that is active in the target tissue. However, in a few cases metabolic conversion in peripheral tissues results in the final active form of the hormone. For instance, testosterone, the major product of the testis, is converted to dihydrotestosterone in peripheral tissues (Chap. 16). The latter steroid is responsible for many (but not all) androgenic actions. Vitamin D, originating from the skin or diet, undergoes sequential hydroxylations in the liver and kidney to produce the final active hormone, 1,25-dihydroxycholecalciferol (Chap. 23). The major active thyroid hormone is triiodothyronine (T_3); the thyroid gland produces some T_3, but most of it comes from monodeiodination of thyroxine (T_4) to T_3 in the peripheral tissues (Chap. 10).

CIRCULATION OF HORMONES

The released hormone may circulate free or bound (Chap. 4). Some hormones circulate predominantly free or loosely associated with other proteins, whereas others circulate mostly bound to proteins (Chap. 4). In the latter case, transport proteins that bind the hormone with a high affinity sequester them. Thyroxine-binding globulin (TBG) binds thyroxine (Chap. 10), corticosteroid-binding globulin (CBG, or transcortin) binds cortisol (Chap. 12), sex hormone–binding globulin (SHBG) binds estradiol and testosterone (Chaps. 16 and 17), and several different IGF (insulin-like growth factor) binding proteins bind IGF (Chaps. 4 and 26). Much of the growth hormone (GH) in the circulation is bound by a GH binding protein that is identical to the extracellular portion of the GH receptor (Chaps. 8 and 26). For the tightly bound hormones, $>$ 90 percent of the total hormone in the circulation is ordinarily bound. By contrast, for a hormone such as aldosterone (Chap. 12), for which there is no specific transport protein, about 50 percent of the hormone is free in the circulation; the remainder is mostly loosely bound to albumin. The levels of the transport proteins can change under a variety of circumstances. For example, both TBG and CBG levels can be increased by estrogens. These changes can affect the total hormone levels, with important consequences for the clinical interpretation of measured hormone levels. Most of the other polypeptide hormones circulate predominantly in the free state (Chap. 4). A unique form of transport is observed with epidermal growth factor (EGF) and platelet-derived growth factor (PDGF), which are transported in platelets and released locally with platelet activation conditions (Chap. 4).

In general, the free rather than the plasma-bound hormones are biologically active. Further, control systems that regulate hormone levels do so by adjusting the free hormone, with only secondary effects on the plasma-bound hormone. The functions of the plasma binding proteins are just beginning to be understood (Chap. 4 and individual chapters). In general, they are not required for the transport of the hormones which are sufficiently soluble at physiologically active concentrations. An exception is cholesterol (usually not considered a hormone) that is transported in the plasma lipoproteins. That hormone transport proteins are generally important is suggested by the fact that they are present in numerous species (even if their levels vary) and that whereas genetic deficiencies in the proteins do occur, they tend not to result in a complete disappearance of the protein. A major function for them may be to regulate hormone distribution to the various tissues. For example, their sequestration of the hormones may prevent excessive hormone uptake as blood flows through proximal portions of the tissues; this will allow subsequent dissociation of bound hormone for uptake more distally. These proteins may also be important for the delivery of hormones to specialized sites. For example, CBG may help deliver cortisol to sites of inflammation (Chap. 12). IGF binding proteins may facilitate a continuous slow release of IGF-I that allows for IGF-I action without excessively down regulating the IGF-I receptors (Chap. 4). Plasma proteins also have a major effect in that they decrease the rate of clearance of the hormone from the plasma; this may be important for stabilizing hormone levels when this is desired. For example, this may be advantageous with thyroxine that has a half-life in the plasma of over 7 days because of its tight association with TBG (Chaps. 4 and 10).

HORMONE METABOLISM

Mechanisms for the clearance of released hormones from the circulation are critical for the regulation of hormone levels in response to various needs. Details of hormone metabolism are given in Chap. 4 and in the sections on individual hormones. The rate of clearance of different hormones varies enormously (Chap. 4), with half-lives ranging from a few minutes for polypeptide hormones such as angiotensin II (Chap. 14), insulin (Chap. 19), ACTH (Chap. 12), and epinephrine (Chap. 13), to minutes to hours for steroid and glycoprotein hormones (Chap. 4), to days for thyroxine (Chaps. 4 and 10). The time required for reaching a new steady state in response to changes in hormone release is dependent on the half-life of the hormone in the circulation. Therefore, a sudden release of a hormone will have much more marked effects if the hormone is cleared rapidly than it will if the hormone is cleared more slowly. For example, thyroxine, with its long plasma half-life, is involved in more long-term responses than are many hormones, and it may not be advantageous for the levels of this hormone to swing widely. Conversely, hormones such as angiotensin II and the catecholamines participate in more rapid responses, and their short half-lives in plasma facilitate the ability to achieve wide swings in their levels. The peptide hormones are mostly cleared by proteolytic destruction after their uptake by cells through internalization mechanisms (Chap. 4). Thyroid hormones, steroids, and catecholamines are metabolically altered inside tissues in which the products are recycled into general metabolic pathways (thyroid and catecholamine hormones) or excreted by the kidneys or the gastrointestinal tract (steroid hormones). Although hormone metabolism can be affected by a variety of factors, this in general is not regulated as extensively as are hormone synthesis and release. Nevertheless, such perturbations in hormone metabolism are sometimes clinically important. For example, the administration of drugs, such as barbiturates, that enhance steroid metabolism can influence the dose of administered glucocorticoid (Chap. 12), and the administration of thyroid hormone, which increases steroid clearance, can precipitate latent adrenal insufficiency (Chap. 12). Decreased clearance of insulin contributes to a decreased need for insulin in diabetes with renal failure (Chap. 19).

REGULATION OF HORMONE LEVELS

A variety of mechanisms regulate circulating hormone levels (Fig. 1-3), as discussed in the individual sections on specific hormones. Thus, there are mechanisms for (1) spontaneous, or basal, hormone release, (2) feedback inhibition by hormones of their synthesis and/or release, (3) stimulation or inhibition of hormone release by substances that may or may not be regulated by the same hormones, (4) establishment of circadian rhythms for hormone release by systems such as the brain, and (5) brain-mediated stimulation or inhibition of hormone release in response to anxiety anticipation of a specific activity, or other sensory inputs.

In some cases complex regulatory networks are present, whereas in other cases the endocrine cells are more independent. The first situation is illustrated by the axis that constitutes the hypothalamus, the anterior pituitary or adenohypophysis, and the target endocrine gland (Chaps. 8 and 12). Thus, the hypothalamus produces CRH, which travels down the portal vessels through the hypothalamic stalk to the anterior pituitary, where it stimulates ACTH release. ACTH then travels to the adrenal gland, where it stimulates the release of cortisol. Cortisol in turn inhibits both CRH and ACTH release (feedback inhibition). The brain establishes circadian rhythms and can trigger increased CRH release in response to stress. The pancreatic islets are an example of a more independent system (Chap. 19). Insulin release is regulated primarily by the levels of blood glucose, decreasing with hypoglycemia and increasing with glucose ingestion. However, hormones such as gastric inhibitory peptide and other substances such as specific amino acids (e.g., arginine) can also affect insulin release, as can stress

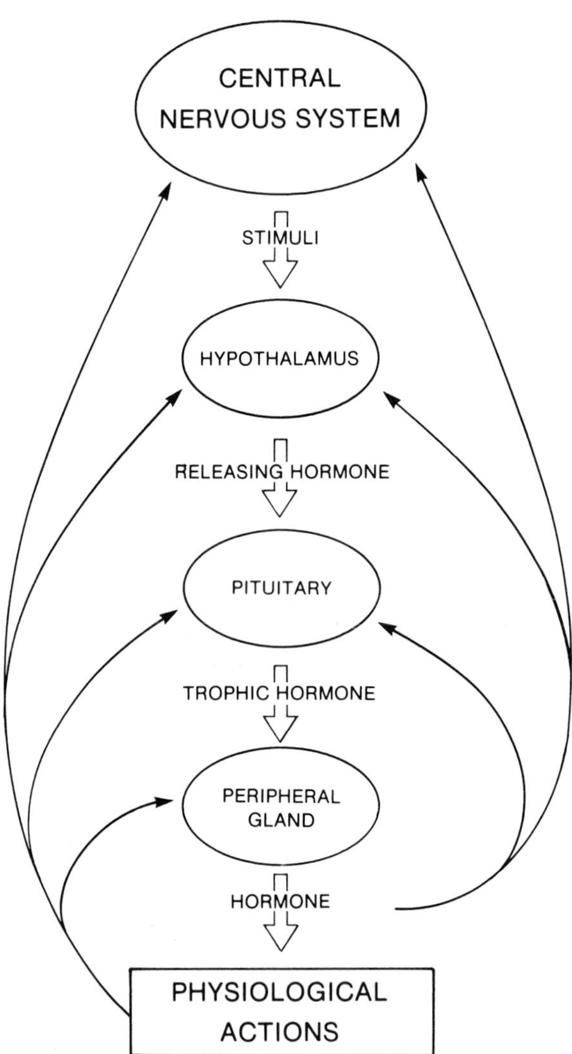

FIGURE 1-3 Organization of a set of endocrine glands, with interrelated regulatory elements. Shown is the flow of information from the central nervous system through the hypothalamus to the pituitary and then to the peripheral glands. Also indicated is that either the hormone product of the peripheral gland or the physiologic actions induced by the hormone can produce feedback inhibition of the stimuli to hormone release at any of several loci. As a rule, all the potential regulatory influences do not operate with respect to a given set of glands, nor do all the components shown operate for all endocrine glands. [*From Baxter JD, in Wyngaarden JB, Smith LH Jr (eds): Cecil's Textbook of Medicine. Philadelphia, Saunders, 1985, p 1221.*]

and trauma via signals from the autonomic nervous system.

HORMONE UPTAKE AND INTERNALIZATION

Various mechanisms account for the uptake of the different hormones by peripheral tissues. These mechanisms are discussed extensively in Chap. 5 and in the sections on individual hormones. The polypeptide and catecholamine hormones and the prostaglandins bind to receptors on the cell surface and are internalized (Chap. 5). The cell surface receptor–hormone interactions initiate the actions of these hormones (Chap. 5).

The internalization mechanism also serves to deliver some regulatory ligands into the cell for intracellular actions. Cholesterol is transported into the cell bound to lipoproteins and there inhibits cholesterol uptake (Chap. 22). Thyroid hormones also bind to surface sites and are internalized (Chaps. 5 and 10). Once inside the cell, the hormone binds to nuclear receptors and affects the transcription of particular genes. However, it is not known whether the internalization accounts for most or all of the uptake of thyroid hormones. The question of whether polypeptide hormones are internalized to act inside the cell is a subject of active inquiry, and proof that this is the case has not been provided (Chap. 5). Steroid hormones that act inside the cell appear to be capable of readily penetrating cells and do not require a specific internalization mechanism; the hydrophobic nature of these molecules may allow them essentially to dissolve in the cell membrane and reappear in the internal milieu of the cell.

MECHANISMS OF HORMONE ACTION

The mechanisms of hormone action are discussed in detail in Chap. 5. Peptide and catecholamine hormones and prostaglandins bind to receptors on the cell surface, where the hormone-receptor interactions affect intracellular mediators, or *second messengers*. The most extensively studied mechanism is the activation of the enzyme adenylyl cyclase by hormones such as beta-adrenergic agonists, ACTH, glucagon, and PTH. This enzyme catalyzes the conversion of adenosine triphosphate (ATP) to adenosine 3′,5′-monophosphate (cyclic AMP, or cAMP), which activates a particular serine and threonine kinase (A kinase). Phosphorylations induced by A kinase then alter the conformations of a diverse number of molecules, with consequent metabolic effects on cells. For example, such phosphorylations activate glycogenolysis through effects on specific enzymes and activate gene transcription by affecting particular transcription factors. Other hormone-receptor interactions, such as those involving insulin, alpha-adrenergic agents, and β-endorphin, can inhibit adenylyl cyclase. Tyrosine kinase can be activated by the action of hormones such as EGF and insulin. Many hormones promote an increase in intracellular calcium. This occurs with alpha-adrenergic agonists and angiotensin II. The calcium comes either from the extracellular fluid or from intracellular stores in organelles such as mitochondria or the sarcoplasmic reticulum. The calcium so released binds to calmodulin and other calcium-binding proteins, activating them to induce other metabolic effects, as on glycogenolysis, transport processes, steroidogenesis, and muscle contraction. In many cases, hormones stimulate the production and/or turnover of phospholipids. These effects can influence and cause increased calcium influx into the cytosol and can activate another serine and threonine kinase termed *C kinase*. Thus, these hormones utilize a variety of intracellular mediators, and a given hormone may utilize more than one of these (and other) pathways.

As was indicated earlier, steroid and thyroid hormones act for the most part by binding to intracellular receptors. Thyroid hormone receptors are associated with chromatin in the presence or absence of the hormone; the hormone-receptor interaction induces changes in the transcription of specific genes. Steroid receptors are either loosely associated or unassociated with chromatin in the absence of the hormone; steroid binding induces the receptor-steroid complexes to bind to specific sites on the DNA or to other transcription factors, where they affect the initiation of transcription of specific genes. The translation products of the steroid- or thyroid hormone–regulated mRNAs in turn have or represent metabolic effects on the cells. For example, thyroid hormones can increase the levels of beta-adrenergic receptors, with consequent effects on beta-adrenergic sensitivity, and glucocorticoids increase the levels of gluconeogenic enzymes, with subsequent increases in glucose production.

REGULATION OF HORMONE RESPONSIVENESS

Hormone responsiveness is regulated extensively (Chap. 5). A common pattern is down regulation resulting from the homologous hormone's induction of a decrease in the levels of its own receptors; this occurs with most polypeptide hormones, catecholamine-responsive systems, and prostaglandin responses and occurs occasionally with steroid and thyroid hormones. Less commonly, hormones may increase responsiveness to themselves by increasing their receptors (angiotensin II and its adrenal receptors). Hormones also regulate responsiveness by influencing postreceptor aspects of the response, and there are numerous situations in which hormones antagonize or enhance the responses to other hormones by affecting receptors or postreceptor responses. For example, estrogens increase progesterone receptors, and glucocorticoids in the liver affect the actions of epinephrine and glucagon at postreceptor loci. Thus, in the clinical assessment of a given state, not only hormone levels but also hormone responsiveness must be considered.

CLASSIFICATION OF HORMONE ACTION

Considered superficially, it might seem simple to classify hormone action. Glucocorticoid action would include all actions of glucocorticoids; insulin action would include all actions of insulin, etc. However, using these hormones as examples, it will be seen that the situation is not so simple. Many glucocorticoid actions *are* typical of glucocorticoids, such as the induction of gluconeogenesis and glycogen deposition in liver, but in other cases glucocorticoids can affect sodium transport in a manner similar to aldosterone (Chap. 12). Similarly, many of the actions of insulin are typical for insulin, such as those which lower the blood sugar, but in other cases insulin can act analogously to IGF-I (Chaps. 5 and 19). These apparent paradoxes occur because cortisol can bind to the mineralocorticoid receptors that have a higher affinity for aldosterone and more typically mediate aldosterone action, and insulin can bind to IGF-I receptors that have a higher affinity for IGF-I.

Fortunately, pharmacologists have dealt with this problem and have developed a simple basis for classifying drugs that is also applicable to hormones. This classification is based on the receptors rather than the hormone. A given glass of action is defined as those actions which are mediated through a given type of receptor. Thus, epinephrine action, rather than including all actions mediated by epinephrine, is defined by the type of receptor that mediates the effect. Epinephrine can have actions through β_1- or β_2-adrenergic receptors or through α_1 or α_2 receptors (Chaps. 5 and 13). Similarly, cortisol can have actions mediated through glucocorticoid or mineralocorticoid receptors, and insulin can have actions mediated through insulin or IGF-I receptors.

EVOLUTION OF THE ENDOCRINE SYSTEM

The evolution of each of the various endocrine systems has involved the assimilation of a number of individual components whose functioning is coordinated in an effective manner (Fig. 1-2). These components include the hormone itself and means for regulating its concentrations and responding to it. It is likely that the roots of these systems are found in simpler regulatory systems that preceded them. The discussions that follow, although speculative, provide a conceptual framework for further thinking on the subject.

Simple and Complex Regulation

Tomkins classified regulation within cells as simple or complex.[7] With simple regulation, the reactants or products in a metabolic pathway regulate enzymatic or other processes important for that pathway. Such regulation is illustrated by feedback inhibition of an enzyme by products of the reaction. If regulation were limited to simple mechanisms, survival might be tenuous, since the regulatory ligands themselves are important intermediaries, and large changes in their concentrations might imperil the organism. Thus, there was a need for more complex regulation involving the use of regulatory ligands that are neither reactants nor products of the processes they regulate. Such ligands therefore may not have any obvious relation to the chemicals involved in the pathway. For example, cAMP regulates the metabolism of glucose and glycogen (Chaps. 5 and 19) but differs chemically from these carbohydrates.

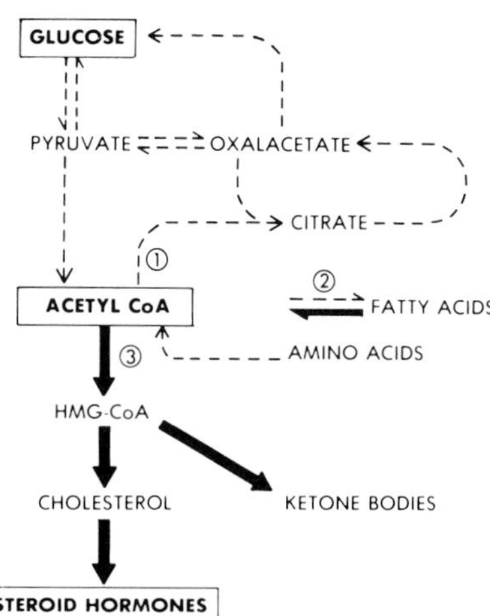

FIGURE 1-4 Metabolic interrelations of glucose, acetyl CoA, and steroid hormones. Numbers indicate the three major fates of acetyl CoA. The bold and dashed arrows indicate, respectively, the more dominant and the minor metabolic pathways under conditions of glucose starvation. HMG CoA = hydroxymethylglutaryl CoA. [*From Baxter and Rousseau.*[8]]

Origin of Hormones and Other Regulatory Ligands

Regulatory ligands of the endocrine system include hormones, second-messenger mediators of hormone-receptor interactions (Chap. 5), and extraneous factors. For a ligand to assume a role in complex regulation, its concentration should change in response to conditions that would benefit from its actions. Tomkins proposed that the concentrations of regulatory ligands such as cAMP can be varied in response to such conditions because they are by-products rather than important intermediates.[7] As such, their production rates can vary when other factors affected the major pathways. ATP is ordinarily converted to ADP or AMP. This reaction is frequently linked to other reactions, such as the conversion of glucose to glucose-6-phosphate. Tomkins speculated that glucose deprivation might therefore diminish both phosphorylation of glucose and conversion of ATP to ADP. In this circumstance, more ATP might be degraded by alternative pathways, as by conversion to cAMP. As a consequence, cAMP could become a "symbol" of insufficient glucose availability in that it would accumulate when levels of the sugar decreased.

The production of hormones may also have been first regulated in response to changes in cellular conditions.[8] For example, steroid hormone production may have been affected when cellular events altered the synthesis, metabolism, or utilization of cholesterol, which is a precursor to all the steroid hormones.[8] The incorporation of cholesterol into membranes is associated with cell growth. When growth is affected, there is altered utilization of cholesterol and potential changes in its conversion to other molecular species such as the steroid hormones. Thus steroids might have evolved into symbols for regulating cell growth. Other factors might also have increased steroid production. For instance (Fig. 1-4), it is possible that with decreased carbohydrate utilization and consequent decreased generation of pyruvate, there would be impaired utilization of acetyl CoA for oxidation through the citric acid cycle and for lipogenesis.[8] This might affect the pathway acetyl CoA → cholesterol → steroids. Such events might explain how glucocorticoids came to symbolize glucose deprivation and take on roles such as enhancing the production and availability of glucose (Chap. 12).

Analogous speculations can be extended to the other hormones. Thyroid and catecholamine hormones are by-products of tyrosine (Chaps. 10 and 13), and their production may have first been regulated by circumstances that affected the metabolism of this amino acid or amino acids in general. Many of the polypeptide hormones and thyroid hormones are derived from the cleavage of large proteins, and variations in their production may have had their origins in events that affected the metabolism of proteins in general or the specific precursor proteins. The genes for these precursor proteins may have evolved from genes that encoded proteins critical for cellular structure or metabolism (Fig. 1-2). Similarly, the genes encoding polypeptide hormones that make up an entire gene may have been derived from an evolutionary precursor gene that served an essential cellular function.

Of course, not all symbols for metabolic control are regulated by simply increasing their synthesis. Ions such as Ca^{2+}, Mg^{2+}, K^{+}, and Cl^{-} are used extensively in the regulation of homeostasis (Chap. 5). In these cases, rather than creating the ions, changes in metabolism could alter their concentrations in specific cellular compartments (cytosol, mitochondria, sarcoplasmic reticulum, etc.). For instance, lack of glucose or other substrate could result in a lack of ATP or other substances which would affect the activity of transport systems involved in the maintenance of ion-concentration gradients across membranes. The ions could then take on regulatory functions by interacting with proteins that evolved as described above.

Origin of Receptors and Other Mediators of Regulatory Ligand Actions

Once mechanisms were established to regulate the concentrations of a ligand by means of appropriate stimuli, there was a need for the ligand to develop means to affect the appropriate metabolic pathway(s). To do this, the ligand must interact with other molecules in the cell. Binding proteins for products such as cAMP were probably already present by the time these ligands appeared, since enzymes that bound their precursors had to be present to form the ligand.[7] If these proteins could be modified to have activities that affected the metabolic pathway and if these activities were stimulated by binding of the ligand, elements for the complex regulation would be established. Genetic events such as mutation, deletion of gene sequences, and the insertion of additional gene sequences would allow the genes for such proteins ultimately to produce a molecule with the needed regulatory properties. These mechanisms are described in more detail in Chap. 3. There would be a selective advantage for any cells containing such regulatory proteins, as they would help the cell respond to overcome the original problem (e.g., glucose deprivation) that stimulated the production of the regulatory ligand. For example, in *Escherichia coli* cAMP accumulates when there is a low concentration of glucose.[7] The nucleotide binds to a regulatory protein, and the complex then stimulates the production of enzymes that metabolize other carbohydrates, such as galactose and lactose. These actions provide the organism an alternative carbohydrate source in the absence of glucose. Thus cAMP, a key mediator in hormone action and neurotransmission in humans, developed as a regulator of metabolism in much lower species.

In mammals, cAMP binds to regulatory subunits that in the absence of cAMP associate with and inhibit the activity of a specific protein kinase (Chap. 5). The binding of cAMP promotes dissociation of the regulatory subunits from the catalytic subunits, which are then active.

Regulatory proteins, or receptors in this case, have also evolved to bind hormones specifically and to transmit this information into postreceptor events. For example, the binding of steroid hormones to their receptors induces conformational changes that stimulate the receptors to bind to specific DNA sequences and influence the transcription of specific genes (Chap. 5).

To gain such specialized and highly specific functions, the genes encoding these proteins have had to evolve to obtain the critical structures (Chap. 3). In some cases, other genes evolved to express products that modify these proteins (e.g., through glycosylation, phosphorylation, or proteolysis). Since the evolution of genes has apparently occurred by mechanisms such as mutation of preexisting genes and recombination of pieces from different genes (mentioned above), some constraints are placed on the way proteins can evolve. Therefore, it has probably been simpler evolutionarily to modify preexisting structures than to create entirely new genes. It may not then be surprising that there is some homology in the amino acid sequences of diverse proteins, because their genes may have arisen by evolution from common precursor genes. Since, as pointed out earlier, binding sites on proteins for regulatory ligands such as cAMP and steroids or their analogues must have existed by the time these ligands appeared, it is easy to see how modification of the genes for these proteins could result in other proteins with high binding specificity for the regulatory ligand.

Diversification of Families of Hormones

Once a given regulatory molecule became established, there was probably evolutionary pressure to preserve it. There might also be an opportunity for the molecule to extend its domain. For example, a hormone that increased in concentration in response to stress might be recruited to elicit additional responses that would relieve the stress. These responses would be recruited by mechanisms similar to those described in the preceding sections. Thus, angiotensin II stimulates not only vascular constriction but also aldosterone release, with consequent effects that conserve sodium (Chap. 12). Conversely, variants of the initial hormone might be produced, and with time they might take on one set of the responses while leaving other responses to the original hormone. Thus, cortisol and aldosterone are both released in response to stress, yet they elicit different sets of responses that help in the adjustment to stress (Chap. 12). These influences would therefore result in the diversification of hormones and their responses.

EVOLUTION OF THE ENDOCRINE GLANDS

As multicellular organisms evolved, cells began to secrete proteins and other ligands that could act on other cells. In many circumstances communication between cells in close proximity was adequate. However, as more complex forms of life evolved, it became necessary to have the more elaborate diversification that now exists for the specialized cells of the nervous and endocrine systems; these cells release regulatory signals that act at more distant sites.

The central nervous system (CNS) has emerged as dominant in regulating and coordinating bodily functions; many processes are regulated by direct nerve-to-cell contact. In simpler forms of life (invertebrates) the CNS communicates directly with all peripheral cells.[9,10] This mechanism is inadequate for survival of the more complex and highly developed species.

The next step in complexity, the release of regulatory molecules to act at more distant loci, apparently became necessary as direct nerve-to-cell contact became impractical. The first process to evolve may have been direct neurosecretion of hormones from the CNS or from specialized effectors developed as outgrowths of nerve endings. The former is represented by the direct release of neurosecretory granules from invertebrate nerve cells as described by Ernst Scharrer,[10] and the latter by cells of the posterior pituitary which secrete vasopressin (Chap. 9) and cells of the adrenal medulla that secrete epinephrine (Chap. 13). In a parallel manner, cells of neural crest origin with neurosecretory elements migrated to various other parts of the body, generally in association with the foregut and midgut and their outpouchings, resulting in CNS-like cells secreting the same neurotransmitters or peptides.[11,12] This provides an explanation of the presence of somatostatin, vasoactive intestinal peptide (VIP), neurotensin, substance P, etc., in both the CNS (Chap. 7) and the gut and pancreas (Chap. 27), the neurosecretory granule-containing Kulchitsky's cells in the bronchi, and the paraendocrine amine precursor uptake and decarboxylation (APUD) cells (Chap 7).[11]

The possible need for higher concentrations of many hormones at particular locations—cortisol acting on phenylethanolamine *N*-methyl transferase (PNMT) in the adrenal medulla (Chap. 13), testosterone acting on spermatogenesis in the testis (Chap. 16), estrogen acting on corpus luteum formation (Chap. 17), and insulin and glucagon regulating hepatic glucose regulation (Chap. 19)—may have required the location of glands that secrete them in areas distant from the CNS. An additional means for the control of these glands evolved with those hormones which could be produced near the CNS and be more readily placed under its control. Thus, the anterior pituitary developed in close proximity to the CNS so that its hormones could be under the control of the releasing-factor hormones synthesized in the brain (Chaps. 7 and 8).

Two other evolutionary processes occurred which helped integrate the endocrine system. First, the appearance of portal vascular systems, hepatic (Chap. 27) and hypophyseal (Chaps. 7 and 8), permitted the localization of hormone action on the basis of concentration as well as the specificity of tissue receptors. Second, varying degrees of susceptibility of hormones to degradation by plasma played an important role in limiting or extending the duration of their effects (discussed above).

INTEGRATION OF THE ENDOCRINE SYSTEM

The maintenance of homeostasis in multicellular organisms requires simultaneous and coordinated monitoring of a number of functions. For instance, a fright response that may involve muscular activity requires recruitment of the musculoskeletal system. To support this, the pulmonary and cardiovascular systems must also be prepared. For all this, energy sources must be mobilized in a manner that does not compromise critical functions. Thus, mechanisms have evolved to release glucose from glycogen, increase glucose production, stimulate alternative pathways to obtain energy (e.g., through mobilization of stored fat), and decrease glucose consumption by tissues that are not in immediate need of the substrate. The endocrine system contributes to these types of controls through (1) integrated sets of responses to each hormone, (2) coordination of simultaneous responses by several hormones, (3) counterbalancing influences by other hormones, and (4) mechanisms for terminating or attenuating the response.

Integrated Actions of a Given Class of Hormone

As discussed earlier, there may be a selective advantage for hormones to regulate simultaneously several different processes that together lead to a given result. Thus, hormones typically stimulate integrated sets of responses. Several simultaneous responses can be stimulated within a given cell, and responses can be stimulated in multiple organs, as was described above for angiotensin II. Glucocorticoids are also illustrative in terms of their fuel-metabolizing and catabolic effects. These steroids enhance gluconeogenesis and glucose production in the liver, decrease glucose uptake in peripheral tissues, enhance protein breakdown, and decrease protein synthesis in fat, muscle, and lymphoid and fibroblastic tissues (Chap. 12). They also stimulate lipolysis (Chap. 12). These actions together increase the blood glucose concentration at the expense of substrate in certain tissues. This glucose is made available for immediate use by other tissues and in particular by the brain, whose continuous function is crucial for survival and is dependent specifically on glucose as a substrate; the brain is not a target for the catabolic actions of the glucocorticoids (Chap. 12).

Hormone Synergisms: Recruitment of Multiple Hormones for Coordinated Responses

The endocrine system has evolved so that particular stimuli can affect more than one hormone simultaneously. The actions of these hormones may be complementary. For example, several classes of hormone (e.g., epinephrine, glucagon, glucocorticoids, growth hormone) are involved in glucose conservation (Chaps. 8, 12, 13, and 19). They increase blood glucose levels by stimulating increases in glucose synthesis, decreases in glucose utilization in certain tissues, and mobilization of substrates that are precursors for glucose synthesis (e.g., glycerol and lactate) or alternative sources of energy (e.g., free fatty acids). The concerted effects of these hormones are greater than those of any single hormone. The plasma concentrations of all these hormones are increased with severe hypoglycemia, although in ordinary physiologic circumstances the blood glucose concentration is not the major regulator of epinephrine, growth hormone, and glucocorticoid production. Catecholamines (Chap. 13), vasopressin (Chap. 9), angiotensin II (Chaps. 12 and 14), glucocorticoids (Chap. 12), mineralocorticoids (Chap. 12), and other hormones are released in response to shock. These hormones increase vascular reactivity, conserve sodium, stimulate cardiac function, and elicit other actions that are useful in compensating for the insult.

Hormone Antagonisms: Fine-Tuning of Metabolism

In many cases responses to hormones are countered by other hormones. This provides capabilities in addition to those derived from the removal of a hormone. For instance, insulin opposes the glucose-elevating properties of epinephrine, glucagon, glucocorticoids, alpha-adrenergic agonists, and growth hormone (Chap. 19). It stimulates glucose uptake in fat and glycogen synthesis. It inhibits glucose synthesis, lipolysis, and glycogenolysis. Further, it stimulates protein synthesis and inhibits protein breakdown. Progesterone inhibits some actions of estrogens (Chap. 17). Calcitonin tends to lower the serum [Ca^{2+}], wherease PTH tends to elevate concentrations of the ion (Chap. 23).

These antagonisms do not always extend to all responses. For instance, although insulin's actions are mostly antagonistic to the actions of the glucocorticoids, both classes of hormones tend to enhance glycogen accumulation (Chaps. 12 and 19). The α- and β-adrenergic agonists both increase glycogenolysis and gluconeogenesis, although the two classes of hormones can have opposing influences on vascular (Chap. 13), muscular (Chap. 13), and hormonal (e.g., insulin) (Chap. 19) secretory responses. The fact that two classes of hormones can be synergistic for some responses and antagonistic for others can commonly be explained in terms of the individual needs the hormones serve.

Mechanisms for Attenuating or Terminating the Response

These responses are attenuated or terminated by a variety of mechanisms. First, most hormones, particularly stress hormones, are cleared rapidly from the circulation so that when secretion ceases, the response disappears rapidly. Second, many hormones exert feedback inhibition of their own release. These inhibitory actions occur typically through actions of other hormones secreted in response to the initial hormone (e.g., blockage of TSH release by thyroid hormone; Chap. 10) or through sequelae of the hormone's action (e.g., PTH-induced increases in Ca^{2+} levels block PTH release). Third, as already discussed, hormones can induce a decrease in sensitivity to their actions. Finally, other hormones secreted simultaneously can blunt the responses; for example, a role of glucocorticoids released in stress may be to blunt the actions or secretions of other hormones (Chap. 12).

ACTIONS OF HORMONES

Hormones affect essentially all types of body processes. Several of the more prominent types of influence among the numerous actions merit particular emphasis.

Intermediary Metabolism and Growth

A number of different hormones regulate intermediary metabolism and growth. Thus, glucocorticoids, catecholamines, prostaglandin E_1, and glucagon tend to promote the availability and/or mobilization of glucose and other fuels and, in some cases, tissue catabolism and antianabolism (Chap. 19). Glucocorticoids (in excess) also inhibit growth (Chap. 12). Insulin and certain growth factors, including IGFs, tend to have varying degrees of growth-promoting and fuel-storing actions (Chap. 19). Androgens, progestins, and estrogens are growth factors (Chaps. 16 and 17), although progesterone at a physiologic level can antagonize the effects of estrogens (Chap. 17). Growth hormone, prolactin, and placental lactogen tend to be growth-promoting, although the growth responses may be due in part to stimulation of the production of growth factors such as IGF-I (Chaps. 8 and 26). In addition, many actions of growth hormone and chorionic somatomammotropin, independent of those mediated secondarily by IGF-I, are more of the fuel-mobilizing type, with a tendency to stimulation of hyperglycemia, increased lipolysis, etc. (Chap. 19). Interestingly, many surface-active hormones of the fuel-mobilizing group activate adenylyl cyclase, whereas those of the growth-stimulating fuel-storage group commonly do not do this (Chap. 5). Thus, as in bacteria, cAMP is used for mobilization of carbohydrate.

Highly Specific Functions

Tropic Actions

Integration of the endocrine system has required the evolution of hormones termed tropic hormones that specifically regulate glands specialized for the production of other hormones. Thus, TSH regulates thyroid hormone production (Chaps. 8 and 10), CG regulates progesterone production (Chap. 17), FSH regulates follicular and Sertoli cell maturation (Chaps. 16 and 17), LH regulates progesterone production in the female (Chap. 17) and testosterone production in the male (Chap. 16), ACTH regulates glucocorticoid production (Chaps. 7, 8, and 12), and angiotensin regulates aldosterone production (Chaps. 12 and 14). Although these tropic hormones may play additional roles (e.g., angiotensin II), for the most part the number of target tissues for these classes of hormones is restricted. In many cases these hormones activate adenylyl cyclase, but some of them (angiotensin II) apparently do not (Chap. 5).

Mineral and Water Metabolism

Aldosterone, vasopressin, PTH, calcitonin, and vitamin D are hormones that have the specialized functions of regulating ion and water concentrations (Chaps. 9, 12, 14, and 23). There is diversity in their mechanisms of action, and the target tissue distribution for each class of these hormones is rather restricted. However, these are not the only hormones that affect fluid and electrolyte metabolism, which is also influenced by insulin, glucagon, glucocorticoids, catecholamines, and others (Chaps. 12–14 and 19).

Cardiovascular Functions

The atrium of the heart devotes more of its protein synthetic efforts to producing a hormone, atrial natriuretic factor, than to producing any other protein, and this hormone has extensive effects on the cardiovascular system (Chap. 14). Numerous other hormones affect cardiovascular function and blood pressure. These include the catecholamines (Chaps. 13 and 14), endothelin, (Chap. 14), thyroid hormone (Chaps. 10 and 14), angiotensin II (Chaps. 12 and 14), mineralocorticoids (Chaps. 12 and 14), bradykinin (Chaps. 14 and 31), and the sex steroids (Chaps. 16 and 17). Most of these hormones also have other important metabolic actions for which they are predominantly known (e.g., glucocorticoids, sex steroids). The fact that they also regulate cardiovascular responses underscores the importance of the endocrine system in responding to numerous physiologic and pathologic perturbations. Further, many elements of these systems are predominantly under CNS control by catecholamines and acetylcholine released at nerve endings.

Reproductive Functions

Hormones are dominant in the control of reproductive functions, as is evidenced by the lack of reproductive capacity in their absence (Chaps. 16–18). Thus, the gonadotropins of pituitary (LH, FSH; Chaps. 8, 16, and 17) or placental origin (CG; Chaps. 8 and 17) play important roles in regulating reproductive organs such as the ovary and testes, which in turn produce hormones such as the sex steroids (androgens, estrogens, and progestins). These steroids control functions critical for pregnancy and for sexual differentiation and development and influence secondary sexual characteristics such as voice, hair, and muscular development as well as sexual behavior to some extent.

Developmental Actions

Hormones play a crucial role in extrauterine growth and development. The sex steroids (Chaps. 16 and 17); insulin (Chap. 19); other growth factors and hormones such as fibroblast growth factor (FGF), PDGF, EGF, and transforming growth factors (TGFs) (Chaps. 4, 5, 7–13, 16, 17, 19, 26–30); thyroid hormone (Chap. 10); and glucocorticoids (Chap. 12) are all important in this respect. Sometimes the effects are predominantly on growth, as illustrated by dwarfism due to growth hormone deficiency and gigantism due to growth hormone excess (Chaps. 8 and 26). In other cases the influences are on development, as illustrated by the pseudohermaphroditism associated with insensitivity to androgens (Chap. 18). In yet others the effects are on growth and development, as illustrated by the lack of growth and brain development in cretinism (Chaps. 10 and 26). In fact, most of the hormones mentioned here are important at some stage for development. In some cases (e.g., growth hormone) it is not clear that the hormone is even needed in the adult, even though its metabolic effects can be classified with those hormones affecting intermediary metabolism.

DISORDERS OF THE ENDOCRINE SYSTEM

Endocrinology has traditionally been signal-level-oriented, concerning itself largely with whether hormones are secreted appropriately or inappropriately (i.e., in excess or deficiency). Most recognizable disorders of the endocrine system are due to an excess or a deficiency of particular hormones, whether caused by abnormalities of endocrine glands, ectopic production of hormones, abnormal conversion of prohormones to their active forms, or iatrogenic factors. However, endocrine abnormalities may also be due to changes in the responses (either enhanced or diminished) of target tissues to hormones. These disorders can occur by a variety of mechanisms (Fig. 1-5).

Hormone Deficiency Syndromes

Hypofunction of Endocrine Glands

Endocrine glands may be injured or destroyed by neoplasia, infections, hemorrhage, autoimmune disorders, and other causes. The destruction may be

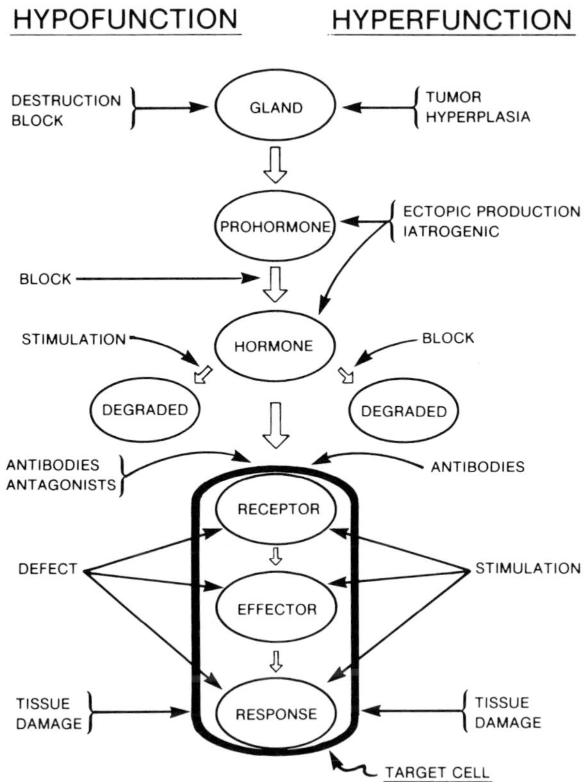

FIGURE 1-5 Causes of hypofunction or hyperfunction of the endocrine system. [*From Baxter JD, in Wyngaarden JB, Smith LH Jr (eds): Cecil's Textbook of Medicine. Philadelphia, Saunders, 1985, p. 1220.*]

acute but is commonly chronic, with normal basal hormone production occurring until late in the disease. The gland is usually compromised in its reserve capacity before the basal level of secretion falls, and it cannot respond normally in circumstances in which an increase in hormone production is needed. Such partial defects may therefore not be detected by measurement of basal hormone levels and may require other testing of the reserve function of the gland. Since many manifestations of endocrine disease require weeks or months to develop, the clinical presentation may vary over a considerable range, depending on the rapidity of glandular destruction.

As would be expected, a deficiency of a hormone that controls the synthesis and release of another hormone may result in a syndrome which simulates a primary deficiency of that target organ. Thus, hypothalamic lesions resulting in impaired secretion of releasing hormones may be manifested by pituitary dysfunction, which in turn may result in abnormalities in the function of its various target organs (gonads, thyroid, adrenals) (Chaps. 7 and 8).

Genetic defects can cause endocrine hypofunction, usually because of abnormalities in hormone synthesis and rarely because of the production of an abnormal hormone (as documented for insulin in rare forms of diabetes mellitus) (Chap. 19). These genetic defects in hormone synthesis may be partial or complete. For example, a rare form of growth hormone deficiency is due to deletion of the growth hormone gene (Chap. 26). A partial defect may be somewhat analogous to incomplete destruction of the gland; i.e., basal hormone production may be normal, but the reserve may be inadequate. In fact, genetic defects sometimes present not with the problems of hormone deficiency but with manifestations of a compensatory adaptation. For example, partial blocks in thyroid hormone biosynthesis may result in an enlarged thyroid gland (goiter) that is due to TSH hypersecretion resulting from low levels of thyroid hormone (Chaps. 10 and 11). In the 17α-hydroxylase deficiency syndrome there is defective cortisol production and consequent ACTH hypersecretion, with excessive production of adrenocorticosteroids that are not 17α-hydroxylated (Chap. 12). One of these, corticosterone, substitutes for cortisol, and so manifestations of cortisol deficiency are not observed. By contrast, excessive compensatory synthesis of corticosterone and deoxycorticosterone leads to a mineralocorticoid excess syndrome with hypertension and hypokalemia.

Hormone Deficiency Secondary to Extraglandular Disorders

Extraglandular disorders can result in hormone deficiency. They may involve defective conversion of prohormones to active forms, enhanced degradation of hormones, or the production of substances (antibodies, hormone antagonists) that block the actions of hormones. Impaired conversion of a prohormone to a hormone occurs in chronic renal failure and in vitamin D–dependent rickets type 1, in which there is defective conversion of 25-hydroxycholecalciferol to 1,25-dihydroxycholecalciferol (Chap. 23). A rare form of androgen deficiency is due to an abnormality in 5α-reductase, which converts testosterone to dihydrotestosterone (Chap. 18). In this condition there is only partial loss of androgenic effects, since testosterone itself is weakly active in some target tissues. Rare forms of diabetes mellitus result from antibodies to the insulin receptor that block insulin action (Chap. 19). Antibodies to insulin develop during insulin therapy for diabetes; when excessive, these antibodies may affect the availability of insulin (Chap. 19). Although no primary disorders are known to be due to enhanced hormone degradation, this may vary with other factors or disease states and may affect the response to exogenously administered hormones; for example, phenytoin and thyroid hormone increase the metabolism of certain glucocorticoids (Chap. 12). Also, such influences may unmask or aggravate a partial hormonal deficiency; for example, the administration of thyroid hormones may unmask latent Addison's disease (Chap. 12).

Hyporesponsiveness to Hormones

Hormone levels may be normal or even elevated in the presence of manifestations of endocrine deficiency. These conditions may be due to some of the problems listed above, e.g., antibodies to the insulin receptor (Chap. 19) and abnormal conversion of testosterone to dihydrotestosterone (Chap. 18). They may also be due to decreased ability of the endocrine target gland to respond to the hormone. Such disorders may be acquired or genetic and may be due to abnormalities at any step in the cascade of the hormone response from the receptor to the effect generated.

Several syndromes are associated with receptor abnormalities. The most commonly recognized abnormality of this type occurs in obese patients with type II diabetes mellitus (Chap. 19). In this case chronic hyperinsulinemia induced by increased food intake induces insulin resistance, in part by down regulating the concentration of insulin receptors. Recognition of this problem also affects the therapy, since treatment is directed not only at correcting the hyperglycemia with insulin or other drugs but also at decreasing insulin need by means of dietary maneuvers that secondarily decrease insulin levels and thus restore tissue sensitivity to the hormones. This form of diabetes also exhibits an additional abnormality by which the pancreatic islets do not release insulin normally in response to glucose. In the testicular feminization syndrome there is unresponsiveness to androgens (Chap. 18). As a consequence, a female phenotype occurs in a person with a male genotype. Most persons with this X-linked disorder have a defect in the androgen receptor.

Hyporesponsiveness may also be due to postreceptor abnormalities. In pseudohypoparathyroidism there is frequently an abnormality in the coupling of hormone-receptor complexes to effector mechanisms. Patients with the disorder have symptoms and chemical derangements of hypoparathyroidism associated with elevated PTH levels and insensitivity to this hormone (Chap. 23). In some of these patients this insensitivity is due to decreased levels of the guanyl nucleotide-binding regulatory protein that couples the PTH receptor complex to adenylyl cyclase because of mutations in the gene encoding the α subunit of this protein. Much of the insulin resistance of type II diabetes mellitus is due to postreceptor abnormalities.

Overall damage to the hormone target tissue may result in insensitivity to hormones. For instance, renal disease may lead to insensitivity to vasopressin (Chap. 9), and liver disease may lead to insensitivity to glucagon (Chap. 19).

Abnormal Production or Administration of Antagonists

Rarely, endogenously produced or exogenously administered substances may produce a hormone-deficient state. Antibodies to the insulin receptor may produce insulin resistance with functional insulinopenia (Chap. 19). Cimetidine given for peptic ulcer disease[13] and spironolactone given for hypertension (Chap. 14) may act as androgen antagonists and produce an androgen-deficient state.

Hormone Excess Syndromes

Hormone excess syndromes may result from hyperfunctioning endocrine glands, from ectopic hormone production by tumors, less commonly from influences on target tissues that enhance hormone sensitivity, from autoimmune disease in which antibodies cause hypersecretion of hormones or act as hormone agonists, from defects in hormone biosynthesis in which precursor hormones produced in excess have deleterious consequences, and from the iatrogenic or therapeutic administration of hormones or substances that act like hormones.

Hyperfunction of Endocrine Glands

The most common cause of hormone excess syndromes is hyperfunction of endocrine glands secondary to tumors of the glands or hyperplasia of several causes. Hyperfunctioning tumors of endocrine glands are usually well-differentiated adenomas (although carcinomas also occur).

Hyperplasia is a cause of the hyperfunctioning of several of the endocrine glands (thyroid, adrenals, parathyroids). The most common form of thyroid hyperplasia appears to be due to an immunologic abnormality in which antibodies stimulate the gland in a manner similar to TSH (Chap. 10). Hyperplasia of the zona fasciculata and zona reticularis of the adrenal with consequent cortisol hypersecretion is usually due to ACTH hypersecretion by a pituitary tumor or an ectopic hormone-secreting tumor (Chaps. 12 and 29). Chief cell hyperplasia of parathyroid glands with PTH hypersecretion most commonly occurs as a genetic defect of an undetermined nature (Chap. 23). The cause in other cases of endocrine gland hyperplasia is less clear, as with hyperplasia of the adrenal zona glomerulosa resulting in excessive aldosterone production (Chap. 14).

Ectopic Hormone Production

Sometimes hormones are produced in excess by cells of endocrine or nonendocrine origin that are not normally the primary source of a hormone (Chap. 29). In most cases, hormones produced ectopically by tumors are those which arise from a single gene (e.g., ACTH, growth hormone, prolactin, PTH, calcitonin, gastrin, erythropoietin) or two genes (CG). This may be due to the fact that the synthesis of other hormones (e.g., steroids, thyroid hormones, catecholamines) requires a large number of genes not ordinarily expressed by the tumor which need to be activated to produce the hormone. Although a large number of different types of tumors can produce hormones, specific cell types are more commonly involved in this process (Chap. 29). For instance, APUD cells are commonly associated with ectopic hormone production. These cells are found in small-cell carcinoma of the lung, carcinoid tumors, thymomas, and other tumors. Although a number of molecular mechanisms are now understood that could explain how genes that are ordinarily not expressed are activated in tumors, those actually causing ectopic hormone production are not well understood.

Hormone Administration

Hormone excess states may occur when hormones are used to treat nonendocrine diseases, hormone replacement therapy is excessive or patients self-administer hormones (or their analogues). Patients sometimes take excessive doses of glucocorticoids (Chap. 12) or thyroxine (Chap. 10) because those hormones produce a feeling of well-being. Rarely, administration of nonhormonal substances can cause hormonelike effects. Licorice ingestion can produce a syndrome mimicking primary aldosteronism, for example (Chap. 14).

Tissue Hypersensitivity

Endocrine excess syndromes caused by hypersensitivity of target tissues are uncommon. Thyroid hormones increase the catecholamine receptors in certain tissues and thus lead to excessive beta-adrenergic stimulation (Chap. 10). In this case, the hyperresponsiveness is actually part of the syndrome of hyperthyroidism. Manifestations of primary aldosteronism occur in a rare syndrome with low plasma renin and aldosterone levels in which the kidney responds as if it were being excessively stimulated by aldosterone (Chap. 14). Finally, disease of the target tissue itself can render it excessively sensitive to a hormone. For instance, cardiac arrhythmias, such as atrial fibrillation in thyrotoxicosis, probably occur most frequently in an already damaged heart (Chap. 10).

A lingering question is whether subtle abnormalities in the sensitivity to hormones contribute to the pathogenesis of disease more often than is generally perceived. With more refined methods for measuring alterations in sensitivity to hormones, it may be possible to detect more subtle abnormalities. For instance, are some forms of essential hypertension due to increased sensitivity to pressor substances or decreased sensitivity to vasodilator substances (Chap. 14)? Are some forms of osteoporosis due to abnormalities in sensitivity to estrogens or to calcium-regulating hormones (Chap. 24)? Why do glucocorticoids increase intraocular pressure (and even precipitate glaucoma) in some persons but not in others (Chap. 12)?

Autoimmune Disease

In addition to endocrine deficiency states which may be precipitated by autoimmune mechanisms (e.g., Schmidt's syndrome, discussed below and in Chap. 12), autoimmune disease can result in the production of antibodies that act as hormones. The most frequent situation in which this occurs is thyrotoxicosis (Graves' disease; Chap. 10). Rarely, antibodies to the insulin receptor are formed that have insulin-like actions (Chap. 19).

Hormone Biosynthetic or Metabolic Defects

Certain adrenal steroid biosynthetic defects (the 21α-and 11β-hydroxylase syndromes) result in overproduction of hormones proximal to the block; these syndromes are discussed in Chap. 12. A defect in the metabolism of cortisol leads to a mineralocorticoid excess state caused by excessive accumulation of cortisol with renal mineralocorticoid receptors (Chap. 14).

Secondary Hormone Hypersecretion

Hypersecretion of hormones may be due to excessive physiologic stimulation of glands that are basically normal. The secondary hyperaldosteronism of hepatic disease and ascites, congestive heart failure, the nephrotic syndrome, and other conditions is illustrative (Chap. 12). The excess aldosterone aggravates the tendency to edema in these conditions. Secondary hyperparathyroidism occurs in azotemia (Chap. 24). Secondary hyperinsulinism occurs in obesity (Chap. 19).

Multiple Endocrine Syndromes

Simultaneous involvement of more than one endocrine gland may result in syndromes of hyper- or hypofunction. The most common syndrome of multiple endocrine deficiences may involve immunologic destruction of the pancreatic islets, thyroid, adrenals, and gonads (Chap. 28). This may result from common antigenic determinants caused possibly by a common developmental origin of the glands.

At least three syndromes of multiple endocrine hyperfunction result from hyperplasia, adenomas, or carcinomas of endocrine tissues, termed *multiple endocrine neoplasia* (MEN) types 1, 2a, and 2b (Chap. 28). Type 1 is associated with hyperfunction of the parathyroids, pancreatic islets, and pituitary. In some cases more than one hormone may be produced by the tumor; islet-cell tumors can produce insulin, glucagon, gastrin, VIP, prostaglandins, ACTH, vasopressin, somatostatin, serotonin, and GRH. Hypersecretion of GRH can produce hyperfunction of the pituitary and acromegaly. MEN type 2a is associated with pheochromocytoma (sometimes bilateral and extraadrenal), medullary carcinoma of the thyroid, and parathyroid hyperplasia. MEN type 2b is associated with medullary thyroid carcinoma, pheochromocytoma, and other features, such as neuromas. These syndromes are often familial, with a dominant transmission, but the basic pathogenesis is unknown.

Abnormalities of Endocrine Glands Not Associated with Hormonal Imbalance

Tumors, nodules, cysts, infiltrative diseases, and other abnormalities may involve endocrine glands without significantly impairing their secretory functions. For instance, nodules of the thyroid gland are common but usually nonfunctioning (Chap. 11). The major problem is that they may become malignant. Sometimes particular processes have a propensity for affecting an endocrine tissue; this is the case with tuberculosis and the adrenals (Chap. 12).

CLINICAL ASSESSMENT OF ENDOCRINE STATUS

The assessment of the endocrine status of a patient relies on findings from the history and physical examination and on laboratory testing. The latter may involve measurements of levels of hormones or their metabolites in plasma or urine either in the basal state or in response to provocative testing. Laboratory tests may also be used to measure abnormalities that result from derangements in hormonal secretion and to evaluate a patient's sensitivity to hormones.

History and Physical Examination

The clinical manifestations of endocrine diseases are summarized in Chap. 2 and in other individual chapters devoted to specific systems. Many syndromes of hormonal excess or deficiency display manifestations that are readily apparent at the time of initial presentation, e.g., severe thyrotoxicosis (Chap. 10) and Cushing's syndrome (Chap. 12). In other instances, the clinical presentation is more subtle and the physician must rely on laboratory testing to establish a diagnosis. This is especially true in the early stages of most endocrine problems, in elderly persons (e.g., with thyrotoxicosis or myxedema) (Chap. 10), or when the disease presents acutely and has not been present long enough for chronic manifestations to develop. Since it is beneficial to treat these diseases early, it is important for the physician to consider endocrine diseases in patients without full-blown manifestations, despite the fact that in the early stages of many of these disorders—e.g., adrenal insufficiency (Chap. 12), hypothyroidism (Chap. 10), Cushing's syndrome (Chap. 12), and hyperparathyroidism (Chap. 23)—the presenting symptoms and signs are sufficiently vague to suggest more common problems. Thus, endocrine diseases should be considered in the differential diagnosis of many common problems, such as weakness, tiredness, vague gastrointestinal discomfort, hypertension, and weight loss or gain (Chap. 2). Once the diagnosis is considered, it is usually relatively easy to establish whether the disorder is present. Since endocrine diseases may be caused by primary processes external to the endocrine systems, the physician should consider these processes in taking the history and performing the physical examination. Sometimes the primary process (e.g., carcinoma of the lung producing ACTH, tuberculosis causing adrenal insufficiency) will so dominate the clinical presentation that hormonal abnormalities are more difficult to detect clinically.

Laboratory Testing

Hormone Levels

Assay of Hormones

Assays are currently available for measuring essentially all the hormones known to be important (Chap. 6). The dominant assays used are immunoassays, which take advantage of the ability to obtain antibodies that bind to specific determinants on hormones with high affinity. The levels of the various hormones are measured by assessing the ability of the hormone in the sample to compete with a labeled hormone or an analogue of it for binding to the antibody. Traditionally, these labels have been radioactive, but increasingly, nonradioactive means for labeling are being used. Certain problems with an immunoassay—for example, when inactive degraded fragments of the hormone give falsely elevated hormone levels (as can occur with PTH in renal failure; Chap. 23)—can be circumvented through the use of two different antibodies, each specific for different parts of the molecule. These assays are described in Chap. 6. Immunoassays have also mostly supplanted competitive protein-binding assays using plasma hormone-binding proteins or receptors, and chemical assays. Some compounds are also measured after passage through high-performance liquid chromatography (HPLC) columns.

Levels of Free Hormone

The level of free rather than total hormone is usually the best index of the effective hormone concentration in plasma. Problems with assessment of total hormone concentrations caused by variations in the concentrations of plasma steroid and thyroid hormone-binding proteins are emphasized earlier in this chapter and in Chaps. 4 and 6.

Levels of free hormone can be assessed by (1) physically separating the free hormone from the plasma-bound hormone and measuring the free hormone directly, (2) measuring the plasma concentration of the binding protein directly (this approach has not been used widely), and (3) assessing the saturation of the binding protein. The latter approach is now used in the case of thyroid hormone (Chap. 10). Thus, the T_3 uptake assay measures the capacity of plasma for T_3 binding, which reflects the extent of saturation of thyroid hormone-binding proteins by T_4. The free hormone concentration is estimated by combining knowledge of the total T_4 levels and the extent of saturation of the proteins (Chap. 10). Both determinations are necessary, since variations in the levels of the binding protein reciprocally affect the total hormone levels and the extent of saturation of the binding proteins (Chaps 6 and 10). The same reasoning is applied to the measurement of free testosterone, used in the evaluation of hirsutism (Chap. 17). As a fourth possibility, an index of the free hormone concentration can sometimes be obtained by measuring the urinary excretion of the free hormone or that of one of its metabolites. For instance, a small fraction (less than 1 percent) of the secreted cortisol is excreted unchanged into the urine (Chap. 12). A measurement of the 24-h urine free cortisol usually provides a reasonable estimate of the integrated levels of free plasma hormone. In essence, this method uses the glomerular basement membrane to separate the free from the bound hormone.

Selective Sampling

Sometimes more accurate indications of a hormone excess state and the site of hormone hypersecretion can be obtained by assaying the venous effluent from a given gland or organ. For example, in renovascular hypertension, peripheral renin levels may be normal but sampling from a catheter inserted into the renal veins may reveal renin hypersecretion from one side and hyposecretion from the other side (Chap. 14). Pituitary venous effluent sampling from the petrosal sinuses can be useful to determine whether ACTH hypersecretion results from a pituitary adenoma or from an ectopic site (Chap. 12).

Clinical Interpretation

The clinician must remember that in both normal subjects and patients with endocrine and other diseases, hormone levels are extensively regulated, and their laboratory measurements thus must be evaluated in this context. For instance, plasma insulin levels should be evaluated in relation to the plasma glucose concentration (Chap. 19) and PTH levels should be considered in relation to serum calcium levels (Chap. 23). Basal hormone secretion may not reflect the functional capacity of the gland, as considered in more detail under Dynamic Testing, below. Hormone levels should be evaluated in relation to target cell sensitivity. For example, in type II diabetes mellitus plasma insulin levels are often elevated but may still be inappropriately low in view of the associated hyperglycemia and insulin resistance (Chap. 19). Since the release of many hormones is not constant, random readings can be particularly misleading. Cortisol, for example, is released episodically (Chap. 12). In Cushing's syndrome, the number of these episodic releases may be increased. Although this commonly results in an elevation of the plasma cortisol throughout the day, the morning plasma levels of this steroid may be in the normal range. Since cortisol production integrated over a 24-h period is increased in Cushing's syndrome, the 24-h urinary free cortisol provides a more accurate index of cortisol hypersecretion.

Urinary measurements can sometimes be more useful than plasma assays for obtaining an integrated assessment of the production of certain hormones (especially steroids). However, the urinary metabolites of steroids can be influenced by changes in renal function and other factors that do not affect the production of the hormone.

Sometimes the significance of hormone levels can be evaluated only by the simultaneous measurement of more than one hormone. For instance, with progressive damage to the thyroid gland and impaired release of thyroid hormones, secretion of TSH increases in a compensatory fashion so that normal plasma levels of the thyroid hormones may be maintained (Chap. 10). When thyroid hormone levels and TSH are measured simultaneously, an indication of the compensatory response can be obtained. Such a simultaneous assessment of linked hormones can also provide an indication of the site of a primary defect. Plasma estrogens are low in ovarian failure (Chap. 17). If ovarian failure is due to disease of the ovary, plasma gonadotropins will be elevated. If ovarian failure is secondary to pituitary or hypothalamic disease, plasma gonadotropin levels will be normal or decreased.

Dynamic Testing

Provocative testing assesses the ability of a gland to respond to stimuli as an index of its reserve capacity. This is especially useful when plasma or urinary hormone measurements are borderline. It can also yield information about the site of an endocrine defect. In some cases, a hormone is administered that stimulates the release of one or more other hormones. For example, the administration of GnRH stimulates LH and FSH release (Chap. 8), and TRH stimulates TSH and prolactin release (Chap. 8). In other cases, hormone production is blocked to interrupt normal feedback inhibition. Metyrapone blocks cortisol production by inhibiting 11β hydroxylation, thus stimulating ACTH release (Chap. 12). The elevated ACTH levels increase the release of adrenal steroids proximal to the block (e.g., 11-deoxycortisol). Sometimes a physiologic stimulus to hormone release is given. Insulin-induced hypoglycemia is used to assess the secretory ability of cells that produce ACTH and growth hormone (Chap. 8). With endocrine hyperfunction, provocative tests can assess the extent to which the normal physiologic mechanisms that control hormone release are suppressed or the degree of autonomy of the hormone-producing tumor or hyperplastic gland. In primary aldosteronism resulting from an aldosterone-producing adenoma, plasma renin levels are suppressed by excessive sodium retention and will not rise with acute postural, salt restriction, or diuretic stimuli (Chap. 14). In Cushing's syndrome resulting from ectopic secretion of ACTH by a tumor, the glucocorticoid dexamethasone ordinarily will not suppress the elevated ACTH levels (Chap. 12).

Tests That Provide Indirect Information

Useful information can frequently be obtained from laboratory tests that provide an index of the actions of hormones (or a lack of them) or an indication of the primary process causing the endocrine disease. Diagnosis of diabetes mellitus and assessment of therapy depend on measurement of plasma glucose rather than insulin levels (Chap. 19). It is helpful to follow the serum calcium levels in hyperparathyroidism (Chap. 23) and the serum potassium levels in primary aldosteronism (Chap. 14). Such tests often provide indexes of the severity of the condition that are even more important than the hormone level. In conditions in which immunologic processes are important, assessment of antibody levels can be helpful. Other tests provide information that is more corroborative but can also be useful. For instance, serum sodium is almost always greater than 139 mEq/liter in patients with an aldosterone-producing adenoma (Chap. 14), plasma cholesterol tends to be high in hypothyroidism and low in hyperthyroidism (Chap. 19), serum potassium tends to be high in Addison's disease (Chap. 12), alkaline phosphatase tends to be elevated in osteomalacia (Chap. 24), and the serum phosphate level tends to be elevated in acromegaly (Chap. 8).

Evaluation of the Sensitivity of Target Cells to Hormones

Suspicion of hyposensitivity to a hormone is raised when the manifestations of a deficiency of that hormone occur in the presence of elevated hormone levels. In type II diabetes mellitus there is hyperglycemia with hyperinsulinism (Chap. 19); in pseudohypoparathyroidism, hypocalcemia is observed in the face of elevated PTH levels (Chap. 23); and pseudohermaphroditism caused by the testicular feminization syndrome is characterized by decreased androgenization with elevated plasma testosterone levels (Chap. 18). The existence of hyposensitivity can be confirmed by administering the hormone in question and determining the presence or extent of response, although commonly it is not necessary to do this. In some cases, as with insulin or androgen resistance, it is possible to obtain further confirmation of the hyposensitivity state by isolating cells from the patient and measuring receptors or responses, although the techniques for this are not generally available. Conversely, hypersensitivity to hormones is characterized by low hormone levels relative to the response. In low-renin essential hypertension the adrenal glomerulosa is excessively sensitive to angiotensin II (Chap. 14). This is reflected by normal to elevated plasma aldosterone levels in the presence of low angiotensin II levels. This sensitivity can be documented by measuring the plasma aldosterone levels after an infusion of angiotensin.

TREATMENT OF ENDOCRINE DISEASES

For endocrine deficiency syndromes, hormones are generally administered to counter the deficiency. In general, the hormone that is deficient is replaced. In some cases this is not possible or expedient, and other hormones are given that help compensate for the defect. For instance, vitamin D is given instead of PTH to treat hypoparathyroidism, since it can increase the extracellular Ca^{2+} (Chap. 23). In cases in which hormone resistance is present, steps are taken when possible to alleviate this, such as through diet restriction in type II diabetes (Chap. 19).

In hormone-excess syndromes, a variety of approaches are used. Hyperfunctioning tumors are removed when possible, and sometimes hyperplastic glands are removed. In other cases drugs are given to block hormone production, such as propylthiouracil for thyrotoxicosis (Chap. 10) and bromocriptine for prolactin-producing adenomas (Chap. 8). Antagonists such as spironolactone can sometimes be useful in primary aldosteronism due to hyperplasia (Chap. 14).

For both excess and deficiency syndromes adjunctive therapy is frequently important. Thus, multiple measures are used to treat the complications of diabetes mellitus, and patients with Addison's disease are cautioned to avoid stress (Chap. 12).

HORMONE AGONIST AND ANTAGONIST THERAPY

Finally, it should be remembered that hormones, which affect so many processes, and their analogues, are also used extensively to treat diseases that do not have a primary endocrine basis. For example, glucocorticoids are used to treat a large number of conditions (Chap. 15), analogues of releasing factors such as GnRH are used to block gonadotropin release (Chap. 17) and treat prostate cancer (Chap. 30), steroid antagonists are used to treat hormone-responsive tumors (Chap. 30), catecholamines are used to treat shock and other cardiovascular problems (Chap. 13), and catecholamine antagonists are used to treat hypertension and other cardiovascular problems.

REFERENCES

1. Erickson N, Quesenberry PJ: Regulation of erythropoiesis: The role of growth factors. *Med Clin North Am* 76:745, 1992.
2. Foxwell BM, Barrett K, Feldmann M: Cytokine receptors: Structure and signal transduction. *Clin Exp Immunol* 90:161, 1992.
3. Rees RC: Cytokines as biological response modifier. *J Clin Pathol* 45:93, 1992.
4. Aaronson SA: Growth factors and cancer. *Science* 254:1146, 1991.
5. Kerr LD, Inoue J, Verma IM: Signal transduction: The nuclear target. *Curr Opinion Cell Biol* 4:496, 1992.
6. Bortner DM, Langer SJ, Ostrowski MC: Non-nuclear oncogenes and the regulation of gene expression in transformed cells. *Crit Rev Oncogenesis* 4:137, 1993.
7. Tomkins GM: The metabolic code. *Science* 189:760, 1975.
8. Baxter JD, Rousseau GG: Glucocorticoids and the metabolic code, in Baxter JD, Rousseau GG (eds): *Glucocorticoid Hormone Action*. Heidelberg, Springer-Verlag, 1979, pp 613–627.
9. Bern HA, Knowles FGW: Neurosecretion, in Martini L, Ganong WF (eds): *Neuroendocrinology*, vol 1. New York, Academic, 1966, pp 139–186.
10. Scharrer E: Principles of neuroendocrine regulation: Endocrines and the central nervous system. *Assoc Res Nerv Ment Dis* 43:1, 1966.
11. Pearse AGE: The cytochemistry and ultrastructure of polypeptide hormone-producing cells of the APUD series and the embryologic, physiologic and pathologic implications of the concept. *J Histochem Cytochem* 47:303, 1969.
12. Pearse AGE: The diffuse neuroendocrine system and the APUD concept: Related "endocrine" peptides in brain, intestine, pituitary placenta and anuran cutaneous glands. *Med Biol* 55:115, 1977.
13. Funder JW, Mercer J: Cimetidine, a histamine H_2-receptor antagonist, occupies androgen receptors. *J Clin Endocrinol* 48:189, 1979.

CHAPTER 2

The Clinical Manifestations of Endocrine Disease

Lawrence A. Frohman
Philip Felig
John D. Baxter

Diseases of the endocrine-metabolic system account for some of the most common disorders encountered in humans: diabetes, obesity, hyperlipedimias, osteoporosis, and thyroid abnormalities. In recent years, a host of laboratory techniques, including radioimmunoassay, receptor methodology, recombinant DNA techniques, hormone stimulative and suppressive procedures, and advances in diagnostic imaging, have markedly enhanced diagnosis and clarified the pathophysiology of such diseases. Nevertheless, in many instances the disorder remains unrecognized until relatively late in its course; symptoms may be attributed to another disease process, and laboratory results may be confusing rather than helpful. Some of the difficulties relate to the complex clinical presentation and the multiplicity of organ systems which may be affected by a given disease process (e.g., thyrotoxicosis may masquerade as an intractable cardiac arrhythmia in an apathetic patient). A second problem concerns the nonspecific nature of some symptoms (e.g., weakness may be the major complaint in Addison's disease).

A further difficulty may arise from the laboratory tests. The striking biochemical and physiologic disturbances which occur in endocrine disease, often with only minimal anatomic changes or physical findings (e.g., diabetes, hyperparathyroidism), tend to focus the physician's attention on the laboratory results, frequently without consideration of the total clinical picture. For a patient with asymptomatic hypercalcemia due to hyperparathyroidism, early diagnosis and treatment based on an elevated serum calcium level obtained during routine multiphasic laboratory screening may prevent the subsequent development of bone disease or renal stones. However, an elevation in the serum thyroxine level of a euthyroid patient may lead to inappropriate use of antithyroid drugs if the physician fails to obtain a history of estrogen use or an assessment of the plasma thyroxine binding capacity. Similarly, the finding of a small adrenal nodule on abdominal computed tomographic evaluation for a specific but unrelated complaint (e.g., abdominal pain) may also lead to confusion and unnecessary diagnostic or therapeutic procedures.

Consequently, the clinical approach which is most successful in diagnosis and management is that which combines a high index of suspicion with knowledge of the various clinical constellations in which endocrine-metabolic disorders may appear, plus an understanding of the indications, interpretations, and inherent weaknesses of various testing procedures. In this chapter the major clinical signs and symptoms which may call attention to a variety of endocrine-metabolic disorders are reviewed. Various testing procedures are considered in Chap. 6.

GENERALIZED SYMPTOMS

Hormones affect the function of all tissues and organ systems. Consequently, the symptoms and signs of endocrine disease are extremely diverse. They may vary from generalized, such as fatigue, to localized, such as weakness of the extraocular muscles. The variable nature of the clinical presentations of many endocrine disorders may result in their going unrecognized for prolonged periods (e.g., the failure to recognize, particularly in the elderly, recurrent supraventricular tachycardia or heart failure as a manifestation of hyperthyroidism). By contrast, there is a tendency (both in the general population and in the medical community) to attribute an endocrine basis to common complaints even when evidence is lacking. For example, hypoglycemia is often invoked to explain weakness and depression, obesity is frequently attributed to a "slow metabolism," and baldness is often ascribed to "glandular dysfunction." While each of these symptoms may in fact be due to an endocrine-metabolic disorder, the diagnosis should rest not on the nature of the symptom but on rigorous clinical and laboratory evaluation.

Weakness and Fatigue

Weakness generally refers to an overall lack of strength (easy fatigability, "loss of pep") which may be persistent or episodic in nature and may be due to an actual loss of strength or only a perceived loss. Persistent weakness may reflect altered muscle function, as in some types of endocrine myopathy, or electrolyte disturbance, dehydration, or the effects of hormonal lack or excess through mechanisms which are poorly understood.

Generalized weakness is a common complaint in patients with Addison's disease or panhypopituitarism. In spontaneous or iatrogenic Cushing's syndrome, weakness secondary to steroid-induced myopathy may be observed. Both hypothyroidism and hyperthyroidism may result in fatigue even when there is hyperactivity and nervousness in the hyperthyroid state.

Hypokalemia accompanying hyperaldosteronism, other mineralocorticoid-excess states, or Bartter's syndrome and hypercalcemia of hyperparathyroidism or malignant disease may result in a generalized decrease in strength. In a poorly controlled diabetic patient or a patient with Addison's disease dehydration may result in or worsen weakness. Furthermore, in some diabetic patients, even in the absence of severe hyperglycemia, postprandial fatigue and somnolence may be reversed by improved regulation of the blood glucose.

Patients with depression, which is common in many endocrine dysfunctions, frequently complain of fatigue or weakness. A distinction between weakness due to organic dysfunction and a feeling of fatigue due to depression can often be made. Patients with depression commonly feel "too weak" to initiate physical activity, whereas those with true weakness generally notice difficulty in the process of exertion or attempted exercise.

Episodic weakness may be caused by hypoglycemia in patients with an insulinoma. Since a marked fall in blood glucose results in a counterregulatory response which restores the blood glucose to normal or in an impairment in brain function (syncope or seizures), persistent generalized weakness lasting days to weeks cannot be ascribed to hypoglycemia. Episodic weakness may also be observed in patients with pheochromocytoma or the carcinoid syndrome as a manifestation of paroxysmal hormonal release and in thyrotoxicosis complicated by periodic paralysis.

Weight Loss

A decrease in body weight in the absence of voluntary or involuntary caloric restriction or a marked increase in exercise generally indicates the presence of an underlying disease process. From a diagnostic standpoint it is useful to differentiate weight loss associated with anorexia from that which occurs in association with hyperphagia or a normal appetite. In the absence of anorexia or diuresis, an increase in metabolic rate, abnormal losses of calorie-containing substrates in urine (e.g., glycosuria or ketonuria), or failure of gastrointestinal absorption must be present in a patient with weight loss. In hyperthyroidism and in decompensated diabetes (in which there is marked glycosuria) weight loss in the presence of hyperphagia is frequently observed. Weight loss due to increased caloric expenditure may also be observed in pheochromocytoma. In patients with severe diabetic neuropathy involving the autonomic nervous system, digestive and absorptive processes may be impaired, resulting in severe cachexia despite seemingly adequate caloric consumption.

Weight loss associated with anorexia is observed in Addison's disease and panhypopituitarism, particularly that following the postpartum state, and in hyperparathyroidism and other hypercalcemic states. Weight loss may occur uncommonly in the presence of hypometabolism in hypothyroidism because of accompanying anorexia. In anorexia nervosa a severe disturbance of appetite (reflecting a psychological and/or hypothalamic disturbance) results in weight loss to the point of cachexia.

Weight Gain

An increase in body weight may reflect an accumulation of interstitial fluid (edema) or an increase in body fat (adiposity). Weight gain due to fluid retention can generally be recognized by palpable edema or rapidity of the increment in weight. A gain in weight of 1 kg or more per day invariably indicates fluid retention.

Weight gain due to an increase in adipose tissue is observed in Cushing's syndrome, where there is a characteristic truncal (rather than peripheral) distribution, a "buffalo hump" (increased fat over the lower part of the back of the neck), and large supraclavicular fat pads. In patients with insulin-producing islet-cell tumors a weight gain of 10 to 15 kg may be observed because of repeated bouts of hypoglycemia resulting in appetite stimulation and increased food intake. Hypometabolism due to hypothyroidism may also result in an increase in body fat. However, fluid retention may also contribute to weight gain in hypothyroidism, as reflected by fluid excess in myxedematous tissues or the presence of ascites or pleural or pericardial effusions.

Obesity is commonly observed in association with non-insulin-dependent diabetes. However, it is the obesity which is the predisposing factor to the development of diabetes, not the reverse. In rare circumstances, disturbances of hypothalamic satiety centers result in weight gain; this may be observed in patients with central nervous system disease (trauma, encephalitis, or tumors) or pituitary tumors with sufficient suprasellar extension to compress the ventral hypothalamus.

It should be noted that primary endocrine-metabolic disorders account for less than 5 percent of all cases of obesity (body weight 30 percent or more above ideal). Furthermore, extreme degrees of weight gain—body weight in excess of 115 to 135 kg (250 to 300 lb)—are almost never due to a primary endocrine disturbance. However, obesity may *secondarily* result in a variety of alterations in endocrine and metabolic processes. In addition, the extent to which an undefined metabolic defect contributes to the pathophysiology of at least some forms of obesity is not known.

Edema may be observed in association with cardiac failure accompanying thyrotoxicosis, myxedema, or acromegaly. In severe anorexia nervosa or in diabetic nephropathy resulting in proteinuria, edema may develop as a consequence of hypoalbuminemia. Edema is generally not observed in patients with primary hyperaldosteronism. By contrast, corticosteroids exhibiting a mineralocorticoid effect may precipitate or exacerbate fluid accumulation when administered to patients with underlying cardiac disease. Mineralocorticoids used in the treatment of Addison's disease rarely cause edema when given in excess in the absence of manifest cardiac disease.

Body Temperature

A mild increase in body temperature may be observed in thyrotoxicosis. In thyroid storm (an acute exacerbation of hyperthyroidism), a fever of 101 °F or more is characteristic. Hyperpyrexia may occur in primary hypothalamic disease, in secondary disturbances of hypothalamic function after pituitary surgery, or in severely decompensated Addison's disease. Cerebral edema, a rare complication of diabetic ketoacidosis, may also result in high fever. Mild increases in temperature may also be seen in untreated Addison's disease. However, caution must be exercised in attributing fever in Addison's disease or diabetic ketoacidosis to the endocrine problem, since infections may be responsible for aggravating these conditions.

Hypothermia is common in hypoglycemia, particularly when induced by alcohol. Severe hypothyroidism (myxedema coma) may also be complicated by hypothermia.

SKIN

Hyperpigmentation of the skin is a characteristic finding in Addison's disease. It is accentuated in the exposed parts of the body. The knuckles, elbows, knees, areolae, genitalia, buccal mucosa, palmar creases, and recent scars are the sites of maximum pigmentation. Similar pigment changes may occur in 15 to 60 percent of patients who undergo bilateral adrenalectomy as treatment for Cushing's disease (bilateral adrenal hyperplasia) and are usually indicative of the presence of an ACTH (adrenocorticotropic hormone)-producing pituitary tumor (Nelson's syndrome). Ectopic production of ACTH by various neoplasms (e.g., lung, pancreas) may also lead to hyperpigmentation. An increase in pigmentation is observed in as many as 40 percent of patients with acromegaly.

Acanthosis nigricans is a syndrome in which there are localized areas of gray-brown hyperpigmentation in the posterior region of the neck and axillae. It is infrequently encountered in uncomplicated obesity, non-insulin-dependent diabetes mellitus, polycystic ovaries, Cushing's syndrome, and acromegaly. Acanthosis nigricans has also been identified in rare diabetic patients with severe insulin resistance associated with a decrease in insulin receptors or the presence of a circulating antibody to or mutation of the insulin receptor.

A generalized decrease in pigmentation occurs in panhypopituitarism. Focal areas of depigmentation (*vitiligo*) are observed in Addison's disease, thyrotoxicosis, and hypoparathyroidism.

Hirsutism, which is defined as an increase in facial hair in women beyond that which is cosmetically acceptable, is observed in a variety of androgen-excess states, including Cushing's syndrome, congenital adrenal hyperplasia, polycystic ovary syndrome, and virilizing ovarian or adrenal tumors. An increase in facial hair may also occur in acromegaly. However, in most cases of hirsutism a specific endocrine cause is not identified.

A decrease in body hair accompanying endocrine disease may be generalized (scalp, axillary and pubic areas, and extremities; *alopecia totalis*), localized to the scalp (*alopecia*), or restricted to the lateral third of the eyebrow. In hypopituitarism and hypothyroidism any of these patterns may be noted. In Cushing's syndrome and virilizing ovarian or adrenal tumors frontal baldness may occur. Hair loss may also be observed in thyrotoxicosis and hypoparathyroidism. Most patients with severe alopecia, however, do not have an endocrine disease.

Coarse, dry skin is found in myxedema and in hypoparathyroidism. In myxedema the changes may be so marked as to resemble ichthyosis. In acromegaly the skin is also coarse and has a leathery texture with enlargement of the sweat glands and a true thickening of the various skin layers.

Excessive sweating occurs in thyrotoxicosis and acromegaly. Acute paroxysms of sweating accompanying adrenergic discharge are observed in pheochromocytoma, during hypoglycemic episodes in patients with insulinomas, and in insulin-treated diabetic patients who are experiencing an insulin reaction.

Acne is observed in men and women with Cushing's syndrome or androgen-producing tumors of the adrenal and in women with congenital adrenal hyperplasia, polycystic ovaries (idiopathic hirsutism, persistent estrus syndrome), and virilizing tumors of the ovary.

Striae, plethora, thinning of the skin, easy bruisability, and ecchymoses may be observed in spontaneous Cushing's syndrome or after glucocorticoid therapy in pharmacologic doses.

NOSE, VOICE, AND TONGUE

The hypertrophy of mucous membranes which occurs in acromegaly results in pale, boggy nasal mucosa, frequently associated with symptoms of nasal and sinus obstruction. Hyperplasia of the membranes of the eustachian tube often results in intermittent middle ear blockage and recurrent episodes of serous otitis media. Pituitary tumors may erode the floor of the sella and extend into the floor of the sphenoid sinus and even into the nose. With rupture of the dura, cerebrospinal rhinorrhea may occur. This can be diagnosed by the presence of glucose in the nasal discharge, which is detected by use of a glucose oxidase–impregnated dipstick.

Loss of olfaction (*anosmia*) can be due to a tumor in the region of the hypothalamus which destroys the olfactory nerve. It can also be seen with Kallman's syndrome, a congenital disorder associated with hypothalamic hypogonadism.

The tongue is increased in size and frequently furrowed in acromegaly. In more severe cases difficulty in articulation can be noted. The tongue, palate, and buccal and gingival mucosa are often hyperpigmented in Addison's disease and with ACTH-producing pituitary tumors, particularly after adrenalectomy (Nelson's syndrome). There are discrete patches of hyperpigmentation in each of these locations, which at times may be confluent. Tongue pigmentation may be present normally in blacks and in this case is of less diagnostic significance.

In hypothyroidism the tongue is enlarged because of myxedematous infiltration, often resulting in slurred speech. In hyperthyroidism a fine rhythmic tremor which is evident in the outstretched fingers is also present in the tongue. Fine fascicular movements of the tongue may occur in hyperparathyroidism.

In acromegaly, hypertrophy of the larynx leads to a huskiness of the voice; an increase in the paranasal sinuses tends to give the voice more resonance. Myxedematous infiltration of the larynx in hypothyroidism results in deepening of the voice and, occasionally, severe hoarseness. Laryngeal examination reveals dullness, thickening, and flabbiness of the free margins of the true vocal cords. With advanced myxedema, smooth edematous polyps may form on the vocal cords. Deepening of the voice frequently occurs in women in the presence of increased androgen secretion, as in Cushing's syndrome, congenital adrenal hyperplasia, and virilizing adrenal or ovarian tumors. In men the influence of excess androgens on the voice cannot be detected clinically unless it occurs during the prepubertal period, as in congenital adrenal hyperplasia. The voice changes do not always completely disappear upon removal of the excess androgen. Large goiters and invasive thyroid carcinomas can also produce hoarseness.

In males in whom pubertal changes fail to occur as a result of androgen deficiency due to a hypothalamic, pituitary, or gonadal disturbance, the voice remains high-pitched. However, once the voice has acquired the typical characteristics of an adult male, loss of androgen does not cause any change in quality.

GASTROINTESTINAL SYSTEM

Anorexia is often observed in primary hyperparathyroidism and other hypercalcemic conditions, Addison's disease, and diabetic ketoacidosis. A reduction in appetite may also occur in hypothyroidism, panhypopituitarism, and apathetic hyperthyroidism. Anorexia nervosa is characterized by abnormal ideation regarding body weight and food intake in addition to loss of appetite. Nausea and vomiting are often seen in diabetic ketoacidosis, hyperparathyroidism and other disorders with significant hypercalcemia, and Addison's disease.

An increase in appetite commonly accompanies hyperthyroidism, diabetes mellitus with moderate hyperglycemia, glucocorticoid therapy, and Cushing's syndrome. It is also seen in about 15 percent of patients with an insulinoma.

Oropharyngeal dysphagia may be caused by a large goiter or by a locally invasive thyroid carcinoma.

Abdominal pain occurs in a variety of endocrine disorders. Nonspecific, diffuse abdominal pain occurs frequently in children with diabetic ketoacidosis. Patients with addisonian crisis often present with diffuse abdominal pain. Less severe pain is a frequent complaint with chronic adrenal insufficiency. In thyroid storm abdominal pain may be a major complaint. However, in all these instances, the physician should consider the possibility that the pain is due to another process that has exacerbated the condition, especially if the pain is unresolved with control of the condition. Ileus with gaseous and colicky pain may be observed in myxedema. Both acute and chronic patterns of abdominal pain occur in patients with the carcinoid syndrome. In primary hyperparathyroidism abdominal pain may be due to peptic ulcer disease or to pancreatitis. In addition, a minority of patients with this disease present with a diffuse and poorly described abdominal pain of uncertain cause which resolves with surgical correction of the hyperparathyroidism. Symptoms of severe or recurrent peptic ulcer are the most characteristic features of the gastrinoma (Zollinger-Ellison) syndrome. Gastrointestinal bleeding may complicate peptic ulceration in primary hyperparathyroidism and in the gastrinoma syndrome. Gastrointestinal bleeding may also occur in Turner's syndrome because of associated intestinal telangiectasia. Patients receiving glucocorticoid therapy in combination with nonsteroidal antiinflammatory agents are at increased risk for developing peptic ulcers, and severely ill patients on high-dose glucocorticoid therapy are at increased risk for developing gastrointestinal hemmorhage.

Constipation occurs frequently in hypothyroidism and in patients with marked hypercalcemia or hypokalemia and may occur with pheochromocytoma. Patients with diabetic autonomic neuropathy may complain of constipation alternating with diarrhea that is often nocturnal and is accompanied by fecal incontinence.

Diarrhea may be prominent in patients with metastatic medullary carcinoma of the thyroid, a metastatic carcinoid tumor, and vasoactive intestinal peptide (VIP)–producing tumors. Approximately one-third of those with the gastrinoma syndrome present with diarrhea; frank steatorrhea may be seen in both the gastrinoma and carcinoid syndromes. Hyperthyroidism is associated with an increased frequency of somewhat poorly formed stools rather than actual diarrhea. Explosive and life-threatening diarrhea dominates the clinical picture in patients with pancreatic cholera due to tumors of the islets that produce VIP or other gastrointestinal neuroendocrine tumors.

Significant hepatic abnormalities are uncommon in endocrine disorders, but liver function tests may be abnormal in both severe thyrotoxicosis and myxedema and also in patients with far-advanced carcinoid tumors. In poorly controlled diabetic patients hepatomegaly due to fatty infiltration may be observed.

HEMOPOIETIC SYSTEM

Anemia occurs frequently in a wide variety of endocrine disorders. The anemia may be a direct consequence of the specific endocrine deficiency or hypersecretion or may result from a complication of endocrine disease such as acute blood loss anemia or iron-deficiency anemia due to peptic ulcer disease in primary hyperparathyroidism or the gastrinoma syndrome.

A mild normocytic normochromic anemia with hypoplastic bone marrow regularly accompanies panhypopituitarism and is corrected by replacement therapy with thyroid, adrenal, and gonadal hormones. Growth hormone deficiency therefore appears not to play a major role in the development of this anemia. The anemia may be partially masked by a coincident contraction in plasma volume.

Pernicious anemia occurs in a small percentage of patients with the polyglandular syndrome of multiple endocrine deficiencies (Schmidt's syndrome); this can result in Addison's disease, insulin-dependent diabetes mellitus, hypothyroidism, and gonadal failure.

A mild to moderate anemia is commonly noted in hypothyroidism. Thyroid hormone deficiency results in a normocytic normochromic anemia with hypoplastic bone marrow, possibly due to a decrease in erythropoietin production, and more commonly in a microcytic hypochromic anemia of iron deficiency. This is due to a high incidence of menorrhagia in female patients and the approximately 50 percent incidence of achlorhydria and iron malabsorption in patients of both sexes. A macrocytic hyperchromic anemia occurs in about 10 percent of patients with hypothyroidism and may be due to deficiency of folic acid or to classic pernicious anemia.

Hyperthyroidism is usually not accompanied by anemia, although severely thyrotoxic patients may display a mild normocytic normochromic or hypochromic anemia. Pernicious anemia with antiparietal cell antibodies occurs in approximately 3 percent of patients with Graves' disease.

Patients with adrenal insufficiency have a mild normocytic normochromic anemia which is often not readily apparent because of the concomitant decrease in plasma volume. Patients with Cushing's disease display a mild erythrocytosis with hemoglobin levels 1 to 2 g/dl higher than normal; this is less often observed with the administration of pharmacologic doses of exogenous steroids.

Androgens have a well-known erythropoietic effect, and pharmacologic doses are employed in treating a variety of refractory anemias. This effect contributes to the anemia in men with severe testosterone deficiency and to the higher hemoglobin values seen in sexually mature males than in females and prepubertal males.

A normocytic normochromic anemia occurring in about 20 percent of patients with primary hyperparathyroidism, particularly in patients with severe hypercalcemia, resolves after surgical correction of the disease. Iron-deficiency anemia may occur in hyperparathyroidism complicated by peptic ulcer disease and gastrointestinal bleeding.

Patients with a pheochromocytoma may display a slight increase in hemoglobin values because of the concomitant contraction in plasma volume. There may also be a direct influence of catecholamines on erythropoietin production.

A relative leukopenia is frequently noted in panhypopituitarism. Approximately 10 percent of patients with thyrotoxicosis present with leukopenia and/or granulocytopenia. Failure to recognize leukopenia before instituting treatment with antithyroid drugs may lead to confusion, since these drugs (e.g., propylthiouracil) may suppress the granulocyte count. The lymphocyte number is normal or slightly increased in hyperthyroid patients, leading to a relative lymphocytosis. No consistent abnormalities in leukocyte values are noted in hypothyroidism. In Cushing's syndrome, mild granulocytosis, lymphopenia, and eosinopenia are commonly observed. Lymphocytosis and eosinophilia are commonly observed in Addison's disease. The latter finding was for many years considered a diagnostic clue to the disorder. A leukocytosis of 15,000 to 30,000 cells per cubic millimeter regularly occurs in diabetic ketoacidosis, and so a leukocyte count is of little value in suggesting infection as the initiating event leading to the ketoacidosis. A marked leukocytosis is also routinely observed in hyperosmolar nonketotic coma. A minority of patients with pheochromocytoma display a mild leukocytosis.

Glucocorticoids may acutely promote a rise in platelets; thrombocytosis may also be observed with chronic glucocorticoid excess.

CARDIOVASCULAR SYSTEM

Tachycardia almost always accompanies hyperthyroidism and pheochromocytoma. Ordinarily this is of sinus origin, but occasionally there may be paroxysmal atrial tachycardia or atrial fibrillation with a rapid ventricular response. An ectopic arrhythmia with these conditions usually signifies underlying heart disease. The tachycardia may give rise to palpitations. Tachycardia also occurs when there is dehydration, as with adrenocortical insufficiency due to destruction of the gland or 21α-hydroxylase deficiency, and in uncontrolled diabetes. There is ordinarily a bradycardia in hypothyroidism. The hypokolemin of primary aldosteronism can result in ventricular ectopy and ventricular tachycardia; rarely, patients with this disorder present with ventricular arrhythmia.

An increased incidence of myocardial infarction and stroke can be observed with any of the syndromes that result in hypercholesterolemia or hypertension. Hypercholesterolemia may be present with hypothyroidism and diabetes. Hypertension is associated with acromegaly, primary aldosteronism, pheochromocytoma, Cushing's syndrome, glucocorticoid therapy (occasionally), renovascular hypertension, and renal disease (as in diabetes or hypercalcemia). An increased incidence of myocardial infarction and stroke is reportedly associated with the use of contraceptive steroids. Although these drugs affect lipid metabolism and can cause hypertension, the reasons for the increase in cardiovascular problems with their use have not been established. The incidence of myocardial infarction, stroke, and peripheral vascular disease is increased with diabetes.

Typically, heart size is smaller than usual in Addison's disease, hypopituitarism, and hyperthyroidism. In hypothyroidism and any conditions associated with hypertension, the heart size may be increased and congestive heart failure may be present. Cardiac failure may accompany hyperthyroidism or pheochromocytoma, presumably because of the excessive demands on the heart due to the increased beta-adrenergic stimulation associated with thyroid hormone or catecholamine excess. In younger people, this rarely leads to congestive failure, but in the elderly with underlying atherosclerotic disease these conditions can lead to serious cardiac decompensation. Heart size is increased in acromegaly and can eventually lead to heart failure.

The causes of edema were discussed earlier in the section on weight gain.

Occasionally toxic reactions or resistance to the drugs used in the treatment of cardiovascular disease may signify or result in endocrine disease. For instance, digitalis toxicity may be precipitated more rapidly in hyperthyroidism and pheochromocytoma and with hypokalemia, as in primary aldosteronism. Insensitivity to the bradycardia and antianginal effects of beta-adrenergic blockers may occur with hyperthyroidism. Amiodarone used in the management of arrhythmias may result in hypothyroidism or, less commonly, hyperthyroidism.

URINARY TRACT

Frequency, polyuria, and nocturia (or enuresis in children) are classically observed in diabetes mellitus and in central or nephrogenic diabetes insipidus. Severe hypercalcemia or hypokalemia may impair renal tubular concentrating ability, and so these symptoms may also be seen in patients with primary hyperparathyroidism and other hypercalcemic disorders and in patients with primary aldosteronism and Bartter's syndrome. Patients with diabetic autonomic neuropathy may complain of frequency, incontinence, or urinary retention.

Diabetes mellitus is associated with an increased incidence of urinary tract and mycotic vaginal and vulvar infections. Patients with diabetes are also prone to the development of papillary necrosis as a complication of pyelonephritis. A number of glomerular lesions occur in diabetes mellitus that are associated with proteinuria and progressive renal impairment. The most specific and important of these lesions is nodular glomerulosclerosis. Mild proteinuria may also be observed in myxedema.

Nephrolithiasis and/or nephrocalcinosis occur in a variety of endocrine disorders. Renal stone formation is a complication of primary hyperparathyroidism. An increased incidence of stones is also observed in a number of other hypercalcemic or hypercalciuric conditions, including sarcoidosis, vitamin D intoxication, idiopathic hypercalciuria, Cushing's syndrome, and acromegaly. Nephrocalcinosis with or without a history of stone or renal impairment occurs in primary hyperparathyroidism, vitamin D intoxication, and the milk-alkali syndrome.

Turner's syndrome may be accompanied by a number of congenital renal abnormalities.

SEXUAL FUNCTION

Endocrine disease must be considered when there is impotence or a change in libido but accounts for only a small proportion of these problems. Changes in libido irregularly accompany hypo- and hyperfunctioning of the adrenal cortex and the thyroid gland, hypokalemia with primary aldosteronism or Bartter's syndrome, hypercalcemia, anorexia nervosa, gonadal failure (ovarian or testicular), poorly controlled diabetes, and hypopituitarism. Impotence can be observed with gonadal failure (primary or secondary), diabetes with autonomic neuropathy, drug therapy for hypertension (especially methyldopa), and hypothyroidism. Hyperprolactinemia of any etiology, but particularly that associated with pituitary tumors, results in decreased libido in both sexes and, frequently, impotence. Any severe illness, including endocrine disease, may be associated with decreased libido, although in such an illness it is unusual for this to be a prominent complaint.

Amenorrhea or oligomenorrhea can be observed in gonadal dysgenesis (e.g., Turner's syndrome), primary ovarian failure, the testicular feminizing and pseudohermaphroditic syndromes, Kallman's syndrome (gonadotropin deficiency associated with anosmia), the adrenogenital syndrome, and menopause. Menstrual disturbances generally occur in hypopituitarism, as in Sheehan's syndrome (panhypopituitarism secondary to pituitary necrosis in women who have suffered postpartum hemorrhagic shock), in patients with prolactin-secreting pituitary tumors, and in Chiari-Frommel syndrome (hyperprolactinemia associated with prolonged lactation and amenorrhea after delivery). Amenorrhea or oligomenorrhea may appear in women after the discontinuation of oral contraceptives, especially if they have a history of prior menstrual irregularities. These problems may also occur in Cushing's syndrome, hyperthyroidism, hypothyroidism, anorexia nervosa, or polycystic ovaries (with increased estrogen and androgen production). When amenorrhea is associated with diabetes, adrenal insufficiency, or hypothyroidism, the syndrome of multiple endocrine deficiency (Schmidt's syndrome) should be considered. Most endocrinopathies in severe form can result in secondary amenorrhea.

Metrorrhagia, or bleeding between menstrual periods, can be present in hyperestrogen states resulting from a number of causes, including high-dose estrogen therapy. Spontaneous causes include anovulation secondary to diverse disorders and excess estrogen production due to tumors. For example, with anovulation associated with polycystic ovarian disease or the period just before and after the menarche, continued gonadotropin secretion results in the formation of a number of estrogen-producing nonovulatory graafian follicles. Tumors causing metrorrhagia may be of ovarian origin (e.g., thecoma, granulosa cell tumor) or of adrenal or pituitary origin. Ectopic production of trophic factors (e.g., ACTH) by tumors may secondarily stimulate estrogen production, leading to metrorrhagia.

Infertility can result from any of the causes of amenorrhea or oligomenorrhea listed above. With oligomenorrhea there may be either oligo-ovulation or anovulation; the distinction is important, since pregnancy can occur in the former case. Infertility may result from a restricted luteal phase leading to defective support of the implantation of the fertilized egg. This situation results from deficient progesterone production due to either defective responsiveness to luteinizing hormone (LH) or inadequate LH production. The latter may result from pituitary disease or from defective hypothalamic function due to psychogenic or neurogenic problems.

In men, endocrine problems resulting in hypothalamic-pituitary or testicular failure account for only a small proportion of cases of infertility or subfertility. Prolactin-producing pituitary tumors have been implicated in some cases of male infertility.

In women, changes due to androgen excess are termed *virilization.* These changes include hirsutism (discussed above), male pattern baldness, deepened voice, acne, and clitoral enlargement. The excess androgens may be of ovarian or adrenal origin or may result from exogenous androgen administration. Ovarian overproduction of androgen may be due to hyperplasia (as in polycystic ovaries or ovarian androgenic dysplasia) or tumor (e.g., arrhenoblastoma, hilar cell tumor, adrenal rest tumor, or gynandroblastoma). Excess adrenal androgen production may be due to Cushing's syndrome, enzyme defects (e.g., 11- or 21-hydroxylase deficiency), or neoplasia and in the absence of glucocorticoid excess may account for some cases of idiopathic hirsutism.

Precocious puberty may be due to a hormone-secreting tumor (most commonly ovarian but less commonly adrenal) or to constitutional, physiologic, or organic disturbances (e.g., postencephalitis, postmeningitis, postcerebral trauma, hypothalamic lesions, pinealoma or other tumors of the central nervous system). It is characterized by early breast development, axillary and pubic hair, onset of menstrual periods, and, in true precocious puberty, fertility. True cyclic menses and fertility are not, however, seen with adrenal or ovarian tumors which suppress gonadotropin secretion and cause precocious pseudopuberty. Sometimes there may be isolated precocious breast development or the appearance of pubic hair. A major problem with this syndrome is that there is premature closure of the epiphyses; as a consequence, many of the subjects are of short stature.

Gynecomastia, or abnormal breast enlargement, occurs physiologically in normal males at puberty, subsiding ordinarily during adolescence. It should be differentiated from breast enlargement due to excess fat tissue rather than ductal tissue (e.g., obesity and lipoma) and from breast tumors.

Gynecomastia may be caused by estrogen-producing tumors that are usually of adrenal origin (usually carcinomas) but may rarely be of chorionic, testicular granulosa cell, or interstitial cell origin. It may also be seen in cirrhosis, presumably because of a decrease in the metabolic clearance of circulating estrogens.

Gynecomastia may occur after estrogen, androgen, digitalis, reserpine, hydralazine, meprobamate, phenothiazine, chorionic gonadotropin, or spironolactone therapy or marijuana use, and it may be seen in hypergonadotropic hypogonadism such as Klinefelter's syndrome or Riefenstein syndrome. Gynecomastia may signify a pituitary or ectopic tumor (usually of pulmonary origin) producing prolactin (occasionally) or gonadotropins (rarely). Gynecomastia is sometimes seen after chronic hemodialysis, in hyperthyroidism, and during recovery from severe malnutrition.

Nonpuerperal lactation (galactorrhea) may occur as a consequence of several types of pituitary disturbance. Commonly, these disturbances are associated with increased prolactin production. Galactorrhea may occur after anesthesia, thoracic surgery, exercise, nipple stimulation, sexual intercourse, chest wall trauma, infection (herpes zoster), spinal cord lesions, and several drugs (phenothiazines, reserpine, methyldopa, and dopaminergic blockade). Galactorrhea is frequently associated with pituitary microadenoma. Galactorrhea is sometimes observed with acromegaly, other pituitary tumors, and destructive lesions of the hypothalamus and pituitary stalk. It may also be seen with hypothyroidism or estrogen therapy and is commonly observed in women with chronic renal failure.

BONES AND JOINTS

Decreased linear growth, dysgenetic epiphyseal centers, and ultimate dwarfing are observed in hypothyroidism that occurs in childhood. Abnormalities in linear growth are also observed in poorly controlled diabetes mellitus, panhypopituitarism, isolated growth hormone deficiency, and endogenous or exogenous glucocorticoid excess. Androgen excess produces an increased *rate* of linear growth, but premature closure of the epiphyseal centers ultimately leads to short stature. Short stature is also observed in Turner's syndrome.

Primary or secondary androgen insufficiency is associated with the development of eunuchoidal skeletal proportions. An unusual pattern of disproportionate growth of the lower extremities occurs in Klinefelter's syndrome.

Increased periosteal bone formation leads to typical facial and acral bone abnormalities in acromegaly. If the disease begins prior to epiphyseal closure, there is increased linear growth leading to gigantism. The various forms of rickets are associated with a number of bone deformities, including bowing of the limbs, frontal bossing, and beading of the ribs. Shortened fourth metacarpals occur regularly in pseudohypoparathyroidism and Turner's syndrome.

Osteoporosis, a feature of a variety of endocrine disorders, occurs in endogenous and exogenous hyperadrenocorticism, adult hypophosphatasia and other metabolic bone diseases, and hypogonadism (including premature ovarian failure). It is particularly severe in Turner's syndrome. Osteopenia is commonly observed in patients with long-standing hyperthyroidism or hyperprolactinemia; bone biopsies in these patients reveal a variable admixture of osteoporosis, osteomalacia, and osteitis fibrosa cystica. Severe calcium deficiency may result in osteoporosis, but there is scant evidence to suggest that calcium deficiency plays a primary role in the osteoporosis commonly encountered in the United States. Mild osteopenia has been reported in both children and adults with diabetes mellitus.

Osteomalacia with diffuse bone pain and tenderness and muscular weakness occurs in simple vitamin D deficiency and in vitamin D and calcium malabsorption due to a number of gastrointestinal diseases. A variety of renal tubular disorders are associated with rickets in children and osteomalacia in adults. Tumor-associated osteomalacia is an unusual and particularly severe form of the disorder which occurs in association with mesenchymal neoplasms.

Significant osteopenia is uncommonly observed in patients receiving anticonvulsant therapy in the United States. Clinically significant osteitis fibrosa cystica may occur with severe primary hyperparathyroidism; clinical or subclinical osteopenia (demonstrable by bone densitometry) in patients with less severe hyperparathyroidism may be due to osteoporosis, osteomalacia, or mild osteitis. Osteoporosis, osteomalacia, or osteitis fibrosa cystica can be present in patients with renal osteodystrophy. In the majority of patients with advanced renal insufficiency, several of these lesions coexist.

In acromegaly, bone overgrowth with distortion of the articular plate leads to degenerative arthritis, which may be severe and disabling. Chronic chondrocalcinosis (pseudogout) may occur in primary hyperparathyroidism; there are questionable associations between acute episodes of pseudogout and diabetes mellitus and between primary gout and primary hyperparathyroidism.

Increased levels of serum uric acid have been reported in primary hyperparathyroidism, myxedema, nephrogenic diabetes insipidus, Bartter's syndrome, and Paget disease. Some reports suggest that episodes of acute gouty arthritis occur with increased frequency in several of these disorders. Marked elevations in serum uric acid may accompany diabetic ketoacidosis but resolve rapidly with control of the ketoacidosis.

CENTRAL NERVOUS SYSTEM

Headache is a common finding in pituitary tumors and is caused by pressure of the expanding tumor on the dura. With rupture of the dura, the headache frequently disappears. Headache is characteristically present in pituitary apoplexy and may be present in tumors of the hypothalamus or the parasellar region. Headache also occurs in pseudotumor cerebri, hypertensive episodes associated with pheochromocytoma, and insulinomas with hypoglycemia. Headache may also be prominent in patients with the "empty sella" syndrome. Although the headaches tend to remain constant in individual patients, no characteristics are specific to the individual disease entities.

Depression, lethargy, apathy, and impaired mentation (disorientation and confusion) can be seen in hyperparathyroidism and other hypercalcemic states, hypothyroidism, hypoglycemia (irrespective of cause), Cushing's syndrome, and severe hyperglycemia (with or without ketoacidosis). Marked changes (either increases or decreases) in serum osmolality such as those seen in severe diabetes insipidus (hypernatremia) and in hyponatremic states due to inappropriately increased vasopressin also lead to a decreased sensorium. In each of theses disorders, if the hormonal or metabolic disturbance is left untreated, a comatose state will develop.

Focal as well as generalized convulsions may occur in patients with severe hypoglycemia, nonketotic hyperglycemia, inappropriately increased vasopressin, Addison's disease, myxedema, hypopituitarism, and hypocalcemia associated with hypoparathyroidism. In the latter case, tetany generally precedes the onset of convulsions by a variable period of time, ranging from days to years. Diabetic ketoacidosis is not accompanied by convulsions, probably because of the anticonvulsive effect of acidosis and/or ketosis.

Central nervous system effects, either direct or indirect, have been demonstrated for virtually every hormone studied. It is therefore not surprising that many abnormalities in endocrine function cause problems ranging from mild to profound depression or anxiety to profound behavioral disorders. In hypopituitarism, depression is common and psychoses are occasionally seen. In hypothyroidism, psychoses (myxedema madness) manifested by hallucinations, paranoid behavior, dementia, and even classic schizophrenic reactions can occur. In general, older patients are more prone than younger ones to develop a typical organic brain syndrome. The response to treatment is usually excellent. However, in elderly patients behavioral aberrations may persist. Hypothyroid patients are generally less aware of exteroceptive stimuli. Consequently, during the initial period of replacement therapy, behavioral problems may worsen until the patient readjusts to the new level of recognizable environmental input signals. Patients with hyperthyroidism show mood fluctuations which may progress to delirium and, as thyroid storm approaches, a florid psychosis. Patients with insulinomas that cause repeated and undiagnosed hypoglycemic episodes may develop bizarre behavioral disturbances due to impaired central nervous system metabolism. The diagnosis of a toxic psychosis is not infrequently made in such patients. In Addison's disease a depressive psychosis can occur. Depression and emotional lability are common in spontaneous Cushing's syndrome. Glucocorticoid therapy commonly results in euphoria. True psychotic behavior occurs uncommonly with both spontaneous and iatrogenic Cushing's syndrome.

NEUROMUSCULAR ABNORMALITIES

Neuropathy is a common long-term complication of diabetes mellitus. In about 15 percent of diabetic patients symptoms of neuropathy are present, while abnormalities of nerve conduction are demonstrable in up to 50 percent of these patients. The spectrum of diabetic neuropathy includes (1) acute mononeuropathy of cranial or peripheral nerves, (2) mononeuropathy multiplex, (3) distal polyneuropathy, and (4) autonomic neuropathy.

In mononeuritis multiplex there is involvement of a mixed sensorimotor nerve or group of nerves, resulting in pain and focal weakness. Frequently the sites of involvement are the hip, knee, and thigh areas, with resultant pain on walking.

In diabetic polyneuropathy there is distal, symmetric involvement primarily of sensory fibers. The feet and legs are affected to a greater extent than are the hands. Numbness and paresthesias are the major complaints. There is loss of the ankle jerk and of various sensory modalities (vibration, position, light touch).

Autonomic neuropathy generally appears in patients who already have severe peripheral neuropathy. The symptoms include loss of sweating, diarrhea which is particularly severe at night and is accompanied by fecal incontinence, orthostatic hypotension, impotence, and an atonic bladder.

Polyneuropathy involving primarily sensory nerves is also occasionally observed in patients with hyperparathyroidism.

A mononeuropathy that involves the distal median nerve and is due to compression at the wrist (*carpal tunnel syndrome*) can be observed in acromegaly and hypothyroidism. This is caused by thickening of connective tissue in acromegaly or increased deposition of mucinous material between connective tissue fibers in myxedema that results in pressure on the median nerve in the carpal tunnel. The symptoms consist of numbness, tingling, and pain in the radial two-thirds of the palmar surface of the hand and fingers. Weakness of abduction and apposition of the thumb may also occur.

A prolongation of the reflex relaxation time ("hung-up reflexes") in the absence of other evidence of neuropathy is a characteristic finding in hypothyroidism. Similar findings may occur in hyponatremic states such as Addison's disease and the syndrome of inappropriate secretion of antidiuretic hormone (SIADH).

Impaired motor function due to myopathic changes may be observed in hyperthyroidism, hypothyroidism, spontaneous or iatrogenic Cushing's syndrome, and disorders of calcium and phosphorus metabolism.

In hyperthyroidism weakness is most marked in the pelvic girdle and thigh muscles and is accompanied by muscle atrophy. The shoulder and hand muscles may also show atrophy. However, tremor rather than weakness is the more prominent symptom in the upper extremities.

Myopathy may also occur in myxedema, in which patients may complain of stiffness and aching in addition to weakness. The muscles may appear hypertrophic because of infiltration with mucinous material.

Corticosteroid myopathy is characterized by weakness that is more prominent in the proximal limb and girdle musculature, resulting in difficulty in arising from a sitting position and in raising the arms.

In hypophosphatemic rickets and osteomalacia, muscle weakness and atrophy are common. In Klinefelter's syndrome, the weakness that commonly occurs is due to androgen deficiency.

Episodic weakness accompanied by hypokalemia is observed in patients with primary hyperaldosteronism or Bartter's syndrome and occasionally in patients with thyrotoxicosis. In the latter group the attacks simulate those observed in familial periodic paralysis, but a family history of episodic paralysis is lacking.

In diabetic amyotrophy, involvement of a peripheral motor nerve or nerve end plate in the neuropathic process results in focal weakness and atrophy in the absence of sensory loss, simulating primary myopathic disease.

Acromegalic neuromyopathy is occasionally seen in patients with long-standing disease. Extreme weakness, primarily of proximal musculature, is the predominant finding.

OPHTHALMIC ABNORMALITIES

Diminished vision occurs with several endocrine diseases as a consequence of pressure on the optic nerve or tract, retinal degeneration, or vascular disease. In pituitary tumors with suprasellar extension, pressure on the optic chiasm typically results in a bitemporal hemianopia, although other specific and often asymmetric field defects can occur. The visual impairment can progress to complete blindness and optic atrophy. The blindness may occur suddenly in association with hemorrhage into the tumor.

Pigmentary optic atrophy has been reported in association with several hereditary syndromes in which obesity, diabetes, mental retardation, and hypogonadism are components. Severe to total visual loss is frequently present. Visual loss may also occur in severe thyroid ophthalmopathy (Graves' disease) as a result of increased orbital pressure leading to compression and ischemia of the optic nerve.

Cataracts and lenticular opacities that can impair vision are seen in hypothyroidism, hypoparathyroidism, and diabetes mellitus. Transient impairment of vision with symptoms of myopia developing over days to weeks accompanies severe hyperglycemic symptoms in approximately one-third of patients with newly discovered or poorly regulated type I diabetes. Hyperopic changes are less frequent but more dramatic in onset, often appearing several days after the onset of insulin treatment. Both symptoms disappear after several weeks of therapy. Blurring of both near and distant vision may develop rapidly during episodes of hyperglycemia in diabetic patients receiving insulin therapy; the visual impairment resolves as the blood glucose concentration returns to normal. These rapid changes in visual acuity due to marked fluctuations in blood glucose must be differentiated from the more permanent and serious visual loss which may occur in diabetic retinopathy. Diabetic retinopathy in its most severe form results in decreased vision by fibrous scar tissue formation in the macular area in association with neovascularization and by hemorrhage into the subhyaloid space or the vitreous humor. Acute, reversible blurring of vision may also occur during attacks of hypoglycemia.

Pain in or about the eye can occur in Graves' ophthalmopathy because of increased intraorbital pressure. It is also seen in diabetes associated with ophthalmoplegia or with rubeosis iridis, a form of neovascularization of the iris which can cause a painful hemorrhagic glaucoma.

Swelling around the eyes or periorbital edema is commonly seen in patients with myxedema, in whom the eyelids and surrounding skin exhibit a nonpitting, puffy swelling which appears boggy. Chemosis and swelling of the lids and periorbital tissue are prominent features of progressive Graves' ophthalmopathy and serve to distinguish the disease from retroorbital tumors, in which these changes are not seen. Increases in lacrimal gland size as well as soft tissue swelling in the periorbital area are frequently seen in acromegaly. Periorbital edema may also occur in diabetic patients with severe renal disease and the nephrotic syndrome.

Loss of the lateral third of the eyebrow is seen in hypothyroidism and in hypopituitarism but is not diagnostic of those diseases. In long-standing hypoparathyroidism, the hair of the eyebrows and eyelids becomes thin and patchy.

Ophthalmoplegia or eye muscle weakness leading to diplopia may be seen with pituitary tumors which extend laterally into the cavernous sinus and impinge on the oculomotor nerves. Slight to moderate impairment of eye movements is extremely common in thyrotoxicosis. In its mildest form, asymptomatic symmetric impairment of elevation of the eyes without diplopia is frequently missed. Unilateral weakness of the superior rectus muscle leading to upper lid retraction may be the first manifestation of Graves' disease. With increasing ophthalmoplegia, diplopia may occur on lateral or superior gaze. Myasthenia gravis can also cause ophthalmoplegia, but ptosis is a more common finding. Diabetic ophthalmoplegia involves the third and sixth nerves with equal frequency, has a rapid onset associated with pain on the ipsilateral side of the face, and, if the third nerve is involved, characteristically spares the pupil. Improvement occurs spontaneously in a few days or weeks, and complete recovery is almost invariable.

Severe protrusion of the eye in Graves' exophthalmos can impair total closure of the lids (*lagophthalmos*), resulting in corneal exposure during sleep and potentially dangerous exposure keratitis. In hypothyroidism discrete gray-colored spots may occur in the central portion of the cornea but do not generally interfere with vision.

In hyperparathyroidism and other hypercalcemic states of long duration, deposition of calcium phosphate crystals, a condition referred to as *band keratopathy,* may be observed at the medial and lateral margins of the cornea close to but separate from the cornea-sclera junction. Slit-lamp examination is frequently required to demonstrate the presence of keratopathy. In hypoparathyroidism there may be severe keratoconjunctivitis. Dilatation of conjunctival venules is seen in patients with diabetes, in parallel with the changes in retinal vessels. The dilatation, which is initially reversible, eventually becomes fixed and exhibits sacculations and even exudation.

Loss of pupillary reflexes may occur with pituitary tumors which invade the cavernous sinus. In diabetic ophthalmoplegia, the pupil is generally spared.

Both flaky and crystalline lenticular opacities are occasionally seen in hypothyroidism, but they generally do not interfere with vision. In contrast, cataracts and lenticular opacities are the most common eye findings in hypoparathyroidism. They may appear as diffuse white opacities separated by fluid clefts or as small and discrete punctate opacities in the lens cortex seen only on slit-lamp examination. The opacities are usually bilateral and frequently do not interfere with vision, though in some cases mature cataracts develop and require extraction. In younger diabetic patients cataracts are classically of the "snowflake" type and appear as bilateral dense bands of white spots situated in the subcapsular region of the lens. In older diabetic patients cataracts are morphologically indistinguishable from the senile cataracts in nondiabetic individuals. Although cataracts are no more frequent in diabetic patients than in nondiabetic individuals, they mature more rapidly and require extraction at an earlier age. Long-term treatment with high-dose glucocorticoids has been associated with posterior capsular cataracts.

Retinal changes characteristic of hypertension can be seen in acromegaly, primary aldosteronism, Cushing's syndrome, pheochromocytoma, and diabetes. Diabetic patients also exhibit a specific retinopathy consisting of capillary, arteriole, and venule microaneurysms appearing as small punctate red dots along the course of small vessels. These lesions may be confused with small hemorrhages but can be differentiated with fluorescein angiography. They are almost always bilateral and tend to be most frequent in the perimacular area. Microaneurysms are seen less frequently with other diseases, such as malignant hypertension, chronic anemias, and central retinal venous thromboses. Coalescence and rupture of microaneurysms lead to hemorrhages; the leakage of protein leads to exudation.

Papilledema is seen in patients with benign intracranial hypertension (pseudotumor cerebri), often associated with the use of oral contraceptives. It also occurs in obesity and in severe Graves' exophthalmos, hypoparathyroidism, the empty sella syndrome, neuroblastoma, and severe hypertension due to pheochromocytoma. It is observed less frequently in Cushing's syndrome and pituitary tumors, and in rare instances it is seen in primary aldosteronism.

Glaucoma can be precipitated or aggravated by spontaneous or iatrogenic hypercorticism. Glaucoma is also observed with increased frequency in diabetes mellitus.

CHAPTER 3

Gene Expression and Recombinant DNA in Endocrinology and Metabolism

David G. Gardner

Barry J. Gertz

Since its advent some 15 years ago, recombinant DNA technology has revolutionized biomedical research. Its application has resulted in a tremendous growth in new information about the structure and function of genes. This information is being used to devise more sophisticated and direct means of diagnosing, preventing, and treating disease. This technology is also providing new approaches to understanding human physiology and its aberrations which result in disease. Particularly exciting is the capacity to produce and purify large quantities of proteins which were previously of limited availability or essentially unobtainable.

Human insulin,[1,2] growth hormone,[3–5] and erythropoietin[6,7] produced by recombinant DNA techniques are currently in clinical use. Many new drugs and vaccines will be developed, the ability to diagnose and predict susceptibility to disease will be greatly expanded, and new types of therapy (including gene transfer) may become available. Physicians should therefore have some understanding of this technology to assess its strengths and weaknesses, to apply it to the management of endocrine and metabolic diseases, and to address certain ethical issues raised by its development. This chapter provides a conceptual framework for understanding the essential aspects of gene expression and regulation and the application of recombinant DNA methodology in endocrinology. Wherever possible, examples are drawn from endocrine systems.

GENES AND THEIR EXPRESSION

The modern era of molecular biology received its greatest impetus in 1953, when Watson and Crick reported the structure of deoxyribonucleic acid (DNA).[8] This finding provided an insight into how, through complementary base pairing, DNA replication could occur and thus how the genetic profile of an organism could be maintained from generation to generation.[9–11] Subsequent breakthroughs have yielded a considerable body of information including (1) how the DNA of a cell evolves and replicates,[9,10] (2) the means by which the DNA is *expressed*,[9–12] i.e., how it is transcribed into ribonucleic acid (RNA) and how those transcripts can be translated into protein—e.g., for messenger RNA (mRNA)—or utilized in other ways [as transfer RNA (tRNA) or ribosomal RNA (rRNA)], and (3) how gene expression is controlled.[9–13] Knowledge in these areas continues to accumulate at an unprecedented pace. A few critical aspects of the structure and function of DNA are described below for purposes of orientation. The references cited offer more detailed information.

DNA Structure and Replication

The structure of DNA is shown in Figs. 3-1 and 3-2. It contains a "backbone" composed of deoxyribose molecules linked together by connecting phosphate groups. These connections occur through the 3′ hydroxyl moiety of the first sugar and the 5′ hydroxyl moiety of the next sugar. Since the 5′ position of the first sugar in the DNA strand is free (i.e., not bound to an adjacent deoxyribose molecule) and the 3′ moiety of the last sugar is free, the direction of the molecule is described as 5′ to 3′. These designations serve as a reference for orientation. Genes are described as being transcribed from 5′ to 3′, since the ribose moieties in the RNA molecule are progressively added in a 5′ to 3′ direction such that the first nucleotide of the initial RNA product has a free 5′ triphosphate group (which may subsequently be modified). The 5′ end of a gene ordinarily refers to the position where transcription is initiated. The portion of the gene farther along in the 5′ direction is designated its *upstream* portion; the 3′ end designates its *downstream* portion, where transcription termination takes place.

Connected to each sugar of the DNA backbone is one of four bases: adenine (A), guanine (G), cytosine (C), or thymine (T). Adenine and guanine are pu-

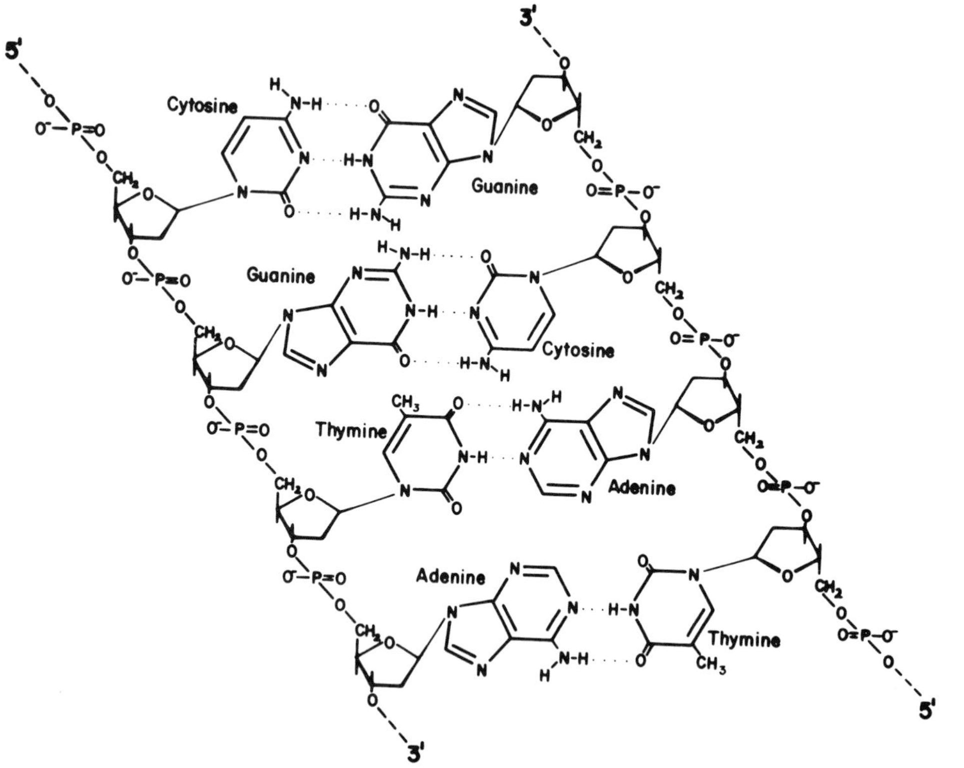

FIGURE 3-1 Structure of DNA. Several structural features of a short stretch of double-stranded DNA are shown. The sugar-phosphate backbones are shown on the outside, running antiparallel to one another: that on the left running 5′ to 3′ and that on the right running from 3′ to 5′. The purines adenine and guanine are shown on the inside, hydrogen-bonded to the pyrimidines thymine and cytosine, respectively.

rines; cytosine and thymine are pyrimidines. *Nucleosides* are bases bound only to the sugar moiety. When the base is coupled to a sugar and phosphate group, it is termed a *nucleotide*. As an example, adenine (a base) bound to ribose is termed *adenosine* (a nucleoside); adenosine coupled to a phosphate group is designated *adenylic acid* (a nucleotide). Several nucleotides linked together in a polymer generate a *nucleic acid*.

DNA is composed of two strands that run antiparallel to each other (i.e., the two strands of nucleotides run in opposite directions such that the 5′

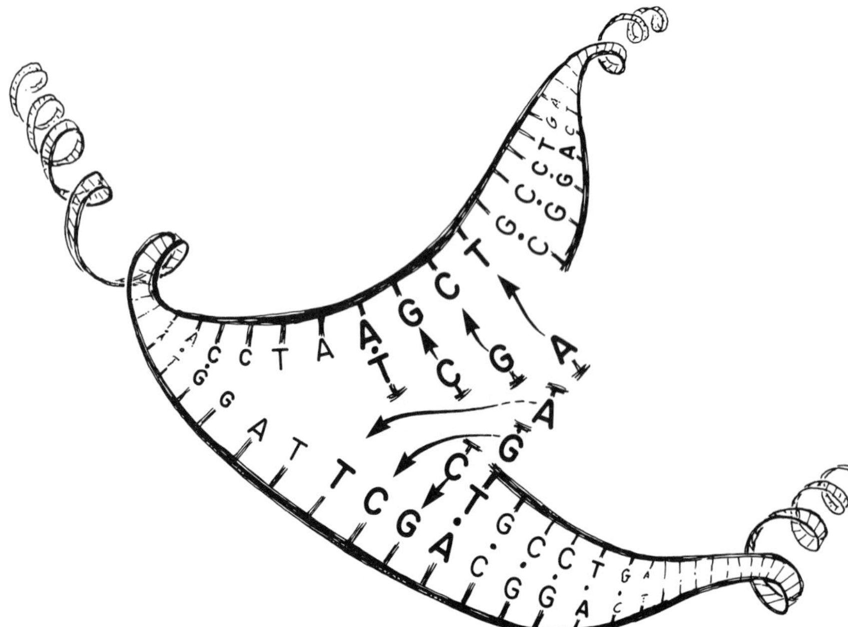

FIGURE 3-2 A highly simplified schematic representation of the essential features of DNA replication. The double helix unwinds, and two daughter strands of DNA are synthesized. Each of the resulting DNA molecules contains one strand of the original parent DNA molecule (semiconservative replication). Complementary base pairing directs the sequence of the addition of nucleoside triphosphates by DNA polymerase (not shown). Each daughter strand of DNA is synthesized in the 5′ to 3′ direction, requiring one strand to be synthesized in a discontinuous fashion. A = adenine; G = guanine; T = thymine; C = cytosine.

terminus of one strand and the 3′ terminus of the second strand lie in close apposition); the purine bases of one strand are hydrogen-bonded to the pyrimidine bases of the complementary strand. A base-pairs with T, and G base-pairs with C. Because of this complementary base pairing, the order of the bases along one strand of the DNA dictates the order along the other strand. This feature is critical in DNA replication and transcription for determining the precise structure of the DNA progeny and the RNA products of genes, respectively. These two strands are wound around each other, generating the well-known *double helix*. The nature of the helix is such that it generates major and minor grooves, or spaces, along its length. These grooves provide regions of contact between the DNA and proteins present in the nucleus. The DNA within the cell is complexed with proteins in a highly ordered, compacted configuration referred to as *chromatin*. As will be described later, these associated chromatin proteins play an important role in determining gene expression.

It is the order of the bases along the DNA strand, along with the feature of precise base pairing, which allows "like to replicate like" and permits information storage. It can be thought of as the body's computer program transmitting a replicate of itself to progeny, directing the developing embryo to differentiate properly into an adult organism, and organizing the enzymatic and other machinery necessary for all the complex metabolic functions of the cell.

When DNA replicates (Fig. 3-2), the individual strands are separated and nucleoside triphosphates are aligned along the sugar-phosphate backbones, with the order determined by complementary base pairing. The sugar moieties are then connected via phosphodiester linkages enzymatically, resulting in complementary DNA strands. Each strand of DNA is copied in the 5′ to 3′ direction; this necessitates that one of the strands be copied in a discontinuous fashion, usually as short fragments (so-called Okazaki fragments) which are then linked together to provide the complete DNA strand. The mechanics of this process are highly complex and outside the scope of this chapter (for a review, see Refs. 9 and 10), but the result is two daughter strands of DNA that are identical to the original DNA. One strand of each daughter DNA molecule is derived from the parent DNA, and the other is newly synthesized (*semiconservative replication*).

Chromatin

The chromosomal DNA in the cell nucleus is packaged into a complex structure termed *chromatin*.[9,10,14] This material contains proteins that serve as a matrix to fold the DNA and participate in replication and transcriptional control activities. One of the major classes of chromatin proteins is the histones, of which there are five major subtypes.[15] The DNA helix is wound twice around a histone octamer (that contains two copies each of histones 2A, 2B, 3, and 4) to form structures called *nucleosomes* (Fig. 3-3). H1, the fifth subtype, is positioned outside the core in a fashion that fosters the packaging of chromatin into higher-order structures. On electron microscopy, the nucleosome, along with the "linker" DNA, has the appearance of "beads on a string." The nucleosomes are further compacted into a structure called the 30-nm chromatin fiber. These fibers in

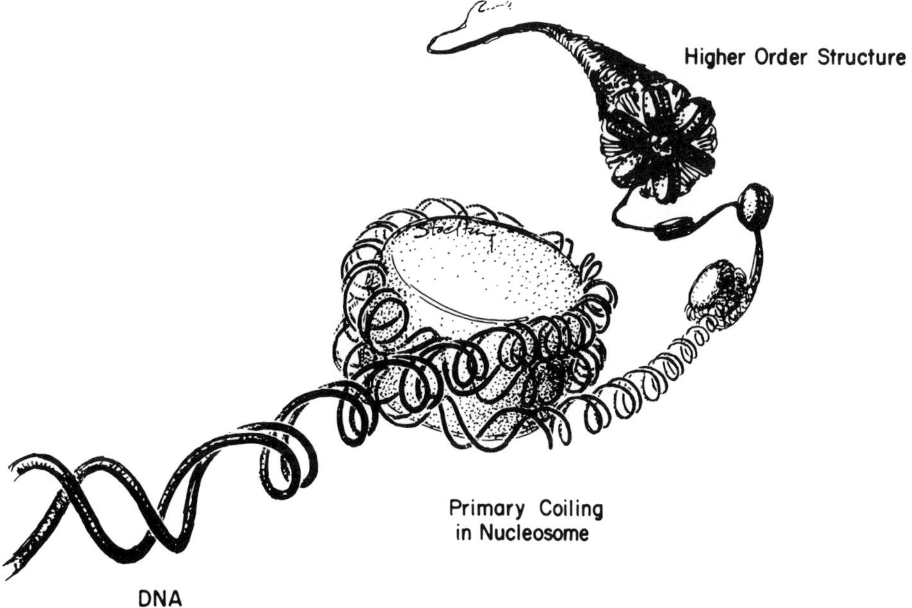

FIGURE 3-3 The fundamental unit of chromatin, the nucleosome, represents two turns of the DNA double helix around a core of histone molecules. The nucleosomes are separated by linker DNA and, under appropriate salt conditions in the presence of H1 histone, will form higher-order structures such as the 30-nm fiber. One possible orientation of the nucleosomes in the 30-nm fiber is depicted here.

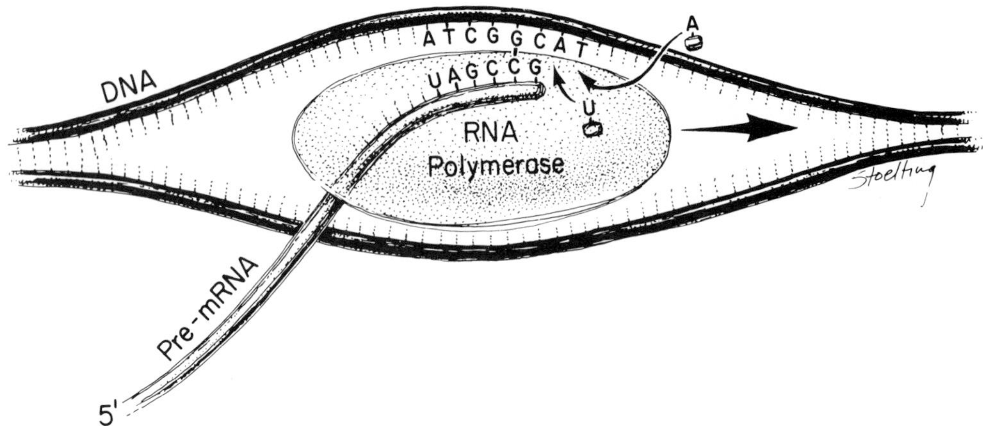

FIGURE 3-4 Synthesis of RNA. Transcription of a precursor species, pre-mRNA, by RNA polymerase is shown diagrammatically. The DNA template is shown to open over the region where transcription is taking place. The enzyme RNA polymerase directs the addition of ribonucleoside triphosphates into the growing pre-mRNA, with the actual sequence determined by complementary base pairing of purines and pyrimidines. The pyrimidine (U) found in RNA is shown as base-pairing with A. Even before transcription of the pre-mRNA is completed, the cap (a methylated guanine nucleotide) will be added to the 5′ end.

turn are organized into chromatin loops. Some investigators believe that these loops represent the structural equivalent of the *replicon,* a fundamental unit involved in DNA replication.[16] Chromatin also contains nonhistone proteins; these include enzymes (e.g., RNA polymerase) and factors that participate in gene transcription, DNA replication, the mediation of hormone action, and tissue-specific expression.[17] A large subgroup of nonhistone proteins, termed high mobility group (HMG) proteins, are concentrated in transcriptionally active chromatin and are believed to participate in transcriptional control.[17,18]

Transcriptionally active chromatin is more sensitive to pertubation with enzymatic reagents such as DNAse I, a nonspecific DNA cleavage enzyme, suggesting that this chromatin may be in a more "open" (accessible) configuration.[18] Such increased sensitivity is seen in the ovalbumin gene region in nuclei from the estrogen-stimulated oviduct but not in nuclei from tissues which do not express the gene.[19] Glucocorticoid activation of gene expression can be associated with an increase in the DNAse sensitivity of the stimulated gene.[20] Glucocorticoid treatment can also affect nucleosome phasing in the regulatory region of hormone-sensitive genes.[21] Together, these data suggest that one result of the interaction of the steroid-receptor complex with DNA is an alteration in chromatin configuration.

Other proteins are organized within a structure termed the *nuclear matrix* that serves as the overall scaffolding which defines nuclear structure.[16] DNA which is active in transcription or replication appears to be selectively associated with this matrix.[22–24] Interestingly, estrogen stimulation of the chicken oviduct results in a reversible association of the ovalbumin gene with the nuclear matrix. The primary transcripts of actively expressed genes, small nuclear RNAs,[25] and a subfraction of nuclear steroid hormone receptors are concentrated in the nuclear matrix.[26,27] Thus, the matrix appears to harbor components of the structural and enzymatic machinery responsible for the replication and transcription of active genes as well as the subsequent processing of their nascent transcripts.[16]

RNA Structure and Function

The first step in gene expression is the transcription of DNA into RNA (Figs. 3-4 and 3-5). RNA is similar in overall structure to DNA except that (1) in RNA the sugar moiety is ribose instead of deoxyribose, (2) the pyrimidine uracil (U) replaces thymine (U then base-pairs with A), and (3) RNA in mammalian cells is ordinarily not double-stranded, although it may fold onto itself (*secondary structure*), resulting in portions that are double-stranded. Some RNA viruses are also double-stranded.[9,10]

The three major classes of RNA are mRNA, tRNA, and rRNA. Other minor RNA species also exist and appear to play important roles in several cellular processes; for example, small RNA molecules are involved in the processing of precursor mRNA into mature mRNA (see below),[28–30] and other small RNAs are components of the *signal recognition particle* involved in the translocation of proteins across the endoplasmic reticulum.[31,32] mRNA contains sequences that are translated into protein (see below). tRNA is involved in protein synthesis, transferring amino acids onto a nascent peptide chain. rRNA, along with associated ribosomal proteins, forms a structure, termed the *ribosome,* that is also

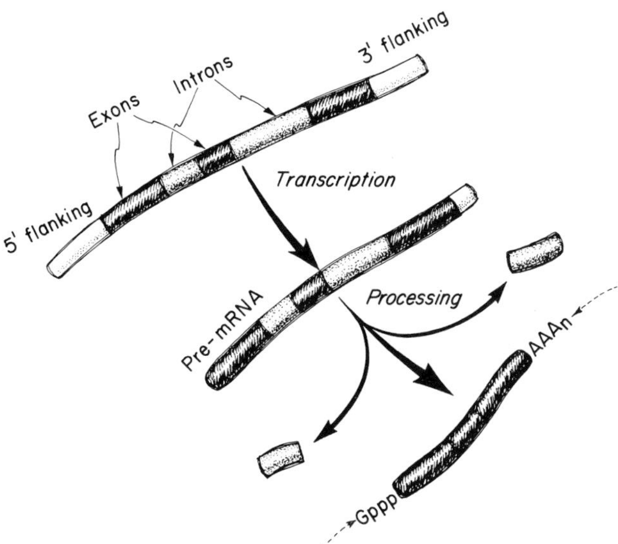

FIGURE 3-5 The initial steps in gene expression of a typical eukaryotic gene encoding a polypeptide. Exons (those regions present in the mature transcript) and introns (those segments destined to be excised from the primary transcript) are distinguished in the parent gene by shading. Both exons and introns are transcribed into the primary gene product, or pre-mRNA. This precursor species then undergoes several processing steps, which include the splicing of the exons associated with removal of the introns, the addition of a cap at the 5′ end, and cleavage and polyadenylation at the 3′ end. This mature transcript is then transported into the cytoplasm.

involved in protein synthesis. The mRNA and tRNA molecules bind to the ribosome during translation, as discussed in Chap. 4. A series of tRNA molecules exists, each one specific for an amino acid. Such "charged" tRNA molecules participate in the addition of amino acids to a growing protein molecule through the formation of peptide bonds.

Gene Expression

In addition to the regions of DNA that are transcribed into RNA, other segments critical for accurate gene expression are present on DNA.[9,10] These DNA segments direct where the enzymes involved in transcription will start and determine how efficiently the gene will be transcribed.[33,34] Other regions of the DNA (control or regulatory sequences) are involved in receiving regulatory signals from the environment (e.g., hormone-receptor complexes) that either inhibit or facilitate gene transcription. Still other sequences may function to determine the tissue-specific expression of a gene, possibly through interaction with factors (e.g., proteins) of limited tissue distribution.[35–37]

Transcription is performed by multisubunit enzymes termed *RNA polymerases* (Fig. 3-4). The region of DNA which determines the basal level of expression and directs where RNA polymerase initiates transcription is termed the *promoter;* the promoter region for mRNA transcription is primarily located just upstream from, i.e., 5′ to the start of transcription.[9,10,34] In contrast, the promoters for tRNA and rRNA genes may be located in part within the gene.[9,10,38,39] For transcription to proceed, the DNA strands are separated and RNA polymerase facilitates base pairing and subsequent polymerization of individual ribonucleoside triphosphates along one of the strands (Figs. 3-2 and 3-4). Transcription termination in eukaryotes is not well understood but appears to occur over a limited region of DNA rather than at a discrete site.[40] The 3′ end of the mRNA is defined by the cleavage and processing of a larger precursor (see below).

The structure of a mammalian gene encoding an mRNA is shown in Fig. 3-5. The DNA upstream from the start of transcription is called the *5′-flanking DNA,* and that downstream from the site directing the addition of the poly A tail in the pre-mRNA is called the *3′-flanking DNA.* The transcribed portion of a gene is composed of exons interrupted by introns, or intervening sequences. The primary transcript, or pre-mRNA, contains both exon and intron sequences. The intron sequences are removed from this precursor, and the exon sequences are spliced together to form a mature RNA product that contains only exon sequences.[12] These processing events involve large RNA-protein complexes, termed *spliceosomes,* which include the primary transcript as well as a number of small ribonucleoprotein particles.[29,41–44] These entities, along with specific processing signals that are present in the sequence of the primary RNA transcript, direct the precise excision of the introns and exon ligation. Consensus splicing signals, which are present in the sequence of the pre-mRNA, include GU/GAGU at the 5′ border of the intervening sequence and $(U/C)_n$ N U/CAG at the 3′ border (N represents any nucleotide, U/C denotes selection of either a uridine or a cytidine residue, and A/G denotes selection of either an adenine or a guanine residue).[45] Mutations at these locations can result in aberrant splicing and an altered gene product.[46,47] Introns are present in most[48] but not all[49] genes encoding mRNA molecules, and their number can vary considerably; for example, there are 2 for the human insulin gene,[50] 9 for the human renin gene,[51] and 17 for the low-density lipoprotein (LDL) receptor gene.[52] Introns are generally not found in bacterial genes. Removal of introns, along with subsequent splicing of the flanking exon sequences, takes place through a complicated mechanism[41–44,53] involving a complex of the mRNA precursor and several small ribonucleoproteins (i.e., snRNPs U_{1-6}) which collectively constitute the spliceosome. A schematic representation of the splicing mechanism is shown in Fig. 3-6. Intron excision involves two successive cleavage steps followed by a single ligation step. The first cleavage takes place at the 5′

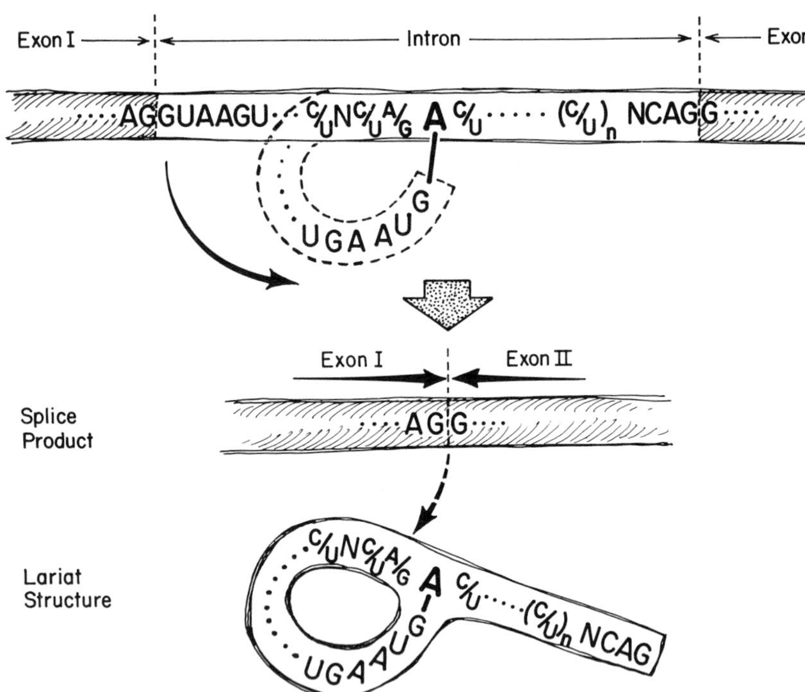

FIGURE 3-6 A schematic of the intro splicing mechanism. The reaction begins with cleavage at the 5″ 2″ phosphodiester linkage between the G residue at the 5″ terminus and an internal A residue. Subsequent cleavage at the 3″ border of the intron is followed by ligation of the upstream exons to the downstream exons, bringing contiguous coding sequences into apposition. The excised intron is released as a lariat structure which is degraded in the nucleus. Consensus sequences for the upstream (splice donor) and downstream (splice acceptor) intron borders as well as those nucleotides surrounding the A residue involved in lariat formation are presented. C/U denotes an alternative of cytidine or uridine in this position; A/G denotes a choice of adenine or guanine; N allows for any ribonucleotide in this position.

border of the intron sequence. The phosphorylated G residue at the 5′ terminus forms a 5′ 2′ phosphodiester linkage with an adenine residue (branch site) located within the intron. Cleavage at the 3′ border of the intron (i.e., to the 3′ side of the consensus G residue) is followed by ligation of the 3′ end of the upstream exon to the 5′ side of the downstream exon to generate the processed RNA product and a lariat-like structure containing only intron sequence. The RNA product is then subjected to further processing of additional intron sequences and readied for transport to the cytoplasm, while the lariat-like structure is turned over rapidly within the nuclear compartment.

RNA processing in lower life-forms appears in some cases to be a property inherent to the RNA molecule itself.[54] The RNA sequences responsible for these autocatalytic processing events, termed *ribozymes,* have attracted considerable attention as a potential modality for inhibiting the expression of selected genes (see below).

The mRNA transcript can also be modified in other ways. A chain of A residues (poly A tail) is added to the 3′ end of most (but not all) mRNA molecules.[12,40] This modification involves the sequence AAUAAA (or minor variants) at the 3′ end which directs, to a major extent, cleavage of the primary transcript approximately 10 to 30 nucleotides downstream.[55] This is followed by the addition of a stretch of A residues catalyzed by the enzyme polyadenylate polymerase. In most cases a "cap" is added to the 5′ end of the mRNA. The cap is a methylated nucleotide, usually a G residue, positioned in an inverted 3′ 5′ orientation.[9,10,56] Thus, the cap site identifies the first nucleotide of the mRNA and, by inference, the transcription start site. The precise function of these structures is unknown, though they appear to play a role in determining the stability and translational efficiency of eukaryotic mRNA molecules.[57,58] The primary transcripts of tRNA and rRNA genes also undergo processing to yield functional RNA molecules.[9,10]

Introns may serve a number of functions: Their presence is sometimes required for mRNA formation in eukaryotes, and DNA structures important for regulating gene expression may on occasion be found within introns. For example, a structure that binds the glucocorticoid receptor and probably mediates responsiveness to these steroids is found in an intron of the human growth hormone gene,[59,60] and a region important in regulating immunoglobulin heavy-chain gene expression is also located within an intron.[61] Similarly, exon sequences within the coding region of a gene may possess regulatory activity in some systems. The first exon of the thyroid-stimulating hormone (TSH) gene harbors a portion of the regulatory element which mediates thyroid hormone–dependent suppression of this gene's transcriptional activity.[62]

The fact that genes are split into introns and exons probably has facilitated the process of gene evolution.[63,64] It is now thought that one mechanism critical for gene evolution involves the movement of DNA segments into existing genes.[48,63,64] Such insertions can result in the addition of amino acid segments which significantly modify the function of the original gene product. One of the best known examples in which the functional domains of the protein product can be traced back to separate exon regions of the gene is the LDL receptor.[52] A highly negatively charged region of the LDL receptor, which appears to be responsible for binding lipoproteins, is composed of seven 40-amino acid repeat segments, 4 of which are encoded by separate exons; the remaining 3 are all on a single exon. The first exon encodes the signal sequence of the protein, while exons 16 and 17 encode the transmembrane domain and exons 17 and 18 encode the cytoplasmic domain of the receptor. Insertions may also bring in domains that contain regulatory structures, conferring on the modified gene new possibilities for control of its expression. The advantage of introns for such rearrangements of DNA lies in the fact that the genetic events can be somewhat imprecise. For example, a recombination event may bring a DNA segment composed of an exon flanked by intervening sequences into an existing gene. If this segment is inserted into an intron of the existing gene with the proper splicing signals, a new exon will be added to the gene that will be expressed in the mRNA product. The protein translated from this modified mRNA will then have an additional segment of amino acids. For this evolutionary event to occur, all that is needed are breaks within the intron in segments that do not contain critical control structures such as those which affect RNA processing; if introns and their removal by processing did not occur, such insertions would have to be much more precise to avoid compromising the coding sequence of the original gene.

The requirement for the removal of intervening sequences from the primary transcript engendered the possibility that differential processing of a pre-mRNA could result in more than one mature mRNA species being derived from a single gene. Such alternative splicing has proved to be more common than was previously anticipated. A prominent example in the endocrine system involves the pre-mRNA of the calcitonin gene, which can undergo differential processing to yield two distinct mRNA species.[65,66] In the brain, the result is an mRNA encoding the calcitonin gene–related peptide (CGRP). In the parafollicular cells of the thyroid gland, the result is predominantly the mRNA for calcitonin. Both of these mRNA species share three exons at the 5′ end which encode the amino-terminal portion common to both the calcitonin and CGRP precursor peptides. However, the mRNA molecules have distinct 3′ ends because differential splicing results in the incorporation of different downstream exons and polyadenylation sites into the two mRNA precursors. It is this region of the mRNA which codes for the distinct carboxy-terminal portions of the respective precursor peptides. These precursor peptides are then proteolytically cleaved to release either calcitonin or CGRP. Other examples of differential splicing include the genes for preprotachykinin[67] and nerve growth factor.[68]

After the mRNA is formed in the cell nucleus, it is transported to the cytoplasm, where it can be translated into protein. The amino acid sequence of the protein is dictated by the sequence of bases along the mRNA, with each set of three nucleotides (a *codon*) specifying an amino acid in accordance with the genetic code. The 5′ end of the mRNA usually includes a region, of variable length, termed the *5′-untranslated region*, which ends at the first codon for the polypeptide. The first codon is always AUG, which codes for methionine; this methionine is sometimes removed from the nascent peptide. In some cases, the initiating AUG lies within a consensus sequence [CCA/GCC*AUG*(G)] which may be of importance in translation initiation.[69,70] Individual amino acids are covalently linked to tRNA molecules specific for that amino acid. These tRNA molecules bind to the mRNA through an *anticodon loop* containing three nucleotides that are complementary to those of the mRNA codon. For example, a methionine tRNA contains UAC in its anticodon loop that base-pairs with the AUG on the mRNA. Whereas each codon is unambiguous in terms of its amino acid specificity, the code is redundant in that except for tryptophan and methionine, more than one codon specifies a given amino acid. Thus, if the nucleic acid sequence of an mRNA is known, the amino acid sequence of its translation product will be known with certainty. Conversely, if the amino acid sequence of a protein is known, the nucleic acid sequence of the mRNA and the gene from which it is transcribed can only be partially known. The ribosome moves along the RNA in the process of protein synthesis until it reaches a "stop," or termination, codon. At this point, translation ceases and the ribosome dissociates from the mRNA. Between the stop codon and the polyadenylation site is a region of highly variable length referred to as the *3′-untranslated region*.

As will be discussed in Chap. 4 the primary translation product, or precursor protein, may undergo extensive modification. For example, the signal peptide sequence which serves to target a protein for secretion is usually but not always[71] removed from the preprotein during the process of the protein translocation into the endoplasmic reticulum (as with preproinsulin) (see Chaps. 4 and 19). Another example is the release of one or more peptides from a larger protein precursor. Corticotropin (ACTH), a 39-amino acid protein, is released from a much larger protein, pro-opiomelanocortin (POMC), by specific proteolytic cleavage events (see Chaps. 7, 8, and 12). Sugars and/or other chemical groups may be also added after translation (see Chap. 4).

Regulation of Gene Expression

During the development of an organism, cells must differentiate to perform numerous specialized functions. This involves the expression of selected genes. Furthermore, both during development and afterward, hormones, neurotransmitters, and other regulatory signals must be capable of controlling the expression of DNA in various tissues in different ways. The molecular mechanisms involved in the regulation of gene expression are beginning to be understood.[19,72,73] The principal control appears to occur at the level of transcription of the DNA into pre-mRNA, although other steps involved in gene expression (e.g., mRNA stability) are also regulated.

The structure of most genes in the germ line cells (the reproductive cells) is essentially identical to that in the various differentiated or somatic cells. However, there are exceptions. The DNA may be modified by methylation of cytosine residues. In general, such methylation is inherited and results in an inhibition of gene expression.[74,75] This mechanism may participate in the transcriptional inactivation of one of the X chromosomes in cells that contain two X chromosomes.[76] Methylation may also be involved in more selective regulation of gene expression. For example, there is a positive correlation between the demethylation of an estrogen/glucocorticoid receptor–binding site and expression of the vitellogenin gene which harbors the site.[77] In other cases, DNA can undergo rearrangement and/or mutation. During the development of antibody-producing cells, there are both rearrangements of large segments of genomic DNA and mutations which are required to generate the expressed immunoglobulin genes. This permits a vast number of different immunoglobulin genes to be formed from a relatively small number of genes in the progenitor cells.[78,79]

The promoter structures for different genes (discussed in the previous section) vary in their capacity to facilitate the initiation of transcription. This affects the genes' basal level of activity. Control or regulatory sequences, in concert with the proteins that interact with them, affect the efficiency of the promoter in initiating transcription. A few examples can illustrate this point.

The growth hormone gene contains regulatory elements in its 5′-flanking region which are important for the expression of this gene. These sequences associate with a number of nuclear proteins. One of these proteins, termed GHF-1 (or Pit 1), binds to the promoter with high specificity and affinity.[35–37] Because the expression of GHF-1 is confined to pituitary cells, it is thought to be especially important for pituitary-specific expression of the growth hormone gene. However, the presence of GHF-1 alone cannot account for somatotrope-specific expression of the growth hormone gene since GHF-1 is also present in pituitary cells (e.g., thyrotropes) that do not express this gene. Emerging models suggest that genes are activated in specific tissues as a result of the combinatorial actions of a set of transcription factors that may be either restricted or generalized in their tissue distribution. Thus, a gene will be expressed in a particular cell type because its regulatory elements represent a composite "best match" for the transcription factors available within that cell.

Hormones and other regulatory molecules also appear to exert their activity through specific DNA sequences. As described in Chap. 5, glucocorticoids bind to intracellular receptors, which in turn associate with a site on DNA termed the *glucocorticoid regulatory element* (GRE) (Fig. 3-7). The steroid-receptor complex binds to the GRE more tightly than it does to random DNA.[80,81] This binding, in an undefined way, then facilitates, or in some cases inhibits, RNA polymerase action at the promoter. These effects probably involve both alterations in chromatin structure, as suggested previously,[20] and protein-protein interaction between the receptors and other transcription factors. A GRE can function as an independent element in that it can be spliced into a gene which is normally not inducible by glucocorticoid and can be shown to confer glucocorticoid responsiveness to the new hybrid gene when it is transferred to a glucocorticoid-responsive cell[59,60,82–84] (see Gene Transfer and Fig. 3-15). Glucocorticoid regulatory elements are found predominantly in the 5′-flanking DNA at a distance of a few to over a thousand nucleotides away from the promoter.[82–84] However, a putative GRE of the human growth hormone gene may be located downstream within an intron.[59,60] Examples in which the glucocorticoid-receptor complex inhibits transcription include the genes encoding POMC,[85–87] the α subunit of the human glycoprotein hormones,[88] and a number of c-jun/c-fos–dependent transcription units.[89,90] In these

FIGURE 3-7 Binding of the glucocorticoid-receptor complex at the GRE. The steroid-receptor complex binds to specific DNA sequences (the GRE). This binding event, in an unknown fashion, enhances (or in some cases inhibits) the interaction of RNA polymerase with the promoter of the glucocorticoid-regulated gene. The result is a stimulation (or inhibition) of the transcription of the gene.

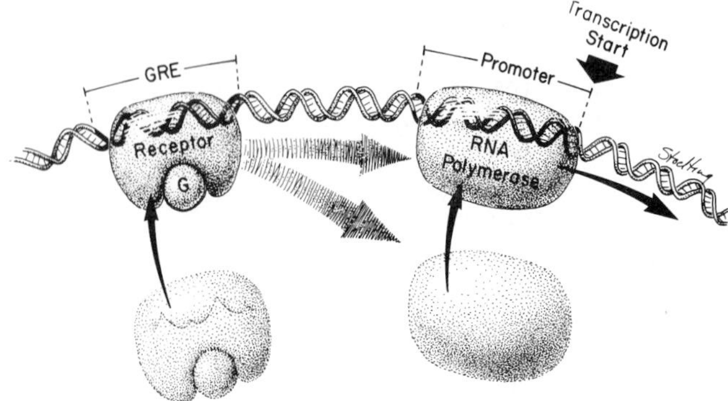

cases, the inhibition appears to result from displacement of a positive transcriptional regulatory factor [i.e., that for the cAMP regulatory element binding (CREB) protein in the case of the α-subunit glycoprotein hormone promoter[88]] from its normal position on the gene by the glucocorticoid receptor complex or through association of the complex with other transcription factors.[89,90] Analogous hormone response elements appear to mediate the actions of other classes of steroid and steroid-like hormones, including estrogen, progesterone, androgen, mineralocorticoid, retinoic acid, vitamin D, and thyroid hormone, each acting through its respective receptors.[91–93]

Hormones which act primarily at the cell surface are also extensively involved in regulating transcription. Agents which increase cellular cAMP levels have been shown to increase the expression of the prolactin,[94] human chorionic gonadotropin,[95] and somatostatin genes,[96] among others. This activation in many cases involves the protein kinase A–dependent phosphorylation of nuclear regulatory proteins; one of these, termed CREB (cAMP regulatory element binding protein), which associates with specific DNA elements in target genes, is activated by phosphorylation to increase the transcription of contiguous coding sequences.[97] Similar mechanisms appear to be involved for hormones which promote phosphoinositide turnover and activate protein kinase C.[98–100] In this case, one of the nuclear protein effectors consists of a heterodimeric complex of the cellular homologues of the c-jun and c-fos oncogene products (termed AP-1). This complex associates with a specific regulatory element, termed the TRE [TPA (phorbol ester) response element, not to be confused with the thyroid hormone response element], within the targeted gene. The details of how protein kinase C activates the complex are only partially understood, but the process appears to involve both increased production of the c-jun and c-fos components of the AP-1 complex[101,102] and posttranslational activation of AP-1, perhaps through dephosphorylation of the protein components[103] or the release of an inhibitory protein factor.[104] Insulin is also known to regulate specific target genes [e.g., the phosphoenolpyruvate kinase (PEPCK) and glyceraldehyde phosphate dehydrogenase (GAPD) genes]. Specific insulin-sensitive regulatory elements have been identified in the 5′ flanking DNA of each of these genes.[105,106]

Hormone response elements (HREs) belong to a larger class of DNA structures termed *enhancers*[107–109] that were described initially in DNA tumor viruses. In most cases, they have the capacity to augment (or enhance) transcriptional activity even if they are located several thousand nucleotides away from a promoter in either orientation relative to the promoter and either upstream or downstream from the gene. In other cases, their activities are more strictly dependent on their placement at a particular position in the gene. These control or regulatory DNA sequences are in effect "cassettes" of information that have been inserted into the DNA in the vicinity of a promoter and that affect promoter function, in some cases in response to regulatory proteins. A gene typically contains several different cassettes that can allow for control of expression by a variety of factors, including those involved in tissue-specific expression or regulation by extrinsic factors such as hormones and neurotransmitters.

Regulatory elements in general acquire their activity by virtue of their ability to associate with specific nuclear regulatory proteins (e.g., the association of the GRE with the liganded glucocorticoid receptor). This association may position these proteins in a fashion which allows them to interact with the core transcriptional apparatus or with other transcription factors. In the case of enhancer elements located at some distance from the promoter, this may involve the formation of a loop in the DNA to permit correct positioning of the enhancer and promoter elements.[110] The precise mechanisms by which enhancers activate transcription remain unknown but probably result from protein-protein interactions involving the enhancer binding protein and proteins of the transcription initiation complex.[111] In many cases one or more additional accessory proteins may be involved in establishing this linkage.[111–113]

Gene expression can also be regulated at the level of RNA processing or turnover. As was discussed above, the pre-mRNA from the calcitonin gene can be processed in two ways: In brain and certain other tissues, the mRNA for CGRP is produced, and in the parafollicular cells of the thyroid gland, calcitonin mRNA is made.[65,66] Presumably, tissue-specific factors regulate this differential RNA processing.[114,115] Variable RNA processing has been described for transcripts of the growth hormone and prolactin genes, although the differences in the resulting mRNA molecules are less striking.[116] Hormones and other factors can also regulate mRNA (and consequently protein) levels by affecting mRNA stability.[117,118] Part of the mechanism by which prolactin stimulates an accumulation of casein in the mouse mammary gland involves a prolactin-mediated decrease in the rate of casein mRNA breakdown with a consequent increase in casein mRNA.[119] In addition, estrogen stimulates the accumulation of ovalbumin mRNA in the chicken oviduct by decreasing the rate of turnover as well as by stimulating the synthesis of the mRNA.[120,121] Similar stabilization of the vitellogenin gene has been demonstrated after estrogen administration.[122] Glucocorticoids have been implicated as playing a role in the regulation of the processing of the α_1-acid glycoprotein gene transcript[123] as well as the growth hormone gene transcript,[124] although the latter implication remains controversial.[125] The means by which hormones accomplish such selective stabilization of mRNA molecules is unknown. Hormones may also regulate the efficiency of processing and/or the stability of a pre-mRNA in the nucleus to alter gene expression.[126]

There are examples in which gene expression may also be regulated at translational and post-translational loci through effects on the efficiency of mRNA translation or covalent modification of protein structure. Steroid and polypeptide hormones may control the translational efficiency of specific mRNAs.[127] However, this probably represents a minor component of their overall activity. For peptides that are cleaved from larger precursor molecules, tissue-specific factors direct which peptides are released. Thus, in the rat, POMC is cleaved to release ACTH and β-lipotropin (β-LPH) in the anterior pituitary and α-melanocyte stimulating hormone (α-MSH) and corticotropin-like intermediate peptide (CLIP) in the intermediate lobe.[128] The extensive control of enzyme activity through the actions of hormones and other regulatory substances is discussed in Chap. 5.

Gene Evolution

Genes are generated during evolution through rearrangements, additions, duplications, and deletions of DNA segments and mutations of individual nucleotides. When genes duplicate, each of the two resulting genes can then evolve independently. This is the probable origin of the so-called gene families whose members share structural similarities. Such families contain from a few to many genes. Gene families are usually identified through comparisons of their members' overall structural organization and homologies (similarities) in their nucleotide sequences.[63,64] Examples of gene families include those encoding growth hormone, prolactin, and placental lactogen (chorionic somatomammotropin); insulin and the somatomedins; the glycoprotein hormones (TSH, human chorionic gonadotropin, luteinizing hormone, and follicle stimulating hormone); and receptors for the steroid and thyroid hormones.

A model for the evolution of the growth hormone gene family is illustrative (Fig. 3-8).[63,129] Initially there was a primitive gene with a promoter and one exon. This exon segment was ultimately duplicated four times to yield the present-day exons 2, 4, and 5, with two of the segments present in exon 5. Apparently an intron between the two duplicated segments constituting exon 5 was removed. Two additional DNA segments were inserted, one encoding what is now exon 3 and another contributing sequences of the 5′-flanking DNA, exon 1, and part of the first intron. The latter insertion brought in a new promoter as well as the putative GRE of the human growth hormone gene; this left a primitive promoter upstream from the current promoter that is still weakly active. This precursor gene underwent several duplications and subsequent mutations to evolve into the genes coding for growth hormone, prolactin, and placental lactogen. Thus, the genes for these three hormones have significant nucleic acid sequence homology and a similar overall structure, with five exons separated by four introns that interrupt the coding sequences at similar locations. Finally, upstream from each gene's dominant promoter is a weakly active promoter element.

Mechanisms of Genetic Disease

There are a number of heritable endocrine disorders in which the genetic defect has been defined at a molecular level. These include pseudohypoparathyroidism,[130] Laron dwarfism,[131,132] congenital adrenal hyperplasia,[133] isolated deficiencies of growth hormone[134,135] and TSH,[136] disorders of lipoprotein metabolism,[137] and selected forms of glucocorticoid,[138] androgen,[139] thyroid hormone,[140] vitamin D,[141] and insulin[142] resistance. A number of mechanisms can account for genetic disease, and these mechanisms have been most clearly elucidated for nonendocrine diseases such as the thalassemias.[143] There can be base change (point) mutations that result in an altered codon (missense mutation). If the subsequent amino acid change in the protein is deleterious, an altered protein that is functionally defective will result. Missense mutations in the insulin gene have been found to be a rare cause of diabetes mellitus.[144,145] Alternatively, a mutation can result in the generation of a translation stop codon (a nonsense mutation), and this can result in the absence of functional protein.[146] In some cases, such changes result in an RNA product which is unstable and does not accumulate normally.[147] Proper processing of pre-mRNA to mature mRNA can be interrupted by a point mutation in a processing site.[148] In addition,

FIGURE 3-8 Evolution of the growth hormone gene family. The ancestral gene with its promoter and single exon undergoes several modifications as a result of exon duplication and DNA insertion events. Finally, as a result of gene duplication and mutation, the members of the growth hormone gene family emerge (growth hormone, prolactin, and human placental lactogen). See text for details.

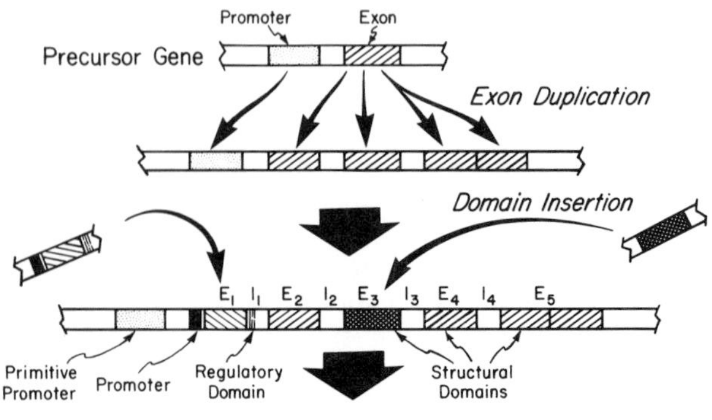

there can be deletions or insertions of DNA segments that disrupt gene function or result in abnormal RNA products. In some cases, the entire gene can be deleted, as has been reported to occur for a rare form of growth hormone deficiency.[134] Finally, mutations or rearrangements in promoter structures can result in abnormalities in the expression of specific genes. This has been shown to occur with some of the thalassemias.[149]

RECOMBINANT DNA TECHNOLOGY

The essence of recombinant DNA technology is that pieces of DNA can be cut or ligated together outside of living cells.[150–152] This *recombinant DNA* can then be inserted back into a living cell, such as a prokaryote (a nonnucleated cell such as a bacterium) or a eukaryote (a nucleated cell such as a yeast or a mammalian cell), in which it can be replicated. In this way, starting from a single molecule of DNA, many new molecules can be obtained. These molecules can be isolated and used to investigate basic biological processes such as how cells regulate gene expression. Alternatively, they can be put to practical uses, such as for the production of hormones or other proteins that cannot be obtained in adequate quantities by other methods.

One of the major developments that led to this new technology resulted from studies of the process of restriction and modification in bacteria.[9,10] Through these processes, organisms destroy DNA they recognize as foreign and simultaneously modify their own DNA to protect it from similar degradation. In effect, the system represents a very primitive "immune system" designed to segregate endogenous from exogenous genetic material. The enzymes responsible for degrading exogenous DNA, termed *restriction enzymes* or *restriction endonucleases,* bind to DNA at specific sequences and cleave it at or in close proximity to these loci. The enzymes are named for the bacteria from which the enzyme is derived. The first restriction enzyme discovered, termed *Eco*RI, was isolated from *Escherichia coli;* its action is depicted in Fig. 3-9. The availability and use of these enzymes has allowed scientists to cleave DNA at specific sites. For example, if a DNA fragment is incubated under appropriate conditions with *Eco*RI, the DNA will be cleaved at all sites containing the sequence shown in Fig. 3-9. In this case the cleavage yields single-stranded overhanging ends that are complementary to each other (*sticky ends*). If one of the resulting pieces is isolated and incubated with a DNA fragment from another source that has been cut with the same enzyme, the complementary ends of each DNA fragment will base-pair (Figs. 3-9 and 3-10). The resulting hybrid DNA molecules can then be ligated together enzymatically to form a new recombinant DNA molecule (Fig. 3-10). Some restric-

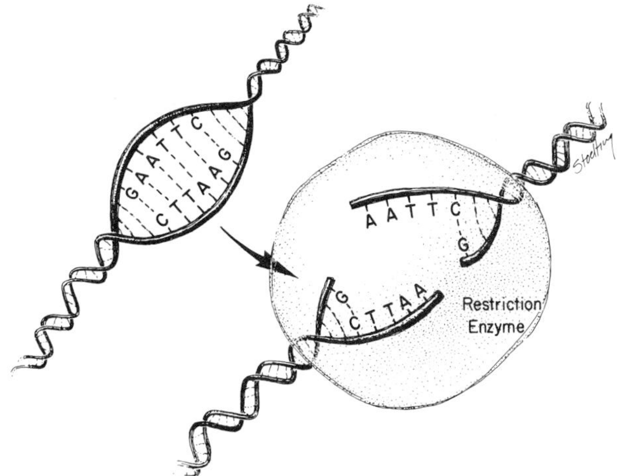

FIGURE 3-9 Endonucleolytic cleavage of DNA by the restriction enzyme *Eco*RI. The six-base-pair sequence recognized by the restriction endonuclease is enlarged for illustration purposes. The result of cleavage is two single-stranded sticky ends, i.e., overhanging, four-nucleotide complementary DNA segments.

tion enzymes yield blunt-ended fragments rather than overhanging or sticky ends; blunt-ended fragments can also be ligated to other blunt-ended fragments. Since blunt ends have no overhanging sequence that require hybridization, they can be ligated to any other blunt-ended molecule regardless of the nature of the enzyme used to produce the cleavage.

The cloning of individual genes involves the isolation of the DNA sequence of interest, the ligation of these sequences into a cloning vector (usually a modified bacterial plasmid or bacteriophage), the introduction of these "recombinant" molecules into the appropriate host cell, and the expansion of this cell lineage in culture. Plasmids are frequently the starting material for constructing recombinant DNA molecules. These are circular pieces of double-stranded DNA which replicate in bacteria as episomes, i.e., extrachromosomally (Fig. 3-10). They frequently transmit antibiotic resistance; for example, they may contain the gene for β-lactamase, whose product confers resistance to ampicillin by cleaving its β-lactam ring. A recombinant plasmid containing inserted foreign DNA (such as that encoding a human gene) may be constructed as shown in Fig. 3-10. The plasmid is then transferred ("transfected") into bacteria, usually *E. coli,* through a treatment which makes the bacteria leaky and thus able to take up foreign DNA (Fig. 3-11). These "transformed" bacteria can then be grown in culture, and the recombinant plasmid will replicate. In practice, when bacteria are transfected with plasmid DNA, only a small percentage of the microorganisms actually take up the plasmid DNA, and on a probability basis only a single plasmid enters per bacterium. If a plasmid containing an antibiotic resistance gene is used, one

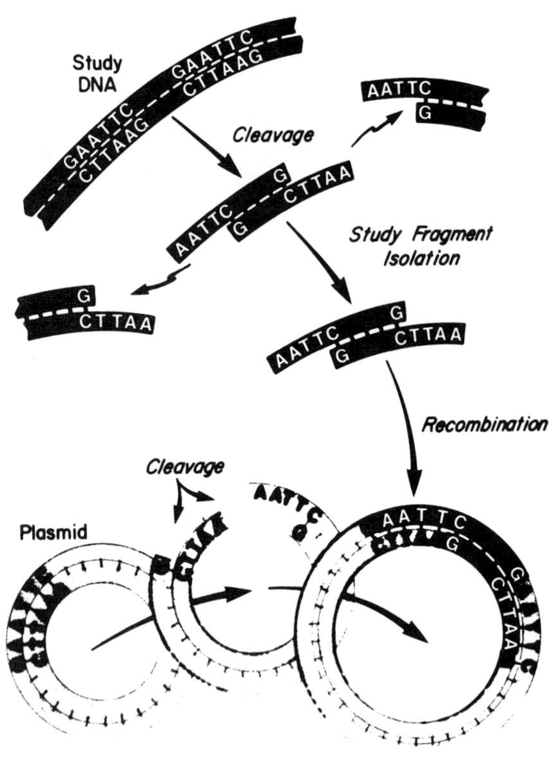

FIGURE 3-10 Generation of a recombinant DNA molecule. The study DNA is cleaved with a restriction enzyme (in this case *Eco*RI), and the released fragment is purified (i.e., separated from the parent DNA on the basis of size by agarose gel electrophoresis). A suitable plasmid containing a unique site for the same enzyme is prepared by cleavage with the enzyme and then mixed together with the purified fragment. The complementary overhanging ends anneal to one another and are then ligated together enzymatically (by DNA ligase) to yield a new recombinant molecule.

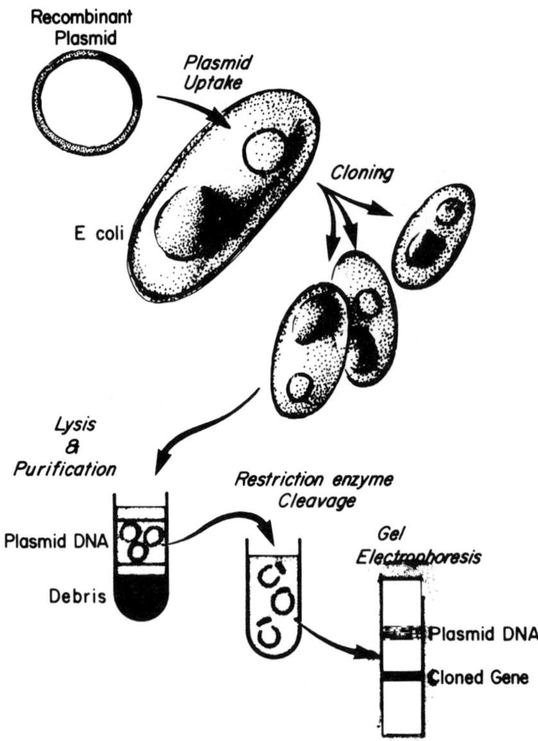

FIGURE 3-11 Cloning of DNA. Bacteria are treated to facilitate the uptake of DNA, often using recombinant plasmids containing a DNA insert of interest. Culturing in the presence of an antibiotic selects for bacteria that harbor a plasmid containing an appropriate antibiotic resistance gene along with the DNA insert. Those bacteria which have failed to take up the plasmid will succumb to the antibiotic. Single colonies (a clone) of the now-resistant bacteria are selected for mass culture. They are then lysed and the cloned plasmid DNA purified. Cleavage with the appropriate restriction enzyme will release the DNA insert, yielding quantities of homogeneous DNA suitable for further experimentation (e.g., sequencing or preparation of specific radiolabeled DNA probes).

can select for the bacteria that harbor these recombinant plasmids by culturing them in the presence of an antibiotic that will kill bacteria that lack plasmid DNA. The population of cells derived from a single parent cell harboring the foreign DNA is said to represent a *clone* of cells, and the DNA insert of the plasmid is said to be cloned (Fig. 3-11). Once a clone is obtained, the bacteria can be grown in large quantities, the plasmid DNA can be isolated from other bacterial constituents, and the DNA insert can be released from the plasmid by cleaving it with the same restriction enzyme utilized for its initial isolation. This DNA can then be separated from the plasmid DNA by electrophoretic techniques and can be characterized. In this fashion, large quantities of homogeneous DNA fragments can be produced for study purposes. One common use for such homogeneous pieces of DNA is in preparing radiolabeled probes for hybridization.

Hybridization

A fundamental property of single-stranded DNA or RNA is its propensity to anneal through base pairing, i.e., hybridize, to a strand of DNA or RNA containing complementary sequences (Fig. 3-12). This very precise process is based on the AT (or AU), GC hydrogen bonding discussed earlier, which permits a single-stranded nucleic acid to find its complement from among millions of noncomplementary competing molecules. Recombinant DNA technology makes extensive use of this property in virtually all its applications. For example, after radiolabeling, a homogeneous population of DNA molecules can be used as a probe to identify a complementary DNA or RNA fragment within a complex mixture or to localize a single colony of bacteria containing a plasmid with complementary DNA sequences from among thousands of bacterial clones, each of which harbors a different plasmid. A standard approach to nucleic acid analysis involves size fractionation of an "un-

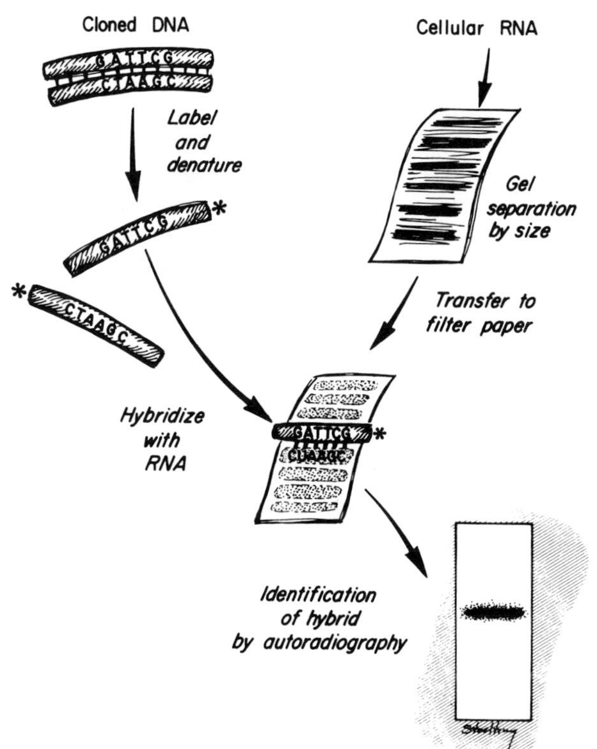

FIGURE 3-12 Use of hybridization to identify specific RNA sequences. A cloned piece of DNA is radiolabeled with ^{32}P nucleoside triphosphates and denatured. Cellular RNA is separated on the basis of size by agarose gel electrophoresis. The RNA is transferred by diffusion blotting onto nitrocellulose filter paper and fixed to the paper. The radiolabeled cDNA probe is incubated with the filter paper. Hybridization with complementary RNA sequences takes place, and the nonhybridized probe is eliminated by washing. Autoradiography of the filter reveals the location (size) of the RNA species, and the strength of the signal is used for quantification.

known" RNA or DNA preparation by gel electrophoresis, transfer (*blotting*) of the nucleic acid onto nitrocellulose filter paper, fixation to the paper, and exposure (hybridization) to the radiolabeled probe. Although this process was originally described for the transfer of DNA molecules (*Southern blotting*),[153] RNA can be similarly transferred if properly treated (commonly referred to as *Northern blotting*.)[154] After elimination of the nonhybridized probe, the strength of the signal from the radiolabeled hybrids can be determined. The level of radioactivity in the hybrid is directly proportional to the amount of specific mRNA in the sample (Fig. 3-12).

DNA Sequencing

Another breakthrough that has facilitated the development of recombinant DNA technology is the design of methods to sequence DNA rapidly. Two general approaches and a multitude of variations are available (for review, see Refs. 150–152 and 155–156). The chemical degradation technique of Maxam and Gilbert[155] relies on the systematic cleavage of homogeneous DNA fragments that are radiolabeled at one end. Chemical reagents and reaction conditions are chosen such that the cleavage process in a given reaction occurs only at one (or two) of the four nucleotides (A residues, for instance) and each susceptible position in a DNA molecule is cleaved at a low frequency. The result is a series of radiolabeled DNA fragments extending from the labeled end to each position of the given nucleotide (i.e., at each A) in the original DNA fragment. These fragments can be visualized after size fractionation of the DNA and radioautography; the size of each band corresponds to the position of the base in the starting DNA (Fig. 3-13).

The more commonly used technique today is the chain termination method of Sanger.[156] For most applications, this technique has used a homogeneous population of single-stranded DNA molecules (often generated in the single-stranded bacteriophage M 13) as templates for complementary DNA synthesis. Newer modifications allow for sequencing of the single-stranded template without prior purification away from its complementary strand.[157] DNA synthesis is initiated at a particular site with the use of

FIGURE 3-13 DNA sequencing by the chemical degradation technique. The radiolabeled DNA is subjected to four separate cleavage reactions, each of which is specific for one (or two) nucleotides. The resulting fragments from each reaction are separated on a gel, and the sequence is read from the autoradiogram. See text for details.

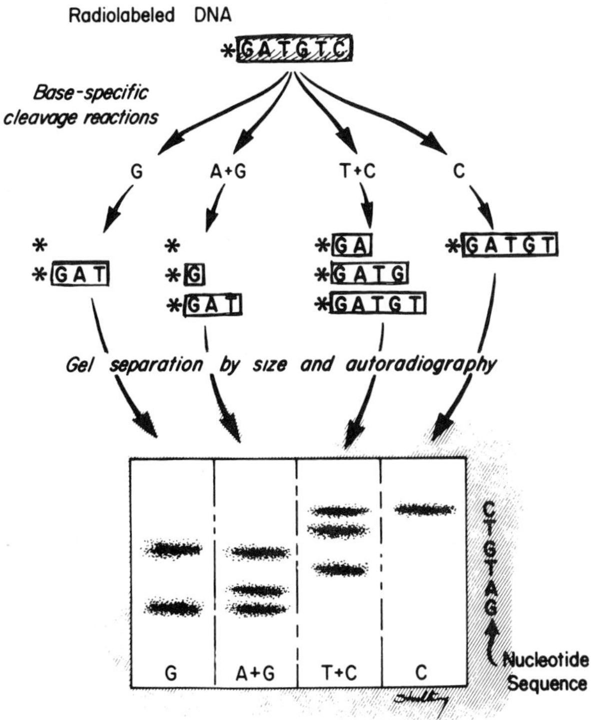

a small "primer" oligonucleotide that hybridizes to a specific DNA sequence. DNA synthesis then is allowed to proceed in the presence of radiolabeled nucleoside triphosphate precursors. The reaction is performed in the presence of an analog of one of the nucleotides, which has a modified 3′-OH group (i.e., converted from the deoxy derivate to the dideoxy derivative with a hydrogen atom at the 3′ position) so that when it is incorporated into a growing DNA chain, further elongation cannot proceed past the analog. Four separate reactions are utilized, with each reaction including one modified nucleotide (dideoxy ATP, for example) in addition to the four unmodified nucleotides. The ratio of deoxy to dideoxy nucleotides in each reaction is chosen so that termination of synthesis of the complementary DNA molecule occurs infrequently at each occurrence of a given base (A in this example). The result is a series of radiolabeled fragments for each reaction that extend from the start site of synthesis to each position occupied by the nucleotide (e.g., deoxyadenosine) under analysis. These are then size-fractionated on gels; as with the chemical degradation technique, the size of each band corresponds to a position of the complementary base in the original template DNA.

Through the use of these methods, even genes that are several thousand nucleotides in length can be sequenced in a reasonable period of time. Thus, once a gene is obtained in pure form, its primary structure, or nucleotide sequence, can be determined rapidly and accurately. Newer automated techniques employing nucleotides labeled with colorimetric tags have brought the sequencing of entire chromosomes within the realm of possibility.[158]

Sources of DNA for Molecular Cloning

Three different sources are ordinarily utilized to obtain the DNA required for molecular cloning. These sources include DNA produced by chemical synthesis, cellular mRNA which can be reverse-transcribed into DNA, and chromosomal DNA.

DNA Synthesis

DNA molecules, particularly those composed of approximately 70 nucleotides or less, can be synthesized within a reasonable time using currently available automated synthesizers.[159,160] When one ligates together a number of oligonucleotides produced in this fashion, an entire gene can be synthesized, provided that its structure or that of the protein it encodes is known. This approach was used for the first synthesis of human insulin by recombinant DNA techniques.[1] When this was done, the human insulin gene had not been isolated. However, the amino acid sequence of human insulin was known, and this information was used to select the nucleotide sequence of the synthetic gene. DNA fragments which would encode the amino acids of the A and B chains of human insulin were inserted into separate plasmids. In each case, the synthetic gene segments were cloned "in phase" (i.e., in the appropriate translational reading frame) into the middle of a bacterial gene. When these plasmids were transformed into (separate) bacteria, the microorganisms synthesized a *fusion protein* containing the amino acids encoded by the bacterial gene linked to the human insulin A or B chain sequences. The A and B chains of human insulin were later cleaved from their respective fusion proteins, purified, and then joined together chemically through the disulfide bonds that ordinarily connect these two chains.

More commonly, however, smaller DNA segments are produced to facilitate the construction of genes or recombinant DNA molecules. For example, small DNA segments containing desired restriction enzyme sites (*linkers*) are frequently added to the ends of DNA fragments to aid in the construction of recombinant molecules. Other small fragments may be employed as adaptor sequences to facilitate the fusion of two DNA segments from independent sources or to provide a critical sequence (e.g., a methionine codon for translation initiation) when this is not available in a cloned DNA fragment from another source. Chemically synthesized fragments are also used commonly as probes to detect complementary nucleic acid sequence in conventional hybridization studies. Finally, as discussed above and in a subsequent section (see Production of Medically Important Proteins by Recombinant DNA Techniques), synthetic DNA may be used to prepare hybrid genes that are combinations of different mammalian or bacterial genes. These genes may be used for protein production in the appropriate host cell.

Reverse Transcription of mRNA

Cells or tissues which selectively express a gene of interest are excellent sources of material for subsequent cloning since they contain mRNAs that encode the products of those genes. Cellular mRNA encoding a particular protein can be isolated from cells that produce the protein product of interest. DNA strands complementary to this mRNA (i.e., cDNA) can be produced from the mRNA template using deoxyribonucleoside triphosphates and reverse transcriptase,[9,10,150–152] an enzyme which is isolated from retrovirus-infected cells. To initiate reverse transcription, the reaction must be "primed" by an oligonucleotide that hybridizes to the RNA being copied. As was described earlier, most mRNA molecules have a polyadenylated, or poly A, tail. Oligomers of polydeoxythymidylate (oligo-dT) can hybridize to this poly A tail and serve to prime the reaction. After the formation of this cDNA, the RNA is destroyed and the single-stranded cDNA is then copied into a double-stranded DNA molecule using the same enzyme (that also copies DNA into DNA) or DNA polymerase.

Several different methods can be utilized to insert the cDNA into a plasmid. For example, chemically synthesized double-stranded DNA linker molecules containing an appropriate restriction site may be ligated to the ends. The entire fragment may then be inserted into a plasmid that was previously cleaved at the same restriction enzyme site (Fig. 3-10).

Since every cell contains thousands of different mRNA molecules, reverse transcription of total cellular mRNA will yield thousands of cDNA molecules. Thus, the investigator must either isolate the mRNA of interest before cDNA synthesis or generate a large number of clones from the mixture of starting cDNA molecules and identify the clone containing the cDNA of interest by using a marker which is relatively specific for the gene sequences of interest. In most cases, the specific mRNA cannot be obtained in homogeneous form before cloning; therefore, some reliance must be placed on the latter approach. However, mixtures of mRNA molecules are sometimes greatly enriched for an mRNA of interest before molecular cloning. This can be accomplished in several ways, including (1) starting with a tissue source which contains a high concentration of the mRNA of interest, (2) employing a physiologic or pharmacologic pertubation in vivo which increases cellular levels of this mRNA (this approach may be employed in combination with a subtraction hybridization[152] technique which selectively reduces the contribution of transcripts unaffected by the pertubation; see below), (3) isolating a limited size range of mRNA molecules using physical separation techniques, and (4) immunoprecipitating polysomes (which contain mRNA and attached nascent protein chains), utilizing antisera that recognize the nascent peptide product of the mRNA.

In any case, all the mRNA molecules present at the time of reverse transcription will serve as templates for cDNA synthesis. This will yield, after cloning, a so-called cDNA library representing from a few to thousands of clones, each harboring the same parent plasmid but a different cDNA insert. This cDNA library must then be screened to identify the clone that contains the plasmid with the cDNA insert of interest.

The screening of a cDNA library may be performed in several ways.[150–152] The most common method—*hybridization screening*—employs radioactively labeled oligonucleotides that are complementary to sequences of the cDNA of interest. If even a portion of the amino acid sequence of the protein encoded by the mRNA is known, this information can be used, through knowledge of the genetic code, to predict a partial DNA sequence for the cDNA. Small oligonucleotide DNA molecules that are complementary to a portion of the nucleotide sequence of the cDNA can be synthesized. Usually a group of such oligonucleotides are made to include all possible sequences in that portion of the cDNA, as determined by the degeneracy in the genetic code; this will compensate for a lack of knowledge of the exact codon usage in the cDNA. If a large stretch of amino acids is known, oligonucleotides are synthesized complementary to that region of the cDNA which has the minimum number of possible codon choices (i.e., degeneracy is most limited). Alternatively, a single large oligonucleotide (50 to 70 mer) may be utilized, with the codon choices determined by their probability of use.[160] DNA from the clones that constitute the cDNA library is transferred to filter paper and then hybridized to the radiolabeled oligonucleotides. Only the DNA from clones carrying plasmids with the correct (complementary) cDNA should hybridize to these oligonucleotide probes; these clones can be readily identified by radioautography. In some cases, a second oligonucleotide (or group of oligonucleotides) probe corresponding to a sequence of amino acids not encoded in the original probe can be used to probe the cDNA library a second time. Identification of clones that hybridize with both the original probes and the secondary probes provides greater assurance that one is dealing with the correct cDNA sequence. Once they are identified as positive, clones can then be isolated for further analysis of the cDNA insert. In some circumstances, one already has available a specific cDNA but wants to isolate the gene or the homologous cDNA in a different species. In this case, the cDNA itself can be radiolabeled and used to probe the appropriate library to identify the clones of interest.

Another approach for screening a cDNA library is to clone the cDNA into a plasmid, or more commonly a bacteriophage,[150–152] in a position which lies within the coding sequences of a gene that encodes a prokaryotic protein. In this case, approximately one of six recombinant molecules will contain a cDNA insert that is in the correct orientation and has its codons in phase with those of the bacterial gene. The bacteria will express this cDNA as part of a fusion protein containing bacterial and cDNA-encoded amino acid sequences. Screening this cDNA expression library with an antibody against the protein product of interest[161,162] will permit the identification of clones that produce the fusion protein and thus harbor the correct cDNA-containing phage.

A second form of "expression" screening has been developed for use in eukaryotic systems. In this case, cDNAs are cloned downstream of a strong eukaryotic enhancer/promoter [e.g., that from the simian virus 40 (SV40)] and transfected into cells in which the promoter is active (e.g., cos cells for the SV40 promoter) but which do not express the endogenous product of the cDNA to be isolated at high levels. Cells are then screened for a specific function (e.g., receptor binding activity) encoded by the cDNA of interest. Such an approach was employed recently to clone the angiotensin II receptor.[163] In an alternative expression screening strategy, mRNA is generated from cDNA templates in the library, and then injected into a eukaryotic host cell (e.g., a *Xenopus* oocyte). Individual oocytes or batches of oocytes are then screened for the activity of interest (e.g., hormone binding or ion transport).[164] Expression screening has been particularly advantageous in identifying cDNAs that encode products for which information about amino acid sequence or antibody reagents are unavailable. In addition, the eukaryotic cell provides a milieu which often is more conducive for obtaining optimal functional activity for expressed proteins with complex cellular compartmentalization or fastidious requirements for cofactors or accessory proteins.

One may also employ the technique of *subtraction screening* to identify cDNA clones of interest. This approach is particularly valuable in identifying cDNAs complementary to mRNAs that are selectively activated or repressed by exogenous hormones, growth factors, neurotransmitters, or other regulatory factors. In one variation of this approach, cDNAs are generated from cells grown in the presence or absence of the regulatory factor. Each cDNA population is then cloned and replicated as a library (see above). Filters generated from each library are then hybridized with radiolabeled cDNA from each of the two cell populations. Clones which are identified with only one of the two cDNA probes represent gene products which are likely to be modulated selectively by the regulatory factor in vivo. For example, hybridization of the untreated cDNA library with radiolabeled cDNA from untreated cells should show positivity in most of the clones, since these clones originated from the same mRNA population used to generate the probe. Failure of a subpopulation of these clones to hybridize with the radiolabeled cDNA from treated cells suggests that the transcripts encoded in these clones are negatively controlled by the regulatory factor. Conversely, hybridization of the cDNA library from treated cells with radiolabeled cDNA from untreated cells may reveal a subpopulation of clones which do not hybridize with the probe, suggesting that these gene products are stimulated by the presence of the regulatory factor. This approach has been employed successfully in the isolation of several differentially regulated gene products.[152]

Another method for screening a cDNA library—*hybrid arrest*—relies on the ability of a cDNA to hybridize specifically to the mRNA from which it was derived and thus block the ability of that mRNA to be translated in a cell-free reaction. Translation of the mRNA of interest is identified through the production of its protein product in the reaction, as detected, for instance, by immunoprecipitation. Plasmid DNA is isolated from each of the clones to be screened and is allowed to hybridize to an RNA sample containing the mRNA of interest. If the group of plasmids being screened contains the desired cDNA, then the mRNA sequestered in the hybrid cDNA-mRNA molecule will not be able to direct the synthesis of protein in the cell-free translation reaction. The converse operation, referred to as *hybrid-selected* or *hybrid release* translation, uses filter-bound, cDNA-containing plasmids to "pull out" a specific mRNA from a mixture of mRNA molecules. The hybridized mRNA is then eluted from the filter and identified by being translated in the cell-free system. These techniques have proved to be cumbersome when employed as primary screening tools, and they are used largely to confirm the identity of a cDNA isolated by another method. To establish rigorously that the cDNA that has been isolated is in fact the correct one, the nucleotide sequence of the cDNA is ordinarily determined. This is then compared to the amino acid sequence of the protein, if known. If the protein sequence is not known, mRNA can be synthesized from the cDNA insert and the encoded protein can be expressed using either an in vivo or an in vitro system (see above). The product can then be examined for the functional or immunologic activity of the naturally occurring protein.

Chromosomal Genes

Using techniques analogous to those used for cDNA cloning described above, it is possible to clone chromosomal genes, i.e., the portions of a chromosome which ultimately code for a protein. Chromosomal DNA isolated from cell nuclei can be physically sheared or, more commonly, cleaved into fragments with restriction enzymes, and the resultant fragments can be ligated into the appropriate restriction site of a bacterial virus (bacteriophage)–based vector.[150–152,165] The use of a bacteriophage to carry the chromosomal DNA inserts is necessitated by their large size (often several thousand nucleotides). The recombinant bacteriophage is used to infect a bacterial host in which its DNA is replicated. The bacteriophage continues to multiply and eventually produces lysis of the host cells which it occupies, generating a macroscopic plaque (clear area) on a background of otherwise normally growing bacteria. A radiolabeled cDNA or a chemically synthesized oligonucleotide may then be used to screen the plaques for the clone that contains the bacteriophage with the chromosomal insert of interest. This is done by transferring the DNA of the phage-lysed bacteria to a nitrocellulose filter and then hybridizing the filter to radioactive cDNA that is known to contain the coding sequence for the gene. The specificity of this hybridization allows one to identify the correct clone or plaque with the desired chromosomal insert. One can then produce this particular bacteriophage in large quantities to obtain sufficient chromosomal DNA for analysis.

Genes can also be cloned into yeasts.[150–152] These organisms have plasmids similar to bacteria and can be used in an analogous fashion. Yeasts have been used to study the mechanisms of regulation of eukaryotic gene expression and to produce medically useful proteins.

Polymerase Chain Reaction

The polymerase chain reaction (PCR) is a powerful method for amplifying DNA; it has revolutionized experimental approaches to problems in modern molecular biology.[166] PCR is based on two basic molecular biological principles: (1) Under suitably stringent conditions, complementary DNA sequences will hybridize selectively to one another as opposed to DNA with more limited sequence homology, and (2) in cases where annealed DNA complements are unequal in length, the shorter of the two can be extended in a 5′→3′ direction with DNA polymerase, deoxyribonucleotide substrate, and appropriate cofactors.

PCR is carried out as follows: Single-stranded oligonucleotide primers (~15 to 30 bases in length), corresponding to DNA sequences present at the opposing extremes of the fragment to be amplified, are synthesized using standard techniques. The primers each contain sequences oriented 5′→3′ so as to point internally from the ends toward the sequence to be amplified. The reaction is begun by the addition of the primers to the appropriate PCR reaction mixture with DNA template and *Taq 1* DNA polymerase (see below). Template DNA can be derived from genomic DNA isolated from tissue or cells, from cloned DNA, or from DNA generated from an RNA template using reverse transcription. The primer and the template DNA are placed in solution and denatured by heating the mixture to approximately 95°C. The mixture is then cooled to a more moderate temperature (55 to 65°C) to permit reannealing of complementary DNA strands. The temperature is chosen empirically to allow homologous base pairing to occur while reducing the probability of the annealing of a mismatched sequence. In cases where annealing of mismatched sequences is desired (e.g., for mutagenesis), the annealing temperature is reduced accordingly. In general, a large excess of primer over template is chosen to favor primer-template vs. template-template reannealing. Once the primer-template association has occurred, the reaction temperature is raised to 72°C. *Taq 1* DNA polymerase, a thermostable enzyme derived from *Thermus aquaticus,* functions optimally at this temperature and extends each of the respective template-annealed primers in a 5′→3′ direction. The reaction is stopped by reheating the mixture to 95°C to denature the newly generated DNA duplexes. The process of annealing the primer and extending with *Taq 1* polymerase is then repeated many times (Fig. 3-14), with the newly synthesized DNA strands serving as templates for subsequent generations of primer-extended products. The net result is a geometric amplification of the DNA sequence bordered by the primer sequence.

PCR has been used to identify single-copy genes in mammalian genomic DNA. These genes may represent the endogenous homologues of genes whose sequences are known to some degree or exogenous sequences integrated into genomic DNA through transgenic manipulation or viral infection. PCR has also been employed to identify and quantify low-abundance mRNA transcripts. In this case, reverse transcripts are used to generate cDNAs for all the transcripts within a given mRNA population. These cDNAs provide the template for subsequent PCR amplification. When certain controls are maintained, these amplified products provide an indirect estimate of the relative levels of the mRNA of interest in the original population. PCR can be used to generate a cDNA or genomic DNA sequence for cloning, regardless of whether the entire sequence or only a portion[167] of the sequence to be amplified is known. It has also been used to introduce additions, deletions, or site-directed mutations into DNA for studies of gene regulation and protein structure.

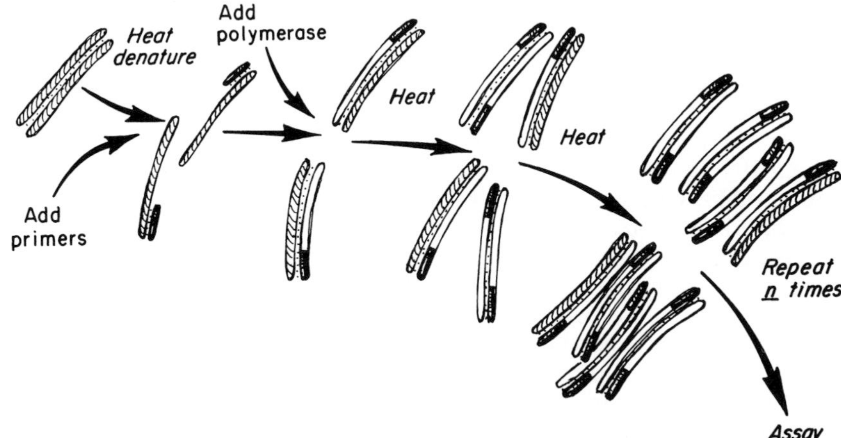

FIGURE 3-14 Polymerase chain reaction. The reaction is begun by annealing primers to denatured template DNA. Primers are then extended with *Taq 1* DNA polymerase, the products are denatured, primers are reannealed, and the process is repeated.

Despite the fact that the PCR technology can be fraught with pitfalls,[168] the continuing interest in new applications suggests that it will continue to play a major role in molecular biological research for years to come.

Transfer of Cloned Genes into Mammalian Cells

Another major advance in molecular biology was the development of methods for transferring cloned genes into mammalian cells where the genes could be expressed. This methodology has had its greatest impact by providing a means to understand gene function, but it is also being used to produce proteins which may be important therapeutically.

DNA can be transferred into mammalian cells in several ways:

1. DNA can be microinjected into the nucleus of a cell.[169]
2. Calcium phosphate precipitates of DNA can be prepared which will be phagocytosed by cells, providing access to the intracellular compartment.[170]
3. DNA complexed with DEAE dextran can be introduced into cells.[171]
4. Cells can be subjected to an electric discharge which temporarily disrupts the plasma membrane and facilitates the transfer of DNA into the cell (i.e., electroporation).[172]
5. Cells can be infected with the DNA of recombinant viruses provided that the host cells possess the requisite receptors for these viruses on their surfaces.[173]

If an experiment requires only a relatively brief examination of the function of the transferred DNA, this can be studied shortly (usually 48 to 72 h) after the transfer (transient expression assays).[174] Acute transfection is relatively efficient and permits the investigator to address questions which require neither long-term expression nor the integration of the transfected gene into the host cell genome. Most of the transfected DNA does not integrate into the host chromosome and will be destroyed after a few days. A small percentage of the transfected DNA, however, will integrate into the host chromatin at low frequency, replicate along with it, and be expressed chronically (stable transfection). The relatively small number of cells in which this has occurred can be isolated in several ways. For example, the DNA of interest can be "cotransfected" with DNA containing a "selectable" gene, i.e., a gene whose product confers on the cell some new property allowing for its selective survival, such as the gene that encodes resistance to neomycin.[175] In this case, when the cells are cultured in the presence of neomycin (or usually an analog of it), only cells that both integrate and express the neomycin resistance gene will survive and propagate. Fortunately, in most instances the selected gene (i.e., neomycin resistance) and the gene of interest will be incorporated into the host genome together; hence, expression of the selectable gene will serve to protect cells that harbor the gene of interest.

These gene transfer techniques have been utilized to study, among other things, the mechanisms of the hormonal regulation of gene expression. The first breakthrough in this area occurred when the cloned α_2-euglobulin gene was transferred into mouse fibroblasts and its expression was found to be glucocorticoid-regulated.[176] This experiment indicated that all the information necessary for a response to glucocorticoids was present on the cloned gene fragment that was transferred. Additional studies to localize the glucocorticoid-sensitive regions (or regulatory elements) in a number of different target genes (Fig. 3-15) have involved deleting successive portions of a gene (e.g., progressively deleting increasing amounts of the 5′-flanking DNA), transferring the truncated gene, and assaying for a loss of steroid responsiveness. Subsequently, selected nucleotides in the regulatory elements were replaced (mutated), using site-directed mutagenesis[177] to define the hormonal regulatory element with confidence. An additional approach involves isolating or synthesizing the DNA segment whose deletion resulted in the extinction of the hormonal response and testing its ability to confer hormonal responsiveness on a gene which normally is not hormonally regulated (Fig. 3-15). The identity of the GRE was confirmed in this way by splicing it upstream from a heterologous promoter that ordinarily is not responsive to glucocorticoids and demonstrating that the transferred hybrid promoter was glucocorticoid-responsive.[60,83,178] Similar combined addition/deletion approaches have been employed to identify hormonally responsive regulatory elements for progesterone,[178] estrogen,[179] androgen,[180] mineralocorticoid,[181] thyroid,[182] and vitamin D[183] receptors. Additional elements have been shown to respond to increases in protein kinase A (i.e., cAMP-dependent protein kinase[184]) or protein kinase C[98,99] activity within the cell. DNA sequences involved in conferring tissue-specific expression on a target gene (e.g., expression of the growth hormone or prolactin gene in the anterior pituitary gland[35–37]) have also been identified using this approach.

Transient and stable transfections have been employed to overexpress cloned gene sequences to provide gene products for biochemical analysis (see below) and to assess the effects of the overproduction of particular genes on target cell functions. In general, this is done by placing the relevant coding sequence (i.e., cDNA or more rarely genomic sequence) of the gene of interest downstream from a strong eukaryotic promoter. In many instances, the viral promot-

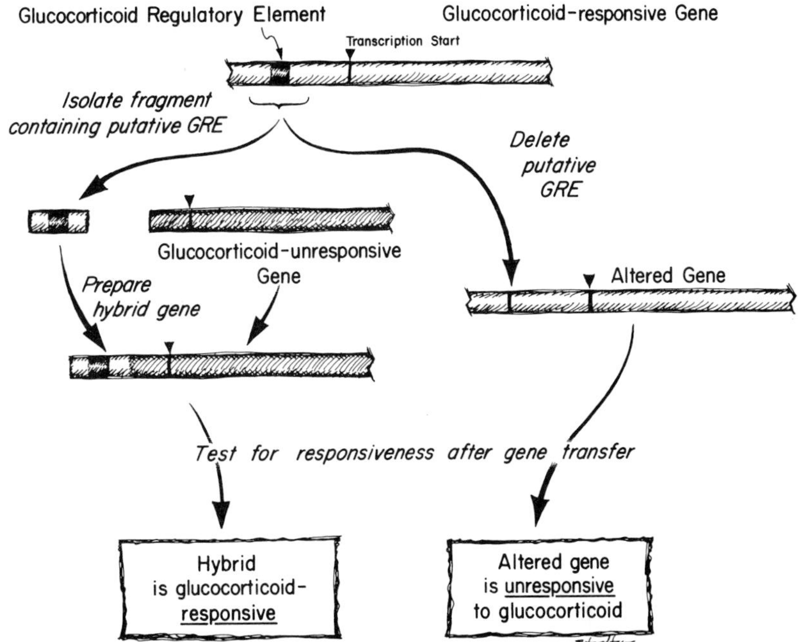

FIGURE 3-15 Identification of the DNA sequences required for glucocorticoid responsiveness. Two separate types of experiments are illustrated. In one experiment (*left*), the DNA containing the GRE is isolated and tested for its ability to confer glucocorticoid responsiveness on a normally nonregulated gene after gene transfer. In the other experiment (*right*), the putative GRE is deleted from the 5′-flanking DNA, and the gene is no longer steroid-responsive after gene transfer.

ers from the Rous sarcoma virus, cytomegalovirus, vaccinia virus, or SV40 have been employed. In other cases, inducible promoters such as that for the metallothionein gene, whose expression is stimulated by the presence of cadmium or zinc ion,[185] are employed to regulate expression of the target gene more closely. Overproduction of human renin in cultured Chinese hamster ovary (CHO) cells generated sufficient material for an x-ray crystallographic analysis which provided its structure at 2.5-Å resolution.[186] Similar overexpression of the glucocorticoid receptor has provided some interesting insights into its molecular structure.[187]

Several gene transfer approaches have been used to suppress or eliminate the expression of targeted genes in transfected cells. Overexpression of antisense (i.e., cRNA or cDNA) sequences has been employed as a means of titrating endogenous transcripts. Hybridization of these nucleic acids with genomic DNA or normal mRNA inside the cell interferes with the transcription of the targeted gene or the subsequent translation of the encoded protein, rendering the cell defective with regard to targeted protein activity.[188] Another approach involves the use of autocatalytic RNA molecules (ribozymes[54]); these molecules can be constructed in a fashion which allows them to hybridize to and cleave selected gene transcripts. This approach has been employed successfully to target human immunodeficiency virus, type I (HIV-1) *gag* transcripts in cultured human cells.[189] A third approach involves overexpression of specific mutants of the targeted gene which retain little or no functional activity of the wild-type protein yet inhibit the activity of the endogenous (i.e., wild-type) gene product. Such "dominant negative" mutants have recently been used to inhibit c-fos activity in cultured cells.[190] The v-erbA and c-erbAα_2 protein products may represent naturally occurring dominant negative mutants of the thyroid hormone receptor.[191,192] Finally, the technique of homologous recombination[193,194] has been used to substitute selectively mutated genes for their normal counterparts in the genome. Sequential selection of recombinants for each allele results in a cell which is homozygous for the mutation at the targeted locus. The ability to produce such mutations in embryonic stem cells suggests that this approach, if used in combination with transgenic animal technology (see below), will be an extremely powerful tool in the study of single-gene function in the whole animal.

Transgenic Animals

During the past 10 years, techniques have become available that allow the introduction of cloned DNA sequences into the genomes of fertilized embryos. This is accomplished most commonly by microinjecting small amounts of DNA into one of the pronuclei (usually the male pronucleus) of a fertilized egg. This DNA is subsequently incorporated, in one or more copies, into the genome of the recipient. Division and propagation of cells within the early embryo assure that the injected DNA will be present within each of the somatic cells of the recipient animal. In addition, the presence of the transgene in the germ line of the recipient permits the transmittal of this gene to subsequent offspring with predictable genetics.

The mechanics of producing transgenic animals are conceptually straightforward (Fig. 3-16). Fertilized ova are collected from female donors, microinjected (or infected if a retroviral vector is employed) with the DNA of interest as described above, and then replaced within the uterus of a foster mother for subsequent development. An alternative approach has employed pluripotent embryonic stem cells as transgene recipients. After transgene introduction, these stem cells are replaced in the early embryo for subsequent development. The resultant transgenic animals are usually chimeric (i.e., only a portion of their cells contain the transgene) as a result of variability in the number of embryonic stem cells that take up the transgene with the initial transfection (or infection). After birth, the offspring's DNA is screened for the presence of the transgene using conventional hybridization or PCR analysis. While mice have represented the predominant model system for transgenic work, a number of larger animals have been employed successfully as transgene recipients, including pigs, sheep, rabbits,[195] and, more recently, rats.[196]

The power of transgenic animal technology derives from the fact that the expression of the transgene can be followed in the recipient, as well as its transgene-bearing offspring, for extended periods. This allows the investigator to carry out developmental and chronic physiologic studies of transgene expression and/or function under conditions which only minimally perturb the animal's genome.

FIGURE 3-16 Transgenic mice. After microinjection with the cloned gene, fertilized oocytes are replaced in the womb of a foster mother and the pregnancy is allowed to go to term. Newborn pups are screened for the presence of the transgene, using conventional techniques. Alternatively, early blastocytes may be supplemented with embryonic stem cells transfected, infected, or microinjected in vitro. Since only a portion of the cells in the resultant embryos will have been infected with the exogenous DNA, the progeny are usually chimeric for the transferred gene.

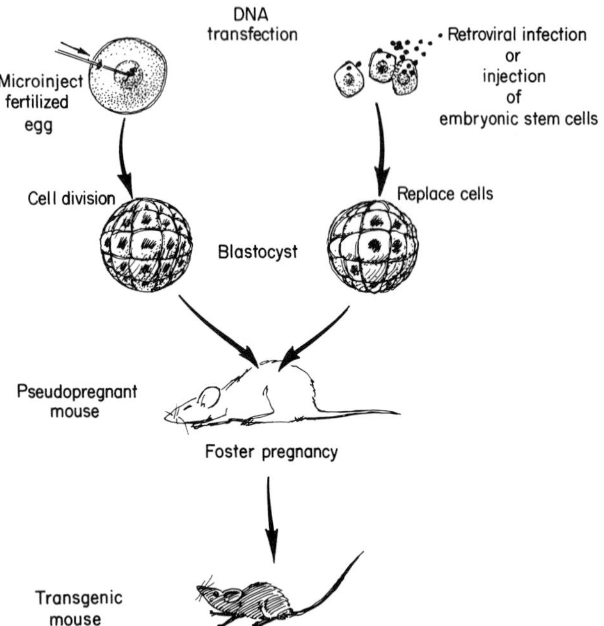

The transgenic approach has been employed to address a number of important questions in endocrine systems, often with exciting results. Transgenic animals have been used to identify the DNA elements responsible for tissue-specific gene expression (e.g., elastase gene expression in pancreatic acinar cells) using an approach somewhat similar to that employed in the in vitro studies described above.[197] They also have been used to locate the genomic regulatory elements responsible for governing target gene sensitivity to hormonal[198,199] or other environmental stimuli.[200] Constructions linking strong heterologous promoters (see above) to coding sequences for selected hormones (e.g., growth hormone, growth hormone releasing factor, renin, angiotensin, and atrial natriuretic factor) have been used to overexpress the encoded proteins, thus generating models of chronic hormone hypersecretion for subsequent study.[196,201–204] In some cases, transgene expression has been employed to correct an intrinsic genetic defect.[205]

Chimeric transgenes linking tissue-specific regulatory elements from genes expressed in endocrine tissues (e.g., insulin) have been linked to oncogene coding sequences (see below) and introduced into mouse embryos. Tissue-specific (i.e., endocrine cell–specific) overexpression of the relevant oncogene in many cases leads to the development of malignancies in the expressing cell. Such an approach has been employed to generate tumors of pancreatic beta cells,[206] gonadotropes,[207] luteinizing hormone releasing factor–producing neurons[208] of the hypothalamus, atrial natriuretic factor–producing atrial cardiocytes,[209] and renin-producing cells of the kidney.[210] In several instances, these tumors have served as a source for the subsequent generation of cell lines capable of expressing the hormones of interest[207,208,210–212] in culture.

Finally, the transgenic approach has been used to produce models of hormone hyposecretion through selected ablation of hormone-producing cells. This has been achieved by linking endocrine cell–specific regulatory elements to toxins,[213] interferon,[214] or major histocompatibility class II gene–coding sequences.[214] Overexpression of these products results in damage, and ultimately death, of the targeted cells. Such losses can result in a state of hormone deficiency (e.g., insulinopenia), creating models of human diseases (e.g., type I diabetes mellitus) which are amenable to detailed metabolic investigation. More recently, two independent groups[215,216] introduced a gene encoding a unique viral protein under the control of the insulin promoter into transgenic mice. This protein is subsequently expressed in pancreatic beta cells. Exposure of these transgenic mice to the intact virus later in life results in progressive damage to the beta cells, leading to insulin-dependent diabetes mellitus (IDDM). These findings suggest that this system may represent a useful model for the investigation of the pathogenesis and pathophysiology of human type I diabetes.

Recent advances in homologous recombination offer the possibility of selectively ablating targeted hormone or other genes without destroying the expressing cell or disrupting the cells' genomic organization. This technique relies on the ability of exogenous, homologous (nearly identical) DNA sequences to recombine, and thus exchange, with targeted sequences in the genome of the host cell. The advantage of this technique is that it allows for mutations in key nucleotide positions without altering the overall spatial configuration of the DNA in the region. This approach, when used in combination with appropriate selection techniques, has permitted the exchange of mutated for wild-type DNA sequences in cultured cells,[193] including embryonic stem cells.[194,217] The return of mutant embryonic cells to the uterus results in the development of an embryo that harbors the mutated gene.[217]

This approach has been employed to correct a hypoxanthine-guanine phosphoribosyl transferase (HGPRT) gene defect in transgenic mice.[218] In this instance, the "corrected" gene was used to replace the endogenous defective gene in embryonic stem cells in vitro. These cells were then introduced into the blastocyst of early mouse embryos. A number of the recipient transgenic animals expressed the "corrected" gene postnatally and successfully transmitted the gene to their offspring. In an alternative approach, Chisaka and Capecchi[219] successfully targeted the homeo box gene *hox-1.5* for disruption in transgenic mice. Mice homozygous for this mutation manifest somatic abnormalities of the thoracic and cervical regions, including the absence of thymic and parathyroid tissue, a phenotype reminiscent of DiGeorge syndrome in humans. More recently, homologous recombination–based "knockouts" have been extended to a number of other genes.[220–222] Taken together, these findings support the viability of the technique and suggest that this approach will provide a powerful tool for future research on transgenic animals.

Production of Medically Important Proteins by Recombinant DNA Techniques

A major use of recombinant DNA technology is in the production of medically useful proteins. Once a gene has been cloned, conditions can often be chosen such that it can be used to produce the protein it encodes, using one of a number of prokaryotic or eukaryotic expression vectors. To date, this is the only means available for producing moderate- to large-size proteins in quantity. Although the methods for synthesizing peptides through chemical techniques have improved considerably in recent years, they have not progressed to the point where large proteins (e.g., over 100 amino acids) can be made efficiently. Whereas some proteins, such as insulin, can be obtained by isolating them from animals, this approach has limitations. It is not practical when large quantities of proteins which are produced naturally in only minute amounts are needed (e.g., interferon and erythropoietin).

As was discussed earlier, genes require control sequences in order to be expressed. Therefore, mammalian DNA sequences inserted randomly into bacteria will commonly not be expressed efficiently. To obtain efficient expression, the sequences that encode the medically relevant protein are inserted into plasmids so that they are placed downstream from bacterial control sequences. Such sequences would include a promoter, the sequences encoding a ribosomal binding site, and an AUG (methionine) codon that is necessary to initiate translation of the mRNA. Ordinarily, a promoter that is highly active in bacteria is chosen to enhance the yields. In this way, bacterial control sequences direct the synthesis of the foreign protein. Utilizing this method of "direct expression," the synthesized protein can frequently be obtained in yields that are several percent of the total bacterial protein.[3,4] These proteins can then be purified from the bacteria with conventional biochemical techniques. This approach was utilized to express methionyl–human growth hormone initially.[3]

The major drawbacks of this approach are that (1) the protein product may be unstable in the bacterial environment, (2) the presence of the initiating methionine may interfere with normal biological activity, and (3) the protein may need to be modified (for example, by glycosylation) to be active. The first two drawbacks can be bypassed by synthesizing a *fusion*, or *hybrid, protein* from which the desired protein can be cleaved (Fig. 3-17). This was described earlier for the example of human insulin, in which the DNA sequences encoding the chains of human insulin were inserted into the coding sequence of a bacterial gene in the appropriate reading frame to allow for translation of the correct (i.e., insulin) sequence at the carboxy terminus of the bacterial protein. In this way, the bacteria synthesize a hybrid protein containing bacterial and mammalian amino acids. These genes are constructed so that a proteolytic or chemically susceptible cleavage site occurs at the junction of the bacterial and mammalian amino acid sequences. This approach was also used for the original bacterial synthesis of human somatostatin, the first mammalian protein to be made by recombinant DNA techniques,[223] and β-endorphin.[224]

Some proteins are produced more efficiently in yeast.[225] The approaches are typically similar to

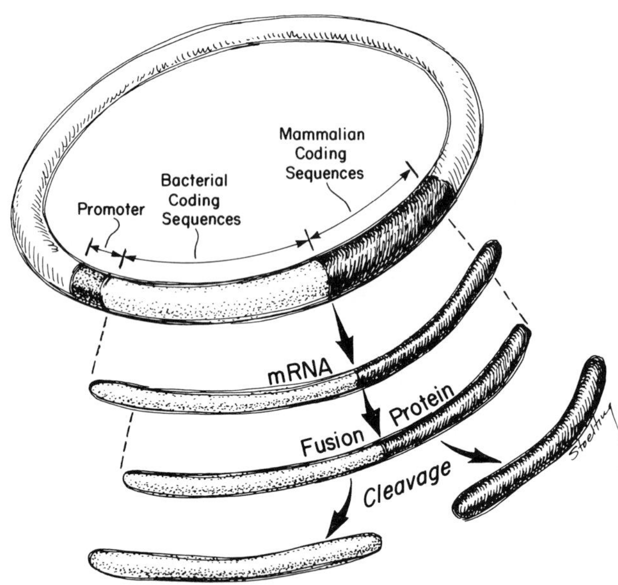

FIGURE 3-17 Expression of a mammalian protein as a fusion protein in bacteria. Sequences coding for a mammalian protein are linked, in phase with respect to the genetic code, to sequences coding for a bacterial protein. The hybrid protein gene is expressed under the control of the bacterial promoter. If engineered properly, the fusion protein can be cleaved chemically or enzymatically to release the mammalian protein, which can then be further purified.

those used in bacteria. One useful feature is that yeasts can be programmed to secrete their expressed proteins, a feature that aids in purification of the protein. In addition, the amino-terminal methionine of these secreted proteins may be removed, eliminating a possibly unwanted amino acid.

Mammalian cells are being used increasingly for the production of recombinant DNA–derived proteins. Increased production yields and the use of more defined media devoid of expensive animal serum have stimulated the use of this approach. The mammalian gene coding sequences are commonly inserted downstream from a highly active promoter to improve yields. The use of mammalian cells has the advantage that they can add important carbohydrate groups to the proteins in a fashion which closely parallels that which takes place in vivo. Often such glycosylation is required for full functional activity. This glycosylation may not be carried out correctly by yeasts and is not performed at all by bacteria. A number of large and fairly complex proteins (e.g., factor VIII) have been successfully expressed in eukaryotic cells.[226]

Products of Recombinant DNA Technology

The human body produces thousands of different proteins, including those which function as hormones or enzymes. A deficiency or excess of many of these proteins has been recognized as contributing to human disease. Recombinant DNA technology, by the means outlined above, will make possible the production of many of these proteins in pure form, which will allow testing of their clinical utility. In addition to providing the natural proteins, this technology should facilitate the production of derivatives which may prove useful as either antagonists or more specific agonists. For example, derivatives which possess a more limited, and thus clinically more specific, range of activities compared with the parent protein may be produced. While a comprehensive review of progress in this area is outside the scope of this chapter, a few examples relevant to endocrinology should be mentioned.

Human insulin prepared by recombinant techniques is now available,[1,2] assuring an unlimited supply of this hormone. Recombinant growth hormone has largely replaced cadaver-derived human growth hormone and the attendant risk of contamination with the Creutzfeldt-Jakob virus.[227] In addition to its use for treating growth hormone–deficient dwarves, the increased supply of recombinant growth hormone has permitted the investigation of its potential efficacy in the management of other clinical disorders, including the negative nitrogen balance associated with the postoperative state,[228] weight reduction in obese subjects,[229] and the muscle-wasting syndrome of the elderly.[230] Thus, this hormone may have considerably broader therapeutic utility in the near future. Recombinant erythropoietin is currently employed for the management of the anemia associated with chronic renal failure,[6] a clinical condition which often is refractory to other forms of treatment. It has also been employed to manage the anemias associated with various malignancies[231,232] as well as AIDS.[7] A number of other growth factors[233,234] and cytokines[235,236] currently under development will in all likelihood increase the importance of recombinant products in clinical medicine.

Recombinant DNA technology lends itself ideally to vaccine production, and a number of different approaches have been employed to this end. Individual genes encoding important antigens can be cloned and expressed; this bypasses the need to give inactivated organisms and may be safer and more specific. Indeed, recent studies have demonstrated that several viral antigens can be inserted into a single benign viral vector to be used for immunization. In early animal studies these "polyvalent" vaccines resulted in antibodies to each of the viral antigens.[237] These vaccines could have an impact greater than that attendant to merely preventing the target disease. For example, it has been postulated that the prevention of certain viral diseases may decrease the incidence of type I diabetes.[238]

As was stated previously, protein derivatives with specific advantages in terms of functional activity may be produced. In addition, hybrid molecules composed of portions of two or more different proteins could theoretically be produced by linking together segments of different genes. Already there has been a major effort to test the activity of hybrid and variant immunoglobulin molecules.[239] Such chimeric proteins would potentially allow for the generation of novel combinations of target cell specificity and functional activity. Such an approach, linking antifibrin antibody fragments to the catalytic portion of plasminogen activator, has been advocated as a potential therapeutic approach for the management of intravascular thromboses.[240]

New Drug Delivery Systems

The products of recombinant DNA technology are largely proteins. They are generally unstable in and poorly absorbed from the gastrointestinal tract. This necessitates their administration by injection, which limits their utility. However, this problem is being bypassed in several ways. As more information is accumulated, it may be possible to determine the critically active structures of these proteins and design orally active drugs that contain only those essential elements which are devoid of protease-sensitive structure. In addition, a number of systems are being developed to facilitate the delivery of these drugs. Microemulsions (i.e., liposomes) may be used which encapsulate and facilitate the movement of a drug through cell membranes and into the intracellular compartment.[241] Implantable devices that release a drug over a prolonged period are also being developed. Another approach involves the intranasal administration of the protein in combination with surface-active agents which promote absorption across the nasal mucosa, bypassing degradation in the intestinal tract.[242,243] Intranasal vasopressin and its analogs have been used for some time. Intranasal luteinizing hormone releasing hormone (LHRH) is now in use,[244] and intranasal calcitonin is being used in Europe in the treatment of osteoporosis and Paget disease.[245] A similar approach is being examined for the delivery of insulin to diabetic patients.[243,246] The insulin is absorbed rapidly into the circulation, mimicking intravenous delivery.

Use of DNA in the Diagnosis of Genetic Disease

In addition to the classic genetic diseases, where defects in particular enzymes, receptors, or other elements in hormone responsiveness are often responsible,[247] more subtle genetic defects contribute to the development of many common diseases, such as diabetes mellitus, hypertension, and predisposition to premature atherosclerosis. The ability to analyze genes in detail now provides the means both to diagnose these diseases and to better understand their pathogenesis. Rapid tests utilizing recombinant DNA probes are now available for diagnosing genetic diseases such as the thalassemias,[248] sickle cell anemia,[249,250] and phenylketonuria.[251]

In several instances, the defective genes contributing to the pathogenesis of a specific disorder are known[248–251] and can be actively searched for in a population at risk. In most cases, however, the exact nature of the defective gene is unknown and other methods of risk identification must be employed.

The most common approach currently used for diagnosing genetic diseases involves the identification of restriction fragment length polymorphisms[252] (Fig. 3-18). *Polymorphisms* are differences in the primary structure of a given gene; they can be observed between the two alleles of a given gene in the same individual or between the genes of two different individuals. Most commonly, the polymorphism reflects single nucleotide differences, but in other cases, they can involve inserted or deleted segments of DNA. These differences can occur in the sequences of the gene that are transcribed or in the flanking DNA. In the process of replication, mutations in the DNA occur at a low frequency. Most of these mutations are "silent" in that they have no effect on the function of the gene or on its products. Once these mutations occur, however, they are inherited and can be used as genetic markers (i.e., polymorphisms).

Assume, for instance, that a given individual develops a single base mutation that results in a genetic trait, for example, a tendency to develop hypertension. In general, such mutations do not generate new sites for restriction endonuclease cleavage and therefore cannot be detected without sequencing the entire gene. However, this individual is likely to have additional differences from other individuals in or around the affected gene. These polymorphic differences are genetically silent but serve as identifiable markers of the underlying genetic abnormality. Occasionally these differences result in the generation or loss of a restriction endonuclease cleavage site (Fig. 3-18). In this case, cleavage of that individual's DNA with the restriction enzyme will result in DNA fragments of a size different from that of fragments from another, presumably unaffected individual. This aberrant fragment can be identified after size-fractionating the DNA fragments on a gel, transferring the DNA to filter paper, and hybridizing to a radiolabeled probe for the gene. If analysis of the DNA from relatives of the test subject indicates that the restriction site polymorphism is inherited along with the mutation that results in disease susceptibility, this polymorphism can be used as a genetic marker for the disease. A pedigree analysis of a hypothetical kindred is shown in Fig. 3-19. All that is required for this type of analysis is an established linkage between a restriction fragment length polymorphism (RFLP) and a disease, and an appropriate probe. It is not necessary to know anything about the gene product or the specific molecular defect that is involved.

In cases where the defective gene is known,[248–251] informative RFLPs in or near the defective gene can be sought. When the defective gene is unknown, in-

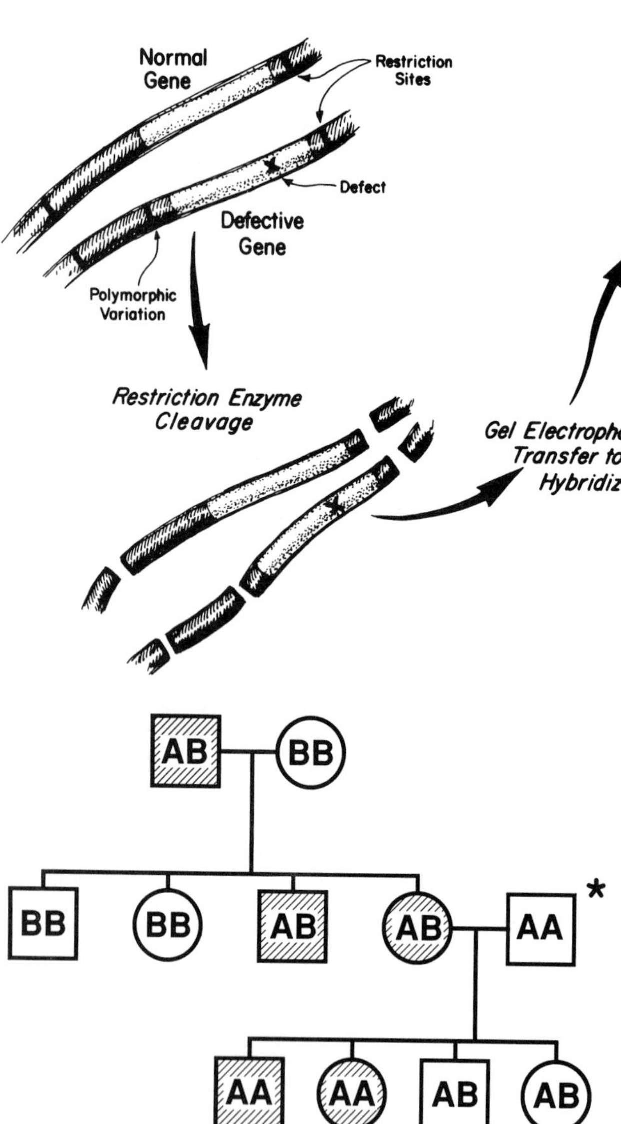

FIGURE 3-18 Use of restriction fragment length polymorphisms as genetic markers of disease. In the case illustrated, a mutation resulting in a defective gene is associated with a polymorphic variation in the 5′-flanking DNA, resulting in the presence of a restriction site that is not present in unafflicted individuals. Cleavage with the appropriate restriction enzyme will yield a smaller fragment for the defective gene than for the normal gene. Subjecting the various fragments to size fractionation on a gel and to hybridization with the radiolabeled gene (or its cDNA) as a probe will allow identification of the aberrant fragment. This obviates the need for isolation and cloning of the genomic DNA to identify the mutation within the gene.

FIGURE 3-19 A hypothetical kindred illustrating the use of RFLPs in assessing the risk for development of a particular disease. In this case, the diseased allele is linked to the A polymorphism in the grandfather (top line); the grandmother carries two B alleles which are not associated with the disease in this kindred. All second-generation progeny carrying the A allele are afflicted with the disease (shaded), while again the BB phenotype is normal (open), suggesting an autosomal dominant pattern of inheritance. Note that when an unaffected male (*) who is homozygous for an A allele not linked to the defect marries into the kindred, the presence of a single A allele no longer indicates disease transmission. Only progeny inheriting the maternal A allele (i.e., AA phenotype) will acquire the disease.

formative RFLPs can be looked for by examining the DNA of individual family members in the affected kindreds, using a large number of probes (50 or more), each complementary to a specific genomic sequence. Such probes are selected to provide markers for as many broadly separated chromosomal loci as possible. The inheritance of a specific RFLP pattern (identified with one of the probes described above) establishes the linkage between the polymorphism and the disease and helps pinpoint the chromosomal location of the defective gene.

In practice, RFLP analysis can be complicated and interpretation must of necessity be cautious. RFLP patterns that are diagnostic for a disease in one family may be found in other unaffected families (Fig. 3-19), confounding population studies. In addition, for many if not most genetic diseases (sickle cell anemia is the exception), a number of different mutations in the affected gene may lead to an identical clinical presentation, and each mutation will be associated with a unique RFLP pattern. For these reasons, in most cases informative diagnostic information can be obtained only by analyzing the DNA of several family members.

In endocrinology, RFLP analysis has been applied to the study of diabetes mellitus,[253–255] hyperlipoproteinemia,[256] congenital adrenal hyperplasia,[257] and multiple endocrine neoplasia types 1,[258] 2A,[259] and 2B.[260]

Potential for Human Gene Therapy

Since genes can be transferred into mammalian cells and function in them (see above), it should be possible to insert genes into the cells of human patients. In fact, the first limited gene transfer experiment has been carried out.[261] In this study, tumor-infiltrating lymphocytes were infected in vitro with a recombinant retroviral vector harboring the gene for neomycin resistance. This gene was then used as a marker to follow the fate of these cells after their reintroduction into patients with malignant melanoma.

The advantages of gene therapy are obvious. For example, if a gene could be transferred to a patient with a particular genetic deficiency and function appropriately, even moderate levels of expression might reduce or eliminate clinical symptoms and thus simplify management. Potential candidates for gene transfer therapy include not only the classical genetic diseases such as adenosine deaminase deficiency, purine nucleoside phosphorylase deficiency, HGPRT deficiency (Lesch-Nyhan syndrome), the thalassemias, and sickle cell anemia,[262,263] but also pathologic states such as hypercholesterolemia and hypertension, where the products of the transferred genes would theoretically act to lower cholesterol levels or blood pressure, respectively, independent of the primary genetic defect. The feasibility of using a transferred LDL receptor gene to lower cholesterol levels has been demonstrated in animals.[264]

Most approaches to human gene therapy have focused on the use of retroviral vectors (Fig. 3-20). Retroviruses are RNA viruses which can infect target cells with a high degree of efficiency. Typically, the gene to be transferred is substituted for a critical gene (usually the envelope gene) within the wild-type viral genome. This recombinant "virus" is no longer competent for infection, since it is defective in the deleted viral envelope gene; however, it can be rendered infective if it is first introduced into a "helper" cell line capable of synthesizing the deleted viral envelope gene but unable to synthesize any virus of its own. This cell line provides the packaging that renders the recombinant virus infective. Virus-rich media from the helper cell line are used to infect target cells in vitro. The recombinant viral DNA, which contains the nonviral gene, is taken up and incorporated into the host cell genome. Expression of the nonviral gene will reconstitute the deficient activity in the recipient cells and retain this activity after reintroduction of these cells into the whole animal. These cells are not capable of manufacturing new virus particles since they lack the envelope packaging function. Therefore, expression in vivo should be confined to cells specifically infected in vitro.

Although most researchers agree that human gene therapy will ultimately be possible, a number of problems must be solved before it becomes generally applicable. For appropriate regulation, the gene must be delivered to the correct tissue, for example, globin genes to erythroid cells. This could be accomplished by infecting erythroid precursor cells taken from the patient's own bone marrow. Often, however, appropriate target cells are not readily accessible (e.g., neuronal cells in HGPRT deficiency). In some instances where only a fixed (nonregulated) level of constitutive expression is required, it may be feasible to transfect heterologous cells (i.e., cells which ordinarily do not express the gene) with DNA containing the relevant gene driven by a promoter capable of functioning in the heterologous cell. Such a transferred gene would need to function at an adequate but not excessive level. Another potential problem is that stably integrated genes are usually established by applying gene transfer techniques to dividing cells, while many targets for gene transfer therapy in vivo are nondividing cells. In addition, since the integration of genes into the chromosome results in an interruption of the cellular DNA at the site of integration, there is a potential risk of mutation and/or malignant transformation in the target cell.

Although these problems are substantial, there are potential approaches to circumventing them. For example, it may be possible to isolate and propagate the relevant cells in culture, transfer the gene to these cells, document that the gene functions properly, and demonstrate that the cells are not malignantly transformed before returning the cells to the patient, ideally in optimal anatomic locations (Fig. 3-20). These cells could also be grown in a permeable capsule or cannula, which would permit transfer of the relevant protein products to the patient but would also be readily accessible for removal if one wants to terminate the treatment. Such "externalization" might also permit the use of heterologous recipient cells for the overexpression of a particular recombinant gene since it would limit the access of cytotoxic lymphocytes to the "graft" and thus forestall rejection.

FIGURE 3-20 Gene transfer in humans. In this simplified schema, somatic cells are removed from the patient and cultured in vitro. Recombinant virus, packaged in an appropriate helper cell line, is used to infect the cells. Cells which have incorporated the recombinant gene into their genomes are then selected and amplified in culture. When enough recombinant cells are available, they are reintroduced into the host organism, preferably in an anatomic location which optimizes the activity of the transfected gene product.

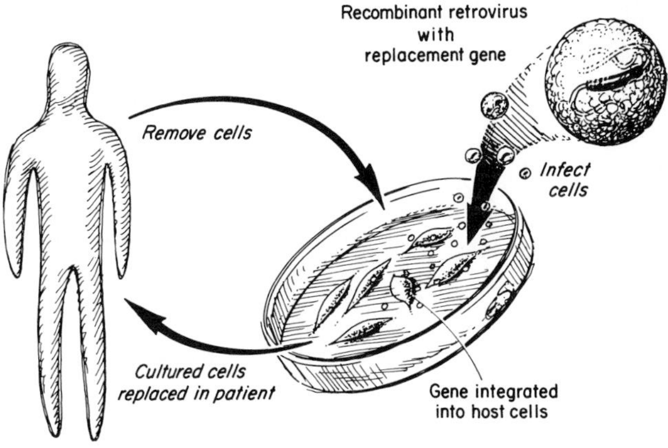

The technology for reintroducing nonhemopoietic cells back into the host animal has also received considerable attention. Recent studies indicate that vascular cells, specifically vascular endothelial cells, can be reseeded in the vascular tree after transfection with a recombinant DNA molecule in vitro.[265] The transfected genes were subsequently expressed by these cells in vivo. A more recent study suggested that vascular cells can also be directly infected with recombinant virus in vivo.[266] The transfected genes were expressed in a distribution which was limited to the site of infection. This approach may have a significant impact on the future use of gene transfer in the management of hypertension or atherosclerosis, diseases where major pathology is often localized to the vascular wall. Preliminary studies suggest that myoblasts may subserve a similar function of introducing transfected genes into skeletal muscle.[267,268,268a]

Impact of Molecular Biology on Medicine

While there have been several important practical applications of recombinant DNA technology, its greatest impact has been in the basic information provided about the structure, function, regulation, and products of eukaryotic genes. In addition, the production of medically useful products has provided means to intensify the investigation of more basic questions. With recombinant production of cytokines, growth factors, and low-abundance hormones, it will be possible to learn much more about their cellular actions, physiologic roles, and potential therapeutic uses.

Recent progress in cancer research illustrates both the impact of molecular biology on medicine and the involvement of the endocrine system in growth control.[269–271] The study of retroviral genes (i.e., genes of RNA viruses that replicate through reverse transcription of RNA into DNA) capable of inducing neoplastic transformation (*oncogenes*) has been particularly instructive. Of special importance was the finding that these oncogenes actually originated from normal cellular genes referred to as proto-oncogenes. This molecular "pirating" of proto-oncogene function affords the retrovirus a selective advantage in promoting its replication and function. While retroviruses have been implicated in a few malignancies (e.g., certain T-cell lymphomas), they are probably not causally related to the majority of human tumors. Instead, many of these tumors harbor abnormalties in the normal cellular homologues of their viral oncogene counterparts. These mutated proto-oncogenes (perhaps generated by chemical, physical, or viral factors) give rise to gene products which do not display the highly regulated activity of the normal proto-oncogene product. This malregulated proto-oncogene activity is believed to promote cell growth and contribute to tumorigenesis.

Elucidation of the nature of retroviral oncogenes and cellular proto-oncogenes has provided important insights into the molecular and cellular biology of eukaryotic cells (Fig. 3-21). Many oncogenes encode proteins related to growth factors. The v-sis (i.e., viral sis) gene product, for example, is similar to one of the two subunits of platelet-derived growth factor.[272,273] In other cases, retroviruses encode protein analogues of growth factor receptors; the v-erb B oncogene, for example, encodes a protein similar to the epidermal growth factor receptor.[274] The proto-oncogene referred to as c-Ha-ras (i.e., cellular Harvey ras, because of its homology to the viral

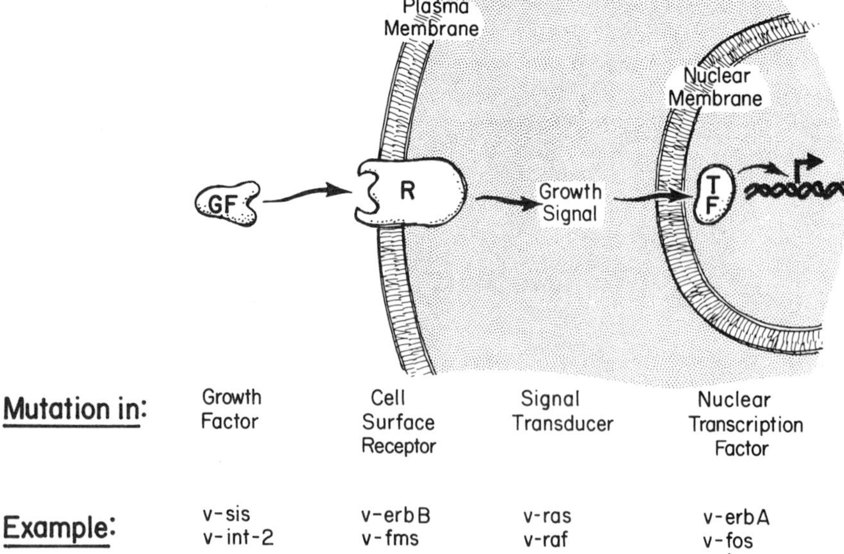

FIGURE 3-21 Relation of known oncogene products to proteins important in the regulation of cellular physiology. In each case, the oncogene product appears to be a mutated variant of an important regulator. For example, v-sis and v-int-2 are highly homologous to the PDGF B chain and FGF, respectively; v-erb B and v-fms are homologous to the receptors for EGF and colony-stimulating factor, respectively; and v-erb A encodes a variant of the thyroid hormone receptor. Cellular homologues for v-ras, v-raf, v-fos, and v-jun have also been identified. Oncogene-dependent malregulation at any point in the cascade may contribute to subsequent unregulated growth.

v-Ha-ras gene) was isolated from a bladder carcinoma and was found to encode a guanyl nucleotide (i.e., GTP)–binding protein.[275,276] Abnormalities in ras gene expression are frequently associated with thyroid neoplasms[277] as well as other solid tumors.[278] Of interest, somatic mutations in G_S and G_i, GTP-binding proteins which are involved directly in the regulation of adenylate cyclase activity,[279,280] have been linked to tumor development in endocrine tissues. Oncogenes also encode a variety of proteins with similarities to eukaryotic nuclear transcription factors (e.g., c-jun, c-fos, c-myc, and c-erb A) which are involved in establishing basal as well as regulated expression for a large number of genes.[270] The endocrine relatedness of these oncogenes is illustrated by the fact that the c-erb A gene is identical to the thyroid hormone receptor.[281] Furthermore, the c-jun and c-fos components of the AP-1 transcription complex have been shown to mediate at least some of the nuclear activities of protein kinase C,[98,99] a second messenger which is activated by a large number of hormones and/or neurotransmitters acting at the cell surface.

Another recent major development in cancer research resulted from the identification of the so-called recessive oncogenes or tumor suppressor genes.[282] Products of these genes antagonize the growth-promoting effects of a number of different oncogenes. It appears that only a single allele harboring a functional tumor suppressor gene is necessary to suppress tumor growth; this explains the recessive nature of the mutation and the need to alter both normal genes to generate the malignant phenotype. Mutations in a tumor suppressor gene have been implicated in the genesis of familial retinoblastomas. In this case, it is thought that the familial defect is a mutation in one of the two alleles that encode the suppressor gene. A subsequent mutation in the other allele, acquired later in life, results in a loss of suppressor gene function and consequent tumorigenesis. Mutations in additional tumor suppressor genes have been implicated in the pathogenesis of neurofibromatosis I,[282] some colon carcinomas,[282] and multiple endocrine neoplasia type I (MEN I).[283,284]

In general, cancer appears not to be a one-step process but requires the sequential activation of two or more events with oncogenic potential.[285,286] Thus, sequential mutation of two proto-oncogenes or a tumor suppressor gene and a proto-oncogene, each possessing unique properties and mechanisms of action, could create the requisite phenotype to produce malignant transformation. The requirement for a multistep process may explain why many malignancies (e.g., postirradiation thyroid cancer and the tumors of the MEN syndromes) occur later in life. With the emergence of models for understanding the fundamental molecular aspects of cancer as well as the control of normal cell growth, scientists can begin to design new approaches toward the prevention, diagnosis, and treatment of endocrine tumors. In particular, as the role of hormones and growth factors in the regulation of cell proliferation becomes better defined, it should be possible to develop specifically targeted strategies to control their activity and limit their contribution to the neoplastic process.

REFERENCES

1. Goeddel DV, Kleid DG, Bolivar F, et al: Expression in Escherichia coli of chemically synthesized genes for human insulin. *Proc Natl Acad Sci USA* 76:106, 1979.
2. Keen H, Glynne A, Pickup JC, et al: Human insulin produced by recombinant DNA technology: Safety and hypoglycemic potency in healthy men. *Lancet:* 2:398, 1980.
3. Goeddel DV, Heyneker HL, Hozumi T, et al: Direct expression in E. coli of a DNA sequence for human growth hormone. *Nature* 281:544, 1979.
4. Martial JA, Hallewell RA, Baxter JD, Goodman HM: Human growth hormone: Complementary DNA cloning and expression in bacteria. *Science* 205:602, 1979.
5. Hintz RL, Rosenfeld RG, Wilson DM, et al: Biosynthetic methionyl human growth hormone is biologically active in adult man. *Lancet* 1:1276, 1982.
6. Eschbach JW, Kelly MR, Haley NR, et al: The treatment of the anemia of progressive renal failure with recombinant human erythropoietin. *N Engl J Med* 321:158, 1989.
7. Fischl M, Galpin JE, Levine JD, Groopman JE, et al: Recombinant human erythropoietin for patients with AIDS treated with Zidovirdine. *N Engl J Med* 322:1488, 1990.
8. Watson JD, Crick FHC: Molecular structure of nucleic acids: A structure for deoxyribose nucleic acid. *Nature* 171:737, 1953.
9. Alberts B, Bray D, Lewis J, et al: *Molecular Biology of the Cell,* 2d ed. New York, Garland, 1989.
10. Lewin B: *Genes II.* New York, Wiley, 1985.
11. Wolpert L: DNA and its message. *Lancet* 2:853, 1984.
12. Nevins JR: The pathway of eukaryotic mRNA formation. *Annu Rev Biochem* 52:441, 1983.
13. Gehring WJ: The molecular basis of development. *Sci Am* 253:152B, 1985.
14. Igo-Kemenes T, Horz W, Zachau HG: Chromatin. *Annu Rev Biochem* 51:89, 1982.
15. McGhee JD, Felsenfeld G: Nucleosome structure. *Annu Rev Biochem* 49:1115, 1980.
16. Getzenberg RH, Pienta KJ, Coffey DS: The tissue matrix: Cell dynamics and hormone action. *Endocr Rev* 11:399, 1990.
17. Weisbrod S: Active chromatin. *Nature* 297:289, 1982.
18. Weintraub H, Groudine M: Chromosomal subunits in active genes have an altered conformation. *Science* 193:848, 1976.
19. O'Malley BW: Steroid hormone action in the eucaryotic cell. *J Clin Invest* 74:307, 1984.
20. Zaret KS, Yamamoto KR: Reversible and persistent changes in chromatin structure accompanying activation of a glucocorticoid-dependent enhancer element. *Cell* 19:527, 1980.
21. Bresnick EH, John S, Berard DS, LeFebvre P, Hager GL: Glucocorticoid receptor-dependent disruption of a specific nucleosome on the mouse mammary tumor virus promoter is prevented by sodium butyrate. *Proc Natl Acad Sci USA* 87:3977, 1990.
22. Pardoll D, Vogelstein B, Coffey DS: A fixed site of DNA replication in eucaryotic cells. *Cell* 19:527, 1980.
23. Robinson SI, Nolkin BD, Vogelstein B: The ovalbumin gene is associated with the nuclear matrix of chicken oviduct cells. *Cell* 28:99, 1982.

24. Ciejek EM, Tsai MJ, O'Malley BW: Actively transcribed genes are associated with the nuclear matrix. *Nature* 306:607, 1983.
25. Nakayasu H, Mori H, Ueda K: Association of small nuclear RNA-protein complex in the nuclear matrix from bovine lymphocytes. *Cell Struct Funct* 7:253, 1982.
26. Alexander RB, Greene GL, Barrack ER: Estrogen receptors in the nuclear matrix: Direct demonstration using monoclonal antireceptor antibody. *Endocrinology* 12:1851, 1987.
27. Mowszowicz I, Doukani A, Giacomini M: Binding of the angrogen receptor to the nuclear matrix of human foreskin. *J Steroid Biochem* 291:715, 1988.
28. Lerner MR, Steitz JA: Snurps and scyrps. *Cell* 25:298, 1981.
29. Padgett RA, Mount SM, Steitz JA, Sharp PA: Splicing of messenger RNA precursors is inhibited by antisera to small nuclear ribonucleoprotein. *Cell* 35:101, 1983.
30. Moore CL, Sharp PA: Site-specific polyadenylation in a cell-free reaction. *Cell* 36:581, 1984.
31. Walter P, Blobel G: Signal recognition particle contains a 7S RNA essential for protein translocation across the endoplasmic reticulum. *Nature* 299:691, 1982.
32. Walter P, Gilmore R, Blobel G: Protein translocation across the endoplasmic reticulum. *Cell* 38:5, 1984.
33. Breathnach R, Chambon P: Organization and expression of eucaryotic split genes coding for proteins. *Annu Rev Biochem* 50:349, 1981.
34. McKnight SL, Kingsbury R: Transcriptional control signals of a eukaryotic protein coding gene. *Science* 217:316, 1982.
35. West BL, Catanzaro DF, Mellon SH, Cattini PA, Baxter JD, Reudelhuber TL: Interaction of a tissue-specific factor with an essential rat growth hormone gene promoter element. *Mol Cell Biol* 7:1193, 1987.
36. Ingraham HA, Chen R, Mangalam HJ, Elsholtz HP, Flynn SE, Lin CR, Simmons DM, Swanson L, Rosenfeld MG: A tissue-specific transcription factor containing a homeodomain specifies a pituitary phenotype. *Cell* 55:519, 1988.
37. Bodner M, Castrillo J-L, Theill LE, Derrinck T, Ellisman M, Karin M: The pituitary-specific transcription factor GHF-1 is a homeobox containing protein. *Cell* 55:505, 1988.
38. Brown DD: The role of stable complexes that repress and activate eucaryotic genes. *Cell* 37:359, 1984.
39. Grummt I, Skinner JA: Efficient transcription of a protein-coding gene from the RNA polmerase I promoter in transfected cells. *Proc Natl Acad Sci USA* 82:722, 1985.
40. Birnstiel ML, Busslinger M, Strub K: Transcription termination and 3′ processing: The end is in site! *Cell* 41:349, 1985.
41. Hernandez N, Keller W: Splicing of in vitro synthesized messenger RNA precursors in Hela cell extracts. *Cell* 35:89, 1983.
42. Padgett RA, Hardy SF, Sharp PA: Splicing of adenovirus RNA in a cell-free transcription system. *Proc Natl Acad Sci USA* 85:5230, 1983.
43. Grabowski PJ, Seiler SR, Sharp PA: A multicomponent complex involved in the splicing of messenger RNA precursors. *Cell* 42:345, 1985.
44. Keller W: The RNA lariat: A new ring to the splicing of mRNA precursors. *Cell* 39:423, 1984.
45. Mount SM: A catalogue of splice junction sequences. *Nucleic Acids Res* 10:459, 1982.
46. Wieringa B, Meyer F, Reiser J, Weissmann C: Unusual splice sites revealed by mutagenic inactivation of an authentic splice site of the rabbit β-globin gene. *Nature* 301:38, 1983.
47. Treisman R, Proudfoot NJ, Shander M, Maniatis T: A single-base change at a splice site in a β-thalassemic gene causes abnormal RNA splicing. *Cell* 29:903, 1982.
48. Gilbert W: Genes in pieces revisited. *Science* 228:823, 1985.
49. Dixon RAF, Kobilka BK, Satrader DJ, Benovic JL, Dohlman HG, Frielle T, Bolanowski MA, Bennett CD, et al: Cloning of the gene and cDNA for mammalian β-adrenergic receptor and homology with rhodopsin. *Nature* 321:75, 1986.
50. Bell GI, Pictet RL, Rutter WJ, et al: Sequence of the human insulin gene. *Nature* 284:26, 1980.
51. Hardman JA, Hort YJ, Catanzaro DF, et al: Primary structure of the human renin gene. *DNA* 3:457, 1984.
52. Sudhof TC, Goldstein JL, Brown MS, Russell DW: The LDL-receptor gene: A mosaic of exons shared with different proteins. *Science* 228:815, 1985.
53. Sharp PA: On the origin of RNA splicing and introns. *Cell* 42:397, 1985.
54. Cech TR: The chemistry of self-splicing RNA and RNA enzymes. *Science* 236:1532, 1987.
55. Proudfoot NJ, Brownlee GG: 3′ Non-coding region sequences in eukaryotic mRNA. *Nature* 263:211, 1976.
56. Shatkin AJ: Capping of eukaryotic mRNAs. *Cell* 9:645, 1976.
57. Furuichi Y, LaFiandra A, Shatkin AJ: 5′-Terminal structure and mRNA stability. *Nature* 266:235, 1977.
58. Darnell JE, Nevins JR, Zeevi MY: The role of poly(A) in mammalian gene expression, in O'Malley B (ed): *Gene Regulation.* UCLA Symposium 26, 1982, p 161.
59. Moore DD, Marks AR, Buckley DI, et al: The first intron of the human growth hormone gene contains a binding site for glucocorticoid receptor. *Proc Natl Acad Sci USA* 82:699, 1985.
60. Slater EP, Rabenau O, Karin M, et al: Glucocorticoid receptor binding and activation of a heterologous promoter by dexamethasone by the first intron of the human growth hormone gene. *Mol Cell Biol* 5:2984, 1985.
61. Gillies SD, Morrison SL, Oi VT, Tonegawa S: A tissue-specific transcriptional enhancer element is located in the major intron of a rearranged immunoglobulin heavy chain gene. *Cell* 33:717, 1983.
62. Wondisford FE, Farr EA, Radovick S, Steinfelder HJ, Oates JM, McClaskey JH, Weintraub BD: Thyroid hormone inhibition of human thyrotropin β-subunit gene expression is mediated by a cis-acting element located in the first exon. *J Biol Chem* 264:14601, 1989.
63. Miller WL, Baxter JD, Eberhardt NL: Peptide hormone genes: Structure and evolution, in Krieger D, Brownstein N, Martin T (eds): *Brain Peptides.* New York, Wiley, 1983, p 15.
64. Doolittle WF: Genes in pieces: Were they ever together? *Nature* 272:581, 1978.
65. Amara SG, Jonas V, Rosenfeld M, et al: Alternative RNA processing in calcitonin gene expression generates mRNAs encoding different polypeptide products. *Nature* 298:240, 1982.
66. Jonas V, Lin CR, Kawashima E, et al: Alternative RNA processing events in human calcitonin/calcitonin gene-related peptide gene expression. *Proc Natl Acad Sci USA* 82:1994, 1985.
67. Nawa H, Kotani H, Nakanishi S: Tissue-specific generation of two preprotachykinin mRNAs from one gene by alternative RNA splicing. *Nature* 312:729, 1984.
68. Edwards RH, Selby MJ, Rutter WJ: Differential RNA splicing predicts two distinct nerve-growth factor precursors. *Nature* 319:784, 1986.
69. Kozak M: Point mutations close to the AUG initiator codon affect the efficiency of translation of rat preproinsulin *in vivo. Nature* 308:241, 1984.
70. Kozak M: Compilation and analysis of sequences upstream from the translational start site in eukaryotic RNAs. *Nucleic Acids Res* 12:857, 1984.
71. Lingappa VR, Lingappa JR, Blobel G: Chicken ovalbumin contains an internal signal sequence. *Nature* 281:117, 1979.
72. Ptashne M, Gann AAF: Activators and targets. *Nature* 346:329, 1990.

73. Mitchell PJ, Tijian R: Transcriptional regulation in mammalian cells by sequence-specific DNA binding proteins. *Science* 245:371, 1989.
74. Bird AP: DNA methylation–how important in gene control? *Nature* 307:503, 1984.
75. Ehrlich M, Wang R: 5-Methylcytosine in eukaryotic DNA. *Science* 212:1350, 1981.
76. Chapman VM, Kratzer PG, Siracusa LD, et al: Evidence for DNA modification in the maintenance of X-chromosome inactivation of adult mouse tissues. *Proc Natl Acad Sci USA* 79:5357, 1982.
77. Saluz HP, Jiricny J, Jost JP: Genomic sequencing reveals a positive correlation between the kinetics of strand-specific DNA demethylation of the overlapping estradiol/glucocorticoid-receptor binding sites and the rate of avian vitellogenin mRNA synthesis. *Proc Natl Acad Sci USA* 83:7167, 1986.
78. Tonegawa S: The molecules of the immune system. *Sci Am* 253:122, 1985.
79. Robberts TH: DNA juggling in the immune system. *Lancet* 2:1086, 1984.
80. Payvar F, DeFranco D, Firestone GL, Edgar B, Wrange O, Okiet S, Gustafsson J, Yamamoto KR: Sequence-specific binding of the glucocorticoid receptor to MTV DNA at sites within and upstream of the transcribed region. *Cell* 35:381, 1983.
81. Scheidereit C, Geisse S, Westphal HM, Beato M: The glucocorticoid receptor binds to defined nucleotide sequences near the promoter of mouse mammary tumor virus. *Nature* 304:749, 1983.
82. Karin M, Haslinger A, Holtgreve H, Richards R, Kravter P, et al: Characterization of DNA sequences through which cadmium and glucocorticoid hormone induce human metallothionein IIA gene. *Nature* 308:513, 1984.
83. Chandler VL, Maler BA, Yamamoto KR: DNA sequences bound specifically by glucocorticoid receptor *in vitro* render a heterologous promoter hormone responsive *in vivo*. *Cell* 33:489, 1983.
84. Ponta H, Kennedy N, Skroch P, Hynes NE, Groner B: Hormonal response regions in the mouse mammary tumor virus long terminal repeat can be dissociated from the proviral promoter and has enhancer properties. *Proc Natl Acad Sci USA* 82:1020, 1985.
85. Eberwine JK, Roberts JL: Glucocorticoid regulation of proopiomelanocortin gene transcription in the rat pituitary. *J Biol Chem* 259:2166, 1984.
86. Israel A, Cohen SN: Hormonally mediated negative regulation of proopiomelanocortin gene transcription in the rat pituitary. *J Biol Chem* 259:2166, 1984.
87. Drouin J, Trifiro MA, Plante RK, Nemer M, Eriksson P, Wrange O: Glucocorticoid receptor binding to a specific DNA sequence is required for hormone-dependent repression of pro-opiomelanocortin gene transcription. *Mol Cell Biol* 9:5305, 1989.
88. Akerblom I, Slater EP, Beato M, Baxter JD, Mellon PL: Negative regulation by glucocorticoids through interference with a cAMP responsive enhancer. *Science* 241:350, 1988.
89. Diamond MI, Miner JN, Yoshinaga SK, Yamamoto KR: Transcription factor interactions: Selectors of positive or negative regulation from a single DNA element. *Science* 249:1266, 1990.
90. Yang-Yen H-F, Chambard J-C, Sun Y-L, Smeal T, Schmidt TJ, Drouin J, Karin M: Transcriptional interference between c-jun and the glucocorticoid receptor: Mutual inhibition of DNA binding due to direct protein-protein interaction. *Cell* 62:1205, 1990.
91. Evans RM: The steroid and thyroid hormone receptor family. *Science* 240:889, 1988.
92. Beato M: Gene regulation by steroid hormones. *Cell* 56:335, 1989.
93. Ozono K, Liao J, Kerner SA, Scott RA, Pike JW: The vitamin D-responsive element in the human osteocalcin gene. *J Biol Chem*265:21881, 1990.
94. Maurer RA: Transcriptional regulation of the prolactin gene by ergocryptine and cyclic AMP. *Nature* 294:94, 1981.
95. Jameson JL, Deutsch PJ, Gallagher GD, Jaffe RC, Habener JF: Trans-acting factors interact with a cyclic AMP response element to modulate expression of the human gonadotrophin α gene. *Mol Cell Biol* 7:3032, 1987.
96. Montminy MR, Sevarino KA, Wagner JA, Mandel G, Goodman RH: Identification of a cyclic-AMP-responsive element within the rat somatostatin gene. *Proc Natl Acad Sci USA* 83:6682, 1986.
97. Yamamoto KK, Gonzalez GA, Biggs WH, Montminy MR: Phosphorylation-induced binding and transcriptional efficacy of nuclear factor CREB. *Nature* 334:494, 1988.
98. Angel P, Imagawa M, Chin R, Stein B, Imbra RJ, Rahmsdorf HJ, Jonat C, Herrlich P, Karin M: Phorbol ester-inducible genes contain a common cis element recognized by a TPA-modulated trans-acting factor. *Cell* 49:729, 1987.
99. Lee W, Mitchell P, Tijian R: Purified transcription factor AP-1 interacts with TPA-inducible enhancer elements. *Cell* 49:741, 1987.
100. Curran T, Franza BR: Fos and Jun: The AP-1 connection. *Cell* 55:395, 1988.
101. Gilman MZ: The c-fos serum response element responds to protein kinase C-dependent and -independent signals but not to cyclic AMP. *Genes Dev* 2:394, 1988.
102. Angel P, Hattori K, Smeal T, Karin M: The Jun protooncogene is positively-autoregulated by its product, jun/AP-1. *Cell* 55:875, 1988.
103. Boyle WJ, Smeal T, Defize LHK, Angel P, Woodgett JR, Karin M, Hunter T: Activation of protein kinase C decreases phosphorylation of c-jun at sites that negatively regulate its DNA-binding activity. *Cell* 64:573, 1991.
104. Auwerx J, Sassone-Corsi P: IP-1: A dominant inhibitor of fos/jun whose activity is modulated by phosphorylation. *Cell* 64:983, 1991.
105. Granner D, Andreone T, Sasaki K, Beale E: Inhibition of transcription of the phosphoenolpyruvate carboxykinase gene by insulin. *Nature* 305:549, 1983.
106. Alexander MC, Lomanto M, Nasrin N, Ramaika C: Insulin stimulates glyceraldehyde-3-phosphate dehydogenase gene expression through *cis*-acting DNA sequences. *Proc Natl Acad Sci USA* 85:5092, 1988.
107. Khoury G, Gruss P: Enhancer elements. *Cell* 33:313, 1983.
108. Parker M: Enhancer elements activated by steroid hormones? *Nature* 304:687, 1983.
109. Gruss P: Magic enhancers? *DNA* 3:1, 1984.
110. Ptashne M: Gene regulation by proteins acting nearby and at a distance. *Nature* 322:697, 1986.
111. Lewin B: Commitment and activation at Pol II promoters: A tail of protein-protein interactions. *Cell* 61:1161, 1990.
112. Tsai SY, Sagami I, Wang H, Tsai M-J, O'Malley BW: Interactions between a DNA-binding transcription factor (COUP) and a non-DNA binding factor (S 300-11). *Cell* 50:701, 1987.
113. Burnside J, Darling DS, Chin WW: A nuclear factor that enhances binding of thyroid hormone receptors to thyroid hormone response elements. *J Biol Chem* 265:2500, 1990.
114. Crenshaw EB, Russo AF, Swanson LF, Rosenfeld MG: Neuron-specific alternative RNA processing in transgenic mice expressing a metallothionein-calcitonin fusion gene. *Cell* 49:389, 1987.
115. Emeson RB, Hedjran F, Yeakley JM, Guise JW, Rosenfeld MG: Alternative production of calcitonin and CGRP mRNA is regulated at the calcitonin-specific splice acceptor. *Nature* 341:76, 1989.
116. Moore DD, Conkling MA, Goodman HM: Human growth hormone: A multigene family. *Cell* 29:285, 1982.

117. Brawerman G: mRNA decay: Finding the right targets. *Cell* 57:9, 1989.
118. Nielsen DA, Shapiro DJ: Insights into hormonal control of messenger RNA stability. *Mol Cell Endocrinol* 4:953, 1990.
119. Guyette WA, Matusik RJ, Rosen JM: Prolactin-mediated transcriptional and post-transcriptional control of casein gene expression. *Cell* 17:1013, 1979.
120. Cell RF: Estrogen withdrawal in chick oviduct: Selective loss of high abundance classes of polyadenylated messenger RNA. *Biochemistry* 16:3433, 1975.
121. McKnight GS, Palmiter RD: Transcriptional regulation of the ovalbumin and conalbumin genes by steroid hormones in chick oviduct. *J Biol Chem* 254:9050, 1979.
122. Brock ML, Shapiro DJ: Estrogen stabilizes vitellogenin mRNA against cytoplasmic degradation. *Cell* 34:207, 1983.
123. Vannice JC, Taylor JM, Ringold GM: Glucocorticoid-mediated induction of α_1-acid glycoprotein: Evidence of hormone-regulated RNA processing. *Proc Natl Acad Sci USA* 81:4241, 1984.
124. Paek I, Axel R: Glucocorticoids enhance stability of human growth hormone mRNA. *Mol Cell Biol* 7:1496, 1987.
125. Gertz BJ, Gardner DG, Baxter JD: Glucocorticoid control of rat growth hormone gene expression: Effect on cytoplasmic messenger ribonucleic acid production and degradation. *Mol Cell Endocrinol* 1:933, 1987.
126. Narayan P, Towle HC: Stabilization of a specific nuclear mRNA precursor by thyroid hormone. *Mol Cell Biol* 5:2642, 1985.
127. Itoh N, Okamoto H: Translation control of proinsulin synthesis by glucose. *Nature* 283:100, 1980.
128. Eberwine JH, Roberts JL: Analysis of pro-opiomelanocortin gene structure and function. *DNA* 2:1, 1983.
129. Slater EP, Baxter JD, Eberhardt NL: Evolution of the growth hormone gene family. *Am Zool* 26:939, 1986.
130. Levine MA, Ahn TG, Klupft SF, Kaufman KD, Smallwood PM, Bourne HR, Sullivan KA, Van Dop C: Genetic deficiency of the subunit of the guanine nucleotide-binding protein G_s as the molecular basis for Albright hereditary osteodystrophy. *Proc Natl Acad Sci USA* 85:617, 1988.
131. Amselem S, Duquesnoy P, Attree O, Novelli G, Bousrina S, Postel-Vinay M-C, Goosens M: Laron dwarfism and mutation of the growth hormone receptor gene. *N Engl J Med* 321:989, 1989.
132. Godowski PJ, Leung DW, Meacham LR, Galgani JP, Hellmiss R, Keret R, Rotwein PS, Parks JS, et al: Characterization of the human growth hormone receptor gene and demonstration of a partial gene deletion in two patients with Laron-type dwarfism. *Proc Natl Acad Sci USA* 86:8083, 1989.
133. White PC: Analysis of mutations causing steroid 21-hydroxylase deficiency. *Endocr Rev* 15:239, 1989.
134. Phillips JA, Hjelle BL, Seeburg PH, Zachmann M: Molecular basis for isolated growth hormone deficiency. *Proc Natl Acad Sci USA* 78:6372, 1981.
135. Vnencak-Jones CL, Phillips JA: Hot spots for growth hormone gene deletions in homologous regions outside Alu repeats. *Science* 250:1745, 1990.
136. Hayashizaki U, Hiraoka Y, Endo Y, Miyai K, Matsubara K: Thyroid stimulating hormone (TSH) deficiency caused by a single base substitution in the CAGYC region of the beta-subunit. *EMBO J* 8:2291, 1989.
137. Brown MS, Goldstein JL: A receptor-mediated pathway for cholesterol homeostasis. *Science* 232:34, 1986.
138. Hurley DM, Accili D, Stratakis CA, Karl M, Vamvakopoulos N, Rorer E, Constantine K, Taylor SI, Chrousos GP: Point mutation causing a single amino acid substitution in the hormone binding domain of the glucocorticoid receptor in familial glucocorticoid resistance. *J Clin Invest* 87:680, 1991.
139. Marcelli M, Zoppi S, Grino PB, Griffin JE, Wilson JD, McPhaul MJ: A mutation in the DNA-binding domain of the androgen receptor gene causes testicular feminization in a patient with receptor-positive androgen resistance. *J Clin Invest* 87:1123, 1991.
140. Takeda K, Balzano S, Sakurai A, DeGroot LJ, Refetoff S: Screening of nineteen unrelated families with generalized resistance to thyroid hormone for known point mutations in the thyroid hormone receptor β gene and the detection of a new mutation. *J Clin Invest* 87:496, 1991.
141. Hughes MR, Malloy PJ, Kieback DG, Kesterson RA, Pike JW, Feldman D, O'Malley BW: Point mutations in the human vitamin D receptor gene associated with hypocalcemic rickets. *Science* 242:1702, 1988.
142. Kadowaki T, Kadowaki H, Rechler MM, Serrano-Rios M, Roth J, Gorden P, Taylor SI: Five mutant alleles of the insulin receptor gene in patients with genetic forms of insulin resistance. *J Clin Invest* 86:254, 1990.
143. Orkin SH, Kazaziain HH: The mutation and polymorphism of the human β-globin gene and its surrounding DNA. *Annu Rev Genet* 18:131, 1984.
144. Shoelson S, Haneda M, Blix P, et al: Three mutant insulins in man. *Nature* 302:540, 1983.
145. Haneda M, Polonsky KS, Bergenstal RM, et al: Familial hyperinsulinemia due to a structurally abnormal insulin. *N Engl J Med* 310:1288, 1984.
146. Chang JC, Kan YW: β^0 Thalassemia, a nonsense mutation in man. *Proc Natl Acad Sci USA* 76:2886, 1979.
147. Marquat LE, Kinniburgh AJ, Rachmileintz EA, Ron J: Unstable β-globin mRNA in mRNA-deficient β^0 thalassemia. *Cell* 27:543, 1981.
148. Treisman R, Orkin SH, Maniatis T: Specific transcription and RNA splicing defects in five cloned β-thalassemia genes. *Nature* 302:591, 1983.
149. Ottolenghi S, Giglioni B, Pulazzini A, Comi P, Camaschella C, Serra A, Guerrasio A, Saglio G: Sardinian delta beta zero-thalassemia: A further example of a C to T substitution at position −196 of the A gamma globin gene promoter. *Blood* 69:1058, 1987.
150. Glover DM (ed): *DNA Cloning,* vols I and II. Oxford, United Kingdom, IRL Press, 1985.
151. Old RW, Primrose SB: *Principles of Gene Manipulation,* 3d ed. Oxford, United Kingdom, Blackwell, 1985.
152. Sambrook J, Fritsch EF, Maniatis T: *Molecular Cloning: A Laboratory Manual,* vols I–III, 2d ed. Cold Spring Harbor, NY, Cold Spring Harbor Laboratory Press, 1989.
153. Southern E: Detection of specific sequences among DNA fragments separated by gel electrophoresis. *J Mol Biol* 98:503, 1975.
154. Thomas PS: Hybridization of denatured RNA and small DNA fragments transferred to nitrocellulose. *Proc Natl Acad Sci USA* 77:5201, 1980.
155. Gilbert W: DNA sequencing and gene structure. *Science* 214:1305, 1982.
156. Sanger F: Determination of nucleotide sequences in DNA. *Science* 214:1205, 1981.
157. Kraft R, Tardiff J, Krauter KS, Leinwand LA: Using miniprep plasmid DNA for sequencing double-stranded templates with sequenase. *Biotechniques* 6:544, 1988.
158. Wilson RK, Chen C, Avdalovic N, Burns J, Hood L: Development of an automated procedure for fluorescent DNA sequencing. *Genomics* 6:626, 1990.
159. Caruthers MH: Gene synthesis machines: DNA chemistry and its uses. *Science* 230:281, 1985.
160. Ullrich A, Bell JR, Chen EY, et al: Human insulin receptor and its relationship to the tyrosine kinase family of oncogenes. *Nature* 313:756, 1985.
161. Kemp DJ, Cowman AF: Direct immunoassay for detecting *Escherichia coli* colonies that contain polypeptides encoded by cloned DNA segments. *Proc Natl Acad Sci USA* 78:4520, 1981.
162. Young RA, Davis RW: Efficient isolation of genes by using antibody probes. *Proc Natl Acad Sci USA* 80:1194, 1983.
163. Murphy TJ, Alexander RW, Griendling KK, Runge MS, Bernstein KE: Isolation of a cDNA encoding the vascular type-1 angiotensin II receptor. *Nature* 351:233, 1991.
164. Williams JA, McChesney DJ, Calayag MC, Lingappa VR,

Logsdon CD: Expression of receptors for cholecystokinin and other Ca^{2+}-mobilizing hormones in Xenopus oocytes. *Proc Natl Acad Sci USA* 85:4939, 1988.

165. Lawn RM, Fritsch EF, Parker RC, et al: The isolation and characterization of linked δ- and β-globin genes from a cloned library of human DNA. *Cell* 15:1157, 1978.
166. Erlich HA: *PCR Technology*. New York, Stockton Press, 1989.
167. Loh EY, Elliott JF, Cwirla S, Lanier LL, Davis MM: Polymerase chain reaction with single-sided specificity: Analysis of T cell receptor δ chain. *Science* 243:217, 1989.
168. Kwok S, Higuchi R: Avoiding false positives with PCR. *Nature* 339:237, 1989.
169. Capecchi MR: High efficiency transformation by direct microinjection of DNA into cultured mammalian cells. *Cell* 22:479, 1980.
170. Pellicer A, Wigler M, Axel R, Silverstein S: The transfer and stable integration of the HSV thymidine kisase gene into mouse cells. *Cell* 14:133, 1978.
171. McCutchan JH, Pagano JS: Enhancement of the infectivity of simian virus 40 deoxyribonucleic acid with diethyl aminoethyl-dextran. *JNCI* 41:351, 1969.
172. Potter H, Weir L, Leder P: Enhancer dependent expression of human k immunoglobulin genes introduced into mouse pre-B lymphocytes by electroporation. *Proc Natl Acad Sci USA* 81:7161, 1984.
173. Doehmer J, Barinaga M, Vale W, et al: Introduction of rat growth hormone gene into mouse fibroblasts via a retroviral DNA vector: Expression and regulation. *Proc Natl Acad Sci USA* 79:2268, 1982.
174. Gorman CM, Moffat L, Howard BH: Recombinant genes which express chloramphenicol acetyl transferase. *Mol Cell Biol* 2:1044, 1982.
175. Southern PJ, Berg P: Transformation of mammalian cells to antibiotic resistance with a bacterial gene under control of the SV40 early promoter. *J Mol Appl Gen* 1:327, 1982.
176. Kurtz DT: Hormone inducibility of rat α2μ-globulin genes in transfected mouse cells. *Nature* 291:629, 1981.
177. Zoller MJ, Smith M: Oligonucleotide-directed mutagenesis using M13-directed vectors: An efficient and general procedure for the production of point mutations in any fragment of DNA. *Nucleic Acids Res* 10:6487, 1982.
178. Von der Ahe D, Janich S, Scheidereit C, Renkawitz R, Schutz G, Beato M: Glucocorticoid and progesterone receptors bind to the same sites in two hormonally regulated promoters. *Nature* 313:706, 1985.
179. Kumar V, Chambon P: The estrogen receptor binds tightly to its responsive element as a ligand-induced homodimer. *Cell* 55:145, 1988.
180. Dabre P, Page M, King RJB: Androgen regulation by the long terminal repeat of mouse mammary tumor virus. *Mol Cell Biol* 6:2847, 1986.
181. Cato ACB, Weinmann J: Mineralocorticoid regulation of transfected mouse mammary tumor virus DNA in cultured kidney cells. *J Cell Biol* 106:2119, 1988.
182. Glass CK, Holloway JM, Devary OV, Rosenfeld MG: The thyroid hormone receptor binds with opposite transcriptional effects to a common sequence motif in thyroid hormone and estrogen response elements. *Cell* 54:313, 1988.
183. Ozono K, Liao J, Kerner SA, Scott RA, Pike JW: The vitamin D-responsive element in the human osteocalcin gene. *J Biol Chem* 265:21881, 1990.
184. Roesler WJ, Vanderbark GR, Hanson RW: Cyclic AMP and the induction of eukaryotic gene transcription. *J Biol Chem* 203:9063, 1988.
185. Duram DM, Palmiter RD: Transcriptional regulation of the mouse metallothionein-I gene by heavy metal. *J Biol Chem* 256:5712, 1981.
186. Sielecki A, Hayakawa K, Fujinaga M, Murphy M, Fraser M, Muir AK, Carilli CT, Lewicki JA, et al: Structure of recombinant human renin, a target for cardiovascular-active drugs, at 2.5 A° resolution. *Science* 243:1346, 1989.
187. Freedman LP, Luisi BF, Korszun ZR, Basauappa R, Sigler PB, Yamamoto KR: The function and structure of metal coordination sites within the glucocorticoid receptor DNA binding domain. *Nature* 334:543, 1988.
188. Van der Krol AR, Mol JNM, Stuitje AR: Modulation of eukaryotic gene expression by complementary RNA or DNA sequences. *Biotechniques* 6:958, 1988.
189. Sarver N, Cantin EM, Chang PS, Zaia JA, Ladne PA, Stephens DA, Rossi JJ: Ribozymes as potential anti-HIV-I therapeutic agents. *Science* 247:1222, 1990.
190. Ransone LJ, Visvader J, Wamsley P, Verma IM: Transdominant negative mutants of fos and jun. *Proc Natl Acad Sci USA* 87:3806, 1990.
191. Damm K, Thompson CC, Evans RM: Protein encoded by v-erbA functions as a thyroid-hormone receptor antagonist. *Nature* 339:593, 1989.
192. Koenig RJ, Lazar MA, Hodin RA, Brent GA, Larsen PR, Chin WW, Moore DD: Inhibition of thyroid hormone action by a non-hormonal binding c-erbA protein generated by alternative RNA splicing. *Nature* 337:659, 1989.
193. Capecchi MR: Altering the genome by homologous recombination. *Science* 244:1288, 1989.
194. Mansour SL, Thomas KR, Capecchi MR: Disruption of the proto-oncogene int-2 in mouse embryo-derived stem cells: A general strategy for targeting mutations to non-selectable genes. *Nature* 336:348, 1988.
195. Hammer RE, Pursel VG, Rexroad CE, Wall RJ, Bolt DJ, Ebert KM, Palmiter RD, Brinster RL: Production of transgenic rabbits, sheep and pigs by microinjection. *Nature* 315:680, 1985.
196. Mullins JJ, Peters J, Ganten D: Fulminant hypertension in transgenic rats harboring the mouse ren-2 gene. *Nature* 344:541, 1990.
197. Ornitz DM, Palmiter RD, Hammer RE, Brinster RL, Swift GH, MacDonald RJ: Specific expression of an elastase-human growth hormone fusion gene in pancreatic acinar cells of transgenic mice. *Nature* 313:600, 1985.
198. Ross SR, Solter D: Glucocorticoid regulation of mouse mammary tumor virus sequences in transgenic mice. *Proc Natl Acad Sci USA* 82:5880, 1985.
199. Hammer RE, Idzerda RL, Brinster RL, McKnight GS: Estrogen regulation of the avian transferrin gene in transgenic mice. *Mol Cell Biol* 6:1010, 1986.
200. Brinster RL, Chen HY, Warren R, Sarthy A, Palmiter RD: Regulation of metallothionein-thymidine kinase fusion plasmids injected into mouse eggs. *Nature* 296:39, 1982.
201. Palmiter RD, Brinster RL, Hammer RE, Trumbauer ME, Rosenfeld MG, Birnberg NC, Evans RM: Dramatic growth of mice that develop from eggs micro-injected with metallothionein-growth hormone fusion genes. *Nature* 300:611, 1982.
202. Hammer RE, Brinster RL, Rosenfeld MG, Evans, RE, Mayo KE: Expression of human growth hormone releasing factor in transgenic mice results in increased somatic growth. *Nature* 315:413, 1985.
203. Ohkubo W, Kawakani H, Kakehi Y, Takumi T, Arai H, Yokota Y, Iwai M, Tanabe Y, et al: Generation of transgenic mice with elevated blood pressure by introduction of the rat renin and angiotensinogen genes. *Proc Natl Acad Sci USA* 87:5153, 1990.
204. Steinhelper ME, Cochrane KL, Field LJ: Hypotension in transgenic mice expressing atrial natriuretic factor fusion genes. *Hypertension* 16:301, 1990.
205. Hammer R, Palmiter RD, Brinster RL: Partial correction of murine hereditary growth disorder by germ-line incorporation of a new gene. *Nature* 311:65, 1984.
206. Hanahan D: Heritable formation of pancreatic β cell tumors in transgenic mice expressing recombinant insulin/simian virus 40 oncogenes. *Nature* 315:115, 1985.
207. Windle JJ, Weiner RI, Mellon PM: Cell lines of the pituitary gonadotrope lineage derived by targeted oncogenesis in transgenic mice. *Mol Cell Endocrinol* 4:597, 1990.

208. Mellon PL, Windle JJ, Goldsmith PC, Padula CA, Roberts JL, Weiner RI: Immortalization of hypothalamic GnRH neurons by genetically targeted tumorigenesis. *Neuron* 5:1, 1990.
209. Field LJ: Atrial natriuretic factor-SV_{40} T antigen transgenes produce tumors and cardiac arrhythmias in mice. *Science* 239:1029, 1988.
210. Sigmund CD, Okuyama K, Ingelfinger J, Jones CA, Mullins JJ, Kane C, Kim V, Wu C, et al: Isolation and characterization of renin-expressing cell lines from transgenic mice containing a renin promoter-viral oncogene fusion construct. *J Biol Chem* 265:19916, 1990.
211. Efrat S, Linde S, Kofod H, Spector D, Delannoy M, Grant S, Hanahan D, Baekkeskov S: Beta-cell lines derived from transgenic mice expressing a hybrid insulin-gene oncogene. *Proc Natl Acad Sci USA* 85:9037, 1988.
212. Steinhelper ME, Lanson NA, Dresdner KP, Delcarpio JB, Wit AL, Claycomb WC, Field LJ: Proliferation *in vivo* and in culture of differentiated adult atrial cardiomyocytes from transgenic mice. *Am J Physiol* 259 (*Heart Circ Physiol* 28):H1826, 1990.
213. Behringer RR, Matthews LS, Palmiter RD, Brinster RL: Dwarf mice produced by genetic ablation of growth hormone expressing cells. *Genes Dev* 2:453, 1988.
214. Sarvetnick N, Liggett D, Pitts SL, Hansen SE, Stewart TA: Insulin-dependent diabetes mellitus induced in transgenic mice by ectopic expression of class II MHC and interferon-gamma. *Cell* 52:773, 1988.
215. Oldstone MBA, Nerenberg M, Southern P, Price J, Lewicki H: Virus infection triggers insulin-dependent diabetes mellitus in a transgenic model: Role of anti-self (virus) immune response. *Cell* 65:319, 1991.
216. Ohashi PS, Oehen S, Buerki K, Pircher H, Ohashi CT, Odermatt B, Malissen B, Zinkernagel RM, Hengartner H: Ablation of "tolerance" and induction of diabetes by virus infection in viral antigen transgenic mice. *Cell* 65:305, 1991.
217. Zimmer A, Gruss P: Production of chimaeric mice containing embryonic stem (ES) cells carrying a homeobox Hox 1.1 allele mutated by homologous recombination. *Nature* 338:150, 1989.
218. Thompson S, Clarke AR, Pow AM, Hooper ML, Melton DW: Germ line transmission and expression of a corrected HGPRT gene produced by gene targeting in embryonic stem cells. *Cell* 56:313, 1989.
219. Chisaka O, Capecchi, MR: Regionally restricted developmental defects resulting from targeted disruption of the mouse homeobox gene hox-1.5. *Nature* 350:473, 1991.
220. Schorle H, Holtschke T, Hunig T, Schimpl A, Horak I: Development and function of T cells in mice rendered interleukin-2 deficient by gene targeting. *Nature* 352:621, 1991.
221. Kitamura D, Roes J, Kuhn R, Rajewsky K: A B cell-deficient mouse by targeted disruption of the membrane exon of the immunoglobulin μ chain gene. *Nature* 350:423, 1991.
222. Mortensen RM, Zubiaur M, Neer EJ, Seidman JG: Embryonic stem cells lacking a functional inhibitory G-protein subunit α_{i2} produced by gene targeting of both alleles. *Proc Natl Acad Sci USA* 88:7036, 1991.
223. Itakura K, Hirose T, Crea R, et al: Expression in *Escherichia coli* of a chemically synthesized gene for the hormone somatostatin. *Science* 198:1056, 1977.
224. Shine J, Fettes I, Lan NC, et al: Expression of cloned β-endorphin gene sequences by *E. coli*. *Nature* 285:456, 1980.
225. Smith RA, Duncan MJ, Moin DT: Heterologous protein secretion from yeast. *Science* 229:1219, 1985.
226. Wood WI, Capon DJ, Simonsen CC, et al: Expression of active human factor VIII from recombinant DNA clones. *Nature* 312:330, 1984.
227. Brown P, Gajdusek C, Gibbs CJ, Asher DM: Potential epidemic of Creutzfeldt-Jakob disease from human growth hormone therapy. *N Engl J Med* 313:728, 1985.
228. Manson JM, Wilmore DW: Positive nitrogen balance with human growth hormone and hypocaloric intravenous feeding. *Surgery* 100:188, 1986.
229. Clemmons DR, Snyder DK, Williams R, Underwood LE: Growth hormone administration conserves lean body mass during dietary restriction in obese subjects. *J Clin Endocrinol Metab* 64:878, 1987.
230. Rudman D, Feller AG, Nagraj HS, Gergans GA, Lalitha PY, Goldberg AF, Schlenker RA, Cohn L, et al: Effects of human growth hormone in men over 60 years old. *N Engl J Med* 323:1, 1990.
231. Oster W, Herrmann F, Gamm N, Zeile G, Lindemann A, Muller G, Brune T, Kraemer H-P, Mertelsmann Z: Erythropoietin for the treatment of anemia of malignancy associated with neoplastic bone marrow filtration. *J Clin Oncol* 8:956, 1990.
232. Ludwig H, Fritz E, Kotzmann H, Hocker P, Gisslinger H, Barnas U: Erythropoietin treatment of anemia associated with multiple myeloma. *N Engl J Med* 322:1693, 1990.
233. Ganser A, Völkers B, Greher J, et al: Recombinant human granulocyte-macrophage colony-stimulating factor in patients with myelodysplastic syndromes: A phase I/II trial. *Blood* 73:31, 1989.
234. Koeffler HP: Colony-stimulating factors: Clinical promises. *Biotechnol Ther* 1:181, 1990.
235. Ozer H: Clinical and biological activities of interferon and hematological malignancies. *Biotechnol Ther* 1:109, 1990.
236. Kaplan LD, Abrams DI, Sherwin SA, Kahn J, Volberding PA: A phase I/II study of recombinant tumor necrosis factor and recombinant interferon gamma in patients with AIDS-related complex. *Biotechnol Ther* 1:229, 1990.
237. Perkus ME, Piccini A, Lipinskas BR, Paoletti E: Recombinant vaccinia virus: Immunization against multiple pathogens. *Science* 229:981, 1985.
238. Albin J, Rifkin H: Etiologies of diabetes mellitus. *Med Clin North Am* 66:1204, 1982.
239. Morrison SL: Transfectomas provide novel chimeric antibodies. *Science* 220:1053, 1983.
240. Haber E, Quertermous R, Matsueda GR: Innovative approaches to plasminogen activator therapy. *Science* 234:51, 1989.
241. Davies SF, Walker IM: Multiple emulsions as targetable delivery systems: Drug and enzyme targeting, in Green R, Widdler KJ (eds): *Methods in Enzymology*. New York, Academic, 1984.
242. Gordon GC, Moses AC, Carey ML, et al: Nasal absorption of insulin: Enhancement by hydrophobic bile salts. *Proc Natl Acad Sci USA* 82:7419, 1985.
243. Moses AC, Gordon GC, Carey ML, et al: Insulin administered intranasally as an insulin-bile salt aerosol: Effectiveness and reproducibility in normal and diabetic subjects. *Diabetes* 32:1040, 1983.
244. DeMuinck Keizer-Schrama SMPF, Hazebroek FWJ, Drop SLS, Molenaar JC, Visser HKA: LH-RH nasal spray treatment for cryptorchidism. *Eur J Pediatr* 146(Suppl 2):535, 1987.
245. Overgaard K, Hansen MA, Nielsen V-AH, Riis BJ, Christiansen C: Discontinuous calcitonin treatment of established osteoporosis—effect of withdrawal of treatment. *Am J Med* 89:1, 1990.
246. Salzman R, Manson JE, Griffing GT, et al: Intranasal aerosolized insulin: Mixed meal and long term use in type I diabetes. *N Engl J Med* 312:1078, 1985.
247. Stanbury JB, Wyngaarden JB, Fredrickson DS, Goldstein JL, Brown MS (eds): *The Metabolic Basis of Inherited Disease,* 5th ed. New York, McGraw-Hill, 1983.
248. Pirastu M, Kan YW, Cao A, et al: Prenatal diagnosis of β-thalassemia: Detection of a single nucleotide mutation in DNA. *N Engl J Med* 309:284, 1983.
249. Chang JC, Kan YW: A sensitive new prenatal test for sickle cell anemia. *N Engl J Med* 307:30, 1982.

250. Saiki RK, Scharf S, Faloona F, et al: Enzymatic amplification of β-globin genomic sequences and restriction site analysis for diagnosis of sickle cell anemia. *Science* 230: 1350, 1985.
251. Woo SLC, Lidsky AS, Guttler F, et al: Cloned human phenylalanine hydroxylase gene allows prenatal diagnosis and carrier detection of classical phenylketonuria. *Nature* 306: 151, 1983.
252. Watkins PC: Restriction fragment length polymorphism (RFLP): Applications in human chromosome mapping and genetic disease research. *Biotechniques* 6:310, 1988.
253. Bell GI, Xiang K-S, Newman MV, Wu SH, Wright LG, Fajans SS, Spielman RS, Cox NJ: Gene for non-insulin-dependent diabetes mellitus (maturity-onset diabetes of the young subtype) is linked to DNA polymorphism on human chromosome 20 q. *Proc Natl Acad Sci USA* 88:1484, 1991.
254. Bell GI, Horita S, Karam JH: A polymorphic locus near the human insulin gene is associated with insulin-dependent diabetes mellitus. *Diabetes* 31:176, 1984.
255. Raffel LJ, Hitman GA, Toyoda H, Karam JH, Bell GI, Rotter JI: The aggregation of the 5′ insulin gene polymorphism in type I (insulin-dependent) diabetes mellitus families. *Am J Hum Genet* (in press).
256. Humphries SE, Horsthemke B, Seed M, Holm M, Wynn V, Kessling AM, Donald JA, Jowett N, et al: A common DNA polymorphism of the low-density lipoprotein (LDL) receptor gene and its use in diagnosis. *Lancet* 1:1003, 1985.
257. White PC, New MI, Dupont B: HLA-linked congenital adrenal hyperplasia results from a defective gene encoding a cytochrome P-450 specific for steroid 21-hydroxylation. *Proc Natl Acad Sci USA* 81:7505, 1984.
258. Larsson C, Skogseid B, Oberg K, et al: Multiple endocrine neoplasia type 1 gene maps to chromosome 11 and is lost in insulinoma. *Nature* 332:85, 1988.
259. Sobol H, Narod SA, Nakamura Y, et al: Screening for multiple endocrine neoplasia type 2A with DNA-polymorphism analysis. *N Engl J Med* 321:996, 1989.
260. Jackson CE, Norum RA, O'Neal LW, et al: Linkage between MEN 2B and chromosome 10 markers. *Am J Hum Genet* 43:A147, 1988.
261. Rosenberg SA, Aebersold P, Cornetta K, Kasid A, Morgan RA, Moen R, Karson EM, Lotze MT, et al: Gene transfer into humans—immunotherapy of patients with advanced melanoma, using tumor-infiltrating lymphocytes modified by retroviral gene transduction. *N Engl J Med* 323:570, 1990.
262. Williams DA, Orkin SH: Somatic gene therapy. *J Clin Invest* 77:1053, 1986.
263. Friedmann T: Progress toward human gene therapy. *Science* 244:1275, 1989.
264. Yokode M, Hammer RE, Ishibashi S, Brown MS, Goldstein JL: Diet-induced hypercholesterolemia in mice: Prevention by over expression of LDL receptors. *Science* 250:1273, 1990.
265. Nabel EG, Plantz G, Boyce FM, Stanley JC, Nabel GJ: Recombinant gene expression *in vivo* within endothelial cells of the arterial wall. *Science* 244:1342, 1989.
266. Nabel EG, Plantz G, Nabel GJ: Site-specific gene expression *in vivo* by direct gene transfer into arterial wall. *Science* 249:1285, 1990.
267. Barr E, Leiden JM: Systemic delivery of recombinant proteins by genetically modified myoblasts. *Science* 254:1507, 1991.
268. Dhawan J, Pan LC, Pavlath GK, Travis MA, Lanctot AM, Blau HM: Systemic delivery of human growth hormone by injection of genetically engineered myoblasts. *Science* 254: 1509, 1991.
268a. Gussoni E, Pavlath GK, Lanctot AM, Sharma KR, Miller RG, Steinman L, Blau HM: Normal dystrophin transcripts detected in Duchenne muscular dystrophy patients after myoblast transplantation. *Nature* 356:435, 1992.
269. Bishop JM: Molecular themes in oncogenesis. *Cell* 64:235, 1991.
270. Lewin B: Oncogenic conversion by regulatory changes in transcription factors. *Cell* 64:303, 1991.
271. Cantley LC, Auger KR, Carpenter C, Duckworth B, Graziani A, Kapeller R, Soltoff S: Oncogenes and signal transduction. *Cell* 64:281, 1991.
272. Doolittle RF, Humhapiller NW, Hood LE, et al: Simian sarcoma virus oncogene, v-sis, is derived from the gene (or genes) encoding a platelet-derived growth factor. *Science* 221:275, 1983.
273. Waterfield MD, Scrace GT, Whittle N, et al: Platelet-derived growth factor is structurally related to the putative transforming protein p28 sis of simian sarcoma virus. *Nature* 304:35, 1983.
274. Downward L, Yarden Y, Mayes E, et al: Close similarity of epidermal growth factor receptor and v-erb B oncogene protein sequences. *Nature* 307:521, 1984.
275. Shih C, Weinberg RA: Isolation of a transforming sequence from a human bladder carcinoma cell line. *Cell* 29:161, 1982.
276. Yoakum GH, Lechner JF, Gabrielson EW, et al: Transformation of human bronchial epithelial cells transfected with Harvey ras oncogene. *Science* 227:1174, 1985.
277. Karga H, Lee JK, Vickery AL, Thor A, Gaz RD, Jameson JL: Ras oncogene mutations in benign and malignant thyroid neoplasms. *J Clin Endocrinol Metab* 73:832, 1991.
278. Meltzer SJ, Ahnen DJ, Battifora H, Yokota J, Cline MJ: Protooncogene abnormalities in colon cancers and adenomatous polyps. *Gastroenterology* 92:1174, 1987.
279. Landis CA, Masters SB, Spada A, Pace AM, Bourne HR, Vallar L: GTPase inhibiting mutations activate the α chain of G_S and stimulate adenylyl cyclase in human pituitary tumors. *Nature* 340:692, 1989.
280. Lyons J, Landis CA, Harsh G, Vallar L, Grunewald K, Feichtinger H, Duh Q-Y, Clark OH, et al: Two G protein oncogenes in human endocrine tumors. *Science* 249:655, 1990.
281. Evans RM: The steroid and thyroid hormone receptor family. *Science* 240:889, 1988.
282. Marshall CJ: Tumor suppressor genes. *Cell* 64:313, 1991.
283. Friedman E, Sakaguchi K, Bale AE, Falchetti A, et al: Clonality of parathyroid tumors in familial multiple endocrine neoplasia type 1. *N Engl J Med* 321:213, 1989.
284. Thakker RV, Bouloux MD, Wooding C, Chotai K, et al: Association of parathyroid tumors in multiple endocrine neoplasia type 1 with loss of alleles on chromosome 11. *N Engl J Med* 321:218, 1989.
285. Lano H, Parada LF, Weinberg RA: Tumorigenic conversion of primary embryo fibrobasts requires at least two cooperating oncogenes. *Nature* 304:596, 1983.
286. Hunter T: Cooperation between oncogenes. *Cell* 64:249, 1991.

CHAPTER 4

Biosynthesis, Secretion, and Metabolism of Hormones

Gordon N. Gill

Endocrinology is the study of hormones, which are allosteric effectors; hormone receptors, which are the allosteric proteins to which they bind; and the biological consequences of their interactions. Although the kinetics of the interactions between hormones and receptor proteins are complex, they can ordinarily be represented as bimolecular reactions:

$$\underset{[\mathrm{H}]}{\text{Hormone}} + \underset{[\mathrm{R}]}{\text{receptor}} \underset{k_2}{\overset{k_1}{\rightleftharpoons}} \underset{[\mathrm{HR}]}{\text{hormone} \cdot \text{receptor}}$$

The binding of hormones to receptor proteins involves primarily hydrophobic interactions with hydrogen bonds, van der Waals forces, and salt bridges but not covalent linkages. Thus, hormone-receptor complex formation is reversible, and allosteric regulation can be terminated quickly once the allosteric effector is reduced in concentration. In the mass action equation shown above, the formation of the active complex [HR] depends on the concentrations of both the hormone and the receptor protein as well as on the intrinsic affinity of the receptor for the hormone. Genetic and acquired endocrine diseases are ultimately expressed as an alteration from normal in one term of this equation.

Extensive control systems regulate all the components of these basic ingredients of the hormone-response system. Synthesis, secretion, transport, and metabolism of hormones determine the hormone concentration term, while synthesis, modification, and metabolism of the receptor protein determine the receptor concentration term in this equation.

Hormones have one of three major chemical structures: peptide, steroid, or amino acid analogue. Although different hormones have distinct biological effects, all hormones of the peptide class and all hormones of the steroid class share common features of biosynthesis, secretion, transport, and mechanism of action with others of the same class. These common features provide a framework in which the unique characteristics of a particular hormone can be understood and comparisons between hormones can be made. Thyroid hormones and catecholamines, which have the amino acid tyrosine as a central structural nucleus, are synthesized and metabolized via pathways which are unique and distinct from peptide or steroid hormones and from each other; these are considered separately (see Chaps. 10 and 13).

PEPTIDE HORMONES

Biosynthesis of Messenger RNA

Because peptide hormones are small secretory proteins, their biosynthesis and secretion occur through the same processes as those which involve larger nonhormonal secretory proteins such as immunoglobulins, albumin, pancreatic enzymes, and egg white proteins. The biosynthetic steps are general ones for all proteins, although there are interesting variations such as multigene families, derivation of different hormones from a common RNA precursor by differential splicing, generation of multiple hormones from a common protein precursor, and synthesis of multisubunit hormones. Gene structure and the steps involved in the initiation and regulation of the transcription of specific genes and the processing of mRNA are also addressed in Chap. 3. The regulation of gene expression by hormones is further addressed in Chap. 5.

In eukaryotes, genes encoding proteins are organized in accordance with the general scheme shown in Fig. 4-1. DNA sequences whose transcripts appear in mature messenger RNA *(exons)* are interrupted by intervening sequences *(introns),* which are transcribed, along with exon and 3′-flanking DNA sequences, into messenger RNA precursors. However, the intron and 3′-flanking DNA sequences are removed during the process of messenger RNA maturation before delivery of the exon-containing messenger RNA to the cytoplasm, where translation into protein occurs. Genes coding for proteins are transcribed by RNA polymerase II, a large multisubunit enzyme which begins transcription at the initiation site upstream from the first amino acid codon (corresponding to AUG) in the messenger RNA. The site of initiation, where capping occurs, is followed by a nontranslated leader sequence of variable length before the sequence which codes for AUG, the messenger RNA translation start signal.

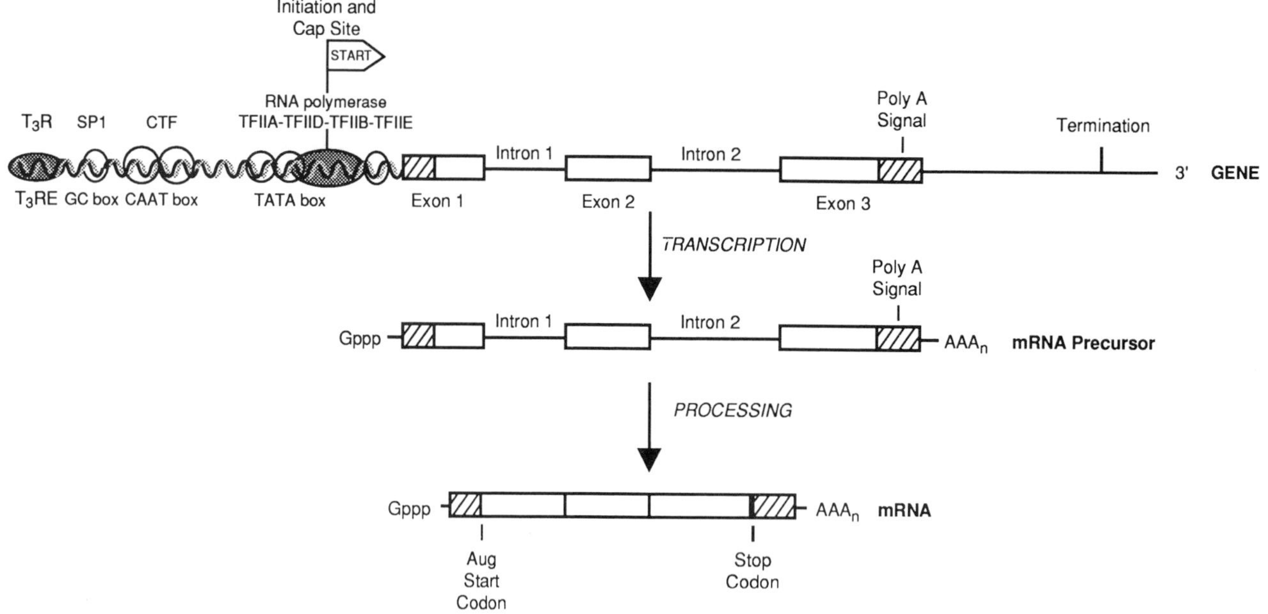

FIGURE 4-1 Messenger RNA synthesis. Exons are indicated by boxes with untranslated regions shaded, and introns and 3′-flanking DNA by single lines. The curved lines denote 5′-flanking DNA. The primary transcript, whose 3′ terminus is cleaved before polyadenylation, is not shown. The principal control of transcription occurs at the initiation step. Basal transcription factors and RNA polymerase II indicated with circles assemble at the TATA box. The rate of initiation of transcription is controlled by transcription regulatory proteins that bind to specific DNA sequences. Shown are examples of such enhancer sequences in the 5′-flanking DNA: T_3RE, GC box, and CAT box. These bind, respectively, the transcription factors thyroid hormone receptor (T_3R), SP1, and CAAT factor (CTF), as indicated by circles. However, enhancer sequences may also be located within the exons, introns, or 3′-flanking DNA.

Capping, which occurs at the site of initiation, begins early during the process of transcription by RNA polymerase II. In the capping reaction, guanylyl transferase adds a 5′-terminal GTP to form a 5′—5′ bond GpppX, and the guanosine is methylated at N_7 by N_7 methylase.[1] Capping stabilizes messenger RNA against degradation and increases the efficiency of translation. The initiator AUG codon is marked for recognition by the 40S ribosome · methionine-tRNA initiation complex by the context of surrounding nucleotides, with the preferred sequence being GCCAC*AUG*G.[2] Secondary structure of downstream RNA may facilitate the initiation of translation which begins at the correct AUG with remarkable fidelity.

The expression of many protein-coding genes is controlled through regulation of the rate of initiation of transcription. In many genes, the sequence TATAA is located 20 to 30 base pairs upstream of the transcription start site. This TATAA box is analogous to the Pribnow box in prokaryotes, where RNA polymerase binds. In eukaryotes a series of basal transcription factors assemble at the TATAA box to facilitate the binding of RNA polymerase II and ensure accurate initiation of transcription at a single downstream start site. The TATAA box binding protein (TBP or TFIID) binds to the DNA sequence and assembles with the general initiation factors TFIIA, TFIIB, and TFIIE.[3] RNA polymerase II selectively binds to this initial complex and, in the presence of additional factors and ATP, forms an active transcription initiation complex.[4] Although the general organization shown in Fig. 4-1 is common, a number of genes lack a TATAA sequence. Many of these genes—such as dihydrofolate reductase, the epidermal growth factor receptor, transforming growth factor α, and *ras*—contain several copies of the sequence GGGCGG, which is recognized by the nuclear protein Sp1.[5] Fidelity of the initiation of transcription of these promoters is less than that of promoters containing a TATAA box, but these promoters can be equally strong and regulated. Because promoters which lack a TATAA box appear to require the same group of basal initiation factors, Sp1 has been proposed to sequester the basal transcription apparatus on these TATAA-less promoters.[6] In some genes, an initiator motif located at the transcription start site is sufficient for initiation.[7]

The rate of initiation of transcription is controlled by a diverse group of proteins which bind to specific DNA sequences to regulate the activity of the basal transcription complex that is assembled at the

TATAA box or its equivalent. The DNA response element to which these regulatory proteins bind is most commonly located in the region 5′ to the TATAA box but may be located 3′ or at quite distal regions. To contact the basal initiation machinery, the DNA to which these proteins are bound must bend, a property of highly compacted DNA in chromosomes.[8] Three types of DNA recognition elements which bind specific transcription factors are illustrated in Fig. 4-1. The CAAT box which binds the nuclear protein NF1 (CTF) is commonly located ~40 base pairs upstream of the TATAA box.[9] Sp1, which appears to be involved in the assembly of the basal transcription complex on non-TATAA promoters, is a strong enhancer of transcription from TATAA promoters. Hormone response elements such as that which specifies thyroid hormone receptor (T_3R) binding, place genes under the regulation of hormone-dependent transcription factors.[10] The biosynthesis of peptide hormones, the biosynthetic enzymes which catalyze the formation of steroid hormones, and hormone receptors is regulated by hormonal signals to elicit and coordinate appropriate responses. The regulatory transcription factors are the targets for the signal transduction pathways which direct these responses, i.e., regulate the regulators.

The transcription regulatory proteins contain discrete functional domains. The DNA binding domain "recognizes" the specific DNA sequences of the response element with an affinity for binding directly related to the extent of DNA contacted, usually by an α-helix contacting the major groove of DNA. The recognition helix can be stabilized in several structures, including the zinc fingers of the steroid receptor superfamily, the helix turn helix motif of the homeodomain proteins, and the leucine zipper-basal region (B-zip) motif.[11,12] Binding to the recognition DNA element positions the transcription factor to regulate a specific gene, but activity requires a second domain in the protein which provides for contact with other proteins. Several activation motifs have been recognized, including amphipathic helices, glutamine-rich domains, and proline-rich domains.[13] These activation domains may be exposed or may become exposed only upon induction.

Induction can be achieved through several mechanisms. A number of peptide hormone and steroid biosynthetic enzymes are regulated via the cyclic AMP second messenger system. Upon activation of cAMP-dependent protein kinase by cAMP, the free catalytic subunit enters the nucleus, where it catalyzes phosphorylation of the transcription factor cAMP response element binder (CREB) at a specific serine residue to induce a conformational change that exposes the activation domain.[14] Triiodothyronine (T_3) binding to the T_3R induces a conformational change, exposing sequences necessary for biological function of the receptor. In the absence of ligand, T_3R binds DNA and may actually decrease transcription.[15]

Decreased synthesis of hormones and receptors is also necessary for the appropriate homeostatic responses that occur in classical negative feedback loops. Principles similar to those involved in inductive responses are operative. Three general mechanisms are proposed[16]:

1. Regulated transcription factors compete with stronger regulatory factors for DNA binding sites. This may be operative where DNA response elements for T_3 receptors are adjacent to the TATAA box of the TSHα gene.
2. Regulated transcription factors form heterodimers with active transcription factors to sequester them from interaction with DNA response elements. This may be operative for cortisol repression of the proliferin and collagenase genes, where glucocorticoid receptors interfere with the action of the AP1 (fos:jun) strong transcriptional activator.[17]
3. There is competition between transcription factors for limiting common factors that serve as a bridge between transcription factors and the basal transcription machinery ("squelching").[18]

Protein · protein interactions are important (1) in forming homodimeric or heterodimeric structures which contact a larger region of DNA and thus have higher affinity and specificity, (2) as bridges for contacting regulatory proteins bound to one region of DNA and the basal transcriptional machinery, and (3) as sequestrators of proteins away from their DNA binding site so that they are released to act only when appropriate environmental signals are received. Chromatin structure is also important in determining which DNA sequences are exposed and whether protein can interact with these sequences to influence the basal transcription machinery.[19]

Regulation occurs not only during the process of transcription but also during RNA processing. The initial RNA polymerase II transcript is a large nuclear RNA which contains both exons and introns. Unlike translation in prokaryotes, which occurs during transcription, translation in eukaryotes occurs only after maturation and transport of messenger RNA to the cytoplasm. Maturation requires the excision of introns and the splicing together of exons.

Newly transcribed RNA is rapidly complexed with small nuclear ribonucleoproteins (snRNPs) which subsequently assemble into a spliceosome where excision of introns occurs and exons are accurately joined together.[20] Genes may contain multiple introns, and the splicing process must be extremely accurate so that the reading frame of the mature exon-containing messenger RNA is maintained. The process must also be sequential to achieve correct ordering of the encoded amino acid sequence. Introns follow the general GT-AG rule that introns begin with GT and end with AG.[21] The snRNPs contain small RNAs and proteins, with the RNAs providing part of the recognition of the splice junctions. In the spliceosome, an A residue in the 3′ end of the intron attacks the 5′ splice site which is cleaved, and the intron forms a lariat structure in which the A is linked to the 5′ end of the intron via a 2′ phosphate.[22] The RNA is then cleaved at the 3′ splice site, and the two exons are accurately joined. The lariat intron is released and degraded in the nucleus.

Termination of transcription occurs 3′ to the final coding exon, in some cases many base pairs downstream. Poly(A) addition (tailing) occurs near points of cleavage in messenger RNA precursors and is dictated by the sequence AAUAAA, which is located 14 to 30 base pairs upstream of the poly(A) tail. The sequence at the start of the poly(A) tail is also similar in many genes. Poly(A) addition is catalyzed by a poly(A) polymerase enzyme.[23,24] Splicing occurs in the nucleus, and snRNPs remain in the nucleus when messenger RNA is transported to the cytoplasm through nuclear pores.

More than one peptide hormone may be encoded in a single gene. Several peptides may be derived by proteolytic processing from a common precursor protein. Alternative RNA processing may also yield different peptide hormones. Many genes are simple transcription units with a single poly(A) addition site and a constant pattern of RNA splicing, but there are also complex transcription units with multiple poly(A) addition sites and alternative RNA splicing sites which can generate multiple messenger RNA species from a single gene. The organization of the calcitonin gene is shown in Fig. 4-2. In C cells of the thyroid, a polyadenylation signal at the end of the calcitonin exon is used. In nervous tissue, a second polyadenylation signal at the end of a downstream exon is used; during processing, the calcitonin exon is removed,[25] so that mature messenger RNA encodes a carboxy-terminal region different from that of the messenger RNA encoding calcitonin. The two precursor protein products have a common amino-terminal region but different carboxy-terminal sequences. In C cells of the thyroid, calcitonin is processed from the precursor protein to function in the regulation of calcium metabolism, whereas in nervous system tissue, a calcitonin gene–related peptide (CGRP) is processed from its precursor protein to function in nociception, ingestive behavior, and the modulation of autonomic responses. Alternative RNA processing thus creates diversity in peptide hormone formation; this process is similar to the alternative RNA processing that occurs in immunoglobulin gene expression and in several other proteins. As described in the following section, alternative protein processing may also create diversity, as with the corticotropin (ACTH) precursor in intermediate and anterior lobe pituitary cells.

Biosynthesis of Peptide Hormones

Because peptide hormones are small proteins, their mature messenger RNAs frequently encode information for initial translation products which are larger than the secretory form of the peptide; that is, messenger RNA is translated into larger protein precursors, which are then processed by a series of proteolytic cleavages to yield the final secreted peptide products.

Messenger RNA translation begins at the AUG codon, specifying methionine, that lies downstream from the cap site. Because peptide hormones are secretory proteins, synthesis occurs on endoplasmic reticulum–bound polyribosomes, with vectorial movement of the growing peptide into the endoplasmic reticulum space (Fig. 4-3). A leader sequence of 15 to 25 largely hydrophobic amino acids is located at the amino terminus of the protein. When this "pre" portion emerges from the ribosome, it binds a signal recognition particle that consists of six proteins and a 7-S RNA.[26] In the absence of endoplasmic reticulum membranes, the signal recognition particle prevents further synthesis of these proteins so that presecretory proteins are not made in the cytoplasm. When the signal recognition particle ribosome complex binds with high affinity to a specific integral membrane protein complex termed the *signal recognition particle receptor,*[27] the signal recognition particle is displaced from the nascent protein chain and its amino-terminal signal sequence in a GTP-dependent reaction.[28] The ribosome, with its growing peptide chain, is now bound to the endoplasmic reticulum, and the growing polypeptide chain is vectorially inserted through a large protein-conducting channel in the endoplasmic reticulum membrane to reach the endoplasmic space.[29] For secretory proteins such as peptide hormones, the completed peptide will ultimately be located completely within the endoplasmic reticulum space, whereas membrane-bound proteins such as hormone receptors will have their amino termini within this space (ultimately to face the outside of the cell), with a portion of the carboxyl terminus of the protein remaining in the membrane and cytoplasm. Stop transfer sequences signal the cessation of transport of the growing polypeptide chain across the endoplasmic membrane, so that membrane proteins such as cell surface hormone receptors are synthesized with their ectodomains inside the endoplasmic reticulum space to ultimately face the exterior of the cell and endodomains are synthesized in the cytoplasm. These proteins must exit the protein channel in the membrane laterally; once outside the protein channel, the positively charged amino acids of the stop transfer sequence prevent protein movement into the hydrophobic membrane.[30] When synthesis is complete, the ribosomes leave the membrane and the protein channel closes. Some peptide hormones, such as epidermal growth

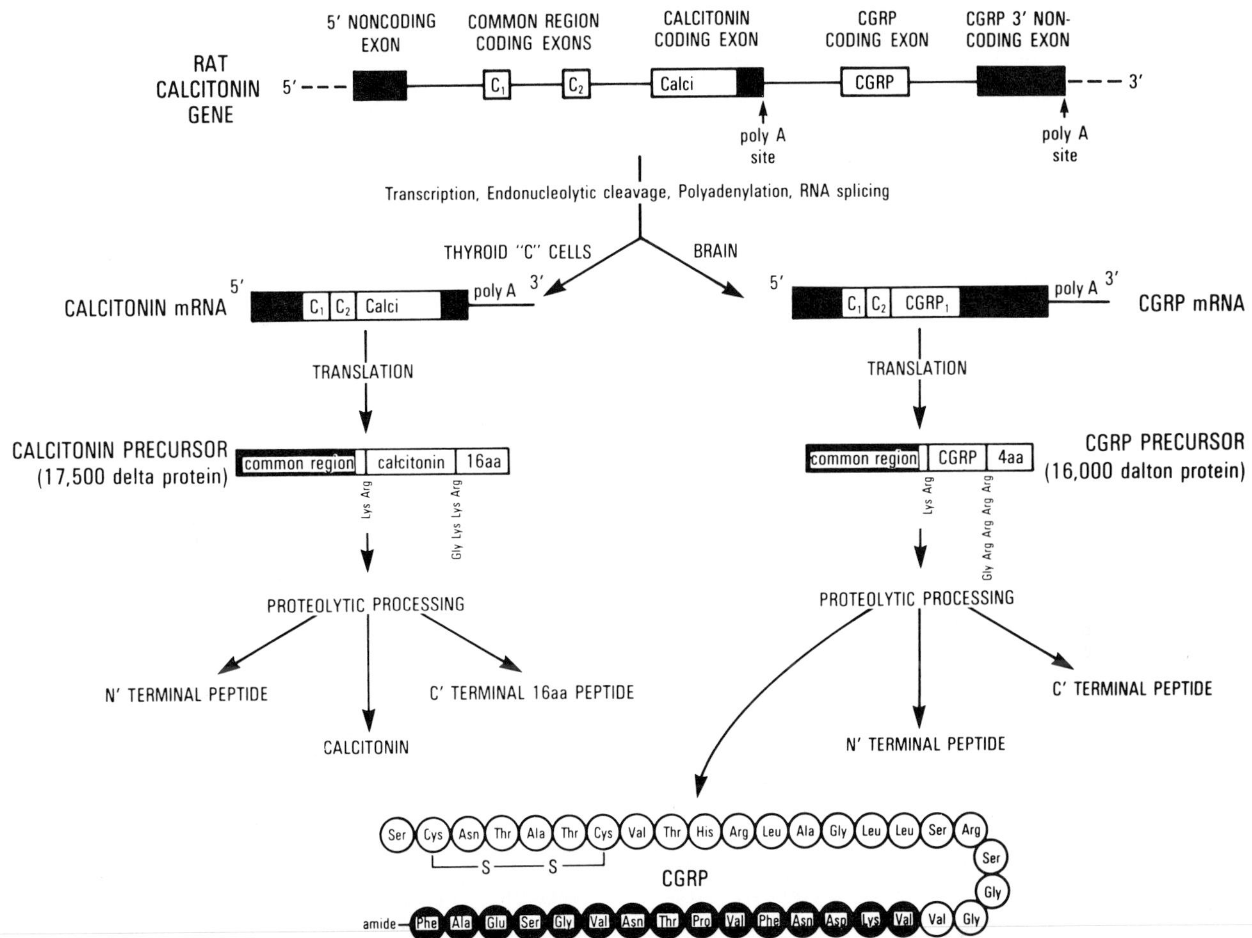

FIGURE 4-2 Generation of peptide hormone diversity by alternative RNA splicing. The rat calcitonin gene contains two common coding exons, a calcitonin exon and a calcitonin gene–related protein (CGRP) exon. Calcitonin is formed when a poly(A) site at the 3′ end of the calcitonin exon is used; CGRP is formed when a poly(A) site in an exon 3′ to CGRP is used. The resulting messenger RNAs have a common 5′ end but divergent 3′ ends. Proteolytic processing results in *N*-terminal peptides, calcitonin or CGRP, and C-terminal peptides. Calcitonin and CGRP have different biological activities. (*From Rosenfeld et al.*[25])

factor, are generated by proteolytic processing from receptor-like precursors.[31]

These general mechanisms do not account for the processing of all peptide hormones and receptors. Some peptide hormones, such as fibroblast growth factor, lack a defined signal sequence but clearly act via cell surface receptors. Alternative mechanisms must exist through which signaling peptides that lack signal sequences exit the cell. Receptors that contain seven membrane-spanning segments and transporter proteins such as the glucose transporters and enzymes such as adenylate cyclase which contain twelve membrane spanning segments must be inserted into the membrane by variations in trafficking which do not stringently depend on stop transfer sequences.

Within the endoplasmic reticulum, the precursor protein is cleaved, may be covalently modified, and is folded into the form which will ultimately be secreted. A signal peptidase first removes the "pre," or leader sequence, portion of the hormone. Larger precursor "pro" hormones are then further processed within this membrane-enclosed space by proteolytic enzymes. Most processing involves trypsin-like activity which recognizes dibasic amino acid residues. For carboxyl-terminal amidation, glycine serves as the donor at the cleavage site.

Peptides generated during the processing of protein precursors may have a variety of functions. The precursors of antidiuretic hormone and oxytocin contain the specific neurophysins which serve as carriers for these two peptides from their site of synthesis in the magnicellular nuclei in the hypothalamus to storage sites in the posterior pituitary (Fig. 4-4*A*; Chap. 9). The ACTH precursor contains information for several peptides, which may all be involved in

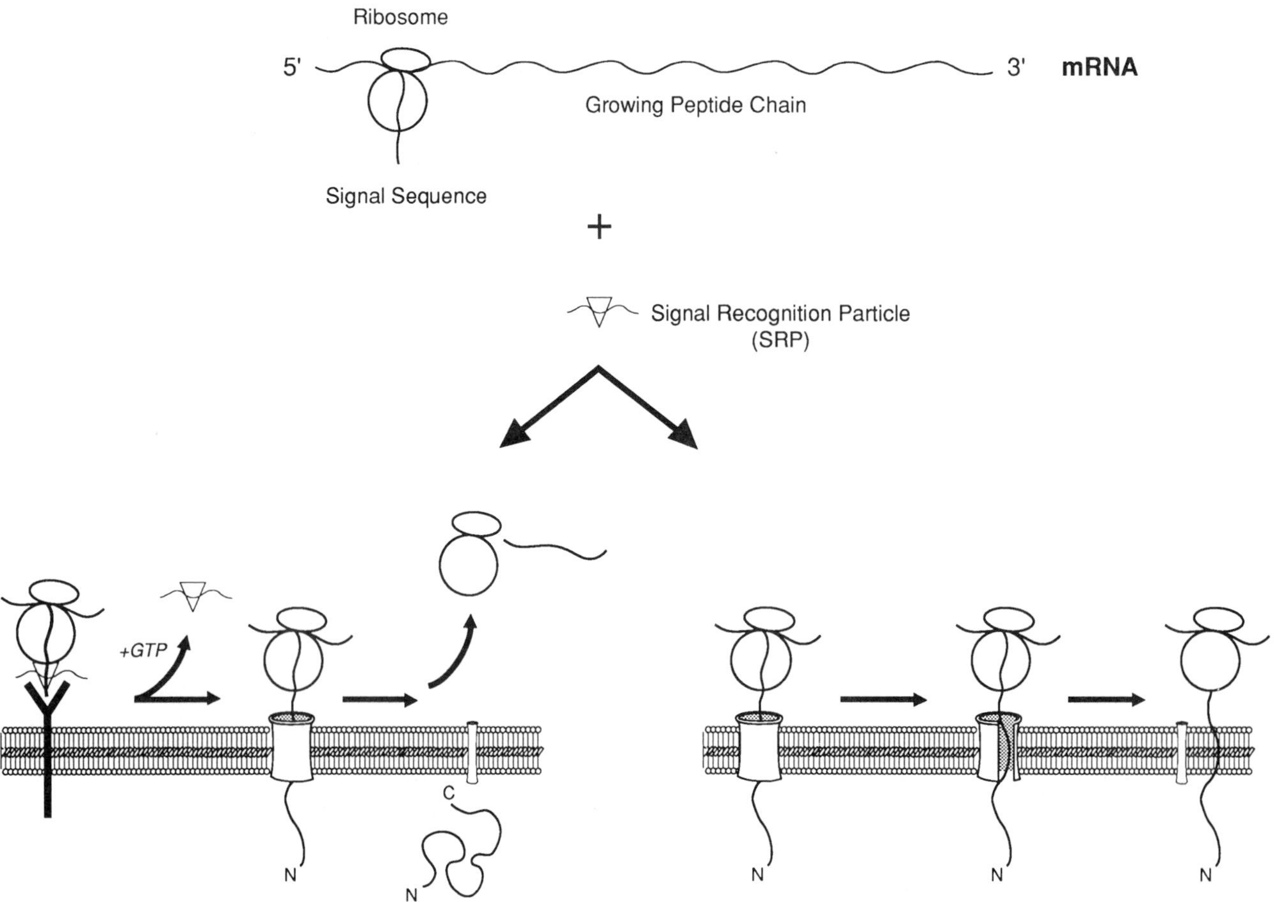

FIGURE 4-3 Synthesis of secretory proteins. The signal sequence at the amino terminus is bound by the signal recognition particle (SRP), which arrests cytoplasmic translation and delivers the complex to a recognition protein intrinsic to the endoplasmic reticulum (ER) membrane. When the SRP binds to the SRP receptor, it is displaced from the signal peptide in a GTP-dependent reaction. The growing polypeptide chain is directed into the ER space through a protein channel. When synthesis is complete, the ribosome dissociates and the protein channel closes. For synthesis of transmembrane receptor proteins, stop transfer sequences arrest vectorial synthesis and completion of synthesis occurs in the cytoplasm. The protein channel has been proposed to open laterally to allow the exit of the transmembrane protein. (*Modified from Simon and Blobel.*[29])

stress responses (Chaps. 8 and 12). Figure 4-4*B* shows the structure of the ACTH precursor molecule predicted from the cDNA sequence. The core sequence for melanocyte stimulating hormone (MSH) is reiterated within the structure of the precursor, suggesting that it arose during evolution by gene duplication. A 16,000 M_r fragment is located on the amino-terminal side, and β-lipotropin is located on the carboxyl-terminal side of the ACTH sequence. Dibasic amino acids serve as recognition signals for proteolytic enzymes which cleave the precursor protein into the final hormonal products. In addition, both glycosylation and phosphorylation of the ACTH precursor occur within the endoplasmic reticulum. There is evidence for different processing of the same precursor in different cells. In the intermediate lobe of the pituitary, ACTH is processed to α-MSH, in which the amino-terminal serine is acetylated and the carboxyl-terminal valine is amidated from the adjacent glycine, and to corticotropin-like intermediate peptide (CLIP; $ACTH_{18-29}$). In the anterior pituitary, the ACTH precursor is processed as shown in Fig. 4-4*B*. The precursor to the enkephalins results in the formation of several peptides with similar activities.[34] Additional information about precursor protein sequences will probably reveal new functions and provide more insight into the evolution of this class of signaling molecules.

The connecting peptide (C peptide) present in the insulin precursor may serve another function—to provide correct folding and alignment of the A and B chains of insulin (see Chap. 19). The insulin precur-

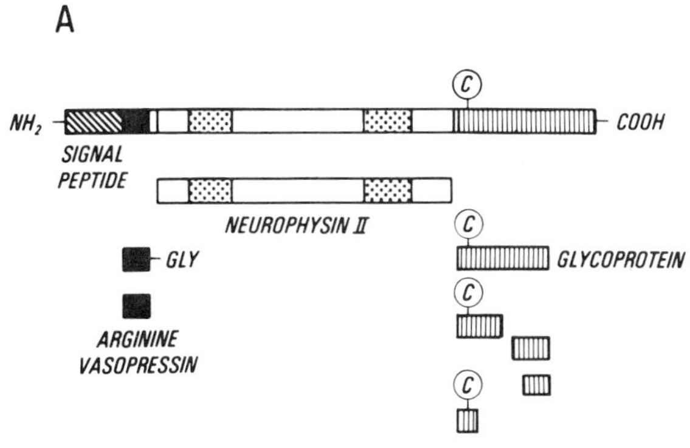

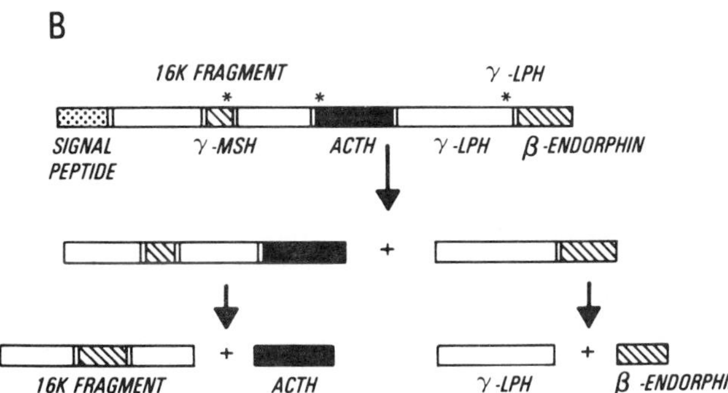

FIGURE 4-4 Proteolytic processing of precursor proteins within the endoplasmic reticulum. (*A*) Structure of the bovine antidiuretic hormone (ADH)–neurophysin II precursor and its proteolytic processing. The 19-amino acid signal peptide is followed by ADH (residues 1 to 9). Neurophysin II begins after processing signals at residue 13 and extends to residue 107; its internal homology is shown by the hatched area. The glycoprotein portion of the precursor is located at the carboxyl terminus. (*From Land et al.*[32]) (*B*) Structure of the bovine ACTH precursor and its proteolytic processing in the anterior pituitary. Reiterated MSH core sequences are indicated by an asterisk. Dibasic amino acid residues, which serve as the recognition signal for proteolytic processing, are indicated by open spaces in the bars. (*From Nakanishi et al.*[33])

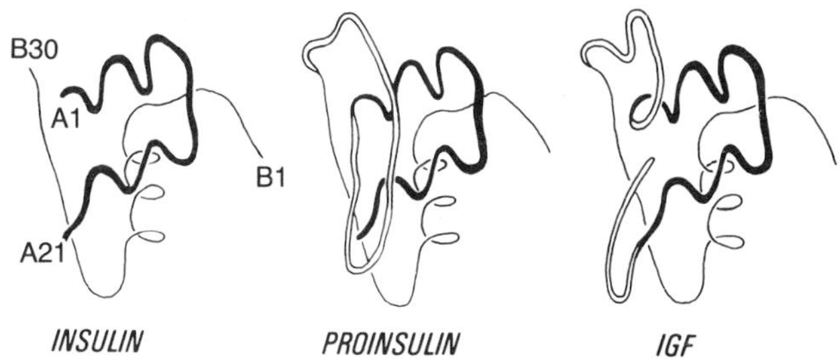

FIGURE 4-5 Schematic representation of three-dimensional structures based on x-ray analysis of insulin and on model building of proinsulin and of insulin-like growth factor 1 (IGF-I). The A chain of insulin is shown by the thickened line, the B chain by the solid line, and the connecting peptide by a double line. Disulfide bridge locations are indicated in the text. (*Modified from Blundell et al.*[35])

sor has the following structure: hydrophobic leader sequence · B chain · C peptide · A chain. The leader sequence is rapidly removed, and the C peptide serves to fold and align the A and B chains of insulin (Fig. 4-5). The disulfide bonds between cysteines A7 and B7, A20 and B19, and A6 and A11 are required for the biological activity of insulin. If the disulfide bonds between the A and B chains of insulin and the intra-A chain disulfide bond are chemically reduced and reoxidized in vitro, random coupling of half-cysteine residues occurs and only a small fraction of biological activity is restored. However, reduced and reoxidized proinsulin (B chain · C peptide · A chain) can generate almost full biological activity.[36] The specific conformation of the proinsulin molecule presumably brings the correct pairs of half-cysteine residues into close approximation for the formation of the mature disulfide-bonded insulin. Under defined in vitro conditions, the A and B chains can efficiently fold to yield native insulin, indicating that the overall structures can align the disulfide bonds correctly, even without the C peptide. During maturation in the endoplasmic reticulum space and Golgi complex, the C peptide, which is flanked by dibasic residues, is removed and mature insulin is secreted by the beta cell with about equimolar amounts of inactive C peptide. Proinsulin has only a small fraction of the activity of insulin, and so removal of C peptide enhances the activity of the final product. A genetic variant proinsulin resistant to proteolytic processing results in the secretion of unprocessed proinsulin.[37]

Active hormones may also be generated outside cells by processing from circulating precursors. The precursor for angiotensin II is a glycoprotein synthesized mainly in the liver. Renin, a proteolytic enzyme made in juxtaglomerular cells of the kidney, cleaves a decapeptide (angiotensin I) from the circulating angiotensin precursor glycoprotein. This decapeptide is then further processed to the octapeptide angiotensin II by the removal of two carboxy-terminal amino acids by a converting enzyme found in the endothelial cells of vascular beds, especially those of the lung (see Chap. 14).

Secretory and membrane proteins which are synthesized in the membrane-enclosed space of the ribosome-bound endoplasmic reticulum (RER) are vectorially transported through cell compartments where covalent modifications occur. These proteins, which always remain enclosed inside membranes, move from the RER to the Golgi complex, which consists of *cis, medial,* and *trans* compartments. Transport vesicles bud from each compartment and fuse with the next to deliver their load of proteins, which are progressively modified by processing enzymes such as glycosyltransferases. The itinerary between compartments is precise and consists of budding followed by the formation of coated vesicles (Fig. 4-6). The coat consists of specific proteins termed COPs

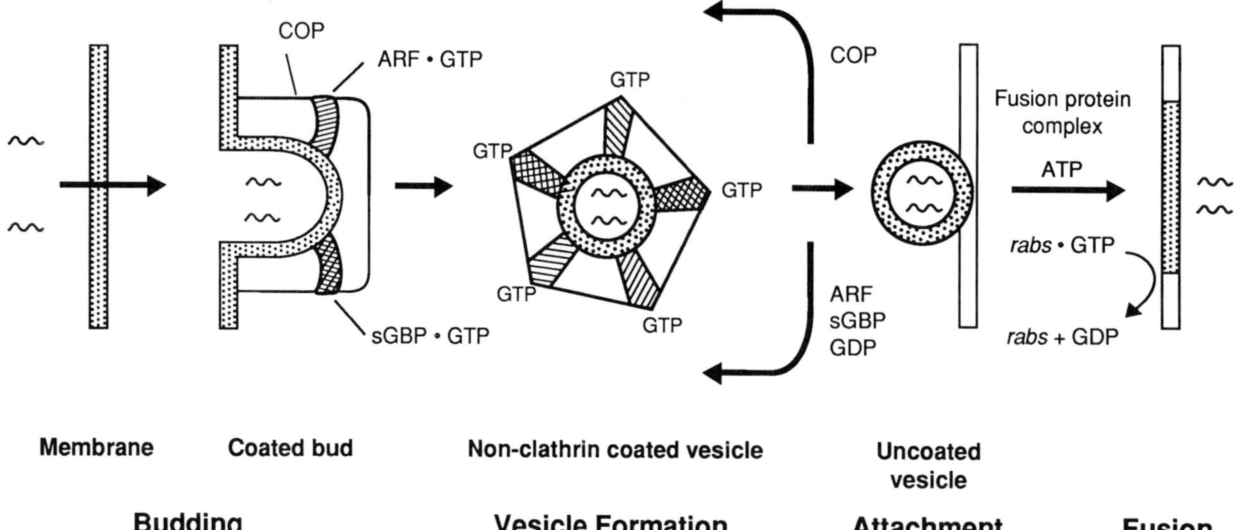

FIGURE 4-6 Subcellular transport of secretory and membrane proteins. Budding of vesicles begins in the RER, where secretory proteins are made. The process of budding, coated vesicle formation, attachment, and fusion is repeated as proteins are moved within membrane-enclosed spaces from RER to *cis* Golgi, to *medial* Golgi, to *trans* Golgi compartments. COP = coat proteins, including α, β, and γ COPs; ARF = ADP ribosylation factors; *rabs* = small GTP binding proteins with sequence homology to *ras*. (*Modified from Rothman and Orci.*[38])

and small GTP-binding proteins (SGBP) such as ADP ribosylation factors (ARFs) and *rabs*.[38] The COP proteins are structurally related to the adapter proteins involved in clathrin coated pit formation.[39] The assembly of the coat and the budding of transport vesicles require ATP. The ARF proteins bind GTP, and it is the ARF · GTP complex which assembles in the vesicle coat. A second group of small GTP-binding proteins termed *rabs* help specify vesicle formation and the compartment to which the coated vesicle docks.[40]

The coated vesicle with its cargo of proteins then binds to the membranes of the next compartment. Whether there is a receptor specific for coated vesicles is not known, but when fusion occurs, the vesicle is uncoated. GTP is hydrolyzed to GDP and COPs, and ARFs/*rabs* are released and recycle to form another coated vesicle. A soluble protein complex catalyzes the fusion of the membranes of the vesicle with the membranes of the recipient compartment in a reaction driven by ATP hydrolysis.[41]

Several covalent modifications may occur during this intracellular journey. Glycosylation is the major modification that affects peptide hormones such as thyroid stimulating hormone (TSH), luteinizing hormone (LH), follicle stimulating hormone (FSH), and human chorionic gonadotropin (hCG). Cell surface receptors for peptide hormones also undergo glycosylation. The initial addition of core oligosaccharide occurs within the endoplasmic reticulum. The predominant glycosylation via nitrogen linkage occurs on asparagine residues found within the sequence asn-x-ser or -thr. This sequence occurs in proteins which are synthesized in the endoplasmic reticulum space but is rare in cytoplasmic proteins, so that glycosylation of intracellular proteins is avoided. Less commonly, oligosaccharides are oxygen-linked via the hydroxyl side-chain group of serine, threonine, or hydroxylysine. The core *N*-linked oligosaccharide contains two *N*-acetylglucosamine residues and three mannose residues. The core oligosaccharide is first formed in the endoplasmic reticulum on an activated lipid molecule, dolichol, via a pyrophosphate bridge and is then transferred intact to the growing polypeptide chain.[42] Complex oligosaccharides are formed within the Golgi complex, where variable numbers of glucosamine-galactose-sialic acid residues are added to the mannose core, through the action of galactosyl transferase enzymes. High-mannose oligosaccharides, which contain additional mannose residues attached to the core, are donated via the dolichol pathway and are trimmed to various degrees by mannosidase enzymes present in the Golgi complex.

The α subunits of the glycoprotein hormones LH, FSH, TSH, and hCG contain two oligosaccharides of the *N*-linked complex type; β subunits contain either one or two similar oligosaccharides. The hCG β subunit, which has a carboxyl-terminal amino acid extension, contains three additional oligosaccharides *O*-linked to serine residues in this extension. In addition to the usual oligosaccharide structures, the pituitary hormones TSH and LH contain peripheral sulfate groups. Glycosylation and sulfation occur as separate processes in Golgi compartments, with sulfation occurring late in the biosynthetic pathway.[43]

Glycosylation of secretory proteins may serve many functions. Glycosylation may favor the protein conformation necessary for optimal intracellular combination of the two subunits which are synthesized on separate messenger RNAs for hormones such as TSH, LH, FSH, and hCG. Glycosylation stabilizes hormones in the circulation. Glycoprotein hormones have circulating half-lives considerably longer than those of nonglycosylated peptide hormones, and desialylation which exposes a β-linked galactose results in a markedly reduced circulating half-life as a result of accelerated clearance via the hepatic asialoglycoprotein receptor. Glycosylation may also be important in receptor recognition through effects on hormone conformation or through interaction with cellular recognition sites.

Secretion, Transport, and Metabolism of Peptide Hormones

Within the Golgi apparatus, proteins which are destined for secretion undergo additional maturation. Modification of carbohydrate, added initially in the rough endoplasmic reticulum, is carried out. Newly synthesized and matured secretory peptides and proteins are then accumulated into condensing vacuoles, which lose water and form mature secretory granules (Fig. 4-7*A*). Mature secretory granules contain large amounts of stored hormone, which can be readily identified by specific immunostaining. In the absence of a secretory stimulus, such granules accumulate; conversely, intensely secreting cells have fewer secretory granules. In response to a secretory stimulus, the stored peptides are discharged by exocytosis, in which the membrane of the secretory granule fuses with the cell membrane. Secretion is directed, occurring at the apical part of the cell, so that the peptide hormone is discharged into the circulation. The membrane of the secretory granule is then reabsorbed into the cell by endocytosis and is reutilized.

Cell surface hormone receptors also reach the plasma membrane via vesicle transport and fusion (Fig. 4-7*B*). In contrast to secretion, which is highly regulated, transport of cell surface proteins is constitutive. In polarized epithelial cells, receptors are

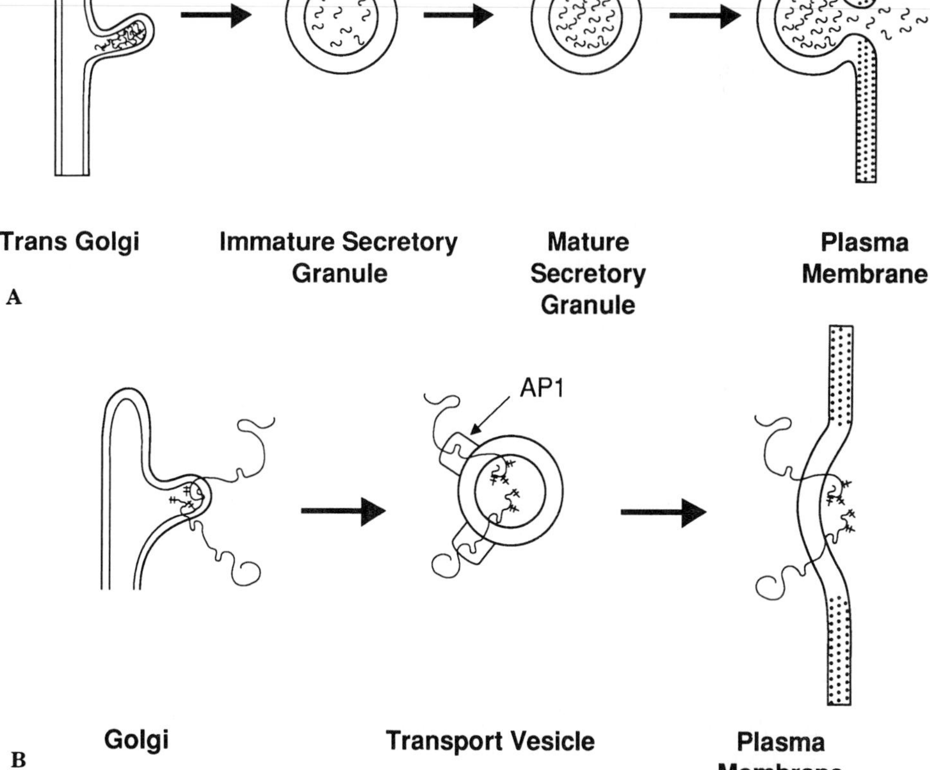

FIGURE 4-7 Transport of peptide hormones and hormone receptors to the cell surface. (*A*) Secretory granules are formed as concentrated granules and bud from the *trans* Golgi. Mature secretory granules exclude water to highly concentrate the hormone. Regulated secretion occurs when the membrane of the secretory granules fuses with the plasma membrane in a process of exocytosis that requires Ca^{2+} and ATP. (*B*) Cell surface receptors are constitutively transported from the *trans* Golgi to the cell surface within vesicles. Signals in the cytoplasmic domain of the receptor direct transport to the basolateral surface in polarized epithelial cells. Branched symbols (‡) represent sites of glycosylation. AP1 adaptor protein 1.

asymmetrically distributed on the cell surface. Vectorial transport from the *trans* Golgi to the basolateral surface requires amino acid sequence codes in the cytoplasmic domain of the receptor.[44] These receptor sequences resemble those which dictate clustering in clathrin coated pits at the cell surface and are thought to form a structure that specifies interaction with the adaptor specific to the *trans* Golgi or with other proteins.[45] In nonpolarized cells, constitutive movement to the cell surface occurs.

Secretion of peptide hormones is regulated by specific signals, many of them hormonal, which couple the rate of secretion to the metabolic needs of the organism.[46] A fundamental action of many hormones is to control the secretion of peptide hormones. Biosynthesis of peptide hormones is coupled to secretion, although the precise biochemical basis of this coupling is poorly defined. Kinetically, two "pools" of hormone have been described, one a rapidly releasable one which reflects hormone stored in secretory granules as well as that being synthesized and the other a slowly releasable one which reflects predominantly newly synthesized hormone.

Once they are secreted, peptide hormones have a short half-life in the circulation. Most peptide hormones, such as ACTH, parathyroid hormone (PTH), insulin, glucagon, antidiuretic hormone (ADH), thyrotropin releasing hormone (TRH), gonadotropin releasing hormone (GnRH), and corticotropin releasing hormone (CRH), act rapidly and are degraded rapidly, having circulating half-lives of 3 to 7 min. Metabolic clearance studies must be interpreted with caution because of the complexity of degrading systems for different hormones in different tissues, but several general principles appear to operate for most peptide hormones. Although peptide hormones may be cleaved by circulating proteases, the initial step leading to the major pathway for peptide hormone degradation consists of binding to receptors in target cells. The receptor does not degrade the hormone but delivers it to degradative enzymes both in the cell membrane and in the interior of target cells. Insulin degradation, for example, is directly related to receptor binding in liver cells, quantitatively the most important site of insulin clearance. Other nonacceptor-binding proteins may also contribute.[47] Peptide hormone degradation is catalyzed by cellular proteases which appear to be somewhat specific. Lysosomal enzymes contribute importantly to degradation of hormone delivered via absorptive endocytosis, but specific enzymes such as an insulin protease which cleaves insulin and glucagon, a postproline cleaving enzyme which cleaves ADH and TRH, and a pyroglutamyl aminopeptidase which cleaves TRH and GnRH appear to first inactivate peptide hormones, which are then further degraded by other cellular proteases (Fig. 4-8). Reduction of disulfide bonds may also be important for the inactivation of certain hormones, such as insulin and ADH.

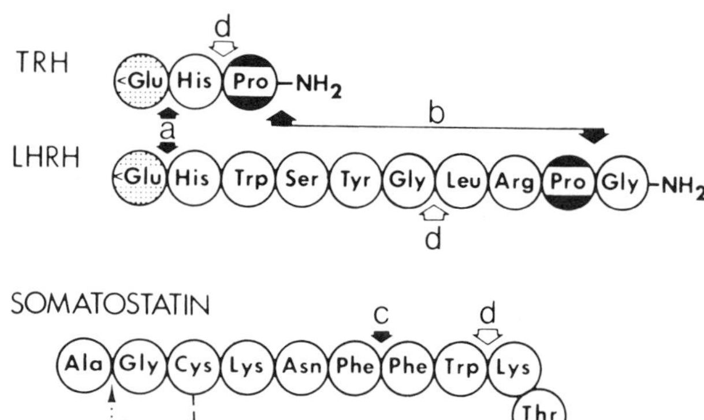

FIGURE 4-8 Sites of proteolytic degradation of three neurohormones. The major sites of cleavage are indicated by arrows: (a) pyroglutamyl peptidase; (b) postproline cleaving enzyme; (c) carboxyl (acid) proteinase; (d) neutral endopeptidase; (e) aminopeptidase. (*From Chertow.*[48])

Glycoprotein hormones have significantly longer circulating half-lives than do unmodified peptide hormones. hCG, the most heavily glycosylated peptide hormone, has a circulating half-life of about 4 h. Removal of terminal sialic acid markedly shortens the half-life of circulating glycoprotein hormones, because the modified proteins are now recognized and cleaved by the asialoglycoprotein receptor that is present in the liver. Although most peptide hormones circulate at low concentrations as unbound species, hormones such as the insulin-like growth factors are bound to carrier proteins in serum.[49] Such binding provides a circulating reservoir and an extended half-life. Platelet-derived growth factor and epidermal growth factor are present in platelet granules and are released locally in high concentrations when platelet activation and release reactions are triggered.[50]

The short circulating half-life of most peptide hormones provides for rapid termination of their biological actions. In normal physiology, synthesis and secretion are regulated to deliver appropriate concentrations of hormone to target tissues. Inactivation of both hormone and receptor buffers tissues against excessive responses. These buffering systems are a barrier to the clinical use of peptide hormones and, with the notable exception of insulin, have limited widespread therapeutic use of most peptide hormones.

STEROID HORMONES

The pathways for the biosynthesis of steroid hormones by the adrenal cortex, ovary, and testis are similar. Many of the biosynthetic enzymes are identical, with specialized enzymes providing modifications which give the final unique steroid structure recognized by target tissue hormone receptors. The rate-limiting step subject to acute hormone regulation is the same in adrenocortical and gonadal tissues; subcellular organization of biosynthetic enzyme pathways is also the same. Enzymes synthesizing the active form of vitamin D are similar to other steroid hydroxylases but are located in different organs (liver and kidney) rather than within a single gland. In addition, the major active androgen, dihydrotestosterone, is formed from testosterone; interconversion of precursors to estrogens occurs in peripheral tissues; and the brain has been shown to be capable of synthesizing several classes of steroid hormones.

Cholesterol Substrate for Steroid Hormone Formation

All steroid hormones are derived from cholesterol, which is provided by de novo synthesis from acetate or by uptake of circulating cholesterol synthesized in the liver and carried in low-density lipoprotein (LDL) particles. In either case, cholesterol may be used immediately for hormone biosynthesis or stored in the gland in lipid droplets as cholesterol esters. The number of LDL receptors in steroidogenic cells is higher than the number in non-steroid-secreting cells, and up to 70 percent of cholesterol utilized for steroid hormone production in the human adrenal cortex is provided from LDL cholesterol. LDL receptors are increased in steroidogenic cells in response to tropic hormones.[51] This increase in LDL receptors results from increased steroid hormone synthesis, which utilizes and reduces cellular cholesterol. A reduction in cellular cholesterol increases LDL receptors to facilitate cholesterol uptake; reduced cellular cholesterol also enhances the activity of 3-hydroxy-3-methylglutaryl coenzyme A synthase (HMG-CoA synthase) and HMG-CoA reductase, the two rate-controlling enzymes of cholesterol synthesis.[52] Cholesterol availability is thus tightly coupled to the metabolic requirements of steroidogenic cells (Fig. 4–9).

Steroidogenic cells contain abundant lipid droplets in which cholesterol esters are stored. In response to tropic hormones, cholesterol esterase is activated via cAMP-dependent phosphorylation to provide free cholesterol as substrate for steroid hormone synthesis. With prolonged stimulation, lipid droplets are depleted of cholesterol, but they are subsequently replenished when stimuli are removed. With prolonged stimulation, most of the cholesterol substrate for steroidogenesis is provided by facilitated uptake of LDL cholesterol. Facilitated uptake from LDL, release from cholesterol ester storage depots, and de novo synthesis provide sufficient cholesterol to sustain the 10-fold increase in adrenal cortisol production which occurs in response to severe stress; when basal conditions are reestablished, reg-

FIGURE 4-9 Provision of cholesterol for steroid hormone formation. The small metabolically active pool of free cholesterol (FC) which is the precursor of steroid hormone formation is maintained in response to stimuli by hydrolysis of cholesterol esters (EC), de novo synthesis from acetyl CoA, and facilitated uptake from circulating lipoproteins (LP). See text for details. (*From Brown et al.*[53])

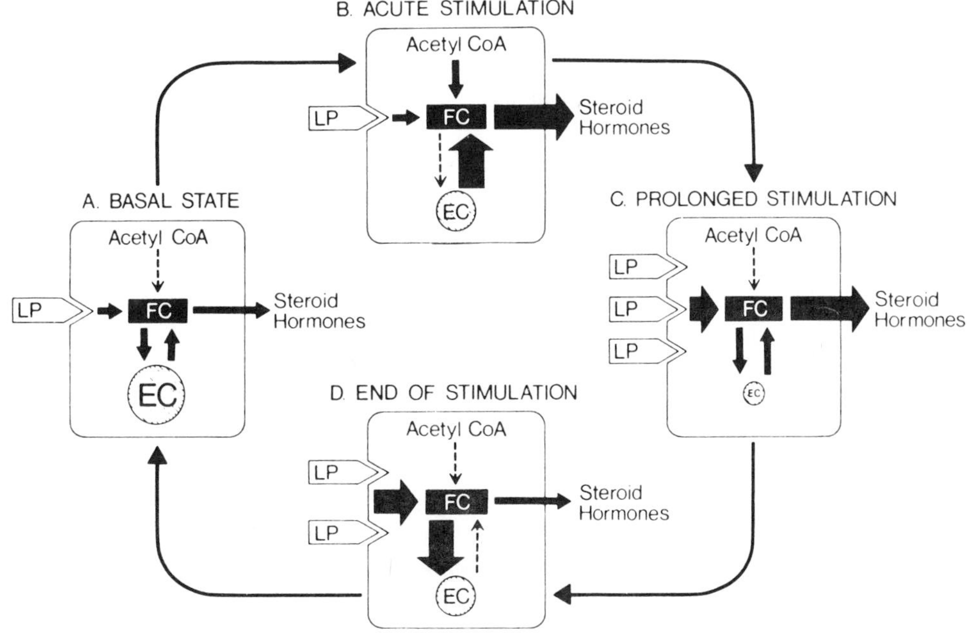

ulatory mechanisms reduce uptake and synthesis to levels appropriate to lower cortisol production rates (Fig. 4-9). Similar changes occur in ovarian and testicular cells stimulated by tropic hormones to produce estrogen, progesterone, and testosterone.

The Rate-Controlling Step in Steroid Hormone Synthesis

The rate-limiting step in total steroid synthesis in steroidogenic tissues is cleavage of the side chain of cholesterol to yield pregnenolone (Fig. 4-10). Cholesterol transformation and subsequent steroid hormone biosynthesis are catalyzed by cytochrome P450 enzymes and dehydrogenases. Stimulation of steroidogenesis in adrenal cortex, ovary, and testis results from accelerated formation of pregnenolone because subsequent enzyme activities are present in relative excess. The cholesterol side-chain cleavage enzyme cytochrome $P450_{scc}$ is located in the inner mitochondrial membrane, and stimulation of steroid hormone formation results from increased interaction of cholesterol with this enzyme.[54] Although hormones such as ACTH, FSH, LH, and hCG increase general cholesterol availability (Fig. 4-9), regulation of the rate of steroidogenesis depends on facilitated interaction of free cholesterol with mitochondrial cytochrome $P450_{scc}$, probably by transfer of cholesterol from the outer to the inner mitochondrial membrane. Because adequate active cytochrome $P450_{scc}$ and fully reduced adrenodoxin are present, the major limitation appears to be transfer of cholesterol to the enzyme. The detailed mechanism through which ACTH, FSH, LH, and hCG, via their intracellular mediator cAMP, increase the interaction of cholesterol with cytochrome $P450_{scc}$ is not fully understood, but it appears to involve synthesis of an activator protein and polyphosphoinositides.[55] Both the activator protein and the polyphosphoinositides are increased in response to elevated concentrations of cAMP, and both increase pregnenolone formation when added to isolated mitochondria. These mediators are envisioned as facilitating delivery of cholesterol to cytochrome $P450_{scc}$ in the inner mitochondrial membrane.

The side-chain cleavage reaction catalyzed by cytochrome $P450_{scc}$ resembles other monoxygenations of cytochrome P450, but three sequential monoxygenations are involved in the scission of the carbon-carbon bond.[56] Mitochondrial cytochrome P450 enzymes such as $P450_{scc}$, involved in synthesis of adrenal and gonadal steroid hormones, $P450_{11\beta}$, involved in cortisol synthesis, $P450_{CMO}$, involved in aldosterone synthesis, and $P450_{1\alpha}$, involved in $1,25(OH)_2$ vitamin D synthesis, utilize a flavoprotein (adrenodoxin reductase) and an iron-sulfur protein (adrenodoxin, a form of ferrodoxin), NADPH (reduced form of nicotinamide adenine dinucleotide phosphate), and molecular oxygen. Microsomal cytochrome P450 enzymes such as 17- and 21-hydroxylases and C17,20-lyase in adrenal cortex and gonads and vitamin D 25-hydroxylase in liver utilize a different flavoprotein, cytochrome P450 reductase, for electron transfer.[57] Cholesterol is first hydroxylated at C22; then it is hydroxylated at C20, and the resulting glycol is cleaved to yield the 20-ketone plus isocapraldehyde. Evidence for dihydroxylation at C22 rather than hydroxylation at C20 has been presented. As in other cytochrome P450 enzymes, the active site region consists of a substrate-binding site and a heme-iron catalytic site. A general model of the reaction cycle of cytochrome P450 includes substrate binding, heme reduction, and oxygen binding (Fig. 4-11). Substrate binding occurs first, and then the iron-oxo hydroxylating complex is formed, followed

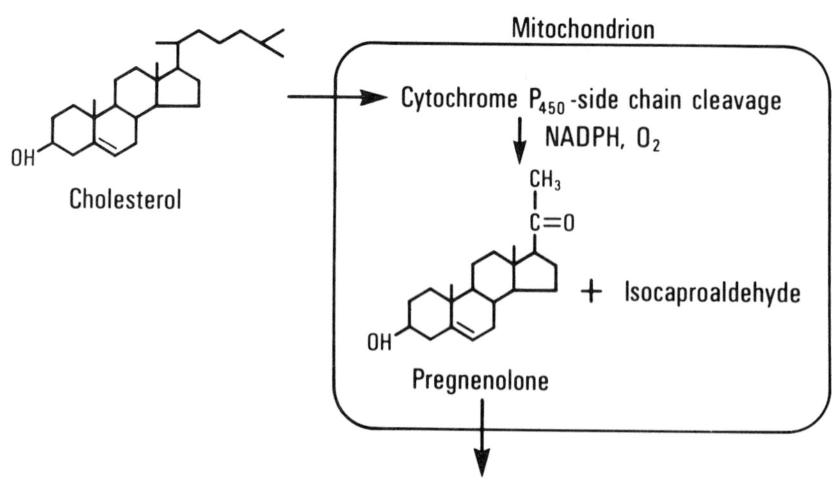

FIGURE 4-10 The rate-limiting step of steroid hormone biosynthesis.

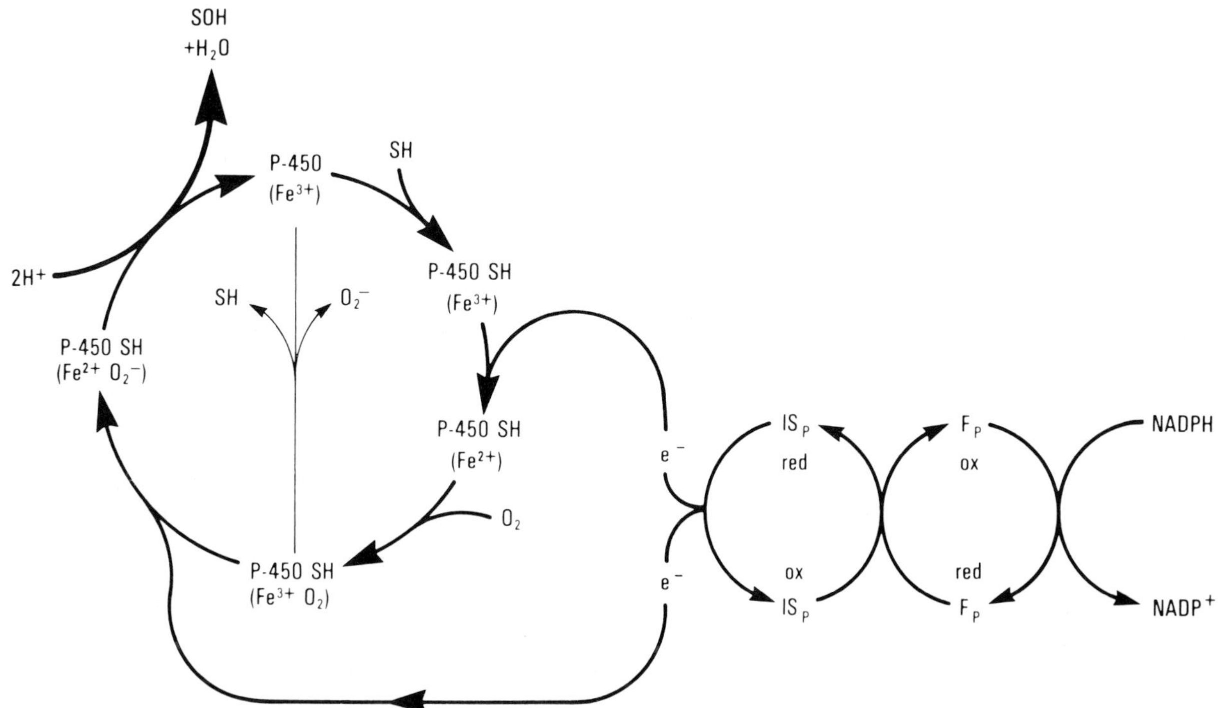

FIGURE 4-11 Model of cytochrome P450 reaction cycle. Electrons are transferred from NADPH via flavoprotein adrenodoxin reductase (Fp) and the iron-sulfur protein adrenodoxin (IS). Substrate (SH) binding to the enzyme brings the portion of the molecule to be modified close to the active center containing porphyrin-bound iron-oxo complex. The cycle is completed with production of product (SOH) and water. When a pseudo substrate is bound, the complex breaks down to form ferric P450 and superoxide (O_2^-) (center).

by product formation. The introduction of activated oxygen into the substrate yields the hydroxylated steroid product which is released along with a molecule of water. Abortive cycles induced by the binding of a pseudosubstrate can result in the production of oxygen-derived radicals which destroy the enzyme.[58] The large antioxidant armamentarium of steroidogenic cells probably evolved as a protective mechanism against such abortive cytochrome P450 cycles.

Steroidogenic tissues contain large numbers of specialized mitochondria and an extensive network of smooth endoplasmic reticulum. The enzymes which progressively modify the cholesterol molecule are located in these two compartments, and substrate flows from mitochondria to endoplasmic reticulum and back to mitochondria as it is progressively modified. The movement of substrate may involve sterol carrier proteins in cytosol or movement on a membrane surface.[59]

Pathway of Steroid Hormone Biosynthesis

Figure 4-12 shows the general pathway for steroid hormone synthesis in the adrenal cortex (see Chap. 12) and other steroid-producing tissues. After cholesterol side-chain cleavage, pregnenolone flows out of mitochondria to the endoplasmic reticulum, where it is sequentially modified. In human adrenal cortex cells, pregnenolone is converted to 17α-OH pregnenolone by cytochrome $P450_{17}$. 17α-OH pregnenolone is converted to 17α-OH progesterone by a 3β-hydroxysteroid dehydrogenase–$\Delta^{4,5}$-isomerase enzyme complex, which converts the 5,6 double bond of cholesterol to a 4,5 double bond and the 3-OH group to a ketone. Cytochrome $P450_{21}$ then adds a hydroxyl group to C21 of 17α-OH progesterone. The product, 11-deoxycortisol, flows back to mitochondria, where cytochrome $P450_{11\beta}$ catalyzes hydroxylation at C11 to yield cortisol, the final active product.

Zona glomerulosa cells contain a specialized mitochondrial cytochrome P450, corticosterone methyl oxidase, which hydroxylates corticosterone at C18 in a double hydroxylation, followed by loss of water to give the aldehyde. Because glomerulosa cells lack cytochrome $P450_{17}$, progesterone is hydroxylated at C21 to yield 11-deoxycorticosterone and then at C11 to yield corticosterone. Mitochondrial cytochrome $P450_{CMO}$ then catalyzes the formation of aldosterone, the active mineralocorticoid.

To produce androgens and estrogens, the C20,21

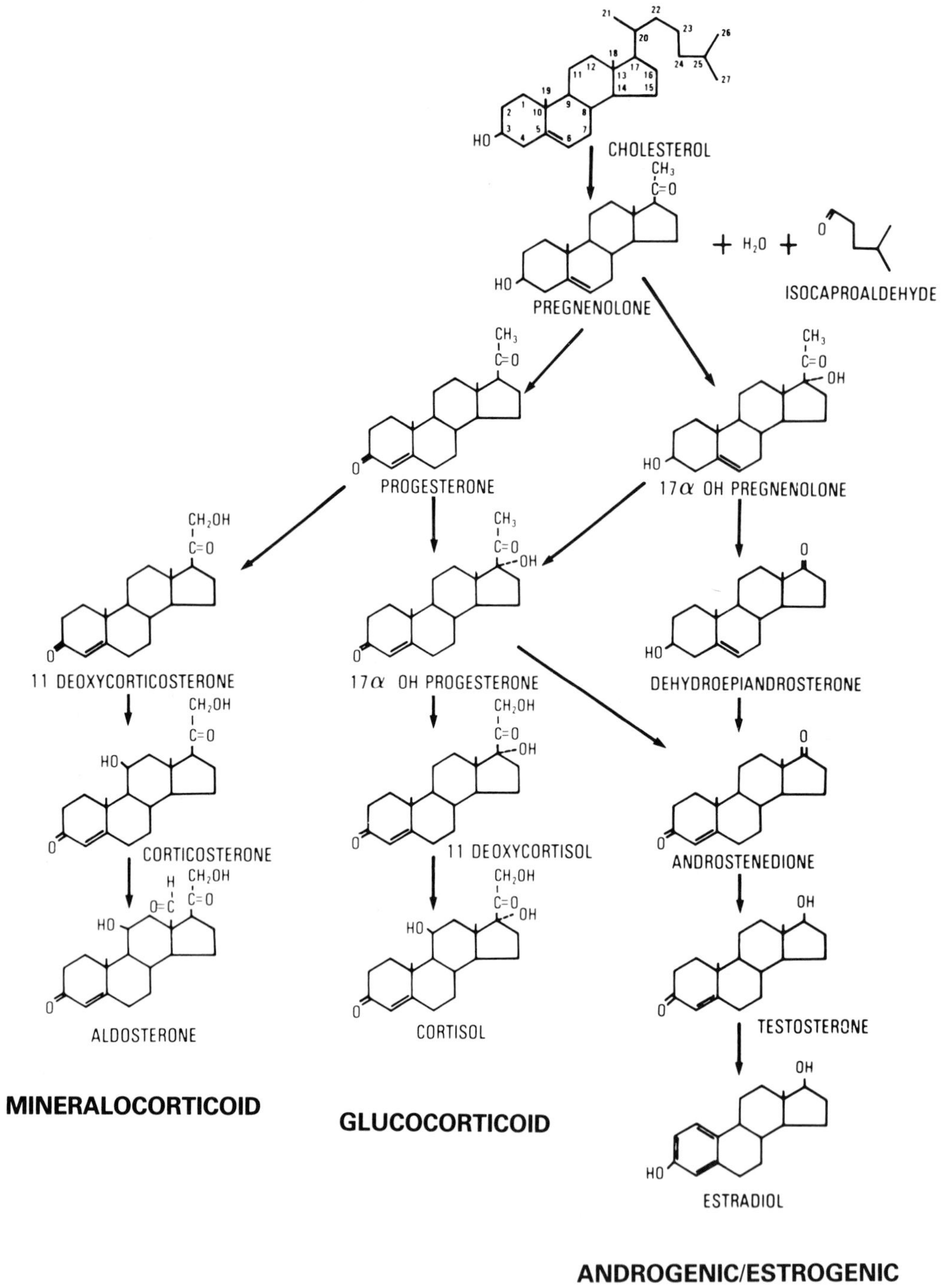

FIGURE 4-12 Pathway for the biosynthesis of steroid hormones. The relative concentrations of the various enzymes determine the flow of reactants through the pathway and the final steroid hormone products.

side chain must be removed. This reaction is catalyzed by C17,20-lyase, an activity intrinsic to cytochrome $P450_{17}$.[60] This enzyme converts 17α-OH pregnenolone to dehydroepiandrosterone (DHEA) and 17α-OH progesterone to androstenedione. In the human fetal zone of the fetal adrenal cortex, 3β-hydroxysteroid dehydrogenase–$\Delta^{4,5}$-isomerase activity is low, and so pregnenolone flows primarily to DHEA, which is then sulfated and transported to the placenta. The human definitive zone of the fetal adrenal cortex and the adult adrenal cortex have increased, though still low, 3β-hydroxysteroid dehydrogenase–$\Delta^{4,5}$-isomerase activity, so C17,20-lyase competes with this enzyme for precursor, and significant amounts of the androgen precursors DHEA and androstenedione are made in addition to cortisol. About half the pregnenolone formed in the human adrenal cortex is metabolized to DHEA. The adrenal cortex produces only minute amounts of testosterone and estradiol as a result of very low concentrations of the relevant enzymes necessary for their production.

Leydig cells of the testis lack cytochrome $P450_{21}$ and $P450_{11\beta}$ activity and thus do not produce significant quantities of mineralocorticoids or glucocorticoids. The androgen pathway shown on the right in Fig. 4-12 thus predominates (see Chap. 16). Androstenedione is converted to the active androgen, testosterone, in these cells through the actions of 17β-hydroxysteroid dehydrogenase. The testis does not produce estradiol in significant quantities.

Estrogen and progesterone are the principal steroid products of the ovary (see Chap. 17). Granulosa cells which are converted to luteal cells during the second half of the menstrual cycle contain low levels of cytochrome $P450_{17}$ and C17,20-lyase and thus convert little pregnenolone or progesterone to androgens. Because these cells also lack cytochrome $P450_{21}$ and $P450_{11\beta}$ activities, progesterone is their major steroid product. Given these enzyme deficiencies, estrogen synthesis must depend on the participation of theca cells with granulosa cells (Fig. 4-13). Theca cells produce androstenedione, which is converted to estrogen by granulosa cells. In granulosa cells, androstenedione is converted to estrone by aromatase, which catalyzes the formation of two additional double bonds in the A ring; aromatase similarly converts testosterone to estradiol. The high activity of aromatase also ensures that most of the testosterone produced is converted to estradiol and that little testosterone is released. Ovarian steroidogenesis thus depends on cooperation between two cell types, theca and granulosa, and two tropic hormones, LH and FSH.[61]

The active steroid hormone $1,25(OH)_2$ vitamin D (1,25-dihydroxycholecalciferol), or $1,25(OH)_2D$, is also synthesized from cholesterol, but the biosynthetic enzymes are located in three separate organs: skin, liver, and kidney (see Chap. 23). Initially vitamin D_3 is formed by ultraviolet irradiation of precursor 7-dehydrocholesterol present in skin (Fig. 4-14). Formation of vitamin D_3 proceeds via a 6,7 cis isomer intermediate, previtamin D. Adequate exposure to ultraviolet light is necessary for this initial step in $1,25(OH)_2D$ formation, with more exposure being required for darker-skinned races. A dietary precursor, ergocalciferol or vitamin D_2, which differs from vitamin D_3 by a double bond between C22 and C23 and a methyl group at C24, is formed in plants from ergosterol. Although most foods have only low amounts of vitamins D_2 and D_3, irradiation can convert precursors to vitamins D_2 and D_3. Intestinal absorption occurs principally in the ileum and requires bile salts.

Vitamins D_3 and D_2 are transported in plasma to liver via a vitamin D transport protein. This transport protein has a greater affinity for vitamin D_3 than for previtamin D, and so the latter remains in skin depots.

In the liver, vitamin D_3 is hydroxylated at C25 by a microsomal enzyme, cytochrome $P450_{25}$; 25(OH)D, which is the major circulating form of vitamin D, is then transported via the α-globulin vitamin D transport protein to proximal tubule cells of the kidney, where the final modification to produce the active species occurs. In the kidney, 1α-hydroxylation of 25(OH)D is catalyzed by mitochondrial cytochrome $P450_{1\alpha}$, a cytochrome P450 enzyme with the proper-

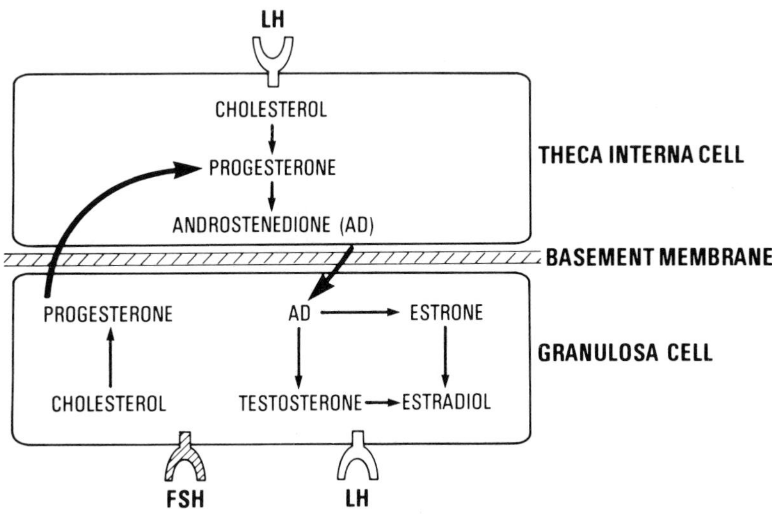

FIGURE 4-13 Two-cell, two-gonadotropin model of ovarian steroid hormone synthesis. Granulosa cells produce principally progesterone but contain aromatase, which converts androstenedione and testosterone to estrone and estradiol, respectively. Androstenedione is synthesized in theca interna cells and diffuses into adjacent granulosa cells.

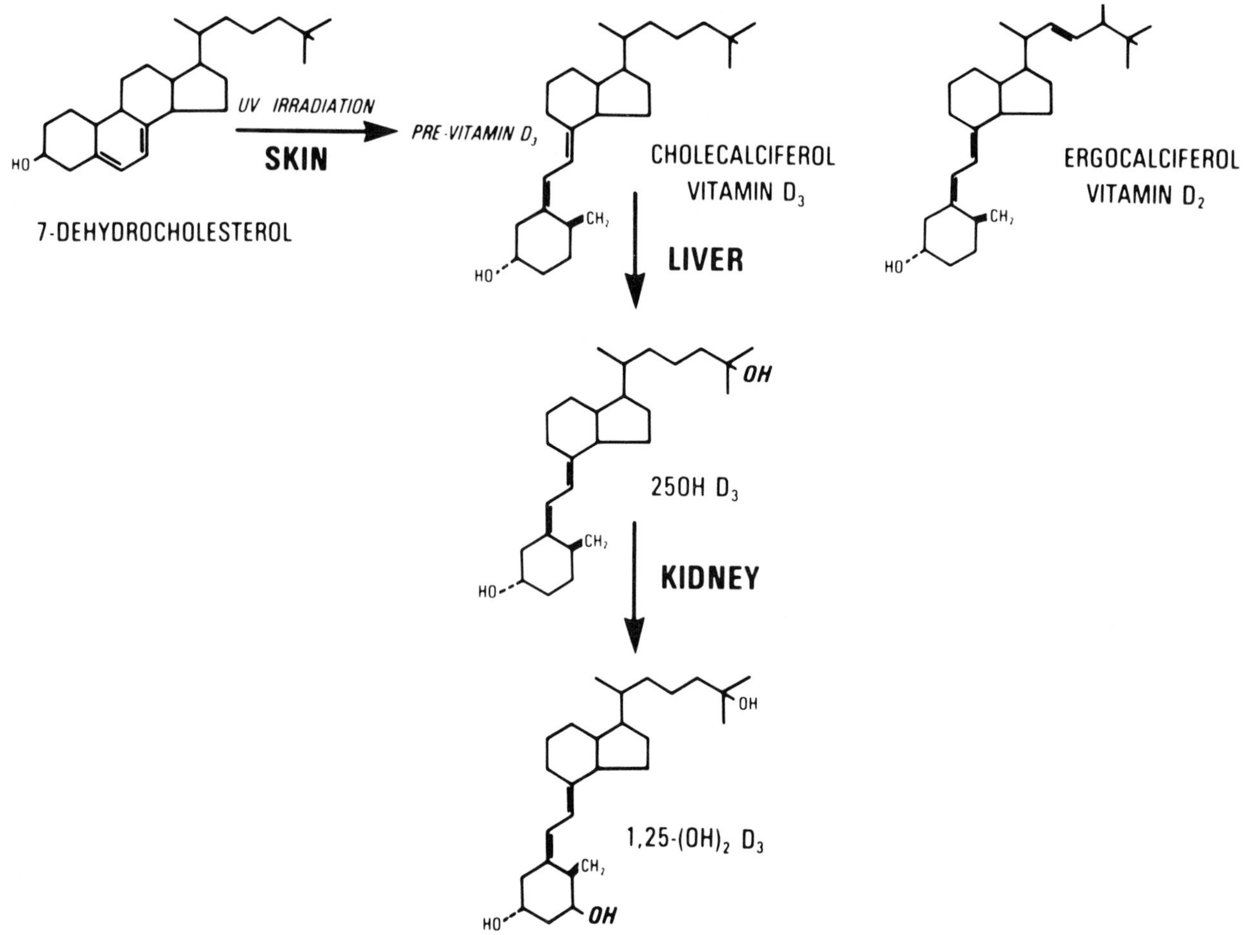

FIGURE 4-14 Biosynthesis of metabolically active 1,25$(OH)_s$D.

ties shown in Fig. 4-12.[62] Biologically active 1,25$(OH)_2$D is secreted and transported to its sites of action.

In this unusual endocrine system with large amounts of precursor present in skin (previtamin D) and circulation [25(OH)D], the major site for synthetic regulation is at the final biosynthetic step in kidney proximal tubule cells. Elevated PTH and decreased serum phosphorus are the major factors known to stimulate cytochrome $P450_{1\alpha}$ activity to increase the formation of 1,25$(OH)_2$D.[63]

Several additional modifications of the 25(OH)D nucleus occur. Hydroxylation at C24 is favored when hydroxylation at C1 is slow, whereas hydroxylation at C24 is low when hydroxylation at C1 is high, suggesting that the formation of 24,25$(OH)_2$D represents a pathway for the inactivation of the steroid. Hydroxylation at C26 may also occur, with or without hydroxylation at C24 and C1.

Tropic Regulation of Steroid Hormone Synthesis

Hormones such as ACTH, FSH, LH, and hCG not only acutely stimulate steroid hormone production but also chronically increase the synthetic capacity of their target glands by inducing synthesis of the enzymes of the biosynthetic pathway. Historically, these tropic effects were recognized from target gland atrophy with hypophysectomy before there was knowledge of the regulation of steroid hormone formation.[64] After hypophysectomy, all the steroid-synthesizing enzymes decrease; administration of tropic hormones restores them to normal by increasing specific messenger RNAs and consequent enzyme protein biosynthesis. In adrenocortical cells, ACTH coordinately increases the synthesis of cytochromes $P450_{scc}$, $P450_{17\alpha}$, $P450_{21}$, $P450_{11\beta}$, adrenodoxin, and adrenodoxin reductase; in granulosa cells, FSH induces aromatase, and increases in most other enzymes also occur.[65,66]

These tropic effects increase the capacity of the adrenal cortex to produce steroids during chronic stress and the capacity of the ovary to produce steroids during the menstrual cycle. Optimal enzyme induction requires increased protein biosynthetic capacity, which is achieved by the coordinate action of growth-promoting factors. The coordinate effects of ACTH and growth factors result in hypertrophied, hyperfunctional adrenocortical cells. The growth factors stimulate cell hypertrophy so that specific inductive effects of ACTH are maximal. ACTH does not directly stimulate cell growth; rather, it blocks cell replication. This coordinate action by two types of signal (ACTH, which induces differentiated function but inhibits replication, and growth factors such as fibroblast growth factor and insulin, which increase cell growth and biosynthetic capacity) provides amplification in response to need and a return to baseline when that need is over. This method of response is well suited to hormone biosynthetic cells, which must frequently change their production capacity, because it permits large changes in this capacity without cell replication or cell death.[67] With continued stimulation, ACTH receptors down regulate and growth factors, probably autocrine under control of ACTH, predominate; cells not only undergo hypertrophy but divide.

Transport and Metabolism of Steroid Hormones

In contrast to peptide hormones, steroid hormones are not stored but are secreted as synthesized. Increased secretion therefore directly reflects increased synthesis. After secretion into the circulation, steroid hormones are bound to transport glycoproteins which are made in the liver. Evidence that transport proteins are not essential for the activity of steroid hormones comes from patients with genetic deficiencies of binding protein who have normal endocrine function and from the observation that some synthetic analogues (e.g., dexamethasone) which are highly active bind poorly to transport proteins. Although deficiencies of steroid carrier proteins are seen in humans who are heterozygous for the protein, homozygous deficiencies are not seen, suggesting that the carrier proteins have an essential function in development and are required for viability. The plasma binding proteins provide a reservoir of hormone, protected from metabolism and renal clearance, which can be released to cells. This reservoir significantly prolongs the circulating half-life of steroid hormones, buffers increases in hormone production, and provides a source of hormone when production decreases. An important function for these proteins may be to ensure acceptable distribution to target tissues, as has been shown for thyroid hormones.[68] For example, when steroid hormones circulate through tissues such as liver, the proximal portion of the tissue may take up an inappropriate proportion of hormone if it is free. By contrast, only a small amount of the total hormone can dissociate from the transport protein in the brief time period while the blood is moving through this tissue, and additional hormone will be available for entering the distal portions of the tissue. The concentration of binding proteins is regulated and affects the concentration of free active hormone.

There are three main steroid hormone transport proteins: corticosteroid-binding globulin (CBG), which binds cortisol and progesterone, sex hormone–binding globulin (SHBG), and vitamin D binding–globulin (DBG). CBG is a 52,000 M_r glycoprotein which binds cortisol and progesterone with about equal affinity (K_d = 30 nM). CBG has homology with the serine proteinase inhibitor superfamily and may act to specifically deliver cortisol to sites of inflammation.[69] CBG contains one high-affinity binding site and is normally present in concentrations sufficient to bind about 250 ng of cortisol per milliliter. When cortisol concentrations exceed this level, the hormone is weakly bound by albumin, and metabolism and excretion of the free hormone increase. Except in the third trimester of pregnancy, when high levels of progesterone occur, cortisol concentrations exceed those of progesterone about 10-fold, and so most binding sites on CBG are filled by cortisol. CBG production is increased by estrogens, so by the third trimester of pregnancy, CBG concentrations are twice those of the nonpregnant state; CBG production is also increased by thyroid hormone.

The affinity of SHBG for testosterone is greater than its affinity for estradiol.[70] In males, the single binding site on the molecule is ordinarily occupied by testosterone and estradiol is weakly bound to albumin. The concentration of SHBG is increased 5- to 10-fold by estrogens and is decreased twofold by androgens; thyroid hormone also increases SHBG. SHBG is closely related to androgen-binding protein (ABP), which is produced in Sertoli cells and secreted into the seminiferous tubules. ABP has been proposed to maintain a high local androgen environment for sperm development and maturation.

DBG, a 56,000 M_r glycoprotein, has a single binding site with a higher affinity for 25(OH)D than for $1,25(OH)_2D$ or previtamin D_3.[71] The relative binding affinities provide a reservoir of circulating 25(OH)D, as well as ready release of active $1,25(OH)_2D$ to target tissues. Like other steroid hormone transport proteins, DBG is synthesized in increased amounts in response to estrogen.

The small fraction of free steroid hormone, which is in equilibrium with that bound to transport protein, binds to intracellular hormone receptors to induce biological responses. The free fraction is also metabolized, principally in the liver, to inactive, water-soluble derivatives. Such metabolic steps are critical because the free hydrophobic steroids, although filtered by the kidney, are mostly reabsorbed and are largely not removed. Cortisol, for example, is inactivated by reduction of the 4,5 double bond of the A ring by converting less polar ketone groups such as those at C3 and C20 to hydroxyl groups and by converting the 11-hydroxyl group to the ketone. The latter reaction converts cortisol to cortisone and appears to be important for keeping cortisol from binding to mineralocorticoid receptors in certain tissues (e.g., kidney; see Chap. 12). Hydroxyl groups, especially at carbon 3, are conjugated with glucuronide and sulfate to render them more water-soluble for effective renal clearance. Hydroxylations of other steroids are also important for increasing solubility and for conjugation with glucuronic acid or sulfate. Estradiol is hydroxylated at either C2 or C16 and can be conjugated at either position, aldosterone can be conjugated via hydroxyls at either C3 or C18, and cortisol can be hydroxylated at C6. More than 50 steroid metabolites, reflecting various combinations or substitutions, have been identified, though most are produced in only small amounts.[72]

Although most metabolic alterations of steroid hormones result in inactivation, there are several which enhance or alter biological activity. The biological activity of testosterone is increased by 5α-reductase, which converts testosterone to 5α-dihydrotestosterone, the major active species in the male reproductive tract and skin. 5α-Reductase is localized in target tissues such as the prostate, so that activation of precursor testosterone occurs at the site of action. Circulating androstenedione, produced in adrenal cortex and gonads, can be converted to testosterone. Aromatase, the cytochrome P450 required for estrogen production, is located in peripheral tissue cells and in producer granulosa cells in the ovary. Significant quantities of estradiol are produced in both men and women by the conversion of circulating androstenedione and testosterone to estrone and estradiol.

THYROID HORMONE

In contrast to many hormones whose concentrations fluctuate rapidly in response to environmental signals, thyroid hormone is remarkably stable. It is synthesized in the largest endocrine gland, stored in large quantities in thyroid follicles as part of the structure of a protein molecule, secreted as a prohormone, transported in the circulation bound to carrier proteins, and converted to its most active form in peripheral tissues (see Chap. 10).

Iodine Metabolism

Thyroid hormones are iodinated derivatives of the amino acid tyrosine (Fig. 4-15). Thyroxine (T_4), the major secretory product of the thyroid gland, consists of two phenyl rings linked via an ether bridge with an alanine side chain on the inner ring. Thyroxine contains four iodine atoms attached to carbons 3 and 5 of the inner ring and 3′ and 5′ of the outer ring. These substitutions impose a three-dimensional structure on the molecule so that the planes of the aromatic rings are perpendicular to each other. 3,5,3′-Triiodothyronine (T_3), the most active form of the hormone, is principally derived from T_4 by removal of one iodine from the outer ring, whereas 3,3′,5′-triiodothyronine (reverse T_3), the major inactive metabolite of T_4, results from the removal of iodine from C5 of the inner ring.

Because iodine is an essential structural component, biosynthesis of thyroid hormone depends on iodine metabolism (see Chaps. 10 and 11). Dietary iodine intake in western cultures is normally about 250 μg per day but may be greater because of the use of iodized salt and iodates in bread and processed foods. In inland mountainous areas of the world iodine intake may be less than 60 μg per day. In these areas, growth of the thyroid gland and enhanced trapping of iodide may maintain a euthyroid state. Although the adaptive capacity of the gland is great, when iodine intake falls below 20 μg per day, thyroid gland compensation may be inadequate and endemic hypothyroidism and cretinism occur.

Under basal conditions, the thyroid uses about 60 μg of iodide daily for thyroid hormone biosynthesis (Fig. 4-16). Of this, 50 μg is of dietary origin and 10 μg is from hormone turnover. Iodide is concentrated from the circulation by active transport via an

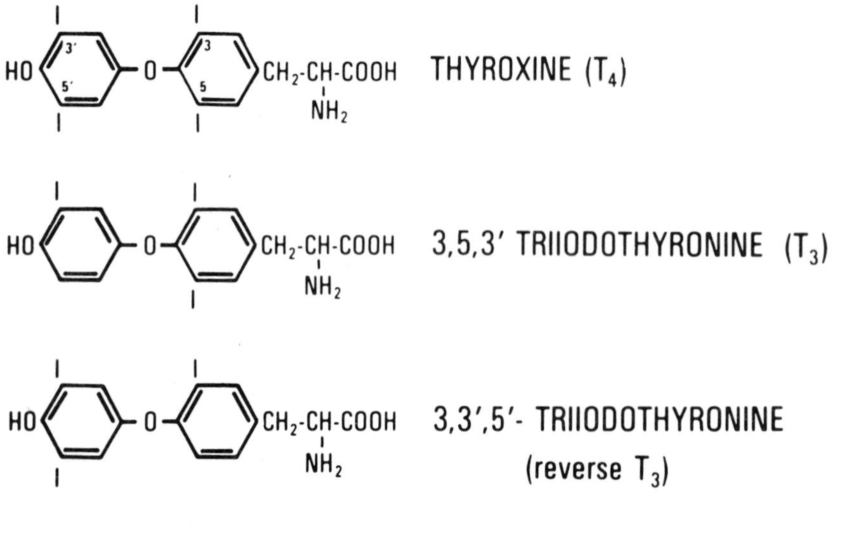

THYROXINE (T_4)

3,5,3′ TRIIODOTHYRONINE (T_3)

3,3′,5′- TRIIODOTHYRONINE (reverse T_3)

FIGURE 4-15 The major circulating thyroid hormones.

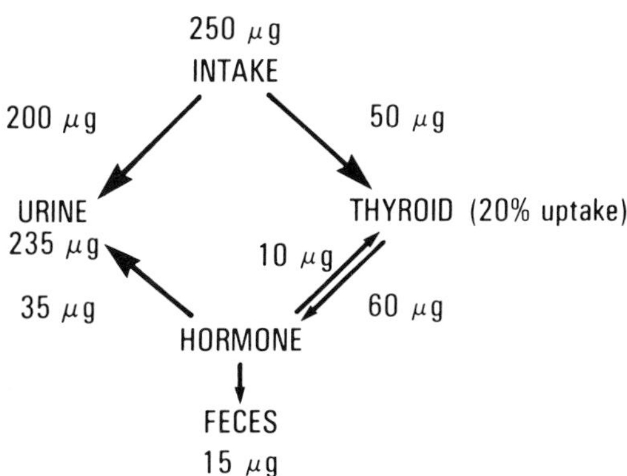

FIGURE 4-16 Average human daily iodine balance in the United States. *(From Robbins.*[73]*)*

iodide pump or trap located at the basal surface of the thyroid cell. The concentrating mechanism requires metabolic energy from ATP and Na^+, K^+-ATPase–mediated sodium transport.[74] The transport process effectively extracts iodide from the circulation and can concentrate it more than 100-fold within the thyroid cell. Other anions, such as perchlorate and pertechnetate, are also concentrated, and these ions have been used for thyroid function tests and for imaging.

Cellular uptake of iodide is regulated by TSH and by local control mechanisms. The local autoregulatory mechanisms help provide adequate iodide for hormone synthesis when circulating levels are low and prevent excessive hormone synthesis when circulating iodide concentrations are high. In response to large quantities of iodine (2 mg or more), there is a sharp decrease in the iodination of tyrosine residues in thyroglobulin.[75] The decreased organification (Wolff-Chaikoff effect) is an acute adaptive response to high intracellular concentrations of iodide. When high iodide concentrations persist, thyroid cells adapt by decreasing active transport of iodide into the cell.[76] Increased cellular concentrations of unbound iodide are then dissipated, and the block to organification is removed. Ingestion of large amounts of iodine thus does not normally affect thyroid hormone synthesis. When these autoregulatory mechanisms are defective, dietary iodine can have marked effects on thyroid hormone synthesis. When inhibition of organification does not occur in response to increased cellular iodide, increased thyroid hormone synthesis and hyperthyroidism may occur (iod-Basedow effect). If organification is inhibited but transport of iodide does not adaptively decrease, high cellular concentrations of iodide will result in decreased thyroid hormone synthesis (iodide goiter and hypothyroidism).

Anatomy of a Distinctive Biosynthetic Pathway

Thyroid cells are organized into follicles with their basal surfaces exposed to the circulation and their apical surfaces facing the lumen of the central follicle, which is filled with thyroglobulin. Iodide is taken up at the basal surface and is rapidly oxidized and incorporated into tyrosine residues in thyroglobulin molecules. In the biosynthetic pathway outlined in Fig. 4-17, both the organification and coupling reactions shown occur at the apical surface of the cell, in microvilli which extend into the colloid space. Thyroid peroxidase is a membrane-bound heme-protein enzyme complex which catalyzes both organification and coupling reactions.[77–79] The proposed reaction scheme for thyroid peroxidase (E) is

(1) Organification:

$$E + H_2O_2 \xrightarrow{\;H_2O\;} EO \longrightarrow [EOI]^- \xrightarrow{+\text{ tyrosine}} \text{iodotyrosine} + OH^- + E$$

(2) Coupling:

$$E + H_2O_2 \xrightarrow{\;H_2O\;} EO \xrightarrow{+\text{ DIT (thyroglobulin)}} T_4 + E$$

The antithyroid drugs (thioureylene compounds) inhibit organification and coupling reactions by inactivating both EO and $[EOI]^-$.

Tyrosines which are iodinated are present in thyroglobulin, a large multisubunit glycoprotein of 660,000 M_r.[80] Thyroglobulin, which accounts for about 50 percent of the total protein made by thyroid cells, has only an average content of tyrosine, but these tyrosines appear to be available for iodination both because of their location in the primary structure and because of the tertiary structure of the mature glycosylated protein. Thyroglobulin is transported in vesicles to the microvilli at the apical surface, where iodination, coupling, and secretion into the follicular lumen occur. Normally iodinated thyroglobulin present in lumen colloid contains about 26 atoms of iodine with 3 to 4 T_4 and 0.2 T_3 residues as well as 6 residues of monoiodotyrosine and 4 residues of diiodotyrosine.[81] Iodide availability affects the proportions of T_3 and T_4, with more T_3 being present when iodide is low.

Large amounts of thyroglobulin are stored as colloid in the lumen of thyroid follicles. The formation of active thyroid hormone requires readsorption of colloid by endocytosis and breakdown of thyroglobulin to T_4 and T_3. Thyroglobulin may be broken down via lysosomal hydrolases, but there is also evidence for cleavage by halogens and peroxidases.[82] If the latter hypothesis is correct, the steps in thyroid hormone synthesis (organification, coupling, and proteolysis) all use one substrate, thyroglobulin, and one enzyme, thyroid peroxidase, and the cellular organization shown in Fig. 4-17 serves to segregate these various reactions.

T_4 and T_3 are secreted in a ratio of about 10:1. The

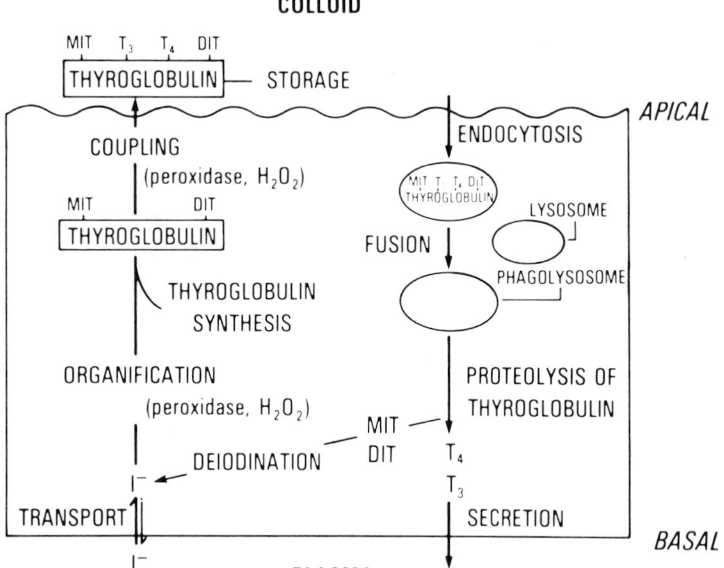

FIGURE 4-17 Pathway for the biosynthesis of thyroid hormones.

iodine in mono- and diiodotyrosine is reclaimed for hormone biosynthesis by a thyroid deiodinase enzyme. This deiodination pathway reclaims about 50 percent of the iodine of thyroglobulin and is quantitatively important in thyroid gland economy, as demonstrated by the fact that congenital defects in deiodinase result in goitrous hypothyroidism.

TSH, which is the major regulator of thyroid gland function, has been reported to increase each step of the biosynthetic pathway. A rate-limiting step analogous to that for steroid hormone synthesis has not been identified, but increased availability of iodide via active transport is among the most rapid responses to TSH.

Transport and Metabolism

T_4, the major secretory product of the thyroid, circulates bound to serum proteins. The binding proteins, like those which transport steroid hormones, are made in the liver, and their synthesis is increased by estrogens and decreased by androgens. More than 99 percent of T_4 is bound to three proteins: thyroid-binding globulin (TBG), thyroid-binding prealbumin (TBPA), and serum albumin. TBG, a 63,000 M_r glycoprotein, which binds about 75 percent of circulating T_4, has the highest affinity, TBPA has a lesser affinity, and serum albumin has the least affinity but the highest capacity. Protein binding provides a large protected reservoir of hormone. Because of extensive protein binding, T_4 has a circulating half-life of about 1 week, while T_3, which is bound less tightly to protein, has a half-life of 1.3 days. The roles of the thyroid hormone transport proteins appear to be similar to those discussed above for the steroid hormone transport proteins.

Thyroxine is a prohormone and is activated in target tissues via 5′-deiodination to metabolically active T_3. 5′-Deiodination is catalyzed by a microsomal enzyme which requires reduced thiols for activity. The type I 5′-deiodinase contains selenocysteine in its active site.[83] Replacement with cysteine results in a less active enzyme, indicating that this unusual amino acid is important for catalytic activity. This enzyme, which is especially prominent in liver and kidney, accounts for more than 80 percent of T_3 production under normal conditions. Its activity, and thus the production of T_3, is influenced by many factors. The first site of control of thyroid hormone synthesis is the thyroid gland, where TSH regulates T_4 production. Under most conditions, conversion of T_4 to T_3 in the periphery is proportional to the concentration of substrate T_4, but a second point of control is present in target organs such as liver and kidney, where under several conditions conversion of T_4 to T_3 is decreased. Fasting, illness, cortisol, propylthiouracil, and other drugs all reduce 5′-deiodinase activity.[84] During fasting, there is a 20 percent decrease in plasma T_3 by the end of the first day and a 50 percent decrease at the end of 3 days. This decrease in T_3 production is thought to be an adaptive response contributing to a decreased metabolic rate and to conservation of body tissues when substrate is unavailable. Use of the circulating pool of prohormone T_4 is thus coupled to metabolic needs.

Type II 5′-deiodinase found in the pituitary and central nervous system differs from that in liver and kidney. It has a lower K_m for T_4, it is not inhibited by propylthiouracil, and its activity increases rather than decreases in hypothyroidism. Type II 5′-deiodinase contains cysteine rather than selenocysteine in the active site.[85] This enzyme is important in feedback effects of T_4 on TSH secretion as well as in biological effects on the nervous system. The type II 5′-deiodinase converts T_4 to T_3 in the pituitary to provide a normal hypothalamic-pituitary-thyroid axis under conditions, such as fasting, where circulating T_3 concentrations are low because of inhibition of liver and kidney 5′-deiodinase. If circulating T_3 were the major feedback regulator of TSH, the reduced circulating concentrations of T_3 in fasting and in systemic illness would remove feedback inhibition to increase TSH and thus thyroid hormone production. The type II 5′-deiodinase of the pituitary allows feedback control via circulating T_4 rather than T_3 and serves to maintain normal thyroid gland production, preventing the thyroid from inappropriately compensating for the physiologically important reduction in circulating T_3 concentrations.

Deiodination of the inner ring of T_4 by 5-deiodinase yields reverse T_3 (rT_3), an inactive metabolite. About equal amounts of T_3 and rT_3 are formed from T_4, but rT_3 is cleared more rapidly, so that circulating concentrations are lower. When 5′-deiodinase activity is reduced, as in fasting, greater amounts of T_4 are metabolized to rT_3.

Inactivation of T_3 occurs by additional deiodinations to give 3,3′-T_2 and 3,5-T_2 and by deamination and decarboxylation of the alanine side chain and conjugation with glucuronic acid and sulfate.

REFERENCES

1. Shatkin, AJ: Capping of eukaryotic mRNAs. *Cell* 9:645, 1976.
2. Kozak M: Structural features in eukaryotic mRNAs that modulate the initiation of translation. *J Biol Chem* 266:19867, 1991.
3. Conaway JK, Conaway RC: Initiation of eukaryotic messenger RNA synthesis. *J Biol Chem* 266:17721, 1991.
4. Sawadogo M, Sentenac A: RNA polymerase B (II) and general transcription factors. *Annu Rev Biochem* 59:711, 1990.
5. Gidoni D, Dynan WS, Tjian R: Multiple specific contacts between a mammalian transcription factor and its cognate promoters. *Nature* 321:409, 1984.
6. Pugh BF, Tjian R: Mechanism of transcriptional activation by Sp1: Evidence for coactivators. *Cell* 61:1187, 1990.
7. Smale ST, Baltimore D: The initiator as a transcription control element. *Cell* 57:103, 1989.
8. Ptashne M, Gann AAA: Activators and targets. *Nature* 346:329, 1990.
9. Jones KA, Kadonaga JT, Rosenfeld PJ, Kelly TJ, Tjian R: A cellular DNA-binding protein that activates eukaryotic transcription and DNA replication. *Cell* 48:79, 1987.
10. Evans RM: The steroid and thyroid hormone receptor superfamily. *Science* 240:889, 1988.
11. Harrison SC: A structural taxonomy of DNA binding domains. *Nature* 353:715, 1991.
12. Pabo CO, Saver RT: Transcription factors: Structural families and principles of recognition. *Annu Rev Biochem* 61:1053, 1992.
13. Frankel AD, Kim PS: Modular structure of transcription factors: Implications for gene regulation. *Cell* 65:717, 1991.
14. Yamamoto KK, Gonzalez GA, Menzel P, Rivier J, Montminy MR: Characterization of a bipartite activator domain in transcription factor CREB. *Cell* 60:611, 1990.
15. Damm K, Thompson CC, Evans RM: Protein encoded by v-erbA functions as a thyroid-hormone receptor antagonist. *Nature* 339:593, 1989.
16. Beato M: Transcriptional control by nuclear receptors. *FASEB J* 5:2044, 1991.
17. Diamond MI, Miner JN, Yoshinaga SK, Yamamoto KR: Transcription factor interactions: Selectors of positive or negative regulation from a single DNA element. *Science* 249:1266, 1990.
18. Gill G, Ptashne M: Negative effect of the transcriptional activator GAL4. *Nature* 334:721, 1988.
19. Laybourn PJ, Kadonaga JT: Role of nucleosomal cores and histone H_1 in regulation of transcription by RNA polymerase II. *Science* 254:238, 1991.
20. Sharp PA: RNA splicing and genes. *JAMA* 260:3035, 1988.
21. Breathnack R, Chambon P: Organization and expression of eukaryotic split genes coding for proteins. *Annu Rev Biochem* 50:349, 1981.
22. Reed R: The organization of 3′ splice-site sequence in mammalian introns. *Genes Dev* 3:2113, 1989.
23. Wickens M: How the messenger got its tail: Addition of poly (A) in the nucleus. *TIBS* 15:277, 1990.
24. Wahle E, Keller W: The biochemistry of 3′-end cleavage and polyadenylation of messenger RNA precursors. *Annu Rev Biochem* 61:419, 1992.
25. Rosenfeld MG, Mermod J-J, Amara SG, Swanson LW, Sawchenko PE, Rivier J, Vale WW, Evans RW: Production of a novel neuropeptide encoded by the calcitonin gene via tissue-specific RNA processing. *Nature* 304:129–135, 1983.
26. Walter P, Blobel G: Signal recognition particle contains a 7S RNA essential for protein translocation across the endoplasmic reticulum. *Nature* 299:691–698, 1982.
27. Gilmore R, Walter P, Blobel G: Protein translocation across the endoplasmic reticulum: Isolation and characterization of the signal recognition particle receptor. *J Cell Biol* 96:470–477, 1982.
28. Connolly T, Gilmore R: The signal recognition particle receptor mediates the GTP-dependent displacement of SRP from the signal sequence of the nascent polypeptide. *Cell* 57:599–610, 1989.
29. Simon SM, Blobel G: A protein conducting channel in the endoplasmic reticulum. *Cell* 65:371–380, 1991.
30. Singer SJ: The structure and insertion of integral proteins in membranes. *Annu Rev Cell Biol* 6:247–296, 1990.
31. Grey A, Dull TJ, Ullrich A: Nucleotide sequence of epidermal growth factor cDNA predicts a 128,000-molecular weight protein precursor. *Nature* 303:722–725, 1983.
32. Land H, Schultz G, Schmale H, Richter D: Nucleotide sequence of cloned cDNA encoding bovine arginine vasopressin-neurophysin II precursor. *Nature* 295:299–303, 1982.
33. Nakanishi S, Inoue A, Kita T, Nakamura M, Chang ACY, Cohen SN, Numa S: Nucleotide sequence of clone cDNA for bovine corticotropin β-lipotropin precursor. *Nature* 278:423–427, 1979.
34. Inayama S, Nakanishi S, Numa S: Cloning and sequence analysis of cDNA for bovine adrenal preproenkephalin. *Nature* 295:202, 1982.
35. Blundell TL, Bedarkar S, Rinderknecht E, Humbel RE: Insulin-like growth factor: A model for tertiary structure accounting for immunoreactivity and receptor binding. *Proc Natl Acad Sci USA* 75:180, 1978.
36. Steiner DS, Clark JL: The spontaneous reoxidation of reduced beef and rat proinsulins. *Proc Natl Acad Sci USA* 60:622, 1968.
37. Gabbay KH, DeLuca K, Fisher JN Jr, Mako ME, Rubenstein AH: Familial hyperproinsulinemia: An autosomal dominant defect. *N Engl J Med* 294:911, 1976.
38. Rothman JE, Orci L: Molecular dissection of the secretory pathway. *Nature* 335:409, 1992.
39. Pearse BMF, Robinson M: Clathrin, adaptors and sorting. *Annu Rev Cell Biol* 6:151, 1990.
40. Bourne HR, Sanders DA, McCormick F: The GTPase super-

family: A conserved switch for diverse cell functions. *Nature* 348:125, 1990.
41. Wilson DW, Wilcox CA, Flynn GC, Chen E, Kuang W-J, Henzel WJ, Block MR, Ullrich A, Rothman JE: A fusion protein required for vesicle-mediated transport in both mammalian cells and yeast. *Nature* 339:355, 1989.
42. Hubbard SC, Ivatt RJ: Synthesis and processing of asparagine-linked oligosaccharides. *Annu Rev Biochem* 50:555, 1981.
43. Sampath D, Varki A, and Freeze HH. The spectrum of incomplete N-linked oligosaccharide synthesis by endothelial cells in the presence of Brefeldin A. *J. Biol Chem* 267:4440, 1992.
44. Hunziker W, Harter C, Matter K, Mellman I: Basolateral sorting in MDCK cells requires a distinct cytoplasmic domain determinant. *Cell* 66:907, 1991.
45. Collawn JF, Stangel M, Kuhn LA, Esekogwu V, Jing S, Trowbridge IS, Tainer JA: Transferrin receptor internalization sequence YXRF implicates a tight turn as the structural motif for endocytosis. *Cell* 63:1061, 1990.
46. Burgess TL, Kelly RP: Constitutive and regulated secretion of proteins. *Annu Rev Cell Biol* 3:243, 1987.
47. Garcia JV, Gehm BD, Rosner MR: An evolutionarily conserved enzyme degrades transforming growth factor-alpha as well as insulin. *J Cell Biol* 109:1301, 1989.
48. Chertow BS: The role of lysosomes and proteases in hormone secretion and degradation. *Endocr Rev* 2:137, 1981.
49. Ooi TF: Insulin-like growth factor-binding proteins (IGFBPs): More than just 1,2,3. *Mol Cell Endocrinol* 71:C39, 1990.
50. Deuel TF, Kawahara RS: Growth factors and wound healing. *Annu Rev Med* 42:567–584, 1991.
51. Kovanen PT, Goldstein JL, Chappell DA, Brown MS: Regulation of low density lipoprotein receptors by adrenocorticotropin in the adrenal gland of mice and rats in vivo. *J Biol Chem* 255:5591, 1980.
52. Brown MS, Anderson RGW, Goldstein JL: Recycling receptors: The round trip itinerary of migrant membrane proteins. *Cell* 32:663, 1983.
53. Brown MS, Kovanen PT, Goldstein JL: Receptor-mediated uptake of lipoprotein cholesterol and its utilization for steroid synthesis in the adrenal cortex. *Recent Prog Horm Res* 35:215, 1979.
54. Jefcoate CR, DiBartolemeos MJ, Williams CA, McNamara BC: ACTH regulation of cholesterol movement in isolated adrenal cells. *J Steroid Biochem* 27:721, 1987.
55. Gill GN: The adrenal gland, in West JW (ed): *Best and Taylor's Physiological Basis of Medical Practice,* 12th ed. Baltimore, Williams & Wilkins, 1990, p. 820.
56. Hall PF, Lewes JL, Lipson ED: The role of mitochondrial cytochrome P-450 from bovine adrenal cortex in side chain cleavage of 20S, *22R*-dihydroxycholesterol. *J Biol Chem* 250:2283, 1975.
57. Gustafsson J-A, Carlstedt-Duke J, Mode A, Rafter J: *Biochemistry, Biophysics and Regulation of Cytochrome P-450.* New York, Elsevier, 1980.
58. Hornsby PJ, Crivello JF: The role of lipid peroxidation and biological antioxidants in the function of the adrenal cortex. *Mol Cell Endocrinol* 30:1, 1983.
59. Lieberman S, Prasad VVK: Heterodox notions on pathways of steroidogenesis. *Endocr Rev* 11:469, 1990.
60. Barnes HJ, Arlotto MP, Waterman MR: Expression and enzyme activity of recombinant cytochrome $P450_{17}$ alpha hydroxylase in Escherichia coli. *Proc Natl Acad Sci USA* 88:5597, 1991.
61. Hseuh AJW, Adashi EY, Jones PBC, Welsh TH Jr: Hormonal regulation of the differentiation of cultured ovarian granulosa cells. *Endocr Rev* 5:76, 1984.
62. DeLuca HF, Schnoes HK: Vitamin D: Recent advances. *Annu Rev Biochem* 52:411, 1983.
63. Caniggia A, Lore F, deCairano G, Nuti R: Main endocrine modulators of vitamin D hydroxylases in human pathophysiology. *J Steroid Biochem* 27:815, 1987.
64. Smith PE: Hypophysectomy and a replacement therapy in the rat. *Am J Anat* 45:205, 1930.
65. Simpson ER, Lund J, Ahlgren R, Waterman MR: Regulation by cyclic AMP of the genes encoding steroidogenic enzymes. *Mol Cell Endocrinol* 70:C25, 1990.
66. Waterman MR, Simpson ER: Regulation of steroid hydroxylase gene expression is multifactorial in nature. *Recent Prog Horm Res* 45:533, 1989.
67. Gill GN, Crivello JF, Hornsby PJ, Simonian MH: Growth, function and development of the adrenal cortex: Insights from cell culture. *Cold Spring Harbor Conf Cell Proliferation* 9:461, 1982.
68. Mendel CM, Cavalieri RR, Weisiser RA: Uptake of thyroxine by the perfused rat liver: Implications for the free hormone hypothesis. *Am J Physiol* 255:410, 1988.
69. Hammond GL: Molecular properties of corticosteroid binding globulin and the sex-steroid binding proteins. *Endocr Rev* 11:65, 1990.
70. Bardin CW, Musto N, Gunsalus G, Kotite N, Cheng SL, Larrea F, Becker R: Extracellular androgen binding proteins. *Annu Rev Physiol* 43:189, 1981.
71. Norman AW, Roth J, Orci L: The vitamin D endocrine system: Steroid metabolism, hormone receptors and biological response (calcium binding proteins). *Endocr Rev* 3:331, 1982.
72. Monder C, Bradlow LH: Cortolic acids: Explorations at the frontier of corticosteroid metabolism. *Recent Prog Horm Res* 36:345, 1980.
73. Robbins J: Iodine deficiency, iodine excess and the use of iodine for protection against radioactive iodine. *Thyroid Today* 3:1, 1980.
74. Nilsson M, Bjorkman U, Ekholm R, Ericson LE: Iodide transport in primary cultured follicle cells: Evidence of a TSH-regulated channel mediating iodide efflux selectively across the apical domain of the plasma membrane. *Eur J Cell Biol* 52:270, 1990.
75. Wolff J, Chaikoff IL: The inhibitory action of iodide upon organic binding of iodine by the normal thyroid gland. *J Biol Chem* 172:855, 1948.
76. Braverman LE, Ingbar SH: Changes in thyroidal function during adaptation to large doses of iodide. *J Clin Invest* 42:1216, 1963.
77. Magnusson RP, Taurog A, Dorris ML: Mechanism of iodide-dependent catalytic activity of thyroid peroxidase and lactoperoxidase. *J Biol Chem* 259:197, 1984.
78. Nakamura M, Yamazaki I, Nakagawa H, Ohtaki S: Steady state kinetics and regulation of thyroid peroxidase-catalyzed iodination. *J Biol Chem* 258:3837, 1983.
79. Morrison M, Schonbaum GR: Peroxidase-catalyzed halogenation. *Annu Rev Biochem* 45:861, 1976.
80. Malthiery Y, Lissitzky S: Primary structure of human thyroglobulin deduced from the sequence of its 8448-base complementary DNA. *Eur J Biochem* 165:491, 1987.
81. Izumi M, Larsen PR: Triiodothyronine, thyroxine and iodine in purified thyroglobulin from patients with Graves' disease. *J Clin Invest* 59:1105, 1977.
82. Alexander NM: Oxidative cleavage of tryptophanyl peptide bonds during chemical- and peroxidase-catalyzed iodinations. *J Biol Chem* 249:1946, 1974.
83. Berry MJ, Banu L, Larsen PR: Type I iodothyronine deiodinase is a selenocysteine-containing enzyme. *Nature* 349:438, 1991.
84. Wartofsky L, Burman KD: Alterations in thyroid function in patients with systemic illness: The "euthyroid sick syndrome." *Endocr Rev* 3:164, 1982.
85. Berry MJ, Kieffer JD, Larsen PR: Evidence that cysteine, not selenocysteine, is in the catalytic site of type II iodothyronine deiodinase. *Endocrinology* 129:550, 1991.

C H A P T E R 5A

Molecular Mechanisms of Hormone Action: Control of Target Cell Function by Peptide and Catecholamine Hormones

Kevin J. Catt

GENERAL ASPECTS OF HORMONE ACTION

Hormones were originally defined as blood-borne molecules that communicate between cells in central and peripheral endocrine organs or within major organ systems such as the gut and its appendages. The current view of hormones as a subset of endocrine regulators within a large group of extracellular messengers is based on the common features shared by hormones, neurotransmitters, growth factors, and cytokines. The major characteristic of hormones and the related chemical messengers is their ability to interact with highly selective receptor sites that activate intracellular signaling pathways within their respective target tissues.

All forms of biological regulation are based on specific interactions between complementary molecular domains or conformations that change the properties and function of one member or both members of the ligand pair. This type of information transfer is highly developed in hormone receptors and regulatory enzymes, which have many features in common. Hormone receptors fall into two major subgroups: those which are membrane-bound at the cell surface and signal primarily into the cytoplasm and those which are intracellular and signal primarily into the nucleus. The cell-surface receptors bind hormones and transmitters and are coupled to plasma membrane enzymes or ion channels that mediate and amplify the effect of ligand binding on subsequent cellular responses. The intracellular receptors bind steroid and thyroid hormones and become associated with specific regulatory domains within the nucleus. Several steroid and peptide hormones also bind to plasma proteins, but these serve largely as reservoirs and/or transport systems for the endogenous hormone and do not usually bind hormone analogues that interact with the cellular receptor sites. This chapter outlines some general aspects of hormone action that apply to both major subgroups of hormone receptors and then describes the cell surface receptors and the mechanisms through which the binding of hormones to these receptors is transmitted into biological responses (see Chap. 5B).

Characteristic features of peptide and steroid hormone receptors include their location and abundance in hormone-responsive tissues, their high specificity and affinity for agonist and antagonist ligands, their finite number and saturability, and their ability to elicit a specific cellular response when activated by the homologous hormone. Endocrine target cells exhibit a wide variety of metabolic, secretory, and growth responses to hormonal stimulation, and most of these responses are mediated by a relatively small group of primary signaling mechanisms that are initiated by receptor activation. Recently, molecular cloning has revealed a great deal of diversity in the components of the receptor-mediated signaling pathways that mediate hormone action. The ability of receptors to both recognize hormonal ligands and activate their target cells implies that they possess two separate structural domains for the transduction of extracellular signals into cellular responses. The existence of specific molecular domains for ligand binding and signal transduction has been demonstrated in many of the plasma membrane and intracellular receptors that mediate hormone action in endocrine target cells.

Classes of Hormone Action and Domains of Hormonal Control

The evolution of hormonal control mechanisms in multicellular organisms has led to the development of two major regulatory systems that integrate the functions of endocrine organs and their target cells. The blood-borne hormones that are secreted by the hypothalamus, pituitary, endocrine glands, gut, and kidney can be broadly subdivided into peptide and steroid hormones (Fig. 5A-1). The first group includes the traditional peptide and protein hor-

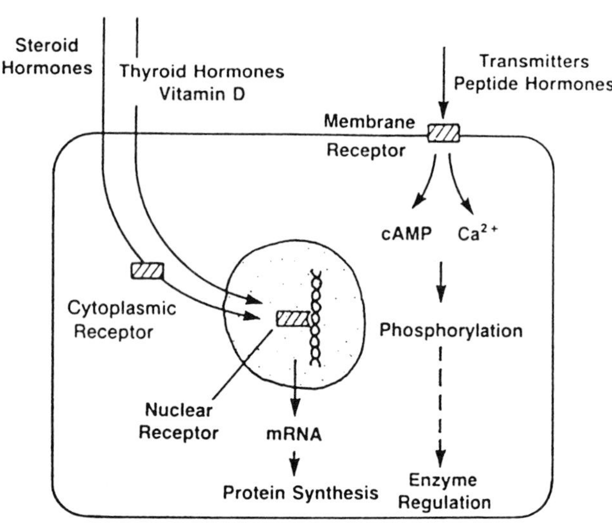

FIGURE 5A-1. Mechanisms of target cell activation by hormones acting on plasma membrane receptors and those acting through cytoplasmic and nuclear receptors. Membrane receptors for peptide hormones and transmitters signal through messengers such as cyclic AMP and calcium to activate the protein kinases that catalyze phosphorylation steps that lead to the phenotypic cell response. The steroid-type hormones, including thyroxine and vitamin D, activate intracellular receptors that in turn bind to chromatin and regulate gene transcription, with increased (or sometimes decreased) production of specific mRNAs that encode regulatory proteins and enzymes.

mones as well as growth factors and neurotransmitters, including the nonpeptide catecholamines. The second group includes the adrenal and gonadal steroid hormones as well as thyroid hormones, retinoids, and vitamin D (see also Chap. 1).

The steroid and thyroid hormones and vitamin D, which are considered in detail in Chap. 5B, regulate the transcription of genes for enzymes and other regulatory proteins that control the biosynthetic and metabolic activities of numerous peripheral tissues.[1] The relatively apolar and hydrophobic steroid molecules usually circulate in association with plasma-binding proteins. The free steroids diffuse readily into cells but exert their metabolic effects only on target tissues that contain their specific receptor proteins. These intracellular receptors bind the respective steroid hormones with high affinity and mediate their effects on gene expression and the synthesis of specific proteins. In many cells, steroid hormone actions are expressed through the synthesis of regulatory enzymes that control metabolic reactions, as exemplified by the effects of glucocorticoids on carbohydrate and protein metabolism in many cell types.[2] In more specialized tissues, steroid hormones induce cellular differentiation and stimulate the synthesis of structural and secreted proteins that may act locally or be transported in the circulation. Such responses are typical of the androgens and estrogens, which control the expression of several proteins that exert their actions in the reproductive tract and promote the growth of their target tissues.[3] The properties and actions of thyroid hormones are in many ways analogous to those of steroids, despite their chemical similarity to peptide hormones and amino acid transmitters. The physical properties of thyroid hormones are also more similar to those of steroids than to those of peptide ligands. Like steroids, circulating thyroid hormones are largely bound to specific plasma proteins and once inside target cells, they interact with nuclear receptor sites that regulate gene expression and protein synthesis.[4] However, their entry into target cells may involve specific transport mechanisms. The molecular cloning of the steroid hormone receptors has led to their recognition as members of a superfamily of transcriptional regulatory proteins that interact with specific DNA sequences (response elements) in the promoter regions of their target genes.[5]

The peptide, protein, and glycoprotein ligands that function as hormones and growth factors, along with transmitters such as catecholamines and acetylcholine, are characterized by their electrically charged and hydrophilic nature. Such ligands typically interact with highly selective cell-surface receptors that are embedded in the plasma membrane of their target cells. The specific binding of hormonal ligands alters the molecular conformation of their receptor sites and changes the activities of plasma membrane enzyme systems and ion channels that produce intracellular signals with transient or long-term effects on target cell function. In certain target tissues, such as the peripheral endocrine glands (adrenal, thyroid, and gonads), the maintenance of cellular differentiation and function is dependent on the trophic actions of the regulatory hormones. Thus, adrenocorticotropic hormone (ACTH), thyroid stimulating hormone (TSH), luteinizing hormone (LH), and follicle stimulating hormone (FSH) are analogous to gonadal steroids and certain growth factors in maintaining the differentiated state and secretory activity of their hormone-dependent target cells. Other peptide hormones, including insulin and catecholamines, are more similar to adrenal steroid hormones in exerting their major actions on metabolic processes rather than on target cell growth and differentiation.

Such generalizations about the major metabolic effects of steroid, thyroid, and peptide hormones are convenient for the broad functional classification of hormone action. In terms of their primary cellular actions, steroid and thyroid hormones act largely as regulators of *nuclear* events, whereas peptide hormones control *plasma membrane* and *cytoplasmic* processes. However, the domains of action of the individual hormones are not exclusive, and the major classes of ligands overlap considerably in their sites and modes of action. Thus, steroid and thyroid hormones exert several rapid extranuclear actions, and peptide hormones often influence gene expression and growth responses in addition to their effects on secretory and other rapid cytoplasmic responses. It is clear that an absolute distinction cannot be drawn between the two major classes of hormonal ligands in terms of their abilities to regulate metabolic and genomic responses to hormonal stimulation. All types of hormones share the ability to elicit genetically programmed target cell responses after binding to their specific plasma membrane or intracellular receptors.

Local Hormonal Regulation: Paracrine and Autocrine Secretion

The systemic actions of blood-borne hormones in controlling peripheral target cell function are often supplemented by the regulatory effects of locally formed messengers that control functional adjustments in response to the prevailing tissue requirements (see Chap. 1). Such local actions are exerted by the products of endocrine/paracrine cells (Fig. 5A-2) and regional neurons, which release amines and peptide hormones that act on adjacent target cells. Paracrine cells are abundant in epithelial structures in the thyroid gland and in the respiratory, gastrointestinal, and genitourinary tracts; local neurons have a similarly wide distribution in many organs and tissues. These central and local regulatory mechanisms are integrated by the neuroendocrine system, which is composed of neurons and endocrine cells that share common pathways of peptide synthesis, processing, and secretion. Their features include the coproduction of amine transmitters and peptides, the processing of large precursors to produce biologically active peptides, the costorage of amines and peptides in secretory granules, and the secretion of such stored products in response to synaptic or hormonal stimulation.[6] While the role of locally released amines in tissue regulation is less clear, the accompanying peptides appear to exert local hormonal actions and serve as neuropeptides by binding to receptors in regional target cells (such as smooth muscle in the intestine and airways) and in the adjacent intramural neuronal systems.

FIGURE 5A-2. The major modes of intercellular communication. The hormonal products of endocrine cells are released into the bloodstream to be carried to distant target cells. Paracrine cells release their products in proximity to neighboring cells, often from long processes with bulbous terminals. Autocrine cells release products which act on their own external receptors to regulate cell growth. Intracrine regulators (not shown) are formed within the target cell and bind directly to response elements without being released from the cell. (*Adapted from Hakanson and Sundler.*[6])

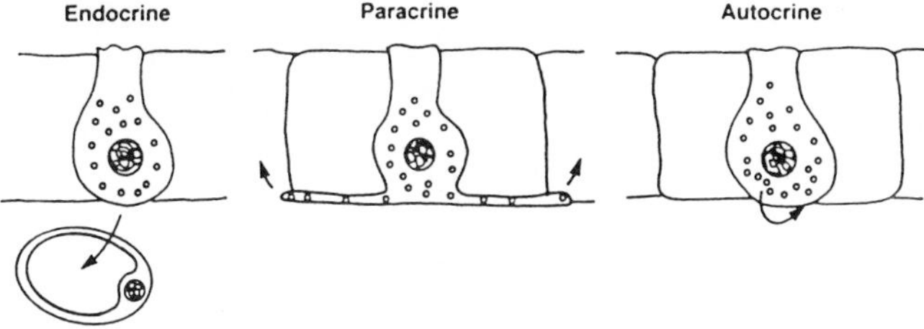

An additional form of local hormonal regulation which appears to be of major importance in the normal and aberrant control of cell proliferation by growth factors is *autocrine* control of cellular growth and differentiation (Fig. 5A-2). Many normal and transformed cells secrete peptides, such as transforming growth factors (TGF-α and TGF-β) and platelet-derived growth factor (PDGF), that bind to receptors in their cells of origin and stimulate or inhibit their proliferation. Such autocrine mechanisms of self-stimulation are probably important in physiologic processes such as wound healing and rapid embryonic growth, and their inappropriate expression in conditions such as atherosclerosis and neoplasia could be related to the pathogenesis of those disorders.[7] Other autocrine mechanisms include changes in the number or affinity of receptors for growth factors and the expression of proteins that subvert the normal pathways of hormone action. For example, the *erbB* oncogene promotes cell transformation by expressing truncated epidermal growth factor (EGF) receptors with unregulated growth activity. Also, several other oncogenes encode major regulatory components of the intracellular signaling pathways that mediate the normal growth response.[8]

Paracrine and autocrine interactions mediated by growth factors, cytokines, and peptide hormones are frequently involved in cell-cell communication in endocrine tissues. Interactions between lactotrophs and gonadotrophs have been established, and some of the hypothalamic releasing hormones [growth hormone releasing hormone (GHRH), gonadotropin releasing hormone (GnRH), and thyrotropin releasing hormone (TRH)] are expressed in the pituitary gland as well as in the hypothalamus. Also, activin is synthesized in gonadotrophs and acts locally on pituitary cells. In the testis, many paracrine factors appear to influence both Leydig cell and seminiferous tubule function, and the ovary is notable for the expression of a variety of growth factors and peptides that are potential modulators of follicle growth and maturation. In addition to these paracrine-type and autocrine-type mechanisms, a novel form of cellular control by internal signals has been proposed. It is based on the potential ability of certain receptor-related proteins [some of which may be receptors for as yet unidentified ligands (Chap. 5B)] to act as transcription factors and control gene expression and has been termed *intracrine* regulation.[9]

PEPTIDE HORMONE RECEPTORS

The ability of peptide hormones and transmitter molecules to generate intracellular signals by binding to receptor sites on the surfaces of their target cells was first demonstrated in 1960 by Sutherland and Robinson,[10] who found that catecholamines stimulate adenylyl cyclase activity in the plasma membrane to produce the second messenger, cyclic AMP. The originally proposed mechanism by which hormones activate the production of second messengers and physiologic responses is shown in Fig. 5A-3.[10] Since then, numerous peptide hormones and other ligands have been shown to interact with cell-surface receptors that influence plasma membrane–associated enzymes and ion channels. Many of these receptors do not activate their effector systems directly but through transducing proteins in the plasma membrane. However, several types of receptors possess intrinsic enzymatic or channel activity, as proposed in the original model for the activation of adenylyl cyclase.

The ability of endocrine target cells to respond to hormonal regulation depends on their expression of highly specific receptors that selectively bind the relevant information-bearing molecules present in the extracellular fluid. The extremely low concentration (about 10^{-10} M) of peptide hormones in the circulation in the presence of a million-fold excess of other proteins requires that target cell receptors possess both high specificity (to recognize the hormone) and high affinity (to bind the hormone at such low concentrations). Most of the receptors for pituitary, parathyroid, and gut hormones and many of those for neurotransmitters, neuropeptides and growth factors have been characterized recently by molecular cloning, and much has been learned about their primary structures and the regions involved in their binding and activation domains. The manner in which receptors and other intrinsic membrane proteins are believed to be embedded in the phospholipid bilayer of the plasma membrane is illustrated in Fig. 5A-4.[11] Another view of this arrangement is shown in Fig. 5A-5, which indicates the way in which the membrane proteins of the erythrocyte are coupled to a submembranous meshwork of spectrin, actin, and associated proteins by ankyrin and protein 4.1. The lipid bilayer is also stabilized by low-affinity interactions between these proteins and the negatively charged phospholipids.[12]

In addition to their extracellular binding domains, peptide hormone receptors possess transmembrane regions and a specialized cytoplasmic domain that mediates intracellular signaling. In many receptors, the signaling domains interact with intermediate regulatory proteins that control plasma membrane enzymes such as adenylyl cyclase and phospholipase C.[13] In others, ligand binding activates enzymes, such as protein kinase and guanylate cyclase, that are intrinsic to the receptor. Through these mechanisms, the binding of hormones to their cell-surface receptors causes rapid changes in cyclic nucleotide production, phospholipid metabolism, calcium mobilization, ion fluxes, protein phosphorylation, and membrane transport systems. These processes lead in turn to the activation or inhibition of cytoplasmic and nuclear signaling pathways that regulate target cell function. Many of these regulatory steps involve phosphorylation of membrane or cytoplasmic proteins, with subsequent changes in

FIGURE 5A-3. Sutherland's classical concept of the hormone as the first messenger and cyclic AMP (or other mediators) as the intracellular second messenger, which is rapidly produced and degraded and through which peptide hormone action is expressed. (*From Sutherland and Robison.*[10])

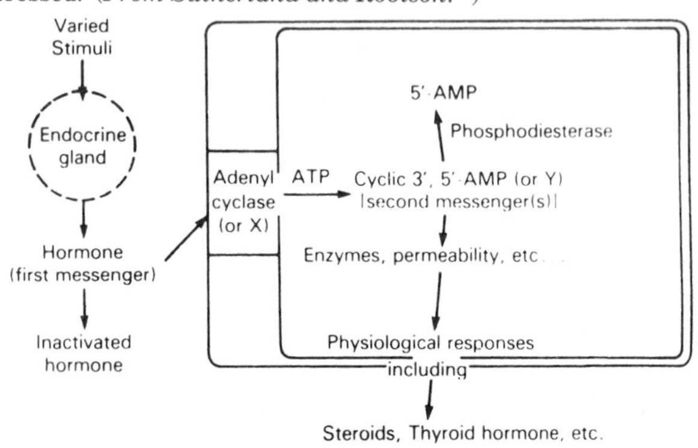

FIGURE 5A-4. The structure of the plasma membrane as proposed by Singer and Nicholson.[11] The proteins of the plasma membrane are visualized as floating within the phospholipid matrix, with some spanning the lipid bilayer and others embedded in the inner or outer surface of the membrane. Proteins protruding on the external surface of the cell are predominantly glycoproteins, as indicated by their attached carbohydrate residues. Many of these proteins function as receptors for extracellular ligands and in turn interact with other membrane-associated proteins during the transmission of hormonal signals to the interior of the cell. Proteins that are associated with the inner surface of the membrane are frequently linked to the lipid bilayers by prenyl groups, which are polyunsaturated hydrocarbons composed of repeating 5-carbon isoprene molecules attached by a thioether bond to cysteine residues.

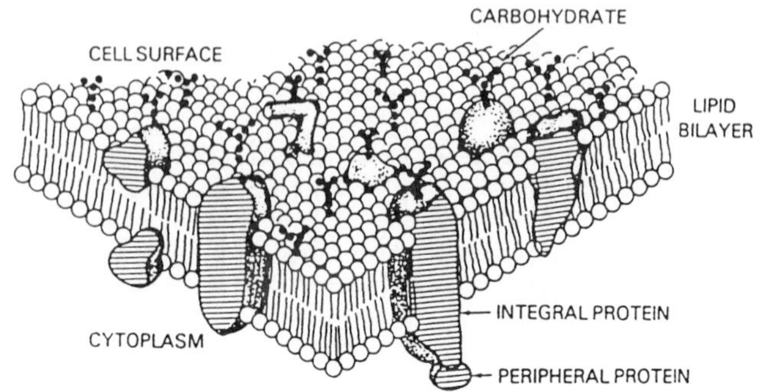

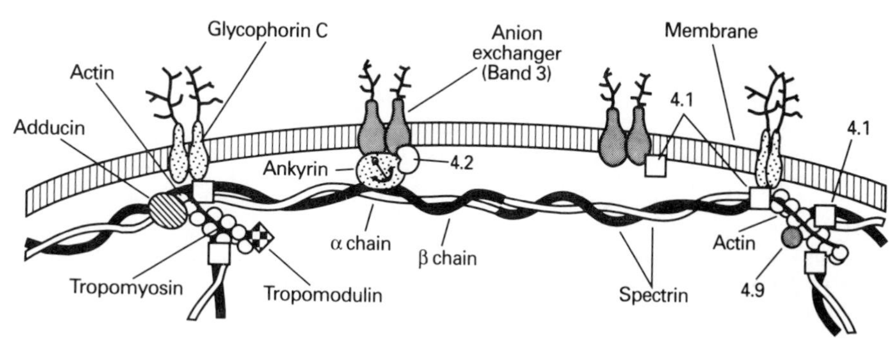

FIGURE 5A-5. Attachments between plasma membrane proteins and the cytoskeleton in erythrocytes. Membrane stability is maintained by the underlying meshwork of spectrin, actin, and other proteins, which is attached to the plasma membrane by ankyrin and protein 4.1. Spectrin and other membrane skeleton components contain specialized domains for interaction with proteins that influence actin polymerization and other processes involved in membrane-cytoskeleton interactions. (*From Luna and Hitt.*[12])

the activities of enzymes responsible for the synthesis, transport, or metabolism of molecules that are essential for cellular activity.[14]

The intermediary proteins that couple receptors to their effector systems are termed G proteins because of their dependence on the guanyl nucleotide guanosine triphosphate (GTP) for their regulatory actions. The G proteins, which are described in detail later in this chapter, are heterotrimers composed of α, β, and γ subunits. During hormone binding to the receptor, the G protein becomes activated by the binding of GTP to its α subunit and dissociates into α-GTP and βγ components. The activated α subunits, and in some cases the βγ subunits, interact with effector enzymes such as adenylyl cyclase and phospholipase C and stimulate or inhibit their activity. The major G proteins involved in signal transduction include G_s and G_i, which couple receptors to the stimulation or inhibition, respectively, of adenylyl cyclase, and G_q, which couples receptors to the stimulation of phospholipase C. The G proteins are also characterized by sensitivity to bacterial toxins. G_s and G_i are sensitive to cholera and pertussis toxins, respectively, and G_q is unaffected by such toxins.

One of the major plasma membrane enzymes regulated by peptide hormones is adenylyl cyclase, which catalyzes the formation of cyclic AMP from ATP. The cyclic nucleotide produced during receptor activation stimulates *cAMP-dependent protein kinase*, a widely distributed cytoplasmic enzyme that initiates many phosphorylation-dependent events involved in target cell regulation.[15] Of equal importance is the group of phospholipases (A_2, C, and D) that catalyze the cleavage and deacylation of membrane phospholipids. These enzymes selectively digest plasma membrane components to generate intracellular messengers (inositol trisphosphate and diacylglycerol) that mobilize calcium and activate Ca^{2+}-dependent enzymes such as Ca^{2+}-calmodulin and Ca^{2+}-phospholipid-dependent protein kinases. Phospholipid hydrolysis also provides arachidonic acid for conversion to prostaglandins (PGs), prostacyclins, leukotrienes, and other active metabolites. Many growth-promoting hormones activate receptor-associated and cytoplasmic tyrosine and serine/threonine protein kinases that mediate signal transduction to the nucleus of the cell. Thus, several distinct enzyme systems and ion channels in the plasma membrane or in the receptor itself participate in the integrated responses of target cells to receptor activation by the homologous hormone (Table 5A-1).

Binding Properties of Peptide Hormone Receptors

A universal feature of hormone receptors is their ability to bind the corresponding chemical messenger or hormone in the presence of a vast excess of other molecular species. There is usually a close relation between hormone binding and the subsequent biochemical responses at the plasma membrane level. For example, receptor occupancy and cyclic AMP production are closely correlated during the actions of ACTH in the adrenal, glucagon in the liver, vasopressin in the kidney, catecholamines in the avian erythrocyte, FSH in the seminiferous tubule, and LH in the testis and ovary. The specific and high-affinity binding of radiolabeled agonist or antagonist ligands provides a valid measure of hormone receptors when appropriate requirements of the binding technique are observed.[16] These include the use of a labeled hormone of demonstrated biological activity (prepared by monoiodination or tritiation), accurate determination of nonspecific binding, and exclusion of binding to metabolizing or degradative enzymes in tissue fractions.

The majority of hormone receptors exhibit high specificity for biologically active hormones and their agonist or antagonist derivatives, high binding affinity with noncovalent and reversible interactions with equilibrium dissociation constants of 10^{-9} to 10^{-11} *M*, and saturability at relatively low hormone concentrations. These properties are consistent with the high selectivity and low concentration of hormone receptors, which usually range from hundreds to tens of thousands of sites per cell in endocrine target tissues. The specific binding of peptide hor-

TABLE 5A-1 Plasma Membrane Receptors and Effector Systems

Receptors	Primary Effector Systems
CRH, GHRH, ACTH, TSH, MSH, LH, FSH, VIP, glucagon, PACAP, PTH, calcitonin, vasopressin V_2, β-adrenergic, dopamine D_1, serotonin $5HT_3$	Adenylyl cyclase: activation
α_2-Adrenergic, somatostatin, opiate, muscarinic M_2 and M_4, adenosine A_1, angiotensin II, serotonin $5HT_1$	Adenylyl cyclase: inhibition
ANP	Guanylyl cyclase: activation
α_1-Adrenergic, muscarinic M_1 and M_3, histamine H_1, vasopressin V_1, TRH, GnRH, angiotensin II, serotonin $5HT_2$, PDGF, thrombin	Phospholipase C: activation Calcium: mobilization
EGF, insulin, IGF-1, PDGF, FGF	Intrinsic receptor tyrosine kinase: activation
Growth hormone, prolactin, other cytokines	Cytoplasmic tyrosine kinase: activation
Activin, TGF-β	Serine/threonine phosphorylation: activation
Nicotinic acetylcholine	Sodium channel: activation
GABA, glycine	Chloride channel: activation
Muscarinic M_2	Potassium channel: inhibition

Abbreviations: ACTH, adrenocorticotropin; ANP, atrial natriuretic peptide; CRH, corticotropin releasing hormone; EGF, epidermal growth factor; FGF, fibroblast growth factor: FSH, follicle stimulating hormone; GABA, γ-aminobutyric acid; GnRH, gonadotropin releasing hormone; GHRH, growth hormone releasing hormone; 5HT, 5-hydroxytryptamine; IGF, insulin-like growth factor; LH, luteinizing hormone; MSH, melanocyte stimulating hormone; PACAP, pituitary adenylate cyclase activating peptide; PDGF, platelet-derived growth factor; PTH, parathyroid hormone; TGF, tranforming growth factor; TRH, thyrotropin releasing hormone; TSH-thyrotropin; VIP, vasoactive intestinal peptide

mones to their receptors is highly temperature-dependent and usualy proceeds rapidly at 37°C in a diffusion-limited manner. In contrast, the rate of dissociation of the hormone-receptor complex varies widely for individual ligand-receptor pairs, and there is sometimes a tightly associated and poorly reversible component of the bound hormone. The rates of ligand binding and dissociation and the turnover of hormone molecules and receptor sites under in vivo conditions of temperature and tissue perfusion are important determinants of the physiologic consequences of hormone-receptor interactions at the target cell level.

The Nature of Hormone-Receptor Interactions

The binding of all classes of hormones to their plasma membrane receptors depends on electrostatic interactions, hydrophobic effects, hydrogen bonds, and van der Waals forces. For many peptides, electrostatic interactions are major determinants of receptor binding. Thus, a basic region of the ACTH molecule is important for binding to adrenal receptors, and the binding of angiotensin II to adrenal receptors is markedly influenced by the basicity of the amino-terminal residue. Hydrophobic effects lead to favorable free energy changes caused by the elimination of the repulsive influences of charges in water through contacts with hydrophobic surfaces. The importance of hydrophobic effects in hormone-receptor binding is indicated by the effects of temperature on the binding process. The role of hydrophobic interactions in receptor binding has been indicated by x-ray diffraction studies on the three-dimensional structures of insulin and glucagon.[17] In the insulin molecule, the relatively constant surface region that determines biological activity contains many hydrophobic residues. Binding of insulin to its receptor has been proposed to occur by a process analogous to dimerization and to depend on hydrophobic effects and hydrogen bonds. In contrast to the relatively rigid structure of insulin, which may determine the spatial arrangement of the amino acids involved in receptor binding, the glucagon molecule has an elongated and fairly flexible structure. It is possible that the biologically active conformation is a helical structure that interacts with the receptor through two hydrophobic regions at each end of the helix.

Although much is known about the mechanisms involved in receptor binding and activation, the processes that terminate hormone-receptor interaction are less well defined. In addition to reversal of the binding reaction by dissociation in accordance with the law of mass action, other mechanisms can determine the duration of receptor activation in an intact cell. Proteolysis of the bound hormone could promote its release, but hormone degradation by isolated target cells is largely unrelated to receptor-binding sites. Indeed, hormones that are specifically bound to target tissues usually retain full biological activity after elution from the receptor sites. An important mechanism for the termination of hormone binding is the fall in receptor affinity that occurs when GTP binds to the inactive guanyl nucleotide-dependent regulatory protein (G protein) during its association with the agonist-activated receptor in the plasma membrane.[18] Such decreases in binding affinity in the presence of GTP are typical of hormones that control the activities of adenylyl cyclase and phospholipase C via transducing G proteins, as will be discussed later in this chapter. In addition to such reversible changes in receptor function, significant numbers of hormone-receptor complexes are cleared from the cell surface by internalization and in some cases are irreversibly inactivated by subsequent intracellular processing.

Hormonal Activation of Receptors

Hormone receptors undergo major changes in molecular conformation and mobility when they are activated by agonist ligands. The agonist-induced conformational changes lead to interaction with other membrane components, including transducing G proteins that activate effector enzymes, and in some cases to dimerization with other receptors of the same type. In these manners, the binding of agonist (but not antagonist) ligands triggers changes to new receptor configurations that permit the information encoded in the receptor to be expressed through its membrane effector systems. Other maneuvers that perturb cell-surface receptors, in particular cross-linking and aggregation by lectins and receptor antibodies, can also cause receptor activation and stimulation of cell responses. For this reason, receptor antibodies, including those to receptors for TSH, insulin, EGF, and prolactin, can exert agonist-like effects on their respective target cells.[19] Similarly, GnRH analogues and deglycosylated human chorionic gonadotropin (hCG) derivatives that act as receptor-blocking antagonists can cause target cell activation when cross-linked by specific antibodies to these ligands. Many growth factor and cytokine receptors undergo dimerization after agonist binding, and this initiates the subsequent phosphorylation cascade that leads to the cellular response. However, there is no evidence that dimerization is necessary for the physiologic activation of other classes of hormone receptors.

Many of the processes involved in cell growth, movement, and recognition are coordinated by a supramolecular complex of cell-surface receptors and submembranous fibrillar structures by which changes in receptor conformation, mobility, and distribution are related to changes in the associated cytoplasmic components.[12] Receptors may be uniformly distributed over the cell surface or arranged in specific regions of the cell, as in polarized cells (e.g., of the renal tubule) and at the neuromuscular junction, where about 10^7 acetylcholine receptors are clustered under the motor end plate. Such clustering favors rapid responses and maximizes signal amplification and may involve specific proteins that link the receptors with the plasma membrane. Structural interactions with submembranous components are probably responsible for the aggregation (clustering, patching, and capping) of receptors induced by divalent antibodies and multivalent lectins. In some cells, binding of hormonal ligands also leads to receptor redistribution in the cell membrane, often with clustering of sites at microdomains that participate in endocytosis, and sometimes to the formation of aggregates on the cell surface. Such clustering is a prelude to internalization of the hormone-receptor complexes but may also be important in the early phase of hormone action. However, the extent to which ligands other than growth factors and cytokines exert their cellular actions via receptor dimerization and clustering is uncertain. Also, the ability of cross-linking maneuvers to mimic hormonal activation by perturbing the receptor does not necessarily reflect the physiologic mechanism by which specific ligand binding elicits target cell responses. The manner in which the several types of cell-surface receptors are activated by their ligands is discussed in detail in subsequent sections.

Receptor Occupancy and Activation of Target Cell Responses

In most endocrine target cells, activation of membrane effector systems and target cell responses by agonist ligands is proportional to the degree of receptor occupancy. However, the hormone concentration at which receptors are half-saturated (K_d) is often lower than the concentration required to elicit a half-maximal biological response (ED_{50}), and maximal cellular responses are evoked by occupancy of only a small proportion of the available receptors (Fig. 5A-6). Also, many hormones can stimulate a much greater degree of intracellular signal generation (e.g., of cyclic AMP) than is necessary to evoke a maximal cellular response. This is attributable to the presence in many hormone-responsive tissues of so-called spare or excess receptors, which were first observed during studies on drug-responsive tissues.[20] Even when present in great excess over the number needed to elicit the maximal cell response,

FIGURE 5A-6. Dose-response relations between hormone binding, cyclic AMP production, steroid production, and agonist concentration in hormone-stimulated gonadal and adrenal cells.

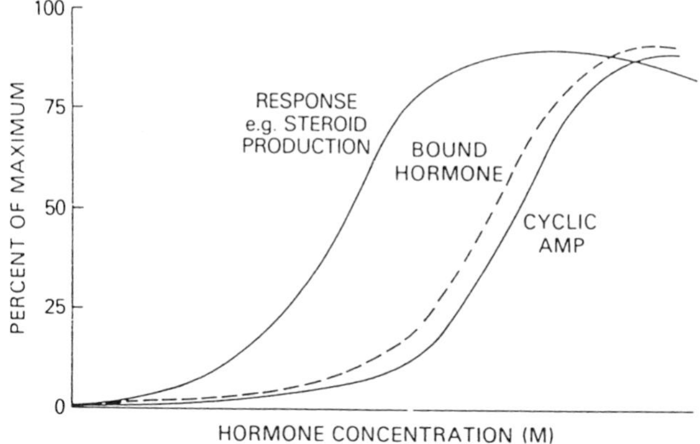

such spare sites are by no means superfluous. Spare receptors serve as a reservoir of surface receptors and also increase the sensitivity of the target cell to activation by low hormone concentrations. Thus, the presence of a high density of plasma membrane receptors would favor greater receptor occupancy at low hormone concentrations and more rapid ligand association to attain the critical level of occupancy that causes target cell activation.

The term *spare receptors* is used in a relative sense, and the degree of receptor excess may differ in accordance with the biological response that is measured.[21] For example, hormone receptors are rarely "spare" for adenylyl cyclase. Thus, ligand binding and adenylyl cyclase activation are closely correlated, even if in a nonlinear manner, and increasing occupancy of hormone receptors is usually accompanied by serial increases in cAMP production. In contrast, measurements of more distal responses such as muscle contraction, steroidogenesis, glucose oxidation, and lipolysis show that the maximum biological response is frequently evoked by occupancy of only a small fraction of the receptor population (Fig. 5A-6). This is attributable to the marked amplification of receptor activation that occurs during the subsequent steps that lead to the final cell response. Clearly, hormonal activation of the small number of receptors needed to elicit the cellular response would be facilitated by the presence of a relatively large pool of receptors at the target cell surface. An additional role for spare receptors is to serve as a reservoir of available sites during the continuous processing and degradation of receptors that occur during the course of hormonal activation of target cell function.

The presence of excess receptors has been demonstrated by direct binding studies with labeled hormones in certain cells and target tissues. For example, in the interstitial cells of the testis, hormone binding to only 5 to 10 LH receptors per cell is sufficient to initiate androgen secretion, and occupancy of only 1 percent of the gonadotropin receptor population is sufficient to elicit maximum testosterone production.[22] Further binding of hormone causes a progressive increase in cAMP production, since most of the receptors are functionally active and are coupled to stimulation of adenylyl cyclase. Similarly, occupancy of less than 0.25 percent of the muscarinic receptors in guinea pig ileum will elicit a half-maximal contractile response. However, in some tissues, hormone binding and the subsequent biological response are closely related over the entire range of receptor occupancy. In the adrenal zona glomerulosa, the binding of angiotensin II to its receptors causes a progressive increase in aldosterone production with increasing receptor occupancy, consistent with the presence of few, if any, spare angiotensin receptors.[23] There is also a close correlation betwen insulin binding and stimulation of amino acid transport in isolated thymocytes. The relation between receptor occupancy and specific cellular responses varies widely among individual target tissues, from the extreme case of Leydig cells with full activation by minimal receptor occupancy to the almost continuous relation between receptor occupancy and response in glomerulosa cells and thymocytes. Within a single cell type, increasing degrees of receptor occupancy can elicit sequential biological responses. In fat cells, occupancy of only a few insulin receptors is sufficient to inhibit lipolysis, whereas glucose metabolism is maximally stimulated when only 2 to 3 percent of the receptors are occupied and amino acid transport and protein synthesis are stimulated at higher degrees of receptor occupancy.[24]

In general, when hormone binding and biological responses are closely related, the receptors are limiting in terms of target cell activation. When abundant or spare receptors are present, the more distal elements are limiting; in the case of adenylyl cyclase–mediated responses, the limiting step is often after the formation of cyclic AMP, which can be produced in much greater amounts than necessary to elicit the target cell response. In many tissues, hormonal stimulation is accompanied by release of cAMP into the surrounding extracellular fluid, sometimes with elevation of blood and/or urinary levels of the cyclic nucleotide. Since this occurs in the kidney during the infusion of parathyroid hormone, the urinary excretion of cAMP provides a diagnostic test for the hormone resistance that occurs in patients with pseudohypoparathyroidism.

Chemical and Physical Properties of Peptide Hormone Receptors

The cell-surface receptors for peptide hormones and transmitters are membrane-spanning proteins and are anchored by one or several hydrophobic membrane-spanning domains that are usually flanked by charged amino acids.[25] Some receptors also possess lipid residues attached to amino acids in their intracellular region that contribute to their attachment to the plasma membrane. Several cell-surface proteins are attached to the plasma membrane by phosphatidylinositol residues that are covalently linked to their carboxy-terminal regions, but this form of attachment has not been found to occur in hormone receptors. Carbohydrate moieties are present in the extracellular domains of peptide hormone receptors and are a common feature of cell-surface recognition sites. Most receptors depend on disulfide groups for the maintenance of their biologically active conformation, in particular in their ligand-binding domains, and some are sensitive to treatment with reducing agents. Peptide hormone receptors, like other membrane proteins, are relatively insoluble in aqueous solutions and must be extracted from tissue homogenates or cell membranes with mild nonionic detergents for physical and biochemical analysis. Several solubilized receptors have been purified and reconstituted into artificial lipid bilayers with their effector systems or into host cell membranes for studies of their activation mechanisms. Solubilized hormone receptors have been purified by conventional fractionation procedures and by affinity chromatography on gel-ligand complexes. In many cases, such procedures have been employed to isolate quantities of receptor protein sufficient for partial sequence analysis, enabling the construction of specific DNA probes for the isolation of receptor clones from cDNA libraries prepared from mRNA extracted from the appropriate target tissues.

RECEPTOR STRUCTURE AND FUNCTION

Major progress has been made in the structural characterization of plasma membrane receptor sites for numerous hormones and other extracellular ligands that regulate cell function. In the last few years, the primary structures of most of the known receptors have been determined by molecular cloning and sequencing of their cDNAs (Chap. 3). The structural analysis of cell membrane receptors for transmitters and peptide hormones has revealed several new aspects of receptor organization and has begun to clarify the manner in which the molecular properties of receptors are related to their ligand-binding and signal-generating functions. The structural and functional properties of several typical receptors for transmitters, hormones, and growth factors are described below. The major subgroups of the cell-surface receptors involved in signal transduction are ligand-gated ion channels, G protein–coupled receptors, and growth factor receptors (Fig. 5A-7).

Ligand-Gated Ion Channels

Neural transmission depends on the appropriate release of chemical transmitters and the operation of two main groups of proteins in neuronal membranes. These are (1) the receptors for neurotransmitters and neuromodulators, many of which are coupled directly or indirectly to ion channels [acetylcholine (ACh), glutamate, γ-aminobutyric acid (GABA), glycine, and others], and (2) voltage-dependent ion channels for sodium, potassium, and calcium. Invertebrate and vertebrate neuroreceptors and ion channels are encoded by multigene superfamilies, members of which have diverged during evolution to produce an impressive variety of subtypes.[26] The simplest receptors, at least in principle, are those in which the receptor and effector components are contained within a single molecule or complex of molecular subunits. Many of the molecular complexes are ionotropic receptors that contain an integral ion channel and are operated by ligands that bind directly to influence channel opening or closing. The superfamily of ligand-gated ion channels includes a number of neurotransmitter receptors (nicotinic, glutamate, GABA, glycine, and $5HT_3$) that are formed of several subunits with common structural features. These include a large amino-terminal extracellular domain, a series of four putative transmembrane domains (M1 to M4), and a carboxy-terminal domain that is also extracellular. The transmitter binding site is located in the large extracellular segment, which contains three loops involved in the binding domain, and the M2 transmembrane domain lines the ion channel. The ligand-gated receptor channels are usually composed of several distinct subunits with considerable amino acid homology. However, some of the individual subunits can form functional channels when expressed as homooligomers in heterologous cells. A typical

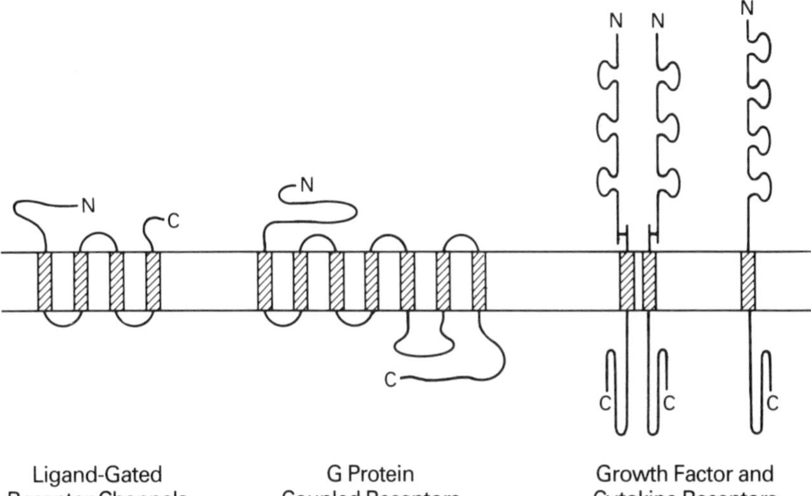

FIGURE 5A-7. Basic structures of the major groups of plasma membrane receptors for transmitters, peptide hormones, growth factors, and cytokines.

ligand-gated channel is the nicotinic receptor for ACh that is present at vertebrate neuromuscular junctions and throughout the central nervous system.

The Nicotinic Acetylcholine Receptor

The nicotinic ACh receptors on muscle and nerve cells form a family of ligand-gated channels that control sodium influx and participate in fast synaptic transmission by depolarizing the cell membrane. As a result of its abundance in the electric organ of certain fish, the nicotinic ACh receptor was the first cell-surface receptor to be extensively characterized and sequenced.[27] The nicotinic receptor of *Torpedo* electric organ and skeletal muscle is a heterooligomer formed of four peptide chains—α, β, γ, and δ—with molecular mass of 40, 50, 60 and 65 kDa, respectively. The subunits have considerable amino acid homology and are combined in the ratio $\alpha_2\beta\gamma\delta$ to form a 250-kDa pentameric receptor that spans the plasma membrane.[28] In adult muscle of some species, the γ subunit is replaced by an ϵ subunit. The receptor binds cholinergic ligands and serves as a ligand-regulated channel through which sodium ions pass when the pore is opened during agonist activation.[29] The α subunit contains the binding site for acetylcholine and other nicotinic agonists, and the other subunits are involved in the formation and function of the ion channel. Neuronal nicotinic receptors are formed mainly of α and β subunits that are encoded by several distinct genes, giving seven α and four β subunits.[30] They also differ from muscle receptors in their higher permeability to calcium and in being modulated by extracellular calcium, which enhances their ion current responses to ACh by increasing the frequency of opening of activated channels.[31]

The holoreceptor molecule is about 8 nm in diameter and 11 nm in length and extends across the plasma membrane to protrude about 5 nm above the cell surface. The outer face of the ACh receptor bears a 2.5-nm pit which leads to an 0.65-nm ion translocation pore through which sodium passes during the ligand-induced gating process. Like most cell membrane receptors, the outer surface of the molecule is glycosylated and generally hydrophilic but also contains hydrophobic domains that interact with corresponding regions of the activating ligand molecule. All subunits are exposed on both sides of the plasma membrane and contain four α-helical transmembrane segments. The ion channel within the transmembrane receptor is lined by a ring of M2 subunits, each of which contributes to the formation of the pore.[32] The vestibules of the holoreceptor contain rings of negatively charged glutamic and aspartic acid residues to exclude anions, and the ion channel is lined by hydrophilic uncharged residues to accommodate the high rate of flow of hydrated cations during the few milliseconds during which the pore remains open after agonist activation. Thus, the 250-kDa pentameric receptor contains the acetylcholine-binding site, the ion channel, and the structural elements involved in the regulation of channel opening by ACh (Fig. 5A-8). The clustering of ACh receptors in the postsynaptic region of the plasma membrane appears to depend on their interaction with a 43-kDa protein that serves as a link between the receptor molecules and the cytoskeleton.[33] Recently, a chimeric channel formed from the α7 subunit of the neuronal ACh receptor and the transmembrane domains of the $5HT_3$ receptor was found to possess the pharmacologic properties of the former receptor and the ion channel properties of the latter.[34] This has clearly assigned the neurotransmitter binding and calcium modulation to the large N-terminal hydrophilic domain, and the ion channel properties to the transmembrane regions of the molecule.

Glutamate Receptors

The principal excitatory neurotransmitter, glutamate, acts on cation-selective receptor channels that are present in most neural and glial cells in vertebrates, often at the neuromuscular junction in invertebrates. Three main subtypes of glutamate receptors have been defined according to their sensitivity to activation by three agonist ligands: AMPA (α-amino-3-hydroxy-5-methyl-isoxazole-4-propionate), kainate, and NMDA (*N*-methyl-D-aspartate).[35] AMPA receptors mainly carry Na^+ ions and small amounts of Ca^{2+} into the cell and are largely responsible for rapid excitatory neurotransmission. They are composed of four related subunits with molecular mass of 108 kDa, each containing four transmem-

FIGURE 5A-8. Structure of the nicotinic acetylcholine receptor of *Torpedo* electric tissue and skeletal muscle. In the adult skeletal muscle of several species, the γ subunit is replaced by an ϵ subunit. The cylinders within each subunit represent the M2 membrane-spanning domains that line the ion channel. (*From Sackman.*[42])

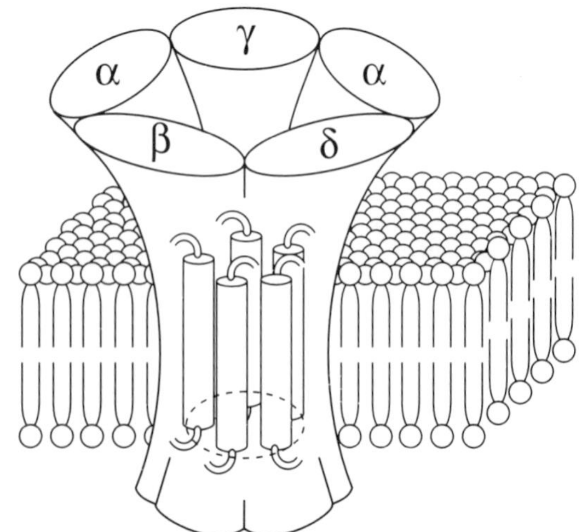

brane domains that contribute to the formation of the central ion channel. Kainate receptors are abundant in the hippocampus and the peripheral neurons of dorsal root ganglia. They are related to AMPA receptors and are composed of five subunits. Kainate receptors can be activated by AMPA, and kainate can activate AMPA receptors, consistent with the overlapping functional properties of those two glutamate receptor subtypes.

NMDA receptors play a major role in many aspects of glutamate transmission in the central nervous system. They are abundant in hippocampal and other neurons and are essential participants in the induction of long-term potentiation, in which synchronously activated neuronal networks are stabilized by selective strengthening of their synaptic connections. Thus, activation of NMDA receptors is involved in learning and memory formation.[36] NMDA receptors are notable for their large calcium conductance, their requirement for glycine as a coagonist, and their voltage-dependent blockade by Mg^{2+}. Also, NMDA receptors exhibit a prolonged opening time of several hundred milliseconds, in contrast to the transient opening of AMPA and kainate receptors. These properties of NMDA receptors are important in their role of synchronizing neural firing and increasing synaptic strength. When neurons are activated by other excitatory synapses, the resulting depolarization relieves the voltage-dependent block by Mg^{2+} and favors activation of NMDA receptors, with a correspondingly increased and prolonged influx of calcium that promotes long-lasting enhancement of synaptic efficacy.[37] The rise in cytoplasmic Ca^{2+} during activation of NMDA receptors is a crucial component not only of neural plasticity but also of glutamate-mediated neuronal toxicity. The major subunit of the NMDA receptors (NR1) shows marked structural similarities with those of AMPA and kainate receptors.[38] These similarities include the presence of four transmembrane domains, one of which (TM2) carries an aspartate residue in place of the glutamine/arginine ($^{Q}/_{R}$) site of the AMPA kainate subunits. This change causes a selective increase in the permeability of the ion channel for Ca^{2+} over Mg^{2+}.[39] The NR1 subunit occurs in several spliced forms that differ in their intracellular amino- and carboxy-terminal regions and have different pharmacologic properties.

In addition to the key subunit of the NMDA receptor (NR1) originally cloned from the rat brain,[38] an additional group of four receptor subunits (NR2A–NR2D) has been isolated from the same source. These subunits show only about 15 percent sequence homology with the NR1 receptor and possess large hydrophilic carboxy-terminal domains in addition to the amino-terminal hydrophilic termini that precede the first transmembrane domain.[39] Whereas the NR1 subunit is expressed in most neurons throughout the brain, the NR2 subunits show overlapping but distinct expression patterns in regions such as the cerebral cortex, hippocampus, forebrain, cerebellum, and diencephalon/brainstem.[40] The NR2 subunits do not form ion channels but appear to modulate the properties of the heteromeric NMDA receptors formed by their assembly with the NR1 subunits. Thus, the functional properties and neural distributions of the subunits are consistent with the concept of heteromeric receptors composed of a common NR1 subunit and a modulatory NR2 subunit.[39] The existence of several distinct forms of the NR1 subunit, along with the formation of heterodimers with the four NR2 subunits, accounts for the functional diversity of the NMDA receptor.

There is also a nonionotropic glutamate receptor subtype, termed the *metabotropic* receptor (mGluR), that is coupled to a pertussis toxin–sensitive G protein which activates phosphoinositide hydrolysis and calcium mobilization. These receptors increase neural firing in hippocampal, thalamic, and spinal neurons and have been implicated in modulation of neuronal plasticity and neuronal degeneration.[37] Metabotropic receptors are 133-kDa proteins that contain seven transmembrane regions and have unusually large extracellular and intracellular domains. The mGluR is activated by L-glutamate and 1S,3R-APCD (1S,3R-1-aminocyclopentyl-1,3-decarboxylate) and is antagonized by MCPG (α-methyl-4-carboxyl-phenylglycine). In addition to activating phospholipase C, mGluR has been proposed to stimulate the production of carbon monoxide and the consequent formation of cGMP by activation of guanylyl cyclase.[41]

GABA Receptors

γ-aminobutyric acid is the most important inhibitory neurotransmitter in the mammalian central nervous system. Its actions are mediated by two types of receptors, of which the classical benzodiazepine-sensitive $GABA_A$ receptors that are coupled to Cl^- channels and mediate rapid inhibitory neurotransmission are the best defined.[42] The more recently identified $GABA_B$ receptors are activated by baclofen and act presynaptically to modulate the release of neurotransmitters and neuropeptides [including GABA, glutamate, noradrenaline, dopamine, 5HT, substance P, cholecystokinin cystokinin (CCK), and somatostatin].[43] Postsynaptic $GABA_B$ receptors appear to be coupled to K^+ channels through G proteins and mediate late inhibitory postsynaptic potentials.

The $GABA_A$ receptor belongs to the superfamily of ligand-gated ion channels and is a heterooligomeric complex of five polypeptide subunits (α, β, γ, δ, ρ) that traverse the membrane and form a chloride ion channel.[44] Each subunit has a large glycosylated extracellular domain linked to four transmembrane segments and a short extracellular carboxy-terminal domain. A large cytoplasmic loop between the third and fourth transmembrane segments contains potential phosphorylation sites that could be involved in the regulation of receptor function. $GABA_A$ receptors are activated by several central nervous system (CNS) depressant drugs, notably the benzodiazepines, that enhance inhibitory neurotransmission by increasing the probability of channel opening by GABA. Conversely, certain convulsants, such as picrotoxin, block chloride channel function by decreasing the mean open time and attenuating inhibitory transmission.

Glycine Receptors

Glycine, like GABA, is a major inhibitory neurotransmitter in the CNS. Whereas GABA is the predominant neuroinhibitory ligand in the brain, glycine is more important in the brainstem and spinal cord. The glycine receptor is a multimeric couple of α and β subunits that forms a glycine-regulated chloride channel in the postsynaptic neuronal membrane. The α-subunit gene can give rise to at least three splice variants, and each subunit contains four transmembrane segments (M1–M4), of which M2 expands to line the ligand-gated channel that conducts chloride ions. The glycine receptor subunits show amino acid sequence homology with the GABA and nicotinic ACh receptors and combine to form a pentameric receptor that contains a central chloride-selective anion channel. The conductance function of the anion channel is blocked by the convulsive alkaloid strychnine, which binds to the α subunit and inhibits chloride transport through the channel. In phospholipid bilayers, synthetic peptides and four-helix bundle proteins containing the amino acid sequence of the M2 transmembrane segment of the α subunit form anion-selective channels that have the properties of the native glycine receptor.[45]

The $5HT_3$ Serotonin Receptor

The actions of serotonin [5-hydroxytryptamine (5HT)] in neural and other cells are mediated by seven types of receptors ($5HT_1$–$5HT_4$), six of which are coupled to G proteins and one of which ($5HT_3$) is a ligand-gated ion channel. Whereas the G protein–coupled 5HT receptors mediate the activation of second messenger systems and modulate the function of ion channels, the $5HT_3$ receptor mediates rapid neuronal depolarization and excitatory responses. It is intriguing that at least four neurotransmitters—5HT, ACh, glutamate, and GABA—activate both ligand-gated ion channels and G protein–coupled receptors. The amino acid sequence of the 50-kDa $5HT_3$ receptor has several similarities with those of other ligand-gated channel subunits, including the presence of four hydrophobic transmembrane domains (M1–M4), a large amino-terminal extracellular domain, and a long cytoplasmic loop between M3 and M4. The expressed $5HT_3$ receptor is a cation-selective channel and is modulated by external Ca^{2+} and Mg^{2+}, like the NMDA and neural nicotinic ACh receptor channels.[46] It is likely that the $5HT_3$ receptor has multiple subtypes formed of several different subunits and that these subtypes account for the different properties of the receptors expressed in various tissues.

G Protein–Coupled Receptors

Many peptide hormones, neurotransmitters, and other regulatory ligands elicit cellular responses by binding to cell-surface receptors that are coupled via heterotrimeric G proteins to a variety of effector enzymes and channels in the plasma membrane. The number of such factors that bind to G protein–coupled receptors is exceeded to a considerable extent by the number of receptors and subtypes that have been identified by pharmacologic studies and molecular cloning (Table 5A-2). Neurotransmitter receptors include 10 types of adrenergic receptors; 5 types of muscarinic and dopamine receptors; several serotonergic, purinergic, and light (rhodopsin) receptors; and a group of odorant receptors.[47] There is also a multiplicity of receptor subtypes for the peptide hor-

TABLE 5A-2 The G Protein–Coupled Seven-Transmembrane Domain Receptor Superfamily

Peptide Hormones	*Neurotransmitters*
Hypothalamic hormones	Adrenergic agents
CRH, GnRH, GHRH, TRH	α_1-adrenergic (α_{1A}–α_{1D})
	α_2-adrenergic (α_{2A}–α_{2c})
Pituitary hormones	β-adrenergic (β_1–β_3)
ACTH, MSH, LH, FSH, TSH	Other amines
	Dopamine (D_1-D_5)
Neurohypophysial peptides	Histamine (H_1-H_3)
	Octopamine
Oxytocin, Vasopressin (V_{1A}, V_{1B}, V_2)	Serotonin ($5HT_{1,2,4-7}$)
	Purines
Vasoactive peptides	Adenosine (A_1, A_2) (P_1)
Angiotensin (AT_1, AT_2)	ATP (P_2)
Endothelin (ET_A, ET_B)	Ion-channel ligands
Atrial natriuretic peptide (ANP B, C)	$GABA_B$
	Metabotropic glutamate
Gut hormones	Muscarinic ACh (M_1–M_5)
Gastrin	Sensory transduction
Glucagon	Olfaction: odorants
Secretin	Taste: tastants
Kinins	Vison: photons
Bradykinin (B_1, B_2)	*Other Ligands*
Tachykinin (NK_1–NK_3)	Lipid derivatives
Calcium-regulating hormones	Platelet-activating factor
	Prostaglandins
Calcitonin	Leukotrienes
Parathyroid hormone	Miscellaneous
Others	Cannabinoids
Bombesin	f-met-leu-phe
Neurotensin	Thrombin
Opiates	Calcium
Somatostatin	

Note: Refer to Table 5A-1 for definitions of acronyms.

mone receptors, although this occurs less frequently for ligands of larger molecular size. Almost all such receptors interact with G proteins after agonist binding and catalyze the exchange of GTP for guanosine diphosphate (GDP) bound to the α subunit, leading to dissociation of the G protein into α and βγ subunits that control the activities of the effector systems of the plasma membrane. The first G protein–coupled receptors to be characterized and sequenced were the visual rhodopsins, a group of seven transmembrane domain molecules that are the photoreceptors of vertebrate rod cells. When rhodopsin is stimulated by the action of photons on its light-sensitive chromophore retinal, it relaxes into its activated form and interacts with transducin, which in turn binds GTP and activates a cyclic GMP–specific phosphodiesterase.[48] The resulting decrease in cGMP causes closure of cation channels in the rod cell plasma membrane, leading to hyperpolarization and neuronal signaling. The subsequent cloning of the β-adrenergic receptor revealed the existence of a superfamily of rhodopsin-like receptors that trigger G proteins to activate a wide variety of signal transduction pathways in response to extracellular stimuli.[49]

About 150 receptors for light, biogenic amines, peptide hormones, alkaloids, and odorants that are structurally related to the visual rhodopsins and are coupled to plasma membrane effector systems via heterotrimeric G proteins have been identified.[47] All such receptors contain seven hydrophobic domains that are believed to form membrane-spanning α helices which anchor the receptor molecule within the plasma membrane. The transmembrane domains are arranged as a group, with their hydrophobic aspects facing the membrane lipids and their hydrophilic surfaces facing centrally toward the active region of the molecule; they are formed of 20 to 28 amino acids and are linked by hydrophilic extracellular and intracellular loops (Fig. 5A-9). The N-terminal region of the receptor is extracellular and varies considerably in size among the various receptors. It usually contains two or three sites for N-linked glycosylation. In β_2-adrenergic and several other receptors, abolition of glycosylation sites has little effect on ligand binding or signal transduction but decreases the number of cell-surface receptors, suggesting a potential role of glycosylation in receptor trafficking and expression. However, since some receptors (eg. α_{2B}-adrenergic) are not glycosylated, carbohydrate residues cannot be a general requirement for receptor expression and function. The intracellular loops and the carboxy-terminal region contain several potential sites for phosphorylation by protein kinases. The third intracellular loop is important for coupling to G proteins and varies in size from tens to hundreds of amio acids. The carboxy-terminal domain sometimes has sites for the attachment of lipid residues that may serve as additional anchorage points to the cell membrane. The protein kinase sites in the cytoplasmic regions of the receptor provide the potential for regulation of its functions by phosphorylation of serine and threonine residues.[50] Tyrosine phosphorylation, in contrast to its frequent role in signaling by growth factor receptors, has not been shown to occur in G protein–coupled receptors.

There is extensive conservation of primary struc-

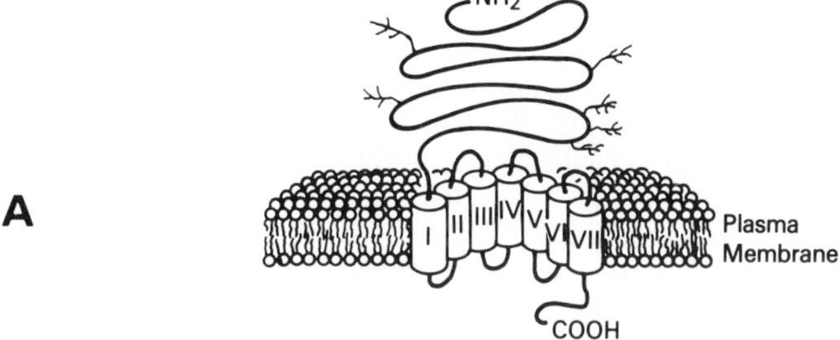

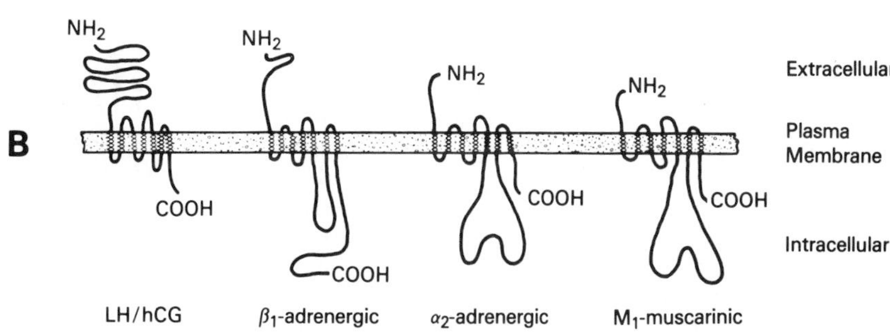

FIGURE 5A-9. Proposed structure of the G protein–coupled receptors, showing the seven transmembrane domains and the extracellular and cytoplasmic domains. (*A*) The LH/hCG receptor, a typical glycoprotein hormone receptor with a characteristically large extracellular domain. (*B*) Comparison of receptors for large (LH/hCG) and small (cationic amine) ligands. Note the wide variation in the size of the third intracellular loop, which is the primary region of coupling to transducing G proteins. In general, the extracellular domains of receptors for peptide hormones are larger than those of receptors for cationic amines and other small ligands.

ture among the G protein–coupled receptors, particularly of amino acid residues in the hydrophobic domains that form their transmembrane regions.[51] Some of these residues are necessary to maintain the conformation of the receptor, and others are involved in ligand binding, receptor activation, and G protein coupling. They include two extracellular cysteine residues that form a disulfide bond which links the second and third extracellular regions in many receptors. Other conserved amino acids include an asparagine in helix I, aspartic acid and leucine in helix II, an arginine at the end of helix III, and proline residues in helices IV through VII. The aspartate residue in the second transmembrane domain appears to be crucial for signal transduction and is present in almost all the G protein–coupled receptors. Another common feature is the presence of an amino acid "signature" sequence that begins in the third transmembrane domain and contains the conserved aspartate-arginine-tyrosine (DRY) sequence at the beginning of the second intracellular loop.[52] Another aspartate residue in the third transmembrane domain has been implicated in the binding and activation functions of adrenergic and related receptors. Proline and tyrosine residues near the cytoplasmic end of the seventh transmembrane domain are conserved in many receptors and appear to be part of a motif (arginine-proline-x-x-tyrosine) that is required for internalization. Analysis of the locations of the conserved amino acids in multiple G protein–coupled receptors has shown that most of the aromatic residues are situated on the external aspects of the helices, whereas the polar residues are displayed on the internal surfaces. The most highly conserved amino acids are probably required for the organization of the basic structure of the receptor. Other residues that are nonidentical but are conserved among the major receptor classes, such as the aspartate residue in the third transmembrane domain of the adrenergic receptors, are more important for their role in the generic binding and/or activation properties of the receptor.[53]

The proposed molecular structure of the G protein–coupled receptors, with seven hydrophobic transmembrane regions forming a bundle of α helices that enclose a ligand-binding pocket, is shown in Fig. 5A-10. This arrangement resembles that of the retinal-binding conformation of rhodopsin,[50] in which retinal is bound as Schiff base to the ϵ-amino group of a lysine residue in the seventh transmembrane domain. The structure of rhodopsin was in turn based on that determined by electron diffraction analysis of the bacterial retinal binding protein bacteriorhodopsin, which pumps protons and is not coupled to a G protein.[54] The proposed structure of the G protein–coupled receptor superfamily has been supported by the results of mutations performed to evaluate the roles of individual residues in binding and activation, which are in general agreement with the serpentine arrangement of the molecule in the plasma membrane. The binding of activating ligands to the intramembrane docking site perturbs the conformation of the bundle of helices and presumably exposes domains in the third intracellular loop and elsewhere that couple with the respective G proteins. Thus, agonist binding releases the receptor from the constraint of the intramolecular forces that maintain it in an inactive basal state.

The interaction of seven transmembrane domain receptors with G proteins occurs largely through regions in the third intracellular loop and in some cases in the carboxy-terminal cytoplasmic domain. Although most of the known G protein–coupled receptors have been cloned and sequenced, the precise features that specify their interaction with the α subunits (and in some cases the β subunits) of the individual G proteins have not been completely identified. Two regions in the third intracellular loop have been found to be involved in signal transduction and are located within the 20 residue sequences adjacent to the fifth and sixth transmembrane domains. Studies with chimeric receptors and deletion mutants have shown that these regions, termed N-III and C-III according to their position at the amino- or carboxy-terminal end of the third loop, participate in determining the coupling of β-adrenergic receptors to G_s and that of α-adrenergic receptors to G_q (Fig. 5A-10). Comparisons of the amino acid sequences of the cytoplasmic third loops have shown that limited structural conservation of specific amino acids or their homologues can be identified,

FIGURE 5A-10. Diagram of the proposed arrangement of the transmembrane domains of G protein–coupled receptors. Agonist binding takes place within a pocket formed by the seven helices, and the interaction with G proteins involves the third intracellular loop and to some extent the carboxy-terminal cytoplasmic domain. (*From Taylor.*[102])

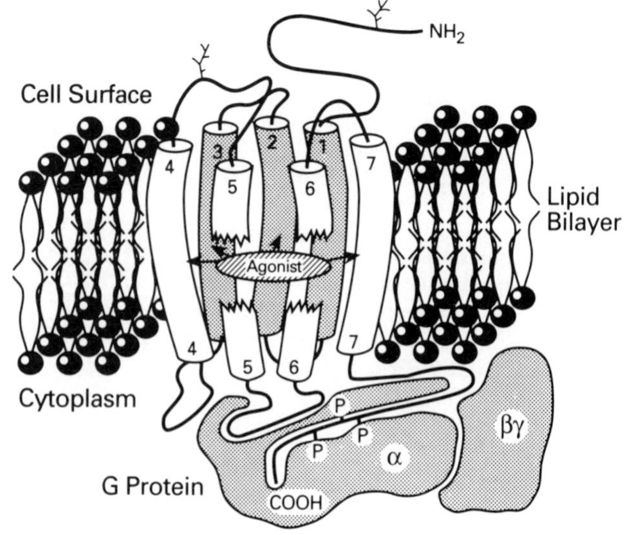

but no unequivocally specific sequences that specify coupling to particular G proteins have been found.[55]

In a few of the seven transmembrane domain receptors, coupling to G proteins appears to be minimal or absent. These include the somatostatin SSTR1 and dopamine D_3 receptors and the recently cloned angiotensin AT_2 receptor. These receptors and a receptor-like *Drosophila* membrane protein possess structural similarities within their third cytoplasmic loops and may be involved in developmental aspects of cell growth and morphogenesis.[56]

Adrenergic Receptors

The traditional subdivision of adrenergic receptors into α and β subtypes on the basis of their pharmacologic properties[57] has been given a structural basis by molecular cloning of the several receptor subtypes that mediate the actions of epinephrine and norepinephrine in their various target tissues. α-adrenoreceptors have a potency rank order of norepinephrine > epinephrine > phenylephrine >> isoproterenol and exist as α_1 and α_2 subtypes that stimulate and inhibit smooth muscle contraction, respectively. α_1 Receptors are coupled through G proteins of the G_q family to stimulation of phospholipase C and calcium mobilization, whereas α_2 receptors are coupled through G_i to inhibition of adenylyl cyclase. β-Receptors have a potency order of isoproterenol > epinephrine ≥ norepinephrine and include three subtypes that are coupled to G_s and the activation of adenylyl cyclase. β_1 Receptors in adipose tissue and cardiac muscle, and β_2 receptors in smooth muscle of the bronchi and blood vessels, differ in their relative potencies for norepinephrine. Specific receptor antagonists for each of the major subtypes include propranolol and phenoxybenzamine for α receptors and propranolol for β receptors and practolol and butoxamine for the β_1 and β_2 receptors, respectively. The adrenergic receptors bind (−) catecholamines with high stereospecificity; their affinity is dependent on the ethanolamine side chain of the catecholamine, and their activation is dependent on the catechol ring.

The cloning of the adrenergic receptors has made it possible to relate these pharmacologic properties to the structural features of the receptor protein and identify the binding and activation domains of the receptor.[47] Conserved cysteine residues in the second and third extracellular loops are essential in maintaining the binding conformation of the receptor, presumably by forming a disulfide bond between the loops to stabilize the transmembrane domains. The ligand-binding site of the adrenergic receptors is located within a pocket formed by the transmembrane helices and involves interactions between the functional groups of the hormone and specific amino acid residues that project into the pocket. These residues include aspartate residues in the second and third transmembrane domains and serine residues in the fifth transmembrane region. The aspartate residue present in the third transmembrane domain of all cationic amine receptors is believed to form a salt bridge with the charged amino groups of catecholamines, dopamine, and serotonin. The serine residues in the fifth transmembrane domain are adjacent to the third intracellular loop, which contains regions that interact with the guanyl nucleotide regulatory proteins that control adenylyl cyclase activity. Consensus sequences for phosphorylation by cAMP-dependent protein kinase are present in the third intracellular loop and the carboxy-terminal domain and have been implicated in heterologous desensitization and down regulation of the receptor. The different properties of the α and β receptors are partly related to sequences in the seventh transmembrane domain.

α-Adrenergic Receptors

The α_1-adrenergic receptor was defined on the basis of its mediation of vascular smooth muscle contraction by catecholamines. It has been found to have four subtypes (α_{1A} through α_{1D}) that differ in their amino acid sequences and affinities for agonists and antagonists. They are coupled through pertussis toxin–insensitive G proteins (G_q, G_{11}) to activation of phospholipase C-β_1, and through pertussis toxin–sensitive G proteins to activation of phospholipase A_2 and L-type calcium channels.[58] Activation of α_1-adrenergic receptors also leads to growth responses in certain cell types. The α_{1A} receptor is present in most tissues and acts through a pertussis-sensitive G protein to activate phospholipase A_2 and increase arachidonic acid production and Ca^{2+} influx. The α_{1B} receptor is abundant in the heart, liver, and spleen and acts through pertussis toxin–insensitive G proteins to activate phospholipase C and calcium signaling. α_1-Adrenergic receptors also stimulate the activity of phospholipase D in the brain, in part by increasing cytoplasmic Ca^{2+}. In some cell types, activation of α_1-adrenergic receptors causes increased cAMP production through an unidentified mechanism.

α_2-Adrenergic receptors were defined as presynaptic receptors inhibitory to norepinephrine release. They include three subtypes (α_{2A} through α_{2C}) that are coupled through pertussis toxin–sensitive G proteins to a wide variety of cell responses, including inhibition of adenylyl cyclase, inhibition of Ca^{2+} channels, and activation of potassium channels.[59] Each of these effects is probably mediated by a separate G protein; coupling to inhibition of adenylyl cyclase is transduced by G_{i1}, and G_o and G_{i2} are involved in coupling to inhibition of Ca^{2+} currents and stimulation of K^+ currents, respectively. The actions of α_2-adrenergic receptor stimulation on ion fluxes are responsible for the inhibition of neuronal firing and neurotransmitter release during activation of these receptors on pre- and postsynaptic neurons, as occurs during agonist treatment with clonidine. α_2-Adrenergic receptors also stimulate phospholipases C and D and exert growth effects in certain cell types. The α_{2A}-adrenergic receptor, which couples to G_{i2} and G_{i3}, has been shown to promote activation of ras and stimulation of the phosphorylation of MAP kinase, which accounts for the mitogenic activity of α_2 agonists in certain cells.[60] It is relevant that the activated α subunit of G_{i2} promotes mitogenic responses in transfected cells. Also, it is possible that the $\beta\gamma$ subunits of G_{i2}, rather than the α subunits, are involved in activation of the ras signaling pathway by the α_{2A} receptor.

The β-Adrenergic Receptor

The β-adrenergic receptor, which mediates the physiologic actions of epinephrine and norepinephrine through the activation of adenylyl cyclase via G_s, has been the most extensively studied G protein–coupled receptor since its cloning in 1986.[49] As was noted above, the β-adrenergic receptor resembles rhodopsin in many of its structural and functional properties. Both molecules possess seven transmembrane regions, share sequence homologies, and act by regulating the activity of GTP-binding proteins, either G_s (β-receptor) or transducin (rhodopsin). The sequence and three-dimensional homologies between the β-adrenergic receptors and rhodopsin are accompanied by several functional similarities in addition to their interaction with nucleotide regulatory proteins. These similarities include homologous densensitization of the β-receptor and light adaptation of rhodopsin. Both responses involve receptor phosphorylation by specific protein kinases termed β-adrenergic receptor kinase (which phosphorylates only the agonist-occupied form of the receptor) and rhodopsin kinase (which phosphorylates only the light-bleached form of rhodopsin).[50] These findings indicate that the mechanisms of regulation of the individual transmembrane signaling systems are basically similar in nature. Both forms of desensitization may represent a general process for controlling the coupling of receptors to guanine nucleotide regulatory proteins and activation of effector systems in the cell membrane.[61] The amino acid sequence of the human β_2-adrenergic receptor and the conserved residues that are present in the majority of the G protein–coupled receptors are shown in Fig. 5A-11.

Other G Protein–Coupled Receptors

The superfamily of G protein–coupled receptors includes several smaller groups of related proteins with variations in their sizes and primary structures. These proteins range in size from the small GnRH receptor, which lacks a carboxy-terminal tail,[62] to the large glycoprotein hormone receptors, which have complex and bulky N-terminal domains.[63] The precise definition of ligand binding sites in the seven transmembrane domain receptors has been more difficult for peptide and protein hormones than for the smaller neurotransmitter molecules. However, amino acid residues in the sixth and seventh transmembrane domains have been found to contribute to ligand binding in many receptors. In peptide hormone receptors, the N-terminal and other extracellular regions, as well as the transmembrane domains, are involved in ligand binding. The N-terminal region is of major importance in receptors for LH, FSH, and TSH, in which the large extracellular domains contain multiple leucine-rich repeats and many cysteine residues that form disulfide bridges and maintain the conformation of the ligand-binding site.[64] The glycoprotein hormones bind with high affinity to this extracellular domain[65] and then interact with a secondary binding site that is located within the bundle of hydrophobic domains that span the plasma membrane.[66] Another type of two-step mechanism is involved in the activation of the thrombin receptor, in which thrombin acts on a cleavage site in the extracellular region to reveal a new N-terminal domain in which the 1-14 peptide acts as a tethered agonist ligand and activates the receptor.[67]

An interesting and valuable development in receptor pharmacology has been the recent introduction of nonpeptide antagonists for several peptide hormone receptors, including those for substance P (NK_1), cholecystokinin-B/gastrin, and angiotensin II (AT_1). In each case, the binding of the respective nonpeptide antagonists has been found to depend on amino acid residues in the fifth and/or sixth transmembrane domains of the receptor, probably close to the outer surface of the membrane. However, these residues do not appear to be important for the binding of the native peptide ligands. These findings indicate that small antagonist molecules, like the adrenergic ligands, interact with a transmembrane binding site that involves the carboxy-terminal helices and may interfere with the packing of those helices within the lipid bilayer.[68] They also suggest that nonpeptide antagonists bind to a site that is distinct from that of the native peptide agonist and may act as allosteric inhibitors of agonist binding. This information will doubtless be of value in the development of additional nonpeptide antagonists with the potential to serve as orally active inhibitors of peptide hormone action.

The G protein–coupled receptor superfamily also includes a large group of recently discovered odorant receptors in the cilia of olfactory neurons that activate second messenger cascades that lead to the modulation of ion channels and the generation of action potentials.[69] At least 150 of these receptors have been cloned, and the size of the olfactory receptor family may be as large as 500 to 1000 in humans and rodents. Several odorant receptors have been found to increase phosphoinositide hydrolysis, and others may activate adenylyl cyclase and ion chan-

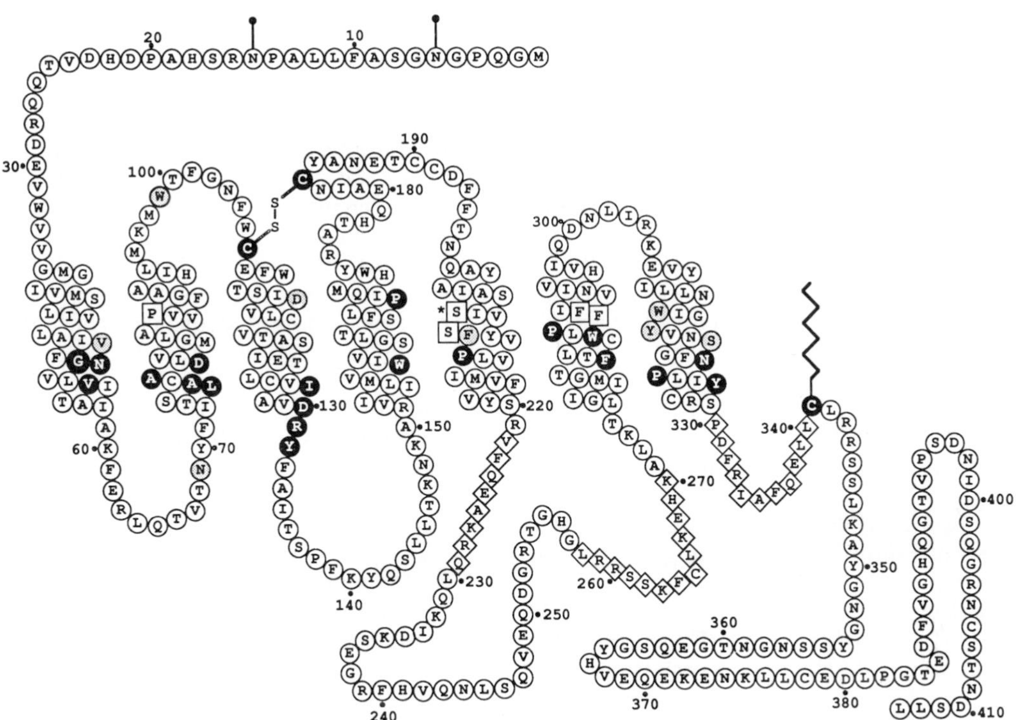

FIGURE 5A-11. Model of a typical G protein–coupled receptor of the seven transmembrane domain family, based on the human beta$_2$-adrenergic receptor. The highly conserved residues are shown in black, and those conserved in cationic amino receptors are stippled. The boxed residues are conserved in all catecholamine receptors, and the asterisk indicates the serine conserved in serotonin receptors. The residues involved in G protein coupling are shown in diamonds. Also shown are the palmitoylated cysteine residue in the carboxy-terminal region, the glycosylation sites in the amino-terminal extracellular domain, and the protein kinase A sites (arrowheads) in the intracellular regions of the receptor. *(Reproduced by permission from Probst et al.*[51]*)*

nels. About 20 odorant-related receptors are expressed in the germ cells of the testis and may be involved in the chemotaxis of sperm migration during fertilization. In the olfactory epithelium, each neuron expresses only a small subset of odorant receptors in their cilial processes. It is of interest that GnRH neurons arise in the nasal placode and migrate to the hypothalamus during embryonic development.[70] Also, GnRH receptors and neural connections are present in the limbic system of the brain, which has evolutionary connections with olfaction as well as the control of reproductive function.[71] The association between olfactory stimuli and reproductive function in several species may be clarified at the molecular level by elucidation of the interactions between the outputs of odorant receptors and the hypothalamic centers that control the episodic secretion of GnRH.

Abnormalities of Receptor Function

The recent cloning of many G protein–coupled receptors and the elucidation of their amino acid sequences has begun to yield valuable insights into the structural requirements for hormone binding and activation of receptor function. The identification of regions involved in ligand binding and coupling to G proteins was followed by a search for receptor mutations that could explain the pathophysiology of several disorders characterized by either hormone resistance or endocrine overactivity in the absence of increased hormone secretion and with no abnormality in G proteins. This has led to the discovery of both inactivating and activating mutations of several G protein-linked hormone receptors. Inactivating mutations have been identified in the vasopressin V_2 receptors of patients with X-linked diabetes insipidus,[72] the ACTH receptor of patients with hereditary glucocorticoid deficiency,[73] and the GHRH receptor in the "little" mouse.[74] Recently, activating mutations have been identified in the LH receptor of patients with familial male precocious puberty[75] and in the TSH receptor of certain thyroid modules.[76] Such mutations have also been found in the melanocyte stimulating hormone (MSH) receptor of mice with inherited hyperpigmentation[77] and in the rhodopsin of patients with certain forms of retinal degeneration.[78] The locations of the mutations that are responsible for these and other forms of constitutive receptor activation are within or adjacent to the transmembrane domains, as shown in Fig. 5A-12. Interestingly, the sites of the activating mutations in the thyrotropin receptor are identical to those found to cause constitutive activation of α- and β-adrenergic receptors, indicating the importance of these residues in maintaining the receptor in its inactive conformation.[79] Further mutations will doubtless be identified in the coding regions of the other G protein–coupled receptors in a variety of disorders of endocrine regulation that involve impaired or excessive hormone secretion and/or action.[80]

Growth Factor Receptors

Growth factors constitute a large group of hormones with prominent actions on cell proliferation, as opposed to the effects on differentiation and secretion that are typical of many other peptide and protein hormones. They include hormones such as insulin and insulin-like growth factor-I (IGF-1) as well as EGF, PDGF, fibroblast growth factor (FGF), and others that promote the growth of specific cell types and target tissues.

The EGF Receptor

The EGF receptor is a 170-kDa glycoprotein that mediates the mitogenic action of EGF and acts as a regulator of proliferation in numerous target cells. The EGF receptor mRNA encodes a precursor consisting of a 24-amino acid signal peptide followed by a 1186-amino acid receptor protein containing regions responsible for hormone binding, membrane attachment, protein tyrosine kinase activity, and autophosphorylation (Fig. 5A-13). The extracellular amino-terminal region of the receptor (621 amino acids) contains the EGF-binding domain and is rich in cysteine residues (for disulfide bond formation) and glycosylation sites.[81] The external binding region is followed by a hydrophobic membrane-spanning domain of 26 amino acids bounded on its cytoplasmic side by a highly basic segment of the 542-residue carboxy-terminal region of the molecule. Phosphorylation of the EGF receptor by protein kinase C at a threonine residue within this basic sequence, between the plasma membrane and the protein kinase domain, causes loss of high-affinity EGF binding and ligand-induced tyrosine phosphorylation.

FIGURE 5A-12. Locations of spontaneous mutations that cause constitutive activation of G protein–coupled receptors and are associated with disorders resulting from persistent receptor activity in the absence of ligand stimulation. 1,2, Melanocyte-stimulating hormone; 3,4, thyrotropin; 5, luteinizing hormone; 6, rhodopsin. (*From Lefkowitz.*[79])

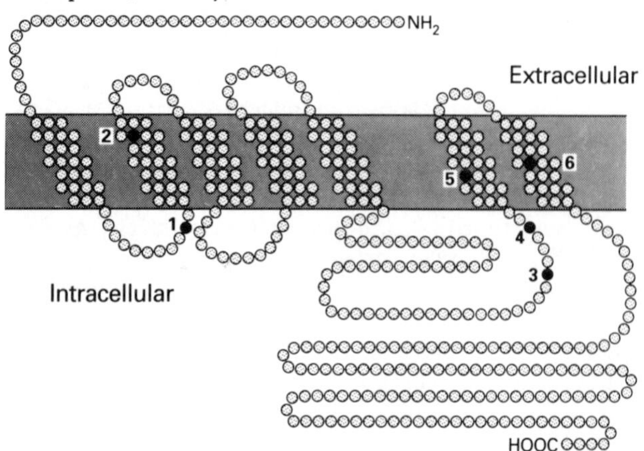

Binding of EGF to the plasma membrane receptor stimulates receptor dimerization that initiates intracellular signaling and gene expression and is followed by clustering and endocytosis of the hormone-receptor complex.[82] The cytoplasmic portion of the receptor contains a tyrosine kinase domain that is activated by ligand binding and receptor dimerization, leading to transphosphorylation of tyrosine residues in the receptor molecules as well as other cellular proteins. The tyrosine autophosphorylation sites on the receptor are located within its cytoplasmic domain, near the carboxy terminus of the molecule. EGF-induced activation of the intrinsic tyrosine kinase activity of the receptor is essential for its signal transduction functions as well as for ligand-induced internalization and down regulation of the receptor. The cytoplasmic region of the receptor adjacent to the tyrosine kinase domain contains several tyrosine residues that undergo autophosphorylation and are important for transducing growth and other signals. One of these, Tyr^{992}, couples the receptor to phospholipase C-γ, leading to phosphoinositide hydrolysis and Ca^{2+} mobilization during EGF action.[83]

In addition to signaling through its tyrosine kinase activity, the EGF receptor is coupled in some manner to G proteins in certain cell types. For example, the stimulation of phospholipase C activity by EGF in hepatocytes is mediated by a pertussis toxin–sensitive G protein. In these cells, EGF has little affect on tyrosine phosphorylation of phospholipase C-γ, in contrast to its prominent activation of the enzyme in tumor cells expressing high levels of EGF receptors.[84] There have also been reports that some of the actions of EGF in various cell types, including Ca^{2+} influx in A431 epidermoid carcinoma cells, appear to be mediated by G_s.[85] Thus, it is possible that the EGF receptor is coupled not only to the defined growth regulatory pathway that is initiated by tyrosine phosphorylation but also to the activation of certain G proteins and their dependent response pathways. The IGF-II receptor also appears to be coupled to a pertussis-sensitive G protein (G_{i2}), through which it activates calcium channels and increases cytoplasmic calcium concentration.

The early cellular responses to EGF include both calcium mobilization by $InsP_3$ and calcium entry

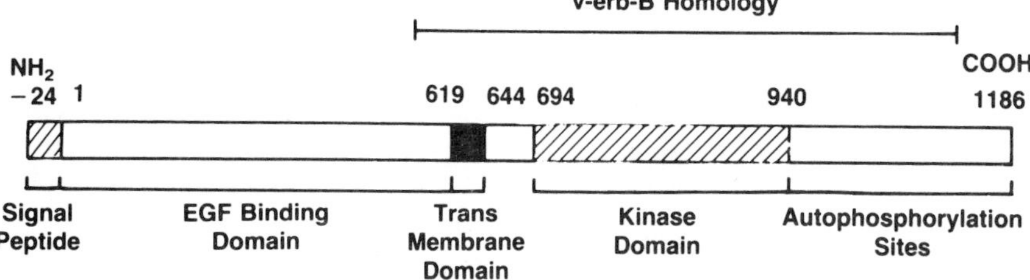

FIGURE 5A-13. Linear structure of the EGF receptor protein. The external EGF-binding domain is on the left, and the cytoplasmic phosphorylation domain is on the right. The region of sequence homologoy with the *erbB* oncogene product is shown above. (*Modified from Hunter.*[88])

through voltage-insensitive Ca^{2+} channels. The calcium influx is mediated in part by leukotriene C_4, a lipoxygenase metabolite of the arachidonic acid formed during activation of phospholipase C and phospholipase A_2.[86] Subsequent responses to EGF include the rapid expression of several early response genes, including *c-fos, c-jun,* and *Jun B.* These are probably induced via the ras/raf protein kinase cascade and activation of mitogen-activated protein kinase (MAP kinase) and are initiated by the tyrosine phosphorylation that follows receptor occupancy by EGF.[87] It is likely that phosphorylation of phospholipase A_2 by MAP kinase contributes to the formation of arachidonic acid and its lipoxygenase metabolites and thus indirectly promotes the activation of plasma membrane Ca^{2+} channels. EGF-induced phosphorylation is also responsible for several early effects of EGF, including activation of Na^+,K^+-ATPase and ornithine decarboxylase, that are not required or are not by themselves sufficient to initiate DNA synthesis.

The carboxy-terminal region of the EGF receptor has marked sequence homology with the *erbB* oncogene, which is located near the EGF receptor gene in human chromosome 7. Their common genomic localization and the 85 percent sequence homology between the relevant regions of the two gene products indicate that the chicken erythroblastosis virus (*v-erbB*) oncogene is derived from the EGF receptor gene, i.e., that the EGF receptor gene is the *c-erbB* gene.[88] The *v-erbB* gene product is a truncated EGF receptor with no external binding site and appears to be constitutively active in cells transformed by the avian erythroblastosis virus. The presence of a similar receptor in *Drosophila* indicates that the coding sequences of the extracellular binding and intracellular kinase domains of the *c-erbB* gene must have arisen over 800 million years ago. In addition to its functions in cellular growth, the EGF receptor serves as a receptor for vaccinia virus. In this regard, it resembles several other cell-surface receptors that act as virus receptors, including the ACh receptor (rabies virus), the beta-adrenergic receptor (reovirus), the complement receptor CR2 (Epstein-Barr virus), and the T4 lymphocyte antigen (HTLV-III).[89] Many tumors and cell lines coexpress EGF receptors and TGF-α, a growth-promoting polypeptide that binds to the EGF receptor. In such cells, activation of EGF receptors by the endogenous ligand can promote cell proliferation by an autocrine feedback action of TGF-α.

The Insulin Receptor

The insulin receptor is composed of two 130-kDa α subunits and two 90-kDa β subunits that are joined by disulfide bonds to form the cross-linked 350- to 400-kDa $(\alpha\beta)_2$ heterotetramer.[90] The holoreceptor has a symmetric immunoglobulin-like structure (β-S-S-α)-S-S-(α-S-S-β) and probably binds more than one molecule of insulin. The α subunits are extracellular and contain the insulin-binding domain, whereas the β subunit is largely intracellular and performs the signaling functions of the receptor. The β subunit has intrinsic tyrosine kinase activity that catalyzes the autophosphorylation of a tyrosine residue within its own structure when the receptor is activated by insulin. The tyrosine kinase activity of the β subunit is inhibited by the unoccupied α subunit. The insulin receptor is derived from a single glycosylated precursor in which disulfide bonds link the future α and β subunit regions. The receptor for IGF-I is similar in subunit composition and intracellular sequence to the insulin receptor but differs in its extracellular region and peptide-binding specificity.

The human insulin receptor precursor deduced from the nucleotide sequence of the cloned cDNA contains 1370 amino acids arranged as a 27-residue signal sequence followed by the α subunit, a precursor processing enzyme cleavage site, and then the β subunit.[91] A single 23-amino acid transmembrane region is present in the β subunit, which also contains sequence homologies with other receptor tyrosine kinase and the *src* oncogene product. The absence of a membrane-spanning region in the α subunit is consistent with its location on the outer surface of the cell, together with 194 residues of the β chain. The α subunit is more heavily glycosylated than the β subunit and is also rich in cysteine residues; it shares sequence homology with the external domain of the EGF receptor, probably reflecting a common feature of the ligand-binding sites. The insulin and EGF receptors both have tyrosine-specific protein kinase domains commencing 50 residues from the end of the transmembrane region (Fig. 5A-14).

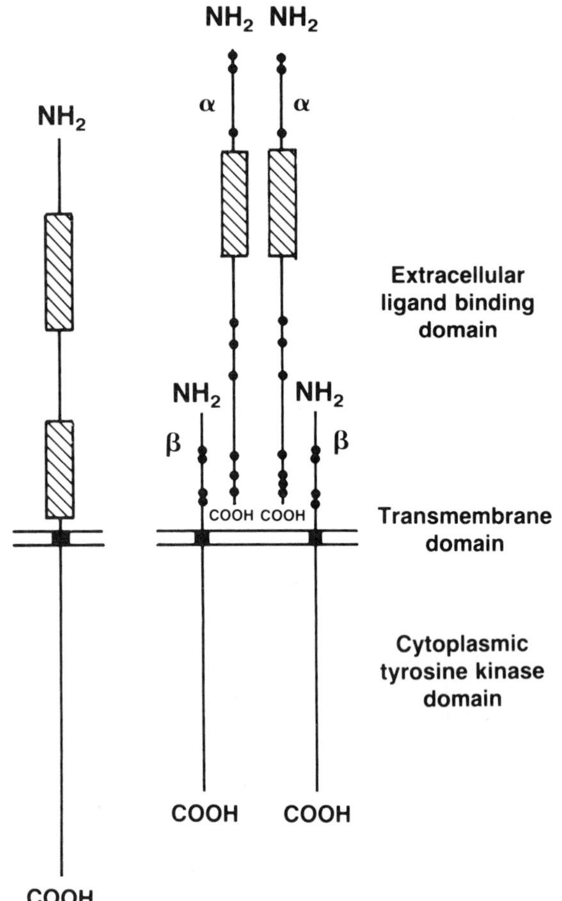

FIGURE 5A-14. Schematic comparison of the insulin receptor (*right*) and the EGF receptor (*left*). Regions of high cysteine content are shown as hatched areas. The single cysteine residues (black circles) may be involved in the formation of the $\alpha_2\beta_2$ insulin receptor complex. Note that the α subunits are completely extracellular, whereas the β subunits, which possess tyrosine kinase activity, are predominantly intracellular. (*From Ullrich et al.*[91])

The intrinsic tyrosine kinase activity of the insulin receptor is an essential component of its signal transduction mechanisms, as in other growth factor receptors, and causes phosphorylation of tyrosine residues in the receptor itself and in other proteins. Insulin binding to the receptor increases the level of ras.GTP and stimulates raf-1 kinase activity and phosphorylation of MAP kinase, with consequent induction of gene expression.[92] The major target of the activated insulin receptor is insulin receptor substrate-1 (IRS-1), a 185-kDa protein that contains several tyrosine phosphorylation sites within motifs that are recognized by proteins containing regions termed SH2 (src homology 2) domains.[93] Several of these proteins become associated with ligand-activated growth factor receptors by binding to their cytoplasmic tyrosine-autophosphorylation domains. When tyrosine-phosphorylated by the insulin receptor, IRS-1 binds to several signal transduction proteins. One of these is growth factor receptor-bound protein 2 (Grb2), an adapter protein that links other receptor tyrosine kinases to the activation of ras. In the case of the insulin receptor, Grb2 binds not to the receptor but to its substrate, IRS-1, and could mediate the activation of ras by the insulin receptor. IRS-1 also binds to phosphatidylinositol-3-kinase (PI-3-kinase), an enzyme that catalyzes the addition of 3-phosphate groups to several phosphoinositides.[94] PI-3-kinase is activated by binding to IRS-1 and is an early and essential component of the insulin-induced signaling pathway that stimulates transcriptional activation of *c-fos* and other early response genes. The precise biological function of PI-3-kinase is not clear, but it appears to operate upstream of ras. In insulin-stimulated cells, it may be involved in the vesicle-mediated translocation of glucose transporters to the cell membrane. Whether its effects on the phosphorylation of phospholipids are related to its growth-signaling action is also unknown, but the enzyme appears to be an important intermediate in the actions of growth factors and mitogens.

Several types of mutations in the insulin receptor gene have been identified in patients with genetic syndromes associated with insulin resistance.[95] These include mutations that decrease the number of receptors expressed at the cell surface and those which interfere with receptor activation and signal transduction. The former can result from mutations that decrease the level of insulin receptor mRNA or cause premature chain termination and thus impair receptor biosynthesis. Receptor number is also reduced by mutations that increase the rate of receptor degradation. Mutations that impair receptor function cause a decrease in the binding affinity of the receptor for insulin or lead to impairment of the intrinsic tyrosine kinase activity of the receptors.

Growth Hormone, Prolactin, and Cytokine Receptors

Growth hormone (GH) and prolactin receptors belong to a recently defined family of single transmembrane domain receptors that share significant amino acid sequence homology in their extracellular hormone-binding domains.[96] Within this family, which includes receptors for GH, prolactin, erythropoietin, colony-stimulating factors, and several interleukins, the individual cytoplasmic domains are highly variable and do not possess sequences associated with tyrosine kinase or other intracellular signaling enzymes. The GH/cytokine receptor family is characterized by the presence of two pairs of cysteine residues and a Trp-Ser-X-Trp-Ser motif in their intracellular domains, and a carboxy-terminal sequence that mediates protein-protein interactions in fibronectin, contactin, and neural adhesion molecules.

In several members of this family, soluble extracellular fragments of the receptors are present in the circulation and bind the respective ligands with almost the same properties as the plasma membrane receptor.[97] The functions of these receptor-derived binding proteins are not known, but they could serve to retard the clearance of the hormone and prolong its actions as well as to compete with the cellular receptor for hormone binding. The GH-binding species has been the most intensively studied of these binding proteins. Its serum level is influenced by developmental, nutritional, and hormonal factors and probably reflects the abundance of GH receptors in tissues. About 50 percent of the circulating GH is associated with the binding protein under normal conditions. As might be expected, no GH-binding activity is detectable in the serum of patients with Laron dwarfism, in which mutations or deletions of the GH receptor abolish its expression or function.

Although the GH/cytokine receptors share considerable amino acid homology, there is little similarity among the sequences of their ligands. However, a common feature shared by this family of hormones and cytokines is a structural motif of four helix bundle folds. Despite this structural resemblance and the similarities between the receptors, there is little cross-reaction between the individual ligands and the heterologous receptors. Thus, the GH molecules of most species are highly specific in their actions on growth and related processes and do not interact with other members of the receptor family, including prolactin. Human GH (hGH) is an exception in this regard and is highly lactogenic in humans and other species as a result of its interaction with prolactin receptors. This property of hGH is highly dependent on the presence of zinc and appears to result from the coordination of Zn^{2+} by a cluster of residues in GH (His^{18}, His^{21}, and Glu^{174}) and one residue (His^{183}) that is conserved in all prolactin receptors but not in GH receptors.[98]

Detailed studies on the interaction between hGH and its receptor-binding protein have identified two functionally distinct but adjacent sites on the hGH molecule that bind to two overlapping sites on the binding protein. This occurs as a sequential reaction in which one molecule of the binding protein associates with site 1 of the GH molecule and another is bound to site 2 to form a trimeric complex.[99] There is also a region of the receptor that forms a binding surface that interacts with a corresponding domain on the second molecule of the binding protein. Since the GH-binding proteins are in fact the extracellular domains of the receptors, their interactions with the GH molecule reflect those of the native holoreceptors, which also form a dimeric complex on the cell surface that is essential for the activation of signal transduction mechanisms that mediate the growth response to GH. Cellular responses mediated by GH and Prl receptors can be elicited by cross-linking the receptors with monoclonal antibodies; this is consistent with the importance of dimerization for the activation of these and probably other members of the cytokine receptor family.

Recently, GH binding to its receptor has been found to cause rapid tyrosine phosphorylation of the receptor itself and in more than a dozen receptor-associated and cytoplasmic proteins. GH also increases the activity of MAP kinase and stimulates the expression of the early response genes *c-fos* and *c-jun*. These responses depend on the GH-induced association of the receptor with a nonreceptor tyrosine kinase, JAK2.[100] The resulting activation of JAK2 causes tyrosine phosphorylation of both the receptor and JAK2, which presumably initiates the GH receptor signaling pathway by phosphorylating other proteins. The recruitment of cytoplasmic tyrosine kinases has been recognized as a common mode of signaling by receptors that do not possess intrinsic tyrosine kinase activity. Several other members of the cytokine/hemopoietin receptor family (erythropoietin, interleukin 3, colony-stimulating factors) have also been found to activate JAK2; this is consistent with its importance as an early signaling molecule in their intracellular transduction pathways. The prolactin receptor has also been found to be coupled to rapid tyrosine phosphorylation of several cellular proteins. One of these is a 120-kDa protein that is associated with the receptor and has been identified as JAK2, which presumably generates the intracellular signaling cascade.[101]

TRANSMEMBRANE SIGNAL TRANSDUCTION MECHANISMS

There are several mechanisms by which hormone-receptor interactions lead to activation or inhibition of specific enzymes or channels that in turn control intracellular signaling pathways. The original proposal that hormone receptors are structurally linked to a signal-generating enzyme (such as adenylyl cyclase) and serve as its regulatory domain was eclipsed by the discovery of G proteins as essential intermediates in the regulation of adenylyl cyclase and phospholipase C activity. Hormone binding to seven transmembrane domain receptors causes conformational changes that increase their affinity for G proteins, which are in turn activated and then control the activities of effector enzymes in the plasma membrane. However, in single transmembrane domain receptors, ligand binding causes activation of intrinsic enzymatic activity (e.g., protein kinase or guanylate cyclase) within the cytoplasmic domain of the receptor and only rarely involves interactions with G proteins. In this group of receptors, the original concept of the receptor as a regulatory domain of its effector enzyme is clearly appropriate.

G Proteins and Signal Transduction

The seven transmembrane domain receptors, including those for photons, peptide and protein hormones, neurotransmitters, eicosanoids, and odorants, are coupled to plasma membrane effector enzymes or ion channels through guanine-nucleotide-binding regulatory proteins (G proteins).[102] These are heterotrimeric complexes composed of three subunit proteins (α, β, and γ) that are tightly associated in the resting state but dissociate into α and $\beta\gamma$ subunits during agonist stimulation. G proteins are interposed between the receptor molecules and their effector systems and undergo repeated cycles of activation and inactivation that are controlled by their interaction with the agonist-occupied receptor. This interaction promotes the exchange of GTP for GDP bound to the α subunit of the G proteins, leading to the formation of a temporarily activated α subunit that in turn regulates the activity of the effector system (Fig. 5A-15). The α subunits of the several signal-transducing G proteins are part of a large family of GTP-binding proteins that participate in the control of diverse cellular functions ranging from signal transduction to protein synthesis and molecular trafficking between subcellular compartments. Their common feature is the ability to shuttle between an unstable transiently activated state and a stable inactive form. This property is conferred by their intrinsic GTPase activity, which catalyzes the hydrolysis of bound GTP to GDP and thus causes reversion to the inactive basal state of the protein.[103]

FIGURE 5A-15. Activation of the G protein cycle by seven transmembrane domain receptors. Hormone binding to the receptor promotes the exchange of GTP for GDP on the α subunit of the inactive heterotrimeric G protein. The consequent dissociation into α-GTP and $\beta\gamma$ provides two regulatory pathways that control the activities of a wide variety of effector systems. The activity of the α subunit is terminated by the hydrolysis of its bound GTP by the intrinsic GTPase activity of the subunit, which then reassociates with $\beta\gamma$ to form the inactive heterotrimeric G protein.

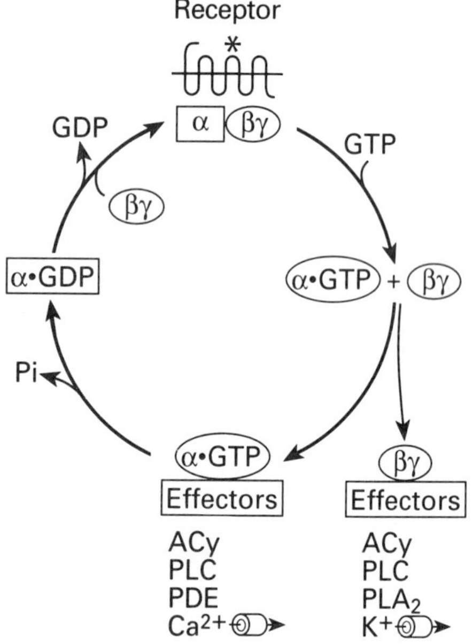

The existence of G proteins, along with their regulatory role in signal transduction, was first indicated by the finding that GTP reduced the binding of glucagon to liver membranes and increased the activity of the adenylyl cyclase system. GTP was subsequently found to exert both stimulatory and inhibitory actions on hormone-sensitive adenylyl cyclase activity and to regulate the binding properties of several receptors, including some that do not operate through the activation of adenylyl cyclase.[18] Some of these receptors proved to be coupled to inhibition of adenylyl cyclase, and others were found to be coupled to phospholipase C and other membrane effector systems. These studies led to the concept that many hormones and other extracellular messengers act by stimulating the binding of GTP to the G protein at a regulatory site in the catalytic region of an intrinsic GTPase domain. This is part of a GTPase regulatory cycle in which hormones promote the exchange of GTP for GDP on the inactive G protein and GTP hydrolysis terminates the transiently activated state of the α subunit and turns off the hormone-stimulated effector system.

The characterization of G protein–regulated processes was facilitated by the use of nonhydrolyzable GTP analogues, including Gpp(NH)p and GTP-γ-S, to activate G proteins and their dependent effectors, and by the recognition that some α subunits are substrates for bacterial toxins that modify their functional activities. Thus, the stable GTP analogues cause irreversible activation of G protein function as a result of their resistance to hydrolysis by the intrinsic GTPase activity of the α subunits. Similarly, the ADP ribosylation of cholera toxin stimulates adenylyl cyclase by preventing GTP hydrolysis and thus promotes continuous activation of the G protein. This action of cholera toxin results from its enzymatic activity as an ADP-ribosyl transferase, leading to covalent modification of the G protein and inhibition of its intrinsic GTPase activity. This effect not only leads to excessive production of cyclic AMP (which underlies the mechanism of cholera-induced fluid loss in the intestinal tract) but also provides a valuable tool for the study of the G protein (G_s) that mediates hormonal activation of the adenylyl cyclase system.

The ability of GTP to exert *inhibitory* as well as stimulatory actions on adenylyl cyclase activity led to the recognition that the enzyme is regulated not only by G_s but also by an inhibitory G protein. G_i is activated by specific receptors for several hormones and transmitters that exert inhibitory effects on adenylyl cyclase, such as opiates, somatostatin, and α_2 agonists. The characterization of G_i and its signaling actions has been aided by the use of *Bordetella pertussis* toxin, which resembles cholera toxin in possessing ADP-ribosyl transferase activity but is specific for the α subunits of G_i and certain other regulatory G proteins. The covalent modification caused by pertussis toxin prevents coupling between G protein and receptors and attenuates the signaling pathways mediated by G_i and other pertussis toxin–sensitive G proteins. G_i was at first regarded simply as an inhibitory counterpart of G_s in the regulation of adenylyl cyclase but is now known to mediate other cellular responses and to exist in three closely related forms. Several additional members of the heterotrimeric G protein family have been identified (G_t, G_o, G_{olf}, and G_α) and are described in more detail below. This group of about 20 G proteins is responsible for coupling to the large number of cell-surface receptors that constitute the seven transmembrane domain superfamily (Table 5A-3). It is important to note that G proteins act as branch points in signal transduction pathways, since one G protein can be acted on by multiple receptors and can modulate the activity of more than one effector system.[104]

Properties of G Proteins

All the G proteins that interact directly with receptors to mediate information transfer through the cell membrane are heterotrimeric structures composed of α, β, and γ subunits. The α subunits are a family of homologous molecules with molecular mass ranging from 40 to 46 kDa and are encoded by about 16 distinct genes.[105] They contain a GDP/GTP-binding site with high (n*M*) affinity for GDP in the basal state. The interaction of agonist-receptor complexes with G proteins promotes the exchange of their bound GDP for $Mg^{2+} \cdot GTP$, leading to activation of the α subunit. This activation process is terminated by the hydrolysis of GTP to GDP by the intrinsic GTPase activity of the α subunit. The α subunits can also be activated by exposure to fluoride ion, which forms a complex with GDP in the presence of Mg^{2+} and Al^{3+}. The Mg • GDP • AIF complex binds to the GTP site to cause prolonged activation similar to that induced by nonhydrolyzable GTP analogues in the presence of hormone.

Under basal conditions, the G protein is in its inactive αβγ form, in which the nucleotide-binding site of the α subnit is empty or is occupied by GDP, which dissociates with a half-time of about 5 min. Since the resting GTPase activity is much higher than the basal rate of nucleotide exchange, most of the G protein is in the inactive form in unstimulated cells. When the receptor is activated by its agonist, its conformation changes to one with high affinity for the inactive G protein. The subsequent interaction of the receptor with the G protein promotes GTP binding to the empty nucleotide site or its exchange with residual bound GDP. The ternary complex formed by the agonist, the receptor, and the inactive G protein is characterized by the high-affinity binding of agonist to the receptor as well as that of the receptor to the G protein. When GTP binds to the nucleotide site on the α subunit, the G protein dissociates from the

TABLE 5A-3. G Proteins: Expression, Receptors, and Signal Transduction Pathways

G Protein	Toxin	Expression	Receptors	Effectors	Signals
G_s	CT	General	Adrenergic (β), glucagon vasopressin V_2, GHRH, VIP, CRF, ACTH, LH/hCG, FSH, TSH	Adenylyl cyclase Ca^{2+} channels	↑cAMP ↑Ca^{2+} influx
G_{olf}	CT	Olfactory	Odorant	Adenylyl cyclase	↑cAMP (olfaction)
C_{t1}	CT/PT	Rods	Rhodopsin	cGMP phosphodiesterase	↓cGMP (vision)
G_{t2}	CT/PT	Cones	Rhodopsin	cGMP phosphodiesterase	↓cGMP (color)
G_{i1}	PT	Neural and	Noradrenaline (α_2), $5HT_1$	Adenylyl cyclase	↓cAMP
G_{i2}	PT	general	muscarinic (M2, M4), opiates, angiotensin AT_1, somatostatin	Phospholipase C Phospholipase A_2	↑$InsP_3$, DAG, Ca^{2+} ↑Arachidonate
G_{i3}	PT	General		K^+ channels	↑Membrane potential
G_o	PT	Neural Endocrine	Not yet defined	Phospholipase C Ca^{2+} channels	↑$InsP_3$, DAG, Ca^{2+} ↑Ca^{2+} influx
G_q	—	General	Adrenergic (α_1), muscarinic	Phospholipase C	↑$InsP_3$, DAG, Ca^{2+}
G_{11}	—	General	(M1, M3), $5HT_2$,		
G_{14}	—	Liver, lung, kidney	histamine, glutamate, vasopressin, oxytocin, GnRH, TRH, angiotensin II, bradykinin, tachykinins thrombin, bombesin, cholecystokinin, leukotrienes		
$G_{15/16}$	—	Blood cells	Not known	?	?
G_z	—	Neural, platelets	Not known	?	?

Abbreviations: CT, cholera toxin; 5HT, serotonin; PT, pertussis toxin; DAG, diacylglycerol. Others are defined in Table 5A-1.

complex into its α-GTP and βγ subunits. At the same time, the receptor returns to its low-affinity state for the agonist, which is then more likely to dissociate from the receptor. The α subunit • GTP complex continues to activate to its effector until the GTP has been hydrolyzed to GDP by the intrinsic GTPase activity of the subunits and then reverts to its inactive form (Fig. 5A-15). This sequence, which is an irreversible first step in the recycling of the receptor to its next interaction with an inactive G protein, or to an inactive resting state if the agonist dissociates and is not replaced by another agonist molecule, can be represented as follows:

$$A \cdot R + \alpha \cdot GDP \cdot \beta\gamma \rightleftharpoons A \cdot R^* \cdot \alpha\beta\gamma \rightarrow A \cdot R + \alpha \cdot GTP + \beta\gamma$$

where R* is the high-affinity state of the receptor.[102]

Several of the α subunits are substrates for ADP ribosylation by cholera toxin or pertussis toxin, which exert marked effects on their functional state. Thus, $G_{s\alpha}$, $G_{t\alpha}$, and $G_{olf\alpha}$ are ADP ribosylated by cholera toxin on arginine residues that are essential for their intrinsic GTPase activity and thus are rendered persistently active in the absence of receptor stimulation. Pertussis toxin catalyzes the ADP ribosylation of several G proteins, including the three forms of G_i as well as G_o and the transducins. In these proteins, the α subunits are ADP ribosylated on cysteine residues in their carboxy-terminal regions. In contrast to the activation that results from ADP ribosylation catalyzed by cholera toxin, the covalent modification caused by pertussis toxin impairs signal transduction by blocking the interaction of the G protein with receptors. This effect is accompanied by a decrease in the binding affinity of the receptors for the cognate ligands. In the adenylyl cyclase system, treatment with pertussis toxin increases the effectiveness of low concentrations of hormones that activate G_s and may cause marked stimulation of cAMP production.

Molecular Structure of G Proteins

The heterotrimeric G proteins are members of a large family of diverse gene products that exist as stable αβγ complexes of 80 to 90 kDa in the unstimulated state. There are at least 16 homologous genes for α subunits, 4 for β subunits, and 8 for γ subunits. The α subunits range in molecular mass from 39 to 50 kDa and contain sequences that are highly homologous with those which are essential for GTP binding and hydrolysis in other important G proteins (e.g., bacterial elongation factor TU and the $p21^{ras}$ proto-oncogene product).[105] These include an 18-amino acid region (identity box) that is present (with minor variations) in all α subunits and another conserved sequence of 7 amino acids that defines specificity for the guanine ring of the G nucleotides. There is also an arginine residue near the center of the G_s sequence that is ADP ribosylated by cholera toxin and a cysteine residue near the carboxy-terminus that is ADP ribosylated in the α subunits that are substrates for pertussis toxin (G_i and G_o). Based on the homologies between the α subunit sequences and that of elongation factor TU and the known crystallographic structure of the latter, a three-dimensional model of a typical G protein α subunit has been constructed and has many features in common with the structure of the *ras* protein.[106] Based on their amino acid sequences and functional properties, the α subunits fall into four classes, as follows: G_s (α_s and α_{olf}: activate adenylyl cyclase); G_i (α_i and α_o: pertussis toxin–sensitive); G_q (α_q, α_{11}, α_{14-16}: activate phospholipase C, pertussis toxin–insensitive); and G_{12} (α_{12} and α_{13}: function unknown). All these classes of G proteins are expressed in species from invertebrates to humans and so must have evolved at least 600 million years ago.[107]

The β and γ subunits of the G proteins, which exist as βγ dimers after GTP-induced dissociation of the heterotrimeric αβγ complex, also occur in several forms and are now receiving increasing attention as potential mediators of agonist-induced signaling.[108] There are at least four genes encoding β subunits (β_1 through β_4) and eight encoding γ subunits (γ_1 through γ_8) of 35 to 36 kDa and 6 to 10 kDa, respectively. The βγ dimers were formerly believed to serve as ligand-independent suppressors of receptor activity and to permit the release of receptors from α-GTP by dissociating from the receptor αβγ-GTP complex. Also, by ultimately reassociating with α-GDP subunits, βγ serves to re-form the heterotrimeric complex needed for further mediation of receptor action. However, the former view that α subunits mediate all the actions of G proteins has been challenged by recent findings that βγ subunits exert regulatory actions on several membrane effector systems.

Roles of β and γ Subunits in Signal Transduction

Although the β and γ subunits are essential for agonist-induced activation of G proteins, they were believed to be less diverse than the α subunits and were thought to be unlikely to be associated with specific modes of signaling. However, this view has changed markedly in the last few years (Table 5A-4). The initial evidence for a role for βγ in transmembrane signaling came from studies on pheromone-induced mating in yeast and activation of phospholipase A_2 in mammalian cells.[109] Also, βγ subunits were found to mediate the M_2-muscarinic receptor activation of a K^+ channel by G_i or G_o (formerly termed G_k) in atrial myocytes.[110] Furthermore, two of the six forms of adenylyl cyclase that have been cloned and expressed were found to be markedly stimulated in vitro by βγ subunits in the presence of activated α subunits, an effect referred to as "conditional" activation of the enzyme.[111] Similar effects were observed in mammalian cells transfected with

TABLE 5A-4. Signaling Functions of G Protein β and γ Subunits

1. βγ is essential for activation of α subunits by receptors.
2. βγ binds to free α to reconstitute αβγ.*
3. βγ mediates pheromone-induced signaling in yeast.
4. βγ stimulates activity of phospholipase A_2.
5. βγ inhibits activity of K^+ channels.
6. βγ stimulates activity of certain isoforms of adenylyl cyclase.
7. $\beta\gamma_t$ enhances phosphorylation of β-adrenergic receptor kinase.
8. βγ stimulates activity of phospholipase C β_2 and β_3.
9. β and γ determine receptor specificity for inhibition of L channels by G_o.
10. γ_1 subunit determines specificity of interaction of α_t with rhodopsin.

*May also mediate the effect of G_i on the inhibition of adenylyl cyclase by quenching the activity of α_s.

the type II adenylyl cyclase and α_2-adrenergic receptors, which normally act through G_i to inhibit adenylyl cyclase. In such cotransfected cells, the activation of α_2-adrenergic receptors causes stimulation rather than inhibition of adenylyl cyclase activity because of the release of βγ subunits from G_i. This effect is prominent during simultaneous activation of G_s in the transfected cells, confirming the ability of βγ to function as a conditional activator of cAMP synthesis by type II adenylyl cyclase in the presence of stimuli that act through G_s. This action of βγ explains a number of apparently paradoxic observations on certain compounds that do not alone activate adenylyl cyclase but sometimes potentiate the action of agents that do.

An important role for βγ subunits in the activation of phospholipase C has been identified recently. The stimulation of phospholipase C activity by βγ subunits is selective for the β_2 isozyme.[112] Furthermore, the receptor-mediated release of βγ from G_i or G_o proteins is probably responsible for mediating the pertussis toxin–sensitive activation of phospholipase C that occurs in certain cell types.[113] A specific role for individual β subunits in signal transduction has been indicated by experiments in which antisense oligonucleotides against mRNAs for the four known β subunits were injected into GH_3 pituitary cells, in which L-type voltage-sensitive calcium channels are inhibited by signaling through G_o from somatostatin and muscarinic receptors.[114] In this system, $\beta_{1\gamma 3}$ and $\beta_{3\gamma 4}$ are selectively involved in signal transduction from somatostatin and muscarinic M_4 receptors, respectively, and β_2 and β_4 do not participate in signaling from either form of receptor.

Recently, the γ subunit has also become established as an important factor in the specificity of receptor–G protein interactions.[115] It is now known that there is a family of at least eight γ subunits that have diverse structures and in some cases are specific to certain tissues or cell types. The γ subunits are isoprenylated at a cysteine residue near their carboxy terminus and are thus tethered to the plasma membrane, together with their associated β subunits. The specific role of a γ subunit in determining the interaction of a receptor with its G protein has been identified in transducin (G_t). Of three γ subunits tested (γ_1, specific to rod outer segments; γ_2, present in many tissues; and γ_3, predominantly present in brain), all interact equally well with the transducin α subunit, but only the γ_1 subunit was able to support interaction of the αβγ complex with rhodopsin.[116] It is likely that the γ subunits are important determinants of the specificity with which receptors bind to individual G proteins, an issue that was hitherto unresolved. It is clear that the former view of G protein action being mediated solely by the respective α subunits was incorrect and that the βγ subunits are important elements in several aspects of the signal transduction process (Table 5A-3).

Abnormalities of G Protein Function

Changes in the function, expression, and structure of G proteins have been identified in several human diseases. In addition to the modifications of G_s and G_i that occur during infection with *Vibrio cholera* and *B. pertussis*, respectively, and contribute to the pathophysiology of these disorders, altered levels of G proteins have been found in diabetes, alcoholism, and heart failure. Recently, G protein mutations that result in decreased expression or constitutive activation of the mutant α subunit have been found in several endocrine disorders.[117] The most common of these disorders are the activating *gsp* mutations present in the α subunit gene in certain somatotroph adenomas and thyroid tumors and in abnormal tissues of patients with the McCune-Albright syndrome.[118] These are single base mutations in the triplets encoding the Arg^{201} and Gln^{227} residues of the α_s subunit. Arg^{201} is the amino acid in α_s that is ADP ribosylated by cholera toxin to inhibit GTPase activity, and Gln^{229} corresponds to the residue in the *ras* proto-oncogene (Gln^{61}) that is necessary for its GTPase activity. Mutations of these amino acids cause a marked decrease in GTPase activity and promote cell proliferation and transformation.

In pituitary somatotrophs, constitutive activation of the mutant α_s subunits causes an overproduction of cyclic AMP that stimulates cell hyperplasia by inducing the expression of the transcriptional regulatory protein Pit-1.[119] In the McCune-Albright syndrome, a form of mosaicism that results from a somatic mutation of α_s in the endocrine glands, melanotrophs, and osteoblasts, overproduction of cyclic AMP leads to cell proliferation and/or overactivity of the affected tissues. In addition to the café au

TABLE 5A-5. The GTP-Binding (GTPase) Superfamily

	Families	Members	Functions
I	Initiation and elongation factors (50–60 kDa)	Initiation factor IF-2	Initiation
		Elongation factor Tu	Proofreading
II	G protein α-subunits (39–52 kDa)	G_s, G_i, G_o, G_q, G_{11}	Signal transduction
		G_{olf}	Odor perception
		G_t	Vision
III	Small GTPases (20–35 kDa)	Ras	Control of growth pathways
		Raf	Activation of MAP kinase
		Rab	Intracellular transport
		Rho	Cytoskeletal organization
		Rac	Actin filamin formation
			Activation of NADPH oxidase
		Ran	Nuclear transport of protein
IV	Microtubule-associated GTPases (~100 kDa)	D100, Mx	

lait spots that reflect the effects of an early somatic mutation on the adult distribution of melanotrophs in the skin, such patients exhibit precocious puberty and hypergonadism as well as hyperthyroidism, adrenal hyperfunction, and sometimes acromegaly. Another type of activating mutation occurs in G_i α subunit (specifically α_{i2}) in some adrenal and ovarian tumors. These mutations (termed *gip2*) are associated with constitutive activation of the G_i protein and inhibition of cAMP production, yet lead to increased cell proliferation.[120] The growth-promoting effects of these mutations probably reflects the fact that certain mitogenic responses to stimulation of G protein–coupled receptors are mediated by G_i proteins and would thus be enhanced by constitutive activation of the α_1 subunit.

In contrast to the stimulatory actions of the *gsp* and *gip2* mutations in endocrine target cells, there is a deficiency of G_s in patients with Albright's hereditary osteodystrophy, or pseudohypoparathyroidism.[121] These patients are resistant to several of the hormones [parathyroid hormone (PTH), TSH, gonadotropins, and glucagon] that stimulate cyclic AMP production by activating G_s and thus adenylyl cyclase. In most cases, the affected tissues contain about 50 percent of the normal level of G_s because of various mutations in the α_s gene. These mutations are often unique to each affected family and may result in altered RNA processing or the expression of a functionally inactive protein.

The GTP-Binding Protein Superfamily

The heterotrimeric G proteins belong to large superfamily of regulatory proteins that bind and hydrolyze GTP, and function as molecular switches that control a wide range of intracellular functions (Table 5A-5).[122] These GTP-binding proteins (or GTPase proteins) are characterized by their ability to assume an active conformation after binding GTP. The bound GTP is subsequently slowly hydrolyzed to GDP, and the protein reverts to its inactive GDP-binding form. The GTP-bound protein interacts with other signaling molecules for a period that depends on the intrinsic GTP-hydrolyzing activity of the protein. Thus, the GDP/GTP cycle controls the activity of the protein and the duration for which it is switched "on" to exert its regulatory actions. The intrinsic GTPase activity of these proteins is relatively weak, and the GDP/GTP cycle is often regulated by additional proteins that influence GTPase activity or the rates of exchange of GDP and GTP (termed guanine nucleotide exchange proteins). In the heterotrimeric G proteins, this function is served by the ligand-activated receptors that promote the exchange of GDP for GTP on the α subunit, leading to dissociation of the complex into α-GTP and βγ subunits. The general mechanism of GTP binding and activation, followed by GTP hydrolysis and inactivation, is utilized by a wide variety of regulatory proteins that control transmembrane signaling, ribosomal protein synthesis, protein translocation into the endoplasmic reticulum, and intracellular vesicular transport, as well as cell differentiation and proliferation (Table 5A-5).

TABLE 5A-6. Formation and Disposition of Intracellular Second Messengers

Derived from abundant precursors
- ATP, GTP
- Membrane phospholipids
- Extracellular Ca^{2+} and internal Ca^{2+} stores

Rapid generated during hormone action, usually in small amounts
- cAMP, cGMP
- $InsP_3$, DAG
- Cytoplasmic Ca^{2+}

Rapidly decreased by enzymatic mechanisms
- Phosphodiesterases
  - cAMP → AMP
  - cGMP → GMP
- Inositol and lipid metabolism
  - $InsP_3 \rightarrow IP_2 \rightarrow$ inositol
  - Calcium pumps in ER and plasma membrane

Abbreviations: DAG, diacylglycerol; $InsP_3$, isositol (1,4,5)-trisphosphate.

Small GTP-Binding Proteins

An important and expanding group of guanine nucleotide regulatory proteins constitutes the so-called GTP-binding proteins (or small GTPases) that have been defined during research on the properties and functions of cellular oncogenes. The prototype of this family is the group of *ras* genes that were originally identified as sites of somatic mutations in human neoplasms and were subsequently found to encode a set of small GTP-binding proteins that participate in the regulation of cell proliferation.[123] Mutations of the *ras* genes that impair the GTPase activity of their protein products are associated with transforming activity and are present in a significant proportion of mammalian tumors. In addition, overexpression of the normal *ras* gene product (ras, or $p21^{ras}$) occurs in certain human tumors, such as breast cancer, and can cause malignant transformation in transfected cells. The mature ras protein is prenylated and palmitoylated at cysteine residues near its carboxy-terminus, and is thus anchored to the cytoplasmic surface of the plasma membrane. The ras proteins and other small GTPases contain four highly conserved regions that participate in guanine nucleotide binding and hydrolysis. It is within these regions that mutations of specific amino acids can endow ras with transforming activity as a result of persistent activation by bound GTP. A critical region of the ras protein, located between residues 32 and 40, is known to interact with other signaling molecules and forms an external loop that changes its conformation when binding GTP versus GDP.

The activity of ras and other small GTPases is controlled by two major factors: the rate of dissociation of the tightly bound GDP from the inactive form of $p21^{ras}$ (which determines its rate of switching by GTP to the "on" conformation) and the rate at which the bound GTP is hydrolyzed to GDP by the intrinsic GTPase activity of the protein, which causes it to assume the "off" conformation. Both reactions are relatively slow in the native ras protein but are regulated by GTPase activating and inhibitory proteins as well as other factors that accelerate or inhibit the release of bound GDP (Fig. 5A-16). Thus, the ras proteins and their relatives can be regulated over a wide range of times to cycle between "on" and "off" conformations in accordance with the extrinsic factors that control the rates of GTP binding and hydrolysis. For this reason, factors such as the GTPase-activating proteins (GAPs) are important regulators of ras activity.[124] GAP is a ubiquitous 120-kDa cytosolic protein that interacts with an effector domain located at residues 32–40 of the ras protein. Ras-GAP appears to act largely as a negative regulator of ras by promoting GTP hydrolysis and keeping $p21^{ras}$ in its inactive form. GAP, together with other cytoplasmic proteins containing SH2 (src homology) domains that interact with phosphotyrosine residues,

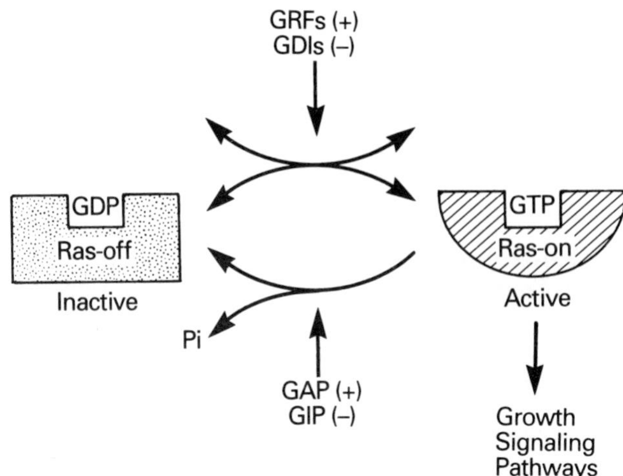

FIGURE 5A-16. Activation of the small GTP-binding protein ras. Binding of GTP switches the molecule to its active conformation, initiating downstream growth signals. The period during which ras remains active depends on the intrinsic GTPase activity and the effects of regulators that influence GTPase activity and nucleotide exchange.

is associated with growth factor receptors (EGF, PDGF, FGF, and others) that possess intrinsic tyrosine kinase activity in their intracellular domains (discussed below). Activation of such receptors increases the active form of ras by inactivation of GAP, which appears to be controlled by products of phospholipid hydrolysis (arachidonic acid, phosphatidic acid, and prostaglandins) that are produced during receptor activation.[125]

In addition to GAP, ras activity is controlled by several other factors that modify the GTPase-driven cycle of this activity. These include proteins that inhibit GTPase activity [GTPase inhibitory proteins (GIPs)] and are regulated by phospholipid breakdown products. In addition, guanine nucleotide releasing factors [GRFs, also termed GTP/GDP dissociation stimulators (GDSs)], which promote the release of GDP from inactive ras and thus increase the rate of association of GTP with the regulatory site, act as exchange proteins to promote the activation of ras. Proteins that inhibit the release of GDP from inactive ras [GDP dissociation inhibitors (GDIs)] have also been found in the cytoplasm and presumably prevent the activation of ras by keeping it in the GDP-associated form.[126] These several forms of regulation interact with the GTPase functions of ras and other small G proteins, which act as molecular switches that operate a variety of effectors for periods that are determined by the rate of hydrolysis or dissociation of their bound GTP.[122] All the ras-related small G proteins undergo several post-translation modifications. These modifications include the attachment of C15 (farnesyl) or C20 (geranyl-geranyl) isoprenoid chains as well as palmitylation, myristylation, carboxymethylation, and phosphorylation.[126] Isoprenylation occurs at specific cysteine-containing motifs at the carboxy-terminal end of the molecule and is required for association with specific intracellular membranes and with the regulatory proteins that control the activity status of the G protein.

Functions of ras and Other Small GTPases

Yeast and Mammalian ras Proteins

In *Saccharomyces cerevisiae*, ras proteins are regulators of adenylyl cyclase activity and serve as a link between the nutritional status of the organism and cAMP production, which controls the growth and division of yeast cells.[127] This process is believed to be mediated by a nutrition-sensing protein that controls the GDP/GTP exchange reaction and thus the proportion of ras in the active form. Ras may also control other pathways that are required for cell growth and viability and in some yeast strains may couple nutrient levels to a pathway that acts in concert with that of the α-mating factor (which reduces adenylyl cyclic activity) to promote conjugation and sexual reproduction.[128]

In mammalian cells, ras proteins are intimately involved in the normal control of cell differentiation and proliferation. Three ras proteins are expressed in virtually all mammalian cells (H-Ras, Ki-Ras, and N-Ras) and are very similar to those present in yeast and other organisms. Their association with the cell membrane, which is essential for their functional activity, is ensured by isoprenylation of the carboxy-terminal cysteine residues and by the addition of palmitic acid (in H-Ras and N-Ras) to an upstream cysteine residue. The importance of ras in growth regulation is indicated by the transforming effects of its constitutively active mutant forms.[123] It is also shown by the ability of ras antibodies to block the cell cycle when injected during the early hours of G_1 and to prevent the actions of several growth factors on cell proliferation. However, the signaling pathways that are utilized by ras for these functions have not been easy to define. Unlike the yeast system, ras does not influence cAMP production in mammalian cells. Also, it has not been shown to act through the phosphoinositide-calcium signaling pathway. Although activation of protein kinase C appears to be essential for the mitogenic action of mutant ras proteins, the manner in which this occurs was not known.

However, recent studies in several species have identified a novel mechanism by which ras couples the growth factor receptor tyrosine kinases to a cascade of serine/threonine protein kinases that activate mitogen-activated protein (MAP) kinase, a central intermediate between cell-surface receptors and signal transduction to the cell nucleus.[129] Activation of receptor tyrosine kinases causes an increase in ras•GTP, which in turn activates Raf-1 and MAP kinase. This pathway, which is explained in detail below, is now recognized as a major signaling route from the cell membrane to the cytoplasm and thence, via MAP kinase, to regulatory substrates in the nucleus, cytoskeleton, and plasma membrane. Activated growth factor receptors have been found to signal to ras via two cytoplasmic proteins, an adapter molecule called Grb2 (growth factor receptor binding protein) and a nucleotide exchange protein called mSos (the mammalian form of a *Drosophila* gene product called "son of sevenless" because it acts downstream of the *sevenless* gene in regulating eye development). The Sos protein promotes GDP/GTP exchange on ras and thus switches it to the active state. During binding of growth factors to their receptors, the Grb2•mSos complex that is present in the cytoplasm of unstimulated cells becomes associated with phosphotyrosine residues in the intracellular domain of the activated receptors. This region binds to Grb2, and the associated Sos protein activates ras by causing it to exchange its bound GDP for GTP.[130] In this way, ras acts as an essential link between external growth signals and the numerous cellular pathways that lead to differentiation, growth, and proliferation.

While ras proteins are specifically responsible for the activation of the growth pathway and the control of cellular proliferation, other small G proteins serve as regulators of numerous intracellular processes, especially those involved in the movement and distribution of cellular components. These processes include the sorting and trafficking of intracellular vesicles, the control of cytoskeletal components, and the importation of proteins into the nucleus. An outline of the localization and functions of the various ras-related small G proteins within the cell is shown in Fig. 5A-17.

Rab and ARF Proteins

About 25 members of the ras superfamily belong to the rab group of small GTP-binding proteins and are localized in the intracellular compartments of the endocytic and exocytic pathways.[126] Rab proteins appear to be involved in all aspects of the regulation of vesicular transport within the cell. Thus, rab1 and rab2 are required for vesicular transport between the endoplasmic reticulum and the Golgi apparatus. In neutrophils, rab1 is associated with a plasma membrane enzyme system that catalyzes the formation of superoxide radicals. Rab3 participates in the regulation of exocytosis and is involved in intracellular vesicle transport during endocytosis and exocytosis. Rab3A is confined to endocrine and other cells with a regulated secretion pathway and is required for neurotransmitter release and calcium-dependent exocytosis by anterior pituitary cells.[131] Rab4 controls the sorting processes that occur in endosomes during recycling of plasma membrane components. Rab5 is present in the plasma membrane and in early endosomes and is a rate-limiting factor in the early endocytic pathway.[132] Rab7 probably controls

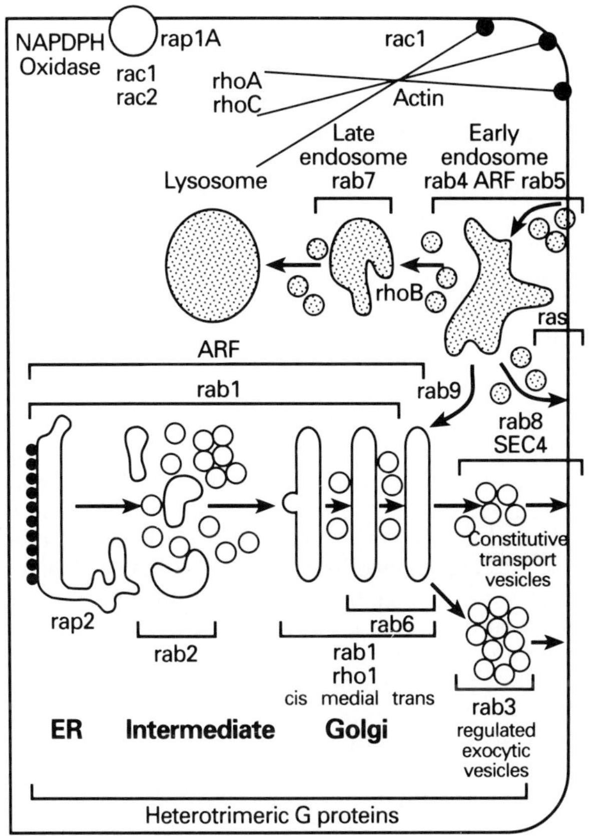

FIGURE 5A-17. Subcellular localization and sites of action of small G proteins of the ras family. In addition to the membrane-associated G proteins of the ras, rab, rap, and ARF varieties, other members of the family (rac and rho) are present in the cytoplasm. Rho1 is a yeast rho homolog located in the Golgi system. *(Modified from Bokoch and Der.*[126]*)*

transport from early to late endosomes and is located in the latter structures. Other small GTPases, the ARF (ADP ribosylation factor) proteins, are involved in the control of transport within the Golgi system and are inhibited by the fungal metabolite brefeldin A.[133] ARF proteins also have been found to be involved in the activation of phospholipase D, leading to the production of lysophosphatidic acid and diacylglycerol from phosphatidylcholine. These actions may be related to the role of ARF in cellular trafficking, since the hydrolysis of phosphatidylcholine and the altered phospholipid content of the membrane could affect the processes of fusion and fission and thus influence vesicular trafficking.[134] Recently, another GTP-binding protein, termed ran4, has been found to be required for the importation of proteins from the cytoplasm to the nucleus.[135] It appears that many of the effects of GTP on vesicular transport and the rates of endocytosis and exocytosis are mediated by the several small GTP-binding proteins that control the individual steps of intracellular transport. However, components of the heterotrimeric G proteins, including the α subunits of G_{i3} and G_q, are present in the Golgi region of pituitary cells and also may be involved in vesicular trafficking through the secretory pathway.[136]

Rho and Rac Proteins

Rho proteins are located in the cytoplasm and are involved in the regulation of actin microfilament organization and assembly. They are also substrates for ADP ribosylation by *Clostridium botulinum* toxin, which causes disassembly of actin filaments and causes marked changes in cell shape. Similar changes are caused by microinjection of activated rho proteins, with contraction and the formation of cytoplasmic extensions. These effects of rho proteins are inhibited by prior ADP ribosylation by botulinus toxin. Rho is also responsible for mediating the effect of serum on actin stress fibers and appears to be required to maintain the organization of the Golgi apparatus.[137]

Rac proteins are also involved in actin filament formation, specifically that which is associated with membrane ruffling and the formation of pinocytic vesicles. Rac appears to mediate the effects of growth factors on these processes, an action that is mimicked by ras and is in turn dependent on the activation of rho. It is likely that ras acts as an intermediate in the actions of growth factors on the cytoskeleton and regulates the activities of rac and rho. The rac protein has an additional action on the generation of superoxide anion by NADPH oxidase in neutrophils and macrophages. In the cytoplasm, rac is present as an inactive complex with a GDI and is activated by factors that dissociate the complex and render it available for GTP binding.[138]

Receptor Phosphorylation and Hormone Action

In addition to the phosphorylation of cytosolic proteins that mediate cellular responses to many forms of hormone action via cAMP-, calcium-, or phospholipid-dependent protein kinases, several plasma membrane proteins are phosphorylated during receptor activation. These proteins include the receptors themselves and some of their transducing proteins, which thus become targets for local regulatory mechanisms in the course of subserving their primary function of transmembrane signaling.[139] The phosphorylation of the β-adrenergic receptor by a specific kinase (βARK) during catecholamine-induced desensitization, as discussed above, may represent a general feature of receptor desensitization by homologous hormones.

An important form of receptor phosphorylation is catalyzed by the protein kinase activity of the receptor itself. Several receptors, including those for the activin/TGF-β group, possess intrinsic serine/threonine kinase domains in their cytoplasmic regions.[140] In contrast, most of the typical receptors for growth factors have intrinsic tyrosine kinase activity and undergo autophosphorylation after activation by their agonist ligands (Table 5A-3). These types of receptors act as ligand-regulated protein kinases and phosphorylate tyrosine residues (as well as serine and threonine) during activation by mitogenic peptides and cytokines. Although tyrosine phosphorylation is relatively minor in most cells, the tyrosine kinase activity of receptors that modify cell growth and proliferation is an essential step in their signal transduction pathway. The importance of tyrosine phosphorylation during insulin action is indicated by the finding of impaired kinase activity and receptor phosphorylation in tissues from patients with mutations of the insulin receptor that cause severe insulin resistance and normal insulin-binding characteristics. One such mutation in the tyrosine kinase domain of the receptor causes impaired tyrosine kinase activity and reduces the ability of insulin to stimulate glucose uptake.[141]

In addition to the frequent occurrence of tyrosine phosphorylation during the regulation of cell growth and metabolism by peptide hormones and growth factors, cell transformation by oncogenic retroviruses is also associated with protein phosphorylation at tyrosine residues. Several of the transforming proteins of oncogenic viruses possess tyrosine-specific protein kinase activity, as exemplified by the protein product ($pp60^{src}$) encoded by the Rous sarcoma virus *src* gene that mediates cellular transformation.[142] Furthermore, the *src* gene product also stimulates phosphorylation of cellular proteins in the same manner in which EGF and other receptors promote tyrosine phosphorylation. These findings have important implications about the role of peptide hormones in the normal control of cellular growth via processes related to tyrosine phosphorylation and about the loss of growth control in transformed and neoplastic cells. The ability of TGF-α to bind to the EGF receptor and activate tyrosine phosphorylation in the receptor illustrates the manner in which receptor phosphorylation can be involved in cell proliferation.[143]

Other examples of ligand-dependent receptor phosphorylation are provided by rhodopsin and the growth factor receptors. As noted earlier, rhodopsin serves as the receptor for photons in retinal rod cells and acts via transducin to stimulate cyclic GMP breakdown and closure of sodium channels. The activated form of rhodopsin is immediately phosphorylated at serine and threonine residues by a cAMP-independent rhodopsin kinase, a reaction which terminates the retinal processes that decrease cGMP levels and modulate sodium flux in the light-sensitive rod cells.[48] In the case of the EGF receptor, ligand binding stimulates the intrinsic kinase activity of the receptor itself, which becomes autophosphorylated at specific tyrosine residues and initiates cell activation. The interaction of EGF with its receptors causes dimerization of the sites, leading to enhanced kinase tyrosine activity and autophosphorylation of the tyrosine residues in the cytoplasmic domain of the receptor.[82] The EGF-stimulated protein kinase phosphorylates adjacent membrane proteins as well as the EGF receptor itself. The manner in which receptor dimerization and autophosphorylation are linked to the mitogenic action of EGF depends on the ability of the tyrosine-phosphorylated domain to interact with other proteins in the growth signaling pathway.

Intrinsic Receptor Signaling Domains

Ligand-Induced Autophosphorylation

An important form of transmembrane signaling is mediated by enzymatic domains in the cytoplasmic regions of many growth factor and cytokine receptors that do not depend on G proteins for the generation of intracellular responses. First observed in the *v-src* oncogene and its cellular homologues, the tyrosine kinase activity of such receptors is responsible for initiating the signaling pathways that lead to growth responses in their target cells. Ligand-induced autophosphorylation occurs at short sequence motifs that serve as specific recognition sites for contact with target proteins that generate intracellular signals or couple tyrosine kinase receptors to a variety of effector pathways. This leads to the formation of multiprotein complexes containing the activated receptor kinases and several signaling molecules, such as phospholipase C-γ, phosphatidylinositol-3-kinase, and ras GTPase-activating protein (ras-GAP).[144] All these receptor-associated proteins have conserved domains of about 100 amino acids that provide phosphorylation-dependent contact regions for the assembly of receptor signaling complexes. These are termed SH2 domains and are present not only in the src family of tyrosine kinases but also in several other cytoplasmic proteins that are involved in cellular signaling.[145] Thus, tyrosine autophosphorylation of activated receptors favors the binding of multiple signaling proteins to form heteromeric complexes around the intracellular domain of the receptor, adjacent to the plasma membrane.

SH2 and SH3 Domains

The *v-src* oncogene product, the first tyrosine protein kinase to be identified, has a cellular homologue (c-src) that belongs to a large family of tyrosine kinases. In addition to the membrane-spanning receptor tyrosine kinases, there is a large group of cytoplasmic tyrosine kinases that are not directly activated by intracellular ligands. These enzymes are exemplified by Src, Fps, Abl, and Fyn, and possess common structural features that enable them to participate in signal transduction.[146] When activated, these tyrosine kinases phosphorylate other intracellular proteins that influence metabolic pathways, cytoskeletal elements, gene expression, and cell division. Although each protein tyrosine kinase has specific structural features, certain sequences occur in all or most members of the family. The catalytic domain of about 260 amino acids, which phosphorylates tyrosine residues in its own sequence and those of other proteins, is common to all members of the family. Adjacent to this primary region of src homology is the SH2 (src homology 2) domain of about 100 residues, which not only modulates the catalytic activity of the kinase domain but also facilitates binding to other proteins that are subsequently phosphorylated on tyrosine residues.[147]

SH2 domains are present in many of the cytoplasmic proteins that participate in intracellular signaling pathways. Major among those are phospholipase C-γ, PI-3-kinase, and ras-GAP as well as Crk and Abl. SH2 domains bring about the tight association of these proteins with activated receptor protein–tyrosine kinases by serving as phosphotyrosine-binding sites. In some receptors, the autophosphorylated region containing phosphotyrosine is located in a segment of the kinase domain, termed the kinase insert, that is not required for catalytic activity but is necessary for signaling responses. Such segments are present in PDGF and colony-stimulating factor (CSF) receptors and probably form a loop that protrudes from the surface of the protein. In the EGF receptor, the same function is performed by an autophosphorylated segment of the carboxy-terminal region of the protein.[148]

An important feature of the SH2 domains is their ability to recognize distinct regions of the receptor so that the several signaling molecules become associated with separate phosphopeptide sequences on its surface. The specificity of binding between individual SH2 domains and an autophosphorylated receptor is determined by the amino acid sequence adjacent to the phosphorylated tyrosine residue. In particular, the three amino acids that are C-terminal to the phosphotyrosine strongly influence the selectivity of the SH2 domains for individual protein regions. Thus, PI-3-kinase and phospholipase C-γ have high affinity for the general sequence pTyr-hydrophobic-x-hydrophobic (e.g., pTyr-Met/Val-x-Met), while other SH2 domain proteins prefer the general motif pTyr-hydrophilic-hydrophilic-Ile-Pro.[149]

Several tyrosine kinases possess an additional src homology domain of about 60 residues (SH3) that is immediately N-terminal to SH2. The SH3 domain does not interact with tyrosine phosphorylated domains but binds to other cellular proteins, such as the GAPs that regulate several of the small G proteins of the Ras and Rho/Rac families.[150] Thus, the SH3 domains can link to both tyrosine kinase– and small G protein–mediated signal transduction pathways. An important element in this process is the recently identified protein Grb2 (growth factor receptor-bound protein 2), which is composed of a single SH2 domain flanked by two SH3 domains.[151] This protein does not become phosphorylated when bound to tyrosine autophosphorylated growth factor receptors but acts as a regulatory subunit of downstream signaling molecules such as ras by influencing GAPs or GDP/GTP exchange factors that modulate ras signaling activity.

In addition to being present in the cytoplasmic tyrosine kinases and signaling molecules such as phospholipase C-γ, Ras-GAP, and PI-3-kinase, SH3 domains are found in other enzymes and in proteins (such as spectrin) with no catalytic activity. Their presence in proteins that are stably or transiently associated with the cell membrane suggests that SH3 domains interact predominantly with plasma membrane or peripheral cytoskeletal elements. The structure of SH3 is distinct from that of the SH2 domain, and its presence in proteins involved in cytoskeleton assembly and membrane rearrangement is consistent with its potential role in intracellular trafficking and structural organization.

Protein Tyrosine Phosphatases

Since the phosphorylation of proteins on tyrosyl residues is a reversible process, the enzymes that catalyze dephosphorylation (protein tyrosine phosphatases or PTPases) are also important in modulating signal transduction. About 30 PTPases have been identified in organisms ranging from bacteria to humans and are involved in the control of cell signaling, cytoskeletal function, cell adhesion, and the cell cycle. These enzymes exist as transmembrane receptor-like molecules, often with an intracellular tandem repeat of PTPhase domains, and also as nontransmembrane forms that contain one catalytic domain. The receptor-like PTPases are very active and possess high affinity for phosphotyrosine substrates. The leukocyte common antigen, CD45, contains PTPase activity in its cytoplasmic domain and has a conserved cysteine-rich sequence that resembles a ligand binding site in its extracellular domain. Such receptor-like PTPases could control transmembrane signaling events by ligand-induced dephosphorylation of phosphotyrosine residues in cell-membrane or cytoplasmic proteins. In addition to the CD45 family, four other groups of receptor-like PTPases have been identified based on the structures of their extracellular domains. The nontransmembrane PTPases are exemplified by PTP1b, the human placental protein that was the first such enzyme to be isolated. Most of the nonreceptor PTPases contain sequences that are related to those of other proteins, and which may target them to specific sites such as the interface between the plasma membrane and cytoskeleton.[152]

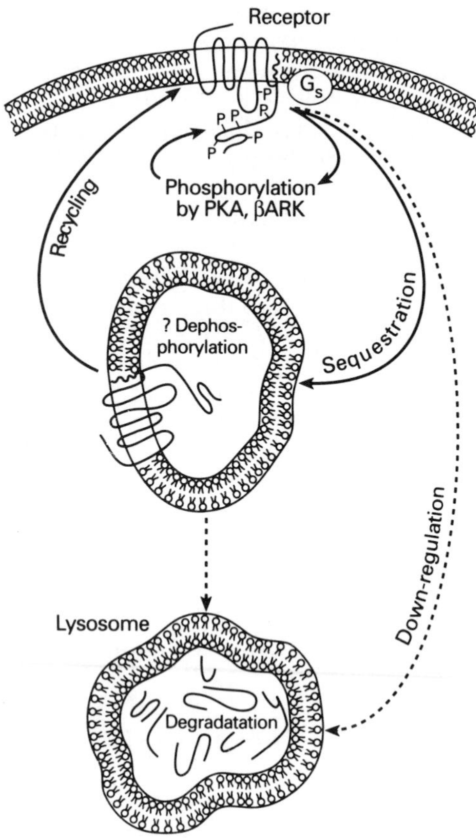

FIGURE 5A-18. Desensitization and internalization of β-adrenergic receptors. Phosphorylation of the agonist-activated receptor by cAMP-dependent protein kinase (PKA) and βARK causes uncoupling of receptors from G_s and desensitization. This is followed by rapid sequestration of receptors into a vesicular compartment adjacent to the plasma membrane. More prolonged exposure to the agonist leads to receptor processing and down-regulation of the total receptor content of the cell. The relation between sequestration and down-regulation is not clear but could be sequential or independent, as shown by the two pathways indicated by dashed lines. (*Modified from Hausdorff et al.*[157])

Hormone Receptors and Target Cell Densensitization

Desensitization of Target Cell Responses

Many receptor-mediated responses in endocrine and other cell types show a marked decline during continuous agonist stimulation or on repeated exposure to the agonist. In many cells, continuous or high-dose agonist treatment causes a rapid initial burst of signaling activity, followed by a fall to nearly basal levels and a temporary loss of responsiveness to further hormonal stimulation. This decrease in responsiveness after agonist treatment is referred to as *desensitization, refractoriness*, or *tachyphylaxis*. Such agonist-induced attenuation of target cell responsiveness is a common feature of hormone-stimulated adenylyl cyclase and other G protein–mediated enzyme responses.[153] In seven transmembrane domain receptors, this transient response to hormonal activation is caused largely by covalent modifications of the receptor that interfere with its interaction with the transducing G protein. Such responses permit rapid cellular activation by the regulatory ligand while preventing the generation of excessively large or sustained rises in second messenger formation.

In many hormone-stimulated cells, desensitization is initiated by the phosphorylation of sites in the intracellular regions involved in coupling to G proteins, and is followed by internalization and subsequently by down-regulation that leads to the loss of cell-surface receptor sites (Fig. 5A-18). A distinction is made between *heterologous* desensitization, in which exposure to one hormone temporarily impairs the ability of the effector system to respond to other ligands, and *homologous* desensitization, in which the attenuation of receptor function is hormone-specific and is limited to the agonist itself.[154] Heterologous desensitization results from phosphorylation of the receptor during agonist-induced signaling by cAMP-dependent protein kinase or protein kinase C. During excessive stimulation of any single hormone receptor system, the overproduction of cyclic AMP or diacylglycerol (DAG) sometimes modifies other systems by promoting the phosphorylation of their receptor sites within the plasma membrane. Another potential cause of heterologous desensitization is increased phosphodiesterase activity, which can cause a general increase in cAMP degradation and thus impair the ability of other cAMP-dependent hormones to elicit their responses.[155]

In homologous desensitization, refractoriness is caused by agonist-induced changes that are specific for the activated receptor sites. These include persistent occupancy by bound hormone, covalent modification and inactivation of the receptors, and internalization with recycling or degradation of the sites. Such changes dampen the cell's response to high or persistent levels of hormonal stimulation. In most cases, the cells continue to respond to the elevated level of hormonal stimulation, although to a lesser degree than would occur in the absence of desensitization. Treatment with superagonist GnRH analogues can cause such marked desensitization that gonadotroph function is selectively inhibited and gonadotropin secretion is suppressed in the face of continued administration of the releasing hormone.[148]

The desensitization of G protein–coupled receptors has been extensively studied in β-adrenergic receptors, in which refractoriness is temporally correlated with increased phosphorylation of the receptor at serine and threonine residues in the third intracellular loop and the carboxy-terminal cytoplasmic tail. Receptor phosphorylation occurs very rapidly during homologous desensitization by β-adrenergic agonists and is mediated by a distinct β-adrenergic receptor kinase (βARK) that phosphorylates sites in the serine- and threonine-rich carboxy-terminus of the agonist-occupied sites.[156] βARK is very similar to rhodopsin kinase and can phosphorylate a specific region of light-bleached rhodopsin. It also phosphorylates the agonist-occupied α_2-adrenergic and muscarinic receptors. Just as phosphorylation of bleached rhodopsin by rhodopsin kinase reduces its interaction with transducin, phosphorylation of agonist-activated β-adrenergic and other receptors by βARK causes uncoupling of the receptor from the regulatory G protein. This action of βARK on the β receptor resembles that of rhodopsin kinase on rhodopsin, which requires an additional protein, retinal arrestin, that binds to and inactivates phosphorylated rhodopsin. A related protein, β-arrestin, binds to the βARK-phosphorylated adrenergic receptor and prevents it from interacting with G_s.

Activation of the cAMP-dependent protein kinase (PKA) pathway is the major cause of β-adrenergic receptor phosphorylation and desensitization at low agonist concentrations.[157] This affects both the activated G_s-coupled receptors and those not currently occupied by hormone, including receptors of the same type and sometimes those for other ligands. This results in a combination of homologous and heterologous desensitization and can involve a variety of receptors in the same cell, including those coupled to phospholipase C. In contrast, βARK phosphorylates only agonist-occupied receptors but is activated at much higher agonist concentrations. Unlike the second messenger–activated protein kinases, its effect can be seen only on the cognate β-adrenergic receptor. Since PKA is always activated at the agonist concentrations needed to stimulate βARK, β-adrenergic stimulation is usually associated with at least two types of phosphorylation that contribute to receptor desensitization.

In addition to undergoing desensitization caused by agonist-induced phosphorylation at specific sites, agonist-activated β receptors are sequestered from the cell surface into a vesicular compartment. This occurs more slowly than does receptor phosphorylation and desensitization and can account for significant loss of plasma membrane receptors during short-term agonist stimulation, but its role in the development of refractoriness is less clear. It is possible that receptors undergo dephosphorylation in the vesicular compartment and subsequently recycle to the cell membrane to participate in further signaling episodes.[158] The relation between the sequestration of receptors into a perimembranal vesicular compartment and their subsequent down-regulation by degradation is not clear. The more well-defined process of receptor down-regulation, with endocytosis and processing of the hormone-receptor complexes, leads to a more substantial and prolonged loss of receptors that occurs within 30 to 60 min and lasts for several hours. In many hormone-receptor systems, such as the interaction of gonadotropins with testicular and ovarian target cells, the phases of desensitization and internalization become merged and the initial period of refractoriness caused by homologous desensitization is followed by a pronounced loss of LH receptors as a result of internalization and degradation of the hormone-receptor complexes.[159]

G Protein–Coupled Receptor Kinases

The rapid desensitization of agonist-activated receptors that primarily involves phosphorylation of the receptor is mediated by two distinct types of serine/threonine protein kinases. In addition to the conventional protein kinases that are activated by the second messengers produced during hormone action (protein kinase A and protein kinase C, discussed later), a recently discovered family of G protein–coupled receptor kinases (GRKs) is specifically involved in receptor phosphorylation and regulation. The archetypal GRKs are rhodopsin kinase and βARKs, which regulate the activities of rhodopsin and β-adrenergic receptors, respectively.[160] They are members of a family of at least six GRKs that phosphorylate activated receptors and thus promote their binding of inhibitory proteins of the arrestin type. These events markedly reduce the ability of receptors to perform functions such as the activation of retinal phosphodiesterase by rhodopsin and activation of the GTPase activity of the G_s α subunit by the β_2-adrenergic receptor. The other GRKs, in addition to GRK1 (rhodopsin kinase) and GRK2 (βARK1), are GRK3 (βARK2), which phosphorylates rhodopsin, β_2, M_2, and substance P receptors and is abundant in the brain; GRK4, which is abundant in the testis and peripheral neurons; and GRK4 and GRK5, which phosphorylate rhodopsin and β_2 receptors and are expressed in several tissues, including the brain. The catalytic domains of the GRK enzymes share primary sequence similarity of 50 to 90 percent and contain several amino acids that are observed in all protein kinases. It is of interest that βARK1 and βARK2 are activated by the βγ subunits of heterotrimeric G proteins. The GRK enzymes generally are located in the cytoplasm but undergo translocation to the plasma membrane during receptor activation, as has been observed for rhodopsin kinase and βARK1. The translocation of rhodopsin kinase to the plasma membrane is dependent on its isoprenylation. However, βARK1 and βARK2 are not isoprenylated and probably depend on their binding to the isoprenylated βγ subunit to become anchored to the membrane-bound receptor.

In the case of G_i-coupled receptors such as the α_2-adrenergic receptor, agonist-induced desensitization is correlated with rapid phosphorylation of sites in the third intracellular loop.[161] This is effected by a βARK-like kinase and leads to major attenuation of the inhibitory effect of epinephrine on adenylyl cyclase activity within 30 min. Unlike the β-adrenergic receptor, there is usually no change in receptor number during desensitization of the α_2-adrenergic receptor. However, there is also a long-term component that results from a 50 percent decrease in the cellular content of G_i after about 24 h. Agonist activation of M_1 muscarinic receptors is also followed by a significant decrease in the level of the G_q/G_{11} α subunits that couple the receptors to phospholipase C, probably resulting from enhanced proteolytic degradation. This decrease in G_q/G_{11} occurs over several hours and may be related to the desensitization of the receptor response.[162]

SYNTHESIS AND REGULATION OF PEPTIDE HORMONE RECEPTORS

Biosynthesis and Expression of Plasma Membrane Receptors

Plasma membrane receptors are synthesized in the same manner as other membrane proteins, by assembly on ribosomes bound to the endoplasmic reticulum (ER), followed by translocation into the lumen of the ER and transfer to the Golgi complex and from there to the plasma membrane (Chap. 4).[163] Like secretory and lysosomal proteins, plasma membrane proteins have a 15- to 20-amino acid leader sequence with a basic amino terminus and an apolar central domain that determines their translocation and passage through the ER-Golgi system. Such sequences are present in many growth factor and other receptors with single transmembrane domains but are not expressed in most of the seven transmembrane receptors (except those for glycoprotein hormones, thrombin, and cannabinoids). The insertion of nascent peptide chains into the ER membrane is mediated by RNA-protein signal recognition particles that "dock" the ribosomal complexes at the ER membrane, and protein synthesis continues only on ribosomes attached to the ER.[164] The proteins transported from the ER to Golgi compartments undergo extensive glycosylation and remodeling of asparagine-linked oligosaccharide chains, followed by the addition of galactose residues before their emergence and sorting for delivery to plasma membrane, lysosomes, and secretory granules.

Several of the signals that determine the destination of each type of protein have been elucidated by studies on the sorting of viral, yeast, and mammalian proteins. For example, terminal mannose-6-phosphate residues on oligosaccharides of lysosomal protein precursors determines their segregation and delivery to lysosomes.[165] Much of the sorting of membrane proteins is performed by clathrin-coated vesicles in the Golgi system, which also participate in the recycling of internalized plasma membrane receptors after their dissociation from bound ligands in endosomes. In some cases, the receptor proteins are associated with secretory granules, which may serve as a route for the recruitment of intracellular receptors to the plasma membrane during ligand-induced exocytosis. This form of transport is a feature of somatostatin receptor regulation in pituitary and pancreatic cells.[166] Other pathways for the migration of cell-surface receptors to the plasma membrane operate in nonsecretory cells, again presumably converging on those involved in the recycling of internalized receptors back to the plasma membrane. The biochemical routing signals of cell-surface receptors may include their characteristic membrane-spanning hydrophobic domains, which range from one to seven in number in the various forms of plasma membrane receptor sites.

These hydrophobic domains of receptors and other integral membrane proteins are composed of about 23 amino acids that are believed to form α helices within the plasma membrane. They are often oriented such that the more positively charged region is facing the cytoplasm.[167] It is possible that the basic amino acids preceding the hydrophobic signal sequences anchor the α helices in the membrane by interacting with the acidic head groups of the lipid bilayer. In the multiple transmembrane-spanning receptors, the orientation of the first transmembrane domain is determined by its charge distribution and is followed by insertion of the succeeding membrane-spanning regions.[168] The occurrence of basic amino acids such as lysine and arginine after the first or second transmembrane domain is seen in some of the helices of the G protein–coupled receptors. However, most of these receptors have a conserved aspartatic acid residue on the cytoplasmic side of the third transmembrane helix. The charge distribution of the hydrophobic domains of the receptor may be an important determinant of its membrane topology. While certain helices are firmly anchored in the membrane, others probably have a degree of flexibility that permits interconversion between more and less constrained forms of the receptor in the absence or presence of the activating ligand. The palmitoylation of receptors on cysteine residues in their carboxy-terminal region provides a further site of membrane insertion that could form an additional cytoplasmic loop and contribute to the stabilization of the receptor within the membrane.

The selection of vesicle-enclosed proteins during intracellular sorting appears to be determined by the coat proteins associated with the cytoplasmic surface of the vesicles. Several signal sequences that interact with the vesicle coats have been identified in the cytoplasmic domains of the sorted proteins. Many of them are short tyrosine-containing motifs that are similar to those which specify the internalization of proteins at the plasma membrane. These sequences determine the distribution of receptors and other proteins among the trans-Golgi network, endosomes, lysosomes, and the plasma membrane.[169] Such signals mediate transport rather than the retention that occurs with the resident proteins of the Golgi complex and the ER. For many proteins, the plasma membrane serves as the destination of a signal-independent default pathway for proteins that are not retained at earlier stations of the vesicular transport pathway.

The generation, movement, and fusion of the vesicles that transport proteins throughout the cell must be regulated by sets of specific proteins that control each of these events. Major among these are three types of GTP-binding proteins that act as switches in the docking and membrane fusion events that occur between vesicles targeted to specific cellular compartments.[170] Of particular importance are the Rab proteins, which belong to the Ras-related family of small GTPases. About 30 individual Rab proteins are involved in all aspects of vesicle transport, together with a host of GAPs and GDIs that control their activities. Several of the Rab proteins are ubiquitously expressed and are probably involved in vesicular transport activities that are common to all mammalian cells. The most important Rab proteins in the transport of proteins to the membrane are Rab 1 and 2, which regulate transport from the ER to the Golgi complex; Rab 6, which is present in the Golgi network; and Rab 8, which is localized in the trans-Golgi network, post-Golgi vesicles, and plasma membrane and regulates trafficking from the Golgi to the cell surface[170] (Fig. 5A-17).

An additional group of small GTP-binding proteins (ARFs, ADP-ribosylation factors), which were first identified by their role as cofactors in the ADP ribosylation of $G_{s\alpha}$ by cholera toxin, have been found to be components of Golgi-derived coated vesicles.[171] ARF is believed to bind to the Golgi membrane by its myristoyl moiety and to promote the assembly of coat proteins and vesicle formation when activated by GTP. After arrival at the target membrane, the interaction of ARF•GTP with a specific GAP causes hydrolysis of the bound GTP and dissociation of the coat proteins before vesicle fusion.[172] Similar types of reaction sequences are thought to occur during the regulation of vesicular trafficking by the Rab proteins. The fungal metabolite brefeldin A disrupts membrane trafficking by inhibiting the activity of a Golgi membrane enzyme that catalyzes the exchange of guanine nucleotide bound to ARF.[128] This effect is responsible for the blockade of coat assembly and vesicle budding that occurs in brefeldin A–treated cells. As noted earlier, ARF also serves as an activator of phospholipase D and could modify the phospholipid content of vesicles reaching the plasma membrane and thus influence their fusion with the lipid bilayer.[134]

The heterotrimeric G proteins have also been implicated in vesicular trafficking, in particular within the secretory pathway leading to exocytosis. Although most of the heterotrimeric G proteins are located in the periphery of the cell, both G_{i3} and G_q α subunits are present in the Golgi cisternae as well as in the plasma membrane.[136] Recently, the G_{i3} α subunit has been found to activate histamine secretion in most cells; it appears to act in conjunction with Rab3 to control the process of regulated exocytosis.[173] It is possible that the $\beta\gamma$ subunits of the G_{i3} protein will also be found to play a role in the control of secretion.

Receptor Regulation in Endocrine Target Cells

Once inserted in the plasma membrane, peptide hormone receptors diffuse freely within the lipid bilayer to interact with their effector systems. In addition, they are distributed between the cell surface and intracellular sites of recycling, synthesis, and degradation. Agonist stimulation often leads to internalization and loss (down-regulation) of specific receptors and in some cases to an increase (up-regulation) of receptors. Such regulation of plasma membrane receptors by the homologous ligand commonly occurs in cells exposed to neurotransmitters, peptide and glycoprotein hormones, and growth factors as well as lectins and immunoglobulins. Thus, the cell-surface receptor population exists in a state of dynamic equilibrium that is readily perturbed by hormonal activation. The depletion of plasma membrane receptors by agonist-induced down-regulation can attenuate target cell responsiveness to subsequent hormonal stimulation. The mechanism of receptor regulation by homologous ligands depends on the mobility of the ligand-receptor complexes within the lipid bilayer and their endocytosis at specialized regions of the plasma membrane. Changes in receptor affinity are rare, but insulin receptors exhibit negative cooperativity on exposure to increasing hormone concentrations and angiotensin II receptor affinity is al-

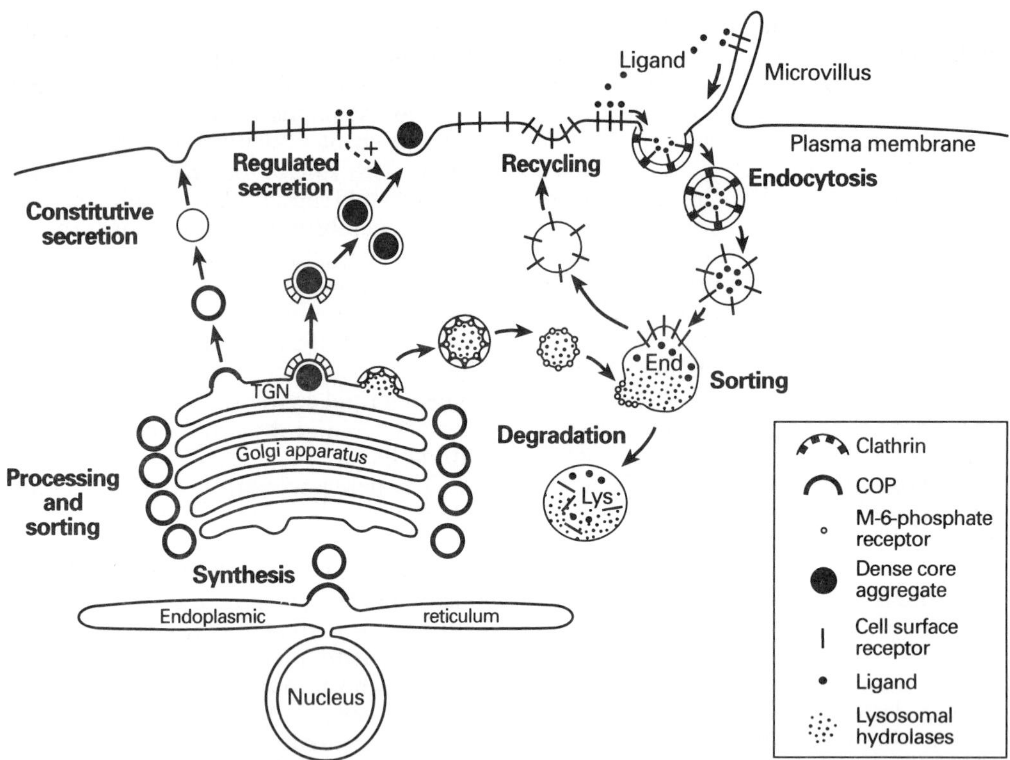

FIGURE 5A-19. Endocytosis and processing of peptide hormone receptors. Hormone-receptor complexes formed at the plasma membrane, often on microvilli, become clustered in clathrin-coated pits and are internalized in clathrin-coated vesicles. After loss of the clathrin coat, the vesicles fuse with endosomes, from which the complexes are dissociated and sorted. Most of the internalized ligand is degraded in lysosomes; a variable and probably small fraction of the receptors is recycled to the plasma membrane. The secretory pathway to constitutive and regulated exocytosis, and the pathway for delivery of lysosomal enzymes from the trans-Golgi network to the lysosome, are also shown. (*Modified from Pley and Parham.*[187])

tered during sodium deficiency. Thus, hormonal stimulation of target cells initiates a sequence of regulatory changes that include alterations in the activity of receptors and other components of the signaling pathway as well as in the metabolic and secretory responses to further hormonal stimulation. Peptide hormone receptors are regulated not only by the homologous hormone but sometimes by other hormones that act on the same target cell, a process known as heterologous regulation.

The cell-surface expression of certain hormone receptors, including those for angiotensin II, GnRH, and prolactin, is increased by exposure to moderately elevated hormone concentrations. This could result from changes in membrane conformation and receptor recruitment from intracellular sites and in some cases from increased receptor synthesis.[174] In the gonads, a transient increase in LH receptors precedes the receptor loss caused by high-dose gonadotropin treatment, suggesting that hormonal stimulation causes new sites to be exposed before the subsequent phase of receptor down regulation.[152] The manner in which testicular gonadotropin receptors are regulated by LH or hCG changes markedly during development. Thus, fetal and neonatal Leydig cells show an increase of LH receptors after hCG treatment, in contrast to the prominent receptor loss and desensitization that occur in the adult testis after gonadotropin administration.[175]

Although the hormone-receptor complex is initially freely reversible, this is often followed by a phase of slow and incomplete dissociation. In many cases, the initial binding reaction leads to a conformational change in the receptor that results in tighter binding of the ligand. This occurs with insulin, EGF, prolactin, and LH and may be a preliminary step in the process of internalization of the hormone-receptor complex. In either case, prolonged occupancy by undissociated agonist ligands leads to functional receptor loss and may increase the probability that hormone-receptor complexes will be processed and destroyed. This could involve occlusion within the cell membrane or shedding from the cell surface, but it usually occurs by endocytosis and subsequent degradation of the internalized hormone-receptor complexes.

Effects of Receptor Regulation on Cell Responses

In hormone-stimulated cells, it is important to distinguish between acute desensitization of the effector system and the development of true receptor loss, which is a more slowly reversible consequence of hormone-receptor interaction. Significant changes in the number of membrane receptors would be expected to influence the sensitivity of the hormone dose-response when there are spare receptors, and to alter the sensitivity and magnitude of the response when the receptor concentration becomes limiting. The general function of receptor regulation as a mechanism to modify target cell sensitivity in the face of altered hormone concentrations could have certain biological advantages. For example, down regulation of insulin receptors and reduced sensitivity of peripheral tissues to insulin would blunt the effect of hyperinsulinemia on the circulating glucose concentration. Similarly, receptor regulation could minimize or buffer cardiovascular responses to excessive levels of angiotensin II and catecholamines. In steroidogenic cells that respond to trophic hormones with cAMP-dependent increases in steroid secretion, it is possible to analyze several levels of response. Leydig cells obtained from the testes of animals that were given desensitizing doses of gonadotropin show marked changes in receptor content and biochemical responses to hormonal stimulation, with decreased cAMP formation and lesions in the steroid biosynthetic pathway.[176] In the pituitary gland, GnRH causes rapid down-regulation of receptors and desensitization of the gonadotroph, with marked suppression of gonadotroph secretion during treatment with potent GnRH agonist analogues.[148]

It is important to note that agonist-induced down regulation of peptide hormone receptors is not necessarily accompanied by decreased cellular responsiveness. For example, adrenalectomy is followed by a marked decrease in pituitary corticotropin releasing factor (CRF) receptors, yet the CRF-induced ACTH responses in corticotrophs are significantly enhanced. Such increased responsiveness to agonist stimulation reflects postreceptor changes in the biosynthetic and secretory pathways of the chronically stimulated target cell.

Fate of the Hormone-Receptor Complex

Peptide hormones and other cell-surface ligands are internalized and degraded at widely differing rates after binding to their plasma membrane receptors (Fig. 5A-19). The two extremes of ligand-receptor activation and processing are associated with two major groups of receptors in accordance with the extent to which the ligand-receptor system primarily subserves information transfer, as in the case of hormone receptors, or mediates ligand uptake and metabolism, as exemplified by low-density lipoprotein (LDL) receptors.[177] The first group of receptors is responsible for binding traditional hormones, neurotransmitters, and other hormonal agents, such as IgE and chemotactic peptides. These receptors often show down-regulation and/or desensitization after binding their agonist ligands; their major function is target cell stimulation and rapid regulation of metabolic processes. Internalization of the hormone-receptor complex often occurs but is not an essential step in the target cell activation mechanism. Disordered function of such receptors is manifested by under- or overstimulation of cellular activity, as discussed earlier. The second group of receptors is mainly responsible for the uptake and internalization of macromolecules, and these receptors are recycled to the cell surface after endocytosis. They do not usually undergo down-regulation except as a secondary response to altered cellular metabolism, as in the case of LDL receptors. Abnormalities of these receptors give rise to inadequate or excessive internalization of the macromolecular ligand.

Internalization and processing of the hormone-receptor complex are frequent consequences of hormonal activation of endocrine target cells. Direct visualization of the internalization of fluorescent derivatives of peptides, including EGF, insulin, hCG, and GnRH, has shown that the hormone-receptor complexes initially are distributed uniformly on the cell surface and then rapidly undergo aggregation into patches that are internalized to form endocytic vesicles within the cytoplasm.[178] Such redistribution and clustering of receptors for hormones and other univalent ligands commonly precede the internalization and subsequent processing of the hormone-receptor complexes. The internalization mechanism for many activated receptors is initiated by their migration into the clathrin-coated pit system responsible for receptor-mediated endocytosis of cell-surface macromolecules such as LDL and transferrin. For example, insulin is rapidly internalized by its target cells, including hepatocytes, adipocytes, fibroblasts, and lymphocytes, and the concomitant uptake of receptor sites accounts for the down-regulation of plasma membrane receptors in insulin-treated cells.[179] Like many other ligands, the receptor-bound insulin is initially located on microvilli and subsequently moves to coated pits on the cell surface. The hormone-receptor complexes pass from the coated pits into transport vesicles for delivery to the endocytic compartment, where sorting occurs before recycling or delivery of the internalized complexes to various locations. The fate of the hormone-receptor complex varies in different cell types but usually involves lysosomal degradation of the ligand and a proportion of the internalized receptor sites. In some cells, internalized receptors may be recycled to the cell surface through a vesicular exocytic mechanism.

The various forms of receptor-mediated endocytosis have been classified according to the four major pathways by which the receptor and ligand are processed after entering the cell.[180] Class I: After dissociation of the receptor-ligand complex, receptors are recycled to the cell membrane and the ligand is degraded in lysosomes. Examples are receptors for LDL, mannose-6-phosphate, α_2-macroglobulin, and asialoglycoproteins. Class II: Both receptor and ligand are recycled to the cell membrane; this is unique to the transferrin receptor. Class III: Both receptor and ligand are degraded in lysosomes. These include most of the signal transduction receptors, such as EGF, insulin, and PDGF, as well as several G protein–coupled receptors. Class IV: The receptor-ligand complexes are transported across polarized cells, with release of the ligand at the opposite side and recycling or degradation of the receptor. These include receptors that mediate the transport of IgG and IgA across renal cells. Several receptors fall into more than one of these categories, depending on the cell type and factors such as ligand concentration and receptor distribution.

The plasma membrane that is internalized during the formation of endocytic vesicles undergoes sorting to separate the vacuolar membrane from its contents. The contents are accumulated or metabolized within the cell, while the membrane components recycle to and from the surface after fusion events with other endocytic vesicles or Golgi components.[181] Agonist-occupied peptide hormone receptors become concentrated in clathrin-coated pits on the cell surface before internalization, a route shared by numerous ligands and viruses. The ability of coated pits to distinguish between occupied and unoccupied receptors implies that hormone binding causes a conformational change in the receptor site that is recognized by the trapping mechanism of the pit. By contrast, receptors that capture macromolecular nutrients, including those for LDL, transferrin, asialoglycoproteins, and α_2-macroglobulin cluster in coated pits in the absence of the ligands and undergo continuous endocytosis and recycling to the plasma membrane.

The receptor-ligand complexes that accumulate in coated pits enter the cell via clathrin-coated vesicles that are pinched off from the base of the invaginated coated pits and pass into the cytoplasm.[182] These vesicles soon lose their clathrin coat and become fused with endosomes, from which receptors are sorted and recycled to the plasma membrane or delivered to lysosomes. Early endosomes are components of a network of vesicles, tubules, and cisternae near the plasma membrane and begin to accumulate internalized ligand-receptor complexes within a few minutes after cell activation. The late endosomes, or multivesiculate bodies, are located near the nucleus and are prelysosomal compartments containing mannose-6-phosphate receptors and several proteolytic enzymes. The pH of the transport vesicles decreases from 6.0 to 6.5 in the early endosomes, to 5.5 to 6.0 in the late endosomes, to 4.5 to 5.5 in the lysosomes. The endosomal compartment provides an acid environment through which the internalized receptor-ligand complexes must pass and is the site from which membrane is returned to the cell surface. Since many ligands are rapidly dissociated from their receptors at low pH, the acidic environment of the endosome favors release of the bound hormone from its receptor sites. Whereas the ligand is usually delivered to lysosomes for degradation, the receptors are often returned to the cell membrane to engage in further cycles of ligand binding and internalization. This series of events is common to the cellular processing of numerous macromolecules, toxins, and viruses. An outline of the vesicular transport pathway is shown in Fig. 5A-19.

Receptors for the transport of nutrients such as LDL and transferrin are normally clustered in coated pits in the plasma membrane and undergo constitutive internalization in the absence or presence of ligand binding. The LDL receptors carry their bound ligand into the endosomes, where they are recycled to the plasma membrane, and the LDL is deposited in lysosomes and further metabolized.[183] In the case of transferrin, the bound iron is released within the endosome and the receptor-transferrin complex is returned to the cell surface.[184] The recycling pathway also provides a route by which receptors reach the plasma membrane via the main exocytic pathway after fusion of sorting endosomes with trans-Golgi elements, especially in cells that are rich in secretory granules.

Several of the constitutively recycling receptors, including those for LDL, transferrin, and mannose-6-phosphate, possess internalization signals of four to six amino acids in their cytoplasmic domains. The tetrapeptide sequence NPXY (Asn-Pro-x-Tyr) is present in LDL receptors and other cell-surface proteins, including the EGF and insulin receptors, and acts as a determinant for migration to coated pits and subsequent internalization.[185] In some cases, other amino acid sequences appear to promote the rapid internalization of receptors (e.g., YTRF), but the sequence patterns are usually similar, either aromatic-x-x-aromatic/large hydrophobic for four-residue signals or aromatic-x-x-x-x-aromatic for six-residue signals.[186] These sequences occur as tight turns in the three-dimensional conformation of the receptor that are exposed on its surface in receptors for LDL and transferrin and presumably are also exposed after activation of receptors of the tyrosine kinase family.

Although receptor domains that promote internalization have been identified for several growth factors and transport poteins, much less is known about the signals that control the endocytosis of the G protein–coupled receptors. Many of these receptors contain amino acid sequences that resemble the tyrosine-containing domains that mediate sequestration of the single transmembrane domain receptors (NPXXY) and have been proposed to function as internalization signals.[151] In contrast to the growth factor receptors, internalization of the G protein–coupled receptor family appears to depend on the phosphorylation of residues in the cytoplasmic regions of the receptor, in particular the third intracellular loop and the carboxy-terminal cytoplasmic domain. Thus, in muscarinic cholinergic receptors, a serine-threonine–rich region in the third loop has been implicated in the internalization process.[188] In β-adrenergic receptors, mutation of serine and threonine residues in the carboxy-terminal domain prevents phosphorylation and sequestration of the sites. However, it is not clear whether such mutations directly prevent agonist-induced changes that trigger internalization or cause a secondary change in conformation that prevents sequestration.[157]

The coated pits in which receptors are concentrated before their internalization exclude other membrane proteins and must possess an efficient sorting mechanism for selection of the appropriate macromolecules.[189] The formation of coated pits involves their assembly from clathrin and adaptor proteins to form a lattice containing an inner layer of adaptor molecules that interact with the cytoplasmic domains of receptors to be concentrated within the pit (Fig. 5A-20). Clathrin molecules are composed of light- and heavy-chain subunits that form triskelions which can pack together into hexagonal lattices. Adaptors are also complex structures that are composed of four proteins and promote the assembly of clathrin as well as forming the inner shell of the coated pit.[190] When the pits are internalized to form coated vesicles, the coat proteins disassemble and recycle through a soluble pool to be reconstituted into new pits in the plasma membrane, while the uncoated vesicles fuse with other vesicular compartments. The dynamic sequence of coat protein assembly, receptor recruitment, coated pit invagination, and vesicle budding depends for its completion on dynamin, a GTP-binding protein that is involved in the early stage of receptor-mediated endocytosis.[191] Another GTP-binding protein, Rab5, which is a member of the Ras family, has also been implicated in the formation of endocytic vesicles.[132]

Most peptide hormones enter their target cells to some degree by receptor-mediated endocytosis, as indicated by the occurrence of receptor down-regulation in many agonist-stimulated cells and tissues. Minor degrees of recycling of receptors for insulin and a few other peptides have been observed and may be a general consequence of the internalization process. The internalized hormone is degraded rapidly after its transfer to lysosomes, but in some cases it is recycled and released from the cell. This occurs during the transit of ligands across renal and vascular endothelial cells and is a prominent feature of the processing of EGF-receptor complexes in epidermoid carcinoma cells.[192] In ovarian granulosa and testicular Leydig cells, gonadotropins bind predominantly to receptors on microvilli, followed by receptor aggregation in coated pits and internalization of the bound hormone. The internalized complexes are partly incorporated into lysosomes and degraded, and some are localized over Golgi elements, from which recycling to the plasma membrane could occur.[193]

Certain plasma membrane transport proteins undergo rapid turnover between the plasma membrane and a microvesicular pool that regulates cellular membrane transport and appears to be derived from the Golgi complex.[194] This mechanism participates in insulin stimulation of glucose transport, histamine stimulation of gastric acid secretion, and vasopressin stimulation of water permeability in bladder and kidney cells. In the adipocyte, recruit-

FIGURE 5A-20. Formation of clathrin-coated pits and vesicles. Clathrin and adaptor protein molecules are assembled from reusable pools to form the characteristic lattice structure at the base of the pit. After internalization, the coat proteins are removed and the contents of the vesicle are transferred to the endosomal compartment for sorting into the degradation or recycling pathways. *(Courtesy of L. Hunyady).*

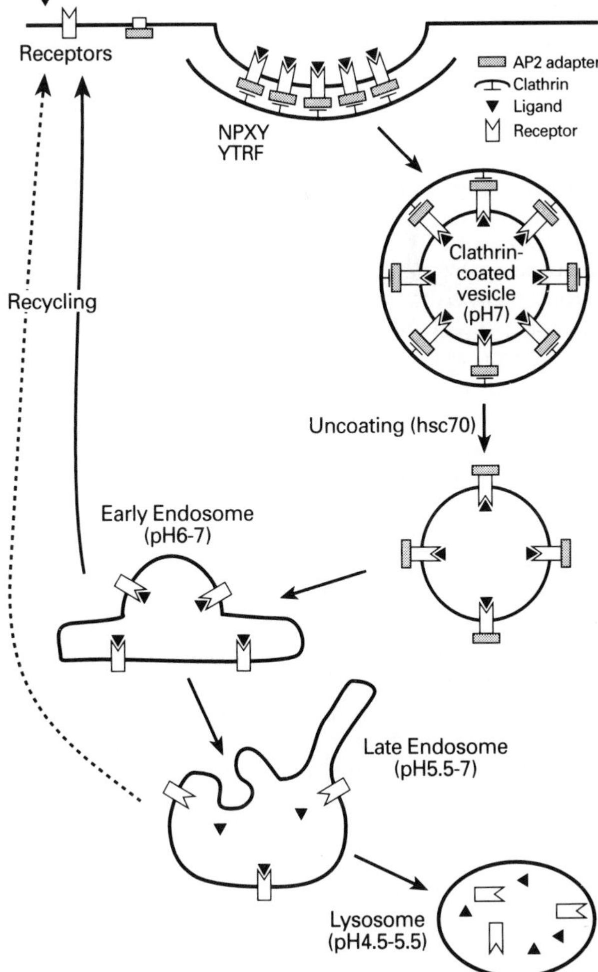

ment of glucose transporter elements from a light membrane (presumably Golgi) fraction to the plasma membrane occurs during insulin action.[195] A similar form of turnover between the plasma membrane and subjacent vesicles may be a general feature of the regulation of cell-surface receptors for peptide hormones. This type of translocation has been well demonstrated for β-adrenergic receptors, which undergo sequestration into a vesicular membrane fraction after occupancy by agonist ligands in several tissues. In this location, the receptors are segregated from their membrane effector systems and are no longer coupled to G_s and adenylyl cyclase.[157] However, other hormone-receptor complexes continue to generate second messengers after internalization and may thus contribute to the maintenance of the agonist-induced cell response.[196]

INTRACELLULAR MEDIATORS OF PEPTIDE HORMONE ACTION

The Second Messenger Hypothesis

The transfer of incoming hormonal signals to the cell interior is performed by a group of second messengers that are generated at the plasma membrane level as a consequence of receptor activation (Table 5A-1). The original formulation of this concept by Sutherland and Robison (Fig. 5A-3) envisaged a general transduction mechanism by which peptide hormones act on the cell surface to stimulate the formation of intracellular messengers such as cyclic AMP. This general scheme of peptide hormone action on membrane receptors and adenylyl cyclase was based on studies with catecholamines, glucagon, and ACTH. It has since been extended to many hormones and transmitters that influence adenylyl cyclase activity either positively or negatively to increase or decrease intracellular cAMP levels. In addition, many hormones and neurotransmitters stimulate the phosphoinositide/calcium signaling pathway and promote the production of inositol 1,4,5-trisphosphate and diacylglycerol from the phospholipids of the plasma membrane. For the growth factors and cytokines, the mechanisms of target cell activation have been clarified only recently and in some cases are still incompletely defined. Several growth factors promote phosphorylation of their homologous receptors via intrinsic kinase domains in their cytoplasmic regions and initiate a cascade of signaling events that extend to the nucleus.[197]

For tissues in which cyclic AMP is the major second messenger of peptide hormone action, the manner in which a single effector system is translated into a spectrum of individual target cell responses was at first difficult to discern. This question is complicated by the dual nature of many peptide and protein hormones, which function both as regulators of rapid target cell responses such as steroidogenesis and hormone secretion and as trophic factors with long-term effects on cell growth and differentiation. The relation between these two aspects of peptide hormone action has been clarified recently and involves new signaling pathways to the nucleus as well as interactions between the recognized activation mechanisms. There is also evidence for the participation of additional messenger systems in target cells that were previously thought to be under the control of one predominant signal pathway, such as cAMP/protein kinase A, calcium/calmodulin, and DAG/protein kinase C. The interactions between these multiple activation systems contribute to many of the immediate and long-term effects of hormones on target cell function. Internalization and processing of the hormone-receptor complex could also generate signals that contribute to both aspects of hormone action.[196]

The intracellular signal molecules generated by hormone-receptor interaction act on membrane and cytoplasmic proteins to alter rate-limiting steps in the effector systems that control target cell responses. The best-characterized mediators are calcium and cyclic nucleotides, which act as intracellular transmitters to adjust target cell metabolism in response to hormones and other ligands. The calcium signal is generated by the mobilization of intracellular calcium stores and the influx of extracellular calcium, with a rise in cytoplasmic calcium that in many cells takes the form of repeated calcium transients or oscillations. Cyclic AMP and cyclic GMP are generated from ATP and GTP by activation of nucleotide triphosphate cyclizing enzymes situated in the plasma membrane and cytoplasm. The formation of cAMP is directly linked to cell-surface receptor occupancy and activation of adenylyl cyclase within the plasma membrane. In contrast, guanylate cyclase activity is intrinsic to certain plasma membrane receptors and is also present as soluble forms in the cytoplasm. Calcium has regulatory actions on both adenylyl cyclase and guanylate cyclase activities and on cyclic nucleotide breakdown by phosphodiesterases. Thus, changes in the intracellular calcium concentration can influence cyclic AMP and cyclic GMP levels. Conversely, in several tissues, including nerve, muscle, and secretory cells, the cyclic AMP pathway can modulate the calcium signaling system.

The essential role of calcium in stimulus-response coupling during activation of contractile and secretory processes has been recognized for many years. However, the manifold actions of cyclic AMP as a second messenger and the slower elucidation of the phosphoinositide/calcium signaling pathway for a time overshadowed the significance of calcium as an intracellular regulator. Over the last several years, the importance of calcium as a second messenger and its interaction with cyclic nucleotides have been

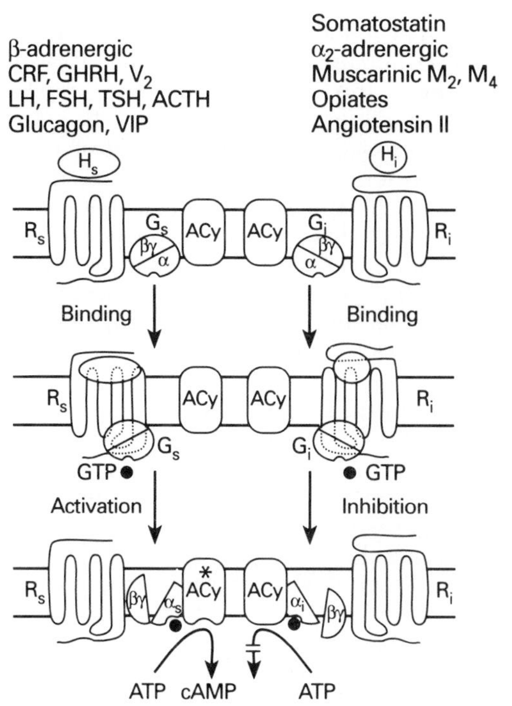

FIGURE 5A-21. Regulation of adenylyl cyclase activity by stimulatory and inhibitory hormones that act through specific receptors (R_s, R_i) which are coupled to the enzyme by G_s and G_i, respectively. G_i probably inhibits adenylyl cyclase via the direct action of α_i as shown, and also by the quenching of α_s by excess $\beta\gamma$ subunits.

demonstrated in many hormone-dependent target tissues.[198]

The Cyclic AMP Signaling System

Numerous peptide hormones and transmitters operate through G protein–coupled receptors to activate or inhibit adenylyl cyclase and cAMP formation (Fig. 5A-21). In some cells, agonist-induced cAMP production reaches high levels and significant amounts of the cyclic nucleotide are released into the extracellular fluid. Such release of cAMP plays a biological role in certain lower organisms (e.g., slime mold) by exerting autocrine actions on its cells of origin but is not thought to act as an intercellular messenger system in higher animals. In mammalian tissues, extracellular cAMP levels are elevated during high or excessive hormone stimulation, as in the kidney during infusion or hypersecretion of PTH. However, the changes in cAMP production in response to physiologic concentrations of peptide hormones are usually quite small, and there sometimes appear to be dissociations between target cell responses and the degree of cAMP production. Such apparent discrepancies have usually been resolved by careful measurements of the cAMP concentration at critical regulatory sites [e.g., bound to the regulatory (R) subunit of protein kinase A]. Using this approach, excellent correlations have been found between R•cAMP levels and the responses of steroidogenic cells to their respective trophic hormones.[16] A summary of the peptide hormones whose receptors are coupled to stimulation or inhibition of cAMP formation is given in Table 5A-1.

Several of the peptide hormones that act primarily through the adenylyl cyclase/cAMP system (e.g., LH, FSH, and TSH) can also activate the phosphoinositide/Ca^{2+} signaling pathway. This results from the coupling of their receptors not only to G_s but also to G proteins that control the activity of phospholipase C. Even when the major actions of a peptide hormone are clearly mediated by cAMP, it is possible that other responses (e.g., cell growth and maintenance of differentiated functions) are dependent on additional messenger systems that act in concert with the primary response pathway. Interactions also occur at loci beyond receptor activation, leading to cross-talk between the signal transduction systems. Thus, some adenylyl cyclases are sensitive to cytoplasmic Ca^{2+}, which thereby modulates cAMP production. Conversely, cAMP-induced phosphorylation of plasma-membrane Ca^{2+} channels influences Ca^{2+} entry in certain cell types.

Cyclic AMP and adenylyl cyclase were discovered during studies of the control of hepatic glycogenolysis by adrenaline and glucagon, which stimulate the activity of glycogen phosphorylase and promote the breakdown of glycogen to glucose phosphates.[10] The activation of glycogen phosphorylase by these hyperglycemic hormones required an intermediate step (later shown to be phosphorylation by protein kinase) that was stimulated by a heat-stable factor generated by the interaction of hormone with the particulate fraction of the liver cell. The latter reaction was dependent on ATP, which in the presence of hormone and magnesium ion was converted to cAMP and inorganic phosphate. The heat-stable factor was found to be cyclic AMP, and the enzyme responsible for its generation was shown to be located on the inner surface of the plasma membrane and to be activated by a wide variety of peptide hormones (Fig. 5A-3). Originally referred to as *adenyl* or *adenylate cyclase*, the plasma membrane enzyme has since been termed *adenylyl cyclase* to more precisely describe its specific cyclizing action on ATP.

The identification of adenylyl cyclase as a membrane-bound enzyme that is regulated by catecholamines and glucagon was followed by the recognition that many hormones which bind to the cell surface, such as peptides and neurotransmitters, activate adenylyl cyclase. The cyclizing enzyme was at first envisaged as a receptor subunit (the recognition site for binding peptide hormones) and a catalytic subunit (to convert ATP to cyclic AMP). Later, these subunits were proposed to exist as separate entities in the lipid bilayer of the cell membrane and to become associated into an active unit during hormonal activation of the receptor site.[199] This concept led to a two-step theory of enzyme activation in which the hormone-receptor complex diffuses laterally within the cell membrane to interact with (and activate) the catalytic subunits on the cytoplasmic surface of the plasma membrane.

This relatively simple model was further elaborated by the recognition that an intermediate process (transduction) intervenes between hormone-receptor interaction and activation of the catalytic subunit. The nature of the intermediate coupling step was indicated by the discovery that guanyl nucleotides enhance the activation of hepatic adenylyl cyclase by glucagon and promote dissociation of the hormone from its receptors. These findings suggested that glucagon does not directly stimulate adenylyl cyclase but facilitates its activation by guanyl nucleotides. The dependence of peptide hormones on guanyl nucleotides for both activation and inhibition of adenylyl cyclase led to the recognition that guanyl nucleotide regulatory proteins (G_s and G_i) mediate the hormonal regulation of adenylyl cyclase and that related G proteins control the activities of other plasma membrane effector systems.[200]

Since hormonal stimulation of target cells is frequently intermittent and transient, intracellular second messengers are subject to rapid turnover (by decay or recycling) so that repetitive and graded external stimuli can be faithfully converted into quantitative cellular responses (Table 5A-6). The dynamic equilibrium between the formation and the removal of cyclic nucleotides controls their intracellular levels in basal and hormone-activated states and permits rapid responses to changes in extracellular regulators. This regulation is largely exerted through activation or inhibition of adenylyl cyclase within the cell membrane, leading to changes in the production and intracellular concentration of cyclic AMP. In some cells, the rate of breakdown of cAMP by specific phosphodiesterases is also under hormonal regulation and can influence the intracellular concentration and actions of the nucleotide (Fig. 5A-3). In eukaryotic cells, most of the actions of cAMP are expressed through the activation of cAMP-dependent protein kinases that catalyze the phosphorylation of specific protein substrates in the target cell. Thus, this major pathway of peptide hormone action is controlled by the hormonal regulation of adenylyl cyclase and phosphodiesterase and by the activation and functions of cAMP-dependent protein kinase (Fig. 5A-22).

Structure and Regulation of Adenylyl Cyclase

Adenylyl cyclases, the enzymes that produce cyclic AMP, are widely distributed in mammalian cells and most organisms and are usually associated with the plasma membrane (Fig. 5A-23). Their activities are regulated by numerous hormones and transmitters acting through G_s and G_i to stimulate or inhibit enzyme activity.

The activation of adenylyl cyclase by G_s is mediated by the dissociated α_s subunit, which binds to the enzyme and promotes its activation. This mechanism is well-defined and is reflected in the impaired cyclase activity of cyc^- mutant lymphoma cells (which lack G_s) and the tissues of patients with inactivation mutations of α_s. However, the mechanism by which G_i attenuates the activity of adenylyl cyclase is less clear, and has been attributed to at least two processes. One of these involves the direct inhibitory action of α_i upon the enzyme, leading to suppression of its activation by α_s. An alternative mechanism is based on the ability of free $\beta\gamma$ subunits to bind to free α subunits to form the inactive $\alpha\beta\gamma$ heterotrimer. Since G_i is present in considerable excess over G_s in many cell types, it is probable that its free $\beta\gamma$ subunits could serve as a reservoir to trap α_s subunits

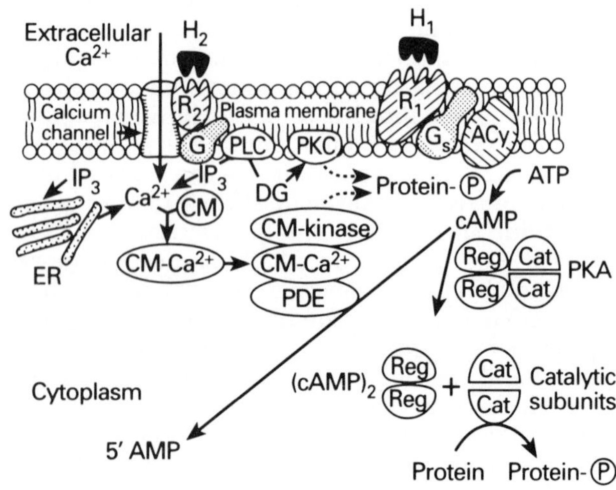

FIGURE 5A-22. Interrelations between calcium mobilization and cAMP formation and degradation in cells stimulated by hormones coupled to phospholipase C and adenylyl cyclase.

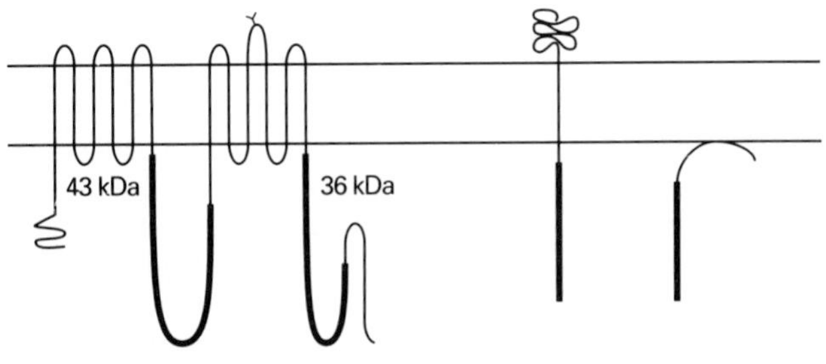

FIGURE 5A-23. Structure of eukaryotic adenylyl cyclases. The regions of similarity are indicated by bold lines. The mammalian enzymes are characterized by multiple membrane-spanning domains and have a short N-terminal region and two large cytoplasmic domains. (*Modified from Tang and Gilman.*[202])

and thus prevent activation of adenylyl cyclase. It is also possible that specific βγ combinations could contribute to the inhibitory regulation of adenylyl cyclase. Based on biochemical studies, three types of adenylyl cyclase were recognized in animal cells: membrane-bound calmodulin-sensitive and calmodulin-insensitive forms and a soluble calmodulin-sensitive enzyme in the testis. After the cloning and sequencing of adenylyl cyclases from bacteria and yeast, a mammalian calmodulin-sensitive neural enzyme was purified and cloned from bovine brain.[201] This enzyme (type I adenylyl cyclase) has two hydrophobic domains each composed of six transmembrane helices that are associated with the plasma membrane and two large cytoplasmic domains of about 40 kDa, one linking the hydrophobic domains and the other constituting the carboxy-terminus of the molecule (Fig. 5A-23). Regions of the large cytoplasmic domains of the adenylyl cyclase molecule are conserved among the several mammalian enzymes and share sequence similarity with the catalytic domains of the membrane-bound guanylyl cyclases and yeast adenylyl cyclases. Both halves of the type I enzyme are necessary for its catalytic activity, which is manifested even when the two portions are expressed together in transfected cells.[202] The site at which the enzyme is activated by forskolin is probably located in the hydrophobic region of the molecule.

Several other mammalian adenylyl cyclases have since been cloned and sequenced, along with related forms from *Drosophila* and *Dictostelium*. Of the mammalian enzymes, type II is expressed in brain and lung, type III in olfactory tissue, type IV in the brain and elsewhere, and types V and VI in heart, brain, and other tissues. All six enzymes are stimulated by $G_{s\alpha}$ and forskolin, and types I and III are also activated by Ca^{2+}-calmodulin. The Ca^{2+}-calmodulin forms of adenylyl cyclase are abundant in neural tissue and are sensitive to the changes in cytoplasmic calcium concentration that occur during stimulation of neurons by neurotransmitters and neuropeptides. Such agents can thus cause significant increases in cyclic AMP in neuronal cells by activating the type I and III enzymes as well as by potentiating the activity of the type II and IV enzymes through G protein βγ subunits, as described below. An opposite form of regulation by Ca^{2+} is its direct inhibitory action on adenylyl cyclase in certain cell types, including pituitary somatotrophs and neuroblastoma cells. This effect occurs at submicromolar Ca^{2+} concentrations and does not involve calmodulin; it is a feature of the type III enzyme. The presence of this enzyme in the heart could provide a negative feedback system for regulating the sympathetic control of cardiac contractility, which involves cAMP-dependent increases in Ca^{2+} influx.[203] The elevation of cAMP that stimulates Ca^{2+} influx into cardiac tissue would be terminated by inhibition of Ca^{2+}-sensitive adenylyl cyclase as well as through Ca^{2+}-induced activation of phosphodiesterase. This could lead to interdependent oscillations in cyclic AMP and Ca^{2+} that control cardiac contractility and rhythmicity in a frequency-encoded manner.

The activities of most of the adenylyl cyclase enzymes are regulated by heterotrimeric G proteins, which act predominantly through their α subunits and in some cases through their βγ subunits. Early studies suggested that effectors such as adenylyl cyclase, phospholipase C, and ion channels are activated by α subunits and that the role of βγ is mainly to be an inactivator through sequestration of α subunits. However, several examples of effector regulator by βγ subunits have been described. In the case of adenylyl cyclases, an interesting and unexpected finding was the sensitivity of three of the mammalian enzymes to regulation by βγ subunits. Type I adenylyl cyclase activity, when stimulated by $G_{s\alpha}$ or Ca^{2+}-calmodulin, is inhibited by βγ.[111] Conversely, βγ subunits markedly potentiate the stimulation of both type II and type IV enzymes by $G_{s\alpha}$. The source of the βγ subunits that modulate adenylyl cyclase activity is probably G_i and G_o, which are abundant in brain and several other tissues. For this reason, activation of adenylyl cyclases by G_s can be potentiated or inhibited by concomitant activation of other receptor-mediated pathways that operate through G_i, G_o, or G_q in the same cell type.

The ubiquitous role of cAMP as a signaling molecule is reflected in the expression of adenylyl cyclases in organisms from bacteria to mammals. In addition to the composite of two large hydrophobic domains containing transmembrane segments and two large hydrophilic domains that is found in higher eukaryotes, the slime mold *Dictostelium* contains an adenylyl cyclase with a single transmembrane segment, and membrane-associated forms are present in yeast and *Escherichia coli*. The single transmembrane domain enzyme of *Dictostelium* is essential for the secretion of cAMP, which then acts on the cell surface to control differentiation and aggregation.[204] The enzyme product of the *Drosophila* rutabaga gene is an adenylyl cyclase that resembles the mammalian type I enzyme in its regulation and structure and has a long (~100 kDa) carboxy-terminal extension. The catalytic activity of the rutabaga enzyme is abolished by a mutation that appears to cause learning impairment in the affected flies. Thus, the structure, regulatory properties, and functional role of the enzyme are conserved to an extraordinary degree across species. It is also noteworthy that the adenylyl cyclase of *S. cerevisiae* is activated by the small GTP-binding protein *ras*, analogous to the role of heterotrimeric G proteins in the activation of the mammalian adenylyl cyclases.

Cyclic Nucleotide Phosphodiesterases

The cyclic AMP produced during hormonal activation of receptors coupled to adenylyl cyclase is inactivated largely by phosphodiesterase (PDE) and to some extent by extrusion from the cell. In agonist-stimulated cells, cyclic nucleotide levels are determined by the balance between biosynthesis and degradation to 5′ AMP. Although cyclic AMP levels are usually governed by the activation of adenylyl cyclase, the activation of PDEs is sometimes responsible for mediating responses to external stimuli. This is exemplified by the retinal PDE that hydrolyzes cyclic GMP by transduction during the activation of rhodopsin by light.[205] Another important function of PDEs is to coordinate the activities of the cyclic nucleotide and phosphoinositide signaling pathways, largely through the regulatory actions of calcium/calmodulin (Fig. 5A-22).

Mammalian cells contain about 20 PDEs that are classified into five main groups according to their physical and functional properties.[206] All mammalian PDEs possess a central catalytic domain of about 270 amino acids and an N-terminal regulatory domain that binds Ca^{2+}/calmodulin and also contains binding sites for cyclic GMP. The major subgroups of PDEs and their properties are as follows: Type I PDEs are stimulated by Ca^{2+}/calmodulin and are activated by several calcium-mobilizing agonists (muscarinic, GnRH) and inhibited by IBMX. Type II PDEs are stimulated by cGMP and are activated by atrial natriuretic peptides. Type III PDEs are inhibited by cyclic guanosine monophosphate (cGMP), which competes with cAMP at the catalytic site, and are regulated by insulin, glucagon, and dexamethasone. Type IV PDEs are specific for cAMP, and are activated by cAMP-stimulating agonists and inhibited by rolipram; they include the enzymes encoded by the *Drosophila* gene *dunce*. Type V PDEs are specific for cGMP and include rod and cone isoforms that are essential components of the visual transduction system; they are activated by transducin during stimulation by light and are inhibited by zaprinest.

Increases in cAMP during hormonal stimulation are accompanied by stimulation of the activity of the cGMP-inhibited PDEs as a result of cAMP-dependent phosphorylation and by a transient decrease in the activity of the Ca^{2+}/CaM PDEs. Also, hormones that stimulate cAMP production often cause a delayed increase in the expression of the high-affinity cAMP-specific PDEs. Such changes can lead to alterations in target cell sensitivity to hormonal stimulation, as in the reduced responsiveness of Sertoli cells to FSH after long-term treatment with the hormone.[207] In cells treated with calcium-mobilizing hormones, increases in cytoplasmic Ca^{2+} activate the Ca^{2+}/CaM–responsive enzyme and thus regulate the concomitant levels of cAMP (Fig. 5A–22). Insulin and other growth factors of the tyrosine kinase group can stimulate cAMP hydrolysis by increasing the activity of cGMP-inhibited PDEs, an effect that may account for the antilipolytic action of insulin. Finally, elevation of cGMP levels, as in cells stimulated with atrial natriuretic peptide (ANP), activates the cGMP-stimulated PDEs and can in turn inhibit cAMP-mediated responses in the same cell. This may be responsible for the inhibitory action of ANP on aldosterone production by zona glomerulosa cells, which contain a high concentration of this enzyme.[208]

Cyclic AMP–Dependent Protein Kinases

All cells contain numerous types of protein kinases, of which the cAMP-dependent enzymes were the first to be discovered, that participate in cellular signaling and metabolic control mechanisms. Cyclic AMP–dependent phosphorylation and activation of regulatory enzymes, first observed for phosphorylase kinase in the liver, exemplify the manner in which the actions of cAMP are expressed through phosphorylation of protein substrates. Cyclic AMP–dependent protein kinases are present in all eukaryotic cells and are the major mediators of the effects of cAMP on cellular function.[209] In contrast, the actions of cAMP in prokaryotes are expressed through the direct interaction of cAMP-binding protein (CAP) with regulatory regions of the genome. Recently, additional types of cyclic AMP receptors have been identified, including cyclic nucleotide–gated ion channels, cGMP-binding phosphodiesterases, and slime mold receptors for extracellular cyclic AMP.

In animal tissues, cAMP-dependent protein kinases catalyze the transfer of γ-phosphate groups from ATP to specific serine and threonine residues of numerous protein substrates. These include enzymes such as phosphorylase kinase, glycogen synthase, and hormone-sensitive lipase as well as nonenzymatic proteins, including histones, nuclear nonhistone proteins, ribosomal proteins, microtubules, and membranes.[210] Most of the enzyme substrates exist in either phosphorylated or dephosphorylated forms and are interconverted between

TABLE 5A-7. Classification of Protein Kinases

Cyclic nucleotide-dependent kinases
cAMP-dependent protein kinases, types I and II
cGMP-dependent protein kinases
Calcium-dependent kinases
Calcium/calmodulin-dependent protein kinases: types I, II, and III
Calcium/phospholipid-dependent protein kinase (protein kinase C): nine isozymes
Cyclic nucleotide– and calcium-independent kinases
Casein kinases
Pyruvate dehydrogenase kinase
Glycogen synthase kinase 3
Rhodopsin kinase; β-adrenergic receptor kinase
Tyrosine-specific kinases
Growth factor receptors
Nonreceptor tyrosine kinases

their active and inactive states by the concerted actions of protein kinases and phosphatases. This cycle of phosphorylation and dephosphorylation is a ubiquitous mechanism of cellular regulation not only for metabolic enzymes but also in the control of contractile mechanisms, membrane activities, and nuclear processes. Each protein substrate is believed to control a specific metabolic or physiologic process, the rate of which is increased or decreased by phosphorylation of the regulatory protein.

The several forms of protein kinase can be broadly divided according to their nucleotide dependence or independence (Table 5A-7). Cyclic nucleotide–independent protein kinases are present in all regions of the cell and are regulated by several other intracellular signals. Major classes of protein kinase that depend on calcium-calmodulin or calcium and phospholipid for activation are intimately involved in transmembrane control systems that are regulated by calcium. Many of the hormonally controlled protein kinases in endocrine target cells are dependent on cyclic AMP or, less often, cyclic GMP. Such

FIGURE 5A-24. Linear structures of cAMP-dependent (PKA) and cGMP-dependent (PKG) protein kinases and the catabolite gene activator protein CAP. D, dimerization domain; I, autoinhibitory domain. The cyclic nucleotide and ATP-binding domains and the catalytic domains of the two kinases are indicated.

	Regulatory Subunit — Catalytic Subunit
PKA	D | I | cAMP | cAMP — ATP | Substrate
	Regulatory Domain — Catalytic Domain
PKG	D | I | cGMP | cGMP | ATP | Substrate
CAP	cAMP | DNA

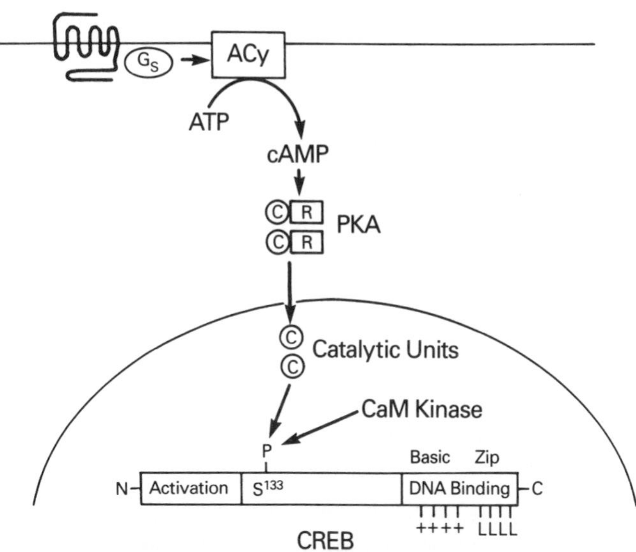

FIGURE 5A-25. Activation of cyclic AMP–dependent protein kinase by cAMP generated during receptor-mediated stimulation of adenylyl cyclase and the ensuing phosphorylation and activation of CREB by the catalytic subunits. (*Modified from Karin and Smeal.*[304])

cyclic nucleotide–dependent protein kinases are abundant in the cytosol but also occur in plasma membranes and other cell organelles. They are activated by micromolar concentrations of cyclic purine nucleotides (cAMP and cGMP) and are rapidly stimulated by the rises in cyclic nucleotide production that follow hormone action on the cell membrane. Both types of cyclic nucleotide–dependent protein kinase are activated by binding of the nucleotide to a specific regulatory site on the enzyme. These enzymes share several common structural features, as shown in Fig. 5A-24. In the case of cAMP-dependent protein kinase (PKA), the regulatory and catalytic domains are expressed as two separate molecules that associate to form the inactive holoenzyme complex. In the cyclic GMP–dependent enzyme (PKG), these domains are present in a single molecule.

Cyclic AMP–dependent protein kinase exists in its inactive form as a tetramer ($R_2 \cdot C_2$) composed of two regulatory (R) subunits and two catalytic (C) subunits (Fig. 5A-25). Binding of cAMP to the R subunits causes the inactive holoenzyme to dissociate, with release of active C subunits that can then phosphorylate intracellular substrates.[211] This sequence can be represented by the equation:

$$\underset{\text{(inactive)}}{R_2 \cdot C_2 + 4\text{cAMP}} \quad \underset{\text{(active)}}{R_2 \cdot \text{cAMP}_4 + 2\text{C}}$$

Once formed, the free C subunit is functionally similar to a cyclic AMP–independent protein kinase and can be distinguished by its characteristic size (38 kDa) and reactivity with a heat-stable inhibitory protein that blocks its catalytic activity and prevents recombination with the regulatory subunit.[212] The catalytic subunit is common to both major forms of cAMP-dependent protein kinase, whereas the regulatory subunits show several differences. The regulatory subunits released on dissociation of protein kinase remain as an R_2 dimer and later undergo reassociation with free catalytic subunits. In the absence of cAMP, the regulatory and catalytic subunits bind to each other with high affinity, and at physiologic concentrations they are mainly present as the inactive holoenzymes.

Two major types of mammalian cAMP-dependent protein kinases can be distinguished by their chromatographic, structural, and functional properties. The type I enzyme is less acidic and is readily dissociated by substrate (histone) or high salt concentration; it re-forms slowly after dissociation by cAMP. The type II enzyme is more acidic and is slowly dissociated by histone and salt but reassociates rapidly to form the inactive holoenzyme. The two forms of protein kinase are present in most tissues, but their proportions vary in each cell type. Thus, the type I enzyme predominates in rabbit skeletal muscle, whereas the type II enzyme is present in bovine cardiac muscle. The two holoenzymes are generally similar in subunit composition ($R_2 \cdot C_2$) and molecular mass (about 170 kDa). The regulatory subunits differ in their molecular masses, R_I being smaller (49 kDa) and more uniform in size than R_{II} (52 to 56 kDa), but the catalytic subunits are more similar (39 kDa). Both R_I and R_{II} contain a sequence that is similar to the consensus phosphorylation site of protein substrates (-Arg-Arg-X-Ser-). This region serves as an autoinhibitory domain by interacting with the catalytic site and maintains the holoenzymes in their inactive state in the absence of cyclic AMP.[213]

The main distinguishing features between the two enzymes are that the type I kinase binds $Mg^{2+} \cdot$ATP whereas the type II kinase catalyzes the phosphorylation of its own regulatory subunit by ATP. Binding of ATP by the type II enzyme reduces its affinity for cAMP and presumably favors the inactive state of the enzyme. The type I subunit is not phosphorylated while binding ATP, in contrast to the autophosphorylation shown by the type II enzyme. This difference reflects the replacement of the *serine* residue that is autophosphorylated in the -Arg-Arg-Val-Ser- sequence of the type II regulatory subunit by an *alanine* residue in the type I subunit (to give -Arg-Arg-Val-Ala-).[214] Both subunits contain two allosteric activator binding sites with high affinity for cyclic AMP, either one of which can activate the holoenzymes. The phosphorylation of type II protein kinase is accompanied by a decrease in the rate of reassociation of the dissociated R and C subunits. Thus, autophosphorylation may control the activity of the dissociated enzyme by regulating its rate of return to the inactive form. Increased dephosphorylation of R would favor recombination to the $R_2 \cdot C_2$ holoenzyme, followed by release and degradation of cAMP. In this way, the proportions of active and inactive enzyme could be regulated in the absence of changes in cAMP concentration. It is possible that type II enzymes concerned with rapid cycling of metabolic processes, as in cardiac and nerve tissue, have acquired the capacity for more highly regulated inactivation by the ultrashort feedback effect of a phosphorylation/dephosphorylation step on the regulatory subunit.[215] The roles of autophosphorylation in the functions of cAMP-dependent and other protein kinases are summarized in Table 5A-8.

TABLE 5A-8. Autophosphorylation and Protein Kinase Activity

Autophosphorylated protein kinases
Regulatory (R) subunit of cAMP-dependent protein kinase
Receptor tyrosine kinases: EGF, insulin, PDGF, FGF
Protein kinase C
Ca^{2+}/calmodulin-dependent protein kinase type II
Effects of autophosphorylation of enzyme activity
Diminished reassociation of holoenzyme
Activation of enzyme
Regulation of membrane association (?)
Decreased affinity for calmodulin, increased substrate phosphorylation

Abbreviations: EGF, epidermal growth factor; PDGF, platelet-derived growth factor; FGF, fibroblast growth factor.

In addition to its role in the phosphorylation of defined enzymes such as phosphorylase kinase, cAMP-dependent protein kinase phosphorylates many basic proteins (including histones, casein, and protamine) as well as many denatured proteins that are not substrates in their native states. Small basic peptides are also phosphorylated by the enzyme, as are synthetic peptide sequences similar to the phosphorylated regions of native and denatured protein substrates. Although the phosphorylation reaction is not highly selective for individual protein sequences, it has relatively high specificity for serine residues in defined regions of the primary sequence of many proteins. The structural requirements for phosphorylation of peptide substrates include the presence of two adjacent basic amino acids, one of which is arginine; the pair is situated two to five residues to the amino-terminal side of the target serine residue.[216]

The physiologically important substrates for cAMP-dependent protein kinase contain one of two consensus amino acid sequences at their phosphorylation sites: -Lys-Arg-X-X-Ser-X-X- and -Arg-Arg-X-Ser-X-. In these sequences, X stands for any amino acid, of which those immediately adjacent to the serine residue usually have hydrophobic side chains. The first type of phosphorylation site, in which the basic amino acids are separated from serine by two residues, occurs in the β subunit of phosphorylase kinase and in glycogen synthase. The second type, with one intervening residue, occurs in pyruvate kinase and the regulatory subunit of type II cAMP-dependent protein kinase. Because the rate of phosphorylation depends on a relatively common primary sequence around the phosphorylated site, the substrate specificity of individual proteins must depend on their secondary and tertiary (i.e., three-dimensional) conformations to restrict the accessibility of potentially phosphorylated regions to the catalytic enzyme units. A proposed role for such higher structures in substrate specificity is the location of the phosphorylated serine at the hydrophilic surface of substrate proteins in a hydrogen-bonded β-bend structure that is recognized by the protein kinase.[217]

The RI and RII subunits are relatively heterogeneous, and each exists in α and β forms that are present in various species and tissues and range in size from 52 to 56 kDa.[218] The α isoforms are expressed constitutively in many tissues, but the β isoforms are most highly expressed in the nervous system and, to a lesser extent, in a few other tissues. Thus, the RIIβ isoform is abundant in the brain and is also expressed in adrenal, testis, ovary, bone marrow, and adipose tissue. The RIβ isoform has a more restricted expression in the brain and the germ cells of the testis. The selective regulation of these isoforms of RII during differentiation and hormonal stimulation could mediate specific responses to signaling via the cAMP–kinase A pathway. In some tissues, free RI and RII subunits are present in considerable excess over the catalytic subunit and interact with other cellular proteins or structures. Several cAMP-mediated hormones stimulate a selective increase in the RII subunit in their target tissues when inducing differentiation, as in the maturing rat granulosa cell under the influence of FSH.[219] It is possible that much of the type II holoenzyme exists in the autophosphorylated form in situ and becomes dephosphorylated after dissociation of the enzymes by cAMP. The C subunits are also encoded by multiple genes, giving rise to α, β, and γ isoforms (the latter confined to the testis) as well as additional forms of Cα and Cβ by alternative splicing. Since each R subunit can associate with any of the α subunits and since RIα and R1β may form heterodimers, a wide variety of $R_2 \cdot C_2$ holoenzymes could exist in various tissues. The presence of at least 12 forms of cAMP-dependent protein kinase provides for a considerable degree of diversity in the tissue-specific expression, intracellular localization, and activation properties of the individual enzymes. For example, the brain-abundant RIβ isoform associates with either Cα or Cβ to form a holoenzyme that is more sensitive to cAMP than the RIα-containing enzyme and may increase the sensitivity of neurons to transmitters that act through cAMP.[220]

Guanylate Cyclase, Cyclic GMP, and cGMP-Dependent Protein Kinase

Cyclic GMP

While the second messenger concept of hormone action has been extensively validated for cyclic AMP, cyclic GMP plays a more restricted role in target cell regulation by hormones. The actions of several hormones that increase phospholipid turnover are accompanied by a rise in cGMP, probably reflecting activation of guanylate cyclase by protein kinase C and/or in association with stimulation of phospholipase A_2 and the formation of arachidonic acid metabolites. A major physiologic role of cGMP has been defined in vascular smooth muscle during the action of ANP (or atriopeptin), which activates membrane-associated guanylate cyclase and causes marked increases in cGMP concentrations in smooth muscle, kidney, endothelial cells, and adrenal glands.[221] Such increases in the cGMP concentration are responsible for smooth muscle relaxation and vasodilation, changes that are mediated by activation of cGMP-dependent protein kinase and phosphorylation of specific proteins involved in the contractile mechanism.

In vertebrates, cGMP has an important function as the intracellular messenger mediating visual transduction and acts by modulating the activity of a cation channel in the plasma membrane of rod photoreceptors of the retina.[222] This action depends on the binding of cGMP to a regulatory site on the channel to maintain it in the open state, leading to an inward (predominantly sodium) current in the dark. The absorption of light by rhodopsin stimulates the activity of cGMP phosphodiesterase via the guanyl nucleotide regulatory protein transducin (G_t). Each photolyzed rhodopsin complex activates hundreds of transducin molecules, and each α_t subunit stimulates a phosphodiesterase molecule to hydrolyze hundreds of molecules of cGMP. In this process, a single photon causes the hydrolysis of about 10^5 cGMP molecules. The resulting light-induced depletion of intracellular cGMP causes the ion channel to close, reducing the influx of sodium (and calcium) and leading to hyperpolarization of the cell membrane. Subsequently, the resulting fall in cytoplasmic calcium releases guanylate cyclase from inhibition by calcium, leading to increased synthesis of cGMP and reopening of the channel.

Guanylyl Cyclase

The formation of cGMP from GTP is catalyzed by a family of guanylate cyclases that are present in most mammalian cells and exist in membrane-associated and soluble forms.[223] The membrane-associated enzymes are regulated by extracellular ligands and are integral domains of the cytoplasmic regions of peptide receptor molecules with a single transmembrane domain and an extracellular hormone-binding domain. The hormones that activate the receptors include sea urchin egg peptides (speract and resact) that stimulate sperm motility, ANPs, and heat-stable *E. coli* enterotoxins. In the retina, membrane-associated guanylate cyclase is under the inhibitory control of calcium, as noted above. Three forms of receptor-controlled guanylyl cyclase termed GC-A, GC-B, and GC-C have been defined by molecular cloning and are glycoproteins of molecular mass 130 to 160 kDa. Each contains a cysteine-rich extracellular domain for ligand binding and two enzymatic domains in its intracellular portion. A protein kinase domain is located near the plasma membrane, as in the receptor tyrosine kinases, but does not appear to be enzymatically active. It is followed by the adjacent catalytic guanylyl cyclase domain of about 250 amino acids, a region that is highly conserved in guanylyl and adenylyl cyclase families.[224] The mammalian guanylyl cyclase receptors are activated by the ANPs produced by the heart and brain, which act on GC-A and GC-B receptors, and by enterotoxins that probably act on the GC-C receptor.

The soluble guanylyl cyclases are present in most tissues and are abundant in lung and smooth muscle. They contain no membrane-spanning or protein kinase–like domains and are activated by nitric oxide, which interacts with a potential heme-binding region of the molecule.[225] This effect of nitric oxide is responsible for the vasodilator actions of nitroglycerin and related compounds and also for the effects of endogenous vasodilators such as acetylcholine, bradykinin, and substance P. The latter agents stimulate nitric oxide synthesis in endothelial cells, and the gas diffuses into vascular smooth muscle cells and activates soluble guanylate cyclase, leading to muscle relaxation.[226]

Cyclic GMP–dependent protein kinases are abundant in insects and arthropods but have a more limited distribution in mammalian tissues, where they function in a manner different from that of the cAMP-dependent enzyme. Their affinity for cAMP is much lower than that for cGMP, and their enzyme activity is usually less than that of the cAMP-dependent form. Whereas the cAMP-dependent kinases mediate the regulation of major metabolic pathways, including lipolysis, glycogenolysis, and steroidogenesis, the cGMP-dependent enzyme is involved in the actions of cGMP on processes, including gene expression, neuronal function, vascular tone, and platelet aggregation. The cGMP-dependent kinase is activated by the binding of cGMP to a regulatory site on the enzyme, without the subunit dissociation that is characteristic of the cAMP-dependent enzyme. There are marked amino acid sequence homologies between cGMP- and cAMP-dependent protein kinases, suggesting a common evolutionary origin of the enzymes from a primitive ancestral phosphotransferase.

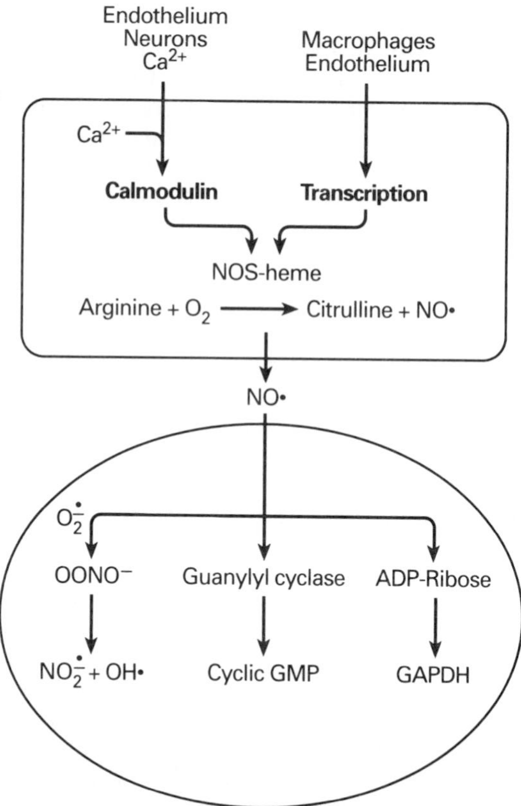

FIGURE 5A-26. Synthesis and actions of nitric oxide (NO) in blood vessels, neurons, and macrophages. NO acts as an intracellular messenger in some cells and acts in others as an intercellular messenger, as shown above. NOS, NO synthase; GAPDH, glyceraldehyde-3-phosphate dehydrogenase. (*Modified from Lowenstein and Snyder.*[227])

Nitric Oxide: A New Signaling Molecule

Nitric oxide (NO) is one of the most interesting of the recently identified molecules that serve as messengers in cellular signaling.[227] NO, which is formed by the enzymatic oxidation of the terminal guanidine-nitrogen atoms of L-arginine, is a free radical gas of limited solubility in water and is degraded by tissues within a few seconds.[228] However, it rapidly diffuses across cell membranes and into other cells and acts as both an intracellular and an intercellular messenger to elicit diverse biological responses, in particular in the vascular, immune, and neural systems. These incude vasodilation, cytotoxic and cytostatic actions, host defense mechanisms, and neurotransmission. One of the best-defined actions of NO is activation of the soluble forms of guanylate cyclase, leading to increased production of cGMP (Fig. 5A-26). NO was first identified in blood vessels as the factor [endothelium-derived relaxation factor (EDRF)] that mediates the actions of vasodilators such as acetylcholine and bradykinin on vascular smooth muscle. Such agents act primarily on endothelial cells to stimulate the production of NO, which in turn promotes relaxation of adjacent smooth muscle cells by increasing cGMP formation.[225] NO is now regarded as a major regulator of blood flow in peripheral vessels. It is also formed in platelets and macrophages and inhibits platelet aggregation through activation of guanylate cyclase and elevation of intraplatelet cGMP levels. NO is released by macrophages and has toxic actions on bacteria, parasites, and tumor cells.[229] In addition to mediating the control of vascular tone and platelet aggregation, NO acts as a neurotransmitter in the central and peripheral nervous systems. Thus, many of its actions are related to intercellular communication of a paracrine or autocrine nature.

The formation of nitric oxide from L-arginine is catalyzed by nitric oxide synthase (NOS), which includes a group of several NADPH-dependent enzymes that oxidize arginine to citrulline and exist in both cytosolic and membrane-associated forms. NOS enzymes are of primitive evolutionary origin and are structurally related to cytochrome P450 reductase, which provides electrons for the activities of the microsomal P450 enzymes.[230] The NOS isoforms range in size from 130 to 160 kDa and include constitutive enzymes in neurons and endothelial cells that are regulated by Ca^{2+}/calmodulin, and inducible calcium-independent enzymes that are regulated at the transcriptional level. The expression of the Ca^{2+}-independent forms of NOS is induced by endotoxins and cytokines such as interleukin 1 (IL-1), tumor necrosis factor (TNF-α), and INF-γ and is important in immune and inflammatory responses in macrophages, endothelial cells, platelets, smooth muscle cells, and hepatocytes (Fig. 5A-26).

In the nervous system, NO is an important messenger molecule in the brain and serves as a transmitter in the peripheral tissues. It is released in response to activation of NMDA receptors and the consequent elevations of cytoplasmic Ca^{2+} that stimulate NO synthase activity. The Ca^{2+}-calmodulin-dependent neural NO synthase is expressed at high concentrations in the cerebellum, hippocampus, and olfactory lobe and is very similar to (or identical to) neural NADPH diaphorase.[230] In the brain, the distribution of the enzyme and that of NO-stimulated cGMP are closely correlated in several regions. NO could exert more prolonged actions than the traditional neurotransmitters and might thus act to mediate slow synaptic transmission as well as retrograde transmission to presynaptic neurons. NO has also been implicated in long-term depression in the cerebellum and long-term potentiation in the hippocampus. In the cerebellum, NO synthase is highly concentrated in the basket cells and in their processes that are in contact with Purkinje cells.[231] In regions where NO synthase is not in close apposition to guanylyl cyclase–containing cells, it may act through other transmitters. For example, NO has been found to mediate NMDA-stimulated release of glutamate and norepinephrine in the cerebral cortex and may thus link NMDA receptor activation to chemical signaling in surrounding synaptic terminals.[232]

In addition to its actions as a neurotransmitter in the brain, NO exerts neurotoxic actions that may account for the neuronal death associated with overstimulation of NMDA receptors, as occurs in cerebral ischemia.[225] These toxic actions of NO, and its bactericidal and tumoricidal effects, are attributed to free radical formation and energy depletion. NO can react with superoxide anions ($O_2^{\cdot}$) to form peroxynitrite anions ($ONOO^-$) that decompose to nitrogen dioxide and highly damaging hydroxyl (OH^-) free radicals, the strongest oxidants in biological systems. NO also inhibits key enzymes in the mitochondrial electron transport chain, the citric acid cycle, and DNA synthesis by binding to the reactive thiol groups in their iron-sulphur centers.[233] An important aspect of NO toxicity is its *S*-nitrosylation and ADP ribosylation of glyceraldehyde-3-phosphate dehydrogenase (GAPDH). This effect of NO is additive to its recently observed action to activate poly(ADP-ribose) synthase (PARS), a nuclear enzyme that is also activated by DNA damage and adds multiple ADP-ribose units to nuclear proteins. Excessive activation of PARS by NO could lead to cell death by depletion of NAD, the source of ADP ribose. The combination of free radical damage caused by NO and the specific depletion of cellular energy sources could account for both the neurotoxicity and the macrophage-mediated cytotoxic action of NO.[234]

Recently, another toxic gas—carbon monoxide—has been found to act as a neural messenger and to regulate the intracellular levels of cGMP in cultured olfactory neurons by stimulatory guanylyl cyclase activity.[235] CO is formed by the action of heme oxygenase-2, which is constitutively expressed in many of the same brain regions that express the soluble guanylyl cyclase. Most of these regions would account for the activation of guanylyl cyclase in areas in which NOS is not expressed, so that much of the regulation of cGMP production in brain could be accomplished by the two gaseous messengers. Like NO, CO is a candidate for the retrograde messenger that is believed to be important in the learning-related process of long-term potentiation in the hippocampus. CO may also have a function in peripheral vascular regulation, since it can activate guanylyl cyclase and relax vascular smooth muscle. Whether CO mimics the other actions of NO, including its mediation of the effects of nonadrenergic, noncholinergic neuron activity on vasodilation in the corpora cavernosa and penile erection,[236] has not been determined.

Calcium and Calcium-Dependent Enzyme Systems

The importance of calcium as an activator of cell

responses was first revealed by Ringer's discovery of its requirement in contractility of the isolated frog heart. In addition to its major roles in muscle contraction and neuromuscular transmission, calcium is an essential intermediate in secretory processes and is involved in many aspects of intracellular regulation. The general function of calcium as an intracellular messenger was predicted by the *stimulus-secretion hypothesis*, which proposed that calcium ions serve as the primary link between cell stimulation and secretion.[237] Subsequent evidence has emphasized the importance of both positive and negative interactions between calcium and cyclic nucleotides as the major components of an intracellular signaling system that regulates target cell function in response to external stimuli.[238] These messengers undergo rapid changes in hormone-stimulated cells, and their intracellular concentrations represent dynamic equilibriums between their rates of production and removal. The high rate of turnover of messenger molecules permits rapid cellular responses to hormone activation and (usually) prompt termination of such a response on withdrawal of the stimulus. During hormone action, the intracellular levels of second messengers are controlled largely by changes in the rates of signal generation, as when adenylyl cyclase activity or calcium influx is stimulated or inhibited by extracellular ligands. However, changes in rates of signal removal are also important determinants of these intracellular levels, as when cAMP and cGMP are regulated by changes in phosphodiesterase activity and cytoplasmic calcium is regulated by membrane-bound calcium pumps. The interactions between calcium and cyclic nucleotide generation and metabolism are particularly important in this regard, since the enzymes responsible for both the synthesis and the degradation of cAMP and cGMP are influenced by calcium-dependent feedback mechanisms that integrate the activities of the second messengers during hormonal stimulation.[239]

Regulation of Intracellular Calcium Concentration

The primary event in the activation of calcium-mediated responses to external stimuli is the movement of calcium ions into the cell cytoplasm. The calcium involved in such movements is derived from two major sources: the extracellular fluid, in which the free calcium concentration is about 1200 μM, and intracellular stores in microsomes, mitochondria, and plasma membrane. The cytosolic free calcium concentration is very low (about 100 nM) under basal conditions and does not usually exceed 1 μM during hormonal stimulation. Plasma membranes contain an appreciable amount of bound calcium both on the inner surface and in the glycocalyx of the external surface of the cell. Although calcium entry is favored by the large calcium gradient across the plasma membrane and the transmembrane electric gradient, the rate of calcium influx is usually low in the absence of cell stimulation. Such restricted membrane permeability and the presence of an external perimembranous pool of bound calcium render most cells relatively unresponsive to changes in ambient calcium concentration, particularly in the basal state. However, the increased sensitivity to calcium that frequently accompanies hormonal stimulation indicates that altered membrane permeability is an essential step in cell activation.[240] The initial rapid increases in cytoplasmic calcium concentration $[Ca^{2+}]_i$ during cell activation by hormonal ligands result from redistribution of the intracellular calcium stores. However, increased entry of calcium across the plasma membrane is the main source of the calcium signal during sustained hormonal stimulation.

The agonist-stimulated release of Ca^{2+} from intracellular stores is mediated by the immediate formation of Ins(1,4,5)P_3 during hydrolysis of the plasma membrane polyphosphoinositide phosphatidylinositol 4,5-biphosphate (PtdInsP_2). This process, which is described in detail below, leads to the activation of specific Ins(1,4,5)P_3 receptor channels in the ER. The consequent release of Ca^{2+} into the cytoplasm activates several enzymatic mechanisms that mediate secretory and other cell responses and indirectly promotes the influx of Ca^{2+} from the extracellular fluid. The influx of calcium through the plasma membrane during agonist-induced changes in membrane permeability is a complex process that depends on the activation of specific sets of ion channels. These include receptor-operated and second messenger–activated calcium channels and voltage-sensitive calcium channels that are activated by changes in membrane potential. The latter mechanism is a feature of excitable cells (neural, muscle, pituitary) that generate action potentials and is sometimes involved in peptide hormone action. It is responsible for the stimulatory effect of high potassium concentrations on secretory cells in vitro caused by depolarization of the plasma membrane and increased calcium entry through voltage-sensitive channels.

Elevations of the intracellular calcium concentration, whether caused by influx or mobilization of calcium, are rapidly corrected by increases in calcium sequestration and efflux. Much of the Ca^{2+} that is released into the cytoplasm during agonist stimulation is returned to the intracellular stores by a specific Ca^{2+}-ATPase that is localized in the ER and is inhibited by the tumor promoter, thapsigargin. Calcium efflux is achieved by active extrusion of excess cytosolic calcium from neuromuscular cells by exchange with sodium and from nonexcitable cells by the plasma membrane calcium pump, Ca^{2+}, Mg^{2+}-ATPase. Hormonal stimuli that cause mobilization of intracellular calcium are frequently accompanied

TABLE 5A-9. Calcium- and Calmodulin-Regulated Enzymes

Cyclic nucleotide metabolism
Adenylyl cyclase
Cyclic nucleotide phosphodiesterase
Protein phosphorylation
Myosin light-chain kinase: smooth muscle and other cell types
Phosphorylase kinase: phosphorylase, glycogen synthase
CaM-dependent protein kinase I: synapsin I, site I
CaM-dependent protein kinase II: synapsin I, site II; glycogen synthase; MAP 2; tryptophan monooxygenase
CaM-dependent protein kinase III: 100,000-Mr protein in many tissues
Protein dephosphorylation
Calcineurin: multifunctional phosphoprotein phosphatase; acts on many brain and other phosphoproteins, including tyrosylphosphoproteins
Calcium transport
Ca^{2+}, Mg^{2+}-dependent ATPase (plasma membrane Ca^{2+} pump)
Sarcoplasmic (Ca^{2+}) ATPase (sarcoplasmic Ca^{2+} transport)
Other
NAD kinase (plants)

Abbreviations: CaM, calmodulin; MAP, microtubule-associated protein

by increased calcium efflux caused by activation of the plasma membrane calcium pump by calcium-calmodulin. This aids in the restoration of the normal cytoplasmic calcium concentration, but the consequent loss of intracellular Ca^{2+} must be compensated by subsequent increases in Ca^{2+} entry through the plasma membrane via calcium channels and other influx mechanisms.

Mechanisms of Calcium's Action as a Second Messenger

The biological actions of calcium are largely mediated by its interaction with binding proteins such as calmodulin and troponin C (Table 5A-9) and regulatory enzymes such as protein kinase C. The calcium-calmodulin complex participates in the regulation of biosynthetic, metabolic, and transport enzymes, including adenylyl and guanylyl cyclase, cyclic nucleotide phosphodiesterase, and Ca^{2+}, Mg^{2+}-ATPase. It therefore influences the cytoplasmic levels of both cyclic nucleotides and links the intracellular messenger systems by feedback mechanisms that integrate their biological activities as well as controlling enzymes involved in signaling, secretion, and contractility.

Calcium-Calmodulin and Enzyme Activation

The calcium-dependent protein calmodulin is structurally and functionally similar to troponin C and other calcium-binding proteins and subserves numerous regulatory functions in eukaryotic cells.[241] During muscle contraction, calcium is bound by troponin C to form a complex that facilitates the interaction between actin and myosin and activates the myosin ATPase necessary for repetition of the actin-myosin reaction. In smooth muscle, calmodulin also activates myosin light-chain kinase and promotes the phosphorylation of regulatory light chains that is an essential step in the initiation of the contractile response to calcium-mobilizing stimuli.[242] The presence of actin in noncontractile cells suggested that similar contractile elements participate in cell mobility and movement of organelles, granule release, and endocytosis. Many cells have extensive arrays of actin-like and myosin-like filament proteins attached to the inner surface of the plasma membrane and often to the membranes of secretory granules. Such actin-containing microfilaments could mediate the effects of calcium on cell motility, membrane fluidity, and rearrangements or internalization of membrane-associated proteins and their bound extrinsic ligands. Although the troponin component of muscle was not initially detected in noncontractile cells, the later discovery of troponin-like calcium-binding proteins in many cell types led to the recognition of calmodulin as a general calcium-dependent regulatory protein.[243]

Calmodulin is one of a family of small, acidic calcium-binding proteins that have evolved from a single ancestral calcium-binding protein and contain multiple copies of a helix-loop-helix motif that binds calcium with high affinity. These domains, which are also termed EF-hand motifs, consist of two α helices that are linked by a loop of 12 amino acids, 5 of which have carboxyl or hydroxyl groups that coordinate the calcium molecule. This calcium-binding structure was first observed in parvalbumin and is present as two to eight copies in calmodulin, troponin C, myosin light chains, calcineurin, and at least 200 other calcium-binding proteins, many of unknown function. Although several of these proteins are widely distributed and are present in all cell types, most of them are expressed in a tissue-specific manner in a wide variety of organisms.[244] Several of them (parvalbumin, troponin C, intestinal calcium-binding protein) subserve specific functions that are restricted to certain tissues. In contrast, calmodulin-like proteins are widely distributed in animal and plant tissues and mediate many of the physiologic actions of calcium by controlling the activities of specific enzymes. The functional role of calmodulin in noncontractile tissues is thus analogous to that of troponin C in muscle, i.e., to mediate the actions of calcium on regulatory enzyme systems. Calmodulin is sometimes associated with the array of microfilaments and in other cases is intimately associated with calcium-regulated enzymes as a tightly bound subunit or congener. By serving as an intracellular calcium receptor, calmodulin modifies calcium transport, the calcium-dependent regulation of cyclic nucleotide and glycogen metabolism, and processes such as secretion and cell motility. Calmodulin is also a dynamic component of the mitotic apparatus, where it can regulate microtubule polymerization, actomyosin, and membrane-bound calcium pumps. Many of the effects of calmodulin on cellular processes are mediated through its activation of enzymes involved in protein phosphorylation and dephosphorylation.

Calmodulin is a 17-kDa protein of 148 amino acids and contains four calcium-binding sites of the helix-loop-helix configuration. The Ca^{2+} binding loops of calmodulins are characterized by the presence of aspartate and glutamate at the first and twelfth positions, respectively.[245] The protein contains a high proportion of phenylalanine and acidic residues and shows considerable sequence homology with troponin C from skeletal and cardiac muscle. The calmodulin molecule possesses significant α helicity, and this increases markedly after calcium binding. The resulting conformational change in the calmodulin molecule favors its binding to enzymes and other regulatory proteins and to drugs such as the phenothiazines. Crystallographic analysis of the three-dimensional structure of calmodulin shows it to consist of two linked globular regions, each of which binds two calcium ions.[246] The two calcium-binding domains are connected by an eight-turn stretch of α helix that is buried in the absence of calcium and becomes exposed when calcium is bound (Fig. 5A-27). This long exposed region of α helix is involved in the calcium-dependent interaction of calmodulin with various proteins and drugs. The DNA sequence of the calmodulin gene contains eight exons and seven introns. The sequences encoding three of the four calcium-binding domains are interrupted by introns; this is consistent with the view that introns separate regions to be displayed on the surface of the protein molecule.

The importance of calmodulin as a mediator of the actions of calcium was first recognized in the brain, where it is required for the activation of a major calcium-dependent phosphodiesterase. The many enzymes that depend on calmodulin for activation by calcium include certain types of adenylyl cyclase and phosphodiesterase, plasma membrane Ca^{2+}, Mg^{2+}-ATPase, and a series of calcium-calmodulin (CaM)-dependent protein kinases (Table 5A-9). The latter enzymes include protein kinases of strict or limited substrate specificity, such as phosphorylase kinase and myosin light-chain kinase, and a multifunctional enzyme (CaM kinase II) that is abundant in the brain and phosphorylates a variety of substrates (synapsin 1, glycogen synthase, microtubule-associated protein 2, and tyrosine hydroxylase). The physiologic functions of CaM kinase II include regulation of neurotransmitter synthesis and release and possibly a role in synaptic plasticity.[247] It is activated by binding Ca^{2+}/CaM, which causes a change in conformation that results in the separation of an autoinhibitory domain from the catalytic site of the enzyme, analogous to the activation of protein kinase A by cyclic AMP. CaM kinase II is also activated by autophosphorylation, which converts the enzyme to a partially Ca^{2+}-independent form.[248] Other calmodulin-regulated phosphokinases include CaM kinase I, with specificity for synapsin-1, and CaM kinase III, which phosphorylates a 100-kDa protein that is present in many mammalian tissues. CaM kinase IV is a multifunctional protein kinase that is widely distributed and has structural and functional features in common with CaM kinase II. However, unlike CaM kinase II, it is a monomeric enzyme and does not become rapidly autophosphorylated and CaM-independent.[249]

Enzyme activation by calmodulin and binding of calmodulin to the enzyme are both dependent on the presence of calcium. Upon binding Ca^{2+}, calmodulin undergoes a conformational change to its active state, which then associates with the enzyme and enhances its catalytic activity. The degree of occupancy of the four calcium-binding sites probably varies among the systems regulated by calmodulin and may explain its diverse biological actions. The role of calmodulin in the phosphorylation of myosin light-chain kinase may be related to the regulation of

FIGURE 5A-27. Conformation and Ca^{2+}-binding domains of the calmodulin molecule. (*Left*) The molecule is composed of α helices (shaded regions) linked by calcium-binding loops, arranged as a bipolar structure with two calcium (C)-binding domains at each each. (*Right*). The amino acids of the connecting loops (light circles) between those forming the α helices (dark circles) contain calcium-binding amino acid residues (D, Asp; N, Asn; Y, Tyr; S, Ser; E, Glu) and sequences (shaded) that favor the formation of β turns. (*Modified from Babu et al.*[246])

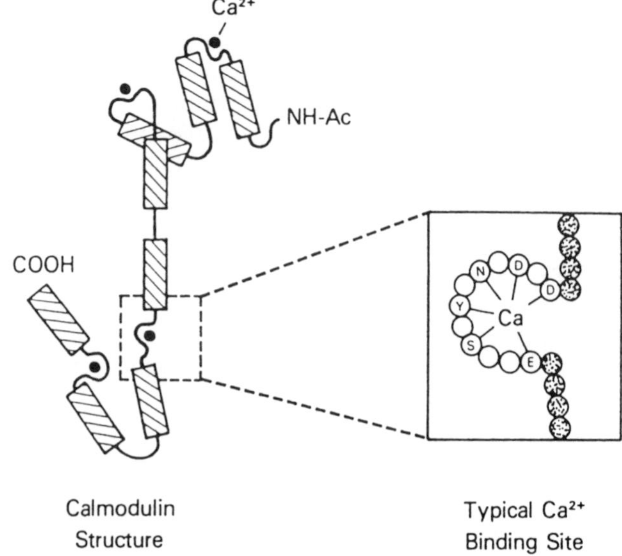

smooth muscle contraction by determining the balance of activity between phosphorylated (inactive) and dephosphorylated (potentially active) myosin kinase. β-Adrenergic stimulation of cAMP formation by epinephrine leads to the activation of protein kinase and the phosphorylation of myosin kinase. The phosphorylated kinase binds calmodulin with lower affinity than the unphosphorylated enzyme. At low levels of calcium-calmodulin, the myosin kinase is less active and phosphatase activity may predominate, causing fewer myosin molecules to be in the phosphorylated state. Then actin-myosin interaction would not occur, resulting in relaxation of smooth muscle.[238]

Several proteins have been found to bind calmodulin in various tissues, and some of them are potential modulators of calmodulin activity. However, most have proved to be calmodulin-regulated enzymes such as calcineurin, which binds calmodulin in the nervous system. Calcineurin was first discovered as an inhibitor of phosphodiesterase in the brain and is now known to be a multifunctional phosphoprotein phosphatase with broad specificity for neuronal and other phosphoproteins, including tyrosyl phosphoproteins such as the EGF receptor. Recently, calcineurin was found to be the intracellular target for immunosuppressive drugs such as cyclosporin, and appears to be involved in signal transduction pathways that regulate IL-2 gene expression in T cells.[250]

Calcium-Dependent Regulatory Enzymes: Protein Kinase C

In addition to acting through calcium receptor proteins that bind to regulatory enzymes and control metabolic pathways, calcium binds directly to several calcium-dependent enzymes without the intervention of calmodulin or other receptor proteins. The most important enzyme in this category is protein kinase C, a calcium- and phospholipid-dependent phosphokinase that depends for its activity on calcium and phosphatidylserine (PS).[251] Under physiologic conditions, protein kinase C is activated by the DAG that is produced from plasma membrane phospholipids in response to extracellular stimuli. Free DAG is present in extremely low concentrations in the membranes of unstimulated cells, but its concentration rises rapidly during receptor-activated hydrolysis of phosphoinositides by phospholipase C. Small amounts of DAG markedly increase the affinity of protein kinase C for calcium and can activate the enzyme in the absence of a change in the cytosolic calcium concentration (Fig. 5A-28).

Protein kinase C was first detected in the brain and was later shown to be activated by thrombin in platelets in the absence of a rise in the cytoplasmic calcium concentration. The calcium- and phospholipid-dependent enzyme is present in numerous tissues and organisms, and its activity frequently exceeds that of cAMP-dependent protein kinase. Protein kinase C is activated by the binding of many

FIGURE 5A-28. Receptor-mediated activation of phospholipase C in the plasma membrane, with production of Ins(1,4,5)P_3 and diacylglycerol and stimulation of calcium mobilization and activation of Ca^{2+}/calmodulin kinase and protein kinase C.

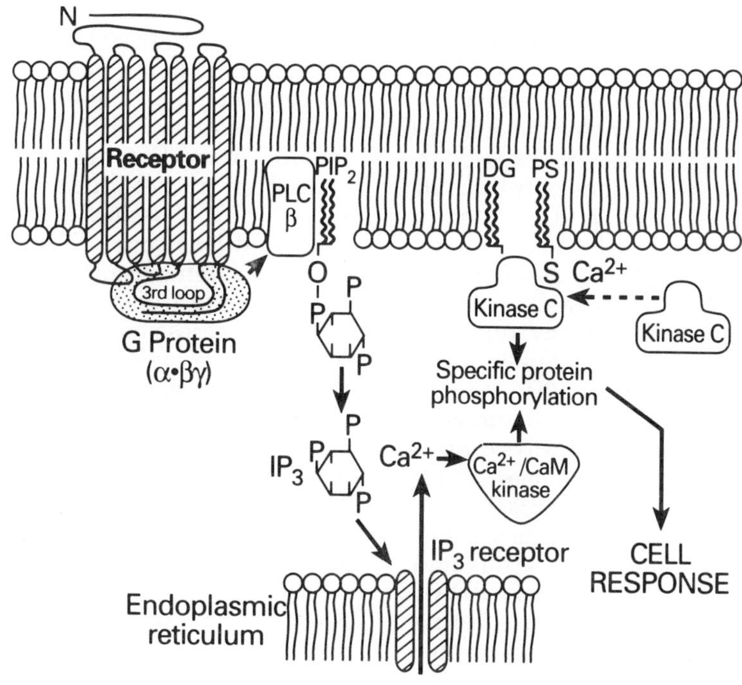

extracellular ligands to their plasma membrane receptors. It is also activated by tumor promoters such as tetradecanoylphorbol acetate (TPA) and cell-permeant DAG derivatives, which bind directly to the enzyme and substitute for DAG in causing its activation.[252] Most of the protein kinase C in unstimulated cells is located in the cytoplasm, but the enzyme undergoes redistribution to the plasma membrane (translocation) in most cells during treatment with phorbol esters. The effects of phorbol esters on protein kinase C differ from those of DAG mainly in terms of their potency and duration, since the endogenous lipid is rapidly metabolized by DAG kinase and diglyceride lipase, whereas phorbol esters become highly bound to the enzyme and cause its prolonged activation and association with the plasma membrane. Several synthetic diglycerides, such as dioctanoyl glycerol, which penetrate the cell membrane and activate the enzyme are also potent stimuli of protein kinase C activity in intact cells.

Structure and Properties of Protein Kinase C Protein kinase C (PKC) was originally defined as a single polypeptide chain of 77 kDa with two functional regions—a hydrophobic membrane-binding domain and a hydrophilic catalytic domain—that are cleaved by calcium-dependent proteases. The hydrophilic segment is enzymatically active in the absence of calcium, phospholipid, and DAG and has been termed *M-kinase*. Once activated by DAG or phorbol esters, PKC phosphorylates serine and threonine residues in numerous cell proteins. The primary structure of the enzyme includes an amino-terminal cysteine-rich domain followed by a calcium-binding domain and a carboxy-terminal region with homology to other protein kinases that represents the 50-kDa catalytic fragment released by proteolysis.[251]

Many of the receptors that stimulate DAG production and activate kinase C also elevate the cytosolic calcium level, which usually potentiates the activation of the enzyme. Thus, in platelets exposed to individually ineffective concentrations of a calcium ionophore and synthetic DAG, PKC is stimulated to the maximal extent elicited by ligands such as thrombin and platelet-activating factor as a result of the synergism between elevated cytosolic calcium and DAG. Hormonal responses in many cells are largely controlled by calcium changes but in some cells are dominated by activation of PKC, and in others require both mechanisms for maximum activation. It is also likely that the two pathways control different phases of the response to hormonal stimulation in certain cells. Since the calcium response is relatively small and transient in many cells because of the compensatory increase in calcium efflux and sequestration, sustained activation of PKC by DAG would serve to prolong the cellular response during sustained hormonal stimulation. This could involve factors such as secondary activation of phospholipase D and phospholipase A_2, the former by increased formation of DAG and the latter by phosphorylation of lipocortin and suppression of its inhibitory action on the enzyme, with increased production of arachidonic acid.

In addition to its numerous stimulatory actions, PKC sometimes acts as a negative feedback regulator of target cell responses.[253] In several cell types, activation of PKC attenuates agonist-induced elevations of cytosolic calcium concentration through two mechanisms: (1) inhibition of phosphoinositide hydrolysis and $InsP_3$ formation, leading to reduced calcium mobilization, and (2) stimulation of calcium extrusion by activation of plasma membrane calcium pumps. Such effects probably contribute to the decreased duration of the calcium signal and the attenuation of secretory responses that may occur during epxosure of target cells to high hormone concentrations. Another inhibitory effect of PKC on signal transduction can result from its actions on the receptor site itself. Thus, phorbol esters promote kinase C–dependent phosphorylation of several peptide hormone receptors, including those for EGF and insulin. In the EGF receptor, phosphorylation of a cytoplasmic threonine residue by PKC causes a decrease in tyrosine kinase activity and a decrease in receptor affinity. The long-term effects of phorbol esters include loss of receptors and, in some cases, impairment of the coupling between receptors and adenylyl cyclase, possibly through an action on the G protein. There is now abundant evidence that PKC plays a bidirectional role in cellular regulation and may participate in the termination as well as the prolongation of agonist-induced responses.

The PKC Superfamily In 1986, PKC was shown by biochemical studies[254] and molecular cloning[255] to exist in three major forms—α, β, and γ—that could be separated by ion-exchange chromatography. These isozymes of PKC exhibit generally similar enzymatic properties but differing cellular distributions. More recent studies have extended the PKC gene family of serine/threonine protein kinases to include at least nine different isoenzymes detected by cDNA cloning from various tissues and cell types. These several isoforms of PKC differ in their structure and expression in different tissues as well as in their mode of activation and substrate specificities. It is possible that each member of the PKC family has a distinct function in signal transduction and subsequent cellular responses, including metabolism, secretion, differentiation, and proliferation. The PKC enzymes are highly abundant in the brain, where multiple isoforms exist in individual neurons, and are involved in modulation of neurotransmitter release and long-term responses related to synaptic plasticity and the processes of learning and memory.[256]

The several PKC isozymes can be divided into

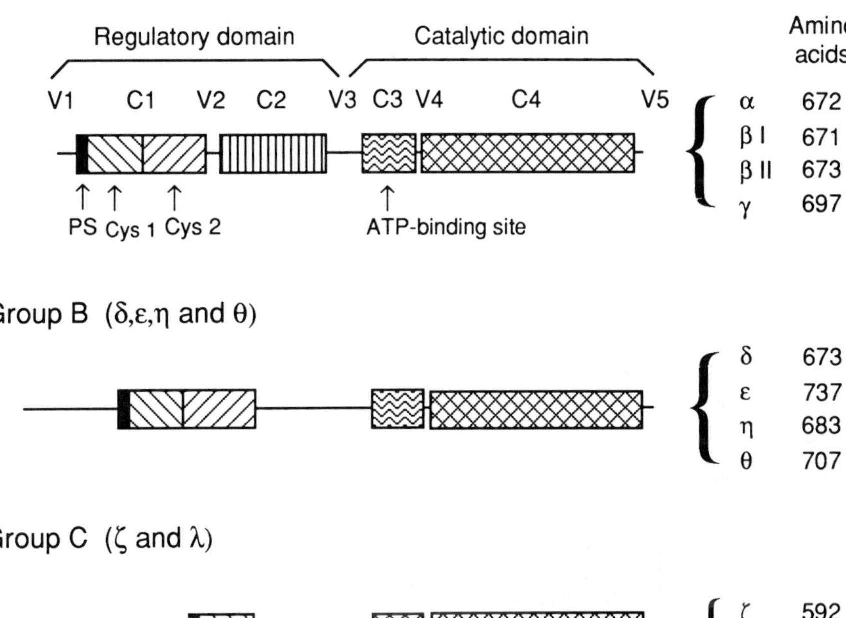

FIGURE 5A-29. Domain structures of the enzymes of the protein kinase C family. *(Courtesy of K.P. Huang.)*

two major groups: the conventional Ca^{2+}-dependent isoforms (α, βI, βII, and γ) and the novel Ca^{2+}-independent isoforms (δ, ϵ, ζ, η, and θ).[257] The genes for PKCs α, β, and γ are located on different chromosomes. All the enzymes are single polypeptide chains containing several conserved functional domains (C1–C4) separated by variable regions (V1–V4) of unknown function. The catalytic domains containing the ATP and substrate binding sites are located in the carboxy-terminal half of the molecule, and the regulatory domains containing the Ca^{2+}, phospholipid, and DAG/phorbol ester binding sites are in the amino-terminal half, separated by the V3 domain or hinge region (Fig. 5A-29). The catalytic domains of the isoenzymes are of similar structure, whereas the regulatory domains are similar among the conventional αβγ group but differ considerably between the recently defined Ca^{2+}-independent δ-θ group. The N-terminal V1 region is only about 20 amino acids in the conventional enzymes but is longer in the Ca^{2+}-independent enzymes and may influence the function of the conserved domains. The latter enzymes lack the C2 domain, which contains many acidic residues that participate in the formation of the Ca^{2+}-binding site and is present in the conventional enzymes. This domain has sequence homologies with other Ca^{2+}-binding proteins including phospholipase A_2 and phospholipase C-γ, and with the synaptic vesicle–specific protein synaptotagmin.[258]

The C1 region of all PKCs contains a modified phosphorylation sequence similar to that present in PKC substrates (-X-Arg-X-X-Ser/Thr-X-Arg-X-) in which the serine or threonine residue is replaced by alanine. This acts as a pseudosubstrate site that cannot be phosphorylated and appears to maintain the enzyme in an inactive state by blocking the substrate-binding sites of the catalytic domain. The C1 domain also contains an important cysteine-rich region that forms two adjacent zinc finger motifs, similar to the DNA-binding sequences of the steroid hormone receptor superfamily and other transcription factors. This region is responsible for binding DAG and phorbol esters and is stabilized by the binding of four Zn^{2+} ions that interact with one histidine nitrogen and three cysteine sulfur atoms.[259] PKC ζ, which is constitutively active and is not activated by PKC, contains only one cysteine-rich region and is presumably regulated by factors other than DAG and Ca^{2+}. The presence of zinc fingers is not necessarily associated with DNA-binding activity, and PKCs have not been found to bind to DNA. Similar motifs are present in other non-DNA-binding proteins, including DAG kinase and the Raf protein kinases.

The hinge region (V3) located between the regulatory and catalytic domains of PKCs contains protease-sensitive sites that are cleaved by trypsin or Ca^{2+}-dependent neutral proteases (calpains). Such cleavage generates a constitutively active protein kinase fragment and a phorbol ester–binding fragment. This region is important for the folding that maintains the pseudosubstrate domain in contact with the catalytic site in the inactive enzyme and for the intramolecular autophosphorylation of three regions in the regulatory and catalytic domains.[260] It may also be involved in the nuclear targeting of PKC α, which is translocated to the nucleus by phorbol ester and IGF-I. The C3 and C4 regions contain the ATP-binding site and the catalytic domain, respectively. ATP binds to the conserved sequence -X-Gly-X-Gly-X_2-Gly-X_{16}-Arg-X- that is present in the C3 region and in most of the protein phosphokinases. Within the catalytic region, about 100 amino acids C-terminal to the ATP-binding site, is the phosphate transfer region with the highly conserved DFG sequence that mediates substrate phosphorylation in protein kinases.

Lipid Activators of PKC

The major lipid activator of PKCs is DAG, acting in conjunction with phosphatidylserine as a cofactor. In ligand-stimulated cells, the Ca^{2+} mobilized from $InsP_3$-sensitive stores binds to the C2 region of conventional PKC isozymes and promotes their translocation to the plasma membrane. There, the C1 region is activated by the phosphatidylserine (PS) present in the lipid bilayer and by the DAG produced from phosphoinositide hydrolysis, and the catalytic domain phosphorylates membrane-associated proteins. In the case of the Ca^{2+}-independent PKCs, phosphatidylserine and DAG or other lipid derivatives are required for activation. Phorbol esters act by mimicking the action of DAG; they bind to the C2 region and lower the Ca^{2+} requirement for kinase activation. Typically, phorbol esters cause marked and prolonged translocation to the plasma membrane, with protracted enzyme activation, ultimately followed by protease degradation that can substantially deplete cellular levels of PKC. For this reason, treatment with phorbol esters has been employed to evaluate the proposed role of PKC in various cellular responses. This maneuver has been useful for those members of the PKC family which are sensitive to phorbol esters, but such down-regulation varies with the cell type and may not provide unambiguous results when applied to processes mediated by some of the PKC isoenzymes.[261]

Other products of phospholipid metabolism have been found to activate several members of the PKC family. These include cardiolipin, *cis*-unsaturated fatty acids, arachidonic acid and its lipoxygenase metabolite lipoxin A, and phosphatidylinositol biphosphate. The ability of several lipid derivatives to activate PKCs and their distinctive sensitivities to the various endogenous activators as well as to phorbol esters suggest that the PKC isozymes could be differentially activated by the individual messengers generated by specific hormonal stimuli. Another means for differential activation by specific stimuli is the generation of DAG from phosphatidylcholine rather than phosphoinositide hydrolysis, as occurs during the action of certain cytokines (interferon-α, IL-1, and IL-3). Thus, IFN-α causes selective activation of the β and ϵ isozymes of PKC, and the PIP_3 formed during stimulation of growth factor receptors has been found to potently and selectively activate PKC ζ.[262] Thus, it is likely that the several PKCs are differentially regulated by various stimuli at different cellular locations, where they preferentially phosphorylate their adjacent substrates.

Mechanism of Activation of PKC Activation of the conventional (α, β, γ) PKCs is dependent on the phosphatidylserine and Ca^{2+} and is stimulated by DAG and phorbol esters. Under physiologic conditions, the PKCs bind Ca^{2+} (up to eight atoms per molecule) during ligand-induced elevations of $[Ca^{2+}]_i$ and then interact with PS to form an active PKC•Ca^{2+}•PS complex. The enzyme becomes fully activated only in the presence of Ca^{2+}, PS, and DAG or phorbol esters; each PKC molecule requires four molecules of PS, one of DAG or phorbol ester, and at least one of Ca^{2+}. The binding of additional Ca^{2+} molecules may promote the association of conventional PKCs with the plasma membrane.

PS is the most effective of the acidic phospholipids in interacting with PKC and supporting DAG binding and enzyme activation. Its interaction with PKC is highly cooperative, and binding of multiple PS molecules is required for maximum enzymatic activity. Each PKC molecule probably makes three or more contacts with carboxy, amino, and phosphate groups of PS in a stereospecific manner. The alignment of carboxyl groups of PKC and the acidic phospholipid may generate Ca^{2+}-binding sites at which the chelated Ca^{2+} molecules serve as a bridge to stabilize the PS•PKC complex.[263] Activation of PKC by DAG is also stereospecific and requires three points of contact with its hydroxy and two ester regions. Active DGs contain saturated fatty acids at the 1 position and unsaturated fatty acids at the 2 position of sufficient hydrophobicity to permit insertion into the lipid bilayer of the plasma membrane. As was noted above, the combined presence of PS and DAG lowers the Ca^{2+} requirement for PKC activation to the micromolar range. Although an increase in Ca^{2+} is not required for activation by phorbol esters, its presence reduces the concentrations of those esters required for maximum enzyme activation. The various tumor promoters that can activate PKC are structurally diverse but appear to contain at least three hydrophilic regions that interact stereospecifically with PKC, as well as hydrophobic regions that are inserted into the plasma membrane.

PKC, like most other protein kinases, is rapidly and extensively autophosphorylated during activation by its allosteric regulator, DAG. This occurs at serine and threonine residues in the regulatory and catalytic domains and is a concomitant of activation rather than a requirement for enzymatic activity. The phosphorylated sites are located in variable rather than conserved regions of the enzyme; this is consistent with the lack of involvement of autophosphorylation in PKC activity. Although autophosphorylation does not appear to have an important function in the activation of PKC, the presence of a basal degree of phosphorylation of PKC seems to be necessary for its activation by DAG and other regulators.[264]

Hormone Action and Phospholipid Metabolism

Plasma membrane phospholipids, in particular the inositol phospholipids known as phosphoinositides, participate in several major aspects of the signal transduction pathway for hormones and other ligands that regulate cellular function. These agents promote the receptor-mediated activation of several enzymes that hydrolyze the phospholipid constituents of the plasma membrane to produce a variety of intracellular signaling molecules with diverse actions on cell metabolism, secretion, transmission, and growth. There are three major mechanisms by which phospholipids are metabolized during hormone-induced activation of phospholipase activity:

1. As a source of arachidonic acid, the precursor of several eicosanoids (prostaglandins, leukotrienes) that exert secondary effects on several target tissues.
2. As sources of diacylglycerol and inositol phosphates, as occurs during the hydrolysis of phosphoinositides by phospholipase C.
3. As sources of phosphatidic acid, which is produced by the action of phospholipase D on phosphatidylcholine. Phosphatidic acid is in turn metabolized to lysophosphatidic acid or is converted to DAG by phosphatidic acid phosphohydrolase.

Naturally occurring phospholipids are derivatives of glycerol phosphate or sphingosine phosphate, containing two fatty acids and a hydrophilic substituent such as choline, ethanolamine, inositol, or serine. They are major constituents of lipoproteins and cell membranes and are abundant in nerve tissue and brain. The phosphoglycerides have the general structure shown in Fig. 5A-30, formed by esterification of glycerol phosphate with two long-chain fatty acids and a hydrophilic component. An important feature of phospholipids is their ability to interact with both hydrophobic and hydrophilic domains and to occupy the interface between organic and aqueous environments. Thus, in lipoproteins they serve as the bond between the protein fraction and the transported neutral lipid, and in the cell membrane they form the characteristic lipid bilayer that defines the intracellular space.

FIGURE 5A-30. Structures of the major plasma membrane phospholipids. R_1 and R_2, Fatty acids; R_3, choline, ethanolamine, inositol, serine.

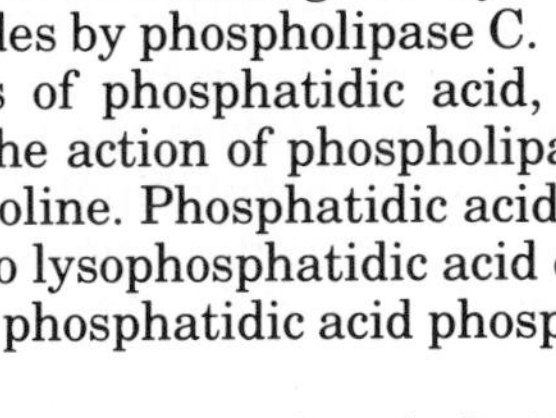

```
                  O
                  ‖
          CH2-O-C-R1
   O       |
   ‖       |
R2-C-O-CH
           |      O
           |      ‖
          CH2-O-P-O-R3
                  |
                  O
```

In the plasma membrane, about 60 percent of the phospholipid is phosphatidylcholine; lesser quantities of phosphatidylinositol and phosphatidylserine are present, and the fatty acid constituents vary in length and degree of saturation in various tissues. Phosphatidylcholines, or *lecithins*, are synthesized by three pathways in animal tissues. In the major pathway, choline is phosphorylated by ATP to form phosphocholine. This combines with cytidine triphosphate (CTP) to form cytidine diphosphate (CDP) choline, which reacts with DAG in the presence of phosphocholine transferase to yield phosphatidylcholine. Other pathways of phosphatidylcholine synthesis are the acylation of lysophosphatidylcholine (formed by hydrolysis of lecithin by phospholipase A_2) and the sequential methylation of phosphatidylethanolamine molecules within the cell membrane. Phosphoinositides are synthesized by sequential phosphorylation of phosphatidylinositol to form phosphatidylinositol 4-phosphate and phosphatidylinositol 4,5-biphosphate. The latter compound constitutes only a small fraction of the total inositol phospholipids but is of major importance in the activation of cells by calcium-mobilizing hormones.

Stimulation of Release and Metabolism of Arachidonic Acid

Many peptide hormones stimulate the production of arachidonic acid and its oxygenated metabolites by their target tissues, often with secondary effects on vascular and cellular responses during hormone action. Although PGs rarely act as mediators of peptide hormone action, stimulation of these locally formed tissue hormones during target cell activation is an important component of the cellular response to peptide hormone–receptor interaction. Prostaglandins and the related prostacyclins and thromboxanes are rapidly synthesized from polyunsaturated fatty acid precursors, in particular arachidonic acid, during target cell stimulation. The unsaturated fatty acids in cells are present as phosphoglyceride, which must be deacylated by phospholipases to provide the substrate for metabolism to PGs and other active intermediates. Arachidonic acid is the most abundant unsaturated fatty acid in tissue phospholipids and undergoes metabolism to several active products (eicosanoids) by two major routes: the *cyclooxygenase* and *lipoxygenase* pathways. The immediate products of the cyclooxygenase pathway are endoperoxides (PGG_2 and PGH_2), which are converted to prostaglandins ($PGE_2\alpha$, PGF_2Q, and PGD_2) by enzymes termed "prostaglandin synthetase" as well as

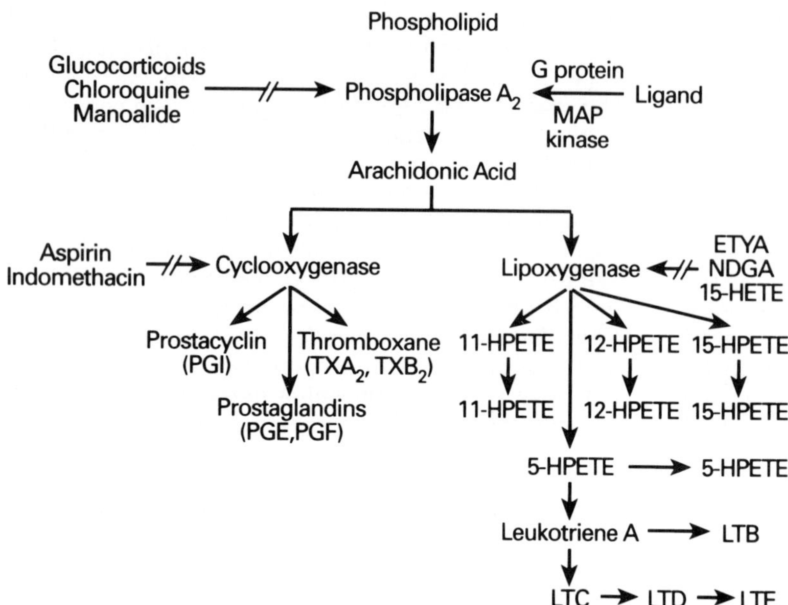

FIGURE 5A-31. Pathways of formation and metabolism of arachidonic acid. The unsaturated fatty acid is released from membrane phospholipids by activated phospholipase A_2 and also by the sequential actions of phospholipase C and diacylglyceride lipase. Arachidonic acid is converted to active derivatives by the enzymes of the lipoxygenase, cyclooxygenase, and prostaglandin synthase pathways. The sites of action of several inhibitors of arachidonate metabolism are indicated.

to thromboxanes (TXA_2 and TXB_2) and prostacyclins (PGI_2) by corresponding synthetases (Fig. 5A-31). The classification of these endoperoxidase metabolites depends on the degree of unsaturation of their precursor fatty acids: Eicosatetraenoic acid is converted to class I products (PGE, PGF, TXA, etc.), and arachidonic acid to class 2 products, including PGE_2, PGF_2Q, TXA_2, TXB_2, and PGI_2.

The thromboxanes and prostacyclins, which are also formed by further metabolism of the endoperoxides produced by the cyclooxygenase pathway, serve as important regulators of platelet and vessel wall interactions. PGI_2 is produced in large amounts by vascular endothelium and smooth muscle cells, where its formation is modulated by hydroperoxide metabolites of the lipooxygenase pathway. PGI_2 is a highly potent inhibitor of platelet aggregation, and its production in endothelial cells is stimulated by thrombin and inhibited by LDLs. There is also evidence that a decreased capacity of vascular smooth muscle cells to produce PGI_2 may contribute to the development of atherosclerosis. The lipoxygenase pathway converts arachidonic acid to hydroxy fatty acids, including hydroperoxyeicosatetraenoic acids (HPETEs), which are then metabolized to hydroxyeicosatetraenoic acids (HETEs). The HETEs and their leukotriene metabolites are important mediators of inflammatory responses, including neutrophil chemotaxis and other consequences of platelet cyclooxygenase and PGI_2 production in vascular tissue. The lipoxygenase metabolites of arachidonic acid participate in the secretory responses to GnRH and several other ligands and peptide hormones. A pathway leading to the formation of epoxide derivatives of arachidonic acid has also been implicated in ligand-stimulated secretion in several tissues.

Each of these pathways for the production of active eicosanoid metabolites depends on an adequate supply of arachidonic acid from the hydrolysis of membrane phospholipids. Many forms of receptor-mediated cell activation involve membrane-bound phospholipases which catalyze the hydrolysis of ester linkages in glycerophospholipids. Phospholipase A_2, which cleaves fatty acids at position 2 of diacylglycerophospholipids to yield the lysophospholipid and an unsaturated fatty acid, commonly arachidonic acid, is particularly important in this regard. The deacylated phospholipid is rapidly reacylated by the transfer of a coenzyme A–activated fatty acid. Arachidonic acid is also produced by the action of diglyceride lipase on the diacylglycerol released during hydrolysis of phosphoinositides by phospholipase C. This source of the fatty acid may be especially important in hormone-regulated secretory cells such as those responsible for the production of gonadotropins and prolactin. Ligand-stimulated turnover of membrane phospholipids provides arachidonic acid for metabolism by the cyclooxygenase and lipooxygenase pathways (Fig. 5A-28) and may influence membrane permeability and the activities of other membrane-bound enzymes.

Phospholipase A_2

The phospholipase A_2 (PLA_2) group of enzymes release arachidonic acid that is esterified in the *sn*-2 position of membrane phospholipids and serves as the precursor of several eicosanoid mediators. The formation of arachidonic acid is the rate-limiting step in the synthesis of prostaglandins, leukotrienes, lipoxins, and platelet-activating factor. The PLA_2 enzymes exist in numerous forms that are divided into two main groups: the extracellular small forms of 14 to 18 kDa (secretory or nonpancreatic) termed $sPLA_2$ and the cellular forms with a molecular mass of 30 to 110 kDa termed $cPLA_2$.[265] The $sPLA_2$ enzymes are present in pancreatic juice and the venom of snakes and bees as well as in synovial fluid and inflammatory exudates. They are rigid molecules containing several disulfide bonds and are activated by calcium in the millimolar range. The $sPLA_2$ enzymes are present in low concentrations in their cells of origin and can be induced by cytokines and suppressed by glucocorticoids. Mammalian $sPLA_2$ genes contain four exons and possess cyclic cAMP and cytokine response elements in their 5′ promoter regions.

The large intracellular $cPLA_2$ enzymes contain several potential sites for phosphorylation by serine/threonine and tyrosine kinases and are activated by micromolar concentrations of calcium. They contain Ca^{2+}/lipid-binding domains similar to those present in PKC and PLC-γ and undergo translocation from the cytoplasm to the plasma membrane in stimulated cells. The small $cPLA_2$ enzymes are regulated by G proteins, and appear to be activated by βγ rather than α subunits. They are also activated by serine phosphorylation by PKC and by tyrosine phosphorylation. The latter form of regulation is exerted by growth factors and platelet-activating factor (PAF) and during the responses of several cell types to inflammatory stimuli. The production of eicosanoids is prevented by inhibition of protein synthesis, possibly resulting from suppression of a PLA_2 activator protein that is rapidly synthesized in stimulated cells.[266] The inhibitory effect of glucocorticoids on inflammatory responses is partly attributable to its suppression of cyclooxygenase gene expression[267] and also to its stimulation of lipocortin production. Lipocortins belong to the annexin family of Ca^{2+}/phospholipase-binding proteins and probably inhibit the action of PLA_2 by reducing its access to the lipid substrate. While the role of the $sPLA_2$ enzymes in inflammatory disorders has not been clarified, the cellular PLA_2 forms are clearly important in signal transduction and other physiologic processes, including several forms of hormone action mediated by growth factor and G protein–coupled receptors.

Stimulation of Phosphoinositide Turnover

Inositol phospholipids make up a minor but important proportion of the plasma membrane phospholipids in eukaryotic cells. The major inositol lipid in most cells is phosphatidyl inositol, in which myoinositol phosphate is attached by a diester linkage to the DAG moiety. Much smaller amounts of the polyphosphoinositides [PtdIns(4)P and PtdIns(4,5)P_2] bearing one or two phosphates on the inositol hydroxyl groups are present in the plasma membrane. The inositol phospholipids are interconverted by ATP-dependent kinases and phosphomonoesterases and are cleaved by phosphodiesterases to inositol phosphates and DAG. The cyclical pathways involved in the breakdown and resynthesis of polyphosphoinositides in agonist-stimulated cells are shown in Fig. 5A-32.

The metabolism of inositol phospholipids has been known for many years to be enhanced during agonist stimulation of certain secretory cells, with increased incorporation of radioactive phosphate into PtdIns and its precursor, phosphatidic acid.[268] This so-called PI response, which is a reflection of phosphoinositide breakdown and resynthesis, is a general feature of cell activation by calcium-mobilizing receptors.[269] Its frequent association with receptor-mediated increases in the cytoplasmic calcium concentration led to the recognition that increased PtdIns turnover is part of the mechanism by which receptor activation increases the intracellular calcium concentration. Thus, the PI response is not simply a general response of cells to activation of their surface receptors but a specific feature of hormones that mobilize calcium as a primary component of the target cell response.[270] Conversely, hormones that cause receptor-mediated increaes in the intracellular cyclic AMP concentration usually have little or no effect on phosphoinositide metabolism.

The link between phosphoinositide turnover and increased cytoplasmic calcium during activation of receptors is inositol 1,4,5-trisphosphate [Ins(1,4,5)P_3], which is formed during the hydrolysis of phosphatidylinositol 4,5-bisphosphate (PIP_2) by phospholipase C.[271] The cellular site of receptor-mediated phosphoinositide hydrolysis is the plasma membrane, where Ins(1,4,5)P_3 is released and causes rapid mobilization of stored calcium into the cytoplasm (Fig. 5A-33). Hormone-stimulated production of Ins(1,4,5)P_3 leads directly or indirectly to the opening of cell-surface calcium channels as well as promoting the release of calcium from intracellular stores.[272] The highly charged polyphosphoinositides undergo extremely rapid metabolic turnover and are broken down within a few seconds during cell stimulation by calcium-mobilizing ligands. The hydrolysis of PIP_2 to Ins(1,4,5)P_3 and DAG constitutes a major signal transduction system for controlling diverse cellular responses, since the mobilization of calcium by Ins(1,4,5)P_3 is integrated with the activation of PKC by DAG. Once released into the cell, Ins(1,4,5)P_3 binds to receptor channels in the ER[273] and is rapidly degraded in a stepwise manner to inositol 1,4-bisphosphate, inositol monophosphate, and inositol. The breakdown of inositol monophosphate to inositol is inhibited by lithium, which is sometimes employed to amplify the agonist-induced accumulation of inositol phosphates during studies on hormone-dependent phosphoinositide metabolism.

Many peptide hormones and transmitters increase PIP_2 hydrolysis and act through Ins(1,4,5)P_3 to mobilize calcium from intracellular pools. In addition to its role in secretory, contractile, and neural cells, Ins(1,4,5)P_3 serves as a calcium-mobilizing signal in the visual system during photoreceptor transduction in invertebrates. The receptors that stimulate phosphoinositide hydrolysis are coupled to phospholipase C by G proteins. In most cells, the G proteins involved in phosphoinositide breakdown belong to the G_q/G_{11} group, but in some cases they are related to G_i and are sensitive to pertussis toxin. In addition to the potential synergistic actions of $InsP_3$ and DAG formed during hormone-stimulated PIP_2 hydrolysis, stimulation of PKC by DAG or phorbol esters can lead to inhibition of $InsP_3$ formation. This suggests that activation of PKC may attenuate receptor coupling to phospholipase C by phosphorylation of the receptor or the nucleotide regulatory protein.

Complexity of Inositol-Phosphate Metabolism

The receptor-stimulated hydrolysis of PtdIns(4,5)P_2 to produce two intracellular messengers, Ins(1,4,5)P_3 and DAG, has been shown to operate in numerous ligand-regulated cells. However, the phosphoinositide signal transduction system has proved to be far more complicated than was originally realized (Fig. 5A-34). This was first indicated by the observation that most of the $InsP_3$ accumulating in agonist-stimulated cells is not the Ca^{2+}-mobilizing (1,4,5) isomer but an inactive form identified as Ins(1,3,4)P_3. The origin of Ins(1,3,4)P_3 was clarified by the discovery of a metabolic pathway through which Ins(1,4,5)P_3 is phosphorylated to inositol 1,3,4,5-tetrakisphosphate [Ins(1,3,4,5)P_4], which is then converted to Ins(1,3,4)P_3 by the same 5-phosphatase that dephosphorylates Ins(1,4,5)P_3. The discovery of the conversion of Ins(1,4,5)P_3 to Ins(1,3,4,5)P_4 led to the proposal that the concerted actions of these two messengers could be responsible for the full development of the cytoplasmic Ca^{2+} signal.[274] This was supported by evidence that Ins(1,3,4,5)P_4 acts in conjunction with Ins(1,4,5)P_3 to elicit Ca^{2+}-dependent responses in certain cell types. Also, Ins(1,3,4,5)P_4 binding sites distinct from those of Ins(1,4,5)P_4 have been identified, and in some cells Ins(1,3,4,5)P_4 elicits Ca^{2+} mobilization by a mechanism distinct from the $InsP_3$ receptor. However, the extent to which Ins(1,3,4,5)P_4 participates in calcium mobilization in most cells remains a moot point.

The activity of the $InsP_3$-kinase enzyme is increased by Ca^{2+}-calmodulin, a property that would accelerate the removal of Ins(1,4,5)P_3 by its conversion to Ins(1,3,4,5)P_4 during agonist-induced elevations of cytoplasmic Ca^{2+}. The enzyme has recently been purified from brain extracts, and its cDNA has been cloned. The $InsP_3$-kinase enzyme can be phosphorylated by both cAMP-dependent protein kinase and PKC, with the former increasing and the latter decreasing its activity.[275]

Mammalian cells have been found to contain several additional Ins-phosphate isomers, including the

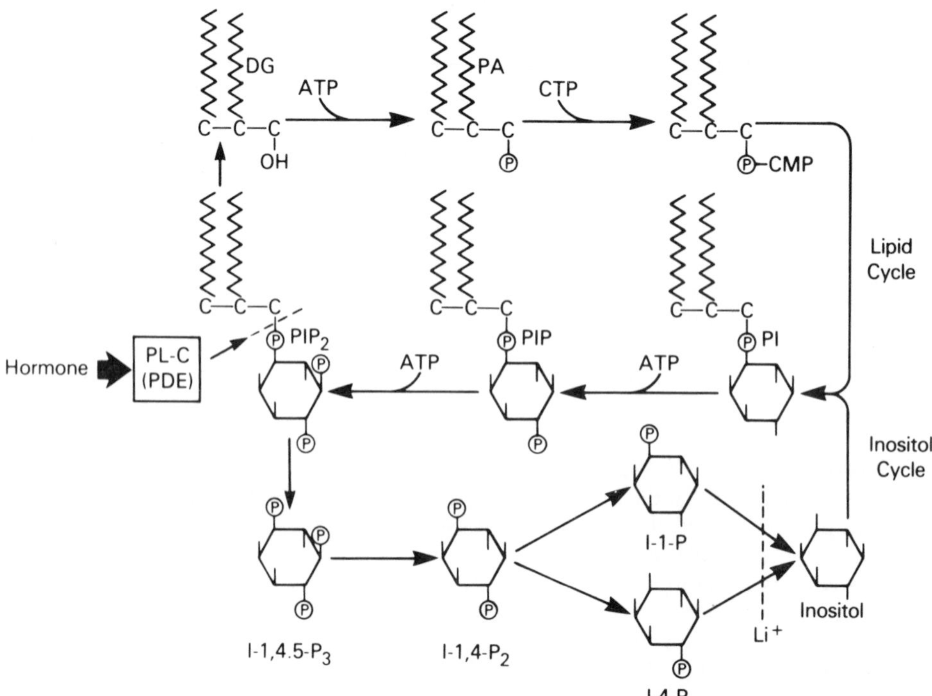

FIGURE 5A-32. Hormone-stimulated breakdown of inositol phospholipids, and the subsequent metabolism of inositol phosphates and lipids followed by resynthesis of polyphosphoinositides in the plasma membrane. The ligand-induced cleavage of PIP_2 into Ins(1,4,5)P_3 and DG by phospholipase C (a phosphodiesterase) is followed by the metabolism of these second messengers through lipid and inositol cycles to re-synthesize the plasma-membrane phosphoinositides. It is during the agonist activated lipid cycle that ^{32}P-phosphate is incorporated into the membrane phospholipids, forming the basis of the "PI effect" originally observed by Hokin and Hokin.[268] Inositol phosphate production and metabolism is studied after incorporation of [^3H]inositol into phosphoinositides to steady-state over 24–48 h. Lithium blocks the dephosphorylation of certain inositol phosphates and increases their leves, but does not cause accumulation of Ins(1,4,5)P_3.

highly phosphorylated inositols $InsP_4$, $InsP_5$, and $InsP_6$. Several $InsP_2$ and InsP isomers are produced by enzymes that remove phosphate groups from specific positions of Ins(1,4,5)P_3 and Ins(1,3,4)P_3 and their metabolites. In addition, the Ins-monophosphate ultimately produced after the degradation of Ins(1,4,5)P_3 to Ins(1,4)P_2 is Ins(4)P rather than Ins(1)P. The Ins(4)P metabolite thus reflects the rate of polyphosphoinositide hydrolysis, whereas Ins(1)P is derived primarily from the breakdown of phosphatidylinositol. Li^+ ions inhibit the Ins-monophosphate and several other phosphatases, most notably the Ins-polyphosphate-1-phosphatase that converts Ins(1,4)P_2 to Ins(4)P as well as converting Ins(1,3,4)P_3 to Ins(3,4)P_2.[276] In general, the use of Li^+ ions to enhance the accumulation of Ins-phosphates is not recommended in studies of inositol phosphate metabolism, since it causes major distortions in their relative proportions in agonist-stimulated cells.

There has been relatively slow progress in defining the origins of the highly phosphorylated inositols; a summary of the current views about their formation and actions is shown in Fig. 5A-34. It is clear that the phosphorylation product of Ins(1,4,5)P_3, Ins(1,3,4,5)P_4, is not further phosphorylated to $InsP_5$ and $InsP_6$. However, at least two additional $InsP_4$ isomers have been detected in mammalian cells and avian erythrocytes and are increased in agonist-stimulated adrenal cells. One of these isomers, Ins(1,3,4,6)P_4, is produced by the phosphorylation of Ins(1,3,4)P_3 by a distinctive 6-kinase and serves as a distant precursor of $InsP_5$. The structure of a third $InsP_4$ isomer, which is increased during agonist stimulation, is Ins(3,4,5,6)P_4. This $InsP_4$ isomer is converted to $InsP_5$ by a specific 1-kinase. Ins(3,4,5,6)P_4 may be a breakdown product of $InsP_5$, but the complete pathways of its formation have not been clarified. Although the levels of these compounds change only moderately during acute stimulation, they are increased substantially after prolonged exposure to agonists and during the maturation of *Xenopus* oocytes, suggesting that they may be involved in the regulation of long-term cellular responses. In this regard, it is interesting that the level of Ins(3,4,5,6)P_4 is greatly increased in fibroblasts transformed with the *v-src* oncogene. Some of the more highly phosphorylated inositols ($InsP_5$ and $InsP_6$) have been proposed to serve as extracellular signals that evoke complex neuronal responses in the CNS, but otherwise there is little evidence for specific roles of the higher inositol phosphates in cellular regulation.[277]

FIGURE 5A-33. Comparison of the mechanisms by which receptors for hormones and neurotransmitters (G protein–coupled receptors) and growth factor (tyrosine kinase) receptors activate phospholipase C and stimulate the phosphoinositide-calcium signal transduction pathways. Ligands that bind the receptors of the seven membrane-spanning or rhodopsin type promote coupling through a G protein to phospholipase C, probably the β isoform of the enzyme. In contrast, growth factors that bind to tyrosine kinase—containing receptors (EGF, PDGF, FGF, and CSF-I) promote the association of the activated intracellular receptor domain with several cytoplasmic proteins, including phospholipase C-γ as well as PI-3-kinase, the GTP-activating protein of *ras* (GAP) and Grb2. These dissimilar types of stimuli cause hydrolysis of PIP_2 and generation of Ins(1,4,5)P_3 and DAG, with mobilization of intracellular calcium and influx of extracellular calcium.

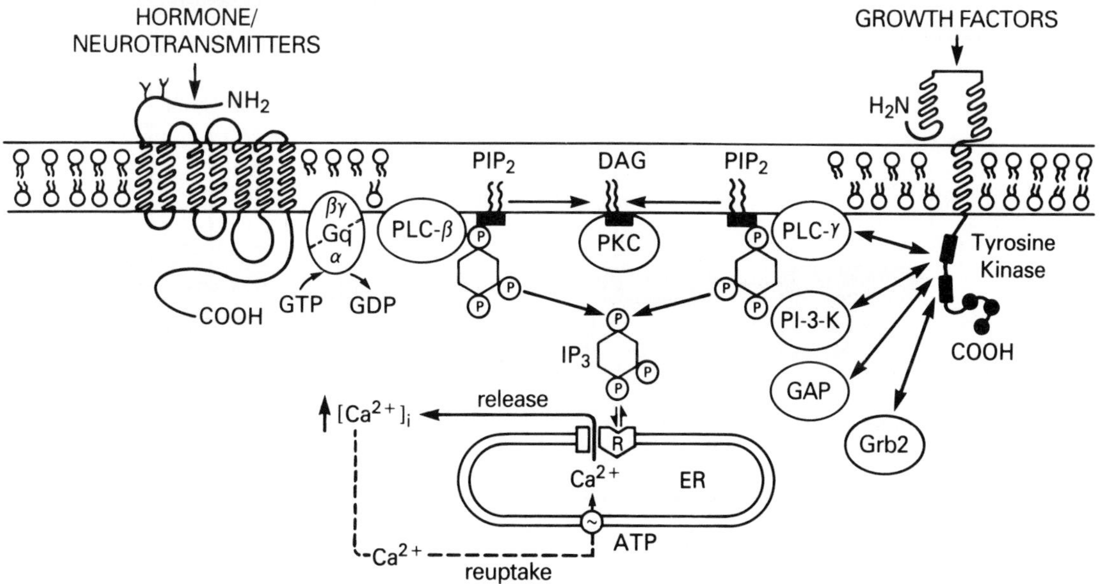

Phosphoinositide-Specific Phospholipase C

The breakdown of plasma membrane phospholipids during receptor activation is catalyzed by phospholipase C (also termed phosphoinositidase C), a family of membrane-bound and cytoplasmic enzymes that hydrolyze phosphoinositides on the inner aspect of the plasma membrane. This reaction leads to the production of DAG and several inositol phosphates, including Ins(1)P, Ins(1,4)P_2, and Ins(1,4,5)P_3. The major substrate for phospholipase C during agonist-stimulated phospholipid hydrolysis is PtdIns(4,5)P_2, which is cleaved to form DAG and Ins(1,4,5)P_3, as shown in Fig. 5A-34. Multiple forms of the enzyme have been characterized in various tissues and can hydrolyze all three plasma membrane phosphoinositides. Three phospholipase C isoenzymes of molecular mass 85, 145, and 150 kDa have been isolated from bovine brain and are structurally and immunologically distinct from the enzymes present in liver, seminal vesicle, and uterus.[278]

The phospholipase C enzymes have been designated by Greek letters for their primary structures and by numerals to indicate products of alternative splicing or proteolysis. The major phospholipases identified by cDNA cloning are distinct polypeptides of molecular mass 57 (PLC-α), 138 (PLC-β), 148 (PLE-γ), and 86 kDa (PLC-δ). The four enzymes show little overall amino acid sequence homology, consistent with their lack of immunologic cross-reactivity, but the β, γ, and δ enzymes contain two domains of 150 and 120 amino acids (termed X and Y) with 54 and 42 percent identity, respectively (Fig. 5A-35). These conserved domains may be involved in the catalytic site of the enzyme or in its interactions with the receptors and/or regulatory proteins that control enzyme activation. The largest enzyme, phospholipase C-γ, has a relatively long variable region which contains sequences homologous to the noncatalytic domain of *src* and other nonreceptor tyrosine kinases. Phospholipase C-γ becomes physically associated with activated growth factor receptors and is tyrosine-phosphorylated during stimulation of phospholipid hydrolysis by growth factors, including EGF, PDGF, and FGF.[279]

Mechanism of Ins(1,4,5)P_3-Induced Ca^{2+} Release

The mechanism by which Ins(1,4,5)P_3 acts as the link between cell-surface receptor activation and intracellular Ca^{2+} mobilization involves binding to specific $InsP_3$ receptor channels in the endoplasmic reticulum. These receptors were detected by studies with radiolabeled Ins(1,4,5)P_3 as specific high-affinity binding sites in subcellular membrane fractions and permeabilized cells. The relative binding affini-

FIGURE 5A-34. Pathways of formation of inositol phosphates and diacylglycerol (DAG) in response to agonist-induced activation of phospholipase C (PLC) by hormones (H) and other ligands. The metabolic pathways linking Ins(1,4,5)P_3 to its dephosphorylated and phosphorylated metabolites, the formation of higher inositol phosphates, and the regeneration of phospholipid precursors in the endoplasmic reticulum (ER) are shown. The major signaling molecules are shown in black.

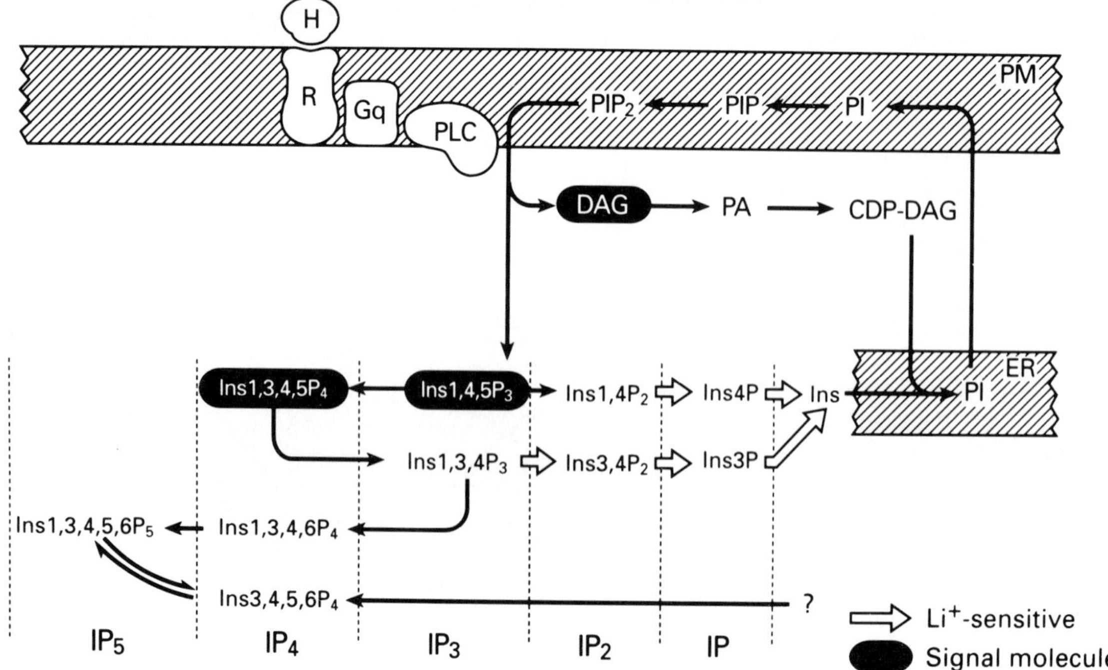

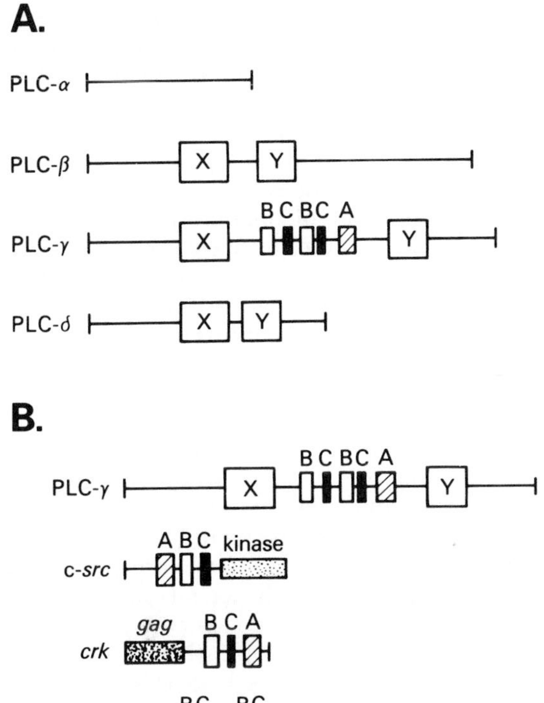

FIGURE 5A-35. (*A*) Linear structures of the major phospholipase C isozymes. The open boxes (X and Y) indicate common sequences of ~20 and ~150 amino acids, respectively, that occur in phospholipases β, γ, and δ. (*B*) Structural similarities between PLC-γ and *c-src, crk,* and GAP. Boxes A, B, and C indicate similar sequences of ~50, ~40, and ~15 amino acids, respectively. (*Modified from Rhee and Choi.*[278])

ties of various inositol phosphates for the Ins(1,4,5)P_3 receptor are in good agreement with their Ca^{2+}-releasing activities. However, the K_d of the binding sites for Ins(1,4,5)P_3 (1 to 30 n*M*) is significantly lower than the ED_{50} for Ca^{2+} release (50 n*M* to 1 μ*M*). This discrepancy between binding and activation constants could reflect the need for the binding of more than one $InsP_3$ molecule to evoke Ca^{2+} release. GTP is also able to release Ca^{2+} from intracellular pools under certain conditions, suggesting that G proteins mediate communication and Ca^{2+} transfer between different vesicular compartments within the cell.[280] The physiologic significance of these observations is not known, but such communication may occur during agonist-stimulated influx of intracellular Ca^{2+} by a recently proposed vesicular uptake mechanism that depends on receptor-mediated endocytosis.

Calcium Oscillation in Agonist-Stimulated Cells

The elevations in cytoplasmic Ca^{2+} concentration that result from activation of Ca^{2+}-mobilizing receptors in many cell types are often evident as a series of oscillations when analyzed in single cells. For this reason, the early peak and subsequent plateau that are commonly observed when cytoplasmic Ca^{2+} levels are measured in cell suspensions usually represent an averaged profile of the more complex changes that occur at the single cell level. Such oscillations are dependent on the release and reuptake of calcium by intracellular stores and are triggered by the action of Ins(1,4,5)P_3 on its receptor channels in the endoplasmic reticulum. In some cells, entry of Ca^{2+} through the plasma membrane is also involved in the generation of Ca^{2+} oscillations. In general, the frequency of Ca^{2+} oscillations is related to the agonist concentration, whereas their amplitude is not. Such frequency modulation, with an increasing rate of oscillation with increasing receptor activation, is now known to be a common mode of Ca^{2+} signaling in endocrine and other cell types.

The Inositol (1,4,5)-Trisphosphate Receptor

Ins(1,4,5)P_3 receptors are present in particulate fractions of many tissues (adrenal, liver, salivary gland, brain, and platelets) and are highly specific for Ins(1,4,5)P_3 and related calcium-mobilizing compounds such as Ins(2,4,5)P_3. The receptors are associated with calcium-mobilizing activity in vesicular structures that are enriched in the plasma membrane fraction in several tissues. Ins(1,4,5)P_3 has been proposed to act on a specific calsequestrin-containing organelle, the calciosome, but the current view is that Ins(1,4,5)P_3 mobilizes calcium from specialized regions of the ER. An action of Ins(1,4,5)P_3 at the plasma membrane level has also been suggested, based on immunolocalization studies and its ability to stimulate inward calcium currents in lymphocytes.[281] The $InsP_3$ receptor is abundant in the brain, particularly the cerebellum, and is highly concentrated in Purkinje cells. The receptor isolated from the cerebellum is a 260-kDa glycoprotein that is inhibited by heparin and can be phosphorylated by cAMP-dependent protein kinase; its binding affinity for Ins(1,4,5)P_3 is increased at alkaline pH and reduced by Ca^{2+}. The receptor is a tetramer of identical subunits, and is located on vesicles associated with the ER. The purified Ins(1,4,5)P_3 receptor protein from brain membranes can be reconstituted into lipid vesicles and mediates calcium influx stimulated by Ins(1,4,5)P_3 and other inositol phosphates with the potencies and specificities that they exhibit in brain microsomes. These findings demonstrated that the brain binding protein is the physiologic intracellular receptor for Ins(1,4,5)P_3 and that a single protein mediates both ligand binding and calcium flux.[282] The tetrameric Ins(1,4,5)P_3 receptor is a ligand-operated ion channel and shares structural features with the tetrameric ryanodine receptor of skeletal muscle and with the nicotinic, GABA, and glycine receptors, in which the associated (dissimilar) subunits contain the ligand-binding site and the respective ion channel.

Molecular cloning revealed the Ins(1,4,5)P_3 receptor to be identical with a previously known 250-kDa membrane glycoprotein (termed P_{400}) that is highly concentrated in Purkinje cells and is deficient in cerebellar ataxic mice with Purkinje cell degeneration.[283] The receptor is a protein of 2749 amino acids and has a molecular mass of 131 kDa. The protein sequence contains six membrane-spanning regions so that its N- and C-terminal regions are both oriented within the cytoplasm. Two potential sites for serine phosphorylation are located within the large N-terminal cytoplasmic domain of the receptor. The mRNA for the Ins(1,4,5)P_3 receptor is highly abundant in Purkinje cells and is present at much lower levels in the cerebrum and peripheral tissues. The expression product of the cloned receptor cDNA has high affinity for Ins(1,4,5)P_3 (K_d = 22 nM) and relative binding potencies for inositol phosphates of Ins(1,4,5)P_3 > Ins(2,4,5)P_3 > Ins(1,3,4,5)P_4 > Ins(1,4)P_2.

The Ins$(1,4,5)_3$ receptor bears a striking resemblance to the ryanodine receptor, which mediates calcium release from the sarcoplasmic reticulum in skeletal and cardiac muscle. The ryanodine receptor also has a large cytoplasmic N-terminal domain and several C-terminal membrane-spanning regions which form the calcium channel that is gated by the voltage-sensing dihydropyridine receptor in the T tubule of the muscle fiber.[284] Both receptors are localized in the ER or its derivatives and form tetramers that have a square shape on electron microscopy. The 260-kDa Ins(1,4,5)P_3 receptor is highly enriched in the cerebellum, is present in most peripheral tissues, and has several isoforms arising from separate genes and their splice variants. The Ins(1,4,5)P_3 receptor shows marked amino acid sequence similarities with the transmembrane regions of the ryanodine-sensitive calcium channel, suggesting that the ion channel is also intrinsic to the Ins(1,4,5)P_3 receptor protein. The otherwise dissimilar regions of the two related calcium-release channels are presumably responsible for the specific recognition of their different activating ligands.

The general structure of the Ins(1,4,5)P_3 receptor is highly conserved in mouse, rat, human, and *Drosophila* tissues. The cloned rat receptor is a 260-kDa protein containing more than 2700 amino acids and forms tetramers similar to the native receptor. The large N-terminal cytoplasmic portion of the receptor contains about 650 conserved residues that are essential for Ins(1,4,5)P_3 binding. The carboxy-terminal 600 amino acids contain six putative transmembrane regions, the last four of which are flanked by net negative charges and show significant homology with the ryanodine receptor. The InsP_3 receptor has four independent binding sites, and each 260-kDa subunit probably binds InsP_3 at an amino-terminal cytoplasmic site that regulates the Ca^{2+} channel formed by the last four of the six carboxy-terminal transmembrane domains (Fig. 5A-36).

The Ins(1,4,5)P_3 receptor is located predominantly in the smooth ER and is also found in the rough ER and outer nuclear membrane. Receptors are also present in the plasma membrane of several cell types and are located in caveolae and possibly in endocytic vesicles. The presence of Ins(1,4,5)P_3 receptors in the plasma membrane could be relevant to the mechanism of calcium influx during sustained responses to agonist stimulation, at least in certain cell types. Several isoforms of the receptor can result from the expression of different genes and from alternative RNA splicing of portions (termed SI and SII) of the coding regions for the ligand-binding and regulatory domains. The SI segment of 45 nucleotides is in the middle of the ligand-binding domain, and the SII segment of 120 nucleotides is located between the two phosphorylation sites in the regulatory domain. It contains three splicing subsegments (A,B,C) that give rise to four possible isoforms of the receptor. The SII(ABC)$^-$ form is expressed in all tissues, and forms containing one or more subsegments are confined to the nervous system. The Ins(1,4,5)P_3 receptors have been divided into two general types: the original cerebellar (type 1) receptor and the type 2 receptor, which is of higher affinity for Ins(1,4,5)P_3. The existence of several receptor isoforms with different binding and regulatory properties could provide for a range of calcium-signaling profiles in specific tissues and cell types.[285]

Ryanodine Receptors

Ryanodine receptors are closely related to Ins(1,4,5)P_3 receptors in their structure and function and have been recognized for several years as the intracellular Ca^{2+} release channels that mediate the contraction of skeletal and cardiac muscle. They were originally defined on the basis of their ability to bind the plant alkaloid ryanodine and to regulate Ca^{2+} release from the sarcoplasmic reticulum (SR). Their function is to release Ca^{2+} from the SR in response to depolarization of skeletal muscle fibers or increased cytoplasmic Ca^{2+} in the heart. The latter process of Ca^{2+}-induced Ca^{2+} release also occurs in smooth muscle cells and in a number of other tissues. Ryanodine receptors are now known to be present in neurons and other cell types, and their localization is distinct from that of the InsP_3 receptors. There are probably at least three types of ryanodine receptors, including skeletal (RYR1), cardiac (RYR2), and a recently discovered form (RYR3) that is widely distributed in the brain and several other tissues.[284]

In skeletal muscle, the ryanodine receptor is a homotetramer of four large (565 kDa) proteins, each containing 5035 amino acids and having a short cytoplasmic C-terminal region and several (4 to 10) transmembrane domains. Most of the molecule makes up a large cytoplasmic foot region that spans the transverse tubule–sarcoplasmic reticulum junction and is closely adjacent to the voltage-sensing dihydropyridine (DHP) receptor in the T-tubule membrane. The DHP receptor is a complex structure composed of four subunits, each with four internal repeats that contain several transmembrane regions, some of which act as voltage sensors.[286] The receptor has structural features in common with calcium channels but is believed to act as a voltage sensor rather than a source of calcium influx. A third protein, triadin, has been proposed to participate in the interaction between the DHP and ryanodine receptors, but it is more likely to act as a link between the ryanodine receptor and the calcium-binding protein sequestrin in the lumen of the SR.

The activity of the ryanodine receptor is regulated by several compounds, including calcium, ryanodine, caffeine, procaine, calmodulin, and dantrolene, which influence channel opening and calcium conductance. The channels are activated by low concentrations of calcium and ryanodine and by caffeine and adenine nucleotides. High concentrations of calcium and ryanodine are inhibitory, as are calmodulin, dantrolene, and procaine. A mutation in the foot region of the ryanodine receptor is responsible for some cases of malignant hyperthermia, a rare inherited myopathy in which certain anesthetic induce muscle rigidity and hyperthermia.[287]

It has become clear that the ryanodine and $InsP_3$ receptors each constitute a large and heterogeneous group of receptors with diverse tissue distributions and regulated functions. The RYR3 receptor channel is probably as ubiquitous as the $InsP_3$ receptor and may operate in many tissues, possibly in combination with the $InsP_3$ receptor, to regulate calcium release from intracellular stores. In particular, the RYR3 channel is likely to mediate the process of calcium-induced calcium release that has been proposed to drive some of the oscillatory calcium response observed in agonist-stimulated cells. Apart from the autoregulatory action of calcium, the nature of the endogenous ligand for the ryanodine receptor channel has not been identified. However, recent evidence has suggested that cyclic ADP-ribose may serve this function in certain cell types as part of its action on calcium regulation.[288]

Growth Factors and Phosphoinositide Hydrolysis

In addition to mediating many of the rapid responses of cells to hormonal stimulation, the products of phosphoinositide hydrolysis participate in the regulation of intracellular events involved in cell growth and proliferation. Several growth factors, including PDGF and EGF, activate phospholipase C and cause changes in intracellular calcium and pH that depend on the signals ($InsP_3$ and DAG) produced by the hydrolysis of PtdIns(4,5)P.[279] In some

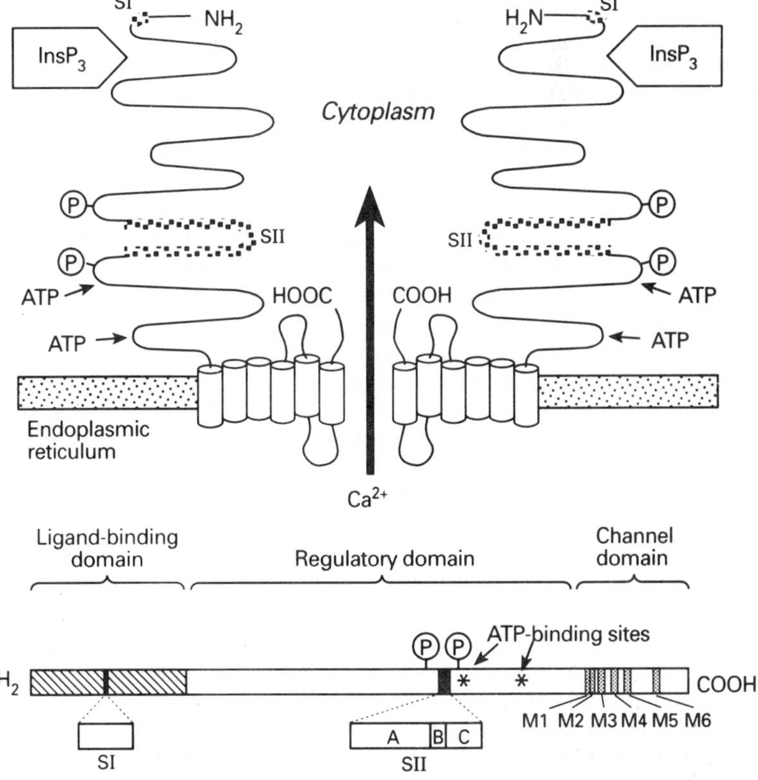

FIGURE 5A-36. Domain structure of the $Ins(1,4,5)P_3$ receptor protein (*below*) and its arrangement in the membrane of the endoplasmic reticulum (above) to form a ligand-regulated calcium channel that conveys Ca^{2+} into the cytoplasm when activated by $InsP_3$. The upper part of the Figure shows a cross-section through two of the four subunits that form the receptor channel, and illustrates the several sites at which the channel is regulated. Each subunit contains an $InsP_3$ binding site in its N-terminal region, located about 1400 amino acids away from the channel-forming transmembrane domains. Sites for ATP binding and cAMP-dependent phosphorylation are located in the large region between the ligand binding site and the transmembrane domains, and regulate the opening state of the channel. RNA splicing sites (SI and SII) are indicated by the shaded areas. (*Modified from Mikoshiba.*[285])

tissues, these effects appear to be mediated by a pertussis-sensitive G protein, but this is not a common feature of growth factor–induced inositol lipid hydrolysis. The activation of phospholipase C by hormones and growth factors occurs by two distinct mechanisms (G proteins and tyrosine phosphorylation) that stimulate the β and γ enzymes, respectively (Fig. 5A-33).

An important step in elucidating the mechanism of growth factor–induced $PtdInsP_2$ hydrolysis was the finding that EGF-stimulated phospholipase C activity could be precipitated from A431 cell extracts by antibodies to phosphotyrosine. This indicated that tyrosine phosphorylation of the enzyme, or of a tightly associated protein, is required for EGF-stimulated $PtdInsP_2$ hydrolysis. Both EGF and PDGF induce phosphorylation of phospholipase C-γ at two identical tyrosine residues. Furthermore, inhibitors of tyrosine phosphorylation block growth factor–induced phosphorylation and activation of phospholipase C-γ as well as the EGF-stimulated Ca^{2+} response. In contrast, inhibitors of tyrosine phosphorylation have no effect on the Ca^{2+} release induced by bradykinin and bombesin, which act through G proteins to activate phospholipase C-β.

The FGF receptor and the HER2/*neu* protein also phosphorylate and associate with phospholipase C-γ. However, not all growth factors act in this manner, since insulin and CSF-I do not promote the tyrosine phosphorylation of phospholipase C-γ. Activation of the T cell antigen receptor stimulates phospholipase C and tyrosine phosphorylation, and inhibitors of tyrosine kinase suppress phospholipase C activity and T cell proliferation. Tyrosine phosphorylation is an early and essential requirement for T cell activation and results from the interaction between its associated regulatory proteins (CD4 and CD8) with $p56^{lck}$, a member of the *src* family of tyrosine kinases.[289]

Several growth factors and oncogene products with tyrosine kinase activity are associated with a novel PtdIns kinase that catalyzes the synthesis of small amounts of unusual phosphoinositides in the plasma membrane. This enzyme, which is termed PtdIns 3-kinase, produces a phospholipid that is phosphorylated in the 3-position of the inositol ring to form phosphatidylinositol-3-phosphate [PtdIns(3)P] instead of the phosphatidylinositol-4-phosphate [PtdIns(4)P] previously thought to be the only form of $PtdInsP_2$. This new enzyme was identified because of its tight association with several tyrosine kinases, including the middle T/$pp60^{c\text{-}src}$ complex from 3T3 cells transformed with polyoma virus. The middle T antigen of this DNA tumor virus associates with and activates tyrosine kinases of the *src* family, which in turn phosphorylate an 85-kDa protein that corresponds to PtdIns 3-kinase. The PtdIns(3)-kinase activity in 3T3 cells also associates with the ligand-activated PDGF receptor and is immunoprecipitated from extracts of PDGF-stimulated cells by antiphosphotyrosine. The enzyme has been shown to be regulated by receptor activation in several cell types, including fibroblasts, neutrophils, vascular smooth muscle, astrocytes, and platelets, where it is activated by thrombin to produce PtdIns(3)P and PtdIns(3,4)P_2. Cells stimulated with PDGF, EGF, CSF-I, and insulin also show increased levels of PtdIns(3,4)P_3 and sometime PtdIns(3,4,5)P_3. These new inositol lipids are not hydrolyzed to produce inositol phosphates but appear to serve as second messengers or cofactors for other membrane-bound enzymes. The association of the PtdIns(3)-kinase with several receptor-associated tyrosine kinases clearly reflects its potential role in the actions of certain growth factors and oncogenes.[290]

The mechanism of action of insulin also involves several facets of phospholipid production and metabolism, but these do not include the established form of agonist-induced phosphoinositide hydrolysis. Inositol glycans are released from membrane glycophospholipids during insulin action and mimic several of the metabolic effects of insulin when added to intact or broken cells. Such cleavage of plasma membrane glycolipids has been attributed to a specific form of phospholipase C that catalyzes the production of inositol glycans and diacylglycerol during insulin action and may be activated by a G protein that is in turn phosphorylated by the tyrosine-specific kinase of the insulin receptor. DAG levels are increased in insulin-stimulated cells and appear to regulate, through the activation of PKC, the expression of several insulin-sensitive genes. Such insulin-induced increases in DAG production may arise from both increased de novo synthesis of membrane glycerolipids and the cleavage by phospholipase C of the phosphatidylinositol glycan described above. The insulin receptor is also associated with phosphatidylinositol kinase activity and could thus regulate the biosynthesis of phospholipids involved in the transduction of mitogenic signals.

Stimulation of Phospholipid Methylation

The synthesis of phosphatidylcholine from phosphatidylethanolamine in cell membranes occurs in two sequential methylation steps by transfer of methyl groups from *S*-adenosylmethionine under the control of two enzymes, *phosphomethyltransferase* 1 and 2. The first enzyme transfers one methyl group to form phosphatidylmonomethylethanolamine; both the substrate, phosphatidylethanolamine, and the first methyltransferase enzyme are located on the cytoplasmic side of the plasma membrane. The second enzyme transfers two more methyl groups, again derived from *S*-adenosylmethionine, to form phosphatidylcholine. Both the phosphatidylcholine produced and the second methyltransferase are located on the exterior surface of the membrane. The topographic distribution of the enzymes and reactants facilitate the rapid transfer of phospholipids across the plasma membrane by successive methylations.[291] The intramembrane synthesis of the intermediate product, phosphatidylmonomethylethanolamine, causes local changes in membrane fluidity and permits increased lateral mobility of intrinsic membrane proteins. β-Adrenergic stimulation of phospholipid methylation and decreased membrane viscosity in reticulocytes are accompanied by unmasking of cryptic β-adrenergic receptors, with increased lateral movement of the receptors and enhanced coupling between receptors and adenylyl cyclase. Several hormone receptors, including those for prolactin and LH, are increased in number by methylation of membrane phospholipids. Other membrane events influenced by the synthesis and translocation of methylated phospholipid include calcium-dependent ATPase, leukocyte chemotaxis, mast cell histamine secretion, and lymphocyte mitogenesis.

These ligand-induced changes in phospholipid methylation and membrane fluidity probably reflect a general phenomenon that influences membrane structure and function during many forms of cellular regulation by hormones and other ligands. They may also explain the short-lived increase in receptors for the homologous hormone and other hormones which is observed after target cell stimulation. Thus, LH causes a transient increase in both LH and prolactin receptors in the rat testis, and ACTH causes an initial rise in adrenal prolactin sites. In each case, these elevations in receptor number precede the well-recognized process of receptor loss (down-regulation) that begins several hours after occupancy in vivo. In the Leydig cell, activation of LH receptors is rapidly followed by a cAMP-dependent increase in phospholipid methyltransferase activity which may be related to changes in receptor exposure and other membrane-associated events in gonadotropin action.[292] The extent to which increased membrane fluidity controls receptor-cyclase coupling in endocrine target cells is not known, but this mechanism may be an important component in the regulation of cellular sensitivity and responsiveness to hormonal stimulation.

SIGNAL TRANSDUCTION TO THE NUCLEUS

As described earlier, tyrosine phosphorylation of plasma-membrane receptors or their associated proteins is the primary event in signal transduction by extracellular stimuli that regulate cell growth, differentiation, and proliferation. Many of these responses are mediated by a small group of tyrosine-phosphorylated protein kinases [known as mitogen-activated (MAP) or extracellular signal regulated (ERK) kinases]. These 42- to 45-kDa enzymes are activated by tyrosine and threonine phosphorylation, and phosphorylate serine and threonine residues in a variety of cytoplasmic and nuclear proteins.[293] Their activities are increased during cell stimulation by growth factors and mitogens, and during germinal vesicle breakdown in oocytes. In quiescent cells, activation of MAP kinase occurs during re-entry into the cell cycle. Tumor-promoting phorbol esters also stimulate the phosphorylation and activation of MAP kinase, consistent with their stimulatory actions on growth responses.[294]

The MAP kinases, which are activated within minutes by growth factors and mitogens, are located in the cytoplasm and nucleus and are central intermediates in the growth response pathways utilized by mitogenic stimuli. Their activation is mediated by a sequence of protein kinases that lead to phosphorylation of both tyrosine and threonine residues in their catalytic domain. In this process, ras proteins provide the link between the cell-surface receptor tyrosine kinases that mediate the actions of growth factors and a casade of serine-threonine protein kinases that extend the signal pathway into the nucleus.[295] Once activated, MAP kinases cause phosphorylation of several proteins in the cytoplasm, cytoskeleton, and plasma membrane, as well as transcriptional regulatory proteins in the nucleus.

The activity of MAP kinase is regulated by a series of protein kinases that are activated by ras• GTP. The first of these is raf-1, a protein kinase that phosphorylates and activates a threonine kinase termed mek (MAP kinase kinase). This takes place within a complex formed between raf-1, mek, and activated ras. In this manner, the formation of ras • GTP by the action of a receptor tyrosine kinase that is linked to Grb2 • 505 triggers a chain of protein kinases that relay growth signals to all regions of the cell.[130] An outline of this signal transduction pathway is shown in Fig. 5A-37. In this sequence, raf-1 acts as a MAP kinase kinase kinase to activate mek, which in turn phosphorylates threonine and tyrosine residues in the active domain of MAP kinase. Activation of PKC by hormones and phorbol esters also leads to phosphorylation of raf-1, which thus integrates signals from the tyrosine phosphorylation and Ca^{2+}/phosphoinositide pathways that regulate MAP kinase activity.

Map kinase is a proline-directed protein kinase with a phosphorylation site sequence of XY (Ser/Thr)Pro, where X is often Pro. It is located in the cytoplasm and nucleus and phosphorylates substrates in both cellular compartments.[296] MAP kinase is translocated into the nucleus during mitogenic stimulation and thus acts as a physical transducer in the signaling pathway from the cell membrane to the nucleus. The signaling molecules that are phosphorylated and activated by MAP kinase are mediated by both protein kinases and protein phosphatases. The former include S6 kinase (or p90[rsk]) and a kinase (MAPKAP-2) that phosphorylates glycogen synthase and small heat shock proteins (hsp25 and hsp27). Once activated, S6 kinase phosphorylates the glycogen-binding subunit of protein phosphatase I, which binds more avidly to its catalytic subunit and thus increases glycogen synthase phosphatase activity. Some of the protein kinases that cause activation of MAP kinase (raf 1, mek) are also substrates for the enzyme, an action that may be involved in regulation of the activity of the mitogen-activated pathway.

The other major extranuclear targets of MAP kinase action include substrates in the plasma membrane and the cytoskeleton. Those associated with the cell surface are the EGF receptor and cytoplasmic phospholipase A_2. The latter is activated when phosphorylated by MAP kinase during growth factor stimulation, leading to increased production of arachidonic acid and its eicosanoid metabolites. An action of MAP kinase on the cytoskeleton is mediated by its phosphorylation of the microtubule-associated protein tau. This may account for the effect of MAP kinase on microtubule dynamics, including the rearrangement of the microtubular network that occurs during the cell cycle.

The most interesting actions of MAP kinase are exerted on nuclear substrates that are involved in the control of gene expression.[297] These include the proto-oncogenes *c-myc* and *c-jun*, in which phosphorylation increases the transactivation of gene expression by the former and possibly by the latter.

FIGURE 5A-37. The pathway of growth factor signaling to the nucleus. The binding of growth factors to their receptors, along with the ensuing autophosphorylation of tyrosine residues in the cytoplasmic domain, is followed by recruitment of Grb2 and the ras exchange factor, Sos. The main downstream target of ras is the enzyme raf, which phosphorylates mek (MAP kinase kinase). Mek subsequently phosphorylates and activates MAP kinase, which in turn signals to the cell nucleus through phosphorylation of transcription factors. *(Modified from Marx.[295])*

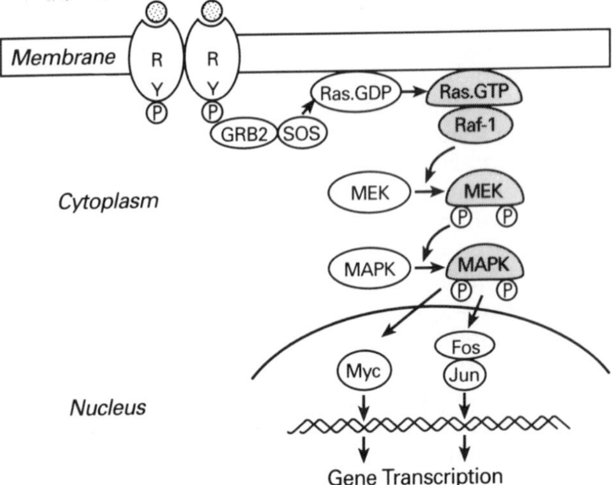

Other transcriptional regulatory substrates of MAP kinase include one of the transactivating factors (p62[TCR]) for the serum response element that controls the expression of *c-fos* and one of the activating fators (ATF-2) for the cAMP response element (CRE). Although the extent to which MAP kinase regulates the expression of *c-jun* is not certain, it is clearly involved in the control of *c-myc* and *c-fos* expression, in the latter case through activation of both the serum response element (SRE) and the CRE in its promoter domain.

Cytokine Receptor Signaling

In addition to the recently defined Ras-mediated signal transduction pathway of the growth factor receptors, leading through MAP kinase to the activation of transcription factor AP-1 (*fos/jun*), a more direct nuclear signaling pathway has been identified for interferons (IFNs) and other cytokines.[298] Whereas the Ras pathway leads to the activation and translocation of cytoplasmic protein kinases that phosphorylate and activate transcription factors, IFNs cause tyrosine phosphorylation and activation of cytoplasmic transcription factor subunits that undergo nuclear translocation and induce the expression of specific IFN-responsive genes. Thus, IFN-α and IFN-γ control the tyrosine phosphorylation of transcription factors containing the p91 subunit of interferon-stimulated gene factor-3 (ISGF3), a complex of cytoplasmic proteins that is translocated to the nucleus in cells stimulated by IFNs. This effect of IFNs is caused by receptor-induced activation of cytoplasmic tyrosine kinases (JAK1, JAK2, and Tyk2) that may be required for the correct assembly of interferon-receptor complexes.[299] In the case of IFN-γ, phosphorylation of a single tyrosine residue in p91 is required for nuclear translocation, DNA binding, and gene activation. The tyrosine kinase substrates that are activated by IFNs and translocated to the nucleus have been termed STAT (signal transducer and activation of transcription) proteins.[300]

A similar pathway has been found to be utilized by certain growth factors and acts as a more direct route to the nucleus than the Ras signal transduction cascade. Thus, several growth factors, including EGF, PDGF, CSF-I, and IL-10, stimulate tyrosine phosphorylation and DNA binding of p91, apparently at the same site that is phosphorylated by INF-γ.[301] Since p91 contains an SH2 domain, it can rapidly and directly interact with autophosphorylated growth factor receptors. Whether p91 is activated directly at the receptor or by an intermediate cytoplasmic tyrosine kinase is not yet known. However, the convergent activation of p91 by several cytokines and growth factors indicates its potential role in targeting various transcriptional regulatory complexes to their nuclear binding sites.

Hormonal Regulation of Early Response Genes

Until recently, surprisingly little was known about the mechanisms by which peptide hormones, growth factors, and transmitters influence long-term responses such as cell hypertrophy and proliferation. There is now evidence for the existence of several growth response pathways through which the activation of plasma membrane receptors by mitogens and other extracellular stimuli can stimulate DNA synthesis. An early step in such pathways is increased expression of genes that encode transcription factors which in turn regulate the expression of other (so-called downstream) genes that control cell growth and mitogenesis. Many growth factors as well as growth-stimulating hormones and transmitters that are coupled to phosphoinositide hydrolysis have been found to stimulate the expression of a large group of *immediate early response genes* (also called primary response genes) that are transcribed within minutes of hormonal activation and are active for only a few hours.[302] Several of the proteins that are encoded by the 100 or so early response genes act as transcription factors to regulate the expression of downstream genes that promote DNA synthesis and cell proliferation and those which encode several peptide hormones, including proenkephalin, insulin, and prolactin. Two important early response genes are the proto-oncogenes *c-fos* and *c-jun*, which encode nuclear proteins (Fos and Jun) that function as dimeric complexes and bind to a specific nucleotide sequence termed the AP-1 site [TPA-responsive element (TRE)] of target genes to promote their transcription (Fig. 5A-38). These and many other early response genes are characterized by their rapid and transient expression in many cell types in response to stimuli of growth or differentiation and their lack of a requirement for new protein synthesis during transcriptional induction. These features are consistent with the initiation of their expression by rapidly formed second messengers produced during receptor activation and the mediation of this expression by posttranslational modification of preexisting regulatory proteins.[303]

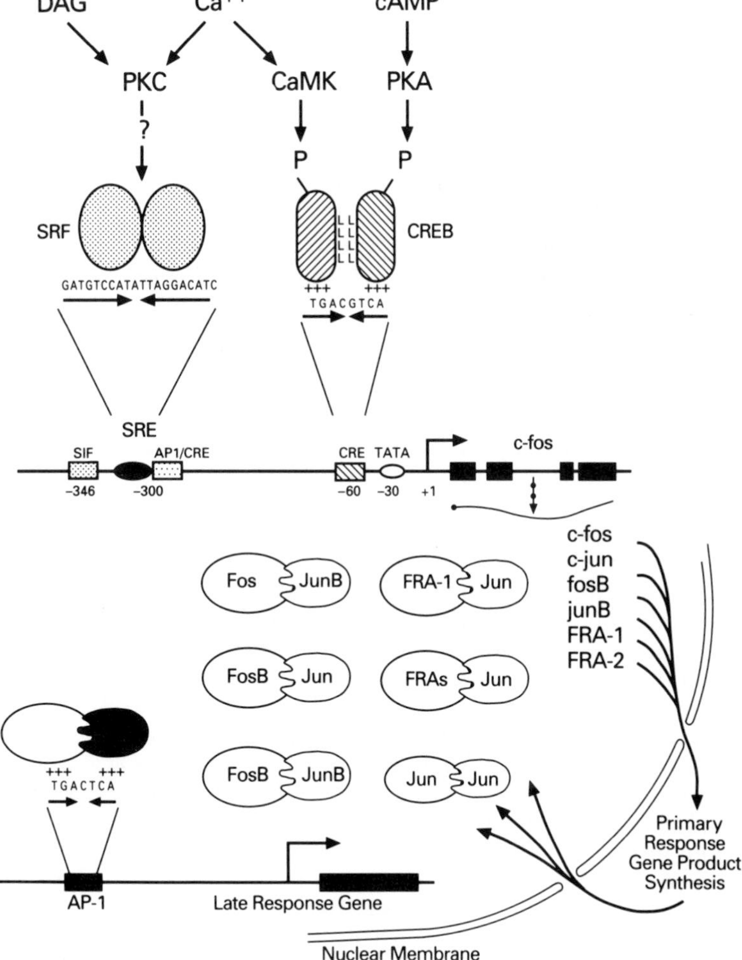

FIGURE 5A-38. Activation of the expression of early response genes (exemplified by *c-fos*) by receptor-mediated signaling pathways. Phosphorylation of the transcriptional regulatory proteins CREB and SRF stimulates the expression of the *c-fos* gene(s), whose protein products form heterodimers with *c-jun* and bind to AP-1 sites in the promoter regions of late response genes. *(Courtesy of S.S. Stojilkovic.)*

The expression of many early response genes is triggered by the actions of second messengers on protein kinases that in turn phosphorylate proteins involved in the regulation of early gene transcription (Fig. 5A-38). Thus, hormone-induced elevations of cAMP and calcium, acting through protein kinase A and Ca^{2+}/calmodulin-dependent protein kinases, cause phosphorylation of a common transcription factor, the cAMP response element binding protein (CREB). Once phosphorylated, CREB activates transcription of the *c-fos* proto-oncogene after binding to the CRE, a regulatory sequence in its 5′ upstream region.[304] Another major transcription factor, the serum response factor (SRF), is a comlex of two proteins ($p67^{SRF}$ and $p62^{TCF}$) that is activated by PKC during stimulation by serum and growth factors and binds to a separate regulatory sequence (the SRE) in the 5′ upstream region of the early response genes. The $p62^{TCF}$ component of the SRF is phosphorylated and activated by MAP kinase, which thus also contributes to mitogen-stimulated activation of the SRE.[305] Since Ca^{2+} is involved in the phosphorylation of both CREB and the SRF, acting through Ca^{2+}/calmodulin-dependent protein kinase and PKC (in conjunction with DAG), respectively, it is a potent stimulus for the expression of early response genes in cells regulated by calcium-mobilizing hormones and growth factors.

The CREB, Fos, and Jun proteins belong to the BZip family of transcriptional regulatory proteins that possess a basic DNA-binding domain and a hydrophobic leucine-rich domain (the leucine zipper), an α helix that contains leucine residues at every seventh amino acid (i.e., at each turn). The leucine zipper region of the Fos family engages in protein-protein interactions with members of the Jun family to form stable heterodimers that are major components of the AP-1 complex. The basic binding domains of the dimeric complexes interact with the TRE, a *cis*-acting transcriptional regulatory sequence that is present in many genes for hormones, receptors, enzymes, and growth-related proteins. The dimerization domains of the Fos and Jun proteins possess a coiled-coil structure formed from two parallel α-helical regions with a hydrophobic contact interface at which the leucine residues are located.[306] By combining through these hydrophobic domains, the Fos and Jun proteins form stable heterodimers containing two DNA-binding domains that can interact specifically with the TRE consensus sequence (5′-TGA$^{C}/_{G}$TAC-3′). In the presence of this nucleotide sequence, the DNA-binding domains undergo a conformational transition to form a DNA contact region of high α-helical content that lies within the major grove of the DNA helix.

The *c-fos* nuclear proto-oncogene is the cellular homologue of the *v-fos* oncogene first identified in murine osteogenic sarcoma viruses. It is now known to belong to a multigene family (*c-fos, fosB, fra-1*, and *fra-2*) that encodes several transcriptional regulatory proteins that contain the hydrophobic leucine zipper domain and form heterodimers with proteins encoded by members of the *jun* gene family (c-jun, jun-B, jun-D).[307] The *c-jun* proto-oncogene is the cellular homologue of the *v-jun* oncogene carried by an avian sarcoma virus. The Jun protein, in addition to forming heterodimers with Fos, also forms homodimers with less stability than Fos-Jun heterodimers but with comparable affinity for the AP-1 site. In contrast, Fos forms only heterodimers with Jun proteins and does not homodimerize. In addition to forming the dimers that constitute the AP-1 complex, Fos and Jun are also phosphorylated by protein kinases that regulate their abilities to modulate the transcription of other genes by transactivation or transrepression. The expression of *c-fos* by growth factors is mediated by the SRE located −300 bp upstream of the transcription start site, whereas the actions of hormones that increase intracellular cAMP and Ca^{2+} are mediated largely by the CRE located at −60 bp from the start site (Fig. 5A-38). The *c-fos* 5′ flanking region also contains other promoter and expression elements; in addition, sequences that control elongation of the *c-fos* transcript are present within at least one intron of the gene. Thus, expression of the *c-fos* gene is controlled by both positive and negative regulatory factors, acting not only to switch on transcription but also to regulate the production of the full-length mRNA transcripts that encode the Fos protein.[308]

The *c-jun* proto-oncogene, unlike *c-fos*, contains no introns and does not possess the CRE and SRE promoter elements that mediate regulation by CREB and SRF, respectively. However, *c-jun* contains a 5′ TRE that binds Jun homodimers and Fos-Jun heterodimers (AP-1) and is the major promoter for gene expression. Thus, *c-jun* is positively autoregulated by its own product and that of the *c-fos* gene. (There is also a TRE in the promoter region of *c-fos*, but the functional role of this sequence and its potential for positive autoregulation have not been established.) In addition to being mediated by the TRE in its promoter region, the induction of *c-jun* requires the presence of preformed Jun protein and is more prolonged than the transient expression of *c-fos*. In contrast to the low or negligible levels of Fos proteins in unstimulated cells, preexisting Jun proteins are relatively abundant in most quiescent cells and contribute to their basal AP-1 activity. The autoregulation of *c-jun* expression by the 5′ TRE probably accounts for its slower induction compared with *c-fos* by stimuli of AP-1 activity and for its more prolonged expression.[309]

The Fos and Jun proteins are also subject to posttranslational modifications, largely by phosphorylation of serine and threonine residues, that influence their activities and contribute to the diversity of the AP-1 response. Thus, phosphorylation of the carboxy-terminal region of Fos by PKC is involved in the negative regulation of *c-fos* expression, which does not require dimerization with Jun. Although this region of Fos also contributes to the activation of AP-1–dependent transcription, its phosphorylation leads to transrepression of the *c-fos* promoter that depends on the presence of a functional SRE. Thus, phosphorylation of Fos by PKC tends to extinguish its expression and probably is responsible for its transient production during ligand-induced activation of the early gene response.

In contrast to the negative effects of phosphorylation of Fos on *c-fos* expression, Jun undergoes more complex regulation that includes both positive and negative changes in its activity. Phosphorylation of the N-terminal activation domain of Jun, which is already functional in the absence of phosphorylation, causes a 10-fold increase in activity by changing its conformation. The kinase that phosphorylates the activation domain of Jun appears to be related to the MAP kinase family and to be regulated by growth factor–regulated tyrosine kinases and Ras proteins (see below). Jun is also phosphorylated at carboxyterminal serine and threonine residues adjacent to the basic DNA-binding domain, resulting in inhibition of its ability to bind to the TRE. This region of Jun is phosphorylated constitutively by casein kinase II and by MAP2 kinases in an inducible manner. In intact cells, carboxy-terminal sites are rapidly dephosphorylated by TPA treatment or Ras activation, probably by a specific phosphatase that reverses the constitutive phosphorylation caused by CKII. Such dephosphorylation increases the DNA-binding affinity of Jun for the TRE of the *c-jun* promoter, thus increasing *c-jun* gene expression and promoting the production of more Jun protein. This is accompanied by an increase in AP-1–binding activity that results from both increased activation of Jun and increased production of Jun-Jun and Jun-Fos dimers.[310]

REFERENCES

1. Yamamoto KR: Steroid regulated transcription of specific genes and gene networks. *Annu Rev Genet* 19:209, 1985.
2. Gronemeyer H: Transcription activation by estrogen and progesterone receptors. *Annu Rev Genet* 25:89, 1991.
3. Funder JW: Glucocorticoid receptors. *J Steroid Biochem Mol Biol* 43:389, 1992.
4. Brent GA, Moore DD, Larsen PR: Thyroid hormone regulation of gene expression. *Annu Rev Physiol* 53:17, 1991.
5. O'Malley BW, Tsai SY, Bagchi M, Weigel NL: Molecular mechanism of action of a steroid hormone receptor. *Recent Prog Horm Res* 47:1, 1991.
6. Hakanson R, Sundler F: The design of the neuroendocrine system: A unifying concept and its consequences. *Trends Pharmacol Sci* 4:41, 1985.
7. Sporn MB, Roberts AB: Autocrine growth factors and cancer. *Nature* 313:745, 1985.
8. Smith MR, Matthews NT, Jones KA, Kung HF: Biological actions of oncogenes. *Pharmacol Ther* 58:211, 1993.
9. O'Malley BW, Conneely OM: Orphan receptors: In search of a unifying hypothesis for activation. *Mol Endocrinol* 6:1359, 1992.
10. Sutherland EW, Robison GA: The role of cyclic-3′,5′-AMP in responses to catecholamines and other hormones. *Pharmacol Rev* 18:145, 1966.
11. Singer SJ, Nicholson G: The fluid mosaic theory of the structure of cell membrane. *Science* 175:721, 1972.
12. Luna EJ, Hitt AL: Cytoskeleton-plasma membrane interactions. *Science* 258:955, 1992.
13. Simon MI: Diversity of G proteins in signal transduction. *Science* 252:802, 1991.
14. Krebs EG, Beavo JA: Phosphorylation-dephosphorylation of enzymes. *Annu Rev Biochem* 48:923, 1979.
15. Scott JD: Cyclic AMP-dependent protein kinases. *Pharmacol Ther* 50:123, 1991.
16. Dufau ML, Catt KJ: Gonadotropin receptors and regulation of steroidogenesis in the testis and ovary. *Vitam Horm* 36:462, 1978.
17. Blundell TL, Humbel RE: Hormone families: Pancreatic hormones and homologous growth factors. *Nature* 287:781, 1980.
18. Birnbaumer L: G proteins in signal transduction. *Annu Rev Pharmacol Toxicol* 30:675, 1990.
19. Taylor SI, Grunberger G, Marcus-Samuels B, Underhill LH, Dons RF, Ryan J, Roddam RF, Rupe CE, Gorden P: Hypoglycemia associated with antibodies to the insulin receptor. *N Engl J Med* 307:1422, 1982.
20. Stephenson RP: A modification of receptor theory. *Br J Pharmacol* 11:379, 1956.
21. Goodford PJ: Receptors, spare receptors and other binding sites. *Trends Pharmacol Sci* 5:90, 1984.
22. Huhtaniemi IT, Clayton RN, Catt KJ: Gonadotropin binding and Leydig cell activation in the rat testis in vivo. *Endocrinology* 111:982, 1982.
23. Douglas J, Saltman S, Fredlund P, Kondo T, Catt KJ: Receptor binding of angiotensin II and antagonists: Correlation with aldosterone production by isolated adrenal glomerulosa cells. *Circ Res* 38(Suppl 2):108, 1976.
24. Kono T: Actions of insulin on glucose transport and cAMP phosphodiesterase in fat cells; Involvement of two distinct molecular mechanisms. *Recent Prog Horm Res* 39:519, 1983.
25. Petty HR: Receptors and responses, in *Molecular Biology of Membranes: Structure and Function*. New York, Plenum, 1993, pp 223–296.
26. Pichon Y, Lunt GG: Invertebrates: Witnesses to the evolution of neuroreceptors and ion channels in the nervous system. *New Biologist* 3:937, 1991.
27. Numa S: A molecular view of neurotransmitter receptors and ionic channels. *Harvey Lect* 83:121, 1989.
28. Changeux JP, Giraudat J, Dennis M: The nicotinic acetylcholine receptors: Molecular architecture of a ligand-regulated ion channel. *Trends Pharmacol Sci* 8:459, 1987.
29. Galzi J-L, Revah F, Bessis A, Changeux J-P: Functional architecture of the nicotinic acetylcholine receptor: From electric organ to brain. *Annu Rev Pharmacol Toxicol* 31:37, 1991.
30. Deneris ES, Connoly J, Rogers S, Duvoison R: Pharmacological and functional diversity of neuronal nicotinic acetylcholine receptors. *Trends Pharmacol Sci* 12:34, 1991.
31. Vernino S, Amador M, Leutje CW, Patrick J, Dani JA: Calcium modulation and high calcium permeability of neuronal nicotinic acetylcholine receptors. *Neuron* 8:127, 1992.
32. Oblatt-Montal M, Bühler LK, Iwamoto T, Tomich JM, Montal M: Synthetic peptides and four-helix bundle proteins as model systems for the pore-forming structure of channel proteins: I. Transmembrane segment M2 of the nicotinic cholinergic receptor channel is a key pore-lining structure. *J Biol Chem* 268:14601, 1993.
33. Phillips WD, Kopta C, Blount P, Gardner PD, Steinbach JH, Merlie JP: ACh receptor-rich membrane domains organized

in fibroblasts by recombinant 43-kilodalton protein. *Science* 251:568, 1991.

34. Eiselé J-L, Bertrand S, Galzi J-L, Devillers-Thiéry A, Changeux J-P, Bertrand D: Chimaeric nicotinic-serotonergic receptor combines distinct ligand binding and channel specificities. *Nature* 366:479, 1993.
35. Monaghan DT, Bridges RJ, Cotman CW: The excitatory amino acid receptors: Their classes, pharmacology, and distinct properties in the function of the central nervous system. *Annu Rev Pharmacol Toxicol* 29:365, 1989.
36. Collingridge GL, Singer W: Excitatory amino acid receptors and synaptic plasticity. *Trends Pharmacol Sci* 11:290, 1990.
37. Gasic GP, Hollman M: Molecular neurobiology of glutamate receptors. *Annu Rev Physiol* 54:507, 1992.
38. Moriyoshi K, Masu M, Ishii T, Shigemoto R, Mizuno N, Nakanishi S: Molecular cloning and characterization of the rat NMDA receptor. *Nature* 354:31, 1991.
39. Seeburg PH: The molecular biology of mammalian glutamate receptor channels. *Trends Pharmacol Sci.* 14:297, 1993.
40. Ishii T, Moriyoshi K, Sugihara H, Sakurada K, Kadotani H, Yokoi M, Akazawa C, Shigemoto R, et al: Molecular characterization of the family of the N-methyl-D-aspartate receptor subunits. *J Biol Chem* 268:2836, 1993.
41. Bashir ZI, Henly JM: The French connection: A magnum of excitatory amino acids in Marseilles. *Trends Pharmacol Sci* 14:387, 1993.
42. Sackmann B: Elementary steps in synaptic transmission revealed by current through single ion channels. *Neuron* 8:613, 1992.
43. Bittiger H, Froestl W, Mickel SJ, Olpe H-R: $GABA_B$ receptor antagonists: From synthesis to therapeutic applications. *Trends Pharmacol Sci* 14:391, 1993.
44. DeLorey TM, Olsen RW: γ-aminobutyric $acid_A$ receptor structure and function. *J Biol Chem* 267:16747, 1992.
45. Reddy GL, Iwamoto T, Tomich JM, Montal M: Synthetic peptides and four-helix bundle proteins as model systems for the pore-forming structure of channel proteins: II. Transmembrane segment M2 of the brain glycine receptor is a plausible candidate for the pore-lining structure. *J Biol Chem* 268:14608, 1993.
46. Maricq AV, Peterson AS, Brake AJ, Myers RM, Julius D: Primary structure and functional expression of the $5HT_3$ receptor, a serotonin-gated ion channel. *Science* 254:432, 1991.
47. Saverese TM, Fraser CM: In vitro mutagenesis and the search for structure-function relationships among G protein-coupled receptors. *Biochem J* 283:1, 1992.
48. Applebury ML: Molecular determinants of visual pigment function. *Curr Opin Neurobiol* 1:263, 1991.
49. Dixon RAF, Kobilka BK, Strader DJ, Benovic JL, Dohlman HG: Cloning of the gene and cDNA for mammalian β-adrenergic receptor and homology with rhodopsin. *Nature* 321:75, 1986.
50. Collins S, Lohse MJ, O'Dowd B, Caron MG, Lefkowitz RJ: Structure and regulation of G protein-coupled receptors: The beta-2 adrenergic receptor as a model. *Vitam Horm* 49:1, 1991.
51. Probst WC, Snyder LA, Schuster DI, Brosius J, Sealfon S: Sequence alignment of the G-protein coupled receptor superfamily. *DNA Cell Biol* 11:1, 1992.
52. Bairoch A: The PROSITE dictionary of sites and patterns in proteins, its current status. *Nucleic Acids Res* 21:3097, 1993.
53. Attwood TK, Eliopoulos EE, Findlay JB: Multiple sequence alignment of protein families showing low sequence homology: A methodological approach using database pattern-matching discriminators for G-protein-linked receptors. *Gene* 98:153, 1991.
54. Khorana HG: Bacteriorhodopsin, a membrane protein that uses light to translocate protons. *J Biol Chem* 263:7439, 1988.
55. Hedin KE, Duerson K, Clapham DE: Specificity of receptor-G protein interactions: Searching for the structure behind the signal. *Cell Signal* 5:505, 1993.
56. Mukoyama M, Nakajima M, Horiuchi M, Sasamura H, Pratt RE, Dzau VJ: Expression cloning of type 2 angiotensin II receptor reveals a unique class of seven-transmembrane receptors. *J Biol Chem* 268:24539, 1993.
57. Ahlquist RP: Development of the concept of alpha and beta adrenotropic receptors. *Ann NY Acad Sci* 139:549, 1967.
58. Garcia-Sainz JA: α_1-Adrenergic action: Receptor subtypes, signal transduction, and regulation. *Cell Signal* 5:539, 1993.
59. Limbird L: *The Alpha-2 Adrenergic Receptors*, Clifton, NJ, Humana Press, 1988.
60. Ablas J, van Corven EJ, Hordijk PL, Milligan G, Moolenaar WH: G_i-mediated activation of the $p21^{ras}$-mitogen-activated protein kinase pathway by α_2-adrenergic receptors expressed in fibroblasts. *J Biol Chem* 268:22235, 1993.
61. Lefkowitz RJ, Caron MG: Molecular and regulatory properties of adrenergic receptors. *Recent Prog Horm Res* 43:469, 1987.
62. Reinhart J, Mertz LM, Catt KJ: Molecular cloning and expression of cDNA encoding the murine gonadotropin-releasing hormone receptor. *J Biol Chem* 267:21281, 1992.
63. Dias JA: Recent progress in structure-function and molecular analyses of the pituitary/placental glycoprotein hormone receptors. *Biochem Biophys Acta* 1135:287, 1992.
64. Sprengel R, Braun T, Nikoliks K, Segaloff DL, Seeburg PH: The testicular receptor for follicle stimulating hormone: Structure and functional expresion of cloned cDNA. *Mol Endocrinol* 4:525, 1990.
65. Tsai-Morris CH, Buczko E, Wang W, Dufau ML: Intronic nature of the rat luteinizing hormone receptor gene defines a soluble receptor subspecies with hormone binding activity. *J Biol Chem* 265:19385, 1990.
66. Ji I, Ji TH: Human choriogonadotropin binds to a lutropin receptor with essentially no N-terminal extension and stimulates cAMP synthesis. *J Biol Chem* 226:13076, 1991.
67. Tapparelli C, Metternich R, Cook NS: Structure and function of thrombin receptors. *Trends Pharmacol Sci* 14:426, 1993.
68. Gether V, Johanson TE, Snider RM, Low JA, Nakanishi S, Schwartz TW: Different binding epitopes on the NK_1 receptor for substance P and a non-peptide antagonist. *Nature* 362:345, 1993.
69. Nef P: Early events in olfaction: Diversity and spatial patterns of odorant receptors. *Receptors Channels* 1:259, 1993.
70. Schwanzel-Fukuda M, Pfaff DW: Origin of luteinizing hormone-releasing hormone neurons. *Nature* 338:161, 1989.
71. Millan M, Aguilera G, Wynn PC, Mendelsohn FAO, Catt KJ: Autoradiographic localization of brain receptors for peptide hormones: Angiotensin II, corticotropin-releasing factor, and gonadotropin-releasing hormone. *Methods Enzymol* 124:590, 1985.
72. Pan Y, Metzenberg A, Das S, Jing B, Gitschier J: Mutations in the V2 vasopressin receptor gene are associated with X-linked nephrogenic diabetes insipidus. *Nat Genet* 2:103, 1992.
73. Clark AJ, McLoughlin L, Grossman A: Familial glucocorticoid deficiency associated with point mutation in the adrenocorticotropin receptor. *Lancet* 341:461, 1993.
74. Godfrey P, Rahal JO, Beamer WG, Copeland NG: GHRH receptor of little mice contains a missense mutation in the extracellular domain that disrupts receptor function. *Nat Genet* 3:227, 1993.
75. Shenker A, Laue L, Kosugi S, Merendino JJ, Minegishi T, Cutler GB: A constitutively activating mutation of the luteinizing hormone receptor in familial male precocious puberty. *Nature* 365:652, 1993.
76. Parma J, Duprez L, Van Sande J, Cochaux P, Gervy C, Mockel J, Dumont J, Vassart G: Somatic mutations in the thyrotropin receptor gene cause hyperfunctioning thyroid adenomas. *Nature* 365:649, 1993.

77. Robbins LS, Nadeau JH, Johnson KR, Kelly MA, Roselli-Rehfuss L, Baack E, Mountjoy KG, Cone RD: Pigmentation phenotypes of variant extension locus alleles result from point mutations that alter MSH receptor function. *Cell* 72:827, 1993.
78. Robinson PR, Cohen GB, Zhukovsky EA, Oprian DD: Constitutively active mutants of rhodopsin. *Neuron* 4:719, 1992.
79. Lefkowitz RJ, Cotecchia S, Samama P, Costa T: Constitutive activity of receptors coupled to guanine nucleotide regulatory proteins. *Trends Pharmacol Sci* 14:303, 1993.
80. Lefkowitz RJ: Turned on to ill effect. *Nature* 365:603, 1993.
81. Carpenter GW: Receptors for epidermal growth factor and other polypeptide mitogens. *Annu Rev Biochem* 56:881, 1987.
82. White MF: Structure and function of tyrosine kinase receptors. *J Bioenerg Biomembr* 23:63, 1991.
83. Carpenter G, Hernandez-Sotomayor T, Jones G: Tyrosine phosphorylation of phospholipase C-gamma 1. *Adv Second Mess Phosphopr Res* 28:179, 1993.
84. Liang M, Garrison JC: Epidermal growth factor activates phospholipid C in rat hepatocytes via a different mechanism from that in A431 or rat1hER cells. *Mol Pharmacol* 42:743, 1992.
85. Kuryshev YA, Naumov AP, Avdonin PV, Mozhayeva GN: Evidence for involvement of a GTP-binding protein in activation of Ca^{2+} influx by epidermal growth factor in A431 cells: Effects of fluoride and bacterial toxins. *Cell Signal* 5:555, 1993.
86. Peppelenbosch MP, Tertoolen LGJ, den Hertog J, de Laat SW: Epidermal growth factor activates calcium channels by phospholipase A_2/5-lipoxygenase-mediated leukotriene C_4 production. *Cell* 69:295, 1992.
87. Campos-Gonzalez R, Glenney JR: Temperature-dependent tyrosine phosphorylation of microtubule-associated protein kinase in epidermal growth factor-stimulated human fibroblasts. *Cell Regul* 2:663, 1991.
88. Hunter T: The epidermal growth factor gene and its product. *Nature* 311:414, 1983.
89. Eppstein DA, Marsh YV, Schreiber AB, Newman SR, Todaro GJ, Nestor JJ: Epidermal growth factor receptor occupancy inhibits vaccinia virus infection. *Nature* 318:663, 1985.
90. Yip CC: Insulin receptor: Aspects of its structure and function. *Adv Exp Med Biol* 334:79, 1993.
91. Ullrich A, Bell JR, Chen EY, Herrera R, Petruzzeli LM, Dull TJ: Human insulin receptor and its relationship to the tyrosine kinase family of oncogenes. *Nature* 313:756, 1985.
92. Draznin B, Chang L, Leitner JW, Takata Y, Olefsky JM: Insulin activates $p21^{ras}$ and guanine nucleotide releasing factor in cells expressing wild type and mutant insulin receptors. *J Biol Chem* 268:19998, 1993.
93. White MF, Kahn CR: The insulin signaling system. *J Biol Chem* 269:1, 1994.
94. Backer JM, Myers MG Jr, Shoelson SE, Chin DJ, Sun XJ, Miralpeix M, Hu P, Margolis B, et al: Phosphatidylinositol-3′-kinase is activated by association with IRS-1 during insulin stimulation. *EMBO J* 11:3469, 1992.
95. Taylor SI, Cama A, Accili D, Barbetti F, et al: Mutations in the insulin receptor gene. *Endocr Rev* 13:566, 1992.
96. Kelly PA, Ali S, Rozakis M, Goujon L, Nagano M, Pellegrini I, Gould D, Djiane J, et al: The growth hormone/prolactin receptor family. *Recent Prog Horm Res* 48:123, 1993.
97. Hochberg Z, Amit T, Youdim MBH: The growth hormone binding protein as a paradigm of the erythropoietin superfamily of receptors. *Cell Signal* 3:85, 1991.
98. Cunningham BC, Bass S, Fuh G, Wells JA: Zinc mediation of the binding of human growth hormone to the human prolactin receptor. *Science* 250:1709, 1990.
99. Cunningham BC, Ultsch M, de Vos AM, Mulkerrin MG, Clauser KR, Wells JA: Dimerization of the extracellular domain of the human growth hormone receptor by a single hormone molecule. *Science* 254:821, 1991.
100. Argetsinger LS, Campbell GS, Yang X, Witthuhn BA, Silvennoinen O, Ihle JN, Carter-Su C: Identification of JAK2 as a growth hormone receptor-associated tyrosine kinase. *Cell* 74:237, 1993.
101. Rui H, Kirken RA, Farrar WL: Activation of receptor-associated tyrosine kinase JAK2 by prolactin. *J Biol Chem* 269:5364, 1994.
102. Taylor CW: The role of G proteins in transmembrane signalling. *Biochem J* 272:1, 1990.
103. Bourne HR, Sanders DA, McCormick F: The GTPase superfamily: Conserved structure and molecular mechanism. *Nature* 349:117, 1991.
104. Hepler JR, Gilman AG: G proteins. *Trends Biochem Sci* 17:383, 1992.
105. Conklin BR, Bourne HR: Structural elements of $G\alpha$ subunits that interact with $G\beta\gamma$, receptors, and effectors. *Cell* 73:631, 1993.
106. Markby DW, Onrust R, Bourne HR: Separate GTPase activating domains of a $G\alpha$ subunit. *Science* 262:1895, 1993.
107. Wilkie TM, Gilbert DJ, Olsen AS, Chen X-N, Amatruda TT, Korenberg JR, Trask BJ, de Jong P, et al: Evolution of the mammalian G protein α subunit multigene family. *Nat Genet* 1:85, 1992.
108. Birnbaumer L: Receptor-to-effector signaling through G proteins: Roles for $\beta\gamma$ dimers as well as α subunits. *Cell* 71:1069, 1992.
109. Axelrod J, Burch RM, Jelsema CL: Receptor-mediated activation of phospholipase A_2 via GTP-binding proteins: Arachidonic acid and its metabolites as second messengers. *Trends Neurosci* 11:117, 1988.
110. Logothetis DE, Kurachi Y, Galper J, Neer EJ, Clapham DE: The $\beta\gamma$ subunits of GTP-binding proteins activate the muscarinic K^+ channel in heart. *Nature* 325:321, 1987.
111. Tang W-J, Gilman AG: Type-specific regulation of adenylyl cyclase by G protein $\beta\gamma$ subunits. *Science* 254:1500, 1991.
112. Camps M, Carozzi A, Schnabel P, Scheer A, Parker PJ, Gierschik P: Isozyme-selective stimulation of phospholipase C-β2 by G protein $\beta\gamma$-subunits. *Nature* 360:684, 1992.
113. Katz A, Wu D, Simon MI: Subunits $\beta\gamma$ of heterotrimeric G protein activate β2 isoform of phospholipase C. *Nature* 360:686, 1992.
114. Kleuss C, Scherübl H, Hescheler J, Schultz G, Wittig B: Selectivity in signal transduction determined by γ subunits of heterotrimeric G proteins. *Science* 259:832, 1993.
115. Cali JJ, Balcueva EA, Rybalkin I, Robishaw JD: Selective tissue distribution of G protein γ subunits, including a new form of the γ subunits identified by cDNA cloning. *J Biol Chem* 267:24023, 1992.
116. Kisselev O, Gautam N: Specific interaction with rhodopsin is dependent on the γ subunit type in a G protein. *J Biol Chem* 268:24519, 1993.
117. Spiegel AM, Shenker A, Weinstein LS: Receptor-effector coupling by G proteins: Implications for normal and abnormal signal transduction. *Endocr Rev* 13:536, 1992.
118. Landis CA, Masters SB, Spada A, Pace AM, Bourne HR, Vallar L: GTPase inhibiting mutations activate the α chain of G_s and stimulate adenylyl cyclase in human pituitary tumours. *Nature* 340:692, 1989.
119. Castrillo J-L, Theill LE, Karin M: Function of the homeodomain protein GHF1 in pituitary cell proliferation. *Science* 253:197, 1991.
120. Lyons J, Landis CA, Harsh G, Vallar L, Grünewald K, Feichtinger H, Duh Q-Y, Clark OH, et al: Two G protein oncogenes in human endocrine tumors. *Science* 249:655, 1990.
121. Carter A, Bardin C, Collins R, Simons C, Bray P, Spiegel A: Reduced expression of multiple forms of the α subunit of the stimulatory GTP-binding protein in pseudohypoparathyroidism type Ia. *Proc Natl Acad Sci USA* 84:7266, 1987.
122. Bourne HR, Sanders DA, McCormick F: The GTPase superfamily: A conserved switch for diverse cell functions. *Nature* 348:125, 1990.
123. Barbacid M: Ras genes. *Annu Rev Biochem* 56:779, 1987.
124. Polakis P, McCormick F: Structural requirements for the

interaction of p21[ras] with GAP, exchange factors, and its biological effector target. *J Biol Chem* 268:9157, 1993.
125. Macara IG: The ras superfamily of molecular switches. *Cell Signal* 3:179, 1991.
126. Bokoch GM, Der CJ: Emerging concepts in the Ras superfamily of GTP-binding proteins. *FASEB J* 7:750, 1993.
127. Broek D, Samiy N, Fasano O, Fujiyama A, et al: Differential activation of yeast adenylate cyclase by wild-type and mutant RAS proteins. *Cell* 41:763, 1985.
128. Hall A: The cellular functions of small GTP-binding proteins. *Science* 249:635, 1990.
129. Satoh T, Nakafuku M, Kaziro Y: Function of ras as a molecular switch in signal transduction. *J Biol Chem* 267:24149, 1992.
130. Egan SE, Weinberg R: The pathway to signal achievement. *Nature* 365:781, 1993.
131. Lledo P-M, Vernier P, Vincent J-D, Mason WT, Zorec R: Inhibition of Rab3B expression attenuates Ca^{2+}-dependent exocytosis in rat anterior pituitary cells. *Nature* 364:540, 1993.
132. Bucci C, Parton RG, Mather IH, Stunnenberg H, Simons K, Hoflack B, Zerial M: The small GTPase rab5 functions as a regulatory factor in the early endocytic pathway. *Cell* 70:715, 1992.
133. Donaldson JG, Finazzi D, Klausner RD: Brefeldin A inhibits Golgi membrane-catalysed exchange of guanine nucleotide onto ARF protein. *Nature* 360:350, 1992.
134. Cockcroft S, Thomas GMH, Fensome A, Geny B, Cunningham E, Gout I, Hiles I, Totty NF, et al: Phospholipase D: A downstream effector of ARF in granulocytes. *Science* 263:523, 1994.
135. Moore MS, Blobel G: The GTP-binding protein Ran/TC4 is required for protein import into the nucleus. *Nature* 365:661, 1993.
136. Wilson BS, Komuro M, Farquhar MG: Cellular variations in heterotrimeric G protein localization and expression in rat pituitary. *Endocrinology* 134:233, 1994.
137. Ridley AJ, Hall A: The small GTP-binding protein rho regulates the assembly of focal adhesions and actin stress fibers in response to growth factors. *Cell* 70:389, 1992.
138. Hart MJ, Maru Y, Leonard D, Witte ON, Evans T, Cerione RA: A GDP dissociation inhibitor that serves as a GTPase inhibitor for the ras-like protein CDC42Hs. *Science* 258:812, 1992.
139. Huganir Rl, Greengard P: Regulation of receptor function by protein phosphorylation. *Trends Pharmacol Sci* 8:472, 1987.
140. Cama A, Quon MJ, de la Luz Sierra M, Taylor SI: Substitution of isoleucine for methionine at position 1153 in the β-subunit of the human insulin receptor. *J Biol Chem* 267:8383, 1992.
141. Matthews LS, Vale WW: Expression cloning of an activin receptor, a predicted transmembrane serine kinase. *Cell* 65:973, 1991.
142. Hunter T, Cooper JA: Protein-tyrosine kinases. *Annu Rev Biochem* 54:897, 1985.
143. Massague J: Transforming growth factor-α: A model for membrane-anchored growth factors. *J Biol Chem* 265:21393, 1990.
144. Cadena DL, Gill GN: Receptor tyrosine kinases. *FASEB J* 6:2332, 1992.
145. Cantley LC, Auger KR, Carpenter C, Duckworth B, Graziani A, Kapeller R, Soltoff S: Oncogenes and signal transduction. *Cell* 64:281, 1991.
146. Samelson LE, Klausner RD: Tyrosine kinases and tyrosine-based activation motifs. *J Biol Chem* 267:24913, 1992.
147. Koch CA, Anderson D, Moran MF, Ellis C, Pawson T: SH2 and SH3 domains: Elements that control interactions of cytoplasmic signaling proteins. *Science* 252:668, 1991.
148. Clayton RN, Catt KJ: Gonadotropin-releasing hormone receptors: Characterization, physiological regulation, and relationship to reproductive function. *Endocr Rev* 2:186, 1981.
149. Songyang Z, Shoelson SE, Chaudhuri M, Gish G, Pawson T, Haser WG, King F, Roberts T, et al: SH2 domains recognize specific phosphopeptide sequences. *Cell* 72:767, 1993.
150. Pawson T, Gish GD: SH2 and SH3 domains: From structue to function. *Cell* 71:359, 1992.
151. Lowenstein EJ, Daly RJ, Batzer AG, Li W, Morgolis B, Lammers R, Ullrich A, Skolnik EY, Bar-Sagi D, Schlessinger J: The SH2 and SH3 domain-containing protein GRB2 links receptor tyrosine kinases to ras signaling. *Cell* 70:431, 1992.
152. Tonks NK, Flint AJ, Gebbink MFBG, Sun H, Yang Q: Signal transduction and protein tyrosine dephosphorylation, in Brown BL, Dobson PRM (eds): *Advances in Second Messenger and Phosphoprotein Research*. New York, Raven, 1993, p 203.
153. Su Y-F, Harden TK, Perkins JP: Isoproterenol-induced desensitization of adenylate cyclase in human astrocytoma cells. *J Biol Chem* 254:38, 1979.
154. Sibley DR, Benovic JL, Caron MG, Lefkowitz RJ: Regulation of transmembrane signaling by phosphorylation. *Cell* 48:913, 1987.
155. Swinner JV, D'Souza B, Conti M, Ascoli M: Attenuation of cAMP-mediated responses in MA-10 Leydig tumor cells by genetic manipulation of a cAMP-phosphodiesterase. *J Biol Chem* 266:14383, 1991.
156. Palczewski K, Benovic JL: G protein-coupled receptor kinases. *Trends Biochem Sci* 16:387, 1991.
157. Hausdorff WP, Caron MG, Lefkowitz RJ: Turning off the signal: Desensitization of β-adrenergic receptor function. *FASEB J* 4:2881, 1990.
158. Barak LS, Tiberi M, Freedman NJ, Kwatra MM, Lefkowitz RJ, Caron MG: A highly conserved tyrosine residue in G protein-coupled receptors is required for agonist-mediated β_2-adrenergic receptor sequestration. *J Biol Chem* 269:2790, 1994.
159. Chan V, Katikineni M, Davies TF, Catt KJ: Hormonal regulation of testicular luteinizing hormone and prolactin receptors. *Endocrinology* 108:1607, 1981.
160. Inglese J, Freedman NJ, Koch WJ, Lefkowitz RJ: Structure and mechanism of the G protein-coupled receptor kinases. *J Biol Chem* 268:23735, 1993.
161. Liggett SB, Ostrowski JO, Chesnut LC, Kurose H, Raymond JR, Caron MG, Lefkowitz RJ: Sites in the third intracellular loop of the α_{2a}-adrenergic receptor confer short term agonist-promoted desensitization. *J Biol Chem* 267:4740, 1992.
162. Mitchell FM, Buckley NJ, Milligan G: Enhanced degradation of the phosphoinositidase C-linked guanine-nucleotide-binding protein $G_q\alpha/G_{11}\alpha$ following activation of the human M_1 muscarinic acetylcholine receptor expressed in CHO cells. *Biochem J* 293:495, 1993.
163. Rothman JE, Lenard J: Membrane traffic in animal cells. *Trends Biochem Sci* 10:176, 1985.
164. Simon SM, Blobal G: Mechanisms of translocation of proteins across membranes. *Subcell Biochem* 21:1, 1993.
165. Griffiths G, Hoflack B, Simons K, Mellman I, Kornfeld S: The mannose 6-phosphate receptor and the biogenesis of lysosomes. *Cell* 52:329, 1988.
166. Draznin B, Mehler PS, Leitner JW, Sussman KE, et al: Localization of somatostatin receptors in secretion vesicles in anterior pituitary cells and pancreatic islets. *J Recept Res* 5:83, 1985.
167. Von Heijne G: Control of topology and mode of assembly of a polytopic membrane protein by positively charged residues. *Nature* 341:456, 1989.
168. Hartmann E, Rapaport TA, Lodish HL: Predicting the orientation of eukaryote membrane-spanning proteins. *Proc Natl Acad Sci USA* 86:5786, 1989.
169. Pelham HRB, Munro S: Sorting of membrane proteins in the secretory pathway. *Cell* 75:603, 1993.
170. Simons K, Zerial M: Rab proteins and the road maps for intracellular transport. *Neuron* 11:789, 1993.
171. Moss J, Vaughan M: ADP-ribosylation factors, 20,000 M_r guanine nucleotide-binding protein activators of cholera

toxin and components of intracellular vesicular transport systems. *Cell Signal* 5:367, 1993.
172. Serafini T, Orei L, Amherdt M, Brunner M, Kahn RA, Rothman JE: ADP-ribosylation factor is a subunit of the coat of Golgi-derived COP-coated vesicles: A novel role for a GTP-binding protein. *Cell* 67:239, 1991.
173. Aridor M, Rajmilevich G, Beaven MA, Sagi-Eisenberg R: Activation of exocytosis by the heterotrimeric G protein G_{i3}. *Science* 262:1569, 1993.
174. Bauer-Dantoin AC, Hollenberg AN, Jameson JL: Dynamic regulation of gonadotropin-releasing hormone receptor mRNA levels in the anterior pituitary gland during the rat estrous cycle. *Endocrinology* 133:1911, 1993.
175. Huhtaniemi IT, Nozu K, Warren DW, Dufau ML, Catt KJ: Acquisition of regulatory mechanisms for gonadotropin receptors and steroidogenesis in the maturing rat testis. *Endocrinology* 111:1711, 1982.
176. Dufau ML: Endocrine regulation and communicating functions of the Leydig cell. *Annu Rev Physiol* 50:483, 1988.
177. Kaplan J: Polypeptide-binding membrane receptors: Analysis and classification. *Science* 212:14, 1981.
178. Pastan IH, Willingham MC: Journey to the center of the cell: Role of the receptosome. *Science* 214:504, 1981.
179. Gorden P, Carptentier J-L, Freychet P, Orci L: Internalization of polypeptide hormones. *Diabetologia* 18:263, 1980.
180. Brown VI, Greene MI: Molecular and cellular mechanisms of receptor-mediated endocytosis. *DNA Cell Biol* 10:399, 1991.
181. Steinman RM, Mellman IS, Muller WA, Cohn ZA: Endocytosis and the recycling of plasma membrane. *J Cell Biol* 96:1, 1983.
182. Helenius A, Mellman I, Wall D, Hubbard A: Endosomes. *Trends Biochem Sci* 8:245, 1983.
183. Brown MS, Goldstein JL: Receptor-mediated endocytosis: Insights from the lipoprotein receptor system. *Proc Natl Acad Sci USA* 76:3330, 1980.
184. Klausner RD, Ashwell G, Van Renswoude J, Harford JE, Bridges KR: Binding of apotransferrin to K562 cells: Explanation of the transferrin cycle. *Proc Natl Acad Sci USA* 80:2263, 1983.
185. Chen W-J, Goldstein JL, Brown MS: NPXY, a sequence often found in cytoplasmic tails, is required for coated pit-mediated internalization of the low density lipoprotein receptor. *J Biol Chem* 265:3116, 1990.
186. Trowbridge IS, Collaun JF, Hopkins CR: Signal-dependent membrane protein trafficking in the endocytic pathway. *Annu Rev Cell Biol* 9:129, 1993.
187. Pley U, Parham P: Clathrin: Its role in receptor-mediated vesicular transport and specialized functions in neurons. *Crit Rev Biochem Mol Biol* 28:431, 1993.
188. Moro O, Lameh J, Sadée W: Serine- and threonine-rich domain regulates internalization of muscarinic cholinergic receptors. *J Biol Chem* 268:6862, 1993.
189. Pearse BMF, Robinson MS: Clathrin, adaptors, and sorting. *Annu Rev Cell Biol* 6:151, 1990.
190. Schmid S: The question of receptor-mediated endocytosis: More questions than answers. *Bioessays* 14:589, 1992.
191. Herskovits JS, Burgess CC, Obar RA, Vallee RB: Effects of mutant rat dynamin on endocytosis. *J Cell Biol* 122:565, 1993.
192. Sorkin A, Waters CM: Endocytosis of growth factor receptors. *Bioassays* 15:375, 1993.
193. Amsterdam A, Naor Z, Knecht M, Dufau ML, Catt KJ: Hormone action and receptor distribution in endocrine target cells: Gonadotropins and gonadotropin-releasing hormone, in Middlebrook JL, Kohn LD (eds): *Receptor-Mediated Binding and Internalization of Toxins and Hormones*. New York, Academic, 1981, p 283.
194. Lienhard GE: Regulation of cellular membrane transport by the exocytotic insertion and endocytic retrieval of transporters. *Trends Biochem Sci* 8:107, 1983.
195. Karnieli E, Zarnowski MJ, Hissin PJ, Simpson IA, Salans LB, Cushman SW: Insulin-stimulated translocation of glucose transport systems in the isolated rat adipose cell. *J Biol Chem* 256:4772, 1981.
196. Hunyady L, Merelli F, Baukal AJ, Balla T, Catt KJ: Agonist-induced endocytosis and signal generation in adrenal glomerulosa cell. *J Biol Chem* 266:2783, 1991.
197. Pazin MJ, Williams LT: Triggering signaling cascades by receptor tyrosine kinases. *Trends Biochem Sci* 17:374, 1992.
198. Cohen P: Signal integration at the level of protein kinases, protein phosphatases and their substrates. *Trends Biochem Sci* 17:408, 1992.
199. De Meyts P, Rousseau GG: Receptor concepts: A century of evolution. *Circ Res* 46(Suppl 1):3, 1980.
200. Rodbell M: The role of hormone receptors and GTP-regulatory proteins in membrane transduction. *Nature* 284:17, 1980.
201. Krupinski J, Coussen F, Bakalyar HA, Tang W-J, Feinstein PG, Orth K, Slaughter C, Reed RR, Gilman AG: Adenylyl cyclase amino acid sequence: Possible channel- or transporter-like structure. *Science* 244:1558, 1989.
202. Tang W-J, Gilman AG: Adenylyl cyclases. *Cell* 70:869, 1992.
203. Debernardi MA, Munshi R, Yoshimura M, Cooper DM, Brooker G: Predominant expression of type-VI adenylate cyclase in C6-2B rat glioma cells may account for inhibition of cyclic AMP accumulation by calcium. *Biochem J* 293:325, 1993.
204. Pitt GS, Milona N, Borleis J, Lin KC, et al: Structurally distinct and stage-specific adenylyl cyclase genes play different roles in Dictyostelium development. *Cell* 69:305, 1992.
205. Hurley JB: Molecular properties of the cGMP cascade of vertebrate photoreceptors. *Annu Rev Physiol* 49:793, 1987.
206. Conti M, Jin SL, Monaco L, Repaske DR, Swinnen JV: Hormonal regulation of cyclic nucleotide phosphodiesterases. *Endocr Rev* 12:218, 1991.
207. Conti M, Toscano MV, Petrelli L, Geremia R, Stefanini M: Involvement of phosphodiesterase in the refractoriness of the Sertoli cell. *Endocrinology* 113:1845, 1983.
208. MacFarland RT, Zelus BD, Beavo JA: High concentrations of a cGMP-stimulated phosphodiesterase mediate ANP-induced decreases in cAMP and steroidogenesis in adrenal glomerulosa cells. *J Biol Chem* 266:136, 1991.
209. Taylor SS: cAMP-dependent protein kinase: Model for an enzyme family. *J Biol Chem* 264:8443, 1989.
210. Krebs EG, Beavo JA: Phosphorylation-dephosphorylation of enzymes. *Annu Rev Biochem* 48:923, 1979.
211. Hanks SM, Quinn AM, Hunter T: The protein kinase family: Conserved features and deduced phylogeny of the catalytic domains. *Science* 241:42, 1988.
212. Whitehouse S, Walsh DA: Purification of a physiological form of the inhibitor protein of the cAMP-dependent protein kinase. *J Biol Chem* 257:6028, 1982.
213. Taylor CW: The role of G proteins in transmembrane signalling. *Biochem J* 272:1, 1990.
214. Hoppe J: cAMP-dependent protein kinases: Conformational kinases during activation. *Trends Biochem Sci* 10:29, 1985.
215. Yonemoto W, Garrod SM, Bell SM, Taylor SS: Identification of phosphorylation sites in the recombinant catalytic subunit of cAMP-dependent protein kinase. *J Biol Chem* 268:18626, 1993.
216. Kemp BE, Pearson RB: Protein kinase recognition sequence motifs. *Trends Biochem Sci* 15:342, 1990.
217. Feramisco JR, Glass DB, Krebs EG: Optimal spatial requirements for the location of basic residues in peptide substrates for the cyclic AMP-dependent protein kinase. *J Biol Chem* 255:4240, 1982.
218. Døskeland SO, Maronde E, Gjertsen BT: The genetic subtypes of cAMP-dependent protein kinase—functionally different or redundant? *Biochim Biophys Acta* 1178:249, 1993.
219. Darbon J-M, Knecht M, Ranta T, Dufau ML, Catt KJ: Hormonal regulation of cyclic AMP-dependent protein kinase in cultured ovarian granulosa cells. *J Biol Chem* 259:14778, 1984.
220. Cadd GG, Uhler MD, McKnight GS: Holoenzymes of cAMP-dependent protein kinase containing the neural form of type

I regulatory subunit have an increased sensitivity to cyclic nucleotides. *J Biol Chem* 265:19502, 1990.
221. Inagami T: Atrial natriuretic factor. *J Biol Chem* 264:3043, 1989.
222. Lolley RN, Lee RH: Cyclic GMP and photoreceptor function. *FASEB J* 4:3001, 1990.
223. Schulz S, Yuen PST, Garbers DL: The expanding family of guanylyl cyclases. *Trends Pharmacol Sci* 12:116, 1991.
224. Garbers DL: Guanylyl cyclase receptors and their endocrine, paracrine, and autocrine ligands. *Cell* 71:1, 1992.
225. Moncada S, Palmer RMJ, Higgs EA: Nitric oxide: physiology, pathophysiology, and pharmacology. *Pharmacol Rev* 43:109, 1991.
226. Ignarro LJ: Biosynthesis and metabolism of endothelium-derived nitric oxide. *Annu Rev Pharmacol Toxicol* 30:535, 1990.
227. Lowenstein CJ, Snyder SH: Nitric oxide, a novel biologic messenger. *Cell* 70:705, 1992.
228. Marletta MA: Nitric oxide synthase structure and mechanism. *J Biol Chem* 268:12231, 1993.
229. McCall T, Vallance P: Nitric oxide takes center stage with newly defined roles. *Trends Pharmacol Sci* 13:1, 1992.
230. Bradt DS, Hwang PM, Glatt CE, Lowenstein C, Reed RR, Snyder SH: Cloned and expressed nitric oxide synthase structurally resembles cytochrome P-450 reductase. *Nature* 351:714, 1991.
231. Snyder SH, Bredt DS: Nitric oxide as a neuronal messenger. *Trends Pharmacol Sci* 12:125, 1991.
232. Montague PR, Gancayco CD, Winn MJ, Marchase RB, Friedlander MJ: Role of NO production in NMDA receptor-mediated neurotransmitter release in cerebral cortex. *Science* 263:973, 1994.
233. Garthwaite J: Glutamate, nitric oxide and cell-cell signalling in the nervous system. *Trends Neurosci* 14;60:1991.
234. Zhang J, Dawson VL, Dawson TM, Snyder SH: Nitric oxide activation of poly(ADP-ribose) synthetase in neurotoxicity. *Science* 263:687, 1994.
235. Verma A, Hirsch DJ, Glatt CE, Ronnett GV, Snyder SH: Carbon monoxide: A putative neural messenger. *Science* 259:381, 1993.
236. Burnett AL, Lowenstein CJ, Bredt DS, Chang TSK, Snyder SH: Nitric oxide: A physiologic mediator of penile erection. *Science* 257:401, 1992.
237. Rubin RP: The role of calcium in the release of neurotransmitter substances and hormones. *Pharmacol Rev* 22:389, 1970.
238. Adelstein RS, Klee CB, Rodbell M (eds): Sixth International Conference on Cyclic Nucleotides, Calcium, and Protein Phosphorylaton. *Advances in Second Messenger and Phosphoprotein Research*. New York, Raven, 1988, p. 222.
239. Stoclet JC, Boulanger-Saunier C, Lassegue B, Lugnier C: Cyclic nucleotides and calcium regulation in heart and smooth muscle cells. Ann NY Acad Sci 522:106, 1988.
240. Berridge MJ: The interaction of cyclic nucleotides and calcium in the control of cellular activity. *Adv Cyclic Nucleotide Res* 6:1, 1975.
241. Cheung WY: Calmodulin plays a pivotal role in cellular regulation. *Science* 207:19, 1980.
242. Sweeney HL, Bowman BF, Stull JT: Myosin light chain phosphorylation in vertebrate striated muscle: Regulation and function. *Am J Physiol* 264:1085, 1993.
243. Cohen P, Klee CB: *Calmodulin: Molecular Aspects of Cellular Regulation*, vol 5. Amsterdam, Netherlands, Elsevier, 1988.
244. Heizmann CW, Hunziker W: Intracellular calcium-binding proteins: More sites than insights. *Trends Biochem Sci* 16:98, 1991.
245. Geiser JR, van Tuinen D, Brockerhoff SE, Neff MM, Davis TN: Can calmodulin function without binding calcium? *Cell* 65:949, 1991.
246. Babu YS, Sack JS, Greenbough TJ, Bugg CE, Means AR, Cook WI: Three-dimensional structure of calmodulin. *Nature* 315:37, 1985.
247. Colbran RJ, Fong YL, Schworer CM, Soderling TR: Regulatory interactions of the calmodulin-binding, inhibitory, and autophosphorylation domains of the Ca^{2+}/calmodulin-dependent protein kinase II. *J Biol Chem* 263:18145, 1988.
248. Soderling TR: Protein kinases: Regulation by autoinhibitory domains. *J Biol Chem* 265:1823, 1990.
249. Cruzalegui FH, Means AR: Biochemical characterization of the multifunctional Ca^{2+}/calmodulin-dependent protein kinase type IV expressed in insect cells. *J Biol Chem* 268: 26171, 1993.
250. Fruman DA, Klee CB, Bierer BE, Burakoff SJ: Calcineurin phosphatase activity in T lymphocytes is inhibited by FK 506 and cyclosporin A. *Proc Natl Acad Sci USA* 89:3686, 1992.
251. Nishizuka Y: The molecular heterogeneity of protein kinase C and its implications for cellular regulation. *Nature* 334:661, 1988.
252. Huang K-P: The mechanism of protein kinase C activation. *Trends Neurosci* 12:425, 1989.
253. Drummond AH, Macintyre DE: Protein kinase C as a bidirectional regulator of cell function. *Trends Pharmacol Sci* 6:233, 1985.
254. Huang K-P, Nakabayashi H, Huang FL: Isozymic forms of rat brain Ca^{2+}-activated and phospholipid-dependent protein kinase. *Proc Natl Acad Sci USA* 83:8535, 1986.
255. Coussens L, Parker PJ, Rhee L, Yang-Fen TL, Chen E, Waterfield MD, Francke U, Ullrich A: Multiple, distinct forms of bovine and human protein kinase C suggest diversity in cellular signaling pathways. *Science* 233:859, 1986.
256. Olds JL, Alkon DL: A role for protein kinase C in associative learning. *New Biologist* 3:27, 1991.
257. Hug H, Sarre TF: Protein kinase C isoenzymes: Divergence in signal transduction? *Biochem J* 291:329, 1993.
258. Perin MS, Fried VA, Mignery GA, Jahn R, Sudhof TC: Phospholipid binding by a synaptic vesicle protein homologous to the regulatory region of protein kinase C. *Nature* 345:260, 1990.
259. Hubbard SR, Bishop WR, Kirschmeier P, George SJ, Cramer SP, Hendrickson WA: Identification and characterization of zinc binding sites in protein kinase C. *Science* 254:1776, 1991.
260. Huang K-P, Huang FL: How is protein kinase C activated in CNS. *Neurochem Int* 22:417, 1993.
261. Wilkinson SE, Hallam TJ: Protein kinase C: Is its pivotal role in cellular activation overstated? *Trends Pharmacol Sci* 15:53, 1994.
262. Nakanishi H, Brewer KA, Exton JH: Activation of the ζ isozyme of protein kinase C by phosphatidylinositol 3,4,5-triphosphate. *J Biol Chem* 268:13, 1993.
263. Bell RM, Burns DJ: Lipid activation of protein kinase C. *J Biol Chem* 266:4661, 1992.
264. Pears C, Stabel S, Cazaubon S, Parker PJ: Studies on the phosphorylation of protein kinase C-alpha. *Biochem J* 283:515, 1992.
265. Glaser KB, Mobilio D, Chang JY, Senko N: Phospholipase A_2 enzymes: Regulation and inhibition. *Trends Pharmacol Sci* 14:92, 1993.
266. Bomalaski JS, Steiner MR, Simon PL, Clark MA: IL-1 increases phospholipase A_2 activity, expression of phospholipase A_2-activating protein, and release of linoleic acid from the murine T helper cell line EL-4. *J Immunol* 148:155, 1992.
267. Raz A, Wyche A, Needleman P: Temporal and pharmacological division of fibroblast cyclooxygenase expression into transcriptional and translational phases. *Proc Natl Acad Sci USA* 86:1657, 1989.
268. Hokin MR, Hokin LE: Enzyme secretion and the incorporation of P^{32} into phospholipids of pancreas slices. *J Biol Chem* 203:967, 1953.
269. Michell RH: Inositol phospholipids and cell surface receptor functions. *Biochim Biophys Acta* 415:81, 1975.
270. Berridge MJ: Phosphatidylinositol hydrolysis: A multifunc-

tional transducing mechanism. *Mol Cell Endocrinol* 24:115, 1981.
271. Berridge MJ, Dawson RMC, Downes CP, Heslop JP, Irvine RF: Changes in the levels of inositol phosphates after agonist-dependent hydrolysis of membrane phosphoinositides. *Biochem J* 212:473, 1983.
272. Burgess GM, Godfrey PP, McKinney JS, Berridge MJ, Irvine RF, Putney JW: The second messenger linking receptor activation to internal Ca release in liver. *Nature* 309:63, 1984.
273. Streb H, Heslop JP, Irvine RF, Schulz I, Berridge MJ: Relationship between secretagogue-induced Ca^{2+} release and inositol polyphosphate production in permeabilized pancreatic acinar cells. *J Biol Chem* 260:7309, 1985.
274. Boynton AL, Dean NM, Hill TD: Inositol 1,3,4,5-tetrakisphosphate and regulation of intracellular calcium. *Biochem Pharmacol* 40:1933, 1990.
275. Choi KY, Kim HK, Lee SY, Moon KH, Sim SS, Kim JW, Chung H, Rhee SH: Molecular cloning and expression of a complementary DNA for inositol 1,4,5-triphosphate 3-kinase. *Science* 248:64, 1990.
276. Majerus PW, Connolly TM, Bansal VS, Inhorn RC, et al: Inositol phosphates: Synthesis and degradation. *J Biol Chem* 263:3051, 1988.
277. Mennitis FS, Oliver KG, Putney JW, Shears SB: Inositol phosphates and cell signaling: New views of $InsP_5$ and $InsP_6$. *Trends Biochem Sci* 18:53, 1993.
278. Rhee SG, Choi KD: Multiple forms of phospholipase C and their activation mechanisms. *Adv Second Mess Phosphopr Res* 26:11, 1992.
279. Whitman M, Cantley L: Phosphoinositide metabolism and the control of cell proliferation. *Biochim Biophys Acta* 948:327, 1988.
280. Gill DL, Ghosh TK, Mullaney JM: Calcium signalling mechanisms in endoplasmic reticulum activated by inositol 1,4,5-triphosphate and GTP. *Cell Calcium* 10:363, 1989.
281. Khan AA, Steiner JP, Klein MG, Schneider MF, Snyder SH: IP_3 receptor: Localization to plasma membrane of T cells and cocapping with the T cell receptor. *Science* 257:815, 1992.
282. Ferris CD, Snyder SH: Inositol 1,4,5-triphosphate-activated channels. *Annu Rev Physiol* 54:469, 1992.
283. Furuichi T, Yoshikawa S, Miyawaki A, Wada K, Maeda N, Mikoshiba K: Primary structure and functional expression of the inositol 1,4,5-triphosphate binding protein P400. *Nature* 342:32, 1989.
284. Sorrentino V, Volpe P: Ryanodine receptors: How many, where and why? *Trends Pharmacol Sci* 14:98, 1993.
285. Mikoshiba K: Inositol 1,4,5-triphosphate receptor. *Trends Pharmacol Sci* 14:86, 1993.
286. McPherson PS, Campbell KP: The ryanodine receptor/Ca^{2+} release channel. *J Biol Chem* 268:13765, 1993.
287. Duefel T: Golla A, Iles D, Meindl A, Meitinger T, Schindelhaver D, DeVries A, et al: Evidence for genetic heserogeneity of malignant hyperthermia susceptibility. *Am J Hum Genet* 50:1151, 1992.
288. Galione A: Cyclic ADP-ribose: A new way to control calcium. *Science* 259:325, 1993.
289. Ettehadieh E, Sanghera JS, Pelech SL, Hess-Bienz D, Watts J, Shastri N, Aebersold R: Tyrosyl phosphorylation and activation of MAP kinases by $p56^{lck}$. *Science* 255:853, 1992.
290. Stephens L, Jackson T, Hawkins PT: Agonist-stimulated synthesis of phosphatidylinositol (3,4,5)-trisphosphate: A new intracellular signalling system? *Biochim Biophys Acta* 1179:27, 1993.
291. Hirata F, Axelrod J: Phospholipid methylation and transmission of biological signals through membranes. *Science* 209:1082, 1980.
292. Nieto A, Catt KJ: Hormonal activation of phospholipid methyltransferase in the Leydig cell. *Endocrinology* 113:758, 1983.
293. Cobb MH, Boulton TG, Robbins DJ: Extracellular signal-related kinases: ERKs in progress. *Cell Regulation* 2:965, 1991.
294. Rossomando A, Wu J, Weber MJ, Sturgell TW: The phorbol ester-dependent activation of the mitogen-activated protein kinase $p42^{mapk}$ is a kinase with specificity for threonine and tyrosine residues. *Proc Natl Acad Sci USA* 89:5221, 1992.
295. Marx J: Forging a path to the nucleus. *Science* 260:1588, 1993.
296. Davis RJ: The mitogen-activated protein kinase signal transduction pathway. *J Biol Chem* 268:14553, 1993.
297. Pulverer BJ, Kryiakis JM, Avruch J, Nikolakaki E, Woodgett JR: Phosphorylation of c-jun mediated by MAP kinases. *Nature* 353:670, 1991.
298. Hunter T: Cytokine connections. *Nature* 366:114, 1993.
299. Müller M, Briscoe J, Laxton C, Guschin D, Ziemiecki A, Silvennoinen O, et al: Protein tyrosine kinase JAK1 complements defects in interferon-α/β and-γ signal transduction. *Nature* 366:129, 1993.
300. Shuai K, Stark GR, Kerr IM, Darnell JE: A single phosphotyrosine residue of Stat91 required for gene activation by interferon-γ. *Science* 261:1744, 1993.
301. Montminy M: Trying on a new pair of SH2s. *Science* 261:1694, 1993.
302. McMahon SB, Monroe JG: Role of primary response genes in generating cellular responses to growth factors. *FASEB J* 6:2707, 1992.
303. Meek DW, Street AJ: Nuclear protein phosphorylation and growth control. *Biochem J* 287:1, 1992.
304. Karin M, Smeal T: Control of transcription factors by signal transduction pathways: the beginning of the end. *Trends Biochem Sci* 17:418, 1992.
305. Gille H, Sharrocks AD, Shaw PE: Phosphorylation of transcription factor $p62^{TCF}$ by MAP kinase stimulates ternary complex formation at *c-fos* promoter. *Nature* 358:414, 1992.
306. Kerppola TK, Curran T: Fos-Jun heterodimers and Jun homodimers bend DNA in opposite orientations: implications for transcription factor cooperativity. *Cell* 66:317, 1991.
307. Lewin B: Oncogenic conversion by regulatory changes in transcription factors. *Cell* 64:303, 1991.
308. Collart MA, Tourkine N, Belin D, Vassali P, Jeanteur P, Blanchard JM: *c-fos* gene transcription in murine macrophages is modulated by a calcium-dependent block to elongation in intron 1. *Mol Cell Biol* 11:2826, 1991.
309. Angel P, Hattori K, Smeal T, Karin M: The *jun* proto-oncogene is positively autoregulated by its product, Jun/AP-1. *Cell* 55:875, 1988.
310. Hunter T, Karin M: The regulation of transcription by phosphorylation. *Cell* 70:375, 1992.

CHAPTER 5B

Molecular Mechanisms of Hormone Action: Regulation of Target Cell Function by the Steroid Hormone Receptor Supergene Family

Jan Carlstedt-Duke
Anthony Wright
Martin Göttlicher
Sam Okret
Jan-Åke Gustafsson

As introduced in Chap. 5A, the mechanisms of action of the steroid hormones are generally similar to those of thyroid hormone, vitamin D, and retinoic acid and its analogues. Therefore, these hormones are discussed here as a group. These similarities have been appreciated for some time; however, recent analyses of the genes that encode the receptors for these hormones have provided a more detailed understanding of the receptors. These genes share many structural similarities and apparently have evolved from a common evolutionary precursor. Their products have common activities that regulate the expression of specific genes at the transcriptional level. In addition to the known receptors for hormones and retinoids, this gene family encodes transcription factors that are not hormone receptors and probably encodes receptors whose ligands have not been identified. The family is called by different names that refer to the ligands that bind to its products; in this chapter, it is termed the *steroid hormone receptor supergene family*.

In spite of the overall functional and structural similarities of these gene products, there are differences in how the various hormones interact with these receptors and the steps that lead to effects on the transcription of specific genes. For these reasons, the products of the superfamily are described under categories such as steroid hormone receptors and thyroid hormone receptors. The mechanisms of actions of the steroid hormones have been studied the most extensively and are described first, although they are also compared to the receptors that are discussed subsequently.

MECHANISMS OF ACTION OF STEROID HORMONES

There are five major classes of steroid hormones (Table 5B-1). These hormones are classified on the basis of the receptors through which their actions are mediated. Whereas glucocorticoid receptors are present in most human tissues, the receptors for androgens, estrogens, mineralocorticoids, and vitamin D have a more limited distribution. The receptor content in general is several thousand molecules per cell, although considerable variations are found. Table 5B-1 also lists the major hormones responsible for actions through the various receptors and other properties. More information about the actions of the individual steroid hormones is provided in the specific chapters on the respective glands. Whereas the active component of vitamin D, 1,25-dihydroxycholecalciferol, is not strictly a steroid, its receptor is ordinarily considered a steroid receptor, and information about 1,25-dihydroxycholecalciferol and its receptor is included.

Figure 5B-1 shows the structures of representative hormones of the group, along with agonist analogues and antagonists. Additional structures of various steroids are described in individual chapters on the various glands that secrete them (see Chaps. 10, 12, 16, and 17), and the structures of vitamin D and its metabolites are discussed in Chap. 23. As indicated in Table 5B-1, in most cases a single steroid mediates most of the actions of a given class of receptors, although with androgen and mineralocorticoid receptors, for example, more than one steroid is in-

TABLE 5B-1 Classes of Steroid Hormones

Receptor	Major Steroid in Humans	Other Steroids That Act through the Receptor	Antagonist Examples	Major Action	Sites of Production
Glucocorticoid	Cortisol	Corticosterone Prednisone Dexamethasone	RU-486	Most tissues; carbohydrate and intermediary metabolism, stress and immune responses	Adrenal fasciculata, reticularis
Mineralocorticoid	Aldosterone Cortisol	Deoxycorticosterone	Spironolactone	Na^+, K^+ balance	Adrenal glomerulosa
Androgen	Dihydrotestosterone Testosterone		Spironolactone Cyproterone	Male sexual, reproductive functions	Testis, adrenal
Estrogen	Estradiol	Estrone Estriol	Tamoxifen	Female sexual, reproductive functions	Ovary, follicle
Progestin	Progesterone		RU-486	Female sexual, reproductive functions	Ovary, corpus luteum
Vitamin D	1,25-Dihydroxy-cholecalciferol			Mineral metabolism	Kidney

volved. In addition, other steroids are important in certain physiologic or pathologic circumstances or with steroid therapy; some examples of these are listed. The table also lists examples of antagonists that block or partially block (partial antagonists) ligand actions through that particular class of receptors and that have important research and/or clinical uses.

After the synthesis of radioactively labeled estradiol with a high specific activity 30 years ago,[1] the basic mechanism of action of steroid hormones was rapidly established during the following decade.[2] Specific intracellular receptor proteins for each of the five major classes of steroid hormones were demonstrated and isolated with the aid of radioactively labeled ligands. A common mechanism of action postulated at an early stage involved first the binding of hormone by the receptor and then interaction of the hormone-receptor complex with the genome, with consequent influences on the transcription of specific genes. The details of these overall stages have been clarified greatly during recent years, and we are now beginning to understand these processes at the molecular level.

The basic mechanism of action of the steroid hormones and other ligands of the family is shown in Fig. 5B-2. Steroids are lipophilic compounds and as such can freely diffuse through the cell membrane. Although some studies have suggested that a facilitated uptake of glucocorticoids can occur,[3] the consensus is that the majority of steroid hormones enter the target cell by passive diffusion. Within the target cell, a soluble receptor protein binds the steroid with high affinity, and the presence of a specific type of receptor protein within a cell is critical for determining whether that cell can respond to the corresponding steroid. Each of the five major steroid hormone receptors, along with the vitamin D receptor, is the product of a single gene. These receptors have molecular weights of around 90,000. In general, one form of each receptor is produced, except that two forms of the progesterone receptors (the A and B forms) are produced; these forms differ in their amino termini and are formed through differential splicing of RNA. However, a multitude of biological effects are elicited by a given steroid hormone in different tissues. This pleiotropy of response to a steroid is determined by events subsequent to the binding of a steroid.

Before the binding of ligand, the steroid hormone and vitamin D receptors are associated with *chaperone proteins* that are *heat shock proteins (hsp)*. Steroid receptors have been shown to be associated with hsp90, hsp70, and hsp56.[4–9] The result of this association is a large receptor complex of up to several hundred thousand in molecular weight that sediments through a glycerol or sucrose gradient at around 8 S. The complex can be demonstrated in vitro after the binding of steroid to the receptor under conditions of low temperature and low ionic strength. The complex is stabilized by the addition of molybdate to the buffer.[10–14] Under physiologic conditions, binding of the steroid hormone to the receptor results in the dissociation of the chaperone proteins from the receptor, enabling the receptor to interact with the genome by binding to DNA. Under physiologic conditions, it is only after the binding of the steroid hormone (or in special circumstances in response to other effector substances, as described later) that the receptor protein can bind to DNA. The steroid receptors apparently bind to DNA as homodimers, with dimerization occurring after the dissociation of the chaperone proteins[15–18] (see below).

After the steroid-induced dissociation of the chaperone proteins, the androgen, glucocorticoid, mineralocorticoid, and progestin receptors sediment at a rate of 4 S in apparently monomeric forms. However, the estrogen receptor complex sediments at an

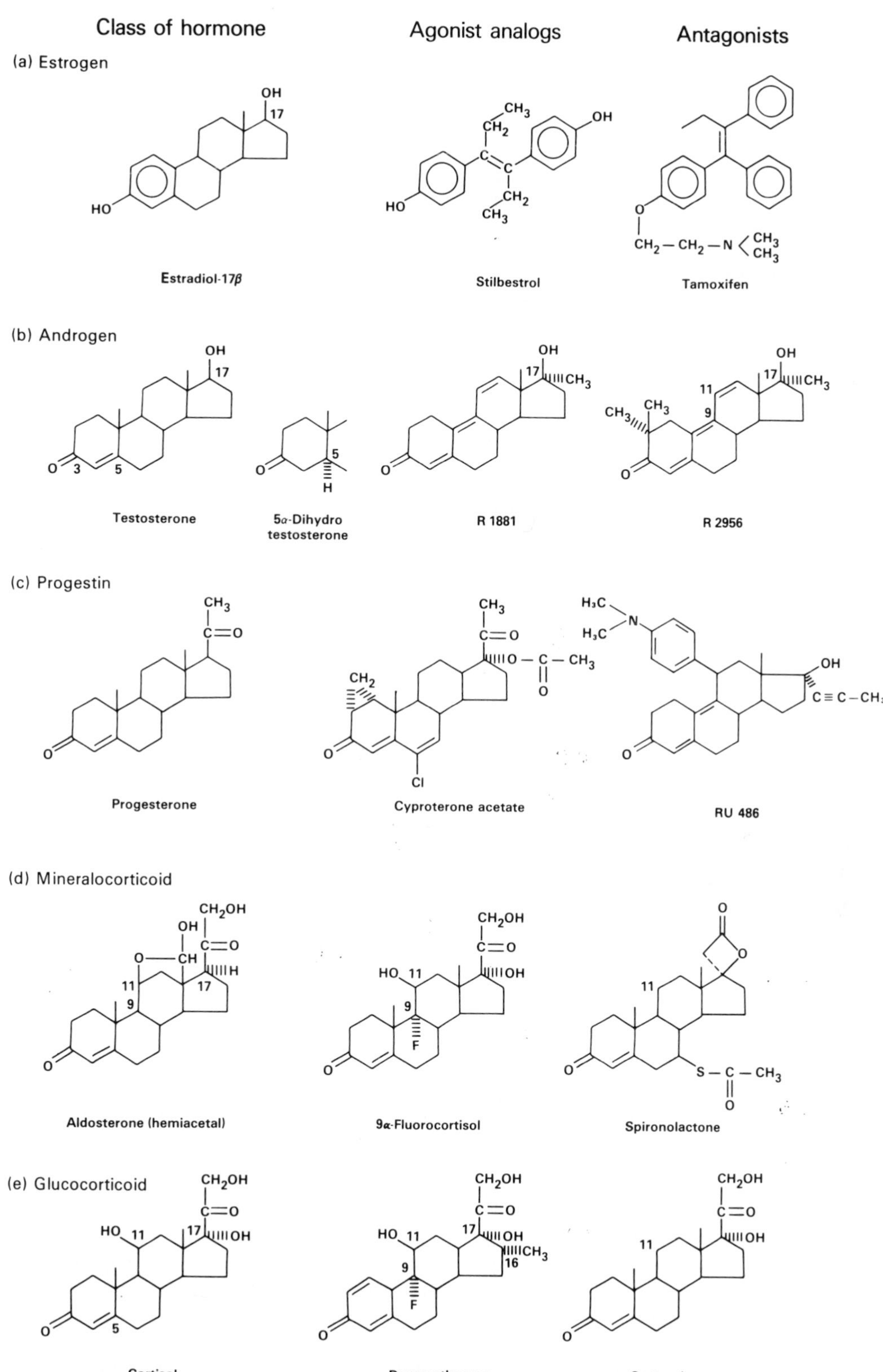

FIGURE 5B-1 Structures of the major classes of steroid hormones.

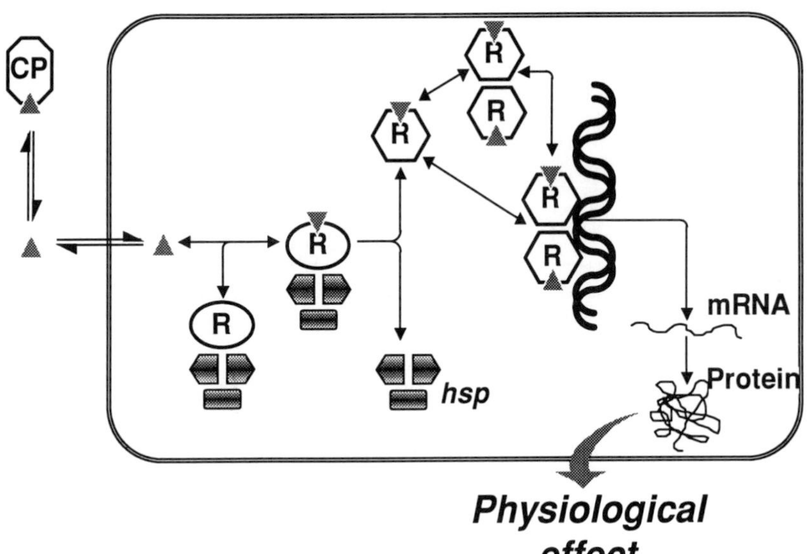

FIGURE 5B-2 Mechanism of action of the steroid hormone receptors (R). The steroid (Δ) reaches the target cell bound to a carrier protein (CP). The receptors are soluble proteins that interact with DNA in a hormone-dependent manner. The intracellular location of the receptor proteins before DNA binding (i.e., cytoplasmic or nuclear) has been a matter of debate in some cases. Before hormone binding, the steroid receptor proteins are associated with chaperone proteins [heat shock proteins (hsp)]. This is not the case for some other members of this superfamily, e.g., the retinoic acid and thyroid hormone receptors.

intermediate rate of 5.4 S[15] and appears to be a homodimer. More recently, it has been shown that the glucocorticoid and progestin receptors also bind to DNA as homodimers[16–21]; it would seem that the estrogen receptor forms more stable homodimers than do the other steroid receptors.

The process by which the chaperone proteins dissociate from the receptor after steroid binding, resulting in the acquisition of the ability of the receptor to bind to DNA, has been termed *activation* or *transformation*. This has been postulated to result from a steroid-dependent conformational change of the receptor protein. However, the molecular basis of this step in steroid action has not been clarified. After activation/transformation and dimerization, the receptor binds tightly to specific DNA sequences in the proximity of genes regulated by the steroid in question. (The receptor also can bind to nonspecific DNA sequences, but with a much lower affinity.) Binding of the receptor protein to the specific DNA sequence, termed the *hormone response element (HRE)*,[22] results in the interaction of the steroid receptor with other transcriptional factors and the basic transcriptional complex. These interactions affect the rate of initiation of transcription of the gene in either a positive or a negative manner. Although the receptor protein for a specific steroid hormone is identical in all target cells within an organism, the network of genes that can be regulated through binding by the receptor to HREs varies from cell type to cell type and results from differentiation. These differences in hormone-regulated gene networks determine the various biological effects of hormones in different target cells.

It was subsequently shown that thyroid hormone, vitamin D, and retinoic acid and its analogues act through a similar mechanism of action, with some variation in the details. In contrast to steroid receptor proteins that are products of single genes, several different genes encode both the thyroid hormone and retinoic acid receptors (see below). Furthermore, the receptors for these two classes of ligands do not form complexes with chaperone proteins but apparently bind to DNA in the absence of hormone/vitamin.[23,24] Although thyroid hormone and retinoic acid receptors can form homodimers, they preferentially bind to DNA as heterodimers with retinoid X receptors or unknown proteins (see below).

In addition to the specific receptor proteins, target cells have been shown to contain other proteins that bind steroid and thyroid hormones, vitamin D, and retinoic acid with high affinity and specificity.[25,26] The affinity of these proteins for the corresponding ligand is in general lower than that of the corresponding receptor protein. The function of these proteins is in most cases unknown. It has been speculated that the proteins that bind thyroid hormone and retinoic acid are intracellular transport proteins that deliver the ligand to the DNA-bound receptor in the nucleus. The retinoid-binding proteins also may play an active role in regulating the level of biologically active retinoic acid in cells during morphogenesis.[27,28] In some cases, the "nonreceptor" hormone-binding proteins may act to regulate hormone availability. For example this may be the case with the androgen-binding protein in the testis and a glucocorticoid-binding protein in the kidney (see Chap. 12). In other cases, these proteins are enzymes involved in hormone metabolism.

Plasma Binding of Steroid Hormones

In the circulation, the steroid hormones are present both free and bound to plasma proteins. Plasma binding is discussed in more detail in Chap. 4 and the chapters that address the individual glands that produce these hormones. The binding involves both specific high-affinity interactions with proteins such as corticosteroid-binding globulin and sex hormone–binding globulins and lower-affinity interactions with proteins such as albumin. It appears that it is the free steroid that is available for entering the cell and binding to the receptors. The plasma-bound steroid probably serves mostly as a reservoir for the hormone that can assure a more even delivery of the hormone to the target tissues as the blood circulates through them. In general, the rates of dissociation of steroids from albumin are much faster than the rates from the specific high-affinity plasma-binding proteins. Therefore, these proteins may be more effective than albumin in providing steroid for the distal portions of the tissue. In this context, both the free and the albumin-bound steroids are taken up through the blood-brain barrier whereas the globulin-bound steroid is not transported into the brain. In rat plasma, this would account for 60 percent of the progesterone, 40 percent of the testosterone, and 15 percent of the corticosteroid (corticosterone), in contrast to the 2 to 8 percent of the hormone that is free. For all these reasons, it is critical to be aware of influences on plasma binding in evaluating disorders of steroid hormone secretion and considering the actions and pharmacokinetics of endogenous or administered steroids.

Structures of Steroid Hormone Receptors

A schematic overview of the structures of the steroid hormone receptors is given in Fig. 5B-3. Other details of these structures are described in subsequent sections. Overall, these molecules have three domains. The amino-terminal domain is usually referred to as the transactivation domain; this domain enhances the transcriptional regulatory activities of the receptors. The region $\tau 1$ shown in Fig. 5B-3 contains the residues that are critical for this function. This region is also heavily phosphorylated. The middle portion of the molecule (indicated by the dark bar) contains the DNA-binding domain (DBD) that is responsible for the specific DNA-binding activities of the receptors and contains weak dimerization, nuclear localization, and transcriptional transactivation functions. The carboxy-terminal portion of the molecule contains the hormone-binding function. This portion of the molecule also contains residues that interact with hsp90, a nuclear localization signal, dimerization functions, and transcriptional transactivation activity.

The various structures of the steroid receptors function in a modular manner. Thus, if the steroid-binding domain of the glucocorticoid receptor is inserted to replace that of the estrogen receptor, the resulting chimeric receptor will respond to glucocorticoids but act on an estrogen response element. The amino-terminal transactivation domain of one receptor can replace that of another receptor, although with some difference in activity.

Steroid Binding

Steroids bind reversibly and with high affinity to their receptors. The thermodynamics of the binding generally resemble bimolecular reactions, as shown in Fig. 5B-4; in this case, the concentration of free steroid that half-maximally saturates the receptors equals the equilibrium dissociation constant, K_d, for binding. In general, the concentrations of free steroids in the plasma are below the equilibrium dissociation constants (K_d) for binding to the receptors. This implies that changes in the concentrations of active steroids in plasma will result in changes in the occupancy of the receptor by the steroids and consequently in the biological responses. Although there are a number of exceptions, in many cases the magnitude of a steroid hormone response parallels the relative saturation of the receptor by that steroid (Fig. 5B-4). This implies that the receptor is relatively limiting for steroid hormone responses, and when receptor levels are increased through the use of gene transfer techniques (see Chap. 3), steroid responses can be obtained that are much greater than those obtained with endogenous receptors.

In general, under physiologic conditions, the rate of association of the steroid with the receptor is rapid, with binding occurring within minutes. Similarly, the rate of dissociation of the steroid from the receptor is usually relatively rapid, with half-lives for dissociation generally in the order of minutes. Thus, the kinetics of steroid association with the receptors do not usually limit steroid responses; conversely, whereas the dissociation of the steroid from the receptors results in a rapid termination of the signal, the biological responses ordinarily persist for a significant period after the dissociation has occurred because the steroid-induced mRNAs and proteins take more time to be degraded.

The steroid hormone–binding domain recognizes a particular three-dimensional configuration. These domains have evolved such that, for example, the progesterone receptor binds progesterone with a high affinity and has almost no affinity for estradiol. However, there can be some overlap in binding such that the receptors for one class of steroid sometimes can bind other steroids. For example, the mineralocorticoid receptors can bind the glucocorticoid cortisol with a high affinity so that they use cortisol predominantly in some tissues (see Chap. 12), and cortisol in excess can lead to mineralocorticoid hypertension (see Chap. 14).

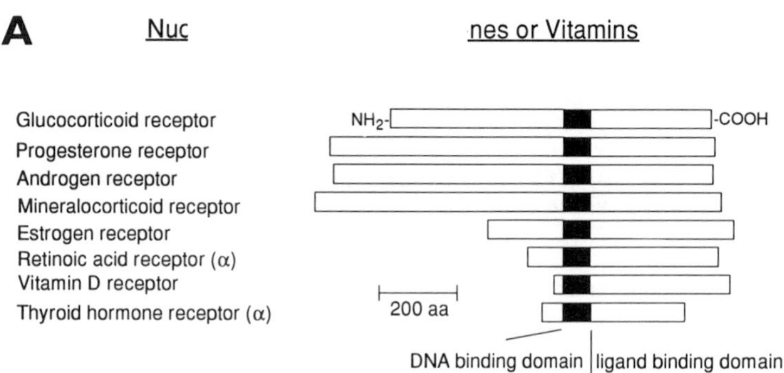

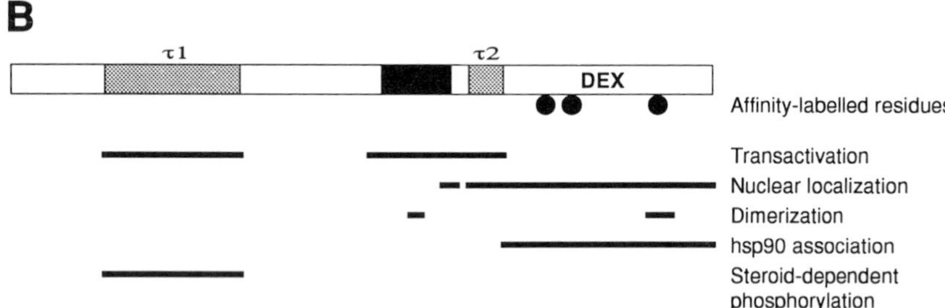

FIGURE 5B-3 (*A*) Comparison of the primary structures of the nuclear receptors for hormones and vitamins. The primary structures are depicted by the open bars in proportion to the size of the proteins. The most highly conserved region of the members of this superfamily of proteins is the DNA-binding domain (filled region). (*B*) Functional regions of the glucocorticoid receptor based on analysis of human, mouse, and rat receptors. For details of the functions listed, see text.

The C-terminal ligand-binding domain of the steroid receptors is less well conserved in the estrogen and vitamin D receptors than in the other four steroid receptor proteins. Affinity labeling of the estrogen (ER), progestin (PR), and glucocorticoid (GR) receptors has identified three different segments within the 200- to 250-residue steroid-binding domain (Fig. 5B-5).[29–33] One segment (containing Cys-638 in human GR) specifically recognizes the side-chain structure of glucocorticoids, as it can be affinity-labeled by dexamethasone 21-mesylate.[30–33]

The other two segments identified interact with the A-ring structure of the steroid, as they can be affinity-labeled by photoactivation of the A ring.[30,31] In the first segment, a common Met residue in both GR and PR (Fig. 5B-5) can be labeled by either a synthetic glucocorticoid or a synthetic progestin.[30] The third segment, the most C-terminal of the three, displays clear differences in the affinity labeling with the three different receptors (Fig. 5B-5). A Cys residue was labeled in both ER and GR,[29–31] whereas a Met residue was labeled in PR,[30] and the positions of the residues do not correspond in the three receptors after sequence alignment (Fig. 5B-5). The differences in this region probably play a role in determining the specificity of binding by the various steroids. Each of the three segments is predominantly hydrophobic in nature.[31] Hydrophobic interactions play an important role in steroid binding, and it would seem that the steroid-binding domain folds to form a hydrophobic steroid-binding surface. Insertions or point mutations almost anywhere within this domain disrupt steroid binding.[34–39]

Chaperone Proteins

As described above, unliganded steroid receptors exist in a high-molecular-weight-complex form. Studies using antibodies against hsp90 and physicochemical analyses of the complex with the GR and the proteins after dissociation indicate that the complex consists of one subunit receptor protein (monomeric) and two subunits of hsp90.[40–42] More recently, there have been reports of other members of the heat shock family associated with the receptor, hsp70 and hsp56. Hsp90 and hsp56 have been reported only in association with the nonactivated (non-DNA-binding) form of receptor proteins.[4–9] Hsp70, by contrast, has been found in association with PR and GR even after activation.[43,44] The role of the different heat shock proteins in steroid hormone action is unclear.

Analysis of complex formation of deletion mutants of GR in the presence of molybdate has indicated that the primary site of interaction between receptor and heat shock protein occurs within the steroid-binding domain[45,46] (Fig. 5B-3). In fact, deletion of this region results in a receptor that has weak constitutive activity, i.e., is capable of inducing transcriptional activation in the absence of steroid.[34–39] Also, treatment of the cytosolic receptor with high salt in the absence of steroid results in dissociation of the chaperone proteins and activation of the recep-

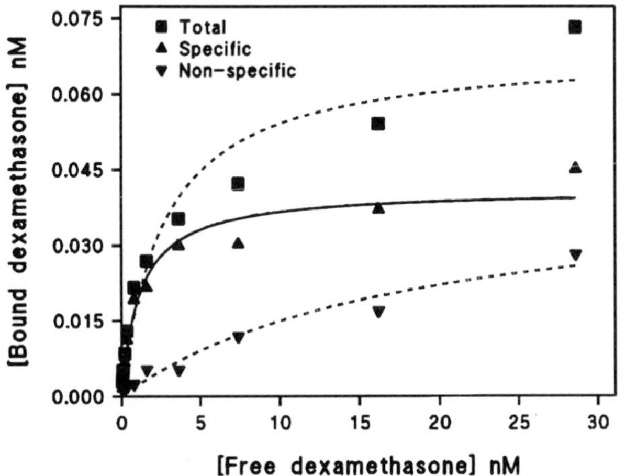

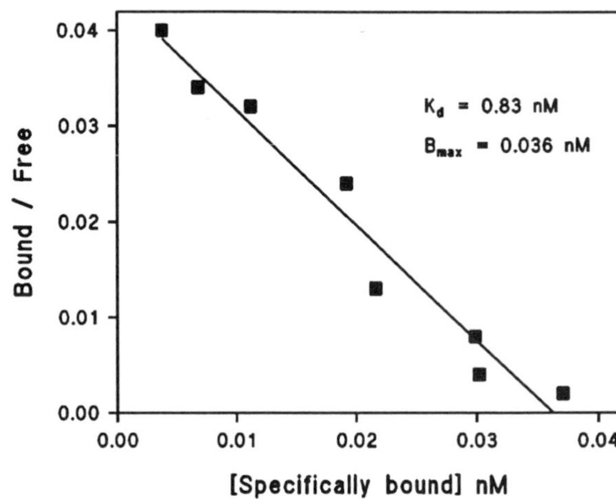

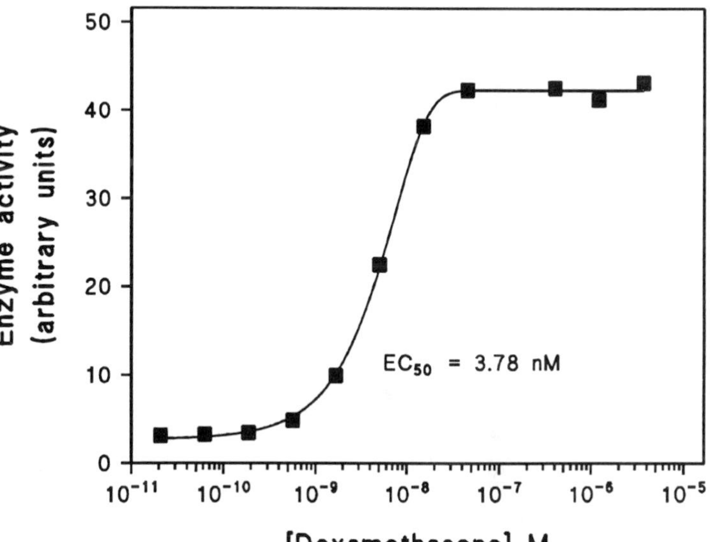

FIGURE 5B-4 Dose-response data for receptor-mediated steroid binding and transcriptional regulation. The human glucocorticoid receptor was expressed in Chinese hamster ovary (CHO) cells together with a reporter gene, alkaline phosphatase, under transcriptional regulation by the glucocorticoid receptor. In the upper left panel, equilibrium binding of ^{3}H-dexamethasone (whole cell binding assay) in the absence (total binding, ■---■) or presence (nonspecific binding ▼----▼) of 200-fold radioinert dexamethasone is shown. Specific binding (▲—▲) is calculated by subtracting nonspecific binding from the total binding. Scatchard analysis of the specific binding is shown in the upper right panel. The equilibrium constant for dissociation (K_d) is calculated from the slope of the line. Dose-response data for dexamethasone on glucocorticoid receptor-mediated regulation of alkaline phosphatase activity are shown in the lower panel. *(Data by courtesy of Stefan Nilsson, KaroBio AB, Huddinge, Sweden.)*

tor's specific DNA-binding activity.[47] Thus, one probable role of the heat shock proteins is to mask the DNA-binding site of the receptor protein, thus blocking any interaction with the genome in the absence of steroid. Fusion of the GR steroid-binding domain with other DNA-binding proteins results in a chimeric protein that binds DNA in a steroid-dependent manner.[48,49] The suppressive effect of the steroid-binding domain in the fusion protein is relatively independent of position, which would indicate that it is not a direct interaction between the two domains that blocks DNA binding. Rather, it is more likely that the suppressive effect is mediated by another factor, such as binding of the chaperone proteins.

At least in the case of the glucocorticoid receptor, the association of hsp90 with the receptor has been shown to play a role in steroid binding. Dissociation of the chaperone proteins by exposure to high ionic strength results in a decrease in affinity for steroid by at least 100-fold.[50] Expression of the GR steroid-binding domain in bacteria results in a product that does not appear to be associated with heat shock proteins with the same low affinity as in the previous case.[51] However, expression of exactly the same constructions by in vitro translation in a rabbit reticulocyte lysate system results in a complex with heat shock proteins that binds steroid with normal affinity.[51] The chaperone proteins appear to play a role in maintaining the correct folding in the GR that is necessary to maintain a normal steroid-binding function.

Dimerization

As was stated earlier, the estrogen-receptor complexes occur in solution as dimers,[15] and more recently GRs have been shown to occur less stably as dimers in solution.[17] In any case, the steroid receptors ultimately bind to the DNA as dimers, and the formation of dimers increases the affinity of the recep-

hGR	597	QYSW*M*FL**M**AFALGWR
hPR	752	QYSWMSL**M**VFGLGWR
hAR	738	QYS*W*MGLMVF*AM*GW*R*
hMR	803	QYSWMCLSSFALSWR
hER	380	ECAWLEILMIGLVWR

hGR	631	EQRMTLP**C**MY*D*QCKH
hPR	786	EQRMKESSFYSLCLT
hAR	772	*E*Y*R*MHKSR*M*YSQCV*R*
hMR	837	EEKMHQSAMYELCQG
hER	413	NQGKCVEGMVEIFDM

hGR	729	VENLLNY***C***FQTFLDK.TMSIEFPEMLAEII
hPR	884	VKQLHLYCLNTFIQSRALSVEFPEM**M**SEVI
hAR	870	A*R*ELHQF*T*FDLLI*K*SHMVS*V*DFPEMMEAII
hMR	935	VSDLLEFCFYTFRESHALKVEFPAMLVEII
hER	518	SNKGME...HLYSMK**C**KNVVPLYDLLLEML

FIGURE 5B-5 Steroid-binding amino acid residues identified in the human (h) glucocorticoid receptor (GR) and the human progestin (hPR), mineralocorticoid (hMR), androgen (hAR), and estrogen receptor (ER) using affinity labeling with radioactive steroids and radiosequence analysis of the complex. The amino acids (in bold) have been affinity-labeled. Mutations of the amino acids (in italic) have been reported to affect steroid binding and receptor function.

tor proteins for their respective HREs,[20] presumably by increasing the size of the contact surface with DNA. It has been shown for the estrogen[16] and progesterone[52] receptors that the major dimerization interactions are mediated by residues within the steroid-binding domain. In the case of the estrogen receptor, the residues involved in the primary contact surfaces for the dimerization interaction have been narrowed down to a 22-amino acid segment close to the C-terminal end of the protein.[20] This segment is characterized by a heptad repeat of hydrophobic amino acids with additional hydrophobic residues at intermediate positions and is conserved in all members of the nuclear receptor family, suggesting that it may represent a common dimerization mechanism for all the receptor proteins. This conservation suggests that dimerization interactions occur between different members of the receptor family, and such heterodimers have been shown between the thyroid hormone and retinoic acid receptors.[53,54] The primary structure of this dimerization region is reminiscent of the leucine zippers that form dimerization interfaces with other proteins,[55,56] but the extent of its relation to this structure remains to be determined. The repetitive hydrophobic nature of this region is more or less conserved between the different members of the steroid receptor family,[20,57] and it has been postulated that the equivalent region may play a role in the dimerization of the other steroid receptors.

A second dimerization interaction has been identified within the DBD of the estrogen[16] and glucocorticoid[58] receptors. In the case of the glucocorticoid receptor DBD, this interaction is mediated by a 5-amino acid loop close to the C-terminal zinc ion[59] (Fig. 5B-6*A*). However, mutagenesis studies suggest that this interaction is responsible for restricting DNA binding by the glucocorticoid receptor to HREs in which the palindromic hexameric sequences are separated by three base pairs[60] (see DNA Binding by Nuclear Receptors below). It is likely that a similar interaction occurs for the other steroid receptors but that it differs or is absent in other members of the family (e.g., the thyroid and retinoic acid receptors) which can bind to palindromic sequences irrespective of the spacing between the constituent hexameric sequences[61] (see DNA Binding by Nuclear Receptors below).

Phosphorylation

Phosphorylation of steroid receptor proteins has been reported in numerous studies over the years (for a review, see ref. 62). However, the nature and function of the phosphorylation have been unclear. Receptor phosphorylation/dephosphorylation has been associated with the ability to bind steroid, agonist/antagonist action, and receptor inactivation, and there are conflicting data in the published reports. The estrogen receptor is reported to be phosphorylated at Tyr residues, whereas GR and PR are phosphorylated at Ser and Thr.[62]

Phosphorylation does not appear to be required for steroid binding or DNA binding of the glucocorticoid receptor, as nonphosphorylated recombinant proteins expressed in bacteria retain these functions. Phosphorylation of GR occurs predominantly in the N-terminal region (transactivation domain) (Fig. 5B-3). The mouse GR contains six phosphoserine residues and one phosphothreonine residue.[63] All seven sites occur within the transactivating region τ_1 previously identified by Giguère and associates.[34] Phosphorylation of this region increases two- to threefold after agonist binding but not antagonist binding.[64] Presumably, the steroid-dependent phosphorylation of this region plays a role in transactivation. Steroid-dependent phosphorylation of the progestin receptor has also been described.[65] In this instance, the primary site of phosphorylation (Ser) occurred in a region between the DNA-binding and steroid-binding domains.

Intracellular Localization

In early studies, cellular fractionation indicated that the steroid receptors are cytosolic before steroid binding and translocate to the nucleus after the binding of steroid and subsequent activation.[2] Later, immunocytochemistry and enucleation experiments

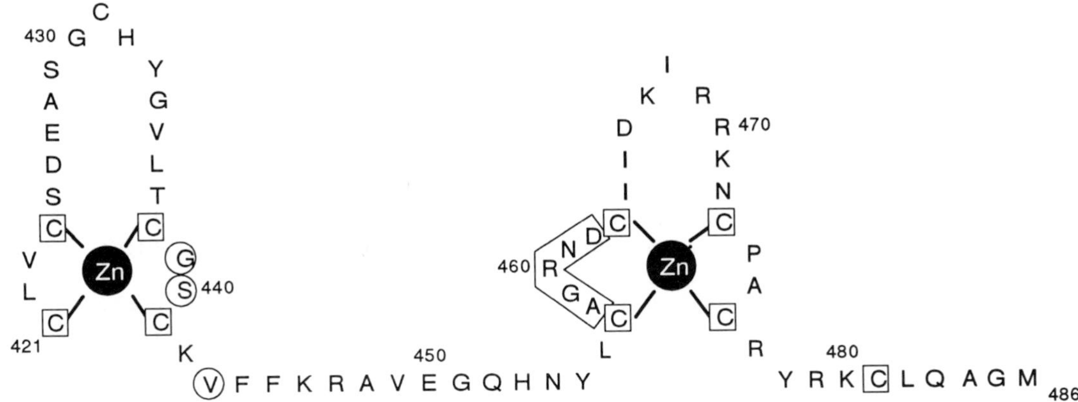

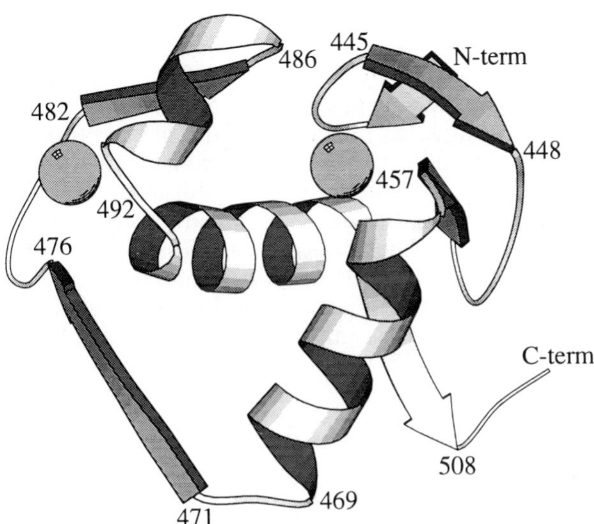

FIGURE 5B-6 (*A*) DNA-binding domain of the human glucocorticoid receptor, showing the coordination of zinc ions by cysteine residues. Cysteine residues conserved within the nuclear receptor family are indicated by square boxes. Circled residues are involved in determining specific binding to a GRE as opposed to an ERE. The boxed residues (458-462) mediate interactions between the two DNA-binding domains within a dimer which restrict binding to GREs in which the two hexanucleotide half sites are separated by three base pairs. (*B*) Three-dimensional structure of the DNA-binding domain of the glucocorticoid receptor. The numbers refer to the sequance of the rat receptor (+19 compared to the human glucocorticoid receptor).

indicated the nuclear localization of estrogen, androgen, and progestin receptors even in the absence of steroid.[66–71] However, most studies of the glucocorticoid receptor indicate predominantly a cytoplasmic localization before the addition of steroid.[72–77] In most in vivo studies, there is a clear concentration of receptor in the nucleus after the addition of steroid. Whether the receptor is weakly associated with the nucleus or cytoplasmic structures before steroid binding remains controversial. At any rate, in all cases there is a two-step mechanism with steroid binding occurring before tight DNA binding.

Picard and Yamamoto[78] have identified two nuclear localization signals within the glucocorticoid receptor, one constitutive and one steroid-dependent. The steroid-dependent nuclear localization signal sequence is dominant over the constitutive signal sequence (located at the C-terminal end of the DBD). The constitutive signal sequence is a very basic region similar to other published nuclear localization signal sequences.[78] The steroid-dependent nuclear localization signal is contained within the steroid-binding domain but has not been analyzed in detail. Fusion of either of these two localization signals with large cytoplasmic proteins such as β-galactosidase and transferrin results in the nuclear localization of the chimeric protein, either constitutively or in a steroid-dependent manner, respectively.

Steroid Hormone Antagonists

Over the years, a number of synthetic steroids with agonist, partial agonist, or antagonist activity have been synthesized. Examples of such steroids are given in Table 5B-1 and Fig. 5B-1. Although many details of steroid hormone action have been clarified in recent years, it is still unclear how many steroids exert an antagonistic action. Furthermore, there is an overlap in the specificity of steroid binding within the subfamily consisting of the androgen, glucocorticoid, mineralocorticoid, and progestin receptors, resulting in mixed effects of some steroids with variations in function in different tissues. For instance, the most potent antiandrogens act as progestin agonists. Occasionally, drugs that are used for other purposes can exhibit steroid agonist or antagonist activities. For example, cimetidine, which is used to diminish gastric acid secretion, can exhibit antiandrogen activity at high concentrations.

Steroid antagonists bind to the appropriate receptor protein and compete for agonist occupancy of the steroid-binding site. Some antagonists, such as the estrogen antagonist ICI 164 384, act by inhibiting DNA binding by interfering with the dissociation of chaperone proteins or receptor dimerization.[79]

Other antagonists, such as the antiestrogen tamoxifen and the antiprogestin/antiglucocorticoid RU-486, activate the receptor to a form that can interact specifically with DNA.[16,80–83] However, there have been several reports on the poor efficiency of activation and dissociation of the chaperone proteins after the binding of these ligands.[84] In transactivation studies, these ligands have low intrinsic activity, and it is believed that their agonist effect is due mainly to insufficient modification of the receptor protein necessary for stimulating transactivation after the interaction with DNA. One example is the difference in phosphorylation of the transactivation region of the glucocorticoid receptor, τ_1, induced by agonists and antagonists.[64] The antiglucocorticoid RU-486 does not induce phosphorylation of this region, and this may correlate with its poor transactivating function.

Activation by Nonsteroidal Entities

It has recently been shown that the steroid receptors can be activated by nonsteroid entities. This has been demonstrated for the progesterone receptor that can be activated by dopamine.[85] Presumably, in this case the dopamine activates a "second messenger" that modifies the receptor by a direct or indirect mechanism that results in the same conformational change that is activated by steroid binding. It is not known how extensively this mechanism is used. However, it may explain previously unclear phenomena such as why there are estrogen and progesterone receptors in the male that produce only minute amounts of estradiol and progesterone.

Regulation of Steroid Receptor Levels and Responsiveness

The levels of the steroid hormone receptors are not as extensively regulated by the homologous ligand as is the case with the polypeptide and catecholamine hormones discussed in the first part of this chapter. However, such regulation is observed in some cases, with significant influences on steroid responsiveness.[86] Sometimes other steroids regulate the levels of receptors. For example, estradiol can induce increases in the levels of the progesterone receptors.[87] In breast cancer, the levels of the estrogen receptors vary considerably and show a general correlation with the estrogen responsiveness of the tumor (see Chap. 30). In this case, the factors that regulate the receptor levels are unknown.

Regulation of responsiveness to the steroid hormones also occurs through mechanisms that are distal to the hormone-receptor interaction. Examples of how other transcription factors influence glucocorticoid responsiveness are described in Synergistic Transactivation by Nuclear Receptors and Negative Regulation by Nuclear Receptor Proteins, below. Such interactions may explain the so-called permissive actions of other hormones and the synergisms and antagonisms between various hormones and steroid hormone actions that are commonly observed.

MECHANISM OF GENE REGULATION BY NUCLEAR RECEPTORS

Once a receptor has been transformed into an activated state by the binding of its cognate ligand, it functions to alter the spectrum of levels of proteins in the target cell and thus alters the cell's function. The dominant mechanism by which the receptors achieve this is modulation of the rate of mRNA transcription from target genes, leading to a change in the level of proteins encoded by such genes. This is generally achieved by binding of the receptor protein to specific DNA-binding sites in the proximity of the regulated genes, followed by subsequent events which modulate the rate of transcriptional initiation from the promoter of the target gene. In addition, there are some cases in which nuclear receptors act to modulate the stability of mRNA rather than its production rate,[88–90] but the mechanism or mechanisms by which this occurs is not known and will not be discussed here.

DNA Binding by Nuclear Receptors

The specific DNA sequences in the proximity of target genes to which nuclear receptors bind and mediate influences on transcription are called hormone response elements (HREs). Within the nuclei of living cells, DNA is packaged together with histones and other proteins in a regularly repeating complex called *chromatin* (see Chap. 3). The repeating units of chromatin are called *nucleosomes,* each of which contains about 150 base pairs of DNA. Binding of nuclear receptors to HREs can be observed in vivo since this causes disruption of the chromatin structure, producing a region of "naked" DNA which is sensitive to nuclear digestion.[91,92] This has also been shown using in vivo footprinting techniques in which binding of the protein within living cells protects the DNA-binding site from chemical modification and cleavage agents.[93] HREs defined in this way also bind their cognate receptors when used in DNA-binding assays in vitro. When cloned upstream of a heterologous promoter, HREs bring expression from the promoter under hormonal control, again indicating binding of receptor protein to the HRE in a functional form within intact cells.

Comparison of HREs defined using these techniques, primarily for the glucocorticoid and estrogen receptors, as well as in vitro mutagenesis studies, has resulted in the determination of consensus HREs for the different receptors (Fig. 5B-7). The con-

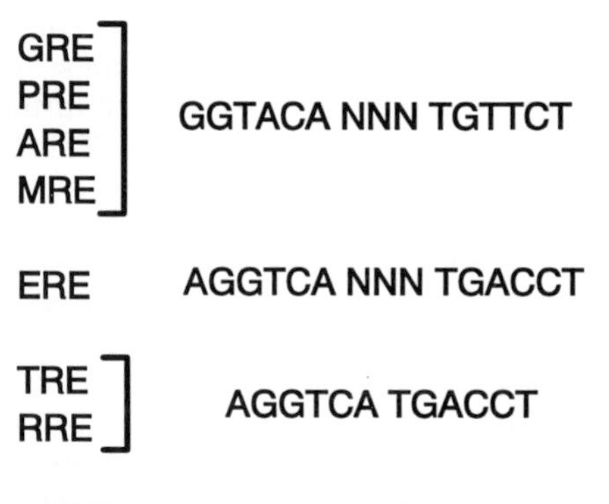

FIGURE 5B-7 Consensus hormone response elements for nuclear receptors.

sensus HREs are characterized by two identical or nearly identical 6-base pair sequences which are oriented palindromically with respect to each other.[94] For steroid hormone receptors, the hexameric sequences are separated by three base pairs, and if this distance is changed, the elements are no longer functional. Surprisingly, the response elements for the glucocorticoid, progesterone, mineralocorticoid, and androgen receptors appear to be identical. Although it is still possible that some of these receptors interact with different aspects of the response element, possibly with different affinities, this does not seem to be the case for the glucocorticoid and progesterone receptors, on which careful studies have been performed.[95,96] This suggests that the presence of the receptors rather than the primary DNA-binding specificity of these receptors is the major determinant of the hormone-specific response. The consensus estrogen response element (ERE) differs from the response elements for the other steroid receptors at the two central base pairs of each hexameric sequence and is functionally distinct. The response element shown in Fig. 5B-7 for the thyroid hormone and retinoic acid receptors can be identical to the ERE except that no base pairs separate the two palindromes. However, this sequence was derived by experimental manipulation of an ERE[61,97] and is not commonly found in naturally occurring thyroid hormone– and retinoic acid–responsive elements.

The region of receptor proteins which is most highly conserved within the nuclear receptor family is the DNA-binding domain. This domain consists of 66 to 68 amino acids and contains nine conserved cysteine residues and a high proportion of basic amino acids. The basic amino acids are thought to form electrostatic interactions with the negatively charged DNA, thus stabilizing DNA binding.[98] The arrangement of the cysteine residues (Fig. 5B-6*A*) is reminiscent of the zinc finger structure, first suggested for the *Xenopus laevis* protein TFIIIA, and it has been shown that the DBD of the glucocorticoid receptor contains two zinc ions tetrahedrally coordinated by cysteine residues.[99] Functional[100] and biochemical[101] studies on the glucocorticoid receptor show that the N-terminal eight conserved cysteines coordinate the zinc ions, as shown in Fig. 5B-6*A*. It has been shown for the glucocorticoid and estrogen receptors that three amino acids in an alpha helix at the end of the first zinc finger are mainly responsible for distinguishing between glucocorticoid and estrogen response elements (see below). The three-dimensional structure of the glucocorticoid receptor DBD (Fig. 5B-6*B*)[98] and the estrogen receptor DBD[102] have been determined. The two structures are very similar, suggesting a highly conserved structure for the DBDs of all members of the nuclear receptor family.

As was described in the section on dimerization, the estrogen,[16,103] glucocorticoid,[19,104] and progesterone[18] receptors interact with their respective response elements as homodimers. That this occurs is also suggested by the palindromic nature of the HREs.[105,106] Also discussed earlier was the fact that the various receptors differ in their tendencies to form dimers in solution, that dimer formation increases the affinities of the receptors for the HREs, and that dimer formation mediated by specific domains on the receptors influences the specificity for binding to specific sequences, particularly with respect to the spacing between the palindromic half sites. In addition, dimer binding on the DNA probably enhances the strength of the dimeric interactions.

The family of nuclear receptors can be divided into two specificity groups with respect to the interaction of the DBD with its hexameric recognition sequence within an HRE. The first group consists of the glucocorticoid, progesterone, mineralocorticoid, and androgen receptors which recognize the TGTTCT sequence. The second group, which includes the estrogen, thyroid hormone, and retinoic acid and retinoid X receptors, recognizes the TGACCT sequence. Studies of the DNA-binding specificity of hybrid receptors constructed using sequences from the glucocorticoid and estrogen receptors have shown that the N-terminal part of the DBD contains the determinants for sequence-specific DNA recognition.[107] Subsequently, the specificity determinants were narrowed down further to three amino acids which are located close to the N-terminal zinc ion on the solvent-exposed surface of the recognition alphahelix (Fig. 5B-6).[60,108,109] However, in DNA-binding experiments using variants of the purified glucocorticoid receptor DBD in which these residues were mutated to their equivalents in the estrogen receptor, the specificity switch to ERE recognition was incomplete.[110] Therefore, other determinants of specific binding-site recognition may remain to be identified.

Mechanism of Transcriptional Transactivation by Nuclear Receptors

Transcription of a gene to produce mRNA requires binding of RNA polymerase II and additional auxiliary transcription factors (e.g., the so-called TATA box factors, which include TFIIA, TFIIB, TFIID, TFIIE, and TFIIF) to the promoter of the gene to form a preinitiation complex[111] (see Chap. 3). In vitro, such a complex has the capacity to initiate transcription when ribonucleotides are added to the reaction. It appears that regulatory transcription factors such as nuclear receptor transactivate transcription by stabilizing the assembly of the preinitiation complex at the promoter, thus increasing the frequency of transcriptional initiation.[112] This stabilization is thought to result from protein-protein interactions between the regulatory transcription factor and one or more factors within the preinitiation complex (Fig. 5B-8). Regions within regulatory transcription factor proteins which are required for transactivation of transcription but not DNA binding have been identified and are termed *transactivation domains*. The transactivation domains of a number of transcription factors are enriched with certain amino acids, particularly acidic, threonine/serine, glutamine, and/or proline residues.[113] These transactivation domains are thought to contact factors in the preinitiation complex either by direct interactions or indirectly via adaptor or coactivator proteins which do not themselves bind to the DNA. For example, the Sp1 protein, which contains glutamine-rich and serine/threonine-rich transactivation domains, appears to interact with TFIID indirectly via an adaptor protein.[114] In the case of the strong acidic transactivation domain of the *Herpes simplex* virus VP16 protein, there have been reports suggesting either indirect interactions with the preinitiation complex[115,116] or direct interactions with the basal transcription factors TFIIB[117] and TFIID.[118,119] It is unclear which of these mechanisms predominates for the nuclear receptors.

FIGURE 5B-8 Hypothetical schemes for the mechanism of transcriptional transactivation by nuclear receptors. Stabilizing protein contacts between receptor proteins, bound to the HRE, and basic transcription factors and/or RNA polymerase II are represented by the filled arrows. (a) Indicates one possible mechanism in which the receptor interacts with basal factors indirectly via a coactivator or adaptor protein. (b) Indicates an alternative mechanism in which the receptor contacts the basal factors directly. The hatched box represents the transcribed region of a gene, the inner boxes represent protein-binding sites within the promoter of the gene, and the open arrow represents a newly initiated transcript.

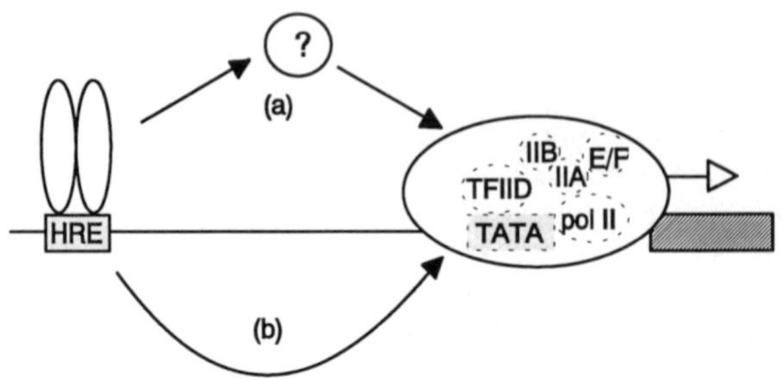

Nuclear receptors appear to function by a general mechanism similar to other known transactivating factors, such as VP16 and Sp1, since the glucocorticoid,[120,121] progesterone,[122,123] and estrogen[124] receptors transactivate transcription in vitro. Also, overexpression of receptor transactivation domains causes a reduction in the expression of other genes, presumably as a result of titration of limiting transcription factors by the overexpressed domain,[125,126] a process which has been called *squelching*. All receptors tested contain a transactivating domain within the ligand-binding domain. In addition, the glucocorticoid,[127] progesterone,[83] and estrogen[128] receptors have been shown to contain a transactivation domain in the N-terminal part of the receptor protein. In the glucocorticoid receptor, these transactivation domains are acidic in nature and are contained between residues 77-262 and 526-556 of the human receptor protein. The transactivation domains of the estrogen and progesterone receptors are less well defined but do not appear to be acidic in nature. In the case of the glucocorticoid receptor, it has been reported that the DBD has weak transactivation activity and that amino acids in the C-terminal part of the DBD may be involved in making contacts with other proteins.[129]

The identity of the proteins contacted by the transactivation domains of nuclear receptors remains to be established. Squelching studies have suggested that the transactivation domains of the estrogen and glucocorticoid receptors may interact with more than one class of proteins.[125] Other squelching experiments suggest that the major transactivation domain of the glucocorticoid receptor (residues 77-262) interacts with one or more factors which are needed for basal transcription.[126] The N-terminal transactivation domain of the estrogen receptor shows variable activity in different cell types, suggesting that it interacts with cell-specific factors.[128] The equivalent region of the progesterone receptor has different transactivation activities for different promoters, suggesting that other aspects of the promoter context are important for activity.[83] The bound ligand also appears to play a role in transactivation since several receptors bound by antagonist hormones have been shown to bind to DNA but fail to transactivate transcription.[81,130]

In addition to the mechanism of transactivation described above, receptors have been shown to use other methods to transactivate gene activity. At least part of the transactivation by the glucocorticoid receptor from the mouse mammary tumor virus (MMTV) long terminal repeat (LTR) appears to be due to modulation of chromatin structure. In several cases, packaging of genes in chromatin has been shown to have a negative effect on the level of basal transcription,[131–133] and this also appears to be the case for the MMTV LTR.[134] The nucleosomes which cover the MMTV LTR are positioned in a sequence-specific manner on the DNA, and it has been shown that binding of the glucocorticoid receptor in vivo causes displacement of one of these nucleosomes.[135] This causes exposure of a binding site for the transcription factor NF1, which was previously occluded by the nucleosome, and it seems that it is NF1 which subsequently transactivates transcription.[136] Thus, in this case the receptor protein transactivates indirectly by modulating chromatin structure and thereby allowing access to other transactivating factors. The generality of this mechanism of receptor action remains to be established, although there is evidence that a similar mechanism may apply to regulation of the tyrosine aminotransferase gene by the glucocorticoid receptor.[137]

Synergistic Transactivation by Nuclear Receptors

In naturally occurring promoters, binding sites for regulatory factors are not found in isolation. They are often present in more than one copy and are interspaced and in some cases overlap with binding sites for other factors.[138] Thus, the activity of the promoter results from the interaction between many regulatory proteins. These interactions are often synergistic, leading to a level of transactivation from the combined sites that is greater than the sum of the activities of each of the sites tested individually. This synergism can cause a large increase in transactivation as a result of only a very small change in the level of a regulatory factor, or alternatively, it can impose a requirement for the presence of more than one regulatory factor before the gene will be significantly induced.

All the glucocorticoid,[139,140] progesterone,[141] and estrogen[142,143] receptors synergize with themselves from two appropriately positioned HREs. For the glucocorticoid[75] and progesterone[141] receptors, synergism results from cooperative binding of receptor dimers to DNA, thus increasing their affinity of binding and thereby their occupancy of the regulated promoter. In the case of the glucocorticoid receptor, the N-terminal transactivation domain is the sole determinant of synergism between glucocorticoid receptor dimers and is involved in direct protein contacts between dimers.[144,145] For the estrogen receptor, the picture is less clear since both cooperative and noncooperative DNA-binding mechanisms have been reported in different systems.[142,143] Synergism also occurs between the glucocorticoid, progesterone, and estrogen receptors. Different parts of the receptors are involved in the various synergistic interactions. For example, the C-terminal part of the estrogen receptor synergizes with the N terminus of both the glucocorticoid and progesterone receptors, while the N-terminal part of the estrogen receptor synergizes only with the N terminus of the progesterone receptor.[146] Nuclear receptors also synergize with other classes of transcription factors. The glucocorticoid receptor, for example, synergizes with the NF1, CP1, Sp1, OTF, CACCC, and octamer factors.[139,140,147] Synergistic interaction between the glucocorticoid receptor and Oct-1 appears to involve a cooperative binding mechanism.[148] Interactions between the estrogen receptor and NF1 result in synergism by a post-DNA-binding mechanism that does not involve cooperative DNA binding.[149] However, the mechanisms underlying most synergistic interactions both between nuclear receptors and between nuclear receptors and other factors have not been determined.

Negative Regulation by Nuclear Receptor Proteins

Although most documented cases of transcriptional regulation involve induction of gene expression, the receptor proteins do act to inhibit transcription. Several different mechanisms are employed to achieve negative regulation.

Comparison of a limited number of binding sites from genes that are negatively regulated by the glucocorticoid receptor has led to the deduction of a consensus sequence for negative GREs (nGREs) which differs slightly from the normal GRE consensus.[94] In a mechanism that has been suggested to account for the inhibition of prolactin gene expression by the glucocorticoid receptor, the receptor protein adopts an altered conformation when bound to the nGRE.[150] A negative TRE has also been described in the chicken lysozyme gene which mediates negative regulation by the thyroid hormone receptor.[151]

A different mechanism has been suggested for inhibition by glucocorticoids of the α-subunit gene of chorionic gonadotropin. The receptor DNA-binding site upstream of the promoter overlaps with a site required for cAMP-mediated induction of transcription, and it has been suggested that the receptors compete with the CRE protein that mediates cAMP responsiveness for binding to the site, with the result that the cAMP response is blunted in the presence of glucocorticoids.[152] A similar mechanism may apply to the pro-opiomelanocortin[153] and osteocalcin[154] genes, where glucocorticoid receptor binding sites overlap with binding sites for the CAAT-box binding factor and the TATA-box binding factor, TFIID, respectively.

Nuclear receptors can also inhibit transcription by forming heterodimers with each other. This has been shown for the thyroid hormone and retinoic acid receptors, which, at least in some cell lines, inhibit each other's activity by forming heterodimers.[54]

Interactions have recently been shown between nuclear receptors and the AP1 transcription factor which is composed of the c-jun and c-fos proteins. The proliferin gene contains a composite GRE which also contains a binding site for AP1 and functions both as a positive and a negative GRE. In the presence of c-jun, it mediates positive glucocorticoid-dependent regulation, whereas if c-jun is replaced by c-fos, glucocorticoids produce a negative effect.[155] The glucocorticoid receptor has been shown to inhibit the activity of AP1 by interacting with c-jun and c-fos, thus preventing DNA binding by AP1.[156–159] This appears to be the mechanism by which the collagenase gene is inhibited by glucocorticoids. A similar mechanism involving interaction between AP1 and the retinoic acid receptor has been implicated in repression of the stromolysin gene by retinoic acid.[160]

GENETIC DEFECTS IN RECEPTOR FUNCTION

Genetic defects have been described for the androgen (see Chap. 16), glucocorticoid (see Chap. 12), and vitamin D (see Chap. 23) receptors. These defects and their clinical consequences are described in the referenced chapters.

The most commonly recognized steroid receptor defect concerns the androgen receptor associated with various degrees of androgen insensitivity from complete testicular feminization to infertility.[161–163] The molecular basis of this syndrome has been characterized for numerous patients, and the syndrome usually results from limited mutations of the gene, which is situated on the X chromosome.[162–171] The mutations described include splicing defects or premature termination resulting in the apparent lack of receptor protein, mutations within the steroid-binding domain resulting in the loss or reduction of affinity for androgen or thermolability in steroid binding, and mutations within the DBD resulting in a receptor that binds steroid but does not transactivate. Similar mutations have been described for the vitamin D receptor in vitamin D–resistant rickets,[172–174] the glucocorticoid receptor in primary cortisol resistance,[175–179] and one of the thyroid hormone receptors in generalized thyroid hormone resistance[180–184] (see below).

The inheritance of vitamin D and glucocorticoid resistance differs from that of androgen resistance. Vitamin D–resistant rickets is inherited in an autosomal recessive pattern, and in the reported cases, subjects with one normal allele do not have clinically detectable disease.[163] Glucocorticoid resistance presents with manifestations caused by compensatory adrenal overactivity (see Chap. 12): androgen excess in the milder cases and both androgen and mineralocorticoid excess in more severely affected individuals.[174,178] The more prominent manifestations of either androgen excess or androgen and mineralocorticoid excess are observed in subjects with homozygous defects in both receptor alleles; the defects reported in heterozygotes have been minor.[174,178] This need to have mutations in both alleles may explain why major glucocorticoid and vitamin D resistance is less common than androgen resistance. Thus, the products of the mutated allele tend not to interfere with those of the normal allele; this is in striking contrast to the dominant negative mode of inheritance in the thyroid hormone resistance syndromes discussed below. However, dominant negative mutations in which the mutant receptor interferes with the function of the normal receptors, have been reported with estrogen receptors in breast cancer.[179] Complete resistance to glucocorticoids, mineralocorticoids, estrogens, and progestins has not been reported; presumably, major disturbances of these four hormone systems will not allow the continuation of life.

STEROID RECEPTORS AND ONCOGENESIS

In tissues in which growth is normally stimulated or repressed by steroid hormones, endocrine therapy plays a major role in the treatment of tumors derived from these cells. The occurrence and function of steroid receptors in such tumor cells are thus of primary interest. The classical example is the role of estrogens in breast cancer (see Chap. 30). Estrogens and progestins play an important role in the regulation and development of normal breast tissue (see Chap. 17). As a result, breast cancer cells also respond to estrogens in many cases, with a resulting stimulation of cell growth. This effect is dependent on the presence of a functional estrogen receptor in the tumor cell. As in normal cells, estrogen action in a tumor cell can be blocked by antiestrogens, and treatment with tamoxifen plays a central role in breast cancer therapy. However, tumors lacking the estrogen receptor do not respond to endocrine therapy, and the determination of receptor content in breast tumors is routine today in many countries[185–187] (see Chap. 30). A number of different types of estrogen receptor defects have been described in these tumors. These receptors can be functionally defective, exhibit dominant negative inhibitory influences on the normal receptors (discussed above), and be constitutively active, i.e., exhibit estrogen receptor influences even without binding estrogen.[332]

Another example of a neoplastic tissue that responds to steroids and in which endocrine therapy plays a major role is acute lymphoblastic leukemia. These cells are inhibited by glucocorticoids, and this has been shown to be related to the level of glucocorticoid receptor in the leukemia cells.[188] However, glucocorticoid receptor content is not generally used to steer therapy in these cases, although it can be used as a prognostic indicator.

Members of the steroid/thyroid hormone superfamily or their derivatives can also play a role in other oncogenic processes. The oncogene v-*erbA* plays a role in avian erythroblast leukemia, blocking the differentiation of the transformed erythroblast cells.[189] The thyroid hormone receptor is the protooncogene of v-*erbA* and a member of the steroid receptor gene superfamily[190] (see Thyroid Hormone Receptors). Another member of the steroid/thyroid hormone receptor family, the retinoic acid receptor β, was cloned through its association with hepatitis B–associated hepatocarcinomas. In the great majority of these cancers, the virus was integrated in the genome at a specific point of insertion, HAP.[191] After cloning of the gene at this site of insertion and characterization, it could be shown that the gene product was very closely related to the retinoic acid receptor β and that it mediated transactivation by retinoids.[192] In acute promyelocytic leukemia, a chromosomal translocation gives rise to a chimeric protein consisting of the retinoic acid receptor α and the transcription factor PML[193–196]; this chimeric protein probably plays a role in leukemogenesis and myelocytic differentiation.[195,196] Both of the oncogenic retroviruses—mouse mammary tumor virus (MMTV) and mouse sarcoma virus (MSV)—have acquired glucocorticoid response elements within the long terminal repeat regions, and transcription of the provirus and propagation of the virus are stimulated by glucocorticoids.

ORPHAN RECEPTORS: NOVEL MEMBERS OF THE STEROID RECEPTOR GENE SUPERFAMILY

Common Characteristics of Orphan Receptors

A number of genes have been found that have striking similarities to the known members of the steroid receptor gene superfamily.[197–217] The encoded proteins present the conserved features of the nuclear receptors. Particularly, the DNA-binding domain and the carboxyl-terminal region show homology with the classical steroid receptors. Since these receptors bind ligands, it appears possible that at least some of the newly discovered proteins represent novel receptors for unidentified ligands. The search for these low-molecular-weight activating compounds has been successful in only two cases so far,[205,218,219] but nevertheless, this group of proteins has been called *orphan receptors*, implying that there might be ligands or low-molecular-weight activators to some more, if not most, of them.[188,197,198,220–223]

Table 5B-2 lists orphan receptors grouped by the method by which they were cloned. The most direct approach, termed *low stringency screening*, was based on their homology to known steroid/vitamin receptors. Probes, mostly derived from the part of the cDNA coding for the DNA-binding domain, were used to identify receptor genes in cDNA libraries. In a second approach, termed *classical cloning*, proteins which attracted attention for other reasons were purified, and after cloning of the corresponding genes, these proteins turned out to be members of the nuclear receptor superfamily. A third strategy, called *southwestern cloning*, was applied for the isolation of genes for DNA-binding proteins with known recognition motifs. Screening of expression libraries with radiolabeled fragments of target DNA led to the cloning of numerous DNA-binding proteins, which in some cases were homologous to the steroid receptors.

TABLE 5B-2 Orphan Receptors Grouped by the Method by Which They Were Cloned

Low stringency screening	
ERR1, ERR2	Estrogen receptor–related genes[197]
ear-1, ear-2, ear-3	Oncogene erb A–related genes[198,199]
hRXR	Retinoid X receptor[200–203, 219]
XR2C	Gene at the *ultraspiracle* locus homologous to RXR (*Drosophila*)[204]
PPAR	Peroxisome proliferator-activated receptor[205,218]
NAK1	Human gene homologous to rat NGFI-B and mouse nur/77[206]
knrl and *egon*	Genes related to the *Drosophila* genes *knirps*[207]
Classical cloning	
COUP-TF	Chicken oviduct upstream promoter-binding factor[208]
HNF-4	Hepatocyte nuclear factor 4[209]
Southwestern cloning	
FTZ-F1	*Fushi-tarazu*–activating factor (*Drosophila*)[210]
ARP-1	Apolipoprotein A-I regulatory protein[211]
Genes which are activated by stimulation of cell growth	
NGFI-B	Nerve growth factor–inducible gene (rat)[212]
nur/77	Growth factor–inducible gene (mouse)[213]
Chromosomal walking	
E75	Ecdysone inducible gene at the 75B puff locus (*Drosophila*)[214]
tll	Gene at the *tailless* locus in *Drosophila*[215]
kni	Gene at the *knirps* locus in *Drosophila*[216]
Others	
svp	Gene at the *seven-up* locus required for eye development (*Drosophila*)[217]

A fourth group of orphan receptors was isolated during the search for genes which are activated under certain conditions of cell growth. A fifth strategy, termed *chromosomal walking,* revealed that the genes at certain genetically defined loci in *Drosophila* are members of the nuclear receptor superfamily.

Homology in the Overall Domain Structure with Classical Nuclear Receptors

Alignment of the amino acid sequence of the orphan receptors clearly demonstrates the homology to classical steroid receptors.[190] In particular, a characteristic Cys_4-zinc finger DNA-binding domain can be discerned. The variability in length and the sequence of the amino-terminal domain(s) of the classical nuclear receptors also characterize the newly discovered members of this gene superfamily (Fig. 5B-9).

The carboxyl-terminal domain shows substantial similarity between the different orphan receptors as well as between orphan and classical receptors. Amino acid homologies range from 10 percent to more than 50 percent, which is in good agreement with the homology between different classical nuclear receptors (reviewed in refs. 224 and 225). In classical steroid receptors, this domain harbors the functions of ligand binding, association with hsp90, protein-protein interaction, and nuclear translocation, although a nuclear translocation signal is also present in the DNA-binding domain. Thus, based on the similarities in the carboxyl-terminal domain, it has been speculated that at least some of the novel members represent true receptors with regard to ligand binding and activation of transcription.

FIGURE 5B-9 Primary structure of orphan receptors predicted from the cDNA sequence. The structures of the estrogen and glucocorticoid receptors are given for comparison and domain assignment.

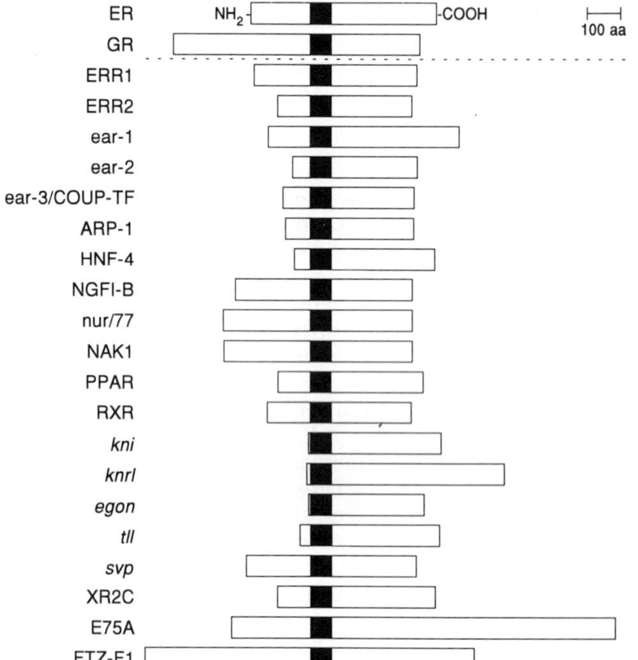

Primary Structure of the Conserved Zinc Finger DNA-Binding Domain

The DNA-binding domain—namely, the 66-68 amino acids constituting the two zinc finger motifs—is the most conserved region among the steroid receptors. This homology also exists between orphan receptors themselves as well as between orphan receptors and classical steroid receptors. As was mentioned earlier, three amino acids in the alpha helix at the end of the first zinc finger in the glucocorticoid and estrogen receptors are mainly responsible for specific recognition of the DNA response element (Fig. 5B-6*A*). According to the combination of amino acids at these discriminatory-positions, orphan receptors may be assigned to different subgroups (Table 5B-3).

None of the orphan receptors characterized thus far contains the amino acid combination in the DBD typical of estrogen or glucocorticoid receptors. The majority of the orphan receptors presents the combination of the thyroid/vitamin A/D receptors (group A in Table 5B-3) or the related v-*erbA* gene product (group B in Table 5B-3). Thus, similarities in the mechanism of target element–specific DNA recognition might be expected between orphan receptors and the classical receptors for thyroid hormone or retinoic acid. Indeed, the prediction of a palindromically symmetric thyroid response element was successfully applied on the retinoid X receptor.[219] However, further analysis revealed that recognition of DNA motifs is complex in the case of retinoic acid/thyroid hormone and orphan receptors. Whereas

TABLE 5B-3 Orphan Receptors Grouped by the Combination of the Three Discriminatory Amino Acids Determining DNA Response Element Specificity

Group	Position 1	Position 2	Position 3	Orphan Receptors
A	Glutamate	Glycine	Glycine	EAR-1, XR2C(*usp*), NGFI-B, nur/77, NAK1, RXR, mPPAR, E75A
B	Glutamate	Glycine	Serine	EAR-2, COUP/EAR-3, *kni, knrl, egon, svp,* ARP-1
C	Glutamate	Alanine	Alanine	ERR1, ERR2
D	Aspartate	Glycine	Glycine	*tll,* HNF-4
E	Glutamate	Serine	Glycine	FTZ-F1

classical steroid receptors preferentially bind as homodimers to palindromically arranged half-site binding motifs, the receptors for retinoic acid, vitamin D, and thyroid hormone recognize DNA motifs, which rather resemble direct repeat arrangements of the half-site binding motifs[226,227] (reviewed in ref. 228). Furthermore, there is increasing evidence that those receptors utilize accessory protein factors for binding to their cognate response elements,[229] and a number of laboratories have shown that retinoid X receptors (RXR), discussed in the section on receptors for retinoic acid and its analogues) are a prevailing heteromerization partner.[230]

Novel combinations of three discriminatory amino acids different from those found in classical steroid/vitamin receptors are presented by some of the orphan receptors (groups C through E in Table 5B-3). Thus, further research might find these novel combinations of discriminatory amino acids reflected in a widely broadened spectrum of DNA motifs recognized by members of this nuclear receptor superfamily.

Properties of Specific Orphan Receptors

Genes Homologous to the Estrogen Receptor or v-*erbA*

When the first genes for steroid receptors were cloned, the search for homologous cDNA sequences was successfully exploited to identify the genes for ERR1, ERR2, ear-1, ear-2, and ear-3, using probes derived from the ligand-binding domain of the estrogen receptor or the viral *erbA* oncogene, respectively. The gene for ear-1 is found at the same chromosomal locus as that for the authentic thyroid hormone receptor α, but the two genes are transcribed in opposite directions. Thus, part of the carboxyl-terminal domain of ear-1 is encoded by a DNA sequence complementary to that coding for the thyroid hormone receptor. Binding of potential ligands has been shown only in the case of ear-1, which binds thyroid hormones, although with low affinities. The ear-3 gene has been independently isolated as the gene for the COUP-TF.

RXR: Dual Function as Retinoid Receptor and Partner for Other Nuclear Receptors

A novel protein which first looked like just another receptor mediating a retinoid response turned out to serve a dual role as a retinoid receptor and an auxiliary factor which complements the function of other receptors for hormones or vitamins. The function of the retinoid X receptor as a ligand-dependent transcription factor mediating retinoid response was first shown utilizing the prediction of a putative response element from the primary structure of the DBD. An expression vector for RXR and a reporter gene with the predicted response element were transfected into mammalian or insect cells, and the testing of a number of putative ligand pools revealed retinoids to be activators of the reporter gene.[219] The suggestion from the initial experiments that classical retinoid receptors and RXR differ in their affinity for different retinoid derivatives was later confirmed by the identification of 9-*cis*-retinoic acid as the authentic ligand to RXR,[231,232] whereas the retinoic acid receptors preferentially bind all-*trans*-retinoic acid. In continuation of the observation that the receptors for thyroid hormone and retinoic acid recognize their DNA targets as complexes with other proteins,[229] many laboratories identified RXR isoforms (α, β, or γ) as heteromerization partners for classical receptors[201–203,228,233,234] or orphan receptors.[202,235] Response elements for RXR heteromeric complexes follow with some degeneracy a common architecture in that they all may be viewed as elements that contain AGGTCA half-site motifs oriented as direct repeats or palindromes, spaced by intervening nucleotides. Direct repeats with different numbers of intervening nucleotides constitute binding sites with differential affinity for RXR complexes with various receptors, such as those for retinoic acid, vitamin D, and thyroid hormone.[230] However, the half-site spacing and orientation requirements for directing specific hormonal signals to their respective target genes remain to be established.[236]

PPAR: Activation by Peroxisome Proliferators and Fatty Acids

The peroxisome proliferator-activated receptor (PPAR) obtained its name after a chimeric receptor encompassing the putative ligand-binding domain of this novel receptor fused to the amino-terminal and DNA-binding domains of the estrogen receptor was shown to activate transcription from an estrogen-responsive promoter upon stimulation by peroxisome proliferation-inducing drugs.[218] A similar approach utilizing chimeric receptors identified fatty acids as the potentially physiologic activators of PPAR, suggesting a pivotal role of PPAR in lipid homeostasis.[205] However, the broad spectrum of activating fatty acids and drugs does not easily comply with the highly discriminative recognition of steroid hormones by their respective receptors. Thus, it appears possible that fatty acids or peroxisome proliferation-inducing drugs cause the accumulation of a common signaling compound rather than bind to PPAR themselves. With regard to the search for the ultimate and physiologically relevant ligands, PPAR is similar to the Ah receptor for aromatic hydrocarbons and polyhalogenated dioxins.[237] This receptor had been suspected for a long time to be a member of the steroid receptor gene superfamily but finally turned out to have a DNA-binding domain constituted by the basic region/helix-loop-helix motif rather than the Cys_4-zinc finger domain.[85]

COUP-TF, ARP-1, and HNF-4: Orphan Receptors with Known Target Genes

The genes for chicken ovalbumin upstream promoter transcription factor COUP-TF and for the apolipoprotein-A-I regulatory protein ARP-1 code for highly similar, although distinct, proteins. Both ARP-1 and COUP-TF are ubiquitously expressed. COUP-TF may be activated by a protein kinase A–dependent signal transduction pathway, indicating a complex regulation and possibly "cross-talk" between different gene-activating signals.[238] In the case of ARP-1, a role in cholesterol homeostasis has been proposed. In contrast, HNF-4 might easily serve a function without the apparent need for low-molecular-weight activators since it is clearly enriched in liver, kidney, and intestine, implying a potential role in tissue/cell-specific gene expression.[209] This view is further supported by the finding that the expression of HNF-4 plays an important role in determining the hepatocyte-specific phenotype of certain subclones of a hepatoma cell line.[239]

Growth Factor–Induced Orphan Receptors

NGFI-B, nur/77, and NAK1 appear to be homologous genes from rat, mouse, and human, respectively. NGFI-B is induced in a pheochromocytoma-derived cell line by nerve growth factor. Similarly, nur/77 is induced by serum or purified growth factors in a mouse fibroblast cell line. The human homologue NAK1 is expressed in liver, brain, thyroid gland, and fetal muscle but not in kidney, placenta, spleen, tonsil, or prostate. In cultured cells, expression of the gene is inducible by growth stimuli appropriate for the cell type used. NGFI-B, nur/77, and NAK1 may represent so-called early immediate genes, i.e., genes which are turned on early during cell proliferation and may play a role in controlling this process.

Orphan Receptors in Embryonal Development of *Drosophila*

A number of genes were characterized first by their role in the embryonal development of *Drosophila,* while subsequent cloning and sequence analysis revealed the homology of the encoded proteins to the steroid receptors. *kni, knrl, egon, tll, svp,* XR2C, E75, and FTZ-F1 play important roles in the early pattern organization of the embryo and neuronal development.

The genes *kni, knrl,* and *egon* constitute a subgroup in that they share a conserved stretch of 19 amino acids carboxyl-terminally to the zinc finger motif of the DBD. The genes for E75 and FTZ-F1 constitute regulatory cascades. The expression of E75 is induced by the *Drosophila* steroid hormone ecdysone that acts via a member of the nuclear receptor superfamily, the ecdysone receptor.[240] The expression of E75 as an early response is a prerequisite for the late responses to ecdysone. The product of the FTZ-F1 gene appears to participate in *Drosophila* development by regulating the expression of the *fushi tarazu* gene, which itself is a member of a different family of DNA-binding proteins (the homeodomain-containing transcription factors).

The *svp* gene product is homologous to the mammalian COUP-TF (over 90 percent amino acid homology in the encoded DNA- and putative ligand-binding domains). Similarly, the *Drosophila* XR2C, which is encoded at the *usp* locus, corresponds to RXR (86 percent and 49 percent homology in the DNA- and putative ligand-binding domains, respectively).[203] The XR2C protein heterodimerize with the *Drosophila* ecdysone receptor, analogously to the case with mammals, where RXR forms heterodimers with members of the steroid receptor superfamily.[241] Thus, structural homology between *Drosophila* and mammalian proteins extends into functional aspects, and it is interesting to speculate how the role of members of the steroid receptor superfamily in the embryonal development of *Drosophila* is represented in the development of mammals.

Physiologic Roles of Orphan Receptors

Three main functions of novel members of the steroid receptor gene superfamily have been shown so far. First, some of them, e.g., RXR and PPAR, actually have been proved to mediate the response to low-molecular-weight activators such as 9-*cis*-retinoic acid, peroxisome proliferators, and fatty acids. Thus, RXR may no longer be called an orphan receptor, considering that 9-*cis*-retinoic acid has been identified as an authentic ligand. Further analysis might identify other unknown activators for novel receptors. A second group of orphan receptors includes genes which are expressed during certain stages of cell proliferation or differentiation, and it appears possible that those orphan receptors function without the need for low-molecular-weight activators. The mitogen-induced genes NAK, NGFI-B, and nur77; the hepatocyte-specific HNF-4; and most of the orphan receptor genes from *Drosophila* provide examples of that group. A third type of orphan receptor function is heteromerization with other receptors; examples of those proteins are RXR and USP, which are homologous proteins in mammals and in *Drosophila,* respectively. Chimeric proteins with classical steroid receptors or reporter genes containing responsive elements which are predicted from the structure of an orphan receptor provide tools to analyze individual gene products. However, it is still a major challenge to identify the mechanism of action of any novel orphan receptor. One might find functions which follow one of the discussed examples or even find several functions covered by a single orphan receptor.

THYROID HORMONE RECEPTORS

Thyroid Hormones and Their Mechanism of Action

Thyroid hormones (THs) have effects on nearly every cell and influence general metabolic homeostasis, growth, differentiation, and development (see Chap. 10 and refs. 242–245 for reviews). Most of these effects are mediated via binding of the THs to intranuclear thyroid hormone receptors (TRs). TRs regulate the expression of TH-sensitive genes by modulating transcriptional activity in a similar way to that described for steroid hormones and their receptor proteins.[246,247] Many of these aspects of thyroid receptor function have been mentioned in the sections on steroid hormone and orphan receptors. However, some effects of THs may be due to direct effects on mitochondria and cell membranes on which binding proteins have been identified.[248–250]

The thyroid gland mainly secretes thyroxine [3,3′,5,5′-tetraiodo-L-thyronine, (T_4)] and to a lesser extent the highly active T_3 [3,5,5′-triiodo-L-thyronine (triiodothyronine)]. Additional T_3 is produced by deiodination of T_4 in the peripheral tissues (see Chap. 10). T_3 is the major intracellular TH and has an approximately 10-fold higher affinity for binding to the TRs ($K_d \sim 0.1$ nM) than T_4. It is thought that THs cross cell membranes through transport processes; in addition, internalization of T_3 bound to plasma membranes via endocytosis has been described.[251,252] An active transport of T_3 from the cytosol to the nucleus has also been suggested.[253]

The TRs are widely distributed in different tissues.[254] The number of receptor molecules per nucleus is around 2000 to 10,000, with the highest concentration found in TH-responsive tissues such as the pituitary, brown fat, liver, heart, and kidney. Low levels are also found in peripheral mononuclear cells. TRs are rare or absent in the spleen and testes. The absence or low level of TRs correlates with the inability of these tissues to increase their oxygen consumption in response to THs.[255] In contrast, the brain is similarly unresponsive to TH regulation of oxygen consumption even though the TR levels are comparable to those of TH-responsive tissues[256]; this may be due to the high expression in this tissue of a TR splicing variant with repressive effects on TH-responsive genes (see below).

TRs are exclusively nuclear and, in contrast to steroid receptors, bind chromatin tightly in the presence or absence of hormone[257,258]; this may be explained by the fact that they do not interact with hsp90.[23]

Structure of TRs

The TRs are encoded by two separate genes, both of which are c-*erbA* proto-oncogenes, the cellular homologues of v-*erbA* (derived from the avian erythroblastosis virus).[259,260] One of the genes, TRα, is located on human chromosome 17, while the other, TRβ, is located on chromosome 3.[260–262]

The overall modular structure of the TRs is similar to that of the steroid receptors; that is, there is a strong conservation of the zinc finger–containing central DNA-binding domain and a less well conserved C-terminal ligand-binding domain (Fig. 5B-3A). TRs have a much shorter N-terminal domain than do the steroid receptors, with the absence of a strong transactivation function in this region.[246] The specificity-determining 3′ knuckle of the first zinc finger in the DNA-binding domain of TRs shows more homology to the receptors for estrogens (ER), vitamin D3 (VD3R), and retinoic acid (RAR) than to receptors for glucocorticoids (GR), mineralocorticoids (MR), progestins (PR), and androgens (AR),[106,107] and there is a close relation of DNA recognition sequences for TRs, RARs, and ER[61,97] (see below for possible functional consequences). The human TRα is a 410-amino acid protein (molecular weight 47,000), while human TRβ is a 456-amino acid protein (molecular weight 57,000).[263,264] These two TRs differ mainly in the N-terminal domain both in length and amino acid homology.[246,248] A short segment of the second zinc finger in the DNA-binding domain (D-box) also differs.[60] The overall amino acid homology in the DNA-binding domain of TRα and TRβ is approximately 86 percent. It is not yet clear whether this leads to differential recognition or binding affinity by the two TR forms to various thyroid hormone response elements (TREs).

The TRα shares the highest homology with the v-*erbA* protein. However, v-*erbA* lacks the ability to bind THs.[260] Since TRs in the absence of THs or TRs incapable of binding TH can act as constitutive dominant repressors of TH-responsive genes (see below), it has been speculated that overexpressed v-*erbA* could be involved in the oncogenic transformation of avian erythroblasts by suppressing gene activation.[189]

Several splicing variants of TRα have been identified.[265–269] In addition to the fully active α1, two non-T3-binding forms, α2 and α3, have been found. The latter two are identical to TRα1 in the N-terminal and DNA-binding domains but diverge in the carboxyl-terminal part of the ligand-binding domain. This explains their inability to bind T_3. In addition, a variant arising from transcription from the noncoding DNA strand in the TRα gene has been described.[199,270,271] The function of this protein, termed rev-erbAα, which does not bind T_3 or TRE, is unknown, but the protein may have postranscriptionally important regulatory properties.[272] In the rat, the TRβ gene also encodes a second form termed TRβ2, which is found only in the pituitary.[273] It is not known whether TRβ2 exists in humans. TRβ2, which binds T_3, is identical to TRβ1 in the ligand-

and DNA-binding domains but differs in the N-terminal domain. Interestingly, its autoregulation in response to THs differs from that of TRβ1, suggesting that it may arise from an alternative pituitary-specific promoter or alternative splicing.[274] Thus, at least three non-T_3-binding TR isoforms exist in addition to the three T_3-binding isoforms. So far, all of them except rev-erbA, whose recognition sequence is unknown, recognize the same TREs, possibly with slightly different affinities.[275–277] The T_3-binding isoforms show similar affinities for various THs, but small distinctions have been reported.[278] However, the physiologic role of all the variants, although largely unknown, is probably important given their high degree of structural conservation.

TRs as Dominant Repressors

An important functional difference between TRs and steroid receptors is the ability of TRs to bind to TREs in the absence of liganded T_3 and constitutively regulate genes in a negative or positive fashion.[279–282] The function of the TH on the TR activity therefore can be both to release suppression and to transactivate target genes. This observation may be of great functional importance in relation to the forms of the TR incapable of binding T_3 (see above). In fact, cotransfection experiments have demonstrated that these non-T_3-binding TR isoforms as well as v-*erbA,* which all interact with the same TRE, may act as dominant repressors of TR isoforms which bind T_3 and thereby stimulate transcription.[276,280,282] This negative effect could be obtained by direct competition for the same TRE, the formation of inactive heterodimers, or competition for binding to a common transcription factor. Thus, the differential expression in a given cell of the different TR isoforms may yield mutually antagonistic proteins.

Possible Functional Significance of Multiple TR Forms and Subtypes

A major question concerns the role of the multiple TRs in the cell. The TR isoforms are expressed in a tissue-specific and developmentally controlled fashion.[259,273,274,283–289] For example, TRα1 is expressed in nearly all tissues but predominantly in brain, brown fat, adipose tissue, heart, and other muscle types, while the non-T_3 binding TRα2 is also found in a number of tissues but is the major TR form in the testes. While TRβ1 is preferentially expressed in the liver and kidney, TRβ2 is found exclusively in the pituitary gland.[273] In the brain, regional variations in the expression of TR isoforms suggest defined roles for the different receptors in regulating brain function.[287,289] The high expression of the non-T_3-binding TRα2 in brain could explain the very modest response of this organ to THs when measured as oxygen consumption and glucose uptake, despite the abundant cellular T_3-binding capacity.[256] During avian development, TRα is expressed more or less ubiquitously from very early on,[287] whereas TRβ is subjected to both temporal and tissue-specific controlled expression. Furthermore, THs can variably regulate TR mRNA isoforms in a tissue-specific way.[273,274,290,291] In addition, the ratio of T_3 binding to TR mRNA shows both tissue and developmental variations,[292] implying that posttranscriptional control mechanisms may also affect TR expression and T_3-binding capacity. One function of rev-erbA or its mRNA may be to regulate TR levels by influencing TR gene expression. All these variations in the relative abundance in a given cell of the various TRs probably are of physiologic relevance in regulating tissue sensitivity toward THs and possibly in the control of gene expression of individual target genes. This notion, however, requires further experimental support.

Heterodimers with TRs and Other Proteins

The complexity of TR-regulated control of gene expression is further illustrated by the observation that TRs can heterodimerize with RXRs and RARs[53,54] and with other transcription factors. Interestingly, these heterodimers regulate gene activation differently depending on the TRE and host cell studied. While TR stimulates RAR effects on a palindromic TRE from the growth hormone gene, it antagonizes the effect of the myosin heavy-chain gene TRE.[53] Given the similarity of TREs, especially to EREs (the ERE has the same consensus hexamer half sites, separated by a different number of nucleotides), identical TREs could be recognized by different members of the nuclear receptor superfamily. The pleiotropy in responses could be further regulated by the ability of TRs to heterodimerize with other proteins, preferentially RXR (see below). As was already mentioned, RAR is capable of recognizing TREs. It has also been shown that TR can interact with an ERE but without giving rise to a TH response, whereas it can negatively influence estrogen responsiveness.[61] The TRE also shows similarity to the vitamin D_3 response element.[227] Functional interference between these receptors or hormone response elements could be physiologically very important, although it has not been demonstrated to occur in a natural situation.

Familial Thyroid Hormone Resistance and TRs

The syndrome of familial thyroid hormone resistance (FTHR) is discussed in Chap. 10. It generally is transmitted in an autosomal dominant fashion.[293] The clinical manifestations vary considerably between kindreds, suggesting that the mutations that give rise to this disease are heterogeneous in nature. In some cases, the molecular mechanisms behind FTHR have been elucidated.

Generalized resistance to thyroid hormone[294] results in elevated levels of thyroid hormone without suppression of the levels of thyroid stimulating hormone (TSH), goiter, and variable manifestations of euthyroidism, hypothyroidism, and hyperthyroidism[295] (see Chap. 10). The syndrome is generally transmitted in an autosomal dominant fashion.[251,295] In almost all the reported cases that have been studied, the mutations have been in the ligand-binding domain of one of the two TRβ genes.[295] Mutations in the TRα gene have not been described.[295] The mutant TRβ's appear to be capable of inhibiting the function of normal TRs, activities that have been demonstrated in gene transfer experiments.[295] Thus, unlike the cases described earlier for androgen, vitamin D, and glucocorticoid receptors, the resistance in these cases is due to inhibition of normal receptor activity by mutant receptors and the phenotypic expression conforms to a dominant negative recessive mode of inheritance.[295]

RECEPTORS FOR RETINOIC ACID AND ITS ANALOGUES

Biology of Retinoids

Retinoids are small lipophilic molecules that, like steroids and thyroid hormones, affect cell proliferation and differentiation (for reviews, see refs. 296–299). Three biologically important retinoids exist: retinol (vitamin A), retinal, and retinoic acid (RA) (Fig. 5B-10). Retinoic acid can induce differentiation in epithelial cells, may have an inhibitory effect in tissue regeneration, and may induce teratogenic changes in embryos.[300–302] Retinoids also act as morphogens, inducing changes in pattern formation, as has best been demonstrated with the chick limb bud and amphibian limb regeneration, where retinoids have produced effects such as pattern duplication, skeletal truncations, and deletions.[303–305]

Vitamin A, an essential nutrient for humans and animals, can be converted by oxidation into retinal and RA.[306] Vitamin A, retinal, and RA have separate biological effects. For example, RA is unable to replace vitamin A or retinal for proper night vision or reproduction, and RA in the concentrations occurring in vivo has an effect on differentiation.[307] Interestingly, differentiation and regeneration are affected differentially by various RA concentrations; for example, when undifferentiated P19 teratocarcinoma cells are exposed to a low concentration of RA (10^{-9} *M*), mainly cardiac muscle is formed.[308] At a higher concentration (10^{-8} *M*) skeletal muscle develops, and at very high concentrations (10^{-7} to 10^{-5} *M*) neurons and glial cells are formed. This may be explained by a different affinity of RA for various RARs (see below) and various threshold levels for activation of target genes. Hox-2 genes are also activated sequentially by RA.[309] These homeobox-containing genes are thought to regulate morphogenesis. RA also can elicit both positive effects on proliferation and negative effects on differentiation. Thus, it seems that RA can induce a variety of different effects that are dependent on cell type and RA concentration.[310–312]

Retinoic Acid Receptors and Their Possible Functional Significance

Receptors for RA (RARs) were initially cloned through their strong homology to the DNA-binding domains of other members in the steroid/thyroid hormone receptor supergene family[313,314] (Fig. 5B-3*A*).

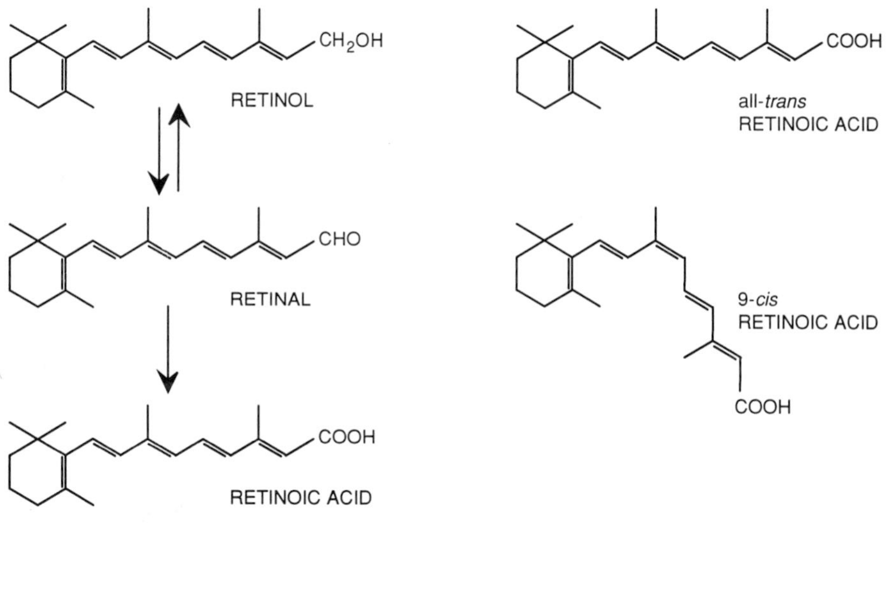

CH$_2$OH
RETINOL
CHO
RETINAL
COOH
RETINOIC ACID
COOH
all-*trans*
RETINOIC ACID
9-*cis*
RETINOIC ACID
COOH

FIGURE 5B-10 (*A*) Structural relation between the various retinoids, retinol (vitamin A), retinal, and retinoic acid. (*B*) The relation between all-*trans*-retinoic acid and 9-*cis*-retinoic acid.

RARs function as RA-activated transcriptional enhancer factors in a similar way to other members of this family. So far three RARs have been identified, termed α, β, and γ, respectively.[192,193,313–317] An alternative RAR has been identified in the newt and termed δ.[318] In addition, three nuclear receptors known as retinoid X receptors (RXRs), α, β, and γ, that are distantly related to RARs have also been cloned[219] (Fig. 5B-9). These receptors do not bind RA, suggesting that RA is not the natural ligand for RXR. More recently, these receptors have been found to bind 9-*cis*-retinoic acid with high affinity (9-*cis*) (Fig. 5B-10*B*). This may be the natural ligand for one or more of these receptors, although there is active inquiry into whether other retinoids also play this role (see below).

The overall structure of the RARs and RXRs is the same as the modular structure of the other members of the steroid receptor superfamily (Figs. 5B-3*A* and 5B-9). The three forms of RARs and RXRs from different species are more highly homologous to each other than to the different forms of RARs and RXRs, respectively, within the same species, suggesting that the individual forms of RAR are functionally distinct and thus may regulate the expression of different sets of RA-responsive genes. The retinoid receptor forms differ mainly in the N-terminal domain and the C-terminal portion of the molecule. Some small but evolutionarily conserved differences are also found in the DBD.

In addition to the three major RAR forms described above, there are multiple splicing variants of all three RARs that differ mainly within their N-terminal sequences.[319–321] For the mouse RARα, at least seven isoforms have been identified.[319] These alternative 5′ sequences may be functionally important in differential activation of target genes, as has been shown for other members of the steroid receptor superfamily.[322] All the RAR types and isoforms appear to be differentially expressed as well as autoregulated by RA.[319,320,323] In the case of RARβ, alternative promoters have also been thought to be responsible for the generation of multiple isoforms.[320] Alternative 5′ ends of the mRNAs may also give rise to differential regulation at the posttranscriptional or translational level.

RARα is expressed more or less ubiquitously, whereas the expression of RARβ and RARγ shows considerable spatial and temporal regulation with partially different tissue distribution.[316,317,323,324] Because of its high level of expression in the brain, RARβ may be important in the development of the central nervous system.[325] The β2 isoform is expressed mainly in RA-treated embryonic stem cells and thus may be particularly important during early development.[320] RARγ is expressed mainly in the skin, neural crest, and mesenchyme and may be involved in RA modulation of craniofacial development.[323]

RARα, β, and γ may also differ in their affinities for various retinoids. This issue is further complicated because of the presence of a cytoplasmic RA-binding protein (CRABP), which also binds RA with high affinity.[326] CRABP may act as a buffer for RA[304] and influence the accessibility of RA for the receptor. Differential recognition of various RA-responsive elements may also be influenced by differences in the DNA-binding domain of the RARs and by heterodimerization of different RAR forms or between different receptors, as exemplified by the RAR-TR or RAR-RXR heterodimer formation (see below). However, the function of individual RAR types or isoforms awaits further clarification.

A Role for RXR in RAR and Other Nuclear Receptor Functions

As mentioned above, a second retinoid transduction pathway, which is mediated by the RXRs, has been described. The cognate ligand for all three RXRs (α, β, and γ) is the RA isomer 9-cis-RA.[231,232,327] This isomer is 40-fold more potent in activating genes via the RXRs than is all-*trans*-RA. In contrast, 9-*cis*-RA and all-*trans*-RA bind and activate RARs with equal efficiency. Since 9-*cis*-RA is found in mammalian tissues along with all-*trans*-RA, the two isomers may function as specific receptor ligands and RA isomerization may be involved in controlling RA-mediated signal transduction. The high expression of RXRs in metabolic organs such as the liver, kidney, and intestine further supports a role for RXRs in retinoid function.[328] The RXRs regulate distinct target genes such as the cellular retinol-binding protein type II (CRBPII),[329] but they also, in combination with other transcription factors such as the RARs, TRs, and VD3Rs, regulate common target genes.[202,228,234,330] This is accomplished by heterodimerization between RXR and one of these receptor molecules. While RARα and RXRβ are more or less ubiquitously expressed, the other forms show a more restricted distribution. The fact that RXR expression is high in liver, kidney, spleen, and a variety of visceral tissues while some RAR subtypes are low in the same tissues suggests a role for RXR in retinoid and lipid metabolism. In fact, CRBPII and apolipoprotein A-I are RXR-responsive genes.[329,331] The role of RXR as partner in heterodimeric complexes with the RAR, TR, or vitamin D receptor as well as for some orphan receptors such as PPAR (see above) is to act as a coregulator of receptor function by synergistically increasing the DNA-binding ability of the receptors.[202,228,234,330] The heterodimerization occurs in solution before DNA binding. Interestingly, the synergistic effect on DNA binding and transactivation of target genes does not require the cognate ligand for RXR, but it does for RAR or TR.[328] This is in contrast to the synergistic effect observed for the RAR/TR heterodimeric complex, which requires both ligands.[52] Although RXR predominantly binds to the AGGTCA direct repeat motif with one base pair spacing (see above), heterodimerization with the other receptors allows interaction with the same motif in the form of palindromic sequences or as direct repeats with three (vitamin D receptor), four (TR), or five (RAR) base pair spacing (see above). The flexibility is further underlined by the observation that this rule is not absolute and that a given complex can have different effects on transcription when bound to different response elements.[236] In addition, the hormones themselves may differentially influence homodimer vs. heterodimer binding to a given response element.[202] The heterodimerization seems to occur between the C-terminal domains, and the heterodimers involving RXRs seem to be particularly stable, so that RXR-RAR and RXR-TR are formed in preference to homodimers and RAR-TR heterodimers.

The many subtypes of RXR and RAR and their differential expression, as well as their ability to heterodimerize and be activated by different retinoid metabolites, provide the possibility for a complex regulation and enhanced combinatorial diversity and versatility in gene regulation both during development and in differentiated tissues. Thus, the response of a specific retinoid target gene depends on the characteristics of the particular response element involved as well as the relative level of RAR, RXR, and all-*trans*- vs. 9-*cis*-RA.

REFERENCES

1. Jensen EV, Jacobson HI: Basic guides to the mechanism of hormone action. *Recent Prog Horm Res* 18:387, 1962.
2. King RJB, Mainwaring WIP: *Steroid-Cell Interactions*. Butterworths, London, 1974.
3. Allera A, Rao GS: Characteristics and specificity of the glucocorticoid "carrier" of rat liver membrane, in Chrousos GP (ed): *Steroid Hormone Resistance*. New York, Plenum, 1986, p 53.
4. Catelli MG, Binart N, Jung-Testas L, Renoir JM, Baulieu EE, Feramisco JR, Welsh WJ: The common 90-kd protein component of non-transformed "8S" steroid receptors is a heat shock protein. *EMBO J* 4:3131, 1985.
5. Sanchez ER, Toft DO, Schlesinger MJ, Pratt WB: Evidence that the 90-kDa phosphoprotein associated with the untransformed L-cell glucocorticoid receptor is a murine heat shock protein. *J Biol Chem* 260:12398, 1985.
6. Tai PKK, Maeda Y, Nakao K, Wakim NG, Duhring JL, Faber LE: A 59-kilodalton protein associated with progestin, estrogen, androgen, and glucocorticoid receptors. *Biochemistry* 25:5269, 1986.
7. Baulieu E-E, Binart N, Cadepond MG, Catelli MG, Chambraud J, Garnier J, Gasc JM, Groyer-Schweizer G, et al: Do receptor-associated nuclear proteins explain earliest steps of steroid hormone function? in Gustafsson J-Å, Eriksson H, Carlstedt-Duke J (eds): *The Steroid/Thyroid Hormone Receptor Family and Gene Regulation*. Birkhäuser, Basel, 1989, p 301.
8. Sanchez ER, Hirst M, Scherrer LC, Tang H-Y, Welsh MJ, Harmon JM, Simons SS, Ringold GM, Pratt WB: Hormone-free mouse glucocorticoid receptors overexpressed in chinese hamster ovary cells are localized to the nucleus and are associated with both hsp 70 and hsp 90. *J Biol Chem* 265:20123, 1990.
9. Sanchez ER: Hsp56: A novel heat shock protein associated with untransformed steroid receptor complexes. *J Biol Chem* 265:22067, 1990.
10. Leach KL, Dahmer MK, Hammond ND, Sando JJ, Pratt WB: Molybdate inhibition of glucocorticoid receptor inactivation and transformation. *J Biol Chem* 254:11884, 1979.
11. Dahmer MK, Housley PR, Pratt WB: Effects of molybdate and endogenous inhibitors on steroid-receptor inactivation, transformation, and translocation. *Annu Rev Physiol* 46:67, 1984.
12. Joab I, Radanyi C, Renoid JM, Buchou T, Catelli MG, Binart N, Mester J, Baulieu E-E: Common non-hormone binding component in non-transformed chick oviduct receptors of four steroid hormones. *Nature* 308:850, 1984.
13. Housley PR, Sanchez ER, Westphal HM, Beato M, Pratt WB: The molybdate stabilized L-cell glucocorticoid receptor isolated by affinity chromatography or with a monoclonal antibody is associated with a90-92 kDa nonsteroid-binding phosphoprotein. *J Biol Chem* 260:13810, 1985.
14. Mendel DB, Bodwell JE, Gametchu B, Harrison RW, Munck A: Molybdate-stabilized nonactivated glucocorticoid-receptor complexes contain a 90 k-Da non-steroid binding phosphoprotein that is lost on activation. *J Biol Chem* 261:3758, 1986.
15. Notides AC, Nielsen S: Estradiol-binding kinetics of the activated and nonactivated estrogen receptor. *J Biol Chem* 257:8856, 1977.
16. Kumar V, Chambon P: The estrogen receptor binds tightly to its responsive element as a ligand-induced homodimer. *Cell* 55:145, 1988.
17. Wrange Ö, Eriksson P, Perlmann T: The purified activated glucocorticoid receptor is a homodimer. *J Biol Chem* 265:5253, 1989.
18. DeMarzo AM, Beck CA, Onate SA, Edwards DP: Dimerizaton of mammalian progesterone receptors occurs in the absence of DNA and is related to the release of the 90-kDa heat shock protein. *Proc Natl Acad Sci USA* 88:72, 1991.
19. Tsai S, Carlstedt-Duke J, Weigel N, Dahlman K, Gustafsson J-Å, Tsai M-J, O'Malley BW: Molecular interactions of steroid hormone receptors with its enhancer element: Evidence for receptor dimer formation. *Cell* 55:361, 1988.
20. Fawell SE, Lees JA, White R, Parker MG: Characterization and colocalization of steroid binding and dimerization activities in the mouse estrogen receptor. *Cell* 60:953, 1990.
21. Chalepakis G, Schauer M, Cao X, Beato M: Efficient binding of glucocorticoid receptor to its responsive element requires a dimer and DNA flanking sequences. *DNA Cell Biol* 9:355, 1990.
22. Yamamoto KR: Steroid regulated transcription of specific genes and gene networks. *Annu Rev Genet* 19:209, 1985.
23. Dalman FC, Koenig RJ, Perdew GH, Massa E, Pratt WB: In contrast to the glucocorticoid receptor, the thyroid hormone receptor is translated in the DNA binding state and is not associated with Hsp90. *J Biol Chem* 265:3615, 1990.
24. Dalman FC, Sturzenbecker LJ, Levin AA, Lucas DA, Perdew GH, Petkovich M, Chambon P, Grippo JF, Pratt WB: Retinoic acid receptor belongs to a subclass of nuclear receptors that do not form docking complexes with hsp90. *Biochemistry* 30:5605, 1991.
25. Kato H, Fukuda T, Parkinson C, McPhie P, Cheng SY: Cytosolic thyroid hormone-binding protein is a monomer of pyruvate kinase. *Proc Natl Acad Sci USA* 86:7861, 1989.
26. Chytil F, Ong DE: Intracellular vitamin A-binding proteins. *Annu Rev Nutr* 7:321, 1987.
27. Dolle P, Ruberte E, Leroy P, Morriss-Kay G, Chambon P: Retinoic acid receptors and cellular retinoid binding proteins. I. A systematic study of their differential pattern of transcription during mouse organogenesis. *Development* 110:1133, 1990.

28. Boylan JF, Gudas LJ: Overexpression of the cellular retinoid acid binding protein-I (CRABP-I) results in a reduction in differentiation-specific gene expression in F9 teratocarcinoma cells. *J Cell Biol* 112:965, 1991.
29. Harlow KW, Smith DN, Katzenellenbogen JA, Greene GL, Katzenellenbogen BS: Identification of cysteine-530 as the covalent attachment site of an affinity-labeling estrogen (ketononestrol aziridine) and antiestrogen (tamoxifen aziridine) in the human estrogen receptor. *J Biol Chem* 264:17476, 1989.
30. Strömstedt P-E, Berkenstam A, Jörnvall H, Gustafsson J-Å, Carlstedt-Duke J: Radiosequence analysis of the human progestine receptor charged with [^{3}H]promegestone: A comparison with the glucocorticoid receptor. *J Biol Chem* 265:12973, 1990.
31. Carlstedt-Duke J, Strömstedt P-E, Persson B, Cederlund E, Gustaffson J-Å, Jörnvall H: Identification of hormone-interacting amino acid residues within the steroid-binding domain of the glucocorticoid receptor in relation to other steroid hormone receptors. *J Biol Chem* 263:6842, 1988.
32. Simons SS, Pumphrey JG, Rudikoff S, Eisen HJ: Identification of cystein 656 as the amino acid of hepatoma tissue culture cell glucocorticoid receptors that is covalently labeled by dexamethasone 21-mesylate. *J Biol Chem* 262:9676, 1987.
33. Smith LI, Bodwell JE, Mendel DB, Ciardelli T, North WG, Munck A: Identification of cystein-644 as the covalent site of attachment of dexamethasone 21-mesylate to murine glucocorticoid receptor in WEHI-7 cells. *Biochemistry* 27:3747, 1988.
34. Giguère V, Hollenberg SM, Rosenfeld MG, Evans RM: Functional domains of the human glucocorticoid receptor. *Cell* 46:645, 1986.
35. Hollenberg SM, Giguère V, Segui P, Evans RM: Colocalization of DNA-binding and transcriptional activation functions in the human glucocorticoid receptor. *Cell* 49:39, 1987.
36. Godowski PJ, Rusconi S, Miesfeld R, Yamamoto KR: Glucocorticoid receptor mutants that are constitutive activators of transcriptional enhancement. *Nature* 325:365, 1987.
37. Miesfeld R, Godowski PJ, Maler BA, Yamamoto KR: Glucocorticoid receptor mutants that define a small region sufficient for enhancer activation. *Science* 236:423, 1987.
38. Rusconi S, Yamamoto KR: Functional dissection of the hormone and DNA binding activities of the glucocorticoid receptor. *EMBO J* 6:1309, 1987.
39. Danielsen M, Northrop JP, Jonklaas J, Ringold GM: Domains of the glucocorticoid receptor involved in specific and nonspecific deoxyribosenucleic acid binding, hormone activation, and transcriptional enhancement. *Mol Endocrinol* 1:816, 1987.
40. Okret S, Wikström A-C, Gustafsson J-Å: Molybdate-stabilized glucocorticoid receptor: Evidence for a receptor heterodimer. *Biochemistry* 24:6581, 1985.
41. Denis M, Wikström A-C, Gustafsson J-Å: The molybdate-stabilized nonactivated glucocorticoid receptor contains a dimer of M_r 90,000 non-hormone-binding protein. *J Biol Chem* 262:11803, 1987.
42. Mendel DB, Orti E: Isoform composition and stoichiometry of the 90-kDa heat shock protein associated with glucocorticoid receptors. *J Biol Chem* 262:6695, 1988.
43. Smith DF, Schowalter DB, Kost SL, Toft DO: Reconstitution of progesterone receptor with heat shock proteins. *Mol Endocrinol* 4:1704, 1990.
44. Wrange Ö, Okret S, Radójcic M, Carlstedt-Duke J, Gustafsson J-Å: Characterization of the purified activated glucocorticoid receptor from rat liver cytosol. *J Biol Chem* 259:4534, 1984.
45. Pratt WB, Jolly DJ, Pratt DV, Hollenberg SM, Giguere V, Capedon FM, Schweizer-Groyer G, Catelli MG, et al: A region in the steroid binding domain determines formation of the non-DNA-binding, 9S glucocorticoid receptor complex. *J Biol Chem* 263:267, 1988.
46. Howard KJ, Holley SJ, Yamamoto KR, Distelhorst CW: Mapping the Hsp90 binding region of the glucocorticoid receptor. *J Biol Chem* 265:11928, 1990.
47. Nemoto T, Mason GGF, Wilhelmsson A, Cuthill S, Hapgood J, Gustafsson J-Å, Poellinger L: Activation of the dioxin and glucocorticoid receptors to a DNA binding state under cell-free conditions. *J Biol Chem* 265:2269, 1990.
48. Picard D, Salser SJ, Yamamoto KR: A movable and regulable inactivation function within the steroid binding domain of the glucocorticoid receptor. *Cell* 54:1073, 1988.
49. Godowski PJ, Picard D, Yamamoto KR: Signal transduction and transcriptional regulation by glucocorticoid receptor-LexA fusion proteins. *Science* 241:812, 1988.
50. Nemoto T, Ohara-Nemoto Y, Denis M, Gustafsson J-Å: The transformed glucocorticoid receptor has a lower steroid-binding affinity than the nontransformed receptor. *Biochemistry* 29:1880, 1990.
51. Ohara-Nemoto Y, Strömstedt P-E, Dahlman-Wright K, Nemoto T, Gustafsson J-Å, Carlstedt-Duke J: The steroid-binding properties of recombinant glucocorticoid receptor: A putative role for heat shock protein hsp 90. *J Steroid Biochem Mol Biol* 37:481, 1990.
52. Guiochon-Mantel A, Loosfelt H, Lescop P, Sar S, Atger M, Perrot-Applanat M, Milgrom E: Mechanism of nuclear localisation of the progesterone receptor: Evidence for interaction between monomers. *Cell* 57:1147, 1989.
53. Glass CK, Lipkin SM, Devary OV, Rosenfeld MG: Positive and negative regulation of gene transcription by a retinoic acid-thyroid hormone receptor dimer. *Cell* 59:697, 1989.
54. Forman BM, Yang C-R, Au M, Casanova J, Ghysdael J, Samuels HH: A domain containing leucine-zipper-like motifs mediates novel *in vivo* interactions between the thyroid hormone and retinoic acid receptors. *Mol Endocrinol* 3:1610, 1989.
55. Landschulz WH, Johnson PF, McKnight SL: The leucine zipper: A hypothetical structure common to a new class of DNA binding proteins. *Science* 240:1759, 1988.
56. Rasmussen R, Benvegnu D, O'Shea EK, Kim PS, Alber T: X-ray scattering indicates that the leucine zipper is a coiled coil. *Proc Natl Acad Sci USA* 88:561, 1991.
57. Lees JA, Fawell SE, White R, Parker MG: A 22-amino-acid peptide restores DNA-binding activity to dimerization-defective mutants of the estrogen receptor. *Mol Cell Biol* 10:5529, 1990.
58. Dahlman-Wright K, Siltala-Roos H, Carlstedt-Duke J, Gustafsson J-Å: Protein-protein interactions facilitate DNA binding by the glucocorticoid receptor DNA-binding domain. *J Biol Chem* 265:14030, 1990.
59. Dahlman-Wright K, Wright APH, Gustafsson J-Å, Carlstedt-Duke J: Interaction of the glucocorticoid receptor DNA-binding domain with DNA as a dimer is mediated via a short segment of five amino acids. *J Biol Chem* 266:3107, 1991.
60. Umesono K, Evans RM: Determinants of target gene specificity for steroid/thyroid hormone receptors. *Cell* 57:1139, 1989.
61. Glass CK, Holloway JM, Devary OV, Rosenfelt MG: The thyroid hormone receptor binds with opposite transcriptional effects to a common sequence motif in thyroid hormone and estrogen response elements. *Cell* 54:313, 1988.
62. Moudgil VK: Phosphorylation of steroid hormone receptors. *Biochim Biophys Acta* 1055:243, 1990.
63. Bodwell JE, Orti E, Coull JM, Pappin DJC, Smith LI, Swift F: Identification of phosphorylated sites in the mouse glucocorticoid receptor. *J Biol Chem* 266:7549, 1991.
64. Hoeck W, Groner B: Hormone-dependent phosphorylation of the glucocorticoid receptor occurs mainly in the amino-terminal transactivation domain. *J Biol Chem* 265:5403, 1990.
65. Denner LA, Schrader WT, O'Malley BW, Weigel NL: Hormonal regulation and identification of chicken progesterone receptor phosphorylation sites. *J Biol Chem* 265:16548, 1990.
66. Gasc J-M, Renoir J-M, Radanyi C, Joab I, Tuohimaa P, Baulieu E-E: Progesterone receptor in the chick oviduct: An im-

munohistochemical study with antibodies to distinct receptor components. *J Cell Biol* 99:1193, 1984.

67. Perrot-Applanat M, Logeat A, Groyer-Picard MT, Milgrom E: Immunocytochemical study of mammalian progesterone receptor using monoclonal antibodies. *Endocrinology* 116:1473, 1985.
68. King WJ, Greene GL: Monoclonal antibodies localize oestrogen receptor in the nuclei of target cells. *Nature* 307:745, 1984.
69. Gorski J, Welshons W, Sakai D: Remodeling the estrogen receptor model. *Mol Cell Endocrinol* 36:11, 1984.
70. Welshons W, Lieberman ME, Gorski J: Nuclear localization of unoccupied oestrogen receptors. *Nature* 307:747, 1984.
71. Sar M, Lubahn DB, French FS, Wilson EM: Immunohistochemical localization of the androgen receptor in rat and human tissues. *Endocrinology* 127:3180, 1990.
72. Fuxe K, Wikström A-C, Okret S, Agnati LF, Härfstrand A, Yu Z-Y, Granholm L, Zoli M, et al: Mapping of glucocorticoid receptor immunoreactive neurons in the rat tel- and diencephalon using a monoclonal antibody against rat liver glucocorticoid receptor. *Endocrinology* 117:1803, 1985.
73. Wikström A-C, Bakke O, Okret S, Brönnegård M, Gustafsson J-Å: Intracellular localization of the glucocorticoid receptor: Evidence for cytoplasmic and nuclear localization. *Endocrinology* 120:1232, 1987.
74. Govindan MV: Immunofluorescence microscopy of the intracellular translocation of glucocorticoid-receptor complexes in rat hepatoma (HTC) cells. *Exp Cell Res* 127:293, 1980.
75. Papamichail M, Tsokos G, Tsawdaroglou N, Sekeris CE: Immunocytochemical demonstration of glucocorticoid receptors in different cell types and their translocation from the cytoplasm to the cell nucleus in the presence of dexamethasone. *Exp Cell Res* 125:490, 1980.
76. Berbard PA, Joh TH: Characterization and immunocytochemical demonstration of glucocorticoid receptor using antisera specific to transformed receptor. *Arch Biochem Biophys* 229:466, 1984.
77. Antakly T, Eisen HJ: Immunocytochemical localization of glucocorticoid receptor in target cells. *Endocrinology* 115:1984, 1984.
78. Picard D, Yamamoto KR: Two signals mediate hormone-dependent nuclear localization of the glucocorticoid receptor. *EMBO J* 6:3333, 1987.
79. Fawell SE, White R, Hoare S, Sydenham M, Page M, Parker MG: Inhibition of estrogen receptor DNA binding by the pure antiestrogen ICI-164,384 appears to be mediated by impaired receptor dimerization. *Proc Natl Acad Sci USA* 87:6883, 1990.
80. Webster NJG, Green S, Jin JR, Chambon P: The hormone binding domains of the estrogen and glucocorticoid receptors contain an inducible transcription activation function. *Cell* 54:199, 1988.
81. Metzger D, White JH, Chambon P: The human oestrogen receptor functions in yeast. *Nature* 334:31, 1988.
82. Lees JA, Fawell SE, Parker MG: Identification of two transactivation domains in mouse oestrogen receptor. *Nucleic Acids Res* 17:5477, 1989.
83. Meyer ME, Pornon A, Ji JW, Bocquel MT, Chambon P, Gronemeyer H: Agonistic and antagonistic activities of RU486 on the functions of the human progesterone receptor. *EMBO J* 9:3923, 1990.
84. Renoir J-M, Radanyi C, Baulieu E-E: The antiprogesterone RU486 stabilizes the heterooligomeric, non-DNA-binding, 8S-form of the rabbit uterus cytosol progesterone receptor. *Steroids* 53:1, 1989.
85. Burbach KM, Poland A, Bradfield CA: Cloning of the Ah-receptor cDNA reveals a distinctive ligand-activated transcription factor. *Proc Natl Acad Sci USA* 89:8185, 1992.
86. Dong Y, Aronsson M, Gustafsson J-Å, Okret S: The mechanism of cAMP-induced glucocorticoid receptor expression. *J Biol Chem* 264:13679, 1989.
87. Horwitz KB, Mockus MB, Pike AW, Fennessey PV, Sheridan RL: Progesterone receptor replenishment in T47D human breast cancer cells. *J Biol Chem* 258:7603, 1983.
88. Paek I, Axel R: Glucocorticoids enhance stability of human growth hormone mRNA. *Mol Cell Biol* 7:1496, 1987.
89. Diamond DJ, Goodman HW: Regulation of growth hormone mRNA synthesis by dexamethasone and triiodothyronine: Transcriptional rate and mRNA stability changes in pituitary tumour cells. *J Mol Biol* 181:41, 1985.
90. Peterson DD, Koch SR, Granner DK: 3′ non-coding region of phosphoenolpyruvate carboxykinase mRNA contains a glucocorticoid-responsive mRNA-stabilizing element. *Proc Natl Acad Sci USA* 86:7800, 1989.
91. Becker PB, Renkawitz R, Schütz G: Tissue specific DNAse I hypersensitive sites in the 5′ flanking sequences of the tryptophan oxygenase and tyrosine aminotransferase genes. *EMBO J* 3:2015, 1984.
92. Zaret KS, Yamamoto KR: Reversible and persistent changes in chromatin structure accompany activation of a glucocorticoid-dependent enhancer element. *Cell* 38:29, 1984.
93. Becker PB, Gloss B, Schmid W, Strähle U, Schütz G: *In vivo* protein-DNA interactions in a glucocorticoid response element require the presence of the hormone. *Nature* 324:686, 1986.
94. Beato M: Gene regulation by steroid hormones. *Cell* 56:335, 1989.
95. Truss M, Chalepakis G, Beato M: Contacts between steroid hormone receptors and thymines in DNA: An interference method. *Proc Natl Acad Sci USA* 87:7180, 1990.
96. Cairns C, Gustafsson J-Å, Carlstedt-Duke J: Identification of protein contact sites within the glucocorticoid/progestin response element. *Mol Endocrinol* 5:598, 1991.
97. Umesono K, Giguère V, Glass CK, Rosenfeld MG, Evans RM: Retinoic acid and thyroid hormone induce gene expression through a common response element. *Nature* 336:262, 1988.
98. Härd T, Kellenbach E, Boelens R, Maler B, Dahlman K, Freedman LP, Carlstedt-Duke J, Yamamoto KR, et al: Solution structure of the glucocorticoid receptor DNA-binding domain. *Science* 249:157, 1990.
99. Freedman LP, Luisi BF, Korszun ZR, Basavappa R, Sigler PB, Yamamoto KR: The function and structure of the metal coordination sites within the glucocorticoid receptor DNA-binding domain. *Nature* 334:543, 1988.
100. Severene Y, Wieland S, Shaffner W, Rusconi S: Metal binding "finger" structures in the glucocorticoid receptor defined by site-directed mutagenesis. *EMBO J* 7:2503, 1988.
101. Zilliacus J, Dahlman-Wright K, Carlstedt-Duke J, Gustafsson J-Å: Zinc coordination scheme for the C-terminal zinc binding site of nuclear hormone receptors. *J Steroid Biochem Mol Biol* 42:131, 1992.
102. Schwabe JWR, Neuhaus D, Rhodes D: Solution structure of the DNA-binding domain of the oestrogen receptor. *Nature* 348:458, 1990.
103. Notides AC, Nielsen S: The molecular mechanism of the *in vitro* 4S to 6S transformation of the uterine estrogen receptor. *J Biol Chem* 249:1866, 1974.
104. Cairns W, Cairns C, Pongratz I, Poellinger L, Okret S: Assembly of a glucocorticoid receptor complex prior to DNA binding enhances its specific interaction with a glucocorticoid response element. *J Biol Chem* 266:11221, 1991.
105. Scheidereit C, Beato M: Contacts between hormone receptor and DNA double helix within a glucocorticoid regulatory element of mouse mammary tumour virus. *Proc Natl Acad Sci USA* 81:3029, 1984.
106. Klein-Hitpass L, Ryffel GU, Heitlinger E, Cato ACB: A 13 base pair palindrome is a functional estrogen responsive element and interacts specifically with estrogen receptor. *Nucleic Acids Res* 16:647, 1988.
107. Green S, Kumar V, Theulaz I, Wahli W, Chambon P: The N-terminal DNA-binding "zinc-finger" of the oestrogen and glucocorticoid receptors determines target gene specificity. *EMBO J* 7:3037, 1988.
108. Mader S, Kumar V, de Verneuil H, Chambon P: Three amino acids of the oestrogen receptor are essential to its ability to

distinguish an oestrogen from a glucocorticoid responsive element. *Nature* 338:271, 1989.
109. Danielsen M, Hinck L, Ringold GM: Two amino acids within the knuckle of the first zinc finger specify DNA response element activation by the glucocorticoid receptor. *Cell* 57:1131, 1989.
110. Zilliacus J, Dahlman-Wright K, Wright A, Gustafsson J-Å, Carlstedt-Duke J: DNA binding specificity of mutant glucocorticoid receptor DNA-binding domains. *J Biol Chem* 266:3101, 1991.
111. Sawadogo M, Sentenac A: RNA polymerase B (II) and general transcription factors. *Annu Rev Biochem* 59:711, 1990.
112. Ptashne M: How eukaryotic transcriptional activators work. *Nature* 335:683, 1988.
113. Mitchell PJ, Tjian R: Transcriptional regulation in mammalian cells by sequence specific DNA binding proteins. *Science* 245:371, 1989.
114. Pugh BF, Tjian R: Mechanism of transcriptional activation by SP1: Evidence for coactivators. *Cell* 61:1187, 1990.
115. Berger SL, Cress WD, Cress A, Treizenberg SJ, Guarente L: Selective inhibition of activated but not basal transcription by the acidic activation domain of VP16: Evidence for transcriptional adaptors. *Cell* 61:1199, 1990.
116. Kelleher RJ, Flanagan PM, Kornberg RD: A novel mediator between activator proteins and the RNA polymerase II transcription apparatus. *Cell* 61:1209, 1990.
117. Lin Y-S, Green MR: Mechanism of cation of an acidic transcriptional activator *in vitro*. *Cell* 64:971, 1991.
118. Stringer KF, Ingles CJ, Greenblatt J: Direct and selective binding of an acidic transcriptional activation domain to the TATA-box factor TFIID. *Nature* 345:783, 1990.
119. Ingles CJ, Shales M, Cress WD, Treizenberg SJ, Greenblatt J: Reduced binding of TFIID to transcriptionally compromised mutants of VP16. *Nature* 351:588, 1991.
120. Freedman PL, Yoshinaga SK, Vanderbilt JN, Yamamoto KR: *In vitro* transcription enhancement by purified derivatives of the glucocorticoid receptor. *Science* 245:298, 1989.
121. Tsai SY, Srinivasan G, Allan GF, Thompson EB, O'Malley BW, Tsai M-J: Recombinant human glucocorticoid receptor induces transcription of hormone response genes *in vitro*. *J Biol Chem* 265:17055, 1990.
122. Klein-Hitpass L, Tsai SY, Weigel NL, Allan GF, Riley D, Rodriguez R, Schrader WT, Tasai M-Y, O'Malley BW: The progesterone receptor stimulates cell-free transcription by enhancing the formation of a stable preinitiation complex. *Cell* 60:247, 1990.
123. Kalff M, Gross B, Beato M: Progesterone receptor stimulates transcription of the mouse mammary tumour virus in a cell-free system. *Nature* 344:360, 1990.
124. Elliston JF, Fawell SF, Klein-Hitpass L, Tsai SY, Tsai M-Y, Parker MG, O'Malley BW: Mechanism of estrogen dependent transcription in a cell-free system. *Mol Cell Biol* 10:6607, 1990.
125. Tasset D, Tora L, Fromental C, Scheer E, Chambon P: Distinct classes of transcriptional activating domains function by different mechanisms. *Cell* 62:1177, 1990.
126. Wright APH, McEwan IJ, Dahlman-Wright K, Gustafsson J-Å: High level expression of the major transactivation domain of the human glucocorticoid receptor in yeast cells inhibits endogenous gene expression and cell growth. *Mol Endocrinol* 5:1366, 1991.
127. Hollenberg SM, Evans RM: Multiple and cooperative transactivation domains of the human glucocorticoid receptor. *Cell* 55:899, 1988.
128. Tora L, White J, Brou C, Tasset D, Webster N, Scheer E, Chambon P: The human estrogen receptor has two independent non-acidic transcriptional activation functions. *Cell* 59:477, 1989.
129. Schena M, Freedman LP, Yamamoto KR: Mutations in the glucocorticoid receptor zinc finger region that distinguish interdigitated DNA binding and transcriptional enhancement activities. *Genes Dev* 3:1590, 1989.
130. Guiochon-Mantel A, Loosfelt H, Ragot T, Bailly A, Atger M, Misrahi M, Perricaudet M, Milgrom E: Receptors bound to antiprogestin form abortive complexes with hormone responsive elements. *Nature* 336:695, 1988.
131. Gottesfeld J, Bloomer LS: Assembly of transcriptionally active 5S RNA gene chromatin *in vitro*. *Cell* 28:781,1982.
132. Matsui T: Transcription of the adenovirus 2 major late and peptide XI genes under conditions of *in vitro* nucleosome assembly. *Mol Cell Biol* 7:1401, 1987.
133. Workman JL, Roeder RG: Binding of transcription factor TFIID to the major late promoter during *in vitro* nuclear assembly potentiates subsequent initiation by RNA polymerase II. *Cell* 51:613, 1987.
134. Perlmann T, Wrange Ö: Inhibition of chromatin assembly in *Xenopus laevis* oocytes correlates with derepression of the MMTV promoter. *Mol Cell Biol* 11:5259, 1991.
135. Richard-Foy H, Hager GL: Sequence-specific positioning of nucleosomes over the steroid inducible MMTV promoter. *EMBO J* 6:2321, 1987.
136. Cordingly MG, Riegel AT, Hager GL: Steroid-dependent interaction of transcription factors with the inducible promoter of mouse mammary tumour virus *in vivo*. *Cell* 48:261, 1987.
137. Carr KD, Richard-Foy H: Glucocorticoids locally disrupt an array of positioned nucleosomes on the rat tyrosione aminotransferase promoter in hepatoma cells. *Proc Natl Acad Sci USA* 87:9300, 1990.
138. Roesler WJ, Park EA, Klemm DJ, Liu J, Gurney AL, Vandenbark GR, Hanson RW: Modulation of hormone response elements by promoter environment. *Trends Endocrinol Metab* 1:347, 1990.
139. Strähle U, Schmid W, Schütz G: Synergistic action of the glucocorticoid receptor with transcription factors. *EMBO J* 7:3389, 1988.
140. Schüle R, Muller M, Kaltschmitt C, Renkawitz R: Many transcription factors interact synergistically with steroid receptors. *Science* 242:1418, 1988.
141. Tsai SY, Tsai M-Y, O'Malley BW: Cooperative binding of steroid hormone receptors contributes to transcriptional synergism at target enhancer elements. *Cell* 57:443, 1989.
142. Martinez E, Wahli W: Cooperative binding of the estrogen receptor to imperfect estrogen-responsive DNA elements correlates with their synergistic hormone-dependent enhancer activity. *EMBO J* 8:3781, 1989.
143. Ponglikitmongkol M, White JH, Chambon P: Synergistic activation of transcription by the human estrogen receptor bound to tandem response elements. *EMBO J* 9:2221, 1990.
144. Schmid W, Strähle U, Schütz G, Schmitt J, Stunnenberg H: Glucocorticoid receptor binds cooperatively to adjacent recognition sites. *EMBO J* 8:2257, 1989.
145. Wright APH, Gustafsson J-Å: Mechanism of synergistic transcriptional transactivation by the human glucocorticoid receptor. *Proc Natl Acad Sci USA* 88:8283, 1991.
146. Cato ACB, Ponta H: Different regions of the estrogen receptor are required for synergistic action with the glucocorticoid and progesterone receptors. *Mol Cell Biol* 9:5324, 1989.
147. Schatt M, Rusconi S, Shaffner W: A single DNA-binding transcription factor is sufficient for activation from a distant enhancer and/or from a promoter position. *EMBO J* 9:481, 1990.
148. Brüggemeier U, Kalff M, Franke S, Scheidereit C, Beato M: Ubiquitous transcription factor OTF-1 mediates induction of the MMTV promoter through synergistic interaction with hormone receptors. *Cell* 64:565, 1991.
149. Martinez E, Dusserre Y, Wahli W, Mermod N: Synergistic transcriptional activation by CTF/NF-1 and the estrogen receptor involves stabilised interactions with a limiting target factor. *Mol Cell Biol* 11:2937, 1991.
150. Sakai DD, Helms S, Carlstedt-Duke J, Gustafsson J-Å, Rottman FM, Yamamoto KR: Hormone mediated repression: A negative glucocorticoid response element from the bovine prolactin gene. *Genes Dev* 2:1144, 1988.

151. Baniahmad A, Steiner C, Köhne AC, Renkawitz R: Modular structure of a chicken lysozyme silencer: Involvement of an unusual thyroid receptor binding site. *Cell* 61:505, 1990.
152. Akerblom IE, Slater EP, Beato M, Baxter JD, Mellon PL: Negative regulation by glucocorticoids through interference with a cAMP responsive enhancer. *Science* 241:350, 1988.
153. Drouin J, Trifiro MA, Plante RK, Nemer M, Eriksson P, Wrange Ö: Glucocorticoid receptor binding to a specific DNA sequence is required for hormone-dependent repression of pro-opiomelanocortin gene transcription. *Mol Cell Biol* 9:5305, 1989.
154. Strömstedt P-E, Poellinger L, Gustafsson J-Å, Carlstedt-Duke J: The glucocorticoid receptor binds to a sequence overlapping the TATA-box of the human osteocalcin promoter: A potential mechanism for negative regulation. *Mol Cell Biol* 11:3379, 1991.
155. Diamond MI, Miner JN, Yoshinaga SK, Yamamoto KR: Transcription factor interactions: Selectors of positive or negative regulation from a single DNA element. *Science* 249:1266, 1990.
156. Jonat C, Rahmsdorf HJ, Park K-K, Cato ACB, Gebel S, Ponta H, Herrlich P: Antitumor promotion and antiinflammation: Down-modulation of AP1 (Fos/Jun) activity by glucocorticoid hormone. *Cell* 62:1189, 1990.
157. Yang-Yen H-F, Chambard A-C, Sun Y-L, Smearl T, Schmidt TJ, Drouin J, Karin M: Transcriptional interference between c-Jun and the glucocorticoid receptor: Mutual inhibition of DNA binding due to direct protein-protein interaction. *Cell* 62:1205, 1990.
158. Schüle R, Rangarajan P, Kliewer S, Ransone LJ, Bolado J, Yang N, Verma IM, Evans RM: Functional antagonism between oncoprotein c-Jun and the glucocorticoid receptor. *Cell* 62:1217, 1990.
159. Lucibello FC, Slater EP, Jooss KU, Beato M, Müller R: Mutual transrepression of Fos and the glucocorticoid receptor: Involvement of a functional domain in Fos which is absent in Fos-B. *EMBO J* 9:2827, 1990.
160. Nicholson RC, Mader S, Nagpal S, Leid M, Rochette-Egly C, Chambon P: Negative regulation of the rat stromolysin gene promoter by retinoic acid is mediated by an AP1 binding site. *EMBO J* 9:4443, 1990.
161. Griffin JE, Wilson JD: The androgen resistance syndromes, in Scriver CR, Beaudet AL, Sly WS, Valle D (eds): *The Metabolic Basis of Inherited Disease.* New York, McGraw-Hill, 1989, pp 1919–1944.
162. McPhaul M, Marcelli M, Zoppi S, Griffin J, Wilson J: Genetic basis of endocrine disease 4: The spectrum of mutations in the androgen receptor gene that causes androgen resistance. *J Endocrinol Metab* 76:17, 1993.
163. Griffin JE: Androgen resistance—the clinical spectrum. *N Engl J Med* 326:611, 1992.
164. Charest NJ, Zhou ZX, Lubahn DB, Olsen KL, Wilson EM, French FS: A frameshift mutation destabilizes androgen receptor messenger RNA in the tfm mouse. *Mol Endocrinol* 5:573, 1991.
165. Lubahn DB, Brown TR, Simental JA, Higgs HN, Migeon CJ, Wilson EM, French FS: Sequence of the intron exon junctions of the coding region of the human androgen receptor gene and identification of a point mutation in a family with complete androgen insensitivity. *Proc Natl Acad Sci USA* 86:9534, 1989.
166. Marcelli M, Zoppi S, Grino PB, Griffin JE, Wilson JD, McPhaul MJ: A point mutation in the DNA-binding domain of the androgen receptor gene causes complete testicular feminization in a patient with receptor-positive androgen resistance. *J Clin Invest* 87:1123, 1991.
167. McPhaul MJ, Marcelli M, Tilley WD, Griffin JE, Isidrogutierrez RF, Wilson JD: Molecular basis of androgen resistance in a family with a qualitative abnormality of the androgen receptor and responsive to high-dose androgen therapy. *J Clin Invest* 87:1413, 1991.
168. Risstalpers C, Kuiper GGJM, Faber PW, Schweikert HU, van Rooij HCJ, Zegers ND, Hodgins MB, Degenhart HJ, et al: Aberrant splicing of androgen receptor messenger RNA results in synthesis of a nonfunctional receptor protein in a patient with androgen insensitivity. *Proc Natl Acad Sci USA* 87:7866, 1990.
169. Sai T, Seino S, Chang C, Trifiro M, Pinsky L, Mhatre A, Kaufman M, Lambert B, et al: An exonic point mutation of the androgen receptor gene in a family with complete androgen insensitivity. *Am J Hum Genet* 46:1095, 1990.
170. Veldscholte J, Risstalpers C, Kuiper GGJM, Jenster G, Berrevoets C, Claassen E, Vanrooij HCJ, Trapman J, et al: A mutation in the ligand binding domain of the androgen receptor of human LNCaP cells affects steroid binding characteristics and response to anti-androgens. *Biochem Biophys Res Commun* 173:534, 1990.
171. Yarbrough WG, Quarmby VE, Simental JA, Joseph DR, Sar M, Lubahn DB, Olsen KL, French FS, Wilson EM: A single base mutation in the androgen receptor gene causes androgen insensitivity in the testicular feminized rat. *J Biol Chem* 265:8893, 1990.
172. Ritchie HH, Hughes MR, Thompson ET, Malloy PJ, Hochberg Z, Feldman D, Pike JW, O'Malley BW: An ochre mutation in the vitamin-D receptor gene causes hereditary 1,25-dihydroxyvitamin-D_3-resistant rickets in 3 families. *Proc Natl Acad Sci USA* 86:9783, 1989.
173. Hughes MR, Malloy PJ, O'Malley BW, Pike JW, Feldman D: Genetic defects of the 1,25-dihydroxyvitamin-D_3 receptor. *J Recept Res* 11:699, 1991.
174. Yagi H, Ozono K, Miyake H, Nayashima K, Kuroume T, Pike W: A new point mutation in the deoxyribonucleic acid-binding domain of the vitamin D receptor in a kindred with hereditary 1,24-dihydroxyvitamin D-resistant rickets. *J Clin Endocrinol Metab* 76:509, 1993.
175. Danielsen M, Hinck L, Ringold GM: Mutational analysis of the mouse glucocorticoid receptor. *Cancer Res* 49:S2286, 1989.
176. Dieken ES, Meese EU, Miesfeld RL: NTI glucocorticoid receptor transcripts lack sequences encoding the amino-terminal transcriptional modulatory domain. *Mol Cell Biol* 10:4574, 1990.
177. Hurley DM, Accili D, Stratakis CA, Karl M, Vamvakopoulos N, Rorer E, Constantine K, Taylor SI, Chrousos GP: Point mutation causing a single amino acid substitution in the hormone binding domain of the glucocorticoid receptor in familial glucocorticoid resistance. *J Clin Invest* 87:680, 1991.
178. Karl M, Lamberts S, Detera-Wadleigh S, Encio I, Stratakis C, Hurley D, Chrousos G: Familial glucocorticoid resistance caused by a splice site deletion in the human glucocorticoid receptor gene. *J Clin Endocrinol Metab* 76:683, 1993.
179. Malchoff D, Brufsky A, Reardon G, McDermott P, Javier E, Bergh C-H, Rowe D, Malchoff C: A mutation of the glucocorticoid receptor in primary cortisol resistance. *J Clin Invest* 91:1918, 1993.
180. Sakurai A, Takeda K, Ain K, Ceccarelli P, Nakai A, Seino S, Bell GI, Refetoff S, De Groot LJ: Generalized resistance to thyroid hormone associated with a mutation in the ligand-binding domain of the human thyroid hormone receptor-β. *Proc Natl Acad Sci USA* 86:8977, 1989.
181. Takeda K, Balzano S, Sakurai A, De Groot LJ, Refetoff A: Screening of 19 unrelated families with generalized resistance to thyroid hormone for known point mutations in the thyroid hormone receptor-β gene and the detection of a new mutation. *J Clin Invest* 87:496, 1991.
182. Usala SJ, Menke JB, Watson TL, Berard J, Bradley WEC, Bale AE, Lash RW, Weintraub BD: A new point mutation in the 3,5,3′-triiodothyronine-binding domain of the c-erbAβ thyroid hormone receptor is tightly linked to generalized thyroid hormone resistance. *J Clin Invest* 72:32, 1991.
183. Usala SJ, Tennyson GE, Bale AE, Lash RW, Gesundheit N, Wondisford FE, Accili D, Hauser P, Weintraub BD: A base mutation of the c-erbA-β thyroid hormone receptor in a kindred with generalized thyroid hormone resistance—molecu-

lar heterogeneity in 2 other kindreds. *J Clin Invest* 85:93, 1990.
184. Usala SJ, Wondisford FE, Watson TL, Menke JB, Weintraub BD: Thyroid hormone and DNA binding properties of a mutant c-erbA-β receptor associated with generalized thyroid hormone resistance. *Biochem Biophys Res Commun* 171:575, 1990.
185. King RJB, Stewart JF, Millis RR, Rubens RD, Hayward JL: Quantitative comparison of estradiol and progesterone receptor contents of primary and metastatic human breast tumors in relation to response to endocrine treatment. *Breast Cancer Res Treat* 2:339, 1982.
186. Stewart J, King R, Hayward JL, Rubens RD: Estrogen and progesterone receptor: Correlation of response rates, site and timing of receptor analysis. *Breast Cancer Res Treat* 2:243, 1982.
187. Clark GM, McGuire WL: Steroid receptors and other prognostic factors in primary breast cancer. *Semin Oncol* 15:20, 1988.
188. Konior Yarbro GS, Lippman ME, Johnson GE, Leventhal BG: Glucocorticoid receptors in subpopulations of childhood acute lymphocytic leukemia. *Cancer Res* 37:2688, 1977.
189. Beug H, Vennström B: Avian erythroleukemia: Possible mechanisms involved in v-*erbA* oncogene function, in Parker MG (ed): *Nuclear Hormone Receptors: Molecular Mechanisms, Cellular Functions, Clinical Abnormalities*. London, Academic, 1991, pp 355–375.
190. Evans RM: The steroid and thyroid hormone receptor superfamily. *Science* 240:889, 1988.
191. de Thé H, Marchio A, Tiollais P, Dejean A: A novel steroid/thyroid hormone receptor-related gene in appropriately expressed in human hepatocellular carcinoma. *Nature* 330: 667, 1987.
192. Brand N, Petkovich M, Krust A, Chambon P, de Thé H, Marchio A, Tiollais P, Dejean A: Identification of a second human retinoic acid receptor. *Nature* 332:850, 1988.
193. De Thé H, Chomienne C, Lanotte M, Degos L, Dejean A: The t(15,17) translocation of acute promyelocytic leukemia fuses the retinoic acid receptor α gene to a novel transcribed locus. *Nature* 347:558, 1990.
194. Chang KS, Trujillo JM, Ogura T, Castiglione CM, Kidd KK, Zhao SR, Freireich EJ, Stass SA: Rearrangement of the retinoic acid receptor gene in acute promyelocytic leukemia. *Leukemia* 5:200, 1991.
195. Kakizuka A, Miller WH, Umesono K, Warrell RP, Frankel SR, Murty VVVS, Dmitrovsky E, Evans RM: Chromosomal translocation t(15;17) in human acute promyelocytic leukemkia fuses RARa with a novel putative transcription factor, PML. *Cell* 66:663, 1991.
196. De Thé H, Lavau C, Marchio A, Chomienne C, Degos L, Dejean A: The PML-RARa fusion mRNA generated by the t(15;17) translocation in acute promyelocytic leukemia encodes a functionally altered RAR. *Cell* 66:675, 1991.
197. Giguère V, Yang N, Segui P, Evans RM: Identification of a new class of steroid hormone receptors. *Nature* 331:91, 1988.
198. Miyajima N, Kdowaki Y, Fukushige S, Shimizu S, Semba K, Yamanashi Y, Matsubara K, Toyoshima K, Yamamoto T: Identification of two novel members of *erbA* superfamily by molecular cloning: The gene products of the two are highly related to each other. *Nucleic Acids Res* 16:11057, 1988.
199. Miyajima N, Horiuchi R, Shibuya Y, Fukushige S, Matsubara K, Toyoshima K, Yamamoto T: Two *erb*A homologs encoding proteins with different T3 binding capacities are transcribed from opposite DNA strands of the same genetic locus. *Cell* 57:31, 1989.
200. Hamada K, Gleason SL, Levi B-Z, Hirschfeld S, Appella E, Ozato K: H-2RIIBP, a member of the nuclear hormone receptor superfamily that binds to both the regulatory element of major histocompatibility class I genes and the estrogen response element. *Proc Natl Acad Sci USA* 86:8289, 1989.
201. Leid M, Kastner P, Lyons R, Nakshatri H, Saunders M, Zacharewski T, Chen J-Y, Staub A, et al: Purification, cloning, and RXR identify of the HeLa cell factor with which RAR or TR heterodimerizes to bind target sequences efficiently. *Cell* 68:377, 1992.
202. Bugge TH, Pohl J, Lonnoy O, Stunnenberg HG: RXRα, a promiscuous partner of retinoic acid and thyroid hormone receptors. *EMBO J* 11:1409, 1992.
203. Gearing K, Göttlicher M, Teboul M, Widmark E, Gustafsson J-Å: Interaction of the peroxisome proliferator activated receptor and retinoid X receptor. *Proc Natl Acad Sci USA* 90:1440, 1993.
204. Oro AE, McKeown M, Evans RM: Relationship between the product of the *Drosophila ultraspiracle* locus and the vertebrate retinoid X receptor. *Nature* 347:298, 1990.
205. Göttlicher M, Li Q, Widmark E, Gustafsson J-Å: Fatty acids activate a chimera of the clofibric acid-activated receptor and the glucocorticoid receptor. *Proc Natl Acad Sci USA* 89:4653, 1992.
206. Nakai A, Kartha S, Sakurai S, Toback FG, DeGroot LJ: A human early response gene homologous to murine nur77 and rat NGFI-B, and related to the nuclear receptor superfamily. *Mol Endocrinol* 4:1438, 1990.
207. Rothe M, Nauber U, Jäckle H: Three hormone receptor-like *Drosophila* genes encode an identical DNA-binding finger. *EMBO J* 8:3087, 1989.
208. Wang L-H, Tsai SY, Cook RG, Beattie WG, Trai M-J, O'Malley BW: COUP transcription factor is a member of the steroid receptor superfamily. *Nature* 340:163, 1989.
209. Sladek FM, Zhong W, Lai E, Darnell JE: Liver-enriched transcription factor HNF-4 is a novel member of the steroid hormone receptor superfamily. *Genes Dev* 4:2353, 1990.
210. Lavorgna G, Ueda H, Clos J, Wu C: FTZ-F1, a steroid hormone receptor-like protein implicated in the activation of *fushi tarazu*. *Science* 252:848, 1991.
211. Ladias JA, Karathanasis SK: Regulation of the apolipoprotein A1 gene by ARP-1, a novel member of the steroid receptor superfamily. *Science* 251:561, 1991.
212. Watson MA, Milbrandt J: The NGFI-B gene, a transcriptionally inducible member of the steroid receptor gene superfamily: Genomic structure and expression in rat brain after seizure induction. *Mol Cell Biol* 9:4213, 1989.
213. Hazel TG, Nathans D, Lau LF: A gene inducible by serum growth factors. *Proc Natl Acad Sci USA* 85:8444, 1991.
214. Segraves W, Hogness DS: The E75 ecdysone-inducible gene responsible for the 75B early puff in *Drosophila* encodes two new members of the steroid receptor superfamily. *Genes Dev* 4:204, 1990.
215. Pignoni F, Baldarelli RM, Steingrimsson E, Diaz RJ, Patapoutian A, Merriam JR, Lengyel JA: The Drosophila gene *tailless* is expressed at the embryonic termini and is a member of the steroid receptor superfamily. *Cell* 62:151, 1990.
216. Nauber U, Pankratz MJ, Kienlin A, Seifert E, Klemm U, Jäckle H: Abdominal segmentation of the *Drosophila* embryo requires a hormone receptor-like protein encoded by the gap gene *knirps*. *Nature* 336:489, 1988.
217. Mlodzik M, Hiromi Y, Weber U, Goodman CS, Rubin GM: The Drosophila *seven-up* gene, a member of the steroid receptor gene superfamily, controls photoreceptor cell fates. *Cell* 60:211, 1990.
218. Isseman I, Green S: Activation of a member of the steroid hormone receptor superfamily by peroxisome proliferators. *Nature* 347:645, 1990.
219. Mangelsdorf DJ, Ong ES, Dyck JA, Evans RM: Nuclear receptor that identifies a novel retinoic acid response pathway. *Nature* 345:224, 1990.
220. O'Malley BW: The steroid receptor superfamily: More excitement predicted for the future. *Mol Endocrinol* 4:363, 1990.
221. Nebert DW: Growth signal pathways. *Nature* 347:709, 1990.
222. O'Malley BW: Did eucaryotic steroid receptors evolve from intracrine gene regulators? *Endocrinology* 125:1119, 1989.
223. Oro AE, McKeown M, Evans RM: The Drosophila nuclear receptors: New insight into the actions of nuclear receptors in development. *Curr Opin Genet Dev* 2:269, 1992.

224. Segraves WA: Something old, some things new: The steroid receptor superfamily in Drosophila. *Cell* 67:225, 1991.
225. Laudet V, Hänni C, Coll J, Catzeflis F, Stéhelin D: Evolution of the nuclear receptor superfamily. *EMBO J* 11:1003, 1992.
226. Sucov HM, Murakami KK, Evans RM: Characterisation of an autoregulated response element in the mouse retinoic acid receptor type β gene. *Proc Natl Acad Sci USA* 87:5392, 1990.
227. Demay MB, Gerardi JM, De Luca HF, Kronenberg HM: DNA sequences in the rat osteocalcin gene that bind the 1,25-dihydroxyvitamin D3 receptor and confer responsiveness to 1,25-dihydroxyvitamin D3. *Proc Natl Acad Sci USA* 87:369, 1990.
228. Marks MS, Hallenbeck PL, Nagata T, Segars JH, Appella E, Nikodem VM, Ozato K: H-2RIIBP (RXRβ) heterodimerization provides a mechanism for combinatorial diversity in the regulation of retinoic acid and thyroid hormone responsive genes. *EMBO J* 11:1419, 1992.
229. Glass KC, Orly VD, Rosenfeld MG: Multiple cell type-specific proteins differentially regulate target sequence recognition by the retinoic acid receptor. *Cell* 63:729, 1990.
230. Umesono K, Murakami KK, Thompson CC, Evans RM: Direct repeats as selective response elements for the thyroid hormone, retinoic acid, and vitamin D3 receptors. *Cell* 65:1255, 1991.
231. Heyman RA, Mangelsdorf DJ, Dyck JA, Stein RB, Eichele G, Evans RM, Thaller C: 9-Cis retinoic acid is a high affinity ligand for the retinoid X receptor. *Cell* 68:397, 1992.
232. Levin AA, Sturzenbecker LJ, Kazmer S, Bosakowski T, Huselton C, Allenby G, Speck J, Kratzeisen C, et al: 9-*Cis* retinoic acid steroisomer binds and activates the nuclear receptor RXRα. *Nature* 355:359, 1992.
233. Yu VC, Delsert C, Andersen B, Holloway JM, Devary OV, Näär AM, Kim SY, Boutin J-M, et al: RXRβ: A coregulator that enhances binding of retinoic acid, thyroid hormone, and vitamin D receptors to their cognate response elements. *Cell* 67:1251, 1991.
234. Zhang X-K, Hoffmann B, Tran PB-V, Graupner G, Pfahl M: Retinoid X receptor is an auxiliary protein for thyroid hormone and retinoic acid receptors. *Nature* 355:441, 1992.
235. Kliewer SA, Umesono K, Noonan DJ, Heyman RA, Evans RM: Convergence of 9-*cis*-retinoic acid and peroxisome proliferator signaling pathways through heterodimer formation of their receptors. *Nature* 358:771, 1992.
236. Durand B, Saunders M, Leroy P, Leid M, Chambon P: All-trans and 9-cis retinoic acid induction of CRABPII transcription is mediated by RAR-RXR heterodimers bound to DR1 and DR2 repeated motifs. *Cell* 71:73, 1992.
237. Poellinger L, Göttlicher M, Gustafsson J-Å: The dioxin and peroxisome proliferator-activated receptors: Nuclear receptors in search of endogenous ligands. *Trends Pharmacol Sci* 13:241, 1992.
238. Power RF, Lydon JP, Conneely OM, O'Malley BW: Dopamine activation of an orphan of the steroid receptor superfamily. *Science* 252:1546, 1991.
239. Kuo CJ, Conley PB, Chen L, Sladek FM, Darnell JE, Crabtree GR: A transcriptional hierarchy involved in mammalian cell-type specification. *Nature* 355:457, 1992.
240. Koelle MR, Talbot WS, Segraves WA, Bender MT, Cherbas P, Hogness DS: The Drosophila *EcR* gene encodes an ecdysone receptor, a new member of the steroid receptor superfamily. *Cell* 67:59, 1991.
241. Yao T-P, Segraves WA, Oro AE, McKeown M, Evans RM: Drosophila ultraspiracle modulates ecdysone receptor function via heterodimer formation. *Cell* 71:63, 1992.
242. Eberhardt NL, Apriletti JW, Baxter JD: The molecular biology of thyroid hormone action, in Litwack G (ed): *The Biochemical Actions of Hormones*. New York, Academic, 1980, vol 7, p 311.
243. Schwartz HL: Effects of thyroid hormone on growth and development, in Oppenheimer JH, Samuels JH (eds): *Molecular Basis of Thyroid Hormone Action*. New York, Academic, 1983, p 413.
244. Dussault JH, Ruel J: Thyroid hormones and gene development. *Annu Rev Physiol* 49:321, 1987.
245. Oppenheimer JH, Schwartz HL, Mariash CN, Kinlaw WB, Wong NCW, Freake HC: Advances in our understanding of thyroid hormone action at the cellular level. *Endocrinol Rev* 8:288, 1987.
246. Brent GA, Moore DD, Larsen PR: Thyroid hormone regulation of gene expression. *Annu Rev Physiol* 53:17, 1991.
247. Chin WW: Nuclear thyroid hormone receptors, in Parker MG (ed): *Nuclear Hormone Receptors*. London, Academic, 1991, p 79.
248. Segal J, Ingbar SH: Plasma membrane-mediated effects of thyroid hormones, in Cumming IA, Funder JW, Mendelsohn FAO (eds): *Endocrinology*. New York, Elsevier/North-Holland, 1980, p 405.
249. Leonard JL, Silva JE, Kaplan MM, Mellen SA, Visser TJ, Larsen PR: Acute posttranscriptional regulation of cerebrocortical and pituitary iodothyronine 5′-diodinases by thyroid hormone. *Endocrinology* 114:998, 1984.
250. Alderson R, Pastan I, Cheng S-Y: Characterization of the 3, 3′, 5-triiodo-L-thyronine-binding sites on plasma membranes from human placenta. *Endocrinology* 116:2621, 1985.
251. Cheng S-Y, Maxfield FR, Robbins J, Willingham MC, Pastan IH: Receptor-mediated uptake of 3, 3′,5-triiodo-L-thyronine by cultured fibroblasts. *Proc Natl Acad Sci USA* 77:3425, 1980.
252. Krenning EP, Docter R, Visser TJ, Hennemann G: Plasma membrane transport of thyroid hormone: Its possible pathophysiological significance. *J Endocrinol Invest* 6:59, 1983.
253. Oppenheimer JH, Schwartz HL: Stereospecific transport of triiodothyronine from plasma to cytosol and from cytosol to nucleus in rat liver, kidney, brain, and heart. *J Clin Invest* 75:147, 1985.
254. Oppenheimer JH, Schwartz HL, Surks MI: Tissue differences in the concentration of triiodothyronine nuclear binding sites in the rat: Liver, kidney, pituitary, heart, brain, spleen and testis. *Endocrinology* 5:897, 1974.
255. Barker SB, Klitgaard HM: Metabolism of tissues excised from thyroxine injected rats. *Am J Physiol* 170:81, 1952.
256. Oppenheimer JH: The nuclear receptor-triiodothyronine complex: Relationship to thyroid hormone distribution, in Oppenheimer JH, Samuels JH (eds): *Molecular Basis of Thyroid Hormone Action*. New York, Academic, 1983, p 1.
257. Spindler BJ, MacLeod KM, Ring J, Baxter JD: Thyroid hormone receptors: Binding characteristics and lack of hormonal dependency for nuclear localization. *J Biol Chem* 250:4113, 1975.
258. Perlman AJ, Stanley F, Samuels HH: Thyroid hormone nuclear receptor: Evidence for multimeric organization in chromatin. *J Biol Chem* 257:930, 1982.
259. Weinberger C, Thompson CP, Ong ES, Lebo R, Gruol DJ, Evans JM: The c-*erb*-A gene encodes a thyroid hormone receptor. *Nature* 324:641, 1986.
260. Sap J, Munoz A, Damm K, Goldberg Y, Ghysdael J, Leutz A, Beug H, Vennström B: The c-*erb*-A protein is a high-affinity receptor for thyroid hormone. *Nature* 324:635, 1986.
261. Dayton AI, Selden JR, Laws G, Dorney DJ, Finan J, Tripputi P, Emanuel BS, Rovcera G, et al: A human c-*erb*-A oncogene homologue is closely proximal to the chromosome 17 breakpoint in acute promyelocytic leukemia. *Proc Natl Acad Sci USA* 81:4495, 1984.
262. Drabkin H, Kao F-T, Hartz J, Hart I, Gazdar A, Weinberger C, Evans R, Gerber M: Localization of human ERBA2 to the 3p22-3p24.1 region of chromosome 3 and variable deletion in small cell lung cancer. *Proc Natl Acad Sci USA* 85:9258, 1988.
263. Horowitz Z, Sahnoun H, Pascual A, Casanova J, Samuels HH: Analysis of photoaffinity label derivatives to probe thyroid hormone receptor in human fibroblasts, GH_1 cells and soluble receptor preparations. *J Biol Chem* 263:6636, 1988.
264. Nakai A, Sakurai A, Bell GI, DeGroot LJ: Characterization

of a third human thyroid hormone receptor coexpressed with other thyroid hormone receptors in several tissues. *Mol Endocrinol* 2:1087, 1988.

265. Benbrook D, Pfahl M: A novel thyroid hormone receptor encoded by a cDNA clone from a human testis library. *Science* 238:788, 1987.
266. Nakai A, Seino S, Sakurai A, Sziiak I, Bell GI, DeGroot LJ: Characterization of a thyroid hormone receptor expressed in human kidney and other tissues. *Proc Natl Acad Sci USA* 85:2781, 1988.
267. Izumo S, Mahdavi V: Thyroid hormone receptor α isoforms generated by alternative splicing differentially activate myosin HC gene transcription. *Nature* 334:539, 1988.
268. Lazar MA, Hodin RA, Chin WW: Human carboxyl-terminal variant of α type c-*erb*-A inhibits trans-activation by thyroid hormone receptors without binding thyroid hormone. *Proc Natl Acad Sci USA* 86:7771, 1989.
269. Mitsuhashi T, Tennyson GE, Nikodem VM: Alternative splicing generates messages encoding rat c-*erb*-A proteins that do not bind thyroid hormone. *Proc Natl Acad Sci USA* 85:5804, 1988.
270. Lazar MA, Hodin RA, Darling DS, Chin WW: A novel member of the thyroid/steroid hormone receptor family is encoded by the opposite strand of the rat c-*erb*-A-alpha transcriptional unit. *Mol Cell Biol* 9:1128, 1989.
271. Lazar MA, Jones KE, Chin WW: Isolation of a cDNA encoding human Rev.erbα: Transcription from the non-coding DNA stand of a thyroid hormone receptor gene results in a related protein which does not bind thyroid hormone. *DNA Cell Biol* 9:77, 1990.
272. Lazar MA, Hodin RA, Cardona G, Chin WW: Gene expression from the c-*erb*-Aα/*Rev-erb*Aα genomic locus: Potential regulation of alternative splicing by opposite strand transcription. *J Biol Chem* 265:12 859, 1990.
273. Hodin RA, Lazar MA, Wintmann BI, Darling DS, Koenig RJ, Larsen PR, Moore DD, Chin WW: Identification of a thyroid hormone receptor that is pituitary-specific. *Science* 244:76, 1989.
274. Hodin RA, Lazer MA, Chin WW: Differential and tissue-specific regulation of multiple rat c-*erb*A messenger RNA species by thyroid hormone. *J Clin Invest* 85:101, 1990.
275. Lazar MA, Hodin RA, Darling DS, Chin WW: Identification of a rat c-*erb*-Aα-related protein which binds DNA but does not bind thyroid hormone. *Mol Endocrinol* 2:893, 1988.
276. Koenig RJ, Lazar MA, Hodin RA, Brent GA, Larsen PR, Chin WW, Moore DD: Inhibition of thyroid hormone action by a non-hormone binding c-*erb*-A protein generated by alternative splicing. *Nature* 337:659, 1989.
277. Thompson CC, Evans RM: Trans-activation by thyroid hormone receptors: Functional parallels with steroid hormone receptors. *Proc Natl Acad Sci USA* 86:3494, 1989.
278. Schueler PA, Schwartz HL, Strait KA, Mariash CN, Oppenheimer JH: Binding of 3,4,3′-triiodothyronine (3) and its analogs to the *in vitro* translational products of c-*erb*-A protooncogenes: Differences in the affinity of the α- and β-forms for the acetic acid analog and failure of the human testis and kidney products to bind T3. *Endocrinology* 4:234, 1990.
279. Brent GA, Dunn MK, Harney JW, Gulick T, Larsen PR, Moore DD: Thyroid hormone aporeceptor represses T3-inducible promoters and blocks activity of the retinoic acid receptor. *New Biologist* 1:329, 1989.
280. Damm K, Thompson CC, Evans RM: Protein encoded by v-*erb*A functions as a thyroid-hormone receptor antagonist. *Nature* 339:593, 1989.
281. Graupner G, Wills KN, Tzukerman M, Zhang XK, Pfahl M: Dual regulatory role for thyroid-hormone receptors allows control of retinoic-acid receptor activity. *Nature* 340:653, 1989.
282. Sap J, Munoz A, Schmitt J, Stunnenberg H, Vennström B: Repression of transcription mediated at a thyroid hormone response element by the v-*erb*A oncogene product. *Nature* 340:242, 1989.
283. Thompson CC, Weinberger C, Lebo R, Evans RM: Identification of a novel thyroid hormone receptor expressed in the mammalian central nervous system. *Science* 37:1610, 1987.
284. Muray MB, Zilz ND, McCreary NL, MacDonald MJ, Towle HC: Isolation and characterization of rat cDNA clones for two distinct thyroid hormone receptors. *J Biol Chem* 263:12770, 1988.
285. Santos A, Freake HD, Rosenberg ME, Schwartz HL, Oppenheimer JH: Triiodothyronine nuclear binding capacity in rat tissues correlates with a 6.0 kilobase (kb) and not a 2.6 kb messenger ribonucleic acid hybridization signal generated by a human c-*erb*A probe. *Mol Endocrinol* 2:992, 1988.
286. Sakurai A, Nakai A, DeGroot LJ: Expression of three forms of thyroid hormone receptor in human tissues. *Mol Endocrinol* 3:392, 1989.
287. Forrest D, Hallbook F, Persson H, Vennström B: Distinct functions for thyroid hormone receptors alpha and beta in brain development indicated by differential expression of receptor genes. *EMBO J* 10:269, 1991.
288. Yaoita Y, Brown DD: A correlation of thyroid hormone receptor gene expression with amphibian metamorphosis. *Genes Dev* 4:1917, 1990.
289. North D, Fisher DA: Thyroid hormone receptor and receptor-related RNA levels in developing rat brain. *Pediatr Res* 28:622, 1990.
290. Lazar MA, Chin WW: Regulation of two c-*erb*A messenger ribonucleic acids in rat GH_3. *Mol Endocrinol* 2:479, 1988.
291. Mitsuhashi T, Nikodem VM: Regulation of expression of the alternative mRNAs of the rat alpha-thyroid hormone receptor gene. *J Biol Chem* 264:8900, 1989.
292. Strait KA, Schwartz HL, Perez-Castillo A, Oppenheimer JH: Relationship of c-*erb*-A mRNA content to tissue triiodothyronine nuclear binding capacity and function in developing and adult rats. *J Biol Chem* 25:10514, 1990.
293. Usala SJ, Weintraub BD: Thyroid hormone resistance syndromes. *Trends Endocrinol Metab* 2:140, 1991.
294. Refetoff S, Weiss R, Usala S: The syndromes of resistance to thyroid hormone. *Endocr Rev* 14:340, 1991.
295. McGuire W, Chamness G, Fugua S: Abnormal estrogen receptor in clinical breast cancer. *J Steroid Biochem Molec Biol* 43:243, 1992.
296. Brockes JP: Retinoids, homeobox genes, and limb morphogenesis. *Neuron* 2:1285, 1989.
297. Eichele G: Retioids and vertebrate limb pattern formation. *Trends Genet* 5:246, 1989.
298. Brockes JP: Reading the retinoid signal. *Nature* 345:766, 1990.
299. Summerbell D, Maden M: Retinoic acid, a development signalling molecule. *Trends Neurosci* 13:142, 1990.
300. Pitt GAJ: Vitamin A, in Isler O (ed): *Carotenoids*. Basel and Stuttgart, Birkhauser-Verlag, 1971, p 717.
301. Alles AJ, Sulik KK: Retinoic-acid-induced limb-reduction defects: Perturbation of zones of programmed cell death as a pathogenetic mechanism. *Teratology,* 40:163, 1989.
302. Satre MA, Kochhar DM: Elevations in the endogenous levels of the putative morphogen retinoic acid in embryonic mouse limb buds associated with limb dysmorphogenesis. *Dev Biol* 133:529, 1989.
303. Tickle C, Summerbell D, Wolpert L: Positional signalling and specification of digits in chick limb morphogenesis. *Nature* 254:199, 1975.
304. Maden M: Vitamin A and pattern formation in the regenerating limb. *Nature* 295:672, 1982.
305. Summerbell D: The effect of local application of retinoic acid to the anterior margin of the developing chick limb. *J Embryol Exp Morph* 78:269, 1983.
306. Napoli JL, Race KR: The biosynthesis of retinoic acid from retinol by rat tissues *in vitro*. *Arch Biochem Biophys* 255:95, 1987.
307. Dowling JE, Wald G: The biological function of vitamin A acid. *Proc Natl Acad Sci USA* 46:587, 1960.
308. Edwards MKS, McBurney MW: The concentration of retinoic

acid determines the differentiated cell types formed by a teratocarcinoma cell line. *Dev Biol* 98:187, 1983.
309. Simeone A, Acampora D, Arcioni L, Andrews PW, Boncinelli E, Mavilio F: Sequential activation of HOX2 homeobox genes by retinoic acid in human embryonal carcinoma cells. *Nature* 346:763, 1990.
310. Kochhar DM: Cellular basis of congenital limb deformity induced in mice by vitamin A, in Bersma D, Lenz W (eds): *Morphogenesis and Malformation of the Limb*. New York, Liss, 1977, p 111.
311. Ide H, Aono H: Retinoic acid promotes proliferation and chondrogenesis in the distal mesodermal cells of chick limb bud. *Dev Biol* 130:767, 1988.
312. Paulsen DF, Langille RM, Dress V, Solrush M: Selective stimulation of *in vitro* limb-bud chondrogenesis by retinoic acid. *Differentiation* 39:123, 1988.
313. Giguere V, Ong ES, Segui P, Evans RM: Identification of a receptor for the morphogen retinoic acid. *Nature* 330:624, 1987.
314. Petkovich M, Brand NJ, Krust A, Chambon P: A human retinoic acid receptor which belongs to the family of nuclear receptors. *Nature* 330:444, 1987.
315. Benbrook D, Lernhardt E, Pfahl M: A new retinoic acid receptor identified from a hepatocellular carcinoma. *Nature* 333:669, 1988.
316. Zelent A, Krust A, Petkovich M, Kastner P, Chambon P: Cloning of murine retinoic acid receptor alpha and beta cDNAs and of a novel third receptor gamma predominantly expressed in skin. *Nature* 339:714, 1989.
317. Krust A, Kastner P, Petkovich M, Zelent A, Chambon P: A third human retinoic acid receptor, hRAR-gamma. *Proc Natl Acad Sci USA* 86:5310, 1989.
318. Ragsdale CW, Petkovich M, Gates PB, Chambon P, Brockes JP: Identification of a novel retinoic acid receptor in regenerative tissues of the newt. *Nature* 341:654, 1989.
319. Leroy P, Krust A, Zelent A, Mendelsohn C, Garnier J-M, Kastner P, Dierich A, Chambon P: Multiple isoforms of the mouse retinoic acid receptor α are generated by alternative splicing and differential induction by retinoic acid. *EMBO J* 10:59, 1991.
320. Zelent A, Mendelsohn C, Kastner P, Krust A, Garnier J-M, Ruffenach F, Leroy P, Chambon P: Differentially expressed isoforms of the mouse retinoic acid receptor β are generated by usage of two promoters and alternative splicing. *EMBO J* 10:71, 1991.
321. Lehmann JM, Hoffmann B, Pfahl M: Genomic organization of the retinoic acid receptor gamma gene. *Nucleic Acids Res* 19:573, 1991.
322. Tora L, Gronemeyer H, Turcotte B, Gaub M-P, Chambon P: The N-terminal region of the chicken progesterone receptor specifies target gene activation. *Nature* 333:185, 1988.
323. Ruberte E, Dolle P, Krust A, Zelent A, Morriss-Kay G, Chambon P: Specific spatial and temporal distribution of retinoic acid receptor gamma transcripts during mouse embryogenesis. *Development* 108:213, 1990.
324. Dolle P, Ruberte E, Kastner P, Petkovich M, Stoner CM, Gudas LJ, Chambon P: Differential expression of genes encoding alpha, beta and gamma retinoic acid receptors and CRABP in the developing limbs of the mouse. *Nature* 342:702, 1989.
325. Rees JL, Daly AK, Refern CPF: Differential expression of the alpha and beta retinoic acid receptors in tissues of the rat. *Biochem J* 259:917, 1989.
326. Goodman DS: Retinoids and retinoid-binding proteins. *Harvey Lect* 81:111, 1985–1986.
327. Mangelsdorf DJ, Borgmeyer U, Heyman RA, Zhou JY, Ong ES, Oro AE, Kakizuka A, Evans RM: Characterization of three RXR genes that mediate the action of 9-*cis* retinoic acid. *Genes Dev* 6:329, 1992.
328. Mangesldorf DJ, Ong ES, Dyck JA, Evans RM: Nuclear receptor that identifies a novel retinoic acid response pathway. *Nature* 345:224, 1990.
329. Mangelsdorf DJ, Umesono K, Kliewer, Borgmeyer U, Ong ES, Evans RM: A direct repeat in the cellular retinol-binding protein type II gene confers differential regulation by RXR and RAR. *Cell* 66:555, 1991.
330. Kliewer SA, Umesono K, Mangelsdorf AJ, Evans RM: Retinoid X receptor interacts with nuclear receptors in retinoic acid thyroid hormone and vitamin D3 signalling. *Nature* 355:446, 1992.
331. Rottman JN, Widom RL, Nadal-Ginard B, Mahdavi V, Karathanasis SK: A retinoic acid-responsive element in the apolipoprotein AI gene distinguishes between two different retinoic acid response pathways. *Mol Cell Biol* 11:3814, 1991.
332. Fugua SAW, Chamness GC, McGuire WL: Estrogen receptor mutations in breast cancer. *J Cell Biochem* 51:135, 1993.

CHAPTER 6

Hormone Assays

A. Eugene Pekary

Jerome M. Hershman

The variety and range of applications of hormone assay methodology have expanded greatly since 1987, when the last edition of this book was published.[1] Because it is not possible to review in one chapter the literature describing the many remarkable developments during this period, we have selected representative examples based on their heuristic value and current and anticipated clinical utility. Automation utilizing a broad range of these new immunoassay technologies has become commonplace, particularly in large clinical laboratories.[2] This process should accelerate as the cost of labor and quality control rise. Safety and environmental concerns will also influence future assay developments.[3]

BIOASSAYS

Results from hormone assays performed in different laboratories must be reported in terms of a common standard. Bioassay results are usually reported in units of an *international standard* distributed by the World Health Organization. They may also be reported in units of a *reference preparation* distributed to laboratories over a more restricted geographic area.[4] Conversion factors for units of reference and units of established international standards should be provided along with assay results. Although polypeptide hormones are highly purified, small but significant contamination of reference preparations may occur and can obviate the reporting of bioassay or other assay results in terms of mass of hormone. The increasing availability of hormonal preparations derived from recombinant DNA expression in bacteria or mammalian cells should greatly simplify the development and maintenance of international protein hormone standards.[5]

Bioassays may be carried out in vivo or in vitro, using graded doses of an appropriate reference preparation or standard against which one interpolates the physiologic effect induced by the hormone contained in an unknown sample.[6]

In Vivo Assays

The McKenzie mouse bioassay exemplifies an in vivo bioassay for thyroid-stimulating activity. Mice are maintained on a low-iodine diet for 10 days to enhance their uptake of radioiodine and then are injected with $Na^{125}I$ and thyroxine or triiodothyronine.[7] On day 14, the mice receive varying doses of the thyrotropic standards and unknown preparations intravenously. Two hours later, blood is drawn for measurement of ^{125}I. A comparison of the effects of pretreatment with T_4 and T_3 on the sensitivity of this bioassay is given in Fig. 6-1. Thyrotropin, a pituitary hormone, and human chorionic gonadotropin (hCG), a placental hormone, both stimulate the release of ^{125}I-labeled thyroid hormones from the thyroid glands of these mice, although the thyrotropic activity of hCG is only one one-thousandth that of thyrotropin.

The dose-response curves of the reference preparation and unknown samples must be parallel to achieve valid assay results. Since the slopes of the thyroid stimulating hormone (TSH) and hCG dose-response curves may vary considerably from bioassay to bioassay, even for the same hormone preparation, statistical analysis for parallelism between the slopes and the homogeneity of variance of the dose-response curve for the assay standard and the unknown is imperative for each assay.[8] This TSH bioassay can detect elevated TSH concentrations in the sera of patients with myxedema, but it is not sufficiently sensitive for the measurement of normal serum TSH levels.

In vivo bioassays remain important tools in basic and pharmaceutical laboratory research.[9] They are generally very labor-intensive, however, in part because of the complexities of preparing the animal subject and administering the test substance, perhaps in divided doses over several days or weeks, along with the large number of replications needed to compensate for the substantial variability of the response. More recently developed in vitro bioassays are usually more precise, sensitive, and specific and require less test substance.

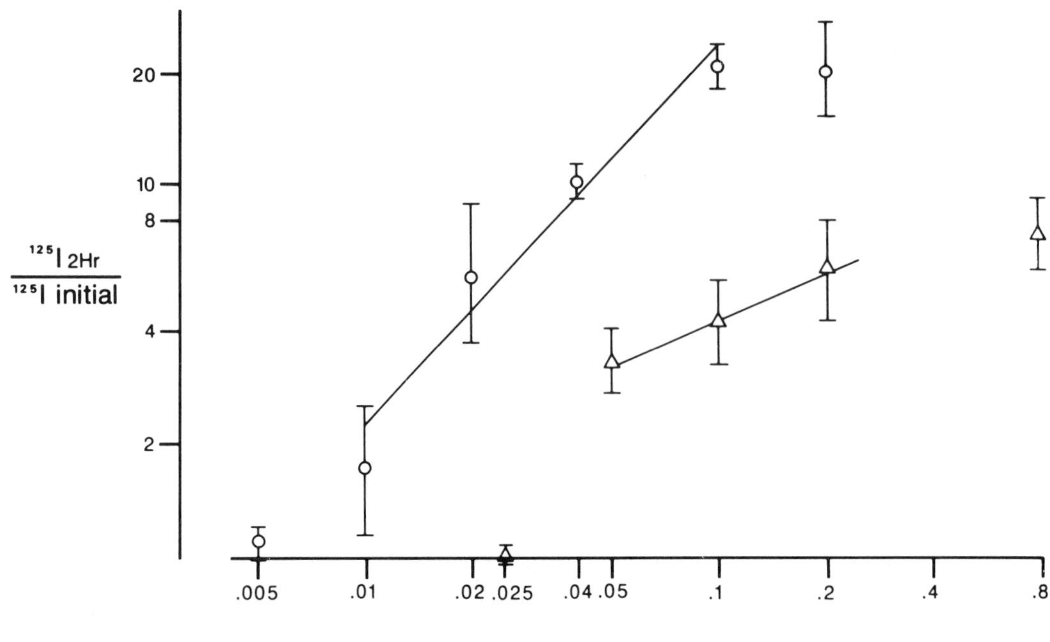

FIGURE 6-1. Dose-response curves of bovine TSH in the McKenzie bioassay using mice pretreated with T_3 (open circles) and T_4 (open triangles). Note the greater sensitivity with the former method. *(From Hershman et al.*[7]*)*

In Vitro Assays

Graded doses of a characterized reference preparation are used to produce a standard curve relative to which the response produced by an unknown substance can be compared for homogeneity of variance, parallelism, and potency. The stimulation of cyclic AMP generation by FRTL-5 rat thyroid cells in response to thyrotropin (TSH) is an example of an in vitro bioassay.[10,11] FRTL-5 cells require TSH-containing media for growth in vitro. After these cells become nearly confluent, they are maintained with TSH-free media for 7 days. During this period, the number of TSH receptors on the plasma membrane of these cells increases, resulting in an increased biological response when TSH or a TSH-like substance is reintroduced into the culture medium. The cyclic AMP released in response to TSH is measured by radioimmunoassay (RIA). This assay is currently used for measuring the thyroid-stimulating immunoglobulin in patients with Graves' hyperthyroidism.[12] Several other biological responses of normal thyroid cells to TSH are retained by FRTL-5 cells, including iodide uptake, incorporationof [^{3}H]-thymidine into DNA, activation of protein kinases, and synthesis of prostaglandin E_2. These effects can also be used with FRTL-5 cells for bioassays of TSH (Fig. 6-2).

Cytochemical Assays

The cytochemical assay is a variant of the bioassay. Cytochemical bioassay responses are quantitated from histologic sections with a special device, a microdensitometer.[13] Histologic sections are prepared from specific hormone target tissues or cells previously exposed to graded concentrations of a standard

FIGURE 6-2. Effect of TNF-α on ^{125}I uptake by FRTL-5 cells stimulated by incubation with bovine TSH (±SD of triplicate wells). *(From Pang, Hershman, Mirell, and Pekary, Endocrinology 125:76, 1989.)*

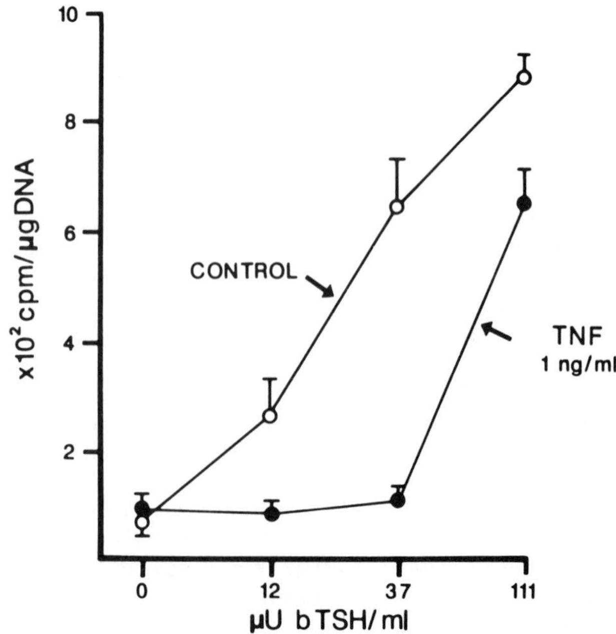

hormone and unknowns. Several cytochemical assays are based on the chromogenic reaction resulting from a change in redox state that is induced by hormone stimulation. Histologic stains that are sensitive to those changes are used for quantitation.[14] A cytochemical bioassay for TSH has been described which quantitates the endocytosis of colloid by thyroid follicle cells.[15] The colloid vesicles fuse with lysosomes, resulting in an increase in the permeability of the lysosomal membrane. The lysosomes are then able to take up the added leucyl-β-naphthylamine substrate which is hydrolyzed by the lysosomal enzymes. The tissue segments are chilled in *n*-hexane at −70°C, cryostat sections are cut, and the visible reaction product is quantitated by scanning densitometry.[16] Cytochemical assays are not practical for routine clinical purposes and serve primarily as sensitive research tools.

Complementarity of in Vivo and in Vitro Assays

In vivo and in vitro bioassays of a given hormonal substance can provide information about its in vivo transport, clearance, and enzymatic transformation prior to binding to its cellular receptor.[17,18] The comparison of the ratio of biological to immunologic activity for a hormonal preparation to that of a well-characterized hormonal standard is useful for the detection of chemical or conformational alterations which can in principle affect these two measurements independently.[19] Some hormones are released into the circulation in a precursor form and acquire a biologically active form only after enzymatic modification in either the circulation or the peripheral tissues. The conversion of T_4 to T_3 by 5′-deiodination in the liver and other tissues is an example. While T_3 has at least 10 times the thyromimetic effect of T_4 as measured with in vitro bioassays,[20] its clearance from the circulation is much faster than that of T_4.[17] This pattern of a relatively stable prohormone or transport form which is enzymatically modified either before or upon release, during circulatory transport, or after binding with a receptor, producing a derivative hormone with altered specific biological activity, is shared by other hormones.

For example, glycoprotein hormones such as TSH undergo major alterations in the composition of glycosylated side chains during biosynthesis and secretion in respcnse to hormonal stimulation. The glycosylation reaction promoted by thyrotropin releasing hormone (TRH) apparently enhances the ratio of biological to immunologic activity of the secreted TSH.[21] Rapid changes in pH, ionic strength, and the activity of associated proteolytic enzymes accompany the exocytosis of hormone-containing secretory granules. These secretion-associated events may explain the observation that the high-molecular-weight precursor form of atrial natriuretic polypeptide (ANP) is found only inside cells while the processed form is entirely extracellular.[22] After secretion, further intravascular modifications of circulating hormones may occur. Parathyroid hormone, for example, is cleaved to smaller forms during passage through the kidney.[23] Most peptide hormones require alpha-amidation of a C-terminal amino acid residue for biological activity. While this reaction occurs predominantly within the secretory vesicle, significant alpha-amidation of TRH-Gly, a TRH precursor peptide, occurs after secretion.[24]

NOMENCLATURE

Immunoassay nomenclature consists of combinations and permutations of a small number of prefixes which designate the type of label used, such as radioactive (*radio*), enzyme (*enzymatic*), fluorometric (*fluoro*), and chemiluminescent (*lumino*), and the labeling of the analyte (e.g., *radioimmuno*) or antibody (e.g., *immunoradio*). Acronyms are also used to identify types of assays, such as ELISA (*e*nzyme-*l*inked *i*mmuno*s*orbent *a*ssay), which utilizes antibody-coated microtiter plates and an enzyme-labeled reporter antibody. Because of the large number of available reagents and their possible combinations for hormone measurement, the nomenclature has become confused. Reference to relevant commercial or scientific literature is the only certain way to determine the methodologic details for any given assay.

TYPES OF IMMUNOASSAYS

Labeled Analyte and Reagent Limiting

Immunoassays using labeled antigen or hapten are equivalent to the classical RIA.[25] They require a very dilute high-affinity antibody which can be immobilized on the surface of a test tube, polystyrene bead, or paramagnetic particle or left in solution for later precipitation with a second antibody.[26] The hormone-antibody reaction can be represented by the following reactions:

$$\mathrm{Ag} + \mathrm{Ab} \underset{k_{-1}}{\overset{k_1}{\rightleftharpoons}} \mathrm{AgAb} \qquad {}^*\mathrm{Ag} + \mathrm{Ab} \underset{k_{-1}}{\overset{k_1}{\rightleftharpoons}} {}^*\mathrm{AgAb}$$

$$K_a = \frac{k_1}{k_{-1}} \qquad K_d = 1/K_a$$

where Ag = antigen or hormone; Ab = antibody to the antigen or hormone; *Ag = radiolabeled antigen or hormone; k_1 = association rate constant; k_{-1} = dissociation rate constant; K_a = equilibrium association constant; K_d = equilibrium dissociation constant.

The labeled hormone may differ substantially from the hormone being measured, particularly if radioiodine, a radioiodinated "tagging" compound, an enzyme, or a fluorescent or chemiluminescent derivative of the analyte is used.[27] The attendant structural modifications can be avoided through the use of the naturally occurring hormone labeled with ^3H or ^{14}C. However, the maximum specific activities attainable with these long-half-life isotopes is very low, resulting in self-displacement of the tracer when the total mass of the label added to each tube is high enough for accurate counting. The detection limit can be improved by adding the label some time after the mixing of the analyte and antibody, the so-called nonequilibrium assay.[25,28] The approach to equilibrium of binding between the antibody, the analyte, and the tracer is slowed by the use of the minimum concentration of antibody required for maximum assay sensitivity. Free label and antibody-bound label are separated, and usually the bound fraction is quantitated. The plot of bound label on a linear scale versus the total antigen concentration on a log scale gives a sigmoid-shaped standard curve with negative slope values.[25] Another representation frequently used in reagent limiting assays is the log-logit plot, which usually produces a linear profile for the standard curve. Unknown results are more readily obtained with linear least-squares analysis of this form of the standard curve than with the sigmoidal form, which is shown in Fig. 6-3 superimposed on the corresponding log-logit plot.

Reagent Excess and Labeled Antibody

The advent of monoclonal antibodies[29] made feasible the "sandwich" assay methodology.[30] With this technique, one monoclonal antibody is adsorbed or chemically bonded to a solid surface such as a test tube or a polystyrene bead. Hormone standards or serum samples are then added, followed by a labeled antibody with binding specificity for a region of the hormone analyte which is different from that of the immobilized antibody.[31] The amount of the labeled antibody which binds to the solid phase should be proportional to the amount of hormone in the sample resulting from the formation of the sandwich complex:

$$\text{SP-Ab-Ag-Ab}^*$$

where SP-Ab is the solid-phase antibody, Ag is the hormone analyte, and Ab* is the labeled antibody.

The addition of a large excess of the immobilized antibody can lead to nearly quantitative binding of any available analyte. A high concentration of a second, labeled "reporter" monoclonal antibody binds in direct proportion to the total analyte concentration. The advantage of this type of assay is that the minimum detectable dose is not limited by the affinity constants of the antibodies used.[32] The only limits on sensitivity are the detectability of the tracer and the extent to which the tracer that is nonspecifically bound to the surfaces of the reaction tube and separation matrix can be minimized by the washing procedure. The analyte must be large enough that two antigen determinants can be bound simultaneously by two different antibody molecules without steric interference.[33] Such a requirement excludes simple steroids and small peptides with fewer than 15 to 20 amino acid residues.

The binding affinity and specificity of the large, stable, bivalent monospecific immunoglobulin molecule are not usually perturbed significantly by the attachment of tracer molecules, whether radioactive, enzymatic, fluorescent, or chemiluminescent. Labeled antibody generally has a greater storage stability than do many labeled polypeptide hormones.[34]

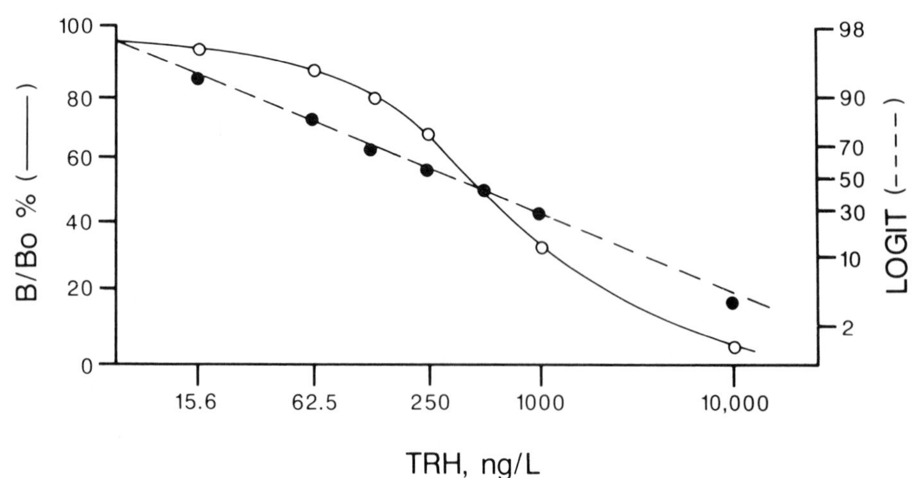

FIGURE 6-3. Standard curve for the thyrotropin releasing hormone radioimmunoassay. Comparison of the sigmoidal and linear log-logit representations.

Free and Total Hormone Measurements

Serum contains binding or transport proteins for thyroid and steroid hormones. The free hormone hypothesis states that the biological action of a hormone is proportional to the concentration of the unbound (free) hormone. The trend in assays for these hormones has been to develop methods which can measure the free hormone directly. Recently, a controversy has arisen concerning the participation of the hormone-binding proteins in hormone transport across the capillary endothelium and the underlying mechanisms of this transport. Both experimental and theoretical aspects of hormone transport have been reviewed.[35] The concept that only the free fraction of plasma hormones is bioavailable and is regulated by negative feedback was based on the observation that free thyroid hormone levels were normal in euthyroid subjects who either lacked the high-affinity thyroxine-binding globulin (TBG deficiency) or had excess serum TBG as a result of a genetic defect, with very low or very high total thyroid hormone levels, respectively.[36]

Ekins has pointed out that in the case of very rapid tissue uptake, the free hormone concentration along the endothelial cell surface may be depleted. Rapid dissociation of hormones from the binding proteins would have the effect of increasing the diffusional flux of the hormone into cells.[37] Pardridge has proposed an alternative model called the *enhanced dissociation hypothesis* in which the dissociation constant of the serum-binding proteins increases within the capillary epithelium and thus facilitates the transit of their bound hormones.[38] While the debate concerning the mechanisms which facilitate hormone transport continues, recent autoradiographic experiments with liver lobules subjected to a single-pass perfusion with radiolabeled T_4, in the absence of thyroid hormone–binding proteins, have emphasized their physiologic significance. Virtually all the T_4 in the perfusate was taken up by the first cells with which it came in contact and was unavailable to cells farther along the sinusoid.[39] When the perfusion was carried out in the presence of thyroid hormone–binding proteins, the fractional extraction was decreased and uniform uptake of T_4 was observed in all the cells of the lobule.

A number of commercial assays for free thyroid hormone are available. They may be divided into three general categories: analog, competitive binding, and ultrafiltration or equilibrium dialysis (ED) combined with immunoassay.[37] The analog assays use a labeled T_4 derivative which is designed to minimize binding to the major thyroid hormone–binding proteins, TBG and thyroxine-binding prealbumin (TBPA); however, the analog does bind to the corresponding thyroid hormone antibody. The assumption is made that the thyroid hormone antibody and the analog tracer added in vitro to the serum sample do not perturb the concentrations of free thyroid hormone. If this assumption is not valid, the measured free hormone value may not correspond to the in vivo concentration, particularly if the thyroid hormone–binding proteins are abnormal. Abnormal free T_4 (FT_4) values are sometimes obtained with this assay method in samples from pregnant women, for example, as a result of the estrogen-induced elevation of TBG values.[40]

The competitive FT_4 assay uses a high-specific-activity labeled monoclonal antibody to T_4 and a suspension of magnetizable particles with T_4 ligands attached. The FT_4 concentration determines the proportion of labeled T_4 antibody which will be precipitated by the magnetic particles. Again, the assumption is made that FT_4 concentration is not affected by the added T_4 antibody and ligand-containing particles.

ED has been considered the gold standard for determining free hormone levels. This method, however, has also produced results, particularly for diluted serum samples from patients with nonthyroid illness,[41] which are difficult to interpret, in part because of a postulated inhibitor of T_4 binding that has not been characterized.[37] In principle, the dilution of serum before or during ED should not have a significant effect on the dializable or "free" T_4 level since 99.97 percent of the total T_4 level should be in the bound form. The decrease in ED-measured FT_4 in the serum of severely ill patients with dilution has been attributed to high free fatty acid (FFA) levels. The in vitro addition of FFA, however, to levels several times higher than the levels seen in even the most severe illness is not sufficient to affect ED values.[35] In vitro artifacts such as heparin-induced release of FFA from frozen plasma during ED may explain some of the discrepant results.[42]

Measurement by immunoassay of total thyroid hormone values requires that all these hydrophobic molecules be displaced from their serum binding proteins. This is usually done by means of the in vitro addition of sodium salicylate or 8-anilino-1-naphthalenesulfonic acid.[43]

Most steroid hormones are associated with serum binding proteins. These include corticosteroid-binding globulin (CBG), which is the major binding protein for progesterone, cortisol, and other glucocorticoids, and sex hormone–binding globulin (SHBG), which binds the gonadal steroids, testosterone and estradiol, with high affinity.[35] These binding proteins interfere with immunoassay measurements. Solvent extraction is a dependable but labor-intensive method for eliminating the effects of steroid-binding proteins prior to immunoassay. Methods have been developed for the direct assay of progesterone, for example, which use acidification and displacing compounds such as cortisol to reduce the binding of label and hormone by CBG.[44]

The immunoassay field remains exceedingly active, with new technologies being rapidly incorpo-

TABLE 6-1 Commercial Hormone Assays Listed in the College of American Pathologists (CAP) Ligand Assay Series 1 and 2 for 1991

Peptide	Thyroid	Steroid
FSH (49)*	T_4 (63)	Aldosterone (7)
Gastrin (10)	FT_4 (25)	Androstenedione (7)
Growth hormone (12)	T_3 (41)	Cortisol (37)
hCG (55)	FT_3 (8)	Deoxycortisol (2)
Insulin (19)	T Uptake (3)	Dehydroepiandrosterone sulfate (11)
LH (48)	T Uptake % (60)	Estradiol (20)
Renin (5)		Estriol (15)
TSH (69)		Estriol (unconjugated) (19)
		17-Hydroxyprogesterone (7)
		Progesterone (21)
		Testosterone (18)

* The numbers in parentheses represent the total number of all kits for each hormone listed in the surveys.

rated into commercial "kit" assays with improved speed, sensitivity, safety, and reproducibility. The commercial assays, listed by hormonal category, which are currently on the College of American Pathologists Ligand Assay Surveys 1 and 2, are listed in Table 6-1.

IMMUNOASSAY REAGENTS

Binding Proteins

Production of Antibodies

The Nature and Structure of Antibodies

Antibodies belong to the class of immunoglobulins and are predominantly gamma globulins (IgG). The IgG molecule is composed of four polypeptide chains: two heavy chains and two light chains symmetrically arranged and covalently bound by disulfide bonds. The molecule is shown schematically in Fig. 6-4.

The interaction of antigen or ligand with antibody may be considered a "lock and key" arrangement. The shape of the antibody combining site is complementary to that of the antigen. The antigen-antibody interaction is a combination of electrostatic, hydrogen-binding, van der Waals, and hydrophobic interactions.[45,46] The amino acid sequence of the binding portion of the IgG molecule determines the "shape" of the binding site and, consequently, the affinity and specificity of the combining site for the desired antigen.[47]

The immune response can be divided into the primary and secondary phases. After the first exposure to a given immunogen and a relatively long lag period, IgM antibodies begin to appear in serum. A second exposure to the immunogen results in a much stronger response, consisting primarily of IgG antibodies, which declines more slowly. Moreover, antibodies of the secondary response generally have much higher affinities for the immunogen.[30] The IgM-IgG transition involves IgG class switching in which the gene coding for the immunogen-recognizing segment of the antibody—the paratope—is combined with the gene coding for the rest of the IgG molecule. With repeated immunization, the affinity of the antiserum may increase. This involves the selection of B cell clones producing antibodies with high affinity for the immunogen. This process is usually facilitated by increasing the interval between immunizations so that the time-averaged tissue concentration of the immunogen is low enough to result in the occupation of only those B-cell-associated antibodies with the highest affinity constant for the antigen.

Polyclonal Antibodies

Polyclonal antisera contain a very heterogeneous mixture of antibodies, only a small fraction of which may be specific for the antigen or hapten of interest. Rabbits, guinea pigs, sheep, and goats are generally

FIGURE 6-4. Schematic representation of a gamma globulin (antibody) molecule. The hormone recognition sites contain the variable amino acid regions of the light and heavy immunoglobulin chains. The light chains are covalently linked to the heavy chains through a disulfide bond (s), and a single disulfide bond exists between the two heavy chains. The immunoglobulin molecule assumes a Y conformation, with the antibody combining sites occupying the top portions of the Y.

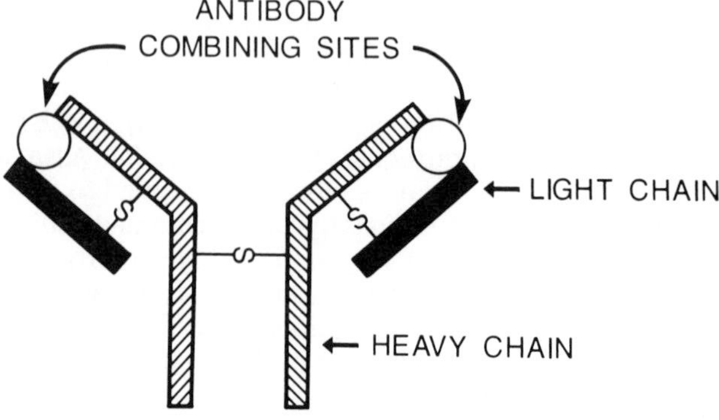

used for polyclonal antibody production. The volume of antiserum required, the quantity of immunogen available, and the degree of structural difference between the endogenous hormone and the immunogen are relevant criteria for selecting the species to be immunized.[48]

Hormonal immunogens generally fall into three antigenic classes: large proteins, small peptides, and steroids. The glycoprotein hormones, such as TSH, luteinizing hormone (LH), follicle stimulating hormone (FSH), and hCG, if foreign to the immunized animal and available in purified form, will suffice as immunogens without further modification.[49] Small peptide hormones such as TRH, by contrast, are not intrinsically immunogenic because of their small size and ubiquitous occurrence in vertebrate and invertebrate species.[50] For these small polypeptides (haptens) to be rendered immunogenic, they must be chemically linked to larger, highly immunogenic proteins such as keyhole limpet hemocyanin, bovine serum albumin, and thyroglobulin.[51] The chemistry used for this coupling reaction is determined in large measure by the available reactive groups on the polypeptide or its derivative that will be used as a haptenic group for the carrier protein. The ratio of hapten to carrier protein is important, since it has a substantial influence on the overall antigenicity of the conjugate.[52] If a small haptenic peptide is derived from an exposed region of a larger protein, the resulting polyclonal antibodies will generally cross-react with the corresponding epitope in the intact protein, providing an alternative to the epitope-specific monoclonal antibody.

Similar recognition constraints apply to the conjugation of steroid haptens to proteins. The cross-linking reagent bridging the hapten with the carrier protein will influence the specificity of the resulting antibody.[53] If appropriate sites for cross-linking to the peptide hapten for iodination are not available, solid-phase synthesis of an analog with the desired characteristics is a convenient option. The judicious combination of coupling chemistry and iodinatable haptenic analogs has facilitated the development of steroid RIAs, such as that for cortisol, that use more conveniently counted ^{125}I tracers.[54,55]

Monoclonal Antibodies

Monoclonal antibodies are usually produced in mice or rats through in vitro transformation of antibody-producing B cells by oncogenic viruses or, more commonly, by fusion of antibody-producing cells with mutant myeloma cells to confer immortality on the B cells.

A frequently used technique for generating antibody-producing hybridomas relies on the use of myeloma cells that lack hypoxanthine guanine phosphoribosyltransferase (HGPRT). HGPRT-deficient myeloma cells are selected by growing them in media containing 6-thioguanine or 8-azaguanine. Cells with HGPRT integrate these base analogs into DNA, resulting in a lethal interference with transcription, while HGPRT-deficient cells can produce nucleic acids only by de novo synthesis.[30]

Lymphocytes do not multiply in vitro but contain the enzymes for both the de novo and salvage pathways for DNA base synthesis. The folic acid antagonist aminopterin, which blocks the de novo synthesis pathway, is used to select for myeloma cells which have fused with lymphocytes. The salvage pathway of the surviving hybridoma cells is stimulated by the addition of hypoxanthine and thymidine [hypoxanthine, aminopterin, and thymidine (HAT) medium]. Only a small proportion of the hybridoma cells will produce useful antibodies. Unless proper precautions are taken, such cells will be rapidly overgrown by more rapidly dividing but nonproducing (revertant) cells. Feeder cells are needed during the first few days of the culture to increase the survival rate of the newly produced hybridomas. Revertant cells can be eliminated by culturing the hybridomas two to three times per year in 8-azaguanine.[30]

Immunization for the production of monoclonal antibodies may be carried out either in vitro or, more commonly, in vivo. The advantages of in vitro immunization are a short (5 days) immunization time and the ability to use self antigens; also, the immunogen concentration can be regulated, and antibody production can be monitored conveniently. The principal disadvantage is that only a primary (IgM) immune response can be elicited unless a complex protocol is followed involving the addition of factors for growth and differentiation to also elicit 10 to 20 percent IgG-producing hybridomas.[56]

Monoclonal antibodies have lower apparent affinity constants because they can bind only to a single region, or epitope, of the antigen; therefore, they are less useful for reagent limiting assays. Polyclonal antibodies, by contrast, can bind to a multitude of different antigenic sites simultaneously and, as a result of the bivalent nature of the IgG molecule, can form complex, highly cooperative interactions.[57] Mixtures of two or more monoclonal antibodies with different binding specificities for a given large antigen can also result in the formation of complexes involving two (or more) antibody molecules and two (or more) antigens in highly cooperative circular or chainlike arrays.

Nonimmunologic Molecular Recognition Systems: Avidin/Biotin

Avidin, a 4-subunit protein derived from egg white, has an exceptionally high affinity for biotin (10^{15} M^{-1}), one of the water-soluble components of the vitamin B complex. Four binding sites for biotin arranged as two pairs of closely juxtaposed, deeply penetrating binding sites occur in avidin.[58] Each paired binding site can accept only a single biotin molecule because of steric effects which perturb the neighboring binding site. The avidin/biotin system has been used for the development of new nonradioisotopic methods for hormone assay. Avidin is a very basic glycoprotein (pI = 10.5) which is stable over a wide range of pH and temperature and is resistant to proteolytic enzymes. Analogs or small fragments of biotin such as urea, glycol, tetrahydrofuran, and caproic acid may bind to or compete in the interaction with avidin. The most advantageous use of avidin is as a bridge between two biotinylated molecules such as a biotinylated enzyme and a biotinylated immunoreactant.

Labels

Radioactive Tracers

The convenience of radiochemical iodination and gamma counter detection of ^{125}I-labeled peptide and protein hormones is being outweighed by the increasingly stringent regulatory burden which accompanies the use of radioisotopes. Nonradioactively labeled tracers for immunoassays are generally obtained as part of commercially prepared kit assays, since their preparation generally involves the use of proprietary methods. For clinical applications, the high cost per tube of such assays is compensated by the maintenance of appropriate quality controls in the manufacturing process and the savings in technician time and labor achieved by using automated assay systems.

Iodination

Oxidationof Na^{125}I to form $^{125}I_2$ through the use of the oxidizing agent chloramine-T remains the most popular method for radiochemically labeling peptides and proteins.[59] The molecular iodine spontaneously reacts with tyrosyl and histidyl residues on the exposed surfaces of proteins. The major drawbacks to this method are that chloramine-T may cause oxidative damage to the substrate protein and that the reactive $^{125}I_2$ is volatile, necessitating the use of specialized fume hoods to minimize the biohazard. An enzymatic method for producing reactive $^{125}I_2$ involves the use of lactoperoxidase and hydrogen peroxide. This method generally results in less oxidative damage to the substrate protein and greater preservation of its initial biological and immunologic potency, provided that reaction-limiting amounts of hydrogen peroxide are used.[59] Because of their electronegativity and large size, iodine atoms incorporated into peptides and proteins alter their chemical and steric properties. The introduction of more than one iodine atom per host polypeptide also results in accelerated radiolytic damage during storage. Optimization of the conditions used for storing and repurification of iodinated proteins which are particularly susceptible to radiolytic damage may be as important as the method selected for the initial iodination to maintain tracer binding for several weeks or months.[28] Iodogen, a water-insoluble form of chloramine-T, was developed as another method for minimizing the exposure of proteins to the damaging effects of this oxidizing agent during the radioiodination procedure.[60] A less popular method of ^{125}I labeling proteins involves the radioiodination of the Bolton-Hunter reagent, 3-(*p*-hydroxyphenyl) propionic acid *N*-hydroxysuccinimide ester, which then is reacted with the amino groups of the polypeptide hormone.[61] Iodination with ^{131}I is infrequently used because of its short half-life of 8 days, compared with 59 days for ^{125}I, and its hazardous, high-energy gamma emission spectrum.

[^{3}H] Labeling

Small antigens, such as steroid hormones, generally cannot accommodate large iodo groups incorporated during radiochemical iodination without a substantial change in their antibody-binding specificity.[54] The incorporation of [^{3}H] into the substrate molecule does not change any chemical or immunologic properties but does necessitate the use of beta counting methods, which are more labor-intensive than the direct gamma counting of ^{125}I. The preparation of [^{3}H]-labeled antigens for immunoassay requires specialized facilities and is usually carried out in a radiolabeling facility on a contract basis if the labeled compound is not commercially available. Environmental concerns connected with the disposal of scintillation vials make this a costly alternative.

Nonradioactive Tracers

Enzyme

Enzyme immunoassays (EIA) may be broadly subdivided into two categories: activity amplification assays and activity modulation assays. Activity amplification assays and activity modulation assays are analogous to reagent excess and reagent limiting immunoassays, respectively. A large excess of immunoreactant is used in activity amplification assays to obtain a maximum signal for the analyte to be tested. From the law of mass action, which states that the rate of complex formation is proportional to the product of the analyte and antibody concentrations, a rapid and nearly quantitative reaction of all the available analyte molecules will occur in an activity amplification assay.[30] A description and examples of activity modulation enzymes assays are given in Homogeneous Assay Systems, below.

Fluorescence

A photon of appropriate energy (wavelength) can excite an atom, molecule, or fluorescent labeling group from its ground state to a higher electronic state. The return to the ground state may occur through nonradiative processes or emission of light at a longer wavelength. The difference between the incident (excitation) wavelength and the emission wavelength is known as the Stokes shift.[62] In fluorescence polarization assays, the path of the filtered or monochromated incident light beam is directed at right angles to the frequency-selected light path to the detector.[63] To minimize the amount of the excitation light which reaches the detector as a result of light scattering from molecules (Rayleigh scattering), particles (Tyndall scattering), and the rotational and vibrational energy of the solvent molecules (Raman scattering), a fluorescent label with a large Stokes shift is selected.[62,64]

One of the advantages of fluorometric methodology is the large dynamic range of the measured response. Endogenous fluorophores of serum, especially hemoglobin and bilirubin, however, interfere with the detection of commonly used fluorescent tags such as fluoroscein, which have similar emission wavelengths. The quantum yield (ratio of emitted to incident quanta) of fluorescent probes is also sensitive to changes in temperature, pH, and solvent polarity and to trace oxidizing agents or dissolved oxygen. Interactions of the fluorophore with quenching agents such as tryptophan, iodine-containing molecules, specific antibody, or nonspecific albumin binding can also reduce the quantum yield.[62,64]

Time-resolved fluorescence spectroscopy has been developed to eliminate the interfering endogenous fluorescence of serum. When europium chelates are used as the labeling reagent, with a fluorescence lifetime longer than that of hemoglobin or bilirubin, the start of fluorescence detection can be delayed or "gated" until these serum fluorophores have decayed completely.[62,64]

Luminescence

The fluorescence phenomenon, as described above, is photo-induced luminescence: the transiting of an electron from a high-energy orbital of an atom or molecule, induced by an initial absorption of electromagnetic radiation, to a lower-energy orbital with the release of a photon of light.[62] *Chemiluminescence*—the excitation of a molecule to a higher-energy state by a chemical reaction followed by the release of a photon—has the potential to be as sensitive as radiochemical labeling without the radiation hazard.[65] Unlike fluorescent compounds, which can be excited repeatedly, chemiluminescent molecules can be activated only once, though all molecules are potentially available for detection. In one study, a chemiluminescent assay for TSH was 10-fold more sensitive than a sensitive immunoradiometric assay and permitted more accurate measurement of subnormal serum TSH levels.[66]

Particle

Latex particle agglutination assays, which were most frequently used in qualitative kits for pregnancy and serology testing, have evolved into fully automated, high-sensitivity quantitative methods for measuring a variety of hormones. Antibody-coated latex particles are mixed with serum or another body fluid sample, resulting in sample antigen-induced aggregation of some of the particles. The mixture is passed through a particle counter, which counts the number of unagglutinated particles remaining. The expanding use of this method has resulted from rapid improvements in its sensitivity and reproducibility, elimination of specific and nonspecific self-agglutination, and extension of the range of application, most importantly to the measurement of small molecules.[67]

Vesicle

Vesicle assays consist of lipid bilayer spheres (micelles) which encapsulate a solution of reporter molecules. Incorporated into the micelle are antigenic molecules which have been chemically combined with phospholipids which "anchor" the antigen to the bilayer surface. The solutions within the micelles may include dyes, fluorescent compounds, hemoglobin, spin-labeled molecules, or enzymes. Because of the high turnover rate of enzymes, amplification of a spectrophotometric or fluorescent signal produced by vesicle lysis is possible. Competitive, reagent excess, two-phase, and homogeneous assay methodologies have been reported.[68,69] A vesicle assay for digoxin uses digoxin antibody–coated tubes which bind either the free digoxin in the patient serum and assay standards or the digoxin-coated micelle. After incubation and washing, the vesicles which remain attached to the test tube are ruptured with detergent and the optical density of the released dye is measured spectrophotometrically.[68]

Multianalyte

Simultaneous measurement of several analytes in the same serum sample has also become an established technique.[70–72] The use of radioactive or nonradioactive tracers which can be detected separately because of differences in spectral energy of emission or absorption saves both sample and labor costs. Simplification of the assay methodology not only saves expense but improves accuracy, since each manipulation represents a potential source of error. Examples are commercial kits for the simultaneous measurement of TSH and FT_4 through the use of ^{125}I and ^{51}Cr labels[70] and for the measurement of LH and FSH.[72]

SEPARATION SYSTEMS

Most assay systems require measurement of the proportion of the total hormonal analyte which is bound or free. Usually this determination is made after the hormone-antibody complex has been separated from the unbound hormone.

Liquid-Phase Precipitation

The addition of nonimmune IgG and anti-IgG antiserum (second antibody) is still a very common method for separating the bound and free hormone fractions, particularly in RIAs.[73,74] This reaction can be greatly accelerated by the addition of polyethylene glycol.[75] The kinetics of this acceleration, however, is highly dependent on the concentration and type of protein in the reaction mixture.

Solid-Phase Adsorption

The RIA, which is a reagent limiting, labeled antigen type of hormone assay, initially dominated the immunoassay field. Adsorption of the first antibody to the assay test tube greatly simplified the separation of the bound hormone but required long incubation times because of the slow kinetics for the antigen-antibody interaction. The use of monoclonal antibodies adsorbed to plastic test tubes, macroporous polystyrene beads with a large surface area, microwells, dipsticks, slides, electrodes, or fiber filters in reagent excess immunoradiometric assays has solved the kinetic limitations of the solid-phase adsorption method for separating the bound and free hormone fractions.[76]

Solid-Phase Precipitation

Another rapid separation method which allows a large amount of a first or second antibody to maintain intimate contact with the analyte-containing sample utilizes antibody-coated magnetizable particles. After binding of the hormone is complete, the tray of assay tubes is placed in a special, permanently magnetized rack which draws the particles toward the sides or bottom of the test tube. The supernatant can then be aspirated or decanted.[77] Clinical assays for cortisol, TSH, LH, FSH, hCG, T_4, FT_4, T_3 and FT_3, progesterone, and unconjugated estriol which utilize this method of separation are widely available.

HOMOGENEOUS ASSAY SYSTEMS

If the bound fraction of a hormone can be measured in the presence of the free fraction, physical separation is not necessary. Such homogeneous assays avoid separation error, one of the major sources of experimental variability in immunoassays. Most separation-free assays, however, have been limited to low-molecular-weight analytes.

Methods for the detection of antigen-antibody complexes without the addition of a second antibody, centrifugation, and separation of the pellet and supernatant continue to proliferate. Fluorescence polarization and amplitude-modulated immunoenzymatic assays are recent strategies for minimizing the errors in determining the bound/free ratio.

Fluorescence Polarization

Molecules in solution rotate in response to collisions with the surrounding solvent molecules which are undergoing rapid, chaotic movements termed *Brownian motion*. The average rotational rate for a given molecule is proportional to 1/V, where V is the volume of the molecule with the fluorescent label. If a small fluorescent-labeled hormone is excited with a polarized beam of light, the excited molecule will rotate through a large angle relative to the orientation of the incident beam before the polarized excitation is reemitted as a polarized fluorescence. If some of the fluorescent hormones are bound to large antibody molecules, these complexes will rotate much more slowly and will reemit their polarized fluorescence at nearly the same angle as the incident beam. If the emitted light is detected with a polarizer alternating between the parallel orientation and the perpendicular orientation of the incident beam, more emitted light will be detected in the parallel orientation as the extent of complexation of labeled hormone with antibody increases. The potential sensitivity of this method depends on the difference in hydrodynamic mobility of the bound hormone and the free hormone. For this reason, fluorescence polarization can be utilized only for small molecules, such as steroid and thyroid hormones, and therapeutic and abused drugs.[78]

Amplitude-Modulated Enzyme Assays

Amplitude-modulated assays can lead to either activation or inhibition of the end product signal, depending on the enzymatic reaction which is modulated and the epitopic specificity of the antibodies used. The first of this general class of assays (Fig. 6-5*A*) was developed by Rubenstein et al.[79] for the detection of morphine, using an enzyme-hapten conjugate. The activity of the conjugated enzyme was modulated by antihapten antibody through steric hindrance or allosteric alteration of the enzyme. Free hapten decreased this modulatory effect by competitively binding with antibody. This method is known by the commercial name EMIT (Syva Co.). If substrate is conjugated to antigen, the reaction of antibody to this conjugate will block the use of the substrate by the enzyme. The addition of free antigen as the standard or unknown leaves some conjugate free to enter the active site of the enzyme (Fig. 6-5*B*). Conjugation of antigen to an enzyme cofactor results in a third type of amplitude-modulated assay (Fig. 6-5*C*). The addition of free antigen leads to an increase in cofactor availability for the enzyme. Enzyme may also be conjugated directly to antibody so

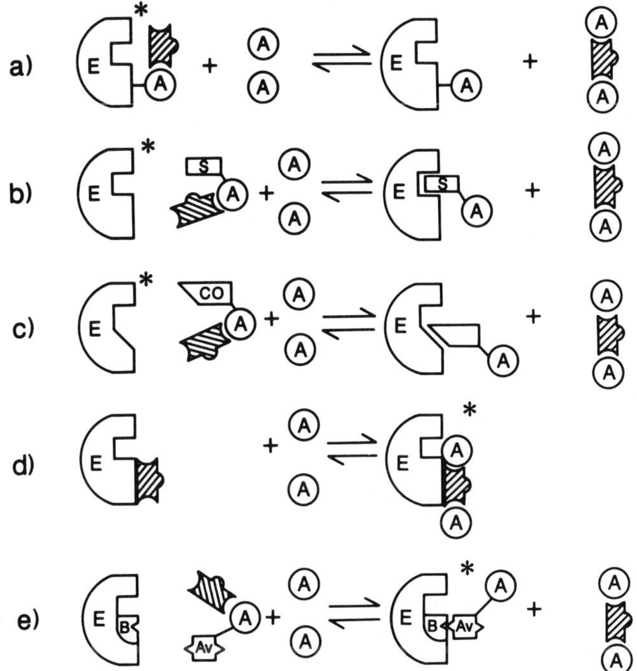

FIGURE 6-5. Competitive, homogeneous (separation-free) enzymatic immunoassays. E = enzyme; A = antigen or hapten; S = substrate; CO = enzyme cofactor; Av = avidin; B = biotin. Enzymes with an asterisk have "modulated" (increased or decreased) activities. *(From Tijssen,*[30] *by permission of Elsevier Science Publishers.)*

that substrate access to the enzyme active site is blocked by antigen binding (Fig. 6-5*D*). The high affinity of avidin-conjugated hapten for biotinylated enzyme has also been utilized for hormone assay (Fig. 6-5*E*). Binding of antibody to hapten sterically hinders access of the avidin to the biotinylated enzyme. The addition of free hapten results in increased avidin/biotin complex formation and enzyme inactivation.[30]

RECEPTOR ASSAYS

The principles underlying receptor assays are very similar to those underlying immunoassays. Instead of antibody molecules, specific hormone receptors from the plasma membranes or nuclei of hormonally responsive tissues are used to bind labeled and unlabeled hormone. Receptors for peptide and protein hormones are found on the cellular plasma membrane,[80] while the steroid, thyroid, and retinoic acid receptors, which are members of the same supergene family,[81] occur in or are translocated to the nucleus, where they associate with chromosomal DNA and other nuclear proteins.[82] Purified plasma membrane receptors tend to be unstable in the absence of bound hormone and detergent or other stabilizing factors.[83] Other problems which occur with many receptor assays are heterogeneity in the binding characteristics of the receptors, with the most abundant form having a low affinity constant, and complex positive and negative cooperativity effects, which complicate dose interpolation from the standard curve.[84]

The major protein, peptide, steroid, 1,25-dihydroxyvitamin D_3, thyroid, and retinoic acid receptors have been cloned, sequenced, and overexpressed in bacterial or mammalian cell systems.[80,85,86] Detailed structural information should lead to the availability of homogeneous, stable high-affinity-constant receptors in quantities useful for basic research and clinical assays.

CHROMATOGRAPHIC ASSAYS

Recent advances in chemical separation technology for peptides, biogenic amines, and steroids combined with immunoassay or physical chemical detection have greatly increased the specificity of hormone assay methods. While many closely related compounds may cross-react with a given antibody or receptor, these molecules can usually be separated according to differences in their tendency to bind to various chromatographic media. Quantitation of the resulting chromatographic fractions allows the measurement of several hormones within the same clinical sample. The combined use of chromatography and immunoassay or direct detection methods has recently been reported for the simultaneous measurement of serum prednisone, prednisolone, and cortisol[87]; unconjugated estriol and estradiol[88]; glucocorticoids[89]; adrenal delta 4-steroids[90]; testosterone in female patients[91]; dehydroepiandrosterone sulfate[92]; and catecholamines, vitamin D, opioid peptides, and gastrointestinal hormones.[93]

Chromatography

The chromatographic method used most frequently in conjunction with hormone measurement is high-pressure liquid chromatography (HPLC). The chromatographic medium usually consists of microspheres of silica gel which have been chemically modified to render them hydrophobic (lipophilic). Molecules are separated on this "reverse-phase" column using a high-pressure flow of an aqueous solution with an increasing concentration of an organic solvent such as acetonitrile.[93,94] Exclusion HPLC, which separates according to effective molecular size, and ion-exchange HPLC, which separates according to the electric charge on the hormone, can also be used.

Detection

A variety of detection methods are being used to quantitate serum and tissue hormones as they emerge from the HPLC column. These include immunoassays, refractometry to measure changes in refractive index, electrochemical conductance, light scattering, ultraviolet spectrometry, fluorometry, chemiluminescence, and mass spectrometry.[93]

IMMUNOASSAY OPTIMIZATION AND VALIDATION

General Considerations

The trend in hormone assays has been toward progressive improvement in detection limits, labor costs, reagent stability, and assay variability. A parallel development has been the institution of laboratory quality assessment programs which distribute pooled or fully characterized samples for interlaboratory comparison. These two processes tend toward the ultimate but never fully attainable goal of providing absolutely precise and reproducible measurement of clinically important hormonal substances.[95]

Detection Limits

Detection and precision limits for competitive or reagent limiting assays are a function of the affinity constant for the antigen-antibody reaction. Selection of the optimal concentrations for the antibody and tracer concentrations and tracer specific activity on a trial-and-error basis is extremely tedious. Graphic representations of RIA detection and precision limits as a function of antibody concentration and affinity constant, labeled antigen concentration, and specific activity have recently been reported.[96] These representations provide valuable insights into the appropriate adjustments to be made in the reagent parameters to provide the greatest assay sensitivity and precision. The important point that optimal assay sensitivity can often be attained at initial binding (B_0/T) values < 30 to 50 percent if a labeled antigen of high specific activity is used has been well illustrated. For competitive assays, the detection limit is proportional to $1/K_a$.[25] Selection of the antiserum with the highest K_a value is conveniently made by comparison of Scatchard plots for each antiserum obtained in the same assay (Fig. 6-6).

Specificity

Many hormonal analytes have similar or identical antigenic binding sites or epitopes. A good example is the α subunit of the glycoprotein hormones LH, FSH, TSH, and hCG, which is the product of a single gene.[97] Polyclonal antibodies produced against any one of these hormones will produce antibodies which will cross-react with the α subunit of other glycoprotein hormones of the same species and possibly related species. One method for suppressing this cross-reactivity is to add a great excess of one of the glycoprotein hormones which is not being analyzed, such as hCG, resulting in nearly complete saturation of the α-subunit-reacting antibodies and greatly reduced cross-reaction with additional hCG (Fig. 6-7).[28] With the advent of monoclonal antibodies, much greater selectivity of the epitopic sites being recognized is possible. Any given protein hormone analyte may in fact represent a large family of chemically distinct but highly cross-reactive species produced by alternative splicing of the corresponding mRNA, variations in posttranscriptional glycosyla-

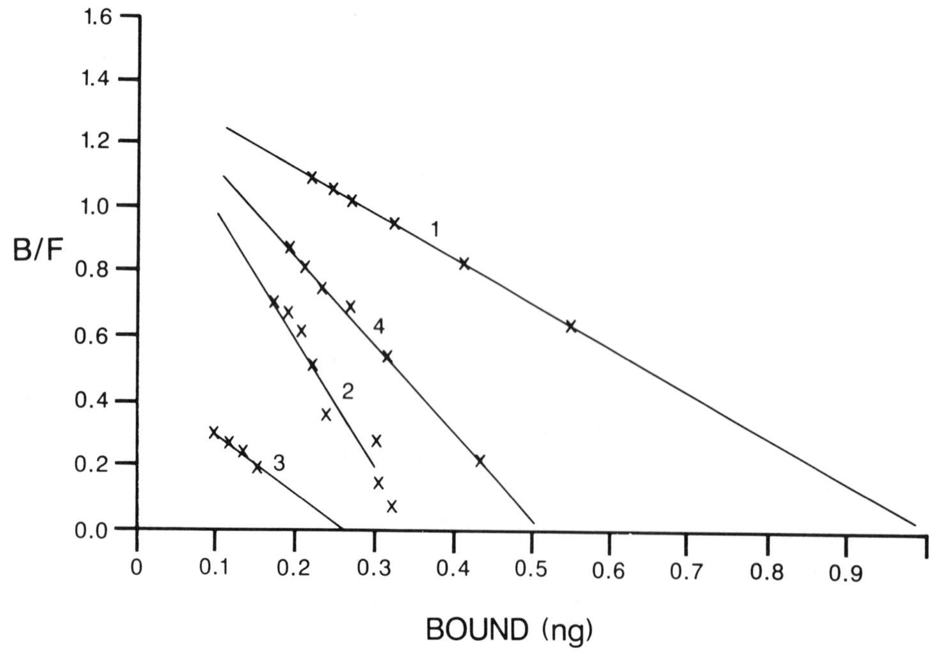

FIGURE 6-6. Scatchard plot comparison of four different rabbit antisera against human TSH. Curve 2 has the steepest slope (equal to $-k_a$) and should provide the most sensitive reagent limiting immunoassay after proper assay optimization. (*From Pekary and Hershman, unpublished results.*)

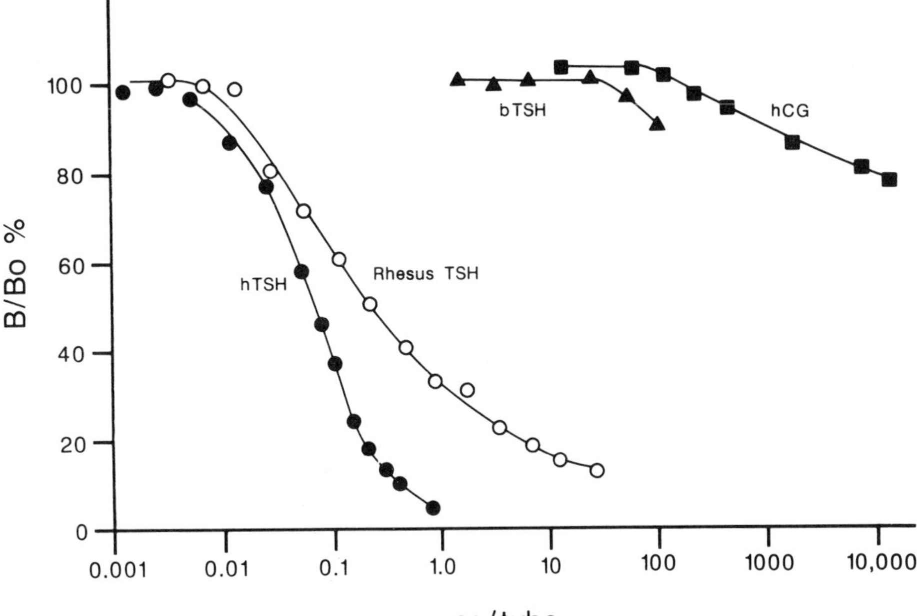

FIGURE 6-7. Saturation curves for the "high-affinity" (curve 2 in Fig. 6-6) human TSH antibody: human chorionic gonadotropin, 2980 IU/mg (solid squares); bovine TSH, 40 mU/μg (solid triangles); Rhesus monkey pituitary homogenate (units in terms of wet weight of tissue/tube are 10^4 times the indicated ng/tube) (open circles); and the 68/38 human TSH standard assuming 10 μU = 1 ng (solid circles). (*From Pekary, Hershman, and Parlow.*[28])

tion, acetylation, methylation, sulfation, and partial enzymatic fragmentation by serum- and membrane-associated enzymes. The biological activity of each analyte may vary from totally inactive to greatly increased effectiveness as assessed by a bioassay. This heterogeneity in the ratio of biological to immunologic activity (B/I ratio) may contribute significantly to such puzzling phenomena as the normal TSH levels in patients with hypothalamic hypothyroidism. Lack of TRH results in secretion of TSH with altered glycosylation and reduced bioactivity.[21] A number of approaches have proved useful in minimizing the interference of biologically irrelevant but highly cross-reactive species in hormonal assays. These include chromatographic separation, protein binding, ultrafiltration, protein precipitation, change in incubation time or temperature, selection of antibodies specific for epitopes unique to the relevant hormonal species, and the use of dual-site assays.[98]

INTERFERENCE

Sample Matrix Effects

The antigen-antibody reaction is very rapid, being limited only by the rate of diffusion of the reacting species. The effective diffusion rate, however, can be greatly reduced if other macromolecules occur in the same reaction mixture. Hormone assay measurements are most often made in undiluted, unextracted human serum or plasma in which serum proteins such as albumin, gamma globulins, lipoproteins, α_2-macroglobulin, and fibrinogen (plasma) occur in great excess compared to the trace levels of the hormonal analyte of interest. Because of the complex structure of proteins which have many different classes of interactive chemical groups exposed on their surfaces, complexes of these proteins with hormonal analyte and antibody, with widely varying stabilities, inevitably form. These interactions greatly retard the diffusional processes leading to the formation of the hormone-antibody complex and reduce the apparent affinity constant of hormone-antibody binding at equilibrium. For competitive or reagent limiting assays, these effects are manifested by a retarded forward rate constant for antigen-antibody binding and a reduction in the tracer bound/total (B/T) ratio for serum-containing samples compared to equivalent samples in protein-free buffer.[28,99] This "serum" or "matrix" effect can usually be compensated for by using the same amount of hormone-free serum to prepare the assay calibrators.

Heterophilic Antibodies

Mouse monoclonal antibodies are sometimes used in various therapeutic modalities, resulting in the production of human antibodies to mouse gamma globulins. The mixing of serum from such patients with the mouse monoclonal antibodies commonly used in commercial kit assays may result in a significant interference with the monoclonal antibody-hormone reaction.[100] Such interfering antibodies can also occur in "naive" (untreated) patients[101] and should be considered as possible explanations for unexpected assay results. The direction of bias caused by the presence of patient antibodies reacting with some component of the assay system can lead to either high or low values depending on the assay method and the specificity of the heterophilic antibody. Inappropriately elevated levels of TSH in a reagent excess assay were traced to patient antibodies to mouse IgG which sandwiched between the immobilized and labeled monoclonal antibodies of the assay, leading to a diagnosis of hypothyroidism and inappropriate therapy.[102]

Complement and Rheumatoid Factors

Immunoassays which use a second antibody for the separation of bound and free antigen can fail because the complement-fixation reaction enzymes in the serum sample destroy the complexes of the first and second antibodies.[103,104] Rheumatoid factor is an IgM molecule which can also fix and activate complement. This potential problem is usually prevented by the addition of a calcium chelator such as edetic acid (ethylenediaminetetraacetic acid, or EDTA) which binds the ionized calcium which is essential for the complement-fixation reaction.[28,103–105]

Enzyme Contaminants

Microbial growth in blood or serum samples may result from an infection in the patient or improper handling and storage of the specimen. In vitro degradation of one or more of the assay reagents or of the analyte itself by the proteolytic enzymes of the contaminated sample may result in a serious measurement error. The addition of a bacteriostatic agent, such as sodium azide, to all hormonal assay reagents retards this process. Rapid sample processing and storage in a −20°C freezer is usually sufficient to avoid this problem. Many hormones, such as β-endorphin, glucagon, and ACTH, may be rapidly degraded by proteases in normal serum. The addition of proteolytic enzyme inhibitors such as aprotinin (Trasylol) or benzamidine combined with special handling of the samples is required for the accurate measurement of these hormones.[106]

Drug Interference

Drug therapy has the potential for biasing the results of a hormone assay. An example is the effect of heparin on the measurement of free T_4; heparin can stimulate the release of FFA in vivo and in vitro, leading to the displacement of T_4 from the thyroid hormone–binding proteins of serum.[41] A number of therapeutic drugs cross-react in hormone assays. For example, prednisolone may cross-react with hydrocortisone and spironolactone may cross-react with aldosterone. Insulin and growth hormone therapy can lead to hormone-specific antibody production which can interfere in the corresponding immunoassays.[101,107] The sera of such patients have high levels of hormone bound to the corresponding antibodies. Autoantibodies to insulin can occur spontaneously. Growth hormone–binding proteins occur normally in patient sera. The affinity constants for these proteins have been shown to be much lower than those for typical monoclonal or polyclonal antibodies used in commercial assays, resulting in dissociation of growth hormone from these binding proteins during incubation and minimal interference.[107] Hormone autoimmunity presents two major complications in immunoassay measurements: (1) the high levels of antibody-associated hormone present in the serum and (2) the competition of the antibodies derived from the patient serum with those of the assay for binding to the corresponding serum hormone. A method for high-performance protein-G affinity chromatography for quantitating hormonal antibodies in patient sera has recently been reported.[108]

Hemodynamic Effects

A substantial increase in blood pressure occurs in normal subjects during the transition from the supine, resting position to normal upright activity. Changes in blood pressure between supine and upright postures may cause fluid shifts that result in changes of blood volume and concentration of hormones which are not freely diffusible across the capillary endothelium. A substantial (one-third) increase in serum T_4 values was measured in subjects engaged in normal activity compared with a 3-h baseline study involving the drawing of blood at 15-min intervals while the subjects were completely supine and motionless. This increase, which would be clinically significant in evaluating borderline T_4 levels, was almost quantitatively abolished by dividing each serum T_4 value by its corresponding total serum protein concentration to normalize for fluid shifts related to physical activity.[109]

QUALITY CONTROL

The standardization of hormonal assay measurements is a complex problem because the substance being measured may be structurally and functionally heterogeneous and may occur in an extremely complex mixture of other compounds whether the source is blood, urine, cerebrospinal fluid, saliva, semen, or tissue.[110] Additional problems have arisen because of a lack of universally accepted and widely available reference preparations and the rapidly increasing variety of assay methodologies to be compared. The advent of legislatively mandated participation in interlaboratory quality control programs has discouraged the clinical use of unique "in-house" assays which do not have an equivalent at other institutions. However, the reliance on commercial kit assays leaves the clinical laboratory dependent on the manufacturer's quality control department and field representatives when problems with assay performance cannot be traced to instrumentation problems or reagent deterioration.[95]

The development of an effective intralaboratory quality control program begins with proper selection and validation of the commercial assay methodology. This process should be influenced strongly by the reputation of the assay and its manufacturer for long-term stability and dependability. The complexity of the assay, the number of "hands-on" manipulations, accuracy, sensitivity, reproducibility, safety, and the cost of the instrumentation and reagents are all relevant to the selection process. The trend toward full automation of the assay methodology, which permits much better control of pipetting accuracy and the temperature and time of incubation, along with computerized diagnosis of instrument and reagent problems, has been driven by high personnel costs and the increasingly stringent regulatory environment.[2]

An understanding of the distinction between the statistical concepts of accuracy and precision is essential to the maintenance of hormone assay performance. Using the analogy of a person firing a rifle at a target with concentric circles, if the bullet holes on the target are widely but evenly distributed about the bull's-eye, we say that the shooter is accurate (unbiased) but imprecise. If the bullet holes are tightly clustered but away from the target center, then the shooter is precise but inaccurate (biased). The goal of a quality control program is to maintain both the accuracy and the precision of hormone assay results. This requires the accumulation of data which characterize the assay standard curve—maximum binding, nonspecific counts, dose at 50 percent curve displacement, and slope—and interassay controls which monitor assay performance across the useful measurement range of the assay standard curve. Criteria for the rejection of both individual data and entire assays must be set. A variety of models for intralaboratory quality control have been proposed.[95,111]

Because of the large number of commercial hormone assays available (Table 6-1) and the continuing introduction of "new and improved" versions of these assays, decisions about when to convert to a new methology must frequently be faced. Improvements in accuracy and reproducibility should be the first criterion when one is considering a change, given the increasingly stringent regulatory environment and the relatively mature state of current assay methodology and support by manufacturers. An improvement in assay sensitivity should be considered as a selection factor only if it is clinically relevant, as it is for TSH measurements in patients who are receiving thyroid hormone suppressive therapy. Labor and materials costs should not be considered unless the new assay is at least comparable to the current assay in all other performance categories.

Frequent changes in methodology should be discouraged since diagnostic cutoff values are dependent on the selection criteria used for the normal population and on the characteristics of the assay used for determining these values. The development and dissemination of these values are time-consuming and must be revised with every significant change in assay procedure. A committee consisting of clinical and laboratory staff members should supervise the introduction of new and replacement assays to facilitate communication between clinic and laboratory when unexpected results arise with the new method.

FUTURE TRENDS

Recombinant DNA technology will have a major impact on the development of future hormone assays. Recombinant proteins will be designed for binding to unique epitopes on specific hormones.[112] Structural characterization of hormones in solution[113] should lead to the development of reagents and assay conditions which further reduce between-assay variability. One can envision the evolution of assays which utilize synthetic "cells" with recombinant hormone receptors and quantitatively monitored "second messengers." Laboratory safety issues will have been resolved. For example, a recently reported assay system employing a pH-sensitive photo-induced current detection system uses urea as the substrate and carbon dioxide and ammonia as the reaction products.[114] Biosensors are currently under development,[115,116] with the potential for continuous endocrine monitoring of ambulatory patients or experimental subjects. In situ measurement of hormones will have many important advantages, including the avoidance of sample storage and processing artifacts, the avoidance of immobilization and venipuncture stress, and the ability to correlate from moment to moment the signal inputs and physiologic responses to hormone secretion.[117]

REFERENCES

1. Gosling JP: A decade of development in immunoassay methodology. *Clin Chem* 36:1408, 1990.
2. Flore M, Mitchell J, Doen T, Nelson R, Winter G, Grandone C, Zeng K, Haraden R, et al: The Abbott IMx™ automated benchtop immunochemistry analyzer system. *Clin Chem* 34:1726, 1988.
3. Patrick JW: Radiation safety in the performance of radioimmunoassay, in Abraham GE (ed): *Handbook of Radioimmunoassay*. New York, Dekker, 1977, pp 1–25.
4. Bangham DR: Standardization and standards, in Thorell JI (ed): *Radioimmunoassay Design and Quality Control*. Oxford, Pergamon, 1983, pp 59–67.

5. Wittliff JL, Wenz LL, Dong J, Nawaz Z, Butt TR: Expression and characterization of an active human estrogen receptor as a ubiquitin fusion protein from *Escherichia coli. J Biol Chem* 265:22016, 1990.
6. Pekary AE: Parallel line and relative potency analysis of bioassay and radioimmunoassay data using a desk top computer. *Comput Biol Med* 9:355, 1979.
7. Hershman JM, Kenimer JG, Kojima A, Saunders RL: Thyroid-stimulating hormone, in Antoniades HN (ed): *Hormones in Human Blood*. Cambridge, MA, Harvard University Press, 1976, pp 464–487.
8. Finney DJ: *Statistical Method in Biological Assay*. London, Charles Griffin, 1964.
9. Bangham DR: What's in a bioassay? in Chayen J, Bitensky L (eds): *Cytochemical Bioassays*. New York, Dekker, 1983, pp 7–43.
10. Vitti P, Rotella CM, Valente WA, Cohen J, Aloj SM, Laccetti P, Ambesi-Impiombato FS, Grollman EF, et al: Characterization of the optimal stimulatory effects of Graves' monoclonal and serum immunoglobulin G on adenosine 3′,5′-monophosphate production in FRTL-5 thyroid cells: A potential clinical assay. *J Clin Endocrinol Metab* 57:782, 1983.
11. Pang X-P, Hershman JM, Smith VP, Pekary AE, Sugawara M: The mechanism of action of tumour necrosis factor-α and interleukin 1 on FRTL-5 rat thyroid cells. *Acta Endocrinol (Copenh)* 123:203, 1990.
12. Morris JC, III, Hay ID, Nelson RE, Jiang N-S: Clinical utility of thyrotropin-receptor antibody assays: Comparison of radioreceptor and bioassay methods. *Mayo Clin Proc* 63: 707, 1988.
13. Loveridge N: The techniques of cytochemical bioassays, in Chayen J, Bitensky L (eds): *Cytochemical Bioassays: Techniques and Clinical Applications*. New York, Dekker, 1983 pp. 45–82.
14. Chayen J, Bitensky L: General introduction to cytochemical bioassay, in Chayen J, Bitensky L (eds): *Cytochemical Bioassays: Techniques and Clinical Applications*. New York, Dekker, 1983, pp 1–6.
15. Dohler K-D, von zur Muhlen A, Wagner TOF, Lucke C, Weitzel HK, Hashimoto T: Thyroid-stimulating hormone, in Chayen J, Bitensky L (eds): *Cytochemical Bioassays: Techniques and Clinical Applications*. New York, Dekker, 1983, pp 107–134.
16. Petersen V, Smith BR, Hall R: A study of thyroid stimulating activity in human serum with the highly sensitive cytochemical assay. *J Clin Endocrinol Metab* 41:199, 1975.
17. DiStefano JJ III, Feng D: Comparative aspects of the distribution, metabolism, and excretion of six iodothyronines in the rat. *Endocrinology* 123:2514, 1988.
18. DiStefano JJ III, Sternlicht M, Harris DR: Rat enterohepatic circulation and intestinal distribution of enterally infused thyroid hormones. *Endocrinology* 123:2526, 1988.
19. Weintraub BD, Stannard BS, Magner JA, Ronin C, Taylor T, Joshi L, Constant RB, Menezes-Ferreira MM, et al: Glycosylation and posttranslational processing of thyroid-stimulating hormone: Clinical implications. *Recent Prog Horm Res* 41:577, 1985.
20. Oppenheimer JH, Schwartz HL, Mariash CN, Kinlaw WB, Wong NCW, Freake HC: Advances in our understanding of thyroid hormone action at the cellular level. *Endocr Rev* 8:288, 1987.
21. Taylor T, Weintraub BD: Altered thyrotropin (TSH) carbohydrate structures in hypothalamic hypothyroidism created by paraventricular nuclear lesions are corrected by in vivo TSH-releasing hormone administration. *Endocrinology* 125:2198, 1989.
22. Vuolteenaho O, Arjamaa O, Ling N: Atrial natriuretic polypeptides (ANP): Rat atria store high molecular weight precursor but secrete processed peptides of 25-35 amino acids. *Biochem Biophys Res Commun* 129:82, 1985.
23. D'Amour P, Lazure C, Labelle F: Metabolism of radioiodinated carboxy-terminal fragments of bovine parathyroid hormone in normal and anephric rats. *Endocrinology* 117:127, 1985.
24. Pekary AE, Stephens R, Simard M, Pang X-P, Smith V, DiStefano JJ III, Hershman JM: Release of thyrotropin and prolactin by a thyrotropin-releasing hormone (TRH) precursor, TRH-Gly: Conversion to TRH is sufficient for in vivo effects. *Neuroendocrinology* 52:618, 1990.
25. Feldman H, Rodbard D: Mathematical theory of radioimmunoassay, in Odell WD, Daughaday WH (eds): *Principles of Competitive Protein Binding Assay*. Philadelphia, Lippincott, 1971, pp 158–203.
26. Ratcliffe JG: Requirements for separation methods in immunoassay, in Hunter WM, Corrie JET (eds): *Immunoassays for Clinical Chemistry*, 2d ed. Edinburgh, Churchill Livingstone, 1983, pp 135–138.
27. Hunter WM: The preparation and assessment of labelled antigen: Outline of requirements, in Hunter WM, Corrie JET (eds): *Immunoassays for Clinical Chemistry*, 2d ed. Edinburgh, Churchill Livingstone, 1983, pp 263–266.
28. Pekary AE, Hershman JM, Parlow AF: A sensitive and precise radioimmunoassay for human thyroid-stimulating hormone. *J Clin Endocrinol Metab* 41:676, 1975.
29. Kohler G, Milstein C: Continuous culture of fused cells secreting specific antibody. *Nature* 256:495, 1975.
30. Tijssen P: *Practice and Theory of Enzyme Immunoassay*, Vol. 15: *Laboratory Techniques in Biochemistry and Molecular Biology*. Amsterdam, Elsevier, 1985.
31. Pekary AE, Turner LF Jr, Hershman JM: New immunoenzymatic assay for human thyrotropin compared with two radioimmunoassays. *Clin Chem* 32:511, 1986.
32. Ekins R, Chu F, Biggart E: Fluorescence spectroscopy and its application to a new generation of high sensitivity, multi-microspot, multianalyte, immunoassay. *Clin Chim Acta* 194:91, 1990.
33. Wide L: Labelled ligand versus labelled ligate and competitive versus non-competitive binding assays, in Thorell JI (ed): *Radioimmunoassay Design and Quality Control*. Oxford, Pergamon, 1983, pp 37–44.
34. Hunter WM, Bennie JG, Budd PS, van Heyningen V, James K, Micklem RL, Scott A: Immunoradiometric assays using monoclonal antibodies, in Hunter WM, Corrie JET (eds): *Immunoassays for Clinical Chemistry*, 2d ed. Edinburgh, Churchill Livingstone, 1983, pp 531–544.
35. Mendel CM: The free hormone hypothesis: A physiologically based mathematical model. *Endocr Rev* 10:232, 1989.
36. Refetoff S: Inherited thyroxine-binding globulin abnormalities in man. *Endocr Rev* 10:232, 1989.
37. Ekins R: Measurement of free hormones in blood. *Endocr Rev* 11:5, 1990.
38. Pardridge WM. Plasma protein-mediated transport of steroid and thyroid hormones (editorial review). *Am J Physiol* 252:E157, 1987.
39. Mendel CM, Weisiger RA, Jones AL, Cavalieri RR: Thyroid hormone-binding proteins in plasma facilitate uniform distribution of thyroxine within tissues: A perfused rat liver study. *Endocrinology* 120:1742, 1987.
40. Ain KB, Mori Y, Refetoff S: Reduced clearance of thyroxine-binding globulin (TBG) with increased sialylation: A mechanism for estrogen induced elevation of serum TBG concentration. *J Clin Endocrinol Metab* 65:689, 1987.
41. Nelson JC, Weiss RM. The effect of serum dilution on free thyroxine (T_4) concentration in the low T_4 syndrome of nonthyroidal illness. *J Clin Endocrinol Metab* 61:239, 1985.
42. Wang YS, Hershman JM, Smith V, Pekary AE: Effect of heparin on free thyroxin as measured by equilibrium dialysis and ultrafiltration. *Clin Chem* 32:700, 1986.
43. Larsen PR: Quantitation of triiodothyronine and thyroxine in human serum by radioimmunoassay, in Antoniades HN (ed): *Hormones in Human Blood*. Cambridge, MA, Harvard University Press, 1976, pp 679–697.
44. Ratcliffe WA: Direct (non-extraction) serum assays for ste-

roids, in Hunter WM, Corrie JET (eds): *Immunoassays for Clinical Chemistry*, 2d ed. Edinburgh, Churchill Livingstone, 1983, pp 401–409.
45. Davies DR, Padlam EA, Segal DM: Three-dimensional structure of immunoglobulins. *Annu Rev Biochem* 44:639, 1975.
46. Poljak RJ, Amzel LM, Chen BL, Chiu YY, Phizackerley RP, Saul F, Yserm X: Three-dimensional structure and diversity of immunoglobulins. *Cold Spring Harbor Symp Quant Biol* 41:639, 1976.
47. Padlam EA, Davies DR, Pecht I, Givol D, Wright C: Model building studies of antigen-binding sites: The hapten-binding site of MOPC-315. *Cold Spring Harbor Symp Quant Biol* 41:627, 1976.
48. Monro AC, Chapman RS, Templeton JG, Fatori D: Production of primary antisera for radioimmunoassay, in Hunter WM, Corrie JET (eds): *Immunoassays for Clinical Chemistry*, 2d ed. Edinburgh, Churchill Livingstone, 1983, pp 447–455.
49. Vaitukaitis JL, Robbins JB, Nieschlag E, Ross GT: A method for producing specific antisera with small doses of immunogen. *J Clin Endocrinol Metab* 33:988, 1971.
50. Pekary AE, Sharp B, Briggs J, Carlson HE, Hershman JM: High concentrations of p-Glu-His-Pro-NH_2 (thyrotropin-releasing hormone) occur in rat prostate. *Peptides* 4:915, 1983.
51. Visser TJ, Klootwijk W, Docter R, Hennemann G: A new radioimmunoassay of thyrotropin-releasing hormone. *FEBS Lett* 83:37, 1977.
52. Corrie JET: Production of anti-hapten sera in rabbits, in Hunter WM, Corrie JET (eds): *Immunoassays for Clinical Chemistry*, 2d ed. Edinburgh, Churchill Livingstone, 1983, pp 469–472.
53. Webb WA, Brooks RV: Some factors influencing antiserum specificity, in Hunter WM, Corrie JET (eds): *Immunoassays for Clinical Chemistry*, 2d ed. Edinburgh, Churchill Livingstone, 1983, pp 474–486.
54. Thorell JI, Ekman R, Malmquist M: Technical aspects of the production and application of iodinated steroids for radioimmunoassay, in *Radioimmunoassay and Related Procedures in Medicine 1982*. Vienna, International Atomic Energy Agency, 1982, pp 147–160.
55. Sugii A, Ogawa N, Kawanishi T, Umeda T, Sato T: One-step synthesis of a cortisol derivative for radioiodination and application of the ^{125}I-labeled cortisol to radioimmunoassay. *Chem Pharm Bull (Tokyo)* 35:5000, 1987.
56. Moller SA, Borrebaeck CAK: Development of an in vitro immunization technique for the production of murine monoclonal antibodies using small amounts of antigen and weak immunogens, in Borrebaeck CAK (ed): *In Vitro Immunization in Hybridoma Technology. Progress in Biotechnology*, vol. 5. Amsterdam, Elsevier, 1988, pp 3–22.
57. Ehrlich PH, Moyle WR: Cooperative immunoassays: Ultrasensitive assays with mixed monoclonal antibodies. *Science* 221:279, 1983.
58. Wilchek M, Bayer EA: Avidin-biotin mediated immunoassays: Overview. *Methods Enzymol* 184:467, 1990.
59. Brown NS, Abbott SR, Corrie JET: Some observations on the preparation, purification and storage of radioiodinated protein hormones, in Hunter WM, Corrie JET (eds): *Immunoassays for Clinical Chemistry*, 2d ed. Edinburgh, Churchill Livingstone, 1983, pp 263–266.
60. Bolton AE, Hunter WM: The labelling of proteins to high specific radioactivity by conjugation to a ^{125}I-containing acylating agent: Application to radioimmunoassay. *Biochem J* 133:529, 1973.
61. Thean ET: Comparison of specific radioactivities of human alpha-lactoalbumin iodinated by three different methods. *Anal Biochem* 188:330, 1990.
62. Kricka LJ: *Ligand-Binder Assays*. New York, Dekker, 1985.
63. Watanabe F, Miyai K: Fluorescence polarization immunoassay: Theory and application, in Ngo TT (ed): *Nonisotopic Immunoassay*. New York, Plenum, 1988, pp 199–209.
64. Soini E, Lovgren T: Time-resolved fluoroimmunoassay, in Ngo TT (ed): *Nonisotopic Immunoassay*. New York, Plenum, 1988, pp 231–243.
65. Kricka LJ, Thorpe GHG: Bioluminescent and chemiluminescent detection of horseradish peroxidase labels in ligand binder assays, in Van Dyke K, Van Dyke R (eds): *Luminescence Immunoassay and Molecular Applications*. Cleveland, CRC Press, 1990, pp 77–98.
66. Ross DS, Ardisson LJ, Meskell MJ: Measurement of thyrotropin in clinical and subclinical hyperthyroidism using a new chemiluminescent assay. *J Clin Endocrinol Metab* 69:684, 1989.
67. Wilkins TA, Brouwers G, Mareschal JL, Limet J, Masson PL: Immunoassay by particle counting, in Collins WP (ed): *Complementary Immunoassays*. Chichester, Wiley, 1988, pp 227–240.
68. O'Connell JP, Campbell RL, Fleming BM, Mercolino MD, Johnson MD, McLaurin DA: A highly sensitive immunoassay system involving antibody-coated tubes and liposome-entrapped dye. *Clin Chem* 31:1424, 1985.
69. Canova-Davis E, Redemann CT, Vollmer YP, Kung VT: Use of a reversed-phase evaporation vesicle formulation for a homogeneous liposome immunoassay. *Clin Chem* 32:1687, 1986.
70. Smith VP, Pekary AE, Hershman JM: Evaluation of a simultaneous TSH and free T_4 radioimmunoassay. *J Clin Immunoassay* 10:50, 1987.
71. Blake C, Al-Bassam MN, Gould BJ, Marks V, Bridges JW, Riley C: Simultaneous enzyme immunoassay of two thyroid hormones. *Clin Chem* 28:1469, 1982.
72. Beinlich CJ, Piper JA, O'Neal JC, White OD: Evaluation of dual-labeled simultaneous assays for lutropin and follitropin in serum. *Clin Chem* 31:2014, 1985.
73. Coxon RE, Rae C, Gallagher G, Landon J: Development of a simple fluoroimmunoassay for paraquat. *Clin Chim Acta* 175:297, 1988.
74. Power MJ, Gosling JP, Fottrell PF: Radioimmunoassay of osteocalcin with polyclonal and monoclonal antibodies. *Clin Chem* 35:1408, 1989.
75. Edwards R: The development and use of PEG assisted second antibody as a separation technique in RIA, in Hunter WM, Corrie JET (eds): *Immunoassays for Clinical Chemistry*, 2d ed. Edinburgh, Churchill Livingstone, 1983, pp 139–146.
76. Rasmussen SE: Solid phases and chemistries, in Collins WP (ed): *Complementary Immunoassays*. Chichester, Wiley, 1988, pp 43–55.
77. Forrest GC, Rattle SJ: Magnetic particle radioimmunoassay, in Hunter WM, Corrie JET (eds): *Immunoassays for Clinical Chemistry*, 2d ed. Edinburgh, Churchill Livingstone, 1983, pp 147–162.
78. Williams ATR: Fluorescence polarization immunoassay, in Collins WP (ed): *Complementary Immunoassays*. Chichester, Wiley, 1988, pp 135–147.
79. Rubenstein KE, Schneider RS, Ullman EF: "Homogeneous" enzyme immunoassay: A new immunochemical technique. *Biochem Biophys Res Commun* 47:846, 1972.
80. Straub RE, Frech GC, Joho RH, Gershengorn MC: Expression cloning of a cDNA encoding the mouse pituitary thyrotropin-releasing hormone receptor. *Proc Natl Acad Sci USA* 87:9514, 1990.
81. Yavita Y, Shi Y-B, Brown DD: Xenopus laaevis alpha and beta thyroid hormone receptors. *Proc Natl Acad Sci USA* 87:7090, 1990.
82. Steinsapir J, Evans AC, Mulroy M, Mahesh VB: Interactions of estrogen receptor with a monoclonal antibody: Localization with electron and light microscope and probing of various molecular forms. Paper presented at the Endocrine Society, 72nd Annual Meeting, Atlanta, June 20–23, 1990, Abst. 929.
83. Phillips WJ, Enyeart JJ, Hinkle PM: Pituitary thyrotropin-releasing hormone receptors: Local anesthetic effects on binding and responses. *Mol Endocrinol* 3:1345, 1989.

84. Azukizawa M, Kurtzman G, Pekary AE, Hershman JM: Comparison of the binding characteristics of bovine thyrotropin and human chorionic gonadotropin to thyroid plasma membranes. *Endocrinology* 101:1880, 1977.
85. Wang LH, Tsai SY, Cook RG, Beattie WG, Tsai M-J, O'Malley BW: COUP transcription factor is a member of the steroid receptor superfamily. *Nature* 340:163, 1989.
86. Power RF, Connelly OM, McDonnell DP, Clark JH, Butt TR, Schrader WT, O'Malley BW: High level expression of a truncated chicken progesterone receptor in *Escherichia coli*. *J Biol Chem* 265:1419, 1990.
87. McBride JH, Rodgerson DO, Park SS, Reyes AF: Rapid liquid-chromatographic method for simultaneous determination of plasma prednisone, prednisolone, and cortisol in pediatric renal-transplant recipients. *Clin Chem* 37:643–646, 1991.
88. Kondo Z, Makino T, Iizuka R: Measurement of serum unconjugated estriol and estradiol by high-performance liquid chromatography. *J Clin Lab Anal* 4:410, 1990.
89. Takeda M, Maeda M, Tsuji A: Chemiluminescence high performance liquid chromatography of corticosteroids using lucigenin as post-column reagent. *Biomed Chromatog* 4:119, 1990.
90. Saisho S, Shimozawa K, Yata J: Changes of several adrenal delta 4-steroids measured by HPLC-UV spectrometry in neonatal patients with congenital adrenal hyperplasia due to 21-hydroxylase deficiency. *Horm Res* 33:27, 1990.
91. Oka K, Hirano T, Noguchi M: Changes in the concentration of testosterone in serum during the menstrual cycle, as determined by liquid chromatography. *Clin Chem* 34:557, 1988.
92. Shackleton CH, Kletke C, Wudy S, Pratt JH: Dehydroepiandrosterone sulfate quantification in serum using high-performance liquid chromatography/mass spectrometry and a deuterated internal standard: A technique suitable for routine use or as a reference method. *Steroids* 55:472, 1990.
93. Makin HLJ, Newton R (eds): *High Performance Liquid Chromatography in Endocrinology. Monographs on Endocrinology*, vol. 30. Berlin, Springer-Verlag, 1988.
94. Pekary AE, Lukaski HC, Mena I, Hershman JM: Processing of TRH precursor peptides in rat brain and pituitary is zinc dependent. *Peptides* 12:1025, 1991.
95. Jeffcoate SL: *Efficiency and Effectiveness in the Endocrine Laboratory*. London, Academic, 1981.
96. Ezan E, Tiberghien C, Dray F: Practical method for optimizing radioimmunoassay detection and precision limits. *Clin Chem* 37:226, 1991.
97. Cos GS, Cosgrove DE, Sullivan TT, Haas MJ: Induction by cycloheximide of the glycoprotein hormone α-subunit gene in human tumor cell lines and identification of a possible negative regulatory factor. *J Biol Chem* 265:13190, 1990.
98. Miller JJ, Valdes R Jr: Approaches to minimizing interference by cross-reacting molecules in immunoassays. *Clin Chem* 37:144, 1991.
99. Berzofsky JA, Berkower IJ: Antigen-antibody interaction, in Paul WE (ed): *Fundamental Immunology*. New York, Raven, 1984, pp 595–644.
100. Boscato LM, Stuart MC: Heterophilic antibodies: A problem for all immunoassays. *Clin Chem* 34:27, 1988.
101. Wasada T, Eguchi Y, Takayama T, Yao K, Hirata Y: Reverse phase high performance liquid chromatographic analysis of circulating insulin in the insulin autoimmune syndrome. *J Clin Endocrinol Metab* 66:153, 1988.
102. Kahn BB, Weintraub BD, Csako G, Zweig MH: Factitious elevation of thyrotropin in a new ultrasensitive assay: Implications for the use of monoclonal antibodies in "sandwich" immunoassay. *J Clin Endocrinol Metab* 66:526, 1988.
103. Brown EJ, Joiner KA, Frank MM: Complement, in Paul WE (ed): *Fundamental Immunology*. New York, Raven, 1984, pp 645–668.
104. Klein J: *Immunology: The Science of Self-Nonself Discrimination*. New York, Wiley, 1982.
105. Buckler JMH: A comparison of the effects of human serum in two double antibody radioimmunoassay systems for the estimation of luteinizing hormone, in Kirkham KE, Hunter WM (eds): *Radioimmunoassay Methods*. Edinburgh, Churchill Livingstone, 1971, pp 273–283.
106. Vaitukaitis JL: Hormone assays, in Felig P, Baxter JD, Broadus AE, Frohman LA (eds): *Endocrinology and Metabolism*, 2d ed. New York, McGraw-Hill, 1986, pp 165–181.
107. Jan T, Shaw MA, Baumann G: Effect of growth hormone-binding proteins on serum growth hormone measurements. *J Clin Endocrinol Metab* 72:387, 1991.
108. Riggin A, Regnier FE, Sportman JR: Quantitation of antibodies to human growth hormone by high-performance protein-G affinity chromatography with fluorescence detection. *Anal Chem* 63:468, 1991.
109. Azukizawa M, Pekary AE, Hershman JM: Plasma thyrotropin, thyroxine, and triiodothyronine relationships in man. *J Clin Endocrinol Metab* 43:533, 1976.
110. Seth J: Laboratory management and quality control, in Hunter WM, Corrie JET (eds): *Immunoassays for Clinical Chemistry*, 2d ed. Edinburgh, Churchill Livingstone, 1983, pp 3–24.
111. Ekins RP: The precision profile: Its use in assay design, assessment and quality control, in Hunter WM, Corrie JET (eds): *Immunoassays for Clinical Chemistry*, 2d ed. Edinburgh, Churchill Livingstone, 1983, pp 76–105.
112. Moore GP: Genetically engineered antibodies. *Clin Chem* 35:1849, 1989.
113. Kay LE, Clore GM, Bax A, Grovenborn A: Four-dimensional heteronuclear triple-resonance NMR spectroscopy of interleukin-1β in solution. *Science* 249:411, 1990.
114. Briggs J, Kung VT, Gomez B, Kasper KC, Nagainis PA, Masino RS, Rice LS, Zuk RF, Ghazarossian VE: Sub-femtomole quantitation of proteins with Threshold®, for the biopharmaceutical industry. *Biotechniques* 9:598, 1990.
115. Barnard SM, Walt DR: Chemical sensors based on controlled-release polymer systems. *Science* 251:927, 1991.
116. Graff G. Polymer scientists work to beef up biosensors. *Science* 253:1097, 1991.
117. O'Byrne KT, Thalabard J-C, Grosser PM, Wilson RC, Williams CL, Chen M-D, Ladendorf D, Hotchkiss J, Knobil C: Radiotelemetric monitoring of hypothalamic gonadotropin-releasing hormone pulse generator activity throughout the menstrual cycle of the rhesus monkey. *Endocrinology* 129:1207, 1991.

PART II

Neuroendocrinology and the Pituitary

CHAPTER 7

Neuroendocrinology

Mark E. Molitch

GENERAL CONCEPTS IN NEUROENDOCRINOLOGY

Neuroendocrinology refers to the general area of endocrinology in which the interactions of the nervous system with the endocrine system are studied. As both systems transmit information from one part of the body to another, their integration links aspects of cognitive and noncognitive neural activity with metabolic and hormonal homeostatic activity. This linkage involves the direct and indirect neural regulation of hormone secretion, the effects of hormones on neuronal action, and the interaction between the two systems in regulating how the body interacts with the environment. Some of the distinctions between the neural and endocrine systems are blurring, however, as we discover the wide range of what were formerly thought of exclusively as hormones (substances secreted directly into the blood) serving as *neurotransmitters* (substances that mediate the synaptic interaction between two neurons). Similarly, classical neurotransmitters may also function as hormones. Furthermore, neurons may have hormone receptors distinct from the area of the synapse, so that neuropeptide hormones may function in a neuromodulatory role. Adding to this complexity is the discovery of the presence of these hormones and neurotransmitters in a wide variety of tissues not thought to be either endocrine or neural, such as the gastrointestinal tract, lung, placenta, and thymus, and the subsequent discovery that the functions of these substances may vary widely depending on the tissue in which they are found.

The primary neuroendocrine interface is that of the hypothalamus and the pituitary. Of critical importance in the early understanding of this interface was the recognition and demonstration by Scharrer and Scharrer of neural cells that can secrete hormones, i.e., *neurosecretory cells*.[1] These cells can propagate action potentials and can be influenced by other neurons with their neurotransmitters, hormones, and metabolites. As such, they serve as the final common pathway linking the brain with the endocrine system. The two types of neurosecretory cells involved in hypothalamic-pituitary regulation are (1) the *neurohypophyseal* neurons, which originate from the paraventricular and supraoptic nuclei, traverse the hypothalamic-pituitary stalk, and release vasopressin and oxytocin from nerve endings in the posterior pituitary (see Chap. 9), and (2) the *hypophysiotropic* neurons, which also originate from hypothalamic nuclei and release their peptide and bioamine products into the median eminence end of the hypothalamic-pituitary portal vessels (Fig. 7-1).

OVERVIEW OF BRAIN-HYPOTHALAMIC-PITUITARY-TARGET ORGAN REGULATION

Neuron-Neuron Interactions

The primary neuron-to-neuron interaction occurs at the *synapse*. Bioamine or peptide neurotransmitters which have been synthesized within the cell body and transported down the axon are stored in synaptic vesicles for release by exocytosis upon depolarization (Fig. 7-2). The bioamines are synthesized enzymatically, a process that often involves several steps, but the peptide neurotransmitters are synthesized in standard fashion for proteins, often necessitating cleavage from larger precursors. The neurotransmitters bind to specific receptors on the postsynaptic neuron, and any neurotransmitter remaining in the synapse is rapidly inactivated by enzymatic degradation or, for bioamines, reuptake by the proximal neuron or uptake into other surrounding neurons or glial tissue.[2] These receptors are specific for the neurotransmitter, and several of them have been sequenced and cloned, including the cholinergic muscarinic, the α and β adrenergic, the serotoninergic, the dopaminergic, and the γ-aminobutyric acid (GABA) receptors.[3] Binding studies have demonstrated a number of different receptor subtypes, such as the muscarinic and nicotinic cholinergic subtypes and the α and β adrenergic receptors, which can be further divided into α_1 and α_2 and β_1 and β_2 subtypes. The recognition of these multiple receptor subtypes has resulted in advances in our knowledge of neural regulation and has allowed the development of neuroactive medications which are highly

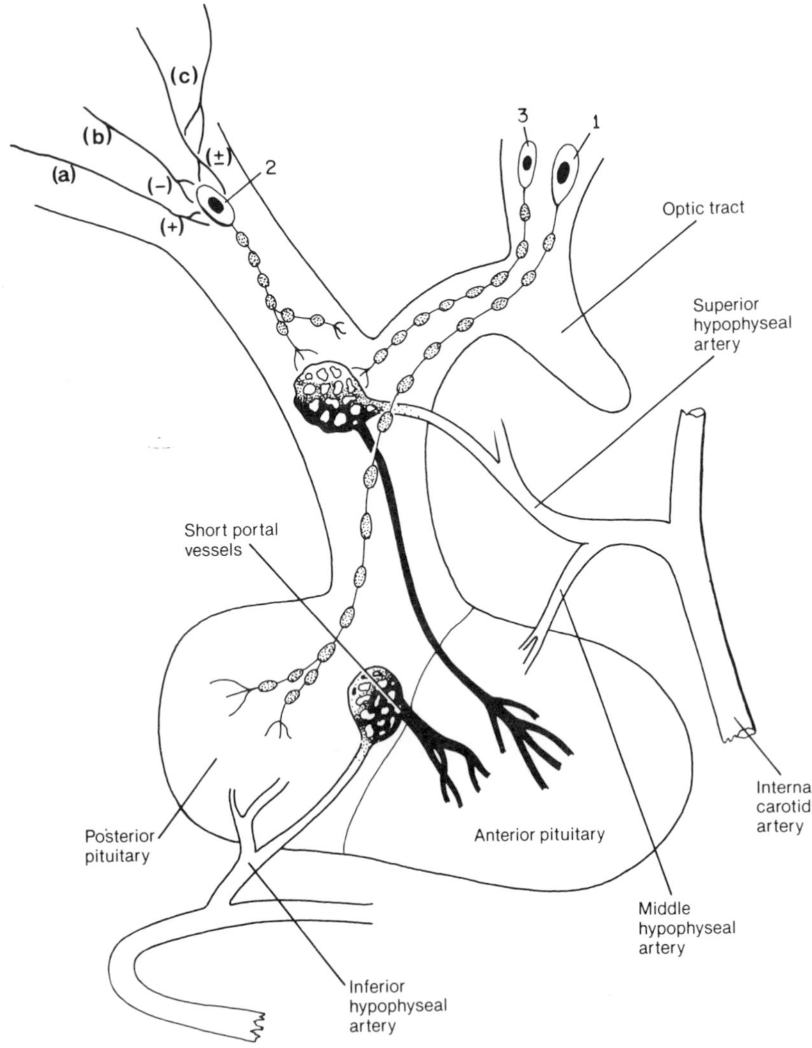

FIGURE 7-1. Neuroendocrine organization of the hypothalamus and pituitary gland. The posterior pituitary is fed by the inferior hypophyseal artery and the hypothalamus is fed by the superior hypophyseal artery, both of which are branches of the internal carotid artery. A small portion of the anterior pituitary also receives arterial blood from the middle hypophyseal artery. Most of the blood supply to the anterior pituitary is venous by way of the long portal vessels, which connect the portal capillary beds in the median eminence to the venous sinusoids in the anterior pituitary. Hypophysiotropic neuron 3 in the parvocellular division of the paraventricular nucleus and neuron 2 in the arcuate nucleus are shown to terminate in the median eminence on portal capillaries. These neurons of the tuberoinfundibular system secrete hypothalamic releasing and inhibiting hormones into the portal veins for conveyance to the anterior pituitary gland. Neuron 2 is innervated by monoaminergic neurons. Note that the multiple inputs to such neurons, using neuron 2 as an example, can be (a) stimulatory, (b) inhibitory, or (c) neuromodulatory, in which another neuron may affect neurotransmitter release. Neuron 1 represents a peptidergic neuron originating in the magnocellular division of the paraventricular nucleus or supraoptic nucleus and projects directly to the posterior pituitary by way of the hypothalamic-neurohypophyseal tract. *(Courtesy of Ronald M. Lechan, M.D., and modified from Lechan [26] with permission.)*

selective in their actions, thus avoiding adverse effects.[2] In addition, it has been found that certain receptor subtypes are more important in some areas of the brain than they are in others. For example, the D_2 dopamine receptor is the primary type in the pituitary lactotrophs that responds to the hypophysiotropic bioamine dopamine, whereas it is primarily the D_1 dopamine receptor that is active in the nigrostrial system.

The precise nature of the mechanisms that transduce the signal sent by the occupied receptor, such as activation of sodium and calcium ion channels, the adenylate cyclase–cAMP cascade, the phosphoinositide–protein kinase C systems, and the calcium-calmodulin system, are currently under investigation (see Chap. 4). The transduction mechanisms for most neurotransmitters are multiple and often redundant and may involve both stimulatory (G_s) and inhibitory (G_s) guanine nucleotide-binding proteins.

A given neuron may have multiple inputs via multiple synapses with different neurotransmitters at each synapse and therefore may have potential for considerable interaction of transduction mechanisms. These multiple inputs can be synergistic or antagonistic (Fig. 7-1). These types of interactions have the potential for a rapid on-off dynamic regulatory system.[3] The same neuron may have its neurotransmitter output modulated by other neurons at a location near the synapse of its axon, an effect referred to as *neuromodulation*. A neuromodulator may augment or block release of the neurotransmitter or alter its turnover.

A single neuron may also secrete more than one neurotransmitter, and the effects of the two neurotransmitters are usually synergistic or complementary. This type of combination generally involves a bioamine and a neuropeptide. Examples include parasympathetic nerves that control the sweat

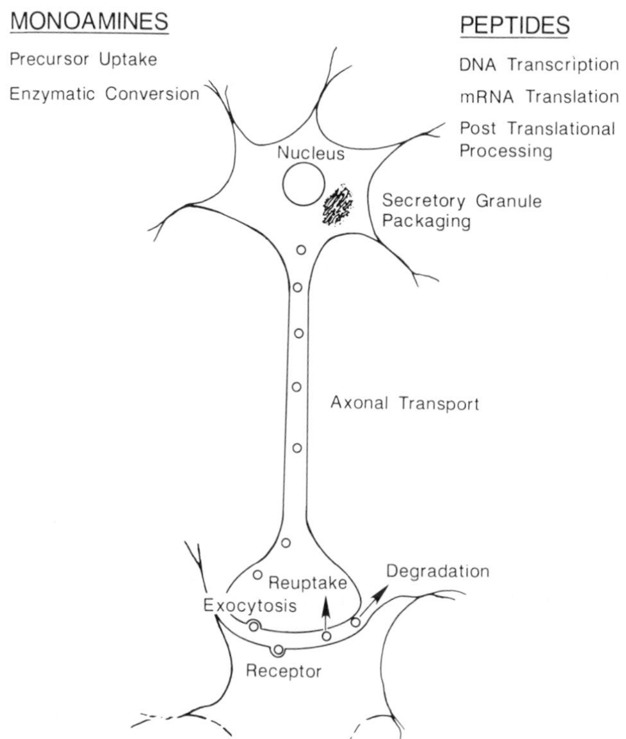

FIGURE 7-2. Schematic diagram of the neuron. For monamines, there is uptake of precursors into the neuronal cell body (perikarya) with subsequent enzymatic conversion into the active monoamine neurotransmitter. Biosynthesis of peptide neurotransmitters includes initial DNA transcription, mRNA translation, and posttranslational processing. The final products are packaged into neurosecretory granules in the cell body. The neurotransmitter reaches the nerve terminal via axonal transport. At the nerve terminal, depolarization results in fusion of the secretory granule membrane with the synaptic membrane and exocytosis with liberation of the neurotransmitter into the synaptic cleft. This liberated neurotransmitter binds to specific receptors on the postsynaptic neuron, with extra neurotransmitter being degraded by enzymes or taken back up into the proximal nerve terminal by specific reuptake mechanisms.

glands and contain both acetylcholine and vasoactive intestinal polypeptide (VIP); the released acetylcholine causes sweat production, while VIP increases blood flow. Conversely, sympathetic nerves to the salivary glands contain norepinephrine and neuropeptide Y; neuropeptide Y causes direct vasoconstriction and potentiates norepinephrine-evoked vasoconstriction.[4] However, two peptides may also be released, such as the corticotropin releasing hormone (CRH) and vasopressin released by neurons of the paraventricular nucleus in times of stress.[5] In this circumstance, this axon terminal is not in the posterior pituitary but rather is in the median eminence, where it releases both substances, which then have synergistic action in stimulating the secretion of adrenocorticotropic hormone (ACTH) from the pituitary.

Hypophysiotropic Hormones

Although it has been known since the beginning of this century that the hypothalamus is involved in hormone regulation, the precise nature of this involvement was not appreciated until the work of Harris[6] and others in the 1940s and 1950s. In 1901, Fröhlich reported a patient with adipsogenital dystrophy due to a pituitary tumor compressing the optic chiasm and hypothalamus.[7] Shortly thereafter, Erdheim reported that obesity and hypogonadism can be caused by hypothalamic lesions that do not involve the pituitary.[8] The hypothalamic-pituitary connection was clarified in a number of experiments in which pituitary function could be enhanced by electric stimulation of the hypothalamus[6] and pituitary function was shown to cease after transplantation to other locations in the body but to remain intact after transplantation to beneath the median eminence.[9,10]

The innervation of the anterior pituitary is negligible.[11] Popa and Fielding initially described the presence of the hypothalamic-pituitary portal vessels but reported that the primary route of blood flow is from the pituitary to the hypothalamus.[12] Subsequent experiments showed that the primary flow of blood is from the hypothalamus to the pituitary,[11,13] although later experiments confirmed that there is a small amount of reverse flow that may carry hormones from the pituitary to the hypothalamus.[14,15] In 1947, on the basis of their physiologic experiments and studies of pituitary stalk blood flow, Green and Harris wrote, "It is suggested that the central nervous system regulates the activity of the adenohypophysis by means of a humoral relay through the hypophysial portal vessels."[11]

Although many experiments carried out over the next two decades confirmed this neurohumoral hypothesis and although extensive efforts were made to isolate these substances, it was not until 1969 that laboratories led by Schally and Guillemin simultaneously elucidated the structure of thyrotropin releasing hormone (TRH).[16,17] Over the subsequent 20 years it was determined that the hypothalamus controls the pituitary not only through neurosecretory substances that stimulate the release of pituitary hormones but also through substances which inhibit the release of pituitary hormones. The releasing hormones not only stimulate release but also stimulate gene transcription and new synthesis of pituitary hormones, as documented by a demonstration of the incorporation of precursors and the stimulation of the production of specific mRNAs.

The releasing and inhibitory hormones have been referred to as *hypophysiotropic hormones* for many years, dating back to a time when it was not known that the hypothalamus contains specific inhibitory substances. However, this name has persevered and is used to refer to both hormone types. Another convention widely adopted for these substances is that a releasing or inhibiting substance is referred to as a factor until it is structurally characterized, after which it is referred to as a hormone. Thus, TRF became TRH, etc.

The hypophysiotropic hormones are synthesized in specific neuronal cell groups (nuclei) within the hypothalamus, and their axons project inferiorly to abut the proximal capillary plexus of the portal vessels in the median eminence (Fig. 7-1). Neurons from other nuclei within the hypothalamus and other parts of the brain influence pituitary hormone secretion by interacting with these specific hypophysiotropic neurons. Pituitary hormone secretion thus is regulated by the release of one or more of these hypophysiotropic hormones into the portal system.

Feedback Loops

One of the major functions of the endocrine system as a whole and of the neuroendocrine system in particular is to help maintain body homeostasis in the face of changes in the environment. This is done in part through a series of feedback loops that control pituitary and target organ hormone levels rather precisely (Fig. 7-3). Physiologic feedback systems require a controller function (in this case the pituitary hormone) and a controlled function (the target organ hormone level). The feedback loops are adjusted to maintain this target organ hormone level within a narrow range. This relation between the pituitary stimulating hormone and the target organ hormone is often referred to as the set point. This set point is analogous to setting the temperature on a thermostat. When the ambient temperature falls, the lower temperature activates the thermostat, which then causes the furnace to go on, raising the ambient temperature level. Similarly, the circulating levels of the target hormone constitute a negative feedback on the pituitary. Therefore, when the target organ hormone level falls, production and secretion of the specific pituitary hormone increase, stimulating additional production and secretion of the target organ hormone. This system is made more complex, however, by the imposition of another controller—the hypothalamus—which in turn controls the pituitary. Target organ hormones can feed back at both the hypothalamic and pituitary levels to complete the loop, and efferent controller factors from the hypothalamus may include both stimulatory and inhibitory substances.

FIGURE 7-3. The hypothalamic-pituitary-target organ feedback loop. The hypothalamus influences pituitary hormone secretion via releasing and inhibiting factors. The pituitary hormone in turn stimulates target organ hormone secretion. The target organ hormone can feed back at both the pituitary and hypothalamic levels, and such feedback can be both negative and positive. The feedback may affect the secretion of the releasing factors as well as the inhibiting factors. The pituitary hormone can also feed back negatively on the hypothalamus, decreasing the secretion of releasing hormone and/or increasing the secretion of inhibiting hormone, a process referred to as short-loop feedback.

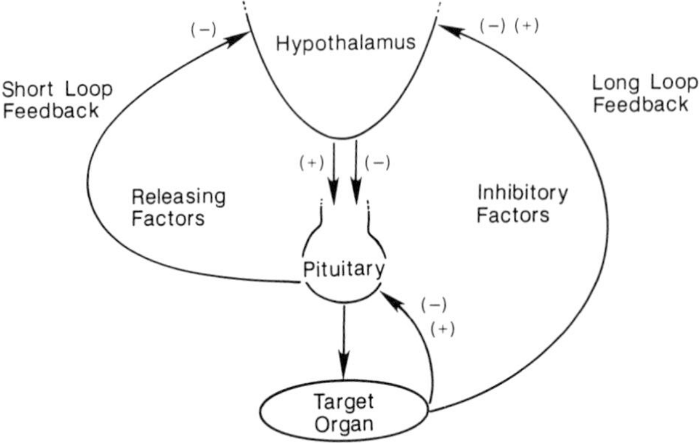

An example of how these feedback loops work is primary thyroid failure due to chronic thyroiditis: A fall in blood thyroxine (T_4) levels results in less negative feedback, causing an increase in thyroid stimulating hormone (TSH) release into the circulation. This increase in TSH then stimulates the failing thyroid gland, resulting in thyroid enlargement (goiter) and an increase in thyroid hormone levels, which may only be temporary if the gland continues to fail. TSH itself is stimulated by TRH and is inhibited by another hypophysiotropic hormone, somatostatin. Lowered thyroid hormone levels affect not only feedback on the pituitary, increasing its sensitivity to TRH in the hypothalamic-pituitary portal blood, but also feedback at the level of the hypothalamus to increase TRH production.[18] Furthermore, the low levels of thyroid hormone decrease hypothalamic somatostatin release.[19] The thyroid hormone responsible for this negative feedback at the intracellular nuclear locus in the hypothalamus and pituitary is triiodothyroinine (T_3), which is derived from plasma T_3 and intracellular deiodination from T_4.[20] The reverse happens if thyroid hormone levels are increased in the circulation as a result of the administration of exogenous thyroid hormone or the autonomous production of thyroid hormone by the thyroid itself (Graves disease). Thus, for a given hormonal axis such as the hypothalamic-pituitary-thyroidal axis, there are multiple feedback loops with considerable built-in redundancy.

Each pituitary hormone has unique aspects to its regulation (Table 7-1). Luteinizing hormone (LH) and follicle stimulating hormone (FSH) have as target organs the ovary in the female and the testes in the male, and their feedback loops are complex. The gonads produce steroid hormones which in the male feed back negatively but in the female feed back both negatively and positively, depending on the phase of the menstrual cycle. In addition, the gonads produce peptides, some of which inhibit (inhibin, follistatin) and some of which stimulate (activin) LH and FSH

TABLE 7-1 Components of the Feedback Loops for Pituitary Hormones

Hypophysiotropic Hormone	Pituitary Effect	Pituitary Hormone	Target Organ Hormone	Feedback Effect
TRH	+	TSH	T_4, T_3	−
Somatostatin	−			
GnRH	+	LH	Estradiol	−, +
			Testosterone	−
GnRH	+	FSH	Inhibin	−
			Activin	+
			Follistatin	−
CRH	+	ACTH	Cortisol	−
Vasopressin	+		Androgens	
GHRH	+	GH	IGF-I	−
Somatostatin	−			
Dopamine	−	PRL	?	?
GAP (?)	−			
TRH	+			
VIP	+			

release. However, there is only one releasing hormone—gonadotropin releasing hormone (GnRH)—and no hypophysiotropic inhibitory hormones for LH and FSH. The differential release of LH and FSH during various phases of the menstrual cycle depends on the interactive feedback effects of these steroid and peptide feedback loops at both the pituitary and hypothalamic levels.

ACTH has no inhibitory hypophysiotropic hormone but probably has two releasing hormones: CRH and vasopressin. Its primary feedback loop involves the adrenal glucocorticosteroid cortisol (hydrocortisone), which has inhibitory effects at both the pituitary and hypothalamic levels.

Growth hormone (GH) and prolactin (PRL) are different in that they have no target organs to supply feedback hormones. However, GH does stimulate the production of insulin-like growth factor-I (IGF-I, also known as somatomedin C), a 7000-dalton protein, from a number of tissues. As discussed in Chap. 8, IGF-I mediates many of the GH's growth-stimulating actions. IGF-I feeds back negatively on GH production,[21,22] and there are both stimulatory [growth hormone releasing hormone (GHRH)] and inhibitory (somatostatin) hypophysiotropic hormones that regulate GH. PRL, unlike other anterior pituitary hormones, has a primary neural stimulus in the form of suckling by the neonate. However, in the absence of a suckling stimulus, PRL levels are maintained at fairly stable levels, though the feedback loops necessary for this maintenance are unknown. Unlike all the other pituitary hormones, the primary influence of the hypothalamus on PRL secretion is inhibitory rather than stimulatory. Therefore, if the hypothalamus and pituitary are disconnected, PRL levels rise while the levels of other pituitary hormone levels fall.

The feedback loops discussed so far are designated as long-loop feedback, referring to the long-distance nature of the target organ feedback. Short-loop feedback involves direct action of the pituitary hormones on hypophysiotropic hormone production or direct action on their own production. Although there is considerable experimental evidence for the existence of short-loop feedback in animal models, evidence for such feedback in humans is only indirect for hormones other than GH.[23]

The feedback loops for the various hormones maintain hormone levels within a narrow range. The loops can be perturbed in a number of ways, resulting in temporary or prolonged alterations of set points. One of the most fundamental of these perturbations is the change in hormone levels that occurs during the course of the day: circadian periodicity. These circadian rhythms are quite regular, resulting in highly reproducible changes in hormone levels at similar times from day to day. The sensitivity of each feedback loop can vary from day to day and even hour to hour and can even switch from negative to positive. This complex type of changing feedback loop is operative for the gonadotropins LH and FSH in women, in whom there is negative feedback by estrogen through most of the menstrual cycle but a switch to positive feedback at the time of the midcycle ovulatory surge of gonadotropins. Yet another type of long-term alteration of the set point has been postulated to occur at the time of puberty, when an increase in the gonadotropin set point results in increased gonadotropin and sex steroid levels.

Stress, nutritional status, and systemic illness are other factors which may perturb the system, resulting in both acute and chronic changes in hormone levels that are not related to specific organ dysfunction. Acute physical stress may result in an increase in ACTH, GH, and PRL, along with epinephrine and glucagon. Malnutrition may cause suppression of the hypothalamic-pituitary-thyroid and hypothalamic-pituitary-gonadal axes. Diseases such as renal failure and hepatic cirrhosis may increase GH levels through interruption of the GH-IGF-I axis, increase PRL levels, and alter the TRH-TSH-thyroid axis; this is referred to as the euthyroid sick syndrome.[24] Often the precise alterations in neurotransmitter and hypothalamic hypophysiotropic hormones that engender such changes are not known.

ANATOMIC ASPECTS

Hypothalamus

The hypothalamus is the most ventral portion of the diencephalon, located beneath the thalamus and subthalamus (Fig. 7-4). Anteriorly, it is bounded by the optic chiasm, lamina terminalis, and anterior commissure. Posteriorly, it is bounded by the midbrain and the posterior commissure. Laterally, it is bounded by the optic nerves, the sulci formed with the temporal lobes, and the internal capsule. When it is viewed from the inferior aspect, several features are apparent. Posteriorly there are the mammillary bodies, which contain the mammillary nuclei. They are so named because of their resemblance to miniature mammary glands. Anterior to the mammillary bodies is a bulging of the hypothalamus known as the tuber cinereum, and arising from it in the midline is the median eminence, which becomes the infundibulum, or the proximal part of the hypothalamic-pituitary stalk (Fig. 7-5). The third ventricle extends ventrally into the middle of the hypothalamus and projects into the hypothalamus above the optic chiasm (supraoptic recess) and down into the infundibulum (infundibular recess).

The fornix, a neuronal fiber bundle that passes through the hypothalamus, divides the hypothalamus into medial and lateral areas (Fig. 7-6). The lateral area contains few neuronal cell bodies (perikarya) and many fibers that connect the hypothalamus and midbrain to the limbic system. The medial area contains many neuronal perikarya clustered together into nuclei, only a small portion of which subserve a neuroendocrine function. Most of the cells of the hypothalamus are involved in other functions, including memory, temperature regulation, sleep, regulation of food intake, sexual behavior, cardiovascular function, and emotions.[25,26] There are a number of connections between the medial and lateral hypothalamic areas which connect hypothalamic nuclei to the rest of the limbic system. The

FIGURE 7-4. Anatomic relations of the human hypothalamus. The MRI scan and the diagram of the midline human hypothalamus are seen in sagittal orientation. The lamina terminalis and anterior commissure constitute the anterior boundary; the posterior commissure and midbrain, the posterior boundary; and the thalamus, the dorsal boundary. *(Courtesy of Ronald M. Lechan, M.D., and reproduced from Lechan[26] with permission.)*

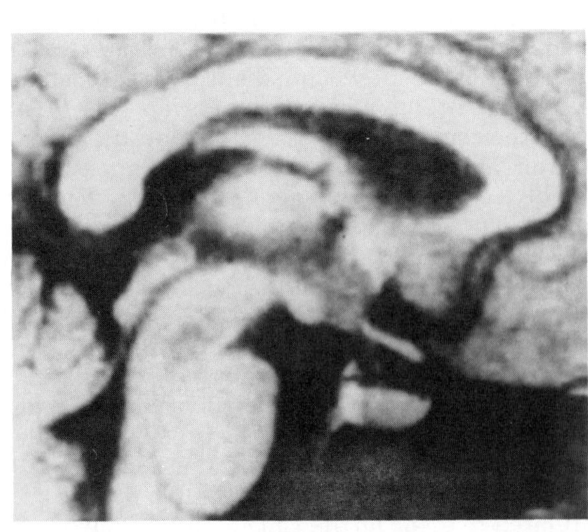

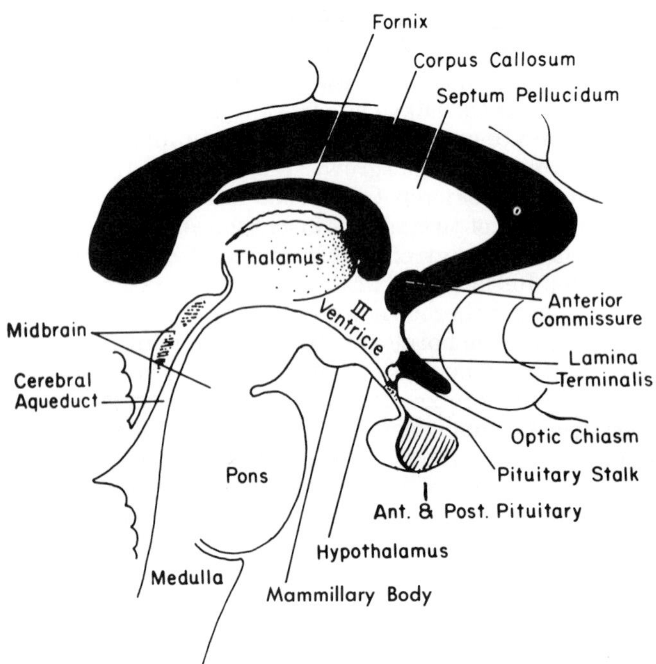

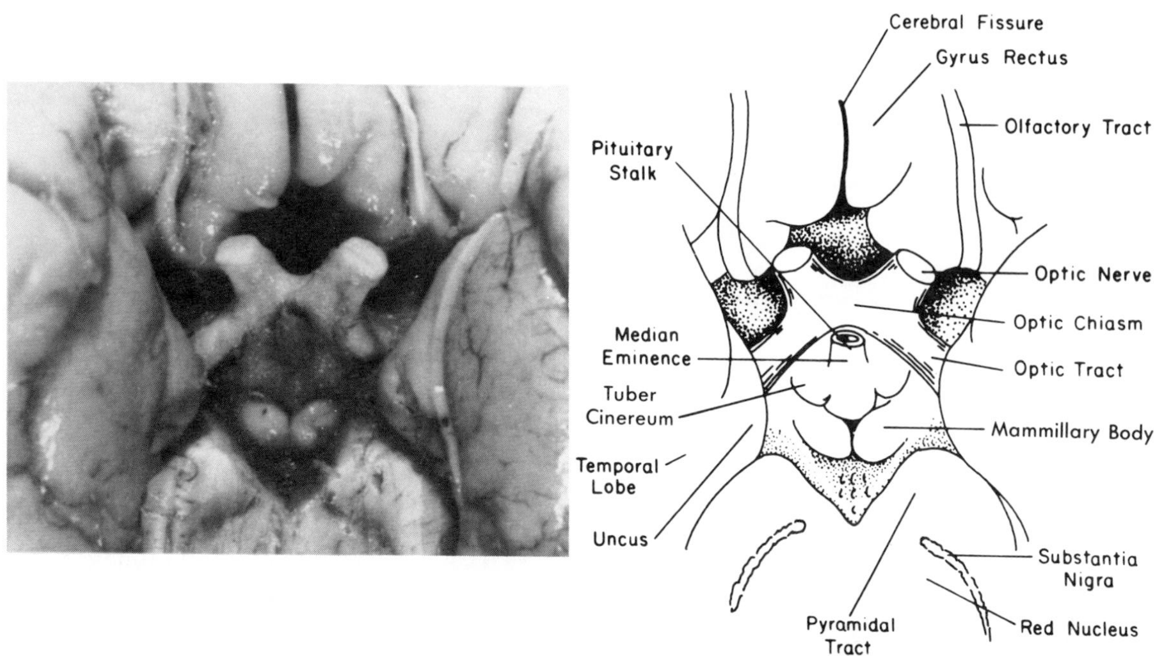

FIGURE 7-5. The ventral surface of the brain showing the tuber cinereum of the hypothalamus and pituitary stalk bordered by the optic chiasm anteriorly, the uncus of the temporal lobes laterally, and the mammillary bodies and the midbrain posteriorly. The location of the neurovascular zone, or median eminence, is shown. *(Courtesy of Ronald M. Lechan, M.D., and reproduced from Lechan[26] with permission.)*

anterior and middle portions of the medial hypothalamus are important areas in neuroendocrine regulation.

Within the anterior portion of the medial area of the hypothalamus are the preoptic, suprachiasmatic, and supraoptic nuclei. The preoptic area and portions of the basal hypothalamus are the sites of neurons which synthesize GnRH[27] and project to the median eminence as part of the tuberoinfundibular tract (see below). The suprachiasmatic nuclei, which are located just above the optic chiasm, are important in regulating the circadian rhythms of the body, receiving neural input from the retina via the retinohypothalamic tract, and sending neuronal output to many areas of the hypothalamus.[28] The supraoptic nuclei are located just above the optic tracts and just behind the chiasm, and most of their neurosecretory magnocellular (large) neurons make vasopressin, although a small number make oxytocin (see Chap. 9).

The midportion of the medial hypothalamus contains the majority of the nuclei that give rise to the tuberoinfundibular tract, i.e., the neurons whose axons project to the external zone of the median eminence.[26,29] This system has been defined by injecting a lectin such as wheat germ agglutinin into the external zone of the median eminence and, because of retrograde transport along axons, determining the neuronal perikarya from which these axons originate.[30] As the various hypophysiotropic hormones were characterized and antihormone antibodies were developed, their immunoreactive neuronal pathways were elucidated and compared with the results of earlier retrograde transport studies. Important nuclei contributing axons to the tuberoinfundibular tract include the ventromedial, arcuate, periventricular, dorsomedial, and the parvocellular (small) division of the paraventricular nucleus. These nuclei contain an ever-expanding list of peptides, the functions of which are not understood in every case (Table 7-2). Within each of the nuclei the specific peptides that are secreted are organized into separate regions. For example, in the paraventricular nucleus the somatostatin-containing neurons are grouped medially, the CRH-containing neurons are found laterally, and the TRH-containing neurons are located between these neurons,[26] (Fig. 7-7). The specific hypophysiotropic hormone distribution among these nuclei will be discussed below. These nuclei also receive input from a variety of other neuronal areas of the brain, including brainstem autonomic centers, and thus mediate the effects of the extrahypothalamic brain on neuroendocrine function.[31]

Median Eminence and Hypothalamic-Pituitary Portal System

The median eminence constitutes the medial portion of the tuber cinereum and, as the infundibulum, constitutes the beginning of the pituitary stalk. Located just below the third ventricle, it can be considered a circumventricular organ and is an interface between

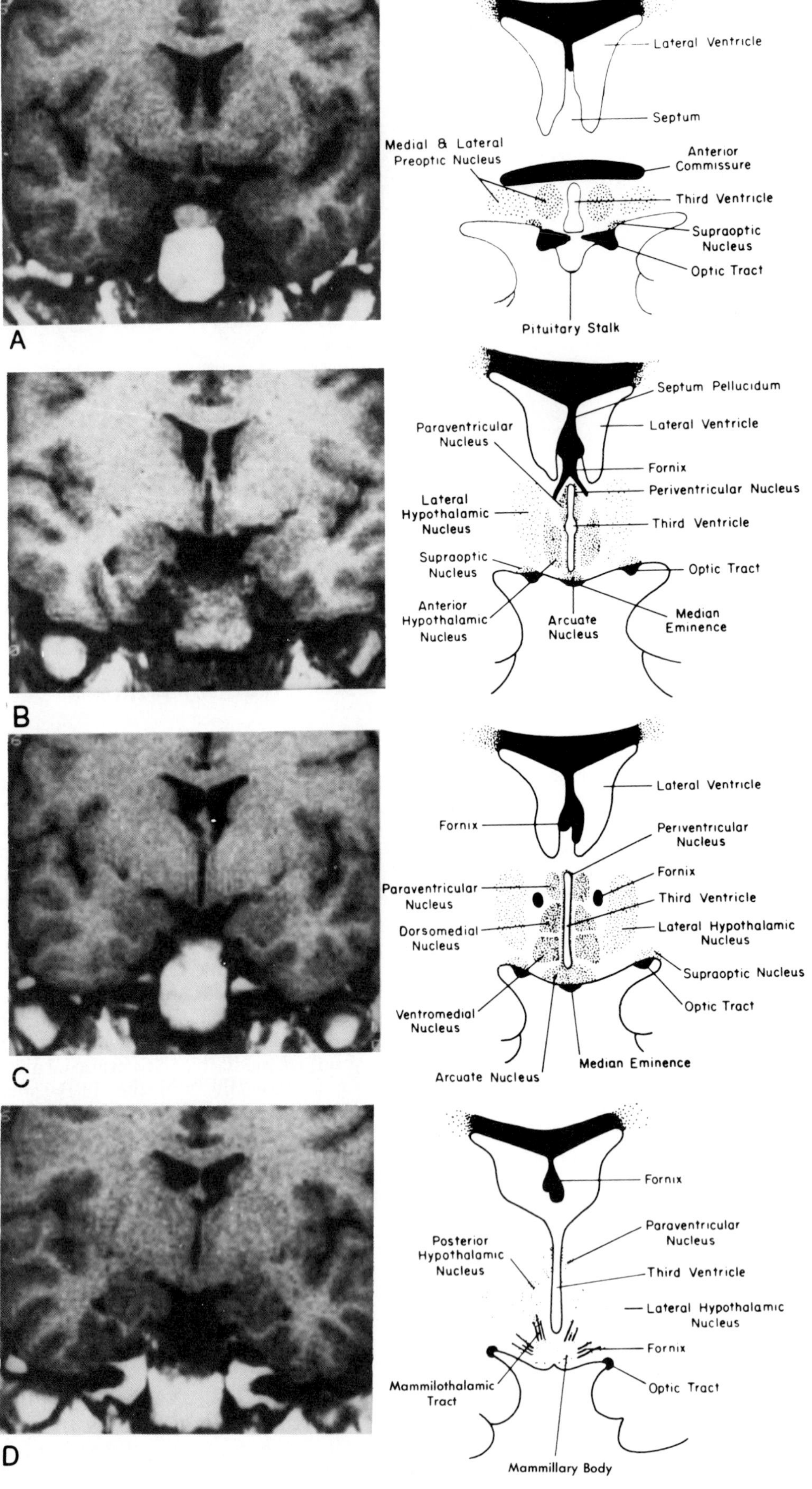

A
Lateral Ventricle
Septum
Medial & Lateral Preoptic Nucleus
Anterior Commissure
Third Ventricle
Supraoptic Nucleus
Optic Tract
Pituitary Stalk
B
Septum Pellucidum
Lateral Ventricle
Paraventricular Nucleus
Fornix
Periventricular Nucleus
Lateral Hypothalamic Nucleus
Third Ventricle
Supraoptic Nucleus
Optic Tract
Anterior Hypothalamic Nucleus
Arcuate Nucleus
Median Eminence
C
Lateral Ventricle
Fornix
Periventricular Nucleus
Fornix
Paraventricular Nucleus
Third Ventricle
Dorsomedial Nucleus
Lateral Hypothalamic Nucleus
Supraoptic Nucleus
Ventromedial Nucleus
Optic Tract
Median Eminence
Arcuate Nucleus
D
Fornix
Paraventricular Nucleus
Posterior Hypothalamic Nucleus
Third Ventricle
Lateral Hypothalamic Nucleus
Fornix
Mammilothalamic Tract
Optic Tract
Mammillary Body

TABLE 7-2 Neuroactive Substances in Paraventricular and Arcuate Nucleus Neurons

Paraventricular nucleus	Arcuate nucleus
Magnocellular division	Acetylcholine
Angiotensin II	Dopamine
Cholecystokinin	Galanin
Glucagon	GABA
Oxytocin	GHRH
Peptide 7B2	Neuropeptide Y
Proenkephalin B (dynorphin, rimorphin, α-neoendorphin)	Neurotensin
	Pancreatic polypeptide
	Proenkephalin A (met-enkephalin, leu-enkephalin)
Parvocellular division	
Angiotensin II	Prolactin
Atrial natriuretic peptide	Pro-opiomelanocortin (ACTH, β-LPH, β-endorphin)
Cholecystokinin	
CRH	Somatostatin
Dopamine	Substance P
GABA	
Galanin	
Glucagon	
Neuropeptide Y	
Neurotensin	
Peptide 7B2	
Proenkephalin A (met-enkephalin, leu-enkephalin)	
Somatostatin	
TRH	
VIP/PHM	

Source: Modified from Lechan.[26]

the cerebrospinal fluid (CSF) and the blood. The median eminence is outside the blood-brain barrier, and systemic hormones and other substances pass freely into the periventricular extracellular space.[30,32] However, there are tight junctions between the tanycyte processes serving as a blood-brain barrier between the lateral margin of the median eminence and the adjacent portions of the basal hypothalamus.[30,32] The location of this barrier has obvious functional significance in that peptides secreted by neurosecretory cells into the perivascular space in the median eminence cannot diffuse out to affect other areas of the hypothalamus.[30]

The median eminence is divided into an internal ependymal zone, a middle internal zone (zona interna), and an external zone (zona externa) (Fig. 7-8). The ependymal cells form the lining of the third ventricle and have microvilli but not cilia on the ventricular surface.[33] Some of these ependymal cells, called tanycytes, are specialized in that they have long cytoplasmic processes on the inner surface that extend into the internal zone of the median eminence. Tight junctions connect the ependymal cells, preventing direct diffusion of substances between the CSF and the interior of the median eminence. The extent to which tanycytes provide a route of neuroendocrine communication between the CSF and the neurosecretory, tuberoinfundibular, and hypothalamic-neurohypophyseal tracts is unknown.[33] The internal zone consists primarily of supportive structures and neurons in passage from the hypothalamus to the posterior pituitary, i.e., the magnocellular hypothalamic-neurohypophyseal tract, or to the capillary plexus of the external zone of the median eminence, i.e., the hypophysiotropic neurons.

The external zone of the median eminence is the contact zone in which the hypophysiotropic neurosecretory axons terminate on or near the capillaries which form the proximal portion of the hypothalamic-pituitary portal vessels. As was discussed above, some axon terminals may end near other axon terminals, playing a neuromodulatory role. The nerve endings are rich in secretory granules, which, upon stimulation, are released into the external zone to be taken up through the fenestrations in the capillaries. True neuron-neuron synapses are not present. The axon terminals containing a given hypophysiotropic peptide tend to cluster in a specific region: GnRH and GRH axon terminals are present in lateral portions of the median eminence, and TRH and somatostatin are present in both the medial and lateral portions (Fig. 7-9).[26]

The median eminence receives its blood supply from the superior hypophyseal artery, which arborizes into a rich capillary bed (Fig. 7-1). The capillary loops extend into the internal and external zones of the median eminence and coalesce to form the long portal veins that traverse the pituitary stalk and end in the pituitary.[11,13,34] Within the external zone the capillary walls are "fenestrated," allowing the entry of peptides secreted by the axon terminals. These fenestrations stop at the level where the blood-brain barrier is reconstituted lateral to the median eminence. At the pituitary end of the stalk the portal vessels again branch to form an extensive capillary plexus. In addition to these *long* portal vessels there is a similar *short* portal system between the posterior and anterior lobes, with the direction of flow being primarily posterior to anterior.[11,34] The resultant blood flow to the anterior pituitary is the highest of any organ in the body, being on the order of 0.7 ml/g per min.[34] By far the predominant direction of blood flow is from the hypothalamus to the pituitary, but at least in some species, there is evidence of retrograde flow.[14,34] Using direct observation or Doppler flow studies, no retrograde flow has been demonstrable in pigs[35] or rhesus monkeys,[36] and no direct observations have been made in hu-

FIGURE 7-6. MRI scans and diagrams of coronal sections through the human hypothalamus. The approximate locations of the hypothalamic nuclear groups and fiber tracts are shown in the illustrations. *(Courtesy of Ronald M. Lechan, M.D., and reproduced from Lechan[26] with permission.)*

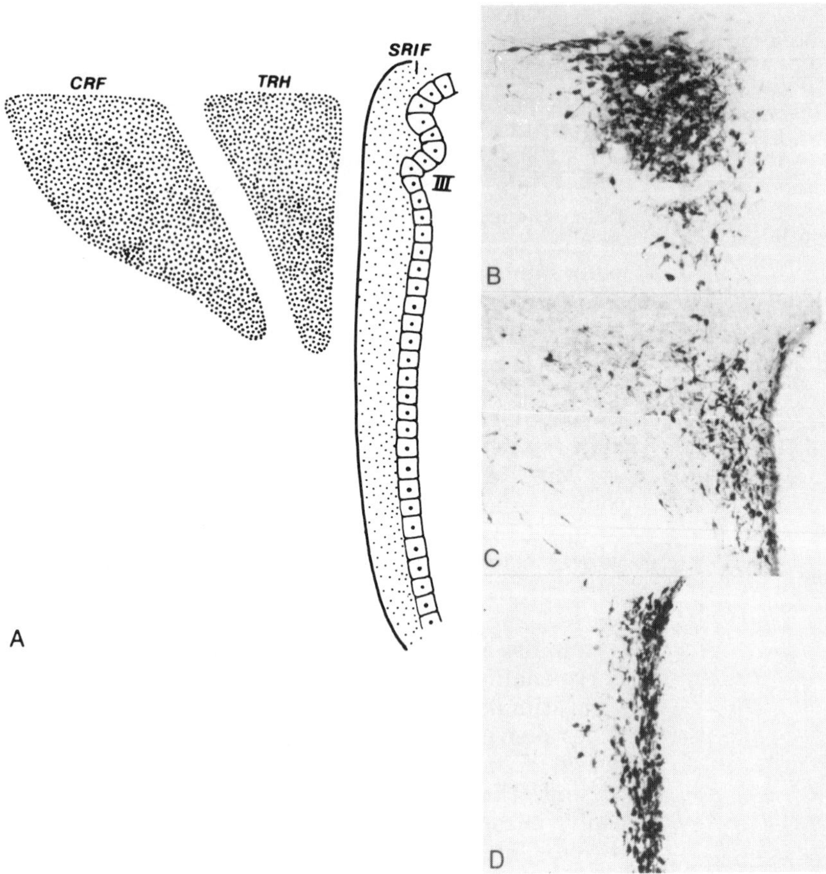

FIGURE 7-7. Organization of hypophysiotropic neurons in the medial parvocellular division of the paraventricular nucleus. *(A)* Schematic illustration of the relative distribution of neurons containing corticotropin releasing hormone (CRH), thyrotropin releasing hormone (TRH), and somatostatin (SRIF). Each of these peptides is shown by immunocytochemical techniques in *B* through *D* (*B*=CRH; C=TRH; D=SRIF). III =third ventricle. *(Courtesy of Ronald M. Lechan, M.D., and reproduced from Lechan[26] with permission.)*

mans. High concentrations of pituitary hormones have been found in the portal vessels in rats,[15] presumably as a result of such retrograde flow. Such flow might be a route for short-loop negative feedback in addition to the systemic circulation.

Pituitary

The pituitary will be discussed in detail in Chap. 8. It is located within a bony pocket in the sphenoid bone referred to as the sella turcica. The pituitary (hypophysis) has two lobes: a glandular anterior lobe (also known as the anterior pituitary or adenohypophysis) and a neural posterior lobe (also known as the posterior pituitary or neurohypophysis). Embryologically, the anterior lobe originates from Rathke's pouch, which is an ectodermal structure that results from an outpouching of the oropharynx. The posterior pituitary is essentially neural tissue and is an extension of the hypothalamus; it is the site of the nerve terminals of the hypothalamic-neurohypophyseal tract (see Chap. 9).

Specialized cell types in the anterior lobe produce the various pituitary hormones. A number of other peptides are present in the pituitary, such as gastrin, renin, angiotensin, human chorionic gonadotropin (hCG), and proteins without clearly defined functions, such as neuromedin B, chromogranin A, and galanin. The physiologic roles of these additional substances are unknown. Interestingly, some substances primarily thought of as hypophysiotropic hormones, such as TRH and VIP, are also produced by the pituitary.[37,38] This fact raises the interesting question of the relative roles of hypothalamic vs. pituitary hypophysiotropic hormones and endocrine vs. paracrine or even autocrine effects. At present, the pituitary production of such hormones is of uncertain significance.

In addition to the hypothalamic-neurohypophyseal tract containing vasopressin and oxytocin, a number of other neural pathways from the mediobasal hypothalamus also project to the posterior pituitary and contain a variety of peptides, including GnRH, TRH, somatostatin, CRH, neurotensin, and dopamine.[26] In various experimental preparations, some of these peptides have been shown to affect vasopressin secretion, but their roles in humans are unknown. As was mentioned above, there are short portal vessels between the anterior and posterior lobes. It has been postulated that the posterior lobe may play a role in the regulation of anterior pituitary hormone secretion either by means of vasopressin

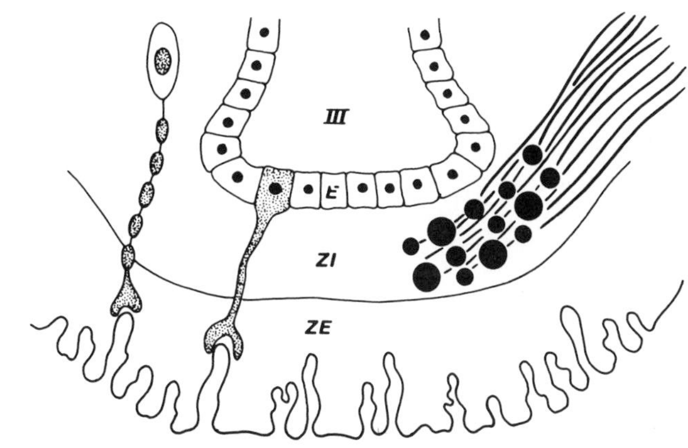

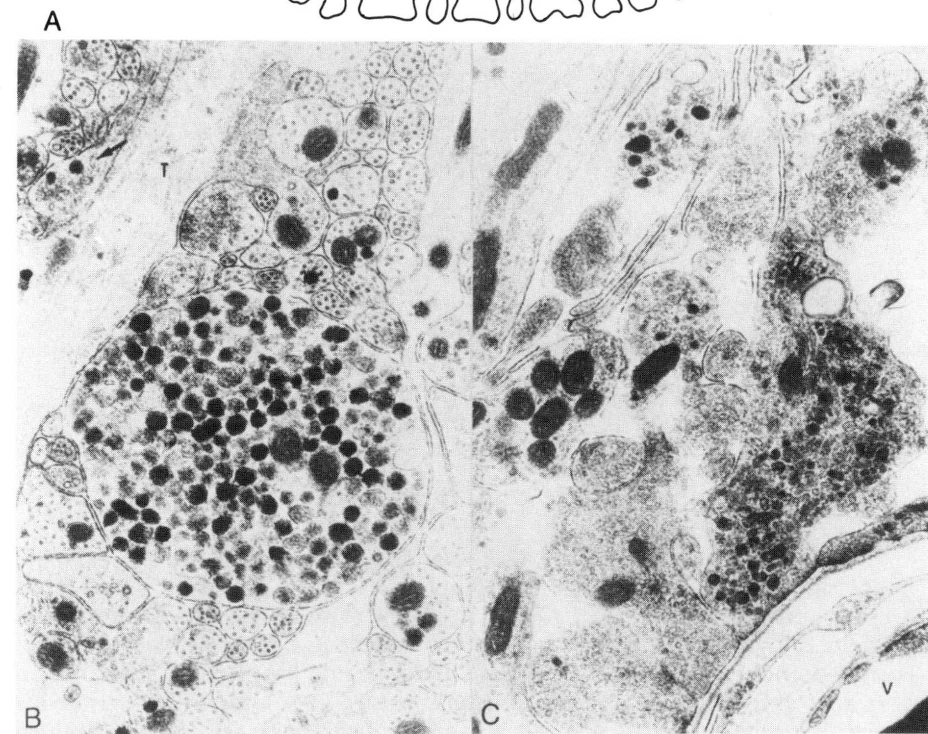

FIGURE 7-8. Diagram of the median eminence showing the location of its three major zones: the ependymal zone (E), the internal zone (ZI), and the external zone (ZE). The ZE is invaginated by portal capillaries which are contacted by axon terminals of the tuberoinfundibular system and by processes of specialized ependymal cells, tanycytes. The Zl contains numerous axons of the hypothalamic neurohypophyseal tract en route to the posterior pituitary. *(B)* Electron micrograph of the Zl showing a Herring body containing neurosecretory granules surrounded by axons of passage. Some of these axons contain dense-core vesicles (arrow) that are considerably smaller than the neurosecretory granules. T = tanycyte process. *(C)* Electron micrograph of the ZE showing axon terminals containing dense-core vesicles and small, clear vesicles abutting a fenestrated capillary of the portal system (v). *(Courtesy of Ronald M. Lechan, M.D., and reproduced from Lechan[26] with permission.)*

and oxytocin or by means of the additional peptides mentioned above.[26,34] This is separate from and in addition to the known effects of vasopressin on ACTH secretion mediated by vasopressinergic neurons whose axons pass directly from the paraventricular nucleus to the external zone of the median eminence to release vasopressin there.[5] At present, the precise role of the posterior pituitary in the regulation of anterior pituitary hormone secretion is unknown.

HYPOPHYSIOTROPIC HORMONES

The elucidation of the structure of TRH in 1969[16,17] was a major milestone in the development of neuroendocrinology and was the culmination of years of effort by many investigators. Guillemin has estimated that it took 270,000 sheep hypothalami weighing 50 tons to yield 1 mg of pure TRH.[39] Interestingly, the subsequent characterization of the entire 255-amino acid precursor was performed with an expression library prepared from only 65 rat hypothalami,[40] a testimony to technological progress. Subsequently, the structures of GnRH, somatostatin, CRH, and GHRH were determined (Fig. 7-10) and their roles in the regulation of the various pituitary hormones were investigated. These investigations have shown that the regulation of each pituitary hormone, as well as the effects of each hypophysiotropic hormone, is unique. Furthermore, other peptides within the hypothalamus, such as VIP, have hypophysiotropic functions under physiologic circumstances, and simple neurotransmitters such as dopamine also serve as hypophysiotropic factors.

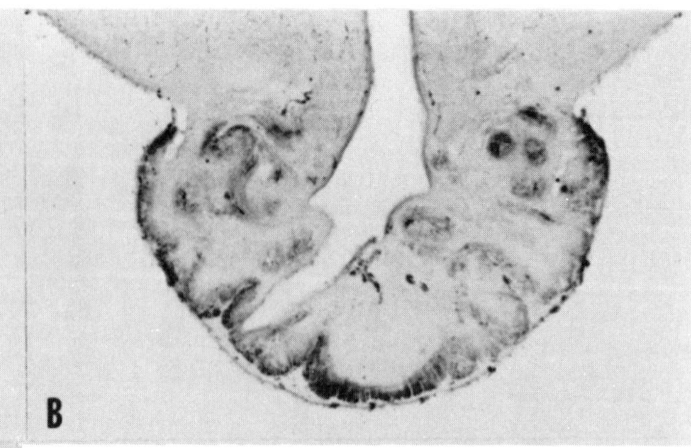

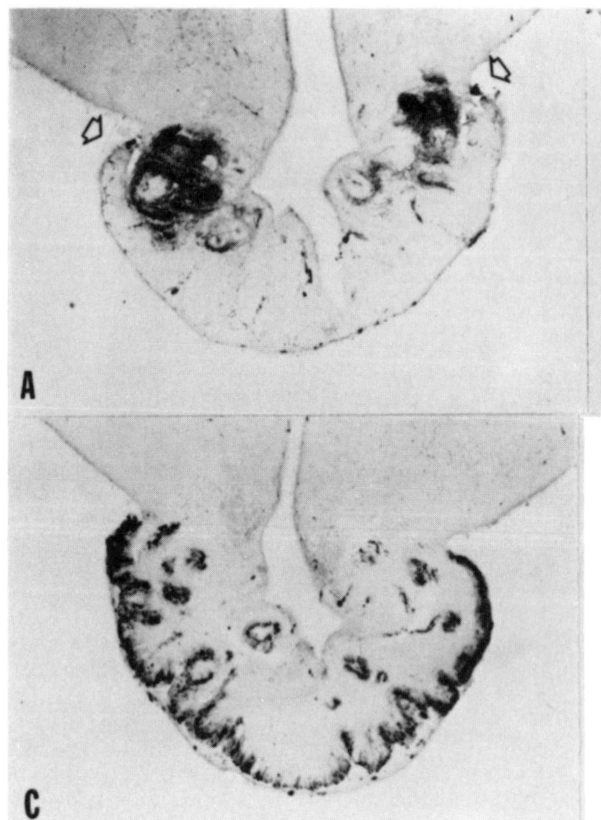

FIGURE 7-9. Immunocytochemical distribution of axon terminals containing growth hormone releasing hormone (GHRH) *(A)*, somatostatin (SRIF) *(B)*, and thyrotropin releasing hormone (TRH) *(C)* in the external zone of the median eminence of the rhesus monkey. Note the tendency for GHRH to organize in lateral portions of the median eminence near the tuberoinfundibular sulci (arrowheads). *(Courtesy of Ronald M. Lechan, M.D., and reproduced from Lechan[26] with permission.)*

The regulation of the pituitary hormones by the hypophysiotropic hormones is quite complex, in part because of the multiplicity of substances present in the hypothalamus that can affect pituitary hormone secretion and in part because of the redundancy and overlapping nature of the feedback loops alluded to above. In addition, some of these hypophysiotropic hormones exert effects on more than one pituitary hormone. While it seems appropriate for GnRH to stimulate the release of LH and FSH, it has also been found that TRH stimulates not only TSH but also PRL and that somatostatin inhibits not only GH but also TSH. Furthermore, a 56-amino acid portion of the precursor to GnRH, referred to as GnRH-associated peptide (GAP), both stimulates gonadotropins and inhibits PRL.

Some of the hypophysiotropic hormones are also found elsewhere in the body, particularly in the gastrointestinal tract and placenta, where they may have significant physiologic functions. For example, somatostatin is present in the pancreatic islets, where it inhibits the secretion of insulin and glucagon. It is also present in the stomach, where it inhibits gastric acid and gastrin secretion. In contrast, VIP, which is thought of primarily as a gut hormone, may serve as a physiologic stimulator of PRL release.

All the hypophysiotropic hormones are also present in the extrahypothalamic brain and subserve different functions as neurotransmitters. For some, such as TRH and GnRH, there may be behavioral effects, but in general, their physiologic functions as neurotransmitters are unknown. The highest concentrations of all these hormones are within the hypothalamus.[41] Several hormones can occur in the same hypothalamic nucleus and even within the same secretory granule of a single cell.[41]

Thyrotropin Releasing Hormone

As was mentioned above, TRH was the first of the hypophysiotropic hormones to be identified.[16,17] It is a tripeptide (Glu-His-Pro) in which the N-terminal glutamine is cyclized and the proline is amidized via the donation of an amide group from the adjacent glycine in the precursor. These latter two posttranslational changes result in the final product, pyroGlu-His-ProNH$_2$, which has a molecular weight of 362. The TRH precursor and gene structure were initially characterized partially in the frog,[42] fully in the rat,[40] and finally in the human,[43] where the prepro-TRH gene has been found to encode six copies of the TRH sequence and has a predicted peptide structure of 242 amino acids (Fig 7-11). Ultrastructural analy-

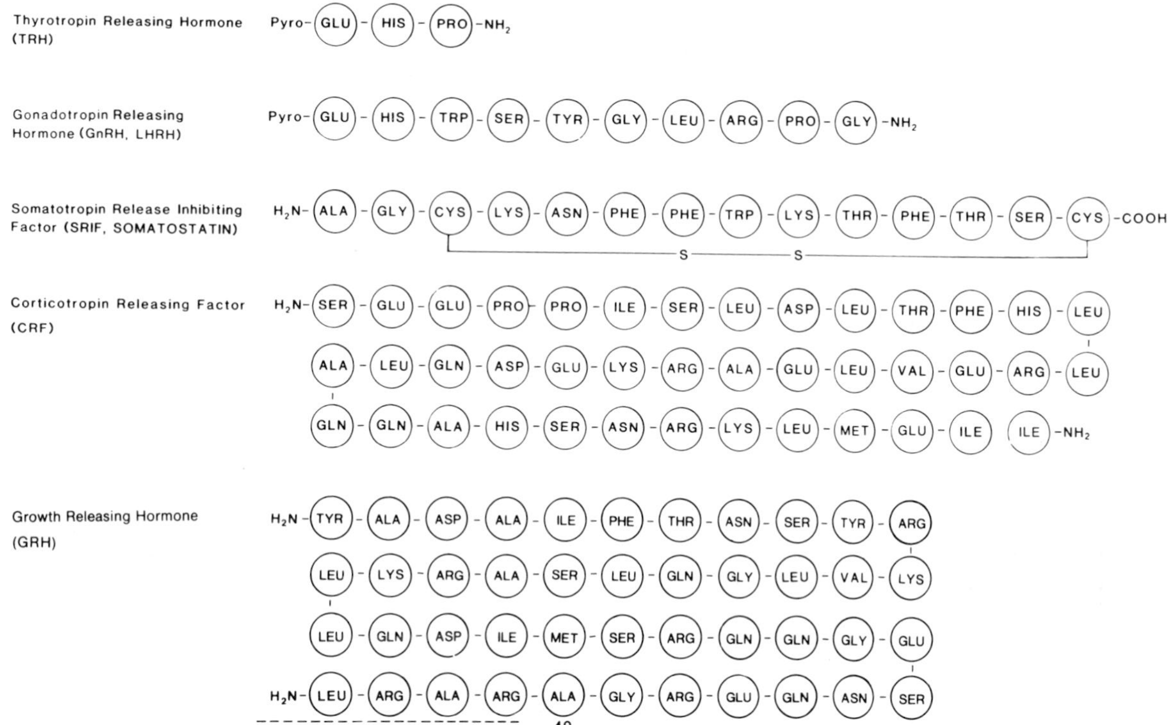

FIGURE 7-10. Structures of hypothalamic releasing and inhibiting hormones. The sequence of TRH, GnRH, and somatostatin are identical in all mammalian species studied. The sequence of human CRH, as shown in the figure, differs by 7 amino acids from ovine CRH. Two forms of GHRH have been identified which differ only by the additional COOH-terminal tetrapeptide indicated by the broken line. Porcine and rat GHRH differ by 3 and 14 amino acids, respectively.

FIGURE 7-11. Schematic diagram of the structures of the human TRH gene, mRNA, and precursor peptide. Note that six copies of TRH are generated from the precursor. The sites of cleavage of each copy are indicated by arrows in the precursor structure. 5'UT = 5' untranslated region; 3'UT = 3' untranslated region.

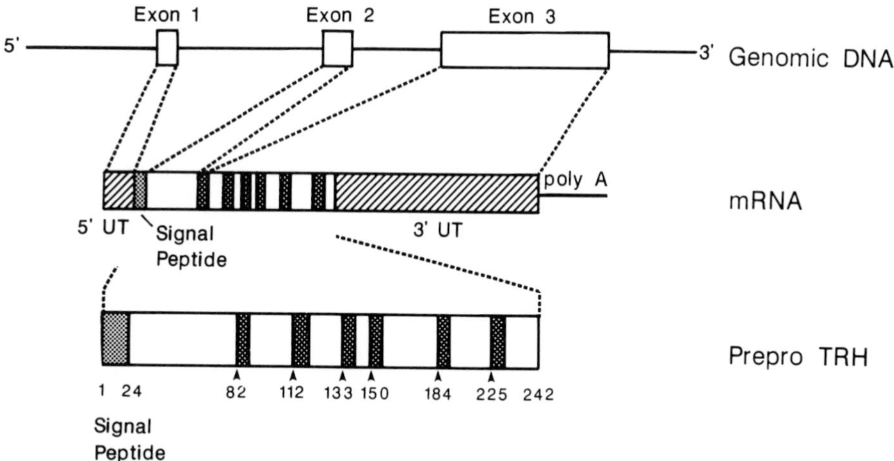

sis has shown that the processing of precursor to mature TRH occurs within the neuronal perikarya, and it is TRH itself that is transported to axon terminals, not proTRH.[40]

TRH is metabolized and inactivated rapidly. One of the metabolites, cycloHis-Pro-diketopiperazine (His-Pro-DKP), has been found to inhibit PRL secretion and reverse ethanol-induced sleep.[44] However, the concentrations of TRH and His-Pro-DKP vary considerably anatomically,[40] and it is possible that His-Pro-DKP arises, at least in part, separately from TRH degradation.

The primary areas containing the TRH neuronal perikarya that project to the median eminence are the anterior, medial, and periventricular regions of the paraventricular nucleus and the anterior portion of the periventricular nucleus.[40] However, TRH-containing neuronal cell bodies are also abundant in the suprachiasmatic subdivision of the preoptic nucleus, the dorsomedial nucleus, and the perifornical region and basolateral hypothalamus.[40] TRH-containing fibers may be found not only in the median eminence but also in the organum vasculosum of the lamina terminalis (OVLT), in the posterior pituitary, and scattered throughout other portions of the brain.[40] In humans, substantial amounts of immunoreactive TRH are found in the thalamus and cerebral cortex.[45] Indeed, over 70 percent of brain TRH is extrahypothalamic.[40] Specific binding sites for TRH have been found in adult human brains in high quantities in the amygdala and hippocampus and in lesser quantities in the cortex, basal ganglia, hypothalamus, and cerebellum,[46] suggesting that this extrahypothalamic TRH is biologically active. The location of TRH receptors contrasts with the location of TRH itself. Low levels of receptors are present in the hypothalamus, which has the highest TRH concentrations, and high levels of receptors are present in the amygdala and hippocampus, which have low TRH concentrations.[46]

Interestingly, a number of areas of the brain stain immunohistochemically for proTRH but not for TRH, such as the reticular nucleus of the thalamus, portions of the hippocampus, the preoptic area, the supraoptic nucleus, the caudate-putamen complex, the substantia nigra, the periaqueductal gray matter, the pontine nuclei, and the dorsal motor nucleus of the vagus.[40] In situ hybridization histochemistry using RNA probes complementary to proTRH mRNA and antisera directed against putative peptides coded for by proTRH confirmed these findings, suggesting a role for both TRH and other non-TRH peptides coded for by the TRH precursor elsewhere in the brain.[40] In some areas, it appears that proTRH is processed preferentially to non-TRH peptides.[40]

TRH is also present in many areas outside the brain. Within the spinal cord, TRH-containing axons descending from the raphe nuclei are found in association with motor nuclei in the ventral gray and preganglionic sympathetic neurons in the intermediolateral column.[47] TRH is present in the mucosa of the gastrointestinal (GI) tract,[48] pancreatic islets,[49] retina,[50] placenta,[51] milk,[52] and prostate, testes, epididymis, and seminal vesicles.[53] All these tissues contribute to peripheral blood and urine TRH levels, making these levels inaccurate with respect to reflecting concentrations in the hypothalamic-pituitary portal vessels.

The primary neuroendocrine function of TRH is to stimulate the synthesis and release of TSH and PRL. Intracellular transduction mechanisms that mediate this function include activation of phosphoinositide–protein kinase C pathways and increasing intracellular calcium through the mobilization of intracellular stores and transport across calcium channels[54,55] (see Chap. 4). TSH is secreted in small-amplitude pulses by the pituitary, presumably as a result of the release of TRH from the hypothalamus in a pulsatile fashion.[56] It has been estimated that a single molecule of TRH, through its TSH-releasing effect, induces the release of over 100,000 molecules of thyroxine from the thyroid.[57]

The fundamental role of TRH in stimulating TSH secretion was shown initially in hypothalamic ablation studies in which the paraventricular nucleus, the primary source of TRH, was lesioned, resulting in hypothyroidism.[58] Electric stimulation of this area causes a rapid release of TSH.[58] More specific experiments have shown that the administration of anti-TRH antibodies results in decreased basal and electrically stimulated TSH levels acutely and in decreased levels of TSH, T_4, and T_3 levels chronically.[59–62]

A number of different experimental approaches have failed to clarify the physiologic role of TRH as a PRL-releasing factor, however. The smallest dose of TRH that releases TSH also releases PRL in humans.[63] Immunoneutralization of endogenous TRH with TRH antisera caused a suppression of basal PRL levels in rats in some studies[59] but not in others.[62] Such immunization also does not affect the PRL response to electric stimulation of the paraventricular nucleus or suckling,[62] and it delays but does not affect the magnitude of the spontaneous surge of PRL at proestrus.[64] Active, chronic immunization of ewes with TRH conjugated to albumin results in only minimal decreases in PRL levels basally and after stimulation by stress, suckling, and estrus, although reductions in TSH and thyroid hormone levels are more marked.[61]

Suckling causes an increase in hypothalamic and portal vessel TRH levels as well as a decrease in dopamine (DA) levels.[65] If TRH mediates the PRL response to suckling even in part, it ought to be accompanied by an increase in TSH unless there is a concomitant increase in somatostatin. Studies of serum levels of PRL and TSH after suckling in humans have not shown any elevations of TSH.[66,67] Very small doses of TRH given systemically were effective in releasing PRL and TSH in lactating women, however, and so it is unlikely that the failure to show a rise in TSH was due to an increase in somatostatin.

In hypothyroidism, TRH synthesis is increased[18] and the amount of TRH in the median eminence is increased.[68] In addition, pituitary TRH binding is increased because of an increased number of TRH receptors, but it is not clear whether there is also an effect on binding affinity.[69] Basal TSH and PRL levels are increased in human hypothyroidism, as are their responses to injected TRH.[70] Correction of the hypothyroidism with thyroid hormones decreases both the elevated TSH and PRL levels and their responses to TRH, although the decrease is more rapid for TSH.[70] Conversely, in hyperthyroidism, portal vessel TRH levels are decreased,[71] basal and TRH-stimulated TSH levels are markedly suppressed, and basal PRL levels are not low, but the PRL response to TRH is markedly blunted and returns to normal with correction of the hyperthyroidism.[70] The feedback effects of thyroid hormones therefore occur at the level of both the hypothalamus and the pituitary.

These conflicting data from passive immunization studies, observation of TSH levels during lactation, and examination of PRL levels in various thyroid states support a role for TRH as a physiologic PRL releasing factor, albeit not the primary one, nor perhaps even one of major importance.

In addition to the feedback effects of thyroid hormones on TRH release, somatostatin, which inhibits TSH secretion directly (see below), also inhibits TRH secretion.[72] The roles of various hypothalamic bioamines on TRH secretion alone are difficult to determine in vivo as they also have effects on somatostatin release and direct effects on the pituitary thyrotrophs. Dopamine decreases the TSH and PRL responses to TRH, implicating action at the pituitary level, although there may be some effect in decreasing TRH secretion.[73] Alpha-adrenergic agonists and serotonin stimulate, and GABA suppresses, TRH and TSH secretion.[74,75]

In various disease states, the stimulatory effect of administered TRH in humans is not limited to TSH and PRL. TRH can stimulate GH secretion in patients with acromegaly and in several states in which there is decreased IGF-I feedback on GH secretion, such as hepatic cirrhosis, renal insufficiency, anorexia nervosa, poorly controlled insulin-dependent diabetes mellitus, and malnutrition.[24] However, such responses are also seen in patients with depression and schizophrenia, which may be associated with disordered central bioaminergic regulation.[24] TRH can also stimulate FSH secretion in most patients with gonadotroph cell adenomas but not in normal individuals.[76] Obviously, somatotroph and gonadotroph cells must have TRH receptors, but there is "activation" of such receptors, which may involve alteration of intracellular transduction mechanisms, only in special circumstances.

In addition, TRH has a number of nonendocrine effects. As a neurotransmitter, TRH has generally been found to be excitatory, causing increased motor activity, tremor, arousal, and peripheral sympathetic neural activity with shivering, hypertension, tachycardia, diaphoresis, and nausea.[77] Early reports suggesting a beneficial effect of TRH on depression have not been confirmed.[77] Because of the association of TRH nerve terminals with motor neurons, TRH has been tried as therapy for amyotrophic lateral sclerosis. Despite early provocative results, subsequent studies have not shown definitive benefit with either intramuscular or intrathecal administration.[77] Early reports also suggested that TRH may be beneficial in septic shock and spinal cord shock after spinal cord trauma, but the role of TRH in the treatment of these conditions is uncertain despite several trials.[78,79]

Gonadotropin Releasing Hormone

GnRH was the second hypophysiotropic hormone to be characterized; it consists of 10 amino acids with a molecular weight of 1182.[80] The single gene encoding the sequence for GnRH was subsequently isolated from human placenta and hypothalamus and was found to encode a 92-amino acid precursor which contains a 23-amino acid signal peptide, the 10-amino acid GnRH, followed by a Gly-Lys-Arg sequence necessary for enzymatic processing and carboxy-terminal amidation of GnRH, and a 56-amino acid peptide that has been termed GAP (Fig. 7-12).[81,82] In contrast to TRH, in which the processing of the precursor occurs in the neuronal perikarya, the processing of the GnRH precursor occurs in the axonal processes and terminals, and both GnRH and GAP are located in nerve terminals.[83,84]

Immunohistochemical studies have localized GnRH-containing neurons to three major areas: (1) the preoptic/lamina terminalis area with projections to the OVLT, (2) the mediobasal hypothalamus just anterior to the mammillary bodies and extending toward the infundibulum with axonal projections to the median eminence (tuberoinfundibular tract) and posterior pituitary, and (3) neurons in the septum, the pericommissural area, and the rostral mesencephalon with projections toward the extrahypothalamic brain, especially to portions of the limbic system such as the amygdala and hippocampus.[27] Studies in which the preoptic area and the mediobasal hypothalamic GnRH area have been surgically interrupted in rats resulted in loss of the midcycle surge of LH and FSH, which is thought to be in part caused by positive estrogen feedback but not negative steroid feedback.[85] Destruction of the anterior hypothalamic area in rhesus monkeys, however, does not abolish this midcycle surge, and it appears

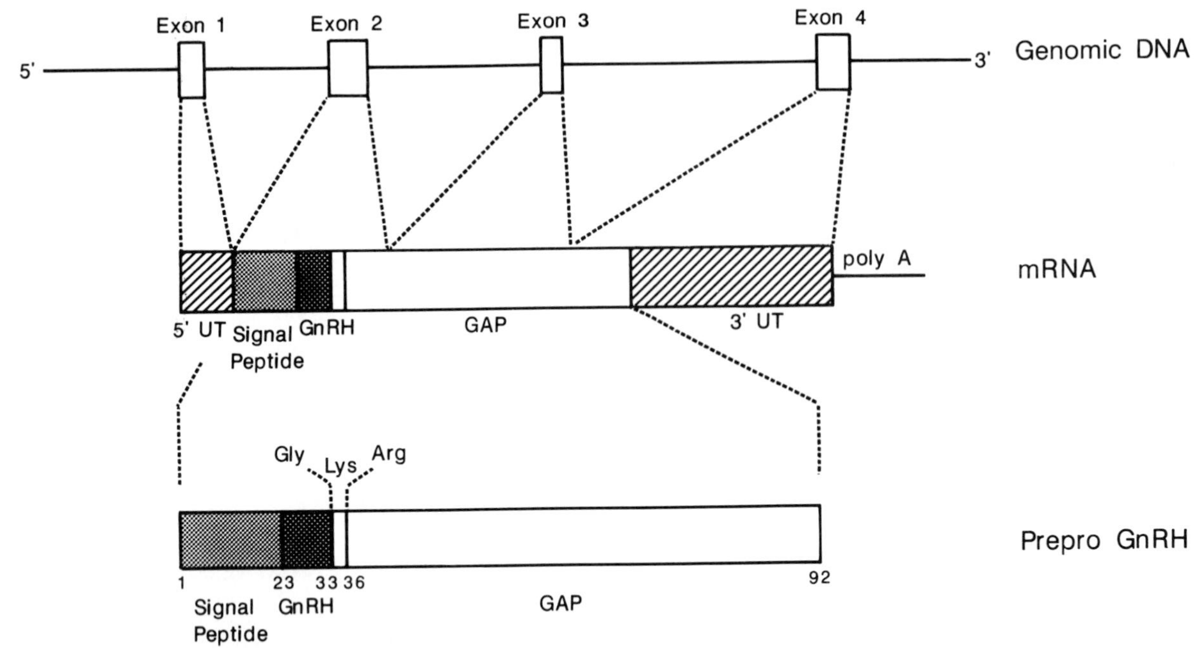

FIGURE 7-12. Schematic diagram of the structures of the human GnRH gene, mRNA, and precursor peptide. Both GnRH and GnRH-associated peptide (GAP) are generated from the precursor. 5'UT = 5' untranslated region; 3'UT = 3' untranslated region.

that in primates the arcuate nucleus is the primary structure involved in positive feedback.[86]

Anatomic embryologic studies performed in mice suggest that GnRH neurons originally develop in the epithelium of the medial part of the olfactory placode, including the part that forms the anlage of the vomeronasal organ. During fetal development, these cells migrate across the nasal septum, enter the forebrain with the nervus terminalis and vomeronasal nerves, travel medial to the olfactory bulbs, and eventually enter the septal-preoptic region of the hypothalamus.[87] This demonstration of the origin of GnRH-producing neurons from olfactory epithelia is of clinical interest with respect to Kallman's syndrome, in which gonadotropin deficiency, presumably due to GnRH deficiency, is associated with anosmia caused by agenesis of the olfactory bulbs (see below).

GnRH is also found in significant quantities in the placenta, where its synthesis has been demonstrated,[82] and in milk.[52] GnRH-like substances but not GnRH itself have been found in testicular interstitial cells [88] and ovaries.[89]

The primary function of GnRH is to stimulate the secretion of LH and FSH. The transduction mechanisms that mediate the action of GnRH involve the phosphoinositide–protein kinase C pathway as well as increases in intracellular calcium via mobilization from intracellular calcium stores and subsequent entry through a voltage-dependent calcium channel [90] (see Chap. 8). GnRH also directly up regulates its own receptors (i.e., it causes an increase in GnRH receptor number), a function shared with estradiol.[91] By contrast, continuous administration of GnRH is associated with down regulation of gonadotropin synthesis and secretion as a result of decreased receptor numbers as well as postreceptor mechanisms.[91]

Although early studies suggested the presence of separate LH and FSH releasing factors,[92] it appears that there is only one GnRH and that the differential secretion of LH and FSH is due to variations in sensitivity of the feedback effects of steroid and peptide hormones and variations in sensitivity to GnRH. For example, slower GnRH pulse frequencies result in a greater FSH/LH ratio,[85,93] inhibin has a much greater inhibitory effect on FSH than on LH,[94] and there is a more marked positive feedback effect of estrogen on LH compared to FSH.[85] When endogenous GnRH is immunoneutralized, the pulsatile secretion of LH is eliminated but FSH secretion is maintained in the short term and decreases in the long term.[93] Similarly, when a specific GnRH antagonist is given to castrate rats, serum levels of LH, FSH, and the α subunit rise, as well as gonadotroph cell mRNA levels of FSHβ, LHβ, and the α subunit.[95]

The concept that exposure to a stimulating hormone in a pulsatile or episodic compared to a continuous manner results in increased target organ response was initially demonstrated for GnRH and gonadotropin secretion.[96] In experiments in rhesus monkeys in which the ovaries had been removed and hypothalamic lesions had been placed, GnRH was given in equal quantities either continuously intravenously or via pulses once per hour. Only the pulsatile administration of GnRH resulted in a reestablishment of normal gonadotropin secretion (Fig. 7-13).[96] The human pituitary secretes gonadotropins in frequent (every 15 min) pulses of small amplitude when cultured in vitro,[97] and frequent sampling can detect these pulses in vivo as well.[98] The pulsatile release of GnRH then superimposes pulses of LH and FSH secretion of larger amplitude about every 70 to 96 min in humans.[99] The fact that these latter pulses are due to GnRH has been shown by means of simultaneous measurement of pituitary portal blood GnRH and peripheral blood LH and FSH concentrations in animals (Fig. 7-14).[100–102] Whether the more frequent pulses of smaller amplitude are due to GnRH or to the intrinsic secretory ability of the pituitary is not clear.[103] The exposure to pulsatile (every 1 h) vs. continuous GnRH also has effects on gonadotropin synthesis and release. Recent studies in rat pituitaries showed that α subunit mRNA increases with either mode but that FSHβ subunit mRNA increases only with pulsatile GnRH and is suppressed with continuous GnRH.[104]

Steroid hormone feedback regulation of the hypothalamic-pituitary-gonadal axis occurs at both the pituitary and hypothalamic levels. Gonadectomy results in increased GnRH secretion into the portal system,[105] with a decrease in hypothalamic GnRH content[106] and hypothalamic GnRH precursor mRNA levels[107] as well as an increase in the pituitary responsiveness to GnRH. As estrogen receptors on GnRH neurons are quite sparse, it is likely that the effect of estrogen on GnRH release is mediated through effects on other neurotransmitter-containing neurons that have synaptic contact with GnRH neurons.[108] Estrogens have a variable feedback effect in vivo, with short-term administration causing an initial decrease in response to GnRH, longer-term administration causing a positive feedback effect, and chronic administration also causing a negative feedback effect.[108] In pituitary cell cultures, estradiol suppresses the gonadotropin response to GnRH added to the medium.[109] However, other studies have shown that short-term incubation of pituitary

FIGURE 7-13. Suppression of plasma LH and FSH concentrations after the initiation on day 0 of continuous GnRH (1μg/min) in an ovariectomized rhesus monkey with a radiofrequency lesion in the hypothalamus; gonadotropin secretion had been reestablished before the intermittent (pulsatile) administration of the decapeptide (1 μg/min for 6 min once per h). The inhibition of gonadotropin secretion was reversed after reinstitution of the intermittent mode of GnRH stimulation on day 20. The vertical lines beneath the LH data points on days 10 and 13 of the continuous infusion regimen indicate values below the sensitivity of the radioimmunoassay. *(Reproduced with permission from Belchetz et al.[96])*

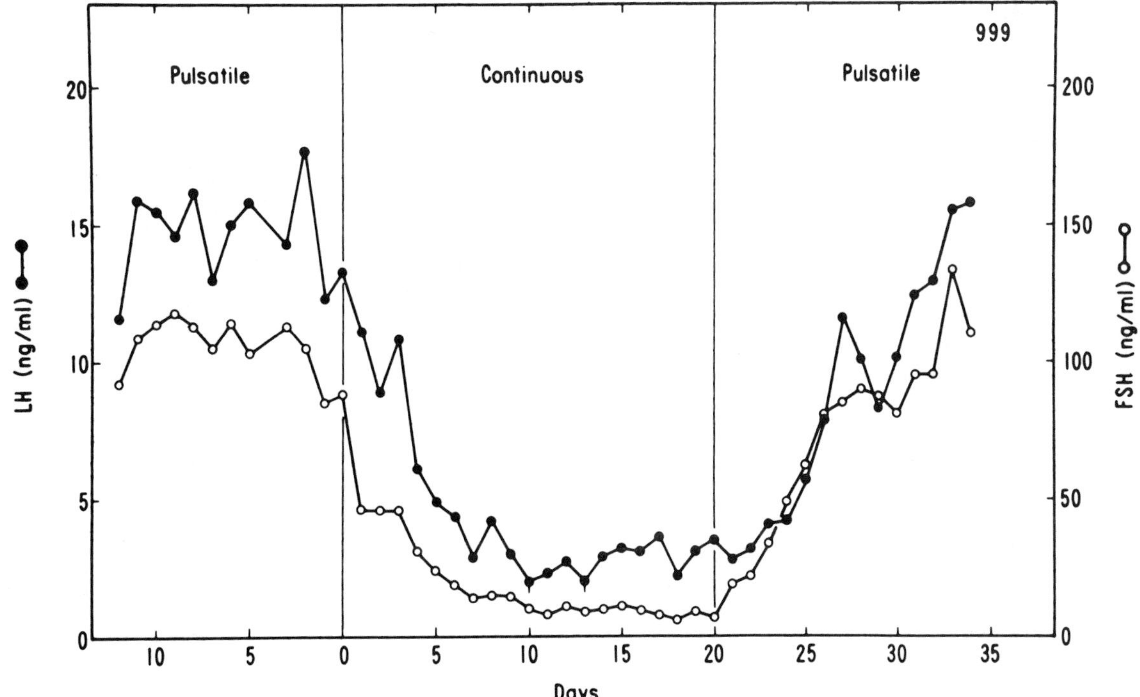

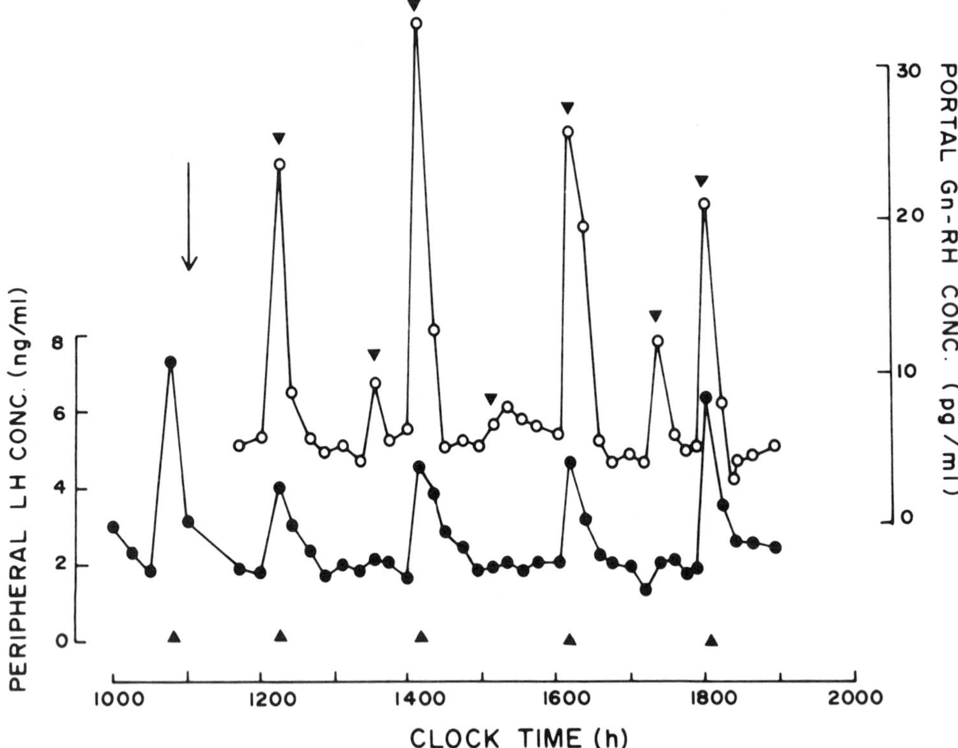

FIGURE 7-14. Concentrations of GnRH in the hypothalamo-hypophyseal portal plasma and LH in the jugular venous (peripheral) plasma of an ovariectomized ewe. The arrow indicates the time at which the portal vessels were cut. Pulsatile secretory episodes (▲ for LH and ▼ for GnRH) were defined as having occurred when the value in a given sample exceeded that of the previous sample by three times the standard deviation of the previous sample. No LH pulses occur without concomitant GnRH pulses, although GnRH pulses sometimes occur without any change in LH secretion. *(Reproduced with permission from Clark and Cummins.[100] Copyright The Endocrine Society.)*

cell cultures with estradiol in the absence of GnRH results in no effect on transcription of α subunit or FSHβ genes, but LHβ mRNA synthesis is increased.[110] This suggests that at least part of the positive feedback effect of estrogen that occurs at midcycle may be due to a direct effect at the pituitary level, but as other studies have shown increased GnRH levels in portal blood at the time of the ovulatory gonadotropin surge,[111] part of the positive feedback effect of estrogen also occurs at the hypothalamic level. The negative effects of estrogen probably occur at both the hypothalamic and pituitary levels, with the hypothalamic effects being the reduction of GnRH pulse amplitude and frequency and the pituitary effects being the modulation of the gonadotropin response to GnRH.[108,110]

Progesterone also has both stimulatory and inhibitory effects on gonadotropin release through effects at both the pituitary and hypothalamic levels, [108,110,112] with the differences probably due to concurrent estrogen levels and the phase of the cycle, as the early preovulatory rise in progesterone augments the ovulatory gonadotropin surge while the later rise of progesterone in the luteal phase is inhibitory.[108] Several experiments have shown that testosterone can inhibit gonadotropin secretion directly, without first having to be aromatized to estrogen.[113] Because testosterone decreases gonadotropin pulse amplitude and frequency as well as the gonadotropin response to exogenous GnRH, it probably acts at both the hypothalamic and pituitary levels.[114]

The negative feedback effects of inhibin are predominantly on FSH and predominantly on the pituitary. Inhibin causes a dose-related decrease in the sensitivity of gonadotrophs to GnRH which may involve a decrease in the number of GnRH receptors [115,116] as well as a direct effect on the synthesis of FSH, as shown by demonstrating effects on α subunit and FSHβ but not LHβ subunit mRNA levels in a pituitary cell culture system.[117] However, the administration of crude inhibin preparations into the dorsal anterior hypothalamus also suppresses FSH levels, and so there may also be a hypothalamic site of action.[118] The related ovarian protein activin stimulates FSH release from the pituitary[94] as well as synthesis.[117] It appears to bind to a receptor separate from the GnRH receptor and acts additively to GnRH in stimulating FSH release.[94] Another go-

gans, which are areas outside the blood-brain barrier through which interaction of peripheral blood-borne substances with the CNS may occur.[157] Recent studies have shown that tumors of cells of glial and neuroblastic origin in humans, such as meningiomas, astrocytomas, and medulloblastomas, retain somatostatin receptors.[158] The binding of somatostatin to its receptor on the cell membrane[159] is coupled to adenylate cyclase by an inhibitory guanine nucleotide-binding regulatory protein, resulting in a decrease in intracellular cAMP levels.[160]

After somatostatin was discovered, its subsequent characterization was based on its ability to inhibit GH secretion.[132,133] When somatostatin is given to humans, it blocks the rise in GH that occurs with all stimuli in a dose-dependent fashion.[161,162] Active immunization against somatostatin or the administration of antisomatostatin antiserum eradicates endogenous somatostatin activity, resulting in a rise in basal and stimulated GH levels in rats and baboons,[163,164] and restores the pulse amplitude of GH that has been decreased by stress[165] or starvation.[166]

The interaction of somatostatin and GRH on GH secretion is complex. Both somatostatin and GRH are secreted episodically into the portal system in rats and sheep in an independent manner in which the secretory bursts are often asynchronous. Thus, GH secretory episodes are associated with increased GRH secretion accompanied by low somatostatin levels and basal or trough GH levels associated with low GRH levels and more elevated somatostatin levels (Fig. 7-16).[164,167,168] Furthermore, somatostatin may also partially inhibit GRH secretion, and somatostatin receptors have been found on GRH neuronal perikarya in the arcuate nucleus.[146,169] Conversely, GRH may stimulate somatostatin release.[170] Because GH responses to exogenous GRH are variable, hypothalamic somatostatin secretion in humans may also be intermittent.[171]

The second major neuroendocrine function of somatostatin is the inhibition of basal and stimulated TSH secretion.[161] In the rat, somatostatin-depleting lesions which increase GH secretion also increase TSH secretion.[172] Neutralization of endogenous somatostatin by means of the administration of antisomatostatin serum raises basal and stimulated TSH levels, as it does with GH levels, as indicated above.[173] Thyroid hormone levels also feed back positively on hypothalamic somatostatin secretion[19] just as they feed back negatively on TRH secretion and the TSH response to TRH (see above), integrating the hypothalamic-pituitary-thyroid feedback loop. Somatostatin has even been found to inhibit directly

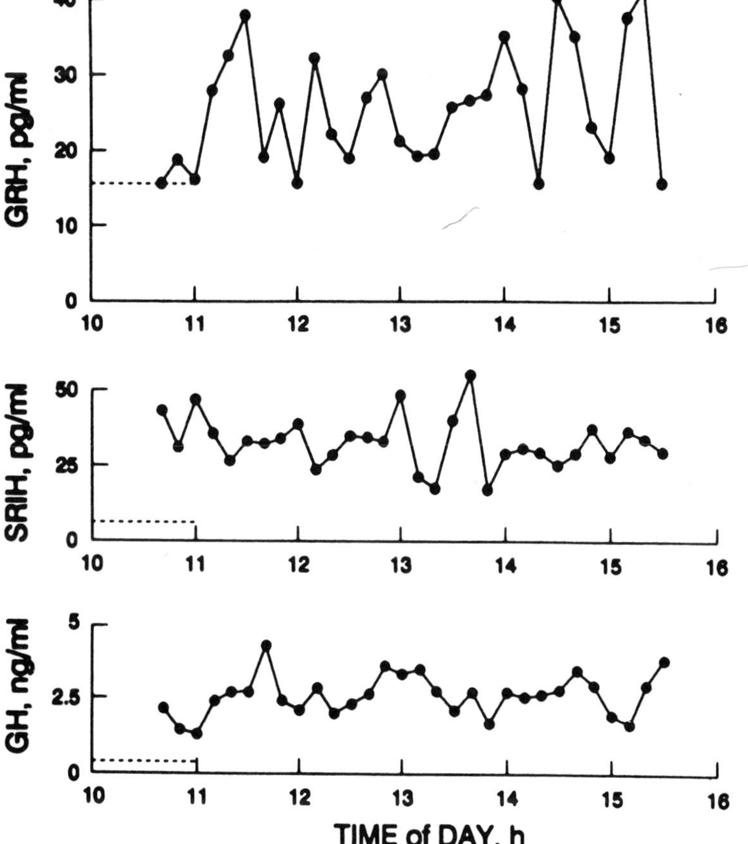

FIGURE 7-16. GHRH (GRH) and somatostatin (SRIH) levels in the hypothalamic-pituitary portal plasma and GH levels in the jugular plasma of an unanesthetized ovariectomized ewe. The interrupted horizontal lines indicate the least detectable value for each assay. Although there is an association between GHRH and GH secretory peaks, there is no association between GHRH and somatostatin secretion or between somatostatin and GH secretion. These data in sheep are compatible with independent neural rhythmicity of GHRH and somatostatin secretion, with a primary role of GHRH in determining pulsatile GH secretion. *(Reproduced with permission from Frohman et al.[168] Copyright The American Society for Clinical Investigation, Inc.)*

the release of TRH from rat hypothalamic cultures.[72] Despite this evidence, questions remain about the physiologic role of somatostatin as an inhibitor of TSH secretion. Careful dose-response studies in humans, using somatostatin infusions that achieved serum somatostatin levels in the range that have been reported to be in rat portal vessels, have shown that GH is about 10-fold more sensitive to inhibition by somatostatin than is TSH.[162,174] On the basis of these studies, it has been suggested that if there is a role of somatostatin in inhibiting TSH secretion and that it is limited to conditions associated with marked somatostatin-mediated suppression of GH.[174]

Hypothalamic somatostatin is itself subject to feedback regulation as well as regulation by a number of bioaminergic and peptidergic neurotransmitters. Growth hormone can itself directly increase somatostatin secretion, as can its target organ hormone, IGF-I (also known as somatomedin C).[21] Experiments which have addressed the issue of the specific regulation of somatostatin secretion and not just GH secretion have by necessity been quite unphysiologic, depending on in vitro hypothalamic explant or culture systems or intraventricular injections and measuring somatostatin in severed portal vessels. Such studies have found that dopamine, norepinephrine, and acetylcholine stimulate somatostatin secretion,[175] as do glucagon,[176] neurotensin,[177] VIP and the closely related peptide-histidine-isoleucine (PHI),[178] interleukin-1β,[179] and the amino acid taurine,[180] although it is thought that arginine causes a decrease in somatostatin release.[181] By contrast, serotonin,[175] substance P, β-endorphin, and met-enkephalin[177] had no effects on somatostatin secretion when injected intraventricularly, but β-endorphin and met-enkephalin decreased K^+-induced somatostatin release from perfused hypothalami in vitro.[182]

One of the intracellular transduction messengers responsible for somatostatin gene transcription is cAMP. In fact, it is in the somatostatin gene system that the interaction of the cAMP response element (CRE) with a specific CRE *trans*-activating binding protein (CREB) has been most completely elucidated.[183,184] In this system, a stimulus activates adenylate cyclase, generating cAMP, which activates cAMP-dependent protein kinase A, which then phorphorylates CREB, which binds to the CRE of the 5′-flanking region of the somatostatin gene, thus stimulating somatostatin gene transcription. The rise in cAMP also stimulates the release of somatostatin. There is also some evidence that voltage-gated calcium channels may be involved in somatostatin secretion, but this requires further definition.

Little is known about the regulation or function of somatostatin in the rest of the brain. In general, somatostatin appears to have an inhibitory function.[161] The number of receptors for somatostatin and somatostatin content are decreased in the cortex of patients with Alzheimer's disease,[185] but somatostatin is increased in the basal ganglia in patients with Huntington's disease.[186] Whether such changes are part of the pathogenesis of these disorders or are merely epiphenomena is not known.

Recently, analogs of somatostatin have been developed for the treatment of acromegaly (see Chap. 8). One analog, octreotide, is in current clinical use and has been found to have efficacy in a wide number of areas besides GH-secreting tumors, including the treatment of carcinoid tumors, VIP-secreting tumors, TSH-secreting tumors, islet-cell tumors, and diarrhea of a number of etiologies (see Chaps. 8 and 27). An interesting side benefit of treatment has been a rapid analgesic effect for headaches that is characterized by significant tolerance. It is likely that this analgesic effect is mediated by an interaction of the analog with opiate receptors elsewhere in the brain.[187]

Corticotropin Releasing Hormone

CRH was the first of the hypophysiotropic hormones for which evidence of bioactivity was demonstrated in hypothalamic extracts[188,189] and one of the last to be completely characterized. It was initially characterized in sheep and was found to have 41 amino acids (molecular weight of 4670).[190] Subsequent studies have shown that human CRH has seven amino acids different from those of ovine CRH[191] and that rat CRH is identical to human CRH. The human gene for CRH has been characterized, and the deduced sequence of preproCRH consists of 192 amino acids with a 24-amino acid leader sequence (Fig. 7-17).[191]

Immunoreactive CRH is found throughout the human hypothalamus, with the highest concentrations in the paraventricular, supraoptic, and infundibular (arcuate) nuclei.[192] However, immunohistochemical studies have shown that most human CRH neuronal perikarya are located in the parvocellular region of the paraventricular nucleus and that most neurons project to the median eminence, where CRH is released into the portal plexus, although a few also project to the posterior pituitary.[193] CRH has been demonstrated in hypothalamic-hypophyseal portal blood in concentrations known to stimulate ACTH from pituitaries in vitro.[194] In rats, lesions of the paraventricular nucleus result in a marked decrease in median eminence CRH and in ACTH released by ether stress.[195] CRH has been found in the human thalamus, cortex, cerebellum, pons, medulla, and spinal cord,[196] where it can be released by depolarizing agents, suggesting a functional role as a neurotransmitter in those areas.[197] It is also present in the adrenal cortex and medulla, lung, liver, stomach, duodenum, pancreas, and placenta, but its functions in these tissues are poorly

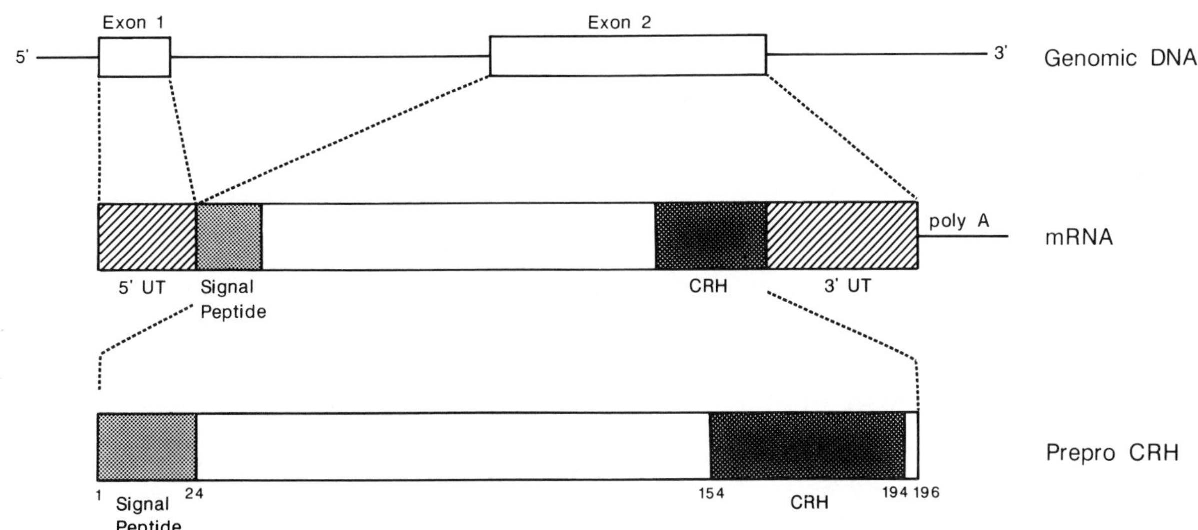

FIGURE 7-17. Schematic diagram of the structures of the human CRH gene, mRNA, and precursor peptide. 5' UT = 5' untranslated region. 3' UT = 3' untranslated region.

understood.[127,196,198] CRH in peripheral blood is derived from both hypothalamic and extrahypothalamic sources[199] and is bound to a binding protein.[200]

CRH receptors have been demonstrated in normal and adenomatous pituitary corticotroph cells[201] and, in rats at least, are widely distributed in the CNS.[202] The transduction mechanisms by which CRH binding to the CRH receptor results in ACTH release involve the activation of adenylate cyclase, the generation of cAMP, and the activation of cAMP-dependent protein kinases as well as less well understood calcium-mediated mechanisms.[203]

CRH releases ACTH, β-endorphin, β-lipotropin, melanocyte stimulating hormone (MSH), and other peptides generated from pro-opiomelanocortin (POMC) in equimolar amounts without releasing other pituitary hormones.[203] There is no difference in the ACTH response between repetitive and continuous administration of CRH, unlike the desensitization seen with GnRH.[204]

The physiologic role of CRH in the regulation of ACTH has been established by the finding that the immunoneutralization of endogenous CRH by anti-CRH antibodies blocks the ACTH response to stress by 75 percent.[205] Furthermore, immunoneutralization studies of endogenous CRH show that CRH is responsible for the augmentation of the amplitude of an underlying CRH-independent rhythm that results in the nocturnal rise in blood ACTH levels.[206] In rats, insulin-induced hypoglycemia causes not only a release of CRH from the median eminence in parallel with the increase in ACTH secretion by the pituitary but an increase in hypothalamic CRH mRNA levels, implying increased CRH gene transcription.[207] The remaining 25 percent of stress-induced secretion is primarily due to vasopressin, which also has very potent ACTH-releasing activity.[208] CRH and vasopressin appear to have synergistic effects on ACTH release[209] (Fig. 7-18). In fact, CRH and vasopressin coexist in about half the CRH-containing parvocellular and paraventricular neurons and even in the same neurosecretory granules.[5,210] Elegant studies in conscious sheep have shown parallel secretion of CRH and vasopressin into the portal circulation coinciding with the release of the POMC peptides ACTH, β-endorphin, and α-MSH into the systemic circulation.[211] CRH and vasopressin are not always released coordinately, however, and stress has been shown to selectively activate the vasopressin-containing subset of CRH neurons.[5] Furthermore, at least in the rat, not all pituitary cells that respond to CRH also respond to vasopressin.[212] In contrast to CRH, which uses the adenylate cyclase–cAMP system for signal transduction, vasopressin appears to use the phosphotidylinositol–diacylglycerol (DAG)–protein kinase C system for signal transduction.[203,213]

Glucocorticoid negative feedback also does not affect all the CRH neurons equally. Adrenalectomy causes an increase in the number of neurons containing both CRH and vasopressin and a decrease in the number containing only CRH,[214] an increase in paraventricular nucleus CRH mRNA[215] (implying increased gene transcription), an increase in portal vessel CRH and vasopressin levels, and an increase in peripheral ACTH levels.[216] All these effects are blocked by concomitant glucocorticoid replacement. Adrenalectomy has no effect on CRH mRNA levels in

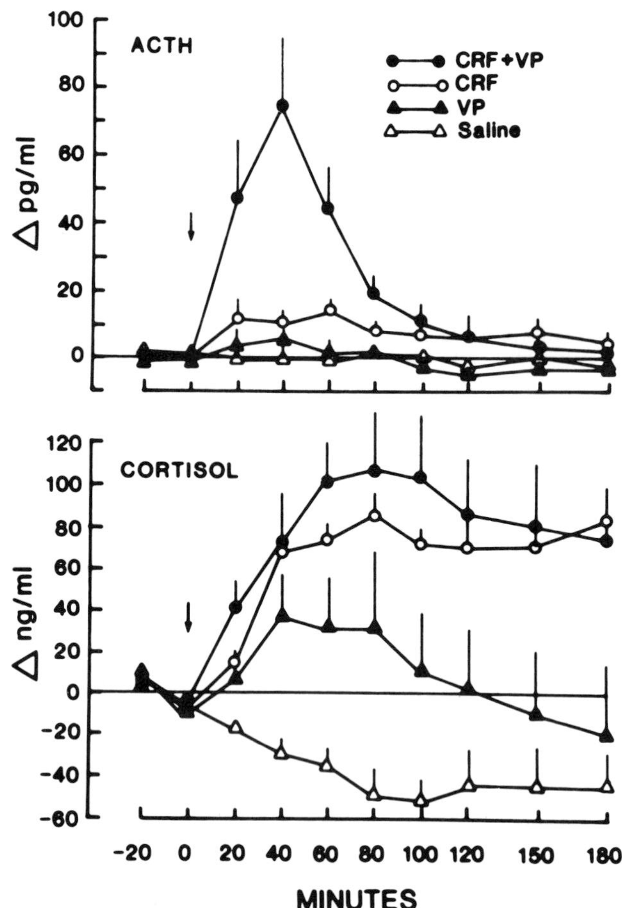

FIGURE 7-18. Net change (± SE) of ACTH and cortisol concentrations in six women in response to the administration of CRH (CRF), vasopressin (VP), or CRH with vasopressin at time 0. Note the marked synergistic effects of CRH and vasopressin on ACTH release. *(Reproduced with permission from Liu et al.[209] Copyright The Endocrine Society.)*

CRH-producing cells elsewhere in the brain.[215] Glucocorticoids can also inhibit the hemorrhage-induced release of CRH into the portal vessels[217] as well as the CRH-induced rise in intracellular cAMP and ACTH release from pituitary cells in vitro.[218]

The more direct products of CRH stimulation also exert negative feedback. ACTH may feed back negatively on its own secretion,[219] at least in part by decreasing CRH release by the hypothalamus.[220] Another product of POMC processing, β-endorphin, also feeds back negatively on ACTH secretion.[221] Although the results from animal studies have been conflicting, morphine suppresses the ACTH response to CRH in humans,[222] presumably acting through opioid μ receptors (see below).

Central bioamines and peptides also influence CRH secretion. Norepinephrine and epinephrine stimulate hypothalamic CRH secretion via α_1 and α_2 receptors and both adenylate cyclase and protein kinase C second messenger systems.[223–225] Norepinephrine and epinephrine also stimulate pituitary ACTH secretion directly and are additive to the stimulatory effect of CRH.[225] Acetylcholine also stimulates CRH secretion via both muscarinic and nicotinic receptors,[225,226] and dopamine has a mild stimulatory effect[224] whereas GABA is inhibitory.[223,224] Under various experimental circumstances, angiotensin II, cholecystokinin, VIP, oxytocin, and atrial natriuretic peptide all have ACTH-releasing properties, but their interactions with CRH are unknown.[203]

Monokines released by inflammatory tissue also exert effects on CRH and ACTH secretion. Interleukin 1 (IL-1, previously known as endogenous pyrogen), a product of mononuclear phagocytes that mediates many of the inflammatory responses, stimulates the synthesis and release of CRH from the hypothalamus and the release of ACTH by the pituitary.[227,228] Although it had been thought that IL-1 exerts its influence on CRH after entry into the hypothalamus via one of the circumventricular organs, the OVLT, recent studies have found nerve fibers that stain immunohistochemically for IL-1β in the magnocellular and parvocellular parts of the human paraventricular nucleus; the preoptic, supraoptic, and arcuate nuclei; and the external zone of the median eminence.[229] It is not clear whether it is these IL-1-containing neurons or other neurons that mediate the CRH-releasing and other central effects of systemic IL-1 that enters via the OVLT.[229] Other cytokines, such as IL-2 and thymosins, have also been found to elicit secretion of ACTH, but their mechanisms of action have not been clarified.[227] ACTH and other POMC-derived peptides are produced by monocytes, but it is not known whether they interact with the central IL-1–CRH–ACTH system.[227]

A number of actions of extrahypothalamic CRH have been postulated. In particular, CRH has been proposed to activate biological systems within the brain in response to stress. For example, CRH administered to dogs via intracerebroventricular cannulae causes increased plasma levels of epinephrine, norepinephrine, glucagon, and glucose and an increase in heart rate and mean arterial blood pressure.[230] In addition, CRH may have central effects of suppressing the release of LH and GH, gastric acid secretion, sexual activity, and feeding activity while stimulating respiration and behavioral arousal even to the point of seizures.[231] CRH is decreased in the cerebral cortex of patients with Alzheimer's disease and in the basal ganglia in patients with Huntington's disease.[198]

Both ovine and human CRH have been given to humans in a variety of experimental paradigms, although CRH has not been approved by the U.S. Food and Drug Administration for commercial use. These preparations have been found to be of some use in stimulating ACTH secretion during petrosal sinus sampling in the differential diagnosis of Cushing's disease vs. ectopic ACTH syndrome[232] (see Chaps. 8 and 12). In patients with hypothalamic hypopituitarism, the ACTH response to CRH is increased and somewhat delayed and prolonged, but the response is markedly blunted in patients with the defect clearly localized to the pituitary, as in Sheehan's syndrome[231] (see Chap. 8). CRH testing has also been used diagnostically in psychiatric disorders in a fashion similar to the dexamethasone suppression test, but the responses have not been highly specific.[231]

Growth Hormone Releasing Hormone

Although GH-releasing activity had been found in hypothalamic extracts since 1964,[233] GH releasing hormone (GHRH or GRH, also referred to as somatocrinin in some laboratories) was finally isolated and characterized in 1982 in two separate laboratories virtually simultaneously not from the hypothalamus but from two pancreatic tumors that produced this substance ectopically, resulting in acromegaly.[234,235] The two peptides isolated from these tumors differed in their lengths, however, one having a length of 44 amino acids and an amidated COOH terminus[236] and the other having a length of 40 amino acids and a free COOH terminus[237]; their molecular weights are 5040 and 4545, respectively. Subsequent analysis of hypothalamic extracts confirmed the presence of both moieties, with about two-thirds being the 1-44 moiety and the remaining one-third being 1-40.[238] A 1-37-amino acid GHRH exists in significant quantities in some pancreatic tumors but is not present in significant quantities in the hypothalamus.[238] Bioactivity resides in the first 27 amino acids.[236] Structurally, GHRH belongs to the secretin-VIP-glucagon family.[237]

The gene for human GHRH has been characterized[239,240] and codes for two mRNAs which differ slightly in the splice site of the fifth exon, resulting in two GHRH precursors of 107 and 108 amino acids, respectively, that vary in the presence or absence of a serine near the 3′ end. The precursors consist of a 20-amino acid signal peptide, a 10-amino acid N-terminal peptide, a 44-amino acid GHRH, and a 30- or 31-amino acid C-terminal peptide[239,240] (Fig. 7-19). GHRH is inactivated quickly in the circulation by a dipeptidylpeptidase, which cleaves the amino terminal two peptides, resulting in a bioinactive $GHRH_{3-44}$.[241]

Early studies with large lesions of the medial basal hypothalamus showed that this region is crucial for growth of rats, and it is thought to be the source of GHRH.[131] In subsequent studies, rats with lesions confined to the ventromedial nucleus had reduced growth and lower pituitary and plasma GH levels.[242] Conversely, electric stimulation of the ventromedial and arcuate area resulted in a pronounced surge of GH.[243] Radioimmunoassays using specific GHRH antibodies have confirmed that very high concentrations of GHRH are found in the median eminence and the infundibular (arcuate) and lower portions of the ventromedial nuclei in the rat and the human, with smaller amounts elsewhere in the hypothalamus and virtually no GHRH in the extrahypothalamic brain.[244–246] Immunohistochemical studies of monkey and human brains have shown GHRH immunoreactive perikarya in the arcuate and ventromedial nuclei with axonal projections terminating in the median eminence,[247,248] with a small number of fibers terminating in the anterior hypothalamus and the arcuate and ventromedial nuclei.[248] GHRH has also been found in a number of other tissues in humans, including the pancreas, thyroid, lung, stomach, duodenum, ileum, colon, adrenal, and kidney.[244] Although GHRH has been found in mouse and rat placentas, it has not been identified in the human placenta.[127] Plasma GHRH levels rise with meals at a time when GH levels are suppressed, even in subjects with idiopathic GH deficiency, suggesting that circulating plasma GHRH is largely gut-derived and is not reflective of hypothalamic function.[249]

$GHRH_{1-40}$ and $GHRH_{1-44}$ are essentially equipotent in stimulating GH secretion in humans in a dose-dependent fashion, with the GH rise beginning within about 5 min and with peak levels occurring about 30 to 60 min after injection.[250,251] Although most studies found GHRH to be specific for releasing only GH, other studies found that in some individuals GHRH is capable of eliciting a small increase in PRL as well.[252] Prolonged infusion of GHRH results in a gradual decrease in the amount of GH released despite maintenance of GHRH levels in the blood, i.e., somatotroph desensitization, which is thought to be due to down regulation of GHRH binding sites or to a depletion of a readily releasable pool of GH.[252,253] With repetitive administration every 3 h, GHRH can cause the release of sufficient GH in children with GHRH deficiency to result in an increase in IGF-I levels and an acceleration of growth.[254] Not only does GHRH stimulate release, it also stimulates GH gene transcription.[255] The critical importance of GHRH to normal GH secretion and growth was demonstrated when monoclonal antibodies to GHRH were shown to inhibit the pulsatile secretion of GH[256] and somatic growth in rats.[257] The primary transduction mechanism mediating the stimulatory effect of GHRH on GH secretion is the adenylate cyclase–cAMP system, but GHRH also stimulates the influx of calcium via calcium channels with activation of the intracellular calcium-calmodulin system.[258]

Considerable evidence in rats has documented the existence of negative feedback regulation of both IGF-I and GH in GH secretion mediated by both a decrease in GHRH synthesis and secretion and an increase in somatostatin synthesis and secretion.[21–23, 259–263] In rats, the large increases in GH

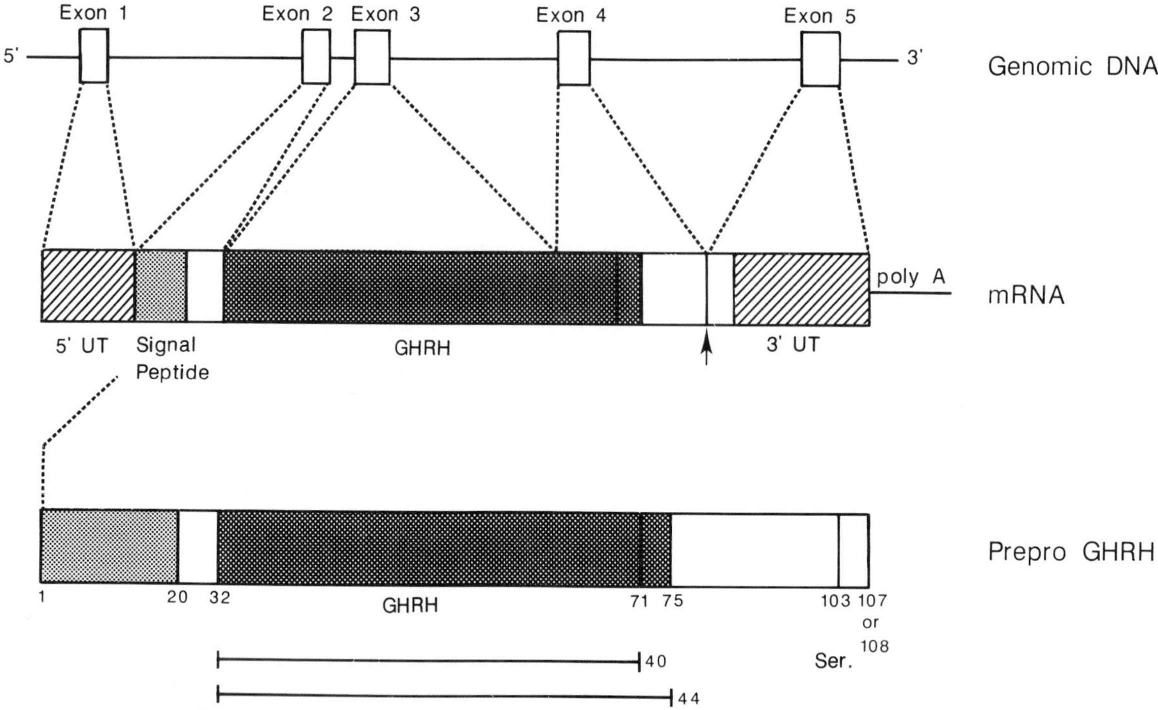

FIGURE 7-19. Schematic diagram of the structures of the GHRH gene, mRNA, and precursor peptide. The gene codes for two mRNAs which differ slightly in the splice site of the fifth exon (denoted by the arrow in the mRNA structure), resulting in two GHRH precursors of 107 and 108 amino acids, respectively, that vary in regard to the presence or absence of a serine at position 103. Both $GHRH_{1-40}$ and $GHRH_{1-44}$ are generated from the precursor. 5' UT = 5' untranslated region; 3' UT = 3' untranslated region.

that occur with each spontaneous GHRH-mediated episodic surge may serve to stimulate somatostatin release, contributing to the trough of GH that follows the surge.[261] Thus, this GH "autoregulation" may prevent somatotroph densensitization.[262] In humans, GH administered acutely can block the GHRH-induced rise of GH.[23] IGF-I is also important, as documented by the high circulating GH levels that occur in IGF-I-deficient states, such as Laron dwarfism (see Chap. 8), renal insufficiency, and cirrhosis.[24] Interactions between GHRH and somatostatin neurons within the hypothalamus have been documented in the rat, but these interactions have not been established in humans. GH short-loop negative feedback may have additional clinical importance in that children who are GH-deficient and receive exogenous GH may develop hypothyrotropic hypothyroidism with a blunting of the TSH response to TRH.[262] It was hypothesized that this was due to an increase in hypothalamic somatostatin generation with subsequent inhibition of TSH secretion, but later studies found a normal TSH response to TRH with short-term GH infusions in normal humans.[263] However, it is likely that GH is considerably more sensitive to the inhibitory effects of somatostatin compared to TSH[162,174] so that small acute changes in somatostatin may have differential effects but long-term changes may have effects on both hormones.

In addition to these negative effects of GH and IGF-I on GHRH secretion, other factors influence GHRH secretion. Adrenergic α_2 receptors and serotonin activate GHRH and GH secretion,[264] but GABA inhibits GHRH secretion.[265] Preliminary studies suggest that the transduction mechanisms mediating GHRH secretion include the adenylate cyclase–cAMP system, the phosphoinositide–protein kinase C system, and the transport of calcium through calcium channels.[265]

GHRH has been used clinically as a test to help determine the GH secretory reserve and the site of the defect in patients who are GH-deficient,[266] although the specificity of GHRH testing in this regard has not been fully established. As was mentioned above, GHRH can cause somatic growth in humans when given chronically,[254] but a clear benefit over standard GH therapy in this regard has not been established.

Prolactin Inhibiting Factor

It was found over 35 years ago that the luteotropic properties of the pituitary (caused by PRL) were increased when pituitaries were transplanted to beneath the renal capsule, a site distant from regulation by the hypothalamus, thus demonstrating the predominance of the inhibitory component of hypothalamic regulation of PRL secretion.[267] Subsequent experiments showed initially that hypothalamic extracts suppress PRL secretion from pituitaries in vitro[268] and then that DA can suppress PRL release from pituitaries in vitro.[269] A number of experiments have firmly established that DA is the predominant physiologic prolactin inhibiting factor (PIF), including the demonstration that the concentration of DA found in the pituitary stalk plasma is sufficient to decrease PRL levels in rats and is 5 to 10 times higher than levels found in peripheral plasma[270] and the finding that stimuli which result in an acute release of PRL usually also result in an acute decrease in portal vessel DA levels.[271] However, in many experiments it has been found that the PRL increase obtained by simply reducing DA is considerably lower than the elevation of PRL achieved by means of simultaneous stimulation by a substance with PRL-releasing activity [PRL releasing factor (PRF)]; similarly, the PRL level achieved with stimulation by a PRF simultaneously with the reduction in DA is usually greater than that achieved by a PRF alone.[272,273] It is likely that in most physiologic circumstances that cause a PRL rise, such as lactation, there is a simultaneous fall in DA along with a rise in a PRF, such as VIP.[274]

Although much of the direct evidence of DA in hypothalamic-pituitary portal vessels and of the effects of DA on PRL release in vitro are derived from animals, it is clear that DA is the primary PIF in humans as well. Infusion of DA causes a rapid suppression of basal PRL levels that can be reversed by metoclopramide, a DA receptor blocker.[275] Dopamine also blocks the increase in PRL release induced by such stimuli as hypoglycemia,[276] arginine,[277] and TRH.[278] Studies with low-dose DA infusions in humans have shown that DA blood concentrations similar to those found in rat and monkey hypothalamic-pituitary portal blood[270,279] are able to suppress PRL secretion.[280] Blockade of endogenous DA receptors by a variety of drugs, including phenothiazines, butyrophenones, metoclopramide, and domperidone, causes a rise in PRL.[281]

The axons responsible for the release of DA into the median eminence originate in perikarya in the dorsomedial portion of the arcuate nucleus and the inferior portion of the ventromedial nucleus of the hypothalamus.[26,282] This pathway is known as the tuberoinfundibular DA (TIDA) pathway, and DA axon terminals constitute about a third of all axon terminals in the zona externa of the median eminence.[282] Some TIDA neurons do not terminate in the median eminence but project to the posterior and intermediate lobes.[282]

The DA that traverses the TIDA pathway binds to DA D_2 receptors[283] on the lactotroph cell membrane.[284] Activation of this receptor results in (1) inhibition of adenyl cyclase with lowered intracellular cAMP levels, (2) inhibition of phosphoinositide metabolism, and (3) decreased intracellular calcium mobilization and inhibition of calcium transport through calcium channels. It has recently been proposed that these different actions of DA may be mediated by multiple similar D_2 receptors that are produced by alternative RNA splicing.[285]

A number of experiments have suggested that there may be other peptide PIFs in addition to DA. The primary candidate for this putative PIF appears to be GAP, the 56-amino acid portion of the precursor to GnRH that was discussed above. In initial studies, GAP was found to have a potency on a molar basis four times that of DA with respect to PIF activity.[128] Immunization of rabbits against GAP results in neutralization of endogenous GAP and a rise in basal PRL levels.[128] GAP_{1-13} also has minimal PRL-lowering properties in the rat.[129] Studies in sheep show no effect of GAP on either gonadotropin or PRL secretion.[286] Limited in vitro studies of GAP_{1-13} in baboon and human pituitary cell cultures have shown no PRL inhibitory effect.[130,287] Whether GAP or a metabolic product is the peptidergic PIF long postulated to exist remains to be determined, and its physiologic importance in PRL regulation in humans has not been defined.

Another potential candidate for PIF activity is GABA. GABA and muscimol, a GABA receptor agonist, have been shown to inhibit PRL synthesis and release in vitro in rats, but blockade of this inhibition with GABA receptor antagonists such as picrotoxin and bicuculline has given variable results.[288,289] A tuberoinfundibular GABAergic system has been described, with perikarya located in the arcuate nucleus and nerve endings demonstrated in the median eminence.[290] GABA is also present in portal blood.[291]

Studies of the GABA system in humans have yielded conflicting results in studies with widely differing experimental designs. Bioactive metabolites of GABA, such as γ-hydroxybutyric acid and γ-amino-β-hydroxybutyric acid and muscimol, cause modest increases in PRL levels when injected into humans.[292,293] However, GABA itself causes a modest decrease in PRL levels when given to humans for several days,[294] and activation of the endogenous GABAergic system with sodium valproate causes a suppression in the PRL rise induced by mechanical breast stimulation in puerperal women.[295] The physiologic role of GABA, like that of GAP, remains to be fully elucidated in humans as well as in various animal species.

Prolactin Releasing Factor

The role of TRH as a PRF is discussed extensively above. A number of other peptides have also been shown to have PRF activity in a variety of experimental situations. VIP stimulates PRL release.[296] VIP neuronal perikarya are present in the parvocellular region of the paraventricular nucleus and suprachiasmatic nucleus with axons terminating in the external zone of the median eminence.[297] Its effects are selective for PRL and additive to TRH[298] at concentrations found in hypothalamic-pituitary portal blood.[299] In addition to stimulating PRL release, VIP increases pituitary PRL mRNA content and PRL synthesis.[300] In conditions of increased PRL synthesis, such as lactation, hypothalamic VIP mRNA levels are also increased.[301] In addition to these studies in rats, intravenously administered VIP has been shown to increase PRL levels in humans[302] at serum levels similar to those demonstrated in rat portal blood.

A number of experiments have been performed using passive immunoneutralization techniques to determine the physiologic role of VIP as a PRF. Anti-VIP antisera administered to rats have been shown to inhibit partially the PRL responses to suckling, ether-induced stress,[274] and estrogen administration[303] and to suppress PRL pulsatile secretion in dopamine receptor–blocked rats.[304]

Part of the 20-kDa 170-amino acid VIP precursor is another similarly sized peptide known as peptide histidine methionine (PHM).[305] VIP has 28 amino acid residues, and PHM has 27. The terminal amino acid in the porcine equivalent of PHM is isoleucine, and therefore the peptide of porcine origin is known as PHI. PHM and VIP colocalize in the hypothalamus and median eminence.[306] Interestingly, PHI is of similar potency to VIP in releasing PRL from rat pituitaries in vitro and in vivo.[307] Furthermore, passive immunoneutralization with anti-PHI plus anti-VIP antisera causes a greater suppression of the PRL responses to the serotonin precursor 5-hydroxytryptophan and ether than does either anti-PHI or anti-VIP antiserum alone.[308] PHM given to humans has caused increases in PRL levels in some experiments[306] but not in others.[302] Further complicating the role of VIP as a PRF is the finding that VIP is actually synthesized by anterior pituitary tissue.[38] Antisera to VIP inhibit basal PRL secretion from dispersed pituitary cells in vitro,[309] suggesting a local "autocrine" role for VIP in PRL regulation within the pituitary. The physiologic role of VIP as a PRF appears to be warranted by the experimental data. The precise roles of VIP vs. PHM and hypothalamic VIP vs. pituitary VIP are not clear. How VIP and PHM interact with other PRFs such as TRH are additional areas requiring clarification. A number of other peptides have PRF activity in various experimental situations, including GHRH, the opioid peptides, oxytocin, vasopressin, GnRH, angiotensin II, neurotensin, substance P, cholecystokinin, secretin, gastrin, bombesin, epidermal growth factor, fibroblast growth factor, and galanin. However, their importance in regulating PRL in humans has not been established.

NEUROTRANSMITTERS

Neurotransmitters may be simple amino acids, bioamines, or peptides. As was noted previously, neurotransmitters may function differently in the synapses of one neuron compared with another, depending on the stage of activity of the cell, other neural inputs, and other hormonal influences, including the feedback effects of target hormones. For example, the inhibitory effect of dopamine on pituitary lactotrophs may be considerably altered by the estrogen milieu at that particular point in time; a high estrogen state, such as pregnancy, causes a considerable blunting of this inhibition. Furthermore, as can be seen from the previous discussions about the nature of neuron-neuron interactions and the characteristics of the specific hypophysiotropic hormones, various neurotransmitters can affect pituitary hormone secretion by direct action at the pituitary and indirect action through modulation of the actions of the various hypophysiotropic hormones, which themselves may be stimulatory or inhibitory. Thus, pituitary hormone secretion reflects the integration of all these inputs.

Biosynthesis and Metabolism of Bioaminergic Neurotransmitters

Bioaminergic neurotransmitters are synthesized within the neuronal perikarya. After initial uptake of specific amino acid precursors, enzymatic synthesis occurs and the monoamines are stored in neurosecretory granules (Fig. 7-2). Upon release into the synapse after neuronal depolarization, the neurotransmitter either binds to the specific receptor on the postsynaptic neuron or is inactivated by degradation or uptake into neuronal tissue. The specific biochemical steps for the synthesis and degradation of the major bioaminergic neurotransmitters are shown in Fig. 7-20.

Anatomic Pathways of Bioaminergic Neurotransmitters

Dopamine

As was discussed above, TIDA has its origins in the arcuate and ventromedial nuclei, with axons projecting inferiorly to the median eminence. Some of these axons also project to the intermediate and posterior lobes.[282,310] It is important to stress that the tuberoinfundibular dopaminergic system so impor-

1. Acetylcholine

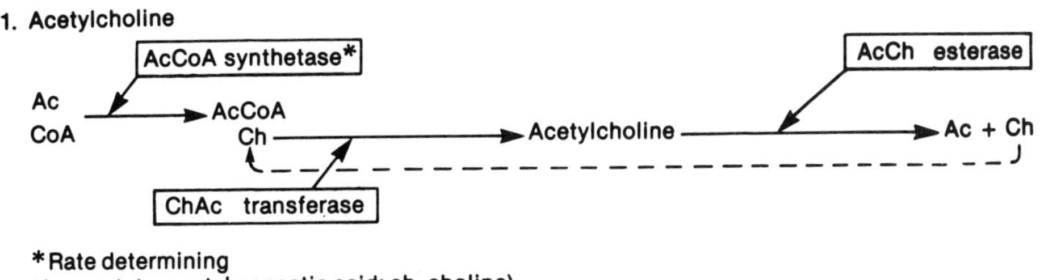

*Rate determining
(Ac, acetate, acetyl or acetic acid; ch, choline)

2. Serotonin

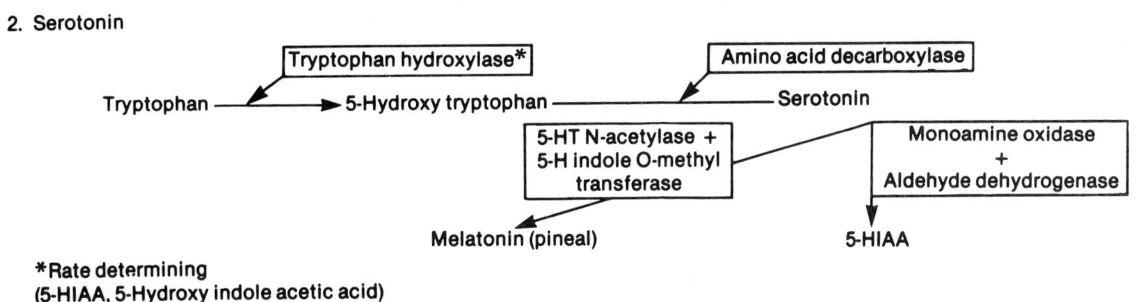

*Rate determining
(5-HIAA, 5-Hydroxy indole acetic acid)

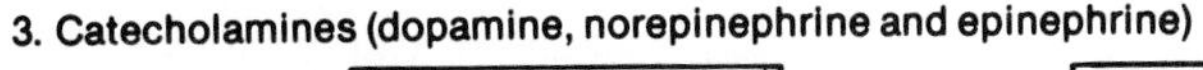

3. Catecholamines (dopamine, norepinephrine and epinephrine)

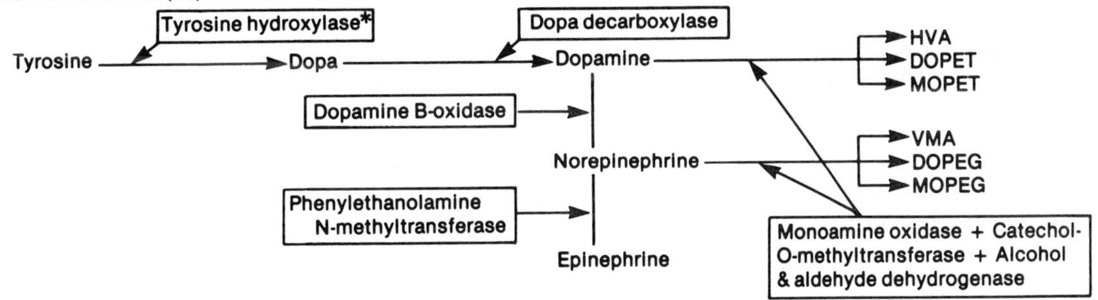

*Rate determining
(HVA, 4-Hydroxy 3-methoxyphenylacetic acid; DOPET, 3, 4 Dihydroxyphenylethanol; MOPET, 4-Hydroxy 3-methoxyphenylethanol; VMA, 4-Hydroxy 3-methoxy D-mandelic acid; DOPEG, 3, 4 Dihydroxyphenylglycol; MOPEG, 4-Hydroxy 3-methoxyphenylglycol)

4. Amino acids

a. γ-Amino butyric acid and glutamine

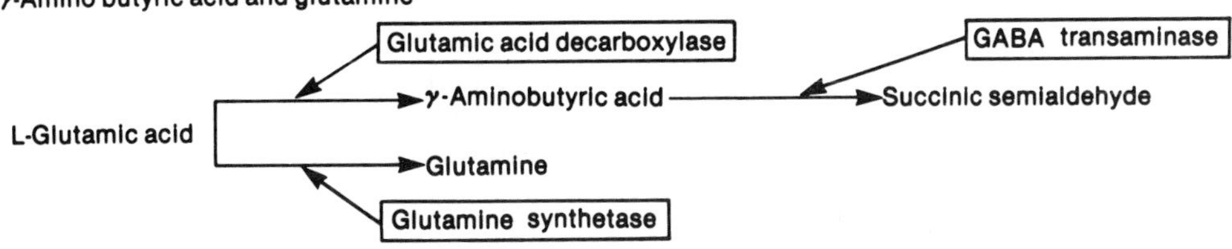

b. Miscellaneous amino acids, peptides and related compounds
(Glycine, taurine, histamine, substance P. endorphins, and vasopressin)

FIGURE 7-20. Neurotransmitters in the mammalian brain and their associated enzymes and major brain metabolites. *(From Samorajski T, J Am Geriatr Soc 25:337, 1977.)*

tant for neuroendocrine regulation is quite separate from the nigrostriatal (mesolimbic) dopaminergic system involved in Parkinson's disease and the cortical (mesocortical) dopaminergic system that has been postulated to be involved in schizophrenia. Nonetheless, medications which are dopaminergic agonists and antagonists may affect all these systems, causing unwanted side effects in one and therapeutic effects in another. For example, dopamine receptor blockers such as the phenothiazines, which may be quite beneficial in the treatment of the psychosis of schizophrenia, commonly block the inhibitory effect of dopamine of PRL, resulting in hyperprolactinemia.

Norepinephrine

Hypothalamic norepinephrine originates in specific brainstem regions: the locus ceruleus, the ventrolateral medulla, and the dorsal vagal complex, which includes the nucleus of the solitary tract.[310,311] Axons project to the hypothalamus via the ventral noradrenergic bundle.[310,311] Because the nucleus of the solitary tract is the major recipient of primary visceral afferent information carried by the vagus and glossopharyngeal nerves, this noradrenergic projection to the hypothalamus is important in the coupling of neuroendocrine and autonomic responses to visceral stimuli.[311] All hypothalamic nuclei contain noradrenergic fibers and terminals, especially the paraventricular and supraoptic nuclei.[311] However, noradrenergic fibers project only to the internal zone, not the external zone, of the median eminence.[312] Thus, noradrenergic neurons serve an integrative function, coupling neuroendocrine with autonomic systems rather than playing a direct role at the pituitary level.

Epinephrine

The cells of origin of adrenergic neural fibers are located primarily in the lateral reticular nucleus of the medulla and the nucleus of the solitary tract,[312] although some are also located within the hypothalamus.[310] They project to the dorsomedial and arcuate nuclei and the medial parvocellular portion of the paraventricular nucleus.[312] Few fibers are found in the external zone of the median eminence,[312] but there is some evidence that there is direct adrenergic influence on the pituitary, including the presence of $beta_2$-adrenergic receptors of pituitary cell membranes[313] and a stimulatory effect of epinephrine on GH secretion from pituitary cell cultures.[314]

Serotonin

Most serotoninergic neuronal perikarya are in the dorsal and median raphe nuclei of the pons and upper medulla, and their axons project forward to the hypothalamus and other limbic and cortical areas.[315] The hypothalamic area most heavily innervated with serotoninergic fibers is the suprachiasmatic nucleus, suggesting a role for serotonin in the generation of circadian rhythms.[315] Since hypothalamic serotonin is reduced by only 60 percent when all afferent nerve fibers are cut, it is likely that a considerable amount of this neurotransmitter is also generated within the hypothalamus, although the specific sources are not known.[315] Serotonin is also present within the anterior pituitary.[316] The pituitary contains tryptophan hydroxylase, the rate-limiting enzyme in serotonin synthesis,[316] suggesting in situ synthesis. High affinity S_2 serotonin receptors are present in the anterior pituitary,[317] and uptake of labeled serotonin has been demonstrated.[318] The results of direct tests of the effects of serotonin on pituitary hormone release, however, have been conflicting.

Acetylcholine

Acetylcholine, acetylcholinesterase, and choline acyltransferase are all present in the hypothalamus, with the highest concentrations occurring in the median eminence.[312] However, the neuronal perikarya and their fiber distribution within the hypothalamus are not known.[319] Acetylcholine has also been found within the pituitary,[320] but its functional significance there is uncertain.

γ-Aminobutyric Acid

Recent studies suggest that GABA is numerically the dominant neurotransmitter in the hypothalamus, being present in half of all synapses.[321] This fact alone emphasizes the importance of inhibitory circuits in neuroendocrine regulation, as GABA can be thought of primarily as an inhibitory neurotransmitter. GABA fibers are widely distributed throughout the hypothalamus and are also present in the median eminence and the posterior pituitary.[290] GABA neuronal perikarya are located primarily in the arcuate nucleus and the posterior hypothalamus, although small numbers are found in many other areas of the hypothalamus.[290] The posterior hypothalamic GABAergic neurons also project to the cortex.[322] Short GABAergic interneurons also exist within all brain areas and act locally as inhibitors within neural circuits unrelated to projections from the hypothalamus.[323]

Histamine

Histamine neuronal perikarya are present in the posterior hypothalamic region, and axons project to almost all the nuclei of the hypothalamus as well as the median eminence.[324] Both H_1 and H_2 receptors are present in the brain,[325] and agonists and antagonists of these receptors can alter hormone secretion in some circumstances.

Neuropharmacology of Bioaminergic Neurotransmitters

Bioaminergic neurotransmitters can affect pituitary hormone secretion via direct action on the pituitary or indirectly via effects on the releasing and inhibiting factors that affect that hormone's secretion. An example of the complexity of this interaction is provided by an examination of the components that result in dopamine stimulating GH secretion: (1) Dopamine appears to inhibit somatostatin secretion in indirect experiments in humans,[325] (2) the GH rise induced by L-dopa is accompanied by increased GHRH levels in plasma, implying that GHRH is the intermediary,[326] (3) dopamine causes an increase in somatostatin release and a decrease in GHRH release from rat hypothalamic slices in vitro,[327] (4) dopamine alone stimulates GH secretion in pituitary cell cultures,[328] and (5) dopamine inhibits the GH response to GHRH in pituitary cell cultures.[329] Table 7-3 lists the overall composite effects of the bioaminergic neurotransmitters on the various pituitary hormones as generally understood. However, depending on the hormonal status and metabolic milieu at any point in time, other effects can be seen. Furthermore, pharmacologic agents which are said to be specific for one class of effects on bioamines rarely are so and, depending on the hormonal and metabolic status, may have different effects at different times (Fig. 7-21).

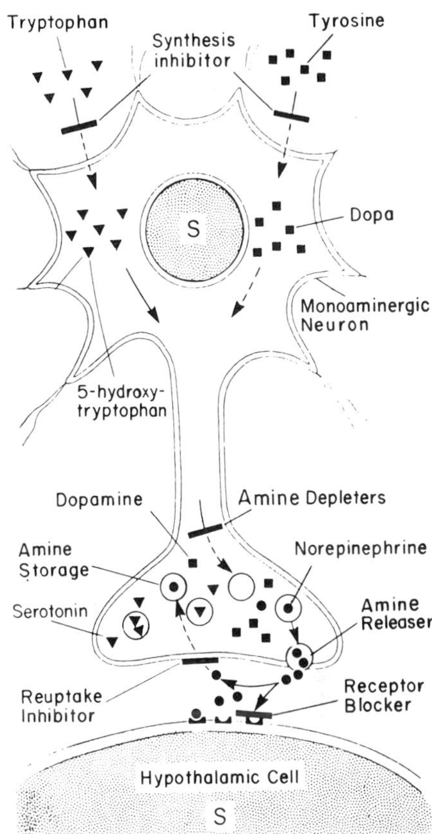

FIGURE 7-21. Schematic showing sites and modes of actions of various categories of drugs (including many agents used therapeutically) that alter neurotransmitter function. Depending on a particular drug's mode of action, the result is a net increase or decrease in the secretion of a releasing or inhibiting factor by the hypothalamic cell. *(Modified from Frohman L, Hosp Pract 10:54, 1975.)*

Amino Acid Neurotransmitters

Glutamate functions as an excitatory neurotransmitter in synapses throughout the mediobasal hypothalamus, including the magnocellular and parvocellular regions of the paraventricular nucleus and the supraoptic and arcuate nuclei.[329] Glutamate and aspartate are also present in the hippocampus, cerebellum, auditory nerve, and spinal cord.[323] Glycine functions as an inhibitory neurotransmitter in the brainstem, the spinal cord, and possibly the hypothalamus.[323] Despite the widespread presence of amino acids as neurotransmitters, little is known about their possible roles in neuroendocrine regulation.

Neuropeptides

Vasoactive Intestinal Peptide

VIP is synthesized by hypothalamic and cerebrocortical tissue[330] and the pituitary[38] and can be found throughout the cortex, amygdala, striatum, hippocampus, midbrain, spinal cord, and sympathetic ganglia and in autonomic nerves such as the vagus.[331] In addition to its effects as a PRF, it stimulates the release of ACTH and GH and has variable effects on LH and FSH, though it has no effect on TSH secretion.[331,332] In other areas of the brain, VIP is excitatory, causing cerebrovascular vasodilatation and stimulating adenylate cyclase.[331,332]

TABLE 7-3 Neurotransmitter Regulation of Pituitary Hormone Secretion

Neurotransmitter	GH	PRL	LH/FSH	TSH	ACTH
Norepinephrine	↑	0	↑	↑	↑↓
Dopamine	↑	↓	↓	↓	↓?
Serotonin	↑	↑	↓?	↑↓	↑
GABA	↑	↓	↑	0	↓
Histamine	0	↑	↑	↑	↑
Acetylcholine	↑	↑↓	↑	0	↑

↑ = increase; ↓ = decrease; 0 = no effect; ↑↓ = increase or decrease in different circumstances.

Substance P

Substance P–containing nerve terminals are abundant in the substantia nigra, amygdala, and hypothalamus, including the median eminence, but their site of origin is not known.[333] Little is present in the cortex or cerebellum.[333] Substance P stimulates PRL release in some experimental situations but not in others[334,335] and inhibits CRF- or vasopressin-stimulated but not basal ACTH release.[336] Its effects on TSH and gonadotropin secretion are not known. The major known physiologic action of substance P is as a sensory neurotransmitter for pain in peripheral nerves and in the spinal cord, and some studies suggest a role in stimulating behavioral arousal.[333] Depletion of substance P with capsaicin, the irritant isolated from hot peppers, results in decreased pain, and this substance has been used therapeutically to treat painful diabetic peripheral neuropathy with varying success.[337]

Neurotensin

Neurotensin causes vasodilation, hypotension, and increased vascular permeability after systemic injection.[338] Within the brain, the highest concentrations are in the hypothalamus, thalamus, preoptic area, interpeduncular nucleus, and brainstem, with little in the cortex or cerebellum.[339] However, most neurotensin is located in the endocrine cells of the GI tract mucosa.[338] In experimental studies, hormonal effects vary with variations in the method of administration. For example, intracerebroventricular administration results in increased somatostatin in portal blood and decreased secretion of GH and PRL, but peripheral injection increases the secretion of GH and PRI.[340] In contrast to these results in rats, intravenous administration of neurotensin to humans has no effect on PRL, GH, LH, or TSH levels.[341] Other central effects of neurotensin include hypothermia, antinociception, and antidopaminergic activity.[338] An important peripheral hormonal effect of neurotensin is its ability to increase glucagon secretion, causing hyperglycemia.[338]

Renin-Angiotensin System

Renin, angiotensinogen, and angiotensin converting enzyme (ACE) are present in the thalamus, basal ganglia, cortex, cerebellum, hypothalamus, median eminence, and pituitary.[342] Renin and angiotensinogen mRNAs have been found in some of these areas, implying local synthesis.[342] In situ hybridization studies have shown that angiotensinogen mRNA is present in the magnocellular neurons of the hypothalamic paraventricular nucleus.[343] In the human pituitary, renin, ACE, and angiotensinogen have been detected in normal lactrotroph cells and in PRL-secreting adenomas.[344] However, when the generation of endogenous angiotensin II is blocked in humans by inhibition of ACE with enalapril, basal levels of PRL, GH, and ACTH and the PRL and TSH rises induced by TRH and metoclopramide are unchanged, and the PRL response to hypoglycemia is decreased only minimally.[345,346] It is therefore unlikely that the endogenous renin-angiotensin system of the hypothalamus and pituitary has significant physiologic effects on pituitary hormone regulation in humans. Angiotensin has also been found in various experimental preparations to have pressor effects, thirst-stimulating capabilities, and vasopressin-releasing properties,[347] but its role in these effects in humans is not well understood.

Cholecystokinin

Cholecystokinin is present in the cortex, thalamus, basal ganglia, and hypothalamus. It increases PRL release in vitro in the rat[298,348] but not from human pituitary cultures.[298] Intravenous administration in rats has provided both positive[348] and negative results[349] with respect to PRL stimulation. Intracerebroventricular cholecystokinin results in a marked PRL release that can be antagonized with antisera to VIP,[349] implying that its action may require the activation of VIPergic systems. The reasons for these varying results and their relevance to humans are unknown. Cholecystokinin has also been implicated in causing satiety, possibly by augmenting vagal afferent neural signals, and studies in humans have shown that intravenous infusions of cholecystokinin result in decreased eating.[350]

Endogenous Opioid Peptides

In the mid-1970s, the discovery of the opiate receptors and the fact that some of the endogenous opioid peptide ligands for those receptors are present within the precursor to ACTH, POMC, prompted widespread speculation about the importance of this system in neuroendocrine regulation as well as the interactions of neuroendocrinology, mental illness, and opiate addiction. Most data now suggest, however, at most a modest role for the endogenous opioid peptides in neuroendocrine regulation.[351]

There are three major opioid peptide receptors and three major groups of opioid peptides, but the correspondence is not one for one. The μ receptor mediates most of the endocrine effects and analgesia, morphine is its prototypic agonist, and naloxone is its prototypic antagonist. The primary peptide ligand for the μ receptor is β-endorphin, which is derived from POMC, although β-endorphin also binds to the δ receptor and the enkephalins also can bind to the μ receptor. The δ receptor mediates behavioral, analgesic, and some endocrine effects and has as its primary peptide ligands met- and leu-enkephalins, which are derived from proenkephalin A. It is much less well blocked by naloxone than is the μ receptor. The κ receptor mediates sedation and ataxia and binds primarily dynorphin and the neoendorphins, which are derived from proenkephalin B (prodynorphin). The importance of the other opioid receptors, σ and ϵ, is not clear.

The β-endorphin opioid system has been the most intensively studied neuroendocrinologically because of the derivation of β-endorphin from POMC. POMC is a 31,000-dalton precursor peptide which harbors within it ACTH, β-lipotropin (β-LPH), and β-endorphin; the last corresponds to the C-terminal 31 amino acids of β-lipotropin (Fig. 7-22). POMC undergoes tissue-specific posttranslational processing: In the anterior pituitary, the major cleavage products are β-LPH and ACTH, with a significant proportion

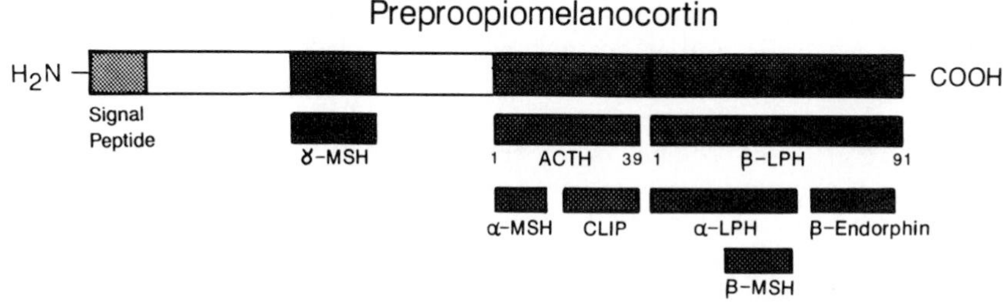

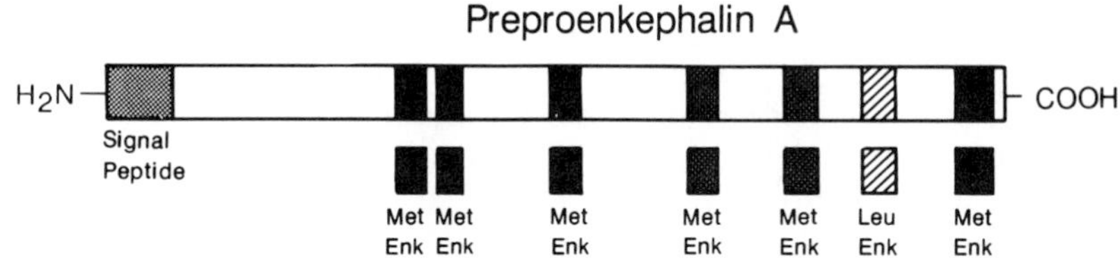

Preproenkephalin B
(Preprodynorphin)
H2N
COOH
Signal Peptide
α-neoendorphin
Dynorphin 1-32
β-neoendorphin
Dynorphin 1-17
Rimorphin
Dynorphin 1-8

FIGURE 7-22. Structures of the precursors of the endogenous opioid peptides. Prepro-opiomelanocortin (POMC) generates several peptides, including β-lipotropin (β-LPH), β-endorphin, ACTH, α-MSH, β-MSH, γ-MSH and corticotropin-like intermediate lobe peptide (CLIP). Preproenkephalin A generates six copies of methionine enkephalin (met-enk) and one copy of leucine enkephalin (leu-enk). Preproenkephalin B (preprodynorphin) generates α- and β-neoendorphins; dynorphins 108, 1–17, and 1–32; and rimorphin.

of β-LPH being further processed to β-endorphin, but in the pituitary intermediate lobe, the major products are α-MSH, corticotropin-like intermediate peptide (CLIP), β-endorphin, and γ-LPH.[352] Brain POMC, however, is processed primarily to β-endorphin, γ-LPH, and ACTH, with most of the ACTH being further processed to CLIP and α-MSH.

All neuronal perikarya containing POMC-derived peptides are located in the arcuate nucleus, from which fibers containing β-endorphin and α-MSH project to the median eminence, and the ventromedial, dorsomedial, paraventricular, and periventricular nuclei of the hypothalamus as well as to the amygdala, preoptic area, periaqueductal gray matter, reticular formation, stria terminalis, locus ceruleus, striatum, and hippocampus.[352] The projection to the median eminence results in significant quantities of β-endorphin being found in portal blood.[352] POMC-derived peptides are also found in the placenta, thyroid C cells, pancreas, testes, ovaries, adrenal medulla, gastric antrum, and macrophages.[352] Anterior pituitary β-endorphin is secreted with ACTH after CRH and vasopressin stimulation (see above), but the only factors known to decrease hypothalamic β-endorphin are dopamine and estradiol.[352]

The pentapeptide enkephalins derive from the 28K precursor, proenkephalin A, which contains six copies of the met-enkephalin sequence and one copy of the leu-enkephalin sequence.[353] Other extended cleavage products with biological activity may also exist, and the ratio of met-enkephalin to leu-enkephalin ranges between 5:1 and 10:1 in various places in the brain, possibly representing evidence of differences in tissue-specific cleavage and/or degradation. Neuronal perikarya containing the enkephalins are widely distributed throughout the brain, as are fiber networks.[353,354] Most enkephalinergic neurons are short, having the characteristics of interneurons.[353] Rich enkephalinergenic neural fiber networks can be found in the globus pallidus, amygdala, and midbrain, with specific areas of innervation including the origin of the central noradrenergic system, the locus ceruleus, the origin of the central serotoninergic system, the raphe nuclei, and the origin of the striatal dopaminergic system, the substantia nigra.[354] Enkephalinergic neurons in the magnocellular portion of the paraventricular and supraoptic nuclei project to the posterior pituitary.[354] Within the pituitary, enkephalins have been detected primarily in the posterior pituitary.[353] Enkephalins have also been found in the adrenal medulla, gut, sympathetic ganglia, vagus, and retina.[353]

Dynorphin is a 17-amino acid peptide derived from a 28K precursor called proenkephalin B or prodynorphin. Shorter peptides termed α- and β-neoendorphin, with 10 and 9 amino acids, respectively, have also been isolated.[353] These peptides react almost exclusively with the κ receptor. Dynorphin-containing cells also project from the magnocellular neurons of the paraventricular nucleus to the posterior pituitary. Other tissues containing dynorphin include the gut, lungs, and adrenal medulla.[353]

The μ receptors are located predominantly in the thalamus, hippocampus, periaqueductal gray matter, and neocortex, and the δ receptors are located primarily in the amygdala, nucleus accumbens septi, and hypothalamus.[353] Dynorphin receptors have been localized to the cerebral cortex, the thalamus, and the caudate nucleus.[353] The anterior pituitary itself is poor in opioid receptors, but the hypothalamus is quite rich, and it has been suggested that the effects of opioid peptides on anterior pituitary hormone secretion occur via modulation of hypothalamic bioamines and hypophysiotropic factors.[353,354]

The specific functions of the various opioid peptides and opioid receptors are not completely understood, although evidence links them to a number of bodily functions, including stress, mental illness, narcotic tolerance and dependence, eating, drinking, GI function, learning, memory, cardiovascular responses, respiration, thermoregulation, seizures, brain electric activity, locomotor activity, pregnancy, and neuroimmune activity.[355] More specific functions of neuroendocrine regulation have been documented, however. In general, endogenous opioids have an inhibitory influence on gonadotropin secretion through their action on GnRH secretion, probably by inhibiting noradrenergic neuronal input.[351] Exogenous β-endorphin and enkephalin analogs increase serum GH and PRL levels,[351] but blockade of endogenous opioid pathways with naloxone does not alter basal or stimulated GH and PRL levels.[351,356] Opioids feed back negatively on ACTH and β-endorphin secretion, and naloxone can increase basal and stimulated ACTH levels.[351] Opioids have virtually no effect on TSH secretion.[351] Overall, the effects of the endogenous opioids on normal physiologic regulation of the various pituitary hormones appear to be minimal. It is possible that increased opioid peptidergic tone is present in some states of pathologic gonadotropin dysfunction, but this appears to be somewhat inconsistent.

Other Peptides

Atrial natriuretic peptide (ANP) is a 28-amino acid peptide derived from a 126-amino acid precursor originally isolated from cardiac tissue and found to stimulate renal water and salt excretion, stimulate vasodilation, and inhibit vasopressin and aldosterone secretion (see Chap. 14). Recent studies have found that atrial natriuretic peptide (ANP) or a cleaved derivative is present in a number of areas of rat brain, with the highest concentrations in the hypothalamus and septum.[357] Substantial numbers of neuronal perikarya are found in the parvocellular part of the paraventricular nucleus with projections to the median eminence, but cell bodies and fibers also occur elsewhere in the brain. Central ANP appears to be active in inhibiting thirst and vasopressin and CRH release, and ANP reaching the pituitary may inhibit ACTH release but stimulate gonadotropin release.[357] A related but separate peptide, *brain natriuretic peptide* (BNP), is present at higher concentrations in the brain than ANP but exists at only 2 percent of the concentration of ANP in cardiac atria.[358] Both peptides have equal affinity for the same receptors. Intravenous infusion of BNP causes a suppression of plasma renin activity and aldosterone secretion, with an increase in urinary sodium excretion.[358]

Galanin is a 29-amino acid peptide of the gut and brain, with neuronal perikarya in the supraoptic, paraventricular, and arcuate nuclei of the hypothalami and fiber projections to the medial basal hypothalamus.[359] Galanin releases GH by means of an effect on GHRH in the hypothalamus.[359] Although galanin augments the GH response to GHRH, suggesting an effect on somatostatin in humans,[360] it has no effect on somatostatin secretion from hypothalamic slices.[359] Galanin also inhibits basal and stress-induced ACTH secretion[361] and is localized to corticotroph cells in human pituitaries.[362]

Endothelins are 21-amino acid vasoconstrictor peptides produced by endothelial cells that are also produced by the supraoptic and paraventricular nuclei, with projections to the posterior pituitary.[363] Water deprivation results in a depletion of neurohypophyseal endothelin.[363] Endothelins also stimulate gonadotropin secretion[364] and inhibit PRL secretion[365] from pituitary cell cultures. Another vasoactive neuropeptide, *neuropeptide Y* (NPY), is important in the regulation of central catecholaminergic mechanisms involved in blood pressure and temperature regulation and food intake. NPY axons innervate portions of the parvocellular division of the paraventricular nucleus in contact with TRH-containing neurons,[366] and central NPY administration reduces serum TSH levels.[367] NPY also enhances the LH-releasing effects of GnRH.[368]

THE PINEAL GLAND

Anatomy

The pineal belongs to the family of *circumventricular organs* of the brain that provide a blood-brain barrier–free interface between the brain, the cerebral circulation, and the CSF of the ventricular system; these organs also include the median eminence, the OVLT, the subcommissural organ, the subfornical organ, and the neurohypophysis. Embryologically, the pineal arises as an outgrowth of the roof of the third ventricle and is an epithalamic structure that is still attached to the posterior roof of the third ventricle, between the posterior commissure and the dorsal habenular commissure, sitting on top of and between the superior colliculi.[369] It is derived phylogenetically from photoreceptor cells that were photosensitive and could generate electric activity. However, these properties have been lost in mammals.[369] The arterial supply is via the posterior choroidal arteries, and the venous drainage is via the internal cerebral veins.[369]

After birth, the pineal loses almost all direct neural connections with the brain. Although it has lost photoreceptor activity, it still receives photosensory information through a very indirect route (Fig. 7-23). Light perceived by the retinal photoreceptors is transduced to electric impulses which go to the suprachiasmatic nucleus (SCN) via the retinohypothalamic tract, although some of these impulses reach the SCN by way of the primary optic tract via the lateral geniculate bodies.[369] From the SCN, this information travels to the lateral hypothalamus and then down through the brainstem via the median forebrain bundle and through the intermediolateral column of the cervical spinal cord, eventually reaching the superior cervical ganglion. Postganglionic noradrenergic fibers from the superior cervical ganglion enter the pineal via the nervi conarii.[369] An undetermined amount of neural input may also arise from the habenular and posterior commissures and sympathetic pathways.[369]

FIGURE 7-23. Neural innervation of the mammalian pineal gland. RHT = retinohypothalamic tract; SCN = suprachiasmatic nuclei; MFB = medial forebrain bundle; SCG = superior cervical ganglion. *(Reproduced with permission from Erlich and Apuzzo.[369])*

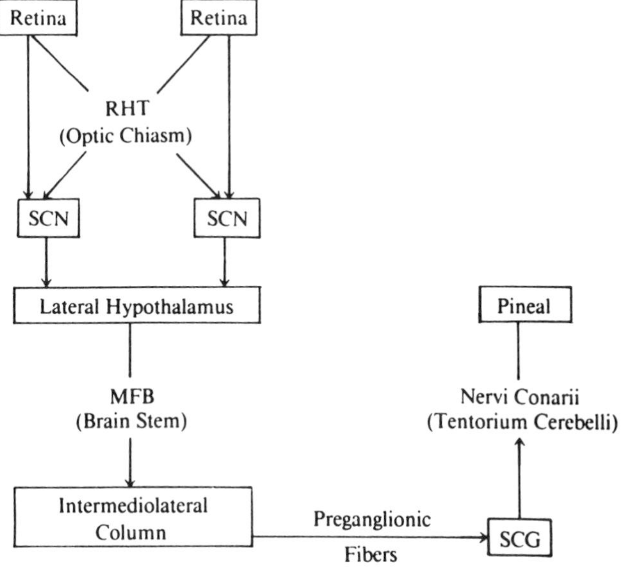

There are two major cell types within the pineal: (1) the parenchymal cell, or pinealocyte, and (2) interstitial cells, which are probably glial. The sympathetic postganglionic nerve fiber terminals end freely in the parenchyma or in the pericapillary spaces rather than in true synapses, so that norepinephrine reaches the pinealocytes by way of diffusion.[369]

Pineal Hormones and Neurotransmitters

Melatonin is the major secretory product of the pineal. It is synthesized from tryptophan through a series of steps, including serotonin (Fig. 7-24). The enzyme *N*-acetyltransferase, which converts serotonin to *N*-acetylserotonin, is the rate-limiting step.[370] The last step—conversion to melatonin—is mediated by hydroxyindole-*O*-methyltransferase. The absence of light, i.e., darkness, rapidly activates the series of neural steps outlined above. The final step is the adrenergic activation of adenylate cyclase in the membranes of the pinealocytes, which causes an increase in *N*-acetyltransferase activity and melatonin synthesis. Melatonin is not stored but is immediately secreted into the blood and possibly also in the CSF, where it crosses into the blood via the choroid plexus.[369,370] Because of this lack of storage and the rapid activation of synthesis, melatonin levels change twofold to 10-fold in blood in synchrony with the dark-light cycle.[370] In humans, increased production of melatonin does not continue throughout the dark cycle but gradually begins to fall over time so that low levels are found by daylight. However, an increase in the duration of the dark period increases the duration of the elevated melatonin levels. The signal that melatonin conveys to other tissues is dependent on both the amplitude and the duration of the melatonin pulse. Furthermore, this signal may change as the dark-light signal changes over days to weeks. In addition, there may be varying sensitivity of organs to melatonin that changes with the dark-light signal.[370]

High-affinity binding sites for melatonin have been described in many tissues of the body, with the highest concentrations occurring in the pituitary, hypothalamus, epididymis, and adrenals.[370] Melatonin has also been localized to the retina, the optic nerve, the SCN, and throughout the GI tract. The primary action of melatonin is antireproductive, although the site of this activity is not certain. Melatonin is able to suppress the LH response to GnRH in pituitary cell cultures, but antigonadotropic effects via modulation of central dopaminergic, serotoninergic, and GABAergic neurotransmission have also been postulated.[370] The exact site of action of melatonin and the importance of melatonin in the human in this regard are not known with certainty.[370] Although increased nocturnal melatonin levels have been observed in patients with hypothalamic amen-

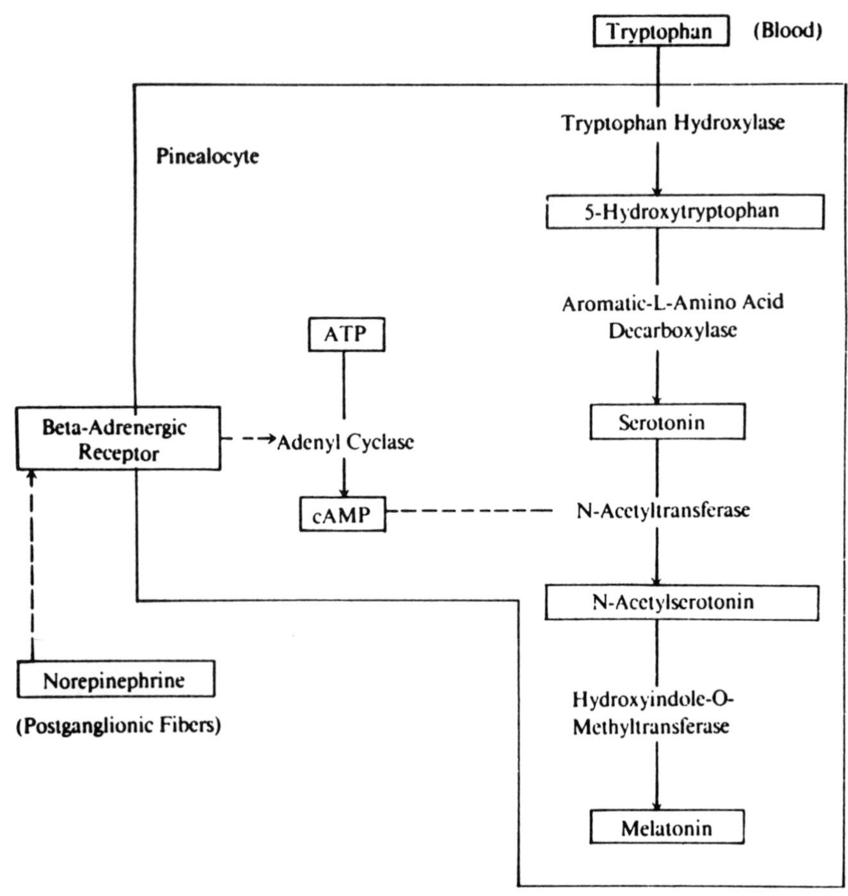

FIGURE 7-24. Stages of melatonin synthesis. ATP = adenosine triphosphate; cAMP = cyclic adenosine 3',5'-monophosphate. *(Reproduced with permission from Erlich and Apuzzo.[369])*

orrhea, anorexia nervosa, delayed puberty, stress, and excessive exercise and decreased melatonin levels have been found in some patients with depression, schizophrenia, manic-depressive illness, and delayed sleep phase syndrome, the importance of melatonin changes in these disorders has not been established.[370]

Other nonmelatonin pineal substances have also been postulated to be of importance in regulating the reproductive axis, including vasotocin, a nonapeptide which differs from vasopressin in that isoleucine is substituted for phenylalanine and differs from oxytocin in that arginine is substituted for leucine. However, none of these other substances have been proved to have more effects on reproduction or other endocrine function than does melatonin.[371] Somatostatin, TRH, and GnRH are also present in the pineal, but there is no evidence for their synthesis there and their functions there are unknown.

Melatonin and the pineal have also been investigated for other neuroendocrine activities. Although melatonin inhibits glucocorticoid secretion at the hypothalamic/pituitary and adrenal levels, GH secretion, and TSH secretion,[371] it is not clear that melatonin is significant in this regard in humans. The effects of melatonin and the pineal on PRL secretion have been quite variable in animal models, although oral melatonin has been shown to cause an increase in PRL levels.[372]

Pineal and Biological Rhythms

The retinal-SCN-pineal link probably serves as the primary mechanism by which light-dark cycles synchronize the reproductive axis on both a short-term and a long-term basis.[373] Variations in exposure to light result in variations in the amount, duration, and phase of the daily melatonin signal, which then alters other functions, especially reproduction; on a long-term basis, this can coordinate seasonal breeding cycles.[373] In animals, other physiologic changes may also be similarly coordinated, such as changes in body weight and coat color.[373] Experimental alteration of the melatonin signal by means of pinealectomy, superior cervical ganglionectomy, or implantation of melatonin constant-release capsules results in a loss of synchronization of reproductive function with the environment. The timing of puberty may also be affected. In animals blinded from birth, there is a delay in the onset of puberty.[374] In humans, one study suggested that the onset of menarche is actually earlier in blind women,[375] but this was not confirmed in another study.[376] Although other studies have shown a modest decrease in serum cortisol and urinary 17-ketosteroid levels in blind women[377] but no changes in testosterone or gonadotropins in blind men,[378] studies with newer methods of documenting gonadal function, such as gonadotropin pulse analysis, have not been performed.

CNS RHYTHMS AND NEUROENDOCRINE FUNCTION

Pituitary hormones are secreted in a pulsatile fashion, with a number of rhythms superimposed. When samples are obtained every 1 to 5 min, frequent pulses of secretion may be detected using computerized algorithms which discriminate secretory pulses that exceed a threshold related to measurement error.[98] Critical to the interpretation of such pulse analyses are the necessity of sampling frequently enough[155] and the use of a hormone assay with sufficient sensitivity to eliminate "undetectable" samples. As has been demonstrated for GH, conventional assays with a lower limit of sensitivity of about 0.5 ng/ml reveal only 4 to 6 pulses of GH per day, whereas an assay with a sensitivity of 10 pg/ml reveals 12 to 14 pulses of GH per day.[379] With sensitive assays and frequent sampling, most analyses reveal that virtually all the hormone is released with each secretory burst and that almost none is released "tonically" between secretory bursts.[380] The actual sustained level of hormone achieved is dependent on the amplitude of the secretory burst, the frequency of the secretory bursts, and the metabolic clearance rate of the hormone. The pulse amplitude of a pituitary hormone reflects the amount of releasing hormone as well as factors that may alter the cell's responsivity to that releasing hormone. Thus, the amplitude can be altered by the presence of inhibitory factors (e.g., GHRH vs. somatostatin), nutritional factors, feedback effects of target organ hormones, and prior stimulation that might have depleted a readily releasable pool of hormone.[380] The frequency is generally governed by the frequency of release of the hypophysiotropic factor, which is regulated by the hypothalamic pulse generator system (see below).

The pituitary appears to have an intrinsic rhythm of small amplitude with a frequency of every 2 to 10 min.[381] Such a rhythm can be discerned from studies in which pituitaries are placed in culture and frequent samples are obtained with a flow-through system.[381] Superimposed on this intrinsic rhythm is the rhythm that is due to the pulsatile release of hypophysiotropic releasing factors, with or without the withdrawal of a corresponding inhibiting factor. For LH, the pulses that are detected every 20 to 25 min have a 1:1 correspondence with GnRH released by the hypothalamus, as determined by simultaneous sampling from portal and peripheral vessels.[100–102] By contrast, the pulses of GH, at least in the rat and probably in the human, are due to an increase in GHRH which often coincides with a decrease in somatostatin.[167,168] Rhythms which are shorter than a day are referred to as *ultradian* rhythms.

The next layer of rhythmicity is the *circadian* rhythm, i.e., rhythms with approximately 24-h periodicity. These rhythms are usually synchronized with the 24-h period by a periodic environmental cue, such as the dark/light cycle. This external cue has been referred to as a *zeitgeber* (time giver). The SCN appears to be important in many mammals, including humans, as an "internal clock" which functions as a circadian pacemaker.[28] Experiments in which the SCN is ablated result in a loss of circadian rhythms.[28] The SCN has extensive projections to and receives projections from multiple hypothalamic nuclei involved in hypophysiotropic hormone production. The SCN will give an approximate 24-h rhythm without the influence of a zeitgeber, but it may vary as much as 3 h from the 24-h periodicity. To maintain a 24-h periodicity, it must synchronize with the zeitgeber. This involves the transmission of light-induced electrical impulses from the retina to the SCN via the retinohypothalamic tract and the transmission of electrical impulses from the SCN to the pineal and then conversion of those impulses into hormonal signals (Fig. 7-23) (see the previous section). As discussed below, all the pituitary hormones have circadian rhythms, but the methods by which increases and decreases in hormone levels occur differ. The circadian increase in all hormone levels is caused by an increase in the amplitude of the secretory pulses; however, for TSH and GH there is also an increase in the frequency of secretory pulses, though this is not true for ACTH, PRL, or LH.[380]

The zeitgeber for a rhythm with a periodicity longer than 24 h, i.e., an *infradian* rhythm, may be the gravitational influence of the moon, which gives rise to a menstrual cycle of approximately the duration of the moon rotating around the earth. Longer-term cycles include responses to seasonal changes such as hibernation and breeding cycles, the timing of the onset of puberty, and perhaps death. Obviously, these rhythms operate differently in different species, and humans may be less tied to these rhythms for some bodily functions than are lower species. Humans have no specific breeding season, for example. However, the menstrual cycle clearly is a monthly rhythm, and the pituitary hormones generally have a well-defined circadian rhythm.

A number of factors may influence circadian and infradian rhythms. One of the most important is the sleep-wake cycle. GH, TSH, PRL, pubertal LH, and ACTH secretion are all entrained more to the sleep-wake cycle than to the dark-light cycle (Fig. 7-25). Each has an increase and a maximal level that occur

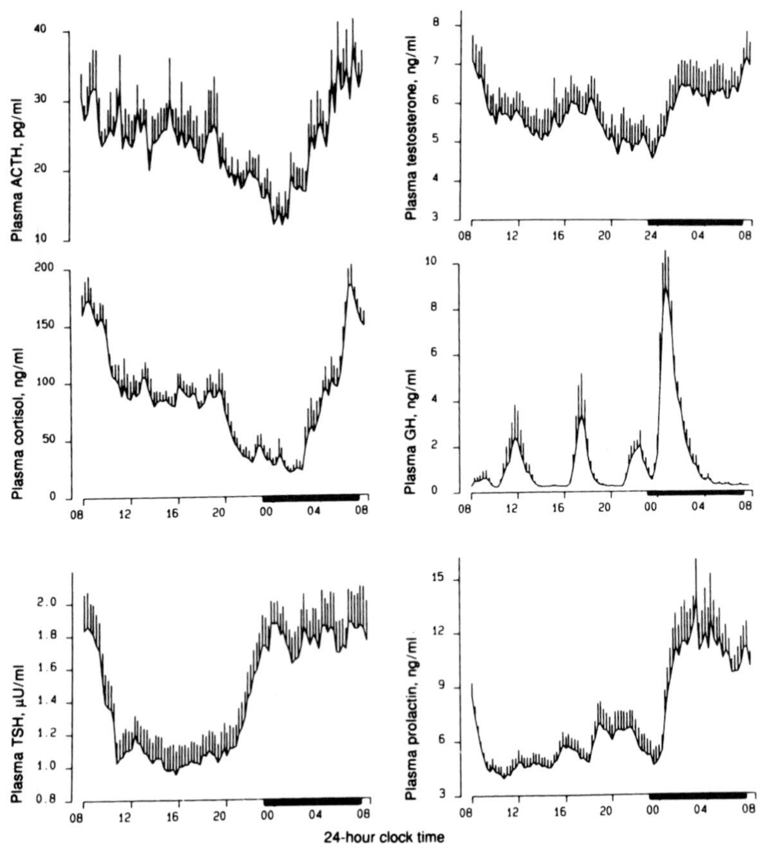

FIGURE 7-25. Mean (±SEM) profiles of plasma levels of ACTH, cortisol, TSH, testosterone, GH, and PRL from a group of 8 to 12 normal men studied at 15-min intervals for 24 h. The sleep times are indicated by black bars. *(Reproduced with permission from Van Cauter.[382])*

at specified times after sleep onset. For all but ACTH, shifting the time of onset of sleep immediately shifts the hormone peak. This shift also occurs for ACTH, but not until 5 to 10 days after the shift.[382] Sleep onset itself, however, appears to be synchronized loosely with the light-dark cycle and the release of melatonin. When melatonin is given orally, it advances the time of sleep onset and waking.[383] Obviously, this cue to the internal clock can be overridden voluntarily.

One of the most striking pituitary rhythms is that of ACTH. Levels rise in the early morning hours to peak at about 0700 to 0800 hours, assuming a sleep time from midnight to 0730 hours.[382] Levels then gradually fall over the course of the day and evening, only to begin rising again 2 to 4 h after the onset of sleep.[382] Cortisol levels follow the ACTH levels with minimal lag time. This ACTH-cortisol rhythm persists despite considerable perturbation of the normal endogenous and exogenous environment, including sleep deprivation, fasting, continuous feeding, constant glucose infusion, and constant lighting.[382] The profound diurnal variation of cortisol and ACTH is often used as an index of the "normality" of the system. Loss of this diurnal rhythm occurs with disordered regulation by CRH, which may be due to endogenous depression or excessive alcohol intake, as well as autonomous secretion of ACTH in Cushing's disease. In fact, this loss of diurnal rhythm of cortisol has been used as a diagnostic test for Cushing's syndrome (see Chap. 8).

TSH secretion is generally low throughout the day but then may double, with the rise occurring at about 2000 hours, substantially before sleep onset. These levels stay elevated through the night and then fall at about 0800 hours.[56,382]

Interesting changes in gonadotropin secretion occur as a child passes through puberty into adulthood. Before puberty, the amplitude of the gonadotropin pulses is low. Early in puberty, the amplitude of the pulses increases during sleep at night, especially for LH, but in adulthood, this nocturnal rise is lost.[384] Testosterone levels tend to rise at night as well.[382] In patients with anorexia nervosa, the pattern of gonadotropin secretion often reverts to this pubertal pattern, only to deviate from the pattern again with weight gain.[384] This suggests that body composition may in some way affect the regulation of the pulsatile secretion of the gonadotropins. In fact, the percentage of body composition that is fat has been proposed to be important in the timing of the onset of puberty.[385]

Although it once was thought that there are only 2 to 6 secretory episodes of GH per day, more sensitive assays have revealed that there are 12 to 14 episodes per day with a large nighttime surge.[379] The largest nighttime surge occurs shortly after the onset of sleep, in association with the first phase of slow-wave sleep.[382] Most episodes of GH secretion correlate with the onset of periods of slow-wave sleep, but later episodes of slow-wave sleep may not be associated with GH release.[384] Although this synchronization with sleep is very strong for GH, the experimental introduction of a 5-h delay in sleep onset results in a rise in GH during wakefulness within 1 h of the expected bedtime in most shifted nights.[382] This implies a circadian rhythm that is independent of sleep per se. Episodic secretion during sleep occurs even in blind individuals, suggesting that entrainment of GH secretion with the light-dark cycle is not very important.[384]

Prolactin shows a similar pattern to GH in that there is a substantial rise with sleep and 13 to 14 peaks per day.[386] An increase in the amplitude of the PRL secretory pulses begins about 60 to 90 min after the onset of sleep; the secretory pulses increase with non-REM sleep and fall before the next period of REM sleep.[386] When subjects are kept awake to reverse the sleep-wake cycle, PRL levels do not rise until sleep begins.[387] Thus, the diurnal variation of PRL secretion is not an inherent rhythm but depends on the occurrence of sleep. Interestingly, the diurnal variation of PRL with the sleep-induced rise persists despite powerful physiologic influences such as breast-feeding.[388]

Endocrine rhythms appear to reflect a rather primitive organizing influence that helps animals adapt to the environment. The circadian synchronization with the light-dark cycle and sleep and the infradian synchronization with seasonal changes are present very early phylogenetically. Even at the top of the evolutionary scale, in humans, these rhythms are of fundamental importance in the maintenance of normal hormonal functioning. However, because humans are able to alter the light-dark cycle, they are less tied to environmental changes. This has led to new problems with these rhythms, such as jet lag, which involves the rapid resynchronization of the rhythms with several-hour time-zone displacements. Because not all rhythms resynchronize at the same rates, some of the disorientation and other symptoms associated with jet lag may be due to abnormal phase relations of various body rhythms with each other and with the dark-light cycle.

NEUROENDOCRINE DISEASE

Diseases of the Hypothalamus

Diseases may affect the hypothalamus by being localized to the hypothalamus, by being part of more generalized CNS disease such as neurosarcoidosis, or by indirect means, such as by causing hydrocephalus. Furthermore, hormonal changes may occur in a variety of psychiatric disorders and are mediated by alterations in hypothalamic regulation (see Chap. 32).

The locations of the neuronal perikarya whose axons project to the median eminence and contain the various hypophysiotropic factors are well established. Most are concentrated in the basal portion of the hypothalamus in the area surrounding the third ventricle, and their axonal pathways all come together in the medial basal hypothalamus as they converge on the median eminence. Thus, lesions within this final common pathway might be expected to cause significant impairment of the hypothalamic regulation of pituitary function for all the pituitary hormones. Other functions of the hypothalamus are more diffuse, such as the regulation of temperature, which occurs in a large region of the preoptic anterior hypothalamus. Hypothalamic dysfunction can be grouped into three major categories: (1) anterior pituitary dysfunction, (2) neurohypophyseal dysfunction, and (3) nonpituitary dysfunction, including disorders of temperature regulation, thirst, eating behavior, sleep, autonomic nervous system regulation, memory, emotional behavior, and cognition.

Symptoms due to hypothalamic dysfunction are related to size of the lesion and, consequently, the area of the hypothalamus involved as well as the rapidity of increase in the size of the lesion. Tumors in this area, such as pituitary adenomas and craniopharyngiomas, can often grow quite large (8 to 10 cm in diameter) over many years with few symptoms. Slowly growing lesions tend to cause problems of hormone dysregulation rather than present with dramatic symptoms. However, a hemorrhage into even a small tumor of 1-cm diameter that causes it to increase rapidly to a 2- to 3-cm diameter can cause major disruption of hypothalamic function, including decreased levels of consciousness, temperature dysregulation, and disturbance of cardiovascular function. Large, slowly growing lesions can cause more acute problems, however, when a slight increment in growth results in the elimination of remaining vestiges of vasopressin or ACTH secretion or completely occludes the aqueduct of Sylvius or the foramen of Monro, causing hydrocephalus. Rarely, such tumors may cause mental dysfunction and symptoms and signs due to increased intracranial pressure, such as nausea, vomiting, headache, and papilledema.

A large number of disorders can affect the hypothalamus. The frequency of these disorders varies with age (Table 7-4). Because anterior pituitary regulation is incompletely developed at birth, certain types of hypothalamic damage that affect pituitary function may not be clinically recognized in the newborn. Magnetic resonance imaging (MRI) with gadolinium enhancement currently represents the best

TABLE 7-4 Etiology of Hypothalamic Disease

Neonates
- Intraventricular hemorrhage
- Meningitis: bacterial
- Tumors: glioma, hemangioma
- Trauma
- Hydrocephalus, hydranencephaly, kernicterus

1 month–2 years
- Tumors: glioma, especially optic glioma, histiocytosis X, hemangiomas
- Hydrocephalus, meningitis
- "Familial" disorders: Laurence-Moon, Barder-Biedel, Prader-Labhart-Willi, etc.

2–10 years
- Tumors: craniopharyngioma, glioma, dysgerminoma, hamartoma, histiocytosis X, leukemia, ganglioneuroma, ependymoma, medulloblastoma
- Meningitis: bacterial, tuberculous
- Encephalitis: viral and demyelinating, various viral encephalitides and exanthematous demyelinating encephalitides, disseminated encephalomyelitis
- "Familial" disorders: diabetes insipidus, etc.
- Damage from nasopharyngeal radiation therapy

10–25 years
- Tumors: craniopharyngioma, pituitary tumors, glioma, hamartoma, dysgerminoma, histiocytosis X, leukemia, dermoid, lipoma, neuroblastoma
- Trauma
- Subarachnoid hemorrhage, vascular aneurysm, arteriovenous malformation
- Inflammatory diseases: meningitis, encephalitis, sarcoid, tuberculosis
- Associated with midline brain defects: agenesis of corpus callosum
- Chronic hydrocephalus or increased intracranial pressure

25–50 years
- Nutritional: Wernicke's disease
- Tumors: glioma, lymphoma, meningioma, craniopharyngioma, pituitary tumors, angioma, plasmacytoma, colloid cysts, ependymoma, sarcoma, histiocytosis X
- Inflammatory: sarcoid, tuberculosis, viral encephalitis
- Subarachnoid hemorrhage, vascular aneurysms, arteriovenous malformation
- Damage from pituitary radiation therapy

>50 years
- Nutritional: Wernicke's disease
- Tumors: sarcoma, glioblastoma, lymphoma, meningioma, colloid cysts, ependymoma, pituitary tumors
- Vascular: infarct, subarachnoid hemorrhage, pituitary apoplexy
- Inflammatory: encephalitis, sarcoid, meningitis

Source: Adapted from Plum and Van Uitert.[25]

way of discerning lesions that affect the hypothalamus and any consequent distortion of other hypothalamic structures. The relation of the hypothalamus, pituitary, and infundibulum (stalk) to routine MRI are shown in Fig. 7-4. Computed tomographic (CT) scanning with intravenous contrast is also quite good at delineating these lesions. Formal visual field testing may discern an impingement of the optic nerves and chiasm by hypothalamic lesions, including the suprasellar extension of a pituitary tumor. The lack of a visual field defect does not exclude suprasellar disease, however, and very large lesions may be present which can be documented to distort the chiasm on MRI scan but may not cause visual field defects. Detailed testing of hypothalamic-pituitary function (see Chaps. 8 and 9) may reveal evidence of functional hypothalamic disruption with great sensitivity.

Congenital Embryopathic Disorders

The most common embryopathic disorders that affect the hypothalamus are the midline cleft syndromes, which cause varying degrees of defects of midline structures, especially the optic and olfactory tracts, the septum pellucidum, the corpus callosum, the anterior commissure, the hypothalamus, and the pituitary. The clinical presentation of patients with midline cleft defects varies in severity from cyclopia to cleft lip. Patients with severe lesions such as holoprosencephaly (failure of cleavage of the prosencephalon into two lateral ventricles) have been reported to have defective hypothalamic structures and absent pituitaries.[389] The combination of an absent septum pellucidum and optic nerve hypoplasia is referred to as septo-optic dysplasia; several patients with these findings have been reported with abnormalities of hypothalamic and other diencephalic structures and varying degrees of anterior and posterior pituitary deficiency.[390] Some patients with septo-optic dysplasia and hypothalamic hypopituitarism have sexual precocity, presumably caused by a lack of inhibitory influences from other parts of the hypothalamus and intact GnRH-producing structures.[391]

Children with very mild midline cleft defects consisting of just a cleft lip or palate or both have been found to have a markedly increased risk of having GH and other pituitary hormone deficiencies.[392] A recent evaluation of 35 patients with "idiopathic" growth hormone deficiency with MR scanning showed that in 43 percent the neurohypophysis (which shows as a bright spot) was adjacent to the median eminence and that there was an absence of the infundibulum (Fig. 7-26). Most of those with an absent infundibulum also had other pituitary hormone deficiencies.[393] It is possible that this group of patients has a very mild variant of the midline cleft syndrome.

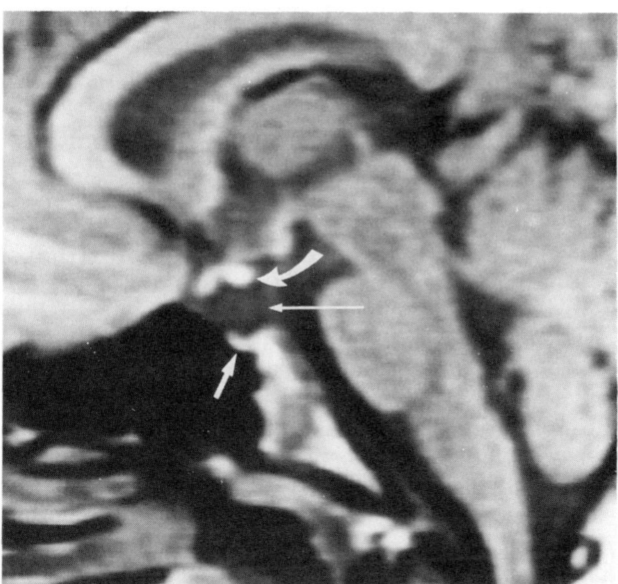

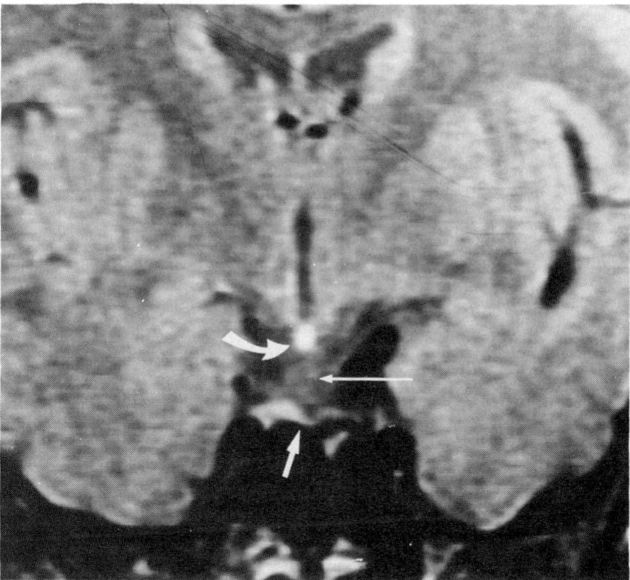

FIGURE 7-26. Small anterior pituitary gland associated with an ectopic neurohypophysis in a patient with idiopathic growth hormone deficiency. (*A* and *B*) Sagittal *(A)* and coronal *(B)* MR images show the absence of the infundibulum (long arrow) and an area of bright signal in the median eminence (curved arrow) which is the ectopic neurohypophysis. *(Reproduced with permission from Abrahams et al.[393])*

Congenital defects in the base of the skull that result in herniation of the pituitary and stalk through the floor of the sella (basal encephalocele) can also cause hypopituitarism and diabetes insipidus.[394] In these cases, such dysfunction could be due to the distortion of the normal hypothalamic-pituitary structures rather than to primary abnormalities of the hypothalamus.[394] However, some of these patients also have evidence of other midline facial defects (cleft lip and palate) and optic nerve abnormalities,[394] so that these dysfunctions may also be considered to be variants of the midline cleft syndrome.

Kallman's syndrome is an autosomal dominant condition characterized by anosmia or hyposmia and hypogonadotropic gonadism (see Chap. 16). It is now known to be due to gene mutations that result in defective proteins normally responsible for facilitating the migration of the GnRH and olfactory neurons from the olfactory placode to their final positions during embryogenesis.[87,394a] MR scanning reveals partial to complete absence of the olfactory sulci.[395] The pituitary is usually intact, and treatment with pulsatile GnRH therapy or gonadotropins results in spermatogenesis and normal gonadal function.[90,396] In some patients, other neurologic abnormalities may be present, including cerebellar ataxia, nerve deafness, color blindness, cleft lip and palate, and mental retardation.[396] Furthermore, in a series of seven subjects with Kallman's syndrome, three had abnormalities of thirst, one had a decreased osmotic threshold for vasopressin release, and one had an increased osmotic threshold for vasopressin release.[397] Thus, there may be more diffuse hypothalamic dysfunction than was formerly thought.

Tumors

The most common tumors affecting the hypothalamus are pituitary adenomas that have a significant suprasellar extension. These tumors can cause varying degrees of hypopituitarism and diabetes insipidus by compressing the normal pituitary (20 to 25 percent) or, more commonly, by affecting the pituitary stalk and mediobasal hypothalamus (75 to 80 percent).[398] Hyperprolactinemia occurs in about half of these tumors, caused primarily by disinhibition by the hypothalamus, with decreased dopamine reaching the pituitary.[398,399] Evidence that hypopituitarism results from pituitary compression includes a low serum PRL level and a lack of TSH response to TRH; pituitary function in such cases usually does not improve after treatment.[398] In patients with normal or elevated PRL levels, pituitary function often returns after therapy.[398] Specific treatments for the different types of pituitary tumors are discussed in Chap. 8.

Craniopharyngiomas are the next most common tumors that affect the hypothalamus. Microscopically, craniopharyngiomas consist of cysts alternating with stratified squamous epithelium. The cyst fluid is usually thick and dark, and the material is often calcified. It is thought that the craniopharyngiomas arise from remnants of Rathke's pouch. A variant or closely related lesion is the Rathke's cleft cyst, which develops from the space between the anterior and rudimentary intermediate lobes. Rathke's cleft cysts are lined with cuboidal as opposed to squamous epithelium, and the cyst fluid is usually a white mucoid fluid.[400] Clinically, the distinction is often impossible, although craniopharyngiomas are more commonly found in a suprasellar location while Rathke's cleft cysts are usually intrasellar.[400] However, craniopharyngiomas sometimes recur postoperatively, while Rathke's cleft cysts rarely recur.[400] Only about 4 percent of this group of tumors are Rathke's cleft cysts.[401] Craniopharyngiomas most commonly present during childhood but also occur in adults and even in the elderly.[401] These tumors present because of mass effects, including headache, vomiting, visual disturbance, seizures, hypopituitarism, and polyuria. Careful endocrine testing reveals varying degrees of hypopituitarism in 50 to 75 percent and modest hyperprolactinemia in 25 to 50 percent.[402–404] Some patients present with galactorrhea, amenorrhea, and hyperprolactinemia, suggestive of a prolactinoma.[404] Surgical extirpation of craniopharyngiomas commonly causes a worsening of pituitary function, often resulting in complete panhypopituitarism and diabetes insipidus because of stalk section.[402–404] Irradiation may be helpful, especially in children.[402]

Suprasellar dysgerminomas are said to arise from primitive germ cells that have migrated to the CNS during fetal life and structurally are identical to germ cell tumors of the gonads.[405] They usually present in children, in whom they most commonly cause decreased growth because of hypopituitarism, diabetes insipidus, and visual problems.[405,406] Hyperprolactinemia occurs in over 50 percent, and 10 percent have precocious puberty caused by the production of hCG by the tumor.[406] As opposed to craniopharyngiomas, these tumors are very radiosensitive, and radiotherapy is the preferred treatment.

Other tumors and space-occupying lesions that occur in the suprasellar area include arachnoid cysts, meningiomas, gliomas, astrocytomas, chordomas, infundibulomas, cholesteatomas, neurofibromas, lipomas, and metastatic cancer (particularly of the breast and lung).[407] These lesions may present with varying degrees of hypopituitarism, diabetes insipidus, and hyperprolactinemia, and surgical therapy often worsens the hormonal deficit.

Hamartomas

A hypothalamic hamartoma is a nodule of growth of hypothalamic neurons attached by a pedicle to the hypothalamus between the tuber cinereum and the mammillary bodies and extending into the basal cistern. Asymptomatic hamartomas may be present in up to 20 percent of random autopsies.[408] Rarely, these lesions may enlarge, causing disruption of hypothalamic function because of compression of adjacent tissue. A variant of the hamartoma consisting of similar tissue present within the anterior pituitary but without a neural attachment to the hypothalamus is called a choristoma or gangliocytoma. These neuronal tumors are of particular endocrine interest because they can produce hypophysiotropic hormones.

A number of cases associated with precocious puberty in which hamartomas produce GnRH have been reported. Electron microscopy with immunohistochemistry reveals GnRH to be present in secretory granules in the nerve endings.[409,410] Within the abnormal tissue, the neurons surround blood vessels which have a fenestrated capillary endothelium, enabling the released GnRH to enter the blood vessels and eventually be transported to the pituitary by vessels of the tuber cinereum.[409] The fact that these lesions cause precocious puberty suggests that the regulation of GnRH and gonadotropins is not normal, and several studies have recorded failure of appropriate negative feedback suppression of gonadotropins or stimulation with clomiphene.[409] Successful treatment has been reported with surgery[410] and with the administration of a long-acting GnRH analog which suppresses gonadotropin secretion but does not affect the tumor.[411] Medical therapy with the GnRH analog may be the best choice, as surgery can be noncurative or even fatal if the hamartoma does not cause other problems from mass effects.

Some gangiocytomas have been reported which produce GHRH and acromegaly.[412] In some of these tumors, there is direct contact between the gangiocytoma GHRH-containing neuronal cells and the pituitary GH-secreting cells, suggesting a paracrine effect.[412] Similarly, a patient with Cushing's disease due to an intrasellar gangliocytoma producing CRH and causing corticotroph cell hyperplasia has been reported.[413]

Inflammatory Disorders

Sarcoidosis

CNS involvement in sarcoidosis occurs in 1 to 5 percent of patients as determined on clinical grounds and in up to 16 percent of cases at autopsy.[414] Isolated CNS sarcoidosis is quite uncommon, however.[414] When sarcoidosis does involve the CNS, the hypothalamus is involved in 10 to 20 percent of cases.[414] Sarcoid granulomas can involve the hypothalamus, stalk, or pituitary[415] and may be infiltrative or present as a mass lesion.[416] Rarely, sarcoid granulomas present as an expanding intrasellar mass mimicking a pituitary tumor.[417] The most common endocrine findings are varying degrees of hypopituitarism, diabetes insipidus, and hyperprolactinemia.[414,415,418] Obesity due to hypothalamic involvement by sarcoidosis has also been reported.[416] In patients with isolated CNS sarcoidosis, the diagnosis may be extremely difficult. Examination of the

CSF usually shows elevated protein levels, low glucose levels, and a pleiocytosis. Biopsy is often necessary. Although corticosteroid therapy has been reported to reverse the thirst disorders at least partially, anterior pituitary hormone deficits usually do not respond to this therapy.[415,418]

Eosinophilic Granuloma (Histiocytosis X)

Eosinophilic granulomatous infiltration of the hypothalamus may cause diabetes insipidus, varying degrees of hypopituitarism, and hyperprolactinemia.[419] Often this infiltration appears on CT as a mass lesion of the hypothalamus[420] (Fig. 7-27) or even the pituitary.[421] Osteolytic lesions may be present in the jaw or mastoid, and x-rays of the jaw are a worthwhile part of the diagnostic evaluation of an unknown suprasellar mass or diabetes insipidus for this reason. Therapy consists of local surgery, focal irradiation, or chemotherapy with alkylating reagents and high-dose corticosteroids.

Other Inflammatory Lesions

A number of other inflammatory lesions can rarely cause hypothalamic dysfunction, including abscesses,[407,422] viral meningoencephalitis,[423] and tuberculous meningitis.[424]

Vascular Disease

Enlarging aneurysms may present as a mass lesion of the hypothalamic-pituitary area and may cause hypopituitarism and visual field defects.[407] Obviously, the distinction must be made before surgery. Tumors and aneurysms may also coexist, and careful radiologic evaluation with MRI is necessary to discern this. Hypothalamic disease due to vascular infarction is extremely rare.

Trauma

Head trauma can cause defects ranging from isolated ACTH deficiency to panhypopituitarism with diabetes insipidus.[425] Within the first 72 h of trauma, GH, LH, ACTH, TSH, and PRL levels may be elevated in blood, perhaps as a result of an acute release.[426] With more prolonged observation, these levels fall and patients either return to normal or develop hypopituitarism, except for a persistent PRL elevation in many cases.[425] These patients may or may not have associated loss of consciousness, but

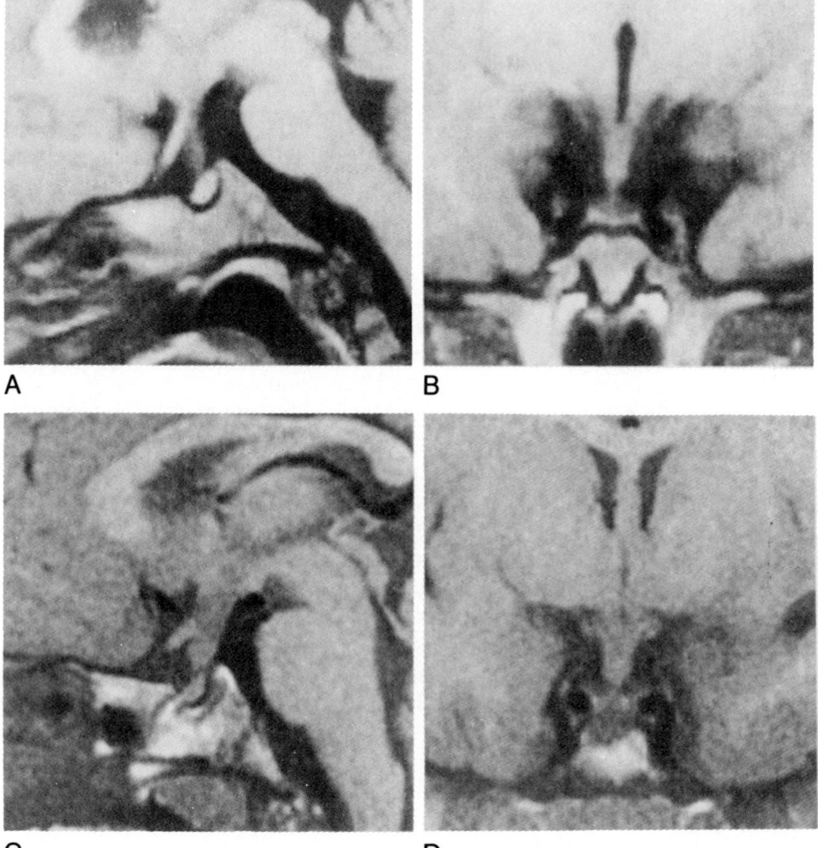

FIGURE 7-27. MR scan in a patient with diabetes insipidus due to hypothalamic infiltration with histiocytosis X. (*A* and *B*) Sagittal *(A)* and coronal *(B)* T_1-weighted images show a symmetric, slightly thickened pituitary stalk and the absence of normal high signal intensity in the posterior pituitary lobe. (*C* and *D*) Sagittal *(C)* and coronal *(D)* T_1-weighted images 2 years later reveal a more markedly thickened pituitary stalk and the absence of high signal intensity in the posterior pituitary lobe. *(Reproduced with permission from Tien et al.[420])*

other neurologic abnormalities are common, such as blindness and cranial nerve palsies.[425] In patients dying of head injury, anterior pituitary infarction has been found in 16 percent of cases, posterior pituitary hemorrhages in 34 percent, and hypothalamic hemorrhages or infarction in 42 percent.[427] The paraventricular and supraoptic nuclei and median eminence are particularly involved with microhemorrhages, resulting in the high frequency of panhypopituitarism with diabetes insipidus.[427] With frontal injuries, the brain travels backward but the pituitary cannot move, and so the pituitary stalk becomes avulsed, with interruption of the portal vessels.[425] Most patients with head injury are hyperprolactinemic, confirming clinically that the hypothalamus and/or stalk is the primary site of injury.[425]

Irradiation

Whole-brain irradiation for intracranial neoplasms results in hypothalamic dysfunction in 1.25 percent of patients, as evidenced by endocrine abnormalities and behavioral changes.[428] The most common endocrine abnormality is hyperprolactinemia, but more severe hypopituitarism can occur.[428] When radiotherapy is targeted to the hypothalamic area, hypopituitarism occurs more frequently. Thus, in patients receiving radiotherapy for nasopharyngeal carcinoma, impairment of pituitary function is common and progressive; 19 percent of these patients become hypopituitary within 2 years, and 100 percent have hyperprolactinemia.[429] When radiotherapy is targeted to the pituitary, by 10 years clinically significant losses of function are quite high: 50 percent for gonadotropins, 20 to 40 percent for ACTH, and 15 to 20 percent for TSH.[430] These frequencies of loss of pituitary function are so high that all patients who have had their pituitary and hypothalamic areas irradiated must be followed closely to detect these deficits when they occur.

Polyostotic Fibrous Dysplasia (McCune-Albright Syndrome)

A number of endocrine disorders have been associated with polyostotic fibrous dysplasia, the most common being precocious puberty and acromegaly associated with hyperprolactinemia.[431–433] In these cases, pituitary histology has shown mammosomatotroph cell hyperplasia or a normal pituitary.[432] A few other patients have had goiters, and one has had Cushing's syndrome due to bilateral micronodular hyperplasia.[434] Although it was hypothesized 20 years ago that the endocrine dysfunction is due to the overproduction of hypothalamic releasing factors,[434] direct measurement of GHRH in peripheral blood has not shown markedly elevated levels.[433] However, if this were due to local overproduction by the hypothalamus with high levels in portal vessels, only slight elevations would be detected in peripheral blood. At present, the etiology of this syndrome remains an enigma, along with its possible relation to hypothalamic dysfunction. Recent studies have demonstrated an activating mutation of the gene for the α subunit of the guanine nucleotide binding G protein that stimulates cAMP formation in the endocrine and other tissues of these patients.[434a] The relationship of this abnormality to the various manifestations of the disorder still needs clarification, however.

Effects of Hypothalamic Disease on Pituitary Function

Hypothalamic disease can cause pituitary hyperfunction and hypofunction in varying degrees of severity. Although severe disease can cause absolute deficiencies of the various hormones, more mild disease may cause a subtle alteration of feedback loops and timing such that, for example, the integration of signals necessary for menstrual cycling is lost, resulting in "hypothalamic" amenorrhea. Furthermore, the hypothalamic defects may be interrelated, so that the rather common finding of hyperprolactinemia occurring with hypothalamic dysfunction causes a hypogonadotropic hypogonadism that is reversible when the elevated PRL levels are brought down to normal. Detailed testing of hypothalamic-pituitary function now can detect such hormonal abnormalities with greater sensitivity and precision and at earlier points in the course of disease compared with early descriptions of hypothalamic disease, which were limited to detecting precocious puberty, hypogonadism, and diabetes insipidus. Whenever hypothalamic lesions are suspected, detailed evaluation of hypothalamic-pituitary function is indicated. Often, however, dynamic testing of pituitary function will not differentiate between the hypothalamus and the pituitary as the specific primary locus of the defect, and neuroradiologic imaging with MRI or CT is almost always necessary.[435]

Growth Hormone

Growth Hormone Deficiency

Loss of normal GH secretion is the most common hormonal defect that occurs with structural hypothalamic disease.[398,402,406,425] However, hypogonadotropic hypogonadism follows closely behind, so that most subjects with hypothalamic disease who are found to be GH-deficient also have deficient levels of sex steroid hormones. It is recognized that an adequate level of sex steroids is necessary for a normal GH response,[436] and sex hormone replacement was not performed in these series before GH testing, so that the prevalence of GH deficiency may have been overestimated. Furthermore, since only about 60 to 80 percent of normal individuals have an adequate GH response to most traditional stimuli of GH secretion and as multiple stimulation tests were not performed in these series, the frequency of GH deficiency may have been overestimated. Therefore, it is not known whether GH deficiency is truly the most common hormone deficiency in patients with hypothalamic disease.

As was discussed above, patients with obvious as well as subtle midline cleft defects often have GH deficiency. Among children with no obvious structural disease, i.e., patients thought to have idiopathic growth hormone deficiency (IGHD), recent studies using MR scanning have found that 43 percent have an absent infundibulum with a small to normal anterior pituitary and a posterior pituitary adjacent to the median eminence[393] (Fig. 7-22). Such patients often have abnormalities of other pituitary hormone functioning[393] as well and should be regarded as having congenital structural defects rather than IGHD. The remaining patients with IGHD studied with MRI had normal infundibula, small to normal anterior pituitaries, and normal posterior pituitaries.[393]

It is likely that IGHD is a heterogeneous disorder that consists of hypothalamic and pituitary defects. Between 5 and 30 percent of IGHD patients have an affected relative, and thus their defect is thought to have a genetic basis.[437] One autosomal dominant form of complete GH deficiency has been found to be associated with a deletion of the GH gene.[438] Evaluations of larger numbers of patients with IGHD with the techniques of polymerase chain reaction amplification of GH genomic DNA and determination of other structural gene abnormalities detectable by linkage to restriction fragment length polymorphisms (RFLP) have shown that such gene defects account for at most a minority of cases.[439,440] A preliminary RFLP linkage analysis of the GHRH gene in such cases has not revealed any abnormalities.[440]

The etiology of the GH deficiency in nongenetic cases of IGHD is not known, but it is thought in most cases to be due to disordered hypothalamic regulation, such as a neurotransmitter abnormality. In many children with IGHD, stimulation with GHRH results in varying GH responses, implying that their pituitaries are capable of producing GH and responding to GHRH, and in some of these patients repeated injections of GHRH can cause greater increases.[266] The initial GH response to a single dose of GHRH and the later response to repetitive doses of GHRH occur primarily in children with documented hypothalamic lesions as the cause of their GH deficiency. However, a prolonged course of repeated injections of GHRH in such children can restore a normal growth pattern in only some cases.[441] Stimulation of GH secretion by dopamine agonists such as bromocriptine has been found to result in normal growth in some patients, implying a possible underlying defect in dopaminergic neurotransmission.[442] Similarly, some studies[443] but not others[444] have found that clonidine, an α-adrenergic agonist, can stimulate normal growth in some children, implying a defect in noradrenergic neurotransmission.

Children with IGHD begin to manifest decreased growth after the first year of life. Prompt treatment with human GH injections usually results in close to normal growth (see Chap. 26).

Growth Hormone Excess

GH excess results in gigantism if it occurs before puberty and in acromegaly if it occurs after epiphyseal closure. As was discussed above, these conditions may develop from a specific lesion, a GHRH-producing gangliocytoma.[412] Although an excess of hypothalamic GHRH has been postulated to cause the acromegaly associated with polyostotic fibrous dysplasia (see above), this has never been proved. The role of the hypothalamus in the etiology of the usual pituitary GH-secreting adenoma is discussed fully in Chap. 8. Depending on the interpretation of the data, conclusions can be reached on both sides of this issue.[445]

Gonadotropins

Hypothalamic Hypogonadism

The primary defect in this group of disorders is thought to involve the secretion of GnRH, with resultant impairment in pituitary gonadotropin secretion and gonadal function. The disorders causing these conditions may be primary (congenital defects) or acquired. Depending on the time of onset, they present either as delayed puberty, interruption of pubertal progression, or loss of adult gonadal function. The lesions causing these disorders may cause a loss of other hormones or may be isolated to GnRH. Loss of gonadotropin secretion as a result of hypothalamic structural damage is the second most common defect after GH deficiency.[398,402,406,425] However, a substantial number of these defects are due to hyperprolactinemia and are reversible with correction of the hyperprolactinemia. Thus, estimates of hypogonadotropic hypogonadism may be excessive.

Prepubertal Lesions presenting prepubertally result in failure of the onset of puberty or incomplete progression of puberty if the defect is partial. If the disorder is limited to GnRH and the gonadotropins, prior growth and development will be normal. However, the growth spurt occurring at puberty will be lost.

The most common congenital lesion causing prepubertal GnRH deficiency is Kallman's syndrome, which is seen in 50 percent of males who present with isolated gonadotropin deficiency.[446] In Kallman's syndrome, there is hyposmia or anosmia due to hypoplasia of the olfactory bulb along with absent GnRH secretion (see above). Patients with other midline cleft defects usually have GH deficiency along with GnRH deficiency. Undescended testes are present in 50 percent of patients with GnRH deficiency, probably as a result of the absence of gonadotropins during fetal development.[446]

In patients with idiopathic GnRH deficiency, the GnRH gene appears to be normal.[447] However, indirect measures of functional GnRH secretion have shown that it is not secreted normally. Detailed study of LH pulsatile secretion in such patients shows that over 90 percent have no detectable LH pulsations, some have episodic LH secretion only during sleep (similar to that described for pubertal subjects[384]), some have normal pulse frequency but decreased amplitude, and some have normal pulse amplitude but decreased frequency.[448] These patterns run true within families with more than one affected sibling.[448] Stimulation with a single dose of GnRH causes a minimal rise in gonadotropins in individuals with absolutely no pubertal development but a normal rise in those with some pubertal development, presumably reflecting prior GnRH exposure.[446]

Among females with primary amenorrhea due to GnRH deficiency, 37 percent have been found to have associated anosmia and therefore have Kallman's syndrome.[448] When 12 women with euosmic primary amenorrhea were studied with respect to gonadotropin pulsatile secretion, 11 were found to have no pulsations.[448]

The ideal therapy for patients with GnRH deficiency consists of the replacement of GnRH. In males, the subcutaneous administration of 25 to 200 ng/kg of GnRH every 2 h with a portable pump causes a rapid rise in the LH and FSH responses to the GnRH, a rise in testosterone to normal, and the development of normal spermatogenesis.[448] Similar studies in women have revealed ovulatory cycles in 80 percent.[448] The success of such therapy confirms the original hypothesis of a primary defect of GnRH secretion. In men, comparable results can be obtained with exogenous gonadotropins given three times per week.[449] However, replacement with testosterone alone does not result in an increase in testicular size or in spermatogenesis.

Hyperprolactinemia can cause a decrease in GnRH secretion and gonadotropin pulsatile secretion.[123,124] When it occurs before puberty, it can prevent the onset of puberty, and it must always be looked for in this setting.

Postpubertal Loss of formerly normal GnRH secretion may be due to structural hypothalamic damage such as a tumor, a functional change unassociated with a detectable lesion, or hyperprolactinemia. Structural disease must be excluded in such patients by means of CT or MR scanning.

Most but not all cases of functional hypogonadotropic hypogonadism occur in women, with the most common causes being weight loss, excessive exercise, and psychogenic stress.[385,450,451] In some cases, the exercise results in a loss of body fat not detected with total body weight measures, and it is unclear whether the hypogonadism is directly due to the loss of body fat or to the exercise per se.[385,451] Studies of pulsatile gonadotropin secretion in such patients reveal absent pulses.[448] Usually there is a normal gonadotropin response to injected GnRH. Regain of weight and cessation of the exercise result in a resumption of normal gonadal function.[385,451] The neurotransmitter mediation of this functional state is not known with certainty, although responses to naloxone and dopamine antagonists suggest that excessive opioid peptidergic and dopaminergic tone may be involved.[452]

As was indicated above, hyperprolactinemia can decrease GnRH and the pulsatile secretion of LH and FSH.[123,124] As gonadotropin responses to GnRH are normal in hyperprolactinemia, it appears that elevated PRL levels act at the hypothalamic level.[453] Hyperprolactinemia also inhibits positive estrogen feedback.[454] Whether these are direct effects of the elevated PRL levels or are mediated via a PRL-induced increase in central dopaminergic tone via short-loop feedback is unknown. This inhibitory effect of PRL on GnRH secretion occurs in both sexes.

Therapy should be directed at the underlying process, if possible. Efforts at weight gain and restriction of exercise should be made when appropriate. In patients with idiopathic, functional hypogonadotropic amenorrhea, there are two goals: (1) restoration of normal estrogen status to promote well-being and prevent osteoporosis and (2) facilitation of ovulation to achieve fertility. The former can generally be achieved with cyclic estrogen and progesterone, while the latter may require clomiphene, GnRH, or gonadotropin therapy.

Hypothalamic Hypergonadism (Precocious Puberty)

Precocious puberty is defined as the onset of puberty before age 8 in girls and age 9 in boys.[455] "True" precocious puberty is due to central causes with increased gonadotropins. "Pseudo" precocious puberty is due to peripheral (gonadal or adrenal) causes (see Chap. 26). Central "true" or GnRH-dependent precocious puberty is characterized by hormonal changes similar to those which occur at the time of normal puberty: an increase in the pulsatile release of LH, an increase in the gonadotropin response to GnRH, and an increase in gonadal steroid secretion.[455] Conceptually, the normal prepubertal childhood condition can be viewed as a "restraint" of the GnRH pulse generator, and puberty can be viewed as a lifting of that restraint so that GnRH secretion increases, with a resultant increase in gonadotropin secretion.[455] GnRH-dependent precocious puberty therefore represents a premature activation of this GnRH pulse generator by a variety of lesions; it may also be idiopathic.

Less than one-quarter of cases of central precocious puberty occur in boys, but boys tend to have more serious underlying disease. In boys with central GnRH-dependent precocious puberty, hypothalamic hamartomas account for 38 percent of cases, other CNS lesions represent 31 percent, familial disease accounts for 23 percent, and idiopathic disease accounts for only 8 percent.[456] The picture is quite different in girls, however, as hypothalamic hamartomas account for only 15 percent of cases, other CNS lesions represent 14 percent, the McCune-Albright syndrome (polyostotic fibrous dysplasia) accounts for 6 percent, and fully 65 percent are idiopathic.[456] CNS lesions other than GnRH-secreting hamartomas that have been reported to trigger precocious puberty include neurofibromatosis, astrocytomas, gliomas, arachnoid cysts, hydrocephalus, neuroblastomas, head trauma, subdural hematomas, and cranial irradiation.[456,457] Dysgerminomas in the suprasellar or pineal region can produce hCG, which acts like LH in stimulating gonadal function.[406] Usually such tumors cause increased sex steroid formation but fail to cause ovulation.

Therapy for central GnRH-dependent precocious puberty consists of surgical removal of the tumor or medical therapy with a long-acting GnRH analog. The latter can suppress gonadotropin and sex steroid hormone levels and cause a stabilization or even regression of secondary sex characteristics and a slowing of growth and bone maturation in most cases with the exception of the McCune-Albright syndrome and familial male precocious puberty.[456,457] When therapy is discontinued at the normal time of puberty, sex steroid levels increase, secondary sexual characteristics again develop, growth increases, and regular menses develop spontaneously.[457] Thus, the GnRH analog has turned out to be an ideal therapy in that it can turn off abnormal precocious puberty for years and then allow puberty to resume at the normal time when it is discontinued. For patients who do not respond to the GnRH analogs, treatment with medroxyprogesterone acetate or testolactone, an aromatase inhibitor, is indicated.[455]

Prolactin

Hypothalamic Hyperprolactinemia

As was discussed previously, PRL is under tonic inhibition by the hypothalamus. Thus, structural or infiltrative lesions of the hypothalamus such as those discussed above can affect hypothalamic function, causing modest hyperprolactinemia. PRL elevations caused by such lesions rarely rise to greater than 150 ng/ml and usually are below 100 ng/ml.[399] Similar elevations are also seen in patients with an empty sella.[399] It is very important to differentiate nonsecreting pituitary adenomas with extensive suprasellar extension causing PRL elevations in this range from PRL-secreting adenomas which, when of such a large size, usually cause PRL elevations 5 to 50 times higher,[399,458] as the therapy is quite different (see Chap. 8). It is interesting that PRL levels can be increased in patients with hypothalamic lesions while other hypothalamic-pituitary function (i.e., ACTH and TSH) is normal, although GH levels and gonadotropin levels are also often suppressed.[399] This means that there is enough destruction or distortion of the stalk and/or mediobasal hypothalamus to cause a deficiency of dopamine while permitting sufficient CRH and TRH secretion.

Some patients with hypothalamic lesions have PRL levels over 100 ng/ml that fall to levels in the range of 35 to 50 ng/ml after surgery to remove the lesion has caused a complete stalk section.[399] Thus, the degree of PRL elevation may depend not only on the degree of defect of dopamine but also on whether the PRL-releasing activity of the hypothalamus (caused by VIP, TRH, etc.) is intact or perhaps even increased. Evidence in favor of possible increased PRL-releasing activity in such patients includes the finding that normal individuals who are given a pharmacologic blockade of dopamine activity with medications such as neuroleptics and who have intact prolactin-releasing activity have PRL elevations only in the range of 30 to 60 ng/ml.[281]

Therapy is generally directed at the underlying cause. The hyperprolactinemia itself may impair gonadal function and so efforts may also be made to lower PRL levels with bromocriptine or another dopamine agonist. PRL levels usually fall readily in such patients. Restoration of gonadal function is not automatic, however, as the primary hypothalamic lesion may also directly impair the release of GnRH. In that circumstance, both bromocriptine and sex steroid replacement may be necessary.

Idiopathic Hyperprolactinemia

Idiopathic hyperprolactinemia is defined as hyperprolactinemia that occurs in the absence of any recognized pituitary, hypothalamic, or other cause; i.e., it is a diagnosis of exclusion. PRL levels in this condition are usually below 100 ng/ml. In such cases, small pituitary or hypothalamic tumors can exist that are beyond the resolution of current imaging techniques. Nonetheless, when such patients are followed for many years, it is very uncommon for tumors to be visualized later.[459] Idiopathic hyperprolactinemia can cause amenorrhea, galactorrhea, impotence, infertility, and loss of libido as occurs with hyperprolactinemia of other causes and therefore may need to be treated. Premature osteoporosis related to the estrogen deficiency may also occur.[460] The only possible treatment is bromocriptine or another dopamine agonist, and these agents are successful in over 90 percent of cases.[461]

Galactorrhea can occur with normal PRL levels and with normal menses and has been attributed to increased sensitivity of the breast to normal circulating levels of PRL.[461] Lowering of the normal PRL levels to very low levels with a dopamine agonist is generally successful in eliminating the galactorrhea.

TSH

Hypothalamic Hypothyroidism

This disorder is also referred to as tertiary hypothyroidism and is due to a central lesion that impairs the secretion of TRH. It occurs considerably less commonly than do hypothalamic GH and gonadotropin deficiency and with about a similar frequency to ACTH deficiency.[398,402,406,425] TSH levels in this syndrome generally are normal or even slightly elevated, and the response to TRH is delayed, peaking at 60 to 120 min rather than at 20 to 30 min.[462] TSH in these patients is biologically less active than normal[462] and binds to the TSH receptor less well.[463] The defective bioactivity and the receptor-binding activity appear to be due to altered glycosylation as a result of the TRH deficiency.[464]

ACTH

Hypothalamic ACTH Deficiency

ACTH deficiency due to hypothalamic lesions occurs less frequently than do GH or gonadotropin deficiencies and with a similar frequency to TSH deficiency.[398,402,406,425] It may also appear as an isolated deficiency. In the absence of CNS lesions or a history of trauma, most cases of isolated ACTH deficiency appear to have a pituitary autoimmune basis[465] (see Chap. 8). Patients without hypothalamic disease do not respond to either hypoglycemia or single or repetitive injections of CRH.[466] However, in patients with hypothalamic disease as the etiology, basal ACTH levels are low and the ACTH response to injected CRH may be prolonged and exaggerated,[466] much as is the case with the TSH reponse to TRH.[462] The best test remains the comparison of the ACTH response to hypoglycemia, which is clearly mediated by the hypothalamus, and to CRH. The ACTH response is low in response to hypoglycemia but is increased and delayed in response to CRH in most patients with hypothalamic CRH deficiency.

Cushing's Disease

As was discussed above, Cushing's disease may develop from a CRH-producing gangliocytoma.[413] The role of the hypothalamus in the etiology of the usual pituitary ACTH-secreting adenoma is discussed fully in Chap. 8.

Vasopressin

Diabetes insipidus can develop as a result of destructive lesions in the supraoptic and paraventricular nuclei or in the mediobasal hypothalamus in the path of neural fibers containing vasopressin that are passing on to the posterior pituitary. Irritative lesions can trigger the release of vasopressin in an unregulated fashion, resulting in the syndrome of inappropriate ADH (vasopressin) secretion (SIADH). These entities are discussed in Chap. 9.

Effects of Hypothalamic Disease on Other Neurometabolic Functions

A number of functions which affect the internal milieu as well as anterior and posterior pituitary function are regulated, at least in part, by the hypothalamus, including temperature regulation, behavior, consciousness, memory, sleep, food intake, and carbohydrate metabolism. Furthermore, the hypothalamus affects cardiovascular, GI, pulmonary, and renal function through the autonomic nervous system. Although clinically obvious disturbances of these functions which occur with lesions of the hypothalamus are far less common than disturbances of hypothalamic-pituitary function, detailed evaluations of subclinical defects in these functions have not been performed to ascertain their frequency and effects on the quality of life.

Alterations in Food Intake

Body weight is kept relatively constant in nonobese individuals through an integration of a number of factors relating to the intake of nutrients, including the total amount of food eaten and the composition of that food and the output of energy, which is affected by hormonal, environmental, and genetic factors[467] (see Chap. 21). As with the regulation of hormone secretion, the regulation of food intake can be conceptually regarded as an adjustment of food intake and energy expenditure around set points which may be different for body weight, total body fat, lean body mass, etc.[467–470] A number of areas of the hypothalamus are involved in the regulation of energy balance.

Destruction of the ventromedial nucleus (VMN) inhibits satiety and results in hyperphagia and hypothalamic obesity.[467–469] The hyperphagia is due to destruction of noradrenergic fibers originating in the paraventricular nucleus (PVN), and the hyperinsulinemia that occurs with hypothalamic obesity is due to destruction of the VMN itself.[469] Lesions of the PVN can also cause hyperphagia and weight gain.[467–469] Normally, the VMN exerts an inhibitory effect on efferent impulses from the dorsal motor nucleus of the vagus, but when the VMN is destroyed, this inhibition is lost and vagal activity is increased.[469] Vagotomy reverses the obesity in VMN-lesioned rats that are fed a chow diet but not a palatable diet.[467–469] Lesions of the lateral hypothalamus, which destroy the nigrostriatal dopaminergic fibers that pass through this area, produce hypophagia along with an increase in the peripheral norepinephrine turnover and metabolic rates. In contrast, stimulation of the VMN inhibits food intake and stimulation of the lateral hypothalamus stimulates food intake.[467–469]

In states of negative energy balance, there is inhibition of the PVN satiety neurons, causing activation of the PVN-VMN noradrenergic system, which results in increases in ingestion of carbohydrate, meal size, and the rate of meal ingestion but not the frequency of meals.[470] Neuropeptide Y is also released from the PVN along with norepinephrine and appears to have an independent role in stimulating food intake, although the site of action is not clear.[470] The endogenous opioid peptides may also act at multiple hypothalamic sites to stimulate eating behavior.[470] Dopamine, epinephrine, and norepinephrine have inhibitory effects on food intake at a site in the lateral hypothalamus.[470] Medications which release or enhance the synthesis of endogenous catecholamines, such as amphetamines, are more effective at this lateral site than they are in the PVN, resulting in a decrease in food intake.[468,470] Serotonin has inhibitory effects at the PVN in opposition to the effects of norepinephrine.[470] Cholecystokinin and CRH also have inhibitory actions on food intake at the PVN.[350,467–470] In addition, peripheral glucocorticoids appear to upregulate hypothalamic noradrenergic receptors, potentiating PVN norepinephrine, decreasing CRH release, and resulting in increased food intake.[468,470]

Hypothalamic Obesity

Destruction of the ventromedial area of the hypothalamus results in obesity in humans as well as in animals. Because the mediobasal hypothalamus is the final common pathway for the hypophysiotropic factors as they travel to the median eminence and for the fibers that go to the posterior pituitary, such lesions commonly also produce hypopituitarism and diabetes insipidus. In one series of eight patients with well-characterized hypothalamic obesity, the lesions included trauma, dermoid tumor, tuberculosis, chordoma, lipoma, craniopharyngioma, aneurysm, and meningioma.[471] Seven of these patients had hypogonadotropic hypogonadism and decreased GH levels, one was also hypothyroid and hypoadrenal, and another had diabetes insipidus and galactorrhea. As the lesion grows, various hypothalamic abnormalities may appear sequentially (Fig. 7-28). In patients with hypothalamic obesity, the weight gain tends to be rapid and eventually stabilizes, with the total gain usually being under 50 kg and the final body weight usually being under 140 kg.[471] The weight gain is due to hypertrophy of existing adipocytes rather than to hyperplasia. The basal metabolic rate and the rate of lipolysis are not different from those of other obese patients or normal individuals. However, patients with hypothalamic obesity are even more insulin-resistant than are idiopathic obese patients, but it is not clear whether this is of pathogenetic importance.[471]

There are a number of rare syndromes in which obesity is a major part for which a hypothalamic etiology has been postulated (Table 7-5). Prader-Willi syndrome is the most common of these syndromes, occurring in 1 in 25,000 births. It is characterized by hypotonia, obesity, short stature, mental deficiency, hypogonadism, and small hands and feet.[472,473] About half these patients have a chromosome 15 deletion. The short stature is associated with low basal and stimulatable GH levels along with an absent pubertal growth spurt.[472,473] The hypogonadism is due to gonadotropin insufficiency that is unresponsive to standard GnRH stimulation tests. However, if patients are pretreated with clomiphene, the gonadotropin responses normalize.[472] Thyroid and adrenal functions are normal.[472] In the few cases studied at autopsy, no discernible hypotha-

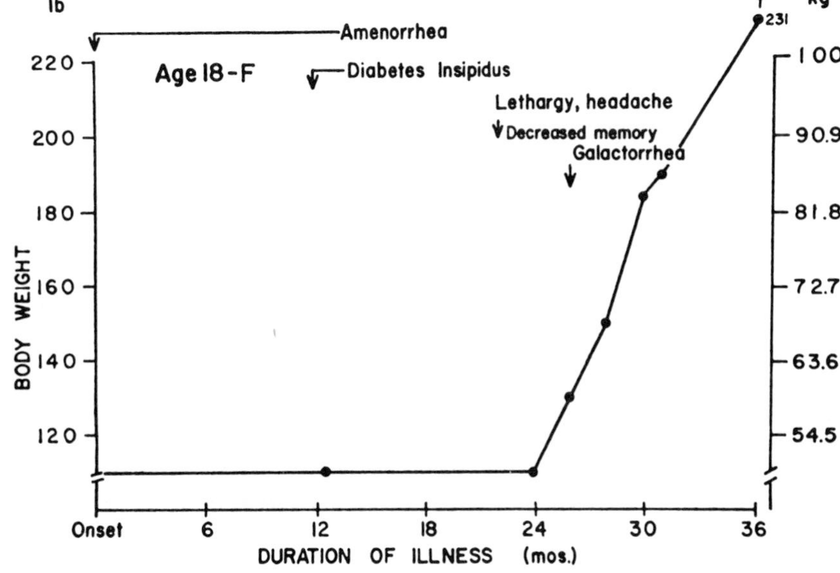

FIGURE 7-28. Clinical sequence in an 18-year-old woman with hypothalamic tuberculosis which progressed despite antituberculosis therapy. Her initial endocrine symptom was amenorrhea, which was followed over several months by the development of diabetes insipidus, lethargy, headache, decreased memory, and galactorrhea and culminated in a massive weight gain over the year before death. *(Reproduced with permission from Bray and Gallagher.[471])*

TABLE 7-5 Syndromes of Hypothalamic Obesity

Syndrome	Clinical features	Etiology
Babinski-Froehlich	Obesity and hypogonadism	Craniopharyngioma or other tumor involving the ventromedial hypothalamus and median eminence
Kleine-Levin	Episodic hyperosmia, hyperphagia, hyperactivity when awake, hypersexuality	Preceding viral infection in some patients; disorder seen primarily in teenage males; usually disappears by mid-twenties; no histologic examinations performed; possible paroxysmal limbic system or hypothalamic disease
Laurence-Moon	Pigmentary retinal degeneration, mental deficiency, spastic paraplegia, hypogonadism, obesity	Autosomal dominant inheritance; no gross or microscopic lesions of hypothalamus seen
Bardet-Biedl	Pigmentary retinopathy, mental deficiency, polydactylism, hypogonadism, obesity	No anatomic lesions seen
Allstrom-Hallgren	Pigmentary retinopathy, hypogonadism, deafness, obesity, diabetes	No anatomic lesions seen
Edwards	Pigmentary retinopathy, hypogonadism, gynecomastia, mental retardation, deafness, obesity, diabetes	Autosomal recessive inheritance; no histologic examinations performed
Prader-Willi	Hypogonadism, diabetes, short stature, obesity, temperature intolerance, loss of diurnal rhythms	No anatomic lesions seen

Sources: Adapted from Edwards et al,[472] Plum and Van Uitert,[25] Bray et al,[472] and McKusick VA: Mendelian Inheritance in Man: Catalogs of Autosomal Dominant, Autosomal Recessive, and X-Linked Phenotypes. Baltimore, The Johns Hopkins University, 1975.

lamic lesions were detected.[473] In the other syndromes listed in Table 7-5, no specific hypothalamic lesions have been found.[25,474]

Hypothalamic Anorexia

This syndrome is very rare, probably owing to the requirement for bilateral lesions. As opposed to a lesion in the midline, which could easily damage both ventromedial nuclei, a single lesion damaging both sides of the hypothalamus in its lateral aspects would have to be very large and cause a great deal of other hypothalamic dysfunction, including panhypopituitarism in most cases.[25] The hormonal changes that occur in anorexia nervosa all appear to be secondary to the weight loss, and there is no evidence for a primary hypothalamic disorder in this syndrome (see Chap. 32).

Diencephalic Syndrome

This syndrome consists of a diencephalic tumor associated with emaciation and minimal neurologic signs and symptoms occurring in infants and children.[475] In most cases the tumor is located in the third ventricle, but some are optic nerve gliomas and others occur in the fourth ventricle. Most of these tumors are gliomas and astrocytomas, although a small number of dysgerminomas have been reported. Although the characteristic clinical feature is emaciation with anorexia and vomiting, these children appear inappropriately alert, hyperactive, and even euphoric.[475] The alert appearance is due to lid retraction rather than true alertness. In addition to these features, a number of neurologic signs may be present if looked for carefully, including nystagmus, optic pallor, irritability, tremor, and excessive sweating. Endocrine features include a loss of cortisol diurnal variation, an increase in basal GH levels, and a paradoxic rise of GH with a glucose load and diabetes insipidus.[475] Most children die of the primary tumor within 2 years of the diagnosis. In those who live longer, there may be a progression of the primary symptoms of emaciation and wasting[475] or there may rarely be a reversal to hypothalamic obesity.[476] These tumors do not specifically affect the lateral hypothalamus and, if anything, tend to cause destruction of the mediobasal hypothalamus. Why the immature ventromedial area should respond differently to destruction compared to that of older individuals with regard to the regulation of food intake is not known.[25]

Hyperglycemia

Hypothalamic activation as part of the generalized response to stress can cause a release of GH, PRL, and ACTH, which serve as counterregulatory hormones with respect to insulin. These hormones serve to promote lipolysis, gluconeogenesis, and insulin resistance, resulting in glucose elevation (see Chaps. 19 and 20). Of more importance in the acute response to stress, this hypothalamic response results in sympathetic activation with release of catecholamines which inhibit insulin secretion and stimulate glycogenolysis. In rare circumstances of acute hypothalamic injury from trauma, stroke, or infection, severe hyperglycemia can occur which is similar to the hyperglycemia seen in animals when the floor of the fourth ventricle is pricked with a needle, a phenomenon referred to as "piqûre" diabetes by Bernard.[477]

Temperature Regulation

The anterior hypothalamus and preoptic area contain temperature-sensitive neurons that respond to internal temperature changes by initiating certain thermoregulatory responses that are necessary to restore a constant temperature.[478] Measures that dissipate heat include cutaneous vasodilation, sweating, panting, and behavioral changes which result in attempts to alter the environment. Measures that increase body heat include increasing metabolic heat production, shivering, cutaneous vasoconstriction, and similar behavioral changes.[478] In humans, much of the increase in metabolic heat production occurs via sympathetic activation. The thermosensitive neurons are affected by endogenous pyrogens and drugs which alter thermoregulation as well as by input from thermoreceptors in the skin and spinal cord.[478]

Rare patients have been reported with anterior hypothalamic lesions which caused sustained hypothermia as a result of failure of heat generation by shivering and vasoconstriction but who had intact heat dissipation[479] or resetting of the temperature set point lower.[480] Paroxysmal hypothermia lasting for minutes to days caused by the sudden onset of sweating, vasodilation, and a fall in core temperature has been reported in a number of patients in association with demonstrated lesions such as tumors and agenesis of the corpus callosum. Some of these patients had evidence of other hypothalamic dysfunction, including diabetes insipidus, hypogonadism, and precocious puberty.[481]

Fever as a manifestation of hypothalamic disease is uncommon but has been reported in relation to trauma or bleeding into the region of the anterior hypothalamus.[25] Such fevers rarely persist more than 2 weeks.[25] Paroxysmal hyperthermia due to hypothalamic dysfunction also occurs. One patient had episodes of fever that recurred in regular 3-week cycles.[482] Some cases of paroxysmal hypo- and hyperthermia respond to anticonvulsant medications, suggesting that the neuronal discharges that cause the temperature changes are seizure-like.[25]

Poikilothermia results from the inability to dissipate or generate heat to keep the body temperature constant in the face of varying ambient temperatures. This condition results from bilateral lesions in the posterior hypothalamus and rostral mesencephalon, which are the areas responsible for the final integration of thermoregulatory neural efferents.[25] Patients with this condition do not feel discomfort with temperature changes and are unaware of having a problem. Depending on the ambient temperature, they may present with life-threatening hypo- or hyperthermia. Poikilothermia is normally present in infants and frequently occurs in elderly individuals.

Neuroendocrine Alterations in Systemic Disease

Systemic diseases have widespread effects on neuroendocrine regulation. In most cases, the only knowledge available is of alterations in pituitary function which reflect the integration of combined stimulatory and inhibitory hypothalamic influences. In many systemic illnesses reported changes in pituitary function have not been distinguished satisfactorily from the changes known to be associated with "stress" due to the illness, and so the effects of such illnesses may be considered nonspecific. In very few circumstances have the alterations in neurotransmitters that cause the changes in hormone secretion been demonstrated.

Stress

Since the early studies of Hans Selye, stress has been known to play an important role in modifying the hormonal regulation of the internal milieu. Although a distinction can be made between physical and mental stress, it is clear that when physical stress occurs, there is a considerable emotional component that must also be considered.

Physical Stress

ACTH and cortisol levels rise within 15 min of the onset of a severe physical stress such as surgery and return to normal 8 to 10 h after surgery.[483] The corticosteroid production rate increases 10-fold during surgery,[483] giving rise to the common clinical practice of administering exogenous steroids in doses 10 times normal during surgery or other severe stress in patients with adrenal insufficiency. It is the triggering of neural afferents to the hypothalamus by the surgery that is responsible for the output of ACTH and cortisol; in patients with spinal cord transection, surgery below the level of the cord lesion does not produce a rise in steroid levels.[483] If the stress is maintained, cortisol secretion stays modestly elevated for as long as the patient is ill.[484] Both cholinergic and serotoninergic pathways probably mediate the release of CRH during stress, and the endogenous opioid pathways probably have little influence in this regard.[356]

Severe illness also causes a rise in GH[485] and PRL levels,[486] but more persistent, less acute illness does not, despite a persistent increase in cortisol.[484] The stress-induced rise in GH is probably mediated by noradrenergic pathways, resulting in an increase in GHRH, as alpha-adrenergic blockade can inhibit this response.[487] By contrast, stress results in a reduction of TSH levels as part of the euthyroid sick syndrome[488] (see Chap. 10) and gonadotropin levels.[489] These hormonal changes may be viewed teleologically as beneficial in that they increase vascular tone, provide increased energy substrate, decrease the basal metabolic rate, and shunt energy away from temporarily unneeded activities. These changes are presumably due to alterations in hypophysiotropic hormone release and/or the pituitary responses to such hormones, and in turn, these alterations result from changes in neurotransmitter turnover and the effects of stress-induced high levels of cortisol.

Psychological Stress

Acute psychological stress can raise ACTH, GH, and PRL levels, and a number of changes in pituitary hormones occur with chronic psychiatric diseases such as depression and schizophrenia. These changes are discussed in Chap. 32.

Metabolic Disorders

Fasting and Malnutrition

Short-term dieting can cause a reduction in gonadotropin levels sufficient to cause amenorrhea, but the LH and FSH responses to GnRH are normal, implying a hypothalamic site of action.[450] A similar blunting of basal and TRH-stimulated TSH secretion occurs.[450,488] With such dieting, basal GH levels become modestly elevated but there is no change in ACTH or PRL levels.[450] Although prolonged protein-calorie malnutrition results in decreased cortisol production, the metabolic clearance rate is also reduced, so that serum cortisol levels are minimally elevated and are only partially suppressible with dexamethasone.[490] Basal GH levels are elevated and IGF-I levels are decreased in protein-calorie malnutrition but not in marasmus,[491] suggesting that it is the decreased IGF-I feedback that causes the increased GH levels. Thyroid hormone levels remain low in protein-calorie malnutrition and basal TSH levels are normal, but the response to TRH is delayed and sometimes exaggerated.[492] With prolonged malnutrition, amenorrhea persists. The hormonal changes in patients with anorexia nervosa are similar to those in patients with simple weight loss (Chap. 32). Again, these hormonal changes may be regarded as being adaptive to conserve energy, as with physical stress.

Obesity

ACTH and cortisol levels are usually normal in obesity, but the normal diurnal rhythm may be disrupted and the cortisol production rate may be increased.[493] Although the overnight dexamethasone suppression test may not fully suppress morning cortisol levels in obese patients, a full 2-day low-dose test usually will.[493] Basal GH levels are low to normal, and the GH response to a variety of stimuli such as hypoglycemia, L-dopa, arginine, and exercise, as well as GHRH itself, are all markedly blunted in the obese.[493] This blunting of the GH response appears to be due to a defect of cholinergic tone, resulting in an excess of somatostatin, as treatment with the cholinesterase inhibitor pyridostigmine restores most of these responses.[494] Basal PRL and TSH levels and the PRL and TSH responses to TRH are usually normal.[493]

The onset of menarche frequently occurs at a younger age in obese girls than in girls of normal weight. It has been proposed that puberty and menstruation are initiated in females when body weight or the percentage of body fat reaches a critical level[385] (see Chap. 26). Obese women often show menstrual irregularity. Analysis of the pattern of hormone secretion during the course of the cycle in obese women reveals that FSH levels do not rise normally during the midfollicular phase and that there is deficient progesterone secretion by the corpus luteum, resulting in a short luteal phase.[494] The mechanisms underlying these changes are not clear, and gonadotropin pulsatile secretion and responses to GnRH are normal in obesity.[493]

It is clear that these hormonal alterations are consequent to and in no way causative of the obesity, since experimental studies have shown that they do not exist prior to the obesity.[495] The hormonal and other consequences of obesity are discussed in Chap. 21.

Diabetes Mellitus

In poorly controlled diabetes mellitus of all types, intracellular glucose metabolism is disrupted. Basal and stimulated GH levels are increased in patients with poorly controlled diabetes and return toward normal with improved control.[496] The elevated GH levels are associated with low IGF-I levels in some studies.[496] The increased GH levels are at least in part mediated by a decrease in somatostatinergic tone. Treatment with the cholinergic agonist pirenzepine, which increases central somatostatin release, causes the elevated GH levels to return to normal.[497] Few data are available on other hormone levels.

Cirrhosis

Cirrhosis of all etiologies may cause abnormalities of neuroendocrine function. However, most of the information has been obtained in patients with Laënnec's cirrhosis, and in many circumstances, the effects of cirrhosis are difficult to separate from the changes induced by the alcohol.

About 25 percent of chronic alcoholics have reduced cortisol responses to insulin-induced hypoglycemia.[498] However, alcoholic patients may uncommonly present with cushingoid features and may have elevated cortisol levels that do not suppress normally in response to dexamethasone within the first few days of admission but return to normal over subsequent weeks.[499]

In patients with cirrhosis, GH levels are elevated both basally and after stimulation with arginine, hypoglycemia, and GHRH.[500,501] GH responses to TRH are found in about 75 percent of such patients.[500] IGF-I levels are decreased.[501] Basal PRL levels are increased in 15 to 20 percent of patients with alcoholic cirrhosis and 5 to 15 percent of those with nonalcoholic cirrhosis.[502] TSH levels, by contrast, are usually normal or decreased despite low to normal thyroid hormone levels, a picture compatible with the euthyroid sick syndrome.[503]

Cirrhosis of all causes has long been known to cause androgen and estrogen deficiency with altered steroid metabolism and a defect in the testicular generation of testosterone.[504] However, despite this apparent primary testicular defect, gonadotropin levels are not usually elevated and the response to GnRH is low to normal and is not increased.[505] The gonadotropin response to clomiphene is markedly blunted in men with Laënnec's cirrhosis even after abstention from alcohol for several weeks, implying that the defect is at the hypothalamic level. LH pulse analysis shows a decrease in the frequency and amplitude of LH pulses.[505]

Excessive alcohol intake in normal volunteers initially causes a decrease in testosterone levels with a rise in LH but not FSH levels. After 1 to 2 weeks of heavy alcohol intake, the testosterone levels remain low, the LH levels become subnormal, but there is no change in FSH levels.[506] Thus, in alcoholic cirrhosis the effects of alcohol and cirrhosis may be additive.

Renal Failure

Basal cortisol levels in renal failure have been reported to be both normal[507] and high.[508] Although ACTH levels are high, the ACTH response to CRH is blunted[507] and the suppression of cortisol by dexamethasone is impaired.[508] Treatment with erythropoietin causes a return to normal of elevated ACTH and cortisol levels. After treatment, these levels are lower than in patients not treated with erythropoietin, but the hematocrits are similar.[509] Thus, the erythropoietin-caused changes are not due exclusively to an improvement in the anemia.

Basal GH levels are increased in patients with chronic renal failure.[510] The GH response to GHRH is increased,[510] and there are paradoxic GH responses to TRH and glucose. Serum IGF-I levels are normal if uremic samples are processed with acid-ethanol extraction and acid chromatography,[511] but uremic children are short and bioassayable IGF-I levels tend to be low, suggesting that the IGF-I has a decreased ability to stimulate mitogenic pathways in growth plate chondrocytes.[511] It has been postulated that there are low-molecular-weight compounds that interfere with the biological activity of IGF-I.[512] If the elevated GH levels are due to decreased feedback of IGF-I, this decreased biological activity of IGF-I also pertains to the feedback effects. As with ACTH, treatment with erythropoietin causes a reduction in GH levels, with at least some of the reduction being independent of the correction of the anemia.[509]

Hyperprolactinemia occurs in 73 to 91 percent of women and 25 to 57 percent of men with end-stage renal disease.[513,514] PRL suppression by dopamine infusion is decreased,[513] but this may be at least in part a result of delayed degradation of PRL in renal failure since the long-term use of bromocriptine results in suppression of PRL levels. Although PRL metabolism is reduced in renal failure, there is also increased production.[515] Therefore, there is disordered regulation of PRL secretion and possibly short-loop feedback, although the exact nature of the defect has not been defined. About one-quarter of individuals with renal insufficiency who do not require dialysis (serum creatinine 2.0 to 12.0 ng/ml) have PRL levels in the range of 25 to 100 ng/ml.[514] When such patients take medications known to alter hypothalamic regulation of PRL, such as methyldopa and metoclopramide, PRL levels may rise to over 2000 ng/ml.[514] Correction of the renal failure with transplantation causes a return of PRL levels to normal.[513] Hyperprolactinemia plays a role in the hypogonadism of chronic renal failure but probably does not explain all the abnormalities in every case. Return of normal menses has occurred in some women and correction of impotence has occurred in some men treated with bromocriptine,[513] but reports of restored ovulation are rare.[513]

Basal levels of TSH are low or normal, TSH responses to TRH are blunted, and thyroid hormone levels are low, compatible with the euthyroid sick syndrome.[516] After renal transplantation, thyroid hormone levels and TSH levels return to normal, but the TSH response to TRH remains blunted, presumably because of corticosteroid administration.[516]

In renal failure there is a primary gonadal failure, but gonadotropin levels are inappropriately low for the degree of hypogonadism.[517] The gonadotropin response to GnRH is normal, but the lack of an exaggerated response suggests blunted pituitary responsiveness.[517] Negative estrogen feedback is preserved, as shown by normal responses to clomiphene, but positive estrogen feedback is impaired. With renal transplantation, ovulatory cycles return in 60 percent of women.[518]

Other CNS Disorders

Pineal Region Tumors

There are a number of different types of pineal region tumors. The term *pinealoma* is incorrect, and tumors should be referred to by their specific tissue types. Tumors of the pineal parenchyma are called pineocytomas or pineoblastomas, depending on the maturity of the cells. Tumors of the supporting pineal glial tissue are gliomas, astrocytomas, or ependymomas. Pineal cell and glial tumors account for nearly 50 percent of these tumors.[519] The most common tumor, called a germinoma, arises from primitive, undifferentiated germ cells.[519] These germ cells appear to migrate aberrantly from the yolk sac to this region during early embryonic development.[405] About one-third of germinomas produce hCG, leading to precocious puberty,[519] and about 10 percent metastasize via the CSF. Some germinomas can affect the hypothalamus by direct infiltration, but others arise there (see above). The germinomas that arise in the suprasellar area were referred to as ectopic pinealomas in the past. A small portion of germ cell tumors are true teratomas, containing cell types originating from each of the three layers that differentiate to form various somatic structures, such as hair and teeth. These teratomas can be benign or malignant, giving rise to choriocarcinomas which can secrete hCG. Among a total of 389 intracranial germ cell tumors, 65 percent were germinomas, 18 percent were teratomas, 5 percent were embryonal carcinomas, 7 percent were endodermal sinus tumors, and 5 percent were choriocarcinomas.[520] Thus, intracranial germ cell tumors are similar to those which occur in the mediastinum and other locations.

Symptoms depend on the site of presentation of the tumor. Suprasellar germinomas classically present with the triad of diabetes insipidus, visual disturbance, and hypogonadism (see above). Pineal region tumors can compress the aqueduct of Sylvius, giving rise to hydrocephalus with associated headaches, vomiting, and loss of consciousness. Pineal region tumors may also compress the quadrigeminal plate, interrupting fibers passing from the cortex to the superior colliculi, giving rise to Parinaud's syndrome (paralysis of conjugate upward gaze and ptosis).

Pineal region tumors have long been associated with the syndrome of precocious puberty. However, it is now known that these tumors account for only a small percentage of such cases (see above), and only a small percentage of pineal region tumors cause precocious puberty. Most cases of precocious puberty associated with pineal region tumors occur because of reasons similar to those for other intracranial neoplasms causing precocious puberty, i.e., a disinhibition of GnRH secretion.[455] Because the pineal tumors that cause precocious puberty are mostly nonparenchymal, destruction of the pineal may result in a decrease of a pineal antigonadotropin substance such as melatonin or another peptide.[521] Some hCG-secreting tumors may produce enough hormone to mimic puberty, and this probably accounts for a number of the cases of precocious puberty associated with pineal region tumors.[522]

HCG or α fetoprotein produced by tumors is often detectable in the CSF and allows an easy diagnosis; α fetoprotein is specific for malignant teratomas.[522] Occasionally malignant cells in the CSF may stain positively for these substances. The germinomas tend to be radiosensitive, and radiotherapy can be given if such markers are found.[522] Otherwise biopsy is necessary, and surgery or radiotherapy may be needed, depending on the tissue type. Chemotherapy may be indicated in some tumors of germ cell origin.[522]

Pseudotumor Cerebri

In this condition there is a chronic increase in intracranial pressure, giving rise to headache as the most common presenting feature, although visual symptoms may also occur. These symptoms mimic those of an intracranial tumor, although no tumor is present—thus the name and the alternative name, *benign intracranial hypertension*. An association with endocrine disease has been suggested in some cases, as it may occur with pregnancy, oral contraceptive use, hypoparathyroidism, or Addison's disease; after glucocorticoid withdrawal and the cure of Cushing's syndrome; and after the institution of thyroid hormone replacement in hypothyroidism.[523] However, with pseudotumor cerebri itself there is no hormonal deficit, although GH responses may be decreased as is expected in a syndrome in which patients are overweight.

In some patients, however, there is an associated partially empty sella. About 10 to 15 percent of patients with pseudotumor cerebri have empty sellas, and 25 to 50 percent of patients with empty sellas who present because of headaches or visual symptoms are found to have increased intracranial pressure. In this circumstance, there is usually a defect in the diaphragm sella with transmission of the increased intracranial pressure to the sella. Varying degrees of hypopituitarism and hyperprolactinemia have been found in patients with empty sellas, and so a brief screening evaluation is usually necessary[524] (see Chap. 8).

Cerebral Gigantism

This rare syndrome is associated with an increased early growth rate, mild mental retardation, and dilated cerebral ventricles unaccompanied by increased GH levels.[525] Other clinical features include a typical facies characterized by hypertelorism, prominent supraorbital ridge, high-arched palate, and prognathism; large hands and feet; advanced bone age; and nonprogressive cerebral dysfunction. In addition to the normal GH levels, bioactive IGF-I levels are also normal. The mean birth weight is between the 75th and 97th percentiles, and the mean birth length is at the 97th percentile, suggesting that the process started during gestation.[526] The children display moderate psychomotor retardation and behavioral difficulties.[526] The etiology of the condition is not known and no identifiable endocrine abnormalities have been found.

REFERENCES

1. Scharrer E, Scharrer B: Secretory cells within the hypothalamus, in *The Hypothalamus.* Res Publ Assoc Res Nerve Ment Dis vol. XX. New York, Hafner, 1940, p 170.
2. Snyder SH: Drug and neurotransmitter receptors in the brain. *Science* 224:22, 1984.
3. Bloom FE: Neurotransmitters: Past, present, and future directions. *FASEB J* 2:32, 1988.
4. Håkanson R, Böttcher G, Ekblad E, Grunditz T, Sundler F: Functional implications of messenger coexpression in neurons and endocrine cells, in Schwartz TW, Hilsted LM, Rehfeld JF (eds): *Neuropeptides and Their Receptors.* Copenhagen, Munksgaard, 1990, p 211.
5. Whitnall MH: Stress selectively activates the vasopressin-containing subset of corticotropin-releasing hormone neurons. *Neuroendocrinology* 50:702, 1989.
6. Harris GW: Neural control of the pituitary gland. *Physiol Rev* 28:139, 1948.
7. Fröhlich A: Ein Fall von Tumor der Hypophysis ceribri ohne Akromegalie. *Klin Rundsch* 15:883, 1901.
8. Erdheim J: Uber hypophysenganggeschwulste and Hirncholesteratome. *Sitzber Akad Wien* 113:537, 1904.
9. Harris GW, Jacobsohn D: Functional grafts of the anterior pituitary gland. *Proc R Soc Lond* 139:263, 1952.
10. Nikitovitch-Winer M, Everett JW: Functional restitution of pituitary grafts retransplanted from kidney to median eminence. *Endocrinology* 63:916, 1958.
11. Green JD, Harris GW: The neurovascular link between the neurohypophysis and adenohypophysis. *J Endocrinol* 5: 136, 1947.
12. Popa G, Fielding U: A portal circulation from the pituitary to the hypothalamic region. *J Anat* 65:88, 1930.
13. Wislocki GB, King LS: The permeability of the hypophysis and hypothalamus to vital dyes, with a study of the hypophyseal vascular supply. *J Anat* 58:421, 1936.
14. Török B: Structure of the vascular connections of the hypothalamo-hypophysial region. *Acta Anat (Basel)* 59:84, 1964.
15. Oliver C, Mical RS, Porter JC: Hypothalamic-pituitary vasculature: Evidence for retrograde blood flow in the pituitary stalk. *Endocrinology* 101:598, 1977.
16. Bøler J, Enzmann F, Folkers K, Bowers CY, Schally AV: The identity of chemical and hormonal properties of the thyrotropin releasing hormone and pyroglutamyl-histidyl-proline amide. *Biochem Biophys Res Commun* 37:705, 1969.
17. Burgus R, Dunn T, Desiderio D, Guillemin R: Structure moleculaire du facteur hypothalamique hypophysiotrope TRF d'origine ovine: Mise en evidence par spectrometre de masse de la sequence PCA-His-Pro-NH_2. *CR Acad Sci (Paris)* 269:1870, 1969.
18. Segerson TP, Kauer J, Wolfe HC, Mobtaker H, Wu P, Jackson IMD, Lechan RM: Thyroid hormone regulates TRH biosynthesis in the paraventricular nucleus of the rat hypothalamus. *Science* 238:78, 1987.
19. Berelowitz M, Maeda K, Harris S, Frohman LA: The effect of alterations in the pituitary-thyroid axis on hypothalamic content and *in vitro* release of somatostatinlike immunoreactivity. *Endocrinology* 107:24, 1980.
20. Larsen PR: Thyroid-pituitary interaction: Feedback regulation of thyrotropin secretion by thyroid hormones. *N Engl J Med* 306:23, 1982.
21. Berelowitz M, Szabo M, Frohman LA, Firestone S, Chu L: Somatomedin-C mediates growth hormone negative feedback by effects on both the hypothalamus and the pituitary. *Science* 212:1279, 1981.
22. Abe H, Molitch ME, Van Wyk JJ, Underwood LE: Human growth hormone and somatomedin C suppress the spontaneous release of growth hormone in unanesthetized rats. *Endocrinology* 113:1319, 1983.
23. Rosenthal SM, Hulse JA, Kaplan SL, Grumbach MM: Exogenous growth hormone inhibits growth hormone-releasing factor-induced growth hormone secretion in normal men. *J Clin Invest* 77:176, 1986.
24. Molitch ME, Hou SH: Neuroendocrine alterations in systemic disease. *Clinics Endocrinol Metab* 12:825, 1983.
25. Plum F, Van Uitert R: Nonendocrine diseases and disorders of the hypothalamus, in Reichlin S, Baldessarini RJ, Martin JB (eds): *The Hypothalamus.* New York, Raven Press, 1978, p 415.
26. Lechan RM: Neuroendocrinology of pituitary hormone regulation. *Endocrinol Metab Clin North Am* 16:475, 1987.
27. King JC, Anthony ELP, Fitzgerald DM, Stopa EG: Luteinizing hormone-releasing hormone neurons in human preoptic/hypothalamus: Differential intraneuronal localization of immunoreactive forms. *J Clin Endocrinol Metab* 60:88, 1985.
28. Moore RY: Organization and function of a central nervous system circadian oscillator: The suprachiasmatic hypothalamic nucleus. *Fed Proc* 42:2783, 1983.
29. Hoffman GE, Phelps CJ, Khachaturian H, Sladek JR Jr: Neuroendocrine projections to the median eminence. *Curr Top Neuroendocrinol* 7:161, 1986.
30. Wiegand SJ, Price JL: Cells of origin of the afferent fibers to the median eminence in the rat. *J Comp Neurol* 192:1, 1980.
31. Swanson LW, Sawchenko PE: Paraventricular nucleus: A site for the integration of neuroendocrine and autonomic mechanisms. *Neuroendocrinology* 31:410, 1980.
32. Krisch B, Leonhardt H, Buchheim W: The functional and structural border of the neurohemal region of the median eminence. *Cell Tissue Res* 192:327, 1978.
33. McKinley MJ, McAllen RM, Mendelsohn FAO, Allen AM, Chai SY, Oldfield BJ: Circumventricular organs: Neuroendocrine interfaces between the brain and the hemal milieu. *Front Neuroendocrinol* 11:91, 1990.

34. Page RB: Pituitary blood flow. *Am J Physiol* 243:E427, 1982.
35. Page RB: Directional pituitary blood flow: A microcinephotographic study. *Endocrinology* 112:157, 1983.
36. Antunes JL, Muraszko K, Stark R, Chen R: Pituitary portal blood flow in primates: A doppler study. *Neurosurgery* 12:492, 1983.
37. Le Dafniet M, Lefebvre P, Barret A, Mechain C, Feinstein MC, Brandi AM, Peillon F: Normal and adenomatous human pituitaries secrete thyrotropin-releasing hormone *in vitro:* Modulation by dopamine, haloperidol, and somatostatin. *J Clin Endocrinol Metab* 71:480, 1990.
38. Arnaout MA, Garthwaite TL, Martinson DR: Vasoactive intestinal polypeptide is synthesized in anterior pituitary tissue. *Endocrinology* 119:2052, 1986.
39. Guillemin R: Biochemical and physiological correlates of hypothalamic peptides: The new endocrinology of neuron, in Reichlin S, Baldessarini RJ, Martin JB (eds): *The Hypothalamus.* New York, Raven Press, 1978, p 155.
40. Jackson IMD, Lechan RM, Lee SL: TRH prohormone: Biosynthesis, anatomic distribution, and processing. *Front Neuroendocrinol* 11:267, 1990.
41. Palkovits M: Neuropeptides in the brain, in Martini L, Ganong WF (eds): *Frontiers in Neuroendocrinology.* New York, Raven Press, 1988, vol. 10, p. 1.
42. Richter K, Kawashima E, Egger R, Kreil G: Biosynthesis of thyrotropin releasing hormone in the skin of Xenopus laevis: Partial sequence of the precursor deduced from cloned cDNA. *EMBO J* 3:617, 1984.
43. Yamada M, Radovick S, Wondisford FE, Nakayama Y, Weintraub BD, Wilber JF: Cloning and structure of human genomic DNA and hypothalamic cDNA encoding human prepro thyrotropin-releasing hormone. *Mol Endocrinol* 4:551, 1990.
44. Peterkofsky A, Battaini F: The biological activities of the neuropeptide histidyl-proline diketopiperazine. *Neuropeptides* 1:105, 1980.
45. Koch Y, Okon E: Localization of releasing hormones in the human brain. *Int Rev Exp Pathol* 19:45, 1979.
46. Manaker S, Eichen A, Winokur A, Rhodes CH, Rainbow TC: Autoradiographic localization of thyrotropin releasing hormone receptors in human brain. *Neurology* 36:641, 1986.
47. Lechan RM, Snapper SB, Jacobson S, Jackson IMD: The distribution of thyrotropin-releasing hormone (TRH) in the rhesus monkey spinal cord. *Peptides* 5:185, 1984.
48. Dolva LO, Hanssen KF, Aadland E, Sand T: Thyrotropin-releasing hormone immunoreactivity in the gastrointestinal tract of man. *J Clin Endocrinol Metab* 56:524, 1983.
49. Kawano H, Daikoku S, Saito S: Location of thyrotropin-releasing hormone-like immunoreactivity in rat pancreas. *Endocrinology* 112:951, 1983.
50. Schaeffer JM, Brownstein MJ, Axelrod J: Thyrotropin-releasing hormone-like material in the rat retina: Changes due to environmental lighting. *Proc Natl Acad Sci USA* 74:3579, 1977.
51. Shambaugh G III, Kubek M, Wilber JF: Thyrotropin-releasing hormone activity in the human placenta. *J Clin Endocrinol Metab* 48:483, 1979.
52. Amarant T, Fridkin M, Koch Y: Luteinizing hormone-releasing hormone and thyrotropin-releasing hormone in human and bovine milk. *Eur J Biochem* 127:647, 1982.
53. Pekary AE, Meyer NV, Vaillant C, Hershman JM: Thyrotropin-releasing hormone and a homologous peptide in the male rat reproductive system. *Biochem Biophys Res Commun* 95:993, 1980.
54. Kolesnick RN, Gershengorn MC: Thyrotropin-releasing hormone and the pituitary. *Am J Med* 79:729, 1985.
55. Gershengorn MC: Mechanism of thyrotropin releasing hormone stimulation of pituitary hormone secretion. *Annu Rev Physiol* 48:515, 1986.
56. Greenspan SL, Klibanski A, Schoenfeld D, Ridgway EC: Pulsatile secretion of thyrotropin in man. *J Clin Endocrinol Metab* 63:661, 1986.
57. Martin JB, Reichlin S: *Clinical Neuroendocrinology,* 2d ed. Philadelphia, Davis, 1987.
58. Reichlin S, Martin JB, Mitnick M, Boshans R, Grimm-Jorgensen Y, Bollinger J, et al: The hypothalamus in pituitary-thyroid regulation. *Recent Prog Horm Res* 28:229, 1972.
59. Koch Y, Goldhaber G, Fireman I, Zor U, Shani J, Tal E: Suppression of prolactin and thyrotropin secretion in the rat by antiserum to thyrotropin-releasing hormone. *Endocrinology* 100:1476, 1977.
60. Szabo M, Kovathana N, Gordon K, Frohman LA: Effect of passive immunization with an antiserum to thyrotropin (TSH)-releasing hormone on plasma TSH levels in thyroidectomized rats. *Endocrinology* 102:799, 1978.
61. Fraser HM, McNeilly AS: Effect of chronic immunoneutralization of thyrotropin-releasing hormone on the hypothalamic-pituitary-thyroid axis, prolactin, and reproductive function in the ewe. *Endocrinology* 111:1964, 1982.
62. Sheward WJ, Fraser HM, Fink G: Effect of immunoneutralization of thyrotrophin-releasing hormone on the release of thyrotrophin and prolactin during suckling or in response to electrical stimulation of the hypothalamus in the anaesthetized rat. *J Endocrinol* 106:113, 1985.
63. Noel GL, Dimond RC, Wartofsky L, Earll JM, Grantz AG: Studies of prolactin and TSH secretion by continuous infusion of small amounts of thyrotropin-releasing hormone (TRH). *J Clin Endocrinol Metab* 39:6, 1974.
64. Horn AM, Fraser HM, Fink G: Effects of antiserum to thyrotrophin-releasing hormone on the concentrations of plasma prolactin, thyrotrophin and LH in the pro-oestrous rat. *Endocrinology* 104:205, 1985.
65. De Greef WJ, Visser TJ: Evidence for the involvement of hypothalamic dopamine and thyrotrophin-releasing hormone in suckling-induced release of prolactin. *J Endocrinol* 91:213, 1981.
66. Gautvik KM, Tashjian AH Jr, Kourides IA, Weintraub BD, Graeber CT, Maloof F, et al: Thyrotropin-releasing hormone is not the sole physiologic mediator of prolactin release during suckling. *N Engl J Med* 290:1162, 1974.
67. Jeppsson S, Rannevik KON, Wide L: Influence of suckling and of suckling followed by TRH or LH-RH on plasma prolactin, TSH, GH and FSH. *Acta Endocrinol (Copenh)* 82:246, 1976.
68. Mori M, Yamada M: Thyroid hormones regulate the amount of thyrotrophin-releasing hormone in the hypothalamic median eminence of the rat. *J Endocrinol* 114:443, 1987.
69. Perrone MH, Hinkle PM: Regulation of pituitary receptors for thyrotropin releasing hormone by thyroid hormones. *J Biol Chem* 253:5168, 1978.
70. Snyder PJ, Jacobs LS, Utiger RD, Daughaday WH: Thyroid hormone inhibition of the prolactin response to thyrotropin-releasing hormone. *J Clin Invest* 52:2324, 1973.
71. Rondeel JMM, DeGreef WJ, Schoot PVD, Karels B, Klootwijk W, Visser TJ: Effect of thyroid status and paraventricular area lesions on the release of thyrotropin-releasing hormone and catecholamines into hypophyseal portal blood. *Endocrinology* 123:523, 1988.
72. Hirooka Y, Hollander CS, Suzuki S, Ferdinand P, Juan S-I: Somatostatin inhibits release of thyrotropin releasing factor from organ cultures of rat hypothalamus. *Proc Natl Acad Sci USA* 75:4509, 1978.
73. Scanlon MF, Rodriguez-Arnao, Pourmand M, Shale DJ, Weightman DR, Lewis M, Hall R: Catecholaminergic interactions in the regulation of thyrotropin (TSH) secretion in man. *J Endocrinol Invest* 3:125, 1980.
74. Terry CL: Regulation of thyrotropin secretion by the central epinephrine system. *Neuroendocrinology* 42:102, 1986.
75. Smythe GA, Bradshaw JE, Cai WY, Symons RG: Hypothalamic serotoninergic stimulation of thyrotropin secretion and related brain-hormone and drug interactions in the rat. *Endocrinology* 111:1181, 1982.

76. Daneshdoost L, Gennarelli TA, Bashey HM, Savino PJ, Sergott RC, Bosley TM, et al: Recognition of gonadotroph adenomas in women. *N Engl J Med* 324:589, 1991.
77. Reichlin S: Neural functions of TRH. *Acta Endocrinol (Copenh) (suppl)* 276:21, 1986.
78. Holaday JW, D'Amato RJ, Faden AI: Thyrotropin-releasing hormone improves cardiovascular function in experimental endotoxic and hemorrhagic shock. *Science* 213:216, 1981.
79. Faden AI, Jacobs TP, Holaday JW: Thyrotropin-releasing hormone improves neurologic recovery after spinal trauma in cats. *N Engl J Med* 305:1063, 1981.
80. Matsuo H, Baba Y, Nair RMG, Arimura A, Schally AV: Structure of the porcine LH- and FSH-releasing hormone: I. The proposed amino acid sequence. *Biochem Biophys Res Commun* 43:1334, 1971.
81. Adelman JP, Mason AJ, Hayflick JS, Seeburg PH: Isolation of the gene and hypothalamic cDNA for the common precursor of gonadotropin-releasing hormone and prolactin release-inhibiting factor in human and rat. *Proc Natl Acad Sci USA* 83:179, 1986.
82. Radovick S, Wondisford FE, Nakayama Y, Yamada M, Cutler GB Jr, Weintraub BD: Isolation and characterization of the human gonadotropin-releasing hormone gene in the hypothalamus and placenta. *Mol Endocrinol* 4:476, 1990.
83. Phillips HS, Nikolics K, Branton D, Seeburg PH: Immunocytochemical localization in rat brain of a prolactin release-inhibiting sequence of gonadotropin-releasing hormone prohormone. *Nature* 316:542, 1985.
84. Rubin BS, King JC, Millar RP, Seeburg PH, Arimura A: Processing of luteinizing hormone-releasing hormone precursor in rat neurons. *Endocrinology* 121:305, 1987.
85. Chappel SC: Neuroendocrine regulation of luteinizing hormone and follicle stimulating hormone: A review. *Life Sci* 36:97–103, 1985.
86. Plant TM, Krey LC, Moossy J, McCormack JT, Hess DL, Knobil E: The arcuate nucleus and the control of gonadotropin and prolactin secretion in the female rhesus monkey (Macaca mulatta). *Endocrinology* 102:52, 1978.
87. Schwanzel-Fukuda M, Pfaff DW: Origin of luteinizing hormone-releasing hormone neurons. *Nature* 338:161, 1989.
88. Paull WK, Turkelson CM, Thomas CR, Arimura A: Immunohistochemical demonstration of a testicular substance related to luteinizing hormone-releasing hormone. *Science* 213:1263, 1981.
89. Aten RF, Ireland JJ, Weems CW, Behrman HR: Presence of gonadotropin-releasing hormone-like proteins in bovine and ovine ovaries. *Endocrinology* 120:1727, 1987.
90. Conn PM, Crowley W Jr: Gonadotropin-releasing hormone and its analogues. *N Engl J Med* 324:93, 1991.
91. Clayton RN: Gonadotrophin-releasing hormone: Its actions and receptors. *J Endocrinol* 120:11, 1989.
92. McCann SM, Mizunuma H, Samson WK, Lumpkin MD: Differential hypothalamic control of FSH secretion: A review. *Psychoneuroendocrinology* 8:299, 1983.
93. McNeilly AS: The control of FSH secretion. *Acta Endocrinol (Copenh)* 288:31, 1988.
94. Ying SY: Inhibins, activins, and follistatins: Gonadal proteins modulating the secretion of follicle-stimulating hormone. *Endocr Rev* 9:267, 1988.
95. Wierman ME, Rivier JE, Wang C: Gonadotropin-releasing hormone-dependent regulation of gonadotropin subunit messenger ribonucleic acid levels in the rat. *Endocrinology* 124:272, 1989.
96. Belchetz PE, Plant TM, Nakai Y, Keogh EJ, Knobil E: Hypophysial responses to continuous and intermittent delivery of hypothalamic gonadotropin-releasing hormone. *Science* 202:631, 1978.
97. Gambacciani M, Liu JH, Swartz WH, Tueros VS, Yen SSC, Rasmussen DD: Intrinsic pulsatility of luteinizing hormone release from the human pituitary in vitro. *Neuroendocrinology* 45:402, 1987.
98. Veldhuis JD, Evans WS, Johnson ML, Wills MR, Rogol AD: Physiological properties of the luteinizing hormone pulse signal: Impact of intensive and extended venous sampling paradigms on its characterization in healthy men and women. *J Clin Endocrinol Metab* 62:881, 1986.
99. Filicori M, Santoro N, Merriam GR, Crowley WF: Characterization of the physiological pattern of episodic gonadotropin secretion throughout the human menstrual cycle. *J Clin Endocrinol Metab* 62:1136, 1986.
100. Clarke IJ, Cummins JT: The temporal relationship between gonadotropin releasing hormone (GnRH) and luteinizing hormone (LH) secretion in ovariectomized ewes. *Endocrinology* 111:1737, 1982.
101. Urbanski HF, Pickel RL, Ramirez VD: Simultaneous measurement of gonadotropin-releasing hormone, luteinizing hormone, and follicle-stimulating hormone in the orchidectomized rat. *Endocrinology* 123:413, 1988.
102. Van Vugt DA, Diefenbach WD, Alston E, Ferin M: Gonadotropin-releasing hormone pulses in third ventricular cerebrospinal fluid of ovariectomized rhesus monkeys: Correlation with luteinizing hormone pulses. *Endocrinology* 117:1550, 1985.
103. Murdoch AP, Diggle PJ, Whites MC, Harris M, Kendall-Taylor P, Dunlop W: Luteinizing hormone in women is secreted in superimposed pulse patterns. *Clin Sci* 76:125, 1989.
104. Weiss J, Jameson JL, Burrin JM, Crowley WF Jr: Divergent responses of gonadotropin subunit messenger RNAs to continuous versus pulsatile gonadotropin-releasing hormone *in vitro*. *Mol Endocrinol* 4:557, 1990.
105. Carmel PW, Araki S, Ferin M: Pituitary stalk portal blood collection in rhesus monkeys: Evidence for pulsatile release of gonadotropin-releasing hormone (GnRH). *Endocrinology* 99:243, 1976.
106. Culler MD, Valenca MM, Merchenthaler I, Flerko B, Negro-Vilar A: Orchidectomony induces temporal and regional changes in the processing of the luteinizing hormone-releasing hormone prohormone in the rat brain. *Endocrinology* 122:1968, 1988.
107. Toranzo D, Dupont E, Simard J, Labrie C, Couet J, Labrie J, et al: Regulation of pro-gonadotropin-releasing hormone gene expression by sex steroids in the brain of male and female rats. *Mol Endocrinol* 3:1748, 1989.
108. Brann DW, Mahesh VB: Regulation of gonadotropin secretion by steroid hormones. *Front Neuroendocrinol* 12:165, 1991.
109. Frawley LS, Neill JD: Biphasic effects of estrogen on gonadotropin-releasing hormone-induced luteinizing hormone release in monolayer cultures of rat and monkey pituitary cells. *Endocrinology* 114:659, 1984.
110. Gharib SD, Wierman ME, Shupnik MA, Chin WW: Molecular biology of the pituitary gonadotropins. *Endocr Rev* 11:177, 1990.
111. Clarke IJ, Cummins JT: Increased gonadotropin-releasing hormone pulse frequency associated with estrogen-induced luteinizing hormone surges in ovariectomized ewes. *Endocrinology* 116:2376, 1985.
112. Steele PA, Judd SJ: Positive and negative feed-back effect of progesterone on luteinizing hormone secretion in postmenopausal women. *Clin Endocrinol (Oxf)* 20:1, 1988.
113. Santen RJ: Is aromatization of testosterone to estradiol required for inhibition of luteinizing hormone secretion in men? *J Clin Invest* 56:1555, 1975.
114. Sheckter CB, Matsumoto AM, Bremner WJ: Testosterone administration inhibits gonadotropin secretion by an effect directly on the human pituitary. *J Clin Endocrinol Metab* 68:397, 1989.
115. Farnworth PG, Robertson DM, de Kretser DM, Buger HG: Effects of 31 kDa bovine inhibin on FSH and LH in rat pituitary cells *in vitro:* Antagonism of gonadotrophin-releasing hormone agonists. *J Endocrinol* 119:233, 1988.
116. Wang QF, Farnworth PG, Findlay JK, Burger HG: Effect of purified 31K bovine inhibin on the specific binding of gona-

dotropin-releasing hormone to rat anterior pituitary cells in culture. *Endocrinology* 123:2161, 1988.

117. Carroll RS, Corrigan AZ, Gharib SD, Vale W, Chin WW: Inhibin, activin, and follistatin: Regulation of follicle-stimulating hormone messenger ribonucleic acid levels. *Mol Endocrinol* 3:1969, 1989.
118. Condon TP, Leipheimer RE, Curry JJ: Preliminary evidence for a CNS site of action for ovarian inhibin. *Life Sci* 32:1691, 1983.
119. DePaolo LV, Shimonaka M, Schwall RH, Ling N: *In vivo* comparison of the follicle-stimulating hormone-suppressing activity of follistatin and inhibin in ovariectomized rats. *Endocrinology* 128:668, 1991.
120. Lachelin GCL, Leblanc H, Yen SSC: The inhibitory effect of dopamine agonists on LH release in women. *J Clin Endocrinol Metab* 44:728, 1977.
121. Rasmussen DD, Liu JH, Wolf PL, Yen SSC: Gonadotropin-releasing hormone neurosecretion in the human hypothalamus: *In vitro* regulation by dopamine. *J Clin Endocrinol Metab* 62:479, 1986.
122. Kaufman JM, Kesner JS, Wilson RC, Knobil E: Electrophysiological manifestation of luteinizing hormone-releasing hormone pulse generator activity in the rhesus monkey: Influence of α-adrenergic and dopaminergic blocking agents. *Endocrinology* 116:1327, 1985.
123. Selmanoff M, Shu C, Petersen SL, Barraclough A, Zoeller RT: Single cell levels of hypothalamic messenger ribonucleic acid encoding luteinizing hormone-releasing hormone in intact, castrated, and hyperprolactinemic male rats. *Endocrinology* 128:459, 1991.
124. Stevenaert A, Beckers A, Vandalem JL, Hennen G: Early normalization of luteinizing hormone pulsatility after successful transsphenoidal surgery in women with microprolactinomas. *J Clin Endocrinol Metab* 62:1044, 1986.
125. Hsueh AJW, Jones PBC: Gonadotropin releasing hormone: Extrapituitary actions and paracrine control mechanisms. *Annu Rev Physiol* 45:83, 1983.
126. Hsueh AJW, Liu YX, Cajander S, Peng XR, Dahl K, Kristensen P, Tor NY: Gonadotropin-releasing hormone induces ovulation in hypophysectomized rats: Studies on ovarian tissue-type plasminogen activator activity, messenger ribonucleic acid content, and cellular localization. *Endocrinology* 122:1486, 1988.
127. Petraglia F, Volpe A, Genazzani AR, Rivier J, Sawchenko PE, Vale W: Neuroendocrinology of the human placenta. *Front Neuroendocrinol* 11:6, 1990.
128. Nikolics K, Mason AJ, Szönyi E, Ramachandran J, Seeburg PH: A prolactin-inhibiting factor within the precursor for human gonadotropin-releasing hormone. *Nature* 316:511, 1985.
129. Yu WH, Seeburg PH, Nikolics K, McCann SM: Gonadotropin-releasing hormone-associated peptide exerts a prolactin-inhibiting and weak gonadotropin-releasing activity *in vivo*. *Endocrinology* 123:390, 1988.
130. Millar RP, Wormald PJ, de L Milton RC: Stimulation of gonadotropin release by non-GnRH peptide sequence of the GnRH precursor. *Science* 232:68, 1986.
131. Reichlin S: Growth and the hypothalamus. *Endocrinology* 67:760, 1960.
132. Krulich L, Dhariwal APS, McCann SM: Stimulatory and inhibitory effects of purified hypothalamic extracts on growth hormone release from rat pituitary *in vitro*. *Endocrinology* 83:783, 1968.
133. Brazeau P, Vale W, Burgus R, Ling N, Butcher M, Rivier J, Guillemin R: Hypothalamic polypeptide that inhibits the secretion of immunoreactive pituitary growth hormone. *Science* 179:77, 1972.
134. Böhlen P, Brazeau P, Esch F, Ling N, Guillemin R: Isolation and chemical characterization of somatostatin-28 from rat hypothalamus. *Regu Pept* 2:359, 1981.
135. Rodriguez-Arnao MD, Rainbow SJ, Comaru-Schally AM, Meyers CA, Gomez-Pan A, Woodhead S, et al: Effects of prosomatostatin on growth hormone and prolactin response to arginine in man. *Lancet* 1:353, 1981.
136. Benoit R, Ling N, Bakhit C, Morrison JH, Alford B, Guillemin R: Somatostatin-28(1-12)-like immunoreactivity in the rat. *Endocrinology* 111:2149, 1982.
137. Shen LP, Rutter WJ: Sequence of the human somatostatin I gene. *Science* 224:168, 1984.
138. Goodman RH, Aron DC, Roos BA: Rat pre-prosomatostatin. *J Biol Chem* 258:5570, 1983.
139. Lechan RM, Goodman RH, Rosenblatt M, Reichlin S, Habener JF: Prosomatostatin-specific antigen in rat brain: Localization by immunocytochemical staining with an antiserum to a synthetic sequence of preprosomatostatin. *Proc Natl Acad Sci USA* 80:2780, 1983.
140. Charpenet G, Patel YC: Characterization of tissue and releasable molecular forms of somatostatin-$28_{1\text{-}12}$-like immunoreactivity in rat median eminence. *Endocrinology* 116: 1863, 1985.
141. Patel YC, Reichlin S: Somatostatin in hypothalamus, extrahypothalamic brain, and peripheral tissues of the rat. *Endocrinology* 102:523, 1978.
142. Epelbaum J, Willoughby JO, Brazeau P, Martin JB: Effects of brain lesions and hypothalamic deafferentation on somatostatin distribution in the rat brain. *Endocrinology* 101: 1495, 1977.
143. Delfs J, Robbins R, Connolly JL, Dichter M, Reichlin S: Somatostatin production by rat cerebral neurones in dissociated cell culture. *Nature* 283:676, 1980.
144. Alpert LC, Brawer JR, Patel YC, Reichlin S: Somatostatinergic neurons in anterior hypothalamus: Immunohistochemical localization. *Endocrinology* 98:255, 1976.
145. Chihara K, Arimura A, Kubli-Garfias C, Schally A: Enhancement of immunoreactive somatostatin release into hypophysial portal blood by electrical stimulation of the preoptic area in the rat. *Endocrinology* 105:1416, 1979.
146. Katakami H, Downs TR, Frohman LA: Inhibitory effect of hypothalamic medial preoptic area somatostatin on growth hormone-releasing factor in the rat. *Endocrinology* 123: 1103, 1988.
147. Ishikawa K, Taniguchi Y, Kurosumi K, Suzuki M, Shinoda M: Immunohistochemical identification of somatostatin-containing neurons projecting to the median eminence of the rat. *Endocrinology* 121:94, 1987.
148. Pierotti AR, Harmar AJ: Multiple forms of somatostatin-like immunoreactivity in the hypothalamus and amygdala of the rat: Selective localization of somatostatin-28 in the median eminence. *J Endocrinol* 105:383, 1985.
149. Delfs JR, Zhu CH, Dichter MA: Coexistence of acetylcholinesterase and somatostatin-immunoreactivity in neurons cultured from rat cerebrum. *Science* 223:61, 1984.
150. Rorstad OP, Senterman MK, Hoyte KM, Martin JB: Immunoreactive and biological active somatostatin-like material in the human retina. *Brain Res* 199:488, 1980.
151. Van Leeuwen FW, de Raay C, Swaab DF, Fisser B: The localization of oxytocin, vasopressin, somatostatin and luteinizing hormone releasing hormone in the rat neurohypophysis. *Cell Tissue Res* 202:189, 1979.
152. Sundler F, Alumets J, Håkanson R, Björklund L, Ljungberg O: Somatostatin-immunoreactive cells in medullary carcinoma of the thyroid. *Am J Pathol* 88:381, 1977.
153. Di SantAgnese PA, de Mesy Jensen KL: Somatostatin and/or somatostatin like immunoreactive endocrine-paracrine cells in the human prostate gland. *Arch Pathol Lab Med* 108:693, 1984.
154. Sasaki A, Yoshinaga K: Immunoreactive somatostatin in male reproductive system in humans. *J Clin Endocrinol Metab* 68:996, 1989.
155. Patel YC, Rao K, Reichlin S: Somatostatin in human cerebrospinal fluid. *N Engl J Med* 296:529, 1977.
156. Sørensen KV, Christensen SE, Hansen AP, Ingerslev J, Pedersen E, Ørskov H: The origin of cerebrospinal fluid

somatostatin: Hypothalamic or dispersed central nervous system secretion? *Neuroendocrinology* 32:335, 1981.
157. Patel YC, Baquiran G, Srikant CB, Posner BI: Quantitative *in vivo* autoradiographic localization of [^{125}I-Tyr^{11}] Somatostatin-14-and [Leu^{8}, D-trp^{22}-^{125}I-tyr^{25}] somatostatin-28-binding sites in rat brain. *Endocrinology* 119:2262, 1986.
158. Reubi JC, Lang W, Maurer R, Koper JW, Lamberts SWJ: Distribution and biochemical characterization of somatostatin receptors in tumors of the human central nervous system. *Cancer Res* 47:5758, 1987.
159. Schonbrunn A, Tashjian AH Jr: Characterization of functional receptors for somatostatin in rat pituitary cells in culture. *J Biol Chem* 253:6473, 1978.
160. Koch BD, Schonbrunn A: The somatostatin receptor is directly coupled to adenylate cyclase in GH_4C_1 pituitary cell membranes. *Endocrinology* 114:1784, 1984.
161. Reichlin S: Somatostatin. *N Engl J Med* 309:1495, 1983.
162. Skamene A, Patel YC: Infusion of graded concentrations of somatostatin in man: Pharmacokinetics and differential inhibitory effects on pituitary and islet hormones. *Clin Endocrinol (Oxf)* 20:555, 1984.
163. Wehrenberg WB, Ling N, Böhlen P, Esch F, Brazeau P, Guillemin R: Physiological roles of somatocrinin and somatostatin in the regulation of growth hormone secretion. *Biochem Biophys Res Comm* 109:562, 1982.
164. Plotsky PM, Vale W: Patterns of growth hormone-releasing factor and somatostatin secretion into the hypophysial-portal circulation of the rat. *Science* 230:461, 1985.
165. Terry LC, Willoughby JO, Brazeau P, Martin JB: Antiserum to somatostatin prevents stress-induced inhibition of growth hormone secretion in the rat. *Science* 192:565, 1976.
166. Tannenbaum GS, Epelbaum J, Colle E, Brazeau P, Martin JB: Antiserum to somatostatin reverses starvation-induced inhibition of growth hormone but not insulin secretion. *Endocrinology* 102:1909, 1978.
167. Tannenbaum GS, Ling N: The interrelationship of growth hormone (GH)-releasing factor and somatostatin in generation of the ultradian rhythm of GH secretion. *Endocrinology* 115:1952, 1984.
168. Frohman LA, Downs TR, Clarke IJ, Thomas GB: Measurement of growth hormone-releasing hormone and somatostatin in hypothalamic-portal plasma of unanesthetized sheep. *J Clin Invest* 86:17, 1990.
169. Epelbaum J, Moyse E, Tannenbaum GS, Kordon C, Beaudet A: Combined autoradiographic and immunohistochemical evidence for an association of somatostatin binding sites with growth hormone-releasing factor-containing nerve cell bodies in the rat arcuate nucleus. *J Neuroendocrinol* 1:109, 1989.
170. Aguila MC, McCann SM: Evidence that growth hormone-releasing factor stimulates somatostatin release *in vitro* via β-endorphin. *Endocrinology* 120:341, 1987.
171. Martha PM Jr, Blizzard RM, McDonald JA, Thorner MO, Rogol AD: A persistent pattern of varying pituitary responsivity to exogenous growth hormone (GH)-releasing hormone in GH-deficient children: Evidence supporting periodic somatostatin secretion. *J Clin Endocrinol Metab* 67:449, 1988.
172. Urman S, Critchlow V: Long term elevations in plasma thyrotropin, but not growth hormone, concentrations associated with lesion-induced depletion of median eminence somatostatin. *Endocrinology* 112:659, 1983.
173. Arimura A, Schally AV: Increase in basal and thyrotropin-releasing hormone (TRH)-stimulated secretion of thyrotropin (TSH) by passive immunization with antiserum to somatostatin in rats. *Endocrinology* 98:1069, 1976.
174. Williams TC, Kelijman M, Crelin WC, Downs TR, Frohman LA: Differential effects of somatostatin (SRIH) and a SRIH analog, SMS 201-995, on the secretion of growth hormone and thyroid-stimulating hormone in man. *J Clin Endocrinol Metab* 66:39, 1988.
175. Chihara K, Arimura A, Schally AV: Effect of intraventricular injection of dopamine, norepinephrine, acetylcholine, and 5-hydroxytryptamine on immunoreactive somatostatin release into rat hypophyseal portal blood. *Endocrinology* 104:1656, 1979.
176. Abe H, Kato Y, Chiba T, Taminato T, Fujita T: Plasma immunoreactive somatostatin levels in rat hypophysial portal blood: Effect of glucagon administration. *Life Sci* 23:1647, 1978.
177. Abe H, Chihara K, Chiba T, Matsukura S, Fujita T: Effect of intraventricular injection of neurotensin and other various bioactive peptides on plasma immunoreactive somatostatin levels in rat hypophysial portal blood. *Endocrinology* 108: 1939, 1981.
178. Tapia-Arancibia L, Reichlin S: Vasoactive intestinal peptide and PHI stimulate somatostatin release from rat cerebral cortical and diencephalic cells in dispersed cell culture. *Brain Res* 336:67, 1985.
179. Scarborough DE, Lee SL, Dinarello CA, Reichlin S: Interleukin-1β stimulates somatostatin biosynthesis in primary cultures of fetal rat brain. *Endocrinology* 124:549, 1989.
180. Aguila MC, McCann SM: Stimulation of somatostatin release from median eminence tissue incubated *in vitro* by taurine and related amino acids. *Endocrinology* 116:1158, 1985.
181. Alba-Roth J, Müller OA, Schopohl J, von Werder K: Arginine stimulates growth hormone secretion by suppressing endogenous somatostatin secretion. *J Clin Endocrinol Metab* 67:1186, 1988.
182. Drouva SV, Epelbaum J, Henry M, Tapia-Arancibia L, Laplante E, Kordon C: Ionic channels involved in the LHRH and SRIF release from rat mediobasal hypothalamus. *Neuroendocrinology* 32:155, 1981.
183. Montminy MR, Sevarino KA, Wagner JA, Mandel G, Goodman RH: Identification of a cyclic-AMP-responsive element within the rat somatostatin gene. *Proc Natl Acad Sci USA* 83:6682, 1986.
184. Andrisani OM, Dixon JE: Somatostatin gene regulation. *Annu Rev Physiol* 52:793, 1990.
185. Beal MF, Mazurek MF, Tran VT, Chattha G, Bird ED, Martin JB: Reduced numbers of somatostatin receptors in the cerebral cortex in Alzheimer's disease. *Science* 229:289, 1985.
186. Aronin N, Cooper PE, Lorenz LJ, Bird ED, Sagar SM, Leeman SE, et al: Somatostatin is increased in the basal ganglia in Huntington disease. *Ann Neurol* 13:519, 1983.
187. Pelton JT, Gulya K, Hruby VJ, Duckles S, Yamamura HI: Somatostatin analogs with affinity for opiate receptors in rat brain binding assay. *Peptides* 6:159, 1985.
188. Guillemin R, Rosenberg B: Humoral hypothalamic control of anterior pituitary: A study with combined tissue cultures. *Endocrinology* 57:599, 1955.
189. Saffran M, Schally AV, Benfey BG: Stimulation of the release of corticotrophin from the adenohypophysis by a neurohypophysial factor. *Endocrinology* 57:439, 1955.
190. Vale W, Spiess J, Rivier C, Rivier J: Characterization of a 41-residue ovine hypothalamic peptide that stimulates secretion of corticotropin and β-endorphin. *Science* 213:1394, 1981.
191. Shibahara S, Morimoto Y, Furutani Y, Notake M, Takahashi H, Shimizu S, et al: Isolation and sequence analysis of the human corticotropin-releasing factor precursor gene. *EMBO J* 2:775, 1983.
192. Favrod-Coune CA, Gaillard RC, Langevin H, Jaquier MC, Doci W, Muller AF: Anatomical localization of corticotropin-releasing activity in the human brain. *Life Sci* 39:2475, 1986.
193. Ohtani H, Mouri T, Sasaki A, Sasano N: Immunoelectron microscopic study of corticotropin-releasing factor in the human hypothalamus and pituitary gland. *Neuroendocrinology* 45:104, 1987.
194. Gibbs DM, Vale W: Presence of corticotropin releasing fac-

tor-like immunoreactivity in hypophysial portal blood. *Endocrinology* 111:1418, 1982.
195. Bruhn TO, Plotsky PM, Vale WW: Effect of paraventricular lesions on corticotropin-releasing factor (CRF)-like immunoreactivity in the stalk-median eminence: Studies on the adrenocorticotropin response to ether stress and exogenous CRF. *Endocrinology* 114:57, 1984.
196. Suda T, Tomori N, Tozawa F, Mouri T, Demura H, Shizume K: Distribution and characterization of immunoreactive corticotropin-releasing factor in human tissues. *J Clin Endocrinol Metab* 55:861, 1984.
197. Smith MA, Bissette G, Slotkin TA, Knight DL, Nemeroff CB: Release of corticotropin-releasing factor from rat brain regions *in vitro*. *Endocrinology* 118:1997, 1986.
198. Linton EA, Lowry PJ: Corticotrophin releasing factor in man and its measurement: A review. *Clin Endocrinol (Oxf)* 31:225, 1989.
199. Sasaki A, Sato S, Murakami O, Go M, Inoue M, Shimizu Y, et al: Immunoreactive corticotropin-releasing hormone present in human plasma may be derived from both hypothalamic and extrahypothalamic sources. *J Clin Endocrinol Metab* 65:176, 1987.
200. Behan DP, Linton EA, Lowry PJ: Isolation of the human plasma corticotrophin-releasing factor-binding protein. *J Endocrinol* 122:23, 1989.
201. Grino M, Guillaume V, Boudouresque F, Margioris AN, Grisoli F, Jaquet P, et al: Characterization of corticotropin-releasing hormone receptors on human pituitary corticotroph adenomas and their correlation with endogenous glucocorticoids. *J Clin Endocrinol Metab* 67:279, 1988.
202. Souza EB, Insel TR, Perrin MH, Rivier J, Vale WW, Kuhar MJ: Corticotropin-releasing factor receptors are widely distributed within the rat central nervous system: An autoradiographic study. *J Neurosci* 5:3189, 1985.
203. Antoni FA: Hypothalamic control of adrenocorticotropin secretion: Advances since the discovery of 41-residue corticotropin-releasing factor. *Endocr Rev* 7:351, 1986.
204. Schopohl J, Hauer A, Kaliebe T, Stalla GK, von Werder K, Müller OA: Repetitive and continuous administration of human corticotropin releasing factor to human subjects. *Acta Endocrinol (Copenh)* 112:157, 1986.
205. Rivier C, Rivier J, Vale W: Inhibition of adrenocorticotropic hormone secretion in the rat by immunoneutralization of corticotropin-releasing factor. *Science* 218:377, 1982.
206. Carnes M, Lent SJ, Goodman B, Mueller C, Saydoff J, Erisman S: Effects of immunoneutralization of corticotropin-releasing hormone on ultradian rhythms of plasma adrenocorticotropin. *Endocrinology* 126:1904, 1990.
207. Suda T, Tozawa F, Yamada M, Ushiyama T, Tomori N, Sumitomo T, et al: Insulin-induced hypoglycemia increases corticotropin-releasing factor messenger ribonucleic acid levels in rat hypothalamus. *Endocrinology* 123:1371, 1988.
208. Plotsky PM, Bruhn TO, Vale W: Hypophysiotropic regulation of adrenocorticotropin secretion in response to insulin-induced hypoglycemia. *Endocrinology* 117:323, 1985.
209. Liu JH, Muse K, Contreras P, Gibbs D, Vale W, Rivier J, et al: Augmentation of ACTH-releasing activity of synthetic corticotropin releasing factor (CRF) by vasopressin in women. *J Clin Endocrinol Metab* 57:1087, 1983.
210. Whitnall MH, Mezey E, Gainer H: Co-localization of corticotropin-releasing factor and vasopressin in median eminence neurosecretory vesicles. *Nature* 317:248, 1985.
211. Engler D, Pham T, Fullerton MJ, Ooi G, Funder JW, Clarke IJ: Studies of the secretion of corticotropin-releasing factor and arginine vasopressin into the hypophysial-portal circulation of the conscious sheep. *Neuroendocrinology* 49:367, 1989.
212. Jia LG, Canny BJ, Orth DN, Leong DA: Distinct classes of corticotropes mediate corticotropin-releasing hormone and arginine vasopressin-stimulated adrenocorticotropin release. *Endocrinology* 128:197, 1991.
213. Oki Y, Nicholson WE, Orth DN: Role of protein kinase-C in the adrenocorticotropin secretory response to arginine vasopressin (AVP) and the synergistic response to AVP and corticotropin-releasing factor by perifused rat anterior pituitary. *Endocrinology* 127:350, 1990.
214. Whitnall MH, Key S, Gainer H: Vasopressin-containing and vasopressin-deficient subpopulations of corticotropin-releasing factor axons are differentially affected by adrenalectomy. *Endocrinology* 120:2180, 1987.
215. Beyer HS, Matta SG, Sharp BM: Regulation of the messenger ribonucleic acid for corticotropin-releasing factor in the paraventricular nucleus and other brain sites of the rat. *Endocrinology* 123:2117, 1988.
216. Plotsky PM, Sawchenko PE: Hypophysial-portal plasma levels, median eminence content, and immunohistochemical staining of corticotropin-releasing factor, arginine vasopressin, and oxytocin after pharmacological adrenalectomy. *Endocrinology* 120:1361, 1987.
217. Plotsky PM, Vale W: Hemorrhage-induced secretion of corticotropin-releasing factor-like immunoreactivity into the rat hypophysial portal circulation and its inhibition by glucocorticoids. *Endocrinology* 114:164, 1984.
218. Bilezikjian LM, Vale WW: Glucocorticoids inhibit corticotropin-releasing factor-induced production of adenosine 3',5'-monophosphate in cultured anterior pituitary cells. *Endocrinology* 113:657, 1983.
219. Halász B, Szentágothai: Control of adrenocorticotrophic function by direct influence of pituitary substance on the hypothalamus. *Acta Morphol Hung* 9:251, 1960.
220. Suda T, Yajima F, Tomori N, Sumitomo T, Nakagami Y, Ushiyama T, et al: Inhibitory effect of adrenocorticotropin on corticotropin-releasing factor release from rat hypothalamus *in vitro*. *Endocrinology* 118:459, 1985.
221. Taylor T, Dluhy RG, Williams GH: β-endorphin suppresses adrenocorticotropin and cortisol levels in normal human subjects. *J Clin Endocrinol Metab* 57:592, 1983.
222. Rittmaster RS, Cutler GB Jr, Sobel DO, Goldstein DS, Koppelman MCS, Loriaux DL, et al: Morphine inhibits the pituitary-adrenal response to ovine corticotropin-releasing hormone in normal subjects. *J Clin Endocrinol Metab* 60:891, 1985.
223. Plotsky PM, Otto S, Sutton S: Neurotransmitter modulation of corticotropin releasing factor secretion into the hypophysial-portal circulation. *Life Sci* 41:1311, 1987.
224. Calogero AE, Gallucci WT, Chrousos GP, Gold PW: Catecholamine effects upon rat hypothalamic corticotropin-releasing hormone secretion *in vitro*. *J Clin Invest* 82:839, 1988.
225. Tsagarakis S, Holly JMP, Rees LH, Besser GM, Grossman A: Acetylcholine and norepinephrine stimulate the release of corticotropin-releasing factor-41 from the rat hypothalamus *in vitro*. *Endocrinology* 123:1962, 1988.
226. Calogero AE, Gallucci WT, Bernardini R, Saoutis C, Gold PW, Chrousos GP: Effect of cholinergic agonists and antagonists on rat hypothalamic corticotropin-releasing hormone secretion in vitro. *Neuroendocrinology* 47:303, 1988.
227. Bateman A, Singh A, Kral T, Solomon S: The immune-hypothalamic-pituitary-adrenal axis. *Endocr Rev* 10:92, 1989.
228. Suda T, Tozawa F, Ushiyama T, Sumitomo T, Yamada M, Demura H: Interleukin-1 stimulates corticotropin-releasing factor gene expression in rat hypothalamus. *Endocrinology* 126:1223, 1990.
229. Breder CD, Dinarello CA, Saper CB: Interleukin-1 immunoreactive innervation of the human hypotholamus. *Science* 240:321, 1988.
230. Lenz HJ, Raedler A, Greten H, Brown MR: CRF initiates biological actions within the brain that are observed in response to stress. *Am J Physiol* 21:34, 1987.
231. Taylor AL, Fishman LM: Corticotropin-releasing hormone. *N Engl J Med* 319:213, 1988.

232. Oldfield EH, Doppman JL, Nieman LK, Chrousos GP, Miller DL, Katz DA, Cuttler GB, Loriaux DL: Petrosal sinus sampling with and without corticotropin-releasing hormone for the differential diagnosis of Cushing's syndrome. *N Engl J Med* 325:897, 1991.
233. Deuben RR, Meites J: Stimulation of pituitary growth hormone release by a hypothalamic extract *in vitro*. *Endocrinology* 74:408, 1964.
234. Thorner MO, Perryman RL, Cronin MJ, Rogol AD, Draznin M, Johanson A, et al: Somatotroph hyperplasia: Successful treatment of acromegaly by removal of a pancreatic islet tumor secreting a growth hormone-releasing factor. *J Clin Invest* 70:965, 1982.
235. Sassolas G, Chayvialle JA, Partensky C, Berger G, Trouillas J, Berger F, et al: Acromégalie, expression clinique de la production de facteurs de libération de l'hormone de croissance (G.R.F.) par une tumeur pancréatique. *Ann Endocrinol (Paris)* 44:347, 1983.
236. Guillemin R, Brazeau P, Böhlen P, Esch F, Ling N, Wehrenberg WB: Growth hormone-releasing factor from a human pancreatic tumor that caused acromegaly. *Science* 218:585, 1982.
237. Rivier J, Spiess J, Thorner M, Vale W: Characterization of a growth hormone-releasing factor from a human pancreatic islet tumour. *Nature* 300:276, 1982.
238. Sasaki A, Sato S, Yumita S, Hanew K, Miura Y, Yoshinaga K: Multiple forms of immunoreactive growth hormone-releasing hormone in human plasma, hypothalamus, and tumor tissues. *J Clin Endocrinol Metab* 68:180, 1989.
239. Gubler U, Monahan JJ, Lomedico PT, Bhatt RS, Collier KJ, Hoffman BJ, et al: Cloning and sequence analysis of cDNA for the precursor of human growth hormone-releasing factor, somatocrinin. *Proc Natl Acad Sci (USA)* 80:4311, 1983.
240. Mayo KE, Cerelli GM, Lebo RV, Bruce BD, Rosenfeld MG, Evans RM: Gene encoding human growth hormone-releasing factor precursor: Structure, sequence, and chromosomal assignment. *Proc Natl Acad Sci USA* 82:63, 1985.
241. Frohman LA, Downs TR, Chomczynski P, Brar A, Kashio Y: Regulation of growth hormone-releasing hormone gene expression and biosynthesis. *Yale J Biol Med* 62:427, 1989.
242. Frohman LA, Bernardis LL: Growth hormone and insulin levels in weanling rats with ventromedial hypothalamic lesions. *Endocrinology* 82:1125, 1968.
243. Frohman LA, Bernardis LL, Kant KJ: Hypothalamic stimulation of growth hormone secretion. *Science* 162:580, 1968.
244. Shibasaki T, Kiyosawa Y, Masuda A, Nakahara M, Imaki T, Wakabayashi I, et al: Distribution of growth hormone-releasing hormone-like immunoreactivity in human tissue extracts. *J Clin Endocrinol Metab* 59:263, 1984.
245. Kita T, Chihara K, Abe H, Minamitani N, Kaji H, Kodama H, et al: Regional distribution of rat growth hormone releasing factor-like immunoreactivity in rat hypothalamus. *Endocrinology* 116:259, 1985.
246. Leidy JW, Robbins RJ: Regional distribution of human growth hormone-releasing hormone in the human hypothalamus by radioimmunoassay. *J Clin Endocrinol Metab* 62:372, 1986.
247. Bloch B, Baillard RC, Brazeau P, Lin HD, Ling N: Topographical and ontogenetic study of the neurons producing growth hormone-releasing factor in human hypothalamus. *Regul Pept* 8:21, 1984.
248. Lechan RM, Lin HD, Ling N, Jackson IMD, Jacobson S, Reichlin S: Distribution of immunoreactive growth hormone releasing factor (1-44) NH_2 in the tuberoinfundibular system of the rhesus monkey. *Brain Res* 309:55, 1984.
249. Kashio Y, Chihara K, Kita T, Okimura Y, Sato M, Kadowaki S, et al: Effect of oral glucose administration on plasma growth hormone-releasing hormone (GHRH)-like immunoreactivity levels in normal subjects and patients with idiopathic GH deficiency: Evidence that GHRH is released not only from the hypothalamus but also from extrahypothalamic tissue. *J Clin Endocrinol Metab* 64:92, 1987.
250. Rosenthal SM, Schriock EA, Kaplan SL, Guillemin R, Grumbach MM: Synthetic human pancreas growth hormone-releasing factor ($hpGRF_{1-44}$-NH2) stimulates growth hormone secretion in normal men. *J Clin Endocrinol Metab* 57:677, 1983.
251. Thorner MO, Spiess J, Vance ML, Rogol AD, Kaiser DL, Webster JD, et al: Human pancreatic growth-hormone-releasing factor selectively stimulates growth-hormone secretion in man. *Lancet* 1:24, 1983.
252. Goldman JA, Molitch ME, Thorner MO, Vale W, Rivier J, Reichlin S: Growth hormone and prolactin responses to bolus and sustained infusions of GRH-1-40-OH in man. *J Endocrinol Invest* 10:397, 1987.
253. Vance ML, Kaiser DL, Evans WS, Thorner MO, Fulanetto R, Rivier J, et al: Evidence for a limited growth hormone (GH)-releasing hormone (GHRH)-releasable quantity of GH: Effects of 6-hour infusions of GHRH on GH secretion in normal man. *J Clin Endocrinol Metab* 60:370, 1985.
254. Thorner MO, Reschke J, Chitwood J, Rogol AD, Furlanetto R, Rivier J, et al: Acceleration of growth in two children treated with human growth hormone-releasing factor. *N Engl J Med* 312:4, 1985.
255. Barinaga M, Yamonoto G, Rivier C, Vale W, Evans R, Rosenfeld MG: Transcriptional regulation of growth hormone gene expression by growth hormone-releasing factor. *Nature* 306:84, 1983.
256. Wehrenberg WB, Brazeau P, Luben R, Böhlen P, Guillemin R: Inhibition of the pulsatile secretion of growth hormone by monoclonal antibodies to the hypothalamic growth hormone releasing factor (GRF). *Endocrinology* 111:2147, 1982.
257. Wehrenberg WB, Bloch B, Phillips BJ: Antibodies to growth hormone-releasing factor inhibit somatic growth. *Endocrinology* 115:1218, 1984.
258. Lussier BT, French MB, Moor BC, Kraicer J: Free intracellular CA^{2+} concentration and growth hormone (GH) release from purified rat somatotrophs: III. Mechanism of action of GH-releasing factor and somatostatin. *Endocrinology* 128: 592, 1991.
259. Chomczynski P, Downs TR, Frohman LA: Feedback regulation of growth hormone (GH)-releasing hormone gene expression by GH in rat hypothalamus. *Mol Endocrinol* 2:236, 1988.
260. Müller EE: Clinical implications of growth hormone feedback mechanisms. *Horm Res* 33:90, 1990.
261. Sato M, Chihara K, Kita T, Kashio Y, Okimura Y, Kitajima N, et al: Physiological role of somatostatin-mediated autofeedback regulation for growth hormone: Importance of growth hormone in triggering somatostatin release during a trough period of pulsatile growth hormone release in conscious male rats. *Neuroendocrinology* 50:139, 1989.
262. Lippe BM, Van Herle AJ, LaFranchi SH, Uller RP, Lavin N, Kaplan SA: Reversible hypothyroidism in growth hormone-deficient children treated with human growth hormone. *J Clin Endocrinol Metab* 40:612, 1975.
263. Kelijman M, Frohman LA: β-adrenergic modulation of growth hormone (GH) autofeedback on sleep-associated and pharmacologically induced GH secretion. *J Clin Endocrinol Metab* 69:1187, 1989.
264. Conway S, Richardson L, Speciale S, Moherek R, Mauceri H, Krulich L: Interaction between norepinephrine and serotonin in the neuroendocrine control of growth hormone release in the rat. *Endocrinology* 126:1022, 1990.
265. Baes M, Vale WW: Growth hormone-releasing factor secretion from fetal hypothalamic cell cultures is modulated by forskolin, phorbol esters, and muscimol. *Endocrinology* 124:104, 1989.
266. Schriock EA, Hulse JA, Harris DA, Kaplan SL, Grumbach

MM: Evaluation of hypothalamic dysfunction in growth hormone (GH)-deficient patients using single versus multiple doses of GH-releasing hormone (GHRH-44) and evidence for diurnal variation insomatotroph responsiveness to GHRH in GH-deficient patients. *J Clin Endocrinol Metab* 65:1177, 1987.
267. Everett JW: Luteotrophic function of autografts of the rat hypophysis. *Endocrinology* 54:685, 1954.
268. Pasteels JL: Administration d'extraits hyothalamiques à l'hypophyse de rat *in vitro* dans le but d'en controler la secretion de prolactine. *C R Acad Sci Paris* 254:2664, 1962.
269. Birge CA, Jacobs LS, Hammer CT, Daughaday WH: Catecholamine inhibition of prolactin secretion by isolated rat adenohypophyses. *Endocrinology* 86:120, 1970.
270. Gibbs DM, Neill JD: Dopamine levels in hypophysial stalk blood in the rat are sufficient to inhibit prolactin secretion *in vivo*. *Endocrinology* 102:1895, 1978.
271. De Greef WJ, Plotsky PM, Neill JD: Dopamine levels in hypophysial stalk plasma and prolactin levels in peripheral plasma of the lactating rat: Effects of a simulated stimulus. *Neuroendocrinology* 32:229, 1981.
272. Plotsky PM, Neill JD: Interactions of dopamine and thyrotropin-releasing hormone in the regulation of prolactin release in lactating rats. *Endocrinology* 111:168, 1982.
273. Mogg RJ, Samson WK: Interactions of dopaminergic and peptidergic factors in the control of prolactin release. *Endocrinology* 126:728, 1990.
274. Abe H, Engler D, Molitch ME, Bollinger-Gruber J, Reichlin S: Vasoactive intestinal peptide is a physiological mediator of prolactin release in the rat. *Endocrinology* 116:1383, 1985.
275. Quigley ME, Judd SJ, Gilliland GB, Yen SC: Functional studies of dopamine control of prolactin secretion in normal women and women with hyperprolactinemic pituitary microadenoma. *J Clin Endocrinol Metab* 50:994, 1980.
276. Leebaw WF, Lee LA, Woolf PD: Dopamine affects basal and augmented pituitary hormone secretion. *J Clin Endocrinol Metab* 47:480, 1978.
277. Bansal S, Lee LA, Woolf PD: Dopaminergic modulation of arginine mediated growth hormone and prolactin release in man. *Metabolism* 30:649, 1981.
278. Burrow CN, May PB, Spaulding SW, Donabedian RK: TRH and dopamine interactions affecting pituitary hormone secretion. *J Clin Endocrinol Metab* 45:65, 1977.
279. Neill JD, Frawley S, Plotsky PM, Tindall GT: Dopamine in hypophysial stalk blood of the rhesus monkey and its role in regulating prolactin secretion. *Endocrinology* 108:489, 1981.
280. Serri O, Kuchel O, Nguyen BU, Somma M: Differential effects of a low dose dopamine infusion on prolactin secretion in normal and hyperprolactinemic subjects. *J Clin Endocrinol Metab* 56:255, 1983.
281. Langer G, Sachar EJ: Dopaminergic factors in human prolactin regulation: Effects of neuroleptics and dopamine. *Psychoneuroendocrinology* 2:373, 1977.
282. Ben-Jonathan N: Dopamine: A prolactin-inhibiting hormone. *Endocr Rev* 6:564, 1985.
283. Creese I, Sibley DR, Leff SE: Agonist interactions with dopamine receptors: Focus on radioligand-binding studies. *Fed Proc* 43:2779, 1984.
284. Brown GM, Seeman P, Lee T: Dopamine/neuroleptic receptors in basal hypothalamus and pituitary: *Endocrinology* 99:1407, 1976.
285. Monsma FJ Jr, McVittie LD, Gerfen CR, Mahan LC, Sibley DR: Multiple D_2 dopamine receptors produced by alternative RNA splicing. *Nature* 342:926, 1989.
286. Thomas GB, Cummins JT, Doughton BW, Griffin N, Millar RP, de L Milton RC, Clarke IJ: Gonadotropin-releasing hormone associated peptide (GAP) and putative processed GAP peptides do not release luteinizing hormone or follicle stimulating hormone or inhibit prolactin secretion in the sheep. *Neuroendocrinology* 48:342, 1988.
287. Wormald PJ, Abrahamson MJ, Seeburg PH, Nikolics K, Millar RM: Prolactin-inhibiting activity of GnRH associated peptide in cultured human pituitary cells. *Clin Endocrinol (Oxf)* 30:149, 1989.
288. Schally AV, Redding TW, Arimura A, DuPont A, Linthicum GL: Isolation of gamma-aminobutyric acid from pig hypothalami and demonstration of its prolactin release-inhibiting (PIF) activity in vivo and in vitro. *Endocrinology* 100:681, 1977.
289. Grossman A, Delitala G, Yeo T, Besser GM: GABA and muscimol inhibit the release of prolactin from dispersed rat anterior pituitary cells. *Neuroendocrinology* 32:145, 1981.
290. Vincent SR, Hokfelt T, Wu JY: GABA neuron systems in the hypothalamus and the pituitary gland. *Neuroendocrinology* 34:117, 1982.
291. Mulcahey JJ, Neill JD: Gamma-aminobutyric acid (GABA) levels in hypophyseal stalk plasma of rats. *Life Sci* 32:453, 1982.
292. Tamminga CA, Neophytides A, Chase TN, Frohman LA: Stimulation of prolactin and growth hormone secretion by muscimol, a gamma aminobutyric acid agonist. *J Clin Endocrinol Metab* 47:1348, 1978.
293. Fioretti P, Melis GB, Paoletti AM, Pardo G, Caminiti F, Corsini GU, Martini L: Gamma-amino-β-hydroxy butyric acid stimulates prolactin and growth hormone release in normal women. *J Clin Endocrinol Metab* 47:1336, 1978.
294. Cavagnini F, Benetti G, Invitti C, Ramella G, Pinto M, Lazza M, et al: Effect of gamma aminobutyric acid on growth hormone and prolactin secretion in man: Influence of pimozide and domperidone. *J Clin Endocrinol Metab* 51:789, 1980.
295. Melis GB, Fruzzetti F, Paoletti AM, Mais V, Kemeny A, Strigíny F, et al: Pharmacological activation of γ-aminobutyric acid-system blunts prolactin response to mechanical breast stimulation in puerperal women. *J Clin Endocrinol Metab* 58:201, 1984.
296. Kato Y, Iwasaki Y, Iwasaki J, Abe H, Yanaihara N, Imura H: Prolactin release by vasoactive intestinal polypeptide in rats. *Endocrinology* 103:554, 1978.
297. Mezey E, Kiss JZ: Vasoactive intestinal peptide-containing neurons in the paraventricular nucleus may participate in regulating prolactin secretion. *Proc Natl Acad Sci USA* 82:245, 1985.
298. Malarkey WB, O'Dorisio TM, Kennedy M, Cataland S: The influence of vasoactive intestinal polypeptide and cholecystokinin on prolactin release in rat and human monolayer cultures. *Life Sci* 28:2489, 1981.
299. Said SI, Porter JC: Vasoactive intestinal polypeptide: Release into hypophyseal portal blood. *Life Sci* 24:227, 1979.
300. Carrillo AJ, Pool TB, Sharp ZD: Vasoactive intestinal peptide increases prolactin messenger ribonucleic acid content in GH_3 cells. *Endocrinology* 116:202, 1985.
301. Gozes I, Shani Y: Hypothalamic vasoactive intestinal peptide messenger ribonucleic acid is increased in lactating rats. *Endocrinology* 119:2497, 1986.
302. Yiangou Y, Gill JS, Chrysanthou BJ, Burrin J, Bloom SB: Infusion of prepro-VIP derived peptides in man: Effect on secretion of prolactin. *Neuroendocrinology* 48:615, 1988.
303. Lasaga M, Debeljuk L, Afione S, Aleman IT, Duvilanski B: Effects of passive immunization against vasoactive intestinal peptide on serum prolactin and LH levels. *Neuroendocrinology* 49:547, 1989.
304. Lopez FJ, Dominguez JR, Sanchez-Franco F, Negro-Vilar A: Role of dopamine and vasoactive intestinal peptide in the control of pulsatile prolactin secretion. *Endocrinology* 124:527, 1989.
305. Itoh N, Obata K, Yanaihara N, Okamoto H: Human preprovasoactive intestinal polypeptide contains a novel PHI-27-like peptide, PHM-27. *Nature* 304:547, 1983.
306. Sasaki A, Sato S, Go M, Shimizu Y, Murakami O, Hanew K, et al: Distribution, plasma concentration, and in vivo pro-

lactin-releasing activity of peptide histidine methionine in humans. *J Clin Endocrinol Metab* 65:683, 1987.
307. Ohta H, Kato Y, Tojo H: Further evidence that peptide histidine isoleucine (PHI) may function as a prolactin releasing factor in rats. *Peptides* 6:708, 1985.
308. Kaji, H, Chihara C, Abe H, Kita T: Effect of passive immunization with antisera to vasoactive intestinal polypeptide and peptide histidine isoleucine amide on 5-hydroxy-l-tryptophan-induced prolactin release in rats. *Endocrinology* 117:1914, 1985.
309. Hagen TC, Arnaout MA, Scherzer WJ, Martinson DR: Antisera to vasoactive intestinal polypeptide inhibit basal prolactin release from dispersed anterior pituitary cells. *Neuroendocrinology* 43:641, 1986.
310. Palkovits M: Catecholamines in the hypothalamus: An anatomical review. *Neuroendocrinology* 33:123, 1981.
311. Sawchenko PE, Swanson LW: Central noradrenergic pathways for the integration of hypothalamic neuroendocrine and autonomic responses. *Science* 214:685, 1981.
312. Hökfelt TH, Elde R, Fuxe K, Johansson O, Ljungdahl Å, Goldstein M, et al: Aminergic and peptidergic pathways in the nervous system with special reference to the hypothalamus, in Reichlin S, Baldessarini RJ, Martin JB (eds): *The Hypothalamus*. New York, Raven Press, 1978, p 69.
313. De Souza EB: Beta-2 adrenergic receptors in pituitary: Identification, characterization, and autoradiographic localization. *Neuroendocrinology* 41:289, 1985.
314. Perkins SN, Evans WS, Thorner MO, Gibbs DM, Cronin MJ: β-adrenergic binding and secretory responses of the anterior pituitary. *Endocrinology* 177:1818, 1985.
315. Palkovits M, Saavedra JM, Jacobowitz DM, Kizer JS, Záborszky L, Browstein MJ: Serotonergic innervation of the forebrain: Effect of lesions on serotonin and tryptophan hydroxylase levels. *Brain Res* 130:121, 1977.
316. Saavedra JM, Palkovits M, Kizer JS, Brownstein M, Zivin JA: Distribution of biogenic amines and related enzymes in the rat pituitary gland. *J Neuroendocrinol* 25:257, 1975.
317. De Souza EB: Serotonin and dopamine receptors in the rat pituitary gland: Autoradiographic identification, characterization and localization. *Endocrinology* 119:1534, 1986.
318. Johns MA, Azmitia EC, Krieger DT: Specific *in vitro* uptake of serotonin by cells in the anterior pituitary of the rat. *Endocrinology* 110:754, 1982.
319. Armstrong DM, Saper CB, Levey AI, Wainer BH, Terry RD: Distribution of cholinergic neurons in rat brain: Demonstrated by the immunocytochemical localization of choline acetyltransferase. *J Comp Neurol* 216:53, 1983.
320. Carmeliet P, Denef C: Synthesis and release of acetylcholine by normal and tumoral pituitary corticotrophs. *Endocrinology* 124:2218, 1989.
321. Decavel C, Van Den Pol AN: GABA: A dominant neurotransmitter in the hypothalamus. *J Comp Neurol* 302:1019, 1990.
322. Vincent SR, Hökfelt T, Skirboll LR, Wu JY: Hypothalamic γ-aminobutyric acid neurons project to the neocortex. *Science* 220:1309, 1983.
323. Fagg GE, Foster AC: Amino acid neurotransmitters and their pathways in the mammalian central nervous system. *Neuroscience* 9:701, 1983.
324. Knigge UP: Histaminergic regulation of prolactin secretion. *Dan Med Bull* 37:109, 1990.
325. Vance ML, Kaiser DL, Frohman LA, Rivier J, Vale WW, Thorner MO: Role of dopamine in the regulation of growth hormone secretion: Dopamine and bromocriptine augment growth hormone (GH)-releasing hormone-stimulated GH secretion in normal man. *J Clin Endocrinol Metab* 64:1136, 1987.
326. Chihara K, Kashio Y, Kita T, Okimura Y, Kaji H, Abe H, Fujita T: L-Dopa stimulates release of hypothalamic growth hormone-releasing hormone in humans. *J Clin Endocrinol Metab* 62:466, 1986.
327. Kitajima N, Chihara K, Abe H, Okimura Y, Fujii Y, Sato M, et al: Effects of dopamine on immunoreactive growth hormone-releasing factor and somatostatin secretion from rat hypothalamic slices perifused *in vitro*. *Endocrinology* 124: 69, 1989.
328. Serri O, Deslauriers N, Brazeau P: Dual action of dopamine on growth hormone release *in vitro*. *Neuroendocrinology* 45:363, 1987.
329. Van Den Pol AN, Wuarin JP, Dudek FE: Glutamate, the dominant excitatory transmitter in neuroendocrine regulation. *Science* 250:1276, 1990.
330. Lorenzo MJ, Sànchez-Franco F, de los Frailes MT, Reichlin S, Fernandez G, Cacicedo L: Synthesis and secretion of vasoactive intestinal peptide by rat fetal cerebral cortical and hypothalamic cells in culture. *Endocrinology* 125:1983, 1989.
331. Said SI: Vasoactive intestinal peptide. *J Endocrinol Invest* 9:191, 1986.
332. Rostène WH: Neurobiological and neuroendocrine functions of the vasoactive intestinal peptide (VIP). *Prog Neurobiol* 22:103, 1984.
333. Iversen LL: Substance P. *Br Med Bull* 38:277, 1982.
334. Rivier C, Brown M, Vale W: Effect of neurotensin, substance p and morphine sulfate on the secretion of prolactin and growth hormone in the rat. *Endocrinology* 100:751, 1977.
335. Arisawa M, Snyder GD, Yu WH, Palatis LRD: Physiologically significant inhibitory hypothalamic action of substance P on prolactin release in the male rat. *Neuroendocrinology* 52:22, 1990.
336. Jones MT, Gillham B, Homes MC, Hodges JR, Buckingham JC: Influence of substance P on hypothalamo-pituitary-adrenocortical activity in the rat. *J Endocrinol* 76:183, 1978.
337. Chad DA, Aronin N, Lundstrom R, McKeon P, Ross D, Molitch M, et al: Does capsaicin relieve the pain of diabetic neuropathy? *Pain* 43:387, 1990.
338. Brown DR, Miller RJ: Neurotensin. *Br Med Bull* 38:239, 1982.
339. Kataoka K, Mizuno N, Frohman LA: Regional distribution of immunoreactive neurotensin in monkey brain. *Brain Res Bull* 4:57, 1979.
340. Maeda K, Frohman LA: Dissociation of systemic and central effects of neurotensin on the secretion of growth hormone, prolactin, and thyrotropin. *Endocrinology* 103:1903, 1978.
341. Blackburn AM, Fletcher DR, Adrian TE, Bloom SR: Neurotensin infusion in man: Pharmacokinetics and effect on gastrointestinal and pituitary hormones. *J Clin Endocrinol Metab* 51:1257, 1980.
342. Moffett RB, Bumpus FM, Husain A: Cellular organization of the brain renin-angiotensin system. *Life Sci* 41:1867, 1987.
343. Aronsson M, Almasan K, Fuxe K, Cintra A, Härfstrand A, Gustafsson JÅ, Ganten D: Evidence for the existence of angiotensinogen mRNA in magnocellular paraventricular hypothalamic neurons. *Acta Physiol Scand* 132:585, 1988.
344. Saint-Andre J, Rohmer V, Alhenc-Gelas F, Menard J, Bigorgne J-C, Corvol P: Presence of renin, angiotensinogen, and converting enzyme in human pituitary lactotroph cells and prolactin adenomas. *J Clin Endocrinol Metab* 63:231, 1986.
345. Anderson PW, Malarkey WB, Salk J, Kletsky OA, Hsueh WA: The effect of angiotensin-converting enzyme inhibition on prolactin responses in normal and hyperprolactinemic subjects. *J Clin Endocrinol Metab* 69:518, 1989.
346. Winer LM, Molteni A, Molitch ME: Effect of angiotensin-converting enzyme inhibition on pituitary hormone responses to insulin-induced hypoglycemia in humans. *J Clin Endocrinol Metab* 71:256, 1990.
347. Phillips MI: Biological effects of angiotensin in the brain. In Gross F, Vogel G (eds): *Enzymatic Release of Vasoactive Peptides*. New York, Raven, 1980, p. 335.
348. Vijayan E, Samson WK, McCann SM: *In vitro* and *in vivo*

effects of cholecystokinin on gonadotropin, prolactin, growth hormone and thyrotropin release in the rat. *Brain Res* 172:295, 1979.

349. Tanomoto K, Tamminga CA, Chase TN: Intracerebroventricular injection of cholecystokinin octapeptide elevates plasma prolactin levels through stimulation of vasoactive intestinal polypeptide. *Endocrinology* 121:127, 1987.
350. Gibbs J, Smith GP: Satiety: The roles of peptides from the stomach and intestine. *Fed Proc* 45:1391, 1986.
351. Morley JE: Neuroendocrine effects of endogenous opioid peptides in human subjects: A review. *Psychoneuroendocrinology* 8:361, 1983.
352. Smith AI, Funder JW: Proopiomelanocortin processing in the pituitary, central nervous system, and peripheral tissues. *Endocr Rev* 9:159, 1988.
353. Beaumont A: Putative peptide neurotransmitters: The opioid peptides. *Int Rev Exp Pathol* 25:279, 1983.
354. Bloom FE: The endorphins: A growing family of pharmacologically pertinent peptides. *Ann Rev Pharmacol Toxicol* 23:151, 1983.
355. Olson GA, Olson RD, Kastin AJ: Endogenous opiates: 1988. *Peptides* 10:1253, 1989.
356. Spiler IJ, Molitch ME: Lack of modulation of pituitary hormone stress response by neural pathways involving opiate receptors. *J Clin Endocrinol Metab* 50:516, 1980.
357. Ma LY, Zhang ML, Yang XD, Tian DR, Qi JS, Zhang DM: Neuroendocrinology of atrial natriuretic polypeptide in the brain. *Neuroendocrinology* 53:12, 1991.
358. McGregor A, Richards M, Espiner E, Yandle T: Brain natriuretic peptide administered to man: Actions and metabolism. *J Clin Endocrinol Metab* 70:1103, 1990.
359. Kitajima N, Chihara K, Abe H, Okimura Y, Shakutsui S: Galanin stimulates immunoreactive growth hormone-release factor secretion from rat hypothalamic slices perifused *in vitro*. *Life Sci* 47:2371, 1990.
360. Davis TME, Burrin JM, Bloom SR: Growth hormone (GH) release in response to GH-releasing hormone in man is 3-fold enhanced by galanin. *J Clin Endocrinol Metab* 65:1248, 1987.
361. Hooi SC, Maiter DM, Martin JB, Koenig JI: Galaninergic mechanisms are involved in the regulation of corticotropin and thyrotropin secretion in the rat. *Endocrinology* 127: 2281, 1990.
362. Vrontakis ME, Sano T, Kovacs K, Friesen HG: Presence of galanin-like immunoreactivity in nontumorous corticotrophs and corticotroph adenomas of the human pituitary. *J Clin Endocrinol Metab* 70:747, 1990.
363. Yoshizawa T, Shinmi O, Giaid A, Yanagisawa M, Gibson SJ, Kimura S, et al: Endothelin: A novel peptide in the posterior pituitary system. *Science* 247:462, 1990.
364. Stojilkovic SS, Merelli F, Iida T, Krsmanovic LZ, Catt KJ: Endothelin stimulation of cytosolic calcium and gonadotropin secretion in anterior pituitary cells. *Science* 248:1663, 1990.
365. Samson WK, Skala KD, Alexander BD, Steven Huang FL: Pituitary site of action of endothelin: Selective inhibition of prolactin release *in vitro*. *Biochem Biophys Res Commun* 169:737, 1990.
366. Toni R, Jackson IMD, Lechan RM: Neuropeptide-Y-immunoreactive innervation of thyrotropin-releasing hormone-synthesizing neurons in the rat hypothalamic paraventricular nucleus. *Endocrinology* 126:2444, 1990.
367. Härfstrand A: Brain neuropeptide Y mechanisms: Basic aspects and involvement in cardiovascular and neuroendocrine regulation. *Acta Physiol Scand* 131:565, 1987.
368. Crowley WR, Hassid A, Kalra SP: Neuropeptide Y enhances the release of luteinizing hormone (LH) induced by LH-releasing hormone. *Endocrinology* 120:941, 1987.
369. Erlich SS, Apuzzo MLJ: The pineal gland: Anatomy, physiology, and clinical significance. *J Neurosurg* 63:321, 1985.
370. Reiter RJ: Pineal melatonin: Cell biology of its synthesis and of its physiological interactions. *Endocr Rev* 12:151, 1991.
371. Relkin R: Pineal-hormonal interactions, in Relkin R (ed): *The Pineal Gland*. New York, Elsevier, 1983, p 225.
372. Waldhauser F, Leberman HR, Lynch HJ, Waldhauser M, Herkner K, Frisch H, et al: A pharmacological dose of melatonin increases PRL levels in males without altering those of GH, LH, FSH, TSH, testosterone or cortisol. *Neuroendocrinology* 46:125, 1987.
373. Tamarkin L, Baird CJ, Almeida OFX: Melatonin: A coordinating signal for mammalian reproduction? *Science* 227:714, 1985.
374. Vaughan GM, Meyer GG, Reiter RJ: Evidence for a pineal-gonad relationship in the human. *Prog Reprod Biol* 4:191, 1978.
375. Zacharias L, Wurtman RJ: Blindness: Its relation to age of menarche. *Science* 144:1154, 1964.
376. Thomas JB, Pizzarello DJ: Blindness, biologic rhythms, and menarche. *Obstet Gynecol* 30:507, 1967.
377. Hollwich F, Dieckhues B: Endokrines systems und erblindung. *Dtsch Med Wochenschr* 96:363, 1971.
378. Bodenheimer S, Winter JSD, Faiman C: Diurnal rhythms of serum gonadotropins, testosterone, estradiol and cortisol in blind men. *J Clin Endocrinol Metab* 37:472, 1973.
379. Winer LM, Shaw MA, Baumann G: Basal plasma growth hormone levels in man: New evidence for rhythmicity of growth hormone secretion. *J Clin Endocrinol Metab* 70:1678, 1990.
380. Veldhuis JD, Iranmanesh A, Johnson ML, Lizarralde G: Twenty-four-hour rhythms in plasma concentrations of adenohypophyseal hormones are generated by distinct amplitude and/or frequency modulation of underlying pituitary secretory bursts. *J Clin Endocrinol Metab* 71:1616, 1990.
381. Stewart JK, Clifton DK, Koerker DJ, Rogol AD: Pulsatile release of growth hormone and prolactin from the primate pituitary *in vitro*. *Endocrinology* 116:1, 1985.
382. Van Cauter E: Diurnal and ultradian rhythms in human endocrine function: A minireview. *Horm Res* 34:45, 1990.
383. Dahlitz M, Alvarez B, Vignau J, English J, Arendt J, Parkes JD: Delayed sleep phase syndrome response to melatonin. *Lancet* 1:1121, 1991.
384. Weitzman ED, Boyar RM, Kapen S: The relationship of sleep and sleep stages of neuroendocrine secretion and biological rhythms in man. *Recent Prog Horm Res* 31:399, 1975.
385. Frisch RE: Body fat, menarche, and reproductive ability. *Semin Reprod Endocrinol* 3:45, 1985.
386. Veldhuis JD, Johnson L: Operating characteristics of the hypothalamo-pituitary-gonadal axis in men: Circadian, ultradian, and pulsatile release of prolactin and its temporal coupling with luteinizing hormone. *J Clin Endocrinol Metab* 67:116, 1988.
387. Sassin JF, Frantz AG, Kapen S, Weitzman ED: The nocturnal rise of human prolactin is dependent upon sleep. *J Clin Endocrinol Metab* 37:436, 1973.
388. Stern JM, Reichlin S: Prolactin circadian rhythm persists throughout lactation in women. *Neuroendocrinology* 51:31, 1990.
389. Hintz RL, Menking M, Sotos JF: Familial holoprosencephaly with endocrine dysgenesis. *J Pediatr* 72:81, 1968.
390. Arslanian SA, Rothfus WE, Foley TP, Becker DJ: Hormonal, metabolic, and neuroradiologic abnormalities associated with septo-optic dysplasia. *Acta Endocrinol (Copenh)* 107:282, 1984.
391. Huseman CA, Kelch RP, Hopwood NJ, Zipf WB: Sexual precocity in association with septo-optic dysplasia and hypothalamic hypopituitarism. *J Pediatr* 92:748, 1978.
392. Rudman D, Davis GT, Priest JH, Patterson JH, Kutner MH, Heymsfield SB, et al: Prevalence of growth hormone deficiency in children with cleft lip or palate. *J Pediatr* 93:378, 1978.
393. Abrahams JJ, Trefelner E, Boulware SD: Idiopathic growth hormone deficiency: MR findings in 35 patients. *AJNR* 12:155, 1991.

394. Lieblich JM, Rosen SW, Guyda H, Reardan J, Schaaf M: The syndrome of basal encephalocele and hypothalamic-pituitary dysfunction. *Ann Intern Med* 89:910, 1978.
394a. Franco B, Guioli S, Pragliola A, Incerti B, Bardoni B, Tonlorenzi R, et al: A gene deleted in Kallman's syndrome shares homology with neural cell adhesion and axonal path-finding molecules. *Nature* 353:529, 1991.
395. Klingmüller D, Dewes W, Krahe T, Brecht G, Schwekert HU: Magnetic resonance imaging of the brain in patients with anosmia and hypothalamic hypogonadism (Kallmann's syndrome). *J Clin Endocrinol Metab* 65:581, 1987.
396. Lieblich JM, Rogol AD, White BJ, Rosen SW: Syndrome of anosmia with hypogonadotropic hypogonadism (Kallmann syndrome). *Am J Med* 73:506, 1982.
397. Hochberg Z, Moses AM, Miller M, Benderli A, Richman RA: Altered osmotic threshold for vasopressin release and impaired thirst sensation: Additional abnormalities in Kallmann's syndrome. *J Clin Endocrinol Metab* 55:779, 1982.
398. Arafah BM: Reversible hypopituitarism in patients with large nonfunctioning pituitary adenomas. *J Clin Endocrinol Metab* 62:1173, 1986.
399. Molitch ME, Reichlin S: Hypothalamic hyperprolactinemia: Neuroendocrine regulation of prolactin secretion in patients with lesions of the hypothalamus and pituitary stalk, in MacLeod RM, Thorner MO, Scapagnini U (eds): *Prolactin Basic and Clinical Correlates*. Padua, Italy, Liviana Press, 1985, p 709.
400. Diengdoh JV, Griffiths D, Crockard HA: Rathke-cleft cyst. *Clin Neuropathol* 3:72, 1984.
401. Banna M: Craniopharyngioma: Based on 160 cases. *Br J Radiol* 49:206, 1976.
402. Thomsett MJ, Conte FA, Kaplan SL, Grumbach MM: Endocrine and neurologic outcome in childhood craniopharyngioma: Review of effect of treatment in 42 patients. *J Pediatr* 97:728, 1980.
403. Landolt AM, Zachmann M: Results of transsphenoidal extirpation of craniopharyngiomas and Rathke's cysts. *Neurosurgery* 28:410, 1991.
404. Kapcala LP, Molitch ME, Post KD, Biller BJ, Prager RJ, Jackson I, et al: Galactorrhea, oligo/amenorrhea, and hyperprolactinemia in patients with craniopharyngiomas. *J Clin Endocrinol Metab* 51:798, 1980.
405. Simson LR, Lampe I, Abell MR: Suprasellar germinomas. *Cancer* 22:533, 1968.
406. Sklar CA, Grumbach MM, Kaplan SL, Conte FA: Hormonal and metabolic abnormalities associated with central nervous system germinoma in children and adolescents and the effect of therapy: Report of 10 patients. *J Clin Endocrinol Metab* 52:9, 1981.
407. Post KD, McCormick PC, Bello JA: Differential diagnosis of pituitary tumors. *Endocrinol Metab Clin North Am* 16:609, 1987.
408. Sherwin RP, Grassi JE, Sommer SC: Hamartomatous malformation of the posterolateral hypothalamus. *Lab Invest* 11:89, 1962.
409. Judge DM, Kulin HE, Page R, Santen R, Trapukdi S: Hypothalamic hamartoma: A source of luteinizing-hormone-releasing factor in precocious puberty. *N Engl J Med* 296:7, 1977.
410. Price RA, Lee PA, Albright AL, Ronnekleiv OK, Gutai JP: Treatment of sexual precocity by removal of a luteinizing hormone-releasing hormone secreting hamartoma. *JAMA* 251:2247, 1984.
411. Comite F, Pescovitz OH, Rieth KG, Dwyer AJ, Hench K, McNemar A, et al: Luteinizing hormone-releasing hormone analog treatment of boys with hypothalamic hamartoma and true precocious puberty. *J Clin Endocrinol Metab* 59:888, 1984.
412. Asa SL, Scheithauer BW, Bilbao JM, Horvath E, Ryan N, Kovacs K, et al: A case for hypothalamic acromegaly: A clinicopathological study of six patients with hypothalamic gangliocytomas producing growth hormone-releasing factor. *J Clin Endocrinol Metab* 58:796, 1984.
413. Asa SL, Kovacs K, Tindall GT, Barrow DL, Horvath E, Vecsei P: Cushing's disease associated with an intrasellar gangiocytoma producing corticotrophin-releasing factor. *Ann Intern Med* 101:789, 1984.
414. Chapelon C, Ziza JM, Piette JC, Levy Y, Raguin G, Wechsler B, et al: Neurosarcoidosis: Signs, course and treatment in 35 confirmed cases. *Medicine (Baltimore)* 69:261, 1990.
415. Stuart CA, Neelon FA, Lebovitz HE: Hypothalamic insufficiency: The cause of hypopituitarism in sarcoidosis. *Ann Intern Med* 88:589, 1978.
416. Vesely DL: Hypothalamic sarcoidosis: A new cause of morbid obesity. *South Med J* 82:758, 1989.
417. Capellan JIL, Olmedo LC, Martin M, Marin Del Mar MA, Villanueva MG, Zarza FM, et al: Intrasellar mass with hypopituitarism as a manifestation of sarcoidosis. *J Neurosurg* 73:283, 1990.
418. Stuart CA, Neelon FA, Lebovitz HE: Disordered control of thirst in hypothalamic-pituitary sarcoidosis. *N Engl J Med* 303:1078, 1980.
419. Braunstein GD, Kohler PO: Pituitary function in Hand-Schüller-Christian disease: Evidence for deficient growth-hormone release in patients with short stature. *N Engl J Med* 286:1225, 1972.
420. Tien RD, Newton TH, McDermott MW, Dillon WP, Kucharczyk J: Thickened pituitary stalk on MR images in patients with diabetes insipidus and Langerhans cell histiocytosis. *AJNR* 11:703, 1990.
421. Goodman RH, Post KD, Molitch ME, Adelman LS, Altemus LR, Johnston H: Eosinophilic granuloma mimicking a pituitary tumor. *Neurosurgery* 5:723, 1979.
422. Mohr PD: Hypothalamic-pituitary abscess. *Postgrad Med J* 51:468, 1975.
423. Lichtenstein MJ, Tilley WS, Sandler MP: The syndrome of hypothalamic hypopituitarism complicating viral meningoencephalitis. *J Endocrinol Invest* 5:111, 1982.
424. Udani PM, Parekh UC, Dastur DK: Neurological and related syndromes in CNS tuberculosis. *J Neurol Sci* 14:341, 1971.
425. Edwards OM, Clark JDA: Post-traumatic hypopituitarism. *Medicine (Baltimore)* 65:281, 1986.
426. King LR, Knowles HC Jr, McLaurin RL, Brielmaier J, Perisutti G, Piziak VK: Pituitary hormone response to head injury. *Neurosurgery* 9:229, 1981.
427. Crompton MR: Hypothalamic lesions following closed head injury. *Brain* 94:165, 1971.
428. Mechanick JI, Hochberg FH, LaRocque A: Hypothalamic dysfunction following whole-brain irradiation. *J Neurosurg* 65:490, 1986.
429. Huang KE: Assessment of hypothalamic-pituitary function in women after external head irradiation. *J Clin Endocrinol Metab* 49:623, 1979.
430. Eastman RC, Gorden P, Roth J: Conventional supervoltage irradiation is an effective treatment for acromegaly. *J Clin Endocrinol Metab* 48:931, 1979.
431. Albright F, Butler AM, Hampton AO, Smith P: Syndrome characterized by osteitis fibrosa disseminata, areas of pigmentation and endocrine dysfunction, with precocious puberty in females. *N Engl J Med* 216:727, 1937.
432. Kovacs K, Horvath E, Thorner MO, Rogol AD: Mammosomatotroph hyperplasia associated with acromegaly and hyperprolactinemia in a patient with the McCune-Albright syndrome. *Virchous Arch* 403:77, 1984.
433. Cuttler L, Jackson JA, Uz-Zafar MS, Levitsky LL, Mellinger RC, Frohman LA: Hypersecretion of growth hormone and prolactin in McCune-Albright syndrome. *J Clin Endocrinol Metab* 68:1148, 1989.
434. Hall R, Warrick C: Hypersecretion of hypothalamic releasing hormones: A possible explanation of the endocrine manifestations of polyostotic fibrous dysplasia (Albright's syndrome). *Lancet* 1:1313, 1972.

434a. Weinstein LS, Shenker A, Gejman PV, Merino MJ, Friedman E, Spiegel AM: Activating mutations of the stimulatory G protein in the McCune-Albright syndrome. *N Engl J Med* 325:1688, 1991.
435. Loes DJ, Barloon TJ, Yuh WTC, DeLaPaz RL, Sato Y: MR anatomy and pathology of the hypothalamus. *AJR* 156:579, 1991.
436. Lippe B, Wong SLR, Kaplan SA: Simultaneous assessment of growth hormone and ACTH reserve in children pretreated with diethylstilbestrol. *J Clin Endocrinol Metab* 33:949, 1971.
437. Rona RJ, Tanner JM: Aetiology of idiopathic growth hormone deficiency in England and Wales. *Arch Dis Child* 52:197, 1977.
438. Phillips JA III, Hjelle BL, Seeburg PH, Zachmann M: Molecular basis for familial isolated growth hormone deficiency. *Proc Natl Acad Sci USA* 78:6372, 1981.
439. Vnencak-Jones CL, Phillips JA III, De-Fen W: Use of polymerase chain reaction in detection of growth hormone gene deletions. *J Clin Endocrinol Metab* 70:1550, 1990.
440. Mullis P, Patel M, Brickell PM, Brook CGD: Isolated growth hormone deficiency: Analysis of the growth hormone (GH)-releasing hormone gene and the GH gene cluster. *J Clin Endocrinol Metab* 70:187, 1990.
441. Ross RJ, Tsagarakis S, Grossman A, Preece MA, Rodda C, Davies PS, et al: Treatment of growth-hormone deficiency with growth-hormone-releasing hormone. *Lancet* 1:5, 1987.
442. Huseman CA, Hassing JM: Evidence for dopaminergic stimulation of growth velocity in some hypopituitary children. *J Clin Endocrinol Metab* 58:419, 1984.
443. Pintor C, Cella SG, Loche S, Puggioni R, Corda R, Locatelli V, Muller EE: Clonidine-treatment for short stature. *Lancet* 1:1226, 1987.
444. Pescovitz OH, Tan E: Lack of benefit of clonidine treatment for short stature in a double-blind, placebo-controlled trial. *Lancet* 2:874, 1988.
445. Molitch ME: Pathogenesis of pituitary tumors. *Endocrinol Metab Clin North Am* 16:503, 1987.
446. Van Dop C, Burstein S, Conte FA, Grumbach MM: Isolated gonadotropin deficiency in boys: Clinical characteristics and growth. *J Pediatr* 111:684, 1987.
447. Weiss J, Crowley WF Jr., Jameson JL: Normal structure of the gonadotropin-releasing hormone (GnRH) gene in patients with GnRH deficiency and idiopathic hypogonadotropic hypogonadism. *J Clin Endocrinol Metab* 69:299, 1989.
448. Santoro N, Filicori M, Crowley WF Jr: Hypogonadotropic disorders in men and women: Diagnosis and therapy with pulsatile gonadotropin-releasing hormone. *Endocr Rev* 7:11, 1986.
449. Liu L, Banks SM, Barnes KM, Sherins RJ: Two-year comparison of testicular responses to pulsatile gonadotropin-releasing hormone and exogenous gonadotropins from the inception of therapy in men with isolated hypogonadotropic hypogonadism. *J Clin Endocrinol Metab* 67:1140, 1988.
450. Vigersky RA, Andersen AE, Thompson RH, Loriaux DL: Hypothalamic dysfunction in secondary amenorrhea associated with simple weight loss. *N Engl J Med* 297:1141, 1977.
451. Shangold MM: Causes, evaluation, and management of athletic oligo/amenorrhea. *Med Clin North Am* 69:83, 1985.
452. Quigley E, Sheenan KL, Casper RF, Yen SSC: Evidence for increased dopaminergic and opioid activity in patients with hypothalamic hypogonadotropic amenorrhea. *J Clin Endocrinol Metab* 50:949, 1980.
453. Biller BJ, Boyd AE III, Molitch ME, Post KD, Wolpert SM, Reichlin S: Galactorrhea syndromes. In Post KD, Jackson IMD, Reichlin S (eds): *The Pituitary Adenoma.* New York, Plenum, 1980, p 65.
454. Glass MR, Shaw RW, Butt WR, Edwards RL, London DR: An abnormality of oestrogen feedback in amenorrhoea-galactorrhoea. *Br Med J* 3:274, 1975.
455. Kaplan SL, Grumbach MM: Pathophysiology and treatment of sexual precocity. *J Clin Endocrinol Metab* 71:785, 1990.
456. Pescovitz OH, Comite F, Hench K, Barnes K, McNemar A, Foster C, et al: The NIH experience with precocious puberty: Diagnostic subgroups and response to short-term luteinizing hormone releasing hormone analogue therapy. *J Pediatr* 108:47, 1986.
457. Manasco PK, Pescovitz OH, Feuillan PP, Hench KD, Barnes KM, Jones J, et al: Resumption of puberty after long term luteinizing hormone-releasing hormone agonist treatment of central precocious puberty. *J Clin Endocrinol Metab* 67:368, 1988.
458. Bevan JS, Burke CW, Esiri MM, Adamas CBT: Misinterpretation of prolactin levels leading to management error in patients with sellar enlargement. *Am J Med* 82:29, 1987.
459. Martin TL, Kim M, Malarkey WB: The natural history of idiopathic hyperprolactinemia. *J Clin Endocrinol Metab* 60:855, 1985.
460. Klibanski A, Biller BMK, Rosenthal DI, Schoenfeld DA, Saxe V: Effects of prolactin and estrogen deficiency in amenorrheic bone loss. *J Clin Endocrinol Metab* 67:124, 1988.
461. Molitch ME, Reichlin S: Hyperprolactinemic disorders. *Dis Mon* 28(9):1, 1982.
462. Faglia G, Peccoz PB, Ambrosi B, Ferrari C, Neri V: Prolonged and exaggerated elevations in plasma thyrotropin (HTSH) after thyrotropin releasing factor (TRF) in patients with pituitary tumors. *J Clin Endocrinol Metab* 33:999, 1971.
463. Beck-Peccoz P, Amr S, Menezes-Ferreira MM, Faglia G, Weintraub BD: Decreased receptor binding of biologically inactive thyrotropin in central hypothyroidism. *N Engl J Med* 312:1085, 1985.
464. Taylor T, Weintraub BD: Altered thyrotropin (TSH) carbohydrate structures in hypothalamic hypothyroidism created by paraventricular nuclear lesions are corrected by *in vivo* TSH-releasing hormone administration. *Endocrinology* 125:2198, 1989.
465. Stacpoole PW, Interlandi JW, Nicholson WE, Rabin D: Isolated ACTH deficiency: A heterogeneous disorder. *Medicine (Baltimore)* 61:13, 1982.
466. Tsukada T, Nakai Y, Koh T, Tsujii S, Inada M, Nishikawa M, et al: Plasma adrenocorticotropin and cortisol responses to ovine corticotropin-releasing factor in patients with adrenocortical insufficiency due to hypothalamic and pituitary disorders. *J Clin Endocrinol Metab* 58:758, 1984.
467. Harris RB: Role of set-point theory in regulation of body weight. *FASEB J* 4:3310, 1990.
468. Morley JE: Neuropeptide regulation of appetite and weight. *Endocr Rev* 8:256, 1987.
469. Bray GA: Autonomic and endocrine factors in the regulation of energy balance. *Fed Proc* 45:1404, 1986.
470. Leibowitz SF: Brain monoamines and peptides: Role in the control of eating behavior. *Fed Proc* 45:1396, 1986.
471. Bray GA, Gallagher TF Jr: Manifestations of hypothalamic obesity in man: A comprehensive investigation of eight patients and a review of the literature. *Medicine (Baltimore)* 54:301, 1975.
472. Bray GA, Dahms WT, Swerdloff RS, Fiser RH, Atkinson RL, Carrel RE: The Prader-Willi syndrome: A study of 40 patients and a review of the literature. *Medicine (Baltimore)* 62:59, 1983.
473. Butler MG: Prader-Willi syndrome: Current understanding of cause and diagnosis. *Am J Med Genet* 35:319, 1990.
474. Edwards JA, Seihi PK, Scoma AJ, Bannerman RM, Frohman LA: A new familial syndrome characterized by pigmentary retinopathy, hypogonadism, mental retardation, nerve deafness and glucose intolerance. *Am J Med* 60:23, 1975.
475. Burr IM, Slonim AE, Danish RK, Gadoth N, Butler IJ: Diencephalic syndrome revisited. *J Pediatr* 88:439, 1976.
476. Gemstorp I, Kjellman B, Palmgren B: Diencephalic syndrome of infancy. *J Pediatr* 70:383, 1967.

477. Bernard C: Chiens rendus diabetiques. *Compt Rend Soc Biol* 1:60, 1849.
478. Boulant JA: Hypothalamic mechanisms in thermoregulation. *Fed Proc* 40:2843, 1981.
479. Fox RH, Davies TW, Marsh FP, Urich H: Hypothermia in a young man with an anterior hypothalamic lesion. *Lancet* 2:185, 1970.
480. Johnson RH, Delahunt JW, Robinson BJ: Do thermoregulatory reflexes pass through the hypothalamus? Studies of chronic hypothermia due to hypothalamic lesion. *Aust N Z J Med* 20:154, 1990.
481. Shapiro WR, Williams GH, Plum F: Spontaneous recurrent hypothermia accompanying agenesis of the corpus callosum. *Brain* 92:423, 1969.
482. Wolff SM, Adler RC, Buskirk ER, Thompson RH: A syndrome of periodic hypothalamic discharge. *Am J Med* 36:956, 1964.
483. Hume DM, Bell CC, Bartter F: Direct measurement of adrenal secretion during operative trauma and convalescence. *Surgery* 52:174, 1962.
484. Korpassy A, Stoeckel H, Vecsei P: Investigation of hydrocortisone secretion and aldosterone secretion in patients with severe prolonged stress. *Acta Anaesthesiol Scand* 16:161, 1972.
485. Cornil A, Blinder D, Leclercq R, Copinschi G: Adrenocortical and somatotropic secretions in acute and chronic respiratory insufficiency. *Am Rev Respir Dis* 112:77, 1975.
486. Corenblum B, Taylor PJ: Mechanisms of control of prolactin release in response to apprehension stress and anesthesia-surgery stress. *Fertil Steril* 36:712, 1981.
487. Martin JB: Functions of central nervous system neurotransmitters in regulation of growth hormone secretion. *Fed Proc* 39:2902, 1980.
488. Wartofsky L, Burman KD: Alterations in thyroid function in patients with systemic illness: The 'euthyroid sick syndrome.' *Endocr Rev* 3:164, 1982.
489. Aono T, Kurachi K, Miyata M, Nakasima A, Koshiyama K, Uozumi T, et al: Influence of surgical stress under general anesthesia on serum gonadotropin levels in male and female patients. *J Clin Endocrinol Metab* 42:144, 1976.
490. Smith SR, Bledsoe T, Chhetri MK: Cortisol metabolism and the pituitary adrenal axis in adults with protein-caloric malnutrition. *J Clin Endocrinol Metab* 40:43, 1975.
491. Mohan PS, Jaya RKS: Plasma somatomedin activity in protein calorie malnutrition. *Arch Dis Child* 54:62, 1979.
492. Pimstone B, Becker D, Hendricks A: TSH response to synthetic thyrotropin-releasing hormone in human protein-calorie malnutrition. *J Clin Endocrinol Metab* 36:779, 1973.
493. Glass AR, Burman KD, Dahms WT, Boehm TM: Endocrine functions in human obesity. *Metabolism* 30:89, 1981.
494. Cordido F, Dieguez C, Gasanueva FF: Effect of central cholinergic neurotransmission enhancement by pyridostigmine on the growth hormone secretion elicited by clonidine, arginine, or hypoglycemia in normal and obese subjects. *J Clin Endocrinol Metab* 70:1361, 1990.
495. Sims EAH, Danforth E Jr, Horton ES, Bray GA, Glennon JA, Salans LB: Endocrine and metabolic effects of experimental obesity in man. *Recent Prog Horm Res* 29:457, 1973.
496. Schaper NC: Growth hormone secretion in type I diabetes: A review. *Acta Endocrinol (Copenh)* 122:7, 1990.
497. Martina V, Maccario M, Tagliabue M, Corno M, Camanni F: Chronic treatment with pirenzepine decreases growth hormone secretion in insulin-dependent diabetes mellitus. *J Clin Endocrinol Metab* 68:392, 1989.
498. Merry J, Marks V: Hypothalamic pituitary adrenal function in chronic alcoholics, in Gross MM (ed): *Alcohol Intoxication and Withdrawal: Experimental Studies. Advances in Experimental Medicine and Biology*. New York: Plenum, 1973, p 167.
499. Rees LH, Besser GM, Jeffcoate WJ, Goldie DJ, Marks V: Alcohol-induced pseudo-Cushing's syndrome. *Lancet* 1:726, 1977.
500. Van Thiel DH, Gavaler JS, Wight C, Smith WI Jr., Abuid J: Thyrotropin-releasing hormone (TRH)-induced growth hormone (HGH) responses in cirrhotic men. *Gastroenterology* 75:66, 1978.
501. Salerno F, Locatelli V, Müller EE: Growth hormone hyperresponsiveness to growth hormone-releasing hormone in patients with severe liver cirrhosis. *Clin Endocrinol (Oxf)* 27:183, 1987.
502. Morgan MY, Jakobovits AW, Gore MBR, Wills MR, Sherlock S: Serum prolactin in liver disease and its relationship to gynecomastia. *Gut* 19:170, 1978.
503. Chopra IJ, Solomon DH, Chopra U, Young RT, Chua Teco GN: Alterations in circulating thyroid hormones and thyrotropin in hepatic cirrhosis: Evidence for euthyroidism despite sub-normal serum triiodothyronine. *J Clin Endocrinol Metab* 39:501, 1974.
504. Baker HWG, Burger HG, De Kretser DM, Dulmanis A, Hudson B, O'Connor S, et al: A study of the endocrine manifestations of hepatic cirrhosis. *Q J Med* 45:145, 1976.
505. Bannister P, Handley T, Chapman C, Losowsky MS: Hypogonadism in chronic liver disease: Impaired release of luteinising hormone. *Br Med J* 293:1191, 1986.
506. Gordon GG, Southren AL, Liever CS: The effects of alcoholic liver disease and alcohol ingestion on sex hormone levels: Alcoholism. *Clin Exp Res* 2:259, 1978.
507. Luger A, Lang I, Kovarik J, Stummvoll HK, Templ H: Abnormalities in the hypothalamic-pituitary-adrenocortical axis in patients with chronic renal failure. *Am J Kidney Dis* 9:51, 1987.
508. Wallace EZ, Rosman P, Toshav N, Sacerdote A, Balthazar A: Pituitary-adrenocortical function in chronic renal failure: Studies of episodic secretion of cortisol and dexamethasone suppressibility. *J Clin Endocrinol Metab* 50:46, 1980.
509. Kokot F, Wiecek A, Grzeszczak W, Klin M: Influence of erythropoietin treatment on function of the pituitary-adrenal axis and somatotropin secretion in hemodialyzed patients. *Clin Nephrol* 33:241, 1990.
510. Bessarione D, Perfumo F, Giusti M, Ginevri F, Mazzocchi G, Gusmano R, et al: Growth hormone response to growth hormone-releasing hormone in normal and uraemic children: Comparison with hypoglycaemia following insulin administration. *Acta Endocrinol (Copenh)* 114:5, 1987.
511. Powell DR, Rosenfeld RG, Baker BK, Liu F, Hintz RL: Serum somatomedin levels in adults with chronic renal failure: The importance of measuring insulin-like growth factor I (IGF-I) and IGF-II in acid-chromatographed uremic serum. *J Clin Endocrinol Metab* 63:1186, 1986.
512. Phillips LS, Fusco AC, Unterman TG, DelGreco F: Somatomedin inhibitor in uremia. *J Clin Endocrinol Metab* 59:764, 1984.
513. Lim VS, Kathpalia SC, Frohman LA: Hyperprolactinemia and impaired pituitary response to suppression and stimulation in chronic renal failure: Reversal after transplantation. *J Clin Endocrinol Metab* 48:101, 1979.
514. Hou SH, Grossman S, Molitch ME: Hyperprolactinemia in patients with renal insufficiency and chronic renal failure requiring hemodialysis or chronic ambulatory peritoneal dialysis. *Am J Kidney Dis* 6:245, 1985.
515. Sievertsen GD, Lim VS, Nakawatase C, Frohman LA: Metabolic clearance and secretion rates of human prolactin in normal subjects and in patients with chronic renal failure. *J Clin Endocrinol Metab* 50:846, 1980.
516. Lim VS, Fang VS, Katz AI, Refetoff S: Thyroid dysfunction in chronic renal failure: A study of the pituitary-thyroid axis and peripheral turnover kinetics of thyroxine and triiodothyronine. *J Clin Invest* 60:522, 1977.
517. Lim VS, Henriquez C, Sievertsen G, Frohman LA: Ovarian function in chronic renal failure: Evidence suggesting hypothalamic anovulation. *Ann Intern Med* 93:21, 1980.

518. Bierman M, Nolan GH: Menstrual function and renal transplantation. *Obstet Gynecol* 49:186, 1977.
519. DeGirolami U, Schmidek H: Clinicopathological study of 53 tumors of the pineal region. *J Neurosurg* 39:455, 1973.
520. Jennings MT, Gelman R, Hochberg F: Intracranial germ-cell tumors: Natural history and pathogenesis. *J Neurosurg* 63:155, 1985.
521. Kitay JI: Pineal lesions and precocious puberty: Review. *J Clin Endocrinol Metab* 14:622, 1954.
522. Jooma R, Kendall BE: Diagnosis and management of pineal tumors. *J Neurosurg* 58:654, 1983.
523. Donaldson JO: Endocrinology of pseudotumor cerebri. *Neurol Clin* 4:919, 1986.
524. Molitch ME: The empty sella, in Bardin CW (ed): *Current Therapy in Endocrinology and Metabolism,* 4th ed. Philadelphia, B.C. Decker, Inc. 1991, p 32.
525. Sotos JF, Dodge PR, Muirhead D, Crawford JD, Talbot NB: Cerebral gigantism in childhood: A syndrome of excessively rapid growth with acromegalic features and a nonprogressive neurologic disorder. *N Engl J Med* 271:109, 1964.
526. Jaeken J, Van Der Schueren-Lodeweyckx M, Eeckels R: Cerebral gigantism syndrome. *Z Kinderheilk* 112:332, 1972.

CHAPTER 8

Diseases of the Anterior Pituitary

Lawrence A. Frohman

PITUITARY GLAND

Anatomy

The pituitary gland is located at the base of the skull in a saddle-shaped bone-lined cavity, the *sella turcica*, which forms a portion of the sphenoid bone. The anterior portion of the sella consists of the midline *tuberculum sellae* and the *anterior clinoid processes*, which are posterior projections from the sphenoid wings. Posteriorly, the sella is limited by the *dorsum sellae*, the lateral angles of which form the *posterior clinoid processes*. A thickened reflection of the dura mater, the *diaphragma sellae*, is attached to the clinoid processes and forms the roof of the sella. The external layer of the dura mater continues into the sella to form the periosteum of the pituitary fossa. As a consequence, the pituitary is extradural and normally is not in contact with cerebrospinal fluid (CSF). The pituitary stalk and its associated blood vessels pass through a foramen in this membrane which may be incomplete or fenestrated (Fig. 8-1).

The shape of the pituitary gland varies from an ovoid to a true spheroid configuration. The shape of the sella turcica conforms to that of the pituitary, making the normal dimensions somewhat variable. Both age and sex influence the size of the sella. Thus, the frequently used dimensions of 10 by 13 by 6 mm must be regarded as only average figures.[1–5] Estimations of pituitary volume based on radiographic measurements have led to a suggested mean value of about 600 mm^3, though there is considerable variation. Measurements of size based on computed tomography (CT) and magnetic resonance imaging (MRI)[3–5] tend to be smaller than those obtained at autopsy.[6] The pituitary weight varies from 0.4 to 0.9 g, being slightly greater in women than in men. During pregnancy, the weight of the anterior lobe, which normally constitutes about 75 percent of the pituitary, increases up to twofold, primarily because of an increase in lactotroph size and number.

Blood and Nerve Supply

Scanning electron microscopy of digested vascular casts, together with direct observation of the direction of blood flow through portal vessels and measurement of pituitary hormone concentrations in these channels, has provided a greater understanding of the blood supply of the pituitary. The arterial blood supply of the pituitary originates from the internal carotid arteries via interconnecting branches of the circle of Willis and the superior, middle, and inferior hypophyseal arteries (Fig. 8-2). This network of vessels forms a unique portal circulation connecting the median eminence and the pituitary. Tiers from the first three vessels coalesce to form coiled capillary loops (*external plexus*) in the outer portion of the median eminence (*infundibulum*) and the upper portion of the pituitary stalk. These loops, along with capillaries from the inner median eminence (*internal plexus*), drain into a series of long portal vessels which traverse the pituitary stalk primarily on its anterior surface and terminate in a dense network of sinusoidal capillaries within the anterior lobe. The middle and inferior hypophyseal arteries, which provide the blood supply to the pituitary stalk and posterior pituitary, do not penetrate the substance of the anterior pituitary en route. Thus, the anterior pituitary receives no direct arterial blood supply, and all arterial blood flow first passes through the portal plexus.[7]

Venous drainage from the pituitary may follow one of several routes. There are sparse and probably insignificant lateral veins draining the anterior pituitary. Other veins join with the posterior pituitary veins and extend to the cavernous sinus. Venous blood from the anterior pituitary also enters the posterior pituitary capillary bed, which is connected to both the long and short portal vessels on the posterior portion of the pituitary stalk. Retrograde blood flow from the posterior pituitary toward the median eminence has been observed in these vessels, and the concentrations of anterior pituitary hormones greatly exceed those in the systemic circulation.[8] Thus, a portion of the adenohypophyseal venous effluent appears to be carried toward the brain by vessels along the pituitary stalk.

The direction of the blood flow from the hypothalamus to the pituitary forms the basis for the portal vessel–chemotransmitter hypothesis of hypotha-

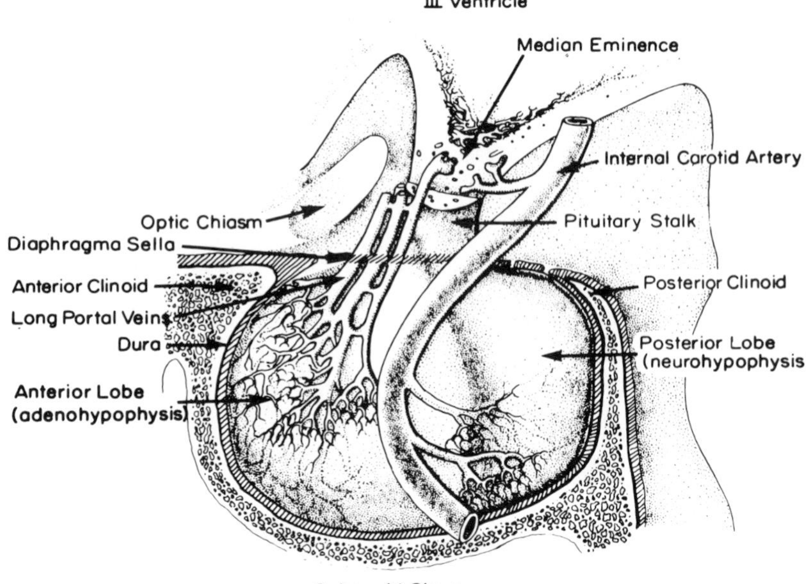

FIGURE 8-1 Schematic representation of the human pituitary gland in relation to its surrounding structures. Refer to text for detailed description.

FIGURE 8-2 Vasculature of the rhesus monkey pituitary (posterior view), as constructed from photographs of digested vascular cast after intravenous injection of methyl methacrylate. I = infundibulum; IS = infundibular stem; IP = infundibular process; HYP = hypothalamus; SHA = superior hypophyseal arteries; MHA = middle hypophyseal artery; IHA = inferior hypophyseal artery; ICA = internal carotid artery; LPV = long portal vein; CS = cavernous sinus. The absence of a direct arterial supply to the anterior lobe and the paucity of venous drainage from the pituitary by a route other than via the stalk (infundibular stem) are evident. (*From Berlund and Page.*[7])

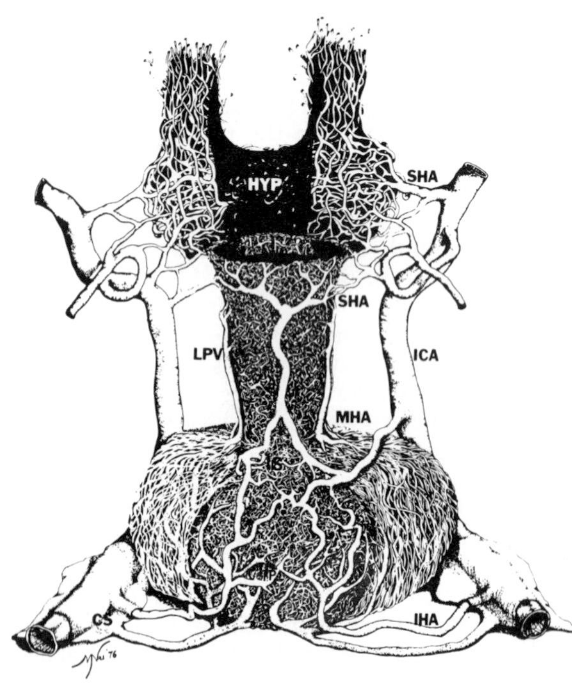

lamic control of anterior pituitary function (see Chapter 7). Although the reverse blood flow provides a theoretical route for the direct feedback of pituitary hormones on the hypothalamus, the reverse flow is restricted to a distance of less than half the length of the stalk and thus does not reach the hypothalamus.[9,10] Blood flow to the anterior pituitary has been estimated to be 0.8 ml/g per min, which is the highest flow rate of any mammalian tissue.

The nerve supply of the anterior pituitary is quite sparse and represents almost exclusively postganglionic sympathetic fibers which accompany arteriolar branches and terminate on blood vessels. There is, however, little evidence to suggest that alterations in sympathetic nervous system activity affect the blood flow rate in the pituitary. Nerve fibers connecting the posterior and anterior lobes have also been described, though their function is unknown.

Embryology

An appreciation of the pattern by which the pituitary gland is formed is important for an understanding of the anatomic distribution of pituitary cell types and the various types of congenital anomalies which occur as well as the origin and potential directions in which pituitary tumors may grow. The glandular portion of the pituitary, or *adenohypophysis*, originates from Rathke's pouch, an ectodermal evagination of the oropharynx which eventually associates with an outpouching of the third ventricle region of the diencephalon of the developing embryo. This portion of the diencephalon subsequently differentiates into the *neurohypophysis*, or posterior lobe. The portion of Rathke's pouch that does not come into contact with the diencephalon enlarges to form the anterior lobe, or *pars anterior*. Early in development, two lateral outgrowths of tissue from the anterior lobes fuse across the midline and extend forward along the hypophyseal stalk. This structure, known as the *pars tuberalis*, forms a complete collar surrounding the stalk in some species; in humans, it is limited to a group of cells along the anterior region of the stalk. The portion of Rathke's pouch that directly contacts the neurohypophysis develops less extensively than the opposite wall of the pouch and forms the intermediate lobe, or *pars intermedia*. In some species, such as the rat, this lobe remains a distinct anatomic region in adult life and can be easily recognized as such. In contrast, the cells of the pars intermedia in humans become intermingled with the anterior lobe, and the combined structure has been referred to as the *pars distalis*.

Cells of the pars intermedia develop the capacity to secrete corticotropin, or adrenocorticotropic hormone (ACTH), melanocyte stimulating hormone (MSH), lipotropin (LPH), and endorphins, whereas those in the pars anterior eventually secrete growth hormone (GH), prolactin, ACTH, LPH, thyroid stimulating hormone (TSH), luteinizing hormone (LH), and follicle stimulating hormone (FSH). Information gained from microsurgical removal of pituitary tumors indicates that the location of hormone-secreting tumors can to some extent be predicted on the basis of the embryogenesis of the cell type involved.

The lumen of Rathke's pouch in humans is obliterated by the developing pituitary gland. Remnants of the pouch may persist at the boundary of the neurohypophysis either as a cleft or as small colloid-filled cysts and are more prominent in children than in adults. The connection of the pouch to the oropharynx is disrupted quite early in development by a mesenchymal ingrowth which forms the sphenoid bone. A few cells of the lower portion of the pouch may persist into adult life within or beneath the sphenoid bone and are known as the *pharyngeal pituitary*. These cells contain secretory granules in which at least GH and prolactin are present, and it is possible that this structure could exhibit a significant endocrine function subsequent to removal or destruction of the pars distalis. These cells may also become neoplastic and develop into extrasellar hormone-secreting pituitary tumors.[11]

The human fetal pituitary anlage is first recognizable at 4 or 5 weeks of gestation, and cytologic differentiation occurs rapidly, with basophilic cells apparent by the seventh week and acidophilic cells apparent by the ninth to tenth week. Similar changes occur in the hypothalamus, with monoamine fluorescence noted in the median eminence by 13 weeks, followed shortly thereafter by the development of the primary plexus of the portal vascular system. By the twentieth week, the anatomic maturation of the hypothalamic-pituitary unit appears to be complete.

Secretory granules occur as early as the end of the first trimester, and immunochemical measurements of hormones occur as early as the seventh week of gestation. There is considerable evidence for the importance of both the secretion of anterior pituitary hormones and their control by the central nervous system early in gestation, primarily on the basis of the decreased adrenal weight observed in anencephalic infants and the genital deformities associated with excessive ACTH and adrenal androgen secretion in the adrenogenital syndrome. True functional maturation, however, is a continuously developing phenomenon, and many aspects of feedback regulation are not developed until well into postnatal life.

Recent studies have identified a nuclear transcription factor, *pit-I*, that is essential for the expression of GH and GH-releasing hormone receptor genes and for the development of several cell types in the pituitary. Deletion of or a mutation in the gene for this protein is associated with failure of development of somatotrophs, lactotrophs, and thyrotrophs in animals[12,13] and humans.[14,15]

Cell Types

The anterior pituitary is composed of numerous cell types, most of which have as their predominant function the synthesis, storage, and release of a specific hormone or hormones. Methods used to identify the cells in the anterior pituitary include histochemical staining techniques, electron microscopy, and, more important, immunocytochemistry. Classic staining methods revealed the presence of acidophil, basophil, and chromophobe cell types. The introduction of histochemical stains revealed the glycoprotein nature of the basophilic cells, and a combination of these techniques demonstrated that both basophils and acidophils consist of distinct classes of cells.[16] Detailed comparisons of the techniques used for distinguishing the morphologic characteristics of anterior pituitary cells are available.[17]

Among the problems with standard light microscopy is the frequent inability to discriminate between the various chromophobe cells, which represent more than half the cells in the anterior lobe. Thus, using light microscopy, it is very difficult to distinguish between corticotropin-secreting cells, whose granules are too small and widely dispersed to be recognized, and other cell types in a state of active secretion which have become degranulated. Electron microscopy has made it possible to recognize that (1) secretory granules and the structure of certain cellular organelles, particularly the rough endoplasmic reticulum, vary greatly between cell types and (2) the size of secretion granules within a single cell type can vary considerably in accordance with the functional state of the cell. Immunocytochemistry, using antisera specific for individual hormones or subunits, is currently the best available technique for the identification of individual cell types. For hormones which share common subunits, e.g., the three glycoprotein hormones, which contain identical α subunits (see the following section), antisera specific for the individual β subunits are required to distinguish between thyrotrophs and gonadotrophs. The use of these techniques has resulted in considerable uncertainty as to the validity of previous morphologic classifications because of the frequent lack of concordance between immunocytochemical and older histochemical procedures.[18] Characteristics of each of the recognized anterior pituitary cell types follow.

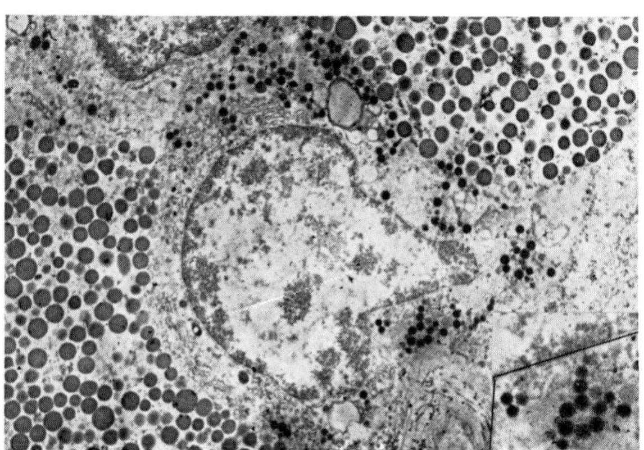

FIGURE 8-3 Immunohistochemical staining of a normal human lactotroph with anti-human-prolactin serum. The small size of the prolactin granules (mean diameter, 185 nm), which appear black, contrasts with the nonstaining granules in the upper right and lower left of the field. The *inset* shows that only the small granules are covered with the immunochemical (peroxidase-antiperoxidase) stain; the others are stained by osmium tetroxide only. (*Courtesy of T. Duello, Colorado State University.*)

Somatotrophs: Growth Hormone-Secreting Cells

Somatotrophs can be recognized as acidophilic in standard hematoxylin and eosin preparations. Their association with GH secretion was originally proposed on the basis of their predominance in pituitary adenomas of patients with acromegaly. The presence of GH has been confirmed by immunochemical stains, and electron microscopy reveals the granules to be approximately 300 to 400 nm in diameter. The somatotroph cells are located predominantly in the lateral portions of the anterior lobe.

Lactotrophs: Prolactin-Secreting Cells

The lactotrophs are a second class of acidophilic cell. They can be differentiated from somatotrophs by their irregular and coarse granulation on light microscopy. Immunologic techniques using antiprolactin serum have confirmed the presence of prolactin in the secretion granules, which electron microscopy shows to be smaller in size than those of GH (Fig. 8-3). Lactotrophs are also located in the lateral portion of the anterior lobe and generally develop peripherally to the somatotrophs. The percentage of lactotrophs in pregnancy and during fetal life is increased, reflecting the effects of elevated estrogen levels in pregnancy. Virtually all the increase in pituitary size during pregnancy is a consequence of lactotroph proliferation.

Thyrotrophs: TSH-Secreting Cells

The thyrotrophs, which are intensely basophilic-staining and polyhedral, tend to occur around the anterior edge of the pituitary near the midline, though they can also be found in deeper portions of the gland. The thyrotroph secretory granules, which are 50 to 100 nm in diameter, are smaller than GH and prolactin granules and exhibit greater heterogeneity in density.[19] Under normal conditions, thyrotrophs constitute about 6 percent of the anterior lobe cells. However, in primary hypothyroidism the cells undergo marked hypertrophy and exhibit the characteristic ultrastructural changes associated with increased secretory activity, including enlarged endoplasmic reticulum and hypertrophy of the Golgi apparatus. The number of secretory granules decreases markedly, indicating the depletion of intracellular hormone storage. These histologic characteristics of the cell have led to its being named the "thyroidectomy cell." After long periods of thyroid hormone deficiency, TSH-secreting tumors can also occur.[20]

Gonadotrophs: LH- and FSH-Secreting Cells

LH and FSH were originally believed to be produced by separate basophilic cells. On the basis of immunocytochemical results using antiserum specific for the β subunits of the individual gonadotropins, however, it is clear that they originate from the same cells. These cells are located deep in the lateral portion of the lateral lobes in association with acidophilic, primarily lactotroph, cells. Hyperplasia of the gonadotrophs and, rarely, even tumor formation occur in association with primary hypogonadism,[21] whereas a decrease is observed during pregnancy in association with chorionic gonadotropin production.

Corticotrophs: ACTH-Secreting Cells

ACTH, MSH, and β-endorphin are all derived from the same precursor, pro-opiomelanocortin (POMC),[22] and thus are produced by the same cell type, the corticotroph. This cell type was originally considered chromophobic and later was shown to be basophilic in its staining characteristics. Corticotrophs have been shown to be embryologically of intermediate lobe origin but reside most commonly in the medial mucoid region of the anterior lobe. A second group of corticotrophs appears to have migrated during development into regions of the posterior lobe which are in contact with the anterior lobe and also into the pars tuberalis. Ultrastructural studies have revealed that the granules are quite variable in size. The cells in the anterior lobe exhibit sparse granulation and relatively poor staining, while those in the intermediate and posterior lobe region contain large electron-dense granules. Differences in the specific peptides found in the corticotrophs located in the anterior and intermediate lobes reflect differences in the processing enzymes present in individual corticotrophs that are responsible for converting the precursor to the mature hormone.[23]

The presence of increased glucocorticoids, whether endogenous or exogenous, produces a degranulation and microtubular hyalinization of corticotrophs known as *Crooke's hyaline degeneration*. The areas of hyaline deposits are associated with diminished immunostaining with anti-ACTH serum. In adrenal insufficiency, the sparsely granulated basophilic cells in the anterior lobe increase in number and the intensely staining basophilic cells of the intermediate and posterior lobe region decrease, suggesting that the former rather than the latter are of physiologic importance in the secretion of ACTH. Similar conclusions have been reached from laboratory studies in animals involving selective pituitary ablation or in situ hybridization.

Other Cell Types

Depending on the staining method used, some anterior pituitary cells, varying from 15 to 40 percent, appear to be chromophobic by light microscopy. Many of these cells resemble either basophils or acidophils, depending on the stain, and have been termed *amphophils*. Although a few secretory granules can be demonstrated by electron microscopy, no identifiable hormone secretory role has been established for these cells. It is possible that they represent actively secreting or even resting degranulated cells or that they are undifferentiated primitive secretory cells. Cells of this type have been associated with hypersecretory pituitary tumors.

A small fraction of cells in the pituitary contain both GH and prolactin secretory granules and are called *somatomammotrophs*.[24] Although there is speculation that these cells may serve as precursors for both somatotrophs and lactotrophs, there is no convincing experimental evidence to support this possibility. These cells may, however, develop into bihormonal-secreting tumors.[25] A small percentage of adenohypophyseal cells remain unidentified after immunohistochemical staining with antibodies to all the recognized pituitary hormones. Some of these cells may be responsible for the secretion of other, yet to be characterized, pituitary hormones such as ovarian growth factor, fibroblast growth factor, and aldosterone stimulating factor.

Finally, a few cells exhibit a stellate shape, with cellular processes that often appear to extend into the perivascular spaces in an arrangement suggestive of primitive follicle formation. Secretory granules are uncommon in these cells, and their function also is unknown. These cells have recently been reported to secrete a peptide with potent angiogenic properties called endothelial stimulating factor.[26]

ANTERIOR PITUITARY HORMONES

There are six well-recognized hormones of the anterior pituitary whose structures have been identified, whose functions have been characterized, and for each of which precise measurements in tissues and biological fluids are available. The hormones are polypeptide in nature and can be divided into three general categories, each of which exhibits unique characteristics: the corticotropin family of peptides (ACTH, MSH, LPH, β-endorphin, and related peptides), the glycoprotein hormones (LH, FSH, TSH, and the related chorionic gonadotropin), and the somatomammotropin hormones (GH, prolactin, and the related placental lactogen). A comparison of the chemical characteristics of these hormones is given in Table 8-1.

Corticotropin-Related Peptides

Chemistry

Adrenocorticotropic hormone (corticotropin, ACTH) is a 39-amino acid single-chain peptide. The NH_2-terminal (the end of the molecule containing the free amino group, conventionally designated as position 1) 24 amino acids are identical in all species studied to date, while there are minor species differences in the COOH-terminal (the end of the molecule containing the free carboxyl group) region. The biologically active portion of the molecule is contained in the NH_2-terminal portion, with the first 18 amino acids being required for full biological activity. Rapid degradation of synthetic $ACTH_{1-18}$ in vivo, however, has necessitated the synthesis of a longer amino acid sequence, $ACTH_{1-24}$, for use in humans.

ACTH is only one of several peptides that are derived from a common precursor molecule, POMC, which has a molecular weight of approximately 29,000 and is glycosylated (Fig. 8-4).[27,28] The POMC gene is located on chromosome 2.[29] Differential processing of this molecule occurs in various cell types, resulting in differing spectra of peptides in brain, posterior pituitary, and anterior pituitary. In addition, peptides once believed to be the final processing product, including ACTH itself, may be further cleaved to fragments that are secreted and bioactive.

TABLE 8-1 Classification of Anterior Pituitary Hormones

Class	Members	Molecular Weight	Amino Acids	Carbohydrate	Other Features
Corticotropin-lipotropin	ACTH	4500	39		All members of this class are derived from a single precursor
	α-MSH	1800	13		NH_2-terminal 13 amino acids of ACTH; in humans, found only in fetal life and in tumors
	β-Lipotropin	11,200	91		
	β-Endorphin	4000	31		COOH-terminal (amino acids 61–91) portion of β-LPH
Glycoprotein	LH	29,000	α subunit: 89 β subunit: 115	1% sialic acid	All have two subunits, with the α subunit being identical or nearly identical and the β subunit conferring biological specificity
	FSH	29,000	α subunit: 89 β subunit: 115	5% sialic acid	
	TSH	29,000	α subunit: 89 β subunit: 112	1% sialic acid	
	Chorionic gonadotropin*	46,000	α subunit: 92 β subunit: 139	12% sialic acid	
Somato-mammotropin	Growth hormone	21,800	191		All single-chain proteins with two to three disulfide bridges
	Prolactin	22,500	198	†	
	Placental lactogen*‡	21,800	191		

* Of placental origin and included for comparison purposes.

† Glycoprotein forms of prolactin have recently been identified which appear to have reduced biological activity.[30]

‡ Although detectable in the pituitary at very low concentrations, its only physiologic effects are a consequence of its secretion from the placenta.

Two of these peptides are derived from the ACTH molecule: α-melanocyte stimulating hormone (α-MSH), which is identical to $ACTH_{1-13}$ with an acetylated NH_2 terminus, and corticotropin-like intermediate lobe peptide (CLIP), which is identical to $ACTH_{18-39}$. α-MSH and CLIP are found primarily in species in which the intermediate lobe is more fully developed (e.g., rat and sheep). In the human, they

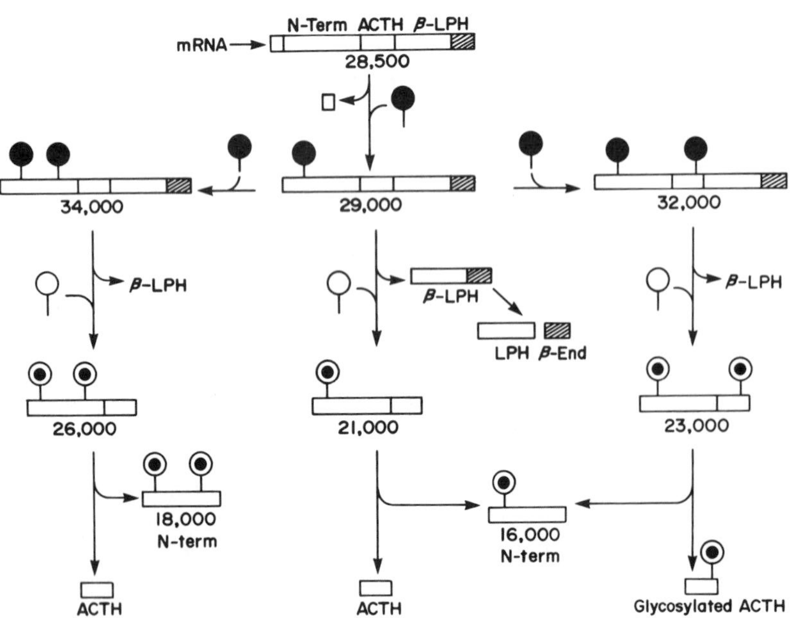

FIGURE 8-4 Biosynthetic pathway of ACTH- and β-LPH-related hormones. A single messenger RNA directs the translation of a precursor polypeptide which contains the amino acid sequences of an NH_2-terminal fragment (which has been proposed to be a hormone but whose function has yet to be detected), ACTH, α-, β-, and γ-MSH, CLIP ($ACTH_{18-38}$), β-LPH, met-enkephalin, and β-endorphin. The earliest form of the molecule detected in the cell is one of molecular weight 29,000 containing carbohydrate in the positions indicated by the black circles. This molecule is further processed by additional glycosylation, yielding forms of 34,000 and 32,000 molecular weight. Subsequent modifications of the carbohydrate side chain are indicated by the white circles. The first proteolytic step involves cleavage of β-LPH from the COOH-terminal portion of the precursor. β-LPH can then be further processed to β-endorphin. Proteolysis of forms remaining after removal of the β-LPH fragment results in removal of the NH_2-terminal fragment, the molecular weight of which depends on its sugar content, and ACTH which is also present in glycosylated (13,000 mol wt) or nonglycosylated (4500 mol wt) forms. (*From Herbert E et al.*[23])

are normally found only during fetal life, when a distinct pars intermedia can be recognized. Neither appears to be secreted in humans.

A second hormone contained within POMC is β-lipotropin (β-LPH), which contains a heptapeptide sequence (β-LPH_{47-53}) that is identical to $ACTH_{4-10}$. This sequence is also present in several peptides derived from cleavage of β-LPH: γ-LPH (β-LPH_{1-58}) and β-MSH (β-LPH_{41-58}). The structures of these peptides are shown in Fig. 7-13. β-MSH does not appear to be present in the human pituitary. Previous reports of a chemically distinct β-MSH (consisting of a 22-amino acid sequence) have been shown to be incorrect, caused by an artifact resulting from postmortem proteolysis during the extraction procedures employed for its purification. Moreover, the immunologic reactivity ascribed to β-MSH in human plasma has been shown to be of a molecular size consistent with β-LPH and/or γ-LPH.[31] The presence of a true β-MSH thus appears to be restricted to species that possess a distinct pars intermedia.

Two other β-LPH fragments, γ-LPH and β-endorphin, have been identified in postnatal human pituitary and are secreted. β-Endorphin itself can be further cleaved to yield the biologically active peptides α-endorphin and γ-endorphin. Although the structure of met-enkephalin is identical to that of the NH_2-terminal pentapeptide sequence of β-endorphin, a separate biosynthetic pathway exists for this peptide (see Chap. 7).

ACTH

Action

The primary effects of ACTH are exerted on the adrenal cortex, where the hormone stimulates the secretion of glucocorticoids, mineralocorticoids, and androgenic steroids. ACTH binds to specific high-affinity receptors on adrenocortical cell membranes and stimulates steroidogenesis by enhancing the conversion of cholesterol to pregnenolone through an adenylate cyclase-mediated mechanism. ACTH also stimulates protein synthesis, leading to adrenocortical hypertrophy and hyperplasia (see Chap. 12 for details).

Extraadrenal Effects

In addition to its effects on the adrenal, ACTH exhibits a lipolytic effect on adipose tissue and a hypoglycemic effect attributed to a direct insulin-releasing action on the pancreatic beta cell. Large doses of ACTH also stimulate GH secretion, enhance glucose and amino acid transport into muscle cells, and, in hypophysectomized animals, impair the hepatic degradation of cortisol, which prolongs its half-life in plasma. Except for patients with ACTH-secreting pituitary tumors, it is unlikely that plasma ACTH levels sufficient to achieve these effects ever occur.

The effects of ACTH on pigmentation have been well recognized for many years. Because ACTH is less effective as a melanin-dispersing agent than is either α-MSH or β-MSH, it had been presumed that ACTH contributes relatively little to the hyperpigmentation seen in states of marked ACTH hypersecretion such as Addison's disease and ACTH-secreting pituitary tumors (Nelson's syndrome) (Table 8-2). However, with the recent data suggesting that neither α-MSH nor β-MSH exists in humans, the role of ACTH may well be greater than was previously believed. In fact, even β-LPH may have significant pigmentation-enhancing effects in conditions where its blood level is markedly increased, e.g., chronic renal failure (see below).[32]

Measurement

Since the levels of plasma cortisol are directly related to those of ACTH under steady-state conditions, the measurement of cortisol serves as a functional bioassay of ACTH when adrenal function is normal. From a practical standpoint, plasma cortisol measurements are less expensive, more reliable, and generally more readily available for assessing ACTH function.

Radioimmunoassay The radioimmunoassay for plasma ACTH, although associated with technological problems in the past, is currently a highly sensitive and reliable assay for clinical use, provided that the samples are properly collected and stored to prevent destruction of the hormone by circulating peptidases.[33] The limitations of the assay relate to the cross-reactivity of both ACTH precursors ("big ACTH") and fragments in the sera of patients with ectopic ACTH-secreting tumors.[34] Molecular sieve chromatography and/or immunoradiometric assays may be used to increase the specificity of the assay for true ACTH.

Other Assays Other techniques for measuring ACTH include in vivo and in vitro bioassays, radioreceptor assays, and cytochemical assays. Each of these assays is used only for research purposes because of the complexity and cost. While the sensitivity of the in vivo and early in vitro bioassays was a limiting factor, the others have sufficient sensitivity to measure circulating ACTH levels, and the cytochemical assay has a sensitivity of 5 fg/ml (10^{-15} *M*), which far exceeds that of all the other assays, and also has excellent specificity.[35]

TABLE 8-2 Pigmenting Effects of ACTH and Related Peptides

Hormone	Potency
α-MSH	100
β-MSH	50
ACTH	1
α-LPH	0.5
β-LPH	0.2

Pituitary and Plasma Levels

The total pituitary content of ACTH is about 0.6 mg. Plasma levels of ACTH in healthy adults vary from less than 10 pg/ml (the lower limit of detection by radioimmunoassay in most laboratories) to 80 pg/ml. ACTH is secreted episodically with a distinct diurnal rhythm. Peak ACTH levels occur in the early morning (5 to 8 A.M.), while the lowest levels occur at about midnight. Changes in plasma cortisol levels closely parallel those in plasma ACTH, with a short lag period. During stress, plasma ACTH levels can rise to 10 times the normal values.

Metabolism

Although ACTH is bound selectively by the adrenal cortex, most of the hormone disappears from circulation by other mechanisms, including intravascular enzymatic degradation. The disappearance rate (half-life) varies according to whether measurements are made by bioassay or radioimmunoassay (RIA), with bioactive ACTH disappearing more rapidly from circulation (half-life 3 to 9 min) than does immunoreactive ACTH (half-life 7 to 12 min).[36] On the basis of the disappearance rate, a presumed tissue distribution equal to that of extracellular space, and a plasma level of 25 pg/ml, the daily secretory rate can be estimated to be 25 μg per day, which represents approximately 5 percent of the pituitary hormone content.

Control of Secretion

There are three major components of the control of ACTH secretion: an inherent diurnal rhythmicity (Fig. 8-5), a closed-loop feedback system which responds to changes in the levels of circulating cortisol, and an open-loop component relating to numerous neurally mediated stimuli commonly referred to as *stress*.

FIGURE 8-5 Concordance between ACTH and cortisol secretion during the early morning. The changes in plasma cortisol levels can be seen to follow those of ACTH with a relatively short lag period. (*From Gallagher TF et al: J Clin Endocrinol Metab 36:1058, 1973.*)

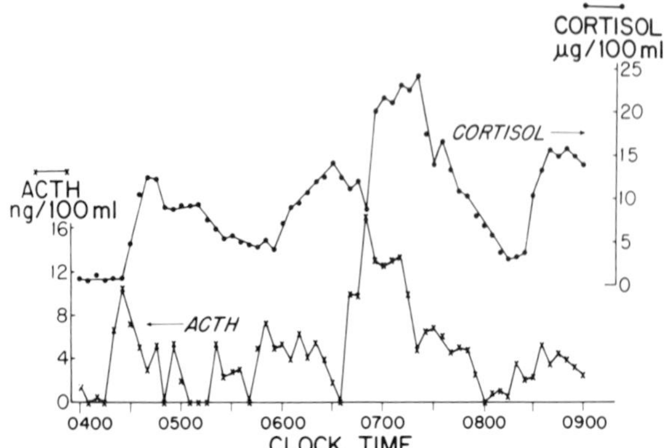

ACTH is secreted in a pulsatile manner which reflects its neural control. A diurnal rhythmicity can be observed in both ACTH and cortisol secretion, which peaks in the morning at about the time of normal awakening and then gradually decreases, reaching a trough at around midnight. Reversal of the normal sleep-wake pattern, as occurs with transoceanic plane travel, is followed by a corresponding change in the diurnal pattern of ACTH secretion.[37] The responsiveness of the hypothalamic-pituitary-adrenal axis to stimulation is therefore greatest in the late evening and lowest in the morning.

The closed-loop feedback control of ACTH secretion is mediated primarily by cortisol, which exhibits inhibitory effects on both the central nervous system (CNS) and the pituitary. The stimulation of the hypothalamic-pituitary-adrenal axis which occurs with a decrease in circulating cortisol levels is sensitive to both the absolute level and the rate of change. Electrophysiologic and binding studies indicate that there are both hypothalamic and extrahypothalamic sites of cortisol feedback which serve to suppress the release of corticotropin releasing hormone (CRH). In addition, cortisol exhibits an inhibitory effect on the pituitary by suppressing the response of the corticotroph to CRH. The evidence currently available suggests that the inhibitory effects of cortisol at the level of the pituitary constitute the most important component of cortisol negative feedback in the physiologic regulation of ACTH secretion.

The open-loop component may be initiated by numerous stimuli, all of which represent types of physical or emotional stress, e.g., pain, fever, anxiety, depression, and hypoglycemia. The trigger sites for these stimuli are undoubtedly different, though they all result in a release of CRH, which also serves as mediator of many stress responses within the CNS. Evidence for a peripheral beta-adrenergic mechanism in the stimulation of ACTH secretion has been observed, though the importance of this pathway in humans is unclear. While none of these stimuli is specific for ACTH (i.e., several lead to the release of GH and/or prolactin), the ACTH responses are mediated by separate neural pathways and are frequently dissociated from those of the other pituitary hormones. These responses are to a large extent unaffected by circulating cortisol levels, though with long-term high-dose glucocorticoid therapy they can be suppressed. Diurnal variation also frequently disappears during periods of stress. A full discussion of the neuroendocrine regulation of ACTH secretion appears in Chap. 7.

β-LPH and Related Peptides

It is currently believed that the LPHs (primarily β-LPH) are present in normal human serum in the range of 10 to 40 pg/ml, that their secretory dynamics can be tested with the same stimuli used for evaluating ACTH secretion (insulin hypoglycemia, metyrapone, vasopressin), and that there is probably equimolar secretion of ACTH and the lipotropins in response to each of these stimuli.[38,39] The presence of both ACTH and LPH in the same parent molecule with enzymatic cleavage immediately before or concomitant with the secretory process explains these observations. In many aspects, the relation between ACTH and LPH is analogous to that between insulin and C peptide (see Chap. 19).

Dissociation of ACTH and LPH levels has been observed in two pathologic conditions. In patients on maintenance hemodialysis, elevated LPH-MSH levels have been reported[40] and correlate with both the extent of pigmentation and the length of time on dialysis.[32] This dissociation may be explained by the facts that LPH, in contrast to ACTH, is stable in plasma (i.e., not subject to intravascular enzymatic degradation) and that its clearance in chronic renal failure is markedly prolonged. It also implies that LPH probably exerts relatively little feedback effect on its own secretion or that of ACTH. In patients with Addison's disease or Nelson's syndrome, the decrease in LPH levels in response to acute hydrocortisone administration is much slower than that in ACTH, again reflecting the differences in metabolic clearance rates.[41]

Endorphins and Enkephalins

The discovery of the existence of synaptosomal receptors in mammalian brain which bound opiates in a stereospecific manner led to a search for endogenous opiates and to the isolation of two pentapeptides, *leu-enkephalin* and *met-enkephalin*,[42] and the observation that the structure of the former was identical to residues 61 to 65 of β-LPH. Somewhat larger pituitary peptides with opiate activity were subsequently found,[43] and three endorphin peptides (α-, β-, and γ-endorphin) have been identified, each consisting of part or all of the COOH-terminal portion of β-LPH beginning with residue 61 (Fig. 7-8).[44,45] On the basis of studies demonstrating cleavage by pituitary enzymes, β-LPH is recognized as the precursor of the endorphins. However, the absence of comparable enzymes in the brain and the difference in the anatomic distribution of endorphins and enkephalins within discrete regions of brain and pituitary make it unlikely that the endorphins serve as precursors of the enkephalins, for which a separate precursor has been identified (see Chap. 7). In the pituitary, β-endorphin has been localized primarily to the cells of the pars intermedia and to a small extent to the adenohypophisis and, using immunohistochemical techniques, has been demonstrated in the same cells as ACTH.

β-Endorphin is measured by RIA,[46,47] and its release into the circulation, along with γ-MSH, another peptide with the MSH sequence contained in the NH_2-terminal portion of POMC, parallels that of ACTH under nearly all conditions (following CRH,[48] metyrapone,[49] and insulin hypoglycemia[50] and in patients with Addison's disease and Nelson's syndrome).[51] The physiologic role of pituitary endorphin remains to be clarified. The peptide cannot cross the blood-brain barrier and does not produce analgesic or other clinical effects when infused systemically at concentrations leading to much higher blood levels than have been observed with endogenous endorphins. Altered states of pain perception (hypalgesia) have also not been associated with clinical states of β-endorphin hypersecretion.

Extrapituitary ACTH and Related Peptides

ACTH, β-endorphin, and γ-MSH are also located in numerous sites distant from the pituitary and CNS, including gastric mucosa,[52] pancreas,[53] semen,[54] and placenta.[55,56] No physiologic function has been evident to date for these peptides in any of the locations. However, a possible role for placental ACTH has been proposed to explain the increase in plasma cortisol levels during pregnancy, particularly with approaching parturition. This extrapituitary source of ACTH, which is unresponsive to normal feedback, could explain the rising total and free cortisol levels seen during pregnancy (above and beyond that explained by the increase in cortisol-binding globulin), which are resistant to dexamethasone suppression.

Glycoprotein Hormones

Chemistry

The glycoprotein hormones of the pituitary include TSH (thyrotropin), LH, and FSH. In addition, a placental chorionic gonadotropin (CG) with both structural and biological similarities to LH is included in this class of hormones.

The glycoprotein hormones are composed of two subunits, α and β, each consisting of a peptide core with branched carbohydrate side chains which contribute from 15 to 30 percent of the weight of the hormone. The sugars include fucose, galactose, galactosamine, glucosamine, mannose, and sialic acid, the presence of which is necessary for the hormones' biological activity. In particular, deglycosylation of the α subunit impairs activation of the glycoprotein receptor once binding has occurred.[57] The sialic acid moiety serves to reduce the rate of metabolic degradation of the glycoprotein hormones but is probably not required for their recognition by target cell receptors.

Within a single species, including humans, the α subunits of the glycoprotein hormones are identical or nearly identical, whereas the β subunits vary, providing biological specificity to each hormone. Even the β subunits exhibit considerable homology within a species. Human CG consists of human LH β with an extended 30-amino acid residue at the COOH terminus.[58,59] Both α and β subunits also exhibit considerable cross-species homology: 70 percent identity exists between human and bovine TSH α subunits, and 90 percent identity exists between the corresponding β subunits.[60] For these reasons, it is not surprising that the biological activity of the glycoproteins is not species-specific and that hormones of bovine or ovine origin are active in humans. The isolated subunits are devoid of the biological activity of the intact hormone, though there have been suggestions that they may have some intrinsic activity of their own.[61] It is the β subunit which determines the biological action of the hormone, since its combination with almost any homologous or heterologous α subunit will provide a biologically active hybrid molecule characteristic of the hormone.

Evidence for hormonal heterogeneity has been uncovered in preparations of LH from individual pituitaries and appears to be related to variations in the carbohydrate content (termed *microheterogeneity*). It has been proposed by some investigators that the type of glycoprotein secreted (with different carbohydrate-containing forms possessing varying biological activity) may be modified by changes in the endocrine milieu. There is evidence for altered forms of glycoprotein hormones for both LH and TSH (see below).

Biosynthesis

The gene for the α subunit is located on chromosome 6, and the genes for all the β subunits are on chromosome 19.[62] Expression of the individual subunit genes is independently regulated.[63,64] The glycoprotein peptide subunits are individually synthesized and posttranslationally glycosylated. Since the concentration of the free α subunit in the pituitary greatly exceeds that of the free β subunit, glycoprotein hormone synthesis is regulated primarily by the level of β-subunit gene expression. Glycoprotein hormone glycosylation is selectively enhanced by releasing hormones.[65]

TSH

Action

The effects of thyrotropin (TSH) on the thyroid gland are to a large extent analogous to those of corticotropin on the adrenal cortex. TSH binds to a membrane receptor that is coupled to adenlyl cyclase through a guanine nucleotide regulatory protein. Increased cAMP production leads to enhanced iodine transport and binding to protein, increased thyroglobulin and thyroid hormone synthesis, and increased proteolysis of thyroglobulin with the release of thyroid hormones. In addition, cell proliferation is stimulated, leading to an increase in thyroid size and the vascularity of the gland. The effects of TSH are discussed in greater detail in Chap. 10.

Measurement

Immunoassays Standard RIAs for TSH, which have been in use for more than two decades, have been largely replaced by immunoradiometric[66] and, more recently, immunochemiluminescent[67] assays (see Chap. 6) that greatly enhance sensitivity (by more than one log order of magnitude) and are highly specific, eliminating previous problems of cross-reactivity with other glycoprotein hormones and free subunits. They also permit, for the first time, a distinction between normal and subnormal values.

Other Assays The MacKenzie bioassay is based on the release of radiolabeled thyroid hormones from the mouse thyroid into the blood. Although a useful assay and one which provided the first documentation of the long-acting thyroid stimulator (LATS, or thyroid-stimulating immunoglobulins), the technique is relatively insensitive and incapable of quantitating levels of TSH in the circulation of normal subjects. The radioligand assay and, in particular, the cytochemical assay for TSH possess sufficient sensitivity for measurement of plasma TSH levels, and values obtained by the latter correlate well with those determined by RIA. Because of technical complexities, however, the cytochemical assay remains a research procedure.

Pituitary and Plasma Levels

Pituitary The human pituitary content of TSH, determined by bioassay, is approximately 0.4 IU.[68] Although most of the TSH is stored as intact hormone, both the free α subunit and TSH β are present, with concentrations of the former exceeding those of the latter. The free subunits are present in the circulation of patients with hypothyroidism and are increased in response to TRH.

Plasma Immunoreactive TSH levels in normal human plasma have been recently redefined on the basis of the newer-generation immunoassays. Although the normal range varies slightly with individual assays, the upper limit of normal is generally 4 to 5 μU/ml and the lower limit is 0.3 to 0.5 μU/ml.[67,69,70] With the most sensitive assays, which exhibit a sensitivity as low as 0.01 μU/ml, TSH levels are detectable in most hypopituitary and hyperthyroid patients and can be readily differentiated from those in normals. The free α subunit is detectable in plasma in about 80 percent of normal men and premenopausal women with levels of 0.5 to 2.0 ng/ml,[71] and the levels rise dramatically in response to thyrotropin releasing hormone (TRH).[72] TSH β is undetectable in the plasma of normal subjects both under basal conditions and in response to TRH. In primary hypothyroidism, the level of the α subunit is increased severalfold (~5 ng/ml), TSH β can be detected (~1.5 ng/ml), and the levels of both subunits rise in response to TRH stimulation.[73]

Immunologically detectable TSH in circulation is presumed to represent biologically active hormone. Where comparisons have been made (i.e., using the cytochemical bioassay), good correlations have been observed.[74] In some children with hypothyroidism that is believed to be due to primary hypothalamic disease, slightly elevated plasma levels of immunoreactive TSH have been found.[75] Administration of TRH results in an exaggerated rise in plasma TSH but a subnormal increase in T_3, suggesting that the TSH secreted under basal conditions and in the absence of endogenous TRH may have reduced biological activity.[76] This hypothesis has been confirmed by two separate bioassay methods[77,78] and is probably attributable to the altered glycosylation of TSH found in states of TRH deficiency.[65] A large-molecular-size form of TSH with reduced bioactivity has also been reported in a patient with hypothyroidism.[79]

Metabolism

The distribution space of TSH is just slightly greater than the plasma volume. The half-life of TSH in plasma is 75 to 80 min, and the secretion rate of the hormone is about 100 to 200 mU per day.[80] In hypothyroidism, a small decrease in the metabolic clearance rate of the hormone is more than offset by the high plasma levels as a result of secretion rates of up to 10 to 15 times that in normal persons. Only small amounts of TSH are found in the urine, in contrast to the large quantities of gonadotropins that are present. There is also no evidence that the TSH subunits dissociate intravascularly.

Control of Secretion

TSH secretion is controlled by two major factors: (1) the feedback effects of the thyroid hormones and (2) stimuli mediated by the CNS and the secretion of TRH, somatostatin, and possibly dopamine. A fine-tuned feedback of thyroid hormones on the thyrotroph is responsive not only to the gross alterations in thyroxine (T_4) and triiodothyronine (T_3) observed in hypo- or hyperthyroidism but also to minor changes of these hormones within the normal range. The feedback affects both basal and TRH-stimulated TSH secretion through an inhibitory mechanism which involves both hormone synthesis and hormone release. The administration of small amounts of thyroxine which do not increase plasma T_4 levels above the normal range can inhibit the TSH response to TRH, and the small decrease in thyroid hormones caused by short-term oral iodide administration is sufficient to increase both basal and TRH-stimulated TSH secretion. Both T_4 and T_3 are potent as feedback hormones on the thyrotroph, which contains deiodinase activity. Thus, normal TSH levels are observed in patients with a variety of chronic illnesses in whom plasma T_4 levels are normal and plasma T_3 levels are decreased because of diminished peripheral deiodinase activity. Conversely, TSH secretion can be readily suppressed by the administration of T_3 in the presence of normal plasma T_4 levels.

Maintenance of the normal pituitary-thyroid axis is also CNS-dependent. Interruption of the normal hypothalamic-pituitary relation, whether by hypothalamic destruction or by stalk section, impairs the ability of the thyrotroph to secrete TSH in response to decreasing thyroid hormone levels. This is mediated by a direct effect of thyroid hormone on the TRH-secreting neurons in the paraventricular hypothalamic nucleus.[81] In addition to this tonic role of the hypothalamus, there is a centrally mediated effect of temperature. In response to decreases in either environmental or core temperature, a neurally mediated rise in TSH occurs which leads to increased thyroid hormone secretion and enhanced thermogenesis. Cold-stimulated increases in TSH secretion are readily demonstrable in the rat but in humans are seen only in newborns in response to the decrease in ambient temperature upon removal from the intrauterine environment and in infants subjected to hypothermia in association with cardiac surgery.[82] With increasing age and maturity of the sympathetic nervous system, the pituitary-thyroid axis appears to participate less in the acute metabolic adaptation to cold.

The participation of TRH in cold-induced TSH secretion has been shown by passive immunization studies in which the injection of anti-TRH serum blocks the rise in plasma TSH in the rat.[83] Studies in hypothyroid rats suggest that the acute removal of TRH only partially inhibits the secretion of TSH in response to decreases in thyroid hormone levls.[84] The acute role of TRH on the pituitary-thyroid axis can therefore be considered to be that of modulating the set point and the intensity of the TSH secretory response to decreasing thyroid hormone levels. Since TRH is also a trophic hormone for the thyrotroph, long-term effects on the axis also include modulation of TSH synthesis and storage. Hypothalamic somatostatin secretion, in contrast, is enhanced by thyroid hormone and suppressed in hypothyroidism,[85] thereby serving to augment the direct effect of thyroid hormones on the pituitary.

The secretion of TSH is also influenced by glucocorticoids, estrogens, and growth hormone.[86] Cortisol exhibits suppressive effects on basal and TRH-stimulated TSH, and a rebound in TSH secretion occurs after the withdrawal of glucocorticoid treatment. There is indirect evidence that a suppressive effect of glucocorticoids on TRH secretion may also occur.

Estrogen does not modify basal levels of TSH but does enhance the TSH response to TRH. This is reflected in the greater response seen (1) in women compared with men, (2) during the late follicular phase of the menstrual cycle at the time of high estradiol levels, and (3) in men pretreated with estrogen.

Somatostatin (SRIF, somatotroph release inhibiting factor) inhibits TSH secretion through an action on the thyrotroph. A physiologic role for this peptide has been provided by the demonstration of increased TSH levels after the injection of anti-SRIF serum in animals.[87] Somatostatin has been shown to inhibit the nocturnal rise in TSH in normal humans and the elevated levels of TSH in patients with primary hypothyroidism. Treatment of children with GH-deficiency of presumed hypothalamic origin with GH has occasionally been complicated by the development of hypothyroidism associated with decreased TSH secretion in response to TRH. The inhibitory effect of GH is believed to be based on a stimulation of SRIF secretion, which in turn would inhibit the TSH response to TRH.[88] The infrequency with which this occurs can be explained by the fact that the thyrotroph is less sensitive to suppression by SRIF in vivo than is the somatotroph.[89]

Several neurotransmitters have also been shown to modulate TSH release.[86] Dopamine inhibits TSH secretion and has its major site of action on the thyrotroph; norepinephrine exhibits a stimulatory effect that is mediated through the alpha$_1$-adrenergic receptor; serotonin has a stimulatory effect mediated through TRH release. A physiologic role for the latter two monoamines in humans, however, remains to be demonstrated. The secretion of TSH also exhibits an ultradian rhythm, with peak levels occurring just before midnight.[90] This rhythm is in part under dopaminergic control, at least in women.[91]

Gonadotropins: LH and FSH

Action

The two pituitary hormones which regulate gonadal function are FSH, which stimulates ovarian follicular growth and testicular growth and spermatogenesis, and LH, which promotes ovulation and luteinization of the ovarian follicle, stimulates testicular interstitial (Leydig) cell function, and enhances steroid production in both ovary and testis. On the basis of its function in the male, LH was once also called interstitial cell stimulating hormone (ICSH). A third pituitary hormone which also exhibits effects on the ovary is prolactin (previously called luteotropic hormone), which in rats assists in maintaining secretory activity and viability of the corpus luteum after ovulation.

FSH and LH bind to membrane-associated receptors in the ovary and testis and exert their effects through the adenylyl cyclase system. In the ovary, the target cell for FSH is the follicular granulosa cell, whose growth and maturation are enhanced. Among its many actions, FSH induces LH receptors, the aromatase enzyme that converts androgen to estrogen, and cholesterol side-chain enzyme, which catalyzes the rate-limiting step in progesterone biosynthesis. The effects of LH on granulosa, theca, and interstitial cells are also mediated through a cAMP-mediated mechanism. LH is the primary regulator of ovarian steroid biosynthesis, stimulating estradiol and progesterone in mature granulosa cells and androgens in theca and interstitial cells by regulating the availability of steroidogenic substrates. Further details of gonadotropin actions on the ovary are described in Chap. 17. In the testis, FSH exerts its actions primarily on Sertoli cells and, together with testosterone, stimulates androgen-binding proteins and the development of seminiferous tubule epithelium. The primary target cell of LH is the Leydig cell, where testosterone production is stimulated. The androgen-binding protein serves to bring a high concentration of testosterone into the tubular cells in the vicinity of the developing spermatogonia and thus promotes their development. Details of the effects of the gonadotropins and testosterone on the testis are provided in Chap. 16.

Measurement

Radioimmunoassay Sensitive RIAs are available for measuring LH and FSH. The specificity of these assays is dependent on the particular antigenic determinants recognized by the antisera used. Although most assays discriminate between the two gonadotropins, cross-reactivity between the intact hormone and its individual subunits may occur. From a practical viewpoint, this does not generally present a problem. Because of the great similarity between the structures of LH and chorionic gonadotropin, significant cross-reactivity is observed in some assays for the intact hormones. To measure low levels of CG to aid in the early diagnosis of pregnancy, an assay for the β subunit of CG is used which exhibits only minimal cross-reactivity with LH.

Measurement of LH and FSH in urine by RIA, although less frequently performed because of the inherent advantages of plasma measurements in evaluating secretory dynamics, is still a useful procedure under certain circumstances, such as quantitating gonadotropin secretion during the early stages of puberty (see Chap. 26). The same RIAs used for plasma can be utilized for the measurement of urinary gonadotropins, though there is evidence for some immunologic dissimilarity of urinary and plasma LH and FSH, presumably on the basis of chemical alteration (e.g., desialation) of the hormones during excretion.

Bioassay

Many bioassays for LH have been described, including the induction of ovulation, ovarian ascorbic acid depletion and progesterone secretion, and prostatic growth. FSH was measured initially by its enhancing effect on the size of female reproductive organs and its potentiating effect on LH. The limited sensitivity and precision of these assays restricted their usefulness to the measurement of urinary (and pituitary) gonadotropins. Furthermore, alterations in the chemical structure of the gonadotropins could lead to underestimation of the actual quantities secreted. More sensitive bioassays have been developed and are important as investigative techniques, though not for routine clinical measurements.

Radioligand assays have been developed for both LH and FSH in parallel with the other pituitary hormones. The receptor assays are highly specific[92,93] and possess sufficient sensitivity for the measurement of circulating levels of the gonadotropins. Together with the RIA, they have been valuable in investigating the secretion of biologically altered forms of gonadotropins. Increases in plasma LH bioassay/immunoassay ratios have been observed at the time of puberty[94] and in response to GnRH during the luteal phase of the menstrual cycle.[95] These differences have been attributed to variations in the carbohydrate content of LH.

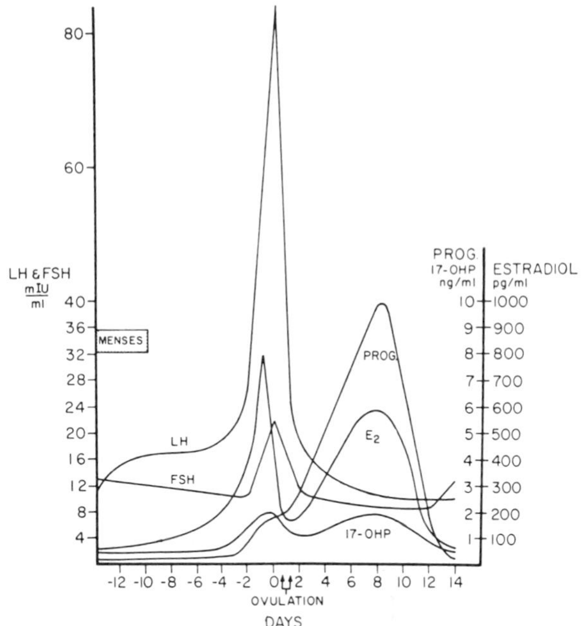

FIGURE 8-6 Changes in pituitary and ovarian hormones during a normal female menstrual cycle. The late follicular rise followed by a decline in estradiol levels can be seen to precede the midcycle surge of LH and FSH which triggers ovulation. *(From Speroff L et al: Am J Obstet Gynecol 109:234, 1971.)*

Pituitary and Plasma Levels

Pituitary The gonadotropin content of the pituitary in men and premenopausal women is about 700 IU LH and 200 IU FSH. Postmenopausally, gonadotropin content increases more than twofold.

Plasma Plasma levels of both LH and FSH rise shortly after birth to reach a peak at 1 to 4 months, with FSH levels in female infants exceeding those in males and the reverse being true for LH.[96] Values of both hormones subsequently decline to low levels until the time of puberty. A nocturnal rise in plasma LH and testosterone associated with non-REM sleep occurs in boys during puberty[97] and results in a marked increase in urinary LH. In girls, cyclic secretion of FSH and to a lesser extent LH can be detected even before the menarche.

The pattern of LH and FSH secretion in the mature ovulating female is shown in Fig. 8-6. During the early follicular phase of the cycle, FSH levels rise slightly and then show a progressive decline. At the same time LH levels are generally stable or rise slightly. At midcycle an abrupt rise in LH, initiated by increasing estrogen secretion by the developing follicle, and to a lesser extent in FSH occurs which triggers ovulation. LH and FSH levels both decline during the luteal phase.

The levels of LH and FSH in males are similar to those in females during the follicular phase, with the exception of the ovulatory surge. A rise in FSH and LH associated with decreasing gonadal function occurs in both sexes. In women the rise occurs at menopause, whereas in men there is a gradual increase during the sixth to eighth decades. Episodic secretion of LH is present in postpubertal men and women, with peaks occurring every 2 to 3 h. Secretory bursts of FSH are less marked and more difficult to detect, in part because of the more prolonged survival of FSH in the circulation. They may or may not coincide with the pulses of LH. The pulses of LH and FSH are triggered by pulsatile secretory bursts of gonadotropin releasing hormone (GnRH). Alteration of the pattern of GnRH exposure to the gonadotrophs markedly alters the quantity of secreted gonadotropins, and either the absence of GnRH or a continuous high level of the hormone (as occurs with continuous infusions) dramatically reduces gonadotropin secretion.

Free glycoprotein α subunit levels in normal plasma are considerably greater in women after menopause. In response to GnRH, an increase occurs in both the α subunit and the LH β subunit.[98]

Urine Urinary gonadotropin measurements generally reflect those in plasma, with the notable exception of the prepubertal period, when urinary LH and FSH levels are disproportionately low in relation to their plasma values. The quantity of LH and FSH in a 3-h urine sample has been shown to correlate well with the integrated value of plasma gonadotropins during the same period[99] and can therefore provide a useful index of gonadotropin secretion.

Metabolism and Secretion Rate

Despite the similarities in structure, the metabolic clearance rates of the individual gonadotropins from plasma exhibit considerable variation.[100] The half-life of LH is approximately 50 min, while that of FSH is about 3 to 4 h and that of chorionic gonadotropin is even longer. The difference is attributed to the varying sialic acid content of the three hormones, since desialation markedly shortens the half-life in plasma. The secretion rate of LH has been estimated at 500 to 1000 IU per day and that of FSH at 50 to 100 IU per day in adults with normal gonadal function. Since the metabolic clearance rates are not altered in the postmenopausal period, the relative change in secretion rates is reflected by the plasma gonadotropin levels.

Control of Secretion

Gonadotropin secretion in the ovulating female is controlled by a complex and integrated circuitry involving the hypothalamus and the gonads. Gonadotropin levels and responses to GnRH in various clinical states are shown in Table 8-3. A progressive rise in estrogen secretion by the developing follicle, which is under the influence of both FSH and LH, exerts a stimulatory effect on the hypothalamus, leading to increased GnRH secretion. There is considerable evidence to suggest that the secretion of estrogen is to some extent under the influence of an intrinsic cyclicity of the ovary itself. Estrogen also sensitizes the gonadotrophs to the effect of GnRH, culminating in the ovulatory surge of LH and FSH. Progesterone secretion by the corpus luteum also enhances the gonadotropin response to GnRH in the presence of estrogen but appears to have a negative feedback effect on the hypothalamus. The estrogen feedback effects are actually considerably more complex in that both stimulatory and inhibitory effects on the pituitary can be demonstrated, depending on both the dose and the duration of exposure. Short-term effects of estrogen on basal LH release and the LH response to GnRH are suppressive.[101] With longer exposure to estrogen, particularly at lower doses, the gonadotropin response is enhanced.[102] More prolonged estrogen therapy will again inhibit the response. Gonadotropin secretion following GnRH is also enhanced by prior exposure to the releasing hormone itself, and this self-priming effect of GnRH is estrogen-dependent. Thus, the FSH and particularly the LH response to GnRH is increased with successive injections of the peptide, a process which is also enhanced by estrogen. In the absence of prior exposure to GnRH such as occurs after pituitary stalk section or in association with certain hy-

TABLE 8-3 Gonadotropin Responses in Disorders of the Hypothalamic-Pituitary-Gonadal Axis

	Basal		Response to GnRH	
	LH	FSH	LH	FSH
Both sexes				
Pituitary destruction	N or ↓	N or ↓	N → 0	N → 0
Primary hypothalamic disease	N or ↓	N or ↓	N or ↓ *	N or ↓ *
Isolated FSH deficiency	N	↓	N	↓ → 0
Precocious puberty	N	N	N	N
Males				
Primary gonadal disease, complete	↑	↑	↑	↑
Azoospermia with normal testosterone	N	↑	N	↑
Testicular feminization	↑	↑	↑	↑
Kleinfelter's syndrome	↑	↑	↑	↑
Estrogen or GnRH agonist administration	↓	↓	↓	↓
Females				
Postmenopausal state	↑	↑	↑	↑
Primary ovarian failure	↑	↑	↑	↑
Anorexia nervosa	N	N	N → ↓	N → ↑
Hyperprolactinemia	N	N	N	N → ↑
Polycystic ovary syndrome	N → ↑	N	N → ↑	N
Estrogen or GnRH agonist administration	N	N	↑ (early) ↓ (late)	↑ (early) ↓ (late)
GnRH antagonist administration	N	N	↓	↓

0 = absent; N = normal; * = normalized with repeated stimulation.

pothalamic diseases, LH and FSH responses to an acute challenge with GnRH may be absent.

The sites of estrogen action on the hypothalamus are still open to debate, but there appear to be two distinct loci, at least from a functional view. The positive feedback effect, that which enhances GnRH secretion, is seen only in females and is believed to occur in the portion of the anterior hypothalamus which participates in the cyclicity of reproductive function. The negative feedback of estrogen occurs in the mediobasal hypothalamus and is most readily demonstrable after menopause or surgical castration, when estrogen therapy results in a reduction of LH and FSH to premenopausal levels.

In males, the regulation of gonadotropin secretion appears to be unaffected by the cyclic function of either the hypothalamus or the testis. The feedback effects of testosterone appear to be primarily negative and can be shown to occur in both the hypothalamus and the pituitary. The elevated levels of LH and FSH often seen after the sixth decade as well as after castration are reduced by testosterone treatment. In contrast to the effects observed in women, estrogen exhibits only an inhibitory effect on gonadotropin secretion in men.

While it is well recognized that testosterone is the primary hormone involved in the feedback control of LH, its role in the control of FSH has been difficult to document. Although both androgens and estrogens undoubtedly play a role in modulating FSH secretion, another hormone, *inhibin*, is primarily responsible for the negative feedback effects. This 32-kDa protein contains two dissimilar subunits that are linked by disulfide bonds. The α subunit is approximately 20 kDa, and the smaller β subunit exists in two forms, β_A and β_B, leading to two forms of inhibin, known as inhibin A ($\alpha\beta_A$) and inhibin B ($\alpha\beta_B$).[103] Inhibin is produced in granulosa cells of the ovary and Sertoli cells in the testis under the stimulation of both FSH and testosterone and is believed to have a paracrine-like modulatory effect on gonadal function.[104] Inhibin suppresses FSH secretion by the pituitary both basally and in response to GnRH.[105] During the menstrual cycle, inhibin levels rise during the late follicular phase, peak before the midcycle surge of FSH and LH, fall slightly, and then rise to an even greater height during the midluteal phase before declining at the end of the cycle. Circulating inhibin levels are inversely related to those of FSH.[106]

In addition to the feedback effects of gonadal hormones, the secretion of LH and FSH is influenced by prolactin. The inhibitory effects of prolactin may occur directly or through an intermediary compound such as dopamine at both the pituitary and hypothalamic levels. Examples of prolactin's effects include anovulation during physiologic postpartum lactation and in patients with prolactin-secreting pituitary tumors. The LH response to GnRH is diminished by glucocorticoid administration and in patients with Cushing's syndrome, indicating an inhibitory effect of glucocorticoids on LH secretion.

Other Glycoprotein Hormones

Several reports have suggested the existence of an aldosterone stimulating factor. One group has partially purified a glycoprotein of 26-kDa size from human urine and identified a similar material in human pituitary.[107,108] Evidence for biological activity of peptides contained in the NH_2-terminal and COOH-terminal regions of POMC has also been reported.[109,110] However, definitive proof for the existence of such a hormone is lacking.

Somatomammotropic Hormones

Chemistry

The somatomammotropic hormones include two pituitary hormones, GH and prolactin, and one hormone of placental origin, placental lactogen or chorionic somatomammotropin, each consisting of a single peptide chain with interchain disulfide linkages. There is extensive interspecies similarity of both GH and prolactin (e.g., 73 percent of the amino acid residues in human and sheep prolactin are identical,[111]as are 64 percent of the residues in human and sheep GH),[112] suggesting relatively limited changes in gene duplication during vertebrate evolution.[113] Despite this similarity, subprimate growth hormones are biologically inactive in humans. There is considerable homology between the primary structure of GH and placental lactogen; 159 (83 percent) of the 191 amino acid residues are identical. In contrast, there is only 16 percent residue identity between prolactin and GH and 13 percent identity between prolactin and placental lactogen. GH and placental lactogen each contain two disulfide bonds, whereas prolactin, which is seven amino acids longer than the other two, contains three. Despite the differences in their structures, each of the three hormones has intrinsic lactogenic and growth-promoting activity.

There are multiple copies of both the GH and placental lactogen genes.[114] The gene complex, consisting of five related genes, is located on chromosome 17,[115] while the prolactin gene, which has only a single copy, is on chromosome 6.[116] Only one of the GH genes (GH-N) is expressed in the pituitary and is responsible for directing GH synthesis. A second GH gene (GH-V) is expressed only in the placenta and results in the secretion of a variant form of GH that differs by 13 amino acids from pituitary GH[117] (see also Chap. 26). This GH form is biologically active[118,119] and is capable of exerting feedback effects on pituitary GH secretion during pregnancy.[120,121] Two of the placental lactogen genes are also expressed.

Extensive structure-function studies have been carried out with GH in an attempt to find the biologically active core of the molecule. Growth-promoting activity has been found to reside in fragments from several different areas of the molecule, most frequently in those containing part or all of residues 80 to 140. Activity has also been observed in synthetic fragments encompassing this region.

Biosynthesis

Cell-free translation studies of GH and prolactin mRNAs have indicated that both hormones are synthesized as higher-molecular-weight species than the secreted hormones. The size of the precursor hormones is approximately 28 kDa, which is due primarily to a 30-amino acid leader sequence at the NH_2 terminus.[122] This sequence is highly hydrophobic and is important in the transportation of newly synthesized protein into the cisternae of the endoplasmic reticulum for subsequent packaging. Enzymes capable of removing the precursor segment from the hormone are present in the endoplasmic membranes.

In addition to the monomeric forms of these hormones, immunoreactive species of approximately twice the size of the monomer have been detected in pituitary extracts and in plasma ("big" GH, "big" prolactin, and "big" placental lactogen). Studies of all three hormones indicate that the big hormone may represent a dimer attached by interchain disulfide linkages rather than by peptide bonds.[123,124] Big GH has been shown to be secreted directly by the pituitary,[125] and there is a suggestion that its amino acid composition may differ from that of monomeric GH. Big GH binds to and displaces the GH monomer from hepatic membrane receptors,[126] though the biological activity of the big moiety is less than that of the monomer and its physiologic significance remains to be determined.

One variant of GH, the 20-kDa fragment, has been extensively studied.[127] It differs from native GH by the absence of residues 32 to 46 and is a consequence of alternative splicing of nascent mRNA to its mature form.[128,129] The variant constitutes up to 30 percent of pituitary GH but is secreted only at low rates.[130] It is not selectively secreted in response to stimuli such as insulin hypoglycemia and GRH, and its levels in acromegaly are not increased. Its biological activity is similar to that of native (22-kDa) GH.

Forms of GH and prolactin with higher molecular weights have also been observed in the pituitary gland and in circulation. Much of this material in the pituitary can be explained by aggregation of the hormone during the processes of extraction, purification, and analysis, though in one report, noncovalent aggregation of endogenous GH appeared to be responsible for impaired growth.[131] A small portion of GH within the pituitary also represents the nascent hormone, still bound to the ribosome.

Nearly two-thirds of GH in circulation is associated with a 29-kDa binding protein that is identical to the extracellular domain of the GH receptor[132–134] and is generated by enzymatic cleavage of the GH receptor. The function of the circulating GH-binding protein is not completely understood at present, but the protein does prolong the half-life of GH in circulation.

A glycosylated form of prolactin has also been described in pituitary extracts.[135] It is presumed to originate from altered processing of prolactin mRNA, since only one copy of the prolactin gene is present in humans. It has a molecular size of 26 kDa and exhibits reduced biological activity. A larger glycosylated form of prolactin has also been detected in the peripheral plasma of pregnant women[136] and may be related to a large and physiologically inactive form of prolactin in the circulation of women with idiopathic hyperprolactinemia but otherwise normal reproductive function.[137]

Growth Hormone

Action

Growth hormone was named for its ability to produce an increase in linear growth which can be detected after a few days of treatment in hypophysectomized animals. The hormone also plays an important role in the regulation of metabolic processes. The interrelation between the metabolic effects of GH and the increase in body mass is only partially understood. The physiologic effects of GH can be categorized by tissue, by time of effect (acute vs. delayed), and by the type of metabolic effect produced (anabolic vs. diabetogenic). At a biochemical level, GH stimulates the activity of numerous enzymes (e.g., ornithine decarboxylase, hepatic drug-metabolizing enzymes) as well as several hormone receptors (epidermal growth factor, prolactin), including its own. The mechanism of its effects on gene expression is incompletely understood but may be associated with its stimulation of a tyrosine kinase and of the nuclear transcription factors *c-fos* and *c-jun*.

Administration of GH to hypophysectomized animals and to GH-deficient humans is followed in a few days by a positive nitrogen balance, a decrease in urea production, a decrease in body fat, and a reduced rate of carbohydrate utilization, reflected by a decrease in the respiratory quotient. The effects observed after a single injection of GH are biphasic. Initially, decreases in concentrations of blood glucose, free fatty acids, and amino acids occur. Within a few hours, blood glucose and amino acid levels return to normal and free fatty acids rise above normal. Most of these effects can also be observed in normal persons, although to a lesser extent.

The mechanism responsible for these changes has been studied extensively by exposing isolated tissues and cultured cells to GH in vitro or by excising and examining tissues at various times after in vivo administration of the hormone.[138] Many of the acute effects of GH in isolated tissues resemble those of insulin. In muscle and liver, GH increases amino acid uptake and incorporation into protein. This process is independent of new RNA synthesis, although that is also stimulated. In muscle and adipose tissue, GH stimulates glucose uptake and enhances glucose utilization. In adipose tissue, GH antagonizes the lipolytic effect of catecholamines and stimulates RNA and mitochondrial protein synthesis.

With the exception of muscle protein synthesis, all these insulin-like effects of GH can be demonstrated at nearly physiologic concentrations of the hormone, have a lag period of 10 to 30 min, and exhibit a characteristic refractory phenomenon. Within 3 to 4 h of their onset, the effects disappear and cannot be reinitiated by additional hormone. The refractoriness, which is specific for GH, requires both RNA and protein synthesis.

Concomitant with the disappearance of the acute effects of GH, a series of delayed effects appear. They include (1) increased mobilization of free fatty acids from adipose tissue as a consequence of increased triglyceride lipolysis, (2) increased sensitivity to the lipolytic effects of catecholamines, and (3) inhibition of both glucose uptake and glucose utilization, the latter on the basis of a decrease in pyruvate decarboxylation. All the late effects persist for many hours, are additive with additional exposure to GH, and form the basis of the diabetogenic effects of GH on carbohydrate and lipid metabolism.

The effect of GH administration on insulin secretion are complex and appear to be triphasic. There is initially an increase in insulin release which appears to be a direct effect of GH on the beta cell and can be observed within 5 min of injection in both normal and GH-deficient subjects.[139] During the subsequent 1 to 5 h, a slight inhibition of insulin secretion can be detected, the basis of which is not fully understood.[140] A more profound and persistent rise observed after longer periods of time is indirect and represents a secondary response to the impairment of carbohydrate utilization. With treatment of sufficient duration, and particularly in the presence of other factors such as glucocorticoids or an appropriate genetic background, overt diabetes may develop. The process is reversible upon the removal of the GH influence, provided that the secretory capacity of the beta cell has not been unduly compromised.

It has been recognized for some time that many of the effects of GH observed after its injection into intact animals cannot be produced by exposure of tissues in vitro to the hormone. Furthermore, although GH binding to membrane receptors in a variety of tissues, including liver, breast, and circulating monocytes, can be readily demonstrated, correlation with its biological effects is less evident than with other hormone-receptor interactions. The demonstration that GH stimulates the incorporation of radiolabeled sulfate into cartilage proteoglycans by inducing a secondary "sulfation factor"[141] led to the recognition that normal plasma contains a number of GH-dependent growth factors which stimulate cellular processes involved with the growth of both skeletal and extraskeletal tissues. The term *somatomedin* was subsequently introduced to denote the more widespread spectrum of biological activity involved. Investigators using differential experimental models found a close similarity between somatomedin C and non-(antibody-) suppressible insulin-like activity, soluble (in ethanol) (NSILA-s), a peptide that shares many properties with insulin, including binding to chick fibroblast insulin receptors, GH dependency, and sulfation activity in cartilage. Their identity has now been confirmed. The currently accepted name for these peptides, insulin-like growth factors (IGFs), reflects their overall biological effects.[142,143]

IGF-I (somatomedin C and NSILA-s) has a molecular size of 7.5 kDa and a structure similar to that of proinsulin. It circulates in plasma primarily in association with a binding protein but also in a free form. It binds to specific receptors as well as (weakly) to insulin receptors and mediates many of the effects of GH. IGF-I stimulates growth in hypophysectomized rats,[144] and anabolic effects virtually identical to those of GH have been observed in a growth-retarded child with GH insensitivity due to a mutation in the GH receptor (Laron-type dwarfism)[145] (see Chap. 26). IGF-I is produced by many cell types, including liver, cartilage, kidney, and pituitary. Furthermore, there is evidence that IGF-I serves as a locally produced intracellular messenger of GH action rather than as a classic hormone.[146,147] For example, direct injection of GH into the tibial growth plate of a rat enhances cartilaginous growth to a greater extent than does a subcutaneous injection, indicating that the effect of GH is local rather than systemic. In fact, there is now considerable question as to whether circulating IGF-I represents a source of tissue IGF activity rather than a reflection of it.

IGF-II (identical to fibroblast multiplication factor) has also been sequenced and found to have a molecular size similar to that of IGF-I. It binds to a different receptor and exhibits tissue growth-promoting activity, particularly in the fetus. However, its GH dependency has been less well established. Somatomedin A, a neutral protein, remains to be fully characterized but appears to be similar to somatomedin C. Somatomedin B is probably identical with epidermal growth factor.

GH has numerous effects on organ growth (e.g., cardiac and renal hypertrophy) and on specific hormone production and metabolism (e.g., aldosterone and renin production and thyroxine conversion to triiodothyronine,[148] the latter of which is discussed in greater detail in subsequent chapters).

Measurement

Radioimmunoassay The standard technique for measuring GH in circulating fluids is the RIA. Antibodies to human GH are readily generated in rabbits, and the assay is reproducible from one laboratory to the next. The sensitivity of the assay, generally less than 10 pg, is more than adequate for measuring basal circulating levels of the hormone for routine clinical purposes, though for studies of spontaneous secretory patterns of GH, even more sensitive assays have been developed.[149] There is no significant cross-reactivity with any of the other pituitary hormones, though most antibodies exhibit cross-reactivity with placental lactogen, which is structurally very similar. Because of the high levels of placental lactogen in pregnancy, measurement of GH levels by routine RIA is unreliable in pregnant women. Many laboratories currently use an immunoradiometric assay to measure GH. The plasma values measured by this technique are slightly lower than those observed with RIA.

Radioreceptor Assay Biologically active human GH can be measured by a radioreceptor assay using mid-pregnancy rabbit hepatic plasma membranes. This assay, though less sensitive than the RIA, is capable of measuring plasma GH levels. It is also less specific, since prolactin exhibits considerable cross-reactivity. The radioreceptor assay has been of use in searching for biologically altered GH molecules.

Bioassay The original methods for assaying GH utilized its ability to increase linear growth in hypophysectomized rats. A more sensitive technique was subsequently developed which involved the measurement of tibial-epiphyseal cartilage width in hypophysectomized rats. This assay ("tibia test") remains useful for determining the biological activity of GH extracted from pituitaries, but it has limited sensitivity (about 10 μg), making it impractical for the measurement of plasma levels. It is also affected by numerous other factors, making it relatively nonspecific for crude extracts of pituitary.

Pituitary and Plasma Levels

Pituitary The GH content of human pituitaries is approximately 2 percent of the wet weight, or 10 to 15 mg.[150] Males and females exhibit similar levels, and no significant changes in content occur with age. Less than 5 percent of the pituitary GH content is released each day, and it is believed that a considerable portion of the hormone in the pituitary undergoes destruction without ever being secreted.

Plasma Plasma GH levels in a fasting, resting adult are generally less than 1 ng/ml, with levels occasionally at the lower limit of sensitivity. GH levels are slightly higher in women than in men, and the differences become more marked upon exercise, when levels increase in both sexes. GH levels are very high at the end of fetal life and during the first few days after birth (often more than 50 ng/ml). They rapidly decrease during the subsequent few weeks to levels just slightly higher than those in adults. GH is secreted episodically, with a periodicity of 3 to 4 h, and occasional values of 50 ng/ml or more may be observed, particularly in young adult males. The use of a high-sensitivity GH assay has revealed an even shorter periodicity (~2 h), with many pulses occurring in a range undetectable by standard assays.[149] Secretory bursts are less common after the fourth decade and rarely occur after the sixth decade.

Only a small fraction of GH in plasma is excreted by the kidneys in an immunologically recognizable form. Urinary concentrations of GH reflect serum levels, being increased in states of GH hypersecretion and decreased in hypopituitarism; however, this measurement is of little practical clinical value in the diagnosis of GH secretory disorders.

Metabolic Clearance and Secretion

GH is cleared from plasma primarily by the liver and to a lesser extent by the kidney. The half-life of GH in serum is 20 to 25 min,[151] and the metabolic clearance rate is approximately 110 ml/m^2 per minute, with little variation in states of GH over- or underproduction.[152] Decreased metabolic clearance rates have been reported in hypothyroidism and in diabetes. With these exceptions, therefore, the measurement of plasma GH provides an accurate reflection of the secretory rate of the hormone. GH secretion in normal men has been estimated at approximately 350 μg/m^2 per 24 h; in premenopausal women, a value of about 500 μg/m^2 per 24 h is found.[153]

Control of Secretion

The regulation of GH secretion is mediated by both a releasing hormone [growth hormone releasing hormone (GRH)] and an inhibiting hormone (SRIF) of hypothalamic origin. Alterations in the secretion of these two hormones represent the mechanism by which neural and extraneural factors regulate GH secretion under normal physiologic conditions. Since the secretion of these factors from the hypothalamus in vivo cannot be determined under physiologic conditions in man, their net effect on GH secretion is measured. The recent availability of GRH has provided new insights into the regulation of GH secretion (see also Chap. 7). Its injection is followed by a rapid increase in GH release (Fig. 8-7). Although reports suggest interactions of drugs affecting neurotransmitter action with GRH at the pituitary,[154,155] possible effects on SRIF secretion provide an equally plausible alternative explanation.

Factors affecting the secretion of GH are summarized in Table 8-4. Because basal GH levels are so

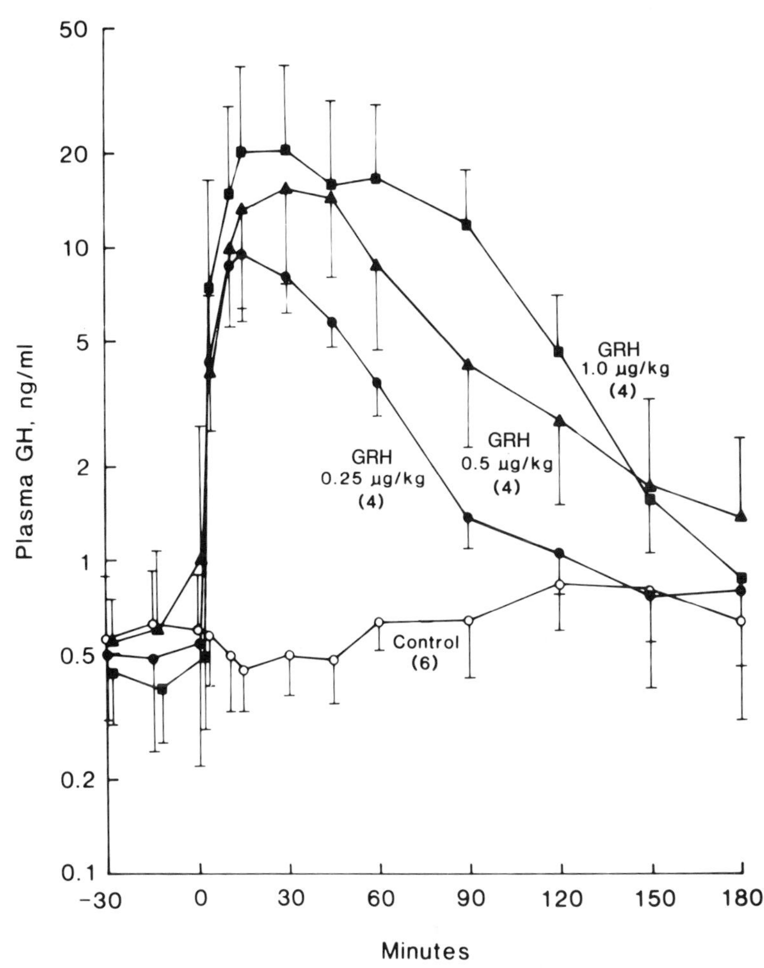

FIGURE 8-7 Plasma GH responses to increasing doses of GRH ($hGRH_{1-44}$-NH_2) given as a single intravenous injection in normal males. The dose of 1 μg/kg produces a maximal response.

frequently near the lower limit of detectability, the demonstration of suppressive effects often requires the concomitant use of a stimulatory agent.

Neural Neural stimuli affecting GH release include both psychic and physical stress and episodic secretion unrelated to stress or recognizable metabolic events.[156] Sleep-associated bursts of GH secretion are most pronounced in infants, in whom they are seen during daytime naps as well as at night, and gradually decrease with age (Fig. 8-8). Nearly 70 percent of total GH secretion occurs during the night. These GH secretory episodes appear to be entrained by deep sleep, since they will not occur if sleep stage III or IV is prevented by awakening the subject. However, a close inspection of this relation in individual normal subjects, in disease states associated with alterations in slow-wave sleep and GH secretion, and in the presence of pharmacologic agents (e.g., imipramine, flurazepam, methylscopolamine, and medroxyprogesterone) which can block the GH response has led to the conclusion that nocturnal GH secretion is frequently concomitant with sleep but is not closely linked to the neural processes required for slow-wave sleep.

Metabolic Changes in the levels of circulating and, more important, intracellular fuels play an important role in regulating GH secretion.[121] Elevations of blood glucose by oral or intravenous glucose administration suppress GH secretion, a phenomenon which has been used extensively in confirming the diagnosis of acromegaly. In contrast, decreasing levels of blood glucose (and more specifically intracellular glucose metabolism), whether occurring as a result of insulin hypoglycemia, during the descending portion of an oral glucose tolerance test, or several hours after a meal, stimulate GH release. The importance of intracellular metabolism is illustrated by the stimulatory effect of 2-deoxyglucose, which produces hyperglycemia with intracellular glucopenia by interfering with glucose phosphorylation. To date, insulin hypoglycemia has proved to be the most reliable stimulus for the evaluation of GH secretory capacity. Both the absolute glucose level and the rate of fall of the glucose concentration are important deter-

TABLE 8-4 Factors Affecting Growth Hormone Secretion

Stimulative	Suppressive*
Physiologic	
Sleep	Postprandial hyperglycemia
Exercise	Elevated free fatty acids
Stress (physical or psychological)	
Postprandial hyperaminoacidemia	
Postprandial hypoglycemia (relative)	
Pharmacologic	
Hypoglycemia	Hormones
Absolute: insulin or 2-deoxyglucose	Somatostatin
Relative: postglucagon	IGF-I (somatomedin C)
Hormones	Growth hormone
Peptides (GRH, ACTH, α-MSH, vasopressin)	Progesterone
Estrogen	Glucocorticoids
Neurotransmitters, etc.	Neurotransmitters, etc.
α-Adrenergic agonists (clonidine)	α-Adrenergic antagonists (phentolamine)
β-Adrenergic antagonists (propranolol)	β-Adrenergic agonists (isoproterenol)
Serotonin precursors(5-hydroxytryptamine)	Serotonergic antagonists (methysergide)
Dopaminergic agonists (L-dopa, apomorphine, bromocriptine)	Dopaminergic antagonists (phenothiazines)
Cholinergic agonists (pyridostigmine, an acetylcholinesterase inhibitor)	Cholinergic (muscarinic) antagonists (pirenzepine)
GABA agonists (muscimol)	
Galanin	
Enkephalin analogues (GHRP-6)	
Pathologic	
Protein depletion and starvation	Obesity
Anorexia nervosa	Hypo- and hyperthyroidism
Chronic renal failure	Acromegaly: dopaminergic agonists
Acromegaly	
TRH	
GnRH	

* Suppressive effects of some factors can be demonstrated only in the presence of a stimulus.

minants of the GH response, since a rapid decrease in glucose levels from hyperglycemic to normoglycemic levels can also cause GH release. Glucose-sensitive neurons in the ventral hypothalamus of rodents and primates have been demonstrated, and these neurons trigger (directly or indirectly) the release of GRH.[156] However, in humans, insulin hypoglycemia enhances the GH response to GRH, suggesting that it may inhibit the release of somatostatin.[157]

Oral administration or intravenous infusions of single amino acids (arginine, lysine, leucine, etc.), mixed amino acids, or proteins stimulate GH re-

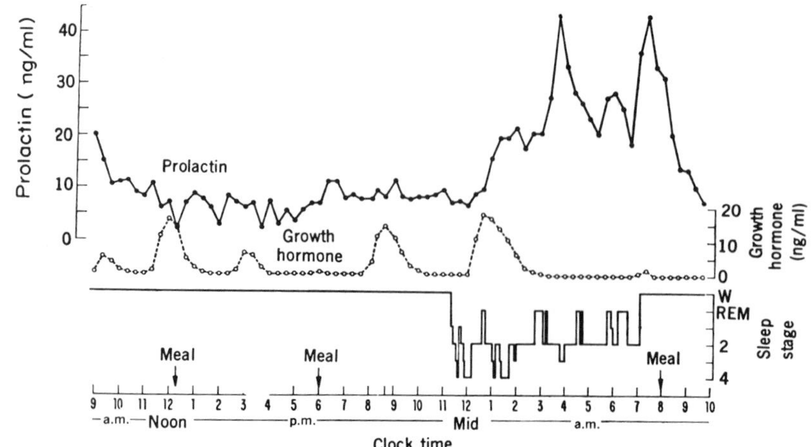

FIGURE 8-8 Sleep-associated changes in GH and prolactin secretion. The rise in GH accompanies the onset of slow-wave (EEG stages III and IV) sleep, which usually occur 90 to 120 min after sleep begins. The rise in prolactin secretion shows a sawtooth pattern, with peak values occurring at the end of the sleep period or shortly after awakening. (*From Sassin J et al: Science 177:1205, 1973.*)

lease. Elevations of plasma free fatty acids produced by infusions of a fat emulsion plus heparin (to activate lipoprotein lipase) acutely suppress GH secretion, while rapid decreases in plasma free fatty acids stimulate GH release. The mechanism of action, as well as the specific CNS site involved in the effect of amino acids and free fatty acids, remains to be determined.

Hormonal GH secretion is affected by numerous hormones. Estrogen enhances the growth hormone secretory response to many stimuli, as it does with prolactin, gonadotropins, and TSH. Progesterone is believed to suppress GH secretion, but the evidence is quite limited. GH responses to stimulation are suppressed by glucocorticoid therapy, endogenous hypercortisolism, hyperthyroidism, and hypothyroidism. Although steroids and thyroxine have both been shown to act directly on the somatotroph in rodents, their effects are clearly more complex and also involve actions on the hypothalamus and on the generation of IGF-I (which is inhibited by both estrogens and glucocorticoids). GH exerts a negative feedback effect on its own secretion, in part mediated through IGF-I.[158] Both GH and IGF-I stimulate SRIF secretion[159,160] and inhibit GRH.[161] Clinical evidence of a feedback role for IGF-I is suggested by the elevated GH levels present in Laron-type dwarfism, where IGF-I levels are markedly depressed.[162] However, the altered GH receptor in this disorder also prevents direct GH feedback effects.

Several peptide hormones (vasopressin, ACTH and some of its fragments, and α-MSH) stimulate GH release acutely. Their effects, for the present, must be considered pharmacologic, perhaps caused by an interaction with the GRH receptor on the somatotroph. Glucagon's effects on GH secretion, by contrast, are delayed and are most likely mediated by changes in carbohydrate metabolism.

Neurotransmitters and Neuropharmacologic Agents Studies on the neurochemical mediation of GH secretion and the effects of neuropharmacologically active agents are extensive and have been reviewed in detail elsewhere.[121,163] The numerous reports which relate to GH secretion in normal humans can be summarized as follows: Irrespective of the nature of the extraneural stimuli, the mediation of the responses in the CNS and specifically within the hypothalamus involves one or more neurotransmitters and eventually results in alterations in the release of GRH or SRIF. The fact that these neurotransmitters are released locally and that two or more neurons involving more than a single neurotransmitter may be required for the response (see Chap. 7) can probably explain some of the apparent contradictions in the literature. It also follows that a neurotransmitter mediating a stimulatory response in one set of neurons can also mediate an inhibitory response in another.

There is, in general, evidence for the role of nearly all the classic monoamine neurotransmitters [norepinephrine, epinephrine, dopamine, serotonin, γ-aminobutyric acid (GABA), and acetylcholine] in the control of GH secretion. The beta-adrenergic receptor appears to be inhibitory, and the alpha receptor appears to be stimulatory. Thus, beta receptor antagonists (e.g., propranolol) will enhance and alpha receptor antagonists (e.g., phentolamine) will suppress a variety of stimuli. Stimulation of the alpha receptor by clonidine also enhances GH release. Because of the lack of specificity of most of the receptor antagonists used clinically, however, caution is required in interpreting individual reports. The dopaminergic receptor is stimulatory, and agents such as L-dopa (the immediate precursor of dopamine), apomorphine, and bromocriptine (dopamine receptor agonists) all stimulate, while chlorpromazine and pimozide (dopamine receptor antagonists) impair, GH responses to numerous stimuli. Serotonergic receptors are also stimulatory with respect to metabolic signals and possibly sleep-associated GH secretion, although the latter is still controversial. Cholinergic mechanisms also appear to be involved in sleep-associated GH release. There is, in addition, evidence for a stimulatory effect of GABAergic neurons on GH secretion.[164]

Although several neuropeptides stimulate GH secretion in animal models, there is evidence only for enkephalins and α-MSH in humans. Enkephalin analogues capable of penetrating the blood-brain barrier stimuluate GH secretion,[165] though the role of endogenous enkephalins in the regulation of GH is still unknown. GHRP-6, a hexapeptide enkephalin analogue (his-*D*-trp-ala-trp-*D*-phe-lys), stimulates GH release in vivo and in vitro through combined actions at the pituitary and hypothalamic levels.[121,166,167] It binds to a pituitary receptor, the endogenous ligand of which is currently unknown, and enhances the GH-releasing effects of GRH.

Prolactin

Action

The primary site of action of prolactin is the breast, where, in conjunction with other hormones, it stimulates mammary tissue development and lactation. Prolactin is required for normal breast development in many species, although an essential role has not been demonstrated in humans. Pathologic elevations of prolactin may be but usually are not associated with an increase in breast size; in men, gynecomastia usually occurs in the presence of normal prolactin levels. During pregnancy, prolactin, in conjunction with estrogen, progesterone, and placental lactogen and in the presence of insulin and cortisol, results in additional mammary tissue growth, leading eventually to milk formation. Prolactin specifically stimulates the synthesis of milk proteins, including lactalbumin, and of lipids and carbohydrates. Prolactin receptors in normal mammary tissue are located on the alveolar surfaces of cells. Prolactin receptors are also present in liver and kidney tissue, and prolactin appears to be capable of increasing the number of its own receptors.

After parturition, the abrupt decrease in estrogen and progesterone of placental origin permits the initiation of lactation. Thus, estrogen, which plays a synergistic role in promoting breast development, antagonizes the effects of prolactin on lactation. This phenomenon forms the basis for the previous use of estrogens to inhibit lactation in the postpartum period and also explains the frequent appearance of galactorrhea in hyperprolactinemic women subsequent to discontinuation of oral contraceptives.

Continued secretion of prolactin is required to maintain lactation once it has begun. Inhibition of prolactin secretion by pharmacologic or surgical means is followed by a cessation of lactation. Prolactin secretion, which is stimulated by suckling, gradually diminishes to normal levels during the postpartum period. The actual milk "let-down" reflex, however, is mediated not by prolactin but by the release of oxytocin from the posterior pituitary. Oxytocin stimulates the contraction of myoepithelial cells around the terminal acinar lobules which expel their milk into the lobular ducts.

In the rat, prolactin is required for the maintenance of the secretory activity of the corpus luteum and is therefore important in maintaining pregnancy during the early stages. This effect does not appear to be important in humans, although small amounts of prolactin are required for progesterone production by human granulosa cells.[168] Higher levels of prolactin are associated with progressive inhibition of progesterone secretion. Prolactin, along with FSH and LH, is present in follicular fluid, and there is evidence that prolactin may block the stimulating effect of FSH on estrogen secretion by the developing graafian follicle.

In addition to these effects on reproductive physiology, prolactin has effects on behavior and on fluid and electrolyte metabolism in several animal species, though evidence of these effects in humans is still unconvincing. In birds and in mice, prolactin enhances maternal nurturing behavior, an action important in the life cycle of these species. Although prolactin levels increase in association with numerous psychic stimuli in humans (see below), the increased secretion of the hormone appears to be in response to, rather than the cause of, the stimuli. Prolactin also stimulates the retention of sodium, potassium, and water by the kidneys in several mammalian species and potentiates the effects of aldosterone and vasopressin. Attempts to demonstrate these actions in humans have been unsuccessful.

The metabolic effects of prolactin in hypophysectomized animals resemble those of GH and include stimulation of protein synthesis, calorigenesis, and the formation of chondroitin sulfate in cartilage. In humans, the administration of ovine prolactin to GH-deficient subjects produces nitrogen retention, hypercalciuria, lipid mobilization, carbohydrate intolerance, and limited skeletal growth. Hyperinsulinemia, reflecting insulin resistance, can also be demonstrated in patients with hyperprolactinemia and can be eliminated by suppressing prolactin secretion.[169]

Measurement

Radioimmunoassay Prolactin is measured by a homologous RIA. Antibodies are raised in rabbits, and the sensitivity is sufficient to measure basal levels of the hormone. The assay is quite specific and exhibits no significant cross-reactivity with either GH or placental lactogen.

Radioreceptor Assay Radioligand assays for prolactin most commonly utilize pregnant rabbit mammary gland membranes.[170] Although this assay has sufficient sensitivity to measure prolactin levels in plasma, the binding of GH by the membrane and its displacement of radiolabeled prolactin have limited the usefulness of this technique. Comparison of RIA and receptor assay potency may be important to distinguish between biologically active and inactive circulating prolactin in certain conditions. A large-molecular-size prolactin in serum has been reported to exhibit reduced biological activity.[171]

Bioassay The stimulatory effect of prolactin on the crop sac of the pigeon provided the basis for a bioassay which was used for many years. Increased sensitivity was subsequently achieved by measuring lactose or casein synthesis in midpregnancy mouse mammary glands. Much of the early information on plasma prolactin levels was obtained through the use of these assays, though they have been replaced by the RIA.

Pituitary and Plasma Levels

Pituitary Measurement of prolactin content in the human pituitary by RIA indicates levels of approximately 100 μg per pituitary. This concentration is considerably lower than that of GH (approximately 10 percent of the GH content) and also is lower with respect to GH than in most mammalian pituitaries. There is some question about the validity of this figure, possibly related to incomplete extraction techniques, since the estimated daily secretion rate of prolactin is several times that of the pituitary content (see below), and this is unique among the anterior pituitary hormones.

Plasma Mean prolactin levels are approximately 5 ng/ml in men and 8 ng/ml in women, and most laboratories report an upper limit of about 15 ng/ml. Plasma prolactin values are detectable in all normal subjects.

Plasma prolactin levels are very high in the fetus and after the twentieth week of gestation may exceed 300 ng/ml. At term, umbilical vein levels are greater than those in maternal blood, indicating that the levels are due to fetal secretion. Similar levels are seen in anencephalic infants, indicating that the hypothalamus is not necessary for fetal prolactin secretion. Prolactin is also secreted by the chorion-decidua tissue of the placenta, and high concentrations of the hormone are present in amniotic fluid.[172]

Plasma prolactin levels in newborn infants decrease during the first few months of life to the values observed in adults. Levels in females begin to exceed those in males at puberty, primarily on the basis of estrogen effects. Prolactin levels in women decrease at menopause. Responses to almost all stimuli of prolactin secretion are greater in women than in men and are also increased in men by estrogen treatment. During pregnancy, prolactin levels rise continuously from early gestation to term.[173] After parturition, levels begin to decline and, even with continued nursing, often return to the nonpregnant range after a few months.

Metabolic Clearance and Secretion

The limited availability of human prolactin has prevented extensive studies of the metabolic clearance rate of the hormone. Data obtained using radiolabeled prolactin indicate the metabolic clearance of prolactin to be about 40 ml/m^2 per minute, or about one-third that of GH.[174] A preliminary report using unlabeled prolactin gave similar findings.[175] The kidney is responsible for approximately 25 percent of prolactin clearance, and the remainder is removed by the liver. The half-life of prolactin in the circulation is approximately 50 min, or about three times that of GH. The prolactin secretion rate, based on metabolic clearance studies, is about 400 μg per day.

Control of Secretion

In contrast to the other anterior pituitary hormones, the neuroendocrine control of prolactin is predominantly inhibitory. Interruption of the integrity of the hypothalamic-pituitary axis, whether by pituitary stalk section or hypothalamic destruction or, in experimental animals, by transplantation of the pituitary to another region of the body, results in increased prolactin secretion. The major physiologic inhibitor [prolactin inhibiting factor (PIF)] has appeared to this point to be dopamine. Dopamine has been identified in portal hypophyseal blood of rats at concentrations greater than in systemic blood and binds to specific receptors on the lactotroph, resulting in direct suppression of prolactin release. A peptide with prolactin-inhibiting activities is present within the COOH-terminal extension of the GnRH precursor.[176,177] This GnRH-associated peptide (GAP) is 56 amino acids in length, was initially reported to exhibit greater potency than dopamine in inhibiting prolactin secretion, and stimulated LH and FSH secretion in vitro. These findings, however, have not been widely confirmed, and the significance of GAP in human physiology and disease is unknown.

As with GH, there is a dual control of prolactin secretion consisting of a stimulatory as well as an inhibitory component. The hypothalamic stimulatory factor, which is influenced by serotonergic mechanisms, was at first believed to be TRH, which exhibits as great a stimulatory effect on prolactin as it does on TSH secretion. TRH binds to lactotroph receptors, activates the phosphatidyl inositol pathway, and increases prolactin synthesis as well as secretion. However, neuroendocrine-mediated secretion of prolactin and TSH is more frequently discordant than concordant; that is, TSH, though not prolactin secretion, is increased by cold, and prolactin, though not TSH secretion, is increased by nursing and stress. These findings suggest that the prolactin stimulatory factor is not TRH. Several hypothalamic factors distinct from TRH also stimulate prolactin release, including vasoactive intestinal polypeptide (VIP) and peptide histidine methionine (PHM). VIP has been shown to play a physiologic role in lactation in the rat.[178] These two peptides are also derived from a common precursor.[179] Recently, a prolactin-releasing factor from the posterior pituitary has been described that is more potent than TRH.[180] Its importance in humans remains to be determined.

Factors influencing prolactin secretion are listed in Table 8-5. Physiologic stimuli, in addition to those of pregnancy and nursing which were described above, include nipple stimulation, which can be demonstrated in both men and women, and sexual intercourse (in part also related to nipple stimulation). Sleep-associated rises in prolactin secretion can be readily demonstrated and begin about 60 to 90 min after the onset of sleep. Secretory bursts of prolactin continue throughout the sleep period, resulting in peak levels at 5 to 8 h after the onset of sleep. In contrast to GH secretion, sleep-associated prolactin secretion is not related to deep (stage III or IV) sleep (Fig. 8-8). Strenuous exercise also stimulates prolactin secretion, possibly by the same mechanisms involved in GH secretion, since, like GH release, prolactin release is stimulated by hypoglycemia and frequently is suppressed by hyperglycemia. Oral protein also stimulates prolactin secretion,[181] though the mediation of this response is not yet understood.

Prolactin secretion is influenced by many hormones. The effects of estrogen are exerted directly on the lactotroph, enhancing both basal and stimulated

TABLE 8-5 Factors Affecting Prolactin Secretion

Stimulative	Suppressive
Physiologic	
Pregnancy	
Nursing	
Nipple stimulation	
Sexual intercourse (women only)	
Exercise	
Sleep	
Stress	
Pharmacologic	
Hypoglycemia	Hyperglycemia*
Hyperaminoacidemia	
Hormones	Hormones:
Estrogen	Glucocorticoids*
TRH	Thyroxine
Neurotransmitters, etc.	Neurotransmitters, etc.
Dopaminergic antagonists (phenothiazine, butyrophenones, metoclopramide)	Dopaminergic agonists (L-dopa, apomorphine, dopamine, bromocriptine)
Catecholamine depletors and synthesis inhibitors (reserpine, α-methyldopa)	Serotonin antagonists (methysergide)
Serotonin precursors (5-hydroxytryptophan)	
GABA agonists (muscimol)	
Histamine H_2 antagonists (cimetidine)	
Opiates, etc. (morphine, enkephalin analogues)	
Pathologic	
Chronic renal failure	
Cirrhosis	
Hypothyroidism*	
Intercostal nerve stimulation (chest wall burns, herpes zoster, postmastectomy)	

* Occasionally observed.

release, and can be seen within 2 to 3 days. Glucocorticoids diminish the prolactin response to TRH by an effect that also occurs at the level of the pituitary. Thyroid hormone administration is not followed by changes in basal prolactin levels but suppresses the response to TRH. This response is increased in hypothyroidism and diminished in hyperthyroidism, and it reverts to normal with appropriate treatment. A minority of patients with primary hypothyroidism have hyperprolactinemia, and some exhibit galactorrhea.

A wide spectrum of agents with neuropharmacologic actions modify prolactin levels.[121] Agents which enhance dopaminergic activity, e.g., L-dopa (precursor), bromocriptine and apomorphine (dopaminergic agonists), and dopamine itself, all suppress prolactin secretion. The effects of dopamine and dopamine agonists are exerted directly on the pituitary and mediated by dopamine D_2 receptors, whereas those of dopamine precursors involve both pituitary and central mechanisms. Dopaminergic receptor antagonists, represented primarily by phenothiazine (chlorpromazine, prochlorperazine) and butyrophenone (haloperidol) neuroleptics, elevate prolactin levels and occasionally produce galactorrhea. The prolactin-elevating effects of these agents correlate well with their antipsychotic potency,[182] even though the maximal prolactin-stimulating effects are achieved at doses below those required for psychotropic effects and despite evidence suggesting that the pituitary dopaminergic receptors are different from those in the CNS.[183] Reserpine, a central catecholamine depletor, has similar stimulatory effects. GABA does not affect prolactin secretion directly, but muscimol, a GABA analogue that crosses the blood-brain barrier after systemic administration, stimulates prolactin release.[164] The effects of histamine on prolactin secretion are incompletely understood. Histamine stimulates prolactin secretion by a central mechanism. The histamine H_2-receptor blockers cimetidine and ranitidine exhibit similar effects (though the latter is less potent),[184,185] indicating a complex role for this neurotransmitter. Serotoninergic mechanisms have been implicated in both stress and nursing-associated prolactin secretion on the basis of the suppression of these responses by serotonin receptor blockers. Prolactin secretion is also increased by opiates and endorphins.[165] The mechanism of this effect is related to the inhibitory action of opiates and endorphins on central dopamine release.

Prolactin secretion is increased with surgical stress, most dramatically during operations performed under general anesthesia, and some though not all of the response may be due to the anesthetic agent. The rise in prolactin secretion seen after chest wall trauma, burns, and thoracic operations may also be stress-mediated and is related to stimulation of afferent intercostal nerves from the area of the nipple.

Hyperprolactinemia is present in up to 65 percent of patients with chronic renal failure who are maintained on hemodialysis, and in women galactorrhea is frequently present.[186] Such patients exhibit impaired responses to short-term dopaminergic suppression and to TRH and chlorpromazine stimulation. Though the metabolic clearance of prolactin is decreased in uremia, the actual hormone secretion rate is increased, suggesting an impairment in feedback inhibition.[174] Renal transplantation is generally associated with a return of prolactin levels to the normal range.

HYPOPITUITARISM

Hypopituitarism is a disorder of diverse etiology that results in a partial or total loss of anterior and posterior pituitary hormone function. The clinical manifestations vary greatly according to the age of the subject, the rapidity of onset, the particular hormones involved, and the extent of their impaired secretion as well as the nature of the primary pathologic process. Complete loss of hormonal secretion can rapidly become life-threatening and require immediate therapy.

Hypopituitarism does not become clinically evident until about 70 to 75 percent of the adenohypophysis is destroyed, though with currently available pituitary hormone function testing, a diminished reserve is likely to be detected with less destruction. Total loss of pituitary secretion requires at least 90 percent destruction of the gland. In many patients with pituitary destruction, minimal clinical evidence of hypopituitarism may escape detection for long periods and may never be recognized.

Etiology

Hypopituitarism can be divided into two general categories: *primary* and *secondary*. Primary hypopituitarism is due to the absence or destruction of the hormone-secreting cells of the pituitary, and secondary hypopituitarism is due to a lack of stimulation of pituitary hormone secretion caused by organic or functional disorders of the vascular and/or neural connections with the brain at the level of the pituitary stalk, hypothalamus, or extrahypothalamic central nervous system (CNS). Deficient anterior pituitary hormone secretion under such conditions is a result of lack of the appropriate releasing factors or excessive release of inhibiting hormones, while diminished posterior pituitary hormone secretion is due to lack of synthesis and axonal transport of the hormones from their site of origin in the anterior hypothalamus, as is discussed in detail in Chap. 9.

Table 8-6 lists the various diseases associated with hypopituitarism. Because of the many ways in which patients with hypopituitarism may present, the specific underlying pathologic process cannot always be reliably demonstrated.

Primary Hypopituitarism

Simmonds, in his classic case of hypopituitarism following necrosis of the pituitary in a woman with severe puerperal sepsis,[187] was the first to associate the clinical disorder of hypopituitarism with ischemic necrosis of the pituitary, although the first report of acute pituitary necrosis appeared the previous year.[188] Simmonds emphasized the term *cachexia*, and for several decades this feature was erroneously considered an important feature of the disease. In fact, one emaciated patient whose picture appeared in several textbooks was subsequently shown at autopsy to have a normal pituitary gland and most probably had anorexia nervosa. The extensive work by Sheehan provided the first clear distinction between pituitary necrosis and hypopituitarism.[189] He demonstrated that fibrosis of the pituitary was a consequence of the ischemic necrosis and infarction that often occurred in association with postpartum hemorrhage and vascular collapse. He also provided convincing proof that cachexia is not an obligatory or even a common feature of the disease.

The mechanism of acute ischemic necrosis is not entirely clear, but the condition is believed to be due to vasospasm of the hypophyseal vessels. Whether the changes in the pituitary during pregnancy associated with its marked increase in size under the influence of increased estrogen secretion result in enhanced sensitivity to vasoconstrictive stimuli or whether the gland becomes more sensitive to hypoxia is not known. However, the most frequent setting in which necrosis of the pituitary occurs is the immediate postpartum period in association with severe hemorrhage and hypotension. Up to 32 percent of women experiencing hemorrhage and vascular

TABLE 8-6 Etiologic Factors in Hypopituitarism

I. Primary
  A. Primary tumors
    1. Primary intrasellar (adenoma, craniopharyngioma)
    2. Parasellar (meningioma, optic nerve glioma)
    3. Metastatic (breast, lung, melanoma)
  B. Ischemic necrosis of the pituitary
    1. Postpartum (Sheehan's syndrome)
    2. Diabetes mellitus
    3. Other systemic diseases (temporal arteritis, sickle cell disease and trait, arteriosclerosis, eclampsia)
  C. Aneurysm of intracranial internal carotid artery
  D. Pituitary apoplexy (almost always related to a primary pituitary tumor)
  E. Cavernous sinus thrombosis
  F. Infectious disease (tuberculosis, syphilis, malaria, meningitis, fungal disease)
  G. Infiltrative disease (hemochromatosis)
  H. Immunologic (granulomatous or lymphocytic hypophysitis)
  I. Iatrogenic
    1. Irradiation of nasopharynx
    2. Irradiation of sella
    3. Surgical destruction
  J. Primary empty sella syndrome
  K. Metabolic disorders (chronic renal failure)
  L. Genetic (*pit-1* gene mutation, deletion, GH gene deletions, β-LH mutation, other familial forms)
  M. Idiopathic (frequently monohormonal)
II. Secondary
  A. Destruction of pituitary stalk
    1. Trauma
    2. Compression by tumor or aneurysm
    3. Iatrogenic (surgical)
  B. Hypothalamic or other central nervous system disease
    1. Inflammatory (sarcoid or other granulomatous disease)
    2. Infiltrative (lipid storage diseases)
    3. Trauma
    4. Toxic (vincristine)
    5. Hormone-induced (glucocorticoids, gonadal steroids)
    6. Tumors (primary, metastatic, lymphoma, leukemia)
    7. Iatrogenic (surgical or irradiation)
    8. Infectious (HIV)
    9. Idiopathic (frequently congenital or familial, often restricted to one or two hormones, and possibly reversible)
    10. Nutritional (starvation, obesity)
    11. Anorexia nervosa
    12. Psychoneuroendocrine (psychosocial dwarfism, stress-associated amenorrhea)

collapse during delivery will develop some degree of hypopituitarism.[190] The extent of pituitary necrosis and the subsequent hypopituitarism are related to the severity of the hemorrhage. A most important clue that pituitary necrosis has occurred is an inability to lactate in the postpartum period and a failure of cyclic menstruation to be reestablished. However, because of the slowly developing picture of hypopituitarism and its frequently incomplete clinical manifestations, the presence of postpartum lactation cannot be used to exclude the existence of at least partial pituitary insufficiency. The relatively large reserve capacity of the anterior pituitary is evident from the discrepancy between the incidence of ischemic pituitary necrosis and that of hypopituitarism.

With the improvement in obstetric care during the past half century, the syndrome of pituitary necrosis has become much less common. It must be emphasized, though, that significant hemorrhage and shock, while important predisposing factors, are not absolutely essential for its development. Ischemic necrosis of the pituitary can be seen in association with numerous other diseases, although the frequency is quite low. In diabetes mellitus a 2 percent incidence at autopsy has been reported,[191] though in most of the patients evidence of clinical hypopituitarism was lacking. When present, hypopituitarism can lead to a marked reduction in insulin requirement primarily as a result of the lack of glucocorticoids. Pituitary necrosis has been reported in epidemic hemorrhagic fever, but the rapid death of patients precluded assessment of their pituitary function. It has also been seen in association with a large variety of other diseases, including malaria, temporal arteritis, hemochromatosis, sickle cell disease, meningitis, eclampsia, and severe vitamin deficiency, and occasionally it occurs without any predisposing illness.[192] In some patients, there is sufficient destruction of the pituitary to result in signs and symptoms of hypopituitarism, whereas in others, detailed testing is required to document the impairment in hormone secretion.

Pituitary tumor is today the most common cause of hypopituitarism involving multiple hormone deficiencies in the adult population. A full discussion of this subject is provided in the following section. Parasellar mass lesions can also invade the sella turcica and cause sufficient destruction of the pituitary to produce hypopituitarism. Similar destruction can be caused by aneurysms of the intracavernous portion of the internal carotid artery.

Hypopituitarism may be secondary to an intrapituitary hemorrhage (*pituitary apoplexy*), which occurs in at least 10 percent of pituitary tumors.[193] The signs and symptoms may vary considerably. If bleeding occurs gradually, leading to pituitary compression, the symptoms of hypopituitarism will predominate, while if the hemorrhage is sudden, the presenting symptoms will be those of an expanding intra- and extrapituitary mass: headache, ophthalmoplegia, and subarachnoid irritation. Patients typically present with features of sudden expansion of a preexisting pituitary adenoma. However, with the ability to make the diagnosis by MRI, many patients with totally asymptomatic intrapituitary hemorrhages are being identified (Fig. 8-9).[194,195] Most patients recover without acute surgical intervention, though in some it may be necessary to correct visual abnormalities. In most patients, some anterior pituitary function is lost,[196] though posterior pituitary function is almost always preserved. During the acute period, glucocorticoid therapy should be provided. While conservative therapy has been recommended if no neurologic deficits are present, evacuation of the hemorrhagic mass in patients who experience acute apoplexy has been associated with at least partial recovery of pituitary function.[197]

The classic examples of hypopituitarism found in diseases such as tuberculosis and syphilis have become exceedingly rare. However, at the time of autopsy, 12 percent of patients with AIDS were found to have pituitary involvement with opportunistic diseases, primarily cytomegalus virus.[198] The extent of pituitary destruction in most cases was limited, consistent with the clinical observation that pituitary insufficiency is uncommon in this disorder.

Nearly 50 percent of patients with hemochromatosis, in whom decreased gonadal function is a common and early manifestation, have evidence of impaired gonadotropin secretion.[199] In some patients, adenocortical insufficiency due to impaired ACTH secretion also occurs. The cause of the hypofunction re-

FIGURE 8-9 Coronal (*left*) and midsagittal (*right*) MRI views of a pituitary tumor with a recent hemorrhage (*pituitary apoplexy*), indicated by the high signal intensity. Rapid suprasellar expansion of the mass has produced bowing of the optic chiasm and the sudden appearance of bitemporal visual field defects.

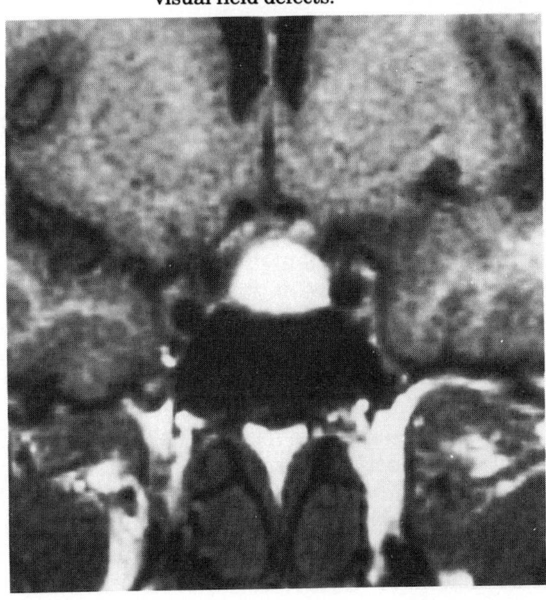

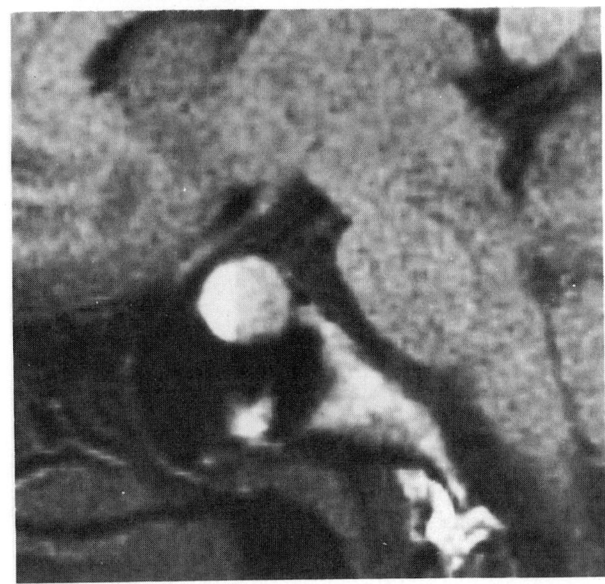

lates to the iron deposition in the pituitary which commonly occurs in this disease. In some patients, however, hypopituitarism may be secondary to a disturbance of hypothalamic function.[200]

Hypopituitarism can also occur on an immunologic basis. There have been several reports of women in the peripartum period who developed hypopituitarism associated with a presumed pituitary tumor,[201,202] though this disease can also occur in men.[203] At surgery, the pituitary tissue is mucoid, partially necrotic, and extensively infiltrated with lymphocytes. The pathogenesis of this disorder is unknown, as is its relation to giant-cell granulomatous hypophysitis, a rare disorder seen primarily in middle-aged or older women.[204] The latter condition is distinct from pituitary sarcoidosis, which most commonly involves the posterior pituitary and is associated with diabetes insipidus. Isolated gonadotropin failure has also been reported in association with polyglandular failure, suggesting that autoimmune hypophysitis may also occur.[205]

The use of ionizing radiation for the treatment of malignant disease in the head and neck (nasopharyngeal carcinomas, brain tumors, leukemia treated with prophylactic cranial irradiation) is being recognized with increasing frequency as a cause of hypopituitarism on both a primary and a secondary basis.[206,207] In children, the most common manifestation has been growth retardation or absence of the onset of puberty, while in adults, symptoms of gonadotropin deficiency have been most prominent. Hypopituitarism can be detected within 6 to 12 months after a dose of about 3000 rad. The normal pituitary gland appears to be more susceptible to irradiation damage in children than in adults, in whom considerably higher doses (10,000 to 18,000 rad) are required to destroy the anterior pituitary in patients with breast cancer or diabetic retinopathy. The dose of irradiation used for the treatment of pituitary tumors is approximately 4500 to 5000 rad, and the short-term incidence of hypopituitarism is relatively low, as is discussed in the following section. However, long-term evaluation of irradiated patients will be required to determine the true incidence of iatrogenic disease.

Surgical excision of the pituitary, which occasionally occurs during removal of a pituitary tumor or, in the past, intended therapy for breast cancer or diabetic retinopathy, produces panhypopituitarism that requires immediate therapy.

The primary empty sella syndrome, described under Pituitary Tumors, below, is infrequently associated with hypopituitarism. Although most reported series of patients with this disorder include a small percentage in whom endocrine function testing reveals a defect in one or more pituitary hormones, the incidence of clinical (symptomatic) hypopituitarism is less than 10 percent.[208] An empty sella can occur secondary to Sheehan's syndrome,[209] sarcoidosis,[210] or other pituitary diseases in which varying degrees of hypopituitarism are present.

Hypopituitarism may occur without any detectable underlying disease and most frequently involves deficiencies in a single hormone or a few rather than in all hormones. Although it is generally sporadic, there are reports of both autosomal and X-linked recessive varieties of hypopituitarism with small, normal, or even slightly enlarged sellae.[211–213]

Recently, a familial form of hypopituitarism associated with absent GH, prolactin, and TSH secretion has been shown to be caused by a mutation in the *pit-1 (GHF-1)* gene.[14,15] *Pit-1* is a nuclear transcription factor required for both the expression of the GH gene and the proliferation of somatotrophs, lactotrophs, and thyrotrophs. A deletion or a point mutation in the *pit-1* gene results in a single amino acid substitution in the protein's DNA-binding region that is similar to the mutation initially recognized as responsible for the combined hormonal deficiencies in Snell and Snell-Jackson mice.[214]

Gene mutations also cause several isohormonal deficiencies. Children with growth retardation in whom GH is undetectable in plasma have been shown to have deletions in the GH gene.[215,216] Hypogonadism has been described in a patient with a point mutation in the LH-β gene resulting in a single amino acid substitution of the β subunit, which interferes with it receptor binding.[217] A single amino acid mutation in the TSH β subunit that interferes with its dimerization with the α subunit and results in hypothyroidism has also been described.[218]

Impaired secretion of TSH and gonadotropins has been documented in chronic renal failure due to a combination of defects at both the pituitary and hypothalamic levels.[219,220] Though the specific factor or factors responsible remain to be identified, the abnormalities appear to be reversible with renal transplantation.

Secondary Hypopituitarism

Secondary hypopituitarism can be caused by numerous central nervous system disorders, all of which have in common disruption of the normal delivery of releasing or inhibiting factors to the pituitary. Primary hypopituitarism can be differentiated from secondary hypopituitarism in the absence of anatomically defined disease of the pituitary or the CNS in some but not all patients by the use of hypothalamic releasing hormones. In addition, diabetes insipidus is more common in secondary than in primary hypopituitarism.

Pathologic processes involving the pituitary stalk are most frequently due to trauma. Basilar skull fractures occasionally lead to tearing of the stalk with rupture of both the neural and vascular connections. Parasellar tumors or aneurysms can also cause sufficient compression of the stalk to impair blood flow to the portal vessels, resulting in hypopituitarism. The sequelae differ from those following hypophysectomy in that (1) prolactin levels frequently rise and remain elevated owing to the loss of hypothalamic prolactin inhibiting factor, provided that sufficient blood flow remains to ensure lactotroph viability, and (2) neovascularization will occasionally lead to reestablishment of the hypophyseal portal vasculature and recovery of pituitary hormone function.

Diseases of the CNS, primarily of the hypothalamus, which impair releasing factor secretion also produce hypopituitarism. Inflammatory diseases such as sarcoidosis; infiltrative processes, including the lipid storage diseases, hemochromatosis, and eosinophilic granuloma; and infectious diseases such as HIV may result in impaired TSH, gonadotropin, GH, and less commonly ACTH and vasopressin secretion. Prolactin levels are frequently elevated, confirming the suprasellar origin of the disease. The frequency of multiple hormone deficiencies in these and other hypothalamic diseases depends on the size of the pathologic process and its location. The closer the location to the median eminence, where the funneling effect of the hypothalamus occurs, the greater the possibility of multiple hormone deficiencies.

Trauma to the hypothalamus frequently occurs in serious head injuries. Evidence for hypopituitarism is often observed in patients with prolonged coma,[221,222] and recovery of pituitary function usually but not invariably parallels the improvement in neurologic status, though residual impairment is not uncommon.

Drugs used in therapy for malignant disease (e.g., vincristine) may also have toxic effects on the hypothalamus, resulting in impaired pituitary hormone secretion. Functional impairment of ACTH and the gonadotropins can also occur as a result of prolonged treatment with glucocorticoids, even with alternate-day therapy,[223] and with oral contraceptives as a result of continuous suppression of the specific releasing factors in an exaggeration of the normal negative feedback mechanism. Recovery of function usually occurs, though often with long delays. Recovery of the hypothalamic-pituitary-adrenal axis after the removal of an adrenocortical adenoma may require 12 to 24 months, and restoration of cyclic ovulation after discontinuation of oral contraceptives may take as long. Although impaired TSH reserve can be demonstrated transiently after prolonged treatment with exogenous thyroid hormone in euthyroid persons, clinical evidence of hypothyroidism is rare.

Tumors of the hypothalamus and third ventricle or hypothalamic involvement with lymphomatous or leukemic infiltrates can result in impaired pituitary function. With successful treatment of the underlying disease, some recovery may occur.

As with primary hypopituitarism, diminished pituitary hormone secretion may occur on the basis of central nervous system disorders which are unassociated with other subjective or objective findings. Single or multiple hormone deficiencies may be involved, and the disease may become evident at any age. The most frequent disorder observed in adults is impaired gonadotropin secretion (hypothalamic hypogonadism or hypothalamic amenorrhea). In both children and adults, hypothalamic hypopituitarism may be secondary to an emotional disturbance and thus may be reversible.

Hypothalamic dysfunction resulting in impaired gonadotropin secretion may occur as a result of marked changes in body weight. Both malnutrition and marked obesity are often associated with amenorrhea, which persists until there is a return to nearly normal body weight. Amenorrhea also occurs with strenuous exercise, particularly in untrained women but also in professional athletes and ballet dancers.[224–226] In patients with anorexia nervosa, secretion of gonadotropin and occasionally TSH may be diminished. Although weight loss contributes to the pathogenesis of the endocrine disorder, other unknown factors are involved, since amenorrhea frequently precedes weight loss and can persist after weight is regained.[227] Stress, such as that associated with severe illness not affecting the CNS, also results in hypogonadism which is reversible upon recovery.[228]

Pinealomas are associated with both precocious puberty and hypogonadism. The secretion of a gonadotropin inhibitor by the tumor has been postulated, but the chemical nature of this substance is not known. These disorders are discussed in some detail in Chap. 7.

Clinical Features

The signs and symptoms of hypopituitarism vary according to the extent of diminished secretion of individual pituitary hormones and the rapidity of onset. Both factors are greatly influenced by the etiology of the disease. In the most extensive form of total absence of pituitary secretion, or *panhypopituitarism*, as is seen after surgical hypophysectomy, severe pituitary apoplexy, or withdrawal of hormone therapy in hypophysectomized subjects, clinical features can develop within a few hours (diabetes insipidus) to a few days (adrenal insufficiency). In partial hypopituitarism, which is more commonly seen with tumors or infiltrative diseases, the signs and symptoms progress slowly and may be vague and nonspecific, with the diagnosis unsuspected for long periods. In general, the most common presenting manifestations are caused by gonadotropin deficiency in adults and GH deficiency in children. The spectrum of clinical features is best described by considering first the effects of deficiencies of the individual pituitary horones and then their interrelations.

ACTH

A deficiency of ACTH is manifested by diminished adrenocortical function, and many of the signs and symptoms of adrenal insufficiency are similar whether caused by pituitary or by adrenal disease. Weakness, postural hypotension, and dehydration commonly occur during stress, although true addisonian crisis is infrequent because of the partial independence of the renin-angiotensin-aldosterone system from the secretion of ACTH. Thus, aldosterone secretion is diminished in hypopituitarism, but to a lesser extent than in primary adrenal insufficiency. Nausea, vomiting, and severe hypothermia may also occur. Hypoglycemia is occasionally seen, particularly after a prolonged fast and/or moderate alcohol ingestion, because of impaired gluconeogenesis. In patients with isolated ACTH deficiency this may be the only symptom of the disease. Unlike patients with primary adrenal insufficiency, in whom ACTH secretion is increased, those with ACTH deficiency show no hyperpigmentation; in fact, there may be hypopigmentation and diminished tanning after exposure to sunlight. Since impairment of ACTH secretion is frequently incomplete, patients may experience symptoms only during periods of stress (e.g., surgery, trauma, severe infections), and ACTH deficiency may thus remain undiagnosed for prolonged periods. The inability to excrete a water load that is seen in Addison's disease also occurs in ACTH deficiency but is less pronounced and often is masked by a concomitant vasopressin deficiency (see below). The loss of adrenal androgens in males is of little consequence if testicular function is preserved. In females, however, it can contribute to decreased libido and is largely responsible for the loss of axillary and pubic hair. Calcification of auricular cartilage, which was once thought to be specific for Addison's disease, may also be seen with ACTH deficiency.[229]

TSH

Secondary or *pituitary hypothyroidism* is a term used to describe the thyroid deficiency state caused by diminished TSH secretion. Primary and secondary hypothyroidism are in general clinically indistinguishable from each other except in regard to their severity. Patients with TSH deficiency exhibit cold intolerance, constipation, dry skin, pallor, mental slowing, bradycardia, and hoarseness. True myxedema occurs infrequently, and hypercholesterolemia and carotenemia are uncommon. Both increased and decreased menstrual flow may be observed. TSH deficiency occurring during childhood results in severe growth retardation that is unresponsive to treatment with GH. Isolated TSH deficiency has been observed on a familial basis[230] and in association with pseudohypoparathyroidism.[231]

LH and FSH

Gonadotropin deficiency in adult women is manifested by amenorrhea and clinical features of estrogen deficiency, including breast atrophy, dryness of skin, and a decrease in vaginal secretions that often results in dyspareunia. A decrease in libido may also occur. In adult males, the loss of gonadotropins results in testes which are decreased in size, soft, and relatively nontender to pressure and in manifestations of decreased androgen production, consisting in diminished libido and potency, a decreased rate of secondary sexual hair growth, and reduced muscular strength. Gonadotropin deficiency occurring before or during the period of sexual maturation results in total or partial impairment of secondary sexual development. In isolated gonadotropin deficiency or when GH secretion is unimpaired, the failure of sex steroid–induced epiphyseal closure in the long bones results in excessive growth of the limbs, leading to a eunuchoid appearance. Although both gonadotropins are usually deficient, an occasional patient has been reported to lack only FSH.[232]

Growth Hormone

Impaired secretion of GH in an adult does not result in easily recognizable clinical symptoms. Although the metabolic effects of GH deficiency can be readily demonstrated, other compensatory mechanisms presumably obscure clinical abnormalities. Impaired carbohydrate tolerance associated with hypoinsulinemia is present in GH-deficient subjects, but this disorder is distinguishable from diabetes mellitus, particularly by the absence of microangiopathy.[233] Adults with GH deficiency have been reported to exhibit an increased risk of cardiovascular mortality, although the mechanism is not known.[234] Muscle strength and performance are also decreased, although the extent to which this impairs normal life activities is debatable.[235–238] At present, there is insufficient information to determine whether wound healing and repair of bone fractures are impaired in GH-deficient subjects. GH also influences immune function, stimulating thymic growth and T and B cell and macrophage function, including natural killer cell activity.[239–241] However, no evidence currently exists for an increase in immune disorders as a consequence of GH deficiency. In children, GH deficiency is associated with growth retardation, as is discussed in detail in Chap. 26. Fasting hypoglycemia occasionally occurs in GH-deficient children and is almost invariably present when there is associated ACTH deficiency.[242]

Prolactin

Prolactin deficiency is associated with only one clinical manifestation: the absence of lactation in the postpartum state.

Vasopressin

Decreased antidiuretic hormone secretion results in diabetes insipidus, as is described in detail in Chap. 9. The inability of the kidneys to reabsorb water leads to polyuria and polydipsia, and if fluid intake is not maintained, as occurs frequently in states of altered consciousness, severe dehydration can result. Patients exhibit extreme thirst, which is preferentially relieved by ice water. In the presence of ACTH deficiency, polyuria may not occur because of the requirement of glucocorticoids for the excretion of free water. The appearance of polyuria during the course of an ACTH test or after the institution of glucocorticoid therapy is highly suggestive of combined vasopressin and ACTH deficiency.

Oxytocin

The absence of oxytocin does not lead to any signs or symptoms in humans. Women with panhypopituitarism who become pregnant are able to initiate labor and experience normal parturition despite the absence of this hormone.

General Features

In hypopituitary patients, the skin frequently exhibits a loss of normal turgor, and in hypopituitarism of long duration, it assumes a waxy character. Wrinkling, particularly around the mouth and eyes, leading to a prematurely aged appearance, is also common. Nutrition is in general well preserved. A moderate anemia is often present and is generally normocytic and normochromic but may also be hypochromic or macrocytic. Thyroid hormone deficiency is the most important contributory factor, though decreased testosterone secretion and impaired erythropoietin production also appear to be involved. Psychiatric disturbances are well recognized in hypopituitarism, with mental slowing or apathy being observed in nearly half the patients reported by Sheehan and Summers.[243] Other psychiatric symptoms include delusions and occasionally paranoid psychoses. These behavioral changes have been attributed to glucocorticoid deficiency.

Carbohydrate metabolism is usually not markedly altered in nondiabetic hypopituitary patients. In contrast, hypopituitarism in insulin-requiring diabetic patients leads to a dramatic reduction in the insulin dosage, frequently to 20 to 50 percent of the original level, and an increased tendency to hypoglycemic reactions. These changes persist even with full glucocorticoid replacement therapy, suggesting an important role of GH and also of epinephrine. The synthesis of epinephrine is decreased because of the absence of high levels of cortisol in the adrenal, required for normal levels of phenylethanolamine-*N*-methyl transferase, the enzyme that converts norepinephrine to epinephrine (see Chap. 13).

The relative frequency of the various features of hypopituitarism varies with the etiology of the disorder. Most recent series relate to patients with a pituitary tumor, which is today the most frequent cause of hypopituitarism. Although some disagreement exists among reports, loss of GH followed by loss of gonadotropins appears to be the earliest and thus the most frequent pattern encountered. ACTH and TSH deficiency occur less frequently and are also seen later in the natural history of the disease. The existence of single or selected hormonal deficiencies, however, precludes the evaluation of pituitary function on the basis of only one or two hormones.

Isolated Hormonal Deficiencies

Deficiencies of individual pituitary hormones frequently occur in the absence of detectable anatomic disease of the pituitary. The signs and symptoms associated with these disorders are described in the preceding section. TSH and gonadotropin deficiencies often cannot be distinguished clinically from decreased secretion of target organ hormones, whereas the absence of hyperpigmentation and salt craving generally serves to differentiate ACTH deficiency from primary adrenal insufficiency. The most common form of isolated pituitary hormone deficiency is GH deficiency, which is a disease of childhood and adolescence and is discussed in greater detail in Chap. 26. The site of the primary disorder in isolated pituitary hormone deficiencies, i.e., the CNS or the pituitary, can usually but not always be determined by detailed testing.

Differential Diagnosis

Hypopituitarism can be confused with two other disease categories. The first includes disorders of hormone hypofunction involving target glands or the region of the CNS (the hypothalamus) involved in neuroendocrine regulation. The second includes diseases that share some of the generalized signs and symptoms of hypopituitarism but are not associated with endocrine hypofunction.

Target Organ and Hypothalamic Hypofunction

Primary failure of the thyroid, adrenals, or gonads must be differentiated from isolated pituitary hormone deficiencies. As indicated above, the signs and symptoms may be indistinguishable from those of hypopituitarism. In particular, the presence of multiple target gland (polyglandular) failure must be considered as a possibility. The diagnosis may be suggested by features of autoimmune disease; the presence of diabetes mellitus, moniliasis, or hypoparathyroidism; or a familial pattern, though none of these may be present. Although the severity of hormone deficiency in primary target organ disease is frequently greater than in hypopituitarism, this is not a distinguishing feature, since partial target organ failure can also occur.

Primary adrenal insufficiency is characteristically associated with hyperkalemia due to diminished aldosterone secretion. In hypopituitarism, partial preservation of aldosterone secretion is sufficient to prevent elevations in serum potassium. The hyperpigmentation and salt craving of Addison's disease are also absent in hypopituitarism. In some patients with primary gonadal failure, there may be a discrepancy between the loss of gonadal steroid (androgen or estrogen) secretion and the loss of spermatogenesis or ovulation. In hypopituitarism, both aspects of gonadal function tend to be diminished to the same extent. The presence of hot flashes may be seen with primary ovarian failure, hypopituitarism, and GnRH deficiency.[244]

Hypopituitarism must also be distinguished from CNS disorders which affect releasing factor secretion. The presence of nonendocrine disturbances such as anosmia in Kallman's syndrome and progressive obesity may suggest the extrapituitary origin of these diseases. Laboratory studies are, however, crucial to distinguish this group of disorders (see Chap. 7).

Nonendocrine Disorders

The possibility of hypopituitarism is frequently raised in patients with chronic malnutrition or liver disease who exhibit weakness, lethargy, cold intolerance, and decreased libido. As stressed above, cachexia is *not* a characteristic finding of hypopituitarism, and its presence should suggest another disease. Anorexia nervosa, a disorder primarily of young adult females, is often confused with hypopituitarism. The severe weight loss, characteristic psychiatric symptoms, and preservation of axillary and pubic hair are all useful in distinguishing anorexia nervosa from hypopituitarism. In chronic malnutrition and anorexia nervosa, GH and ACTH secretion are intact and are often increased. This disorder is discussed in Chap. 7.

Diagnostic Procedures

The diagnosis of hypopituitarism must be established by appropriate and carefully conducted studies of pituitary hormone secretion, since these studies provide the basis on which decisions are made concerning lifelong hormone replacement therapy. The studies must address two questions: (1) Is pituitary hormone secretion diminished? and (2) Is the disorder of pituitary or nonpituitary origin? In addition, nonendocrine (neuroanatomic) studies are required to determine the etiology of hypopituitarism. The latter procedures are discussed under Pituitary Tumors, below.

Diagnostic studies that evaluate the function of anterior pituitary hormones have undergone considerable change during recent years, reflecting the change from indirect tests of pituitary function such as indexes of carbohydrate metabolism or assessment of target organ function by injection of pituitary hormones to direct measurement of circulating levels of pituitary hormones in relation to those of target hormones and the response to releasing hormone stimulation. The availability of certain tests varies from one laboratory to the next, though most can be performed by regional reference laboratories if not in individual hospitals.

This section considers the evaluation of the six major anterior pituitary hormones and the differentiation of pituitary from extrapituitary sites of the primary disorder. The rationale for the various tests, their advantages, and their limitations are discussed here, while the specific details are provided at the end of the chapter under Details of Hypothalamic-Pituitary Testing.

ACTH

ACTH secretion is evaluated by the measurement of plasma ACTH and cortisol levels. Cortisol measurement is a more useful screening procedure since it can be performed rapidly, is less expensive, and does not fluctuate as greatly as does ACTH. Morning values of < 10 μg/dl or values of < 20 μg/dl under conditions of stress are suggestive of hypopituitarism. In contrast to patients with primary adrenal insufficiency, patients with hypopituitarism may exhibit no appreciable clinical symptoms and yet have nearly undetectable circulating cortisol levels.

Simultaneous measurement of plasma ACTH (which is warranted when there is a high index of suspicion of the diagnosis) provides important information. A low or even normal ACTH level in the presence of a low cortisol level is highly suggestive of total or partial ACTH deficiency, whereas a high ACTH level is indicative of primary adrenal disease. Conclusive evidence of hypopituitarism is provided by demonstrating that the administration of ACTH (250 μg synthetic $ACTH_{1-24}$) is capable of eliciting a plasma cortisol response (measured at 30 min) while stimuli requiring the participation of the entire hypothalamic-pituitary-adrenal axis or of the pituitary-adrenal component are ineffective. Patients with prolonged ACTH deficiency usually develop adrenal atrophy and may not respond to an acute ACTH challenge. This lack of response has been used by some physicians for an indirect assessment of ACTH secretion and has been reported to correlate with the response to insulin hypoglycemia (see below).[245] However, a response does not necessarily indicate an axis that will respond normally to surgical stress.[246]

If cortisol levels are normal and an intact response to ACTH is present, the hypothalamic-pituitary axis can be evaluated by (1) stimulation with CRH, (2) an insulin tolerance test, which measures the response to hypoglycemic stress, or (3) metyrapone (Metopirone) administration, which measures the response to the interruption of the negative feedback effects of cortisol.

The most specific stimulus is CRH, which causes

a rapid release of ACTH from the pituitary, followed by cortisol secretion by the adrenal. The plasma cortisol response to CRH is more reproducible than is the response of ACTH,[247,248] in part because of the short half-life of ACTH. The response to an intravenous injection of 100 μg CRH in normal subjects is a plasma cortisol increase of at least 10 μg/dl which peaks at 30 to 60 min. Side effects of CRH are minimal, consisting of facial flushing that may last for up to an hour. Ovine rather than human CRH is preferred because of its longer half-life in circulation, which results in a greater and more consistent ACTH response.[249–251] At the time of writing, CRH is still an investigational drug in the United States.

The stimulus of insulin hypoglycemia is based on the normal activation of the hypothalamic-pituitary-adrenal axis in response to central glucopenia (Fig. 8-10). An adequate stimulus requires that the blood glucose be reduced by 50 percent (or to 40 mg/dl). Normal subjects will experience adrenergic symptoms of hypoglycemia (diaphoresis, tachycardia, mild anxiety, headache), indicating that sufficient decrease in blood glucose has occurred. The standard dose of 0.1 U/kg IV may need to be increased (to 0.15 or 0.2 U/kg) in patients with obesity, maturity-onset diabetes, acromegaly, or other states of insulin resistance, while in patients strongly suspected of having hypopituitarism, a reduction of the dose to 0.05 U/kg is recommended. The test should *not* be performed in patients with suspected Addison's disease, those manifesting obvious clinical signs and symptoms of adrenal insufficiency, elderly patients, or those with coronary artery or cerebrovascular disease.

FIGURE 8-10 Plasma GH and cortisol responses to hypoglycemia produced by insulin (0.1 U/kg IV) in normal subjects. Blood glucose should decrease by 50 percent (or to 40 mg/dl) to ensure an adequate stimulus.

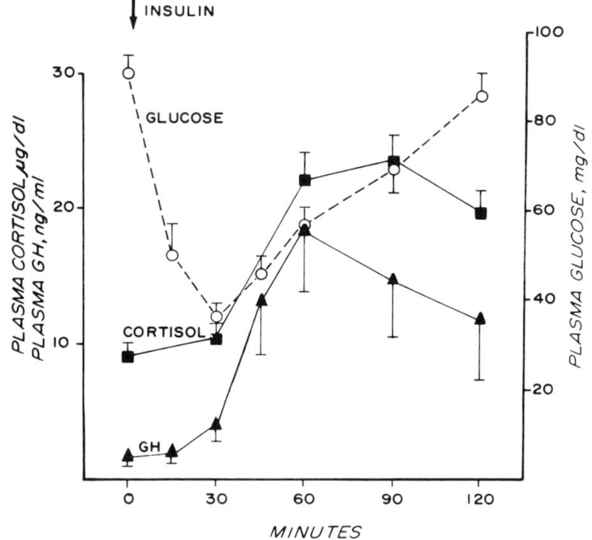

Metyrapone impairs cortisol biosynthesis in the adrenal cortex by blocking the hydroxylation of 11-deoxycortisol and interrupts the negative feedback effect of cortisol on the CNS and pituitary. The administration of metyrapone therefore leads to an activation of the hypothalamic-pituitary axis and an accumulation of 11-deoxycortisol in the blood and tetrahydro-11-deoxycortisol in the urine. The latter is a 17-OH corticoid. Metyrapone (2.0 g for patients weighing < 70 kg, 2.5 g for patients 70 to 90 kg, 3.0 g for patients > 90 kg) is given orally at midnight, and plasma cortisol and 11-deoxycortisol are measured at 8 A.M.[252] In persons with a normal pituitary-adrenal axis, plasma 11-deoxycortisol should be < 7 μg/dl, whereas in patients with hypothalamic or pituitary disease, varying degrees of impairment are present. Variations in gastrointestinal absorption of the drug and increased degradation in patients on phenytoin (Dilantin) may interfere with the inhibition of 11-β-hydroxylase, and a plasma cortisol of < 10 μg/dl is required to confirm adequate enzyme inhibition. As with insulin hypoglycemia, the test is contraindicated in patients suspected of having primary adrenal insufficiency until this diagnosis has been excluded. It is important to emphasize that the patient must not be receiving any glucocorticoid therapy, since the basis of the test is the creation of short-term adrenocortical insufficiency.

In determining which test(s) to use, it is important to consider the practical implications. The test is performed to identify patients with suspected relative adrenal insufficiency, i.e., those in whom a possible inadequate response to stress may occur. If the suspected disease is in the pituitary, CRH or, as a second choice, insulin hypoglycemia should be used. The cortisol response to insulin hypoglycemia correlates well with the response to surgical stress. It also allows simultaneous evaluation of a second pituitary hormone,[253] as is described below. The metyrapone response has a fairly high degree of concordance with that of insulin hypoglycemia, and therefore, until CRH is widely available, it remains a suitable alternative in patients in whom the risk of inducing hypoglycemia is not justified.

The diagnosis of primary adrenal insufficiency is relatively easy to establish whether or not the patient is receiving replacement therapy when first seen, but prior glucocorticoid therapy, with its suppressive effects on the hypothalamus and pituitary, can complicate the work-up of a patient with suspected hypopituitarism. The suppressive effects are most pronounced on metyrapone stimulation but can occur with other stimuli as well. A subnormal or absent response to any stimulus in a patient with a history of prolonged glucocorticoid therapy must therefore be interpreted with reservation. Glucocorticoids should be discontinued for at least 1 month, if possible, before definitive testing. Short-term glucocorticoid therapy, such as that provided during a perioperative period, does not significantly interfere with testing procedures if it is discontinued for 24 to 48 h before testing.

TSH

Basal plasma TSH levels in normal subjects can be differentiated from those in patients in whom TSH secretion is suppressed by exogenous thyroid hormone administration and as a result of thyrotoxicosis. In patients with hypopituitarism, however, basal values may be in the low-normal range, particularly if some residual function is present. Therefore, a combination of TSH and T_4 levels provides the best initial assessment of thyrotroph function. If the T_4 level is normal, it excludes a total, though not necessarily a partial, defect in TSH secretion. A decreased T_4 level associated with an elevated TSH level is indicative of intact TSH function (primary hypothyroidism). Simultaneously decreased T_4 and TSH levels, in the absence of severe systemic illness or cachexia, indicate pituitary (secondary hypothyroidism) or hypothalamic (tertiary hypothyroidism) dysfunction. Pituitary disease and hypothalamic disease can generally be differentiated from each other by determining the TSH response to a maximal stimulatory dose of TRH (200 μg or greater) (Fig. 8-11). In normal subjects, peak TSH values occur at 15 to 30 min after TRH and generally reach a level of at least twice the upper limit of normal basal values. An impaired or absent response is indicative of decreased pituitary reserve. In patients in whom a hypothalamic disorder is responsible for the decreased TSH secretion, the response to TRH is often enhanced and the peak may be delayed, occurring at 60 to 120 mm.[254] However, normal or impaired responses may also be seen, limiting the discriminating ability of this test. It is important that patients undergoing TRH testing be withdrawn from thyroid hormone therapy for at least 1 month before the study to eliminate any suppressive effects of thyroid hormones on the TSH response to TRH.

FIGURE 8-11 Plasma TSH and prolactin responses to TRH (500 μg IV) in normal men and women. The dose used produces a maximal response. Delayed TSH responses are occasionally observed in patients with hypothalamic disease. (*Modified from Hershman JM, Pittman JA Jr: J Clin Endocrinol Metab 31:457, 1970; and from Jacobs L et al: J Clin Endocrinol Metab 36:1069, 1973.*)

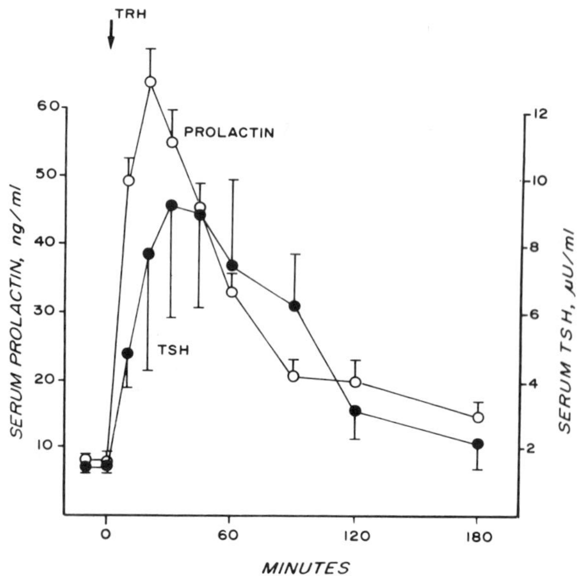

LH and FSH

Basal levels of plasma LH and FSH in hypopituitary patients are often indistinguishable from those in the lower part of the normal range for men and for women in the follicular phase. In a clinically hypogonadal female with low (< 30 pg/ml) or undetectable estradiol values or in a hypogonadal male with low plasma testosterone levels (< 3 ng/ml) associated with primary gonadal disease, plasma LH and FSH levels are elevated. The diagnosis of hypopituitarism can therefore be suspected in hypogonadal patients with levels of LH and FSH in the normal range. The differentiation between pituitary and suprapituitary causes of diminished gonadotropin secretion, however, is more difficult and cannot always be achieved with certainty. Three types of studies may be used: (1) direct stimulation of the pituitary with GnRH, (2) interference with the negative feedback of estrogen, using clomiphene, and (3) stimulation in women of the positive feedback effects of estrogen on GnRH secretion, using exogenous hormone.

Injection of GnRH (100 μg IV) results in a rise of plasma LH to at least 3 times and often to 10 times basal levels, with peak values occurring within 15 to 30 min (Fig. 8-12). The FSH response, which is of lesser magnitude, exhibits a similar temporal pattern, though it is occasionally delayed.[255] In patients with hypopituitarism, a full range of gonadotropin responses may be seen despite clinical hypogonadism; i.e., there may be normal, diminished, or absent responses, depending on the extent of gonadotroph destruction. In contrast, patients with primary hypogonadism exhibit an enhanced LH and FSH response to GnRH as well as elevated basal gonadotropin levels. The loss of the LH response tends to occur more frequently than the loss of the FSH response in patients with nonfunctioning pituitary tumors.[256] Repeated administration of GnRH to such patients does not enhance the LH or FSH response, indicating impaired functional residual capacity of the gonadotrophs. With isolated FSH deficiency, the LH response to GnRH is normal while the FSH response is impaired or absent.

In patients with gonadotropin deficiency of hypothalamic origin, the LH and FSH responses to GnRH may also be normal, diminished, absent, or even exaggerated. LH responses are usually absent in patients with congenital or prepubertal GnRH defi-

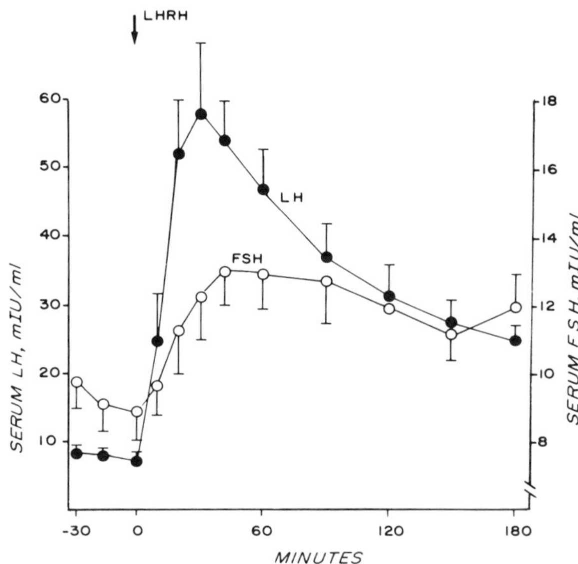

FIGURE 8-12 Plasma LH and FSH responses to GnRH (250 μg IV) in normal men. The peak response of LH is greater and occurs earlier than that of FSH. LH (but not FSH) responses in normal women are affected by the stage of the menstrual cycle, with the greatest responses occurring at the time of ovulation. (*Modified from Snyder P et al: J Clin Endocrinol Metab 41:938, 1975.*)

ciency, whereas in those with adult-onset disorders, the response is intact. The LH response pattern in particular appears to be in part a reflection of endogenous GnRH secretion, and repeated injections of GnRH frequently restore a previously diminished or absent response to normal. Thus, while an impaired or absent LH and FSH response to GnRH cannot be used to distinguish hypothalamic from pituitary disease, the appearance of a response after repeated injections of GnRH indicates an intact pituitary functional reserve and points to the hypothalamus as the cause of the disorder.[257]

Evaluation of the hypothalamic component of the neuroendocrine regulation of gonadotropin secretion involves assessment of the negative and positive feedback effects of estrogen in women and the negative feedback effects of estrogen and testosterone in men. Clomiphene citrate, a weak estrogen, is capable of competing with estradiol for binding to receptors in the uterus, pituitary, and hypothalamus. When administered to adult women with nearly normal estrogen levels, clomiphene acts as an estrogen antagonist and stimulates the release of endogenous GnRH, resulting in gonadotropin secretion. If gonadotropin secretion has been shown to be intact (by a normal response to GnRH), the absence of a gonadotropin response to clomiphene (100 mg per day for 5 days) indicates an impaired hypothalamic response to interruption of the negative feedback effect of estrogen.

The positive feedback effects of estrogen, which can be demonstrated by elevating estradiol levels for at least 24 h (by injection of a long-acting estrogen preparation such as estradiol benzoate or estradiol valerate or by the continuous infusion of estradiol), are followed by a rise in LH but generally not in FSH, presumably mediated by a release of GnRH, which is maximal at 4 to 5 days. The inability of an anovulatory patient with intact gonadotropins to respond normally to exogenous estradiol administration indicates a hypothalamic defect related to the positive feedback effect of estrogen. This defect is characteristically seen in patients with hyperprolactinemia.

In men, estrogens have only inhibitory effects on LH secretion and are of no value as diagnostic agents. Clomiphene, however, is useful as a probe of the negative feedback effect of testosterone. After a dose of 100 or 200 mg per day for 6 to 7 days, LH increases to at least twice basal levels in normal men. Clomiphene is thus useful as a test of the hypothalamic-pituitary axis, provided that endogenous testosterone levels are at least 1 ng/ml.

Growth Hormone

Documentation of GH deficiency is important in children with short stature in whom therapy with exogenous hormone is under consideration. In adults, its importance relates to providing evidence for acquired hypopituitarism, such as that typically occurring with pituitary tumors. Many different methods have been advocated for documenting GH deficiency, though no single one is universally accepted. In children, nonresting levels of GH or those obtained from 60 to 90 min after the onset of sleep are often capable of distinguishing GH-deficient from normal subjects because of the frequent secretory bursts of the hormone. A plasma level of 6 ng/ml or more provides evidence of normal GH secretion. Postexercise GH values of the same magnitude are also useful, as are age-adjusted serum IGF-I levels (see also Chap. 26). In adults, in whom basal levels are lower and secretory bursts are fewer, normal and GH-deficient subjects generally cannot be distinguished without the aid of stimulation tests.

There are two types of stimuli for evaluating GH secretion: GRH, which acts directly on the somatotroph, and agents (insulin, arginine, L-dopa, clonidine, and pyridostigmine) which evaluate the hypothalamic-pituitary axis and probably require the participation of endogenous GRH. The choice of the stimulus is determined by whether the physician wishes to assess pituitary GH reserves or the etiology of unexplained GH deficiency.

GRH is the most reliable stimulus for evaluating pituitary GH secretory capacity. The two forms of this hormone, GRH_{1-44}-NH_2 and GRH_{1-40}-OH, and a GH fragment, GRH_{1-29}-NH_2, are equipotent in humans, and comparable response curves have been observed.[258,259] The intravenous injection of GRH produces a rapid increase in the plasma GH level

(Fig. 8-7), which peaks at 15 to 30 min and is dose-dependent. The most commonly employed dose is 1 μg/kg, which is a maximal stimulus and is unaccompanied by any significant side effects. The response is variable, and peak GH values in normal subjects range from 10 to 100 ng/ml. In patients with hypopituitarism, the response is impaired or absent. In patients with hypothalamic disease, i.e., deficiency of endogenous GRH, GH responses to GRH appear to be intact, though reduced responses are seen in some patients with GH deficiency of unknown cause or long duration.[260] In general, about half of patients with idiopathic GH deficiency exhibit a normal GH response to GRH.[260] At the time of writing, GRH_{1-29}-NH_2 (Sermolin) has been approved for clinical use in the United States.

The most effective indirect stimulus for GH secretion is insulin hypoglycemia, which is described under ACTH, above (Fig. 8-10). GH levels peak at 60 to 90 min and should equal or exceed 10 ng/ml. Approximately 20 percent of normal subjects exhibit a subnormal response, and a second stimulus must be used. The infusion of arginine (0.5 g/kg to a maximum of 30 g) is effective in raising GH to similar levels in 70 percent of normal persons, with a majority of the nonresponders usually being male. Although estrogen pretreatment will enhance the response, it is seldom used for practical reasons. The effects of insulin hypoglycemia and arginine are believed to be mediated in part by inhibition of somatostatin secretion, based on indirect evidence.[157,261] L-Dopa (0.5 g PO) stimulates GH secretion in 60 to 70 percent of normal subjects to a level of at least 6 ng/ml, peaking at 60 to 150 min. Mild to moderate symptoms of nausea and vomiting occur in 15 to 20 percent of subjects because of concomitant stimulation of the emesis center. Clonidine (0.15 mg/m^2 or 25 μg PO), a centrally active $alpha_2$-adrenergic agonist, also stimulates GH secretion.[262,263] The mechanism of clonidine action is stimulation of endogenous GRH release. Pyridostigmine, an acetylcholinesterase inhibitor that enhances cholinergic tone, also stimulates GH secretion, presumably by inhibiting somatostatin.[264] However, its side effects detract from its overall usefulness. Either L-dopa or arginine therefore serves as the most useful second-choice stimulus if no response occurs with insulin. It should be noted that responses are generally absent in obesity, irrespective of whether the stimulus is direct (GRH)[265] or indirect[266] and even in obese children with normal linear growth. They are also impaired in hypothyroidism[267,268] and often are restored to normal by thyroxine treatment.

Prolactin

The lower limit of plasma prolactin values in normal subjects extends to the lowest levels of detectability in many assays. Demonstration of prolactin responsiveness to TRH stimulation is the simplest and most useful method of documenting intact lactotroph function. Prolactin levels increase at least twofold after TRH and peak at the same time as TSH levels (15 to 30 min), permitting both hormones to be assessed by use of the same stimulus. An alternative method of testing prolactin reserves is by injection of metoclopramide (10 mg IV), a D_2-dopaminergic receptor antagonist which is almost completely excluded from the CNS by the blood-brain barrier. Peak levels of 100 ng/ml or more are seen at 30 to 60 min in normal subjects. An impaired response is seen in pituitary disease with diminished lactotrophs, pituitary tumors, and disorders of neuroendocrine regulation (see Chap. 7); thus, the test is not particularly helpful in the differential diagnosis. The prolactin response to insulin hypoglycemia also provides an index of the hypothalamic-pituitary axis.[269]

Combined Pituitary Hormone Testing

All four of the hypothalamic releasing hormones (TRH, GnRH, CRH, and GRH) can be injected simultaneously without altering the individual pituitary hormone responses.[270] This reduces substantially the time and effort required to assess pituitary function. Alternatively, insulin hypoglycemia may be combined with TRH and GnRH in a single injection to provide slightly different information, as was indicated above.

Treatment

Replacement therapy in hypopituitarism must be considered for each individual hormone, and the treatment goals must be specifically defined. The therapeutic use of anterior pituitary hormones is currently limited to GH for correcting problems of growth retardation and gonadotropins for inducing ovulation or spermatogenesis, as is described below. The use of hypothalamic releasing hormones and/or their synthetic analogues is currently restricted to GnRH for hypothalamic hypogonadism (including anovulation and infertility), though GnRH agonists and antagonists are effective in treating precocious puberty and non-pituitary-related disorders (endometriosis and prostatic carcinoma). GRH is also currently under investigation as therapy for certain types of GH deficiency. For the most part, however, therapy consists of replacing the target organ secretions by the use of natural hormones or synthetic analogues.

ACTH

ACTH deficiency is treated with adrenal glucocorticoids. Either cortisone (25 mg per day) or hydrocortisone (20 mg per day) given as a divided dose will provide adequate therapy for most patients under normal conditions. Because of the partial independence of aldosterone secretion from the pituitary, supplemental mineralocorticoid therapy is unnecessary. As a result, the physician can nearly always use prednisone (5 mg per day), which is considerably less expensive, instead of the natural glucocorticoids. Occasionally patients require full glucocorticoid replacement therapy (37.5 mg cortisone or 7.5 mg prednisone), though many will develop signs of steroid overdose (Cushing's syndrome) at these doses. Under conditions of stress (acute febrile illness, moderate to severe trauma, etc.), the dose should be increased two- to threefold and then gradually tapered as the stress subsides. If the patient is unable to retain oral medication, injectable hydrocortisone must be used (50 mg IM or IV q 6 h). The acute treatment of all severely ill hypopituitary patients requires the same dose of hydrocortisone (100 to 300 mg per day) that is used for primary adrenal insufficiency. Since some patients with hypopituitarism of long duration exhibit euphoric or even psychotic behavior with full replacement or larger doses of glucocorticoids, the minimal dose necessary should be used. Patients should take with them a supply of injectable steroids for emergency treatment if they plan to travel in areas where good medical care may not be immediately available. Preoperatively, patients should be treated as though primary adrenal insufficiency were present: hydrocortistone hemisuccinate 50 mg IM q 6 h before surgery and continuing through the immediate postoperative period, followed by a gradual tapering to maintenance by the second or third day.

The decision to treat a patient with glucocorticoids should be based on a low basal cortisol level or on signs or symptoms of adrenal insufficiency associated with normal cortisol levels but an absent or impaired response to stimulation. A more difficult decision relates to patients with partial ACTH deficiency without signs or symptoms in the nonstressed states. With adequate education, many patients in this category do not need maintenance glucocorticoid replacement and require therapy only in times of stress. Good medical practice dictates that these patients in particular, as well as all patients on maintenance glucocorticoid therapy, wear an appropriate medical identification tag.

The response to therapy is quite rapid and often dramatic, and many patients will recognize only in retrospect their malaise and weakness before therapy. The initiation of glucocorticoid therapy may also permit the clinical appearance of diabetes insipidus, manifested by polyuria and polydipsia. Treatment of diabetes insipidus is discussed in Chap. 9.

TSH

Treatment of patients with TSH deficiency is similar to that of patients with primary hypothyroidism. The indications for treatment are not based primarily on the TSH reserve, since patients with absent or impaired TSH responses to TRH may have normal serum thyroxine levels. Rather, they relate to the presence of a decreased serum thyroxine. The preferred treatment is with L-thyroxine, 0.10 to 0.125 mg per day, though in occasional patients an even lower dose may suffice. The clinical assessment of the patient, supplemented at appropriate intervals by measurement of serum thyroxine levels, is used to establish the appropriate dose. In this condition, unlike primary hypothyroidism, the measurement of plasma TSH is of no value.

It is most important to correct overt adrenal insufficiency before the institution of thyroid hormone therapy, and patients with partial adrenal insufficiency may require glucocorticoid replacement therapy after thyroid hormone replacement is started. In severe or long-standing hypothyroidism, therapy should be initiated with a small dose of thyroxine (0.05 mg per day) and increased slowly until a maintenance dose is achieved. Long-term maintenance with triiodothyronine is not recommended, because its shorter biological half-life will result in the earlier appearance of symptoms of thyroid deficiency if therapy is omitted.

LH and FSH

Restoration of gonadal function requires consideration of two components: gonadal steroid replacement and treatment of infertility. These subjects are considered briefly here and discussed in greater detail in Chaps. 16 and 17.

Women

In premenopausal women, estrogen replacement therapy is indicated for many reasons, including the maintenance of secondary sex characteristics, i.e., breast size and vaginal and vulvar turgor and lubrication; reduction of the risk factors for osteoporosis and coronary artery disease; and preservation of a sense of well-being. A variety of estrogenic preparations can be used, including ethinyl estradiol 5 to 20 μg per day, conjugated estrogens (Premarin) 0.625 to 1.25 mg per day, and an estradiol transdermal patch (Estraderm), which delivers 50 to 100 μg per day of the hormone. The lowest possible dose which produces the desired clinical effects should be used. Because of the occasional development of cystic breast changes and, more important, the frequent breakthrough bleeding that occurs with continuous estrogen therapy, the hormone should be given for only 20 to 25 days each month and should be accompanied on the last 5 to 10 days by a progestational agent such as medroxyprogesterone acetate 5 to 10 mg per day, which will induce menstrual bleeding and prevent endometrial hyperplasia. Alternatively, one of the oral contraceptive preparations containing no more than the equivalent of 25 μg estradiol per day may be used. It is not known whether the increased risks of thromboembolism, hyperlipidemia, and carbohydrate intolerance associated with the use of oral contraceptives by normal women also occur in hypopituitary patients. However, the benefits of restoring normal physiologic function in these women warrant the use of replacement estrogen therapy. It is still controversial whether the advantages of replacement therapy persist after the time of the expected menopause, i.e., mid- to late forties. The possible mitigating effects of progestational agents on those of estrogen are also not fully resolved. The potential risks (endometrial carcinoma) and benefits (diminished rate of bone loss and clinically significant osteoporosis and reduced coronary heart disease) should be frankly discussed with the patient in order to make an appropriate decision (see also Chap. 25).

Although dyspareunia and diminished satisfaction from sexual activity in hypopituitary women, attributable to local tissue changes, are usually corrected by estrogen therapy, the decreased libido due to the absence of adrenal androgens may not be. Libido can be restored by the injection of a small dose of a long-acting androgen such as testosterone enanthate, 50 mg every 1 to 2 months, or by orally active fluoxymesterone, 5 to 10 mg once or twice weekly. The lowest effective dose should be used to avoid the development of hirsutism. Inquiry regarding the patient's libido is important, since this information may not be volunteered and the patient may believe that no treatment is available.

Restoration of fertility is possible in a high percentage of gonadotropin-deficient women. In many patients with gonadotropin deficiency of hypothalamic etiology, clomiphene citrate therapy results in ovulation. If this is unsuccessful, GnRH administered every 3 h by an intermittent infusion pump will frequently be effective.[271] In the presence of primary pituitary disease, combined therapy with FSH-LH preparations is successful in up to 75 percent of patients. Treatment is initiated with daily injections of menotropins (Pergonal), an FSH-rich preparation of urine from postmenopausal women, to initiate follicular growth and maturation, which is monitored by measurement of plasma estradiol levels. When the estradiol value exceeds 1200 ng/ml (usually after 2 weeks), human chorionic gonadotropin is injected to induce ovulation. In contrast to GnRH therapy, gonadotropin injections may cause ovarian hyperstimulation and superovulation, leading to multiple births.

Men Testosterone replacement therapy in adult males consists of the intramuscular injection of a long-acting testosterone preparation such as testosterone enanthate or cypionate, 200 mg every 3 weeks. Treatment with an oral preparation (fluoxymesterone) is less effective than is injected testosterone because of variation in absorption and is associated with the development of cholangiolitic hepatitis in a small percentage of patients. The goal of testosterone therapy is the restoration of full androgenization, which includes beard growth, generalized improvement in muscular strength, libido, and potency. Overdosage is associated with salt and fluid retention leading to edema, excessive sexual stimulation, priapism, nightmares, and occasionally gynecomastia, acne, and overaggressive behavior. The presence of testosterone is required for the development of baldness in a genetically predisposed person, and this may occur in hypopituitary males as a result of therapy. Androgen therapy should be withheld as long as possible in adolescents with growth retardation to avoid premature epiphyseal closure and limitation of potential for further linear growth (see Chap. 26).

Testosterone therapy may need to be given for many months before libido and performance are fully restored, depending on the duration of hypogonadism. In some patients in whom gonadotropin deficiency has developed before puberty, full androgenization may never occur. In other patients, the reverse problem may be seen. With long-standing hypogonadism, psychosocial behavioral changes develop which may pattern a patient's entire lifestyle, including occupation and choice of a marital partner. The changes in libido and generalized behavior patterns which occur in response to replacement therapy can lead to major adjustment problems in both sexual and nonsexual relationships. This possibility must be carefully considered before the initiation of replacement therapy.

The treatment of infertility follows the same principles in men as in women. If the disease is of hypothalamic origin, intermittent therapy with GnRH (2 μg q 2 h) using an infusion pump will frequently result in full androgenic stimulation and spermatogenesis.[272,273] Alternatively, or in patients with gonadotropin insufficiency of pituitary origin, human chorionic gonadotropin (hCG), alone or in combination with menotropins, will produce similar results. In patients with postpubertal onset of hypogonadism, an increase in sperm count occurs with hCG alone, while in those with prepubertal hypogonadism, menotropins must also be used.[274] The presence of prior cryptorchism, however, precludes normalization of the sperm count. Each form of therapy may be required for up to 3 months and possibly longer, and overall success (i.e., induction of fertility) occurs in only about 60 percent of patients in whom sperm counts become normal. It has also been suggested that fertile men who are about to undergo potentially destructive surgery to the hypothalamic-pituitary region consider the advisability of placing sperm in a sperm bank. Stored under the appropriate conditions, sperm can be kept viable for several years.

Growth Hormone

Treatment of GH deficiency is at present limited to children with significant growth retardation before the age of long-bone epiphyseal closure, which occurs at puberty. This consists primarily of classic idiopathic GH deficiency but recently has been expanded on an investigational basis to children with Turner syndrome, chronic renal failure, and osteogenesis imperfecta. In adults, there is considerable interest in the possible therapeutic efficacy of GH in patients with GH deficiency, obesity, or severe catabolism associated with burns; patients receiving parenteral nutrition; and in aging.[236,237,275–278]

At the present time, however, such use must still be considered experimental. Two forms of therapy for GH deficiency are currently available—GH and GRH—although only GH has been approved in the United States. In addition, IGF-I is currently being investigated as a potential alternative agent. The one condition in which IGF-I is uniquely effective is in children with GH receptor mutations who are GH-resistant (Laron-type dwarfism).[145]

Until mid-1985 the only available form of GH used in therapy was the natural hormone extracted from pituitaries removed at autopsy. This was discontinued because of the discovery of several cases of Creutzfeldt-Jakob disease, a degenerative and invariably fatal CNS disease related to kuru and believed to be attributable to the prion particle, in children who received pituitary GH during the 1970s.[279] At about the same time, recombinant DNA–derived GH became available and today is the only form of the hormone in use. Two preparations are currently available, one of which, methionine-GH, contains a single amino acid carboxyl-terminal extension. The two are equipotent and equally efficacious. The dose in children with idiopathic GH deficiency is 0.2 to 0.3 mg/kg on a weekly basis, given in divided daily injections. In other forms of short stature, such as Turner syndrome, larger doses are required (see Chap. 26). A major controversy exists concerning the use of GH therapy in children with short stature who show only minimal or no GH deficiency on testing. Short-term studies confirm the enhancement of growth, though long-term effects are unknown, the ethical issues have been fiercely debated, and a consensus has not been reached.

Since many children with GH deficiency are believed to have adequate stores of GH but lack an appropriate releasing mechanism, it is anticipated that as many as half may be responsive to therapy with GRH.[280,281] The route of administration (subcutaneous or intranasal), the dose required, and the possible use of GRH analogues are currently under active investigation.

More recently, a synthetic GH-releasing hexapeptide (GHRP-6), which is an enkephalin-like analogue, has been shown to stimulate GH release and to act synergistically with GRH.[167] The potential utility of this peptide and an even more recently described nonpeptide GH-releasing agent that is orally active[282] requires further study.

The potential value of GH in adult hypopituitary patients who receive thyroid, adrenal, and gonadal replacement therapy is an area of great interest. Several studies in adult hypopituitary subjects and endocrinologically intact elderly subjects have reported increases in nitrogen retention, improved muscle performance, and an enhanced sense of well-being.[236,237,276,283] It remains to be determined whether such therapy is justified on the basis of the cost/benefit ratio, particularly when the issue of enhancement of the quality of life is considered.

GH has also been subject to abuse in muscle-building programs and among athletes. The relative difficulty in detecting its use has helped it supplant anabolic steroids in such arenas. Its enhancement of athletic performance is unproven, and its potential side effects, as described in the section on acromegaly, below, justify strong condemnation of this practice.

Prolactin

The unavailability of recombinant DNA–derived human prolactin has precluded the therapeutic use of this hormone in humans for investigational purposes. With the exception of an absence of postpartum lactation, disorders of prolactin deficiency, if they exist, are currently unrecognized. In women with impaired postpartum lactation, repeated administration of TRH has been reported to enhance milk production.[284]

PITUITARY TUMORS

Classification

Tumors of the pituitary gland can be classified by histologic characteristics and by functional activity. Both are important and reflect the spectrum of problems to be considered in evaluating a patient with a suspected pituitary tumor. There are two major histologic types of pituitary tumor: adenomas and craniopharyngiomas. In addition, tumors originating in the parasellar region, such as meningiomas, optic nerve gliomas, and sphenoid wing sarcomas, as well as metastatic tumors can be found within the sella turcica and must be differentiated from primary pituitary tumors. Although tumors originating within the pituitary can be locally invasive, truly malignant tumors are rare, and concern over a possible malignant tumor need not influence decisions concerning diagnosis and treatment. Pituitary tumors can also be divided into those associated with hormone hypersecretion *(functioning)* and those that are not *(nonfunctioning)*. The relative frequency of each type has changed considerably in the past decade as more functioning tumors have been recognized by measurement of circulating hormone levels and immunohistochemical analyses rather than by clinical manifestations. Some tumors may synthesize hormones but, because of alterations in intracellular secretory mechanisms or degradative processes, may not release the hormones into the circulation.[285] Others may synthesize only the portions of a hormone (e.g., the glycoprotein α subunit) which are biologically inactive.[286]

Pituitary Adenomas

Pituitary adenomas originate from one of the adenohypophyseal cell types and make up more than 90 percent of all pituitary neoplasms. They were for many years subdivided into chromophobic (originally synonymous with nonfunctioning) and chromophilic types, the latter being either eosinophilic (associated with acromegaly) or basophilic (associated with Cushing's syndrome). With the recognition that tumor histology frequently varied in different sections of individual tumors, that tumors from patients with acromegaly and Cushing's syndrome were frequently chromophobic, and that prolactin hypersecretion was often present in patients with chromophobic tumors, this cytochemical differentiation has ceased to be useful. At present, the significance of a chromophobic appearance in an adenoma is merely that the tumor does not contain recognizable secretion (stored hormone) granules. Thus, the adenoma either is not producing a hormone, is storing a hormone in an altered chemical form which does not stain with the techniques used, or, most likely, is secreting the hormone immediately after synthesis without storage. Electron microscopy and immunohistochemical stains have provided evidence to support the latter possibility.

In several large neurosurgical series, pituitary tumors accounted for 6 to 18 percent of all brain tumors,[287,288] and in an unselected autopsy series, microadenomas were found in one-third of patients, with 41 percent revealing immunohistochemical evidence of functional (prolactin) activity.[289]

There is no evidence to suggest that the growth pattern or biological behavior of functioning tumors is different from that of nonfunctioning tumors. Both may grow extremely slowly or may exhibit rapid enlargement. Slow-growing tumors which are nonfunctioning may never produce clinical manifestations and may be detected coincidentally at autopsy or during neuroradiologic investigations for unrelated causes. In a series of 941 pituitary adenomas, over 50 percent were first discovered at autopsy.[290] Rapidly enlarging pituitary tumors are usually recognized because of the consequence of an enlarging intrasellar mass lesion, and the hormone hypersecretion either is incidental or contributes in a minor way to the overall clinical problem. In contrast, a slow-growing functioning pituitary tumor allows for full development of the manifestations of hormone hypersecretion. On the basis of the currently available RIAs for the anterior pituitary hormones, 70 to 80 percent of pituitary adenomas are believed to be functioning tumors, with the majority secreting prolactin.[291] The peak incidence of tumors in most series has been reported to be between 40 and 50 years,[290,292] though with earlier recognition now possible, the age at peak incidence has decreased. Most series consisting of macroadenomas report a similar incidence in men and women, though the majority of prolactin-secreting microadenomas occur in women.

Pituitary adenomas are generally solid tumors. They may on occasion be cystic, with evidence of hemorrhage within the tumor. At times the center of the cyst may communicate with the subarachnoid space and contain CSF, giving rise to an empty sella. Calcification, if present, represents the end stage of organization of a previous hemorrhage and usually occurs in a diffuse pattern.

Craniopharyngiomas

Craniopharyngiomas are benign tumors of congenital origin which may be partly or entirely cystic. Histologically they consist of bands of interwoven epithelium, often similar to tumors of the enamel organ of the teeth. The most superficial cells of the tumor often give rise to micro- or macrocysts, which frequently contain a brown fluid with a high cholesterol content and which develop calcifications in 50 percent of patients. The appearance of the tumor may vary, and it is often difficult to distinguish it from an ependymoma or epidermoid cyst. The tumor grows at a variable rate and may eventually cease to grow entirely. Half the patients develop symptoms during childhood, one-fourth between ages 20 and 40, and the rest later in life.[293] The site of origin for most tumors appears to be in the midline at the upper end of the pituitary stalk, though some originate lower in the stalk and about 15 percent involve the upper part of the anterior lobe and are thus intrasellar (Fig. 8-13). Large tumors push the chiasm upward and displace the hypothalamus and third ventricle. Downward pressure tends to compress the anterior lobe but more frequently results in atrophy of the posterior lobe because of damage to the stalk. Though it was previously believed that the tumor originated from remnants of Rathke's pouch, this has now been questioned because of the infrequency of a primary intrasellar site and the rarity of the tumor along the embryologic migration tract through bone.

Signs and Symptoms

The initial manifestations of pituitary tumors as well as their subsequent clinical features can be divided into three general categories: neuroanatomic, radiologic, and endocrinologic. The following sections are concerned primarily with those manifestations which relate to all pituitary tumors; the individual features of hormone-secreting tumors are considered separately.

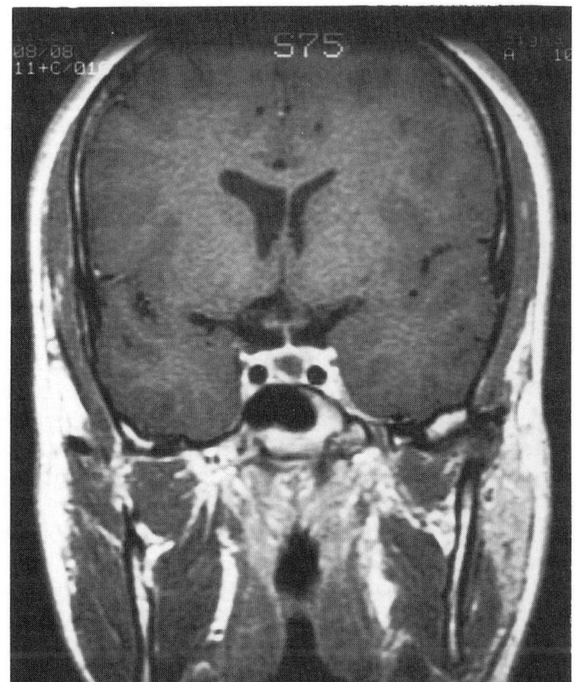

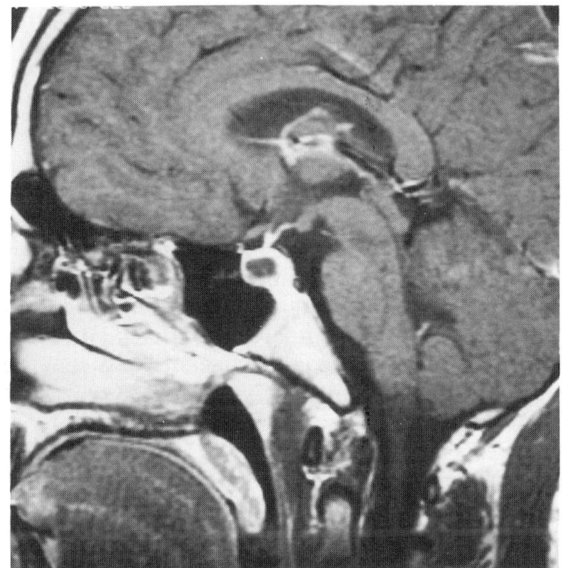

FIGURE 8-13 Coronal (*left*) and midsagittal (*right*) MRI views of an intrasellar craniopharyngioma in a 17-year-old male. The large nonhomogeneous and irregularly shaped tumor occupies more than half the sella. The normal-appearing optic chiasm and pituitary stalk are seen just above the tumor.

The presenting symptoms of pituitary tumors have undergone a marked change in distribution frequency during the past 2 decades as refinements in neuroradiologic procedures and pituitary hormone function testing have permitted their progressively earlier diagnosis and treatment. For example, whereas nearly 90 percent of patients in a large series of pituitary tumors diagnosed in the 1940s and 1950s exhibited visual disturbances,[292] subsequent series indicate visual abnormalities to be present in only about 25 percent.[294,295] This percentage can be expected to decrease further. Visual field defects are particularly common in craniopharyngiomas and other tumors with suprasellar extension.[296] In contrast, abnormalities in endocrine function, most frequently amenorrhea, decreased libido, or infertility associated with prolactin-secreting pituitary tumors, now represent the most common presenting symptoms, whereas in earlier series only 25 to 35 percent of patients presented in this manner. The accidental discovery of a pituitary tumor during neuroradiologic investigation continues to account for a small percentage of each reported series.

Endocrinologic Manifestations

Two types of endocrine symptoms are observed in patients with pituitary tumors: (1) hypofunction due to destruction of normal adenohypophyseal tissue by tumor compression, interference with the delivery of portal blood, or secondary disturbances in hypothalamic function and (2) hyperfunction due to tumor and/or hyperplasia. The tumors involved in such hyperfunction, primarily GH-, prolactin-, and ACTH-secreting tumors but also TSH- and FSH-secreting tumors, are described below. In addition, a combination of the two types of symptoms may be present, as in hypogonadism secondary to hyperprolactinemia.

The signs and symptoms of endocrine hypofunction were described in the previous section. The most frequent symptoms relate to decreased gonadal function followed by symptoms of adrenal and thyroid insufficiency. The frequency of growth hormone deficiency is intermediate, but unless it occurs before the completion of the growth process, it is of little clinical significance. Posterior pituitary dysfunction (diabetes insipidus) is quite uncommon with pituitary adenomas until the tumor is very large but occurs frequently with craniopharyngiomas or malignant disease metastatic to the pituitary.

Neuroanatomic Manifestations

The increase in size of an intrasellar tumor leads to compression of the surrounding pituitary tissue and pressure on the overlying dura which makes up the diaphragma sellae. This in turn results in headaches which are variable in nature and may be frontal, temporal, or retroorbital in location, generally dull in quality, unassociated with nausea or visual symptoms, unaltered by change in position, and inconsistently relieved by analgesics. With rupture of the dura, the headaches often disappear. Many patients with pituitary tumors have headaches which are not attributable to the tumor and are not relieved by tumor removal. These are most readily differentiated in patients with microadenomas in whom the diaphragma sellae is normal.

Once the tumor has expanded in a suprasellar direction, the first structures encountered are the optic nerves, optic chiasm, or optic tracts. Most commonly it is the optic chiasm on which the tumor exerts its upward pressure, leading to the classic findings of bitemporal hemianopsia. If examined just after chiasmal pressure begins, the patient may exhibit only a superior temporal field defect, and asymmetric changes are frequently seen. With continued expansion of the tumor, visual loss may progress toward complete blindness, and optic atrophy will eventually develop. On occasion, tumor growth occurs primarily anterior to the chiasm, resulting in visual impairment limited to one eye. This is most common with a postfixed chiasm. When the chiasm is fixed anteriorly (prefixed), the pattern of visual field loss will reflect optic tract involvement. Papilledema is uncommon in pituitary adenomas but occurs in 27 percent of craniopharyngiomas.[293] With continued upward expansion of the tumor, symptoms of ventral hypothalamic compression may occur, including temperature fluctuations, hyperphagia, alterations in sleep pattern, and emotional disturbances. With pressure on the third ventricle, internal hydrocephalus may be seen. Rarely, there is compression of the temporal or frontal lobes causing behavioral changes and seizures, midbrain compression resulting in long tract signs, or cerebellar compression. Compression of extrahypothalamic structures occurs more frequently with craniopharyngiomas that have an extrasellar origin than with pituitary adenomas. Expansion of the tumor in a lateral direction may lead to compression of cranial nerves III, IV, and VI as they pass through the cavernous sinus, resulting in ophthalmoplegia and diplopia. Tumor growth in an inferior direction results in rupture of the sellar floor and expansion into the clivus or the sphenoid sinus, which may result in CSF rhinorrhea. The reason for the variations in the direction of tumor growth is not known.

Although tumor growth is usually slow and the progression of symptoms is gradual, the sudden appearance of symptoms in a patient with a pituitary tumor may be caused by hemorrhage into the tumor, or *pituitary apoplexy*.[196] This complication of pituitary tumors was initially recognized only in its most dramatic form and often carried a very poor prognosis. However, it is now apparent that hemorrhage within the tumor mass occurs fairly frequently. In its mildest form it may cause no symptoms whatever or may be associated with the sudden onset of headache of varying intensity which subsides after a few days. The diagnosis is readily established by magnetic resonance imaging. The bleeding often causes rapid expansion of the tumor, which can lead, if intrasellar, to the development of hypopituitarism and, if extrasellar, to sudden visual impairment or blindness. It may also result in the "spontaneous cure" of a hormone-secreting tumor and may result in an empty sella.

The factors responsible for tumor growth are not entirely understood. Large doses of estrogen will cause pituitary tumors to develop in rats, but there is no evidence to date that this occurs in humans. It is important to recognize, however, that tumor growth may be accelerated during pregnancy. Women with evidence of a pituitary tumor who become pregnant have an increased risk of developing the symptoms of chiasmal compression during the second or third trimester. Whether this represents growth of the tumor or only of the normal pituitary is unclear, since the symptoms generally regress spontaneously after parturition. Craniopharyngiomas have on occasion appeared to increase in size in children receiving GH therapy, though a causal relation remains to be proved.

Neuroradiologic Presentation

A small percentage (5 to 15 percent) of pituitary tumors are initially discovered from skull x-rays obtained for unrelated purposes which reveal an enlarged or deformed sella. Because of the sensitivity of magnetic resonance imaging,[297] a greater number of intrasellar abnormalities are currently being recognized, and the differentiation of tumors from other nonneoplastic conditions must be carefully considered. The presence of endocrine symptoms and/or hormonal abnormalities thus becomes of great importance in the differential diagnosis (see below; see also Table 8-7).

Diagnostic Procedures

The diagnostic procedures routinely employed are required to (1) differentiate between pituitary tumors and other parasellar disorders, (2) determine the tumor size and the extent of sellar and extrasellar destruction, (3) define the hormone(s) hypersecreted, and (4) determine the degree of hormone deficiency present. In addition, certain procedures are used to define precisely the anatomic boundaries of the tumor and the extent of distortion of surrounding normal structures to aid in decisions concerning therapy.

The endocrine evaluation of pituitary hypofunction is described elsewhere in this chapter and in Chap. 9, and that of hyperfunction follows in the next section. It is important that an assessment of endocrine function be performed before definitive therapy, since the degree of hypopituitarism may

TABLE 8-7 Presence of Clinical Symptoms in Patients with an Enlarged Sella

Clinical Symptom	Primary Intrasellar Tumor [27], %	Extrasellar Disease [13], %	Empty Sella Syndrome [25], %	Undiagnosed [10], %
Headache	85 (18)	100 (69)	48 (24)	80 (80)
CSF rhinorrhea	0	0	8 (8)	0
Endocrine	67 (67)	54 (31)	0	0
Visual	0	31 (0)	0	0
Asymptomatic	15 (15)	0	44 (44)	20 (20)

Note: The number of patients in each group is indicated in brackets in the column heads; the percentage of patients with each symptom at the time of diagnosis is indicated in each column, followed in parentheses by the percentage of patients in whom it was a presenting symptom.

Source: Modified from Weisberg et al.[300] This series excluded 22 patients presenting with visual symptoms.

influence the type and extent of therapy. There are circumstances in which delays must be minimized, e.g., in a patient with rapidly deteriorating vision or with other progressive neurologic symptoms which necessitate immediate surgical intervention. Under such circumstances, the patient must be considered panhypopituitary and must be treated with steroids before invasive diagnostic procedures and surgery. However, even in these patients, it is imperative to exclude a prolactin-secreting tumor, since the therapeutic approach in that disorder differs markedly.

Radiographic Evaluation

Initial Studies

The initial radiographic study to be obtained in a patient with a suspected tumor is determined by the degree of suspicion, based on the history and physical examination, and the type of tumor for which the physician is searching. An initial screening study consists of a lateral view of the skull—or possibly a "coned-down" view of the sella. This is the least expensive study and will detect evidence of nearly all large tumors, such as overt enlargement or destruction of the sella (Fig. 8-14). Using a standard lateral view, the upper limit of the anteroposterior diameter, measured as the maximum distance from the anterior concavity of the sella to the anterior rim of the dorsum sellae, is 17 mm and the upper limit of the depth of the pituitary fossa, measured as the greatest distance between the floor to a perpendicular line between the top of the dorsum sellae and the tuberculum sellae, is 13 mm.[298] However, measurement of sellar dimensions provides limited help in the diagnosis of pituitary tumors,[299] since there is generally other evidence of a sellar abnormality when the normal dimensions are exceeded, and sellae obviously abnormal by other criteria frequently have normal dimensions. Assessment of the shape of the sella involves a more subjective approach, and terms such as *bulging* and *ballooning* have been used to indicate the impression of minimal enlargement. None of these changes, however, is pathognomonic of a pituitary tumor. They can be seen with the empty sella syndrome, parasellar masses which have invaded the pituitary fossa, increased intracranial pressure, and, in their mildest forms, in patients with no endocrinologic or neurologic evidence of pituitary disease.

Intrasellar and extrasellar calcifications may also be seen on the lateral view of the sella. The presence of calcification, particularly in the suprasellar region, is highly suggestive of a craniopharyngioma, in which this change occurs in 50 percent of cases. No more than 5 percent of pituitary adenomas are associated with calcification. When seen, calcifi-

FIGURE 8-14 Lateral views of skull, demonstrating an enlarged sella with destruction of the floor and dorsum in a patient with a GH-secreting pituitary tumor. Note also the increased size of the sinuses.

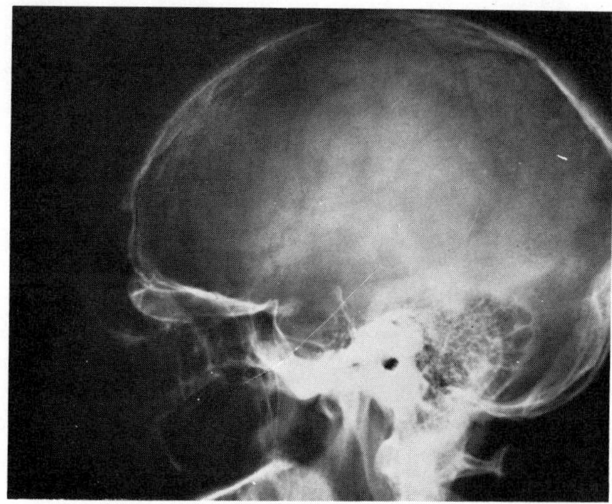

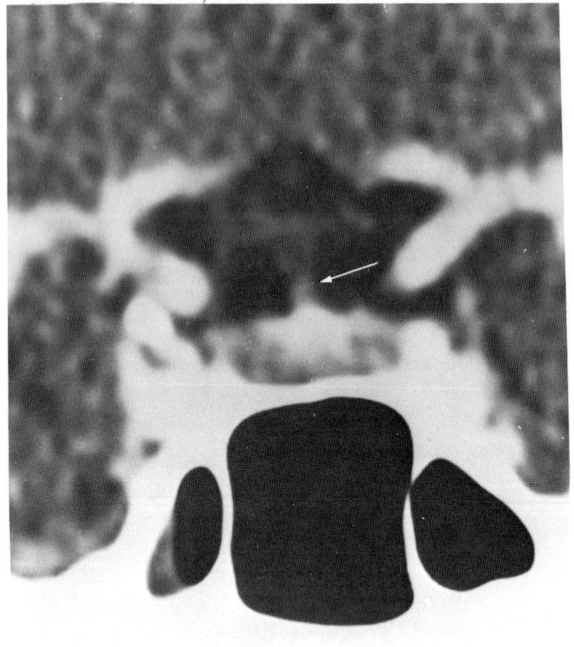

A

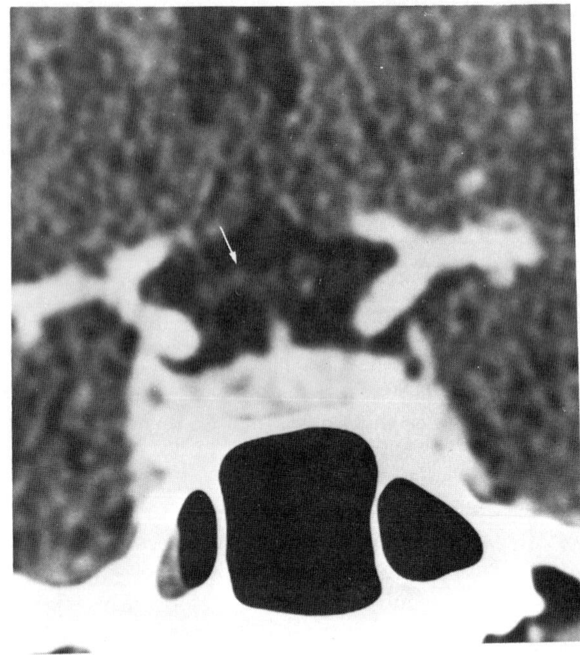

B

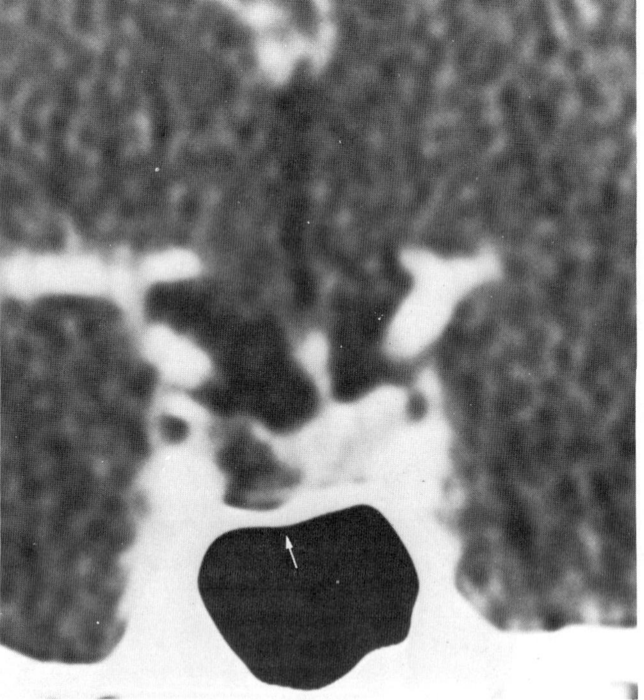

C

FIGURE 8-15 Computed tomography (coronal views) of the normal and abnormal pituitary. (*A*) Dynamic contrast scan of the normal pituitary. Shortly after the injection of contrast material, the pituitary stalk (arrow) and the vascular tuft at its base can be visualized. (*B*) Same, 3 s later. The stalk is still visible, and the entire pituitary appears to be enhanced compared with the brain. Some nonhomogeneity is commonly present. The horizontal structure above the stalk (arrow) is the optic chiasm. (*C*) Pituitary microadenoma. A hypodense area is present in the left side of the pituitary, associated with slight depression (arrow) of the sellar floor. The pituitary stalk is displaced to the contralateral side. (*D*) Pituitary macroadenoma. A large homogeneous mass extending in a suprasellar direction is evident without erosion of the sellar floor. (*E*) Empty sella. Contrast material outlines a rim of pituitary tissue in the inferior portion of the sella (arrow), the remainder of which exhibits low contrast comparable to that of cerebrospinal fluid. (*Courtesy of R. Lukin, University of Cincinnati Hospital.*)

cation is usually intrasellar, almost always curvilinear, and located in the tumor capsule or the wall of a cystic tumor.

Previously, numerous other diagnostic procedures were used for more detailed examination, including hypocycloidal tomography, pneumoencephalography, and carotid angiography. These procedures have been replaced by CT scanning and more recently by magnetic resonance imaging (MRI) (Fig. 8-15).

Computed Tomography

The resolution that is possible with fourth-generation CT scanners permits the recognition of tumors

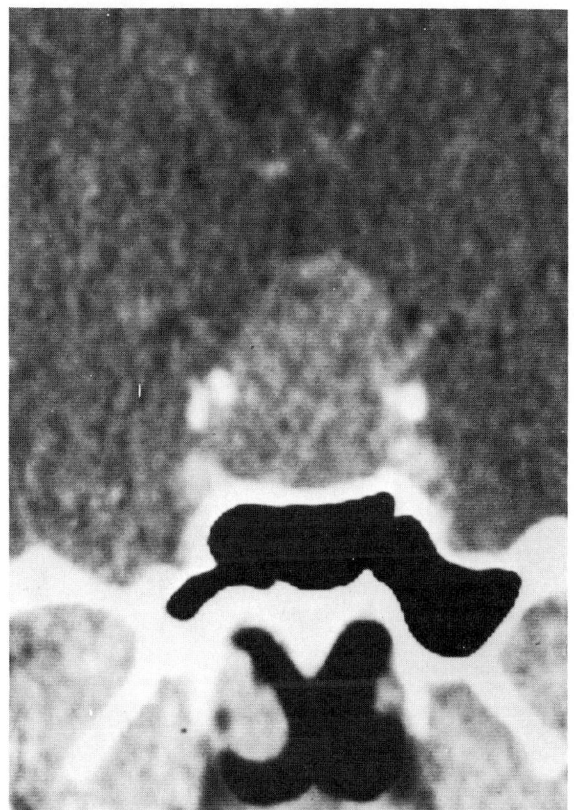

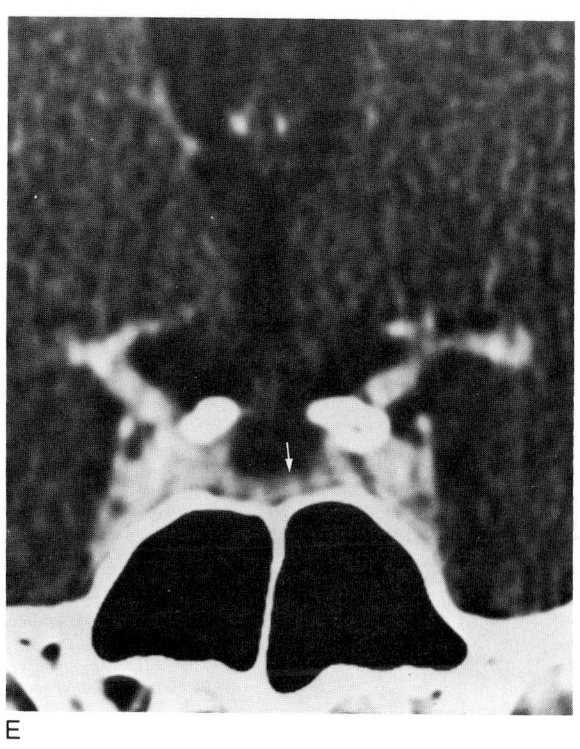

E

D **FIGURE 8-15** *(Continued)*

3 to 4 mm in diameter, and the use of intravenous contrast material with dynamic scanning has further improved diagnostic accuracy. The preferred technique for the evaluation of suspected pituitary tumors is coronal scanning of the pituitary region in conjunction with contrast injection. The pituitary gland is outside the blood-brain barrier and thus is enhanced by the contrast material. Shortly after injection, the portal vessels and the tuft of vessels at the inferior end of the stalk are visualized, and then the contrast material spreads to the entire pituitary. The maximal height of the normal pituitary gland, as determined from coronal scanning of women of childbearing age, has been estimated to be between 9 and 10 mm (95 percent confidence limits),[301,302] though occasional values above 10 mm are encountered. In postpartum women, this value increases to 11.5 mm.[303] In men, the upper limit of normal is 6.0 to 6.5 mm. The upper contour of the pituitary is most commonly flat, but up to 44 percent of normal subjects exhibit convexity, resulting in an upward bulge that was previously believed to be indicative of a tumor.[302] The distribution of contrast material within the gland is usually homogeneous, but nonhomogeneity has been found in 40 to 75 percent of normal subjects. For the diagnosis of a pituitary microadenoma by CT, there should be a region of diminished uptake of contrast in conjunction with evidence of either bony erosion of the sellar floor on the ipsilateral side or lateral displacement of the pituitary vascular tuft or stalk to the contralateral side.[304,305] It is important to emphasize that the early changes of pituitary tumors on CT may be nonspecific, and differentiation from nonneoplastic changes is often impossible by radiographic techniques alone.[306]

CT readily demonstrates extrasellar extension of a pituitary macroadenoma. In the suprasellar region, macroadenomas often appear enhanced in relation to the surrounding brain tissue. The position of the intracranial segments of the carotid artery can be determined, and their displacement, if any, is easily demonstrated. Differentiation of pituitary tumors from carotid aneurysms can usually be made without difficulty.

Diminished density within the sella (comparable to the density of CSF), seen in unenhanced scans, is suggestive of the empty sella syndrome. The diagnosis can be confirmed by repeat scanning after intrathecal injection of metrizamide, though this invasive technique is seldom required. The limitations of CT scanning lie in its resolution and, more important, the dose of radiation administered, specifically that received by the lens during coronal imaging. Repeat studies raise the risk of radiation-induced cataracts. In addition, the use of this procedure during pregnancy in women with suspected tumors should be avoided if possible.

Magnetic Resonance Imaging

Magnetic resonance imaging has added a new dimension to the evaluation of the pituitary gland and its surrounding structures. It is currently the definitive radiologic procedure for identifying pituitary tumors as well as other intrasellar and parasellar lesions (Fig. 8-16). The ability to scan in many different planes, elimination of the requirement that the patient remain in awkward positions during the procedure, and noninterference by dental fillings result in satisfactory imaging in virtually all studies.[297] The absence of any radiation exposure also provides a great advantage for repeated examinations. As with CT, contrast agents have been found to be of great value in increasing the information provided by MRI. The agent currently being used, gadolinium pentetic acid (DTPA), provides a greater visual contrast between the higher signal intensity of a normal pituitary and the less dense signal of a pituitary adenoma in T_1-weighted images.[307] The only contraindication is the presence of aneurysm clips, because of their potential movement, or of other metallic implants, including pacemakers. The major disadvantage of the procedure is its cost, which is generally three times that of a CT scan.

The value of MRI in distinguishing between pitu-

FIGURE 8-16 Magnetic resonance imaging of the pituitary. (*A*) Sagittal view of the normal adult female pituitary. The pituitary appears round (arrow) and isodense with the brainstem and the frontal lobes. The CSF appears black and demarcates the superior surface of the gland. (*B*) In the coronal view, the pituitary appears rectangular and contrasts superiorly with CSF and laterally with the circular low densities (arrows) of the intracavernous carotid arteries. (*C*) Macroadenoma of the pituitary. The right side of the gland reveals a slightly convex enlarged superior surface (arrow) and a pronounced downward enlargement. The higher (lighter) signal beneath the gland represents cancellous bone in the basisphenoid. (*From Kaufman.*[310])

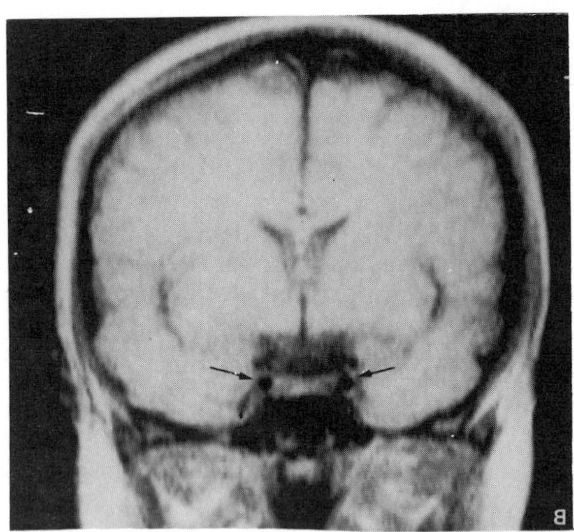

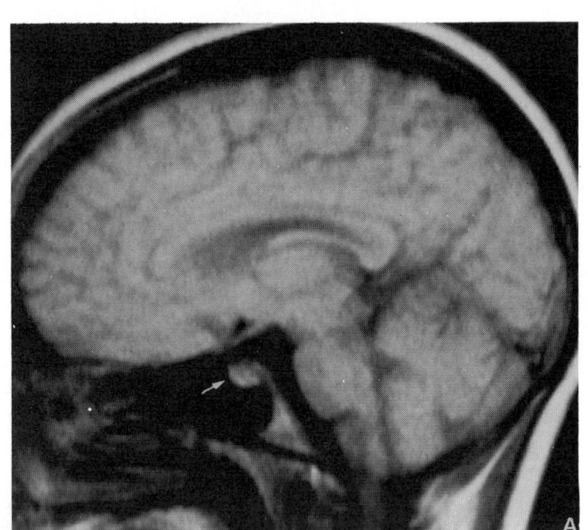

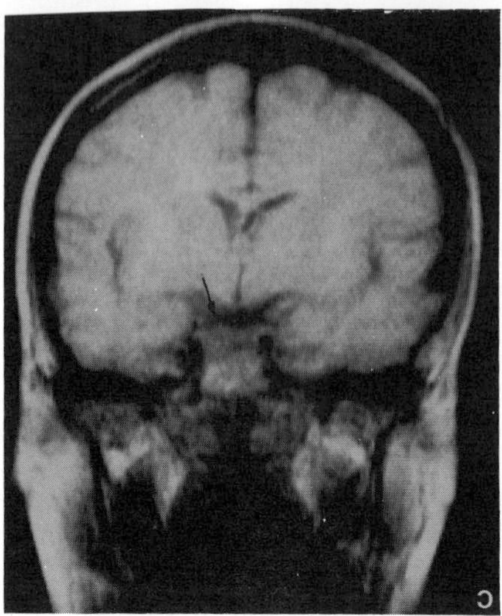

itary tumors and nontumorous dyshomogeneity of the pituitary requires further study, as has been necessary for CT evaluation. At present, specific changes in an "abnormal" pituitary gland which differentiate tumors have not been established, and the need for a careful and complete endocrinologic evaluation is essential to avoid potentially unnecessary therapy.[308] However, the ability to follow the response of tumors to specific therapy and its use as a primary screening procedure in suspected tumors are among the greatest advantages of MRI.

Positive emission tomography (PET) has also been found to be useful in identifying pituitary macroadenomas. While PET is not more sensitive than MRI, positive PET results have been seen in 70 percent of surgically proven microadenomas that were not detected on MRI.[309]

Neuroophthalmologic Studies

Visual Fields

A visual field examination performed at the bedside is a useful screening procedure. Because subtle defects are often missed with this technique, however, all patients with evidence of a suprasellar lesion should have formal visual field testing by perimetry. This procedure is currently performed by an automated method and provides an excellent assessment of both the central and peripheral visual fields. Its reproducibility and sensitivity make it extremely useful in following patients for serial changes (Fig. 8-17).

Though chiasmal compression with bitemporal field defects is the characteristic finding in pituitary tumors with suprasellar extension, this is neither specific for pituitary tumors nor the only change seen. In addition to pituitary tumors, bitemporal field defects may be seen with parasellar tumors, vascular abnormalities, demyelinating plaques in the chiasm, focal (sector) retinitis pigmentosa, adhesive arachnoiditis, and CNS sarcoidosis as well as after irradiation of the chiasm and, rarely, with prolapse of the chiasm into the sella in association with the empty sella syndrome. Similarly, in a patient in whom the chiasm is fixed anteriorly (prefixed) or posteriorly (postfixed), the predominant visual field defect may relate to one eye (optic nerve) or one field (optic tract). Finally, there are occasional patients with atypical field defects (asymmetric or even suggestive of superior pressure) associated with pituitary tumors in whom the defect disappears after removal of the tumor.

The importance of visual field examinations in diagnosing suprasellar extension of pituitary tumors has diminished with the availability of improved radiologic techniques. However, all such patients require evaluation as a baseline for comparison with findings during and after various forms of therapy.

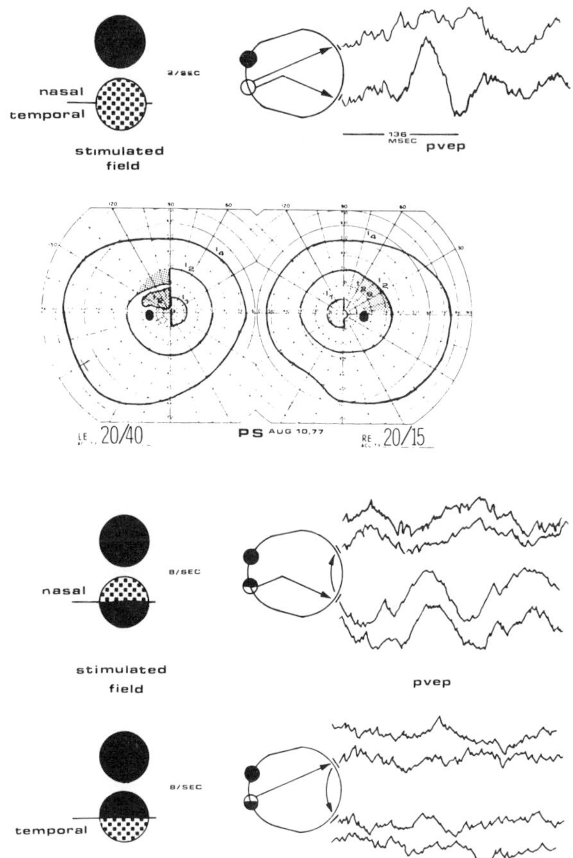

FIGURE 8-17 Visual fields and pattern visual evoked potential (PVEP) in a patient with suprasellar extension of a pituitary tumor. (*Top*) Stimulation of complete visual field (left eye) by a reversing checkerboard pattern. A large PVEP is elicited in the left occipital lobe, which receives input from the nasal field via uncrossed pathways in the chiasm. A low-amplitude distorted PVEP is produced in the right occipital lobe from the temporal field via crossed fibers in the chiasm. (*Middle*) Visual fields of the patient demonstrating low-grade upper temporal defects in both eyes. Fields were normal when all but the smallest targets were used. (*Bottom*) Separate stimulation of nasal and temporal fields of the left eye. A large sinusoidal PVEP occurs in the left hemisphere via uncrossed chiasmal pathways when the nasal field is stimulated. A low-amplitude response 180° out of phase is recorded over the right occipital lobe, which represents either volume conduction within the cranium or conducted activity across the corpus callosum (arrow). Stimulation of the temporal field fails to evoke a response at the right occiput. (*Courtesy of J. Goodwin, Michael Reese Hospital.*)

Visual Evoked Response

Measurement of the visual evoked response is a very sensitive technique for detecting early chiasmal compression by pituitary tumors (Fig. 8-17). The procedure measures the pattern and latency of the electrical response from the occipital cortex produced by photic stimulation of the eyes. Portions of the individual fields can be evaluated selectively, and effects on crossed and uncrossed pathways can be distinguished. With chiasmal pressure, a delayed response and/or a reduction in the response can be seen in crossed compared with uncrossed pathways. This technique is highly reliable and reproducible, although it seldom provides information critical to decision making in the management of patients with pituitary tumors.

Other Studies

Pituitary hormones have been demonstrated in the CSF, and it has been observed that the levels, which normally are lower than in peripheral blood, are increased in patients with primary tumors in the presence of suprasellar extension but not in patients whose tumors are entirely intrasellar in location, irrespective of whether the tumor is functional.[311,312] The single exception to this rule occurs with prolactin-secreting tumors, where increased prolactin levels in the CSF can be present even without suprasellar extension.[313] The elevated CSF hormone concentrations do not appear to be due to a loss of the normal blood-CSF barrier but most likely occur because of direct secretion by the pituitary.[312] Measurement of pituitary hormones in the CSF has not, however, proved to be of particular use in the evaluation of pituitary tumors.

Differential Diagnosis

The diagnosis of a pituitary tumor is made on the basis of two types of evidence: neuroanatomic confirmation of a tumor mass and, if present, hormone or hormone fragment hypersecretion. If both exist, the diagnosis is established. The differential diagnosis of hormonal hypersecretion in the absence of neuroanatomic abnormalities is considered in the following section. If the tumor is hormonally inactive, the frequent lack of specificity of the neuroanatomic studies and clinical findings requires careful consideration of other diagnostic possibilities. It should be emphasized that hypopituitarism, whether partial or complete, in the presence of neuroradiologic evidence of sellar enlargement does not necessarily indicate the presence of a pituitary tumor.

The differential diagnosis of decreased pituitary function has already been presented. That of an enlarged sella is listed in Table 8-8 according to the frequency of occurrence. Among a series of patients with an enlarged sella without visual symptoms, the frequency of primary intrasellar tumors and that of the empty sella syndrome were similar (36 and 33 percent, respectively), extrasellar disease (including both tumors and granulomatous disease) was less

TABLE 8-8 Differential Diagnosis of Nonfunctioning Pituitary Tumors

Diagnosis	Sella Size	Sella Deformity	Pituitary Function	Other Features
Empty sella syndrome	Generally increased	May be present Low-density contents	Almost always normal	Endocrine function testing may show mild abnormalities, obesity and benign intracranial hypertension may occur
Parasellar tumor	Normal or increased	Usually present	Normal or decreased	Headache pattern different; extraocular nerve involvement frequent; visual field defects atypical
Intrasellar aneurysm	Normal or increased	Usually present	Normal or decreased	Throbbing headaches with vomiting may occur; extraocular nerve involvement common; symptoms begin suddenly and are often periodic
Immunologic or granulomatous disease	Increased	May be present	Usually normal except for hyperprolactinemia	Decreased endocrine function, if present, is on hypothalamic basis; diabetes insipidus present
Primary hypothyroidism	Increased	May be present	Usually normal but may be decreased and prolactin may be increased	Elevated TSH and prolactin suppressed by thyroxine
Primary hypogonadism	Increased	May be present	Normal with increased gonadotropins	Gonadotropins suppressed by gonadal steroids
Familial hypopituitarism	Increased	None	Decreased GH and TSH; gonadotropins may also be decreased	Asymptomatic except for hormone deficiency

common (17 percent), and no diagnosis could be established in the remaining 14 percent.[300] With newer neuroradiologic techniques, this percentage has decreased. The other disorders listed in Table 8-8 are relatively uncommon but necessitate markedly different diagnostic and therapeutic considerations.

Empty Sella Syndrome

Empty sella is a term applied to all sellae which exhibit low density on CT (Fig. 8-15*E*) comparable to that of CSF. The use of MRI has made the diagnosis even more simplified, since the actual content of the sella, or the absence thereof, is easily identifiable (Fig. 8-18). It results from an extension of the subarachnoid space into the intrasellar region and is often associated with flattening of the pituitary gland, usually along the posterior portion of the floor and dorsum. The sella turcica is generally, though not invariably, enlarged. The term *primary empty sella syndrome* has been used for cases unassociated with prior surgery, irradiation, or pharmacotherapy for a pituitary tumor. A primary empty sella has been found in up to 24 percent of autopsy series with no history of endocrine disease.[314]

The etiology of the primary empty sella syndrome is multifold. An increasing number of patients with this syndrome are being recognized in childhood, many with single or multiple hormonal deficiencies. In particular, 60 percent of children with GH deficiency unassociated with birth trauma have evidence of a partial empty sella by MRI.[315] In some, associated hypothalamic defects suggest secondary hypopituitarism, though in others, impaired somatotroph development is suspect. Circulating antibodies directed against corticotroph or somatotroph cells have been reported in 75 percent of patients, though it is not known whether they exert a pathogenic role.[316] Patients with Sheehan's syndrome invariably demonstrate a partially or totally empty sella, with the extent of the pituitary remnant inversely related to the degree of hypopituitarism.[317] In most patients, however, it is likely that a preexisting pituitary tumor underwent spontaneous necrosis, leading to loss of volume within the sella. This is consistent with the occasional finding of a coexistent pituitary adenoma, usually a microadenoma. It has also been postulated that an incompletely formed diaphragma sellae permits CSF pressure to be transmitted to the contents of the sella, gradually leading to a herniation of the arachnoid with flattening of the adenohypophysis and remodeling of the sella.

Nearly all patients with primary empty sella syndrome are asymptomatic. Although headache is frequently noted, it is probably unrelated and merely leads to the neuroradiographic procedure and the subsequent diagnostic evaluation. The syndrome is frequently seen in obese women and is associated with an increased frequency of systemic hypertension, benign intracranial hypertension (pseudotumor cerebri), and CSF rhinorrhea, as indicated in Table 8-9.[207,208] Visual disturbances, which are more common in the secondary form of the syndrome (after surgery or radiotherapy), occur in the primary empty sella syndrome and include generalized peripheral field constriction, bitemporal hemianopsia, and papilledema.

FIGURE 8-18 Coronal (*left*) and midsagittal (*right*) MRI views of an empty sella. The signal intensity of the sella is that of the cerebrospinal fluid directly above it, with the exception of a very thin rim of tissue at the sellar floor, which is depressed. The optic chiasm can be seen to be retracted (prolapsed) into the sella.

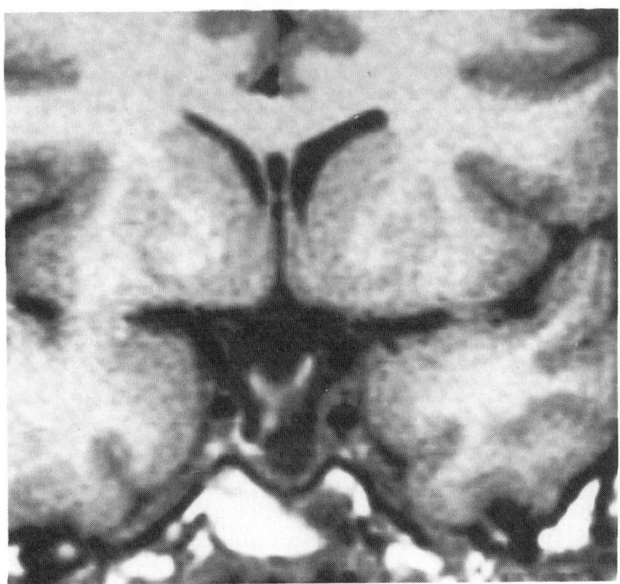

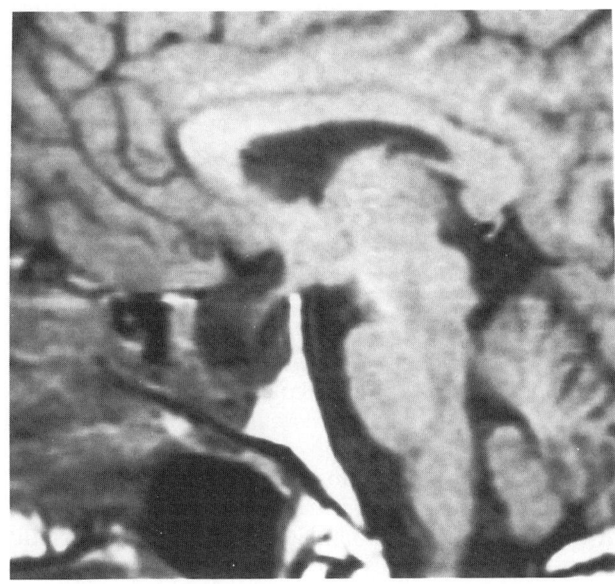

TABLE 8-9 Features Commonly Associated with the Primary Empty Sella Syndrome

Feature	Frequency, %
Female sex	83.7
Obesity	78.4
Systemic hypertension	30.5
Benign intracranial hypertension (pseudotumor cerebri)	10.5
CSF rhinorrhea	9.7

Source: Modified from Jordan et al.[208]

The sella is usually symmetrically enlarged or ballooned (84 percent of patients) and may also be deformed (42 percent), most commonly showing a straightening of the dorsum with demineralization and less frequently showing asymmetry of the floor and erosion of the clinoids. The bony changes can be indistinguishable from those of pituitary tumors.

Endocrine function tests in the majority of patients with the primary empty sella syndrome are normal,[318] though hyperprolactinemia is common, and occasional patients exhibit diminished TSH and gonadotropin reserves, ACTH deficiency, and, rarely, panhypopituitarism and diabetes insipidus.[318–320]

The diagnosis of the primary empty sella syndrome is usually made during the course of a work-up for a pituitary tumor. It should be suspected in a patient with an enlarged sella who has no clinical symptoms or minimal symptoms and normal endocrine function. Most such patients can be followed without the need for invasive procedures, and the symptoms of headache frequently disappear without therapy. However, the presence of an empty sella does not exclude the coexistence of a pituitary tumor. GH-, prolactin-, and ACTH-secreting tumors have all been reported in patients with the primary empty sella syndrome.[207,321,322] Fortunately, the diagnostic evaluation of such patients is guided by the hypersecretory features, and the presence of the empty sella syndrome, if discovered preoperatively, should not alter the planned therapy.

Parasellar Diseases

A number of diverse disorders arising in the parasellar area are associated with signs and symptoms which mimic those of pituitary tumors. They include inflammatory and granulomatous diseases (sarcoidosis, eosinophilic granuloma, arachnoiditis), degenerative disorders (aneurysms), and neoplasms (meningiomas, gliomas, sarcomas, hamartomas, and rarely metastatic tumors). By invading the sella, these disorders can cause enlargement and deformity of the bony structure and varying degrees of hypopituitarism in addition to their suprasellar manifestations. They must be distinguished from primary pituitary tumors if appropriate therapy is to be provided.

Suprasellar tumors usually present with predominantly neurologic manifestations: severe headache often associated with nausea and vomiting, asymmetric visual disturbances, papilledema, and extraocular nerve involvement. Tumors of the hypothalamus or third ventricle often produce symptoms of hypothalamic dysfunction and increased intracranial pressure.

In parasellar tumors, unlike pituitary tumors, endocrine manifestations often follow rather than precede the neurologic symptoms. Radiologic manifestations of suprasellar tumors frequently provide clues to their origin, e.g., suprasellar calcification in craniopharyngiomas and meningiomas and erosion of the anterior clinoids with an otherwise intact sella. These manifestations are readily identified on MRI.

Aneurysms of the internal carotid artery siphon or the anterior communicating artery can expand into the sella and, like suprasellar tumors, mimic a pituitary tumor.[322a] Headaches, which are frequently throbbing and fluctuate in severity, are the predominant symptoms, and involvement of cranial nerves III, IV, and VI is also common. The diagnosis can be established by MRI.

Sarcoidosis and other granulomatous diseases affect primarily the hypothalamus, though pituitary involvement may also occur, leading to increased sellar size. Giant-cell granulomatous hypophysitis, a disorder localized to the pituitary, cannot be distinguished from a pituitary adenoma except by tissue examination.[323] Patients may exhibit varying degrees of hypopituitarism and/or hyperprolactinemia.

Pituitary Enlargement Associated with Other Endocrine Diseases

The presence of long-standing primary hypothyroidism or primary hypogonadism has been associated with the development of sellar enlargement, increased TSH or gonadotropin secretion, and in some patients, TSH-secreting pituitary tumors.[20,21,324] As can be shown in laboratory animals, long-standing target organ insufficiency results in hyperplasia of the tropic hormone-producing cells, leading eventually to tumor formation. Occasionally there is some overlap in hormone hypersecretion in that long-standing juvenile hypothyroidism has been associated with premature puberty. It is extremely important to recognize this syndrome, though it is quite uncommon, in its early stages, since the hypersecretion and hyperplastic changes can be reversed with appropriate therapy, i.e., thyroxine or gonadal steroids (Fig. 8-19).

A syndrome of familial hypopituitarism involving growth hormone, TSH, and possibly gonadotropin secretion associated with an enlarged sella has also been described.[325] The basis for the enlarged but not

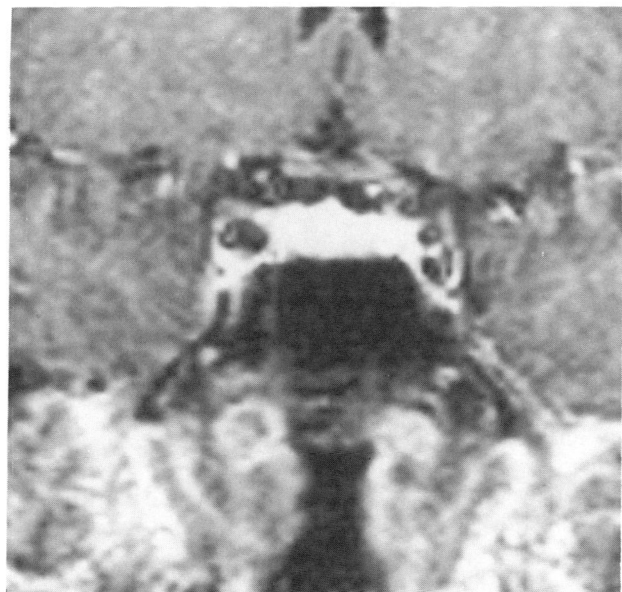
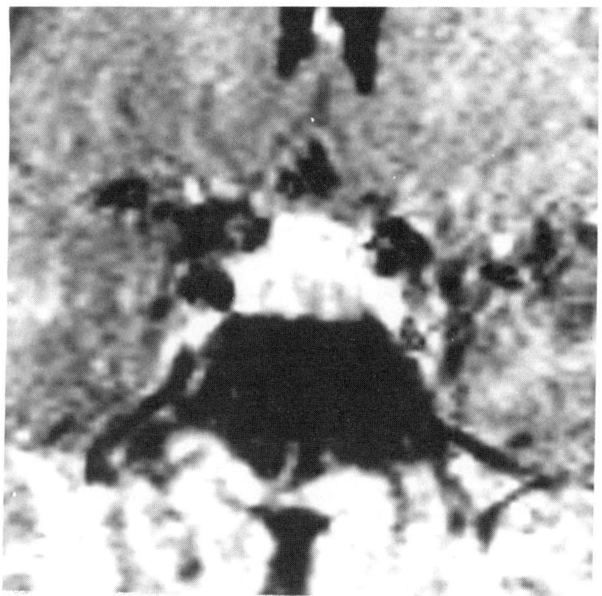

FIGURE 8-19 Coronal MRI views of the sellar region, demonstrating massive thyrotroph hyperplasia resembling a pituitary tumor (*left*) in a patient with long-standing primary hypothyroidism and a plasma TSH of > 400 μU/ml. The pituitary mass shows marked suprasellar extension with encroachment on the optic chiasm. After 4 months of thyroxine treatment and normalization of the plasma TSH level, the pituitary size returned to normal (*right*).

deformed sella is not known, and the possibility of tumor formation has not been excluded, since surgical exploration has not been carried out in the patients described.

Therapy

Therapy for nonfunctional pituitary tumors is necessary to prevent or limit loss of pituitary function and the consequences of suprasellar extension on the optic chiasm and hypothalamus. Although an occasional patient with a nonfunctioning pituitary tumor will respond to bromocriptine,[326] most will not.[327] The routine use of this agent is therefore not indicated, and the choice of therapy is between surgery and irradiation.

Surgery

Pituitary surgery has for many years been the conventional therapy for nonfunctioning pituitary tumors. The frontal approach remains the technique of choice for most parasellar tumors and craniopharyngiomas arising outside the sella and for primary pituitary tumors with extensive suprasellar extension, particularly when they are separated from the intrasellar portion by a narrow neck. Tumors that have encircled the optic nerves can also be removed only by this approach. The operative mortality of frontal surgery has ranged from 1.2 percent to 10 percent, depending on the type of cases included.[328,329]

Transsphenoidal microsurgery, which was popularized by Guiot[330] and Hardy,[331] has been the procedure of choice during the past two decades for all but very large tumors. It is associated with a mortality rate below 1 percent.[332] Tumors with moderate suprasellar extension can be removed transsphenoidally, and even tumors which require a frontal approach are often removed in a two-stage procedure, with the intrasellar portion of the tumor excised by the transsphenoidal route after removal of the suprasellar portion. There are no absolute contraindications to the transsphenoidal approach, though an inadequately pneumatized sinus and anatomic variations in the position of the carotid siphon can make the procedure more difficult.

The preoperative endocrine evaluation of patients is helpful in deciding on the extent of the surgical resection to be performed. If the patient has intact target organ function, a somewhat more conservative approach is indicated to preserve the remaining pituitary hormone-secreting tissue. If, however, hypopituitarism is documented preoperatively, there is little reason to be concerned with preservation of the contents of the sella. In practice, a small rim of adenohypophyseal tissue at the periphery of the sella is often sufficient to maintain pituitary function.

It is essential to provide steroid coverage for the surgical period even in patients with an intact pituitary-adrenal axis because of the possibility that more normal tissue will be removed than is anticipated preoperatively. Parenteral hydrocortisone, 50 mg q 6 h, beginning the morning of surgery or, if the patient is hypopituitary, at least 24 h before surgery, provides adequate coverage, and the dosage is rapidly tapered postoperatively over a 3- to 4-day period. Pituitary function should be evaluated in the postoperative period to assess the need for replacement therapy.

Postoperatively, the patient must be carefully observed for the development of diabetes insipidus, particularly since an obtunded patient may not perceive thirst. Polyuria and increasing plasma osmolality commonly occur during the immediate postoperative period if there has been even mild trauma to the pituitary stalk. Persistence of these findings beyond the first 48 h usually indicates destruction of the stalk or posterior pituitary and some permanent impairment of function. However, most patients have clinical recovery. In some patients, a recovery phase occurs which is followed by permanent return of symptoms. Although infrequent, delayed recovery of posterior pituitary function can be observed for up to at least 1 year postoperatively. The recovery period has been attributed to the release of vasopressin from degenerating posterior pituicytes. Because the course of events during the first few postoperative days is unpredictable, fluid balance must be monitored carefully and the patient must be treated with desmopressin (DDAVP) 1 to 2 μg IM or aqueous vasopressin 5 U IM as necessary. A full discussion of the treatment of diabetes insipidus is provided in Chap. 9.

If rhinorrhea develops after transsphenoidal surgery, a glucose oxidase-impregnated strip (e.g., Dextrostix) should be used to determine whether the fluid is CSF. Postoperative CSF rhinorrhea frequently subsides spontaneously within 7 to 10 days. If it does not, surgical repair of the defect in the floor of the sella is required.

Radiation Therapy

As an alternative to surgical excision of pituitary adenomas, a variety of radiotherapeutic procedures have been used. Patients considered to be candidates for radiotherapy are those without or with only limited suprasellar extension. In the presence of marked visual field defects, the use of external radiation carries an increased risk of further visual impairment because of the initial inflammatory response which occurs within the tumor. In addition, a larger field of radiation is required for tumors with marked suprasellar extension, leading to increased risk of damage to surrounding neural structures.

The dose of radiation currently used for most patients is 4500 to 5000 rad, which is an effective tumoricidal dose and is less than the 8000 to 9000 rad used to destroy normal pituitary tissue. The therapy is given in multiple divided doses with rotating ports and usually produces only minimal side effects, with little or no hair loss. Long-term follow-up of patients receiving such therapy, however, reveals that up to 25 percent develop at least partial hypopituitarism, and the incidence is dose-dependent.[333,334]

Conventional irradiation employing high-energy sources (supervoltage) is the most commonly employed procedure. Stereotaxic implantation of ^{90}Y pellets was initially found to be an effective alternative, but the frequency of complications, including improper placement of pellets and CSF rhinorrhea, led to discontinuation of the procedure. Heavy-particle (proton beam and alpha particle) irradiation is also an effective technique but is currently available in only the few locations with a cyclotron.[335–337] The dose can be administered within a few hours and produces results at least comparable with and possibly better than those of conventional irradiation. Neurologic complications, including oculomotor nerve palsies, visual field defects, and temporal lobe necrosis, are uncommon today because of increased precision in directing the therapeutic beam. Pituitary function, at least in the short term, is preserved in 80 to 85 percent of patients.

A combination surgical-radiation technique known as the "gamma knife" has recently been used successfully for the treatment of pituitary tumors.[338] Long-term follow-up of patients treated in this manner is still needed to compare the therapeutic efficacy and complications of this technique with those of conventional irradiation.

Craniopharyngiomas, unlike chromophobe adenomas, were initially considered to be radioresistant tumors. However, there are numerous reports of the efficacy of postoperative irradiation,[339,340] and most patients are now being treated in this manner.

Factors Relating to the Choice of Therapy

Many patients with pituitary tumors are candidates for either surgical or radiation therapy as the primary treatment. The major advantages of surgery are (1) the immediate results, which are at times necessary in terms of visual symptoms and hormone hypersecretion (discussed below), and (2) the ability to obtain a tissue diagnosis and treat effectively tumors which are relatively radioresistant (e.g., cystic tumors and craniopharyngiomas). The disadvantages of surgery relate to the rare operative mortality and occasional morbidity, consisting primarily of damage to the frontal lobe, optic nerves, or pituitary stalk; pituitary hemorrhage; infection; and, particularly with the transsphenoidal procedure, CSF rhinorrhea.

Radiotherapy avoids the acute surgical complications and is a far simpler procedure for the patient. The disadvantages of radiotherapy include (1) unsuccessful outcome in the occasional patient with a radioresistant tumor (some radiotherapists insist on a histologic diagnosis before therapy), (2) slow response, coupled with the risk of acute swelling of the tumor, (3) occasional occurrence of pituitary apoplexy after therapy, (4) very infrequent episodes of damage to surrounding neural tissue, and (5) long-term development of hypopituitarism as a result of irradiation of normal adenohypophyseal tissue. Both surgery and radiotherapy share the problem of the occasional development of an empty sella syndrome with visual disturbances caused by prolapse of the optic chiasm.

The major determining factors in the treatment of nonfunctioning pituitary tumors which meet the criteria for treatment by either modality relate to the long-term results with respect to preservation and/or restoration of vision, the maintenance of endocrine function, and the frequency of recurrence. Although most series do not distinguish between functioning and nonfunctioning pituitary tumors, the recurrence rates after surgery and radiotherapy appear to be similar.[340,341] It is encouraging that the recurrence rates reported in the past few years have been lower than those of one or two decades earlier for both procedures. It is also important to recognize, however, that the diagnostic criteria, therapeutic techniques, and posttherapy evaluation methods vary enormously among reports; thus, the patient populations are in many respects not comparable. Nevertheless, the prognosis with respect to improvement of visual symptoms and recurrence appears excellent for most patients with other than extremely large pituitary tumors.

The relative frequency of hypopituitarism as a consequence of surgery or of pituitary macroadenomas (> 10 mm in diameter) is also roughly comparable (about 15 percent), although a difference exists with respect to time of onset: Hypopituitarism following surgery is immediate, whereas that following irradiation tends to be delayed by up to several years. The use of irradiation as primary therapy for a nonfunctioning pituitary tumor does not interfere with subsequent surgical therapy in the event of recurrence, nor does initial surgery preclude subsequent irradiation. A most important use of radiation therapy is as an adjunct to surgery. Most, and in some series nearly all, tumors showing mass effects will recur within 5 years after surgical treatment alone.[342] Postoperative irradiation will prevent tumor regrowth in 90 to 95 percent of patients. It is therefore the author's practice to recommend surgery as the primary therapy for nonfunctioning tumors except when medically inadvisable and to use radiation therapy postoperatively except in unusual circumstances.

PITUITARY TUMORS ASSOCIATED WITH HORMONE HYPERSECRETION

Most pituitary tumors (> 70 percent) are associated with hypersecretion of one or more hormones,[343] although in some patients the elevated hormone levels do not produce any clinical symptoms and thus serve only as biochemical tumor markers. The hormones secreted, in decreasing order of frequency, are prolactin, GH, ACTH, TSH, FSH, and LH. While the tumors are commonly of a single cell type and are associated with overproduction of a single hormone, prolactin hypersecretion is commonly seen in combination with GH and, to a lesser extent, TSH and ACTH hypersecretion. Pancreatic islet, carcinoid, and parathyroid tumors may also occur in association with hyperfunctioning pituitary tumors as part of the multiple endocrine neoplasia (type I) syndrome (see Chap. 28).

Therapeutic considerations of hormone-secreting pituitary tumors also differ from those of nonfunctioning tumors in that treatment sufficient to arrest the growth of the tumor may be inadequate to inhibit the excessive secretion of hormone. In addition, medical (pharmacologic) therapy directed at the hormone hypersecretion and reduction in tumor size is available as an alternative mode of treatment. This section describes the features unique to hormone-secreting tumors and stresses the differences in the management of these tumors compared with nonfunctioning tumors.

Growth Hormone–Secreting Pituitary Tumors: Acromegaly

GH hypersecretion is usually associated with a pituitary tumor composed of somatotrophs or somatomammotrophs. In about 20 percent of patients, the tumor cells contain eosinophilic-staining granules, while in the remainder, the cells are chromophobic. If one uses electron microscopy together with immmunochemical staining techniques, however, GH-containing secretory granules can be demonstrated in almost all chromophobic tumors associated with acromegaly.[344] The presence or absence of abundant GH secretory granules in tumor cells does not correlate with plasma GH levels but is merely a reflection of hormone storage capacity compared with its synthesis and release. The absence of storage granules does, however, indicate a relatively less differentiated tumor, which in turn is reflected in its growth rate. Thus, adenomas with intense GH staining tend to be smaller, grow more slowly, and permit signs and symptoms of GH hypersecretion to develop for a prolonged period, whereas poorly staining tumors frequently exhibit a more rapid growth rate and produce symptoms of an expanding tumor mass, with those of GH hypersecretion being less pronounced. In somatotroph tumors, GH and prolactin are both present in the same cell and frequently the same secretory granule. Acromegaly can also rarely (less than 1 percent of cases) be caused by somatotroph hyperplasia,[345,346] which is seen in association with GRH overproduction. Excessive GRH secretion may also lead to somatotroph adenoma formation, generally seen as nests of adenomatous transformation superimposed on the hyperplasia.[347]

Signs and Symptoms

The classic manifestations of GH-secreting tumors are produced by one or more of three factors: mass effects of the expanding tumor, pituitary hormone deficiencies, and GH hypersecretion. The clinical findings due to the first two have already been described, and their frequency in patients with GH-secreting tumors was once considerable. With earlier diagnosis, they are becoming less common.

Signs and symptoms of GH hypersecretion are a function of both the plasma GH concentration and the duration of hypersecretion. They may begin at any age, and the interval from onset to diagnosis may range from 1 to 2 years to several decades. In an extensive epidemiologic survey, however, the mean age at onset was 36 years and the age of clinical diagnosis was 46 years.[348] The earliest recognizable findings are soft tissue swelling and hypertrophy involving the extremities and the face (Fig. 8-20). Photographs taken over a one- or two-decade span will frequently document the progressive changes in appearance. The acral changes are most prominent in the hands and feet, where spadelike changes develop in the fingers and increased soft tissue volume results in the need for progressively larger rings, gloves, and shoes. The skin becomes thickened and leathery, and the prominence of skin folds increases. Generalized hirsutism and increased pigmentation may develop. Fibroma molluscum is seen in one-fourth of patients, and acanthosis nigricans is occasionally present. Sebaceous gland hypersecretion leading to oiliness of the skin and cyst formation is common, as is furrowing of the tongue. Most active acromegalic patients exhibit increased sweating, which is a sensitive clinical indicator of the activity of the disease. The bony changes develop more slowly and include cortical thickening, osteophyte proliferation, and tufting of the terminal phalanges. Hypertrophic arthropathy associated with thickened and eventually degenerated articular cartilages and ligamentous hypertrophy cause symptoms ranging from mild arthralgias to deforming and crippling arthritis. The mandible undergoes marked enlargement, leading to prognathism and a significant overbite of the lower incisors. In addition, there is often increased spacing between the teeth. The bony ridges of the calvarium are thickened, and there is often overgrowth of the frontal, malar, and nasal bones. The sinuses are generally increased in size, and this, along with hypertrophy of the vocal cords, leads to a deepening of the voice. Mucosal hypertrophy occasionally results in eustachian tube obstruction and serous otitis media.

FIGURE 8-20 Facial appearance of a 43-year-old woman with acromegaly whose disease had been present for 15 years. Soft tissue overgrowth about the eyes, nose, and mouth resulted in coarsening of the features. Lacrimal overgrowth is evident, as is thickening of the skin folds and the presence of fibroma molluscum (acrochordon).

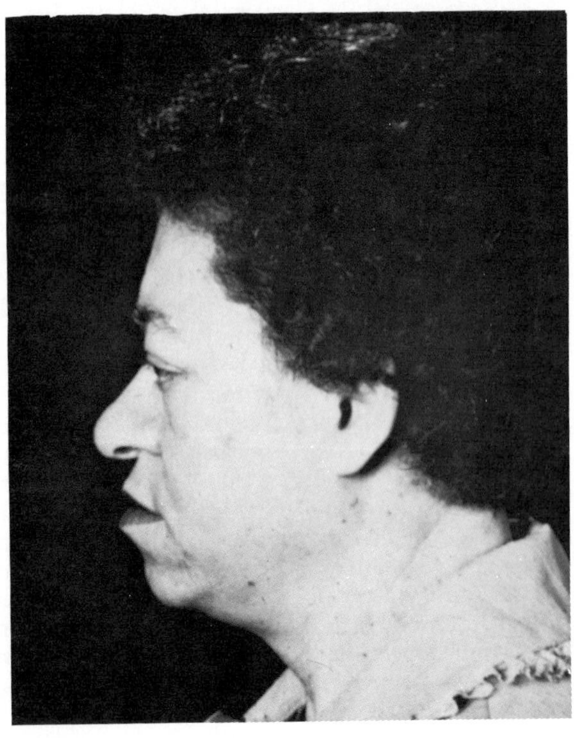

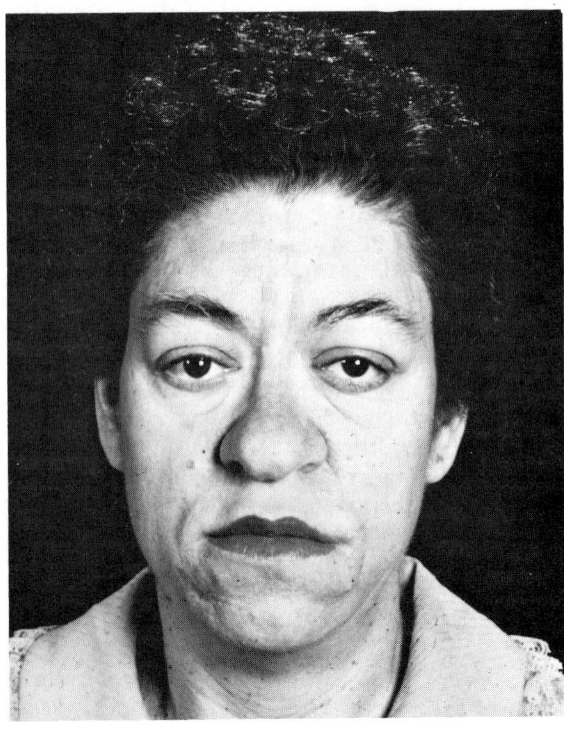

When GH hypersecretion begins during childhood before fusion of the epiphyseal plates, the increase in skeletal growth tends to be proportional and leads to true gigantism. Because of the hypogonadism that is frequently present, epiphyseal closure is delayed and the period available for growth is prolonged. The most celebrated pituitary giant (the Alton giant) reached a height of nearly 9 ft. It is more usual to see patients with the features of both gigantism and acromegaly, reflecting persistence of GH hypersecretion in adult life. GH-secreting tumors constitute 20 percent of all pituitary adenomas diagnosed during childhood.[349]

Peripheral neuropathy is common and is due to a combination of (1) nerve entrapment due to overgrowth of the surrounding ligamentous and fibrous tissue, most commonly affecting the median nerve (e.g., carpal tunnel syndrome) and less frequently the spinal nerves and the cauda equina, and (2) segmental paranodal and internodal demyelination of small (early)- and large (late)-diameter fibers.[350] Complete axonal demyelination occurs at a late stage and is associated with a proliferation of the perineurial and subepineurial elements, resulting in palpable nerves.[351] Acromegalic patients exhibit paresthesia and sensory losses and characteristic proximal muscle weakness, which is usually not severe but may become debilitating. Muscle histology is relatively normal in most patients, although a few exhibit evidence of muscle degeneration.

Prolonged GH hypersecretion results in generalized visceromegaly that includes salivary glands, liver, spleen, and kidneys. Salivary gland enlargement is clinically apparent, while enlargement of the other organs is generally not. Thus, significant hepatosplenomegaly usually implies the presence of a coexisting disease.[352] Renal hypertrophy is associated with an increase of both secretory and reabsorptive functions. Several types of neoplasms, including gastrointestinal cancers (carcinoma of the esophagus, stomach, and colon), colonic polyps, and thyroid cancer are increased in patients with acromegaly. The risk is even greater in patients with a positive family history of colonic carcinoma.[353–355]

Enlargement and hyperfunction of other endocrine glands are common in acromegaly. Thyromegaly with adenomatous change is frequently seen, though true hyperfunction occurs infrequently. The presence of decreased thyroid-binding globulin and increased thyroid-binding prealbumin complicates the interpretation of thyroid function tests. Parathyroid hyperplasia and adenoma formation are common along with pancreatic islet tumors and carcinoid tumors as part of the multiple endocrine neoplasia (type 1) syndrome (though otherwise rare in acromegaly) and explain the occasional hypercalciuria and nephrolithiasis. A more specific role of carcinoid and islet tumors in the pathogenesis of acromegaly, as a result of their ectopic production of GRH, is discussed below. Galactorrhea, amenorrhea, and decreased libido, when they occur, are usually due to associated prolactin hypersecretion by a somatomammotroph tumor, which may occur in up to one-third of patients.[356] The pathophysiology is discussed in the section on prolactin-secreting tumors. Mild hyperprolactinemia may, however, be seen in pure somatotroph tumors for reasons that are currently unclear.[357] Plasma testosterone levels are occasionally decreased, secondary to the hyperprolactinemia and reduced levels of testosterone-binding globulin.

The effect of GH on the cardiovascular system has been extensively described, but there is still controversy about whether acromegaly causes a unique form of heart disease or merely aggravates disorders such as hypertensive and coronary heart disease. Heart disease is seen in 25 percent of patients with acromegaly, cardiac deaths occur in 25 to 30 percent, and the risk of cardiovascular death is increased 2.7-fold.[234,348,358] However, acromegalic heart disease is rare in the absence of other forms of heart disease.[359] There is a high frequency of increased left ventricular mass, much of which represents fibrous connective tissue hyperplasia. Clinically, the heart is enlarged, ECG changes of left ventricular hypertrophy are present, and arrhythmias occur. Echocardiography reveals decreased left ventricular function even when the blood pressure is normal. Blood pressure elevations are not well tolerated, and eventually impaired left ventricular wall motion occurs. The effects are seen in patients with acromegaly of long duration and may continue to progress even after GH is normalized. Improvement is readily seen in asymptomatic patients with only echocardiographic findings but is infrequent in end-stage disease. Hypertension occurs in one-third of patients with acromegaly, though the pathogenesis is unclear. Renin levels are low, and aldosterone levels are not increased. The antinaturetic effect of GH is believed to contribute to this process.

Respiratory disease in acromegaly consists primarily of upper airway obstruction caused by nasopharyngeal mucosal hypertrophy, bone and cartilage enlargement, and reduced nasopharyngeal muscle tone. It occurs in half of all acromegalic patients.[360] About one-fourth of these patients exhibit nocturnal hypoxemia. Although classical sleep apnea syndrome occurs only rarely, most patients with acromegaly snore, which often interferes with the sleep of the patient or the patient's spouse.

Weight gain is not a common feature of acromegaly. Fewer than one-third of these patients are obese. However, carbohydrate metabolism is altered as a consequence of the diabetogenic effects of GH. Glucose intolerance and hyperinsulinemia are common, and diabetes (defined as fasting hyperglycemia) is seen in about 25 percent of patients, primarily those with a positive family history of diabetes, suggesting that acromegaly may precipitate the expression of an underlying genetic potential for type II diabetes. Although the diabetes is generally non-insulin-dependent, large doses of insulin are frequently required because of insulin resistance, and occasional patients are ketosis-prone. Despite these alterations, the vascular complications of diabetes are extremely uncommon.[361] Although subtle evidence of retinopathy may be present, significant visual loss, renal failure due to diabetic nephropathy, peripheral diabetic neuropathy, and vascular insufficiency are extremely rare, even in long-standing disease.

In evaluating patients with acromegaly both before and after therapy, one occasionally encounters patients with typical acral and facial features of long duration but with little evidence of recent metabolic activity. Such patients may have truly inactive diseases due to infarction of the tumor (with or without clinically evident pituitary apoplexy) or may have very mild GH hypersecretion of long duration. Assessment of plasma hormone levels is necessary to distinguish between these alternatives.

Laboratory Studies

Direct

The diagnosis of acromegaly is established by the demonstration of an elevated plasma GH level which does not respond normally to stimulatory and suppressive agents. Plasma GH levels in patients with acromegaly may range from 3 to 5 ng/ml, well within the normal range, to more than 1000 ng/ml. The levels in general reflect the secretory activity of the tumor but not necessarily the duration of the disease or the severity of the clinical manifestations. Because normal children and younger adults may sporadically exhibit elevated GH levels of more than 50 ng/ml, dynamic studies of GH secretion are indicated unless the basal GH considerably exceeds this value or the clinical and radiologic features are unequivocal. GH secretion in acromegaly is qualitatively distinct from that in normal subjects by many parameters. The suppressive effect of oral glucose administration in normal persons (to less than 2 ng/ml) is absent in acromegaly, and assessment of this response is the most reliable method of confirming the diagnosis. It must be recognized, however, that plasma GH levels in patients with acromegaly can decrease, remain unchanged, or even increase paradoxically in response to oral glucose. Changes in GH levels in response to glucose are seen in 70 to 80 percent of acromegalic patients.[362] When suppression occurs, however, GH levels do not decrease to the normal range.

IGF-I levels are uniformly elevated in acromegaly. There are conflicting data concerning the utility of plasma IGF-I levels in providing a better correlation with the clinical manifestations of GH hypersecretion than with the GH level itself.[363–365] Since IGF-I levels are influenced by many factors other than GH (see Chap. 26) and are one step removed from the hormone (GH) being hypersecreted, they can provide only ancillary help. In patients with only minimal elevations of plasma GH initially and while one is monitoring the effects of therapy, IGF-I measurements are useful in assessing the activity of the disease.

Plasma GH levels increase in response to TRH administration in 70 to 80 percent of acromegalic patients (but not in normal subjects), and this stimulus has been as reliable as glucose for establishing the diagnosis.[366] TRH administration is particularly useful when the response to glucose suppression is borderline. Plasma GH increases after GnRH administration,[367] although the magnitude and frequency of the response are generally lower than is the case after TRH. GRH stimulates GH release in most (> 90 percent) acromegalic patients, and in some the response is exaggerated.[368,369] A reduced response has been reported in patients with the Gsp mutation[370] (see the section on pathogenesis). This finding, however, is of little diagnostic help. Although initial reports suggested that patients with acromegaly secondary to ectopic GRH secretion fail to respond to exogenous GRH,[371,372] subsequent experience has indicated heterogeneity of responses.[347] Some patients with acromegaly also respond, occasionally in a paradoxic manner, to insulin hypoglycemia or arginine, but these stimuli are not useful in establishing the diagnosis. L-Dopa administration suppresses GH levels in most acromegalic subjects,[373] in contrast to normals. This effect can be duplicated by apomorphine and by systemic dopamine infusion and is due to a direct dopaminergic inhibitory effect on the tumor. Other differences in GH secretory patterns between acromegalic and normal subjects include a lack of deep sleep-associated GH secretion and a tendency to wide spontaneous fluctuations in GH levels, indicating a preservation of pulsatile secretory activity.[374]

Indirect

Numerous indirect measurements of GH hypersecretion are no longer used or are obtained only as ancillary information because of the current reliance on measurements of circulating GH levels. Serum inorganic phosphorus is often elevated, as is the tubular reabsorption of phosphate. Hyperinsulinemia with or without glucose intolerance is usually present, and IGF-I levels, irrespective of the type of assay used, are also elevated. Radiographic changes include tufting of the terminal phalanges, enlargement of the sinuses, and an increased thickness of the heel pad. Hypercalcemia, if present, suggests the presence of hyperparathyroidism and the multiple endocrine neoplasia syndrome.

Differential Diagnosis

The clinical features of acromegaly are not readily confused with those of any other disease.

Rather, one is more often confronted with the question of whether a patient's features (primarily facial and acral) are due to acromegaly or whether the disease may have been present at one time and is now inactive. Dynamic studies of GH secretion with more than one agent (glucose, TRH, GRH, or L-dopa) may be required to establish a diagnosis of "inactive" acromegaly. Gigantism during childhood has been reported to occur in the absence of GH hypersecretion (cerebral gigantism) and in some patients may be associated with increased IGF-I production.

GH levels are elevated in patients with chronic renal failure, cirrhosis, starvation, anorexia nervosa, diabetes,[375] and protein-calorie malnutrition, and there is often a stimulatory response to TRH. Differential diagnosis presents no problem, however, because of the absence of the clinical features of acromegaly. Elevated levels of GH are also present in Laron-type dwarfism,[162] in association with mutation(s) of the GH receptor.[376] However, these children have decreased IGF-I levels and clinical signs of GH deficiency rather than GH excess. GH responses to TRH are also seen in some tall adolescents,[377] but clinical features of acromegaly are not present and there is normal GH suppression with glucose.

Increased GH levels and features of acromegaly have been observed with CNS tumors (e.g., ependymomas of the third ventricle, hypothalamic hamartomas, intrapituitary gangliocytomas)[378,379] and in association with carcinoid and pancreatic islet tumors and small-cell lung carcinomas.[345] These tumors have been shown to secrete GRH ectopically, and tumor removal has often led to restoration of normal GH secretion. In tumors secreting GRH into the systemic circulation, measurement of plasma GRH levels, which range from 0.4 to 50 ng/ml, compared with 20 pg/ml or less in normals,[380] will confirm the diagnosis. Although the frequency of ectopic GRH secretion as a cause for acromegaly is quite low (<1 percent),[381,382] the implications for therapy are sufficient to warrant a plasma GRH measurement in each newly diagnosed acromegalic patient. Plasma GRH levels are not elevated in patients with CNS or pituitary GRH-secreting tumors, as might be expected, since GRH either is secreted into the portal system or acts in a paracrine manner.

GH itself has been reported to be secreted ectopically, though rarely, by lung carcinomas,[383] carcinoid tumors,[384,385] and a pancreatic islet tumor,[386] alone or in combination with GRH. However, in only one report has acromegaly unequivocally been attributed to extrapituitary GH production.[386]

Pathogenesis of Acromegaly: Hypothalamic versus Pituitary Disease

There has been a long-standing controversy as to whether acromegaly is a primarily pituitary disease due to de novo tumor formation or is of hypothalamic (or other CNS) origin occurring as a consequence of excessive secretion of GRH or possibly decreased secretion of somatostatin (Fig. 8-21).

The evidence for possible hypothalamic etiology is as follows:

1. GH secretion in most acromegalic patients is not autonomous but exhibits pulsatility[374] and responds to stimuli mediated through the hypothalamus, such as glucose, insulin hypoglycemia, and arginine. This implies that the somatotrophs, even though neoplastic, are capable of responding to hypothalamic signals.
2. Nearly all GH-secreting pituitary tumors respond to GRH with normal to excessive GH secretion.[368,369]
3. GH responses to glucose suppression and insulin stimulation, when examined after the removal of a GH-secreting adenoma, frequently remain abnormal, even when basal GH levels are normal.[387]
4. GH secretion in acromegaly is altered by neuropharmacologic agents (alpha-adrenergic antagonists and beta-adrenergic agonists stimulate GH secretion)[388] that are believed to act within the CNS.
5. Some acromegalic subjects exhibit relative resistance to the inhibitory effects of somatostatin,[389] a phenomenon consistent with excessive stimulation by a releasing factor. However, the demonstration of decreased or absent somatostatin receptors in some GH-secreting tumors provides an alternative explanation for this finding.[390,391]
6. Most important, ectopic GRH secretion, whether from a pancreatic islet or carcinoid tumor with transport by the systemic circulation or from a pituitary tumor, results in not only GH overproduction but also somatotroph hyperplasia and eventually tumor formation. Thus, GRH acts not only as a releasing factor but also as a mitogenic factor.

These arguments support a hypothalamic etiology for acromegaly and are consistent with the eventual development of an autonomous pituitary tumor.

The evidence that GH-secreting pituitary tumors are caused by a primary pituitary disease was originally based on two observations: (1) in a few selected cases, restoration not only of normal GH levels but of normal secretory responses to neurally mediated signals has been seen after complete excision of the tumor,[392] and (2) adenohypophyseal tissue surrounding most GH tumors, when examined histologically, does not appear to exhibit evidence of somatotroph hyperplasia.[393]

Recently, two additional types of studies have provided strong evidence for a pituitary origin. The first is based on X-chromosome inactivation analysis. Using restriction fragment length polymorphism with a marker for genes on the X chromosome together with a restriction endonuclease for methylated DNA cytosine residues, one can define a popula-

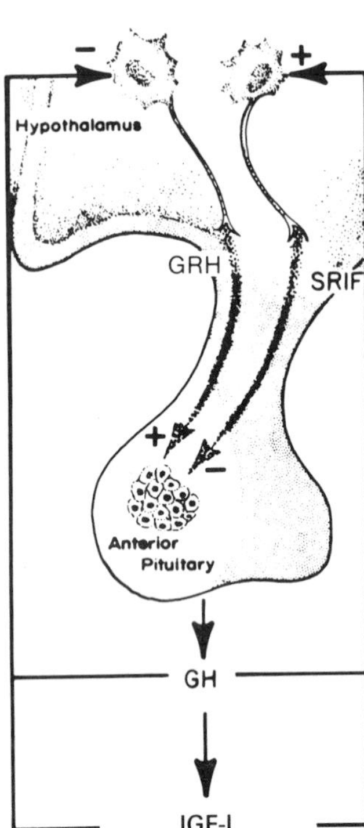

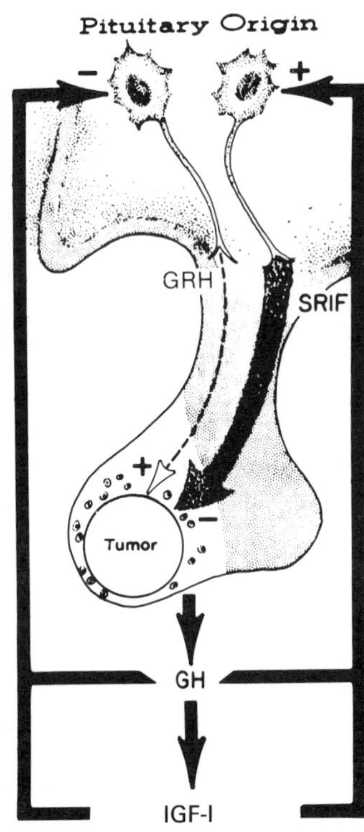

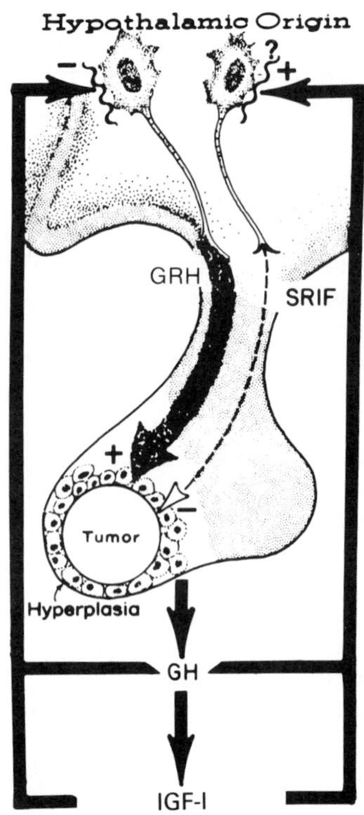

FIGURE 8-21 Possible neuroendocrine disturbances in the pathogenesis of GH-secreting pituitary tumors. (*Left*) Normal feedback regulation of GH secretion, which is mediated by both GH and IGF-I and involves both a stimulatory effect on somatostatin (SRIF) release and an inhibitory effect on GRH release. (*Middle*) Alterations which would occur if the pituitary tumor arose de novo. Enhanced GH secretion would lead to suppression of GRH and stimulation of SRIF release, resulting in hypofunction of the normal somatotrophs. It follows that the pituitary tumor must exhibit some resistance to the suppressive effects of SRIF for GH hypersecretion to occur. GH release in acromegaly is suppressed by exogenous SRIF, but the relative sensitivity compared with normal subjects is reduced.[391] (*Right*) Alterations which would occur with a hypothalamic etiology. The primary disturbance proposed is that of GRH hypersecretion leading to somatotroph hyperplasia and eventually tumor formation. Also implied are (1) an impairment of the negative feedback effect on GRH release and (2) a similar impairment of SRIF release or (3) a relative resistance to the effects of SRIF.

tion of cells as being polyclonal (exhibiting both maternal and paternal markers) or monoclonal (derived from the progeny of either a maternal or paternal cell). Such analyses performed on GH-secreting tumors have revealed that all are monoclonal, pointing to clonal expansion of a single transformed somatotroph.[394,395]

A molecular basis for such a transformation has now been demonstrated in 40 percent of patients with GH-secreting tumors. The mutations consist of a single base change in the guanine nucleotide-binding protein α subunit ($G_s\alpha$) that results in an amino acid substitution at position 201 or 227.[370,396] The former is at the cholera toxin–binding site, and the latter is within the GTP-binding region. The consequence of both mutations is to inhibit the molecule's intrinsic GTPase activity, which maintains $G_s\alpha$ in a constitutively activated state, leading to increased cyclic AMP, protein kinase activity, GH secretion, and mitogenic activity.

Somatotroph hyperplasia and GH hypersecretion also occur in transgenic mice with somatotroph-specific cholera toxin gene overexpression,[397] supporting the critically important role of the signal transducing protein $G_s\alpha$ in pituitary neoplasia. Comparison of patients with and without the $G_s\alpha$ mutation (Gsp) reveals that the former tend to have smaller tumors with intense GH staining and lesser responses to exogenous GRH, although other parameters of hormone secretion and the natural history of the disease are similar.

Somatotroph hyperplasia and tumors are seen in a subset of patients with the McCune-Albright syndrome. This disorder has recently been shown to result from a similar somatic $G_s\alpha$ mutation that occurs early in development, leading to mosaicism.[398] If somatotrophs exhibit the defect, they develop hyperplastic changes and eventually tumor formation. These changes occur during childhood, leading to gigantism with or without signs of acromegaly. GH responses to GRH are preserved in these patients, indicating that the mutated $G_s\alpha$ is still capable of stimulation.[399]

Thus, in nearly half of the GH-secreting pituitary tumors, an activating mutation in the GH signal transduction pathway can explain the pathogenesis of the disorder. Other mutations in the pathway will probably be found in the near future. However, the persistence of GH responses to GRH in patients with the $G_s\alpha$ mutation (*gsp* oncogene) and the presence of GH-secreting tumors in GRH transgenic mice[400,401] preclude the exclusion of a contributing role of the hypothalamus in at least some phase of tumor development.

Therapy

Three forms of therapy must be considered in patients with acromegaly: surgery, irradiation, and pharmacotherapy. As in patients with nonfunctioning pituitary tumors, consideration must be given to the consequences of an expanding intracranial mass, the need to preserve residual pituitary function, and replacement therapy for hormone deficiencies. The presence of GH hypersecretion by the tumor does not alter the rationale for the therapy of pituitary tumors already presented. The present section is concerned primarily with the effectiveness of the various therapeutic modalities in reducing GH levels to normal and alleviating the clinical manifestations of hormone hypersecretion. The goals of the therapy are to correct the metabolic disturbances, reverse as much as possible the soft tissue changes, and to arrest the progression of the musculoskeletal complications. Slight regression of bony changes can occur, though this is relatively uncommon. The reduction of GH levels has been reported to improve existing cardiovascular disease in some but not all patients. Therapy for acromegaly does not at present depend on whether the disease is of pituitary or hypothalamic origin. However, before initiating therapy directed at the pituitary, one should consider the possibility of an extrapituitary (carcinoid or pancreatic islet) GRH- or GH-secreting tumor, the removal of which may reverse the GH hypersecretion.

Surgery

Surgical excision of GH-secreting tumors is a rapid and effective treatment for acromegaly. The surgical considerations, including the risks, are similar to those in nonfunctioning tumors, with the exception that once a diagnosis of acromegaly is established, surgical intervention is warranted even in the presence of only minimal radiographic findings. The success rate varies in different series,[332,402] depending on the size of the tumor and the criteria used for a "cure." Based on current standards, a GH value of 2 ng/ml or less and normalization of IGF-I levels must be achieved for the disease to be fully inactive. Fewer than 50 percent of postoperative patients fulfill these criteria. The best results are seen in tumors restricted entirely within the sella and those with preoperative GH levels <20 ng/ml. The success in restoring GH levels to normal is inversely related to the size of the tumor, with considerably less favorable results occurring with tumors greater than 2 cm or extending beyond the sella,[403] where complete removal of the tumor is not generally feasible. Although tumor size is not necessarily related to the level of circulating GH, the likelihood of normalization of plasma GH levels is substantially lower when the initial value is more than 40 ng/ml. Remission of clinical symptoms and metabolic alteration of acromegaly occur in nearly all patients in whom a moderate reduction of GH levels occurs. The rapidity with which these symptoms (e.g., diaphoresis and soft tissue swelling) remit is at times striking. However, these parameters do not always correlate with the degree of GH hypersecretion, and in some patients clinical features may disappear completely even with persistence of elevated GH levels. Thus, the levels of plasma GH are the most objective means of evaluating the effects of therapy. Tumor recurrence in patients whose GH and IGF-I levels have been normalized is infrequent but can be seen for up to 6 years and perhaps longer.[404] Postoperative testing with TRH may help define that subgroup of patients in whom the tumor is most likely to recur.[405] In the larger tumors where nearly the whole adenohypophysis may need to be removed for GH levels to revert to normal, it is preferable to leave sufficient residual tissue to retain anterior pituitary function and treat the patient postoperatively with radiotherapy and/or pharmacotherapy. Repeat surgery is indicated only if tumor tissue is identified on MRI scan, and then only by an experienced surgeon.

Radiation Therapy

Two forms of external radiation are currently in use as primary therapy for acromegaly. Conventional (supervoltage) irradiation, which is available at most large medical centers, involves the use of 1 MeV or higher-energy photon beams with radiation doses to the pituitary of 4000 to 5000 rad. Therapy is given in divided doses over a 4- to 6-week interval. Heavy-particle therapy (proton beam) provides a much higher energy particle (340 to 900 MeV), and a slightly greater dose of radiation (4500 to 6500 rad) can be delivered in a single treatment. Heavy particle radiation is not indicated for tumors with more than minimal suprasellar extension because of the greater risk of damage to the optic nerves.

Improvement in clinical features and reduction in GH levels are comparable with the two techniques, though GH is normalized in less than 20 percent of patients after 2 years. Additional improvement has been claimed with heavy-particle and conventional irradiation after 5 and 10 years,[406] with 50 percent of patients exhibiting GH levels below 2.5 ng/ml by 5 years.[406a]

Recently, the "gamma knife" has begun to be used for the treatment of pituitary tumors. Stereotaxic placement of the radiation-emitting probes allows for restriction of the radiation effects to the sella (or to a larger area if indicated by tumor size) with less exposure of surrounding tissue.[338] A comparison of the efficacy of this form of therapy with that of conventional radiotherapy has not been performed.

A direct comparison of irradiation with surgery for the treatment of GH-secreting tumors is difficult because of the differences in the patient populations treated by each method, though the overall impression is that the two methods are comparable. Normalization of GH levels occurs in nearly all patients with initial values of 15 ng/ml or less. However, patients with initial GH values greater than 15 ng/ml are infrequently normalized.[406a] Another major difference is the rapidity with which GH values are normalized and the frequency of loss of other anterior pituitary function. Mono- or pleurihormonal deficiency is seen in up to 50 percent of patients, depending on the intensity of the investigative procedures utilized.[333,334] A comparison of the frequency of recurrence is also difficult because of the recent change in the size of the tumors being removed at surgery and the relatively shorter period of follow-up in most recent surgical series. The use of irradiation after surgical removal of GH-secreting tumors has been recommended as a means of decreasing the frequency of recurrence.[341] This suggestion should be followed in most patients whenever there is persistence of GH hypersecretion postoperatively. In patients in whom GH levels return to normal after surgery, radiotherapy is probably unnecessary. The use of pharmacotherapy as an alternative to postoperative irradiation is currently receiving considerable attention.

At the present time, the use of irradiation as primary therapy should be reserved for patients whose tumors are too extensive for removal without producing neurologic deficits or who are not surgical candidates of coexisting medical diseases.

Pharmacologic Therapy

Pharmacologic therapy for acromegaly was initiated with the use of hormones which were presumed to act by antagonizing the peripheral effects of GH (estrogen) or by some incompletely defined action inhibiting the release of GH by the tumor (progesterone). Some regression of the clinical features of the disease was occasionally seen, though most patients responded minimally if at all.

The observation that orally administered L-dopa acutely suppressed GH secretion in acromegaly[373] was followed by attempts to use the drug for chronic suppression. Partial suppression was achieved, though the drug's short duration of action and frequency of side effects at the doses required precluded its general acceptance. However, bromocriptine, an ergot derivative with strong dopamine agonist activity that was initially evaluated as a prolactin suppressant, was found to exhibit potent GH suppressive effects in acromegaly.[407] Although bromocriptine can cross the blood-brain barrier and exert central dopaminergic activity, its effects on GH secretion in acromegaly occur directly on the tumor and are demonstrable in vitro.

The frequency with which acromegalic patients respond to bromocriptine or to a related drug, pergolide, with a reduction of GH to normal levels has varied considerably in different series,[407–409] with the average range being 25 to 50 percent, and is dependent on the concentration (density) of dopamine receptors on the tumor cells. Thus, somatomammotroph tumors which secrete both GH and prolactin (about one-third) are more likely to respond. The dose of bromocriptine required is generally greater than that used for the treatment of prolactinomas, with daily doses commonly ranging from 15 to 60 mg in two to three divided doses. Mild hypotensive symptoms and nausea (both caused by central actions of the drug) are occasionally seen but often disappear with time and usually can be prevented by initiating therapy with a small dose in the evening and gradually increasing the dose until the desired effect is achieved. Many patients, however, may be intolerant of the large doses required to suppress GH levels. Long-term experience with bromocriptine in a few patients indicates that it can be given for more than 10 years with continued effectiveness. Discontinuation of the drug is associated with the return of GH hypersecretion, and therapy must therefore be continued indefinitely. Bromocriptine decreases the size of experimentally induced tumors in rats[410] and exhibits antitumor effects as well as hormone suppressive activity in acromegaly. Reduction of GH levels to normal occurs in less than 25 percent of patients, and a reduction in tumor size can be expected in only about 25 percent of patients whose GH levels have been normalized.[411]

Somatostatin has been shown to suppress GH secretion in acromegaly,[412] but the effects require continuous intravenous administration of the peptide. However, octreotide, an octapeptide analogue of somatostatin, is moderately effective in reducing GH levels in 70 to 90 percent of patients with acromegaly (Fig. 8-22).[413,414] The drug is currently given by subcutaneous injection 3 to 4 times a day at a dose of 300 μg per day and reduces GH levels to < 5 ng/ml in 50 percent of patients.[413] Normalization of GH and IGF-I levels was achieved in nearly all acromegalic patients with initial GH levels of 20 ng/ml or less. The combination of octreotide and bromocriptine

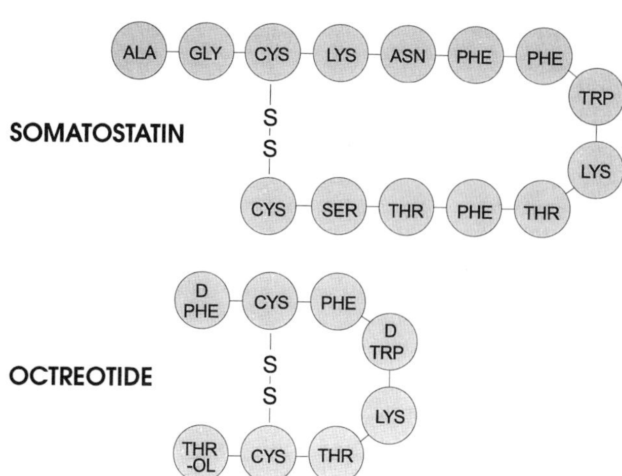

FIGURE 8-22 Primary sequences of somatostatin and its long-acting analogue octreotide (Sandostatin). Octreotide binds to the pituitary somatostatin receptor with an affinity greater than that of native somatostatin. It also has a plasma half-life of 1 h after intravenous injection, compared with 1 to 2 min for somatostatin, as a consequence of substitution of *D*-amino acids at sites of peptidase cleavage of the native hormone.

may be beneficial in some patients, particularly those with both GH and prolactin hypersecretion, whose tumors contain both somatostatin and dopamine receptors.

Improvement has been noted in symptomatic arthropathy,[415] cardiac disease,[416] sleep apnea,[417] and carbohydrate tolerance.[418] Tumor shrinkage occurred in up to 37 percent of patients,[413] though despite occasional dramatic effects in selected patients, the reduction in size was only moderate.

The side effects of octreotide include acholic stools, gastritis, occasional impaired carbohydrate tolerance, and cholestasis leading to cholelithiasis. Cholelithiasis occurs in about 25 percent of acromegalic patients and approaches 50 percent in some series.[419,420] It does not preclude continued use of the drug, since nearly all gallstones are silent and obstructive symptoms are very infrequent. Dissolution of the gallstones occurs with discontinuation of octreotide.

Prolactin-Secreting Tumors: Amenorrhea-Galactorrhea Syndrome

The clinical manifestations of prolactin-secreting tumors were well recognized long before prolactin was identified as a separate hormone. Galactorrhea and amenorrhea were initially classified on the basis of whether they occurred during the postpartum period (Chiari-Frommel syndrome) or not (Ahumada-del Castillo or Forbes-Albright syndrome). Long-term follow-up of both groups of patients, particularly the latter, revealed that a large percentage eventually developed signs of a pituitary tumor. With the development of the prolactin RIA, it was recognized not only that high levels of circulating prolactin were present in patients without demonstrable evidence of pituitary tumors but also that considerable numbers of patients with pituitary tumors and hyperprolactinemia did not exhibit galactorrhea. In fact, the incidence of elevated prolactin levels in pituitary adenomas ranges from 60 to 80 percent. The finding of unexplained hyperprolactinemia in a patient with amenorrhea, menstrual irregularity, or infertility warrants a work-up for a pituitary tumor, which will frequently be found. Many patients previously diagnosed as having idiopathic hyperprolactinemia were shown to have pituitary tumors when they were restudied using MRI.

Prolactin-secreting pituitary tumors often appear chromophobic with routine stains, and this is why most pituitary tumors were originally believed to be nonfunctioning. With immunohistochemical staining techniques, prolactin can be demonstrated in almost all these tumors.[344]

Prolactin-secreting tumors can be divided into two major types: microadenomas (< 10 mm in diameter) and macroadenomas. Studies of the natural history of microadenomas have revealed that 5 percent or possibly less progress to macroadenomas.[421–424] Moreover, a different pathogenesis is suggested, based on the duration of symptoms and the age of onset of patients with microadenomas and macroadenomas. A third subgroup of patients with macroadenomas and only minimally elevated prolactin levels have tumors that stain poorly or not at all for prolactin. These tumors are termed *pseudoprolactinomas*, and their natural history and management closely parallel those of nonfunctioning tumors. In addition, some macroadenomas exhibit aggressive behavior, become invasive,[425] and can rarely progress to carcinomas, with both intracranial and systemic metastases.[426]

Signs and Symptoms

Women with hyperprolactinemia present with galactorrhea, abnormalities of menstrual function, or infertility. The development of galactorrhea requires the presence of gonadal steroids as well as prolactin and therefore is not necessarily seen in all patients. It commonly occurs in association with oral contraceptives, either during their use or, more frequently, after their discontinuation. It is believed that the sudden decrease in estrogen and progesterone levels in a patient whose breasts have been prepared by the combination of gonadal steroids and hyperprolactinemia is responsible for the onset of galactorrhea, as occurs physiologically in the immediate postpartum period. The incidence of galactorrhea in patients with prolactin-secreting pituitary tumors varies from 50 to 90 percent[427–429] and reflects the changing spectrum of hyperprolactinemia caused by earlier recognition of the disorder.

Amenorrhea or oligomenorrhea with loss of normal cyclicity occurs in 60 to 90 percent of women with hyperprolactinemia and in nearly all with radiologic evidence of a pituitary tumor. The order of appearance of amenorrhea and galactorrhea can vary, with either symptom preceding the other by months to years. Hyperprolactinemia can interfere with the normal hypothalamic-pituitary-ovarian axis at three locations. First, prolactin suppresses progesterone production by ovarian granulosa cells.[430] However, the ovary of a hyperprolactinemic woman is capable of responding to exogenous gonadotropins, suggesting that ovarian function is intact. Second, prolactin can act within the pituitary to suppress the gonadotropin response to GnRH. This is unlikely, since numerous studies have demonstrated normal or increased gonadotropin responses to GnRH in hyperprolactinemic women.[431,432] Finally, hyperprolactinemia inhibits the ultradian secretion of LH, which requires a pulsatile release of endogenous GnRH.[433] It also inhibits the positive feedback response of exogenous estrogen on gonadotropin secretion[434,435] and possibly the negative feedback response as well. Thus, the most likely explanation for the hypogonadism of hyperprolactinemia is a derangement of hypothalamic GnRH secretion due either to an effect of prolactin itself or, more likely, to enhanced tuberoinfundibular dopaminergic tone secondary to the enhanced prolactin secretion (see below). In addition to anovulation, patients with hyperprolactinemia usually exhibit hypoestrogenemia accompanied by a decrease in vaginal secretion and dyspareunia, which may be responsible for a diminished libido. Many women with hyperprolactinemia have also noted mild hirsutism accompanied by an increase in dehydroepiandrosterone sulfate production by the adrenals.[436] Elevations of plasma free testosterone also occur and are attributed to decreased testosterone (estrogen)-binding globulin.[437] Decrease in bone density is present, though there is controversy about whether it is caused by hypoestrogenemia or is an independent effect of hyperprolactinemia.[438,439] It is also not known to what extent this osteopenia predisposes hyperprolactinemic women to symptomatic osteoporosis, since bone loss is negligible, unlike that seen after oophorectomy and menopause.[440]

The major clinical features of hyperprolactinemia in men are impotence and loss of libido and performance.[441] Prolactin-secreting tumors in men are usually quite large by the time medical attention is sought, unlike those in women, in whom the features of hyperprolactinemia often occur in the presence of microadenomas. Both gynecomastia and galactorrhea may be seen in men, though these findings are uncommon. Testosterone levels are uniformly depressed, and, as in women, the defect lies within the hypothalamus, since Leydig cell function is intact when stimulated by hCG administration, as are the pituitary LH and FSH responses to GnRH. The absence of a rise in LH in the presence of low testosterone levels under these conditions points to a defect in endogenous GnRH secretion analogous to the findings in women. Impotence is in part related to factors other than decreased testosterone production, since testosterone replacement therapy alone is often ineffective in restoring potency.[441] Oligospermia is also seen in some but not all hyperprolactinemic men.[436,442,443] Reduction of prolactin levels to the normal range usually restores both libido and sperm counts to normal.[443]

Laboratory Studies

Plasma prolactin levels in patients with prolactin-secreting tumors vary from just above the upper limit of normal (15 to 20 ng/ml) to values greater than 10,000 ng/ml. Prolactin levels greater than 200 ng/ml are almost always indicative of a pituitary tumor. Repeated sampling in individual patients reveals considerable variation in prolactin levels, suggesting, as in acromegaly, inconstant hormone secretion by the tumor. Since prolactin is a stress-responsive hormone, two or three separate plasma samples should be obtained for prolactin determination to confirm pathologic hyperprolactinemia when values are <100 ng/ml.

Dynamic studies of prolactin secretion have revealed several differences between normal subjects and patients with tumors but are not generally useful in distinguishing between pituitary tumors and other causes of hyperprolactinemia. The absolute prolactin responses to TRH in patients with tumors may be absent or indistinguishable from normal responses and probably reflect the degree to which TRH receptors are preserved in the tumor cells. Although proposed as a diagnostic procedure in the past, TRH testing is not currently believed to be helpful in making the diagnosis.

The prolactin response to dopamine receptor blockers is almost always reduced or absent in patients with tumors. This impaired response is not a consequence of hyperprolactinemia, since normal to enhanced responses are seen in postpartum hyperprolactinemic women.[444] Since agents excluded from the CNS (e.g., metoclopramide) and those with CNS activity (e.g., chlorpromazine and haloperidol) produce similar results, the site of the abnormal response must be at or beyond the lactotroph dopamine receptor. The absence of an increase in prolactin therefore suggests that the tumor is not responding to the suggestive signal (dopamine) or that the signal itself is decreased or absent. The lack of prolactin response to dopamine antagonists, however, is also found in patients with hypothalamic disorders and is not of diagnostic help. L-Dopa and dopamine suppress prolactin secretion in most patients with pituitary tumors to an extent similar to that in normal subjects,[431,445] though in occasional patients reduced or no suppression is observed.[446–448]

Unfortunately, the patients in whom the most clearly abnormal responses to all agents are observed are those with markedly elevated prolactin values and unmistakable radiologic evidence of a pituitary tumor, whereas in patients with only moderately elevated levels (less than 100 ng/ml) and normal radiologic findings, the responses are generally inconclusive.

Administration of L-dopa combined with the dopa-decarboxylase inhibitor carbidopa results in an inhibition of peripheral dopa decarboxylation and an enhanced uptake of L-dopa by the CNS. In normal subjects and in postpartum hyperprolactinemia, the persistence of prolactin suppression by the combination of these agents indicates a CNS-mediated suppressive action of L-dopa. In contrast, prolactin suppression is markedly attenuated in patients with prolactin-secreting tumors, suggesting a loss of the central L-dopa effect.[445] Overall, neither stimulation tests nor suppression tests are useful in the differential diagnosis of prolactin-secreting tumors, and their use has generally been discontinued.

Differential Diagnosis

Prolactin-secreting tumors are likely to be present in most patients with persistent hyperprolactinemia in whom no other obvious cause can be found. An unequivocal diagnosis of a prolactin-secreting tumor requires neuroradiologic evidence of a tumor as well as hyperprolactinemia, and this is found with the greatest frequency in the patients with the most pronounced elevations of prolactin values. In patients with prolactin levels greater than 200 ng/ml, MRI examination almost always provides evidence of a tumor. With levels below 200 ng/ml, radiologic findings may be nondiagnostic, though many patients previously considered to have idiopathic hyperprolactinemia on the basis of polytomography and CT examination are currently diagnosed by MRI as having prolactinomas.

In a patient with hyperprolactinemia who does not exhibit radiographic evidence of a pituitary tumor, other causes must be considered (Table 8-10). Careful questioning may uncover a history of ingestion of drugs which can cause hyperprolactinemia. These drugs include primarily agents affecting central dopamine regulation or estrogen-containing medications. The most common drugs in use today include psychotropic dopamine receptor antagonists (phenothiazines, butyrophenones, thioxanthenes) and tricyclic antidepressants, antihypertensives (α-methyldopa, reserpine medroxalol), phenothiazine antihistaminics (meclizine) and antiemetics (metoclopramide, prochlorperazine), and some histamine receptor blockers (cimetidine) and oral contraceptives. Galactorrhea has also been reported in heroin addicts and may be caused by stimulation of CNS enkephalin receptors.

Primary disorders of the CNS which interfere with the integrity of the hypothalamic-pituitary axis can also produce hyperprolactinemia by decreasing the inhibitory CNS influence on prolactin secretion. Hyperprolactinemia and galactorrhea are occasionally seen in association with granulomatous lesions of the hypothalamus such as those which occur in sarcoidosis. The abnormalities generally respond to treatment with anti-inflammatory agents. Infiltrative disorders such as eosinophilic granuloma are

TABLE 8-10 Differential Diagnosis of Hyperprolactinemia

Prolactin-secreting pituitary tumor
Pharmacologic agents
- Monoamine synthesis inhibitors (α-methyldopa)
- Monoamine depletors (reserpine)
- Dopamine receptor antagonists (phenothiazines, butyrophenones, thioxanthenes
- Adrenergic receptor antagonists (medroxalol)
- Monoamine uptake inhibitors (tricyclic antidepressants)
- Estrogens (oral contraceptives)
- Narcotics (morphine, heroin)

Central nervous system disorder
- Inflammatory/infiltrative (sarcoidosis, histiocytosis)
- Traumatic (stalk section)
- Neoplastic (hypothalamic or parasellar tumors)
- Stress

Other
- Hypothyroidism
- Renal failure
- Cirrhosis
- Polycystic ovarian disease
- Autoimmune or granulomatous hypophysitis
- Chest wall diseases (burns, *Herpes zoster*)
- Spinal cord lesions
- Empty sella

often associated with hyperprolactinemia. Other evidence of hypothalamic dysfunction usually includes diabetes insipidus, which is rare in small pituitary tumors. Head injuries associated with basal skull fractures of penetrating wounds can cause trauma to the pituitary stalk, leading to hyperprolactinemia. Similarly, parasellar tumors (meningiomas, optic gliomas, craniopharyngiomas) or tumors arising within the hypothalamus (ependymomas) can produce hyperprolactinemia along with evidence of hypopituitarism.

Patients with nonfunctioning pituitary macroadenomas may also exhibit hyperprolactinemia, usually less than 100 ng/ml. In some, suprasellar extension of the tumor with compression of the stalk or hypothalamus can explain the findings, while in others such an explanation is lacking. While it is always possible that a few prolactin-secreting cells may have escaped detection, an alternative explanation is that the tumor may have so altered intrapituitary blood flow as to eliminate the normal hypothalamic inhibitory tone. Such tumors are more appropriately termed *pseudoprolactinomas*.

Patients with hypothyroidism frequently exhibit breast tenderness and, on occasion, galactorrhea. While prolactin levels are usually normal, they may be elevated, though rarely to more than 100 ng/ml. With long-standing hypothyroidism, pituitary enlargement may occur and lead to the erroneous diagnosis of a pituitary tumor. In contrast to prolactin-secreting tumors, the prolactin response to TRH is increased in hypothyroidism.

Prolactin levels are increased in 60 to 70 percent of patients with chronic renal failure to values as high as 150 ng/ml. The prolactin response to TRH is impaired, but L-dopa and dopamine are ineffective in decreasing prolactin levels acutely, suggesting a receptor or postreceptor defect in the lactotroph.[186] These abnormalities, as well as the hyperprolactinemia, are unaltered by hemodialysis but are reversed by renal transplantation.

Hyperprolactinemia of two to three times normal levels has been observed in cirrhosis, particularly in patients with hepatic encephalopathy,[449] and has been attributed to the presence of false neurotransmitters, which have also been implicated in other CNS manifestations of the disease.

Galactorrhea and hyperprolactinemia can be seen after spinal cord lesions and injuries to the chest wall (burns, thoracic incisions, herpes zoster) involving the fourth to sixth intercostal nerves, stimulation of which produces nonpuerperal lactation.[450,451] Anesthesia of the intercostal nerves will suppress the prolactin levels and frequently the lactation.[451]

If none of the above disorders is present and there is no history of drug ingestion, a patient with elevated prolactin levels and a normal MRI is considered to have idiopathic hyperprolactinemia. This disorder is often seen after the discontinuation of oral contraceptives or for prolonged periods in the postpartum state. Galactorrhea may or may not be present. The differentiation between a "functional" disorder and an occult prolactin-secreting tumor is often difficult or impossible at this stage. A few patients have been reported with hyperprolactinemia, no evidence of a tumor, preservation of normal menstrual function, retained fertility, and minimal lactation. Size fractionation of their serum has shown the presence of a large-molecular-mass (150 kDa) prolactin which is believed to have markedly reduced biological activity.[452]

In patients with galactorrhea who have normal prolactin levels, dynamic studies of prolactin secretion are usually normal, the likelihood of a pituitary tumor is small, and continued ovulatory menstrual cycles and normal fertility can be predicted. This group of patients probably represents the most common type of nonpuerperal galactorrhea, termed *normoprolactinemic galactorrhea*, which is probably due to an enhanced sensitivity of the breast to normal circulating prolactin levels. This form of galactorrhea is commonly seen as a persistence of postpartum galactorrhea or after the discontinuation of oral contraceptives.

Pathogenesis of Prolactin-Secreting Tumors: Hypothalamic vs. Pituitary Disease

There is general agreement that CNS (hypothalamic) dysfunction is probably responsible for the hyperprolactinemia seen after the discontinuation of oral contraceptives and that persisting for excessive time periods in the postpartum state. Idiopathic hyperprolactinemia has also been attributed to an alteration of hypothalamic-pituitary dopaminergic mechanisms.[452a] Whether the dopaminergic defect is in the hypothalamic tuberoinfundibular system or at the lactotroph receptors and whether a separate nondopaminergic abnormality exists are areas of disagreement (Fig. 8-23). With respect to pituitary tumors, however, the role of the hypothalamus has taken on less importance with the increasing recognition of specific molecular defects in prolactin-secreting tumors.

A hypothalamic etiology is supported by the following evidence:

1. Prolactin-secreting tumors often show diminished sensitivity to dopamine receptor antagonists in vivo[447,448] though not in vitro,[453,453a] suggesting an extrapituitary factor that stimulates prolactin release and antagonizes the effects of dopamine. Both VIP and PHM, which are hypothalamic peptides with physiologic stimulatory effects on prolactin secretion,[178,454] have been proposed though not proved.
2. Abnormalities related to dopaminergic regula-

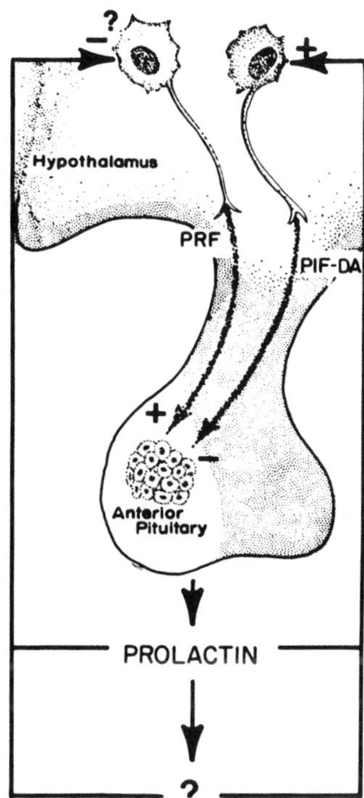

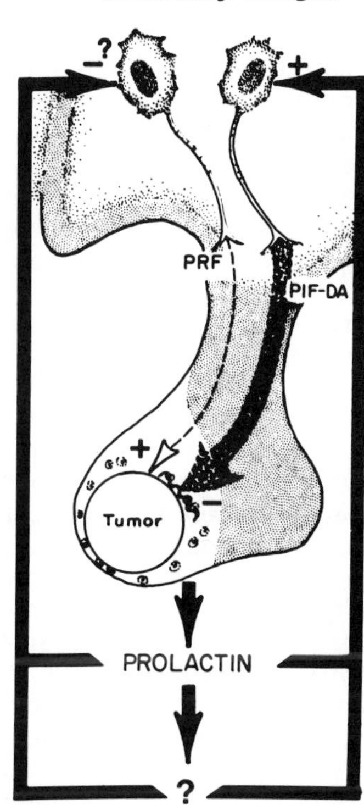

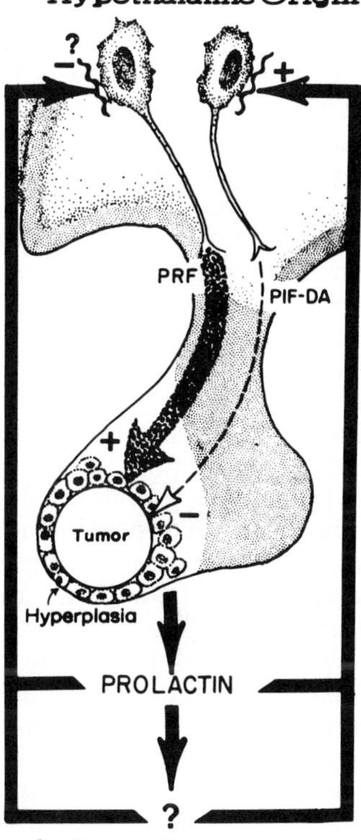

FIGURE 8-23 Possible neuroendocrine disturbances in the pathogenesis of prolactin-secreting pituitary tumors. (*Left*) Normal feedback regulation of prolactin secretion, which is mediated by prolactin itself or by some undefined intermediary and involves a stimulatory effect on dopamine (DA) and/or a separate prolactin inhibiting factor (PIF) and an inhibitry effect on a prolactin releasing factor (PRF). (*Middle*) Alterations which would occur if the pituitary tumor arose de novo. Increased prolactin secretion would lead to suppression of PRF and stimulation of DA-PIF, resulting in hypofunction of the normal lactotrophs. It follows that the pituitary tumor must exhibit some resistance to the suppressive effects of DA or PIF for prolactin hypersecretion to occur. Since prolactin-secreting tumors respond normally to exogenous dopaminergic suppression, this model would require that PIF be distinct from DA. (*Right*) Alterations which would occur with a hypothalamic etiology. The primary disturbance proposed is that of PRF hypersecretion or of DA-PIF hyposecretion leading to lactotroph hyperplasia and eventually tumor formation. Also implied are (1) an impairment of the negative feedback effect on PRF release and (2) a similar impairment of DA-PIF release or (3) a relative resistance to the effects of PIF.

tion persist postoperatively in some patients whose basal prolactin levels have returned to normal.[455,456] This argues for a continuation of the pathogenic mechanism even though the specific adenoma is no longer present.

3. A decrease in circulating dopamine, norepinephrine, and epinephrine levels occurs in response to bromocriptine in normal subjects through a CNS-mediated mechanism.[457] In patients with prolactin-secreting tumors, however, no decrease is observed either preoperatively or possibly postoperatively after the reduction of prolactin levels to normal. Thus, although hyperprolactinemia causes an alteration of hypothalamic dopamine turnover,[458] abnormalities in central dopaminergic function appear to be in part independent of hyperprolactinemia.
4. Lactotroph hyperplasia has been found in up to one-third of patients with prolactin-secreting adenomas, supporting the hypothesis that a hyperfunctional disorder eventually leads to tumor formation.[459]
5. Prolactin-releasing activity has been described in the serum of patients with prolactin-secreting tumors.[460] The activity has been reported to be peptide in nature, but its identity is unknown.
6. Most important, recurrence of prolactinomas, as indicated by the reappearance of hyperprolac-

tinemia, is seen in about 25 percent (range, 17 to 50 percent in various series) of patients previously considered as cured.[461–463]

The most important evidence for a pituitary origin of prolactinomas is derived from clonality studies in which prolactinomas have been shown to be monoclonal in origin.[394,395] Unlike GH-secreting tumors, only an occasional prolactinoma has been reported to contain a mutation in a known oncogene,[464] although transforming DNA sequences related to the human fibroblast growth factor gene have been identified in two of five prolactin-secreting tumors examined.[465] It is likely that a specific mutation will be identified in the near future.

The high success rate of restoring reproductive endocrine function after adenomectomy also supports a pituitary pathogenesis, although a substantial recurrence of hyperprolactinemia raises the possibility of a hypothalamic contribution. In addition, the histology of the pituitary tissue surrounding the prolactinoma rarely shows evidence of hyperplasia.

Overall, therefore, evidence is accumulating that prolactin-secreting tumors are of pituitary origin. However, it remains a distinct possibility that at some stage in the development of the tumor, excessive hypothalamic stimulation may play a contributing role.

Therapy

Therapy for prolactin-secreting tumors has undergone considerable change over the past two decades, and there is now general agreement among internists, gynecologists, and neurosurgeons about the use of the various modalities of therapy. Much of this change is based on extensive information concerning the natural history of prolactin-secreting tumors, the recurrence rate after surgery, long-term experience with pharmacotherapy, and the risks of observation alone. A general set of guidelines can therefore be proposed for microadenomas (including the few patients still classified as having idiopathic hyperprolactinemia) and macroadenomas.

Microadenomas

Continued follow-up of untreated patients with idiopathic hyperprolactinemia indicates that only a small percentage will develop identifiable tumors over a 5- to 10-year period and that only a few patients with microadenomas will progress to macroadenomas over a similar period of time.[421–424] The initial decision should be based on the extent to which the pathophysiologic consequences of hyperprolactinemia are of concern to the patient. If the patient is desirous of becoming pregnant or there is a need to eliminate galactorrhea or relieve other symptoms of hypoestrogenism, pharmacotherapy is indicated. If these problems are not of concern, therapy may be withheld and the patient can be followed periodically, using prolactin levels to monitor disease activity. An area of controversy involves the osteopenia frequently seen in hyperprolactinemic patients. One school of thought is that this represents a significant risk factor in the subsequent development of symptomatic osteoporosis and that therapy is therefore warranted.[438] However, there is an absence of reports demonstrating an increased frequency of pituitary tumors or previous symptoms of hyperprolactinemia in patients with osteoporosis, and bone turnover does not appear to be increased in such patients.[440] Furthermore, hyperprolactinemia spontaneously remits with time in some patients.

The primary mode of therapy is pharmacologic (Fig. 8-24). All the agents currently in use are ergoline derivatives. They bind with high affinity to the dopamine D_2 receptor in both pituitary and brain and act as potent agonists, though some newer agents have antagonist properties within the brain (see Pharmacotherapy, below). Surgery is limited to patients in whom pharmacotherapy is unsuccessful (generally <5 percent of treated patients). While the "cure" rate, variously defined as normalization of prolactin levels or resumption of ovulatory menses, ranges from 80 to 90 percent, the recurrence rate, generally defined as the reappearance of hyperprolactinemia over a 3- to 5-year period, is about 15 to 20 percent.[462,466]

Microadenomas do not constitute a significant risk during pregnancy.[467] Only 3 to 5 percent of patients have symptomatic enlargement of the tumor while pregnant, and they respond to pharmacologic treatment. In addition, up to 30 percent of patients will experience a remission of hyperprolactinemia after bromocriptine-induced pregnancies.[468]

Macroadenomas

Treatment of macroadenomas encompasses all the indications for the treatment of microadenomas and, in addition, the problem of the tumor mass itself.[469] Pharmacotherapy is the preferred method of treatment of macroadenomas even if the tumor is extrasellar and causes optic tract compression or other neurologic dysfunction. The response is rapid, and functional improvement is often seen even before anatomic shrinkage can be documented. Maximum tumor shrinkage takes many months and sometimes even years. Headache appearing in a patient with a macroadenoma treated with bromocriptine may be an indication of an intratumoral hemorrhage (pituitary apoplexy).[470] While most patients can be managed medically, surgical intervention may be required if visual impairment or other neurologic sequelae develop.

Surgical therapy for patients with macroadenomas is reserved primarily for patients in whom pharmacotherapy is unsuccessful in reducing tumor size. These patients have tumors with relatively few

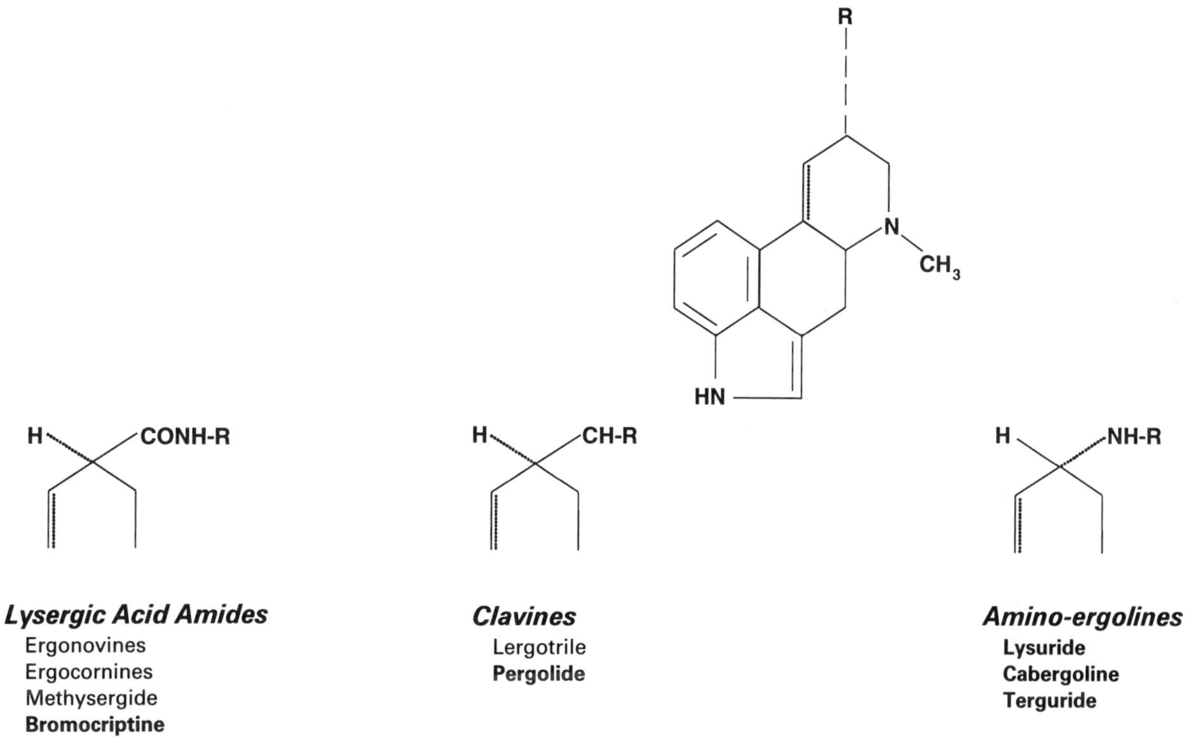

R
N
CH_3
HN

H CONH-R
H CH-R
H NH-R

Lysergic Acid Amides
Ergonovines
Ergocornines
Methysergide
Bromocriptine

Clavines
Lergotrile
Pergolide

Amino-ergolines
Lysuride
Cabergoline
Terguride

FIGURE 8-24 Ergoline compounds with dopamine D_2-receptor agonist activity. Shown is the basic erogline structure along with its three subclasses, each of which contains clinically useful prolactin-lowering drugs (indicated in bold type). Only bromocriptine is currently approved in the United States for the treatment of hyperprolactinemia, though pergolide is also available and has similar effects, though they have been less extensively documented. Other agents that are available elsewhere are also effective and have fewer side effects or a longer duration of action.

dopamine receptors. Most tumors can be approached transsphenoidally, though a few large tumors require a transfrontal approach. Total removal of tumors with extrasellar extension occurs in 30 percent or less of patients. Postoperative pharmacotherapy should be used, if feasible, in patients with residual tumor; if it is not, radiation therapy should be given. This is particularly important in tumors that exhibit invasive or other aggressive behavior.

In patients with macroadenomas who become pregnant, there is a risk of about 25 percent that the tumor will expand and produce symptoms.[467] Thus, many physicians favor surgical tumor removal before a woman becomes pregnant. The risks of surgery, compared with those of no treatment, must be discussed with the patient who has a macroadenoma. If tumor expansion occurs during pregnancy, pharmacotherapy with bromocriptine can be reinstituted safely and effectively.

Pharmacotherapy

For nearly two decades, pharmacologic therapy has centered on one drug, bromocriptine (2-bromo-α-ergocriptine).[471] This agent is currently the only approved drug for treatment of hyperprolactinemia in the United States, although pergolide, another related compound, is also effective[409] and is considerably less expensive. Other ergot derivatives are available elsewhere in the world (Fig. 8-24) and appear to have advantages over bromocriptine because of greater pituitary selectivity (terguride)[472] and/or longer duration of action (cabergoline).[473–474] Bromocriptine binds to the dopamine receptor with 5 to 10 times greater affinity than does dopamine, has a long half-life in plasma, and is effective when administered every 8 to 12 h. The most marked effect of bromocriptine is in decreasing prolactin levels to subnormal values in normal subjects and into the normal range in patients with prolactinomas, at times representing a decrease of more than 99 percent in prolactin secretion. The effects are rapid in onset (1 to 2 h), and the rate of fall is exponential; i.e., the greatest decrease in prolactin levels occurs at the start of therapy, and normalization may take weeks or months. Nearly all patients with prolactinomas respond to the prolactin-lowering effects, although the dose required varies from 5 to 15 mg per day. Occasional patients fail to respond or respond only partially because of reduced or absent dopamine receptors on the cell membrane of the tumor.

The biological half-life of bromocriptine is similar to its plasma half-life. Discontinuation of the drug is followed in nearly all patients by a return of hyperprolactinemia, though in some patients not to the initial values. Galactorrhea is eliminated or improved in many patients even if prolactin levels remain slightly elevated. Similarly, cyclic menses and fertility may be restored without complete normalization of prolactin levels. The drug is also used for interruption of postpartum lactation.

An injectable form of bromocriptine that is effective for 4 to 6 weeks is available in Europe.[475,476] In addition to its prolonged duration of action, it appears to have fewer side effects. A newer-generation nonergot drug, octahydrobenzquinolone (CV 205-502), is currently in investigational status in the United States.[477] Its efficacy appears to be comparable to that of bromocriptine, though there are some patients whose response to this agent is better than their response to bromocriptine and vice versa.

Bromocriptine therapy is initiated with 1.25 mg given at bedtime, and the dose is increased at 3- to 4-day intervals to minimize the symptoms of nausea, vomiting, and postural hypotension which may otherwise occur. In most patients these side effects disappear within a few days, though in some they persist and in a few they may preclude continued use of the drug.

The dose should be increased until the desired effect is achieved or side effects become the limiting factor. Intolerance to oral therapy may be overcome by means of vaginal administration of the drug at the same dose.[478] Patients should be advised about the restoration of fertility, and mechanical contraception should be used, if appropriate, to prevent pregnancy. Bromocriptine is not teratogenic in humans. The frequency of fetal loss and of congenital malformation in infants of women receiving bromocriptine at the time of conception is not increased.[479] Nevertheless, women who become pregnant should be advised to discontinue the drug. Bromocriptine is equally effective in decreasing prolactin levels in men with prolactinomas and, as a result, in restoring normal testosterone levels, libido, and potency. Treatment of such patients with testosterone alone, without reducing prolactin levels to normal, may be insufficient to restore sexual function.[441]

Bromocriptine produces tumor shrinkage in 60 to 75 percent of prolactinomas, with size reduction averaging 50 to 70 percent.[469,480,481] The onset of action is extremely rapid, with effects apparent within 48 h, as manifested by improvement in visual fields. Size reduction may at times be dramatic. Large suprasellar tumor components may disappear, and a partial empty sella may even occur (Fig. 8-25). Histologic examination of bromocriptine-treated adenomas reveals a decrease in both nuclear and cytoplasmic size, a reduction in prolactin storage granules, and other changes indicative of a reduction of cell metabolic activity.[482] With long-term treatment, cytolysis has been noted in some tumors.[483] Although escape from the drug's effects does not occur even after many years, discontinuation of the drug after short treatment periods may lead to rapid reexpansion of tumor size. Therapy can be maintained for many years, often at doses lower than those initially required.[480] After several years of therapy, most patients will not exhibit tumor reexpansion after discontinuation of therapy, though hyperprolactinemia often recurs.[484] Although the effects are frequently linked, drug efficacy in reducing prolactin levels does

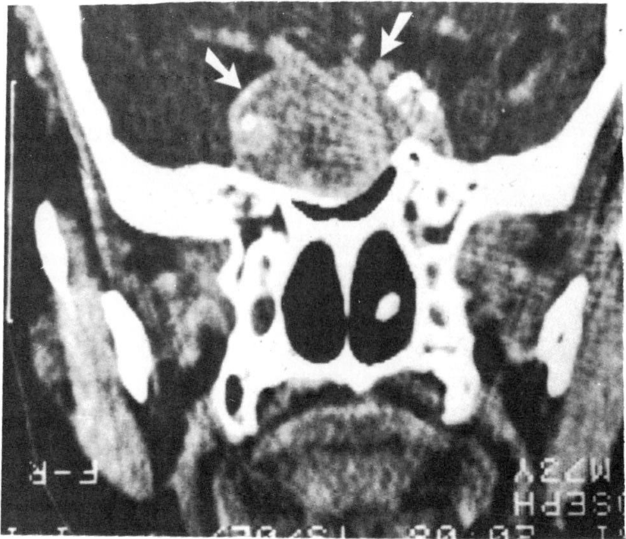

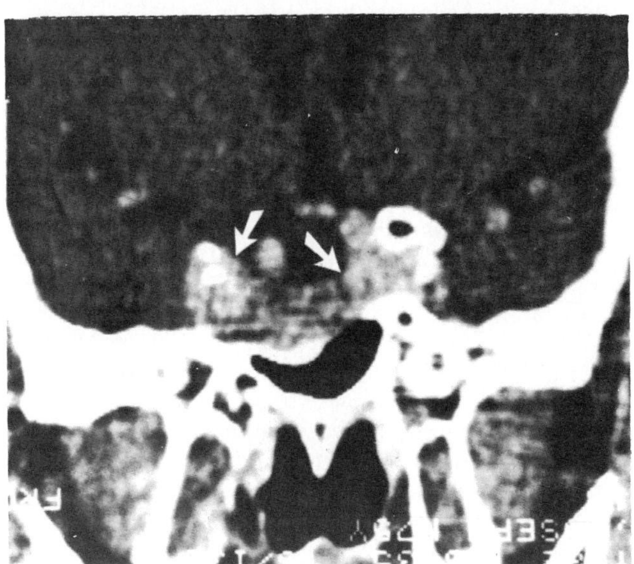

FIGURE 8-25 Effect of bromocriptine on reduction of prolactinoma size. (*Upper panel*) Pretreatment scan of a large macroadenoma with extensive suprasellar extension. (*Lower panel*) Effect of 1 year of treatment. The upper border of the tumor is indicated by the arrows. (*From Molitch et al.*[481])

not necessarily predict tumor size reduction. Tumor shrinkage is seen even when prolactin levels are not normalized, and normalization of prolactin levels is not invariably accompanied by a decrease in size. The tumors most likely to respond are those which have the highest prolactin levels and are not combined prolactin- and GH-secreting tumors. A macroadenoma with only modest hyperprolactinemia (less than 100 ng/ml) is less likely to exhibit size reduction. Histologic examination of such tumors often reveals moderate cystic or hemorrhagic changes and relatively few prolactin-secreting lactotrophs.

Surgical Therapy

Although surgical treatment of macroadenomas was at one time the therapy of choice, it is now used primarily in two circumstances: (1) patients who are intolerant of pharmacologic agents or show an inadequate response, and (2) patients who prefer to have surgical therapy before becoming pregnant. Reduction in tumor size by the preoperative use of bromocriptine is believed to improve the surgical success rate,[485] though prospective studies have not been performed. The results of preoperative treatment of microadenomas with bromocriptine are still controversial, with some but not all reports suggesting that the drug causes the shrunken tumor to adhere to adjacent normal pituitary tissue,[486–489] making total removal more difficult. This has been noted primarily in tumors treated for more than 12 months.

Most prolactinomas can be resected transsphenoidally, and many can readily be dissected away from the surrounding tissue. However, some tumors, particularly macroadenomas, are adherent to the surrounding normal pituitary tissue, contain necrotic or hemorrhagic centers, or have cystic components. The cyst may even communicate with the subarachnoid space and give the appearance of a partially empty sella.

The frequency of a surgical cure, defined as a return of prolactin levels to the normal range or the spontaneous resumption of menses, varies greatly between series owing to a difference both in the selection of patients and in surgical technique. It is generally agreed that the smaller tumors (less than 10 mm in size or with preoperative prolactin levels of less than 200 ng/ml) yield the best results.[294,295,490] Cure rates as high as 94 percent have been described in this group,[295] although in most series the numbers are somewhat lower. With the larger tumors, the outcome is less favorable, with only 20 to 30 percent of patients exhibiting a return of prolactin to normal levels, even though reductions of 70 to 80 percent are commonly seen. It is not uncommon for the entire tumor to appear to be removed, only to have the postoperative prolactin value remain elevated. Whether this represents residual or multicentric tumor, surrounding hyperplasia, or altered blood flow to normal lactotrophs is frequently difficult to determine. Residual hyperprolactinemia is readily corrected with bromocriptine. Recurrence rates of up to 80 percent, as defined by the reappearance of hyperprolactinemia, have been observed.[462]

Radiotherapy

Primary treatment of prolactin-secreting tumors with external irradiation has received less attention than has surgery but is also effective in reducing prolactin levels.[491] However, the reduction in prolactin levels occurs more slowly and less completely than is the case after surgery. Radiotherapy has been suggested as an alternative to surgery in patients with hyperprolactinemia and minimal radiologic abnormalities of the sella who desire to become pregnant, before the institution of pharmacotherapy.[492] Concern for damage to the residual normal anterior pituitary, however, limits the enthusiasm for such therapy, which is best reserved for use postoperatively in tumors which show signs of aggressive behavior.

ACTH-Secreting Tumors: Cushing's Disease

The association of bilateral adrenocortical hyperplasia and the clinical features of hypercortisolism with pituitary adenomas was first described by Cushing.[493] The small size of the tumors and the infrequency with which they were detected at the time patients presented with signs and symptoms of adrenal hyperplasia resulted in attention being focused on the adrenal cortex as the site of the primary disease. On the basis of the results obtained with transsphenoidal surgery, it is now accepted that ACTH-secreting pituitary tumors coexist in nearly all patients with adrenal cortical hyperplasia (Cushing's disease). The appearance of pituitary tumors after bilateral adrenalectomy in patients with Cushing's disease was first described by Nelson et al., who demonstrated increased ACTH activity in plasma and postulated that an ACTH-secreting tumor could develop as a consequence of adrenalectomy.[494]

Pituitary tumors in patients with Cushing's disease and Nelson's syndrome may exhibit basophilic staining (about 80 percent) or may be chromophobic. It is now known that POMC, the 31-kDa ACTH precursor, is a glycoprotein and that the capacity of tumor cells to stain with basic dyes is dependent on the presence of this glycoprotein. With the use of immunohistochemical stains, both basophilic and chromophobic tumors can be shown to contain ACTH. In addition, β-LPH and β-endorphin may be present in tumor tissue and in the circulation of patients with ACTH-producing tumors.

Basophilic adenomas are found in about 5 percent of pituitaries at autopsy in patients without evidence of ACTH hypersecretion during life. Nonfunctioning tumors of this type may biosynthesize

ACTH which is never released and undergoes intracellular (lysosomal) degradation, possibly owing to a defect in precursor processing or the secretory mechanism of the tumor cell.[495] ACTH-secreting tumors are usually benign but can exhibit true malignant potential on rare occasions and metastasize both within and outside the CNS.[496,497] Mixed ACTH- and prolactin-secreting tumors may also be seen. In a small percentage of patients with pituitary-dependent Cushing's disease, diffuse corticotroph hyperplasia rather than an adenoma is found.

Signs and Symptoms

The clinical features of ACTH-secreting tumors can be divided into two components: those related to adrenocortical hyperplasia and hypercortisolism and those involving extraadrenal effects of ACTH and associated peptides. Signs and symptoms of hypercortisolemia are similar irrespective of whether they are due to pituitary or extrapituitary ACTH hypersecretion, adrenocortical adenomas, or exogenous cortisol, as discussed in detail in Chap. 12. The major features include centripetal obesity, hypertension, diabetes, amenorrhea, hirsutism, acne, osteoporosis and compression fractures, muscular wasting, violaceous striae, capillary fragility, impaired wound healing, decreased resistance to infection, and behavioral changes such as mania and psychosis.

The increased secretion of ACTH and probably β-LPH results in increased pigmentation similar to that seen in Addison's disease. Skin darkening occurs over the pressure points (knees, elbows, knuckles, belt and brassiere strap regions); in the areolae, genitalia, and mucous membranes; and at the sites of new scar formation. Because ACTH secretion by pituitary tumors is not entirely autonomous but is partially suppressed by hypercortisolemia, hyperpigmentation is not pronounced in the early stages of the disease and is most prominent after adrenalectomy, when ACTH levels may increase markedly. It is a major feature of Nelson's syndrome and of extrapituitary ACTH-producing tumors. Although ACTH fragments and endorphins exert profound effects on the CNS, the behavioral changes seen in patients with Cushing's disease (euphoria, decreased sleep requirements, and occasionally true psychoses) can be explained by the elevated levels of plasma cortisol.

While once common, symptoms due to the expanding pituitary tumor itself (headache, visual disturbances, hypopituitarism) are seen only infrequently, owing to earlier diagnosis and therapy.

Laboratory Findings

A full discussion of the laboratory tests used in the differential diagnosis of adrenocortical hyperfunction appears in Chap. 12. This section relates primarily to the studies which are used to diagnose ACTH-secreting tumors. Patients with these tumors exhibit an increase in plasma ACTH and cortisol levels, elevated urinary excretion of cortisol and adrenocortical steroid metabolites, evidence of altered negative feedback of cortisol, and disturbances in the neuroendocrine regulation (primarily periodicity) of GH and prolactin as well as ACTH.

Plasma ACTH values are elevated in about 50 percent of patients with Cushing's disease.[41,498] The upper limit of normal is in the range of 80 to 100 pg/ml. Diurnal variation is absent, and even the values in the normal range are relatively elevated in relation to circulating cortisol levels. Morning plasma cortisol values are elevated in most but not all patients with Cushing's disease. The upper limit of plasma cortisol is 25 μg/dl in the morning and 15 μg/dl in the evening. The diurnal variation observed in normal subjects is absent in patients with Cushing's disease; therefore, elevation of plasma cortisol levels is more common in the late afternoon. The 24-h secretion of free cortisol is the most reliable urinary measurement for distinguishing between normal and increased adrenocortical function.[499] The upper limit of the normal range in most laboratories is less than 100 μg/24 h, though an even lower limit (less than 60 μg/24 h) is used by some, based on more precise extraction and assay techniques. Urinary 17-OH corticoid or corticosteroid (17-OHCS) measurements are less discriminating and should not be performed. Though a 24-h urine collection has advantages over a single plasma sample in that it provides an integrated assessment of cortisol secretion, the completeness of collection when used as a screening procedure in ambulatory patients is at times questionable. In obese patients, however, it is a more discriminating screening procedure. Measurements of urine volume and creatinine are useful indicators of the reliability of the collection.

Assessment of the alteration in negative feedback control of the hypothalamic-pituitary-adrenal axis is the most reliable procedure available for distinguishing between normal subjects and those with Cushing's disease or adrenal tumors. The basis for this test is the characteristic decreased sensitivity of ACTH secretion by pituitary tumors to cortisol suppression. The screening procedure of choice is the overnight (rapid) dexamethasone suppression test. Dexamethasone, 1 mg, is given at 11 P.M., and the plasma cortisol level is measured at 8 A.M. the following day. Plasma cortisol levels < 5 μg/dl exclude the diagnosis, whereas values above this level warrant further study. The standard dexamethasone suppression test involves the measurement of serial morning cortisol levels and/or 24-h urine samples before and after 2 days of dexamethasone treatment at 2 mg/day and 8 mg/day, respectively.[500] In normal subjects, the low dose of dexamethasone decreases urinary free cortisol to < 20 μg/24 h and plasma cortisol to < 5 μg/dl at 4 P.M. of the second day.[501] In patients with ACTH-secreting tumors, suppression of urinary steroid secretion is impaired with the low dose but should be at least 50 percent with the high dose. Plasma cortisol should be ≤ 10 μg/dl at 4 P.M. of the second day.[501] Lack of suppression at the high dose is suggestive of an adrenal tumor. It must be emphasized, however, that exceptions to this pattern exist. Some patients with ACTH-secreting tumors show no suppression until 32 mg per day of dexamethasone is administered.

Stimulation of the hypothalamic-pituitary axis with metyrapone reveals an increased adrenocortical response in patients with Cushing's disease, reflecting the hyperresponsiveness of the entire axis to both CNS-mediated signals and the removal of the negative feedback. The cortisol response to exogenous ACTH administration is also increased. These procedures are particularly helpful when responses to dexamethasone suppression are atypical. The cortisol response to insulin hypoglycemia is decreased.

Patients with ACTH-secreting tumors exhibit a hyperresponsiveness to CRH. After successful tumor removal, the response returns to normal. The greatest utility of this procedure, however, lies in its ability to distinguish between ACTH-secreting pituitary tumors and ectopic ACTH secretion, in which CRH does not stimulate ACTH release.[502] Ovine rather than human CRH is preferred because of its longer half-life in plasma. The sensitivity and specificity of the CRH test are about 95 percent.

MRI of the pituitary in patients with ACTH-secreting tumors identifies the tumor in about 70 percent.[503] As in other functioning tumors, however, MRI is useful as a localizing procedure after the diagnosis has been made on the basis of hormonal measurements.

Bilateral inferior petrosal sinus sampling for ACTH (and other pituitary hormone) measurements has recently been advocated as an alternative means of distinguishing between pituitary and peripheral sources of ACTH production.[504,505] Ratios of basal inferior petrosal sinus to peripheral ACTH of 2.0 or greater are indicative of a pituitary source, with a sensitivity of 95 percent and a specificity of 100 percent. A ratio of inferior petrosal sinus to peripheral ACTH of 3.0 or greater after CRH identified 100 percent of patients with pituitary disease, with no false positives.[504] It is necessary to sample both petrosal sinuses to achieve this degree of accuracy. The use of this technique to lateralize the tumor, however, has been less successful. Correct prediction of laterality occurs in only 60 to 70 percent of patients and is not improved by comparing ratios to those of other pituitary hormones.[504,506] The need to perform this procedure in all patients with suspected Cushing's disease is controversial, in part because of the cost. Given the sensitivity of the CRH test and the MRI, petrosal sinus sampling can generally be reserved for patients in whom the diagnosis is unclear on the basis of noninvasive studies.

Differential Diagnosis

In approximately 80 percent of patients with Cushing's syndrome (excluding those secondary to exogenous hormone administration), the abnormality is due to an ACTH-secreting pituitary tumor or to corticotroph hyperplasia. In about 10 percent an adrenal tumor is present, and in the remainder the abnormality is due to ACTH production by an ectopic source.[504] The diagnosis is made on the basis of increased cortisol secretion, altered dexamethasone suppressibility, elevated plasma cortisol levels, detectable or elevated plasma ACTH levels, and hyperresponsiveness of the hypothalamic-pituitary-adrenal axis in the absence of any evidence of another neoplasm and irrespective of findings on sellar tomography. There are two major steps in establishing the diagnosis. The first is to differentiate patients with hyperadrenocorticism from those with clinical features of the disease but with normal steroid secretion; the second is to differentiate mechanisms not dependent on the hypothalamic-pituitary axis for the hyperadrenocorticism. These topics are discussed further in Chap. 12. One entity deserving special emphasis is the ectopic ACTH syndrome (see also Chap. 29). ACTH is most commonly produced by small-cell lung carcinomas, carcinoids, and pancreatic islet tumors. The disease can mimic pituitary-dependent Cushing's disease in its clinical and biological features, though in patients with malignant tumors, the weight gain is often absent and severe hypokalemia is a prominent feature. The results of dexamethasone suppression tests indicate a variable degree of suppressibility. Some of these tumors have been shown to secrete CRH rather than or in addition to ACTH,[507,508] and this may explain the similarity in the dynamic responses. Removal of such tumors completely reverses the biochemical and clinical abnormalities.

Loss of periodicity of cortisol secretion and dexamethasone suppressibility and frequently mild elevations in plasma cortisol levels are seen in patients under stress, with alcoholism,[509] during periods of bereavement, and with emotional disorders, typically depressive illnesses.[510] Such patients, in contrast to those with Cushing's disease, may respond to insulin hypoglycemia with an increase in cortisol levels. While it may be impossible to distinguish these patients from those with ACTH-secreting tumors on a biochemical basis, the clinical features of the latter are generally absent.

Etiology of ACTH-Secreting Tumors: Hypothalamic vs. Pituitary Disease

Cushing originally attributed the origin of the disease to the pituitary. Subsequent observations suggested that the cause, at least in some patients, resided within the CNS (Fig. 8-26).[511] More recently, however, molecular studies have refocused attention on the pituitary.

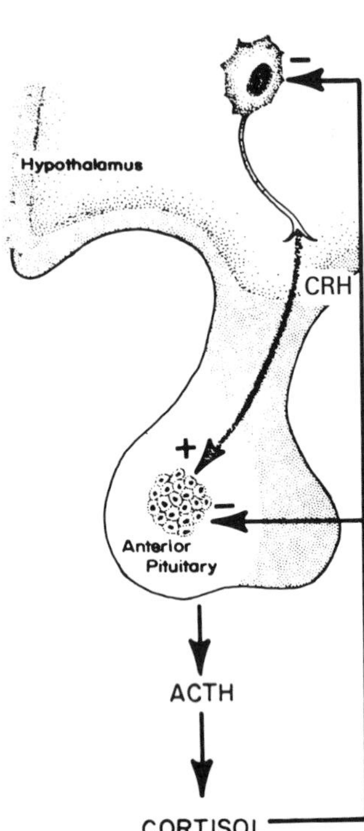

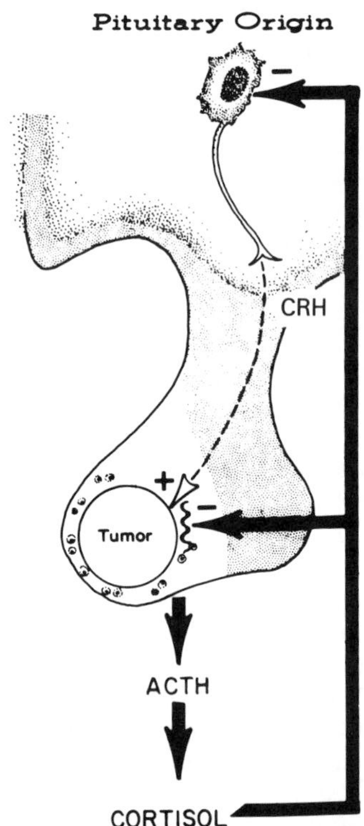

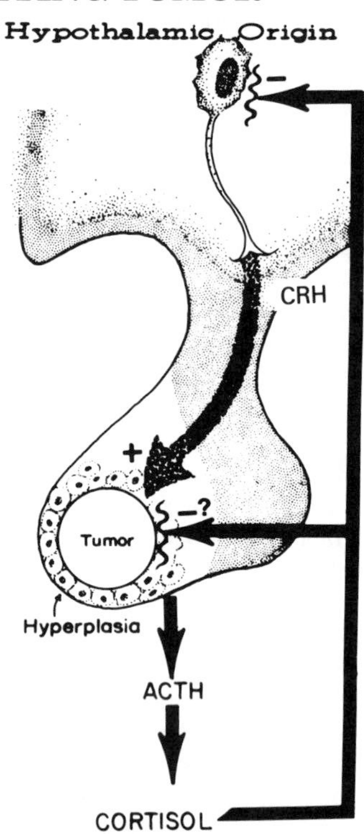

FIGURE 8-26 Possible neuroendocrine disturbances in the pathogenesis of ACTH-secreting tumors. (*Left*) Normal feedback regulation of ACTH secretion, which is mediated by cortisol and involves an inhibitory effect on both the pituitary and the hypothalamus (and possibly other CNS loci). The hypothalamic effects inhibit the release of corticotropin releasing hormone (CRH), and the pituitary effects suppress the effects of CRH on ACTH release. (*Middle*) Alterations which would be expected if the pituitary tumor arose de novo. Increased ACTH and cortisol secretion would lead to suppression of CRH secretion and of its effects on the tumor. It follows that the pituitary tumor must exhibit some resistance to the suppressive effects of cortisol, for which there is abundant evidence. (*Right*) Alterations which would be expected with a primary hypothalamic disturbance. An increase in CRH secretion would lead to corticotroph hyperplasia and eventual tumor formation. Also implied are (1) an impairment of the negative feedback effects of cortisol on CRH release and (2) possibly a resistance to the suppressive effects of cortisol on the action of CRH.

The hypothesis of a hypothalamic etiology is based on the following:

1. Lesions have been noted at autopsy in the hypothalamic paraventricular and supraoptic nuclei of patients with Cushing's disease,[512] and there have been case reports of Cushing's disease associated with CNS tumors and increased intracranial pressure in which symptoms regressed after tumor removal. In particular, CRH-producing gangliocytomas of the pituitary as well as other ectopic CRH-producing tumors can cause corticotroph hyperplasia and tumor formation.[253]
2. A 10 to 25 percent incidence of basophil hyperplasia has been found in the pituitaries of patients with Cushing's disease at autopsy, and in one series, 87 perent of pituitaries removed transsphenoidally for the treatment of Cushing's disease exhibited diffuse or nodular corticotroph hyperplasia, while tumors were found in 73 percent.[393] Similar changes were present in pituitaries from patients with Nelson's syndrome.
3. Analysis of the pulsatility of ACTH secretion in patients with Cushing's disease has revealed both hypopulsatile and hyperpulsatile subgroups which respond differently to surgical treatment, with the latter exhibiting a lower success rate.[513] It has been proposed that the hyperpulsatile subgroup may represent disturbed hypothalamic function.
4. ACTH-secreting tumors in the intermediate lobe of the pituitary have been reported to contain nests of hyperplastic corticotrophs and exhibit bromocriptine suppression and relative cortisol insensitivity, in contrast to anterior lobe tumors.[514,515] There is, however, disagreement about the frequency of tumors in this location, with some believing it to be relatively uncommon.[516]

5. Some patients with Cushing's disease respond to neuropharmacologic agents such as the serotonin receptor blocker cyproheptadine,[517] valproic acid (a GABA agonist),[518] and bromocriptine,[514] which have been shown to affect CNS control of ACTH secretion in animals. The responses include restoration of normal glucocorticoid suppressibility of ACTH secretion[519] and amelioration of the clinical manifestations of the disease.[511]

The major evidence for a pituitary etiology of Cushing's disease is based on the results of X-chromosome inactivation analysis studies which show that most if not all corticotroph tumors are monoclonal.[394,520,521] This suggests that clonal expansion of the tumor cells was preceded by somatic mutations. In support of this finding is the observation that after selective adenomectomy there is initially a deficiency of ACTH secretion followed by a recovery of the hypothalamic-pituitary axis.[498,522,523] The impairment in ACTH secretion is secondary to a suppression of the normal corticotrophs by the ACTH-secreting tumors, analogous to that seen after the removal of an adrenal cortical adenoma. The reestablishment not only of cortisol secretion but also of normal diurnal periodicity and glucocorticoid suppressibility supports the argument for a pituitary origin of the disease. Since glucocorticoids can suppress ACTH secretion at the level of the pituitary as well as by CNS-mediated mechanisms, the altered feedback sensitivity observed in ACTH-secreting tumors remains consistent with a pituitary etiology.

The occasional patient with corticotroph hyperplasia and the clinical characterization of the various subgroups still, however, support the possibility that in some patients with Cushing's disease, an excess of CRH secretion is a significant pathogenetic factor, at least at some stage of tumor development. Identification of specific oncogenes and their characterization in the various clinical and pathologic subgroups will be required to resolve this question.

Therapy

Among all the hyperfunctioning pituitary tumors, those secreting ACTH provide the clearest indication for definitive therapy because of the problems associated with prolonged adrenocortical hypersecretion. Although the effectiveness of therapy directed at the pituitary was initially demonstrated by Cushing, subsequent attention was given to the adrenals, and the return to a pituitary focus occurred only after the reintroduction of transsphenoidal surgery. While improvement in the agents available for pharmacotherapy directed at the adrenals has provided the physician with alternative options, primary therapy should be directed at the pituitary. Before initiating therapy to the pituitary, adrenals, or even the CNS, it is essential to exclude (or at least minimize) the possibility of an extrapituitary ACTH- or CRH-secreting tumor.

Surgery

The current procedure of choice is a transsphenoidal approach with adenomectomy.[524–526] In ACTH-secreting tumors, unlike other hyperfunctioning pituitary tumors, operations are warranted for patients in whom the diagnosis has been established even in the presence of a normal MRI. The tumors may be externally small (2 to 3 mm) and may be located throughout the anterior lobe as well as in the midline as originally described.[331] Although a total anterior hypophysectomy has been favored by one group because of the frequency of multicentric areas of hyperplasia,[393] most prefer simple adenomectomy as the initial procedure. Cure rates with this technique, based on a postoperative reduction in cortisol hypersecretion of 80 to 90 percent, have been reported for microadenomas,[524,525] though overall experience appears closer to 60 to 75 percent.[526–528] After surgery, there is generally evidence of adrenocortical hypofunction, requiring glucocorticoid replacement therapy, which has been attributed to suppression of the hypothalamic-pituitary axis, as is seen after the removal of an adrenal adenoma. The time required for recovery of the axis is usually 9 to 12 months but may extend to 2 years, and the frequency of recurrence remains to be determined. Patients may also experience steroid withdrawal syndrome (see Chap. 15). The surgical results in patients with Nelson's syndrome are not as encouraging, with reduction in hyperpigmentation and ACTH levels being seen in only 30 percent.[498]

Assessment of factors predictive of surgical success has indicated that small tumor size and the location of a tumor in the anterior lobe are important. The success rate is lower if no definitive tumor is found, and in such a patient a total anterior hypophysectomy should be performed if the patient does not have a desire for future reproductive capability. In the postoperative period, the presence of a low plasma cortisol level (<4 μg/dl)[527] and suppressed urinary free cortisol (<40 μg/24 h)[528] are predictors of a cure. However, recurrence rates of about 25 percent have been reported over a 4- to 6-year period.[526,527,529]

Bilateral adrenalectomy is an alternative procedure that has been used successfully for many decades. It is very effective in eliminating the hypercortisolism and the signs and symptoms of Cushing's disease. Its major disadvantages are (1) the need for permanent glucocorticoid and mineralocorticoid replacement postoperatively and (2) the failure to address the pituitary tumor. Postoperatively, ACTH levels increase because of the reduction of glucocorticoid feedback, leading to increases in pigmentation. In addition, about 10 percent of patients will develop large, often invasive, and even metastatic ACTH-secreting tumors.[497,530] The latency of tumor appearance after adrenalectomy is highly variable (1 to 16 years) and cannot be completely prevented by the use of postoperative irradiation.[497]

Radiation Therapy

Conventional radiotherapy has been used, together with pharmacotherapy, for the treatment of ACTH-secreting tumors. Radiation doses of about 45 Gy (4500 rad) have been associated with a cure rate of only 57 percent in 10 years[531] and therefore should only be considered as a second-choice therapy. Its use is best reserved for patients in whom surgical removal of ACTH-secreting tumors cannot be accomplished.

Pharmacologic Therapy

Pharmacologic agents used in the treatment of Cushing's disease are directed at either cortisol biosynthesis by the adrenals (ketoconazole, aminoglutethimide, metyrapone, mitotane, or trilostane), the glucocorticoid receptor (RU-486), or neurotransmitter metabolism within the CNS. Differences in the mechanism of action, doses, effectiveness, and side effects of the steroid synthesis inhibitors are described in Chap. 12. They were initially used as primary therapy directed to the adrenals and subsequently as an adjunct to radiation therapy to the pituitary. At present they are in use as alternative therapy when surgery is contraindicated or unsuccessful and in the normalization of cortisol levels before surgery. The latter, while theoretically of value, has not been very popular because of the low morbidity associated with surgery for ACTH-secreting pituitary tumors.

The addition of steroid biosynthesis inhibitors improves the rapidity with which cortisol secretion is normalized after radiation therapy, particularly in patients with moderately severe clinical symptoms. However, this combination is still considered to be a secondary form of treatment.

Ketoconazole (Nizoral), an imidazole broad-spectrum antimycotic, is very effective in reducing cortisol secretion in patients with Cushing's disease.[532–534] The drug impairs cortisol biosynthesis by inhibiting P_{450} enzymes associated with cholesterol side-chain cleavage[535] and inhibiting $C_{17\text{-}20}$ lyase.[536] The absence of a rise in ACTH levels after cortisol secretion is normalized is unexplained.[533] A dose of 600 to 800 mg per day is generally required to suppress cortisol secretion to the normal range, though higher doses may be needed. The drug may be combined with other steroid biosynthesis inhibitors to eliminate side effects, which are primarily gastrointestinal.

Metyrapone (Metopirone) is a competitive 11-hydroxylase inhibitor and blocks the conversion of 11-deoxycortisol to cortisol. At higher doses, it also inhibits 21-hydroxylation. At its usual dose of 3 to 4 g per day, metyrapone exhibits a rapid onset of action and reduces circulating cortisol levels to normal.[537] The reduction of the negative feedback effect of cortisol leads to an increase in ACTH secretion which often overrides the block unless other drugs are also used. Metyrapone also occasionally causes hirsutism.

Aminoglutethimide (Cytadren) inhibits the conversion of cholesterol to 20 α-hydroxy cholesterol, an early step in cortisol biosynthesis. The usual dose range is from 1 to 2 g per day in divided doses. This drug is frequently used in combination with metyrapone.

Trilostane (Modrastane) is a hydroxyandrostane derivative that is an inhibitor of 3β-hydroxysteroid dehydrogenase, one of the early steps in cortisol biosynthesis. At doses of 120 to 360 mg per day, it is an effective inhibitor of glucocorticoid synthesis. Since escape occurs, it may have to be combined with other agents.

Mitotane (Lysodren) is a cytotoxic agent, the action of which is limited to the mitochondria of the adrenal cortex. Its cortisol-lowering effects are also produced by the inhibition of steroid biosynthesis. Reduction of cortisol secretion into the normal range generally occurs in 3 to 4 months. Although some patients are rendered permanently euadrenal, many become permanently adrenocortically insufficient within a year or so and require glucocorticoid replacement therapy. The dose of mitotane generally ranges from 2 to 4 g per day. Side effects include primarily gastrointestinal symptoms.

Mefipristone (RU-486) is a progesterone receptor antagonist that also exhibits potent glucocorticoid receptor antagonism. It has been shown to inhibit the effects of glucocorticoids at an oral dose of 5 to 22 mg/kg per day. The clinical manifestations of non-pituitary-dependent Cushing's syndrome are reversed despite high levels of plasma cortisol. However, in pituitary-dependent disease, the interference with glucocorticoid action leads to an increase in ACTH and cortisol secretion.[538] The possibility of its use in conjunction with cortisol biosynthesis inhibitors remains to be evaluated.

As the understanding of the neurotransmitter control of ACTH secretion increased, and during the time when the pathogenic role of the hypothalamus was considered paramount, neuropharmacologic agents that affected CNS control of ACTH secretion were evaluated in the treatment of Cushing's disease. Bromocriptine, valproic acid (a GABA antagonist), and cyproheptadine (a serotonin antagonist) were reported to exhibit beneficial results in some patients, including those with Nelson's syndrome.[517,539,540] However, the response rate has been small and enthusiasm for these agents has not persisted. They may be considered when other forms of therapy have been unsuccessful.

Glycoprotein-Secreting Tumors

TSH-Secreting Tumors

The number of TSH-secreting tumors reported to date is under 150, making this a relatively uncommon tumor.[541–543] Most of these tumors are macroadenomas (>90 percent), many exhibit extensive suprasellar extension, and, rarely, metastases may occur.[544] Molecular studies have not revealed any specific abnormalities. Nearly all these patients have a goiter which is usually but not invariably nonnodular. The disease should be suspected in patients with thyrotoxicosis who do not exhibit completely suppressed TSH levels on the high-sensitivity assay. TSH levels may not be elevated above the normal range. Unless there is a serum thyroid hormone–binding abnormality or thyroid hormone resistance (in both circumstances the patient should not be hyperthyroid), the diagnosis of a TSH-secreting tumor can be made. Another entity that should not be confused with a TSH-secreting tumor is the pituitary enlargement associated with thyrotroph hyperplasia that occurs with long-standing hypothyroidism, where MRI changes can be mistaken for a tumor. In such patients, treatment of the hypothyroidism rapidly suppresses TSH levels and, with time, restores the pituitary size to normal (Fig. 8-19). Most patients also have α-subunit levels that are greater than TSH levels (on a molar basis), but this measurement is unnecessary unless the patient has a negative MRI. With the availability of highly sensitive TSH assays, it is anticipated that more TSH-secreting microadenomas will be identified, and thus specific biochemical markers will assume greater importance. Growth hormone and prolactin levels are each elevated in about 25 percent of patients with tumors. Histologic examination of the tumors has revealed tumors composed both of separate cell types secreting TSH and GH and of a single cell type secreting both hormones with or without the α subunit. Although TSH responses to stimulation by TRH and suppression by thyroid hormone, dopamine agonists, glucocorticoids, and octreotide vary from those with nontumorous elevation of TSH, the distinctions are not sufficiently clear to consider any of these procedures as definitive at the present time.[542]

Therapy for TSH-secreting tumors requires correlation of both the hyperthyroidism and the tumor mass. Hyperthyroidism can be controlled by radioiodine ablation or antithyroid drugs. However, the treatment of the pituitary tumor is more difficult. Only 38 percent of patients treated by surgery alone have been cured, probably because of the size of the tumors. Irradiation by itelf has not been effective and, when combined with surgery, has not resulted in a greater cure rate, although the follow-up period may at present not be of sufficient duration to resolve this issue completely. Octreotide has been shown to suppress TSH levels in > 90 percent of patients, with a mean reduction of about 75 percent. Tumor size has also been reduced in half these patients. Dopamine agonists decrease TSH levels in about 30 percent of patients, though their effect on tumor size is unknown.

Gonadotropin- and α-Subunit-Secreting Tumors

A subset of clinically "nonfunctioning" tumors have been identified which secrete FSH, LH (less commonly), and/or the glycoprotein α or β subunits. These tumors are seen most commonly in men over age 50 years, though they are also being recognized in postmenopausal women and, rarely, in premenopausal women. Intact glycoprotein hormones or their subunits are produced by the majority of these tumors, which constitute about 25 percent of all pituitary tumors. Despite the fact that the secreted gonadotropins are biologically active,[545] most of these tumors are associated with hypogonadism. In some patients, long-standing hypogonadism preceded tumor formation and has raised the possibility of a causative role.[546] However, since most patients with glycoprotein-secreting tumors do not have evidence of prior gonadal failure and since the incidence is quite low in postmenopausal women, the overall frequency of gonadal failure as a cause for these tumors is very low. Because of the variety of glycoprotein forms that can be found in these tumors, ratios of intact hormone to individual subunits are quite variable and strict diagnostic criteria are not available. Nevertheless, high levels of the free subunits in circulation strongly point to the diagnosis.

From a clinical standpoint, the approach to therapy is similar to that for truly nonfunctioning tumors, with surgical removal being the first line of treatment. Since most of these tumors are large, total tumor removal is infrequent and postoperative therapy is indicated. At present, irradiation is still the most common form of adjunct therapy. However, the wish to avoid the undesired effects of irradiation has led to numerous attempts to treat these tumors medically.[547] A few tumors have responded to bromocriptine.[548,549]

DETAILS OF HYPOTHALAMIC-PITUITARY TESTING

The list of testing procedures described below is not intended to constitute an exhaustive list but includes those which have been found to have the greatest utility in diagnosing disorders of pituitary hormone secretion. The rationale for their use and a detailed interpretation of the results are provided in the preceding sections.

ACTH

Basal Measurements

Plasma ACTH RIAs are now reliably performed by many laboratories. Normal values range from 20 to 80 pg/ml, though their interpretation requires a simultaneous cortisol determination. Measurement of plasma cortisol still provides, for practical purposes, a reliable index of ACTH secretion when pituitary function is being evaluated, provided that adrenocortical function is intact. The normal range is 5 to 25 μg/dl. The normal diurnal variation is at least 5 μg/dl. The 24-h urinary excretion of free cortisol is 20 to 100 μg in normal adults in most laboratories, though it is lower in a few.

Stimulation Tests

Corticotropin Releasing Hormone

At the time of writing, CRH is available only as an investigational agent in the United States.

Method Ovine CRH, 100 μg, is injected intravenously, and blood samples are obtained at 0, 15, 30, 60, and 120 min. This test may be combined with GRH, TRH, and GnRH testing.

Normal Values The increase in cortisol should be at least 10 μg/dl. Peak values should occur by 30 to 60 min. Measurement of ACTH levels gives more variable results, and peak increments at 15 to 30 min may range from 20 to 50 pg/ml.

Interpretation In both hypothalamic and pituitary disease, the cortisol response is decreased. However, the ACTH response is intact if the cause of diminished function is in the hypothalamus. More extensive evaluation of this test in hypothalamic-pituitary disease is needed to define the reliability of the test in separating the two disease categories. Patients with ACTH-secreting pituitary tumors respond to CRH with a supranormal response, while those with ectopic ACTH secretion are unresponsive.

Risks There are no significant risks. Immediately after injection, patients experience facial flushing which may last for several minutes.

Insulin Hypoglycemia

Method This study should be performed in the morning after an overnight fast. An indwelling needle is inserted into a forearm vein and is kept patent with heparinized saline. Regular insulin is injected intravenously at a dose sufficient to decrease the blood glucose by 50 percent or to at least 40 mg/dl. The standard dose is 0.1 U/kg, though this is increased to 0.15 U/kg in states of presumed insulin resistance, e.g., obesity, acromegaly, and Cushing's syndrome, and is reduced to 0.05 U/kg when hypopituitarism is strongly suspected. If signs and symptoms of adrenergic discharge occur, the hypoglycemic stimulus is adequate even if the full extent of glucose reduction is not achieved. If none of these criteria is met, the test may need to be repeated with a larger dose of insulin. Dextrose (50%) should be immediately available in case of unexpectedly severe hypoglycemia. Blood glucose is measured at 0, 15, 30, 45, 60, 90, and 120 min. Plasma cortisol is measured at 0, 30, 60, 90, and 120 min. The insulin hypoglycemia test can be performed simultaneously with the TRH and GnRH tests if indicated.

Normal Values The minimal glucose value should occur at 30 to 45 min. A normal cortisol response consists of a rise of at least 10 μg/dl and a value of at least 20 μg/dl.

Interpretation A normal response indicates an intact hypothalamic-pituitary-adrenal axis. An impaired response does not identify the site of the abnormality. An ACTH stimulation test should be used to document intact adrenocortical function, and a CRH test to evaluate the pituitary-adrenal axis. The response to insulin hypoglycemia may be blunted or absent if the initial cortisol level is high, as often occurs in patients under stress. It is also reduced in patients who are receiving exogenous glucocorticoids at the time of testing or have received it in the recent past, in patients with Cushing's syndrome or Cushing's disease, and in patients with depressive illness.

Risks All subjects should be under the direct observation of a physician until the time of maximal hypoglycemia has passed. The test should not be performed in patients with clinical evidence of adrenocortical insufficiency and should be performed only with caution in elderly individuals or when a history of coronary or cerebrovascular insufficiency is present.

Metyrapone

Metyrapone stimulation was originally performed by administering the drug orally and collecting and measuring urine for four sequential 24-h periods. This time-consuming procedure has been shortened by the substitution of plasma for urine steroid measurements.

Method Metyrapone, 0.75 g, is given PO at midnight (patient weight $<$ 70 kg, 2.0 g; 70 to 90 kg, 2.5 g; $>$ 90 kg, 3.0 g), and plasma cortisol and 11-deoxycortisol are measured at 8 A.M. the next day.

Normal Values Plasma cortisol levels should be less than 10 μg/dl to ensure adequate suppression of hormone biosynthesis. Plasma 11-deoxycortisol value should equal or exceed 7 μg/dl.

Interpretation Adequate suppression of plasma cortisol confirms the reduction of the negative feedback effect. A normal 11-deoxycortisol rise indicates the ability of the hypothalamic-pituitary system to respond to interruption of the steroid feedback effect. An impaired response does not distinguish the site of the defect. Enhanced responses are seen in Cushing's disease, whereas the response is impaired in patients receiving exogenous steroids or with adrenocortical adenomas.

Risks The procedure is generally safe. However, in patients with only minimal residual cortisol secretion, irrespective of etiology, mild to moderate symptoms of adrenocortical insufficiency may occur during the course of the test and may require its interruption. The test cannot be performed if the patient is receiving glucocorticoid therapy and should not be performed in patients with primary adrenal insufficiency.

Suppression Tests

Overnight "Screening" Dexamethasone Test

Method The subject is given 1 mg dexamethasone PO at 11 P.M., and plasma cortisol is measured at 8 A.M. the following day.

Normal Values The plasma cortisol level should be 5 μg/dl or less.

Interpretation This is the most commonly used screening test to exclude Cushing's syndrome. A lack of suppression requires that the standard dexamethasone suppression test be performed. Acutely ill or depressed patients and those who are under stress or are obese may also lack suppression.

Standard Dexamethasone Test

Method This test requires the collection of six consecutive 24-h urine samples for free cortisol measurement or, alternatively, daily morning plasma samples for cortisol determinations. Dexamethasone, 0.5 mg every 6 h PO, is given on days 3 and 4, 2.0 mg every 6 h is given on days 5 and 6.

Normal Values In normal subjects, urinary free cortisol is decreased to less than 20 μg per 24 h on the low dose (2 mg per day) of dexamethasone. Plasma cortisol at 48 h should be < 5 μg/dl.

Interpretation A normal response excludes the diagnosis of Cushing's syndrome or Cushing's disease. In patients with Cushing's disease, there is failure of adequate suppression on the low-dose dexamethasone, but a suppression of 50 percent is observed with the high dose. Patients with adenocortical tumors characteristically do not show suppression even with the high dose. Lack of low-dose suppression can also be seen in patients with acute illness or stress. Occasionally, patients with Cushing's disease require larger doses of dexamethasone (up to 32 mg per day) for suppression. Urinary free cortisol measurement provides the best discrimination between normal and abnormal responses.

Overnight High-Dose Dexamethasone Test

Method This is a brief version of the standard high-dose dexamethasone test. The subject is given 8 mg dexamethasone PO at 11 P.M., and plasma cortisol is measured at 8 A.M. the following day.

Normal Values A positive response (normal suppressibility) consists of a cortisol value that is 50 percent or less of the baseline value.

Interpretation A positive response (suppression) occurs in pituitary-dependent Cushing's disease, while a negative response (failure of suppression) is seen in adrenal and ectopic ACTH-secreting tumors.

TSH

Basal Measurements

Using the new third-generation TSH assays, it is possible to distinguish between normal and low TSH values. The normal range in most laboratories is from 0.5 to 6.0 μU/ml. Elevated values are occasionally seen in children with hypothalamic hypothyroidism. Low values (<0.5 μU/ml) are seen in hypopituitary patients, and even lower levels (<0.1 μU/ml) are present in thyrotoxicosis or in patients receiving fully suppressive doses of thyroxine.

Stimulation Tests

Thyrotropin Releasing Hormone Test

Method TRH, 500 μg, is injected intravenously, and blood samples are obtained for TSH at 0, 15, 30, 60, and 120 min.

Normal Values The increase in TSH should be at least 6 μU/ml in females and in males under 40 years and at least 2 μU/ml in males over 40 years of age. Peak values should occur by 30 min.

Interpretation Occasionally, normal subjects may show a slightly decreased response, and differentiation from patients with a partial deficiency of TSH reserve may be difficult. In primary hypothyroidism the response to TRH is increased, whereas in hyperthyroidism or in patients receiving thyroxine, triiodothyronine, or pharmacologic doses of glucocorticoids and frequently in euthyroid Graves' disease it is absent. In hypothalamic hypothyroidism, the TSH response to TRH is increased and the peak is often delayed to 60 min. The delayed response is, however, occasionally seen in patients with pituitary disease. Impaired responses are seen in patients with chronic renal failure.

Risks There are no significant risks. Immediately after injection, subjects experience a sensation of warmth, nausea, a strange taste, and an urge to micturate, which persists for 30 to 60 s and then disappears.

LH and FSH

Basal Measurements

FSH and LH determinations vary with the methods and standards used by the individual laboratory. Most values are reported in relation to the Second IRP/HMG. FSH levels in postpubertal females are approximately 4 to 15 mIU/ml in the follicular and luteal phases, 10 to 50 mIU/ml at midcycle, and 30 to 200 mIU/ml postmenopausally. LH levels are 4 to 30 mIU/ml in the follicular phase, 30 to 150 mIU/ml at midcycle, 4 to 40 mIU/ml in the luteal phase, and more than 40 mIU/ml postmenopausally. Levels in males are similar to those in the follicular phase until the seventh or eighth decade, when increased values occur. Though it is usually not possible to distinguish low from normal values, the absence of elevated LH or FSH levels in patients with clinical and biochemical evidence of hypogonadism is indicative of hypothalamic or pituitary hypofunction.

Stimulation Tests

Gonadotropin Releasing Hormone Test

Method GnRH, 100 μg, is injected intravenously and blood samples are obtained for LH and FSH at 0, 15, 30, and 60 min.

Normal Values The normal response varies considerably between laboratories. In general, an LH response of more than 12 mIU/ml and an FSH response of more than 3 mIU/ml in females and an LH response of more than 8 mIU/ml and an FSH response of more than 3 mIU/ml in males are considered normal. In females, the LH responses vary with the phase of the menstrual cycle, with the greatest response being seen at midcycle. Peak values for LH occur within the first 30 min, though those of FSH may be delayed in some subjects.

Interpretation In patients with hypopituitarism, the responses to GnRH may be normal, impaired, or absent, and the same is true of patients with hypothalamic disease. Thus, an intact response can exclude a pituitary etiology for hypogonadism, but an impaired or absent response cannot be used to define the anatomic site of the abnormality. The test does, however, reflect the functional capacity of the gonadotrophs, and if pituitary function is otherwise intact, an impaired response is suggestive of lack of exposure to endogenous GnRH. Repeat testing after 3 to 7 days of intermittent GnRH therapy permits the differentiation of hypothalamic from pituitary disease. Estrogen deficiency generally decreases the LH response more than the FSH response, resulting in a reversed FSH/LH response ratio. In women with secondary amenorrhea of hypothalamic origin (e.g., anorexia nervosa), the FSH response may be increased.

Clomiphene Test

Clomiphene citrate, a synthetic steroid with weak estrogen activity, binds to estrogen receptors in the hypothalamus, where it exhibits antiestrogenic activity and in adults stimulates the secretion of GnRH and consequently LH and FSH. In prepubertal children, in whom no estrogen levels are present, clomiphene at low doses suppresses gonadotropin secretion. In early puberty a resistance to the effect is noted, and by mid- to late puberty the adult pattern of stimulation is seen.

Method for Women A dose of 100 mg is given PO each day for 5 days (beginning on day 5 of the cycle if the patient is menstruating). Blood samples for LH and FSH are obtained on days 0, 5, 7, 10, and 13.

Method for Men A dose of 100 mg per day is given for 1 to 4 weeks. Blood samples for LH and FSH are obtained twice weekly.

Normal Values In women, FSH and LH should rise and peak on the fifth day of treatment at a level usually above the normal range. After the last dose, the levels should decrease, with a secondary rise in LH between days 9 and 14. In men, a doubling of LH values is seen by 1 week, and the response increases with time. FSH levels rise similarly, but to a lesser extent.

Interpretation A normal rise in gonadotropins indicates an intact hypothalamic response to interruption of the negative feedback effect of estrogen. An absent response coupled with a normal response to GnRH points to a hypothalamic origin for the gonadotropin deficiency. In the presence of an abnormal GnRH response, the clomiphene test is usually abnormal and does not distinguish between hypothalamic and pituitary disease. Responses are generally absent in anorexia nervosa and in hyperprolactinemic states.

Growth Hormone

Basal Measurements

GH deficiency in adults is difficult to establish by basal GH measurements, since values in normals overlap with those in the hypopituitary range. Furthermore, values are age-dependent and are also influenced by nutritional status. Measurement of IGF-I levels can assist, primarily by excluding the diagnosis if the levels are normal. For criteria used during childhood, see Chap. 26. In a patient with suspected acromegaly, a single sample obtained without preparation, preferably 2 h after a meal, is adequate to exclude active disease if the value is < 2 ng/ml.

Stimulation Tests

GRH stimulation directly assesses the capacity of the pituitary to secrete GH. All other available stimulation tests require the presence of an intact hypothalamic-pituitary axis and therefore cannot be used to distinguish the anatomic site of an abnormality. With nearly all the stimuli, an elevated basal GH level usually results in an impaired or absent response. However, for diagnostic purposes, the elevated initial value is sufficient to exclude GH deficiency. An absent or decreased response to each of the tests is seen with sufficient frequency in normal subjects that a deficient response to at least two stimuli is needed to make a definitive diagnosis of GH deficiency.

Growth Hormone Releasing Hormone

Method GRH, 1 μg/kg IV, is injected, and blood samples are obtained at 0, 15, 30, and 60 min. The test may be combined with CRH, TRH, and GnRH tests.

Normal Values GH responses in normal subjects are quite variable, with peak levels occurring at 15 to 30 min and ranging from 10 to > 50 ng/ml in normal young adults. Responses in women are slightly higher than those in men, and responses decrease with age.

Interpretation Diminished responses are seen in hypothyroidism and obesity. Patients with GH deficiency secondary to hypothalamic disease should respond to initial GRH stimulation.

Risks Mild and transient facial flushing is seen occasionally at the recommended dose and is seen more commonly at higher doses.

Insulin Tolerance Test

Hypoglycemia stimulates the secretion of GH in normal subjects, and this test is the most frequently used method of evaluating GH reserve.

Method The details of testing, including dosage, criteria for adequate hypoglycemia, and times of blood sampling, are as described under ACTH testing. GH is measured at 0, 30, 60, 90, and 120 min.

Normal Values A peak value of 9 ng/ml or more, which usually occurs at 60 or 90 min, is considered a normal response. Responses in females are higher than those in males, but this difference is of no diagnostic importance.

Interpretation A normal response excludes GH deficiency. However, up to 20 percent of normal subjects exhibit an impaired or absent response. Such responses are seen frequently but not exclusively when the initial value is elevated. Impaired or absent responses are also seen in obesity, depression, hypothyroidism, hyperthyroidism, Cushing's syndrome (including exogenous steroids), and chronic renal failure and frequently occur in acromegaly.

Risks The risks are as described under ACTH testing.

L-Dopa Test

L-Dopa stimulates GH secretion by enhancing CNS dopaminergic transmission, which in turn is believed to enhance GRH secretion. This test is often used as a secondary procedure for evaluating GH reserve.

Method L-Dopa, 0.5 g PO, is given to a fasting, resting subject, and blood samples for GH are obtained at 0, 60, 90, 120, 150, and 180 min.

Normal Values A normal response consists of a peak value of 6 ng/ml or more, usually between 90 and 150 min. Reduced or absent responses are more frequently observed when initial values are elevated.

Interpretation An intact response excludes GH deficiency but is seen in only 65 to 75 percent of normal subjects, particularly in older persons. Reduced or absent responses occur in obesity and hypothyroidism and in patients receiving α-methyldopa and neuroleptics. In most acromegalic patients, GH levels decrease after the administration of L-dopa owing to a direct dopaminergic action on the neoplastic somatotroph.

Risks The major side effects of L-dopa are nausea and vomiting, which are due to stimulation of a dopamine-sensitive, CNS-mediated mechanism. They are seen in 20 to 25 percent of subjects, usually during the second hour, and while often mild can cause moderate discomfort. Symptoms are generally self-limited but can be controlled by the administration of a dopamine receptor antagonist (e.g., perphenazine, 5 mg) after completion of the study.

Arginine Infusion Test

L-Arginine stimulates GH secretion by an undefined CNS-mediated mechanism.

Method L-Arginine hydrochloride, 0.5 g/kg to a maximum dose of 30 g, is infused intravenously over a 30-min period to an overnight-fasted, resting subject. Blood samples for GH are obtained at 0, 30, 60, 90, and 120 min.

Normal Values A normal response consists of a peak value of at least 9 ng/ml, which usually occurs at 60 to 90 min. Responses are higher in females than in males.

Interpretation A normal response is seen in 65 to 75 percent of normal subjects. The response is decreased or absent in obesity and hypothyroidism, while in acromegaly it is variable and is of no diagnostic significance.

Risks The test has virtually no risks or side effects except in patients with severe liver or renal failure, in whom it should not be used.

Clonidine

Clonidine is a central alpha$_2$-adrenergic agonist that stimulates GH secretion by augmenting the release of endogenous GRH.

Method Clonidine is administered orally (25 μg), and plasma GH is measured at 0 and 75 min.

Normal Values A GH rise of at least 7 ng/ml is seen in normal subjects.

Interpretation A normal response is indicative of an intact hypothalamic-pituitary GH axis. The test has been evaluated more extensively in children than in adults.

Risks Because of its central adrenergic actions, clonidine administration may be associated with postural hypotension and drowsiness, though at the dose recommended these effects are minimal.

Suppression Tests

Glucose Suppression Test

This test is based on the suppression of GH secretion, which normally occurs in response to hyperglycemia.

Method A standard oral glucose tolerance test is performed (75 g of partially hydrolyzed carbohydrate or 100 g of glucose PO), and blood samples for GH are obtained at 0, ½, 1, 2, and 3 h. Additional samples at 4 and 5 h are often useful to demonstrate a GH rebound.

Normal Values Normal subjects will exhibit a decrease in GH levels to less than 2 ng/ml within 2 h. At 4 and 5 h, a rebound of GH to more than 7 ng/ml is common.

Interpretation This test is used to evaluate patients suspected of having acromegaly. Absence of suppression, incomplete suppression, or even paradoxic stimulation is seen in acromegalic patients; normal suppression excludes the diagnosis. Patients with anorexia nervosa who exhibit increased GH levels may have only partial suppression of GH secretion. After a period of refeeding, however, normal suppression is regained.

Prolactin

Basal Measurements

Plasma prolactin values vary among laboratories according to the method and the reference standard utilized. The upper limit of normal is 15 ng/ml in men and 15 to 20 ng/ml in women. The lower limit is generally about 3 ng/ml. Levels in children are similar, though neonates exhibit levels as high as 150 ng/ml during the first few weeks of life. When a single determination is used as a screening tool to exclude hyperprolactinemia, more than one normal value may be required because of the intermittent elevations which are occasionally observed. Plasma prolactin values can be detected in all normal subjects, though in some, the values are near the lower limit of the assay sensitivity. Therefore, a distinction between normal and hypopituitary values is not always possible. Stimulation and suppression tests are not routinely used for clinical purposes.

Stimulation Tests

Stimuli for prolactin secretion can be divided into those which act on the lactotroph dopamine or TRH receptors.

TRH Test

TRH stimulates prolactin secretion via a direct action of the lactotroph.

Methods The dosage and the times of blood sampling are as described under TSH testing.

Normal Values A prolactin rise of at least three times basal values and a peak level of more than 20 ng/ml at 15 or 30 min are seen in normal persons. The rise is greater in females than in males.

Interpretation A reduced or absent response in a patient with low basal levels indicates a deficient prolactin reserve and implies a primary pituitary disorder. A reduced or absent response in patients with hyperprolactinemia may be seen with prolactin-secreting tumors, drug-induced hyperprolactinemia, chronic renal failure, and idiopathic hyperprolactinemia. Furthermore, some patients with pituitary tumors exhibit a normal response to TRH. Thus, the test cannot be used to distinguish between prolactin-secreting tumors and other forms of hyperprolactinemia with any degree of certainty.

Metoclopramide

Prolactin secretion is increased after metoclopramide administration as a result of blockade of pituitary dopaminergic receptors.

Method Metoclopramide, 10 mg IV, is injected, and blood samples are obtained for prolactin at 0, 30, 60, and 120 min.

Normal Values An increase of prolactin to levels of at least 50 ng/ml should be observed, with the peak value occurring at 60 min.

Interpretation This test is useful in evaluating the lactotroph responsiveness to alterations in dopaminergic tone. Nearly all patients with prolactin-secreting tumors as well as those with hypothalamic disorders have a reduced or absent response to metoclopramide; consequently, the usefulness of the test is limited.

Risks Metoclopramide has no side effects and involves no risks.

Insulin Hypoglycemia

The mechanism by which insulin hypoglycemia stimulates prolactin secretion is not known. Prolactin is measured at the same time intervals as is GH. A normal response consists of a rise of 10 ng/ml or more and is seen in 70 percent of normal subjects. A decreased or absent response is seen in patients with pituitary tumors and hypopituitarism, but the test is not discriminatory.

Suppression Tests

Prolactin secretion can at present be suppressed only by stimulation of dopaminergic receptors. This can be done by administration of dopamine itself or of a dopamine agonist. The most commonly used agent is the dopamine precursor L-dopa.

L-Dopa Test

Method The dosage and the times of blood sampling are as described under GH testing.

Normal Values Prolactin levels are suppressed by at least 50 percent in normal subjects at 2 or 3 h.

Interpretation Prolactin suppression is seen in most patients with hyperprolactinemia. A few patients with prolactin-secreting tumors have impaired suppression, but prolongation of the observation period is usually associated with evidence of normal suppression. Thus, L-dopa, like other tests, does not distinguish patients with prolactin-secreting tumors. Patients with chronic renal failure do not show acute suppression with L-dopa.

Risks Risks are as described under GH testing.

REFERENCES

1. DiChiro G, Nelson KB: The volume of the sella turcica. *AJR* 87:989, 1962.
2. Swartz JD, Russell KB, Basile BA, O'Donnell PC, Popky GL: High-resolution computed tomographic appearance of the intrasellar contents in women of childbearing age. *Radiology* 147:115, 1983.
3. Lurie SN, Doraiswamy PM, Husain MM, Boyko OB, Ellinwood EH Jr, Figiel GS, Krishnan KRR: In vivo assessment of pituitary gland volume with magnetic resonance imaging: The effect of age. *J Clin Endocrinol Metab* 71:505, 1990.
4. Kaufman B: Magnetic resonance imaging of the pituitary gland. *Radiol Clin North Am* 22:795, 1984.
5. Glaser B, Sheinfeld M, Benmair J, Kaplan N: Magnetic resonance imaging of the pituitary gland. *Clin Radiol* 37:9, 1986.
6. Wolpert SM, Molitch ME, Goldman JA, Wood JB: Size, shape, and appearance of the normal female pituitary gland. *AJR* 143:377, 1984.
7. Berglund RM, Page RB: Can the pituitary secrete directly to the brain? (Affirmative anatomical evidence). *Endocrinology* 102:1325, 1978.
8. Oliver C, Mical RS, Porter JC: Hypothalamic-pituitary vasculature—evidence for retrograde blood flow in pituitary stalk. *Endocrinology* 101:598, 1977.
9. Mezey E, Palkovits M: Two-way transport in the hypothalamo-hypophyseal system, in Ganong WF, Martini L (eds): *Frontiers in Neuroendocrinology*. New York, Raven, 1982, vol 7, p 1.
10. Page RB: Directional pituitary blood flow: A microcinephotographic study. *Endocrinology* 112:157, 1983.
11. Warner BA, Santen RJ, Page RB: Growth of hormone and prolactin secretion by a tumor of the pharyngeal pituitary. *Ann Intern Med* 96:65, 1982.
12. Bodner M, Castrillo J-L, Theill LE, Deerinck T, Ellisman M, Karin M: The pituitary-specific transcription factor GHF-1 is a homeobox-containing protein. *Cell* 55:505, 1988.
13. Ingraham HA, Chen R, Mangalam HJ, Elsholtz HP, Flynn SE, Lin CR, Simmons DM, Swanson L, Rosenfeld MG: A tissue-specific transcription factor containing a homeodomain specifies a pituitary phenotype. *Cell* 55:519, 1988.
14. Tatsumi K, Miyai K, Notomi T, Kaibe K, Amino N, Mizuno Y, Kohno H: Cretinism wih combined hormone deficiency caused by a mutation in the PIT1 gene. *Nature Gen* 1:56, 1992.
15. Pfaffle RW, DiMattia GE, Parks JS, Brown MR, Wit JM, Jansen M, VanderNat H, VandenBrande JL, et al: Mutation of the POU-specific domain of Pit-1 and hypopituitarism without pituitary hypoplasia. *Science* 257:1118, 1992.
16. Kovacs K, Horvath E, Ryan N: Immunocytochemistry of the human pituitary, in Delellis RA (ed): *Diagnostic Immunocytochemistry*. New York, Masson, 1981, p 17.
17. Baker BL: Functional cytology of adenohypophyseal pars distalis and pars intermedia, in Greep RO (ed): *Handbook of Physiology*. Washington, D.C., American Physiological Society, 1974, vol 4, p 45.
18. Duello TM, Halmi NS: Ultrastructural-immunocytochemical localization of growth hormone and prolactin in human pituitaries. *J Clin Endocrinol Metab* 49:189, 1979.
19. Moriarty GC, Tobin RB: Ultrastructural immunocytochemical characterization of the thyrotroph in rat and human pituitaries. *J Histochem Cytochem* 24:1131, 1976.

20. Samaan NA, Osborne BM, MacKay B, Leavens ME, Duello TM, Halmi NS: Endocrine and morphologic studies of pituitary adenomas secondary to primary hypothyroidism. *J Clin Endocrinol Metab* 45:903, 1977.
21. Bower BF: Pituitary enlargement secondary to untreated primary hypogonadism. *Ann Intern Med* 69:107, 1968.
22. Roberts JL, Herbert E: Characterization of a common precursor to corticotropin and beta-lipotropin: Cell-free synthesis of the precursor and the identification of corticotropin peptides in the molecule. *Proc Natl Acad Sci USA* 74:4826, 1977.
23. Herbert E, Roberts J, Phillips M, Allen R, Hinman M, Budarf M, Policastro P, Rosa P: Biosynthesis, processing and release of corticotropin, β endorphin, and melanocyte stimulating hormone in pituitary cell culture systems, in Martini L, Ganong WF (eds): *Frontiers in Neuroendocrinology*. New York, Raven, 1980, vol 6, p 67.
24. Lloyd RV, Anagnostou D, Cano M, Barkan AL, Chandler WF: Analysis of mammosomatotropic cells in normal and neoplastic human pituitary tissues by the reverse hemolytic plaque assay and immunocytochemistry. *J Clin Endocrinol Metab* 66:1103, 1988.
25. Melmed S, Braunstein GD, Horvath E, Ezrin C, Kovacs K: Pathophysiology of acromegaly. *Endocr Rev* 4:271, 1983.
26. Ferrara N, Henzel WJ: Pituitary follicular cells secrete a novel heparin-binding growth factor specific for vascular endothelial cells. *Biochem Biophys Res Commun* 161:851, 1989.
27. Mains RE, Eipper BA: Biosynthesis of adrenocorticotropic hormone in mouse pituitary tumor cells. *J Biol Chem* 251:4115, 1976.
28. Eipper BA, Mains RE, Guenzi D: High molecular weight forms of adrenocorticotropic hormone are glycoproteins. *J Biol Chem* 251:4121, 1976.
29. Owerbach D, Rutter WJ, Roberts JL, Whitfeld P, Shine J, Seeburg PH, Shows TB: The proopiocortin (adrenocorticotropin/beta-lipotropin) gene is located on chromosome 2 in humans. *Somatic Cell Genet* 7:359, 1981.
30. Markoff E, Sigel MB, Lacour N, Seavey BK, Friesen HG, Lewis UJ: Glycosylation selectively alters the biological activity of prolactin. *Endocrinology* 123:1303, 1988.
31. Tanaka K, Nicholson WE, Orth DN: The nature of the immunoreactive lipotropins in human plasma and tissue extracts. *J Clin Invest* 62:94, 1978.
32. Gilkes JJH, Eady RAJ, Rees LH, Munro DD, Moorhead JF: Plasma immunoreactive melanotrophic hormones in patients on maintenance hemodialysis. *Br Med J* 1:656, 1975.
33. Berson SA, Yalow RS: Radioimmunoassay of ACTH in plasma. *J Clin Invest* 47:2725, 1968.
34. Yalow RS: Heterogeneity of peptide hormone. *Recent Prog Horm Res* 30:597, 1974.
35. Chayen J, Daly JR, Loveridge N, Bitensky L: The cytochemical bioassay of hormones. *Recent Prog Horm Res* 32:33, 1976.
36. Krieger DT, Allen W: Relationship of bioassayable and immunoassayable plasma ACTH and cortisol concentrations in normal subjects and in patients with Cushing's disease. *J Clin Endocrinol Metab* 10:675, 1975.
37. Desir D, Van Cauter E, Fang V, Martino E, Jadot C, Spire J-P, Noel P, Refetoff S, et al: Effects of "jet lag" on hormonal patterns: I. Procedures, variations in total plasma proteins and disruption of adrenocorticotropin-cortisol periodicity. *J Clin Endocrinol Metab* 52:628, 1981.
38. Gilkes JJH, Bloomfield GS, Scott AP, Lowry PJ, Ratcliffe JG, Landon J, Rees LH: Development and validation of a radioimmunoassay for peptides related to a melanocyte-stimulating hormone in human plasma: The lipotropins. *J Clin Endocrinol Metab* 40:450, 1975.
39. Krieger DT, Liotta AS, Suda T, Goodgold A, Condon E: Human plasma immunoreactive lipotropin in normal subjects and in patients with pituitary/adrenal disease. *J Clin Endocrinol Metab* 48:566, 1979.
40. Bertagna XY, Stone WJ, Nicholson WE, Mount CD, Orth DN: Simultaneous assay of immunoreactive β-lipotropin, γ-lipotropin, and β-endorphin in plasma of normal human subjects, patients with ACTH/lipotropin hypersecretory syndromes, and patients undergoing chronic hemodialysis. *J Clin Invest* 67:124, 1981.
41. Rees LH: ACTH, lipotrophin, and MSH in health and disease, in Besser GM (ed): *Clinics in Endocrinology and Metabolism: The Hypothalamus and Pituitary*. London, Saunders, 1977, vol 6, p 137.
42. Hughes J, Smith TW, Fothergill LA, Morgan BA, Morris HR: Identification of two related pentapeptides from the brain with potent opiate agonist activity. *Nature* 258:577, 1975.
43. Goldstein A: Opioid peptides (endorphins) in pituitary and brain. *Science* 193:1081, 1976.
44. Guillemin R, Ling N, Lazarus L, Burgus R, Minick S, Bloom F, Nicoll R, Siggins G, Segal D: The endorphins, novel peptides of brain and hypophyseal origin, with opiate-like activity: Biochemical and biologic studies, in Krieger DT, Ganong WF (eds): *ACTH and Related Peptides: Structure, Regulation, and Action*. New York Academy of Science, 1977, p 131.
45. Li CH, Yamashiro D, Chung D, Doneen BA, Loh HH, Tseng L: Isolation, structure, synthesis and morphine-like activity of beta-endorphin from human pituitary glands, in Krieger DT, Ganong WF (eds): *ACTH and Related Peptides: Structure, Regulation, and Action*. New York Academy of Science, 1977, p. 158.
46. Wilkes MM, Stewart RD, Bruni JF, Quigley ME, Yen SS, Ling N, Chretien M: A specific homologous radioimmunoassay for human beta-endorphin: Direct measurement in biologic fluids. *J Clin Endocrinol Metab* 50:309, 1980.
47. Nakao K, Oki S, Tanaka I, Nakai Y, Imura H: Concomitant secretion of σ-MSH with ACTH and beta-endorphin in humans. *J Clin Endocrinol Metab* 51:1205, 1980.
48. Jackson RV, DeCherney GS, DeBold CR, Sheldon WR, Alexander AN, Rivier J, Vale W, Orth DN: Synthetic ovine corticotropin-releasing hormone: Simultaneous release of proopiomelanocortin peptides in man. *J Clin Endocrinol Metab* 58:740, 1984.
49. Nakao K, Nakai Y, Oki S, Horii K, Imura H: Presence of immunoreactive β-endorphin in normal human plasma: A concomitant release of β-endorphin with adrenocorticotropin after metyrapone administration. *J Clin Invest* 63:1395, 1978.
50. Nakao K, Nakai Y, Jingami H, Oki S, Fukuta J, Imura H: Substantial rise of plasma beta-endorphin levels after insulin-induced hypoglycemia in human subjects. *J Clin Endocrinol Metab* 49:838, 1979.
51. Suda T, Liotta AS, Krieger DT: β-Endorphin is not detectable in plasma from normal human subjects. *Science* 202:221, 1978.
52. Tanaka I, Nakai Y, Nakao K, Oki S, Masaki N, Ohtsuki H, Imura H: Presence of immunoreactive gamma-melanocyte-stimulating hormone, adrenocorticotropin, and beta-endorphin in human gastric antral mucosa. *J Clin Endocrinol Metab* 54:1982, 1982.
53. Bruni JF, Watkins WB, Yen SS: Beta-endorphin in the human pancreas. *J Clin Endocrinol Metab* 49:649, 1979.
54. Sharp B, Pekary AE: Beta-endorphin 61–91 and other beta-endorphin-immunoreactive peptides in human semen. *J Clin Endocrinol Metab* 52:586, 1981.
55. Liotta AS, Krieger DT: In vitro biosynthesis and comparative posttranslational processing of immunoreactive precursor corticotropin/β-endorphin by human placental and pituitary cells. *Endocrinology* 106:1504, 1980.
56. Genazzani AR, Fraioli F, Hurlimann J, Fioretti P, Felber JP: Immunoreactive ACTH and cortisol plasma levels during pregnancy: Detection and partial purification of corticotrophin-like placental hormone. The human chorionic corticotrophin (HCC). *Clin Endocrinol (Oxf)* 4:1, 1975.

57. Sairam MR, Bhargavi GN: A role for glycosylation of the alpha subunit in transduction of biologic signal in glycoprotein hormones. *Science* 229:65, 1985.
58. Carlsen RB, Bahl OP, Swaminathan N: Human chorionic gonadotropin. *J Biol Chem* 248:6810, 1973.
59. Shome B, Parlow AF: Human follicle stimulating hormone: First proposal for the amino acid sequence of the hormone specific beta-subunit (hFSH-β). *J Clin Endocrinol Metab* 39:203, 1974.
60. Sairam MR, Li CH: Human pituitary thyrotropin: The primary structure of the α and β subunits. *Can J Biochem* 55:755, 1977.
61. Begeot M, Hemming FJ, Dubois PM, Combarnous Y, Dubois MP, Aubert ML: Induction of pituitary lactotrope differentiation by luteinizing hormone α subunit. *Science* 226:566, 1984.
62. Naylor SL, Chin WW, Goodman HM, Lalley PA, Grzeschik KH, Sakaguchi AY: Chromosome assignment of genes encoding the alpha and beta subunits of glycoprotein hormones in man and mouse. *Somatic Cell Genet* 9:757, 1983.
63. Chin WW: Hormonal regulation of thyrotropin and gonadotropin gene expression. *Clin Res* 36:484, 1988.
64. Mercer JE: Pituitary gonadotropin gene regulation. *Mol Cell Endocrinol* 73:C63, 1990.
65. Weintraub BD, Gesundheit N, Taylor T, Gyves PW: Effect of TRH on TSH glycosylation and biological action. *Ann NY Acad Sci* 553:205, 1989.
66. Odell WD, Griffin J, Zahradnik R: Two-monoclonal antibody sandwich-type assays for thyrotropin with use of an avidin-biotin separation technique. *Clin Chem* 32:1873, 1986.
67. Spencer CA, LoPresti JS, Patel A, Guttler RB, Eigen A, Shen D, Gray D, Nicoloff JT: Applications of a new chemiluminometric TSH assay to subnormal assessment. *J Clin Endocrinol Metab* 70:453, 1990.
68. Van Helaelst L, Bonnyns M, Golstein-Golaire J: Pituitary TSH in normal subjects and in patients with asymptomatic atrophic thyroiditis: Evidence for its immunological heterogeneity. *J Clin Endocrinol Metab* 41:115, 1975.
69. Nicoloff JT, Spencer CA: The use and misuse of sensitive thyrotropin assay. *J Clin Endocrinol Metab* 71:553, 1990.
70. Blunt S, Woods CA, Joplin GF, Burrin JM: The role of a highly sensitive amplified enzyme immunoassay for thyrotrophin in the evaluation of thyrotroph function in hypopituitary patients. *Clin Endocrinol (Oxf)* 29:387, 1988.
71. Kourides IA, Weintraub RD, Ridgway EC, Maloof F: Pituitary secretion of free alpha and beta subunits of human thyrotropin in patients with thyroid disorders. *J Clin Endocrinol Metab* 40:872, 1975.
72. Edmonds M, Molitch M, Pierce J, Odell WD: Secretion of alpha and beta subunits of TSH by the anterior pituitary. *Clin Endocrinol (Oxf)* 4:525, 1975.
73. Kourides IA, Weintraub BD, Ridgway EC, Maloof F: Pituitary secretion of free alpha and beta subunits of human thyrotropin in patients with thyroid disorders. *J Clin Endocrinol Metab* 40:872, 1975.
74. Peterson V, Smith BR, Hall R: A study of thyroid stimulating activity in human serum with the highly sensitive cytochemical bioassay. *J Clin Endocrinol Metab* 41:199, 1975.
75. Illig R, Krawczynska H, Torresani T, Prader A: Elevated plasma TSH and hypothyroidism in children with hypothalamic hypopituitarism. *J Clin Endocrinol Metab* 41:722, 1975.
76. Faglia G, Ferrari C, Paracchi A, Spada A, Beck-Peccoz P: Triiodothyronine response to thyrotropin-releasing hormone in patients with hypothalamic-pituitary disorders. *Clin Endocrinol (Oxf)* 4:585, 1975.
77. Faglia G, Bitensky L, Pinchera A, Ferrari C, Paracchi A, Beck-Peccoz P, Ambrosi B, Spada A: Thyrotropin secretion in patients with central hypothyroidism: Evidence for reduced biological activity of immunoreactive thyrotropin. *J Clin Endocrinol Metab* 48:989, 1979.
78. Beck-Peccoz P, Amr S, Menezes-Ferreira M, Faglia G, Weintraub BD: Decreased receptor binding of biologically inactive thyrotropin in central hypothyroidism: Effect of treatment with thyrotropin-releasing hormone. *N Engl J Med* 312:1085, 1985.
79. Spitz IM, LeRoith D, Hirsch H, Carayon P, Pekonen F, Liel Y, Sobel R, Chorer Z, Weintraub B: Increased high-molecular weight thyrotropin with impaired biologic activity in a euthyroid man. *N Engl J Med* 304:278, 1981.
80. Kuku SF, Harsoulis P, Kjeld M, Fraser TR: Human thyrotrophic hormone kinetics and effects in euthyroid males. *Horm Metab Res* 7:54, 1975.
81. Segerson TP, Kauer J, Wolfe HC, Mobtaker H, Ping W, Jackson IMD, Lechan RM: Thyroid hormone regulates TRH biosynthesis in the paraventricular nucleus of the rat hypothalamus. *Science* 238:78, 1987.
82. Fisher DA, Dussault JH, Sack J, Chopra IJ: Ontogenesis of hypothalamic-pituitary-thyroid function and metabolism in man, sheep and rat. *Recent Prog Horm Res* 33:59, 1977.
83. Szabo M, Frohman LA: Suppression of cold-stimulated thyrotropin secretion by antiserum to thyrotropin-releasing hormone. *Endocrinology* 101:1023, 1977.
84. Szabo M, Kovathana N, Gordon K, Frohman LA: Effect of passive immunization with an antiserum to TRH on plasma TSH levels in thyroidectomized rats. *Endocrinology* 102:799, 1978.
85. Berelowitz M, Maeda K, Harris S, Frohman LA: The effect of alterations in the pituitary-thyroid axis on hypothalamic content and *in vivo* release of somatostatin-like immunoreactivity. *Endocrinology* 107:24, 1980.
86. Peters JR, Foord SM, Dieguez C, Scanlon MF: TSH neuroregulation and alterations in disease states. *Clin Endocrinol Metab* 12:669, 1983.
87. Ferland L, Labrie F, Jobin M, Arimura A, Schally AV: Physiological role of somatostatin in the control of growth hormone and thyrotropin secretion. *Biochem Biophys Res Commun* 68:149, 1976.
88. Cobb WE, Reichlin S, Jackson IM: Growth hormone secretory status is a determinant of the thyrotropin response to thyrotropin-releasing hormone in euthyroid patients with hypothalamic pituitary disease. *J Clin Endocrinol Metab* 52:324, 1981.
89. Williams TC, Kelijman M, Crelin WC, Downs TR, Frohman LA: Differential effects of somatostatin and a somatostatin analog, SMS 201-995, on the secretion of growth hormone and thyroid-stimulating hormone in man. *J Clin Endocrinol Metab* 66:39, 1988.
90. Weeke J: Circadian variation of serum thyrotropin level in normal subjects. *Scand J Clin Lab Invest* 31:337, 1973.
91. Rossmanith WG, Mortola JF, Laughlin GA, Yen SSC: Dopaminergic control of circadian and pulsatile pituitary thyrotropin release in women. *J Clin Endocrinol Metab* 67:560, 1988.
92. Reichert LE Jr, Ramsey RB, Carter EB: Application of a tissue receptor assay to measurement of serum follitropin (FSH). *J Clin Endocrinol Metab* 41:634, 1975.
93. Catt KJ, Dufau ML, Tsuruhara T: Radioligand-receptor assay of luteinizing hormone and chorionic gonadotropin. *J Clin Endocrinol Metab* 34:123, 1972.
94. Lucky AW, Rich BH, Rosenfield RG, Fang VS, Roche-Bender N: LH bioactivity increases more than immunoreactivity during puberty. *J Pediatr* 97:205, 1980.
95. Dufau ML, Beitins IZ, McArthur JW, Catt KJ: Effects of luteinizing hormone releasing hormone (LHRH) upon bioactive and immunoreactive serum LH levels in normal subjects. *J Clin Endocrinol Metab* 43:658, 1976.
96. Winter JSD, Faiman C, Hobson WC, Prasad AV, Reyes FI: Pituitary-gonadal relations in infancy: I. Patterns of serum gonadotropin concentrations from birth to 4 years of age in man and chimpanzee. *J Clin Endocrinol Metab* 40:545, 1975.
97. Boyar RM, Finkelstein J, Roffwarg H, Kapen S, Weitzman

E, Hellman L: Synchronization of augmented luteinizing hormone secretion with sleep during puberty. *N Engl J Med* 287:582, 1972.

98. Hagen C, McNeilly AS: Changes in circulating levels of LH, FSH, LH beta- and alpha-subunit after gonadotropin-releasing hormone, and of TSH, LH beta- and alpha-subunit after thyrotropin-releasing hormone. *J Clin Endocrinol Metab* 41:466, 1975.
99. Kulin HE, Bell PM, Santen RJ, Ferber AJ: Integration of pulsatile gonadotropin secretion by timed urinary measurements: An accurate and sensitive 3-hour test. *J Clin Endocrinol Metab* 40:783, 1975.
100. Cobel YD, Kohler PO, Cargille CM, Ross GT: Production rates and metabolic clearance rates of human follicle-stimulating hormone in premenopausal and postmenopausal women. *J Clin Invest* 48:359, 1969.
101. Keye WR Jr, Jaffe RV: Modulation of pituitary gonadotropin response to gonadotropin-releasing hormone by estradiol. *J Clin Endocrinol Metab* 38:805, 1974.
102. Lasley BL, Wang CF, Yen SSC: The effects of estrogen and progesterone on the functional capacity of the gonadotrophs. *J Clin Endocrinol Metab* 41:820, 1975.
103. McLachlan RI, Robertson DM, deKrester DM, Berger HG: Advances in the physiology of inhibin and inhibin-related peptides. *Clin Endocrinol (Oxf)* 29:77, 1988.
104. Ying S-Y: Inhibins, activins and follistatins: Gonadal proteins modulating the secretion of follicle-stimulating hormone. *Endocr Rev* 9:267, 1988.
105. Baker HWG, Bremmer WJ, Burger HG, de Kretser DM, Eddie LW, Hudson B, Keogh EJ, Lee WK, Rennie CG: Testicular control of follicle stimulating hormone secretion. *Recent Prog Horm Res* 32:429, 1976.
106. McLachlan RI, Cohen NL, Dahl KD, Bremner WJ, Soules MR: Serum inhibin levels during the periovulatory interval in normal women: Relationships with sex steroid and gonadotrophin levels. *Clin Endocrinol (Oxf)* 32:39, 1990.
107. Sen S, Valenzuela R, Smeby R, Bravo EL, Bumpus FM: Localization, purification, and biological activity of a new aldosterone-stimulating factor. *Hypertension* 3 (Suppl 1):81, 1981.
108. Sen S, Bumpus FM, Oberfield S, New MI: Development and preliminary application of a new assay for aldosterone-stimulating factor. *Hypertension* 5 (Suppl 1):27, 1983.
109. Lis M, Hamet P, Gutkowska J, Maurice G, Seidah NG, LaRiviere N, Chretien M, Genest J: Effect of N-terminal portion of proopiomelanocortin on aldosterone release by human adrenal adenoma in vitro. *J Clin Endocrinol Metab* 52:1053, 1981.
110. Matsuoka H, Mulrow PJ, Franco-Saenz R, Li CH: Effects of β-lipotropin-derived peptides on aldosterone production in the rat adrenal gland. *J Clin Invest* 68:752, 1981.
111. Shome B, Parlow AF: Human pituitary prolactin: The entire linear amino acid sequence. *J Clin Endocrinol Metab* 45:1112, 1977.
112. Li CH: The chemistry of human pituitary growth hormone: 1967–1973, in Li CH (ed): *Hormonal Proteins and Peptides*. New York, Academic, 1975, vol 3, p 1.
113. Niall HD, Hogan ML, Traeger GW, Segre GV, Hwang P, Friesen HG: The chemistry of growth hormone and the lactogenic hormones. *Recent Prog Horm Res* 29:387, 1973.
114. Miller WL, Eberhardt NL: Structure and evolution of the growth hormone gene family. *Endocr Rev* 4:97, 1983.
115. Owerbach D, Martial JA, Baxter JD, Rutter WJ, Shows TB: Genes for growth hormone, chorionic somatomammotropin and a growth hormone–like gene are located on chromosome 17 in humans. *Science* 209:289, 1980.
116. Owerbach D, Rutter WJ, Cooke NE, Martial JA, Shows TB: The prolactin gene is located on chromosome 6 in humans. *Science* 212:815, 1981.
117. Cooke NE, Ray J, Watson MA, Estes PA, Kuo BA, Liebhaber SA: Human growth hormone gene and the highly homologous growth hormone variant gene display different splicing patterns. *J Clin Invest* 82:270, 1988.
118. Goodman HM, Tai LR, Ray J, Cooke NE, Liebhaber SA: Human growth hormone variant produces insulin-like and lipolytic responses in rat adipose tissue. *Endocrinology* 129:1779, 1991.
119. MacLeod JN, Worsley I, Ray J, Friesen HG, Liebhaber SA, Cooke NE: Human growth hormone-variant is a biologically active somatogen and lactogen. *Endocrinology* 128:1298, 1991.
120. Eriksson L, Frankenne F, Eden S, Hennen G, Von Schoultz B: Growth hormone 24-h serum profiles during pregnancy—lack of pulsatility for the secretion of the placental variant. *Br J Obstet Gynaecol* 96:949, 1989.
121. Frohman LA, Downs TR, Chomczynski P: Regulation of growth hormone secretion. *Front Neuroendocrinol* 13:344, 1992.
122. Maurer RA, Gorski J, McKean DJ: Partial amino acid sequence of rat preprolactin. *Biochem J* 161:189, 1977.
123. Benveniste R, Stachura M, Szabo M, Frohman LA: Big growth hormone: Conversion to small growth hormone without peptide bond cleavage. *J Clin Endocrinol Metab* 41:422, 1975.
124. Lewis UJ, Peterson SM, Bonewald LF, Seavey BK, VanderLaan WP: An interchain disulfide dimer of human growth hormone. *J Biol Chem* 252:3697, 1977.
125. Stachura ME, Frohman LA: Growth hormone: Independent release of big and small forms from rat pituitary in vitro. *Science* 187:447, 1975.
126. Soman V, Goodman AD: Studies of the composition and radioreceptor activity of "big" and "little" human growth hormone. *J Clin Endocrinol Metab* 44:569, 1977.
127. Lewis UJ, Dunn JT, Bonewald LF, Seavey BNK, VanderLaan WP: A naturally occurring structural variant of human growth hormone. *J Biol Chem* 253:2679, 1978.
128. DeNoto FM, Moore DD, Goodman HM: Human growth hormone DNA sequence and mRNA structures: Possible alternative splicing. *Nucleic Acids Res* 9:3719, 1981.
129. Estes PA, Cooke NE, Liebhaber SA: A native RNA secondary structure controls alternative splice-site selection and generates two human growth hormone isoforms. *J Biol Chem* 267:14902, 1992.
130. Baumann G, MacCart JG, Amburn K: The molecular nature of circulating growth hormone in normal and acromegalic man: Evidence for a principal and minor monomeric form. *J Clin Endocrinol Metab* 456:946, 1983.
131. Valenta LJ, Sigel MB, Lesniak MA, Elias AN, Lewis UJ, Friesen HG, Kershnar AK: Pituitary dwarfism in a patient with circulating abnormal growth hormone polymers. *N Engl J Med* 312:214, 1985.
132. Baumann G: Growth hormone binding proteins in plasma—An update. *Acta Paediatr Scand* 79:142, 1990.
133. Hocquette JF, Postel-Vinay MC, Djiane J, Tar A, Kelly PA: Human liver growth hormone receptor and plasma binding protein: Characterization and partial purification. *Endocrinology* 127:1665, 1990.
134. Matthews LS: Molecular biology of growth hormone receptors. *Trends Endocrinol Metab* 2:176, 1991.
135. Lewis UJ, Sinha YN, Markoff E, VanderLaan WP: Multiple forms of prolactin: Properties and measurement, in Muller EE, MacLeod RM, Frohman LA (eds): *Neuroendocrine Perspectives*. Amsterdam, Elsevier, 1985, vol 4, p 43.
136. Shoupe D, Montz FJ, Kletzky DA, Di Zerega GS: Prolactin molecular heterogeneity: Response to TRH stimulation of concanavalin-A bound and unbound immunoassayable prolactin during human pregnancy. *Am J Obstet Gynecol* 147:482, 1983.
137. Jackson RD, Wortsman J, Malarkey WB: Characterization of a large molecular weight prolactin in women with idiopathic hyperprolactinemia and normal menses. *J Clin Endocrinol Metab* 61:258, 1985.
138. Isaksson OGP, Eden S, Jansson J-O: Mode of action of

pituitary growth hormone on target cells. *Annu Rev Physiol* 47:483, 1985.
139. Frohman LA, MacGillivray M, Aceto T Jr: Acute effects of human growth hormone on insulin secretion and glucose utilization in normal and growth hormone deficient subjects. *J Clin Endocrinol Metab* 27:561, 1967.
140. Adamson U, Cerasi E: Acute effects of exogenous growth hormone in man: Time- and dose-bound modification of glucose tolerance and glucose-induced insulin release. *Acta Endocrinol (Copenh)* 80:247, 1975.
141. Salmon WD Jr, Daughaday WH: A hormonally controlled serum factor which stimulates sulfate incorporation by cartilage in vitro. *J Lab Clin Med* 49:825, 1957.
142. Froesch ER, Schmid C, Schwander J, Zapf J: Actions of insulin-like growth factors. *Annu Rev Physiol* 47:443, 1985.
143. Zapf J, Froesch ER, Humbel RE: The insulin-like growth factors (IGF) of human serum: Chemical and biological characterization and aspects of their possible physiological role. *Curr Top Cell Regul* 19:257, 1981.
144. Schoenle E, Zapf J, Humbel RE, Froesch ER: Insulin-like growth factor I stimulates growth in hypophysectomized rats. *Nature* 296:252, 1982.
145. Walker JL, Ginalska-Malinowska M, Romer TE, Pucilowska JB, Underwood LE: Effects of the infusion of insulin-like growth factor I in a child with growth hormone insensitivity syndrome (Laron dwarfism). *N Engl J Med* 324:1483, 1991.
146. Isaksson OGP, Jansson J-O, Gause IAM: Growth hormone stimulates longitudinal bone growth directly. *Science* 216: 1237, 1982.
147. Russell SM, Spencer EM: Local injections of human or rat growth hormone or of purified human somatomedin-C stimulate unilateral tibial epiphyseal growth in hypophysectomized rats. *Endocrinology* 116:2563, 1985.
148. Rezvani I, DiGeorge AM, Doroshen SA, Bourdony CJ: Action of human growth hormone on extrathyroidal conversion of thyroxine to triiodothyronine in children with hypopituitarism. *Pediatr Res* 15:6, 1981.
149. Winer LM, Shaw MA, Baumann G: Basal plasma growth hormone levels in man: New evidence for rhythmicity of growth hormone secretion. *J Clin Endocrinol Metab* 70:1678, 1990.
150. Raiti S: The National Hormone and Pituitary Program: Achievements and current goals, in Raiti S, Tolman RA (eds): *Human Growth Hormone*. New York, Plenum, 1986, p 1.
151. Parker ML, Utiger RD, Daughaday WH: Studies in human growth hormone: II. The physiologic disposition and metabolic fate of human growth hormone in man. *J Clin Invest* 41:262, 1962.
152. MacGillivray MH, Frohman LA, Doe J: Metabolic clearance and production rates of human growth hormone in subjects with normal and abnormal growth. *J Clin Endocrinol Metab* 30:632, 1970.
153. Thompson RG, Rodriguez A, Kowarski A, Blizzard RM: Growth hormone: Metabolic clearance rates, integrated concentrations and production rates in normal adults and the effect of prednisone. *J Clin Invest* 51:3193, 1972.
154. Imaki T, Shibisaki T, Shizume K, Masuda A, Hotta M, Kiyosawa Y, Jibiki K, Demura H, et al: The effect of free fatty acids on growth hormone (GH)-releasing hormone mediated GH secretion in man. *J Clin Endocrinol Metab* 60:290, 1985.
155. Massara F, Ghigo E, Goffi S, Molinatti GM, Muller EE, Camanni F: Blockade of hpGRF-40-induced GH release in normal men by a cholinergic muscarinic antagonist. *J Clin Endocrinol Metab* 59:1025, 1984.
156. Sato M, Frohman LA: Differential sensitivity of growth hormone-releasing hormone and somatostatin release from perifused mouse hypothalamic fragments in response to glucose deficiency. *Neuroendocrinology* 57:1097, 1993.
157. Kelijman M, Frohman LA: Discordant effects of insulin-hypoglycemia on growth hormone-releasing hormone-stimulated growth hormone and thyrotropin-releasing hormone-stimulated thyrotropin secretion. *J Clin Endocrinol Metab* 66:872, 1988.
158. Berelowitz M, Szabo M, Frohman LA, Firestone S, Chu L, Hintz RL: Somatomedin-C mediates growth hormone negative feedback by effects on both the hypothalamus and the pituitary. *Science* 212:1279, 1981.
159. Berelowitz M, Firestone SL, Frohman LA: Effects of growth hormone excess and deficiency on hypothalamic somatostatin content and release and on tissue somatostatin distribution. *Endocrinology* 109:714, 1981.
160. Tannenbaum GS: Evidence for autoregulation of growth hormone secretion via the central nervous system. *Endocrinology* 107:2117, 1980.
161. Sato M, Frohman LA: Differential effects of central and peripheral administration of growth hormone (GH) and insulin-like growth factor on hypothalamic GH-releasing hormone (GRH) and somatostatin gene expression in GH-deficient dwarf rats. *Endocrinology* 133:793, 1993.
162. Laron Z: Laron-type dwarfism (hereditary somatomedin deficiency): A review, in Frick P, Harnack G-A, Kochsiek K, Martini GA, Prader A (eds): *Advances in Internal Medicine and Pediatrics*. Berlin, Springer-Verlag, 1984, p 117.
163. Muller EE: Neural control of somatotropic function. *Physiol Rev* 67:962, 1987.
164. Tamminga CA, Neophytides A, Chase TN, Frohman LA: Stimulation of prolactin and growth hormone secretion by muscimol, a gamma-amino-butyric acid agonist. *J Clin Endocrinol Metab* 47:1348, 1978.
165. Stubbs WA, Jones A, Edwards CRW, Delitala G, Jeffcoate WJ, Ratter SJ, Besser GM, Bloom SR, Alberti KGMM: Hormonal and metabolic responses to an enkephalin analogue in normal man. *Lancet* 2:1225, 1978.
166. Bowers CY, Momany FA, Reynolds GA, Hong A: On the *in vitro* and *in vivo* activity of a new synthetic hexapeptide that acts on the pituitary to specifically release growth hormone. *Endocrinology* 114:1537, 1984.
167. Bowers CY, Reynolds GA, Durham D, Barrera CM, Pezzoli SS, Thorner MO: Growth hormone (GH)-releasing peptide stimulates GH release in normal men and acts synergistically with GH-releasing hormone. *J Clin Endocrinol Metab* 70:975, 1990.
168. McNatty KP, Sawers RS: Relationship between the endocrine environment within the graafian follicle and the subsequent rate of progesterone secretion by human granulosa cells in vitro. *J Endocrinol* 66:391, 1975.
169. Landgraf R, Landgraf-Leurs MMC, Weissmann A, Horl R, Von Werder K, Scriba PC: A diabetogenic hormone. *Diabetologia* 13:99, 1977.
170. Shiu RPC, Kelly PA, Friesen HG: Radioreceptor assay for prolactin and other lactogenic hormones. *Science* 180:968, 1973.
171. Soong YK, Ferguson KM, McGarrick G, Jeffcoate SL: Size heterogeneity of immunoreactive prolactin in hyperprolactinemic women. *Clin Endocrinol (Oxf)* 16:259, 1982.
172. Golander A, Hurley T, Barrett J, Hizi A, Handwerger S: Prolactin synthesis by human chorion-decidual tissue: A possible source of prolactin in the amniotic fluid. *Science* 202:311, 1978.
173. Rigg LA, Lein A, Yen SSC: Pattern of increase in circulating prolactin levels during human gestation *Am J Obstet Gynecol* 129:454, 1977.
174. Sievertsen G, Lim VS, Nakawatase C, Frohman LA: Metabolic clearance and secretion of human prolactin in normal subjects and in patients with chronic renal failure. *J Clin Endocrinol Metab* 50:846, 1980.
175. Molitch ME, Raiti S, Baumann G, Belknap S, Reichlin S: Pharmacokinetic studies of highly purified human prolactin in normal human subjects. *J Clin Endocrinol Metab* 65:299, 1987.
176. Phillips HS, Nikolics K, Branton D, Seeburg PH: Immuno-

cytochemical localization in rat brain of a prolactin release-inhibiting sequence of gonadotropin-releasing hormone prohormone. *Nature* 316:542, 1985.
177. Nikolics K, Mason AJ, Szonyi E, Ramachandran J, Seeburg PH: A prolactin-inhibiting factor within the precursor for human gonadotropin-releasing hormone. *Nature* 316:511, 1985.
178. Abe H, Engler D, Molitch ME, Bollinger-Gruber J, Reichlin S: Vasoactive intestinal peptide is a physiological mediator of prolactin release in the rat. *Endocrinology* 116:1383, 1985.
179. Bloom SR, Christofides ND, Delemarter J, Buell G, Kawashima E, Polak JM: Diarrhea in vipoma patients associated with cosecretion of a second active peptide (peptide histidine isoleucine) explained by single coding gene. *Lancet* 2:1163, 1983.
180. Ben-Jonathan N, Arbogast LA, Hyde JF: Neuroendocrine regulation of prolactin release. *Prog Neurobiol* 33:399, 1989.
181. Carlson HE, Wasser HL, Levin SR: Prolactin stimulation by meals is related to protein content. *J Clin Endocrinol Metab* 57:334, 1983.
182. Langer G, Sachar EJ, Gruen PH, Halpern F: Human prolactin responses to neuroleptic drugs correlate with antischizophrenic potency. *Nature* 266:639, 1977.
183. Rick J, Szabo M, Payne P, Kovathana N, Cannon JG, Frohman LA: Prolactin-suppressive effects of two aminotetralin analogs of dopamine: Their use in the characterization of the pituitary dopamine receptor. *Endocrinology* 104:1234, 1979.
184. Gonzalez-Villalpado C, Szabo M, Frohman LA: Central nervous system–mediated stimulation of prolactin secretion by cimetidine, a histamine H_2-receptor antagonist: Impaired responsiveness in patients with prolactin-secreting tumors and idiopathic hyperprolactinemia. *J Clin Endocrinol Metab* 51:1417, 1980.
185. Knigge U, Wollesen F, Dejgarrd A, Theusen B: Comparison between dose-responses of prolactin, thyroid stimulating hormone and growth hormone to two different histamine H-2 rceptor antagonists in normal men. *Clin Endocrinol (Oxf)* 15:585, 1981.
186. Lim VS, Kathpalia S, Frohman LA: Hyperprolactinemia and impaired pituitary responses to suppression and stimulation in chronic renal failure: Reversal following transplantation. *J Clin Endocrinol Metab* 48:101, 1979.
187. Simmonds M: Uber hypophysisschwund mit todlichem Ausgang. *Dtsch Med Wochenschr* 40:322, 1914.
188. Glinski LK: Anatomische Veranderungen der Hypophyse. *Dtsch Med Wochenschr* 39:473, 1913.
189. Sheehan HL: Postpartum necrosis of the anterior pituitary. *J Pathol Bacteriol* 45:189, 1937.
190. Sheehan HL, Murdoch R: Postpartum necrosis of the anterior pituitary: Pathological and clinical aspects. *J Obstet Gynecol Br Empire* 45:456, 1938.
191. Brennan CF, Malone RGS, Weaver JA: Pituitary necrosis in diabetes mellitus. *Lancet* 2:12, 1956.
192. Kovacs K: Necrosis of anterior pituitary in humans. *Neuroendocrinology* 4:170, 1969.
193. Cardoso ER, Peterson EW: Pituitary apoplexy: A review. *Neurosurgery* 14:363, 1984.
194. Ostrov SG, Quencer RM, Hoffman JC, Davis PC, Hasso AN, David NJ: Hemorrhage within pituitary adenomas: How often associated with pituitary apoplexy syndrome. *Am J Roentgenol Radium Ther Nucl Med* 153:153, 1989.
195. Onesti ST, Wisniewski T, Post KD: Clinical versus subclinical pituitary apoplexy: Presentation, surgical management, and outcome in 21 patients. *Neurosurgery* 26:980, 1990.
196. Pelkonen R, Kuusisto A, Salmi J, Eistola P, Raitta C, Karonen S-L, Aro A: Pituitary function after apoplexy. *Am J Med* 65:773, 1978.
197. Arafah BM, Harrington JF, Madhoun ZT, Selman WR: Improvement of pituitary function after surgical decompression for pituitary tumor apoplexy. *J Clin Endocrinol Metab* 71:323, 1990.
198. Sano T, Kovacs K, Scheithauer BW, Rosenblum MK, Petito CK, Greco CM: Pituitary pathology in acquired immunodeficiency syndrome. *Arch Pathol Lab Med* 113:1066, 1989.
199. Stocks AE, Powell LW: Pituitary function in idiopathic hemochromatosis and cirrhosis of the liver. *Lancet* 2:298, 1972.
200. Williams T, Frohman LA: Hypothalamic dysfunction associated with hemochromatosis. *Ann Intern Med* 103:550, 1985.
201. Asa SL, Bilbao JM, Kovacs K, Josse RG, Kreines K: Lymphocytic hypophysitis of pregnancy resulting in hypopituitarism. *Ann Intern Med* 95:166, 1981.
202. Baskin DS, Townsend JJ, Wilson CB: Lymphocytic adenohypophysitis of pregnancy simulating a pituitary adenoma: A distinct pathologic entity. *J Neurosurg* 56:148, 1982.
203. Guay AT, Agnello V, Tronic BC, Gresham DG, Freidberg SR: Lymphocytic hypophysitis in a man. *J Clin Endocrinol Metab* 64:631, 1987.
204. Rickards AG, Harvey PW: "Giant cell granuloma" and other pituitary granulomata. *Q J Med* 23:425, 1954.
205. Barkan AL, Kelch RP, Marshall JC: Isolated gonadotrope failure in the polyglandular autoimmune syndrome. *N Engl J Med* 312:1535, 1985.
206. Samaan NA, Bakdesh MM, Caderao JB, Cangir A, Jesse RH Jr, Ballantyne AJ: Hypopituitarism after external irradiation: Evidence for both hypothalamic and pituitary origin. *Ann Intern Med* 83:771, 1975.
207. Romshe CA, Zipf WB, Miser A, Miser J, Sotos JF, Newton WA: Evaluation of growth hormone release and human growth hormone treatment in children with cranial irradiation–associated short stature. *J Pediatr* 104:177, 1984.
208. Jordan RM, Kendall JW, Kerber CW: The primary empty sella syndrome. *Am J Med* 62:569, 1977.
209. Fleckman AM, Schubart UK, Danziger A, Fleischer N: Empty sella of normal size in Sheehan's syndrome. *Am J Med* 75:585, 1983.
210. Chiang R, Marshall MC Jr, Rosman PM, Hotson G, Mannheimer E, Wallace EZ: Empty sella turcica in intracranial sarcoidosis. *Arch Neurol* 41:662, 1984.
211. Schimke RN, Spaulding JJ, Hollowell JG: X-linked congenital panhypopituitarism. *Birth Defects* 7:21, 1971.
212. Ferrier PE, Stone EF Jr: Familial pituitary dwarfism associated with an abnormal sella turcica. *Pediatrics* 43:858, 1969.
213. Parks JS, Tenore A, Bongiovanni AM, Kirkland RT: Familial hypopituitarism with large sella turcica. *N Engl J Med* 298:698, 1978.
214. Li S, Crenshaw EB III, Rawson EJ, Simmons DM, Swanson LW, Rosenfeld MG: Dwarf locus mutants lacking three pituitary cell types result from mutations in the POU-domain gene pit-1. *Nature* 347:528, 1990.
215. Phillips JA III, Vnencak-Jones CL: Genetics of growth hormone and its disorders. *Adv Hum Genet* 18:305, 1989.
216. Parks JS: Molecular biology of growth hormone. *Acta Paediatr Scand* 78:127, 1989.
217. Weiss J, Alexrod L, Whitcomb RW, Harris PE, Crowley WF, Jameson JL: Hypogonadism caused by a single amino acid substitution in the B subunit of luteinizing hormone. *N Engl J Med* 326:179, 1992.
218. Hayashizaki Y, Hiraoka Y, Endo Y, Miyai K, Matsubara K: Thyroid-stimulating hormone (TSH) deficiency caused by a single base substitution in the CAGYC region of the beta-subunit. *EMBO J* 8:2291, 1989.
219. Lim VS, Fang VS, Katz AJ, Refetoff S: Thyroid dysfunction in renal failure: A study of the pituitary axis and peripheral turnover kinetics of thyroxine and triiodothyronine. *J Clin Invest* 60:522, 1977.
220. Lim VS, Henriquez C, Sievertsen G, Frohman LA: Ovarian function in chronic renal failure: Evidence suggesting hypothalamic anovulation. *Ann Intern Med* 93:21, 1980.

221. Rudman D, Fleischer AS, Kutner MH, Raggio JF: Suprahypophyseal hypogonadism and hypothyroidism during prolonged coma after head trauma. *J Clin Endocrinol Metab* 45:747, 1977.
222. Yuan XQ, Wade CE: Neuroendocrine abnormalities in patients with traumatic brain injury. *Front Neuroendocrinol* 12:209, 1991.
223. Schurmeyer TH, Tsokos GC, Avgerinos PC, Balow JE, D'Agata R, Loriaux DL, Chrousos GP: Pituitary-adrenal responsiveness to corticotropin-releasing hormone in patients receiving chronic alternate day glucocorticoid therapy. *J Clin Endocrinol Metab* 61:22, 1985.
224. Bullen BA, Skrinar GS, Beitens IZ, von Mering G, Turnbull BA, McArthur JW: Induction of menstrual disorders by strenuous exercise in untrained women. *N Engl J Med* 312:1349, 1985.
225. Pirke KM, Schweiger U, Broocks A, Tuschl RJ, Laessle RG: Luteinizing hormone and follicle stimulating hormone secretion patterns in female athletes with and without menstrual disturbances. *Clin Endocrinol (Oxf)* 33:345, 1990.
226. Brooks GJ, Warren MP, Hamilton LH: The relation of eating problems and amenorrhea in ballet dancers. *Med Sci Sports Exerc* 19:41, 1987.
227. Vigersky R (ed): *Anorexia Nervosa*. New York, Raven, 1977.
228. Woolf PD, Hamill RW, McDonald JV, Lee LA, Kelly M: Transient hypogonadism caused by critical illness. *J Clin Endocrinol Metab* 60:444, 1985.
229. Barkan A, Glantz I: Calcification of auricular cartilages in patients with hypopituitarism. *J Clin Endocrinol Metab* 55:354, 1982.
230. Miyai K, Azukizawa M, Kumahara Y: Familial isolated thyrotropin deficiency with cretinism. *N Engl J Med* 285:1043, 1971.
231. Zisman E, Lotz M, Jenkins ME, Bartter FC: Studies in pseudohypoparathyroidism: Two new cases with a probable selective deficiency of thyrotropin. *Am J Med* 46:464, 1969.
232. Bell J, Benveniste R, Spitz I, Rabinowitz D: Isolated deficiency of follicle-stimulating hormone: Further studies. *J Clin Endocrinol Metab* 40:790, 1975.
233. Merimee TJ: A follow-up study of vascular disease in growth hormone–deficient dwarfs with diabetes. *N Engl J Med* 298:1217, 1978.
234. Rosen T, Bengtsson B-A: Premature mortality due to cardiovascular disease in hypopituitarism. *Lancet* 336:285, 1990.
235. Jorgensen JOL, Pedersen SA, Thuesen L, Jorgensen J, Ingemann-Hansen T, Skakkebaek NE, Christiansen JS: Beneficial effects of growth hormone treatment in GH-deficient adults. *Lancet* 1:1221, 1989.
236. Salomon F, Cuneo RC, Hesp R, Sonksen PH: The effects of treatment with recombinant human growth hormone on body composition and metabolism in adults with growth hormone deficiency. *N Engl J Med* 321:1797, 1989.
237. Degerblad M, Almkvist O, Grunditz R, Hall K, Kaijser L, Knutsson E, Ringertz H, Thoren M: Physical and psychological capabilities during substitution therapy with recombinant growth hormone in adults with growth hormone deficiency. *Acta Endocrinol (Copenh)* 123:185, 1990.
238. Haeger A: Should adults with growth hormone deficiency be maintained on growth hormone substitution therapy? *Acta Paediatr Scand* 78:72, 1989.
239. Kelley KW: The role of growth hormone in modulation of the immune response. *Ann NY Acad Sci* 594:95, 1990.
240. Mocchegiani E, Paolucci P, Balsamo A, Cacciari E, Fabris N: Influence of growth hormone on thymic endocrine activity in humans. *Front Endocrinol* 33:248, 1990.
241. Gala RR: Prolactin and growth hormone in the regulation of the immune system. *Proc Soc Exp Biol Med* 198:513, 1991.
242. Goodman HG, Grumbach MM, Kaplan SL: Growth and growth hormone: II. A comparison of isolated growth hormone deficiency and multiple pituitary hormone deficiencies in 35 patients with idiopathic hypopituitary dwarfism. *N Engl J Med* 278:57, 1968.
243. Sheehan HL, Summers VK: The syndrome of hypopituitarism. *Q J Med* 18:319, 1949.
244. Gambone J, Meldrum DR, Laufer L, Chang RJ, Lu JKH, Judd HL: Further delineation of hypothalamic dysfunction responsible for menopausal hot flashes. *J Clin Endocrinol Metab* 59:1097, 1984.
245. Lindholm J, Kehlet H, Blichert-Toft M, Dinesen B, Riishede J: Reliability of the 30-min ACTH test in assessing hypothalamic-pituitary-adrenal function. *J Clin Endocrinol Metab* 47:272, 1978.
246. Borst GC, Michenfelder HJ, O'Brian JT: Discordant cortisol response to exogenous ACTH and insulin-induced hypoglycemia in patients with pituitary disease. *N Engl J Med* 306:1462, 1982.
247. Grossman A, Kruseman AC, Perry L, Tomlin S, Schally AV, Coy DH, Rees LH, Comaru-Schally AM, Besser GM: New hypothalamic hormone, corticotropin-releasing factor, specifically stimulates the release of adrenocorticotropic hormone and cortisol in man. *Lancet* 1:921, 1982.
248. Orth DN, Jackson RV, DeCherney GS, DeBold CR, Alexander AN, Island DP, Rivier J, Rivier C, et al: Effect of synthetic ovine corticotropin-releasing factor: Dose response of plasma adrenocorticotropin and cortisol. *J Clin Invest* 71:587, 1982.
249. Nicholson WE, DeCherney GS, Jackson RV, DeBold CR, Uderman H, Alexander AN, Rivier J, Vale W, Orth DN: Plasma distribution, disappearance half-time, metabolic clearance rate, and degradation of synthetic ovine corticotropin-releasing factor in man. *J Clin Endocrinol Metab* 57:1263, 1983.
250. Schurmeyer TH, Avgerinos PC, Gold PW, Gallucci WT, Tomai TP, Cutler GB Jr, Loriaux DL, Chrousos GP: Human corticotropin-releasing factor in man: Pharmacokinetic properties and dose response of plasma adrenocorticotropin and cortisol secretion. *J Clin Endocrinol Metab* 59:1103, 1984.
251. Nieman LK, Loriaux DL: Corticotropin-releasing hormone: Clinical applications. *Annu Rev Med* 40:331, 1989.
252. Spiger M, Jubiz W, Meikle AW, West CD, Tyler FJ: Single-dose metyrapone test: Review of a four-year experience. *Arch Intern Med* 135:698, 1975.
253. Asa SL, Kovacs K, Tindall GT, Barrow DL, Horvath E, Vecsei P: Cushing's disease associated with an intrasellar gangliocytoma producing corticotrophin-releasing factor. *Ann Intern Med* 101:789, 1984.
254. Costom BH, Grumbach MM, Kaplan SL: Effect of thyrotropin-releasing factor on serum thyroid-stimulating hormone. *J Clin Invest* 50:2219, 1971.
255. Besser GM, McNeilly AS, Anderson DC, Marshall JC, Harsoulis P, Hall R, Ormston BJ, Alexander L, Collins WP: Hormonal responses to synthetic luteinizing hormone and follicle stimulating hormone releasing hormone in man. *Br Med J* 3:267, 1972.
256. Mortimer CH, Besser GM, McNeilly AS, Marshall JC, Harsoulis P, Tunbridge WNG, Gomez-Pan A, Hall R: Luteinizing hormone and follicle stimulating hormone releasing hormone test in patients with hypothalamic-pituitary-gonadal dysfunction. *Br Med J* 4:73, 1973.
257. Snyder PJ, Rudenstein RS, Gardner DF, Rothman JG: Repetitive infusion of gonadotropin-releasing hormone distinguishes hypothalamic from pituitary hypogonadism. *J Clin Endocrinol Metab* 48:864, 1979.
258. Vance ML, Borges JCL, Kaiser DL, Evans WS, Furlanetto R, Thominet JL, Frohman LA, Rogol AD, et al: Human pancreatic tumor growth hormone releasing factor (hpGRF-40): Dose response relationships in normal man. *J Clin Endocrinol Metab* 58:838, 1984.
259. Gelato MC, Pescovitz OH, Cassorla F, Loriaux DL, Merriam GR: Dose-response relationships for effects of growth

hormone releasing factor-(1–44)-NH_2 in young adult men and women. *J Clin Endocrinol Metab* 59:107, 1984.
260. Schriock EA, Lustig RH, Rosenthal SM, Kaplan SL, Grumbach MM: Effect of growth hormone (GH)-releasing hormone (GRH) on plasma GH in relation to magnitude and duration of GH deficiency in 26 children and adults with isolated deficiency or multiple pituitary hormone deficiencies: Evidence for hypothalamic GRH deficiency. *J Clin Endocrinol Metab* 58:1043, 1984.
261. Alba-Roth J, Mueller OA, Schopohl J, Von Werder K: Arginine stimulates growth hormone secretion by suppressing endogenous somatostatin secretion. *J Clin Endocrinol Metab* 67:1186, 1988.
262. Gil-Ad I, Topper E, Laron Z: Oral clonidine as a growth hormone stimulation test. *Lancet* 2:278, 1979.
263. Laron Z, Gil-Ad I, Topper E, Kaufman H, Josefsberg Z: Low oral dose of clonidine an effective screening test for growth hormone deficiency. *Acta Paediatr Scand* 71:847, 1982.
264. Massara F, Ghigo E, Demislis K, Tangolo D, Mazza E, Locatelli V, Muller EE, Molinatti GM, Camanni F: Cholinergic involvement in the growth hormone releasing hormone-induced growth hormone release: Studies in normal and acromegalic subjects. *Neuroendocrinology* 43:670, 1986.
265. Williams T, Berelowitz M, Joffe SN, Thorner MO, Rivier J, Vale W, Frohman LA: Impaired growth hormone responses to growth hormone-releasing factor in obesity: A pituitary defect reversed with weight reduction. *N Engl J Med* 311:1403, 1984.
266. Sims EAH, Danforth E Jr, Horton ES, Bray GS, Glennon JA, Salans LB: Endocrine and metabolic effects of experimental obesity in man. *Recent Prog Horm Res* 29:457, 1973.
267. MacGillivray MH, Aceto T, Frohman LA: Plasma growth hormone response and growth retardation of hypothyroidism. *Am J Dis Child* 115:273, 1968.
268. Williams T, Maxon H, Thorner MO, Frohman LA: Blunted growth hormone response to growth hormone-releasing hormone in hypothyroidism resolves in the euthyroid state. *J Clin Endocrinol Metab* 61:454, 1985.
269. Woolf PH, Lee LA, Leebaw WF: Hypoglycemia as a provocative test of prolactin release. *Metabolism* 27:869, 1978.
270. Sheldon WR Jr, DeBold CR, Evans WS, DeCherney GS, Jackson RV, Island DP, Thorner MO, Orth DN: Rapid sequential intravenous administration of four hypothalamic releasing hormones as a combined anterior pituitary function test in normal subjects. *J Clin Endocrinol Metab* 60:623, 1985.
271. Hurley DM, Brian R, Outch K, Stockdale J, Fry A, Hackman C, Clarke I, Burger HG: Induction of ovulation and fertility in amenorrheic women by pulsatile low-dose gonadotropin-releasing hormone. *N Engl J Med* 310:1069, 1984.
272. Hoffman AR, Crowley WF Jr: Induction of puberty in men by long-term pulsatile administration of low-dose gonadotropin-releasing hormone. *N Engl J Med* 307:1237, 1982.
273. Skarin G, Nillius SJ, Wibell L, Wide L: Chronic pulsatile low dose GnRH for induction of testosterone production and spermatogenesis in a man with secondary hypogonadotropic hypogonadism. *J Clin Endocrinol Metab* 55:723, 1982.
274. Finkel DM, Phillips JL, Snyder PJ: Stimulation of spermatogenesis by gonadotropins in men with hypogonadotropic hypogonadism. *N Engl J Med* 313:651, 1985.
275. Gore DC, Honeycutt D, Jahoor F, Wolfe RR, Herndon DN: Effect of exogenous growth hormone on whole-body and isolated-limb protein kinetics in burned patients. *Arch Surg* 126:38, 1991.
276. Marcus R, Butterfield G, Holloway L, Gilliland L, Baylink DJ, Hintz RL, Sherman BM: Effects of short term administration of recombinant human growth hormone to elderly people. *J Clin Endocrinol Metab* 70:519, 1990.
277. Snyder DK, Clemmons DR, Underwood LE: Treatment of obese, diet-restricted subjects with growth hormone for 11 weeks: Effects on anabolism, lipolysis, and body composition. *J Clin Endocrinol Metab* 67:54, 1988.
278. Ziegler TR, Young LS, Manson JM, Wilmore DW: Metabolic effects of recombinant human growth hormone in patients receiving parenteral nutrition. *Ann Surg* 208:6, 1988.
279. Brown P, Gajdusek DC, Gibbs CJ Jr, Asher DM: Potential epidemic of Creutzfeldt-Jakob disease from human growth hormone therapy. *N Engl J Med* 313:728, 1985.
280. Thorner MO, Reschke J, Chitwood J, Rogol AD, Furlanetto R, Rivier J, Vale W, Blizzard RM: Acceleration of growth in two children treated with human growth hormone-releasing factor. *N Engl J Med* 312:4, 1985.
281. Gelato MC, Ross JL, Malozowski S, Peskovitz OH, Skerda M, Cassorla F, Loriaux DL, Merriam GL: Effects of pulsatile administration of growth hormone (GH)-releasing hormone on short term linear growth in children with GH deficiency. *J Clin Endocrinol Metab* 61:444, 1985.
282. Smith RG, Cheng K, Schoen WR, Pong SS, Hickey G, Jacks T, Butler B, Chan WWS, et al: A nonpeptidyl growth hormone secretagogue. *Science* 260:1640, 1993.
283. Rudman D, Feller AG, Cohn L, Shetty KR, Rudman IW, Draper MW: Effects of human growth hormone on body composition in elderly men. *Horm Res* 36:73, 1991.
284. Tyson JE, Perez A, Zanartu J: Human lactational response to oral thyrotropin releasing hormone. *J Clin Endocrinol Metab* 43:760, 1976.
285. Kovacs K, Horvath E, Bayley TA, Hassaram ST, Ezrin C: Silent corticotroph cell adenoma lysosomal accumulation and crinophagy. *Am J Med* 64:492, 1978.
286. Kourides IA, Weintraub BD, Rosen SW, Ridgway EC, Kliman B, Maloof F: Secretion of alpha subunit of glycoprotein hormones by pituitary adenomas. *J Clin Endocrinol Metab* 43:97, 1976.
287. Younghusband OZ, Horax G, Hurxthal LM, Hare HF, Poppen JL: Chromophobe pituitary tumors: I. Diagnosis. *J Clin Endocrinol Metab* 12:611, 1952.
288. Bakay L: The results of 300 pituitary adenoma operations. *J Neurosurg* 7:240, 1950.
289. Burrow GN, Wortzman G, Rewcastle NB, Holgate RC, Kovacs K: Microadenomas of the pituitary and abnormal sellar tomograms in unselected autopsy series. *N Engl J Med* 304:156, 1981.
290. Earle JM, Dillard SH Jr: Pathology of adenomas of the pituitary gland, in Kohler PO, Ross GT (eds): *Diagnosis and Treatment of Pituitary Tumors*. Amsterdam, Excerpta Medica, 1973, p 3.
291. Wilson CB, Dempsey LC: Transsphenoidal microsurgical removal of 250 pituitary adenomas. *J Neurosurg* 48:13, 1978.
292. Furst E: On chromophobe pituitary adenoma. *Acta Med Scand* 180(Suppl 452):1, 1966.
293. Bartlett JR: Craniopharyngiomas—a summary of 85 cases. *J Neurol Neurosurg Psychiatry* 34:37, 1971.
294. Wilson CB, Dempsey LC: Transsphenoidal microsurgical removal of 250 pituitary adenomas. *J Neurosurg* 48:13, 1978.
295. Tindall GT, McLanahan CS, Christy JC: Transsphenoidal microsurgery for pituitary tumors associated with hyperprolactinemia. *J Neurosurg* 48:849, 1981.
296. Crane TB, Yee RD, Hepler FS, Hallinan JM: Clinical manifestations and radiologic findings in craniopharyngiomas in adults. *Am J Ophthalmol* 94:220, 1982.
297. Kucharczyk W, Davis DO, Kelly WM, Sze G, Norman D, Newton TH: Pituitary adenomas: High resolution MR imaging at 1.5T. *Radiology* 161:761, 1986.
298. Taveras JM, Wood EH: *Diagnostic Neuroradiology*. Baltimore, Williams & Wilkins,1964, p 1.101.
299. McLachlan MSF, Wright AD, Doyle FH: Plain film and tomographic assessment of the pituitary fossa in 140 acromegalic patients. *Br J Radiol* 43:360, 1970.
300. Weisberg LA, Zimmerman EA, Frantz AG: Diagnosis and evaluation of patients with an enlarged sella turcica. *Am J Med* 61:590, 1976.

301. Brown SB, Irwin KM, Enzmann DR: CT characteristics of the normal pituitary gland. *Neuroradiology* 24:259, 1983.
302. Swartz MD, Russell KB, Basile BA, O'Donnell PC, Popky GL: High-resolution computed tomographic appearance of the intrasellar contents in women of childbearing age. *Radiology* 145:115, 1983.
303. Hinshaw DB Jr, Hasso AN, Thompson JR, Davidson BJ: High resolution computed tomography of the postpartum pituitary gland. *Neuroradiology* 26:299, 1984.
304. Hemminghytt S, Kalkhoff DK, Daniels DL, Williams AL, Grogan JP, Haughton VM: Computed tomographic study of hormone-secreting microadenomas. *Radiology* 146:65, 1983.
305. Chambers AL, Turski PA, LaMasters D, Newton TH: Regions of low density in the contrast-enhanced pituitary gland: Normal and pathologic processes. *Radiology* 144: 109, 1982.
306. Taylor CR, Jaffe CC: Methodological problems in clinical radiology research: Pituitary microadenoma detection as a paradigm. *Radiology* 149:279, 1983.
307. Dwyer AJ, Frank JA, Doppman JL, Oldfield EH, Hickey AM, Cutler GB, Loriaux DL, Schiable TF: Pituitary adenomas in patients with Cushing disease: Initial experience with Gd-DTPA-enhanced MR imaging. *Radiology* 163:421, 1987.
308. Molitch ME, Russell EJ: The pituitary "incidentaloma." *Ann Intern Med* 112:925, 1990.
309. De Souza B, Brunetti A, Fulham MJ, Brooks RA, DeMichele D, Cook P, Nieman L, Doppman JL, et al: Pituitary microadenomas: A PET study. *Radiology* 177:39, 1990.
310. Kaufman B: Magnetic resonance imaging of the pituitary gland. *Radiol Clin North Am* 22:795, 1984.
311. Linfoot JA, Garcia JF, Wei W, Fink R, Sarin R, Born JL, Lawrence JH: Human growth hormone levels in cerebrospinal fluid. *J Clin Endocrinol Metab* 31:230, 1970.
312. Jordan RM, Kendall JW, Seaich JL, Allen JP, Paulsen A, Kerber CW, VanderLaan WP: Cerebrospinal fluid hormone concentration in the evaluation of pituitary tumors. *Ann Intern Med* 85:49, 1976.
313. Schroeder LL, Johnson JC, Malarkey WB: Cerebrospinal fluid prolactin: A reflection of abnormal prolactin secretion in patients with pituitary tumors. *J Clin Endocrinol Metab* 43:1255, 1976.
314. Bergland RM, Ray BS, Torack RM: Anatomical variations in the pituitary gland and adjacent structures in 225 human autopsy cases. *J Neurosurg* 28:93, 1968.
315. Marwaha R, Menon PS, Jena A, Pant C, Sethi AK, Sapra ML: Hypothalamo-pituitary axis by magnetic resonance imaging in isolated growth hormone deficiency patients born by normal delivery. *J Clin Endocrinol Metab* 74:654, 1992.
316. Komatsu M, Kondo T, Yamauchi K, Yokokawa N, Ichikawa K, Ishihara M, Aizawa T, Yamada T, et al: Antipituitary antibodies in patients with the primary empty sella syndrome. *J Clin Endocrinol Metab* 67:633, 1988.
317. Bakiri F, Bendib SE, Maoui R, Bendib A, Benmiloud M: The sella turcica in Sheehan's syndrome: Computerized tomographic study in 54 patients. *J Endocrinol Invest* 14:193, 1991.
318. Buchfelder M, Brockmeier S, Pichl J, Schrell U, Fahlbusch R: Results of dynamic endocrine testing of hypothalamic pituitary function in patients with a primary "empty" sella syndrome. *Horm Metab Res* 21:573, 1989.
319. Gharib H, Frey HM, Laws ER Jr, Randall RV, Scheithauer BW: Coexistent primary empty sella syndrome and hyperprolactinemia. *Arch Intern Med* 143:1383, 1983.
320. Gallardo E, Schachter D, Caceres E, Becker P, Colin E, Martinez C, Henriquez C: The empty sella: Results of treatment in 76 successive cases and high frequency of endocrine and neurological disturbances. *Clin Endocrinol (Oxf)* 37:529, 1992.
321. Domingue JN, Wing SD, Wilson CB: Coexisting pituitary adenomas and partially empty sellas. *J Neurosurg* 48:23, 1978.
322. Ganguly A, Stanchfield JB, Roberts TS, West CD, Tyler FH: Cushing's syndrome in a patient with an empty sella turcica and a microadenoma of the adenohypophysis. *Am J Med* 60:306, 1976.
322a. Arseni C, Chitescu M, Cristescu A, Mihaila G: Intrasellar aneurysms simulating hypophyseal tumors. *Eur Neurol* 3:321, 1970.
323. Scanarini M, D'Avella D, Rotilio A, Kitromilis N, Mingrino S: Giant-cell granulomatous hypophysitis: A distinct clinicopathological entity. *J Neurosurg* 71:681, 1989.
324. Valenta LJ, Tamkin J, Sostrin R, Elias AN, Eisenberg H: Regression of a pituitary adenoma following levothyroxine therapy of primary hypothyroidism. *Fertil Steril* 40:389, 1983.
325. MacCarty CS, Hanson EJ Jr, Randall RV, Scanlon PW: Indications for and results of surgical treatment of pituitary tumors by the transfrontal approach, in Kohler PO, Ross GT (eds): *Diagnosis and Treatment of Pituitary Tumors*. Amsterdam, Excerpta Medica, 1973, p 139.
326. Van Schaardenburg D, Roelfsema F, Van Seters AP, Vielvoye GJ: Bromocriptine therapy for non-functioning pituitary adenoma. *Clin Endocrinol (Oxf)* 30:475, 1989.
327. Grossman A, Ross R, Charlesworth M, Adams CBT, Wass JAH, Doniach I, Besser GM: The effect of dopamine agonist therapy on large functionless pituitary tumors. *Clin Endocrinol (Oxf)* 22:679, 1985.
328. Ray BS, Patterson RH Jr: Surgical experience with chromophobe adenomas of the pituitary gland. *J Neurosurg* 34:726, 1971.
329. Wirth FP, Schwartz HG, Schwetschenau PR: Pituitary adenomas: Factors in treatment. *Clin Neurosurg* 21:8, 1974.
330. Guiot G, Thibaut B: L'Extirpation des adenomas hypophysiaire par voie transsphenoidale. *Neurochirurgie* 1:133, 1959.
331. Hardy JJ: Transsphenoidal surgery of hypersecreting pituitary tumors, in Kohler PO, Ross GT (eds): *Diagnosis and Treatment of Pituitary Tumors*. Amsterdam, Excerpta Medica, 1973, p 179.
332. Ross DA, Wilson CB: Results of transsphenoidal microsurgery for growth hormone-secreting pituitary adenoma in a series of 214 patients. *J Neurosurg* 68:854,1988.
333. Littley MD, Shalet SM, Beardwell CG, Ahmed SR, Applegate G, Sutton ML: Hypopituitarism following external radiotherapy for pituitary tumours in adults. *Q J Med* 70:145,1989.
334. Littley MD, Shalet SM, Beardwell CG, Robinson EL, Sutton ML: Radiation-induced hypopituitarism is dose-dependent. *Clin Endocrinol (Oxf)* 31:363, 1989.
335. Kjelberg RM, Kliman B: Bragg peak proton treatment for pituitary-related conditions. *Proc R Soc Med* 67:32, 1974.
336. Braunstein CG, Loriaux DL: Proton-beam therapy. *N Engl J Med* 284:332, 1971.
337. Lawrence JA, Chong CY, Lyman JT, Tobias CA, Born JL, Garcia JF, Manougian E, Linfoot JA, Connell GM: Treatment of pituitary tumors with heavy particles, in Kohler PO, Ross GT (eds): *Diagnosis and Treatment of Pituitary Tumors*. Amsterdam, Excerpta Medica, 1973, p 297.
338. Thoren M, Rahn T, Guo WY, Werner S: Stereotactic radiosurgery with the cobalt-60 gamma unit in the treatment of growth hormone-producing pituitary tumors. *Neurosurgery* 29:663, 1991.
339. Fischer EQ, Welch K, Belli JA, Wallman J, Shillito JJ: Treatment of craniopharyngiomas in children: 1972–1981. *J Neurosurg* 62:496, 1985.
340. Manaka S, Teramoto A, Takakura K: The efficacy of radiotherapy for craniopharyngioma. *J Neurosurg* 62:648, 1985.
341. Sheline GE: Treatment of chromophobe adenomas of the pituitary gland and acromegaly, in Kohler PO, Ross GT

(eds): *Diagnosis and Treatment of Pituitary Tumors*. Amsterdam, Excerpta Medica, 1973, p 201.

342. Bakay L: The results of 300 pituitary adenoma operations. *J Neurosurg* 7:240, 1950.
343. Randall RV, Laws ER Jr, Trautmann JC: Results of transsphenoidal microsurgery for pituitary adenoma in 892 patients, in Camanni P, Muller EE (eds): *Pituitary Hyperfunction: Pathophysiology and Clinical Aspects*. New York, Raven, 1984, p 417.
344. Zimmerman EA, Defendini R, Frantz AG: Prolactin and growth hormone in patients with pituitary adenomas: A correlative study of hormone in tumor and plasma by immunoperoxidase technique and radioimmunoassay. *J Clin Endocrinol Metab* 38:577, 1974.
345. Frohman LA: Ectopic hormone production by tumors: Growth hormone releasing factor, in Muller EE, MacLeod RM (eds): *Neuroendocrine Perspectives*. Amsterdam, Elsevier, 1984, p 201.
346. Thorner MO, Perryman RL, Cronin ML, Rogol AD, Draznin J, Johanson A, Vale W, Horvath E, Kovacs K: Somatotroph hyperplasia: Successful treatment of acromegaly by removal of a pancreatic islet tumor secreting a growth hormone-releasing factor. *J Clin Invest* 70:965, 1982.
347. Zimmerman D, Young WF, Ebersold MJ, Scheithauer BW, Kovacs K, Horvath E, Whittaker MD, Eberhardt NL, et al: Congenital gigantism due to growth hormone releasing hormone excess and pituitary hyperplasia with adenomatous transformation. *J Clin Endocrinol Metab* 76:216, 1993.
348. Bengtsson B-A, Eden S, Ernest I, Oden A, Sjoegren B: Epidemiology and long-term survival in acromegaly: A study of 166 cases diagnosed between 1955 and 1984. *Acta Med Scand* 223:327, 1988.
349. Richmond IL, Wilson CB: Pituitary adenomas in childhood and adolescence. *J Neurosurg* 49:163, 1978.
350. Dinn JJ, Dinn EI: Natural history of acromegalic peripheral neuropathy. *Q J Med* 57:833, 1985.
351. Low PA, McLeod JG, Turtle JR, Donnelly P, Wright RG: Peripheral neuropathy in acromegaly. *Brain* 97:139, 1974.
352. Sober AJ, Gorden P, Roth J, AvRuskin TW: Visceromegaly in acromegaly: Evidence that clinical hepatomegaly or splenomegaly (but not sialomegaly) are manifestations of a second disease. *Arch Intern Med* 134:415, 1974.
353. Brunner JE, Johnson CC, Zafar S, Peterson EL, Brunner JF, Mellinger RC: Colon cancer and polyps in acromegaly: Increased risk associated with family history of colon cancer. *Clin Endocrinol (Oxf)* 32:65, 1990.
354. Ron E, Gridley G, Hrubec Z, Page W, Arora S, Fraumeni JF: Acromegaly and gastrointestinal cancer. *Cancer* 68:1673, 1991.
355. Barzilay J, Heatley GJ, Cushing GW: Benign and malignant tumors in patients with acromegaly. *Arch Intern Med* 151:1629, 1991.
356. Melmed S, Braunstein GD, Horvath E, Ezrin C, Kovacs K: Pathophysiology of acromegaly. *Endocr Rev* 4:271, 1983.
357. Basetti M, Arosio M, Spada A, Brina M, Bazzoni N, Faglia G, Giannattasio G: Growth hormone and prolactin secretion in acromegaly: Correlations between hormonal dynamics and immunocytochemical findings. *J Clin Endocrinol Metab* 67:1195, 1988.
358. Rodrigues EA, Caruana MP, Lahiri A, Nabarro JDN, Jacobs HS, Raftery EB: Subclinical cardiac dysfunction in acromegaly: Evidence for a specific disease of heart muscle. *Br Heart J* 62:185, 1989.
359. Hayward RP, Emanuel RW, Nabarro JDN: Acromegalic heart disease: Influence of treatment of the acromegaly on the heart. *Q J Med* 62:41, 1987.
360. Trotman-Dickenson B, Weetman AP, Hughes JMB: Upper airflow obstruction and pulmonary function in acromegaly: Relationship to disease activity. *Q J Med* 290:527, 1991.
361. Ballantine EJ, Foxman S, Gorden P, Roth J: Rarity of diabetic retinopathy in patients with acromegaly. *Arch Intern Med* 141:1625, 1981.
362. Lawrence AM, Goldfine ID, Kirsteins L: Growth hormone dynamics in acromegaly. *J Clin Endocrinol Metab* 31:239, 1970.
363. Clemmons DR, Van Wyk JJ, Ridgway EC, Kliman B, Kjelberg RN, Underwood LE: Evaluation of acromegaly by radioimmunoassay of somatomedin-C. *N Engl J Med* 301:1138, 1979.
364. Stonesifer LD, Jordan RM, Kohler PO: Somatomedin C in treated acromegaly: Poor correlation with growth hormone and clinical response. *J Clin Endocrinol Metab* 53:931, 1981.
365. Rieu M, Girard F, Bricaire H, Binoux M: The importance of insulin-like growth factor (somatomedin) measurements in the diagnosis and surveillance of acromegaly. *J Clin Endocrinol Metab* 55:147, 1982.
366. Irie M, Tsushima P: Increase of serum growth hormone concentration following thyrotropin-releasing hormone injection in patients with acromegaly or gigantism. *J Clin Endocrinol Metab* 35:97, 1972.
367. Faglia G, Beck-Peccoz P, Travaglini P, Paracchi A, Spada A, Lewin A: Elevations in plasma growth hormone concentration after luteinizing hormone-releasing hormone (LRH) in patients with active acromegaly. *J Clin Endocrinol Metab* 37:338, 1973.
368. Gelato MC, Merriam GR, Vance ML, Goldman JA, Webb C, Evans WS, Rock J, Oldfield EH, et al: Effects of growth hormone-releasing factor upon growth hormone secretion in acromegaly. *J Clin Endocrinol Metab* 60:251, 1985.
369. Wood SM, Ch'ng JLC, Adams EF, Webster JD, Joplin GR, Mashiter K, Bloom SR: Abnormalities of growth hormone release in response to human pancreatic growth hormone releasing factor (GRF 1–44) in acromegaly and hypopituitarism. *Br Med J* 286:1687, 1983.
370. Spada A, Arosio M, Bochicchio D, Bazzoni N, Vallar L, Bassetti M, Faglia G: Clinical, biochemical, and morphological correlates in patients bearing growth hormone-secreting pituitary tumors with or without constitutively active adenylyl cyclase. *J Clin Endocrinol Metab* 71:1421, 1990.
371. Ch'ng JLC, Christofides ND, Kraenzlin ME, Keshavarzian A, Burrin JM, Woolf IL, Hodgson HJF, Bloom SR: Growth hormone secretion dynamics in a patient with ectopic growth hormone-releasing factor production. *Am J Med* 79:135, 1985.
372. Schulte HM, Benker G, Windeck R, Olbricht T, Reinwein D: Failure to respond to growth hormone releasing hormone (GHRH) in acromegaly due to a GHRH secreting pancreatic tumor: Dynamics of multiple endocrine testing. *J Clin Endocrinol Metab* 61:585, 1985.
373. Liuzzi A, Chiodini PG, Botalla L, Cremascoli G, Silvestrini F: Inhibitory effects of L-dopa on GH release in acromegalic patients. *J Clin Endocrinol Metab* 35:941, 1971.
374. Barkan AL, Stred SE, Reno K, Markovs M, Hopwood NJ, Kelch RP, Beitins IZ: Increased growth hormone pulse frequency in acromegaly. *J Clin Endocrinol Metab* 69:1225, 1989.
375. Kaneko K, Komine S, Maeda T, Ohta M, Tsushima T, Shizume K: Growth hormone responses to growth-hormone-releasing hormone and thyrotropin-releasing hormone in diabetic patients with and without retinopathy. *Diabetes* 34:710, 1985.
376. Amselem S, Duquesnoy P, Attree O, Novelli G, Bousnina S, Postel-Vinay M-C, Goossens M: Laron dwarfism and mutations of the growth hormone-receptor gene. *N Engl J Med* 321:989, 1989.
377. Evain-Brion D, Garnier P, Schimpff RM, Chaussain JL, Job JC: Growth hormone response to thyrotropin-releasing hormone and oral glucose-loading tests in tall children and adolescents. *J Clin Endocrinol Metab* 56:429, 1983.
378. Asa SL, Scheithauer BW, Bilbao JM, Horvath E, Ryan N, Kovacs K, Randall RV, Laws ER Jr, et al: A case for hypo-

thalamic acromegaly: A clinicopathological study of six patients with hypothalamic gangliocytomas producing growth hormone-releasing factor. *J Clin Endocrinol Metab* 58:796, 1984.

379. Asa SL, Bilbao JM, Kovacs K, Linfoot JA: Hypothalamic neuronal hamartoma associated with pituitary growth hormone cell adenoma and acromegaly. *Acta Neuropathol (Berl)* 52:231, 1980.
380. Frohman LA, Jansson J-O: Growth hormone-releasing hormone. *Endocr Rev* 7:223, 1986.
381. Thorner MO, Frohman LA, Leong DA, Thominet J, Downs T, Hellman P, Chitwood J, Vaughn JM, Vale W: Extrahypothalamic growth hormone-releasing factor (GRF) secretion is a rare cause of acromegaly: Plasma GRF levels in 177 acromegalic patients. *J Clin Endocrinol Metab* 59:846, 1984.
382. Penny ES, Penman E, Price J, Rees LH, Sopwith AM, Wass JAH, Lytras N, Besser GM: Circulating growth hormone-releasing factor concentrations in normal subjects and patients with acromegaly. *Br Med J* 289:453, 1984.
383. Greenberg PB, Beck C, Martin PJ, Burger HG: Synthesis and release of human growth hormone from lung carcinoma in cell culture. *Lancet* 1:350, 1972.
384. Dabek JT: Bronchial carcinoid tumor with acromegaly in two patients. *J Clin Endocrinol Metab* 38:329, 1974.
385. Leveston SA, McKeel DW Jr, Buckley PJ, Deschryver K, Greider MH, Jaffe BM, Daughaday WH: Acromegaly and Cushing's syndrome associated with foregut carcinoid tumor. *J Clin Endocrinol Metab* 53:682, 1981.
386. Melmed S, Ezrin C, Kovacs K, Goodman RS, Frohman LA: Acromegaly due to secretion of growth hormone by an ectopic pancreatic islet-cell tumor. *N Engl J Med* 312:9, 1985.
387. Decker RE, Epstein JA, Carras R, Rosenthal AD: Transsphenoidal microsurgery for pituitary tumors: Experience with 45 cases. *Mt Sinai J Med* 34:565, 1976.
388. Cryer PE, Daughaday WH: Adrenergic modulation of growth hormone secretion in acromegaly: Suppression during phentolamine and phentolamine-isoproterenol administration. *J Clin Endocrinol Metab* 39:658, 1974.
389. Pieters GFFM, Romeijn JE, Smals AGH, Kloppenborg PWC: Somatostatin sensitivity and growth hormone responses to releasing hormones and bromocriptine in acromegaly. *J Clin Endocrinol Metab* 54:942, 1982.
390. Reubi JC, Landolt AM: The growth hormone responses to octreotide in acromegaly correlate with adenoma somatostatin receptor status. *J Clin Endocrinol Metab* 68:844, 1989.
391. Kelijman M, Williams TC, Downs TR, Frohman LA: Comparison of the sensitivity of growth hormone secretion to somatostatin in vivo and in vitro in acromegaly. *J Clin Endocrinol Metab* 67:958, 1988.
392. Hoyte KM, Martin JB: Recovery from paradoxical growth hormone response in acromegaly after transsphenoidal selective adenomectomy. *J Clin Endocrinol Metab* 41:656, 1975.
393. Ludecke D, Kautzky R, Saeger W, Schrader D: Selective removal of hypersecreting pituitary adenomas. *Acta Neurochir (Wien)* 35:27, 1976.
394. Herman V, Fagin J, Gonsky R, Kovacs K, Melmed S: Clonal origin of pituitary adenomas. *J Clin Endocrinol Metab* 71:1427, 1990.
395. Jacoby LB, Hedley-Whyte ET, Pulaski K, Seizinger BR, Martuza RL: Clonal origin of pituitary adenomas. *J Neurosurg* 73:731, 1990.
396. Landis CA, Harsh G, Lyons J, Davis RL, McCormick F, Bourne HR: Clinical characteristics of acromegalic patients whose pituitary tumors contain mutant Gs protein. *J Clin Endocrinol Metab* 71:1416, 1990.
397. Burton FH, Hasel KW, Bloom FE, Sutcliffe JG: Pituitary hyperplasia and gigantism in mice caused by a cholera toxin transgene. *Nature* 350:74, 1991.
398. Schwindinger WF, Francomano CA, Levine MA: Identification of a mutation in the gene encoding the alpha subunit of the stimulatory G protein of adenyl cyclase in McCune-Albright syndrome. *Proc Natl Acad Sci USA* 89:5152, 1992.
399. Cuttler L, Jackson J, Zafar MS, Levitsky LL, Mellinger RC, Frohman LA: Hypersecretion of growth hormone and prolactin in McCune-Albright Syndrome. *J Clin Endocrinol Metab* 68:1148, 1989.
400. Asa SL, Kovacs K, Stefaneanu L, Horvath E, Billestrup N, Gonzalez-Manchon C, Vale W: Pituitary mammosomatotroph adenomas develop in old mice transgenic for growth hormone-releasing hormone. *Proc Soc Exp Biol Med* 193:232, 1990.
401. Lloyd RV, Jin L, Chang A, Kulig E, Camper SA, Ross BD, Downs TR, Frohman LA: Morphological effects of hGRH gene expression on the pituitary, liver, and pancreas of MT-hGRH transgenic mice: An in situ hybridization analysis. *Am J Pathol* 141:895, 1992.
402. Fahlbusch R, Honneger J, Buchfelder M: Surgical management of acromegaly. *Endocrinol Metab Clin North Am* 21:669, 1992.
403. Baskin DS, Boggan JE, Wilson CB: Transsphenoidal microsurgical removal of growth hormone-secreting pituitary adenomas. *Neurosurg* 56:634, 1982.
404. Arafah BM, Rosenzweig JL, Fenstermaker R, Salazar R, McBride CE, Selman W: Value of growth hormone dynamics and somatomedin C (insulin-like growth factor I) levels in predicting the long-term benefit after transsphenoidal surgery for acromegaly. *J Lab Clin Med* 109:346, 1987.
405. Arosio M, Giovanelli MA, Riva E, Nava C, Ambrosi B, Faglia G: Clinical uses of pre- and postsurgical evaluation of abnormal GH responses in acromegaly. *J Neurosurg* 59:402, 1983.
406. Eastman RC, Gorden P, Roth J: Conventional supervoltage irradiation is an important treatment for acromegaly. *J Clin Endocrinol Metab* 48:931, 1979.

406a. Littley MD, Shalet SM, Swindell R, Beardwell CG, Sutton ML: Low-dose pituitary irradiation for acromegaly. *Clin Endocrinol (Oxf)* 32:261, 1990.

407. Liuzzi A, Chiodini PG, Botalla L, Cremascoli G, Muller E, Silvestrini F: Decreased plasma growth hormone levels in acromegalics following CB 154 (2-Br-α-ergocryptine) administration. *J Clin Endocrinol Metab* 38:910, 1974.
408. Moses AS, Molitch ME, Sawin CT, Jackson IM, Biller BJ, Furlanetto R, Reichlin S: Bromocriptine therapy in acromegaly: Use in patients resistant to conventional therapy and effect on serum levels of somatomedin-C. *J Clin Endocrinol Metab* 53:772, 1981.
409. Kleinberg DL, Boyd AE III, Wardlaw S, Frantz AG, George A, Bryan N, Hilal S, Greising J, et al: Pergolide for treatment of pituitary tumors secreting prolactin or growth hormone. *N Engl J Med* 309:704, 1983.
410. MacLeod RM, Lehmeyer JE: Suppression of pituitary tumor growth and function by ergot alkaloids. *Cancer Res* 33:849, 1973.
411. Oppizzi G, Liuzzi A, Chiodini P, Dallabonzana D, Spelta B, Silvestrini F, Borghi G, Tanon C: Dopaminergic treatment of acromegaly: Different effects on hormone secretion and tumor size. *J Clin Endocrinol Metab* 58:988, 1984.
412. Hall R, Besser GM, Schally AV, Coy DH, Evered D, Goldie DJ, Kastin AJ, McNielly BS, et al: Action of growth hormone-release inhibitory hormone in healthy men and in acromegaly. *Lancet* 2:581, 1973.
413. Ezzat S, Snyder PJ, Young WF, Boyajy LD, Newman C, Klibanski A, Molitch M, Boyd AE, et al: Octreotide treatment of acromegaly: A randomized, multicenter study. *Ann Intern Med* 117:711, 1992.
414. Vance ML, Harris AG: Long-term treatment of 189 acromegalic patients with the somatostatin analog octreotide: Results of the International Multicenter Acromegaly Study Group. *Arch Intern Med* 151:1573, 1991.
415. Layton MW, Fudman EJ, Barkan A, Braunstein EM, Fox IH: Acromegalic arthropathy: Characteristics and response to therapy. *Arthritis Rheum* 31:1022, 1988.

416. Lim MJ, Barkan AL, Buda AJ: Rapid reduction of left ventricular hypertrophy in acromegaly after suppression of growth hormone hypersecretion. *Ann Intern Med* 117:719, 1992.
417. Main G, Borsey DQ, Newton RW: Successful reversal of sleep apnoea syndrome following treatment for acromegaly, confirmed by polygraphic studies. *Postgrad Med J* 64:945, 1988.
418. Ho KK, Jenkins AB, Furler SM, Borkman M, Chisholm DJ: Impact of octreotide, a long-acting somatostatin analogue, on glucose tolerance and insulin sensitivity in acromegaly. *Clin Endocrinol (Oxf)* 36:271, 1992.
419. Catnach SM, Anderson JV, Fairclough PD, Trembath RC, Wilson PA, Parker E, Besser GM, Wass JA: Effect of octreotide on gall stone prevalence and gall bladder motility in acromegaly. *Gut* 34:270, 1993.
420. Shi YF, Zhu XF, Harris AG, Zhang JX, Dai Q: Prospective study of the long-term effects of somatostatin analog (octreotide) on gallbladder function and gallstone formation in Chinese acromegalic patients. *J Clin Endocrinol Metab* 76:32, 1993.
421. March CM, Kletzky OA, Davajan V, Teal J, Weiss J, Apuzzo MLJ, Marrs RP, Mishell DR Jr: Longitudinal evaluation of patients with untreated prolactin-secreting pituitary adenomas. *Am J Obstet Gynecol* 139:835, 1981.
422. Von Werder K, Eversmann T, Fahlbusch R, Muller OA, Rjosk H-K: Endocrine-active pituitary adenomas: Long-term results of medical and surgical treatment, in Camanni P, Muller EE (eds): *Pituitary Hyperfunction: Pathophysiology and Clinical Aspects.* New York, Raven, 1984, p 385.
423. Martin TL, Kim A, Malarkey WB: The natural history of idiopathic hyperprolactinemia. *J Clin Endocrinol Metab* 60:855, 1985.
424. Schlechte J, Dolan K, Sherman B, Chapler F, Luciano A: The natural history of untreated hyperprolactinemia: A prospective analysis. *J Clin Endocrinol Metab* 68:412, 1989.
425. Davis JRE, Sheppard MC, Heath DA: Giant invasive prolactinoma: A case report and review of nine further cases. *Q J Med* 74:227, 1990.
426. Popovic EA, Vattuone JR, Siu KH, Busmanis I, Pullar MJ, Dowling J: Malignant prolactinomas. *Neurosurgery* 29:127, 1991.
427. Jacobs HS, Frank S, Murray MAF, Hull MGR, Steele SJ, Nabarro JDN: Clinical and endocrine features of hyperprolactinaemic amenorrhoea. *Clin Endocrinol (Oxf)* 5:439, 1976.
428. Jaquet P, Grisli F, Guibout M, Lissitzky J-C, Carayon P: Prolactin secreting tumors: Endocrine studies before and after surgery in 33 women. *J Clin Endocrinol Metab* 64:459, 1978.
429. Antunes JL, Housepian EM, Frantz AG, Holub DA, Hui RM, Carmel PW, Quest DO: Prolactin-secreting pituitary tumors. *Ann Neurol* 2:148, 1977.
430. McNatty KP, Sawers RS, McNeilly AS: A possible role for prolactin in control of steroid secretion by the human graafian follicle. *Nature* 250:653, 1974.
431. Boyd AE III, Reichlin S, Turksoy RN: Galactorrhea-amenorrhea syndrome: Diagnosis and therapy. *Ann Intern Med* 87:165, 1977.
432. Spark RF, Pallota J, Naftolin F, Clemens R: Galactorrhea-amenorrhea syndromes: Etiology and treatment. *Ann Intern Med* 84:532, 1976.
433. Boyar RM, Capen S, Finkelstein JW, Perlow M, Sassin JF, Fukushima DK, Weitzman ED, Hellman L: Hypothalamic-pituitary function in diverse hyperprolactinemic states. *J Clin Invest* 53:1588, 1974.
434. Aono T, Miyaki A, Shioji T, Kinugasa T, Onishi T, Kurachi K: Impaired LH release following exogenous estrogen administration in patients with amenorrhea-galactorrhea syndrome. *J Clin Endocrinol Metab* 42:696, 1976.
435. L'Hermite M, Delogne-Desnoeck J, Michaux-Duchene A, Robyn C: Alteration of feedback mechanism of estrogen on gonadotropin by sulpiride-induced hyperprolactinemia. *J Clin Endocrinol Metab* 47:1132, 1978.
436. Carter JN, Tyson JE, Warne GL, McNeilly AS, Faiman C, Friesen HG: Adrenocortical function in hyperprolactinemic women. *J Clin Endocrinol Metab* 45:973, 1977.
437. Glickman SP, Rosenfield RL, Bergenstal RM, Helke J: Multiple androgenic abnormalities, including free testosterone, in hyperprolactinemic women. *J Clin Endocrinol Metab* 55:251, 1982.
438. Klibanski A, Neer RM, Beitens IZ, Ridgway EC, Zervas NT, McArthur JW: Decreased bone density in hyperprolactinemic women. *N Engl J Med* 303:1511, 1980.
439. Schlechte JM, Sherman B, Martin R: Bone density in amenorrheic women with and without hyperprolactinemia. *J Clin Endocrinol Metab* 56:1120, 1983.
440. Schlechte J, Walkner L, Kathol M: A longitudinal analysis of premenopausal bone loss in healthy women and women with hyperprolactinemia. *J Clin Endocrinol Metab* 75:698, 1992.
441. Carter JN, Tyson JE, Tolis G, Van Vliet S, Faiman C, Friesen HG: Prolactin-secreting tumors and hypogonadism in 22 men. *N Engl J Med* 299:847,1978.
442. Segal LS, Polishuk WZ, Ben-David M: Hyperprolactinemic male infertility. *Fertil Steril* 26:1425, 1976.
443. Said K, Wenn RV, Sharif F: Bromocriptine for male infertility. *Lancet* 1:250, 1977.
444. Rao R, Scommegna A, Frohman LA: Integrity of central dopaminergic system in women with postpartum hyperprolactinemia. *Am J Obstet Gynecol* 143:883, 1982.
445. Fine SA, Frohman LA: Loss of central nervous system component of dopaminergic inhibition of prolactin secretion in patients with prolactin-secreting pituitary tumors. *J Clin Invest* 61:973, 1978.
446. Kleinberg DL, Noel GL, Frantz AG: Galactorrhea: A study of 235 cases, including 48 with pituitary tumors. *N Engl J Med* 296:589, 1977.
447. Webb CB, Thominet JL, Barowsky H, Berelowitz M, Frohman LA: Evidence for lactotroph dopamine resistance in idiopathic hyperprolactinemia. *J Clin Endocrinol Metab* 56:1089, 1983.
448. Bansal S, Lee LA, Woolf PD: Abnormal prolactin responsiveness to dopaminergic suppression in hyperprolactinemic patients. *Am J Med* 71:961, 1981.
449. McLain CJ, Kromhout J, Van Thiel D: Prolactin levels in portal systemic encephalopathy. *Clin Res* 26:664A, 1978.
450. Boyd AE III, Spare S, Bower B, Reichlin S: Neurogenic galactorrhea-amenorrhea. *J Clin Endocrinol Metab* 47:1374, 1978.
451. Morley JE, Dawson M, Hodgkinson H, Kalk WJ: Galactorrhea and hyperprolactinemia associated with chest wall injury. *J Clin Endocrinol Metab* 45:931, 1977.
452. Jackson RD, Wortsman J, Malarkey WB: Characterization of large molecular weight prolactin in women with idiopathic hyperprolactinemia and normal menses. *J Clin Endocrinol Metab* 61:258, 1985.
452a. Bression D, Brandi AM, Martres MP, Nousbaum A, Cesselin F, Radacot J, Peillion F: Dopaminergic receptors in human prolactin-secreting adenomas: A quantitative study. *J Clin Endocrinol Metab* 51:1037, 1980.
453. Lachelin GCL, Abu-Fadil S, Yen SSC: Functional delineation of hyperprolactinemia-amenorrhea. *J Clin Endocrinol Metab* 44:1163, 1977.
453a. Cronin MJ, Cheung CY, Wilson CB, Jaffe RB, Weiner RI: ^{3}H-Spiperone binding to human anterior pituitaries secreting prolactin, growth hormone, and adrenocorticotropic hormone. *J Clin Endocrinol Metab* 50:387, 1980.
454. Kato Y, Shimatsu A, Matsushita N, Ohta H, Tojo K, Kabayama Y, Inoue T, Imura H: Regulation of pituitary hor-

mone secretion by VIP and related peptides, in Labrie F, Proulx L (eds): *Endocrinology*. Amsterdam, Elsevier, 1984, p 175.
455. Tucker HS, Grubb SR, Wigand JP, Taylor A, Lankford HV, Blackard WG, Becker SP: Galactorrhea-amenorrhea syndrome: Followup of forty-five patients after pituitary tumor removal. *Ann Intern Med* 94:303, 1981.
456. Frohman LA, Berelowitz M, Gonzalez C, Barowsky H, Rao R, Lim VS, Frohman MA, Thominet JL: Studies of dopaminergic mechanisms in hyperprolactinemic states, in Crosignani P, Rubin B (eds): *Serono Clinical Symposia on Reproduction*. London, Academic, 1981, vol 2, p 39.
457. VanLoon GR: A defect in catecholamine neurones in patients with prolactin-secreting pituitary adenoma. *Lancet* 2:868, 1978.
458. Hokfelt T, Fuxe K: Effects of prolactin and ergot alkaloids on the tuberoinfundibular dopamine neurones. *Neuroendocrinology* 9:100, 1972.
459. McKeel DW Jr, Fowler M, Jacobs LS: The high prevalence of prolactin cell hyperplasia in the human adenohypophysis. *Endocrinology* 102:353A, 1978.
460. Garthwaite TL, Hagen TC: Plasma prolactin-releasing factor-like activity in the amenorrhea-galactorrhea syndrome. *J Clin Endocrinol Metab* 47:885, 1978.
461. Rodman EF, Molitch ME, Post KD, Biller BJ, Reichlin S: Long-term follow-up of transsphenoidal selective adenomectomy for prolactinoma. *JAMA* 252:921, 1984.
462. Serri O, Rasio E, Beauregard H, Hardy J, Somma M: Recurrence of hyperprolactinemia after selective transsphenoidal adenomectomy of women with prolactinoma. *N Engl J Med* 309:280, 1983.
463. Schlechte J, Sherman B, VanGilder J, Chapler F: Recurrence of hyperprolactinemia after transsphenoidal surgery for prolactin-secreting pituitary tumors. *Clin Res* 33:828A, 1985.
464. Karga HJ, Alexander JM, Hedley-Whyte ET, Klibanski A, Jameson JL: Ras mutations in human pituitary tumors. *J Clin Endocrinol Metab* 74:914, 1992.
465. Gonsky R, Herman V, Melmed S, Fagin J: Transforming DNA sequences present in human prolactin-secreting pituitary tumors. *Mol Endocrinol* 5:1687, 1991.
466. Ciccarelli E, Ghigo E, Miola C, Gandini G, Muller EE, Camanni F: Long-term follow-up of "cured" prolactinoma patients after successful adenomectomy. *Clin Endocrinol (Oxf)* 32:583, 1990.
467. Molitch ME: Pregnancy and the hyperprolactinemic woman. *N Engl J Med* 312:1364, 1985.
468. Mornex R, Hugues B: Remission of hyperprolactinemia after pregnancy. *N Engl J Med* 324:60, 1991.
469. Bevan JS, Webster J, Burke CW, Scanlon MF: Dopamine agonists and pituitary tumor shrinkage. *Endocr Rev* 13:220, 1992.
470. Yousem DM, Arrington JA, Zinreich SJ, Kumar AJ, Bryan RN: Pituitary adenomas: Possible role of bromocriptine in intratumoral hemorrhage. *Radiology* 170:239, 1989.
471. Hokfelt B, Nillius SJ: The dopamine agonist bromocriptine: Theoretical and clinical aspects. *Acta Endocrinol (Copenh)* (Suppl) 88:1, 1978.
472. Dallabonzana D, Liuzzi A, Oppizzi G, Cozzi R, Verde G, Chiodini P, Rainer E, Dorow R, Horowski R: Chronic treatment of pathological hyperprolactinemia and acromegaly with the new ergot derivative terguride. *J Clin Endocrinol Metab* 63:1002, 1986.
473. Ferrari C, Mattei A, Melis GB, Paracchi A, Muratori M, Faglia G, Sghedoni D, Crosignani PG: Cabergoline: Long-acting oral treatment of hyperprolactinemic disorders. *J Clin Endocrinol Metab* 68:1201, 1989.
474. Ferrari C, Paracchi A, Mattei AM, de Vincentiis S, D'Alberton A, Crosignani P: Cabergoline in the long-term therapy of hyperprolactinemic disorders. *Acta Endocrinol (Copenh)* 126:489, 1992.
475. Ciccarelli E, Camanni F, Miola C, Besser GM, Avataneo T, Grossman A: Long-term treatment with a new repeatable injectable form of bromocriptine, Parlodel LAR, in patients with tumorous hyperprolactinemia. *Fertil Steril* 52:930, 1989.
476. Schettini G, Lombardi G, Merola B, Colao A, Miletto P, Caruso E, Lancranjan I: Rapid and long-lasting suppression of prolactin secretion and shrinkage of prolactinomas after injection of long-acting repeatable form of bromocriptine (Parlodel LAR). *Clin Endocrinol (Oxf)* 33:161, 1990.
477. Vance ML, Lipper M, Klibanski A, Biller BMK, Samaan NA, Molitch ME: Treatment of prolactin-secreting pituitary macroadenomas with the long-acting non-ergot dopamine agonist CV 205-502. *Ann Intern Med* 12:668, 1990.
478. Katz E, Schran HF, Adashi EY: Successful treatment of a prolactin-secreting pituitary macroadenoma with intravaginal bromocriptine: A novel approach to interance of oral therapy. *Obstet Gynecol* 73:517, 1989.
479. Turkalj I, Braun P, Krupp P: Surveillance of bromocriptine in pregnancy. *JAMA* 247:1589, 1982.
480. Liuzzi A, Dallabonzana D, Oppizzi G, Verde GG, Cozzi R, Chiodini P, Luccarelli G: Low dose dopamine agonists in the long-term treatment of macroprolactinomas. *N Engl J Med* 313:656, 1985.
481. Molitch M, Elton RL, Blackwell RE, Caldwell B, Chang J, Jaffe R, Joplin G, Robbins RJ, et al, and the Bromocriptine Study Group: Bromocriptine as primary therapy for prolactin-secreting macroadenomas: Results of a prospective multicenter study. *J Clin Endocrinol Metab* 60:698, 1985.
482. Tindall GT, Kovacs K, Horvath E, Thorner MO: Human prolactin-producing adenomas and bromocriptine: A histological, immunocytochemical, ultrastructural and morphometric study. *J Clin Endocrinol Metab* 55:1178, 1982.
483. Gen M, Uozumi T, Ohta M, Ito A, Kajiwara H, Moro S: Necrotic changes in prolactinomas after long term administration of bromocriptine. *J Clin Endocrinol Metab* 59:463, 1984.
484. Johnston DG, Hall K, Kendall-Taylor P, Patrick D, Watson M, Cook DB: Effect of dopamine agonist withdrawal after long-term therapy in prolactinomas. *Lancet* 2:187, 1984.
485. Perrin G, Treluyer C, Trouillas J, Sassolas G, Goutelle A: Surgical outcome and pathological effects of bromocriptine preoperative treatment in prolactinomas. *Pathol Res Pract* 187:587, 1991.
486. Fahlbusch R, Buchfelder M: Transsphenoidal operations for prolactinomas, in Auer LM, Leb G, Tscherne G, Urdl W, Walter GF (eds): *Prolactinomas*. Berlin, de Gruyter, 1985, p 209.
487. Landolt AM, Osterwalder V: Perivascular fibrosis in prolactinomas: Is it increased by bromocriptine? *J Clin Endocrinol Metab* 58:1179, 1984.
488. Watanabe K, Fukushima T: Transsphenoidal microsurgical treatment of 77 prolactinomas. *J Clin Endocrinol Metab* 58:235, 1984.
489. Faglia G, Moriondo, P, Travaglini P, Giovanelli MA: Influence of previous bromocriptine therapy on surgery for microprolactinomas. *Lancet* 1:133, 1983.
490. Sherman BM, Harris CE, Schlechte J, Duello TM, Halmi NS, VanGlider J, Chapler FK, Granner DK: Pathogenesis of prolactin-secreting adenomas. *Lancet* 2:1019, 1978.
491. Tsagarakis S, Grossman A, Plowman PN, Jones AE, Touzel R, Rees LH, Wass JAH, Besser GM: Megavoltage pituitary irradiation in the management of prolactinomas: Long-term follow-up. *Clin Endocrinol (Oxf)* 34:399, 1991.
492. Thorner MO, Besser GM, Jones A, Dacie J, Jones AE: Bromocriptine treatment of female infertility: Report of 13 pregnancies. *Br Med J* 4:694, 1975.
493. Cushing H: The basophil adenomas of the pituitary body and their clinical manifestations (pituitary basophilism). *Bull Johns Hopkins Hosp* 50:137, 1932.

494. Nelson DH, Meakin JW, Dealy JB Jr, Matson DD, Emerson K Jr, Thorn GW: ACTH-producing tumor of the pituitary gland. *N Engl J Med* 259:161, 1958.
495. Nagaya T, Seo H, Kuwayama A, Sakurai T, Tsukamoto N, Nakane T, Sugita K, Matsui N: Pro-opiomelanocortin gene expression in silent corticotroph-cell adenoma and Cushing's disease. *J Neurosurg* 72:262, 1990.
496. Scholz DA, Gastineau CF, Harrison EG Jr: Cushing's syndrome with malignant chromophobe tumor of the pituitary and extra-cranial metastasis: Report of a case. *Proc Staff Meet Mayo Clin* 37:31, 1962.
497. Moore TJ, Dluhy RG, Williams GH, Cain JP: Nelson's syndrome: Frequency, prognosis and effect of prior pituitary irradiation. *Ann Intern Med* 85:731, 1976.
498. Tyrrell JB, Brooks RM, Fitzgerald PA, Cofoid PB, Forsham PH, Wilson CG: Cushing's disease: Selective transsphenoidal resection of pituitary microadenomas. *N Engl J Med* 298:753, 1978.
499. Eddy RL, Jones AL, Gilliland PF, Ibarra JD Jr, Thompson JQ, McMurray JF Jr: Cushing's syndrome: A prospective study of diagnostic methods. *Am J Med* 55:621, 1973.
500. Liddle GW: Tests of pituitary-adrenal suppressibility in the diagnosis of Cushing's syndrome. *J Clin Endocrinol Metab* 20:1539, 1960.
501. Ashcraft MW, Van Herle AJ, Vener SL, Geffner DL: Serum cortisol levels in Cushing's syndrome after low- and high-dose dexamethasone suppression. *Ann Intern Med* 97:21, 1982.
502. Chrousos GP, Schulte HM, Oldfield EH, Gold PW, Cutler GB Jr., Loriaux DL: The corticotropin-releasing factor stimulation test. *N Engl J Med* 310:622, 1984.
503. Peck WW, Dillon WP, Norman D, Newton TH, Wilson CB: High-resolution MR imaging of pituitary microadenomas at 1.5 T: Experience with Cushing disease. *Am J Roentgenol Radium Ther Nucl Med* 152:145, 1989.
504. Oldfield EH, Doppman JL, Nieman LK, Chrousos GP: Petrosal sinus sampling with and without corticotropin-releasing hormone for the differential diagnosis of Cushing's syndrome. *N Engl J Med* 325:897, 1991.
505. Findling JW, Kehoe ME, Shaker JL, Raff H: Routine inferior petrosal sinus sampling in the differential diagnosis of adrenocorticotropin (ACTH)-dependent Cushing's syndrome: Early recognition of the occult ectopic ACTH syndrome. *J Clin Endocrinol Metab* 73:408, 1991.
506. Tabarin A, Greselle JF, San Galli F, Leprat F, Caille JM, Latapie JL, Guerin J, Roger P: Usefulness of the corticotropin-releasing hormone test during bilateral inferior petrosal sampling for the diagnosis of Cushing's disease. *J Clin Endocrinol Metab* 73:53, 1991.
507. Upton GV, Amatruda TT Jr: Evidence for the presence of tumor peptides with corticotropin-releasing factor-like activity in the ectopic ACTH syndrome. *N Engl J Med* 285:419, 1971.
508. Carey RM, Varma SK, Drake CR Jr, Thorner MO, Kovacs K, Rivier J, Vale W: Ectopic secretion of corticotropin-releasing factor as a cause of Cushing's syndrome. *N Engl J Med* 311:13, 1984.
509. Lamberts SWJ, Klijn JGM, de Jong FH, Birkenhager JC: Hormone secretion in alcohol-induced pseudo-Cushing's syndrome: Differential diagnosis with Cushing's disease. *JAMA* 242:1640, 1979.
510. Carroll BJ, Curtis GC, Mendels J: Neuroendocrine regulation in depression: I. Limbic system-adrenocortical dysfunction. *Arch Gen Psychiatry* 33:1039, 1976.
511. Krieger DT: Pathophysiology of Cushing's disease. *Endocr Rev* 4:22, 1983.
512. Heinbecker P: Pathogenesis of Cushing's syndrome. *Medicine (Baltimore)* 23:225, 1944.
513. Van Cauter E, Refetoff S: Evidence for two subtypes of Cushing's disease based on the analysis of episodic cortisol secretion. *N Eng J Med* 312:1343, 1985.
514. Lamberts SWJ, Klijn JGM, de Quijada M, Timmermans HAT, Uitterlinden P, de Jong FH, Birkenhager JC: The mechanism of the suppressive action of bromocriptine on adrenocorticotropin secretion in patients with Cushing's disease and Nelson's syndrome. *J Clin Endocrinol Metab* 51:307, 1980.
515. Lamberts SWJ, de Lange SA, Stefanko SZ: Adrenocorticotropin-secreting pituitary adenomas originate from the anterior or the intermediate lobe in Cushing's disease: Differences in the regulation of hormone secretion. *J Clin Endocrinol Metab* 54:286, 1982.
516. McNicol AM, Teasdale GM, Beastall GH: A study of corticotroph adenomas in Cushing's disease: No evidence of intermediate lobe origin. *Clin Endocrinol (Oxf)* 24:715, 1986.
517. Krieger DT, Amorosa L, Linick F: Cyproheptadine-induced remission of Cushing's disease. *N Engl J Med* 293:893, 1975.
518. Jones MT, Gillham B, Beckford U, Dornhorst A, Abraham RR, Seed M, Wynn V: Effect of treatment with sodium valproate and diazepam on plasma corticotropin in Nelson's syndrome. *Lancet* 1:1179, 1981.
519. Lankford HV, Tucker HTS, Blackard WG: A cyproheptadine-reversible defect in ACTH control presenting after removal of the pituitary tumor in Cushing's disease. *N Engl J Med* 305:1244, 1981.
520. Schulte HM, Oldfield EH, Allolio B, Katz DA, Berkman RA, Ali IU: Clonal composition of pituitary adenomas in patients with Cushing's disease: Determination by X-chromosome inactivation analysis. *J Clin Endocrinol Metab* 73:1302, 1991.
521. Gicquel C, Le-Bouc Y, Luton JP, Girard F, Bertagna X: Monoclonality of corticotroph macroadenomas in Cushing's disease. *J Clin Endocrinol Metab* 75:472, 1992.
522. Lagerquist LW, Meikle AW, West CD, Tyler FH: Cushing's disease with cure by resection of a pituitary adenoma: Evidence against a primary hypothalamic defect. *Am J Med* 57:826, 1974.
523. Bigos ST, Robert F, Pelletier G, Hardy J: Cure of Cushing's disease by transsphenoidal removal of a microadenoma from a pituitary gland despite a radiographically normal sella turcica. *J Clin Endocrinol Metab* 45:1251, 1977.
524. Ludecke DK: Transnasal microsurgery of Cushing's disease 1990: Overview including personal experiences with 256 patients. *Pathol Res Pract* 187:608, 1991.
525. Tindall GT, Herring CJ, Clark RV, Adams DA, Watts NB: Cushing's disease: Results of transsphenoidal microsurgery with emphasis on surgical failures. *J Neurosurg* 72:363, 1990.
526. Guilhaume B, Bertagna X, Thomsen M, Bricaire C, Vila-Porcile E, Olivier L, Racadot J, Derome P, et al: Transsphenoidal pituitary surgery for the treatment of Cushing's disease: Results in 64 patients and long term follow-up studies. *J Clin Endocrinol Metab* 66:1056, 1988.
527. Pieters GFFM, Hermus ARMM, Meijer E, Smals AGH, Kloppenborg PWC: Predictive factors for initial cure and relapse rate after pituitary surgery for Cushing's disease. *J Clin Endocrinol Metab* 69:1122, 1989.
528. Arnott RD, Pestell RG, McKelvie PA, Henderson JK, McNeill PM, Alford FP: A critical evaluation of transsphenoidal pituitary surgery in the treatment of Cushing's disease: Prediction of outcome. *Acta Endocrinol (Copenh)* 123:423, 1990.
529. Fahlbusch R, Buchfelder M, Muller O: Transsphenoidal surgery for Cushing's disease. *J R Soc Med* 79:262, 1986.
530. Scholz DA, Gastineau CF, Harrison EG Jr: Cushing's syndrome with malignant chromophobe tumor of the pituitary and extracranial metastasis: Report of a case. *Mayo Clin Proc* 37:31, 1962.
531. Howlett TA, Plowman PN, Wass JAH, Rees LH, Jones AE, Besser GM: Megavoltage pituitary irradiation in the management of Cushing's disease and Nelson's syndrome: Long-term follow-up. *Clin Endocrinol (Oxf)* 31:309, 1989.
532. Sonino N, Boscaro M, Merola G, Mantero F: Prolonged

treatment of Cushing's disease by ketoconazole. *J Clin Endocrinol Metab* 61:718, 1985.
533. Loli P, Berselli ME, Tagliaferri M: Use of ketoconazole in the treatment of Cushing's syndrome. *J Clin Endocrinol Metab* 63:1365, 1986.
534. Tabarin A, Navarranne A, Guerin J, Corcuff JB, Parneix M, Roger P: Use of ketoconazole in the treatment of Cushing's disease and ectopic ACTH syndrome. *Clin Endocrinol (Oxf)* 34:63, 1991.
535. Loose DS, Kan PB, Hirst MA, Marcus RA, Feldman D: Ketoconazole blocks adrenal steroidogenesis by inhibiting cytochrome P450-dependent enzymes. *J Clin Invest* 71:1495, 1983.
536. Santen RJ, Van den Bossche H, Symoens J, Brugmans J, de Costar R: Site of action of low dose ketoconazole on androgen biosynthesis in men. *J Clin Endocrinol Metab* 57:732, 1983.
537. Jeffcoate WJ, Rees LH, Tomlin S, Jones AE, Edwards CRW, Besser GM: Metyrapone in long-term management of Cushing's disease. *Br Med J* 2:215, 1977.
538. Bertagna X: L'action antiglucocorticoide du RU 486. *Ann Endocrinol (Paris)* 50:208, 1989.
539. Lamberts SWJ, Timmermans HAT, DeJong FH, Birkenhager JC: The role of dopaminergic depletion in the pathogenesis of Cushing's disease and the possible consequences for medical therapy. *Clin Endocrinol (Oxf)* 7:185, 1977.
540. Loli P, Berselli ME, Vignati F, De Grandi C, Tagliaferri M: Size reduction of an ACTH-secreting pituitary macroadenoma in Nelson's syndrome by sodium valproate: Effect of withdrawal and re-institution of treatment. *Acta Endocrinol (Copenh)* 119:435, 1988.
541. Weintraub BD, Gershengorn MC, Kourides IA, Fein H: Inappropriate secretion of thyroid-stimulating hormone. *Ann Intern Med* 95:339, 1981.
542. Smallridge RC: Thyrotropin-secreting tumors, in Mazzaferri EL (ed): *Endocrine Tumors*. Oxford, Blackwell, 1993, pp 136–151.
543. Wynne AG, Gharib H, Scheithauer BW, Davis DH, Freeman SL, Horvath E: Hyperthyroidism due to inappropriate secretion of thyrotropin in 10 patients. *Am J Med* 92:15, 1992.
544. Mixson AJ, Friedman TC, Katz DA, Feuerstein I, Doppman J, Oldfield E, Weintraub BD: Thyrotropin-secreting pituitary carcinoma. *J Clin Endocrinol Metab* 76:529, 1993.
545. Galway AB, Hseuh AJW, Daneshdoost L, Zhou M-H, Pavlou SN, Snyder PJ: Gonadotroph adenomas in men produce biologically active follicle-stimulating hormone. *J Clin Endocrinol Metab* 71:907, 1990.
546. Nicolis G, Shimshi M, Allen C, Halmi NS, Kourides IA: Gonadotropin-producing pituitary adenoma in a man with long-standing primary hypogonadism. *J Clin Endocrinol Metab* 66:237, 1988.
547. Oppenheim DS, Klibanski A: Medical therapy of glycoprotein hormone-secreting pituitary tumors. *Endocrinol Metab Clin North Am* 18:339, 1989.
548. Vance ML, Ridgway EC, Thorner MO: Follicle-stimulating hormone and α-subunit-secreting pituitary tumor treated with bromocriptine. *J Clin Endocrinol Metab* 61:580, 1985.
549. Comtois R, Bouchard J, Robert F: Hypersecretion of gonadotropins by a pituitary adenoma: Pituitary dynamic studies and treatment with bromocriptine in one patient. *Fertil Steril* 52:569, 1989.

CHAPTER 9

Posterior Pituitary

Gary L. Robertson

POSTERIOR PITUITARY HORMONES

Anatomy

The *neurohypophysis* is an elongated extension of the ventral hypothalamus which attaches to the dorsal and caudal surface of the adenohypophysis (Fig. 9-1). In adult men and women it weighs approximately 100 mg and is divided into two parts by the diaphragm of the sella. The upper part is variously referred to as the *infundibulum* or *median eminence,* and the lower part is referred to as the *infundibular process* or *pars nervosa.* The two parts are supplied with blood by branches from the superior and inferior hypophyseal arteries which arise from the posterior communicating and intracavernous portion of the internal carotid. In the pars nervosa, the arterioles break up into localized capillary networks which drain directly into the jugular vein via the sellar, cavernous, and lateral venous sinuses. In the infundibulum, the primary capillary networks coalesce into another system, the portal veins, which perfuse the adenohypophysis before discharging into the systemic circulation.

Microscopically, the neurohypophysis appears as a densely interwoven network of capillaries, pituicytes, and nonmyelinated nerve fibers containing many electron-dense neurosecretory granules.[1,2] These neurosecretory neurons terminate as bulbous enlargements on capillary networks scattered throughout all parts of the neurohypophysis, including the stalk and infundibulum. The neurosecretory neurons that form the pars nervosa originate primarily in the large cells of the supraoptic nuclei and probably provide most if not all of the vasopressin and oxytocin in plasma.[2–6] Those which terminate in the median eminence originate primarily in the small cells of the paraventricular nucleus or other hypothalamic nuclei and release their hormones into the portal blood supply of the anterior pituitary. Some of these cells also contain corticotropin releasing factor and appear to participate in the regulation of ACTH secretion by cells of the anterior pituitary.[7] Another and somewhat smaller division of vasopressin- or oxytocin-containing neurons projects caudally from the paraventricular nucleus to the medulla and spinal cord, where it appears to terminate on neurons in the nucleus tractus solitarii, substantia gelatinosa, and other areas thought to be involved in the regulation of autonomic function.[3–6] A third vasopressin-containing division of the paraventricular nucleus projects through the stria terminalis to the lateral amygdala,[4] and a fourth appears to terminate on the walls of the lateral and third ventricles, where the neurons probably secrete directly into the cerebrospinal fluid.[8] Multipolar cell bodies containing vasopressin or its associated neurophysin also have been identified in the suprachiasmatic nuclei of humans as well as other primates and most laboratory animals.[3–5] The neurons that arise in this nucleus are of relatively fine caliber and appear to project exclusively to other neurons in the amygdala, lateral septum, and mediodorsal thalamus.[3,4] The widespread distribution of vasopressin in the central nervous system has also been demonstrated by direct radioimmunoassay of tissue extracts.[9]

Oxytocinergic cell bodies appear to be less numerous than those containing vasopressin and are found primarily in discrete areas in or around the paraventricular and, to a lesser extent, supraoptic nuclei.[3] Most of these neurons project to the pars nervosa, but many also terminate in the lamina terminalis or the median eminence. In addition, a relatively large paraventricular division runs in parallel with vasopressinergic fibers to the medulla and spinal cord, where it terminates on or near the same neural elements.

Chemistry

The neurohypophysis contains several peptides which probably serve as neurohormones, but the only ones which have been extensively studied are vasopressin and oxytocin. Their structures were first established by du Vigneaud and coworkers more than 30 years ago.[10] Each is a nonapeptide composed of a six-member disulfide ring and a three-member tail on which the carboxy-terminal group is amidated (Fig. 9-2). Vasopressin differs from oxytocin

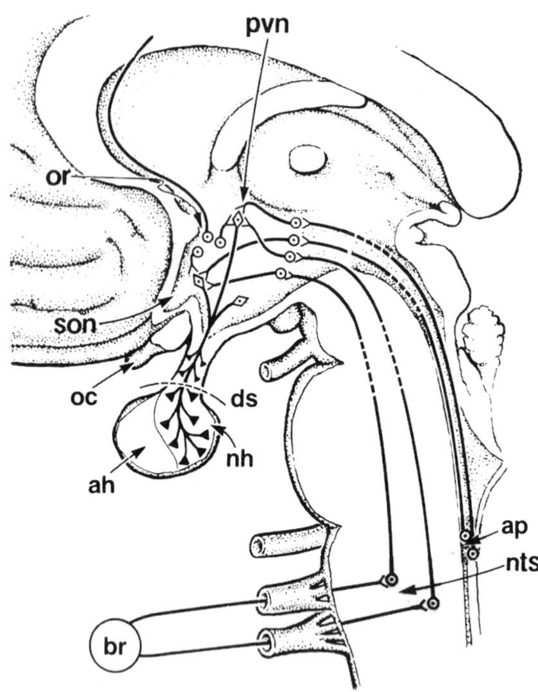

FIGURE 9-1 The neurohypophysis and its principal regulatory afferents. Key: nh = neurohypophysis; ah = adenohypophysis; ds = diaphragm of the sella; oc = optic chiasm; son = supraoptic nucleus; pvn = paraventricular nucleus; or = osmoreceptor; br = volume sensor and baroreceptor; nts = nucleus tractus solitarii; ap = area postrema (emetic center). Shading indicates areas which lack a blood-brain barrier and contain receptors for plasma insulin.

only in the substitution of phenylalanine for isoleucine in the ring and of arginine for leucine in the tail. These two hormones have been found in all mammals except the suborder Suina, several species of which make a variant of vasopressin containing lysine instead of arginine in position 8.[11] Oxytocin also occurs in many birds, reptiles, amphibians, and bony fishes. Instead of vasopressin, however, the pituitaries of nonmammalian vertebrates contain arginine vasotocin, which differs structurally from vasopressin only by the presence of isoleucine at position 3 and has similar biological effects. Because it is the only nonapeptide hormone found in some older vertebrate phyla, vasotocin is thought to be the precursor from which oxytocin and vasopressin evolved by genetic mutation and duplication.

The synthesis of a large number of structural analogues of vasopressin and oxytocin has made it possible to define more precisely the relation between conformation and biological activity.[12] The ratio of antidiuretic to pressor effects of vasopressin is increased markedly by substituting D-arginine for L-arginine at position 8. This modification, as well as removal of the terminal amino group from cystine, yields desamino-8-D-arginine vasopressin (DDAVP) (Fig. 9-2), a clinically useful analogue with prolonged and enhanced antidiuretic activity.[13] A number of analogues that antagonize selectively the antidiuretic or pressor action of vasopressin have also been synthesized.[14] They have been used effectively to help define the role of vasopressin in the regulation of water balance or blood pressure in health and disease and may also prove to be clinically useful in treating certain types of osmoregulatory or baroregulatory dysfunction.

Vasopressin and oxytocin are stored in the neurohypophysis as insoluble complexes with carrier proteins known as *neurophysins*. Separation of these neurophysins from the active hormones was first achieved by Acher and his colleagues over 30 years ago.[15] However, it has been possible to isolate individual neurophysins in a form sufficiently pure to define their physicochemical characteristics.[16] In humans and most other mammals, two major types of neurophysin have been identified by both immunologic and chromatographic methods. One type is found exclusively in granules containing oxytocin; the other, in granules containing vasopressin. Both appear to be single-chain polypeptides which have a basic molecular weight of approximately 10,000 but readily form dimers and tetramers in concentrated solutions. Each type of neurophysin binds oxytocin and vasopressin equally well, indicating that the specific hormonal associations found in vivo are a function of anatomic compartmentalization. Binding of the hormones to neurophysin exhibits a pH optimum around 5.2 to 5.8 and a binding constant (K°) of approximately 2×10^4 *M*. These values favor complete dissociation of the neurophysin-hormone complex in plasma. The amino acid sequence of several neurophysins has been determined and has been found to have a considerable degree of internal homology in a part of the molecule thought to be the hormone-binding site.

Biosynthesis and Release

Vasopressin and oxytocin are synthesized in the cell bodies of the supraoptic and paraventricular nuclei, packaged in granules with their respective neurophysins, and transported down the axons to be stored in terminal dilatations until their release.[2,17] Both hormones are synthesized via macromolecular precursors or prohormones which, in addition to the hormone residue on the amino terminus, include its associated neurophysin and, in the case of vasopressin, a glycosylated peptide known as copeptin (Fig. 9-3*A*).[18] The genes for these prohormones have been cloned and sequenced.[18,19] That for the vasopressin precursor is composed of three exons which code, respectively, for (1) vasopressin, a short linking peptide, and the variable, amino-terminal part of neurophysin, (2) the central, highly conserved portion of neurophysin, and (3) the variable, carboxy-terminal part of neurophysin, another linking pep-

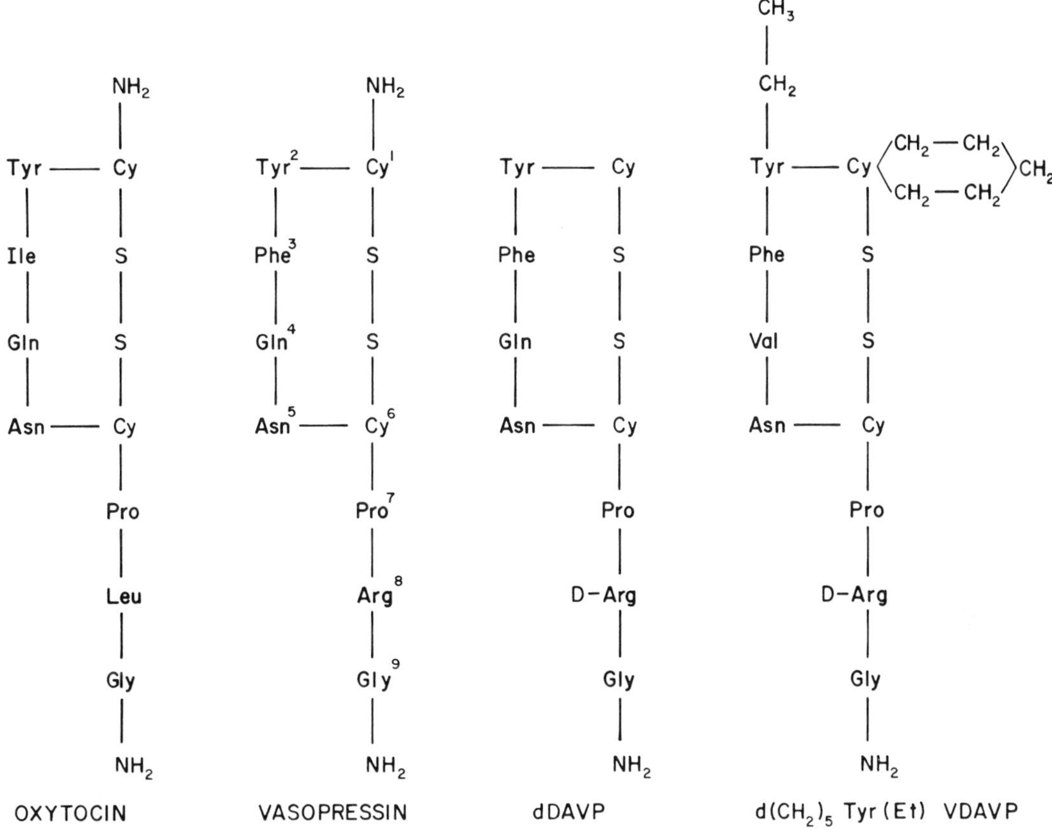

FIGURE 9-2 The amino acid sequence of oxytocin and vasopressin as well as a synthetic agonist, 1-desamino-8-D-arginine vasopressin (DDAVP), and an antagonist, $d(CH_2)_5$ Tyr(Et) (vDAVP), of vasopressin.

tide, and copeptin (Fig. 9-3*B*). The gene for the oxytocin precursor is arranged similarly, but the third exon contains a stop codon after the region that encodes the carboxy terminus of its neurophysin. The two genes are located in close proximity on opposing strands of DNA[18,19] and in humans are on chromosome 20.[20] Despite their proximity, however, the genes for oxytocin and vasopressin are expressed differentially by distinct subsets of neurons.[21]

The synthesis of vasopressin and vasopressin mRNA is increased by stimuli, such as dehydration, which also increase secretion.[17,22] At least in rats, however, this compensatory response develops only gradually and may never completely match the increased rate of release. As a consequence, the neurohypophyseal stores of vasopressin tend to be severely depleted by a chronic stimulus such as prolonged water deprivation.[23]

The process by which the prohormones are packaged in granules, and transported down the axon has not been completely defined. The granules are membrane-bound and appear in some species to arise from the Golgi apparatus in the perikaryon. Transport may be effected by the kind of axon flow phenomenon demonstrated for other nervous tissue or by some more rapid mechanism involving the microtubules.

The hormone and its associated neurophysin appear to be secreted by a calcium-dependent exocytotic process similar to that described for other neurosecretory systems.[24] According to this view, secretion is triggered by propagation along the neuron of an electric impulse which causes depolarization of the cell membrane, an influx of calcium, fusion with the membranes of secretory granules, and extrusion of their contents.

Regulation of Secretion

Vasopressin

Osmotic Factors

The secretion of vasopressin is known to be influenced by a number of variables.[25–29] Probably the most important under physiologic conditions is the effective osmotic pressure of plasma. Its influence on vasopressin is mediated by specialized neurons, known collectively as *osmoreceptors,* which appear to be concentrated in the anterolateral hypothalamus

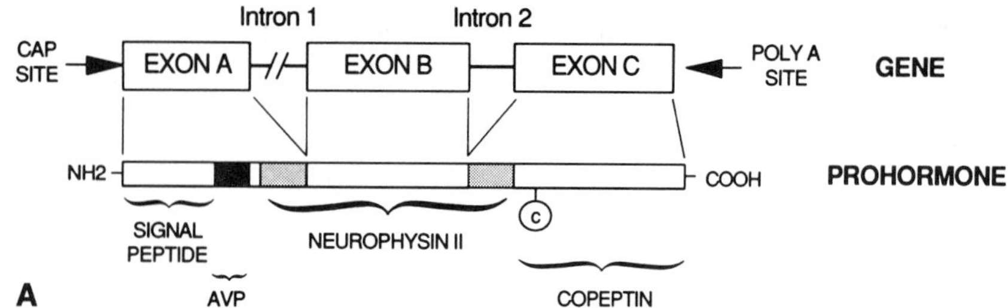

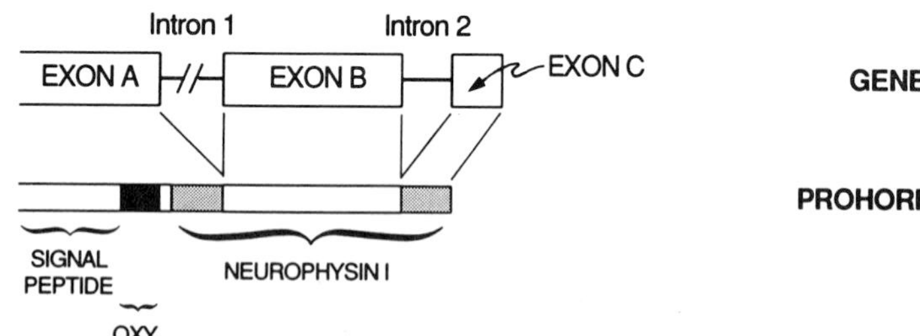

FIGURE 9-3 The structure of the vasopressin and oxytocin prohormones and the genes that encode them. The shaded areas at the ends of the neurophysin II and neurophysin I moieties in both prohormones represent the variable portions encoded by exons A and C, and the clear area in the middle represents the highly conserved portion encoded by exon B. © indicates the glycosylation site on the copeptin moiety.

near but separate from the supraoptic nuclei (Fig. 9-1).[30–34] This part of the brain receives its blood supply from small perforating branches of the anterior cerebral and/or communicating arteries.[35]

The functional properties of the osmoregulatory mechanism resemble those of a discontinuous or "set point" receptor (Fig. 9-4*A*). Thus, at plasma osmolalities below a certain minimum or threshold level, plasma vasopressin is suppressed to low or undetectable concentrations. Above this point, plasma vasopressin rises steeply in direct proportion to plasma osmolality. The slope of this relation indicates that a change in plasma osmolality of only 1 percent will change plasma vasopressin by an average of 1 pg/ml (1 pmol/L), an amount sufficient to significantly alter urinary concentration and flow (Fig. 9-4*B*). This extraordinary sensitivity confers on the osmoreceptor the primary role in mediating the antidiuretic response to changes in water balance.

The sensitivity of the osmoregulatory system varies appreciably from person to person.[27] In a healthy adult population, as much as 10-fold differences in slope have been observed. In the most sensitive people, physiologically significant changes in vasopressin can be induced by changes in plasma osmolality as small as 0.5 mosmol/kg (0.17 percent), an amount far too low to be detected by even the best available laboratory osmometers. At the other extreme of normal, comparable changes in plasma vasopressin may require changes in plasma osmolality

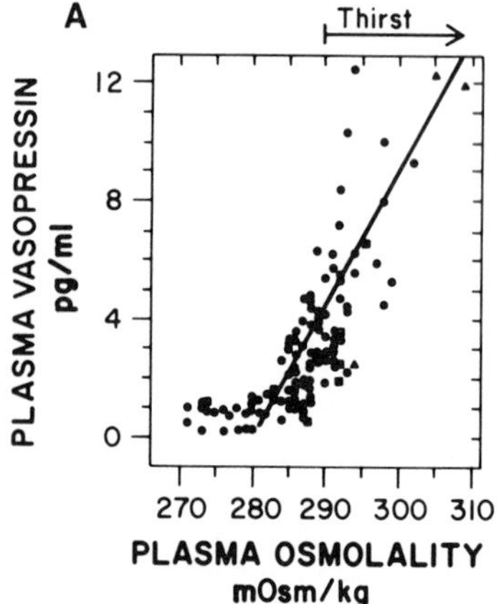

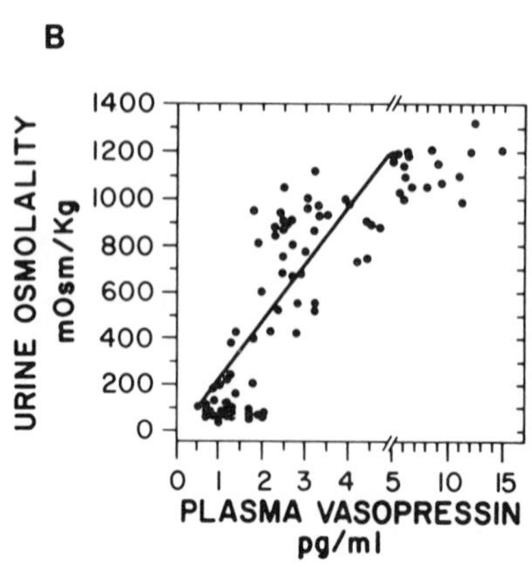

FIGURE 9-4 The relation of plasma vasopressin to plasma and urine osmolality in healthy adults in various states of hydration. (*Redrawn from Robertson et al.*[27])

of up to 5 mosmol/kg (1.7 percent). These individual differences in osmoregulatory sensitivity are constant over prolonged periods and appear to be determined largely by genetic factors.[36] However, this property of the system is not totally immutable, since hypovolemia, angiotensin, glucopenia, hypercalcemia, insulinopenia, and lithium all increase the slope of the plasma vasopressin-osmolality relation (see below). The sensitivity of the osmoregulatory system also appears to increase with age, at least in men.[37] The effect of sex and/or gonadal hormones on vasopressin secretion is controversial. One study found no differences in osmoregulatory function in adult males and females,[27] while others observed increased sensitivity in females and estrogen-treated males[38,39] and in estrogen-treated rats.[40]

The "set" of the osmoregulatory system also varies from person to person. In healthy adults, the osmotic threshold for vasopressin secretion ranges from 275 to 290 mosmol/kg, with an average of about 285 mosmol/kg.[36] These interindividual differences in the "set" of the osmoregulatory system are also genetically determined[36] but can vary over time, possibly as a result of changes in blood volume and/or pressure. The set of the osmoregulatory system is also reduced during pregnancy[41] and during the luteal phase of the menstrual cycle.[42,43] The mechanism is unknown.

It is uncertain whether the threshold concept accurately represents the operation of the osmoreceptor at its most fundamental level.[44–46] Some analyses of the relation between plasma vasopressin and osmolality suggest that it may be described better by an exponential rather than a linear threshold model, while others find no significant difference in the fit of the data. Indeed, it is uncertain whether current methods are sufficiently precise to distinguish between the two models or, if they could, whether the distinction would be important. Moreover, there is reason to think that vasopressin secretion reflects the balance of inhibitory as well as stimulatory input from a bimodal system of osmoreceptors.[29] If this is so, both types probably have a common set or null point that corresponds closely to the normal basal effective osmotic pressure of body water. For practical purposes, however, the concept of an osmotic threshold for vasopressin secretion remains for the present a useful if not valid way of describing many aspects of normal and abnormal osmoregulatory function in intact animals and humans.

It is also uncertain whether vasopressin is secreted continuously or episodically in response to osmotic stimulation. When nonosmotic stimuli such as posture, activity, and blood pressure are controlled or constant, the infusion of hypertonic saline in humans usually produces a smooth progressive rise in systemic venous plasma vasopressin that correlates closely with the rise in plasma osmolality.[29,36,46] However, when samples are obtained from animals at a point nearer the source of the hormone, e.g., from the right atrium or internal jugular vein, large fluctuations in plasma vasopressin have been observed during osmotic stimulation.[47] Whether these fluctuations reflect an intrinsic property of the neurohypophysis or are artifacts of the experimental conditions is unknown. Irregular phasic firing of neurosecretory neurons has been observed by unit recording techniques,[48,49] but this activity is unlikely to be related to episodic fluctuations in plasma vasopressin, since the discharge cycles have a much shorter periodicity and are not synchronized from cell to cell.

The osmoregulatory mechanism is not equally sensitive to all plasma solutes (Fig. 9-5).[50] Sodium and its anions, which normally contribute more than 95 percent of the osmotic pressure of plasma, are the most potent solutes known in terms of their capacity to stimulate vasopressin release.[51] However, certain sugars, such as sucrose and mannitol, are also very effective when infused intravenously.[25,51,52] In fact, particle for particle, mannitol appears to be nearly as potent as sodium chloride.[51] In this respect, therefore, the control mechanism behaves like a true osmoreceptor. However, a rise in plasma osmolality due to urea or glucose causes little or no increase in plasma vasopressin in healthy adults or animals.[27,51,52] These differences in the response to various plasma solutes are independent of any recognized nonosmotic influence and are probably a

FIGURE 9-5 The relation of plasma vasopressin to elevations in plasma osmolality induced by various solutes in healthy adults. Each oblique line represents the mean regression function obtained during intravenous infusion of hypertonic solutions of the specified solutes. (*From Robertson.*[50])

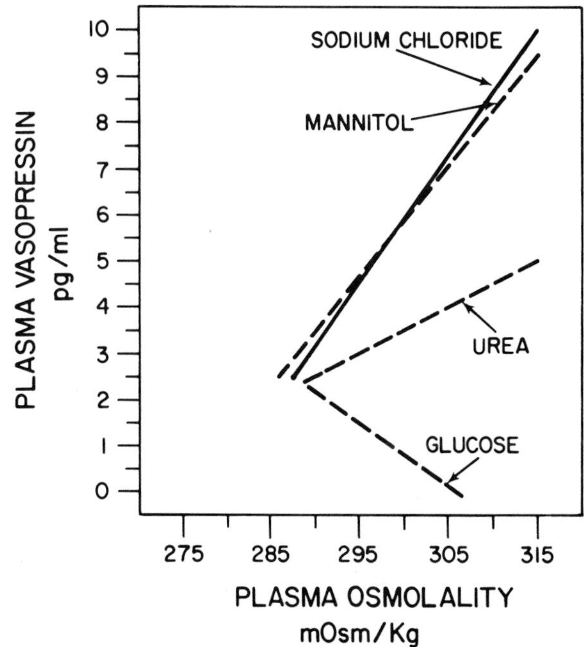

property of the osmoregulatory mechanism per se. Precisely how and why the osmoreceptor discriminates so effectively between different kinds of plasma solutes is unsettled. According to current concepts, the signal which stimulates the osmoreceptor is an osmotically induced decrease in the water content of the cell. If this hypothesis is correct, the ability of a given solute to stimulate vasopressin secretion ought to be inversely related to the rate at which it passes from plasma into the osmoreceptor neuron.[25] This concept agrees well with the observed inverse relation between the effect of solutes such as sodium, mannitol, and glucose on vasopressin secretion and the rate at which they penetrate the blood-brain barrier. The latter observations are also consistent with the view that the osmoreceptors are actually sodium receptors located within the blood-brain barrier.[53,54] However, the sodium receptor theory is difficult to reconcile with the behavior of urea, which penetrates the blood-brain barrier quite slowly yet causes little or no stimulation of thirst or vasopressin release.[51,52] This singular disparity suggests that most if not all of the osmoreceptors are located outside the blood-brain barrier and that another factor, most likely the permeability of the osmoreceptor neuron per se, determines the specificity of the system.

The sensitivity of the osmoreceptors to stimulation by plasma glucose appears to be critically dependent on the level of plasma insulin. Thus, hyperglycemia stimulates thirst and vasopressin secretion in patients with insulin-deficient diabetes mellitus[55] but has no effect on either variable in healthy adults[51] or in patients with insulin-treated diabetes.[56] These observations probably explain the hyperdipsia and some of the hypervasopressinemia that occur in uncontrolled patients with diabetes mellitus[57,58] and indicate that glucose uptake by osmoreceptor neurons is probably dependent on the action of insulin. This concept is supported by other evidence that high-affinity receptors for plasma insulin are present in an area of the anterior hypothalamus that is thought to contain the osmoreceptors.[59]

Oropharyngeal Factors

Water intake may also inhibit the secretion of vasopressin via receptors located in the oropharynx or upper gastrointestinal tract.[60–64] This effect occurs rapidly but is transient unless it is followed by a decrease in plasma osmolality or sodium. The kind of receptor involved is unknown, and the effect may depend more on the temperature than on the tonicity of the fluid ingested.

Hemodynamic Factors

The secretion of vasopressin is also affected by changes in blood volume and/or pressure.[25,26,28] These hemodynamic influences are mediated largely if not exclusively by neurogenic afferents that arise in pressure-sensitive receptors in the cardiac atria and large arteries, travel via the vagal and glossopharyngeal nerves, and synapse in the nucleus of the solitary tract (Fig. 9-1).[64,65] From there, postsynaptic pathways ascend to the lateral parabranchial nucleus, the A1 region of the ventrolateral medulla, and the vicinity of the paraventricular and supraoptic nuclei.[66,67] The input from these pathways appears to be predominantly negative, or inhibitory, under basal normovolemic, normotensive conditions, since their elimination results in an acute rise in plasma vasopressin as well as arterial pressure.[68]

The functional properties of this baroregulatory system are exemplified in Fig. 9-6. In healthy adult humans, monkeys, and rats, acutely lowering blood pressure by any of several methods increases plasma vasopressin by an amount that is roughly proportional to the degree of hypotension achieved.[29,69,70] However, this stimulus-response relation follows a distinctly exponential pattern. Thus, small decreases in blood pressure of the order of 5 to 10 percent usually have little effect on plasma vasopressin, while decreases in blood pressure of 20 to 30 percent result in hormone levels many times those required to produce maximum antidiuresis. The vasopressin response to changes in blood volume has not been so well defined but appears to be quantitatively and qualitatively similar to the response to blood pres-

FIGURE 9-6 The relation of plasma vasopressin to percent fall in blood pressure in healthy adults and patients with idiopathic postural hypotension. In healthy adults, blood pressure was reduced by the infusion of trimethaphan (Arfonad) (solid circle) or by orthostasis immediately after phlebotomy (open circle). In patients with orthostatic hypotension, blood pressure was reduced by tilting (triangle). *(From Robertson.[50])*

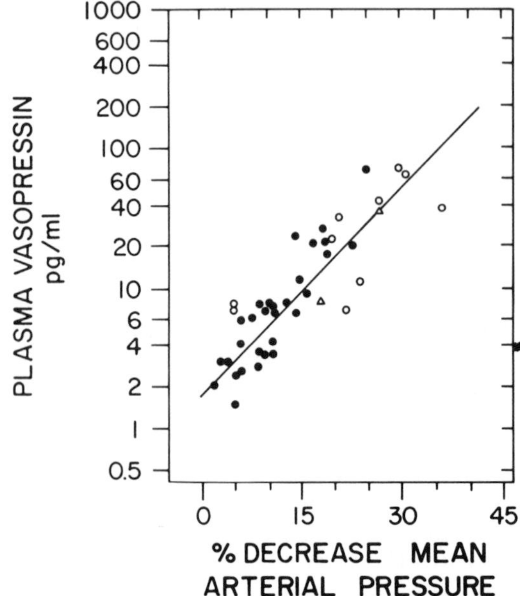

sure. In rats, plasma vasopressin increases as an exponential function of the degree of hypovolemia.[71] Thus, little or no rise in plasma vasopressin can be detected until blood volume falls by 6 to 8 percent. Beyond that point, plasma vasopressin begins to rise at a rapidly increasing rate in relation to the degree of hypovolemia and usually reaches levels 20 to 30 times normal when blood volume is reduced by 20 to 30 percent. The volume-vasopressin relation in humans and other animals has not been so thoroughly characterized but appears to follow a similar pattern.[26,71–73] Thus, in healthy adults, plasma vasopressin is unchanged by a fall in blood volume of up to 7 percent, is doubled by a reduction of 10 to 15 percent, and increases markedly if the hypovolemia exceeds 20 percent.

The minimal effect of small changes in blood volume and pressure on vasopressin secretion contrasts sharply with the extraordinary sensitivity of the osmoregulatory system. Recognition of this difference is essential for understanding the relative contribution of each system to the control of the hormone under physiologic and pathologic conditions. Since day-to-day variations of total body water rarely exceed 2 to 3 percent, their effect on vasopressin secretion must be mediated largely, if not exclusively, by the osmoregulatory system.[71,74] This concept is consistent with the observation that patients with destruction of the osmoreceptor exhibit a markedly subnormal vasopressin response to changes in water balance even though baroregulatory mechanisms are completely intact.[32] However, baroregulatory input may be responsible for the increase in plasma vasopressin that normally occurs during sleep.[75] Hence, hemodynamic and osmotic influences may be equally active under physiologic conditions, even though their determinants and effect on salt and water balance are quite different.

The baroreceptor also appears to mediate the effects of a large number of pharmacologic and pathologic influences (Table 9-1). Among the pharmacologic influences are diuretics, isoproterenol, nicotine, prostaglandins, nitroprusside, trimethaphan, histamine, morphine, and bradykinin, all of which stimulate vasopressin at least in part by lowering blood volume or pressure, and norepinephrine, which suppresses vasopressin by raising blood pressure. In addition, upright posture, sodium depletion, congestive heart failure, cirrhosis, and nephrosis probably stimulate vasopressin by reducing total or effective blood volume,[76–78] while orthostatic hypotension, vasovagal reactions, and other forms of syncope markedly stimulate the hormone by reducing blood pressure.[69,79,80] This list probably could be extended to include almost every other hormone, drug, or condition known to affect blood volume or pressure. The only recognized exception is a form of orthostatic hypotension associated with the loss of afferent baroregulatory function.[81]

TABLE 9-1 Variables That Influence Vasopressin Secretion

Osmotic
Plasma osmolality
Changes in water balance
Infusion of hypertonic or hypotonic solutions
Deficiency of insulin and hyperglycemia
Hemodynamic
Blood volume (total or effective)
Posture
Hemorrhage
Aldosterone deficiency or excess
Gastroenteritis
Congestive heart failure
Cirrhosis
Nephrosis
Positive pressure breathing
Diuretics
Blood pressure
Orthostatic hypotension
Vasovagal reaction
Drugs (isoproterenol, norepinephrine, nicotine, nitroprusside, trimethaphan, histamine, bradykinin, morphine)
Emetic
Nausea
Drugs (apomorphine, morphine, nicotine)
Motion sickness
Glucopenic
Drugs (insulin, 2-deoxyglucose)
Other
Angiotensin
P_{CO_2}, P_{O_2}, pH
Stress (?)
Temperature (?)

Changes in blood volume or pressure large enough to affect vasopressin secretion do not necessarily interfere with osmoregulation of the hormone. Instead, they appear to act by shifting the set of the system in a way that increases or decreases the effect on vasopressin of a given osmotic stimulus (Fig. 9-7).[27,82–87] Thus, in the presence of a hemodynamic stimulus, plasma vasopressin can still be fully suppressed if plasma osmolality falls below the new, lower set point.[85] This aspect of the interaction is important because it ensures that the capacity to osmoregulate is not lost even in the presence of hemodynamic stimuli. It also indicates that the osmoregulatory and baroregulatory systems, though different in location and function, ultimately converge and act on the same population of neurosecretory neurons.[27]

Emetic Factors

Nausea is an extremely potent stimulus for vasopressin secretion in humans.[88,89] The pathway that mediates this effect has not been defined but probably involves the chemoreceptor trigger zone in the area postrema of the medulla (Fig. 9-1). It can be

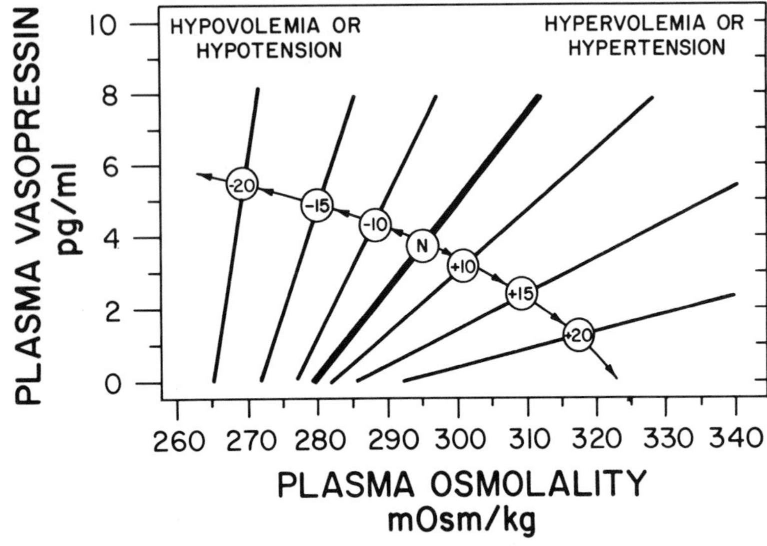

FIGURE 9-7 Schematic representation of the relation between plasma vasopressin and plasma osmolality in the presence of differing states of blood volume and/or pressure. The line labeled N represents normovolemic, normotensive conditions. Negative numbers to the left indicate percent fall and positive numbers to the right indicate percent rise in blood volume or pressure. (*From Robertson.*[50])

activated by a variety of drugs and conditions, including apomorphine, morphine, nicotine, alcohol, and motion sickness. Its effect on vasopressin is instantaneous and extremely potent (Fig. 9-8). Increases of 100 to 1000 times basal levels are not unusual even when the nausea is transient and unaccompanied by vomiting or changes in blood pressure. Pretreatment with fluphenazine, haloperidol, or promethazine in doses sufficient to prevent nausea completely abolishes the vasopressin response. The inhibitory effect of these dopamine antagonists is specific for emetic stimuli, since they do not alter the vasopressin response to osmotic and hemodynamic stimuli. Water loading blunts but does not abolish the effect of nausea on vasopressin release, suggesting that osmotic and emetic influences interact in a manner similar to the interaction of osmotic and hemodynamic pathways. Emesis is the only vasopressin stimulus known to exhibit significant species differences. In rats, apomorphine has little or no effect on vasopressin[88,90] but produces marked increases in oxytocin.[90]

Emetic stimuli probably mediate many pharmacologic and pathologic effects on vasopressin secretion. They may be responsible at least in part for the increase in vasopressin secretion that has been observed with intravenous cyclophosphamide,[91,92] vasovagal reactions,[79] ketoacidosis,[57,58] acute hypoxia,[93] and motion sickness.[94] Since nausea and vomiting are frequent side effects of many other

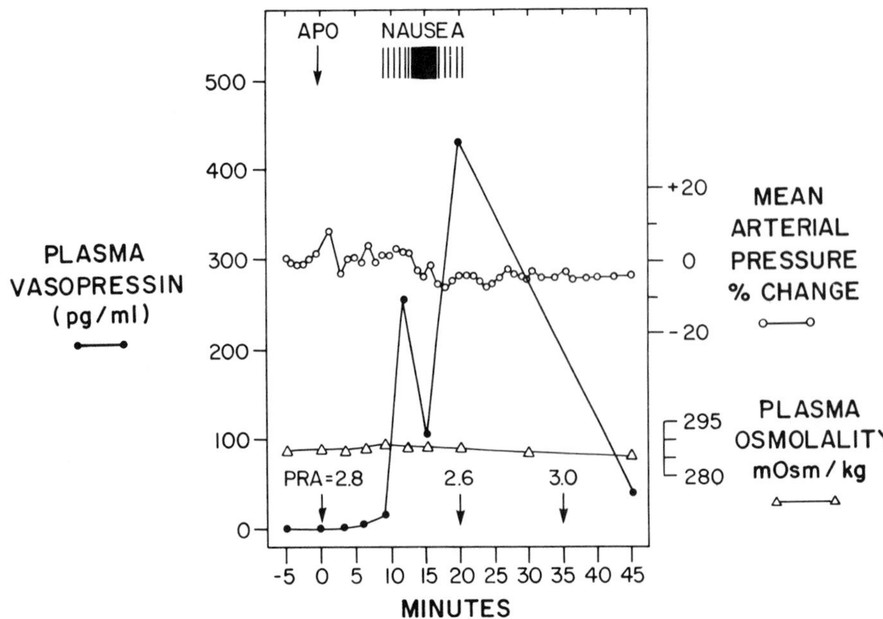

FIGURE 9-8 Relation of nausea to vasopressin secretion. Apomorphine (APO) was injected at the point indicated by the vertical arrow. Note that the rise in plasma vasopressin coincided with the occurrence of nausea and was not associated with detectable changes in plasma osmolality or blood pressure. (*From Robertson.*[50])

drugs and diseases, additional examples of emetically mediated vasopressin secretion undoubtedly will be demonstrated. The potency and ubiquity of emetic stimuli create special problems for research studies of vasopressin secretion in animals and unconscious subjects, since the occurrence of nausea is difficult to ascertain except by verbal report.

Glucopenic Factors

Acute hypoglycemia is also a stimulus for vasopressin release,[95–98] but the effect is much less potent than that of nausea. The receptor and pathway that mediate this effect are unknown. However, they seem to be separate from those of other recognized stimuli, since hypoglycemia stimulates vasopressin secretion in patients who have lost selectively the capacity to respond to osmotic, hemodynamic, or emetic stimuli. The effect of hypoglycemia is not due to nonspecific stress, since it can occur in the absence of symptoms and is more pronounced in rats,[96] a species in which vasopressin secretion appears to be completely unresponsive to pain and other noxious stimuli (see below). The variable that actually triggers the release of vasopressin may be an intracellular deficiency of glucose or one of its metabolites, since 2-deoxyglucose is also an effective stimulus.[99,100]

The stimulus-response relations to hypoglycemia appears to be exponential.[97] Thus, in healthy adults, a drop in plasma glucose of as much as 10 to 20 percent usually has little or no effect, whereas a decrease of 50 percent increases plasma vasopressin about threefold. The rate of fall in glucose is probably the critical determinant, however, since the rise in plasma vasopressin is not sustained even when the hypoglycemia persists.[96] In addition, the vasopressin response to hypoglycemia is accentuated by dehydration and abolished by water loading.[96] Thus, glucopenic stimuli probably act in concert with osmotic influences even though the osmoreceptors per se are unnecessary for the response.

Glucopenic stimuli are probably of little importance in clinical disorders of vasopressin secretion. Apart from acute hyperinsulinemia, few drugs or conditions lower plasma glucose quickly enough to stimulate release of the hormone. Moreover, even if secretion were increased, it would not be expected to influence perceptibly the regulation of water balance, since the effect tends to be transient and is prevented completely by a small decrease in plasma osmolality.

Renin-Angiotensin

The renin-angiotensin system has also been implicated in the control of vasopressin secretion.[101] The precise site and mechanism of action have not been defined, but central receptors seem likely, since angiotensin is most effective when injected directly into brain ventricles or cranial arteries.[102] Moreover, intraventricular administration of angiotensin antagonists inhibits the vasopressin response to osmotic and hemodynamic stimuli.[103] The levels of plasma renin and/or angiotensin required to stimulate vasopressin release have not been determined but probably are quite high. When given intravenously, pressor doses of angiotensin increase plasma vasopressin only about two- to fourfold. The magnitude of the vasopressin response may depend on the concurrent osmotic stimulus, since angiotensin has been observed to increase the sensitivity of the osmoregulatory system.[104] Hence, the effect of angiotensin on vasopressin may be imperceptible when plasma osmolality is depressed and exaggerated when plasma osmolality is high. This dependency on osmotic influences resembles that seen with glucopenic stimuli and may account for the failure of some investigators to demonstrate stimulation by exogenous angiotensin.[105]

Stress and Temperature

Nonspecific stress caused by factors such as pain, emotion, and physical exercise has long been thought to cause the release of vasopressin.[106] However, it has never been determined whether this effect is mediated by a separate pathway or is secondary to another stimulus, such as the hypotension and/or nausea that usually accompanies stress-induced vasovagal reactions. In rats and humans, a variety of noxious stimuli capable of activating the pituitary adrenal axis and sympathetic nervous system do not stimulate vasopressin secretion unless they also lower blood pressure or alter blood volume.[26,107–109] The same stresses may stimulate the release of oxytocin,[109] but the role of other nonosmotic stimuli in the response has not been excluded. The marked rise in plasma vasopressin elicited by manipulation of the abdominal viscera in anesthetized dogs has been attributed to nociceptive influences,[110] but mediation by emetic pathways cannot be excluded in this setting.

Environmental temperature can also influence vasopressin secretion.[76] In healthy adults, exposure to cold for a relatively short period depresses plasma vasopressin, while a hot environment has the opposite effect. These changes occur independently of changes in plasma osmolality but cannot be disassociated from changes in effective blood volume or blood pressure. Hence, it is unclear whether there is a distinct thermoregulatory system for vasopressin secretion. Clarification of the possible role of nociceptive and thermal influences in vasopressin secretion is particularly important in view of the frequency with which painful or febrile illnesses are associated with osmotically inappropriate secretion of the hormone.

Hypoxia-Hypercapnia

Acute hypoxia and hypercapnia also stimulate vasopressin release.[93,111–114] In conscious humans, however, the stimulatory effect of moderate hypoxia (Pa_{O_2} > 35 mmHg) is inconsistent[93,111] and seems to occur only in subjects who develop nausea or hypotension.[93] In conscious dogs, more severe hypoxia (Pa_{O_2} < 35 mm Hg) consistently increases vasopressin secretion without reducing arterial pressure.[113] Studies in anesthetized dogs suggest that the vasopressin response to acute hypoxia depends on the level of hypoxemia achieved. At a Pa_{O_2} of 35 mmHg or below, plasma vasopressin is markedly elevated despite the absence of change or even an increase in arterial pressure.[112,114] However, less severe hypoxemia (Pa_{O_2} > 40 mmHg) has no effect on vasopressin.[112] These results indicate a hypoxemic threshold for vasopressin release and suggest that severe acute hypoxemia per se may also stimulate vasopressin secretion in humans. If this is so, it may be responsible, at least in part, for the osmotically inappropriate hormonal elevations noted in some patients with acute respiratory failure.[115] In conscious or anesthetized dogs, acute hypercapnia per se, independent of hypoxia or hypotension, also increases vasopressin secretion.[112,113] It has not been determined whether this response also exhibits threshold characteristics or otherwise depends on the degree of hypercapnia. It is also unknown whether hypercapnia has similar effects on vasopressin secretion in humans or other animals.

TABLE 9-2 Drugs and Hormones That Affect Vasopressin Secretion or Action

Secretion	
Stimulate/potentiate	Inhibit
Acetylcholine	Norepinephrine
Nicotine	Fluphenazine (emetic)
Apomorphine	Haloperidol (emetic)
Morphine (high doses)	Promethazine
Epinephrine	Opioid agonists
Isoproterenol	mu, e.g., morphine (low doses)
Histamine	kappa, e.g., oxilorphan, butorphanol, U50488H
Bradykinin	delta, e.g., DAMME, met-enkephalin
Prostaglandins	Opiod antagonists
Insulin	Nonselective: diprenorphine (hypovolemic)*
2-Deoxyglucose	Alcohol
Angiotensin	Carbamazepine
Cyclophosphamide (IV)	Glucocorticoids
Vincristine	Clonidine
Lithium	Muscimol
? Chlorpropamide	
? Clofibrate	
Opioid antagonists	
mu, naloxone, naltrexone	
Action	
Potentiate	Inhibit
Chlorpropamide	Barbiturates
Indomethacin	Lithium
Acetaminophen	Tetracyclines
? Clofibrate	Methoxyflurane
? Carbamazepine	Glyburide
	Ifosfamide
	Vinca alkaloids
	Vasopressin antagonists
	Platinum
	? Glucocorticoids

* Experimental drug provided by National Institute of Drug Abuse.

Pharmacologic Factors

A large number of drugs and hormones have also been shown to influence vasopressin secretion (Table 9-2).[116,117] Many stimulants, such as isoproterenol, nicotine, and high doses of morphine, undoubtedly act at least in part by lowering blood pressure or producing nausea.[116–118] Others, such as substance P, histamine, bradykinin, and prostaglandin, have not been studied sufficiently to define their mechanism of action but probably act the same way.[118,119] As discussed elsewhere, insulin and 2-deoxyglucose seem to act by producing intracellular glucopenia, while angiotensin has an undefined but probably independent central effect. Vincristine may act by a direct effect on the neurohypophysis or the peripheral neurons involved in the regulation of vasopressin secretion.[120] Lithium, which antagonizes the antidiuretic effect of vasopressin, also increases secretion of the hormone.[121–123] This effect is independent of changes in water balance and appears to result from an increase in the sensitivity of the osmoregulatory system.[121] The stimulatory effects of chlorpropamide and clofibrate are still controversial.[124–127] Carbamazepine inhibits vasopressin secretion by diminishing the sensitivity of the osmoregulatory system.[128–130] This effect occurs independently of changes in blood volume, blood pressure, or blood glucose, suggesting that the ability of carbamazepine to produce antidiuresis in patients with neurogenic diabetes insipidus is due to an action on the kidney. Opioid antagonists selective for mu receptors may potentiate the vasopressin response to certain stimuli,[131–133] presumably by blocking the inhibitory influence of some endogenous opioid, such as β-endorphin. Vasopressin secretion can be inhibited indirectly by drugs or hormones, such as norepinephrine, which raise arterial pressure.[116,117]

Dopaminergic antagonists such as fluphenazine, haloperidol, and promethazine probably act by suppressing the emetic center, since they inhibit the vasopressin response to emetic and not to osmotic or hemodynamic stimuli. In low doses, a variety of opioids, including morphine, inhibit vasopressin secretion in rats[134–137] and humans.[138–141] The inhibition by morphine, butorphanol, and oxilorphan is due to an increase in the osmotic threshold for vasopressin release[134,136] but is independent of changes in blood volume or pressure.[134] The inhibitory action of these opioids has not been completely defined but would appear to be an agonistic effect, since it is blocked completely by naloxone.[134–136] The nonselective opioid antagonist diprenorphine inhibits the vasopressin response to hypovolemic but not osmotic or hypotensive stimuli.[132] This specific inhibitory effect occurs in the lateral parabrachial nucleus[142] and cannot be reproduced with more selective antagonists of mu or delta receptors. Presumably, therefore, it blocks synaptic transmission of some type of endogenous kappa agonist in the neuronal pathway that mediates the volume control of vasopressin secretion. The inhibitory effect of alcohol[143,144] may be mediated at least in part by endogenous opiates, since it also is due to an elevation in the osmotic threshold for vasopressin release and can be blocked in part by treatment with naloxone.[145] Other drugs which have the capacity to inhibit vasopressin secretion include clonidine,[146,147] which appears to act via both central and peripheral adrenoreceptors,[146] and muscimol,[148] which is postulated to act as a γ-aminobutyric acid (GABA) agonist.

Vasopressin and oxytocin may also feed back to inhibit or facilitate their own secretion.[149–151] In the case of vasopressin, at least, the feedback effect occurs after systemic as well as central administration and is not mediated by osmotic or hemodynamic influences.[149,150] The importance of local feedback effects on the physiology or pathophysiology of vasopressin secretion is uncertain because the phenomenon has been demonstrated only after exogenous administration of relatively large doses of the hormone.

Oxytocin

The regulation of oxytocin secretion has not been well defined because simple and specific assays have been lacking. Bioassays, direct as well as indirect, have often been employed, but their specificity is suspect because vasopressin and possibly other peptides possess oxytocin activity. Radioimmunoassays have also been developed and used to characterize secretion of the hormone. However, even this information must now be viewed with caution, because some oxytocin and vasotocin assays have been found to cross-react with one or more plasma components other than oxytocin.[152] To further complicate matters, the ovary also synthesizes oxytocin or oxytocin-like peptides,[153] and this material may be the source of some of the immunoreactivity in plasma.

Studies employing specific assays have confirmed that nursing, mechanical stimulation, or manual stimulation of nipples is a stimulus for oxytocin release in women during lactation or certain phases of the menstrual cycle.[152] In men as well as women, oxytocin secretion may also be stimulated by insulin-induced hypoglycemia.[154] However, contrary to previous findings using less specific assays, it now appears that pregnancy and/or high levels of estrogen do not result in increased secretion of oxytocin but do cause an increase in the plasma level of a novel peptide which may be structurally related to oxytocin.[152] The source and biological action, if any, of this novel peptide are unknown. In rats but not in humans, oxytocin is also released in response to osmotic and emetic stimuli.[90]

Distribution and Clearance

The concentration of vasopressin and oxytocin in plasma is determined by the difference between the rates of production and removal from the vascular compartment. In healthy adults, intravenously injected vasopressin distributes rapidly into a space roughly equivalent in size to the extracellular compartment.[26,155] In this initial, or "mixing," phase, the vasopressin has a half-life of 4 to 8 min, and the process is virtually complete in 10 to 15 min. The rapidity with which vasopressin diffuses across capillary membranes approximates that of many other small peptides and is consistent with its lack of binding to neurophysin or other macromolecular components of plasma. The rapid mixing phase is followed by a second, slower decline that probably corresponds to the metabolic, or irreversible, phase of vasopressin clearance. Studies with one immunoassay yielded mean values of 10 to 20 min by both steady-state and non-steady-state techniques.[26,149,156,157] The rate of decline in urine osmolality after water loading is consistent with these estimates.[155] It should be noted that smaller animals such as the rat clear vasopressin much more rapidly than humans do because their cardiac output is also much higher relative to their body weight and surface area.[155]

Although many tissues have the capacity to inactivate vasopressin in vitro, most metabolism in vivo appears to occur in the liver and kidney.[155] The enzymatic processes by which the liver and kidney inactivate vasopressin have not been established with certainty but appear to involve an initial reduction of the disulfide bridge followed by aminopeptidase cleavage of the bond between amino acid residues 1 and 2. The extent of further degradation and the peptide products, if any, that escape into plasma and urine are currently unknown. In pregnant women, the metabolic clearance of vasopressin is increased three- to fourfold because the placenta produces a vasopressinase that rapidly degrades the hormone in vivo as well as in vitro.[157]

Some vasopressin is excreted intact in the urine, but the amounts are quite small relative to total metabolic clearance. In healthy, normally hydrated adults, the urinary clearance of vasopressin ranges from 0.1 to 0.6 ml per kilogram of body weight per minute under basal conditions and has never been found to exceed 2 ml per kilogram of body weight per minute even in the presence of a solute diuresis.[26] The mechanisms involved in the excretion of vasopressin have not been defined with certainty, but the hormone is probably filtered at the glomerulus and variably reabsorbed at one or more sites along the tubule. The latter process may be linked in some way to the handling of sodium in the proximal nephron, since the urinary clearance of vasopressin varies as much as 20-fold in direct relation to solute clearance.[26] Consequently, measurements of vasopressin excretion in humans do not provide a consistently reliable index of changes in plasma vasopressin and must be interpreted cautiously when glomerular filtration and/or solute clearance are inconstant or abnormal.

The distribution and metabolic clearance of oxytocin appear to be similar to those of vasopressin.[152]

Extrahypophyseal Pathways

Little is known about the regulation of secretion by vasopressin- or oxytocin-containing neurons that project to areas other than the pars nervosa. The parvicellular division that projects from the paraventricular nucleus to the median eminence and portal veins contains corticotropin releasing factor (CRF) as well as vasopressin and appears to be stimulated by general anesthesia, surgery, and glucocorticoid deficiency but not by osmolality.[7] In contrast, the oxytocin-containing neurons in this pathway appear to be unaffected by adrenal insufficiency.[7] The vasopressinergic magnicellular neurons that arise in the suprachiasmatic nucleus and project to other areas of the hypothalamus also appear to be unresponsive to osmotic stimuli.[158]

The regulation of vasopressin and oxytocin secretion into spinal fluid is understood only slightly better. Most if not all of the vasopressin in CSF probably derives from direct secretion rather than diffusion from plasma.[8] In humans, the concentration of vasopressin in CSF appears to be slightly lower than the concentration in plasma,[8,159] although the opposite has also been reported in humans as well as animals.[160,161] Secretion into CSF seems to be influenced by some if not all of the same variables that stimulate release from the pars nervosa, since CSF concentrations correlate with those in plasma[8,159] and change appropriately during dehydration or rehydration in humans[8] or dogs,[161] during the infusion of hypertonic saline,[161] and during hemorrhage.[161] In humans, unlike in some lower species, CSF vasopressin does not show diurnal variation but oxytocin, which is also present, shows a distinct diurnal rhythm, with the peak occurring at about noon.[162] The function of the vasopressin in CSF is unknown, but it may play a role in regulating brain hydration,[8] thirst,[163] or intellectual function.[164] CSF vasopressin is abnormal in the syndrome of inappropriate antidiuresis,[8] diabetes insipidus,[8] dementia,[165] affective disorders,[166] and benign intracranial hypertension,[167] but the role of the abnormalities in the pathophysiology of these disorders is unknown.

Biological Action

The most important action of vasopressin is to conserve body water by reducing the rate of urine output. This antidiuretic effect is achieved by promoting the reabsorption of solute-free water in the distal and/or collecting tubules of the kidney (Fig. 9-9).[168] In the absence of vasopressin, the membranes lining this portion of the nephron are uniquely resistant to the diffusion of water as well as solutes. Hence, hypotonic filtrate formed in the more proximal part of the nephron passes unmodified through the distal tubule and collecting duct. In this condition, which is referred to as *water diuresis,* urine osmolality and flow in a healthy adult usually approximate 60 to 70 mosmol/kg and 15 to 20 ml/min, respectively. In the presence of vasopressin, the hydroosmotic permeability of the distal and collecting tubules increases, allowing water to diffuse back down the osmotic gradient that normally exists between tubular fluid and the isotonic or hypertonic milieu of the renal cortex and medulla (Fig. 9-9). Because water is reabsorbed without solute, the urine that remains has an increased osmotic pressure as well as decreased volume or flow rate.

The amount of water reabsorbed in the distal nephron—and thus the degree of urinary concentration—varies as a function of the plasma vasopressin concentration (see Fig. 9-4*B*). In healthy adults, this stimulus-response relation is extremely sensitive, since the full range of urinary concentration and dilution is covered by a 10-fold or smaller change in plasma vasopressin. At maximally effective levels of vasopressin, urine osmolality and flow approximate 1200 to 1400 mosmol/kg and 0.3 to 0.6 ml/min, respectively. Certain other species, particularly rodents, can achieve much higher levels of urinary concentration, apparently because of longer renal papillae and correspondingly higher levels of hypertonicity in the medulla.

The effect of vasopressin on urinary concentration and/or flow can be markedly influenced by changes in the volume of filtrate presented to the distal tubule. In a normal adult, 85 to 90 percent of the approximately 200 L of plasma filtered daily by the glomerulus is reabsorbed isoosmotically with salts and glucose in the proximal part of the nephron. The remaining 20 L is made hypotonic by selective reabsorption of sodium and chloride in the ascending limb of Henle's loop and then presented to the distal nephron, where, depending on the level of vasopressin activity, additional water up to a maximum of 19 L a day may be selectively reabsorbed. In situations in which the intake of salt is high or a poorly reabsorbed solute such a mannitol, urea, or glucose is present in increased amounts, considerably more than 10 to 15 percent of the filtrate may escape the proximal tubule. The resultant increase in the volume of fluid delivered to the distal nephron may overwhelm its limited capacity to reabsorb water and electrolytes. As a conseqence, urine osmolality falls and the rate of flow rises even in the presence of supranormal levels of vasopressin. This type

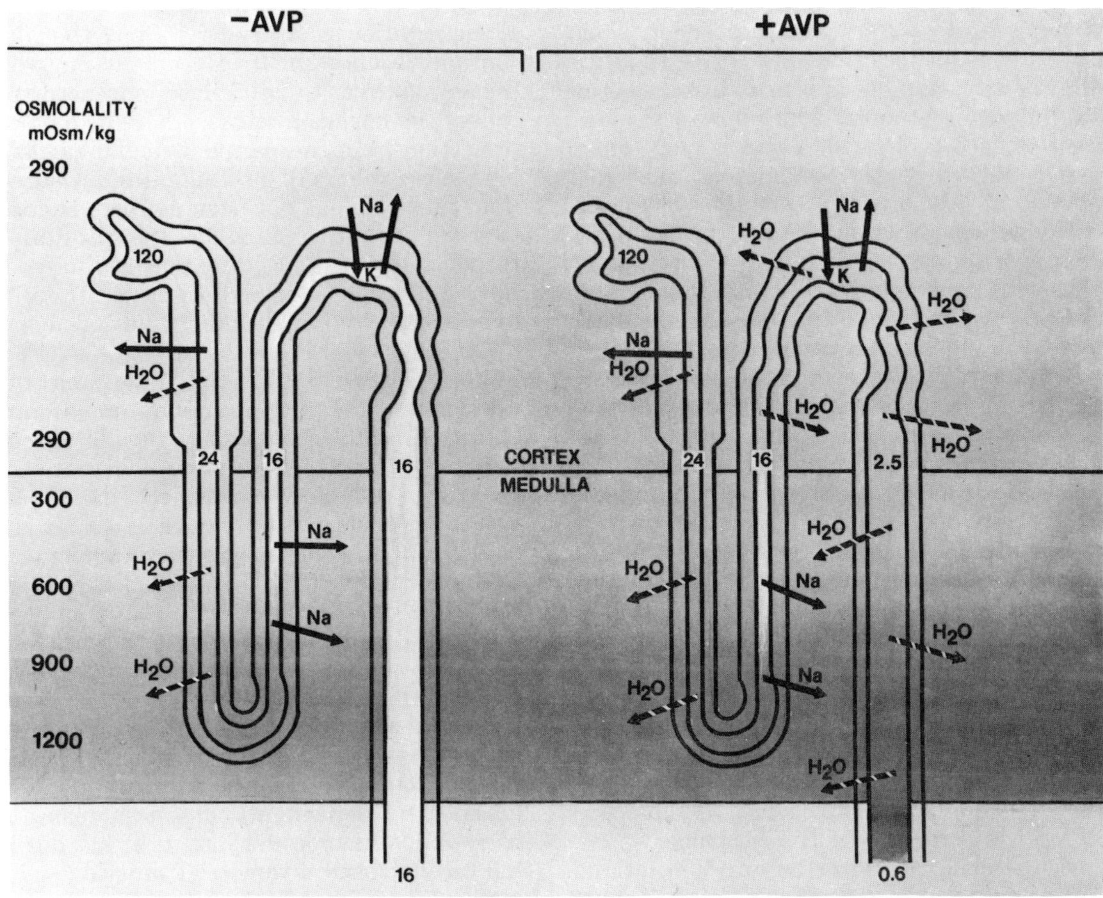

FIGURE 9-9 Schematic representation of the effect of vasopressin on the formation of urine by the nephron. The osmotic pressure of tissue and tubular fluid is indicated by the density of the shading. The numbers within the lumen of the nephron indicate typical rates of flow in milliliters per minute. Solid arrows indicate reabsorption of sodium (Na) or water (H_2O) by active mechanisms; broken arrows indicate reabsorption by passive mechanisms. Note that vasopressin acts only on the distal nephron, where it increases the hydroosmotic permeability of tubular membranes. The fluid which reaches this part of the nephron normally amounts to 10 to 15 percent of the total filtrate and is hypotonic because of selective reabsorption of sodium in the ascending limb of Henle's loop. In the absence of vasopressin the membranes of the distal nephron remain relatively impermeable to water as well as solute, and the fluid issuing from Henle's loop is excreted essentially unmodified as urine. With maximum vasopressin action, all but 5 to 10 percent of the water in this fluid is reabsorbed passively down the osmotic gradient which normally exists with the renal medulla.

of polyuria is referred to as *solute diuresis* to distinguish it from that due to a deficiency of vasopressin action. Conversely, in clinical situations such as congestive failure, where the proximal nephron reabsorbs increased amounts of filtrate, the capacity to excrete solute-free water is greatly reduced even in the absence of vasopressin action.

The antidiuretic effect of vasopressin also may be inhibited by breakdown in the medullary concentration gradient. This may result from causes as diverse as chronic water diuresis, reduced medullary blood flow, and protein deficiency. However, probably because the bulk of the fluid issuing from Henle's loop can still be reabsorbed isotonically in the distal convoluted tubule and/or proximal collecting duct, loss of the medullary concentration gradient alone rarely results in marked degrees of polyuria.

The cellular mechanism by which vasopressin alters the hydroosmotic permeability of the distal nephron has not been fully determined. However, there is abundant evidence that it binds to receptors on the serosal surface of tubular epithelia. This receptor, which has been designated V_2 to distinguish it from those which mediate the extrarenal actions of vasopressin (see below), has been cloned and sequenced and mapped to the distal long arm of the X chromosome.[169,170] It has a transmembrane topography characteristic of G-protein-coupled receptors and uses cyclic AMP as a second messenger. The exact nature and sequence of events triggered by the cyclic AMP are unknown but appear to involve activation of cellular microtubules which open pores on the mucosal surface of the cell. There is also some evidence suggesting that the prostaglandins operate as a kind of local or short-loop feedback system to modulate the actions of vasopressin on the kidney. Thus, it has been shown that vasopressin stimulates the synthesis of prostaglandin E and that prostaglandin E in turn can inhibit the effect of the hormone on adenyl cyclase and hydroosmotic flow. Conversely, inhibitors of prostaglandin synthesis such as indomethacin and chlorpropamide potentiate the antidiuretic effect of the hormone. Renal prostaglandin synthesis can also be stimulated by angiotensin, bradykinin, and hypertonicity, suggesting that a variety of factors may be capable of influencing water balance by modifying the effects of vasopressin on the kidney. The antidiuretic effect of vasopressin can also be inhibited by barbiturates, lithium, tetracyclines, and several other drugs (Table 9-2), as well as by hypokalemia and hypercalcemia.

As its name implies, vasopressin can also raise blood pressure by constricting vascular smooth muscle.[169] The pressor and antidiuretic effects of vasopressin are mediated by different parts of the molecule, since the two effects can be selectively altered by modifying the structure of the hormone[12,13] or treating with specific V_1 (vascular) or V_2 (antidiuretic) antagonists.[14] In dogs and some other quadrupeds, the pressor effect of vasopressin begins at plasma concentrations of around 50 pg/ml,[171] i.e., about 10 times that required to produce maximum antidiuresis. However, healthy humans appear to be more refractory to the pressor effects of vasopressin[172,173] and at high concentrations of the hormone may actually have a depressor response, at least in some vascular beds.[174] Thus, although vasopressin may play a role in the physiology or pathophysiology of baroregulation in some animals,[175,176] most of the evidence indicates that it is relatively unimportant in humans. Patients with severe diabetes insipidus do not have appreciable defects in baroregulation, and neither the secretion nor the pressor action of vasopressin is increased in essential hypertension.[70,172,177,178] However, some patients with postural hypotension due to autonomic dysfunction appear to be supersensitive to the pressor effects of vasopressin,[179] and in some of them, failure to secrete the hormone normally in response to hypotension[81] may contribute to the baroregulatory defects.

Vasopressin, administered alone or in combination with CRF, also stimulates the release of ACTH.[180,181] This effect requires concentrations of the hormone 100 to 1000 times the normal peripheral level and is mediated at least in part by a distinct class of V_1 receptors on ACTH-producing cells of the anterior pituitary.[182,183] Since the portal veins contain vasopressin in concentrations well within those required to stimulate adrenocorticotrophic cells,[19] the hormone released here by a parvicellular projection from the paraventricular nucleus probably plays a role in regulating pituitary adrenal function. This role has not been defined. It does not appear to be important for the pituitary-adrenal response to stress[184,185] and may be limited to potentiating the effects of certain other stimuli, such as hypovolemia[186] and glucocorticoid deficiency.[19]

At physiologic concentrations, vasopressin also inhibits water loss from skin, lungs, and other extrarenal sites.[187,188] Other actions of vasopressin include inhibition of pancreatic flow,[189] stimulation of hepatic glycogenolysis,[190] and aggregation of platelets,[191] but the role of these effects in human physiology and pathology is unknown.

The major biological action of oxytocin is to facilitate nursing by stimulating the contraction of myoepithelial cells in the lactating mammary gland.[192] The blood levels required to produce milk ejection are unknown but probably are comparable to those achieved by mammary stimulation.[152] It is unclear, however, whether oxytocin is necessary for nursing.[192] Oxytocin may also aid in parturition by stimulating contraction of the uterus.[192] This effect apparently is dependent not on increased oxytocin secretion (which occurs late, if at all, during labor) but on increased myometrial sensitivity to the hormone. When oxytocin is infused to treat hypocontractile labor, the plasma oxytocin concentration at which adequate uterine contractility occurs varies markedly from one patient to the next but usually lies within the range 1 to 5 μU/ml (2.5 to 12.5 pM).[193] As with nursing, however, it is still unclear whether the hormone is necessary for labor and delivery.[192] It is also unknown whether oxytocin has any significant effect in males. In humans[194] as well as rats[195] with neurohypophyseal diabetes insipidus, oxytocin can cause concentration of the urine, but the blood levels required to produce this antidiuretic effect are 10 to 100 times the normal basal level.

The neurophysins have no recognized biological action apart from complexing oxytocin and vasopressin in neurosecretory granules of the neurohypophysis. Although present in plasma, they do not serve as binding or transport proteins, because the high pH and low concentration of the reactants favor complete dissociation.[16]

Thirst

In terrestrial animals, the thirst mechanism provides an indispensable adjunct to the antidiuretic control of water balance.[196,197] When used in a physiologic sense, *thirst* is defined as a conscious inner desire to drink and must be distinguished from nondipsetic determinants of water intake such as social custom and the circumstance of eating. As might be expected, thirst is stimulated by many of the same variables that cause vasopressin release.[196–199] Of these, hypertonicity appears to be the most potent. In healthy adults, a rise in effective plasma osmolality of only 2 to 3 percent above basal levels produces a strong desire to drink. This response is not dependent on changes in extracellular volume, since it occurs when plasma osmolality is raised by the infusion of hypertonic saline as well as by water deprivation. The absolute level of plasma osmolality at which a desire for water is first perceived may be termed the *osmotic threshold* for thirst. It varies appreciably from one person to the next, but among healthy adults it averages about 295 mosmol/kg. This level is well above the osmotic threshold for vasopressin release and closely approximates that at which maximum concentration of the urine is normally achieved (Fig. 9-4). The sensitivities of the thirst and vasopressin osmoreceptors cannot be compared precisely but probably are equivalent. Thus, in healthy adults, intensity of thirst increases rapidly in direct proportion to plasma sodium or osmolality and generally becomes almost intolerable at levels only 3 to 5 percent above the threshold level. Water consumption also appears to be proportional to the intensity of the thirst and under conditions of maximum osmotic stimulation may reach rates approximating 20 to 25 L/day. This response is so effective that it can present the development of dehydration even under conditions of maximal renal and extrarenal water loss. Thirst can also be osmotically inhibited by a sensation that is best described as "satiety."[199] This mechanism is normally so effective that it can prevent overhydration even when the capacity of the kidneys to excrete water is maximally inhibited by the administration of high doses of antidiuretic hormone.[200] Thus, in patients on ad libitum water intake, the development of hyper- or hyponatremia almost always signals the existence of an underlying abnormality in the osmoregulation of thirst.

The neuronal pathways that mediate the osmoregulation of thirst have not been totally defined but appear to involve osmoreceptors located in the anterior hypothalamus, near but not totally coincident with those which regulate vasopressin secretion.[201,202] The solute specificities of the two osmoreceptors also appear to be similar since plasma solutes such as urea and glucose, which have little or no effect on vasopressin secretion, are equally ineffective as dipsogens.[51,52]

Hypovolemia and/or hypotension are also dipsogenic.[196–199] The degree of hypovolemia and/or hypotension required to produce thirst has not been defined for humans but appears to be greater even than that needed to effect vasopressin release. Thus, upright posture often induces a small but significant rise in plasma vasopressin but does not produce thirst. Hypovolemia may be a more potent dipsogen in rats, but even in that species reductions of less than 15 percent have little or no effect on water intake. The pathways by which hypovolemia and/or hypotension produce thirst are uncertain, but they are different from those which mediate osmotic dipsogenesis[203] and probably are close to if not identical with those which mediate the baroregulation of vasopressin. Hemodynamic stimuli also reset the osmotic threshold for thirst as they do for vasopressin.[204] The effects of hypovolemia on thirst and vasopressin may also be mediated partially via the renin-angiotensin system. The latter is a potent dipsogen in rats[205,206] but has not been shown to affect thirst in humans.

Thirst may also be affected by changes in plasma or CSF vasopressin and a variety of other hormones.[205,206] Since osmotic and hemodynamic stimuli cause release of vasopressin into CSF as well as plasma (see above), the dipsogenic effect of dehydration may be mediated in part by increases in endogenous vasopressin secretion. However, the hormone probably does not play an essential or even a major role in the regulation of thirst, since dipsogenesis is normal in Brattleboro rats which lack the capacity to make vasopressin. The mechanism and site at which the various osmotic, hemodynamic, and hormonal influences are integrated to regulate thirst have not been defined.[207]

Maintenance of Salt and Water Balance

Water is by far the largest constituent of the human body.[208] In lean, healthy adults, it makes up 55 to 65 percent of body weight, and it accounts for an even larger proportion in infants and young children. About two-thirds of body water is intracellular (Fig. 9-10). The rest is extracellular and is divided further into the intravascular (plasma) and extravascular (interstitial) compartments. Plasma is much the smaller of the two, accounting for only about one-fourth of total extracellular volume. The solute compositions of intracellular and extracellular fluid differ markedly, because most cell membranes possess an array of transport systems that actively accumulate or expel specific solutes.[209] Thus, sodium and chloride are confined largely to extracellular fluid, whereas potassium, magnesium, and various organic acids or phosphates are predominantly intracellular. Glucose, which requires an insulin-activated transport system to enter most somatic cells and is rapidly converted in those cells to glycogen or other metabolites, is present in significant amounts only in extracellular fluid. Bicarbonate is present in both compartments but is about three times more concentrated in extracellular fluid. Urea is unique among the major naturally occurring solutes in that it diffuses freely across most cell membranes and is therefore present in similar concentrations in virtually all body fluids.

Despite marked differences in the concentration

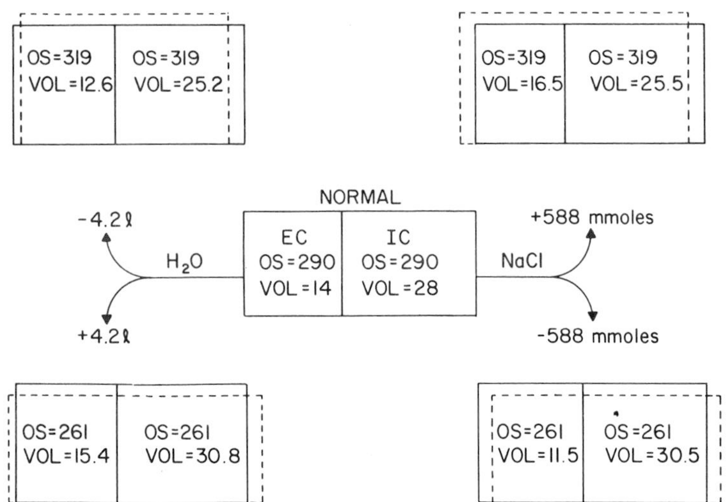

FIGURE 9-10 The osmolality and volume of intracellular and extracellular fluid under different conditions of salt and water balance. The vertical and horizontal dimensions of each box represent, respectively, the osmolality (OS) in milliosmols per kilogram and volume (VOL) in liters of the intracellular (IC) and extracellular (EC) compartments. The box in the center depicts the values in a typical 70-kg human. The values depicted with dotted lines to the left and right represent the changes that occur when total body water or sodium is altered by the amounts specified. Note that a 10 percent decrease in total body water and a 30 percent increase in total exchangeable sodium increase osmolality and decrease intracellular volume by about the same amount (10 percent) but have opposite and unequal effects on extracellular volume. The same is true for an increase in body water or a decrease in sodium, except that all the changes in osmolality and volume are reversed. (*From Robertson and Berl.*[209])

of particular solutes in extracellular and intracellular fluid, the total solute concentration is almost everywhere the same (Fig. 9-10). This osmotic equilibrium is due to the fact that most of the membranes that separate the various compartments are freely permeable to water.[210,211] Consequently, if the total solute concentration of one compartment becomes higher than that of the others, the difference in osmotic pressure induces a rapid influx of water from the neighboring compartments until equilibrium is restored. The osmolality determined by measurement of freezing point or vapor pressure of a fluid[212] must be distinguished from biologically effective osmolality. The former is a physicochemical property and is a function of all the solutes present, regardless of their ability to penetrate biological membranes. The effective osmolality of body fluid is a biological property and is a function only of those solutes which can generate osmotic pressure—i.e., a concentration gradient for water—across the membranes of living cells. Thus, solutes, such as sodium and chloride, which are actively excluded from the intracellular compartment are osmotically effective. In contrast, urea is osmotically ineffective because it diffuses rapidly across most cell membranes. Normally, the difference between the effective osmolality of body fluids and that determined by freezing point or vapor pressure osmometry is too small to be important, because most of the solute of plasma and extracellular fluid is composed of osmotically effective solutes such as sodium and its anions. However, in certain situations, such as chronic renal failure, effective osmolality may be considerably less than that determined by conventional osmometry because the concentration of ineffective solutes such as urea is much higher than normal.

Because most cell membranes are freely permeable to water, any changes in the effective osmolality of one compartment also changes its volume as well as the volume and osmolality of the other compartments (Fig. 9-10).[213] For example, a rise in extracellular osmolality induced by dehydration causes water to flow from the intracellular to the extracellular compartment. As a result, the water deficit distributes evenly throughout the body, causing a proportionally equal decrease in volume and increase in osmolality in each of the compartments. Conversely, a fall in extracellular osmolality induced by overhydration causes water to flow in the opposite direction, redistributing the excess to all compartments. However, if osmolality is changed by a gain or loss of solute, intracellular and extracellular volume change in opposite directions (Fig. 9-10). In each of these acute situations, the cells as a whole behave essentially like perfect osmometers; that is, the observed changes in the volume and osmolality of extracellular fluid conform closely to theoretical expectations. However, deviations from this kind of ideal behavior may occur when the disturbance in salt and water balance is particularly severe and/or prolonged. Under these conditions, many cells appear to be able to counteract osmotically induced changes in volume by reversibly activating or deactivating intracellular solute.[214] In addition, these acute disturbances in the osmolality and volume of body fluids bring into play a variety of other homeostatic mechanisms which, by altering total body content of salt and/or water, gradually restore the balance to normal (see below).

Both body water and solutes are in a state of continuous exchange with the environment. Ordinarily, the intake of water and solute is determined not only by fluid and electrolyte requirements but also by cultural influences and/or nutritional needs. In contrast, the excretion of water and solute is geared quite closely to the physiologic control of fluid and electrolyte balance. Normally, most water is excreted via the kidneys and is under the control of

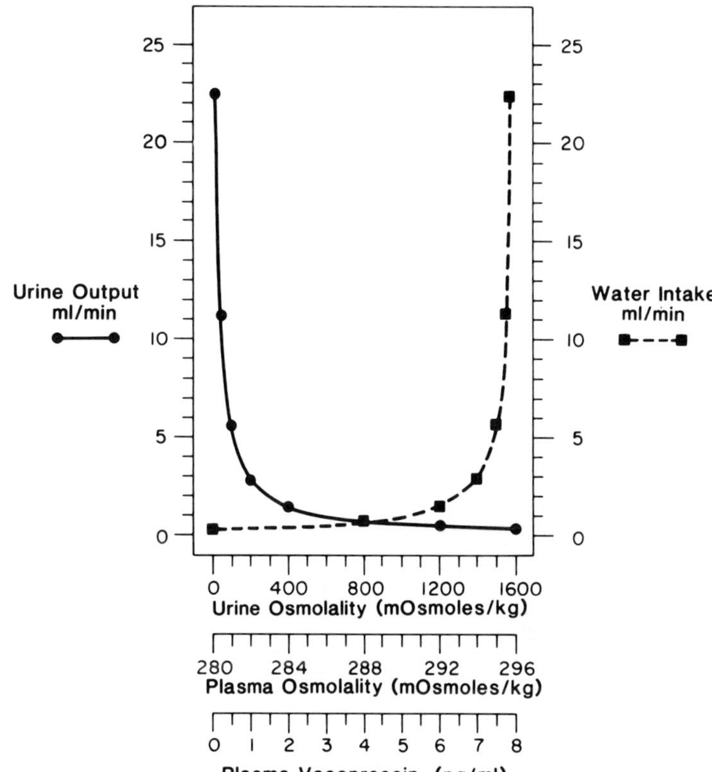

FIGURE 9-11 The relation of renal excretion or oral intake of water to urine osmolality, plasma osmolality, and plasma vasopressin in a typical 70-kg human. The line describing urine flow was calculated assuming a solute load of 800 mosmol/day. The line describing water intake was obtained by analyzing the relation of water intake to plasma osmolality in 12 healthy adults after infusion of hypertonic saline. The contributions of insensible loss and dietary water to total output and intake usually approximate 1.4 L/day (1 ml/min). Neither is included in these calculations. (*From Robertson and Berl.*[209] *Water intake–plasma osmolality data courtesy of R. L. Zerbe and G. L. Robertson.*)

antidiuretic hormone. However, the rate of urine output is also influenced significantly by the rate of solute excretion and cannot be reduced below a certain minimum or obligatory level required to carry the solute load. The volume required for this purpose depends on the level of antidiuresis and the size of the load (Fig. 9-11). The amount of water lost by evaporation from skin and lungs also varies markedly, depending on several factors, including dress, humidity, temperature, and exercise,[215] as well as antidiuretic activity.[187,188] Under the conditions typical of modern urban life, insensible water loss in a healthy 70-kg man or woman approximates 1 L/day (14 ml/kg). However, if antidiuretic hormone is absent or environmental temperature or activity increases, the rate of insensible water loss increases significantly and under extreme conditions may approximate the maximum rate of free water excretion by the kidney (Fig. 9-12). Thus, in quantitative terms, insensible loss and the factors that influence it are just as important to the economy of water balance as are the factors that regulate urine output.

In healthy adults, plasma osmolality and its principal determinant, plasma sodium concentration, are maintained within a remarkably narrow range. This stability is achieved largely by adjusting total body water to keep it in balance with sodium. The most important element in this homeostatic process is the threshold or set point of the osmoreceptors, which regulates thirst and vasopressin secretion. Through their ability to effect large increases in the

FIGURE 9-12 The effect of activity and temperature on insensible water loss in a typical 70-kg human. The solid lines indicate insensible loss for different activities in healthy adults. (*Redrawn from Adolph.*[215]) The broken line indicates insensible loss during minimal activity in a typical patient with neurogenic diabetes insipidus. (*Courtesy of G. L. Robertson.*)

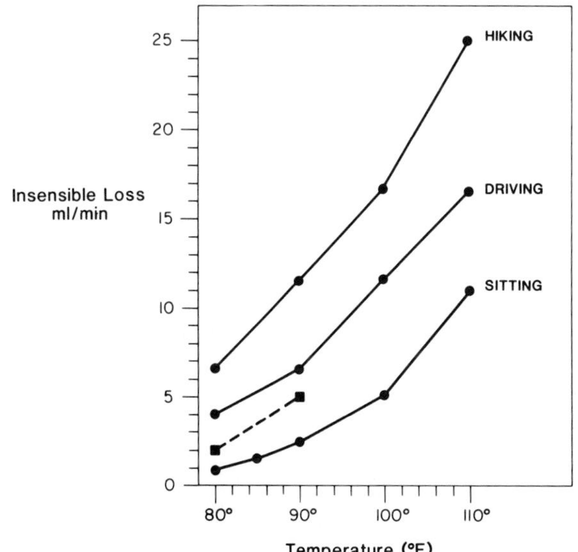

rate of water intake or excretion, these two control functions provide almost insurmountable barriers to extreme over- or underhydration. The capacity of this osmoregulatory system to cope with disturbances in water balance is enormous. Because of the inverse exponential relation between urinary osmolality and flow (Fig. 9-11), the suppression of plasma vasopressin to levels that permit maximum urinary dilution normally increases the rate of water excretion to more than 10 ml/min. Since outputs of this magnitude equal or surpass all but the most pathologically excessive rates of water intake, maximum suppression of vasopressin secretion normally provides an almost insurmountable barrier against water intoxication. Consequently, the osmotic threshold for vasopressin secretion effectively determines the lower limit for the osmotic pressure of body fluids. The upper limit is established by the osmotic threshold for thirst. Provided that access to fresh water is unrestricted, a rise in plasma osmolality above the threshold for thirst will increase the rate of water intake to levels sufficient to offset all but the most extraordinary rates of loss. To appreciate the effectiveness of this defense mechanism, it is necessary only to recall that many patients with severe neurogenic or nephrogenic diabetes insipidus excrete as much as 16 L of urine per day for years yet maintain their plasma osmolality at or only slightly above the upper limit of normal. Between the limits imposed by the osmotic threshold for thirst and vasopressin release, plasma osmolality may be regulated more precisely still by small osmoreceptor-mediated adjustments in urine concentration and flow. The exact level at which stabilization occurs depends on individual differences in the rate of water loss from skin and lungs relative to the rate of gain from eating, nondipsetic drinking, and the metabolism of fat. On the average, however, overall intake and output come into balance at a plasma osmolality around 288 mosmol/kg, or about halfway between the thresholds for thirst and vasopressin release. From this position, minor deviations in free water balance can be promptly counteracted by appropriate adjustments in vasopressin secretion and urine flow.

In humans and possibly other mammals, the operation of this osmoregulatory system is complicated somewhat by the superimposition of intermittent hemodynamic stimuli generated by standing and other activity. As was noted previously, however, these influences do not interfere significantly with the control of vasopressin secretion by the osmoreceptor. Instead, they merely shift the set of the mechanism a few percent to the left or right, depending on whether blood pressure and/or effective blood volume are rising or falling. This constant resetting has the effect of widening slightly the allowable fluctuations in plasma osmolality but does not jeopardize the essential homeostatic function of the osmoregulatory system. It should be noted that the effects of vasopressin and thirst on the regulation of blood volume and pressure are normally trivial and occur largely as an indirect consequence of efforts to preserve osmolality. Indeed, in situations characterized by an abnormal increase in total body sodium, thirst and vasopressin act in a way that aggravates instead of ameliorates the underlying hypervolemia. The responsibility for coping with disturbances in volume per se rests primarily with those elements of the renal and endocrine systems which regulate sodium excretion. This distinction is useful to bear in mind when one is considering the role of the hypothalamic-neurohypophyseal system in the pathogenesis of clinical disorders of salt and water balance.

PATHOLOGY

Decreased Secretion

Etiology

Diabetes Insipidus

Deficient secretion of vasopressin may result in a syndrome variously referred to as neurogenic, neurohypophyseal, hypothalamic, central, or vasopressin-responsive diabetes insipidus. It is almost always due to destruction of neurosecretory neurons by any of a variety of pathologic processes (Table 9-3).[216] Probably the best-studied cause is hypophysectomy, or section of the pituitary stalk.[217–219] Autopsy studies after such procedures have revealed not only extensive destruction of the pars nervosa but also a loss of the large neurosecretory cells in the supraoptic and, to a lesser extent, paraventricular nuclei of the hypothalamus.[217] This hypocellularity requires 4 to 6 weeks to develop fully and presumably results from retrograde degeneration of axonal processes sectioned during the surgery. Because these axons normally terminate at all levels along the neurohypophyseal tract (Fig. 9-1), the extent of the degeneration depends on how high the damage extends. To destroy more than 80 percent of the supraoptic nucleus, the minimum required to produce significant polyuria, the stalk must be sectioned at the level of the infundibulum or above. This fact probably explains why tumors and other pathologic conditions confined to the sella turcica rarely result in clinically apparent diabetes insipidus.

In addition to surgical interruption of the pituitary stalk, neurogenic diabetes insipidus also results commonly from head trauma,[220,221] a variety of primary, metastatic, or hematologic neoplasms,[222,223] generalized granulomatous diseases that also can involve the brain[224–226] (Table 9-3). Except for head trauma, most of these diseases are readily identified by a standard history and physical and radiologic examinations, including magnetic resonance imaging of the pituitary hypothalamic area. Infectious and vascular etiologies are distinctly less common except for Sheehan's syndrome.[227]

TABLE 9-3 Causes of Diabetes Insipidus

- Vasopressin deficiency (neurogenic diabetes insipidus)
  - Acquired
    - Trauma (accidental, surgical)
    - Neoplasm
      - Primary (craniopharyngioma, dysgerminoma, meningioma, adenoma)
      - Metastatic (lung, breast)
      - Hematologic (lymphoma, granulocytic leukemia)
    - Granuloma (sarcoid, histiocytosis, xanthoma disseminatum)
    - Infectious (meningitis, encephalitis)
    - Vascular (Sheehan's syndrome, aneurysm, aortocoronary bypass)
    - Idiopathic
  - Familial (autosomal dominant)
- Excessive water intake (primary polydipsia)
  - Acquired
    - Dipsogenic (downward resetting of the thirst osmostat)
    - Psychogenic
  - Familial (?)
- Vasopressin insensitivity (nephrogenic diabetes insipidus)
  - Acquired
    - Infectious (pyelonephritis)
    - Postobstructive (prostatic, ureteral)
    - Vascular (sickle cell disease, trait)
    - Infiltrative (amyloid)
    - Cystic (polycystic disease)
    - Metabolic (hypokalemia, hypercalcemia)
    - Granuloma (sarcoid)
    - Toxic (lithium, demeclocycline, methoxyflurane)
    - Solute overload (glucosuria, postobstructive)
  - Familial (X-linked recessive)

In many patients, the deficiency of vasopressin is idiopathic. The few neuropathologic studies performed on these patients also have revealed atrophy of the pars nervosa in association with a marked deficiency of neurosecretory cells in the supraoptic nuclei.[228–230] Not infrequently, idiopathic diabetes insipidus occurs on a familial basis. The classical and more common form is inherited in an autosomal dominant mode with virtually complete penetrance.[231–243] The deficiency of vasopressin can be partial or severe,[235–239,243] does not develop until several months to several years after birth, and usually increases in severity throughout childhood and early adolescence.[243] It appears to be due to postnatal degeneration of the neurons which make vasopressin because autopsy studies in four patients with familial neurogenic diabetes insipidus (FNDI) showed gliosis and a marked deficiency of magnicellular neurosecretory neurons in the supraoptic and, to a lesser extent, paraventricular nuclei of the hypothalamus.[228–230] For unknown reasons, some adults with the disease eventually regain the capacity to concentrate urine, even though they continue to have a severe deficiency of vasopressin.[243] Oxytocin secretion has not been characterized in this disease, but it may be normal since it is produced by a different population of neurosecretory neurons.[21] The mutation responsible for FNDI maps to chromosome 20, very near the genes that code for oxytocin and vasopressin.[240] Consistent with this location, three different missense mutations in one allele of the vasopressin-neurophysin gene have been identified in the affected members of three apparently unrelated kindreds from Japan,[241] Holland,[242] and America.[243] These mutations occur in highly conserved parts of exon 2 or exon 1 that code, respectively, for the midportion of the neurophysin moiety or the carboxyterminal amino acid of the signal peptide in the vasopressin-neurophysin II-copeptin precursor (Fig. 9-13). The way in which these mutant alleles destroy the neurons that express them is unknown, but they probably direct the production of an abnormal prohormone that is cytotoxic as a result of inefficient or abnormal processing.[243]

There is another form of neurogenic diabetes insipidus that is associated with diabetes mellitus, optic atrophy, deafness, and other abnormalities.[244] It is sometimes referred to as DIDMOAD or Wolfram syndrome and may show a familial predisposition suggestive of autosomal recessive transmission. However, almost nothing is known about the pathogenesis or genetics of this disorder. An X-linked form of vasopressin-responsive diabetes insipidus also has been reported in humans,[245] but there is reason to suspect that those patients actually had a recently discovered form of partial nephrogenic diabetes insipidus.[246]

Brattleboro rats also have a form of hereditary

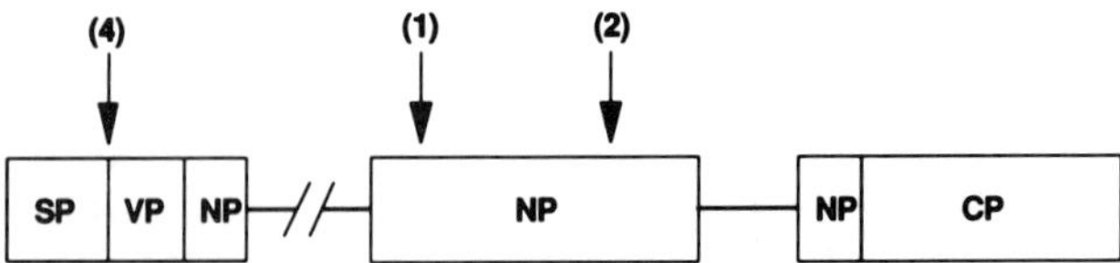

FIGURE 9-13 Map of missense mutations in the vasopressin gene associated with familial neurogenic diabetes insipidus in seven unrelated kindreds. The mutation found most frequently (four kindreds) is a G to A transition at base 55 in exon A which predicts the substitution of threonine for alanine at the −1 position of the signal peptide. In two other kindreds, the disease was associated with a substitution at nucleotide 1859 in exon B, but in one it was a G to A transition which predicted the replacement of glycine with serine at amino acid 57 in neurophysin; in the other, it was a G to C transition which predicted the substitution of arginine for glycine at the same position. In one kindred, the mutation was a G to T transition which predicted the replacement of glycine with valine at amino acid 17 in neurophysin. SP = signal peptide; VP = vasopressin; NP = neurophysin; CP = copeptin coding regions of gene.

diabetes insipidus which follows an autosomal, semirecessive mode of inheritance.[18] However, the defect in these animals is different, because it is present from birth and is due to a genetic failure in biosynthesis of vasopressin rather than a loss of neurosecretory neurons.

Osmoreceptor Ablation

Deficient secretion of vasopressin can also result from a lesion which selectively destroys the osmoreceptors without involving either the neurohypophysis or its other regulatory afferents.[247–249] This kind of lesion can be induced by a variety of hypothalamic disorders (Table 9-4), including tumors, granulomas, vascular occlusion, trauma, hydrocephalus, nonspecific inflammation, degenerative disorders, and developmental defects. In a few patients, no anatomic lesions have been identified. In all the patients studied to date, the deficient vasopressin response to osmotic stimulation has been associated with a deficiency in the osmoregulation of thirst, presumably because the osmoreceptors involved in the two functions are in overlapping areas of the anterior hypothalamus. Rarely, however, hypodipsia can occur without any deficiency in vasopressin secretion.[250] Autopsy studies delineating the precise location and histologic appearance of these lesions have not been reported. However, experiments in animals have shown that similar defects in vasopressin secretion can be produced by a lesion in an area of the anterolateral hypothalamus near the supraoptic nuclei.[33,34,201]

TABLE 9-4 Causes of Osmoreceptor Destruction

Tumors
- Craniopharyngioma
- Pinealoma
- Meningioma
- Metastatic

Granuloma
- Histiocytosis
- Sarcoidosis

Vascular
- Occlusion of anterior communicating artery

Tramua
- Penetrating
- Closed

Other
- Hydrocephalus
- Developmental
- Cysts
- Inflammation
- Degenerative

Idiopathic

Primary Polydipsia

Reduced secretion of vasopressin can also result from excessive water intake. This condition, which is often referred to as *primary polydipsia*, can result from a primary defect in the osmoregulation of thirst, a syndrome that has been called dipsogenic diabetes insipidus,[251,252] or, more commonly, as part of a general cognitive defect associated with schizophrenia or other mental disorders, a syndrome referred to as psychogenic polydipsia.[253–257] In humans, little is known about the precise location or nature of the lesions responsible for either type of polydipsia. However, organic lesions may be directly responsible in some cases, since dipsogenic diabetes insipidus has been associated with tuberculous meningitis,[251] multiple sclerosis,[251] and neurosarcoid.[251,252] In addition, hyperdipsia can be produced experimentally in rats by making lesions in the midbrain,[258] septal nuclei,[259] and nucleus medianus.[260]

Nocturnal Enuresis

Absence of the normal nocturnal rise in plasma vasopressin is associated with a condition known as monosymptomatic nocturnal enuresis.[75] This defect is not associated with any detectable pathology in the brain or elsewhere and is of unknown etiology.

Impaired Action

Nephrogenic Diabetes Insipidus

Polyuria and polydipsia can also result from insensitivity to the antidiuretic actions of vasopressin. This syndrome, which is commonly referred to as *nephrogenic diabetes insipidus*, was first recognized as a familial disorder that is carried by females and is expressed most fully in their male offspring.[261] Consistent with this X-linked mode of inheritance, the disease cosegregates with markers from the distal long arm of the X chromosome.[262–264] In each of 13 apparently unrelated kindreds with familial nephrogenic diabetes insipidus, the disease was linked to a different marker, indicating that it was not passed on from a common progenitor but resulted from independent mutations.[264] Consistent with this finding, the disease has now been linked to eight different mutations in the gene that codes for the renal, V_2 receptor, with no two kindreds having the same mutation.[265a–c] Nephrogenic diabetes insipidus can also be caused by various drugs[266] or other diseases (Table 9-2).

Increased Metabolism

Gestational Diabetes Insipidus

A unique form of vasopressin-deficient diabetes insipidus can also develop during pregnancy as a result of overproduction of the placental hormone that rapidly degrades vasopressin.[267] In some cases at least, there is also an underlying, subclinical deficiency in vasopressin secretion[268] that may predispose to the syndrome by limiting the capacity to compensate for the increased rate of metabolism.

Pathophysiology

Decreased Secretion

Diabetes Insipidus

When sufficiently severe, destruction of vasopressin-producing neurons results in a decrease in urinary concentration and an increase in urine flow.[217] As a consequence of the dehydration, there is a rise in plasma osmolality which stimulates the thirst mechanism and induces polydipsia. The resultant increase in body water restores the balance between intake and output and stabilizes the tonicity of blood fluids at a new, slightly higher level which closely approximates the osmotic threshold for thirst.

It is important to note that the deficiency of vasopressin need not be complete for polyuria and polydipsia to occur.[217,268–277] *It is necessary only that the maximum plasma vasopressin concentration achievable at or below the osmotic threshold for thirst be inadequate to concentrate the urine.* The degree of neurohypophyseal destruction at which such failure occurs varies considerably from person to person, largely because of individual differences in the solute load or the set and the sensitivity of the osmoregulatory system.[36,272] However, an average value can be estimated from the known relation between urine flow, urine osmolality, plasma vasopressin, plasma osmolality, and thirst in a typical healthy adult (Fig. 9-11). At an average rate of solute excretion, urine flow does not rise to symptomatic levels (>2.5 L/day) until urine osmolality falls below 300 mosmol/kg. Thus, if renal sensitivity to vasopressin is normal, polyuria should not begin until the level of plasma vasopressin achievable at the osmotic threshold for thirst falls below 1.5 pg/ml, the amount required to maintain urinary concentration above 300 mosmol/kg (Fig. 9-4*B*). For this degree of deficiency to occur, secretory capacity must be reduced by at least 75 percent (Fig. 9-14). This estimate agrees relatively well with that obtained by neuroanatomic

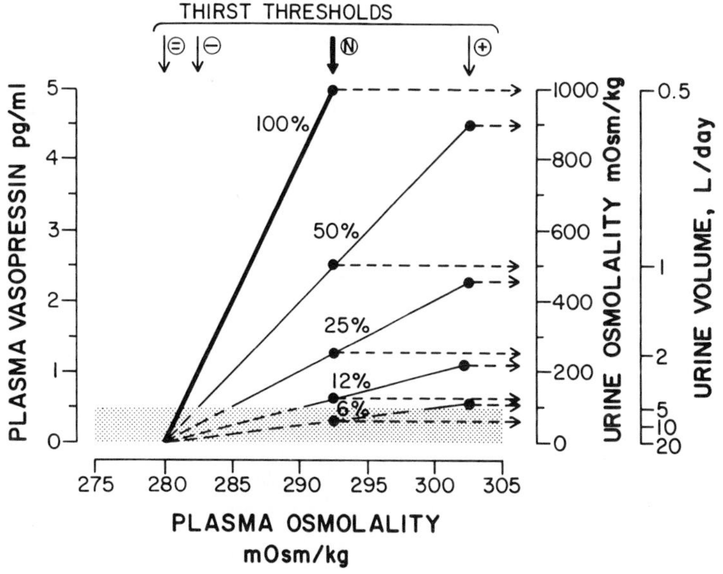

FIGURE 9-14 Plasma vasopressin and urine osmolality as a function of plasma osmolality in a typical healthy adult and in patients with various defects in thirst and/or hormone secretion. Each oblique line depicts schematically the relation between plasma vasopressin and plasma osmolality when secretory capacity is reduced to a specific percentage of normal. The vertical arrows indicate the osmotic threshold for thirst as it occurs in a typical healthy adult (N) and in patients in whom it is abnormally high (+), low (−), or very low (=). The solid circles on each oblique line indicate the highest level to which plasma osmolality and vasopressin are normally allowed to rise at each thirst setting. The broken horizontal arrows indicate the daily urine osmolalities that result when plasma vasopressin is limited to the specified levels. The shaded area indicates undetectable concentrations of plasma vasopressin. These figures assume a normal renal sensitivity to vasopressin. Note that the degree of impairment of vasopressin secretory capacity that results in urinary dilution depends on the "set" of the thirst mechanism. If the thirst threshold is normal, a significant water diuresis does not begin until secretory capacity falls to 15 to 25 percent of normal. However, if the thirst threshold is set 10 mosmol/kg higher, secretory capacity must be reduced to 12 percent of normal for the same concentrating defect to occur. Conversely, if the thirst threshold is set 10 mosmol/kg below normal, polyuria occurs even if vasopressin secretory capacity is normal. (*From Robertson and Berl.*[209])

studies of cell loss in the supraoptic nuclei after pituitary surgery[217] and is also consistent with functional tests of secretory capacity in a large series of patients with diabetes insipidus of variable severity, duration, and etiology.[271]

Recognition of the fact that almost all patients with neurogenic diabetes insipidus retain a limited capacity to secrete vasopressin is the key to understanding many otherwise perplexing features of the disorder. For example, in many patients, restricting water intake long enough to raise plasma osmolality by only 1 to 2 percent will induce the release of enough vasopressin to concentrate the urine (Figs. 9-15 and 9-16). This response illustrates the relative nature of the vasopressin deficiency and underscores the importance of the thirst mechanism in preventing the use of residual secretory capacity under basal conditions of ad libitum water intake. Even in patients who are unable to respond appreciably to hypertonicity, a more potent stimulus such as severe hypotension (Fig. 9-6) or nausea (Fig. 9-8) may evoke an increase in vasopressin secretion sufficient to concentrate the urine. Consequently, when interpreting diagnostic or therapeutic procedures in these patients, it is necessary to be circumspect about the presence of drugs or associated diseases that can modify vasopressin secretion via nonosmotic mechanisms.

FIGURE 9-15 The relation of plasma vasopressin to concurrent plasma osmolality in patients with polyuria of diverse etiology. All measurements were made at the end of a standard dehydration test.[270,271] The shaded area represents the range of normal. In patients with severe (◆) or partial (▲) neurogenic diabetes insipidus, plasma vasopressin was almost always subnormal relative to plasma osmolality. In contrast, the values from patients with dipsogenic (○) or nephrogenic (■) diabetes insipidus were consistently within the above-normal range. Normal subjects are represented by the plus (+) symbol. *(From Robertson.[277])*

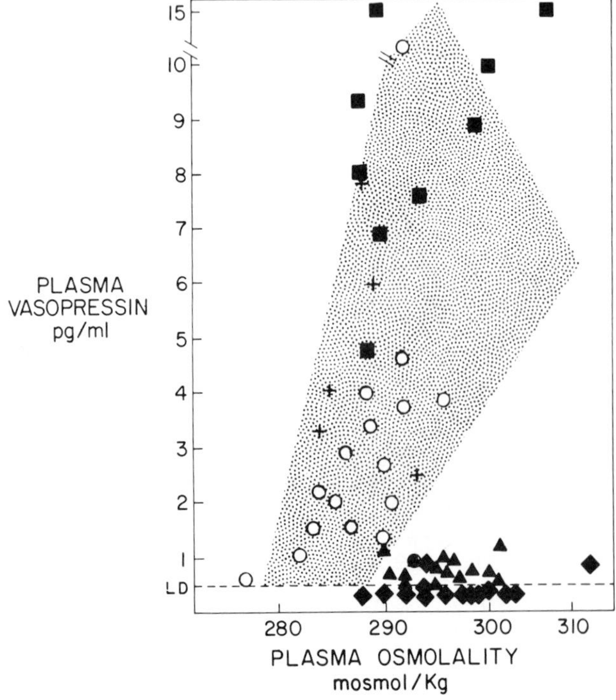

The development of diabetes insipidus in the period immediately after surgical or traumatic injury to the neurohypophysis can follow any of several different patterns.[218] In some patients, polyuria develops 1 to 4 days after injury and continues permanently. In others, the polyuria is transient and is followed in 4 to 7 days by a decline in urine volume to normal. In some of the latter patients, polyuria never recurs. In others, however, the interphase lasts only a few days and is followed by a second and permanent phase of polyuria. The functional and anatomic basis for the triphasic pattern of response is unknown. Presumably, however, the initial phase of polyuria reflects a kind of paralysis of vasopressin secretion secondary to neurohypophyseal damage. The interphase period during which urine output is normal may reflect degeneration and death of neurosecretory neurons, with release of stored vasopressin into the circulation. The final permanent phase of polyuria reflects degradation of released vasopressin and inability of the surviving neurons to produce adequate amounts of the hormone.

Neurogenic diabetes insipidus also is associated with changes in the renal response to vasopressin (Figs. 9-16 and 9-17). The most obvious change is a reduction in maximum concentrating capacity which is due to washout of the medullary concentration gradient caused by the chronic polyuria.[273–276] The severity of this defect is proportional to the magnitude of the polyuria and is independent of its cause.[271] Because of this defect, the levels of urinary concentration achieved at maximally effective levels of plasma vasopressin are reduced in all three types of diabetes insipidus (Fig. 9-17). In patients with neurogenic diabetes insipidus, this concentrating abnormality is offset to some extent by an increase in renal sensitivity to low levels of plasma vasopressin (Figs. 9-16 and 9-17). In this range, urine osmolality is usually supranormal for the amount of hormone present. The cause is unknown, but the supersensitivity may reflect upward regulation of vasopressin receptors secondary to a chronic deficiency of the hormone.

Osmoreceptor Dysfunction

The deficiency of vasopressin secretion that results from loss of osmoregulatory input usually produces a constellation of clinical abnormalities very different from that due to neurohypophyseal damage. Because the osmoreceptors for thirst and vasopressin secretion are located in overlapping if not identical areas of the hypothalamus (see above), destruction of one almost always results in equally serious damage to the other. Consequently, the pre-

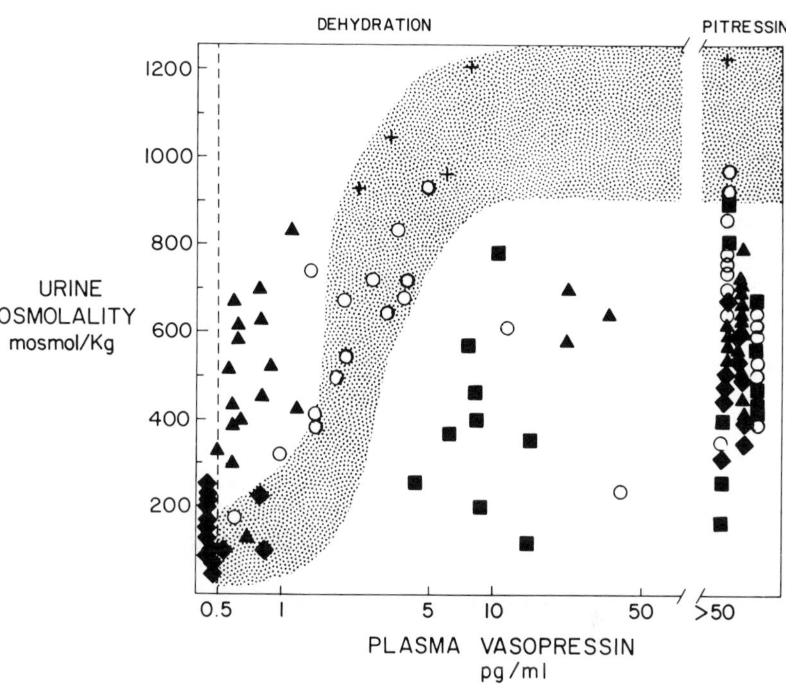

FIGURE 9-16 The relation of urine osmolality to concurrent plasma vasopressin in patients with polyuria of diverse etiology. All measurements were made at the end of a standard dehydration test.[270] The shaded area represents the range of normal. In patients with severe (◆) or partial (▲) neurogenic diabetes insipidus, urine osmolality is normal or supranormal relative to plasma vasopressin when the latter is submaximal. In patients with nephrogenic diabetes insipidus (■), urine osmolality is always subnormal relative to plasma vasopressin. In patients with dipsogenic diabetes insipidus (○), the relation is often normal, but urine osmolality may be subnormal when plasma vasopressin is supramaximal because of blunting of concentrating capacity. Normal subjects are represented by the plus (+) symbol. (*From Robertson.*[277])

dominant clinical manifestation of osmoreceptor destruction is chronic or recurrent hypernatremia in association with hypodipsia and a *relative* deficiency of vasopressin. Except under certain conditions, polyuria is *not* a prominent feature of the syndrome and usually is not a major or even a contributing cause of the recurrent episodes of severe hypertonic dehydration. The primary and, in many cases, the only cause is a failure of the thirst mechanism to maintain water intake at a level sufficient to replenish normal obligatory renal and extrarenal losses.[196,278] If sufficiently severe, the hypertonic dehydration may result in a variety of complications, including orthostatic hypotension, azotemia, hypokalemia, chorea, confusion, coma, convulsions, and paralysis, with or without rhabdomyolysis.[279–282]

Although polyuria is not a prominent feature of osmoreceptor ablation, defects in vasopressin secre-

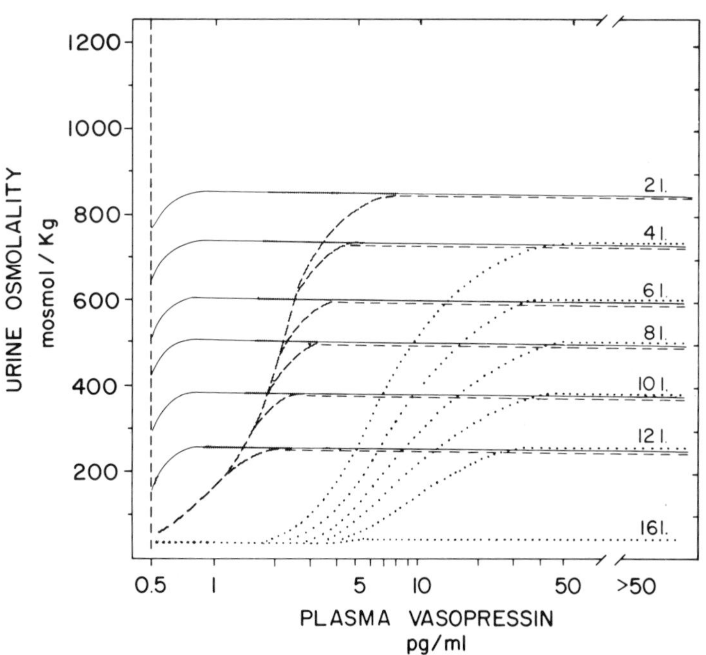

FIGURE 9-17 Schematic diagram of the relation between urine osmolality and plasma vasopressin in patients with diabetes insipidus of diverse etiology and severity. The shaded area represents the range of normal. The number at the common terminus of each family of lines indicates the magnitude of the basal polyuria. Note that for any given level of urine output, maximum concentrating capacity is reduced to the same extent in all three kinds of diabetes insipidus. However, at submaximal or physiologic levels of plasma vasopressin, urine osmolality is above normal in neurogenic (——), normal in dipsogenic (- - -), and subnormal in nephrogenic (· · · ·) diabetes insipidus. (*From Robertson.*[277])

tion are a frequent if not constant feature of the syndrome. In most cases, however, these defects are not recognized clinically until efforts are made to correct the hypernatremia by water loading. At that time, one of two abnormalities appears. Most often, patients begin to form dilute urine and develop frank polyuria before rehydration succeeds in restoring plasma osmolality to normal. Originally, this abnormality was attributed to upward resetting of the osmostat, an entity sometimes referred to as *essential hypernatremia*.[283] However, regression analysis of the relation between plasma osmolality and urine osmolality or plasma vasopressin has shown that this abnormality in antidiuretic function can result from a marked reduction in the slope or sensitivity of the system (Fig. 9-18).[32,247–249,278] Since none of the patients reported to have essential hypernatremia was studied by the kind of regression methods needed to distinguish true from apparent resetting of the osmostat, it is possible that all of them actually had a normal threshold with reduced sensitivity of the system.

In some patients with hypodipsic hypernatremia, forced hydration results in hyponatremia in association with an inability to dilute the urine maximally (Fig. 9-18).[32,247–249,278] This paradoxic defect resembles that seen in the syndrome of inappropriate antidiuresis and appears to result from two different mechanisms. One is a continuous or fixed secretion of vasopressin due to a total loss of osmoregulatory function (Fig. 9-18). In these patients, plasma vasopressin continues to circulate in small but biologically effective amounts irrespective of increases or decreases in hydration. In the other type of dilutional defect, urine osmolality remains high even when plasma vasopressin is suppressed to undetectable levels. The cause of this abnormality is unknown but may involve supersensitivity of the kidney to low levels of vasopressin.

In many, if not most, patients with adipsic hypernatremia the deficient or absent vasopressin response to changes in hydration is due to selective loss of osmoreceptor function. The neurohypophysis and its other regulatory afferents appear to be totally intact, since vasopressin responds normally or even supranormally to hemodynamic, emetic, and glucopenic stimuli.[247–251,278]

Primary Polydipsia

Excessive intake of water causes expansion and dilution of body fluids. The resultant fall in plasma osmolality suppresses vasopressin secretion, thereby inducing dilution of the urine. As a consequence, the rate of water excretion rises to balance intake and the osmolality of body water stabilizes at a new, slightly lower level approximating the osmotic threshold for vasopressin secretion. The magnitude of the polyuria and polydipsia varies considerably, depending on the nature and/or intensity of the stimulus to drink. In some patients, it is motivated by true thirst and appears to be due to an underlying abnormality in the osmoregulatory mechanism.[251] In such cases, the polyuria and polydipsia are usually moderate (4 to 10 L/day) and relatively constant from day to day. In most patients, however, the polydipsia is not attributed to thirst but appears to be due to a more general cognitive defect associated with psychosis or another serious mental disorder.[253–257] Typically, these patients explain their water intake by other motives, such as an effort to cleanse the body of poison, relieve anxiety, or prevent kidney disease. In these patients, the amount of water ingested tends to fluctuate widely from day to day and at times may be incredibly large. Rarely, it

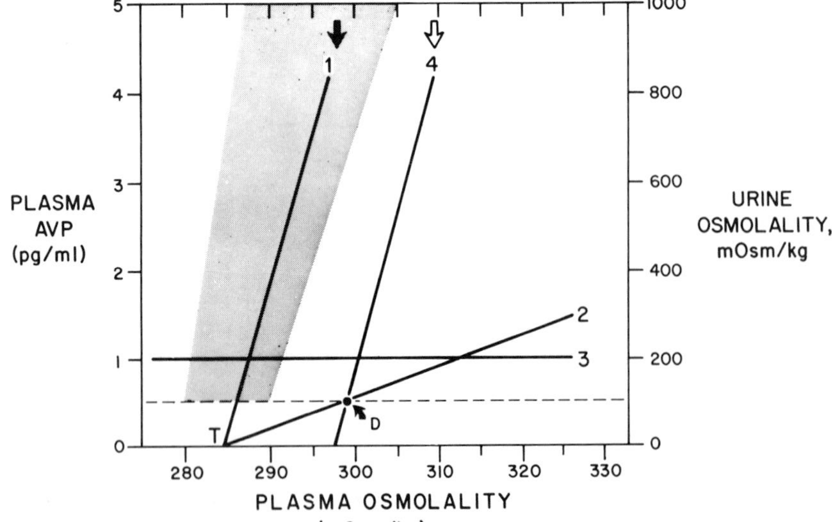

FIGURE 9-18 Schematic diagram of the relation of plasma osmolality to plasma vasopressin or urine osmolality in healthy adults and in patients with hypernatremia of diverse etiology. Line 1 represents a healthy adult. Lines 2 and 3 represent patients with partial and complete osmoreceptor destruction, respectively. Line 4 indicates the relation for a patient with the hypothetical entity of reset osmostat. The open and the solid arrows indicate the osmotic thirst threshold in the patient with resetting of the osmostat and in the healthy adult, respectively. The level of vasopressin at which urinary dilution occurs is indicated by D. Note that dilution of the urine at inappropriately high levels of plasma osmolality can result either from partial osmoreceptor destruction or resetting of the osmostat. (*From Robertson and Aycinena.*[278])

rises to such extraordinary levels that it exceeds the excretory capacity of the kidney.[284] More often, however, the development of water intoxication in psychogenic polydipsia is due to an associated abnormality in the osmoregulation of vasopressin secretion.[285–287] Inappropriate secretion of the hormone can take any of several forms,[32] but most often it is due to resetting of the osmostat.[285] Patients with this condition often present with hyponatremia and maximum urinary dilution, suggesting that their water intoxication was caused by excessive drinking alone. However, if tested serially during water restriction, they begin to concentrate their urine before plasma osmolality and/or sodium return to normal. Since this diagnostic approach was not used in most previous studies, many patients in whom hyponatremia was attributed to polydipsia per se probably had resetting of the osmostat as an unrecognized contributory factor.[288] Studies in rats suggest that this resetting could be a consequence of the polydipsia per se.[289] However, the chronic suppression of vasopressin secretion that occurs in primary polydipsia does not impair the hormonal response to a subsequent osmotic stimulus[251,257,289] even if the condition is associated with significant chronic or recurrent hypoosmolemia.

Nocturnal Enuresis

In patients with nocturnal enuresis, the failure of plasma vasopressin to rise normally during sleep results in a decrease in urine osmolality and an increase in urine output at night.[75] During the day, urinary concentration and flow are normal. Consequently, polyuria and polydipsia are absent but the patient has nocturia and/or enuresis, depending on the degree of control of the urinary bladder. For unknown reasons, a larger proportion of daily solute is also excreted at night, exacerbating the effect of the relative deficiency of vasopressin. Overall fluid and electrolyte balance appear to be normal.

Impaired Action

Nephrogenic Diabetes Insipidus

Renal insensitivity to the antidiuretic effect of vasopressin also results in the excretion of increased volumes of dilute urine. The resultant decrease in body water causes a rise in plasma osmolality, which, by stimulating the thirst mechanism, induces a compensatory increase in water intake. As a consequence, the osmolality of body fluid stabilizes at a new and higher level which approximates the osmotic threshold for thirst. As in patients with neurogenic diabetes insipidus, the magnitude of the polyuria and polydipsia varies greatly, depending on a number of factors, including individual differences in solute load. It is important to note that the renal insensitivity to vasopressin need not be complete for polyuria to occur.[246,277,290] It is necessary only that the defect be great enough to prevent concentration of the urine at plasma vasopressin levels achievable under ordinary conditions of ad libitum water intake, i.e., at plasma osmolalities near the osmotic threshold for thirst. Calculations analogous to those used for vasopressin deficiency indicate that this requirement will not be met until the renal sensitivity to vasopressin is reduced more than 10-fold. Studies of the relation between urine osmolality and plasma vasopressin in patients with familial and acquired forms of partial nephrogenic diabetes insipidus are consistent with these calculations.[246,277,290] When renal insensitivity to the hormone is incomplete, patients with nephrogenic diabetes insipidus are able to concentrate their urine when deprived of water or given large doses of vasopressin.[246,277,290] In all likelihood, the X-linked form of familial vasopressin-responsive diabetes insipidus described by Forssman was really an example of partial nephrogenic rather than neurogenic diabetes insipidus.[245]

Increased Metabolism

Gestational Diabetes Insipidus

The deficiency of vasopressin caused by increased metabolic clearance during pregnancy results in the same disturbances in water balance that occur in patients with the more conventional type of neurogenic diabetes insipidus. The only differences are that the polyuria and polydipsia of gestational diabetes insipidus respond differently to therapy (see below) and almost always remit spontaneously several weeks after delivery.[267,268]

Diagnosis

Neurogenic Diabetes Insipidus

The diagnosis of neurogenic diabetes insipidus requires that it be differentiated from other causes of polyuria and polydipsia (Table 9-5). Confusion with diabetes mellitus is not a problem, since routine urinalysis usually reveals the glucosuria which is responsible for the solute diuresis. Differentiation from dipsogenic or nephrogenic diabetes is also relatively easy when the disorders are severe and present in the classic way. More often than not, however, this distinction cannot be made by conventional indirect tests,[270] because many patients with neurogenic or nephrogenic diabetes insipidus have a partial defect in vasopressin secretion or action and as a consequence are able to concentrate their urine during a standard dehydration test.[246,269–271,277] To make matters worse, maximum concentrating capacity is reduced to variable degrees in all three forms of diabetes insipidus.[271–277] As a result, the absolute level of urine osmolality achieved during water deprivation or vasopressin treatment can be similarly subnormal in all three types of polyuria (Fig. 9-17). This diagnostic dilemma usually cannot

Table 9-5 Diagnostic Evaluation of Nonglucosuric Polyuria

1. Measure plasma osmolality and/or sodium concentration under conditions of ad libitum fluid intake.
   A. If they are above 295 mosmol/kg and 143 mEq/L, respectively, primary polydipsia is excluded and the work-up should proceed directly to a therapeutic trial of DDAVP (step 4) to distinguish between neurogenic and nephrogenic diabetes insipidus.
   B. If they are below 295 mosmol/kg and 143 mEq/L, the work-up should proceed to step 2.
2. Perform a dehydration test.
   A. If urinary concentration does not occur before plasma osmolality and sodium reach 295 mosmol/kg and 143 mEq/L, primary polydipsia is excluded and the work-up should proceed directly to step 4.
   B. If urinary concentration occurs during the dehydration test, measure plasma vasopressin and plasma osmolality and proceed to step 3.
3. Perform a hypertonic saline infusion and measure plasma vasopressin and osmolality (or sodium).
   A. If the plasma vasopressin value is subnormal relative to plasma osmolality and/or sodium, the diagnosis of neurogenic diabetes insipidus is established and therapy may be started.
   B. If the relation of plasma vasopressin to osmolality and/or sodium is normal, neurogenic diabetes insipidus is excluded. Differentiation between primary polydipsia and nephrogenic diabetes insipidus can be effected by examining the relation of urinary osmolality to plasma vasopressin during the dehydration test or by proceeding to step 4.
4. Perform a therapeutic trial of DDAVP
   A. If the polyuria and polydipsia are eliminated and hyponatremia does not develop, the diagnosis of neurogenic diabetes insipidus is established and antidiuretic treatment can be continued in the standard manner.
   B. If urinary output decreases and osmolality increases but polydipsia persists and/or dilutional hyponatremia and hypoosmolality develop, the diagnosis of primary polydipsia is likely and therapy should be discontinued until additional studies of vasopressin secretion and action can be performed.
   C. If urinary volume and osmolality do not change, the diagnosis of nephrogenic diabetes insipidus is established and appropriate therapy may be initiated.

be resolved by other criteria, such as measurements of basal plasma osmolality or sodium, because these values also overlap considerably in the various kinds of diabetes insipidus.[259,277]

To cope with this diagnostic problem, several auxiliary criteria have been proposed. One approach is to determine the ratio of urine to plasma osmolality at the end of a brief period of fluid restriction.[291] Because most patients with diabetes insipidus can concentrate only in the face of supranormal dehydration, the ratio tends to be higher in normal subjects or patients with primary polydipsia. In a significant number of patients, however, the ratio falls between 1.8 and 2.2, a borderline zone which does not permit a clear distinction. The other indirect approach is a variation on that originally proposed by Barlow and de Wardener, in which a comparison is made of the maximum urine osmolalities achieved after fluid restriction and vasopressin injection.[270] Although this test is sometimes helpful, it is tedious and cumbersome to perform and often gives ambiguous or erroneous results.[271–277]

A simpler and more definitive diagnostic approach is to measure plasma or urinary vasopressin after a suitable osmotic stimulus such as fluid restriction or hypertonic saline infusion.[271,277,292–294] For this method to be useful, the vasopressin values must be plotted as a function of the concurrent plasma osmolality (Fig. 9-15). With this approach, even patients with mild, partial defects in vasopressin secretion can be differentiated easily from those with other forms of diabetes insipidus. The diagnostic accuracy of this method also benefits from the fact that the functional properties of the osmoregulatory system do not seem to be appreciably depressed by chronic dehydration or overhydration.[251,257,289] Hence, the relation of plasma vasopressin to osmolality is usually within or slightly above normal limits in both dipsogenic and nephrogenic diabetes insipidus. In most cases, the latter two disorders can be distinguished by measuring urine osmolality at the end of the dehydration test and relating it to the concurrent plasma vasopressin concentration (Fig. 9-16). However, this distinction is sometimes problematic, because maximum concentrating capacity is often severely blunted in patients with dipsogenic diabetes insipidus.[271] In such cases, the correct diagnosis usually can be made by examining the relation at submaximal levels of plasma vasopressin (Fig. 9-17).[277,290] Under these conditions, patients with dipsogenic diabetes will almost always fall within the normal range, while those with nephrogenic diabetes insipidus will be clearly subnormal.

Occasionally, the measurement of vasopressin after fluid restriction does not provide a clear distinction between neurogenic and dipsogenic diabetes insipidus. This problem usually arises in patients who, because of excessive thirst and/or prompt antidiuretic response, fail to increase their plasma osmolality to 295 mosmol/kg, the lowest level at which a clear separation of normal and subnormal vasopressin values can be made. In this situation, it may be necessary to give a short intravenous infusion of hypertonic saline and obtain one or more additional measurements of plasma vasopressin. Patients with neurogenic diabetes insipidus may exhibit a further rise in plasma vasopressin, but it is always distinctly subnormal relative to the increment in plasma osmolality. In contrast, the slope of the response is normal in patients with dipsogenic or nephrogenic diabetes insipidus. Because of the solute diuresis, measurements of urine osmolality and/or vasopressin excretion during the infusion of hypertonic saline are unreliable indicators of changes in hormone secretion and are of no diagnostic value.

As might be expected, most patients with diabetes insipidus also exhibit a subnormal rise in vasopressin secretion after hemodynamic, emetic, and glucopenic stimuli.[293] For diagnostic purposes, however, these nonosmotic tests of neurohypophyseal function do not appear to provide any particular advantage over dehydration and/or hypertonic saline infusion. Part of the problem is that orthostatic, emetic, and glucopenic stimuli are difficult to control and/or quantitate and normally result in a highly variable vasopressin response. Drug-induced hypotension permits more precise definition of the stimulus-response relation, but the procedure is cumbersome and potentially hazardous to perform. A more fundamental disadvantage with all nonosmotic stimuli is the real possibility of false-positive as well as false-negative results. A few patients have been found who exhibit little or no rise in vasopressin after hypotension or emesis yet lack polyuria and have a normal response to osmotic stimuli.[81] Conversely, there are rare patients with polyuria who exhibit little or no rise in plasma vasopressin during the infusion of hypertonic saline but have a relatively normal response to hypotensive, emetic, and glucopenic stimuli.[293] The latter observations suggest that diabetes insipidus may result rarely from a lesion which selectively damages the osmoreceptor that controls vasopressin release.

It has been reported that neurogenic diabetes insipidus also can be diagnosed by demonstrating the absence of the posterior pituitary "bright spot" on T_1-weighted, midsagittal MRI images of the pituitary and hypothalamus.[295,296] However, the utility of this method in the differential diagnosis of diabetes insipidus is still unclear because it has not been validated against an established method and because the exact source of the signal in the vicinity of the neurohypophysis is still controversial. In addition, recent studies suggest that the bright spot is absent in a large proportion of healthy people[297,298] and is not reproducible on repeat studies in the same subjects.[298]

Osmoreceptor Dysfunction

Differentiating adipsic hypernatremia from other causes of vasopressin deficiency or hypernatremia is usually a simple clinical exercise (Table 9-6). In conscious adults, a lack of thirst when plasma osmolality and sodium concentration are greater than 310 mosmol/kg and 150 mEq/L, respectively, is almost always diagnostic of adipsic hypernatremia due to osmoreceptor dysfunction. In doubtful situations, thirst and plasma vasopressin can be monitored during dehydration or a standard infusion of hypertonic saline.[32,196]

Nocturnal Enuresis

Monosymptomatic nocturnal enuresis due to a nocturnal deficiency of vasopressin has to be differentiated from bladder abnormalities and other causes of the syndrome. This differentiation can be achieved most easily by aerodynamic tests and a measurement of the ratio of the day/night urine volume (7 a.m. to 11 p.m./11 p.m. to 7 a.m.). If the ratio is less than 2.0, a nocturnal deficiency of antidiuretic function is likely. Measurements of plasma vasopressin are not recommended because the nocturnal

TABLE 9-6 Differential Diagnosis of Hypernatremia

- I. Deficiency of body water
  - A. Inadequate intake
    - 1. Loss of thirst (adipsia)
      - a. Tumor (craniopharyngioma, pinealoma, germinoma, meningioma)
      - b. Granuloma (histiocytosis)
      - c. Vascular (ligation of anterior communicating artery or internal carotid artery)
      - d. Other (hydrocephalus, cysts, trauma)
    - 2. Physical limitation
      - a. Exogenous (desert, ocean)
      - b. Endogenous (coma, paresis)
  - B. Excessive loss
    - 1. Renal (neurogenic or nephrogenic diabetes insipidus)
    - 2. Extrarenal (lungs, perspiration)
- II. Excess of body sodium
  - A. Excessive intake (accidental substitution in infant formula)
  - B. Excessive retention (hyperaldosteronism)

values are normally variable and only slightly higher than the anytime mean. The diagnosis can be confirmed by a therapeutic trial of DDAVP or LVP (lypressin, Diapid) at bedtime (see below).

Therapy

Decreased Secretion

Neurogenic Diabetes Insipidus

Recovery of vasopressin secretion is extremely rare once the deficiency has been established for a week or two. After that time, any spontaneous improvement in the polyuria almost always indicates progression of the underlying disease to involve the pituitary-adrenal axis[299,300] or the thirst mechanism. Rarely, it may indicate the development of a malignant condition with ectopic production of vasopressin.[301] Although persistent polyuria and polydipsia do not pose a serious hazard for most patients, they are an annoying and embarrassing inconvenience and should be treated whenever possible. Fortunately, there are several safe, simple, and effective treatment methods.

For many years, the standard treatment for neurogenic diabetes insipidus was Pitressin tannate in oil, a partially purified extract of vasopressin prepared from animal pituitaries. Intramuscular injection of 5 to 10 USP units every 2 to 3 days produces satisfactory relief of the polyuria and polydipsia in most patients. Resistance due to the development of antibodies has been observed but is relatively rare.[302] A poor or erratic antidiuretic response is usually due to a failure to adequately emulsify the mixture by manually shaking and warming the vial immediately before use. Adverse reactions to the drug are uncommon and are usually allergic in nature. The major disadvantage of Pitressin therapy is the need for lifelong injections. Because its duration of action is only a few hours, aqueous Pitressin is not suitable for long-term treatment of diabetes insipidus, but it is useful for certain diagnostic tests.

Diapid (lypressin) is a preparation of synthetic lysine vasopressin which may be given by nasal spray. Since the antidiuretic effect of each spray lasts a maximum of only 4 to 6 h, it is generally used only as an adjunct to other forms of therapy.

A synthetic analogue of vasopressin, DDAVP (desmopressin) (Fig. 9-2), is now widely available for use in the United States.[303] Extensive experience indicates that it has many advantages in the treatment of diabetes insipidus. The modifications in positions 1 and 8 of the molecule double its antidiuretic therapy, eliminate its pressor actions, and increase significantly its resistance to metabolic degradation. Consequently, it has a much longer duration of action than does the native molecule and can be given either parenterally or by nasal insufflation. In most patients, administration of 10 to 25 μg intranasally twice a day or 1 to 2 μg parenterally once a day affords prompt and complete relief of polyuria and polydipsia. Secondary failures are uncommon and usually are due to poor absorption of the nasal preparation caused by rhinitis or sinusitis. A poor initial response to DDAVP, particularly the parenteral form, almost always indicates that the patient has nephrogenic rather than neurogenic diabetes insipidus. Resistance due to antibody production has not been observed. Toxic side effects of DDAVP are also uncommon. An occasional patient with severe or long-standing neurogenic diabetes insipidus may develop water intoxication when first started on DDAVP therapy. However, the effect is usually transient and will subside with continued treatment. Severe or sustained hyponatremia constitutes a reason to stop treatment and repeat diagnostic studies, since it usually indicates that the patient has dipsogenic diabetes insipidus or some associated defect in thirst regulation.

Largely by chance, several oral drugs have also been found to be efficacious in treating neurogenic diabetes insipidus. Chlorpropamide (Diabinese), a drug more commonly used to treat hyperglycemia, is the most potent. At conventional doses of 250 to 500 mg per day, it reduces polyuria by 25 to 75 percent in patients with neurogenic diabetes insipidus.[124,126–127,304,305] Contrary to long-held views,[303] this effect is independent of the severity of the disease.[124,277] It is associated with a proportionate rise in urine osmolality, correction of dehydration, and a reduction in drinking similar to that caused by small doses of vasopressin or DDAVP (Fig. 9-19). Chlorpropamide may also cause inappropriate antidiuresis in some patients with other diseases.[304–308] Like vasopressin, chlorpropamide has no effect in patients with nephrogenic diabetes insipidus,[303] a fact suggesting that the drug and the hormone act via a similar mechanism. Potentiation of the renal tubular effects of small subthreshold amounts of vasopressin is probably the major mechanism of action,[124,126,277,309–313] although one study suggests that chlorpropamide may also stimulate release of the hormone.[126] A prolonged deficiency of vasopressin may be necessary for the antidiuretic effect of chlorpropamide to manifest, because its onset of action is slower in patients recently treated with vasopressin, and its antidiuretic effects can be reversed acutely by simultaneous administration of the hormone.[314]

Clofibrate (Atromid-S), a drug more commonly used to treat hyperlipidemia, also reduces polyuria and polydipsia in patients with diabetes insipidus.[125,315] At a maximum dose of 1 g tid, its antidiuretic effect is usually less than that of chlorpropamide,[316] although in a few patients it is more effective. Its mechanism of action is also uncertain. Like chlorpropamide, it is ineffective in patients with nephrogenic diabetes insipidus, and it has little if any antidiuretic action in normal subjects or patients with primary polydipsia. However, it has been

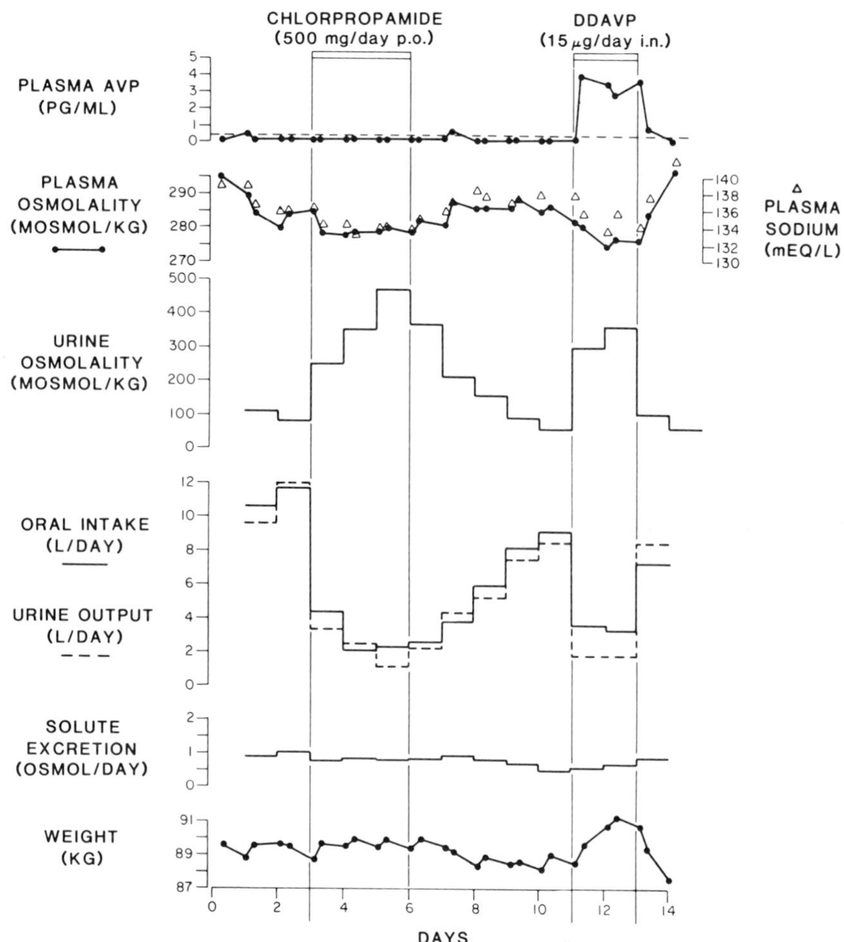

FIGURE 9-19 Effect of chlorpropamide and DDAVP on water metabolism in neurogenic diabetes insipidus. The patient was a 32-year-old woman with severe familial diabetes insipidus and no detectable vasopressin secretion even during stimulation with apomorphine. (*From Robertson.*[277])

difficult to show that clofibrate potentiates the renal actions of vasopressin, and there is evidence suggesting that the drug increases hormone secretion.[125]

Several other measures may be helpful in reducing polyuria in neurogenic diabetes insipidus. Restricting salt intake reduces urine output by reducing solute load. A similar effect may be achieved with thiazide diuretics, which deplete body sodium by inhibiting its reabsorption in the ascending limb of Henle's loop.[317] Because this step is necessary for maximum urinary dilution, the thiazides also raise urine osmolality and impair the ability to excrete a water load. Thus, if given to a patient with primary polydipsia, they may precipitate water intoxication.

The proper role of oral drugs in the management of diabetes insipidus is currently uncertain. Used alone or in combination with thiazide diuretics, they can reduce polyuria to asymptomatic levels in virtually all patients with the disorder. However, they also have some undesirable side effects, such as hypoglycemia[305] and myalgia,[318] and the long-term safety, particularly of chlorpropamide, is open to question. When Pitressin tannate in oil was the only real alternative, many patients preferred those disadvantages to the discomfort and inconvenience of frequent injections. However, the advent of the long-acting analogue DDAVP probably will relegate the oral agents to a secondary therapeutic role.

The management of patients with diabetes insipidus also requires a careful search for its cause. At a minimum, this search should include x-rays of the chest and skull, visual field examination, and computed tomography and/or magnetic resonance imaging of the pituitary-hypothalamic area. In some cases, a lumbar puncture may also be needed to establish the presence or absence of treatable disease such as germinoma. Because of the possible coinvolvement of hypothalamic release factors, anterior pituitary function also should be evaluated even if there is no other evidence of intrasellar disease.

The management of diabetes insipidus in comatose and/or postoperative patients poses special problems, because medication cannot be given orally or intranasally and water intake is not regulated by the thirst mechanism. In this situation, the easiest and most effective approach is to maintain a relatively fixed level of antidiuresis by means of parenteral administration of DDVAP (1 μg IM or IV once or twice daily) and concentrate on adjusting fluid intake to match renal and extrarenal losses. Urine output and gastrointestinal losses, if any, should be measured during each nursing shift, and the total volume plus approximately 500 ml (to cover insensible losses) should be replaced with half-normal saline or dextrose and water during the succeeding 8-h shift. In addition, the effectiveness of the regimen should be monitored by measuring plasma osmolality or sodium at least twice a day. A rise in either variable indicates dehydration and should be treated by administering supplemental fluid. The amount will depend on the level of hypertonicity or hypernatremia and can be estimated by the formulas

$$H_2O = \frac{P_{os} - 295}{295} \times 0.6\ \text{BW}$$

or

$$H_2O = \frac{P_{Na} - 145}{145} \times 0.6\ \text{BW}$$

where

P_{os} = plasma osmolality in milliosmol per kilogram
P_{Na} = plasma sodium in milliequivalents per liter
BW = body weight in kilograms
H_2O = total water in liters

An excessive decrease in plasma osmolality or sodium indicates overhydration. It should be treated by reducing fluid intake by an amount estimated with the same formulas. Attempting to regulate water balance by altering the dose of antidiuretic hormone is not recommended, because the resultant changes in urine flow are impossible to control precisely and often lead to large and rapid fluctuations in salt and water balance.

Osmoreceptor Dysfunction

The treatment of adipsic hypernatremia is largely a matter of patient education. A regular schedule of water intake adjusted according to changes in hydration as determined by changes in body weight[196] will usually suffice to maintain plasma osmolality and sodium within 5 percent of normal. This regimen is particularly important in patients with impaired urinary dilution, since these patients are prone to over- as well as underhydration. In patients in whom the development of polyuria interferes with the achievement or maintenance of normonatremia, the use of vasopressin or one of the oral agents to promote antidiuresis may be helpful. The latter drugs may also slightly increase drinking, although this effect is mild at best and cannot be relied on to replace other measures for maintaining water intake.

Dipsogenic Diabetes Insipidus

At present, there is no satisfactory treatment for dipsogenic diabetes insipidus. Administration of antidiuretic hormone or thiazides is hazardous because these agents diminish water excretion without reducing intake. The resultant water intoxication may develop rapidly and cause confusion, convulsions, coma, and even death. For this reason, any therapeutic trial in a patient in whom the cause of the polyuria is in doubt should always be conducted in the hospital with close monitoring of fluid balance. A few patients with dipsogenic diabetes insipidus due to resetting of the thirst osmostat can be managed effectively with antidiuretic therapy, because a fall in plasma osmolality inhibits thirst before significant water retention occurs.[277] In addition, the disruption of sleep that results from nocturia can almost always be eliminated by administering intranasal DDAVP or Diapid at bedtime. The dose must be carefully titrated to ensure that the antidiuretic effect does not persist into the following day, when drinking resumes and water intoxication can develop.

Nocturnal Enuresis

The enuresis associated with low plasma vasopressin and high urinary output at night also can be controlled completely by means of intranasal administration of DDAVP at bedtime.[75]

Impaired Action

Nephrogenic Diabetes Insipidus

Some patients with nephrogenic diabetes insipidus can be treated by eliminating the drug or disease responsible for the disorder. In many others, however, the only practical form of treatment is to restrict sodium intake and/or administer thiazide diuretics.[317] The latter will generally reduce polyuria by about 50 percent and improve dehydration in all forms of nephrogenic diabetes insipidus. Thiazides work by a vasopressin-independent mechanism that involves inhibition of sodium reabsorption in the diluting segment of the nephron followed by increased reabsorption of glomerular filtrate in the proximal tubule.[317] Some patients with partial nephrogenic diabetes insipidus can be treated successfully with high doses of DDAVP. However, the great expense of this approach currently makes it an impractical form of treatment.

Increased Metabolism

Gestational Diabetes Insipidus

The deficiency of vasopressin that is caused by increased metabolic clearance during pregnancy can be treated successfully with conventional or slightly increased doses of DDAVP.[267,268] Pitressin tannate in oil is usually ineffective because the vasopressinase degrades the native hormone much more readily than does the DDAVP analogue. Chlorpropamide and clofibrate are contraindicated because of possible teratogenic effects.

PATHOLOGIC HYPERFUNCTION

Increases in thirst and/or vasopressin secretion occur in many clinical conditions. Often they are an appropriate homeostatic response to some form of hyperosmolar dehydration. Not infrequently, however, they result from some other stimulus and are inappropriate for the osmolality of body fluids. These osmotically inappropriate increases in thirst and/or vasopressin secretion are customarily divided into three categories, based on the nature of the stimulus and the state of intravascular and extracellular fluid volume.[249] Category 1 includes patients in whom total and/or effective blood volume is reduced but interstitial volume is increased as evidenced by the presence of generalized edema. Category 2 includes patients in whom interstitial as well as total and/or effective blood volume or blood pressure is reduced. Category 3, which is often referred to as the *syndrome of inappropriate secretion of antidiuretic hormone* (SIADH), includes patients in whom blood and extracellular volume and blood pressure are normal or slightly increased. The major clinical manifestation of all three categories is hyponatremia with impaired water excretion. However, the etiology, pathophysiology, and treatment of the underlying disturbance in salt and water balance are quite different in each category.

Etiology and Pathophysiology

Hypervolemic Hyponatremia

Severe low-output congestive failure is a common cause of abnormal retention of water and sodium.[319] This retention is thought to be secondary to low cardiac output or effective hypovolemia, which acts via several incompletely defined mechanisms to stimulate proximal tubular reabsorption of filtered electrolytes and water. As a consequence, less filtrate is delivered to the distal tubular sites where free water is formed and the ability to excrete a water load is correspondingly diminished. In many cases, this deficiency is complicated by impaired urinary dilution, which is usually due to increased secretion of vasopressin.[319–322] Studies of osmotic stimulation and suppression indicate that this defect in vasopressin secretion is due to downward resetting of the osmostat,[320–322] probably as a consequence of the effective hypovolemia. If this is so, however, it probably is not mediated by the usual volume receptors, because left ventricular failure usually produces atrial distension, which suppresses vasopressin secretion.[319] For unknown reasons, some patients have impaired urinary dilution in the absence of detectable increases in vasopressin. In addition, thirst and/or water intake appear to be increased inappropriately in some patients. This combination of excessive intake and reduced excretion of water leads to the development of hyponatremia even though total body sodium is usually increased by more than 25 percent.

Patients with advanced cirrhosis and ascites also develop hyponatremia as a consequence of impaired water excretion.[319] The classic view suggests that the avid retention of salt and water characteristic of this disorder is also secondary to effective hypovolemia, although other explanations have been advanced.[319] In any event, osmotically inappropriate secretion of vasopressin also occurs in humans[319] as well as animals with advanced cirrhosis. Earlier indirect studies anticipated this finding and suggested that the increase in vasopressin secretion may also be due to downward resetting of the osmostat secondary to effective hypovolemia.[323]

The nephrotic syndrome is also associated with hyponatremia, impaired water excretion, and increased secretion of vasopressin.[319] These abnormalities may also be due to a reduction in total or effective blood volume, since they are often associated with elevations in plasma renin and can be corrected at least in part by maneuvers which expand central blood volume. However, in some patients total blood volume may be expanded, suggesting some other cause for the antidiuretic defects.

The clinical hallmark of all patients with the defect of hypervolemic hyponatremia is generalized edema. It may be associated with various signs of volume depletion, including tachycardia, orthostatic hypotension, azotemia, hypokalemia, hyperaldosteronism, hyperreninemia, and low urinary sodium. In addition, if sufficiently severe, the hyponatremia may cause lethargy, anorexia, nausea, headache, confusion, seizures, and even coma.

Hypovolemia Hyponatremia

Perhaps the most common form of hypovolemic hyponatremia is that due to abuse of thiazide diuretics. The thiazides act primarily by interfering with sodium reabsorption in the diluting segment of the nephron.[317] As a consequence, maximum urinary dilution is impaired and urine flow decreases because of compensatory increases in the reabsorption of salt and water in the proximal tubule. This impairment in water excretion does not result in hyponatremia unless water intake is abnormally increased.[324,325] The cause of the polydipsia in these patients has not been determined, but in some cases at least, it could be secondary to potassium depletion.[324,326] Bioassays indicate that plasma vasopressin is also increased in this syndrome,[324] but the cause is unclear because the degree of volume depletion is very small and potassium depletion inhibits rather than stimulates vasopressin secretion.[327] The more potent loop diuretics can also produce hyponatremia, apparently by producing enough hypovolemia to lower the osmotic thresholds for both thirst and vasopressin secretion.[85]

Adrenal insufficiency can also result in hyponatremia and impaired water excretion.[328] In primary adrenal insufficiency in which cortisol and aldosterone are both deficient, the defect in water excretion appears to be due to a variety of factors, including decreased glomerular filtration and solute excretion, increased vasopressin secretion, and possibly a vasopressin-independent form of urinary concentration.[328–337] Probably because of their aldosterone deficiency, these patients develop hyperkalemia, azotemia, and other signs of hypovolemia which are responsible in part for the abnormalities in vasopressin and/or water excretion.[324,328,331,335] Indeed, these same abnormalities occur in isolated mineralocorticoid deficiency.[335,336,338] As in other forms of hypovolemia, the increase in vasopressin secretion in the face of hypoosmolality is due to resetting of the osmostat,[278] and volume expansion alone is sufficient to correct the abnormalities in water metabolism.[336] Isolated deficiency of cortisol also causes hyponatremia and impaired water excretion,[339] but the mechanism of the defect is somewhat more complex and controversial.[328,330,332,333,335,339–345] While it is clear that plasma vasopressin is usually elevated in secondary (pituitary) or isolated glucocorticoid deficiency,[333,341–344] water excretion may also be impaired in the absence of detectable elevations in the hormone.[332,335] The cause of the increase in vasopressin secretion is also uncertain. It cannot be attributed to hypovolemia but may be due to reduced cardiac output[341,343] or a direct effect on the neurohypophysis.[333,346] The cause of the vasopressin-independent defect in water excretion is also unsettled and may be due to a change in renal hemodynamics or a direct effect of glucocorticoid deficiency that increases the hydroosmotic permeability of the collecting tubules. The role of the thirst mechanism in producing the increase in water intake necessary to produce hyponatremia is also unclear.[345] Whatever the precise mechanism of the fluid and electrolyte imbalance, however, it is important to remember that patients with isolated glucocorticoid deficiency do not have hyperkalemia or signs of hypovolemia or edema. Therefore, they are virtually impossible to differentiate from patients with the syndrome of inappropriate antidiuresis except by measurements of plasma cortisol.

Diarrhea, bulimia, renal tubular acidosis, medullary cystic disease of the kidney, and many other disorders associated with sodium depletion also result in hypovolemia, hyponatremia, and impaired water excretion. Although not studied extensively, the pathophysiology of these two defects is probably similar to those seen with diuretic abuse, mineralocorticoid deficiency, and other forms of chronic hypovolemia and/or hypotension.

Euvolemic Hyponatremia

The syndrome of inappropriate antidiuresis is also characterized by hyponatremia and impaired water excretion. However, it is distinguished by the fact that blood volume and pressure are normal or slightly increased and edema is absent. SIADH was first described in two patients with bronchogenic carcinoma.[347] Since then, it has been recognized with increasing frequency in association with a great many other diseases and drugs (Table 9-7). For reasons not altogether clear, these diseases usually involve the lungs or nervous system. Among the latter, patients with schizophrenia or other psychosis are noteworthy for the frequency and severity of the syndrome,[285–288] possibly because they also have a high incidence of psychogenic polydipsia.[288] Polydipsia alone is rarely capable of inducing water intoxication, because the excretory capacity of the kidneys is normally so great. However, by stressing the system, polydipsia probably brings out many subtle defects in vasopressin secretion that would otherwise go unrecognized. SIADH also occurs in some patients with myxedema.[348,349] However, water excretion is usually normal in uncomplicated hypothyroidism in humans, and those defects which can be demonstrated are usually mild and unrelated to inappropriate secretion of vasopressin.

A large number of drugs have also been implicated in the pathogenesis of SIADH. In most cases, however, it is difficult to distinguish an effect of the drug from that of the disease for which it was given. Moreover, certain drugs, such as the phenothiazines and haloperidol, may stimulate vasopressin release by producing orthostatic hypotension, while others probably impair water excretion by vasopressin-independent mechanisms. Nevertheless, the clinical aspects of the hyponatremic disorders with which these drugs are associated are sufficiently similar to warrant inclusion in the category of SIADH.

In most patients with SIADH, secretion of the hormone is inappropriately high relative to the hypotonicity of body fluids (Fig. 9-20). Only rarely, however, is plasma vasopressin above the range found in normally hydrated recumbent adults. Consequently, hypersecretion can be identified with certainty only by measuring vasopressin under conditions of overhydration and relating it to plasma osmolality and/or sodium concentration.

Dynamic studies of vasopressin secretion in patients with SIADH have shown that it is a heterogeneous disorder which encompasses at least four distinct types of osmoregulatory defect (Fig. 9-21).[249,350–352] Each behaves in a characteristic way during water loading and/or hypertonic saline infusion and probably reflects a basically different pathogenetic mechanism. Type A is characterized by large and erratic fluctuations in plasma vasopressin which bear no relation whatever to changes in plasma osmolality. It is found in about 25 percent of all patients with SIADH and appears to be due to a total loss of osmoreceptor control or intermittent stimulation by some unrecognized nonosmotic pathway. In the type B defect, plasma vasopressin remains fixed at an inappropriately high level until

TABLE 9-7 Causes of the Syndrome of Inappropriate Antidiuretic Hormone

Neoplastic	
1. Bronchogenic carcinoma	6. Carcinoma of ureter
2. Carcinoma of duodenum	7. Lymphoma
3. Carcinoma of pancreas	8. Ewing's sarcoma
4. Thymoma	9. Carcinoma of the prostate
5. Mesothelioma	10. Carcinoma of the bladder
Nonneoplastic	
1. Trauma	
2. Pulmonary disease	
a. Pneumonia, bacterial or viral	e. Abscess
b. Cavitation (aspergillosis)	f. Asthma
c. Tuberculosis	g. Pneumothorax
d. Positive pressure breathing	h. Cystic fibrosis
3. Central nervous system disorders	
a. Meningitis, bacterial or viral	i. Psychosis
b. Head trauma	j. Delirium tremens
c. Brain abscess	k. Cerebral atrophy
d. Encephalitis, bacterial or viral	l. Cavernous sinus thrombosis
e. Guillain-Barré syndrome	m. Hydrocephalus
f. Subarachnoid hemorrhage	n. Rocky Mountain fever
g. Acute intermittent porphyria	o. Cerebrovascular accident
h. Peripheral neuropathy	p. Multiple sclerosis
4. Endocrine disease: myxedema	
5. Idiopathic	
Pharmacologic	
1. Vasopressin and DDAVP	8. Nicotine
2. Oxytocin (Pitocin)	9. Phenothiazines
3. Vincristine	10. Cyclophosphamide
4. Chlorpropamide	11. Haloperidol
5. Thiazide diuretics	12. Tricyclic antidepressants
6. Clofibrate (Atromid-S)	13. Monoamine oxidase inhibitors
7. Carbamazepine	

plasma osmolality rises into the normal range. At that point, plasma vasopressin begins to rise appropriately in close association with a further increase in plasma osmolality. This pattern also occurs in about 25 percent of all patients with SIADH. It appears to reflect a constant, nonsuppressible leak of vasopressin in the presence of otherwise normal osmoregulatory function. The type C defect is the most common, occurring in at least 35 percent of all patients. It is characterized by plasma vasopressin lev-

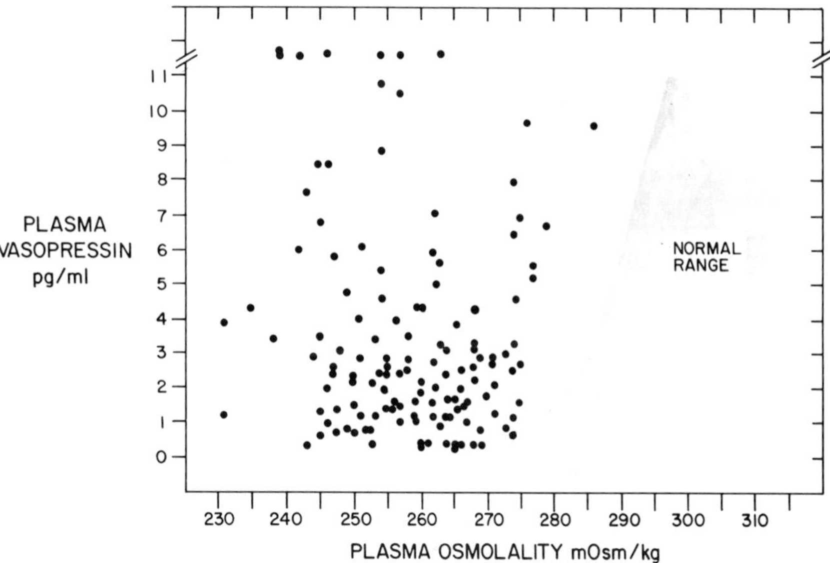

FIGURE 9-20 The relation of plasma vasopressin to plasma osmolality in the syndrome of inappropriate antidiuresis. Each value represents a single patient. (*From Robertson and Aycinena.*[278])

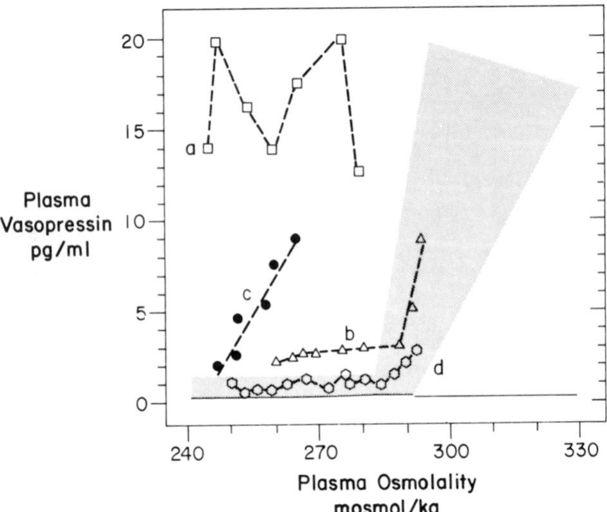

FIGURE 9-21 The relation of plasma vasopressin to osmolality during hypertonic saline infusion in four patients with the clinical syndrome of inappropriate antidiuresis. (*From Robertson.*[29])

els that rise and fall in close correlation with changes in plasma osmolality. Regression analysis of the relation between these two variables shows that the precision and sensitivity of the response are normal but that the extrapolated threshold value is subnormal. Patients with this type of defect have resetting of the osmostat and exhibit clinical characteristics slightly different from those found in other forms of SIADH. Type D is much less common than the other three and probably represents a basically different defect in antidiuretic function. In these unusual patients, vasopressin secretion is stimulated and suppressed normally but urine osmolality remains fixed at a hypertonic level. The reason for this apparent dissociation between plasma vasopressin and urinary concentration has not been determined.

Except in those cases in which the hormone is produced ectopically by malignant disease or released from the neurohypophysis in response to emetic stimuli, the cause of the vasopressin secretion is unknown. There appears to be no relation between the type of osmoregulatory defect and the underlying disease.[350] Thus, it may be that the diseases most commonly associated with the syndrome can stimulate vasopressin secretion by any of several different mechanisms. It is particularly noteworthy in this regard that bronchogenic carcinoma has been associated with every type of osmoregulatory defect, including type C, the rest osmostat.[353] Since it is highly unlikely that anaplastic cells could acquire the normally separate capacities of osmoregulation and vasopressin synthesis, many malignant diseases probably produce the syndrome by some mechanism other than ectopic production.

With the exception of the type C defect, the pathophysiology of the fluid and electrolyte disturbance in patients with SIADH is probably similar in most respects to that observed when healthy volunteers are treated with vasopressin.[200,354] If the subjects are allowed to drink ad libitum[200] or are restricted to a total intake of 1 to 2 L a day,[352] the administration of Pitressin or DDAVP in doses sufficient to maintain a fixed, maximum antidiuresis causes little or no increase in total body water or a decrease in plasma osmolality because the combination of low intake with continued insensible loss and minimal obligatory urine output is sufficient to maintain water balance. However, if fluid intake is maintained at a level above 2 liters a day, a commensurate increase in output does not occur because urine concentration is not suppressed normally by the fall in plasma osmolality. As a consequence, the excess water ingested accumulates, causing progressive dilution of solute concentration in all compartments of the body. When the expansion of body water reaches about 10 percent, the excretion of sodium begins to increase as a result of both decreased reabsorption in the proximal tubule and suppression of the renin-angiotensin-aldosterone system. This natriuresis has the effect of ameliorating the hypervolemia and increasing urinary dilution and flow slightly, but it also aggravates the hyponatremia and hypotonicity of body fluids. At this point, a new steady state may be achieved and plasma osmolality and sodium may stabilize unless some further change in intake occurs. If intake increases again, another cycle of water retention and natriuresis ensues, causing a further decline in plasma osmolality and sodium concentration. By contrast, if water intake is sharply curtailed, the entire series of events reverses as water is lost, sodium is retained, and plasma osmolality and sodium gradually return to their original levels.

It should be noted that the clinical consequences of hypersecretion of vasopressin depend almost solely on the rate of water intake. If it is regulated normally, inappropriate secretion will be clinically inapparent no matter how high plasma vasopressin may rise. If water intake is high, an increase in hormone secretion above the minimum level required to concentrate the urine will cause no appreciable worsening of the salt and water imbalance, because the rate of urine output falls only slightly when urine osmolality increases from 400 to 1200 mosmol/kg (Fig. 9-11). Once antidiuresis is established, only a change in intake can appreciably alter the salt and water balance. In a real sense, therefore, hypersecretion of vasopressin plays only a permissive role in the series of events which leads to water intoxication. This role contrasts sharply with that of many other hormones, such as insulin and parathormone, whose hypersecretion per se is sufficient to cause clinical abnormalities.

The pathophysiology of the fluid and electrolyte imbalance is much the same when vasopressin is produced endogenously. One important difference occurs in patients with the type C defect, the reset osmostat. Because their threshold function is retained, increasing water intake leads eventually to maximum urinary dilution[355–357] and, consequently, a rate of water excretion sufficient to prevent further overhydration. As a consequence, plasma osmolality may stabilize, albeit at a markedly subnormal level. This variant constitutes an important exception to the rule that patients with SIADH are unable to excrete a maximally dilute urine. Most cases of reset osmostat probably go unrecognized, because the water loading and/or vasopressin studies necessary to demonstrate the condition are not employed routinely for diagnosis. A second difference is that many patients with endogenous SIADH have associated abnormalities in the thirst mechanism.[249,358] Because of the slight volume expansion induced by water retention, plasma renin activity and aldosterone tend to be suppressed,[359] but blood pressure is not elevated.[360]

Patients with SIADH usually manifest few clinical symptoms and signs other than the neurologic abnormalities due to hyponatremia.[361] These include lethargy, confusion, muscle cramps, anorexia, pathologic reflexes, pseudobulbar palsy, coma, Cheyne-Stokes respiration, and seizures. These symptoms and signs are probably due to a swelling of brain cells that results from the decrease in extracellular osmolality (Fig. 9-10). Postmortem studies in patients who died with hyponatremia show cerebral edema, herniation of the brain, and, in a few cases, central myelinolysis.[362] The severity of the neurologic defects depends on several factors, including the degree of hyponatremia, the rate of decline, and the age of the patient.[361] Unless the patient has epilepsy or another preexisting brain disease, seizures and coma usually do not occur until plasma sodium falls below 120 mEq/L. If hyponatremia is chronic or slow to develop, cerebral swelling and symptoms appear to be less severe, probably because brain cells are able to inactivate or otherwise rid themselves of solute.[363]

Diagnosis

In evaluating a patient with hyponatremia, the first step is to rule out factitious causes.[364] If plasma sodium is measured with a flame photometer, its concentration will appear to be low in any disease in which plasma proteins or lipids are markedly elevated. This effect is an artifact caused by a relative decrease in the sodium-containing aqueous portion of the plasma. Since the *concentration* of sodium and its anions in plasma water is unaffected by the addition of lipid or protein, plasma osmolality and sodium as determined by an ion-specific electrode are normal in the presence of hyperproteinemia or hyperlipidemia. A rise in the plasma concentration of glucose or mannitol will also produce hyponatremia. In this case, however, the fall in plasma sodium concentration is real, since it is due to an osmotically induced shift of water from the intracellular to the extracellular space. Therefore, plasma sodium will be low when measured by an ion-specific electrode or flame photometer, but plasma osmolality will be normal or slightly increased. Thus, the sine qua non for true hyponatremia is a commensurate reduction in the osmolality and sodium concentration of heparinized plasma. Serum or edetic acid (EDTA) plasma should not be used for these measurements, since both are subject to significant artifacts in the osmolality measurements.

Differentiation between the three major categories of true hyponatremia is based largely on clinical assessment of the extracellular volume (Table 9-8). Generalized edema and/or association with a disease known to cause edema is pathognomonic of hypervolemic hyponatremia. In these patients, urinary sodium is usually low (<20 mEq/day), and plasma renin activity, aldosterone, and urea may be elevated because of a reduction in effective blood volume and glomerular filtration. The cardiac, hepatic, and nephrotic causes of this category of hyponatremia are differentiated by the usual clinical methods.

Hypovolemic hyponatremia is characterized by signs and symptoms of volume depletion *without* edema. Urinary sodium is usually low, but it may be increased if the condition is due to renal sodium wasting (e.g., adrenal insufficiency, diuretic abuse, or sponge kidney). Some degree of hypokalemia is the rule, except in patients with Addison's disease or isolated aldosterone deficiency, in whom serum potassium is usually elevated. Normokalemia or hypokalemia does not exclude secondary adrenal insufficiency, and so plasma cortisol should be measured in all cases and treated the same as SIADH.

Euvolemic hyponatremia, or the syndrome of inappropriate antidiuresis, is distinguishable by the lack of any clinical signs of edema, hypovolemia, or hypotension. Thus, in contrast to the other two forms of hyponatremia, plasma urea, urate, and renin tend to be low while urinary sodium is high. The latter may be misleading, however, since the natriuresis can reverse quickly when the excess body water begins to decline.

Measurements of plasma vasopressin are of no help in distinguishing between the various types of hyponatremia, since it is usually elevated to the same extent in all three. However, plasma vasopressin levels may determine whether the hormone contributes to the impairment in urinary dilution and, if it does, which type of osmoregulatory defect is responsible. At present this information is of no clinical utility, since the therapy is essentially the same in any case. However, diagnostic studies of this type may prove more useful when and if more specific and effective methods for inhibiting the secretion or action of vasopressin come into general clinical use.

TABLE 9-8 Diagnostic Evaluation of Hyponatremia

1. Measure plasma osmolality.
   A. If it is decreased in proportion to plasma sodium (1 mEq/L = 2 mosmol/kg), true hyponatremia is present and the work-up should proceed directly to step 2.
   B. If it is not depressed, factitious hyponatremia should be suspected and evaluated by measuring plasma protein, lipids, and glucose. If they are normal, the presence of some abnormal osmogenic solute such as alcohol should be sought.
2. Examine the patient for evidence of edema, congestive heart failure, cirrhosis, nephrosis, hypotension, hypovolemia, adrenal insufficiency, or hypothyroidism.
   A. If any of these abnormalities is present, the diagnosis of SIADH is excluded and therapy to correct the underlying disease should be started.
   B. If these abnormalities are absent, proceed to step 3.
3. Measure urine osmolality.
   A. If it is more than 100 mosmol/kg, the work-up should proceed directly to step 4.
   B. If it is less than 100 mosmol/kg, perform a dehydration test and repeat the measurement at hourly intervals. If urine concentration occurs before plasma osmolality and sodium reach 270 mosmol/kg and 130 mEq/L, respectively, the diagnosis of reset osmostat is likely and the work-up should proceed to step 4. However, if urine concentration does not occur prematurely, a persistent defect in water excretion is excluded and the clinical history should be reviewed, looking for evidence of severe polydipsia (> 20 L/day) and/or some transient antecedent stimulus to vasopressin release.
4. Measure urinary sodium.
   A. If it is less than 20 mEq/day, the diagnosis of SIADH is unlikely and further studies should be performed to determine whether there is evidence of diuretic abuse, chronic diarrhea, vomiting, or subclinical cardiac or hepatic failure.
   B. If it is more than 20 mEq/day, proceed to step 5.
5. Measure plasma vasopressin and renin activity while the patient is hyponatremic.
   A. If plasma vasopressin is inappropriately high and renin is low, the diagnosis of SIADH is established and appropriate therapy should be started.
   B. If both plasma vasopressin and renin are suppressed, a vasopressin-independent form of SIADH should be suspected.
   C. If plasma vasopressin and renin activity are both elevated, diuretic abuse, adrenal insufficiency, or some other cause of sodium wasting should be sought.
6. A water load test may be performed if the hyponatremia remits before the other diagnostic studies are performed.
   A. If the load is excreted normally, SIADH and all other forms of impaired water excretion are excluded.
   B. If the load is not excreted normally, steps 1 through 4 should be performed to determine the cause of the defect.

Therapy

Hypervolemic Hyponatremia

In patients with edema and hyponatremia, the ideal treatment would be to correct the cardiac, hepatic, or renal defect that is responsible for the impairment in water excretion. Indeed, some improvement in water excretion and/or hyponatremia may occur when cardiac output is increased[365] or ascitic fluid is shunted into the vascular space.[366] Usually, however, the basic hemodynamic defect cannot be completely rectified, and other methods must be used to correct the edema and hyponatremia. Since patients in this category have a greater increase in total body water than in sodium, the most rational and effective therapy is to combine fluid restriction with the administration of an osmotic or loop diuretic.[367,368] Initially, infusion of mannitol will expand extracellular volume and increase hyponatremia by osmotically extracting cellular water. However, the fall in plasma sodium is inconsequential, because it is more than offset by the osmotic effect of the mannitol, and the hypervolemia and hyponatremia usually disappear in a few hours when the mannitol is excreted. Hypertonic saline should not be used in these patients, because they retain the sodium and develop more severe edema.

Hypovolemic Hyponatremia

These patients are usually the simplest to treat, since it is necessary only to expand blood and extracellular volume by oral or parenteral administration of salt and water. Since their sodium deficit is greater than their water deficit, the ideal combination is hypertonic; i.e., the ratio of sodium chloride to water should exceed 150 mEq/L. However, this approach is necessary only if the hyponatremia is severe and must be corrected quickly. In such a situation, an infusion of 3% saline at a rate of 0.1 ml/kg per minute for 2 h will raise plasma sodium by almost 10 mEq/L, an amount that is usually sufficient to eliminate the threat of serious neurologic complications. In using this approach, it is important not to raise the plasma sodium too far or too fast (see below). In most cases of hypovolemic hyponatremia, it is sufficient and probably preferable simply to infuse isotonic saline with or without supplementary potassium. In addition, the cause of the sodium loss should be identified and, if possible, corrected. If the patient's pituitary-adrenal status is in question, parenteral cortisol should be administered pending completion of steroid measurements. If sodium wasting cannot be stopped (e.g., in a patient with chronic diarrhea due to bowel disease), intake of sodium and other electrolytes should be supplemented orally as needed to maintain balance. In no case should patients in this category be treated by water restriction, since these measures only aggravate the underlying hypovolemia.

Euvolemic Hyponatremia

In patients with SIADH, the most rational therapy would be to correct the underlying abnormality in vasopressin secretion. However, it is rarely possible to do this except in cases where the hormone is produced ectopically or secreted in response to emetic stimuli. Therefore, it is usually necessary to employ other methods to reduce the excess of body water which is responsible for the hyponatremia. The traditional method is to restrict water intake. To be effective, however, the *total* intake of water must be at least 500 ml a day less than the total of urinary and insensible output. Since the amount of water provided by food normally approximates insensible loss, discretionary intake of water must be kept at least 500 ml a day below urine output. In many patients, the requisite restriction is difficult to achieve because their urine is concentrated and/or their thirst is also inappropriately increased. And even if restriction is successful, the rate of decrease in body water and rise in plasma osmolality is only about 1 to 2 percent a day. Therefore, additional measures are almost always needed, particularly if the hyponatremia is symptomatic.

Infusion of hypertonic saline provides more rapid correction and is almost always indicated when the hyponatremia is sufficiently severe to cause neurologic abnormalities. When given IV as 3% saline at a rate of 0.1 ml/kg per minute, it will increase plasma sodium and osmolality at a rate of approximately 2 percent an hour. Since it acts both by producing a water-depleting solute diuresis and by correcting the sodium deficit, this approach is rational as well as rapid. In our experience and that of others, it is also safe.[369–371] However, there is some question as to whether in certain patients rapid correction of hyponatremia with hypertonic saline may be associated with central pontine myelinolysis,[372] a rare and often fatal neurologic disorder characterized by quadriparesis, dysphagia, and dysarthria. Therefore, hypertonic saline should be used cautiously in patients with SIADH and only to the extent necessary to raise plasma sodium to asymptomatic levels. This caveat applies particularly to patients in whom the hyponatremia has been present for more than 48 h. Generally speaking, it is usually unnecessary and probably imprudent to raise plasma sodium by more than 2 percent an hour or 12 mEq/L per day or to levels above 130 mEq/L in the first 24 to 48 h.

Body water can also be reduced by inhibiting the antidiuretic effects of vasopressin. Among the drugs that have been used for this purpose, demeclocycline (Declomycin) is probably the best.[373,374] At conventional doses of up to 1.2 g per day, it causes a reversible form of nephrogenic diabetes insipidus in almost all patients with SIADH. Its mechanism of action has not been defined precisely but appears to involve a step distal to the generation of cyclic AMP.[375] Because of other catabolic as well as nephrotoxic effects, it may cause a rise in plasma urea, which is reversible when the drug is stopped. However, demeclocycline can have serious or potentially lethal side effects in patients with edema and hyponatremia.[376,377] Hence, its use should be monitored closely and probably restricted to SIADH patients in whom the hyponatremia is chronic and symptomatic, strict fluid restriction is not feasible, and significant underlying cardiac, renal, or hepatic disease is not present. Lithium carbonate also causes a form of reversible nephrogenic diabetes insipidus. At conventional doses, however, it has a much less consistent inhibitory effect on urinary concentration and is even more prone to produce undesirable side effects.[378] For these reasons, its use to treat SIADH or other forms of hyponatremia is not recommended.

Other measures which can be useful in the treatment of chronic SIADH include the administration of oral sodium chloride with or without furosemide.[379] This regimen works much like an osmotic diuretic in that it increases free water excretion by increasing solute load. Much the same result can be obtained by giving salt or urea per os,[380] but the latter is unpalatable and may not be well accepted by patients.

TESTS USED IN DIAGNOSIS

Hypofunction

Fluid Restriction

This test is basic to the differential diagnosis of polyuria. It should not be used when basal osmolality and sodium concentration are above 295 mosmol/kg and 143 mEq/L because in that situation it does not provide additional information of diagnostic value and may cause the patient unnecessary discomfort. If basal urine output is less than 6 liters per day, the test should be started at bedtime. Otherwise, it should be started early in the morning after an overnight fast. After initial samples of urine and plasma for the measurement of osmolality have been obtained, the patient is weighed and instructed to stop all intake of fluids. The use of tobacco and unnecessary drugs is also prohibited, but lemon drops or other hard candy may be taken to assuage thirst or hunger. Every hour for the next 3 to 6 h, urine and plasma are collected for osmometry and the patient is reweighed. If urine osmolality does not rise above 300 mosmol/kg *before* plasma osmolality and sodium concentration reach 295 mosmol/kg and 143 mEq/L, the test is abnormal and a diagnosis of primary polydipsia is excluded. A measurement of vasopressin in the final plasma or urine sample or a therapeutic trial of DDAVP may then be used to differentiate neurogenic from nephrogenic diabetes insipidus.

If urine osmolality rises above 300 mosmol/kg before plasma osmolality or sodium reaches the prescribed level, the dehydration test is inconclusive and should be supplemented with measurements of plasma vasopressin during hypertonic saline infusion to distinguish neurogenic diabetes insipidus from primary polydipsia.

If the urine remains dilute but plasma osmolality and sodium do not reach 295 mosmol/kg and 145 mEq/L within 3 to 4 h, surreptitious drinking should be suspected. If this is confirmed by a finding that the changes in body weight or plasma osmolality are not commensurate with total urine output, the test is invalid and should be repeated under closer observation or replaced by a hypertonic saline infusion.

Hypertonic Saline Infusion

This test is used to distinguish between primary polydipsia and neurogenic diabetes insipidus when the fluid restriction test is not followed or results in urinary concentration before plasma osmolality and sodium reach 295 mosmol/kg and 145 mEq/L, respectively. At the conclusion of the fluid restriction test, 3% saline is infused via intravenous catheter at a rate of 0.1 ml/min per kilogram of body weight for 1 to 2 h. Plasma samples for osmometry and vasopressin assay was collected from the opposite antecubital vein before and at 30-min intervals during the infusion. The results should be interpreted by plotting on a nomogram such as Fig. 9-15.

Therapeutic Trial of DDAVP

This test can be used to differentiate between primary polydipsia and neurogenic diabetes insipidus. The patient should be hospitalized in an environment where intake, output, body weight, and plasma electrolytes can be closely monitored. After at least 2 days of observation to determine basal values, DDAVP is given by intramuscular injection (1 to 2 μg bid) or nasal insufflation (25 μg bid) for 1 to 3 days. Body weight and plasma sodium should be measured in the morning and late afternoon while daily intake and output continue to be monitored. If this treatment reduces polydipsia as well as polyuria and does not produce water intoxication, the patient probably has neurogenic diabetes insipidus. However, if DDAVP has no effect on water balance, the patient probably has nephrogenic diabetes insipidus and should be tried on a 10-fold higher dose of DDAVP to determine whether the renal resistance is partial or complete. However, if the standard dose of DDAVP reduces urine output without reducing intake or produces other signs of water intoxication (such as a gain in weight or fall in plasma sodium of more than 5 percent), the patient probably has some form of primary polydipsia, and all antidiuretic therapy should be discontinued until a definitive diagnosis is obtained.

Vasopressin Assay

Plasma or urinary vasopressin should be measured concurrently with plasma and urine osmolality during the dehydration test to verify the diagnosis of diabetes insipidus and differentiate the neurogenic and nephrogenic forms. The results should be interpreted by plotting on appropriate nomograms such as those in Figs. 9–15 and 9–16.

Hyperfunction

Vasopressin Assay

Measurements of plasma or urinary vasopressin can be used to verify the cause of impaired water excretion. However, they should be obtained only when plasma osmolality and sodium concentration are below 270 mosmol/kg and 130 mEq/L, respectively, and the results should be plotted on a nomogram like that in Fig. 9–20. Inadequate suppression of vasopressin is indicative of SIADH only if hypovolemia, hypotension, and certain other abnormalities are excluded (Table 9–8). Urinary sodium excretion or plasma renin activity may be measured concurrently as an indicator of blood volume status.

Water Load Test

This test is used primarily to verify suspected defects in water excretion at a time when plasma osmolality and sodium concentration are within normal limits. It may also be used in the presence of hypotonicity to test for resetting of the osmostat.

The test should be started in the morning 2 h after a light breakfast. After initial plasma and urine samples are obtained for osmometry, the patient is weighed and instructed to drink 20 ml of cool tap water per kilogram of body weight within 15 to 30 min. If necessary, lightly salted crackers may be eaten to overcome distate for the water. The patient is then placed in a semirecumbent position. Each hour for the next 4 h, a sample of plasma is obtained and the total urine output is collected for the measurement of osmolality and volume.

Normally this procedure should result in a fall in plasma osmolality of at least 5 mosmol/kg, a decrease in urine osmolality to less than 100 mosmol/kg, and excretion of 90 percent of the water load or more within 5 h (Fig. 9-22). Failure to achieve either of the latter criteria in the presence of good absorption (i.e., a normal decline in plasma osmolality) is

FIGURE 9-22 The effect of a standard water load on renal function. Shaded areas indicate the range of values obtained in 24 healthy adults. A water load of 20 ml per kilogram of body weight was given between 0 and 30 min. The bottom panel indicates cumulative excretion expressed as a percentage of the total load.

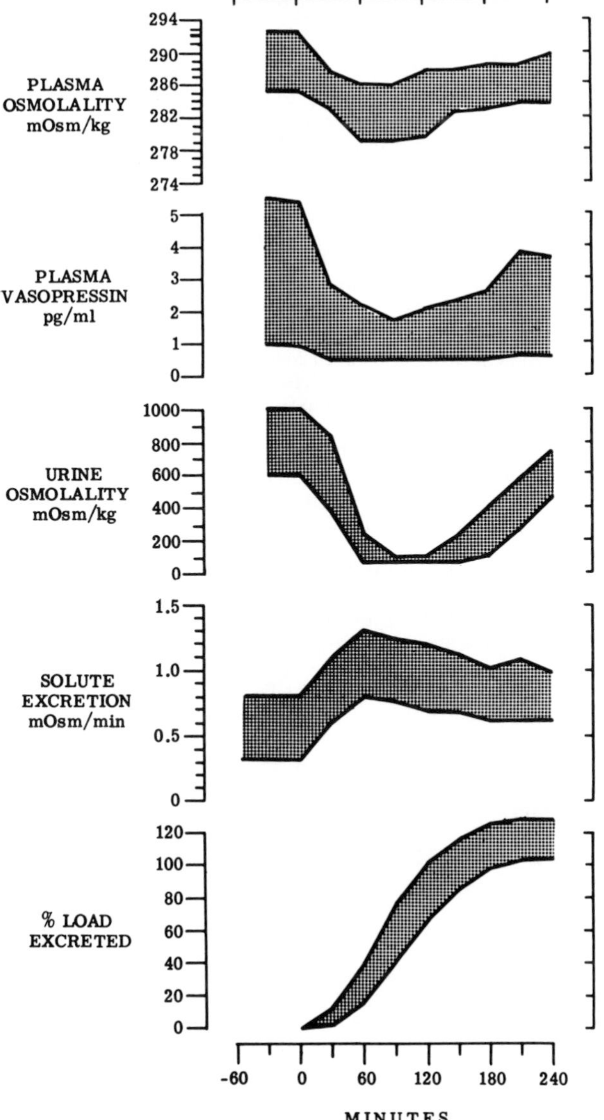

diagnostic of a defect in water and/or solute excretion. Some indication of the case may be obtained by calculating the solute excretion rate (urine flow in liters per minute times urine osmolality in milliosmols per kilogram) and plotting it along with urine osmolality on a suitable nomogram such as that in Fig. 9-22. A defect in distal delivery of filtrate is indicated by a subnormal rate of solute excretion. SIADH is characterized by a normal or supranormal rate of solute excretion in association with a less than maximum dilution of the urine. Measurements of plasma or urinary vasopressin on samples obtained 90 to 120 min after the load may be used to confirm the diagnosis.

General Considerations

The use of nicotine, caffeine, and all unnecessary drugs should be prohibited during any study of vasopressin function. The patient should also be monitored for symptoms of nausea or changes in blood pressure, which may confuse interpretation of the results.

Plasma for osmometry should always be collected in heparin with as little stasis as possible. Serum or EDTA produces relatively large artifactual increases in osmolality[381] which make interpretation of most vasopressin tests impossible. Osmometry should be performed only by freezing-point depression on equipment calibrated with a 290-mosmol/kg standard as well as 100- and 500-mosmol/kg standards. If the accuracy of the osmometry is poor or doubtful, measurements of plasma sodium should be substituted.

Samples of plasma and urine for vasopressin assay should always be collected, processed, and transported according to the specifications of the laboratory that is to carry out the test. The results should always be compared with normal values supplied by the same laboratory, since not all laboratories use the same reference standards.

REFERENCES

1. Haymaker W: Hypothalamo-pituitary neural pathways and the circulatory system of the pituitary, in Haymaker W, Anderson E, and Nauta W (eds): *The Hypothalamus*. Springfield, Charles C Thomas, 1969, p 219.
2. Scharrer E, Scharrer B: Hormones produced by neurosecretory cells. *Recent Prog Horm Res* 10:183, 1954.
3. Zimmerman EA: The organization of oxytocin and vasopressin pathways, in Martin JB, Reichlin S, Bick KL (eds): *Neurosecretion and Brain Peptides*. New York, Raven, 1981, pp 63–75.
4. Sofroniew MV, Weindl A, Schrell U, Wetzstein R: Immunohistochemistry of vasopressin, oxytocin and neurophysin in the hypothalamus and extrahypothalamic regions of the human and primate brain. *Acta Histochem [Suppl]* 24:79, 1982.
5. Dierickx K, Vandesande F: Immunocytochemical localization of the vasopressinergic and the oxytocinergic neurons in the human hypothalamus. *Cell Tissue Res* 184:15, 1977.

6. Rhodes CH, Morrell JI, Pfaff DW: Immunohistochemical analysis of magnocellular elements in rat hypothalamus: Distribution and numbers of cells containing neurophysin, oxytocin and vasopressin. *J Comp Neurol* 198:45, 1981.
7. Plotsky PM, Sawchenko PE: Hypophysial-portal plasma levels, median eminence content, and immunohistochemical staining of corticotropin-releasing factor, arginine vasopressin, and oxytocin after pharmacological adrenalectomy. *Endocrinology* 120:1361, 1987.
8. Luerssen TG, Robertson GL: Cerebrospinal fluid vasopressin and vasotocin in health and disease, in Wood JH (ed): *Neurobiology and Cerebrospinal Fluid.* New York, Plenum, 1980, vol 1, pp 613–623.
9. Glick SM, Brownstein MJ: Vasopressin content of rat brain. *Life Sci,* 27:1103, 1980.
10. Du Vigneaud V: Hormones of the posterior pituitary gland: Oxytocin and vasopressin, in *Harvey Lectures, 1954–1955.* New York, Academic, 1956.
11. Sawyer WW: Evolution of antidiuretic hormones and their functions. *Am J Med* 42:678, 1967
12. Walter R, Smith CW, Mehta PK, Boonjarern S, Arruda JAL, Kurtzman N: Conformational considerations of vasopressin as a guide to development of biological probes and therapeutic agents, in Andreoli TE, Grantham JJ, and Rector FC (eds): *Disturbances in Body Fluid Osmolality.* Bethesda, American Physiological Society, 1977, pp 1–36.
13. Vavra I, Machova A, Holecek V, Cort JH, Zaoral M, Sorm F: Effect of a synthetic analogue of vasopressin in animals and in patients with diabetes insipidus. *Lancet* 1:948, 1968.
14. Sawyer WH, Manning M: The development of potent and specific vasopressin antagonists. *Kidney Int* 34(Suppl 26):S–34, 1988.
15. Acher R, Chauvet J, Olivry G: Sur l'existence éventuelle d'une hormone unique hypophysaire: I. Relations entre l'oxytocine, la vasopressine et la protein de Van Dyke extraites de la neurohypophyse du boeuf. *Biochim Biophys Acta* 22:421, 1956.
16. Breslow E: The neurophysins. *Adv Enzymol* 40:271. 1974.
17. Sachs H, Fawcett P, Takabatake Y, Portanova R: Biosynthesis and release of vasopressin and neurophysin. *Recent Prog Horm Res* 25:447, 1969.
18. Schmale H, Fehr S, Richter D: Vasopressin biosynthesis—from gene to peptide hormone. *Kidney Int* 32(Suppl 21):S–8, 1987.
19. Sausville E, Carney D, Battey J: The human vasopressin gene is linked to the oxytocin gene and is selectively expressed in a cultured lung cancer cell line. *J Biol Chem* 260:10236, 1985.
20. Riddell DC, Mallonee R, Phillips JA, Parks JS, Sexton LA, Hamerton JL: Chromosomal assignment of human sequences encoding arginine vasopressin-neurophysin II and growth hormone releasing factor. *Somatic Cell Mol Genet* 11:189, 1985.
21. Mohr E, Bahnsen U, Kiessling C, Richter D: Expression of the vasopressin and oxytocin genes in rats occurs in mutually exclusive sets of hypothalamic neurons. *FEBS Lett* 242:144, 1988.
22. Carrazana EJ, Pasieka KB, Majzoub JA: The vasopressin mRNA poly (A) tract is unusually long and increases during stimulation of vasopressin gene expression in vivo. *Mol Cell Biol* 8:2267, 1988.
23. Moses AM, Miller M: Accumulation and release of pituitary vasopressin in rats heterozygous for hypothalamic diabetes insipidus. *Endocrinology* 86:34, 1970.
24. Douglass WW: How do neurons secrete peptides? Exocytosis and its consequences including synaptic vesicle formation in the hypothalamo-neurohypophyseal system. *Prog Brain Res* 39:21, 1973.
25. Verney EB: Antidiuretic hormone and the factors which determine its release. *Proc R Soc Lond* [Biol] 135:25, 1947.
26. Robertson GL: The regulation of vasopressin function in health and disease. *Recent Prog Horm Res* 33:333, 1977.
27. Robertson GL, Athar S, Shelton RL: Osmotic control of vasopressin function, in Andreoli TE, Grantham JJ, and Rector FC (eds): *Disturbances in Body Fluid Osmolality.* Bethesda, American Physiological Society, 1977, p 125.
28. Schrier RW, Berl T, Anderson RJ: Osmotic and nonosmotic control of vasopressin release. *Am J Physiol* 236(4):F321, 1979.
29. Robertson GL: Thirst and vasopressin function in normal and disordered states of water balance. *J Lab Clin Med* 101(3):351, 1983.
30. Jewell PA, Verney EB: An experimental attempt to determine the site of the neurohypophyseal osmoreceptors in the dog. *Philos Trans R Soc Lond* [Biol] 240:197, 1957.
31. Andersson B: Thirst and brain control of water balance. *Am Sci* 59:408, 1971.
32. Robertson GL: Physiopathology of ADH secretion, in Tolis G, Labrie F, Martin JB, Naftolin F (eds): *Clinical Neuroendocrinology: A Pathophysiological Approach.* New York, Raven, 1979, pp 247–260.
33. Gardiner TW, Verbalis JG, Stricker EM: Impaired secretion of vasopressin and oxytocin in rats after lesions of nucleus medianus. *Am J Physiol* 249 (*Regulatory Integrative Comp Physiol* 18):R681, 1985.
34. Thrasher TN, Keil LC: Regulation of drinking and vasopressin secretion: Role of organum vasculosum laminae terminalis. *Am J Physiol* 253 (*Regulatory Integrative Comp Physiol* 22):R108, 1987.
35. Strong OS, Elwyn A: *Human Neuroanatomy.* Baltimore, Williams & Wilkins, 1948, p. 398.
36. Zerbe RL, Miller JZ, Robertson GL: The reproducibility and heritability of individual differences in osmoregulatory function in normal human subjects. *J Lab Clin Med* 117:51, 1991.
37. Helderman JH, Vestal RE, Rowe JW, Tobin JD, Andres R, Robertson GL: The response of arginine vasopressin to intravenous ethanol and hypertonic saline in man: The impact of aging. *J Gerontol* 33:39, 1978.
38. Legros LL, Govaerts A, Demoulin A, Franchimont P: Interactions entre un dérive progestatif et l'ethinyl oestradiol sur l'élimination urinaire de neurophysine d'oxytocine et de vasopressine immunoactives et sur le taux de neurophysine sérique I et II chez l'homme normal. *C R Soc Biol (Paris)* 167(11):1668, 1973.
39. Vallotton MB, Merkelbach U, Gaillard RC: Studies of the factors modulating antidiuretic hormone exretion in man in response to the osmolar stimulus: Effects of oestrogen and angiotensin II. *Acta Endocrinol (Copenh)* 104:295, 1983.
40. Skowsky WR, Swan L, Smith P: Effects of sex steroid hormones on arginine vasopressin in intact and castrated male and female rats. *Endocrinology* 104:105, 1979.
41. Barron WM: Water metabolism and vasopressin secretion during pregnancy. *Br J Obstet Gynaecol* 1:853, 1987.
42. Vokes TJ, Weiss NM, Schreiber J, Gaskill MB, Robertson GL: Osmoregulation of thirst and vasopressin during normal menstrual cycle. *Am J Physiol* 254 (*Regulatory Integrative Comp Physiol* 23):R641, 1988.
43. Spruce BA, Baylis PH, Burd J, Watson MJ: Variation in osmoregulation of arginine vasopressin during the human menstrual cycle. *Clin Endocrinol (Oxf)* 22:37, 1985.
44. Rodbard D, Munson PJ: Editorial comment. *Am J Physiol* 234:E340, 1978.
45. Wade CE, Bie P, Keil LC, Ramsay DJ: Osmotic control of plasma vasopressin in the dog. *Am J Physiol* 243:E287, 1982.
46. Hammer M, Ladefoged J, Olgaard K: Relationship between plasma osmolality and plasma vasopressin in human subjects. *Am J Physiol* 238:E313, 1980.
47. Weitzman RE, Fisher DA, DiStefano JH III, Bennett CM: Episodic secretion of arginine vasopressin. *Am J Physiol* 233:E32, 1977.
48. Brimble MJ, Dyball REJ: Characterization of the responses

of oxytocin- and vasopressin-secreting neurones in the supraoptic nucleus to osmotic stimulation. *J Physiol (Lond)* 271:253, 1977.
49. Poulain DA: Electrophysiology of the afferent input to oxytocin- and vasopressin-secreting neurones: Facts and problems. *Prog Brain Res* 60:39, 1983.
50. Robertson GL: Regulation of vasopressin secretion, in Seldin DW, Giebisch G (eds): *The Kidney: Physiology and Pathophysiology*. New York, Raven, 1985, pp 869–884.
51. Zerbe RL, Robertson GL: Osmoregulation of thirst and vasopressin secretion in human subjects: Effect of various solutes. *Am J Physiol* 224:E607, 1983.
52. Thrasher TN, Brown CJ, Keil LC, Ramsay DJ: Thirst and vasopressin release in the dog: An osmoreceptor or sodium receptor mechanism? *Am J Physiol* 238:R333, 1980.
53. McKinley MJ, Denton DA, Weisinger RS: Sensors of antidiuresis and thirst: Osmoreceptors or CSF sodium detectors? *Brain Res* 141:89, 1978.
54. Olsson K, Kolmodin R: Dependence of basic secretion of antidiuretic hormone on cerebrospinal fluid [Na]. *Acta Physiol Scand* 91:286, 1974.
55. Vokes TP, Aycinena PR, Robertson GL: Effect of insulin on osmoregulation of vasopressin. *Am J Physiol* 252 (*Endocrinol Metab* 15):E538, 1987.
56. Zerbe RL, Vinicor F, Robertson GL: The regulation of plasma vasopressin in insulin dependent diabetes mellitus. *Am J Physiol* 249(3):E317, 1985.
57. Zerbe RL, Vinicor F, Robertson GL: Plasma vasopressin in uncontrolled diabetes mellitus. *Diabetes* 28(5):503, 1979.
58. Walsh CH, Baylis PH, Malins JM: Plasma arginine vasopressin in diabetic ketoacidosis. *Diabetologia* 16:93, 1979.
59. Van Houten M, Posner BI, Kopriwa BM, Brawer JR: Insulin binding sites in the rat brain: In vivo localization to the circumventricular organs by quantitative radioautography. *Endocrinology* 105(3):666, 1979.
60. Greelen G, Keil LC, Kravik SE, Wade CE, Thrasher TN, Barnes PR, Pyka G, Nesvig C, Greenleaf JE: Inhibition of plasma vasopressin after drinking in dehydrate humans. *Am J Physiol* 247 (*Regulatory Integrative Comp Physiol* 16):R968, 1984.
61. Seckl JR, Williams TDM, Lightman SL: Oral hypertonic saline causes transient fall of vasopressin in humans. *Am J Physiol* 251 (*Regulatory Integrative Comp Physiol* 20): R214, 1986.
62. Salata RA, Verbalis JG, Robinson AG: Cold water stimulation of oropharyngeal receptors in man inhibits release of vasopressin. *J Clin Endocrinol Metab* 65:561, 1987.
63. Thompson CJ, Burd JM, Baylis PH: Acute suppression of plasma vasopressin and thirst after drinking in hypernatremic humans. *Am J Physiol* 352 (*Regulatory Integrative Comp Physiol* 21):R1138, 1987.
64. Kirchheim HR: Systemic arterial baroreceptor reflexes. *Physiol Rev* 56(1):100, 1976.
65. Goetz KL, Bond GC, Bloxham DD: Atrial receptors and renal function. *Physiol Rev* 55:157, 1975.
66. Herbert H, Moga MM, Saper CB: Connections of the parabrachial nucleus with the nucleus of the solitary tract and the medullary reticular formation in the rat. *J Comp Neurol* 293:540, 1990.
67. Jhamandas JH, Harris KH, Krukoff TL: Parabrachial nucleus projection towards the hypothalamic supraoptic nucleus: Electrophysiological and anatomical observations in the rat. *J Comp Neurol* 308:42, 1991.
68. Thames MD, Schmid PG: Cardiopulmonary receptors with vagal afferents tonically inhibit ADH release in the dog. *Am J Physiol* 237:H299, 1979.
69. Fumoux F, Czernichow P, Arnauld E, Du Pont J, Vincent JD: Effect of hypotension induced by sodium nitrocyanoferrate (III) on the release of arginine-vasopressin in the unanaesthetized monkey. *J Endocrinol* 78:449, 1978.
70. Robertson GL, Ganguly A: Osmoregulation and baroregulation of plasma vasopressin in essential hypertension. *J Cardiovasc Pharmacol* 8(Suppl 7):S87, 1986.
71. Dunn FL, Brennan TJ, Nelson AE, Robertson GL: The role of blood osmolality and volume in regulating vasopressin secretion in the rat. *J Clin Invest* 52:3212, 1973.
72. Goldsmith SR, Francis CS, Crowley AW, Cohn JN: Response of vasopressin and norepinephrine to lower body negative pressure in humans. *Am J Physiol* 243:H970, 1982.
73. Goetz KL, Wang BC, Sundet WD: Comparative effects of cardiac receptors and sinoaortic baroreceptors on elevations of plasma vasopressin and renin activity elicited by haemorrhage. *J Physiol (Lond)* 79:440, 1984.
74. Wade CE, Keil LC, Ramsay DJ: Role of volume and osmolality in the control of plasma vasopressin in dehydrated dogs. *Neuroendocrinology* 37:349, 1983.
75. Rittig S, Knudsen UB, Norgaard JP, Pedersen EB, Djurhuus JC: Abnormal diurnal rhythm of plasma vasopressin and urinary output in patients with enuresis. *Am J Physiol* 256 (*Renal Fluid Electrolyte Physiol* 25):F664, 1989.
76. Segar WE, Moore WW: The regulation of antidiuretic hormone release in man. *J Clin Invest* 47:2143, 1968.
77. Szatalowicz VL, Arnold PE, Chaimovitz C, Bichet D, Berl T, Schrier RW: Radioimmunoassay of plasma arginine vasopressin in hyponatremic patients with congestive heart failure. *N Engl J Med* 305:263, 1981.
78. Riegger GAJ, Liebau G, Kochsie K: Antidiuretic hormone in congestive heart failure. *Am J Med* 72:49, 1982.
79. Wiggins RC, Basar I, Slater JDH, Forsling M, Ramage CM: Vasovagal hypotension and vasopressin release. *Clin Endocrinol (Oxf)* 6:387, 1977.
80. Baylis PH, Heath DA: Influence of presyncope and postural change upon plasma vasopressin concentration in hydrated and dehydrated man. *Clin Endocrinol (Oxf)* 7:79, 1977.
81. Zerbe RL, Henry DP, Robertson GL: Vasopressin response to orthostatic hypotension: Etiological and clinical implications. *Am J Med* 74(2):265, 1983.
82. Quillen EW Jr, Crowley AW Jr: Influence of volume changes in osmolality-vasopressin relationships in conscious dogs. *Am J Physiol* 244:H73, 1983.
83. Leimbach WN, Schmid PG, Mark AL: Baroreflex control of plasma arginine vasopressin in humans. *Am J Physiol* 247 (*Heart Circ Physiol* 16):H638, 1984.
84. Wang BC, Sundet WD, Hakumaki MOK, Geer PG, Goetz KL: Cardiac receptor influences on the plasma osmolality–plasma vasopressin relationship. *Am J Physiol* 246(15):-H360, 1984.
85. Weiss NM, Robertson G, Byun K: The effect of hypovolemia on the osmoregulation of thirst and AVP. *Clin Res* 32(4):786A, 1984.
86. Moses AM, Miller M, Streeten DHP: Quantitative influence of blood volume expansion on the osmotic threshold for vasopressin release. *J Clin Endocrinol Metab* 27:655, 1967.
87. Moses AM, Miller M: Osmotic threshold for vasopressin release as determined by saline infusion and by dehydration. *Neuroendocrinology* 7:219, 1971.
88. Rowe JW, Shelton RL, Helderman JH, Vestal RE, Robertson GL: Influence of the emetic reflex on vasopressin release in man. *Kidney Int* 16:729, 1979.
89. Coutinho EM: Oxytocic and antidiuretic effects of nausea in women. *Am J Obstet Gynecol* 105:127, 1969.
90. Verbalis JG, McHale CM, Gardiner TW, Stricker EM: Oxytocin and vasopressin secretion in response to stimuli producing learned taste aversions in rats. *Behav Neurosci* 100:466, 1986.
91. DeFronzo RA, Braine H, Colvin OM, Davis PJ: Water intoxication in man after cyclophosphamide therapy: Time course and relation to drug activation. *Ann Intern Med* 78:861, 1973.
92. Steele TH, Serpick AA, Block JB: Antidiuretic response to cyclophosphamide in man. *J Pharmacol Exp Ther* 185:245, 1973.

93. Heyes MP, Farber MO, Manfredi F, Robertshaw D, Weinberger M, Fineberg N, Robertson G: Acute effects of hypoxia on renal and endocrine function in normal man. *Am J Physiol* 243:R265, 1982.
94. Eversmann T, Guttsmann M, Uhlich E, Ulbrecht G, von Werder K, Scriba PC: Increased secretion of growth hormone, prolactin, antidiuretic hormone and cortisol induced by the stress of motion sickness. *Aviat Space Environ Med* 49:53, 1978.
95. Baylis PH, Heath DA: Plasma-arginine-vasopressin response to insulin-induced hypoglycemia. *Lancet* 2:428, 1977.
96. Baylis PH, Robertson GL: Rat vasopressin response to insulin-induced hypoglycemia. *Endocrinology* 107:1975, 1980.
97. Baylis PH, Zerbe RL, Robertson GL: Arginine vasopressin response to insulin-induced hypoglycemia in man. *J Clin Endocrinol Metab* 53:935, 1981.
98. Keller-Wood ME, Wade CE, Shinsako J, Keil LC, Van Loon GR, Dallman MF: Insulin-induced hypoglycemia in conscious dogs: Effects of maintaining carotid arterial glucose levels on the adrenocorticotropin, epinephrine and vasopressin responses. *Endocrinology* 112(2):624, 1982.
99. Baylis PH, Robertson GL: Vasopressin response to 2-deoxy-D-glucose in the rat. *Endocrinology* 107:1970, 1980.
100. Thompson DA, Cambell RG, Lilavivat U, Welle SL, Robertson GL: Increased thirst and plasma arginine vasopressin levels during 2-deoxy-D-glucose-induced glucoprivation in humans. *J Clin Invest* 67:1083, 1981.
101. Bonjour JP, Malvin RL: Stimulation of ADH release by the renin-angiotensin system. *Am J Physiol* 218:1555, 1970.
102. Mouw D, Bonjour JP, Malvin RL, Vander A: Central action of angiotensin in stimulating ADH release. *Am J Physiol* 220:239, 1971.
103. Yamaguchi K, Sakaguchi T, Kamoi K: Central role of angiotensin in the hyperosmolality- and hypovolaemia-induced vasopressin release in conscious rats. *Acta Endocrinol (Copenh)* 101:524, 1982.
104. Shimizu K, Share L, Claybaugh JR: Potentiation of angiotensin II of the vasopressin response to an increasing plasma osmolality. *Endocrinology* 93:42, 1973.
105. Cadnapaphornchai P, Boykin J, Harbottle JA, McDonald KM, Schrier RW: Effect of angiotensin II on renal water excretion. *Am J Physiol* 228:155, 1975.
106. Rydin H, Verney EB: The inhibition of water-diuresis by emotional stress and by muscular exercise. *Q J Exp Physiol* 27:343, 1938.
107. Edelson JT, Robertson GL: The effect of the cold pressor test on vasopressin secretion in man. *Psychoneuroendocrinology* 11:307, 1986.
108. Punnonen R, Teisala K, Hakkinen V, Viinamaki O, Pystynen P: Vasopressin and prolactin as stress hormones. *Gynecol Obstet Invest* 21:76, 1986.
109. Lang RE, Heil JWE, Ganten D, Hermann K, Unger T, Rascher W: Oxytocin unlike vasopressin is a stress hormone in the rat. *Neuroendocrinology* 37:314, 1983.
110. Ukai M, Moran WH, Zimmerman B: The role of visceral afferent pathways in vasopressin secretion and urinary excretory patterns during surgical stress. *Ann Surg* 168:16, 1968.
111. Baylis PH, Stockley RA, Heath DA: Effect of acute hypoxemia on plasma arginine vasopressin in conscious man. *Clin Sci Mol Med* 53:401, 1977.
112. Raff H, Shinsako J, Keil LC, Dallman MF: Vasopressin, ACTH, and corticosteroids during hypercapnia and graded hypoxia in dogs. *Am J Physiol* 244:E453, 1983.
113. Rose CE Jr, Anderson RJ, Carey RM: Antidiuresis and vasopressin release with hypoxemia and hypercapnia in conscious dogs. *Am J Physiol* 247:R127, 1984.
114. Raff H, Shinsako J, Keil LC, Dallman MF: Vasopressin, ACTH, and blood pressure during hypoxia induced at different rates. *Am J Physiol* 245:E489, 1983.
115. Farber MO, Weinberg MH, Robertson GL, Fineberg NS, Manfredi F: Hormonal abnormalities affecting sodium and water balance in acute respiratory failure due to chronic obstructive lung disease. *Chest* 85(1):49, 1984.
116. Miller M, Moses AM: Drug-induced states of impaired water excretion. *Kidney Int* 10:96, 1976.
117. McDonald KM, Miller PD, Anderson RJ, Berl T, Schrier RW: Hormonal control of renal water excretion. *Kidney Int* 10:38, 1976.
118. Rockhold RW, Crofton JT, Wang BC, Share L: Effect of intracarotid administration of morphine and naloxone on plasma vasopressin levels and blood pressure in the dog. *J Pharmacol Exp Ther* 224(2):386, 1982.
119. Ukai M, Nagase T, Hirohashi M, Yanaihara N: Antidiuretic activities of substance P and its analogs. *Experientia* 37:521, 1981.
120. Robertson GL, Bhoopalam N, Zelkowitz LJ: Vincristine neurotoxicity and abnormal secretion of antidiuretic hormone. *Arch Intern Med* 132:717, 1973.
121. Gold PW, Robertson GL, Post RM, Kaye W, Ballenger J, Rubinow D, Goodwin FK: The effect of lithium on the osmoregulation of arginine vasopressin secretion. *J Clin Endocrinol Metab* 56(2):295, 1983.
122. Miller PD, Dubovsky SL, McDonald KM, Katz FJ, Robertson GL, Schrier RW: Central, renal and adrenal effects of lithium in man. *Am J Med* 66:797, 1979.
123. Padfield PL, Park SJ, Morton JJ, Braidwood AE: Plasma levels of antidiuretic hormone in patients receiving prolonged lithium therapy. *Br J Psychiatry* 130:144, 1977.
124. Byun KY, Gaskill MB, Robertson GL: The mechanism of chlorpropamide antidiuresis in diabetes insipidus. *Clin Res* 32:483A, 1984.
125. Moses AM, Howanitz J, van Gemert M, Miller M: Clofibrate-induced antidiuresis. *J Clin Invest* 52:535, 1973.
126. Moses AM, Numann P, Miller M: Mechanism of chlorpropamide-induced antidiuresis in man: Evidence for release of ADH and enhancement of peripheral action. *Metabolism* 22:59, 1973.
127. Pockracki FJ, Robinson AG, Seif SM: Chlorpropamide effect: Measurement of neurophysin and vasopressin in humans and rats. *Metabolism* 30:72, 1978.
128. Gold PW, Robertson GL, Ballenger JC, Kaye W, Chen J, Rubinow DR, Goodwin FK, Post RM: Carbamazepine diminishes the sensitivity of the plasma arginine vasopressin response to osmotic stimulation. *J Clin Endocrinol Metab* 57(5):952, 1983.
129. Stephens WP, Coe JY, Baylis PH: Plasma arginine vasopressin concentrations and antidiuretic action of carbamazepine. *Br Med J* 1:1445, 1978.
130. Thomas TH, Ball SG, Wales JK, Lee MR: Effect of carbamazepine on plasma and urine arginine-vasopressin. *Clin Sci Mol Med* 54:419, 1978.
131. Knepel W, Nutto D, Anhut H, Hertting G: Vasopressin and β-endorphin release after osmotic and non-osmotic stimuli: Effect of naloxone and dexamethasone. *Eur J Pharmacol* 77:299, 1982.
132. Robertson GL, Oiso Y, Vokes TP, Gaskill MB: Diprenorphine inhibits selectively the vasopressin response to hypovolemic stimuli. *Trans Assoc Am Physicians* XCVIII:322, 1985.
133. Forsling ML, Matziari C, Aziz L: A comparison of the vasopressin response of rats to intraperitoneal and intravenous administration of hypertonic saline, and the effect of opioid and aminergic antagonists. *J Endocrinol* 116:217, 1988.
134. Kamoi K, White K, Robertson GL: Opiates elevate the osmotic threshold for vasopressin (VP) release in rats. *Clin Res* 27:254A, 1979.
135. Miller M: Inhibition of ADH release in the rat by narcotic antagonists. *Neuroendocrinology* 19:241, 1975.
136. Van Wimersma Greidanus TB, Thody TJ, Verspaget H, deRotte GA, Goedemans HJH, Croiset G, van Ree JM: Effects of morphine and β-endorphin on basal and elevated

plasma levels of α-MSH and vasopressin. *Life Sci* 24:579, 1979.

137. Summy-Long JY, Keil LC, Deen K, Severs WB: Opiate regulation of angiotensin-induced drinking and vasopressin release. *J Pharmacol Exp Ther* 217:630, 1981.
138. Brownell J, del Pozo E, Donatsch P: Inhibition of vasopressin secretion by a met-enkephalin (FK 33-824) in humans. *Acta Endocrinol (Copenh)* 94(3):304, 1980.
139. Grossman A, Besser GM, Milles JJ, Baylis PH: Inhibition of vasopressin release in man by an opiate peptide. *Lancet* 2:1108, 1980.
140. Zerbe RL, Henry DP, Robertson GL: A new met-enkephalin analogue suppresses plasma vasopressin in man. *Peptides* 1:199, 1981.
141. Miller M: Role of endogenous opioids in neurohypophyseal function in man. *J Clin Endocrinol Metab* 50:1016, 1980.
142. Iwasaki Y, Gaskill MB, Robertson GL: Diprenorphine microinjected into parabrachial nucleus inhibits the vasopressin response to hypovolemic stimuli. *Clin Res* 38:86A, 1990.
143. Kleeman CR, Rubini ME, Lamdin E, Epstein FH: Studies on alcohol diuresis: II. The evaluation of ethyl alcohol as an inhibitor of the neurohypophysis. *J Clin Invest* 34(3):448, 1955.
144. Helderman JH, Vestal RE, Rowe JW, Tobin JD, Andres R, Robertson GL: The response of arginine vasopressin in intravenous ethanol and hypertonic saline in man: The impact of aging. *J Gerontol* 33:339, 1978.
145. Oiso Y, Robertson GL: Effect of ethanol on vasopressin secretion and the role of endogenous opioids, in Schrier R (ed): *Vasopressin*. New York, Raven, 1985, p 265–269.
146. Reid IA, Ahn JN, Trinh T, Schackelford R, Weintraub M, Keil LC: Mechanism of suppression of vasopressin and adrenocorticotropic hormone secretion by clonidine in anesthetized dogs. *J Pharmacol Exp Ther* 229(1):18, 1984.
147. Roman RJ, Cowley AW Jr, Lechene C: Water diuretic and natriuretic effect of clonidine in the rat. *J Pharmacol Exp Ther* 211:385, 1979.
148. Iovino M, De Caro G, Massi M, Steardo O, Poenaru S: Muscimol inhibits ADH release induced by hypertonic sodium chloride in rats. *Pharmacol Biochem Behav* 19:335, 1983.
149. Engel P, Rowe J, Minaker K, Robertson GL: Effect of exogenous vasopressin release. *Am J Physiol* 246(9):E202, 1984.
150. Wang BC, Share L, Crofton JT: Central infusion of vasopressin decreased plasma vasopressin concentration in dogs. *Am J Physiol* 243(6):E365, 1982.
151. Moos F, Freund-Mercier MJ, Guerne Y, Guerne JM, Stoeckel ME, Richard P: Release of oxytocin and vasopressin by magnocellular nuclei in vitro: Specific facilitatory effect of oxytocin on its own release. *J Endocrinol* 102:63, 1984.
152. Amico JA, Ervin MG, Leake RD, Fisher DA, Finn FM, Robinson AG: A novel oxytocin-like and vasotocin-like peptide in human plasma after administration of estrogen. *J Clin Endocrinol Metab* 60(1):5, 1985.
153. Fehr S, Ivell R, Koll R, Schams D, Fields M, Richter D: Expression of the oxytocin gene in the large cells of the bovine corpus luteum. *FEBS Lett* 210:45, 1987.
154. Nussey SS, Ang VTY, Finer N, Jenkins JS: Responses of neurohypophysial peptides to hypertonic saline and insulin-induced hypoglycaemia in man. *Clin Endocrinol (Oxf)* 24:97, 1986.
155. Lausen HD: Metabolism of the neurohypophyseal hormones, in Greep RO, Astwood EB, Knobil E, Sawyer WH, Geiger SR (eds): *Handbook of Physiology*. Washington, American Physiological Society, 1974, vol 4, pp 287–393.
156. Robertson GL, Mahr EA, Athar S, Sinha T: Development and clinical application of a new method for the radioimmunoassay of arginine vasopressin in human plasma. *J Clin Invest* 52(9):2340, 1973.
157. Davison JM, Sheills EA, Barron WM, Robinson AG, Lindheimer MD: Changes in the metabolic clearance of vasopressin and in plasma vasopressinase throughout human pregnancy. *J Clin Invest* 83:1313, 1989.
158. Sherman TG, McKelvy JF, Watson SJ: Vasopressin mRNA regulation in individual hypothalamic nuclei: A northern and in situ hybridization analysis. *J Neurosci* 6:1685, 1986.
159. Jenkins JS, Mather HM, Ang V: Vasopressin in human cerebrospinal fluid. *J Clin Endocrinol Metab* 59(2):364, 1980.
160. Dogterom J, van Wimersma Greidanus TB, de Weid D: Vasopressin in cerebrospinal fluid and plasma of man, dog and rat. *Am J Physiol* 234(5):E463, 1978.
161. Szczepanska-Sadowska E, Gray D, Simon-Opperman C: Vasopressin in blood and third ventricle CSF during dehydration, thirst and hemorrhage. *Am J Physiol* 245:R549, 1983.
162. Amico JA, Tenicela R, Robinson AG: Neurohypophysial hormones in cerebrospinal fluid of adults: Absence of arginine vasotocin and of a diurnal rhythm of arginine vasopressin. *J Clin Endocrinol Metab* 61:794, 1985.
163. Szczepanska-Sadowska E, Sobocinska J, Sadowski B: Central dipsogenic effect of vasopressin. *Am J Physiol* 242: R372, 1982.
164. De Wied D: Behavioral effects of intraventricularly administered vasopressin and vasopressin fragments. *Life Sci* 19:685, 1976.
165. Sorensen PS, Hammer M, Vorstrup S, Gjerris F: CSF and plasma vasopressin concentration in dementia. *J Neurol Neurosurg Psychiatry* 46:911, 1983.
166. Gold PW, Goodwin FK, Ballenger JC, Post RM, Weingartner H, Robertson GL: Central vasopressin function in affective illness. *Int J Ment Health* 9(3–4):91, 1981.
167. Sorensen PS, Hammer M, Gjerris F: Cerebrospinal fluid vasopressin in benign intracranial hypertension. *Neurology* 32:1255, 1982.
168. Teitelbaum I, Berl T, Kleeman CR: The physiology of the renal concentrating and diluting mechanisms, in Maxwell MH, Kleeman CR, Narins RG (ed): *Clinical Disorders of Fluid and Electrolyte Metabolism*. New York, McGraw-Hill, 1987 pp 79–103.
169. Lolait SJ, O'Carroll AM, McBride OW, Konig M, Morel A, Brownstein MJ: Cloning and characterization of a vasopressin V_2 receptor and possible link to nephrogenic diabetes insipidus. *Nature* 357:336, 1992.
170. Birnbaumer M, Seibold A, Gilbert S, Ishido M, Barberis C, Antaramian A, Brabet P, Rosenthal W: Molecular cloning of the receptor for human antidiuretic hormone. *Nature* 357:333, 1992.
171. Montani JP, Liard JF, Schoun J, Mohring J: Hemodynamic effects of exogenous and endogenous vasopressin at low plasma concentrations in dogs. *Circ Res* 47:346–355, 1980.
172. Graybiel A, Glendy RE: Circulatory effects following the intravenous administration of pitressin in normal persons and in patients with hypertension and angina pectoris. *Am Heart J* 21:481, 1941.
173. Bussien JP, Waeber B, Nussberger J, Schaller MD, Gavras H, Hofbauer K, Brunner HR: Does vasopressin sustain blood pressure of normally hydrated healthy volunteers? *Am J Physiol* 246 (*Heart Circ Physiol* 15):H143, 1984.
174. Suzuki S, Takeshita A, Imaisumi T, Hirooka Y, Yoshida M, Ando S, Nakamura M: Biphasic forearm vascular responses to intraarterial arginine vasopressin. *J Clin Invest* 84:427, 1989.
175. Cowley AW, Quillen EQ, Skelton MM: Role of vasopressin in cardiovascular regulation. *Fed Proc* 42:3170, 1983.
176. Share L, Crofton JT: The role of vasopressin in hypertension. *Fed Proc* 43:106, 1984.
177. Davies R, Forsling M, Bulger G, Phillips T: Plasma vasopressin and blood pressure studies in normal subjects and in benign essential hypertension at rest and after postural challenge. *Br Heart J* 49:428, 1983.
178. Thibonnier M, Sassano P, Daufresne S, Corvol P, Menard J:

Osmoregulation and renal effects of vasopressin in normal and mildly hypertensive subjects. *Kidney Int* 25:411, 1984.
179. Mohring J, Glanger K, Maciel JA, Dusing R, Kramer HJ, Arbogast R, Koch-Weser J: Greatly enhanced pressor response to antidiuretic hormone in patients with impaired cardiovascular reflexes due to idiopathic orthostatic hypotension. *J Cardiovasc Pharmacol* 2:367, 1980.
180. Liu JH, Muse K, Contreras P, Gibbs D, Vale W, Rivier J, Yeu SSC: Activation of ACTH-releasing activity of synthetic corticotropin releasing factor (CRF) by vasopressin in women. *J Clin Endocrinol Metab* 57:1087, 1983.
181. Rivier C, Vale W: Interaction of corticotropin releasing factor and arginine vasopressin on adrenocorticotropin secretion in vivo. *Endocrinology* 113:939, 1983.
182. Spinedi E, Negro-Vilar A: Angiotensin II and ACTH release: Site of actin and potency relative to corticotropin releasing factor and vasopressin. *Neuroendocrinology* 37:446, 1983.
183. Jard S, Gaillard RC, Guillon G, Marie J, Schoenenberg P, Muller AF, Manning M, Sawyer WH: Vasopressin antagonists allow demonstration of a novel type of vasopressin receptor in the rat adenohypophysis. *Mol Pharmacol* 30:171, 1986.
184. McCann SM, Antunes-Rodrigues J, Nallar R, Valtin H: Pituitary adrenal function in the absence of vasopressin. *Endocrinology* 76:1058, 1966.
185. Arimura A, Saito T, Bowers CY, Schally AV: Pituitary adrenal activation in rats with hereditary hypothalamic diabetes insipidus. *Acta Endocrinol (Copenh)* 54:155, 1967.
186. Carlson DE, Gann DS: Effect of vasopressin antiserum on the response of adrenocorticotropin and cortisol to hemorrhage. *Endocrinology* 114:317, 1984.
187. Dicker SE, Nunn JE: The role of the antidiuretic hormone during water deprivation in rats. *J Physiol* 136:235, 1957.
188. Gaskill MB, Reilly M, Robertson GL: Vasopressin decreases insensible water loss. *Clin Res* 31:780A, 1983.
189. Schapiro H: Inhibiting action of antidiuretic hormone on canine pancreatic exocrine flow. *Am J Digest Dis* 20:853, 1975.
190. Heims DA, Whitton PD, Ma GY: Metabolic actions of vasopressin, glucagon and adrenalin in the intact rat. *Biochim Biophys Acta* 411:155, 1975.
191. Grant JA, Scrutton MC: Positive interaction between agonists in the aggregation response of human blood platelets: Interaction between ADP, adrenaline and vasopressin. *Br J Haematol* 44:109, 1980.
192. Amico JA: Diabetes insipidus and pregnancy. *Front Horm Res* 13:266, 1985.
193. Amico JA, Seitchik J, Robinson AG: Studies of oxytocin in plasma of women during hypocontractile labor. *J Clin Endocrinol Metab* 58:274, 1984.
194. Kelley S, Robertson GL, Amico JA: Antidiuretic action of oxytocin in humans. *Clin Res* 40:711A, 1992.
195. Edwards BR, LaRochelle T: Antidiuretic effect of endogenous oxytocin in dehydrated brattleboro homozygous rats. *Am J Physiol* 247 (*Renal Fluid Electrolyte Physiol* 16):F453, 1984.
196. Ramsay DJ: Water: Distribution between compartments and its relationship to thirst, in Ramsay DJ, Booth DA (eds): *Thirst—Physiological and Psychological Aspects*. London, Springer-Verlag, 1990, pp 23–52.
197. Robertson GL: Disorders of thirst in man, in Ramsay DJ, Booth DA (eds): *Thirst—Physiological and Psychological Aspects*. London, Springer-Verlag, 1990, pp 453–475.
198. Rolls BJ: Physiological determinants of fluid intake in humans, in Ramsay DJ, Booth DA (eds): *Thirst—Physiological and Psychological Aspects*. London, Springer-Verlag, 1990, pp 391–398.
199. Verbalis JG: Inhibitory controls of drinking: Satiation of thirst, in Ramsay DJ, Booth DA (eds): *Thirst—Physiological and Psychological Aspects*. London, Springer-Verlag, 1990, pp 313–330.
200. Kovacs L, Rittig S, Robertson GL: Effects of sustained antidiuretic treatment on plasma sodium concentration and body water homeostasis in healthy humans on ad libitum-fluid intake. *Clin Res* 40:165A, 1992.
201. McKinley MJ: Osmoreceptor for thirst, in Ramsay DJ, Booth DA (eds): *Thirst—Physiological and Psychological Aspects*. London, Springer-Verlag, 1990, pp 77–91.
202. Johnson AK, Edwards GL: Central projections of osmotic and hypovolaemic signals in homeostatic thirst, in Ramsay DJ, Booth DA (eds): *Thirst—Physiological and Psychological Aspects*. London, Springer-Verlag, 1990, pp 149–168.
203. Thrasher TN: Volume receptors and the stimulation of water intake, in Ramsay DJ, Booth DA (eds): *Thirst—Physiological and Psychological Aspects*. London, Springer-Verlag, 1990, pp 93–107.
204. Kozlowski S, Szczepanska-Sadowska E: Antagonistic effects of vasopressin and hypervolemia on osmotic reactivity of the thirst mechanism in dogs. *Pflugers Arch* 353:59, 1975.
205. Szczepanska-Sadowska E: Hormonal inputs to thirst, in Ramsay DJ, Booth DA (eds): *Thirst—Physiological and Psychological Aspects*. London, Springer-Verlag, 1990, pp 110–125.
206. Oldfield BJ: Neurochemistry of the circuitry subserving thirst, in Ramsay DJ, Booth DA (eds): *Thirst—Physiological and Psychological Aspects*. London, Springer-Verlag, 1990, pp 176–188.
207. Stricker EM: Central control of water and sodium chloride intake in rats during hypovolaemia, in Ramsay DJ, Booth DA (eds): *Thirst—Physiological and Psychological Aspects*. London: Springer-Verlag, 1990, pp 194–203.
208. Altman PL, Dittmer DS (eds): *Blood and Other Body Fluids*. Washington, American Society of Experimental Biology, 1961.
209. Robertson GL, Berl T: Water metabolism, in Brenner BM, Rector FC (eds): *The Kidney*, 3d ed. Philadelphia, Saunders, 1985, pp 385–432.
210. Leaf A, Chatillon JY, Wrong O, Tuttle EP Jr: The mechanism of the osmotic adjustment of body cells as determined in vivo by the volume of distribution of a large waterload. *J Clin Invest* 33:1261, 1954.
211. Wolf AV, McDowell ME: Apparent and osmotic volumes of distribution of sodium, chloride, sulfate and urea. *Am J Physiol* 176:207, 1954.
212. Hendry EB: Osmolarity of human serum and of chemical solutions of biologic importance. *Clin Chem* 7:156, 1961.
213. Darrow DC, Yanett H: Changes in distribution of body water accompanying increase and decrease in extracellular electrolytes. *J Clin Invest* 14:266, 1935.
214. Arieff AI, Guisado R, Lazarowitz VC: Pathophysiology of hyperosmolar states, in Andreoli TE, Grantham JJ, and Rector FC (eds): *Disturbances in Body Fluid Osmolality*. Bethesda, American Physiological Society, 1977, pp 227–250.
215. Adolph EF: *Physiology of Man in the Desert*. New York, Hafner, 1969.
216. Coggins CH, Leaf A: Diabetes insipidus. *Am J Med* 42:807, 1967.
217. Maccubbin DA, Van Buren JM: A quantitative evaluation of hypothalamic degeneration and its relation to diabetes insipidus following interruption of the human hypophyseal stalk. *Brain* 46:443, 1963.
218. Randall RV, Clark EC, Dodge HW Jr, Love JG: Polyuria after operation for tumors in the region of the hypophysis and hypothalamus. *J Clin Endocrinol Metab* 20:1614, 1960.
219. Timmons RL, Dugger GS: Water and salt metabolism following pituitary stalk section. *Neurology* 19:790, 1969.
220. Notman DD, Mortek MA, Moses AM: Permanent diabetes insipidus following head trauma: Observations on ten patients and an approach to diagnosis. *J Trauma* 20(7):599, 1980.

221. Kern KB, Meislin HW: Diabetes insipidus: Occurrence after minor head trauma. *J Trauma* 24:69, 1984.
222. Kimmel DW, O'Neill BP: Systemic cancer presenting as diabetes insipidus. *Cancer* 52:2355, 1983.
223. De Le Chapelle A, Lahtinen R: Monosomy 7 predisposes to diabetes insipidus in leukaemia and myelodysplastic syndrome. *Eur J Haematol* 39:404, 1987.
224. Winnacker JL, Becker KL, Katz S: Endocrine aspects of sarcoidosis. *N Engl J Med* 278(9):483, 1968.
225. Halprin KM, Lorincz AL: Disseminated xanthosiderohistiocytosis (Xanthoma disseminatum). *Arch Dermatol* 82(2):171, 1960.
226. Greger NG, Kirkland RT, Clayton GW, Kirkland JL: Central diabetes insipidus. *Am J Dis Child* 140:551, 1986.
227. Iwasaki Y, Oiso Y, Yamauchi K, Takatsuki K, Kondo K, Hasegawa H, Itatsu T, Niinomi M, Tomita A: Neurohypophyseal function in postpartum hypopituitarism: Impaired plasma vasopressin response to osmotic stimuli. *J Clin Endocrinol Metab* 68:560, 1989.
228. Blotner H: Primary or idiopathic diabetes insipidus: A system disease. *Metabolism* 7:191, 1958.
229. Braverman LE, Mancini JP, McGoldrick DM: Hereditary idiopathic diabetes insipidus: A case report with autopsy findings. *Ann Intern Med* 63(3):503, 1965.
230. Green JR, Buchan GC, Alvord EC Jr, Swanson AG: Hereditary and idiopathic types of diabetes insipidus. *Brain* 90(3):707, 1967.
231. Forssman H: On hereditary diabetes insipidus. *Acta Med Scand* 159(suppl):1, 1945.
232. Martin FIR: Familial diabetes insipidus. *Q J Med* 28:573, 1959.
233. Meinders AE, Bijlsma JB: A family with congenital hypothalamic neurohypophyseal diabetes insipidus. *Folia Med Neerl* 13:68, 1970.
234. Andersson KE, Arner B, Furst E, Hedner P: Antidiuretic responses to hypertonic saline infusion, water deprivation and a synthetic analogue of vasopressin in patients with hereditary, hypothalamic diabetes insipidus. *Acta Med Scand* 195:17, 1974.
235. Baylis PH, Robertson GL: Vasopressin function in familial cranial diabetes insipidus. *Postgrad Med J* 57:36, 1981.
236. Kaplowitz PB, D'Ercole AJ, Robertson GL: Radioimmunoassay of vasopressin in familial central diabetes insipidus. *Pediatrics* 100:76, 1982.
237. Toth EL, Bowen PA, Crockford PM: Hereditary central diabetes insipidus: Plasma levels of antidiuretic hormone in a family with a possible osmoreceptor defect. *Can Med Assoc J* 131:1237, 1984.
238. Aakesson IOI, Enger E: Plasma vasopressin in hereditary cranial diabetes insipidus. *Acta Med Scand* 217:429, 1985.
239. Pedersen EB, Lamm LU, Albertsen K, Madsen M, Bruunpetersen G, Henningsen K, Friedrich U, Magnusson K: Familial cranial diabetes insipidus: A report of five families: Genetic, diagnostic and therapeutic aspects. *Q J Med* 57:883, 1985.
240. Repaske DR, Phillips III JA, Kirby LT, Tze WJ, D'Ercole AJ, Battey J: Molecular analysis of autosomal dominant neurohypophyseal diabetes insipidus. *J Clin Endocrinol Metab* 70:752, 1990.
241. Ito M, Mori Y, Oiso Y, Saito H: A single base substitution inthe coding region for neurophysin II associated with familial central diabetes insipidus. *J Clin Invest* 87:725, 1991.
242. Bahnsen U, Oosting P, Swaab DF, Nahke P, Richter D, Schamale H: A missense mutation in the vasopressin–neurophysin precursor gene cosegregates with human autosomal dominant neurohypophyseal diabetes insipidus. *EMBO J* 11:19, 1992.
243. Kovacs L, McLeod JF, Rittig S, Gaskill MB, Bradley G, Cox N, Robertson GL: A single base substitution in exon 1 of the vasopressin-neurophysin II gene is linked to familial neurogenic diabetes insipidus in a caucasian kindred, abstract 111. *Am J Hum Genet* 51(suppl):30A, 1992.
244. Cremers CWRJ, Wijdeveld PGAB, Pinckers AJLG: Juvenile diabetes mellitus, optic atrophy, hearing loss, diabetes insipidus, atonia of the urinary tract and bladder, and other abnormalities (Wolfram syndrome). *Acta Paediatr Scand* 264:3, 1977.
245. Forssman H: Two different mutations of X-chromosome causing diabetes insipidus. *Am J Hum Genet* 7:21, 1955.
246. Robertson GL, Scheidler JA: A newly recognized variant of familial nephrogenic diabetes insipidus distinguished by partial resistance to vasopressin (type II). *Clin Res* 29:555A, 1981.
247. Schaff-Blass E, Robertson GL, Rosenfield RL: Chronic hypernatremia resulting from a congenital defect in osmoregulation of thirst and vasopressin. *J Pediatr* 102(5):703, 1983.
248. Yamamoto T, Shimizu M, Fukuyama J, Yamaji T: Pathogenesis of extracellular fluid abnormalities of hypothalamic hypodipsia-hypernatremia syndrome. *Endocrinol Jpn* 35:915, 1988.
249. Kovacs L, Robertson GL: Disorders of water balance—hyponatraemia and hypernatraemia. *Br Clin Endocrinol Metab* 6:107, 1992.
250. Hammond DN, Moll GW, Robertson GL, Chelmicka-Schorr E: Hypodipsic hypernatremia with normal osmoregulation of vasopressin. *N Engl J Med* 315:433, 1986.
251. Robertson GL: Dipsogenic diabetes insipidus: A newly recognized syndrome caused by a selective defect in the osmoregulation of thirst. *Trans Assoc Am Physicians* C:241, 1987.
252. Stuart CA, Neelon FA, Lebovitz HE: Disordered control of thirst in hypothalamic-pituitary sarcoidosis. *N Engl J Med* 303:1078, 1980.
253. Sleeper FH, Jellinek EM: A comparative physiologic, psychologic and psychiatric study of polyuric and nonpolyuric schizophrenic patients. *J Nerv Ment Dis* 83:557, 1936.
254. Barlow ED, de Wardener HED: Compulsive water drinking. *Q J Med* 28:235, 1959.
255. Kirch DG, Bigelow LB, Weinberger DR, Lawson WB, Wyatt RJ: Polydipsia and chronic hyponatremia in schizophrenic inpatients. *J Clin Psychiatry* 46:179, 1985.
256. Illowsky BP, Kirch DG: Polydipsia and hyponatremia in psychiatric patients. *Am J Psychiatry* 145:675, 1988.
257. Goldman MB, Luchins DJ, Robertson GL: Mechanisms of altered water metabolism in psychotic patients with polydipsia and hyponatremia. *N Engl J Med* 318:397, 1988.
258. Coscina DV, Grant LD, Balagura S, Grossman SP: Hyperdipsia after serotonin-depleting midbrain lesions. *Nature [New Biol]* 235:53, 1972.
259. Blass EM, Nussbaum AI: Specific enhancement of drinking to angiotensin in rats. *J Comp Physiol Psychol* 87(3):422, 1974.
260. Gardiner TW, Stricker EM: Hyperdipsia in rats after electrolytic lesions of nucleus medianus. *Am J Physiol* 248 (*Regulatory Integrative Comp Physiol* 17):R214, 1985.
261. Bode HH, Crawford JD: Nephrogenic diabetes insipidus in North America—the Hopewell hypothesis. *N Engl J Med* 280(14):750, 1969.
262. Knoers N, Van der Heyden H, van Oost BA, Ropers HH, Monnens L, Willems J: Nephrogenic diabetes insipidus: Close linkage with markers from the distal long arm of the human x chromosome. *J Hum Genet* 80:31, 1988.
263. Kambouris M, Dlouhy SR, Trofatter JA, Conneally PM, Hodes ME: Localization of the gene for x-linked nephrogenic diabetes insipidus to xq28. *Am J Med Genet* 29:239, 1988.
264. Bichet DG, Hendy GN, Lonergan M, Arthus MF, Ligier S, Pausova Z, Kluge R, Zingg H, et al: X-linked nephrogenic diabetes insipidus: From the ship Hopewell to RFLP studies. *Am J Hum Genet* 51:1089, 1992.
265a. Rosenthal W, Seibold A, Antaramian A, Lonergan M,

Arthus MF, Hendy GN, Birnbaumer M, Bichet DQ: Molecular identification of the gene responsible for congenital nephrogenic diabetes insipidus. *Nature* 359:233, 1992.
265b. Pan Y, Metzenberg A, Das S, Jing B, Gitschier J: Mutations in the V2 vasopressin receptor gene are associated with x-linked nephrogenic diabetes insipidus. *Nature Genet* 2:103, 1992.
265c. Davies K: Diabetes defect defined. *Nature* 359:434, 1992.
266. Singer I, Forrest JN Jr: Drug-induced states of nephrogenic diabetes insipidus. *Kidney Int* 10:82, 1976.
267. Dürr JA, Hoggard JG, Hunt JM, Schrier RW: Diabetes insipidus in pregnancy associated with abnormally high circulating vasopressinase activity. *N Engl J Med* 316: 1070, 1987.
268. Iwasaki Y, Oiso Y, Kondo K, Takagi S, Takatsuki K, Hasegawa H, Ishikawa F, Fujimura Y, et al: Aggravation of subclinical diabetes insipidus during pregnancy. *N Engl J Med* 324:522, 1991.
269. Lipsett MB, Pearson OH: Further studies of diabetes insipidus following hypophysectomy in man. *J Lab Clin Med* 49:190, 1957.
270. Miller M, Dalakos T, Moses AM, Fellerman H: Recognition of partial defects in antidiuretic hormone secretion. *Ann Intern Med* 73:721, 1970.
271. Zerbe RL, Robertson GL: A comparison of plasma vasopressin measurements with a standard indirect test in the differential diagnosis of polyuria. *N Engl J Med* 305:1539, 1981.
272. Robertson GL: Osmoregulation of thirst and vasopressin secretion: Functional properties and their relationship to water balance, in Schrier R (ed): *Vasopressin*. New York, Raven, 1985, pp 202–212.
273. Epstein FH, Kleeman CR, Hendrikx A: The influence of bodily hydration on the renal concentrating process. *J Clin Invest* 36:629, 1957.
274. De Wardener HE, Herxheimer A: The effect of high water intake on the kidney's ability to concentrate the urine in man. *J Physiol (Lond)* 139:42, 1957.
275. Alexander CS, Filbin DM, Fruchtman SA: Failure of vasopressin to produce normal urine concentration in patients with diabetes insipidus. *J Lab Clin Med* 54:566, 1959.
276. Harrington AR, Valtin H: Impaired urinary concentration after vasopressin and its gradual correction in hypothalamic diabetes insipidus. *J Clin Invest* 47:502, 1968.
277. Robertson GL: Differential diagnosis of polyuria. *Annu Rev Med* 39:425, 1988.
278. Robertson GL, Aycinena P: Neurogenic disorders of osmoregulation. *Am J Med* 72:339, 1982.
279. Opas LM, Adler R, Robinson R, Lieberman E: Rhabdomyolysis with severe hypernatremia. *J Pediatr* 90(5):713, 1977.
280. Zierler KL: Hyperosmolarity in adults: A critical review. *J Chronic Dis* 7(1):1, 1958.
281. Simon RP, Freedman DD: Neurologic manifestations of osmolar disorders. *Geriatrics* p 71, June 1980.
282. Sparacio RR, Anziska B, Schutta HS: Hypernatremia and chorea: A report of two cases. *Neurology* 26:46, 1976.
283. Welt LG: Hypo- and hypernatremia. *Ann Intern Med* 56(1):161, 1962.
284. Smith WO, Clark ML: Self-induced water intoxication in schizophrenic patients. *Am J Psychiatry* 137(9):1055, 1980.
285. Hariprasad MK, Eisinger RP, Nadler IM, Padmanabhan CS, Nidus BD: Hyponatremia in psychogenic polydipsia. *Arch Intern Med* 140:1639, 1980.
286. Rosenbaum JF, Rothman JS, Murray GB: Psychosis and water intoxication. *J Clin Psychiatry* 40:287, 1979.
287. Raskind MA, Orenstein H, Christopher TG: Acute psychosis, increased water ingestion and inappropriate antidiuretic hormone secretion. *Am J Psychiatry* 132(9):907, 1975.
288. Robertson GL: Psychogenic polydipsia and inappropriate antidiuresis. *Arch Intern Med* 140:1574, 1980.
289. Verbalis JG, Dohanics J: Vasopressin and oxytocin secretion in chronically hyposmolar rats. *Am J Physiol* 261 (*Regulatory Integrative Comp Physiol* 30):R1028, 1991.
290. Weiss NM, Robertson GL: Effect of hypercalcemia and lithium therapy on the osmoregulation of thirst and vasopressin secretion, in Schrier R (ed): *Vasopressin*. New York, Raven, 1985, pp 281–289.
291. Dashe AM, Cramm RE, Crist CA, Habener JF, Solomon DH: A water deprivation test for the differential diagnosis of polyuria. *JAMA* 185(9):699, 1963.
292. Miller M, Moses AM: Urinary antidiuretic hormone in polyuric disorders and in inappropriate ADH syndrome. *Ann Intern Med* 77:715, 1972.
293. Baylis PH, Gaskill MB, Robertson GL: Vasopressin secretion in primary polydipsia and cranial diabetes insipidus. *Q J Med* 199:345, 1981.
294. Milles JJ, Spruce B, Baylis PH: A comparison of diagnostic methods to differentiate diabetes insipidus from primary polyuria: A review of 21 patients. *Acta Endocrinol (Copenh)* 104:410, 1983.
295. Fujisawa I, Nishimura K, Asato R, Togashi K, Itoh K, Noma S, Kawamura Y, Sago T, et al: Posterior lobe of the pituitary in diabetes insipidus: MR findings. *J Comput Assist Tomogr* 2:221, 1987.
296. Tien R, Kucharczyk J, Kucharczyk W: MR imaging of the brain in patients with diabetes insipidus. *AJNR* 12:533, 1991.
297. Brooks BS, Gammal TE, Allison JD, Hoffman WH: Frequency and variation of the posterior pituitary bright signal on MR images. *AJNR* 10:943, 1989.
298. Cox TD, Elster AD: Normal pituitary gland: Changes in shape, size, and signal intensity during the 1st year of life at MR imaging. *Pediatr Radiol* 179:721, 1991.
299. Skillern PG, Corcoran AC, Scherbel AL: Renal mechanisms in coincident Addison's disease and diabetes insipidus: Effects of vasopressin and hydrocortisone. *J Clin Endocrinol Metab* 16(2):171, 1956.
300. Martin MM: Combined anterior pituitary and neurohypophyseal insufficiency: Studies of body fluid spaces and renal function. *J Clin Invest* 38(6):882, 1958.
301. Takeda R, Hiraiwa Y, Hayashi T, Yasuhara S, Yanase E, Sakoto T, Nakabayashi H, Takegoshi T, et al: Spontaneous remission of cranial diabetes insipidus due to concomitant development of ADH-producing lung cancer—an autopsied case. *Acta Endocrinol (Copenh)* 104:417, 1983.
302. Vokes TJ, Gaskill MB, Robertson GL: Antibodies to vasopressin in patients with diabetes insipidus: Implications for diagnosis and therapy. *Ann Intern Med* 108:190, 1988.
303. Richardson DW, Robinson AG: Desmopressin. *Ann Intern Med* 103:228, 1985.
304. Arduino F, Ferraz FPJ, Rodriques J: Antidiuretic action of chlorpropamide in idiopathic diabetes insipidus. *J Clin Endocrinol Metab* 26:1325, 1966.
305. Webster B, Bain J: Antidiuretic effect and complications of chlorpropamide therapy in diabetes insipidus. *J Clin Endocrinol Metab* 30(2):215, 1970.
306. Weissman PN, Shenkman L, Gregerman RI: Chlorpropamide hyponatremia: Drug-induced inappropriate antidiuretic-hormone activity. *N Engl J Med* 284(2):65, 1971.
307. Hayes JS, Kaye M: Inappropriate secretion of antidiuretic hormone induced by chlorpropamide. *Am J Med* 263(3):137, 1972.
308. Garcia M, Miller M, Moses AM: Chlorpropamide-induced water retention in patients with diabetes mellitus. *Ann Intern Med* 75:549, 1971.
309. Mendoza SA, Brown CF Jr: Effect of chlorpropamide on osmotic water flow across toad bladder and the response to vasopressin, theophylline and cyclic AMP. *J Clin Endocrinol Metab* 388:883, 1974.
310. Berndt WO, Miller M, Kettyle M, Valtin H: Potentiation of the antidiuretic effect of vasopressin by chlorpropamide. *Endocrinology* 86(5):1028, 1970.

311. Miller M, Moses AM: Potentiation of vasopressin action by chlorpropamide in vivo. *Endocrinology* 86(5):1024, 1970.
312. Murase T, Yoshida S: Mechanism of chlorpropamide action in patients with diabetes insipidus. *J Clin Endocrinol Metab* 36:174, 1973.
313. Ingelfinger JR, Hays RM: Evidence that chlorpropamide and vasopressin share a common site of action. *J Clin Endocrinol Metab* 29:738, 1969.
314. Meinders AE, Van Leeuwen AM, Borst JGG, Cejka V: Paradoxical diuresis after vasopressin administration to patients with neurohypophyseal diabetes insipidus treated with chlorpropamide, carbamazepine or clofibrate. *Clin Sci Mol Med* 49:283, 1975.
315. de Gennes JL, Bertrand C, Bigorie B, Truffert J: Etudes preliminaires de l'action antidiuretique du clofibrate (ou atromid S) dans le diabète insipide pitressonsensible. *Ann Endocrinol (Copenh)* 31:300, 1970.
316. Thompson P Jr, Earll JM, Schaaf M: Comparison of clofibrate and chlorpropamide in vasopressin-responsive diabetes insipidus. *Metabolism* 26(7):749, 1977.
317. Earley LE, Orloff J: The mechanism of antidiuresis associated with administration of hydrochlorothiazide to patients with vasopressin resistant diabetes insipidus. *J Clin Invest* 41:1988, 1962.
318. Sekowski J, Samuel P: Clofibrate-induced acute muscular syndrome. *Am J Cardiol* 30:572, 1972.
319. Bichet D, Schrier RW: Water metabolism in edematous disorders. *Semin Nephrol* 4:325, 1984.
320. Takasic T, Lasker N, Shalhouh RJ: Mechanisms of hyponatremia in chronic congestive heart failure. *Ann Intern Med* 55:368, 1961.
321. Pruszczynski W, Vahanian A, Ardaillou R, Acar J: Role of antidiuretic hormone in impaired water excretion of patients with congestive heart failure. *J Clin Endocrinol Metab* 58:599, 1984.
322. Uretsky BF, Verbalis JG, Generalovich T, Valdes A, Reddy PS: Plasma vasopressin response to osmotic and hemodynamic stimuli in heart failure. *Am J Physiol* 248:H396, 1985.
323. Earley LE, Sanders CA: The effect of changing serum osmolality on antidiuretic hormone release in certain patients with decompensated cirrhosis of the liver and low serum osmolality. *J Clin Invest* 38:545, 1959.
324. Fichman MP, Vorherr H, Kleeman CR, Tefler N: Diuretic induced hyponatremia. *Ann Intern Med* 75:853, 1971.
325. Friedman E, Shadel M, Halkin H, Farfel Z: Thiazide-induced hyponatremia: Reproducibility by single dose rechallenge and an analysis of pathogenesis. *Ann Intern Med* 110:24, 1989.
326. Berl T, Linas SL, Aisenbrey GA, Anderson RJ: On the mechanism of polyuria in potassium depletion: The role of polydipsia. *J Clin Invest* 60:620, 1977.
327. Rutecki GW, Cox JW, Robertson GL, Francisco LL, Ferris TF: Urinary concentrating ability and antidiuretic hormone responsiveness in the potassium depleted dog. *J Lab Clin Med* 100:53, 1982.
328. Kleeman CR, Maxwell MH, Rockney RE: Mechanisms of impaired water excretion in adrenal and pituitary insufficiency: I. The role of altered glomerular filtration rate and solute excretion. *J Clin Invest* 37:1799, 1958.
329. Dingman JF, Despointes RH: Adrenal steroid inhibition of vasopressin release from the neurohypophysis of normal subjects and patients with Addison's disease. *J Clin Invest* 39:1851, 1960.
330. Cutler RE, Kleeman CR, Koplowitz J, Maxwell MH, Dowling JT: Mechanisms of impaired water excretion in adrenal and pituitary insufficiency: III. The effect of extracellular or plasma volume expansion, or both, on the impaired diuresis. *J Clin Invest* 41:1524, 1962.
331. Gill JR, Gann DS, Bartter FC: Restoration of water diuresis in Addisonian patients by expansion of the volume of extracellular fluid. *J Clin Invest* 41:1078, 1962.
332. Kleeman CR, Czaczkes JW, Cutler R: Mechanisms of impaired water excretion in adrenal and pituitary insufficiency: IV. Antidiuretic hormone in primary and secondary adrenal insufficiency. *J Clin Invest* 43:1641, 1964.
333. Ahmed ABJ, George BC, Gonzalez-Auvert C, Dingman JF: Increased plasma arginine vasopressin in clinical adrenocortical insufficiency and its inhibition by glucosteroids. *J Clin Invest* 46:111, 1967.
334. Share L, Travis RH: Plasma vasopressin concentration in the adrenally insufficient dog. *Endocrinology* 86:196, 1970.
335. Green HH, Harrington AR, Valtin H: On the role of antidiuretic hormone in the inhibition of acute water diuresis in adrenal insufficiency and the effects of gluco- and mineralocorticoids in reversing the inhibition. *J Clin Invest* 49:1724, 1970.
336. Ufferman RC, Schrier RW: Importance of sodium intake and mineralocorticoid hormone in the impaired water excretion in adrenal insufficiency. *J Clin Invest* 51:1639, 1972.
337. Seif SM, Robinson AG, Zimmerman EA, Wilkins J: Plasma neurophysin and vasopressin in the rat: Response to adrenalectomy and steroid replacement. *Endocrinology* 103: 1009, 1978.
338. Boykin J, deTorrente A, Robertson GL, Erickson A, Schrier RW: Persistent plasma vasopressin levels in the hypoosmolar state associated with mineralocorticoid deficiency. *Miner Electrolyte Metab* 2:310, 1979.
339. Bethune JE, Nelson DH: Hyponatremia in hypopituitarism. *N Engl J Med* 272:771, 1965.
340. Ackerman GL, Miller CL: Role of hypovolemia in the impaired water diuresis of adrenal insufficiency. *J Clin Endocrinol Metab* 30:252, 1970.
341. Boykin J, deTorrente A, Erickson A, Robertson GL, Schrier RW: Role of plasma vasopressin in impaired water excretion of glucocorticoid deficiency. *J Clin Invest* 62:738, 1978.
342. Mandell IN, DeFronzo RA, Robertson GL, Forrest JN: Role of plasma arginine vasopressin in the impaired water diuresis of isolated glucocorticoid deficiency in the rat. *Kidney Int* 17:186, 1980.
343. Linas SL, Berl T, Robertson GL, Aisenbrey GA, Schrier RW, Anderson RJ: Role of vasopressin in the impaired water excretion of glucocorticoid deficiency. *Kidney Int* 18:58, 1980.
344. Oelkers W: Hyponatremia and inappropriate secretion of vasopressin (antidiuretic hormone) in patients with hypopituitarism. *N Engl J Med* 321:492, 1989.
345. Robertson GL: Syndrome of inappropriate antidiuresis. *N Engl J Med* 321:538, 1989.
346. Silverman AJ, Hoffman D, Gadde CA, Krey LC, Zimmerman EA: Adrenal steroid inhibition of the vasopressin-neurophysin neurosecretory system to the median eminence of rat: Differential effects of corticosterone and desoxycorticosterone administration after adrenalectomy. *Neuroendocrinology* 32:129, 1981.
347. Bartter FC: The syndrome of inappropriate secretion of antidiuretic hormone (SIADH). *Dis Mon*, November 1973, 1–47.
348. Skowsky WR, Kikuchi TA: The role of vasopressin in the impaired water excretion of myxedema. *Am J Med* 64:613, 1978.
349. De Rubertis FR, Michelis MF, Bloom ME, Mintz DU, Fidd JB, Davis BD: Impaired water excretion in myxedema. *Am J Med* 51:41, 1971.
350. Zerbe RL, Stropes L, Robertson GL: Vasopressin function in the syndrome of inappropriate antidiuresis. *Annu Rev Med* 31:315, 1980.
351. Thomas TH, Morgan DB, Swaminathan R, Gall SG, Lee MR: Severe hyponatræmia: A study of 17 patients. *Lancet* I(8065):661, 1978.
352. Hammer M: Defects in osmoregulation of vasopressin secretion. *Acta Med Scand* 211:133, 1982.
353. Robertson GL: Cancer and inappropriate antidiuresis, in

Rudden RW (ed): *Biological Markers of Neoplasia: Basic and Applied Aspects.* New York, Elsevier North-Holland, 1978, pp 277–293.

354. Leaf A, Bartter FC, Santos RF, Wrong O: Evidence in man that urinary electrolyte loss induced by pitressin is a function of water retention. *J Clin Invest* 32:868, 1953.
355. Michelis MF, Fusco RD, Bragdon RW, Davis BB: Reset of osmoreceptors in association with normovolemic hyponatremia. *Am J Med Sci* 267:267, 1974.
356. DeFronzo RA, Goldberg M, Agus ZS: Normal diluting capacity in hyponatremic patients. *Ann Intern Med* 84:538, 1976.
357. Assadi FK, Agrawal R, Jocher C, John EG, Rosenthal IM: Hyponatremia secondary to reset osmostat. *J Pediatr* 108:262, 1986.
358. Whitaker MD, McArthur RG, Corenblum B, Davidman M, Haslam RH: Idiopathic, sustained, inappropriate secretion of ADH with associated hypertension and thirst. *Am J Med* 67:511, 1979.
359. Fichman MP, Michelakis AM, Horton R: Regulation of aldosterone in the syndrome of inappropriate antidiuretic hormone secretion (SIADH). *J Clin Endocrinol Metab* 39:136, 1974.
360. Padfield PL, Brown JJ, Lever AF, Morton JJ, Robertson JIS: Blood pressure in acute and chronic vasopressin excess: Studies of malignant hypertension and the syndrome of inappropriate antidiuretic hormone secretion. *N Engl J Med* 304:1067, 1981.
361. Arieff AI, Llach F, Massry SG: Neurological manifestations and morbidity of hyponatremia: Correlation of brain water and electrolytes. *Medicine (Baltimore)* 55:121, 1976.
362. Messert B, Ornson WW, Hawkins MJ: Central pontine myelinolysis. *Neurology* 29:147, 1979.
363. Covey CM, Arieff AI: Disorders of sodium and water metabolism and their effects on the central nervous system, in Brenner BM, Stein JH (eds): *Sodium and Water Homeostasis. Contemporary Issues in Nephrology,* vol. I. New York, Churchill Livingston, 1978, pp 212–241.
364. Smithline N, Gardner K: Gaps—anionic and osmolal. *JAMA* 236:1594, 1976.
365. Dzau VJ, Colucci WS, Williams GH, Curfman G, Meggs L, Hollenberg NK: Sustained effectiveness of converting enzyme inhibition in patients with severe congestive heart failure. *N Engl J Med* 302:1373, 1980.
366. Yamahiro HW, Reynolds TB: Effects of ascitic fluid infusion on sodium excretion, blood volume and creatinine clearance in cirrhosis. *Gastroenterology* 40:497, 1961.
367. Schedl HP, Bartter FC: An explanation for an experimental correction of the abnormal water diuresis in cirrhosis. *J Clin Invest* 39:248, 1960.
368. Schrier RW, Lehman D, Zacherle B, Early LE: Effect of furosemide on free water excretion in edematous patients with hyponatremia. *Kidney Int* 3:30, 1973.
369. Ayus JC, Olivero JJ, Fromer JP: Rapid correction of severe hyponatremia with intravenous hypertonic saline solution. *Am J Med* 72:43, 1982.
370. Ayus JC, Krothapalli RK, Arieff AI: Treatment of symptomatic hyponatremia and its relation to brain damage. *N Engl J Med* 317:1190, 1987.
371. Cheng JC, Zikos D, Skopicki HA, Peterson DR: Long-term neurologic outcome in psychogenic water drinkers with severe symptomatic hyponatremia: The effect of rapid correction. *Am J Med* 88:561, 1990.
372. Sterns RH: The treatment of hyponatremia: First, do no harm, editorial. *Am J Med* 88:557, 1990.
373. Cherrill DA, Stote RM, Birge JR, Singer I: Demeclocycline treatment in the syndrome of inappropriate antidiuretic hormone secretion. *Ann Intern Med* 83:654, 1975.
374. deTroyer A: Demeclocycline: Treatment of syndrome of inappropriate antidiuretic hormone secretion. *JAMA* 237:2723, 1977.
375. Dousa TP, Wilson DM: Effect of demethylchlortetracycline on cellular action of antidiuretic hormone in vitro. *Kidney Int* 5:279, 1974.
376. Miller PD, Linas SL, schrier RW: Plasma demeclocycline levels and nephrotoxicity: Correlation in hyponatremic cirrhotic patients. *JAMA* 243:2513, 1980.
377. Oster JR, Epstein M, Ulano HB: Deterioration of renal function with demeclocycline administration. *Curr Ther Res* 20:794, 1976.
378. Forrest JN, Cox M, Hong C, Morrisson G, Bia M, Singer I: Superiority of demeclocycline over lithium in the treatment of chronic syndrome of inappropriate secretion of antidiuretic hormone. *N Engl J Med* 298:173, 1978.
379. Decaux G, Waterlot Y, Genette F, Mockel J: Treatment of the syndrome of inappropriate secretion of antidiuretic hormone with furosemide. *N Engl J Med* 304:329, 1981.
380. Decaux G, Genette F: Urea for long term treatment of syndrome of inappropriate secretion of antidiuretic hormone. *Br Med J* 283:1081, 1981.
381. Redetzki HM, Hughes JR, Redetzki JE: Difference between serum and plasma osmolalities and their relationship to lactic acid values. *Proc Soc Exp Biol Med* 139:315, 1972.

PART III

Thyroid Disease

CHAPTER 10

The Thyroid: Physiology, Thyrotoxicosis, Hypothyroidism, and the Painful Thyroid

Robert D. Utiger

Thyroid hormones are the only iodine-containing compounds with biological activity. In maturing mammals, they are crucial determinants of normal development. In adults, their major role is to maintain metabolic stability; in so acting, they affect the function of virtually every organ system. These actions require that thyroid hormone be constantly available. To maintain constant hormone availability, there is a large reservoir of thyroid hormone in the circulation, and thyroid hormone biosynthesis and secretion by the thyroid are maintained within narrow limits by a hypothalamic-pituitary regulatory mechanism that is very sensitive to small changes in circulating hormone concentrations.

Thyroid diseases are relatively common. They occur in the form of abnormalities of the size and shape of the thyroid gland (goiter) and abnormalities of thyroid secretion that can exist alone or in combination. Moreover, nonthyroidal illness is accompanied by many different alterations in thyroid physiology, which can complicate the evaluation of thyroid status.

ANATOMY AND PHYSIOLOGY

Clinical Anatomy

The normal adult thyroid gland is composed of two encapsulated lobes, one on either side of the trachea (Fig. 10-1*A*), connected by a thin isthmus that crosses the trachea anteriorly below the cricoid cartilage. The right lobe is often somewhat larger than the left lobe. Sometimes a pyramidal lobe is found extending superiorly from the isthmus in the midline, indicating the embryologic path along which the thyroid developed. The mean thyroid weight in groups of men and women of different ages in the United States ranges from 15 to 20 g.[1] Thyroid volume, which is normally 10 to 30 ml, is slightly greater in men than women, increases slightly with age and weight, and decreases with increasing iodine intake.[2]

The thyroid develops as a thickening in the pharyngeal floor that elongates inferiorly as the thyroglossal duct and becomes bilobar as it descends through the neck. Rarely, one or both thyroid lobes will fail to develop.[3] The thyroid may remain at the base of the tongue (lingual thyroid), may be found at other locations between the base of the tongue and the lower neck (thyroglossal duct remnants), or may follow the developmental path of the heart into the thorax, where, decades later, it may become manifest as a substernal goiter, compressing the trachea, a recurrent laryngeal nerve, or even the superior vena cava. Some of these anomalies of development are shown in Figure 10-1. The arterial supply of the thyroid is derived primarily from paired superior and inferior thyroid arteries. The venous drainage is more complex and variable, but usually there are paired superior, middle, and inferior thyroid veins. Normally, two parathyroid glands lie behind the upper and lower poles of each lobe of the thyroid. The recurrent laryngeal nerves run along the trachea, medially and behind the thyroid lobes.

Physical Examination

The patient should always be sitting, as it is impossible to examine the thyroid adequately when the patient is supine. The patient's neck should first be inspected from the front while the patient swallows with the head slightly extended. The thyroid lobes may be seen, and any lobar enlargement or thyroid nodules noted. The examiner should then move behind the patient to palpate the neck. Both sides of the neck should be palpated while the patient swallows, first with the examiner's hands on the same side of the patient's neck and then by palpation of the left side of the neck with the right hand and vice versa. This maneuver allows lateral displacement of the sternomastoid muscle and thus better delineation of the outline of each lobe.

The thyroid is palpable in most normal individuals, with the lobes being up to 3 cm long. Its surface may be slightly irregular. Both the size and the consistency of the gland should be recorded, in addition

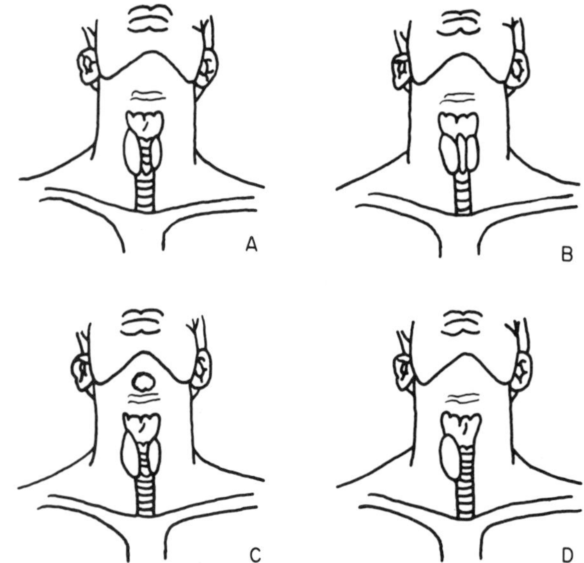

FIGURE 10-1 The normal thyroid gland and variations in thyroid anatomy. (*A*) Normal thyroid gland. (*B*) Pyramidal lobe between two normal thyroid lobes. (*C*) Thyroglossal remnant above the larynx. (*D*) Agenesis of the left lobe of the thyroid.

to any local irregularities. In addition to the isthmus and the pyramidal lobe, several lesions may be found in the midline, and other masses in addition to the thyroid lobes and abnormalities of the lobes may be palpable in the lateral neck regions (Table 10-1). Most, however, can be distinguished from thyroid masses by their position or failure to move with swallowing.

The most practical way to assess the size of thyroid lobes and nodules is to measure their vertical and horizontal dimensions. An outline of the thyroid can be traced on thin flexible paper. Estimates based on degree of enlargement or weight are so subjective as to be of little value at another time or to another examiner. Furthermore, the correlation between estimates of thyroid size by palpation and by ultrasonography is poor.[2]

TABLE 10-1 Differential Diagnosis of Neck Masses

Midline mass
Thyroid isthmus, pyramidal lobe
Thyroglossal duct cyst
Pretracheal lymph nodes
Lateral neck mass
Thyroid lobes and intrathyroidal lesions
Anterior cervical lymphadenopathy
Branchial cleft cyst
Arterial aneurysm
Carotid body tumor
Parathyroid masses

Histology

Microscopically, thyroid tissue consists of spherical thyroid follicles. Each follicle is composed of a single layer of cuboidal follicular cells surrounding a lumen filled with a homogeneous material called *colloid*. When stimulated, the follicular cells become columnar and the follicles are depleted of colloid; when suppressed, the follicular cells become flat and colloid accumulates. The luminal surface of each follicular cell is covered with microvilli extending into the colloid. The cytoplasm is filled with membrane-bound microsomes and a large Golgi apparatus. Near the apex of the cell are both exocytotic vesicles (secretory droplets) and endocytotic vesicles (colloid droplets), which are formed by the invagination of part of the luminal membrane.

Between the follicles and impinging on their surface are capillaries and adrenergic, cholinergic, and peptidergic nerve terminals, including terminals containing vasoactive intestinal peptide, neuropeptide Y, substance P, and somatostatin. These nerve terminals abut both capillaries and follicles, and their activation may alter thyroid secretion as well as thyroid blood flow.[4] The thyroid also contains parafollicular, or C, cells in the interfollicular connective tissue and, in lesser numbers, within thyroid follicles that produce calcitonin.

Chemistry of Thyroid Hormones

The structures of the two thyroid hormones—thyroxine (T_4) and triiodothyronine (T_3)—their precursor iodotyrosines, thyronine, and several metabolites of T_4 and T_3 are shown in Figure 10-2. T_4, T_3, and many of their metabolites are iodinated thyronines; they are composed of a phenyl ring attached via an ether linkage to tyrosine and contain from one to four iodine atoms. T_4 is 3,5,3′,5′-L-tetraiodothyronine, whereas T_3 is 3,5,3′-L-triiodothyronine, having one less iodine atom on its outer ring. The compound formed if an iodine atom is removed from the inner ring of T_4 is 3,3′,5′-triiodothyronine [reverse T_3 (rT_3)]. Diiodothyronine, or T_2, can exist in three forms: two iodine atoms on the outer ring (3′,5′-T_2), two on the inner ring (3,5-T_2), or one on each ring (3,3′-T_2). Oxidative deamination and decarboxylation of T_4 result in the formation of tetraiodothyroacetic acid (tetrac); triiodothyroacetic acid (triac) is formed from T_3 in the same way. Of the compounds shown in Fig. 10-2, only T_4, T_3, tetraiodothyroacetic acid, and triiodothyroacetic acid have biological activity. The latter two are produced in such small amounts that they contribute little if at all to thyroid hormone action in vivo.

Thyroid Hormone Biosynthesis

T_4 is produced only by the thyroid gland, whereas T_3 is produced both by the thyroid and by deiodination

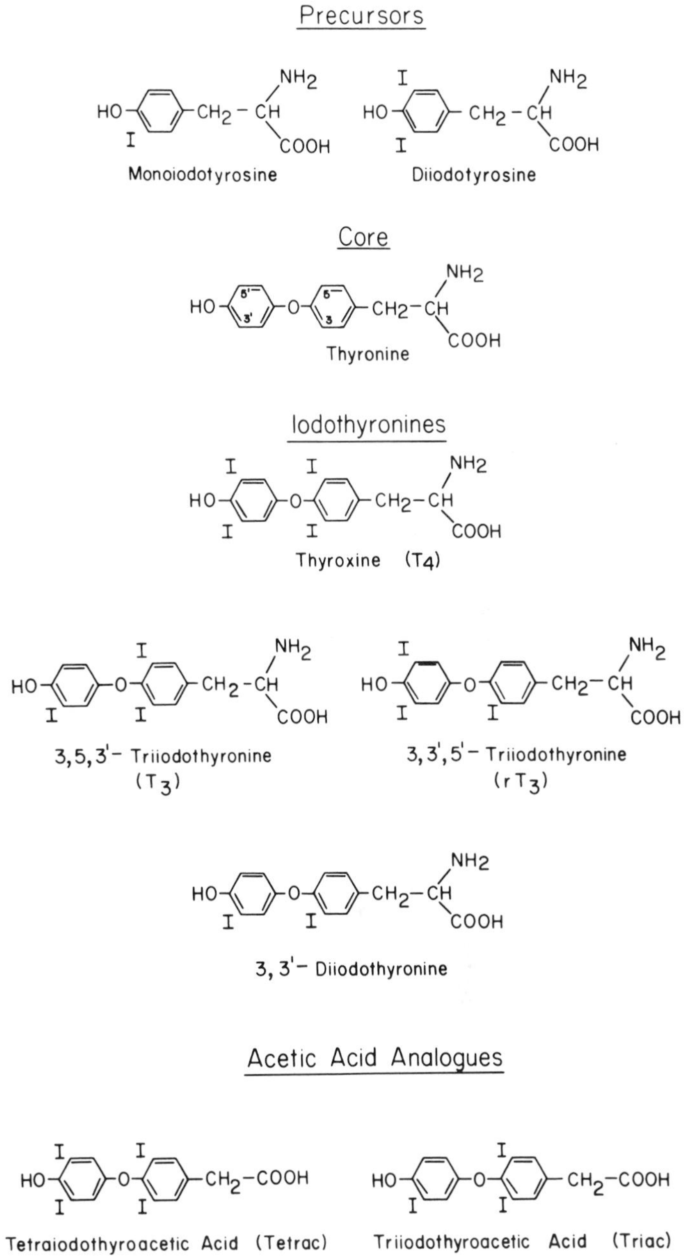

Precursors

Monoiodotyrosine

Diiodotyrosine

Core

Thyronine

Iodothyronines

Thyroxine (T_4)

3,5,3′- Triiodothyronine (T_3)

3,3′,5′- Triiodothyronine (rT_3)

3, 3′- Diiodothyronine

Acetic Acid Analogues

Tetraiodothyroacetic Acid (Tetrac)

Triiodothyroacetic Acid (Triac)

FIGURE 10-2 Structural formulas of various iodothyronines and iodothyronine analogs.

of T_4 at extrathyroidal sites. The thyroid gland contains large amounts of T_4 and T_3 incorporated in thyroglobulin, the unique protein within which the two hormones are synthesized and stored. Because of these stores, T_4 and T_3 can be secreted rapidly without the need for new hormone synthesis. The overall process of hormone production within the thyroid gland is shown in Figure 10-3.

Iodine Economy

An adequate supply of iodine is essential for normal thyroid function. Iodine intake varies greatly as a result of both varying iodine content of food and water and dietary preferences and in many regions of the world is inadequate or barely adequate (see Chap. 11). In the United States, the daily intake of iodine ranges from 300 to 1000 μg because iodide is added to salt and iodate is added to flour. The recommended minimum intake is 100 to 150 μg daily, although the minimum amount required to prevent goiter due to iodine deficiency in adults is about 50 μg daily. Dietary iodine is absorbed rapidly and is distributed in the extracellular fluid, in which the iodide concentration is about 1 μg/dl (80 nmol/liter). This pool receives not only dietary iodine but also iodide that is released from the thyroid and iodide derived from the peripheral deiodination of iodothyronines. Iodide leaves this pool mostly by transport

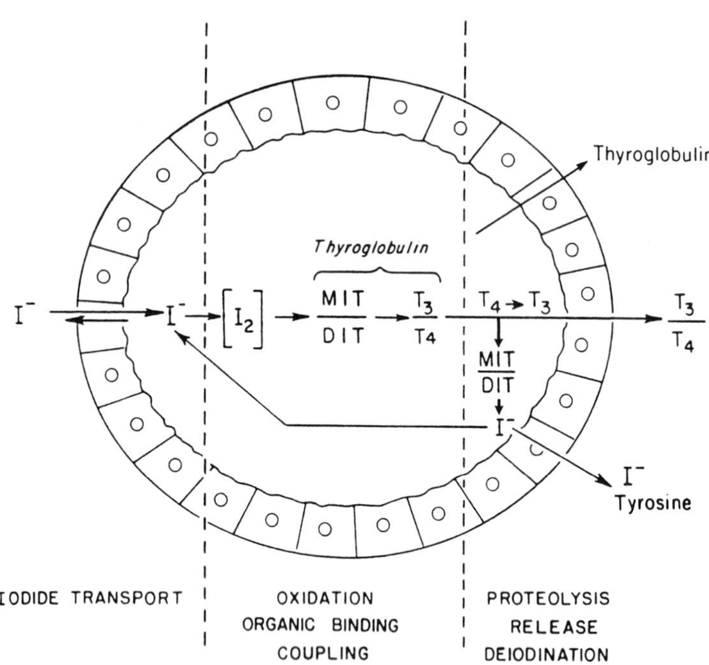

FIGURE 10-3 Outline of a thyroid follicle and the major steps in thyroid hormone biosynthesis and release. MIT = monoiodotyrosine; DIT = diiodotyrosine.

into the thyroid or excretion in the urine. The normal renal iodide clearance is about 30 ml/min, while thyroid clearance ranges from 10 to 20 ml/min, resulting in an absolute thyroid iodide uptake rate of about 150 μg/day (1200 nmol/day).

Thyroidal Hormonogenesis

Thyroid Iodide Transport

Iodide is transported into thyroid follicular cells against a chemical and electrical gradient; it then rapidly diffuses into the follicular lumen.[5] Iodide transport is a critical step in thyroid hormonogenesis; sufficient iodide to sustain normal T_4 and T_3 synthesis cannot be provided by diffusion from the extracellular fluid. Iodide transport occurs at the basal membrane of the follicular cell, is energy-dependent and saturable, and requires oxidative metabolism. It is linked to sodium transport and may involve a protein or phospholipid carrier. Iodide transport is stimulated by thyroid-stimulating hormone (TSH; thyrotropin). In addition, it is inhibited by excess iodide and increased by iodide deficiency, independent of TSH.

Ions of similar size, shape, and charge, such as perchlorate and pertechnetate, can serve as substrates for the transport system and therefore as competitive inhibitors of iodide transport. The ability of the thyroid to transport pertechnetate is useful clinically; $^{99m}TcO_4$, a gamma-emitting radioisotope with a short half-life, is used for thyroid scanning.

Tyrosyl Iodination and Coupling

In the thyroid, iodide is very rapidly oxidized and then covalently bound (organified) to some of the tyrosyl residues of thyroglobulin.[5] These two reactions occur in exocytotic vesicles fused with the apical cell membrane, in effect at the cell-lumen interface. Iodide oxidation is catalyzed by thyroid peroxidase, a heme-containing glycoprotein that is bound to the walls of the exocytotic vesicles. The oxidized form of the iodine atom is not known. Hydrogen peroxide is required for iodide oxidation; it is probably generated by NADPH–cytochrome c reductase. This process results in mono- or diiodination of about 15 of the 134 tyrosine residues of thyroglobulin.

T_4 is formed by the coupling of two diiodotyrosyl residues, and T_3 is formed by the coupling of one monoiodotyrosyl residue and one diiodotyrosyl residue within individual thyroglobulin molecules. The coupling reaction is an oxidative one, and it too is catalyzed by thyroid peroxidase.[5] The most likely mechanism involves the oxidation of two iodotyrosyl residues, followed by their ether linkage, leaving a dehydroalanyl residue at the site of the iodotyrosyl residue contributing the outer ring of the iodothyronine.

Thyroglobulin Synthesis

Thyroglobulin constitutes about 75 percent of the protein content of the thyroid gland, and almost all of it is within the follicular lumen.[6] It is a 660-kilodalton (kDa) glycoprotein composed of two identical noncovalently linked subunits and contains about 10 percent carbohydrate. A 8.5-kilobase (kb) messenger RNA (mRNA) coding for the subunit peptide has been isolated from human thyroid tissue, from which complementary DNA has been prepared and the protein's amino acid sequence has been deduced. Thyroglobulin mRNA is translated by large polyribosomes attached to the rough endoplasmic reticulum. Glycosylation and subunit combination are initiated before the release of the thyroglobulin from the endoplasmic reticulum and continue during its transfer to the Golgi apparatus and incorporation into the exocytotic vesicles that fuse with the apical cell membrane (Figure 10-4). Only then do iodination and coupling occur. Fully glycosylated, iodinated, and iodothyronine-containing thyroglobulin is found only in the follicular lumen.

The unique feature of thyroglobulin that favors iodotyrosyl coupling is its primary structure. Its content of 134 tyrosyl residues is rather low among proteins, and tyrosyl residues in all proteins can be iodinated. However, coupling occurs only in thyroglobulin. It is not random; rather, T_4 and T_3 are formed in limited domains that are located near the ends of each subunit of the molecule and have unique amino acid sequences.[6]

The iodoamino acid content of thyroglobulin is dependent on iodide availability. Normal thyroglobulin contains about 6 residues of monoiodotyrosine, 4 residues of diiodotyrosine, 2 residues of T_4, and 0.2 residue of T_3 per molecule. Poorly iodinated thyroglobulin has a lower total iodide content and higher monoiodotyrosine/diiodotyrosine and T_3/T_4 ratios.[6]

Colloid Endocytosis and Hormone Release

Thyroglobulin not only is the site of formation of T_4 and T_3 but also is the storage form of the two hormones. The process of T_4 and T_3 secretion requires the reuptake of thyroglobulin into the thyroid follicular cells and its enzymatic hydrolysis (Figure 10-5). Thyroglobulin in the follicular lumen is engulfed by pinocytotic extensions of microvilli from the apical membrane, forming endocytotic vesicles *(colloid droplets)*. These vesicles fuse with lysosomes to form phagolysosomes. As these particles migrate toward the base of the cell, the thyroglobulin is selectively cleaved by several endo- and exopeptidases to form hormone-containing peptide intermediates that are then cleaved to form the individual hormones. The T_3 and T_4 diffuse into the extracellular fluid and enter the circulation. During this process, some of the T_4 is deiodinated by a T_4-5′-deiodinase to form T_3, so that thyroidal T_3 secretion is greater than expected on the basis of its content in thyroglobulin.[7] The iodotyrosines liberated by thyroglobulin hydrolysis are rapidly deiodinated by a specific iodotyrosine deiodinase. Most of the iodide formed as a result of these deiodinations is reutilized in the thyroid, but some is released. Iodotyrosine deiodination provides more iodide for new hormone formation than does new iodide transport and thus is of critical importance in maintaining iodothyronine synthesis. A small amount of thyroglobulin is not hydrolyzed and is released into the circulation.[8]

FIGURE 10-4 Schematic drawing of the pathway of thyroglobulin biosynthesis and iodination in a thyroid follicular cell. The apical cell surface is at the top, and the extracellular space is at the bottom.

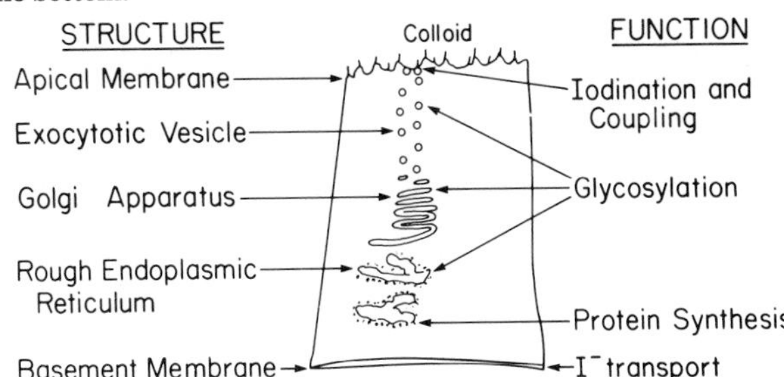

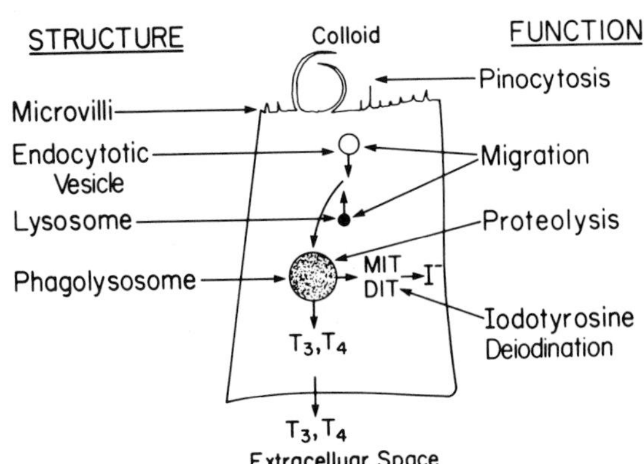

FIGURE 10-5 Schematic drawing of the pathway of thyroglobulin proteolysis and T_4 and T_3 release in a thyroid follicular cell. MIT = monoiodotyrosine; DIT = diiodotyrosine.

Extrathyroidal Hormonogenesis

Most of the T_3 produced each day is formed by the extrathyroidal 5′-deiodination (outer ring deiodination) of T_4. This reaction is catalyzed by T_4-5′-deiodinase, a microsomal enzyme that requires reduced sulfhydryl groups as a cofactor. The liver and kidney have the highest T_4-5′-deiodinase activity per unit tissue,[9,10] and these tissues are probably the largest sources of circulating T_3. However, some 5′-deiodination of T_4 occurs in most if not all tissues. There are two types of T_4-5′-deiodinase, distinguished by their location, structure, kinetic properties, sensitivity to inhibition by propylthiouracil (PTU), substrate preference, and responses to physiologic stimuli.[10,11] Type I T_4-5′-deiodinase is the predominant T_4-deiodinating enzyme in the liver, kidney, and thyroid. Its K_m for T_4 is high (μM), it is PTU-sensitive, and it contains a selenocysteine residue near its active site. The order of substrate preference is $rT_3 > T_4 > T_3$. Human liver and thyroid T_4-5′-deiodinase has similar properties.[12,13] The type II enzyme is the predominant T_4-5′-deiodinase in brain, pituitary, and skin. Its K_m for T_4 is low, it is not inhibited by PTU, and it

TABLE 10-2 Serum Concentrations and Production Rates of Various Iodothyronines

	Serum Concentration		Production Rate	
Compound	ng/dl	nmol/liter	μg/day	nmol/day
Thyroxine (T_4)	5,000–11,000	65–140	80–100	100–130
3,5,3′-Triiodothyronine (T_3)	75–200	1.1–3.0	30–40	45–60
3,3′,5′-Triiodothyronine (rT_3)	20–50	0.3–0.8	30–40	45–60
3,3′-Diiodothyronine (T_2)	2–10	0.04–0.20	25–35	48–67
3,5-Diiodothyronine (T_2)	1–10	0.02–0.20	2–5	4–10
3,5′-Diiodothyronine (T_2)	2–6	0.04–0.12	5–20	10–40
Tetraiodothyroacetic acid	20–50	0.26–0.65	1–2	1–4
Triiodothyroacetic acid	2–8	0.03–0.12	4–8	6–12

Conversion factors: Thyroxine, 1 nmol = 777 ng; triiodothyronine, 1 nmol = 651 ng; diiodothyronine, 1 nmol = 525 ng; tetraiodothyroacetic acid, 1 nmol = 748 ng; triiodothyroacetic acid, 1 nmol = 622 ng.

Source: Engler and Burger[9] and Koehrle et al.[10]

contains cysteine near the active site; its order of substrate preference is $T_4 > rT_3$.[10,11]

Reverse T_3 is produced at extrathyroidal sites by 5-deiodination (inner ring deiodination) of T_4. The enzyme that catalyzes this reaction, T_4-5-deiodinase (type III deiodinase), is widely distributed throughout the body. The properties of T_4-5-deiodinase in human liver are very similar to those of type I T_4-5′-deiodinase, and they may be the same enzyme.[12]

Thyroid Hormone Production and Metabolism

The total daily production rate of T_4 is 80 to 100 μg (100 to 130 nmol), all derived from thyroidal secretion (Table 10-2 and Fig. 10-6). The extrathyroidal T_4 pool contains 800 to 1,000 μg (1000 to 1300 nmol), most of which is extracellular. The T_4 turnover rate is 10 percent per day. Thus, T_4 remains available for several weeks in the absence of any thyroidal secretion. Approximately 80 percent is metabolized by deiodination, with about 40 percent being converted to T_3 and 40 percent to rT_3. The remaining 20 percent is metabolized by conjugation with sulfate and glucuronide, oxidative deamination and decarboxylation to form tetraiodothyroacetic acid, and ether-link cleavage.[10] Deiodination of T_4 to T_3 leads to enhanced biological activity, but all the other metabolites of T_4 have little if any biological activity. The extrathyroidal conversion of T_4 to T_3 is regulated by a variety of factors, so that production of T_3, the most active thyroid hormone, may be altered independently of changes in pituitary-thyroid function.

T_3 is produced primarily (80 percent) by extrathyroidal deiodination of T_4; the remainder comes from the thyroid. The total daily production rate is 30 to 40 μg (45 to 60 nmol).[10,11] The extrathyroidal T_3 pool contains about 50 μg (75 nmol), most of which is intracellular. T_3 is much more rapidly degraded than is T_4, its turnover rate being about 75 percent per day. Hence, alterations in T_3 production readily alter its availability. After being sulfated, somewhat more than half of the T_3 produced each day is deiodinated to 3,3′-diiodothyronine by T_4-5-deiodinase. A small amount is deiodinated to 3,5-diiodothyronine (Fig. 10-7), and the remainder (about 10 percent) is metabolized to triiodothyroacetic acid.

FIGURE 10-6 Sources and production rates of circulating T_4, T_3, and rT_3 in normal adults. The diagonally lined area of each bar represents production in the thyroid gland; the clear area represents production in the periphery from T_4. The daily production rates are given in μg (nmoles), and the serum concentrations in ng/dl or μg/dl (nmol/liter). The T_4/T_3 and T_4/rT_3 ratios shown at the top are those in thyroglobulin. See Table 10-2 for ranges of production rates and serum T_4, T_3, and rT_3 concentrations in normal subjects.

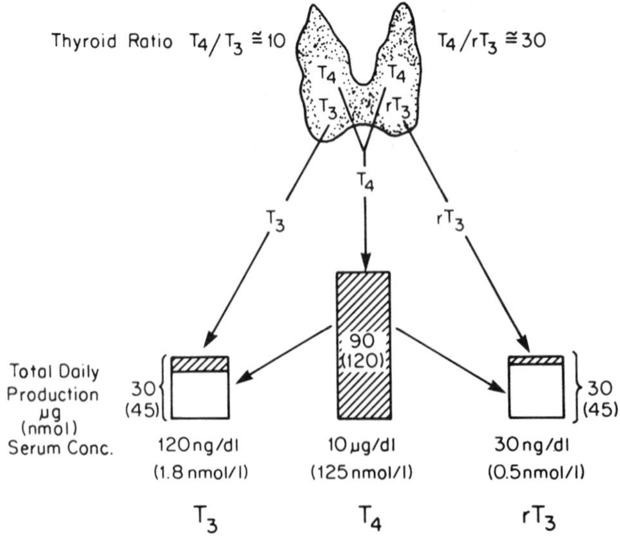

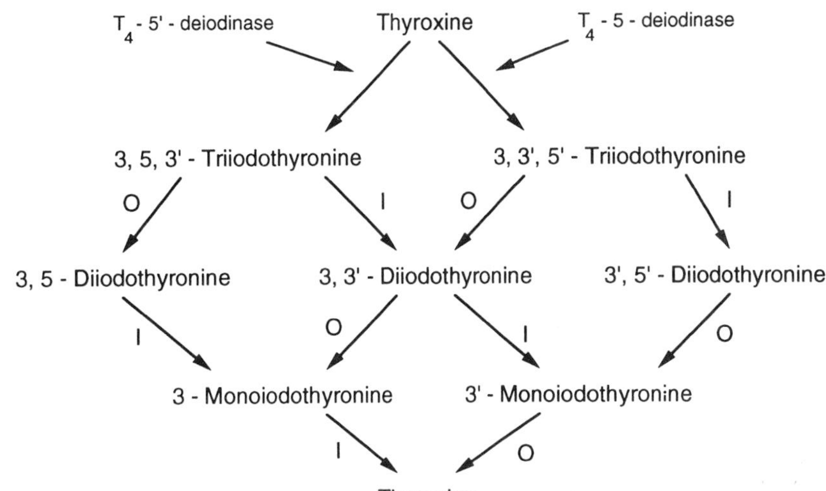

FIGURE 10-7 Pathways of deiodination of T_4 and its metabolites. O = outer ring deiodination (5′-deiodination); I = inner ring deiodination (5-deiodination).

The daily production rate of rT_3 is 30 to 40 μg (45 to 60 nmol); over 95 percent is produced at extrathyroidal sites.[10,11] It is cleared from the circulation even more rapidly than is T_3. Most is deiodinated by type I T_4-5′-deiodinase to 3,3′-diiodothyronine (Fig. 10-7), but some is deiodinated to 3′,5′-diiodothyronine or metabolized by nondeiodinative pathways.

The various diiodothyronines also are very rapidly metabolized to monoiodothyronines and ultimately to thyronine, but little is known about the sites and regulation of these conversions. Table 10-2 shows the serum concentrations and production rates of most of these compounds. The serum concentrations of 3′-T_2 and 3-T_2 are less than 2 ng/dl (4 pmol/liter). Tetraiodothyroacetic acid, triiodothyroacetic acid, and the conjugates of T_4 and T_3 also are metabolized largely by deiodination.

Monoiodotyrosine and diiodotyrosine are present in the circulation in low concentrations. They are derived both from dietary sources and from the thyroid gland. Both iodotyrosines are degraded rapidly by tyrosine deiodinase in peripheral tissues.

About 100 μg of thyroglobulin is released from the thyroid each day. This is a tiny fraction of the 25 mg that must be hydrolyzed to yield the 100 μg (130 nmol) of T_4 that is secreted each day. The serum half-life of thyroglobulin is 30 h.[14]

Transport and Cellular Binding of Thyroid Hormones

Serum Binding Proteins

Very little of the T_4 and T_3 in the circulation is free; more than 99.95 percent of the T_4 and 99.5 percent of the T_3 are bound in reversible physicochemical equilibrium to several serum proteins (Fig. 10-8). These proteins are thyroxine-binding globulin (TBG), transthyretin [TTR, formerly called thyroxine-binding prealbumin (TBPA)], albumin, and lipoprotein. In normal subjects, approximately 75 percent of the T_4 in serum is bound to TBG, 10 percent to TTR, 12 percent to albumin, and 3 percent to lipoprotein. In comparison, about 80 percent of the T_3 in serum is bound to TBG, 5 percent to TTR, and 15

FIGURE 10-8 *(Top)* Origin, circulating forms, and degradation of T_4. *(Bottom)* Origin, circulating forms, and degradation of T_3. Only the liver is shown as a site of T_4 conversion to T_3, but the conversion occurs in many tissues. TBG = thyroxine-binding globulin; TTR = transthyretin.

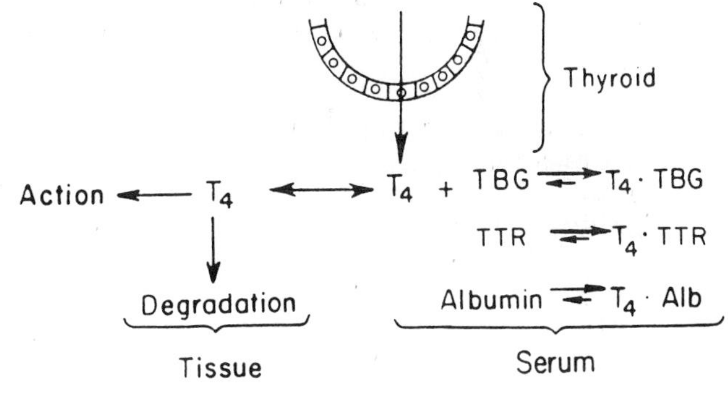

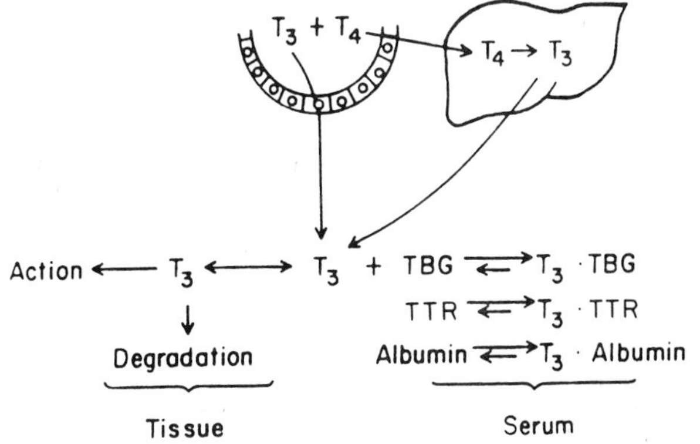

percent to albumin and lipoprotein. Approximately 0.05 percent of the total serum T_4, or about 2 ng/dl (26 pmol/liter), is free; the free T_3 concentration is about 0.4 ng/dl (6 pmol/liter). Because so much of the T_4 and T_3 in serum is bound, changes in serum concentrations of binding proteins have a large effect on serum total T_4 and T_3 concentrations and fractional T_4 and T_3 metabolism, but they do not alter free hormone concentrations or the absolute rates of T_4 and T_3 metabolism. These proteins also bind other iodothyronines, but much less avidly.

It is the serum free T_4 and T_3 concentrations that determine the hormones' biological activity (see Chaps. 4 and 5). The overall effect of the binding proteins is to maintain serum free T_4 and T_3 concentrations within narrow limits yet ensure that the hormones are continuously and immediately available to tissues. They have, therefore, both storage and buffer functions. The storage function serves to facilitate a uniform distribution of T_4 and T_3 within tissues, particularly large solid organs. For example, when the liver is perfused through the portal vein with T_4 alone, the hormone is taken up only by the hepatocytes in the periportal areas; perfusion with T_4 and TBG, TTR, or albumin results in the distribution of T_4 throughout the liver.[15] In the longer term, if thyroid secretion ceases, the T_4 stored in serum serves to delay the appearance of thyroid deficiency greatly, whereas if only free T_4 were available, its supply would be exhausted within hours. Conversely, the binding proteins serve to buffer the free T_4 and T_3 concentrations in serum from sudden increases in thyroid secretion or extrathyroidal hormone release.

Thyroxine-Binding Globulin

Thyroxine-binding globulin (TBG) is a 54-kDa glycoprotein that is synthesized in the liver. It has one binding site for T_4. While the affinity constant of TBG for T_4 is high, about $10^{10}\ M^{-1}$ (Table 10-3), the rate of dissociation is rapid ($t_{1/2}$ of 40 s). T_3 binds to TBG considerably less avidly than does T_4.[16] The carbohydrate content of TBG in serum is about 20 percent, but the content of individual TBG molecules varies, primarily as a result of differences in sialic acid content.[17] The serum TBG concentration in normal subjects is about 1.5 mg/dl (0.27 μmol/liter). This amount is capable of binding about 20 μg T_4 (26 nmol), but only about one-third of the TBG in serum normally contains T_4.

Transthyretin

Transthyretin (TTR) is a 55-kDa tetrameric protein composed of four identical subunits. It is synthesized in the liver and also in pancreatic islets and choroid plexus. Each molecule has two identical T_4 binding sites, but occupation of one site by T_4 greatly decreases the affinity of the second site for T_4. The affinity constant of TTR for binding of T_4 is about $7 \times 10^7\ M^{-1}$, its affinity for T_3 is considerably less, and the T_4-TTR complexes dissociate very rapidly (Table 10-3).[16,17] The serum concentration of TTR is about 25 mg/dl (4.6 μmol/liter), an amount capable of binding up to 200 μg T_4 (260 nmol).

TTR also binds retinol-binding protein, which in turn binds retinol (vitamin A). The binding of T_4 and of retinol-binding protein to TTR is independent, so that T_4 binding to TTR is not influenced by changes in retinol-binding protein concentrations. The serum half-life of TTR is considerably shorter than is that of TBG, so that serum TTR concentrations change rapidly when its production rate changes, for example, during malnutrition.

Albumin

Albumin has one strong binding site (affinity constant $7 \times 10^5\ M^{-1}$) and several weaker binding sites for T_4. There are four T_4-binding albumin isoforms, and their relative affinity for T_4 and T_3 varies.[17] Since only about 12 percent of the T_4 in serum is bound to albumin, changes in serum albumin concentrations have little effect on serum T_4 concentrations.

Lipoproteins

A small percentage of the T_4 and T_3 in serum is bound to lipoproteins.[16] Among them, high-density lipoproteins, mostly their apoprotein A-I component, bind the most T_4 and T_3. The apoprotein B-100 component of low-density and very low density lipoproteins also binds some T_4 and T_3.

Cellular Hormone Entry and Binding

Serum free T_4 and free T_3 are available for cellular uptake at any instant, and the rates of dissociation of T_4 and T_3 from their binding proteins are so

TABLE 10-3 Properties of Serum Thyroid Hormone–Binding Proteins

	Affinity Constant M^{-1}		Serum Concentration		Serum Half-Life,	T_4-Binding Capacity	
Protein	T_4	T_3	mg/dl	μmol/liter	Days	μg/dl	nmol/liter
Thyroxine-binding globulin	1×10^{10}	5×10^8	1.5	0.27	5	20	260
Transthyretin	7×10^7	2×10^7	25	4.6	2	200	2,600
Albumin	7×10^5	1×10^5	4,000	640	15	2,000	26,000

Source: Robbins.[16]

rapid that additional T_4 and T_3 become available very rapidly. The primary mechanism of cellular uptake of T_4 and T_3 is simple diffusion (Fig. 10-9), but uptake by the liver and some other tissues also may be mediated by a carrier-mediated plasma membrane transport system.[18] The role of this mechanism in hormone entry is probably limited, since tissue uptake of T_4 approximates the rate of dissociation of the hormone from its binding proteins.[19] Other factors, such as vascular flow and permeability and intracellular binding, also are important in determining T_4 and T_3 entry into cells. Ultimately, if the intracellular free hormone concentrations decline sufficiently, virtually all the protein-bound T_4 and T_3 in serum become free and may enter cells.

T_3 is also available to cells as a result of its production from T_4 within the cells (Fig. 10-9). Some of the locally produced T_3 must diffuse out of the cells, since serum free (and total) T_3 concentrations are normal in hypothyroid patients who take T_4 in doses that raise their serum T_4 concentrations to normal. Much is not exported, however, since in many tissues local production of T_3 provides much of the T_3 that is bound to nuclear and perhaps other receptors linked to hormone action. Overall, about 90 percent of the total extrathyroidal T_3 pool of 50 μg (75 nmol) in humans is in the intracellular compartment.

The distribution of T_4 and T_3 in different tissues is not uniform. Neither is the fraction of the T_3 that is produced locally from T_4 or the contribution of locally produced T_3 to the amount of T_3 bound to its receptors. For example, locally produced T_3 accounts for about 20 percent of the nuclear T_3 in rat liver, 50 percent in the pituitary, and 80 percent in cerebral cortex but $<$10 percent in other tissues.[20]

T_4 and T_3 exist within cells both free and bound to cytosol, microsomes, mitochondria, and nuclei.[21] The cytosol binding proteins probably have buffering and storage functions like those of the iodothyronine-binding proteins in serum. The nature and importance of T_4 and T_3 binding to the other nonnuclear constituents are not known. Their affinity and specificity for T_4 and T_3 are much lower than are those of the nuclear receptors, and their overall binding capacity is much higher. Nevertheless, some may be receptors mediating hormone action.

FIGURE 10-9 Schematic outline of extracellular and intracellular translocations of T_4 and T_3 and their actions in target cells. Hormone binding to nuclear receptors and the subsequent activation of RNA synthesis results in increased synthesis of mRNAs that direct the synthesis of membrane proteins, secreted proteins, and lipogenic and other enzymes.

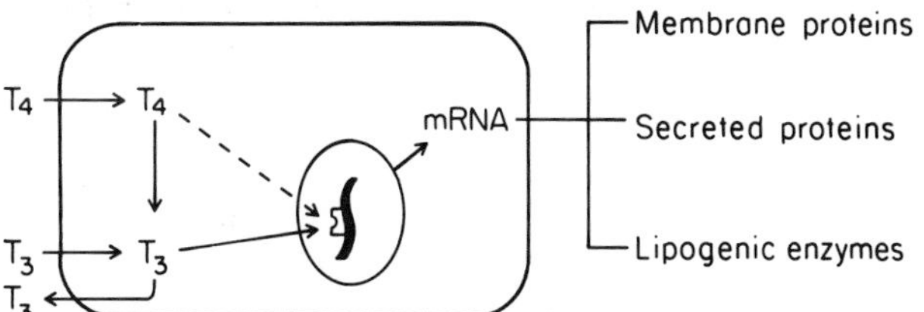

Biochemical Actions of Thyroid Hormones

T_3 Nuclear Receptors

Thyroid hormone receptors in the nuclei of most tissues (Fig. 10-9) mediate nearly all the known physiologic actions of thyroid hormone.[21,22] These receptors are members of a superfamily that includes the receptors for steroid hormones, vitamin D, and retinoids; the molecular biology of this superfamily is described in Chap. 5. T_3 enters nuclei directly from the cytosol by diffusion or via a transport system in the nuclear membrane and then binds to the chromatin-localized receptors; no cytosol or soluble nuclear T_3-binding protein is required. The T_3 nuclear receptors are acidic proteins that bind T_3 10-fold more avidly than T_4 in vitro; in vivo, T_3 constitutes nearly all the nuclear-bound hormone. T_4 can thus be considered largely a prohormone, although it may have some intrinsic biological activity.

The general structure of the T_3 nuclear receptors is shown in Fig. 10-10.[21–23] The receptors are coded by two genes that are the cellular homologues *(c-erbA)* of the avian erythroblastosis virus oncogene *v-erbA*. One of these genes—the T_3 nuclear receptor alpha gene—is located on chromosome 17, and the other—the T_3 nuclear receptor beta gene—is located on chromosome 3. Each of these two genes codes for mRNAs that can be alternatively spliced, and so there are at least three products of the T_3 nuclear receptor alpha gene and two products of the T_3 nuclear receptor beta gene. These gene products are linear polypeptides that range in molecular weight from 47 to 57 kDa; the differences among them are due to differences in their amino- and carboxyl-terminal regions. They contain separate highly conserved DNA and T_3-binding regions, and each receptor binds to DNA in the absence of T_3. Two of the products of the alpha gene—the $alpha_2$ and $alpha_3$ receptors—do not bind T_3 and hence are not strictly speaking T_3 receptors; at least one of them, the $alpha_2$ receptor, inhibits the action of T_3-T_3 nuclear receptor complexes either by forming heterodimers with the other receptors or by inhibiting their binding to the thyroid response elements of DNA. The distribution of the different receptors among tissues

FIGURE 10-10 Schematic drawing of the structure of the T_3 nuclear receptor. NH_2 = amino-terminal end of the receptor; DNA = region of the receptor that binds to DNA; T_3 binding = region that binds T_3; COOH = carboxyl-terminal end. See also Chap. 5.

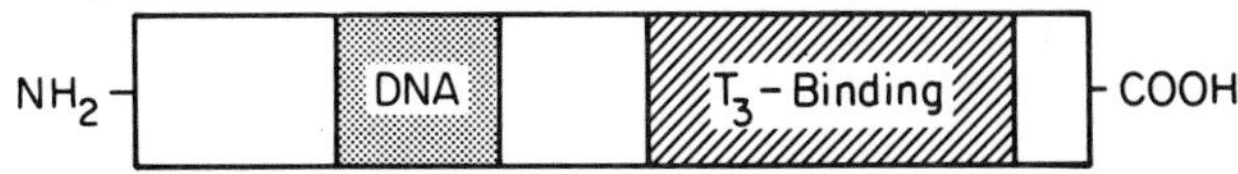

also varies. For example, the beta$_1$ and beta$_2$ receptors are concentrated, respectively, in brain, heart, liver, and kidney and in pituitary and hypothalamic tissue, and the alpha$_2$ receptor is much more abundant in brain than in other tissues.[24] The relative importance of the alpha and beta forms of the receptors is not evident from their tissue distribution.

The T_3 response elements on DNA (Chap. 5) are usually located upstream of the transcription start sites of the responsive genes, but some are located near those sites or even in exons. Most appear to contain at least two half-sites, to which the T_3 receptors may bind as dimers or heterodimers. The elements differ somewhat among T_3-responsive genes, especially between genes on which the action of T_3 is stimulatory and those on which it is inhibitory. Any individual response element can bind either alpha or beta receptors, but its affinity for the different receptors may vary. The consequences of these interactions are activation or inhibition of DNA transcription.

The extent to which different tissues are affected by T_3 varies widely. In some tissues many genes and cellular functions are affected, whereas in others only a few of each are affected. In some tissues, such as the pituitary and heart, there is a linear correlation between the relative saturation of these nuclear sites by T_3 and the relative response. In other tissues, increases in receptor occupancy result in nonlinear, amplified responses. For example, in the liver, an increase in T_3 receptor occupancy from 50 to 100 percent results in a 10-fold increase in the rate of synthesis of some enzymes.[21]

Several factors underlie these differences. They include the diversity of the T_3 nuclear receptors themselves, the variations in their distribution among tissues, the fact that receptors containing ligand and those not containing ligand have biological activity, the possibility of the formation of heterodimers between different forms of the receptor and other transcription factors, and the tissue content of these transcription factors. Hence, there is an opportunity for many different alterations of gene expression, both qualitatively and quantitatively.

The cell content of T_3 nuclear receptors is generally high in tissues that are most responsive to thyroid hormone, such as the pituitary and liver, and low in poorly responsive tissues, such as the spleen and testes. There is tissue-specific regulation of the mRNAs for the different forms of the T_3 nuclear receptor by thyroid hormone.[25] In animals, hepatic T_3 nuclear receptor content per cell is reduced by starvation, diabetes, uremia, and partial hepatectomy.[26–28] Such changes, if they occurred in humans, could be an additional mechanism serving to limit the impact of thyroid hormone in patients with nonthyroidal illness.

Tissue Responses to Thyroid Hormones

Thyroid hormones modulate a large number of metabolic processes (Fig. 10-9) by regulating the production and activity of many enzymes, the production and metabolism of other hormones, and the utilization of substrates, vitamins, and minerals. Not all of these actions are due to effects on transcription. Among the nonnuclear actions are stimulation of amino acid and sugar transport in lymphoid cells and calcium-ATPase activity in red blood cells.[29] Thus, either T_3 nuclear receptors mediate extranuclear events or there are undetected high-affinity T_3 receptors in other cellular locations.

Thermogenic Actions

Energy released by the oxidation of substrate is stored by the formation of ATP or liberated as heat. The utilization of ATP for ion transport, synthesis of cell constituents, and muscle contraction results in the formation of ADP, and its rephosphorylation to form ATP requires augmented mitochondrial oxidative metabolism. The single largest requirement for ATP in resting cells is for Na/K-dependent ATPase-mediated sodium transport; thus, changes in transport should have a substantial overall effect on oxidative metabolism.

Thyroid hormone stimulation of thermogenesis can be demonstrated both in vivo and in isolated tissues such as muscle, liver, and kidney.[30] The degree of stimulation correlates with the number of T_3 nuclear receptors in most tissues, except in the brain, in which there are receptors but no thermogenic response. There is a latent period of hours to days before T_3-induced increases in oxygen consumption occur. The increase correlates with increased sodium transport as measured by increases in Na/K-dependent ATPase activity and is prevented by inhibition of ATPase activity with ouabain.[30] The increase in sodium transport results from an increase in cellular Na/K-dependent ATPase mRNA and enzyme production, i.e., an increase in sodium pump units.[31] Thus, thyroid hormone augmentation of thermogenesis can be explained at least in part by increased mitochondrial oxidative metabolism driven by the increase in ATP utilization that occurs as a result of increased Na/K-dependent ATPase activity. In cardiac muscle, T_3 stimulates the transcription of both the myosin heavy-chain alpha gene, leading to an increase in a myosin isoenzyme that has a high level of ATPase activity, and calcium ATPase; these effects lead to increases in both cardiac contractility and oxygen consumption.[32] There also is evidence for actions of thyroid hormone on mitochondria that could mediate some of the hormone's thermogenic actions. T_3 stimulates mitochondrial protein synthesis; inward transport of ADP, inorganic phosphate, and fuels; and ATP production and oxygen consumption.[29]

Lipolysis and Lipogenesis

Thyroid hormones stimulate lipolysis in adipose tissue by increasing the activity of hormone-sensitive lipase. The increase in lipolysis provides fatty acids that can be oxidized to generate the ATP used for thermogenesis.[33] Thyroid hormones also stimulate the synthesis of mRNAs for malic enzyme and other enzymes that are involved in lipogenesis in the liver and adipose tissue. The increase in lipogenesis serves to maintain the lipid stores needed to provide the fatty acids used to fuel thermogenesis and other energy-consuming reactions.[34]

Effects on Carbohydrate Metabolism

The thermogenic effects of thyroid hormone are accompanied by increased peripheral and splanchnic utilization of glucose.[35] The increased need for glucose is balanced by increases in hepatic glucose output. These increases are due to increases in both gluconeogenesis and glycogenolysis.[36]

Effects on Protein Synthesis

Thyroid hormones stimulate the synthesis of many structural proteins, enzymes, and hormones. The consequences of this action are most obvious in the decreased neural and somatic growth that accompanies hypothyroidism in infants and children. The biochemical bases for increased protein synthesis are increased production of mRNA resulting from augmented gene transcription, proliferation of the ribosomal constituents involved in protein synthesis, increased translational efficiency, and perhaps increased amino acid transport. One of the most closely studied responses is that of malic enzyme in liver. Increases in malic enzyme activity can be correlated with nuclear T_3 occupancy, followed after a lag period by increases in the appropriate mRNA, and subsequently proportionate increases in enzyme protein and catalytic activity.[21] However, not all thyroid hormone actions on synthetic processes are stimulatory. For example, thyroid hormones inhibit TSH secretion primarily by inhibiting the expression of the genes for its subunits,[37] and they inhibit the synthesis of glycosaminoglycan and fibronectin in fibroblasts.[38]

Thyroid Hormone–Catecholamine Interactions

Many of the signs and symptoms of thyrotoxicosis appear to reflect increased sympathetic nervous system activity, and those of hypothyroidism reflect decreased activity. The efficacy of beta-adrenergic antagonist drugs in ameliorating some of the clinical manifestations of thyrotoxicosis illustrates the apparent enhancement of adrenergic activity induced by thyroid hormone. However, serum concentrations and production rates of norepinephrine are normal or decreased in thyrotoxicosis and increased in hypothyroidism, while those of epinephrine are not altered by either condition.[39] Thyroid hormones do have actions by which the apparent increase in sympathetic activity could be explained. They increase the number of beta-adrenergic receptors in cardiac and skeletal muscle and adipose tissue and decrease myocardial alpha-adrenergic receptors.[40] These changes do not, however, result in increased in vivo sensitivity to beta-adrenergic agonists.[41]

Regulation of Thyroid Hormone Production

Thyroid hormone production is regulated in two ways (Fig. 10-11). First, thyroidal T_4 and T_3 biosynthesis and secretion are stimulated by TSH. The secretion of TSH in turn is inhibited by circulating T_4 and T_3 and is stimulated by thyrotropin-releasing hormone (TRH). Second, extrathyroidal T_3 production from T_4 is regulated by a variety of nutritional, hormonal, and illness-related factors, and the effect of these regulatory factors differs in different tissues. The first mechanism provides a sensitive defense against alterations in thyroid secretion. The second provides for the rapid alterations in tissue thyroid hormone availability in response to nonthyroidal illness that constitute an important adaptation to illness (see Nonthyroidal Illness).

Control of Thyroid Secretion

Thyroid-Stimulating Hormone

TSH, a 28-kDa glycoprotein, is synthesized and secreted by the thyrotrophs of the anterior pituitary,

FIGURE 10-11 The hypothalamic-pituitary-thyroid axis. TSH regulates the thyroid glandular synthesis and secretion of T_4 and T_3; T_3 is also produced in many other tissues by deiodination of T_4. TSH secretion is regulated by serum T_4, serum T_3, T_3 produced from T_4 within the pituitary, and thyrotropin-releasing hormone (TRH). T_4 and T_3 probably also regulate TRH secretion. (−) = inhibitory effect; (+) = stimulatory effect.

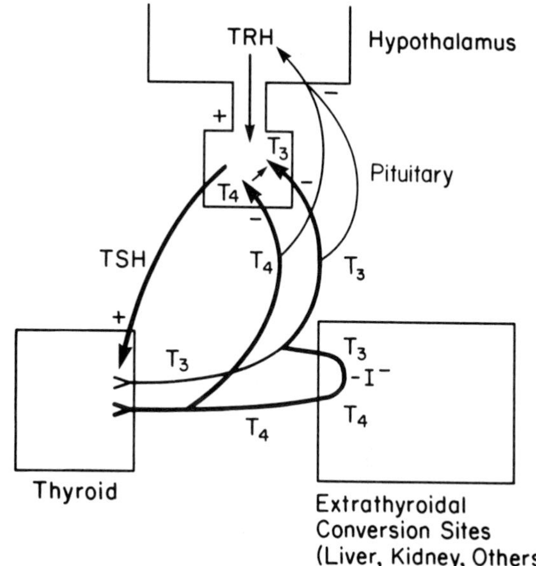

as described in greater detail in Chaps. 4 and 8. TSH is composed of two noncovalently linked peptide subunits, an alpha subunit and a beta subunit, and contains about 15 percent carbohydrate. The alpha subunit of TSH is the same as that of luteinizing hormone, follicle-stimulating hormone, and chorionic gonadotropin. The beta subunit of TSH is unique, and it thus determines the hormone's biological specificity. The synthesis of each subunit is directed by separate mRNAs that are coded by separate genes on different chromosomes.[37] After synthesis, the subunits are glycosylated and linked together to form TSH, which is then packaged into granules. During the linkage and packaging steps, the carbohydrate components of the subunits are converted from components rich in mannose residues to complex oligosaccharides containing acetylated sugars, sialic acid, and sulfate.[42]

The estimated TSH secretion rate in normal subjects ranges from 75 to 150 mU/day (15 to 30 μg/day, 0.5 to 1 nmol/day). The pattern of TSH secretion is both circadian and pulsatile. Its plasma half-life ranges from 50 to 80 min, and its clearance rate ranges from 40 to 60 ml/min. Small amounts of the individual subunits are found in the thyrotrophs and in the circulation, and their secretion is regulated in the same way as is that of intact TSH.[42]

Thyroid Hormone Regulation of TSH Secretion

T_4 and T_3 directly inhibit TSH secretion, and a deficiency of T_4 and T_3 increases it (Fig. 10-12). The sensitivity of the thyrotrophs is great, so that very small changes in serum T_4 and T_3 concentrations have large effects on TSH secretion, when the changes in serum T_4 and T_3 are due to changes in thyroid secretion (Fig. 10-13). Both T_4 and T_3 participate in this regulation, which serves to maintain thyroid secretion within very narrow limits. In contrast, the substantial decrease in serum T_3 concentrations that occurs in many patients with nonthyroidal illness results in little change in TSH secretion (see Nonthyroidal Illness). The probable reason is that circulating T_4 contributes more to the nuclear T_3 content of the pituitary than it does in many other tissues because the pituitary has considerable T_4-5′-deiodinase activity.[10,20] The relatively smaller contribution of circulating T_3 to pituitary nuclear T_3 content also allows increased TSH secretion and thus increased thyroid secretion in patients with abnormal thyroid glands or iodine deficiency, in whom T_3 is produced and secreted by the thyroid in relatively more normal amounts than is T_4.[7]

FIGURE 10-12 Factors regulating TSH secretion by the thyrotrophs of the pituitary. (−) = inhibitory effect; (+) = stimulatory effect; SRIH = somatostatin.

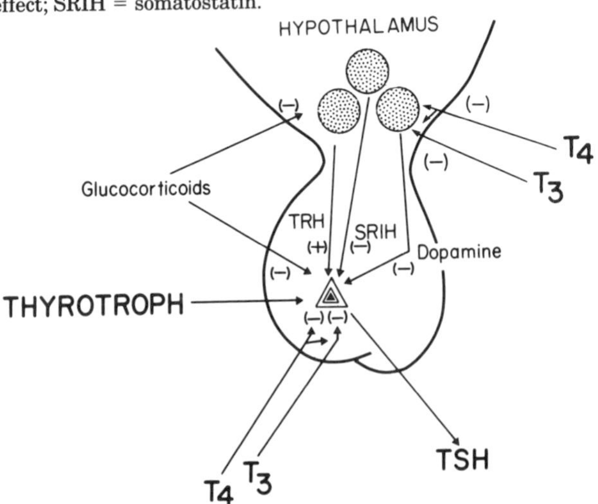

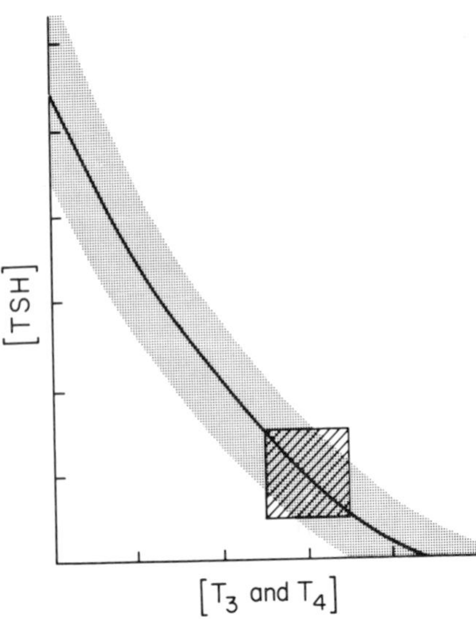

FIGURE 10-13 Diagram of the interrelation between serum TSH concentrations and serum T_4 and T_3 concentrations. The diagonally lined box encloses the respective normal ranges, and the shaded region indicates the pattern of changes in serum TSH concentrations that follow changes in thyroid secretion.

T_4 and T_3 inhibit TSH secretion by decreasing both the biosynthesis and the release of TSH and to a lesser extent by decreasing the secretion of TRH (Fig. 10-12).[37,43] The first action is achieved primarily by thyroid hormone regulation of the transcription of the TSH subunit genes and correlates with the extent of T_3 nuclear binding. The rapidity with which T_4 and T_3 administration can acutely lower TSH secretion suggests that the hormones also directly inhibit TSH release. Thyroid hormones also decrease the glycosylation of TSH, which reduces TSH bioactivity, and the number of thyrotroph receptors for TRH.[42] The rate and extent of thyroid hormone inhibition of TSH secretion are dependent on the initial serum TSH concentration, the hormone given, and its dose. Serum TSH concentrations decline, but not to normal, within hours after the administration of single doses of 400 to 500 μg or more of T_3 or T_4 to hypothyroid patients. The maximum inhibition of TSH secretion occurs much later than the peak serum T_4 or T_3 concentrations. When given in the usual therapeutic doses, T_3 decreases serum TSH to normal in approximately a week, but the response to T_4 is considerably slower. In normal subjects, even smaller doses of T_4 or T_3, doses not sufficient to cause thyrotoxicosis, inhibit TSH secretion in a few days. When given chronically, T_3 has about three times the potency of T_4 as an inhibitor of TSH secretion.[44] Recovery of suppressed TSH secretion, by contrast, takes at least several weeks or longer after the treatment of thyrotoxicosis or discontinuation of thyroid therapy.

Thyrotropin-Releasing Hormone

Thyrotropin-releasing hormone (TRH) is the tripeptide pyroglutamyl-histidyl-prolineamide (see Chap. 8). The content of TRH is highest in the median eminence and paraventricular nuclei of the hypothalamus, but some TRH is found in most hypothalamic nuclei.[45] Most of the TRH entering the hypothalamic-pituitary portal circulation comes from the paraventricular nuclei. These nuclei therefore are considered the thyrotrophic areas of the hypothalamus. Lesser amounts of TRH are found throughout the central nervous system and in the pituitary gland, gastrointestinal tract, pancreatic islets, and reproductive tract.[46] Its physiologic functions in these sites are unknown, but it may serve as a local neuromodulator.

TRH is synthesized as a 26-kDa protein (proTRH) that contains five copies of the sequence glutamine-histidine-proline-glycine flanked by proteolytic cleavage sites; TRH is formed from proTRH by the action of peptidases followed by cyclization of the glutamine residue to form a pyroglutamyl residue.[47] The production of proTRH mRNA and proTRH itself in the paraventricular nuclei is increased in hypothyroid rats and decreases after local or systemic injection of T_4 or T_3.[43] Presumably, TRH secretion from these neurons is regulated in a similar fashion. TRH is metabolized very rapidly, its plasma half-life being about 5 min.

TRH stimulates TSH secretion (Fig. 10-12) by binding to receptors on thyrotroph cell membranes that are linked to phospholipase C. The phosphoinositides formed by the action of this enzyme stimulate the release of calcium from intracellular storage sites, and this in turn stimulates exocytosis of TSH.[48] More chronic actions of TRH include the stimulation of TSH subunit biosynthesis and TSH glycosylation; the latter action results in the secretion of TSH with enhanced biological activity.[42] The number of TRH receptors on the thyrotrophs is down regulated by TRH as well as by thyroid hormones.

TRH secretion is probably pulsatile, accounting for the pulsatility of TSH secretion, and surges of TRH secretion are responsible for the surges of TSH secretion that occur in newborn infants and cold-exposed children. TRH is required for maintenance of normal TSH secretion, and it determines the set point about which thyroid hormones regulate TSH secretion. Administration of anti-TRH serum and lesions of the paraventricular nuclei reduce serum TSH and thyroid hormone concentrations in animals. In some patients with low serum TSH concentrations and hypothyroidism, repeated TRH administration restores serum TSH, T_4, and T_3 concentrations to normal. Moreover, in patients or animals with TRH deficiency, thyroid deficiency results in smaller increases in TSH secretion, and thyroid hormones more readily inhibit TSH secretion than is the case in normal subjects or animals.

Exogenously administered TRH causes a dose-dependent increase in serum TSH concentrations in normal subjects. TRH administered continuously for several days stimulates the release of more TSH than does the same dose given intermittently, although in both situations serum TSH concentrations decline after about 1 day.[49] Administration of TRH for several months results in sustained increases in serum TSH of only 100 percent and in serum T_4 and T_3 concentrations of only 50 percent, providing further testimony to the ability of small increases in serum thyroid hormone concentrations to inhibit TSH secretion directly.[50]

Exogenous TRH administration also stimulates prolactin release in normal subjects and most hyperprolactinemic patients and growth hormone secretion in elderly normal subjects and patients with various disorders, including acromegaly, chronic liver disease, and diabetes mellitus. However, endogenous TRH is not a physiologic regulator of either prolactin or growth hormone secretion.

Other Factors Altering TSH Secretion

Several other factors, in addition to thyroid hormones and TRH, alter TSH secretion (Fig. 10-12). One is somatostatin.[51] Infusions of somatostatin and its long-acting analog octreotide reduce basal serum TSH concentrations and inhibit the serum TSH response to exogenous TRH. Both are less potent inhibitors of TSH than of growth hormone secretion; patients receiving long-term treatment with octreotide do not become hypothyroid.[52] Conversely, infusions of somatostatin antiserum increase basal serum TSH concentrations, and hypothalamic lesions that reduce median eminence somatostatin content are accompanied by increased serum TSH concentrations. Thus, somatostatin may be a physiologically important tonic inhibitor of TSH secretion.

Dopamine also may be a physiologically important inhibitor of TSH secretion.[51] Serum TSH concentrations decline during infusions of dopamine and increase acutely after the administration of dopaminergic antagonists such as metoclopramide and domperidone in both normal and hypothyroid subjects. Since domperidone does not cross the blood-brain barrier and dopamine infusions decrease TSH pulse amplitude but not pulse frequency, dopamine most likely has a direct action on the thyrotrophs.[53]

Glucocorticoids also can inhibit TSH secretion.[51] Their major action is to decrease pulsatile TSH secretion, suggesting that they inhibit TRH secretion, but they also inhibit serum TSH responses to exogenous TRH. Conversely, metyrapone-induced decreases in glucocorticoid production are accompanied by increases in serum TSH concentrations.

The overall importance of the effects of somatostatin, dopamine, and glucocorticoids on TSH secretion in the long term is probably small. Transient increases in endogenous dopamine, somatostatin, or glucocorticoid secretion may transiently decrease TSH secretion. However, sustained increases in the endogenous production of these agents do not lead to decreases in TSH secretion sufficient to cause hypothyroidism. The reason for this is that the direct stimulatory effect on TSH secretion of any initial decreases in thyroid hormone secretion overcomes the inhibition of TSH secretion induced by these agents.

Mechanism of Action of TSH

TSH stimulates virtually every aspect of thyroid hormone biosynthesis and secretion by the thyroid. It also stimulates many steps in intermediary metabolism and the expression of many genes in thyroid tissue and causes thyroid hyperplasia and hypertrophy. The actions of TSH are initiated by its binding to specific plasma membrane receptors. It is the beta subunit of TSH that binds to the receptor, but high-affinity binding and signal transduction require the presence of the alpha subunit as well.[54] The receptor is an 85-kd glycoprotein with an extracellular domain of approximately 400 amino acids, seven transmembrane domains of about 250 amino acids, and an intracytoplasmic domain of about 100 amino acids.[55] The binding of TSH to its receptors activates adenylate cyclase, increasing cyclic AMP formation, which then activates several protein kinases. How this process is linked to specific steps of iodide metabolism or other thyroid metabolic processes is not known. TSH regulates the production of its receptor in a positive way,[56] a not unexpected finding in view of clinical evidence that sustained increases in TSH secretion cause sustained increases in thyroid gland function. TSH also stimulates phospholipase C activity in thyroid tissue, probably via the same receptor, thus increasing phosphoinositide turnover, intracellular calcium ion concentrations, and protein kinase C activity.[55] This action of TSH on phospholipase C is slower and requires more TSH than does stimulation of adenylate cyclase activity, and its physiologic importance is not known.

TSH stimulates most if not all aspects of intrathyroidal iodide and thyroglobulin metabolism.[5,55] The stimulation of iodide transport is slow, requiring 24 h of exposure to TSH, and is due to the production of additional transport units. The TSH-induced increase of iodothyronine formation is rapid and occurs in the absence of measurable increases in H_2O_2 production or thyroid peroxidase activity. Stimulation of colloid endocytosis and thyroglobulin proteolysis is even more rapid, occurring within minutes after TSH exposure. TSH stimulation of thyroidal T_4-5′-deiodinase activity increases the proportion of T_3 that is secreted, thus helping conserve iodine stores.[7] Most if not all of these TSH actions are mimicked by cyclic AMP. Physiologically, TSH stimulates the secretion of thyroglobulin as well as that of T_4 and T_3, although more slowly. It is more effective when its secretion is pulsatile than when it is continuous.[49]

TSH stimulates many other facets of thyroid cell function.[55] It increases oxygen consumption, glucose and fatty acid utilization, phospholipid turnover, and the content of NADPH, which is utilized for H_2O_2 generation as well as iodotyrosine and perhaps iodothyronine deiodination. A clinically obvious and important chronic action of TSH is stimulation of thyroid hypertrophy and hyperplasia, i.e., goiter formation (see Chap. 11). This growth reflects the ability of TSH to stimulate the synthesis of DNA, RNA, and structural proteins.

Other factors that may be involved in the growth of the thyroid include insulin-like growth factor-I (IGF-I), epidermal growth factor (EGF), interleukin-1, and tumor necrosis factor (see Chap. 11). Thyroid cells produce and have receptors for IGF-I and EGF, and IGF-I augments the stimulatory effect of TSH on thyroidal DNA synthesis. Interleukin-1 and tumor necrosis factor, which may be produced by thyroid cells as well as intrathyroidal mononuclear cells, stimulate thyroid cell growth but inhibit differentiated functions in thyroid cells.[57,58]

Regulation of Thyroid Secretion by Iodide

The thyroid gland utilizes iodide most efficiently when it is scarce, and much less efficiently when it is abundant. Much of this regulation is achieved by TSH, but iodide also participates in this process.[5] When little iodide is available, iodide transport and T_4 and especially T_3 synthesis are increased, even in the absence of TSH. With increasing iodide availability, the synthesis of T_4 increases more than does that of T_3; at high concentrations, iodide inhibits the synthesis of both hormones. The dose of iodine at which this inhibition occurs in humans is about 5 mg daily. Surges in iodine intake therefore do not result in increases in thyroid hormone synthesis.

When iodide intake is chronically increased, there is adaptation to the antithyroid effect of iodide so that hormone formation is not chronically inhibited. This adaptation results from inhibition of iodide transport; therefore, intracellular iodide concentrations sufficient to maintain the block in hormone synthesis and thus cause thyroid deficiency do not develop. Iodide excess also inhibits thyroglobulin proteolysis and thus the release of T_4 and T_3 from the thyroid. This is its most rapid effect, occurring within hours, and is the principal mechanism for the antithyroid effect of iodide in patients with hyperthyroidism.

Regulation of Extrathyroidal Triiodothyronine Production

The activities of the extrathyroidal T_4-5′-deiodinases that catalyze the conversion of T_4 to T_3 are altered by a number of factors (Fig. 10-14). The activity of type I T_4-5′-deiodinase, the enzyme that predominates in liver and kidney and appears to produce most of the circulating T_3, is decreased in tissues from animals that are selenium-deficient, pointing to the key role of the selenocysteine residue in enzyme activity.[11,59] Type I T_4-5′-deiodinase activity is also decreased in fetal animals and animals that are starved, hypothyroid, diabetic or uremic, or have other nonthyroidal illnesses (Table 10-4).[9–11,26,27,60–62] It is also decreased by PTU, glucocorticoids, beta-adrenergic antagonist drugs, and various iodothyronine analogues, notably rT_3. Conversely, type I T_4-5′-deiodinase activity is increased by thyroid hormone administration, glucose plus insulin, and a high caloric intake.[63,64] The biochemical mechanisms that might cause alterations in tissue T_4-5′-deiodinase activity include alterations in substrate (T_4) production, transfer of T_4 into cells, intracellular distribution of T_4, enzyme activity or mass, and cofactor availability. The drugs that reduce T_4-5′-deiodinase activity bind to the enzyme, whereas starvation may decrease hepatic T_3 production by decreasing T_4 uptake into the liver.[65] In other situations, alterations of enzyme mass or activity are the likely causes of decreased T_3 production, but the specific nutritional, hormonal, or toxic factors or cytokines that cause the alterations are not known.

TABLE 10-4 Conditions Altering Thyroxine 5′-Deiodinase Activity

Condition	Enzyme Type Affected*	
	Type 1	Type 2
Fetus	Decreased	Decreased
Hypothyroidism	Decreased	Increased†
Thyrotoxicosis	Increased	Decreased†
Starvation	Decreased	Normal
Diabetes mellitus	Decreased	Normal
Uremia	Decreased	Normal
Selenium deficiency	Decreased	Decreased‡
Administration of		
Propylthiouracil	Decreased	Normal
Iopanoic acid	Decreased	Decreased
Amiodarone	Decreased	Decreased
Propranolol	Decreased	?

* Type 1 predominates in the liver and kidneys; type 2, in the brain and pituitary gland.

† Excluding the thyrotrophs of the pituitary gland.

‡ Secondary effect caused by hyperthyroxinemia resulting from decreased type I T_4-5′-deiodinase activity.

Source: Refs. 9–11, 26, 59, 60–62, 148, 149.

FIGURE 10-14 Effect of various nonthyroidal disorders and drugs on T_4 conversion to T_3 in the organs (liver and kidney) that are the predominant sites of extrathyroidal T_3 production. Conversion is low in fetal tissues; is inhibited by illness, starvation, and some drugs; and is augmented by overnutrition.

The regulation of the T_4-5′-deiodinase (type II) that predominates in the brain and pituitary is different (Table 10-4). Its activity is increased by thyroid deficiency, is little affected by nutritional deficiency and PTU, and is decreased by thyroid hormone.[9–11,61,62,66] Such regulation serves to reduce the impact of systemic thyroid deficiency in these tissues by increasing the availability of T_3 for the maintenance of neural growth and function and pituitary function. The increase in pituitary T_4-5′-deiodinase activity that occurs in thyroid deficiency and the decrease that occurs with thyroid hormone excess probably do not include the thyrotrophs, since alterations in T_3 production in these cells would blunt the changes in TSH secretion needed to defend against changes in thyroidal T_4 and T_3 secretion.

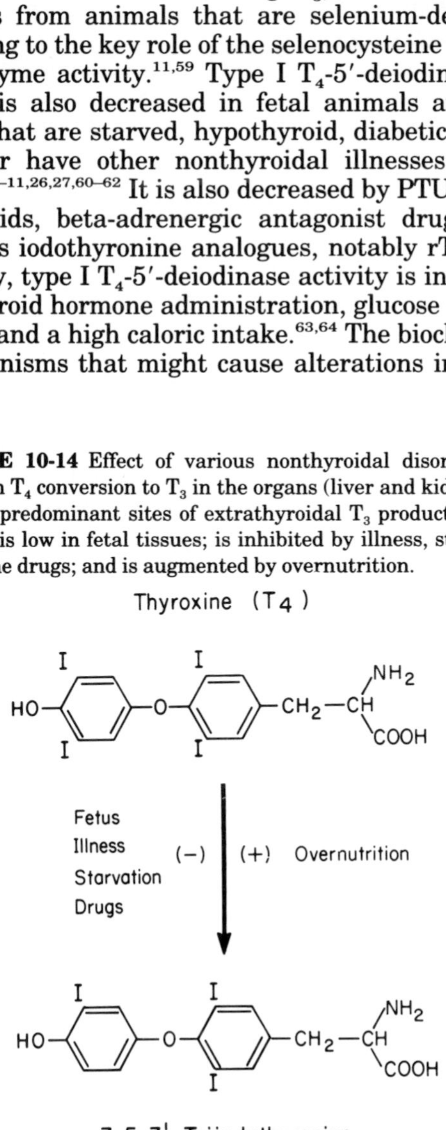

Overall, these findings indicate that T_3 production in various tissues is regulated in different ways and that changes in thyroidal or extrathyroidal thyroid hormone production, as manifested by their circulating concentrations, are not the only, and perhaps not the major, determinants of intracellular T_3 availability. Local regulation of T_3 production may

TABLE 10-5 Strategies for Testing Thyroid Function

Subject	Possible Thyroid Dysfunction	Serum Test
Clinically euthyroid, healthy		
Solitary nodule	Thyrotoxicosis	TSH
Multinodular goiter	Thyrotoxicosis	TSH
Diffuse goiter	Thyrotoxicosis or hypothyroidism	TSH
Clinically euthyroid, nonthyroidal illness*	Thyrotoxicosis or hypothyroidism	TSH, free T_4 index
Suspected thyrotoxicosis		TSH, free T_4 index
Suspected hypothyroidism		TSH, free T_4 index
Thyrotoxicosis, during treatment	Thyrotoxicosis, euthyroid, or hypothyroidism	TSH, free T_4 index
Hypothyroidism, during treatment		TSH

* May include patients admitted to nursing homes and psychiatric services.

be particularly important in limiting the effects of thyroid deficiency in tissues such as the brain and pituitary and undoubtedly leads to differences in T_3 availability in different tissues in patients with nonthyroidal illness.

Evaluation of Thyroid Function

Sensitive and specific tests are available for the evaluation of patients suspected of having abnormalities in thyroid secretion and identifying whether the abnormality is thyroidal or hypothalamic-pituitary (central) in origin. The single most important question in an individual patient is, What is the level of thyroid secretion? The best way to answer this question is to measure the serum TSH concentration, the serum free T_4 index (or free T_4 concentration), or both. Measurement of the serum TSH concentration is seemingly less direct; its value lies in the fact that TSH secretion is such a sensitive indicator of changes in serum free T_4 concentrations. In general, the costs of the two tests are roughly similar, although there are wide local variations. The choice of tests depends on the circumstances in which the testing is done. Both tests should be done in patients strongly suspected of having thyrotoxicosis or hypothyroidism and in hospitalized patients with nonthyroidal illness. Only one test needs to be done initially for case finding in patients not suspected of having any abnormality in thyroid secretion. For these purposes, the single best test is measurement of the serum TSH concentration (Table 10-5), although the serum free T_4 index is a satisfactory substitute. Screening of healthy people for thyroid disease (except newborn infants) is not warranted.[67]

Serum TSH Concentrations

Measurements of serum TSH provide a very precise indication of the availability of T_4 and T_3 to the pituitary in healthy subjects and patients with thyroid disease (Fig. 10-15). Serum TSH concentrations in normal subjects range from approximately 0.3 to 3.0 mU/liter. The assays now in use have a sensitivity of about 0.02 to 0.05 mU/liter (in some instances 0.005 mU/liter), and so subnormal serum TSH values can be identified readily.[68,69] Most of these assays utilize two rodent monoclonal antibodies, one against an epitope of the beta subunit of TSH and the other against an epitope on the common alpha subunit of the glycoprotein hormones. To be detected, a molecule must have both epitopes, and so the assays are very specific. The normal range for serum TSH concentrations largely encompasses the circadian and pulsatile variation in TSH secretion that occurs in normal subjects (see below).

Serum TSH concentrations are increased in patients with hypothyroidism when it is due to thyroid disease and are normal or low when it is due to hypothalamic or pituitary disease (central hypothyroidism) (Fig. 10-15). Serum TSH concentrations are low or undetectable in patients with thyrotoxicosis. The change in serum TSH concentrations in patients with thyroid disease is continuous, so that they range from very high in patients with overt hypothyroidism to very low in patients with overt thyrotoxicosis (Fig. 10-13). Changes in serum T_4 concentrations of as little as 15 to 20 percent that occur as a result of changes in thyroid secretion (as opposed to nonthyroidal illness) are sufficient to raise or lower serum TSH concentrations outside the normal range. Thyroid secretion and serum T_4 concentrations therefore need not be outside the normal range for serum TSH concentrations to be abnormal.

Because of the sensitivity of TSH secretion to small changes in thyroid secretion, an abnormal serum TSH concentration usually indicates the presence of an abnormality in thyroid secretion. Conversely, a normal serum TSH concentration provides strong evidence against the presence of any abnormality of thyroid secretion.[68,70] Serum TSH concentrations are normal in most patients with nonthyroidal illness who have decreased serum thyroid hormone concentrations but can be either low or high (see Nonthyroidal Illness). Some seemingly healthy subjects have low values that cannot be related to any thyroid disease and that do not persist[71]; whether such changes are due to wider than usual variations in pulsatile TSH secretion or to transient, clinically unrecognized nonthyroidal illness is not known.

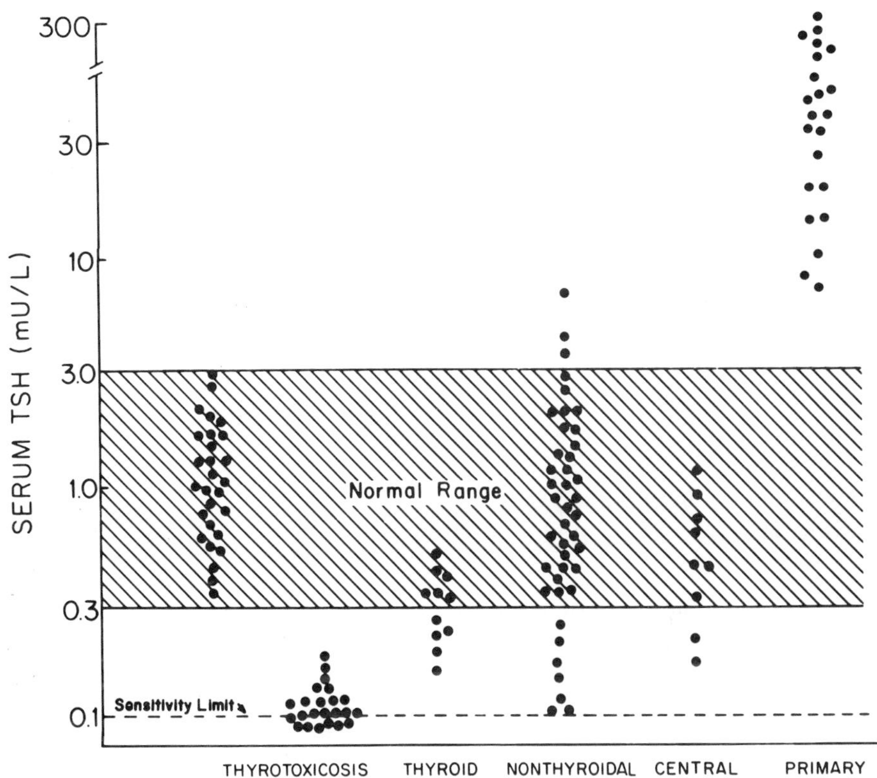

FIGURE 10-15 Serum TSH concentrations in normal subjects and patients with thyrotoxicosis, thyroid autonomy (euthyroid, some of whom have subclinical thyrotoxicosis), nonthyroidal illness, and central and primary hypothyroidism. The diagonally lined area indicates the normal range. Note the logarithmic scale of the y-axis.

The results of serum TSH measurements can be misleading in patients in whom serum thyroid hormone concentrations change abruptly, because the impact of such changes on TSH secretion may not be manifested for several days or occasionally weeks. Spurious elevations are very rare and have so far been identified only in patients with antibodies that react with mouse or other animal immunoglobulins; most such patients have autoimmune disease or have been extensively exposed to animals.[72]

Serum Thyroxine Concentrations

Serum total T_4 concentrations are measured by radioimmunoassays that use specific anti-T_4 antibodies and require the use of an agent to block T_4 binding to the serum T_4-binding proteins so that all the T_4 is available for reaction with the anti-T_4 antibody. The normal range in adults is about 5 to 11 μg/dl (64 to 140 nmol/liter). The terms *hyperthyroxinemia* and *hypothyroxinemia* are used to define values above and below this range, respectively. Serum T_4 concentrations are determined primarily by thyroid secretion of T_4 and serum concentrations of the thyroid hormone-binding proteins (Table 10-6). Therefore, serum T_4 concentrations are high in patients with thyrotoxicosis and those with increased serum concentrations of TBG and other binding proteins (see Alterations in Serum Thyroid Hormone Binding). Rarer causes of raised T_4 concentrations include the presence of autoantibodies that bind T_4 and decreases in T_4 clearance. Thus, the serum T_4 concentration can be high in patients who are euthyroid or even hypothyroid.

Conversely, serum T_4 concentrations are low in patients with hypothyroidism. They also are low in patients who have decreased serum concentrations of TBG and other binding proteins or who are receiving drugs that inhibit the binding of T_4 to TBG, patients receiving T_3, and those who have serious nonthyroidal illness (Table 10-6).

Misinterpretation usually can be avoided by simultaneous determination of serum T_4-binding capacity or direct measurement of serum free T_4 concentrations.

Serum T_4-Binding Capacity (Thyroid Hormone–Binding Ratio) and Free Thyroxine Index

Since nearly all the T_4 in serum is bound to TBG or other proteins, the extent of protein binding must be determined to interpret the results of serum T_4 measurements properly. This is done most simply by determination of the thyroid hormone–binding ratio (THBR), also known as the T_3-resin uptake. This test measures the number of unoccupied protein-binding sites for T_4. It is done by mixing radiolabeled T_3 with serum, adding a resin or another particulate substance, and then determining the amount of radiola-

TABLE 10-6 Conditions Altering Serum Thyroxine Concentrations, Thyroid Hormone–Binding Ratios (THBR), and Serum Free Thyroxine Index Values

	Serum T_4 Concentration	THBR	Free T_4 Index
Thyrotoxicosis	Increased	Increased	Increased
Increased serum TBG*	Increased	Decreased	Normal
Familial dysalbuminemic hyperthyroxinemia	Increased	Normal	Increased
Hypothyroidism	Decreased	Decreased	Decreased
Decreased serum TBG	Decreased	Increased	Normal
Inhibitors of TBG binding	Decreased	Increased	Normal
T_3 treatment	Decreased	Decreased	Decreased
Nonthyroidal illness	Normal, decreased or increased	Normal or increased	Normal, decreased or increased

* TBG = thyroxine-binding globulin.

beled T_3 bound to the resin (Fig. 10-16). In normal serum, the unoccupied protein-binding sites, primarily TBG, take up about 55 to 75 percent of the radiolabeled T_3, and 25 to 45 percent is bound to the resin, i.e., is the T_3-resin uptake, depending on the amounts of serum and particulate substance used. The results also may be expressed as the ratio of the amount of radiolabeled T_3 bound to the resin in the presence of the test serum to that bound in the presence of normal serum (normal range, 0.80 to 1.20). The THBR determination is not a measurement of the serum T_3 concentration. Moreover, since the affinity of TBG for T_3 is low in comparison with its affinity for T_4, the test is altered little by alterations in serum T_3 concentrations. Serum TBG can be measured directly, but such measurements are needed only when the specific cause of a binding abnormality is being sought.

There are three ways in which the number of unoccupied T_4-binding sites in serum may be decreased, resulting in a high THBR: (1) when more binding sites are occupied with T_4, as in thyrotoxicosis, (2) when binding sites are occupied by a ligand that competes with T_4 for binding to TBG, such as salicylate, and (3) when there is a decrease in the number of binding sites, as occurs when serum concentrations of TBG or another binding protein are decreased (Table 10-6). There are two ways in which the number of unoccupied T_4-binding sites in serum may be increased, resulting in a low THBR: (1) when fewer binding sites are occupied by T4, as in hypothyroidism, and (2) when there is an increase in

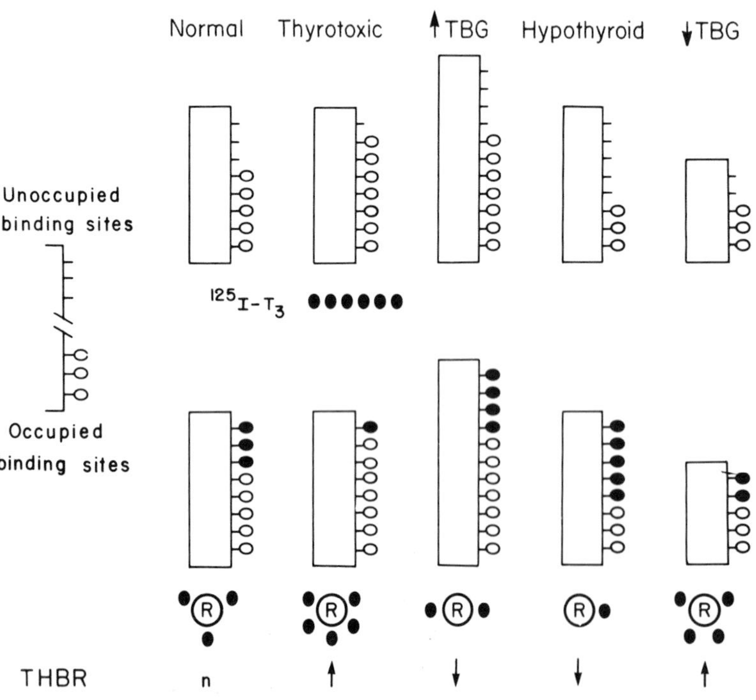

FIGURE 10-16 The thyroid hormone–binding ratio (THBR) test (T_3-resin uptake test). For clarity of representation, the proportion of the total number of binding sites occupied by endogenous hormone is underrepresented in this figure. R = resin or other inert substance added to bind the $[^{125}I]T_3$ that is not bound to serum protein.

the number of binding sites, as occurs when serum concentrations of TBG or another binding protein are increased.

Thus, a serum T_4 value must be examined in conjunction with the THBR; if both the THBR and the serum T_4 concentration are high or if both are low, thyroid secretion is altered. If the two results are discordant, an abnormality of binding protein is likely. The product of the serum T_4 value and THBR is the free T_4 index (Table 10-6). This value generally correlates well with direct measurements of serum free T_4 concentrations, although it may underestimate the degree of abnormality in protein binding in patients with nonthyroidal illness, those with very large increases or decreases in serum TBG concentrations, and those with familial dysalbuminemic hyperthyroxinemia.

Serum Free Thyroxine Concentrations

Serum free T_4 concentrations can be measured directly by equilibrium dialysis, ultrafiltration, and radioimmunoassay. Although the first two methods are thought to provide the closest approximation to the serum free T_4 concentration in vivo, they are technically difficult and not widely available. Normal values range from 1 to 3 ng/dl (13 to 39 pmol/liter). The radioimmunoassays for free T_4 provide accurate estimates of serum free T_4 concentrations in patients with thyroid disease, but the results may not be accurate in patients with nonthyroidal illness and those with abnormalities in binding proteins, particularly the results of assays that use a T_4 analog that may not inhibit the binding of T_4 to the binding protein.[73] As a practical matter, serum free T_4 measurements provide information comparable to that provided by serum free T_4 index measurements, which are more widely available and less expensive.

Serum Triiodothyronine Concentrations

Serum T_3 concentrations are measured by radioimmunoassay. The normal range is 75 to 200 ng/dl (1.1 to 3.0 nmol/liter). Serum T_3 concentrations, like those of T_4, are altered by changes in thyroid secretion and changes in serum thyroid hormone–binding proteins. In patients with thyrotoxicosis, they usually are increased to a greater degree than are serum T_4 concentrations; in patients with hypothyroidism, they are more often within the normal range than are serum T_4 concentrations. Serum T_3 concentrations are low in most patients with nonthyroidal illness (see Nonthyroidal Illness). The major if not only indication for measurement of the serum T_3 concentration is in patients with clinical manifestations of thyrotoxicosis who have serum T_4 concentrations that are within the normal range.

Serum Reverse Triiodothyronine Concentrations

Serum reverse T_3 (rT_3) concentrations, also measured by radioimmunoassay, range from 20 to 50 ng/dl (0.3 to 0.8 nmol/liter) in normal subjects. Serum rT_3 concentrations depend primarily on the level of T_4 secretion, since virtually all the rT_3 in serum is produced from T_4 at extrathyroidal sites. Changes in serum thyroid hormone–binding proteins have little effect on serum rT_3 concentrations because the affinity of TBG and other binding proteins for rT_3 is low. Serum rT_3 concentrations are often high in patients with nonthyroidal illness, in whom rT_3 degradation is decreased. Serum rT_3 measurements are not useful clinically because they provide little information about thyroid secretion and because of the wide variations that occur in patients with nonthyroidal illness.

Serum Thyroglobulin Concentrations

Thyroglobulin is found in small amounts [5 to 25 μg/liter (7.5 to 37.5 nmol/liter)] in the circulation of virtually all normal subjects.[8] Thyroglobulin antibodies interfere with the measurement of thyroglobulin; therefore, serum thyroglobulin cannot be measured accurately in patients with such antibodies.

Serum thyroglobulin concentrations are increased in patients with thyrotoxicosis, except those in whom thyrotoxicosis is due to exogenous thyroid administration; they have low serum thyroglobulin concentrations. Thus, measurements of serum thyroglobulin can be used to differentiate spontaneously occurring from exogenous thyrotoxicosis. Serum thyroglobulin concentrations also are increased in some patients with endemic goiter, multinodular goiter, and benign and malignant thyroid tumors, and they may increase transiently after needle-aspiration biopsy of thyroid nodules. In hypothyroid patients, measurements of serum thyroglobulin can be used to distinguish those who have no thyroid tissue from those in whom thyroid hormonogenesis is abnormal but thyroid tissue is present, for example, to distinguish infants with thyroid agenesis from those with thyroid dysgenesis.

Serum thyroglobulin measurements are most useful in the follow-up of patients with thyroid carcinoma who have undergone thyroidectomy and usually also radioiodine ablation of any remaining thyroid tissue. A normal or high value in such a patient provides strong evidence of tumor recurrence.

Antithyroid Peroxidase and Antithyroglobulin Antibodies

Antibodies to thyroid peroxidase, formerly known as thyroid microsomal antigen, can be detected in high titer in the serum of most patients with chronic autoimmune thyroiditis, especially those with the goitrous form of the disease (Hashimoto's disease). They can be detected nearly as often, usually in somewhat lower titer, in patients with Graves' disease. Low titers of these antibodies also are found in patients with most other thyroid diseases; patients with other autoimmune diseases, such as pernicious anemia, idiopathic Addison's disease, and insulin-dependent diabetes mellitus; and in normal subjects, particularly elderly women. These people probably have some degree of chronic autoimmune thyroiditis, and some of them have elevated serum TSH concentrations. The principal value of tests for these antibodies is to confirm a suspected diagnosis of chronic autoimmune thyroiditis.

Circulating antibodies to thyroglobulin are also found in the serum of many patients with autoimmune thyroid disease, and less often in patients with other thyroid diseases and normal subjects. Tests for antithyroglobulin antibodies have little clinical value.

Thyrotropin-Releasing Hormone Stimulation Tests

TRH testing is usually done by the administration of 400 or 500 μg given as an intravenous bolus dose. In normal subjects, serum TSH concentrations increase 2- to 8-fold, to peak values of 5 to 25 mU/liter, 20 to 30 min after TRH administration. The intravenous injection of TRH is often followed by transient nausea and an urge to urinate and occasionally by hypertension. The serum TSH response to TRH is characteristically increased in patients with primary hypothyroidism and is subnormal, delayed, or both in those with TSH or TRH deficiency; the test cannot be used to distinguish between TSH deficiency and TRH deficiency. The response is inhibited by very small increases in serum T_4 and T_3 concentrations, so that TRH fails to increase serum TSH in euthyroid patients with autonomous thyroid secretion as well as in patients with thyrotoxicosis. The use of various drugs and nonthyroidal illness also result in subnormal serum TSH responses to TRH.

The serum TSH response to TRH correlates directly with the level of basal TSH secretion.[68] The TRH stimulation test therefore provides no information beyond that obtained by measurement of the basal serum TSH concentration. The only important clinical uses of TRH testing now are in patients with TSH-induced hyperthyroidism and those suspected of having gonadotroph adenomas (see Chap. 8).

Radionuclide Tests

The various radionuclides useful for thyroid studies and their characteristics are shown in Table 10-7. As discussed in detail in Chap. 11, concern about the radiation exposure from ^{131}I makes ^{123}I the iodine isotope of choice for nearly all clinical tests.

Measurement of thyroid radioiodine uptake as the proportion of administered isotope concentrated in the thyroid per unit of time can occasionally be useful as an index of thyroid function. In the United States, the normal thyroid radioiodine uptake is 5 to 15 percent 4 h and 10 to 25 percent 24 h after oral administration of the isotope. The values are low in hypothyroid patients; they are high in thyrotoxic patients, except those who have some type of thyroiditis or exogenous thyrotoxicosis.

The most common cause of a low radioiodine uptake is not hypothyroidism but an expanded extracellular iodine pool resulting from oral, parenteral, or cutaneous use of inorganic iodine or iodine-containing drugs. At least a week should elapse between the use of inorganic iodine and measurement of radioiodine uptake, and 2 or more weeks after the use of organic iodine compounds. Radionuclides should not be administered to pregnant women.

Thyroid radioisotope imaging (scan) studies are useful for the detection of anatomic variations and ectopic location of thyroid tissue and for assessing regional function within the thyroid gland. In patients with nodular thyroid disease, scans determine whether nodules can concentrate radioisotope and the extent to which the function of extranodular tissue is suppressed. Scanning may be done with either ^{123}I-iodide or pertechnetate-99m ($^{99m}TcO_4$). The latter, like iodide, is transported into the thyroid, but unlike iodide, it is not organified and diffuses back into the circulation rapidly. The peak pertechnetate uptake therefore is 20 to 30 min after its administration. Although it must be given intravenously, it has favorable detection and safety features, it costs less than ^{123}I, and it is more convenient for the patient because the thyroid scan can be done soon after its administration. In contrast, peak radioiodine uptake occurs 18 to 24 h after its administration, so that a second visit is required. All these features make

TABLE 10-7 Radiation Exposure from Isotopes Used for Thyroid Studies

				Radiation Exposure			
		Usual scanning dose		Total Body		Thyroid*	
Isotope	Half-Life	uCi	MBq	mrad	Gy	rads	Gy
^{123}I	13 h	200	7.4	6	0.0006	2.6	0.026
^{131}I	8 days	50	1.8	36	0.0036	65	0.65
$^{99m}TcO_4^-$	6 h	3000	110	15	0.0015	1	0.01

* Based on 25 percent 24-h uptake.

^{123}I and ^{131}I are given orally, and $^{99m}TcO_4^-$ is given intravenously.

Bq = becquerel; Gy = gray.

pertechnetate the isotope of choice for thyroid imaging in most patients. In either instance, proper interpretation of the scan requires that both the patient's thyroid gland and the scan be examined at the same time.

Ultrasonography and Needle Biopsy

These tests are useful principally in patients with thyroid nodular disease (see Chap. 11).

Tests of Thyroid Hormone Action in Tissue

Thyroid hormones alter the function of many tissues, and measurements reflecting their impact on tissues might be expected to be useful adjuncts for the diagnosis of thyrotoxicosis or hypothyroidism. However, the tests available for this purpose, such as measurements of serum cholesterol or sex hormone–binding globulin concentrations and basal metabolic rate and tests of myocardial contractility (systolic and diastolic time intervals), are neither sensitive nor specific indicators of the impact of thyroid hormones on their target tissues.

Physiologic Variables Affecting Pituitary-Thyroid Function and Tests

Daily Variations

TSH secretion is pulsatile, with 6 to 12 secretory episodes per 24 h (Fig. 10-17). The daytime and nighttime pulse frequencies are similar, but the pulse amplitude is greater at night, with the peaks of greatest magnitude occurring at the time of sleep onset.[53,74] There is therefore a circadian pattern of TSH secretion, so that mean serum TSH concentrations throughout the night are about 50 to 100 percent higher than during the day. Infants older than 1 month and children have a similar nocturnal increase in TSH secretion, but it is diminished in elderly subjects.[75] The normal pattern of nocturnal TSH secretion persists in patients who have small increases or decreases in thyroid secretion.[76] There is no circadian variation in serum T_4 and T_3 concentrations.

FIGURE 10-17 Serum TSH concentrations measured at frequent (10-min) intervals for 24 h in a normal man. The lines at the top indicate the number of pulses of TSH secretion as detected by the computer programs Desade and Cluster. 0 hours = midnight. *(Reproduced with modification from J Clin Endocrinol Metab 70:403, 1990, with permission of the publisher.)*

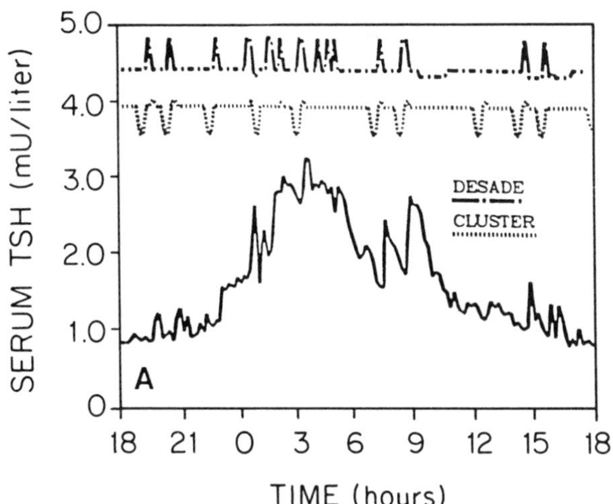

Pregnancy

Serum T_4 and T_3 concentrations increase progressively throughout the first half of pregnancy to values 30 to 50 percent higher than those in nonpregnant women and in men. They then remain constant during the latter half of pregnancy.[77] This increase is due to an increase in serum TBG concentrations. Serum free T_4 and T_3 concentrations rise transiently, largely within the normal range, at the end of the first trimester. This rise coincides with the period of highest serum chorionic gonadotropin concentrations and is due to its weak thyroid-stimulating activity. Serum TSH concentrations decrease slightly, by about 30 to 40 percent, when the serum free T_4 and T_3 concentrations rise during the first trimester but then gradually increase, within the normal range, during the remainder of gestation. These changes tend to be exaggerated in women with hyperemesis gravidarum (see Thyrotoxicosis during Pregnancy). Serum TBG and therefore T_4 and T_3 concentrations fall to their respective normal ranges 4 to 6 weeks after delivery.

Pregnancy increases the need for iodine, because maternal thyroid hormone synthesis and renal iodide clearance are increased and the fetal thyroid must be provided with iodine. Thyroid size changes little in pregnant women whose iodine intake is as large as it is in the United States,[78] but it increases in those whose iodine intake is low.

Fetal Thyroid Function

Thyroid function begins at about the tenth week of fetal life, and T_4 secretion begins soon afterward.[79] Fetal serum T_4 concentrations are initially very low and rise progressively so that at term the concentrations are similar to those in maternal serum. The pattern of increase in serum free T_4 concentrations is similar, but the increment is somewhat greater because the increase in serum TBG concentrations is not as large as that in T_4 secretion. Therefore, serum free T_4 concentrations in newborn infants are slightly higher than are those in maternal serum, whereas serum TBG concentrations are somewhat lower (although higher than in normal subjects). The progressive rise in serum free T_4 concentrations is due to a progressive rise in TSH secretion and maturation of the fetal thyroid. TSH can be detected in serum by 12 weeks, and its serum concentration rises progressively to between 4 and 10 mU/liter at term.[80] This increase, in the face of increasing serum free T_4 concentrations, indicates that pituitary sensitivity to T_4 during fetal life is limited. TRH is detectable in the hypothalamus in the first trimester, but its role in fetal pituitary-thyroid function is limited. The pituitary in the fetus responds in a qualitatively normal way to hypothyroidism and thyrotoxicosis with increases and decreases, respectively, in TSH secretion.[81]

In contrast to serum T_4, fetal serum T_3 concentrations are low and serum rT_3 concentrations are high throughout gestation. Fetal tissues have little T_4-5′-deiodinase activity and placental tissue is rich in T_4-5′-deiodinase activity,[10] explaining the low fetal serum T_3 concentrations. The high placental T_4-5′-deiodinase activity also results in rapid conversion of maternal or fetal T_4 to rT_3, explaining the high fetal serum rT_3 concentrations.

Iodide crosses the placenta freely. Some maternal T_4 also crosses the placenta, since infants who cannot synthesize any T_4 have serum T_4 concentrations at birth that are about 25 to 40 percent of those of normal infants.[82] This is enough T_4 to allow some T_3 production in fetal tissues, particularly the central nervous system, and therefore to provide some protection against fetal hypothyroidism.[83] Maternal T_3 does not reach the fetus in appreciable amounts, presumably because of the high placental level of T_4-5′-deiodinase activity. Similarly, little maternal TSH or TRH reaches the fetus.

Amniotic fluid contains small amounts of T_4, T_3, and TSH and large amounts of rT_3. The concentrations vary rather widely, and amniotic fluid measurements have not proved useful for the diagnosis of fetal thyroid disease.[84]

Infants and Children

Serum TSH concentrations increase abruptly soon after birth, reaching 50 to 100 mU/liter 60 to 120 min after delivery, and then decline to near adult values by the third or fourth day of life.[79] Thereafter, they decline very gradually, reaching adult values at the end of puberty.[85] The neonatal surge in TSH secretion results in an increase in T_4 secretion, so that serum total and free T_4 concentrations increase 1.5- to 2-fold during the first day of life. Serum T_3 concentrations increase fourfold- to sixfold at the same time because of increases in thyroidal secretion and extrathyroidal T_3 production. Both serum T_4 and T_3 concentrations then fall but remain slightly higher than in adults throughout infancy and childhood, gradually declining to adult levels at the end of puberty.[86] The decline throughout childhood is a result of declining serum TBG concentrations; free hormone concentrations are similar to those of adults after the neonatal period. Serum rT_3 concentrations decline rapidly after birth, presumably as a result of rapid maturation of 5′-deiodinating pathways.

The clearance of T_4 and T_3 is more rapid in children than in adults and slows progressively throughout childhood. Thus, the production rates of T_4 and T_3 per kilogram of body weight are higher in children, and adequate treatment of hypothyroidism requires relatively larger doses of T_4 in children as compared with adults.

Sex

There are no differences in pituitary-thyroid function in women and men in regard to thyroid secretion, extrathyroidal thyroid hormone metabolism, or serum thyroid hormone–binding proteins. Thus, their serum T_4, T_3, and TSH concentrations are similar. While serum TBG concentrations are increased by excess estrogen and decreased by excess androgen, serum TBG concentrations are similar in normal men and premenopausal and postmenopausal women despite the disparities in gonadal steroid hormone production among these groups.

Aging

Serum total and free T_4 concentrations are similar in young and elderly adults, as are serum T_3 and TSH concentrations for the most part. Some older persons have slightly low serum T_3 concentrations, more likely caused by subtle nonthyroidal illness than by an age-related decrease in extrathyroidal T_4 conversion to T_3. There is no age-related change in serum binding of T_4 and T_3 or in tissue sensitivity to T_4 or T_3. The nocturnal surge in TSH secretion is decreased in elderly subjects, and so their 24-h mean serum TSH concentrations are lower.[75] The clearance and production rates of T_4 and T_3 decrease with age, but in parallel, explaining why serum T_4 and T_3 concentrations do not change even though TSH secretion decreases.

The range of serum TSH concentrations in apparently healthy subjects seems to widen with age. Reports from the United States and the United Kingdom that describe somewhat elevated serum TSH concentrations in the elderly, especially elderly women, probably reflect the inclusion of subjects with mild autoimmune thyroiditis.[87] Subjects with elevated serum TSH concentrations often have positive tests for antithyroid antibodies and histologic evidence of thyroiditis. The frequency of low serum TSH concentrations also seems to be higher in elderly subjects; such low values may reflect some thyroid autonomy, a lower set point for TSH secretion, or the need for less thyroid secretion because of the decrease in T_4 clearance.

Environmental Factors

Serum T_4, T_3, and TSH concentrations vary little when measured at regular intervals for several months. Small variations in serum T_4 and TSH concentrations do occur as a result of climatologic variation, with T_4 being slightly lower and TSH being higher in the winter than in the summer in temperate regions.[88] Cold exposure has small, variable effects on thyroid function, depending on the duration and extent of exposure and the age of the subject. Among workers in cold-storage plants, it can raise serum T_4 and T_3 concentrations slightly.[89] Prolonged residence in Antarctica resulted in a small decline in serum T_3 but no change in T_4 or TSH concentrations.[90] Although increases in serum TSH concentrations cannot be detected in acutely cold-exposed adults, serum TSH concentrations do increase in cold-exposed infants, and the abrupt rise in serum TSH in the first hours after birth is due to cold exposure. Physical stresses such as acute or chronic physical exertion are not accompanied by significant changes in pituitary-thyroid function.

Alterations in Serum Thyroid Hormone Binding

Changes in serum thyroid hormone–binding proteins are important causes of both hyperthyroxinemia and hypothyroxinemia (Table 10-8) but do not usually result in abnormal serum free T_4 concentrations or free T_4 index values. The most important alterations in binding are those due to changes in serum TBG concentrations, because so much of the T_4 and T_3 in serum is bound to it. If TBG or another binding protein is added to serum in vitro, the equilibrium between free and bound T_4 is altered so that more of the T_4 becomes bound, but the total T_4 or T_3 concentration does not change. In vivo, however, the fall in serum free T_4 and T_3 concentrations that follows an increase in serum TBG results in a transient increase in pituitary-thyroid function and a decrease in T_4 and T_3 clearance, so that the free hormone concentrations are restored to normal. Once a new steady state is reached, serum total T_4 concentrations are increased, free T_4 concentrations are normal, and fractional daily clearance is decreased, but total daily clearance and production are normal. The opposite changes occur when serum TBG concentrations decrease.

TABLE 10-8 Causes of Hyperthyroxinemia and Hypothyroxinemia

Hyperthyroxinemia
Thyrotoxicosis
Increased thyroxine binding in serum
Increased thyroxine-binding globulin (TBG) binding
Pregnancy
Endogenous and exogenous estrogen excess
Acute and chronic hepatitis, hepatoma
Human immunodeficiency virus infection
Drugs: opiates, 5-fluorouracil, clofibrate
Inherited TBG excess
Increased albumin binding
Familial dysalbuminemic hyperthyroxinemia
Increased transthyretin binding
Familial increase in transthyretin binding
Islet-cell carcinoma
Nonthyroidal illness
Medical illness
Psychiatric illness
Drug-induced hyperthyroxinemia
Drugs slowing thyroxine clearance*
Amiodarone
Oral cholecystographic agents
Propranolol
Drugs mimicking thyroxine (L-thyroxine)
Generalized thyroid hormone resistance
Hypothyroxinemia
Hypothyroidism
Decreased thyroxine binding in serum
Decreased thyroxine-binding globulin (TBG) binding
Inherited complete and partial TBG deficiency
Exogenous androgen and anabolic steroid hormone excess
Glucocorticoid excess
Drugs: asparaginase, colestipol-niacin
Nonthyroidal illness
Decreased transthyretin binding
Nonthyroidal illness
Familial amyloidotic polyneuropathy
Decreased albumin binding
Nonthyroidal illness
Drug-related inhibition of binding
Salicylates
Furosemide

* Increased thyroxine secretion contributes to hyperthyroxinemia.

Increased Serum Binding

Increased serum TBG concentrations are most commonly caused by estrogen excess, whether due to pregnancy, the administration of estrogen or estrogen-containing medication, or estrogen-secreting tumors (Table 10-8). The increase is due to production of TBG that is more heavily glycosylated and that therefore is cleared from the circulation more slowly than is the TBG produced by normal subjects rather than the production of increased amounts of TBG protein.[91] The response to exogenous estrogen occurs over a period of 4 weeks and is dose-dependent. For conjugated estrogen, the maximal dose is 1.25 mg daily; it results on average in a 50 percent increase in serum TBG concentrations and a 30 percent increase in serum T_4 concentrations.[92] With ethinyl estradiol, 20-μg doses have comparable effects; 50-μg doses raise serum TBG concentrations nearly 100 percent and T_4 concentrations 60 percent.[93] In contrast, vaginal and transdermal estrogen preparations have little effect on serum TBG concentrations. Serum TBG concentrations return to normal about 4 weeks after the termination of estrogen therapy. The amount of estrogen in most oral contraceptive agents now in use ranges from 20 to 30 μg ethinyl estradiol or its equivalent; women taking the lower doses thus do not usually have serum T_4 concentrations above the upper limit of normal, and the increase is less if the progestational component of the preparation has some androgenic activity. Pure progestogens have no effect on serum TBG concentrations. The partial estrogen antagonist tamoxifen raises serum TBG concentrations slightly.

Patients with several liver diseases have increases in serum TBG concentrations. The increases are greatest and occur most frequently in patients with acute hepatitis, but increases also occur in patients with chronic hepatitis, biliary cirrhosis, and hepatoma. Human immunodeficiency virus infection is another cause of increased serum TBG concentrations (see Effects of Specific Disorders on Thyroid Function). A variety of drugs raise serum TBG concentrations. They include methadone, heroin, clofibrate, perphenazine, and 5-fluorouracil.[17,62] The cause of the increase is increased glycosylation of TBG in acute hepatitis and increased synthesis of TBG in patients treated with 5-fluorouracil. Small increases in serum TBG concentrations also occur in patients with acute intermittent porphyria and hypothyroidism.

Increased TBG production occurs as an X-linked inherited disorder.[94] Hemizygous affected males (about 1 in 30,000, based on the results of neonatal screening programs) have a threefold increase in serum TBG concentrations and therefore high serum T_4 concentrations; heterozygous affected females have a twofold increase in serum TBG and a lesser increase in serum T_4. The basic abnormality is increased production of TBG; the composition and binding properties are normal. The production of other transport proteins such as corticosteroid- and sex hormone–binding globulin is not increased in these subjects.

Increased serum T_4 concentrations also occur as a result of increased production of other binding proteins. One such syndrome is known as familial dysalbuminemic hyperthyroxinemia (FDH).[17,95] The affected subjects, who are euthyroid and have normal serum TSH concentrations, produce increased quantities of the albumin isoforms that have a higher affinity for T_4 than for T_3. As a result, their serum T_4 concentrations are increased, whereas their serum T_3 concentrations are usually normal. Serum free T_4 (and T_3) concentrations are normal, but serum free T_4 index values are increased. (The free T_4 index is increased because the serum T_4 concentration is increased, although the THBR is normal. The THBR is normal because the radiolabeled T_3 used in the test binds poorly to the excess albumin binding sites, so that the increased number of unoccupied binding sites is not detected.) This disorder is inherited as an autosomal dominant trait.

Increases in TTR binding of T_4 are rare. They occur on a familial basis (autosomal dominant inheritance) and in some patients with pancreatic islet-cell carcinoma.[96,97] The biochemical findings are similar to those in patients with FDH; they include normal serum T_3 concentrations and THBR test values because of the limited binding of T_3 to TTR. In one family with increased TTR binding, the serum TTR concentrations were normal; the abnormality was an amino acid substitution that resulted in the production of TTR with an increased affinity for T_4. Islet-cell carcinoma patients, by contrast, have increased serum TTR concentrations. The diagnosis of FDH and of disorders of TTR transport can be confirmed by the use of $[^{125}I]T_4$ instead of $[^{125}I]T_3$ in a resin uptake test; in these patients, the resin uptake of $[^{125}I]T_4$ is low because of the increased albumin or TTR binding of $[^{125}I]T_4$.[73]

Hyperthyroxinemia is occasionally due to serum autoantibodies that bind T_4, T_3, or both.[98] Such antibodies raise the serum total T_4 or T_3 concentrations (in most assays) and slow the clearance of the hormones; they serve in effect as a binding protein. These antibodies are antithyroglobulin antibodies for which the immunogenic thyroglobulin epitopes include T_4, T_3, or both. They are usually polyclonal IgG antibodies and are found most often in patients with autoimmune thyroid disease. Most of these patients are euthyroid, but some are hypothyroid or thyrotoxic.

Decreased Serum Binding

Decreased serum binding of thyroid hormones may occur as a result of decreased thyroid hormone–binding protein production or competitive interactions of drugs with the T_4 binding sites (Table 10-8).

The lowest serum TBG concentrations occur in subjects with inherited complete TBG deficiency (X-linked).[94] Hemizygous affected males have no detectable serum TBG (<0.05 percent of normal), whereas heterozygous affected females have serum TBG concentrations that are 50 percent of normal. The disorder occurs in about 1 in 6,000 newborn infants. Other, more common heritable forms of TBG deficiency result in varying reductions in serum TBG and therefore T_4 concentrations that are due either to decreased rates of TBG synthesis or to the production of TBG that has reduced T_4-binding properties or is cleared from the circulation more rapidly than is normal TBG.[94] Some are the result of single amino acid substitutions or deletions.

Serum TBG concentrations may be decreased in patients with acromegaly, Cushing's syndrome, and thyrotoxicosis. They also may be decreased by the administration of androgens, anabolic steroids, large doses of glucocorticoids given chronically, colestipol combined with niacin, and L-asparaginase.[17,62]

Variant forms of TTR are found in patients with familial amyloidotic polyneuropathy, in whom the TTR is an important component of the amyloid fibrils.[17] Some of these forms of TTR have a reduced affinity for T_4, and so affected subjects may have slightly decreased serum T_4 concentrations.

Patients with many acute and chronic nonthyroidal illnesses have decreased serum T_4 and T_3 concentrations (see Nonthyroidal Illness). Among the causes of these changes are decreased serum TBG, TTR, and albumin concentrations. Serum TTR concentrations decrease transiently in patients with many acute illnesses and are low in many chronically ill patients, although the effect on serum T_4 concentrations is small because of the relatively small contribution of TTR to overall T_4 binding in serum. The reduction in serum TBG concentrations that occurs in various nonthyroidal illnesses also is usually small. Some of the TBG in these patients may be desialylated; the affinity of such TBG for T_4 is lower than that of normal TBG, and so the serum T_4 concentration is disproportionately lower than the serum TBG concentration.[99,100] Patients with nonthyroidal illness also often have some degree of hypoalbuminemia, which may contribute slightly to the decrease in serum T_4 concentrations. The proposal that patients with nonthyroidal illness have serum inhibitors of T_4 binding to TBG or other serum proteins could not be confirmed.[100,101] Except perhaps in renal disease, the inhibition of T_4 binding was probably due to the release of fatty acids from triglycerides in vitro (see below). Whatever the specific causes or the degree of deficiency of the various thyroid hormone–binding proteins, there is little doubt that many patients with severe acute or chronic nonthyroidal illness have overall decreases in serum thyroid hormone binding and thus high THBR values. In such patients, the dialyzable fraction of T_4 is often relatively increased, so that serum free T_4 concentrations are more often normal than are serum free T_4 index values.

If substances that compete with T_4 for binding to TBG or other binding proteins are present in sufficient concentration, they alter the equilibrium between free T_4 and bound T_4. The result is an initial increase in serum free T_4 concentrations, which then return toward normal as a result of transient decreases in thyroid secretion, increases in T_4 clearance, or both. Thus, these patients have low serum T_4 concentrations and elevated THBR values, like patients with decreased serum TBG concentrations. Pharmacologic agents that competitively inhibit T_4 binding to TBG or TTR include salicylates, some other nonsteroidal antiinflammatory drugs, and furosemide.[62,73] Phenytoin, phenylbutazone, and sulfonylureas also inhibit T_4 binding, but not at the concentrations achieved when they are used therapeutically. Other substances that have been reported to inhibit T_4 binding to TBG or albumin include free fatty acids and heparin.[102] However, very high free fatty acid concentrations are required.[103] The effect of heparin can be explained by its ability to activate lipoprotein lipase and therefore raise free fatty acid concentrations, and it can be blocked by the in vitro addition of protamine, a heparin inhibitor.[104]

Nonthyroidal Illness

A wide variety of reversible abnormalities of pituitary-thyroid function, serum thyroid hormone binding, and extrathyroidal thyroid hormone metabolism occur in patients with nonthyroidal illness. These abnormalities result in decreased serum T_3 concentrations, less often in decreased serum T_4 concentrations, and occasionally in decreased serum free T_4 concentrations. In general, the degree and extent of the abnormalities correlate with the severity of the nonthyroidal illness, and the nature of the illness is of secondary importance. The changes in serum hormone concentrations are accompanied by changes in T_4 metabolism, in particular by changes in T_4 conversion to T_3 in different tissues, and less often by changes in TSH and thyroid secretion. In addition, illness-related decreases in T_3 nuclear receptors and postreceptor actions of T_3 have been identified in animals.

The two most common abnormalities in patients with nonthyroidal illness are decreased serum T_3 concentrations and decreased serum T_3 and T_4 concentrations; the latter abnormalities thus mimic those of hypothyroidism. These abnormalities are frequently referred to as the *euthyroid sick syndrome,* a term that is inappropriate for several reasons. First, the spectrum of the abnormalities is very broad, and no single set of abnormalities can be designated the euthyroid sick syndrome. Second, while such patients have no overt clinical manifestations of hypothyroidism, the actions of thyroid hormone in some tissues may be diminished. It is more likely that these changes represent adaptive forms of hypothyroidism, serving to reduce the availability and action of thyroid hormones and lessen the physiologic impact of the nonthyroidal illness. They therefore are probably beneficial adaptations to illness. The fact that no overt manifestations of thyroid deficiency occur may reflect the transient nature of the abnormalities, their lack of equal impact in all tissues because of variations in local T_3 production and action, and the modifying effects of the nonthyroidal illness on the responsiveness of different tissues to thyroid deficiency. To confuse matters further, some patients with nonthyroidal illnesses have elevated serum T_4 concentrations. It is tempting to attribute many of these changes to the production of various cytokines, but evidence that cytokines are involved is limited.

These various syndromes are shown schemati-

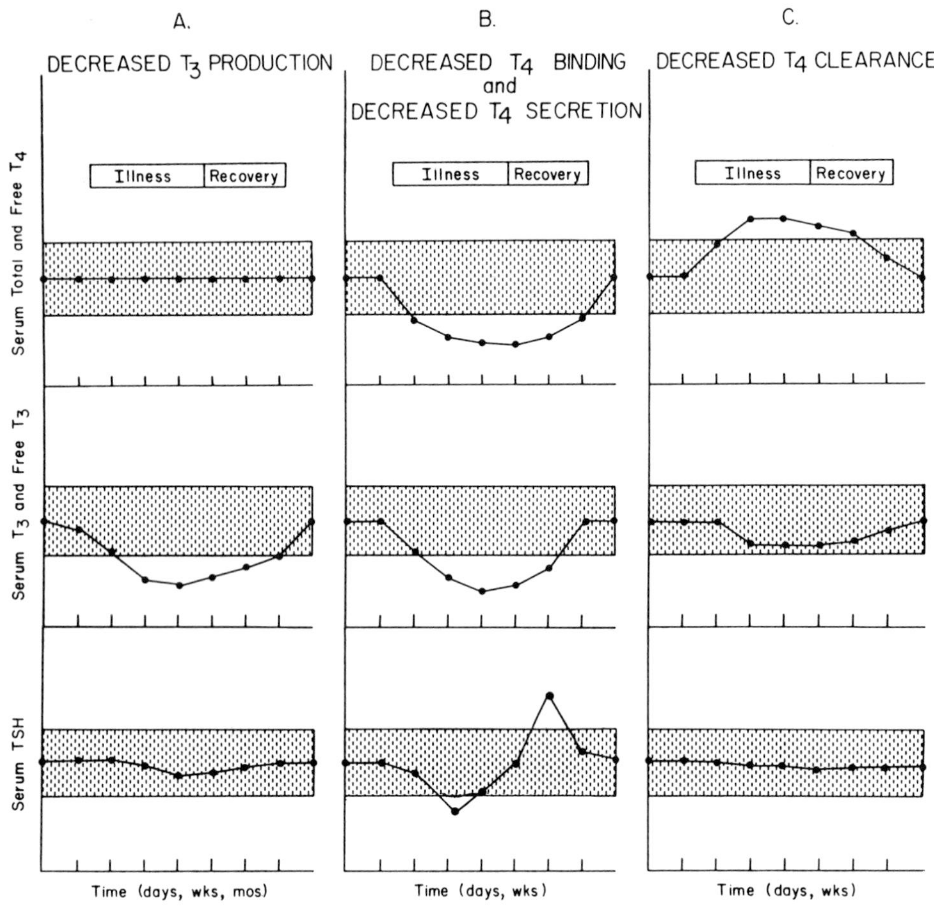

FIGURE 10-18 Patterns of the three major types of abnormalities of pituitary-thyroid function that occur in patients with nonthyroidal illness. (*A*) Decreased extrathyroidal T_3 production. (*B*) Decreased T_4 binding and decreased TSH secretion. (*C*) Decreased T_4 clearance. The shaded areas indicate the normal ranges.

cally in Fig. 10-18, and the derangements that contribute to them are listed in Table 10-9. Each will be discussed in more detail below. The frequency of abnormalities of thyroid function in hospitalized patients is high. In one study of 264 patients admitted to a medical service, 19 percent had decreased serum T_3 concentrations, 8 percent had decreased serum T_4 concentrations, and 15 percent had decreased serum free T_4 concentrations (about 1 percent had increased serum T_4 or free T_4 concentrations).[105] In a study of 1580 hospitalized patients, 17 percent had abnormal serum TSH concentrations (12 percent low and 6 percent high), 12 percent had abnormal serum T_4 concentrations, and 8 percent had abnormal se-

TABLE 10-9 Alterations in Hypothalamic-Pituitary-Thyroid Function in Nonthyroidal Illness

Alteration	Site	Cause
Decreased serum T_3 concentrations	Extrathyroidal tissue	Decreased T_4-5′-deiodinase activity
Decreased serum total T_4 concentrations	Extrathyroidal tissue	Decreased serum binding of T_4
Decreased serum free T_4 concentrations	Thyroid	Decreased TSH secretion
Decreased serum TSH concentrations	Pituitary	Decreased TRH secretion Increased dopamine, somatostatin, or cortisol secretion
Decreased T_3 action	Extrathyroidal tissue	Decreased T_3 receptors or postreceptor action
Increased serum T_4 concentrations	Thyroid Extrathyroidal tissue	Increased TSH secretion Decreased T_4 clearance

rum free T_4 index values.[106] Most of the abnormal serum free T_4 index values were low, and the proportion of patients with low values among the patients with low, normal, and high serum TSH concentrations ranged from 6 to 12 percent. The mean serum T_3 concentrations in these groups were lower than those of T_4, so that the proportion of T_3 values that were low must have been higher. The proportion of patients in either study who proved to have either thyrotoxicosis or hypothyroidism was very low. Even higher frequencies of abnormal test results are found in patients admitted to emergency rooms or intensive care units, and there is an inverse correlation between serum T_4 and T_3 concentrations and survival among patients admitted to intensive care units.[107,108] These abnormalities do not occur in isolated forms, and their extent varies widely in individual patients. Their occurrence also means that it may be very difficult to identify thyrotoxicosis or hypothyroidism in patients who have nonthyroidal illness.

Decreased Extrathyroidal Triiodothyronine Production

Decreased serum T_3 concentrations occur in patients with virtually all acute and chronic illnesses (Fig. 10-18*A*). These include illnesses such as acute infections, which need not be severe; myocardial infarction; pulmonary embolism; sudden decreases in caloric intake; and after trauma, burns, and surgery. Serum T_3 concentrations also are low in patients with chronic illnesses such as diabetes mellitus; chronic liver, renal, cardiac, pulmonary, and rheumatologic disease; cancer; and chronic malnutrition. Caloric deficiency undoubtedly contributes to the decline in serum T_3 concentrations that occurs in many of these illnesses, but is not the sole explanation. Drugs such as glucocorticoids and propranolol may also result in decreased serum T_3 concentrations (see Effects of Various Drugs on Thyroid Function).

The cause of the decreased serum T_3 concentrations in these situations is decreased extrathyroidal conversion of T_4 to T_3. The fall in serum T_3 concentrations may be as great as 40 percent, indicating a roughly 50 percent decrease in extrathyroidal production of T_3 from T_4. Both the fall and the subsequent recovery from it can occur within 24 to 48 h, depending on the cause of the nonthyroidal illness and the rapidity of its onset and reversal. The particular organs in which T_3 production is impaired are not known, but they presumably include the liver and kidneys, since these organs are important sources of circulating T_3.

This decrease in T_4 conversion to T_3 could result from decreased cellular uptake of T_4, cofactor availability or enzyme production, or inhibition of enzyme activity. Which of these mechanisms are operative is not known, nor are the factors that might cause them (see Regulation of Extrathyroidal Triiodothyronine Production). One possible cause is the increase in circulating (or locally produced) cytokines that accompanies many illnesses. Infusions of tumor necrosis factor lower serum T_3 concentrations slightly, and an inverse correlation between serum tumor necrosis factor and T_3 concentrations was found in one study, although not in another.[109–111]

These patients have normal serum total and free T_4 concentrations. Their serum rT_3 concentrations are usually high as a result of decreased extrathyroidal 5′-deiodination of rT_3; rT_3 production is not increased. Serum TSH concentrations are usually within the normal range, although they may be slightly decreased and the nocturnal surge in TSH secretion may be diminished.[112] The lack of increase in serum TSH in the face of decreased serum T_3 concentrations is probably due to the continuing availability of T_4 for intrapituitary T_3 generation; other possibilities include altered thyrotroph sensitivity to T_3 deficiency as a result of decreased TRH or increased somatostatin production and intrinsic changes in the function of the thyrotrophs.

The administration of exogenous T_3 during fasting in normal subjects and to patients with uremia in doses that prevent decreases in serum T_3 concentrations increases urinary nitrogen and 3-methylhistidine excretion.[113–115] Such T_3 administration does not alter the carbohydrate or lipid responses to fasting. The decrease in T_3 production that occurs during illness or fasting should therefore reduce protein catabolism and serve to conserve nitrogen stores; it may also reduce the generation of free radicals, facilitating the repair of injured tissue. The decrease is accompanied by some tissue responses indicative of decreased T_3 action, for example, reductions in cardiac contractility and rate that are reversed by small doses of T_3. In animals, reductions in extrathyroidal T_3 production and T_3 nuclear receptor content are accompanied by decreased production of some liver enzymes and of cardiac beta-adrenergic receptors and myosin ATP isoenzymes. T_3 administration reverses these changes.[26,116,117] All these responses could serve to conserve substrate and maintain tissue integrity, although some could impair organ function.

Decreased Serum Thyroxine Concentrations

Low serum T_4 as well as low serum T_3 concentrations are found in critically ill patients with various infections; cardiac, pulmonary, renal, and other diseases; burns; and severe trauma (Fig. 10-18*B*). The rate at which serum T_4 concentrations decline varies from hours to weeks, depending on the abruptness and severity of the illness. Often, only the serum total T_4 concentrations are decreased and free T_4 concentrations are normal.[118,119] These changes are due to diminished serum T_4 binding resulting from decreased serum concentrations of TBG, TTR, and albumin or from the use of drugs that inhibit T_4-binding in serum (see Alterations in Serum Thyroid Hormone Binding). The overall rate of clearance of T_4 is therefore increased, and the rate of production of T_4 is normal or slightly decreased.[118] These patients have very low serum T_3 concentrations not only because of decreased serum binding of T_3 but also because their illness is always sufficiently severe to inhibit extrathyroidal production of T_3.

Some severely ill patients have low serum free T_4 index values, and a smaller number have low serum free T_4 concentrations.[118–120] These patients are unable to maintain normal thyroid secretion. They have low-normal or low serum TSH concentrations, markedly decreased nocturnal TSH secretion, and subnormal or absent serum TSH responses to TRH,[106,121] and the TSH that is secreted may have diminished biological activity.[122] Many of these patients are receiving dopamine or glucocorticoids, which are recognized inhibitors of TSH secretion. The mechanisms responsible for decreased TSH secretion in others may be direct inhibition of TSH secretion, decreased TRH secretion, or increased endogenous dopamine, somatostatin, or cortisol secretion. Candidate causes include tumor necrosis factor and interleukin-1, which lower serum TSH concentrations in humans and animals and hypothalamic TRH content in animals.[109,123,124] These substances may also inhibit thyroidal responses to TSH. Whatever the causes, the prognosis in such patients with low serum free T_4 values is poor; in one study, for example, more than 60 percent of patients with low serum free T_4 index values died.[107]

These patients are often confused or obtunded, puffy, or hypothermic. They may have poor respiratory function, inappropriately slow pulse rates, and sluggish deep tendon reflexes. These clinical findings could be caused either by the nonthyroidal illness or by thyroid hormone deficiency; it is not usually possible to distinguish between the two at the bedside.

The findings in these patients thus mimic those of central hypothyroidism, with the addition of decreased serum binding of T_4 and T_3. They are indicative of a greater degree of adaptive hypothyroidism than occurs in less ill patients in whom the major change is decreased extrathyroidal conversion of T_4 to T_3. Presumably, the greater reduction in thyroid hormone availability confers some additional benefit beyond that conferred by decreased extrathyroidal T_3 production alone. The administration of T_4 to a group of such patients in an intensive care unit did not lower mortality.[125]

The practical question raised by these findings in an individual patient is, Could the patient have central hypothyroidism that predated the illness and should be treated? The answer is usually no, especially in patients who are receiving dopamine or glucocorticoids, for several reasons. First, low serum TSH and T_4 values are expected in such patients, and the abnormalities disappear during recovery. Second, their serum free T_4 values, whether measured directly or indirectly, are less depressed than are their serum T_4 values, whereas in patients with hypothyroidism the converse is true. Third, central hypothyroidism is rare, whereas illness-related decreases in serum TSH and T_4 concentrations are not. Even so, it is often worthwhile to evaluate pituitary-adrenal function (see Chap. 12) in such patients to provide assurance that cortisol secretion is adequate and further evidence that preexisting hypothalamic-pituitary disease is not present.

When recovery begins, serum TSH concentrations may rise transiently above the normal range for several days (Fig. 10-18*B*).[120] The peak values usually range from 5 to 20 mU/liter but are occasionally higher.[126] This increase in serum TSH indicates that the illness has somehow impaired the ability of the thyrotroph cells to respond to decreased serum free T_4 concentrations; with recovery, that ability returns. The rise in serum TSH is followed by a rise in serum T_4 and T_3 concentrations that is due not only to the action of TSH on the thyroid gland but also to increases in serum binding proteins and in extrathyroidal T_3 production. Occasionally the first recorded serum TSH value in a seriously ill patient is slightly elevated. This could mean that recovery from the illness has already begun or that the patient has primary hypothyroidism. Reevaluation a few days later should provide the information needed to distinguish between these possibilities.

Increased Serum Thyroxine Concentrations

Increased serum T_4 and free T_4 concentrations also may occur in patients with nonthyroidal illness (Fig. 10-18*C*).[62] Such findings have been reported most often in patients with psychiatric disorders, although their frequency in groups of such patients varies widely (see Effects of Specific Disorders on Thyroid Function). They also occur in patients with various acute medical illnesses and in patients who have received drugs such as amiodarone, oral cholecystographic agents, and propranolol (see Effects of Various Drugs on Thyroid Function). Serum T_3 concentrations are usually slightly decreased or normal, and serum TSH concentrations are usually normal. These patients have few clinical manifestations of thyrotoxicosis, and their serum T_4 concentrations decline to normal within 1 or 2 weeks as they recover from the illness (longer in the case of amiodarone).

One cause of these elevations in serum total and free T_4 concentrations is decreased clearance of T_4 without inhibition of TSH secretion. This is clearly the case when one of the drugs listed above has been given. A second cause is a transient increase in TSH and therefore thyroid secretion. This mechanism may be operative in patients with psychiatric disease. An additional abnormality that is probably invariably present is decreased extrathyroidal T_3 production.

In general, patients with elevated serum T_4 concentrations caused by nonthyroidal illness are not severely ill. The diversity of the illnesses and the transient nature of the abnormalities have made prospective study difficult, and the physiologic importance of the changes, if any, is not known. The practical importance, however, is clear: The diagnosis of thyrotoxicosis in patients who are ill must be based on clinical evidence, not merely on elevated serum T_4 and free T_4 values.

Effects of Specific Disorders on Thyroid Function

Caloric Restriction and Fasting

The most widely studied cause of decreased serum T_3 concentrations is caloric deficiency. Normal or obese subjects who eat 600 calories or less a day have a fall in serum T_3 concentrations of approximately 40 percent and a 100 percent increase in serum rT_3 concentrations within 48 h.[127] The abnormalities persist until the subjects are fed either carbohydrate or protein. Similar changes occur in patients with protein-calorie malnutrition and short bowel syndromes who are otherwise healthy. The changes are due to increased extrathyroidal conversion of T_4 to T_3 and of rT_3 to 3,3′-T_2. Serum T_4 concentrations do not change. Basal serum TSH concentrations and nocturnal TSH secretion may decline slightly, but not sufficiently to decrease T_4 production. (The inhibition of TSH secretion is not sufficient to reduce serum TSH concentrations in patients with primary hypothyroidism.[128]) The thyrotroph cells remain exquisitely sensitive to increased amounts of T_3, since the maintenance of normal (fed) serum T_3 concentrations during starvation by exogenous T_3 administration decreases TSH secretion.[113] These cells also remain sensitive to the antithyroid effect of inorganic iodide, since the administration of inorganic iodide during fasting results in the same increase in TSH secretion that occurs during normal food intake.

Renal Disease

Patients with stable chronic renal insufficiency and those treated with hemodialysis or peritoneal dialysis usually have normal or low serum T_4, normal free T_4, low T_3, and normal TSH concentrations.[129,130] The serum T_4 values are lower than those in normal subjects because serum T_4 binding is decreased by the presence of inhibitors of binding or abnormal forms of TBG; serum TBG concentrations are normal. Extrathyroidal production of T_3 from T_4 is decreased. Serum rT_3 concentrations are normal rather than high as in most patients with nonthyroidal illness because extravascular binding of rT_3 is increased, a phenomenon unique to renal disease.[130] Patients with acute renal failure have similar abnormalities, but their magnitude is greater. Serum T_4 and especially T_3 concentrations are more normal after transplantation; any persisting abnormalities are likely to be due to the glucocorticoid these patients receive for immunosuppression.

Patients with the nephrotic syndrome may excrete substantial amounts of T_4 and TBG as well as albumin in their urine.[131] Their serum TBG has a decreased affinity for T_4, and when proteinuria is massive, serum TBG concentrations may be low. Their serum T_4 concentrations are usually decreased, whereas their serum free T_4 values are normal, indicating decreased T_4 binding. Serum T_3 concentrations are low because of decreases in both T_3 binding and extrathyroidal T_3 production. The loss of T_4 in the urine may be large enough to result in increased TSH secretion.[132]

Liver Disease

Patients with acute hepatitis have increased serum TBG and therefore increased T_4 concentrations.[133] Their serum T_3 concentrations are normal, reflecting the counterbalancing effects of decreased extrathyroidal T_3 production and increased serum TBG concentrations. All these changes disappear with recovery. The increase in serum TBG may be due to the release of preformed TBG, slowed clearance of TBG, or increased hepatic synthetic function.

Serum TBG concentrations are increased in some patients with chronic active hepatitis, primary biliary cirrhosis, and hepatoma. In portal cirrhosis, serum T_4 binding is variably decreased, so that serum T_4 concentrations tend to be low, T_3 concentrations are low, and rT_3 concentrations are high.[134] Patients with hepatic coma have the usual findings of severe nonthyroidal illness: low serum T_4 and T_3 concentrations and free T_4 index values and normal or low serum TSH concentrations.

Human Immunodeficiency Virus Infection

Some patients with human immunodeficiency virus (HIV) infection have moderate increases in serum TBG concentrations. In some studies, the concentrations were increased only in patients with the acquired immune deficiency syndrome. In others, however, patients with less advanced infection, including those who were HIV-seropositive but otherwise well, had increased values.[135–137] Possible explanations for these discrepancies include differences in patients, coincident illness, and the methods used to measure TBG, particularly if, as seems likely, the extent of glycosylation of TBG, and therefore its affinity for T_4 and its rate of clearance, vary among patients.

As their illness progresses and opportunistic infections develop, these patients have the abnormalities of thyroid function characteristic of nonthyroidal illness described previously. *Pneumocystis carinii* infections are very common in these patients, and this organism can cause local or generalized thyroid infection and hypothyroidism.[138]

Psychiatric Disease

Surveys of patients who are hospitalized for the treatment of acute psychiatric illness have often revealed abnormalities of thyroid function. The most common is an increased serum T_4 concentration. Its frequency varies widely. In several large series of such patients, 0 to 33 percent had increased serum T_4 concentrations and 0 to 18 percent had increased serum free T_4 index values.[139–141] Serum T_3 concentrations were increased less often, and serum TSH concentrations were usually normal or slightly increased. The hyperthyroxinemia and increased TSH secretion, when present, usually subsided in a week or so.

The simplest explanation for these findings is that acute psychiatric illness results in a transient increase in TSH and therefore thyroid secretion. The greater frequency of high serum T_4 as compared with high free T_4 or T_3 values argues for the presence of some slowing of T_4 clearance or the mobilization of T_4 from extrathyroidal stores. The abnormalities are not diagnosis-specific, since they occur in patients with all forms of acute psychosis, nor can they be related to the use of particular psychotropic drugs.

Abnormalities of TSH secretion are found in 20 to 30 percent of patients with depression.[142] A few of these patients have slightly increased serum TSH concentrations, indicative of mild hypothyroidism. The most common abnormality, however, is an impaired serum TSH response to TRH, and both daytime and nocturnal TSH secretion may be decreased. Serum T_4 and T_3 concentrations are usually normal. The impaired TSH secretion may be due to increased ACTH and cortisol secretion, although the correlation between decreased serum TSH responses to TRH and abnormal pituitary-adrenal responses to dexamethasone in depressed patients is poor. Patients with alcoholism or anorexia nervosa have similar abnormalities and also may have decreased serum T_3 concentrations because of nutritional deficiency.

Effects of Various Drugs on Thyroid Function

Dopamine

Infusions of dopamine in doses of 5 to 10 μg/min result in an immediate reduction of TSH secretion.[118] This drug reduces the amplitude of pulsatile TSH secretion so that nocturnal TSH secretion decreases more than daytime TSH secretion.[53] The decrease is sufficient to decrease thyroid secretion and lower serum T_4 and T_3 concentrations in 48 h in normal subjects. Dopamine is widely used in very sick patients in intensive care units, and its use contributes substantially to the abnormalities in thyroid function that are found in such patients.[143] It (and severe illness) can decrease TSH secretion to normal in a patient with primary hypothyroidism. None of the other drugs used to increase blood pressure or cardiac output in critically ill patients are known to alter TSH or thyroid secretion.

Glucocorticoids

Endogenous or exogenous glucocorticoid excess has multiple effects on pituitary-thyroid function,[62] and increased endogenous cortisol production may account for some of the changes that occur in patients with nonthyroidal illness. Moderate glucocorticoid excess inhibits pulsatile TSH secretion, the nocturnal surge in serum TSH concentrations, and serum TSH responses to exogenous TRH, indicating an inhibition of both TSH and TRH secretion.[144,145] Large doses inhibit extrathyroidal T_3 production and increase extrathyroidal rT_3 production and therefore decrease serum T_3 concentrations and increase rT_3 concentrations, respectively, within several days. Finally, chronic glucocorticoid excess decreases serum TBG and increases TTR concentrations.[146] The net result of these various actions of glucocorticoids in patients with spontaneous or iatrogenic Cushing's syndrome is low-normal serum T_4, normal free T_4, low T_3, increased rT_3, and low-normal TSH concentrations. Glucocorticoids also directly inhibit thyroid radioiodine uptake and thyroidal T_4, T_3, and thyroglobulin release in patients with hyperthyroidism caused by Graves' disease.[147]

Adrenergic Antagonists

When given in large doses, the beta-adrenergic antagonist propranolol is a weak inhibitor of extrathyroidal T_4 conversion to T_3. Large doses reduce serum T_3 concentrations about 20 to 30 percent.[148] Serum T_4 concentrations increase modestly in an occasional patient. Other beta-adrenergic antagonist drugs reduce serum T_3 concentrations to a lesser extent or not at all. All these drugs inhibit T_3 production from T_4 in rat liver homogenates, but propranolol is the most potent.[149] Their ability to inhibit T_3 production is not related to their adrenergic antagonist properties, since D-propranolol, which is not an adrenergic antagonist, is equally active as an inhibitor of 5′-deiodination of T_4.

Propylthiouracil and Methimazole

Propylthiouracil and methimazole are commonly used antithyroid drugs. Both inhibit thyroid hormone biosynthesis (see Treatment of Thyrotoxicosis). In addition, PTU inhibits type I T_4-5′-deiodinase activity.[10,11,62,148] It therefore slows the clearance of T_4 and inhibits the extrathyroidal conversion of T_4 to T_3. When it is given to T_4-treated hypothyroid patients, serum T_3 concentrations fall by about 30 percent in 24 h and stay at that level until the drug is discontinued.[150] Serum TSH concentrations increase slightly, providing evidence that PTU has little effect on T_4 deiodination in the thyrotrophs.

Iodine

The administration of iodine or iodide formed in vivo by the deiodination of iodide-containing drugs alters thyroid hormone production in several ways (see Regulation of Thyroid Secretion by Iodide). Inorganic iodide in doses of 500 μg daily or more, in addition to the usual dietary iodine intake, has a weak, unsustained antithyroid action in normal subjects.[151] The administration of iodide can induce overt hypothyroidism in iodide-sufficient patients who were previously treated with ^{131}I or surgery for hyperthyroidism or who have chronic autoimmune thyroiditis. Conversely, the administration of iodide may cause thyrotoxicosis in patients with iodine deficiency or those with autonomously functioning thyroid tissue that concentrates iodide poorly. Either hypothyroidism or thyrotoxicosis may also occur occasionally in apparently normal subjects after iodine administration.

Amiodarone

The antiarrhythmic drug amiodarone is an iodine-containing drug that has many effects on pituitary-thyroid function.[148] It is an inhibitor of both type I and type II T_4-5′-deiodinase and may also inhibit the binding of T_3 to its nuclear receptors. In normal subjects, it inhibits both extrathyroidal T_3 production and rT_3 deiodination, so that serum T_3 concentrations decrease and those of rT_3 increase. During the first several months of treatment, serum TSH concentrations increase, T_4 clearance decreases, and both absolute thyroidal iodine uptake and T_4 secretion increase. Therefore, serum T_4 concentrations increase, sometimes to above the normal range. Thereafter, serum TSH and T_4 concentrations return to normal, but the changes in serum T_3 and rT_3 persist as long as the drug is given and for several months afterward, because it is stored in adipose tissue and is metabolized or excreted very slowly.

Amiodarone contains 37 percent iodine and is in part metabolized by deiodination. The iodide that is formed can cause either hypothyroidism or thyrotoxicosis in appropriately susceptible persons (see the preceding section).[152] Thyrotoxicosis may occur at any time during amiodarone therapy, but hypothyroidism usually occurs during the first several months. Amiodarone may also initiate thyroid autoimmune disease.

Patients with amiodarone-induced hypothyroidism have the typical biochemical findings of hypothyroidism: low-normal or low serum T_4 and increased TSH concentrations. It may be difficult to confirm a suspected diagnosis of thyrotoxicosis in a patient taking amiodarone, because some increase in serum T_4 concentrations is a regular occurrence in patients taking the drug. The key finding indicative of thyrotoxicosis in such a patient is a subnormal serum TSH concentration.

Iodinated Radiographic Contrast Agents

Iodinated radiographic agents, such as iopanoic acid and sodium ipodate, that are used for oral cholecystography have effects that are similar to those of amiodarone, except that they are short-lived, because only single doses are given and the drugs are not stored as amiodarone is.[148] They reduce serum T_3 and raise serum rT_3 concentrations for up to 2 weeks, and serum TSH and T_4 concentrations increase, sometimes to slightly above the normal range. Persistent changes can be induced by weekly administration.

The water-soluble iodinated contrast agents used for arteriography, pyelography, and computed tomography do not alter pituitary-thyroid function. All these agents contain large amounts of iodide and are deiodinated in vivo, and so the changes in thyroid secretion that can be induced by iodide in appropriately susceptible patients may follow their use (see above).

Lithium

Lithium is concentrated by the thyroid and inhibits the formation and release of thyroid hormones. It is thus goitrogenic, although only weakly so. Elevations in serum TSH concentrations occur in about 20 percent of patients receiving therapeutic doses of lithium carbonate, but overt clinical and biochemical hypothyroidism is rare.[153] Decreases in thyroid secretion are most likely to occur in patients treated for long periods and in those with thyroid antibodies, who presumably also have autoimmune thyroid disease. Lithium also slows the rate of T_4 degradation but does not decrease extrathyroidal T_3 production.

Phenytoin, Carbamazepine, and Rifampin

Phenytoin, carbamazepine, and rifampin accelerate the nondeiodinative clearance of T_4 and, to a lesser extent, that of T_3 because of their ability to increase the activity of hepatic microsomal oxidative enzymes.[148,154] In addition, phenytoin has weak T_4 agonist properties.[155] As a result, serum T_4 and free T_4 concentrations decline by about 20 percent, while serum T_3 concentrations decrease somewhat less. Serum TSH concentrations increase slightly, as does the volume of the thyroid gland. Phenytoin impairs T_4 absorption in addition to increasing T_4 clearance, thus decreasing serum T_4 concentrations somewhat more in T_4-treated hypothyroid patients as compared with normal subjects.

THYROTOXICOSIS

Thyrotoxicosis is the clinical, physiologic, and biochemical syndrome that results when tissues are exposed to excessive concentrations of thyroid hormones. The term *hyperthyroidism,* although often used synonymously with *thyrotoxicosis,* refers to excessive T_4 and T_3 synthesis and secretion by the thyroid gland and is used in this context here. Hence, hyperthyroid patients have thyrotoxicosis, but thyrotoxicosis has causes other than hyperthyroidism.

Thyrotoxicosis may result in abnormalities of widely varying severity in virtually all tissues. Many patients have overt clinical and biochemical disease that may be life-threatening, but others have what is called subclinical thyrotoxicosis. This is defined biochemically as normal serum T_4 and T_3 and decreased TSH concentrations; these patients have few or no symptoms and signs of thyrotoxicosis. The onset of thyrotoxicosis may be gradual or sudden, and its course may be transient or persistent. The diagnosis may be obvious and may be confirmed readily by a few simple laboratory tests or difficult, requiring repeated investigation or prolonged observation.

Thyrotoxicosis is a rather common disorder. Surveys in Europe and New Zealand in the 1970s and 1980s revealed annual incidence rates of 0.2 to 0.3 per 1000 people.[87,156,157] Most of these surveys were based on tests ordered by physicians in the community and performed in centralized laboratories. A community survey in Great Britain in the 1970s revealed a prevalence rate of 19 per 1000 women and 1.6 per 1000 men; about 30 percent of the cases were previously unrecognized.[87] The annual incidence rate was estimated to be 3 per 1000 women. In other community surveys and in groups of patients undergoing periodic health examinations, unsuspected overt thyrotoxicosis has been found in from less than 1 to 10 persons per 1000.[67] These variations mostly reflect differences in study methodology. The proportion of persons with subclinical thyrotoxicosis is as high or higher.

Among patients with thyrotoxicosis, women outnumber men by from 4 to 10 to 1, largely independent of the cause. The peak age incidence varies from the fifth to the seventh decade; patients with Graves' disease are on average about 10 to 15 years younger than are those with toxic multinodular or uninodular goiter.[158] The cause of thyrotoxicosis is Graves' disease in 60 to 85 percent of these patients, toxic nodular goiter in 10 to 30 percent, toxic thyroid adenoma in 2 to 10 percent, and some form of thyroiditis in the remainder.[156–158] The frequency of toxic multinodular goiter and toxic adenoma varies the most, being higher in areas of lower but not truly deficient iodine intake.[158]

Pathophysiology of Thyrotoxicosis

Thyrotoxicosis is due to the unregulated release of T_4 and T_3 from the thyroid gland or the ingestion of excessive amounts of T_4, T_3, or both. It may be due to increased T_4 and T_3 synthesis and release caused by intrinsic thyroid disease, excessive TSH or theoretically excessive TRH secretion, or the production of other thyroid-stimulating hormones, such as thyroid-stimulating autoantibodies (TSab) and chorionic gonadotropin. It also may be due to destruction of thyroid tissue with excessive release of T_4 and T_3. These situations are all characterized by unregulated hormone release, and thyrotoxicosis, whether overt or subclinical, cannot occur in their absence. Compensatory increases in T_4 and T_3 secretion (secondary hyperthyroidism) may occur in patients who have accelerated degradation or urinary excretion of T_4 and T_3 or peripheral resistance to the actions of T_4 and T_3, but thyrotoxicosis does not occur in such circumstances. Increased extrathyroidal T_4 conversion to T_3 should not cause thyrotoxicosis, since any substantial increase in extrathyroidal T_3 production would be expected to decrease TSH and therefore decrease thyroidal T_4 and T_3 secretion.

Most patients with thyrotoxicosis have increased production of both T_4 and T_3 and increased serum T_4 and T_3 concentrations. The increases in the T_3 production rate and serum T_3 concentrations are characteristically greater than are those in T_4. Figure 10-19 shows a schematic summary of these findings.[159] In one study of hyperthyroid patients, the mean T_4 production rate was increased 3.5-fold, whereas the mean T_3 production rate was increased over sevenfold.[160] There are several causes for the disproportionate increase in T_3 production. First, thyroid tissue from patients with hyperthyroidism has an increased T_3/T_4 ratio, indicating that glandular synthesis of T_3 is increased to a greater extent

FIGURE 10-19 Diagram of thyroidal T_4/T_3 ratios, thyroidal and extrathyroidal production rates of T_4 and T_3, and serum T_4 and T_3 concentrations in normal subjects and patients with thyrotoxicosis. The diagonally lined areas in the T_4 (upper) rectangles indicate the proportion of T_4 converted to T_3 at extrathyroidal sites, and the diagonally lined areas in the T_3 (lower) rectangles indicate the proportion of T_3 formed from T_4 at extrathyroidal sites.

NORMAL

THYROTOXICOSIS

90 µg/day (120 nmol/day)

T4

T4/T3 = 10

10 µg/dl (125 nmol/l)

SERUM

T3

100 ng/dl (1.5 nmol/l)

30 µg/day (45 nmol/day)

300 µg/day (400 nmol/day)

20 µg/dl (250 nmol/l)

SERUM

T4

5 = T4/T3

T3

500 ng/dl (7.5 nmol/l)

200 µg/day (300 nmol/day)

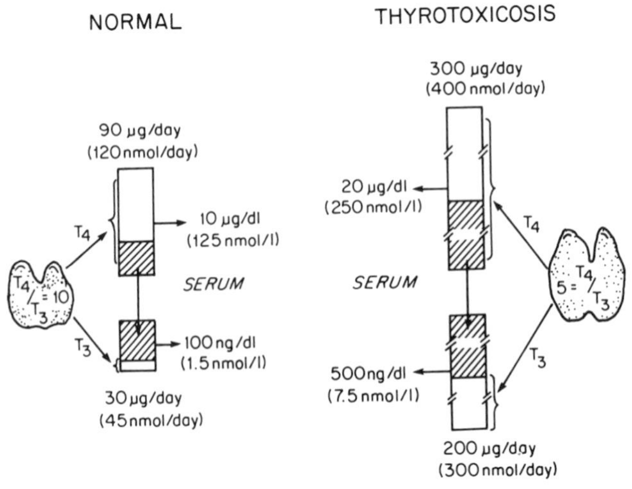

than is that of T_4. Second, the rates of both thyroidal and extrathyroidal T_4 conversion to T_3 are increased.

Some patients with thyrotoxicosis have increased serum T_3 concentrations but normal serum T_4 concentrations. This is called T_3 thyrotoxicosis and results from a disproportionate increase in the amount of T_3 produced relative to T_4. There are no characteristic clinical manifestations of T_3 thyrotoxicosis. It tends to occur in patients whose thyrotoxicosis is due to a toxic adenoma or recurrent Graves' disease but may be due to hyperthyroidism of any cause. T_3 thyrotoxicosis is rare in the United States but more common in regions where iodine intake is limited. The abnormality responsible for it is probably relative intrathyroidal iodide deficiency.

A few patients with thyrotoxicosis have elevated serum T_4 but normal T_3 concentrations (T_4 thyrotoxicosis).[9,161] In addition to thyrotoxicosis, these patients have another serious illness or have recently received a drug that inhibits extrathyroidal conversion of T_4 to T_3. The biochemical findings of T_4 thyrotoxicosis therefore are a result of excessive thyroidal T_4 and T_3 secretion and concomitantly impaired extrathyroidal T_3 production.

Causes of Thyrotoxicosis

The causes of thyrotoxicosis are listed in Table 10-10. An attempt should always be made to distinguish among them, since they differ in their natural history and may require different forms of therapy. The cause of thyrotoxicosis usually can be identified by history and physical examination. The most important findings concern the duration of symptoms, the degree and pattern of thyroid enlargement, and the presence or absence of thyroid pain and tenderness and of the extrathyroidal manifestations of Graves' disease. Laboratory procedures such as measurements of thyroid radioiodine uptake, thyroid scans, and thyroid antibody tests occasionally may be helpful but are usually unnecessary.

TABLE 10-10 Causes of Thyrotoxicosis

Graves' disease
Thyroiditis
Subacute thyroiditis
Painless (silent) thyroiditis
Radiation-induced thyroiditis
Exogenous thyrotoxicosis
Iatrogenic thyrotoxicosis
Factitious thyrotoxicosis
Iodide-induced thyrotoxicosis
Toxic multinodular goiter
Toxic uninodular goiter (toxic adenoma)
Ectopic thyrotoxicosis
Thyroid carcinoma
TSH hypersecretion
Trophoblastic tumors

Graves' Disease

By far the single most common cause of thyrotoxicosis, Graves' disease most often occurs in women 30 to 60 years old but may occur in children and in adult men and women of any age. It is not fundamentally a thyroid disease but rather a multisystem autoimmune disorder consisting of one or more of the following: hyperthyroidism, diffuse thyroid enlargement, infiltrative ophthalmopathy (exophthalmos), localized myxedema, and thyroid acropachy (see Extrathyroidal Manifestations of Graves' Disease). The clinical features and treatment of the extrathyroidal manifestations of Graves' disease are described later in this chapter. Most patients with Graves' disease have both thyrotoxicosis and diffuse goiter, and many have ophthalmopathy as well, whereas localized myxedema and especially thyroid acropachy are rare. The extrathyroidal manifestations of Graves' disease can occur in the absence of thyroid disease.

Thyroid-Stimulating Antibodies in Graves' Disease

Hyperthyroidism in patients with Graves' disease is caused by autoantibodies that stimulate thyroid secretion. These thyroid-stimulating antibodies (TSab) are IgG immunoglobulins that bind to and activate the TSH receptors on thyroid follicular cells; they are therefore TSH receptor antibodies that cause hyperthyroidism by mimicking the action of TSH. They are neither monoclonal nor polyclonal antibodies, but their clonality is restricted, so that the TSab in an individual patient usually belong to a single class of IgG and have a single type of light chain.[162,163] Peripheral blood and thyroid lymphocytes from patients with Graves' disease produce TSab in vitro.[164]

TSab can be detected in serum by both bioassay and receptor assay. The bioassays are based on the ability of TSab to stimulate thyroidal adenylate cyclase activity, iodide uptake, and T_4 and T_3 synthesis and release in animal or human thyroid cells and homogenates in vitro or various facets of thyroid radioiodine metabolism in animals.[165,166] The receptor assays are based on the ability of TSab to inhibit the binding of TSH to plasma membranes of animal or human thyroid cells or recombinant TSH receptors[167]; such activity is referred to as TSH-binding inhibitory activity. The assays that are based on the measurement of a biological response are the most specific but also the most cumbersome. TSab receptor assays are less specific because patients with other thyroid diseases, notably chronic autoimmune thyroiditis, may have serum autoantibodies that inhibit the binding and action of TSH in thyroid tissue.

TSab can be detected in the serum of nearly all patients with hyperthyroidism due to Graves' disease and may be found in the thyroid even when not present in serum.[165–168] The presence of TSab correlates well with the presence of thyrotoxicosis in untreated patients with Graves' disease and with the presence of thyroid autonomy, as reflected by low serum TSH concentrations, in patients who have received antithyroid therapy. Similarly, their presence in the serum of newborn infants of mothers with Graves' disease correlates well with the presence of hyperthyroidism in these infants. TSab can be detected in some patients before they develop thyrotoxicosis and in others who are euthyroid after completing a course of antithyroid drug therapy. Therefore, the presence of TSab does not invariably indicate the presence of thyrotoxicosis; TSab can be produced in amounts just sufficient to substitute for normal amounts of TSH.

TSab stimulate thyroid growth as well as thyroid function, acting primarily via receptors linked to adenylate cyclase.[169] There also may be separate thyroid growth-stimulating immunoglobulins, that is, IgGs that stimulate thyroid growth, at least as measured in vitro by stimulation of thymidine incorporation, but not thyroid adenylate cyclase, in thyroid tissue.[170] Their existence is controversial but could explain the wide variations in thyroid enlargement that occur in patients with hyperthyroid Graves' disease.[171] Variations in the degree of lymphocytic infiltration undoubtedly also contribute to the variation in enlargement.

Pathogenesis of Graves' Disease

If the hyperthyroidism of Graves' disease is caused by the production of TSab, what factors initiate and maintain their production? The disease could be initiated by exposure to an infectious agent or other agent that causes production of antibodies that cross-react with thyroid tissue.[162] The best-studied candidate agent is *Yersinia enterocolitica*. Some subtypes of this organism have membrane-binding sites for TSH, and some patients with Graves' disease have anti-*Yersinia* antibodies, but the association is weak. Graves' disease does not often follow *Yersinia* infections, and there is little evidence that the anti-*Yersinia* antibodies are present before the appearance of Graves' disease. A second possibility is that TSab production is initiated by an injury that alters a normal thyroid component, presumably a portion of the TSH receptor, so that it becomes antigenic, serving as a stimulus for TSab production. No known thyroid injury, however, whether due to an infectious agent, a toxin, or a drug, is followed by sustained TSab production; no thyroid tissue abnormality unique to Graves' disease has been found; and thyroid tissue from patients with Graves' disease behaves normally after transplantation into nude mice.[172,173] Moreover, normal thyroid tissue stimulates TSab production by lymphocytes in vitro. A third possibility is that TSab production results from the activation of B lymphocytes capable of producing TSab that were not clonally deleted in utero.

The ability of B cells to produce TSab therefore may be newly acquired or inherent; the limited structural heterogeneity of TSab provides evidence for the latter possibility. However B cells acquire the capability to produce TSab, they must be stimulated to expand and differentiate into antibody-secreting cells and then persistently stimulated so that antibody production is maintained. Their activation, expansion, and persistence probably result from stimulation by interleukins and other cytokines produced by T helper-inducer cells.

The process by which T helper-inducer (CD4) cells are activated to expand and to produce cytokines involves the binding of intracellularly processed antigen in combination with HLA (human leukocyte antigen) class II (HLA-D) molecules to the antigen receptors on T cells. HLA class II molecules are expressed on thyroid cells from patients with Graves' disease but not on normal thyroid cells; TSH and interferon and other cytokines can induce their expression on normal thyroid cells.[162,174] By acquiring class II molecules, thyroid cells can present their own components, such as portions of the TSH receptor, to T helper-inducer cells without the antigens being released into the interstitial fluid and taken up and processed by macrophages or other cells that normally express class II molecules and have the ability to process and present antigens. The binding of the thyroid cell class II molecule–thyroid antigen complex to the T-cell antigen receptor may be augmented by heat shock proteins or various adhesion molecules.[175]

Figure 10-20 shows a hypothetical scheme for the development of Graves' disease that is based on these considerations. The disease could be initiated in a susceptible host by some agent, perhaps a low-grade viral infection or toxin, that localizes in the thyroid gland and induces, respectively, interferon secretion by lymphocytes (or macrophages), which in turn induces class II molecule expression on the thyroid cells, and antigenic processing of nascent TSH receptors in thyroid cells. The class II molecule–TSH receptor antigen complexes then bind to the antigen receptors of T helper-inducer cells, thereby activating these T cells. The cytokines produced by the activated T cells stimulate B cells that were not clonally deleted to produce TSab. The thyroid cells cannot be injured by the initiating agent to the point where their function and growth capacity are impaired. The process could also be initiated by presentation by macrophages of an exogenous antigen that shared epitopes with the TSH receptor (molecular mimickry), in conjunction with HLA class II molecules (normally expressed on macrophages), to T helper-inducer cells. There is also evidence for a defect in T helper-suppressor cells in Graves' disease[176]; such a defect could contribute to continued activation of T helper-inducer cells. Even so, the process does not persist indefinitely, as TSab production ceases and

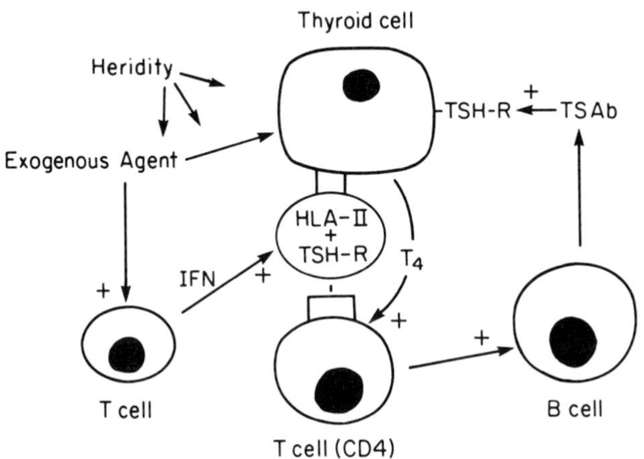

FIGURE 10-20 Hypothetical mechanisms for the development of Graves' disease and the hyperthyroidism it causes. In a subject with inherited susceptibility to the disease, an exogenous agent (virus or toxin) activates intrathyroidal T cells (or macrophages) to secrete cytokines, shown here as interferon (IFN), which then induce the expression of HLA class II (HLA-II) molecules on the thyroid cells. The agent also affects thyroid cells so that components of the TSH receptor (TSH-R) are processed as antigen. The class II molecules and TSH receptor antigens form complexes that bind to the antigen receptors of T helper-inducer (CD4) cells, inducing the secretion of other cytokines by the T cells. These cytokines stimulate B cells to expand and secrete thyroid-stimulating autoantibodies (TSab) that bind to and activate the TSH receptors of thyroid cells, thus inducing thyroid hypersecretion. T-cell function may be enhanced by T_4 (and T_3).

hyperthyroidism disappears in some patients. TSH and T_4 may help perpetuate the autoimmune process by stimulating the production of TSH receptors and augmenting T-cell activation, respectively.[177,178]

Although the overall number of B and T lymphocytes in peripheral blood is normal in patients with Graves' disease, variable decreases in the proportion of T suppressor cells have been reported. The thyroid tissue of such patients contains increased numbers of T lymphocytes; either T helper-inducer or T suppressor-cytotoxic cells may predominate.[162] The antigen receptors of these T cells are less structurally diverse than are those of circulating T cells, suggesting that these cells accumulate in response to specific intrathyroidal stimuli.

There are several risk factors for Graves' disease. One is female sex; a second is heredity. Evidence for heredity includes the high concordance rate (50 percent) in monozygotic twins (compared with less than 10 percent in dizygotic twins) and the increased frequency of thyroid antibodies, abnormalities in thyroid regulation, and Graves' disease or chronic autoimmune thyroiditis in the relatives of patients with Graves' disease.[162] The pattern of inheritance is probably polygenic. Compared with the general population, patients with Graves' disease have a predominance of certain HLA haplotypes, especially HLA-DR3, although the specific haplotype associations vary among different ethnic groups, and linkage analysis indicates that there must be other loci of susceptibility.[179] Other risk factors for the disease include smoking and perhaps stressful life events.[180–182] The occurrence of Graves' disease in the spouses of patients points to the existence of other environmental factors.[183]

Natural History of Graves' Disease

The natural history of Graves' disease varies considerably (Fig. 10-21). Some patients have a single episode of Graves' disease and therefore of thyrotoxicosis that subsides spontaneously after months or years. In others, both are persistent, perhaps lifelong. Still others have repeated episodes. The patterns of change in thyroid secretion are paralleled by changes in TSab production. In patients who are treated with an antithyroid drug, the occurrence of a remission of Graves' disease means that prolonged therapy is not required. The proportion of patients who have a remission of the first episode of Graves' hyperthyroidism varies widely, ranging from less than 10 to over 80 percent (see Treatment of Thyrotoxicosis).[177,184] The reasons for this very wide variability are not known. One important factor is time, since the rate of remission is higher among patients treated with an antithyroid drug for longer intervals.[185,186] Another factor may be the patient's HLA

FIGURE 10-21 Variation in the natural history of Graves' disease as exemplified by variations in either serum TSab (thyroid-stimulating autoantibody) or T_4 concentrations. *(Top panel)* Single episode of production of TSab and therefore of increased serum T_4 concentrations and thyrotoxicosis followed by disappearance of TSab and decline of the serum T_4 concentration to normal. *(Middle panel)* Persistent production of TSab and therefore persistently increased serum T_4 concentrations and persistent thyrotoxicosis. *(Bottom panel)* Multiple episodes of TSab production and increased serum T_4 concentrations with an intervening remission.

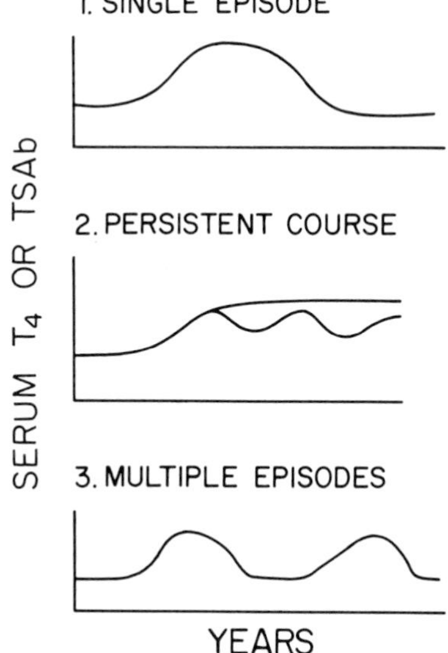

haplotype; patients with HLA-DR3 are less likely to have a remission than are those with other haplotypes. The antithyroid drugs methimazole and PTU may have immunosuppressive actions; if so, their use could contribute to the occurrence of remissions, but remissions also occur in patients treated with propranolol or potassium perchlorate and those not treated at all.[162,187] Finally, effective amelioration of thyrotoxicosis combined with inhibition of TSH secretion increases the likelihood of remission.[177]

Some patients who have a remission of hyperthyroidism have normal pituitary-thyroid regulation, a finding that suggests that their Graves' disease has disappeared. In others, however, abnormalities of pituitary-thyroid regulation persist, suggesting that the Graves' disease continues, but at a subclinical level.[188] Such patients probably have persistent TSab production, but the amount produced is too small to cause thyrotoxicosis. Thus, there is a pathophysiologic, although not clinical, distinction between remission of thyrotoxicosis alone and remission of Graves' disease. Approximately 10 percent of these patients develop hypothyroidism or at least chronic autoimmune thyroiditis after being in remission for many years, suggesting that Graves' disease can evolve into chronic autoimmune thyroiditis.[189] Conversely, hypothyroidism occasionally precedes the development of hyperthyroidism due to Graves' disease, indicating that a converse evolution can occur.[190]

TSab usually gradually disappear from the serum of patients treated with radioactive iodine or subtotal thyroidectomy, although there are transient increases in the first several weeks after thyroidectomy and more prolonged increases, lasting up to a year, after radioiodine therapy. These decreases provide evidence of the natural tendency of Graves' disease to subside.

The major pathologic finding of Graves' disease is diffuse thyroid enlargement. Microscopic examination reveals hypertrophy and hyperplasia of the thyroid follicular cells. The thyroid follicles are small, contain decreased quantities of colloid, and are lined by columnar epithelium, which often projects into the follicular lumen. The individual follicular cells have increased numbers of mitochondria, a hypertrophic Golgi apparatus, and increased microvilli at the apical surface. The interfollicular spaces are richly vascular, often containing foci of lymphocytes and occasionally lymphoid germinal centers.

Pathogenesis of Ophthalmopathy and Localized Myxedema

The causes of the extrathyroidal manifestations of Graves' disease—ophthalmopathy, localized myxedema, and thyroid acropachy—are poorly understood. The most prominent pathologic abnormality in patients with ophthalmopathy is enlargement of the extraocular muscles. This enlargement is caused by edema, infiltration of mononuclear cells, and proliferation of fibroblasts; the muscle cells appear normal. The muscle enlargement causes proptosis, the characteristic clinical finding of ophthalmopathy, and can impair venous drainage and compress the optic nerve. The inflammatory process may begin with the accumulation of T cells sensitized to antigens shared by orbital connective tissue or muscle cells and thyroid cells.[191] The cytokines secreted by these T cells may then damage the fibroblasts or muscle cells, causing inflammation and edema, or stimulate the synthesis of glycosaminoglycans by fibroblasts. They also may induce the fibroblasts to express class II molecules, rendering the cells capable of presenting antigen and therefore of perpetuating the activation of T cells, and produce heat shock proteins, which have immunomodulatory actions.[192]

The retroorbital inflammatory process may be enhanced by the actions of systemically or locally produced autoantibodies to fibroblasts or muscle cells. The local production of such antibodies could be augmented by the stimulatory action on B cells of the cytokines secreted by the activated T cells. Antibodies that have been found in the serum of patients with ophthalmopathy include antibodies that react with eye muscle cells and their plasma membranes, antibodies that are cytotoxic to eye muscle cells, and antibodies that react with orbital fibroblasts and stimulate the synthesis of glycosaminoglycans and protein by these cells as well as their proliferation.[193,194] Like thyroid disease, therefore, the pathogenesis of ophthalmopathy probably involves abnormalities in cell- and antibody-mediated immunity, and the antibodies and sensitized T cells are probably primarily thyroid-directed. The well-defined thyroid antibodies, such as antithyroid peroxidase antibodies and TSab, do not react with orbital tissue.

Very little is known about the pathogenesis of localized myxedema and thyroid acropachy, although they too probably have an autoimmune basis. The basic pathologic abnormalities of localized myxedema are proliferation of fibroblasts and subcutaneous accumulation of glycosaminoglycans, most often in the pretibial region.[38] The simplest explanation for localized myxedema is that it is caused by antibodies, presumably primarily thyroid-directed, that react with an antigen shared with fibroblasts, stimulating both their function and their proliferation. The serum of patients with localized myxedema contains antibodies that react with a 23-kd fibroblast protein and stimulate glycosaminoglycan synthesis by fibroblasts, and fibroblasts from affected regions have increased sensitivity to interferon-γ in terms of HLA class II molecule expression and decreased sensitivity to T_3.[195,196] The predilection for the pretibial region is unexplained.

Thyroiditis

The thyrotoxicosis that occurs in all the forms of thyroiditis is caused by the release of stored hormone as a result of thyroid inflammation and follicular disruption. Because the stores of thyroglobulin are limited and new T_4 and T_3 synthesis ceases, the thyrotoxicosis is transient.

Subacute Thyroiditis

Clinical manifestations of thyrotoxicosis occur in approximately 50 percent of patients with subacute thyroiditis, although nearly all of these patients have elevated serum T_4 and T_3 concentrations. The illness, however, is dominated by the nonspecific systemic manifestations of inflammation, such as fever, malaise, and myalgia, and by thyroid pain and tenderness, both of which may be severe. About half of these patients have a history of a recent upper respiratory infection. The thyroid is usually slightly or moderately enlarged. Any manifestations of thyrotoxicosis are modest and short-lived, lasting 4 to 6 weeks or less. The inflammatory and thyrotoxic phase is often followed by transient hypothyroidism, but permanent hypothyroidism is rare.[197] This disorder is discussed in more detail in the Painful Thyroid.

Painless (Silent) Thyroiditis

Thyroiditis without pain or tenderness may be the second or third most common cause of thyrotoxicosis in the United States. It occurs in more nearly equal numbers of men and women, in contrast to Graves' disease.[197] In women, it is particularly well recognized as a component of postpartum thyroid disease. Characteristically, the thyrotoxicosis is of recent onset and is mild, and there is no recent history of upper respiratory infection. The thyroid gland is not painful or tender and is not enlarged or is only slightly enlarged. There are none of the extrathyroidal manifestations of Graves' disease. The thyroid radioiodine uptake is low, and the sedimentation rate is usually normal. Thyroid antibodies are not present or are present in low titer, except in women with postpartum thyroiditis, in whom the titers are higher. The thyrotoxicosis lasts 2 to 6 weeks and is followed by either recovery or transient hypothyroidism that lasts 2 to 8 weeks. About 50 percent of these patients later develop goitrous autoimmune thyroiditis or hypothyroidism. Painless thyroiditis with thyrotoxicosis is most likely a variant form of chronic autoimmune thyroiditis (see Transient Hypothyroidism in Autoimmune Thyroiditis.

Other Forms of Thyroiditis

Radiation-induced thyroid follicular necrosis and inflammation occur regularly after ^{131}I therapy and occasionally are sufficiently intense to cause exacerbations of thyrotoxicosis, thyroid pain and tenderness, or both. These complications of ^{131}I therapy occur in the first 1 to 2 weeks after treatment, last a week or two, and then subside. Transient thyrotoxicosis has also been reported after thyroid trauma, surgical or otherwise, and tumor infiltration.

Exogenous Thyrotoxicosis

Thyroid Hormone–Induced Thyrotoxicosis

Thyrotoxicosis occurs as a result of the prescription of excessive doses of thyroid hormone by physicians, the use of large doses by patients on their own initiative, and the ingestion of food containing thyroid hormone. It is likely to occur in patients receiving thyroxine in doses of 0.2 mg/day or more, triiodothyronine in doses of 0.075 mg/day or more, or desiccated thyroid in doses of 180 mg/day or more (or the equivalent as combinations of synthetic T_4 and T_3). Somewhat smaller doses can cause subclinical and occasionally overt thyrotoxicosis. Single large doses of T_4, for example, 0.5 mg/kg or more, taken accidentally by children or with suicidal intent by adults can cause transient thyrotoxicosis.[198]

Thyroid hormone–induced thyrotoxicosis is especially likely to develop when T_3 alone or combinations of T_4 and T_3 (as desiccated thyroid or combinations of synthetic T_4 and T_3) are used, because serum T_4 measurements underestimate the total dose of thyroid hormone administered, particularly when T_3 alone is used. In euthyroid patients with autonomous (TSH-independent) thyroid function, such as a multinodular goiter, even usual doses of thyroid hormone, e.g., 0.1 mg T_4/day, may cause thyrotoxicosis.

Patients receiving thyroid therapy may increase the dose to alleviate symptoms thought to be due to hypothyroidism or in an effort to lose weight or treat menstrual irregularities. Other patients, particularly health care workers, surreptitiously take large doses of thyroid hormone because of psychological disturbances. They usually deny use and decline psychiatric care.[199]

Exogenous thyrotoxicosis has occurred as a result of improper meat-packing practices that resulted in the inclusion of thyroid tissue in neck muscle that was removed for consumption as ground meat.[200,201]

Important clues to the presence of exogenous thyrotoxicosis are the absence of thyroid enlargement, the failure of thyroid enlargement to regress much if the treatment was given for this purpose, and normal or low serum T_4 concentrations if the patient is taking T_3 or preparations containing T_3. Most patients with exogenous thyrotoxicosis also have low thyroid radioiodine uptake values and low serum thyroglobulin concentrations.

Iodine-Induced Thyrotoxicosis

Iodine supplementation for inhabitants of endemic goiter regions decreases the size of the goiter in most of the population. In some people, however, it induces thyrotoxicosis,[202] so that the incidence of thyrotoxicosis transiently increases twofold to fourfold. For thyrotoxicosis to occur, the patient must have a preexisting thyroid abnormality, for example, Graves' disease or a nodular goiter, but insufficient iodine intake to permit excessive production of T_4 and T_3 (see Chap. 11).

Iodine-induced thyrotoxicosis also occurs in nonendemic goiter regions.[202] Most of these patients have autonomously functioning thyroid tissue, such as a multinodular goiter or a thyroid adenoma, that transports iodide poorly. They become thyrotoxic several weeks or months after receiving pharmacologic doses of inorganic iodide, iodine-containing radiographic contrast agents, or iodine-containing drugs. Whatever the source of iodine, serum iodide concentrations must increase sufficiently that enough iodide can enter the thyroid by diffusion to allow excessive thyroid hormone synthesis and secretion by the autonomous thyroid tissue.

Toxic Multinodular Goiter

Thyrotoxicosis may be a late development in the natural history of multinodular goiter, usually in women 60 years old or older (see Chap. 11). The usual patient has a long history of gradually increasing thyroid enlargement and develops subclinical and then overt thyrotoxicosis insidiously. There is no ophthalmopathy or localized myxedema and no spontaneous remission; thyrotoxicosis persists until the autonomous thyroid tissue is destroyed. The number of palpable nodules varies from one to many, and sometimes they are so numerous and small that the thyroid seems to be diffusely enlarged. Even so, the hyperfunctioning regions usually account for only a portion of the total thyroid mass; other regions are composed of hyperplastic but inactive thyroid follicles, atrophic follicles, or fibrous tissue. This process starts as local areas of hyperplastic follicular cells capable of autonomous iodine metabolism. As these areas grow and replicate, they account for an increasing proportion and eventually all thyroid secretion, and there is a concomitant gradual decline in TSH secretion.[203] Such a formulation, based largely on autoradiographic and pathologic studies, explains the very gradual development of toxic nodular goiter, the fact that most patients with multinodular goiter never become thyrotoxic, and the varied pathology of the disorder.[204]

Toxic Uninodular Goiter (Toxic Thyroid Adenoma)

Thyrotoxicosis occurs in some patients with an autonomously functioning thyroid adenoma; its frequency in patients with this lesion is about 20 percent (see Chap. 11).[205] Although thyroid adenomas occur in adults of all ages and occasionally in children, most patients with thyrotoxicosis are in the older age groups. The adenomas in thyrotoxic patients are nearly always greater than 3 cm in diameter. Thyrotoxicosis develops infrequently during follow-up of euthyroid patients with an autonomously functioning thyroid adenoma who are not treated. It may also occur transiently as a result of hemorrhagic infarction of such an adenoma.[206]

The characteristic finding in patients with a toxic thyroid adenoma is a solitary nodule. Thyroid radioisotope scans show intense uptake of isotope in the location of the palpable nodule and nearly complete absence of uptake in the remainder of the thyroid gland. Pathologically, these lesions are well-encapsulated masses of hyperplastic thyroid tissue, although they may be cystic. They are generally considered to be true tumors, in contrast to the nodules found in patients with multinodular goiter.

Ectopic Thyrotoxicosis (Struma Ovarii)

The only recognized causes of thyrotoxicosis due to excessive ectopic thyroid hormone secretion are dermoid tumors and teratomas of the ovary (struma ovarii).[207] Most patients with thyrotoxicosis and struma ovarii have Graves' disease or multinodular goiter. Thus, they have one of the common causes of thyrotoxicosis, affecting both the thyroid gland and the thyroid tissue within the ovarian tumor. The ectopic thyroid tissue is the sole source of excessive thyroid hormone only when it contains a toxic thyroid adenoma or the patient has Graves' disease and all of the thyroid was removed earlier; these are both very rare events.

Thyroid Carcinoma

Few thyroid carcinomas can transport iodide, and therefore they cannot synthesize T_4 and T_3, even though most do synthesize thyroglobulin. For this reason, thyrotoxicosis is very rare in patients with thyroid carcinoma. When it occurs, it is in patients with follicular carcinoma, usually many years after the initial appearance of the tumor and when the tumor burden is very large.

Thyroid-Stimulating Hormone Excess

Pituitary TSH Hypersecretion

Excessive TSH secretion is a rare cause of thyrotoxicosis. Such patients have a diffuse goiter but no ophthalmopathy. The majority have a macro- or microadenoma of the pituitary; the remainder have no tumor and are said to have pituitary resistance to T_4 and T_3.[208,209] The serum TSH concentrations vary widely in these patients from normal to many-fold above normal, indicating that the biological activity of the TSH that is secreted varies widely.[210] There may be concomitant hypersecretion of growth hormone or other pituitary hormones as well. The tumoral and nontumoral forms of TSH-induced thyrotoxicosis are best distinguished by radiologic studies rather than by biochemical tests. As a general rule, however, patients with a TSH-secreting pituitary tumor have increased serum TSH and especially glycoprotein hormone alpha subunit concentrations, so that the ratio of alpha subunit to TSH is high. Patients with no demonstrable tumor usually have normal basal serum alpha subunit concentrations, so that the molar ratio of the alpha subunit to TSH is normal or low. Patients with TSH-secreting tumors should have the tumors removed surgically. If that is not possible or if there is no tumor, treatment with octreotide or occasionally bromocriptine may be effective.[208,209]

Trophoblastic Tumors

Tumors of trophoblastic origin—hydatidiform mole, choriocarcinoma, and embryonal carcinoma of the testes—may cause thyrotoxicosis. It is due to secretion of human chorionic gonadotropin (hCG) by the tumor. These patients usually have serum hCG concentrations greater than 300 × 10^3 units/liter, higher than is found in euthyroid patients with the same tumors.[211] Furthermore, purified hCG has thyroid-stimulating activity, and there is a rough correlation between the hCG concentration and the bioassayable thyroid-stimulating activity in the serum of these patients. Other patients with these tumors, while not overtly thyrotoxic, have elevated serum T_4 and T_3 concentrations and decreased TSH secretion. The lack of overt thyrotoxicosis may be due to the short duration of excess thyroid secretion or masking of the symptoms and signs of thyrotoxicosis by those of the trophoblastic disease.

Clinical Manifestations of Thyrotoxicosis

Thyrotoxicosis is usually first suggested by evidence of increased thyroid hormone actions on one or more organ systems. However, it may be discovered coincidentally in patients who seek care for thyroid enlargement or ophthalmopathy. The symptoms and signs of thyrotoxicosis usually reflect accelerated organ system function or the inability of an organ system to meet the demands imposed by thyrotoxicosis. The most common symptoms and signs are listed in Table 10-11.[212–216] The frequency and severity of the symptoms and signs of thyrotoxicosis vary substantially among patients, and the correlation between clinical severity and serum T_4 and T_3 concentrations is poor.

Factors that influence the clinical severity of the disorder include the rate of onset, the age of the patient, and the vulnerability of different organ systems to excessive thyroid hormone action. The clinical manifestations of thyrotoxicosis tend to be less severe when its onset is gradual, and it is often tolerated well, particularly by younger patients. Indeed, some patients may feel better than when they were euthyroid; for example, they have more energy, can eat more without gaining weight, and are more comfortable in cool weather. Careful questioning usually reveals undesirable changes such as tremor, muscle weakness, emotional lability, and fatigue on exertion. However, thyrotoxicosis is fundamentally a catabolic process, and sooner or later more disabling manifestations are likely to develop. The symptoms and signs in children and adolescents are similar to those in young adults.

TABLE 10-11 Common Symptoms and Signs of Thyrotoxicosis

	Frequency in Thyrotoxic Patients, %
Symptom	
Nervousness	69–99
Increased sweating	45–91
Heat intolerance	41–89
Palpitations	63–89
Dyspnea	66–81
Fatigue and weakness	44–88
Weight loss	52–85
Increased appetite	11–65
Hyperdefecation	12–33
Sign	
Thyroid enlargement	37–100
Lid retraction	34–80
Hyperactivity	39–80
Tremor	40–97
Tachycardia (>90 beats/min)	58–100
Atrial fibrillation	3–38

Source: Refs. 212–216.

Compared with younger adults, elderly patients more often have weight loss, atrial fibrillation, and cardiovascular symptoms, whereas increased appetite, heat intolerance, and tremor are less frequent; these patients tend to have fewer symptoms and signs overall.[215,216] The terms *apathetic thyrotoxicosis* and *masked thyrotoxicosis* are sometimes used in describing older patients because of their lack of the symptoms and signs of neural activation, but there is no evidence that apathetic or masked thyrotoxicosis is pathophysiologically different from "ordinary" thyrotoxicosis, and careful evaluation will often elicit the presence of the symptoms and signs of neural activation. Death is usually due to cardiac failure.[217] The most life-threatening form of thyrotoxicosis—thyroid storm—is discussed below.

General Appearance

Figure 10-22 shows a woman with thyrotoxicosis. Her appearance alone should suggest the diagnosis. She appears to have lost weight and has a pained or apprehensive expression. Her skin is shiny and smooth, her eyelids are retracted, and her goiter is obvious. She is probably unable to sit quietly and talk calmly but rather is restless and unable to concentrate and speaks rapidly.

Skin and Appendages

The skin is warm and moist, and its texture is smooth or velvety; erythema and pruritis may be present. Perspiration is increased. The hair may become thin and fine in texture, and alopecia can occur. The nails may be soft and separated from the nail bed (onchyolysis). Other occasional findings are hyperpigmentation and vitiligo, the latter occurring

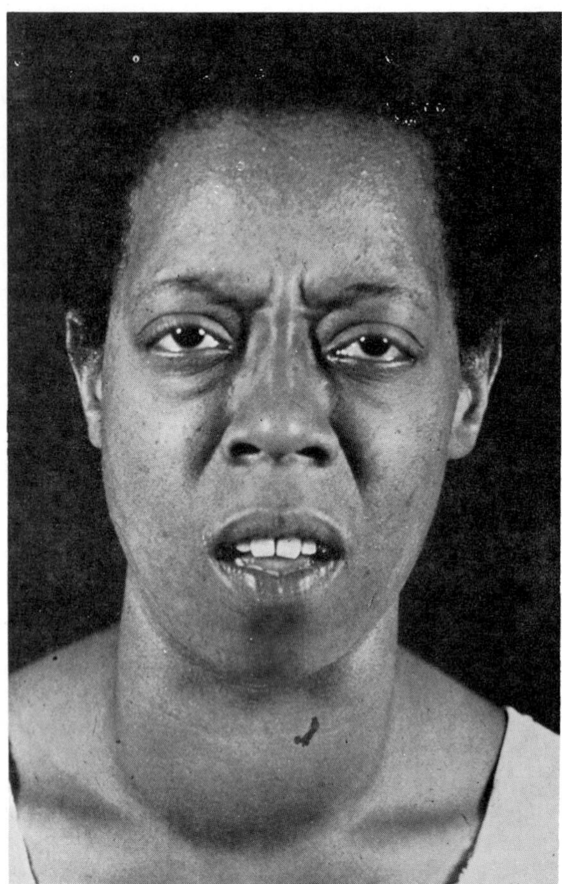

FIGURE 10-22 Photograph of a woman with thyrotoxicosis and ophthalmopathy caused by Graves' disease. Note the anxious expression, prominent eyes, periorbital edema, and diffuse goiter.

mostly in patients with Graves' disease. Localized myxedema, not a manifestation of thyrotoxicosis per se, is described in Extrathyroidal Manifestations of Graves' Disease.

Eyes

Two types of ocular abnormalities occur in thyrotoxic patients: noninfiltrative and infiltrative. The noninfiltrative signs of lid retraction and lid lag occur in patients with thyrotoxicosis of any cause. Usually the upper lids are symmetrically retracted so that some sclera is visible, but lid retraction may be asymmetric or may involve the lower lids as well. Lid retraction results in apparent proptosis but not in actual forward protrusion of the eyes and is often accompanied by symptoms of conjunctival irritation. Lid lag is a common but less reliable finding. Infiltrative ophthalmopathy is discussed in Extrathyroidal Manifestations of Graves' Disease.

Thyroid Gland

Thyroid enlargement of some type is a common finding. It may be the initial or only clue to the presence of thyrotoxicosis and usually indicates its cause. In Graves' disease, both thyroid lobes are usually diffusely, more or less symmetrically enlarged; the right lobe tends to be somewhat larger, as it is in normal subjects. The goiter is usually moderate; i.e., the thyroid is twofold to fourfold enlarged. The thyroid gland is sometimes slightly tender, its consistency varies from soft to firm, and the surface is usually smooth, although it can be irregular or lobulated. There may be a thyroid bruit or thrill caused by greatly increased thyroid blood flow. However, about 20 percent of these patients have no thyroid enlargement; the proportion is higher among elderly patients.[218] Thyroiditis usually results in slight diffuse thyroid enlargement, and the thyroid is tender in subacute thyroiditis. Toxic multinodular goiters tend to be large and asymmetric and uneven in consistency. A thyroid adenoma causing thyrotoxicosis is usually at least 3 cm in diameter, and no other thyroid tissue should be palpable.

Nervous System and Muscle

Most thyrotoxic patients have symptoms of central nervous system dysfunction. Common complaints are nervousness, physical hyperactivity, emotional lability, anxiety, and irritability. Lability of mood is often striking; these patients are easily angered and prone to episodes of anxiety or even paranoia. They often are restless, are unable to remain still for any length of time, and sleep fitfully. Their ability to concentrate decreases, and complaints of memory loss are common. Objective testing may show some impairment of cognitive function. These changes often result in impairment of work or school performance and disturbances in home and family life. Most of the patients are aware of these changes, but their extent often becomes more clear when a family member or friend is interviewed. At the other extreme, depression and withdrawal may occur in older patients. These striking clinical findings occur in the absence of gross abnormalities of cerebral oxygen consumption or substrate utilization.

The most prominent neuromuscular symptoms are tremor and muscle weakness. The tremor is usually limited to the hands and fingers and is most evident when the hands are extended, but it may involve the arms, legs, tongue, and head. The movements are rapid and uniform and of low amplitude. Although the tremor is not worsened by voluntary movement, the performance of skills requiring fine coordination, such as threading a needle and writing, becomes difficult. The pathophysiology of the thyrotoxic tremor is unclear. It is not a manifestation of muscle weakness, although that may aggravate it, and it is decreased by propranolol.

Some evidence of myopathy is evident in nearly all thyrotoxic patients. Muscle weakness usually develops gradually and varies from mild to severe; it is due to both muscle wasting and decreased efficiency of muscle contraction.[219] It affects the strength and endurance of both proximal and distal muscles, thus causing difficulty in reaching above the head, rising from a lying or sitting position, and gripping objects.[220] Deep tendon reflexes are hyperactive, with both contraction and relaxation phases being accelerated, despite muscle weakness, and unsustained clonus may be present. Myopathy can also involve the respiratory and oropharyngeal musculature, causing difficulty in swallowing or hoarseness. Ophthalmoplegia, most commonly limitation of upward gaze, may occur but is a manifestation of infiltrative ophthalmopathy rather than extraocular muscle weakness caused by thyrotoxicosis. Serum concentrations of creatine kinase and myoglobin are normal or low, but it is possible that increased release from muscle is overshadowed by increased clearance.

A syndrome of periodic muscle weakness that is clinically and pathophysiologically very similar to familial hypokalemic periodic paralysis occurs in patients with thyrotoxicosis. Nearly all these patients are men, and most are of Asian origin.[221] As in hypokalemic periodic paralysis, the attacks may follow exercise or may be induced by food or alcohol ingestion. They respond to potassium therapy and also to propranolol, and they invariably disappear after antithyroid treatment. These patients have no family history of periodic paralysis.

Cardiovascular System

Heart rate, cardiac contractility, stroke volume, and cardiac output are all increased in thyrotoxicosis, and peripheral resistance is decreased.[222–224] These changes are due both to direct inotropic and chronotropic effects of thyroid hormone and to an increased need for peripheral oxygen delivery. Although cardiac output is increased, regional blood flow is not uniformly increased; skin, muscle, cerebral, and coronary flow are increased, whereas hepatic flow is not. Another adaptive mechanism augmenting peripheral oxygen delivery is an increase in red blood cell mass.[225]

These changes in cardiovascular function may result in palpitation, tachycardia, atrial fibrillation, and heart failure. Atrial fibrillation may be the sole manifestation of thyrotoxicosis in elderly patients, although the percentage of patients with idiopathic atrial fibrillation who have thyrotoxicosis is low.[224] The pulse pressure is increased, arterial pulsations are bounding, and systolic hypertension may be present. A jugular venous hum is often heard. Examination of the heart reveals a prominent apical impulse, accentuated heart sounds, systolic ejection or other murmurs, and occasionally cardiac enlargement. Other than disturbances of rhythm, electrocardiographic changes are limited to nonspecific ST- and T-wave abnormalities. Noninvasive studies reveal shortened systolic and diastolic time intervals, increased systolic and diastolic function, increased ventricular mass, and reductions in the left ventricular ejection fraction during exercise.

The question of whether thyrotoxicosis alone causes cardiac failure is controversial. Most of these patients have intrinsic heart disease; their cardiac function decompensates because of vasodilatation, increased blood volume, and rhythm-related decreases in diastolic filling. Cardiac failure can occur, however, especially in association with atrial fibrillation, in younger patients who have no evidence of cardiac disease when studied after treatment. Dynamic studies in these patients have shown higher systemic vascular resistance both at rest and during exercise compared with those with no cardiac symptoms.[222] Their resting cardiac output may be normal or increased, and it does not change or decrease during exercise, changes indicative of cardiomyopathy. Symptomatic coronary artery disease is aggravated by thyrotoxicosis.

Respiratory Function

Abnormalities in respiratory function described in thyrotoxicosis include decreased vital capacity, decreased pulmonary compliance, and increased minute ventilation.[226] Alveolar and arterial oxygen and carbon dioxide content and airway resistance are usually normal, although thyrotoxicosis can aggravate asthma.[227] Ventilatory responses to hypoxemia or hypercapnea are increased. Dyspnea during exercise is a common symptom and is probably multifactorial, being due to respiratory muscle weakness, decreased lung compliance, increased ventilation, and occasionally cardiac dysfunction.

Renal Function and Fluid and Electrolyte Metabolism

Renal blood flow, glomerular filtration rate, and renal tubular reabsorptive and secretory capacities are increased, but sodium balance and serum electrolyte concentrations are normal.[228] Serum atrial natriuretic hormone concentrations are increased and aldosterone secretion is decreased, presumably because of the increase in plasma volume, although renin activity is often increased, probably as a result of adrenergic stimulation.[229,230] Renin, aldosterone, and renal responses to sodium restriction and volume expansion are normal.[231] Polydipsia and polyuria may be prominent symptoms. In such patients, serum osmolality tends to be lower than normal, indicating primary thirst stimulation,[232] which is not surprising in view of the heat sensitivity and physical and emotional lability that so often occur. Urine-concentrating ability may be impaired after both dehydration and vasopressin administration.

Gastrointestinal System

The major abnormality in gastrointestinal function is more rapid small and large intestinal transit.[233] The most common symptom is increased frequency of bowel movements, although frank diarrhea may occur. Intestinal hypermotility and increased dietary fat intake may result in steatorrhea; absorption of most other nutrients is normal. Occasional patients have nausea, vomiting, or abdominal pain, possibly as a result of gastric stasis or chemoreceptor activation.[234]

Some abnormalities in hepatic function are found in the majority of patients. These include mild increases in serum alanine and aspartate aminotransferase, alkaline phosphatase, and bilirubin concentrations; occasionally jaundice is clinically evident.[134] Liver histology is normal or shows mild hepatocellular injury.

Hematopoietic System

Both red cell mass and plasma volume tend to be increased, with the increase in plasma volume predominating.[225] Thus, some patients have a modest reduction in hematocrit and hemoglobin values. Red cell survival is normal or slightly shortened. Serum vitamin B_{12}, folate, and iron concentrations and iron stores may be low. Iron clearance and serum erythropoetin tend to be increased. The bone marrow shows erythroid hyperplasia and occasionally megaloblastic changes. These findings, which are indicative of increased iron utilization and increased red cell production, are the expected responses to the need for increased peripheral oxygen delivery. A few patients are truly anemic, as a result of deficiency of one or more hematopoietic nutrients. About 1 percent of patients with Graves' disease have pernicious anemia, although not necessarily in a close chronologic relation to their thyroid disease, and parietal cell antibodies are found in about 10 percent.

Granulocyte and lymphocyte counts are usually normal, although some patients have mild lymphocytosis or granulocytopenia.[235] Lymphadenopathy, thymic enlargement, and splenomegaly are rare findings; whether they are manifestations of thyrotoxicosis per se or of Graves' disease is not clear. Some patients have easy bruising and thrombocytopenia; their platelets contain increased amounts of IgG and aggregate abnormally.[236]

Energy, Nutrient, and Drug Metabolism

A major consequence of thyrotoxicosis is increased oxygen consumption and substrate utilization, and maintenance of basic physiologic functions and mechanical work are less efficient than normal. To counterbalance these changes, food intake, utilization of stored energy, and oxygen consumption all increase, with an attendant increase in heat production. Increases in appetite and food intake are therefore a very common feature of thyrotoxicosis. In most of these patients, however, compensation is inadequate and some weight loss occurs. The loss in weight averages 15 percent, but the variation is large.[237] It tends to be greater in elderly patients and those who are obese. By contrast, in some young patients the increase in appetite and food intake is sufficient to cause modest weight gain; such patients probably eat to satisfy emotional needs.

Major changes occur in the metabolism of carbohydrate, lipid, and protein. The absorption of glucose is increased, as is gluconeogenesis and glycogenolysis.[35] Peripheral insulin sensitivity is normal or decreased, and hepatic insulin sensitivity may be decreased.[238] Muscle, adipose tissue, and splanchnic glucose utilization is increased. Serum glucose and insulin responses to an oral glucose load are usually normal. In about one-third of these patients, however, oral glucose tolerance is impaired, insulin responses are inadequate, and glucagon secretion is not suppressed normally by glucose. Thus, thyrotoxicosis, like pregnancy and Cushing's syndrome, may uncover an insulin secretory deficiency. In patients with preexisting diabetes mellitus, requirements for exogenous insulin increase because of accelerated insulin catabolism.[239]

Both the synthesis and the clearance of cholesterol are increased in thyrotoxicosis, with the increase in clearance predominating. This probably results from an increase in low-density lipoprotein (LDL) receptors. Thus, modest reductions in serum total and LDL cholesterol concentrations are the usual findings[240]; serum high-density lipoprotein (HDL) cholesterol and lipoprotein(a) may be reduced as well. Serum triglyceride concentrations are usually normal. Hepatic lipase activity is increased, but lipoprotein lipase activity is normal. The mobilization of adipose tissue lipid stores also is accelerated, resulting in increased plasma free fatty acid concentrations.

Protein synthesis and catabolism are also increased, the latter to a greater extent. The net overall result is excessive protein catabolism, resulting in loss of muscle mass, negative nitrogen balance, and increased urinary amino acid excretion. Serum concentrations of proteins secreted by the liver—for example, albumin, TBG, TTR, and some other transport proteins—are normal or slightly decreased. An exception is sex hormone–binding globulin (SHBG). Its production is stimulated by T_3 and T_4, and its serum concentrations are elevated in thyrotoxic patients. The serum concentrations of proteins of endothelial origin, such as fibronectin, von Willebrand factor, and angiotensin-converting enzyme, also are increased.[241]

The metabolism and clearance of some drugs, including digoxin and propranolol, are increased in thyrotoxic patients, and so larger doses may be needed.[242] By contrast, thyrotoxic patients may need less warfarin (Coumadin), because the clearance of vitamin K–dependent clotting factors is increased. The metabolism of methimazole and PTU is normal.

Endocrine System

Pituitary Hormone Secretion

Linear growth in children with thyrotoxicosis is increased, as are mean 24-h serum growth hormone (GH) concentrations and growth hormone secretion rates (in adults).[243] Serum GH responses to growth hormone–releasing hormone or other stimuli are normal or slightly decreased. Serum insulin-like growth factor-I concentrations are within the normal range. Serum prolactin concentrations are normal or slightly decreased.

Adrenal Function

Thyrotoxicosis results in an acceleration of cortisol clearance. As a result, ACTH secretion, the number of cortisol secretory episodes, the cortisol secretion rate, and urinary 17-hydroxycorticosteroid excretion are increased. Serum cortisol concentrations and urinary cortisol excretion are normal, as are adrenal responses to ACTH and hypoglycemia. The development of thyrotoxicosis, however, can unmask subclinical adrenal insufficiency (see Chap. 12).

Circulating levels and secretion rates of epinephrine and norepinephrine are normal.[39]

Gonadal Function

Menstrual cycles are normal in most women with thyrotoxicosis, although they may have oligomenorrhea or amenorrhea. An increase in serum SHBG concentrations results in increased serum total estradiol and estrone concentrations but low-normal or low serum free estradiol and estrone concentrations.[244,245] Serum luteinizing hormone (LH) and follicle-stimulating hormone (FSH) concentrations are slightly increased during most of the cycle, probably as a result of the reduced serum free estrogen levels. The midcycle serum LH and FSH peaks are subnormal in regularly cycling or oligomenorrheic thyrotoxic women, but these peaks usually are followed by increases in serum progesterone, indicating that the cycles were ovulatory.[244] Thus, infertility should occur only in women with amenorrhea. In postmenopausal women, serum LH and FSH concentrations are appropriately elevated.

In men, thyrotoxicosis results in decreased potency and occasionally loss of libido and gynecomastia. Sperm density and motility may be decreased. Serum SHBG concentrations are increased, resulting in increased serum total testosterone concentrations; serum free testosterone concentrations are normal.[245,246] Extragonadal conversion of androgen to estrogen is increased, resulting in increased serum total and free estradiol concentrations. The increased serum estradiol concentrations cause the gynecomastia and seminiferous tubule dysfunction and increase serum LH and FSH concentrations modestly.

Parathyroid-Vitamin D-Bone System

Thyrotoxicosis results in an increase in bone resorption through a direct effect on osteoclastic activity. Bone formation increases secondarily, but less than bone resorption.[247,248] Both trabecular and cortical bone density therefore tend to be decreased, but no increase in the fracture rate has been reported, perhaps because of the usually short duration of thyrotoxicosis. Mild hypercalcemia caused by the increase in bone resorption is an occasional finding[249]; another cause should be sought if the hypercalcemia is severe. Serum phosphate concentrations are usually normal, and concentrations of skeletal alkaline phosphatase and osteocalcin may be increased. Serum parathyroid hormone and 1,25-dihydroxycholecalciferol concentrations and gastrointestinal calcium absorption are decreased as a consequence of the augmented skeletal calcium resorption.

Laboratory Diagnosis of Thyrotoxicosis

The biochemical hallmarks of thyrotoxicosis are increased serum total and free T_4 and T_3 concentrations and decreased serum TSH concentrations (Fig. 10-15). The correlation between the clinical and biochemical severity of thyrotoxicosis is poor,[250] and therefore judgments about its severity should be based on clinical findings.

Serum TSH Concentrations

Serum TSH concentrations are low not only in nearly all patients with thyrotoxicosis but also in many patients who are euthyroid and have normal serum T_4 and T_3 concentrations. Many of these euthyroid patients have some autonomous thyroid secretion or are receiving T_4 therapy (see Subclinical Thyrotoxicosis). Others have no evident thyroid disease and may not have persistently low serum TSH concentrations (see Aging).[71,87,251,252] However, as a group these patients tend to have serum T_4 and T_3 concentrations in the upper part of the normal range, and their serum TSH concentrations are not usually as low as are those in patients with overt thyrotoxicosis (Fig. 10-15). Serum TSH concentrations may also be low in patients with nonthyroidal illness or central hypothyroidism. The only patients with increased serum free T_4 values who have normal or high serum TSH concentrations are those with FDH, TSH-induced thyrotoxicosis, or generalized resistance to thyroid hormone.

Serum Thyroxine and Triiodothyronine Concentrations

Serum total and free T_4 concentrations and free T_4 index values are increased in most patients with thyrotoxicosis. Since serum total T_4 concentrations are increased in many other situations (Table 10-8), confirmation of the diagnosis of thyrotoxicosis must be based on the finding of a high serum free T_4 index or free T_4 concentration. Even these are not completely specific indicators of thyrotoxicosis, since the results of one or both of these tests may be high in patients with FDH, nonthyroidal illness, or generalized resistance to thyroid hormone.

Serum total (and free) T_3 concentrations also are increased in nearly all patients with thyrotoxicosis. The values usually are more abnormal than are serum T_4 values, especially in younger patients.[253] Serum T_3 measurements thus may help confirm or exclude a suspected diagnosis of thyrotoxicosis in patients who have serum T_4 and free T_4 index values within the normal range (T_3 thyrotoxicosis), and their principal value is for this purpose. Increases in serum TBG concentrations raise serum T_3 concentrations just as they raise those of T_4, and isolated elevations, with or without thyrotoxicosis, occur in patients who are taking T_3 or desiccated thyroid.

Conversely, some patients with thyrotoxicosis, especially elderly patients, have increased serum T_4 but normal serum T_3 concentrations (T_4 thyrotoxicosis).[9,161] Its occurrence provides evidence that impaired extrathyroidal conversion of T_4 to T_3 caused by nonthyroidal illness or pharmacologic agents can impair extrathyroidal T_3 production even in thyrotoxic patients. In other patients with various nonthyroidal illnesses, serum T_4 concentrations may be elevated and serum T_3 concentrations may be normal or low initially, but both return to normal during recovery (see Nonthyroidal Illness).

Thyroid Radioiodine Uptake and Scanning

Thyroid radioiodine uptake is increased in most patients with thyrotoxicosis; that is, these patients have thyroid gland hyperfunction. The exceptions are patients with subacute thyroiditis, painless thyroiditis, and exogenous thyrotoxicosis. Among thyrotoxic patients, thyroid radioiodine uptake measurements should be done only to distinguish between Graves' disease and painless thyroiditis and to confirm a suspected diagnosis of exogenous thyrotoxicosis when it is denied by the patient.

Thyroid radioisotope scans may be helpful in identifying a thyroid adenoma or multinodular goiter as a cause of thyrotoxicosis. In patients with diffuse thyroid enlargement, a thyroid scan provides little information beyond that obtained by careful palpation of the thyroid gland.

Thyroid-Stimulating Antibodies

The cause of thyrotoxicosis in most patients is Graves' disease, and TSab are detectable in the serum of most of them (see Causes of Thyrotoxicosis).[165–167,184] However, TSab may be found during or after treatment when the patient is euthyroid or hypothyroid and occasionally in seemingly normal subjects. Thus, a positive test does not necessarily indicate the presence of thyrotoxicosis. Moreover, the tests for TSab that are the most widely available are receptor assays that can detect either thyroid-stimulating or thyroid-inhibiting antibodies.

Thyrotropin-Releasing Hormone Stimulation Test

Serum TSH concentrations increase promptly after the intravenous administration of TRH in normal subjects. In thyrotoxicosis, the inhibition of TSH secretion resulting from T_4 and T_3 overproduction is accompanied by subnormal or absent serum TSH responses to TRH. This is a sensitive test of pituitary suppression, but no more so than measurement of the basal serum TSH concentration using the TSH assays that are now available (Fig. 10-15).

Summary: Laboratory Diagnosis of Thyrotoxicosis

A scheme for the evaluation of patients with suspected thyrotoxicosis is shown in Fig. 10-23. The initial step should be measurement of the serum TSH concentration and the serum free T_4 index. If the

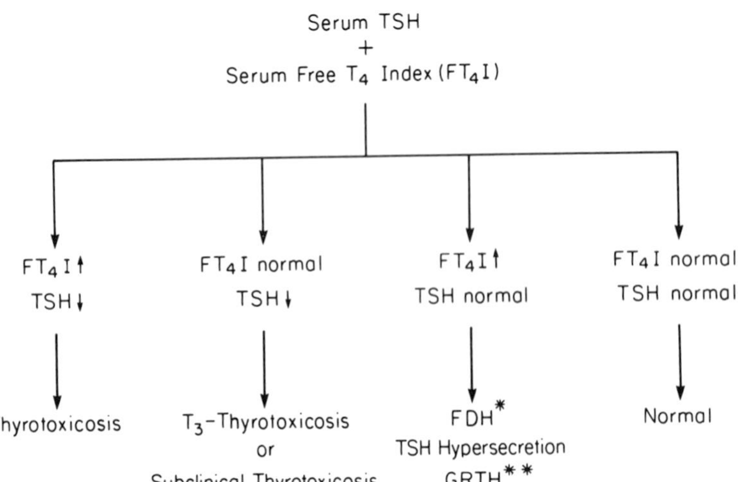

FIGURE 10-23 Diagnostic scheme for the evaluation of patients with suspected thyrotoxicosis. *, Familial dysalbuminemic hyperthyroxinemia; **, generalized resistance to thyroid hormone.

serum free T_4 index value is high and the serum TSH concentration is low, the diagnosis of thyrotoxicosis is confirmed and no further tests are needed. If the serum free T_4 index value is normal and the serum TSH concentration is low, the patient may have T_3 thyrotoxicosis or subclinical thyrotoxicosis; these two possibilities can be distinguished by measurement of the serum T_3 concentration.

A high serum free T_4 index and a normal serum TSH concentration indicate the presence of FDH, primary TSH hypersecretion, or generalized resistance to thyroid hormone. FDH is probably the most common of these disorders, but all are rare. Among them, only primary TSH hypersecretion results in thyrotoxicosis. FDH may be confirmed by finding a normal or nearly normal serum T_3 concentration, a low THBR if $[^{125}I]T_4$ instead of $[^{125}I]T_3$ is used in the test, and a high serum free T_4 index and normal TSH concentration in a family member.[73] Generalized resistance to thyroid hormone is discussed in Hypothyroidism.

Other Laboratory Manifestations of Thyrotoxicosis or Diseases Causing Thyrotoxicosis

Many other physiologic, biochemical, and serologic abnormalities may be found in patients with thyrotoxicosis. Some result from excessive thyroid hormone action in various tissues, and others reflect the various diseases that cause thyrotoxicosis. The most sensitive tests of tissue thyroid hormone action are probably measurements of cardiac systolic time intervals and serum SHBG concentrations.[222,245]

Tests indicative of thyroid disease include measurements of serum thyroglobulin and thyroid antibodies. Serum thyroglobulin concentrations are increased in most patients with thyrotoxicosis, except those in whom it is due to exogenous thyroid hormone administration.[8] Antithyroid peroxidase (thyroid microsomal) and antithyroglobulin antibodies are present in the serum of most patients with Graves' disease, although not usually in the high titers found in patients with chronic autoimmune thyroiditis. However, these antibodies are not specific for thyroid autoimmune disease (see Evaluation of Thyroid Function).

Treatment of Thyrotoxicosis

The most important treatments that are available for patients with thyrotoxicosis are listed in Table 10-12. The ideal therapy is elimination of its cause so that the thyrotoxicosis disappears and normal pituitary-thyroid function is restored. However, for most patients, the fundamental cause is not known and no truly curative treatment is available.

The following sections deal with the treatment of thyrotoxicosis due to Graves' disease, thyroiditis, multinodular goiter, and thyroid adenoma. The treatment of many of the rarer causes of thyrotoxicosis listed in Table 10-10 is obvious. For patients with any of them, therapy with drugs that decrease thyroidal production of T_4 and T_3 or relieve the peripheral manifestations of thyrotoxicosis may be needed before or during more specific and permanent therapy. The considerations pertaining to the use of these drugs are the same as when they are given to patients with Graves' disease, as discussed below. Not all patients with overt thyrotoxicosis need treatment. In particular, treatment is not needed when the thyrotoxicosis is mild and can be expected to subside soon, for example, in patients with painless thyroiditis.

TABLE 10-12 The Major Forms of Therapy for Thyrotoxicosis

Treatment of the cause of thyrotoxicosis
Antithyroid therapy
Drugs
Methimazole
Propylthiouracil
Iodide
Radioactive iodine (^{131}I)
Subtotal thyroidectomy
Amelioration of thyroid hormone action
Beta-adrenergic antagonist drugs

There are wide geographic variations in treatment practices. Antithyroid drug therapy is preferred in Europe and Japan, whereas ^{131}I therapy is preferred in the United States.[254] These differences reflect differences in the opinions of both physicians and patients regarding the efficacy, convenience, side effects, and costs of these treatments.

Thyrotoxicosis Caused by Graves' Disease

An antithyroid drug and radioactive iodine (^{131}I) are the two best treatments for this disorder. Both are effective, safe, and relatively inexpensive. They are treatments for hyperthyroidism rather than for Graves' disease itself, although antithyroid drugs may have some immunosuppressive action. The major reason to choose antithyroid drug therapy is that a spontaneous remission of Graves' disease may occur, allowing therapy to be discontinued and leaving the patient with normal, and often normally regulated, thyroid function. Remissions are often said to occur in 40 to 50 percent of these patients. In fact, the reported variation in the frequency of remission is much larger, ranging from less than 10 percent to over 80 percent in patients treated for 1 year or more.[177,184–186,255–258] The clinical features of Graves' disease that have been associated with remission are a recent onset, mild or moderate severity of thyrotoxicosis, and little or no goiter. Treatment factors that have been associated with remissions include a longer duration of treatment, lower dietary iodine intake, the use of larger doses of antithyroid drug, and the concomitant use of thyroxine.

The uncertainty concerning remission does not apply to ^{131}I therapy, since it is destructive and its effects are ongoing. The hazards and expense of subtotal thyroidectomy are greater than are those of either an antithyroid drug or ^{131}I, and it should be used rarely in patients of any age.

The choice between an antithyroid drug and ^{131}I therapy depends on several theoretical and practical considerations. A rough comparison of their features is shown in Table 10-13. Antithyroid drug therapy is more rapidly effective, does not cause permanent thyroid damage, may not have to be given indefinitely, and is less expensive. For these reasons, an antithyroid drug is the initial treatment of choice for most patients, both children and adults of all ages. If a remission does not occur and the patient tires of taking medication or if the thyrotoxicosis is difficult to control, ^{131}I can always be given then. ^{131}I treatment is simple, though not as rapidly effective, and hypothyroidism usually develops subsequently. With either form of treatment, no matter how effective it is in the early months, indefinite follow-up is necessary to ensure that thyrotoxicosis has not recurred, that hypothyroidism has not developed, or, if it has, that replacement therapy is continued. Whatever the physician's preference, the recommendations for therapy must be acceptable to the patient.

Antithyroid Drugs

Thionamide Antithyroid Drugs

The thionamide drugs used in the United States are methimazole (MMI) and PTU. In Europe, carbimazole, which is rapidly metabolized to MMI, is used instead of MMI. These drugs inhibit thyroid hormone biosynthesis by inhibiting the oxidation and organification of iodine and the coupling of iodotyrosines, reactions that are catalyzed by thyroid peroxidase.[5] Both drugs are concentrated and metabolized by the thyroid by reactions involving this peroxidase. Thus, these drugs are less effective when iodine intake and intrathyroidal iodine stores are plentiful. PTU also inhibits the extrathyroidal conversion of T_4 to T_3.[148] Both MMI and PTU are absorbed rapidly and nearly completely from the gastrointestinal tract, and peak serum concentrations are reached about 1 h after their ingestion.[259,260] MMI is metabolized more slowly than is PTU; the plasma half-life of MMI is 4 to 6 h, whereas that of PTU is 1 to 2 h. Both drugs are concentrated in the thyroid, and intrathyroidal concentrations, especially of MMI, remain high for considerably longer than do serum concentrations.[261]

Both drugs have immunosuppressive actions and may ameliorate Graves' disease directly. For example, they may inhibit thyroid autoantibody production, and high-dose regimens may be accompanied by more frequent remissions.[162,262,263] Antithyroid drugs also reduce the number of intrathyroidal T cells and inhibit lymphocyte function and viability in vitro, although the latter actions require high concentrations.

The initial goal of antithyroid drug therapy is to inhibit thyroidal T_4 and T_3 synthesis completely. Even if this is achieved, release of intrathyroidal hormone stores, which may be substantial, continues until they are depleted. The usual initial dose of MMI is 10 to 20 mg per day, and it can be given once daily.[264,265] The usual initial dose of PTU is 300 to 450 mg per day, best given in divided doses.[266] Patients treated with MMI become euthyroid more rapidly than do those treated with PTU.[267] The larger doses are usually given to patients who have more severe clinical thyrotoxicosis, a large goiter, or both.

TABLE 10-13 Comparison of Features of Antithyroid Drug and ^{131}I Therapy for Hyperthyroidism Caused by Graves' Disease

	Drug Therapy	^{131}I
Dosage	Daily	Single dose
Initial response	2–6 weeks	8–12 weeks
Side effects*	Uncommon	Rare
Hypothyroidism	Uncommon	Common
Therapy inadequate	Uncommon	Rare
Cost of medication	$60/year	$1000/treatment†
Need for chronic or repeated courses of therapy	Common	Rare
Long-term outcome	Euthyroidism or hyperthyroidism	Hypothyroidism
Outcome dependent on continued TSab production	Yes	No
Use during pregnancy	Acceptable	Never

* Toxic drug effects and radiation thyroiditis.

† Excludes costs of follow-up examinations, serum hormone assays, and treatment of subsequent hypothyroidism in ^{131}I-treated patients.

The greater potency of MMI is due to its slower metabolism, its greater accumulation in thyroid tissue, and its greater potency as an inhibitor of thyroid peroxidase. Failure of antithyroid drug therapy to control thyrotoxicosis effectively may result from inadequate dosage or noncompliance, usually the latter.[268] Noncompliance can be minimized by careful explanation of the need for therapy and its goals to the patient. In some patients, thyrotoxicosis persists and the thyroid may enlarge further despite a fall in serum T_4 concentrations; such patients have persistently high serum TSab and T_3 concentrations.[269] They do become euthyroid when the dose of antithyroid drug is increased, but doses as high as 100 mg MMI and 1000 mg PTU daily may be required and such patients are unlikely to have a remission.

The patient should be reevaluated 4 to 6 weeks after the initiation of therapy. Some clinical and biochemical improvement is usually apparent after 1 or 2 weeks, and it is usually substantial after 4 to 6 weeks, especially in patients treated with MMI; many patients have normal serum T_4 and T_3 concentrations by this time. If considerable improvement has occurred, the antithyroid drug dose should be reduced 25 to 50 percent. Further follow-up visits should take place at about 8-week intervals. Once the patient has become euthyroid, the goal of continued therapy is partial rather than complete inhibition of thyroid hormone biosynthesis so that hypothyroidism does not occur. Patients treated with PTU can be changed to a once-daily regimen. Biochemical monitoring during the early months of therapy should be done with measurements of serum T_4 concentrations, because serum TSH concentrations may remain low for several months after the initiation of antithyroid drug therapy, even if thyroid secretion falls to below normal levels, as a result of prior suppression of TSH secretion.

Several programs for long-term therapy have been advocated. One is treatment with gradually decreasing doses of antithyroid drug, with the goal of withdrawal as soon as possible. As improvement occurs, the dosage of the antithyroid drug is reduced at approximately 8-week intervals. If the patient remains euthyroid while receiving 5 mg MMI or 50 mg PTU daily for 8 weeks, the drug is discontinued. It may be possible to discontinue therapy in as little as 4 months with such a regimen. If thyrotoxicosis recurs after the dose is reduced or discontinued, remission obviously has not occurred and treatment is increased or resumed until the euthyroid state is achieved, at which time the dose may again be reduced. In such a pragmatic program, decisions are made largely on clinical grounds, supported when necessary during the early months of therapy by serum T_4 and less often TSH determinations; later, serum TSH concentrations alone are sufficient. Figure 10-24 shows the results of this type of program in a patient treated with MMI for 7 months who remained euthyroid after it was discontinued.

A second treatment program consists simply of continued therapy with the initial dose of antithyroid drug until the patient is clinically and biochemically euthyroid, at which time therapy is discontinued. In the study describing this program, the mean duration of therapy was 4.8 months and the sustained remission rate was 29 percent.[270]

A third program consists of prolonged treatment for 1 to 2 years. Such a program requires one or more reductions in dosage after the first several months of treatment. Prolonged antithyroid drug therapy results in higher remission rates, probably because remissions continue to occur as a function of time.[185,186] The program of treatment for a fixed interval is probably the most widely used, but it results in the treatment of some patients for longer periods than necessary.

Prevention of hypothyroidism and further thyroid enlargment during antithyroid drug therapy are best achieved by means of a judicious reduction in drug dosage; the addition of thyroid hormone has not been thought necessary or desirable. The results of a recent study challenge this view.[177] Among a group of patients treated with MMI for 18 months and another group treated similarly with MMI plus 0.1 mg T_4 daily for 4 years, starting after 6 months, the rates

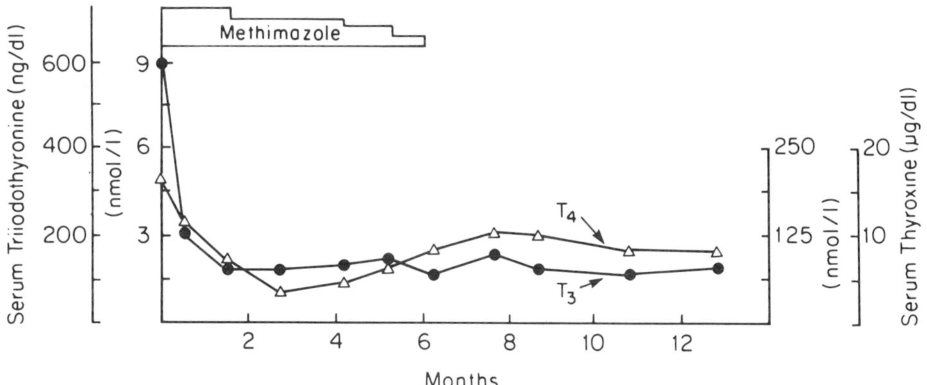

FIGURE 10-24 Serum T_3 and T_4 concentrations in a patient with thyrotoxicosis caused by Graves' disease during and after treatment with methimazole. Note the prompt fall in serum hormone concentrations after the initiation of treatment and the lack of change after treatment was discontinued.

of relapse were 37 and 2 percent, respectively. This is a remarkably low rate of relapse and makes this a regimen worthy of serious consideration.

Several tests have been proposed to determine if a remission of Graves' disease has occurred and therefore if antithyroid drug therapy is no longer needed. They include measurements of TSab and serum thyroglobulin concentrations, tests for antithyroid peroxidase antibodies, and determination of serum TSH and T_3 responses to TRH stimulation. Patients who remain euthyroid after the withdrawal of therapy tend to have negative tests for the various antibodies, normal serum thyroglobulin concentrations, and normal serum TSH responses to TRH (the antithyroid drug must be discontinued before this test). Neither the specificity nor the sensitivity of these tests for this purpose is high.[184]

Thus, whatever therapeutic program is used, it is simpler merely to discontinue the drug at the end of the initial treatment period and reexamine the patient in 6 to 8 weeks and subsequently less often if thyrotoxicosis does not recur. Most recurrences develop in the first few months after drug withdrawal and may be treated with an antithyroid drug. However, many patients choose ablative therapy if thyrotoxicosis recurs after drug withdrawal. Patients whose thyrotoxicosis is easily controlled with small doses of drug may prefer to continue treatment for many years, and there are no contraindications to such a program.[271]

Toxic reactions to antithyroid drugs are uncommon, and there is little evidence that one drug is more toxic than the other. Pruritis, urticaria or other rashes, arthralgia or myalgia, and fever occur in 2 to 5 percent of patients taking either drug,[260] and PTU may cause abnormal taste sensation. The most feared side effect is agranulocytosis [<500 cells/mm^3 ($<0.5 \times 10^9$/liter)], generally cited as occurring in 0.2 to 0.5 percent of patients, but in two large recent surveys the risks were estimated to be 10-fold or more lower.[272,273] Very rare side effects include aplastic anemia, thrombocytopenia, hepatocellular (PTU) or cholestatic (MMI) hepatitis, vasculitis (PTU), and the insulin-autoimmune syndrome (MMI). These side effects, which presumably are immunologic in origin, usually occur during the first several months of treatment, when the dose of drug is higher, and also can occur for the first time during a subsequent course of therapy.[273] Agranulocytosis has been reported to be more common in older patients and when higher doses (30 mg/day or more) of MMI are used, but no dose relation for PTU has been found.[274] It usually develops rapidly, and precautionary white blood cell counts are generally thought not to be useful, although this view was recently challenged.[275]

To minimize the severity and consequences of the side effects of antithyroid drugs, patients must be warned about the symptoms of these side effects and instructed to discontinue therapy and contact the physician immediately if any symptoms occur. Hematologic or liver function testing may then be indicated. The minor side effects may subside with no treatment or with antihistamine therapy in the case of urticaria and generally do not require the discontinuation of therapy. The drug should be discontinued in patients who have a more severe reaction, which then will subside. Patients with granulocytopenia and fever should be hospitalized and given antibiotic therapy. Administration of granulocyte colony-stimulating factor may hasten recovery from agranulocytosis.[276] Patients who have had a severe reaction to an antithyroid drug may then tolerate the other drug, but they are more appropriately treated with ^{131}I.

Of the two drugs, MMI is preferable for several reasons. Its action is more prolonged, and so single daily doses are nearly always effective.[264,265,277] The number of pills needed is lower, since MMI is available in 5- and 10-mg tablets and PTU is available only in 50-mg tablets. It may have fewer side effects, and it is cheaper. Since PTU also inhibits extrathyroidal T_3 production, it causes a somewhat more rapid reduction in serum T_3 concentrations during the first week of therapy, but MMI lowers both serum T_4 and T_3 concentrations more rapidly.

Inorganic Iodide

Iodide inhibits thyroid hormone secretion, primarily by inhibiting thyroglobulin proteolysis, and also inhibits thyroidal iodide transport, oxidation, and organification.[5] These actions require only 5 to 10 mg iodide daily, although it is usually given in far greater doses, such as 5 to 10 drops of a saturated solution of potassium iodide (50 mg iodide/drop) several times daily. The major limitation of iodide as antithyroid therapy is escape from its antithyroid effects. When it is given alone, serum T_4 and T_3 concentrations usually decrease about 50 to 75 percent, reaching a nadir in 2 to 3 weeks, and may then increase.[278] Therefore, iodide should not be used as sole therapy. Iodide given after ^{131}I therapy results in more rapid amelioration of thyrotoxicosis, and escape does not occur in this setting. Iodide is also used in preparation for thyroidectomy, both for its antithyroid action and because it reduces thyroid vascularity. Iodide produced by the metabolism of organic iodine compounds has the same antithyroid actions.

There are three indications for iodide therapy: in preparation for subtotal thyroidectomy, for which it is given for 7 to 10 days before surgery; in severe thyrotoxicosis or thyroid storm (see below); and occasionally for several weeks or months in patients recently treated with ^{131}I. It is used in conjunction with an antithyroid drug in the first two situations and alone in the third.

Other Antithyroid Drugs

The oral cholecystographic agents sodium ipodate and iopanoic acid are iodine-rich compounds that are metabolized in part by deiodination. The iodide that is formed inhibits T_4 and T_3 secretion, and the intact compound inhibits extrathyroidal T_3 production.[148] Administration of either agent in doses of 0.25 or 0.5 g daily is therefore accompanied by prompt reductions in both serum T_4 and T_3 concentrations.[279,280] In the majority of patients, however, the benefit is not sustained and serum T_4 and T_3 concentrations do not become normal. These drugs may be useful for short-term therapy for patients who cannot be given MMI, PTU, or ^{131}I.

Lithium carbonate has antithyroid actions similar to those of iodide and has proved effective in doses of 300 mg three or four times daily.[281] Some escape from its actions occurs, and it has many side effects. It may nevertheless be useful in an occasional patient who cannot tolerate MMI or PTU and in whom ^{131}I therapy is planned but cannot be given immediately because of previous iodine exposure.

Potassium perchlorate is a competitive inhibitor of thyroidal iodide transport. It is not widely used because of its toxicity (aplastic anemia) and the need for multiple daily doses. It may be useful in patients with iodine- and amiodarone-induced thyrotoxicosis.[282]

Drugs Inhibiting Extrathyroidal T_3 Production

Drugs that inhibit extrathyroidal T_3 production decrease serum T_3 concentrations and thus might be expected to ameliorate thyrotoxicosis. While this is a reasonable expectation, there is no evidence that such amelioration occurs. Drugs that have both thyroidal and extrathyroidal actions, such as PTU and sodium ipodate, are no more effective clinically than is MMI, which acts only on the thyroid.

Propranolol and other beta-adrenergic antagonists cause a 20 to 30 percent reduction in serum T_3, but not serum T_4, concentrations after several weeks of therapy.[148] This modest and gradual fall in serum T_3 does not explain the clinical benefits of propranolol in patients with thyrotoxicosis.

Drugs Ameliorating Peripheral Thyroid Hormone Action

Beta-adrenergic antagonist drugs ameliorate many of the symptoms and signs of thyrotoxicosis. The administration of propranolol in doses of 80 to 180 mg daily results in improvement in many of the common symptoms of thyrotoxicosis, including palpitation, increased perspiration and heat intolerance, nervousness, tremor, and weakness, within several days. However, such symptoms do not disappear completely even during prolonged therapy.[220,283,284] The pulse rate slows, and myocardial contractility decreases. Nitrogen balance, oxygen consumption, and cardiac output improve but do not become normal. Thus, propranolol alone is an inadequate treatment for thyrotoxicosis, and it has no beneficial effect when used in conjunction with an antithyroid drug.[285] It is contraindicated in patients with asthma and heart failure due to intrinsic cardiac disease. Other beta-adrenergic antagonist drugs have similar actions in thyrotoxic patients, even though they differ in the degree of selectivity as beta-adrenergic antagonists, potency as inhibitors of extrathyroidal T_3 production, and duration of action. These variables are not known to be important, except that compliance may be better with the use of the longer-acting analogs.

Beta-adrenergic antagonist drugs should not be used routinely in patients treated with an antithyroid drug or ^{131}I and should never be used alone in patients with thyrotoxicosis caused by Graves' disease. They are useful for the amelioration of thyrotoxic symptoms before and for several weeks after ^{131}I therapy, before subtotal thyroidectomy, in thyroiditis, and in thyroid storm.

Radioactive Iodine Therapy

The goal of ^{131}I therapy is to reduce the amount of functioning thyroid tissue. The effect of this therapy is independent of whether a spontaneous remission of Graves' disease occurs. Although the occurrence of such a remission after ^{131}I therapy would contribute to the effectiveness of the therapy, in fact, TSab production often increases within the first year after ^{131}I therapy. The major advantages of ^{131}I therapy are that usually only a single dose is needed, it is safe, and its cost is relatively low (Table 10-13). One disadvantage is that the amelioration of thyrotoxicosis is slower. For markedly symptomatic patients, therefore, a period of antithyroid drug therapy before ^{131}I therapy is often advisable. The drug therapy then must be discontinued 3 to 4 days before thyroid radioiodine uptake is determined and the therapeutic dose of ^{131}I is given. Antithyroid drug therapy may then be resumed several days later, if indicated. Alternatively, propranolol can be given continuously for relief of symptoms both before ^{131}I therapy is given and until its effects become apparent. Iodide should not be given before therapy, and care should be taken to avoid iodine-containing drugs or contrast agents if ^{131}I therapy is planned. Iodide administration may be beneficial after ^{131}I therapy.[286]

Various methods for determining ^{131}I dosage have been used, but all are subject to considerable error because it is difficult to estimate the size of the thyroid gland, isotope retention within the thyroid is variable, and radiation sensitivity is not predictable.[258] Many clinicians now believe that a fixed dose of 8 to 12 mCi (296 to 444 MBq) is appropriate for the treatment of nearly all patients, with small increments if thyroid radioiodine uptake is nearly normal or if thyroid enlargement is substantial.[287] Such doses deliver approximately 100 to 200 μCi/g (3.7 to 7.4 MBq/g) estimated thyroid weight or 10,000 to 20,000 rad (100 to 200 Gy) to the thyroid. They result in clinical and biochemical improvement and reduction in thyroid size in 6 weeks to 3 months, and most patients are euthyroid, if not hypothyroid, in 4 to 6 months. Patients who receive ^{131}I therapy should be advised to use contraception for several months and to avoid close contact with very young children for several days.

There are two important untoward effects of ^{131}I therapy—persistent thyrotoxicosis and hypothyroidism—and several rare ones. Among the latter are acute temporary exacerbations of thyrotoxicosis and the development of thyroid pain and tenderness. Both are due to radiation thyroiditis, and the risk of each is reduced by prior antithyroid drug therapy. Hypoparathyroidism is an even rarer consequence of ^{131}I therapy. Persistent thyrotoxicosis results from inadequate ^{131}I therapy and, not surprisingly, is more common when lower doses of ^{131}I are given.[258,287,288] Even a large dose may be inadequate in an occasional patient.

Hypothyroidism is not so much a complication of ^{131}I treatment as an almost inevitable consequence of it. It may occur in the first few months after therapy, in which case it may be transient, or at any time thereafter. Early hypothyroidism, defined as that occurring within a year after treatment, is caused by the acute destructive effects of ^{131}I. Its frequency ranges from 40 to as high as 80 percent in patients treated with 8 to 12 mCi (296 to 444 MBq) ^{131}I.[258,289] Smaller doses result in early hypothyroidism less often and persistent thyrotoxicosis more often. The larger doses are more appropriate, since the primary goal of therapy should be the permanent amelioration of thyrotoxicosis as expeditiously as possible.

After 1 year, hypothyroidism develops in additional patients (0.5 to 2 percent) each year for at least 10 years, whether the treatment dose was large or small.[258,288,290] Thus, late hypothyroidism is independent of the dose of ^{131}I given; it is due to damage to the replicative ability of thyroid follicular cells and perhaps autoimmune thyroid injury. It usually develops very slowly, with many patients having elevated serum TSH concentrations but normal serum T_4 and T_3 concentrations (subclinical hypothyroidism) for several years before they develop overt hypothyroidism.[291]

Many physicians have been reluctant to use ^{131}I therapy in young adults and especially in adolescents and children. The reasons for this reluctance are that (1) ^{131}I might cause thyroidal or other tumors, (2) ^{131}I might cause gonadal damage, and (3) the patient may be pregnant. Fears that ^{131}I therapy is a risk factor for thyroid or other tumors have proved unfounded.[292–294] The gonadal radiation dose after ^{131}I is no more than that which results from several diagnostic radiologic procedures, and follow-up of children and adolescents treated with ^{131}I has revealed neither impaired fertility nor an increase in birth defects in their offspring.[292] ^{131}I crosses the placenta and can destroy the fetal thyroid, and so pregnancy is an absolute contraindication to its use.

Subtotal Thyroidectomy

The simplicity, safety, and low cost of antithyroid drug and ^{131}I therapy have led to a declining use of subtotal thyroidectomy for the treatment of Graves' hyperthyroidism. The goal of thyroidectomy, like that of ^{131}I, is reduction of the functioning mass of thyroid tissue. Subtotal thyroidectomy has little perioperative morbidity and mortality in properly prepared children and young adults. Preoperative treatment is generally accomplished by antithyroid drug treatment for 6 to 8 weeks and iodide treatment for 7 to 10 days. Treatment with a beta-adrenergic antagonist drug for several weeks, with or without concomitant iodide therapy for 10 to 14 days, also has proved to be a safe and effective preoperative therapy.[295]

Postoperative problems after thyroidectomy include transient or permanent hypocalcemia, vocal cord paralysis, recurrent thyrotoxicosis, and transient or permanent hypothyroidism. The frequency of nonthyroid complications is low. Transient hypocalcemia may be due to temporary hypoparathyroidism or healing of thyrotoxic osteopenia. Permanent hypoparathyroidism occurs in less than 5 percent of patients. Recurrent thyrotoxicosis occurs now in less than 10 percent of patients.[288,296] It usually develops several years or even decades after thyroidectomy and is due to persistent Graves' disease. The long lag time reflects the time required for regrowth of sufficient thyroid tissue to sustain hyperthyroidism.

Overt or subclinical hypothyroidism may occur in the first 1 to 2 months after surgery in as many as 30 percent of patients, but in some of these patients thyroid secretion later returns to normal as a result of TSH-stimulated growth of the thyroid remnant. Therefore, a diagnosis of permanent hypothyroidism should not be made for at least 4 to 6 months after surgery. Currently, permanent hypothyroidism develops in the first year after surgery in 25 to 75 percent of patients because of more aggressive surgery intended to reduce the frequency of recurrent hyperthyroidism.[258,288,296] Subsequently, hypothyroidism occurs in 0.5 to 1 percent/year. These data indicate that postoperative hypothyroidism is now nearly as common as is post-^{131}I hypothyroidism, and for the same reason, namely, the intent to reduce the frequency of recurrent thyrotoxicosis. Because subtotal thyroidectomy has nonthyroid hazards, its overall risks relative to benefit and its expense render it unacceptable for occasional patients who have marked thyroid enlargement or are pregnant and cannot tolerate antithyroid drugs.

Treatment of Thyrotoxicosis Caused by Thyroiditis

The diagnosis and treatment of subacute thyroiditis are discussed in The Painful Thyroid. Painless thyroiditis is more difficult to recognize; clues to its presence were described previously. Since it is transient and usually mild, most patients need no therapy, but they can be given propranolol if necessary. Glucocorticoids and other, less toxic anti-inflammatory drugs reduce serum T_4 and T_3 concentrations rapidly in patients with painless thyroiditis,[297] but their use is not warranted because of the mild nature and limited duration of thyrotoxicosis in most patients.

Treatment of Thyrotoxicosis Caused by Toxic Multinodular Goiter

^{131}I is the treatment of choice for patients with thyrotoxicosis due to a multinodular goiter, since spontaneous remissions do not occur in this disease. Large doses, e.g., 25 to 30 mCi (925 to 1110 MBq), should be given because thyroid ^{131}I uptake is usually only moderately increased and the risk of persistent thyrotoxicosis should be minimized in these patients, who are usually elderly. Multiple doses may be required. Hypothyroidism is an unusual sequela of treatment because the thyroid gland contains tissue that is subnormally functioning but autonomous or tissue that is appropriately suppressed but can regain its function as needed.[298] Since most patients with thyrotoxicosis due to toxic multinodular goiter are elderly and have serious cardiovascular manifestations of the disease, a period of treatment with an antithyroid drug before and after ^{131}I administration is often indicated. Such a regimen accelerates recovery, since antithyroid drugs are more rapidly effective than ^{131}I, and minimizes the chances of an exacerbation of thyrotoxicosis after ^{131}I therapy.

Treatment of Thyrotoxicosis Caused by Thyroid Adenoma

These tumors cause permanent thyrotoxicosis, and so the most appropriate therapy is ^{131}I (see Chap. 11). The dose used should be relatively large [25 mCi (925 MBq)] so that the nodule is destroyed, its size decreases, and the likelihood of recurrent thyrotoxicosis is low. Smaller doses may be as effective, but some patients have recurrent thyrotoxicosis.[299] Transient hypothyroidism may occur until TSH secretion recovers. The risk of permanent hypothyroidism is low, as the suppressed extranodular tissue does not concentrate appreciable quantities of ^{131}I and recovers function as TSH secretion resumes.

Special Situations

Subclinical Thyrotoxicosis

Patients with subclinical thyrotoxicosis—normal serum T_4 and T_3 and low TSH concentrations—are by definition clinically euthyroid. Their low serum TSH concentrations reflect the effects of small increases in TSH-independent thyroid secretion. This condition may be due to a multinodular goiter, an autonomously functioning thyroid adenoma, Graves' disease, or exogenous thyroid hormone administration.

While asymptomatic, some of these patients have manifestations of thyroid hormone excess in addition to low serum TSH concentrations. Some but not other studies of women treated with thyroid hormone for long periods have demonstrated modest decreases in both cortical and trabecular bone density compared with age-matched normal women.[300–302] These patients may also have an increase in cardiac rate and contractility and may be prone to arrhythmias.[302]

Patients with subclinical thyrotoxicosis due to exogenous thyroid hormone administration should be treated by reduction of the dose of thyroid hormone. Those in whom it is due to a thyroid disease are not usually treated, for several reasons. First, subclinical thyrotoxicosis is a biochemical diagnosis, and the decrease in serum TSH may not be persistent.[251,252,291] Second, there is no clear evidence that rates of fracture or arrhythmia are increased. Third, none of the available treatments are simple, safe, and inexpensive, and there is no evidence that lowering thyroid secretion in these patients is beneficial. For patients with large goiters, thyroidectomy, administration of ^{131}I, or injection of prominent functioning nodules with ethanol may be considered.[303,304] The administration of T_4 is not likely to decrease goiter size but is very likely to induce overt thyrotoxicosis.

Thyroid Storm

Thyroid storm is severe, life-threatening thyrotoxicosis. There are no fixed criteria for its diagnosis and no evidence that its pathophysiology differs from that of thyrotoxicosis in general. It usually occurs in a thyrotoxic patient who has another major problem, such as an acute infection or other medical illness, injury, or surgery, situations that do not increase serum T_4 and T_3 concentrations. However, it may occur after ^{131}I therapy, discontinuation of antithyroid drug therapy, or spontaneously.[305] Thyrotoxicosis may or may not have been diagnosed previously, but the symptoms nearly always have been present for months. The key clinical findings are fever (>38.5°C) and tachycardia, but the patient may have anorexia, nausea, vomiting, abdominal pain, and cardiac failure as well as any of the manifestations of less severe thyrotoxicosis. There is usually marked anxiety, agitation, and restlessness and occasionally acute psychosis, but confusion and coma may develop terminally. Signs such as fever and tachycardia may be due either to the thyrotoxicosis or to the accompanying illness, making it difficult to gauge the severity of the thyrotoxicosis. A decision concerning therapy must usually be made with the recognition that there are no pathognomonic symptoms or signs as well as before any laboratory test results are available.

There also are no characteristic laboratory abnormalities in patients with thyroid storm, emphasizing that it is a clinical diagnosis. Serum T_4 and T_3 concentrations are elevated, but no more so than in ordinary thyrotoxicosis. Since acute illness can decrease TBG and TTR production and thus decrease serum total T_4 and T_3 concentrations, the free T_4 and T_3 concentrations may be relatively higher in these patients than in most patients with thyrotoxicosis.

Treatment of thyroid storm should be directed toward decreasing thyroidal production of T_4 and T_3, peripheral production of T_3, and the peripheral actions of thyroid hormone as well as providing general supportive measures and treatment needed to deal with any coexisting illness. MMI or PTU should be given in large doses, such as 10 mg or 250 mg, respectively, every 6 h, by nasogastric tube or even rectally if necessary. Some physicians prefer PTU, based on the possibility that it may be more rapidly beneficial because it inhibits extrathyroidal production of T_3 as well as thyroidal synthesis of T_4 and T_3. Sodium iodide should be given orally or intravenously in a dose of 500 mg daily to inhibit the release of T_4 and T_3 from the thyroid. The iodide should be given 1 to 2 h after MMI or PTU so that the iodide content of the thyroid gland is not increased before T_4 and T_3 synthesis is blocked. Propranolol given orally or intravenously is the most effective treatment for the cardiac and neuromuscular manifestations of thyroid storm. The oral dose is 20 to 40 mg every 4 to 6 h or more if necessary. The intravenous dose is 0.5 to 1 mg per min for 5 to 10 min, followed by doses of 2 to 3 mg given 5 to 10 min every 2 to 4 h as needed. Glucocorticoids are usually given in large doses, such as 50 mg hydrocortisone or its equivalent of a synthetic glucocorticoid intravenously every 8 h. The rationale for their use is the possibility that ACTH and cortisol secretion may not increase sufficiently to meet cortisol requirements in a situation of increased need superimposed on accelerated cortisol degradation. Glucocorticoids also inhibit thyroid secretion (in patients with Graves' disease[147]) and extrathyroidal T_3 production. These measures usually result in clinical improvement and reduction in serum T_4 and T_3 concentrations in 24 to 48 h. Supportive therapy should include treatment to reduce hyperpyrexia and appropriate parenteral fluid and electrolyte therapy. Combined with aggressive treatment of coexisting illness, these measures collectively have reduced mortality from thyroid storm.

Thyrotoxicosis during Pregnancy

The occurrence of thyrotoxicosis during pregnancy introduces additional considerations relating to the effect of the thyrotoxicosis, which is nearly always caused by Graves' disease, and its management on the mother and her fetus. In some women, the thyrotoxicosis precedes the pregnancy. In others, thyrotoxicosis may first develop during pregnancy, usually being recognized in the first trimester or early in the second. Relapses of thyrotoxicosis also occur during pregnancy in women who were in remission before becoming pregnant.[306] In general, no matter when it begins, thyrotoxicosis caused by Graves' disease tends to subside during the third trimester, and so treatment can be withdrawn in up to half of these patients.

Thyrotoxicosis may be hard to recognize in a pregnant woman because pregnancy is characterized normally by increases in oxygen consumption, heat production, and cardiovascular activity and by anxiety or nervousness. Findings that are particularly indicative of thyrotoxicosis include marked tachycardia, muscle weakness, weight loss, and thyroid enlargement. Thyrotoxicosis is usually tolerated well by pregnant women, as it is by nonpregnant women of the same age, and there is no increase in maternal mortality or morbidity in untreated patients.[307]

The situation with regard to the fetus is different. If the mother is not treated, there is an increase in congenital anomalies and increased fetal loss resulting from spontaneous abortion and premature delivery.[307,308] These are probably direct effects of maternal thyrotoxicosis, as they do not occur in mothers who receive antithyroid treatment. Some fetuses have thyrotoxicosis manifested by growth retardation, tachycardia (pulse rate greater than 160 beats/min), and hyperactivity.[309] The most conspicuous findings in fatal cases are cardiac and thyroid enlargement and congestion of the viscera.[310] Fetal thyrotoxicosis is caused by the transplacental passage of TSab and perhaps also T_4 and T_3 from the mother. It also occurs in mothers who have TSab but are euthyroid as a result of earlier ^{131}I therapy or thyroidectomy. It can be proved by measurements of serum TSH and T_4 concentrations in blood samples collected by cordocentesis.[311] Treatment of the mother with an antithyroid drug reduces fetal tachycardia, and such therapy may be indicated even in mothers with previously treated Graves' disease who are euthyroid.

The diagnosis of thyrotoxicosis in a pregnant woman is confirmed by the finding of an unequivocally low serum TSH concentration; a serum total T_4 concentration that is above the normal range for pregnancy, which is about 50 percent higher than normal; and an elevated serum free T_4 index. If the diagnosis is not established by these tests, the wisest course is continued observation. Women with hyperemesis gravidarum tend to have higher serum T_4, T_3, and hCG and slightly lower TSH concentrations than normal pregnant women at comparable stages of gestation. They do not have thyroid enlargement, there is no evidence that antithyroid therapy is benefical, and their serum T_4 concentrations decline as the hyperemesis subsides.[312]

Antithyroid drug therapy is the most appropriate treatment for pregnant women with thyrotoxicosis. Both PTU and MMI cross the placenta, although the fractional transplacental transfer of PTU is lower.[259,260] For this reason, PTU has been preferred, at least in the United States, but the relation between maternal and fetal serum T_4 concentrations at delivery in mothers treated with either drug is the same.[313] Whatever drug is used, only doses sufficient to ameliorate the clinical manifestations of thyrotoxicosis and lower the serum free T_4 index value to near or just within the normal range should be given. An appropriate initial dose is 15 mg MMI or 300 mg PTU daily. The patient should be evaluated at 3- to 4-week intervals and the dose reduced as necessary to maintain this thyroid secretory level, and attempts should be made to discontinue therapy. The rationale for this approach is that mild thyrotoxicosis is tolerated well by pregnant women and that the fetus is exposed to as little antithyroid drug as possible consistent with preventing overt thyrotoxicosis in the mother. However, pregnant women with severe thyrotoxicosis should be treated vigorously because serious maternal illness threatens fetal development and survival.

Both PTU and MMI may cause fetal goiter, hypothyroidism, or both, which subside soon after birth.[313] Transplacental passage of these drugs is variable, as evidenced by the finding of these abnormalities in only one of the twins of mothers treated during pregnancy.[314] Infants exposed to these drugs do not have an increase in congenital anomalies, and their postnatal growth and development are normal.[308,315,316] The use of T_4 in addition to an antithyroid drug is not warranted, since it increases the amount of antithyroid drug required to control thyrotoxicosis in the mother and does not protect the fetus because of the limited transplacental transfer of T_4 and T_3. The fetal thyroid is sensitive to the antithyroid actions of iodine, but small (5 to 40 mg) doses may be used safely.[317] Propranolol should not be administered to pregnant women with thyrotoxicosis.[318]

While subtotal thyroidectomy has been used for the treatment of hyperthyroidism during pregnancy, it should be done only when the previously mentioned side effects of antithyroid drugs preclude their continuation. Surgery is safe only after a period of drug treatment. This may have been achieved with MMI or PTU before the side effects developed or may necessitate short-term treatment with iodide and propranolol. Additional hazards of subtotal thyroidectomy during pregnancy include abortion, premature labor, and fetal anoxia. ^{131}I therapy is absolutely contraindicated in pregnant women.

T_4 and T_3 are present in breast milk in low concentrations; the iodide concentration is about 10 μg/dl (0.8 μmol/liter). The concentrations of MMI in milk are similar to those in serum, whereas the concentrations of PTU in milk are lower than those in serum.[259,319] Limited data indicate that milk does not contain enough of either drug to cause hypothyroidism in a nursing infant.[319,320] A mother wishing to nurse may do so, but the infant's thyroid function should be evaluated periodically.

Neonatal Graves' Disease

Neonatal Graves' disease, manifested primarily as thyrotoxicosis, occurs in a small fraction (less than 10 percent) of the infants of mothers with Graves' disease. It is caused by the transplacental passage of TSab and occurs only in infants whose mothers have high levels of TSab,[321,322] indicating that the extent of transplacental passage of TSab is limited. The mothers of about half of these infants have a history of thyrotoxicosis during the pregnancy; the others were euthyroid, having received antithyroid therapy earlier.

TSab is detectable in the serum of these infants at birth, and it disappears within weeks. The duration of the thyrotoxicosis is a function of the initial concentration of TSab and its rate of metabolism, which is about 3 to 4 percent/day (half-life of 10 to 14 days).

Some infants are thyrotoxic at the time of delivery. In others, thyrotoxicosis develops several days after delivery; their mothers usually received antithyroid therapy during pregnancy. These infants tend to be small for gestational age and are hyperactive, tremulous, and irritable. Other problems include tachycardia, tachypnea, hyperphagia, feeding problems, diarrhea, cardiac failure, thyroid enlargement, and proptosis.

Infants with neonatal thyrotoxicosis have high serum T_4 and T_3 concentrations, although the hormone levels may not be elevated at birth if the infant's mother was taking an antithyroid drug just before delivery. They also have low serum TSH concentrations. The results of serum T_4 and T_3 measurements in neonates must be interpreted in relation to norms that differ markedly from adult values and change rapidly after birth (see Physiologic Variables Affecting Pituitary-Thyroid Function and Tests).

Neonates with thyrotoxicosis should be treated with an antithyroid drug, for example, 5 mg MMI or 50 mg PTU daily. If the thyrotoxicosis is clinically severe, iodide and propranolol should be given as well. The drugs subsequently should be gradually withdrawn as indicated by clinical evaluation and serum T_4 measurements. Therapy can usually be discontinued within 6 to 8 weeks and is rarely followed by recurrence, but subsequent intellectual and physical development may be subnormal.

Postpartum Thyrotoxicosis

Thyrotoxicosis may occur in the first several months after delivery. Three forms of postpartum thyrotoxicosis are recognized.[306,323] One is the new development of Graves' hyperthyroidism. A second is recurrence of Graves' hyperthyroidism, which may be persistent or transient and may be minimized by the administration of thyroxine during and after pregnancy.[324] In all these patients, thyroid radioiodine uptake is high. Third and most commonly, thyrotoxicosis occurs as part of the syndrome of postpartum thyroiditis.

Postpartum thyroiditis is a clinically heterogeneous disorder; some women have only transient thyrotoxicosis, others have transient thyrotoxicosis followed by transient hypothyroidism, and still others have only transient hypothyroidism.[323,325–327] It occurs in 1 to 6 percent of postpartum women; among this group, about half have thyrotoxicosis. The characteristics of the thyrotoxic phase of this syndrome are similar to those of the thyrotoxic phase of painless thyroiditis as it occurs in men and in women who did not recently deliver a baby. The thyrotoxicosis is mild and transient, there is little or no thyroid enlargement, and thyroid radioiodine uptake is low. Indeed, many patients have no symptoms; modestly elevated serum T_4 concentrations and subclinical thyrotoxicosis are the only abnormalities. The thyrotoxicosis usually develops 2 to 6 months postpartum, lasts 2 to 6 weeks, and in about half of patients is followed by transient hypothyroidism. Because postpartum thyrotoxicosis is mild as well as transient, most patients need no treatment. Propranolol may be useful in patients with many symptoms. Postpartum thyroiditis is discussed further in Hypothyroidism.

Extrathyroidal Manifestations of Graves' Disease

Infiltrative Ophthalmopathy

Clinical evidence of ophthalmopathy is present in 20 to 40 percent of patients with hyperthyroidism caused by Graves' disease, although measurements of orbital protrusion and orbital radiographic studies indicate that it is present to some degree in nearly all of them.[328,329] It usually develops concurrently with thyrotoxicosis and between 18 months before and 18 months after it in about 80 percent of patients.[330] There is little correlation between the severity of the thyrotoxicosis and that of the ophthalmopathy, and some euthyroid and even hypothyroid patients have ophthalmopathy that is clinically indistinguishable (euthyroid Graves' disease). For this reason, the disorder is also called thyroid-associated ophthalmopathy. Smoking is an even greater risk factor for ophthalmopathy than it is for Graves' hyperthyroidism.[180] The pathogenesis of infiltrative ophthalmopathy is poorly understood (see Graves' Disease).

Clinical Manifestations

The clinical manifestations of Graves' ophthalmopathy reflect the fact that the orbital cavity is nearly filled with the eye so that a small increase in the contents of the cavity results in forward displacement of the eye, known as proptosis or exophthalmos. All the other components of the eye may be involved as well, leading to the problems listed in Table 10-14.[331]

The most common complaint among these patients is proptosis. Other symptoms that may be present include periorbital puffiness, eye discomfort or pain, a gritty or burning sensation in the eyes, excessive tearing, and photophobia.[332] There also may be intermittent or persistent diplopia and blurring or loss of vision. The onset is usually gradual but may be abrupt. Even when asymptomatic, ophthalmopathy may be very distressing to the patient for cosmetic reasons.

The major sign is the proptosis, which is usually bilateral and symmetric, although the extent of protrusion can vary by several millimeters. It is important to distinguish proptosis from lid retraction, which is caused by thyrotoxicosis itself. Lid retraction gives the appearance of proptosis and may be accompanied by tearing, eye discomfort, conjunctival injection, and photophobia. Lid retraction and proptosis can usually be distinguished with an exophthalmometer, a device that measures the distance from the lateral orbital notch to the anterior surface of the cornea. True proptosis—exophthalmometer readings greater than 20 mm in whites and greater than 24 mm in blacks—is thus distinguished from apparent proptosis by lid retraction alone.

TABLE 10-14 Clinical Classification of Eye Changes of Infiltrative Ophthalmopathy (NOSPECS)*

Class	Finding
0	No symptoms or signs
1	Only thyrotoxic signs and mild proptosis (<2 mm)
2	Soft tissue involvement
3	Proptosis
4	Extraocular muscle involvement
5	Corneal involvement
6	Sight loss

* Useful as a reminder of the clinical manifestation of ophthalmopathy but not for evaluating severity or the efficacy of therapy.

Source: Werner.[331]

The other principal signs of ophthalmopathy are periorbital edema, conjunctival congestion and edema (chemosis), and limitation of ocular mobility (Fig. 10-25). Extraocular muscle involvement most often results in limitation of upward gaze, but movement in any direction may be limited. It is due to inflammatory restriction of the muscles rather than muscle weakness. Interstitial keratitis and corneal ulceration caused by marked proptosis and decreased visual acuity or visual field defects due to optic neuropathy from compression of the optic nerve are fortunately rare. Finally, intraocular pressure is often increased, especially on upward gaze.

The diagnosis of infiltrative ophthalmopathy when thyrotoxicosis is or was present is usually not difficult. Except when it is minimal, the patient should have a complete ophthalmologic examination. Orbital computed tomography or magnetic resonance imaging is indicated in patients with severe proptosis, loss of vision, or marked asymmetry. The characteristic finding is enlargement of the extraocular muscles (Fig. 10-26), and the retroorbital fat content may be increased as well.[329]

Euthyroid Graves' Disease

This term is applied to euthyroid patients who have infiltrative ophthalmopathy that is clinically and pathologically indistinguishable from that occurring in thyrotoxic patients with Graves' disease. Such patients account for less than 10 percent of all patients with opthalmopathy.[330] While these patients are by definition euthyroid and have little or no thyroid enlargement, nearly all have some biochemical evidence of thyroid dysfunction or autoimmune thyroid disease. Their serum TSH concentrations may be either low (subclinical thyrotoxicosis) or high (subclinical hypothyroidism), or they have antithyroid peroxidase or other antithyroid antibodies. Hence, they have many manifestations of Graves' thyroid disease; they are euthyroid because they do not produce much TSab or because they have

FIGURE 10-25 Photographs of three patients with ophthalmopathy caused by Graves' disease. (*A, B*) A young woman with moderate asymmetric proptosis and marked retraction of the left eyelid. This patient has few manifestations of ocular inflammation. (*C*) A young woman with marked periorbital edema, bilateral lid retraction, and proptosis. (*D*) A middle-aged woman with marked infraorbital edema, conjunctival injection and chemosis, and muscle restriction of the right eye but little proptosis.

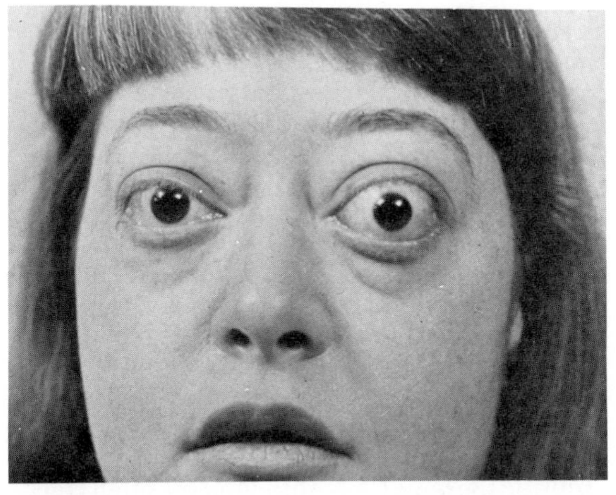

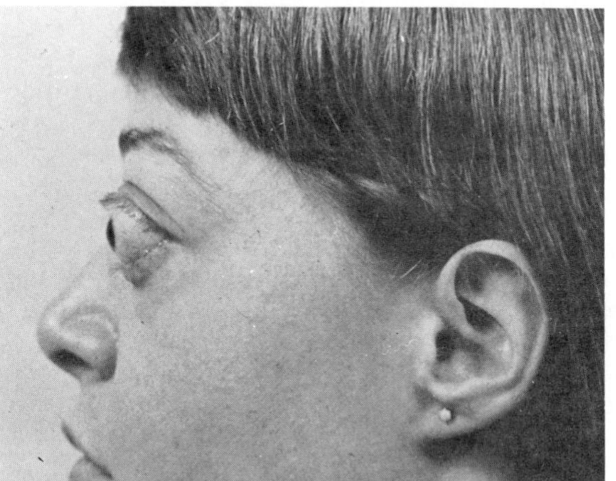

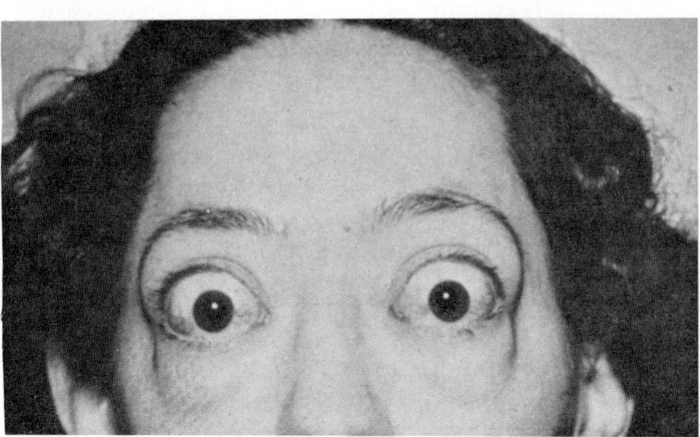

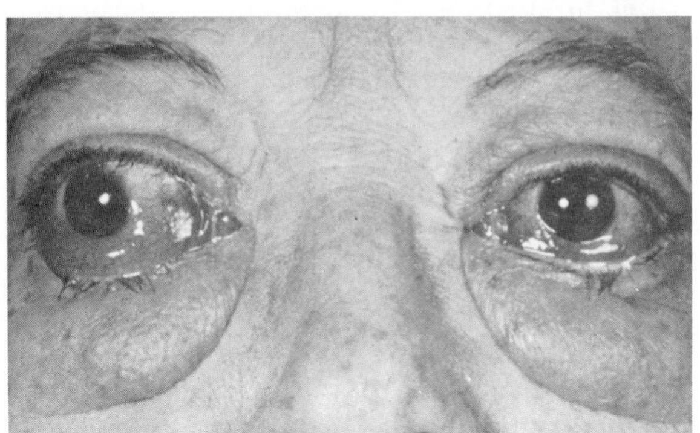

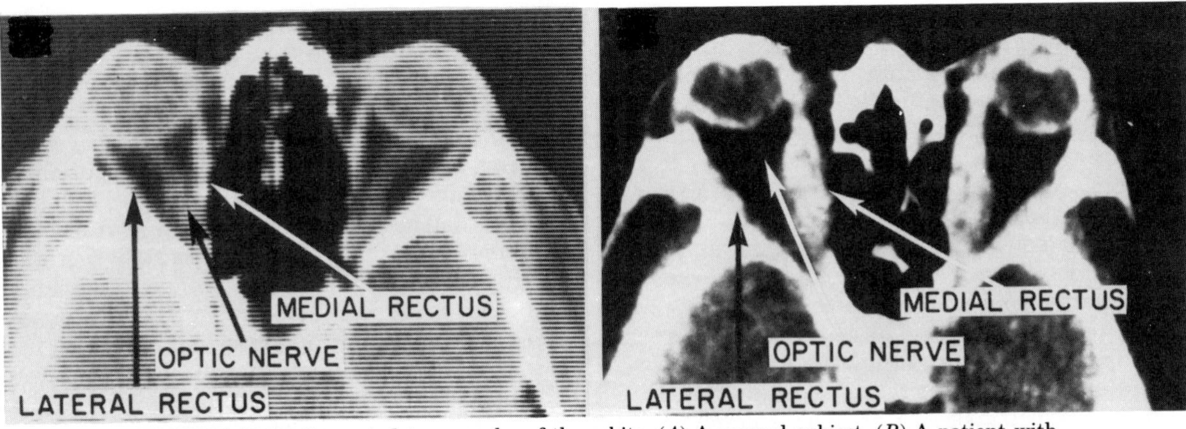

FIGURE 10-26 Computed tomography of the orbits. (*A*) A normal subject. (*B*) A patient with ophthalmopathy caused by Graves' disease. Note the enlarged medial rectus muscle in *B*.

some other thyroid problem, so that thyroidal responsiveness to TSab is limited.

The diagnosis of Graves' ophthalmopathy is less certain in these euthyroid patients even when the clinical manifestations are characteristic of it. Their evaluation should include measurements of serum TSH and T_4 to confirm that they are euthyroid, a complete ophthalmologic examination, and an imaging procedure. The imaging procedure will not only confirm the presence of Graves' ophthalmopathy but also exclude other causes of ophthalmopathy. Among them are pseudotumor of the orbit, orbital myositis, histiocytosis X, granulomatous diseases (sarcoidosis, Wegener's granulomatosis), arteriovenous malformations, lymphoma and leukemia, and metastatic cancer. Tumors, vascular abnormalities, and pseudotumor of the orbit are the usual causes of unilateral ophthalmopathy.

Course and Management

The natural history of Graves' ophthalmopathy is one of persistent proptosis, but the symptoms and signs of ocular inflammation gradually subside. This course is independent of the type of antithyroid treatment that is given, but restoring normal thyroid secretion does seem important, as ophthalmopathy more often persists or worsens in patients with persistent thyroid dysfunction.[333]

The role of antithyroid therapy in the development or worsening of ophthalmopathy has been studied both retrospectively and, more recently, prospectively. In a group of 218 patients followed for up to 11 years, ophthalmopathy worsened in about 20 percent, independently of whether they had been treated with an antithyroid drug, ^{131}I, or thyroidectomy.[334] In only 8 percent did it worsen enough to require glucocorticoid or surgical therapy, and then only within the first 2 years after antithyroid therapy. Ophthalmopathy improved in 12 to 14 percent of the patients in the three treatment groups. It became clinically evident after treatment for hyperthyroidism in only 6 percent of 288 patients who did not have it initially. In a study of 122 patients followed for up to 19 years after antithyroid therapy, proptosis did not change in 79 percent, worsened in 16 percent, and improved in 6 percent.[335] In a much smaller prospective study, ophthalmopathy developed or worsened in more patients treated with ^{131}I than patients treated with MMI or surgery (33 vs. 10 vs. 16 percent, respectively).[336] The slight worsening that occurs after surgery or ^{131}I can be prevented by glucocorticoid therapy,[337] but its routine use is not warranted.

Many patients with ophthalmopathy need no treatment, and most of the others need only conservative treatment. For patients who have thyrotoxicosis, antithyroid drug therapy is probably preferable to ^{131}I therapy. Patients can be told that their ophthalmopathy is not likely to worsen, that control of thyrotoxicosis should result in the disappearance of lid retraction and some eye symptoms, and that their conjunctival and periorbital edema should subside later.

Simple measures that can be used to relieve discomfort, diminish periorbital and conjunctival edema, and provide protection for the eyes include the use of dark glasses and artificial tears, sleeping with the head elevated, cessation of smoking, and diuretic therapy.[332,338] Mild diplopia often can be corrected with prism lenses. The few patients with severe, progressive ophthalmopathy can be treated with glucocorticoids, orbital radiation, or surgical decompression of the orbits. The indications for the use of these treatments are not clearly defined but include severe local eye symptoms and, less often, threatened or actual loss of vision. All three treatments are most effective when the ophthalmopathy is of recent onset, but none are uniformly effective and all have side effects.

Glucocorticoid therapy is most effective in relieving periorbital and conjunctival edema, so that eye discomfort, tearing, and photophobia diminish, usually within several days after the initiation of therapy. Proptosis may diminish a few millimeters, and optic neuropathy and vision may improve, but diplopia is not usually altered.[332,338] The usual initial dose is 60 to 80 mg/day of prednisone for a week or two, followed by gradual reductions in dosage and discontinuation of treatment in 6 to 8 weeks. Unfortunately, the ophthalmopathy often worsens when the dose of prednisone is reduced or discontinued. Short courses of large doses of glucocorticoids given intravenously and retrobulbar injections of glucocorticoids have proved beneficial in some patients.[332,338] Azathioprine and cyclosporine have not proved useful in small numbers of patients, but the combination of prednisone and cyclosporine was beneficial in some patients who had responded poorly to prednisone alone.[339]

Orbital radiation may be used in patients who do not respond to glucocorticoids, have intolerable side effects, or relapse after dose reduction or discontinuation. Radiotherapy usually results in improvement in periorbital and conjunctival edema and the symptoms they cause but does not often relieve proptosis or diplopia.[338] It is therefore a second-line anti-inflammatory therapy and is not suitable for patients with threatened or actual loss of vision. The dose of radiation is usually 2000 rad (20 Gy), given in a 2-week period and delivered so as to spare the lens and to some extent the retina. A few patients, however, develop retinopathy several years later.

Surgical decompression of the orbits is the treatment of choice for any patient in whom vision is threatened or impaired by optic neuropathy or who has corneal involvement or severe proptosis. It relieves periorbital and conjunctival edema and may be indicated for those problems alone in patients who do not respond to or relapse after glucocorticoid therapy. The orbit may be surgically decompressed by transantral, transfrontal, or lateral approaches; transantral decompression is the most satisfactory.[338] Proptosis usually diminishes by 3 to 5 mm; diplopia may worsen. Other surgical procedures done occasionally are tarsorrhaphy to protect the cornea from exposure and muscle operations to correct diplopia.

Localized Myxedema and Thyroid Acropachy

Localized myxedema is rare, occurring in perhaps 2 percent of patients with Graves' disease. It usually occurs several years or more after treatment for thyrotoxicosis in patients who also have severe ophthalmopathy. Localized myxedema consists of circumscribed areas of accumulation of glycosaminoglycans, just as occurs in a generalized distribution in hypothyroidism, but worse.[38] The lesions nearly always involve the pretibial regions but can appear on the hands, arms, trunk, or face. They are usually asymptomatic but may be pruritic and rarely are painful. The lesions initially appear as nontender, erythematous or hyperpigmented, slightly scaly indurated plaques or papules 10 to 20 mm in diameter, with an orange peel appearance (Fig. 10-27). Although often unilateral when first detected, they usually become bilateral and symmetric. They ultimately regress, although in a few patients they become bullous or ulcerated. A few patients have a diffuse form of localized myxedema characterized by generalized painless, nonpitting induration of the lower leg and foot; some plaques or nodular lesions may be superimposed on the diffuse swelling.

Most of these patients require no therapy. For those with extensive bullous or ulcerated lesions, topical application of 0.2 percent fluocinolone or another fluorinated glucocorticoid cream covered by an occlusive dressing has proved effective.[340] It should initially be used nightly or every other night, but when improvement occurs, the frequency of use can be reduced to once weekly or biweekly.

Thyroid acropachy is the rarest manifestation of Graves' disease. Nearly all reported patients have had localized myxedema as well as hyperthyroidism (usually previously treated) and ophthalmopathy.[38]

FIGURE 10-27 Photograph of localized myxedema. Note the raised, slightly hyperpigmented plaques on both anterolateral pretibial regions.

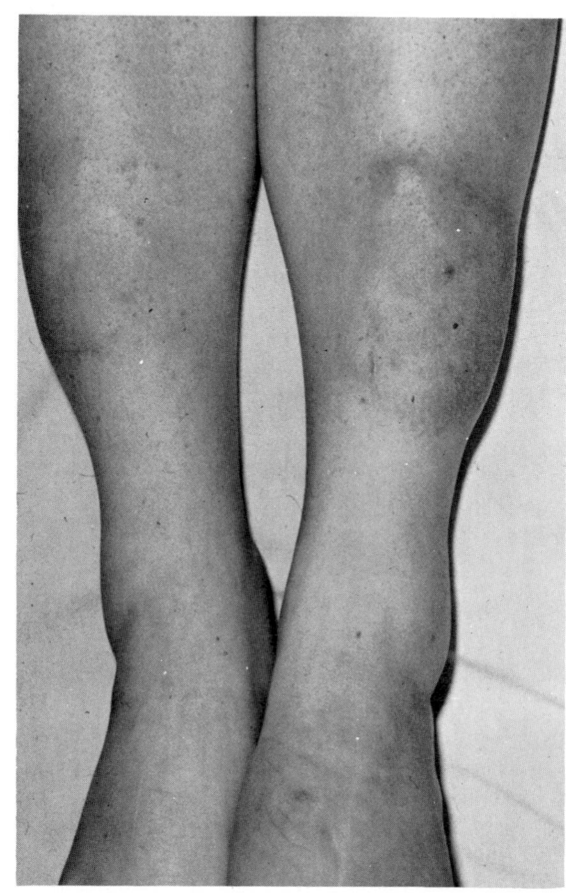

Its manifestations are clubbing of the fingers and toes, subcutaneous edema and fibrosis of the hands and feet, and periosteal bone formation involving the phalanges and metacarpal and metatarsal bones. It usually causes no symptoms or deformity, but contractures may occur. The pathogenesis is not known, and there is no effective therapy.

HYPOTHYROIDISM

Hypothyroidism is the clinical and biochemical syndrome that results from decreased thyroid hormone production by the thyroid gland. The term *adaptive hypothyroidism* is used (see Nonthyroidal Illness) to describe the reductions in extrathyroidal T_3 and less often thyroidal T_4 and T_3 production that occur in patients with nonthyroidal illness. While adaptive hypothyroidism results from decreased thyroid hormone production, it is transient and is not accompanied by clinical manifestations of hypothyroidism, and so thyroid hormone treatment is not indicated. This section is devoted to a discussion of the causes, symptoms and signs, diagnosis, and management of hypothyroidism as traditionally defined.

The severity of hypothyroidism varies widely. Some patients have no symptoms and normal serum T_4 and T_3 concentrations but elevated serum TSH concentrations; this is defined as *subclinical hypothyroidism*. In other patients, hypothyroidism is overt, with low serum T_4 as well as high serum TSH concentrations; these patients have symptoms and signs that reflect abnormal function of one or many organ systems. Rarely, hypothyroidism constitutes a medical emergency (myxedema coma).

The frequency of hypothyroidism also varies considerably, depending on the population studied. The prevalence rate of overt hypothyroidism is 1 to 2 per 1000 in community surveys[67,87] and 5 to 20 per 1000 in patients seeking medical care. Subclinical hypothyroidism is found in from 20 to 120 per 1000 persons in the community. The higher rates occur in older women, most of whom have antithyroid antibodies.[87] The ratio of women to men with either overt or subclinical hypothyroidism ranges from 2 to 1 to 8 to 1 and increases with age.

Pathophysiology of Hypothyroidism

A comparison of thyroidal and extrathyroidal production of T_4 and T_3 in normal subjects and patients with hypothyroidism is shown in Fig. 10-28. The daily rate of T_4 production in patients with overt hypothyroidism is about 25 percent of normal. The daily T_3 production rate is decreased less, and the proportion of T_3 that originates in the thyroid is increased and the proportion that originates in extrathyroidal sites is decreased.[160,341]

There are several defenses against the development of hypothyroidism. The most important is increased TSH secretion, which increases in response to very small decreases in thyroid secretion and may restore thyroid secretion to nearly normal by stimulating thyroid hyperplasia and hypertrophy. TSH also stimulates the synthesis of T_3 in preference to that of T_4, and it stimulates thyroidal T_4-5′-deiodinase activity.[7,13] Therefore, thyroidal T_3 secretion is decreased less than is that of T_4, and the thyroidal contribution to overall T_3 production is increased. Other mechanisms that minimize the development of hypothyroidism include an increase in the fraction of T_4 that is converted to T_3 at extrathyroidal sites, particularly in tissues rich in type II T_4-5′-deiodinase.[342] All these changes serve to limit the decrease in the availability of T_3, the more efficiently produced and more active thyroid hormone, and therefore to minimize the impact of thyroid deficiency.

Causes of Hypothyroidism

Hypothyroidism is caused by thyroid disease (primary hypothyroidism) in more than 98 percent of patients, but it can be caused by pituitary or hypothalamic disease (central hypothyroidism). The ma-

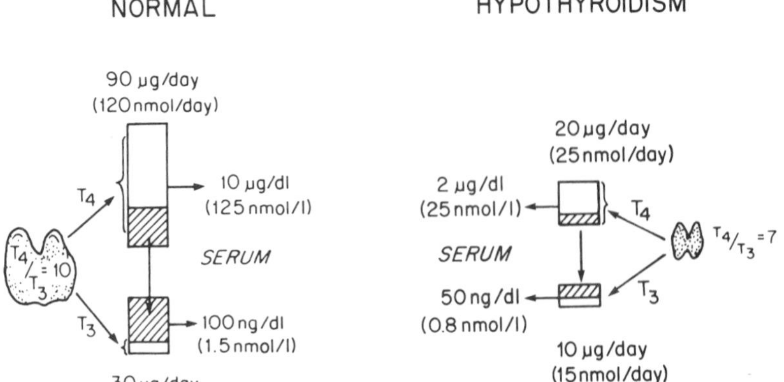

FIGURE 10-28 Diagram of thyroidal T_4/T_3 ratios, extrathyroidal production rates of T_4 and T_3, and serum T_4 and T_3 concentrations in normal subjects and patients with hypothyroidism. The diagonally lined areas in the T_4 (upper) rectangles indicate the proportion of T_4 converted to T_3 at extrathyroidal sites, and the diagonally lined areas in the T_3 (lower) rectangles indicate the proportion of T_3 formed from T_4 at extrathyroidal sites. *(Reproduced with modification from DeGroot LJ (ed): Endocrinology, 2d ed. Philadelphia, Saunders, 1989, p. 703, with permission of the publisher.)*

jor causes of hypothyroidism are listed in Table 10-15. An attempt should always be made to distinguish among them, particularly since hypothyroidism may be the predominant or only manifestation of serious hypothalamic or pituitary disease. History and physical examination alone may be sufficient for this purpose, with particular attention being paid to whether the patient has had thyroid disease or has received antithyroid treatment, current drug history, and palpation of the thyroid gland.

The single most common cause of hypothyroidism throughout the world is undoubtedly iodine deficiency (see Chap. 11). Where it is not a problem, the most common causes are chronic autoimmune thyroiditis and previous ^{131}I therapy.

Chronic Autoimmune Thyroiditis

Chronic autoimmune thyroiditis is the most common cause of hypothyroidism in persons living in iodine-replete areas. It most often occurs in women in the fourth decade or later but can occur in men and children. Also known as chronic lymphocytic thyroiditis, it exists in an atrophic (nongoitrous) form and a goitrous form. The atrophic form was previously called idiopathic hypothyroidism, primary myxedema, or primary thyroid atrophy, and the goitrous form is also known as Hashimoto's disease. The two forms differ clinically only in the presence or absence of goiter. Pathologically, the atrophic form is characterized by thyroid follicular atrophy, lymphocytic infiltration, and fibrosis and the goitrous form is characterized by thyroid follicular hyperplasia, lymphocytic and plasma cell infiltration, lymphoid germinal centers, and fibrosis.

Patients with either atrophic or goitrous autoimmune thyroiditis may be euthyroid or have subclinical or overt hypothyroidism; the hypothyroidism is often but not always permanent. The extent of thyroid enlargement, when present, varies greatly, and the goiter is occasionally tender.[343] Painless thyroiditis with thyrotoxicosis and postpartum thyroiditis are probably part of the spectrum of autoimmune thyroiditis.

All forms of chronic autoimmune thyroiditis probably result from both antibody- and cell-mediated thyroid dysfunction and destruction.[162] Table 10-16 lists the antibodies that have been found in these patients and their functions. The information concerning biological activity is based largely on in vitro tests, and the extent to which different activities reside in the same antibody molecule is not known.[344–347] At least some antibodies, however, inhibit the binding of TSH to its receptors or TSH biological activity in vivo. Some newborn infants of mothers with chronic autoimmune thyroiditis have antibodies that block the binding and the action of TSH and are hypothyroid, and they become euthyroid as the antibodies disappear.[348] Similarly, in some adult hypothyroid patients the presence and disappearance of the same antibodies correlate with the patient's need for T_4 therapy.[347] Thus, variations in the types and amounts of antibodies produced are probably important determinants of the degree of thyroid dysfunction, the degree to which the thyroid gland is atrophic or enlarged, and the natural history of the disorder. The proportion of hypothyroid patients with either atrophic or goitrous autoimmune thyroiditis who have these presumably functional antibodies is about 20 percent.[346,347]

Like Graves' disease, thyroid cells from patients with goitrous autoimmune thyroiditis express HLA class II molecules. Therefore, the thyroid cells, along with other antigen-presenting cells, may activate T helper-inducer (CD4) cells, which then stimulate B cells to produce the various antithyroid antibodies described above.

The permanent thyroid injury that occurs in most patients with autoimmune thyroiditis is more likely to result from disordered cellular immunity. These

TABLE 10-15 Causes of Hypothyroidism

Primary (thyroidal) hypothyroidism
Insufficient functional thyroid tissue caused by
Chronic autoimmune thyroiditis*
^{131}I therapy
Thyroidectomy
Thyroid dysgenesis
Infiltrative disease*
Defective thyroid hormone biosynthesis
Congenital defects*
Iodine deficiency*
Antithyroid agents*
Iodine excess*
Central (hypothyrotropic) hypothyroidism
TSH deficiency
TRH deficiency
Generalized resistance to thyroid hormone

* Goiter often present.

TABLE 10-16 Types of Thyroid Autoantibodies Found in Patients with Chronic Autoimmune Thyroiditis

Antibody	Biological Activity of Antibody
Thyroid peroxidase	Inhibits peroxidase activity
TSH-binding inhibiting	Inhibits TSH receptor binding
TSH-bioactivity inhibiting	Inhibits TSH action
Growth-stimulating	Stimulates thyroid growth
Cytotoxic	Cytotoxic to thyroid cells
Thyroglobulin	No activity on thyroid cells

patients have activated intrathyroidal B and T cells, although the nature of the T cells is uncertain, since increased proportions of suppressor-cytotoxic, helper-inducer, and cytolytic T cells have been described in different studies.[162,349,350] Antigens are presented to T suppressor-cytotoxic (CD8) cells in combination with HLA class I molecules, which are expressed constitutively on thyroid as on most other cells. Once activated by the binding of complexes of HLA class I molecules and thyroid antigens to their antigen receptors, the activated T suppressor-cytotoxic cells secrete cytokines that have cytotoxic actions—for example, interleukin-2—or differentiate into so-called natural killer cells. Thus, cytokines, cytotoxic T cells, or both are probably responsible for the thyroid injury that occurs in chronic autoimmune thyroiditis.

Figure 10-29 shows an outline of the processes by which cell- and antibody-mediated immune mechanisms, once activated, may result in chronic autoimmune thyroiditis. The initiating factors are not known but may be an infectious agent or toxin, as in Graves' disease (see Graves' Disease). Exogenously administered interleukin-2 and interferon-α, but not interferon-γ, have been reported to induce autoimmune thyroiditis.[351–353]

There are several known risk factors for autoimmune thyroiditis.[354] One is female sex; a second is heredity. Thyroid autoantibodies are found in up to 50 percent of the siblings of patients and with lesser but still substantial frequency in other relatives; the frequency of Graves' disease in siblings and relatives may be increased. The predominance of certain HLA haplotypes, notably HLA-DR3 and HLA-DR5, has been reported in some ethnic groups. Patients with autoimmune thyroiditis and their relatives may have autoantibodies to other endocrine tissues and occasionally other hormonal deficiency syndromes indicative of the presence of the autoimmune polyglandular syndromes (see Chap. 28).

The natural history of autoimmune thyroiditis is quite variable. In patients with atrophic thyroiditis and subclinical hypothyroidism, overt hypothyroidism develops in 5 to 20 percent per year[71,355], but in occasional patients thyroid autoantibodies disappear, serum TSH declines to normal, or both changes occur. Hypothyroidism also develops in time in the majority of patients with goitrous autoimmune thyroiditis who are not hypothyroid initially.[356] Treatment with T_4 results in decreases in goiter size in about half these patients. Repeated biopsies show little change with time, and withdrawal of thyroid therapy usually results in recurrence of hypothyroidism.[357,358] Thus, either form of chronic autoimmune thyroiditis tends to cause progressive and persistent thyroid failure, although remissions do occur,[348] and Graves' disease has occurred later in a few patients.[190] Chronic autoimmune thyroiditis is a major risk factor for thyroid lymphoma.[359]

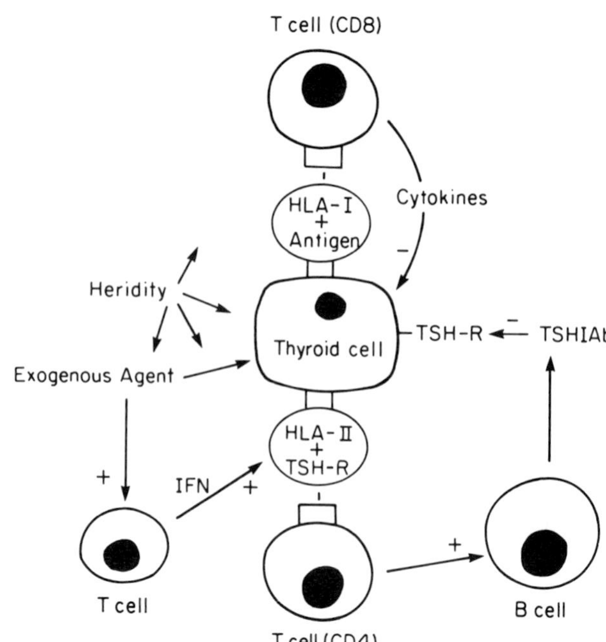

FIGURE 10-29 Hypothetical mechanisms for the development of chronic autoimmune thyroiditis. In a subject with inherited susceptibility to the disease, an exogenous agent (virus or toxin) activates intrathyroidal T cells (or macrophages) to secrete cytokines, shown here as interferon (IFN), which then induce HLA class II (HLA-II) molecule expression on thyroid cells. The exogenous agent also affects the thyroid cells so that TSH receptors (TSH-R) and other thyroid proteins are processed as antigens. The HLA class II molecules and antigens form complexes that bind to the antigen receptor of T helper-inducer (CD4) cells, inducing the secretion of other cytokines by the T cells. These cytokines stimulate B cells to expand and secrete antibodies that inhibit the receptor binding and action of TSH (TSHIab) so that thyroid secretion declines, or antibodies that are cytotoxic (not shown) so that the thyroid cells are destroyed. The same exogenous agent induces the processing of other thyroid proteins to form antigens that bind to constitutively expressed HLA class I (HLA-I) molecules. The binding of these antigen-HLA class I complexes to the antigen receptors of T suppressor-cytotoxic (CD8) cells stimulates the cells to differentiate into natural killer cells or secrete cytokines that damage or kill thyroid cells.

Transient Hypothyroidism in Autoimmune Thyroiditis

Transient hypothyroidism is an integral part of the syndromes of painless thyroiditis with thyrotoxicosis and postpartum thyroiditis. Among patients with painless thyroiditis, about 50 percent become hypothyroid several weeks after the thyrotoxic phase subsides.[197] The hypothyroid phase is usually asymptomatic and lasts 2 to 8 weeks, but some patients have permanent hypothyroidism or develop it later.

Postpartum thyroiditis occurs in 1 to 6 percent of women after pregnancy.[323,327] About 80 percent have hypothyroidism, preceded in about half by thyrotoxicosis (see Postpartum Thyrotoxicosis). Whether preceded by thyrotoxicosis or not, the hypothyroidism usually develops 4 to 8 months after delivery and lasts 2 to 8 weeks. The patient may have a small diffuse goiter, and the hypothyroidism is often subclinical. This syndrome may be associated with postpartum depression.[360]

Painless thyroiditis with thyrotoxicosis and postpartum thyroiditis appear to be variant forms of chronic autoimmune thyroiditis. The thyroid inflammation and injury are more intense than in chronic autoimmune thyroiditis, but thyroid follicular cells are not destroyed. Immune activation seemingly develops more rapidly, but tolerance is regained more quickly. Thyroid biopsies show lymphocytic thyroiditis, but the cellular infiltration is less intense than in chronic autoimmune thyroiditis, and there are no germinal centers or fibrosis. The two disorders differ in that women with postpartum thyroiditis more often have antithyroid antibodies before, during, and after their thyroid illness and are more likely to have recurrences and develop chronic autoimmune thyroiditis.[197,327,361]

Hypothyroidism after Radioiodine Therapy for Thyrotoxicosis and External Radiotherapy

Hypothyroidism occurs within a year after therapy in a substantial number of patients treated with ^{131}I for thyrotoxicosis (see Treatment of Thyrotoxicosis), and thereafter it occurs at a rate of 0.5 to 2 percent per year.[258,288–290] Its occurrence within the first year, but not later, is dependent on the size of the dose of ^{131}I. Late hypothyroidism is preceded by a long period of subclinical hypothyroidism,[291] attesting to the ability of TSH hypersecretion to maintain nearly adequate thyroid secretion if the thyroid is not badly damaged. Among patients with subclinical hypothyroidism after ^{131}I therapy, only about 5 percent become hypothyroid each year. Late post-^{131}I hypothyroidism probably occurs because the thyroid follicular cells that survive acute radiation injury can maintain their function but cannot replicate. However, autoimmune thyroid cell injury may occur, just as it may occur long after antithyroid drug treatment for hyperthyroidism due to Graves' disease. Hypothyroidism is unusual after ^{131}I therapy for toxic uninodular or multinodular goiter, since some of the thyroid tissue in these patients is atrophic at the time ^{131}I is given and thus does not concentrate the radioisotope.

External neck irradiation therapy in doses of 2500 rad (25 Gy) or more, as used in the treatment of patients with lymphoma, laryngeal carcinoma, and nasopharyngeal carcinoma, also causes hypothyroidism in children and adults.[362,363] Its effect is dose-dependent; 50 percent of patients who receive 4000 rad (40 Gy) ultimately develop hypothyroidism. Hypothyroidism also occurs in patients with posterior fossa tumors who are treated with radiation, and in patients who receive total body radiation for bone marrow transplantation. External irradiation-induced overt hypothyroidism, like that occurring 1 or more years after ^{131}I therapy, is usually preceded by months or years of subclinical hypothyroidism.

Postoperative Hypothyroidism

Total thyroidectomy results in an increase in serum TSH concentrations within 1 week and overt hypothyroidism within 1 month.[364] The frequency of hypothyroidism after subtotal thyroidectomy for hyperthyroid Graves' disease is now high, ranging from 25 to 75 percent in the first year after surgery.[258,288,296] This high rate of postoperative hypothyroidism is a result of aggressive surgery undertaken to reduce the frequency of recurrent thyrotoxicosis after surgery. Hypothyroidism developing in the first months after subtotal thyroidectomy is not invariably permanent; in some patients, the remaining thyroid mass is sufficient to maintain normal thyroid secretion after a period of stimulation by TSH.

Hypothyroidism also may develop later than 1 year after surgery, at a rate of about 0.5 to 1 percent per year. Late postoperative hypothyroidism is probably due to destruction of the thyroid remnant by autoimmune processes, since it is more likely to occur in patients whose excised thyroid tissue had histologic evidence of autoimmune thyroiditis.

Thyroid Dysgenesis (Sporadic Nongoitrous Cretinism)

Developmental defects of the thyroid gland are the most common cause of hypothyroidism in the newborn. Some patients have virtually complete thyroid agenesis, but in about half thyroid tissue is detectable by thyroid radioisotope scan.[79] The thyroid tissue may be located in the midline anywhere from the base of the tongue to below the thyroid cartilage or in the normal location on one or both sides of the neck. The cause of abnormal thyroid development is not known. One possibility is that it is due to transplacental passage of maternal thyroid autoantibodies that are cytotoxic, but such antibodies are found with similar frequency in normal and hypothyroid neonates.[365]

Transplacental passage of autoantibodies that inhibit TSH binding or action causes transient but not permanent neonatal hypothyroidism.[348] These antibodies have been found only in infants whose mothers had chronic autoimmune thyroiditis.

Hypothyroidism Due to Infiltrative Disease of the Thyroid

A variety of infiltrative diseases may rarely result in thyroid damage sufficient to cause hypothyroidism. They include amyloidosis, sarcoidosis, scleroderma, cystinosis, iron deposition, leukemia, fibrous invasive thyroiditis (Riedel's thyroiditis), and various infections.[366]

Biosynthetic Defects in Thyroid Hormonogenesis

Thyroid hormone biosynthesis and secretion depend on the availability of iodine and the ability of thyroid tissue to carry out the multiple reactions needed to synthesize and secrete T_4 and T_3. The entire process is dependent on the responsiveness of thyroid tissue to TSH. It is not surprising, therefore, that there are multiple genetic, nutritional, and pharmacologic causes of decreased thyroid hormone production.

Congenital Defects

While rare, the several congenital defects in thyroid hormone biosynthesis have provided insight into the normal mechanisms of thyroid hormone biosynthesis and release.[367] Most of these disorders are inherited as autosomal recessive traits. In homozygotes, hypothyroidism is severe and becomes apparent early in life. The compensatory increase in TSH secretion leads to thyroid enlargement, which may be minimal early in life but becomes marked in childhood or later. In presumed heterozygotes, the abnormality is usually mild and results only in a moderate degree of thyroid enlargement.

1. *Iodide concentration defect.* This very rare abnormality is characterized by partial or complete lack of ability of thyroid tissue to transport iodide.[5] Thus, thyroid radioiodine uptake is very low despite the presence of goiter. Treatment with iodide in doses of 5 mg or more daily restores thyroid hormone secretion to normal as a result of passive diffusion of iodide into the thyroid, but treatment with T_4 is more convenient.
2. *Iodide organification defects.* Several different defects in iodine oxidation and organification have been described. They include quantitative deficiency of thyroid peroxidase, qualitative abnormalities such as defective binding of heme prosthetic groups to the enzyme and abnormal intracellular localization of the enzyme, and deficient hydrogen peroxide generation. Thyroid iodide transport is increased, but little further intrathyroidal iodide metabolism occurs, so that inorganic iodide accumulates in the thyroid. This accumulation can be detected by a perchlorate discharge test; when iodide transport is inhibited by perchlorate, the outward diffusion of inorganic iodide that has accumulated can be detected. Perchlorate discharge tests are done by administration of 500 mg $KClO_4$ 1 h after a tracer dose of ^{123}I; a fall in thyroid radioactivity of 10 percent or more 1 h after $KClO_4$ administration indicates defective iodide oxidation and organification.

   In some families, goiter, usually with only minimal hypothyroidism, occurs along with congenital sensorineural deafness (Pendred's syndrome). These patients have a positive perchlorate discharge test, and so they are considered to have an organification defect. However, their thyroid tissue usually has normal peroxidase activity, and it forms iodotyrosines but not iodothyronines normally in vitro. The deafness usually precedes the development of goiter and may occur in patients with no thyroid abnormality.
3. *Thyroglobulin biosynthetic defects.* Thyroglobulin production may be inadequate even though its structure is normal. It may be produced in adequate quantities but may be structurally abnormal, so that organification or iodotyrosyl coupling within it is poor or it cannot be secreted into the thyroid follicular lumen. The latter abnormalities may result from synthesis of thyroglobulin that is abnormal in either amino acid or carbohydrate composition.
4. *Iodotyrosine deiodinase defect.* Thyroid iodotyrosine deiodinase plays an important role in the recirculation of iodide and thus in its conservation. Deiodinase deficiency results in the release of large quantities of mono- and diiodotyrosine from the thyroid gland. Since extrathyroidal iodotyrosine deiodinase also is lacking in these patients, the iodotyrosines are excreted in the urine. Thus, iodide that normally becomes available for reuse within the thyroid is lost, resulting in secondary iodide deficiency.
5. *Thyroid insensitivity to TSH.* Congenital hypothyroidism can also be caused by thyroidal unresponsiveness to TSH. The patients have no goiter and their thyroid does not respond to either endogenous or exogenous TSH. In vitro studies demonstrate TSH binding but poor cyclic AMP or other responses to TSH in thyroid tissue, suggesting a postreceptor defect. Thyroidal resistance to TSH also occurs in patients with pseudohypoparathyroidism, although this does not usually result in overt hypothyroidism.

These disorders can be differentiated in a general way by the presence or absence of goiter, measurements of serum thyroglobulin and thyroid radioiodine uptake, and perchlorate discharge testing. The identification of specific defects requires detailed in vitro studies of thyroid iodine metabolism or thyroglobulin structure, or DNA analysis.

Iodine Deficiency

The presence of hypothyroidism (cretinism) in some inhabitants of regions where iodine deficiency is endemic has long been recognized (see Chap. 11). Many more of these subjects have thyroid enlargement, abnormalities in thyroid iodide metabolism and secretion, and elevated serum TSH concentrations, although the frequency of these abnormalities varies greatly depending on the degree of iodine deficiency. A daily iodine intake of 25 to 50 μg or less is associated with a goiter prevalence of 15 to 30 percent; when intake is lower, the prevalence of goiter is higher and overt hypothyroidism occurs frequently. Other variables, such as dietary and waterborne goitrogens and genetic factors, may be important contributory factors in some regions. Iodine deficiency persists worldwide, not just in underdeveloped areas, despite the fact that it can be readily prevented by supplementation of salt or other foods with iodine or by oral or parenteral treatment with iodized oil.

Antithyroid Agents

A variety of inorganic and organic compounds, both naturally occurring and synthetic, have antithyroid actions. Since these compounds inhibit thyroidal T_4 and T_3 synthesis and secretion, usually by inhibiting iodide transport or iodide organification and coupling, they can cause both hypothyroidism and goiter. PTU and MMI are the most potent antithyroid drugs; their use should usually be evident. The most commonly used drug that may cause hypothyroidism and goiter is lithium carbonate (see Effects of Various Drugs on Thyroid Function). Many other drugs, chemicals, and constituents of naturally occurring foodstuffs have antithyroid effects and occasionally have been implicated as the cause of hypothyroidism or goiter in individual patients.[366] They are not, however, important causes of hypothyroidism. Most are very weak antithyroid agents and probably cause hypothyroidism only if there is preexisting subclinical thyroid disease. Furthermore, other than lithium carbonate, none are widely used.

Interferon-α and interleukin-2 can induce autoimmune thyroiditis and hypothyroidism.[351,352]

Iodine Excess

Iodine excess also may result in subclinical or overt hypothyroidism. The iodine may be used as either inorganic iodide or organic iodine compounds in the form of dietary supplements, drugs, radiographic contrast agents, or disinfectants. Patients susceptible to iodide-induced hypothyroidism are those who have abnormal thyroid tissue as a result of chronic autoimmune thyroiditis or previous ^{131}I or surgical therapy for Graves' thyrotoxicosis.[5] In such patients, escape from the antithyroid action of iodide does not occur as it does in normal subjects and untreated patients with Graves' hyperthyroidism, and thus the action of iodide is sustained (see Effects of Various Drugs on Thyroid Function).

Central (Hypothyrotrophic) Hypothyroidism

Pituitary Hypothyroidism

TSH is required for normal thyroid secretion, and decreased thyroid secretion and thyroid atrophy follow TSH deficiency. This condition is much less common than primary (thyroidal) hypothyroidism. TSH deficiency may be caused by destruction of the thyrotrophs by hormone-secreting or nonsecreting pituitary adenomas (see Chap. 8). Nearly all patients with pituitary microadenomas are euthyroid, whereas 10 to 25 percent of those with macroadenomas are hypothyroid. If not present initially, TSH deficiency may result from surgical or radiation therapy for such tumors. Conversely, some initially hypothyroid patients may become euthyroid after treatment of their tumors. TSH deficiency may also result from postpartum pituitary necrosis (Sheehan's syndrome), craniopharyngioma, carotid aneurysm, trauma, hemochromatosis, and infiltrative processes such as lymphocytic hypophysitis, metastatic cancer, tuberculosis, and histiocytosis. In any of these situations, TSH deficiency may occur in association with other tropic hormone deficiencies or as an isolated abnormality. In infants and children, TSH deficiency may be caused by many of the same diseases and also by inherited structural defects in the gene for the beta subunit of TSH.[368]

Pituitary enlargement and hypothyroidism do not invariably indicate the presence of a primary pituitary tumor and pituitary hypothyroidism. Pituitary enlargement is present in some patients with severe primary hypothyroidism.[369,370] It is due to compensatory hyperplasia and hypertrophy of the thyrotroph cells and occasionally is sufficient to cause radiologically and even clinically evident pituitary enlargement, even visual field defects.[370] Recognition that pituitary enlargement can occur in patients with primary hypothyroidism is very important so that they do not undergo unnecessary pituitary surgery. The serum TSH concentrations in patients with secondary pituitary enlargement are usually very high (200 to 500 mU/liter). The concentrations decline during thyroid hormone therapy, indicating that TSH secretion is not autonomous, and the pituitary gland diminishes in size.

Hypothalamic Hypothyroidism

TRH deficiency also causes hypothyroidism (see Chaps. 7, 8). TRH deficiency may be isolated or may coexist with other hypothalamic hormone deficiencies. Hypothalamic hypothyroidism occurs predominantly in children, in whom it is not usually accompanied by any anatomic abnormality. In adults and children, it may occur as a result of cranial radiation therapy; traumatic, infiltrative, and neoplastic diseases of the hypothalamus; or pituitary lesions that interrupt the hypothalamic-pituitary portal circulation.

TSH Secretion in Central Hypothyroidism

Most hypothyroid patients with pituitary or hypothalamic disease have low or normal serum TSH concentrations (Fig. 10-15). Even when the concentrations are normal, nocturnal TSH secretion is usually decreased.[371] Characteristically, there is little increase in serum TSH after TRH administration in patients with pituitary hypothyroidism and a normal or delayed response in those with hypothalamic hypothyroidism, but the responses are too variable for these tests to be useful in an individual patient. Rare patients with central hypothyroidism have elevated basal serum TSH concentrations.[372] Their TSH is immunoreactive but biologically inactive, and its biological activity increases when they are given TRH, probably because of changes in TSH glycosylation.

Generalized Resistance to Thyroid Hormone

Generalized resistance to thyroid hormones is a rare hereditary disorder characterized by few or no symptoms and signs of thyroid dysfunction, thyroid enlargement, elevated serum total and free T_4 and T_3 concentrations, and normal or slightly elevated TSH concentrations.[373] It is caused by mutations in the T_3 nuclear receptor. A few of these patients have had physical findings, such as deafness, stippled epiphyses, and short stature, indicative of hypothyroidism in infancy. Others have had tachycardia or hyperactivity suggestive of excessive thyroid hormone action, presumably because the receptors mediating these actions of thyroid hormone are normal. Hypothyroidism may be evident in patients mistakenly treated for thyrotoxicosis by ^{131}I or surgical therapy; recurrent goiter in a hypothyroid or euthyroid patient with such a history is a clue to the presence of generalized thyroid hormone resistance.

Most reported patients have been adolescents or adults, but the disorder can be recognized soon after birth. Men and women are affected in equal numbers. The pattern of inheritance is autosomal recessive in most families and autosomal dominant in a few. These patients are euthyroid because they produce increased amounts of T_4 and T_3; the pituitary is resistant to the same extent as other tissues, and the resistance is not complete in any tissue. Additional thyroid hormone evokes little additional response unless very large doses are given.[374]

A variety of defects in T_3 nuclear receptors have been identified in families with this syndrome. Most of them have consisted of point mutations of the gene for the beta form of the receptor on chromosome 3 that resulted in amino acid substitutions in the T_3-binding region of the receptor (see Biochemical Actions of Thyroid Hormones), but large segments of the gene were deleted in another family.[375] Defects in the alpha form of the receptor have not been found. The mutant receptors not only may have reduced affinity for T_3, but may also inhibit the actions of the normal receptors on the T_3 response elements of DNA, thus explaining the dominant effect of the mutation (dominant recessive mutation).[376] The differences in phenotype among the patients with this syndrome are probably due to differences in the extent to which the abnormal receptors interact with the normal receptors and interfere with their actions.

Clinical Manifestations of Hypothyroidism

The clinical manifestations of hypothyroidism are highly variable, depending on its cause, duration, and severity. The spectrum of hypothyroidism extends from subclinical hypothyroidism to overt hypothyroidism to myxedema coma. The characteristic change in organ system function in hypothyroid patients is slowing; thus, there is slowing of physical and mental activity and of cardiovascular, gastrointestinal, and neuromuscular function.

The clinical manifestations of overt hypothyroidism and their frequency in older studies are listed in Table 10-17.[377–379] Among these symptoms and signs, the most discriminating are slow movements, decreased sweating, hoarseness, paresthesia, cold intolerance, periorbital edema, and delayed reflexes.[379] Their frequency in patients who are found to have hypothyroidism today is undoubtedly considerably lower. A history of events that might cause it, such as previous ^{131}I therapy, thyroid surgery, or the use of iodine-containing drugs or lithium carbonate, may suggest its presence.

Spontaneously occurring hypothyroidism, for example, that due to chronic autoimmune thyroiditis, usually develops slowly, and as thyroid secretion declines, the resulting rise in TSH secretion limits the decline in thyroid secretion. Thus, the symptoms and signs of hypothyroidism develop very slowly. When

TABLE 10-17 Symptoms and Signs of Hypothyroidism

	Frequency in Overtly Hypothyroid Patients, %
Symptom	
Dry skin	60–100
Cold intolerance	60–95
Hoarseness	50–75
Weight gain	50–75
Constipation	35–65
Decreased sweating	10–65
Paresthesia	50
Decreased hearing	5–30
Weakness and fatigue	90
Sign	
Slow movements	70–90
Coarse skin and hair	70–100
Cold skin	70–90
Periorbital puffiness	40–90
Bradycardia	10–15
Slow reflex relaxation	50

Source: Refs. 377–379.

they develop more rapidly, for example, within the first year after ^{131}I therapy or subtotal thyroidectomy, patients recognize the changes more readily, and symptoms such as muscle cramps and weakness are more prominent. Hypothyroidism due to hypothalamic or pituitary disease is less likely to be associated with periorbital and peripheral edema, hoarseness, and weight gain.

The characteristic pathologic finding in patients with hypothyroidism is the accumulation of glycosaminoglycans, primarily hyaluronic acid, in interstitial tissue.[38] They accumulate because their synthesis is increased, and, as a consequence of their hydrophilic properties, they lead to the mucinous edema that is characteristic of the disorder. This is myxedema. Mucinous edema of the dermis produces some of the most obvious clinical manifestations of hypothyroidism, and in fatal cases, mucinous edema has been found in the interstitial tissue of most organ systems.[380]

General Appearance

A patient with hypothyroidism may appear normal, have obvious myxedema of the face and extremities, or be comatose. The major presenting manifestations often are subjective. The patient complains of being tired and weak, becomes fatigued easily, and may be unable to continue normal physical or mental activities. Too often such behavior is attributed to aging by the patient or the patient's relatives. Cold intolerance may be marked, with the patient using extra clothing even in the summer.

Skin and Appendages

The characteristic but now rare appearance of a patient with overt hypothyroidism (Fig. 10-30) is primarily a reflection of the nonpitting periorbital and peripheral mucinous edema. The facial features are coarse, blepharoptosis is present, and the skin becomes rough, scaly, and thickened. More often the patient's appearance is less altered. The skin is dry and scaly, but it is not thickened or particularly rough, and periorbital and peripheral edema is mild. At times, the edema is pitting, particularly in the legs; such a finding need not indicate the presence of cardiac or other disease. There is often pallor caused by the thickened dermis and epidermis, decreased cutaneous blood flow, and sometimes anemia. The yellowish hue of carotenemia may be evident. The skin feels cold as a result of both thickening and decreased blood flow.

Decreased sebaceous and sweat gland secretions add to the dryness of the skin. The hair may be coarse, dry, and brittle, and hair growth may slow or cease. Hair may be lost on the scalp, the extremities, or the eyebrows. The nails also grow slowly and may be thickened and brittle.

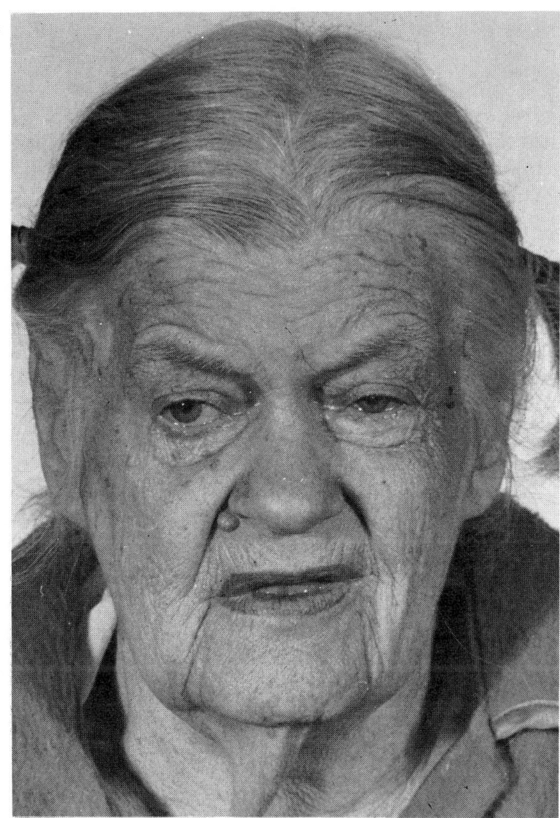

FIGURE 10-30 Photograph of a woman with severe chronic hypothyroidism, showing facial puffiness and periorbital edema.

Thyroid Gland

The size of the thyroid may provide a valuable clue to the cause of hypothyroidism and even to its presence, since thyroid enlargement may be the first objective sign of hypothyroidism. Goitrous autoimmune thyroiditis is characterized by diffuse thyroid enlargement, although the surface may be irregular or even nodular. The consistency of the thyroid gland is often described as firm or rubbery. The thyroid gland also is diffusely enlarged in patients with hypothyroidism caused by iodide deficiency, congenital defects in thyroid hormone biosynthesis, or any antithyroid agent but eventually becomes irregular or even nodular. It is not palpable in atrophic autoimmune thyroiditis or central hypothyroidism.

Nervous System

Hypothyroid patients have many symptoms of mental dysfunction. While central nervous system glucose and oxygen consumption are normal, cerebral vascular resistance is increased and cerebral blood flow is reduced in proportion to the decrease in cardiac output. The reduced delivery of oxygen to tissue utilizing it at a normal rate should result in some degree of cerebral hypoxia.

The psychological and behavioral symptoms of hypothyroidism include lethargy and fatigue, decreased attention span, loss of ambition, slowing of movement and thought, and memory loss. The patient becomes complacent, less alert, mentally slow, and physically clumsy. Speech is slow and hesitant as well as hoarse. There may be some cognitive impairment,[381] and occasional patients have overt dementia. Often the patient describes significant limitations of activity with inappropriate amusement, and such limitations may be accepted with equanimity; in other patients, these problems lead to anxiety and depression. Headache and hearing loss may be prominent complaints. The patient may sleep longer at night or may fall asleep frequently during the day. Rarely, there is severe anxiety and agitation ("myxedema madness").

Hypothyroid patients often complain of paresthesia, but few have objective neurologic findings other than slow deep tendon reflexes. Both the contraction and relaxation phases of the reflexes are prolonged, the latter more than the former. Several neurologic syndromes that are reversible may occur, however; they include the carpal tunnel syndrome due to mucinous edema of the flexor retinaculum of the wrist, a symmetric sensorimotor polyneuropathy, and cerebellar dysfunction with signs such as ataxia, intention tremor, and nystagmus.[382,383]

Musculoskeletal System

Subjective muscle dysfunction manifested by myalgia and muscle cramps and stiffness occurs in many hypothyroid patients.[384] Movements may be slow and clumsy, and complaints of muscle weakness and fatigability are common. There may be objective muscle weakness. Rarely, chronic hypothyroid myopathy results in increased muscle mass (pseudohypertrophy), muscle spasms, and pseudomyotonia. Elevated serum creatine kinase (MM fraction) concentrations are common in hypothyroidism, even in the absence of muscle symptoms.[134,385] The elevation is due to release from skeletal muscle, presumably as a result of increased sarcolemmal permeability, and also slowed clearance. Serum lactate dehydrogenase and aminotransferase concentrations may be increased as well. Muscle biopsies show interstitial edema and muscle fiber enlargement, loss of striations, and sarcoplasmic degenerative changes.

Hypothyroid patients may complain of arthralgia and joint stiffness. Some have synovial thickening and synovial effusions, usually of the knees.

Cardiovascular-Pulmonary System

Hypothyroidism results in decreases in the rate and force of cardiac contractility and in peripheral oxygen needs.[223] Peripheral resistance increases, and cerebral, cutaneous, and renal blood flow and blood volume are reduced. The physiologic consequences are decreased cardiac output, but ventricular end-diastolic pressure and peripheral arteriovenous oxygen differences are normal. During exercise, cardiac output increases and peripheral resistance decreases appropriately, indicating a normal cardiac reserve. In fatal cases, the myocardial fibers are edematous and vacuolated.[380]

The symptoms and signs of cardiovascular dysfunction include bradycardia, evidence of poor peripheral circulation such as pallor and cold skin, dyspnea on exertion, decreased exercise tolerance, fatigability, and distant heart sounds. The lethargy, puffiness, edema, and diminished cardiac activity may suggest cardiac failure, but this is rare. When cardiac failure occurs, it is most likely due to the hemodynamic changes of hypothyroidism superimposed on preexisting cardiac disease, but T_4-reversible hypothyroid cardiomyopathy has been described.[386] There may be clinical and radiographic evidence of cardiac enlargement, and a few patients have pericardial effusion; the cholesterol- and protein-rich effusions have little hemodynamic effect. The electrocardiogram shows bradycardia and low-amplitude P waves and QRS complexes and, less often, conduction disturbances and nonspecific QRS and T-wave abnormalities. Echocardiography reveals pericardial effusion, varying degrees of septal and wall thickening, and diminished myocardial relaxation.[387]

About 20 percent of hypothyroid patients have hypertension.[222] It is undoubtedly coincidental in many but is aggravated by the increase in peripheral resistance that occurs in hypothyroidism. By contrast, some patients become hypertensive as they become hypothyroid, and the hypertension disappears with T_4 treatment.

The coexistence of angina pectoris and hypothyroidism in some patients warrants special mention. Although hypercholesterolemia occurs as a result of hypothyroidism, there is no compelling evidence that hypothyroidism is accompanied by accelerated atherogenesis. The development of hypothyroidism may ameliorate angina pectoris, whether directly because cardiac work and thus myocardial oxygen requirements are reduced or simply because the patient becomes less active. Hypothyroid patients should not be denied T_4 treatment because of the possibility that they might develop symptoms of ischemic heart disease, but should be treated cautiously. In a series of 55 patients with angina and hypothyroidism, the angina improved or disappeared during thyroid hormone therapy in 21 patients, did not change in 25, and worsened in 9.[388] Among about 1400 other hypothyroid patients, new-onset angina appeared in 6 patients during the first month of thyroid therapy, in another 6 within the first year, and in 23 after that. Antianginal therapy can be added if necessary. However, coronary revascularization, if otherwise indicated, can be done safely in untreated hypothyroid patients.[389,390]

Complaints referable to the airways and respiratory system include chronic nasal congestion, hoarseness, shortness of breath, and sleep apnea. Nasal congestion and hoarseness are due to mucinous edema of the nasal mucosa and larynx, respectively. Shortness of breath may reflect cardiac disease, the presence of pleural effusion, or generalized impairment of pulmonary function.

Most hypothyroid patients have normal lung volumes, vital capacity, and arterial P_{O_2}, P_{CO_2}, and pH values. Maximum breathing capacity, compliance, and ventilatory drive may be reduced[391] because of respiratory muscle weakness or depression of the respiratory center. Pleural effusions may be present without other evidence of lung disease.[392]

Some hypothyroid patients have symptoms of sleep apnea, and it can be demonstrated by polysomnography in many others. It is due largely to enlargement of the tongue and pharyngeal muscles but has a central component in some patients.[393,394]

Fluid and Electrolyte Metabolism and Renal Function

Hypothyroid patients often appear puffy or even edematous, and total body water and sodium content are increased as a result of the accumulation of hydrophilic glycosaminoglycans in extravascular tissue, increased vascular permeability, and decreased lymph flow.[395] Plasma volume is decreased, and serum atrial natriuretic hormone and aldosterone concentrations and plasma renin activity are normal or slightly decreased.[229,230,396,397]

In regard to renal function, renal blood flow is reduced in proportion to the decrease in cardiac output, and the glomerular filtration rate is usually slightly reduced. Serum concentrations of urea, creatinine, and electrolytes are usually normal; there may be hyperuricemia and modest proteinuria.

Free water clearance is decreased, as is the ability to excrete a water load, resulting in hyponatremia in some patients. Vasopressin secretion, both basally and in response to saline infusion, is normal in most of these patients but may be increased.[397,398]

Gastrointestinal System

The tongue is often enlarged. Decreased gastric emptying may result in nausea and vomiting, and decreased intestinal motility may result in constipation and abdominal distension, especially constipation. Hypomotility may be severe enough to produce paralytic ileus or megacolon, with the clinical picture of intestinal obstruction.[399] Liver size and function are usually normal, although the elevated serum creatine kinase, lactate dehydrogenase, and aminotransferase concentrations mentioned previously may be due in part to reduced hepatic enzyme clearance. Ascites is occasionally present; it is probably due to abnormal capillary permeability and reduced hepatic lymph flow. The gallbladder may be dilated and may empty poorly.

Intestinal absorption is usually normal. Gastric atrophy and achlorhydria can occur and may be associated with vitamin B_{12} malabsorption. About 25 percent of patients with chronic autoimmune thyroiditis have antiparietal cell antibodies. Defects in gastric acid secretion and vitamin B_{12} malabsorption are more frequent in patients with this type of hypothyroidism, some of whom have or later develop pernicious anemia.

Hematopoietic System

A substantial proportion of hypothyroid patients have a low red cell mass because of the decreased oxygen requirements and therefore decreased erythropoietin secretion.[225] Some of these patients are truly anemic, but the condition is usually mild. The anemia may be normocytic, microcytic, or macrocytic; the hemoglobin concentration is rarely less than 100 g/liter. Serum iron, iron binding capacity, and vitamin B_{12} and folate concentrations usually are normal. The bone marrow is hypocellular, and kinetic studies indicate slowed iron clearance and incorporation. Occasional patients have iron, folic acid, or vitamin B_{12} deficiency with the appropriate peripheral blood and bone marrow findings. Iron deficiency may result from excessive menstrual bleeding or poor iron absorption secondary to decreased gastric acid production. Megaloblastic anemia may be due to malabsorption of folic acid or vitamin B_{12} caused by hypothyroidism or by pernicious anemia in patients with chronic autoimmune thyroiditis.

Leukocyte, lymphocyte, and platelet counts are normal in hypothyroidism. Platelet function or aggregation may be abnormal, bleeding time may be prolonged, and the concentrations of some clotting factors may be slightly decreased.[225,399] Some patients may bruise easily, but the abnormalities in platelet function and clotting factors do not correlate well with clinical bleeding.

Energy, Nutrient, and Drug Metabolism

The decrease in energy expenditure and oxygen consumption in hypothyroidism is accompanied by decreased utilization of a variety of substrates. The result is decreased heat production, probably the major cause of the cold intolerance that is so characteristic of hypothyroidism. Decreased metabolic activity and substrate utilization, as well as physical inactivity and mental depression, also result in decreased appetite and food intake. Body weight may increase modestly, but marked increases in weight are unusual. When it occurs, weight gain is due to retention of salt and water in interstitial tissue as well as fat deposition.

Patients with hypothyroidism have normal carbohydrate tolerance, although glucose absorption may be delayed. Blood glucose does not fall excessively in the postabsorptive state, and hepatic glycogen stores are normal. Overall glucose utilization is normal. Insulin responses to oral glucose are appropriate for the rise in glucose that occurs. Glucose administered intravenously is utilized more slowly than normal because of decreased insulin secretion. In insulin-dependent diabetic patients, exogenous insulin is degraded more slowly than normal; thus, sensitivity to exogenous insulin may increase.

The synthesis of secreted, functional, and structural proteins in many tissues is impaired, most obviously in hypothyroid children, in whom growth is very poor (see Hypothyroidism in Newborn Infants and Children). Protein catabolism also is impaired. For several proteins, such as lipoproteins and albumin, degradation is impaired more than is synthesis. Since blood volume is reduced and serum albumin concentrations are normal, the excess albumin is largely in the interstitial space.

The serum concentrations of total and LDL cholesterol and, less often, triglycerides and lipoprotein(a) are elevated in hypothyroidism.[240,400,401] The synthesis of triglycerides is decreased, but so is their metabolism, since the activity of adipose tissue and probably hepatic lipase is decreased. The increase in serum LDL cholesterol concentrations and those of its apoprotein B constituent are due primarily to decreases in the concentration of LDL receptors and consequently in receptor-mediated clearance and conversion of cholesterol to bile acids. Serum HDL cholesterol concentrations are usually normal but may be increased or decreased.[240,401] They do not change in a consistent way in response to T_4 treatment, whereas serum LDL cholesterol concentrations decrease. Carotene also is transported by LDL, and thus carotenemia may occur.

The metabolism or renal clearance of many drugs, including digoxin and morphine, is slowed by hypothyroidism.[242] Hence, their actions may be prolonged or exaggerated. The action of warfarin (Coumadin) is decreased because the catabolism of vitamin K–dependent clotting factors is decreased.

Endocrine System

Hypothyroidism results in changes in the dynamics of other endocrine systems and in some patients causes clinically important abnormalities in endocrine function. Rates of hormone degradation are decreased, resulting in compensatory reduction in rates of hormone secretion; thus, serum hormone concentrations usually are normal.

Pituitary Function

Nocturnal growth hormone secretion and growth hormone responses to a provocative stimuli such as growth hormone-releasing hormone, insulin-induced hypoglycemia, and arginine infusion are reduced. Serum insulin-like growth factor-I values are low but increase normally in response to exogenous growth hormone.[402,403] These data suggest that hypothyroid patients have decreases in 24-h growth hormone secretion sufficient to decrease insulin-like growth factor-I production, partially explaining the short stature that occurs in hypothyroid children. In addition, thyroid deficiency directly impairs bone formation.

Basal serum prolactin concentrations are normal or slightly elevated but may be as high as 200 μg/liter.[404] Hyperprolactinemia is most likely to occur in patients with chronic hypothyroidism and may result in amenorrhea and galactorrhea, as it does in other women with hyperprolactinemia.

These abnormalities of pituitary hormone secretion are functional ones and are reversed by treatment of hypothyroidism. Trophic hormone deficiencies may also occur as a result of any of the hypothalamic or pituitary diseases that cause hypothyroidism.

Adrenal Function

Twenty-four-hour mean serum cortisol concentrations may be slightly increased.[405] Cortisol clearance is slowed, but cortisol production is nearly normal, suggesting that the sensitivity of ACTH secretion to inhibition by cortisol is decreased. The urinary excretion of cortisol is normal, whereas that of steroid metabolites tends to be low. Pituitary-adrenal responses to metyrapone, insulin-induced hypoglycemia, corticotropin-releasing hormone (CRH), and ACTH are normal or, in the case of CRH, increased.[406] Serum cortisol concentrations increase normally in hypothyroid patients who have other illnesses.

Hypothyroidism due to chronic autoimmune thyroiditis and adrenal insufficiency due to autoimmune adrenalitis may occur in the same patient (autoimmune polyglandular syndromes). Elevated serum TSH concentrations and sometimes overt hypothyroidism also can occur in patients with adrenal insufficiency from other causes.[407] Glucocorticoid replacement alone may result in the restoration of normal thyroid function, indicating the sensitivity of autoimmune disease mechanisms to glucocorticoids.

Circulating levels and production rates of norepinephrine are increased, whereas those of epinephrine are normal.[39]

Gonadal Function

Women with hypothyroidism tend to have low serum estradiol concentrations because hepatic production of SHBG is decreased, but free estradiol concentrations are normal. The secretion of estradiol and progesterone is decreased, as is their clearance. FSH and LH secretion is usually in the normal range for the follicular phase of the cycle, but there is no ovulatory surge. These women therefore tend to have anovulatory and irregular cycles and excessive menstrual bleeding. In postmenopausal women, serum FSH and LH concentrations may be somewhat lower than expected.

In men, serum testosterone concentrations may be low because SHBG production is decreased, but serum free testosterone concentrations are usually normal.[408] Serum FSH and LH concentrations are usually normal. Little is known about reproductive capacity, but impotence, probably not due specifically to hypothyroidism, is common.

Parathyroid-Vitamin D-Bone System

Serum calcium and phosphate concentrations are normal, whereas those of parathyroid hormone and 1,25-dihydroxyvitamin D may be increased.[247] Calcium absorption is decreased, as are bone formation and resorption, suggesting the presence of some resistance to the actions of PTH and 1,25-dihydroxyvitamin D. Further supporting the presence of such resistance are reports of delayed recovery from induced hypocalcemia and amelioration of primary hyperparathyroidism by hypothyroidism. Calcitonin deficiency also would be expected because of the destruction or removal of thyroid parafollicular cells, and recovery from induced hypercalcemia is slowed in hypothyroid patients. Lumbar, femoral, and radial bone density is normal.

Pregnancy in Hypothyroidism

Infertility is increased among women with hypothyroidism, but these women can become pregnant. Its outcome can be normal, but the likelihood of abortion, stillbirth, or premature delivery is increased.[409] Even if the pregnancy is successful, the growth of the fetus and the subsequent growth and development of the child may be retarded.[410] The frequency of subclinical hypothyroidism and antithyroid peroxidase antibodies among pregnant women in the first trimester is about 2 percent, similar to that among women of the same age who are not pregnant,[411] but the presence of these antibodies alone early in pregnancy may be a risk factor for spontaneous abortion.[412]

Illness and Surgery in Hypothyroid Patients

The extent to which hypothyroidism alters the course or outcome of nonthyroidal illness is not known. Serum T_3 concentrations decline in hypothyroid patients who have nonthyroidal illness as they do in normal individuals.[128] Serum TSH concentrations do not change during mild nonthyroidal illness, although they may fall during febrile illnesses or when a glucocorticoid or dopamine is given.[118] Such a change could make it more difficult to diagnose hypothyroidism.

The overall morbidity or mortality of surgery do not appear to be increased in hypothyroid patients, although some complications of surgery, such as hypotension, cardiac failure, and gastrointestinal dysfunction, may be more common.[413,414] Nonetheless, hypothyroid patients should be given anesthetic, analgesic, and sedative drugs very cautiously.

Laboratory Diagnosis of Hypothyroidism

Serum TSH and Thyroid Hormone Concentrations

Measurement of the serum TSH concentration is an indispensable test for the recognition of primary hypothyroidism and the differentiation of primary from central hypothyroidism, whether due to pituitary or hypothalamic disease (Fig. 10-15). Serum TSH concentrations are elevated in all patients with overt primary hypothyroidism and, by definition, in all patients with subclinical hypothyroidism. The elevations are due primarily to increased TSH secretion, although TSH clearance also is decreased. Rare patients with central hypothyroidism have increased serum TSH concentrations, and transient increases (rarely to more than 20 mU/liter) occur in some patients recovering from nonthyroidal illness.

In contrast, serum TSH concentrations are normal or low in most patients with hypothyroidism due to pituitary or hypothalamic disease (see TSH Secretion in Central Hypothyroidism). Measurement of serum TSH therefore not only is an exquisitely sensitive test for the recognition of primary hypothyroidism but also may represent the first indication that hypothyroidism in an individual patient is due to pituitary or hypothalamic disease, indicating the need for neuroradiologic studies and other tests of pituitary function. Moreover, even if the patient has manifestations of pituitary disease or enlargement, such as hyperprolactinemia, sellar enlargement, and visual impairment, serum TSH must be measured since all those findings may result from primary hypothyroidism and improve with T_4 therapy alone.[369,370] Serum TSH concentrations also are normal or low in patients with severe nonthyroidal illness who have low serum T_4 and T_3 concentrations,[105,106] so that TSH measurements cannot be used to differentiate between central hypothyroidism and illness-related decreases in TSH secretion.

Most patients with symptomatic hypothyroidism have decreased serum total and free T_4 concentrations. By contrast, low serum T_4 concentrations do not invariably indicate the presence of hypothyroidism. Serum total T_4 concentrations may be reduced as a result of decreased production of TBG or by agents, such as salicylate, that competitively inhibit the binding of T_4 to TBG or other binding proteins (see Alterations in Serum Thyroid Hormone Binding). In the latter situations, THBR (T_3-resin uptake) tests indicate decreased numbers of unoccupied T_4 binding sites; therefore, serum free T_4 concentrations and free T_4 index values are normal. Decreased serum total T_4 and sometimes free T_4 concentrations also occur in patients who are seriously ill as a result of nonthyroidal illness (see Nonthyroidal Illness).

Since most of the T_3 in serum is produced as a

result of extrathyroidal deiodination of T_4, serum T_3 concentrations are usually low in patients with hypothyroidism. However, measurement of serum T_3 is neither a specific nor a sensitive test for hypothyroidism. About 20 to 30 percent of patients with hypothyroidism and low serum T_4 concentrations have normal serum T_3 concentrations[401] as a result of both TSH-induced stimulation of thyroidal T_3 secretion and an increase in the fractional conversion of T_4 to T_3 at extrathyroidal sites. Conversely, serum T_3 concentrations are low in patients with a wide variety of nonthyroidal illnesses and those receiving various drugs who are euthyroid and have normal serum T_4 and TSH concentrations (see Nonthyroidal Illness).

Summary: Laboratory Diagnosis of Hypothyroidism

A scheme for the evaluation of patients with clinically suspected hypothyroidism is shown in Fig. 10-31. The initial step should be measurement of the serum TSH concentration and free T_4 index. If the serum TSH concentration is high and the serum free T_4 index value is low, the diagnosis of primary hypothyroidism is confirmed. If the serum TSH concentration is normal or low and the serum free T_4 index value is low, the diagnosis is central hypothyroidism or adaptive hypothyroidism. Reliable differentiation between these two disorders in a seriously ill patient at a single point in time may be impossible. The distinction must be based on the presence or absence of symptoms and signs of hypothyroidism and of hypothalamic or pituitary disease, the results of THBR measurements (low in hypothyroidism and normal or high in nonthyroidal illness), and knowledge that central hypothyroidism is rare (see Nonthyroidal Illness).

FIGURE 10-31 Diagnostic scheme for the evaluation of patients with suspected hypothyroidism.

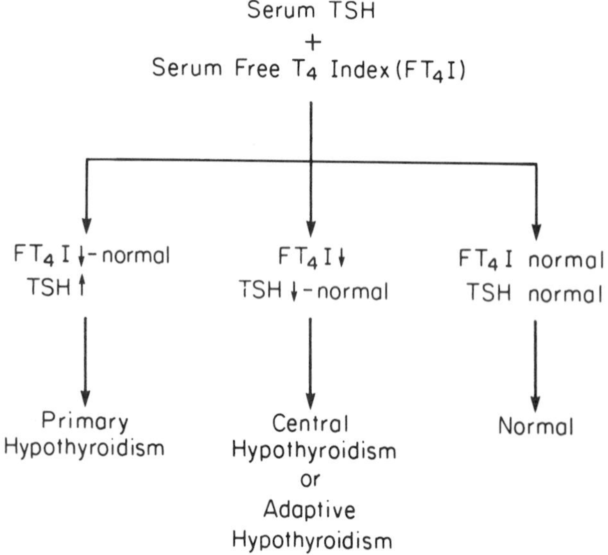

Other Laboratory Procedures

Serum thyroglobulin concentrations are usually low but may be increased in patients with goitrous hypothyroidism or may be artifactually high because of the presence of antithyroglobulin antibodies. The presence of antithyroid peroxidase or other autoantibodies indicates the presence of autoimmune thyroiditis but provides no information about thyroid secretion. Thyroidal radioiodine uptake is reduced in most patients with hypothyroidism but can be normal or supranormal in patients with chronic autoimmune thyroiditis, iodine deficiency, and inherited defects of thyroid hormone biosynthesis.

Treatment of Hypothyroidism

The treatment of hypothyroidism is simple and effective. Occasionally, all that is required is discontinuation of iodide, lithium, or another medication. Consideration also should be given to the possibility that hypothyroidism is transient (see Causes of Hypothyroidism). For most patients, however, lifelong thyroid hormone replacement is required. The general principle is simple: to restore and maintain the euthyroid state. Besides the prescription of medication, patients must be educated about the need for lifelong replacement and periodic follow-up to evaluate the response to therapy, confirm compliance, and reinforce the need for therapy.

L-Thyroxine is the proper treatment. The initial dose should be 0.075 to 0.1 mg/day orally in young or middle-aged adults. For elderly patients, the initial dose should be smaller, 0.05 mg/day, because of the small risk of precipitation of angina, cardiac arrhythmia, or cardiac failure, and it should be 0.025 mg/day if the patient is known to have ischemic heart disease or cardiac arrhythmias. Increases in well-being and pulse rate and diuresis occur within 1 to 2 weeks. An appropriate time for the first follow-up visit is 4 to 6 weeks. The dose should not be increased sooner, because this period of time is needed for an individual oral dose to become fully effective; even this period may not be sufficient to obtain the full effect on TSH secretion if the baseline serum TSH concentration was very high. Most symptoms and signs of hypothyroidism disappear within 1 to 2 months, although some neuropsychological and biochemical abnormalities may persist for 4 to 6 months.

While about 80 percent of an oral dose of T_4 is absorbed,[415] absorption is slow and the distribution volume is large; therefore, serum T_4, T_3, and TSH concentrations do not change appreciably between doses.[416] There may be small variations in the potency or bioavailability of different T_4 preparations, but these variations are so small that they are rarely of clinical importance. A very rare patient has cutaneous allergy to T_4 or to the dye used to color the tablets.

Adequate replacement, i.e., normal serum TSH concentrations, in most young or middle-aged adults requires a daily oral dose of 0.075 to 0.125 mg T_4 daily. Several factors may alter the dose needed for adequate replacement (Table 10-18). Slightly lower doses are usually adequate in older patients because of their slower clearance of T_4.[417] Patients with hypothyroidism caused by ablative therapy for Graves' hyperthyroidism or toxic multinodular goiter also may require slightly less T_4 if they have some remaining autonomous thyroid tissue.[418] Conversely, pregnant women and obese patients may require larger doses.[419] Patients with various intestinal disorders and those taking various drugs that bind T_4 within the gastrointestinal tract also may need larger doses because of decreased absorption, as may younger patients and those taking phenytoin, carbamazepine, and rifampin because of more rapid clearance.[148,420–423] Patients with no intestinal disease who are suspected of having T_4 malabsorption usually prove to be noncompliant.[424]

Patients receiving therapy chronically should be seen at 6-month intervals. Assessment of the adequacy of therapy should be based on the clinical response and the serum TSH concentrations; no other test is as sensitive an indicator of over- or undertreatment.[425] The goal of treatment is to maintain both well-being and normal serum TSH concentrations (0.3 to 3.0 mU/liter). When that is done, most patients have normal serum T_4 and T_3 concentrations. In the absence of symptoms, minor increases (for example, values of 10 mU/liter or less) or decreases (values of 0.1 or 0.2 mU/liter) in serum TSH concentrations do not necessitate changes in T_4 dosage; if greater abnormalities are encountered, the serum T_4 concentration should be measured and a change in dose may be needed. An elevated serum TSH concentration indicates that the dose of T_4 is inadequate or that compliance is poor. In the former situation, the serum T_4 concentration should be low. In the case of poor compliance, the serum T_4 concentration may be either low or high depending on whether the patient had taken little or no T_4 or a large dose, for example, 0.6 to 0.8 mg, before visiting the physician.[426] A low serum TSH concentration indicates that treatment is excessive. One must rely entirely on serum T_4 measurements in patients with central hypothyroidism.

How important is it to maintain normal serum TSH concentrations in a hypothyroid patient? Inadequate therapy may be associated with hypercholesterolemia, and excessive therapy with decreased bone density.[300–302,401] There is, however, no evidence of an increased risk of ischemic vascular disease in undertreated patients or of an increased fracture rate in those who are overtreated. Because these risks are largely hypothetical and because frequent changes in the dose of T_4 are inconvenient and lead to overzealous testing, the dosage should not be changed merely because a patient has a slightly abnormal serum TSH concentration at the time of a follow-up visit.

A patient who cannot take T_4 orally, for example, because of illness or an operation, need not be given T_4 for 5 to 7 days. If oral treatment cannot then be resumed, 50 to 75 percent of the usual T_4 dose should be given intravenously each day.

Other thyroid hormone preparations are avail-

TABLE 10-18 Factors Altering Thyroxine (T_4) Dosage Needed for Adequate Replacement Therapy in Hypothyroid Patients

- Decreased dosage requirement
  - Decreased T_4 clearance
    - Older age
  - Remaining autonomous thyroid tissue
    - Graves' disease
    - Toxic multinodular goiter
- Increased dosage requirement
  - Increased T_4 production
    - Pregnancy
    - Obesity
  - Decreased gastrointestinal absorption of T_4
    - Malabsorption and short bowel syndromes
    - Therapy with agents that bind T_4 in the gastrointestinal tract: sucralfate, bile acid–sequestering drugs, ferrous sulfate, aluminum hydroxide
  - Increased T_4 clearance
    - Younger age
    - Therapy with phenytoin, carbamazepine, rifampin
  - Decreased extrathyroidal T_4 conversion to T_3
    - Therapy with amiodarone
- Apparent increase in dosage requirement (pseudomalabsorption)
  - Noncompliance

Source: Refs. 417–424.

able for the treatment of hypothyroidism. They include T_3, combinations of T_4 and T_3, desiccated thyroid, and thyroglobulin. Serum T_3 concentrations fluctuate widely in patients treated with T_3, while serum T_4 remains low; similar although less marked changes occur in patients receiving the other preparations. Treatment with such preparations can be monitored with serum TSH measurements, but serum T_4 measurements greatly underestimate the dosage and low serum T_4 values often lead to excessive treatment. These preparations therefore have important disadvantages and no advantages in comparison with T_4 and should not be used.

Special Situations

Subclinical Hypothyroidism

Patients with subclinical hypothyroidism have normal serum T_4 and increased TSH concentrations and are by definition clinically euthyroid. Their increased serum TSH concentrations reflect the effects of small decreases in thyroid secretion. These decreases may be due to any of the causes of hypothyroidism (Table 10-15); the most common causes are chronic autoimmune thyroiditis, prior ^{131}I therapy for thyrotoxicosis, and iodine deficiency.

Some of these patients have thyroid enlargement and may have some nonspecific symptoms of hypothyroidism, such as fatigue and loss of energy. They may also have slightly increased serum total and LDL cholesterol and creatine kinase concentrations, diminished cardiac contractility, and decreases in hearing.[401,427–429]

Whether patients with subclinical hypothyroidism should be treated is controversial.[427] Treatment is not necessary just to forestall the development of overt hypothyroidism, because that is not inevitable and progression to it is slow (5 to 20 percent per year).[291,355] Treatment may reduce thyroid enlargement or vague symptoms if they are present. In controlled trials of T_4 therapy, these symptoms improved more during therapy with T_4 than during therapy with placebo, as did cardiac contractility in one study, but serum cholesterol concentrations changed little.[428,429] These results lead to the conclusion that T_4 therapy is indicated for patients with subclinical hypothyroidism who have thyroid enlargement or nonspecific symptoms, but not merely because their serum TSH concentrations are increased.

Thyroid Hormone Withdrawal

Patients receiving thyroid hormone therapy or their physicians may question whether the therapy is needed because documentation of hypothyroidism is not available or the hypothyroidism is thought to have been transient. Assuming that the patient's serum TSH concentration is not high, the question can be answered only by discontinuation of therapy. Normal persons recover pituitary and thyroid function within 1 month after thyroid withdrawal, although they may have symptoms of hypothyroidism and subnormal serum T_4 concentrations for a few weeks after thyroid withdrawal.[430,431] In contrast, virtually all patients who are hypothyroid develop symptoms and unequivocal biochemical evidence of the condition within 1 month.

Hypothyroidism in Newborn Infants and Children

Hypothyroidism in neonates may result in respiratory difficulty, cyanosis, persistent jaundice, umbilical hernia, lethargy, somnolence, poor feeding, hoarse crying, constipation, or the presence of large anterior or open posterior fontanels. More often, however, their appearance and behavior are normal despite severe biochemical hypothyroidism.[79,432] Because hypothyroidism during the first months of life is hard to recognize yet results in irreversible mental and physical retardation, newborn screening is now widespread; this is usually done by measuring T_4 in blood collected on filter paper in the first days of life. Permanent hypothyroidism is found in about 1 of every 4000 infants in North America; additional infants have transient hypothyroidism due to maternal antithyroid drug therapy or transplacental passage of maternal TSH inhibitory antibodies.[348,432] Properly run screening programs miss few infants later found to have hypothyroidism in the first year or so of life, indicating that it rarely develops within this period, and infants identified by screening who are treated promptly develop and grow normally.[433]

When hypothyroidism develops later in infancy or childhood, little permanent mental or physical retardation results. These older children have some form of acquired hypothyroidism, usually chronic autoimmune thyroiditis. Their symptoms and signs of hypothyroidism are similar to those in adults; they also have impaired skeletal growth and development and delayed epiphyseal maturation and dental development. Both growth hormone and insulin-like growth factor-I production are decreased.[403,434] The age of onset of hypothyroidism may be dated by determining when growth slowed from school or other records and by the appearance of the epiphyses; those formed before its onset are normal, whereas those appearing after its onset are delayed or abnormal in appearance (epiphyseal stippling). Sexual maturation in some children is accelerated, with serum gonadotropin concentrations being increased in relation to maturational if not chronologic age.[434] In other children, however, sexual maturation is delayed because gonadotropin secretion is decreased.

Hypothyroid infants and children also should be treated with T_4, with the recognition that inadequate treatment is more hazardous in these patients since it may result in some impairment of mental and physical growth even in the absence of symptoms of hypothyroidism. Since the clearance rate of T_4 is about 50 percent greater in infants and children than in adults, the dose of T_4 should be relatively higher. Doses of 0.025 to 0.05 mg T_4 daily (6 to 10 μg/kg) are usually adequate in young infants, and older children should receive 0.1 to 0.15 mg T_4 daily (3 to 6 μg/kg). Despite the more rapid turnover of T_4 in children, these doses often result in some degree of thyrotoxicosis, but it is better to err on the side of over- than undertreatment. As in adults, the goal should be normal serum TSH concentrations; the doses of T_4 that achieve this should result in serum T_4 concentrations near the upper limit of the normal range in adults.

Myxedema Coma

The development of coma in a patient with primary or central hypothyroidism constitutes a life-threatening emergency. It occurs most often in the winter in elderly patients. Coma may develop spontaneously as the end stage of severe prolonged hypothyroidism, as a result of progressive respiratory center depression and decreased cardiac output and cerebral blood flow. It also may be precipitated by cold exposure, infection, cardiovascular or respiratory disease, and inappropriate administration of narcotic and analgesic drugs.[435,436]

Patients with myxedema coma usually have overt hypothyroidism. In addition to progressive stupor and coma, nearly all have hypothermia, and they may also have seizures, hyponatremia, hypotension, hypoglycemia, and hypoventilation with hypercapnia and respiratory acidosis. The hypothermia is due to severe hypometabolism and may precede the development of coma; any situation that hastens heat loss will hasten the development of coma in these patients. Its severity may be overlooked or underestimated if the thermometer that is used does not register more than 1 to 2 degrees below normal. Hypoventilation may be caused by respiratory muscle weakness, upper airway obstruction from the large tongue, or impairment in respiratory center function. Hyponatremia and water intoxication are due to excess vasopressin secretion or a direct renal effect of thyroid hormone deficiency. Hypoglycemia suggests the presence of accompanying cortisol deficiency but may result from impaired gluconeogenesis caused by the severe hypothyroidism alone.

Patients with myxedema coma must be treated aggressively with T_4 and other measures. Blood for serum T_4, TSH, and cortisol determinations should be obtained, and T_4 should be given promptly. While the administration of large doses can be hazardous, the mortality of myxedema coma is such that aggressive therapy is justified. T_4 should be given intravenously in an initial dose of 0.3 to 0.4 mg followed by 0.1 mg daily because of the possibility of gastric retention or malabsorption. Such a large initial dose should rapidly restore the serum T_4 concentration to normal, and substantial quantities of unbound T_4 thus should be available to the tissues.[437] With the use of large doses of T_4, pulse rate, blood pressure, and temperature increase and mental status improves within 24 h.[436] T_3, which is now available for parenteral use, has been advocated because it acts more rapidly and because extrathyroidal conversion of T_4 to T_3 is decreased in such seriously ill patients. However, there is some evidence that rapid increases in serum T_3 are more likely to be accompanied by a fatal outcome.[435] Hydrocortisone or a synthetic glucocorticoid should be given intravenously, since the patient may have concomitant adrenal insufficiency due to hypopituitarism or adrenal disease or impaired ACTH or adrenal responses to stress as a result of severe primary hypothyroidism. However, most hypothermic hypothyroid patients have appropriately elevated serum cortisol concentrations.[438] Supportive therapy is as important as hormonal treatment. Ventilatory assistance may be required. Infection should be sought and treated appropriately. Fluid replacement may be needed but should be given cautiously, as insensible loss is decreased and water loads are excreted poorly. Water intoxication and hyponatremia, if present, should be treated by fluid restriction. Further heat loss should be prevented by adequate covering, but active rewarming is unwise since it may result in vasodilatation and vascular collapse. These measures result in the recovery of a substantial proportion of patients with myxedema coma.

THE PAINFUL THYROID

The thyroid is an encapsulated organ; therefore, acute thyroid enlargement results in pain and tenderness in the thyroid region. The pain may be confined to the thyroid region or referred to the ears, throat, jaws, or laterally in the neck. The thyroid diseases that cause these findings characteristically develop rapidly and include subacute thyroiditis, hemorrhage into a thyroid nodule, radiation thyroiditis, and acute (suppurative) thyroiditis. Patients with many other thyroid diseases, such as Graves' disease, chronic autoimmune thyroiditis, and thyroid carcinoma, occasionally complain of discomfort in the thyroid region and have some thyroid tenderness. However, in these patients thyroid pain and tenderness are usually mild, their illnesses (and thyroid enlargement) do not develop rapidly, and manifestations of thyroid dysfunction or a mass lesion rather than inflammation predominate. A variety of nonthyroid diseases, such as musculoskeletal disorders, pharyngeal and laryngeal inflammatory diseases, and globus hystericus, also cause neck pain and tenderness, but these disorders do not cause localized thyroid tenderness or thyroid enlargement.

Subacute Thyroiditis

Subacute thyroiditis, also known as granulomatous thyroiditis, de Quervain's thyroiditis, and acute nonsuppurative thyroiditis, is the most common cause of thyroid pain and tenderness. Its onset is usually sudden and is accompanied by malaise, myalgia, fatigue, and fever. About half of these patients have had a recent upper respiratory infection.[439] The pain typically radiates to the upper neck, ears, throat, or jaws. Slight to moderate thyroid enlargement is nearly always present; the goiter is commonly diffuse, but the enlargement, pain, and tenderness may be confined to one thyroid lobe or may shift from one lobe to the other during the course of the illness. The thyroid is usually firm in consistency and may be quite hard. Cervical lymphadenopathy is rare. Although serum T_4 and T_3 concentrations are increased in nearly all these patients, only about half have clinical manifestations of thyrotoxicosis, and they are usually overshadowed by the thyroid pain and tenderness. The thyroid pain and tenderness and thyrotoxicosis usually subside within 4 to 6 weeks, but some patients have recurrent or persistent thyroid symptoms. There may be a transient (2 to 8 weeks) period of subclinical or occasionally overt hypothyroidism after the inflammation subsides, but permanent hypothyroidism is rare.[197]

Considerable indirect evidence suggests that subacute thyroiditis is a viral illness, but conclusive proof is lacking. The disease has been associated with mumps, influenza, adenovirus, and other viral infections; small epidemics have been reported; and about 50 percent of patients have increases in titers of several antiviral antibodies after recovery.[440,441] These increases in antibody titers, however, are probably anamnestic responses rather than responses to specific infection. The disease is closely associated with the HLA-Bw35 haplotype,[197] suggesting that HLA-Bw35 molecules react uniquely with antigens from one or more viruses to initiate the thyroiditis.

Pathologically, subacute thyroiditis is characterized by disruption of thyroid follicles; infiltration of polymorphonuclear, mononuclear, and giant cells; microabscess formation; and fibrosis. This process results in thyroid follicular disruption and thyroglobulin proteolysis and therefore increased serum T_4, T_3, thyroglobulin, and iodide concentrations and increased urinary iodide excretion. Thyroid radioiodine uptake is low early in the illness as a result of the follicular damage, decreased TSH secretion, and increased serum iodide. Other common laboratory findings are mild anemia and an elevated erythrocyte sedimentation rate; leukocytosis is uncommon. Antithyroid peroxidase and antithyroglobulin antibodies may appear in the serum transiently during the latter stages of the illness or after recovery, but subacute thyroditis does not result in persistent autoimmunization.

Both the inflammatory and the thyrotoxic components of subacute thyroiditis may be so mild and transient that no therapy is necessary. More often, thyroid pain and tenderness result in sufficient discomfort to warrant anti-inflammatory therapy. Salicylates in doses of 2.4 to 3.6 g daily usually provide effective relief. Patients with severe thyroid pain and tenderness and those who do not improve rapidly with salicylates may be treated effectively with prednisone 40 to 60 mg daily. Treatment should be continued for 2 to 3 weeks and then withdrawn gradually to minimize the likelihood of recurrence. Adequate anti-inflammatory therapy not only relieves the symptoms of subacute thyroiditis but also probably reduces thyroid hormone release, thus accelerating recovery from thyrotoxicosis. The thyrotoxicosis usually requires no therapy, but propranolol in doses of 20 to 40 mg three or four times daily may be given if clinically indicated. When hypothyroidism occurs during the recovery phase, it is usually mild as well as transient and rarely requires therapy.

Hemorrhage in a Thyroid Nodule

The sudden development of pain, tenderness, and a localized thyroid mass is indicative of hemorrhage into a thyroid nodule, and the local symptoms may be accompanied by transient thyrotoxicosis.[206] The nodule may or may not have been recognized previously. The distinction between this process and subacute thyroiditis may be difficult, but findings localized to the region of a nodule and lack of the systemic manifestations of inflammatory disease and of thyrotoxicosis favor the former diagnosis. A thyroid radioisotope scan will show little isotope uptake in the region of the painful nodule but some uptake elsewhere. The pain and swelling may subside spontaneously or require needle aspiration.

Radiation Thyroiditis

Clinically important thyroiditis, with or without exacerbation of thyrotoxicosis, is an occasional complication of ^{131}I therapy for hyperthyroidism. It develops 1 to 2 weeks after therapy and then subsides spontaneously.

Suppurative Thyroiditis

Bacterial, fungal, and protozoal infections of the thyroid are rare. The routes of entry of organisms into the thyroid include the circulation, a persistent thyroglossal duct, a fistula from the piriform sinus, and direct trauma.[439,442,443] The thyroidal infection may develop acutely or gradually, depending on the organism, and usually is asymmetric. Staphylococcal, streptococcal, and anaerobic species are the organisms most commonly recovered from thyroid tissue, but mycobacteria, other bacteria, or fungi may be found; *Pneumocystis* infections have been identified in several patients with the acquired immune deficiency syndrome.[138,444]

Patients suspected of having suppurative thyroiditis should undergo immediate ultrasonography and needle aspiration of any regions that contain fluid. In patients with no evidence of systemic infection, and particularly in those with recurrent thyroid infections, a search for a piriform sinus fistula should be undertaken.

REFERENCES

1. Pankow BG, Michalak J, McGee MK: Adult human thyroid weight. *Health Phys* 49:1097, 1985.
2. Hegedus L: Thyroid size determined by ultrasound. *Dan Med Bull* 37:249, 1990.
3. Meinick JC, Stemkowski PE: Thyroid hemiagenesis (hockey stick sign): A review of the world literature and a report of four cases. *J Clin Endocrinol Metab* 52:247, 1981.
4. Ahren B: Regulatory peptides in the thyroid gland—a review on their localization and function. *Acta Endocrinol (Copenh)* 124:225, 1991.
5. Taurog A: Hormone synthesis, in Braverman LE, Utiger RD (eds): *The Thyroid: A Fundamental and Clinical Text,* 6th ed. Philadelphia, Lippincott, 1991, pp 51–97.
6. Dunn JT: Thyroglobulin: Chemistry and biosynthesis, in Braverman LE, Utiger RD (eds): *The Thyroid: A Fundamental and Clinical Text,* 6th ed. Philadelphia, Lippincott, 1991, pp 98–110.
7. Laurberg P: Mechanisms governing the relative proportions of thyroxine and 3,5,3′-triiodothyronine in thyroid secretion. *Metabolism* 33:379, 1984.
8. Van Herle AJ, Vassart G, Dumont JE: Control of thyroglobulin synthesis and secretion. *N Engl J Med* 301:239, 1979.
9. Engler D, Burger AG: The deiodination of the iodothyronines and of their derivatives in man. *Endocr Rev* 5:151, 1984.
10. Koehrle J, Hesch RD, Leonard JL: Intracellular pathways of iodothyronine metabolism, in Braverman LE, Utiger RD (eds): *The Thyroid: A Fundamental and Clinical Text,* 6th ed. Philadelphia, Lippincott, 1991, pp 144–189.
11. Berry MJ, Larsen PR: The role of selenium in thyroid hormone action. *Endocr Rev* 13:207, 1992.
12. Visser TJ, Kaptein E, Terpstra OT, Krenning EP: Deiodination of thyroid hormone by human liver. *J Clin Endocrinol Metab* 67:17, 1988.
13. Ishii H, Inada M, Tanaka K, Mashio Y, Naito K, Nishikawa M, Matsuzuka F, Kuma K, Imura H: Induction of outer and inner ring monodeiodinases in human thyroid gland by thyrotropin. *J Clin Endocrinol Metab* 57:500, 1983.
14. Izumi M, Kubo I, Taura M, Yamashita S, Morimoto I, Ohtakara S, Okamoto S, Kumagai L, et al: Kinetic study of immunoreactive human thyroglobulin. *J Clin Endocrinol Metab* 62:410, 1986.
15. Mendel CR, Weisiger RA, Jones AL, Cavalieri R: Thyroid hormone-binding proteins in plasma facilitate uniform distribution of thyroxine within tissues: A perfused rat liver study. *Endocrinology* 120:1742, 1987.
16. Robbins J: Thyroid hormone transport proteins and the physiology of hormone binding, in Braverman LE, Utiger RD (eds): *The Thyroid: A Fundamental and Clinical Text,* 6th ed. Philadelphia, Lippincott, 1991, pp 111–125.
17. Bartalena L: Recent achievements in studies on thyroid hormone-binding proteins. *Endocr* Rev 11:47, 1990.
18. Krenning EP, Docter R: Plasma membrane transport of thyroid hormone, in Henneman G (ed): *Thyroid Hormone Metabolism.* New York, Marcel Dekker, 1986, pp 107–131.
19. Mendel CR, Weisiger RA: Thyroxine uptake by perfused rat liver: No evidence for facilitation by five different thyroxine-binding proteins. *J Clin Invest* 86:1840, 1990.
20. Larsen PR, Silva JE, Kaplan MM: Relationships between circulating and intracellular thyroid hormones: Physiological and clinical implications. *Endocr Rev* 2:87, 1981.
21. Oppenheimer JH: Thyroid hormone action at the cellular level, in Braverman LE, Utiger RD (eds): *The Thyroid: A Fundamental and Clinical Text,* 6th ed. Philadelphia, Lippincott, 1991, pp 204–224.
22. Lazar MA, Chin WW: Nuclear thyroid hormone receptors. *J Clin Invest* 86:1777, 1990.
23. Brent GA, Moore DD, Larsen PR: Thyroid hormone regulation of gene expression. *Annu Rev Physiol* 53:17, 1991.
24. Strait KA, Schwartz HL, Perez-Castillo A, Oppenheimer JH: Relationship of c-erbA mRNA content to tissue triiodothyronine nuclear binding capacity and function in developing and adult rats. *J Biol Chem* 265:10514, 1990.
25. Hodin RA, Lazar MA, Chin WW: Differential and tissue-specific regulation of the multiple rat c-erbA messenger RNA species by thyroid hormone. *J Clin Invest* 85:101, 1990.
26. Lim VS, Passo C, Murata Y, Ferrari E, Nakamura H, Refetoff S: Reduced triiodothyronine content in liver but not pituitary of the uremic rat model: Demonstration of changes compatible with thyroid hormone deficiency in liver only. *Endocrinology* 114:280, 1984.
27. Grajower MM, Surks MI: Effect of decreased hepatic nuclear L-triiodothyronine receptors on the response of hepatic enzymes to L-triiodothyronine in tumor-bearing rats. *Endocrinology* 104:697, 1979.
28. Jolin T: Diabetes decreases liver and kidney nuclear 3,5,3′-triiodothyronine receptors in rats. *Endocrinology* 120:2144, 1987.
29. Davis PJ: Cellular actions of thyroid hormones, in Braverman LE, Utiger RD (eds): *The Thyroid: A Fundamental and Clinical Text,* 6th ed. Philadelphia, Lippincott, 1991, pp 190–203.
30. Guernsey DL, Edelman IS: Regulation of thyroid thermogenesis by thyroid hormones, in Oppenheimer JH, Samuels HH (eds): *Molecular Basis of Thyroid Hormone Action.* New York, Academic Press, 1983, pp 293–312.
31. Chaudhury S, Ismail-Beigi F, Gick GG, Levenson R, Edelman IS: Effect of thyroid hormone on the abundance of Na,K-adenosine triphosphatase a-subunit messenger ribonucleic acid. *Mol Endocrinol* 1:83, 1987.
32. Dillmann WH: Biochemical basis of thyroid hormone action in the heart. *Am J Med* 88:626, 1990.
33. Beylot M, Martin C, Laville M, Riou JP, Cohen R, Mornex R: Lipolytic and ketogenic fluxes in human hyperthyroidism. *J Clin Endocrinol Metab* 73:42, 1991.
34. Freake HC, Schwartz HL, Oppenheimer JH: The regulation of lipogenesis by thyroid hormone and its contribution to thermogenesis. *Endocrinology* 125:2868, 1989.
35. Sandler MP, Robinson RP, Rabin D, Lacy WW, Abumrad NN: The effect of thyroid hormones on gluconeogenesis and forearm metabolism in man. *J Clin Endocrinol Metab* 56:479, 1983.
36. Karlander S-G, Khan A, Wajngot A, Torring O, Vranic M, Efendic S: Glucose turnover in hyperthyroid patients with normal glucose tolerance. *J Clin Endocrinol Metab* 68:780, 1989.
37. Shupnik MA, Ridgway EC, Chin WW: Molecular biology of thyrotropin. *Endocr Rev* 10:459, 1989.
38. Smith TJ, Bahn RS, Gorman CA: Connective tissue, glycosaminoglycans, and diseases of the thyroid. *Endocr Rev* 10:366, 1989.
39. Levey GS: Catecholamine-thyroid hormone interactions and the cardiovascular manifestations of hyperthyroidism. *Am J Med* 88:642, 1990.
40. Bilezikian J, Loeb JN: The influence of hyperthyroidism ana hypothyroidism on α- and β-adrenergic receptor systems and adrenergic responsiveness. *Endocr Rev* 4:378, 1983.

41. Liggett SB Shah SD, Cryer PE: Increased fat and skeletal muscle β-adrenergic receptors but unaltered metabolic and hemodynamic sensitivity to epinephrine in vivo in experimental human thyrotoxicosis. *J Clin Invest* 83:803, 1989.
42. Magner JA: Thyroid-stimulating hormone: Biosynthesis, cell biology, and bioactivity. *Endocr Rev* 11:354, 1990.
43. Dyess EM, Segerson TP, Liposits Z, Paull WK, Kaplan MM, Wu P, Jackson IMD, Lechan RM: Triiodothyronine exerts direct cell-specific regulation of thyrotropin-releasing hormone gene expression in the hypothalamic paraventricular nucleus. *Endocrinology* 123:2291, 1988.
44. Sawin CT, Hershman JM, Chopra IJ: The comparative effect of T4 and T3 on the TSH response to TRH in young adult men. *J Clin Endocrinol Metab* 44:273, 1977.
45. Kubek M, Wilber JF, George JM: The distribution and concentration of thyrotropin-releasing hormone in discrete human hypothalamic nuclei. *Endocrinology* 105:537, 1979.
46. Jackson IMD: Thyrotropin-releasing hormone. *N Engl J Med* 306:145, 1982.
47. Wu P, Lechan RM, Jackson IMD: Identification and characterization of thyrotropin-releasing hormone precursor peptides in rat brain. *Endocrinology* 121:108, 1987.
48. Gershengorn MC: Mechanism of action of thyrotropin-releasing hormone. *Thyroid Today* 9:1, 1986.
49. Shulkin BL, Pruitt RE, Utiger RD: TSH and thyroidal responses to continuous and intermittent TRH administration, in Medeiros-Neto G, Gaitan E (eds): *Frontiers in Thyroidology*. New York, Plenum, 1986, pp 285–290.
50. Kaplan MM, Taft JA, Reichlin S, Munsat TL: Sustained rises in serum thyrotropin, thyroxine and triiodothyronine during long term, continuous thyrotropin-releasing hormone treatment in patients with amyotrophic lateral sclerosis. *J Clin Endocrinol Metab* 63:808, 1986.
51. Scanlon MF: Neuroendocrine control of thyrotropin secretion, in Braverman LE, Utiger RD (eds): *The Thyroid: A Fundamental and Clinical Text,* 6th ed. Philadelphia, Lippincott, 1991, pp 230–256.
52. Williams TC, Kelijman M, Crelin WC, Downs TR, Frohman LA: Differential effects of somatostatin (SRIH) and a SRIH analog, SMS 201-995, on the secretion of growth hormone and thyroid-stimulating hormone in man. *J Clin Endocrinol Metab* 66:39, 1988.
53. Brabant G, Prank K, Hoang-Vu C, Hesch RD, von zur Muhlen A: Hypothalamic regulation of pulsatile thyrotropin secretion. *J Clin Endocrinol Metab* 72:145, 1991.
54. Endo Y, Tetsumoto T, Nagasaki H, Kashiwai T, Tamaki H, Amino N, Miyai K: The distinct roles of α- and β-subunits of human thyrotropin in the receptor-binding and postreceptor events. *Endocrinology* 127;149, 1990.
55. Vassart G, Dumont JE: The thyrotropin receptor and the regulation of thyrocyte function and growth. *Endocr Rev* 13:596, 1992.
56. Huber GK, Concepcion ES, Graves PN, Davies TF: Positive regulation of human thyrotropin receptor mRNA by thyrotropin. *J Clin Endocrinol Metab* 72:1394, 1991.
57. Kawabe Y, Eguchi K, Shimomura C, Mine M, Otsubo T, Ueki Y, Tezuka H, Nakao H, et al: Interleukin-1 production and action in thyroid tissue. *J Clin Endocrinol Metab* 68:1174, 1989.
58. Sato K, Satoh T, Shizume K, Ozawa M, Han DC, Imamura H, Tsushima T, Demura H, et al: Inhibition of ^{125}I organification and thyroid hormone release by interleukin-1, tumor necrosis factor-α, and interferon-γ in human thyrocytes in suspension culture. *J Clin Endocrinol Metab* 70:1735, 1990.
59. Chanoine J-P, Safran M, Farwell AP, Tranter P, Ekenbarger DM, Dubord S, Alex S, Arthur JR, et al: Selenium deficiency and type II 5′-deiodinase regulation in the euthyroid and hypothyroid rat: Evidence of a direct effect of thyroxine. *Endocrinology* 130:479, 1992.
60. Kaplan MM, Utiger RD: Iodothyronine metabolism in rat liver homogenates. *J Clin Invest* 61:459, 1978.
61. Santini F, Chopra IJ: A radioimmunoassay of rat type I iodothyronine 5′-monodeiodinase. *Endocrinology* 131:2521, 1992.
62. Griffin JE: The dilemma of abnormal thyroid function tests—is thyroid disease present or not? *Am J Med Sci* 289:76, 1985.
63. Gavin LA, Cavalieri RR, Moeller M: Glucose and insulin reverse the effects of fasting on 3,5,3′-triiodothyronine neogenesis in primary cultures of rat hepatocytes. *Endocrinology* 121:858, 1987.
64. Danforth E, Horton ES, O'Connell M, Sims EAH, Burger AG, Ingbar SH, Braverman L, Vagenakis AG: Dietary-induced alterations in thyroid hormone metabolism during overnutrition. *J Clin Invest* 64:1336, 1979.
65. Van der Heyden JTM, Docter R, van Toor H, Wilson JHP, Henneman G, Krenning EP: Effects of caloric deprivation on thyroid hormone tissue uptake and generation of low-T_3 syndrome. *Am J Physiol* 251:E156, 1986.
66. Silva JE, Leonard JL: Regulation of rat cerebrocortical and adenohypophyseal type II 5′-deiodinase by thyroxine, triiodothyronine and reverse triiodothyronine. *Endocrinology* 116:1627, 1985.
67. Helfand M, Crapo LM: Screening for thyroid disease. *Ann Intern Med* 112:840, 1990.
68. Toft AD: Use of sensitive immunoradiometric assay for thyrotropin in clinical practice. *Mayo Clin Proc* 63:1035, 1988.
69. Nicoloff JT, Spencer CM: The use and misuse of the sensitive thyrotropin assays. *J Clin Endocrinol Metab* 71:553, 1990.
70. Ross DS, Daniels GH, Gouveia D: The use and limitations of a chemiluminescent thyrotropin assay as a single thyroid function test in an out-patient endocrine clinic. *J Clin Endocrinol Metab* 71:764, 1990.
71. Parle JV, Franklyn JA, Cross KW, Jones SC, Sheppard MC: Prevalence and follow-up of abnormal thyrotrophin (TSH) concentrations in the elderly in the United Kingdom. *Clin Endocrinol (Oxf)* 34:77, 1991.
72. Kahn BB, Weintraub BD, Csako G, Sweig MH: Factitious elevation of thyrotropin in a new ultrasensitive assay: Implications for the use of monoclonal antibodies in "sandwich" immunoassay. *J Clin Endocrinol Metab* 66:526, 1988.
73. Stockigt JR: Serum thyrotropin and thyroid hormone measurements and assessments of thyroid hormone transport, in Braverman LE, Utiger RD (eds): *The Thyroid: A Fundamental and Clinical Text,* 6th ed. Philadelphia, Lippincott, 1991, pp 463–485.
74. Brabant G, Prank K, Ranft U, Schuermeyer Th, Wagner TOF, Hauser H, Kummer B, Feistner H, et al: Physiological regulation of circadian and pulsatile thyrotropin secretion in normal man and woman. *J Clin Endocrinol Metab* 70:403, 1990.
75. Greenspan SL, Klibanski A, Rowe JW, Elahi D: Age-related alterations in pulsatile secretion of TSH: Role of dopaminergic regulation. *Am J Physiol* 260:E486, 1991.
76. Evans PJ, Weeks I, Jones MK, Woodhead JS, Scanlon MF: The circadian variation of thyrotrophin in patients with primary thyroidal disease. *Clin Endocrinol (Oxf)* 24:343, 1986.
77. Glinoer D, De Nayer P, Bourdoux P, Lemone M, Robyn C, Van Steirteghem A, Kinthaert J, Lejeune B: Regulation of maternal thyroid during pregnancy. *J Clin Endocrinol Metab* 71:276, 1990.
78. Nelson M, Wickus GG, Caplan RH, Beguin EA: Thyroid gland size in pregnancy: An ultrasound and clinical study. *J Reprod Med* 32:88, 1987.
79. Fisher DA, Klein AH: Thyroid development and disorders of thyroid function in the newborn. *N Engl J Med* 304:702, 1981.
80. Thorpe-Beeston JG, Nicolaides KH, Felton CV, Butler J, McGregor AM: Maturation of the secretion of thyroid hormone and thyroid-stimulating hormone in the fetus. *N Engl J Med* 324:532, 1991.
81. Roti E: Regulation of thyroid-stimulating hormone (TSH) secretion in the fetus and neonate. *J Endocrinol Invest* 11:145, 1988.

82. Vulsma T, Gons MH, de Vijlder JJM: Maternal-fetal transfer of thyroxine in congenital hypothyroidism due to a total organification defect or thyroid agenesis. *N Engl J Med* 321:13, 1989.
83. Calvo R, Obregon MJ, de Ona CR, Escobar del Rey F, Morreale de Escobar G: Congenital hypothyroidism, as studied in rats: Crucial role of maternal thyroxine but not of 3,5,3'-triiodothyronine in the protection of the fetal brain. *J Clin Invest* 86:889, 1990.
84. Hollingsworth DR, Alexander NM: Amniotic fluid concentrations of iodothyronines and thyrotropin do not reliably predict fetal thyroid status in pregnancies complicated by maternal thyroid disorders or anencephaly. *J Clin Endocrinol Metab* 57:349, 1983.
85. Penny R, Spencer CA, Frasier SD, Nicoloff JT: Thyroid-stimulating hormone and thyroglobulin levels decrease with chronological age in children and adolescents. *J Clin Endocrinol Metab* 56:177, 1983.
86. Fisher DA, Sack J, Oddie TH, Pekary AE, Hershman JM, Lam RW, Parslow ME: Serum T4, TBG, T3 uptake, T3, reverse T3, and TSH concentrations in children 1 to 15 years of age. *J Clin Endocrinol Metab* 45:191, 1977.
87. Tunbridge WMG, Caldwell G: The epidemiology of thyroid diseases, in Braverman LE, Utiger RD (eds): *The Thyroid: A Fundamental and Clinical Text,* 6th ed. Philadelphia, Lippincott, 1991, pp 578–587.
88. Konno N, Morikawa K: Seasonal variation of serum thyrotropin concentration and thyrotropin response to thyrotropin-releasing hormone in patients with primary hypothyroidism on constant replacement dosage of thyroxine. *J Clin Endocrinol Metab* 54:1118, 1982.
89. Solter M, Brkic K, Petek M, Posavec L, Sekso M: Thyroid hormone economy in response to extreme cold exposure in healthy factory workers. *J Clin Endocrinol Metab* 68:168, 1989.
90. Reed HL, Burman KD, Shakir KMM, O'Brien JT: Alterations in the hypothalamic-pituitary-thyroid axis after prolonged residence in Antarctica. *Clin Endocrinol (Oxf)* 25:55, 1986.
91. Ain KB, Mori Y, Refetoff S: Reduced clearance rate of thyroxine-binding globulin (TBG) with increased sialylation: A mechanism for estrogen-induced elevation of serum TBG concentration. *J Clin Endocrinol Metab* 65:689, 1987.
92. Geola FL, Frumar AM, Tataryn IV, Lu KH, Hershman JM, Eggena P, Sambhi MP, Judd HL: Biological effects of various doses of conjugated equine estrogens in postmenopausal women. *J Clin Endocrinol Metab* 51:620, 1980.
93. Mandel FP, Geola FP, Lu JKH, Eggena P, Sambhi MP, Hershman JM, Judd HL: Biologic effects of various doses of ethinyl estradiol in postmenopausal women. *Obstet Gynecol* 59:673, 1982.
94. Refetoff S: Inherited thyroxine-binding globulin abnormalities in man. *Endocr Rev* 10:275, 1989.
95. Ruiz M, Rajatanavin R, Young RA, Taylor C, Brown R, Braverman LE, Ingbar SH: Familial dysalbuminemic hyperthyroxinemia: A syndrome that can be confused with thyrotoxicosis. *N Engl J Med* 306:635, 1982.
96. Moses AC, Rosen HN, Moller DE, Tsuzaki S, Haddow JE, Lawlor J, Liepnieks JJ, Nichols WC, et al: A point mutation in transthyretin increases affinity for thyroxine and produces euthyroid hyperthyroxinemia. *J Clin Invest* 86:2025, 1990.
97. Rajatanavin R, Liberman C, Lawrence GD, D'Arcangues CM, Young RA, Emerson CH: Euthyroid hyperthyroxinemia and thyroxine-binding prealbumin excess in islet cell carcinoma. *J Clin Endocrinol Metab* 61:17, 1985.
98. Benvenga S, Trimarchi F, Robbins J: Circulating thyroid hormone antibodies. *J Endocrinol Invest* 10:605, 1987.
99. Reilly CP, Wellby ML: Slow thyroxine binding globulin in the pathogenesis of increased dialysable fraction of thyroxine in nonthyroidal illnesses. *J Clin Endocrinol Metab* 57:15, 1983.
100. Mendel CM, Laughton CW, McMahon FA, Cavalieri RR: Inability to detect an inhibitor of thyroxine-serum protein binding in sera from patients with nonthyroid illness. *Metabolism* 40:491, 1991.
101. Chopra IJ, Huang T-S, Beredo A, Solomon DH, Chua Teco GN: Serum thyroid hormone binding inhibitor in nonthyroidal illnesses. *Metabolism* 35:152, 1986.
102. Chopra IJ, Chua Teco GN, Mead JF, Huang T-S, Beredo A, Solomon DH: Relationship between serum free fatty acids and thyroid hormone binding inhibitor in nonthyroid illnesses. *J Clin Endocrinol Metab* 60:980, 1985.
103. Mendel CM, Frost PH, Cavalieri RR: Effect of free fatty acids on the concentration of free thyroxine in human serum: The role of albumin. *J Clin Endocrinol Metab* 63:1394, 1986.
104. Mendel CM, Frost PH, Kunitake ST, Cavalieri RR: Mechanism of the heparin-induced increase in the concentration of free thyroxine in plasma. *J Clin Endocrinol Metab* 65:1259, 1987.
105. Gow SM, Elder A, Caldwell G, Bell G, Seth J, Sweeting VM, Toft AD, Beckett GJ: An improved approach to thyroid function testing in patients with non-thyroidal illness. *Clin Chim Acta* 158:49, 1986.
106. Spencer CA, Eigen A, Shen D, Duda M, Qualls S, Weiss S, Nicoloff J: Specificity of sensitive assays of thyrotropin (TSH) used to screen for thyroid disease in hospitalized patients. *Clin Chem* 33:1391, 1987.
107. Kaptein EM, Weiner JM, Robinson WJ, Wheeler WS, Nicoloff JT: Relationship of altered thyroid hormone indices to survival in nonthyroidal illnesses. *Clin Endocrinol (Oxf)* 16:565, 1982.
108. Maldonado LS, Murata GH, Hershman JM, Braunstein GD: Do thyroid function tests independently predict survival in the critically ill? *Thyroid* 2:119, 1992.
109. Van der Poll T, Romijn JA, Wiersinga WM, Sauerwein HP: Tumor necrosis factor: A putative mediator of the sick euthyroid syndrome in man. *J Clin Endocrinol Metab* 71:1567, 1990.
110. Mooradian AD, Reed RL, Osterweil D, Schiffman R, Scuderi P: Decreased serum triiodothyronine is associated with increased concentrations of tumor necrosis factor. *J Clin Endocrinol Metab* 71:1239, 1990.
111. Chopra IJ, Sakane S, Chua Teco GN: A study of the serum concentration of tumor necrosis factor-α in thyroidal and nonthyroidal illnesses. *J Clin Endocrinol Metab* 72:1113, 1991.
112. Romijn JA, Wiersinga WM: Decreased nocturnal surge of thyrotropin in nonthyroidal illness. *J Clin Endocrinol Metab* 70:35, 1990.
113. Gardner DF, Kaplan MM, Stanley CA, Utiger RD: Effect of triiodothyronine replacement on the metabolic and pituitary responses to starvation. *N Engl J Med* 300:579, 1979.
114. Burman KD, Wartofsky L, Dinterman RE, Kesler P, Wannemacher RW Jr: The effect of T3 and reverse T3 administration on muscle protein catabolism during fasting as measured by 3-methyihistidine excretion. *Metabolism* 28:805, 1979.
115. Lim VS, Tsalikian E, Flanigan MJ: Augmentation of protein degradation by L-triiodothyronine in uremia. *Metabolism* 38:1210, 1989.
116. Lim VS, Henriquez C, Seo H, Refetoff S, Martino E: Thyroid function in a uremic rat model: Evidence suggesting tissue hypothyroidism. *J Clin Invest* 66:946, 1980.
117. Dillmann WH, Berry S, Alexander NM: A physiological dose of triiodothyronine normalizes cardiac myosin adenosine triphosphatase activity and changes myosin isoenzyme distribution in semistarved rats. *Endocrinology* 112:2081, 1983.
118. Kaptein EM, Spencer CA, Kamiel MB, Nicoloff JT: Prolonged dopamine administration and thyroid hormone economy in normal and critically ill subjects. *J Clin Endocrinol Metab* 51:387, 1980.
119. Surks MI, Hupart KH, Pan C, Shapiro LE: Normal free

thyroxine in critical nonthyroidal illnesses measured by ultrafiltration of undiluted serum and equilibrium dialysis. *J Clin Endocrinol Metab* 67:1031, 1988.
120. Hamblin PS, Dyer SA, Mohr VS, Le Grand BA, Lim C-F, Tuxen DV, Topliss DJ, Stockigt JR: Relationship between thyrotropin and thyroxine changes during recovery from severe hypothyroxinemia of critical illness. *J Clin Endocrinol Metab* 62:717, 1986.
121. Arem R, Deppe S: Fatal nonthyroidal illness may impair nocturnal thyrotropin levels. *Am J Med* 88:258, 1990.
122. Lee H-Y, Suhl J, Pekary AE, Hershman JM: Secretion of thyrotropin with reduced concanavalin-A-binding activity in patients with severe nonthyroid illness. *J Clin Endocrinol Metab* 65:942, 1987.
123. Pang X-P, Hershman JM, Mirell CJ, Pekary AE: Impairment of hypothalamic-pituitary-thyroid function in rats treated with human recombinant tumor necrosis factor-α (cachectin). *Endocrinology* 125:76, 1989.
124. Dubuis J-M, Dayer J-M, Siegrist-Kaiser CA, Burger AG: Human recombinant interleukin-1B decreases plasma thyroid hormone and thyroid stimulating hormone levels in rats. *Endocrinology* 123:2175, 1988.
125. Brent GA, Hershman JM: Thyroxine therapy in patients with severe nonthyroidal illnesses and low serum thyroxine concentration. *J Clin Endocrinol Metab* 63:1, 1986.
126. Brent GA, Hershman JM, Braunstein GD: Patients with severe nonthyroidal illness and serum thyrotropin concentrations in the hypothyroid range. *Am J Med* 81:463, 1986.
127. O'Brian JT, Bybee DE, Burman KD, Osburne RC, Ksiazek MR, Wartofsky L, Georges LP: Thyroid hormone homeostasis in states of relative caloric deprivation. *Metabolism* 29:721, 1980.
128. Shulkin BL, Utiger RD: Caloric restriction does not alter thyrotropin secretion in hypothyroidism. *J Clin Endocrinol Metab* 60:1076, 1985.
129. Lim VS, Fang VS, Katz AI, Refetoff S: Thyroid function in chronic renal failure: A study of the pituitary-thyroid axis and peripheral turnover kinetics of thyroxine and triiodothyronine. *J Clin Invest* 60:522, 1977.
130. Kaptein EM, Feinstein EI, Nicoloff JT, Massry SG: Serum reverse triiodothyronine and thyroxine kinetics in patients with chronic renal failure. *J Clin Endocrinol Metab* 57:181, 1983.
131. Gavin LA, McMahon FA, Castle JN, Cavalieri RR: Alterations in serum thyroid hormones and thyroxine-binding globulin in patients with nephrosis. *J Clin Endocrinol Metab* 46:125, 1978.
132. Fonseca V, Thomas M, Katrak A, Sweny P, Moorhead JF: Can urinary thyroid hormone loss cause hypothyroidism? *Lancet* 338:475, 1991.
133. Gardner DF, Carithers RL Jr, Utiger RD: Thyroid function tests in patients with acute and resolved hepatitis B virus infection. *Ann Intern Med* 96:450, 1982.
134. Salata R, Klein I, Levey GS: Thyroid hormone homeostasis and the liver. *Semin Liver Dis* 5:29, 1985.
135. LoPresti JS, Fried JC, Spencer CA, Nicoloff JT: Unique alterations of thyroid hormone indices in the acquired immunodeficiency syndrome (AIDS). *Ann Intern Med* 110:970, 1989.
136. Lambert M, Zech F, De Nayer P, Jamex J, Vandercam B: Elevation of serum thyroxine-binding globulin (but not of cortisol-binding globulin and sex hormone-binding globulin) associated with the progression of human immunodeficiency virus infection. *Am J Med* 89:748, 1990.
137. Feldt-Rasmussen U, Sestoft L, Berg H: Thyroid function tests in patients with acquired immune deficiency syndrome and healthy HIV_1-positive out-patients. *Eur J Clin Invest* 21:59, 1991.
138. Battan R, Mariuz P, Raviglione MC, Sabatini MT, Mullen MP, Poretsky L: Pneumocystis carinii infection of the thyroid in a hypothyroid patient with AIDS: Diagnosis by fine needle aspiration biopsy. *J Clin Endocrinol Metab* 72:724, 1991.
139. Kramlinger KG, Gharib H, Swanson DW, Maruta T: Normal serum thyroxine values in patients with acute psychiatric illness. *Am J Med* 76:799, 1984.
140. Chopra IJ, Solomon DH, Huang T-S: Serum thyrotropin in hospitalized psychiatric patients: Evidence for hyperthyrotropinemia as measured by an ultrasensitive thyrotropin assay. *Metabolism* 39:538, 1990.
141. Spratt DI, Pont A, Miller MB, McDougall IR, Bayer MF, McLaughlin WT: Hyperthyroxinemia in patients with acute psychiatric disorders. *Am J Med* 73:41, 1982.
142. Loosen PT: Thyroid function in affective disorders and alcoholism. *Endocrinol Metab Clin North Am* 17:55, 1988.
143. Faber J, Kirkegaard C, Rasmussen B, Westh H, Busch-Sorensen M, Jensen IW: Pituitary-thyroid axis in critical illness. *J Clin Endocrinol Metab* 65:315, 1987.
144. Benker G, Raida M, Olbricht T, Wagner R, Reinhardt W, Reinwein D: TSH secretion in Cushing syndrome: Relation to glucocorticoid excess, diabetes, goitre, and the "sick euthyroid syndrome." *Clin Endocrinol (Oxf)* 33:777, 1990.
145. Bartalena L, Martino E, Petrini L, Velluzzi F, Loviselli A, Grasso L, Mammoli C, Pinchera A: The nocturnal serum thyrotropin surge is abolished in patients with adrenocorticotropin (ACTH)-dependent or ACTH-independent Cushing's syndrome. *J Clin Endocrinol Metab* 72:1195, 1991.
146. Gamstedt A, Jarnerot G, Kagedal B: Dose related effects of betamethasone on iodothyronines and thyroid hormone-binding proteins in serum. *Acta Endocrinol (Copenh)* 96:484, 1981.
147. Williams DE, Chopra IJ, Orgiazzi J, Solomon DH: Acute effects of corticosteroids on thyroid activity in Graves' disease. *J Clin Endocrinol Metab* 41:354, 1975.
148. Burger AG: Effects of pharmacologic agents on thyroid hormone metabolism, in Braverman LE, Utiger RD (eds): *The Thyroid: A Fundamental and Clinical Text,* 6th ed. Philadelphia, Lippincott, 1991, pp 335–346.
149. Shulkin BL, Peele ME, Utiger RD: β-Adrenergic inhibition of hepatic 3′,3,5-triiodothyronine production. *Endocrinology* 115:858, 1984.
150. Saberi M, Sterling FH, Utiger RD: Reduction in extrathyroidal triiodothyronine production by propylthiouracil in man. *J Clin Invest* 55:218, 1975.
151. Chow CC, Phillips DIW, Lazarus JH, Parkes AB: Effect of low dose iodide supplementation on thyroid function in potentially susceptible subjects: Are dietary iodide levels in Britain acceptable? *Clin Endocrinol (Oxf)* 34:413, 1991.
152. Trip MD, Wiersinga W, Plomp TA: Incidence, predictability, and pathogenesis of amiodarone-induced thyrotoxicosis and hypothyroidism. *Am J Med* 91:507, 1991.
153. Perrild H, Hegedus L, Baastrup PC, Kayser L, Kastberg S: Thyroid function and ultrasonically determined thyroid size in patients receiving long-term lithium treatment. *Am J Psychiatry* 147:1518, 1990.
154. Curran PG, DeGroot LJ: The effect of hepatic enzyme-inducing drugs on thyroid hormones and the thyroid gland. *Endocr Rev* 12:135, 1991.
155. Smith PJ, Surks MI: Multiple effects of 5,5′-diphenylhydantoin on the thyroid hormone system. *Endocr Rev* 5:514, 1984.
156. Berglund J, Borup Christensen S, Hallengren B: Total and age-specific incidence of Graves' thyrotoxicosis, toxic nodular goitre and solitary toxic adenoma in Malmo 1970–74. *J Intern Med* 227:137, 1990.
157. Brownlie BEW, Wells JE: The epidemiology of thyrotoxicosis in New Zealand: Incidence and geographical distribution in North Canterbury, 1983–1985. *Clin Endocrinol (Oxf)* 33: 249, 1990.
158. Reinwein D, Benker G, Konig MP, Pinchera A, Schatz H, Schleusener A: The different types of hyperthyroidism in Europe: Results of a prospective survey of 924 patients. *J Endocrinol Invest* 11:193, 1988.
159. Kaplan MM, Utiger RD: Diagnosis of hyperthyroidism. *Clin Endocrinol Metab* 7:97, 1978.
160. Nicoloff JT, Low JC, Dussault JH, Fisher DA: Simultaneous

measurement of thyroxine and triiodothyronine peripheral turnover kinetics in man. *J Clin Invest* 51:473, 1972.

161. Caplan RH, Pagliara AS, Wickus G: Thyroxine toxicosis: A common variant of hyperthyroidism. *JAMA* 244:1934, 1980.
162. De Groot LJ, Quintans J: The causes of autoimmune thyroid disease. *Endocr Rev* 10:537, 1989.
163. Weetman AP, Yateman ME, Ealey PA, Black CM, Reimer CB, Williams RC Jr, Shine B, Marshall NJ: Thyroid-stimulating antibody activity between different immunoglobulin G subclasses. *J Clin Invest* 86:723, 1990.
164. McLachlan SM, Pegg CAS, Atherton MC, Middleton SL, Clark F, Rees Smith B: TSH receptor antibody synthesis by thyroid lymphocytes. *Clin Endocrinol (Oxf)* 24:223, 1986.
165. Rees Smith B, McLachlan SM, Furmaniak J: Autoantibodies to the thyrotropin receptor. *Endocr Rev* 9:106, 1988.
166. McKenzie JM, Zakarija M: The clinical use of thyrotropin receptor antibody measurements. *J Clin Endocrinol Metab* 69:1093, 1989.
167. Filetti S, Foti D, Costante G, Rapoport B: Recombinant human thyrotropin (TSH) receptor in a radioreceptor assay for the measurement of TSH receptor autoantibodies. *J Clin Endocrinol Metab* 72:1096, 1992.
168. Sugenoya A, Kobayashi S, Kasuga Y, Masuda H, Fujimori M, Komatsu M, Takahashi S, Yokoyama S, et al: Evidence of intrathyroidal accumulation of TSH receptor antibody in Graves' disease. *Acta Endocrinol (Copenh)* 126:416, 1992.
169. Zakarija M, Jin S, McKenzie JM: Evidence supporting the identity in Graves' disease of thyroid-stimulating antibody and thyroid growth-promoting immunoglobulin G as assayed in FRTL5 cells. *J Clin Invest* 81:879, 1988.
170. Dumont JE, Roger PP, Ludgate M: Assays for thyroid growth immunoglobulins and their clinical implications: Methods, concepts, and misconceptions. *Endocr Rev* 8:448, 1987.
171. Zakarija M, McKenzie JM: Do thyroid growth-promoting immunoglobulins exist? *J Clin Endocrinol Metab* 70:308, 1990.
172. De Bruin TWA, Bussemaker JK, Heidema J, Hermans J, van der Heide D: Thyrotropin (TSH) receptor modulation by specific TSH receptor antibodies in Graves' disease. *J Clin Endocrinol Metab* 67:676, 1988.
173. Kasuga Y, Matsubayashi S, Akasu F, Miller N, Jamieson C, Volpe R: Effects of recombinant human interleukin-2 and tumor necrosis factor-α with or without interferon-γ on human thyroid tissues from patients with Graves' disease and from normal subjects xenografted into nude mice. *J Clin Endocrinol Metab* 72:1296, 1991.
174. Migita K, Eguchi K, Otsubo T, Kawakami A, Nakao H, Ueki Y, Shimomura C, Kurata A, et al: Cytokine regulation of HLA on thyroid epithelial cells. *Clin Exp Immunol* 82:548, 1990.
175. Heufelder AE, Goellner JR, Wenzel BE, Bahn RS: Immunohistochemical detection and localization of a 72-kilodalton heat shock protein in autoimmune thyroid disease. *J Clin Endocrinol Metab* 74:724, 1992.
176. Iitaka M, Aguayo JF, Iwatani Y, Row VV, Volpe R: Studies of the effect of suppressor T lymphocytes on the induction of antithyroid microsomal antibody-secreting cells in autoimmune thyroid disease. *J Clin Endocrinol Metab* 66:708, 1988.
177. Hashizume K, Ichikawa K, Sakurai A, Suzuki S, Takeda T, Kobayashi M, Miyamoto T, Arai M, et al: Administration of thyroxine in treated Graves' disease: Effects on the level of antibodies to thyroid-stimulating hormone receptors and on the risk of recurrence of hyperthyroidism. *N Engl J Med* 324:947, 1991.
178. Volpe R, Karlsson A, Jansson R, Dahlberg PA: Evidence that antithyroid drugs induce remissions in Graves' disease by modulating thyroid cellular activity. *Clin Endocrinol (Oxf)* 25:453, 1986.
179. Roman SH, Greenberg D, Rubinstein P, Wallenstein S, Davies TF: Genetics of autoimmune thyroid disease: Lack of evidence for linkage to HLA within families. *J Clin Endocrinol Metab* 74:496, 1992.
180. Prummel M, Wiersinga WM: Smoking and risk of Graves' disease. *JAMA* 269:479, 1993.
181. Gray J, Hoffenberg R: Thyrotoxicosis and stress. *Q J Med* 54:153, 1985.
182. Winsa B, Adami H-O, Bergstrom R, Gamstedt A, Dahlberg PA, Adamson U, Jansson R, Karlsson A: Stressful life events and Graves' disease. *Lancet* 338:1475, 1991.
183. Ebner SA, Badonnel M-C, Altman LA, Braverman LE: Conjugal Graves' disease. *Ann Intern Med* 116:479, 1992.
184. Schleusener H, Schwander J, Fischer C, Holle R, Holl G, Badenhoop K, Hensen J, Finke R, et al: Prospective multicentre study on the prediction of relapse after antithyroid drug treatment in patients with Graves' disease. *Acta Endocrinol (Copenh)* 120:689, 1989.
185. Tamai HT, Nakagawa T, Fukino O, Ohsako N, Shinzato R, Suematsu H, Kuma K, Matsuzuka F, et al: Thionamide therapy in Graves' disease: Relation of relapse rate to duration of therapy. *Ann Intern Med* 92:488, 1980.
186. Allannic H, Fauchet R, Orgiazzi J, Madec AM, Genetet B, Lorcy Y, Le Guerrier AM, Delambre C, Derennes V: Antithyroid drugs and Graves' disease: A prospective randomized evaluation of the efficacy of treatment duration. *J Clin Endocrinol Metab* 70:675, 1990.
187. Davies TF, Yang C, Platzer M: The influence of antithyroid drugs and iodine on thyroid cell MHC class II antigen expression. *Clin Endocrinol (Oxf)* 31:125, 1989.
188. Murakami M, Koizumi Y, Aizawa T, Yamada T, Takahashi Y, Watanabe T, Kamoi K: Studies of thyroid function and immune parameters in patients with hyperthyroid Graves' disease in remission. *J Clin Endocrinol Metab* 66:103, 1988.
189. Tamai H, Kasagi K Takaichi Y, Takamatsu J, Komaki G, Matsubayashi S, Konishi J, Kuma K, et al: Development of spontaneous hypothyroidism in patients with Graves' disease treated with antithyroidal drugs: Clinical, immunological, and histological findings in 26 patients. *J Clin Endocrinol Metab* 69:49, 1989.
190. Takasu N, Yamada T, Sato A, Nakagawa M, Komiya I, Nagasawa Y, Asawa T: Graves' disease following hypothyroidism due to Hashimoto's disease: Studies of eight cases. *Clin Endocrinol (Oxf)* 33:687, 1990.
191. Weetman AP: Thyroid-associated eye disease: Pathophysiology. *Lancet* 338:25, 1991.
192. Bahn RS, Heufelder AE: Retroocular fibroblasts: Important effector cells in Graves' ophthalmopathy. *Thyroid* 2:89, 1992.
193. Hiromatsu Y, Fukazawa H, Wall JR: Cytotoxic mechanisms in autoimmune thyroid disorders and thyroid-associated ophthalmopathy. *Endocrinol Metab Clin North Am* 16:269, 1987.
194. Bahn RS, Gorman CA, Johnson CM, Smith TJ: Presence of antibodies in the sera of patients with Graves' disease recognizing a 23 kilodalton fibroblast protein. *J Clin Endocrinol Metab* 69:622, 1989.
195. Heufelder AE, Smith TJ, Gorman CA, Bahn RS: Increased induction of HLA-DR by interferon-γ in cultured fibroblasts derived from patients with Graves' ophthalmopathy and pretibial dermopathy. *J Clin Endocrinol Metab* 73:307, 1991.
196. Shishiba Y, Imai Y, Odajima R, Ozawa Y, Shimizu T: Immunoglobulin G of patients with circumscribed pretibial myxedema of Graves' disease stimulates proteoglycan synthesis in human skin fibroblasts in culture. *Acta Endocrinol (Copenh)* 127:44, 1992.
197. Nikolai TF: Silent thyroiditis and subacute thyroiditis, in Braverman LE, Utiger RD (ed): *The Thyroid: A Fundamental and Clinical Text*, 6th ed. Philadelphia, Lippincott, 1991, pp 710–727.
198. Litovitz TL, White JD: Levothyroxine ingestions in children: An analysis of 78 cases. *Am J Emerg Med* 3:297, 1985.
199. Gorman CA, Wahner HW, Tauxe WH: Metabolic malingerers. *Am J Med* 48:708, 1970.
200. Hedberg CW, Fishbein DB, Janssen RS, Meyers B, McMillen

JM, MacDonald KL, White KE, Huss LJ, et al: An outbreak of thyrotoxicosis caused by the consumption of bovine thyroid gland in ground beef. *N Engl J Med* 316:993, 1987.

201. Kinney JS, Hurwitz ES, Fishbein DB, Woolf PD, Pinsky PF, Lawrence DN, Anderson LJ, Holmes GP, et al: Community outbreak of thyrotoxicosis: Epidemiology, immunogenetic characteristics, and long-term outcome. *Am J Med* 84:10, 1988.
202. Fradkin JE, Wolff J: Iodide-induced thyrotoxicosis. *Medicine (Baltimore)* 62:1, 1984.
203. Berghout A, Wiersinga WM, Smits NJ, Touber JL: Interrelationships between age, thyroid volume, thyroid nodularity and thyroid function in patients with sporadic nontoxic goiter. *Am J Med* 89:602, 1990.
204. Studer H, Gerber H: Pathogenesis of nontoxic diffuse and nodular goiter, in Braverman LE, Utiger RD (eds): *The Thyroid: A Fundamental and Clinical Text,* 6th ed. Philadelphia, Lippincott, 1991, pp 1107–1113.
205. Hamburger JI: Evolution of toxicity in solitary nontoxic autonomously functioning thyroid nodules. *J Clin Endocrinol Metab* 50:1089, 1980.
206. Hamburger JI, Taylor CL: Transient thyrotoxicosis associated with acute hemorrhagic infarction of autonomously functioning thyroid nodules. *Ann Intern Med* 91:406, 1979.
207. Lazarus JH, Richards AR, MacPherson MJ, Dinnen JS, Williams ED, Owen GM, Wade JSH: Struma ovarii: A case report. *Clin Endocrinol (Oxf)* 27:715, 1987.
208. Gesundheit N, Petrick PA, Nissim M, Dahlberg PA, Doppman JL, Emerson CH, Braverman LE, Oldfield EH, et al: Thyrotropin-secreting pituitary adenomas: Clinical and biochemical heterogeneity. *Ann Intern Med* 111:827, 1989.
209. Beck-Peccoz P, Mariotti S, Guillausseau PJ, Medri G, Piscitelli G, Bertoli A, Barbarino A, Rondena M, et al: Treatment of hyperthyroidism due to inappropriate secretion of thyrotropin with the somatostatin analog SMS 201-995. *J Clin Endocrinol Metab* 68:208, 1989.
210. Magner J, Klibanski A, Fein H, Smallridge R, Blackard W, Young W Jr, Ferriss JB, Murphy D, et al: Ricin and lentil lectin-affinity chromatography reveals oligosaccharide heterogeneity of thyrotropin secreted by 12 human pituitary tumors. *Metabolism* 41:1009, 1992.
211. Kennedy RL, Sheridan E, Darne J, Griffiths H, Davies R, Price A, Cohn M: Thyroid function in choriocarcinoma: Demonstration of a thyroid-stimulating activity in serum using FRTL-5 and human thyroid cells. *Clin Endocrinol (Oxf)* 33:227, 1990.
212. Oddie TH, Boyd CM, Fisher DA, Hales IB: Incidence of signs and symptoms in thyroid disease. *Med J Aust* 2:981, 1972.
213. Vaidya VA, Bongiovanni AM, Parks JS, Tenore A, Kirkland RT: Twenty-two years' experience in the medical management of juvenile thyrotoxicosis. *Pediatrics* 54:565, 1974.
214. Crooks J, Murray IPC, Wayne EJ: Statistical methods applied to the clinical diagnosis of thyrotoxicosis. *Q J Med* 28:211, 1959.
215. Davis PJ, Davis FB: Hyperthyroidism in patients over the age of 60 years. *Medicine (Baltimore)* 53:161, 1974.
216. Nordyke RA, Gilbert FI Jr, Harada ASM: Graves' disease: Influence of age on clinical findings. *Arch Intern Med* 148:626, 1988.
217. Parker JLW, Lawson DH: Death from thyrotoxicosis. *Lancet* 2:894, 1973.
218. Greenwood RM, Daly JG, Himsworth RL: Hyperthyroidism and the impalpable thyroid gland. *Clin Endocrinol (Oxf)* 22:583, 1985.
219. Zurcher RM, Horber FF, Grunig BE, Frey FJ: Effect of thyroid dysfunction on thigh muscle efficiency. *J Clin Endocrinol Metab* 69:1082, 1989.
220. Olson BR, Klein I, Benner R, Burdett R, Trzepacz P, Levey GS: Hyperthyroid myopathy and the response to treatment. *Thyroid* 1:137, 1991.
221. Ober KP: Thyrotoxic periodic paralysis in the United States: Report of 7 cases and review of the literature. *Medicine (Baltimore)* 71:109, 1992.
222. Klein I: Thyroid hormone and the cardiovascular system. *Am J Med* 88:631, 1990.
223. Ladenson PW: Recognition and management of cardiovascular disease related to thyroid dysfunction. *Am J Med* 88:638, 1990.
224. Woeber KA: Thyrotoxicosis and the heart. *N Engl J Med* 327:94, 1992.
225. Das KC, Mukherjee M, Sarkar TK, Dash RJ, Rastogi GK: Erythropoiesis and erythropoietin in hypo- and hyperthyroidism. *J Clin Endocrinol Metab* 40:211, 1975.
226. Kendrick AH, O'Reilly JF, Laszlo GA: Lung function and exercise performance in hyperthyroidism before and after treatment. *Q J Med* 68:615, 1988.
227. White NW, Raine RI, Bateman ED: Asthma and hyperthyroidism: A report of 4 cases. *S Afr Med J* 78:750, 1990.
228. Ford HC, Lim WC, Chisnall WN, Pearce JM: Renal function and electrolyte levels in hyperthyroidism: Urinary protein excretion and the plasma concentrations of urea, creatinine, uric acid, hydrogen ion and electrolytes. *Clin Endocrinol (Oxf)* 30:293, 1989.
229. Rolandi E, Santaniello B, Bagnasco M, Cataldi A, Garibaldi C, Franceschini R, Barreca T: Thyroid hormones and atrial natriuretic hormone secretion: Study in hyper- and hypothyroid patients. *Acta Endocrinol (Copenh)* 127:23, 1992.
230. Hauger-Klevene JH, Brown H, Zavaleta J: Plasma renin activity in hyper- and hypothyroidism: Effect of adrenergic blocking agents. *J Clin Endocrinol Metab* 34:625, 1972.
231. Cain JP, Dluhy RG, Williams GH, Selenkow HA, Milech A, Richmond S: Control of aldosterone secretion in hyperthyroidism. *J Clin Endocrinol Metab* 36:365, 1973.
232. Harvey JN, Nagi DK, Baylis PH, Wilkinson R, Belchetz PE: Disturbance of osmoregulated thirst and vasopressin secretion in thyrotoxicosis. *Clin Endocrinol (Oxf)* 35:29, 1991.
233. Wegener W, Wedmann B, Langhoff T, Schaffstein J, Adamek R: Effect of hyperthyroidism on the transit of a calorie solid-liquid meal through the stomach, the small intestine, and the colon in man. *J Clin Endocrinol Metab* 75:745, 1992.
234. Harper MB: Vomiting, nausea and abdominal pain: Unrecognized symptoms of thyrotoxicosis. *J Fam Pract* 29:382, 1989.
235. Reddy J, Brownlie BEW, Heaton DC, Hamer JW, Turner JG: The peripheral blood picture in thyrotoxicosis. *N Z Med J* 93:143, 1981.
236. Hymes K, Blum M, Lackner H, Karpatkin S: Easy bruising, thrombocytopenia, and elevated platelet immunoglobulin G in Graves' disease and Hashimoto's thyroiditis. *Ann Intern Med* 94:27, 1981.
237. Hoogwerf BJ, Nuttal FQ: Long-term weight regulation in treated hyperthyroid and hypothyroid subjects. *Am J Med* 76:963, 1984.
238. Shen D-C, Davidson MB, Kuo S-W, Sheu WH-H: Peripheral and hepatic insulin antagonism in hyperthyroidism. *J Clin Endocrinol Metab* 66:565, 1988.
239. Cooppan R, Kozak GP: Hyperthyroidism and diabetes mellitus: An analysis of 70 patients. *Arch Intern Med* 140:370, 1980.
240. Heimberg M, Olubadewo JO, Wilcox HG: Plasma lipoproteins and regulation of hepatic metabolism of fatty acids in altered thyroid states. *Endocr Rev* 6:590, 1985.
241. Graninger W, Pirich KR, Speiser W, Deutsch E, Waldhausl WK: Effect of thyroid hormones on plasma protein concentrations in man. *J Clin Endocrinol Metab* 63:407, 1986.
242. O'Connor P, Feely J: Clinical pharmacokinetics and endocrine disorders: Therapeutic implications. *Clin Pharmacokinet* 13:345, 1987.
243. Iranmanesh A, Lizarralde G, Johnson ML, Veldhuis JD: Nature of altered growth hormone secretion in hyperthyroidism. *J Clin Endocrinol Metab* 72:108, 1991.
244. Akande ED, Hockaday TDR: Plasma concentration of gonadotrophins, oestrogen, and progesterone in thyrotoxic women. *Br J Obstet Gynaecol* 92:541, 1975.

245. Aoki N, Maruyama Y, Imamura M, Ohno Y, Saika T, Yamamoto T, Suzuki Y, Sinohara H: Studies of sex hormone-binding plasma protein (SBP) in Graves' disease before and under antithyroid drug therapy. *Acta Endocrinol (Copenh)* 113:249, 1986.
246. Hudson RW, Edwards AL: Testicular function in hyperthyroidism. *J Androl* 13:117, 1992.
247. Benker G, Breuer N, Windeck R, Reinwein D: Calcium metabolism in thyroid disease. *J Endocrinol Invest* 11:61, 1988.
248. Lee MS, Kim SY, Lee MC, Cho BY, Lee HK, Koh C-S, Min HK: Negative correlation between the change in bone mineral density and serum osteocalcin in patients with hyperthyroidism. *J Clin Endocrinol Metab* 70:766, 1990.
249. Daly JG, Greenwood RM, Himsworth RL: Serum calcium concentration in hyperthyroidism at diagnosis and after treatment. *Clin Endocrinol (Oxf)* 19:397, 1983.
250. Trzepacz PT, Klein I, Roberts M, Greenhouse J, Levey GS: Graves' disease: An analysis of thyroid hormone levels and hyperthyroid signs and symptoms. *Am J Med* 87:558, 1989.
251. Sawin CT, Geller A, Kaplan MM, Bacharach P, Wilson PWF, Hershman JM: Low serum thyrotropin (thyroid-stimulating hormone) in older persons without hyperthyroidism. *Arch Intern Med* 151:165, 1991.
252. Sundbeck G, Jagenburg R, Johansson P-M, Eden S, Lindstedt G: Clinical significance of low serum thyrotropin concentration by chemiluminometric assay in 85-year-old women and men. *Arch Intern Med* 151:549, 1991.
253. Aizawa T, Ishihara M, Hashizume K, Takasu N, Yamada T: Age-related changes of thyroid function and immunologic abnormalities in patients with hyperthyroidism due to Graves' disease. *J Am Geriatr Soc* 37:944, 1989.
254. Wartofsky L, Glinoer D, Solomon B, Nagataki S, Lagasse R, Nagayama Y, Izumi M: Differences and similarities in the diagnosis and treatment of Graves' disease in Europe, Japan, and the United States. *Thyroid* 1:129, 1991.
255. Hedley AJ, Young RE, Jones SJ, Alexander WD, Bewsher PD, and Scottish Automated Follow-up Register Group: Antithyroid drugs in the treatment of hyperthyroidism of Graves' disease: Long-term follow-up of 434 patients. *Clin Endocrinol (Oxf)* 31:209, 1989.
256. Young ET, Steel NR, Taylor JJ, Stephenson AM, Stratton A, Holcombe M, Kendall-Taylor P: Prediction of remission after antithyroid drug treatment in Graves' disease. *Q J Med* 66:175, 1988.
257. Lippe BM, Landaw EM, Kaplan SA: Hyperthyroidism in children treated with long term medical therapy: Twenty-five percent remission every two years. *J Clin Endocrinol Metab* 64:1241, 1987.
258. Orgiazzi J: Management of Graves' hyperthyroidism. *Endocrinol Metab Clin North Am* 16:365, 1987.
259. Kampmann JP, Hansen JM: Clinical pharmacokinetics of antithyroid drugs. *Clin Pharmacokinet* 6:401, 1981.
260. Cooper DS: Antithyroid drugs. *N Engl J Med* 311:1353, 1984.
261. Jansson R, Dahlberg PA, Johansson H, Lindstrom B: Intrathyroidal concentrations of methimazole in patients with Graves' disease. *J Clin Endocrinol Metab* 57:129, 1983.
262. McGregor AM, Petersen MM, McLachlan SM, Rooke P, Smith BR, Hall R: Carbimazole and the autoimmune response in Graves' disease. *N Engl J Med* 303:302, 1980.
263. Romaldini JH, Bromberg N, Werner RS, Tanaka LM, Rodrigues HF, Werner MC, Farah CS, Reis LCF: Comparison of effects of high and low dosage regimens of antithyroid drugs in the management of Graves' hyperthyroidism. *J Clin Endocrinol Metab* 57:563, 1983.
264. Shiroozu A, Okamura K, Ikenoue H, Sato K, Nakashima T, Yoshinari M, Fujishima M, Yoshizumi T: Treatment of hyperthyroidism with a small single daily dose of methimazole. *J Clin Endocrinol Metab* 63:125, 1986.
265. Messina M, Milani P, Gentile L, Monaco A, Brossa C, Porta M, Camanni F: Initial treatment of thyrotoxic Graves' disease with methimazole: A randomized trial comparing different dosages. *J Endocrinol Invest* 10:291, 1987.
266. Gwinup G: Prospective randomized comparison of propylthiouracil. *JAMA* 239:2457, 1978.
267. Okamura K, Ikenoue H, Shiroozu A, Sato K, Yoshinari M, Fujishima M: Reevaluation of the effects of methylmercaptoimidazole and propylthiouracil in patients with Graves' hyperthyroidism. *J Clin Endocrinol Metab* 65:719, 1987.
268. Cooper DS: Propylthiouracil levels in hyperthyroid patients unresponsive to large doses: Evidence of poor patient compliance. *Ann Intern Med* 102:328, 1985.
269. Takamatsu J, Sugawara M, Kuma K, Kobayashi A, Matsuzuka F, Mozai T, Hershman JM: Ratio of serum triiodothyronine to thyroxine and the prognosis of triiodothyronine-predominant Graves' disease. *Ann Intern Med* 100:372, 1984.
270. Bouma DJ, Kammer H, Greer MA: Follow-up comparison of short-term versus one year antithyroid drug therapy for the thyrotoxicosis of Graves' disease. *J Clin Endocrinol Metab* 55:1138, 1982.
271. Slingerland DW, Burrows BA: Long-term antithyroid treatment in hyperthyroidism. *JAMA* 242:2408, 1979.
272. International Agranulocytosis and Aplastic Anaemia Study: Risk of agranulocytosis and aplastic anaemia in relation to use of antithyroid drugs. *Br Med J* 297:262, 1988.
273. Tamai H, Takaichi Y, Morita T, Komaki G, Matsubayashi S, Kuma K, Walter RM Jr, Kumagai LF, et al: Methimazole-induced agranulocytosis in Japanese patients with Graves' disease. *Clin Endocrinol (Oxf)* 30:525, 1989.
274. Cooper DS, Goldminz D, Levin AA, Ladenson PW, Daniels GH, Molitch ME, Ridgway EC: Agranulocytosis associated with antithyroid drugs: Effects of patient age and drug dose. *Ann Intern Med* 98:26, 1983.
275. Tajiri J, Noguchi S, Murakami T, Murakami N: Antithyroid drug-induced agranulocytosis: The usefulness of routine white blood cell count monitoring. *Arch Intern Med* 150:621, 1990.
276. Heinrich B, Gross M, Goebel FD: Methimazole-induced agranulocytosis and granulocyte-colony stimulating factor. *Ann Intern Med* 111:621, 1989.
277. Cooper DS: Which antithyroid drug? *Am J Med* 80:1165, 1986.
278. Philippou G, Koutras DA, Piperingos G, Souvatzoglou A, Moulopoulos SD: The effect of iodide on serum thyroid hormone levels in normal persons, in hyperthyroid patients, and in hypothyroid patients on thyroxine replacement. *Clin Endocrinol (Oxf)* 36:573, 1992.
279. Shen D-C, Wu S-Y, Chopra IJ, Huang H-W, Shian L-R, Bian T-Y, Jeng C-Y, Solomon DH: Long term treatment of Graves' hyperthyroidism with sodium ipodate. *J Clin Endocrinol Metab* 61:723, 1985.
280. Wang Y-S, Tsou C-T, Lin W-H, Hershman JM: Long term treatment of Graves' disease with iopanoic acid (Telepaque). *J Clin Endocrinol Metab* 65:679, 1987.
281. Kristensen O, Andersen HH, Pallisgaard G: Lithium carbonate in the treatment of thyrotoxicosis: A controlled trial. *Lancet* 1:603, 1976.
282. Reichert LJM, de Rooy HAM: Treatment of amiodarone induced hyperthyroidism with potassium perchlorate and methimazole during amiodarone treatment. *Br Med J* 298:1547, 1989.
283. Klein I, Trzepacz PT, Roberts M, Levey GS: Symptom rating scale for assessing hyperthyroidism. *Arch Intern Med* 148:387, 1988.
284. Codaccioni JL, Orgiazzi J, Blanc P, Pugeat M, Roulier R, Carayon P: Lasting remissions in patients treated for Graves' hyperthyroidism with propranolol alone: A pattern of spontaneous evolution of the disease. *J Clin Endocrinol Metab* 67:656, 1988.
285. Kvetny J, Frederikesen PK, Jacobsen JG, Haas V, Feldt-Rasmussen U, Date J: Propranolol in the treatment of thyrotoxicosis: A randomized double-blind study. *Acta Med Scand* 209:389, 1981.
286. Ross DS, Daniels GH, De Stefano P, Maloof F, Ridgway EC: Use of adjunctive potassium iodide after radioactive iodine

(^{131}I) treatment of Graves' hyperthyroidism. *J Clin Endocrinol Metab* 57:250, 1983.
287. Nordyke RA, Gilbert FI Jr: Optimal iodine-131 dose for eliminating hyperthyroidism in Graves' disease. *J Nucl Med* 32:411, 1991.
288. Sridama V, McCormick M, Kaplan EL, Fauchet R, DeGroot LJ: Long-term follow-up study of compensated low-dose ^{131}I therapy for Graves' disease. *N Engl J Med* 311:426, 1984.
289. Cunnien AJ, Hay ID, Gorman CA, Offord KP, Scanlon PW: Radioiodine-induced hypothyroidism in Graves' disease: Factors associated with the increasing incidence. *J Nucl Med* 23:978, 1982.
290. Franklyn JA, Daykin J, Droic Z, Farmer M, Sheppard MC: Long-term follow-up of treatment of thyrotoxicosis by three different methods. *Clin Endocrinol (Oxf)* 34:71, 1991.
291. Davies PH, Franklyn JA, Daykin J, Sheppard MC: The significance of TSH values measured in a sensitive assay in the follow-up of hyperthyroid patients treated with radioiodine. *J Clin Endocrinol Metab* 74:1189, 1992.
292. Graham GD, Burman KD: Radioiodine treatment for Graves' disease: An assessment of its potential risks. *Ann Intern Med* 105:900, 1986.
293. Holm L-E, Hall P, Wiklund K, Lundell G, Berg G, Bjelkengren G, Cederquist E, Ericsson U-B, et al: Cancer risk after iodine-131 therapy for hyperthyroidism. *JNCI* 83:1072, 1991.
294. Hall P, Boice JD Jr, Berg G, Bjelkengren G, Ericsson U-B, Hallquist A, Lidberg M, Lundell G, et al: Leukaemia incidence after iodine-131 exposure. *Lancet* 340:1, 1992.
295. Peek CM, Sawers JSA, Irvine WJ, Beckett GJ, Ratcliffe WA, Toft AD: Combination of potassium iodide and propranolol in preparation of patients with Graves' disease for thyroid surgery. *N Engl J Med* 302:883, 1980.
296. Maier WP, Derrick BM, Marks AD, Channick BJ, Au FC, Caswell HT: Long-term follow-up of patients with Grave's disease treated by subtotal thyroidectomy. *Am J Surg* 147:266, 1984.
297. Nikolai TF, Coombs GJ, McKenzie AK, Miller RW, Weir J Jr: Treatment of lymphocytic thyroiditis with spontaneously resolving hyperthyroidism (silent thyroiditis). *Arch Intern Med* 142:2281, 1982.
298. Kinser JA, Roesler H, Furrer T, Grutter D, Zimmermann H: Nonimmunogenic hyperthyroidism: Cumulative hypothyroidism incidence after radioiodine and surgical treatment. *J Nucl Med* 30:1960, 1989.
299. Hamburger JI: The autonomously functioning thyroid nodule: Goetsch's disease. *Endocr Rev* 8:439, 1987.
300. Greenspan SL, Greenspan FS, Resnick NM, Block JE, Friedlander AL, Genant HK: Skeletal integrity in premenopausal and postmenopausal women receiving long-term L-thyroxine therapy. *Am J Med* 91:5, 1991.
301. Franklyn JA, Betteridge J, Daykin J, Holder R, Oates GD, Parle JV, Lilley J, Heath DA, et al: Long-term thyroxine treatment and bone mineral density. *Lancet* 340:9, 1992.
302. Ross DS: Subclinical hyperthyroidism, in Braverman LE, Utiger RD (eds): *The Thyroid: A Fundamental and Clinical Text,* 6th ed. Philadelphia, Lippincott, 1991, pp 1249–1255.
303. Verelst J, Bonnyns M, Glinoer D: Radioiodine therapy in voluminous multinodular non-toxic goitre. *Acta Endocrinol (Copenh)* 122:417, 1990.
304. Livraghi T, Paracchi A, Ferrari C, Bergonzi M, Garavaglia G, Raineri P, Vettori C: Treatment of autonomous thyroid nodules with percutaneous ethanol injection: Preliminary results. *Radiology* 175:827, 1990.
305. McDermott MT, Kidd GS, Dodson LE Jr, Hofeldt FD: Radioiodine-induced thyroid storm: Case report and literature review. *Am J Med* 75:353, 1983.
306. Amino N, Tanizawa O, Mori H, Iwatani Y, Yamada T, Kurachi K, Kumahara Y, Miyai K: Aggravation of thyrotoxicosis in early pregnancy and after delivery in Graves' disease. *J Clin Endocrinol Metab* 55:108, 1982.
307. Davis LE, Lucas MJ, Hankins CDV, Roark ML, Cunningham FG: Thyrotoxicosis complicating pregnancy. *Am J Obstet Gynecol* 160:63, 1989.
308. Momotani N, Ito K, Hamada N, Ban Y, Nishikawa Y, Mimura T: Maternal hyperthyroidism and congenital malformation in the offspring. *Clin Endocrinol (Oxf)* 20:695, 1984.
309. Cove DH, Johnston P: Fetal hyperthyroidism: Experience of treatment in four siblings. *Lancet* 1:430, 1985.
310. Page DV, Brady K, Mitchell J, Pehrson J, Wade G: The pathology of intrauterine thyrotoxicosis: Two case reports. *Obstet Gynecol* 72:479, 1988.
311. Wenstrom KD, Weiner CP, Williamson RA, Grant SS: Prenatal diagnosis of fetal hyperthyroidism using funipuncture. *Obstet Gynecol* 76:513, 1990.
312. Goodwin TM, Montoro M, Mestman JH: Transient hyperthyroidism and hyperemesis gravidarum: Clinical aspects. *Am J Obstet Gynecol* 167:648, 1992.
313. Momotani N, Noh J, Oyanagi H, Ishikawa N, Ito K: Antithyroid drug therapy for Graves' disease during pregnancy: Optimal regimen for fetal thyroid status. *N Engl J Med* 315:24, 1986.
314. Refetoff S, Ochi Y, Selenkow HA, Rosenfield RL: Neonatal hypothyroidism and goiter in one infant of each of two sets of twins due to maternal therapy with antithyroid drugs. *J Pediatr* 85:240, 1974.
315. Khoury MJ, Becerra JE, d'Almada PJ: Maternal thyroid disease and risk of birth defects in offspring. A population-based case-control study. *Pediatr Perinat Epidemiol* 3:402, 1989.
316. Messer PM, Hauffa BP, Olbricht T, Benker G, Kotulla P, Reinwein D: Antithyroid drug treatment of Graves' disease in pregnancy: Long-term effects on somatic growth, intellectual development and thyroid function of the offspring. *Acta Endocrinol (Copenh)* 123:311, 1990.
317. Momotani N, Hisaoka T, Noh J, Ishikawa N, Ito K: Effects of iodine on thyroid status of fetus versus mother in treatment of Graves' disease complicated by pregnancy. *J Clin Endocrinol Metab* 75:738, 1992.
318. Sherif IH, Oyan WT, Bosairi S, Carrascal SM: Treatment of hyperthyroidism in pregnancy. *Acta Obstet Gynecol Scand* 70:461, 1991.
319. Cooper DS: Antithyroid drugs: To breast-feed or not to breast-feed. *Am J Obstet Gynecol* 157:234, 1987.
320. Momotani N, Yamashita R, Yoshimoto M, Noh J, Ishikawa N, Ito K: Recovery from foetal hypothyroidism: Evidence for the safety of breast-feeding while taking propylthiouracil. *Clin Endocrinol (Oxf)* 31:591, 1989.
321. Mortimer RH, Tyack SA, Galligan JP, Perry-Keene DA, Tan YM: Graves' disease in pregnancy: TSH receptor binding inhibiting immunoglobulins and maternal and neonatal thyroid function. *Clin Endocrinol (Oxf)* 32:141, 1990.
322. Tamaki H, Amino N, Aozasa M, Mori M, Iwatani Y, Tachi J, Nose O, Tanizawa Q, et al: Universal predictive criteria for neonatal overt thyrotoxicosis requiring treatment. *Am J Perinatol* 5:152, 1988.
323. Gerstein HC: How common is postpartum thyroiditis? A methodologic overview of the literature. *Arch Intern Med* 150:1397, 1990.
324. Hashizume K, Ichikawa K, Nishii Y, Kobayashi M, Sakurai A, Miyamoto T, Suzuki S, Takeda T: Effect of administration of thyroxine on the risk of postpartum recurrence of hyperthyroid Graves' disease. *J Clin Endocrinol Metab* 75:6, 1992.
325. Jansson R, Bernander S, Karlsson A, Levin K, Nilsson G: Autoimmune thyroid dysfunction in the postpartum period. *J Clin Endocrinol Metab* 58:681, 1984.
326. Rajatanavin R, Chailurkit L, Tirarungsikul K, Chalayondeja W, Jittivanich U, Puapradit W: Postpartum thyroid dysfunction in Bangkok: A geographical variation in the prevalence. *Acta Endocrinol (Copenh)* 122:283, 1990.
327. Learoyd DL, Fung HYM, McGregor AM: Postpartum thyroid dysfunction. *Thyroid* 2:73, 1992.
328. Amino N, Yuasa T, Yabu Y, Miyai K, Kumahara Y: Exoph-

thalmos in autoimmune thyroid disease. *J Clin Endocrinol Metab* 51:1232, 1980.

329. Forbes G, Gorman CA, Brennan MD, Gehring DG, Ilstrup DM, Earnest F IV: Ophthalmopathy of Graves' disease: Computerized volume measurements of the orbital fat and muscle. *Am J Neuroradiol* 7:651, 1986.
330. Marcocci C, Bartalena L, Bogazzi F, Panicucci M, Pinchera A: Studies on the occurrence of ophthalmopathy in Graves' disease. *Acta Endocrinol (Copenh)* 120:473, 1989.
331. Werner SC: Modification of the classification of the eye changes of Graves' disease: Recommendations of the ad hoc committee of the American Thyroid Association. *J Clin Endocrinol Metab* 44:203, 1977.
332. Fells P: Thyroid-associated eye disease: Clinical management. *Lancet* 338:29, 1991.
333. Prummel MF, Wiersinga WM, Mourits MPh, Koornneef L, Berghout A, van der Gaag R: Effect of abnormal thyroid function of the severity of Graves' ophthalmopathy. *Arch Intern Med* 150:1098, 1990.
334. Sridama V, DeGroot LJ: Treatment of Graves' disease and the course of ophthalmopathy. *Am J Med* 87:70, 1989.
335. Streeten DHP, Anderson GH Jr, Reed GF, Woo P: Prevalence, natural history and surgical treatment of exophthalmos. *Clin Endocrinol (Oxf)* 27:125, 1897.
336. Tallstedt L, Lundell G, Torring O, Wallin G, Ljunggren J-G, Blomgren H, Taube A, and the Thyroid Study Group: Occurrence of ophthalmopathy after treatment for Graves' hyperthyroidism. *N Engl J Med* 326:1733, 1992.
337. Marcocci C, Bartalena L, Bogazzi F, Bruno-Bossio G, Pinchera A: Relationship between Graves' ophthalmopathy and type of treatment of Graves' hyperthyroidism. *Thyroid* 2:171, 1992.
338. Bahn RS, Gorman CA: Choice of therapy and criteria for assessing treatment outcome in thyroid-associated ophthalmopathy. *Endocrinol Metab Clin North Am* 16:391, 1987.
339. Prummel MF, Mourits MPh, Berghout A, Krenning EP, van der Gaag R, Koornneef L, Wiersinga WM: Prednisone and cyclosporine in the treatment of severe Graves' ophthalmopathy. *N Engl J Med* 321:1353, 1989.
340. Kriss JP, Pleshakov V, Rosenblum A, Sharp G: Therapy with occlusive dressings of preribial myxedema with fluocinolone acetonide. *J Clin Endocrinol* 27:595, 1967.
341. Bianchi R, Pilo A, Mariani G, Molea N, Cazzuola F, Ferdeghini M, Bertelli P: Comparison of plasma and urinary methods for the direct measurement of the thyroxine to 3,5,3′-triiodothyronine conversion rate in man. *J Clin Endocrinol Metab* 58:993, 1984.
342. Lum SM, Nicoloff JT, Spencer CA, Kaptein EM: Peripheral tissue mechanism for maintenance of serum triiodothyronine values in a thyroxine-deficient state in man. *J Clin Invest* 73:570, 1984.
343. Zimmerman RS, Brennan MD, McConahey WM, Goellner JR, Gharib H: Hashimoto's thyroiditis: An uncommon cause of painful thyroid unresponsive to corticosteroid therapy. *Ann Intern Med* 104:355, 1986.
344. Okamoto Y, Hamada N, Saito H, Ohno M, Noh J, Ito K, Morii H: Thyroid peroxidase activity-inhibiting immunoglobulins in patients with autoimmune thyroid disease. *J Clin Endocrinol Metab* 68:730, 1989.
345. Bogner U, Kotulla P, Peters H, Schleusener H: Thyroid peroxidase/microsomal antibodies are not identical with thyroid cytotoxic antibodies in autoimmune thyroiditis. *Acta Endocrinol (Copenh)* 123:431, 1990.
346. Chiovato L, Vitti P, Santini F, Lopez G, Mammoli C, Bassi P, Giusti L, Tonacchera M, et al: Incidence of antibodies blocking thyrotropin effect *in vitro* in patients with euthyroid or hypothyroid autoimmune thyroiditis. *J Clin Endocrinol Metab* 71:40, 1990.
347. Takasu N, Yamada T, Takasu M, Komiya I, Nagasawa Y, Asawa T, Shinoda T, Aizawa T, et al: Disappearance of thyrotropin-blocking antibodies and spontaneous recovery from hypothyroidism in autoimmune thyroiditis. *N Engl J Med* 326:513, 1992.
348. Takasu N, Mori T, Koizumi Y, Takeuchi S, Yamada T: Transient neonatal hypothyroidism due to maternal immunoglobulins that inhibit thyrotropin-binding and postreceptor processes. *J Clin Endocrinol Metab* 59:142, 1984.
349. Jansson R, Totterman TH, Sallstrom J, Dahlberg PA: Thyroid-infiltrating T lymphocyte subsets in Hashimoto's thyroiditis. *J Clin Endocrinol Metab* 56:1164, 1983.
350. Del Prete GF, Maggi E, Mariotti S, Tiri A, Vercelli D, Parronchi P, Macchia D, Pinchera A, et al: Cytolytic T lymphocytes with natural killer activity in thyroid infiltrate of patients with Hashimoto's thyroiditis: Analysis at a clonal level. *J Clin Endocrinol Metab* 62:52, 1986.
351. Atkins MB, Mier JW, Parkinson DR, Gould JA, Berkman EM, Kaplan MM: Hypothyroidism after treatment with interleukin-2 and lymphokine-activated killer cells. *N Engl J Med* 318:1557, 1988.
352. Ronnblom LE, Alm GV, Oberg KE: Autoimmunity after alpha-interferon therapy for malignant carcinoid tumors. *Ann Intern Med* 115:178, 1991.
353. Kung AWC, Jones BM, Lai CL: Effects of interferon-γ therapy on thyroid function, T-lymphocyte subpopulations and induction of autoantibodies. *J Clin Endocrinol Metab* 71:1230, 1990.
354. Weetman AP: Autoimmune thyroiditis: Predisposition and pathogenesis. *Clin Endocrinol (Oxf)* 36:307, 1992.
355. Tunbridge WMG, Brewis M, French JM, Appleton D, Bird T, Clark F, Evered DC, Evans JG, et al: Natural history of autoimmune thyroiditis. *Br Med J* 282:258, 1981.
356. Maagoe H, Reintoft I, Christensen HE, Simonsen J, Mogensen EF: Lymphocytic thyroiditis: II. The course of the disease in relation to morphologic, immunologic and clinical findings at the time of biopsy. *Acta Med Scand* 202:469, 1977.
357. Hayashi Y, Tamai H, Fukata S, Hirota Y, Katayama S, Kuma K, Kumagai LF, Nagataki S: A long term clinical, immunological, and histological follow-up study of patients with goitrous chronic lymphocytic thyroiditis. *J Clin Endocrinol Metab* 61:1172, 1985.
358. Takasu N, Komiya I, Asawa T, Nagasawa Y, Yamada T: Test for recovery from hypothyroidism during thyroxine therapy in Hashimoto's thyroiditis. *Lancet* 336:1084, 1990.
359. Holm L-E, Blomgren H, Lowhagen T: Cancer risks in patients with chronic lymphocytic thyroiditis. *N Engl J Med* 312:601, 1985.
360. Harris B, Othman S, Davies JA, Weppner GJ, Richards CJ, Newcombe RG, Lazarus JH, Parkes AB, et al: Association between postpartum thyroid dysfunction and thyroid antibodies and depression. *Br Med J* 305:152, 1992.
361. Othman S, Phillips DIW, Parkes AB, Richards CJ, Harris B, Fung H, Darke C, John R, et al: A long-term follow-up of postpartum thyroiditis. *Clin Endocrinol (Oxf)* 32:559, 1990.
362. Schimpff SC, Diggs CH, Wiswell JG, Salvetore PC, Wiernik PH: Radiation-related thyroid dysfunction: Implication for treatment of Hodgkin's disease. *Ann Intern Med* 92:91, 1980.
363. Hancock SL, Cox RS, McDougall IR: Thyroid diseases after treatment of Hodgkin's disease. *N Engl J Med* 325:599, 1991.
364. Tamai H, Suemastu H, Kurokawa N, Esaki M, Ikemi T, Matsuzuka F, Kuma K, Nagataki S: Alterations in circulating thyroid hormones and thyrotropin after complete thyroidectomy. *J Clin Endocrinol Metab* 48:54, 1979.
365. Dussault JH, Letarte J, Guyda H, Laberge C: Lack of influence of thyroid antibodies on thyroid function in the newborn infant and on a mass screening program for congenital hypothyroidism. *J Pediatr* 96:385, 1980.
366. Barsano CP: Other forms of primary hypothyroidism, in Braverman LE, Utiger RD (eds): *The Thyroid: A Fundamental and Clinical Text,* 6th ed. Philadelphia, Lippincott, 1991, pp 956–967.
367. Stanbury JB: Inherited metabolic disorders of the thyroid system, in Braverman LE, Utiger RD (eds): *The Thyroid: A Fundamental and Clinical Text,* 6th ed. Philadelphia, Lippincott, 1991, pp 934–941.

368. Hayashizaki Y, Hiraoka Y, Tatsumi K, Hashimoto T, Furuyama J-I, Miyai K, Nishijo K, Matsuura M, et al: Deoxyribonucleic acid analyses of five families with familial inherited stimulating hormone deficiency. *J Clin Endocrinol Metab* 71:792, 1990.
369. Katevuo K, Valimaki M, Ketonen L, Lamberg B-A, Pelkonen R: Computed tomography of the pituitary fossa in primary hypothyroidism: Effect of thyroxine treatment. *Clin Endocrinol (Oxf)* 22:617, 1985.
370. Yamamoto K, Saito K, Takai T, Naito M, Yoshida S: Visual field defects and pituitary enlargement in primary hypothyroidism. *J Clin Endocrinol Metab* 57:283, 1983.
371. Caron PJ, Nieman LK, Rose SR, Nisula BC: Deficient nocturnal surge of thyrotropin in central hypothyroidism. *J Clin Endocrinol Metab* 62:960, 1986.
372. Beck-Peccoz P, Amr S, Menezes-Ferreira MM, Faglia G, Weintraub BD: Decreased receptor binding of biologically inactive thyrotropin in central hypothyroidism: Effect of treatment with thyrotropin-releasing hormone. *N Engl J Med* 312:1085, 1985.
373. Refetoff S, Weiss RE, Usala SJ: The syndromes of resistance to thyroid hormone. *Endocrine Reviews* 14:348, 1993.
374. Sarne DH, Refetoff S, Rosenfield RL, Farriaux JP: Sex hormone-binding globulin in the diagnosis of peripheral tissue resistance to thyroid hormone: The value of changes after short term triiodothyronine administration. *J Clin Endocrinol Metab* 66:740, 1988.
375. Takeda K, Balzano S, Sakurai A, DeGroot LJ, Refetoff S: Screening of nineteen unrelated families with generalized resistance to thyroid hormone for known point mutations in the thyroid hormone receptor β gene and the detection of a new mutation. *J Clin Invest* 87:496, 1991.
376. Chatterjee VKK, Nagaya T, Madison LD, Datta S, Rentoumis A, Jameson JL: Thyroid hormone resistance syndrome: Inhibition of normal receptor function by mutant thyroid hormone receptors. *J Clin Invest* 87:1977, 1991.
377. Wayne EJ: Clinical and metabolic studies in thyroid disease. *Br Med J* 1:1, 78, 1960.
378. Watanakunakorn C, Hodges RH, Evans TC: Myxedema: A study of 400 cases. *Arch Intern Med* 116:183, 1965.
379. Billewicz WZ, Chapman RS, Crooks J, Day ME, Gossage J, Wayne E, Young JA: Statistical methods applied to the diagnosis of hypothyroidism. *Q J Med* 38:255, 1969.
380. Douglas RC, Jacobson SD: Pathologic changes in adult myxedema: Survey of 10 necropsies. *J Clin Endocrinol* 17:1354, 1957.
381. Osterweil D, Syndulko K, Cohen SN, Pettler-Jennings PD, Hershman JM, Cummings JL, Tourtellotte WW, Solomon DH: Cognitive function in non-demented older adults with hypothyroidism. *J Am Geriatr Soc* 40:325, 1992.
382. Swanson JW, Kelly JJ Jr, McConahey WM: Neurologic aspects of thyroid dysfunction. *Mayo Clin Proc* 56:504, 1981.
383. Beghi E, Delodovici M, Bogliun G, Crespi V, Paleari F, Gamba P, Capra M, Zarrelli M: Hypothyroidism and polyneuropathy. *J Neurol Neurosurg Psychiatry* 52:1420, 1989.
384. Khaleeli AA, Griffith DG, Edwards RHT: The clinical presentation of hypothyroid myopathy and its relationship to abnormalities in structure and function of skeletal muscle. *Clin Endocrinol (Oxf)* 19:365, 1983.
385. Goldman J, Matz R, Mortimer R: High elevations of creatine phosphokinase in hypothyroidism. *JAMA* 238:325, 1977.
386. Ladenson PW, Sherman SI, Baughman KL, Ray PE, Feldman AM: Reversible alterations in myocardial gene expression in a young man with dilated cardiomyopathy and hypothyroidism. *Proc Natl Acad Sci USA* 89:5251, 1992.
387. Shenoy MM, Goldman JM: Hypothyroid cardiomyopathy: Echocardiographic documentation of reversibility. *Am J Med Sci* 294:1, 1987.
388. Keating FR Jr, Parkin TW, Selby JB, Dickinson LS: Treatment of heart disease associated with myxedema. *Prog Cardiovasc Dis* 3:364, 1961.
389. Becker C: Hypothyroidism and atherosclerotic heart disease: Pathogenesis, medical management, and the role of coronary artery bypass surgery. *Endocr Rev* 6:432, 1985.
390. Sherman SI, Ladenson PW: Percutaneous transluminal coronary angioplasty in hypothyroidism. *Am J Med* 90:367, 1991.
391. Zwillich CW, Pierson DJ, Hofeldt FD, Lufkin EG, Weil JV: Ventilatory control in myxedema and hypothyroidism. *N Engl J Med* 292:662, 1975.
392. Gottehrer A, Roa J, Stanford GG, Chernow B, Sahn SA: Hypothyroidism and pleural effusions. *Chest* 98:1130, 1990.
393. Rajagopal KR, Abbrecht PH, Derderian SS, Pickett C, Hofeldt F, Tellis CJ, Zwillich CW: Obstructive sleep apnea in hypothyroidism. *Ann Intern Med* 101:491, 1984.
394. Grunstein RR, Sullivan CE: Sleep apnea and hypothyroidism: Mechanisms and management. *Am J Med* 85:775, 1988.
395. Parving HH, Hansen JM, Nielsen SL, Rossing N, Munck O, Lassen NA: Mechanism of edema formation in myxedema–increased protein extravasation and relatively slow lymphatic drainage. *N Engl J Med* 301:460, 1979.
396. Zimmerman RS, Gharib H, Zimmerman D, Heublein D, Burnett JC Jr: Atrial natriuretic peptide in hypothyroidism. *J Clin Endocrinol Metab* 64:353, 1987.
397. Iwasaki Y, Oiso Y, Yamauchi K, Takatsuki K, Kondo K, Hasegawa H, Tomita A: Osmoregulation of plasma vasopressin in myxedema. *J Clin Endocrinol Metab* 70:534, 1990.
398. Skowsky WR, Kikuchi TA: The role of vasopressin in the impaired water excretion of myxedema. *Am J Med* 64:613, 1978.
399. Tachman MC, Guthrie GP Jr: Hypothyroidism: Diversity of presentation. *Endocr Rev* 5:456, 1984.
400. Kuusi T, Taskinen M-R, Nikkila EA: Lipoproteins, lipolytic enzymes, and hormonal status in hypothyroid women at different levels of substitution. *J Clin Endocrinol Metab* 66:51, 1988.
401. Staub J-J, Althaus BU, Engler H, Ryff AS,Trabucco P, Marquardt K, Burckhardt D, Girard J, et al: Spectrum of subclinical and overt hypothyroidism: Effect on thyrotropin, prolactin, and thyroid reserve, and metabolic impact on peripheral target tissues. *Am J Med* 92:631, 1992.
402. Chernausek SL, Turner R: Attenuation of spontaneous, nocturnal growth hormone secretion in children with hypothyroidism and its correlation with plasma insulin-like growth factor I concentrations. *J Pediatr* 114:968, 1992.
403. Valcavi R, Dieguez C, Preece M, Taylor A, Portioli I, Scanlon MF: Effect of thyroxine replacement therapy on plasma insulin-like growth factor I levels and growth hormone responses to growth hormone releasing factor in hypothyroid patients. *Clin Endocrinol (Oxf)* 27:85, 1987
404. Contreras P, Generini G, Michelsen H, Pumarino H, Campino C: Hyperprolactinemia and galactorrhea: Spontaneous versus iatrogenic hypothyroidism. *J Clin Endocrinol Metab* 53:1036, 1981.
405. Iranmanesh A, Lizarralde G, Johnson ML, Veldhuis JD: Dynamics of 24-hour endogenous cortisol secretion and clearance in primary hypothyroidism assessed before and after partial thyroid hormone replacement. *J Clin Endocrinol Metab* 70:155, 1990.
406. Kamilaris TC, DeBold CR, Pavlou SN, Island DP, Hoursanidis A, Orth DN: Effect of altered thyroid hormone levels on hypothalamic-pituitary-adrenal function. *J Clin Endocrinol Metab* 65:994, 1987.
407. Topliss DJ, White EL, Stockigt JR: Significance of thyrotropin excess in untreated primary adrenal insufficiency. *J Clin Endocrinol Metab* 50:52, 1980.
408. Wortsman J, Rosner W, Dufau ML: Abnormal testicular function in men with primary hypothyroidism. *Am J Med* 82:207, 1987.
409. Davis LE, Leveno KJ, Cunningham FG: Hypothyroidism complicating pregnancy. *Obstet Gynecol* 72:108, 1988.
410. Glinoer D, Soto MF, Bourdoux P, Lejeune B, Delange F,

Lemone M, Kinthaert J, Robijn C, et al: Pregnancy in patients with mild thyroid abnormalities: Maternal and neonatal repercussions. *J Clin Endocrinol Metab* 73:421, 1991.
411. Klein RZ, Haddow JE, Faix JD, Brown RS, Hermos RJ, Pulkkinen A, Mitchell ML: Prevalence of thyroid deficiency in pregnant women. *Clin Endocrinol (Oxf)* 35:41, 1991.
412. Stagnaro-Green A, Roman SH, Cobin RH, El-Harazy E, Alvarez-Marfany M, Davies TF: Detection of at-risk pregnancy by means of highly sensitive assays for thyroid autoantibodies. *JAMA* 264:1422, 1990.
413. Weinberg AD, Brennan MD, Gorman CA, March HM, O'Fallon WM: Outcome of anesthesia and surgery in hypothyroid patients. *Arch Intern Med* 143:893, 1983.
414. Ladenson PW, Levin AA, Ridgway EC, Daniels GH: Complications of surgery in hypothyroid patients. *Am J Med* 77:261, 1984.
415. Fish LH, Schwartz HL, Cavanaugh J, Steffes MW, Bantle JP, Oppenheimer JH: Replacement dose, metabolism, and bioavailability of levothyroxine in the treatment of hypothyroidism: Role of triiodothyronine in pituitary feedback in humans. *N Engl J Med* 316:764, 1987.
416. Sturgess I, Thomas SH, Pennell DJ, Mitchell D, Croft DN: Diurnal variation in TSH and free thyroid hormones in patients on thyroxine replacement. *Acta Endocrinol (Copenh)* 121:674, 1989.
417. Griffin JE: Hypothyroidism in the elderly. *Am J Med Sci* 299:334, 1990.
418. Burmeister LA, Goumaz MO, Mariash CN, Oppenheimer JH: Levothyroxine dose requirements for thyrotropin suppression in the treatment of differentiated thyroid cancer. *J Clin Endocrinol Metab* 75:344, 1992.
419. Kaplan MM: Monitoring thyroxine treatment during pregnancy. *Thyroid* 2:147, 1992.
420. Utiger RD: Therapy of hypothyroidism: When are changes needed: *N Engl J Med* 323:126, 1990.
421. Havrankova J, Lahaie R: Levothyroxine binding by sucralfate. *Ann Intern Med* 117:445, 1992.
422. Campbell NRC, Hasinoff BB, Stalts H, Rao B, Wong NCW: Ferrous sulfate reduces thyroxine efficacy in patients with hypothyroidism. *Ann Intern Med* 117:1010, 1992.
423. Sperber AD: Evidence for interference with the intestinal absorpton of levothyroxine sodium by aluminum hydroxide. *Arch Intern Med* 152:183, 1992.
424. Ain KB, Refetoff S, Rein HG, Weintraub BD: Pseudomalabsorption of levothyroxine. *JAMA* 266:2118, 1991.
425. Helfand M, Crapo LM: Monitoring therapy in patients taking levothyroxine. *Ann Intern Med* 113:450, 1990.
426. England ML, Hershman JM: Serum TSH concentration as an aid to monitoring compliance with thyroid hormone therapy in hypothyroidism. *Am J Med Sci* 292:264, 1986.
427. Drinka PJ, Nolten WE: Subclinical hypothyroidism in the elderly: To treat or not to treat? *Am J Med Sci* 295:125, 1988.
428. Cooper DS, Halpern R, Wood LC, Levin AA, Ridgway EC: L-Thyroxine therapy in subclinical hypothyroidism: A double-blind, placebo-controlled trial. *Ann Intern Med* 101:18, 1984.
429. Nystrom E, Caidahl K, Fager G, Wikkelso C, Lundberg P-A, Lindstedt G: A double-blind cross-over 12-month study of L-thyroxine treatment of women with "subclinical" hypothyroidism. *Clin Endocrinol (Oxf)* 29:63, 1988.
430. Vagenakis AG, Braverman LE, Azizi F, Portnay GI, Ingbar SH: Recovery of pituitary thyrotropic function after withdrawal of prolonged thyroid-suppression therapy. *N Engl J Med* 293:681, 1975.
431. Krugman LG, Hershman JM, Chopra IJ, Levine GA, Pekary AE, Geffner DL, Chua Teco GN: Patterns of recovery of the hypothalamic-pituitary-thyroid axis in patients taken off chronic thyroid therapy. *J Clin Endocrinol Metab* 41:70, 1975.
432. Fisher DA: Management of congenital hypothyroidism. *J Clin Endocrinol Metab* 72:523, 1991.
433. New England Congenital Hypothyroidism Collaborative: Elementary school performance of children with congenital hypothyroidism. *J Pediatr* 116:27, 1990.
434. Buchanan CR, Stanhope R, Adlard P, Jones J, Grant DB, Preece MA: Gonadotropin, growth hormone and prolactin secretion in children with primary hypothyroidism. *Clin Endocrinol (Oxf)* 29:427, 1988.
435. Hylander B, Rosenqvist U: Treatment of myxoedema coma—factors associated with fatal outcome. *Acta Endocrinol (Copenh)* 108:65, 1985.
436. Arlot S, Debussche X, Lalau J-D, Mesmacque A, Tolani M, Quichaud J, Fournier A: Myxoedema coma: Response of thyroid hormones with oral and intravenous high-dose L-thyroxine treatment. *Intensive Care Med* 17:16, 1991.
437. Ridgway EC, McCammon JA, Benotti J, Maloof F: Acute metabolic responses in myxedema to large doses of intravenous L-thyroxine. *Ann Intern Med* 77:549, 1972.
438. Sprunt JG, Maclean D, Browning MCK: Plasma-corticosteroid levels in accidental hypothermia. *Lancet* 1:324, 1970.
439. Levine SN: Current concepts of thyroiditis. *Arch Intern Med* 143:1952, 1983.
440. Volpe R, Row VV, Ezrin C: Circulating viral and thyroid antibodies in subacute thyroiditis. *J Clin Endocrinol* 27:1275, 1967.
441. De Bruin TWA, Riekhoff FPM, de Boer JJ: An outbreak of thyrotoxicosis due to atypical subacute thyroiditis. *J Clin Endocrinol Metab* 70:396, 1990.
442. Berger SA, Zonszein J, Villamena P, Mittman N: Infectious diseases of the thyroid gland. *Rev Infect Dis* 5:108, 1983.
443. Miyauchi A, Matsuzuka F, Kuma K, Takai S-I: Piriform sinus fistula: An underlying abnormality common in patients with acute suppurative thyroiditis. *World J Surg* 14:400, 1990.
444. Drucker DJ, Bailey D, Rotstein L: Thyroiditis as the presenting manifestation of disseminated extrapulmonary *Pneumocystis carinii* infection. *J Clin Endocrinol Metab* 71:1663, 1990.

CHAPTER 11

The Thyroid: Nodules and Neoplasia

Gerard N. Burrow

Interest in the thyroid gland has centered on goiter and nodule formation. Goiter may be defined as a thyroid gland that is twice normal size, or about 40 g for an adult. Endemic goiter is the major thyroid disease worldwide, probably affecting more than 200 million people. Many goitrous glands contain one or more nodules.[1] The use of iodized salt has eliminated goiter as a medical problem in developed countries, although it continues to be a major problem in developing countries whose geographic location makes them susceptible to iodine deficiency. In North America and other developed areas, sporadic nodular goiter and the possibility of associated thyroid carcinoma cause problems in diagnosis and management. The concern about "lumps" and cancer seems particularly acute with respect to the thyroid, where a nodule is easily palpable and is often observable by the patient.

GOITER

Classification of Goiter and Thyroid Neoplasia

To bring order out of chaos in the classification of goiter, the American Thyroid Association has suggested the terminology in Table 11-1 for nontoxic goiter. This system of classification is based on whether the goiter is diffuse or nodular. Goiters are further subdivided according to whether they are endemic, sporadic, or compensatory and, if nodular, whether they are uninodular or multinodular and functional or nonfunctional.

Historical Overview

The thyroid gland was first described in detail by Vesalius in the sixteenth century. Thomas Wharton (1614–1673) named the gland from the Greek word *thureos* ("shield"). He noted:

> It contributes much to the rotundity and beauty of the neck filling up the vacant spaces around the larynx and making its protuberant parts almost to subside, and become smooth, particularly in females to whom for this reason a larger gland has been assigned, which renders their necks more even and beautiful.[2]

Goiter once was prevalent in Switzerland, Austria, and southern Germany as well as in northern Spain, southernmost France, and northern Italy. As a consequence, some of the earliest descriptions of goiter and cretinism came from these regions.[3]

Endemic cretinism was described by the Swiss German physician Paracelsus (1493–1541) in the region around Salzburg.[4] Paracelsus pointed out that cretinism occurred together with endemic goiter. Felix Platter (1536–1614), a Swiss physician who was a professor of medicine in Basel, also described cretinism and associated mental deficiency and noted that affected individuals "frequently have a struma at the throat."

Swellings of the neck, particularly those caused by the thyroid and glandular tuberculosis, had been treated for centuries with iodine-containing substances such as seaweed and burned sponge. In 1817, Bernard Courtois, a French manufacturer of saltpeter, discovered iodine. Subsequent research on iodine and iodine compounds led Jean François Coindet to introduce tincture of iodine for the treatment of goiter. In 1820, Coindet reported to the Swiss Scientific Society that he had administered an iodine solution to 150 goiter patients without ill effects. Coindet's work strongly influenced other physicians, among them J. G. A. Lugol, who used an aqueous solution of iodine and potassium iodide which later was named for him. Awareness of the potential problems associated with iodine eventually led to the limitation of its use, especially after 1910, when Kocher described the production of toxic goiter (iod-Basedow) in goitrous patients treated with iodine. Marine popularized the use of iodized salt in North America for the prevention of simple endemic goiter beginning in 1917.[5]

Sporadic cretinism, as opposed to the endemic form, was described by Fagge, a physician at Guy's Hospital in London, before the Royal Medical and Surgical Society in 1871. Fagge expressed the view that sporadic cretinism is caused by absence of a thyroid gland.

TABLE 11-1 Classification of Nontoxic Goiter

Nontoxic diffuse goiter
Endemic, induced by
Iodine deficiency
Iodine excess
Dietary goitrogens
Sporadic, caused by
Congenital defect in thyroid hormone biosynthesis
Chemical agents, e.g., lithium, thiocyanate, *p*-aminosalicylic acid
Iodine deficiency
Compensatory, following subtotal thyroidectomy
Nontoxic nodular goiter caused by causes listed above
Uninodular or multinodular
Functional and/or nonfunctional

Source: Modified from Werner SC: *J Clin Endocrinol* 29:860, 1969.

Etiology of Goiter

In 1924, Marine first developed the concept that periods of iodide deficiency and repletion result in cyclic hyperplasia and involution of thyroid follicular cells, with the eventual development of nodular hyperplasia.[5]

Whatever the specific cause, goitrogenesis involves the generation of new follicular epithelial cells and new follicles. Goitrogenic stimuli occurring over a long period produce the macroscopic, microscopic, and functional heterogeneity characteristic of simple goiter.[6] In contrast, a more short-term potent goitrogenic stimulus can result in follicular hypertrophy with less generation of new follicular cells and follicles, i.e., Graves' goiters.

The suggestion has also been made that thyroid nodules are caused by the shunting of blood to a particular area of the thyroid, with a subsequent increase in tissue growth. Thyroid follicles are bound together to form a lobule; a single artery supplies each lobule. In long-standing goiters, the blood supply may be greatly increased.

There has been increasing interest in the idea that growth factors in addition to thyroid stimulating hormone (TSH) play a role in the etiology of goiter.[7] The insulin-like growth factors are pleiotropic growth factors that affect DNA synthesis and differentiated cellular function in thyroid cells in culture and are produced by thyroid cells.[8,9] Epidermal growth factor (EGF) may affect the thyroid gland.[10] Immunoglobulin fractions capable of stimulating thyroid growth in a cytochemical assay based on DNA determinations have been reported in patients with nontoxic goiter.[11,12] In addition to growth factors, there are also inhibitory factors. Transforming growth factor β (TGFβ) has an inhibitory action on thyroid cell growth and is also produced by the thyroid.[13] Interleukin 1 (IL-1) may suppress responsiveness to TSH.[14] Further, it has been suggested that iodine stimulates TGFβ production, which could partially explain the effect of iodine on the size of goiter.[15]

TSH Secretion

As discussed in more detail in Chap. 10, TSH secretion is controlled by the serum thyroid hormone concentration. As the concentration of thyroid hormone falls, TSH secretion increases; TSH secretion declines as the thyroid hormone concentration rises. Feedback control of TSH secretion by thyroid hormone occurs at the level of the pituitary. The hypothalamus modulates information from the rest of the central nervous system and provides the set point for TSH secretion in response to thyrotropin releasing hormone (TRH)[16] and other hormones, including estrogens, dopamine, and somatostatin (see Chap. 10).

Each individual appears to possess his or her own unique TSH set point that may be anywhere in the normal range. With the advent of second- and third-generation sensitive TSH assays, TSH responses to TRH have been found to be proportional to the basal value, with an approximate tenfold increase.[17]

There appear to be substantial variations between individuals in the relations of serum thyroid hormone concentration to TSH concentration; these variations may reflect variations in the cellular sensitivity of the pituitary to thyroid hormone, the degree of TRH release, or other factors.

As discussed in Chap. 10, the actions of thyroid hormone appear to be due to triiodothyronine (T_3); thyroxine (T_4) serves as a prohormone. This function is particularly important in the case of the pituitary, where T_4 5′-deiodinase is most active.[18] This feature allows the gland to respond more readily to changes in T_4 release than do peripheral tissues (Fig. 11-1).

TSH Stimulation of the Thyroid Gland

TSH is essential for the maintenance of normal thyroid hormone synthesis, although hypophysectomized animals secrete thyroid hormone to a very limited degree. The secretion of thyroid hormone is particularly sensitive to TSH and is proportional to the dose of administered TSH over a particular range. Under most physiologic conditions, TSH secretion maintains a stable serum concentration of thyroid hormone. However, the growth response of the thyroid to TSH has fixed limits; the thyroid is not capable of enlarging infinitely, and eventually a growth plateau is reached.

Evidence that goiter can be due to increased TSH stimulation has come mainly from studies of endemic goiter. In a study of 285 patients from endemic goiter regions of New Guinea, mean serum TSH concentrations were found to be increased [16 μunits per milliliter (μU/ml)] compared with normal values in North America (1.2 μU/ml).[19] However, within the group from the endemic goiter region, there was no difference in serum TSH concentration between go-

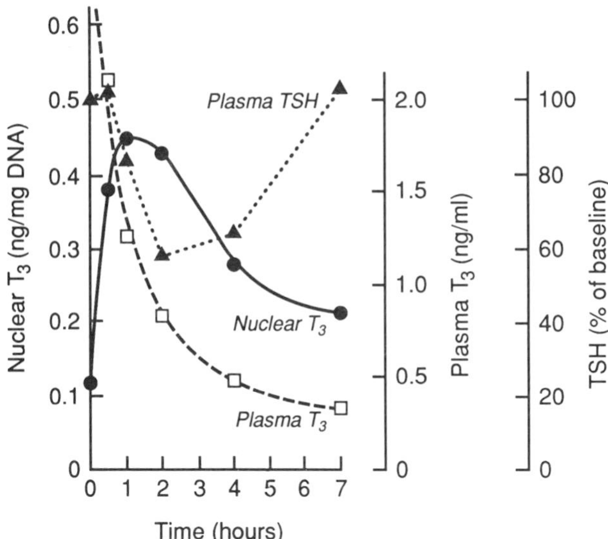

FIGURE 11-1 Time course of changes in pituitary nuclear T_3 and plasma T_3 and TSH levels. A single intravenous dose of T_3 was administered to thyroidectomized rats. The data suggest that the rapid inhibitory effect of T_3 on pituitary TSH release occurs through T_3 binding to receptors with kinetics similar to those of nuclear receptor binding. (*From Silva JE, Larsen PR: Science 198:617, 1977.*)

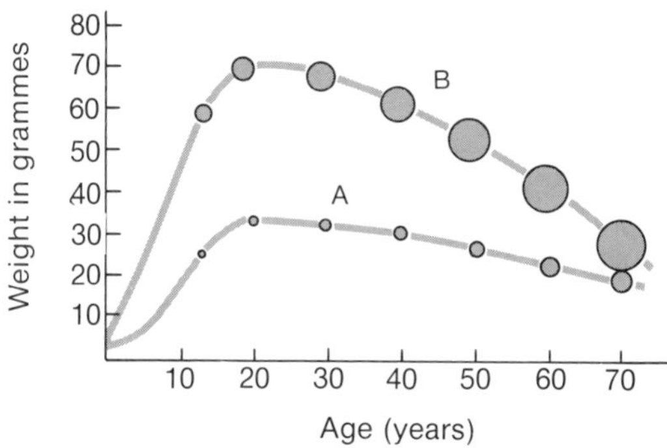

FIGURE 11-2 Goiter formation as a function of age. The size of the thyroid in grams is shown as a function of age for both nonendemic goiter areas (*A*) and endemic goiter areas (*B*). The circles represent the relative size of thyroid nodules throughout life in both groups. (*From Farris, in Deficiency Diseases. Springfield, IL, Charles C Thomas, 1958.*)

itrous and nongoitrous patients, suggesting that a factor in addition to TSH contributes to goitrogenesis. Perhaps that factor is the differential sensitivity of the cells of the thyroid gland to TSH.[6] In endemic goiter areas of Brazil, serum TSH concentrations were higher in goitrous patients from iodine-deficient areas than in goitrous patients from iodine-replete areas.[20] Furthermore, there was a higher peak TSH response to TRH (see Chap. 10) in the iodine-deficient goitrous group. The authors suggested that there may have been an increase of the set point so that TSH secretion continued at a higher level. However, studies from Greece, another endemic goiter area, suggested that an iodine-deficient thyroid is more sensitive to the stimulatory effect of TSH.[21,22] All these studies were done before the introduction of the sensitive TSH assay.

Studies of sporadic nontoxic goiter are even more complicated because the etiology is so diverse, ranging from thyroiditis to goitrogen ingestion. Serum TSH concentrations have been found to be increased slightly, and patients with sporadic nontoxic goiter often have an increased TSH response to TRH.[23] Patients with nodular goiter more often have an impaired or absent response to TRH compared with those with diffuse goiter. This impaired TSH response may indicate that there are areas of autonomy in the nodular gland, so that some thyroid hormone production is not under pituitary control; this would act to suppress the sensitivity of the pituitary to TRH. Serum TSH concentrations were higher in individuals who had goiters for less than a year.[24] Growth of the thyroid is more rapid early in life; the gland actually regresses later on (Fig. 11-2). TSH values also increase during the early decades of life. Subsequently, TSH secretion and reserve progressively decrease.[25] The prevalence of thyroid nodules, however, may increase with age (Fig. 11-3).

The variability in TSH concentrations associated with goiter may be explained by the natural progression of the disease. Overall, in the early stages of goiter formation there may be a relative thyroid hormone deficiency; this results in increased TSH release, which then stimulates thyroid hypertrophy and hyperplasia. Enlargement in thyroid size augments the ability of the gland to produce thyroid hormone, which in turn results in a suppression of TSH levels toward normal. Further, in some cases, serum TSH stimulation may result in relatively autonomous foci of thyroid hormone–producing tissue within the gland, which could lead to depressed TSH levels. Thus, depending on the stage of the disease, TSH levels can be elevated, normal, or de-

FIGURE 11-3 Prevalence of thyroid nodules with age. (*After Maxon et al.*[143])

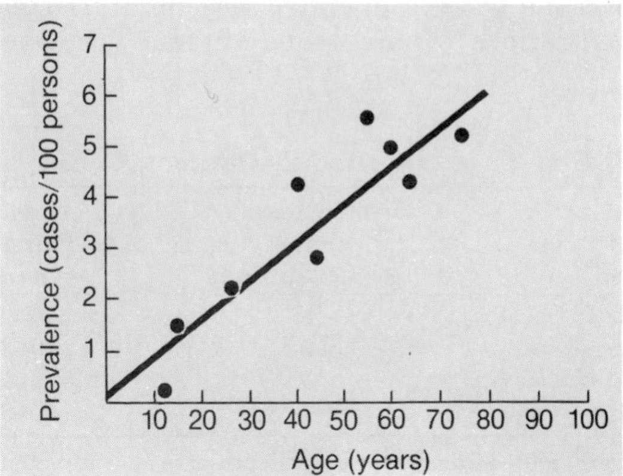

pressed.[19–25] However, individual variations in the sensitivity of the gland to TSH and other growth or inhibitory factors may be capable of stimulating thyroid gland growth[11,26,27] and may also participate in these variations.

Endemic Goiter

When the incidence of goiter in a population rises above 10 percent, the goiter becomes "endemic." Clearly, this is not a stringent criterion. However, there is an implication that an environmental factor is the causative agent. Worldwide, iodine deficiency is the major cause of goiter, but other goitrogens have been described which affect entire populations, usually in association with iodine deficiency.

Geography, Diet, and Iodine Abundance

Although Noah might have saved the animals from extinction, the flood left their descendants susceptible to goiter. In areas subjected to flooding or intense glaciation in the last ice age, iodine was leached out of the soil. Newly formed soils are relatively iodine-deficient, although they are enriched by airborne iodine, the major source of which is seawater deposited in rain.[28]

Although individual requirements vary, most people require more than 50 μg of iodine daily to replace iodine excreted in the urine (Table 11-2).[29] Diets that do not supply this amount of iodine are most often found in areas where the soil is poor in iodine. Individuals who live in villages in these areas and eat predominantly local food have iodine-deficient diets. Iodine deficiency is less likely in larger cities because the food there comes from a much wider geographic area. Similarly, members of upper socioeconomic classes are less apt to have goiter because they eat a more varied diet. In developed countries, iodine added to salt makes a major contribution to the iodine intake. With the exception of saltwater fish, there is relatively little iodine in natural food.

Development of Endemic Goiter

The development of endemic goiter presumably follows the pattern of goiter in general. Decreased concentrations of circulating thyroid hormone resulting from iodine deficiency lead to increased TSH secretion and hyperplasia of the gland. As was discussed above, factors other than TSH (such as cellular sensitivity to TSH and growth factors) also play a role in goiter formation.[30] It is necessary to invoke these factors to explain, for instance, why goiter is present only in certain individuals in areas of endemic goiter and the heterogeneity of the follicles within a goitrous gland (see below). There is no characteristic histologic picture that distinguishes endemic goiter. With the initial stimulation, hypertrophy of the follicular cells occurs, followed by hyperplasia of the follicles and a concomitant increase in the vascularity of the gland. All the follicles in an endemic goiter are not affected equally; radioautographic studies have shown an unequal distribution of radioiodine within the individual follicles.[31] This heterogeneity, combined with an overall increase in the size of the gland, may explain why some endemic goiters contain a higher than average total amount of iodine.[32] Also, some of this thyroidal iodine may be outside the hormonally active pool. Nodular goiter may therefore be considered an extreme variant of this heterogeneity. Part of the thyroid irregularity leading to nodule formation may be due to the accumulation of connective tissue, which, during periods of further stimulation, may serve as a focus of retraction and may hinder the function of adjacent follicles.[6]

The human thyroid is limited in its ability to adapt to iodine deficiency compared with iodine excess. In severe iodine deficiency, there is an inability of the thyroid to compensate completely for the low plasma inorganic iodide concentration by proportionally increasing the iodide clearance rate.[33] In a euthyroid patient with endemic goiter, total thyroid iodine stores may be normal, although the iodine concentration in the hormonally active pool is low. With less iodine, less iodothyronine is synthesized. Iodine deficiency also increases the monoiodotyrosine/diiodotyrosine ratio. These changes do not occur early in goiter formation but are often found in nodular glands. Iodine deficiency and perhaps the increased stimulation from TSH also result in a high T_3/T_4 ratio in these goiters. This adaptive effect results in the production of the more potent T_3 despite a deficiency of iodine.

TABLE 11-2 Urinary Iodide Content, Goiter, and Development

Severity of Goiter	Urinary Iodide Excretion, μg/g Creatinine	Percent with Palpable Goiter	Clinical Spectrum
Mild	>50	10–20	Normal
Moderate	25–50	20–30	Occasional deafness and retardation; serum TSH elevated in 10–20%
Severe	<25	40–90	Cretinism in 1–10%; elevated serum TSH in 30–50%

Source: Modified from Ibbertson.[29] Represents approximate relations in endemic goiter areas.

Clinical Findings in Endemic Goiter

In areas of severe iodine deficiency, virtually everyone is goitrous regardless of sex or age. In less severely affected areas, surveys have shown that the thyroid gland may be moderately enlarged in early childhood but that the incidence of goiter is usually at its height in pubertal children. The goiter of puberty is one of the more sensitive indicators of iodine lack in a particular region. A difference in gland size between the two sexes appears during puberty. After puberty, the thyroid gland frequently diminishes in size in males but not in females. Why females are more affected than males is not clear. In the endemic goiter area of New Guinea, thyroid enlargement was found to be related to breast development but not to pregnancy, lactation, or parity.[34] The thyroid gland is more difficult to palpate in men, which may account for part of the discrepancy. However, all thyroid disease is more common in females, and the difference does not appear to be due solely to estrogens. The diagnosis and treatment of goiter are discussed later in this chapter.

Relation to Thyroid Cancer

Despite continuing long-term interest in the problem, the relation between endemic goiter and thyroid cancer remains unclear. After the introduction of iodine prophylaxis, the incidence of both nodular goiter and certain adenocarcinomas and sarcomas of the thyroid decreased. Appreciation of this change was complicated by an increase in the incidence of papillary carcinoma of the thyroid. However, when the geographic pattern of goiter prevalence was compared with the geographic patterns of mortality from thyroid cancer, there was no convincing evidence for an association between the two diseases.[35] In contrast, the comparison of the occurrence of goiter with that of hyperthyroidism showed the two to be highly significantly correlated.

Hyperfunction

Although data are not available, hyperthyroidism appears to be more common in areas of endemic goiter, especially after iodine therapy (iod-Basedow). Toxic nodular goiter (Plummer's disease) is common in association with endemic goiter; this may provide an explanation of the iod-Basedow phenomenon.[36] These hyperfunctioning nodules are avid for iodine and respond with a greatly increased production of thyroid hormone.

Cretinism

In areas of mild iodine deficiency, the inhabitants are usually euthyroid. With more profound iodine depletion, hypothyroidism may occur. A much more severe problem is the occurrence of cretinism in this population. Cretinism has been defined as permanent neurologic and skeletal retardation resulting from an inadequate supply of thyroid hormone during fetal and neonatal life, in this case caused by iodine deficiency.[29,32] Endemic cretins may present with neurologic defects, particularly spastic diplegia and mental retardation, deafness, mutism, dwarfism, and hypothyroidism in varying combinations, depending on the locale. Hypothyroidism can be diagnosed clinically by retarded linear growth and maturation of body proportions, myxedematous skin, and a marked delay in sexual development (see Chap. 10).

The various symptoms and signs of cretinism vary with the region. In central Africa, most cretins are athyrotic and myxedematous, while in the Andes, New Guinea, and the Himalayan foothills, the "nervous" type of cretinism predominates. For example, the "myxedematous" type is characterized by hypothyroidism, dwarfism, and epiphyseal dysgenesis consistent with deficient hormone production. In contrast, the "nervous" type is characterized by mental retardation and deaf-mutism. Both groups may have goiter. The prevalence of cretinism observed in these regions also varies markedly, from 1 percent in Zaire to almost 6 percent in endemic goiter districts in Nepal. The clinical picture of endemic cretinism represents a spectrum of clinical and metabolic signs reflecting varying degrees of impairment of the nervous system and thyroid function.[37,38]

The clinical features of endemic cretinism appear to result from the combined effects of hypothyroidism in utero and postnatally.[39] Fetal hypothyroidism during the first half of pregnancy affects the developing nervous system predominantly, whereas postnatal hypothyroidism results in manifestations of myxedema. Congenital hypothyroidism which persists causes stunting of growth and the other characteristic somatic abnormalities. Strict adherence to the classification of myxedematous or neurologic cretinism may obscure the spectrum of abnormalities caused by combined fetal and neonatal hypothyroidism.

Etiology of Cretinism and Iodine Deficiency

Endemic cretinism occurs only in areas where long-standing, severe endemic goiter is present. The prevalence of cretinism appears to be related to the severity of iodine deficiency. However, comparable states of iodine deficiency may be accompanied by cretinism in some areas but not in others.[40] The intrauterine period is important for the development of cretinism,[41] but this can be prevented by means of iodine administration to mothers. In a severely iodine-deficient area in Africa, 40 percent of newborns had elevated TSH concentrations more than 2.5 standard deviations (SD) above those of controls whose mothers had received iodine.[42] In 6 of 34 iodine-deficient neonates, definite biochemical signs of hypothyroidism were encountered.

Endemic Goiter due to Other Causes

Although iodine deficiency represents the major cause of endemic goiter, genetic factors and dietary goitrogens may also participate in endemic goiter formation. For example, a striking difference in the incidence of goiter was found between the inhabitants of two regions of an isolated island in Kivu Lake in Zaire, although the iodine intake in the two areas was the same and the two groups were ethnically similar.[42] Subsequent studies indicated that goiter in this population was related to the consumption of cassava, which, like several other chemical substances, can impair the utilization of iodine by the thyroid gland. However, cassava appears to be active as a goitrogen only in the presence of severe iodine deficiency, since data from Vietnam indicate that the goitrogenic effect of this substance is easily overcome by supplementary iodine.[43]

Protein-calorie malnutrition (PCM) often is present in iodine-deficient areas and may contribute to thyroid abnormalities. Malnutrition causes various alterations in the structure and function of the thyroid gland; a defective thyroid iodine concentration has been found despite adequate hormone secretion, which would further deplete iodine stores.[44] These abnormalities can be corrected by means of adequate protein and calorie intake. Studies from Senegal have suggested that PCM may cause goiter by resulting in defective formation of the mannosyl retinene phosphate complex necessary for normal glycosylation of thyroglobulin.[45] Experimental data suggest that glycosylation is obligatory for the processing of thyroglobulin, including iodination and subsequent thyroid hormone production.[46]

Prophylaxis of Endemic Goiter

One of the strongest pieces of evidence in support of the contention that endemic cretinism is due to iodine deficiency is the disappearance of cretinism when iodine is added to the diet. Supplements of iodine to the daily diet have been widely employed since their efficacy was demonstrated by Marine and Kimball in 1917.[5,47] Similar results have been duplicated throughout the world, but the total impact so far has been small compared with the magnitude of the goiter problem. This apathetic approach may be partly due to the complexity of the etiologic aspects of endemic goiter; for example, the persistent endemic goiter which affects about 20 percent of schoolchildren in Colombia has been attributed to a goitrogenic agent in well water. However, despite these natural goitrogens and the possibility of genetically determined metabolic defects of thyroid hormone, studies have indicated that iodine is a highly effective agent for the prevention of goiter.

Iodizing salt has been the most satisfactory method so far developed to provide populations with an adequate supply of iodine. Iodination of the water supply is effective but requires that everyone use a particular water supply. Iodized oil has been used successfully as an injectable form of goiter prophylaxis that lasts for 3 or more years. This form of prophylaxis is particularly useful in less developed areas of endemic goiter, where the distribution of iodized salt is difficult. The excreted iodine may be recycled in less developed areas.

Iodine is more effective in preventing the development of goiter than in suppressing an already enlarged thyroid gland. Early diffuse hyperplastic goiters may involute, but enlarged glands that have formed nodules and undergone cystic degeneration usually do not. After a diagnosis of cretinism has been made, thyroid hormone therapy ensures an adequate hormone concentration, but the patient may not improve in growth or mentation and his or her behavior pattern may deteriorate.

Surgery may be indicated for large goiters (Fig. 11-4). The most important indication for surgery is the presence of pressure symptoms, which rarely occur in a goiter situated high up in the neck. Goiters that are low in the neck, intrathoracic goiters, and goiters that encircle the trachea are the most likely to produce pressure symptoms.

Sporadic Goiter

Sporadic goiter can perhaps best be defined as goiter occurring in a nonendemic goiter region. Although a number of known goitrogens and errors in thyroid

FIGURE 11-4 Large goiter in a cretin. (*From Merke F: Geschichte von Fropf und Kretinismus. Bern, Hans Huber, 1971.*)

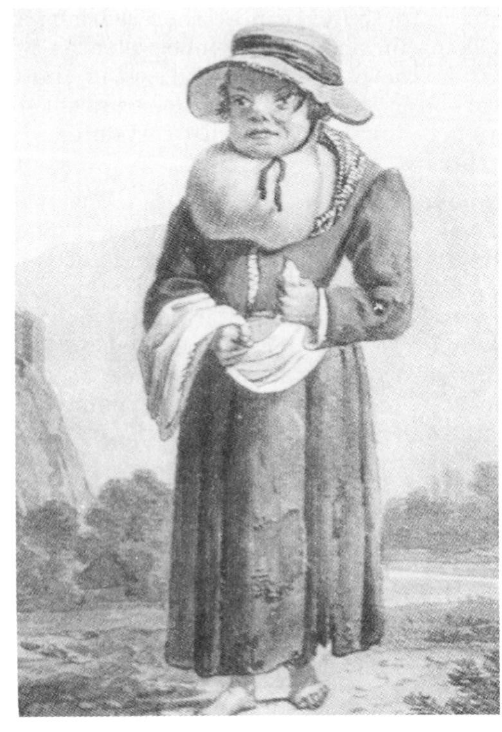

hormone biosynthesis may cause goiter, most cases of sporadic goiter have no known etiology. The pathophysiology of sporadic goiter formation is presumably identical to that of endemic goiter. Population studies have indicated that approximately 4 percent of individuals in a nonendemic area have thyroid nodules.[48] In autopsy studies of unselected patients over 20 years of age, the incidence of nodules 1 cm or larger rose to 50 percent when the thyroid gland was sectioned serially.[49]

Sex and Age in Relation to Goiter

Most types of thyroid dysfunction are approximately four to five times more common in females than in males, and goiter formation is no exception. Estrogens are an obvious source of this difference, but there is no convincing evidence to support this possibility. In an effort to determine the reasons for this sex difference, systematic comparisons were made of the development of the pituitary-thyroid axis in male and female rats.[50] The serum TSH concentration in adult male rats is 2.8 times higher than in females, but the serum T_4 concentration in males is 28 percent lower. Whether these findings are pertinent to the sex differences in human thyroid dysfunction remains to be determined.

Sporadic goiter does not usually occur before puberty. In endemic areas, the highest incidence of goiter is found between ages 10 and 50; the incidence decreases in later decades. In contrast, the incidence of sporadic goiter has no age peak. Frequently, the thyroid gland increases rapidly in size at the time of puberty, especially in girls. Whether this "physiologic" goiter represents relative thyroid hormone deficiency caused by the stress of puberty is not clear, but the goiter tends to disappear subsequently without thyroid hormone therapy.

Goiter during Pregnancy

A physiologic increase in the size of the thyroid appears to occur during some pregnancies. Histologic examination of the typical thyroid gland during gestation reveals large follicles with abundant well-stained colloid and frequent vacuolation. Papillary infolding of thyroid follicles can be seen in 25 percent of cases, and the thyroid follicular cells are columnar rather than flat. All these findings reinforce the impression of thyroid hyperplasia. This histologic picture is one of active formation and secretion of thyroid hormone.

In a study of pregnant women in Scotland, goiter was considered to be present if the thyroid gland was both palpable and visible.[51] By these criteria, 70 percent of pregnant women had goiter, compared with 38 percent of nonpregnant women. The prevalence of goiter did not appear to be affected by previous parity, since goiter occurred in 39 percent of nulliparous women and 35 percent of nongravid parous women. Thyroid enlargement occurred in each trimester with the same frequency, suggesting that goiter appears early and persists during pregnancy. When the same study was repeated in Iceland, no increase in goiter was found during pregnancy.[52] The difference in goiter incidence during pregnancy between the two countries was attributed to differences in dietary iodine content. Renal clearance of iodine is increased during pregnancy as a consequence of the increased glomerular filtration rate. The plasma inorganic iodine concentration decreases because more iodine is excreted in the urine and less is available for thyroid hormone biosynthesis. To compensate, the thyroid gland may enlarge and clear more plasma of iodine to ensure adequate thyroid hormone biosynthesis. Therefore, in areas of marginal iodine intake, pregnancy is more likely to lead to goiter formation.

In a study done in Belgium, an area of marginal iodine intake, there was a progressive increase in thyroid volume during pregnancy.[53] An analysis of 552 ultrasound tests indicated that 73 percent of pregnant women had a significant increase in thyroid volume, with an average increase of 18 percent. True goiter, defined as a total thyroid volume greater than 33 ml, was found in 9 percent of the women in the study at the time of delivery. A study done in the United States did not find a significant difference in iodine balance between pregnant and nonpregnant women.[54] The high-iodine diet in North America may vitiate the increased iodine loss during pregnancy, and goiter is apparently not significantly more common during pregnancy.[55]

Genetic Influences on Goiter Formation

It has been suggested that even in endemic goiter areas, individuals who develop goiter are genetically distinct from nongoitrous individuals from the same area. In an endemic goiter region of Greece, a uniformly high thyroidal uptake of radioiodine occurred, but only certain individuals were goitrous.[56] Since these goiters were grouped within particular families, genetic factors may play a role in goiter formation. Goiter prevalence was compared in monozygotic and dizygotic twin pairs of like sex to obtain an index of the importance of inheritance in the etiology of goiter in healthy people.[57] The data suggested that a genetically determined tendency toward thyroid growth may exist. The suggestion that the goiter of puberty and pregnancy is a consequence of an increased requirement for thyroid hormone during a period of stress does not explain why only a minority of individuals develop this goiter. Nor does this hypothesis explain the results of radioiodine studies or the abundance of colloid found in most goiters of puberty.[58] The familial occurrence of thyroid disease in adolescents with the goiter of puberty again suggests a genetic predisposition.

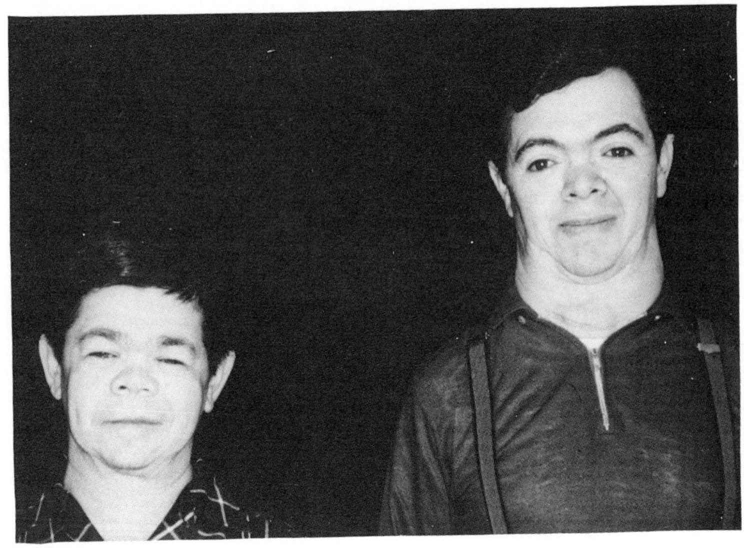

FIGURE 11-5 Two brothers with goitrous cretinism caused by a defect in thyroglobulin synthesis.

Specific Inherited Defects in Thyroid Hormone Biosynthesis

The clearest examples of genetic influences on thyroid function and goiter formation are found in a small group of individuals with hypothyroidism and goiter. These persons have inherited specific autosomal recessive defects in hormone synthesis (Fig. 11-5). These defects lead to inadequate thyroid hormone production, which results in prolonged stimulation of TSH release, in some cases leading to an enlarged sella. The hypersecretion of TSH leads to intense thyroid gland hyperplasia and goiter; the hyperplasia can be mistaken for a malignancy. In fact, thyroid malignancy appears to be no more common in these patients.[59] These conditions apparently occur because of genetic defects of single enzymes or other proteins, presumably corresponding to each step in thyroid hormone biosynthesis (see Chap. 10).

As indicated in Fig. 11-6, there are five major recognized defects in thyroid hormone biosynthesis, but it is almost certain that there are many more:

1. There may be a defect in the ability of the thyroid gland to trap iodine.
2. A defect may exist in the ability of the gland to convert inorganic iodide to an organic form, as an iodotyrosine. This defect is characterized by precipitate discharge of radioactive iodine from the thyroid after the administration of thiocyanate or perchlorate; it may be associated with deafness. This is a heterogeneous group of defects related to the peroxidase system and associated with the various steps in organification.
3. Thyroid hormone is synthesized within the interstices of the very large thyroglobulin molecule. Defects in thyroglobulin synthesis lead to inadequate or absent thyroid hormone synthesis. This probably reflects a large, heterogeneous group of

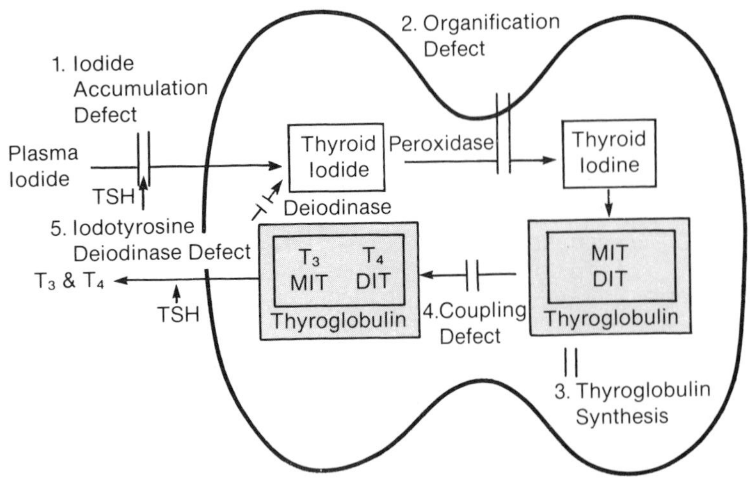

FIGURE 11-6 Defects in thyroid hormone biosynthesis.

defects. Although no proof exists, a number of cases of sporadic goiter may in fact represent minor defects in thyroglobulin synthesis.

4. There may be coupling defects resulting from a variety of defects which impair iodothyronine formation.
5. The iodotyrosine deiodinase defect results in iodine loss from the gland. The enzyme usually deiodinates iodotyrosines which have not coupled to form iodothyronines, allowing the iodine to be reused within the gland.

In addition to the defects listed above, there may be an impaired tissue response to TSH or to thyroid hormones (see Chap. 10). However, the former condition would not cause goiter. Whatever the specific defect, genetic influences lead to inadequate thyroid hormone production and goiter formation. Whether similar but less well defined genetic influences play a role in sporadic goiter remains to be determined.

Specific Goitrogens

Any substance that interferes with the biosynthesis of thyroid hormone can be a goitrogen.[60] This includes a number of chemical compounds that inhibit specific steps of thyroid hormone biosynthesis as well as dietary goitrogens in which the active compound is unknown.

Dietary Goitrogens

The development of antithyroid drug therapy began with the observation that rabbits that were fed cabbage developed goiters and the later finding that goiters developed in rats fed seeds of brassicas (cabbage, turnips, Brussels sprouts, rutabagas, etc.).[61] This finding led to the appreciation of thiourea as a goitrogen and eventually to the introduction of thioamides as valuable therapeutic agents in the treatment of hyperthyroidism. The quantity of the goitrogen and perhaps the quality of the vegetables containing the goitrogen are such that the chance of significant goiter formation in human beings is rare. Soybean milk has been observed to produce goiter in infants. The goitrogenic substance in soybean flour has not been identified, but supplemention of the diet with iodide eliminates the problem. Foods such as cassava contain compounds that on hydrolysis release free cyanide. After ingestion, the cyanide is converted to thiocyanate. Cassava has been suggested as a cause of endemic goiter in central Africa.[42] In Colombia, sulfur-containing compounds found in the water supply, which are derived from sedimentary rocks, are thought to be goitrogenic.[62]

Chemical Goitrogens

Various chemical goitrogens, ranging from salts and minerals to complex nitrogen-containing heterocyclic compounds, interfere with the synthesis of thyroid hormone (Table 11-3). The salts and minerals of interest here include lithium, which has an inhibitory effect on the release of thyroid hormone, and cobalt, the action of which is unclear. Type I iodothyronine deiodinase is a selenocysteine-containing enzyme, and selenium is essential for the conversion of T_4 to T_3.[63]

TABLE 11-3 Chemical Goitrogens

Effect within the Thyroid
Modifiers of iodine transport: complex anions: technetium perchlorate, thiocyanate (active ingredient in *Brassica* spp. and cassava)
Modifiers of iodination of thyroglobulin
Thioamides: propylthiouracil, methimazole, carbimazole
Thiocyanate
Aniline derivatives: sulfonamides, *p*-aminosalicylic acid, amphenone B, aminoglutethimide, phenylbutazone
Effects on iodothyronine formation
Thioamides
Sulfonamides
Influences on secretion of thyroid hormone
Iodide
Lithium
Effect on Peripheral Disposal of Thyroid Hormone
Hormone deiodination: propylthiouracil, iopanoic acid, ipodate, amiodarone
Intestinal absorption of hormones: soy flour, resins (e.g., cholestyramine)
Hormone inactivation: inducers of hepatic drug-metabolizing enzymes (e.g., phenobarbital)

Selenium deficiency occurs in areas of iodine deficiency and may contribute to the development of myxedematous endemic cretinism.[64] The more complex chemical compounds which interfere with thyroid function by blocking iodination and the coupling reaction have some common structural features. None of the nitrogen heterocyclics are as potent as the thioamides, e.g., propylthiouracil, but there is no apparent fundamental difference in their antithyroid action.

Environmental Goitrogens

Pollution of drinking water is known to precipitate goiter in low-iodine areas. McGarrison noted that goiter prevalence increased downstream from the water supply in the group of villages which make up Gilgit in the foothills of the Himalayas.[65] Goiter occurred in 12 percent of the inhabitants at the source, and the prevalence increased to 45 percent at the terminus of the river, which had served as a drinking channel and open sewer for the villages on its banks. McGarrison was able to produce goiter in himself and his colleagues by ingesting suspended matter from those goiter-producing waters.[65] The goiter did not occur if the water was boiled first. In subsequent studies, low urinary iodine excretion (4 to 6 μg/L) was found in residents of this area, but equally low levels were found in both goitrous and nongoitrous individuals.

Nontoxic Goiter

Whatever the cause, both endemic and sporadic goiters present clinically as nontoxic goiter and, depending on duration, may be either diffuse or nodular. Some goiters which may be associated with hyperthyroidism were considered in Chap. 10. More frequently, some of the nodules may be autonomous; i.e., they release hormone constitutively and are no longer responsive to normal pituitary-thyroid regulation.

Incidence

The incidence of nontoxic goiter varies widely depending on whether goiter is endemic in the area. The discussion here centers on nonendemic areas such as North America. The occurrence of goiter has been determined in both autopsy and clinical studies. In an unselected autopsy series of 1000 patients over 20 years old, the prevalence of goiter was 5 percent. When they were sectioned, half the thyroids contained nodules that were at least 1 cm across and would have been palpable if they had been anterior and superficial.[49] The study was carried out in Minnesota, which was an endemic goiter region before the introduction of iodine, and goiter may still be more common in these regions. However, similar results were found in Connecticut, a nonendemic goiter area.[66]

Presentations and Complications

Nontoxic goiter is usually discovered during a routine examination. Occasionally the patient will have noticed a lump in the throat. Rarely, the goiter may be symptomatic and cause pressure symptoms such as coughing, wheezing, dysphagia, and hoarseness. The last presentation is uncommon, and so carcinoma of the thyroid or an unrelated condition should be ruled out. These symptoms, with the exception of carcinoma, are more likely to occur in a long-standing goiter low in the neck which is compressed by the sternum or grows around behind the trachea. X-rays of the trachea may show deviation or even some compression. However, peak inspiratory and expiratory flow studies should be done to determine whether there is a significant decrease in airflow. Upper airway obstruction may actually be more common than is realized.[67] Such obstruction is potentially dangerous because tracheitis with edema can result in severe compromise of the airway.[68] Occasionally the thyroid may suddenly increase in size, accompanied by pain and tenderness. This sudden change is often indicative of hemorrhage into a cystic area of the nodular goiter and usually subsides within several weeks.

Complaints of a "lump in the throat" are most often due to globus hystericus, an anxiety reaction characterized by a constrictive feeling in the throat. This feeling is heightened by the presence of a nontoxic goiter, presenting a difficult problem for physicians. Patients frequently describe fluctuation in goiter size, often related to periods of emotional stress or to the menstrual cycle, but these changes are almost impossible to document. The position and irregular shape of the thyroid have made it difficult to estimate the size of the gland accurately over a period of time. The thyroid does have a rich blood supply, and changes in blood flow may change the volume of the gland. The ancient Romans are reputed to have believed that the thyroid gland swells with sexual excitement; they used to measure a bride's neck to prove that the marriage had been consummated.[69]

Risk of Carcinoma in Multinodular Goiter

One of the undesirable side effects of cancer education programs is that the discovery of a "lump" frequently means cancer to the patient. Thus, a patient with a multinodular goiter is often very anxious, and this may make the physician anxious enough to recommend surgery. If the patient demands that the physician guarantee that the thyroid nodule is not malignant, this can be done only if the nodule is excised and examined histologically. The decision to remove a thyroid nodule is thus a result of both the patient's anxiety and the physician's anxiety. Since as many as 50 percent of thyroid glands in adults may harbor a nodule 1 cm or greater, physicians must know exactly how suspicious they should be about the possibility of carcinoma occurring in a nontoxic multinodular goiter. (Solitary thyroid nodules are considered separately below.)

The questions to be answered are, (1) What is the risk of thyroid carcinoma in the general population? and (2) Does the presence of a nontoxic goiter increase this risk?

In two separate series of unselected autopsies, thyroid carcinoma was found in approximately 3 percent of the patients.[48,65] More recently, autopsy studies in Japan and Minnesota indicated a prevalence of small histologic malignancies in the thyroid as high as 13 percent when serial sections were carefully examined.[70,71] In contrast, the frequency of clinical thyroid cancer is about 39 cases diagnosed annually per 1 million population, or 0.0004 percent.[72] The reason for the marked discrepancy between histologic and clinically apparent thyroid carcinoma can be explained by reference to the concept that cancer is a multistep process. The histologic diagnosis of small thyroid malignancies (minimal papillary thyroid carcinoma) does not appear to correlate with true invasiveness, which is compatible with this concept. Similar relations have been found with prostatic carcinoma, with which the incidence is much higher at autopsy than is clinically apparent during life.

The important question is whether the presence of a nontoxic goiter increases the incidence of clinically important thyroid cancer. The mortality rate for thyroid carcinoma was found to be 10 times higher in Switzerland, where goiter is endemic, than in England.[73] Furthermore, as the use of iodized salt increased in Switzerland, deaths from thyroid carcinoma decreased. The difficulty with this type of study is that a higher rate of thyroid surgery with careful pathologic examination might have resulted in the increased diagnosis of thyroid cancer. If the prevalence of goiter is based on medical examinations of draftees for World War I and World War II and this difference is compared with the prevalence of thyroid carcinoma and hyperthyroidism, an estimate of the effect of goiter on thyroid carcinoma can be made.[35] The reduction in goiter prevalence between World War I and World War II was associated with the introduction of iodized salt. Despite the decrease in goiter frequency, the death rate for thyroid carcinoma changed very little during this period. Hyperthyroidism mortality rates increased immediately after the introduction of iodized salt, perhaps owing to the iod-Basedow phenomenon, and then decreased in parallel with the decrease in goiter. The comparison of goiter prevalence with hyperthyroidism strongly supports that endemic goiter is an important factor in the pathogenesis of hyperthyroidism. In contrast, comparison of thyroid cancer and goiter failed to provide convincing evidence for the existence of an association between these two diseases.

Thyroid malignancy can be induced experimentally in rats by means of prolonged TSH stimulation, but there is no convincing evidence that TSH stimulation is carcinogenic in normal individuals.[74,75] Although there have been several reports on congenital goiters which were intensely hyperplastic and developed carcinomas, an intensely hyperplastic gland may also be mistaken for a malignancy.[76,77] Most of the nodules in goiters are polyclonal; i.e., they have arisen from more than one cell.[78] This situation contrasts with thyroid cancers that are monoclonal in origin, suggesting that some event in a single cell led to the malignant state.[78] However, large nodules in a multinodular goiter can be monoclonal in origin, implying that they may be premalignant.[78] Nevertheless, with the exception of the latter caveat, the evidence seems to indicate that the presence of goiter per se does not predispose a patient to thyroid carcinoma.

Laboratory Evaluation

When a patient presents with a goiter, the first question to be asked is whether the goiter is toxic or nontoxic. If the goiter is nontoxic, is thyroiditis the cause? Is the goiter diffuse or nodular, and is the nodule solitary or multiple? If the gland is nodular, are the nodules autonomous?

Evaluation of thyroid function is described in detail in Chap. 10. Patients with goiter should have a sensitive TSH determination, a serum T_4 determination, a measurement of thyroxine-binding antibodies, and an assay for thyroid antibodies to determine the functional thyroid state and the presence of thyroiditis. A radioisotopic thyroid scan may be helpful in identifying nodularity and autonomy but is not necessary. If the thyroid function tests reveal evidence of hyperthyroidism, hypothyroidism, or thyroiditis, the patient should be managed as described in Chap. 10. If goiter persists once these conditions have resolved, the patient should be treated as described below.

Therapy

Is the presence of goiter in a euthyroid patient a sufficient indication for thyroid hormone suppressive therapy? All goiters probably should be suppressed with thyroid hormone, with the exception of self-limited conditions such as the goiters of puberty and of pregnancy and the goiters of some elderly patients who have an increased risk of osteoporosis (described below). One must be aware of the caveat that autonomous areas of the goiter may not be suppressible, resulting in too much circulating thyroid hormone. Thyroid hormone therapy has a relatively low cost (only pennies per day) and is relatively nontoxic when the dose is adjusted properly. Therapy may decrease the size of the goiter or block a further increase in its size. However, treatment of long-standing goiter may not result in a decrease in gland size because of the presence of fibrosis. Patients who are symptomatic with compression symptoms are candidates for surgery. Some patients with large, symptomatic goiters can best be handled by treatment with 20 to 100 millicuries (mCi) of ^{131}I to decrease the goiter before thyroid hormone suppression therapy. Furthermore, in a double-blind randomized study, solitary benign nodules did not decrease significantly with thyroid hormone therapy.[79] Therapy for solitary nodules is discussed in Solitary Thyroid Nodules below.

Therapy is recommended even if the goiter is not large initially or is fibrotic and probably will not decrease in size. Without therapy, prolonged TSH stimulation of the gland results in dilated capillaries, which may rupture and result in a hemorrhagic cyst, may eventually lead to nodule formation, and may allow the goiter to progress. The presence of a thyroid nodule often makes both the patient and the physician anxious and may lead ineluctably to the operating table.

Results

Despite the large number of patients receiving thyroid hormone suppression, relatively few large, controlled studies have examined the efficacy of such treatment carefully.[80–84] Two hundred thirty patients with nontoxic goiter were treated with 180 mg of desiccated thyroid and were observed at intervals of 1 to 3 months.[80] The goiter was regarded as diffuse if the entire gland was enlarged, even if the two lobes differed in size, or if there was considerable irregularity in the shape of the gland. The goiter was called nodular only when conspicuous nodules were prominent or when a single nodule was found in an enlarged thyroid. A single nodule was diagnosed when there was an isolated nodule in an otherwise normal gland. Regression of the goiter with therapy was considered complete when the thyroid decreased to its normal size. The response to therapy was called "moderate" for any unequivocal regression short of a complete response. The results shown in Table 11-4 indicate that in one-fourth of patients with nodular goiter complete regression occurred and that in one-half there was moderate regression.

The administration of L-thyroxine or placebo to 53 patients in a double-blind manner with a colloid solitary thyroid nodule was evaluated by means of ultrasound of the thyroid.[79] The dose of L-thyroxine was 3 μg per kilogram of body weight per day and was given for 6 months. Despite effective suppression of serum TSH concentrations as determined by TRH tests, there was no significant decrease in nodule size with L-thyroxine compared to placebo.

Questions have been raised whether thyroid hormone suppressive therapy may accelerate bone loss and osteoporosis by producing subclinical hyperthyroidism.[85] For this reason, it is reasonable to withhold therapy in elderly patients with long-standing nodular disease in whom thyroxine treatment carries an increased risk. Large, symptomatic, nontoxic multinodular goiters do not respond to thyroid hormone suppressive therapy, and recurrence after partial thyroidectomy may occur in 10 to 15 percent of patients.[86] For these reasons, 14 patients with large multinodular goiters were treated with 20 to 100 mCi of ^{131}I. There was a significant decrease in goiter size in 11 of the 14 patients. Similar findings have been reported in another study.[87] In the absence of medical complications, surgery may be the preferable choice in view of the radiation dose required.

Thyroid Hormone Therapy

To decrease the size of the thyroid gland, sufficient thyroid hormone has to be given to suppress TSH secretion without inducing hyperthyroidism. Therapy with L-triiodothyronine results in markedly elevated serum levels of the hormone for several hours after ingestion. Although there is no evidence that transient serum elevations of triiodothyronine in an otherwise healthy individual are harmful, it seems best to avoid these elevations if possible. Consequently, L-thyroxine should be used, since the hormone is slowly converted to triiodothyronine and since elevated serum concentrations of T_3 do not occur. Triiodothyronine is less effective in maintaining TSH suppression.[18] Studies of TSH concentrations in hypothyroid women receiving L-thyroxine indicated that 90 percent of the patients were optimally managed, as indicated by normal serum TSH concentration, with the daily administration of 100 to 200 μg of L-thyroxine,[88] but this was not a sensitive TSH determination. As was mentioned previously, the presence of an autonomous nodule may result in excessive circulating thyroid hormone.

With the introduction of the third-generation sensitive TSH assay, it has become clear that TSH suppression is a relative, not an absolute, phenomenon.[17] For benign, nontoxic nodular or diffuse goiter, replacement thyroxine therapy, which usually consists of 0.10 mg/day or less, is appropriate. The goal of therapy should be to use the minimal dose of thyroxine to keep the plasma TSH levels as low as possible without inducing the symptoms of hyperthyroidism. It appears reasonable to attempt to suppress the sensitive TSH value to the range of 0.1 to 0.3 μU/ml.

Initial follow-up after the institution of therapy should be done at 6 to 8 weeks, with repeat thyroid function tests to exclude the possibility of autonomous functioning of the goiter. Once the dose has been adjusted, the patient generally can be followed annually, at which time the status of the goiter and of overall thyroid function can be assessed.

TABLE 11-4 Response of Nontoxic Goiter to Thyroid Hormone Therapy

Usual Dose of 180 μg of Desiccated Thyroid Hormone Administered for Periods Ranging from 1 Month to More Than 24 Months

		Percent with Each Level of Response		
Type of goiter	No. patients	Complete	Moderate	None
Diffuse	115	33	34	23
Nodular	78	24	52	24
Solitary nodule	37	27	27	46

Source: Astwood et al.[80]

SOLITARY THYROID NODULES

Although the risk of thyroid carcinoma does not appear to be increased in patients with a multinodular goiter, the risk is increased with a solitary thyroid nodule. In a series of 300 unselected autopsies of adults, 19 single thyroid nodules (6 percent) were found after sectioning of the gland.[66] The chance that a solitary thyroid nodule in this series would be a benign or malignant neoplasm was almost three times higher than was the case with a multinodular goiter. The frequency of thyroid carcinoma in single nodules was almost four times the frequency in the entire series of unselected thyroid glands. Thus, despite the difficulty in separating single from multiple thyroid nodules clinically, thyroid cancer has been found more frequently in a solitary thyroid nodule. Since thyroid carcinoma usually does not concentrate radioiodine as well as normal tissues does, malignant thyroid nodules commonly appear as hypofunctioning or nonfunctioning ("cold") areas on a radioactive iodine scan of the thyroid gland.[89] However, it must be emphasized that thyroid carcinoma also occurs in functioning nodules and that the presence of a functioning thyroid nodule does not eliminate the possibility of malignancy. In a series of 202 patients with solitary thyroid nodules, there was an overall prevalence of thyroid carcinoma of 29 percent.[90] If cold solitary thyroid nodules had been the sole criterion for selection for surgery, 40 percent of the carcinomas would have been missed.

Factors Predisposing to Thyroid Cancer

If there is an increased risk of malignancy in solitary cold thyroid nodules, are there criteria available to select patients who are at higher risk?

Gender

As was mentioned earlier, most forms of thyroid disease are more common in females; this is true of thyroid malignancy as well. However, females have a higher incidence of nontoxic nodular goiter than males do. As a consequence, a solitary thyroid nodule occurring in a male is three times more likely to be malignant than is a solitary nodule occurring in a female.

Age

It has been estimated that half the thyroid nodules that appear in children may be malignant. The implication is not that thyroid cancer is more common in childhood but that thyroid nodules in general are uncommon in this age group. Eighty percent of the children with carcinoma of the thyroid who formed the basis of this estimate had a history of exposure to radiation.[91,92] The chance of malignancy in the thyroid nodule of a child needs to be reappraised now that this type of irradiation has practically been discontinued.

Among 30 children with solitary thyroid nodules, only 4 had a history of neck irradiation.[93] Nevertheless, there was a 40 percent incidence of carcinoma in the series, including the four irradiated children. These data suggest that thyroid carcinoma continues to be a significant risk in children with solitary thyroid nodules. However, in a study of 5179 schoolchildren in grades 6 through 12, nodularity of the thyroid was found in 93 (1.8 percent).[94] The nodularity represented adolescent goiter in 34 children and thyroiditis in 31. Only two thyroid cancers were found, which raised the question whether all thyroid nodules in children should be removed surgically. However, 5 of 14 children with solitary thyroid nodules operated on in New York over a 10-year period had thyroid cancer without any history of external radiation.[95] Nodules that proved to be neoplasms were usually discrete, solitary, and of firm consistency and were not associated with changes in the rest of the thyroid.

Previous Irradiation of the Head and Neck

Previous irradiation of the head and neck markedly increases the chances of malignancy in a thyroid nodule. The observation in 1950 that 9 of 28 children with carcinoma of the thyroid had received radiotherapy to the thymus in infancy first highlighted this association, which was confirmed in prospective studies.[96,97] Most instances of thyroid malignancy after neck irradiation were reported within 10 years after radiation therapy. Since this type of radiation therapy to the neck has been discontinued, a degree of complacency developed among many physicians. However, reports indicating an increased incidence of thyroid carcinoma an average of 25 years or more after radiation exposure of the head and neck have dispelled this illusion.[98,99] Although irradiation therapy for benign diseases of infancy and childhood was discontinued many years ago, the occurrence of radiation-associated thyroid carcinoma has apparently not declined.

Despite direct questioning, few patients with a thyroid nodule were able to give a history of irradiation during infancy. Public awareness increased dramatically after the relation was featured in a television drama. This increased awareness was largely due to the fact that mothers are more knowledgeable than their children about medical history. (Perhaps all patients, regardless of age, should bring their mothers with them for the initial visit to the physician's office!)

The magnitude of the increase in thyroid carcinoma after irradiation to the neck has not been proved, but the current estimate is that about 14 percent of irradiated patients will develop a malignancy.[100] There has been an increase in benign as well as malignant thyroid nodules, and, importantly, both forms of thyroid nodules have continued to occur with no indication of a decrease with time. There was also an increase in salivary gland tumors and neurilemomas.

Physical Characteristics

Careful examination of the thyroid can be extremely helpful in determining how suspicious to be of the presence of an underlying malignancy. A history of recent thyroid growth, dysphagia, or dyspnea should make the examiner suspicious of malignancy. Palpation of the thyroid should be done carefully, with particular attention to how regular and hard the nodule is, whether the gland is fixed to surrounding structures, and whether there are palpable regional lymph nodes. However, the presence of a multinodular goiter decreases the likelihood of malignancy.

A group of 53 patients with thyroid nodules were first classified clinically as to whether their nodules were benign or malignant, and these results were compared with the findings at surgery.[101] Thyroid cancer was found in 76 percent of cases thought to be malignant nodules clinically; 12 percent of cases thought to be benign clinically but symptomatic as indicated by pain, recent change in goiter size, or dysphagia; and 3 percent of patients whose nodules were thought to be benign and who were asymptomatic. In this study, only two patients with thyroid carcinoma were free of symptoms.

The most important physical sign of thyroid malignancy is the presence of a hard, irregular thyroid nodule. Extreme hardness may be due to hemorrhage into a cyst with subsequent calcification. If the thyroid cancer has spread beyond the capsule and invaded surrounding structures, the clinical diagnosis becomes comparatively simple, although Riedel's struma (see Chap. 10) can also extend beyond the gland. Fixation to the strap muscles, trachea, or larynx is easily detected on physical examination. Recurrent laryngeal nerve paralysis is not a common presenting symptom in thyroid cancer, but it does occur.

Laboratory Diagnosis

The presence of a solitary thyroid nodule raises the question of thyroid malignancy, and the predisposing factors discussed above may strengthen or allay suspicions about an individual patient. The next step in the evaluation of a solitary thyroid nodule is to use the laboratory to further discriminate which nodules may be malignant and which may be benign.

Radioisotopic Scan of the Thyroid

Scanning of the thyroid after the administration of a tracer dose of radioactive iodine or technetium 99m permits the delineation of functioning and nonfunctioning areas of the thyroid (Fig. 11-7). Since

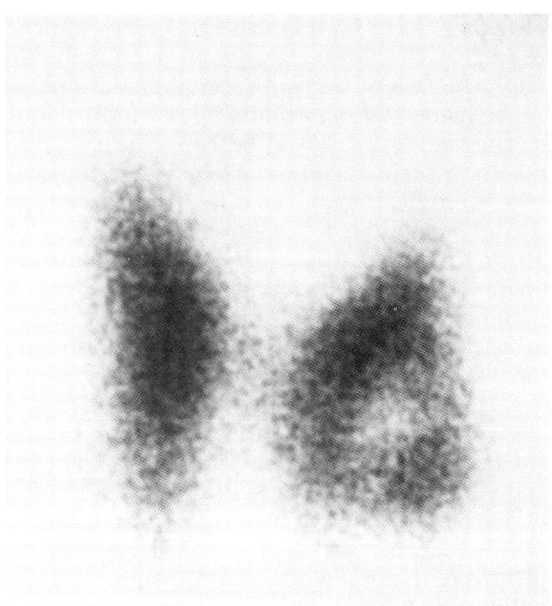

FIGURE 11-7 A radioisotopic scan shows a nonfunctioning solitary nodule in the lower pole of the right lobe of the thyroid.

even well-differentiated thyroid carcinomas do not concentrate iodine as efficiently as the normal thyroid does, hypofunctioning (cold) thyroid nodules have been considered to carry a greater risk of malignancy. This classification is established by assessing the amount of radioactivity within the nodule relative to that in extranodular tissue. To be detectable under optimal conditions, the cold nodule must be at least approximately 1 cm in diameter. Large nodules may produce a well-defined focal defect, marginal indentation, or locally reduced parenchymal activity. The demonstration of a cold thyroid nodule is significant but nonspecific. The majority of clinically significant thyroid nodules are less functional than the extranodular thyroid tissue.[102]

Iodine 131 has been the radionuclide most widely used for thyroid imaging, although the high radiation doses absorbed have been a matter of concern. This concern has heightened with the recurrence of interest in the delayed effects of neck irradiation.[103] The administration of 100 μCi of ^{131}I for a thyroid scan can result in a dose of 80 rads to the thyroid.[104] Since several scans will raise the dose of radiation delivered to the thyroid to a level which has been associated with subsequent thyroid cancer, alternative methods of thyroid imaging are highly desirable.

Iodine 123 is perhaps the ideal isotope for in vivo diagnostic studies of thyroid function and structure. Its short half-life of 13.3 h is suitable for routine uptake tests. Scans superior in resolution to those afforded by ^{99m}Tc or ^{131}I can be obtained with a radiation dose $1/85$ that for a comparable ^{131}I study. Technetium 99m is probably the most readily available isotope of choice for thyroid scanning at present.

Technetium 99m delivers about 0.6 rad to the thyroid during a scanning procedure. The pertechnetate ion ($^{99m}TcO_4^-$) is rapidly trapped by the thyroid but is not organically bound and does not remain in the gland. The difference between technetium and iodine radioisotopes has clinical significance because some thyroid malignancies trap pertechnetate but not ^{131}I as a result of a defect in organification.[105]

The findings in most studies have been consistent with the physiologic considerations discussed above. Most thyroid cancers were found to be cold, but benign thyroid nodules are also predominantly cold. This lack of discrimination makes it difficult to use a thyroid scan to differentiate between benign and malignant thyroid nodules. Certainly no patient with a solitary thyroid nodule should be either selected for surgery or screened from surgical consideration by a thyroid scan, although the scan can be helpful in eliminating the minority of solitary nodules with increased radioisotope uptake from serious consideration of malignancy.

Ultrasound

A cold nodule on thyroid imaging may represent either a solid nodule that does not trap the radionuclide or a cystic area in the gland. Diagnostic ultrasound employs acoustic properties to distinguish different soft tissues by passing ultrahigh sound frequencies into the nodule and analyzing the reflected echoes. The diagnostic principle is based on the partial reflection of ultrasound at boundaries or tissue interfaces. An analysis of ultrasound echoes may permit the distinction of solid from cystic nodules. In solid thyroid nodules, multiple echoes are generated with high sensitivity levels, but this does not occur in a thyroid cyst.

The thyroid gland is not as acoustically dense as the surrounding tissue; tracheal cartilage represents the densest structure in the area (Fig. 11-8).

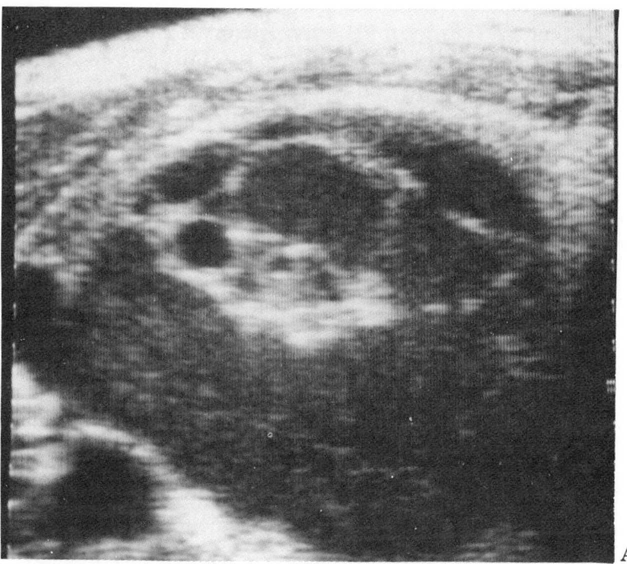

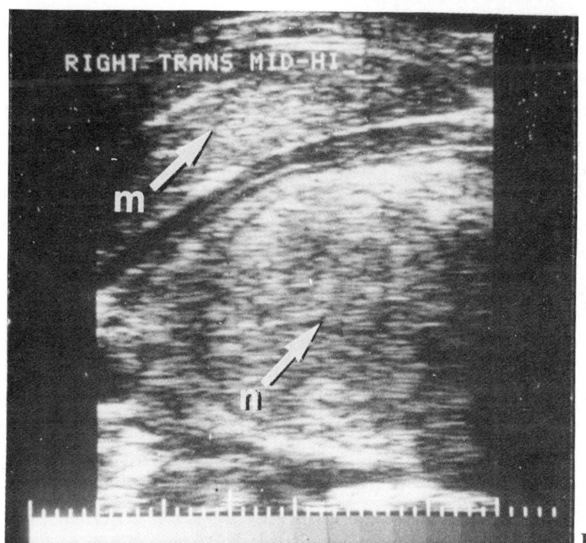

FIGURE 11-8 (*A*) A transverse ultrasound scan of the thyroid showing a 2-cm mass which has numerous septations and a mixture of cystic and solid elements. (*B*) A transverse ultrasound scan of the right lobe of the thyroid. Arrow n indicates a solid nodule that is well defined by its echo-free capsule. Arrow m indicates the sternocleidomastoid muscle.

The typical ultrasound features of a benign thyroid nodule include a large cystic component with a peripheral sonolucent halo, peripheral calcification, and a hyperechoic texture.[106] In contrast, the typical malignant thyroid nodule is an irregular, poorly defined solid mass that is hypoechoic. Not only can solid and cystic thyroid nodules be distinguished, but enlargement of the thyroid caused by tumor growth can be differentiated from enlargement resulting from cystic or hemorrhagic degeneration.[107] The thyroid's volume can also be estimated with ultrasound.[83]

Cysts have been reported to occur in 20 percent of solitary thyroid nodules.[108] Although the possibility of malignancy is significant, particularly in a partially cystic lesion, malignancy is less common than in solid lesions. Thyroid hormone suppression has not been found to be helpful in preventing the recurrence of benign cysts after initial aspiration.[109] Successful sclerosis of a recurrent thyroid cyst with injected tetracycline has been reported but is not indicated in the great majority of cases.[110] The use of ultrasound to evaluate solitary nodules over 4 cm is limited because both solid and cystic lesions give rise to heterogeneous echoes. Small nodules are also difficult, and cystic lesions less than 1 cm in diameter may not be identified. Substernal goiters are difficult to study because the sternum reflects the sound. Despite the useful information that can be obtained, ultrasound does not differentiate between benign and malignant thyroid nodules.

Other Imaging Techniques

Thyroid imaging techniques other than radioisotopic scan and ultrasound are available. The high Z number (i.e., radiographic density) of the thyroid has facilitated the use of the CT scan with or without prior loading with stable iodine.[111] However, the patient receives more radiation to the thyroid, and the resolution of nodules is probably no better than with ultrasound. Magnetic resonance imaging (MRI) techniques can be used for the thyroid gland.[112] The spatial resolution of the MRI approximates that of the CT scan and allows better definition of thyroid nodules, thyroid cysts, and parathyroid tumors. This is a useful, albeit expensive, technique for thyroid imaging.[113] This technique may come into clinical use. Since the thyroid gland has a rich blood supply, angiography can be helpful in conjunction with other findings but is primarily of academic interest.[114]

Thyroid Biopsy

Although various diagnostic procedures may heighten suspicion that a particular solitary thyroid nodule is malignant, only a tissue diagnosis can ultimately diagnose or exclude thyroid cancer. Needle biopsy of the thyroid had been considered an alternative to surgery, but fear that cancer might be disseminated along the track delayed the acceptance of this procedure.[115,116] Spread of malignant cells has proved not to be a problem, and fine-needle aspiration biopsy of the thyroid has gained wide acceptance.[115,116]

Although there are special thyroid biopsy sets, a 10-ml syringe with a 22-gauge needle works well. After the patient is reclining with a pillow under the shoulders to hyperextend the neck, the nodule is palpated and the area is prepped with alcohol. Three biopsies are done with three different syringes and needles. The aspirate is placed on a clear glass slide, and the two slides are "pulled." One slide is put into Papanicolaou fluid, and the other is air-dried. Hank's solution is withdrawn into the syringes and rinsed out. The material from the three syringes is subsequently centrifuged and examined on a block. There are many variations, but an adequate specimen for the cytopathologist is the necessary endpoint. The most difficult thyroid lesions to diagnose are follicular carcinomas, whose identification often depends on the demonstration of vascular and capsular invasion. Lymphomas may be confused with thyroiditis.[117,118] Papillary carcinoma, by contrast, usually is easily identified because of its unique histologic characteristics.[106]

Since the majority of patients who have had a biopsy of the thyroid do not have a subsequent thyroidectomy, comparison of the biopsy specimen with the entire thyroid gland is frequently impossible. In a series of 81 cases in which 93 percent of cutting needle biopsy diagnoses were confirmed by thyroid surgery, errors were found in 7 percent, and half of those errors were due to lymphoma complicating Hashimoto's disease, undifferentiated carcinoma diagnosed as nonspecific thyroiditis, and follicular carcinoma mistaken for follicular adenoma.[116] No serious complications occurred with the needle biopsy procedure, and there was no evidence of tumor implantation in the needle track in any of the primary cancers. There was a single example of seeding in a renal cell carcinoma that was metastatic to the thyroid. If there is significant clinical suspicion of thyroid cancer, a negative needle biopsy should not preclude surgery.

Fine-needle aspiration biopsy avoids the morbidity that may occur with cutting needles like the Vim-Silverman and has become the determining factor in the management of a solitary thyroid nodule (Fig. 11-9).[119] In a review of 1330 patients, all of whom underwent surgery, 22 cases were diagnosed as negative by aspiration biopsy but were found to be malignant at surgery, an incidence of false negatives of 1.7 percent.[120] In the same study, the false-positive incidence was 0.5 percent. The diagnosis of malignancy by fine-needle aspiration biopsy had a specificity of 0.99 and a sensitivity of 0.73[116] (sensitivity measures the fraction of patients with thyroid cancer detected by the biopsy, while specificity measures the fraction of patients correctly identified as having no thyroid malignancy). The results of the various diagnostic techniques for detecting thyroid cancer can be expressed according to Bayes' theorem to give the predictive value of a positive test (Fig. 11-10).[121]

In the same study, three strategies were studied for the diagnosis of thyroid nodules. Two began with a radioisotopic thyroid scan, followed, if the scan was positive, by either aspirate biopsy or ultrasound; the third began with aspiration biopsy followed by a scan.[119] The last strategy was the most cost-effective. Fine-needle aspiration biopsy was the most success-

FIGURE 11-9 A fine-needle biopsy aspirate of papillary carcinoma of the thyroid, demonstrating papillary configuration.

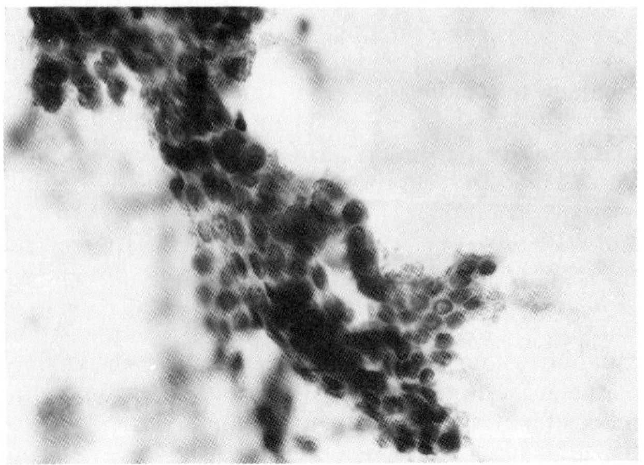

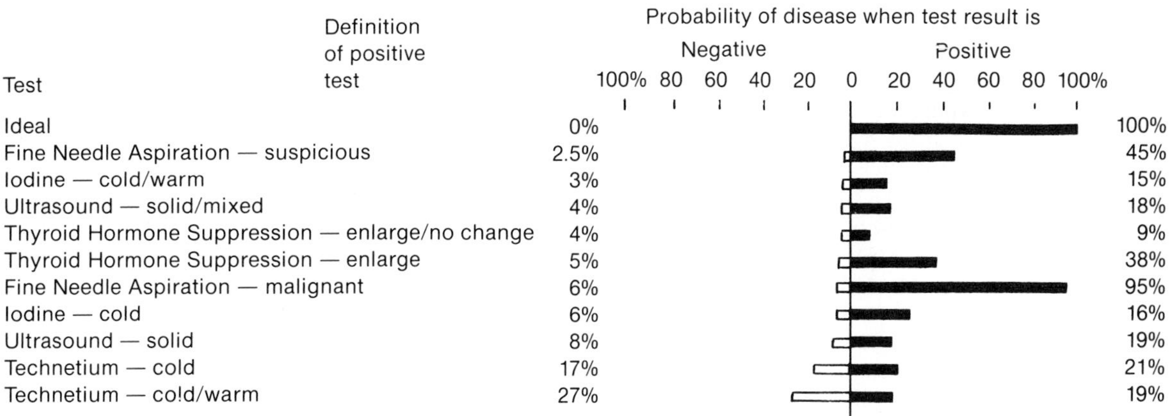

Test
Definition of positive test
Probability of disease when test result is
Negative
Positive
100% 80 60 40 20 0 20 40 60 80 100%
Ideal 0% 100%
Fine Needle Aspiration — suspicious 2.5% 45%
Iodine — cold/warm 3% 15%
Ultrasound — solid/mixed 4% 18%
Thyroid Hormone Suppression — enlarge/no change 4% 9%
Thyroid Hormone Suppression — enlarge 5% 38%
Fine Needle Aspiration — malignant 6% 95%
Iodine — cold 6% 16%
Ultrasound — solid 8% 19%
Technetium — cold 17% 21%
Technetium — cold/warm 27% 19%

FIGURE 11-10 Probability of disease based on test results calculated according to Bayes' theorem. Open bars represent missed malignancies; solid bars represent the percentage of surgeries in which malignancies were found. (*Modified from Van Herle et al.*[119])

ful of the available tests when applied alone. Neither radioisotopic scan of the thyroid nor ultrasound has high specificity. Combining the two procedures yields the highest sensitivity but does not improve specificity.

The use of needle biopsy in a large series of 455 patients with thyroid nodules decreased the number of patients sent to surgery by half and doubled the number of patients who were to be observed.[122] Operation for benign disease decreased 70 percent, while thyroid carcinoma identified at operation increased 75 percent.[123] The accuracy depends on both sampling and the ability to read the cytologic determination.[124] A number of factors critical in assessing the value of thyroid biopsy are shown in Table 11-5.

Although most physicians agree that positive or undeterminable biopsies are indications for surgery, there is concern about whether an apparently negative biopsy rules out the possibility of thyroid cancer. Only 100 to 1000 cells are examined out of perhaps 1 billion in the thyroid; sampling error thus may occur. A negative biopsy should not dissuade the physician from referring for thyroid surgery a patient who has significant risk factors, e.g., a young male with a firm, irregular thyroid nodule. However, this is a subjective decision.

TABLE 11-5 Factors in Assessing Fine-Needle Aspiration Biopsy of the Thyroid

	Percent of Biopsies
Inadequate study	3–11
Undeterminable*	17–30
False negatives	2–4
False positives	0–3

* The frequency of carcinoma in undeterminable cases is 20 to 60 percent.

Source: Block MA: Surgery of thyroid nodules and malignancy, in Ravitch M (ed): *Current Problems in Surgery*. Chicago, Year Book, 1983, vol 20, p 135.

Management of a Solitary Thyroid Nodule

A therapeutic decision must be made about the management of a solitary thyroid nodule. A decision tree for management is outlined in Fig. 11-11. A solitary thyroid nodule occurring in a child or an individual with a history of neck irradiation should be operated on immediately, as should a patient who has a clini-

FIGURE 11-11 Management of a solitary thyroid nodule.

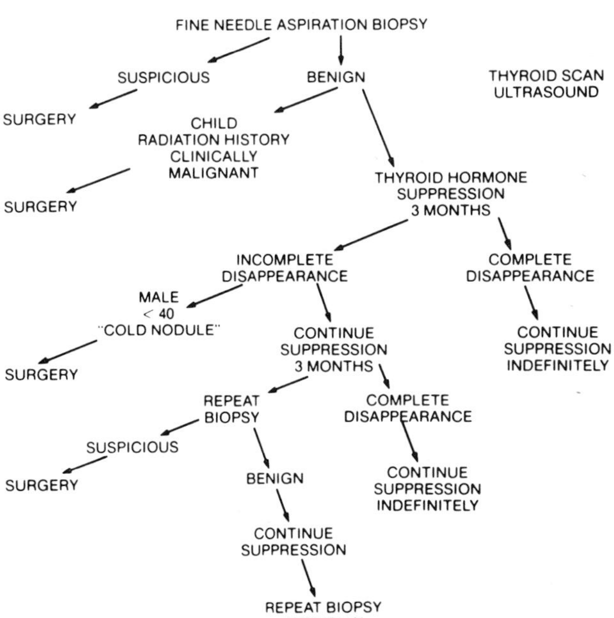

cally "malignant" thyroid on physical examination. Before surgery, it is important to be sure that a solitary nodule does not represent a single thyroid lobe with compensatory hypertrophy. If the other lobe cannot be palpated, a thyroid scan is indicated.

In the absence of immediate indications for surgery, the patient should have a fine-needle biopsy. If the fine-needle aspiration biopsy is not diagnostic, the gland should be suppressed with thyroid hormone for 3 months as described below; disappearance of the nodule is an indication for continued thyroid hormone suppression. A radionuclide scan may be helpful to rule out a hot nodule which may be a follicular adenoma but virtually never a follicular carcinoma. An occasional patient may have an autonomous nodule and become hyperthyroid with thyroid hormone suppression; as was mentioned previously, the presence of an autonomous nodule makes malignancy very unlikely. Therefore, thyroid function tests should be done several weeks after suppressive therapy has been started. If the response is incomplete—i.e., the nodule does not disappear and the patient is a young male—surgery is indicated. Otherwise, thyroid hormone suppression can be continued for another 3-month trial period.

If the solitary thyroid nodule is nonfunctioning, ultrasound may be used to determine whether it is solid or cystic, although this determination can also be made during aspiration. If it is cystic and aspiration does not reveal evidence of malignancy, thyroid hormone suppression can be attempted for 3 months. Complete disappearance of the nodule is an indication for the continuation of thyroid hormone suppression therapy. All solitary thyroid nodules should be biopsied by fine-needle aspiration, even when the decision to operate has already been made. Certain knowledge that the nodule is malignant is helpful to the surgeon. If a malignancy is not found, the gland should be suppressed with thyroid hormone and managed like a functioning nodule; the type of treatment depends on the response.

Should the management of a solitary thyroid nodule be altered in elderly patients? In a study of 100 patients more than 60 years old, two distinct groups could be identified.[125] Sixty-six patients were in the high-risk group, i.e., having a solitary cold nodule, hoarseness, etc.; 11 of those patients had thyroid malignancies, 6 of which were poorly differentiated. There was no operative mortality. Surgery is indicated for elderly patients with thyroid nodules at risk for malignancy.

Thyroid Hormone Suppression

Once the decision not to operate has been made, the patient should be given a course of thyroid hormone suppression in an attempt to shut off TSH secretion and decrease the size of the nodule. Thyroid hormone suppressive therapy for a solitary nodule as opposed to diffuse or multinodular goiter is a matter of degree, keeping in mind the risk of osteoporosis (see Therapy for Nontoxic Goiter above).

Questions have been raised about the practice of employing thyroid hormone suppression in solitary cold nodules, with the idea that "cold" means inactive. Actually, cold nodules have been shown to be more active biochemically than "warm" nodules.[126] They appear to have a defect in iodine trapping, but other parameters, such as glucose oxidation and cAMP levels, are actually increased.[127] In one study, 50 percent of the cold nodules decreased in size with thyroid hormone therapy.[82]

If a patient with a solitary nodule is to have a trial of thyroid hormone suppression, it is important to know how long thyroid hormone should be administered before deciding that the nodule is not going to regress with suppression of circulating TSH. Some goiters did not regress until the treatment was continued for a year or longer.[80] In half the patients receiving thyroid hormone suppression therapy for nontoxic goiter in one series, thyroid nodules decreased in size after 3 months. When patients who had not responded were treated for another 4 months, one-third of the nodules decreased in size; it made no difference whether the dose of thyroid hormone was increased.[82] These data suggest a course of therapy for at least 3 months and preferably 6 months before the thyroid nodule is considered nonsuppressible. Other studies have indicated that no further suppression should be attempted after 3 months.[83] Reevaluation at 3-month intervals allows a management decision to be based on factors such as sex and age in addition to thyroid hormone response.

If the thyroid nodule disappears completely, thyroid hormone suppression should be continued indefinitely. Regression of a solitary nodule does not eliminate the possibility of thyroid cancer but does indicate that the nodule is responsive to TSH. Thyroid hormone administration should be continued as long as there is no change in the size of the nodule; immediate surgery is advised if the nodule enlarges during suppressive therapy. If the nodule does not regress completely, the decision whether to operate depends on the other factors discussed above.

Surgery

If the decision is made to operate, both thyroid lobes should be totally exposed even though the nodule is palpable in only one lobe before surgery. Multiple thyroid nodules are discovered at surgery in up to 60 percent of cases diagnosed as a single nodule preoperatively by means of careful palpation and scan. If multinodular goiter is discovered at operation, the risk of carcinoma in the thyroid nodule is dramatically lower, but the surgeon should probably go on to remove the nodular tissue.

If only a single nodule is discovered at surgery on complete palpation and there are no suspicious signs of extrathyroid involvement, extracapsular lobectomy with removal of the isthmus is indicated. If the thyroid nodule appears benign on frozen section but turns out to be papillary carcinoma after a review of the permanent sections, adequate surgery has probably been performed and reoperation is not indicated. The surgical approach to thyroid cancer is discussed later in this chapter.

THYROID CARCINOMA

The biological behavior of thyroid cancer may vary markedly. Minimal papillary thyroid carcinoma is considered to have a negligible biological risk, while anaplastic carcinoma of the thyroid is one of the most malignant human tumors.

The finding that thyroid follicular cells express a number of nuclear proto-oncogenes, including c-*fos*, c-*myc*, and c-*ras*, that encode for proteins involved in transcription and signal transduction has implications for thyroid cancer.[128–131] In addition, the expression of these proto-oncogenes and their oncogene counterparts has been detected in thyroid cancers.[128–134] Studies suggest that *ras* mutations generally occur in up to 20 to 50 percent of thyroid neoplasms. The prevalence of mutations in specific histologic classes varies widely. A rearranged *ret* proto-oncogene also has been found in papillary carcinomas.[133] As discussed in Goiter (above), thyroid carcinomas seem to be monoclonal in that they appear to have arisen from a cancer-inducing event in a single cell.[135]

Classification

Nearly all thyroid tumors arise from the follicular or parafollicular cells. These epithelial tumors of the thyroid are shown in the classification system in Table 11-6. Thyroid carcinoma may be follicular, forming recognizable thyroid follicles, or these follicular cells may form papillary structures, either pure or mixed with follicles. Alternatively, the follicular cells may be largely undifferentiated and appear as giant spindle cells or small cells. Follicular cells may also grow as squamous cells. Carcinomas arising from parafollicular cells have different histologic subtypes, but these types have no definite clinical significance; all are called medullary. Classification based on the histology of the tumor does have biological significance. In a 5- to 30-year follow-up, 11 percent of patients with papillary carcinoma died of the disease, compared with 25 percent of patients with follicular carcinoma, 50 percent of patients with sporadic medullary carcinoma, and 90 percent of patients with undifferentiated carcinoma.

Thyroid carcinoma may also be classified in regard to biological behavior (Table 11-7). Papillary thyroid cancers occur in all age groups and tend to

TABLE 11-6 World Health Organization Histologic Classification of Thyroid Tumors

- Epithelial tumors
  - Benign
    - Follicular adenoma
    - Others
  - Malignant
    - Follicular carcinoma
    - Papillary carcinoma
    - Squamous cell carcinoma
    - Undifferentiated (anaplastic) carcinoma
      - Spindle cell type
      - Giant cell type
      - Small cell type
    - Medullary carcinoma
- Nonepithelial tumors
  - Benign
  - Malignant
    - Fibrosarcoma
    - Others
  - Miscellaneous tumors
    - Carcinosarcoma
    - Malignant hemangioendothelioma
    - Malignant lymphoma
    - Teratoma
    - Secondary tumors

Source: World Health Organization: *International Histological Classification of Tumors,* no. 11: *Histological Typing of Thyroid Tumors.* Geneva, WHO, 1974.

metastasize to lymph nodes, follicular carcinomas tend to have blood-borne metastases and occur in older age groups, and undifferentiated thyroid cancers occur predominantly in older patients and usually kill by local invasion. Although at present there is no completely satisfactory system for staging thyroid cancer, certain pathologic characteristics relate to therapy and prognosis. The following prognostic factors for papillary and follicular thyroid carcinomas are thought to be of importance: (1) histologic type, (2) age of patient, (3) extent of primary tumor, (4) distant metastases, (5) size of thyroid, (6) blood vessel invasion, (7) multiple foci, and (8) sex.[136] Clinical staging of thyroid carcinoma has also been attempted (Table 11-8). In a more recent study of 14 possible variables, only patient age, tumor histologic grade, and tumor extent (invasion or metastasis and tumor size) (AGE) were significant in predicting mortality from papillary carcinoma.[137,138] Nuclear DNA content as measured by flow cytometry has also been used as a prognostic factor,[139] and DNA nondiploid tumors were associated with a higher risk of mortality.

Incidence of Thyroid Carcinoma

Much of the confusion about the incidence of thyroid carcinoma is due to the presence of minimal papillary thyroid cancer, which can be defined as a tumor

TABLE 11-7 Biological Behavior of Thyroid Tumors According to Histologic Classification

Tumor	Age Group	Growth Rate	Lymph Node Metastases	Distant Metastases
Papillary	All	Slow	Common	Uncommon
Follicular	Middle-aged to old	Slow	Uncommon	Common
Medullary	All	Moderate	Common	Common
Undifferentiated	Older	Rapid	Extensive	Common (with local growth)

Source: Meissner.[136]

less than 1.5 cm in size. The prevalence of these small tumors has been reported to be as high as 28 percent in Japan and 13 percent in the United States.[71] Since the biological risk of minimal papillary carcinoma is probably negligible, these tumors rarely are a cause of death. As a consequence, they are responsible for the disparity between thyroid cancer as a cause of death and thyroid cancer prevalence in some surgical series. The reported prevalence varies widely because diagnosis is exquisitely sensitive to the method of pathologic examination of the thyroid gland. These thyroid tumors may be occult and hence not grossly visible; as many as 300 to 900 slides per gland must be prepared to avoid missing the smallest tumor. If all thyroids were studied in this manner, as many as 10 million to 30 million North Americans might be found to have minimal papillary thyroid carcinoma.[71] The magnitude of this problem is overwhelming but, from the patient's point of view, probably biologically unimportant. However, the presence of such tumors makes it difficult to evaluate incidence carefully. Mortality from thyroid cancer approximates 0.8 death per 100,000 per year in females and 0.4 death per 100,000 per year in males; these data show that deaths from tumors of the thyroid are uncommon compared with deaths from other cancers.

The Effects of Radiation on the Development of Thyroid Carcinoma

External irradiation of the thyroid, as was mentioned earlier, is associated with an increased incidence of thyroid neoplasm, including carcinomas, after a delay of many years. There is no evidence at present that this radiation-associated increase in the incidence of thyroid carcinoma disappears with time, and so exposed individuals must be followed.[140–142]

Fortunately, radiation-associated thyroid carcinomas are almost always well differentiated and have a good prognosis when detected in patients under age 40.

There is a linear relation between the dose of radiation to the thyroid and the incidence of thyroid cancer without a clear threshold up to about 1000 rads (Fig. 11-12). Whether the relation remains linear at very low doses and at high doses is not clear.

When data from several studies were combined, the absolute risk for thyroid cancers was found to be 1.5 cases per million patients per rad per year.[143,144] The failure of therapeutic doses of ^{131}I to result in an increased risk for thyroid carcinoma has also been explained by the destruction of thyroid cells or by the

TABLE 11-8 Clinical Stages of Thyroid Carcinoma

Stage I	Intrathyroidal lesions only
Stage II	Nonfixed cervical metastases
Stage III	Fixed lymph node metastases or invasion into the neck outside the thyroid
Stage IV	Metastases outside the neck

Source: Modified from Smedal ML, Salzman FA, Meissner WA: *AJR* 99:352, 1967.

FIGURE 11-12 Incidence of thyroid cancer as a function of the dose of external radiation. (*After Maxon et al.* [143])

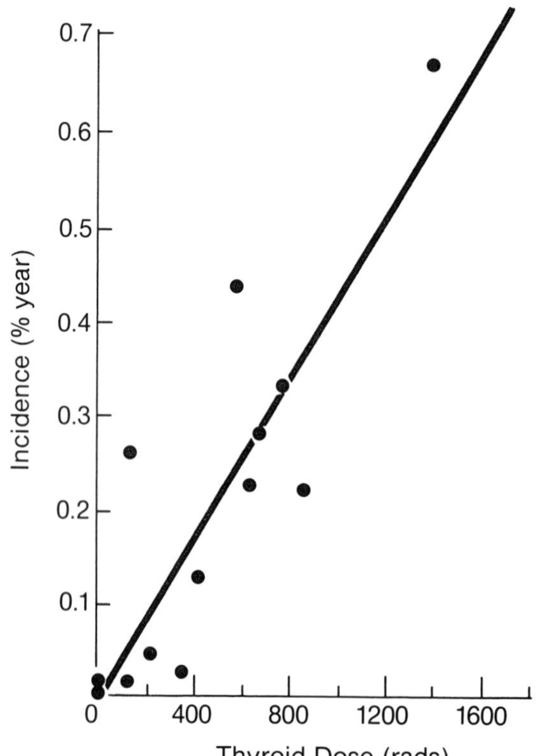

slow radiation dose rate. Therapeutic doses of ^{131}I given for hyperthyroidism result in the delivery of 5000 to 8000 rad to the thyroid.[145] Doses of external radiation as low as 50 rad have been associated with an increased risk of thyroid carcinoma, and it is likely that any amount of radiation represents an increased risk. Since low doses of radiation may induce thyroid carcinoma, the use of ^{131}I for routine thyroid scans should be discouraged.

A characteristic of radiation-associated thyroid carcinoma is multicentricity. In one series, multicentric thyroid cancer was found in 55 percent of operated cases compared with 22 percent in nonirradiated controls.[140]

If progression of the thyroid disease involves hyperplasia, adenoma formation, and eventually malignancy, there should be an age progression of radiation-induced malignancy through the group of irradiated individuals. However, since progression did not continue, the data suggest that irradiation induced an immediate tendency to malignancy which then took several years to become clinically evident.

Benign thyroid nodularity associated with external radiation to the head and neck has a high recurrence rate after subtotal thyroidectomy[146] similar to that reported with benign thyroid nodules in nonirradiated patients. Thyroid hormone suppression decreased the risk of recurrence of benign thyroid nodules, especially in women, but not the recurrence of thyroid cancer.

The great majority of tumors have been papillary thyroid carcinomas. Malignancies found at the time of surgery do not just represent minimal papillary carcinoma. Approximately two-thirds of the carcinomas were greater than 1 cm in size, and 59 percent were multifocal, with lymph node metastases in 25 percent.[99] Although children are two to three times as susceptible as adults are to radiation-induced thyroid nodules, they appear to be equally susceptible to the induction of thyroid carcinoma.[95] Although prophylaxis with thyroid hormone has not been shown to prevent new disease,[99] such suppression will be reasonable in patients exposed to external radiation to the head and neck until further information is available.[147]

Natural History of Thyroid Carcinoma

Carcinoma of the thyroid is three times more common in females than in males.[148] It has an incidence peak in the sixth decade but ranges from infancy to old age. However, death from thyroid cancer has a very different age distribution. Mortality is low in the young, but the prognosis steadily worsens with age.[149] This difference between mortality and incidence rates is related to the fact that most thyroid carcinomas in younger individuals are well differentiated, while anaplastic thyroid carcinoma, with its higher mortality, is predominant in the elderly. The highly malignant anaplastic thyroid carcinoma seldom occurs before the age of 40; after age 40, both mortality and the occurrence of metastases from thyroid carcinoma increase sharply.

Papillary Carcinoma

Papillary carcinoma is the most common form of thyroid carcinoma, accounting for about 75 percent of clinically evident thyroid tumors in adults. It is three times more common in females than in males and represents the greater majority of thyroid cancers in childhood. Although more common, papillary carcinoma has a better prognosis in women and children compared with men. Nevertheless, the overall prognosis is generally good. Less than 10 percent of patients die of papillary thyroid cancer in prolonged follow-up, and only 25 percent have a recurrence.[149]

Histologically, the epithelial cells of the tumor have a definite papillary pattern (Fig. 11-13). Although follicular patterns with colloid-filled vesicles may be found frequently in the tumor, the follicular

FIGURE 11-13 Papillary carcinoma of the thyroid. The papillary bandlike structure is lined by low columnar cells. In the lower panel, optically clear "Orphan Annie nuclei" are seen.

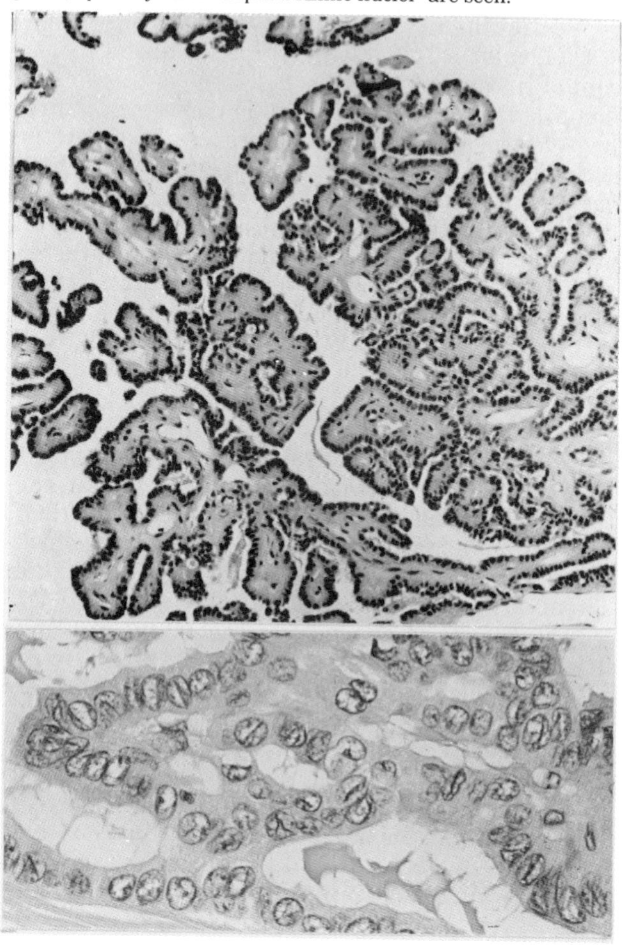

component apparently does not alter the behavior of the tumor, which is still classified as papillary. Approximately 40 percent of cases of papillary carcinoma contain laminated calcific spherules called psammoma bodies. These bodies can sometimes be identified as finely stippled calcifications on a properly exposed x-ray of the neck.[150] Xeroradiography may be particularly helpful but is not necessary. The tumor is slow-growing and usually of low-grade malignancy, which means that long follow-up periods are necessary.[138] Spread occurs characteristically to the cervical lymph nodes; patients may actually present with enlarged cervical nodes rather than with a mass in the thyroid. Interestingly, the presence of metastases to the cervical nodes seems to have little deleterious effect on mortality.[151,152] Metastases to bones and lungs are much less common. Intraglandular metastases in both the same lobe as the primary tumor and the opposite lobe are not uncommon. Papillary carcinomas may remain indolent for long periods even with widespread metastases or may have more aggressive properties. In the latter case, the progression is often associated with a change to a more malignant type of thyroid cancer.

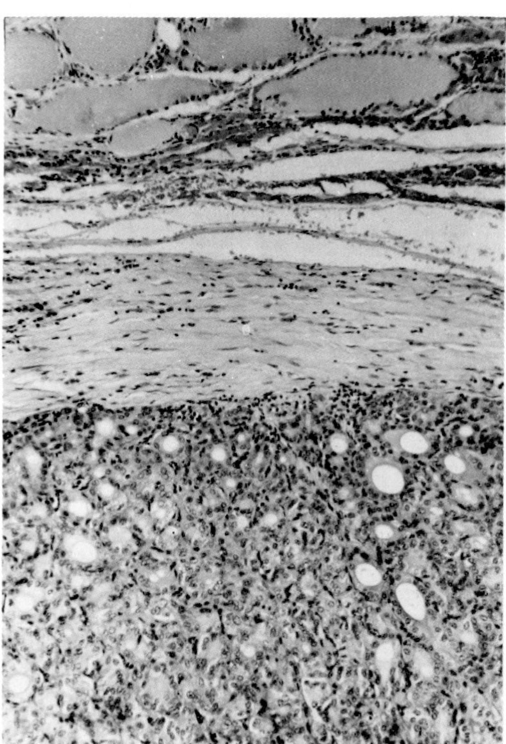

FIGURE 11-14 Follicular carcinoma of the thyroid. The follicles are of uniform size and are distinctly different from the normal follicles in the upper part of the micrograph. The carcinoma is surrounded by a well-defined capsule without signs of invasion in this instance.

Follicular Carcinoma

Follicular carcinoma accounts for about 15 percent of thyroid carcinomas and, like papillary carcinoma, is three times more common in women than in men. However, this tumor occurs less frequently in children; it is more a disease of the middle and later years. Advancing age, extrathyroidal invasion, and distant metastases are associated with a poorer prognosis.[153] Histologically, the tumor is characterized both by the formation of acinar structures with varying colloid content and by the absence of papillary elements (Fig. 11-14). Because of the relatively normal morphology, the tumor may be very difficult to distinguish from follicular adenomas; usually invasion of the capsule, the adjacent thyroid, or blood vessels must be demonstrated. The initial appearance of follicular carcinoma may be as a distant metastasis with no thyroid lesion clinically evident. These tumors tend to metastasize through the bloodstream or invade adjacent structures rather than spread to local lymph nodes.

The prognosis depends on the extent of tumor invasion at the time of surgery. Follicular carcinomas that show minimal invasion and appear grossly similar to adenomas have a very high cure rate. With more extensive invasion, the prognosis becomes progressively poorer. In a study of 18 cases in which the patient died from follicular carcinoma of the thyroid, 56 percent had lung metastases, 89 percent had lymph node metastases, and 17 percent had skeletal, liver, or brain metastases.[154] The development of metastases may be delayed as long as 10 to 20 years.

Anaplastic Carcinoma

Anaplastic carcinomas of the thyroid are those which form neither papillary nor follicular structures and do not have amyloid stroma. The cells tend to be strikingly pleomorphic and devoid of any special arrangement. Bizarre multinucleated giant cells are encountered frequently (Fig. 11-15). A spindle cell growth pattern sometimes predominates; this may be suggestive of fibrosarcoma. Diffuse small cell carcinoma of the thyroid forms a special group which may be difficult to differentiate from lymphosarcoma; lymphosarcoma may be much more common in the thyroid.[155] The ratio of females to males is lower than in papillary or follicular carcinoma, and the mean age—57 years—is older.

Anaplastic carcinomas grow rapidly, infiltrate neck structures, and may spread to regional lymph nodes, lungs, bones, and liver. Death often occurs as a result of rapid local spread before distant metastases appear. In one patient with anaplastic carcinoma of the thyroid, it was necessary to readjust the cord which held the tracheotomy tube in place every 4 h because of tumor growth. Anaplastic thyroid tumors have a grim prognosis, with a 10-year survival rate of only about 1 percent. The symptom cluster of dyspnea, dysphagia, and dysphonia is a bad prognostic sign.[156]

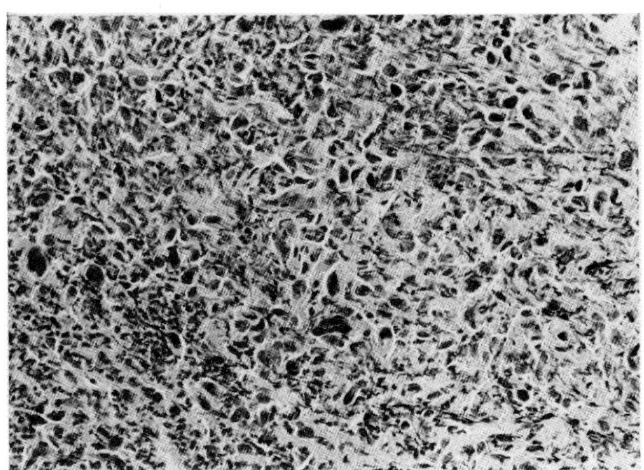

FIGURE 11-15 Anaplastic carcinoma of the thyroid. The cells are bizarre and pleomorphic. The mitotic rate is high.

Evaluation of Thyroid Carcinoma

Thyroid carcinoma usually presents as a mass in the neck. Tumors tend to be harder and more irregular than goiter, and the entire gland may not be enlarged. There can be symptoms and signs associated with local invasion or metastases. In general, the work-up should include a careful history and physical exam, thyroid function studies, fine-needle aspiration of the lesion, an ^{123}I uptake study, a sonogram, and, when appropriate, CT scan or MRI. If the results of fine-needle aspiration are equivocal, open biopsy is indicated in some cases.

Therapy for Thyroid Carcinoma

Surgical resection of a tumor with variable removal of all portions of the thyroid gland is indicated for all but the most advanced differentiated thyroid carcinomas. With such a wide variation in the behavior of differentiated tumors of the thyroid, the extent of the surgery remains controversial.[157] Because of this wide range, methods of treatment can be compared only with difficulty even when cases are matched for age, sex, and histology. The risks of therapy must be weighed carefully against the prognosis for each individual. Radical procedures carry a risk of serious disability, e.g., recurrent laryngeal nerve paralysis and hypoparathyroidism, and should be used with restraint when the prognosis is good. Dangerous and disfiguring operations are virtually never indicated.

Radioactive iodine may be of real benefit in treating surgically inaccessible metastases without damaging the surrounding tissue. The normal thyroid gland is so avid for iodine that radioactive iodine cannot be given for the treatment of any metastases until the thyroid gland has been ablated. Therefore, surgical removal of most of the gland or ablation of the gland with ^{131}I before ^{131}I treatment of the metastases is required. Whether the isotope has a role in the routine ablation of the remaining thyroid gland after partial thyroidectomy for well-differentiated tumors in the absence of extension or metastases remains a subject for debate.[138,149]

Hormone dependence of certain well-differentiated carcinomas of the thyroid is well established. There is good evidence that the induction of hypothyroidism with a concomitant elevated serum TSH concentration has resulted in the growth of thyroid metastases. Certainly avoidance of hypothyroidism and suppression of TSH levels are accepted parts of the therapy for thyroid carcinoma.

Therapy for Papillary Carcinoma

If a lesion is found at surgery to be a minimal papillary carcinoma (< 1 cm), the procedure of choice is thyroid lobectomy on the affected side and removal of the isthmus.[151] Although there is still substantial controversy about the proper treatment of larger lesions, the evidence favors nearly total thyroidectomy, leaving only enough of the gland to preserve the recurrent laryngeal nerve and the parathyroid glands. In one study, residual cancer would have persisted in remaining thyroid tissue in two-thirds of the patients if only a lobectomy had been performed.[157] In a study of 576 patients with carcinoma of the thyroid, there was a significant inverse correlation between the extent of surgery and recurrence of the tumor (Table 11-9).[151,152] The tumor recurred with twice the frequency after subtotal thyroidectomy compared with nearly total thyroidectomy, and the proportion of deaths from thyroid cancer was greater. Cervical lymph node metastases found at initial surgery were associated with higher recur-

TABLE 11-9 Influence of Initial Treatment on Recurrence and Survival in Thyroid Papillary Carcinoma

	Recurrence, %	Deaths, %
Surgical therapy		
Thyroidectomy		
Subtotal	19.2	0.6
Total	10.9*	1.5
Lymphadenectomy		
None	12.3	0.8
Simple	17.9	1.7
Excision	14.7	0.7
Medical therapy after surgery		
None	40.0	10.0
Thyroid	13.1†	0.2
^{131}I and thyroid hormone	6.4	0.9

* The difference in recurrence frequency between patients with total thyroidectomy vs. subtotal thyroidectomy was statistically significant, $p < .01$.

† The difference between patients with thyroid therapy and patients who received no therapy statistically significant, $p < .001$.

Source: Mazzaferri and Young.[152]

rence rates but not higher mortality rates.[149,158] The nodes should be removed with a modified neck dissection, including the lymphatics.[159,160]

The major argument against total thyroidectomy is the increased risk of hypoparathyroidism and recurrent laryngeal nerve involvement.[155,161] If the posterior capsule on the contralateral side is left intact, this risk can be reduced to as low as 5 percent.[162] In one large series, hypoparathyroidism occurred in 13.5 percent of patients who had a total thyroidectomy and was clearly related to the extent of the surgery.[152] Recurrent laryngeal nerve paralysis occurred in 1.2 percent of these patients; it was also related to the extent of surgery. There was no evidence that extensive neck dissection in addition to total thyroidectomy improved survival or lessened recurrence, and major postoperative complications occurred in 44 percent of patients who were treated in this manner. In contrast, major complications occurred in only 13 percent of patients when total thyroidectomy was combined with selective regional lymph node excision.

As indicated in Fig. 11-16, medical therapy also significantly influenced survival and recurrence. The recurrence rate after thyroid hormone therapy was significantly less than that with no therapy but was significantly greater than that with ^{131}I plus thyroid hormone therapy. Differences in recurrence rates among these three subgroups were apparent within the first year after the completion of previous therapy. The indication for therapy with ^{131}I was almost exclusively residual uptake in the neck, particularly in patients with large tumors.[152] The average dose of radioactive iodine was 140 mCi; the dose was less than 200 mCi in 87 percent of the patients.

FIGURE 11-16 Recurrence of papillary thyroid carcinoma after surgery with and without adjunctive medical therapy. (*From Mazzaferri et al.*[152])

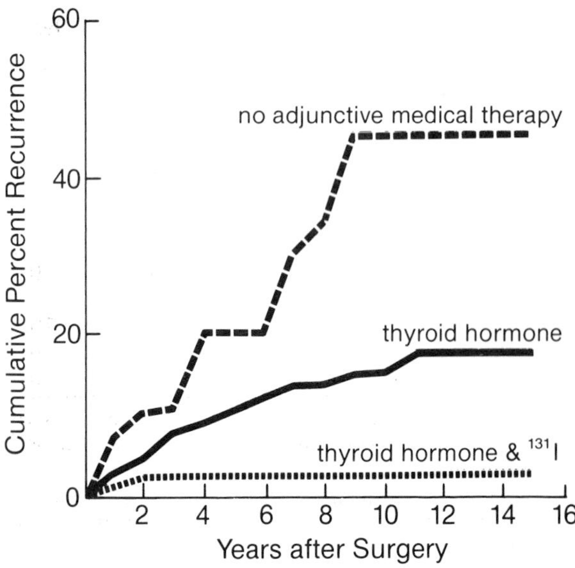

The data suggest that ablative doses of radioactive iodine should be given postoperatively to patients with papillary carcinoma whose lesions are multiple, metastatic, locally invasive, or larger than 2.5 cm.[163] For patients with papillary tumors less than 1.5 cm in diameter, less aggressive therapy, consisting of subtotal thyroidectomy and thyroid hormone suppression, may be adequate.[152] Treatment of these patients resulted in lower recurrence and mortality rates.[151] Therapy should also be administered to patients with local or distant metastases, provided that adequate ^{131}I uptake can be demonstrated.[164,165]

Numerous studies have indicated that thyroid carcinomas may be subject to endocrine control, with depression of serum TSH concentration by thyroid hormone. Thyroid hormone was given to 19 patients with inoperable metastases of papillary carcinoma of the thyroid; this treatment resulted in the regression of metastases in 12 of the patients for periods that averaged 11 years.[166] The aim of thyroid hormone therapy in patients with thyroid carcinoma is not replacement but depression of serum TSH concentration. Total suppression of TSH secretion is difficult regardless of the dose of thyroid hormone; however, TSH secretion should be inhibited as much as possible without the induction of iatrogenic hyperthyroidism. Suppressive hormone therapy should be started as soon as possible, even before surgery if the diagnostic studies have been completed.

Since there is evidence that thyroid hormone suppressive therapy can decrease the recurrence of papillary thyroid cancer, it is reasonable to suppress the sensitive TSH value below 0.1 μU/ml. Whether the patient should be made thyrotoxic, e.g., with suppression of the TSH to below 0.05 μU/ml, depends on the extent of the malignancy.

External irradiation at a moderate dose can eradicate microscopic papillary and follicular carcinoma; gross tumor also responds favorably, but the regression rate is slow.[167] At present, external irradiation is indicated in patients who have been treated surgically and no longer respond to ^{131}I.

Therapy for Follicular Carcinoma

The therapy for follicular carcinoma differs from that for papillary carcinoma for several reasons. Follicular carcinoma is a more aggressive tumor and should be treated more aggressively. Blood-borne metastases are more common, often necessitating radionuclide therapy. Furthermore, patients in whom well-differentiated metastases outside the neck have been ablated are three times more likely to survive than are patients who have not been freed of metastases.[168] Since radioactive iodine is ineffective for the treatment of metastases until the thyroid gland has been ablated, total or nearly total thyroidectomy is indicated even if the diagnosis must be made after a review of the permanent sections, necessitating reoperation.[169] If follicular carcinoma was diagnosed in the distant past and a total thyroidectomy was not done, reoperation does not seem to be indicated. A patient in this situation should be followed carefully.

In some cases the thyroid remnant can be ablated with radioactive iodine, but ablation of a normally functioning remnant may require a large radioactive iodine dose, e.g., 60 mCi, which can contribute to the radiation dose imposed on the patient without significantly affecting the cancer. However, 30 mCi may be sufficient in most cases, providing a lower radiation burden.[170,171]

The immediate postoperative period is often difficult for patients with thyroid carcinoma; making the patients hypothyroid accentuates the problem. Placing patients on suppressive doses of L-thyroxine for 3 months and then switching them to 50 μg of T_3 per day for 4 weeks is preferred. The triiodothyronine is discontinued for 2 weeks, and radioactive iodine is given. This regimen appears to produce optimal radioisotope uptake.[172,173] The patient is put on suppressive therapy during this period, and the risk of malignant growth is minimal. The patient can be kept on thyroid hormone suppressive therapy, and 10 U of bovine TSH can be administered intramuscularly daily for 3 days. However, the administration of bovine TSH may result in the development of antibodies and toxic reactions and should be avoided in most instances.[174,175]

Alternatively, the patient can be allowed to become hypothyroid immediately after surgery, e.g., 2 to 4 weeks after total thyroidectomy. When the serum TSH concentration is elevated to the range of 50 μU/ml, 2 mCi of ^{131}I can be given and a whole-body scan can be performed; the use of ^{123}I, if available, will lower the radiation dose for diagnostic purposes. If any uptake occurs in the thyroid or elsewhere, 100 mCi of ^{131}I should be given. The amount of ^{131}I taken up by the tumor should be maximized by decreasing the iodide pool.[176] This can be accomplished by placing the patient on a low-iodine diet for 3 weeks and administering hydrochlorothiazide 50 mg daily during the week before therapy. The administration of a cathartic and secretagogue on the day of ^{131}I therapy may minimize the retention of radioactive iodine by the bowel and salivary glands.

There is some question whether the serum TSH concentration is as high with exogenous TSH stimulation as it is when the endogenous TSH concentration is allowed to rise as a result of the induction of hypothyroidism.[175] In any case, the patient should not be allowed to remain hypothyroid any longer than absolutely necessary, and thyroid hormone therapy should be restarted as quickly as possible.

Therapy for Anaplastic Carcinoma

For most patients, anaplastic carcinoma of the thyroid has progressed beyond the possibility of cure when they are first seen. A tissue diagnosis is often established by means of needle biopsy. Radical surgery has no role in the treatment of anaplastic carcinoma. Surgical procedures have failed to improve the prognosis; radiotherapy probably provides the best palliation. However, partial excision of the tumor as well as tracheostomy may be needed both to provide relief of tracheal compression and to decrease the amount of tumor to be irradiated. External radiotherapy may be given in a dose of 4000 to 5000 rad to the neck and upper mediastinum through a variety of ports. Shrinkage of the tumor may occur rapidly (hyperfractionation of the radiation dose, 100 rad qid at 3-h intervals, caused complete tumor regression in 6 of 14 patients[177]), but recurrence is the rule. The aim of radiotherapy in these cases is to prevent obstruction, ulceration, and hemorrhage. Although anaplastic carcinomas rarely pick up sufficient iodine to make treatment possible, a radioiodine uptake test and scan should be done before other therapy is attempted. Occasionally, an anaplastic carcinoma of the thyroid takes up enough ^{131}I to make therapy possible.[178]

Chemotherapy has not been very helpful in the treatment of these very aggressive tumors but could be considered an alternative to radiation therapy.[179] A partial remission associated with subjective improvement was achieved in 5 of 19 patients with anaplastic carcinoma treated with doxorubicin (Adriamycin).[180] All histologic cell types responded, although spindle cell and giant cell types appeared to be less responsive. The most significant toxicity encountered was Adriamycin-induced cardiomyopathy. Bleomycin is another antibiotic that has been suggested to be effective in treating thyroid cancer.[181]

Thyroid Lymphoma

Primary thyroid lymphoma accounts for about 1 percent of thyroid cancer and frequently occurs in conjunction with Hashimoto's thyroiditis.[182] Fine-needle aspiration biopsy may confuse the issue. If the lymphoma is localized to the thyroid, there appears to be a benefit from total thyroidectomy.[183] If disseminated disease is present, treatment with radiation or chemotherapy is indicated. Despite aggressive therapy, the mortality rate in patients with thyroid lymphoma is about 50 percent.[184]

Subsequent Follow-Up

General Follow-Up

After surgery for differentiated thyroid carcinoma, residual thyroid tissue and metastases which concentrate radioiodine should be defined by a radioactive iodine scan, as was discussed previously. In addition, chest films should be taken on a yearly basis to rule out the possibility of metastases. Annual or biannual bone scans may also be helpful in checking for possible bone metastases, particularly in patients with follicular carcinoma.[185]

Thyroglobulin Determinations

There has been interest in serum thyroglobulin concentration as an aid in the diagnosis and follow-up of thyroid carcinoma.[186–188] Although the assay is probably not specific in distinguishing benign from malignant thyroid tissue, it is valuable in assessing treatment of thyroid carcinoma during the course of the disease.[189] Circulating thyroglobulin concentrations tend to be high in patients with thyroid tumors but are also increased in a number of other thyroid diseases, including Graves' disease, subacute thyroiditis, and endemic goiter. The major use of the thyroglobulin assay is in the follow-up of patients who have had a thyroid carcinoma removed and in whom postoperative thyroglobulin levels are very low or undetectable. The persistence of elevated thyroglobulin levels or an increase in previously low levels indicates that residual thyroid carcinoma should be searched for carefully.[190,191] Serum thyroglobulin concentration should be determined only if the assay is sufficiently sensitive (limit of detection less than 10 to 15 ng/ml) and no antithyroglobulin antibody has been demonstrated. Thyroid hormone withdrawal and concomitant TSH stimulation may significantly enhance serum thyroglobulin concentrations.[192] However, thyroglobulin concentrations below 10 ng/ml are rarely associated with significant disease, and thyroid hormone withdrawal and TSH are not routinely indicated.

In an effort to screen patients who had received irradiation to the head and neck for thyroid carcinoma, a battery of tests were done, including assays for serum thyroglobulin concentration, antithyroglobulin and antithyroid microsomal antibodies, and carcinoembryonic antigen.[193] Positive results were more frequent in the irradiated population than in the controls; however, with the exception of thyroglobulin, these tests did not clearly differentiate patients with benign vs. malignant lesions. Elevations of the serum thyroglobulin concentration above 300 ng/ml were found only in patients with thyroid cancer, but the diagnosis was usually obvious in such patients.

IgG antibody to human thyroglobulin has been radiolabeled and successfully used to locate thyroid follicular and papillary tumors.[194] The results suggest that ^{131}I antithyroglobulin scanning may be more sensitive than conventional [^{131}I]iodide scanning in locating metastases. However, this test is not generally available.

Medullary Carcinoma of the Thyroid

Although medullary carcinoma accounts for only 5 to 10 percent of all thyroid malignancies, there has been intense interest in this tumor because it has a number of unique properties. Medullary carcinoma of the thyroid (MCT) differs from other thyroid carcinomas in that the cell of origin is the parafollicular C, or light, cell, which is of neural crest origin. As a result, the tumor has endocrine and biochemical properties that provide a distinctive means for early detection and follow-up and possibly for prevention.

Natural History

MCT occurs over an age range from 5 to 80 years without a particular predilection for age or sex. Most of these malignancies are apparently sporadic, in which case the tumors are usually unicentric and are not associated with other endocrine lesions. However, in approximately 20 percent of patients the disease is familial, transmitted as an autosomal dominant trait. The familial form usually occurs as Sipple's syndrome or multiple endocrine neoplasia (MEN) types 2A and 2B (see Chap. 28).

MEN 2A is characterized by the combination of MCT, bilateral adrenal pheochromocytomas, and parathyroid adenomas.[195] It occurs as an autosomal dominant disorder. Genetic linkage studies have localized the MEN 2A gene to chromosome 10. With families of sufficiently large size, genetic screening can estimate the risk of MEN 2A in a new form at 1 to 2 percent if low-risk marker alleles are found or at 97 to 99 percent with high-risk marker alleles.[196] Although this screening is plausible only as a research tool at present, with refinement it may become more generally adaptable and may evolve into an efficient means to predict individuals who have inherited the defective gene. The principles of this type of screening are described in Chap. 3.

MEN 2B is thought to constitute a separate variant of the syndrome in which cutaneous or mucosal neuromas involving the face, lips, and tongue may also occur in association with MCT and bilateral pheochromocytomas.[197] Patients with MEN 2B tend to have a characteristic facial appearance (Fig. 11-17). This syndrome is also inherited in an autosomal dominant mode, and the defect has been mapped to chromosome 10.

The different characteristics of the hereditary and sporadic varieties of MCT may be explained by the two-hit theory proposed by Knudson.[198] In the hereditary form, the first event was postulated to be a germinal mutation resulting in many susceptible cells. This would be followed by a second somatic mutation which would transform the cell into a tumor cell. In the sporadic form, both mutational events were postulated to occur in somatic cells. Comparison of the ages of onset of hereditary and sporadic MCT have been consistent with this theory.[199] Further evidence was provided by studies

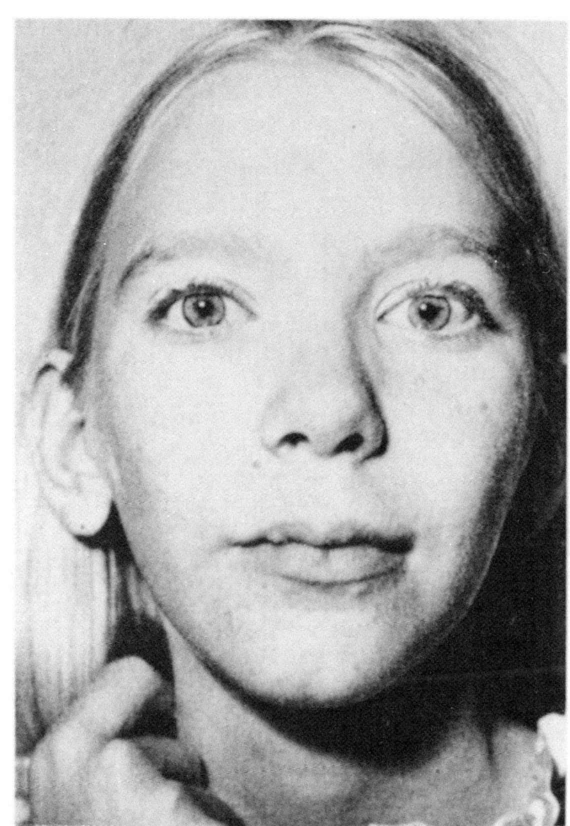

FIGURE 11-17 Typical facies of a patient with MEN 2b syndrome. (*From Khairi et al.*[197])

with glucose-6-phosphate dehydrogenase in heterozygotes, indicating a clonal origin of medullary carcinoma.[200] The finding of C cell hyperplasia in patients with hereditary disease but not in those with sporadic forms is compatible with this theory and suggests that the hyperplasia was the expression of the germ line mutation. The high degree of penetrance of C cell hyperplasia suggests that this mutation is ubiquitous and that cancer occurs when a second somatic mutation converts a hyperplastic cell to the malignant form.

Clinical Course

MCT is intermediate in malignancy between follicular carcinoma and anaplastic carcinoma; the 5-year survival rate is 70 to 80 percent.[201] Characteristically, the tumor runs a slow but progressive course; neck structures are invaded, and metastases go both to cervical lymph nodes and to distant sites. MCT may be sharply demarcated from surrounding normal thyroid or may infiltrate the adjacent thyroid. Smaller tumors are almost invariably located in the upper, posterior portion of the thyroid lobes. Microscopically, the tumor is distinguished by clusters of polyhedral, neoplastic cells (Fig. 11-18) arranged in compartments separated by hyaline amyloid-containing stroma, which is formed by the tumor cells. This organization, together with the absence of neoplastic follicles and papillary elements, is the diagnostic microscopic feature.

Diagnosis

In contrast to the faint homogeneous calcification seen in other thyroid tumors, MCT has a tendency to calcify with a characteristic dense, irregular distribution of calcium throughout the tumor mass in both thyroid primary lesions and metastases.

The parafollicular cells of the thyroid which give rise to MCT secrete the calcium concentration–lowering peptide hormone calcitonin; virtually all patients with MCT have elevated calcitonin levels in their blood.[202] Some patients may have borderline elevated basal calcitonin values but respond with increased calcitonin secretion when calcium, glucagon, or pentagastrin is administered. The use of calcium and pentagastrin in combination appears to be superior to the administration of either agent alone.[203] Normal individuals may have low circulating calcitonin levels (<250 pg/ml) because of a small number of calcitonin-producing C cells in the normal thyroid. There are calcitonin assays available that can measure calcitonin at levels as low as 10 pg/ml.[204]

The pentagastrin stimulation test is performed by administering 0.5 μg/kg of pentagastrin intravenously and measuring the plasma calcitonin levels at 0, 1.5, 5, 10, and 15 min. Normal ranges vary in different laboratories, but basal calcitonin levels are ordinarily less than 24.5 pmol/liter (91 pg/ml) in males and less than 19.2 pmol/liter (71 pg/ml) in females. A positive response is a 1.5-min level of > 51.4 pmol/liter in a male or 21.6 pmol/liter in a female.

Since the tumor secretes large amounts of calcitonin and this secretion can be stimulated, the calcitonin stimulation test has been used for the early diagnosis of MCT. However, in most cases of sporadic MCT, in contrast to the familial type, the disease is unsuspected either until surgery is performed or occasionally until a fine-needle biopsy is done. There is a direct correlation between the basal level of calcitonin and the extent of the tumor. Calcitonin determinations are not indicated in the evaluation of all thyroid nodules. The long-range outcome for patients identified early in the course of the disease must await follow-up studies. When MCT was confined to the thyroid gland, serum calcitonin concentration was unmeasurable in 95 percent of patients for periods up to 3 years after surgery.[202] Other markers, such as carcinoembryonic antigen, have also been studied, but their usefulness is questionable. High levels of histaminase activity have been found in MCT tissue and in the serum of patients with this disease.[205] However, simultaneous measurements of serum histaminase and serum calcitonin levels in MCT patients have indicated that the

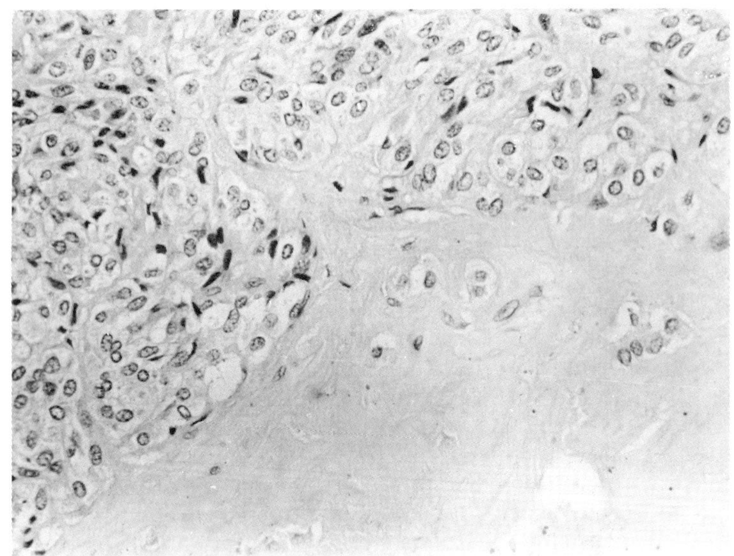

FIGURE 11-18 Medullary carcinoma of the thyroid. Pleomorphic cells are in clumps separated by amyloid.

calcitonin assay is a more sensitive method of identifying the presence of MCT. In addition to calcitonin and histaminase, the tumors may secrete prostaglandins and serotonin, but measurement of these is not generally recommended.

The major use of calcitonin stimulation tests is to identify individuals who are at high risk by virtue of heredity.[206] In kindreds with familial MCT, stimulation tests should be initiated by age 5 years and should continue annually until age 30[207]; after age 30, less frequent testing should be adequate (these recommendations are based on sequential testing of 445 members of 11 kindreds to determine the age-related probability of developing hereditary MCT). With this screening procedure, individuals have been identified with early changes in C cell mass which could represent preinvasive hyperplasia of the C cells. The thyroid glands in these cases were grossly normal. However, microscopic clusters of C cells occurred focally in the middle third of the junction of the middle and upper thirds of the lateral lobe (Fig. 11-19). No microscopic tumors or evidence of vascular or lymphatic invasion were found. If, in fact, parafollicular cell hyperplasia precedes invasive carcinoma in this disease, calcitonin stimulation tests should lead to early recognition of the disease at a stage which is potentially curable. These screening procedures are of much more than academic interest in affected kindreds where half the group is potentially at risk to develop this aggressive neoplasm.

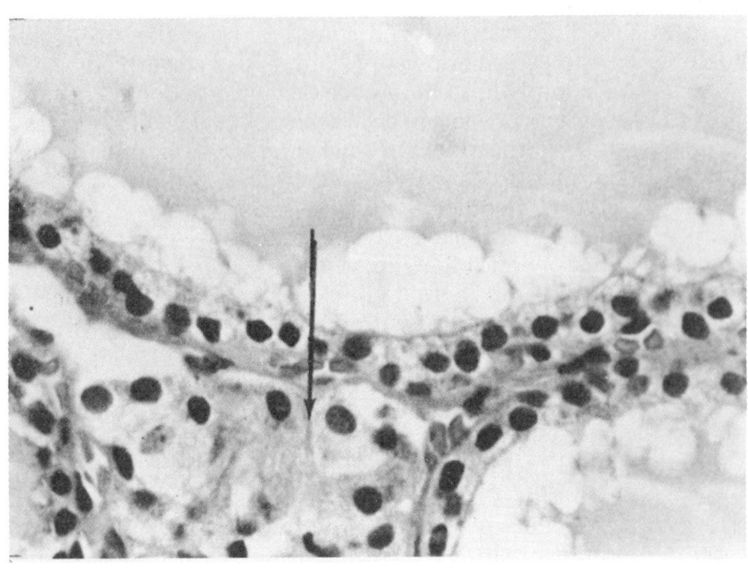

FIGURE 11-19 C cell hyperplasia. Clusters of polygonal to spindle-shaped C cells are seen in a parafollicular location. (*From Tashjian et al.*[202])

Therapy for Medullary Carcinoma

The treatment of MCT is surgical, but metastases have already occurred in more than half the patients with the sporadic form at the time of diagnosis; thus, complete excision of the tumor is difficult. If an affected kindred is followed with calcitonin screening, the presence of tumors will be detected at a much less advanced stage. Because of the frequent occurrence of multicentricity, nearly total thyroidectomy is the procedure of choice. The initial surgical approach to MCT should include thorough central neck dissection of lymph nodes, extending as far substernally as possible.[201] The tumor often shows early aggressive behavior in terms of local metastases; this must be treated promptly. However, an extensive thyroidectomy should not be done at the expense of the recurrent laryngeal nerve and parathyroid glands, and disfiguring neck dissection also should not be done. Since pheochromocytoma is a distinct possibility in these patients, this disease must be ruled out with appropriate tests, such as urinary catecholamine determinations, before thyroid surgery can be considered.

Medullary carcinomas rarely take up radioactive iodine; this modality should not be considered as a possible therapeutic measure. Although there have been reports of temporary responses to thyroid hormone, this form of therapy is not nearly as effective as it is in differentiated thyroid tumors.[208] No good therapy for MCT exists; therefore, a vigorous and effective screening program offers the best chance for patient survival.

After surgery, serum calcitonin levels tend to drop to normal but do not disappear. Patients should be followed at 6-month intervals with physical examinations plus measurements of basal calcitonin levels. If the calcitonin level rises to an abnormal level, further studies such as MRI imaging should be done to localize tumor recurrences.

REFERENCES

1. Kelly FC, Snedden WW: Prevalence and geographical distribution of endemic goitre. *Bull WHO* 18:5, 1958.
2. Wharton T: *Adenographia: Sive, Glandularum Totius Corporis Descriptio.* London, 1656.
3. Burgi H, Supersaxo Z, Selz B: Iodine deficiency diseases in Switzerland one hundred years after Theodor Kocher's survey: A historical review with some new goitre prevalence data. *Acta Endocrinol (Copenh)* 123:577, 1990.
4. Rolleston HD: *The Endocrine Organs in Health and Disease.* London, Oxford University Press, 1936.
5. Marine D: Etiology and prevention of simple goiter. *Medicine (Baltimore)* 3:453, 1924.
6. Studer H, Ramelli F: Simple goiter and its variants: Euthyroid and hyperthyroid multinodular goiters. *Endocr Rev* 3:40, 1982.
7. Eggo MC, Bachrach LK, Fayet G, Errick J, Cohen MF, Kudlow JE, Burrow GN: The effects of growth factors and serum on DNA synthesis and differentiation in thyroid cells in culture. *Mol Cell Endocrinol* 38:141, 1984.
8. Bachrach LK, Eggo MC, Hintz RL, Burrow GN: Insulin-like growth factors in sheep thyroid cells: Action, receptors and production. *Biochem Biophy Res Commun* 154:861, 1988.
9. Maciel RMB, Moses AC, Villone G, Tramontano D, Ingbar SH: Demonstration of the production and physiological role of insulin-like growth factor II in rat thyroid follicular cells in culture. *J Clin Invest* 82:1546, 1988.
10. Tseng Y-CL, Burman KD, Schaudies P, Ahmann AJ, D'avis J, Geelhoed GW, Wartofsky L: Effects of epidermal growth factor on thyroglobulin and adenosine 3′,5′-monophosphate production by cultured human thyrocytes. *J Clin Endocrinol Metab* 69:771, 1989.
11. Drexhage HA, Bottazzo GF, Doniach D, Bitensky L, Chayen J: Evidence for thyroid-stimulating immunoglobulins in some goitrous thyroid diseases. *Lancet* 2:287, 1980.
12. Meinkoth JL, Goldsmith PK, Spiegel AM, Feramisco JR, Burrow GN: Inhibition of TSH-induced DNA synthesis in thyroid follicular cells by microinjection of an antibody to the stimulatory G protein of adenylyl cyclase, G_s. *J Biol Chem* 267:13239, 1992.
13. Grubeck-Loebenstein B, Buchan G, Sadeghi R, Kissonerghis M, Londei M, Turner M, Pirich K, Roka R, et al: Transforming growth factor beta regulates thyroid growth: Role in the pathogenesis of nontoxic goiter. *J Clin Invest* 83:764, 1989.
14. Tetsuya T, Sugawa H, Kosugi S, Inoue D, Toru M, Hiroo I: Prolonged effects of recombinant human interleukin-1α on mouse thyroid function. *Endocrinology* 127:2322, 1990.
15. Yuasa R, Eggo MC, Meinkoth J, Dillmann WH, Burrow GN: Iodine induces transforming growth factor beta 1 (TGF-β1) mRNA in sheep thyroid cells. *Thyroid* 2:141, 1992.
16. Bowers CY, Lee KL, Schally AV: A study on the interaction of the thyrotropin-releasing factor and L-triiodothyronine: Effects of puromycin and cycloheximide. *Endocrinology* 82:75, 1968.
17. Spencer CA, LoPresti JS, Patel A, Guttler RB, Eigen A, Shen D, Gray D, Nicoloff JT: Applications of a new chemiluminometric TSH assay to subnormal measurement. *J Clin Endocrinol Metab* 70:453, 1990.
18. Larsen PR: Thyroid-pituitary interaction: Feedback regulation of thyrotropin secretion by thyroid hormones. *N Engl J Med* 306:23, 1982.
19. Chopra IJ, Hershman JM, Hornabrook RW: Serum thyroid hormone and thyrotropin levels in subjects from endemic goiter regions of New Guinea. *J Clin Endocrinol Metab* 40:326, 1975.
20. Medeiros-Neto GA, Penna M, Monteiro K, Kataoka K, Imai Y, Hollander C: The effect of iodized oil in the TSH response to TRH in endemic goiter patients. *J Clin Endocrinol Metab* 41:504, 1976.
21. Koutras DA, Alexander WD, Buchanan WW, Crooks J, Wayne EJ: Stable iodine metabolism in non-toxic goitre. *Lancet* 2:784, 1960.
22. Vagenakis AG, Koutras DA, Burger A, Malamos B, Ingbar SH, Braverman LE: Studies of serum triiodothyronine, thyroxine and thyrotropin concentrations in endemic goiter in Greece. *J Clin Endocrinol Metab* 37:485, 1973.
23. Dige-Petersen H, Hummer L: Serum thyrotropin concentrations under basal conditions and after stimulation with thyrotropin-releasing hormone in idiopathic non-toxic goiter. *J Clin Endocrinol Metab* 44:1115, 1977.
24. Young RL, Harvey WC, Mazzaferri EL, Reynolds JC, Hamilton CR Jr: Thyroid-stimulating hormone levels in idiopathic euthyroid goiter. *J Clin Endocrinol Metab* 41:21, 1975.
25. Bachtarzi H, Benmiloud M: TSH-regulation and goitrogenesis in severe iodine deficiency. *Acta Endocrinol (Copen)* 103:21, 1983.
26. Brown RS, Jackson IMD, Pohl SL, Reichlin S: Do thyroid-stimulating immunoglobulins cause non-toxic and toxic multinodular goitre? *Lancet* 1:904, 1978.
27. Valente WA, Vitti P, Rotella CM, Vaughan MM, Aloj SM, Grollman EF, Ambesi-Impiombato FS, Kohn LD: Antibodies that promote thyroid growth: A distinct population of thy-

roid-stimulating autoantibodies. *N Engl J Med* 309:1028, 1983.

28. Hetzel BS, Maberly GF: Iodine, in Mertz W (ed): *Trace Elements in Human and Animal Nutrition,* Vol 2. New York, Academic, 1986, p 139.
29. Ibbertson HK: Endemic goitre and cretinism. *J Clin Endocrinol Metab* 8:97, 1979.
30. Van Herle AJ, Chopra IJ, Hershman JM, Hornabrook RW: Serum thyroglobulin in inhabitants of an endemic goiter region of New Guinea. *J Clin Endocrinol Metab* 43:512, 1976.
31. Pitt-Rivers R, Niven JSF, Young MR: Localization of protein-bound radioactive iodine in rat thyroid glands labelled with ^{125}I or ^{131}I. *Biochem J* 90:205, 1964.
32. Stanbury JB, Querido A: Genetic and environmental factors in cretinism: A classification. *J Clin Endocrinol Metab* 16:1522, 1956.
33. Dumont JE, Ermans AM, Bastenie PA: Thyroid function in a goiter endemic: V. Mechanism of thyroid failure in the Uele endemic cretins. *J Clin Endocrinol Metab* 23:847, 1963.
34. McCullagh SF: The Huon Peninsula endemic: III. The effect in the female of endemic goitre of reproductive function. *Med J Aust* 1:844, 1963.
35. Pendergrast WJ, Milmore BK, Marcus SC: Thyroid cancer and thyrotoxicosis in the United States: Their relation to endemic goiter. *J Chronic Dis* 13:22, 1961.
36. Studer H, Hunziker HR, Ruchti C: Morphologic and functional substrate of thyrotoxicosis caused by nodular goiters. *Am J Med* 65:227, 1978.
37. Delange F, Costa A, Ermans AM, Ibbertson HK, Querido A, Stanbury JB: A survey of the clinical and metabolic patterns of endemic cretinism, in Stanbury JB, Kroc RL (eds): *Human Development and the Thyroid Gland: Relation to Endemic Cretinism.* New York, Plenum, 1972, p 175.
38. Editorial: Endemic goitre and cretinism. *Lancet* 2:1165, 1979.
39. Eastman CJ, Phillips DIW: Endemic goitre and iodine deficiency disorders—aetiology, epidemiology and treatment. *Baillieres Clin Endocrinol Metab* 2:719, 1988.
40. Patel YC, Pharoah POD, Hornabrook RW, Hetzel BS: Serum triiodothyronine, thyroxine and thyroid-stimulating hormone in endemic goiter: A comparison of goitrous and nongoitrous subjects in New Guinea. *J Clin Endocrinol Metab* 37:783, 1973.
41. Pretell EA: Role of the placenta and of plasma hormone binding in the pathogenesis of cretinism, in Stanbury JB, Kroc RL (eds): *Human Development and the Thyroid Gland: Relation to Endemic Cretinism.* New York, Plenum, 1972, p 449.
42. Thilly CH, Delange F, Lagasse R, Bourdoux P, Ramioul L, Berquist H, Ermans AM: Fetal hypothyroidism and maternal thyroid status in severe endemic goiter. *J Clin Endocrinol Metab* 47:354, 1978.
43. Hershman JM, Due DT, Sharp B, My L, Kent JR, Binh LN, Reed AW, Phuc LD, et al: Endemic goiter in Vietnam. *J Clin Endocrinol Metab* 57:243, 1983.
44. Gaitan JE, Mayoral LG, Gaitan E: Defective thyroidal iodine concentration in protein-calorie malnutrition. *J Clin Endocrinol Metab* 57:327, 1983.
45. Ingenbleek Y, Luypaert B, De Nayer PH: Nutritional status and endemic goitre. *Lancet* 1:388, 1980.
46. Eggo MC, Burrow GN: Glycosylation of thyroglobulin—its role in secretion, iodination, and stability. *Endocrinology* 113:1655, 1983.
47. Kimball OP: The prevention of simple goiter in man. *Am J Med Sci* 163:634, 1922.
48. Vander JB, Gaston EA, Dawber TR: The significance of nontoxic thyroid nodules. *Ann Intern Med* 69:537, 1968.
49. Mortensen JD, Bennett WA, Woolner LB: Incidence of carcinoma in thyroid glands removed at 1000 consecutive routine necropsies. *Surg Forum* 5:659, 1955.
50. Kieffer JD, Mover H, Federico P, Maloof F: Pituitary-thyroid axis in neonatal and adult rats: Comparison of the sexes. *Endocrinology* 98:295, 1976.
51. Crooks J, Aboul-Khair SA, Turnbull AC, Hytten FE: The incidence of goitre during pregnancy. *Lancet* 2:334, 1964.
52. Crooks J, Tulloch MI, Turnbull AC, Davidsson D, Skulason T, Snaedal G: Comparative incidence of goitre in pregnancy in Iceland and Scotland. *Lancet* 2:625, 1967.
53. Glinoer D, De Nayer P, Bourdoux P, Leome M, Robyn C, Van Steirteghem A, Kinthaert J, Lejeune B: Regulation of maternal thyroid during pregnancy. *J Clin Endocrinol Metab* 71:276, 1990.
54. Dworkin HJ, Jacquez JA, Beierwaltes WH: Relationship of iodine ingestion to iodine excretion in pregnancy. *J Clin Endocrinol Metab* 26:1329, 1966.
55. Levy RP, Newman DM, Rejali LS, Barford DAG: The myth of goiter in pregnancy. *Am J Obstet Gynecol* 137:701, 1980.
56. Malamos B, Miras K, Kostamis P, Mantzos J, Kralios AC, Rigopoulos G, Zerefos N, Koutras DA: Epidemiologic and metabolic studies in the endemic goiter areas of Greece, in Cassano C, Andreoli M (eds): *Current Topics in Thyroid Research.* New York, Academic, 1965, p 851.
57. Greig WR, Boyle JA, Duncan A, Nicol J, Gray MJB, Buchanan WW, McGirr EM: Genetic and non-genetic factors in simple goitre formation: Evidence from a twin study. *Q J Med* 36:175, 1967.
58. Nilsson LR: Adolescent colloid goitre. *Acta Paediatr Scand* 55:49, 1966.
59. Vickery AL: The diagnosis of malignancy in dyshormonogenic goiter. *J Clin Endocrinol Metab* 10:317, 1981.
60. Gaitan E: Goitrens. *Baillieres Clin Endocrinol Metab* 2:683, 1988.
61. Chesney AM, Clawson TA, Webster B: Endemic goitre in rabbits: I. Incidence and characteristics. *Bull Johns Hopkins Hosp* 43:261, 1928.
62. Gaitan E, Wahner HW, Correa P, Bernal R, Jubiz W, Gaitan JE, Llanos G: Endemic goiter in the Cauca Valley: I. Results and limitations of twelve years of iodine prophylaxis. *J Clin Endocrinol Metab* 28:1730, 1968.
63. Berry MJ, Banu L, Larsen PR: Type 1 iodothyronine deiodinase is a selenocysteine-containing enzyme. *Nature* 349:438, 1991.
64. Goyens P, Golstein J, Nsombola B, Vis H, Dumont JE: Selenium deficiency as a possible factor in the pathogenesis of myxedematous endemic cretinism. *Acta Endocrinol (Copenh)* 114:497, 1987.
65. McGarrison R: *The Thyroid Gland in Health and Disease.* London, Bailliere, Tindall and Cox, 1917.
66. Silverberg SG, Vidone RA: Carcinoma of the thyroid in surgical and postmortem material. *Ann Surg* 164:291, 1966.
67. Jauregui R, Lilker ES, Bayley A: Upper airway obstruction in euthyroid goiter. *JAMA* 238:2163, 1977.
68. Cady B: Management of tracheal obstruction from thyroid diseases. *World J Surg* 6:696, 1982.
69. Medvei UC: *A History of Endocrinology.* Lancaster, United Kingdom, MTP, 1982.
70. Sampson RJ, Key CR, Buncher CR, Iijima S: Thyroid carcinoma in Hiroshima and Nagasaki: I. Prevalence of thyroid carcinoma at autopsy. *JAMA* 209:65, 1969.
71. Sampson RJ: Prevalence and significance of occult thyroid cancer, in DeGroot LJ (ed): *Radiation-Associated Thyroid Carcinoma.* New York, Grune & Stratton, 1977, p 45.
72. Cutler SJ, Young JL (eds): *Third National Cancer Survey: Incidence Data.* National Cancer Institute Monograph 41, U.S. DHEW publication (NIH) 75-787, Bethesda, MD, 1975, pp 107, 111.
73. Taylor S, Goolden AWG: Thyroid and thymus, in Kunkler PB, Rains AJH (eds): *Treatment of Cancer in Clinical Practice.* Edinburgh, E & S Livingstone, 1959, p 410.
74. Money WL, Rawson RW: The experimental production of thyroid tumors in the rat exposed to prolonged treatment with thiouracil. *Cancer* 3:321, 1950.
75. Al-Saadi A: Precursor cytogenic changes of transplantable

thyroid carcinoma in iodine-deficient goiters. *Cancer Res* 28:739, 1968.
76. Elman DS: Familial association of nerve deafness with nodular goiter and thyroid carcinoma. *N Engl J Med* 259:219, 1958.
77. McGirr EM, Clement WE, Currie AR, Kennedy JS: Impaired dehalogenase activity as a cause of goitre with malignant changes. *Scott Med J* 4:232, 1959.
78. Namba H, Matsuo K, Fagin JA: Clonal composition of benign and malignant human thyroid tumors. *J Clin Invest* 86:120, 1990.
79. Gharib H, James EM, Charboneau JW, Naessens JM, Offord KP, Gorman CA: Suppressive therapy with levothyroxine for solitary thyroid nodules: A double-blind controlled clinical study. *N Engl J Med* 317:70, 1987.
80. Astwood EB, Cassidy CE, Aurbach GD: Treatment of goiter and thyroid nodules with thyroid. *JAMA* 174:459, 1960.
81. Lamberg BA, Hernberg CA, Hakkila R: Treatment of nontoxic goitre with thyroid preparations. *Acta Endocrinol (Copen)* 33:584, 1960.
82. Shimaoka K, Sokal JE: Suppressive therapy of nontoxic goiter. *Am J Med* 57:576, 1974.
83. Hansen JM, Kampmann J, Madsen SH, Skovsted L, Solgaard S, Grytter C, Grontveldt T, Rasmussen SN: L-thyroxine treatment of diffuse nontoxic goitre evaluated by ultrasonic determination of thyroid volume. *Clin Endocrinol (Oxf)* 10:1, 1979.
84. Clark OH: TSH suppression in the management of thyroid nodules and thyroid cancer. *World J Surg* 5:39, 1981.
85. Paul TL, Kerrigan J, Kelly AM, Braverman LE, Baran DT: Long-term L-thyroxine therapy is associated with decreased hip bone density in premenopausal women. *JAMA* 259:3137, 1988.
86. Geerdsen JP, Frolund L: Recurrence of non-toxic goitre with and without postoperative thyroxine medication. *Clin Endocrinol (Oxf)* 21:529, 1984.
87. Verelst J, Bonnyns M, Glinoer D: Radioiodine therapy in voluminous multinodular nontoxic goitre. *Acta Endocrinol (Copenh)* 122:417, 1990.
88. Stock JM, Surks MI, Oppenheimer JH: Replacement dosage of L-thyroxine in hypothyroidism. *N Engl J Med* 290:529, 1974.
89. Shimaoka K, Sokal JE: Differentiation of benign and malignant thyroid nodules by scintiscan. *Arch Intern Med* 114:36, 1964.
90. Hoffmann GL, Thompson NW, Heffron C: The solitary thyroid nodule. *Arch Surg* 105:379, 1972.
91. Hempelmann LH: Thyroid neoplasms following irradiation in infancy, in DeGroot LJ (ed): *Radiation-Associated Thyroid Carcinoma.* New York, Grune & Stratton, 1977, p 221.
92. Winship T, Rosvoll RV: Childhood thyroid carcinoma. *Cancer* 14:734, 1961.
93. Rallison ML, Dobyns BM, Keating FR Jr, Rall JE, Tyler FH: Thyroid nodularity in children. *JAMA* 233:1069, 1975.
94. Kirkland RT, Kirkland JL, Rosenberg HS, Harberg FJ, Librik L, Clayton GW: Solitary thyroid nodules in 30 children and report of a child with a thyroid abscess. *Pediatrics* 51:85, 1973.
95. Silverman SH, Nussbaum M, Rausen AR: Thyroid nodules in children: A ten-year experience at one institution. *Mt Sinai J Med (NY)* 46:460, 1979.
96. Duffy BJ Jr, Fitzgerald PJ: Cancer of the thyroid in children: A report of 28 cases. *J Clin Endocrinol Metab* 10:1296, 1950.
97. Pifer JW, Hempelmann LH: Radiation-induced thyroid carcinoma. *Ann NY Acad Sci* 114:838, 1964.
98. Refetoff S, Harrison J, Karanfilski BT, Kaplan EL, DeGroot LJ, Bekerman C: Continuing occurrence of thyroid carcinoma after irradiation to the neck in infancy and childhood. *N Engl J Med* 292:171, 1975.
99. DeGroot LJ, Reilly M, Pinnameneni K, Refetoff S: Retrospective and prospective study of radiation-induced thyroid disease. *Am J Med* 74:852, 1983.
100. Schneider AB: Thyroid nodules following childhood irradiation: A 1989 update. *Thyroid Today* 12:1, 1989.
101. Bowens OM, Vander BJ: Thyroid nodules and thyroid malignancy. *Ann Intern Med* 57:245, 1962.
102. Miller JM, Hamburger JI, Mellinger RC: The thyroid scintigram: II. The cold nodule. *Radiology* 85:702, 1965.
103. DeGroot LJ (ed): *Radiation-Associated Thyroid Carcinoma.* New York, Grune & Stratton, 1977.
104. Esser PD: Absorbed radiation doses in adults, in Freeman LM, Johnson PM (eds): *Clinical Scintillation Imaging,* 2d ed. New York, Grune & Stratton, 1975, p 799.
105. Keyes JW, Thrall JH, Carey JE: Technical considerations in in vivo thyroid studies. *Semin Nucl Med* 8:43, 1978.
106. Gharib H, Goellner JR: Evaluation of nodular thyroid disease. *Endocrinol Metab Clin North Am* 17:511, 1988.
107. Blum M: Enhanced clinical diagnosis of thyroid disease using echography. *Am J Med* 59:301, 1975.
108. Miller JM, Zafar SU, Karo JJ: The cystic thyroid nodule. *Radiology* 110:257, 1974.
109. McCowen KD, Reed JW, Fariss BL: The role of thyroid therapy in patients with thyroid cysts. *Am J Med* 68:853, 1980.
110. Treece GL, Georgitis WJ, Hofeldt FD: Resolution of recurrent thyroid cysts with tetracycline instillation. *Arch Intern Med* 143:2285, 1983.
111. Reede DL, Bergeron RT, McCauley DI: CT of the thyroid and of other thoracic inlet disorders. *J Otolaryngol* 11:349, 1982.
112. De Certaines J, Herry JV, Lancien G, Benoist L, Bernard AM, Le Clech G: Evaluation of human thyroid tumors by proton nuclear magnetic resonance. *J Nucl Med* 23:48, 1982.
113. Burman KD, Andersen JH, Wartofsky L, Mong DP, Jelinek JJJ: Management of patients with thyroid carcinoma: Application of thallium-210 scintigraphy and magnetic resonance imaging. *J Nucl Med* 31:1958, 1990.
114. Mojab K, Ghosh BC: Thyroid angiography. *Am J Surg* 132:620, 1976.
115. Maloof F, Wang CA, Vickery AL Jr: Nontoxic goiter—diffuse or nodular. *Med Clin North Am* 59:1221, 1975.
116. Vickery AL Jr: Needle biopsy and the thyroid nodule, in DeGroot LJ (ed): *Radiation-Associated Thyroid Carcinoma.* New York, Grune & Stratton, 1977, p 339.
117. Burke JS, Butler JJ, Fuller LM: Malignant lymphomas of the thyroid: A clinical pathologic study of 35 patients including ultrastructural observations. *Cancer* 39:1587, 1977.
118. Sirota DK, Segal RL: Primary lymphomas of the thyroid gland. *JAMA* 242:1743, 1979.
119. Van Herle AJ, Rich P, Ljung B-ME, Ashcraft MW, Solomon DH, Keeler EB: The thyroid nodule. *Ann Intern Med* 96:221, 1982.
120. Ashcraft MW, Van Herle AJ: Management of thyroid nodules: II. Scanning techniques, thyroid suppressive therapy, and fine-needle aspiration. *Head Neck Surg* 3:297, 1981.
121. McNeil BJ, Keeler E, Adelstein SJ: Primer on certain elements of medical decision making. *N Engl J Med* 293:211, 1975.
122. Miller JM, Hamburger JI, Kini S: Diagnosis of thyroid nodules: Use of fine-needle aspiration and needle biopsy. *JAMA* 241:481, 1979.
123. Miller JM, Hamburger JI, Kini S: The needle biopsy diagnosis of papillary thyroid carcinoma. *Cancer* 48:989, 1981.
124. Chu EW, Hanson TA, Goldman JM, Robbins J: Study of cells in fine-needle aspirations of the thyroid gland. *Acta Cytol* 23:309, 1979.
125. Clark OH, Demling R: Management of thyroid nodules in the elderly. *Am J Surg* 132:615, 1976.
126. Field JB, Larsen PR, Yamashita K, Mashiter K, Dekker A: Demonstration of iodine transport defect but normal iodide organification in nonfunctioning nodules of human thyroid glands. *J Clin Invest* 52:2402, 1973.
127. Shiroozu A, Inoue K, Nakashima T, Okamura K, Yoshinari M, Nishitani H, Omae T: Defective iodide transport and normal organification of iodide in cold nodules of the thyroid. *Clin Endocrinol (Oxf)* 15:411, 1981.

128. Frauman AG, Moses BS: Oncogenes and growth factors in thyroid carcinogenesis. *Endocrinol Metab Clin North Am* 19:479, 1990.
129. Suarez HG, Du Villard JA, Calliou B, Schlumberger M, Tubiana M, Parmentier C, Montier R: Detection of activated ras oncogenes in human thyroid carcinomas. *Oncogene* 2:403, 1988.
130. Terrier P, Sheng Z-M, Schlumberger M, Tubiana M, Caillou B, Travagli JP, Fragu P, Parmentier C, Riou G: Structure and expression of c-myc and c-fos proto-oncogenes in thyroid carcinomas. *Br J Cancer* 57:43, 1988.
131. Yamashita S, Ong J, Fagin JA, Melmed S: Expression of the myc cellular proto-oncogene in human thyroid tissue. *J Clin Endocrinol Metab* 63:1170, 1986.
132. Lemoine NR, Mayaii ES, Wylie FS, Farr CJ, Hughes D, Padua RA, Thurston V, Williams ED, Wynford-Thomas D: Activated ras oncogenes in human thyroid cancers. *Cancer Res* 48:4459, 1988.
133. Grieco M, Santoro M, Berlingeri MT, Meillo RM, Donghi R, Bongarzone I, Piertotti MA, Porta GD, et al: PTC is a novel rearranged form of the ret protooncogene and is frequently detected in vivo in human thyroid papillary carcinomas. *Cell* 60:557, 1990.
134. Karga H, Lee J-K, Vickery AL Jr, Thor A, Gaz RD, Jameson JL: Ras oncogene mutations in benign and malignant thyroid neoplasms. *J Clin Endocrinol Metab* 73:832, 1991.
135. Thomas GA, Williams D, Williams ED: The clonal origin of thyroid nodules and adenomas. *Am J Pathol* 134:141, 1989.
136. Meissner WA: The pathologic classification and staging of thyroid cancer, in DeGroot LJ (ed): *Radiation-Associated Thyroid Carcinoma.* New York, Grune & Stratton, 1977, p. 45.
137. Hay ID, Grant CS, Taylor WF, McConahey WM: Ipsilateral lobectomy versus bilateral lobar resection in papillary thyroid carcinoma: A retrospective analysis of surgical outcome using a novel prognostic scoring system. *Surgery* 102:1088, 1987.
138. Hay ID: Papillary thyroid carcinoma. *Endocrinol Metab Clin North Am* 19:545, 1990.
139. Smith SA, Hay ID, Goellner JR, Ryan JJ, McConahey WM: Mortality from papillary thyroid carcinoma: A case-control study of 56 lethal cases. *Cancer* 62:1381, 1988.
140. Schneider AB: Radiation-induced thyroid tumors. *Endocrinol Metab Clin North Am* 19:495, 1990.
141. DeGroot LJ: Radiation and thyroid disease. *Baillieres Clin Endocrinol Metab* 2:777, 1988.
142. DeGroot LJ: Diagnostic approach and management of patients exposed to irradiation to the thyroid. *J Clin Endocrinol Metab* 69:925, 1989.
143. Maxon HR, Thomas SR, Saenger EL, Buncher CR, Kereiakes JG: Ionizing irradiation and the induction of clinically significant disease in the human thyroid gland. *Am J Med* 63:967, 1977.
144. Maxon HR, Saenger EL, Thomas SR, Buncher CR, Kereiakes JG, Shafer ML, McLaughlin CA: Clinically important radiation-associated thyroid disease: A controlled study. *JAMA* 244:1802, 1980.
145. Holm L-E, Dahlqvist I, Israelsson A, Lundell G: Malignant thyroid tumors after iodine-131 therapy: A retrospective cohort study. *N Engl J Med* 303:188, 1980.
146. Fogelfeld L, Wiviott MBT, Shore-Freedman E, Blend M, Bekerman C, Pinsky S, Schneider AB: Recurrence of thyroid nodules after surgical removal in patients irradiated in childhood for benign conditions. *N Engl J Med* 320:835, 1989.
147. Getaz EP, Shimaoka K, Kazack M, Friedman M: Suppressive therapy for postirradiation thyroid nodules. *Can J Surg* 23:558, 1980.
148. Schimpff SC: Specialty rounds: Well-differentiated thyroid carcinoma: Epidemiology, etiology and treatment. *Am J Med Sci* 278:100, 1979.
149. DeGroot LJ, Kaplan EL, McCormick M, Straus FH: Natural history, treatment, and course of papillary thyroid carcinoma. *J Clin Endocrinol Metab* 71:414, 1990.
150. Margolin FR, Steinbach HL: Soft tissue roentgenography of thyroid nodules. *AJR* 102:844, 1968.
151. Mazzaferri EL, Young RL, Oertel JE, Kemmerer WT, Page CP: Papillary thyroid carcinoma: The impact of therapy in 576 patients. *Medicine (Baltimore)* 56:171, 1977.
152. Mazzaferri EL, Young RL: Papillary thyroid carcinoma: A 10-year follow-up report of the impact of therapy in 576 patients. *Am J Med* 70:511, 1981.
153. Simpson WJ, McKinney SE, Carruthers JS, Gospodarowicz MK, Sutcliffe SB, Panzarella T: Papillary and follicular thyroid cancer: Prognostic factors in 1578 patients. *Am J Med* 83:479, 1987.
154. Silliphant WM, Klinck GH, Levitin MS: Thyroid carcinoma and death: A clinicopathological study of 193 autopsies. *Cancer* 17:513, 1964.
155. Heimann R, Vannineuse A, De Sloover C, Dor P: Malignant lymphomas and undifferentiated small cell carcinoma of the thyroid: A clinicopathological review in the light of the Kiel classification for malignant lymphomas. *Histopathology* 2:201, 1978.
156. Kerr DJ, Burt AD, Boyle P, Macfarlane GJ, Storer AM, Brewin TB: Prognostic factors in thyroid tumors. *Br J Cancer* 54:475, 1986.
157. Clark OH: Total thyroidectomy: The treatment of choice for patients with differentiated thyroid cancer. *Ann Surg* 196:361, 1982.
158. Mazzaferri EL: Papillary thyroid carcinoma: Factors influencing prognosis and current therapy. *Sem Oncol* 14:315, 1987.
159. Demeure MJ, Clark OH: Surgery in the treatment of thyroid cancer. *Endocrinol Metab Clin North Am* 19:663, 1990.
160. Clark OH, Duh Q-Y: Thyroid cancer. *Med Clin North Am* 75:211, 1991.
161. Foster RS Jr: Morbidity and mortality after thyroidectomy for carcinoma. *Surg Gynecol Obstet* 146:423, 1978.
162. Thompson NW, Harness JK: Complications of total thyroidectomy for carcinoma. *Surg Gynecol Obstet* 131:861, 1970.
163. Schlumberger M, Tubiana M, De Vathaire F, Hill C, Gardet P, Travagli J-P, Fragu P, Lumbroso J, et al: Long-term results of treatment of 283 patients with lung and bone metastases from differentiated thyroid carcinoma. *J Clin Endocrinol Metab* 63:960, 1986.
164. Varma VM, Beierwaltes WH, Nofal MM, Nishiyama RH, Copp JE: Treatment of thyroid cancer: Death rates after surgery and after surgery followed by sodium iodide I131. *JAMA* 214:1437, 1970.
165. Leeper RD: The effect of ^{131}I therapy on survival of patients with metastatic papillary or follicular thyroid carcinoma. *J Clin Endocrinol Metab* 36:1143, 1973.
166. Crile G: The endocrine dependency of papillary carcinoma of the thyroid, in Smithers D (ed): *Tumours of the Thyroid Gland.* Edinburgh, E & S Livingstone, 1970, p 269.
167. Simpson WJ, Carruthers JS: The role of external radiation in the management of papillary and follicular thyroid cancer. *Am J Surg* 136:457, 1978.
168. Beierwaltes WH, Nishiyama RH, Thompson NW, Copp JE, Kubo A: Survival time and "cure" in papillary and follicular thyroid carcinoma with distant metastases: Statistics following University of Michigan therapy. *J Nucl Med* 23:561, 1982.
169. Samaan NA, Maheshwari YK, Nader S, Hill CS Jr, Schultz PN, Haynie TP, Hickey RC, Clark RL, et al: Impact of therapy for differentiated carcinoma of the thyroid: An analysis of 706 cases. *J Clin Endocrinol Metab* 56:1131, 1983.
170. DeGroot LJ, Reilly M: Comparison of 30- and 50-mCi doses of iodine-131 for thyroid ablation. *Ann Intern Med* 96:51, 1982.
171. Beierwaltes WH: The treatment of thyroid carcinoma with radioactive iodine. *Semin Nucl Med* 8:79, 1978.
172. Hilts SV, Hellman D, Anderson J, Woolfenden J, Van Ant-

werp J, Patton D: Serial TSH determination after T3 withdrawal of thyroidectomy in the therapy of thyroid carcinoma. *J Nucl Med* 20:928, 1979.
173. Goldman JM, Line BR, Aamodt RL, Robbins J: Influence of triiodothyronine withdrawal time on ^{131}I uptake postthyroidectomy for thyroid cancer. *J Clin Endocrinol Metab* 50:734, 1980.
174. Melmed S, Harada A, Hershman JM, Kirshnamurthy GT, Blahd WH: Neutralizing antibodies to bovine thyrotropin in immunized patients with thyroid cancer. *J Clin Endocrinol Metab* 51:358, 1980.
175. Hershman JM, Edwards CL: Serum thyrotropin (TSH) levels after thyroid ablation compared with TSH levels after exogenous bovine TSH: Implications for ^{131}I treatment of thyroid carcinoma. *J Clin Endocrinol Metab* 34:814, 1972.
176. Hamburger JI: Diuretic augmentation of ^{131}I uptake in inoperable thyroid cancer. *N Engl J Med* 280:1091, 1969.
177. Simpson WJ: Anaplastic thyroid carcinoma: A new approach. *Can J Surg* 23:25, 1980.
178. Smithers D (ed): *Tumours of the Thyroid Gland*. Edinburgh, E & S Livingstone, 1970.
179. Shimaoka K: Adjunctive management of thyroid cancer: Chemotherapy. *J Surg Oncol* 15:283, 1980.
180. Gottlieb JA, Hill CS Jr: Chemotherapy of thyroid cancer with Adriamycin. *N Engl J Med* 290:193, 1974.
181. Harada T, Nishikawa Y, Suzuki T, Ito K, Baba S: Bleomycin treatment for cancer of the thyroid. *Am J Surg* 122:53, 1971.
182. Campagno J, Oertel JE: Malignant lymphoma and other lymphoproliferative disorders of the thyroid gland: A clinicopathologic study of 245 cases. *Am J Clin Pathol* 74:1, 1980.
183. Rosen IB, Sutcliffe SB, Gospodarowicz MK, Chua T, Simpson WJK: The role of surgery in the management of thyroid lymphoma. *Surgery* 104:1095, 1988.
184. Hamburger JI, Miller JM, Kini SR: Lymphoma of the thyroid. *Ann Intern Med* 99:685, 1983.
185. Dewan SS: The bone scan in the thyroid cancer. *J Nucl Med* 20:271, 1979.
186. Charles MA: Comparison of serum thyroglobulin with iodine scans in thyroid cancer. *J Endocrinol Invest* 5:267, 1982.
187. Gebel F, Ramelli F, Burgi U, Ingold U, Studer H, Winand R: The site of leakage of intrafollicular thyroglobulin into the blood stream in simple human goiter. *J Clin Endocrinol Metab* 57:915, 1983.
188. Van Herle AJ, Uller RP, Matthews NL, Brown J: Radioimmunoassay for measurement of thyroglobulin in human serum. *J Clin Invest* 52:1320, 1973.
189. Schneider AB, Favus MJ, Stachura ME, Arnold JE, Ryo UY, Pinsky S, Colman M, Arnold MJ, Frohman LA: Plasma thyroglobulin in detecting thyroid carcinoma after childhood head and neck irradiation. *Ann Intern Med* 86:29, 1977.
190. Charles MA, Dodson LE, Waldeck N, Hofeldt F, Ghaed N, Telepak R, Ownbey J, Burnstein P: Serum thyroglobulin levels predict total body iodine scan findings in patients with treated well-differentiated thyroid carcinoma. *Am J Med* 69:401, 1980.
191. Black EG, Cassoni A, Gimlette TMD, Harmer CL, Maisey MN, Oates GD: Serum thyroglobulin in thyroid cancer. *Lancet* 2:443, 1981.
192. Schneider AB, Line BR, Goldman JM, Robbins J: Sequential serum thyroglobulin determinations, ^{131}I scans and ^{131}I uptakes after triiodothyronine withdrawal in patients with thyroid cancer. *J Clin Endocrinol Metab* 53:1199, 1981.
193. DeGroot LJ, Hoye K, Refetoff S, Van Herle AJ, Asteris GT, Rochman H: Serum antigens and antibodies in the diagnosis of thyroid cancer. *J Clin Endocrinol Metab* 45:1220, 1977.
194. Fairweather DS, Bradwell AR, Watson-James SF, Dykes PW, Chandler S, Hoffenberg R: Detection of thyroid tumours using radio-labelled anti-thyroglobulin. *Clin Endocrinol (Oxf)* 18:563, 1983.
195. Steiner AL, Goodman AD, Powers SR: Study of a kindred with pheochromocytoma, medullary thyroid carcinoma, hyperparathyroidism and Cushing's disease: Multiple endocrine neoplasia, type 2. *Medicine (Baltimore)* 47:371, 1968.
196. Mathew CGP, Easton DF, Nakamura Y, Ponder BA: Presymptomatic screening for multiple endocrine neoplasia type 2a with linked DNA markers: The MEN 2A International Collaborative Group. *Lancet* 337:7, 1991.
197. Khari MRA, Dexter RN, Burzynski NJ, Johnston CC Jr: Mucosal neuroma, pheochromocytoma and medullary thyroid carcinoma: Multiple endocrine neoplasia type 3. *Medicine (Baltimore)* 54:89, 1975.
198. Knudson AG: Mutation and cancer: Statistical study of retinoblastoma. *Proc Natl Acad Sci USA* 68:820, 1971.
199. Jackson CE, Block MA, Greenawald KA, Tashjian AH: The two-mutational-event theory in medullary thyroid cancer. *Am J Hum Genet* 31:704, 1979.
200. Baylin SB, Hsu SH, Gann DS: Inherited medullary thyroid carcinoma: A final monoclonal mutation in one of multiple clones of susceptible cells. *Science* 199:429, 1978.
201. Hill CS Jr, Ibanez ML, Samaan NA, Ahearn MJ, Clark RL: Medullary (solid) carcinoma of the thyroid gland: An analysis of the M.D. Anderson Hospital experience with patients with the tumor, its special features, and its histogenesis. *Medicine (Baltimore)* 52:141, 1973.
202. Tashjian AH Jr, Wolfe HJ, Voelkel EF: Human calcitonin. *Am J Med* 56:840, 1974.
203. Wells SA Jr, Baylin SB, Linehan WM, Farrell RE, Cox EB, Cooper CW: Provocative agents and the diagnosis of medullary carcinoma of the thyroid gland. *Ann Surg* 188:139, 1978.
204. Kaplan MM: Progress in thyroid cancer. *Endocrinol Metab Clin North Am* 19:469, 1990.
205. Baylin SB, Beaven MA, Keiser HR, Tashjian AH Jr, Melvin KEW: Serum histamine and calcitonin levels in medullary carcinoma of the thyroid. *Lancet* 1:455, 1972.
206. Wolfe HJ, Melvin KEW, Cervi-Skinner SH, Al Saadi AA, Juliar JF, Jackson CE, Tashjian AH Jr: C-cell hyperplasia preceding medullary thyroid carcinoma. *N Engl J Med* 289:437, 1973.
207. Gagel RF, Jackson CE, Block MA, Feldman ZT, Reichlin S, Hamilton BP, Tashjian AH: Age-related probability of development of hereditary medullary thyroid carcinoma. *J Pediatr* 101:941, 1982.
208. Wahner HW, Cuello C, Aljure F: Hormone-induced regression of medullary (solid) thyroid carcinoma. *Am J Med* 45:789, 1968.

PART IV

Adrenal Disease

CHAPTER 12

The Adrenal Cortex

Walter L. Miller
J. Blake Tyrrell

EMBRYOLOGY, ANATOMY, AND HISTORY

The adrenal cortex produces three principal categories of steroid hormones. The *mineralocorticoids,* of which aldosterone is most important, regulate renal sodium retention and thus are key components in regulating sodium, potassium, blood pressure, and intravascular volume. Mineralocorticoid excess can cause hypertension and hypokalemia; mineralocorticoid deficiency can cause hyponatremia, hyperkalemia, hypotension, and shock. The *glucocorticoids,* of which cortisol is most important, are named for their role in maintaining serum glucose and regulating carbohydrate metabolism but also play key regulatory roles in a wide variety of physiologic processes, including development, growth, immune responses, cardiovascular function, and responses to stress. Glucocorticoid excess causes weight gain, moon facies, striae, growth arrest, weakness, easy bruisability, and glycosuria; glucocorticoid deficiency causes anorexia, apathy, fatigue, weight loss, hypoglycemia, and hypotension. *Adrenal androgens* play no known physiologic role, although they mediate some female secondary sexual characteristics. Overproduction leads to hirsutism, virilism, ovarian dysfunction, and infertility. Thus, the physiology and biochemistry of the adrenal cortex are of general interest in medicine and biology because of the numerous and diverse effects of the various and rather similar secretions of the cortex. The adrenal cortex secretes over 50 steroids; while many of them are precursors or metabolites of the principal hormones, most have some biological activity. Knowledge about the actions of the various steroids in health and disease also facilitates an understanding of the actions of synthetic steroid hormones (e.g., prednisone and dexamethasone) widely used as pharmacotherapeutic agents.

Diseases of the adrenal cortex are relatively rare but are being recognized with increasing frequency. Addison's disease, Cushing's syndrome, and Conn's (primary aldosteronism) syndrome, which are traditionally regarded as the three principal disorders of the adrenal cortex, are together far less common than genetic disorders of steroid hormone synthesis, which are now recognized with increasing frequency. As the signs and symptoms of adrenal dysfunction are often relatively nonspecific, adrenal disorders must be considered in the differential diagnosis of many common complaints. Furthermore, because synthetic steroids are widely used to treat nonadrenal disorders, physicians often encounter syndromes of iatrogenic steroid excess. This chapter will deal with the biochemistry and physiology of steroid hormone synthesis and disorders of the adrenal cortex. Chap. 15 will discuss steroid hormone therapy, and Chap. 14 will deal in detail with the roles of steroid hormones in hypertension.

History

The history of medical and scientific study of the adrenal cortex closely parallels general advances in medicine, physiology, biochemistry, and molecular biology and has been reviewed in detail.[1] The adrenals were apparently first described by Bartolomeo Eustacchio (better known for the discovery of the eustachian tube of the ear) in 1563, but this work was lost until Lancisi republished it in 1714.[2,3] Scientific interest in the adrenals began with the description by Thomas Addison in 1849 and 1855 of the classic features of adrenocortical deficiency, which included "general languor and debility, remarkable feebleness of the heart's action, irritability of the stomach and a peculiar change in the colour of the skin." In 1856, Brown-Sequard showed that adrenalectomy is incompatible with life, supporting Addison's idea. The syndrome of glucocorticoid excess had been well described in association with adrenal tumors by the turn of the century, long before Harvey Cushing attributed the syndrome that bears his name to "pituitary basophilism." [4]

The roles of the specific products of the adrenal were elucidated with improved surgical approaches to adrenalectomy and hypophysectomy and were clarified further by the development of adrenal extracts that could replace lost function. A role for the adrenal in regulating carbohydrate metabolism was slowly elucidated between 1908 and 1940. Hypoglycemia in adrenal insufficiency was known by 1910, and in 1927 Cori and Cori showed that adrenalectomy decreases hepatic glycogen.[5] Britton and Silvette proposed that the loss of an adrenal carbohydrate-regulating property can cause the debility and mortality in adrenal insufficiency,[6] and Long and associates reported correction of hypoglycemia and decreased hepatic glycogen in adrenalectomized animals that were given adrenal extracts.[7] Additional roles for the adrenal in nitrogen excretion, gluconeogenesis, and lipid metabolism were recognized concurrently.[1,2]

The role of the adrenals in salt and water balance was appreciated somewhat later. In 1927 Banmann and Kurland reported that adrenalectomy causes hyponatremia, hypothermia, and hyperkalemia,[8] and in 1933 Loeb showed that saline can extend the survival of patients with Addison's disease.[9] By 1937 it was understood that sodium is necessary but not sufficient to maintain the life of adrenalectomized rats: Adrenalectomized rats were also found to be susceptible to toxins, trauma, infection, strenuous exercise, drugs, and other forms of stress. In 1946, Hans Selye coined the terms *glucocorticoid* and *mineralocorticoid,* emphasizing that both functions of the adrenal are needed for survival and for responses to stress.[10]

A role for the pituitary in regulating the adrenal was suspected by about 1925 (see Refs. 1 and 2), and by 1930 it was known that hypophysectomy causes adrenal atrophy. Adrenal feedback on pituitary function was reported in 1937, but it was correctly deduced that not all adrenal function is pituitary-dependent because survival after hypophysectomy was longer than survival after adrenalectomy. ACTH was purified in 1943 and its structure was known by 1956, but the origin of ACTH as a proteolytic cleavage product from a larger protein was not established until the late 1970s (see Chap. 8).

Hypothalamic regulation of ACTH release was hypothesized in the late 1940s. Vasopressin stimulation of ACTH release was reported in 1954,[11] and this was quickly followed by studies showing that another factor is also involved.[12,13] However, another 16 years passed before the structure of corticotropin releasing hormone (CRH) was determined.[14]

The functional significance of adrenal zonation, the role of the zona glomerulosa in electrolyte balance, and the independence of the glomerulosa from pituitary regulation emerged in the late 1940s. Aldosterone was identified and characterized in the 1950s,[15] and Conn described hypertension and hypokalemia with aldosterone excess in 1955.[16]

Edward Kendall and Tateus Reichstein independently purified and crystallized the first known glucocorticoid—corticosterone,[17] determined chemical structures, and synthesized numerous steroids, including the first known mineralocorticoid, deoxycorticosterone (DOC).[18] When Philip Hench administered cortisone to 14 arthritic patients in 1949, the results were dramatic.[19] The impact of the discovery that steroids can ameliorate the symptoms of rheumatoid arthritis made cortisone a household word. Kendall, Hench, and Reichstein were rewarded with the Nobel prize in December 1950.

The availability of cortisone led immediately to its use in treating congenital adrenal hyperplasia by Wilkins[20] and Bartter.[21] The success of this experiment stimulated great interest in studying inborn errors of steroid synthesis, leading to our contemporary understanding of the pathways of steroidogenesis. The association of cytochrome P450 with 21-hydroxylase was made in 1965,[22] leading to an active era of enzymologic study. The steroidogenic enzymes were ultimately isolated in the 1970s and 1980s, and their genes were cloned in the 1980s and 1990s.[23] At the same time, studies of steroid hormone action led to the identification of steroid hormone receptors in the 1960s, but it was not until they were studied using recombinant DNA techniques in the 1980s and 1990s that their biology was understood clearly.[24]

Embryology and Development

The adrenal cortex derives from the embryonic mesoderm, in contrast to the ectodermal origin of the medulla.[25,26] Between the fifth and sixth weeks of fetal development, the gonadal ridge, a proliferation of cells in the developing peritoneal epithelium at the base of the dorsal mesentery, develops near the cranial end of the mesonephros. These cells give rise to the steroidogenic cells of both the adrenal cortex and the gonads. The precursors of the adrenal and gonadal cells separate, with the adrenal anlage penetrating the retroperitoneal mesenchyme to form the primitive cortex while the gonadal anlage migrates caudally. The primitive adrenal soon becomes enveloped by a thick layer of more compactly arrayed cells to become the adrenal cortex. Soon thereafter, between the seventh and eighth weeks, the adrenal cortex is invaded by sympathetic neural cells that form the adrenal medulla. By the end of the eighth week, the adrenal has become encapsulated and has taken up residence on the cranial pole of the kidney, which at this time is much smaller than the developing adrenal.[25,26]

The fetal adrenal cortex consists of three zones: the subcapsular "definitive" zone, an ill-defined transitional zone, and the large fetal zone. Recent data suggest that these three fetal zones have steroidogenic potentials analogous to the zonae glomerulosa, fasciculata, and reticularis, respectively.[26a] The fetal zone, which accounts for the overwhelming majority of fetal adrenal cells, makes androgenic

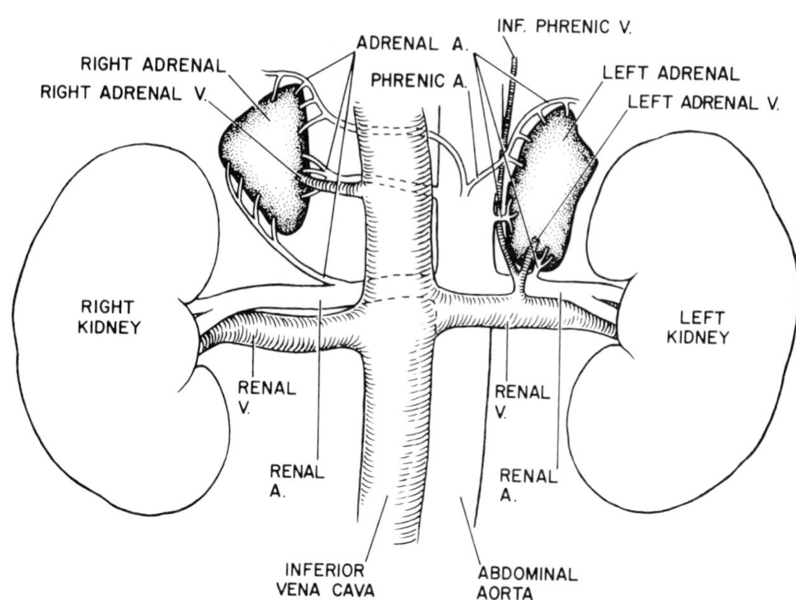

FIGURE 12-1 Location and blood supply of the adrenal glands.

precursors (principally dehydroepiandrosterone) that are used as substrates for the placental synthesis of estrogens. The adrenal is relatively huge in the fetus and newborn. At birth, the adrenals weigh about 8 to 9 g, about twice the weight of adult adrenals, and represent 0.5 percent of total body weight, compared with 0.005 percent in the adult. However, even before birth, the fetal zone begins to involute. By the second week after birth adrenal weight has decreased by one-third, and the fetal zone is no longer detectable by age 1 year. The definitive zone of the fetal adrenal simultaneously develops into the adult adrenal cortex. However, the zona glomerulosa and zona fasciculata are not fully developed until about 3 years of age, and the zona reticularis may not be fully differentiated until age 15 years.

Anatomy

The adrenal glands are extraperitoneal at the upper poles of the kidneys (Fig. 12-1). They are located on the posterior parietal wall, on each side of the vertebral column, lateral to the eleventh thoracic and the first lumbar vertebrae. The average adult gland weighs 4 g irrespective of an individual's sex or size and is 2 to 3 cm wide and 4 to 6 cm long.[27] It enlarges in response to ACTH and becomes smaller when ACTH production decreases. The gland is variably corrugated and nodular; it is surrounded by areolar tissue and a thick fibrous capsule. Unlike the kidneys, the adrenals are not displaced by changes in respiration or posture.[25,27] The right gland tends to be higher and more lateral than the left, which frequently overlaps the abdominal aorta.

The adrenal arteries and veins do not run in parallel (Fig. 12-1), as do those of most other organs. Blood is supplied by several short arteries that are terminal branches of the inferior phrenic artery; the superior, middle, and inferior adrenal arteries; and occasionally the ovarian or left spermatic artery.[25] Because there are several arteries, adrenal infarction is unusual. Arterial blood enters a sinusoidal circulation in the cortex and drains toward the medulla so that medullary chromaffin cells are bathed in very high concentrations of steroid hormones. The adrenal vein empties directly into the vena cava on the right and into the renal vein on the left.[25]

The innervation of the adrenal gland is autonomic.[25] Sympathetic preganglionic fibers are axons of cells in the lower thoracic and upper lumbar segments, whereas the parasympathetic fibers come from the celiac branch of the posterior vagal trunk; the latter may relay in ganglia in or near the adrenal. Most of the nerves are contained in an adrenal (suprarenal) plexus along the medial border of the adrenal gland, enter it as bundles near the hilus, and run through the cortex to the medulla. This innervation may participate in the control of adrenocortical growth and steroid secretion, and an afferent neural pathway from the adrenal to the hypothalamus mediates stress-induced feedback inhibition of ACTH secretion.[28]

In adults, the cortex makes up about 90 percent of the adrenal and surrounds the centrally located medulla.[27] The cortex consists of three histologically distinct zones: the zonae glomerulosa, fasciculata, and reticularis. The zona glomerulosa produces aldosterone but not cortisol. It is located under the capsule in ill-defined foci that constitute about 15 percent of the cortex (Fig. 12-2).[27] Glomerulosa cells have a relatively small cytoplasmic volume, with small amounts of lipid. The zona fasciculata pro-

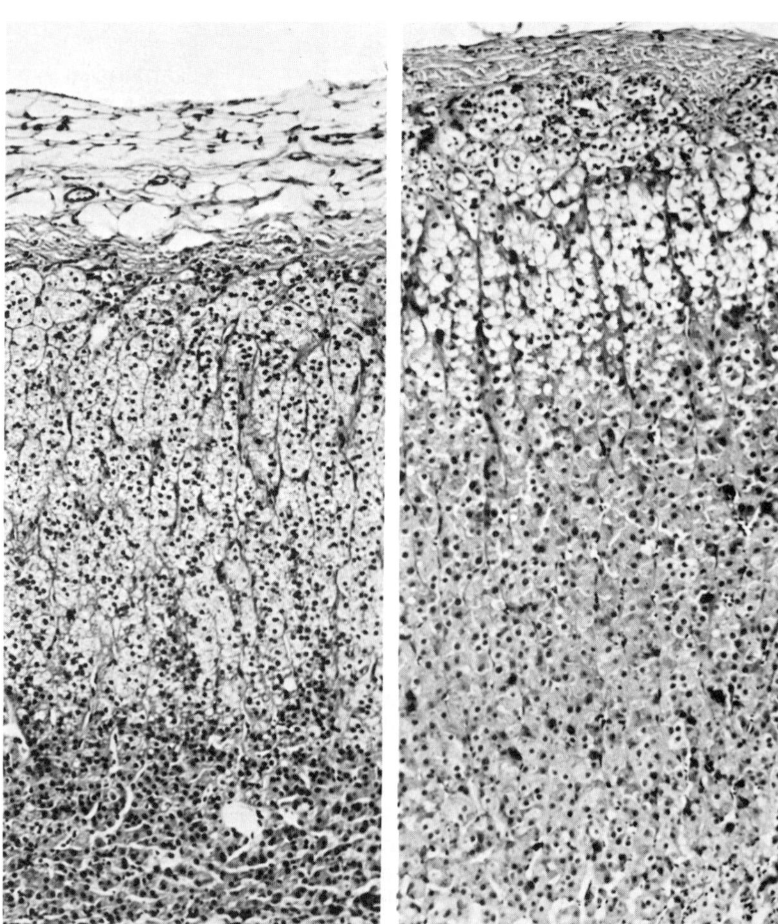

FIGURE 12-2 Normal adrenal cortex *(left)* before and *(right)* after ACTH stimulation. The focal zona glomerulosa under the capsule contains cells with a relatively small cytoplasmic volume. The zona fasciculata in the center contains clear cells, and the zona reticularis at the bottom contains compact cells separated by a clearly demarcated undulating border. After ACTH stimulation, only a narrow rim of clear cells of the fasciculata remains on the outer aspect of the gland; the remainder consists of compact cells. Hematoxylin and eosin stain; 104X. *(From Neville and MacKay.[27])*

duces cortisol but not aldosterone (Fig. 12-2). It is located between the zona glomerulosa and the zona reticularis and constitutes about 75 percent of the cortex. Its cells contain more cholesterol and cholesterol esters, giving them a vacuolated or "clear" appearance on stained sections.[27] The zona reticularis also produces cortisol (albeit at a much lower rate than do the fasciculata cells) and the major adrenal androgens dehydroepiandrosterone (DHEA), DHEA sulfate (DHEA-S), and Δ^4-androstenedione. Cells of the zona reticularis are relatively free of lipids and have a granular, compact appearance.[27] The zonae fasciculata and reticularis also produce most of the DOC and 18-hydroxydeoxycorticosterone (18-OH-DOC) secreted by the adrenal. The three zones of the adrenal cortex cannot be dissected from one another cleanly, as each zone projects "fingers" of cells into the neighboring zones.[29,30]

ACTH has a dramatic effect on the adrenal.[27,28] Within 2 to 3 min after its administration, adrenal blood flow increases and cortisol is released. Within hours, adrenal weight increases; ultimately, the adrenal can double in size. The clear cells at the junction of the zonae fasciculata and reticularis lose their lipid content and become compact. This conversion gradually extends outward, broadening the zona reticularis, which may reach the zona glomerulosa. Meanwhile, the zona fasciculata acquires ultrastructural features of zona reticularis cells. Thus, the two inner zones appear to function as a unit; whereas by light microscopy there appears to be an abrupt structural change between the two zones, electron microscopy reveals cells with intermediate ultrastructural features. Prolonged stimulation by ACTH causes both hypertrophy and hyperplasia,[28] possibly as a result of the actions of insulin-like growth factors,[31,32,99] basic fibroblast growth factor,[33,34] and epidermal growth factor.[34] The adrenal also can regenerate.[28,31,32] This has been observed after enucleation of the rat adrenal[28] and after incomplete adrenalectomy for Cushing's disease. By contrast, ACTH deficiency leads to atrophy of the zonae fasciculata and reticularis. Similarly, when angiotensin II and potassium ion concentrations are elevated, there is hyperplasia of the zona glomerulosa, and when their levels are decreased, there can be atrophy.

Accessory adrenal glands composed of cortical tissue occasionally occur[25]; more rarely, such accessory glands contain both cortical and medullary tissue. By contrast, nests of adrenal "rest cells" are

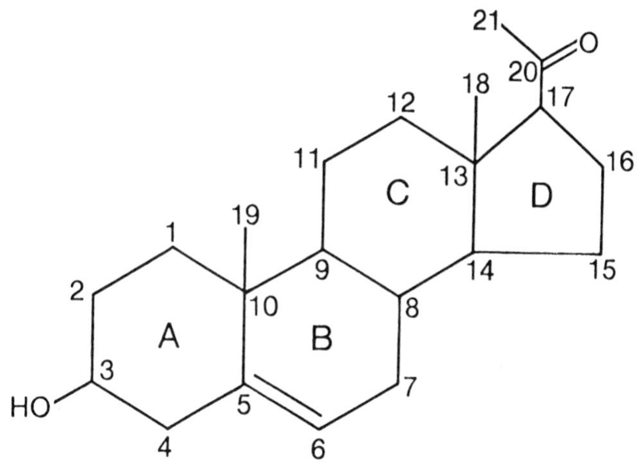

FIGURE 12-3 Structure of pregnenolone. The carbon atoms are indicated by numbers and the rings are designated by letters in accordance with standard convention. Pregnenolone is derived from cholesterol, which has a 6-carbon side chain attached to carbon 21. Pregnenolone is "Δ^5 compound," having a double bond between carbons 5 and 6; the action of 3β-hydroxysteroid dehydrogenase/isomerase moves this double bond from the B ring to carbons 4 and 5 in the A ring, forming Δ^4 compounds. All the major biologically active steroid hormones are Δ^4 compounds.

common in the testis (reviewed in Ref. 35). Adrenal tissue may be present in the celiac plexus, kidney, spleen, or retroperitoneal area below the kidneys; along the aorta, pelvis, spermatic cord, or the broad ligament of the uterus; or attached to the uterus. One adrenal gland may occasionally be absent, but bilateral agenesis is rare.

STEROID HORMONE BIOSYNTHESIS

Studies and discussions of steroid hormone synthesis have traditionally emphasized the complex structural organic chemistry of these hormones. The understanding of their structures led to the determination of precursor-product relation and an understanding of both the pathways of steroidogenesis and the structural requirements for the various steroidal activities. This traditional chemical approach has been largely supplanted by molecular and cellular biological approaches, yet familiarity with both is needed to understand the synthesis, regulation, and pathologic disorders of steroid hormones (see also Chap. 4).

Chemistry of Steroid Hormones

All steroid hormones are derived from pregnenolone, whose structure is shown in Fig. 12-3. Pregnenolone and all its naturally occurring mineralocorticoid and glucocorticoid products contain 21 carbon atoms and hence are termed C-21 steroids (Fig. 12-4). The numbering of each carbon atom facilitates an understanding of how each step in steroid hormone synthesis alters the steroid molecule. 17α-Hydroxypregnenolone, a C-21 steroid, can be cleaved to the C-19 steroid DHEA, which is the precursor of sex steroids. With the exception of the estrogens, which are characterized by an aromatic A ring, all steroid hormones have a single unsaturated carbon-carbon double bond. In pregnenolone and other so-called Δ^5 steroids, this double bond connects carbons 5 and 6 in the B ring (Fig. 12-3). The action of 3β-hydroxysteroid dehydrogenase/isomerase moves this double bond to the A ring between carbons 4 and 5.

A rigorous, logically systematic, and unambiguous chemical terminology has been formulated to describe the structure of the steroid hormones and all their conceivable derivatives. However, this terminology is very cumbersone; for example, cortisol is 11β,17α,21-trihydroxypregn-4-ene-3,20-dione, and dexamethasone is 9α-fluoro-11β,17α,21-trihydroxy-16α-methypregna-1,4,-diene-3,20-dione. Therefore, we shall use the standard "trivial" names in this chapter. The trivial and systematic names are given in Table 12-1. The chemical nomenclature system lists in order the hydroxyl groups, the aldehyde groups, the core ring structure (pregnane, pregnene, androstane, androstene), and the ketones, with the number of the carbon to which each is attached. In the case of carbon-carbon double bonds, the numbers of the two carbons are given with the lower number first; the presence of a double bond is alternatively indicated by the uppercase Greek delta (Δ), with a superscript indicating the lower-numbered carbon atom of the bond. A saturated ring structure is indicated by *-ane* (as in pregnane or androstane), and an unsaturated ring structure by *-ene* (as in pregnene or androstene). The core ring structure for the C-21 steroids is termed *pregnane,* C-19 steroids are *androstanes,* C-18 steroids are *estranes,* and C-27 steroids are *cholestanes*.

Before the structures of the various steroid hormones were known, Reichstein, Kendall, and others identified them as spots on paper chromatograms and referred to them as unknown compounds A, B, C, etc. Unfortunately, many researchers persist in using this archaic and arcane terminology half a century later, so that corticosterone is sometimes termed "compound B," cortisol is termed "compound F," and 11-deoxycortisol is termed "compound S." This outmoded terminology obscures the precursor-product relations among the steroids and should be abandoned.

The biological activities of the various steroid hormones are determined by several factors: the class (or classes) of steroid hormone receptors to which they bind and the affinity of that binding, the plasma proteins to which they bind and the affinity of that binding, their metabolic half-lives, and "peripheral" enzymes that metabolize steroid hormones

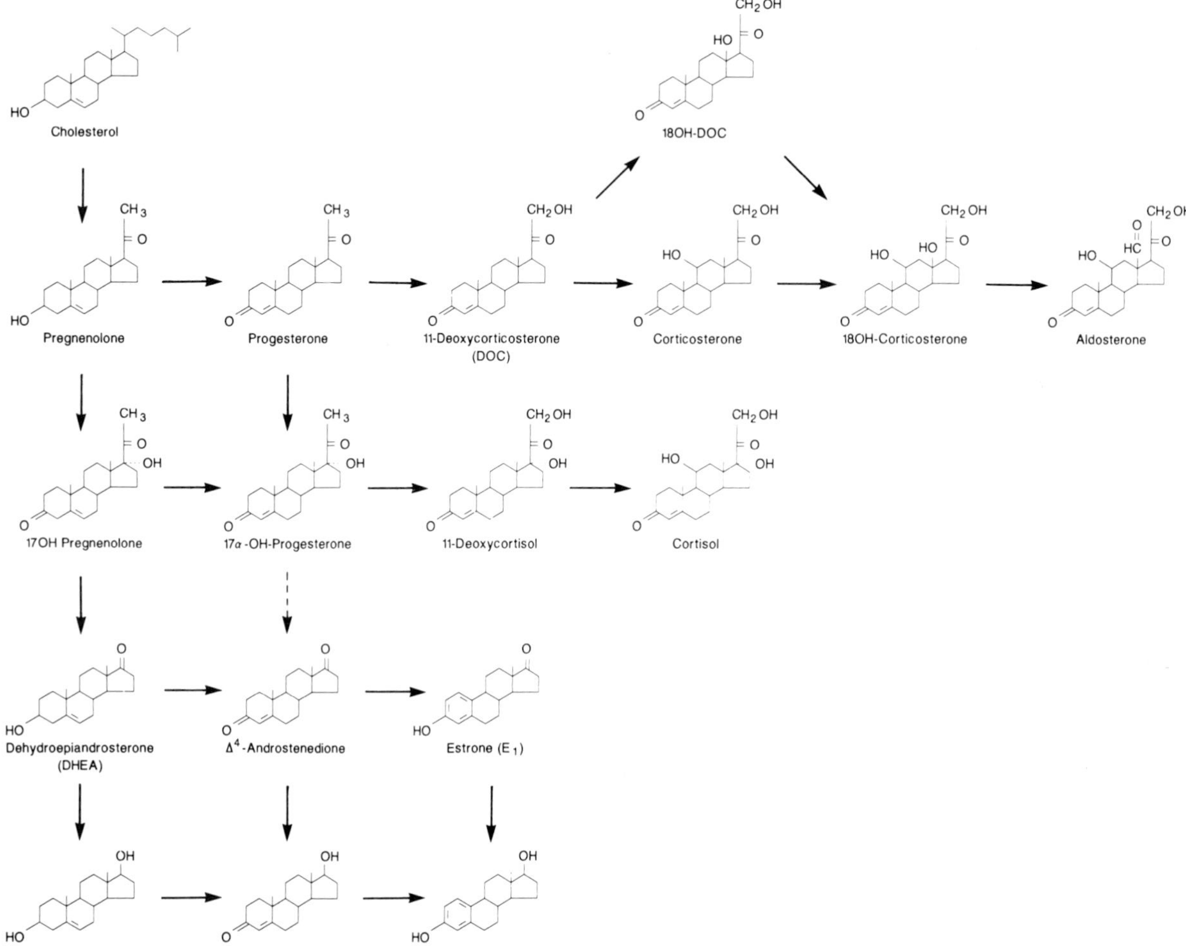

FIGURE 12-4 The principal pathways of adrenal steroidogenesis, showing the structures of the most important steroidal products and intermediates. The enzymes mediating the steroidal interconversions are shown in Fig. 12-7. The steroids in the left vertical column (cholesterol, pregnenolone, 17-OH pregnenolone, DHEA, and androstenediol) are all Δ^5 steroids that have double bond between carbons 5 and 6 (see Fig. 12-3). All the other nonaromatic steroids shown are Δ^4 compounds, having a double bond between carbons 4 and 5. The top horizontal row of compounds, showing the pathway from pregnenolone to aldosterone, is the mineralocorticoid pathway found almost exclusively in the zona glomerulosa; all these compounds have 21 carbon atoms (C-21 steroids). The second row of compounds showing the pathway from 17-hydroxypregnenolone to cortisol is the glucocorticoid pathway, found in the zona fasciculata and, to a lesser extent, the zona reticularis. These are all 17-hydroxy C-21 steroids. The third and fourth rows show the sex steroid pathway, found principally in the gonads but also in the zona reticularis. The 17,20-lyase activity of P450c17 has cleaved off carbon atoms 20 and 21 to yield C-19 steroids. Very little aromatase activity is found in the adrenal; estrone and estradiol are largely synthesized by peripheral conversion of androstenedione and testosterone in the liver and adipose tissues, but are shown here for clarity and completeness.

in target tissues. These variables are determined by the various side groups attached to the four-member cyclopentanophenanthrene ring and the extent of angulation among these four component rings. This angulation is determined by the saturation of the carbon atoms and attached groups. The cyclopentanophenanthrene ring can be visualized as an irregular plane, with groups projecting below the plane (α position) or above it (β position) (Fig. 12-5).

Cholesterol: The Precursor of Steroid Hormones

Cholesterol Synthesis and Uptake

The adrenal readily synthesizes cholesterol from acetyl CoA[36–38] in response to tropic stimulation by ACTH. The activity of 3-hydroxy-3-methylglutaryl coenzyme A reductase (HMGCoA reductase), the rate-limiting enzyme in cholesterol synthesis, gener-

TABLE 12-1 Trivial and Systematic Names of Some Commonly Encountered Naturally Occurring and Synthetic Steroids

Trivial Name	Systematic Name
Aldosterone	11β,21-Dihydroxy-3,20-dioxopregn-en-18-al
Androsterone	3α-Hydroxy-5α-androstan-17-one
Corticosterone (compound B)	11β-21 Dihydroxypregn-4-ene-3,20-dione
Cortisol (hydrocortisone, compound F)	11β-17α,21-trihydroxypregn-4-ene-3,20-dione
Cortisone (compound E)	17α,21-Dihydroxypregn-4-ene-3,1-20-trione
Cortol	5β-Pregnane-3α,11β,17α,20,21-pentol
Cortolone	3α,17α,20α,21-Tetrahydroxy-5β-pregnan-11-one
Dehydroepiandrosterone (prasterone, DHEA)	3β-Hydroxyandrost-5-en-17-one
11-Deoxycorticosterone (DOC)	21-Hydroxypregn-4-ene-3,20-dione
11-Desoxy-17-hydroxycorticosterone (11-deoxycortisol, cortexolone, compound S)	17α,21-Dihydroxypregn-4-ene-3,20-dione
Dexamethasone	9α-Fluoro-11β,17α,21-trihydroxy-16α-methylpregna-1,4-diene-3,20-dione
Estradiol	Estra-1,3,5(10)-triene-3,17β-diol
Etiocholanolone	3α-Hydroxy-5β-androstan-17-one
Fludrocortisone (9α-fluorocortisol)	9α-Fluoro-11β,17α,21-trihydroxypregn-4-ene-3,20-dione
17α-Hydroxypregnenolone	3β,17α-Dihydroxy-5β-pregnen-20-one
17α-Hydroxyprogesterone	17α-Hydroxypregn-4-ene-3,20-dione
Betamethasone	9α-Fluoro-11β,17α,21-trihydroxy-16β-methylpregna-1,4-diene-3,20-dione
Prednisone	17α,21-Dihydroxypregna-1,4-diene-3,11,20-trione
Prednisolone	11β,17α,21-trihydroxypregna-1,4-diene-3,20-dione
Pregnanediol	5β-Pregnane-3α,20α-diol
Pregnanetriol	5β-Pregnane-3α,17α,20α-triol
Pregnenetriol	Pregn-5-ene-3β,17α,20α-triol
Pregnenolone	3β-Hydroxypregn-5-en-20-one
Progesterone	Preg-4-ene-3,20-dione
Testosterone	17β-Hydroxyandrost-4-en-3-one
Tetrahydroaldosterone	3α,11β,21-Trihydroxy-20-oxo-5β-pregnan-18-al
Tetrahydrocortisol	3α,11β,17α,21-Tetrahydroxy-5β-pregnan-20-one
Tetrahydrocortisone	3α,17α,21-Trihydroxy-5β-pregnane-11,20-dione
Triamcinolone	9α-Fluoro-11β,16α,17α,21-tetrahydroxypregna-1,4-diene-3,20-dione

Source: *Biochem J* 113:5, 1969; modified from Brooks.[469]

ally parallels steroidogenic activity. HMGCoA reductase is inactivated by phosphorylation and is activated by dephosphorylation in response to intracellular cAMP elicited by the binding of ACTH to its receptor. However, endogenous synthesis is an important source of cholesterol only in transient situations or during profound stimulation.[36] Similarly, cholesterol stored as intracellular cholesterol esters is a relatively minor source of the cholesterol used for steroidogenesis.[37]

About 80 percent of the cholesterol used for steroid hormone synthesis derives from dietary cholesterol transported in the plasma as low-density lipoprotein (LDL) particles synthesized in the liver.[36,37] Rats and members of other species principally employ high-density lipoproteins (HDL) for this purpose,[37,39] and human ovarian granulosa cells also may be able to take up HDL particles that contain apolipoprotein E,[40] but a clear role for HDL in human adrenal steroidogenesis has not been established. HDL does not stimulate or sustain human adrenal steroidogenesis.[37,39,40] In abetalipoproteine-

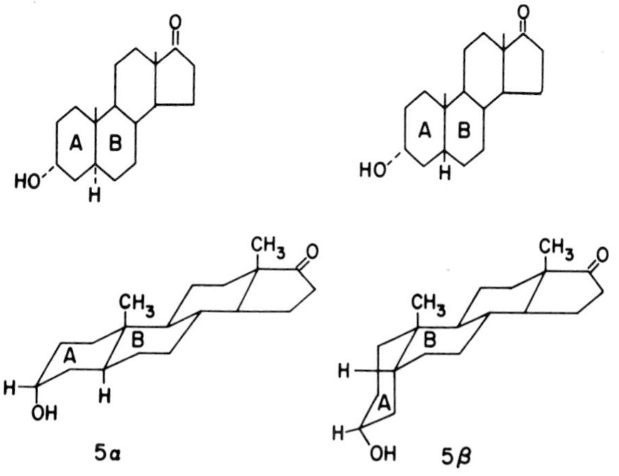

FIGURE 12-5 Effect of the hydrogen at position 6 on the conformation of the steroid molecule. The 5α-hydrogenated molecule is androsterone, and the 5β-hydrogenated molecule is etiocholanolone. The usual outline structural formulas are shown at the top, and the perspective views are shown at the bottom. *(From Bondy.[414])*

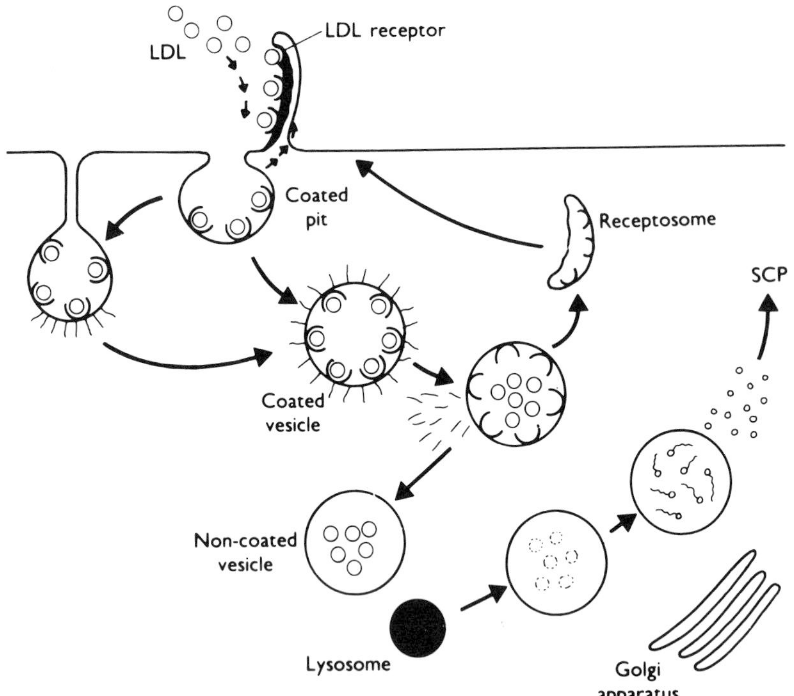

FIGURE 12-6 The LDL pathway of cholesterol uptake by the adrenal. LDL binds to receptors that are internalized in coated vesicles and is then separated from its receptor, which is recycled back to the plasma membrane. LDL then travels in noncoated vesicles to the vicinity of the Golgi apparatus, where lysosomal hydrolases are induced. Acid proteinases degrade LDL apolipoproteins to amino acids, and acid lipase frees cholesterol from esters. Free cholesterol then diffuses out of lysosomes and may be transferred to organelles by sterol carrier proteins (SCP). *(From Strauss and Miller.[40])*

mia, in which LDL particles are absent, the cortisol response to ACTH is blunted, but basal cortisol concentrations are normal and symptomatic adrenal insufficiency does not occur.[41] Thus, in these patients, endogenous synthesis of cholesterol and/or uptake of HDL provides an alternative source of cholesterol.

Adrenal uptake of LDL is regulated coordinately with steroid synthesis. Adequate concentrations of LDL will suppress HMGCoA reductase activity,[42] and blockade of cholesterol synthesis with HMGCoA reductase inhibitors will not suppress the secretion of cortisol in response to ACTH.[43] ACTH stimulates the activity of HMGCoA reductase, LDL receptors, and the uptake of LDL cholesterol.[44] LDL uptake is rapid; radiotracer studies show that plasma LDL cholesterol is nearly equilibrated with the intracellular pool of steroidogenic sterols.[45] In fact, imaging studies of steroidogenic tissues with radiolabeled analogs of cholesterol are not especially effective and are possible only because of the voracious appetite of steroidogenic tissues for plasma cholesterol.[45]

LDL uptake principally entails receptor-mediated endocytosis (Fig. 12-6); less than 10 percent of LDL enters the cell by a receptor-independent mechanism.[36,37] Specific "B-E receptors," which recognize apolipoproteins B and E, are located on microvilli and, upon binding of LDL, become concentrated in "coated pits" at the base of the villi. The coating of these pits is composed of clathrin; changes in the array of clathrin molecules result in the closure of the pit into a vesicle, thus internalizing the LDL. The receptors are separated from the LDL and are recycled back to the cellular surface, while the vesicles bearing LDL fuse with lysosomes.[36,37] Lysosomal proteases degrade the protein moieties, and lysosomal acid lipase cleaves the cholesterol esters to free cholesterol (Fig. 12-6). By contrast, the uptake of HDL entails receptor-independent mechanisms.[46]

Intracellular Cholesterol Storage and Transport

The regulation of the flux of cholesterol into adrenal mitochondria to initiate steroidogenesis is not well understood; however, several factors have been identified in this pathway. Free sterols, including cholesterol, are esterified by acyl coenzyme A cholesterol acyltransferase (ACAT), which is found in the rough endoplasmic reticulum.[40] Sterol esters accumulate and bud off as lipid droplets from the endoplasmic reticulum. The esterification entails linkage of polyunsaturated fatty acids such as linolenic, arachidonic, docosapentanoic, and docosahexanoic acids derived from the circulation or synthesized de novo.[40] It is not clear how the specific unsaturated fatty acids are chosen for esterification, but in ovarian cells the patterns change with the functional status of the cell, suggesting different metabolic roles for each one.[40] Such fatty acid esters are generally hydrolized to free cholesterol by cholesterol esterase (sterol ester hydrolase). However, pregnenolone may be reesterified in the mitochondria to pregnenolone fatty acid esters,[47] which form biosynthetic intermediates in the synthesis of corresponding adrenal steroids.[47] In the uterus, such fatty acid esters are involved in the synthesis of long-acting lipoidal derivatives of estradiol.[48]

Cholesterol storage as cholesterol esters in lipid droplets is controlled by the action of two opposing enzymes: cholesterol ester synthetase and cholesterol ester hydrolase (cholesterol esterase). ACTH or other tissue-specific tropic hormones [e.g., luteinizing hormone (LH) and follicle stimulating hormone (FSH)] stimulate the esterase and inhibit the synthetase, thus increasing the availability of free cholesterol for steroid hormone synthesis.[49,50] The esterase, which is encoded by a gene on chromosome 10,[51] is a soluble protein that is similar to gastric and lingual lipases,[51] and is activated by phosphorylation of serine residues by a cAMP-dependent protein kinase.[52] The synthetase, ACAT, is insoluble and is confined to the membrane of the endoplasmic reticulum. In addition to ACTH, γ3-MSH (melanocyte stimulating hormone) may also activate the esterase by a cAMP-independent mechanism.[53]

Free cholesterol, which is insoluble in the aqueous cytosol, may bind to sterol carrier protein 2 (SCP-2), a 13-kDa basic protein in the cytosol.[54,55] Another 11.3-kDa protein, sometimes termed a sterol carrier protein (SCP), apparently functions principally in fatty acid binding and hence is not truly a sterol carrier protein.[54,56] These two proteins have been found in the mitochondria, cytosol, and endoplasmic reticulum of steroidogenic tissues, and their synthesis responds to tropic hormone stimulation.[56,57] SCP-2 may facilitate the flux of cholesterol more by its action of removing cholesterol from membranes than by acting as a directed transport protein. SCP-2 promotes the flux of cholesterol from lipid droplets to mitochondria and increases pregnenolone synthesis in cell-free systems[56]; antibodies to SCP-2 partially inhibit steroidogenesis.[57] Thus, SCP-2 apparently carries free cholesterol to the mitochondria but does not enter the mitochondria, while SCP is found within the mitochondria. The role of SCP is unclear, but since mitochondria generate ATP by oxidizing fatty acids, SCP may promote steroidogenesis by providing fuel for the steroidogenic machinery.

The flux of cholesterol from lipid droplets to the mitochondria and the subsequent flux of pregnenolone from the mitochondria to the endoplasmic reticulum may be facilitated by changes in the cytoskeleton.[58,59] Agents that disrupt microfilaments and microtubules inhibit cholesterol flux and steroidogenesis. Such agents include cytocholasins, which inhibit the polymerization of microfilaments; vinblastine, which disrupts microtubules; and antibodies to actin. An intact cytoskeleton may simply maintain the various intracellular organelles in their proper spatial arrangement, or it may actively direct the movement of SCP-2 or other factors that promote steroidogenesis.

Numerous experiments indicate that a labile cycloheximide-sensitive factor is needed for steroidogenesis, possibly to promote the flux of cholesterol from the outer to the inner mitochondrial membrane.[60–62] The existence of such a factor was first suggested by a rapid cycloheximide-induced inhibition of steroidogenesis that did not affect P450scc protein.[60,61] Two likely candidates for this labile factor have been identified. One, termed steroidogenesis activator peptide (SAP), is identical to the 30 amino acids from the carboxy terminus of a 78-kDa heat shock protein termed glucose-regulated protein.[63] SAP has a short half-life, is sensitive to cycloheximide and other inhibitors of protein synthesis, and appears to facilitate the flux of cholesterol across the outer mitochondrial membrane[64,65] but does not seem to facilitate the access of cholesterol to P450scc.[66] The other newly described facilitator of steroidogenesis is endozepine, the endogenous ligand of the peripheral benzodiazepine receptor. Endozepine appears to facilitate both transport across the outer mitochondrial membrane and access to P450scc by increasing the concentration of cholesterol in both the outer and inner mitochondrial membranes and by increasing the binding of cholesterol to P450scc.[67,68] The mechanisms by which SAP, endozepine, or any other candidate for the "labile factor" might work are unknown. Such factors might facilitate contact between the inner and outer mitochondrial membranes or regulate a mitochondrial cholesterol translocator system.[69] Recent work suggests that the peripheral-type benzodiazepine receptor may be this long-sought mitochondrial cholesterol translocator (for a review, see Ref. 70). This receptor consists of three components: a 32-kDa voltage-dependent anion channel (VDAC), an 18-kDa protein on the outer mitochondrial membrane, and a 30-kDa adenine nucleotide carrier protein on the inner membrane. The genes for two of these components have been cloned recently.[71,72]

Cytochrome P450

Most steroidogenic enzymes are members of the cytochrome P450 superfamily of oxidases.[23,73] *Cytochrome P450* is a generic term for a large number of oxidative enzymes, all of which have about 500 amino acids and contain a single heme group. They are termed P450 (pigment 450) because they all exhibit a characteristic shift in the Soret absorbance peak from 420 to 450 nm when they are reduced with carbon monoxide.[74] All cytochrome P450 enzymes reduce atmospheric O_2 with electrons donated by NADPH according to the general reaction

$$\mathrm{NADPH} + \mathrm{H}^+ + \mathrm{O}_2 + \mathrm{RH} \xrightarrow{\mathrm{P450}} \mathrm{R-OH} + \mathrm{H_2O} + \mathrm{NADP}^+$$

The electrons from NADPH reach the P450 via one or two electron transport intermediates, one of

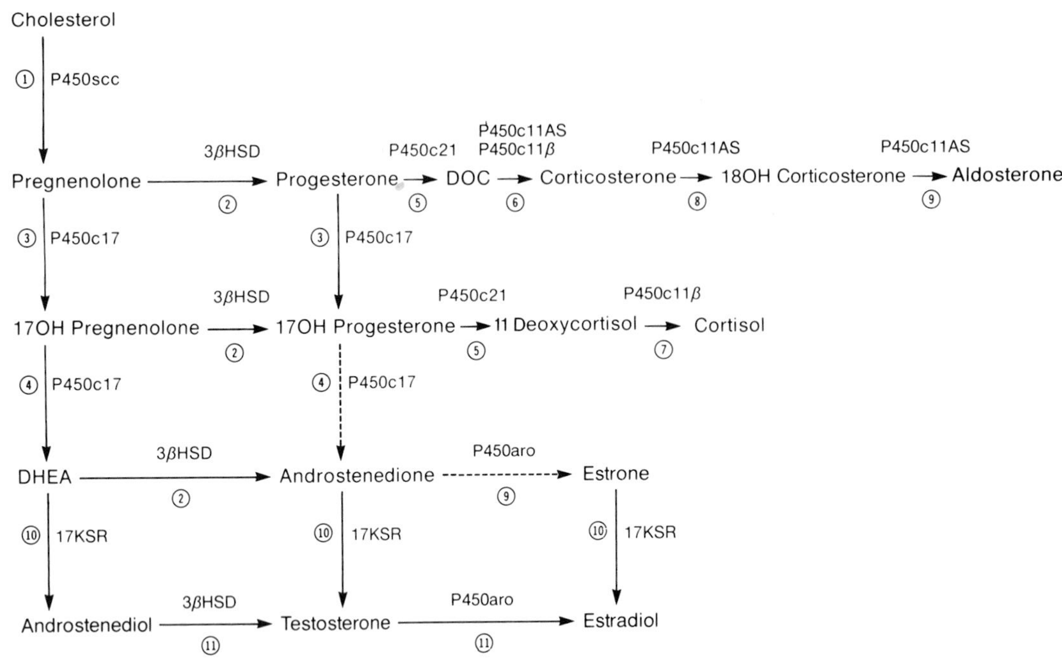

FIGURE 12-7 Principal pathways of human adrenal steroid hormone synthesis. The structures of the steroids named are shown in Fig. 12-4. Other quantitatively and physiologically minor steroids are also produced. The names of the enzymes are shown by each reaction, and the traditional names of the enzymatic activities correspond to the circled numbers. Reaction 1: Mitochondrial cytochrome P450scc mediates 20α-hydroxylation, 22-hydroxylation, and scission of the C20-22 carbon bond, a set of reactions traditionally termed 20,22-desmolase. Reaction 2: 3β-HSD, a non-P450 enzyme bound to the endoplasmic reticulum, mediates 3β-hydroxysteroid deyhdrogenase and isomerase activities, converting Δ^5 steroids to Δ^4 steroids. Reaction 3: P450c17 catalyzes the 17α-hydroxylation of pregnenolone to 17OH-pregnenolone and, to a lesser extent, that of progesterone to 17OH-progesterone. Reaction 4: The 17,20-lyase activity of P450c17 converts 17OH-pregnenolone to DHEA; clinical evidence suggests that some 17-OH-progesterone is similarly converted to Δ^4 androstenedione, but this reaction is not catalyzed by human P450c17 in vitro. Reaction 5: P450c21 catalyzes the 21-hydroxylation of progesterone to DOC and that of 17OH-progesterone to 11-deoxycortisol. Reaction 6: DOC is converted to corticosterone by the 11-hydroxylase activity of P450c11AS in the zona glomerulosa and by P450c11β in the zona fasciculata. Reaction 7: 11-Deoxycortisol is 11-hydroxylated by P450c11 to produce cortisol in the zona fasciculata. Reactions 8 and 9: The 18-hydroxylase and 18-oxidae activities of P450c11AS convert corticosterone to 18-OH-corticosterone and aldosterone, respectively, in the zona glomerulosa. Reactions 10 and 11 are found principally in the testes and ovaries: 17B-HSD, a reversible non-P450 enzyme of the endoplasmic reticulum, mediates both 17-ketosteroid reductase and 17β-hydroxysteroid dehydrogenase activities. Reaction 10: 17-Ketosteroid reductase converts DHEA to androstenediol, androstenedione to testosterone, and estrone to estradiol. The precise nature of this enzyme(s) is still being elucidated. Reaction 11: Testosterone may be converted to estradiol by P450aro (10), another P450 enzyme of the endoplasmic reticulum mediating the aromatization of the A ring of the steroid nucleus.

which is always flavoprotein. The heme-binding sites of all P450 enzymes have certain common amino acids, but these enzymes are otherwise quite heterogeneous.

Certain steroidogenic enzymes are termed "P450-dependent" enzymes, but this is a misnomer, as it implies a generic P450 cofactor to a substrate-specific enzyme. The P450 *is* the enzyme that binds the steroidal substrate and mediates the steroidal conversion on an active site associated with the heme group. Most cytochrome P450 enzymes are found in the endoplasmic reticulum of the liver, where they metabolize innumerable endogenous and exogenous toxins, drugs, xenobiotics, and environmental pollutants.[73,75,76] Despite this huge variety of substrates, it appears that there are only about 200 types of cytochrome P450 enzymes.[73,75,76] Thus, most, if not all, P450 enzymes can metabolize multiple substrates, catalyzing a broad array of oxidations (for a review, see Ref. 76). This theme recurs with each adrenal P450 enzyme. The size and complexity of the cytochrome P450 superfamily led to many conflicting systems of nomenclature; however, a consensus system has found widespread acceptance.[77]

Six distinct P450 enzymes are involved in steroidogenesis (Fig. 12-7). P450scc, which is found in adrenal mitochondria, is the cholesterol side-chain cleavage enzyme that mediates the series of reactions formerly termed "20,22-desmolase." Two forms of P450c11—P450c11β and P450c11AS (aldosterone synthase)—also found in mitochondria mediate 11-hydroxylase activity, while P450c11AS also has 18-hydroxylase and 18-methyl oxidase activities. P450c17, which is found in the endoplasmic reticulum, mediates both 17α-hydroxylase and 17,20-lyase activities, and P450c21 mediates the 21-hydroxylation of both glucocorticoids and mineralocorticoids. In the gonads (and elsewhere), P450aro in the endoplasmic reticulum mediates the aromatization of androgens to estrogens.

The present structural knowledge of steroidogenic cytochromes P450 is based on amino acid and nucleotide sequencing data. Since these enzymes exist in membrane lipid environments, they cannot be readily crystallized; hence, their nascent three-dimensional structures have not been determined. However, a prokaryotic P450—the P450cam of *Pseudomonas putida*—has been crystallized, and its three-dimensional structure has been determined to 1.6-Å resolution.[78,79] The structure of this P450 suggests that the association of a substrate with the P450 and the dissociation of the resulting product entail different conformational changes. The substrate of P450cam appears to enter the substrate-binding pocket through a hydrophobic channel and depart through a different hydrophilic channel.[79] Such a directional structure, if true for steroidogenic P450, might have important implications for directing the flow of steroid molecules among the membranes of the mitochondria and the endoplasmic reticulum, as intact membranes are required for steroidogenesis.[80]

P450scc: Conversion of Cholesterol to Pregnenolone

Enzymology The conversion of cholesterol to pregnenolone in mitochondria is the first and rate-limiting step in the synthesis of steroid hormones (for a review, see Refs. 80 and 40). This involves three distinct chemical reactions: 20α-hydroxylation, 22-hydroxylation, and scission of the cholesterol side chain to yield pregnenolone and isocaproic acid. Early studies suggested that three separate and distinct enzymes were involved: a 20-hydroxylase, a 22-hydroxylase, and a 20,22-lyase. However, protein purification studies and in vitro reconstitution of enzymatic activity showed that a single protein, termed P450scc (scc refers to the side-chain cleavage of cholesterol), is responsible for all the steps between cholesterol and pregnenolone[81–85] on a single active site[86] that is in contact with the hydrophobic bilayer membrane.[74]

Although some data suggest the presence of several isozymes of P450scc,[87,88] protein purification data indicate the existence of a single immunologically identifiable species of P450scc. Thus, any hypothetical alternative enzyme with the same activity as P450scc must have a sufficiently different structure so that it shares no antibody cross-reactivity with P450scc and is encoded by an mRNA that has less than 65 to 70 percent nucleotide identity with P450scc. As discussed below, a single Mendelian autosomal recessive disease, congenital lipoid adrenal hyperplasia, eliminates all adrenal and gonadal steroidogenesis. This strongly argues against a second gene that could encode another protein with the ability to produce pregnenolone.

Mechanism of Action The cholesterol side-chain cleavage reaction consists of three catalytic cycles; the first two hydroxylate the carbon atoms at positions C-22 and C-20, and the third results in cleavage of the bond connecting these two carbons. Each catalytic cycle requires one molecule of NADPH and one molecule of O_2, such that the overall stoichiometry is cholesterol + 3NADPH + $3H^+$ + $3O_2 \rightarrow$ pregnenolone + isocapraldehyde + $4H_2O$ + $3NADP^+$.[74] The reaction intermediates bind to the single active site tightly, and thus one cholesterol molecule is converted to pregnenolone by a single molecule of P450scc. The sterol substrate remains bound to a single active site on cytochrome P450scc because of a tight binding of the reaction intermediates. The K_d for the binding of cholesterol is about 5000 n*M*, whereas the K_d for (22R) 22-hydroxycholesterol and (20R, 22R) 20,22-dihydroxycholesterol are 4.9 and 81 n*M*, respectively. Thus, once cholesterol is bound to the enzyme, it is committed to completing the reaction sequence. The estimated K_d for pregnenolone is 2900 *nM*, which permits the dissociation of the final reaction product from the enzyme.[74]

P450scc is the rate-limiting step in steroidogenesis and is one of the slowest enzymes known, with a V_{max} of ~1 mol cholesterol/mol enzyme per second.[85] The slowest component of this complex reaction appears to be the entry and binding of cholesterol to the active site.[69,89] The composition of the inner mitochondrial membrane may influence the binding of cholesterol, as cardrolipin increases the affinity of purified P450scc for cholesterol. Molecular models derived from the study of cholesterol analogs and purified P450scc suggest that carbon 22 of the cholesterol molecule lies within 0.4 Å of the heme iron of P450scc and that carbon 20 lies 1.54 Å farther away.[90] The first hydroxylation probably occurs at carbon 22 because of its proximity to the heme iron. The introduction of the 22R hydroxyl group may move the substrate slightly to bring carbon 20 closer to the heme iron, thus permitting the second hydroxylation reaction. The third step is the cleavage of the 20,22-dihydroxy cholesterol to yield pregnenolone and isocapraldehyde; this does not involve incorporation of oxygen into either product, but oxygen is required for the reaction.

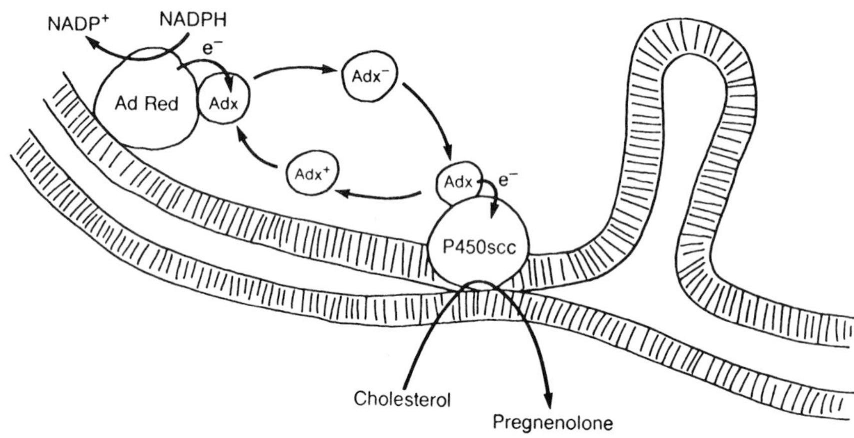

FIGURE 12-8 Electron transport to mitochondrial forms of cytochrome P450. Adrenodoxin reductase (AdRed), a flavoprotein loosely bound to the inner mitochondrial membrane, accepts electrons (e^-) from NADPH, converting it to $NADP^+$. These electrons are passed to adrenodoxin (Adx^+), an iron-sulfur protein loosely associated with the inner mitochondrial membrane that functions as a freely diffusable electron shuttle mechanism. Electrons from charged adrenodoxin (Adx^-) are accepted by any available cytochrome P450, such as P450c11 or P450scc, shown here. The uncharged adrenodoxin (Adx^+) may then be again bound to adrenodoxin reductase to receive another pair of electrons. For P450scc, three pairs of electrons must be transported to the P450 to convert cholesterol to pregnenolone. The inner and outer mitochondrial membranes may become more closely opposed during active steroidogenesis, facilitating the flux of hydrophobic steroid molecules. *(Modified from Miller.[23])*

Genetics Molecular cloning studies, beginning with the cloning of bovine P450scc cDNA,[91] have revealed much about P450scc. The human genome contains only a single gene encoding P450scc.[92,93] It is about 20 kb long, is divided into nine exons,[94] is located on band q23 or q24 of chromosome 15,[93,95] and encodes an mRNA of 2.0 kb. The encoded 521-amino acid protein is proteolytically cleaved to 482 amino acids[93] by an endoprotease[96] that removes the 39-amino acid "leader peptide" that directs the protein to the mitochondria. This single gene is expressed in all the conventional tissues that make steroid hormones, including the adrenal cortex, testis, ovary, and placenta.[92,93,97–100] Extraglandular synthesis of various steroids has been described, and P450scc has been demonstrated in rat kidney[101] and brain[102]; however, the function of this extraglandular P450scc has not been demonstrated.

Transcription of the P450scc gene is regulated by ACTH in the adrenal, by gonadotropins in the testes and ovaries, and by unknown factors in the placenta, all functioning through cAMP as the intracellular second messenger[103–109] (see Chaps. 4 and 5). By contrast, angiotensin II stimulates P450scc gene transcription in the zona glomerulosa through the calcium–protein kinase C system.[105,110] Although experiments in bovine adrenal cells suggested that cAMP stimulates the synthesis of a protein which stimulates the transcription of the P450scc gene,[103] other work in rat and human systems indicates that this is not true for all species.[100,104,105,111,112] The action of ACTH can be rapid, stimulating preexisting steroidogenic machinery, but the effects on transcription, while rapid at the molecular level, have a fairly slow and persistent effect and account for the chronic response of the adrenal to ACTH. For example, in Cushing's disease, chronic stimulation of the adrenal by ACTH results in increased transcription of the genes for P450scc and for all the other steroidogenic enzymes, so that the adrenal stereoidogenic capacity is greatly increased. Angiotensin II also stimulates the adrenal acutely, working through alterations in intracellular calcium and activation of protein kinase C.[110] However, prolonged stimulation with angiotensin II or with agents that activate the protein kinase C pathway represses the quantities and activities of steroidogenic enzymes in cultured adrenal cells.[113–115] This same short-term stimulation followed by long-term repression can be demonstrated at the level of the P450scc gene.[105] The details of the transcriptional regulation of the human P450scc gene differ among Y-1 adrenal cells,[105] JEG-3 cytotrophoblast cells,[107] and MA-10 Leydig cells,[108] consistent with the idea that different cells, employing different nuclear proteins, utilize the promoters of various genes in a tissue- specific fashion (for a review, see Ref. 109).

Transport of Electrons to P450scc: Adrenodoxin Reductase and Adrenodoxin

P450scc functions as the terminal oxidase in a mitochondrial electron transport system. Electrons from NADPH are accepted by a flavoprotein—adrenodoxin reductase—that is loosely associated with the inner mitochondrial membrane.[116–118] Adrenodoxin reductase transfers the electrons to an iron/sulfur protein termed adrenodoxin, which is found either in solution in the mitochondrial matrix[116–119] or loosely associated with the inner mitochondrial membrane.[120] Adrenodoxin then transfers the electrons to P450scc (Fig. 12-8). Adrenodoxin reductase and adrenodoxin serve as generic electron transport proteins for all mitochondrial P450s, not just for those involved in steroidogenesis; hence, these proteins are also termed ferredoxin reductase and ferredoxin.

Adrenodoxin Reductase Adrenodoxin reductase is transcribed from a single-copy gene located on band q24 or q25 of chromosome 17.[95,121,122] The primary RNA transcript of this gene can be alternately spliced into two forms of mRNA that differ by 18 bases.[121] Both forms of this mRNA are expressed in all tissues,[123] but the protein encoded by the longer form is inactive in steroidogenesis.[124]

The adrenodoxin reductase gene is unique among the genes that encode steroidogenic enzymes in two respects. First, it lacks the conventional TATA and CAAT sequences typical of most eukaryotic promoters and instead has six copies of the sequence GGGCGGG, which appear to bind transcription factor Sp-1.[122] Such promoter structures are common in so-called housekeeping genes that are expressed ubiquitously without tissue specificity. Second, cAMP regulates the abundance of adrenodoxin reductase mRNA posttranscriptionally but does not regulate the transcription of the gene.[123] Adrenodoxin reductase is expressed in all human tissues, but its level is 100-fold greater in steroidogenic tissues.[123] By contrast, the gene for adrenodoxin is also expressed ubiquitously and always functions with adrenodoxin reductase, yet it has a classical promoter structure.

Adrenodoxin Adrenodoxin is a small, soluble ionsulfur protein that forms a 1:1 complex with adrenodoxin reductase, then dissociates, and subsequently re-forms an analogous 1:1 complex with P450scc or P450c11, thus functioning as an indiscriminate diffusable electron shuttle mechanism.[86,125–131] Each adrenodoxin molecule contains two iron atoms tetrahedrally coordinated with the thiols of two cysteine residues and two labile sulfur atoms to form an Fe_2S_2 center.[129,130] There are one[132] or two[133] functional adrenodoxin genes encoding indistinguishable mRNAs and proteins[112] lying on band q11 of chromosome 11 and two nonexpressed pseudogenes on band q11 or q12 of chromosome 20.[95,134] There are multiple species of human adrenodoxin mRNA ranging from 1.0 to 1.8 kb in length that arise by the use of three or four different polyadenylylation sites in the 3′ untranslated region.[112,135] A role for this 3′ untranslated region in regulating adrenodoxin mRNA half-life has been ruled out.[136] Adrenodoxin mRNA is found in all human tissues[112] and accumulates in response to tropic stimulation of cultured adrenal cells with ACTH or cAMP or of cultured ovarian granulosa cells with FSH, human chorionic gonadotropin (hCG), or cAMP,[101,137] as does the mRNA for P450scc.

Interactions of P450scc, Adrenodoxin, and Adrenodoxin Reductase

P450scc, adrenodoxin, and adrenodoxin reductase are associated with the inner mitochondrial membrane.[120] Adrenodoxin first accepts electrons from NADPH and then forms a 1:1 complex with adrenodoxin reductase, which catalyzes the reduction of adrenodoxin. Reduced adrenodoxin dissociates from the adrenodoxin reductase and may then form a 1:1 complex with P450scc or with any other available mitochondrial cytochrome P450, such as adrenal P450c11. Upon binding to P450scc, the adrenodoxin is oxidized and then discharged, making it available to bind again to adrenodoxin reductase and repeat the cycle. Adrenodoxin reductase has a greater affinity for oxidized adrenodoxin than for reduced adrenodoxin, favoring productive interactions betweeen these two proteins. Similarly, the binding of cholesterol to P450scc causes a 20-fold increase in the affinity of P450scc for reduced adrenodoxin. These differences in binding affinities promote the flux of electrons from NADPH to P450scc. These three components of the cholesterol side-chain cleavage system appear to be present in varying molar ratios in different tissues,[120] but the different and sensitive control of the transcription of each gene suggests that these ratios can be changed easily. P450scc, adrenodoxin, and adrenodoxin reductase apparently do not form a ternary complex in vivo, because the same surface of the adrenodoxin molecule interacts with both adrenodoxin reductase and P450scc.[138,139] However, a covalently linked trimolecular complex of these three components is functional with an increased V_{max}.[140]

3β-Hydroxysteroid Dehydrogenase/ Δ^5-Δ^4 Isomerase

Once pregnenolone is produced from cholesterol, it may be converted to 17-hydroxypregnenolone or to progesterone by 3β-hydroxysteroid dehydrogenase (3β-HSD). This single microsomal enzyme catalyzes both the 3β-hydroxysteroid dehydrogenation and the isomerization of the double bond from the B ring (Δ^5 steroids) to the A ring (Δ^4 steroids).[141–143] Both 3β-HSD and isomerase activities are found in a single 42-kDa protein,[141] and expression of the cloned cDNA in COS-1 cells confers both activities to the cells.[143,144] Thus, it is clear that both the hydroxysteroid dehydrogenase and isomerase activities lie in a single protein.

There are at least two forms of human 3β-HSD, encoded by different genes. The 3β-HSD type I gene is expressed in the placenta, skin, mammary gland,

and possibly other peripheral tissues.[142–145] A distinct 3β-HSD type II gene is expressed in the adrenals and gonads.[146,147] These genes and several pseudogenes are localized on band p13 of chromosome 1.[144–148] Electron microscopic cytochemistry has localized 3β-HSD activity to the endoplasmic reticulum adjacent to mitochondria, facilitating the rapid metabolism of pregnenolone produced by P450scc.[149] Despite this widespread expression and concentrated activity in steroidogenic glands, the human fetal adrenal gland has relatively little 3β-HSD activity as a result of very low levels of 3β-HSD mRNA.[150] This permits the fetal adrenal to make very large quantities of the Δ^5 steroid DHEA and its sulfate, which are then metabolized to estrogens by the placenta. Even the widespread expression of multiple forms of 3β-HSD may not explain all extraglandular 3β-HSD/$\Delta^5 \rightarrow \Delta^4$ isomerase activity. In the rabbit, such 3β-HSD activity has been found to be associated with hepatic cytochrome P450IIC5,[151] an enzyme which has 21-hydroxylase activity but is structurally unrelated to the adrenal 21-hydroxylase P450c21 (see 21-Hydroxylase, below).

P450c17: 17α Hydroxylase/17,20-Lyase

Genetics and Enzymology

Both pregnenolone and progesterone may undergo 17α-hydroxylation to 17α-hydroxypregnenolone and 17α-hydroxyprogesterone (17-OHP), respectively. These 17-hydroxylated steroids may then undergo scission of the C-17,20 carbon bond to yield DHEA and androstenedione, respectively. These four reactions are mediated by a single enzyme, cytochrome P450c17 (for a review, see Ref. 23), which is bound to the smooth endoplasmic reticulum, where it accepts electrons from a flavoprotein that is different from the adrenodoxin reductase in mitochondria, and without the need of an intermediary iron/sulfur protein. As P450c17 has both 17α-hydroxylase activity and C-17,20-lyase activity, it is a key branch point in steroid hormone synthesis, directing pregnenolone to mineralocorticoids (neither activity), glucocorticoids (17α-hydroxylation but not C-17,20 cleavage), or sex steroids (after both 17α-hydroxylation and C-17,20 cleavage) (Figs. 12-4 and 12-7).

Based on observations of separate regulation of 17α-hydroxylase and 17,20-lyase activities, it was previously thought these were two separate enzymes. The adrenals of prepubertal children synthesize ample cortisol but virtually no sex steroids (i.e., have 17α-hydroxylase activity but not 17,20-lyase activity). Adrenarche, a somewhat mysterious event that slightly precedes puberty but is independent from the GnRH-gonadotropin-gonadal axis, initiates the production of adrenal androgens (i.e., appears to turn on 17,20-lyase activity).[152,153] Exhaustive searches for pituitary-derived adrenal androgen stimulatory factors have been unrewarding.[154–156] Furthermore, patients have been described who lack 17,20-lyase activity but retain normal 17α-hydroxylase activity,[157,158] again suggesting that 17,20-lyase activity can be separated from 17α-hydroxylase activity. However, purification of pig testicular microsomal P450c17 and in vitro reconstitution of enzymatic activity clearly proved that both 17α-hydroxylase and 17,20-lyase activities reside in a single protein, P450c17.[159–162] Any residual doubts about this fact have been dispelled by two definitive genetic experiments. First, when vectors expressing bovine, human, or rat P450c17 cDNA are put into COS-1 cells or yeast, these cells acquire both 17α-hydroxylase and 17,20-lyase activities.[163–166] Second, single mutations in the human gene encoding P450c17 destroy all 17α-hydroxylase and 17,20-lyase activity in both the adrenals and the gonads.[166–168] Thus, differences in 17α-hydroxylase and 17,20-lyase activities are functional and physiologic but not genetic.

The single human gene encoding P450c17 is located on band q24 or q25 of chromosome 10[95,169] and shows a striking structural similarity to the P450c21 gene.[170,171] Of the seven introns dividing the eight exons in the P450c17 gene, the locations of introns 3 to 7 correspond to the nucleotide with the locations of introns 5 to 9 in the gene encoding P450c21. Furthermore, introns 1 and 2 of P450c17 are within a few bases of the locations of introns 2 and 3 of P450c21.[171] Transcriptional regulation of the human P450c17 gene is tropicly stimulated by intracellular cAMP and repressed by phorbol esters through separate segments of DNA in the 5′ flanking region of the gene.[172]

The P450c17 and P450c21 proteins also appear to be very similar despite having only 28.9 percent amino acid identity.[171] Computer-inferred structural analysis shows that they have virtually identical hydropathy. They also have very similar patterns of regions predicted to form α-helix, β-sheets, or random coils. By contrast, the hydropathy profile and predicted α/β regions of P450scc are grossly different. These analyses suggest that the constraints on steroidogenic P450 evolution are confined to maintaining only four things: (1) a P450 heme-binding site, (2) a steroid-binding site, (3) a P450 reductase docking site, and (4) a protein superstructure adequate to keep these three functional regions in an appropriate spatial relation with one another.[171] Computer-graphic molecular modeling of these two enzymes also suggest that their active sites are quite similar.[171a]

Several factors appear to be involved in determining whether a steroid molecule will remain on the single active site of P450c17 and undergo 17,20-bond scission after 17α-hydroxylation or whether it will leave the enzyme as a 17α-hydroxy C-21 steroid. Enzymologic parameters measured in vitro indicate that P450c17 prefers Δ^5 substrates, especially for

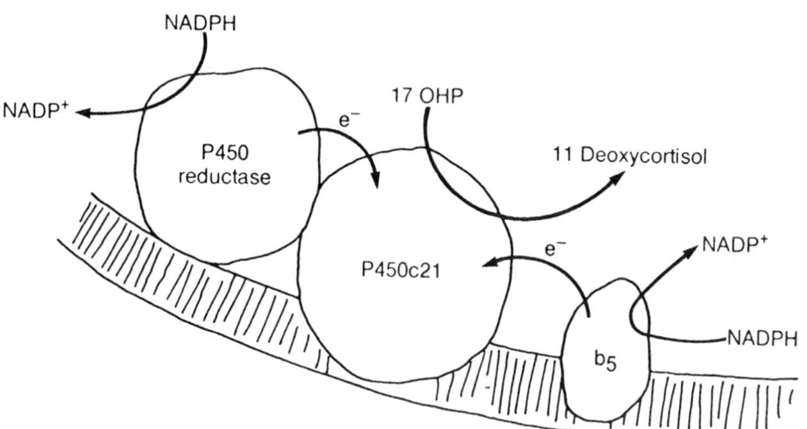

FIGURE 12-9 Electron transport to microsomal cytochromes P450. P450 reductase, a flavoprotein distinct from adrenodoxin reductase, accepts electron pairs from NADPH, converting it to $NADP^+$. These electrons are then passed directly to a cytochrome P450, such as P450c21, shown here. Transfer of the second electron from P450 reductase is slow; hence, this second electron may alternatively be provided by cytochrome b5. *(Modified from Miller.[23])*

17,20-bond scission, consistent with the large amounts of DHEA secreted by both the fetal and adult adrenal. Furthermore, the 17α-hydroxylase reaction occurs more readily (at a lower K_m) than does the 17,20-lyase reaction.[162,163,173] However, perhaps more important than the relative concentrations of steroids and competing enzymes are factors regulating electron transport to P450c17.

Electron Transport to P450c17: P450 Reductase

P450c17 receives electrons from a membrane-bound flavoprotein termed P450 reductase, which is a protein different from mitochondrial adrenodoxin reductase. It appears that there is only one species of P450 reductase, encoded by a single gene on chromosome 7.[174] Each molecule of P450 reductase is 677 amino acids long and contains a molecule of flavin mononucleotide (FMN) and a molecule of flavin adenine dinucleotide (FAD).[174] The enzyme is attached to the endoplasmic reticulum by a hydrophobic amino-terminal peptide so that most of the enzyme lies in the cytosol.[175] P450 reductase receives a pair of electrons from NADPH and transfers them one at a time to the various forms of cytochrome P450 found in the endoplasmic reticulum.[176] In the adrenal, this includes P450c17 and P450c21 (steroid 21-hydroxylase); in other steroidogenic tissues, such as the ovary and placenta, this includes P450aro (aromatase); and in the liver, it includes most of the enzymes involved in drug metabolism, such as those induced by phenobarbital or 3-methylcholanthrene. The first electron is transferred more rapidly than is the second. Alternatively, the second electron may be donated to the P450 by cytochrome b_5[177] (Fig. 12-9). The endoplasmic reticulum in the adrenal contains many more molecules of P450c17 and P450c21 than molecules of P450 reductase; thus, it appears that these P450s compete with one another for the reducing equivalents provided by the reductase. Phospholipids may facilitate the formation of complexes of P450, P450 reductase, and cytochrome b_5, thus increasing the transfer of electrons and consequently increasing enzymatic activity.[178,179] Different phospholipids or other such molecules may influence the choice of which reactions a steroid molecule will undergo (e.g., 17-α vs. 21-hydroxylation of progesterone or 21-hydroxylation vs. 17,20-bond scission of 17-hydroxyprogesterone).

The availability of reducing equivalents from P450 reductase (or cytochrome b_5) appears to be the most important factor in determining whether a 17α-hydroxylated C-21 steroid will undergo subsequent 17,20-bond cleavage to a C-19 steroid. Competition between P450c17 and P450c21 for available 17-OHP does not appear to be important in determining whether 17-OHP undergoes 21-hydroxylation or 17,20-bond scission, as antibodies to P450c21 do not increase the conversion of 17-OHP to androstenedione despite eliminating the possibility of its conversion to 11-deoxycortisol.[180] The testis normally contains three to four times more P450 reductase activity than does the adrenal, consistent with its need for greater 17,20-lyase activity to produce C-19 androgens. Furthermore, increasing the ratio of P450 reductase to P450c17 in vitro[174] or in transfected cells[181] increases 17,20-lyase activity relative to 17α-hydroxylase activity.

P450c21:21-Hydroxylase

After the synthesis of progesterone and 17-OHP, these steroids are hydroxylated at the 21 position to yield DOC and 11-deoxycortisol, respectively (Fig. 12-7). The nature of the 21-hydroxylating step has been of great clinical interest because congenital adrenal hyperplasia (CAH) resulting from 21-hydroxylase deficiency is an extremely common inborn error of metabolism, as discussed below. The clinical manifestations of CAH can vary greatly, and in the most severe form, decreased synthesis of cortisol and aldosterone leads to sodium loss, hypotension, cardiovascular collapse, and, if untreated, death within the first month of life. Decreased cortisol synthesis in utero leads to overproduction of ACTH and consequent stimulation of adrenal steroid synthesis; as the 21-hydroxylase step is impaired, precursor steroids are converted to androstenedione and testosterone, resulting in severe prenatal virilization of female fetuses (for reviews, see Refs. 182 and 183). CAH has been studied extensively at both the clinical and molecular genetic levels. Variations in the manifestations of the disease, especially the presence of many patients without apparent defects in mineralocorticoid activity ("simple virilizing CAH" and "nonclassical CAH"), led to the belief that there are two separate 21-hydroxylating enzymes that are differentially expressed in the zona glomerulosa and zonae fasciculata and reticularis of the adrenal, specifically synthesizing aldosterone or cortisol, respectively. However, characterization of the P450c21 protein from the endoplasmic reticulum and cloning of the gene have shown that there is only one adrenal 21-hydroxylase. P450c21 employs the same P450 reductase used by P450c17 to transport electrons from NADPH. Isolation of P450c21 from bovine adrenals showed a single species of protein that could 21-hydroxylate both progesterone and 17-OHP[184] but it was not until the cDNAs and genes were cloned that it was proved that there is only one functional adrenal 21-hydroxylase gene in human beings.[185–187]

21-Hydroxylase Genes

There are two 21-hydroxylase genes, generally termed P450c21A and P450c21B, and they overlap the newly discovered X and Y genes,[188,189] forming a unique "polygene" array. This complex was duplicated with the adjacent C4A and C4B loci encoding the fourth component of serum complement; this cluster in turn lies in the midst of the HLA locus on human chromosome 6p21.3 (for reviews, see Refs. 190 and 191). The genetic structures of the 21-hydroxylase genes are unusual as a result of the very high rate of crossover and genetic exchange between the two 21-hydroxylase genes.[190,191] As a detailed understanding of the genetics of this locus is required to understand congenital adrenal hyperplasia, the structure and genetics of these genes are discussed in Disorders of Steroid Hormone Synthesis, below, in conjunction with the clinical disorders of steroid hormone synthesis.

Extraadrenal 21-Hydroxylase

21-Hydroxylase activity is found in a broad range of extraadrenal tissues, especially in the fetus and the pregnant woman.[192,193] However, this extraadrenal 21-hydroxylation is not mediated by the P450c21 enzyme found in the adrenal,[194] and this activity persists in congenital adrenal hyperplasia. The nature of the enzyme(s) responsible for extraadrenal 21-hydroxylation is unknown. In the rabbit, hepatic 21-hydroxylase activity is mediated by P450IIC5,[131] but the human homologue of this enzyme lacks significant 21-hydroxylase activity. By contrast, authentic P450c21 mRNA is found in mouse liver,[195] in bovine testis,[196] and in a human testicular tumor.[35] However, human P450c21 mRNA is not found in normal human extraadrenal tissues.[194] The presence of such other 21-hydroxylating enzymes complicates the phenotypic presentation and clinical understanding of 21-hydroxylase deficiency, because even patients who are homozygous for a P450c21 gene deletion may still synthesize some 21-hydroxylated steroids.[197]

P450c11:11β-Hydroxylase/18-Hydroxylase/18-Oxidase

The nature of the enzyme or enzymes that mediate the conversion of DOC to aldosterone has been studied and debated with vigor. Based on clinical studies, it was long thought that 11β-hydroxylase, 18-hydroxylase, and one or more corticosterone methyl oxidases were separate enzymes.[198,199] More recently, studies of bovine P450c11 suggested that a single enzyme mediates all steps in the conversion of DOC to aldosterone as well as converting 11-deoxycortisol to cortisol.[200] While a single bovine enzyme does indeed possess all these activities,[201] the biology of the human and rodent enzymes differs from that in cattle.

P450c11, like P450scc, is found in the inner mitochondrial membrane and, like P450scc, uses adrenodoxin reductase and adrenodoxin as electron transport intermediates to receive electrons from NADPH. Also like P450scc, P450c11 appears to exist as a large, loosely aggregated multimer in vivo (for a review, see Ref. 23). However, unlike P450scc, the genetics of P450c11 are complex.

The sequence of P450c11 is typical of mitochondrial forms of P450.[202] P450c11 and P450scc share 39 percent amino acid identity and are encoded by evolutionarily related genes that have essentially identical intron/exon structures.[203] Like the bovine genome,[204] the human genome also has two P450c11 genes[203] located on chromosome 8 between q13 and q22.[205] These genes encode two P450c11 proteins that have 93 percent amino acid sequence identity. The gene generally termed CYP11B1 is expressed at high levels in the zonae fasciculata and reticularis and encodes an enzyme, generally termed P450c11β, that only has 11β-hydroxylase activity. The related CYP11B2 gene is expressed solely in the zona glomerulosa and at very low levels. It encodes an enzyme generally termed P450c11AS (for aldosterone synthase), which has 11β-hydroxylase, 18-hydroxylase, and 18-oxidase activities.[206–210] This enzyme is also termed P450c11aldo, P450c11cmo, P450c18, and P450c11B. As expected, the CYP11B1 gene encoding the P450c11β needed for cortisol synthesis is regulated by ACTH and suppressed by dexamethasone, while the CYP11B2 gene encoding the P450c11AS needed for aldosterone synthesis is regulated by angiotensin II, salt, and potassium.[210] Patients with classical 11β-hydroxylase deficiency have defects in their genes for P450c11β,[211] while patients with the so-called CMOI and CMOII (18-hydroxylase and 18-oxidase) deficiencies that disrupt aldosterone synthesis have defects in their genes for P450c11AS.[212,213] Thus, the molecular characterization of these genes and their encoded products has greatly clarified this formerly confusing area of steroidogenesis.

17-Ketosteroid Reductase/17β-Hydroxysteroid Oxidoreductase

In the adrenal, DHEA is converted to Δ^5 androstenediol and Δ^4 androsterone is converted to testosterone by 17-ketosteroid reductase (17-KSR), which is also termed 17-oxidoreductase. In the ovary and elsewhere, estrone undergoes a similar 17-ketosteroid reductase reaction to produce estradiol. This is the only readily reversible reaction in steroidogenesis; hence, Δ^5 androstenediol, testosterone, and estradiol may also be converted to DHEA, Δ^4 androstenedione, and estrone, respectively, by the same enzyme, but this "reverse" activity is generally termed 17β-hydroxysteroid dehydrogenase (17β-HSD) activity (Figs. 12-4 and 12-7). While it has been reported that 17-KSR and 17β-HSD activities are mediated by separate enzymes, no such enzymes have been isolated, sequenced, or cloned. The reversibility of this reaction has led to the use of multiple names, incorrectly implying the presence of separate enzymes for each reaction. However, these three 17-KSR/17β-HSD reactions may be catalyzed by more than one enzyme, although the exact number is not known; hence, terms such as *estradiol 17β-dehydrogenase* are also used.

17-KSR is an NADPH-dependent, non-P450 enzyme of about 35,000 daltons bound to the endoplasmic reticulum.[214,215] In the placenta, 17-KSR is found as a 68 to 70-kDa dimer having one NADPH-binding site per monomer.[214,215] 17-KSR is widely distributed in both steroidogenic and nonsteroidogenic tissues.[216,217]

Human cDNAs for placental estradiol 17β-HSD have been cloned.[218,219] While the sequence of this enzyme bears no similarity to that of the steroidogenic cytochrome P450 enzymes, it bears substantial similarity to bacterial dehydrogenases that metabolize compounds with sterol-like configurations,[220] suggesting that 17-KSR and these bacterial enzymes derive from a common evolutionary ancestor that recognized various polyols.[220]

There are two small tandemly linked genes of only 3.25 kb, termed HSD I and HSD II, that encode this placental cDNA.[221] These genes, which lie on band q11 or q12 of chromosome 17,[219,222] have 89 percent nucleotide sequence identity, but it appears that only HSD II can encode the functional protein of 328 amino acids. The HSD II gene apparently can use two different sequences in its 5′ flanking DNA as promoters, resulting in two different mRNAs. These mRNAs are detectable only in estrogenic, but not in androgenic, tissues (adrenal, testis); hence, the enzyme encoded by this mRNA is termed *estrogenic 17-KSR*.[222] The retention of hepatic and other extraglandular 17-KSR activity in 17-ketosteroid reductase deficiency and the different hormonal consequences of this disorder in males and females[223] suggest that more than one 17-KSR/17β-HSD enzyme functions in normal human steroidogenesis.

A very recent report indicates that a second human "type 2 17β-HSD" has been cloned.[224] This enzyme can interconvert testosterone and androstenedione as well as estradiol and estrone and thus has the properties of both an androgenic and an estrogenic 17-KSR. Both the estrogenic and androgenic forms of 17-KSR are found in the placenta, and both also possess 20α-hydroxysteroid dehydrogenase activity. This activity may be involved in maintaining the high progesterone concentrations that occur in pregnancy by oxidizing 20α-dihydroprogesterone.[224]

Other Steroidogenic Enzymes

Several other enzymes are involved in synthesizing and metabolizing various steroids. These enzymes are especially important in the production of sex steroids and in regulating mineralocorticoid activity. However, as their roles are somewhat peripheral to adrenal steroidogenesis, they are considered in less detail here.

P450aro: Aromatase

The aromatization of C-18 estrogenic steroids from C-19 androgens is mediated by P450aro, which is found in the endoplasmic reticulum. P450aro converts androgens to estrogens by two hydroxylations at the C-19 methyl group and a third hydroxylation at C-2, resulting in the loss of carbon 19 and the consequent aromatization of the A ring of the steroid (Fig. 12-4).[225,226] This series of reactions requires three pairs of electrons donated by three molecules of NADPH through P450 reductase, and all occur on a single active site.[227] P450aro has been purified and cloned.[228–233] The single gene for human aromatase[234] is located on band q21.1 of chromosome 15[230] and encodes two mRNAs that differ in the lengths of their 3′ untranslated regions.[231,234] Expression of human aromatase cDNA in COS-1 cells[232] or yeast[233] shows that all the successive oxidation reactions that are needed to aromatize androgens to estrogens are catalyzed by this single form of cytochrome P450. The CYP19 gene encoding P450aro is quite large, encompassing over 75 kb.[235]

Transcription is initiated from two or three alternative untranslated first exons which permit different segments of DNA to function as the regulatory sequences in a tissue-specific fashion in the placenta, the ovary, and adipose tissue.[236] Thus, the same enzyme is produced in different tissues under different regulatory control.

5α-Reductase

Testosterone is converted to the more potent androgen dihydrotestosterone by 5α-reductase, a membrane-bound non-P450 enzyme found primarily in peripheral target tissues such as genital skin and hair follicles rather than in the adrenal or testis.[237–240] The syndrome of 5α-reductase deficiency is a rare autosomal recessive disorder that causes incomplete differentiation of male genitalia but is phenotypically silent in females.[238,239,241]

Cloning and expression of two distinct isozymes of human 5α-reductase have been reported recently.[242,243] The type I enzyme is a hydrophobic protein of about 29 kDa encoded by an mRNA of about 2.4 kb encoded by a large gene of about 35 kb divided into five exons that is located on the distal short arm of chromosome 5.[244]

This gene encodes the enzyme found in the scalp but does not encode the enzyme required for male sexual differentiation.[244,245] The type 2 enzyme is encoded by a gene on band p23 of chromosome 2 that has the same intron/exon structure as the gene for the type 1 enzyme.[246] A wide variety of mutations have been described in this gene that cause the classical syndrome of 5α-reductase deficiency.[246] The type 1 and 2 genes show an unusual pattern of developmental regulation of expression.[247] The type 1 gene is not expressed in the fetus, then is expressed briefly in the skin of the newborn, and then remains unexpressed until its activity and protein are found again after puberty. The type 2 gene is expressed in fetal genital skin, in the normal prostate, and in prostatic hyperplasia and adenocarcinoma. Thus, the type 1 enzyme may be responsible for the pubertal virilization seen in patients with classic 5α-reductase deficiency, and the type 2 enzyme may be involved in male-pattern baldness.[247]

Steroid Sulfotransferase and Sulfatase

Steroid sulfates may be synthesized directly from cholesterol sulfate or may be formed by the sulfation of steroids by cytosolic sulfotransferases. Steroid sulfates may also be hydrolyzed to the native steroid by steroid sulfatase. An estrogen sulfotransferase has recently been cloned from bovine placenta[248] and guinea pig adrenal,[249] and it appears that there are other steroid sulfotransferases as well. Because deletions of this gene are a common cause of steroid sulfatase deficiency with X-linked icthyosis, much more is known about this enzyme.[250] In the fetal adrenal and placenta, diminished or absent sulfatase deficiency reduces the pool of free DHEA available for placental conversion to estrogen, resulting in prolonged gestation and prolonged, delayed labor. The accumulation of steroid sulfates in the stratum corneum of the skin causes the icthyosis.

11β-Hydroxysteroid Dehydrogenase

The conversion of cortisol to cortisone is mediated by 11β-hydroxysteroid dehydrogenase (11β-HSD). The reverse reaction is mediated by an 11-oxidoreductase activity, and whether these two activities are catalyzed by one or two enzymes has been controversial. Enzymologic studies suggested the presence of two enzymes,[251] and purification of a hepatic 34-kDa protein with 11β-dehydrogenase but no 11-oxidoreductase activity has been reported.[252] However, cloning and expression of the cDNA encoding this 11β-dehydrogenase showed that the protein has both 11β-dehydrogenase and 11-oxidoreductase activity.[253] The gene for this hepatic form of 11β-HSD has been cloned from human beings[254] and squirrel monkeys.[255] Assays of enzymatic activity, protein blotting, and RNA blotting all show that this enzyme is widely distributed in many tissues.[253–257]

Although glucocorticoids and mineralocorticoids have been distinguished functionally for 50 years,[10] the cloning of glucocorticoid and mineralocorticoid receptors raised a logical conundrum since the human mineralocorticoid (type I) receptor bound aldosterone, corticosterone, and cortisol with equal affinities.[258] Thus, it was unclear how mineralocorticoids could exhibit tissue-specific effects when the circulating concentrations of cortisol were 100 to 1000 times greater. A proposed explanation for the apparent physiologic specificity of the mineralocorticoid receptor in the presence of the molecular nonspecificity of the receptor came from studies of two disorders of 11β-HSD. In the syndrome of apparent mineralocorticoid excess,[259–261] there is a genetic defect in 11β-HSD so that cortisol is not inactivated to cortisone. Similarly, in liquorice poisoning,[262] glyceyrrhizic acid and its metabolite glyceyrrhetinic acid inhibit 11β-HSD activity, resulting in sodium retention and hypertension. Stewart and associates[262] suggested that both conditions lead to high intrarenal cortisol concentrations that then occupy the mineralocorticoid receptor. Funder and coworkers[257] expanded this idea to suggest that the enzyme "protects" the mineralocorticoid receptor from the action of glucocorticoids. In fact, glyceyrrhetinic acid inhibits 11β-HSD activity but not 11-oxidoreductase activity,[263] and functional data provide evidence for 11β-HSD activity in the renal target cells for aldosterone.[264] However, the protein and mRNA corresponding to the cloned hepatic form of 11β-HSD appear to be absent from the distal nephron, where mineralocorticoids exert their most important functions.[265–267] A distinct 11β-HSD activity dependent on NAD, rather than the NADP dependence characteristic of the hepatic enzyme, has been reported in the rat kidney[268] and human placenta.[269] It appears that this distinct form of 11β-HSD may be the postulated defender of the mineralocorticoid receptor.

Steroid Synthesis in the Fetal Adrenal

Adrenal steroidogenesis begins early in embryonic life, probably by the eighth week of gestation. In fetuses affected with genetic disorders of steroidogenesis such as 21-hydroxylase deficiency, the dysfunctional fetal adrenal can produce enough testosterone to virilize a female fetus to a male appearance (closure of the urogenital sinus, with a urethra traversing part or all of the clitoral phallic shaft).[182,183,238] Testosterone has such effects only between the eighth and thirteenth weeks,[238] indicating that the fetal adrenal is already steroidogenically active during this period. Preliminary experimental attempts to suppress fetal adrenal steroidogenesis in 21-hydroxylase deficiency required the administration of suitable glucocorticoids to the mother before the eighth week of pregnancy (for reviews, see Refs. 189 and 270). Thus, fetal adrenal steroidogenesis begins early.

Fetal adrenal steroidogenesis differs from that in older children or adults. The thin definitive zone of the fetal adrenal produces cortisol, corticosterone, DOC, progesterone, aldosterone, and androstenedione according to the pathways shown in Figs. 12-4 and 12-7.[271] However, this accounts for only about 65 percent of circulating fetal cortisol; the remainder comes from direct placental transfer of cortisol and from fetal conversion of placentally produced cortisone back to cortisol. The placenta has abundant 11β-dehydrogenase activity, so that about 85 percent of maternally produced cortisol crossing the placenta is inactivated by conversion to cortisone; the fetus can convert only very small amounts of this cortisone back to cortisol.[272] The large fetal zone of the fetal adrenal is steroidogenically very active but has very little 3β-HSD activity because of the barely detectable amounts of 3β-HSD mRNA.[150] The fetal zone also has a relatively high ratio of 17,20-lyase to 17α-hydroxylase activity of P450c17, favoring abundant production of DHEA, and also has considerable sulfotransferase activity but little steroid sulfatase activity, favoring conversion of the DHEA to DHEA-S. The resulting DHEA-S cannot be a substrate for 3β-HSD activity and must undergo the sulfatase reaction in the placenta. Placental estrogens also inhibit adrenal 3β-HSD activity, providing a feedback system that further promotes the production of DHEA-S.[273] As a result, the fetal adrenal produces tremendous quantities of DHEA and DHEA-S. These steroids are converted to 16α-OH-DHEA and 16α-OH-DHEA-S in the liver and other tissues and then are converted by placental 3β-HSD, 17-KSR, and aromatase to estriol either directly or after removal of the sulfate by placental sulfatase activity. Alternatively, placental 3β-HSD and aromatase can act on DHEA to produce estrone, or 3β-HSD, aromatase, and 17-KSR can act on DHEA to produce estradiol. Fetal adrenal DHEA and DHEA-S account for about 90 percent of estriol and about 50 percent of estrone and estradiol in the maternal circulation. Thus, measurement of circulating maternal estriol constitutes a useful assay of the health of the fetoplacental unit.

REGULATION OF ADRENAL STEROIDOGENESIS

Steroidogenic tissues do not store appreciable amounts of steroid hormones; therefore, the regulation of steroid hormone secretion occurs primarily at the level of steroid hormone synthesis. The principal regulator of glucocorticoid synthesis is the hypothalamic-pituitary-adrenal axis, and the principal regulator of adrenal mineralocorticoid synthesis is the renin-angiotensin system. The mechanisms regulating adrenal androgens are controversial but clearly involve both ACTH and other factors. The classical physiologic interrelations among the various tissues and factors regulating steroid hormone synthesis, uptake, and metabolism are shown in Fig. 12-10. This complex homeostatic balance allows rapid and sensitive control of the circulating concentrations of steroid hormones in a broad range of normal and abnormal physiologic states.

Regulation of Glucocorticoids

The Hypothalamic-Pituitary-Adrenal Axis

The hypothalamus, pituitary, and adrenal form a neuroendocrine axis whose principal function is to regulate the production of cortisol (Fig. 12-10). Corticotropin-releasing hormone, arginine vasopressin (AVP), and possibly other factors are secreted by the hypothalamus into the hypothalamic portal veins, thus exposing the anterior pituitary to high concentrations of those hypothalamic factors before they are diluted by entry into the general circulation. These factors stimulate the synthesis and release of corticotropin (ACTH) into the general circulation. ACTH in turn stimulates the synthesis and release of adrenal steroids, principally cortisol. The synthesis and release of adrenal steroids may also be mediated centrally by adrenal innervation.

Hypothalamus: CRH and AVP

Two hypothalamic peptides—CRH and AVP—are the principal but not the sole regulators of ACTH synthesis and release. CRH is a 41-amino acid peptide synthesized primarily by the paraventricular nucleus.[274] The same neuronal bodies in the paraventricular nucleus also produce AVP [also

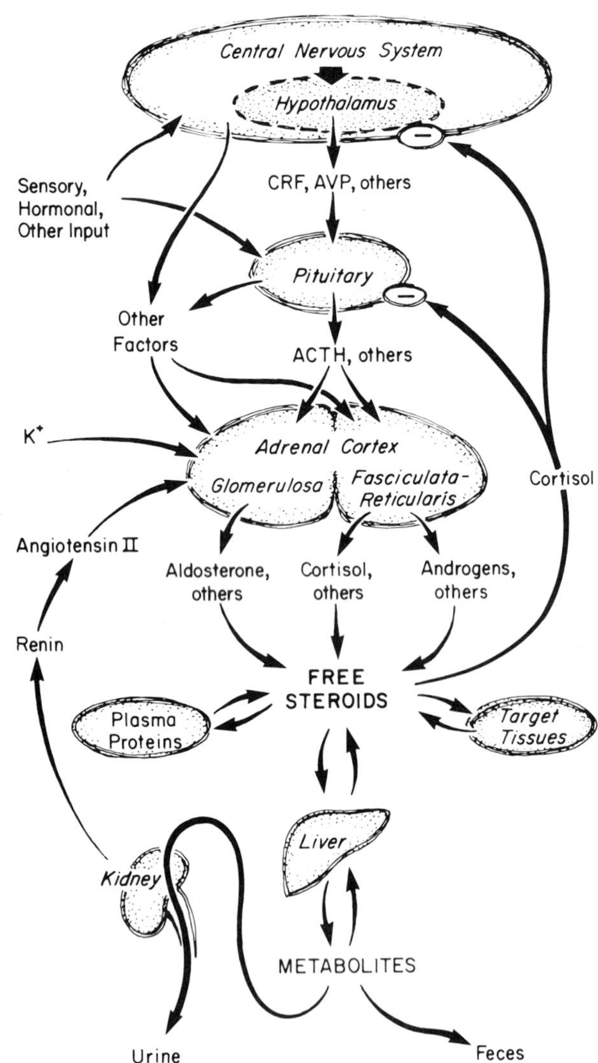

FIGURE 12-10 Interrelations among various tissues and factors involved in adrenal steroid hormone synthesis, uptake, metabolism, and excretion.

known as antidiuretic hormone (ADH)], which is also produced in the supraoptic nucleus.[275,276] Both CRH and AVP are proteolytically cleaved from larger precursors. Prepro-CRH contains no other peptides with a known function. The precursor to AVP, however, also gives rise to neurophysin II, the AVP-binding protein. The gene encoding AVP/ neurophysin II is structurally very similar to the gene for oxytocin; these two evolutionarily duplicated genes lie in a tandemly duplicated tail-to-tail arrangement on chromosome 20 (for a review, see Ref. 277). Both CRH and AVP travel through neurons to the median eminence,[276] which releases them into the pituitary portal circulation, which in turn carries them to the anterior pituitary in high concentrations. These peptides normally occur at undetectably low concentrations in the general venous circulation, except during pregnancy.[278] CRH and AVP stimulate the synthesis and release of ACTH by different mechanisms. CRH acts, at least in part, by interacting with receptors linked to the protein kinase A pathway, stimulating the production of intracellular cyclic AMP.[279] AVP appears to act through other messengers, principally calcium ion.[279] When administered together, CRH and AVP act additively or synergistically, as would be predicted from their independent mechanisms of action,[280–282] and also induce hyperplasia of the ACTH-producing corticotropes.[283]

CRH and its receptor are found throughout the body, notably in the brain and gastrointestinal tract.[284,285] In the brain, CRH is an excitatory neurotransmitter that may be epileptogenic[285a]; it stimulates sympathetic outflow and may modulate blood pressure.[275,286] Thus, CRH appears to be involved in responses to stress; concentrations of CRH in the cerebrospinal fluid (CSF) are increased during depression.[287]

CRH is probably the most important physiologic stimulator of ACTH. CRH is pharmacologically more potent than AVP in vivo and in vitro,[282,288] even though maximally effective doses of AVP can release an equivalent amount of ACTH.[281,282] Antibodies to CRH decrease ACTH release in rats in response to ether, stress, formalin, CRH, or AVP.[282,289–291] The release of CRH can be decreased by AVP[292] and increased by CRH[293] in short feedback loops.

Pituitary release of ACTH is not totally dependent on CRH. Antibodies to CRH block the rise in ACTH only in response to various stimuli; they do not block basal ACTH release.[294] Similarly, AVP can act alone or act synergistically with CRH. Other factors also appear to be important. Oxytocin, which is structurally related to AVP, does not stimulate the release of human ACTH, although it does this in some animals.[295] Both α- and β-adrenergic stimuli, lymphokines, angiotensin II, opiate peptides, and somatostatin may be involved in the regulation of ACTH synthesis and release; however, their importance remains to be established.[296]

Pituitary: POMC and ACTH

ACTH is made primarily in the anterior pituitary, although it is also synthesized in the intermediate lobe of the pituitary as well as the brain, placenta, lymphocytes, and testes. These extrapituitary sources make negligible (if any) contributions to circulating concentrations of immunoreactive ACTH, although huge amounts of "ectopic" ACTH can be produced by some malignancies. This ectopic ACTH derives from pro-opiomelanocortin (POMC) and is identical to pituitary ACTH.[297]

ACTH is a 39-amino acid peptide proteolytically cleaved from a larger 241-amino acid precursor gener-

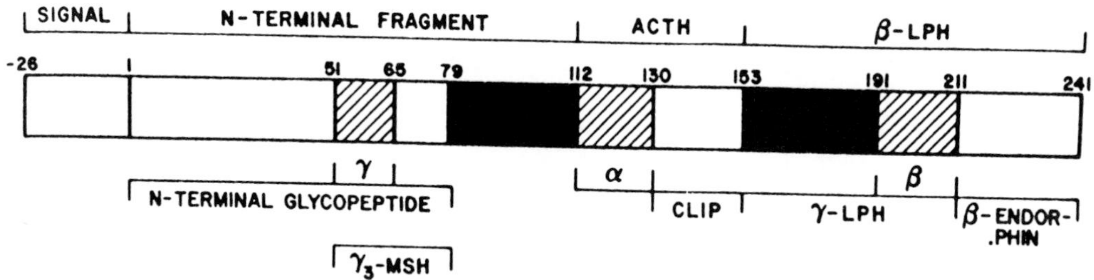

FIGURE 12-11 Structure of human prepro-opiomelanocortin. The numbers refer to amino acid positions, with 1 assigned to the first amino acid of POMC after the 26-amino acid signal peptide. The α-, β- and γ-MSH regions, which characterize the three "constant" regions, are indicated by diagonal lines; the "variable" regions are solid. The amino acid numbers shown refer to the N-terminal amino acid of each cleavage site; because these amino acids are removed, the numbers do not corrrespond exactly with the amino acid numbers of the peptides as used in the text. *(From Miller et al.[299])*

ally termed POMC. POMC is an unusual polyhormonal precursor that is differentially cleaved in various tissues into several hormonally active peptides (Fig. 12-11).[298,299] ACTH consists of amino acids 112 through 150 of POMC. The N-terminal glycopeptide can stimulate steroidogenesis and may function as an adrenal-specific mitogen.[300] POMC 112-126 and POMC 191-207 constitute α- and β-MSH, respectively; POMC 210-241 is β-endorphin, and corticotropin-like intermediate peptide (CLIP) is POMC 129-150. The recent proposal that all or part of the POMC 79-109 region may function as an adrenal androgen stimulating hormone has been rejected convincingly.[154–156] ACTH can stimulate lipolysis in fat cells,[301] an action that may be related to the historical but technically inaccurate naming of the carboxy-terminal POMC peptides POMC 153-241 and POMC 153-191 as β- and γ-LPH (lipotrophic hormone), respectively.

Both ACTH and MSH appear to have neurotransmitter functions. They affect learning and behavior in rats and affect opiate action (see Chap. 8). The melanocyte-stimulating properties of α-, β-, and γ-MSH appear to come from their activities within ACTH, β-LPH, and the N-terminal glycopeptide, respectively, because free MSH peptides have not been found in human circulation. Most MSH activity appears to come from the α-MSH region of ACTH, since α-MSH (in ACTH) is four times more potent than β-MSH (in LPH) and since ACTH and LPH are present in approximately equimolar concentrations. CLIP can stimulate pancreatic exocrine function,[302] and γ-MSH may play a minor natriuretic role.[303] However, essential physiologic roles have not been established for any of the POMC peptides other than ACTH. ACTH can be modified further by phosphorylation and, in rats, by glycosylation, but glycosylation of human ACTH is negligible.[297,304]

Only the amino-terminal half of the ACTH molecule is needed for biological activity, and the first 24 amino acids are identical among all mammals studied to date (Fig. 12-12). ACTH 1-24, 1-23, and 1-20 are all equipotent on a molar basis compared to ACTH 1-39, but the circulating half-life and duration of adrenal stimulation decrease as the molecule is shortened. As a result, synthetic ACTH 1-24 is widely used in diagnostic tests of adrenal function.

ACTH circulates unbound to other proteins and is quickly cleared from the circulation, with a half-life of about 10 min.[305] Biological activity disappears from the circulation even more rapidly than does immunoassayable activity, suggesting that the biologically most important regions, the 10 amino-terminal amino acids, are attacked early, leaving immunoactive but biologically inert peptides. ACTH is catabolized in many tissues, principally the liver and kidneys, and is not excreted in the urine in significant amounts.[305]

Actions of ACTH

ACTH stimulates the synthesis and release of steroids by interacting with cell-surface ACTH receptors that stimulate the production of intracellular cAMP. This increased cAMP in turn mediates both acute and chronic effects on steroidogenesis.

Acute Actions ACTH acutely increases cortisol synthesis and release within 2 to 3 min, principally by stimulating the activity of cholesterol esterase and inhibiting cholesterol ester synthetase.[173,306] ACTH rapidly facilitates the transport of cholesterol across the mitochondrial membranes (see Steroid Hormone Biosynthesis, above), the binding of cholesterol to P450scc, and the release of newly synthesized pregnenolone from mitochondria. Although the concentration of cortisol and other steroids is 100 to 1000 times higher in the adrenal than in the circulation, this constitutes a nearly insignificant reservoir,[307] and the release of preformed steroids is relatively unimportant. The presense of high intraadrenal steroid concentrations suggests an active mechanism to regulate release, but little is known about this sub-

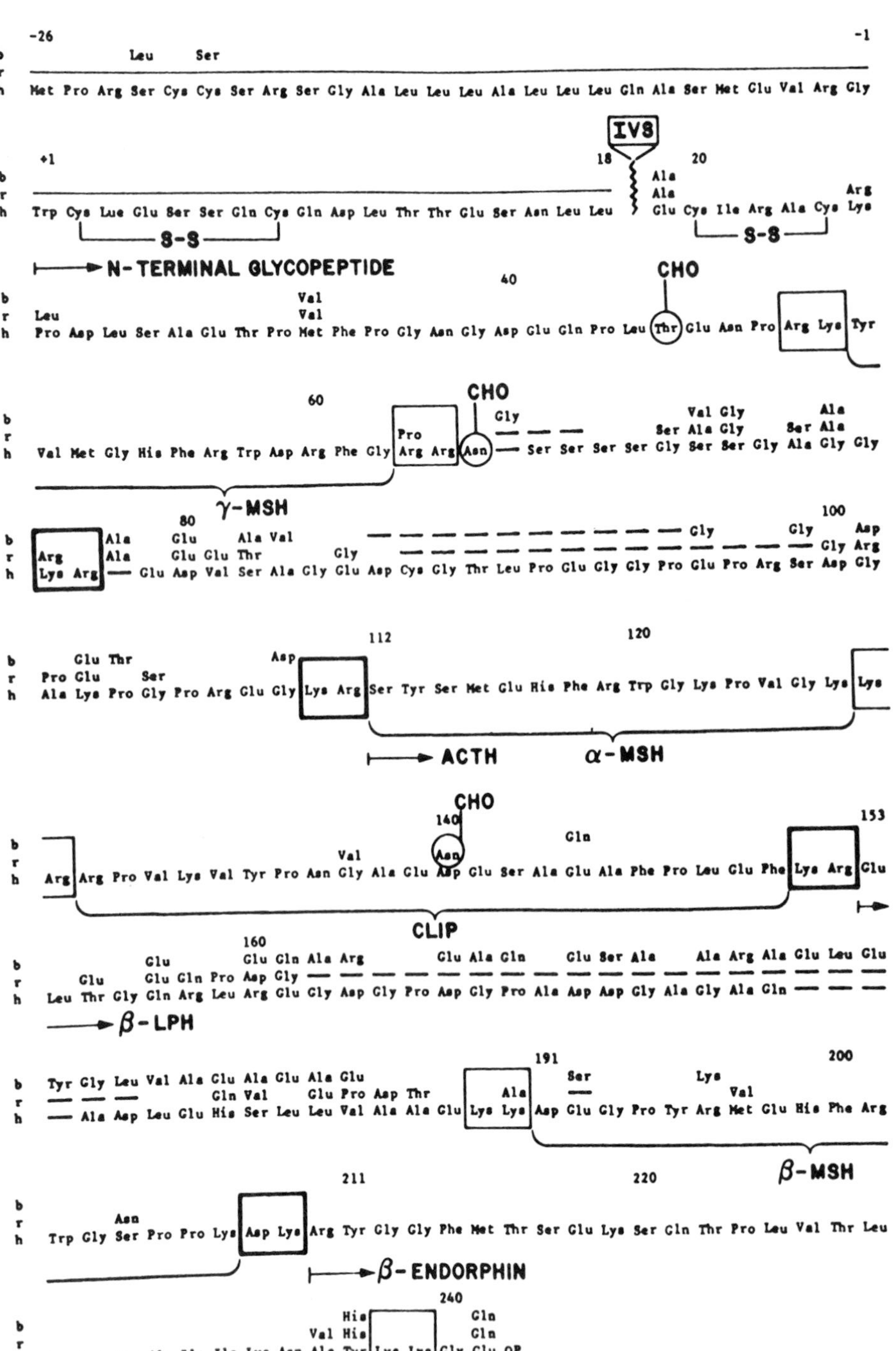

FIGURE 12-12 Bovine, rat, and human POMC. Amino acid sequences were taken from the established gene sequences. Only the complete sequence of human pre-POMC is shown. For the bovine and rat sequences, the amino acids that differ from the human sequence are shown; those which are the same are represented as blanks. Where a sequence lacks a corresponding amino acid, the gap is indicated as a dash. The amino acid numbers correspond only to the human sequence. The various known glycosylation sites are encircled and indicated by "CHO." The pairs of basic amino acids that represent major cleavage sites are enclosed in heavy boxes; other possible cleavage sites are enclosed in light boxes. *(From Miller et al.[299])*

ject. ACTH also facilitates the release of adrenal androgens and mineralocorticoids as well as stimulating the release of various steroidal intermediates. By contrast, when ACTH concentrations fall, steroidogenesis decreases rapidly.

Receptors ACTH receptors are found on the surface of adrenal cortical cells, where they bind ACTH with a K_d (equilibrium dissociation constant) of about $10^{-9} M$.[308,309] It is not clear if there is only one class of ACTH receptor, as some evidence indicates that there may be two binding sites with differing K_d.[310,311] The abundance of ACTH receptors can be suppressed by ACTH.[308,309] Binding of ACTH to its receptor activates adenylate cyclase.[173,305,310] This increases intracellular concentrations of cAMP, which in turn activates a number of protein kinases, but it is not known which specific proteins are phosphorylated in response to ACTH or precisely how they promote steroidogenesis. However, accumulation of cAMP does precede steroidogenesis, and binding of cAMP to the regulatory subunit of protein kinase A correlates well with stimulation of steroidogenesis.[312]

Chronic Actions ACTH exerts chronic actions on both adrenal architecture and steroidogenesis. Prolonged stimulation with ACTH increases adrenal protein and DNA synthesis and net growth.[28] There is both cellular hypertrophy (increased cell size) and hyperplasia (increased cell number). It has been claimed that adrenal cellular hypertrophy and hyperplasia are promoted by distinct regions of the N-terminal glycopeptide of POMC,[300] but synthetic ACTH 1-24 is sufficient by itself to increase the adrenal mass severalfold.[28] The mechanisms by which ACTH promotes adrenal growth are not clear. Antibodies to ACTH inhibit steroidogenesis but do not inhibit adrenal growth in animals,[313] and in primary cultures of animal or human fetal adrenal cells, ACTH inhibits rather than promotes growth. ACTH chronically increases steroidogenesis by promoting the transcription of genes for steroidogenic enzymes (see below), an action apparently not linked to adrenal growth. Physiologic concentrations of ACTH also directly stimulate the synthesis and accumulation of insulin-like growth factor-II (IGF-II) mRNA[31,34,99] and consequently IGF-II peptide.[314] ACTH also promotes the synthesis of basic fibroblast growth factor and epidermal growth factor, which may act with IGF-II to stimulate adrenal growth.[33,34] However, IGF-II mRNA is unchanged in rat adrenals induced to grow by unilateral adrenalectomy and decreases in rat adrenals induced to grow by ACTH.[32]

Conversely, when ACTH concentrations are chronically low, as in hypopituitarism or when suppressed by glucocorticoid therapy, adrenal protein content, steroidogenic activity, and mass decrease substantially. After such long-term privation of ACTH and adrenal atrophy, the adrenal will recover when treated with ACTH. However, stimulation of steroidogenesis may take 24 h, full activity may take 3 days, and recovery of the ability to mount a stress-induced hypercortisolemic response may take weeks to months.

Chronic actions of ACTH on steroidogenesis occur principally by promoting the transcription of the genes that encode steroidogenic enzymes and other factors. Although most experiments in vitro and in cell culture systems show transcriptional responses to ACTH and cAMP within 1 or 2 h, the net effects on steroidogenic capacity take longer. Thus, one can conceptualize the acute action of ACTH as turning on the steroidogenic machinery to maximum capacity, while the chronic action increases that capacity by producing more steroidogenic machinery. ACTH increases the transcription of the genes for P450scc, P450c17, P450c21, P450c11, adrenodoxin reductase, and adrenodoxin[103–108,123,172,210] (for a review, see Ref. 109). Because P450scc is the rate-limiting step in steroidogenesis, much attention has been focused on it. ACTH in the adrenal and gonadotropins in the gonads stimulate the accumulation of human P450scc mRNA and human P450scc activity[97,98] (for a review, see Ref. 315), yet ACTH and cAMP increase the transcription of both the P450scc and P450c17 genes about equally.[105,172] Some but not most of the actions of ACTH (or other tropic peptides) in stimulating steroidogenesis may be blocked by the inhibition of protein synthesis.[100,101,104,111,112] It appears likely that the effects of inhibiting protein synthesis occur largely by inhibiting the synthesis of various factors involved in the transport of cholesterol to the P450scc enzyme rather than by affecting factors that regulate the transcription of the genes that encode the steroidogenic enzymes. Calcium is also important for ACTH- or cAMP-induced steroidogenesis, as it can be blocked by inhibitors of calmodulin,[74] yet calcium ionophores suppress P450scc mRNA accumulation and transcription of the P450scc gene.[105]

ACTH also chronically stimulates LDL uptake and metabolism and the synthesis and accumulation of LDL receptor and HMGCoA reductase and their mRNAs. Furthermore, ACTH also stimulates cholesterol esterase,[49,50] SCP-2,[316] and endozepine,[67] so that it has general tropic effects on all known early steps in steroidogenesis (see Steroid Hormone Biosynthesis, above).

A role for newly synthesized phospholipids in mediating the chronic actions of ACTH has been proposed. The reported actions can be mimicked by cAMP, require calcium, and are blocked by inhibitors of protein synthesis.[306,310,317,318] The mechanism of action of such phospholipids is unknown but may be related to promoting the flux of free cholesterol across the mitochondrial membranes to P450scc.[58,173,306,317]

While chronic treatment with glucocorticoids clearly suppresses the hypothalamic-pituitary axis, thus suppressing the adrenal indirectly through ACTH privation, a direct action of glucocorticoids on the adrenal cortex has also been proposed. Glucocorticoids can inhibit steroidogenesis in primary cultures of human adrenal cells in vitro,[319] and a direct action of suppressing the transcription of the human P450c17 gene has been suggested.[172] However, such direct feedback probably plays a minor role in human physiology, as the hypercortisolism found in syndromes of ACTH excess does not effectively reduce steroidogenesis, and the administration of dexamethasone does not inhibit ACTH-induced cortisol secretion.[320]

Direct Patterns of ACTH and Cortisol Synthesis and Release

Plasma concentrations of ACTH and cortisol tend to be high in the morning and low in the evening. Peak ACTH levels are usually seen at 4 to 6 A.M., and peak cortisol levels follow at about 8 A.M. Both ACTH and cortisol are released episodically in pulses every 30 to 120 min throughout the day, but the frequency and amplitude of these pulses are much greater in

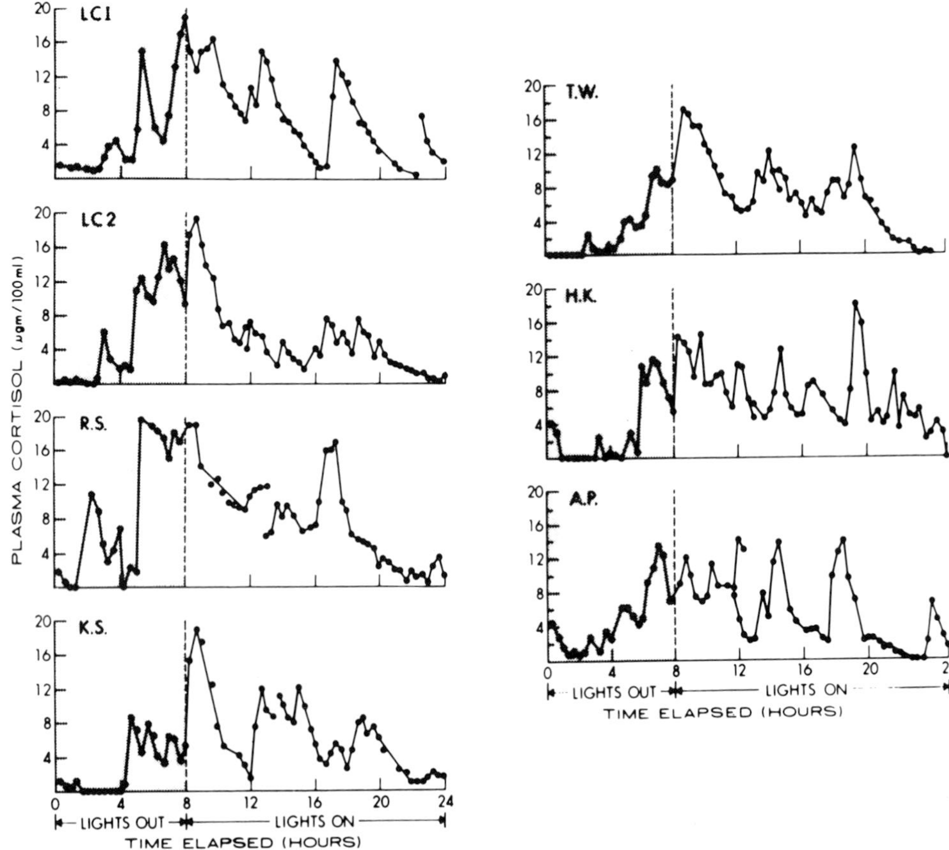

FIGURE 12-13 Plasma cortisol values of normal subjects for 24-h periods of study. Samples were obtained every 20 min. "Lights out" indicates the period available for sleep. LC1 and LC2 refer to studies done on the same subject in two different 24-h periods. *(From Weitzman et al.[321])*

the morning.[321–327] Each pulse of cortisol release is characterized by a very rapid rise in circulating cortisol concentration, followed by a slower, generally smooth decline. Pulses of cortisol release may occur when basal cortisol concentrations are either high or low, resulting in very widely and rapidly fluctuating serum cortisol concentrations. During periods of minimal secretion, especially in the late evening, cortisol can decrease to levels that are unmeasurable in most assays. Pulses of cortisol release occur more frequently in the early morning hours, leading to the characteristic diurnal rhythm of cortisol secretion. The basis of this diurnal rhythm is complex and poorly understood. At least four factors appear to be involved in the rhythm of ACTH and cortisol: (1) intrinsic rhythmicity of the synthesis and secretion of CRH by the hypothalamus, (2) feeding cycles, (3) light/dark cycles, (4) inherent rhythmicity in the adrenal, possibly mediated by adrenal innervation.

Rhythmicity of Hypothalamic CRH Both static measures of CRH content and dynamic measures of CRH synthesis show a diurnal rhythm which appears to be inherent in the hypothalamic cell bodies. There does not appear to be a diurnal rhythm in the responsiveness of the pituitary to CRH,[322] and the diurnal pattern of hypothalamic CRH content persists in hypophysectomized animals that are deprived of ACTH and glucocorticoid feedback.[322] Furthermore, this diurnal pattern is maintained even when CRH is infused continuously,[327] showing insensitivity of this hypothalamic rhythm to ultra–short loop feedback. Thus hypothalamic rhythmicity appears to be neuronal or intrinsic but not hormonal. Furthermore, while the diurnal rhythms of CRH, ACTH, and cortisol are generally correlated, not all peaks of cortisol secretion are associated with pulses of CRH or ACTH and not all pulses of ACTH release are followed by pulses of cortisol.[322,326] Similar inherent rhythmicity of LRF-secreting hypothalamic neurosecretory neurons has been demonstrated in immortalized hypothalamic cell cultures.[328]

Feeding Cycles While diurnal rhythms are generally associated with light/dark cycles, increasing evidence points to a major role for feeding schedules in the diurnal patterns of ACTH and cortisol. Concentrations of cortisol are highest before breakfast, and additional peaks appear to be coincident with lunch and supper,[323,324] although there is great individual variability in these patterns (Fig. 12-13). In rats, the feeding schedule appears to be more important than light/dark cycles in determining the diurnal rhythm of glucocorticoid release.[325,329] However, if rats are fed only during hours of light, the circadian pattern slowly changes so that after about 10 days maximal glucocorticoid concentrations coincide with the start of feeding. Thus, it appears that glucocorticoids tend to be released during fasting and decrease with feeding. This is consistent with their carbohydrate-mobilizing properties, suggesting that the diurnal rhythms either protect against hypoglycemia or are entrained by subclinical hypoglycemia.

Less is known about the effect of eating patterns on human patterns of ACTH and cortisol release. Although preprandial peaks of cortisol are common,[323,324] they are quite variable and do not occur in subjects whose normal patterns of activity do not include these meals.[324]

Light/Dark Cycles The simplest correlation with the circadian rhythms of ACTH and cortisol is light/dark cycles. Nocturnal secretory episodes increase between the third and fifth hours of sleep, followed by the main secretory bursts in the sixth to eighth hours of sleep and the first several hours of wakefulness. Infants do not have diurnal rhythms of sleep or feeding, a behavioral phenomenon that is well known to all parents. However, infants acquire their behavioral rhythms and learn to sleep through the night, presumably in response to their environment, long before they acquire a rhythm of ACTH and cortisol. The diurnal rhythm of ACTH and cortisol does not appear until after the first year of life, may not appear until age 3 years, and may not become solidly established until age 8 years.[322] However, once it is established, this rhythm is not changed easily and persists after prolonged bed rest, continuous feeding, and 2- to 3-day periods of sleep deprivation.[322] It remains unchanged in people who work night shifts but maintain conventional hours on weekends. When individuals shift sleep/walking, light/dark, and feeding schedules congruently, such as by moving to a distant time zone, the circadian rhythm of ACTH and cortisol changes slowly over the course of 2 or 3 weeks.[322]

Inherent Rhythmicity and Other Factors Adrenal activity appears to exhibit some diurnal rhythmicity that is independent of CRH and ACTH; this may reflect inherent rhythmicity or may be regulated via adrenal innervation. Glucocorticoid rhythms are seen in hypophysectomized animals that are given continuous nondiurnal infusions of ACTH.[28] Furthermore, spinal transsection above the level of adrenal innervation or autotransplantation of adrenals freed of neural input will abolish the rhythm.[28] These experiments suggest a direct effect of adrenal innervation on adrenal steroidogenesis or sensitivity to ACTH. A role for factors other than ACTH is indicated by the occasional dissociation between peaks of ACTH and cortisol[322,326] and by the frequent lack of proportionality between the magnitudes of ACTH peaks and cortisol peaks.[326,330]

Changes in the Diurnal Rhythm of Cortisol

A wide variety of physical and psychological factors can alter the complex control of the diurnal variation of ACTH and cortisol secretion. These factors appear to be mediated largely by the central nervous system (CNS), although circulating catecholamines also play a role, as in insulin-induced hypoglycemia.[296] Age does not appear to alter integrated 24-h adrenal function, but maximal and minimal concentrations of cortisol occur somewhat earlier in the day.[331] Seemingly mild fear or psychological stress, such as anticipation of venipuncture,[332] or more severe stress, such as preparation for cardiac surgery,[333] can increase the secretion of cortisol, as can anticipation of athletic competition or university examinations.[327,334] However, responses to ACTH and cortisol to routine daily stresses have not been documented.

Major physical stresses such as severe trauma, major surgery, severe illness, hypoglycemia, fever, burns, exposure to cold, irradiation, hypotension, dehydration, smoking tobacco, and moderate to intensive exercise can increase the secretion of ACTH and cortisol.[327,334,335] The response to surgery is illustrated in Fig. 12-14; such stress can increase cortisol production up to sixfold,[336] and the need for administration of increased doses of glucocorticoids to addisonian patients undergoing surgery is well known. However, minor illnesses such as upper respiratory infections and minor surgery[336,337] have little influence on cortisol secretion.

Chronic illnesses also alter the diurnal rhythm of ACTH and cortisol.[338] Congestive heart failure and primary liver disease alter cortisol disposal, and hypothalamic and limbic system disorders directly affect central control.[339] Patients with major depression have increased basal ACTH, cortisol, and urinary steroid excretion as a result of a blunting of the diurnal rhythm of ACTH and cortisol similar to that seen in Cushing's disease.[340] CRH concentrations are increased in the CSF of depressed patients,[287] and the hypothalamic-pituitary-adrenal axis of such patients is less sensitive to suppression by exogenously administered glucocorticoids. Spinal fluid CRH and circulating cortisol are increased and diurnal variation and sensitivity to dexamethasone are decreased in anorexia nervosa.[341] However, many common drugs, including atropine, phenobarbital, reserpine, chlordiazepoxide, meprobamate, chlorpromazine, and phenytoin, have no detectable affect on the circadian rhythm of cortisol secretion,[322] although cyproheptadine, a serotonin antag-

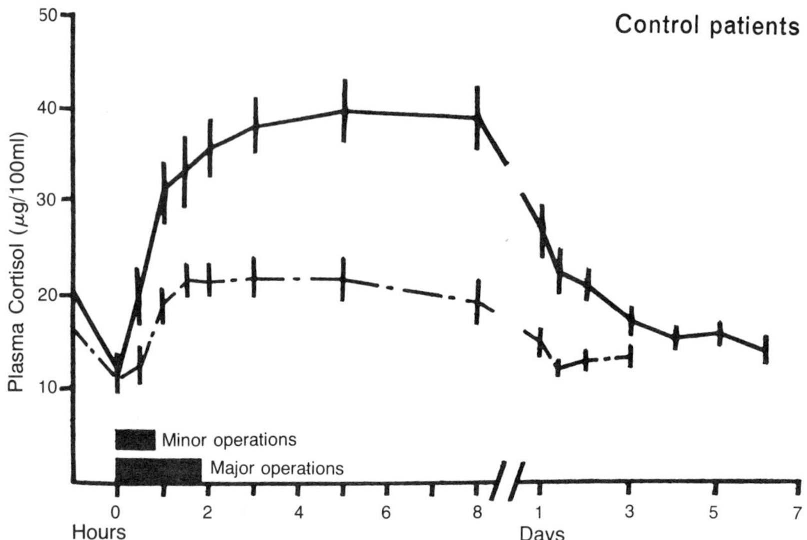

FIGURE 12-14 Plasma cortisol responds to major surgery (continuous line) and minor surgery (broken line) in normal subjects. Mean values and standard errors are shown for 20 patients in each case. *(From Plumpton et al.[336])*

onist, can inhibit rises in ACTH and cortisol induced by hypoglycemia or metyrapone.[342,343]

Glucocorticoid Feedback on ACTH Release

The hypothalamic-pituitary-adrenal axis is a classic example of an endocrine feedback system. ACTH increases the production of cortisol, and cortisol in turn decreases the production of both CRH and ACTH.[335,338,340–345] Disruption of this homeostatic system by adrenal insufficiency can raise concentrations of ACTH 10 to 20 times above normal, yet these profoundly elevated concentrations of ACTH can be suppressed by replacement with physiologic doses of glucocorticoids. Similarly, plasma concentrations of ACTH and ACTH responses to CRH and stress are suppressed by high concentrations of glucocorticoids.

Glucocorticoid feedback on ACTH has been described as consisting of fast, intermediate, and slow components,[344] but as in most physiologic systems, there is a continuum of responses. When patients with Addison's disease are given intravenous cortisol, the concentration of circulating ACTH decreases within 15 min and is substantially suppressed to about 10 percent of the initial value by 90 to 120 min (Fig. 12-15). This initial fast feedback blunts the ACTH response to some stimuli, such as histamine, but not the response to strong stimuli such as endotoxin and major surgery. This initial fast phase of glucocorticoid feedback appears to be exerted more at the level of hypothalamic CRH release than at the level of the pituitary, although both appear to be involved.[346,347] Both fast feedback and intermediate feedback appear to be mediated by inhibition of the release of existing CRH and ACTH rather than by inhibition of their synthesis. Fast feedback and intermediate feedback are distinguished in animals by the effects of certain agents in overcoming glucocorticoid suppression[344] and possibly by a requirement for protein synthesis to maintain intermediate feedback. Increased concentrations of glucocorticoids accelerate the progression from fast to slow feedback. Slow feedback is characterized by decreased or absent synthesis of ACTH, complete suppression of POMC gene transcription, unresponsiveness to the administration of CRH, and a decrease in the pituitary content of ACTH. Glucocorticoids decrease the hypothalamic content of CRH[348] and AVP[275] and also decrease AVP mRNA content[349] but have a lesser effect on CRH mRNA.[350] With increasing dose and duration of glucocorticoid exposure (such as in long-term Cushing's disease and long-term pharmacologic glucocorticoid therapy), the pituitary becomes completely unresponsive even to extreme stimuli.[337,338,344] When glucocorticoid concentrations return to normal, the recovery of the hypothalamic-pituitary axis may be slow and, depending on the dose and duration of glucocorticoid exposure, recovery of fully normal function may take months (see Chap. 15).

Regulation of Mineralocorticoids

Secretion of aldosterone from the zona glomerulosa accounts for most, but not all, mineralocorticoid activity in human plasma. Other glomerulosa steroids secreted in small quantities, such as DOC, 18-OH DOC, 18-OH-corticosterone, 18-OH-cortisol, and 19-oxo-cortisol, also have some mineralocorticoid activity. The secretion of these glomerulosa steroids is regulated primarily by the renin-angiotensin system and by potassium ion and, to a lesser degree, by ACTH, sodium ion, and other factors. The zona fasciculata, under the control of ACTH, also secretes appreciable quantities of DOC.[350] Extraadrenal production of DOC can also contribute appreciable min-

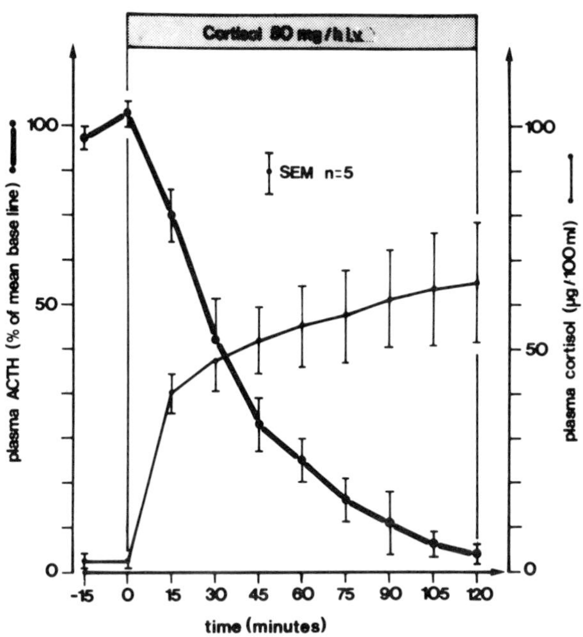

FIGURE 12-15 Time course of ACTH concentrations in response to cortisol constantly infused at 50 mg/h in patients with Addison's disease. ACTH values are given as a percentage of the individual mean starting levels. The difference between ACTH values at 15 min and the starting value was significant ($p < 0.025$). *(From Fehm et al.[346])*

eralocorticoid activity, especially in the fetus and during pregnancy.[192–194] Finally, it is important to remember that cortisol also has appreciable mineralocorticoid activity, especially when present in excess.

The Renin-Angiotensin System

Renin

Renin is a serine protease enzyme synthesized largely by the juxtaglomerular cells of the kidney; this accounts for virtually all circulating renin activity. Renin is also produced in a variety of other tissues, including the glomerulosa cells of the adrenal cortex,[351] and adrenal renin appears to act as a paracrine factor regulating expression of the gene that encodes P450c11AS but not P450c11β.[351,351a] Renin is initially synthesized as a preproprotein of 406 amino acids[352] that is cleaved to 386-amino acid prorenin and then to the mature 340-amino acid form of renin. Both prorenin and renin can be found in the circulation. Hypotension, upright posture, sodium depletion, vasodilatory drugs, kallikrein, opiates, and β-adrenergic stimulation all promote the release of renin from the renal juxtaglomerular cells. Of these, serum sodium concentration is most important (Fig. 12-16). Renin enzymatically attacks angiotensinogen, the renin substrate, in the circulation. Angiotensinogen is a highly glycosolated protein and therefore has a highly variable molecular mass ranging from 50,000 to 100,000 daltons. This renin substrate is regulated in part by estrogens and hence is elevated in pregnancy and in women taking oral contraceptives. Renin proteolytically releases the amino-terminal 10 amino acids of angiotensinogen, referred to as angiotensin I. This decapeptide is biologically inactive until its two carboxy-terminal amino acids are cleaved by the action of converting enzyme to become the octapeptide, angiotensin II. Converting enzyme is found principally in the lungs and blood vessels. Because converting enzyme is a metalloenzyme containing zinc, it can be inhibited by chelating agents and certain metals. However, the only therapeutically useful inhibitors of converting enzyme are analogs of its substrate, angiotensin I, such as captopril. Such agents are useful in the diagnosis and treatment of hyperreninemic hypertension. For a detailed discussion of the renin-angiotensin system, see Chap. 14.

Angiotensin II

The octapeptide angiotensin II (and in some species its amino-terminally cleaved heptapeptide derivative, angiotensin III) has two principal actions, both of which increase blood pressure. It directly stimulates arteriolar vasoconstriction within a few seconds and stimulates the synthesis and secretion of aldosterone within minutes.[110,353] Angiotensin II binds to receptors on the surface of glomerulosa cells with an affinity of about 0.5 n*M*.[354] The number of these receptors increases in response to angiotensin II and potassium ion and decreases in hypokalemia. Angiotensin does not work through cAMP and the protein kinase A pathway[355] but acutely stimulates mineralocorticoid production by hydrolysis of phosphatidyl inositol, mobilization of intracellular Ca^{2+}, influx of extracellular Ca^{2+}, and activation of protein kinase C.[110] Short-term stimulation of adrenal cells with angiotensin II or other activators of protein kinase C will stimulate the production of aldosterone and the enzymes needed for its synthesis. However, prolonged stimulation will repress the production of those enzymes and aldosterone.[113–115,356] It appears that much, if not all, of this biphasic response to angiotensin II is mediated directly at the level of transcription of the genes for the steroidogenic enzymes, especially of the gene for P450scc.[105,357] When the promoter of the human P450scc gene is transfected into mouse adrenal Y-1 cells, both the transfected human promoter and the endogenous mouse P450scc promoter can be stimulated acutely by calcium ionophore and phorbol ester, which are agonists of the protein kinase C pathway. The action of these two agents on P450scc gene transcription is synergistic, rapid, and biphasic, so that prolonged exposure represses transcription of the P450scc gene to levels substantially below baseline.[105] These actions appear to be mediated by several regions of the P450scc gene promoter, but these are clearly differ-

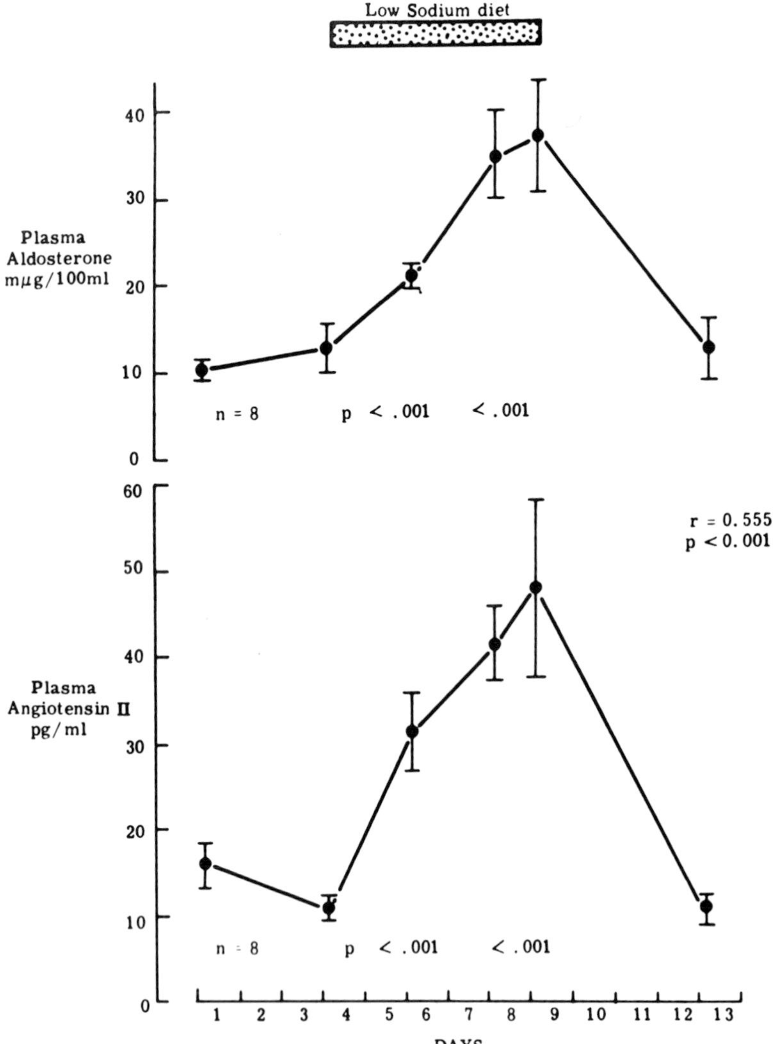

FIGURE 12-16 Effect of a low-sodium diet on plasma angiotensin II and aldosterone concentrations in normal subjects. *(From Brown et al.[374]).*

ent from those which mediate induction by cAMP (stimulated by ACTH).[105] Thus, the hormonal regulation of glucocorticoids (cortisol) and mineralocorticoids (aldosterone) is clearly distinct at all levels: the circulating hormonal stimuli, the intracellular second messengers, and the DNA sequences conferring the regulation to the gene for P450scc.

The potential role of angiotensin II in stimulating the late steps in the synthesis of aldosterone is not clear. Because 18-hydroxylase and 18-methyl oxidase activities are specifically associated with mineralocorticoid production, the potential role of angiotensin II in regulating these activities has been of interest. As was discussed in Steroid Hormone Biosynthesis, above, these activities are mediated by P450c11AS, a glomerulosa-specific enzyme encoded by one of the two duplicated genes for P450c11. The transcriptional regulation of the gene encoding P450c11β has been studied in the mouse,[358–361] showing inducibility by cAMP and both P450c11β and P450c11AS can be induced by cAMP in human adrenal NCI-H295 cells,[358–361] but the transcriptional regulation of the human gene for P450c11AS has not been studied in detail. Similarly, the potential actions of angiotensin II on the earliest steps of steroidogenesis (production of cholesterol and its flux to the mitochondria) have not been studied in detail.

Potassium Ion

Increases in plasma K^+ stimulate aldosterone production, and decreased plasma K^+ decreases aldosterone production and blunts its response to hyponatremia.[362–365] The zona glomerulosa is sensitive to very small changes in K^+, independent of the concentrations of Na^+ and angiotensin II. Prolonged hyperkalemia, prolonged exposure to angiotensin II, and chronic hyponatremia will cause hypertrophy of the adrenal zona glomerulosa and increase its sensitivity to hormonal induction. Although hyperkalemia decreases renin release, its action of stimulating aldosterone secretion predominates.[365] These divergent actions correspond to the different intracellular actions of potassium and angiotensin II on steroidogenesis. Potassium ion probably acts by depolarizing the glomerulosa cell membrane, facilitating increased uptake of extracellular calcium ion. As in the actions of angiotensin II, increased intracellular calcium increases hydrolysis of phosphoinositides. Thus, the similar actions of K^+ and angiotensin II differ in that K^+ primarily stimulates the uptake of calcium ion with secondary effects of decreasing the formation of phosphatidic acid and phosphoinositides, while angiotensin II initially affects the hydrolysis of phosphatidyl inositol. Thus, angiotensin II and potassium work at different levels of the same intracellular second messenger pathway, but they differ fundamentally from the action of ACTH. As with angiotensin II, however, the potential action of potassium on the late steps in aldosterone synthesis has not been studied in depth.

ACTH and Other Factors

POMC Peptides

ACTH and other peptides derived from POMC can influence aldosterone production, although to a much smaller degree than can angiotensin II and potassium ion. Neither acute hypophysectomy nor long-term administration of dexamethasone will lower basal aldosterone secretion or its responsiveness to sodium depletion. However, some patients with long-term hypopituitarism have blunted aldosterone responses, and decreased aldosterone production has been described in isolated ACTH deficiency.[365,366] The effects of ACTH on aldosterone are variable in different species, with relatively lesser effects in human beings, and may be permissive. Alternatively, they may reflect less than complete functional distinction between the zona glomerulosa and the zona fasciculata. Other POMC peptides, such as β-endorphin,[367] β-MSH,[368] and portions of the N-terminal glycopeptide such as γ3-MSH,[369] have all been reported to stimulate mineralocorticoid synthesis. Although there is no definitive evidence that POMC peptides regulate aldosterone production, it appears that cAMP, the second messenger of ACTH action, stimulates the production of the P450c11AS enzyme required for the late steps in aldosterone synthesis.[357]

Sodium Ion, ANP, and Other Factors

Hyponatremia increases and hypernatremia decreases aldosterone secretion, principally by the effects of intravascular volume and sodium ion on the renin-angiotensin system (Fig. 12-16). Small changes in sodium concentration can also have a substantial effect on the angiotensin-induced or potassium-induced secretion of aldosterone. These actions appear to be independent of the osmotic effects of sodium, possibly accounting for blunted aldosterone responses during water deprivation.[370]

Other factors can also influence aldosterone secretion. Ammonium ion can stimulate plasma aldosterone,[371] but it is not clear if this effect is direct or secondary to the effects of acidosis on renin and potassium. Dopamine appears to inhibit the stimulation of aldosterone secretion by other factors,[367,372] possibly by affecting late steps in the mineralocorticoid pathway, but the physiologic relevance of this is unclear, as dopamine infusion does not diminish circulating concentrations of aldosterone or their response to angiotensin II.

Atrial natriuretic peptide (ANP) appears to be a potent inhibitor of aldosterone synthesis but has no detectable effect on cortisol synthesis.[373] ANP is synthesized and possibly secreted by a wide variety of tissues in addition to cardiocytes, including the adrenal medulla, but is not produced by the adrenal cortex.[374] The biologically active 28-amino acid peptide increases with increased intravascular volume and serum sodium[375] and inhibits aldosterone secretion. However, although glucocorticoids regulate ANP secretion,[376,377] no role has been established for mineralocorticoids in ANP regulation.

Regulation of Adrenal Androgens

ACTH is the principal agent regulating adrenal androgen synthesis. Plasma concentrations of DHEA and androstenedione follow the patterns of circadian and episodic secretion of cortisol closely, rise in response to the administration of ACTH, and fall when ACTH secretion is blocked by glucocorticoids. Concentrations of DHEA-S, which is quantitatively the principal secretory product of the human adrenal, do not follow this pattern as clearly because of its very long plasma half-life, yet DHEA-S is increased by chronic elevations of ACTH and suppressed by chronic ACTH deficiency. However, despite the closely parallel secretion of cortisol and adrenal androgens, substantial evidence indicates that factors other than ACTH have a specific effect on adrenal androgens.[153,307,378–385]

Adrenarche

The term *adrenarche,* which was first coined by Fuller Albright,[386] refers to the onset of increased adrenal androgen secretion in children at about 8 years of age. Circulating plasma concentrations of DHEA-S are a simple effective index of adrenarche[153]; DHEA-S has a long plasma half-life and exhibits little diurnal variation.[387–389] Although the gonads produce DHEA and androstenedione as precursors to testosterone and estrogens, they secrete negligible amounts of DHEA and DHEA-S. More than 90 percent of circulating DHEA-S derives either from direct adrenal secretion[390–392] or from peripheral sulfation of DHEA secreted by the adrenals.[390–392] Furthermore, plasma concentrations of DHEA and DHEA-S are essentially the same in boys and girls before puberty and during the early stages of puberty to Tanner stage III.[387,390,393,394]

Because the effects of adrenal androgens are mild and because the onset of adrenarche is usually followed by the onset of puberty within 2 years, endocrinologists often fail to understand that adrenarche is independent of puberty. Whereas puberty is defined as the activation of the hypothalamic-pituitary-gonadal axis [and hence begins with increased secretion of hypothalamic gonadotropin releasing hormone (GnRH)], adrenarche is independent of GnRH and gonadotropins. Children under age 6 years with true central precocious puberty have increased responses of gonadotropins to GnRH and increased serum concentrations of gonadotropins and sex steroids but have DHEA-S concentrations indistinguishable from those of age-matched controls.[153] Similarly, patients with gonadal dysgenesis (Turner's syndrome) have increased responses of gonadotropins to GnRH and increased circulating gonadotropin concentrations but have DHEA-S concentrations indistinguishable from those of age-matched controls.[153] Thus, the increased secretion of adrenal androgens at adrenarche is not regulated by the hypothalamic-pituitary-gonadal axis and is not associated with increased secretion of ACTH or cortisol.

The developmental timing of adrenarche and its independence from gonadotropins, ACTH, and angiotensin II have prompted a search for other mechanisms for the induction of adrenarche. One hypothesis posits the existence of a pituitary hormone that specifically stimulates the zona reticularis, analogous to the action of angiotensin II on the glomerulosa or that of ACTH on the fasciculata. The advocates of this hypothesis generally consider that such a hormone would work synergistically with ACTH to stimulate adrenal androgens.[153,379] In fact, the zona reticularis does exhibit characteristic structural changes at the time of adrenarche.[395] This factor has been termed adrenal androgen stimulating hormone (AASH)[153] or cortical androgen stimulating hormone (CASH).[378] Putative identification of various candidates for CASH has been reported,[396,397] but careful studies have shown these substances to be inactive.[154–156] Thus, there is no chemical evidence for CASH, yet its existence cannot be ruled out or discounted until the mechanisms of adrenarche are delineated.

An alternative explanation of adrenarche posits that increased adrenal DHEA-S secretion at adrenarche is secondary to changes in adrenal mass and architecture and steroid concentrations.[398] This view is based on the ability of estrogens to inhibit 3β-HSD activity and the fact that adrenal 3β-HSD activity changes as a function of age during childhood. Measurements of intraadrenal steroid concentrations correlate well with the corresponding plasma concentrations of DHEA and cortisol throughout life.[398] None of the current hypotheses about adrenarche account for the fact that the 17,20-lyase activity of P450c17 appears to depend on the relative availability of reducing equivalents from P450 reductase[180,181,399] (see Steroid Hormone Biosynthesis, above). We favor the hypothesis that adrenarche is regulated via the abundance of P450 reductase or by a regulated posttranslational change in either P450c17 or P450 reductase that increases the association of those two proteins.

Adrenal versus Ovarian Sex Steroids

Plasma concentrations of androstenedione, testosterone (T), and dihydrotestosterone (DHT) vary during the menstrual cycle as a result of ovarian secretion of androstenedione and its peripheral conversion to T and DHT.[400,401] Plasma androstenedione averages 125 ng/dl and testosterone averages 25 ng/dl during the early follicular phase, and these values rise to 200 ng/dl and 50 ng/dl, respectively, during midcycle.[400] During the follicular phase, the adrenal accounts for about 67 percent of the testosterone, about 50 percent of the DHT (via peripheral conversion of testosterone), 55 percent of the androstenedione, 80 percent of the DHEA, and 96 percent of the DHEA-S.[400] During midcycle, the adrenal contribution to testosterone and androstenedione drops to 40 percent and 30 percent respectively.[400] Small amounts of estradiol and estriol are also synthesized by the adrenal, but most of the adrenal contribution to circulating estrogens is due to conversion of adrostenedione to estrone by 17-KSR in peripheral tissues. In postpubertal males, the adrenal contribution to circulating androgens is quantitatively similar to that in females but is biologically negligible because of the 10- to 20-fold higher levels of testosterone produced by the testes.

Adrenal androgens play no known essential role. However, as was described above, the adrenal contributes most of the circulating androgens in women. These adrenal androgens are thus important in the development of the partial virilization that accompanies development of normal female secondary sexual characteristics. Thus, the development of pubic and axillary hair, body odor, and comedones in pubertal females is due primarily to synergism between ovarian estrogens and adrenal androgens.

PLASMA STEROIDS AND THEIR DISPOSAL

Quantities of Steroids Produced

Several techniques have been devised to estimate the secretion rates of the steroid hormones,[402,403] and despite methodologic problems, reasonable estimates have been obtained[403–409] (Table 12-2). Cortisol is the adrenal steroid secreted in the greatest quantity, and its production has generally been estimated to be 8 to 25 mg/day.[403,406,407] However, in a

TABLE 12-2 Secretion Rates and Plasma Concentrations of Various Steroids*

Steroid	Secretion rate, mg/24 h	Ref.	Plasma concentration, ng/ml	Ref.
Aldosterone	0.15	406	0.15–0.17	Chap. 14
Androstenedione	2.5 (F)	403	1.80 ± 0.21 (F)	404
	2.2 (M)	403	1.14 ± 0.21 (M)	404
Corticosterone	1–4	403, 406, 407	2.4 ± 1.5 (F)†	408
			5.4 ± 2.2 (M)†	408
Cortisol	8–25	403, 406, 407	85 (20–140) (F)	409
	9.9 ± 2.7	410–412	116 (40–180) (M)	409
11-Deoxycorticosterone (DOC)	0.6	403, 406, 407	0.15–0.17	Chap. 14
11-Deoxycortisol	0.4	406	0.95–2.5	406
DHEA	0.7 (F)	406	5.34 ± 1.57 (F)	404
	3.0 (M)	404	5.53 ± 1.78 (M)	404
DHEA-S	6–8	403, 404	1130 ± 280 (F)	404
			1260 ± 340 (M)	404
Etiocholanolone sulfate	—	—	17 ± 6 (F)	404
			15 ± 4 (M)	404
Etiocholanolone glucuronide			15 ± 5 (F)	404
			18 ± 7 (M)	404
Progesterone (M)			0.2 ± 0.09 (F)‡	408
			11.8 ± 7.00 (F)§	408
			0.18 ± 0.10 (M)	408
17α-Hydroxyprogesterone			0.58 ± 0.26 (F)‡	408
			1.96 ± 0.75 (F)	408
			0.18 ± 0.06 (M)	408
Testosterone	0.23 (F)	404	0.48 ± 0.14 (F)	404
			5.59 ± 1.51	404

* Values are for adults and are given as mean values alone, with ranges, or ± SD. F and M denote females and males, respectively. Data on 18-hydroxycorticosterone and 18-hydroxydeoxycorticosterone can be found in Chap. 14. For many of the steroids, plasma concentrations vary with the time of day and, in females, with the menstrual cycle. Levels also change with growth and development and with aging. Estradiol and estrone production in males is extremely low and is not listed. The selection of literature sources is somewhat arbitrary; values vary in different reports.

† Samples taken 8 to 9 A.M.

‡ Follicular phase of the menstrual cycle.

§ Luteal phase of the menstrual cycle.

recent study using stable isotope infusion, the cortisol production rate in normal adult volunteers was considerably lower at 9.9 ± 2.7 mg/24 h (5.7 mg/m^2 per day).[410] A second study using the same method showed virtually identical results in male and female children and adolescents; i.e., the cortisol production rate was 9.5 ± 2.5 mg/day or 6.8 ± 1.9 mg/m^2 per day.[411] An additional study using deconvolution analysis in normal adolescent males demonstrated a cortisol production rate of 5.7 ± 0.3 mg/m^2 per day.[412] The only other major glucocorticoid, corticosterone, has a secretion rate of 1 to 4 mg/24 h.[403,406,407] The adrenal production of cortisone is only about 4 percent that of cortisol.[403] Adrenal production of DHEA-S is also high, i.e., 6 to 8 mg/day; the adrenals secrete 90 percent of this steroid in females[413] and an even greater percentage in males. This gland also makes appreciable quantities of androstenedione (50 percent of the production in females and a higher percentage in males)[413] and its 11-oxygenated derivatives, 11-ketoandrostenedione and 11β-hydroxyandrostenedione.[404,414] Androstenedione is converted to testosterone more readily than is DHEA or DHEA-S (Fig. 12-4). Adrenal testosterone accounts for only a minor fraction of total production in men (Chap. 16). In women, the adrenals and ovaries each contribute about 25 percent of total testosterone by direct secretion.[415] The remaining 50 percent is derived from peripheral conversion of androstenedione and, to a lesser extent, DHEA.[413,415] 17α-Hydroxypregnenolone and progesterone are produced in small quantities by the normal adrenal cortex and in much higher quantities in various pathologic states.[404] Negligible quantities of estradiol are produced by the adrenal. Aldosterone is produced in small quantities, but this steroid is active at low concentrations. Significant quantities of DOC are also produced.

Inhibitors of Adrenal Steroid Biosynthesis

A number of compounds inhibit adrenal steroid biosynthesis by enzymatic inhibition or through a cytotoxic effect on adrenocortical cells (for reviews, see Refs. 414 and 416–422). These compounds have been useful for research and in the diagnosis and treatment of adrenal disorders (discussed below).[420–423]

Mitotane (*o,p'*-DDD) is a derivative of DDT that was first noted to cause adrenal insufficiency in dogs.[421] The compound inhibits the mitochondrial enzymes P450c11 and P450scc, leading to decreased synthesis of glucocorticoids and DHEA in the zona fasciculata and zona reticularis.[421–424] There are relatively minor effects on the zona glomerulosa, and aldosterone production usually remains normal. Mitotane also causes structural damage to mitochondria and thus causes necrosis of the inner two zones of the cortex. It also alters hepatic metabolism of cortisol, leading to decreased urinary excretion of 17-hydroxycorticosteroids.[419,421,423,424] Mitotane is used to treat patients with adrenocortical carcinoma and, to a lesser extent, patients with Cushing's disease (discussed below).

Metyrapone in the usual doses administered to humans is a selective inhibitor of P450c11 in all zones of the adrenal cortex.[421,423] Thus, the lesion is identical to that seen with congenital deficiency of P450c11; i.e., there is inhibition of both cortisol and aldosterone secretion and a secondary rise in ACTH and renin production. Steroids proximal to the inhibited steps increase, leading to increased levels of 11-deoxycortisol, DOC (hypertension and hypokalemia), and adrenal androgens (hirsutism). Metyrapone is useful as a test of pituitary-adrenal reserve and in therapy for Cushing's syndrome.[425]

Aminoglutethimide, which was developed as an anticonvulsant, inhibits P450scc, thus blocking the synthesis of all adrenal steroids.[421–423,426] This drug also blocks the conversion of adrenal androgens to estrogens and is used to inhibit estrogen synthesis in patients with breast carcinoma.[427]

Cyanoketone and trilostane are inhibitors of 3β-hydroxysteroid dehydrogenase and thus decrease the production of all classes of adrenocortical steroids.[421] Cyanoketone has not been used in humans, and there are conflicting reports of the efficacy of trilostane in Cushing's syndrome.[422,428,429]

Ketoconazole, an imidazole antifungal agent, is an inhibitor of cytochrome P450 enzymes.[420,430,431] This inhibition accounts for both its antifungal effects and its inhibition of steroidogenesis. In the adrenal, ketoconazole inhibits P450c11 and P450scc.[420,431] These effects decrease cortisol production when doses greater than 800 mg/day are utilized in the treatment of fungal infections.[420] When doses of 800 to 1200 mg/day are utilized in patients with Cushing's syndrome, the majority have normalization of cortisol secretion.[420,430,431]

Etomidate, an imidazole anesthetic agent, has also been shown to inhibit P450c11 and, to a lesser extent, P450scc.[420,421,432,433] This drug was found to impair cortisol and aldosterone secretion and to inhibit the response of these hormones to ACTH.[420] Its prolonged use to sedate patients in the intensive care unit is associated with increased mortality.[420,432] In one study, etomidate was shown to rapidly reduce the hypercortisolism of Cushing's syndrome, but its clinical role has not been defined.[433]

A number of other compounds also inhibit adrenal steroid biosynthesis. Macromolecular synthesis inhibitors block overall steroidogenesis and have been useful for research.[416] Heparin can inhibit aldosterone biosynthesis in vivo but not in vitro.[416,417] This effect requires several weeks and sometimes occurs with heparin therapy.[434] Spironolactone can block aldosterone biosynthesis,[418,435] predominantly at the 11β-hydroxylation and 18-dehydrogenation steps.[427,435] This may contribute to the antimineralocorticoid actions of this compound (in addition to its antagonist actions, as discussed below) and may explain why the plasma aldosterone response to renin is blunted after spironolactone therapy (see Chap. 14).[435]

Physical State of Steroids in Plasma

Cortisol and Other Glucocorticoids

The cortisol released by the adrenal gland is free. However, approximately 90 to 97 percent of the circulating cortisol is bound by plasma proteins (see also Chap. 4).[436–441] About 90 percent of this binding is with corticosteroid-binding globulin [(CBG), also termed transcortin], which binds cortisol specifically and with a high affinity (i.e., it is saturable at moderately low concentrations of cortisol) (Fig. 12-17). A lesser quantity of cortisol is bound by albumin, and a negligible amount by other plasma proteins (Fig. 12-17).

Corticosteroid-Binding Globulin

Some properties of CBG are listed in Table 12-3. This protein has been detected in all species examined, although the levels vary from about 1 μg/dl in the sheep to 100 μg/dl in the iguana and the squirrel.[436] CBG is produced primarily in the liver,[436,441–445] but it has also been found in a number of other tissues, including brain, pituitary, lung, kidney, muscle, and uterus, and in lymphocytes.[441,442,445,446] Human CBG is a 383-amino acid glycoprotein with a molecular weight of approximately 58,000.[436,441,443] Recent studies have shown that CBG is not structurally related to other steroid-binding proteins or to steroid hormone receptors. However, it is similar to several members of the serine protease inhibitor (SERPIN) superfamily.[443,444] It is most closely related to α1-proteinase inhibitor (A1-PI), α1-chymotrypsin (A1-ACT), and thyroxine-binding globulin (TBG).[443,444] This similarity with the SERPIN family has led to speculation that CBG plays a role in delivering cortisol to sites of inflammation.[443–445,447,448]

At the usual concentrations in humans, CBG can bind up to 25 μg/dl of cortisol[436] at physiologic condi-

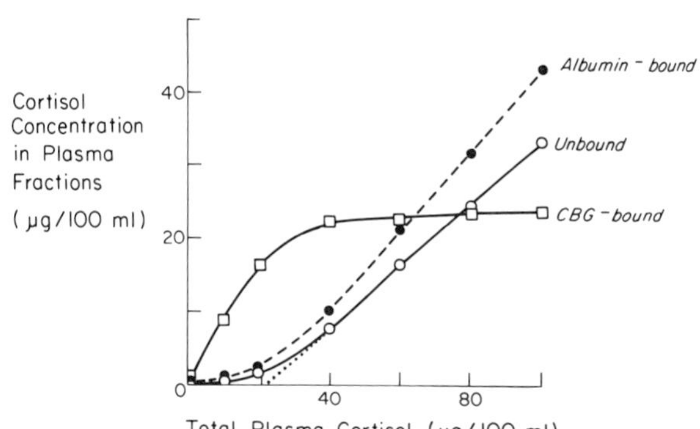

FIGURE 12-17 Distribution of cortisol in plasma. *(From Ballard.[436])*

tions (Fig. 12-17). Cortisol binds to and dissociates rapidly from the protein.[436–438,449] Its affinity for cortisol ($K_d \approx$ 13 to 30 nM)[436–438,449] is such that at a total plasma cortisol of 10 µg/dl the protein is 50 percent saturated, and it is over 90 percent saturated at a total cortisol concentration of 40 µg/dl. Since CBG is the major cortisol-binding protein, the free cortisol in plasma is almost linearly related to the total cortisol at normal concentrations. However, when the total cortisol concentration rises above 25 µg/dl, CBG becomes more saturated with the steroid, and the proportion of the total cortisol that is free increases in a nonlinear fashion (Fig. 12-13). Thus, at a total plasma cortisol concentration of 40 µg/dl, the free cortisol ($\approx$ 10 µg/dl) would be 10-fold higher than it would be at a total plasma cortisol concentration of 10 µg/dl (free cortisol concentration $\approx$ 1 µg/dl).

A number of other endogenous and synthetic steroids also bind to CBG (Table 12-4).[436,439,444,450] However, considering their affinity for CBG and/or their plasma concentrations, the extent of this binding in physiologic circumstances is ordinarily minor and almost all the CBG-bound steroid is cortisol. One exception is third-trimester pregnancy, in which increased progesterone accounts for about 25 percent of the total CBG-bound steroid.[436,437] Also, in congenital adrenal hyperplasia (discussed below and in Chap. 4), several steroids can be elevated enough to occupy CBG to a major extent. These include corticosterone, 17α-hydroxyprogesterone, progesterone, 11-deoxycortisol, DOC, and 21-deoxycortisol. Most of the synthetic glucocorticoids used in therapy (prednisolone is an exception) have a low affinity for CBG (Table 12-5) and therefore bind negligibly to it (see also Chap. 15). Whereas prednisone and cortisone bind weakly, these compounds are converted to prednisolone and cortisol, which bind tightly.

The CBG concentrations in plasma vary between individuals and are also regulated by hormones and other factors.[441,444,445,448] Circulating glucocorticoids at supraphysiologic concentrations decrease CBG concentrations.[445,448] Estrogens increase CBG levels, and elevated concentrations are seen in pregnancy and with estrogen therapy and oral contraceptive use.[436,438] In pregnancy, CBG levels gradually rise and are twice normal in the third trimester.[437] With estrogen treatment, the effect is maximal in about 3 to 5 days, and CBG levels return to normal 2 to 3 weeks after the cessation of therapy.[437] Thyroid hormones increase CBG synthesis[438]; CBG levels are reduced in hypothyroidism and increased in hyperthyroidism.[438] Elevated CBG levels in some cases may have a genetic basis and can be associated with certain HLA types.[438,451,452] Elevated levels also occur in diabetes, chronic active hepatitis,[451,453] and certain hematologic disorders.[451] CBG levels are subnormal in liver disease (decreased protein production), multiple myeloma, obesity, and the nephrotic syndrome (urinary loss of protein).[436,437,444,445,448,454] Complete absence of CBG has not been substantiated, but there is a familial condition in which CBG levels are about 50 percent of normal with normal plasma free cortisol concentrations and no clinical symptoms.[448,455,456]

Albumin and Other Cortisol-Binding Proteins

Cortisol binding to albumin has different characteristics. The kinetics of cortisol association with and dissociation from albumin are much more rapid than is the case with CBG. The affinity of albumin for cortisol is much lower, but the capacity is over 1000-fold higher than that of CBG (Table 12-3).[436,438] At cortisol concentrations below 20 µg/dl, about 7 percent of the plasma cortisol is albumin-bound.[439] With an increasing cortisol level, CBG becomes saturated with the steroid, and a larger proportion of the plasma-bound steroid is associated with albumin (Fig. 12-17).[436]

Synthetic glucocorticoids are bound by albumin with an affinity similar to or slightly exceeding that of cortisol.[436] For instance, 55 percent of the total prednisolone, 62 percent of the betamethasone, and 77 percent of the dexamethasone are bound by human plasma.[436]

Although the proportion of free steroid bound by albumin is relatively independent of the steroid concentration, it is affected by the plasma albumin concentration.[436] Thus, in premature infants and in hypoalbuminemia, the proportion of non-CBG-bound steroid that is free is increased.[436,439]

The α_1 acid glycoprotein that binds progesterone and other steroids also binds cortisol (Table 12-4), but this appears be of minor importance.[436]

Physiologic Role of Plasma Binding

Despite much speculation and intense interest, the precise functions of CBG and other steroid-binding proteins remain obscure (see also Chap. 4).[444,445,448] Traditional and more recent theories are

TABLE 12-3 General Properties of Corticosteroid-Binding Proteins in Human Serum

	CBG	Albumin	α_1 Acid glycoprotein
Molecular weight	58,000	69,000	39,000
Concentration, μM	0.71	550	18
Concentration, g/liter	0.037	38	0.18
Cortisol-binding capacity, μg/dl	25	>20,000	630
Equilibrium dissociation constant for cortisol at 37°C (K_d), M	3×10^{-8}	2×10^{-4}	8.5×10^{-6}
Cortisol-binding sites per molecule	1	1–20	1
Relative distribution of cortisol at 37°C, %	77.3	15.0	0

Source: Modified from Ballard[436]; data from Sandberg and Slaunwhite[437] and Westphal.[438]

TABLE 12-4 Relative Affinities of Steroids for CBG, Cytoplasmic Glucocorticoid Receptor, and Albumin in Humans

	CBG	Relative affinity for receptor*	Albumin
Cortisol	100	100	100
Fluocinolone acetonide	<1	1350	
Methylprednisolone	<1	1190	74
Dexamethasone	<1	710	>100
Betamethasone	<1	540	>100
Fluorometholone	<1	400	
9α-Fluorocortisol	<1	350	
Triamcinolone acetonide	<1	190	
Corticosterone	94	85	100
Prednisolone	58	220	61
Aldosterone	6	38	34
11-Deoxycorticosterone (DOC)	45	39	221
11-Deoxycortisol	77	19	
Progesterone	27	11	244
17α-Hydroxyprogesterone	70	>1	225
Prednisone	6	5	68
Cortisone	6	1	128
Testosterone	5	2	232
Pregnenolone	<1		
Estradiol	<1	5	1600
Estrone	<1		800
Androstenedione	<1	<1	223
Dehydroepiandrosterone (prasterone, DHEA)	<1		506

Note: Data for CBG and receptor obtained at 2°C; however, the relative binding at 37°C is similar overall.

* Human fetal lung.

Source: Ballard.[436]

TABLE 12-5 Urinary Steroid Metabolites of Intravenously Administered Radioactive Cortisol*

Steroid	Percent in extract
Cortols (α and β)	7
Cortolones (α and β)	17
Allocortols and allocortolones	2
Tetrahydrocortisol	14
Tetrahydrocortisone	18
Allotetrahydrocortisol	6
Cortisol	1
6β-Hydroxycortisol	1
Cortisone	1
11β-hydroxyetiocholanolone	4
11-Ketoetiocholanolone	2
11β-Hydroxyandrosterone	<1
Cortoic acids	10

* The data are taken from Peterson[468] and Monder and Bradlow.[470] The precentages of Peterson that did not include the cortoic acids were reduced by 25 percent (and rounded off) to include the contribution of the cortoic acids calculated from the data of Monder and Bradlow as based on the percentage of total cortoic acid relative to the sum of tetrahydrocortisol and tetrahydrocortisone. The numbers reported by different workers show considerable variation, and this table is intended to serve only as a rough estimate. It is also stressed that all the known metabolites have not been included and that there are probably other, unidentified metabolites.

discussed below. One theory is that these proteins serve as a reservoir to sequester steroids in an inactive form, thus influencing the availability of steroids to tissues, their receptors, and steroid-metabolizing enzymes. However, these plasma-binding proteins have not been proved to be essential for transporting steroids in the circulation, as these steroids are sufficiently water-soluble at biologically active concentrations.[436] Further, humans with low CBG levels and animals such as sheep with extremely low CBG levels show no decrement in their responsiveness to glucocorticoids.[436,438,441]

The steroids are inactive when bound by plasma protein.[436,441,449] For example, when tissue culture cells are incubated with cortisol and either CBG or albumin, the glucocorticoid dose response is reduced concomitantly to the extent of cortisol binding.[436,449] Further, the physiologic mechanisms that control the plasma cortisol concentration respond to free rather than total cortisol levels, so that with variations in CBG levels, free cortisol concentrations do not change, even though total cortisol levels do.[436] The CBG-bound cortisol and, to a lesser extent, the albumin-bound cortisol are also protected from metabolic degradation, and when CBG levels are increased, the rate of cortisol clearance is decreased.[436] Thus, the proteins can serve as a reservoir to sequester active steroids.

Whereas in any equilibrium situation the plasma-bound steroids are sequestered in an inactive state, they can become active through dissociation from the proteins. This can occur rapidly. Cortisol can dissociate from albumin with a $t_{1/2}$ of around 5 s at 37°C.[440]

Thus, as the free and protein-bound steroid circulates through the various tissues, the free steroid binds specifically to receptors, steroid-metabolizing enzymes, and other proteins and binds nonspecifically to a number of cellular components. This reduces the free steroid concentration and shifts the equilibrium toward dissociation of plasma protein-steroid complexes. The dissociated steroid is then free for further tissue uptake. Current data are consistent with the hypothesis that tissue uptake of cortisol can be accounted for entirely by the pool of free cortisol. Thus, there is no need to postulate other protein or receptor mechanisms.[457,458] This available fraction depends on both the extent of tissue uptake that shifts the equilibrium and the time of transport.[459] Since the rate of dissociation from albumin is more rapid than that from CBG, steroid bound by albumin is a more readily available source. Since the capillary transit time through tissues such as liver is slower (around 5 s) than it is in tissues such as brain (around 1 s), the former tissues can extract a larger proportion of the cortisol.[459] In fact, brain uptake of corticosterone in the rat approximates the non-CBG-bound (free plus albumin-bound) steroid, whereas in liver it exceeds this fraction by three times and includes CBG-bound steroid.[440,441]

By sequestering the relevant steroid and releasing it more gradually, plasma binding may also serve to dampen the swings in cortisol levels in plasma caused by episodic pulsatile release. This could protect the steroid from metabolic degradation and render changes in receptor occupancy more gradual.

Recent studies have demonstrated that a major role of hormone-binding proteins in plasma may be to ensure uniform delivery and distribution of the hormone to the individual cells of a target tissue.[458,460] Thus, in studies with thyroxine infusion into the perfused rat liver, the absence of binding globulin or prealbumin leads to nonuniform distribution of the hormone, with the major proportion being rapidly taken by the first cells encountered. Conversely, when the thyroxine was infused with its binding proteins, there was uniform uptake and distribution within hepatic cells[458,460] (see also Chap. 4).

CBG is synthesized in the liver.[436,442] However, other tissues have substantial concentrations of CBG or CBG-like proteins, and it is not clear whether these proteins are synthesized locally or taken up from the circulation.[440,444,446]

Additional physiologic roles of CBG are also possible. It has been demonstrated that CBG binds specifically to plasma membranes and leads to increased intracellular cAMP. This binding occurred only when CBG was bound to either cortisol or progesterone.[445,448] The relevance of these observations is unclear. Also, the knowledge that CBG has a structure homologous to that of the SERPIN superfamily led to the observation that the CBG-cortisol complex is cleaved by neutrophil-derived elastase at sites of inflammation.[444,445,447,448] Thus, a possible physiologic role for CBG could be to facilitate the delivery of glucocorticoids to sites of infection and inflammation.[444,445,447,448]

Aldosterone

Aldosterone does not bind to a specific or high-affinity protein, and this steroid weakly binds to plasma proteins, including albumin and CBG.[437,439,459,461,462] It also binds to red cells.[463] At 37°C, about 20 percent of the total aldosterone in plasma is bound to CBG and about 40 percent is bound to other proteins.[439,459] Although high concentrations of cortisol can decrease the total plasma binding of aldosterone slightly, the percentage of free aldosterone in plasma is relatively invariant even with wide fluctuations in the concentrations of this and other steroids.[464]

Although CBG binding of aldosterone is minor relative to total plasma aldosterone, changes in aldosterone binding by this protein can affect the metabolic clearance rate of aldosterone.[461] This occurs, for instance, when cortisol concentrations are low. This greater influence of CBG compared with that of other proteins presumably results from the slower rate of dissociation of aldosterone from CBG than from other plasma-binding proteins, resulting in more of the CBG-bound aldosterone surviving passage through the liver.

Deoxycorticosterone

About 97 percent of circulating DOC is bound by plasma proteins.[439] About 60 percent and 36 percent are associated with albumin and CBG, respectively.[439] The extent of DOC binding by plasma varies little over a wide range of concentrations of this steroid (2 to 200 ng/dl).[464]

Adrenal Androgens and Estrogens

The adrenal androgens, i.e., DHEA, DHEAS, and Δ^4-androstenedione and its 11β-hydroxylated derivatives, are bound extensively to plasma proteins, mostly to albumin.[405,436,439,441,459,465–467] About 98 percent of the testosterone circulating in plasma is bound both to albumin and to a specific testosterone-estradiol-binding globulin (TeBG) whose plasma concentration is increased by estrogens (as in pregnancy) and in hyperthyroidism and is decreased by testosterone and in acromegaly (see Laboratory Evaluation of Adrenocortical Function, below, and Chaps. 16 and 17). Plasma binding of estrogens is discussed in Chap. 17.

Metabolism of Adrenocortical Steroids

The continuous dynamic control of plasma concentrations of the adrenal steroids requires mechanisms for their removal from the body. The hydrophobic steroids are filtered by the kidney but are actively reabsorbed (e.g., about 95 percent of cortisol and 86 percent of aldosterone)[468] and are therefore not excreted into the urine. Thus, the steroids undergo enzymatic modifications that transform them into inactive substances with increased water solubility that can be removed more readily.[468–471] The modifications result largely in the conversion of some of the less polar ketone groups to hydroxyl groups and of the C-21 groups to acid forms. The hydroxyl groups can then be conjugated with glucuronide or sulfate groups, rendering them even more water-soluble. The liver is the major site of metabolic conversion, although most mammalian tissues, including the adrenal, metabolize steroids to some extent, and in pregnancy the placenta is quite active in the metabolism of steroids (see Steroid Synthesis in the Fetal Adrenal, above).[468] These metabolized compounds are then excreted. Illustrative of their enhanced capacity to be excreted is the fact that the renal clearance of a major cortisol metabolite, tetrahydrocortisone glucuronide, is around 70 percent of the creatinine clearance.[468] In most cases, the kidney accounts for over 90 percent of the excretion of metabolized steroids (DOC and corticosterone are exceptions; see below); the remainder are lost in the gut. Most of the metabolized steroids excreted into the gut are reabsorbed; in addition, especially with aldosterone, there can be further metabolism by the intestinal flora before absorption.

Over 50 different metabolites of cortisol and aldosterone have been detected (Fig. 12-18).[468–470] These metabolites are generated by a limited number of metabolic conversions. Since many of the structural differences among the various steroid hormones are eliminated during metabolism, it is often difficult to identify the true precursor(s) of a given metabolite.

Cortisol

Cortisol is cleared with a half-time of 80 to 120 min in various studies (Chap. 15).[468] If radioactively labeled hormone is given, 70 percent of the radioactivity appears in the urine within 24 h and over 90 percent appears by 72 h (Table 12-5).[468] Approximately 3 percent is recovered in the feces.[472] Almost all the radioactivity is present as cortisol metabolites; less than 1 percent appears as unchanged cortisol (Table 12-5).

Cortisol may be modified by several different enzymes. The most important initial reaction is the reduction of the 4,5 double bond by at least two Δ^4-reductases. This reaction is irreversible, inactivates the molecule, and results in dihydrocortisol, which may be an α or a β form depending on the orientation of the hydrogen in the 5 position; the 5α/5β ratio is about 5:1.[468] Dihydrocortisol is rapidly converted by a 3-hydroxysteroid dehydrogenase to tetrahydrocortisol (Table 12-5). Cortisol can be oxidized at the 11β-hydroxyl group by the enzyme 11-β hydroxysteroid dehydrogenase to form the ketone (cortisone); this reaction does not occur after the A ring has been reduced[468] (see Steroid Hormone Biosynthesis, above). The reaction is reversible and may be mediated by two separate enzymes.[473] In general, the equilibrium is shifted to favor the 11-keto form,[473] and thus, there is substantial cortisol-to-cortisone conversion. This conversion increases in hyperthyroidism and is marked in the fetus.[473] Cortisone is in general metabolized similarly to cortisol and therefore is also converted via the dihydro derivative to the tetrahydro metabolite. The net result is that roughly similar quantities of unaltered cortisol and cortisone and their metabolites are excreted (Table 12-5).[470] Cortisol, cortisone, and their tetrahydro derivatives can also be reduced to the cortols and cortolones, respectively, via hydroxysteroid dehydrogenases (Fig. 12-14). There can also be oxidation at C-21 to form cortolic and cortolonic acids (Fig. 12-14) and conversion of the C-17 side chain to the C-20 acid.[470] The conversion to the acidic derivatives renders the steroids even more water-soluble.[470] Reduction of the C-20 keto group of cortisol or cortisone to 20-hydroxycortisol also occurs to a lesser extent. 6β-Hydroxylated or 16α-hydroxylated metabolites of cortisol and other steroids ordinarily are formed in small quantities.[468] However, the 6β-hydroxylation pathway can be of major importance in infants in whom the esterification mechanisms are not fully developed, in some disease states, and after treatment with certain drugs (discussed below).[468,474–476] The 16α-hydroxylation pathway can be important for the conversion of estradiol to estriol. Finally, there can be some oxidative cleavage of the C-17 side chain to C-19 11-oxygenated 17-ketosteroids (5 to 10 percent).[468]

About 96 percent of the C-19 and C-21 metabolites of cortisol and cortisone are excreted as conjugates of cortisol, and less than 1 percent as unchanged cortisol (Table 12-5)[468]; 60 to 70 percent appears as conjugates at the 3α-hydroxyl position with glucuronic acid. A smaller amount of conjugates is formed with the sulfate through the C-21 hydroxyl.[477] The conjugation with glucuronide is due to the glucuronyl transferase, and the glucuronide donor is uridine diphosphoglucuronic acid. Glucuronyl

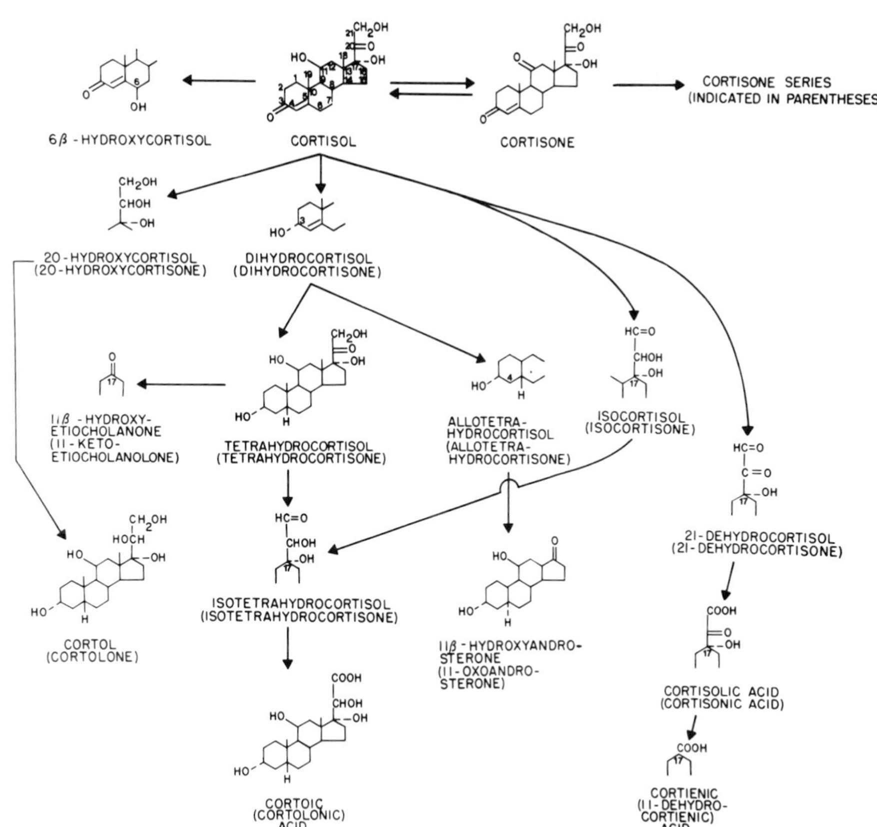

FIGURE 12-18 Pathways of cortisol and cortisone metabolism. Cortisol and cortisone are interconvertible. The steps shown are for cortisol metabolism; however, the metabolism of cortisone is similar. Thus, the name of the 11-keto metabolite resulting from cortisone metabolism is shown in parentheses for each cortisol metabolite. In many cases, only the portion of the steroid affected by the particular metabolic step is shown.

transferase is so active that reduced steroids are almost completely esterified when they leave the liver.[478] Further, this enzyme system differs from that responsible for conjugating bilirubin, because patients defective in the latter enzyme system have a much lesser defect in steroid conjugation.[479]

There are marked variations in cortisol metabolism in various tissues. As was discussed in Steroid Hormone Biosynthesis, above, there is extensive metabolism of cortisol to cortisone in the kidney by 11β-hydroxysteroid dehydrogenase.[252–257] This inactivation is of major physiologic significance since it protects the mineralocorticoid receptor from occupancy by cortisol and thus prevents cortisol from causing a mineralocorticoid excess state.[252–257] The quantitative role of the renal enzyme in total cortisol metabolism is unknown, but plasma cortisone levels are reduced in patients with renal disease.[474,479] In contrast, when cortisone or prednisone (both also have an 11-keto group and no intrinsic glucocorticoid activity) is administered, the steroids are almost completely converted in the liver to cortisol and prednisolone, both of which have 11-hydroxyl groups and thus are biologically active.[252–257]

Corticosterone, 11-Deoxycortisol, and 11-Deoxycorticosterone

The metabolism of corticosterone, 11-deoxycortisol, and DOC is generally similar to that of cortisol except for minor quantitative differences.[468,470] For instance, more corticosterone than cortisol is excreted as the 21-conjugate,[468] its half-time of disappearance is shorter, C-19 metabolites have not been found,[468] and more of the metabolites are excreted into the gut.[470] A much greater proportion of DOC (perhaps 50 percent) is excreted into the gut.[470]

Aldosterone

Aldosterone turns over rapidly,[468,480] with a half-time of 15 min or less; it is almost completely removed by one passage through the liver, and less than 0.5 percent appears in urine in the free state.[468,469,480] About 35 percent of the aldosterone is excreted as tetrahydroaldosterone glucuronide (3 position; see the earlier discussion on cortisol metabolism); up to 20 percent appears as the glucuronide (18 position).[468] This metabolite is termed either the acid-labile conjugate (since free aldosterone can be released from it by hydrolysis at pH 1)[481] or the 3-oxo conjugate (since the 3-oxo group is intact). Determinations of urinary aldosterone usually measure the concentration of this metabolite. The remainder of the aldosterone is metabolized to a variety of other compounds, including a number of polar derivatives such as carboxylic acid and hydroxylated metabolites, and 21-deoxytetrahydroaldosterone.[480] This steroid is probably produced in the gut (after biliary excretion of tetrahydroaldosterone), reabsorbed, and

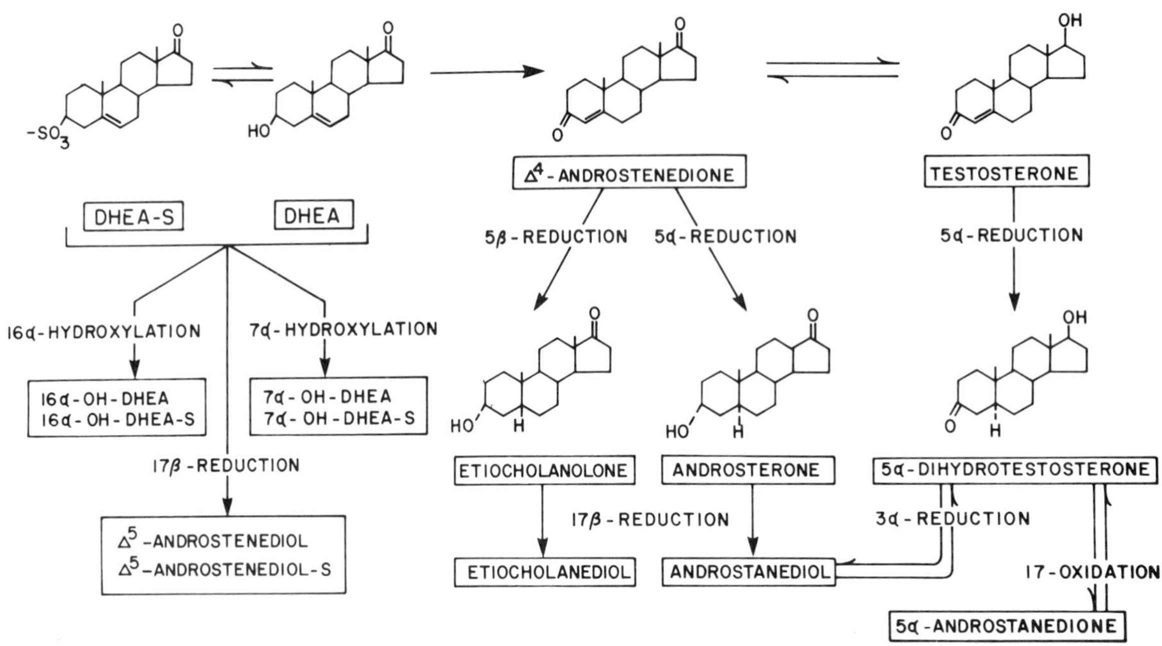

FIGURE 12-19 Major pathways in androgen metabolism. Most of the steps shown are involved in androgen degradation. However, the 5α reduction of testosterone occurs in androgen target tissues to yield the highly active 5α-dihydrotestosterone. See the text for details.

excreted into the urine.[480] There is less metabolic modification of the 11β-hydroxy group of aldosterone than is the case in cortisol because this is protected by the steroid's cyclic 11,18-hemiacetyl form.[469] In the rat, there are significant sex differences in aldosterone metabolism, with a greater proportion of various metabolites being present in male than in female tissues; also, aldosterone metabolism can be affected by both potassium ion and spironolactone.[480]

Androgens and Estrogens[405,415,421,482–484]

The androgens are excreted predominantly as conjugates in the urine; a small fraction is excreted into the gut.[405] Over 80 percent of the androstenedione is removed from the circulation after one passage through the liver.[439] By contrast, only 44 percent of the testosterone is removed.[405] DHEA-S of adrenal origin can be excreted unchanged; DHEA-S is also formed in liver and kidney. Both of these compounds can be further metabolized[439] by either hydroxylation at positions 7 and 16 of transformation of the 17-keto group into a 17β-hydroxyl group (Fig. 12-19). DHEA is also irreversibly converted to androstenedione. As mentioned earlier, androstenedione is converted to testosterone (mostly by extrahepatic tissues) or its 4,5 double bond is reduced, resulting in androsterone or etiocholanolone (Fig. 12-19). These steroids can be further reduced, respectively, to androstenediol and etiocholanediol (Fig. 12-19).[405] Testosterone is also converted in the androgen target tissues to DHT (Chaps. 16 and 18); DHT is reversibly inactivated, mainly by 3α-reduction to 3α-androstenediol[482,483]; a lesser amount is reversibly converted to 5α-androstenedione (Fig. 12-19). Both of these compounds can be converted to androsterone. All these metabolites are further conjugated to glucuronides, and compared with cortisol metabolites, a larger proportion of them are converted to the sulfate derivatives (mostly through the 3 position). The sulfate conjugates are more slowly cleared because they bind more extensively to plasma proteins and are not filtered as well as are the glucuronides.

Testosterone and androstenedione are cleared two to three times more rapidly from plasma in men than in women.[405] Apparently, this is due to an effect of the androgens on their own metabolism, as values more similar to those of females are observed in the testicular feminization syndrome, in which plasma androgen concentrations tend to be elevated and there is peripheral insensitivity to androgens.[405]

Variations in Steroid Metabolism

The rate of metabolism of adrenal steroids is affected by a number of diseases, drugs, and other hormones. Plasma binding was discussed above; agents that increase plasma CBG levels also decrease the rate of cortisol clearance.[436,468] Plasma binding also decreases aldosterone clearance.[461]

In chronic liver disease, the metabolism of cortisol and estrogens is decreased.[468] These effects are relatively specific, since the metabolism of a number of other steroids (e.g., aldosterone, cortisone, and certain cortisol metabolites) is unaffected or minimally affected. This influence may be due to changes in specific metabolizing enzymes and does not result from alterations in hepatic circulation or CBG levels. The decreased metabolism of cortisol tends to decrease cortisol secretion, presumably by feedback inhibition of ACTH release. Thus, urinary excretion of the metabolites of cortisol and other ACTH-dependent steroids (e.g., urinary 17-ketosteroids) is also low in chronic liver disease. However, plasma cortisol is normal unless CBG levels fall. By contrast, the decreased metabolism of estrogens in chronic liver disease results in elevated plasma concentrations of these steroids; such elevations may produce the feminizing features of cirrhosis.

The metabolism of cortisol, aldosterone, and several other adrenal steroids is increased in hyperthyroidism and decreased in hypothyroidism.[468] This apparently is a specific effect of the hormone on biotransformation rather than conjugation and is not due to hypermetabolism per se, as the increase is not observed in other hypermetabolic states. There is also increased secretion of cortisol and aldosterone in hyperthyroidism and decreased secretion in hypothyroidism; these are felt to be compensatory effects on ACTH and renin release that maintain normal plasma steroid levels. They are also reflected by increased urinary 17-hydroxycorticosteroid (17-OHCS) levels in hyperthyroidism and decreased levels in hypothyroidism. The metabolism of progesterone and estrogens is much less affected by alterations in thyroid function, whereas the clearance of the androgens is, if anything, decreased.

The metabolism of corticosteroids is also altered in several other circumstances. Although renal disease affects the clearance of cortisol metabolites, it does not have a major effect on the hepatic metabolism of cortisol.[468] In congestive heart failure, there can be decreased clearance of aldosterone.[468] In general, there are no major differences in cortisol or aldosterone metabolism in chronic diseases, obesity, starvation, stress, anxiety, or depression.[468] In some of these cases, changes in steroid production can alter the amount of steroid excreted.[468] There can also be minor sex differences in the relative metabolic pathways.[480] The clearance of cortisol is decreased in the extremes of old age and infancy[414] but otherwise changes little throughout life.[468] Drugs such as mitotane (*o,p'*-DDD), phenytoin, rifampin, aminoglutethimide, and barbiturates result in differences in the patterns of urinary steroid secretion, including an increase in 6β-hydroxycortisol, but have only a minor influence on the total rate of disappearance of infused cortisol.[414] However, these drugs increase the clearance of synthetic glucocorticoids such as dexamethasone and prednisolone, possibly by affecting the 6β-hydroxy modification and conjugation, which are more important in the metabolism of these steroids.[468,478] The 6β-hydroxycortisol pathway is also increased in patients with liver disease,[476] in hyperestrogenic states,[476] and in cancer or prolonged terminal illness.[475] The antihypertensive agent minoxidil (unlike hydralazine) increases aldosterone clearance, possibly by hemodynamic influences.[485] In pregnancy, the cortisol clearance rate is lowered, probably as a result of increased CBG levels.[468] Finally, there can be some impairment in cortisol clearance in anorexia nervosa and protein-calorie malnutrition.[486]

MOLECULAR MECHANISMS AND PHYSIOLOGIC ACTIONS

Definition of a Glucocorticoid

The term *glucocorticoid* was coined to denote the glucose-regulating properties of these steroids.[487,488] However, glucocorticoids have many actions that do not involve carbohydrate metabolism. Thus, it seems preferable to define adrenal steroid actions in terms of the receptors that mediate them.[488] Thus, a glucocorticoid effect is one that is mediated through a class of receptors termed glucocorticoid receptors. In addition, certain glucocorticoids can act by binding to other classes of receptors, for instance, through mineralocorticoid receptors, in which case the action is termed mineralocorticoid.

Molecular Mechanisms of Glucocorticoid Hormone Action

The molecular events in glucocorticoid hormone action are similar to those of other classes of steroid hormones (Chap. 5).[489–492] In the absence of the steroid, the receptors are predominantly localized in the cytosol (Chap. 5). The receptors are encoded from a single gene, have a molecular weight of about 90,000, and are phosphorylated (Chap. 5).[493,494] There are from 5000 to 100,000 cytoplasmic receptors per cell.[493] They bind cortisol with an affinity constant (K_d) of around 20 to 40 n*M;* this value is close to the free cortisol concentration in plasma, suggesting that saturation of the receptors is probably ordinarily in the range of 10 to 70 percent and that increases or decreases in plasma cortisol will change the receptor occupancy and thus the physiologic responses. These receptors bind a variety of glucocorticoids in proportion to their biological activities.[489]

As described in Chap. 5, the glucocorticoid receptor gene is a member of a much larger family of genes that encode the other steroid hormone receptors, vitamin D receptors, retinoic acid and retinoid X receptors, and a number of other transcription factors. These receptors contain an amino-terminal activation domain that is larger for the glucocorticoid receptor than that of most of the other members of the family, a centrally located DNA-binding domain, and a carboxy-terminal glucocorticoid-binding domain.

This receptor and the receptor-glucocorticoid complex probably mediate almost all the actions of the glucocorticoids on transcription (Chap. 5).[491,495–498] These include both physiologic actions and those in glucocorticoid therapy. However, there are at least two exceptions. First, the fast feedback suppression of ACTH by glucocorticoids occurs too rapidly to be explained by effects on transcription (Fig. 12-5)[499–503]; second, the effects of high-dose glucocorticoids in spinal cord trauma appear to be mediated through other mechanisms (Chap. 15).

Glucocorticoids are also capable of binding to and acting through mineralocorticoid receptors.[256–258,265,504–506] In the kidney, this effect is blocked by the inactivation of glucocorticoids by 11β-hydroxysteroid dehydrogenase.[253–257,507,508] Mineralocorticoid receptors are also present in certain regions of the brain and in the rat are occupied by corticosterone.[257,258] These receptors mediate certain effects of the steroid on brain cell metabolism, serotoninergic neurotransmission, and behavioral adaptation.[505,506] In fact, the affinity of corticosterone for these mineralocorticoid receptors is so high that in the brain they are nearly fully occupied at basal levels of corticosterone.[506] An analogous situation probably occurs in human beings, although most glucocorticoid effects in the brain are mediated through the classic glucocorticoid receptors.

As described in Chap. 5, the unliganded glucocorticoid receptors are associated with at least two heat shock proteins and perhaps with other proteins. Hormone binding induces a conformational change in the receptors termed *activation* (or *transformation*), which results in a dissociation of the heat shock proteins from the receptors. This exposes nuclear translocation sequences on the receptors, resulting in their uptake into the nucleus. It also results in the formation of receptor dimers and exposes DNA- and protein-binding sites on the receptors so that 50 to 70 percent of the hormone-receptor complexes then bind to sites in the chromatin of the nucleus termed *acceptors*.[491]

The receptor-glucocorticoid complexes bind to either DNA sites in the nucleus termed hormone response elements (HREs)[491,492] or proteins involved in transcriptional stimulation. It is of interest that the HREs for the glucocorticoid, mineralocorticoid, progesterone, and androgen receptors are identical (for a review, see Chap. 5 and Refs. 509 and 510). Thus, the specificity of individual hormone action appears to be conveyed by the presence of the receptor and the interaction of the HREs with other factors to form composite response elements.[509,510] The HREs (Chap. 5) contain specific sequences that have a much higher affinity for binding the receptor-glucocorticoid complexes than does random DNA. For the glucocorticoid receptors, these sites tend to be direct palindromes of six base pairs separated by three base pairs (Chap. 5). The protein to which glucocorticoid binding has been most extensively studied is the *jun* component of the *jun* and *fos* complex termed AP1 (see Chap. 5).

Binding of receptor-glucocorticoid complexes to HREs or proteins affects the transcription of nearby genes. The effects can be to either stimulate or inhibit transcription. Thus, the HRE functions as a regulated enhancer element and can function either upstream (with respect to transcription) or downstream (for instance, in an intron), in either orientation, and at a considerable distance away from the promoter for transcriptional initiation.[491,494,511,512] The mechanisms by which these effects occur are not understood, but two types of phenomena are being deciphered. First, different portions of the receptors interact with proteins associated with the proximal promoter and its associated TATA box factors. This could occur directly or through other proteins and ultimately could stimulate or inhibit, directly or indirectly, the initiation of transcription by RNA polymerases. Second, binding of the receptor-glucocorticoid complex to DNA can induce rapid and local influences on chromatin structure that can result in changes in the access of other transcription factors to the DNA, thus influencing transcriptional initiation (Chap. 5).[491,492]

Changes in the production of RNA transcripts in response to the steroid are reflected by consequent influences on the respective mature mRNAs and protein products. The steroid-regulated proteins are responsible for the steroid response. For example, these may be enzymes such as those involved in gluconeogenesis or hormones such as POMC; the latter is an example in which glucocorticoids inhibit transcription.[498] Inhibitory actions can also be mediated by inducing the synthesis of proteins (such as the phospholipase A_2 inhibitor) that block specific cellular functions.

Glucocorticoid receptors have been detected in most tissues.[491] This extensive tissue distribution of receptors contrasts with the much more restricted distribution of the receptors for other classes of steroids (Chap. 5) and is consistent with the notion that glucocorticoids affect most, if not all, mammalian tissues.

There is generally[491] but not exclusively[513] a close correlation between the relative saturation of the receptor by the hormone and the relative magnitude of the glucocorticoid hormone response, suggesting that the receptor concentration limits the magnitude of the steroid hormone response. This contrasts with polypeptide and catecholamine hormones, in which "spare" receptors are present (Chap 5).

A variety of factors can affect glucocorticoid responsiveness.[491,513,514] First, factors in the cell may modulate hormone-binding activity. Second, receptor levels can be regulated by glucocorticoids (ordinarily negatively), the cell cycle, and other factors. However, glucocorticoid receptors are not as extensively regulated as are those for polypeptide hormones. Finally, responsiveness is affected by many of the interrelations with other hormones that were discussed above.

Glucocorticoid action is rapidly reversible. When steroid levels drop, the hormone dissociates from the receptor and the receptor dissociates from the DNA, resulting in a cessation of the effect on gene transcription. The hormone response, however, can be longer-lived because of the persistence of mRNAs and proteins whose levels were increased by the steroid.

The glucocorticoid hormone response is restricted to a small subset of the expressed genes in each cell type. For instance, in cultured pituitary cells, the steroid affects the rate of synthesis of only 1 percent or less of the detectable proteins.[491] In liver, the steroid affects 7 percent of 200 quantifiable proteins.[515] Further, the proteins induced are specific for each cell type; i.e., a given protein may be induced in only one or a few but not all glucocorticoid-responsive tissues. This also indicates that factors other than the presence of the glucocorticoid receptors determine whether the expression of a given gene can be under glucocorticoid hormone control, since the receptors may be similar in the various glucocorticoid-responsive tissues.

Glucocorticoid Agonists and Antagonists

Cortisol, corticosterone, aldosterone, and the synthetic steroids used in steroid therapy (prednisolone, dexamethasone, triamcinolone, etc.) are glucocorticoid agonists and therefore elicit glucocorticoid responses.[489,516] The activity of these compounds depends on their affinity for the receptors and their plasma concentrations. Cortisol and corticosterone have similar affinities for the glucocorticoid receptor (Table 12-4); however, cortisol is the more important glucocorticoid because it circulates at much higher concentrations (Table 12-2). In the syndrome which results when P450c17 is deficient (discussed below and in Chap. 14), corticosterone is the predominant glucocorticoid. Aldosterone is not an important glucocorticoid in humans even in mineralocorticoid excess states, because it does not reach high enough concentrations.

Antagonist steroids can bind to the glucocorticoid receptor; these steroids do not elicit glucocorticoid responses[489,516–518] (Chap. 5) but can compete with agonists for binding to the receptors and thus block the agonist response. Some compounds have partial agonist (partial antagonist) activity such that full receptor occupancy by these steroids results in an intermediate response; when present at a sufficient concentration, they can also block agonist binding, in which case only the intermediate response of the partial agonist will be observed.

Glucocorticoid antagonists are unable to promote the conformational changes in the receptors necessary for subsequent steps in the response[491,519] (Chap. 5). In some cases, antagonist receptor complexes do not bind to the nucleus.[491] However, in other cases they do.[519–522] Relative to cortisol, compounds that have antagonist or partial agonist activity tend to have ketone, hydrogen, or other substitutions of the 11-hydroxyl group; alterations or deletions of the side chain at C-17; C-21 substitutions; reduction of the 4,5 double bond; or bulky 9-position substitutions.[489,516,517,523] Although these substitutions have been studied most extensively in animals, the compound RU-486 (Mifepristone), which contains several changes relative to cortisol, including a (*p*-dimethylamino)phenyl substitution at C-11, has a high affinity for both the glucocorticoid and progesterone receptors[517,518,524,525] and has been shown to be active in humans as an antiglucocorticoid.[526] It has been used to treat patients with Cushing's syndrome due to ectopic ACTH secretion or adrenal carcinomas (see below). Cortisone and prednisone are also antagonists; however, these activities are ordinarily not significant in vivo because their affinities for the glucocorticoid receptor are too low relative to their plasma concentrations in most natural or therapeutic situations.[489]

Structure-Activity Relations of Glucocorticoids: Basis for Biological Activity

The activities of a large number of synthetic and naturally occurring glucocorticoid agonists have been examined. Several factors, such as availability for receptor binding, intrinsic agonist activity, affinity, and clearance, are important. For steroids that are useful for systemic glucocorticoid therapy, two major types of differences relative to cortisol have been found (Chap. 15). First, some compounds are more potent than cortisol because of their increased affinity for the glucocorticoid receptors and/or a decrease in their metabolic clearance rate. Second, some compounds have less mineralocorticoid activity relative to glucocorticoid activity (see Chap. 15), probably because of enhanced glucocorticoid receptor affinity relative to mineralocorticoid receptor affinity. This property results in fewer mineralocorticoid side effects.

In the circulation, affinity is the major immediate determinant of steroid activity at a given time, and the rate of clearance determines the duration of exposure to the steroid. The overall steroid effect is a product of these two parameters. A study with dexamethasone illustrates the need to consider both parameters.[527] This steroid was found to be 17-fold more potent than cortisol when its effect on the suppression of cortisol secretion was extrapolated to zero time. By contrast, dexamethasone was 154 times more potent than cortisol when they were evaluated after 14 h. The early time estimate reflects the intrinsic activity differences between the two steroids but underrates the long-term relative potency of dexamethasone because of the differences in cortisol and dexamethasone clearance. Considerations such as these must be kept in mind when evaluating reports of relative potency. Prednisolone has about a twofold higher affinity for the receptor than does cortisol (Table 12-4) and is cleared more slowly[527]; its net activity is about five times that of cortisol (Chap. 15).

Other factors in evaluating steroid potency are discussed in Chap. 15. In brief, cortisol and the synthetic steroids used in glucocorticoid therapy are readily absorbed in the gut, and their potencies after oral or parental administration are similar. Uptake is a factor, however, when glucocorticoids are given topically or in "depo" injections (Chap. 15). The extent to which variations in the distribution of steroids within body compartments affect activity has not been determined. With the exception of prednisone and cortisone, which are converted to prednisolone and cortisol, respectively, other glucocorticoids do not require metabolic conversion in vivo to be active.

Structural features that promote glucocorticoid activity confer the ability to have agonist (rather than partial agonist or antagonist) activity, enhance the steroid's affinity for the glucocorticoid receptors, and decrease the rate of metabolic inactivation.[489,523] These structural features can be considered in terms of modifications of the progesterone skeleton (substitutions conferring antagonist or partial agonist activity are discussed in the preceding section). Features associated with higher affinity include a reduced 4,5 or 1,2 double bond; a 9α-fluoro or 6α-methyl group; a C-17 side chain; hydroxyl groups at positions 11, 17, and 21; C-3 and C-20 keto groups; and the presence of certain 16- and 17-substitutions (16α- or 16β-methyl, 16,17-acetonide, etc.).

The ways in which such changes affect activity are partly understood.[489,523] Receptor binding involves hydrophobic contact between the surface of the steroid molecule and the receptor protein; removal of hydrophilic water from the steroid via hormone-receptor interaction is perhaps the major force driving the binding reaction, Thus, an increased surface area, such as with 9α-substitution (provided that the substituent is not too large), can increase the strength of binding. Affinity is also enhanced by the presence of key hydroxyl and keto groups that form hydrogen bonds with particular amino acids in the receptor. There is a critical angle between the A and B rings; 9α-substitution and the addition of a 1,2 double bond alter the AB angle to a more optimal position and increase the affinity relative to cortisol. Other substitutions, for instance, the Δ' substitution, render the molecule more resistant to metabolic degradation and decrease its clearance rate.

Actions of Glucocorticoids

The glucocorticoids are ubiquitous as physiologic regulators and play a role in differentiation and development. They are essential for survival, at least to overcome certain stressful insults. Conversely, an excess of these hormones, particularly over a prolonged period, can lead to severe adverse influences (see Cushing's Syndrome, below). Nevertheless, glucocorticoids given in pharmacologic doses can also have useful therapeutic effects (see Chap. 15). Some effects of these steroids are observed only with glucocorticoid excess, as occurs with spontaneous Cushing's syndrome or glucocorticoid therapy.

Intermediary Metabolism

Glucocorticoids were named for their glucose-regulating properties and have extensive influences on carbohydrate, lipid, protein, and nucleic acid metabolism. Although these steroids are secondary to insulin in regulating glucose metabolism in humans, they influence blood sugar levels and play a protective role against glucose deprivation (Chap. 1).[528] This latter role provides an excellent conceptual framework for considering many of the coordinated actions of the glucocorticoids on carbohydrate, lipid, protein, and nucleic acid metabolism (Fig. 12-20).

Carbohydrate Metabolism

Glucocorticoids in excess increase hepatic glycogen and glucose production and decrease glucose uptake and utilization in peripheral tissues.[488,489,529–532] Although the relative importance of these various influences has not been clarified, they result in a tendency to hyperglycemia and decreased carbohydrate tolerance. Conversely, in glucocorticoid deficiency, there is decreased glucose production and hepatic glycogen content and an increased sensitivity to insulin which may result in hypoglycemia. The extent of these effects depends on food intake and on insulin, which opposes many glucocorticoid actions and whose secretion increases in response to steroid-mediated increases in blood glucose concentration. Thus, in a nondiabetic individual exposed to an excess of glucocorticoids, increased insulin secretion counterbalances the glucocorticoid effect so that the fasting blood sugar level, although higher on average, is usually in the normal range even though carbohydrate tolerance is impaired. In a diabetic patient with an inadequate insulin reserve, glucocorticoids in excess exacerbate the carbohydrate intolerance, resulting in an increased insulin require-

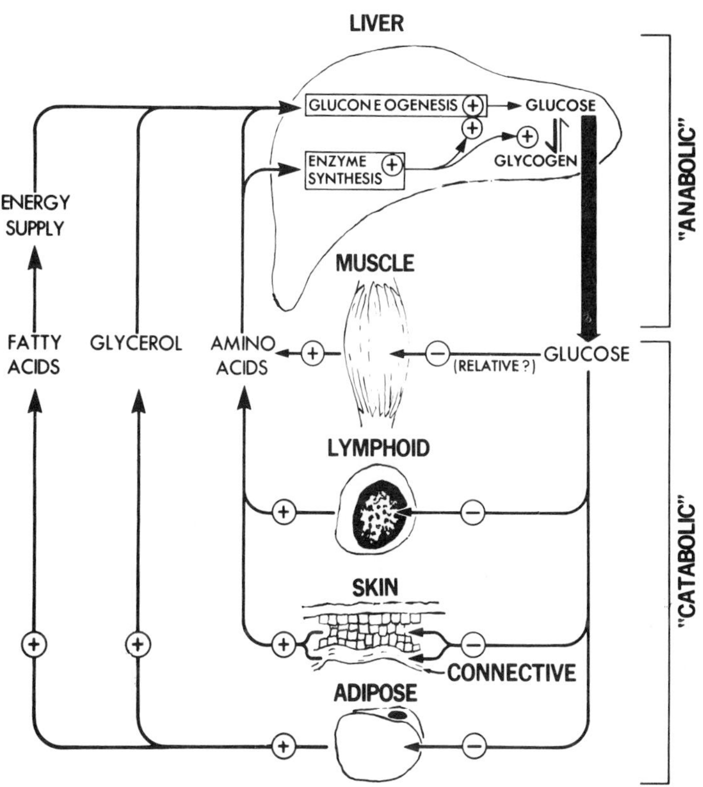

FIGURE 12-20 Glucocorticoid influences on peripheral tissues. Plus signs refer to stimulation, and minus signs to inhibitions. *(From Baxter and Rousseau,[550] modified from Baxter and Forsham, Am J Med 53:573, 1972.)*

ment. Conversely, in an addisonian subject, feeding and a relative decrease in insulin secretion due to the lower blood sugar level blunt the tendency to hypoglycemia so that the fasting blood sugar level is commonly in the normal range.

Glucocorticoids increase glucose production by enhancing hepatic gluconeogenesis, the release of gluconeogenic substrate from peripheral tissues, and the ability of other hormones to stimulate gluconeogenesis.[530] In fed adrenalectomized animals, basal gluconeogenesis is not impaired but there is an impaired response to glucagon or catecholamines (see Chap. 19). In fasted or diabetic animals, adrenalectomy results in a net reduction in hepatic gluconeogenesis which is reversible with cortisol administration. Thus, glucocorticoids are required to maintain gluconeogenesis in fasting and insulin deficiency but not for basal gluconeogenesis in the fed state.

It has been argued that essentially every step in the gluconeogenic pathway is increased by glucocorticoids.[529] Indeed, these steroids increase total hepatic protein synthesis and also increase several of the transaminases, especially alanine aminotransferase.[531,533] These steroids also increase the activity of phosphoenolpyruvate carboxykinase (PEPCK)[533] and possibly glucose-6-phosphatase. However, the changes in PEPCK may be offset by insulin, which depresses the activity of this enzyme.[530] There is little direct information about other gluconeogenic enzymes.

Glucocorticoids also play a permissive role (discussed below) by increasing the sensitivity of the liver to the gluconeogenic actions of glucagon and the catecholamines.[489,529,530,534] For instance, the effect of glucagon or α-adrenergic stimulation on hepatic gluconeogenesis is impaired by adrenalectomy.

Several types of glucocorticoid influences result in an increased release of gluconeogenic substrate from peripheral tissues.[489,529,530,535–537] Perfused muscle from adrenalectomized rats shows a net decrease in the release of amino acids which is reversed by glucocorticoids. The steroids decrease protein synthesis and can increase protein breakdown in several tissues, such as muscle, adipose, and lymphoid, resulting in an increased release of amino acids.[489,529,530,534,536–538] In rats, the inhibition of protein synthesis can be observed in the fed and fasted states and at lower steroid doses, but an enhancement of protein breakdown is observed only in the fasted state and at higher doses.[534,536–538] Although the predominant glucocorticoid effect in muscle may be inhibition of protein synthesis,[530,534,536–538] increased proteolysis from other tissues in response to the steroid may be more prominent.[530,534,536–538] These influences are accompanied by increased urinary excretion of 3-methylhistidine, nitrogen, and plasma amino acids, primarily valine, leucine, isoleucine, tyrosine, phenylalanine, and histidine.[530,534,536–538] These amino acids serve as gluconeogenic precursors, and the conversion of leucine to alanine is increased, as are plasma pyruvate levels.[538] With short exposure, many of these influences can be observed in the absence of changes in plasma insulin and glycogen concentrations.[538] With time, the secondary hyperinsulinism can attenuate the increase in total protein breakdown.[536,537] In humans, the immediate net result of glucocorticoid excess is selective increases in the levels of several amino acids[535,539]; with more prolonged exposure in the fed state, only the alanine concentration is elevated.[537] This is due to the conversion of other amino acids to alanine, which is the major gluconeogenic precursor. Glucocorticoids may also increase the amounts of amino acids available for gluconeogenesis by blocking the stimulatory effects of insulin in peripheral tissues on amino acid uptake and protein synthesis.[530]

Glucocorticoids also increase gluconeogenic substrates by increasing glycerol release from fat cells (by stimulating lipolysis) and lactate release from muscle.[530] The latter effect appears to be due to stimulation of the glycogenolytic actions of the catecholamines. The lipolysis also provides free fatty acids, which cannot themselves contribute to a net increase in gluconeogenesis but can provide energy for gluconeogenesis and spare other substrate that can be converted into glucose.

A second major effect of glucocorticoids on carbohydrate metabolism results from their inhibition of glucose uptake and metabolism in peripheral tissues (Fig. 12-21).[489,538–540] There is a direct inhibition of glucose uptake in adipose tissue,[540,541] fibroblasts,[540] certain lymphoid cells,[540,542] and fat cells.[540] In the last case, they decrease the number of glucose transporter molecules by mechanisms that require protein and RNA synthesis.[540] Even in muscle, the major site of peripheral glucose metabolism, the uptake of glucose (relative to the blood glucose concentration) may be decreased, although a direct effect on glucose uptake has not been demonstrated.[529] The decrease in glucose uptake appears to be the major early influence on carbohydrate tolerance; after cortisol infusion, the blood glucose concentration can rise with no change in glucose output (Fig. 12-21).[538,539]

Glucocorticoids have complex effects on insulin release and action.[532] Glucocorticoid excess results in increased basal and glucose-stimulated insulin levels, and pancreatic beta cell hyperplasia occurs in the long term.[532] These effects are secondary to the glucocorticoid-induced hyperglycemia; reports concerning direct effects of the steroids on the pancreatic islets are in conflict.[532] The elevated glucose and insulin levels imply that insulin resistance is present in the glucocorticoid excess states. This is due primarily to all the anti-insulin actions described above, which are predominantly post-insulin-receptor events.[532,543] In addition, there may be more direct effects on insulin action. It has been reported that glucocorticoids can increase, decrease, or not affect insulin receptor levels; decrease the affinity of the insulin-receptor interaction; and stimulate insulin degradation, although the overall contribution of these influences to glucocorticoid action has not been clarified.[532,543]

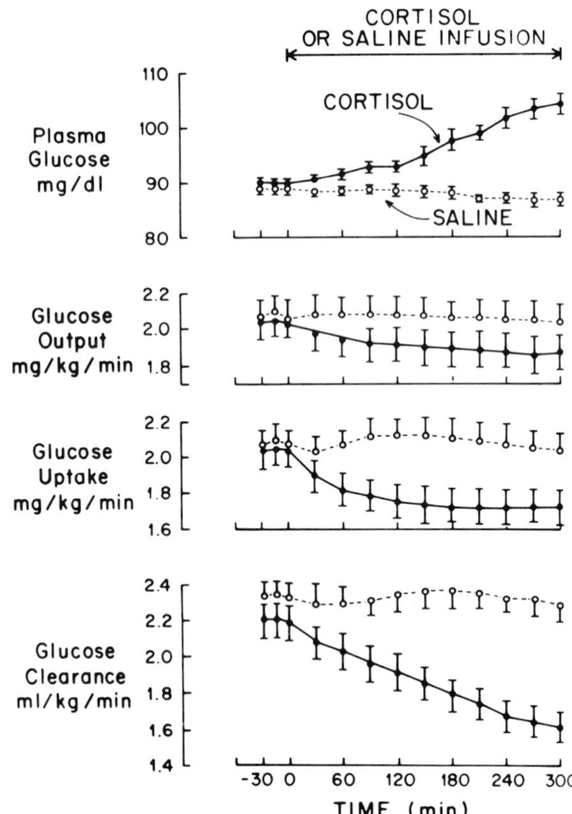

FIGURE 12-21 The effect of cortisol infusion on plasma concentration and glucose kinetics in normal humans. *(From Shamoon et al.[539])*

Glycogen Metabolism

Glucocorticoids increase glycogen deposition in the livers of both fed and fasted animals.[531] After 12 to 24 h, the glycogen content is slightly increased in muscle but not in kidney.[544] Conversely, adrenalectomy impairs hepatic glycogen synthesis; this effect is more prominent in fed than in fasted animals.[531] In this case, glucocorticoids and insulin have similar rather than opposing actions; however, the role of the steroid can be perceived as protecting against long-term food deprivation by promoting glycogen storage, whereas that of insulin is more important for short-term lowering of the blood sugar level by shunting glucose into glycogen.

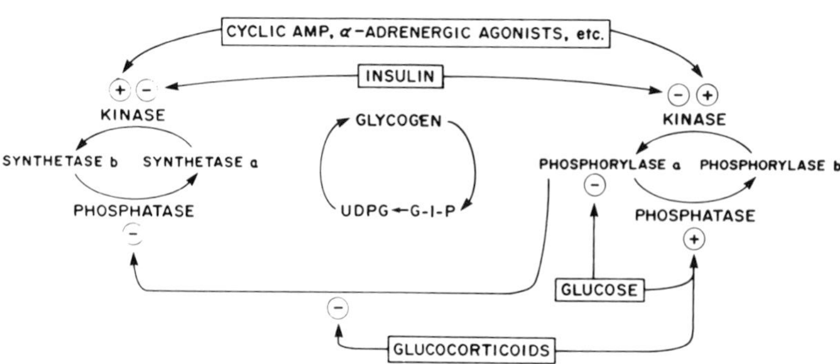

FIGURE 12-22 Actions of glucocorticoids on glycogen accumulation. The dominant effect of the steroid is to induce a factor or factors that block the inhibition by phosphorylase a of glycogen synthetase phosphotase. The steroid also decreases phosphorylase a, but this appears to be of secondary importance. Shown also are the actions of insulin, cAMP (as a mediator of glucagon action), and glucose. Plus signs refer to stimulation; minus signs refer to inhibition. UDPG = uridine diphosphoglucose; G-1-P = glucose-1-phosphate.

Glucocorticoids stimulate glycogen synthetase (UDPG-glycogen transglycosidase) by promoting its conversion from the inactive b form to the active a form[531] (Fig. 12-22). This may be a result of stimulation of glycogen synthetase phosphatase (which activates glycogen synthetase) by blocking the actions of glycogen phosphorylase a, which inhibits the phosphatase.[531] The steroid may induce a protein that inhibits the actions of phosphorylase a.[531]

A second effect of the steroid, probably of less importance, may be to inhibit glycogen breakdown by the inactivation of phosphorylase a, which may occur by simulating by unknown mechanisms its conversion to (inactive) phosphorylase b (Fig. 12-22).[531] This may occur because the phosphatase (activated by glucocorticoids) that stimulates glycogen synthetase activity (Fig. 12-22) also inactivates the enzyme that converts phosphorylase b to phosphorylase a.[531] Such an effect would favor a decrease in the amount of phosphorylase a.

Glucocorticoids also stimulate glycogen production in the fetal liver.[531] In this case, in addition to the mechanisms described above, the steroid may increase the amount of glycogen synthetase itself.[531]

In vivo, glucocorticoid actions on glycogen accumulation appear to be predominantly, although not exclusively, insulin-dependent, since glycogen accumulation is markedly reduced in pancreatectomized animals.[531] Glucocorticoid-stimulated increases in insulin secretion promote further glycogen accumulation.[531]

Lipid Metabolism

Obvious manifestations of the effects of glucocorticoids on lipid metabolism are observed in individuals with Cushing's syndrome who have excess fat in the neck, face, and trunk and loss of fat from the extremities. The steroid also increases plasma free fatty acid and lipoprotein concentrations.

Glucocorticoids increase lypolysis and plasma free fatty acid levels.[536,541,544] Lipolysis and free fatty acid release are increased by the glucocorticoid-induced decrease in glucose uptake and metabolism that reduces the glycerol production necessary for reesterification of fatty acids. The steroids also stimulate lipolysis by increasing the efficiency of other lipolytic factors, such as catecholamines.[541] The increase in free fatty acid release and the possible augmentation of hepatic conversion of free fatty acids to ketones by glucocorticoids cause a tendency to ketosis.[539,541] These effects are ordinarily countered by increased insulin release and glucocorticoid-stimulated gluconeogenesis.

It is not known why in glucocorticoid excess states fat is lost in some areas and increased in others. However, fat deposition in certain areas may be due to lipogenic actions (see Chap. 19) of the increased plasma insulin concentrations. This is consistent with the finding that there can be overall fat loss in diabetic patients with Cushing's syndrome.[489] Increased fat deposition may also be due to stimulation of the appetite by glucocorticoids. Fat loss may be due to direct inhibitory actions of the hormones exerted on adipose tissue.[541] Thus, if different tissues vary in their relative sensitivity to glucocorticoids and insulin, there will be net fat deposition where sensitivity to insulin is dominant and fat loss where the glucocorticoid influence is dominant.

Glucocorticoids have been reported to affect the lipid content of membranes, with influences on cholesterol and sphingomyelin.[545,546] The consequences of these changes are not known, but they could influence the properties of cell membrane–localized receptors, enzymes, and other important molecules.

In glucocorticoid excess states, there is an increase in very low density lipoproteins (VLDL), LDL, and HDL, with consequent elevations of total triglyceride and cholesterol levels.[547] The mechanisms for these changes are probably multifactorial, with influences on VLDL synthesis, free fatty acid production, hepatic endothelial lipase activity, and other components all possibly contributing.[547]

Protein and Nucleic Acid Metabolism

In addition to the actions of glucocorticoid-receptor complexes on the levels of particular RNAs and their protein products (discussed above), the steroids affect protein and RNA synthesis and breakdown and/or DNA synthesis and degradation more generally in a number of tissues.[489,548,549]

The trend with protein and RNA is for the steroid to stimulate synthesis in the liver, to inhibit synthesis and stimulate breakdown in many peripheral tissues, such as muscle, skin, adipose, lymphoid, and fibroblastic (Fig. 12-20); and to have a lesser general influence on brain and cardiac tissue. The general effect on DNA synthesis is inhibitory, although there are some circumstances in which DNA synthesis is stimulated, and rarely DNA breakdown can be stimulated (see below). Overall, this results in net nitrogen loss in the glucocorticoid excess state.[535,538,539,548,549] This pattern may again be perceived as a general attempt by the body to provide substrate for hepatic gluconeogenesis from "less essential" tissues such as muscle and to decrease other types of substrate utilization while sparing certain critical tissues (e.g., brain and heart). However, in glucocorticoid excess states, other deleterious or beneficial effects (osteoporosis, immunosuppression, etc.) are more prominent. Many examples and more details about these effects are provided in the following sections.

Liver The liver is one of the few tissues in which there is an overall stimulatory influence of glucocorticoids on protein and RNA synthesis and in which the steroids cause a slight increase in the total hepatic protein and RNA content.[489,550] Nevertheless, the steroid effects are selective, since certain proteins (e.g., tyrosine aminotransferase and tryptophan oxygenase) are stimulated much more than are others.[489,551] The effects on other gluconeogenic enzymes and glycogen accumulation are discussed above. However, there can be inhibitory glucocorticoid actions in the liver, such as one hepatic DNA synthesis.[548,549]

Muscle Glucocorticoid influences on muscle glucose and protein metabolism have already been discussed. The overall importance of these actions is underscored by the fact that muscle, because of its bulk, is a major source of gluconeogenic precursors and glucose utilization. Glucocorticoids also inhibit muscle DNA and probably RNA synthesis and promote RNA breakdown.[489,529,534–537,549] These effects are partially counteracted by insulin and diet but can lead to frank muscular wasting in glucocorticoid excess states. Glucocorticoids have more pronounced influences on type 2 white glycolytic fibers than on type 1 fibers.[552] The steroid both enhances proteolysis and decreases muscle synthesis; the proteolysis is probably the more important influence and is associated with increases in certain proteolytic enzymes.[552,553]

Immunologic and Inflammatory Responses

Glucocorticoids in excess suppress immunologic and inflammatory responses[489,554–567] and are used extensively to treat diseases in which excessive inflammatory or immunologic activity is damaging (see Chap. 15). These suppressive actions can also be deleterious, and infections increase in frequency and severity in spontaneous Cushing's syndrome and with corticosteroid therapy (see Cushing's Syndrome, below, and Chap. 15).

In contrast to the well-documented immunosuppressive and anti-inflammatory actions of corticosteroids in excess, little is known about the role of basal levels of glucocorticoids in immunologic and inflammatory responses. However, a role seems possible, since glucocorticoids can influence these responses at doses that result in steroid levels equivalent to those which occur physiologically.

The role of increased cortisol secretion during stresses such as infection is also unknown. There is evidence for immunosuppression in postsurgical patients,[558] and inflammatory reactions in these and other "stressed" patients may be blunted by the increased cortisol concentrations. It has been suggested that the increased cortisol in these circumstances may help prevent autoimmune responses to tissue antigens released by cellular injury.[558] The finding that corticosteroids can suppress autologous mixed leukocyte reactions without affecting allogenic reactions is consistent with such a role.[554,557] Nevertheless, the major role of the increased steroid levels in these circumstances may be to prevent a number of host responses recruited during the infection from becoming excessive[560]; this hypothesis is discussed below (see Glucocorticoids and Stress).

Many of the data on glucocorticoids and immunologic responses have come from animal studies. Responses vary among species; for example, the mouse, rat, and rabbit are relatively steroid-sensitive, whereas guinea pigs and humans are more steroid-resistant.[555] Nevertheless, these differences may be more quantitative than qualitative, and in various animal and human systems glucocorticoids have been shown to affect nearly every step in the immunologic and inflammatory responses.[489,542,554–566,568] They affect inflammatory reactions by inhibiting (1) the production and/or activity of vasoactive agents, (2) the movement of leukocytes to inflamed areas, and (3) the function of immunocompetent cells at the site of inflammation. The third effect includes actions on antigen processing by macrophages, specific B and T cell functions, antibody production and clearance, mobilization and functioning of polymorphonuclear and mononuclear cells, the liberation and actions of effector substances (prostaglandins, leukotrienes, interleukins, kinins, proteases such as plasminogen activator, etc.) at the site of cellular injury, and the fibroblastic proliferative response. Interestingly, glucocorticoids do not cause permanent damage to the immunologic system. Thus, the precursor cells are steroid-resistant. This underscores the point that different stages in the response vary markedly in their sensitivity to glucocorticoids. The particular actions that are the most important in the observed responses are commonly unclear. In general, it appears that in humans the steroids affect cellular processes more than humoral processes, leukocyte distribution within body compartments more than function, and macrophages more than polymorphonuclear leukocytes and are more effective if given before or concurrently with a challenge rather than later.

Effects on Vasoactive and Other Inflammatory Agents Early inflammatory changes at a site of injury result in enhanced vascular permeability and edema. These changes are mediated by a variety of inflammatory agents, including prostaglandins (PG), kinins, histamines, and the slow-reacting substance of anaphylaxis (SRS-A).[560–568]

Arachidonic acid is the precursor of a number of molecules collectively called eicosanoids.[560–568] It is derived directly from the actions of phospholipase A_2 or indirectly from phospholipase C. Arachidonic acid can then be converted into prostaglandins, thromboxanes, hydroperoxyeicosatetraenoic acids (HPETE), hydroxyeicosatetraenoic acids (HETE), and leukotrienes.[562–564] A number of these compounds are relevant in inflammatory reactions, and their role is further suggested by the fact that certain nonsteroidal anti-inflammatory agents block the production of some of these substances.[562,563]

Glucocorticoids inhibit PG synthesis in a variety of cell types,[560–568] although this does not occur in all cases, and in certain conditions total prostanoid levels or excretion may not be affected by the steroids.[559–568] These inhibitory actions on production may be due to the actions of a protein, termed lipoprotein or macrocortin, that inhibits phospholipase A_2 and whose levels are increased by glucocorticoids.[559,562,564,565,569] These actions of glucocorticoids in inhibiting phospholipase A_2 result in a more general inhibition of eicosanoid production than is the case with indomethacin and aspirin, and they may help explain the greater anti-inflammatory actions of the steroids in comparison to these other molecules.

Glucocorticoids block the actions of bradykinin, which may also regulate PG synthesis.[563] They also block the release of histamine and SRS-A, which may be leukotrienes.[563]

Leukocyte Movement Glucocorticoid administration to human subjects causes a circulating lymphocytopenia, monocytopenia, and eosinopenia (Table 12-6).[554,570,571] Conversely, these cell types are increased in adrenal insufficiency.[489] The actions on lymphocytes and monocytes are maximal within 4 to 6 h and return to normal by 24 to 48 h but persist with continued steroid administration.[554,563,571] These effects are due to a redistribution of cells, with

TABLE 12-6 Glucocorticoid Effects on Leukocyte Movements in Humans

1. Lymphocytes
   a. Circulating lymphocytopenia caused by redistribution of cells to other lymphoid compartments
   b. Depletion of recirculating lymphocytes
   c. Selective depletion of T lymphocytes (especially T_M subset) more than B lymphocytes
2. Monocyte-macrophages
   a. Circulating monocytopenia, probably caused by redistribution
   b. Inhibition of accumulation of monocyte-macrophages at inflammatory sites
3. Neutrophils
   a. Circulating neutrophilia
   b. Accelerated release of neutrophils from the bone marrow
   c. Blocked accumulation of neutrophils at inflammatory sites, probably caused by reduced adherence
4. Eosinophils
   a. Circulating eosinopenia, probably caused by redistribution
   b. Decreased migration of eosinophils into immediate hypersensitivity skin test sites

Source: Modified from Parrillo and Fauci.[554]

cells moving out of the circulation and into other body compartments, such as bone marrow, spleen, lymph nodes, and thoracic duct.[554,570] In other species, circulating lymphoid cells are also killed by the steroid, but this appears not to be the case with humans.[489,554,555] Although there are effects on both T (thymus-derived) and B (marrow-derived) lymphocytes, the influence is much greater on the T lymphocytes, especially those with an Fc receptor for IgM (TM) compared with those with a receptor for IgG (TG).[554]

Glucocorticoid administration also increases (maximally after 4 to 6 h) the blood polymorphonuclear leukocyte concentration.[489,554,563] This is due to an accelerated release of neutrophils from the bone marrow, an increase in the half-life of circulating neutrophils, and reduced neutrophil egress from the blood.[554]

Glucocorticoids decrease markedly the number of polymorphonuclear leukocytes, monocyte-macrophages, and lymphocytes that accumulate at inflammatory sites; the effect is evident by 2 h.[489,555,558,563] Although decreases are ordinarily similar for both monocytes and polymorphonuclear leukocytes, the effects on mononuclear cells appear to be longer-lived. These actions may be due in part to the fact that glucocorticoids can inhibit chemotactic and other factors, such as plasminogen activator,[563] that affect inflammatory cell accumulation at sites of injury, and may be a major mechanism of the anti-inflammatory actions of the glucocorticoids.[554] Blood basophils are elevated in Addison's disease and depressed in Cushing's disease or with glucocorticoid therapy.[489] Presumably, the same mechanisms that regulate the levels of eosinophils are operative here.

Leukocyte Function Glucocorticoids affect lymphocyte function, and in some animals the steroids at high doses kill lymphocytes and cause involution of lymphoid tissues.[489,542] There are marked variations in the sensitivity of lymphoid cell subpopulations; for instance, in the mouse thymus, about 95 percent of the cells are killed by the steroid, whereas the remaining 5 percent are steroid-resistant.[489,542] This 5 percent must contain the precursor cells for immunologic responses, since steroid treatment does not abolish certain thymic-dependent responses. Although most human lymphocytes are not killed by glucocorticoids, in some cases (e.g., cells of acute lymphocytic leukemia of childhood) there can be lymphoid cell killing (see also Chap. 15).[572] The actions of glucocorticoids on lymphocytes involve stimulation (or blockade) of specific functions; even the killing activity appears to involve specific programming and is associated with an early response in which a discrete set of proteins is induced.[573] One or a few of these ultimately result in cell killing, possibly through direct or indirect actions that induce or enhance the actions of a DNase that digests the cell's DNA.[574]

A number of specific lymphocyte functions are blocked by the steroids without cell death (Table 12-7),[489,542,554,555,560,563] and there are variations in sensitivity. For instance, the lymphocyte-proliferative response to some but not other antigens can be suppressed.[554] The proliferative responses to antigens are more readily suppressed than are those to mitogens.[554] Nevertheless, blockage of some T cell mitogenic responses has been observed; this may be due to steroid actions that block the release of T cell growth factor (interleukin 2).[560,563] This block is secondary to decreased leukotriene B_4 production resulting from the steroid-mediated inhibition of phospholipase A_2.[561] This action may help explain why the steroids are more effective when given early in an immunologic response than they are later, because interleukin 2 is important for clonal expansion of cells early on but not later.[560,563] The steroids also suppress macrophage functions (see below) that affect T cell function. They suppress T lymphocyte production of interferon-γ,[560] with subsequent effects on macrophages (see below), including Fc receptors, activation of macrophages, and enhancement of natural killer cell activity and macrophage activating factor.[560,563] They also block the production of colony-stimulating factor, which stimulates granulocyte and macrophage production,[560] and that of cachectin (tumor necrosis factor), which is involved in tumor rejection.[568] Whereas the steroids generally do not suppress antibody-dependent cell-mediated cytotoxicity of human cells, they can suppress spontaneous toxicity and cutaneous delayed hypersensitivity; the latter effect is probably due to an inhibition of lymphocyte-derived mediators (such as migration inhibition factor) that recruit cells (i.e., macrophages) necessary for the response.[554]

Overall, glucocorticoid effects on B cell functions are more modest. In humans, high-dose corticosteroid therapy causes a small decrease in immunoglobulin levels as a result of both decreased synthesis and increased catabolism,[575] and antibody responses to specific antigens ordinarily are not affected by glucocorticoids.[554] In vitro, the steroids can in some cases even stimulate immunoglobulin production by cultures of B and T lymphocytes.[576] However, immunoglobulin production by B cells results from a series of steps involving early activation, later B cell growth factor–mediated proliferation, and final differentiation to the immunoglobulin-producing state. These steps are affected by suppressor cell and helper cell functions and can be suppressed by glucocorticoids.[489,554,555,563] Studied in vitro, glucocorticoids affect substantially the early activation, have a lesser effect on the B cell growth factor response, and do not affect the final step.[577] Because of varying sensitivities and complex accessory cell effects on B and/or T cell function, it is possible to observe a variety of effects, either stimulatory or inhibitory. Inhibition of suppressor cell function may explain why in sarcoidosis with anergy (that may be due in part to increased suppressor activity), glucocorticoids may increase immune responsiveness.[556]

Macrophage functions are relatively sensitive to glucocorticoid inhibitory actions.[554] The steroids induce a monocytopenia, suppress committed marrow-forming monocyte stem cells, and block the differentiation of monocytes into macrophages.[578] This may explain the effectiveness of glucocorticoids in treating many granulomatous diseases, since the monocyte is felt to be important in granuloma formation.[554] By blocking the production of interferon-γ, glucocorticoids can also decrease the levels of Fc receptors (that bind the Fc portion of immunoglobulin)

TABLE 12-7 Immunologic Mediators Whose Production and/or Actions Can Be Blocked by Glucocorticoids

Bradykinin
Cachectin (tumor necrosis factor)
Collagenase
Colony-stimulating factor
Eicosanoids (prostaglandins, leukotrienes, etc.)
Histamine
γ-Interferon
Interleukin 1 (lymphocyte-activating factor)
Interleukin 2 (T-cell growth factor)
Migration inhibition factor
Plasminogen activator

Note: The inhibitions are not always observed in all tissues. See text for references (see especially Ref. 560).

on monocytes and macrophages[562]; these receptors facilitate the phagocytosis of particulate antigens and other functions of the cells in the inflammatory responses. Steroids can block the ability of the monocytes to bind to antibody-coated cells,[554] elicit bactericidal activity and cytotoxicity,[554] and release neutral proteases, including collagenase, elastase, and plasminogen activator,[563] that participate in the immunologic and inflammatory responses. The steroids suppress the production by macrophages of lymphocyte activating factor, which is involved in T cell mitogenesis,[563] and of lymphocyte-derived macrophage factors that may block the exit of macrophages from inflammatory sites.[563] They block the production of macrophage-activating factor by T cells and its actions on macrophages.[560] However, glucocorticoid actions are not always inhibitory: The steroids can increase the expression of mannose receptors in macrophages, and this has an anti-inflammatory effect by enhancing the uptake and internalization of lysosomal enzymes.[566]

Actions of glucocorticoids on neutrophil functions other than regulating their trafficking are less definite. Suppression of functions such as phagocytosis, chemotaxis, and bactericidal activity has been elicited at steroid concentrations that rarely if ever are achieved in vivo.[554]

Erythroid Cells and Thrombocytes A mild polycythemia can occur in Cushing's syndrome, and there may be normochromic normocytic anemia in Addison's disease.[489] Glucocorticoids may acutely promote a rise in thrombocytes, but thrombocytopenia has also been reported after long-term administration.[489] The mechanisms for these influences are not known.

Fibroblastic and Epithelial Tissues The actions of glucocorticoids on fibroblastic tissues constitute a major drawback to their long-term use in therapy.[489,550,579–581] These actions probably contribute to the thinning of the bone matrix and osteoporosis seen in glucocorticoid excess states (see Chap. 15). The steroids inhibit both specific matrix cell activities such as collagen and glycosaminoglycan formation and overall fibroblast function.[579–584] Inhibitory actions on fibroblasts also lead to easy bruising, poor wound healing, and a tendency to wound dehiscence after surgery in the glucocorticoid excess state. The steroids do not appear to alter the epithelialization of a wound, except indirectly through inhibition of the fibrous scar which serves as a scaffolding for the cells, (3), but they can inhibit epidermal epithelial cell proliferation in other circumstances; this action is useful in the treatment of psoriasis.[585]

Glucocorticoid effects on fibroblast and epithelial cells can be observed in isolated cells in culture. Both stimulation and inhibition of cellular functions have been reported.[579,586] Inhibitory effects lead to decreased uptake and metabolism of glucose, decreased protein and RNA synthesis, and inhibition of DNA synthesis.[587] The steroid can also affect collagen, fibronectin, and glycosaminoglycan formation.[582–584,586] These effects can also be specific and are observed in the absence of major influences on most cellular functions. The effects on collagen involve a selective decrease in collagen mRNA, resulting in decreased collagen synthesis.[581] The steroids can also affect other enzymes involved in collagen metabolism, such as collagen galactosyltransferase and hydroxylase.[581] By contrast, stimulatory effects result in increased cell replication and incorporation of thymidine into DNA.[587] These seemingly paradoxic responses may be due to the fact that glucocorticoids can affect the actions or production of various growth factors either positively or negatively.[588] In humans, the result is predominantly inhibitory.

Cardiovascular System and Fluid and Electrolyte Balance

Glucocorticoids affect the heart, vasculature, regulators of blood pressure, water excretion, and electrolyte balance. Some of these actions are direct; others involve mineralocorticoid-like actions.

In glucocorticoid-deficient states, there is hypotension with decreased responsiveness to pressor stimuli[589,590] and decreased cardiac output[589]; stresses such as surgery, infection, and trauma can precipitate an adrenal crisis with shock. This is only partly due to a loss of the mineralocorticoid functions of the adrenal steroids. However, the importance of glucocorticoids in the maintenance of normal cardiovascular function is emphasized by the finding that the hypotension seen in patients with adrenal insufficiency crisis is not reversed by correction of volume or sodium losses or by the administrationof mineralocorticoids, such as DOC, that do not have glucocorticoid activity (Figs. 12-23 and 12-24).

Conversely, in glucocorticoid excess states there is hypertension, which occurs in almost all patients

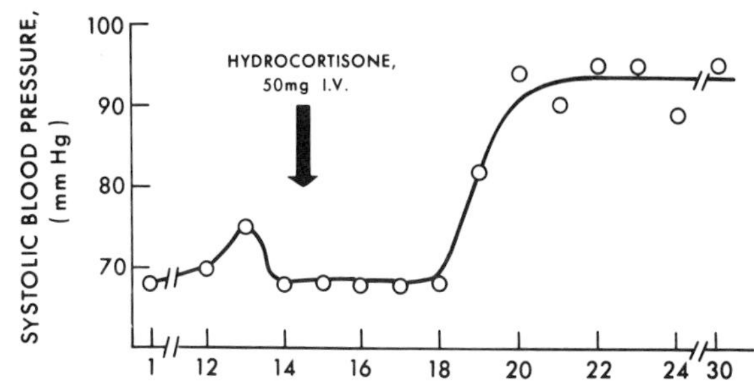

FIGURE 12-23 Effect of cortisol (hydrocortisone) on blood pressure in a patient with Addison's disease. The blood pressure had not responded to fluid replacement and other supportive measures. Cortisol was given when the diagnosis of adrenocortical insufficiency was suspected. *(From Baxter.[489])*

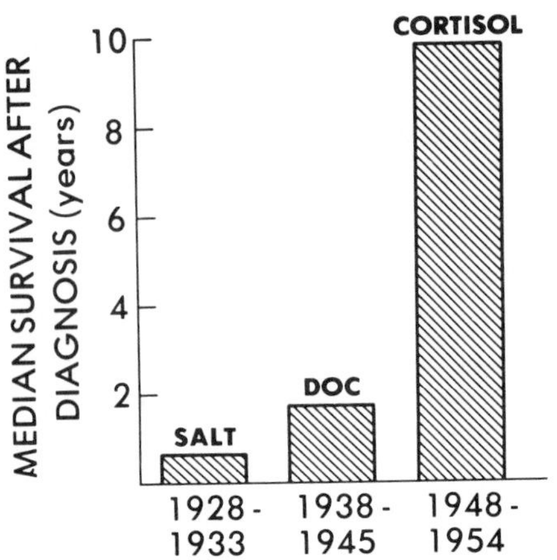

FIGURE 12-24 Median duration of survival of individuals with Addison's syndrome in years after the diagnosis in relation to therapeutic advances. The specific time periods chosen were selected to avoid having patients fall into overlapping therapy categories. However, the survival in the postcortisol era is actually greater than indicated, since most of the individuals in this group were still alive in 1963, when the data were collected, and it is not clear that all the individuals who died actually received cortisol. *(From Baxter and Rousseau[550] based on data from Dunlop.[680])*

with spontaneous Cushing's syndrome[590] and in a lesser proportion of patients on glucocorticoid therapy (see Chaps. 14 and 15), and enhanced responsiveness to pressors such as angiotensin II and norepinephrine.[589,590] The hypertension in spontaneous Cushing's syndrome is not accompanied by frank stigmata of mineralocorticoid excess such as depressed plasma renin levels and hypokalemia, indicating that there are mineralocorticoid-independent effects of the glucocorticoids.[590] Further, in the rat, glucocorticoid-induced hypertension is specifically blocked by glucocorticoid antagonists but not by low salt intake or mineralocorticoid antagonists.[591]

The mechanisms of these vascular effects are complex and multifactorial. The steroids can have direct actions on the heart (discussed below) and enhance the activities of vasoactive substances (as described under Synergistic and Antagonistic Interrelations between Glucocorticoids and Other Hormones, below). They may have direct actions on vascular smooth muscle[592,593] and endothelial cells.[594] The steroids can also suppress the synthesis and actions of vasodilator and cardiac-suppressant substances that are produced in excess in adrenal insufficiency and/or in response to stress. (The role of PGs in this respect is discussed below, but this issue is addressed more comprehensively later, under Glucocorticoids and Stress.) Glucocorticoids can directly affect other components involved in blood pressure control, such as the renin-angiotensin system (see below).

The heart is a direct glucocorticoid target, and in isolated preparations glucocorticoids can induce cardiac protein synthesis, increase the coupling between cardiac beta-adrenergic receptors and adenylate cyclase, and have positive inotropic influences and effects on the left ventricular work index.[595] They have also been reported to induce cardiac ultrastructural damage.[596] Further, they probably have mineralocorticoid-independent effects on cardiac output and stroke volume.[597]

The ability of glucocorticoids to decrease PG production probably contributes to these vascular responses,[559] and although controversial[567] (see also Immunologic and Inflammatory Responses, above), decreased urinary PGE_2 production has been reported in glucocorticoid excess.[590] In glucocorticoid-induced hypertension in the rat, the basal and angiotensin II–stimulated release of this PG from the renal medulla is diminished even though plasma and urinary PGE_2 concentrations are increased.[597] PGE_2 is a potent vasodilator and is the principal product of arachidonic acid in arteries and veins. Its production is stimulated by angiotensin II and norepinephrine.[598] Thus, glucocorticoid inhibition of the production of this vasodilator could contribute significantly to the increased vascular reactivity and blood pressure that occur in glucocorticoid excess states.[598] Conversely, overproduction of this mediator could result in decreased vascular reactivity and hypotension in an addisonian patient. PGE_2 also causes tachycardia, and excess PGE_2 could contribute to the presence of this sign in an addisonian individual.[598] It has been suggested that glucocorticoids stimulate the ability of mitochondria to retain calcium and thus improve vascular responses by enhancing ATP generation.[599]

Glucocorticoids can increase the levels of prorenin 326 and renin substrate 314 and, in isolated cells,[600] the activity of angiotensin-converting enzyme (angiotensinogen) (see Chap. 14).[601] Whereas plasma renin levels are generally in the normal to high normal range in glucocorticoid excess states, this level of elevation is inappropriate in the face of hypertension.[590] Also, the hypertension in Cushing's syndrome is responsive to the administration of inhibitors of converting enzymes (see also Chap. 14).[590,602] Conversely, angiotensin II generation is impaired in adrenal insufficiency in the face of elevated renin and converting enzyme levels, possibly as a result of decreased angiotensinogen, and this could contribute to the refractoriness of addisonian shock to therapy.[601,603]

Although glucocorticoids can affect salt and water excretion by binding to mineralocorticoid receptors (discussed below), they also have other actions that are not elicited through mineralocorticoid receptors. They increase the glomerular filtration rate (GFR).[604,605] Whether this is due to an increase in cardiac output or to direct influences on the kidney is not known. Glucocorticoids can increase the levels of cardiac ANP (see Chap. 14) and its mRNA,[376] and this can increase GFR (Chap. 14). The increase in GFR can enhance the excretion of salt and water, and steroids such as dexamethasone, with much greater glucocorticoid than mineralocorticoid activity, sometimes produce natriuresis rather than sodium retention.[604,605] Glucocorticoids increase Na^+,K^+-ATPase activity in the renal outer medullary tubules,[606] erythrocytes,[607] and colon[608] and prekallikrein in the urine and on the basal membrane of distal tubular cells.[609] Although the physiologic role of these actions has not been established, they imply that the steroid can have direct effects on renal hemodynamics and/or salt excretion.

Glucocorticoid deficiency results in a decreased ability to excrete water.[610] This effect is probably due both to the decreased GFR and to the fact that glucocorticoids can inhibit vasopressin release; in their absence, vasopressin levels are increased, leading to abnormal water retention.[610,611] In fact, water intoxication can occur rarely in panhypopituitarism with glucocorticoid but not mineralocorticoid deficiency.[610]

Glucocorticoids also affect potassium balance.[604,605,612,613] At higher concentrations, steroids such as cortisol can produce hypokalemia through mineralocorticoid actions (see below and Chap. 14). However, their major effect is to produce a transient kaliuresis by increasing urine flow through increases in GRF and, possibly, protein catabolism with release of intracellular K^+. However, the plasma potassium concentration is usually normal or only slightly decreased (see Chap. 14).

Glucocorticoids can increase renal acid output. Thus, in glucocorticoid excess there is a tendency to alkalosis and in glucocorticoid deficiency there is a tendency to acidosis. These effects occur with minimal influences on urinary pH; they are due to stimulation of excretion of buffer as phosphate and ammonia by blocking tubular reabsorption of phosphate and increasing the production of ammonia.[614,615] The latter may occur as a result of a stimulation of Na^+-H^+ exchange in the proximal tubule brush border, which results in ammonia trapping.[614]

Bone and Calcium Metabolism

Glucocorticoids affect bone and calcium dynamics in a variety of ways. In Addison's disease, mild hypercalcemia can occur,[616–618] but glucocorticoid excess does not usually result in lower serum Ca^{2+} levels.[619] Serum phosphate levels are lowered and urinary Ca^{2+} and phosphorus concentrations are elevated in glucocorticoid excess states.[619] Glucocorticoid excess ultimately leads to osteoporosis (see also Chaps. 15 and 24), a major limitation to their long-term use. Several independent actions contribute to these effects.

Glucocorticoids partly block intestinal calcium absorption (Chap. 23).[620,621] This is a direct effect on the gut that is more prominent in the duodenum and jejunum.[622,623] Glucocorticoids apparently do not block vitamin D action in the intestine[622] and do not decrease vitamin D metabolite levels; renal vitamin D 1α-hydroxylase activity is increased by the steroid.[620,621,624] Earlier reports suggested that the steroid promotes a redistribution of calcium from extracellular into intracellular compartments,[599,625,626] but the significance of this is not known.

Glucocorticoids decrease renal reabsorption of calcium and phosphate and in excess cause hypercalciuria and renal calculi.[580,619,627] Hypercalciuria is a consistent effect of glucocorticoids, and a major contributor to the negative calcium balance.[619,626]

The glucocorticoid-induced tendency to hypocalcemia induces a secondary rise in the parathyroid hormone (PTH) level.[580,619,628] There may also be a direct increase of PTH release[619,628]; this action explains why the steroid can increase both serum calcium and PTH levels in primary hyperparathyroidism.[628] However, glucocorticoids cause hypocalcemia in parathyroidectomized animals maintained on a constant dose of PTH and are necessary for the induction of hypocalcemia in animals by thyroparathyroidectomy.[623]

Shortly after glucocorticoid administration, there is enhanced bone accretion, but with continued administration, inhibition is the predominant effect.[580] The inhibitory effects on accretion are probably due to decreased bone cell function and collagen formation; inhibition by glucocorticoids of bone cell proliferation and synthesis of protein, RNA, collagen, and hyaluronate has been demonstrated in vitro.[580,624,626,629] Decreased bone synthesis in glucocorticoid excess states is probably also reflected by lower blood osteocalcin (bone Gla-protein) levels.[630]

Glucocorticoid excess also results in enhanced osteolysis with an increased number of osteoclasts and urinary excretion of hydroxyproline.[578] These steroids in vitro can stimulate the resorptive activity of macrophages, from which osteoclasts are derived, possibly by affecting cell-surface glycoproteins involved in the association of these cells with bone.[578,629] They can inhibit osteoclast function in vitro, but in vivo this function apparently is not predominant.[568,629] Enhanced resorption may also be due to the increased PTH levels and steroid augmentation of the actions of PTH, including its ability to stimulate cAMP accumulation in bone cells.[631,632] However, the increased osteolysis ordinarily is not profound enough to lead to bone changes typical of hyperparathyroidism (i.e., osteitis fibrosa cystica) in glucocorticoid excess states.[580] Glucocorticoids may also increase bone resorption by enhancing the sensitivity of bone cells to 1α-25-$(OH)_2D_3$, possibly by increasing the number of 1α,25-$(OH)_2D_3$ receptors, although in other instances they decrease osteoblast

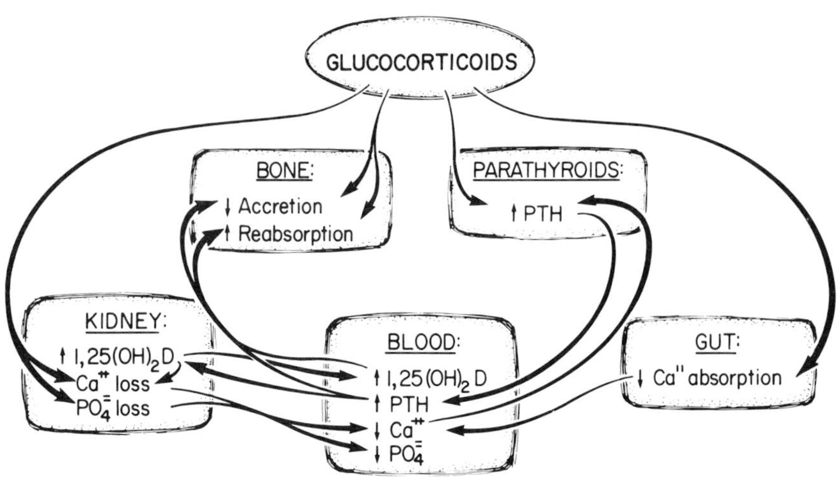

FIGURE 12-25 Effect of glucocorticoids on bone and calcium dynamics. See text.

1α,25-$(OH)_2D_3$ receptors.[633,634] Finally, glucocorticoids may block the inhibitory actions of calcitonin on bone resorption.[633]

These collective actions are summarized in Fig. 12-25. The decreased calcium absorption by the gut and increased urinary calcium and phosphate loss lead to a net negative calcium balance and a tendency to hypocalcemia and hypophosphatemia. This, plus direct steroid actions on the parathyroid gland, results in increased PTH release that in turn results in increased 1α,25-$(OH)_2D_3$ formation. The increased PTH and 1α,25-$(OH)_2D_3$ blunt the hypocalcemic response but also, in combination with direct glucocorticoid effects, decrease bone accretion and increase bone resorption, resulting in an overall loss of bone mineral.

Central Nervous System

Glucocorticoids affect the brain in a number of ways. Thus, behavior, mood, neural activity, and a number of specific biochemical processes can be influenced by these hormones.[636,637] Glucocorticoids can penetrate the blood-brain barrier; their ability to do this is inversely proportional to their polarity, which is largely dependent on the number of hydroxyl groups.[638] They can also regulate the permeability of the blood-brain barrier to other substances and are used for therapy to reduce brain edema[639]; conversely, pseudotumor cerebri is rarely associated with glucocorticoid therapy.[612]

Mood changes (and rarely psychosis) are observed with both glucocorticoid excess and glucocorticoid deficiency.[636,637] Patients receiving glucocorticoid therapy may initially have a feeling of well-being.[612,640,641] By contrast, patients with spontaneous Cushing's syndrome are commonly depressed.[612] Patients with Addison's disease tend to be depressed, negativistic, irritable, seclusive, and apathetic.[640] Several types of psychoses have been reported (particularly in glucocorticoid excess states); these responses were not predicted by the patient's prior psychiatric history or personality traits. Patients with Addison's disease have anorexia,[641] whereas glucocorticoid excess stimulates the appetite.[612,640,641] In addition, high doses of glucocorticoids can affect sleep, with a trend toward increased wakefulness and a reduction in rapid eye movement (REM) sleep, an increase in stage II sleep, and an increase in the time to the first REM sleep.[642]

Conversely, in depressive syndromes there can be excessive glucocorticoid production with blunted circadian rhythm and a decreased ability of glucocorticoids to suppress the hypothalamic-adrenal-pituitary axis (see above).[643,644] These abnormalities occur commonly in both unipolar and bipolar depression and occur particularly frequently in delusional depression.[644] They also occur in schizoaffective disorders, catatonia, borderline character disorders, chronic pain syndromes, and bulimia but are uncommon in schizophrenia and mania.[644] The abnormalities usually abate with clinical improvement; failure to do so is correlated with a high rate of relapse. The contribution of glucocorticoid excess to these problems and the mechanisms of its development are not understood. The fact that dextroamphetamine but not a number of other CNS-active agents can transiently decrease the cortisol hypersecretion in depression has been taken as suggesting that depression may be due to cholinergic excess.[643]

Addisonian subjects can have increased sensitivity to a variety of sensory stimuli, including sound and taste, and impaired judgment and ability to discriminate sensory input.[636,640,645] In animals, bilateral adrenalectomy attenuates the circadian variations in paradoxic sleep.[636] Adrenal steroids can also facilitate the extinction of previously acquired avoidance habits,[636] an effect opposite to that induced by ACTH and other POMC fragments.[636,646] However, this effect may not be glucocorticoid-specific,[636] since it can also be elicited by steroids, such as pregnenolone, that do not have glucocorticoid activity.

Glucocorticoids regulate a variety of developmental and other events in the brain.[637] In excess, they can have detrimental effects on brain development in animals. They regulate the catecholamine biosynthetic pathway (discussed below), transsynaptic induction, the actions of nerve growth factor and epidermal growth factor on brain cells, the development of cholinergic ganglionic properties, glutamine synthetase, α-glycerophosphate dehydrogenase, myelination, γ-aminobutyric acid, and a neuron-specific phosphoprotein, protein 1.[637,647] They can affect brain cell electric activity and the EEG.[636,642] Most of these effects have been elicited at very high steroid concentrations; therefore, their importance is not understood.

Whereas most of these actions on the CNS are probably mediated by the glucocorticoid receptors (see below), some may be mediated through mineralocorticoid receptors. In the brain, cortisol can have ready access to the receptor and in fact may keep it relatively saturated even under nonstimulated conditions.[504,505]

Adrenal Medulla

The adrenal cortex surrounds and is contiguous with the adrenal medulla (Chap. 13), which is also involved in stress responses. The adrenal medulla receives adrenocortical venous effluent and thus is exposed to much higher cortisol concentrations than are other tissues.[637] Glucocorticoids affect adrenal chromaffin cell phenotypic characteristics and the catecholamine biosynthetic pathway.[637] In the latter, they regulate phenylethanolamine *N*-methyl transferase (PNMT), tyrosine hydroxylase, and dopamine β-hydroxylase activities.[637,648] The effects are most prominent on PNMT, which catalyzes the formation of epinephrine. Thus, resting and exercise-stimulated epinephrine levels are reduced in ACTH deficiency states; the physiologic importance of this is not known.[649] Glucocorticoids can also increase adrenal medullary proenkephalin.[650]

Eye

Glucocorticoids in excess can increase the intraocular pressure in certain susceptible individuals, particularly patients with primary open-angle glaucoma.[489,651] This appears to be due to a glucocorticoid effect on the aqueous outflow, perhaps through actions on the trabecular meshwork.[651] The role of the endogenous glucocorticoids in determining intraocular pressure in normal individuals is not known, but the intraocular pressure tends to show a circadian variation that parallels, with about a 3-h lag, the overall fluctuations in plasma cortisol,[651] and an increase in intraocular pressure can be observed in ocular hypertensive patients about 3 h after glucocorticoid administration.[651] Glucocorticoid therapy can stimulate cataract formation after long-term high-dose therapy.[651] Interestingly, this may be due to covalent linkage of the steroid molecules to the lens crystalline proteins.[652] Glucocorticoids decrease the absorption of topical antibiotics, and therapy can result in nonspecific keratitis, refractive changes, papilledema due to intracranial hypertension, limitation of ocular movement, and changes in the aqueous and vitreous compositions.[652]

Gastrointestinal Tract

In animals, glucocorticoids at high doses inhibit DNA synthesis in gastric but not jejunal mucosa,[549] increase acid secretion in response to stimuli such as histamine,[489] and increase the incidence of gastric ulceration.[489] In humans, prolonged steroid treatment may increase acid output slightly.[653] Although the issue has been controversial,[654] the most recent data suggest that glucocorticoids in high doses do not result in an increased incidence of peptic ulcers, except in patients who are concomitantly receiving nonsteroidal anti-inflammatory agents.[655] In glucocorticoid-deficient states there can be nausea and vomiting. The mechanisms for this are not known, but as was discussed above, a deficiency of cortisol may lead to PGE_2 excess, which can produce such symptoms.[598]

Growth and Development

Glucocorticoids in excess inhibit linear growth; this limits their prolonged use in children.[548,549,656] These steroids also inhibit skeletal maturation; the result is that growth potential is maintained during and after therapy, and there can be further growth (sometimes with a growth spurt) after its withdrawal.

Glucocorticoids also inhibit growth (and cell division) in a number of individual tissues.[548,549] The effects on lymphoid, fibroblastic, epithelial, and bone cells have already been discussed. These actions are useful in steroid therapy but can also be detrimental. There are variations in sensitivity; in a growing rat, for instance, liver, heart, muscle, and kidney are more sensitive than gastric and jejunal mucosa, spleen, brain, and testis.[549] More information is needed with respect to humans.

In vitro, glucocorticoids can either stimulate or inhibit cell division of a larger number of cell types.[548,549,551–553,572,581,587,588] Stimulation may occur by a steroid-induced augmentation of the actions of growth factors such as fibroblast growth factor[657] and IGF-I,[658] and the steroid can also increase the levels of IGF-I receptors.[659] Conversely, inhibition could be due to actions of the steroid in blocking growth factor (e.g., PG)[588] production and/or action; it could be due to other inhibitory actions of the glucocorticoids on the cell (discussed in Protein and Nucleic Acid Metabolism and in Carbohydrate Metabolism, above).[489,544,548,555,572] The steroid-induced increase in fibronectin biosynthesis could also inhibit replication, since this extracellular glycoprotein may stimulate cell adhesion, which may inhibit cell replication.[586]

The mechanisms of inhibition of growth in the intact organism are not known.[548,549,656,660] They may in part be due to inhibitory influences on bone cells; for instance, chondrocyte proliferation can be inhibited by steroids. Glucocorticoids also inhibit growth hormone production, but this action probably does not explain the growth-inhibiting effects of the steroid, since they are not overcome by the administration of growth hormone. Although glucocorticoids do not decrease levels of IGF-I in plasma, they increase the levels of an inhibitor of IGF-I.

It is not known whether glucocorticoids at physiologic concentrations play a role in regulating growth. In animals, physiologically equivalent concentrations of glucocorticoids inhibit new cell accretion in several growing tissues.[548,656] It has also been reported that adrenalectomy increases the mitotic index in skin.[549]

Glucocorticoids accelerate developmental events in various species in several fetal and postnatal differentiating tissues, including liver (induce enzymes of intermediary metabolism), intestine (induce digestive enzymes), pancreas (regulate the production of insulin and induce digestive enzymes), stomach (induce pepsinogen), skin (induce epidermal proteins), retina (induce glutamine synthetase), brain (induce Na^+, K^+-ATPase), adrenal medulla (induce PNMT), placenta (induce enzymes for estrogen synthesis), mammary gland, and heart.[661] The endogenous glucocorticoids may act similarly in the developing fetus, since plasma corticosteroid levels increase before term delivery, and this is associated with normal maturation of the tissues. In general, glucocorticoids tend to affect the timing and rate of differentiation but not the sequence of development events. Thus, with adrenal insufficiency in utero, there is continued development of the fetus and of certain specialized functions, but this differentiation is delayed.

Sensitivity to glucocorticoids varies during development, and various proteins may be regulated by the steroids only at certain stages.[661] For instance, corticosteroids regulate surfactant synthesis in the fetal lung but not in the adult. In some instances (e.g., induction of intestinal sucrase activity) the steroid-induced changes are reversible, whereas in other instances (e.g., induction of glutamine synthetase in neural retina) the enzyme does not return to pretreatment levels after the withdrawal of the steroid. There is also an increased sensitivity of certain responses to glucocorticoids just before the endogenous increase in glucocorticoid levels that precedes term delivery.

Little is known about the importance of these developmental influences in children, but glucocorticoid effects on the fetus may prepare it for extrauterine existence. For instance, the actions on hepatic enzymes and the pancreatic islets are probably important for regulating glucose homeostasis, the effects on the adrenal medulla could aid in responsiveness to stress, and the surfactant-inducing actions permit the lung to carry out gas exchange.[661] Some of these functions can be induced by glucocorticoids before the normal increase in steroid levels that precedes delivery. For example, treatment of a mother in spontaneous premature labor increases fetal surfactant levels and reduces the incidence and/or severity of the respiratory distress syndrome (hyaline membrane disease) associated with premature birth.

Production and Clearance of Other Hormones

Glucocorticoids can affect the production and/or clearance of other classes of hormones. In the liver, these steroids induce a specific cytochrome P450 that could participate in oxidative reactions involving a variety of drugs, steroids, bile acids, and other compounds.[662] The influences on ACTH, angiotensin II, vasopressin, IGF-I growth hormone, insulin, glucagon, PTH, vitamin D, epinephrine, and PGs have been mentioned. Glucocorticoids in excess inhibit pancreatic polypeptide production,[663] basal and metoclopramide-stimulated prolactin release,[663] and basal and stimulated gastrin secretion.[663] They can stimulate the production of calcitonin and related peptides.[664]

Glucocorticoids affect thyroid stimulating hormone (TSH) release and thyroxine (T_4) metabolism. In glucocorticoid excess states, there is a blunted TSH response to thyrotropin releasing hormone (TRH).[665] Plasma T_4 concentrations are generally in the low normal range in glucocorticoid excess states, but triiodothyronine (T_3) levels can be subnormal[665] because of decreased conversion of T_4 to T_3 and increased conversion of T_4 to reverse T_3.[666] Glucocorticoids also increase the thyroid hormone–binding prealbumin concentration.[666]

Reproductive Function

The effects of glucocorticoids on reproductive function are predominantly inhibitory, are observed at high levels of the steroids, and may be part of an overall mechanism that delays reproductive function in times of stress. In men, glucocorticoid therapy and spontaneous Cushing's syndrome decrease the plasma testosterone concentration.[667,668] This is probably due both to an inhibition of LH release and to direct actions on the testis.[668,669] In the short term, there can be a decrease in the testosterone concentration without a change in LH levels, whereas long-term testosterone levels are better correlated with depressed LH (but not FSH) levels.[668,670] Glucocorticoids may also increase the ability of testosterone to block gonadotropin release by feedback inhibition.[667] They may also regulate factors that delay the onset of puberty.[671] In females, glucocorticoids in excess suppress basal and gonadotropin releasing hormone–stimulated LH (but not FSH) levels, plasma estrogen and progestin concentrations (variably), ovulation, and the onset of puberty. They result in a slight increase in testosterone clearance and have selective effects on FSH action.[671–673] In fat cells, they increase the levels of aromatase, which converts androgens to estrogens.[674]

Synergistic and Antagonistic Interrelations between Glucocorticoids and Other Hormones

The complex interactions between the actions of glucocorticoids and those of other hormones have already been emphasized. Illustrative of these interrelations are the synergism between glucocorticoids and glucagon or epinephrine and the antagonism between glucocorticoids and insulin. Glucocorticoids can modulate cellular sensitivity to other hormones, regulate the same processes as other hormones, and have indirect influences that affect the overall response to other hormones. Conversely, other hormones can directly or indirectly affect glucocorticoid action.

Glucocorticoids can positively or negatively alter cellular sensitivity to other hormones by shifting the dose-response curve or influencing the maximal response obtained.[489,551,675,676] In some cases, the cellular response to another hormone is amplified by the glucocorticoid and vice versa, effects termed by Ingle "permissive."[489,551,675] Tissue synergistic and antagonistic actions can occur by influencing receptors for the other hormones or, more typically, through postreceptor mechanisms. Influences of the steroid on receptors mediating the actions of insulin and immunologic mediators and on the postreceptor steps in these processes are discussed above. Other permissive actions may explain glucocorticoid effects on blood pressure in addisonian individuals,[489] lipolysis,[541] and PTH action.[631,632] Many of the synergisms occur with hormones that activate adenylate cyclase (epinephrine, glucagon, PTH).[489,675] Occasionally, glucocorticoids increase cAMP levels by decreasing levels of the phosphodiesterase that degrades cAMP.[673] Conversely, cAMP can modulate glucocorticoid receptor action.[677] Glucocorticoids can affect β-adrenergic receptors. In adipocytes, the steroid promotes a loss in β_1- and an increase in β_2-adrenergic receptors[678]; in human neutrophils, glucocorticoids induce a tightened coupling of β-adrenergic receptors and adenylate cyclase and attenuate isoproterenol-induced uncoupling between receptors and cyclase activation.[679] Glucocorticoids increase β-adrenergic receptor density in several other cell types.[679] These actions may contribute to glucocorticoid effectiveness in treating asthma, in which the steroid can return desensitized bronchial tissue to normal.[679]

Glucocorticoids and Stress

The survival rate in patients with untreated adrenocortical insufficieny is decreased (Fig. 12-24).[680] Therapy with mineralocorticoids alone [e.g., with DOC (Fig. 12-24)] increases life expectancy only slightly.[680] However, survival is increased markedly when cortisol is given.[680] Decompensation is usually precipitated by a stressful insult (surgery, infection, injury, etc.) and is associated with a variety of derangements, including an inability to maintain a normal blood pressure (Fig. 12-23). Thus, the view has emerged that these steroids are needed to cope with stress. It is generally thought that glucocorticoid levels higher than basal are required to combat stress. This would be consistent with the fact that glucocorticoid production is generally increased in stress and with the occasional finding of a patient in addisonian crisis who has a normal random plasma cortisol concentration.

The multiple actions of glucocorticoids on the cardiovascular system discussed earlier probably contribute to the steroidal stress-combating effect. Thus, these actions would improve vascular reactivity and cardiac performance.

The actions of glucocorticoids inhibiting the production of mediators active on vascular and other systems may be especially critical in the response to stress.[560] It has been proposed that one of the important physiologic functions of glucocorticoids during stress is protection against the harmful effects of the body's defense mechanisms and the products produced by those mechanisms.[542,560,563] The specific case with prostaglandins was discussed above (see Cardiovascular System and Fluid and Electrolyte Balance). In addition, many stressful stimuli, such as serious infections, result in an increased production of numerous mediator substances, including kinins such as bradykinin; lymphokines such as γ-interferon, which stimulates the release of other inflammatory mediators; serotonin; histamine; collagenase, which causes tissue damage; plasminogen activator, which in excess can cause blood vessel leakage and hemorrhage; catecholamines; immunologic mediators; fever-producing substances such as endogenous pyrogen (interleukin 1); PGs and related substances; vasopressin; myocardial depressant factor; cachectin, which has been implicated in endotoxin-induced shock[568]; and other vasoactive substances. It is possible that the actions of these substances are so profound that they can be harmful if left unchecked. Indeed, these substances could result in excessive vasodilatation, cardiac suppression, edema, fever, hemorrhage, and other deleterious effects. Glucocorticoids suppress the production and/or actions of most of the mediators listed above.

Other specific effects may also contribute to the stress response.[560] For example, the increase in GFR may facilitate the clearance of toxic products and combat excessive fluid retention. The induction of glutamine synthetase in the brain may help lower concentrations of the potentially toxic glutamate and ammonia, which are elevated in stress. The induc-

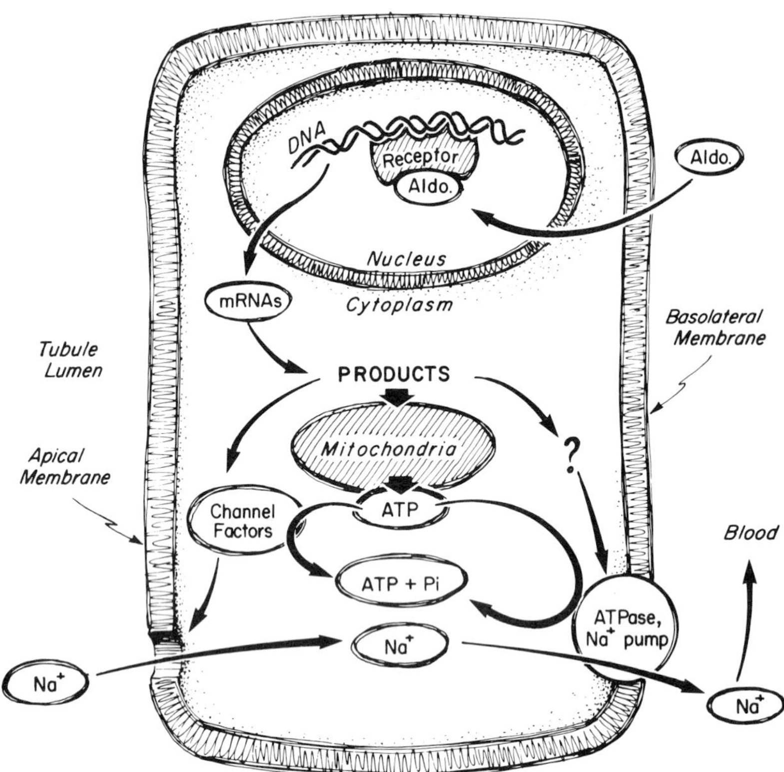

FIGURE 12-26 Steps in mineralocorticoid action. Illustrated are the early molecular events leading to the association of the aldosterone (Aldo)-receptor complex with DNA with consequent induction of mRNA's that encode proteins that could affect the sodium channel, ATP generation, and Na^+ pumping activity.

tion of hepatic cytochrome P450 may help remove toxic foreign chemicals. The induction of metallothionein may help in the elimination of toxic metals such as zinc.

Definition of a Mineralocorticoid

Because both glucocorticoids and mineralocorticoids affect salt balance, it is important to define the term *mineralocorticoid.* As already mentioned, there is a class of binding proteins that appear to mediate the actions of these steroids on ion movement, and these receptors can be distinguished from glucocorticoid receptors. Thus, analogous to the case with glucocorticoids, "mineralocorticoid" actions are referred to as those mediated through these receptors. This would also apply to actions of glucocorticoids on these receptors, for instance, in the brain and pituitary (see above). Also, it is possible that other receptors mediating the actions of sodium-retaining steroids will be found (Chap. 14).

Molecular Mechanisms of Mineralocorticoid Action

The early molecular events in aldosterone action are similar to those of other classes of steroids (see above, Fig. 12-26, and Chap. 5). Thus, specific mineralocorticoid receptors (MR) which bind aldosterone are present in the cytosol of mineralocorticoid-responsive tissues; they have been best characterized in kidney and toad bladder.[681–685] They are similar to glucocorticoid receptors but can be distinguished from them by some differences in their binding characteristics. For example, they have a much higher affinity for mineralocorticoids such as aldosterone and DOC than do glucocorticoid receptors[681] and have a low affinity for certain glucocorticoid receptor–specific compounds, such as RUE-26988.[686] As discussed earlier, they have a relatively high affinity (although lower than that for aldosterone and DOC) for certain "classic" glucocorticoids, such as cortisol and corticosterone.[685] In the kidney, these receptors are located in the branched collecting tubules, the cortical collecting tubules, and the outer medullary collecting tubules.[684] In intact cells, they bind aldosterone and DOC with a K_d of around 0.6 to 1 n*M* and cortisol with a K_d of around 50 n*M*,[685] although in isolated kidney preparations the relative affinity for cortisol is higher.[504–506] The steroid enters the cell and binds to the specific receptor proteins; the receptor-mineralocorticoid complex is then translocated to the nucleus and binds to either specific DNA sequences (HREs) or to other transcription factors[681] (Chap. 5).

As discussed earlier, the glucocorticoid, mineralocorticoid, progesterone, and androgen receptors share a common HRE (Chap. 5). Thus, specificity of mineralocorticoid action is not solely dependent on binding of the MR to DNA, since the other steroid receptors bind equally well. Specificity is multifactorial and is dependent on (1) the presence of the receptor in specific tissues, (2) the ability of certain tissues to inactivate other steroids which bind to the MR, e.g., cortisol inactivation in the kidney (see below), and (3) the interaction of steroid-receptor complexes with "composite response elements," which results in differential transcriptional effects of the MR and glucocorticoid receptors (GR).[509,510] This results in an increase (or decrease) in the transcription of particular genes.[683] Presumably, the protein products of these mineralocorticoid-regulated mRNAs then mediate the mineralocorticoid hormone responses.

As discussed earlier, the kidney is also a glucocorticoid target and contains both glucocorticoid and mineralocorticoid receptors. The free cortisol concentrations in plasma are 100 times those of aldosterone in basal conditions. Thus, left unchecked, cortisol would be the major occupant of the mineralocorticoid receptor. The 50- to 100-fold lower apparent affinity for cortisol relative to aldosterone appears to be due to the fact that cortisol is metabolized to cortisone[256,257]; thus, aldosterone is more available for receptor occupancy and mineralocorticoid actions. Nevertheless, cortisol may occupy the mineralocorticoid receptor to some extent, especially at very high levels.[685]

Sodium bathing the luminal surface passively enters the renal cell through channels in the apical membrane. The intracellular sodium ions are then pumped into the interstitial fluid on the serosal side of the cell by an Na^+, K^+-dependent ATPase. ATP is required to drive the pump and for maintenance of the Na^+ channels in the apical membrane. Aldosterone may act in three ways (Fig. 12-22)[480,681,683]: (1) by increasing the cellular permeability to Na^+ by affecting channels in the apical membrane, (2) by affecting the energy-generating system and thus increasing cellular energy, and (3) by affecting the pump.

Mineralocorticoids increase the number of Na^+ specific apical membrane channels,[681,683] with an increase in the conductance of the apical membrane and an increased number of conducting sodium channels.[687] An aldosterone-regulated protein recruits these channels from a pool of nonconducting channels. This may be the earliest and primary effect. In the toad bladder, aldosterone stimulates phospholipase activity, fatty acid synthesis, and acryltransferase activity.[681] These actions may affect membrane phospholipids and ion transport (Chap. 5) and may thus mediate aldosterone action.

With respect to energy generation, aldosterone increases the renal NADH/NAD^+ ratio and the activities of mitochondrial enzymes involved in ATP generation, in particular citrate synthase,[681,688–690] and, in the toad bladder, cellular ATP levels.[691] These changes have been correlated kinetically with effects on Na^+ transport and may be due to increased enzyme synthesis. Thus, the effect of the hormone in increasing the potential to generate ATP may both drive the Na^+ pump and affect the number of active Na^+ channels.

Aldosterone also increases the incorporation of riboflavin into renal flavin nucleotides, and analogues of riboflavin that inhibit this incorporation also block the antinatriuretic effects of the steroid; more work is needed to determine the significance of these observations.[480]

Aldosterone also increases the Na^+,K^+-ATPase activity of the basolateral membranes of the cortical collecting tubule.[681,688,689,692–695] This may be due to an augmentation of the activity of pump sites rather than an increase in Na^+,K^+-ATPase synthesis. Whether it involves the direct actions of an aldosterone-induced protein or is a secondary effect that occurs after initial effects on the apical membrane and possibly mediated by the increased sodium entry is controversial. Nevertheless, this influence would further enhance sodium transport. These changes in the cortical collecting tubules are also associated with aldosterone-regulated increases in the basolateral cell membrane areas in which the Ka^+,K^+-ATPase enzyme unites are located.

Thus, several aldosterone-regulated proteins appear to act in a coordinated manner to stimulate sodium transport. Several other aldoesterone-regulated proteins have also been identified,[681] and some of them could also affect energy generation, the apical channels, or other processes.

Much less is known about the way aldosterone stimulates potassium or hydrogen ion secretion. The Na^+,K^+-ATPase action affects K^+ excretion by exchanging K^+ for Na^+. However, since effects on Na^+ can occur in the absence of influences on K^+, there might also be effects on a potassium pump or on the permeability of the luminal membrane to K^+.[681]

The effects on hydrogen ion appear to be exerted predominantly in the medullary collecting tubule and in this respect are independent of effects on Na^+, although the factors mentioned above are operative.[681] Suggested targets for aldosterone effects on hydrogen ion include effects on glutamine entry into or exit from mitochondria, on mitochondrial glutaminase, and on cytoplasmic PEPCK.[681]

Mineralocorticoid Agonists and Antagonists

Natural and synthetic steroids have mineralocorticoid agonist activity. Aldosterone, the predominant mineralocorticoid, contains an aldehyde at position 18 that is in equilibrium with the 11-hydroxyl function, forming a cyclic 11,18-hemiacetyl (Fig. 12-27). Cortisol, corticosterone, DOC, 19-nor-DOC, 19-OH-androstenedione, and other 18- and 19-substituted derivatives of these steroids have mineralocorticoid agonist activities (Chap. 14). The synthetic steroid fludrocortisone (9α-fluorocortisol) is extremely po-

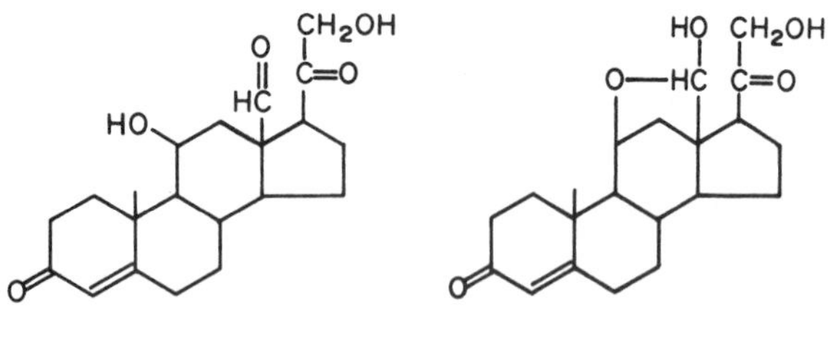

ALDEHYDE FORM HEMIACETAL FORM

FIGURE 12-27 The two forms of aldosterone.

tent and ordinarily is the steroid chosen for replacement mineralocorticoid therapy. Aldosterone and DOC are not useful for oral therapy, since they are rapidly degraded by the liver after absorption (Chap. 14).

A number of compounds have mineralocorticoid antagonist activity. Progesterone, the most potent naturally occurring antagonist, plays a minor physiologic role, except possibly during the third trimester of pregnancy, when progesterone concentrations are extremely high (see Chap. 17). Spironolactone, a steroid analogue, is the compound used clinically as a mineralocorticoid antagonist (Chap. 15). Mineralocorticoid antagonists competitively inhibit the binding of agonists by the receptors.[681]

Radioreceptor assays suggest that under ordinary conditions, almost all the mineralocorticoid activity of human plasma can be accounted for by aldosterone and cortisol.[696,697] As discussed above, the role of cortisol is limited as a result of its metabolism to cortisone. The extent to which cortisol, DOC, 18- and 19-substituted derivatives of these steroids, and 19-OH-androstenedione contribute to mineralocorticoid activity has not been clarified. DOC circulates at concentrations similar to those of aldosterone (see above and Chap. 14) and has equal affinity for mineralocorticoid receptors.[697] However, because less than 5 percent of circulating DOC is free compared with 45 percent of aldosterone,[698] it is likely that this steroid contributes negligibly to mineralocorticoid action under physiologic circumstances. The physiologic importance of 19-nor-DOC and 19-OH-androstenedione is currently under investigation and is potentially significant; since 19-nor-DOC is produced in the kidney, its plasma concentrations may not reflect its levels in the renal target tissue.[699–701] 19-OH-androstenedione is present in the circulation in concentrations about half those of aldosterone, although its plasma binding has not been reported.[699] The role of various steroids in mineralocorticoid excess syndromes is discussed in Chap. 14.

Physiologic Actions of Mineralocorticoids

In humans, mineralocorticoid actions are predominantly due to aldosterone, although cortisol and occasionally DOC may play roles. Mineralocorticoids regulate sodium and potassium balance and act on fewer tissues than do glucocorticoids; mineralocorticoid-responsive tissues include the kidney, gut, salivary glands, sweat glands, vascular endothelium, brain, and possibly mammary gland and pituitary.[480,681,682,686,702,703] The major effect of these actions is to conserve sodium and eliminate potassium and hydrogen ions.

Kidney

The kidney is the most important known site of mineralocorticoid action. Most, if not all, of the physiologically relevant effects occur in the connecting segment, cortical collecting tubules, and medullary collecting tubules.[480,681]

Mineralocorticoids promote the reabsorption of sodium and the secretion of potassium in the cortical collecting tubules and possibly the connecting segment and hydrogen ion secretion in the medullary collecting tubules.[480,681,684,692–695] Aldosterone also has a permissive effect on the osmotic water flux response to vasopressin in the cortical collecting tubule.[681,704] These effects can be observed after a lag of about 30 min to 2 h and require protein and RNA synthesis.[681] In mineralocorticoid deficiency states, there is sodium loss, potassium retention, and decreased renal acid excretion, leading to dehydration, hyponatremia, hyperkalemia, and metabolic acidosis.[705] Conversely, in mineralocorticoid excess states, there is an increase in total body sodium, hypertension, hypokalemia, and a tendency to metabolic alkalosis (Chap. 14).[683]

Only a fraction of the filtered sodium is reabsorbed in response to aldosterone, but this fraction can have marked influences on electrolyte balance. The magnitude of the response to aldosterone is dependent on the amount of solute delivered to the kidney.[683] The amount of sodium retention that can occur in response to an excess of mineralocorticoids in subjects with normal cardiac and renal function is limited[683,701,707]; i.e., such patients do not usually develop edema (Chap. 14).[706] Thus, in primary mineralocorticoid excess states, after an initial period of positive sodium balance, the body adjusts to the excess sodium (the "escape" phenomenon; see Chap. 14) by reabsorbing less of the filtered sodium. This decrease occurs mostly in the proximal tubule, so that sodium intake ultimately equals excretion.[706] Patients with heart failure, cirrhosis of the liver, or nephrosis cannot respond normally and do not escape[707]; thus, secondary aldosteronism contributes to the fluid retention and edema. The mineralocorticoid influence on potassium excretion does not show this escape phenomenon.[706,707]

The escape phenomenon may in part be mediated through secondary increases in ANP levels which produce natriuresis (Chap. 14). ANP levels increase in response to volume expansion, as occurs after mineralocorticoid treatment, and increase in dogs under conditions of escape.[708] Cardiac output also increases under these conditions; this can increase GFR with secondary increases in sodium excretion.[708] A volume increase caused by sodium retention also depresses proximal sodium reabsorption, although this is partly compensated by distal tubular reabsorption.[706] This effect can be independent of increases in GFR[706] and may be due in part to an increase in renal interstitial pressure that lowers the tubular capacity for sodium reabsorption.[706] Urinary PGs and kallikrein increase in concentration after mineralocorticoid administration, have natriuretic actions, and also could conceivably participate in escape.[706] Finally, although escape can occur in the absence of afferent and efferent neural pathways, it is conceivable that the increased vascular volume stimulates volume receptors that decrease renal adrenergic activity and that this decreases sodium transport directly and through renal vasodilatory mechanisms.[706]

Stimulation of potassium loss by mineralocorticoids depends largely on sodium intake.[681,683,707,708] The sodium reabsorbed by the distal tubule increases the electronegativity of the lumen in relation to the peritubular fluid; this is important for passive diffusion of potassium ion into the tubule from which it is excreted. Thus, when there is sufficient delivery of sodium to the distal tubules, a kaliuretic effect of aldosterone is readily observed. By contrast, when sodium intake is restricted, there is minimal delivery of sodium to the distal tubule, since it is mostly reabsorbed in the proximal tubule. In this case, the necessary electronegativity is not generated and potassium excretion is not stimulated. This lack of a prominent kaliuretic effect can be apparent when aldosterone is present in excess in patients with cardiac failure, nephrosis, or cirrhosis who have a decreased GFR and increased proximal tubular reabsorption of sodium.

Changes in sodium and potassium concentrations do not always parallel each other. Further, there is not a stoichiometric relation between sodium reabsorption and potassium excretion.[681,708] Potassium excretion may increase before there is an effect on sodium, and vice versa.[681]

In addition to their role in the ordinary maintenance of potassium balance, mineralocorticoids participate in the defense against chronic hyperkalemia.[681,707,709] Increased aldosterone secretion in response to hyperkalemia increases potassium excretion.

Several factors account for the effects of mineralocorticoids on renal acid production. First, aldosterone produces a net decrease in urinary pH and therefore an increase in urinary acidification without much change in titratable acid.[615,710] This effect is due to an increase in the tubular fluid-to-blood pH gradients across the distal nephron, predominantly across the inner stripe of the outer medulla.[615,710] These effects on hydrogen ion can occur independently of those on sodium and potassium ions. Second, some of the sodium reabsorbed in response to aldosterone is exchanged for hydrogen ion, and this accelerates urinary loss of acid.[710,711] Thus, hydrogen ion loss due to mineralocorticoid excess can be decreased by reducing the intake of sodium and thus its delivery to the distal nephron.[710,711] Third, there is some movement of hydrogen ions into cells in exchange for the potassium lost in the urine.[710,711] Fourth, the potassium deficiency increases hydrogen ion excretion by increasing ammonia production and decreasing the exchange of Na^+ for K^+ that enhances the exchange of Na^+ for H^+.[710,711] The production of alkalosis is blunted by the increased extracellular volume that suppresses bicarbonate reabsorption.[710,711] In adrenal insufficiency, the opposite effect occurs and there are increases in bicarbonate removal and urinary pH and decreased excretion of titratable acid and ammonia.[711]

Mineralocorticoids also influence magnesium and calcium ion excretion.[707] In primary aldosteronism, there is increased urinary excretion of both magnesium and calcium but normal plasma levels are maintained.[707] This effect is probably secondary to sodium retention, which decreases proximal tubular resorption of these ions.

Mineralocorticoids do not directly affect water excretion, GFR, renal plasma flow, or renin production. However, their effects on sodium and water retention with increased extracellular fluid volume indirectly increase GFR and renal plasma flow and suppress the plasma renin concentration (Chap. 14). In addition, these steroids (and also glucocorticoids) enhance vasopressin actions, increasing water permeability.[681]

Mineralocorticoids increase the levels of urinary kallikrein, the enzyme that cleaves bradykinin from kininogen (Chap. 31). The urinary kallikrein level is increased in primary aldosteronism but not in most other forms of hypertension. Although the role of this influence is not known, bradykinin generated as a result of kallikrein action may block sodium reabsorption and serve to blunt aldosterone action.[712]

Extrarenal Tissues

Mineralocorticoid actions on extrarenal tissues also contribute to sodium retention and potassium excretion. Mineralocorticoids decrease sodium excretion and enhance potassium loss in the ileum, colon, skin, and salivary glands.[707,713] Thus, patients with primary aldosteronism lose potassium in the stool, have a decreased level of stool sodium, have an increased potential difference across the colonic epithelium, and have a decreased salivary Na^+/K^+ ratio. In arterial smooth muscle, the steroids stimulate passive and sodium pump–dependent transmembrane movements.[701] Indirect influences of aldosterone outside the kidney (e.g., on blood pressure) are discussed in Chap. 14. Actions of glucocorticoids through mineralocorticoid receptors in brain are discussed under Molecular Mechanisms of Glucocorticoid Hormone Action, above).

Actions of Adrenal Androgens and Estrogens

The biological actions of the androgens are described in Chap. 16. The intrinsic androgenicity of androstenedione, DHEA, and DHEA-S is minimal, and their activity in physiologic and pathologic states is due to their peripheral conversion to testosterone and DHT (Chaps. 4 and 16).[714] The androgenic contribution of the adrenal can be estimated by its contribution to the total production of these two steroids. In men, this is negligible since less than 5 percent of total testosterone production is from sources other than the testicle (see Chap. 16).[715] This small adrenal contribution is due mainly to peripheral conversion of androstenedione and to a lesser extent DHEA and DHEAS. In women, the adrenals contribute significantly to total androgen production.[400,415,715,716] Thus, the adrenals and ovaries each contribute approximately 25 percent of total testosterone production by direct secretion. Peripheral conversion of androstenedione accounts for the other 50 percent; the adrenal and ovarian contributions to androstenedione production vary during the menstrual cycle. After menopause, the adrenal is the major site of androstenedione and testosterone production.

The biological actions of the estrogens are discussed in Chap. 17. The adrenal contribution to plasma estrogens results largely from the peripheral conversion of androstenedione.[717–719] In premenopausal women, this accounts for less than 4 percent of the estrogen supply.[717] However, in postmenopausal women, the adrenal is the major source of estrogens.[715,720] In the male, direct adrenal secretion of estradiol is negligible.[721] About 50 percent of estradiol production is from peripheral conversion of testosterone (of testicular origin), and a minor amount is secreted directly by the testis.[721] The remainder comes from peripheral conversion if androstenedione to estrone and then to estradiol.[721] In the fetus, the adrenal is a major source of estrogen precursors (discussed above and in Chap. 17).

LABORATORY EVALUATION OF ADRENOCORTICAL FUNCTION

Specific plasma assays allow the precise determination of adrenal hormones, including the major glucocorticoids, mineralocorticoids, androgens, and estrogens, and the trophic hormones, i.e., ACTH, angiotensin, and renin, which control adrenal secretion. In many instances, these assays have simplified the evaluation of adrenal dysfunction and have supplanted previously used determinations of urinary metabolites. However, some urinary assays and, in particular, measurement of the 24-h urinary free cortisol can be useful. The plasma steroid methods described measure the total hormone concentration; therefore, alterations in plasma-binding proteins must be considered in their interpretation. The plasma concentrations of the adrenal hormones and their trophic factors vary widely in normal individuals and in both endocrine and nonendocrine disorders (see also Chap. 14). Thus, isolated plasma measurements are frequently not reliable in establishing definitive diagnoses and must be interpreted with regard to the time of the sample and the clinical situation. In general, more precise information is obtained by determining integrated assessments of hormone production and the responses of those hormones to appropriate stimulation and suppression tests (Fig. 12-28).

Plasma Cortisol and Related Steroids

Determination of the plasma cortisol concentration is essential in the evaluation of adrenal function. The current method of choice is radioimmunoassay[722,723];

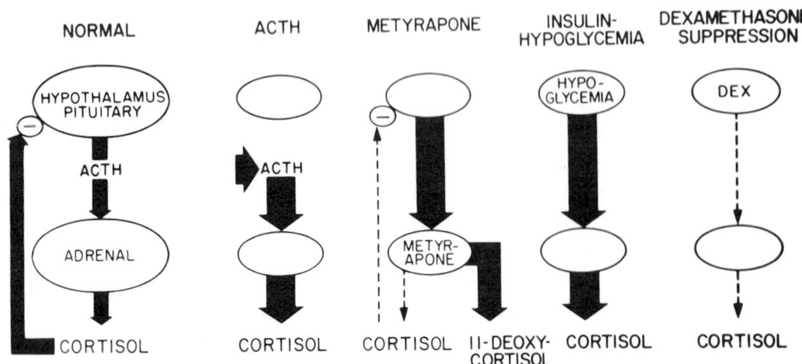

FIGURE 12-28 Tests used to evaluate the hypothalamic-pituitary-adrenal axis. The thickness of the arrow indicates the relative quantities of compounds present if the test is normal. Dotted lines show a blocked pathway. See text for details.

however, cortisol can also be measured by high-performance liquid chromatography (HPLC)[724,725] and by competitive protein-binding radioassay.[726,727] These methods have replaced the classic Porter-Silber method (adapted for plasma), which measures 17,21-dihydroxy-20-ketosteroids,[728,729] the fluorimetric determination of plasma 11-hydroxycorticosteroids.[730,731]

Cortisol

Radioimmunoassay

Radioimmunoassay is the most extensively used assay for the determination of plasma cortisol. Currently available antibodies have limited cross-reactivity with other steroids.[723,732,733] In early assays, the antisera varied greatly in specificity and exhibited cross-reactivity with 11-deoxycortisol, 21-deoxycortisol, 17α-hydroxyprogesterone, corticosterone, DOC, progesterone, cortisone, prednisone, and prednisolone.[704,723,734] Commonly used drugs and medications also do not interfere with the radioimmunoassay.

Liquid Chromatography (HPLC)

In this assay, cortisol is separated from other steroids by liquid chromatography and the concentration of the eluted cortisol is then measured by spectrophotometry or fluorimetry.[724,725] This assay is not interfered with by drugs and medications and does not detect prednisone, prednisolone, cortisone, dexamethasone, or other common natural and synthetic steroids.[725] Although accurate and reliable, this assay has not come into widespread use because the technique is very time consuming.

Competitive Protein-Binding Radioassay

This assay is similar to radioimmunoassay except that CBG is used instead of an antibody to cortisol.[726,727] This assay usually provides a valid estimate of plasma cortisol except when levels of steroids which also have a high affinity for CBG are elevated, e.g., pregnancy (progesterone), congenital adrenal hyperplasia (17α-hydroxyprogesterone, progesterone, corticosterone, DOC, 21-deoxycortisol, or 11-deoxycortisol), and adrenal carcinoma (11-deoxycortisol). The synthetic steroids prednisolone and methylprednisolone also cross-react in this assay system. Modifications of this method to separate the various steroids can circumvent these problems.[726,735] This assay is not interfered with by other hormones and commonly used drugs and medications.[726]

Salivary Cortisol Measurement

The estimation of cortisol in saliva accurately reflects the plasma free cortisol[736] and has been measured by both radioimmunoassay and competitive protein binding.[737,738] This method has proved useful in the assessment of adrenocortical function because of the ease of sample collection and because it allows the collection of multiple or frequent samples in ambulatory outpatients.[738] In one study, normal volunteers had values of 5.6 ± 0.3 ng/ml at 8 A.M. and 1.4 ± 0.1 at 10 P.M., showing the expected normal diurnal variation.[738] Values were markedly elevated after stimulation with ACTH (18.9 ± 0.8) and were suppressed after the administration of 1 mg dexamethasone (0.8 ± 0.4).[738]

Basal salivary cortisol was subnormal in adrenal insufficiency with deficient responses to ACTH administration. In primary adrenal insufficiency, basal salivary cortisol was 1.3 ± 0.2 ng/ml and there was no response to ACTH stimulation (1.5 ± 0.3 ng/ml). In secondary adrenal insufficiency, basal levels were equally low (1.8 ± 0.3 ng/ml); however, in these patients there was an increase (although inadequate) to 3.62 ± 0.8, indicating partial ACTH deficiency and partial adrenal atrophy.[738] In Cushing's syndrome, both 8 A.M. and 10 P.M. salivary cortisol levels were elevated (11.5 ± 1.9 and 13.0 ± 1.8, respectively), demonstrating elevated basal secretion and abnormal diurnal variation. There was no overlap in this series between 10 P.M. salivary cortisol values in normals (range, 0.8 to 1.5 ng/ml) and in patients with Cushing's syndrome (range, 3.3 to 23.9 mg/ml). In addition, patients with Cushing's syndrome had subnormal suppression of salivary cortisol values (range, 2.1 to 24.2) after 1 mg dexamethasone, and there was no overlap with normal subjects (range 0.6 to 1.1 ng/ml). Salivary cortisol levels are also elevated in third trimester pregnancy but maintain a normal diurnal variation.[739]

Interpretation of Plasma Cortisol Determinations

Variations in plasma cortisol levels due to circadian changes, episodic release, and stimulation of the hypothalamic-pituitary-adrenal axis must be considered in evaluating plasma cortisol determinations and limit the usefulness of single measurements.[321,740–742] Subnormal or elevated levels should arouse suspicion of adrenal hypo- or hyperfunction, but in general, more specific testing of the hypothalamic-pituitary-adrenal axis is required. Plasma cortisol levels are not altered with advancing age.[743]

The method used must be considered in interpreting the results of plasma cortisol determinations. Morning (8 A.M.) plasma cortisol levels measured by either radioimmunoassay or competitive protein binding average 10 to 12 μg/dl with a range of 3 to 20 μg/dl,[722,735,742] and values at 4 to 6 P.M. approximate 50 percent of morning levels. In one study using the competitive protein-binding assay, values were 10.4 ± 4 (mean ± SD) at 8 A.M. compared to 4.0 ± 2.0 at 8 P.M. and were less than 3 μg/dl between 10 P.M. and 2 A.M.[742]

Plasma cortisol is appropriately elevated with acute illness, trauma, or surgery,[333,336,744] and levels tend to be elevated in patients with depression, alcoholism, severe anxiety, starvation, anorexia nervosa, and chronic renal failure.[332–334,341,745–748] Since the generally available assays measure total plasma steroid levels, the cortisol concentration is elevated in conditions with increased CBG levels, such as pregnancy and estrogen (including oral contraceptive) therapy.[436,438,745,749] In these instances, plasma cortisol levels may be as high as 40 to 60 μg/dl and may take several weeks to return to normal after delivery or the cessation of estrogen therapy.[437,745] CBG levels may also be increased congenitally and in hyperthyroidism, diabetes, and certain hematologic disorders[438,451]; decreased CBG levels also occur congenitally and in hypothyroidism, liver disease, nephrotic syndrome, multiple myeloma, and obesity.[436–438] CBG binding capacity may be measured in plasma.[436]

Determination of Other Plasma Steroids

Plasma androgen assays are discussed below, and the measurement of aldosterone and DOC is reviewed in Chap. 14. The precursors of both cortisol and aldosterone can be assayed in plasma. These steroids include pregnenolone, 17α-hydroxypregnenolone, progesterone, 17α-hydroxyprogesterone, DOC, corticosterone, and 11-deoxycortisol. The steroids are first separated by solvent extraction and/or chromatography, and their concentrations are then measured by either competitive protein binding or radioimmunoassay[726,735,750,751]; their levels can also be measured by HPLC. Precursors to cortisol include pregnenolone, 17α-hydroxypregnenolone, 17α-hydroxyprogesterone, and 11-deoxycortisol. Steroids of the mineralocorticoid pathway include pregnenolone, progesterone, DOC, and corticosterone as well as 18-hydroxy DOC and 18-hydroxy corticosterone (see Chap. 14).

Measurements of these steroids is most useful in the diagnosis of congenital enzymatic defects of adrenal steroid biosynthesis. Normal ranges and responses to ACTH stimulation are described below in the sections on adrenocortical function testing in children and disorders of steroid hormone biosynthesis. Many of the steroids mentioned above are elevated in patients with adrenocortical carcinoma, and plasma 11-deoxycortisol is measured in assessing the adrenal response to metyrapone (see below).

Plasma ACTH and Related Peptides

Assays of plasma ACTH have simplified the diagnosis of pituitary-adrenal dysfunction.[752,753] Early assays lacked sensitivity and specificity, required extraction of plasma before assay, and were not widely available.[752,753] In addition, ACTH is unstable in plasma, is inactivated at room temperature, and adheres strongly to glass. Careful sample collection and preparation are essential; specimens must be collected with heparin or EDTA in plastic or siliconized tubes on ice, centrifuged in the cold within an hour of collection, and then frozen until assayed. Antisera have been produced which react with the NH_2-terminal or COOH-terminal sequences or against the entire molecule.[754,755] In general, an antiserum should be chosen which reacts with the biologically active 1-24 sequence of human ACTH to reduce the detection of biologically inactive fragments.

A recent radioimmunoassay uses a sensitive and highly specific antiserum which binds to ACTH (5-18) but not to other fragments or precursors.[756] This assay can be performed in unextracted plasma and has a lower limit of detection of 5 pg/ml. In addition, "two-site" or "sandwich" immunoradiometric assays (IRMA) have been developed,[757–761] and one of them is commercially available.[757–761] These methods utilize two antibodies directed at the N- and C-terminal portions of ACTH (1-39) and thus have excellent sensitivity and specificity. These assays can be performed on unextracted plasma, and the detection limit is 2 to 4 pg/ml.[757–761]

When one is evaluating and interpreting ACTH levels, the status of adrenal secretion must be compared and the factors discussed above (in Plasma Cortisol and Related Steroids), such as episodic secretion and circadian variation, must also be considered. The normal range of plasma ACTH concentration with specific radioimmunoassay is 20 to 80 pg/ml in the morning.[756] With the IRMA, the normal range is 10 to 50 pg/ml in the morning; at 4:30 P.M., mean values were 15 pg/ml.[757–761]

Plasma ACTH levels are of the greatest diagnostic utility in the differential diagnosis of spontaneous adrenal disorders. In patients with adrenal insufficiency proved by stimulation testing with exogenous ACTH, elevated plasma ACTH levels confirm primary adrenal insufficiency. In these patients, ACTH levels are usually greater than 200 pg/ml and can be as high as 1000 to 2000 pg/ml. Conversely, plasma ACTH levels below 20 pg/ml are diagnostic of secondary hypoadrenalism (ACTH deficiency).[757–761]

In Cushing's syndrome, a suppressed plasma ACTH level (less than 10 pg/ml) is diagnostic of a primary glucocorticoid-producing adrenal tumor or the rare forms of ACTH-independent micro- or macronodular hyperplasia. In contrast, patients with pituitary ACTH hypersecretion have plasma ACTH levels in the normal to moderately elevated range (20 to 200 pg/ml), and in general, patients with the ectopic ACTH syndrome have markedly elevated plasma ACTH concentrations (200 to >1000 pg/ml).[762,763] However, plasma ACTH levels do not always correctly differentiate pituitary from ectopic sources of ACTH hypersecretion, since a considerable overlap occurs in the range of 100 to 200 pg/ml.[763]

Sensitive bioassays have also been described, but they are technically difficult and have been restricted largely to research use. These bioassays measure plasma ACTH concentration by radioreceptor assay,[764] steroid response of dispersed adrenal cells, or an extremely sensitive cytochemical bioassay.[765]

Radioimmunoassays have also been developed for human β-lipotropin (β-LPH); normal concentrations are 20 to 200 pg/ml.[766–768] β-LPH and ACTH are secreted simultaneously; thus, the circadian variations of β-LPH follow those of ACTH.[768,769] β-LPH levels also respond to hypoglycemia, dexamethasone, and other factors that influence ACTH secretion.[768,769] β-LPH has a longer half-life and greater stability in plasma than does ACTH; in addition, immunoassays are less difficult than those for ACTH. However, this assay is not in general use, and it is not clear that it has any specific advantage over the measurement of plasma ACTH concentration. Similarly, radioimmunoassays for plasma β-endorphin have been developed, but their clinical utility is unknown, and β-LPH cross-reacts with all these assays.[770,771] Thus, precise measurement of the β-endorphin concentration requires prior separation of the peptides by chromatography. An IRMA which measures the ACTH precursors POMC and pro-ACTH has also been described.[772]

Urinary Corticosteroids

Several methods measure levels of urinary cortisol and its metabolites. Traditionally, these methods have involved 24-h urine collections, a feature that can be a disadvantage because of the difficulty of obtaining complete collections. However, these methods provide an integrated assessment of the amount of cortisol produced over a 24-h period, and the problems of episodic release that are present with plasma assays can be bypassed. The 24-h urine sample is collected in a suitable preservative and is then stable when refrigerated. The utility of spot and shorter collections is described below.

Free Cortisol

In spite of the fact that less than 1 percent of the total cortisol secreted by the adrenal is excreted unchanged in the urine (see Variations in Steroid Metabolism, above),[773] a measurement of this fraction can yield useful information. It is especially helpful when cortisol secretion is increased because the unbound plasma cortisol is elevated more than the total level since the capacity of CBG is exceeded.

Urinary free cortisol is measured by extraction of the steroid from the urine and assay of the extract by radioimmunoassay,[722] competitive protein-binding radioassay,[774,775] or HPLC.[776] These assays are rapid and suitable for routine clinical use but have the same limitations of specificity described for the assay of plasma cortisol. In 24-h urine collections, normal values range from 20 to 100 μg/24 h when measured by radioimmunoassay and from 10 to 50 μg/24 h with HPLC.[762,775,776] Elevated levels are nearly always found in spontaneous Cushing's syndrome. In contrast to urinary 17-OHCS, the urinary free cortisol excretion is not elevated in obesity,[774] and this greatly enhances the diagnostic usefulness of this test in Cushing's syndrome. Levels are increased in acute illness and the other stresses discussed above and may be elevated in pregnancy.

In addition, 1-h or 4-h urine collections for free cortisol measurement are useful in assessing dynamic adrenocortical function.[777,778] In one study in normal subjects, urine collections from 7 to 8 A.M. and 10 to 11 P.M. demonstrated normal diurnal variation and suppressibility in response to dexamethasone. In contrast, patients with Cushing's syndrome had absent diurnal variability and lack of suppression with dexamethasone,[777] whereas patients with adrenal insufficiency had very low values in both the morning and evening.[777] In another study, urine cortisol collected from 8 P.M. to 12 midnight clearly separated normal controls from patients with Cushing's syndrome.[778] However, there was some overlap between markedly obese subjects (those >50% above normal weight) and patients with Cushing's syndrome.[778]

Thus, spot and shorter urine collections and the estimation of salivary cortisol are useful methods for assessing free cortisol in ambulatory subjects.

17-Hydroxycorticosteroids and 17-Ketogenic Steroids

Measurements of urinary 17-OHCS and 17-ketogenic steroids (17-KGS) were previously of major importance in the evaluation of adrenal function; these tests also provide an integrated assessment of adrenal function. The response of urinary 17-OHCS level to stimulation or suppression does have clinical utility; however, determination of urinary free cortisol and measurement of plasma cortisol with the rapid dynamic tests discussed below are preferred. Further, urinary 17-KGS determinations are no longer used for the reasons outlined below.

Urinary 17-OHCS are assayed by the Porter-Silber reaction, which is specific for steroids with a 17,21-dihydroxy-20-keto configuration.[728,729] The method ordinarily measures levels of the major urinary metabolites of cortisol and cortisone (discussed above), but with inhibition of 11β-hydroxylase, as with metyrapone testing (see below), it determines the metabolites of 11-deoxycortisol. The normal excretion rate of urinary 17-OHCS is 3 to 10 mg/24 h. Total urinary excretion is elevated in obesity, but this elevation can be compensated for by comparing the result to urinary creatinine excretion (normal range, 2.0 to 6.5 mg per gram of creatinine).[762,779] Urinary 17-OHCS may be decreased in starvation, renal failure, liver disease, pregnancy, and hypothyroidism and may be increased in hyperthyroidism.[779–784] Drugs which induce hepatic microsomal enzymes, such as phenytoin, primidone, phenobarbital, and mitotane, reduce urinary 17-OHCS excretion by increasing steroid metabolism via the 6β-hydroxylation pathway to metabolites that are not measured by the Porter-Silber method.[745,785,786] Other drugs cause direct interference with urinary 17-OHCS determinations, including spironolactone, chlordiazepoxide, hydroxyzine, meprobamate, phenothiazines, quinine, and troleandomycin.[787,788]

The 17-ketogenic steroids are those which are converted to 17-ketosteroids by oxidation and then measured colorimetrically by the Zimmerman reaction (discussed in Urinary Androgens, below).[789] Such steroids include the 17-OHCS (cortisol, cortisone, 11-deoxycortisol), the cortols and cortolones, steroids without a hydroxyl at position 21 (17 α-hydroxyprogestrone and 21-deoxycortisol), pregnanetriol, and certain of their metabolites. In addition, the assay measures levels of the endogenous 17-ketosteroids. However, these levels can be determined separately (see Urinary Androgens, below), and the values can be subtracted from the total of ketogenic steroids to yield the actual level of 17-KGS. Normal values are 6 to 20 mg/24 h in most laboratories.

The assay of 17-KGS does not have any advantages over the other tests and has several disadvantages.[414,787,788] Basal measurements are not reliable in the diagnosis of adrenal insufficiency, Cushing's syndrome, or CAH, and drug interference is common. Thus, this method is no longer used in most centers.

Cortisol Production Rate

Several methods are available for the determination of the production or secretory rate of cortisol.[403] However, technical complexity has largely limited their use to research situations.[403,404] Previous studies have estimated that cortisol production ranges from 8 to 25 mg/day, and most studies have given results in the higher range.[403,404] In recent studies using more specific methods, the cortisol production rate was about 10 mg/day (5.7 to 6.8 mg/m^2 per day) in normal adult volunteers and normal children and adolescents.[410–412] In adult patients with Cushing's syndrome, the cortisol production rate was 30.7 ± 9.3 mg/day (18.1 mg/m^2 per day). These studies suggest that the usual cortisol replacement dose of 20 to 30 mg/day used in adrenal insufficiency may be too high; however, this has not been confirmed. Cortisol production is also increased in obesity, pregnancy, hyperthyroidism, and other circumstances, as discussed earlier; it is decreased in adrenal insufficiency and hypothyroidism.[404]

Dexamethasone Suppression Tests

Low-Dose Tests

Low-dose tests are used in the diagnosis of Cushing's syndrome and assess the integrity of negative feedback control by glucocorticoids of the hypothalamic-pituitary-adrenal axis (see above). Dexamethasone is used since in the small amounts utilized, it is not measured in the plasma and urine corticosteroid assays employed. Thus, in normal individuals, dexamethasone inhibits pituitary ACTH release and consequently adrenal cortisol secretion. In patients with Cushing's syndrome (in whom feedback control is abnormal), secretion is rarely normally suppressible with these tests.[745,762,790–793] These low-dose tests diagnose Cushing's syndrome but do not define the specific etiology.

Overnight Test

The overnight dexamethasone suppression test is a reliable screening test for Cushing's syndrome and requires only one plasma specimen. Dexamethasone (1.0 mg orally) is administered at 11 P.M., and plasma cortisol is measured at 8 A.M. the following morning. A plasma cortisol level below 5 μg/dl excludes Cushing's syndrome with rare exceptions, and patients with Cushing's syndrome have plasma cortisol levels above 10 μg/dl.[762] If the response is abnormal, Cushing's syndrome should be suspected and confirmed with other diagnostic tests.

Less than 2 percent of patients with Cushing's syndrome show normal suppressibility, and only 1.1 percent of outpatient controls have false-positive results.[762] Thus, this test is valuable for outpatient screening. It is less useful in obese individuals, since 13 percent fail to show suppression, and it is of minimal usefulness in hospitalized or chronically ill patients, among whom approximately 25 percent have false-positive results.[762] False-positive responses may also occur in acutely ill patients; in those with severe depression, anorexia nervosa, anxiety, alcoholism, or chronic renal failure; and in high-estrogen states (pregnancy, estrogen therapy, and oral contraceptive administration).[745] Lack of suppression can also occur when accelerated metabolism of dexamethasone caused by phenytoin, barbiturates, or other anticonvulsants results in failure to achieve plasma levels of the steroid sufficient to suppress ACTH secretion.[745]

Two-Day Test

This test, introduced by Liddle in 1960,[793] has been used extensively in the diagnosis of Cushing's syndrome and provides the same information that the overnight 1-mg test provides. In its original form, the test is performed by collecting a 24-h urine sample for baseline determination. Dexamethasone is then given in a dose of 0.5 mg every 6 h for 2 days, with concurrent 24-h urine collections. Although the test can be performed on an outpatient basis, hospitalization may be required to ensure adequate urine collections. A normal urinary 17-OHCS response is suppression to less than 2.5 mg per day on the second day of dexamethasone administration.[762,793]

When these criteria are used, approximately 94 percent of patients with Cushing's syndrome have lack of suppression, and false-positive responses in controls are rare.[762] False-positive results occur rarely in obesity or high-estrogen states,[745,779,794,795] but as is the case with the overnight 1-mg test, false positives occur with acute and chronic illness, depression, alcoholism, and phenytoin therapy.[745,796,797] Since some patients with Cushing's syndrome show normal suppression with this dose, a modification of the test was introduced in which dexamethasone is given in a dose of 20 μg per kilogram of body weight per day.[779] In this study, normal and obese controls had urinary 17-OHCS excretion of less than 1 mg per gram of creatinine whereas none of 15 patients with Cushing's syndrome displayed this degree of suppression.[779]

The response of the urinary free cortisol excretion to the 2-day low-dose dexamethasone test was assessed in two studies; the lower limit was 19 to 25 μg/24 h on the second day.[794,795] Using these criteria, 95.6 percent of patients with Cushing's syndrome failed to suppress normally, and the frequency of false-positive responses in control subjects was 3 percent.[762] In one study, plasma cortisol fell to less than 5 μg/dl in normal subjects in response to low-dose dexamethasone.[798]

High-Dose Tests

High-dose dexamethasone tests are helpful in differentiating Cushing's disease from other types of hypercortisolism once the presence of Cushing's syndrome has been confirmed. These tests depend on the characteristic finding that the hypothalamic-pituitary axis in patients with Cushing's disease is suppressible with glucocorticoids, although pharmacologic doses are required. Thus, ACTH and cortisol secretion decrease when large amounts of dexamethasone are administered.[762,793,799] In contrast, in patients with hypercortisolism secondary to autonomous adrenal tumors or the ectopic ACTH syndrome, high-dose dexamethasone characteristically fails to suppress cortisol hypersecretion, since it is not under the control of the hypothalamic-pituitary axis. Although it is extremely useful, a number of exceptions occur in the use of the high-dose dexamethasone suppression test. These are discussed below (under Diagnosis and Differential Diagnosis and Determining the Etiology and Tumor Localization in the section on Cushing's syndrome) and include Cushing's syndrome with periodic hormonogenesis, nonsuppressible pituitary Cushing's disease, occasional ectopic ACTH-secreting tumors which are suppressible, and nodular adrenal hyperplasia.[745,762]

Overnight 8-mg Test

The overnight high-dose dexamethasone suppression test is more reliable and easier to perform than the standard 2-day test described below (Fig. 12-29). A baseline morning cortisol specimen is obtained, and a single dose of dexamethasone (8.0 mg) is administered orally at 11 P.M. Plasma cortisol is then measured at 8 A.M. the following morning.[800] Among 60 patients with Cushing's disease, plasma cortisol levels were suppressed below 50 percent of baseline in 55 (92 percent), whereas in no patient with either the ectopic ACTH syndrome or glucocorticoid-producing adrenal tumors ($N = 16$) was this degree of suppression achieved. This test had a sensitivity of 92 percent, a specificity of 100 percent, and a diagnostic accuracy of 93 percent.[800] This single-dose test was found to be more reliable than the 2-day test when compared in the same patients, since in only 75 percent of patients with Cushing's disease was urinary 17-OHCS excretion suppressed with the 2-day test.[800] This overnight 8-mg high-dose dexamethasone suppression test is the procedure of choice because of its simplicity and reliability.

Two-Day High-Dose Test

This test first reliably differentiated Cushing's disease from other types of endogenous hypercortisolism.[762,793] A baseline 24-h urine sample is collected, and then dexamethasone (2.0 mg every 6 h for 2 days) is administered with concurrent 24-h urine collection. Again, hospitalization may be required for accurate urine collection. The test is best standardized for urinary 17-OHCS; patients with Cushing's disease show suppression of urinary 17-OHCS level to below 50 percent of baseline levels.[793,800] In patients with adrenal tumors or the ectopic ACTH syndrome, there is usually no decrease in urinary corticosteroid excretion.

The diagnostic accuracy of this procedure is limited because 15 to 30 percent of patients with pituitary-dependent Cushing's disease do not adequately suppress urinary 17-OHCS excretion.[745,762,800,801] The response of urinary free cortisol level has been less extensively studied, but in two series, 16 percent of patients with Cushing's disease did not display 50 percent suppression.[794,795] Measurement of plasma cortisol does not increase diagnostic reliability,[794,795] and measurement of urinary 17-KGS excretion is less reliable than that of urinary 17-OHCS.[762,795]

In a recent study, the responses of both urinary free cortisol and urine 17-OHCS to the 2-day high-dose test were compared.[802] These authors reported that urine cortisol was more profoundly suppressed than was urine 17-OHCS and proposed new criteria for the responses of both measurements. Thus, sup-

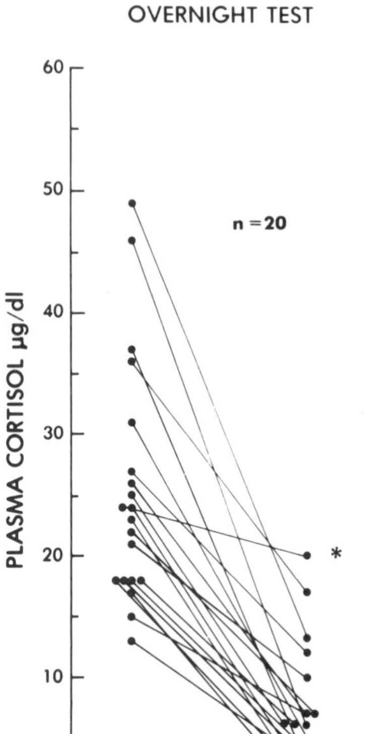

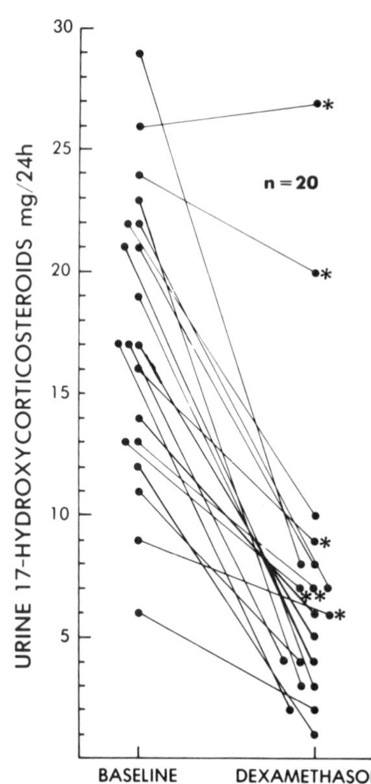

FIGURE 12-29 *(Left)* Plasma cortisol response to the overnight high-dose (8 mg) dexamethasone suppression test. *(Right)* Urinary 17-OHCS response to the standard 2-day, high-dose dexamethasone suppression test in 20 patients with Cushing's disease. Asterisks indicate tests in which the response was not suppressed to <50 percent of the baseline level. *(Based on data of Tyrrell et al.[800])*

pression of urinary cortisol by >90 percent or suppression of urine 17-OHCS by >64 percent correctly established a diagnosis of pituitary disease, and with these criteria no patient with the ectopic ACTH syndrome or an adrenal tumor was incorrectly classified. The sensitivity was 83 percent, the specificity was 100 percent, and the diagnostic accuracy was 86 percent. The disadvantage is that 17 to 31 percent patients with Cushing's disease do not suppress to this extent and will not be correctly identified.

Tests of Pituitary-Adrenal Reserve

Tests of pituitary-adrenal reserve assess the functional capacity of the hypothalamic-pituitary-adrenal axis, its reserve capacity, and its ability to respond to stress. The four most reliable tests use (1) ACTH, which directly stimulates adrenal glucocorticoid secretion, (2) metyrapone, which inhibits adrenal cortisol production and thus indirectly stimulates pituitary ACTH secretion, (3) human or ovine CRF to stimulate ACTH and cortisol release,[803–806] and (4) insulin-induced hypoglycemia, which acts via the pituitary to stimulate ACTH release.[807] Measurement of the adrenal and pituitary responses to these tests is thus used to establish the diagnosis of primary or secondary adrenal insufficiency.

The administration of ACTH directly stimulates adrenal cortisol secretion. In primary adrenocortical insufficiency, the adrenal cortex is destroyed and thus cannot respond. In secondary adrenocortical insufficiency, there is atrophy of the cortex; thus, there is an inadequate acute response to ACTH although cortisol secretion ultimately increases if ACTH stimulation is continued. The rapid ACTH stimulation is usually the first step in evaluating patients with suspected adrenocortical insufficiency.

Rapid ACTH Stimulation Test

This test measures the acute response to ACTH; it is useful in the diagnosis of both primary and secondary adrenal insufficiency. It can be performed on an outpatient basis at any time of the day, does not require fasting, and in emergencies requires only a 30-min delay in the institution of therapy.[808–814] The potent synthetic ACTH derivative cosyntropin (tetracosactrin) is used. It contains the first 24 amino acids of human ACTH and is preferred to previously used animal ACTH preparations, to which there is a greater incidence of allergic reactions.[808] Cosyntropin (250 µg) is administered intramuscularly (IM) or intravenously (IV), and samples for plasma cortisol determination are obtained at 30 min or 60 min after the injection (Fig. 12-30). An additional basal plasma sample is collected before the injection; this is subsequently assayed for plasma ACTH if the response to cosyntropin is subnormal (see Adrenocortical Insufficiency, below).

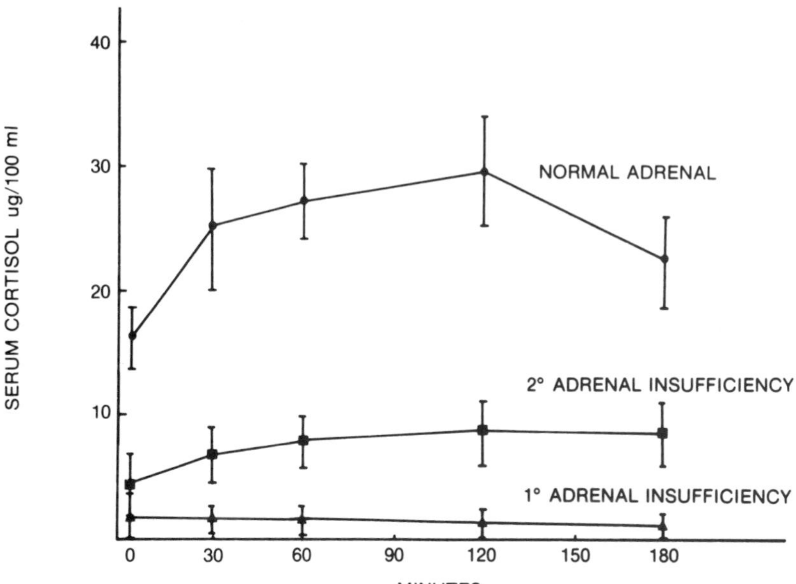

FIGURE 12-30 Serum cortisol response to 0.25 mg cosyntropin in nine normal individuals (normal adrenal), eight patients with hypopituitarism (secondary adrenal insufficiency), and seven patients with Addison's disease (primary adrenal insufficiency). *(From Speckart et al.[809])*

The original normal criteria using the fluorimetric cortisol assay were a basal level of plasma cortisol >5 μg/dl, an ACTH-stimulated increment of >7 μg/dl, and a maximal level of >18 μg/dl at 30 min.[808–810] However, more recent studies have established the fact that the best criteria for a normal response is the maximal plasma cortisol level achieved. In a retrospective study using a cortisol immunoassay, a normal response was defined as a peak cortisol of 20 μg/dl or greater regardless of the increment.[811] This study documented the frequently noted clinical finding that patients with high basal cortisol values may show no further increase in response to acute ACTH stimulation. A recent prospective study in 50 normal patients confirmed that the peak serum cortisol 30 min after ACTH stimulation should exceed 20 μg/dl and that the calculation of the increment is of no value.[812] Another study showed that the 30-min peak cortisol value was most useful and that the response was not related to either the time of day or the basal cortisol level.[813] In an additional study, either IM or IV administration of ACTH resulted in equal adrenal cortisol responsiveness.[814] Thus, the rapid ACTH stimulation test can be performed at any time of the day, the ACTH can be administered either IV or IM, the plasma cortisol response is best assessed at 30 min after ACTH administration, and a normal response is a peak plasma cortisol of 20 μg/dl or greater regardless of the increment.

Subnormal responses to the rapid ACTH stimulation test establish the diagnosis of primary or secondary adrenal insufficiency. In primary adrenal insufficiency, the cortex is damaged; cortisol secretion is reduced, endogenous ACTH secretion is increased, and any remaining cortical tissue is unable to increase cortisol secretion in response to maximal stimulation with exogenous ACTH (decreased adrenal reserve). In secondary adrenal insufficiency, inadequate ACTH secretion leads to atrophy of the zonae fasciculata and reticularis and therefore to adrenal unresponsiveness to brief (but not prolonged) stimulation with exogenous ACTH. In this setting, a subnormal response to exogenous ACTH accurately predicts deficient responsiveness to insulin hypoglycemia, metyrapone, and surgical stress.[811,815–821] The cortisol determinations per se do not differentiate primary from secondary etiology; however, the plasma ACTH concentration is elevated in the primary form but depressed in the second form (see Adrenocortical Insufficiency, below).

A normal response to the rapid ACTH stimulation test excludes the diagnosis of primary adrenal insufficiency, since it provides a direct assessment of adrenal reserve. The response is also abnormal in almost all cases of secondary adrenocortical insufficiency; however, in partial ACTH deficiency, ACTH secretion may be sufficient to maintain adrenocortical function to the extent that atrophy does not occur, and so adrenal responsiveness to exogenous ACTH stimulation remains normal or nearly normal. However, in these patients ACTH secretion is unable to increase further in response to stress because they have a decreased pituitary reserve.[818,819,821] Thus, a normal response to ACTH does not always predict a normal response to direct stimuli such as hypoglycemia and stress and cannot be used to exclude partial secondary adrenal insufficiency with an inadequate pituitary reserve.[820] Such patients are best studied with the overnight metyrapone test, as described below.

The rapid ACTH stimulation test can also be used to measure plasma aldosterone responsiveness.

This modification can be used to differentiate primary and secondary adrenocortical insufficiency.[822] In primary adrenal insufficiency, destruction of all three zones of the cortex leads to deficient responses of both cortisol and aldosterone to exogenous ACTH. However, in most patients with secondary adrenal insufficiency, aldosterone secretion is maintained by the renin-angiotensin system. Therefore, the aldosterone response to exogenous ACTH is normal even though cortisol does not respond. Patients with secondary adrenal insufficiency have an increment in plasma aldosterone of >4 ng/dl, whereas patients with primary Addison's disease have no response.[822]

Three-Day ACTH Stimulation Tests

Three-day ACTH stimulation tests have traditionally been used in the diagnosis of adrenal insufficiency and the differentiation of the primary and secondary forms. These tests are rarely performed at present.

Metyrapone Testing

Metyrapone stimulation assesses both pituitary and adrenal reserve and thus can be used in the diagnosis of both primary and secondary adrenal insufficiency. Metyrapone inhibits adrenal P450c11 and thus blocks cortisol synthesis. The fall in circulating cortisol levels increases a release of ACTH that in turn stimulates increased production of steroids proximal to the site of enzyme inhibition. As a result, plasma levels of 11-deoxycortisol increase, as does urinary 17-OHCS excretion (due to increased excretion of the tetrahydro metabolite of 11-deoxycortisol).[815,823,824] The response to metyrapone correlates well with insulin-induced hypoglycemia,[815,817,824] and a normal metyrapone test predicts a normal response to surgical stress in virtually all patients.[818] Because of its simplicity and low risk, the overnight metyrapone test is preferred to insulin-induced hypoglycemia. This test is not used in patients with suspected primary adrenal insufficiency since the rapid ACTH stimulation test is diagnostic in virtually all patients (see above and the section on adrenocortical insufficiency). The metyrapone test is used to evaluate patients with suspected secondary adrenal insufficiency who have normal or nearly normal responses to ACTH stimulation. In this setting, a subnormal response to metyrapone confirms secondary adrenal insufficiency, and glucocorticoid therapy is required in times of stress.

Overnight Test

The overnight test is performed by administering a single dose of metyrapone at midnight, with a snack to minimize gastrointestinal upset. The dose of metyrapone is 30 mg/kg, i.e., approximately 2.0 g for patients weighing less than 70 kg, 2.5 g for patients weighing 70 to 90 kg, and 3.0 g for patients weighing more than 90 kg.[823] Blood for 11-deoxycortisol and cortisol is drawn at 8 A.M. Patients with a normal pituitary-adrenal axis have a postmetyrapone level of plasma 11-deoxycortisol >7 μg/dl, whereas patients with adrenal insufficiency do not respond.[823] Simultaneous plasma cortisol measurement is useful since 4 percent of normal subjects and patients on phenytoin have a rapid clearance or inactivation of metyrapone, and thus adequate 11 β-hydroxylase inhibition does not occur.[823] An 8 A.M. plasma cortisol level of <10 μg/dl indicates adequate 11β-hydroxylase inhibition. A normal response to the overnight test indicates normal ACTH secretion and adrenal function, since both are required to increase plasma 11-deoxycortisol concentration. A subnormal response indicates primary or secondary adrenal insufficiency but does not differentiate between them.

Three-Day and Intravenous Tests

The original 3-day protocol of the metyrapone test and an intravenous modification are less commonly used. The overnight test described above provides the same information and does not require either urine collections or IV administration of the drug. These procedures are described in Chap. 7.

CRH Testing

Synthetic human CRH and ovine CRH are available for experimental evaluation of the pituitary-adrenal axis.[803–806,825] Ovine CRH is more useful for testing because of its longer duration of action. The peptide is given IV in a dose of 1 μg per kilogram of body weight. CRH directly stimulates pituitary secretion of the products of POMC, e.g., ACTH, β-LPH, and β-endorphin. Reported normal responses of ACTH and cortisol have varied and will have to be established for individual laboratories.

Patients with primary adrenal insufficiency have high basal ACTH levels and subnormal cortisol levels. In response to CRH, ACTH levels increase but cortisol levels do not, reflecting primary adrenal damage. In secondary adrenal insufficiency, plasma cortisol also fails to respond to CRH; however, reported ACTH responses have been very variable and are probably not diagnostically reliable. In general, CRH testing is not required in patients who are being evaluated for adrenal insufficiency since adequate information can be obtained with standard ACTH stimulation and metyrapone tests (see above and Ref. 825).

CRH has also been used to differentiate the various etiologies of Cushing's syndrome. In general, patients with Cushing's disease have normal or exaggerated plasma ACTH and cortisol responses to CRH, although an occasional patient fails to respond. Patients with the ectopic ACTH syndrome do not respond to CRH, although exceptions do occur.[805,826] Patients with adrenal tumors causing Cushing's syndrome have suppressed ACTH levels which do not respond to CRH.

Insulin-Induced Hypoglycemia

The response to insulin-induced hypoglycemia (insulin tolerance test) is the most sensitive and accurate test of the integrity of the hypothalamic-pituitary-adrenal axis[820,821,827,828] and its ability to respond to stress. However, this test is generally limited to the evaluation of patients with suspected hypopituitarism in whom the growth hormone response can be simultaneously evaluated; the test is not commonly used at present (see Chap. 7). Hypoglycemia elicits a potent stress response via pituitary adrenergic receptors[807] and stimulates ACTH release. The test is performed after an overnight fast with measurement of plasma cortisol and glucose (and serum growth hormone, if desired) levels before and at 30, 45, 60, and 90 min after the administration of IV regular insulin. The plasma glucose concentration is measured to assess the adequacy of the hypoglycemia; a value less than 40 mg/dl is considered an adequate stimulus.[820,821,827,829] The usual dose of insulin is 0.15 U/kg of body weight (0.10 U/kg in children) but must be adjusted on the basis of the patient's clinical status and suspected pituitary function. In suspected hypopituitarism or adrenal insufficiency, 0.1 U/kg of body weight is used (0.05 U/kg in children), and the usual dose of 0.15 U/kg is increased by 0.1 U/kg in patients with obesity, diabetes mellitus, Cushing's syndrome, or acromegaly, since these patients exhibit significant insulin resistance. An experienced physician must be in attendance, with careful monitoring of the patient and with IV glucose available. Most patients experience hypoglycemic symptoms, i.e., sweating, tachycardia, and hunger; the test should be terminated with IV glucose if significant symptoms of neuroglycopenia, such as confusion and disorientation, occur. The test is contraindicated in patients with seizure disorders, cardiovascular disease, and cerebrovascular disease and in those greater than 65 years of age. It should not be performed in acutely ill patients with suspected adrenocortical insufficiency since they may be extremely sensitive to insulin. When these precautions are observed, there is little risk to the patient.

With adequate hypoglycemia, plasma cortisol levels peak 60 to 90 min after insulin injection. A normal response is an increment of plasma cortisol of >8 μg/dl and a maximum plasma cortisol level of >18 to 20 μg/dl when cortisol concentration is measured fluorimetrically.[336,821,827,829–831] Normal criteria using the competitive protein-binding assay are an increment of plasma cortisol of >5 μg/dl and a maximal level >15 μg/dl.[815]

A normal plasma cortisol response to hypoglycemia excludes adrenal insufficiency and indicates an intact hypothalamic-pituitary-adrenal axis; these patients do not require glucocorticoid supplementation for stress or surgery.[336] A subnormal response documents adrenal insufficiency and the requirement for glucocorticoid therapy.

Mineralocorticoids

The measurement of aldosterone, DOC, 18-OH-DOC, and other mineralocorticoid levels and the clinical evaluation of the renin-angiotensin-aldosterone axis are discussed in Chap. 14.

Androgens

Dynamic tests such as those described above for studying cortisol excess or cortisol deficiency states have not been as useful in the evaluation of disorders of adrenal androgen production. Thus, greater reliance has been placed on measurement of basal plasma levels of the major adrenal androgens and the active metabolites derived from them (i.e., androstenedione, testosterone, and DHT). These steroids are assayed after extraction and chromatographic separation. Additional techniques that measure the free fraction of testosterone (and other hormones) or the binding capacity of sex hormone–binding globulin (SHBG, TeBG) improve the diagnostic usefulness of the tests. Urinary assays of androgen metabolites are being replaced by more sensitive plasma assays.

Plasma Androgens

Because of similarities in their structures, it has been difficult to assay the individual androgens in unfractionated plasma extracts.[750,751] However, DHEA-S can be measured directly since it is present in plasma in relatively high concentrations.[750] The other androgens and their precursors require separation and purification before assay. This is accomplished by solvent extraction, which fractionates steroids with differing polarity, and then chromatography.[750] After separation, the concentrations of steroids can be accurately measured by radioimmunoassay[750] or competitive protein binding.[832] With these techniques, total plasma levels of DHEA, DHEA-S, androstenedione, testosterone, and DHT can be measured simultaneously.[750,751] The normal plasma levels of these steroids are listed in Table 12-2.

The plasma concentration of free testosterone may also be assayed by methods which include flow dialysis, charcoal adsorption, equilibrium dialysis, steady-stage gel filtration, and ultrafiltration.[832–837] Plasma free testosterone concentrations (mean ± SD) have been reported as follows: normal females, 5.39 ± 2.13 pg/ml (1 to 1.4 percent free); pregnancy, 4.64 ± 1.70 pg/ml (0.6 percent free); hirsute females, 16.1 ± 11.7 pg/ml (1.7 to 2.2 percent free); and normal males, 128 ± 57 pg/ml (1.7 to 2.5 percent free).[832–835] These free levels more clearly reflect the biological activity of circulating testosterone than do total testosterone levels[832–841] (discussed further below). Recent studies have also confirmed the utility of measuring plasma androstenediol and androstenediol glucuronide concentrations in disorders of androgen excess. Levels of these metabolites of DHT are elevated in the majority of women with androgen excess and provide an assessment of the tissue metabolism of androgens.[842]

The binding capacity of SHBG is estimated after its removal from plasma (by adsorption or precipitation) with the use of radiolabeled testosterone or DHT.[841,843] The SHBG binding capacity is higher in normal women than in normal men. It is increased in pregnancy, cirrhosis, and hyperthyroidism and with estrogen (including oral contraceptive) therapy.[838,841,843] SHGB binding capacity is decreased in most females with hirsutism and in acromegaly.[838,841]

Urinary Androgens

Measurement of urinary 17-ketosteroid excretion was the first method of quantification of adrenal hormone levels, but it is a less useful index of androgenicity than are the plasma methods described above.[844] This method measures the levels of urinary metabolites of plasma androgens; the major contribution to urinary 17-ketosteroids is from DHEA and DHEA-S (Table 12-2). Testosterone and DHT constitute less than 1 percent of the total urinary 17-ketosteroids.[844] The ketosteroids are first extracted from urine and then measured by a colorimetric chemical assay (the Zimmerman reaction).[845] Normal excretion is generally in the range of 7 to 17 mg/24 h in males and 5 to 15 mg/24 h in females.[715] Drug interference is a disadvantage; i.e., chlorpromazine, ethinamate, meprobamate, nalidixic acid, penicillin, phenaglycodol, spironolactone, and troleandomycin falsely increase 17-ketosteroid levels, and chlordiazepoxide, etryptamine acetate, progestins, propoxyphene, and reserpine decrease 17-ketosteroid levels.[787]

Clinical Utility

The assays described above are used in the evaluation of hyperandrogenic states. Idiopathic hirsutism and the polycystic ovary syndrome are the most frequent causes of elevated androgen secretion; however, androgen levels are also elevated in Cushing's syndrome, congenital adrenal hyperplasia, adrenal tumors, and ovarian tumors (see below and Chaps. 17 and 18). Hypoandrogenicity (hypogonadism) in the male is discussed in Chap. 16.

The utility of 17-ketosteroid determination is limited since this measurement is unreliable in the diagnosis of Cushing's syndrome[762,801] and androgen excess in hirsutism.[844] The diagnosis of congenital adrenal hyperplasia is best established by an assay of more specific plasma steroids (see below). Plasma androgen assays are more useful; however, serial plasma samples and the assay of several plasma hormones may be required to document androgen excess.[836,840,844,846,847] In addition, assay of the plasma free testosterone concentration is the best single indicator of androgen excess.[832–836,838,841,848]

Adrenocortical Function in Children

Laboratory evaluation of adrenocortical function in children and adolescents should be preceded by a complete clinical evaluation. In addition, the rarity and complexity of these patients usually mandate referral to a pediatric endocrinologist. The laboratory evaluation must take into account the age-related changes in adrenocortical function. As stated above, precise plasma assays are tending to replace urinary steroid determinations, and as is the case with adult patients, interpretation of plasma steroid values must take into account the diurnal and episodic variability of those levels.

Plasma and Urinary Steroids

The normal plasma concentrations of glucocorticoids and mineralocorticoids in children and adolescents are shown in Table 12-8.[394] The concentrations of adrenal precursor steroids and gonadal steroids are shown in Table 12-9.[394]

Current methods include radioimmunoassay and competitive protein-binding radioassay, as discussed above. However, cross-reactivity is a problem with these assays: in the newborn cortisone can cross-react; in patients with CAH elevated levels of adrenal steroid precursors may cross-react. Thus, precise determination of specific steroids requires chromatographic separation procedures or specific measurement by HPLC.[394]

As discussed above, urinary 17-OHCS measures the major metabolites of cortisol; however, this measurement has been largely replaced by the more specific measurement of urine free cortisol. Normal excretion of free cortisol in children is 15 to 20 μg per gram of creatinine and may be up to 40 μg in obese children.[394] Urine cortisol expressed in terms of body surface area is 25 to 75 $\mu g/m^2$ per 24 h in normal children and adolescents.[849] Values above these normal ranges are found in Cushing's syndrome.

Plasma DHEA-S measurements should replace the traditional use of urine 17-ketosteroids to assess the secretion of adrenal androgens (see above). These measurements have their greatest utility in the evaluation of patients with CAH and in rare patients with adrenocortical carcinoma.

Dexamethasone Suppression Tests

In children as in adults, these tests are used to establish the diagnosis of Cushing's syndrome. A

TABLE 12-8 Mean Glucocorticoid and Mineralocorticoid Concentrations

	Cortisol	DOC	Corticosterone	18-OH Corticosterone	Aldosterone	Plasma Renin Activity
Cord blood	12	180	650		85	1800
Prematures	6.5			200	100	8000
Newborns	5		230	350	95	2100
Infants	9	20	545	80	30	1200
Children (8 A.M.)						
1–2 yr	4–20			65	28	535
2–10 yr	As adults	10		45	10→30*	300
10–15 yr	As adults			25	5→20*	120
Adults (8 A.M.)	10–20	7	425	20	7→13*	100→145*
(4 P.M.)	5–10		130			

DOC = deoxycorticosterone.

All values in ng/dl plasma except cortisol (μg/dl) and plasma renin activity (ng/dl/per hr).

* Two values separated by an arrow indicate those in supine and upright posture.

Source: Reproduced with permission from Miller.[394]

modification of the overnight screening test demonstrated that a dose of 0.3 mg/m^2 of dexamethasone could suppress plasma cortisol in normal children.[850]

Traditional low- and high-dose dexamethasone suppression tests are extremely useful and are best performed in a hospital or metabolic ward.[394] After the collection of baseline data, dexamethasone is administered in a dose of 20 μg/kg per day (low-dose) given in divided doses every 6 h for 2 days. For the subsequent 2 days, the patient is given 80 μg/kg per day (high-dose) in divided doses every 6 h. Normal responses to the low-dose test are plasma cortisol

TABLE 12-9 Mean Sex Steroid Concentration in Infants and Children

	PROG	17-OHP	DHEA	DHEA-S μg/dl	Δ^4-A	E_1	E_2	T M	T F	DHT M	DHT F
Cord Blood	36000	1900	600	235	90	1400	810	30	25	6	6
Prematures	350	250	800	400	200			120	10	30	40
Term newborns		35	570	160	150			200	40	25	10
Infants	30	30	110	30	20	<1.5	<1.5	190	<10	40	<3
Children 1–6 yr			30	10	25	<1.5	<1.5	5		<3	
6–8 yr			90	20	25	<1.5	<1.5	5		<3	
8–10 yr			160	50	25	<1.5	<1.5	5		<3	
Males											
Pubertal stage I	20	40	160	35	25	1.1	0.8	5		<3	
II	20	50	300	95	45	1.6	1.1	40		8	
III	25	60	390	120	70	2.1	1.6	190		20	
IV	35	80	400	200	80	3.3	2.2	370		35	
V	40	100	500	230	100	3.2	2.1	550		45	
Adult	35	100	450	270	115	3.0	2.0	620		50	
Females											
Pubertal stage I	20	30	160	40	25	1.3	0.8	5		<3	
II	30	50	330	70	65	2.1	1.6	20		8	
III	40	70	390	90	120	3.0	2.5	25		10	
IV	290	90	430	120	130	3.6	4.7	25		10	
V	160	110	540	150	160	6.1	11.0	30		10	
Adult											
Follicular	30	45	450	150	165	6.0	5.0	30		10	
Luteal	750	165	450	150	165	11.0	13.0	30		10	

PROG = progesterone; 17-OHP = 17-hydroxyprogesterone; DHEA = dehydroepiandrosterone; DHEA-S = DHEA sulfate; Δ^4-A = androstenedione; E_1 = estrone; E_2 = estradiol; T = testosterone; DHT = dihydrotestosterone; M = male; F = female.

All values except DHEA-S are in ng/dl.

Data adapted from Endocrine Sciences, Tarzana, California.

Source: Reproduced with permission from Miller.[394]

TABLE 12-10 Responses of Adrenal Steroids to a 60-Min ACTH Test

	Infants		Prepubertal		Pubertal	
	Basal	Stimulated	Basal	Stimulated	Basal	Stimulated
17-OH-Pregnenolone	225		55	320	120	800
17-OHP	25	190	50	190	60	160
DHEA	40		70	125	260	560
11-Deoxycortisol	80		60	200	60	170
Cortisol (μg/dl)	10	30	13	30	10	25
DOC	20	80	8	55	8	55
Progesterone	35	100	35	125	60	150

All values are mean values in ng/dl of plasma, except cortisol, which is μg/dl.

Data adapted from Endocrine Sciences, Tarzana, California.

Source: Reproduced with permission from Miller.[394]

values less than 5 μg/dl and urine 17-OHCS <1 mg per gram of creatinine. In most patients, normal responses to low-dose dexamethasone exclude Cushing's syndrome; however, some children and adolescents with Cushing's disease have normal responses to this test. In these patients, the diagnosis must be established by elevated urine cortisol values and by the demonstration of abnormal diurnal variation of plasma cortisol.[394]

The responses to high-dose dexamethasone testing are the same as those described above in adults. Patients with Cushing's disease suppress plasma or urine steroids to <50 percent of baseline; patients with adrenal tumors or the ectopic ACTH syndrome show little change in steroid levels.[394]

Plasma ACTH Levels

Plasma ACTH in children measured by sensitive radioimmunoassay or by IRMA has the same utility as in adults (described above). Thus, elevated levels are present in Cushing's disease, Nelson's syndrome, the ectopic ACTH syndrome, primary adrenal failure (Addison's disease), and, most important in children, CAH. Suppressed levels are present with adrenal tumors causing Cushing's syndrome and in hypopituitarism (secondary hypoadrenalism) or after exogenous glucocorticoid therapy.

Adrenal Stimulation Testing

Stimulation of the adrenal cortex with ACTH is the most direct means of testing adrenocortical function. In children, these procedures are of the greatest utility in the diagnosis of primary adrenocortical insufficiency (Addison's disease) (see above) and the syndromes of CAH (see the next section).

The traditional ACTH stimulation test consists of the administration of 0.5 units/kg of ACTH (1-39) given as a 4- to 6-h infusion which results in maximal stimulation of adrenocortical steroids.[394] However, this procedure has been replaced by the plasma corticosteroid response to a single intravenous dose of synthetic ACTH (1-24). With this procedure, the response of plasma cortisol or other steroids is measured 60 min after ACTH injection; the usual doses are 0.1 mg in newborns, 0.15 mg in children less than 2 years of age, and 0.25 mg in older children and adults. Normal responses to this ACTH stimulation test in children are shown in Table 12-10.[394]

The greatest utility of ACTH stimulation testing in childhood is in patients with suspected CAH. In such patients, ACTH markedly stimulates steroids proximal to the enzymatic block. For example, in P450c21 deficiency, the classic and most frequent form of CAH, plasma 17-hydroxyprogesterone increases excessively. The utility of this diagnostic procedure in CAH is described in Disorders of Steroid Hormone Synthesis, below.

Other Pituitary-Adrenal Stimulation Tests

Metyrapone

Metyrapone blocks P450c11 and cortisol secretion, thus stimulating ACTH secretion and increasing adrenal 11-deoxycortisol secretion. In children, metyrapone has been most frequently given in dose of 300 mg/m^2 orally every 4 h for six doses (total dose not to exceed 3.0 g).[394] The normal response is a peak plasma 11-deoxycortisol level of >5 μg/dl. Older children and adults can also be tested with a variation of the overnight test in which 30 mg/kg is given at midnight (see above).[394]

Other Tests

Testing with CRH and insulin hypoglycemia has been used less extensively in the evaluation of adrenal function in childhood. These procedures are described above and in Chap. 7.

DISORDERS OF STEROID HORMONE SYNTHESIS

Introduction

Genetic abnormalities of each of the steps in the biosynthesis of steroid hormones have been described (see Steroid Hormone Biosynthesis, above).

Since the same steroidogenic enzymes are involved in the synthesis of steroid hormones in both the adrenal cortex and the gonads, genetic disorders of steroidogenesis may affect both the adrenals and the gonads. Many of these disorders impair cortisol synthesis, resulting in stimulation of pituitary POMC and secretion of ACTH, which in turn causes adrenal growth. This adrenal enlargement, which was described at autopsy in the nineteenth century, is the basis of the term *congenital adrenal hyperplasia* (CAH), which refers to genetic disorders of cortisol synthesis. Disorders of 21-hydroxylation account for over 90 percent of these genetic disorders, and thus, the term *CAH* generally implies 21-hydroxylase deficiency.

Congenital adrenal hyperplasia is generally considered a rare disease; however, the incidence of severe forms of CAH is probably greater than 1 in 10,000 people and the incidence of the milder forms is probably 10 times higher. Patients with genetic disorders of steroid hormone synthesis may seek medical attention for infertility, impotence, hypertension, menstrual irregularity, hirsutism, and acne as well as coming to medical attention as newborns with ambiguous genitalia and life-threatening cardiovascular collapse.

In theory, the congenital adrenal hyperplasias are easy to understand. A genetic disorder in one of the steroidogenic enzymes interferes with normal steroid hormone synthesis. The signs and symptoms of the disease derive from a deficiency of the steroidal end product and from the effects of the accumulated steroidal precursors proximal to the disordered step. Thus, reference to Figs. 12-4 and 12-7 and a knowledge of the biological actions of the various steroids permit one to deduce and predict the clinical manifestations of the disease.

In practice, the various forms of CAH can be confusing both clinically and scientifically. The principal clinical, laboratory, and therapeutic features of the major forms of CAH are shown in Table 12-11. As discussed in Steroid Hormone Biosynthesis, above, each steroidogenic enzyme has multiple activities, and many extraadrenal tissues contain other enzymes with similar steroidogenic activities. Thus, complete elimination of an adrenal enzyme may not result in the complete elimination of certain steroids from the circulation, making diagnosis difficult. For example, patients with severe salt-losing 21-hydroxylase deficiency can nevertheless have nearly normal levels of serum 21-hydroxylated steroids as adults[851] as a result of an extraadrenal 21-hydroxylase that is different from adrenal P450c21.[192–194] In the past, disorders of steroidogenesis could be studied only by examining steroids in blood or urine because the disordered enzymes and the disordered genes encoding them were not available. This indirect approach, which is analogous to studying hemoglobinopathies by examining O_2 carrying capacity, led to many incorrect conclusions about the nature of the steroidogenic enzymes and their disorders. The cloning of the genes for the various steroidogenic enzymes has recently permitted direct study of these complex disorders. The emerging picture is substantially different from what was understood just a few years ago.

21-Hydroxylase Deficiency

21-Hydroxylase deficiency is one of the most common inborn errors of metabolism. It is due to mutations in the gene encoding adrenal P450c21; recent surveys show that the incidence of the severe form is about 1 in 12,000 and that the mild nonclassical forms affect about 1 in 1000 persons (see incidence of 21-Hydroxylase Deficiency, below). Because of increased success in diagnosis and treatment in infancy, many patients with severe forms of 21-hydroxylase deficiency now live well into the adult age group. Furthermore, there is increasing recognition of the milder forms. Detailed reviews of the complex clinical physiology and molecular genetics of this disorder have appeared recently.[182,183,190,191,852,853]

Pathophysiology

For patients with complete deficiency of P450c21 (for example, a patient with homozygous gene deletion), the resulting clinical manifestations can be deduced from Fig. 12-7. Inability to convert progesterone to DOC results in aldosterone deficiency which causes profound hyponatremia (Na^+ often below 110 mEq/liter), hyperkalemia (K^+ often above 10 mEq/liter), and acidosis (pH often below 7.1) with concomitant hypotension, shock, cardiovascular collapse, and death in an untreated newborn infant. As the control of fluids and electrolytes in the fetus can be maintained by the placenta and the mother's kidneys, this "salt-losing crisis" develops only after birth, usually during the second week of life. In addition, the inability to convert 17-OHP to 11-deoxycortisol results in a glucocorticoid deficiency, which impairs postnatal carbohydrate metabolism and exacerbates cardiovascular collapse. Cortisol deficiency is also manifested prenatally since low concentrations of fetal cortisol result in increased production and secretion of ACTH from the fetal pituitary. ACTH stimulates adrenal hyperplasia and transcription of the genes for all the steroidogenic enzymes, especially for P450scc, the rate-limiting enzyme in steroidogenesis (see Regulation of Adrenal Steroidogenesis, above). This increased gene transcription results in increased enzyme production and activity, with consequent accumulation of non-21-hydroxylated steroids, especially 17-OHP. As the pathways in Fig. 12-7 indicate, these steroids are converted to testosterone.

In the male fetus, the testes produce large amounts of mRNA for the steroidogenic enzymes and

TABLE 12-11 Clinical and Laboratory Findings in Congenital Adrenal Hyperplasia

Enzyme Deficiency	Presentation	Laboratory Findings	Therapeutic Measures
Lipoid CAH	Salt-wasting crisis Male pseudohermaphroditism	Low levels of all steroid hormones, with decreased/absent response to ACTH Decreased/absent response to HCG in male pseudohermaphroditism ↑ ACTH ↑ plasma renin activity (PRA)	Glucocorticoid and mineralocorticoid replacement Sex hormone replacement consonant with sex of rearing Gonadectomy of male pseudohermaphrodite
3β-HSD	*Classical form:* Salt-wasting crisis Male and female pseudohermaphroditism Precocious adrenarche *Nonclassical form:* Precocious adrenarche, disordered puberty, menstrual irregularity, hirsutism, acne, infertility	↑ Baseline and ACTH-stimulated Δ^5 steroids (pregnenolone, 17-OH pregnenolone, DHEA); ↑ Δ^5/Δ^4 serum steroids Suppression of elevated adrenal steroids after glucocorticoid administration ↑ ACTH ↑ PRA	Glucocorticoid and mineralocorticoid replacement Surgical correction of genitalia and sex hormone replacement as necessary, consonant with sex of rearing
P450c21	*Classical form:* Salt-wasting crisis Female pseudohermaphroditism Pre- and postnatal virilization *Nonclassical form:* Precocious adrenarche, disordered puberty, menstrual irregularity, hirsutism, acne, infertility	↑ Baseline and ACTH-stimulated 17-OHP ↑ Serum androgens and urine 17-KS Suppression of elevated adrenal steroids after glucocorticoid administration ↑ ACTH ↑ PRA	Glucocorticoid and mineralocorticoid replacement Vaginoplasty and clitoroplasty in female psudohermaphroditism
P450c11	*Classical form:* Female pseudohermaphroditism Postnatal virilization in males and females Hypertension *Nonclassical form:* Precocious adrenarche, disordered puberty, menstrual irregularity, hirsutism, acne, infertility, hypertension	↑ Baseline and ACTH-stimulated 11-deoxycortisol and DOC ↑ Serum androgens and urine 17-KS Suppression of elevated adrenal steroids after glucocorticoid administration ↑ ACTH ↓ PRA Hypokalemia	Glucocorticoid administration Vaginoplasty and clitorial recession in female pseudohermaphroditism
P450c17	Male pseudohermaphroditism Sexual infantilism Hypertension	↑ DOC, 18-OH-DOC, corticosterone, 18-hydroxycorticosterone Low 17α-hydroxylated steroids and poor response to ACTH Poor response to HCG in male pseudohermaphroditism ↑ ACTH ↓ PRA Hypokalemia	Glucocorticoid administration Surgical correction of genitalia and sex steroid replacement in male pseudohermaphroditism consonant with sex of rearing Sex hormone replacement in female

Source: Reprinted with permission from Miller.[394]

concentrations of testosterone are high in early to midgestation.[854] This testosterone differentiates external male genitalia from the pluripotential embryonic precursor structures. In the male fetus with 21-hydroxylase deficiency, the additional testosterone produced in the adrenals has little if any demonstrable phenotypic effect. In a female fetus, the ovaries lack steroidogenic enzyme mRNAs and are quiescent.[854] No sex steroids or other factors are needed for differentiation of the female external genitalia (i.e., the default phenotype of the human fetus is female) (for a review, see Refs. 182 and 855). In a

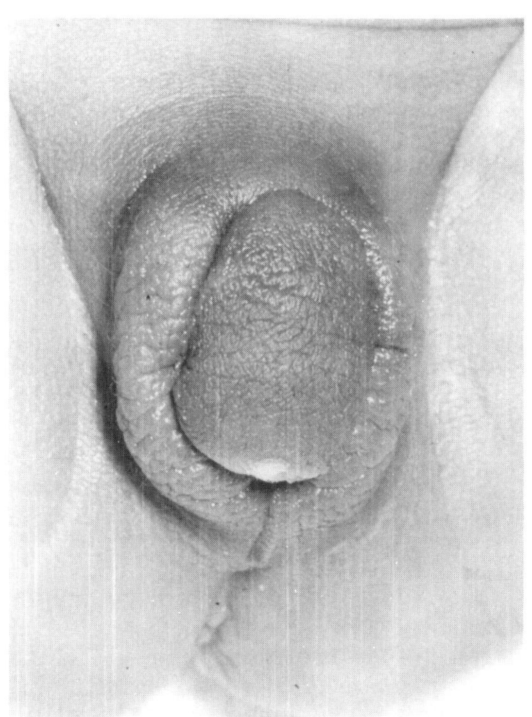

FIGURE 12-31 Genitalia of a severely virilized 2-week-old 46, XX female with severe salt-losing CAH. At birth, this infant was incorrectly thought to be a male with undescended testes and mild hypospadias. Presenting symptoms included vomiting, dehydration, $Na^+ = 107$ mEq/liter, $K^+ = 10.1$ mEq/liter, pH 7.4.

female fetus with 21-hydroxylase deficiency, the testosterone inappropriately produced by the adrenals causes varying degrees of virilization of the external genitalia. This can range from mild cliteromegaly with or without posterior fusion of the labioscrotal folds to complete labioscrotal fusion that includes a urethra traversing the enlarged clitoris (Fig. 12-31). At birth, these female infants, who have normal ovaries, fallopian tubes, and a uterus, may have "ambiguous" genitalia or may be sufficiently virilized so that they appear to be male, resulting in errors of sex assignment at birth. This physiology leads to the other common terms for 21-hydroxylase deficiency: *virilizing adrenal hyperplasia* and *adreno-genital syndrome*.

The diagnosis of 21-hydroxylase deficiency is suggested by genital ambiguity in females, a salt-losing episode in either sex, or rapid growth and virilization in males. Plasma 17-OHP is markedly elevated (>2000 ng/dl after 24 h of age) and hyperresponsive to stimulation with ACTH (Fig. 12-32). Measurement of other steroids, such as 11-deoxycortisol, 17-OHP, DHEA, and androstenedione, is important since certain adrenal or testicular tumors can also produce 17-OHP[35] and high 17-OHP values that rise further after ACTH can also be seen in 3β-HSD and P450c11 deficiencies.[856] 17-OHP is normally high in cord blood but falls to "normal" levels in the newborn after 12 to 24 h (Fig. 12-33) so that assessment of 17-OHP levels should not be made in the first 24 h of life. Endocrinologically normal premature infants and term infants under severe stress (e.g., with cardiac or pulmonary disease) may have persistently elevated concentrations of 17-OHP with normal 21-hydroxylase.

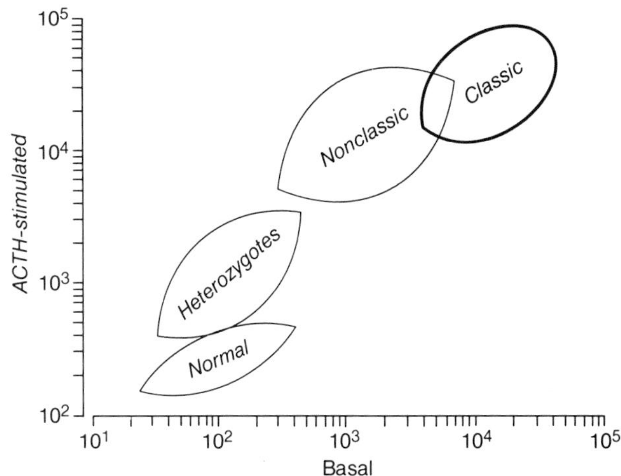

FIGURE 12-32 17-OHP values before and after stimulation with ACTH in normals, patients with CAH, and heterozygotes. *(Redrawn from Miller.[394])*

FIGURE 12-33 Means and ranges of 17-OHP in normal newborns. Note that values can be very high and quite variable for the first 24 h of life. *(Redrawn from Miller.[394])*

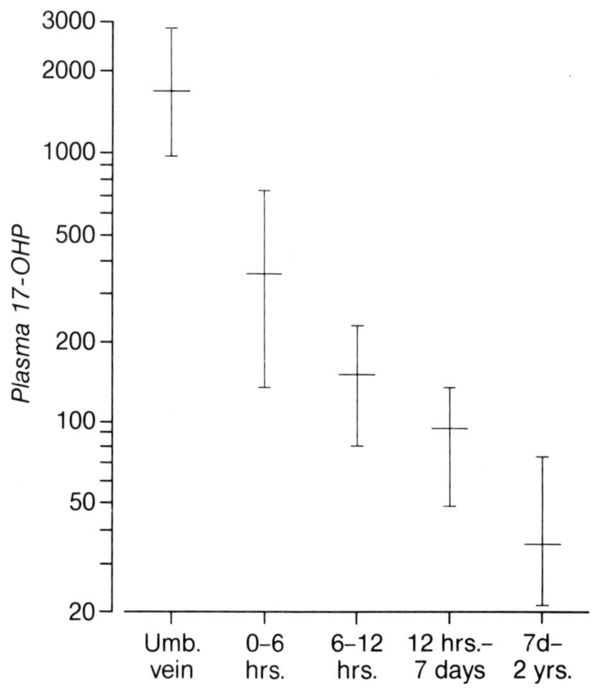

Clinical Forms of 21-Hydroxylase Deficiency

21-Hydroxylase deficiency is characterized by a broad spectrum of clinical manifestations, depending on the genetic disorders of the P450c21 alleles. While these presentations are generally described as different diseases or different forms of 21-hydroxylase deficiency, there is a continuous spectrum of manifestations of this disease, ranging from the severe "salt-wasting form" described above to clinically inapparent forms that may be normal variants. Thus, the disease forms listed below are mainly a clinical convenience.

Salt-Wasting CAH

The clinical phenotype described previously is that of a patient with salt-wasting 21-hydroxylase deficiency. Females with this disorder are frequently diagnosed at birth because of ambiguous development of the external genitalia. After appropriate resuscitation of the cardiovascular collapse, acidosis, and electrolyte disorders, the mineralocorticoids and glucocorticoids can be replaced orally and the ambiguous genitalia can be corrected with a series of plastic surgical procedures. The steroidal replacement management is difficult because of the rapidly changing needs of a growing infant or child. Not only must drug doses be adjusted frequently as the child grows, there is also considerable individual variability in what constitutes "physiologic" replacement. As an underdosage of glucorticoids can be life-threatening, especially during illness, physicians have tended to err on the "safe side" and so these children usually receive inappropriately large doses of glucocorticoids. It is not possible to compensate for the growth lost during the first 2 years of life, when growth is fastest, and so these children inevitably end up shorter than predicted from their genetic potential. Female survivors may have sexual dysfunction, marry with a low frequency, and have decreased fertility.[857] Males with this disorder generally go undiagnosed at birth and either come to medical attention during the salt-losing crisis that follows 5 to 15 days later or die, invariably with an incorrect diagnosis.

Simple Virilizing CAH

Females who are virilized with ambiguous genitalia and increased concentrations of 17-OHP but who do not suffer a salt-losing crisis have long been recognized as having the "simple virilizing" form of CAH. The existence of this clinical variant first led to the incorrect belief that there are two different adrenal 21-hydroxylases, one metabolizing progesterone in the zona glomerulosa and the other metabolizing 17-OHP in the zona fasciculata. Males with this disorder often escape diagnosis until age 4 to 7 years, when they come to medical attention because of inappropriate virilization (pubic, axillary, and facial hair, etc.). An astute physician can readily differentiate boys with sexual precocity caused by CAH from boys with true central precocious puberty: In CAH the testes remain of prepubertal size, while gonadotropic stimulation in true precocious puberty results in pubertal-sized testes. Although these children grow rapidly and are tall for age when diagnosed, their epiphyseal maturation (bone age) advances at a disproportionately rapid rate so that their ultimate adult height is invariably compromised. Untreated or poorly treated children with CAH may fail to undergo normal puberty, and boys may have small testes and azoospermia because of the feedback effects of the adrenally produced testosterone. When treatment is begun at several years of age, suppression of adrenal testosterone secretion may remove tonic inhibition of the hypothalamus, occasionally resulting in true central precocious puberty, requiring treatment with a GnRH agonist. High concentrations of ACTH in some poorly treated boys may stimulate the enlargement of adrenal rests in the testes. These enlarged testes are usually nodular, unlike the homogeneously enlarged testes in central precocious puberty (for review and references, see Ref. 35). Because the adrenal normally produces 100 to 200 times as much cortisol as aldosterone, mild defects (point mutations) in P450c21 are much less likely to affect mineralocorticoid secretion than cortisol secretion. Thus, patients with simple virilizing CAH simply have a less severe disorder of P450c21. This is reflected physiologically by the increased plasma renin activity seen in these patients after moderate salt restriction.

Nonclassic CAH

Many people have very mild forms of 21-hydroxylase deficiency. These forms may be evidenced by mild to moderate hirsutism, virilism, menstrual irregularities, and decreased fertility in adult women (so-called late-onset CAH),[858–860] or there may be no phenotypic manifestations at all other than an elevated response of plasma 17-OHP in response to the administration of ACTH (so-called cryptic CAH).[861] Despite the minimal manifestations of this disorder, these individuals also have hormonal evidence of a mild impairment in mineralocorticoid secretion, as predicted from the existence of a single adrenal 21-hydroxylase.[862]

There has been considerable debate about how to classify patients into these three categories. The difficulty is due principally to the fact that each diagnostic category is not a specific disease but represents a typical picture in a continuous spectrum of disease. As described below, this is due to a broad spectrum of genetic lesions in the P450c21 gene. Furthermore, because many different mutant P450c21 alleles are common in the general population, most patients are compound heterozygotes, carrying a different mutation in the alleles inherited from each parent.

Incidence of 21-Hydroxylase Deficiency

The reported incidence of 21-hydroxylase deficiency varies widely. Perinatal screening for elevated concentrations of serum 17-OHP in several countries yielded an incidence of 1 in 14,000 for "classical" CAH (i.e., salt-wasting and simple virilizing CAH) and 1 in 60 for heterozygous carriers.[863] However, this calculation excluded two groups: the Yupik Eskimos of Alaska, a genetic isolate in which salt-losing CAH occurs in 1 in 280 persons, and the population of Réunion, a French island in the Indian Ocean east of Madagascar, where the incidence is 1 in 2000.[863] Thus, the overall incidence appears to be closer to 1 in 12,000.

Nonclassical CAH is clearly much more common, but these data are also variable. One group has reported very high frequencies: 1 in 27 for Ashkenazi Jews, 1 in 53 for Hispanics, 1 in 63 for Yugoslavs, 1 in 333 for Italians, and 1 in 1000 for other whites.[864–866] These data would indicate that one-third of Ashkenazi Jews, one-fourth of Hispanics, one-fifth of Yugoslavs, one-ninth of Italians, and one-fourteenth of other whites are heterozygous carriers. However, other studies have shown carrier rates of 1.2 percent[860] to 6 percent[867,868] for white populations that were not subdivided further. The considerable differences in the reported incidences reflect differences in the small populations examined and the errors that inevitably arise when hormonal data are used to distinguish individuals with nonclassical CAH from heterozygous carriers of classical CAH. This error can be circumvented by careful measurement of 17-OHP before and after stimulation with ACTH (Fig. 12-32).[183] Furthermore, in homozygotes for both classical and nonclassical CAH, serum concentrations of 21-deoxycortisol rise in response to ACTH, but ACTH-induced 21-deoxycortisol remains normal in heterozygotes for both classical and nonclassical CAH.[869] However, all these studies have classified individuals only by hormonal phenotype; none has examined the P450c21 genes directly to establish these incidences. Therefore, the diagnosis of nonclassical CAH requires family studies, as the hormonal data (17-OHP responses to ACTH) in these individuals may be indistinguishable from those for unaffected heterozygous carriers of the more severe forms. The high incidence, lack of mortality, and lack of decreased fertility in most individuals with nonclassical CAH indicate that this is probably a variant of normal and is not a disease in the classic sense. Nevertheless, patients with nonclassical CAH may seek help for complaints of virilism and menstrual disorders.

Genetics of the 21-Hydroxylase Locus

21-Hydroxylase Genes

There are two 21-hydroxylase loci, a functional gene formally termed CYP21A2 and a nonfunctional pseudogene formally termed CYP21A1P.[77] These are generally termed P450c21B (functional gene) and P450c21A (pseudogene). These two genes are duplicated in tandem with the C4A and C4B genes encoding the fourth component of serum complement[870,871] (Fig. 12-34). The P450c21A gene cannot encode P450c21 because it has three different mutations, each of which prevents the translation of a corresponding mRNA.[185–187] However, the P450c21A locus is transcribed into two alternately spliced, adrenal-specific, polyadenylated mRNAs.[188] It appears that neither of these mRNAs encodes a protein; instead, they may participate in the regulated expression of P450c21B and XB mRNAs.[188,189] Thus, only the P450c21B gene encodes adrenal 21-hydroxylase. P450c21 has a calculated molecular weight of 55,829, and Western blotting studies show a single band of this size.[872] The P450c21 genes consist of 10 exons, are about 3.4 kb long, and differ in only 87 or 88 of these bases.[185,187] This very great degree of sequence similarity indicates that these two genes are evolving in tandem (concerted evolution)[873–875] through intergenic exchange of DNA. The P450c21 genes of mice[876] and cattle[877,878] are also duplicated

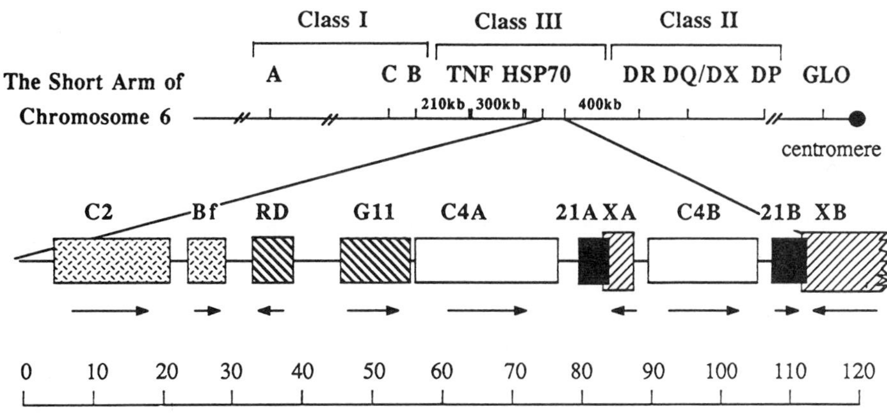

FIGURE 12-34 Genetic map of the region of the HLA locus containing the genes for P450c21 (in black). The scale below is in kilobases (kb). The arrows show transcriptional direction; roles have not been determined for RD and G11. The XB gene coding Tenascin-X is shown truncated; it is about 65 kb long. *(From Morel and Miller.[191])*

and linked to leukocyte antigen loci. However, while only the P450c21B gene functions in human beings, only the P450c21A gene functions in mice[879,880] and both genes function in cattle.[881] Nevertheless, sequencing of the gene duplication boundaries show that this locus duplicated after mammalian speciation,[882] consistent with data that indicate that horses[883] and pigs[884] may have single P450c21 gene copies.

HLA Linkage The diagnosis of 21-hydroxylase deficiency is greatly facilitated by the linkage of the P450c21 gene to the human major histocompatibility complex (MHC).[885] This complex contains genes encoding three major classes of proteins: HLA-A, -B, and -C (class I); HLA-DP, -DQ, and -DR (class II); and serum complement components C2 and C4, properdin factor Bf, and tumor necrosis factors α and β (class III) (Fig. 12-34). HLA typing is now widely used for prenatal diagnosis and to identify heterozygous family members. The P450c21 locus lies about 600 kb from HLA-B and about 400 kb from HLA-DR.[886,887]

Statistical associations (linkage disequilibrium) are well established between CAH and certain specific HLA types. Salt-losing CAH is associated with HLA-B60 and HLA-40 in some populations,[888] and the rare HLA type Bw47 is very strongly associated with salt-losing CAH.[889,890] HLA-Bw51 is often associated with simple virilizing CAH in some populations,[891] and 30 to 50 percent of haplotypes for nonclassical CAH carry HLA-B14.[892] HLA-B14 is often associated with a duplication of the C4B gene.[893,894] By contrast, all HLA-B alleles can be found linked to CAH.

Different individuals in the same family may have markedly different clinical features of CAH despite HLA identity of the affected individuals.[895–898] Such cases can represent extraadrenal 21-hydroxylation, de novo mutations, or double-crossover events. In one family with clinically nonconcordant HLA-identical siblings, the Southern blotting pattern of P450c21 genes digested with *Eco* RI showed a within-generation genetic rearrangement not detectable by other means.[897]

C4 Genes The tandemly duplicated C4A and C4B loci are both functional, and their encoded serum proteins can be distinguished functionally and immunologically. The C4A gene is 22 kb long and encodes a 5-kb mRNA. The C4B gene exists in a long (22 kb) form and a short (16 kb) form as a result of the presence or absence of a 6.8-kb intron at the 5′ end of the gene.[899,900]

Other Genes in the 21-Hydroxylase Locus

Recent studies have shown that the genetic anatomy of the 21-hydroxylase locus is complicated and crowded. In addition to the P450c21 and C4 genes, there are at least 10 and possibly more genes within 100 kb of the P450c21 gene (Fig. 12-34). The genes for complement factor C2 and properdin factor Bf lie 80 to 100 kb 5′ to the P450c21 gene and have the same transcriptional orientation (i.e., lie on the same strand of DNA). Lying just 3′ of the Bf gene is the RD gene, so called because it encodes a protein with a long stretch of alternating arginine (R) and aspartic acid (D) residues.[901] This gene lies on the opposite strand of DNA from the complement and P450c21 genes and is expressed in all tissues, but the function of this gene and its influence, if any, on the genetics of this locus are unknown.[902] Thirteen other putative genes have been identified lying between the gene for tumor necrosis factor (TNF) and C4A, but no functions have been ascribed to any of these genes.[903]

Another pair of genes, termed XA and XB, is duplicated with the C4 and P450c21 genes. These genes lie on the strand of DNA opposite from the C4 and P450c21 genes and overlap the 3′ end of P450c21. The last exon of XA and XB lies within the 3′ untranslated region of exon 10 in P450c21A and P450c21B, respectively.[904] Although the human XA locus was truncated during the duplication of the ancestral C4-P450c21-X genetic unit, the XA gene is abundantly transcribed in the adult and fetal adrenal.[882] By contrast, the XB gene encodes a large extracellular matrix protein—Tenascin X—that is expressed in a wide variety of adult and fetal tissues, especially in cardiac, smooth, and striated muscle.[189] Finally, an additional pair of transcripts, termed YA and YB, arise from the P450c21A and P450c21B promoters, respectively.[188] These transcripts do not appear to encode protein but may interact with the XA and XB transcripts.[188]

P450c21 Gene Lesions Causing 21-Hydroxylase Deficiency

21-Hydroxylase deficiency can be caused by three general categories of mutations in the P450c21B gene: gene deletions, gene conversions, and apparent point mutations (see Chap. 3 for the general principles of molecular biology and DNA analysis of genetic defects). As summarized below and reviewed in detail elsewhere,[190,191] all the point mutations described in the P450c21B gene to date are actually small gene conversion events, so that gene conversions account for about 85 percent of the lesions in 21-hydroxylase deficiency. This highly unusual genetics led to controversy and confusion in this field, but all authorities now agree on the nature of the various genetic lesions causing CAH. Because the P450c21 genes are autosomal, each person has 21-hydroxylase activity encoded by two different alleles, one contributed by the mother and one by the father. As is typical of any autosomal recessive disorder, the severity and clinical manifestations of 21-hydroxylase deficiency are determined by the less severely affected allele. Unlike patients with sickle cell anemia, who are homozygous for a single mutation, most patients with 21-hydroxylase deficiency are compound heterozygotes, having different lesions on their two alleles. Hence, statistical calculations about the causes of CAH must be measured in terms of the frequency of specific alleles rather than in terms of how many patients have which mutation. Because gene deletions and large conversions eliminate all P450c21B gene transcription, in the homozygous state these lesions will always cause salt-losing CAH. Some microconversions, such as those creating premature translational termination, are also associated with salt-losing CAH. Milder forms, such as simple virilizing and nonclassical CAH, are associated with various amino acid replacements in the P450c21 protein caused by other gene microconversion events. Patients with these forms of CAH are usually compound heterozygotes bearing a severely disordered allele (e.g., a gene deletion) and a mildly disordered allele (a microconversion) so that the clinical manifestations are based on the nature of the mildly disordered allele.

Mapping of P450c21 Genes in Normals and in CAH Although the P450c21B and P450c21A loci differ by only 87 or 88 nucleotides, they can be distinguished by restriction endonuclease digestion and Southern blotting. The P450c21A locus is characterized by 3.2- and 2.4-kb *Taq* I fragments and 12-kb *Bgl* II fragments, whereas the functional P450c21B gene is characterized by 3.7- and 2.5-kb *Taq* I fragments and 11-kb *Bgl* II fragments. *Eco* RI digests led to much initial confusion about this locus (for a review, see Refs. 190 and 191) because the sites at the 3′ end of the genes are polymorphic, and the digestion is unpredictable because of variable methylation of these sites. Nevertheless, *Eco* RI digests can be highly informative in family studies.[897] Two unusual and related features of the 21-hydroxylase locus complicate its analysis. First, although gene deletions in this locus are not rare, they are most unusual in that they extend 30 kb from a point in the middle of the P450c21A pseudogene to the precisely homologous point in the P450c21B gene. Thus, the 15 percent of alleles that have gene deletions do not yield a typical Southern blotting pattern with a band of a size different from that of one of the normal bands. This is true irrespective of the restriction endonuclease used to examine the locus, unless one uses very rarely cutting enzymes and analyzes the DNA fragments by pulsed-field gel electrophoresis.[905–909] With this technique, the entire gene complex extending from C4A to P450c21B can be seen as a 110-kb *Bss* HII fragment, with typical P450c21B gene deletions (which also delete C4B) appearing as 80-kb fragments. The second unusual feature of this locus is that gene conversions are extremely common.[881,918]

Gene Conversions The term *gene conversion* refers to a change in which a segment of gene A replaces the corresponding segment of related gene B; thus, the structure of recipient gene B is "converted" to that of donor gene A.[910] A hallmark of gene conversion is that the number of closely related genes remains constant, while their diversity decreases. Gene conversion is thus the key mechanism in concerted evolution.[873–875] The mechanism of gene conversion is unclear, but evidence in yeast favors the creation of double-stranded breaks yielding a double-stranded gap which is repaired by copying both strands of the undamaged homologue.[911–913] Gene conversion–like events have been reported with a broad array of human genes.

Two types of gene conversions commonly cause 21-hydroxylase deficiency: large gene conversions that can be mistaken for gene deletions and small microconversions that resemble point mutations. When a large gene conversion causes 21-hydroxylase deficiency, the *Taq* I digestion pattern of the functional P450c21B gene is converted to that of the P450c21A pseudogene. This gene conversion changes the 5′ end of the P450c21B sequence to the 5′ end of P450c21A, as detected by Southern blotting studies,[894,895,914] oligonucleotide probing,[915] or sequencing.[916] The relative frequency of large gene conversions versus gene deletions in CAH has been controversial,[915–919] principally because initial studies used relatively small groups of patients from single locations or ethnic groups. A study of 68 French patients showed that 12.5 percent of the mutant alleles had large gene conversions, 12.5 percent had gene deletions, and 75 percent had microconversions.[894] A compilation of the world literature on the genetics of CAH found that 19 percent of mutant alleles had gene deletions, 8 percent had large gene conversions, 67 percent had microconversions, and 6 percent had uncharacterized lesions[191] (Fig. 12-35). However, such statistics must be viewed with caution because there is considerable ascertainment bias in favor of the more severely affected patients[894] and because some studies excluded mildly affected patients. Thus, the above statistics are weighted in favor of gene deletions and large conversions, which can only yield a phenotype of salt-wasting CAH.

Point Mutations (Microconversions) Causing CAH About 75 percent of mutated P450c21 genes appear to be structurally intact by Southern blotting and thus appear to carry point mutations.[918] Many such mutant P450c21B genes causing CAH have been cloned and sequenced (Table 12-12), revealing 10 phenotypically expressed changes that cause CAH. All 10 changes are also found in the P450c21A pseudogene. These observations indicate that most CAH alleles bearing apparent point mutations (as inferred from Southern blotting patterns) actually carry microconversions.[190,191] Small localized gene conversions may occur more than once in a single P450c21 gene. Several mutant P450c21B genes have been described as having structures suggesting mul-

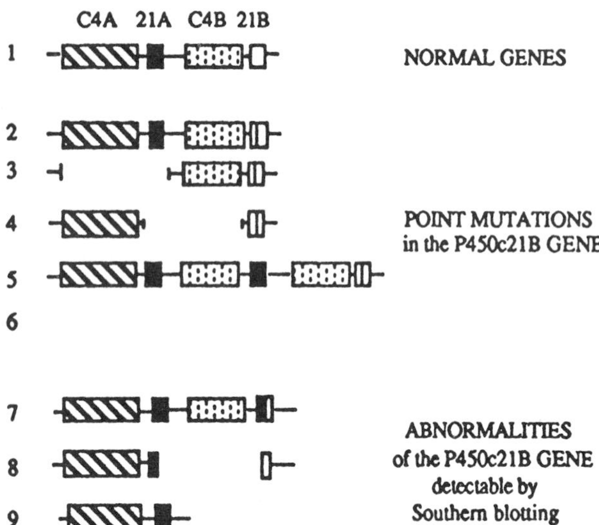

FIGURE 12-35 Classes of genetic rearrangements causing 21-hydroxylase deficiency. Deletions or duplications of the C4A and C4B genes can occur with or without associated lesions in the P450c21B gene. Note that all "point mutations" in P450c21B are actually "microconversions" (see text). *(Modified from Morel and Miller.[191])*

tiple crossover events, i.e., having alternating segments derived from the B and A genes.[920,921]

Effects of Known Point Mutations on 21-Hydroxylase Activity The biochemical consequences of microconversions on 21-hydroxylase activity have been studied by expressing the mutated genes and cDNAs transferred into various cell systems.[872,922,923] There are three changes in the P450c21A pseudogene that render its product nonfunctional. Each change results in an altered reading frame, with a consequent downstream in-phase translational stop codon (nonsense mutation). Each mutation can also be found in the P450c21B gene. The C→T transition at codon 318, the 8-bp deletion in exon 3, and the T insertion in exon 7 have all been found in P450c21B alleles that cause severe salt-losing CAH.[915,921,924–927] Three closely clustered base changes alter the normal amino acid sequence Ile-Val-Glu-Met at codons 236 to 239 in exon 6 to Asn-Glu-Glu-Lys in both P450c21A and a small number of genes causing CAH.[922] The result is severe salt-losing CAH in the patient and absent assayable 21-hydroxylase activity when this gene is transfected into COS cells.

The most common lesion in classical CAH is an A→G change in the second intron, 13 bases upstream from the normal 3′ splice acceptor site of this intron.[922] This mutation, which is found in over 25 percent of severely affected CAH alleles, results in aberrant splicing of the P450c21 mRNA in a cryptic splice site 19 bases upstream from the 5′ end of exon 3. This changes the reading frame, destroying all P450c21 activity. However, a small portion of this mRNA may be spliced normally in some patients. Thus, the phenotypic presentation of this mutation can be somewhat variable; most such patients are salt losers, but some are more typical of non-salt-losing classic CAH. This intronic mutation, which results from another gene microconversion event, is often associated with the Ser→Thr polymorphism at codon 268; this is a true polymorphism as Ser268→Thr does not alter enzymatic activity.[928] This mutation is the most common lesion causing classical simple virilizing CAH in white patients, but it is rare in black and Hispanic patients.[925,926,929–931] In addition to these mutations which grossly alter the structure of the encoded P450c21 protein, the mutation Arg356→Trp, which results from a microconversion, eliminates all detectable activity,[872] apparently because it changes a residue in the steroid-binding site.[932,933] This mutation is found in about 10 percent of severely affected alleles.[928,931]

Missense Mutations Causing Simple Virilizing CAH A change of isoleucine, a nonpolar amino acid, to asparagine, a polar one, at codon 172 is the most common cause of simple virilizing CAH.[872,920,924] Ile 172 is conserved in the other known mammalian P450c21 genes and may contribute to the hydrophobic interactions needed to maintain the correct conformation of the enzyme. This mutation does not appear to affect the abundance or stability of P450c21 mRNA, suggesting that the resulting clinical phenotype is directly due to altered enzyme activity.[920] When Ile 172 was changed to Asn, Leu, Gln, or His and the constructed mutants were expressed in mammalian cells, the mutant constructions yielded only 3 to 7 percent of the 21-hydroxylase activity of normal P450c21.[872,923] Thus, Ile 172 is crucial, but its precise role has not been established.

As mentioned above, the common mutation causing a splicing error in intron 2 has occasionally been associated with simple virilizing CAH. The mutation Pro30→Leu is generally associated with the milder, nonclassical phenotype of CAH. However, the activity of this mutation in vitro is less than that of the common Val281→Leu mutation causing nonclassical CAH and has been reported in some patients with simple virilizing CAH. This emphasizes the fact that the distinctions among salt-losing, simple virilizing, and nonclassical CAH are matters of degree, so that some overlap is to be expected. Similarly, as the Arg356→Trp mutant retains a small degree of activity,[872,924] it would not be surprising if it were described in simple virilizing rather than salt-wasting patients.

Missense Mutations Causing Mild, Nonclassic CAH DNA sequencing and oligonucleotide hybridization studies have established the fact that the most common mutation causing nonclassical CAH is Val281→Leu.[894,928,934] This mutation is seen in all

TABLE 12-12 P450c21 Microconversions Causing 21-Hydroxylase Deficiency

Mutation	Location	Associated Phenotypes	Activity
Pro30 → Leu	Exon 1	NC/SV	30–60%
A → G	Intron 2	SV/SW	Minimal
8 bp deletion	Exon 3	SW	0
Ile 172 → Asn	Exon 4	SV	3–7%
Ile 236 → Asn Val 237 → Glu Met 239 → Lys	Exon 6	SW	0
Val 281 → Leu	Exon 7	NC	18 ± 9%
Gly 292 → Ser	Exon 7	SW	
T insertion @ 306	Exon 7	SW	0
Gly 318 → Stop	Exon 8	SW	0
Arg 339 → His	Exon 8	NC	20–50%
Arg 356 → Trp	Exon 8	SV/SW	2%
Pro 453 → Ser	Exon 10	NC	20–50%
GG → C @ 484	Exon 10	SW	0

Source: Data as compiled by Miller.[853]

patients with the form of nonclassical CAH linked to HLA-B14 and HLA-DR1 but is also found in patients with other HLA types, as is expected from a common gene conversion event. This mutation does not alter the affinity of the enzyme for substrate but drastically reduces its V_{max}.[934]

The second most common mutation causing nonclassical CAH is Pro30→Leu, which is found in about 15 to 20 percent of alleles for this disorder. Both in vitro measurements of the activity of this mutant and some clinical studies have suggested that this mutation is slightly more severe and may also be associated with simple virilizing CAH in some patients.[927,931,935,936] In addition, the mutations Arg339→His and Pro453→Ser have been associated with nonclassical CAH.[937,938] Initial surveys of the mutations in the P450c21A pseudogene failed to reveal these mutations, suggesting that they are bona fide point mutations rather than gene microconversions.[937,938] However, examination of large numbers of P450c21A pseudogenes shows that at least the Pro453→Ser mutation is polymorphic in about 20 percent of P450c21A pseudogenes; hence, its rare association with CAH is probably due to a microconversion event.[937]

Structure-Function Inferences from P450c21 Mutations Each P450c21 missense mutation appears to occur in a functional domain of P450c21. By analogy with the membrane-anchoring domain of hepatic P450IIB,[939] amino acids 167 to 178 of P450c21, including the crucial Ile 172 residue, appear to constitute a similar domain.[872] As mentioned above, Arg 356 may be part of the steroid-binding site,[932] Val 281 appears to participate in coordinating the heme moiety, and Cys 428 is the crucial cystine residue in the heme-binding site found in all cytochrome P450 enzymes.[75,76] All these mutations can arise by gene microconversions. Finally, recent studies suggest that the N-terminal region of P450c21, including Pro30, is required for membrane insertion and enzyme stability.[940]

Finding most mutations in the amino-terminal portion of P450c21 is consistent with finding most gene conversion and gene deletion events occurring in exons 1-8 of the P450c21B gene. Changes in exons 9 and 10 are very rare, probably as a result of evolutionary pressure to retain the 3′ untranslated and 3′ flanking DNA of the P450c21B gene, as this DNA also contains the 3′ end of the XB gene.[189,904]

Prenatal Diagnosis and Treatment of CAH

The prenatal diagnosis of and therapy for 21-hydroxylase deficiency are being actively pursued, but both are complicated by the difficulties described below and must still be considered experimental.[853] Because the fetal adrenal is active in steroidogenesis from very early in gestation, the diagnosis can be made by amniocentesis and measurement of amniotic fluid 17-hydroxyprogesterone.[270,941,942] Concentrations of Δ^4-androstenedione are also elevated in the amniotic fluid of fetuses with CAH, providing a useful adjunctive assay.[943] However, amniotic fluid concentrations of 17-hydroxyprogesterone and Δ^4-androstenedione are reliable only for identifying fetuses bearing a severe salt-losing form of CAH, because these hormones may not be elevated above the broad range of normal in non-salt-losing or nonclassical CAH.[944,945]

If a fetus is known to be at risk because the parents are known heterozygotes (e.g., they have had an affected child previously), 21-hydroxylase deficiency can be diagnosed by HLA typing of fetal amniocytes or by analysis of fetal amniocyte DNA. If the fetus has the same HLA type as the previously affected child, the fetus will be affected; a fetus that shares one parent's HLA type with the index case will be a heterozygous carrier, and a fetus having both haplotypes differing from the index case will be unaffected.

However, such prenatal diagnostic tactics have distinct shortcomings. Informative HLA typing of cultured amniocytes requires the presence of a previously affected child and previous linkage analysis of the affected child and parents. Only HLA-A and HLA-B can be serologically determined with fairly good reliability in cultured amniocytes. However, some HLA-B alleles are expressed weakly in amniocytes; furthermore, there is a relatively high incidence of HLA-B homozygosity among CAH patients, HLA-B loci are frequently identical between parents and patients, and some HLA-B antigens may cross-react, making the results of amniocyte HLA typing difficult to interpret. Also, amniocytes do not express HLA-DR antigens, further limiting the usefulness of HLA typing. Finally, recombination events occur much more frequently in this locus than in other genetic disease loci; hence, inheritance is not always strictly Mendelian.[897]

The possibility of prenatal treatment has increased the need for early and accurate prenatal diagnosis. Female fetuses affected with CAH become virilized at about 8 to 12 weeks gestation, i.e., at the same time that a normal male fetal testis produces large amounts of testosterone, causing fusion of the labioscrotal folds, enlargement of the genital tubercle into a phallus, and the formation of the phallic urethra.[855] The adrenals of female fetuses with CAH can produce concentrations of testosterone that may approach those in a normal male, resulting in varying degrees of masculinization of the external (but not internal) genitalia. If fetal adrenal steroidogenesis is suppressed in a female fetus with CAH, the virilization can theoretically be reduced or eliminated. Some initial studies have reported the successful application of this approach through the administration of dexamethasone to the mother as soon as pregnancy is diagnosed. This approach has been attempted only when the parents are known to be heterozygotes by having already had an affected child. However, even in such pregnancies, Mendelian genetics requires that only one in four fetuses will have CAH. Furthermore, as no prenatal treatment is needed for male fetuses affected with CAH, only one in eight pregnancies of obligate heterozygous parents would harbor a fetus that might potentially benefit from prenatal treatment.

The efficacy, safety, and desirability of such prenatal treatment remain highly controversial.[191,270,853,946,947] The rationale for prenatal treatment is that dexamethasone will suppress fetal ACTH and consequently suppress adrenal steroidogenesis. However, it is not known precisely when the fetal hypothalamus begins to produce CRH, when the fetal pituitary begins to produce ACTH, whether all fetal ACTH production is regulated by CRH, or whether these hormones are suppressible by dexamethasone in the early fetus (for a review, see Ref. 270). While there is considerable evidence that pharmacologic doses of glucocorticoids do not harm pregnant women, no such data exist for the fetus. Pregnant women with diseases such as nephrotic syndrome and systemic lupus erythematosus are generally treated with prednisone, which does not reach the fetus because it is inactivated by placental 11β-hydroxysteroid dehydrogenase/oxidoreductase. Treatment of a fetus with CAH requires the use of fluorinated steroids that escape metabolism by this enzyme, and few data are available about the long-term use of such agents throughout gestation. The available preliminary studies also indicate that the fetal response to treatment is variable and unpredictable; in general, virilization is reduced, but it is generally not eliminated, so that at least one reconstructive surgical procedure is still needed in the infant.[942,947,948] Thus, prenatal treatment of CAH remains an experimental therapy that is done in only a few research centers. Nevertheless, the possibility of eliminating the need for some of the surgical reconstruction of these female infants and the reduction in accompanying emotional trauma to the patient, parents, and family have generated great enthusiasm for prenatal treatment. Thus, accurate, very early prenatal diagnosis is being sought with increasing frequency.

Diagnosis

As discussed earlier, genital ambiguity or a salt-losing crisis will generally alert pediatricians to most cases of severe 21-hydroxylase deficiency. Salt-losing crises generally occur in the second week of life, and the child presents with vomiting, diarrhea, dehydration, hyperkalemia, and hyponatremia. Such infants have on occasion been thought to have viral syndromes or gastrointestinal obstructions; such a failure to make the diagnosis will result in the infant's death. Similarly, boys with simple virilizing CAH often escape diagnosis until they are 4 to 7 years old, when they present with isosexual precocity, advanced bone age, and characteristically prepubertal testes. Teenage and adult females with nonclassical CAH may consult an internist, obstetrician, or dermatologist for virilism, hirsutism, menstrual irregularity, infertility, or acne.

The key diagnostic maneuver in all the various forms of 21-hydroxylase deficiency is the measurement of the 17-OHP response to intravenous synthetic ACTH (cosyntropin), The usual doses are 0.1 mg in newborns, 0.15 mg in children up to 2 years of age, and 0.25 mg in older children and adults. 17-

OHP and cortisol should be measured at 0 and 60 min. Individual patient responses must be compared to age- and sex-matched normative data.[949] Normal responses are shown in Table 12-10 and Fig. 12-32. Both basal and stimulated levels of 17-OHP are markedly elevated in patients with salt-losing and simple virilizing forms of 21-hydroxylase deficiency. Basal levels are usually greater than 2000 ng/dl and increase to more than 5000 to 10,000 ng/dl after ACTH (see Fig. 12-32). Patients with the milder late-onset or cryptic forms typically have normal to mildly elevated basal levels but have supranormal responses to ACTH stimulation, i.e., 1500 to >10,000 μg/dl.[950,951] The cortisol response to ACTH varies from absent to subnormal in patients with the classic severe forms of 21-hydroxylase deficiency and is normal in patients with late-onset and cryptic forms. Basal plasma ACTH levels reflect the extent of 21-hydroxylase and cortisol deficiency; i.e., they are markedly elevated in severe forms (<500 pg/ml) and may be "normal" in patients with the milder forms who are not overtly adrenal-insufficient.

Other ancillary tests are listed in Table 12-11. Urinary excretion of 17-ketosteroids will generally be elevated, but this test is more useful for monitoring the efficacy of suppressive therapy than for initial diagnosis. When urinary steroids are measured, a complete 24-h sample must be obtained, and a concomitant measurement of creatinine excretion is required to monitor the completeness of the collection. Shorter urine collections are not accurate because of diurnal variability of the steroids.

Plasma renin activity and its response to salt-restriction constitute an especially useful test. Most patients with "simple virilizing" 21-hydroxylase deficiency have high plasma renin activity which increases further on sodium restriction, confirming the fact that these patients are partially mineralocorticoid deficient and can maintain a normal serum sodium only by hyperstimulation of the zona glomerulosa. Mineralocorticoid therapy in these patients returns plasma volume to normal and eliminates the hypovolemic drive to ACTH secretion. Thus, mineralocorticoid therapy often permits the use of lower doses of glucocorticoids in patients with simple virilizing CAH, optimizing growth in children and diminishing unwanted weight gain in adults.

Long-term management is difficult to monitor and requires careful clinical and laboratory evaluation. Measurements of growth should be made at 3- to 4-month intervals in children, along with an annual assessment of bone age. Each visit should be accompanied by measurement of urinary 17-KS and serum Δ^4-androstenedione, DHEA, DHEA sulfate, and testosterone. Measurement of 3α-androstenediol glucuronide may also be very useful. In general, plasma 17-OHP is not a useful indicator of therapeutic efficacy because of its great diurnal variation.

Treatment

Although Wilkins[20] and Bartter[21] first demonstrated effective treatment of 21-hydroxylase deficiency with cortisone in 1950, the management of this disorder remains difficult. Overtreatment with glucocorticoids causes delayed growth even when the degree of overtreatment is insufficient to produce signs and symptoms of Cushing's syndrome. Undertreatment results in continued overproduction of adrenal androgens which hastens epiphiseal maturation and closure, again resulting in compromised growth and other manifestations of androgen excess.

Doses of glucocorticoids should be based on the expected normal cortisol secretory rate. Widely cited classical studies have reported that the secretory rate of cortisol is 12.5 ± 3 mg/m^2 per day[472,952,953] and have led most authorities to recommend doses of 10 to 20 mg of hydrocortisone (cortisol)/m^2 per day.[183] However, recent data indicate that the cortisol secretory rate is substantially lower, at 7 ± 2 mg/m^2/per day[411] or even 5 to 6 mg/m^2 per day.[412] While no single formula can be applied to all patients and extensive experience and judgment are needed, we consider the cortisol secretory rate to be about 6 to 8 mg/m^2 per day. It must be stressed, however, that newly diagnosed patients, especially newborns, will require substantially higher initial dosages to suppress their hyperactive CRH-ACTH-adrenal access.

The glucocorticoid used is also important. Most widely used tables of glucocorticoid dose equivalencies are based on their equivalence in anti-inflammatory assays. However, the growth-suppressant equivalences of various glucocorticoids do not parallel their anti-inflammatory equivalencies.[954] Thus, long-acting synthetic steroids such as dexamethasone have a disproportionately greater growth-suppressant effect and hence must be avoided in treating growing children and adolescents (Table 12-13). Most authorities favor the use of oral hydrocortisone or cortisone acetate in three divided daily doses in growing children. However, adults and older teenagers who already have fused their epiphyses may be managed very effectively with 0.25 to 0.5 mg dexamethasone once daily.

Only one oral mineralocorticoid preparation, fludrocortisone (9α-fluorocortisol), is currently available. When the oral route is not available in severely ill patients, mineralocorticoid replacement is achieved through supraphysiologic doses of intravenous hydrocortisone plus sodium chloride. About 20 mg of hydrocortisone has a mineralocorticoid effect of about 0.1 mg of 9α-fluorocortisol (Table 12-13). Mineralocorticoids are unique in pharmacology in that their doses are essentially the same regardless of the size of the patient. In fact, newborns are quite insensitive to mineralocorticoids and often require larger doses than do adults (0.15 to 0.30 mg/day). In older children, the replacement dose of 9α-fluoro-

TABLE 12-13 Potency of Various Therapeutic Steroids (Relative to the Potency of Cortisol)

Steroid	Anti-inflammatory Glucocorticoid Effect	Growth-Retarding Glucocorticoid Effect	Salt-Retaining Mineralocorticoid Effect
Cortisol (hydrocortisone)	1.0	1.0	1.0
Cortisone acetate (oral)	0.8	0.8	0.8
Cortisone acetate (IM)	0.8	1.3	0.8
Prednisone	3.5–4.0	5	0.8
Prednisolone	4		0.8
Methyl prednisolone	5	7.5	0.5
Betamethasone	25–30		0
Triamcinolone	5		0
Dexamethasone	30	80	0
Fludrocortisone (9α-fluorocortisol)	15		200
DOC acetate*	0		20
Aldosterone†	0.3		200–1000

* No longer commercially available.

† Not commercially available. Shown for comparison.

Data compiled from various sources and Styne et al.[954]

cortisol is 0.05 to 0.15 mg daily. It must be emphasized that a mineralocorticoid is essentially useless unless adequate sodium is presented to the renal tubules. Thus, additional salt supplementation, usually 1 to 2 g NaCl/day in the newborn, is also needed. Patients with severe salt-losing congenital adrenal hyperplasia can in some cases discontinue mineralocorticoid replacement and salt supplementation as adults. Perhaps adults become more sensitive to the mineralocorticoid action of hydrocortisone via a developmental decrease in renal 11β-HSD activity, which normally inactivates cortisol to cortisone.

3β-Hydroxysteroid Dehydrogenase Deficiency

Severe deficiency of 3β-HSD activity is a rare cause of glucocorticoid and mineralocorticoid deficiency and is fatal if not diagnosed early in infancy.[955] In its classic form, genetic females have cliteromegaly and mild virilization because the fetal adrenal overproduces large amounts of DHEA, a small portion of which is converted to testosterone by extraadrenal 3β-HSD and other enzymes. Genetic males also synthesize some androgens by peripheral conversion of adrenal and testicular DHEA, but the concentrations are insufficient for complete male genital development, so that these males have a small phallus and severe hypospadias.

There are at least two functional human genes for 3β-HSD: the type I gene is expressed in the placenta and peripheral tissues,[142–145] and the type II gene is expressed in the adrenals and gonads.[146,147] Clinical, genetic, and endocrine studies of 3β-HSD deficiency show that both the gonads and the adrenals are affected as a result of a single mutated 3β-HSD gene expressed in both tissues. However, considerable hepatic 3β-HSD activity persists in the face of complete absence of adrenal and gonadal activity and is presumably due to the enzyme encoded by the type I gene, thus complicating the diagnosis of 3β-HSD deficiency. Not surprisingly, recent genetic studies have shown that the mutations causing 3β-HSD deficiency are all found in the type II gene.[956,957,957a] Some alleles causing the severe, salt-losing form of 3β-HSD deficiency have a nonsense mutation at the position normally occupied by Trp 171. Others have point mutations, including Tyr253→Asn, Glu142→Lys, and the insertion of a single base, causing a frame shift.[957] One patient with a milder, non-salt-losing form of 3β-HSD deficiency was homozygous for the mutation Ala245→Pro.[957] The wide variety of mutations found in the small number of alleles studied to date suggests that a great variety of mutations cause 3β-HSD deficiency.

The presence of peripheral 3β-HSD activity complicates the hormonal diagnosis of this disease; i.e., affected infants should have low concentrations of 17-OHP, the steroid that is typically elevated in 21-hydroxylase deficiency. Yet some newborns with 3β-HSD deficiency have very high concentrations of serum 17-OHP, approaching those of patients with classical 21-hydroxylase deficiency. The high 17-OHP concentrations are due to extraadrenal 3β-HSD activity,[856] presumably encoded by the type I 3β-HSD gene. The adrenal of a patient with 3β-HSD deficiency will secrete very large amounts of the three principal Δ^5 compounds: pregnenolone, 17-hydroxypregnenolone, and DHEA. Some of the secreted Δ^5 17-hydroxypregnenolone is then peripherally converted to 17-OHP. However, in all cases, the ratio of the Δ^5 to the Δ^4 compound is high, consistent with the adrenal and gonadal deficiency of 3β-HSD.[856] Thus, the principal diagnostic test in 3β-HSD deficiency is intravenous administration of ACTH with measurement of the three Δ^5 compounds and the corresponding Δ^4 compounds.

Mild or "partial" defects of adrenal 3β-HSD activity occur without adrenal insufficiency; these patients are typically young girls with premature adrenarche or young women with a history of premature adrenarche and complaints of hirsutism, virilism, and oligomenorrhea.[958–960] This mild form of 3β-HSD deficiency and the mild form of 21-hydroxylase deficiency account for 10 to 15 percent of such patients, many of whom are otherwise classed as having the polycystic ovary syndrome. Patients with mild 3β-HSD deficiency have high basal concentrations of 17-hydroxypregnenolone and DHEA that exceed those seen in hirsute women with nonclassical 21-hydroxylase deficiency. More important, they have abnormally high ratios of Δ^5 to Δ^4 steroids after stimulation with ACTH. In adult women, the hirsutism can be ameliorated and regular menses can be restored by suppressing ACTH with 0.25 to 0.5 mg of dexamethasone given orally each day. The management of children with very mild forms of 3β-HSD deficiency should be more conservative, as unnecessary administration of glucocorticoids has a significant adverse effect on normal growth.

P450c17 (17α-Hydroxylase/17,20-Lyase) Deficiency

P450c17 is the single enzyme, found in both the adrenals and gonads, that has both 17α-hydroxylase and 17,20-lyase activities (see Steroid Hormone Biosynthesis, above). Deficient 17α-hydroxylase activity and deficient 17,20-lyase activity have been described as separate genetic diseases, but it is now clear that they represent different clinical manifestations of different lesions in the same gene.

P450c17 deficiency is fairly rare, although over 120 cases have been reported (for a review, see Ref. 961). Deficient 17α-hydroxylase activity results in decreased cortisol synthesis, overproduction of ACTH, and stimulation of the steps proximal to P450c17. These patients may have mild symptoms of glucocorticoid deficiency, but this is not life-threatening, as the lack of P450c17 results in the overproduction of corticosterone which has glucocorticoid activity. These patients typically overproduce DOC in the zona fasciculata, which causes sodium retention, hypertension, and hypokalemia and also suppresses plasma renin activity and aldosterone secretion from the zona glomerulosa When P450c17 deficiency is treated with glucocorticoids, DOC secretion is suppressed and plasma renin activity and aldosterone concentrations rise to normal.[962]

The absence of 17α-hydroxylase and 17,20-lyase activities prevents the synthesis of adrenal and gonadal sex steroids. As a result, affected females are phenotypically normal but fail to undergo adrenarche and puberty[963] and genetic males have absent or incomplete development of the external genitalia (male pseudohermaphroditism).[964] The classical presentation is that of a teenage female with sexual infantilism and hypertension.[965] The diagnosis is readily made by finding low or absent 17-hydroxylated C-21 and C-19 plasma steroids and low urinary 17-OHCS and 17-KS, which respond poorly to stimulation with ACTH. Serum levels of DOC, corticosterone, and 18-OH-corticosterone are elevated, show hyperresponsiveness to ACTH, and are suppressible with glucocorticoids.

Selective deficiency of the 17,20-lyase activity P450c17 has been reported in about a dozen cases (for a review, see Ref. 961), which initially led to the incorrect conclusion that 17α-hydroxylase and 17,20-lyase are separate enzymes. Such patients have not been characterized in great detail but generally have low concentrations of DHEA and sex steroids that respond subnormally to stimulation with ACTH or hCG. Urinary excretion of the metabolites of cortisol and DOC are normal, while metabolites of 17-OHP are increased.[157] This suggests that essentially normal amounts of cortisol are produced through vigorous stimulation of the zona fasciculata; however, measurements of plasma ACTH have not been reported. Thus, 17,20-lyase deficiency probably represents a mild, partially compensated form of 17α-hydroxylase deficiency, analogous to the "milder" forms of 21-hydroxylase deficiency. It has been suggested that some patients with 17,20-lyase deficiency may have a defect selective for the Δ^4 pathway[966]; however, such patients probably have a general mild defect that appears to be selective for the Δ^4 pathway because the enzyme normally prefers Δ^5 substrates.[163–166]

The single gene for P450c17 has been cloned[171] and localized to chromosome 10q24-q25.[95,169] The molecular basis of 17α-hydroxylase deficiency has been determined in several patients by cloning and sequencing of the mutated gene.[166,168,961,967,967a] The genetic lesions identified include three point mutations that cause premature translational termination, two small duplications of 4 to 7 bp that change the translational reading frame, a 3-bp deletion removing a Phe codon, a 9-bp deletion removing three codons, replacement of a large segment of the gene with foreign DNA, and six point mutations causing single amino acid replacements.[967a] One of these point mutations, Ser106→Pro, was found in a homozygous state in two affected patients from Guam, suggesting that this may be an important lesion in Micronesian people.[166] Thus, a large number of apparently random mutations can cause 17α-hydroxylase deficiency, rendering genetic diagnosis difficult unless a specific ethnic association is identified. Patients with well-documented isolated 17,20-lyase deficiency have not been studied at the molecular level. Since they retain at least some 17α-hydroxylase activity, it is most likely they will have point mutations causing a single amino acid change that disrupts the structure of P450c17 only mildly. Such mutations have already been created by site-directed mutagenesis based on examination of the active site residues.[171a,933]

P450c11 Deficiency

There are two distinct forms of 11-hydroxylase (see Steroid Hormone Biosynthesis, above). P450c11β mediates the 11β-hydroxylation of 11-deoxycortisol to cortisol and that of DOC to corticosterone in the zonae fasciculata and reticularis. P450c11AS, or aldosterone synthase, is found only in the zona glomerulosa and mediates 11β-hydroxylation, 18-hydroxylation, and 18-oxidation; thus, it is the sole enzyme required to convert DOC to aldosterone. Deficient P450c11β activity is a rare cause of CAH in persons of European ancestry but accounts for about 15 percent of cases in both Moslem and Jewish Middle Eastern populations.[968] Severe deficiency of P450c11β results in decreased secretion of cortisol, causing CAH and virilization of affected females, as described above for P450c21 deficiency. However, unlike the typical salt-losing syndrome seen in 21-hydroxylase deficiency, patients with P450c11β are able to retain sodium normally because the substrate for 11β-hydroxylation in the mineralocorticoid pathway DOC, is itself a mineralocorticoid. Although DOC is less potent than aldosterone, it is secreted at higher levels in 11β-hydroxylase deficiency, so that salt is retained and the serum sodium remains normal. Overproduction of DOC frequently leads to hypertension; as a result, 11β-hydroxylase deficiency is often termed "the hypertensive form of CAH". However, newborns often manifest mild, transient salt loss,[968,969] presumably as a result of the normal newborn resistance to mineralocorticoids; this often obscures the diagnosis. Thus, there may be a poor correlation between DOC concentrations, serum potassium, and blood pressure or between the degree of virilization in affected females and the electrolyte and cardiovascular manifestations.[183] The diagnosis is established by demonstrating elevated basal concentrations of DOC and 11-deoxycortisol which hyperrespond to ACTH the normal or suppressed plasma renin activity is a hallmark of this disease.[970]

The genetic lesions causing 11β-hydroxylase deficiency are in the CYP11B1 gene that encodes P450c11β. In a study of Sephardic Jews of Moroccan ancestry, 11 of 12 affected alleles bore the mutation Arg448→His.[211] In several other patients,[971,972] the identified mutations include two frame shifts due to the insertion or deletion of one or two nucleotides, three premature stop codons (nonsense mutations), and four missense mutations that change amino acids: Thr318→Met, Arg374→Glu, Arg384→Gln, and Val441→Gly. All these mutations appear to cluster in exons 6–8 of the CYP11B1 gene, possibly associated with frequent CpG sites.[972]

Some patients have deficiencies of 18-hydroxylase and 18-methyloxidase activities sometimes termed *corticosterone methyl oxidase (CMO) deficiency*, while maintaining a nearly normal capacity for 11-hydroxylation. Type II CMO deficiency affects only 18-oxidation, while type I deficiency affects both 18-hydroxylation and 18-oxidation.[198] Corticosterone secretion is increased and aldosterone secretion is markedly decreased or absent in both disorders, the type I disorder is characterized by low concentrations of 18-hydroxycorticosterone, and the type II disorder is characterized by high concentrations of 18-hydroxycorticosterone. The most valuable diagnostic measurements are the absolute concentration of 18-hydroxycorticosterone and the ratio of corticosterone to 18-hydroxycorticosterone. This ratio is increased in the type I disorder and decreased in the type II disorder.[212]

It is now clear that these two disorders are simply different clinical manifestations of various mutations in the CYP11B2 gene encoding P450c11AS. Jews of Iranian origin have a very high incidence of this defect in aldosterone synthesis, possibly as high as 1 in 4000.[973] These patients are homozygous for two different point mutations: Arg181→Trp and Val386→Ala213. When expressed in transfected cells, the Arg181→Trp mutation alone destroyed nearly all conversion of 18-OH corticosterone to aldosterone and retained nearly normal 11β-hydroxylase activity, while the Val386→Ala mutant was essentially indistinguishable from the normal enzyme. While these studies suggest that the Arg181→Trp mutation alone suffices to confer the disease phenotype, homozygosity for this mutation in the absence of homozygosity for the Val386→Ala mutation did not cause the disease.[213] This study emphasizes that in vitro measurements of enzyme activity do not always correlate well with a clinical phenotype. Mutations causing the more severe type I form of aldosterone deficiency, in which both 18-hydroxylase and 18-oxidase activities are absent, have not been reported. However, it is likely that severe defects such as deletions, frame shifts, and nonsense mutations in the CYP11B2 cause this disorder by destroying all P450c11AS activity. In such cases, one would expect the patient to retain the ability to convert DOC to corticosterone, as is seen in the type I deficiency, because this reaction would continue to be catalyzed by P450c11β.

It is of interest that the genes encoding P450c11β and P450c11AS are a pair of tandemly duplicated genes that have 93 percent nucleotide sequence identity, a genetic anatomy reminiscent of the

P450c21A and P450c21B genes. Although gene conversion can cause CMO II deficiency,[973a] gene convertion appears to be much rarer than in the P450c21 locus. This may be due to the higher recombinational frequency in the HLA region carrying the P450c21 genes, or it may be related to the abundant antisense transcripts produced in the P450c21 locus.[188,189]

While gene conversion events in the P450c11 locus are rare, an unusual gene duplication causes glucocorticoid-suppressible hyperaldosteronism (see also Chap. 14).[974,975] This homologous recombination event creates a third P450c11 gene that fuses the 5′ flanking DNA of the P450c11β gene onto a gene for P450c11AS. In two such patients the genetic crossover occurred in intron 2, and in two other patients it occurred in intron 3 or exon 4.[975] All these hybrid genes produce a hybrid P450c11 that retains aldosterone synthase activity; however, as the hybrid gene has P450c11β regulatory regions, it is turned on by ACTH and cAMP, as is the normal P450c11β gene. Thus, these patients make P450c11AS in response to physiology that should stimulate P450c11β. The excess P450c11AS causes hyperaldosteronism and hypertension; this is then suppressible by glucocorticoid suppression of ACTH.

Congenital Lipoid Adrenal Hyperplasia

Lipoid CAH is the rarest and most severe genetic disorder of steroid hormone synthesis. This disorder is characterized by the absence of significant concentrations of all steroids, high basal concentrations of ACTH and plasma renin activity, an absent steroidal response to long-term treatment with high doses of ACTH or hCG, and grossly enlarged adrenals laden with cholesterol and cholesterol esters.[976–979] These findings indicate a lesion in the first step in steroidogenesis—the conversion of cholesterol to pregnenolone—and have been confirmed by enzymologic studies.[979–983] In fact, these studies have led to other names for lipoid CAH, including *20,22-desmolase deficiency* and *P450scc deficiency*.

Congenital lipoid adrenal hyperplasia might conceivably be caused by a genetic lesion in any of the three components of the cholesterol side-chain cleavage system: P450scc, adrenodoxin, and adrenodoxin reductase. In one autopsied patient, P450scc protein was undetectable,[982] thus implying that the lesion was in P450scc. However, the P450scc gene is structurally intact in these patients,[925,983] and the sequence of the P450scc gene and cDNA from one affected individual were normal.[983] Similarly, a lesion in adrenodoxin reductase or adrenodoxin appears highly unlikely. These proteins serve as electron transport intermediates for all mitochondrial forms of cytochrome P450, not just for P450scc. These include hepatic P450c26/25, which mediates bile acid 26-hydroxylation and vitamin D 25-hydroxylation,[984–986] and the renal vitamin D 1-hydroxylase, yet patients with lipoid CAH who survive to adulthood do not have disorders of vitamin D metabolism or bile acid metabolism.[978,979] Another probability is that lipoid CAH is a disorder of one or more factors involved in the the transport of free cholesterol into the michondria.[71] Thus, it is not clear which gene is disordered in lipoid CAH.[983]

Infants with lipoid CAH are normal at birth, indicating that maternal transplacental steroids suffice for fetal glucocorticoid requirements. It should be noted that fetuses with this disorder, as well as fetuses with 17α-hydroxylase/17,20-lyase deficiency and fetuses with placental aromatase deficiency,[987] survive to term and develop normally in the absence of the high concentrations of estriol normally associated with pregnancy. Thus, if estrogens are needed to maintain pregnancy, the contribution of the mother's ovaries is sufficient. The amniotic fluid of a woman carrying a fetus with lipoid CAH had modest concentrations of pregnenolone and progesterone, contributed by the mother's ovaries, but fetal serum estrogen concentrations were very low.[988]

All the affected infants are phenotypically female. The testes of genetic XY males with lipoid CAH cannot produce testosterone[979] but continue to produce müllerian inhibitory factor, which is a glycoprotein. As a result, affected male fetuses cannot virilize their external genitalia and hence have normal-appearing female external genitalia with a blind vaginal pouch but lack a uterus, fallopian tubes, and cervix. Affected females have normal nonvirilized external genitalia.

Clinical signs of lipoid CAH become apparent in the second week of life, when affected infants have a typical salt-losing crisis, essentially identical to that seen in infants with severe salt-losing 21-hydroxylase deficiency. Clinical signs include poor feeding, lethargy, diarrhea, vomiting, hypotension, dehydration, hyponatremia, hyperkalemia, and acidosis. The outcome is invariably fatal if an early diagnosis is not made. Fluid resuscitation, salt replacement, and appropriate doses of glucocorticoids and mineralocorticoids can lead to normal growth and life to the adult years.[978–979] Genetic males with this disorder are raised as females and should undergo orchiectomy in early childhood.[978,979,983,989]

Only 34 clearly described patients with lipoid CAH have been reported.[979,983] Among these patients, 20 (59 percent) were of Japanese or Korean heritage and 5 (15 percent) were from southern Germany or Switzerland, suggesting that the disorder occurs in genetic clusters. Of the 34 patients, only 13 survived.[979,983] However, it is likely that both the incidence and survivability of this disease are greater than the numbers would imply; several Japanese pediatric endocrinologists have told us that they were caring for several unreported patients with lipoid CAH. Its diagnosis is inherently indirect and presumptive. With each of the other forms of CAH, one can measure both the accumulation of specific precursor steroids and low or absent product steroids in the basal and ACTH-stimulated states, thus readily identifying the enzymatic step involved. By contrast, lipoid CAH is characterized by the absence of all circulating and excreted steroids, enlargement of the adrenals, and the absence of any unique biochemical marker such as increased serum concentrations of the precursor in an enzymatic reaction. In the absence of a defined molecular lesion, congenital lipoid adrenal hyperplasia remains a syndrome. It is possible that some patients will be found with P450scc gene lesions and that such patients will have phenotypic and clinical manifestations indistinguishable from those of lipoid CAH patients with intact P450scc genes. In fact, a deletion of the P450scc gene has been reported in rabbits with a form of CAH that looks exactly like lipoid CAH.[990] It is likely that this rare disorder will continue to attract considerable attention because the finding of normal P450scc genes in at least one patient indicates that other, unidentified factors play a crucial role in the early steps of steroid hormone synthesis.

ADRENOCORTICAL INSUFFICIENCY

Impairment of adrenal function leads to deficient adrenal production of glucocorticoids and/or mineralocorticoids. Such impairment usually results from destruction of or damage to the adrenal cortex (primary adrenocortical insufficiency, Addison's disease) or is secondary to deficient pituitary ACTH secretion (secondary adrenocortical insufficiency) (Fig. 12-36) (see Disorders of Steroid Hormone Biosynthesis, above). Primary adrenocortical insufficiency is an uncommon disorder. However, it must be considered in the differential diagnosis of many common conditions that present with weakness, lassitude, weight loss, anorexia, or gastrointestinal symptoms. Secondary adrenal insufficiency due to natural causes is also uncommon (see Chap. 7); however, iatrogenic secondary adrenocortical insufficiency is more frequent because of the large number of individuals who receive exogenous glucocorticoid therapy which suppresses pituitary ACTH production (see Chap. 15).

FIGURE 12-36 Causes of adrenocortical insufficiency. Secondary insufficiency can be due to lesions of either the hypothalamus or the pituitary, although the most common cause (indicated by the asterisk) is iatrogenic and is due to glucocorticoid therapy. The most common cause of primary adrenocortical insufficiency is idiopathic, also indicated by an asterisk.

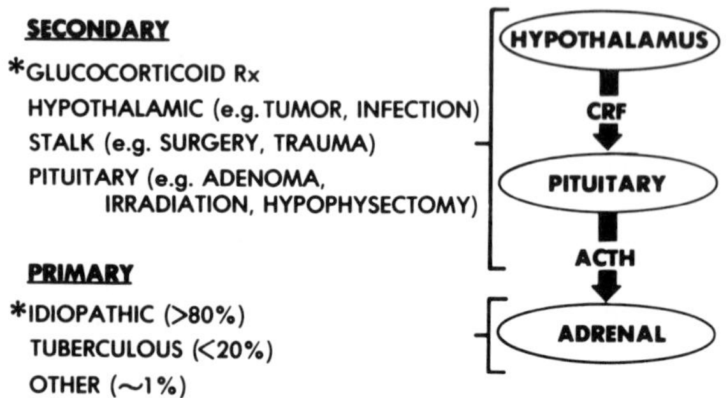

Primary Adrenocortical Insufficiency (Addison's Disease)

Adrenal destruction results from a variety of causes (Fig. 12-36 and Table 12-14); however, excluding CAH, the autoimmune or "idiopathic" atrophic type of Addison's disease (autoimmune adrenal atrophy, autoimmune adrenalitis, lymphocytic adrenalitis) accounts for approximately 75 to 80 percent of cases.[991] These patients have disordered organ-specific immunity, a high incidence of associated immunologic and autoimmune endocrine dysfunction, and disorders of other tissues and organs (Chap. 28).[992–996] In addition, there are two distinct subtypes of these syndromes known as the polyglandular autoimmune syndromes (PGA types I and II) (Chap. 28).[993–995,997–999]

Tuberculosis currently accounts for approximately 20 percent of cases of Addison's disease, with a higher prevalence in populations with poor control of this disease. This current distribution is a marked reversal of the relative frequency in the 1920s and 1930s, when tuberculosis was responsible

TABLE 12-14 Etiology of Primary Adrenocortical Insufficiency

Idiopathic/autoimmune (~80%)
Tuberculosis (~20%)
Miscellaneous causes (~1%)
Vascular
Hemorrhage: sepsis, anticoagulants, coagulopathy, trauma, surgery, pregnancy, neonate
Infarction: thrombosis, embolism, arteritis
Fungal infection: histoplasmosis, paracoccidioidomycosis, blastomycosis, coccidioidomycosis, cryptococcosis
Acquired immune deficiency syndrome (AIDS)
Metastases
Lymphoma
Amyloidosis
Sarcoidosis
Hemochromatosis
Irradiation
Surgery: bilateral adrenalectomy
Enzyme inhibitors: ketoconazole, etomidate, metyrapone, aminoglutethimide, trilostane
Cytotoxic agents: mitotane
Congenital: adrenal hypoplasia, familial glucocorticoid deficiency, adrenal leukodystrophy

Source: Irvine et al.[705] and Irvine and Barnes.[991]

TABLE 12-15 Changing Patterns in Primary Adrenocortical Insufficiency

	Percent*	
	1928–1938	1962–1972
Idiopathic	17	78
Tuberculous	79	21
Other	4	1

* Percent of cases with each of the three classes of adrenocortical insufficiency in each time period.

Source: Dunlop[680] and Irvine and Barnes.[991]

for 70 to 80 percent of reported cases (Table 12-15).[705,991,1000] Adrenal insufficiency is relatively unusual in patients with tuberculosis,[1001,1002] and even with adrenal involvement, the extent of cortical destruction may not be sufficient to impair adrenal function.[1001]

Other etiologies of primary adrenal insufficiency are distinctly unusual in larger published series (Table 12-14).[705,991,1000] However, personal experience suggests that adrenal insufficiency due to invasive and hemorrhagic disorders is becoming more commonly diagnosed. These etiologies include many systemic disorders (e.g., infections, hemorrhagic disorders, neoplasia, trauma) that involve a number of organ systems. The most common cause of adrenal hemorrhage in adults is anticoagulant therapy or spontaneous coagulopathy,[1003–1007] and in childhood it is meningococcal and *Pseudomonas* septicemias.[1008,1009] Adrenal insufficiency may also occur in the acquired immune deficiency syndrome (AIDS); however, the exact cause and incidence are unknown.[1010]

Primary adrenocortical insufficiency due to any cause is a rare disease; the exact incidence and prevalence are unknown. Current reports may underestimate the true incidence, since patients may die in acute crisis without an established diagnosis.[1011] A prevalence of Addison's disease of 39 per 1 million inhabitants in the age group from 25 to 69 years in the United Kingdom was reported, and there were 60 cases per 1 million population in Denmark.[1000,1011] It is difficult to determine whether the dramatic alteration in the relative frequencies of autoimmune and tuberculous Addison's disease is due to an increase in the incidence of autoimmune cases or to a decrease in the number of cases secondary to tuberculosis. However, the series of Dunlop[680] suggests that the total incidence of Addison's disease is declining concomitantly with control of tuberculosis, favoring the idea that the increase in the autoimmune variety is a relative one.

Tuberculous Addison's disease occurs predominantly in male patients, but autoimmune Addison's disease is more frequent in females. Thus, in recent series, the female/male ratio approximates 1.25.[1012] In autoimmune Addison's disease, the female/male ratio is 2/6.[705]

Addison's disease is an unusual diagnosis at the extremes of life; approximately 60 to 70 percent of cases are diagnosed in the third to fifth decade.[705] The autoimmune variety occurs among all age groups, but tuberculous Addison's disease was previously diagnosed in patients over age 40 years.[1000,1012,1013] However, in more recent reports, mean ages were 34 and 38 years.[705,1000,1012]

Only isolated information regarding death rates is available. Guttman estimated in 1930 that the death rate from Addison's disease was 4 per million population in the United States,[1001] and Stuart-Mason and coworkers reported an annual death rate of 1.4 per million population in the United Kingdom in the 1960s.[1011]

Autoimmune Adrenocortical Insufficiency

Etiology, Pathogenesis, and Genetic Aspects

The etiology of the most common form of primary adrenocortical failure appears to be autoimmune in nature. Early in the course of the disease, there is lymphocytic infiltration of the gland. There is a high incidence of associated endocrine disorders as well as of pernicious anemia, vitiligo, and other disorders. There is also a genetic predisposition. Antibodies to the adrenal gland and to other potentially affected organs are commonly present, and there is evidence for abnormal cell-mediated immunity. These aspects are discussed in detail in Chap. 28.

Although circulating antibodies to adrenocortical antigens are present in up to 65 percent of patients at the time of diagnosis,[705,992,993] their role in the pathogenesis of Addison's disease has been obscure. However, recent studies have raised new interest in the possible roles of these circulating antibodies. In one study, serum immunoglobulins from patients with autoimmune Addison's disease were incubated with cultured adrenal cells[1014]; immunoglobulins from 23 of 25 patients blocked the ACTH-induced increases in both cortisol and DNA synthesis.[1014] Thus, such antibodies could inhibit adrenal steroidogenesis early in the course of Addison's disease, before extensive destruction of adrenocortical cells.

Other recent studies have begun to identify the adrenocortical antigens against which circulating antibodies are directed. It has now been demonstrated in PGA type I that P450c17 (17α-hydroxylase) is a major autoantigen.[1015] This finding was not present in two patients with sporadic Addison's disease that was not associated with PGA type I.[1015] In other studies, addisonian patients who had positive immunofluorescence to adrenal cortical tissue were studied.[1016,1017] Patient characteristics were not clearly defined; however, these patients had adult-onset Addison's disease and did not have PGA type I, and so presumably they had either sporadic Addison's disease or PGA type II. In this group of patients a 54- to 55-kDa autoantigen was identified which migrated on Western blots identically with P450c21.[1016,1017] There was no evidence that P450scc, P450c17, or P450c11 was an autoantigen in these patients. Although in theory these autoantibodies could interfere with adrenal steroidogenesis, their exact pathogenetic significance remains unclear.[1018,1019]

Associated Disorders

In 1926, Schmidt described two patients with Addison's disease who had chronic lymphocytic thyroiditis at autopsy.[1020] In 1964, Carpenter and coworkers reviewed this association of hypoadrenalism and hypothyroidism and also noted the association of diabetes mellitus.[399] More recently, an association of Addison's disease with gonadal failure, hyperthyroidism, hypothyroidism, Hashimoto's thyroiditis, vitiligo, hypoparathyroidism, and pernicious anemia has been established (see Chap. 28).[705,991,1000,1012,1013,1021] One or more of these clinical disorders are present in about half the patients with autoimmune Addison's disease, and the presence of organ-specific antibodies is even more common. These disorders are not associated with Addison's disease due to tuberculosis or other invasive or infiltrative processes. Although these associated disorders are common in patients with primary adrenal insufficiency, patients with more commonly occurring conditions such as diabetes mellitus and autoimmune thyroid disease rarely develop Addison's disease. Autoimmune hypoparathyroidism represents an exception, since the two disorders commonly coincide and are frequently familial (see below).[705,1022,1023]

The association of Addison's disease with one or more of these conditions has been referred to by a number of terms, including Schmidt's syndrome, autoimmune endocrine failure, the polyglandular failure syndrome, and the polyglandular autoimmune syndromes (PGA types I and II) (Table 12-16).[993,994,997–999]

TABLE 12-16 Polyglandular Failure Syndromes

Endocrine Disorders	Type I Prevalence, %	Type II Prevalence, %
Adrenal insufficiency	60	100
Hypoparathyroidism	89	—
Mucocutaneous candidiasis	75	—
Gonadal failure	45	5–50
Autoimmune thyroid disease	12	70
Insulin-dependent diabetes mellitus	1	50
Hypopituitarism	Rare	Rare
Diabetes insipidus	Rare	Rare
Nonendocrine Disorders		
Pernicious anemia	16	Rare
Vitiligo	4	5
Alopecia	20	Rare
Malabsorption syndrome	25	—
Chronic active hepatitis	9	—
Myasthenia gravis	—	Rare
Thrombocytopenic purpura	—	Rare
Sjögren's syndrome	—	Rare
Rheumatoid arthritis	—	Rare

Source: Modified and reproduced with permission from Leshin.[994]

PGA Type I Polyglandular autoimmune syndrome type I may occur sporadically but is more commonly familial.[994,995,997–999] It is inherited in an autosomal recessive pattern[995,997,998] with a slight female preponderance, and there is no HLA association. The cardinal manifestations are hypoparathyroidism, mucocutaneous candidiasis, and adrenal insufficiency (Table 12-16).[994] Hypoparathyroidism and mucocutaeous candidiasis occur in about 90 percent and 75 percent of patients, respectively, and are the earliest manifestations, with onset usually occurring in early childhood.[994] The onset of adrenal insufficiency occurs later in 95 percent of patients, with a peak incidence at 10 to 15 years.[994] The overall incidence of gonadal failure is about 45 percent of patients, but it is present in 60 percent of female patients.[994,995,997–999] Autoimmune thyroid disease occurs in 12 percent, but diabetes mellitus is rare. There is a high incidence of hypoplasia of dental enamel, dystrophic nails, and keratopathy; nonendocrine disorders such as vitiligo, alopecia, pernicious anemia, malabsorption, and chronic active hepatitis occur in 4 to 25 percent of these patients.[995]

PGA TYPE II Polyglandular autoimmune syndrome type II is the classic prototype of these disorders and has most frequently been termed Schmidt's syndrome. This syndrome is familial in about half the patients, and its inheritance is linked to the inheritance of the HLA antigens B8 (DW3), DR3, and DR4.[997,998] There is a female/male ratio of 1.8/1, and the age at onset is usually in the range of 20 to 35 years.[1024] The classic manifestations are adrenal insufficiency (in 100 percent of patients) plus either autoimmune thyroid disease (70 percent) or insulin-dependent diabetes mellitus (50 percent) (Table 12-16).[994] The incidence of gonadal failure has been variably reported (5 to 50 percent) and is rare in males.[994,997–999] Ovarian and adrenal failure may occur in the same patient in the absence of thyroid disease or diabetes mellitus.[994] Vitiligo is present in about 5 percent of patients, and other nonendocrine disorders are unusual.

Pathology

In autoimmune adrenal insufficiency, there is early lymphocytic infiltration of the adrenal cortex, thus giving rise to the term *diffuse lymphocytic adrenalitis*. Subsequently, the adrenal cortex is gradually destroyed and the adrenals are small, atrophic, and frequently difficult to locate at autopsy. The capsule is thickened, and the normal cortical architecture is destroyed; however, the adrenal medulla is preserved. The cortical cells of all three zones are largely absent, and those remaining are scattered, show degenerative change, and are surrounded by a fibrous stroma and lymphocytic infiltrates. The degree of lymphocytic infiltration is variable, but its association with the loss of cortical cells is the classic pathologic feature.[705,1001,1025]

Primary Adrenocortical Insufficiency due to Invasive or Hemorrhagic Disorders

Adrenal insufficiency secondary to invasive or hemorrhagic disorders is a consequence of total or nearly total destruction of both glands and is often accompanied by advanced or disseminated systemic disease. Thus, destruction of the adrenal rarely occurs without involvement of other organs by the same disease process. In these conditions, the rate of development of adrenocortical insufficiency can vary markedly, depending on the nature of the primary process. With septicemia or hemorrhage, the adrenal can be rapidly destroyed, whereas with conditions such as tuberculosis, a much longer period may be required.

Invasive Disorders

Adrenal tuberculosis is a consequence of bloodborne infection of the adrenal cortex. It is virtually always accompanied or preceded by tuberculous infection elsewhere in the body, especially of the lung, gastrointestinal tract, or kidney.[1001,1002] Although the adrenals may be involved in 85 percent of patients dying of tuberculosis,[1001] the incidence of clinical adrenal insufficiency is much lower and appears to occur in only a minority of patients.[1001] In one series, adrenal insufficiency was present in 3 percent of patients with extrapulmonary tuberculosis. Since extrapulmonary tuberculosis is present in about 10 percent of all cases of tuberculosis, this would suggest an overall incidence of adrenal insufficiency of about 0.3 percent.[1002] The incidence of adrenal involvement with atypical strains of tuberculosis is unknown; however, *Mycobacterium avium-intracellulare* (MAI) was demonstrated at autopsy in the adrenals of 5 of 41 (12 percent) patients with AIDS[1026] (see below).

In tuberculous Addison's disease, the adrenal glands are totally replaced by caseous necrosis with little or no remaining cortical or medullary tissue. CT scan shows adrenal enlargement in patients with tuberculous Addison's disease of less than 2 years duration,[1027] and in these patients there is typically a central hypodense area of caseous necrosis with contrast enhancement of the periphery of the gland.[1028] In response to therapy, the enlarged adrenals may revert to normal size or become atrophic, and in a few patients there is recovery of adrenal function.[1028] In patients with a longer duration of adrenal insufficiency, the adrenals become atrophic and calcification is radiologically evident in approximately 50 percent of cases.[1012,1027]

Fungal infections can also involve the adrenal glands and cause Addison's disease. This can occur with histoplasmosis, paracoccidioidomycosis (South American blastomycosis), North American blastomycosis, coccidioidomycosis, and cryptococcosis. Histoplasmosis in its rare disseminated form is an important cause of Addison's disease, since as many as 50 percent of these patients develop adrenal insufficiency.[1029] CT scans demonstrate bilateral adrenal enlargement with central necrosis,[1030,1031] and recovery of adrenal function with therapy is unusual.[1032] Paracoccidioidomycosis is also a frequent cause of Addison's disease in endemic areas, and adrenal insufficiency may occur in as many as 10 percent of these patients.[1033] In contrast, North American blastomycosis rarely causes adrenal insufficiency, and only a few cases have been reported.[1034,1035] Coccidioidomycosis and cryptococcosis are also rare causes of Addison's disease.[1036,1037] Syphilis is an additional rare cause of adrenal destruction.[1001]

Metastases to the adrenal are quite common (reviewed in Ref. 1024), but overt adrenal disease requires bilateral involvement and destruction of both cortices. Thus, Addison's disease has been relatively unusual, but more recent studies suggest that it may occur in up to 20 percent of patients with bilateral adrenal metastases[1038,1039] and may occasionally be the presenting feature of malignancy.[1040] Both Hodgkin's and non-Hodgkin's lymphoma may also cause adrenal insufficiency,[1041,1042] and an occasional patient recovers normal function after chemotherapy.[1043]

Other rare invasive etiologies of Addison's disease include amyloidosis and sarcoidosis.[1044–1047] When destruction is due to processes other than tuberculosis, the pathologic findings in the adrenal are characteristic of the particular disorder, with loss of adrenal tissue and scarring, inflammatory changes, or replacement of tissue with abscess, tumor, amyloid, etc. Adrenal calcification is less common than with tuberculosis.

AIDS

Although adrenal insufficiency occurs in only a minority, pathologic abnormalities of the adrenal glands are extremely common in patients dying of AIDS and have been demonstrated in 50 to 78 percent of these patients.[1026,1048–1051] HIV can directly infect adrenocorticol cells,[1051a] but it is not known if this contributes to adrenal dysfunction in AIDS. The most common abnormality at autopsy is that of involvement of the adrenal cortex by cytomegalovirus

(CMV) with typical inclusion bodies and adrenalitis.[1026,1049,1050] However, the adrenal necrosis in these patients is generally not extensive enough to impair adrenal function.[1026] However, other infectious and invasive etiologies of adrenal insufficiency occur, and patients with AIDS have been shown to have adrenal involvement with *Mycobacterium tuberculosis, M. avium-intracellulare,* toxoplasmosis, cryptococcosis, Kaposi's sarcoma, and lymphoma.[1026,1048–1051] Despite this high incidence of adrenal involvement, clinically significant adrenal insufficiency occurs in only a few percent of patients.[1048] However, even this low incidence would make AIDS a more common etiology than the autoimmune and tuberculous forms.

Some patients with AIDS have elevated cortisol levels.[1048] This has been attributed to a stress response to chronic severe illness[1052] or to the development of an acquired form of glucocorticoid resistance with abnormalities of the glucocorticoid receptor.[1053] This latter report has not been confirmed, and there is no evidence that treating patients with elevated cortisol levels is beneficial.

Adrenal Hemorrhage

Bilateral adrenal hemorrhage may cause rapid and total adrenal destruction, leading to acute loss of both glucocorticoid and mineralocorticoid secretion. In adults, adrenal hemorrhage usually occurs in patients over age 50 years, and anticoagulant therapy and spontaneous coagulopathy are the most common contributing factors, being present in most patients.[1003–1007] Adrenal hemorrhage can also occur in patients with either overwhelming infection with sepsis or severe and frequently life-threatening major illnesses.[1006–1009,1054] These include coagulation disorders, adrenal vein thrombosis, adrenal metastases, trauma, major surgery, severe cardiovascular disease, congestive heart failure, pulmonary emboli, acute renal failure, local infection, leukemias, lymphomas, malignancy, trauma, and severe burns.[1006–1009,1054] In children, the most common cause of bilateral adrenal hemorrhage is fulminant meningococcemia or *Pseudomonas* septicemia.[1008–1009] Adrenal hemorrhage may also occur in a neonate after a complicated delivery or in the presence of a coagulation disorder. Adrenal hemorrhage may also occur during a complicated pregnancy or in the postpartum period.

Until recently, the diagnosis of bilateral adrenal hemorrhage was rarely made premortem and was usually established only at autopsy.[1005] However, increased awareness of this syndrome and the availability of modern imaging techniques have led to more frequent recognition.[1055] Survival with adrenal insufficiency is now being reported more frequently,[1007,1055,1056] and recovery of adrenal function occurs in an occasional patient.[1003,1057]

The adrenal glands in this syndrome are enlarged, not infrequently to a massive degree, and the cortex may be totally destroyed.[1007,1027,1058] The hemorrhage usually replaces the medulla and inner cortex; the outer cortex undergoes ischemic necrosis, with only a thin rim of cortical cells remaining.[1054] Venous thrombosis frequently accompanies the hemorrhage. CT and MR imaging studies demonstrate the adrenal enlargement and usually can establish the diagnosis. In surviving patients, the hematomas resolve and the adrenals atrophy and may calcify.[1003,1055]

Other Congenital and Familial Etiologies

Adrenal insufficiency due to inherited disorders of adrenal steroid biosynthesis (CAH) is discussed in the previous section.

Adrenoleukodystrophy

These disorders are inherited in an X-linked recessive pattern, and thus males are most commonly affected. The basic defect is that of abnormal peroxisomal function which leads to defective oxidation of very long chain fatty acids and their accumulation in the brain, spinal cord, adrenal, gonads, and other tissues.[1059,1060] Adrenoleukodystrophy, the classic form of the disorder, which occurs in 60 percent of all cases and has its onset before age 21, is characterized by progressive CNS deterioration and primary adrenal failure.[1059,1060] Over 80 percent of neurologically affected patients have adrenal insufficiency. Adrenomyeloneuropathy is a phenotypic variant of the same genetic lesion which has an onset after age 21 and is characterized by demyelination of the spinal cord and peripheral nerves. Approximately 90 percent of these patients have adrenal insufficiency,[1060] and an additional 20 to 40 percent of adult patients have impaired testicular function.[1059] A few kindreds have been reported with the biochemical defect who have only adrenal insufficiency without any neurologic dysfunction.[1059,1060]

It is important to consider this rare disorder in males with adrenal insufficiency, since adrenal insufficiency precedes neurologic symptoms in 30 to 40 percent of cases of adrenoleukodystrophy and adrenomyeloneuropathy.[1061] In a study of eight male children with Addison's disease without obvious family histories, five were proved to have abnormal plasma amino acid concentrations, and MRI studies showed brain involvement in each one.[1061]

Adrenal Hypoplasia

This rare cause of adrenal insufficiency is due to failure of development of the adult adrenal cortex, and these children thus present with features of adrenal failure shortly after birth.[1062] Several variants of the syndrome have been reported: (1) an X-linked form with glycerol kinase deficiency and muscular dystrophy, (2) an X-linked form with hypogonadotropic hypogonadism, (3) an autosomal recessive form, and (4) a sporadic form with pituitary hypoplasia.[1062]

Familial Glucocorticoid Deficiency

Familial glucocorticoid deficiency (hereditary adrenocortical unresponsiveness to ACTH) is a rare type of adrenal insufficiency which is inherited as an autosomal recessive and which in one family was due to a point mutation in the ACTH receptor.[1063] The disorder is characterized by glucocorticoid and adrenal androgen deficiency with elevated plasma ACTH levels.[1064–1066] Cortisol secretion does not respond to prolonged ACTH stimulation; however, aldosterone is usually normally responsive to posture and sodium deprivation.[1064–1066] The disorder usually presents in childhood and may be accompanied by achalasia, alacrima, and autonomic and motor neuropathy.[1065–1068]

Pathophysiology

The development of the clinical manifestations of adrenocortical insufficiency requires the loss of over 90 percent of both adrenal cortices. In the autoimmune and invasive types, destruction is usually gradual, leading to the manifestations of chronic adrenocortical insufficiency; however, in one-third of cases there is a more rapid course, with a symptom duration less than 3 months.[1012] In addition, approximately 25 percent of these patients are in crisis or impending crisis at the time of diagnosis.[1012] Hemorrhagic destruction of the adrenals results in an abrupt state of adrenal insufficiency with sudden loss of both glucocorticoid and mineralocorticoid secretion.

With gradual destruction, normal regulatory mechanisms are able to compensate temporarily. Decreased cortisol production results in decreased feedback at the hypothalamus and pituitary with increased release of CRH and the POMC-derived peptides ACTH, β-LPH, and the NH_2-terminal fragment. The increased ACTH level results in increased stimulation of the remaining adrenal with normal cortisol production in the early stages but inadequate production as the disease progresses. The MSH sequences within the POMC-derived peptides also lead to increased pigmentation, one of the cardinal signs of the disease (see below). In the minority of patients with more rapid adrenal destruction, prominent hyperpigmentation may not be present. The decreased mineralocorticoid production leads to sodium loss and potassium retention. The sodium loss results in stimulation of renin release and angiotensin II production. The increased potassium and angiotensin II stimulate the remaining glomerulosa to produce more aldosterone, but with progressive adrenal destruction, this mechanism also becomes inadequate.

When adrenal destruction is gradual, there is a phase characterized by normal basal steroid secretion but inability to respond to stress, i.e., a decreased adrenal reserve. This may progress to a state in which overall steroid production is diminished but enough episodic releases of cortisol occur so that basal cortisol determinations can be in the normal range. In this state of partial adrenal insufficiency, the patient may have few complaints, but a history usually discloses symptoms and most of these patients show pigmentation because of increased POMC peptide production. In this state, a crisis can be precipitated by the stress of surgery, trauma, or infection.

As destruction of the adrenal cortex progresses, mineralocorticoid and glucocorticoid secretion become inadequate and even basal cortisol levels are low, leading to all the metabolic derangements described above (see Actions of Glucocorticoids and Physiologic Actions of Mineralocorticoids). These derangements are reflected in manifestations of chronic adrenocortical insufficiency (see below).

Clinical Features

The clinical presentation depends on the rate and degree of adrenocortical destruction and on extraadrenal factors which may precipitate a crisis. Thus, most cases with autoimmune or invasive etiologies are insidious in onset and gradually progressive, but a crisis may be precipitated by intercurrent stress.[1012] Adrenal hemorrhage also presents with acute adrenal insufficiency. Because the presentations of these three subtypes of primary adrenocortical insufficiency differ, the clinical manifestations are discussed separately here.

Chronic Primary Adrenocortical Insufficiency

The gradual development of adrenal insufficiency may go unnoticed by the patient or physician until adrenocortical function is lost to a major extent. However, in retrospect, it is noted that the symptoms were usually present for months or even years before diagnosis or presentation.

Major clinical features and an estimate of their frequency are shown in Table 12-17.[991,1012,1022] These features include weakness and fatigue, weight loss, anorexia, and gastrointestinal symptoms. The most distinctive physical finding is hyperpigmentation. Its presence in association with any of these other manifestations should elicit the suspicion of Addison's disease. Weakness is always present and is accompanied by fatigue and malaise. It is generalized and usually is manifested by an inability to complete routine tasks rather than being restricted to particular muscle groups. Weight loss is also very common, may vary from 2 to 15 kg, and becomes more severe as adrenal failure progresses.[680] It is largely due to tissue loss resulting from anorexia, but dehydration also contributes.

TABLE 12-17 Clinical Features of Chronic Primary Adrenocortical Insufficiency

Feature	Percent with Condition
Weakness and fatigue	100
Weight loss	100
Anorexia	100
Hyperpigmentation	92
Hypotension	88
Gastrointestinal symptoms	56
Salt craving	19
Postural symptoms	12

Source: Adapted from Nerup[1012] and Thorn.[1069]

The majority of these patients have gastrointestinal symptoms. Anorexia is extremely common and contributes to the weight loss. Nausea, vague abdominal discomfort, and vomiting occur more frequently with progressive adrenal failure. Diarrhea may be present but occurs less frequently. Gastrointestinal symptoms may be pronounced as an adrenal crisis supervenes and may lead to the mistaken diagnosis of primary gastrointestinal disease. It is important for the physician to consider Addison's disease in patients with these symptoms, since radiologic studies that require enemas, cathartics, and fasting can precipitate shock and collapse.

Hypotension is common but in many patients may not be profound enough to suggest the diagnosis. Nevertheless, systolic blood pressure is <110 mmHg in over 90 percent of these patients and is frequently associated with complaints of orthostatic dizziness and occasionally[680,991] syncope. In patients in crisis, recumbent hypotension or shock is an almost universal finding.

Hyperpigmentation of the skin and mucous membranes is the single most distinctive sign in chronic primary adrenocortical insufficiency and can be most useful, especially in an acutely ill patient with unexplained hypotension. It may precede other manifestations of adrenal insufficiency (Fig. 12-37). It is generalized, with accentuation in sun-exposed areas and pressure points such as the elbows, knees, knuckles, and toes and around the wrist. Abnormal pigmentation should be suspected when it is present on palmar creases, nail beds, buccal mucosa, nipples, navel, areolae, and the perivaginal or perianal mucosa. Pigmentation of the buccal mucosa and gums is always accompanied by generalized hyperpigmentation.[705] Surgical scars acquired after the onset of Addison's disease are frequently hyperpigmented, whereas previous scars remain unpigmented. The increased pigmentation is frequently accompanied by the appearance of numerous black or brown freckles. In people of dark-skinned races, pigmentation of the mouth, palmar creases, vulva, and anus may be normally present and the diagnosis of hyperpigmentation is frequently difficult. Pigmentation of the tongue is probably abnormal regardless of racial background. The hyperpigmentation is commonly misinterpreted as being due to sun exposure, and the healthy appearance of the patient may lead to dismissal of other symptoms.

Vitiligo occurs in 4 to 17 percent of patients with autoimmune Addison's disease; however, it occurs rarely in those with tuberculosis.[680,1012]

Salt craving is a significant feature in approximately 20 percent of cases[1069]; some patients may actually eat salt by the spoonful despite anorexia.

Although both fasting and postprandial hypoglycemia were frequently reported in older series,[680,1070] they are currently uncommon.[991,1071] The fasting blood sugar level is within the low normal range in most patients; it is unusual for a patient with Addison's disease to present with or have symptomatic complaints of hypoglycemia, and severe hypoglycemia is rare, except in children. Hypoglycemia may be provoked by fasting, fever, infection, or nausea and vomiting and may be present in acute adrenal crisis.[1070] In a patient with preceding diabetes, improvement in blood sugar control and a decrease in insulin requirement tend to occur when Addison's disease emerges.

Amenorrhea is common in untreated Addison's disease patients and may be a manifestation of weight loss and chronic illness or of primary ovarian failure from an associated immunologic cause. Loss of axillary and pubic hair occurs in a minority of female patients as a result of a loss of adrenal androgens.

Patients with autoimmune Addison's disease may also have symptoms of the associated disorders discussed earlier. Similarly, patients with tuberculosis or other invasive diseases causing adrenal insufficiency usually have involvement of other organ systems.

Acute Adrenocortical Insufficiency (Adrenal Crisis)

The most common emergency presentation of primary adrenal insufficiency is that of acute adrenal crisis in a patient with undiagnosed or treated Addison's disease who is exposed to stress such as infection, trauma, surgery, or dehydration as a result of salt deprivation, vomiting, or diarrhea. The requirement for increased glucocorticoid levels during stress has already been emphasized, although addisonian patients usually tolerate minor insults such as upper respiratory infections. Thus, an addisonian patient who does not receive therapy during these stresses may rapidly develop an acute adrenal crisis.

When acute adrenal insufficiency develops (Table 12-18), anorexia becomes profound and there is increased nausea and vomiting; this contributes to volume depletion and dehydration. Abdominal pain occurs frequently and may mimic an acute surgical

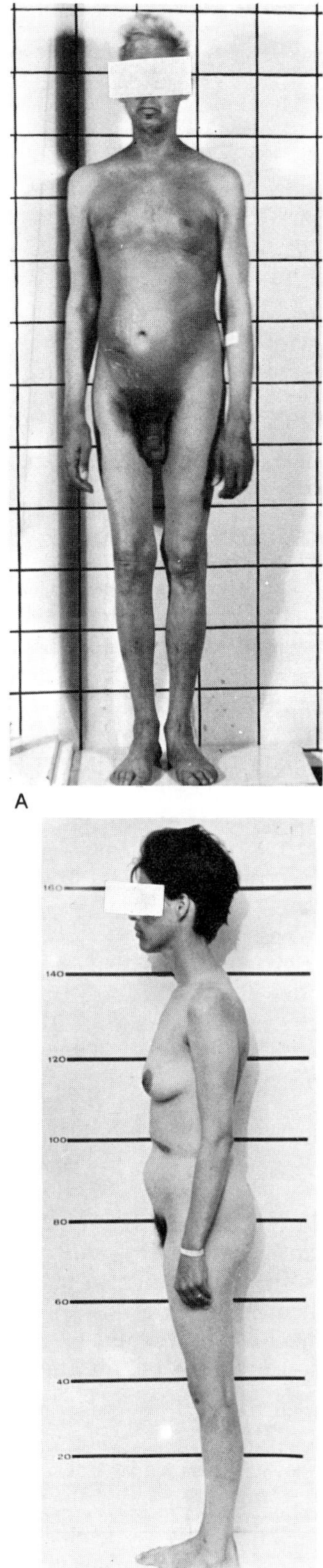

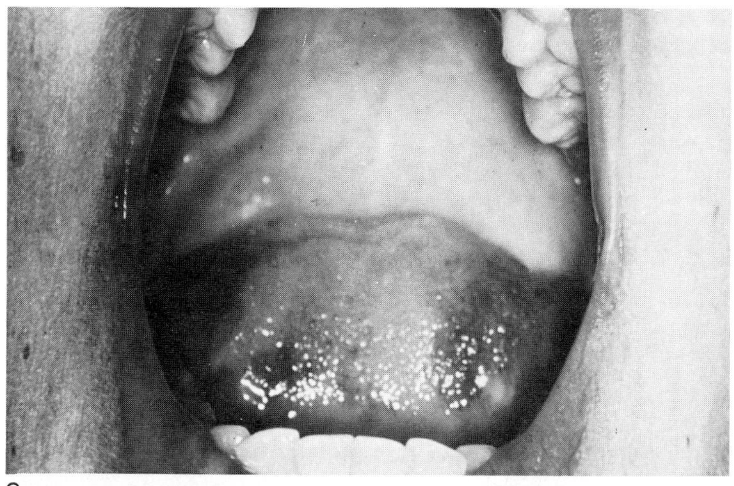

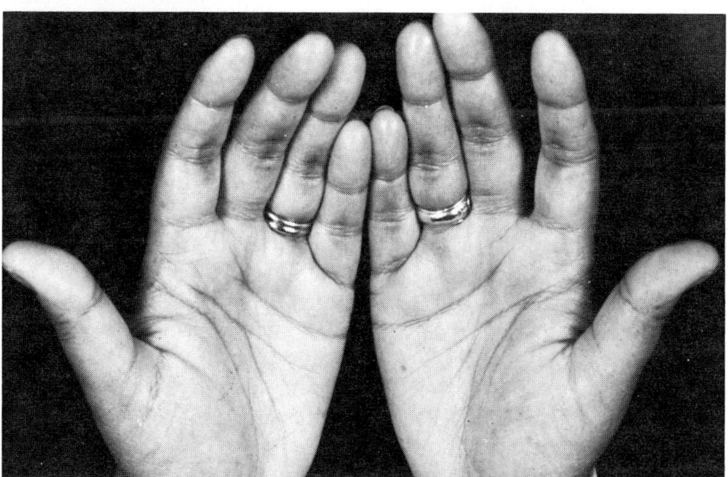

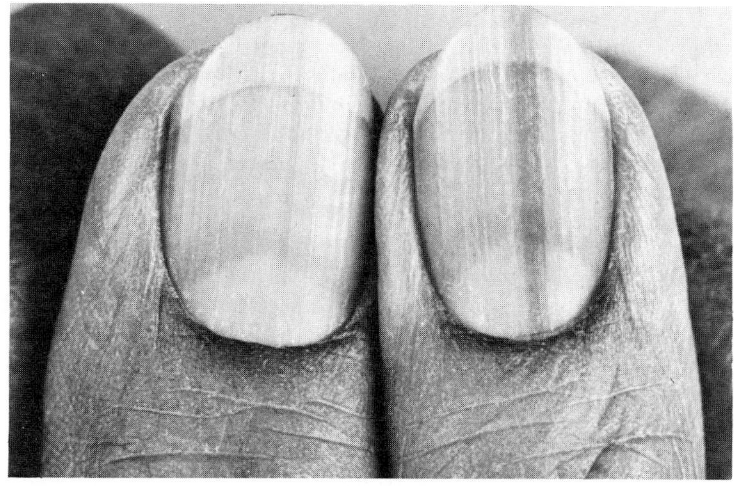

FIGURE 12-37 Abnormal pigmentation due to hypersecretion of ACTH and β-LPH. *(A)* Generalized hyperpigmentation with accentuation over exposed areas. *(B)* Pigmentation in sun-exposed areas, although the abdominal surgical scar is markedly hyperpigmented. *(C)* Hyperpigmentation of the tongue. *(D)* Hyperpigmentation is prominent in skin creases. *(E)* Hyperpigmentation of and around the nails.

TABLE 12-18 Clinical Features of Acute Primary Adrenocortical Insufficiency (Adrenal Crisis)

Hypotension/shock (vascular collapse)
Weakness, apathy, confusion
Nausea, vomiting, anorexia
Dehydration, hypovolemia, hyponatremia, hyperkalemia
Abdominal or flank pain
Hyperthermia
Hypoglycemia

TABLE 12-19 Clinical Features of Adrenal Hemorrhage

Features	Percent
General	
Hypotension/shock	74
Fever	59
Nausea and vomiting	46
Confusion, disorientation	41
Tachycardia	28
Cyanosis/lividity	28
Local	
Abdominal, flank, or back pain	77
Abdominal or flank tenderness	38
Abdominal distension	28
Abdominal rigidity	20
Chest pain	13
Rebound tenderness	5

Source: Adapted from Xarli et al.[1006]

abdomen. Specific localizing features are usually absent, although there may be tenderness and pain on deep palpation. The blood pressure falls farther, and hypovolemic shock develops with extreme weakness, apathy, and confusion. The patient may rapidly develop severe dehydration. Fever is common, and hypoglycemia may be present. The fever may be due either to hypoadrenalism or to a precipitating infection. Hyperpigmentation is usually present in a patient with primary adrenocortical insufficiency and is an important clinical sign. Without appropriate therapy death may occur rapidly, with coma and shock. Hyponatremia, hyperkalemia, lymphocytosis, and eosinophilia should suggest the diagnosis of adrenal crisis, and the possibility of adrenal insufficiency must be considered in any patient with unexplained shock. Since another process commonly precipitates adrenal crises, these manifestations may divert attention from the possibility of Addison's disease. For instance, in a patient with coexisting diabetes mellitus, ketoacidosis can precipitate or be caused by the crisis. In previously undiagnosed patients, it is frequently possible to obtain a history of preceding chronic adrenal insufficiency at the time of acute presentation; however, this is not always the case, because some patients may have enough basal glucocorticoid production to prevent chronic symptoms but the adrenal reserve may be decreased in response to stress.

Adrenal Hemorrhage Causing Acute Adrenal Insufficiency

The typical clinical picture in patients with bilateral adrenal hemorrhage and acute adrenal destruction is that of a progressively deteriorating course in an already complicated patient with a major illness (Table 12-19).[1003–1009,1054] The classic clinical features of Addison's disease—hyperpigmentation, weight loss, and preceding chronic gastrointestinal symptoms—are absent. The patients at greatest risk are those with thromboembolic disease, those with spontaneous or iatrogenic coagulopathy, and those who are postoperative.[1003–1005] The usual presenting symptoms are abdominal, flank, or chest pain with abdominal tenderness.[1006,1007] Fever, hypotensin leading to shock, and electrolyte abnormalities are common, as are nausea, vomiting, confusion, and disorientation. With progression, severe hypotension, volume depletion, dehydration, hyperpyrexia, cyanosis, coma, and death ensue.[1006,1007] The diagnosis of acute adrenal hemorrhage should be considered in a deteriorating patient with thromboembolic disease, with coagulopathy, or in the postoperative period who develops unexplained abdominal or flank pain, vascular collapse, hyperpyrexia, electrolyte abnormality, or hypoglycemia.

Laboratory Features of Primary Adrenocortical Insufficiency

The specific laboratory diagnosis of Addison's disease depends on measurement of plasma cortisol and ACTH levels (see below). However, other laboratory abnormalities which are not diagnostic should suggest the diagnosis (Table 12-20).

Hyponatremia and hyperkalemia secondary to mineralocorticoid deficiency are characteristic manifestations of primary adrenal insufficiency; in the absence of chronic renal failure, their presence should suggest Addison's disease. Hyponatremia is present in 88 percent and hyperkalemia in 64 percent of patients at the time of diagnosis.[1000]

A normocytic normochromic anemia is common but may also be masked by dehydration and hemo-

TABLE 12-20 Laboratory Features of Primary Adrenocortical Insufficiency

Hyponatremia (88%)*	Eosinophilia
Hyperkalemia (64%)*	Lymphocytosis
Azotemia	Hypoglycemia
Anemia	Hypercalcemia

* Percent occurrence from Nerup.[1012]

concentration. Pernicious anemia is present in 4 percent of patients with autoimmune Addison's disease.[991] The differential white cell count shows neutropenia, a relative lymphocytosis, and eosinophilia. Elevations of blood urea nitrogen (BUN) and serum creatinine levels are ascribable to dehydration and hemoconcentration and are frequently accompanied by mild acidosis due to dehydration, hyperkalemia, and the loss of the acid-secreting properties of the mineralocorticoids.

Mild to moderate hypercalcemia occurs in approximately 6 percent of patients[1071] and may be mistaken for the hypercalcemia of dehydration. Hypocalcemia and hyperphosphatemia are present in patients with associated hypoparathyroidism.

The heart can be small and vertical on x-ray. Routine radiographs of the abdomen are usually normal, but adrenal calcification is present in approximately 50 percent of cases because of tuberculosis[680,1071] and can also be present with other invasive etiologies and after hemorrhagic destruction of the gland. With CT of the abdomen, adrenal enlargement and/or calcification is demonstrated with tuberculosis, metastases, adrenal hemorrhage, and other invasive etiologies, whereas in the autoimmune form, the adrenals may be destroyed and thus are small or absent on abdominal scans.[1024,1027,1028,1045,1055,1058]

The electrocardiogram may reveal low voltage with a vertical QRS axis. There may be nonspecific abnormalities due to electrolyte imbalance (e.g., peaked T waves due to the hyperkalemia or a shortened QT segment).

With sudden adrenal destruction, typical laboratory manifestations are usually absent. Hyponatremia and hyperkalemia occur in a minority of patients; however, their presence should suggest the diagnosis.[1006,1007,1054] Azotemia is common, whereas hypoglycemia occurs infrequently.[1007,1054] Increased circulating eosinophils or an increased total eosinophil count may be present and should also arouse the suspicion of acute insufficiency.

Secondary Adrenocortical Insufficiency

Etiology

The causes of secondary adrenocortical insufficiency are reviewed in Chaps. 7 and 8. Therapy with pharmacologic doses of glucocorticoids is the most frequent cause (Chap. 15). If the steroid-treated population is excluded, tumors of the pituitary and/or hypothalamic region are the most common cause of pituitary ACTH deficiency, and surgical or radiation therapy for these tumors may also contribute to panhypopituitarism. In patients with hypothalamic or pituitary tumors, ACTH deficiency is virtually always accompanied by deficiencies of other anterior pituitary hormones, since the ACTH-producing cells are more resistant to pituitary damage. Growth hormone and gonadotropins are usually lost first, followed by the loss of TSH and finally of ACTH (Chap. 8). Other, less common causes of hypothalamic-pituitary dysfunction are discussed in Chaps. 7 and 8.

Isolated ACTH Deficiency

This fascinating disorder is a rare cause of secondary adrenocortical failure. In a recent review of 76 patients, 54 percent were male and 46 percent female; the mean age at diagnosis was 50 years (range, 24 to 79 years).[1072] Thus, in most patients this is an acquired disorder. Current data suggest that the etiology of this disorder is frequently autoimmune in nature and that in many instances it is a sequela of lymphocytic hypophysitis.[1072,1073] Thus, most women of childbearing age who have isolated ACTH deficiency develop it postpartum, and many of these patients have autoimmune thyroid disorders and positive antithyroid and antipituitary antibody titers.[1072,1074] Whether isolated ACTH deficiency in male patients is autoimmune in etiology is less clear. The idea that a primary pituitary defect is responsible in most cases is confirmed by the failure of the pituitary to respond to repeated stimulation with CRH or vasopressin.[1072,1075,1076] Other possible etiologies include congenital defects, birth trauma, and partial pituitary infarction associated with pregnancy.[1072]

Isolated ACTH deficiency is accompanied by numerous endocrine abnormalities which appear to be secondary to the glucocorticoid insufficiency. These include elevations of TSH, prolactin, and LH which are not accompanied by hypothyroidism or hypogonadism and are reversible with glucocorticoid replacement.[1072] In contrast, growth hormone secretion was impaired in about one-third of patients and was also reversible after glucocorticoid therapy.[1072]

In many patients with isolated ACTH deficiency there is decreased plasma renin activity and a decreased plasma aldosterone concentration.[366,1072,1077] These patients may be hypotensive and hyponatremic, but hyperkalemia is rare. A return to normal of plasma renin activity (PRA) and plasma aldosterone concentration (PAC) has been reported after glucocorticoid therapy.[366,1072,1077] Hyponatremia in these patients with glucocorticoid insufficiency may also occur as a result of the inability to excrete a water load, a syndrome which resembles syndrome of inappropriate secretion of ADH (SIADH).

Pathophysiology

The pathogenesis of secondary adrenal insufficiency differs from that of primary adrenocortical destruction since the predominant effect of ACTH deficiency is decreased cortisol and adrenal androgen secretion. With hypothalamic or pituitary tumors, gradual growth of the lesion compresses the normal anterior pituitary, resulting in gradual destruction of corticotrophic cells with impairment of ACTH secretion. Initially, basal ACTH levels are maintained; however, there may be impaired ACTH reserve. Basal cortisol secretion is also normal, but ACTH and cortisol levels cannot increase in response to stress. With progression, basal ACTH secretion becomes deficient, resulting in atrophy of the adrenal zonae fasciculata and reticularis and decreased cortisol secretion in the basal state. When this occurs, not only is there an impaired ability to increase ACTH secretion in response to stress, the atrophic adrenal becomes unable to increase cortisol secretion in response to acute stimulation with ACTH.

Glucocorticoid therapy also suppresses the pituitary-adrenal axis; the effect is both dose- and time-dependent (Chap. 15). Although growth hormone and gonadotropin secretion may be depressed, pituitary function is generally intact (see Actions of Glucocorticoids, above; Cushing's Syndrome, below; and Chap. 15).

The glucocorticoid deficiency present in these conditions results in manifestations similar to those seen in primary adrenocortical insufficiency except that derangements due to mineralocorticoid deficiency are usually absent. The functional status of the zona glomerulosa is initially preserved, and aldosterone secretion, controlled by the renin-angiotensin system, is normal. When ACTH deficiency is long-standing, mineralocorticoid deficiency may develop in a few patients; many of those reported have had isolated ACTH deficiency.[366,1072,1077] The majority of these patients have hyporeninemia, and the renin and aldosterone deficiencies are correctable with glucocorticoid administration.[366,1072,1077,1078]

Clinical Features

The clinical presentation of secondary adrenal insufficiency, like that of the primary type, is usually chronic. However, an acute presentation can occur in undiagnosed patients during stress and in treated patients who do not receive increased steroid dosage during infection, surgery, or trauma. Pituitary apoplexy, i.e., hemorrhagic infarction of a pituitary tumor, may be accompanied by acute secondary adrenocortical insufficiency.

The usual presentation of secondary adrenal insufficiency is similar to that of primary adrenocortical insufficiency, with two important exceptions. First, since pituitary secretion of ACTH and β-LPH is deficient, the characteristic hyperpigmentation of Addison's disease is absent. In fact, patients with hypopituitarism frequently present with pallor of the skin. Second, as discussed above, the clinical features of mineralocorticoid deficiency are usually absent, and therefore volume depletion, dehydration, and hyperkalemia are usually absent. Hypotension is also less severe, except in acute presentations. Hyponatremia can be present and is usually due to water retention and the inability to excrete a water load rather than to sodium loss (see Cardiovascular System and Fluid and Electrolyte Balance under Actions of Glucocorticoids, above). Thus, the clinical features of ACTH and glucocorticoid deficiency are nonspecific and consist predominantly of weakness, lethargy, easy fatigue, anorexia, weight loss, nausea, and occasionally vomiting. Patients may also describe arthralgias, myalgias, and exacerbation of allergic responses. Hypoglycemia is occasionally the presenting feature.[1069,1072] With acute decompensation, severe hypotension or shock may occur and be unresponsive to vasopressors unless glucocorticoids are administered.

Patients with secondary adrenal insufficiency (except those with isolated ACTH deficiency) commonly have associated historical or clinical features which suggest the diagnosis. There may be a history of glucocorticoid therapy or the presence of cushingoid features, suggestive of previous therapy (Chap. 15). Patients with hypothalamic or pituitary tumors usually have loss of other pituitary hormones; i.e., hypogonadism and hypothyroidism are common, and there may be hypersecretion of growth hormone or prolactin. Most patients also have local tumor manifestations such as visual field defects, headache, and enlargement of the sella turcica (see Chaps. 7 and 8).

Laboratory Features

Routine laboratory testing in secondary adrenal hypofunction may reveal a mild normochromic normocytic anemia, neutropenia, relative lymphocytosis, and eosinophilia. The serum sodium concentration may be low, but potassium, BUN, creatinine, and bicarbonate concentrations are usually normal. Hypoglycemia may be present. Cardiac size on x-ray is normal, as is the ECG. MRI studies of the head may reveal a hypothalamic or pituitary tumor.

Diagnosis

Although the clinical suspicion of adrenal insufficiency must be confirmed by definitive laboratory testing, therapy should not be delayed by prolonged diagnostic measures, and the patient should not be subjected to ancillary diagnostic tests which may lead to further volume loss, dehydration, and hypotension. In the acute situation, if rapid diagnostic tests are not available, therapy should be instituted and the diagnosis should be established later.

Measurement of basal levels of urine or plasma cortisol is generally not recommended, since partial degrees of adrenal insufficiency occur. Thus, a normal plasma cortisol level (5 to 20 μg/dl) does not exclude the diagnosis of adrenocortical insufficiency since it is not uncommon to find random cortisol determinations in the normal range with partial adrenal insufficiency. However, the finding of a basal

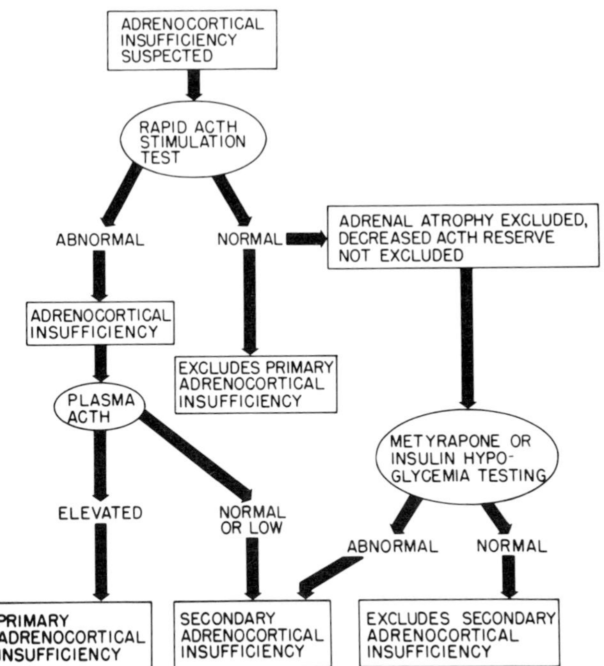

FIGURE 12-38 Evaluation of suspected primary or secondary adrenocortical insufficiency. Boxes enclose clinical decisions; circles enclose diagnostic tests.

plasma cortisol level of 20 μg/dl or greater virtually excludes the diagnosis. Conversely, if plasma cortisol is low or undetectable in a critically ill patient, adrenal insufficiency should be strongly considered. Tests which specifically measure adrenocortical reserve are needed to confirm the diagnosis (Fig. 12-38). These tests, discussed below in the context of their diagnostic utility, are described in Laboratory Evaluation of Adrenocortical Function, above.

The rapid ACTH stimulation test is the procedure of choice in the assessment of patients with possible adrenal insufficiency. This test is used as the initial diagnostic step in all suspected cases, either primary or secondary.[808–810,812–814,1079] Since the procedure requires only 30 min, it usually can be performed even in acute situations. In suspected primary adrenal insufficiency, a normal response (peak plasma cortisol >20 μg/dl at 30 min after ACTH administration) excludes the diagnosis, and these patients do not require further evaluation.[812,1079] However, normal responses do not always exclude secondary adrenal insufficiency, since some patients have a decreased pituitary reserve or decreased responsiveness of the hypothalamic-pituitary-adrenal axis to stress but maintain the ability to respond to exogenous ACTH stimulation (discussed below and under Laboratory Evaluation of Adrenocortical Function, above).[808,817–819,821,1080]

Subnormal responses to the rapid ACTH stimulation test establish the diagnosis of adrenocortical insufficiency and correlate well with subnormal responsiveness of the pituitary-adrenal axis to metyrapone, insulin-induced hypoglycemia, and stress.[808,817–819,821,1080] Three-day ACTH stimulation tests were traditionally used in the diagnosis of adrenocortical insufficiency but are usually unnecessary and give little additional diagnostic information in the presence of a subnormal response to the rapid ACTH stimulation test.

If the rapid ACTH stimulation test indicates adrenal insufficiency, primary and secondary forms are readily differentiated by measurement of the plasma ACTH level. Plasma ACTH levels in patients with untreated primary adrenal insufficiency exceed 200 pg/ml and are usually between 400 and 2000 pg/ml (Fig. 12-39).[1081] In secondary adrenal insufficiency due to pituitary ACTH deficiency, plasma ACTH levels are inappropriately low compared to circulating cortisol levels and are less than 10 to 20 pg/ml.[756–781,1081]

If plasma ACTH assays are unavailable, the plasma aldosterone response to the rapid ACTH stimulation test or the 3-day ACTH stimulation test can be used to differentiate primary from secondary adrenal insufficiency. However, experience with the aldosterone response is less extensive than experi-

FIGURE 12-39 Basal plasma ACTH levels in primary and secondary adrenocortical insufficiency. *(From Irvine et al.[705] based on data from Besser et al.[1081])*

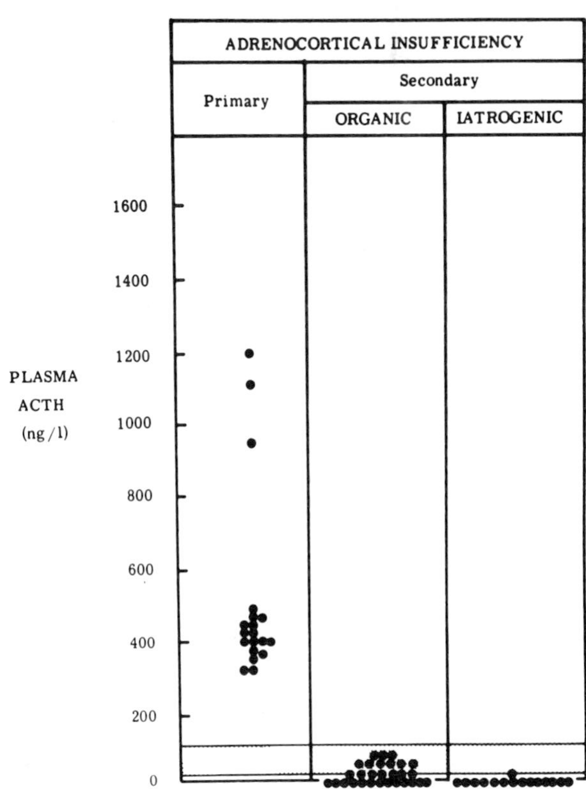

ence with measurement of plasma ACTH levels (see Laboratory Evaluation of Adrenocortical Function, above).

Although a subnormal response to the rapid ACTH stimulation test establishes the diagnosis of adrenal insufficiency, a normal adrenal response to ACTH stimulation does not exclude partial ACTH deficiency. This problem usually arises in patients who have been treated with glucocorticoids (Chap. 15) and patients with partial pituitary or hypothalamic dysfunction. When secondary adrenal insufficiency is still suspected in a patient with a normal response to the rapid ACTH stimulation test, more specific information regarding pituitary responsiveness can be obtained by testing with metyrapone or insulin-induced hypoglycemia. The overnight metyrapone test is preferred because of its simplicity and low risk. A normal response to either metyrapone or hypoglycemia excludes secondary adrenocortical insufficiency (see Laboratory Evaluation of Adrenocortical Function, above). Subnormal responses to these tests establish the diagnosis of secondary adrenal insufficiency, since in these patients the primary form has been excluded by a normal rapid ACTH stimulation test and normal or subnormal plasma ACTH levels.

In patients with primary adrenocortical insufficiency, further evaluation may be required to establish the specific etiology. If the patient has manifestations of or a family history of the PGA I or PGA II syndrome, autoimmune Addison's disease is present with rare exceptions. The presence of adrenal antibodies confirms the diagnosis, but these assays are not generally available. If autoimmune adrenal insufficiency is established, patients and their families should be screened for the associated disorders detailed above. If other endocrine autoimmune disorders are not present and if adrenal antibodies are negative or not available, an adrenal CT scan should be performed. Absent or atrophic adrenals are most consistent with autoimmune adrenal failure, but adrenal atrophy may also occur months or years after adrenal hemorrhage or infections. Bilateral adrenal enlargement in primary adrenal failure can be due to hemorrhage or any of the infectious or invasive etiologies described above.[1024,1027,1028,1045,1048,1055,1058] Hemorrhage can usually be demonstrated by current CT or MRI techniques.[1055,1058] If hemorrhage is not present, further evaluation should be directed to determining the specific cause and a CT-guided adrenal biopsy with appropriate cytology and cultures is indicated to establish the diagnosis and direct specific therapy. Further evaluation should then be directed to determining the extent of dissemination of the primary disease, e.g., extrapulmonary tuberculosis, disseminated fungal infection, AIDS, or metastatic malignancy (see the section on Primary Adrenocortical Insufficiency due to Invasive or Hemorrhagic Disorders, above, and Refs. 1024, 1027, 1045, and 1048).

In secondary adrenocortical insufficiency, the patient should be evaluated for other pituitary deficiencies and for the presence of a hypothalamic or pituitary tumor (see Chap. 7). The evaluation of patients with adrenal insufficiency resulting from steroid therapy is discussed in Chap. 15.

In an acutely ill patient with adrenal insufficiency, it is also imperative to determine the etiology of the condition that precipitates the crisis. For example, whereas fever can be due to glucocorticoid insufficiency, it may also be a manifestation of an underlying infection or another systemic disorder.

A patient who has been treated with glucocorticoids before the establishment of a diagnosis presents a special problem, since the therapy may itself suppress the hypothalamic-pituitary-adrenal axis. This is especially true when high-dose glucocorticoids are given to an acutely ill patient. However, when the steroid is tapered and the patient is placed on maintenance cortisol, normal hypothalamic-pituitary-adrenal responsiveness should return within several weeks and the rapid ACTH stimulation test can be used (see Chap. 15). In the exceptional circumstance in which longer high-dose therapy has been given, the 3-day ACTH stimulation test can be used; the overall management and diagnostic approaches in this case are discussed in Chap. 15.

Treatment

Acute Addisonian Crisis

Therapy for acute addisonian crisis should be instituted immediately if a strong clinical suspicion is present (Table 12-21). The rationale for high-dose glucocorticoids is based on the fact that the adrenal gland responds to serious illness with increased cortisol production. Therapy should include the administration of large doses of a soluble glucocorticoid preparation, the correction of hypovolemia and electrolyte abnormalities, general supportive measures, and treatment of coexisting or precipitating disorders. Since both mineralocorticoid deficiency and glucocorticoid deficiency are present in primary adrenocortical insufficiency, a preparation with so-

TABLE 12-21 Treatment of Acute Adrenocortical Insufficiency (Adrenal Crisis)

1. Cortisol* 100 mg IV, q6 h for 24 h. Reduce to 50 mg q 6 h if progress is satisfactory and then taper to oral maintenance dose by day 4 or 5. Maintain or increase dose to 200 to 400 mg/24 h if complications persist
2. IV saline and glucose
3. Correction of precipitating factors
4. General supportive measures

* As hydrocortisone phosphate or hemisuccinate.

dium-retaining potency is recommended. The drug of choice is a soluble form of injectable cortisol (hydrocortisone hemisuccinate or hydrocortisone phosphate), which should be administered IV in doses of 100 mg q 6 h for the first 24 h. If the patient's progress is satisfactory and no additional complications are present, dose may be reduced to 50 mg q 6 h on the second day and then tapered gradually to oral maintenance doses by the fourth to fifth day. When severe concurrent illnesses are present, a dose of 50 to 100 mg q 6 h should be continued until the patient stabilizes. Intramuscular cortisone acetate should not be used in the treatment of acute adrenal insufficiency since there is poor absorption, failure to achieve adequate blood levels of cortisol, and inadequate biological activity, as evidenced by failure to suppress ACTH levels.[1082] Mineralocorticoid therapy is usually required when the cortisol dose is decreased below 50 to 60 mg per day (see below).

Since patients in adrenal crisis may have profound dehydration, volume depletion, hypotension, and hypoglycemia, adequate replacement with IV glucose and saline must be given. Severe hyperkalemia and/or acidosis may occasionally require specific therapy.

A patient with a crisis due to secondary adrenocortical insufficiency usually does not have the severe electrolyte abnormalities and volume depletion seen in patients with primary adrenocortical insufficiency. Thus, the major requirement is for glucocorticoid replacement; the regimen outlined above is standard, has been proved effective, and will provide adequate mineralocorticoid replacement in the few patients with impaired aldosterone production. The use of other glucocorticoids, such as prednisolone and dexamethasone, is probably equally effective.

Chronic Adrenal Insufficiency

The treatment of chronic primary Addison's disease requires maintenance therapy with both glucocorticoids and mineralocorticoids (Table 12-22). The patient must be taught that a lifetime of therapy is required and that cessation of therapy may endanger life. In the majority of patients, 20 to 30 mg of cortisol per day is sufficient, with two-thirds given in the morning and one-third in the late afternoon. The higher morning dose is given to approximate roughly the normal circadian rhythm of cortisol secretion. Cortisol is ordinarily used; it may have a theoretical advantage over some of the cortisol analogues (prednisone, prednisolone, dexamethasone, etc.), as it has greater mineralocorticoid potency and may therefore serve as partial replacement for the deficient mineralocorticoid function as well. However, an equivalent dose of a steroid such as prednisone, prednisolone, or dexamethasone is also acceptable.[1083] Oral cortisone acetate (approximately 37.5 mg per day) is equally acceptable, since oral absorption is rapid and it is converted to cortisol.[1082]

TABLE 12-22 Treatment of Chronic Primary Adrenocortical Insufficiency

1. Cortisol, 15–20 mg in A.M. and 10 mg at 4–5 P.M.
2. 9α-fluorocortisol 0.05–0.2 mg orally in A.M.
3. Clinical follow-up: maintenance of normal weight, blood pressure, and electrolytes with regression of clinical features
4. Patient education plus identification card or bracelet
5. Increased cortisol dosage during "stress"

Mineralocorticoid replacement is given using 9α-fluorocortisol 0.05 to 0.2 mg daily. A majority of these patients require mineralocorticoid therapy, although a minority do not and can be maintained on cortisol alone.[1084] The major problem with omission of the mineralocorticoid is a tendency to develop hyperkalemia. The natural steroids aldosterone and DOC are not available and are not useful since they are degraded rapidly after ingestion so that adequate plasma concentrations are not achieved.

These doses are satisfactory in the majority of patients; they are accompanied by regression of the classic clinical features, including a return of a general feeling of well-being, weight gain, maintenance of normal blood pressure, improvement in pigmentation, and a return to normal physical activity. Occasional patients who perform heavy manual labor may require up to 40 mg. Many of the subjective complaints of Addison's disease can be reversed within a few days; a somewhat longer period is required before strength returns to normal, and weeks may be required before the abnormal pigmentation subsides.

In an evaluation of the adequacy of glucocorticoid replacement, strong reliance is placed on the patient's subjective assessment. Excessive dosage is usually manifested by excessive weight gain; this is an indication to lower the dose. Since glucocorticoids given in excess can produce euphoria, occasional patients may increase the dose on their own. Such excessive glucocorticoid replacement should be avoided. Inadequate dosage results in continuing manifestation of Addison's disease, especially weakness, fatigue, and excessive pigmentation. Caution should be exercised in the administration of other drugs, since those, such as rifampin, which induce hepatic microsomal enzymes may result in accelerated glucocorticoid metabolism with the induction of an adrenal crisis.[1085] This may also occur with phenytoin and phenobarbital. The timing of the doses can be varied to fit individual needs and activities; i.e., although most patients do well with twice-daily doses, some feel better with three doses. The last dose is usually given at 4 to 5 P.M., since the cortisol may cause insomnia in some patients when given later in the evening. Plasma or urinary cortisol determinations are not usually necessary or helpful, and there is no reliable biochemical method for assessing the adequacy of glucocorticoid therapy. Thus, plasma ACTH levels have not proved useful because of episodic variation in secretion and because therapy with the short-acting glucocorticoids usually does not suppress ACTH levels to normal.[1086–1088]

Adequate mineralocorticoid therapy is indicated by the maintenance of normal blood pressure and sodium, potassium, and plasma renin levels.[1084,1089] Excessive therapy causes hypertension and hypokalemia,[1084] and inadequate therapy may result in persisting fatigue, malaise, orthostatic hypotension, hyponatremia, hyperkalemia, and hyperreninemia.[1089] The dose may be altered using these parameters; the usual dose of 9α-fluorocortisol is 0.05 to 0.2 mg daily. Some patients may require variable doses at different times of the year, e.g., 0.1 to 0.2 mg and increased salt intake during the summer and 0.05 mg in the winter. Measurement of the plasma renin concentration is useful, since an increased level suggests inadequate replacement and a suppressed level may indicate excessive mineralocorticoid therapy.[1084,1089,1090]

Every effort should be made to avoid adrenal crises. This can be achieved by patient education and an appropriate increase in steroid dosage during stress. It is therefore necessary to inform the patient fully of the nature of his or her disorder and the necessity of obtaining prompt medical assistance in the event of illness or injury. Patients should carry an identification card or bracelet to notify the treating physician of the diagnosis of Addison's disease and should be instructed to increase the dose of cortisol in the event of illness. Since it is difficult for the patient to assess the severity of illness, it is best to err on the side of overreplacement rather than underreplacement during acute minor illnesses. Thus, patients are instructed to double or triple the cortisol dose at the onset of minor illnesses such as upper respiratory and viral infections. If the illness is minor, the dose can be reduced to the usual maintenance level in 24 to 48 h; no adverse effects accompany this short-term increase. If more severe or persisting symptoms develop, the patient is instructed to continue the increased cortisol dose and contact a physician. Increased dosage of 9α-fluorocortisol is not required during minor illnesses, provided that adequate cortisol is given. Patients with vomiting, and thus an inability to take oral cortisol, must seek immediate medical attention and receive parenteral cortisol, as must those with diarrhea, who may rapidly develop dehydration, volume depletion, and hypotension. Patients who do not have rapid access to medical attention should be provided with injectable cortisol and instructed in its use (available in preloaded syringes of hydrocortisone phosphate, 100 mg).

In patients with secondary adrenal insufficiency, mineralocorticoid therapy is usually not required and the cortisol doses listed above may be given without 9α-fluorocortisol except in occasional patients with inadequate aldosterone production.

Patients with adrenal insufficiency due to previous high-dose glucocorticoid therapy are ordinarily maintained quite adequately on the same steroid they received for therapy (usually prednisone). The management of these patients is discussed in Chap. 15.

Steroid Coverage for Illness, Surgery, or Trauma

Patients with primary or secondary adrenocortical insufficiency who suffer trauma or an acute illness should be treated according to the protocol described above for acute addisonian crisis. In patients undergoing elective surgery (Table 12-23), electrolyte status, blood pressure, and hydration should be assessed and, if necessary, corrected before the induction of anesthesia. A regimen that has been proved effective for increased steroid coverage includes the administration of 100 mg cortisol IM on call to the operating room, 50 mg IM or IV in the recovery room, and then 50 mg q 6 h for three doses. On the second postoperative day, if the patient is progressing satisfactorily, the dose may be reduced to 25 mg q 6 h. The dose may then be tapered to normal maintenance levels over a period of 3 to 5 days. If fever, hypotension, or other complications occur or persist, the dosage should be maintained at or increased to a total of 200 to 400 mg/24 h.

This protocol, a modification of that described by others,[1091] has been used successfully for the past 20 years in patients with primary, secondary, or glucocorticoid-induced adrenal insufficiency. It is also used routinely in patients undergoing adrenalectomy or pituitary surgery. No instance of acute adrenal insufficiency has been noted, nor have complications of the glucocorticoid therapy occurred. Intramuscular cortisone acetate should not be used (see above), since adequate plasma cortisol concentrations are not achieved even if the cortisone acetate is administered 12 to 24 h before surgery.[1082,1091]

TABLE 12-23 Steroid Coverage for Surgery

1. Correct electrolyte levels, blood pressure, and hydration if necessary.
2. Give cortisol,* 100 mg IM, on call to operating room.
3. Give cortisol, 50 mg IM or IV, in recovery room and q 6 h for first 24 h.
4. If progress is satisfactory, reduce dose to 25 mg q 6 h for 24 h; then taper to maintenance dose over 3 to 5 days. Resume previous 9α-fluorocortisol dose when patient is taking oral medications.
5. Maintain or increase cortisol dose to 200 to 400 mg/24 h if fever, hypotension, or other complications occur.

* As hydrocortisone phosphate or hemisuccinate.

Intraoperative or postoperative shock has been reported in such patients receiving injectable cortisone acetate in preparation for surgery.[1092] Recent studies in animals suggest that such supraphysiologic doses are not required during surgical stress; however, no studies in humans are available, and thus we continue to recommend the above protocol.[1093]

Prognosis and Survival

Before the availability of glucocorticoid therapy, primary adrenocortical insufficiency was a rapidly and uniformly fatal illness, and most patients died within 2 years of the diagnosis (Fig. 12-24).[680] Life expectancy increased somewhat when mineralocorticoid therapy in the form of deoxycorticosterone acetate became available in the late 1930s. However, despite correction of mineralocorticoid deficiency, hypotension, and electrolyte abnormalities, life expectancy was still usually less than 5 years and these patients were still susceptible to stress.[680] The introduction of glucocorticoid therapy in the late 1940s resulted in an immediate and marked increase in survival (Fig. 12-24).[680,1011] Survival in patients with either primary or secondary adrenocortical insufficiency now approximates that of the normal population when appropriate therapy, including patient education and increased coverage for stress, is carried out.[680,1011] Deaths from adrenal insufficiency are rare in diagnosed and appropriately treated patients, and the majority of deaths occur in patients with a more rapid "acute" course, such as those with a massive bilateral adrenal hemorrhage. These patients are frequently not receiving medical care; many die without diagnosis, and the adrenocortical insufficiency is discovered only at autopsy.[1011]

Hypoaldosteronism

Hypoaldosteronism may occur selectively or in association with an impairment in the production of cortisol. Hypoaldosteronism in association with hypocortisolism due to Addison's disease, hypopituitarism, and congenital adrenal biosynthetic defects are discussed in other sections. Selective hypoaldosteronism is commonly associated with a deficiency of renin secretion by the kidney (hyporeninemic hypoaldosteronism). It can also be due to defective adrenal release of aldosterone in association with normal or elevated plasma renin levels.[1094,1095] These primary adrenal causes of selective hypoaldosteronism occur with isolated adrenal biosynthetic defects [corticosterone methyloxidase deficiency which is due to mutations in the gene for P450c11AS (see Disorders of Steroid Hormone Synthesis, above)], with focal dysfunction of the adrenal glomerulosa with absent responsiveness to angiotensin II (hyperreninemic hypoaldosteronism), after resection of an aldosterone-producing adenoma (see Chap. 14), in pseudohypoaldosteronism (unresponsiveness to aldosterone), after heparin administration (discussed in Inhibitors of Adrenal Steroid Biosynthesis, above[416,417,434]), and with potassium deficiency.[1094]

Hyporeninemic Hypoaldosteronism

Hyporeninemic hypoaldosteronism occurs generally in older patients with renal disease who have hyperkalemia and hyperchloremic metabolic acidosis that is disproportionately more severe than expected from the extent of renal impairment.[1094–1097] In a series of 22 patients, the mean creatinine clearance was 33 (range, 11 to 56) ml/min per 1.73 m^2 [1097]; six patients had diabetes mellitus, one had multiple myeloma, and most of the remainder appeared to have interstitial nephritis. The hypoaldosteronism is due to decreased renin release by the kidney.[1094–1097] Plasma renin levels are low and do not increase normally in response to postural changes and sodium restriction. Plasma aldosterone levels are also low and do not increase normally with postural changes and sodium restriction. However, they do increase appropriately relative to the small change in plasma renin levels, suggesting that the adrenal glomerulosa is normal.[1094,1096] In addition, angiotensin II infusion or ACTH administration results in prompt increases in aldosterone release.[1094–1097] In fact, the plasma aldosterone concentration is disproportionately high relative to the plasma renin concentration, possibly because of the associated hyperkalemia.[1094–1097] However, occasional patients with hyporeninemic hypoaldosteronism also have a defect in the late steps in adrenal aldosterone biosynthesis, and plasma aldosterone levels do not respond normally to increased renin concentration (e.g., with diuretic treatment) or ACTH.[1094,1096] This may be due to the hyperreninemic syndrome discussed below.

The pathogenesis of the hyporeninemia is not clear.[1094–1099] It is likely that the renal disease in some way impairs the ability of the kidney to release renin. This could be due to direct damage to the juxtaglomerular or macula densa cells or to an effector mechanism such as the efferent limb of the autonomic nervous supply, the functions that control exposure or responsiveness to ions, and the renal baroreceptor system (Chap. 14). It has also been speculated that there is a defect in the conversion of prorenin to renin or an inhibitor of renin. Others have proposed that increased extracellular fluid volume causes physiologic suppression; indeed, an increase in extracellular fluid volume has been found in some patients, hypertension is present in about a third of cases, and renin and aldosterone concentrations have been shown to increase progressively as the extracellular fluid volume decreases with diuretic therapy, although it is not clear that the renin level increases normally. Another postulated mediator of the hyporeninemia is ANP, which reduces renin levels and inhibits responsiveness to potassium (see above).[373,1100–1102] In addition, a deficiency of renal PG or prostacyclin production has been implicated in the renin deficiency.[1100,1103]

The major consequence of the hypoaldosteronism in these patients is hyperkalemia; the serum potassium concentration is usually between 5.5 and 6.5 mEq/liter.[1094,1096,1098] The extent of hyperkalemia is related to dietary potassium intake and, in diabetic patients, to diabetic control.[1094] Occasional patients have had third-degree heart block.[1094,1096,1097] In fact, this condition appears to be the most common cause of chronic hyperkalemia in patients without severe renal disease (e.g., creatinine clearance less than 15 mg/min per 1.73 m^2).[1094] Most patients do not lose sodium or develop dehydration; increased extracellular fluid volume and hypertension are more common.[1094] This lack of salt wasting may be due to the associated renal disease, to other primary factors, and to the fact that cortisol secretion is normal. However, hyponatremia is occasionally present.[1098]

These patients also develop hypochloremic acidosis,[1094] which is accentuated by the renal insufficiency; the extent of acidosis is related to the degree of glomerular insufficiency. The acidosis is renal in origin and can be differentiated from renal tubular acidosis type 1 by the fact that the urine is acidotic and relatively bicarbonate-free during periods of acidosis; it can be distinguished from type 2 renal tubular acidosis by the fact that the extent of decreased reabsorption of bicarbonate at normal bicarbonate concentrations is not great enough to indicate defective proximal tubular dysfunction and by a lack of aminoaciduria, glucosuria, or increased renal phosphate clearance. Urinary excretion of ammonia is markedly reduced, even with an acidic urine. Thus, these changes, combined with evidence for low potassium clearance, have led to the classification of the dysfunction as type 4 renal tubular acidosis. The acidosis itself appears to be due to both the hyperkalemia that reduces renal ammonia production and the reduced hydrogen secretory capacity.

The initial differential diagnosis includes all the causes of hyperkalemia,[1094–1099] including the hypoaldosterone states mentioned above that have normal or elevated plasma renin levels. Pseudohypokalemia due to abnormal potassium release from clotting when elevated platelet or white blood cell counts are present can be excluded by obtaining heparinized blood with minimal turbulence and measuring the plasma K^+ concentration, which is normal in this condition. The use of drugs that elevate the serum potassium ion concentration (spironolactone, triamterene, amiloride) can be excluded by history and also by the fact that the plasma aldosterone concentration is not abnormally low in these circumstances. Also, hyporeninemic hypoaldosteronism has been reported in association with chronic and massive intake of sodium bicarbonate.[1101] Addison's disease and adrenal biosynthetic deficiency states are usually associated with a high plasma renin concentration and may have the other manifestations described above. However, as mentioned earlier, occasional patients with hyperkalemia and chronic renal disease have hypoaldosteronism with normal plasma renin levels. Oliguric renal failure and other causes of severe acidosis (e.g., diabetic ketoacidosis) can be excluded by the clinical setting. There are rare syndromes with hyperkalemia and lack of responsiveness to aldosterone (pseudohypoaldosteronism; see below); however, these patients have several distinguishing clinical characteristics, including high aldosterone and renin levels.

Patients with hyporeninemic hypoaldosteronism generally respond to 9α-fluorocortisol with amelioration of the hyperkalemia and acidosis.[1096–1098] Doses of around 0.2 mg per day are ordinarily required[1096–1098]; however, in some patients the kidneys appeared to be hyporesponsive to mineralocorticoids, and in these patients higher doses of the steroid are required.[1095] Mineralocorticoid replacement is not the therapy of choice in patients with hypertension and increased fluid volume. In many cases, furosemide therapy can ameliorate both the hyperkalemia and the acidosis.[1104] Further, in patients with severe hypoaldosteronism, the combination of furosemide and small doses of mineralocorticoids can be synergistic.[1098,1104] Thus, diuretics and mineralocorticoids should be used alone or in combination, and the relative doses should be individualized, depending on the clinical setting and the response. Alternative measures depending on the individual patient can include restriction of dietary potassium; oral administration of sodium polystyrene sulfonate, a resin that binds potassium ion and releases sodium ion in the gastrointestinal tract; and the oral administration of sodium bicarbonate.[1095]

Normoreninemic or Hyperreninemic Hypoaldosteronism

Normo- and hyperreninemic hypoaldosteronism appear to result from acquired dysfunction of the adrenal glomerulosa.[1095,1105–1108] This occurs most commonly in critically ill patients with hypotension[1107,1108]; it has been reported in over 50 percent of such patients. These patients have hypoaldosteronism despite markedly increased plasma renin level; aldosterone secretion is subnormally responsive to stimulation with ACTH or angiotensin II.[1107,1108] The mechanism of impaired aldosterone production and the role of ischemia with potential anoxia and adrenal damage are not known, but the frequency of this condition should alert the physician to consider it in such patients. There has been one report of a patient with hyperkalemia and moderate renal insufficiency who had hyperreninemia and subnormal plasma aldosterone responses to ACTH, upright posture, and sodium depletion.[1105]

This patient was shown to have antibodies against the zona glomerulosa, suggesting possible selective autoimmune destruction of the adrenal glomerulosa.[1106]

Pseudohypoaldosteronism (Unresponsiveness to Aldosterone)

There are rare cases in which patients do not exhibit a response to aldosterone.[1094,1095] This has been reported in infants without renal parenchymal disease and in children and adults with azotemia due to renal interstitial disease (salt-wasting nephropathy). These patients have hyperkalemia, metabolic acidosis, and renal sodium wasting with extracellular fluid depletion and hypotension despite elevated plasma aldosterone and renin levels. These abnormalities do not respond to large doses of mineralocorticoids. These patients apparently have a renal defect which leaves them unable to respond to mineralocorticoids, and treatment with sodium chloride and/or bicarbonate is ordinarily required to maintain them.

An additional rare syndrome has been termed *type 2 pseudohypoaldosteronism*.[1095,1109] It has been described in children and young adults and is characterized by hyperkalemia and hyperchloremia, metabolic acidosis with hypertension, hyporeninemia, and hypoaldosteronism. These patients differ from hyporeninemic hypoaldosteronism patients in that they have a normal GFR. As is the case with pseudohypoaldosteronism, their renal potassium excretion fails to increase normally when large amounts of mineralocorticoids are administered, but unlike the case with pseudohypoaldosteronism, pseudohypoaldosteronism type 2 patients have a normal antinatriuretic and antichloriduric response to mineralocorticoids.[1095] It has been suggested that the primary abnormality in this syndrome is a defect in the distal nephron for chloride reabsorption that increases distal NaCl reabsorption, resulting in hyperchloremia, volume expansion, and hypertension that also limits the sodium- and mineralocorticoid-dependent voltage driving force for potassium and hydrogen secretion, resulting in hyperkalemia and hypertension[1095]; the syndrome might also be explained by an isolated collecting tubule defect in potassium secretion.[1095] Restriction of dietary NaCl or administration of a chloruretic diuretic ameliorates the hyperkalemia and acidosis in these patients.[1095]

There can also be other circumstances in which selective unresponsiveness to certain actions of mineralocorticoids occurs. Thus, after several days of mineralocorticoid excess, further sodium retention does not occur (the escape phenomenon) even though responses of potassium and hydrogen loss persist (see above). The lack of response of the kaliuretic actions of the mineralocorticoids occurs in the rare hypertensive syndrome with possibly increased chloride reabsorption (see above), and in pregnancy there is a relative resistance to the kaliuretic responses of the mineralocorticoids (discussed below).

ADRENOCORTICAL HYPERFUNCTION

Hyperfunction of the adrenal cortex can result from excessive activity of the zonae fasciculata and reticularis or the zona glomerulosa and from steroid-producing adenomas or carcinomas. Excessive stimulation of the zonae fasciculata and reticularis by ACTH is due to pituitary hypersecretion of ACTH (usually by a small adenoma), abnormal ACTH release by extrapituitary tumors (ectopic ACTH syndrome), or ACTH therapy. This results in increased secretion of cortisol, adrenal androgens, and DOC. Excessive activity of the zona glomerulosa can be due to primary aldosteronism, with adenomas or hyperplasia resulting from unknown causes (see Chap. 14), or it can be due to activation of the renin-angiotensin system by a variety of causes. Adrenal adenomas usually produced either cortisol or aldosterone and rarely androgens, whereas carcinomas frequently secrete multiple steroids.

Cushing's Syndrome

Cushing's syndrome refers to the manifestations of glucocorticoid excess without regard to specific etiology; there may also be androgen excess. It is most commonly iatrogenic, caused by glucocorticoid therapy (Chap. 15). Cushing's *disease* refers to the disorder resulting from pituitary ACTH hypersecretion. Spontaneous Cushing's syndrome is an uncommon disorder; however, it must be considered in the differential diagnosis of such diverse entities as obesity, hypertension, diabetes, weakness, osteoporosis, hirsutism, and menstrual disorders.

Classification, Occurrence, and Age and Sex Distributions

Spontaneous Cushing's syndrome is either ACTH-dependent or ACTH-independent (Table 12-24). The ACTH-dependent types are Cushing's disease, the ectopic ACTH syndrome, and, more rarely,

TABLE 12-24 Classification and Etiology of Cushing's Syndrome

	Percent
ACTH-dependent	
Cushing's disease	68
Ectopic ACTH syndrome	15
ACTH-independent	
Adrenal adenoma	9
Adrenal carcinoma	8
	100

Source: Huff.[1113]

ectopic CRH production.[1110–1112] In these disorders, chronic ACTH hypersecretion stimulates the zonae fasciculata and reticularis, resulting in bilateral adrenocortical hyperplasia with increased secretion of cortisol, androgens, and DOC. ACTH-independent Cushing's syndrome is due to primary adrenocortical neoplasms, either adenomas or carcinomas; the resulting hypercortisolism suppresses the hypothalamic-pituitary axis. Other rare forms of Cushing's syndrome are discussed below.

Cushing's disease accounts for approximately 70 percent of adult patients in current series,[1113,1114] and the majority of these patients have pituitary microadenomas (see below). There is a distinct female preponderance in Cushing's disease. In older series, the female/male ratio was 3:1,[1115] but it is 8:1 in current experience.[1116,1117] The age range in Cushing's disease is most frequently 20 to 40 years.[1115]

Ectopic ACTH hypersecretion is responsible for approximately 15 percent of reported cases of Cushing's syndrome. This is an underestimate of the true incidence, since many patients lack the classic features of hypercortisolism. They are thus not brought to the attention of an endocrinologist; severe hypercortisolism and rapid death are common.[1118] The tumors causing the ectopic ACTH syndrome are discussed below; oat-cell carcinoma of the lung is the most common, and ectopic ACTH secretion occurs in 0.5 to 2 percent of these patients.[1119] In addition, immunoreactive and bioactive ACTH has been demonstrated in the majority of these tumors, even when clinical evidence of ectopic ACTH hypersecretion is not present.[1120–1122] The ectopic ACTH syndrome is more common in males (female/male ratio = 1:3), and the peak incidence of 40 to 60 years reflects the greater incidence of malignancy in this age group.[1114,1123]

ACTH-independent primary adrenal tumors cause 17 to 19 percent of cases of Cushing's syndrome, with equal frequencies of adenoma and carcinoma in adults.[1113,1114] Adrenal adenomas causing Cushing's syndrome occur more frequently in females.[1114] Adrenocortical carcinoma causing Cushing's syndrome also shows a female preponderance (approximately 66 percent of cases)[1124]; however, the prevalence of all types of adrenal carcinoma is higher in males.[1124] The overall prevalence of adrenal carcinoma is approximately 2 per 1 million population. Approximately 75 percent of cases occur after age 12, with the peak incidence in the fourth to sixth decade; the mean age at diagnosis is 38 years.[1025,1114,1124]

Cushing's syndrome in childhood is distinctly unusual. Cushing's disease is responsible for only 35 percent of cases; the majority of these patients are 10 years old or older at the time of diagnosis,[1114,1125–1128] and the incidence by sex is approximately equal.[1125–1128] Adrenal tumors account for the majority (65 percent) of cases in childhood, with carcinoma responsible for 51 percent and adenoma for 14 percent.[1114] The majority of these tumors occur in girls, and most occur between the ages of 1 and 8 years.[1114]

Pathology

Anterior Pituitary

Pituitary adenomas are found either at surgery or at autopsy in over 90 percent of patients with Cushing's disease[1116,1129–1132] and confirm Cushing's original description of pituitary adenomas in six of his eight autopsied cases (Fig. 12-40). Approximately 80 to 90 percent of these are microadenomas (diameter less than 10 mm); 50 percent are 5 mm or less in diameter, and microadenomas less than 2 mm in diameter have been reported.[1116,1129–1132] Thus, these small adenomas do not result in sellar enlargement, although focal radiologic abnormalities may occur.[1131] The remainder of the pituitary adenomas in Cushing's disease are larger than 10 mm; these adenomas cause sellar enlargement, frequently with extrasellar extension, and invasive tendencies are common.[1133] Malignant tumors have occasionally been reported.[1133]

The adenomas of Cushing's disease are characteristically basophilic, unencapsulated, and located within the anterior pituitary.[1130,1131,1134–1136] Chromophobe adenomas may also occur.[1131] The tumors are composed of compact sheets of uniform, well-granulated cells with a sinusoidal arrangement and a high content of ACTH, β-LPH, and β-endorphin.[1137,1138] The cytoplasm usually contains abundant basophilic granules which, on immunocytochemical staining, are positive for ACTH and β-LPH. These cells frequently show a zone of perinuclear hyalinization known as Crooke's changes which results from exposure of the corticotrophs to hypercortisolism.[1130] Electron microscopy demonstrates considerable heterogeneity of granule size (200 to 700 mm) and variability in the number of granules, which may be scattered throughout the cytoplasm or marginated along the cell membrane.[1130] The hyaline changes seen on light microscopy appear as bundles of perinuclear microfilaments (average 7.0 nm in diameter) which encircle the nucleus.[1130]

The portion of the anterior pituitary not involved by the adenoma has been less well studied. In most cases there is atrophy of the surrounding corticotrophs; however, paraadenomatous hyperplasia has been reported in some cases.[1139–1141] In addition, ACTH content in the paraadenomatous tissue is decreased, in contrast to the increased content in the adenoma cells themselves.[1137,1138]

Patients in the subgroup with Cushing's disease and no demonstrable pituitary adenoma usually have diffuse corticotroph hyperplasia,[1136,1142,1143] although a few patients have no demonstrable pituitary abnormality.[1144,1145] Several patients with corticotroph hyperplasia have been found to have

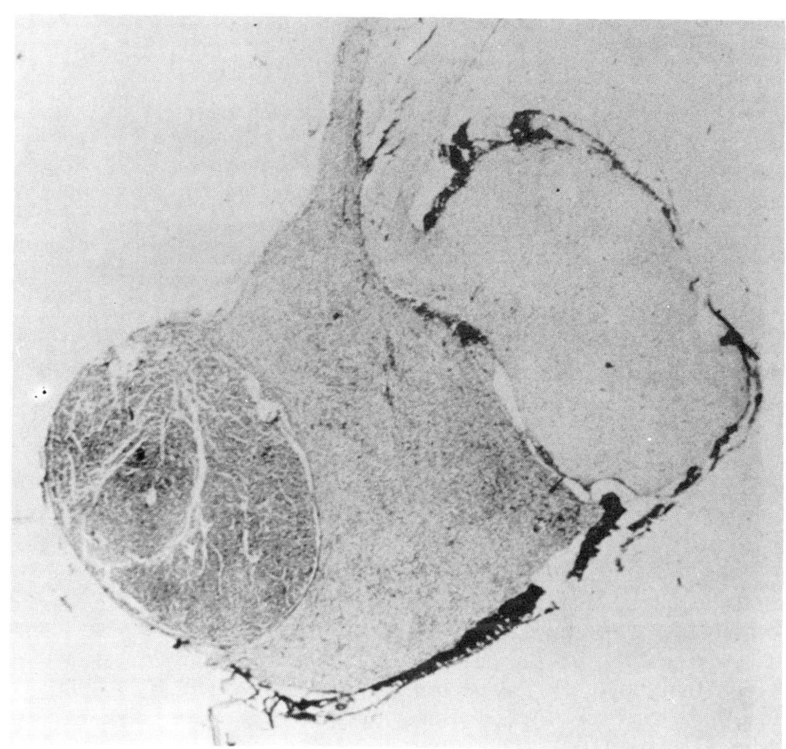

FIGURE 12-40 A basophilic anterior pituitary microadenoma from Cushing's original series. *(From Cushing.[4])*

intrasellar gangliocytomas which secrete CRH,[1110] and a few additional patients have been found to have ectopic tumors that secrete CRH but not ACTH.[1111,1112,1143] Additional patients have been described with ad nomatous hyperplasia postulated to be of intermediate lobe origin[1146]; however, in other series, this type of hyperplasia has been absent or rare.[1135,1147,1148]

In patients with adrenal tumors or the ectopic ACTH syndrome and in those subjected to steroid therapy, the pituitary corticotrophs show prominent Crooke's hyaline changes with perinuclear microfilaments and reduced ACTH content.

Adrenal Cortex

Adrenocortical Hyperplasia Bilateral hyperplasia of the adrenal cortex occurs in patients with ACTH hypersecretion from either pituitary or ectopic sources. Three types of hyperplasia have been described: simple, that associated with the ectopic ACTH syndrome, and bilateral nodular.[1114,1149,1150] With simple hyperplasia (usually secondary to Cushing's disease), the combined adrenal weight is between 12 and 24 g (normal weight, 8 to 10 g; see (Anatomy, above). The enlarged glands have a yellowish-brown color. On microscopic examination, the cortex is thickened because of approximately equal hyperplasia of the compact cells of the zona reticularis and the clear cells of the zona fasciculata, with normal ultrastructural features. The zona glomerulosa is normal.

The adrenals in the ectopic ACTH syndrome are usually much more enlarged, with combined weights of 24 to more than 100 g.[1025,1114,1123,1149,1150] The cut surface of the cortex is generally brownish. Microscopically, there is typically marked hyperplasia of the zona reticularis, with columns of hypertrophied compact cells extending to and into the zona glomerulosa. The clear cells of the zona fasciculata are markedly reduced; however, the zona glomerulosa is normal. These histologic features are consistent with the effects of the markedly elevated ACTH levels typically seen in the ectopic ACTH syndrome.[1025]

Bilateral nodular hyperplasia is present in approximately 20 percent of cases.[1114,1149,1150] The precise etiology of these pathologic subtypes is unclear, although most result from pituitary ACTH excess (see Etiology and Pathogenesis, below). The adrenals are enlarged, and adrenal weight is variable, depending on the number and size of the nodules present. The cut surface reveals at least one and usually multiple macroscopic yellow nodules which are usually bilateral. The nodules resemble both nonfunctioning adenomas and those causing Cushing's syndrome and consist mainly of clear cells which are similar to those of the normal zona fasciculata. The intervening cortex shows the typical features of simple hyperplasia described above.[1114,1150]

Rarely, this condition is associated with adrenal carcinoma.[1151]

Adrenocortical Tumors Benign hyperfunctioning adrenal adenomas causing Cushing's syndrome weigh from 10 to 70 g and range in size from 1 to 6 cm.[1114,1149,1150] They are encapsulated, with a well-delineated margin, and the cut surface is yellow with brown or red areas. Microscopically, clear cells of the zona fasciculata type predominate and make up the yellow areas, whereas the darker areas contain cells resembling those of the compact zone of the zona reticularis. Rarely, these adenomas can be black because of the presence of lipofuscin.[1025]

Adrenal carcinomas are generally quite large (over 100 g), may weigh in excess of several kilograms, and are commonly palpable as abdominal masses.[1114,1149,1150] These tumors are encapsulated; the cut surface reveals a highly vascular tumor with necrosis, hemorrhage and cystic degeneration. Calcification is not uncommon. Adrenal carcinomas may have a benign histologic appearance with a predominance of compact cells, although variable degrees of pleomorphism occur, especially in larger tumors. The histologic features frequently do not predict the clinical behavior of the tumor.[1114,1149,1150] Thus, in many cases, a definite diagnosis of malignancy can be established only if there is vascular invasion, local extension, or metastatic spread. These carcinomas spread by local invasion of the retroperitoneum, kidney, or liver or hematogenously to the liver and lungs.[1124]

With both functioning adrenal adenomas and carcinomas there is atrophy of the cortex contiguous to the tumor and of the contralateral gland.[1149] The capsule of the uninvolved cortex is thickened, and the atrophic cortex is narrow and consists entirely of clear, lipid-containing cells. The zona reticularis is absent, and the zona glomerulosa is normal.[1123]

Etiology and Pathogenesis

Cushing's Disease

Cushing's disease is caused by pituitary ACTH hypersecretion, and pituitary adenomas are present in the great majority of patients (see Pathology, above, and Treatment of Cushing's Syndrome, below). Most cases of Cushing's disease are due to spontaneous ACTH-secreting pituitary adenomas, and hypothalamic abnormalities are secondary to hypercortisolism. However, other researchers feel that this disorder results from a primary CNS abnormality with excessive stimulation of anterior pituitary corticotrophs by CRH or other factors with secondary adenoma formation (see Chaps. 7 and 8).[1131,1152,1153]

Several endocrine abnormalities are characteristic of Cushing's disease. First, there is hypersecretion of ACTH with bilateral adrenocortical hyperplasia and hypersecretion of cortisol (Table 12-25). Second, there is absent circadian periodicity of ACTH and cortisol release; episodic secretion persists at a higher than normal frequency but is sporadic and lacks a diurnal pattern.[1154,1155] Third, there is absent responsiveness of ACTH and cortisol to stresses such as hypoglycemia and major surgery.[763,1156] Fourth, although negative feedback regulation of ACTH secretion by glucocorticoids is present, pharmacologic concentrations are required to suppress ACTH release and there is hyperresponsiveness of ACTH release when cortisol secretion is inhibited.[763] Fifth, abnormalities of other pituitary hormones are present in most of these patients, including subnormal responsiveness of growth hormone, TSH, and gonadotropin release to a variety of stimuli.[1156–1159]

TABLE 12-25 Endocrine Abnormalities in Cushing's Disease

Hypersecretion of ACTH and cortisol
Absent circadian periodicity of ACTH and cortisol
Abnormal ACTH and cortisol responsiveness to stress (hypoglycemia, surgery)
Abnormal negative feedback regulation of ACTH secretion by glucocorticoids
Abnormal suppressibility with dexamethasone
Hyperresponsiveness to inhibition of cortisol synthesis with metyrapone
Subnormal responsiveness of growth hormone, thyrotropin, and gonadotropins to stimulation

That Cushing's disease is a primary pituitary disorder in most patients is based on the high frequency of pituitary adenomas, the response to their removal, and the interpretation of hypothalamic abnormalities as being secondary to hypercortisolism. ACTH hypersecretion from a pituitary adenoma results in hypercortisolism which suppresses the normal hypothalamic-pituitary axis and CRH release; this abolishes hypothalamic regulation of circadian variability and stress responsiveness.[1131,1160] It has been postulated that the feedback control of ACTH secretion is mediated directly on the pituitary tumor and that other pharmacologic agents, such as vasopressin, cyproheptadine, and bromocriptine, directly inhibit an ACTH-secreting adenoma.[1131,1160] In addition, abnormalities of growth hormone, TSH, and gonadotropin secretion are due to hypercortisolism, and not to a primary hypothalamic disorder.[1131,1160] Also, when hypersecreted in rare patients with CRH-secreting tumors or when administered to animals, CRH does not result in pituitary adenomas but instead leads to pituitary corticotroph hyperplasia.[1143,1161]

The response to pituitary microsurgery strongly supports a primary pituitary etiology. Selective removal of pituitary microadenomas by transsphenoidal microsurgery corrects ACTH hypersecretion and hypercortisolism in most patients.[1116,1131,1159,1160,1162–1165] This suggests that the adenoma, not generalized corticotroph hyperplasia, is responsible for ACTH excess. Postoperatively, almost all these patients have transient ACTH deficiency and secondary hypoadrenalism with preservation of other pituitary hormones,[1131,1159,1162–1165] demonstrating that the normal hypothalamic-pituitary axis is suppressed by the hypercortisolism. This is supported by the in vitro demonstration of markedly decreased ACTH content in nonadenomatous pituitary tissue removed from patients with active Cushing's disease.[1137,1138] In cases studied after selective surgical removal of the adenoma, there is a return to normal of (1) the circadian rhythm of ACTH and cortisol secretion, (2) the responsiveness of the hypothalamic-pituitary axis to hypoglycemic stress, (3) suppressibility of cortisol secretion by dexamethasone,[1159,1162–1165] and (4) the formerly suppressed growth hormone, TSH, and gonadotropin responses.[1159,1163–1166] Thus, in these patients, there is no evidence for a persisting hypothalamic abnormality. Recovery of ACTH and growth hormone responsiveness to hypoglycemia also occurs when patients with Cushing's disease are treated with bilateral adrenalectomy.[763,1167] The idea that these abnormalities are due to hypercortisolism rather than to a primary hypothalamic lesion is further supported by the fact that glucocorticoid administration can suppress ACTH responses to hypoglycemia as well as growth hormone, TSH, and gonadotropin responses.[665,1156,1159,1166] Thus, the hypothalamic abnormalities of Cushing's disease are reversed simply by removing the source of hypercortisolism, suggesting again that the preoperative abnormalities were due solely to the pituitary adenoma with resulting hypersecretion of ACTH and cortisol.

The postulate that suppression of ACTH and cortisol secretion by high-dose dexamethasone in Cushing's disease occurs directly at the pituitary level is supported by evidence that the pituitary is an important site of glucocorticoid feedback (see above) and by the demonstration in vitro of a direct suppressive effect of glucocorticoids on ACTH secretion by adenomas removed from patients with Cushing's disease.[1168–1170]

There is also evidence for direct effects of other pharmacologic agents at the pituitary level in Cushing's disease. Vasopressin, which stimulates ACTH release in patients with Cushing's disease and in normal individuals, also stimulates secretion in ACTH-secreting pituitary adenomas in vitro but does not release ACTH in normal nonadenomatous anterior pituitary tissue from these patients.[1168–1170] Evidence that bromocriptine, cyproheptadine, and dopamine directly suppress pituitary ACTH secretion in patients with Cushing's disease is less direct.[1171] In one pituitary adenoma from a patient with Cushing's disease, dopamine inhibited ACTH release,[1168] and in a tumor from a patient with Nelson's syndrome, dopamine and cyproheptadine inhibited ACTH secretion.[1172]

TABLE 12-26 Tumors Most Frequently Causing the Ectopic ACTH Syndrome

Oat-cell carcinoma of the lung
Pancreatic islet-cell carcinoma
Carcinoid tumors (lung, gut, thymus, pancreas, ovary)
Thyroid medullary carcinoma
Pheochromocytoma and related tumors

The Ectopic ACTH Syndrome

The ectopic ACTH syndrome is caused by ACTH hypersecretion from nonpituitary tumors. These tumors contain immunoreactive and bioactive ACTH; they also secrete ACTH in vitro.[1173] They contain the POMC mRNA and secrete β-LPH, β-endorphin, and both large and small ACTH fragments, suggesting that the ACTH is derived from a POMC similar to that of the anterior pituitary.[1174–1176] Ectopic tumors may also contain CRH-like activity[1174]; the biological significance of this is unclear, since most of these tumors also contain and secrete ACTH. It is unlikely that the CRH in these cases is stimulating pituitary ACTH, since the histology of the gland in the ectopic ACTH syndrome shows Crooke's changes that are consistent with its suppression by hypercortisolism.[1176] However, as mentioned above, several tumors have been described which secrete CRH in quantities sufficient to cause pituitary ACTH hypersecretion.[1111,1112,1143]

The majority of cases of the ectopic ACTH syndrome are due to a small number of tumor types (Table 12-26).[1175–1178] Oat-cell carcinoma of the lung is by far the most common type. Other tumors, in order of frequency, are islet-cell tumors of the pancreas; carcinoid tumors of the lung, thymus, gut, pancreas, and ovary; medullary carcinoma of the thyroid; and pheochromocytoma and its related neuroectodermal tumors.[1178] Additional miscellaneous and rare cases include prostate carcinoma, malignant melanoma, adenocarcinoma of the colon, ovarian arrhenoblastoma, parathyroid carcinoma, and nephroblastoma.[1111,1112,1175,1178,1179] Undifferentiated or poorly differentiated carcinomas in the gallbladder, parotid, ovary, and cervix have been described with the ectopic ACTH syndrome, but the exact pathologic classification and site of origin of these carcinomas are difficult to ascertain.[1178]

Adrenal Tumors

Glucocorticoid-producing adrenal tumors, whether adenoma or carcinoma, arise de novo and autonomously secrete adrenocortical steroids. Rarely, adrenal carcinomas occur in patients with nodular adrenal

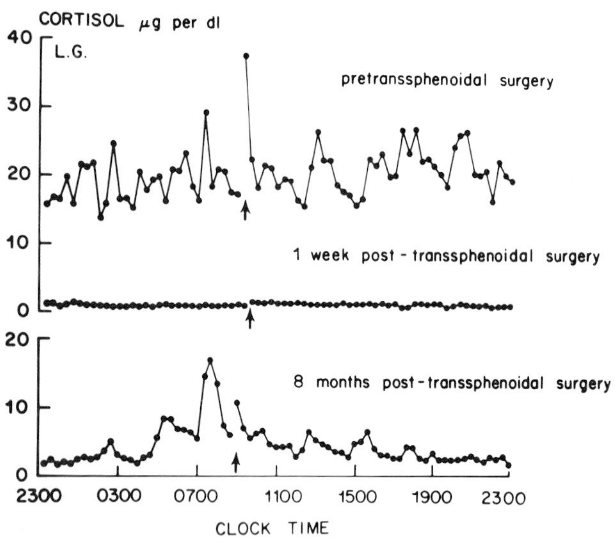

FIGURE 12-41 Twenty-four-h cortisol secretory patterns in a patient with Cushing's disease before treatment *(top)* and 1 week *(middle)* and 8 months *(bottom)* after transsphenoidal adenomectomy. Arrows denote the start of the sampling period. *(From Boyer et al.[1165])*

hyperplasia[1151] or congenital adrenocortical hyperplasia, raising the possibility that in these special circumstances the development of carcinoma is promoted by prolonged ACTH stimulation of the adrenal. However, the majority of adrenal tumors developed spontaneously and are not associated with chronic ACTH excess.

Pathophysiology

Cushing's Disease

In Cushing's disease, pituitary adenomas release ACTH episodically without a circadian pattern,[1154,1155,1165] and since the feedback inhibition of ACTH by glucocorticoids is defective,[799] the elevated cortisol secretion does not adequately decrease ACTH secretion (Fig. 12-41). Thus, a state of glucocorticoid excess persists; it is the number and magnitude of ACTH and adrenal secretory episodes which account for the increase in total cortisol secretion. This episodic secretion results in variable plasma cortisol and ACTH levels, which may at times be moderately or markedly elevated and at other times may be within the normal range.[799,1154,1155,1165] However, measurement of cortisol production rate or urinary free cortisol excretion or multiple plasma cortisol samples over 24 h reveal cortisol hypersecretion (see Laboratory Features and Diagnosis, below, and Refs. 1154,1155,1165). Thus, the major differences in plasma ACTH and cortisol in Cushing's disease occur in the afternoon and at night, when cortisol secretion is usually low in normal individuals. This overall increase in tissue exposure to glucocorticoids is sufficient to cause obvious Cushing's syndrome; however, the modest increase in ACTH secretion usually does not cause increased pigmentation. β-LPH is also hypersecreted.[766–768] In addition to ACTH hypersecretion and resistance to suppression with glucocorticoids, the axis does not respond normally to stressful stimuli such as hypoglycemia and surgery.[763,1156] This is probably due to the relative autonomy of the pituitary adenoma and suppression by glucocorticoids of the normal ability of the hypothalamic-pituitary axis to secrete CRH and ACTH.

The pathophysiologic basis for the clinical abnormalities caused by excess cortisol have already been described (see Actions of Glucocorticoids, above). Thus, cortisol not only inhibits normal pituitary and hypothalamic function, affecting ACTH, TSH, growth hormone, and gonadotropin release, but also causes all the peripheral effects described on most tissues of the body.

The secretion of adrenal androgens (also controlled by ACTH) is increased in patients with Cushing's disease; the extent of hypersecretion is roughly proportional to and parallels that of ACTH and cortisol. DHEA, DHEA-S, and androstenedione are all hypersecreted; they are converted peripherally to testosterone and DHT. Thus, plasma levels of these steroids are moderately increased in Cushing's disease, and a state of androgen excess develops. In the female, this causes the classic manifestations of hirsutism, acne, and amenorrhea. Amenorrhea is in part a consequence of androgen suppression of gonadotropin secretion.[1158] In a male patient with Cushing's disease, testicular production of testosterone is decreased by the glucocorticoid suppression of gonadotropin secretion.[1180] Despite increased adrenal androgen production, the net result is a lowering of circulating testosterone levels, accompanied by decreased libido and impotence.

Aldosterone production is usually not increased in Cushing's disease, and the renin-angiotensin-aldosterone axis usually remains intact. Although there is some increase in DOC production, DOC and cortisol are not elevated enough to produce a frank mineralocorticoid excess state, in contrast to the case with the ectopic ACTH syndrome (Chap. 14).

Ectopic ACTH Syndrome

Patients with this syndrome usually have much more marked ACTH and cortisol hypersecretion than is seen in Cushing's disease. β-LPH and other POMC peptides are also secreted in excess (see Chap. 27).[1174,1175] ACTH and cortisol hypersecretion are also episodic, although at greatly elevated levels. With uncommon exceptions, the secretion of ACTH by an ectopic tumor is not suppressible even with high doses of glucocorticoids.

The marked ACTH hypersecretion results in a greater degree of hyperplasia of the zonae fasciculata and reticularis, and the secretion of cortisol, adrenal androgens, and DOC is higher than in most patients with Cushing's disease.[1114] Thus, plasma levels and urinary excretion of these steroids and their metabolites usually are markedly elevated.[627,1181] However, in spite of the marked elevations of these steroids, the classic features of Cushing's syndrome are commonly absent.[1181] This is presumably due to the rapid onset of hypercortisolism and the associated malignancy. Also, manifestations of androgen excess may not be prominent because most of these patients are male. However, the elevated DOC and cortisol concentrations frequently result in a frank mineralocorticoid excess syndrome with hypertension, hypokalemia, and suppressed plasma renin levels (Chap. 14).

Adrenal Tumors

Glucocorticoid-secreting primary adrenal tumors, whether adenomas or carcinomas, autonomously hypersecrete cortisol and suppress the hypothalamic-pituitary axis, CRH, and circulating plasma ACTH levels.[763] This results in atrophy of the zonae fasciculata and reticularis not involved by the tumor.[1114]

Adrenal adenomas causing Cushing's syndrome usually secrete only cortisol in significant excess; thus, the clinical picture is one of pure glucocorticoid excess. Cortisol secretion is again episodic, but feedback control of cortisol release is lost, and thus these tumors typically show no response to either dexamethasone or metyrapone. The adrenal secretion of androgens is usually subnormal, as manifested by low urinary 17-ketosteroid excretion or plasma DHEA-S levels.[1182]

Adrenal carcinomas frequently secrete multiple steroids in an unpredictable pattern.[1124] However, most commonly, cortisol, DOC, and androgens are secreted in excess; less commonly, there is hypersecretion of aldosterone or estrogens. Concentrations of plasma cortisol and its urinary metabolites frequently are markedly elevated in patients with adrenal carcinomas. In addition, androgen hypersecretion is frequently even more markedly elevated, with very high levels of urinary 17-ketosteroids or plasma DHEA and DHEA-S.[1124] These patients usually have severe and rapidly progressive clinical manifestations of cortisol excess; in females, androgen excess is prominent.[1124] These patients also frequently have mineralocorticoid excess due to cortisol and DOC, with resulting hypertension and hypokalemia.

Clinical and Laboratory Features

Clinical Features

The clinical manifestations of Cushing's syndrome were well described by Cushing himself[4]; the frequencies of these features are listed in Table 12-27.[627,1115] Although the frequency of presenting signs and symptoms has remained remarkably constant, the severity of the condition appears to be less in more recent series, presumably because of earlier clinical recognition and diagnosis.[627,1115]

TABLE 12-27 Clinical Features of Cushing's Syndrome

Feature	Percent with Feature
Obesity	94
Facial plethora	84
Hirsutism	82
Menstrual disorders	76
Hypertension	72
Muscular weakness	58
Back pain	58
Striae	52
Acne	40
Psychological symptoms	40
Bruising	36
Congestive heart failure	22
Edema	18
Renal calculi	16
Headache	14
Polyuria/polydipsia	10
Hyperpigmentation	6

Source: Modified from Plotz et al.[1115] and Ross et al.[627]

Obesity is the most common manifestation (Fig. 12-42), and weight gain is usually the initial symptom. Weight gain is classically central, affecting mainly the face, neck, trunk, and abdomen, with relative sparing of the extremities.[1115] However, generalized obesity is equally frequent and was present in 60 percent of the cases described by Ross and associates.[627] In children with Cushing's syndrome, obesity is invariably present and is usually generalized.[1125–1128] In addition to obesity, 85 percent of children with Cushing's syndrome have short stature and growth failure.[1125] Whether central or generalized, the obesity of Cushing's syndrome has certain features which distinguish it from simple obesity. Accumulation of fat in the face leads to the typical "moon facies," which is present in 75 percent and is accompanied by facial plethora in most patients. Fat accumulation around the neck is prominent in the supraclavicular and dorsocervical fat pads; the fat deposition in the latter is responsible for the "buffalo hump." Adipose tissue accumulates over the thorax and frequently leads to protruberance of the abdomen. A minority of the patients are not obese and do not gain weight; however, they usually have central redistribution of fat and a typical facial appearance.[1115]

Although skin changes are less common, their presence should arouse suspicion of cortisol excess. Atrophy of the epidermis and its underlying connective tissue leads to thinning and a transparent appearance of the skin in advanced cases. This also accounts for the plethoric appearance. Easy bruis-

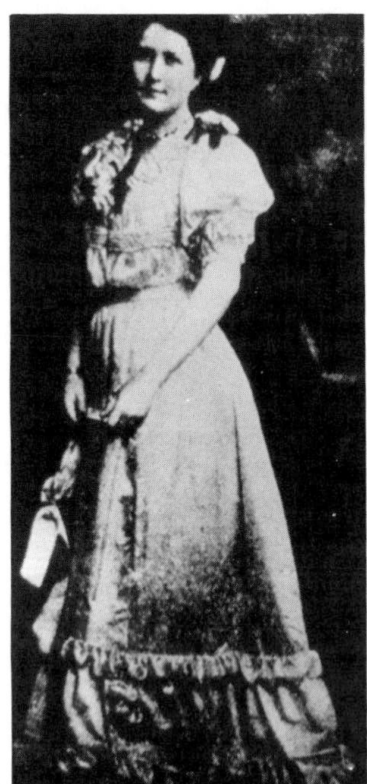
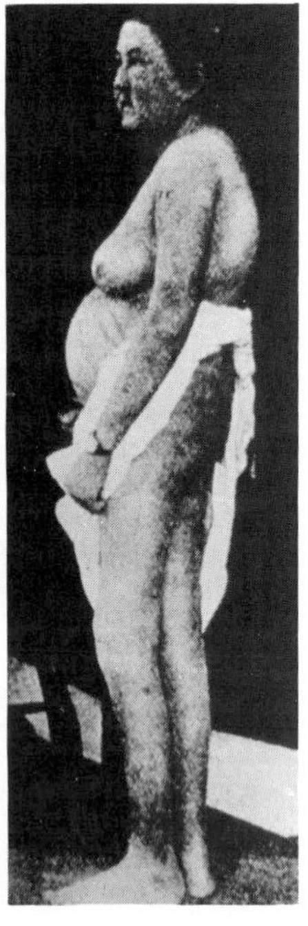
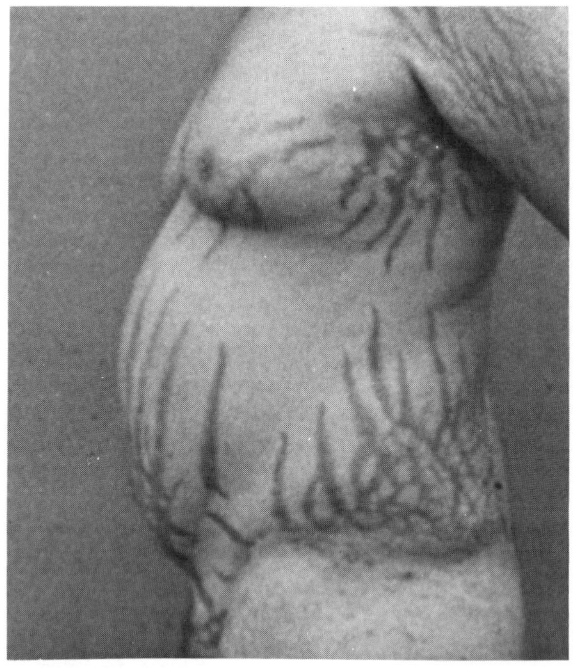

A B

FIGURE 12-42 *(A)* Patient from Cushing's original series before and after the development of clinical features. *(B)* Marked striae in a patient with Cushing's syndrome. *(Panel A from Cushing.[4])*

ability with minimal trauma is present in 40 to 60 percent of patients. Such patients on occasion have been detected after referral for a work-up of a bleeding diathesis. Purple striae occur in 50 to 70 percent of these patients; they are typically red to purple in color, depressed below the skin surface because of loss of underlying connective tissue, and wider (not infrequently 0.5 to 2.0 cm) than the pinkish-white striae seen with pregnancy or rapid weight gain. These striae are most commonly abdominal but also may occur over the breasts, hips, buttocks, thighs, and axillae. Minor wounds and abrasions frequently heal slowly and poorly, as do surgical incisions, which sometimes dehisce.[1115] Mucocutaneous fungal infections occur frequently, including tinea versicolor, involvement of the nails, and oral candidiasis. Hyperpigmentation of the skin occurs rarely in patients with Cushing's disease or adrenal tumors but is more common in the ectopic ACTH syndrome.[627,1182] Hirsutism is present in 65 to 70 percent of female patients as a result of hypersecretion of adrenal androgens; it is generally mild to moderate. Facial hirsutism is most common, but increased hair growth also may occur over the abdomen, breasts, chest, and upper thighs. Virilism is unusual except in adrenal carcinomas, in which it occurs in approximately 20 percent.[1124] Acne, most frequently involving the face, and seborrhea usually accompany hirsutism.

Hypertension, a classic feature of spontaneous Cushing's syndrome, is present in 75 to 85 percent of these patients. The diastolic blood pressure is > 100 mmHg in over 50 percent of patients (see Chap. 14).[627] In one series, 23 of 24 patients over age 40 were hypertensive, and of these, 11 had congestive heart failure.[627] Hypertension and its complications contribute greatly to morbidity and mortality in spontaneous Cushing's syndrome; in the series of Plotz and colleagues, 40 percent of those dying with the syndrome did so directly as a result of hypertension and/or atherosclerosis.[1115] Peripheral edema was frequently described in early series[1115,1182] but was present in only 18 percent of the patients in the series of Ross et al.[627]

Gonadal dysfunction is extremely common because of elevated levels of androgens (in females) and cortisol (in males and, to a lesser extent, females). Amenorrhea occurs in approximately 75 percent of premenopausal females and is usually accompanied by infertility.[627,1115] Patients without amenorrhea have generally had a shorter duration of symptoms.[1182] Male patients frequently have decreased libido, and some have decreased body hair and soft testes.[627,1182] Gynecomastia is unusual in male patients but may be seen in patients with estrogen-producing adrenal carcinomas.

Psychological disturbances occur in approximately two-thirds of these patients.[1115] The presentation and severity of these features are extremely variable. Mild features include emotional lability and increased irritability. Increased anxiety, depression, decreased concentration, and poor memory may also be present. Some patients are euphoric and occasionally may manifest overtly manic behavior. The majority of these patients also have disordered sleep with either insomnia or early morning awakening. A minority of patients exhibit more severe psychological disorders, which may include severe depression, psychosis with delusions or hallucinations, and paranoia, and some have committed suicide.[1115] A patient's premorbid personality or psychiatric history has not been helpful in predicting the types of psychoses which occur.

Muscle weakness occurs in approximately 60 percent; it is most frequently proximal and is usually most prominent in the lower extremities.[627] Thus, patients typically first note difficulty in climbing stairs and in more severe cases may have difficulty arising from a chair.

Approximately 50 percent of these patients have clinically obvious osteoporosis, although the incidence of this probably approaches 100 percent when refined measurements are made (Chap. 15). Back pain is an initial complaint in 40 percent.[627] Pathologic fractures occur frequently in severe cases and most often involve the ribs and vertebral bodies.[627,1182] Compression fractures of the spine are demonstrable radiographically in 16 to 22 percent and may be accompanied by loss of height and kyphosis.[627,1182]

Renal calculi occur in approximately 15 percent of these patients, and renal colic may occasionally be a presenting complaint.[627] These calculi are a consequence of glucocorticoid-induced hypercalciuria, although a few patients have had associated primary hyperparathyroidism.[627] Thirst and polyuria may also occur in an occasional patient with hypercalciuria. Thirst and polyuria ascribable to overt hyperglycemia and diabetes mellitus occur in approximately 10 percent of these patients, whereas glucose intolerance is much more common. Diabetic ketoacidosis is rare, as are diabetic microvascular complications.

Laboratory Features

Routine laboratory examinations are rarely of major diagnostic utility in the diagnosis of Cushing's syndrome, although certain abnormalities may suggest the diagnosis. The specific utility of ACTH and corticosteroid measurements is discussed below.

Patients with Cushing's syndrome frequently have high normal values of hemoglobin, hematocrit, and red cell count, but elevations into the range of polycythemia are rare.[627] The total white cell count is usually normal; however, the percentage of lymphocytes is below 25 in 50 percent of cases and the total lymphocyte count is subnormal in 35 percent.[627] The total eosinophil count is usually below 100/mm^3 and is less than 10/mm^3 in approximately 30 percent of patients. Serum sodium concentration is normal in most patients. In patients with Cushing's disease, serum potassium and bicarbonate concentrations are usually normal, but hypokalemia and alkalosis are common with the ectopic ACTH syndrome and adrenocortical carcinoma.[627,1181] The degree of hypokalemia correlates well with adrenocortical hypersecretion; thus, it is not unexpected that hypokalemic alkalosis occurs most frequently in these latter two conditions, in which steroid levels frequently are markedly elevated.[1181,1183] Renal function is normal in uncomplicated Cushing's syndrome but can be abnormal in patients with long-standing hypertension, renal stones, nephrocalcinosis, or infection. Serum calcium and phosphorus concentrations are normal; however, hypercalciuria occurs in 40 percent of these patients.[627] Fasting hyperglycemia occurs in 10 to 15 percent of cases, and glucose intolerance with associated hyperinsulinemia occurs in the majority.[627,1115,1182] Glycosuria is present in patients with fasting hyperglycemia and may also occur postprandially. Ketosis or ketoacidosis is rare; its presence suggests coexisting insulinopenic diabetes. Plasma lipoprotein (VLDL, LDL, and HDL) concentrations tend to be elevated, with consequent elevations of triglyceride and cholesterol levels,[1184] especially in patients with hyperglycemia.

Routine radiographs may reveal cardiomegaly due to hypertensive or atherosclerotic heart disease; rib or spinal compression features and renal calculi may be noted. The ECG may be abnormal in patients with long-standing disease in whom hypertensive or atherosclerotic myocardial injury has occurred.

Features Suggesting a Specific Etiology

Although a definitive diagnosis of the type of Cushing's syndrome present must be established biochemically, certain features suggest a specific etiology.

Patients with Cushing's disease present with the classic clinical picture. Women predominate, the onset is generally between ages 20 and 40, and the clinical manifestations are usually slowly progressive over several years. Hyperpigmentation and hypokalemic alkalosis are rare. Cortisol and adrenal androgen secretion is increased moderately, and androgenic manifestations are generally limited to acne and mild to moderate hirsutism.[627]

In contrast, the ectopic ACTH syndrome occurs predominantly in males, with the highest incidence in the fifth to seventh decade.[1181] The primary tumor is usually apparent, but the clinical manifestations are frequently limited to weakness, hypertension, and glucose intolerance. Hyperpigmentation, hypokalemia, and alkalosis are common.[1181] Weight loss and anemia due to malignancy are also common. The features of hypercortisolism are of rapid onset. Steroid hypersecretion is frequently severe, with equally elevated levels of glucocorticoids, androgens, and DOC.[1181] Survival in these patients with both metastatic carcinoma and severe hypercortisolism is extremely limited.[1181]

A minority of patients with the ectopic ACTH syndrome have more "benign" tumors, especially bronchial carcinoids, and present with a more slowly progressive course with typical features of Cushing's syndrome. These patients may be clinically identical to those with pituitary-dependent Cushing's disease; the responsible tumor may not be apparent.[745,1185] Hyperpigmentation, hypokalemic alkalosis, and anemia are commonly absent. Further confusion may arise since a number of these patients with occult ectopic tumors may have ACTH and steroid dynamics typical of Cushing's disease (see below).[826,1185,1186]

The clinical picture in patients with adrenal adenomas is usually that of glucocorticoid excess alone. Androgenic effects such as hirsutism are usually absent. The onset is gradual, and the hypercortisolism is mild to moderate. Urinary 17-ketosteroid excretion and plasma androgen concentrations are usually in the low normal or subnormal range.[1187]

With adrenal carcinomas in general, the clinical features of excessive glucocorticoid, androgen, and mineralocorticoid hypersecretion have a rapid onset and are rapidly progressive.[1124] Marked elevations of cortisol, androgens, and DOC are usual. Hypokalemia is common. Abdominal pain, palpable masses, and hepatic and pulmonary metastases are also common at the time of diagnosis.[1124]

Diagnosis and Differential Diagnosis

Diagnosis

The evaluation of Cushing's syndrome must first include a general assessment of the patient regarding the presence of other illnesses, drugs and medications, alcoholism, and depression, since these factors may lead to misleading results (see Laboratory Features, above). In suspected hypercortisolism, either the overnight 1-mg dexamethasone suppression test or the measurement of the 24-hr urine cortisol may be chosen as the initial test.[1188] The overnight 1-mg dexamethasone suppression test is an excellent screening test in an outpatient setting and for many is the initial procedure of choice because of its simplicity. A normal response to the overnight test (plasma cortisol <5 ng/dl) excludes Cushing's syndrome with 98 percent accuracy (Fig. 12-43),[762] and the only exceptions have been rare patients with episodic Cushing's syndrome or abnormal dexamethasone metabolism (see below). The test should not be used in patients with marked obesity, patients receiving estrogen therapy, and those who are on drugs which accelerate dexamethasone metabolism (see below). In these patients, measurement of free urinary free cortisol is preferable.

Measurement of the 24-h urine cortisol (Fig. 12-44) is an equally acceptable initial test and is preferable in the setting of marked obesity, with estrogen therapy, or if the patient is taking drugs which accelerate dexamethasone metabolism.[762,774,794,795] Urine cortisol levels are elevated in more than 90 percent of patients with Cushing's syndrome[762] but may also be elevated in stress, depression, and alcoholism (see below). An abnormal result of either test should be confirmed by the performance of the other, and if both tests are abnormal, hypercortisolism is present and the diagnosis of Cushing's syndrome is established, provided that conditions causing false-positive responses are excluded (see below).

In patients with equivocal or borderline results, the 2-day low-dose dexamethasone suppression test is performed, with measurement of urinary 17-OHCS or free cortisol excretion (normal responses, 11-OHCS ⩾ 2.5 mg/24 h or 1.0 mg per gram of creatinine;[762,779] free cortisol <20 μg/24 h.[762,794,795] In this setting, a normal response excludes Cushing's syndrome and abnormal suppressibility is consistent with the diagnosis, since the incidence of false-positive responses is negligible.[762]

The measurement of late evening (11 P.M. to 2 A.M.) plasma, salivary or urine cortisol level, and the cortisol production rate are also useful in the diagnosis of Cushing's syndrome,[762] but these procedures have not come into general use (see Laboratory Features, above).

Other tests and procedures are less reliable in the diagnosis and are no longer recommended since there is considerable overlap between patients with and without Cushing's syndrome.[762,801] These include basal morning cortisol levels; afternoon or early evening diurnal cortisol level; basal 24-h urinary 17-OHCS, 17-KGS, or 17-ketosteroid excretion; and responsiveness to either ACTH or metyrapone stimulation tests (see Laboratory Evaluation of Adrenocortical Function, above).[762,801]

Problems in Diagnosis

Despite the generally clear separation of patients with and without Cushing's syndrome using a combination of the tests described above, several factors may complicate the diagnosis.[745,762,1188] These include both rare false-negative results and, more commonly, false-positive results.

False-negative responses have been reported in several patients with Cushing's syndrome. First, there may be normal suppression of glucocorticoid secretion with low-dose dexamethasone because of delayed clearance of the steroid and higher than usual plasma levels of dexamethasone.[745,762,790,791] In this situation, urinary free cortisol level should be

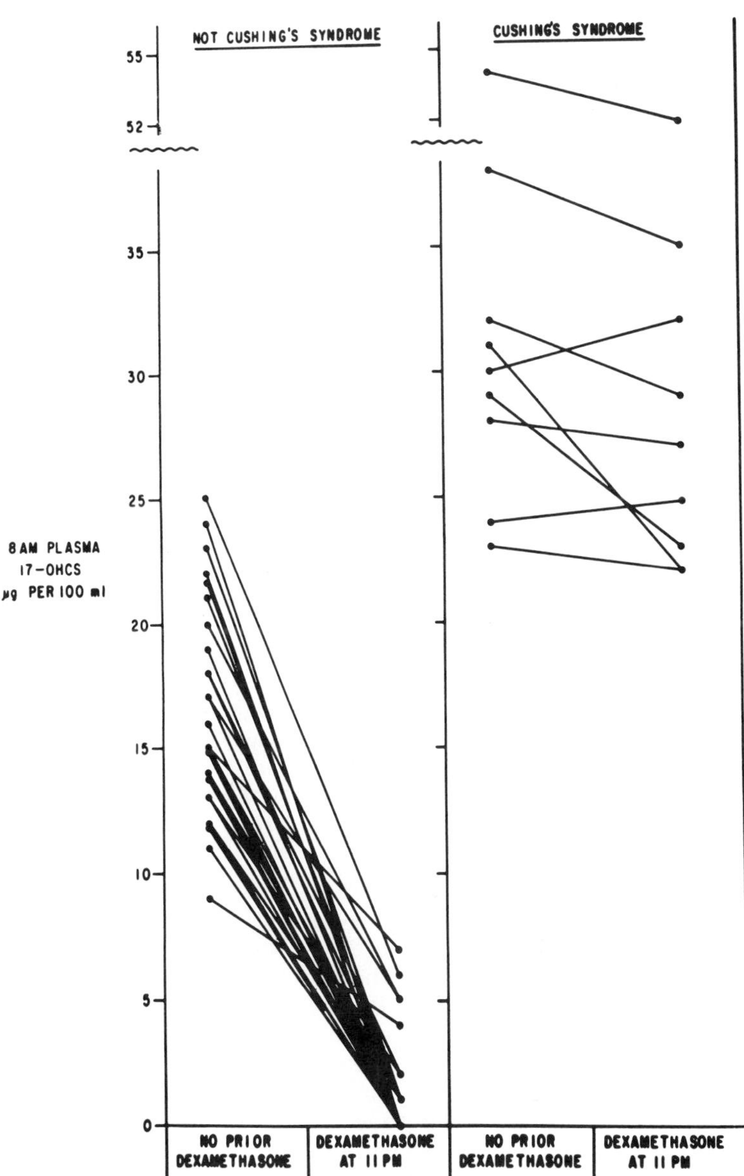

FIGURE 12-43 Plasma cortisol (8 A.M. plasma 17-OHCS) response to the low-dose dexamethasone suppression test (see text) in control subjects ("not Cushing's syndrome") and patients with Cushing's syndrome. *(From Nugent CA, et al., Arch Intern Med 116:172, 1965.)*

elevated and can assist in establishing the diagnosis.[745,791] The measurement of plasma dexamethasone concentrations, if available, will reveal the reason for "normal" suppressibility.[790,791] A second unusual cause of normal suppressibility is periodic or episodic hormonogenesis in Cushing's syndrome.[792,1190,1191] In these patients, hypercortisolism is either cyclic, with a regular period of days to weeks, or episodic, without a regular pattern; cortisol secretion may be normal or nearly normal between cycles or episodes.[792,1190] Thus, in these patients with spontaneously varying cortisol secretion, adrenal function may be normal at times and dexamethasone administration during phases of normal secretion may reveal normal suppressibility.[792] In these patients, repeated evaluation is required to establish the diagnosis of hypercortisolism and additional difficulties may be encountered in the differential diagnosis (see below).

False-positive responses are more common. Patients with acute and/or chronic illnesses, especially those who are hospitalized, may have appropriately elevated glucocorticoid secretion. These patients may have elevated plasma cortisol and urinary free cortisol levels, and their adrenal function is frequently nonsuppressible with the 1-mg overnight suppression test.[762] If Cushing's syndrome is suspected, diagnostic evaluation should be repeated when the acute stress has resolved.

Obesity is the most common differential diagnostic problem since approximately 15 percent of obese patients have abnormal responses to the overnight

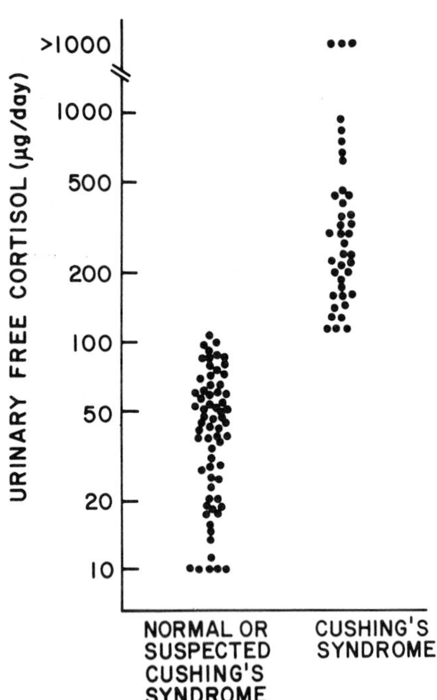

FIGURE 12-44 Urinary free cortisol excretion (measured by the competitive protein-binding assay) in normal individuals, individuals with suspected but not substantiated hypercortisolism, and patients with Cushing's syndrome. *(Based on data of Burke and Beardwell.[795])*

1-mg suppression test.[762] Urinary excretion of 17-OHCS and 17-KGS is also elevated in obese patients and is the major reason for the limited ability of these tests.[745,762,1188] However, the urinary free cortisol excretion is virtually always normal in simple obesity.[774,794,795] In addition, in those with an abnormal overnight test, the 2-day low-dose suppression test will resolve the problem, since normal suppressibility is maintained in obese patients.[745,779]

High-estrogen states (pregnancy, estrogen therapy, and oral contraceptive use) which increase CBG also cause confusion since total plasma cortisol levels may be as high as 40 to 60 μg/dl[745,779] and the overnight 1-mg test may be abnormal; however, urinary free cortisol excretion is normal.

Patients on phenytoin, rifampin, and other anticonvulsants, including phenobarbital and primidone, can have false-positive results on low-dose dexamethasone tests. However, urinary free cortisol excretion is normal, as is the suppressibility of plasma corticosterone levels by oral hydrocortisone.[745]

A number of alcoholic patients have both clinical and biochemical features of Cushing's syndrome ("alcohol-induced pseudo–Cushing's syndrome").[745,1192] These patients have elevated basal plasma cortisol levels with abnormal circadian variation, an increased cortisol production rate, increased urinary corticosteroid excretion, and abnormal suppressibility with dexamethasone, i.e., steroid dynamics consistent with Cushing's syndrome.[745,1192] The steroid dynamics revert to normal after the cessation of alcohol intake; thus, if diagnostic test results are abnormal, testing should be repeated after abstention from alcohol for at least 4 weeks. In view of the frequency of excessive alcohol use, this possibility should be considered whenever hypercortisolism is suspected.

Similarly, patients with depression frequently have abnormal steroid dynamics which suggest Cushing's syndrome.[745] These patients also have increased cortisol secretion with elevated plasma levels, absence of diurnal variation, increased urinary free cortisol excretion, and impaired dexamethasone suppression.[745] The abnormal steroid dynamics revert to normal upon psychological recovery. These patients can be differentiated from those with true Cushing's syndrome, since patients with depression alone do not have clinical manifestations of cortisol excess and retain normal suppressibility in response to the 2-day low-dose dexamethasone suppression test. In addition, these patients have normal cortisol responsiveness to insulin-induced hypoglycemia, whereas in patients with Cushing's syndrome, cortisol levels do not increase further during hypoglycemia.[745,763] CRH testing does not appear to differentiate these etiologies adequately.[1193]

Patients with anorexia nervosa also have cortisol dynamics similar to those of Cushing's disease.[341] However, these patients can be distinguished from Cushing's disease patients by their clinical presentation and from those with the ectopic ACTH syndrome by high-dose dexamethasone suppression.

Determining the Etiology and Tumor Localization

When Cushing's syndrome is present, the specific etiology must be defined, and this diagnosis cannot be completely secure until a tumor is localized and confirmed histologically. Thus, the most common etiology, pituitary ACTH hypersecretion (Cushing's disease), must be differentiated from the ectopic ACTH syndrome and primary adrenal tumors. Less common etiologies account for a few percent of patients with Cushing's syndrome (see above and below). The initial step in establishing the etiology of Cushing's syndrome is the measurement of a plasma ACTH level[762,763] (Fig. 12-45). Subsequent evaluation is directed by the ACTH level and consists of additional endocrine tests such as high-dose dexamethasone suppression and CRH stimulation (see Laboratory Features, above, and Refs. 745, 762, 763, 803–806, 1194, 1195) and radiologic evaluations which may include CT scans of the adrenals, MRI of the pituitary, and venous sampling of the inferior petrosal sinuses to determine whether ACTH hypersecretion is of pituitary origin.

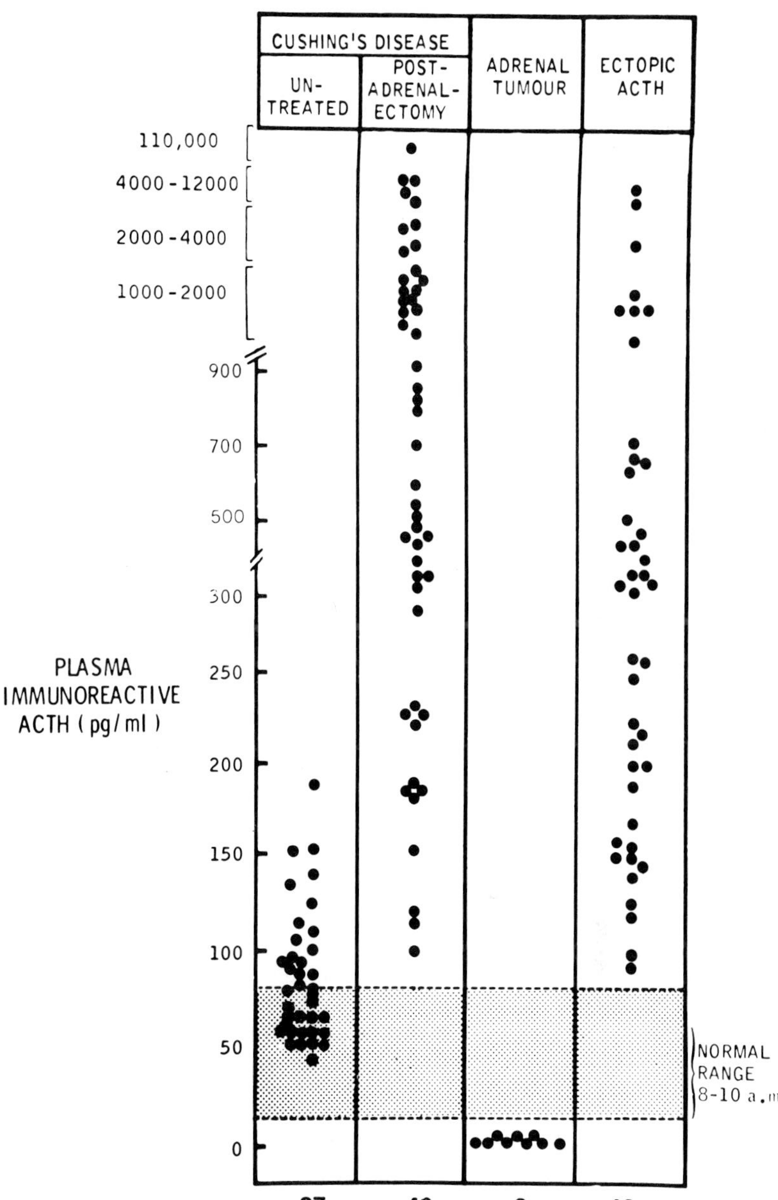

FIGURE 12-45 Basal plasma ACTH levels in patients with Cushing's disease before (untreated) and after bilateral adrenalectomy and with cortisol-producing adrenal adenomas and ectopic ACTH syndrome. *(From Besser and Edwards.[763])*

If the plasma ACTH level is suppressed (<10 pg/ml by IRMA or <20 pg/ml by radioimmunoassay (RIA), the patient has ACTH-independent Cushing's syndrome.[759,761,762] In this case, the next step is to perform a CT scan of the adrenals which will reveal a solitary adrenal tumor with rare exceptions.[1196,1197] Adrenal adenomas are homogenous, 3 to 6 cm in diameter, and secrete only cortisol. Larger tumors, in particular, those which secrete multiple steroids (especially androgens), are likely to be adrenocortical carcinomas. Measurement of DHEA-S levels is useful in this differential diagnosis; i.e., they are suppressed with adrenal adenomas and usually are elevated in patients with adrenal carcinoma.[1124,1187] If adrenal carcinoma is suspected, an evaluation for local and distant spread should be undertaken.

If the CT scan shows "normal" adrenals, the diagnostic possibilities include primary pigmented nodular adrenocortical disease (PPNAD) (described above) and exogenous cortisol or cortisone administration.[1198–1201] The diagnosis of PPNAD is likely if the patient is young and if there is familial Cushing's syndrome or manifestations of the Carney complex.[1198–1201] In addition, careful review of the CT scans or additional MR imaging will reveal irregularity of the adrenals consistent with micronodularity.[1198–1201] If the imaging procedures do not demonstrate nodularity of the adrenals, iodocholesterol scanning should be performed; the demonstration of bilateral function excludes exogenous glucocorticoid administration.[1198–1201]

If the CT scan demonstrates bilateral adrenal enlargement, the patient has macronodular adrenal hyperplasia which may be either ACTH-independent or ACTH-dependent (a variant of Cushing's disease).[1186,1202–1206] The differentiation of these two entities is best substantiated by repeated plasma ACTH determinations and by CRH stimulation testing of ACTH and cortisol.[1202] The rare primary adrenal form of this disorder is characterized by repeatedly and markedly suppressed ACTH levels, failure to respond to CRH administration, and absent responses to high-dose dexamethasone. Patients with ACTH-dependent macronodular hyperplasia have variable ACTH levels; however, the levels are measurable if repeated determinations are obtained, and virtually all these patients have ACTH responsiveness to CRH.[1202] Responses to high-dose dexamethasone are variable; however, about 50 percent of those patients show suppression. If ACTH dependency is confirmed, further evaluation of these patients with pituitary MRI and inferior petrosal sinus sampling should follow the guidelines described below to establish a pituitary source. Ectopic tumors rarely cause macronodular hyperplasia.

If the initial ACTH determination is low normal (10 to 30 pg/ml) but not suppressed, ACTH dependency should be confirmed by repeat ACTH determinations, CRH stimulation, and high-dose dexamethasone. These patients should next undergo CT scans of the adrenals, which may demonstrate macronodular or simple hyperplasia. These patients should then be studied as described below.

If the plasma ACTH level is normal to moderately elevated (40 to 200 pg/ml), Cushing's disease is the most likely etiology. However, about 5 percent of patients will have the occult ectopic ACTH syndrome, primarily as a result of small ACTH-secreting carcinoid tumors.[1185] The next step is to perform high-dose dexamethasone suppression and CRH testing. If these two tests are positive, Cushing's disease is present with rare exceptions[826,1125,1207–1211] and the patient should undergo an MRI study of the pituitary with gadolinium enhancement. If this study demonstrates a definite adenoma, surgery is recommended. However, caution should be exercised if the MRI study revals only minor abnormalities; i.e., 1- to 3-mm lesions may be artifacts or incidental cysts or incidental adenomas. If the MRI is equivocal or normal, inferior petrosal sinus sampling for ACTH determinations should be performed; the demonstration of central ACTH gradients documents Cushing's disease.[1212] If the result of ACTH sampling is negative, further evaluation for an ectopic source is indicated.[1185,1213,1214] If the responses to high-dose dexamethasone and CRH are negative, the ectopic ACTH syndrome is most likely, although a few patients with Cushing's disease do not respond to these procedures. In this setting, venous sampling for ACTH should be performed; the results, if positive, confirm Cushing's disease and, if negative, direct an evaluation to localize an ectopic tumor.

In patients with initial ACTH levels greater than 200 pg/ml, the ectopic ACTH syndrome is probable. ACTH levels frequently are markedly elevated (500–10,000 pg/ml), and in most patients the tumor is either already clinically evident or readily localized by appropriate imaging studies. If no tumor is evident, venous sampling will exclude a pituitary source and CT scans and MRI of the chest and abdomen are employed to localize nonpituitary tumors.[1213,1214]

Problems in Determining the Etiology

Although the procedures described in the preceding section can establish a specific etiology in the majority of cases, enough exceptions occur to warrant discussion.

Problems are encountered in the rare patients with periodic or episodic hormonogenesis who may have Cushing's disease, the ectopic ACTH syndrome, or adrenal tumors.[792,1190,1191] Thus, these patients may show normal suppression with the low-dose test if it is performed during certain periods; when studied at other times, secretion in these patients may be nonsuppressible or even show paradoxic increases during high-dose dexamethasone administration.[792,1190] Repeated evaluations and use of the localizing procedures described below may be necessary to establish the correct etiology in such patients.

About 10 to 20 percent of patients with Cushing's disease fail to suppress with high-dose dexamethasone, and an additional 10 percent do not respond to CRH stimulation; these responses falsely suggest the ectopic ACTH syndrome.[745,762,800,801,1194,1207] Thus, the diagnostic accuracy of either procedure is about 90 percent; however, if both tests are utilized, diagnostic accuracy is close to 100 percent.[1207–1211] Failure of suppression may occur with pituitary macroadenomas and in patients with macronodular adrenal hyperplasia. This variant of Cushing's disease frequently causes diagnostic difficulties since approximately 50 percent of these patients do not suppress with the standard 2-day high-dose dexamethasone suppression test[745,762,1186] and plasma ACTH levels may be undetectable, normal, or elevated.[762,1186] In patients who do not show suppression with high-dose dexamethasone, in whom ACTH levels are not markedly elevated, and who do not have an obvious pituitary or ectopic tumor, selective venous ACTH sampling should be performed (see below).[745,1186] In addition, the diagnosis is supported by the demonstration of nodular hyperplasia by CT scan of the adrenals.[745,1186]

Although the ectopic ACTH syndrome is usually easily diagnosed by markedly elevated ACTH levels and absent responses to high-dose dexamethasone and CRH in the presence of an extrapituitary tumor, there are some cases in which the tumor is occult.[826,1185] In these cases, steroid secretion may be responsive to dexamethasone, CRH, and metyrapone.[745,826,1185] In addition, the tumor may not reveal itself for a number of years after the onset of Cushing's syndrome.[745,1185] These occult tumors are usually bronchial carcinoids, and the plasma ACTH levels can be in the range of those seen with Cushing's disease.[745,1185] These findings may lead to the mistaken diagnosis of Cushing's disease and lead to inappropriate pituitary therapy. Although it is not possible to make this differentiation with certainty in all cases, certain features should increase suspicion of the presence of the ectopic ACTH syndrome; these are male sex, rapid onset, severe hypercortisolism, hypokalemia, and weight loss. If the ectopic ACTH syndrome is suspected but no tumor is obvious, selective venous ACTH sampling is helpful; the demonstration of a pituitary venous ACTH gradient establishes the diagnosis of Cushing's disease.[745,1185,1212,1215–1219] In the absence of a pituitary gradient, the ectopic ACTH syndrome is likely, and selective venous sampling may occasionally localize the ACTH-secreting ectopic tumor.[1175,1217] Additional diagnostic and radiologic procedures should be directed to the common sites of ACTH production: lungs, thymus, pancreas, thyroid, and adrenals.[1213,1214]

Adrenal tumors rarely cause diagnostic difficulties, since the ACTH levels are undetectable and the tumor is easily visualized by CT scan. Reproducible suppressibility by dexamethasone has not been documented[762] but might occur with episodic secretion.[1191] Another rare exception is that of an ACTH-secreting adrenal carcinoma.[1220]

Tumor Localization

These procedures are used to localize tumors in Cushing's syndrome and must be integrated with the biochemical tests described above, since radiologic procedures alone can give misleading results.

In Cushing's disease, MRI of the pituitary is the procedure of choice and is used to define sellar size and anatomy and suprasellar tumor extension. In the 10 to 15 percent of patients with larger tumors (macroadenomas), MRI defines the size of the tumor and may demonstrate extrasellar extension.

The problem of tumor localization in patients with Cushing's disease who have microadenomas has not been solved, and this remains the major difficulty in the differential diagnosis of Cushing's syndrome. MRI is performed with thin sections and gadolinium enhancement, which clearly define normal sellar anatomy. The presence of a convex upper pituitary margin, increased height of the pituitary, deviation of the stalk, and focal "low-intensity" areas are the criteria on which a diagnosis of a pituitary adenoma is based. However, MRI is clearly positive in only approximately 60 percent of patients with Cushing's disease, presumably because adenomas less than 5 mm in diameter are too small to resolve with current techniques. False-positive scans may occur in patients with coincidental nonfunctional pituitary adenomas, intrapituitary cysts, or the empty sella syndrome.[1194,1207]

Selective pituitary venous ACTH sampling is helpful in patients in whom the source of ACTH hypersecretion is in doubt, i.e., when clinical features suggest the ectopic ACTH syndrome, when responses to high-dose dexamethasone or CRH are negative, or when a sellar MRI does not reveal a conclusive adenoma. In these circumstances, venous sampling will establish or exclude the pituitary as the source of ACTH.[1175,1212,1215–1217] The venous system is catheterized by the femoral route; ACTH samples are obtained simultaneously from the inferior petrosal sinuses (a major site of venous drainage of the anterior pituitary) and are compared to simultaneous peripheral vein samples. ACTH gradients are enhanced by CRH stimulation during the procedure.[1212,1218,1219] In patients with Cushing's disease, basal inferior petrosal sinus/peripheral ACTH ratios are usually greater than 2:1 and are greater than 3:1 after CRH administration.[1212,1216] In patients with the ectopic ACTH syndrome, no inferior petrosal/peripheral ACTH gradient is demonstrable. The attempt to lateralize pituitary microadenomas with venous sampling is successful in only about 65 percent of cases, and thus significant exceptions occur.[1207,1212]

CT scans are most commonly used to define adrenal pathology. However, ultrasonography and isotope scanning using radiolabeled cholesterol are also useful.[1045,1196,1197,1221,1222] In patients with ACTH hypersecretion, these procedures exclude an adrenal tumor and confirm bilateral adrenal hyperplasia or nodular adrenal hyperplasia. These procedures also effectively localize adrenal tumors in virtually all cases, since these tumors are usually over 2 cm in diameter (Fig. 12-46). However, nodular hyperplasia of the adrenals with a solitary or dominant nodule can be misinterpreted as an autonomous hyperfunctioning adenoma.[745,1186]

Treatment of Cushing's Syndrome

The treatment of Cushing's syndrome has been improved by advances in pituitary microsurgery and sophisticated radiotherapeutic techniques. Medical therapy is also becoming more effective in controlling ACTH and/or cortisol secretion. The aim of treatment in Cushing's syndrome is to remove or destroy the basic lesion and thus correct hypersecretion of adrenal hormones without inducing permanent pituitary or adrenal deficiencies.[1223]

Cushing's Disease

Treatment of Cushing's disease is currently directed at the pituitary to control ACTH hypersecre-

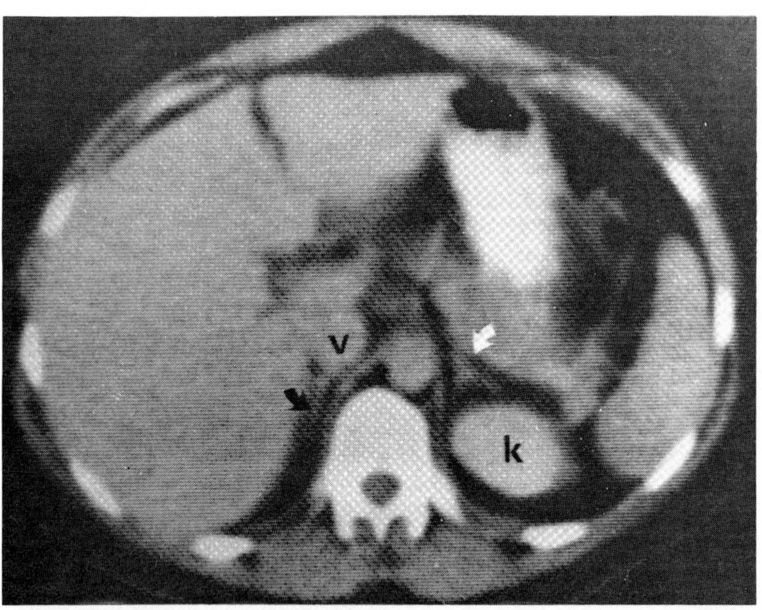

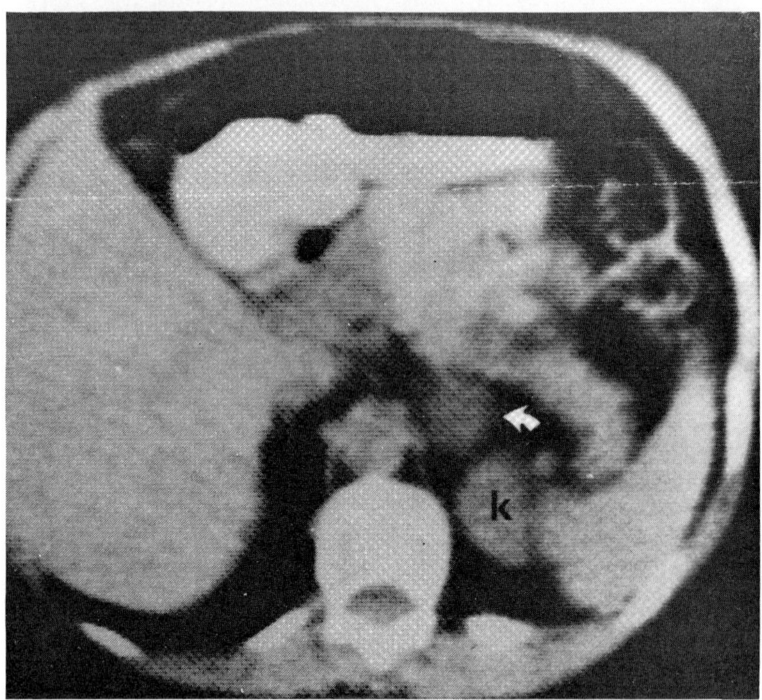

FIGURE 12-46 CT scans in Cushing's syndrome. *(A)* A patient with ACTH-dependent Cushing's syndrome. The adrenal glands are not detectably abnormal by this procedure. The curvilinear right adrenal (black arrow) is shown posterior to the inferior vena cava (v) between the right lobe of the liver and the right crus of the diaphragm. The left adrenal (white arrow) has an inverted Y appearance anteromedial to the left kidney (k). *(B)* A 3-cm left adrenal adenoma (white arrow) anteromedial to the left kidney (k). *(From Korobkin et al.[1045])*

tion; available methods include microsurgery, various forms of radiation therapy, and pharmacologic inhibition of ACTH secretion. Treatment of hypercortisolism per se by surgical or medical adrenalectomy is less commonly used. Since pituitary adenomas in Cushing's disease are frequently not localized by MRI, venous sampling should be used when necessary to confirm the diagnosis.

Transsphenoidal microsurgery is the current procedure of choice for Cushing's disease in both adults and children.[1116,1128,1131,1132,1162–1165] Hypertension and hyperglycemia should be controlled before surgery, and these patients should receive glucocorticoid coverage for surgery according to the protocol described above (see Adrenocortical Insufficiency). Since the pituitary tumors of Cushing's disease are small and are frequently within the anterior lobe tissue, an experienced surgeon and meticulous exploration of the intrasellar contents are required.[1116,1131,1132] Once identified, the micro- or macroadenoma is selectively removed, and the normal gland is left intact.

Among patients with microadenomas (less than 1 cm in diameter), selective microsurgery is successful in correcting the biochemical abnormalities in approximately 85 percent.[1116,1128,1131,1132,1162,1163] Surgical damage to anterior pituitary function is rare, but the majority of successfully treated patients develop transient secondary adrenocortical insufficiency, which is followed by the recovery of normal pituitary-adrenal function (see Etiology and Pathogenesis, above). In approximately 10 percent the tumor is too small to locate at surgery, and in adult patients hemihypophysectomy on the side of lateralization of the venous sampling or total hypophysectomy may be performed.[1116,1131,1132] Patients with corticotroph hyperplasia obviously do not respond to selective pituitary microsurgery and must be treated with other modalities, as is discussed below.[1143] Unfortunately, current diagnostic procedures cannot identify these patients preoperatively.

Transsphenoidal surgery is successful in only 25 percent of the approximately 10 to 15 percent of patients with Cushing's disease with pituitary macroadenomas and in those with extrasellar extension of the tumor.[1116,1132,1163] These patients usually require multiple therapies (see below) and frequently present difficult problems in management. Rare patients with massive tumors and suprasellar extension may require craniotomy to achieve decompression of the optic chiasm and other vital structures.

Postoperatively, steroid coverage is reduced to maintenance doses of hydrocortisone (30 mg/day) by the seventh to tenth day. In these patients, who are accustomed to cortisol excess, the steroid withdrawal syndrome (see Chap. 15) may be prominent and may necessitate increased cortisol dosage and slower tapering to maintenance levels. The pituitary-adrenal axis is reevaluated 4 to 6 weeks after surgery to ensure that hypercortisolism has been corrected; other pituitary hormones are also reevaluated at this time. Since the majority of these patients develop transient secondary adrenal insufficiency,[1159] cortisol therapy is required until there is recovery of normal responsiveness of the pituitary-adrenal axis (see Diagnosis under Adrenocortical Insufficiency, above, and Chap. 15). The complications of selective transsphenoidal microsurgery have been surprisingly few, considering the nature of the metabolic abnormalities in these patients. Transient diabetes insipidus occurs in approximately 20 percent, and there is intra- or postoperative hemorrhage in an occasional patient.[1116,1131,1132,1160,1162,1163] Potential complications such as hypopituitarism, CSF rhinorrhea, infection, meningitis, visual impairment, and oculomotor dysfunction have not materialized in larger series.[1116,1132] Patients undergoing total hypophysectomy develop panhypopituitarism; in these patients, diabetes insipidus may persist. The subsequent management of these patients is discussed in Chaps. 7 and 8 and above (see Treatment under Adrenocortical Insufficiency). Follow-up data in patients with successful surgical removal of microadenomas, although limited, are accumulating; the majority of patients achieve persisting control of Cushing's disease, although in a minority it recurs.[1116,1131,1132,1159,1162–1165] Thus, transsphenoidal microsurgery is an effective therapy for Cushing's disease and corrects hypercortisolism with minimal morbidity in the majority of patients with microadenomas.

Heavy particle irradiation of the pituitary is also an effective initial therapy for Cushing's disease, although this technique is currently available in only one center in the United States.[1224] Since the size of the radiation field is limited, these methods are not applicable to patients with either suprasellar or sphenoid sinus extension of the tumor. Alpha particle radiation is effective in controlling hypercortisolism in 80 percent of patients, with an incidence of hypopituitarism of approximately one-third.[1225] Proton beam therapy is effective in 65 percent of patients, and the incidence of hypopituitarism was reported to be 13 percent, although the follow-up period was not reported.[1224] Neurologic complications, including visual loss and oculomotor paralysis, rarely occur.[1224,1225] With both of these techniques there is a lag period of 6 to 12 months before cortisol secretion returns to normal, and since the effects of radiation are prolonged, the incidence of hypopituitarism may increase with further follow-up.

Conventional pituitary irradiation has been used for many years; however, it is effective in only a minority of adults.[1126,1217,1223] Additional disadvantages include the prolonged period of time (often 12 to 18 months) before it is effective and the occurrence of posttreatment hypopituitarism, which is increasingly being recognized.[1226] In children, conventional irradiation has been reported to be effective in 80 percent;[1126] however, the potential for hypopituitarism and consequent growth failure must be considered. Because of the limitations of conventional radiotherapy in adults, various other maneuvers have been used to increase its efficiency. Pituitary irradiation combined with unilateral adrenalectomy increases the remission rate to 50 percent; however, this rate does not appear to justify the use of both radiation and a major surgical procedure.[1227] Radiation has also been combined with either metyrapone or mitotane.[419,1217,1228,1229] These regimens have the advantage of reducing cortisol secretion more rapidly, although it appears that the ultimate response to radiation will still be unsatisfactory and prolonged drug therapy is required. Thus, conventional pituitary irradiation is not recommended as the primary therapy for adults with Cushing's disease. However, this therapy plays a definite role in patients who have persisting pituitary hypersecretion of ACTH after transphenoidal microsurgery and those with extrasellar extension of the tumor.

Implantation of radioactive seeds within the sella turcica has been used in Cushing's disease, although experience is limited.[1127,1230] In the largest reported series, remission occurred in 65 percent of patients with no radiologic evidence of a pituitary tumor; however, in patients with possible tumors and those with definite tumors, remission occurred in only 50 percent and 14 percent, respectively.[1230,1231] Replacement hormone therapy was required in 55 percent for total or partial hypopituitarism, and 5 percent developed CSF rhinorrhea.[1230] The same group reported successful treatment of juvenile Cushing's disease with pituitary implants; remission was attained in each of nine patients, and partial or complete hypopituitarism developed in only two.[1127]

Pharmacologic inhibition of ACTH secretion in Cushing's disease has been attempted with limited success. Cyproheptadine, a serotonin antagonist, and bromocriptine, a dopamine agonist, have been reported to control both ACTH hypersecretion and hypercortisolism in a few cases.[1152,1171,1217] However, to date these agents have been successful in only a minority of patients and cannot be considered a definitive therapy since relapse occurs after their discontinuation.

Treatment of Cushing's disease by adrenalectomy was the major form of therapy from the early 1950s until the 1970s. This method has now been largely replaced by therapy directed at the pituitary. Although bilateral adrenalectomy rapidly reverses hypercortisolism, it is accompanied by an operative mortality of 5 to 10 percent, a high incidence of postoperative complications (poor wound healing, infection, pancreatic injury, and thromboembolism), permanent glucocorticoid and mineralocorticoid deficiency, and a recurrence rate of approximately 10 percent.[1217,1232] Further, it may be followed by the development of large and progressive pituitary tumors (Nelson's syndrome; see below). Adrenalectomy should be used only in the few patients who cannot be treated successfully by other methods.

Pharmacologic agents which inhibit adrenal cortisol secretion are useful in Cushing's disease but mainly as adjunctive therapy[420,424,426,431,1217,1229,1233] (see Inhibitors of Adrenal Steroid Biosynthesis, above). Ketoconazole is the drug of choice and is effective in most patients in doses of 800 to 1000 mg/day in divided doses.[420,431] Metyrapone and aminoglutethimide inhibit cortisol synthesis, although this is accompanied by increased ACTH levels which may overcome the enzyme inhibition. Adequate data are not available on the long-term use of these agents as the sole treatment of Cushing's disease; relapse occurs after discontinuation. Ketocanazole is generally well tolerated but may cause liver damage. Metyrapone is expensive and causes gastrointestinal side effects. Aminoglutethimide causes somnolence, skin rash, and goiter. Thus, these agents are ordinarily used while one is awaiting a response to therapy or in the preparation of patients for surgery.[1217,1229] More effective control of hypercortisolism with fewer side effects is obtained by the combined use of these agents.[426] The adrenolytic drug mitotane not only inhibits cortisol synthesis but also causes adrenal atrophy, predominantly of the zonae fasciculata and reticularis. It induces remissions in approximately 80 percent of patients with Cushing's disease, but 60 percent relapse after the cessation of therapy.[424] Approximately 60 percent of these patients experience gastrointestinal side effects; other side effects include somnolence, depression, and skin rash. The high rate of relapse after treatment usually necessitates more definitive therapy.[424]

Ectopic ACTH Syndrome

Therapy for the ectopic ACTH syndrome is difficult in the setting of metastatic malignancy and the accompanying severe hypercortisolism. Although therapy is directed at the primary tumor, this is usually unsuccessful and other means must be used to correct the steroid excess state. Since severe hypokalemia may be present, it may be necessary to administer potassium replacement in large doses and spironolactone to block mineralocorticoid effects. Drugs which block steroid synthesis, including ketoconazole, metyrapone, and aminoglutethimide, are more useful in this situation, since in the ectopic ACTH syndrome plasma ACTH levels usually do not increase in response to the lowered cortisol levels.[1233] Since these drugs may produce hypoadrenalism, steroid secretion must be monitored and replacement steroids must be given if necessary. In this setting, mitotane is less useful because of its slow onset of action and because several weeks may be required to control cortisol secretion. Bilateral adrenalectomy rarely may be required if hypercortisolism cannot otherwise be controlled. Cure of the ectopic ACTH syndrome is usually possible only in tumors such as carcinoids or in pheochromocytomas, which are frequently benign.[826,1175,1179,1185]

Adrenal Tumors

Benign adrenal adenomas are successfully treated by unilateral adrenalectomy; the outlook is excellent. Since the hypothalamic-pituitary axis and the contralateral adrenal are suppressed by the prolonged autonomous cortisol secretion, these patients have postoperative adrenal insufficiency.[1234] Thus, they require glucocorticoid but usually not mineralocorticoid therapy both during and after surgery, until the remaining adrenal recovers. This usually requires 6 to 12 months but may take as long as 2 years (see Chap. 15).[1234]

Therapy for adrenocortical carcinoma is less satisfactory; the majority of patients have metastases at the time of diagnosis, usually to the retroperitoneum, liver, and lungs.[1124,1235] Surgery is the first step in therapy. Although surgical cure is rare, it serves to reduce the tumor mass and the degree of steroid hypersecretion. Curative surgery should be accompanied by essentially absent steroid secretion, since the hypothalamic-pituitary axis and the contralateral adrenal are suppressed. Persisting nonsuppressible steroid secretion in the immediate postoperative period indicates a residual or metastatic tumor. When metastatic or residual disease is present, mitotane is the drug of choice.[1236] It is administered in doses of 6 to 12 g per day; however, the dose must be reduced because of side effects in 80 percent of patients (diarrhea, nausea, vomiting, depression, somnolence). Approximately 10 percent of these patients display a reduction of steroid secretion, but only 35 percent show a reduction in tumor size.[1235,1236] Since mitotane reduces urinary 17-OHCS excretion by altering the hepatic metabolism of cortisol, these patients should be followed up with plasma cortisol or urinary free cortisol assays. Ketoconazole, metyrapone, and/or aminoglutethimide are useful in controlling steroid hypersecretion in patients who do not respond to mitotane. Radiotherapy and conventional chemotherapy have not been useful in treating this disease.

Nelson's Syndrome

Nelson's syndrome involves the appearance or clinical progression of an ACTH-secreting pituitary adenoma after bilateral adrenalectomy for Cushing's disease.[1136,1237] Since pituitary adenomas are present in the majority of patients with untreated Cushing's disease, it is presumed that the tumors of Nelson's syndrome are due to progressive growth of preexisting pituitary adenomas. It is possible that the hypercortisolism in untreated patients restrains not only ACTH secretion but also growth of the adenoma. That ACTH secretion in Cushing's disease is restrained by the circulating cortisol levels is demonstrated by its stimulation with metyrapone. Further, the tumors in Nelson's syndrome are dexamethasone-suppressible, although larger doses may be required than with untreated Cushing's disese.[799] Thus, after adrenalectomy, the suppressive effect of cortisol is no longer present, ACTH secretion increases, and the adenoma may progress. Conventional pituitary irradiation before or after adrenalectomy does not prevent the development of Nelson's syndrome, and it may rarely occur after heavy particle irradiation.[1225,1238]

The incidence of Nelson's syndrome ranges from 5 to 78 percent in reported series.[1238–1240] It is higher in series studied with immunoreactive plasma ACTH levels and more sophisticated radiologic techniques.[1239,1240] About 30 percent of patients adrenalectomized for Cushing's disease have been found to develop classic Nelson's syndrome. Another 50 percent develop evidence of a microadenoma without marked progression, and about 20 percent never develop a progressive pituitary tumor. The reasons for these differences in clinical behavior are unknown and have not been predictable. Thus, patients who have undergone bilateral adrenalectomy for Cushing's disease require continuous observation by means of plasma ACTH assay, sellar radiology, and visual field examinations so that pituitary tumors may be diagnosed and treated early.

The tumors in patients with classic Nelson's syndrome are among the most aggressive and rapidly growing of all pituitary tumors.[1133] These patients present with hyperpigmentation similar to but generally more severe than that seen in Addison's disease and the manifestations of an expanding intrasellar mass lesion, usually within months to 2 years after adrenalectomy. Sellar enlargement, extrasellar extension, headache, visual field defects, and hypopituitarism are common.[1133] Invasion of the cavernous sinus or cranial fossae may lead to extraocular muscle palsies and other neurologic defects.[1133] These tumors can occasionally be frankly malignant with local invasion and extracranial metastases, and there is a high incidence of pituitary apoplexy (spontaneous hemorrhagic infarction of the tumor).[1133] The diagnosis is usually obvious from the history of bilateral adrenalectomy followed by hyperpigmentation and the manifestations of an expanding pituitary tumor. Plasma ACTH levels are markedly elevated, usually to more than 1000 pg/ml, and levels not infrequently are higher than 10,000 pg/ml.[763] MRI is used to define the extent of tumor growth and the response to therapy.

These tumors are treated by pituitary surgery and radiotherapy. Larger tumors, especially those with extrasellar extension, are frequently unresectable at surgery by either transsphenoidal or craniotomy approaches. Conventional radiation alone is satisfactory in only a minority of patients but should nonetheless be used postoperatively in patients with residual or extrasellar tumor extension, in whom it may prevent progression.

Patients adrenalectomized for Cushing's disease who develop pituitary microadenomas generally present later and usually have a slower course accompanied by mild to moderate hyperpigmentation and plasma ACTH levels in the range of 500 to 4000 pg/ml.[1239,1240] The sella turcica is usually normal in size; however, MRI reveals a pituitary microadenoma.[1240] Extrasellar extension, visual defects, headache, and panhypopituitarism are unusual.[1240] Spontaneous remission has occurred in such a patient ("silent pituitary apoplexy").[1241] Transsphenoidal microsurgery or heavy particle irradiation is somewhat more successful in these patients with microadenomas. Although hyperpigmentation resolves, plasma ACTH levels frequently remain modestly elevated.

Patients who never manifest evidence of a progressive pituitary tumor after adrenalectomy for Cushing's syndrome do not develop hyperpigmentation or abnormal pituitary function. However, plasma ACTH levels in these patients are mildly elevated in the range of 100 to 500 pg/ml and are not normally suppressible with low doses of dexamethasone.

Prognosis

Untreated Cushing's syndrome is frequently a fatal illness. Mortality may be due to the underlying tumor itself, as in the ectopic ACTH syndrome and adrenal carcinoma. However, in many cases, death is a consequence of sustained hypercortisolism and its complications, including hypertension, cardiovascular disease, stroke, thromboembolism, and susceptibility to infection.[1115,1232] Thus, in a series reported in 1952, 50 percent of the patients died within 5 years of the onset of the disease.[1115]

With current refinements in pituitary microsurgery and heavy particle irradiation, the great majority of patients with Cushing's disease can be treated successfully and the operative mortality and morbidity which attended bilateral adrenalectomy are no longer present. Although there is currently no statistical information regarding survival in these patients, it appears that they live considerably longer. Patients with Cushing's disease who have large pituitary tumors at the time of diagnosis and those with Nelson's syndrome have a considerably less satisfactory prognosis and may die as a consequence of tumor invasion and persisting hypercortisolism.[1133]

The prognosis in adrenal adenomas is excellent, although there is the mortality and morbidity of adrenalectomy in these patients.[1235] In adrenal carcinoma, the prognosis is almost universally poor and the median survival from the onset of symptoms is approximately 4 years.[1124,1235]

The prognosis is also poor in patients with ectopic ACTH syndrome due to malignant tumors. In these patients with severe hypercortisolism, survival is frequently only days to weeks.[1118,1181] However, a minority of patients respond to tumor resection or chemotherapy.[1179] The prognosis is better in those with benign tumors producing the ectopic ACTH syndrome.[745,826,1185]

Hyperaldosteronism

Hyperaldosteronism (aldosteronism) can occur as a "primary" adrenal problem or can be secondary to other metabolic derangements that stimulate its release.

Primary Hyperaldosteronism

Primary hyperaldosteronism (primary aldosteronism) results from adrenal tumors or from a hyperplastic adrenal glomerulosa and leads to hypertension and hypokalemia, as discussed in detail in Chap. 14.

Secondary Hyperaldosteronism

Secondary hyperaldosteronism due to stimulation of the adrenal glomerulosa by extraadrenal factors (usually the renin-angiotensin system) is classified in Table 12-28. It can be physiologic or can contribute to the pathology of disease states.

The factors that stimulate the renin-angiotensin system and the influences of aldosterone are discussed in preceding sections and in Chap. 14. The role of increased aldosterone in chronic hyperkalemia[707,709] has been discussed above (see Physiologic Actions of Mineralocorticoids). Secondary hyperaldosteronism can occasionally occur on an iatrogenic basis as a result of oral contraceptive use (see Chap. 14).

Extrarenal Sodium Loss and Sodium Restriction

In these circumstances (Table 12-28 and Chap. 14), activation of the renin-angiotensin-aldosterone system serves to correct the deficiency by conserving sodium ion with minimal potassium wasting (see above).[1242]

Changes in Aldosterone during the Menstrual Cycle and Pregnancy

Modest increases in plasma renin, angiotensin, and aldosterone concentrations of unknown cause occur during the luteal phase of the menstrual cycle and could be due to the marked increase (10- to 20-fold) in the plasma progesterone level.[1094] The mineralocorticoid antagonist properties of this steroid (discussed above) would block mineralocorticoid action, promoting sodium loss and in turn stimulating renin release.[1095] Levels of estrogens which induce renin substrate (Chap. 14) are also increased, but this has not been shown to be a significant factor.[1095] The increased aldosterone concentration could contribute to the pathogenesis of premenstrual edema, but this is difficult to conceive of if the increased aldosterone concentration is secondary to natriuresis. Further, there is no correlation between the severity of edema and the levels of renin and aldosterone.[1095]

Aldosterone secretion increases progressively during normal pregnancy, although its physiologic significance is not known.[1094,1243] It is of maternal origin, is increased by the fifteenth week of gestation, and reaches levels in the third trimester 10 times those of nonpregnant women. The aldosterone contributes to sodium retention since blockade of aldosterone production by heparin results in natriuresis.[1094] The increased renin levels may be due to the decrease in blood pressure that occurs in early pregnancy because of decreased systemic vascular resistance.[1243] In addition, particularly in late pregnancy, progesterone levels are high and may further in-

TABLE 12-28 Classification of Secondary Hyperaldosteronism

Primary Abnormality	Potassium Loss	Edema	Hypertension	Effect of Sodium Load
Extrarenal sodium loss (e.g., from hemorrhage, thermal stress, or gastrointestinal loss)	Absent	Absent	Absent	Repairs deficit
Sodium restriction	Absent	Absent	Absent	Repairs deficit
Abnormal distribution of sodium excess (e.g., from congestive heart failure, nephrotic syndrome, cirrhosis with ascites, or idiopathic edema)	Present	Present	Absent	Worsens edema
Abnormal renal electrolyte loss (e.g., from salt-losing renal disease,* Bartter's syndrome, diuretic abuse, or renal tubular acidosis)	Present	Absent	Absent	Variable
Other renal lesions (e.g., renal artery stenosis, unilateral renal ischemia, accelerated hypertension, renin-secreting tumor, or chronic renal failure*)	Present	Absent	Present	May worsen hypertension
Excessive potassium intake	Present	Absent	Absent	May facilitate kaliuresis
Luteal phase of menstrual cycle and pregnancy	Absent	May be present	Usually present	Suppresses renin and aldosterone

* Exception; no potassium loss.

Source: Modified from Stockigt.[1242]

crease renin release by the mechanisms discussed above.[1094] However, renin levels are elevated more during the first trimester, whereas plasma aldosterone levels are highest during the third trimester.[1094] This may be due to a progressive increase in the sensitivity of the glomerulosa to angiotensin II, caused by either chronic exposure to angiotensin II (Chaps. 4 and 14) or to unidentified factors. Whereas there is increased sodium retention in pregnancy, potassium loss does not occur.[1094] This suggests that a functional mineralocorticoid excess state is not present and that activation of the renin-angiotensin-aldosterone system is a compensatory response to other changes.

Since the renin-angiotensin-aldosterone axis is activated in pregnancy, there has been considerable interest in whether this contributes to the hypertension, edema, and other manifestations of toxemia.[1094] If anything, levels of the components of the renin-angiotensin-aldosterone axis are decreased rather than increased in toxemia, although this condition is associated with an increased sensitivity to angiotensin II.[1094,1243] However, certain of the changes observed in toxemia (e.g., reduced uterine blood flow) are opposite to those elicited by angiotensin II (which leads to vasodilatation and increased blood flow in the uterine circulation, in contrast to its effects in other vascular beds; Chap. 14).[1094]

Abnormal Distribution of Sodium Excess

The renin-angiotensin-aldosterone system is only one of several factors involved in the pathogenesis of edema.[1094,1242] In untreated patients with congestive heart failure, aldosterone excess is not consistently present, although it might be argued that normal aldosterone levels are inappropriate. In severe congestive failure, aldosterone excess may result from increased production as well as decreased clearance. Overall, aldosterone levels in congestive heart failure result from the counterbalancing influences of decreased renal perfusion due to decreased cardiac output that increases renin and aldosterone release and subsequent sodium retention that tends to suppress renin and aldosterone levels.

Secondary hyperaldosteronism ordinarily occurs when there is significant hypoalbuminemia and decreased plasma oncotic pressure associated with the nephrotic syndrome. Although aldosterone is only one factor, it appears to play a role in the sodium retention that occurs.

In liver disease with ascites, renin and aldosterone concentrations are commonly elevated, but this is unusual in cirrhosis without ascites. There appears to be general agreement that mineralocorticoid excess plays at most a small role in the initial development of ascites. The stimulus to renin release appears to be an effectively decreased arterial volume due to abnormal transudation of fluid from the vascular compartment. The increased renin level promotes aldosterone production; aldosterone levels rise, and this is accentuated by the decreased clearance of aldosterone in this condition. The increased aldosterone concentration further promotes sodium retention and potassium loss; the sodium retention can be more marked than in other circumstances, because escape fails to occur in these patients, probably as a result of the lack of retention of the excess sodium in the intravascular space. Thus, in this condition, the administration of aldosterone antagonists can be particularly beneficial.

Aldosterone has been implicated in the pathogenesis of idiopathic edema, a form of dependent edema that occurs in women who do not have a history of heart, liver, kidney, or venous disease. These patients have an increased incidence of impaired carbohydrate tolerance and may be emotionally disturbed or may have history of allergy, subtle abnormalities in albumin metabolism with slightly low serum albumin concentrations, capillary permeability defects, and occasionally abnormalities in the sympathetic nervous system. The diagnosis is made by exclusion of other causes of edema; these causes are commonly unveiled during the evaluation. Although aldosterone excretion is usually in the normal range, it has been argued that the values found are inappropriate relative to the increased extracellular fluid volume and that these patients do not adequately escape from the sodium-retaining actions of the mineralocorticoids. However, the syndrome has been described in addisonian patients with very low aldosterone levels and no specific mineralocorticoid replacement. Thus, this syndrome may not be a single entity, and the various defects described above could contribute to the pathogenesis. In any event, it is unlikely that aldosterone is primarily responsible, since this syndrome differs significantly from primary aldosteronism, in which edema does not usually occur (Chap. 14). The edema ordinarily responds to conservative measures such as bed rest, use of elastic stockings, limitation of sodium intake, caloric restriction, intermittent diuretic use, and administration of aldosterone antagonists.

Abnormal Renal Electrolyte Loss

The renin-angiotensin-aldosterone system is stimulated by excessive salt loss by the kidney resulting from salt-losing nephropathy, Bartter's syndrome (discussed below), excessive diuretic use, or renal tubular acidosis. In these syndromes, the compensatory increase in aldosterone level does not correct the loss, but because there is increased sodium delivery to the distal nephron, aldosterone can accelerate potassium loss.[1242]

Bartter's Syndrome

Bartter's syndrome is characterized by increased renin, angiotensin II, and aldosterone concentrations; hypokalemia and alkalosis; normal blood pressure; absence of edema; and hyperplasia of the renal juxtaglomerular cells.[1095,1244] In addition, there is decreased pressor responsiveness to angiotensin II, vasopressin-resistant impairment in urinary concentrating ability, variably decreased pressor responsiveness to IV norepinephrine, hypomagnesemia, hyperuricemia, and increased amounts of urinary PGE_2. The pathogenesis of this disorder is discussed in Chap. 29.

Other Renal Lesions

Hyperaldosteronism can occur with renal artery stenosis, unilateral renal ischemia, accelerated hypertension, and renin-secreting tumors. These disorders are associated with hypertension and are discussed in Chap. 14.

REFERENCES

1. Baxter JD: Cortisone and the adrenal cortex. *Trans Assoc Am Physicians* 100:clxvii, 1987.
2. Gaunt R: History of the adrenal cortex, in Greep RO, Astwood EB (eds): *Handbook of Physiology: Endocrinology.* Washington, D.C., American Physiological Society, 1975, section 7, vol 6, p 1.
3. Fine LG: Eustachio's discovery of the renal tubule. *Am J Nephrol* 6:47, 1986.
4. Cushing H: The basophil adenomas of the pituitary body and their clinical manifestations. *Bull Johns Hopkins Hosp* 50:137, 1932.
5. Cori CF, Cori GT: The fate of sugar in the animal body: VII. The carbohydrate metabolism of adrenalectomized rats and mice. *J Biol Chem* 74:473, 1927.
6. Britton SW, Silvette H: The apparent prepotent function of the adrenal glands. *Am J Physiol* 100:701, 1932.
7. Long CNH, Katzin B, Fry EG: The adrenal cortex and carbohydrate metabolism. *Endocrinology* 26:39, 1940.
8. Banmann EJ, Kurland S: Changes in the inorganic constituents of blood in supradrenalectomized cats and rabbits. *J Biol Chem* 71:281, 1927.
9. Loeb EG: Effect of sodium chloride in treatment of a patient with Addison's disease. *Proc Soc Exp Biol* 30:808, 1933.
10. Selye H: The general adaptation syndrome and the diseases of adaptation. *J Clin Endocrinol* 6:117, 1946.
11. McCann SM, Brobeck JR: Evidence for a role of the supraopticohypophyseal system in regulation of adrenocorticotropin secretion. *Proc Soc Exp Biol Med* 87:318, 1954.
12. Saffran M, Schally AV, Benfey BG: Stimulation of the release of corticotropin from the adenohypophysis by a neurohypophysial factor. *Endocrinology* 57:439, 1955.
13. Guillemin R, Rosenberg B: Humoral hypothalamic control of anterior pituitary: A study with combined tissue cultures. *Endocrinology* 57:599, 1955.
14. Spiess J, Rivier J, Rivier C, Vale W: Primary structure of corticotropin-releasing factor from bovine hypothalamus. *Proc Natl Acad Sci USA* 78:6517, 1981.
15. Fasciolo JC: Historical background of the renin angiotensin system, in Genest J, Koiw E, Kuchel E (eds): *Hypertension.* New York, McGraw-Hill, 1977, p 134.
16. Conn JH: Primary aldosteronism. *J Lab Clin Med* 45:661, 1955.
17. Kendall EC, Mason HL, McKenzie BF, Myers CS, Koelsche GA: Isolation in crystalline form of the hormone essential to life from the suprarenal cortex: Its chemical nature and physiologic properties. *Trans Assoc Am Physicians* 49:147, 1934.
18. Steiger M, Reichstein T: Desoxy-cortico-steron (21-oxy-progesterone) aus Δ^5-3-oxy-ätio-cholensäure. *Helv Chim Acta* 20:1164, 1937.
19. Hench PS, Kendall EC, Slocumb CH, Polley HF: The effect of a hormone of the adrenal cortex (17-hydroxy-11-dehydrocorticosterone compound E) and of pituitary adrenocorticotrophic hormone on rheumatoid arthritis. *Proc Staff Meet Mayo Clin* 24:181, 1949.
20. Wilkins L, Lewis RA, Klein R, Rosenberg E: The suppres-

sion of androgen secretion by cortisone in a case of congenital adrenal hyperplasia. *Bull Johns Hopkins Hosp* 86:249, 1950.
21. Bartter FC, Forbes AO, Leaf A: Congenital adrenal hyperplasia associated with the adrenogenital syndrome: An attempt to correct its disordered hormonal pattern. *J Clin Invest* 29:797, 1950.
22. Cooper DY, Levin S, Narasimhulu S, Rosenthal O, Estabrook RW: Photochemical action spectrum of the terminal oxidase of mixed function oxidase systems. *Science* 145: 400, 1965.
23. Miller WL: The molecular biology of steroid hormone synthesis. *Endocr Rev* 9:295, 1988.
24. Evans RM: The steroid and thyroid hormone receptor superfamily. *Science* 240:889, 1988.
25. Netter FH: Endocrine system and selected metabolic diseases, in *Ciba Collection of Medical Illustrations*. Summitt, N.Y., Ciba Pharmaceutical, 1965, vol 4, p 77.
26. Langman J: *Medical Embryology*, Baltimore, Williams & Wilkins, 1963.
26a. Mesiano S, Coulter CL, Jaffe RB: Localization of cytochrome P450 cholesterol side-chain cleavage, cytochrome P450 17α-hydroxylase/17,20 lyase, and 3β-hydroxylsteroid dehydrogenase isomerase steroidogenic enzyme in human and rhesus monkey fetal adrenal glands: Reappraisal of functional zonation. *J Clin Endocrinol Metab* 77:1184, 1993.
27. Neville AM, Mackay AM: The structure of the human adrenal cortex in health and disease. *Clin Endocrinol Metab* 1:361, 1972.
28. Dallman MF: Control of adrenocortical growth *in vivo*. *Endocr Rev* 10:213, 1985.
29. Marusic ET, Mulrow PJ: *In vitro* conversion of corticosterone-4-^{14}C to 18-hydroxycorticosterone by zona fasciculata-reticularis of beef adrenal. *Endocrinology* 80:214, 1967.
30. Oshima T, Suzuki H, Hata JI, Mitani F, Ishimura Y: Zone-specific expression of aldosterone synthase cytochrome P450 and cytochrome P45011b in rat adrenal cortex: Histochemical basis for the functional zonation. *Endocrinology* 130:2971, 1992.
31. Voutilainen R, Miller WL: Coordinate tropic hormone regulation of mRNAs for insulin-like growth factor II and the cholesterol side-chain cleavage enzyme, P450scc in human steroidogenic tissues. *Proc Natl Acad Sci USA* 84:1590, 1987.
32. Townsend S, Dallman MF, Miller WL: Rat insulin-like growth factors-I and -II mRNAs are unchanged during compensatory adrenal growth but decrease during ACTH-induced adrenal growth. *J Biol Chem* 265:22117, 1990.
33. Mesiano S, Mellon SH, Gospodarowicz D, DiBlasio AM, Jaffe RB: Basic fibroblast growth factor expression is regulated by corticotropin in the human fetal adrenal: A model for adrenal growth regulation. *Proc Natl Acad Sci USA* 88:5428, 1991.
34. Mesiano S, Mellon SH, Jaffe RB: Mitogenic action, regulation and localization of insulin-like growth factors in the human fetal adrenal gland. *J Clin Endocrinol Metab* 76:968, 1993.
35. Solish SB, Goldsmith MA, Voutilainen R, Miller WL: Molecular characterization of a Leydig cell tumor presenting as congenital adrenal hyperplasia. *J Clin Endocrinol Metab* 69:1148, 1989.
36. Brown MS, Kovanen PT, Goldstein JL: Receptor-mediated uptake of lipoprotein-cholesterol and its utilization for steroid synthesis in the adrenal cortex. *Recent Prog Horm Res* 35:215, 1979.
37. Gwynne JT, Strauss JF III: The role of lipoproteins in steroidogenesis and cholesterol metabolism in steroidogenic glands. *Endocr Rev* 3:299, 1982.
38. Hechter O, Solomon MM, Zaffaroni A, Pincus G: Transformation of cholesterol and acetate to adrenal cortical hormones. *Arch Biochem Biophys* 46:201, 1953.
39. Ohashi M, Carr BR, Simpson ER: Binding of high density lipoprotein to human fetal adrenal membrane fractions. *Endocrinology* 109:783, 1981.
40. Strauss JF III, Miller WL: Molecular basis of ovarian steroid synthesis, in Hiller SG (ed): *Ovarian Endocrinology*. Oxford, UK, Blackwell, 1991, p 25.
41. Illingworth DR, Keny TA, Orwoll ES: Adrenal function in heterozygous and homozygous hypobetalipoproteinemia. *J Clin Endocrinol Metab* 54:27, 1982.
42. Mason JI, Rainey WE: Steroidogenesis in the human fetal adrenal: A role for cholesterol synthesized de novo. *J Clin Endocrinol Metab* 64:149, 1987.
43. Farnsworth WJ, Hoeg JM, Maher M, Brittain EH, Sherins RJ, Brewer HBJ: Testicular function in type II hyperlipoproteinimic patients treated with lovastatin (mevinolin) or neomycin. *J Clin Endocrinol Metab* 65:546, 1987.
44. Golos TG, Strauss JF III: 8-Bromo adenosine cyclic 3′5′ phosphate rapidly increases 3-hydroxy-3-methylglutaryl coenzyme A reductase mRNA in human granulosa cells: Role of cellular sterol balance in controlling the response to tropic stimulation. *Biochemistry* 27:3503, 1988.
45. Bolte E, Coudert S, Lefebvre Y: Steroid production from plasma cholesterol: II. *In vivo* conversion of plasma cholesterol to ovarian progesterone and adrenal C19 and C21 steroids in humans. *J Clin Endocrinol Metab* 38:394, 1974.
46. Glass C, Pittman RC, Civen M, Steinberg D: Uptake of high-density lipoprotein-associated apoliprotein A-I and cholesterol esters by 16 tissues of the rat *in vivo* and by adrenal cells and hepatocytes *in vitro*. *J Biol Chem* 260:744, 1985.
47. Mellon-Nussbaum S, Ponticorvo L, Lieberman S: Characterization of the lipoidal derivatives of prenenolone prepared by incubation of the steroid with adrenal mitochondria. *J Biol Chem* 254:12500, 1979.
48. Mellon-Nussbaum S, Ponticorvo L, Schatz F, Hochberg RB: Estradiol fatty acid esters: The isolation and identification of the lipoidal derivative of estradiol synthesized in the bovine uterus. *J Biol Chem* 257:5678, 1982.
49. Beins DM, Vining R, Balasubramaniam S: Regulation of neutral cholesterol esterase and acyl-CoA: cholesterol acetyltransferase in the rat adrenal gland. *Biochem J* 202:631, 1982.
50. Suckling KE, Tocher DR, Smelhe CG, Boyd GS: *In vitro* regulation of bovine adrenal cortical acyl-CoA: cholesterol acyltransferase and comparison with rat liver enzyme. *Biochem Biophys Acta* 753:422, 1983.
51. Anderson RA, Sando GN: Cloning and expression of cDNA encoding human lysosomal acid lypase/cholesterol ester hydrolase. *J Biol Chem* 266:22479, 1991.
52. Colbran RJ, Garton AJ, Cordle SR, Yeaman SJ: Regulation of cholesterol ester hydrolase by cyclic AMP-dependent protein kinase. *FEBS Lett* 201:257, 1986.
53. Pedersen RC, Brownie AC, Ling N: Pro-adrenocorticotropin/endorphin derived peptides: Coordinate action on adrenal steroidogenesis. *Science* 208:1044, 1980.
54. Scallen TJ, Noland BJ, Gavey KL, Bass NM, Ockner RK, Chanderbhan R, Vahouny GV: Sterol carrier protein 2 and fatty acid-binding protein: Separate and distinct physiological functions. *J Biol Chem* 260:4733, 1985.
55. Chanderbhan R, Noland BJ, Scallen TJ, Vahouny GV: Sterol carrier protein 2: Delivery of cholesterol from adrenal lipid droplets to mitochondria for pregnenolone synthesis. *J Biol Chem* 257:8928, 1982.
56. Vahouny GV, Chanderbhan RF, Kharroubi A, Noland BJ, Pastuszyn A, Scallen TJ: Sterol carrier and lipid transfer proteins. *Adv Lipid Res* 22:83, 1987.
57. Trzeciak WH, Simpson ER, Scallen TJ, Vahouny GV, Waterman MR: Studies on the synthesis of sterol carrier protein 2 in rat adrenocortical cells in monolayer culture: Regulation by ACTH and dibutyryl cyclic 3′,5′-AMP. *J Biol Chem* 262:3713, 1987.
58. Hall PF: The role of the cytoskeleton in the supply of

cholesterol for steroidogenesis in lipoprotein and cholesterol metabolism in steroidogenic tissues, in Strauss JF III, Menon KMJ (eds): *Lipoprotein and Cholesterol Metabolism in Steroidogenic Tissues*. Philadelphia, George F Stickley, 1985, p 207.

59. Amsterdam A, Rotmensch S: Structure-function relationships during granulosa cell differentiation. *Endocr Rev* 8:309, 1987.
60. Simpson ER, McCarthy JL, Peterson JA: Evidence that the cycloheximide-sensitive site of adrenocorticotropic hormone action is in the mitochondria changes in pregnenolone formation, cholesterol content, and the electron paramagnetic resonance spectra of cytochrome P450. *J Biol Chem* 253:3135, 1978.
61. Toaff ME, Strauss JFI, Flickinger GL, Shattil SJ: Relationship of cholesterol supply to luteal mitochondrial steroid synthesis. *J Biol Chem* 254:3977, 1979.
62. Privalle CT, McNamara BC, Dherwal MS, Jeffcoate CR: ACTH control of cholesterol side-chain cleavage at adrenal mitochondrial cytochrome P450scc: Regulation of intramitochrondrial cholesterol transfer. *Mol Cell Endocrinol* 53:87, 1987.
63. Li X, Warren DW, Gregorie J, Pedersen RC, Lee AS: The rat 78000 dalton glucose regulated protein (GRP-78) as a precursor for the rat steroidogenesis-activator polypeptide (SAP): The SAP coding sequence is homologous with the terminal end of GRP-78. *Mol Endocrinol* 3:1944, 1989.
64. Pedersen RC, Brownie AC: Cholesterol side-chain cleavage in the rat adrenal cortex: Isolation of a cycloheximide-sensitive activator peptide. *Proc Natl Acad Sci USA* 80:1881, 1983.
65. Pedersen RC, Brownie AC: Steroidogenesis-activator polypeptide isolated from a rat Leydig cell tumor. *Science* 236:188, 1987.
66. Privalle CT, Crivello JF, Jefcoate CR: Regulation of intramitochondrial cholesterol transfer to side-chain cleavage cytochrome P-450 in rat adrenal gland. *Proc Natl Acad Sci USA* 80:702, 1983.
67. Yanagibashi K, Ohno Y, Kawamura M, Hall PF: The regulation of intracellular transport of cholesterol in bovine adrenal cells: Purification of a novel protein. *Endocrinology* 123:2075, 1988.
68. Besman MJ, Yanagibashi K, Lee TD, Kawamura M, Hall PF, Shively JE: Identification of des-(Gly-Ile)-endozepine as an effector of corticotropin-dependent adrenal steroidogenesis: Stimulation of cholesterol delivery is mediated by the peripheral benzodiazepine receptor. *Proc Natl Acad Sci USA* 86:4897, 1989.
69. Lambeth JD, Xu XX, Glover M: Cholesterol sulfate inhibits adrenal mitochondrial cholesterol side-chain cleavage at a site distinct from cytochrome P450scc: Evidence for an intramitochondrial cholesterol translocator. *J Biol Chem* 262:9181, 1987.
70. Papadopoulos V: Peripheral-type benzodiazepine/diazepam binding inhibitor receptor: Biological role in steroidogenic cell function. *Endocr Rev* 14:222, 1993.
71. Lin D, Chang YJ, Strauss JF III, Miller WL: The human peripheral benzodiazepine receptor gene: Cloning and characterization of alternative splicing in normal tissues and in a patient with congenital lipoid adrenal hyperplasia. *Genomics* 18:643, 1993.
72. Blachly-Dyson E, Zambronicz EB, Yu WH, Adams V, McCabe ERB, Adelman J, Colombini M, Forte M: Cloning and functional expression in yeast of two human isoforms of the outer mitochondrial membrane channel, the voltage-dependent anion channel. *J Biol Chem* 268:1835, 1993.
73. Nebert DW, Gonzalez FJ: P450 genes: Structure, evolution and regulation. *Annu Rev Biochem* 56:945, 1987.
74. Hall PF: Cytochromes P450 and the regulation of steroid syntheses. *Steroids* 48:131, 1986.
75. Black SD, Coon MJ: P450 cytochromes: Structure and function. *Adv Enzymol Relat Areas Mol Biol* 60:35, 1987.
76. Gonzalez FJ: The molecular biology of cytochrome P450s. *Pharmacol Rev* 40:243, 1989.
77. Nebert DW, Nelson DR, Coon MJ, Estabrook RW, Feyereisen R, Fujii-Kuriyama Y, Gonzalez FJ, Guengerich FP, et al: The P450 superfamily: Update on new sequences, gene mapping, and recommended nomenclature. *DNA Cell Biol* 10:1, 1991.
78. Poulos TL, Finzel BC, Howard AJ: High-resolution crystal structure of cytochrome P450cam. *J Mol Biol* 195:687, 1987.
79. Raag R, Poulos TL: Crystal structure of the carbon monoxide-substrate-cytochrome P450cam ternary complex. *Biochemistry* 28:7586, 1989.
80. Sybert DW, Lancaster JRJ, Lambeth JD, Kamin H: Participation of the membrane in the side-chain cleavage of cholesterol. *J Biol Chem* 254:12088, 1979.
81. Shikita M, Hall PF: Cytochrome P450 from bovine adrenocortical mitochondria: An enzyme for the side-chain cleavage of cholesterol: I. Purification and properties. *J Biol Chem* 248:5596, 1973.
82. Shikita M, Hall PF: Cytochrome P450 from bovine adrenocortical mitochondria: An enzyme for the side-chain cleavage of cholesterol: II. Subunit structure. *J Biol Chem* 248:5605, 1973.
83. Simpson ER: Cholesterol side-chain cleavage, cytochrome P450, and the control of steroidogenesis. *Mol Cell Endocrinol* 13:213, 1979.
84. Kimura T: ACTH stimulation on cholesterol side-chain cleavage activity of adrenocortical mitochondria. *Mol Cell Biochem* 36:105, 1981.
85. Morisaki M, Duque C, Ikekawa N, Shikita M: Substrate specificity of adrenocortical cytochrome P450: I. Effect of structural modification of cholesterol side-chain on pregnenolone production. *J Steroid Biochem* 13:545, 1980.
86. Lambeth JD, Pember SO: Cytochrome P450scc-adrenodoxin complex: Reduction properties of the substrate-associated cytochrome and relation of the reduction states of heme and iron-sulfur centers to association of the proteins. *J Biol Chem* 258:5596, 1983.
87. Wolfson AJ, Lieberman S: Evidence suggesting that more than one steroid side-chain cleavage enzyme exists in mitochondria from bovine adrenal cortex. *J Biol Chem* 254:4096, 1979.
88. Lieberman S, Prasad VVK: Heterodox notions on pathways of steroidogenesis. *Endocr Rev* 11:469, 1990.
89. Iida S, Papadopoulos V, Hall PF: The influence of exogenous free cholesterol on steroid synthesis in cultured adrenal cells. *Endocrinology* 124:2619, 1989.
90. Heyl BL, Tyrrell DJ, Lambeth JD: Cytochrome P450scc-substrate interactions: Role of the 3β- and side-chain hydroxyls in binding to oxidized and reduced forms of the enzyme. *J Biol Chem* 261:2743, 1986.
91. Morohashi K, Fujii-Kuriyama Y, Okada Y, Sogawa K, Hirose T, Inayama S, Omura T: Molecular cloning and nucleotide sequence of cDNA for mRNA of mitochondrial P450scc of bovine adrenal cortex. *Proc Natl Acad Sci USA* 81:4647, 1984.
92. Matteson KJ, Chung B, Urdea MS, Miller WL: Study of cholesterol side-chain cleavage (20,22 desmolase) deficiency causing congenital lipoid adrenal hyperplasia using bovine-sequence P450scc oligodeoxyibonucleotide probes. *Endocrinology* 118:1296, 1986.
93. Chung B, Matteson KJ, Voutilainen R, Mohandas TK, Miller WL: Human cholesterol side-chain cleavage enzyme, P450scc: cDNA cloning, assignment of the gene to chromosome 15, and expression in the placenta. *Proc Natl Acad Sci USA* 83:8962, 1986.
94. Morohashi K, Sogawa K, Omura T, Fujii-Kuriyama Y: Gene structure of human cytochrome P450scc, cholesterol desmolase. *J Biochem* 101:879, 1987.

95. Sparkes RS, Klisak I, Miller WL: Regional mapping of genes encodng human steroidogenic enzymes: P450scc to 15q23-q24; adrenodoxin to 11q22; adrenodoxin reductase to 17q24-q25; and P450c17 to 10q24-q25. *DNA Cell Biol* 10:359, 1991.
96. Matocha MF, Waterman MR: Synthesis and processing of mitochondrial steroid hydroxylases: *In vivo* maturation of the precursor of cytochrome P450scc, cytochrome P450 and adrenotoxin. *J Biol Chem* 260:12259, 1985.
97. Voutilainen R, Tapananinen J, Chung B, Matteson KJ, Miller WL: Hormonal regulation of P450scc (20,22 desmolase) and (17α-hydroxylase/17,20 lyase) in cultured human granulosa cells. *J Clin Endocrinol Metab* 63:202, 1986.
98. DiBlasio AM, Voutilainen R, Jaffe RB, Miller WL: Hormonal regulation of mRNAs for P450scc (cholesterol side-chain cleavage enzyme) and P450c17 (17α-hydroxylase/17,20 lyase) in cultured fetal adrenal cells. *J Clin Endocrinol Metab* 65:170, 1987.
99. Voutilainen R, Miller WL: Developmental and hormonal regulation of mRNAs for insulin-like growth factor II and steroidogenic enzymes in human fetal adrenal and gonads. *DNA* 7:9, 1988.
100. Ringler GE, Kao LC, Miller WL, Strauss JF III: Effects of 8-bromo-cAMP on expression of endocrine functions by cultured human trophoblast cells: Regulation of specific mRNAs. *Mol Cell Endocrinol* 61:13, 1989.
101. Mellon SH, Kushner JA, Vaisse C: Expression and regulation of adrenodoxin and P450scc mRNAs in rodent tissues. *DNA Cell Biol* 10:339, 1991.
102. Mellon SH, Deschepper CF: Neurosteroids are synthesized by adrenal steroidogenic enzymes. *Brain Res* 629: 283, 1993.
103. John ME, John MC, Boggaram V, Simpson ER, Waterman MR: Transcriptional regulation of steroid hydroxylase genes by corticotropin. *Proc Natl Acad Sci USA* 83:4715, 1986.
104. Mellon SH, Vaisse C: CAMP regulates P450scc gene expression by a cycloheximide-insensitive mechanism in cultured mouse Leydig MA-10 cells. *Proc Natl Acad Sci USA* 86:7775, 1989.
105. Moore CCD, Brentano ST, Miller WL: Human P450scc gene transcription is induced by cyclic AMP and repressed by 12-*O*-tetradecanolyphorbol-13-acetate and A23187 through independent cis elements. *Mol Cell Biol* 10:6013, 1990.
106. Ahlgren R, Simpson ER, Waterman MR, Lund J: Characterization of the promoter/regulatory region of the bovine CYP11A (P450scc) gene. *J Biol Chem* 265:3313, 1990.
107. Moore CCD, Hum DR, Miller WL: Identification of positive and negative placental-specific basal elements and a cyclic adenosine 3′,5′-monophosphate response element in the human gene for P450scc. *Mol Endocrinol* 6:2045, 1992.
108. Hum DW, Staels B, Black SM, Miller WL: Basal transcriptional activity and cyclic adenosine 3′,5′-monophosphate responsiveness of the human cytochrome P450scc promoter transfected into mouse Leydig MA-10 cells. *Endocrinology* 132:546, 1993.
109. Hum DW, Miller WL: Transcriptional regulation of human genes for steroidogenic enzymes. *Clin Chem* 39:333, 1993.
110. Barret PQ, Bollag WB, Isales CM, McCarthy RT, Rasmussen H: The role of calcium in angiotensin II-mediated aldosterone secretion. *Endocr Rev* 10:496, 1989.
111. Golos TG, Miller WL, Strauss JF III: Human chorionic gonadotropin and 8-bromo cyclic adenosine monophosphate promote an acute increase in cytochrome P450scc and adrenodoxin messenger RNAs in cultured human granulosa cells by a cycloheximide-insensitive mechanism. *J Clin Invest* 80:896, 1987.
112. Picado-Leonard J, Voutilainen R, Kao L, Chung B, Strauss JF III, Miller WL: Human adrenodoxin: Cloning of three cDNAs and cycloheximide enhancement in JEG-3 cells. *J Biol Chem* 263:3240, 1988.
113. Enyedi P, Szaba B, Spat A: Reduced responsiveness of glomerulosa cells after prolonged stimulation with angiotensin II. *Am J Physiol* 248:E209, 1985.
114. Mason JI, Carr BR, Rainey WE: The action of phorbol ester on steroidogenesis in cultured human fetal adrenal cells. *Endocr Res* 12:447, 1986.
115. Cozza EN, Vila MDC, Acevedo-Duncan M, Farese RV, Gomez-Sanchez CE: Treatment of primary cultures of calf adrenal glomerulosa cells with adrenocorticotropin (ACTH) and phorbol esters: A comparative study of the effects on aldosterone production and ACTH signaling system. *Endocrinology* 126:2169, 1990.
116. Omura T, Sanders S, Estabrook RW, Cooper DY, Rosenthal O: Isolation from adrenal cortex of a non-heme iron protein and a flavoprotein functional as a reduced triphosophopyridine nucleotide-cytochrome P450 reductase. *Arch Biochem Biophys* 117:660, 1966.
117. Nakamura Y, Otsuka H, Tamaoki B: Requirement of a new flavoprotein and a non-heme iron-containing protein in the steroid 11β- and 18-hydroxylase system. *Biochem Biophys Acta* 122:34, 1966.
118. Kimura T, Suzuki K: Components of the electron transport system in adrenal steroid hydroxylase. *J Biol Chem* 242:485, 1967.
119. Gnanaiah W, Omdahl JL: Isolation and characterization of pig kidney mitochondrial ferredoxin: $NADP^+$ oxidoreductase. *J Biol Chem* 261:12649, 1986.
120. Hanukoglu I, Suh BS, Himmelhoch S, Amsterdam A: Induction and mitochondrial localization of cytochrome P450scc enzymes in normal and transformed ovarian granulosa cells. *J Cell Biol* 111:1373, 1990.
121. Solish SB, Picado-Leonard J, Morel Y, Mohandas TK, Honakoglu I, Miller WL: Human adrenodoxin reductase: Two mRNAs encoded by a single gene on chromosome 17cen q25 are expressed in steroidogenic tissues. *Proc Natl Acad Sci USA* 85:7104, 1988.
122. Lin D, Shi Y, Miller WL: Cloning and sequence of the human adrenodoxin reductase gene. *Proc Natl Acad Sci USA* 87:8516, 1990.
123. Brentano ST, Black SM, Harikrishna J, Miller WL: cAMP post-transcriptionally diminishes the abundance of adrenodoxin reductase mRNA. *Proc Natl Acad Sci USA* 89:4099, 1992.
124. Brandt ME, Vickery LE: Expression and characterization of human mitochondrial ferredoxin reductase in Escherichia coli. *Arch Biochem Biophys* 294:735, 1992.
125. Lambeth JD, Seybert D, Kamin H: Ionic effects on adrenal steroidogenic electron transport: The role of adrenodoxin as an electron shuttle. *J Biol Chem* 254:7255, 1979.
126. Lambeth JD, Seybert DW, Kamin H: Phospholipid vesicle-reconstituted cytochrome P450scc: Mutually facilitated binding of cholesterol and adrenodoxin. *J Biol Chem* 255:138, 1980.
127. Hanukoglu I, Jefcoate CR: Mitochondrial cytochrome P450scc: Mechanism of electron transport by adrenodoxin. *J Biol Chem* 255:3057, 1980.
128. Hanukoglu I, Spitsberg V, Bumpus JA, Dus KM, Jefcoate CR: Adrenal mitochondrial cytochrome P450scc: Cholesterol and adrenodoxin interactions at equilibrium and during turnover. *J Biol Chem* 256:4321, 1981.
129. Cupp JR, Vickery LE: Identification of free and $[Fe_2S_2]$-bound cysteine residues of adrenodoxin. *J Biol Chem* 263:17418, 1988.
130. Coghlan VM, Vickery LE: Expression of human ferredoxin and assembly of the [2Fe-2S] center in *Escherichia coli. Proc Natl Acad Sci USA* 86:835, 1989.
131. Cupp JR, Vickery LE: Adrenodoxin with a COOH-terminal deletion (des 116-128) exhibits enhanced activity. *J Biol Chem* 269:1602, 1989.

132. Chang CY, Wu DA, Lai CC, Miller WL, Chung B: Cloning and structure of the human adrenodoxin gene. *DNA* 7:609, 1988.
133. Chang CY, Wu DA, Mohandas TK, Chung B: Structure, sequence, chromosomal location, and evolution of the human ferredoxin gene family. *DNA Cell Biol* 9:205, 1990.
134. Morel Y, Picado-Leonard J, Wu DA, Chang C, Mohandas TK, Chung B, Miller WL: Assignment of the functional gene for adrenodoxin to chromosome 11q13 qter and of adrenodoxin pseudogenes to chromosome 20cen q13.1. *Am J Hum Genet* 43:52, 1988.
135. Okamura T, Kagimoto M, Simpson ER, Waterman MR: Multiple species of bovine adrenodoxin mRNA: Occurrence of two different mitochondrial precursor sequences associated with the same mature sequence. *J Biol Chem* 262:10335, 1987.
136. Brentano ST, Miller WL: Regulation of human cytochrome P450scc and adrenodoxin messenger ribonucleic acids in JEG-3 cytotrophoblast cells. *Endocrinology* 131:3010, 1992.
137. Voutilainen R, Picado-Leonard J, DiBlasio AM, Miller WL: Hormonal and developmental regulation of adrenodoxin messenger ribonucleic acid in steroidogenic tissues. *J Clin Endocrinol Metab* 66:383, 1988.
138. Coghlan VM, Vickery LE: Site-specific mutations in human ferredoxin that affect binding to ferredoxin reductase and cytochrome P450scc. *J Biol Chem* 266:18606, 1991.
139. Coghlan VM, Vickery LE: Electrostatic interactions stabilizing ferredoxin electron transfer complexes: Disruption by "conservative mutations." *J Biol Chem* 267:8932, 1992.
140. Harikrishna JA, Black SM, Szklarz GD, Miller WL: Construction and function of fusion enzymes of the human cytochrome P450scc system. *DNA Cell Biol* 12:371, 1993.
141. Thomas JL, Myers RP, Strickler RC: Human placental 3β-hydroxy-5-ene steroid dehydrogenase and steroid-5-4-ene isomerase: Purification from mitochondria and kinetic profiles, biophysical characterization of the purified mitochondrial and microsomal enzymes. *J Steroid Biochem* 33:209, 1989.
142. Luu-The V, Lachance Y, Labrie C, Leblanc G, Thomas JL, Strickler RC, Labrie F: Full length cDNA structure and deduced amino acid sequence of human 3β-hydroxy-5-ene steroid dehydrogenase. *Mol Endocrinol* 3:1310, 1989.
143. Lorence MC, Murry BA, Trant JM, Mason JI: Human 3β-hydroxysteroid dehydrogenase/Δ^5-Δ^4 isomerase from placenta: Expression in nonsteroidogenic cells of a protein that catalyzes the dehydrogenation/isomerization of C21 and C19 steroids. *Endocrinology* 126:2493, 1990.
144. Lachance Y, Luu-The V, Labrie C, Simard J, Dumont M, Launoit Y, Guerin S, Leblanc G, et al: Characterization of human 3β-hydroxysteroid dehydrogenase/Δ^5-Δ^4 isomerase gene and its expression in mammalian cells. *J Biol Chem* 265:20469, 1990.
145. Lorence MC, Corbin CJ, Kamimura N, Mahendrou MS, Mason JI: Structural analysis of the gene encoding human 3β-hydroxysteroid dehydrogenase/Δ^5-Δ^4 isomerase. *Mol Endocrinol* 4:1850, 1990.
146. Lachance Y, Luu-The V, Verreault H, Dumont M, Leblanc G, Labrie F: Characterization and expression of human type II 3β-hydroxysteroid dehydrogenase/Δ^5-Δ^4 isomerase (3β-HSD) gene, the almost exclusive 3β-HSD species expressed in the adrenals and gonads. *DNA Cell Biol* 10:701, 1991.
147. Rheaume E, Lachance Y, Zhao H, Boeton N, Dumont M, DeLaunoit Y, Trudel C, Luu-The V, et al: Structure and expression of a new cDNA encoding the major 3β-hydroxysteroid dehydrogenase/Δ^5-Δ^4 isomerase present in human adrenals and gonads. *Mol Endocrinol* 5:1147, 1991.
148. Berube D, Luu-The V, Lachance Y, Gagne R, Labrie F: Assignment of the human 3β-hydroxysteroid dehydrogenase gene (HSDB3) to the p13 band of chromosome 1. *Cytogenet Cell Genet* 52:199, 1989.
149. Laffargue P, Chamlian A, Adechy-Senkoel L: Localization probable en microscopie electronique de la 3β-hydroxysteroide dehydrogenase, de la glucose-6-phosphate dehydrogenase et de la NADH diaphorase dans le corps jaune ovarien de la femme. *J Microsc* 13:325, 1972.
150. Voutilanen R, Ilvesmaki V, Miettinen PJ: Low expression of 3β-hydroxy-5-ene steroid dehydrogenase gene in human fetal adrenals *in vivo:* Adrenocorticotropin and protein kinase C-dependent regulation in adrenocortical cultures. *J Clin Endocrinol Metab* 72:761, 1991.
151. Trant JM, Lorance MC, Johnson EF, Shackleton CHL, Mason JI, Estabrook RW: Characterization of the steroid-metabolizing capacity of the hepatic cytochrome P450II5 expressed in COS-1 cells: 3β-hydroxysteroid dehydrogenase/Δ^5 Δ^4 isomerase type activity. *Proc Natl Acad Sci USA* 87:9756, 1990.
152. Parker LN, Sack J, Fisher DA, O'Dell WD: The adrenarche: Prolactin, gonadotropins, adrenal androgens, and cortisol. *J Clin Endocrinol Metab* 46:396, 1978.
153. Sklar CA, Kaplan SL, Grumbach MM: Evidence for dissociation between adrenarche and gonadarche: Studies in patients with idiopathic precocious puberty, gonadal dysgenesis, isolated gonadotropin deficiency, and constitutionally delayed growth and adolescence. *J Clin Endocrinol Metab* 51:548, 1980.
154. Mellon SH, Shively JE, Miller WL: Human proopiomelanocortin (79-96), a proposed androgen stimulatory hormone, does not affect steroidogenesis in cultured human fetal adrenal cells. *J Clin Endocrinol Metab* 72:19, 1991.
155. Penhoat A, Sanchez P, Jaillard C, Langlois D, Begeot M, Saez JM: Human proopiomelanocortin (79-96), a proposed cortical androgen stimulating hormone, does not affect steroidogenesis in cultured human adult adrenal cells. *J Clin Endocrinol Metab* 72:23, 1991.
156. Robinson P, Bateman A, Mulay S, Spencer SJ, Jaffe RB, Solomon S, Bennett HPJ: Isolation and characterization of three forms of joining peptide from adult pituitaries: Lack of adrenal androgen-stimulating activity. *Endocrinology* 129:859, 1991.
157. Zachman M, Vollmin JA, Hamilton W, Prader A: Steroid 17,20 desmolase deficiency: A new cause of male pseudohermaphroditism. *Clin Endocrinol* 1:369, 1972.
158. Goebelsmann U, Zachmann M, Davajan V, Israel R, Mestman JH, Mishell DR: Male pseudohermaphroditism consistent with 17,20-desmolase deficiency. *Gynecol Invest* 7:138, 1976.
159. Nakajin S, Hall PF: Microsomal cytochrome P450 from neonatal pig testis. Purification and properties of a C21 steroid side-chain cleavage system (17α-hydroxylase-C17,20 lyase). *J Biol Chem* 256:3871, 1981.
160. Nakajin S, Hall PF, Onoda M: Testicular microsomal cytochrome P450 for C21 steroid side-chain cleavage. *J Biol Chem* 256:6134, 1981.
161. Nakajin S, Shively JE, Yuan P, Hall PF: Microsomal cytochrome P450 from neonatal pig testis: Two enzymatic activities (17α-hydroxylase and C17,20-lyase) associated with one protein. *Biochemistry* 20:4037, 1981.
162. Nakajin S, Shinoda M, Haniu M, Shively JE, Hall PF: C21 steroid side-chain cleavage enzyme from porcine adrenal microsomes: Purification and characterization of the 17α-hydroxylase/C17,20 lyase cytochrome P450. *J Biol Chem* 259:3971, 1984.
163. Zuber MX, Simpson ER, Waterman M: Expression of bovine 17α-hydroxylase cytochrome P450 cDNA in non-steroidogenic (COS 1) cells. *Science* 234:1258, 1986.
164. Sakaki T, Shibata M, Yabusaki Y, Murakami H, Ohkawa H: Expression of bovine cytochrome P450c17 cDNA in Saccharomyces cerevisiae. *DNA* 8:409, 1989.
165. Fevold HR, Lorence MC, McCarthy JL, Trant JM, Kagimoto M, Waterman MR, Mason JI: Rat P450-17α from

testis: Characterization of a full-length cDNA encoding a unique steroid hydroxylase capable of catalyzing both Δ^4- and Δ^5-steroid-17,20-lyase reactions. *Mol Endocrinol* 3:968, 1989.
166. Lin D, Harikrishna JA, Moore CCD, Jones KL, Miller WL: Missense mutation Serine^{106} Proline causes 17α-hydroxylase deficiency. *J Biol Chem* 266:15992, 1991.
167. Yanase T, Simpson ER, Waterman MR: 17α-hydroxylase/1720 lyase deficiency: From clinical investigation to molecular definition. *Endocr Rev* 12:91, 1991.
168. Fardella CE, Zhang L, Mahachoklertwattana P, Lin D, Miller WL: Deletion of amino acids Asp^{487}-Ser^{488}-Phe^{489} of cytochrome P450c17 causes severe 17α-hydroxylase deficiency. *J Clin Endocrinol Metab* 77:489, 1993.
169. Matteson KJ, Picado-Leonard J, Chung B, Mohandas TK, Miller WL: Assignment of the gene for adrenal P450c17 (17α-hydroxylase/17, 20 lyase) to human chromosome 10. *J Clin Endocrinol Metab* 63:789, 1986.
170. Chung B, Picado-Leonard J, Haniu M, Bienkowski M, Hall PF, Shively JE, Miller WL: Cytochrome P450c17 (steroid 17α-hydroxylase/17,20 lyase): Cloning of human adrenal and testis cDNAs indicate the same gene is expressed in both tissues. *Proc Natl Acad Sci USA* 84:407, 1987.
171. Picado-Leonard J, Miller WL: Cloning and sequence of the human gene for P450c17 (steroid 17α-hydroxylase/17,20 lyase): Similarity to the gene for P450c21. *DNA* 6:437, 1987.
171a. Lin D, Zhang L, Chiao E, Miller WL: Modeling and mutagenesis of the active site of human P450c17: *Mol Endocrinol* 8:392, 1994.
172. Brentano ST, Picado-Leonard J, Mellon SH, Moore CCD, Miller WL: Tissue-specific, cAMP-induced, and phorbol ester repressed expression from the human P450c17 promoter in mouse cells. *Mol Endocrinol* 4:1972, 1990.
173. Jefcoate CR, McNamara BC, DeBartolomeis MS: Control of steroid synthesis in adrenal fasciculata cells. *Endocr Res* 12:35, 1986.
174. Yamano S, Aoyama T, McBride OW, Hardwick JP, Gelboin HV, Gonzalez FJ: Human NADPH-P450 oxidoreductase: Complementary DNA cloning, sequence, vaccinia virus-mediated expression, and localization of the CYPOR gene to chromosome 7. *Mol Pharmacol* 35:83, 1989.
175. Black SD, Coon MJ: Structural features of liver microsomal NADPH-cytochrome P450 reductase: Hydrophobic domain, hydrophilic domain, and connecting region. *J Biol Chem* 257:5929, 1982.
176. Oprian DD, Coon MJ: Oxidation-reduction states of FMN and FAD in NADPH-cytochrome P450 reductase during reduction by NADPH. *J Biol Chem* 257:8935, 1982.
177. Tamburini PP, Gibson GG: Thermodynamic studies of the protein-protein interactions between cytochrome P450 and cytochrome b_5. *J Biol Chem* 258:13444, 1983.
178. French JS, Guengerich FP, Coon MJ: Interactions of cytochrome P450, NADPH-cytochrome P450 reductase, and substrate in the reconstituted liver microsomal enzyme system. *J Biol Chem* 255:4112, 1980.
179. Muller-Enoch D, Churchill P, Fleischer S, Guengerich FP: Interaction of liver microsomal cytochrome P450 and NADPH-cytochrome P450 reductase in the presence and absence of lipid. *J Biol Chem* 259:8174, 1984.
180. Yanagibashi K, Hall PF: Role of electron transport in the regulation of the lyase activity of C21 side-chain cleavage P450 from porcine adrenal and testicular microsomes. *J Biol Chem* 261:8429, 1986.
181. Lin D, Black SM, Nagahama Y, Miller WL: Steroid 17α-hydroxylase and 17,20 lyase activities of P450c17: Contributions of serine 106 and of P450 reductase. *Endocrinology* 132:2498, 1993.
182. Miller WL, Levine LS: Molecular and clinical advances in congenital adrenal hyperplasia. *J Pediatr* 111:1, 1987.
183. New MI, White P, Pang S, Dupont B, Speiser P: The adrenal hyperplasias, in Scriver C, Beaudet A, Sly W, Valle D (eds): *The Metabolic Basis of Inherited Disease*. New York, McGraw-Hill, 1989, p 1881.
184. Kominami S, Ochi H, Kobayashi T, Takemori S: Studies on the steroid hydroxylation system in adrenal cortex microsomes: Purification and characterization of cytochrome P450 specific for steroid 21-hydroxylation. *J Biol Chem* 255:3386, 1980.
185. Higashi Y, Yoshioka H, Yamane M, Gotoh O, Fujii-Kuriyama Y: Complete nucleotide sequence of two steroid 21-hydroxylase genes tandemly arranged in human chromosome: A pseudogene and a genuine gene. *Proc Natl Acad Sci USA* 83:284, 1986.
186. White PC, New MI, Dupont B: Structure of human steroid 21-hydroxylase genes. *Proc Natl Acad Sci USA* 83:5, 1986.
187. Rodriguez NR, Dunham I, Yu CY, Carroll MC, Porter RR, Campbell RD: Molecular characterization of the HLA-linked steroid 21-hydroxylase B gene from an individual with congenital adrenal hyperplasia. *EMBO J* 6:1653, 1987.
188. Bristow J, Gitelman SE, Tee MK, Staels B, Miller WL: Abundant adrenal-specific transcription of the human P450c21A "pseudogene." *J Biol Chem* 268:12919, 1993.
189. Bristow J, Tee MK, Gitelman SE, Mellon SH, Miller WL: Tenascin-X: A novel extracellular matrix protein encoded by the human XB gene overlapping P450c21B. *J Cell Biol* 122:265, 1993.
190. Miller WL, Morel Y: Molecular genetics of 21-hydroxylase deficiency. *Annu Rev Genet* 23:371, 1989.
191. Morel Y, Miller WL: Clinical and molecular genetics of congenital adrenal hyperplasia due to 21-hydroxylase deficiency. *Adv Hum Genet* 20:1, 1991.
192. Casey ML, MacDonald PC: Extraadrenal formation of a mineralocorticoid: Deoxycorticosterone and deoxycorticosterone sulfate biosynthesis and metabolism. *Endocr Rev* 3:396, 1982.
193. Casey ML, Winkel CA, MacDonald PC: Conversion of progesterone to deoxycorticosterone in the human fetus: Steroid 21-hydroxylase activity in fetal tissues. *J Steroid Biochem* 18:449, 1983.
194. Mellon SH, Miller WL: Extra-adrenal steroid 21-hydroxylation is not mediated by P450c21. *J Clin Invest* 84:1497, 1989.
195. Amor M, Tosi M, Duponchel C, Steinmetz M, Meo T: Liver cDNA probes disclose two cytochrome P450 genes duplicated in tandem with the complement C4 loci of the mouse H-2S region. *Proc Natl Acad Sci USA* 82:4453, 1985.
196. Chung B, Matteson KJ, Miller WL: Structure of the bovine gene for P450c21 (steroid 21-hydroxylase) defines a novel cytochrome P450 gene family. *Proc Natl Acad Sci USA* 83:4243, 1986.
197. Speiser PW, Agdere L, Veshiba H, White PC, New MI: Aldosterone synthesis in patients with salt-wasting congenital adrenal hyperplasia (21-hydroxylase deficiency) and complete absence of adrenal 21-hydroxylase (P450c21). *N Engl J Med* 3221:145, 1991.
198. Ulick S: Diagnosis and nomenclature of the disorders of the terminal portion of the aldosterone biosynthetic pathway. *J Clin Endocrinol Metab* 43:92, 1976.
199. Veldhuis JD, Kulin HE, Santen RJ, Wilson TE, Melby JC: Inborn error in the terminal step of aldosterone biosynthesis: Corticosterone methyl oxidase type II deficiency in a North American pedigree. *N Engl J Med* 303:118, 1980.
200. Yanagibashi K, Haniu M, Shively JE, Shen WH, Hall P: The synthesis of aldosterone by the adrenal cortex: Two zones (fasciculata and glomerulosa) possess one enzyme for 11β-18-hydroxylation, and aldehyde synthesis. *J Biol Chem* 261:3556, 1986.
201. Mathew PA, Mason JI, Trant JM, Sanders D, Waterman MR: Amino acid substitutions Phe66→Leu and Ser126→Pro abolish cortisol and aldosterone synthesis by

bovine cytochrome P45011β. *J Biol Chem* 265:20228, 1990.

202. Morohashi K, Yoshioka H, Gotoh O, Okada Y, Yamamoto K, Miyata T, Sogawa K, Fujii-Kuriyama Y, et al: Molecular cloning and nucleotide sequences of DNA of mitochondrial P-450 (11β) of bovine adrenal cortex. *J Biochem* 102:559, 1986.
203. Mornet E, Dupont J, Vitek A, White P: Characterization of two genes encoding human steroid 11β-hydroxylase (P-450-11β). *J Biol Chem* 264:20961, 1989.
204. Kirita S, Morohashi K, Hashimoto T, Yoshioka H, Fujii-Kuriyama Y, Omura T: Expression of two kinds of cytochrome P-450 (11β) mRNA in bovine adrenal cortex. *J Biochem* 104:683, 1988.
205. Chua SC, Szabo P, Vitek A, Grzechik K-H, John M, White PC: Cloning of cDNA encoding steroid 11β-hydroxylase P450c11. *Proc Natl Acad Sci USA* 84:7193, 1987.
206. Kawamoto T, Mitsuuchi Y, Ohnishi T, Ichikawa Y, Yokoyama Y, Sumimoto H, Toda K, Miyahara K, et al: Cloning and expression of a cDNA for human cytochrome P-450aldo as related to primary aldosteronism. *Biochem Biophys Res Commun* 173:309, 1990.
207. Kawamoto T, Mitsuuchi Y, Toda K, Yokoyama Y, Miyahara K, Miura S, Ohnishi T, Ichikawa Y, et al: Role of steroid 11β-hydroxylase and steroid 18-hydroxylase in the biosynthesis of glucocorticoids and mineralocorticoids in humans. *Proc Natl Acad Sci USA* 89:1458, 1992.
208. Carnow KM, Tusie-Luna M, Pascoe L, Natarajan R, Gu J, Nadler JL, White PC: The product of the CYP11B2 gene is required for aldosterone biosynthesis in the human adrenal cortex. *Mol Endocrinol* 5:1513, 1991.
209. Domalik LJ, Chaplin DD, Kirkman MS, Wu RC, Liu W, Howard TA, Seldin MF, Parker KL: Different isozymes of mouse 11β-hydroxylase produce mineralocorticoids and glucocorticoids. *Mol Endocrinol* 5:1853, 1991.
210. Malee MP, Mellon SH: Zone-specific regulation of two distinct messenger RNAs for P450c11 (11/18-hydroxylase) in the adrenals of pregnant and non-pregnant rats. *Proc Natl Acad Sci USA* 88:4731, 1991.
211. White PC, Dupont J, New MI, Lieberman E, Hochberg Z, Rosler A: A mutation in CYP11B1 (Arg448→His) associated with steroid 11β-hydroxylase deficiency in Jews of Moroccan origin. *J Clin Invest* 87:1664, 1991.
212. Ulick S, Wang JZ, Morton DH: The biochemical phenotypes of two inborn errors in the biosynthesis of aldosterone. *J Clin Endocrinol Metab* 72:1415, 1992.
213. Pascoe L, Curnow KM, Slutsker L, Rosler A, White PC: Mutations in the human CYP11B2 (aldosterone synthase) gene causing corticosterone methyloxidase II deficiency. *Proc Natl Acad Sci USA* 89:4996, 1992.
214. Inano H, Tamaoki B: The reaction of 1-ethyl-3-(3-dimethyl aminopropyl) carbodiimide with an essential carboxy group of human placental estradiol 17β-dehydrogenase. *J Steroid Biochem* 21:59, 1984.
215. Engel LL, Groman EV: Human placental 17β-estradiol dehydrogenase: Characterization and structural studies. *Recent Prog Horm Res* 32:139, 1974.
216. Milewich L, Hendricks TS, Romero LH: Interconversion of estrone and estradiol-17β in lung slices of the adult human. *J Steroid Biochem* 17:669, 1982.
217. Fournier S, Brihmat F, Durand JC, Sterkers N, Martin PM, Kutten F, Mauvaris-Jarvis P: Estradiol 17β-hydroxysteroid dehydrogenase, a marker of breast cancer hormone dependency. *Cancer Res* 45:2895, 1985.
218. Peltoketo H, Isomaa V, Mentausta O, Vihkko R: Complete amino acid sequence of human placental 17β-hydroxysteroid dehydrogenase deduced from cDNA. *FEBS Lett* 239:73, 1988.
219. Luu-The V, Labrie C, Zhao H, Couet J, Lachance Y, Simard J, Leblanc G, Cote J, et al: Characterization of cDNAs for human estradiol 17β-dehydrogenase and assignment of the gene to chromosome 17: Evidence of two mRNA species with distinct 5′-termini in human placenta. *Mol Endocrinol* 3:1301, 1989.
220. Baker ME: Human placental 17β-hydroxysteroid dehydrogenase is homologous to Nod G protein of Rhizobium meliloti. *Mol Endocrinol* 3:881, 1989.
221. Luu-The V, Labrie C, Simard J, Lechance Y, Zhao HF, Couet J, Leblanc G, Labrie F: Structure of two in tandem human 17β-hydroxysteroid dehydrogenase genes. *Mol Endocrinol* 4:268, 1990.
222. Tremblay Y, Ringler GE, Morel Y, Mohandas TK, Labrie F, Strauss JF III, Miller WL: Regulation of the gene for estrogenic 17-ketosteroid reductase lying on chromosome 17cen→q25. *J Biol Chem* 264:20458, 1989.
223. Pang S, Softness B, Sweeny WJI, New MI: Hirsutism, polycystic ovarian disease, and ovarian 17-ketosteroid reductase deficiency. *N Engl J Med* 316:1295, 1987.
224. Wu L, Einstein M, Geissler WM, Chan HK, EllisonKO, Andersson S: Expression cloning and characterization of human 17β-hydrosteroid dehydrogenase Type 2, a microsomal enzyme possessing 20α-hydroxysteroid dehydrogenase activity. *J Biol Chem* 268:12964, 1993.
225. Fishman J, Goto J: Mechanism of estrogen biosynthesis: Participation of multiple enzyme sites in placental aromatase hydroxylations. *J Biol Chem* 256:4466, 1981.
226. Fishman J, Rajo MS: Mechanism of estrogen biosynthesis: Stereochemistry of C-1 hydrogen elimination in the aromatization of 2β-hydroxy-19-oxoandrostenedione. *J Biol Chem* 256:4472, 1981.
227. Thompson EAJ, Siiteri PK: The involvement of human placental microsomal cytochrome P450 in aromatization. *J Biol Chem* 249:5373, 1974.
228. Nakajin S, Shinoda M, Hall PF: Purification to homogeneity of aromatase from human placenta. *Biochem Biophys Res Commun* 134:704, 1986.
229. Evans CT, Ledesma DB, Schulz TZ, Simpson ER, Mendelson CR: Isolation and characterization of a complementary DNA specific for human aromatase-system P-450 mRNA. *Proc Natl Acad Sci USA* 83:6387, 1986.
230. Chen S, Besman MJ, Sparkes RS, Zollman S, Klisak I, Mohandas T, Hall PF, Shively JE: Human aromatase: cDNA cloning, Southern blot analysis and assignment of the gene to chromosome 15. *DNA* 7:27, 1988.
231. Harada N: Cloning of a complete cDNA encoding human aromatase: Immunochemical identification and sequence analysis. *Biochem Biophys Res Commun* 156:725, 1988.
232. Corbin CJ, Graham-Lorence S, McPhaul M, Mason JI, Mendelson CR, Simpson ER: Isolation of a full-length cDNA insert encoding human aromatase system cytochrome P-450 and its expression in nonsteroidogenic cells. *Proc Natl Acad Sci USA* 85:8948, 1988.
233. Pompon D, Liu RYK, Besman MJ, Wang PL, Shively JE, Chen S: Expression of human placental aromatase in *Saccharomyces cerevisae*. *Mol Endocrinol* 3:1477, 1989.
234. Means GD, Mahendroo MS, Corbin CJ, Mathis JM, Powel FE, Mendelson CR, Simpson ER: Structural analysis of the gene encoding human aromatase cytochrome P-450, the enzyme responsible for estrogen biosynthesis. *J Biol Chem* 264:19385, 1989.
235. Mahendroo MS, Means GD, Mendelson CR, Simpson ER: Tissue specific expression of human P-450arom: The promoter responsible in adipose tissue is different from that utilized in placenta. *J Biol Chem* 266:11276, 1991.
236. Simpson ER, Mahendroo MS, Means GD, Kilgore MW, Corbin CJ, Mendelson CR: Tissue-specific promoters regulate aromatase cytochrome P450 expression. *Clin Chem* 39:317, 1993.
237. Mooradian AD, Morley JE, Korenman SG: Biological actions of androgens. *Endocr Rev* 8:1, 1987.
238. Saenger P: Abnormal sex differentiation. *J Pediatr* 104:1, 1984.
239. Wilson JD: Disorders of androgen action. *Clin Res* 35:1, 1987.

240. Cunha GR, Donjacour AA, Cooke PS, Mee S, Bigsby RM, Higgins SJ, Sugimora Y: The endocrinology and developmental biology of the prostate. *Endocr Rev* 8:338, 1987.
241. Johnson L, George FW, Neaves WB, Rosenthal IM, Christensen RA, Decristoforo A, Schweikert H, Sauer MV, et al: Characterization of the testicular abnormality in 5α-reductase deficiency. *J Clin Endocrinol Metab* 63:1091, 1986.
242. Andersson S, Russell DW: Structural and biochemical properties of cloned and expressed human and rat steroid 5α-reductases. *Proc Natl Acad Sci USA* 87:3640, 1990.
243. Andersson S, Berman DM, Jenkins EP, Russell DW: Deletion of steroid 5α-reductase 2 gene in male pseudohermaphroditism. *Nature* 354:159, 1991.
244. Jenkins EP, Anderson S, Imperato-McGinley J, Wilson JD, Russell DW: Genetic and pharmacologic evidence for more than one human steroid 5α-reductase. *J Clin Invest* 89:293, 1992.
245. Harris G, Azzolina B, Baginsky W, Cimis G, Rasmussen GH, Tolman RL, Raetz CRH, Ellsworth K: Identification and selective inhibition of an isozyme of steroid 5α-reductase in human scalp. *Proc Natl Acad Sci USA* 89:10787, 1992.
246. Thigpen AE, Davis DL, Milatovich A, Mendonca BB, Imperato-McGinley J, Griffin JE, Franke U, Wilson JD, et al: Molecular genetics of steroid 5 alpha-reductase 2 deficiency. *J Clin Invest* 90:799, 1992.
247. Thigpen AE, Silver RI, Guileyardo JM, Casey ML, McConnell JD, Russel DW: Tissue distribution and ontogeny of steroid 5α-reductase isozyme expression. *J Clin Invest* 92:903, 1993.
248. Nash AR, Glenn WK, Moore SS, Kerr J, Thompson AR, Thompson EOP: Oestrogen sulfotransferase: Molecular cloning and sequencing of cDNA for the bovine placental enzyme. *Aust J Biol Sci* 41:507, 1988.
249. Oeda T, Lee Y, Driscoll W, Chen H, Strott C: Molecular cloning and expression of full-length complementary DNA encoding the guinea pig adrenocortical estrogen sulfotransferase. *Mol Endocrinol* 6:1216, 1992.
250. Yen PH, Allen E, Marsh B, Mohandas T, Shapiro LJ: Cloning and expression of steroid sulfatase cDNA and the frequent occurrence of deletions: Implications for X-Y interchange. *Cell* 49:443, 1987.
251. Lakshmi V, Monder C: Evidence for independent 11-oxidase and 11-reductase activities of 11β-hydroxysteroid dehydrogenase: Enzyme latency, phase transitions and lipid requirements. *Endocrinology* 116:552, 1985.
252. Lakshmi V, Monder C: Purification and characterization of the corticosteroid 11β-dehydrogenase component of the rat liver 11β-hydroxysteroid dehydrogenase complex. *Endocrinology* 123:2390, 1988.
253. Agarwal AK, Monder C, Eckstein B, White PC: Cloning and expression of rat cDNA encoding corticosteroid 11β-dehydrogenase. *J Biol Chem* 264:18939, 1989.
254. Tannin GM, Agarwal AK, Monder C, New MI, White PC: The human gene for 11β-hydroxysteroid dehydrogenase. *J Biol Chem* 26:16653, 1991.
255. Moore CCD, Mellon SH, Murai J, Siiteri PK, Miller WL: Structure and function of the hepatic form of 11β-hydroxysteroid dehydrogenase in the squirrel monkey, an animal model of glucocorticoid resistance. *Endocrinology* 133: 368, 1993.
256. Edwards CRW, Burt D, McIntyre MA, deKloet ER, Stewart PM, Brett L, Sutanto WS, Monder C: Localization of 11β-hydroxysteroid dehydrogenase—tissue specific protector of the mineralocorticoid receptor. *Lancet* 2:986, 1988.
257. Funder JW, Pearce PT, Smith R, Smith AI: Mineralocorticoid action: Target tissue specificity is enzyme, not receptor, mediated. *Science* 242:583, 1988.
258. Arriza JL, Weinberger C, Cerelli G, Glaser TM, Handelin B, Housman DE, Evans RM: Cloning of human mineralocorticoid receptor complementary DNA: Structural and functional kinship with the glucocorticoid receptor. *Science* 237:268, 1987.
259. Ulick S, Levine LS, Gunczler P, Giovanni Z, Ramirez LC, Rauh W, Rosler A, Bradlow HL, et al: A syndrome of apparent mineralocorticoid excess associated with defects in the peripheral metabolism of cortisol. *J Clin Endocrinol Metab* 49:757, 1979.
260. Monder C, Shackleton CHL, Bradlow HL, New MI, Stoner E, Iohan F, Lakshmi V: The syndrome of apparent mineralocorticoid excess: Its association with 11-dehydrogenase and 5α-reductase deficiency and some consequences for corticosteroid metabolism. *J Clin Endocrinol Metab* 63:550, 1986.
261. Stewart PM, Corrie JET, Shackleton CHL, Edwards CRW: Syndrome of apparent mineralocorticoid excess: A defect in the cortisol-cortisone shuttle. *J Clin Invest* 82:340, 1988.
262. Stewart PM, Wallace AM, Valentino R, Burt D, Shackleton CHL, Edwards CRW: Mineralocorticoid activity of liquorice: 11-beta-hydroxysteroid dehydrogenase deficiency comes of age. *Lancet* 2:821, 1987.
263. Monder C, Stewart PM, Lakshmi V, Valentino R, Burt D, Edwards CRW: Licorice inhibits corticosteroid 11β-dehydrogenase of rat kidney and liver. *In vivo* and *in vitro* studies. *Endocrinology* 125:1046, 1989.
264. Naray-Fejes-Toth A, Watlington CO, Fejes-Toth G: 11β-hydroxysteroid dehydrogenase activity in the renal target cells of aldosterone. *Endocrinology* 129:17, 1991.
265. Rundle SE, Funder JW, Lakshmi V, Monder C: The intrarenal localization of mineralocorticoid receptors and 11β-dehydrogenase: Immunochemical studies. *Endocrinology* 125:1700, 1989.
266. Moisan MP, Edwards CRW, Seckl JR: Ontogeny of 11β-hydroxysteroid dehydrogenase in rat brain and kidney. *Endocrinology* 130:400, 1992.
267. Krozowski Z, Stuchberry S, White P, Monder C: Characterization of 11β-hydroxysteroid dehydrogenase gene expression: Identification of multiple unique forms of messenger ribonucleic acid in the rat kidney. *Endocrinology* 127:3009, 1990.
268. Mercer WR, Krozowski ZS: Localization of an 11β-hydroxysteroid dehydrogenase activity to the distal nephron: Evidence for the existence of two species of dehydrogenase in the rat kidney. *Endocrinology* 130:540, 1992.
269. Brown RW, Chapman KE, Edwards CRW, Seckl JR: Human placental 11β-hydroxysteroid dehydrogenase: Evidence for and partial purification of a distinct NAD-dependent isoform. *Endocrinology* 132:2614, 1993.
270. Pang SY, Clark A: Newborn screening, prenatal diagnosis, and prenatal treatment of congenital adrenal hyperplasia due to 21-hydroxylase deficiency. *Trends Endocrinol Metab* 1:300, 1990.
271. Sippell WG, Muller-Holve W, Dorr HG, Bidlingmaier F, Knorr D: Concentrations of aldosterone, corticosterone, 11-deoxy-corticosterone, progesterone, 17-hydroxy-progesterone, 11-deoxycortisol, cortisol, and cortisone determined simultaneously in human amniotic fluid throughout gestation. *J Clin Endocrinol Metab* 52:385, 1981.
272. Pasqualini JR, Nguyen BL, Uhrich F, Wiqvist N, Diczfalvay E: Cortisol and cortisone metabolism in the human fetoplacental unit at midgestation. *J Steroid Biochem* 1:209, 1970.
273. Fujieda K, Faiman C, Feyes FI, Winter JSD: The control of steroidogenesis by human fetal adrenal cells in tissue culture: IV. The effects of exposure to placental steroids. *J Clin Endocrinol Metab* 54:89, 1982.
274. Furutani Y, Morimoto Y, Shibahara S, Noda M, Takahashi H, Hirose T, Asai M, Inayama S, et al: Cloning and sequence analysis of cDNA for ovine corticotropin-releasing factor precursor. *Nature* 301:537, 1983.
275. Sawchenko PE, Swanson LW, Vale WW: Co-expression of

corticotropin-releasing factor and vasopressin immunoreactivity in parvocellular neurosecretory neurons of the adrenalectomized rat. *Proc Natl Acad Sci USA* 81:1883, 1984.

276. Whitnall MH, Mezey E, Gainer H: Co-localization of corticotropin-releasing factor and vasopressin in median eminence neurosecretory vesicles. *Nature* 317:248, 1985.
277. Miller WL: Molecular genetics of familial central diabetes insipidus. *J Clin Endocrinol Metab* 77:592, 1993.
278. Sasaki A, Liotta AS, Luckey MM, Margioris AN, Suda T, Krieger DT: Immunoreactive corticotropin-releasing factor is present in human maternal plasma during the third trimester of pregnancy. *J Clin Endocrinol Metab* 59:812, 1984.
279. Aguilera G, Harwood JP, Wilson JX, Morell J, Brown JH, Catt KJ: Mechanisms of action of corticotropin-releasing factor and other regulators of corticotropin release in rat pituitary cells. *J Biol Chem* 258:8039, 1983.
280. Vale W, Vaughan J, Smith M, Yamamoto G, Rivier J, Rivier C: Effects of synthetic ovine corticotropin-releasing factor, glucocorticoids, catecholamines, neurohypophyseal peptides, and other substances on cultured corticotropic cells. *Endocrinology* 113:1121, 1983.
281. Lamberts SWJ, Verleun T, Oosterom R, de Jong F, Hackeng WHL: Corticotropin-releasing factor (ovine) and vasopressin exert a synergistic effect on adrenocorticotropin release in man. *J Clin Endocrinol Metab* 58:298, 1984.
282. Tilders FJH, Berkenbosh F, Vermes I, Linton EA, Smelik PG: Role of epinephrine and vasopressin in the control of the pituitary-adrenal response to stress. *Fed Proc* 44:155, 1985.
283. Westlund KN, Aquilera G, Childs GV: Quantification of morphological changes in pituitary corticotropes produced by *in vivo* corticotropin-releasing factor stimulation and adrenalectomy. *Endocrinology* 116:439, 1985.
284. Nieuwenhuijzen-Kruseman AC, Linton EA, Lowry PJ, Rees LH, Besser GM: Corticotropin-releasing factor immunoreactivity in human gastrointestinal tract. *Lancet* 2: 1245, 1982.
285. De Souza EB, Perrin MH, Insel TR, Rivier J, Vale WW, Kuhar MJ: Corticotropin-releasing factor receptors in rat forebrain: Autoradiographic identification. *Science* 224: 1449, 1984.
285a. Baram TZ: Pathophysiology of massive infantile spasms: Perspective in the putative role of the brain-adrenal access. *Ann Neurol* 33:231, 1993.
286. Brown MR, Fisher LA, Spiess J, Rivier C, Rivier J, Vale W: Corticotropin-releasing factor: Actions on the sympathetic nervous system and metabolism. *Endocrinology* 111:928, 1982.
287. Nemeroff CB, Widerlov E, Bissette G, Walleus H, Karlsson I, Eklund K, Kilts CD, Loosen PT, et al: Elevated concentrations of CSF corticotropin-releasing factor-like immunoreactivity in depressed patients. *Science* 226: 1342, 1984.
288. Gillies GE, Linton EA, Lowry PJ: Corticotropin releasing activity of the new CRF is potentiated several times by vasopressin. *Nature* 299:355, 1982.
289. Rivier C, Vale W: Interaction of corticotropin-releasing factor and arginine vasopressin on adrenocorticotropin secretion *in vivo*. *Endocrinology* 113:939, 1983.
290. Rivier J, Rivier C, Vale W: Synthetic competitive antagonists of corticotropin-releasing factor: Effect on ACTH secretion in the rat. *Science* 224:870, 1984.
291. Linton EA, Tilders FJH, Hodgkinson S, Berkenbosch F, Vermes I, Lowry PJ: Stress-induced secretion of adrenocorticotropin in rats is inhibited by administration of antisera to ovine corticotropin-releasing factor and vasopressin. *Endocrinology* 116:966, 1985.
292. Plotsky PM, Bruhn TO, Vale W: Central modulation of immunoreactive corticotropin-releasing factor secretion by arginine vasopressin. *Endocrinology* 115:1639, 1984.
293. Ono N, Bedran de Castro JC, McCann SM: Ultrashort-loop positive feedback of corticotropin (ACTH)-releasing factor to enhance ACTH release in stress. *Proc Natl Acad Sci USA* 82:3528, 1985.
294. Ono N, Samson WK, McDonald JK, Lumpkin MD, Bedran De Castro JC, McCann SM: Effects of intravenous and intraventricular injection of antisera directed against corticotropin-releasing factor on the secretion of anterior pituitary hormones. *Proc Natl Acad Sci USA* 82:7787, 1985b.
295. Lewis DA, Sherman BM: Oxytocin does not influence adrenocorticotropin secretion in man. *J Clin Endocrinol Metab* 60:53, 1985.
296. Mezey E, Reisine TD, Brownstein MJ, Palkovits M, Axelrod J: β-Adrenergic mechanism of insulin induced adrenocorticotropin release from the anterior pituitary. *Science* 226:1085, 1984.
297. Miller WL, Johnson LK, Baxter JD, Roberts JL: Processing of the precursor to corticotropin and beta-lipoprotein in man. *Proc Natl Acad Sci USA* 77:5211, 1980.
298. Whitfeld PL, Seeburg PH, Shine J: The human proopiomelanocortin gene: Organization, sequence, and interspersion with repetitive DNA. *DNA* 1:133, 1982.
299. Miller WL, Baxter JD, Eberhardt NL: Peptide hormone genes: Structure and evolution, in Krieger DT, Martin JB (eds): *Brain Peptides*. New York, Wiley, 1983, p 15.
300. Lowry PJ, Silas L, McLean C, Linton EA, Estivariz FE: Pro-γ-melanocyte-stimulating hormone cleavage in adrenal gland undergoing compensatory growth. *Nature* 306:70, 1983.
301. Grunfeld C, Hagman J, Sakin EA, Buckley DI, Jones DS, Ramachandran J: Characterization of adrenocorticotropin receptors that appear when 3T3-L1 cells differentiate into adipocytes. *Endocrinology* 116:113, 1985.
302. Marshall JB, Kapcala LP, Manning LD, McCullough AJ: Effect of corticotropin-like intermediate lobe peptide on pancreatic exocrine function in isolated rat pancreatic lobules. *J Clin Invest* 74:1886, 1984.
303. Lymangrover JR, Buckalew VM, Harris J, Klein MC, Gruber KA: γ-2-MSH in natriuretic in the rat. *Endocrinology* 116:1227, 1985.
304. Miller WL, Johnson LK: Synthesis and glycosylation of proopiomelanocortin by a Cushing tumor. *J Clin Endocrinol Metab* 55:441, 1982.
305. Nicholson WE, Liddle RA, Puett D, Liddle GW: Adrenocorticotrophic hormone biotransformation, clearance and catabolism. *Endocrinology* 103:1344, 1978.
306. Hall PF: Trophic stimulation of steroidogenesis: In search of the elusive trigger. *Recent Prog Horm Res* 41:1, 1985.
307. Dickerman Z, Grant DR, Faiman C, Winter JSD: Intraadrenal steroid concentrations in man: Zonal differences and developmental changes. *J Clin Endocrinol Metab* 59:1031, 1984.
308. Cheitlin R, Buckley DI, Ramachandran J: The role of extra-cellular calcium in corticotropin-stimulated steroidogenesis. *J Biol Chem* 260:5323, 1985.
309. Catalano RD, Stuve L, Ramachandran J: Characterization of corticotropin receptors in human adrenocortical cells. *J Clin Endocrinol Metab* 62:300, 1986.
310. Kojima I, Kojima K, Rasmussen H: Role of calcium and cAMP in the action of adrenocorticotropin on aldosterone secretion. *J Biol Chem* 260:4248, 1985.
311. Gallo-Payet N, Escher E: Adrenocorticotropin receptors in rat adrenal glomerulosa cells. *Endocrinology* 117:38, 1985.
312. Hayashi K, Sala G, Catt KJ, Dufau ML: Regulation of steroidogenesis by adrenocorticotrophic hormone in isolated adrenal cells. *J Biol Chem* 254:6678, 1979.
313. Jagannadha Rao J, Long JA, Ramachandran J: Effects of

antiserum to adrenocorticotropin on adrenal growth and function. *Endocrinology* 102:371, 1978.
314. Ramasharma K, Li CH: Human pituitary and placental hormones control human insulin-like growth factor II secretion in human granulosa cells. *Proc Natl Acad Sci USA* 84:2643, 1987.
315. Miller WL: Regulation of mRNAs for human steroidogenic enzymes. *Endocr Res* 15:1, 1989.
316. Conneely OM, Headon DR, Olson CD, Ungar F, Dempsey ME: Intramitochondrial movement of adrenal sterol carrier protein with cholesterol in response to corticotropin. *Proc Natl Acad Sci USA* 81:2970, 1984.
317. Farese RV, Sabir AM: Polyphosphoinositides: Stimulator of mitochondrial cholesterol side chain cleavage and possible identification as an adrenocorticotropin-induced, cycloheximide-sensitive, cytosolid steroidogenesis factor. *Endocrinology* 106:1869, 1980.
318. Farese RV: Phospholipids as intermediates in hormone action. *Mol Cell Endocrinol* 35:1, 1984.
319. Saito E, Ichikawa Y, Homma M: Direct inhibitory effect of dexamethasone on steroidogenesis of human adrenal *in vivo*. *J Clin Endocrinol Metab* 48:861, 1979.
320. Rosenfield RL, Lucky AW, Helke J: Dexamethasone preparation does not alter corticoid and androgen responses to adrenocorticotropin. *J Clin Endocrinol Metab* 60:585, 1985.
321. Weitzman ED, Fukushima D, Nogeire C, Roffwarg H, Gallagher TF, Hellman L: Twenty four hour pattern of the episodic secretion of cortisol in normal subjects. *J Clin Endocrinol Metab* 33:14, 1971.
322. Krieger DT: Rhythms in CRF, ACTH, and corticosteroids, in Krieger DT (ed): *Endocrine Rhythms*. New York, Raven, 1979, p 123.
323. Goldman J, Wajchenberg BL, Liberman B, Nery M, Achando S, Germek OA: Contrast analysis for the evaluation of the circadian rhythms of plasma cortisol, androstenedione, and testosterone in normal men and the possible influence of meals. *J Clin Endocrinol Metab* 60:164, 1985.
324. Follenius M, Brandenberger G, Hietter B, Simqoni M, Reinhardt B: Diurnal cortisol peaks and their relationships to meals. *J Clin Endocrinol Metab* 55:757, 1982.
325. Dallman MF: Viewing the ventromedial hypothalamus from the adrenal gland. *Am J Physiol* 246:R1, 1984.
326. Fehm HL, Klein E, Holl R, Voigt FH: Evidence for extrapituitary mechanisms mediating the morning peak of plasma cortisol in man. *J Clin Endocrinol Metab* 58:410, 1984.
327. Schulte HM, Chrousos GP, Gold PW, Booth JD, Oldfield ED, Cutler GB Jr, Loriaux DL: Continuous administration of synthetic bovine corticotropin-releasing factor in man. *J Clin Invest* 75:1781, 1985.
328. Mellon PL, Windle JJ, Goldsmith PC, Padula CW, Roberts JL, Weiner RI: Immortalization of hypothalamic GnRH neurons by genetically targeted tumorigenesis. *Neuron* 5:1, 1990.
329. Kato H, Saito M, Suda M: Effect of starvation on the circadian adrenocortical rhythm in rats. *Endocrinology* 106:918, 1980.
330. Brandenberger G, Follqnius M, Muzet A, Simqoni M, Reinhardt B: Interactions between spontaneous and provoked cortisol secretory episodes in man. *J Clin Endocrinol Metab* 59:406, 1984.
331. Sherman B, Wysham C, Pfohl B: Age-related changes in the circadian rhythm of plasma cortisol in man. *J Clin Endocrinol Metab* 61:439, 1985.
332. Davis J, Morrill F, Fawcett J, Upton V, Bondy PK, Spiro HM: Apprehension and serum cortisol levels. *J Psychosom Res* 6:83, 1962.
333. Czeister CA, Ede MCM, Regenstein QR, Kisch ES, Fang US, Ehrlich EN: Episodic 24-hour cortisol secretory patterns in patients awaiting elective cardiac surgery. *J Clin Endocrinol Metab* 42:273, 1976.
334. Sutton JR, Casey JH: The adrenocortical response to competitive athletics in veteran athletes. *J Clin Endocrinol Metab* 40:135, 1975.
335. Dallman MF: Adrenal feedback on stress-induced corticoliberin (CRF) and corticotropin (ACTH) secretion, in Jones MT, Gillham B, Dallman MF, Chattopadahyay S (eds): *Interaction within the Brain-Pituitary Adrenocortical System*. New York, Academic, p 149, 1979.
336. Plumpton FS, Besser GM, Cole PV: Corticosteroid treatment and surgery: I. An investigation of the indications for steroid cover. *Anaesthesia* 24:3, 1969.
337. Dempsher DP, Gann DS: Increased cortisol secretion after small hemorrhage is not attributable to changes in adrenocorticotropin. *Endocrinology* 113:86, 1983.
338. Parker LN, Levin ER, Lifrak ER: Evidence for adrenocortical adaptation to severe illness. *J Clin Endocrinol Metab* 60:947, 1985.
339. Krieger DT: Rhythms of ACTH and corticosteroid secretion in health and disease and their experimental modification. *J Steroid Biochem* 6:785, 1975.
340. Linkowski P, Mendlewicz J, Leclercq R, Brasseur M, Hubain P, Goldstein J, Copinschi G, Van CE: The 24-hour profile of adrenocorticotropin and cortisol in major depressive illness. *J Clin Endocrinol Metab* 61:429, 1985.
341. Hotta M, Shibasaki T, Masuda A, Imaki T, Demura H, Ling N, Shizume K: The responses of plasma adrenocorticotropin and cortisol to corticotropin-releasing hormone (CRH) and cerebrospinal fluid immunoreactive CRH in anorexia nervosa patients. *J Clin Endocriol Metab* 62:319, 1986.
342. Plank J, Feldman JM: Modification of adrenal function by the antiserotonin agent cyproheptadine. *J Clin Endocrinol Metab* 42:291, 1976.
343. Chimara K, Kato Y, Maeda K, Matsukura S, Imura H: Suppression by cyproheptadine of human growth hormone and cortisol during sleep. *J Clin Invest* 57:1393, 1976.
344. Keller-Wood ME, Dallman ME: Corticosteroid inhibition of ACTH secretion. *Endocr Rev* 5:1, 1984.
345. Birnberg NC, Lissitzky J-C, Hinman M, Herbert E: Glucocorticoids regulate pro-opiomelanocortin gene expression *in vivo* at the levels of transcription and secretion. *Proc Natl Acad Sci USA* 80:6982, 1983.
346. Fehm HL, Voigt KH, Kummer G, Lang R, Pfeiffer EF: Differential and integral corticosteroid feedback effects on ACTH secretion in hypoadrenocorticism. *J Clin Invest* 63:247, 1979.
347. Widmaier EP, Dallman MF: The effects of corticotropin-releasing factor on adrenocorticotropin secretion from perfused pituitaries *in vitro:* Rapid inhibition by glucocorticoids. *Endocrinology* 115:2368, 1984.
348. Suda T, Tomori N, Tozawa F, Mouri T, Demura H, Shizume K: Effect of dexamethasone on immunoreactive corticotropin-releasing factor in the rat median eminence and intermediate-posterior pituitary. *Endocrinology* 114:851, 1984.
349. Davis LG, Arentzen R, Reid JM, Manning RW, Wolfson B, Lawrence KL, Baldino FJ: Glucocorticoid sensitivity of vasopressin mRNA levels in the paraventricular nucleus of the rat. *Proc Natl Acad Sci USA* 83:1145, 1986.
350. Tan SY, Mulrow PJ: The contribution of the zona fasciculata and glomerulosa to plasma 18-deoxycorticosterone levels in man. *J Clin Endocrinol Metab* 41:126, 1975.
351. Deschepper CF, Mellon SH, Cumin F, Baxter JD, Ganong WF: Analysis by immunocytochemistry and in situ hybridization of renin and its mRNA in kidney, testis, adrenal, and pituitary of the rat. *Proc Natl Acad Sci USA* 83:7552, 1986.
351a. Sander M, Ganten D, Mellon SH: The role of adrenal renin

in the regulation of adrenal steroidogenesis by ACTH. *Proc Natl Acad Sci USA* 91:148, 1994.

352. Hardman JA, Hort YJ, Catanzaro DF, Telloam JT, Baxter JD, Morris BJ, Shine J: Primary structure of the human renin gene. *DNA* 3:457, 1984.
353. Kramer RE, Gallant S, Brownie AC: Actions of angiotensin II on aldosterone biosynthesis in the rat adrenal cortex. *J Biol Chem* 255:3442, 1980.
354. Catt KJ, Harwood JP, Aquilera G, Dufau ML: Hormonal regulation of peptide receptors and target cell responses. *Nature* 280:109, 1979.
355. Fujita K, Aguilera G, Catt KJ: The role of cyclic AMP in aldosterone production by isolated zona glomerulosa cells. *J Biol Chem* 254:8567, 1979.
356. McAllister JM, Hornsby PJ: Dual regulation of 3β-hydroxysteroid dehydrogenase, 17α-hydroxylase, dehydroepiandrosterone sulfotransferase by adenosine 3′,5′-monophosphate and activators of protein kinase C in cultured human adrenocortical cells. *Endocrinology* 122:2012, 1988.
357. Staels B, Hum DW, Miller WL: Regulation of steroidogenesis in NCI-H295 cells: A cellular model of the human fetal adrenal. *Mol Endocrinol* 7:423, 1993.
358. Wong M, Rice DA, Parker KL, Schimmer BP: The roles of cAMP and cAMP-dependent protein kinase in the expression of cholesterol side-chain cleavage and steroid 11β-hydroxylase genes in mouse adrenocortical tumor cells. *J Biol Chem* 264:12867, 1989.
359. Mouw AR, Rice DA, Meade JC, Chua CS, White PC, Schimmer BP, Parker KL: Structural and functional analysis of the promoter region of the gene encoding mouse steroid 11β-hydroxylase. *J Biol Chem* 264:1305, 1989.
360. Rice DA, Aitkin LD, Vandenbark GR, Mouw AR, Franklin A, Schimmer BP, Parker KL: A cAMP-responsive element regulates expression of the mouse steroid 11β-hydroxylase gene. *J Biol Chem* 264:14011, 1989.
361. Bogerd AM, Franklin A, Rice DA, Schimmer BP, Parker KL: Identification and characterization of two upstream elements that regulate adrenocortical production of steroid 11β-hydroxylase. *Mol Endocrinol* 4:845, 1990.
362. Farese RV, Larson RE, Sabir MA, Gomez-Sanchez CE: Effects of angiotensin II, K^+, adrenocorticotropin, serotonin, adenosine 3′,5′-monophosphate, guanosine 3′,5′-monophosphate, A23187, and EGTA on aldosterone synthesis and phospholipid metabolism in the rat adrenal zona glomerulosa. *Endocrinology* 113:1377, 1983.
363. McKena TJ, Island DP, Nicholson WE, Liddle GW: The effects of potassium on early and late steps in aldosterone biosynthesis in cells of the zona glomerulosa. *Endocrinology* 103:1411, 1978.
364. Fraser R, Mason PA, Buckingham JC, Gordon RD, Morton JJ, Nicholls MG, Semple PF, Tree M: The interaction of sodium and potassium states, of ACTH and of angiotensin II in the control of corticosteroid secretion. *J Steroid Biochem* 11:1039, 1979.
365. Williams GH, Bailey LM: Effects of dietary sodium intake and potassium intake and acute stimulation on aldosterone output by isolated human cells. *J Clin Endocrinol Metab* 45:55, 1977.
366. Merriam GR, Baer L: Adrenocorticotropin deficiency: Correction of hyponatremia and hypoaldosteronism with chronic glucocorticoid therapy. *J Clin Endocrinol Metab* 50:10, 1980.
367. Gullner H-G, Gill JR Jr: Beta-endorphin selectively stimulates aldosterone secretion in hypophysectomized, nephrectomized dogs. *J Clin Invest* 71:124, 1983.
368. Yamakado AM, Franco-Saenz R, Mulrow PJ: Effect of sodium deficiency on β-melanocyte-stimulating hormone stimulation of aldosterone in isolated rat adrenal cells. *Endocrinology* 113:2168, 1983.
369. Seidah NG, Rochemont J, Hamelin J, Lis M, Chretien M: Primary structure of the major human pituitary pro-opiomelanocortin NH_2-terminal glycopeptide: Evidence for an aldosterone-stimulating activity. *J Biol Chem* 256:7977, 1981.
370. Scheider EG, Radke KJ, Ulderich DA, Taylor RE Jr: Effect of osmolality on aldosterone secretion. *Endocrinology* 116:1621, 1985.
371. Perez GO, Oster JR, Vaamondi CA, Katz FH: Effect of NH_4Cl on plasma aldosterone, cortisol and renin activity in supine man. *J Clin Endocrinol Metab* 45:762, 1977.
372. Sowers JR, Berg G, Martin VS, Mayes D: Dopaminergic modulation of aldosterone secretion in the rhesus monkey: Evidence that dopamine affects the late pathway of aldosterone biosynthesis by inhibiting the conversion of corticosterone to 18-hydroxycorticosterone. *Endocrinology* 110:1173, 1982.
373. Atarashi K, Mulrow PJ, Franco-Saenz R: Effect of atrial peptides on aldosterone production. *J Clin Invest* 76:1807, 1985.
374. Brown JJ, Fraser R, Lever AF, Morten JJ, Oelkeis W, Robertson JIS, Young J: Further observations on the relationship between plasma angiotensin II and aldosterone during sodium deprivation. *Excerpta Med Int Cong Ser* 302:148, 1973.
375. Yamaji T, Ishibashi M, Takaku F: Atrial natriuretic factor in human blood. *J Clin Invest* 76:1705, 1985.
376. Gardner DG, Hane S, Trachewsky D, Schenk D, Baxter JD: Atrial natriuretic peptide mRNA is regulated by glucocorticoids *in vivo*. *Biochem Biophys Res Commun* 139:1047, 1986.
377. Gardner DG, Gertz BJ, Deschepper CF, Kim DY: Gene for the rat atrial natriuretic peptide is regulated by glucocorticoids *in vitro*. *J Clin Invest* 82:1275, 1988.
378. Parker LN, Odell WD: Evidence for existence of cortical androgen-stimulating hormone. *Am J Physiol* 236:E616, 1979.
379. Parker LN, Odell WD: Control of adrenal androgen secretion. *Endocr Rev* 1:392, 1980.
380. Hauffa BP, Kaplan S, Grumbach MM: Dissociation between plasma adrenal androgens and cortisol in Cushing's disease and ectopic ACTH-producing tumour: Relation to adrenarche. *Lancet* 1:1373, 1984.
381. Voutilainen R, Riikonen R, Simell O, Perheentupa J: The effect of ACTH on serum dehydroepiandrosterone, androstenedione, testosterone, and 5α-dihydrotestosterone in infants. *J Steroid Biochem* 28:193, 1987.
382. Albertson BD, Hobson WC, Burnett BS, Turner PT, Clark RV, Schiebinger RJ, Loriaux DL, Cutler GB Jr: Dissociation of cortisol and adrenal androgen secretion in the hypophysectomized, adrenocorticotropin-replaced chimpanzee. *J Clin Endocrinol Metab* 59:13, 1984.
383. Rittmaster RS, Loriaux DL, Cutler GB Jr: Sensitivity of cortisol and adrenal androgens to dexamethasone suppression in hirsute women. *J Clin Endocrinol Metab* 61:462, 1985.
384. Zumoff B, Walsh BT, Katz JL, Lerin J, Rosenfeld RS, Kream J, Weiner H: Subnormal plasma dehydroisoandrosterone to cortisol ratio in anorexia nervosa: A second hormonal parameter of ontogenic regression. *J Clin Endocrinol Metab* 56:668, 1983.
385. Winterer J, Gwirtsman HE, George DT, Kaye WH, Loriaux DL, Cutler GB Jr: Adrenocorticotropin-stimulated adrenal androgen secretion in anorexia nervosa: Impaired secretion at low weight with normalization after long-term weight recovery. *J Clin Endocrinol Metab* 61:693, 1985.
386. Albright F, Smith PH, Fraser R: A syndrome characterized by primary ovarian insufficiency and decrease of stature: Report of 11 cases with digression on hormonal control of axillary and pubic hair. *Am J Med Sci* 204:625, 1942.
387. Korth-Schutz S, Levine L, New MI: Dehydroepiandrosterone sulfate (DS) levels, a rapid test for abnormal adrenal

androgen secretion. *J Clin Endocrinol Metab* 42:1005, 1976.

388. Korth-Schutz S, Levine L, New MI: Serum androgens in normal prepubertal and pubertal children and children with precocious adrenarche. *J Clin Endocrinol Metab* 42:117, 1976.
389. Vaitukaitis JL, Dale SL, Melby JC: Role of ACTH in the secretion of free dehydroepiandrosterone and its sulfate ester in man. *J Clin Endocrinol Metab* 29:1443, 1969.
390. Reiter EO, Fuldauer VG, Root AW: Secretion of the adrenal androgen, dehydroepiandrosterone sulfate, during normal infancy, childhood, and adolescence, in sick infants and in children with endocrinologic abnormalities. *J Pediatr* 90:766, 1977.
391. Nieschlag E, Loriaux DL, Ruder HJ, Zucker IR, Kirschner MA, Lipsett MB: The secretion of dehydroepiandrosterone and dehydroepiandrosterone sulphate in man. *J Endocrinol* 57:123, 1973.
392. Abraham GE, Chakmakjian ZH: Serum steroid levels during the menstrual cycle in a bilaterally adrenalectomized woman. *J Clin Endocrinol Metab* 37:581, 1973.
393. DePeretti E, Forest MG: Pattern of plasma dehyroepiandrosterone sulfate levels in humans from birth to adulthood: Evidence for testicular production. *J Clin Endocrinol Metab* 47:572, 1978.
394. Miller WL: The adrenal cortex, in Rudolph AM, Hoffman JIE, Rudolph CR (eds): *Rudolph's Pediatrics*, 19th ed. Norwalk, Conn., Appleton & Lange, 1991, p 1584.
395. Dohm G: The prepubertal and pubertal growth of the adrenal (adrenarche). *Beitr Pathol* 150:357, 1973.
396. Parker LN, Lifrak ET, Odell WD: A 60,000 molecular weight human pituitary glycopeptide stimulates adrenal androgen secretion. *Endocrinology* 113:2092, 1983.
397. Parker L, Lifrak E, Shively J, Lee T, Kaplan B, Walker P, Calaycay J, Florsheim W, et al: Human adrenal gland corticol androgen-stimulating hormone (CASH) is identical with a portion of the joining peptide of pituitary proopiomelanocortin (POMC). 71st Annual Meeting of the Endocrine Society, Seattle, Washington: Abstract 299, 1989.
398. Byrne GC, Perry YS, Winter JSD: Kinetic analysis of adrenal 3β-hydroxysteroid dehydrogenase activity during human development. *J Clin Endocrinol Metab* 60:934, 1985.
399. Carpenter CJ, Solomon N, Silverberg SG, Bledsoe T, Northcutt RC, Klinenberg JR, Bennett IL, McGehee HA: Schmidt's syndrome (thyroid and adrenal insufficiency): A review of the literature and a report of 15 new cases including 10 instances of co-existent diabetes mellitus. *Medicine (Baltimore)* 43:153, 1964.
400. Abraham GE: Ovarian and adrenal contribution to peripheral androgens during the menstrual cycle. *J Clin Endocrinol Metab* 39:340, 1974.
401. Carter JN, Tysen JE, Warne GJ, McNeilly AS, Faiman C, Friesen HG: Adrenocortical function in hyperprolactinemic women. *J Clin Endocrinol Metab* 45:973, 1977.
402. Siiteri PK: Qualitative and quantitative aspects of adrenal secretion of steroids, in Cristy NP (ed): *The Human Adrenal Cortex*. New York, Harper & Row, 1971, p 1.
403. Zumoff B, Fukushima DK, Hellman L: Intercomparison of four methods for measuring cortisol production. *J Clin Endocrinol Metab* 38:169, 1974.
404. Nelson DH: The adrenal cortex: Physiological function and disease, in Smith LH (ed): *Major Problems in Internal Medicine*. Philadelphia, Saunders, 1980, vol 18, p 1.
405. Migeon C: Adrenal androgens in man. *Am J Med* 53:606, 1972.
406. New MI, Seaman MP, Peterson RE: A method for the simultaneous determination of the secretion rates of cortisol, 11-deoxycortisol, corticosterone, 11-deoxycorticosterone and aldosterone. *J Clin Endocrinol Metab* 29:514, 1969.
407. Peterson RE: The miscible pool and turnover rate of adrenocortical steroids in man. *Recent Prog Horm Res* 15:231, 1959.
408. Schoneshofer M, Wagner GG: Sex differences in corticosteroids in man. *J Clin Endocrinol Metab* 45:814, 1977.
409. Zumoff B, Fukushima DK, Weitzman ED, Kream J, Hellman L: The sex difference in plasma cortisol concentration in man. *J Clin Endocrinol Metab* 39:805, 1974.
410. Esteban NV, Loughlin T, Yergey AL, Zawadzki JK, Booth JD, Winterer JC, Loriaux DL: Daily cortisol production rate in man determined by stable isotope dilution/mass spectrometry. *J Clin Endocrinol Metab* 72:39, 1991.
411. Linder BL, Esteban NV, Yergey AL, Winterer JC, Loriaux DL, Cassoria F: Cortisol production rate in childhood and adolescence. *J Pediatr* 117:892, 1990.
412. Kerrigan JR, Veldhuis JD, Leyo SA, Iranmanesh A, Rogol AD: Estimation of daily cortisol production and clearance rates in normal pubertal males by deconvolution analysis. *J Clin Endocrinol Metab* 76:1505, 1993.
413. Stearns HC, Sneeden VD, Fearl JD: A clinical and pathologic review of ovarian stromal hyperplasia and its possible relationship to common diseases of the female reproductive system. *Am J Obstet Gynecol* 119:375, 1974.
414. Bondy PK: The adrenal cortex, in Bondy PK, Rosenberg LE (eds): *Metabolic Control and Disease*. Philadelphia, Saunders, 1979, p 1427.
415. Longcope C: Adrenal and gonadal androgen secretion in normal females. *Clin Endocrinol Metab* 15:213, 1986.
416. Samuels LT, Nelson DH: Biosynthesis of corticosteroids, in Greep RO, Astood EB (eds): *Handbook of Physiology: Endocrinology*. Washington, D.C., American Physiological Society, 1975, vol 6, section 7, p 55.
417. Liddle GW: Regulation of adrenocortical function in man, in Christy NP (ed): *The Human Adrenal Cortex*. New York, Harper & Row, 1968, p 41.
418. Aguilera G, Catt KJ: Loci of action of regulators of aldosterone biosynthesis in isolated glomerulosa cells. *Endocrinology* 104:1046, 1980.
419. Schteingart DE, Tsao HS, Taylor CI, McKenzie A, Victoria R, Therrien BA: Sustained remission in Cushing's disease with mitotane and pituitary irradiation. *Ann Intern Med* 92:613, 1980.
420. Feldman D: Ketoconazole and other imidazole derivatives as inhibitors of steroidogenesis. *Endocr Rev* 7:409, 1986.
421. James VHT, Few JD: Adrenocorticosteroids: Chemistry, synthesis and disturbances in disease. *Clin Endocrinol Metab* 14:867, 1985.
422. Miller JW, Crapo L: The medical treatment of Cushing's syndrome. *Endocr Rev* 14:443, 1993.
423. Schteingart DE: Cushing's syndrome. *Endocrinol Metab Clin North Am* 18:311, 1989.
424. Luton JP, Mahoudeau JA, Bouchard PH, Thiebolt PH, Hautecouverture M, Simon D, Laudat MH, Touitou Y, et al: Treatment of Cushing's disease by o,p′-DDD: Survey of 62 cases. *N Engl J Med* 300:459, 1979.
425. Verheist JA, Trainer PJ, Howlett TA, Perry L, Rees LH, Grossman AB, Wass JAH, Besser GM: Short and long-term responses to metyrapone in the medical management of 91 patients with Cushing's syndrome. *Clin Endocrinol* 35:169, 1991.
426. Child DF, Burke CW, Burley DM, Rees LH, Russell Fraser T: Drug control of Cushing's syndrome: Combined aminoglutethimide and metyrapone therapy. *Acta Endocrinol* 82:330, 1976.
427. Samojlik E, Veldhius JD, Wells SA, Santen RJ: Preservation of androgen secretion during estrogen suppression with aminoglutethimide in the treatment of metastatic breast cancer. *J Clin Invest* 65:602, 1980.
428. Dewis P, Anderson C, Bu'lock DE, Earnshaw R, Kelly WF: Experience with Trilostane in the treatment of Cushing's syndrome. *Clin Endocrinol* 18:533, 1983.
429. Komanicky P, Spark RF, Melby JC: Treatment of Cush-

ing's syndrome with trilostane (WIN 24,250), an inhibitor of adrenal steroid biosynthesis. *J Clin Endocrinol Metab* 47:1024, 1978.

430. Sonino N, Boscaro M, Merola G, Mantero F: Prolonged treatment of Cushing's disease by ketoconazole. *J Clin Endocrinol Metab* 61:718, 1985.
431. Sonino N, Boscaro M, Paoletta A, Mantero F, Ziliotto D: Ketoconazole treatment in Cushing's syndrome: Experience in 34 patients. *Clin Endocrinol* 35:347, 1991.
432. Wagner RL, White PF, Kan PB, Rosenthal MH, Feldman D: Inhibition of adrenal steroidogenesis by the anesthetic etomidate. *N Engl J Med* 310:1415, 1984.
433. Schulte HM, Benker G, Reinwein D, Sippell WG, Allolio B: Infusion of low dose etomidate: Correction of hypercortisolemia in patients with Cushing's syndrome and dose-response relationship in normal subjects. *J Clin Endocrinol Metab* 70:1426, 1990.
434. Wilson ID, Goetz FC: Selective hypoaldosteronism after prolonged heparin administration. *Am J Med* 36:635, 1964.
435. Tuck ML, Sowers JR, Fittingoff DB, Fisher JS, Berg GJ, Asp ND, Mayes DM: Plasma corticosteroid concentrations during spironolactone administration: Evidence for adrenal biosynthetic blockade in man. *J Clin Endocrinol Metab* 52:1057, 1981.
436. Ballard PL: Delivery and transport of glucocorticoids to target cells, in Baxter JD, Rousseau GG (eds): *Glucocorticoid Hormone Action*. New York, Springer-Verlag, 1979, p 25.
437. Sandberg AA, Slaunwhite WR Jr: Physical state of adrenal cortical hormones in plasma, in Christy NP (ed): *The Human Adrenal Cortex*. New York, Harper & Row, 1971, p 69.
438. Westphal U: *Steroid-Protein Interactions*. New York, Springer-Verlag, 1971.
439. Dunn JF, Nisula BC, Rodbard D: Transport of steroid hormones. Binding of 21 endogenous steroids to both testosterone-binding globulin and corticosteroid-binding globulin in human plasma. *J Clin Endocrinol Metab* 53:58, 1981.
440. Partridge WM, Sakiyama R, Judd HL: Protein bound corticosterone in human serum is selectively transported into rat brain and liver *in vivo*. *J Clin Endocrinol Metab* 57:160, 1983.
441. Siiteri PK, Murai JT, Hammond GL, Nisker JA, Raymoure WJ, Kuhn RW: The serum transport of steroid hormones. *Recent Prog Horm Res* 38:457, 1982.
442. Wolf G, Armstrong EG, Rosner W: Synthesis *in vitro* of corticosteroid-binding globulin from rat liver messenger ribonucleic acid. *Endocrinology* 108:805, 1981.
443. Hammond GL, Smith CL, Goping IS, Underhill DA, Harley MJ, Reventos J, Musto NA, Gunsalus GL, et al: Primary structure of human corticosteroid binding globulin, deduced from hepatic and pulmonary cDNAs, exhibits homology with serine protease inhibitors. *Proc Natl Acad Sci USA* 84:5153, 1987.
444. Hammond GL: Molecular properties of corticosteroid binding globulin and the sex-steroid binding proteins. *Endocr Rev* 11:65, 1990.
445. Rosner W: Plasma steroid-binding proteins. *Endocrinol Metab Clin North Am* 20:697, 1991.
446. Perrot-Applanat M, Racodot O, Milgrom E: Specific localization of plasma corticosteroid binding globulin immunoreactivity in pituitary corticotrophs. *Endocrinology* 115: 559, 1984.
447. Hammond GL, Smith CL, Paterson NAM, Sibbald WJ: A role for corticosteroid-binding globulin in delivery of cortisol to activated neutrophils. *J Clin Endocrinol Metab* 71:34, 1990.
448. Rosner W: The functions of corticosteroid-binding globulin and sex hormone-binding globulin: recent advances. *Endocr Rev* 11:80, 1990.
449. Ogawa T, Sudea K, Matsui N: The effect of cortisol, progesterone, and transcortin on phytohemagglutinin-stimulated human blood mononuclear cells and their interplay. *J Clin Endocrinol Metab* 56:121, 1983.
450. Pugeat MM, Dunn JF, Nisula BC: Transport of steroid hormones: Interaction of 70 drugs with testosterone-binding globulin and corticosteroid-binding globulin in human plasma. *J Clin Endocrinol Metab* 53:69, 1981.
451. DeMoor P, Louwagie A, Van Baelen H, Van de Putte I: Unexplained high transcortin levels in patients with various hematological disorders and in their relatives: A connection between these high transcortin levels and HLA antigen B12. *J Clin Endocrinol Metab* 50:421, 1980.
452. Coolens JL, Heyns W: Marked elevation and cyclic variation of corticosteroid-binding globulin: An inherited abnormality. *J Clin Endocrinol Metab* 68:492, 1989.
453. Orbach O, Schussler GG: Increased serum cortisol binding in chronic active hepatitis. *Am J Med* 39, 1989.
454. Kawai S, Ichikawa Y, Homma M: Differences in metabolic properties among cortisol, prednisolone and dexamethasone in liver and renal diseases. Accelerated metabolism of dexamethasone in renal failure. *J Clin Endocrinol Metab* 60:848, 1985.
455. Roitman A, Bruchis S, Bauman B, Kaufman H, Laron Z: Total deficiency of corticosteroid-binding globulin. *Clin Endocrinol* 21:541, 1984.
456. Doe RP, Lohrenz FN, Seal US: Familial decrease in corticosteroid-binding globulin. *Metabolism* 14:940, 1965.
457. Mendel CM, Kuhn RW, Weisiger RA, Cavalieri RR, Siiteri PK, Cunha GR, Murai JT: Uptake of cortisol by the perfused rat liver: Validity of the free hormone hypothesis applied to cortisol. *Endocrinology* 124:468, 1989.
458. Mendel CM: The free hormone hypothesis: A physiologically based mathematical model. *Endocr Rev* 10:232, 1989.
459. Partridge WM: Transport of protein-bound hormones into tissues *in vivo*. *Endocr Rev* 2:103, 1981.
460. Mendel CM, Weisiger RA, Jones AL, Cavalieri RR: Thyroid hormone-binding proteins in plasma facilitate uniform distribution of thyroxine within tissues: A perfused rat liver study. *Endocrinology* 120:1987, 1987.
461. Zager PG, Burtis WJ, Luetscher JA, Dowdy AJ, Sood S: Increased plasma protein binding and low metabolic clearance rate of aldosterone in plasma of low cortisol concentration. *J Clin Endocrinol Metab* 42:207, 1976.
462. Zipser RD, Meidor V, Horton R: Characteristics of aldosterone binding in human plasma. *J Clin Endocrinol Metab* 50:158, 1979.
463. Chanarri M, Luetscher JA, Dowdy AJ, Ganguly A: The effects of temperature and plasma cortisol on distribution of aldosterone between plasma and red blood cells: Influences on metabolic clearance rate and on hepatic and renal extraction of aldosterone. *J Clin Endocrinol Metab* 44:752, 1977.
464. Matulich DT, Morris JA, Bartter FC, Baxter JD: Unpublished data.
465. Plager JE: The binding of androsterone sulfate, etiocholanolone sulfate and dehydroisoandrosterone sulfate by plasma protein. *J Clin Invest* 44:1234, 1965.
466. Forest MG, Rinarola MA, Migeon CJ: Percentage binding of testosterone, androstenedione and dehydroisoandrosterone in human plasma. *Steroids* 12:323, 1968.
467. Pearlman WH, Crepy O, Murphy M: Testosterone-binding levels in the serum of women during the normal menstrual cycle, pregnancy and the post-partum period. *J Clin Endocrinol Metab* 27:1012, 1967.
468. Peterson RE: Metabolism of adrenal cortical steroids, in Christy NP (ed): *The Human Adrenal Cortex*. New York, Harper & Row, 1971, p 87.
469. Brooks RV: Biosynthesis and metabolism of adrenocortical steroids, in James VHT (ed): *The Adrenal Gland*. New York, Raven, 1979, p 67.

470. Monder C, Bradlow LH: Cortoic acids: Exploration at the frontier of corticosteroid metabolism. *Recent Prog Horm Res* 36:345, 1980.
471. Bradlow HL, Monder C, Zumoff B: Metabolism of cortoic acids in man. *J Clin Endocrinol Metab* 54:296, 1982.
472. Peterson KE: The production of cortisol and corticosterone in children. *Acta Paediatr Scand* 281:2, 1980.
473. Abramovitz M, Branchaud CL, Pearson-Murphy BE: Cortisol-cortisone interconversion in human fetal lung: Contrasting results using explant and monolayer cultures suggest that β-hydroxysteroid dehydrogenase (EC 1.1.1.146) comprises two enzymes. *J Clin Endocrinol Metab* 54:563, 1982.
474. Ulstrom RA, Colle E, Burkey J, Gummelle R: Adrenocortical steroid metabolism in newborn infants: II. Urinary excretion of 6β-hydroxycortisol and other polar metabolites. *J Clin Endocrinol Metab* 20:1080, 1961.
475. Werk EE, MacGee J, Sholiton LJ: Altered cortisol metabolism in advanced cancer and other terminal illnesses: Excretion of 6β-hydroxycortisol. *Metabolism* 13:1425, 1964.
476. Katz FH, Lipman MM, Frantz AG, Jailer JW: The physiologic significance of β-hydroxycortisol in human corticoid metabolism. *J Clin Endocrinol Metab* 22:71, 1962.
477. Pasqualini JR, Jayle MR: Corticosteroid 21-sulphates in human urine. *Biochem J* 81:147, 1961.
478. Drucker WD, Sfikakis A, Borowski AJ, Christy NP: On the rate of formation of steroidal glucuronides in patients with familial and acquired jaundice. *J Clin Invest* 43:1952, 1964.
479. Whitworth JA, Stewart PM, Burt D, Atherden SM, Edwards CRW: The kidney is the major site of cortisone production in man. *Clin Endocrinol* 31:355, 1989.
480. Morris DJ: The metabolism and mechanism of action of aldosterone. *Endocr Rev* 2:234, 1981.
481. Luetscher JA, Hancock EW, Camargo CA, Dowdy AJ, Nokes GW: Conjugation of 1,2-^{3}H-aldosterone in human liver and kidneys and renal extraction of aldosterone and labeled conjugates from blood plasma. *J Clin Endocrinol Metab* 25:628, 1965.
482. Parker L: *Adrenal Androgens in Clinical Medicine*. San Diego, Academic Press, 1989.
483. Parker LN: Control of adrenal androgen secretion. *Endocrinol Metab Clin North Am* 20:401, 1991.
484. Meikle AW, Daynes RA, Araneo BA: Adrenal androgen secretion and biologic effects. *Endocrinol Metab Clin North Am* 20:381, 1991.
485. Pratt JH, Grim CE, Parkinson CA: Minoxidil increases aldosterone metabolic clearance in hypertensive patients. *J Clin Endocrinol Metab* 49:834, 1979.
486. Doehr P, Fichter M, Pirke KM, Lund R: Relationship between weight gain and hypothalamic pituitary adrenal function in patients with anorexia nervosa. *J Steroid Biochem* 13:529, 1980.
487. Gaunt R: History of the adrenal cortex, in Greep RO, Astwood EB (eds): *Handbook of Physiology: Endocrinology*. Washington, DC, American Physiological Society, 1975, section 7, vol 6, p 1.
488. Tan SY, Mulrow PJ: Aldosterone in hypertension and edema, in Bondy PK, Rosenberg LE (eds): *Metabolic Control and Disease*. Philadelphia, Saunders, 1979, p 1501.
489. Baxter JD: Glucocorticoid hormone action, in Gill GN (ed): *Pharmacology of Adrenal Cortical Hormones*. Oxford, Pergamon, 1979, p 67.
490. Bloom E, Matulich DT, Higgins SJ, Simons SJ, Baxter JD: Nuclear binding of glucocorticoid receptors: Relations between cytosol binding, activation and the biological response. *J Steroid Biochem* 12:175, 1980.
491. Lan NC, Karin M, Nguyen T, Weisz A, Birnbaum MJ, Eberhardt NL, Baxter JD: Mechanisms of glucocorticoid hormone action. *J Steroid Biochem* 20:77, 1984.
492. Yamamoto KR: Steroid receptor regulated transcription of specific genes and gene networks. *Annu Rev Genet* 19:209, 1985.
493. Singh VB, Moudgil VK: Phosphorylation of rat liver glucocorticoid receptor. *J Biol Chem* 260:3684, 1985.
494. Moudgil VK: Phosphorylation of steroid hormone receptors. *Biochim Biophys Acta* 1055:243, 1990.
495. Duval D, Durant S, Homo-Delarche F: Non-genomic effects of steroids: Interactions of steroid molecules with membrane structures and functions. *Biochim Biophys Acta* 737:409, 1983.
496. Raghow R, Gossage D, Kang AH: Pretranslational regulation of type I collagen, fibronectin, and a 50-kilodalton noncollagenous extracellular protein by dexamethasone in rat fibroblasts. *J Biol Chem* 261:4677, 1986.
497. Fulton R, Birnie DG, Knowler JT: Post-transcriptional regulation of rat liver gene expression by glucocorticoids. *Nucleic Acids Res* 13:6467, 1985.
498. Birnberg NC, Lissitzky J-C, Hinman M, Herbert E: Glucocorticoids regulate pro-opiomelanocortin gene expression *in vivo* at the levels of transcription and secretion. *Proc Natl Acad Sci USA* 80:6982, 1983.
499. Keller-Wood ME, Dallman MF: Corticosteroid inhibition of ACTH secretion. *Endocr Rev* 5:1, 1984.
500. Fehm HL, Voigt KH, Kummer G, Lang R, Pfeiffer EF: Differential and integral corticosteroid feedback effects on ACTH secretion in hypoadrenocorticism. *J Clin Invest* 63:247, 1979.
501. Widmaier EP, Dallman MF: The effects of corticotropin-releasing factor on adrenocorticotropin secretion from perfused pituitaries *in vitro:* Rapid inhibition by glucocorticoids. *Endocrinology* 115:2368, 1984.
502. Jones MT, Gillham B: Factors involved in the regulation of adrenocorticotropic hormone/β-lipotropic hormone. *Physiol Rev* 68:743, 1988.
503. Dallman MF, Akana SF, Cascio CS, Darlington DN, Jacobson L, Levin N: Regulation of ACTH secretion: Variations on a theme of B. *Recent Prog Horm Res* 43:113, 1987.
504. Krozowski ZS, Funder JW: Renal mineralocorticoid receptors and hippocampal corticosterone binding species have identical intrinsic steroid specificity. *Proc Natl Acad Sci USA* 80:6056, 1983.
505. Reul MJH, de Kloet ER: Two receptor systems for corticosterone in rat brain: Microdistribution and differential occupation. *Endocrinology* 117:2505, 1985.
506. Beaumont K, Fanestil DD: Characterizaztion of rat brain aldosterone receptors reveals high affinity for corticosterone. *Endocrinology* 113:2043, 1983.
507. Lakshmi V, Monder C: Evidence for independent 11-oxidase and 11-reductase activities of 11β-hydroxysteroid dehydrogenase: Enzyme latency, phase transitions and lipid requirements. *Endocrinology* 116:552, 1985.
508. Lakshmi V, Monder C: Purification and characterization of the corticosteroid 11β-dehydrogenase component of the rat liver 11β-hydroxysteroid dehydrogenase complex. *Endocrinology* 123:2390, 1988.
509. Funder JW: Mineralocorticoids, glucocorticoids, receptors and response elements. *Science* 259:1132, 1993.
510. Pearce D, Yamamoto KR: Mineralocorticoid and glucocorticoid receptor activities distinguished by nonreceptor factors at a composite response element. *Science* 259:1161, 1993.
511. Ponta H, Kennedy N, Skroch P, Hynes NE, Groner B: Hormonal response region in the mouse mammary tumor virus long terminal repeat can be dissociated from the proviral promoter and has enhancer properties. *Proc Natl Acad Sci USA* 82:1020, 1985.
512. Slater EP, Rabenau O, Karin M, Baxter JD, Beato M: Glucocorticoid receptor binding and activation of a heterologous promoter by dexamethasone by the first intron of the human growth hormone gene. *Mol Cell Biol* 5:2984, 1985.

513. Rousseau GG, van Bohemen GC, Lareau S, Degelaen J: Submicromolar free calcium modulates dexamethasone binding to the glucocorticoid receptor. *Biochem Biophys Res Commun* 106:16, 1982.
514. Holbrook NJ, Bodwell JE, Munck A: Effects of ATP and pyrophosphate on properties of glucocorticoid-receptor complexes from rat thymus cells. *J Biol Chem* 258:14885, 1983.
515. Beyer HS, Carr FE, Mariash CN, Oppenheimer JH: Hepatic messenger ribonucleic acid activity profile of rats subjected to alterations in thyroidal and adrenocortical states: Evidence for significant interaction. *Endocrinology* 116:2669, 1985.
516. Rousseau GG, Baxter JD: Glucocorticoid receptors, in Baxter JD, Rousseau GG (eds): *Glucocorticoid Hormone Action*. New York, Springer-Verlag, 1979, p 49.
517. Chrousos GP, Cutler GB Jr, Sauer M, Simons SS Jr, Loriaux DL: Development of glucocorticoid antagonists. *Pharmacol Ther* 20:263, 1983.
518. Healy DL, Chrousos GP, Schulte HM, Gold PW, Hodgen GD: Increased adrenocorticotropin, cortisol, and arginine vasopressin secretion in primates after the antiglucocorticoid steroid RU 486: Dose response relationshps. *J Clin Endocrinol Metab* 60:1, 1985.
519. Schmidt TJ: Comparison of *in vivo* activation of triamcinolone acetonide- and RU 38486-receptor complexes in the CEM-C7 and IM-9 human leukemic cell lines. *Cancer Res* 49:4390, 1989.
520. Schmidt TJ: *In vitro* activation and DNA binding affinity of human lymphoid (CEM-C7) cytoplasmic receptors labeled with the antiglucocorticoid RU38486. *J Steroid Biochem* 24:1986.
521. Gruol DJ, Wolfe KA: Transformation of glucocorticoid receptors bound to the antagonist RU 486: Effects of aldaline phosphatase. *Biochemistry* 29:7958, 1990.
522. Bourgeois S, Pfahl M, Baulieu E-E: DNA binding properties of glucocorticosteroid receptors bound to the steroid antagonist RU-486. *EMBO J* 3:751, 1984.
523. Wolff ME: Structure-activity relationships in glucocorticoids, in Baxter JD, Rousseau GG (eds): *Glucocorticoid Hormone Action*. New York, Springer-Verlag, 1979, p 97.
524. Baulieu E-E: The antisteroid RU486: Its cellular and molecular mode of action. *Trends Endocrinol Metab* 2:233, 1991.
525. Spitz IM, Bardin CW: Mifepristone (RU486)—a modulator of progestin and glucorticoid action. *N Engl J Med* 329:404, 1993.
526. Nieman LK, Chrousos GP, Kellner C, Spitz IM, Nisula BC, Cutler GB Jr, Merriam GR, Bardin CW, et al: Successful treatment of Cushing's syndrome with the glucocorticoid antagonist RU-486. *J Clin Endocrinol Metab* 61:536, 1985.
527. Meikle AW, Tyler FH: Potency and duration of action of glucocorticoids: Effects of hydrocortisone, prednisone and dexamethasone on human pituitary adrenal function. *Am J Med* 63:200, 1977.
528. Rousseau GG, Baxter JD: Glucocorticoids and the metabolic code, in Baxter JD, Rousseau GG (eds): *Glucocorticoid Hormone Action*. New York: Springer-Verlag, 1979, p 613.
529. Cahill GF: Action of adrenal cortical steroids on carbohydrate metabolism, in Christy NP (ed): *The Human Adrenal Cortex*. New York, Harper & Row, 1971, p 205.
530. Exton JH: Regulation of gluconeogenesis by glucocorticoids, in Baxter JD, Rousseau GG (eds): *Glucocorticoid Hormone Action*. New York, Springer-Verlag, 1979, p 535.
531. Stalmans W, Laloux M: Glucocorticoids and hepatic glycogen metabolism, in Baxter JD, Rousseau GG (eds): *Glucocorticoid Hormone Action*. New York, Springer-Verlag, 1979, p 517.
532. Lenzen S, Bailey CJ: Thyroid hormones, gonadal and adrenocortical steroids and the function of the islets of Langerhans. *Endocr Rev* 5:411, 1984.
533. Coufalik AH, Monder C: Stimulation of gluconeogenesis by cortisol in fetal rat liver in organ culture. *Endocrinology* 108:1132, 1981.
534. Goldberg AL, Tischler M, DeMortino G, Griffin G: Hormonal regulation of protein degradation and synthesis in skeletal muscle. *Fed Proc* 39:31, 1980.
535. Wise JK, Hendler R, Felig P: Influences of glucocorticoids on glucagon secretion and plasma amino acid concentrations in man. *J Clin Invest* 52:2774, 1973.
536. Tomas FM, Munro HN, Young VR: Effect of glucocorticoid administration on the rate of muscle protein breakdown *in vivo* in rats, as measured by urinary excretion of N-methylhistidine. *Biochem J* 178:139, 1979.
537. Odedra B, Millward D: Effect of corticosterone treatment on muscle protein turnover in adrenalectomized rats and diabetic rats maintained on insulin. *Biochem J* 204:663, 1982.
538. Simmons PS, Miles JM, Gerich JE, Haymond MW: Increased proteolysis: An effect of increased plasma cortisol within the physiologic range. *J Clin Invest* 73:412, 1984.
539. Shamoon H, Soman V, Sherwin RS: The influence of acute physiological increments of cortisol on fuel metabolism and insulin binding to monocytes in normal humans. *J Clin Endocrinol Metab* 50:495, 1980.
540. Carter-Su C, Okamoto K: Effect of glucocorticoids on hexose transport in rat adipocytes. *J Biol Chem* 260:11091, 1985.
541. Fain JN: Inhibition of glucose transport in fat cells and activation of lipolysis by glucocorticoids, in Baxter JD, Rousseau GG (eds): *Glucocorticoid Hormone Action*. New York, Springer-Verlag, 1979, p 7.
542. Munck A, Crabtree GR, Smith KA: Glucocorticoid receptors and actions in rat thymocytes and immunologically-stimulated human peripheral lymphocytes, in Baxter JD, Rousseau GG (eds): *Glucocorticoid Hormone Action*. New York, Springer-Verlag, 1979, p 341.
543. Rizza RA, Mandarino LJ, Gerich JE: Cortisol-induced insulin resistance in man: Impaired suppression of glucose production and stimulation of glucose utilization due to a post-receptor defect of insulin action. *J Clin Endocrinol Metab* 54:131, 1982.
544. Gaca G, Bernend K: Plasma glucose, insulin and free fatty acids during long term corticosteroid treatment in children. *Acta Endocrinol (Copenh)* 77:699, 1974.
545. Murray DK, Ruhmann-Wennhold A, Nelson DH: Adrenalectomy decreases the sphingomyelin and cholesterol content of fat cell ghosts. *Endocrinology* 111:452, 1982.
546. Nelson DH: Corticosteroid induced changes in phospholipid membranes as mediators of their action. *Endocr Rev* 1:180, 1980.
547. Taskinen M-R, Nikkila EA, Pelkonen R, Sane T: Plasma lipoproteins, lipolytic enzymes, and very low density lipoprotein triglyceride turnover in Cushing's syndrome. *J Clin Endocrinol Metab* 57:619, 1983.
548. Baxter JD: Mechanisms of glucocorticoid inhibition of growth. *Kidney Int* 14:330, 1978.
549. Loeb JN: Corticosteroids and growth. *N Engl J Med* 295:547, 1976.
550. Baxter JD, Rousseau GG: Glucocorticoid hormone action: An overview, in Baxter JD, Rousseau GG (eds): *Glucocorticoid Hormone Action*. New York, Springer-Verlag, 1979, p 1.
551. Ernest MJ, Feigelsen P: Multihormonal control of tyrosine aminotransferase in isolated liver cells, in Baxter JD, Rousseau GG (eds): *Glucocorticoid Hormone Action*. New York, Springer-Verlag, 1979, p 219.
552. Clark AF, Vignos PJ: Experimental corticosteroid myopathy: Effect on myofibrillar ATPase activity and protein degradation. *Muscle Nerve* 2:265, 1979.

553. Clark AF, Vignos PJ: The role of proteases in experimental glucocorticoid myopathy. *Muscle Nerve* 4:219, 1981.
554. Parrillo JE, Fauci AS: Mechanisms of glucocorticoid action on immune processes. *Annu Rev Pharmacol Toxicol* 19:179, 1979.
555. Glaman NH: How corticosteroids work. *J Allergy Clin Immunol* 55:145, 1975.
556. Saxon A, Stevens RH, Ramer SJ, Clements PJ, Yu DTY: Glucocorticoids administered *in vivo* inhibit suppressor T lymphocyte function and diminish B lymphocyte responsiveness in *in vivo* immunoglobulin synthesis. *J Clin Invest* 61:922, 1978.
557. Fauci AS, Dale DC, Balow JE: Glucocorticoid therapy: Mechanisms of action and clinical considerations. *Ann Intern Med* 84:304, 1976.
558. Craddock CG: Corticosteroid-induced lymphopenia, immunosuppression and body defense. *Ann Intern Med* 88:564, 1978.
559. Casey LM, MacDonald PC, Mitchell MD: Despite a massive increase in cortisol secretion in women during parturition, there is an equally massive increase in prostaglandin synthesis. *J Clin Invest* 75:1852, 1985.
560. Munck A, Guyre PM, Holbrook NJ: Physiological functions of glucocorticoids in stress and their relation to pharmacological actions. *Endocr Rev* 5:25, 1984.
561. Goodwin JS, Atluru D, Sierakowski S, Lianos EA: Mechanism of action of glucocorticosteroids: Inhibition of T cell proliferation and interleukin 2 production by hydrocortisone is reversed by leukotriene B_4. *J Clin Invest* 77:1244, 1986.
562. Larsen GL, Henson PM: Mediators of inflammation. *Annu Rev Immunol* 1:335, 1983.
563. Fahey JV, Guyre PM, Munck A: Mechanisms of anti-inflammatory actions of glucocorticoids, in Weissman G (ed): *Advances in Inflammatory Research*. New York, Raven, 1981, vol 2, p 21.
564. Goetzl EJ: Oxygenation products of arachidonic acid as mediators of hypersensitivity and inflammation. *Med Clin North Am* 65:809, 1981.
565. Flower RJ: The mediators of steroid action. *Nature* 320:20, 1986.
566. Johnson LK, Baxter JD: The mechanism of action of adrenocorticosteroids at the molecular level, in McCarty D (ed): *Landmark Advances in Rheumatology*. New York, Contact Associates, 1985, p 13.
567. Naray-Fejes-Toth A, Fejes-Toth G, Fischer C, Frolich JC: Effect of dexamethasone on *in vivo* prostanoid production in the rabbit. *J Clin Invest* 74:120, 1984.
568. Beutler B, Cerami A: Cachectin and tumour necrosis factor as two sides of the same biological coin. *Nature* 320:584, 1986.
569. Wallner B, Mattalino RJ, Hession L, Cate RL, Tizard R, Sinclair LK, Foeller C, Chow EP, et al: Cloning and expression of human lipocortin, a phospholipase A2 inhibitor with potential anti-inflammatory activity. *Nature* 320:77, 1986.
570. Altman LC, Hill JS, Hairfield WM, Mullarkey MF: Effects of corticosteroids on eosinophil chemotaxis and adherence. *J Clin Invest* 67:28, 1981.
571. Shoenfeld Y, Gurewich Y, Gallant LA, Pinkhas J: Prednisone-induced leukocytosis: Influence of dosage, method and duration of administration on the degree of leukocytosis. *Am J Med* 71:773, 1981.
572. Lippman ME: Glucocorticoid receptors and effects in human lymphoid and leukemic cells, in Baxter JD, Rousseau GG (eds): *Glucocorticoid Hormone Action*. New York, Springer-Verlag, 1979, p 377.
573. Maytin EV, Young DA: Separate glucocorticoid, heavy metal, and heat shock domains in thymic lymphocytes. *J Biol Chem* 258:12718, 1983.
574. Compton MM, Cidlowski JA: Rapid *in vivo* effects of glucocorticoids on the integrity of rat lymphocyte genomic deoxyribonucleic acid. *Endocrinology* 118:38, 1986.
575. Butler WT, Rossen RD: Effects of corticosteroids on immunity in man: I. Decreased serum IgG concentration caused by 3 or 5 days of high doses of methylprednisolone. *J Clin Invest* 52:2629, 1973.
576. Grayson J, Dooley NJ, Koski IR, Blaese RM: Immunoglobulin production induced *in vitro* by glucocorticoid hormones. *J Clin Invest* 68:1539, 1981.
577. Cupps TR, Gerrard TL, Falkoff RFM, Whalen G, Fauci AS: Effects of *in vitro* corticosteroids on B cell activation, proliferation, and differentiation. *J Clin Invest* 75:754, 1985.
578. Bar-Shavit Z, Kahn AJ, Pegg LE, Stone KR, Teitelbaum SL: Glucocorticoids modulate macrophage surface oligosaccharides and their bone binding activity. *J Clin Invest* 73:1277, 1984.
579. Aronow L: Effects of glucocorticoids on fibroblasts, in Baxter JD, Rousseau GG (eds): *Glucocorticoid Hormone Action*. New York, Springer-Verlag, 1979, p 327.
580. Gordan GS: Drug treatment of the osteoporoses. *Annu Rev Pharmacol Toxicol* 18:253, 1978.
581. Cutroneo KR, Rokowski R, Counts DF: Glucocorticoids and collagen synthesis: Comparison of *in vivo* and cell culture studies. *Coll Relat Res* 1:557, 1981.
582. Furcht LT, Mosher DF, Wendelschafter-Crabb G, Woodbridge PA: Dexamethasone induced accumulation of a fibronectin and collagen extracellular matrix in transformed human cells. *Nature* 277:393, 1979.
583. Smith TJ: Dexamethasone regulation of glycosaminoglycan synthesis in cultured human skin fibroblasts. *J Clin Invest* 74:2157, 1984.
584. Sterling KMJ, Harris MJ, Mitchell JJ, DiPetrillo TA, Delaney GL, Cutroneo KR: Dexamethasone decreases the amounts of type I procollagen mRNAs *in vivo* and in fibroblast cell cultures. *J Biol Chem* 258:7644, 1983.
585. Hammarstrom S, Hamberg M, Duell EA, Stawiski MA, Anderson TF, Voorhees JJ: Glucocorticoid in inflammatory proliferative skin disease reduces arachidonic and hydroxyeicosatetraenoic acids. *Science* 197:994, 1977.
586. Oliver N, Newby RF, Furcht LT, Bourgeois S: Regulation of fibronectin biosynthesis by glucocorticoids in human fibrosarcoma cells and normal fibroblasts. *Cell* 33:287, 1983.
587. De Asua LJ, Carr B, Clingan D, Rudland P: Specific glucocorticoid inhibition of growth promoting effects of prostaglandin F2α on 3T3 cells. *Nature* 265:450, 1977.
588. Pratt WB, Aronow L: The effect of glucocorticoids on protein and nucleic acid synthesis in mouse fibroblasts growing *in vitro*. *J Biol Chem* 241:5244, 1966.
589. Christy NP: Adrenal cortical steroids in various types of hypertension, in Manger MW (ed): *Hormones and Hypertension*. Springfield, IL, CC Thomas, 1966, p 169.
590. Saruta T, Suzuki H, Handa M, Igarashi Y, Kondo K, Senba S; Multiple factors contribute to the pathogenesis of hypertension in Cushing's syndrome. *J Clin Endocrinol Metab* 62:275, 1986.
591. Grunfeld J, Eloy L, Moura A, Ganeval D, Ramos-Frendo B, Worcel M: Effects of antiglucocorticoids on glucocorticoid hypertension in the rat. *Hypertension* 7:292, 1985.
592. Nichols NR, McNally M, Campbell JH, Funder JW: Overlapping but not identical protein synthetic domains in cardiovascular cells in response to glucocorticoid hormones. *Hypertension 2* 663:1984.
593. Nichols NR, Tracy KE, Funder JW: Glucocorticoid effects on newly synthesized proteins in muscle and non-muscle cells cultured from neonatal rat hearts. *J Steroid Biochem* 21:487, 1984.
594. Nichols NR, Lloyd CJ, Mendelsohn FAO, Funder JW: Glucocorticoid-induced proteins in bovine endothelial cells. *Mol Cell Endocrinol* 32:245, 1983.
595. Davies AO, De Lean A, Leflkowitz RJ: Myocardial beta-

adrenergic receptors from adrenalectomized rats: Impaired formation of high-affinity agonist-receptor complexes. *Endocrinology* 108:720, 1981.
596. Clark AF, Tandler B, Vignos PJ: Glucocorticoid-induced alterations in the rabbit heart. *Lab Invest* 47:603, 1982.
597. Sambhi MP, Weil MH, Udhoji VN: Acute pharmacologic effects of glucocorticoids: Cardiac output and related hemodynamic changes in normal subjects and patients with shock. *Circ Res* 31:523, 1965.
598. Axelrod L: Inhibition of prostacyclin production mediates permissive effect of glucocorticoids on vascular tone. *Lancet* 2:904, 1983.
599. White BC, Hoehner PJ, Wilson RF: Mitochondrial O_2 use and ATP synthesis: Kinetic effects of Ca^{+2} and HPO_4^{-2} modulated by glucocorticoids. *Ann Emerg Med* 2:396, 1980.
600. Friedland J, Setton C, Silverstein E: Angiotensin converting enzyme induction by steroids in alveolar macrophages in culture. *Science* 197:64, 1977.
601. Stockigt JR, Hewett MJ, Topliss DJ, Higgs EJ, Taft P: Renin and renin substrate in primary adrenal insufficiency: Contrasting effects of glucocorticoid and mineralocorticoid deficiency. *Am J Med* 66:915, 1979.
602. Nasjletti A, Erman A, Cagen LM, Baer PG, Matthews C, Killmar JT: Plasma concentrations, renal excretion, and tissue release of prostaglandins in the rat with dexamethasone-induced hypertension. *Endocrinology* 114: 1033, 1984.
603. Falezza G, Santonactaso CL, Parisi T, Muggeo M: High serum levels of angiotensin-converting enzyme in untreated Addison's disease. *J Clin Endocrinol Metab* 61:496, 1985.
604. Bengele HH, McNamara ER, Alexander ER: Natriuresis after adrenal enucleation: Effect of spironolactone and dexamethasone. *Am J Physiol* 233:F8, 1977.
605. Haack D, Mohring J, Mohring B, Petri M, Hackenthal E: Comparative study on development of corticosterone and DOCA hypertension in rats. *Am J Physiol* 233:F403, 1977.
606. Klein LE, Hsiao P, Bartolomei M, Lo CS: Regulation of rat renal (Na^+K^+)-adenosine triphosphatase activity by triiodothyronine and corticosterone. *Endocrinology* 115: 1038, 1984.
607. Kaji DM, Thakkar U, Kahn T, Torelli JA: Glucocorticoid induced alterations in the sodium potassium pump of the human erythrocyte. *J Clin Invest* 68:422, 1981.
608. Bastl CP, Barnett CA, Schmidt TJ, Litwack G: Glucocorticoid stimulation of sodium absorption in colon epithelia is manifested by corticosteroid IB receptor. *J Biol Chem* 259:1186, 1984.
609. Noda Y, Yamada K, Igic R, Erdos EG: Regulation of rat urinary and renal kallikrein and prekallikrein by corticosteroids. *Proc Natl Acad Sci USA* 80:3059, 1983.
610. Boykin J, deTorrente A, Erickson A, Robertson G, Shrier RW: Role of plasma vasopressin in impaired water excretion of glucocorticoid deficiency. *J Clin Invest* 62:738, 1978.
611. Schwartz J, Keil L, Maselli J, Reid I: Role of vasopressin in blood pressure regulation during adrenal insufficiency. *Endocrinology* 112:234, 1983.
612. Christy NP: Iatrogenic Cushing's syndrome, in Christy NP (ed): *The Human Adrenal Cortex*. New York, Harper & Row, 1971, p 395.
613. Stanton B, Giebisch G, Klein-Robbenhaar G, Wade J, DeFronzo RA: Effects of adrenalectomy and chronic adrenal corticosteroid replacement on potassium transport in rat kidney. *J Clin Invest* 75:1317, 1985.
614. Freiberg JM, Kinsella J, Sacktor B: Glucocorticoids increase the Na^+-H^+ exchange and decrease the Na^+ gradient-dependent phosphate-uptake systems in renal brush border membrane vesicles. *Proc Natl Acad Sci USA* 79:4932, 1982.
615. Wilcox CS, Cemerikic DA, Giebisch G: Differential effects of acute mineralo- and glucocorticosteroid administration on renal acid elimination. *Kidney Int* 21:546, 1982.
616. Cope CL: *Adrenal Steroids and Disease*. London, Pitman, 1972.
617. Nerup J: Addison's disease—clinical studies: A report of 108 cases. *Acta Endocrinol (Copenh)* 76:127, 1974.
618. Downic WW, Gunn A, Paterson CR, Howie GF: Hypercalcaemic crisis as presentation of Addison's disease. *Br Med J* 1:145, 1977.
619. Findling JW, Adams ND, Lemann JJ, Gray RW, Thomas CJ, Tyrrell JB: Vitamin D metabolites and parathyroid hormone in Cushing's syndrome: Relationship to calcium and phosphorus homeostasis. *J Clin Endocrinol Metab* 54:1039, 1982.
620. Hahn TJ, Halstead LR, Baran DT: Effects of short term glucocorticoid administration on intestinal calcium absorption and circulating vitamin D metabolite concentrations in man. *J Clin Endocrinol Metab* 52:111, 1981.
621. Hahn TJ, Halstead LR, Teitelbaum SL: Altered mineral metabolism in glucocorticoid-induced osteopenia. *J Clin Invest* 64:655, 1979.
622. Lee DBN: Unanticipated stimulatory action of glucocorticoids on epithelial calcium absorption. *J Clin Invest* 71:322, 1983.
623. Williams GA, Peterson WC, Bowser EH, Henderson WJ, Hargis GK, Martinez NJ: Interrelationship of parathyroid and adrenocortical function in calcium homeostasis in the rat. *Endocrinology* 95:707, 1974.
624. Manolagas SC, Anderson DC, Lamb GA: Glucocorticoids regulate the concentration of 1,25 dihydroxycholecalciferol receptors in bone. *Nature* 277:314, 1979.
625. Kimura S, Rasmussen H: Adrenal glucocorticoids, adenine nucleotide translocation, and mitochondrial calcium accumulation. *J Biol Chem* 252:1217, 1977.
626. Hansen JW, Gordan GS, Purssin SG: Direct measurement of osteolysis in man. *J Clin Invest* 52:304, 1973.
627. Ross EJ, Marshall-Jones P, Friedman M: Cushing's syndrome: Diagnostic criteria. *Q J Med* 35:149, 1966.
628. Breslau NA, Zerwekh JE, Nicar MJ, Pak CYC: Effects of short term glucocorticoid administration in primary hyperparathyroidism: Comparison to sarcoidosis. *J Clin Endocrinol Metab* 54:824, 1982.
629. Chyun YS, Kream BE, Raisz LG: Cortisol decreases bone formation by inhibiting periosteal cell proliferation. *Endocrinology* 114:477, 1984.
630. Reid IR, Chapman GE, Fraser TRC, Davies AD, Surus AS, Meyer J, Huq NL, Ibbertson HK: Low serum osteocalcin levels in glucocorticoid treated asthmatics. *J Clin Endocrinol Metab* 62:379, 1986.
631. Chen TL, Feldman D: Glucocorticoid potentiation of the adenosine 3′,5′-monophosphate response to parathyroid hormone in cultured rat bone cells. *Endocrinology* 102:589, 1978.
632. Ng B, Hekkelman JW, Heersche JNM: The effect of cortisol on the adenosine 3′,5′-monophosphate response to parathyroid hormone of bone *in vitro*. *Endocrinology* 104:1130, 1979.
633. Wong GL, Kukert BP, Adams JS: Glucocorticoids increase osteoblast like bone cell response to $1,25(OH)_2D_3$. *Nature* 285:254, 1980.
634. Chen TL, Cone CM, Morey-Holton E, Feldman D: Glucocorticoid regulation of $I,25(OH)_2$-vitamin D_3 receptors in cultured mouse bone cells. *J Biol Chem* 257:13564, 1982.
635. Binstock ML, Mundy GR: Effect of calcitonin and glucocorticoids in combination in the hypercalcemia of malignancy. *Ann Intern Med* 93:269, 1980.
636. McEwen BS: Influences of adrenocortical hormones on pituitary and brain function, in Baxter JD, Rousseau GG (eds): *Glucocorticoid Hormone Action*. New York, Springer-Verlag, 1979, p 467.
637. Doupe AJ, Patterson PH: Glucocorticoids and the develop-

ing nervous system, in Ganten D, Pfaff D (eds): *Current Topics in Neuroendocrinology*. New York, Springer-Verlag, 1982, vol 2, p 23.
638. Partridge WM, Mietus LJ: Transport of steroid hormones through the rat blood-brain barrier. *J Clin Invest* 64:145, 1979.
639. Long JB, Holaday JW: Blood-brain barrier: Endogenous modulation by adrenalcortical function. *Science* 27:1580, 1985.
640. Woodbury DM: Relation between the adrenal cortex and the central nervous system. *Pharmacol Rev* 10:275, 1958.
641. Knowlton AI: Addison's disease: A review of its clinical course and management, in Christy NP (ed): *The Human Adrenal Cortex*. New York, Harper & Row, 1971, p 329.
642. Gillin JC, Jacobs LS, Fram DH, Snyder F: Acute effect of a glucocorticoid on normal human sleep. *Nature* 237:398, 1972.
643. Sachar EJ, Asnis G, Halbreich U, Nathan RS, Halpern F: Recent studies in the neuroendocrinology of major depressive disorders. *Adv Psychoneuroendocrinol* 3:313, 1980.
644. Sternberg DE: Biologic tests in psychiatry. *Psychiatry Clin North Am* 7:639, 1984.
645. Bohus B, deKloet ER: Behavioral effects of neuropeptides (endorphins, enkephalins, ACTH fragments) and corticosteroids, in Jones MT, Giliham B, Dallman MF, Chattopadhyay S (eds): *Interaction within the Brain Pituitary-Adrenocortical System*. New York, Academic, 1979, p 7.
646. Sandman CA, George J, McCanne TR, Nolan JD, Kaswan J, Kastin AJ: MSH/ACTH 4-10 influences behavioral and physiological measures of attention. *J Clin Endocrinol Metab* 44:884, 1977.
647. Nestler EJ, Rainbow TC, McEwen BS, Greengard P: Corticosterone increases the amount of protein 1, a neuron-specific phosphoprotein in rat hippocampus. *Science* 212:1162, 1981.
648. Axelrod J, Reisine TD: Stress hormones: Their interaction and regulation. *Science* 224:452, 1984.
649. Rudman D, Moffitt SD, Fernoff PM, Blackston RD, Faraj BA: Epinephrine deficiency in hypocorticotropic hypopituitary children. *J Clin Endocrinol Metab* 53:722, 1981.
650. Naranjo JR, Mocchetti I, Schwartz JP, Costa E: Permissive effect of dexamethasone on the increase of proenkephalin mRNA induced by depolarization of chromaffin cells. *Proc Natl Acad Sci USA* 83:1513, 1986.
651. Polansky JR, Weinreb RM: Anti-inflammatory agents: Steroids as anti-inflammatory agents, in Sears ML (ed): *Handbook of Experimental Pharmacology*. New York, Springer-Verlag, 1984, vol 69, p 459.
652. Manabe S, Bucala R, Cerami A: Nonenzymatic addition of glucocorticoids to lens proteins in steroid-induced cataracts. *J Clin Invest* 74:1803, 1984.
653. Fenster FL: The ulcerogenic potential of glucocorticoids and possible prophylactic measures. *Med Clin North Am* 57:1289, 1973.
654. Conn HO, Blitzer BL: Nonassociation of adrenocorticosteroid therapy and peptic ulcer. *N Engl J Med* 294:473, 1976.
655. Messer J, Reitman D, Sacks HS, Smith H, Chalmers TC: Association of adrenocorticosteroid therapy and peptic-ulcer disease. *N Engl J Med* 309:21, 1983.
656. Daughaday WJ, Herrington AC, Phillips LS: The regulation of growth by endocrines. *Annu Rev Physiol* 37:211, 1975.
657. Gospodarowicz D, Moran J: Stimulation of division of sparse and confluent 3T3 cell populations by a fibroblast growth factor, dexamethasone and insulin. *Proc Natl Acad Sci USA* 71:4584, 1974.
658. Conover CA, Rosenfeld RG, Hintz RL: Aging alters somatomedin-C-dexamethasone synergism in the stimulation of deoxyribonucleic acid synthesis and replication of cultured human fibroblasts. *J Clin Endocrinol Metab* 61:423, 1985.
659. Bennett A, Chen T, Feldman D, Hintz RL: Characterization of insulin-like growth factor I receptors on cultured rat bone cells: Regulation of receptor concentration by glucocorticoids. *Endocrinology* 116:1577, 1984.
660. Unterman TG, Phillips LS: Glucocorticoid effects on somatomedins and somatomedin inhibitors. *J Clin Endocrinol Metab* 61:618, 1985.
661. Ballard PL: Glucocorticoids and differentiation, in Baxter JD, Rousseau GG (eds): *Glucocorticoid Hormone Action*. New York, Springer-Verlag, 1979, p 493.
662. Schuetz EG, Wrighton SA, Barwick JL, Guzelian PS: Induction of cytochrome P-450 by glucocorticoids in rat liver: I. Evidence that glucocorticoids and pregnenolone 16α-carbonitrile regulate de novo synthesis of a common form of cytochrome P-450 in cultures of adult rat hepatocytes and in the liver *in vivo*. *J Biol Chem* 259:1999, 1984.
663. Lantiguce RL, Streck WF, Lockwood DH, Jacobs LS: Glucocorticoid suppression of pancreatic and pituitary hormones: Pancreatic polypeptide, growth hormone, and prolactin. *J Clin Endocrinol Metab* 50:298, 1980.
664. Muszynski M, Birnbaum RS, Roos BA: Glucocorticoids stimulate the production of preprocalcitonin-derived secretory peptides by a rat medullary thyroid carcinoma cell line. *J Biol Chem* 19:11678, 1983.
665. Sowers JR, Carlson HE, Brautbar N, Hershman JM: Effect of dexamethasone on prolactin and TSH responses to TRH and metoclopramide in man. *J Clin Endocrinol Metab* 44:237, 1977.
666. Burr WA, Griffiths RS, Ramsden DB, Black EG, Hoffenberg R, Meinhold H, Wenzel KW: Effect of a single dose of dexamethasone on serum concentration of thyroid hormone. *Lancet* 2:58, 1976.
667. Vreeburg JTM, de Greef WJ, Ooms MP, van Wouw P, Wever RFA: Effects of adrenocorticotropin and corticosterone on the negative feedback action of testosterone in the adult male rat. *Endocrinology* 115:977, 1984.
668. Karpas AE, Rodriguez-Rigau LJ, Smith KD, Steinberger E: Effect of acute and chronic androgen suppression by glucocorticoids on gonadotropin levels in hirsute women. *J Clin Endocrinol Metab* 59:780, 1984.
669. Sapolsky RM: Stress-induced suppression of testicular functionin the wild baboon: Role of glucocorticoids. *Endocrinology* 116:2273, 1985.
670. Cumming DC, Quigley ME, Yen SSC: Acute suppression of circulating testosterone levels by cortisol in men. *J Clin Endocrinol Metab* 57:671, 1983.
671. Novotny M, Jemiolo B, Harvey S, Wiesler D, Marchlewska-Koj A: Adrenal-mediated endogenous metabolites inhibit puberty in female mice. *Science* 231:722, 1986.
672. Schoonmaker JN, Erickson GF: Glucocorticoid modulation of follicle-stimulating hormone-mediated granulosa cell differentiation. *Endocrinology* 113:1356, 1983.
673. Suter DE, Schwartz NB: Effects of glucocorticoids on secretion of luteinizing hormone and follicle-stimulating hormone by female rat pituitary cells *in vitro*. *Endocrinology* 117:849, 1985.
674. Simpson ER, Ackerman GE, Smith ME, Mendelson CR: Estrogen formation in stromal cells of adipose tissue of women: Induction by glucocorticosteroids. *Proc Natl Acad Sci USA* 78:5690, 1981.
675. Granner DK: The role of glucocorticoids as biological amplifiers, in Baxter JD, Rousseau GG (eds): *Glucocorticoid Hormone Action*. New York: Springer-Verlag, 1979, p 593.
676. Harris AW, Baxter JD: Variations in the cellular sensitivity to glucocorticoids: Observations and mechanisms, in Baxter JD, Rousseau GG (eds): *Glucocorticoid Hormone Action*. New York, Springer-Verlag, 1979, p 423.
677. Gruol DJ, Campbell NF, Bourgeois S: Cyclic AMP-dependent protein kinase promotes glucocorticoid receptor function. *J Biol Chem* 261:4909, 1986.

678. Lai E, Rosen O, Rubin CS: Dexamethasone regulates the β-adrenergic receptor subtype expressed by 3T3-L1 preadipocytes and adipocytes. *J Biol Chem* 257:6691, 1982.
679. Davies AO, Lefkowitz RJ: *In vitro* desensitization of beta adrenergic receptors in human neutrophils. *J Clin Invest* 71:565, 1983.
680. Dunlop D: Eighty six cases of Addison's disease. *Br Med J* 2:887, 1963.
681. Marver D, Kakko JP: Renal target sites and the mechanism of action of aldosterone. *Miner Electrolyte Metab* 9:1, 1983.
682. Claire M, Oblin M-E, Steimer J, Nakane H, Misumi J, Michaud A, Corvol P: Effect of adrenalectomy and aldosterone on the modulation of mineralocorticoid receptors in rat kidney. *J Biol Chem* 256:142, 1981.
683. Ludens JH, Fanestil DD: The mechanism of aldosterone function, in Gill GN (ed): *Pharmacology of Adrenal Cortical Hormones*. New York, Pergamon, 1979, p 143.
684. Kurt Lee S-M, Chekal MA, Katz AL: Corticosterone binding sites along the rat nephron. *Am J Physiol (Renal Fluid Electrolyte Physiol 13)* 244:F504, 1983.
685. Lan NC, Graham B, Bartter FC, Baxter JD: Binding of steroids to mineralocorticoid receptors: Implications for *in vivo* occupancy by glucocorticoids. *J Clin Endocrinol Metab* 54:332, 1982.
686. Quirk SJ, Gannell JE, Funder JW: Aldosterone-binding sites in pregnant and lactating rat mammary glands. *Endocrinology* 113:1812, 1983.
687. Park SC, Edelman IS: Dual action of aldosterone on toad bladder: Na^+ permeability and Na^+ pump modulation. *Am J Physiol (Renal Fluid Electrolyte Physiol 15)* 246:F517, 1984.
688. Park SC, Edelman IS: Effect of aldosterone on abundance and phosphorylation kinetics of Na-K-ATPase of toad urinary bladder. *Am J Physiol (Renal Fluid Electrolyte Physiol 15)* 246:F509, 1984.
689. El Mernissi G, Chabardes D, Doucet A, Hus-Citharel A, Imbert-Teboul M, Le Bouffant F, Montegut M, Siaume S, et al: Changes in tubular basolateral membrane markers after chronic DOCA treatment. *Am J Physiol (Renal Fluid Electrolyte Physiol 14)* 245:F100, 1983.
690. Karbowiak Al, Krozowski Z, Funder JW, Adam WR: The mechanism of mineralocorticoid action of carbenoxolone. *Endocrinology* 111:1683, 1982.
691. Cortas N, Abras E, Arnaout M, Mooradian A, Muakasah S: Energetics of sodium transport in the urinary bladder of the toad: Effect of aldosterone and sodium cyanide. *J Clin Invest* 73:46, 1984.
692. Tomita K, Pisano JJ, Knepper MA: Control of sodium and potassium transport in the cortical collecting duct of the rat. *J Clin Invest* 76:132, 1985.
693. Petty KJ, Kokko JP, Marver D: Secondary effect of aldosterone on Na-K-ATPase activity in the rabbit cortical collecting tubule. *J Clin Invest* 68:1514, 1981.
694. Mujais SK, Chekal MA, Jones WJ, Hayslett JP, Katz AI: Modulation of renal sodium-potassium-adenosine triphosphate by aldosterone. *J Clin Invest* 76:170, 1985.
695. Mujais SK, Chekal MA, Jones WJ, Hayslett JP, Katz AL: Regulation of renal Na-K-ATPase in the rat. *J Clin Invest* 73:13, 1984.
696. Speiser PW, Martin KO, Kao-Lo G, New MI: Excess mineralocorticoid receptor activity in patients with dexamethasone-suppressible hyperaldosteronism is under adrenocorticotropin control. *J Clin Endocrinol Metab* 61:297, 1985.
697. Lan NC, Matulich DT, Stockigt JR, Biglieri EG, New MI, Baxter JD: Radioreceptor assay of plasma mineralocorticoid activity. *Circ Res* 46(Suppl.):194, 1980.
698. Dunn JF, Nisula BC, Rodbard D: Transport of steroid hormones: Binding of 21 endogenous steroids to both testosterone-binding globulin and corticosteroid-binding globulin in human plasma. *J Clin Endocrinol Metab* 53:58, 1981.
699. Gomez-Sanchez CE, Gomez-Sanchez EP, Shackleton CHL, Milewick L: Identification of 19-hydroxydeoxycorticosterone, 19-oxo-deoxycorticosterone, and 19-oic-deoxycorticosterone as products of deoxycorticosterone metabolism by rat adrenals. *Endocrinology* 110:384, 1982.
700. Griffing GT, Wilson TE, Melby JC: Unconjugated and conjugated urinary 19-nor-deoxycorticosterone glucosiduronate: Elevated levels in essential hypertension. *Hypertension* 7:112, 1985.
701. Griffing GT, Dale SL, Holbrook MM, Melby JC: Relationship of 19 nor-deoxycorticosterone to other mineralocorticoids in low-renin hypertension. *Hypertension* 5:385, 1983.
702. Moura AM, Worcel M: Direct action of aldosterone on transmembrane ^{22}Na efflux from arterial smooth muscle: Rapid and delayed effects. *Hypertension* 6:425, 1984.
703. Nichols NR, Nguyen HH, Meyer WJ III: Physical separation of aortic corticoid receptors with type I an type II specificities. *J Steroid Biochem* 22:577, 1985.
704. West CD, Mahajan DK, Chavre VJ, Nabors CJ, Tyler FH: Simultaneous measurement of multiple plasma steroids by radioimmunoassay demonstrating episodic secretion. *J Clin Endocrinol Metab* 36:1230, 1973.
705. Irvine WJ, Toft AD, Feek CM: Addison's disease, in James VHT (ed): *The Adrenal Gland*. New York, Raven, 1979, p 131.
706. Knox FG, Burnett JC Jr, Kohan DE, Spielman WS, Strand JC: Escape from the sodium-retaining effects of mineralocorticoids. *Kidney Int* 17:263, 1980.
707. Forman BH, Mulrow PJ: Effect of corticosteroids on water and electrolyte metabolism, in Greep RO, Astwood EB (eds): *Handbook of Physiology: Endocrinology*. Washington, DC, American Physiological Society, 1975, vol 6, p 179.
708. Metzler CH, Gardner DG, Keil LC, Baxter JD, Ramsay DJ: Increased synthesis and release of atrial peptide during mineralocorticoid escape in conscious dogs. *Am J Physiol* 252:R188, 1987.
709. Cox M, Stevens RH, Singer I: The defense against hyperkalemia: The roles of insulin and aldosterone. *N Engl J Med* 299:525, 1978.
710. Seldin DW: Metabolic acidosis, in Brenner B, Rector F (eds): *The Kidney*. Philadelphia, Saunders, 1976, p 615.
711. Sebastian A, Sutton JM, Hulter HM, Schambelan M, Poler SM: Effect of mineralocorticoid replacement therapy on renal acid-base homeostasis in adrenalectomized patients. *Kidney Int* 18:762, 1980.
712. Lieberthal W, Oza NB, Arbeit L, Bernard DB, Levinsky NG: Effects of alterations in sodium and water metabolism on urinary excretion of active and inactive kallikrein in man. *J Clin Endocrinol Metab* 56:513, 1983.
713. Binder HJ: Effect of dexamethasone on electrolyte transport in the large intestine of the rat. *Gastroenterology* 75:212, 1978.
714. Wilson JD: The pathogenesis of benign prostatic hypertrophy. *Am J Med* 68:745, 1980.
715. Migeon C: Adrenal androgens in man. *Am J Med* 53:606, 1972.
716. Carter JN, Tysen JE, Warne GJ, McNeilly AS, Faiman C, Friesen HG: Adrenocortical function in hyperprolactinemic women. *J Clin Endocrinol Metab* 45:973, 1977.
717. Yuen BH, Kelch RP, Jaffe RB: Adrenal contribution to plasma estrogens in adrenal disorders. *Acta Endocrinol (Copenh)* 76:117, 1974.
718. Nimrod A, Ryan KJ: Aromatization of androgens by human abdominal and breast fat tissue. *J Clin Endocrinol Metab* 40:367, 1975.
719. Schweikert HU, Milewich L, Wilson JD: Aromatization of androstenedione by isolated human hairs. *J Clin Endocrinol Metab* 40:413, 1975.
720. Vermeulen A: The hormonal activity of the postmenopausal ovary. *J Clin Endocrinol Metab* 42:247, 1976.

721. MacDonald PC, Madden JD, Brenner PF, Wilson JD, Siiteri PK: Origin of estrogen in normal men and women with testicular feminization. *J Clin Endocrinol Metab* 49:905, 1979.
722. Ruder HJ, Guy RL, Lipsett MB: A radioimmunoassay for cortisol in plasma and urine. *J Clin Endocrinol Metab* 35:219, 1972.
723. Vecsi P: Glucocorticoids: Cortisol, corticosterone and compound S, in Jaffe BM, Behrman HR (eds): *Methods of Hormone Radioimmunoassay*. New York, Academic, 1974, p 393.
724. Kabra PM, Tsai L, Marton LJ: Improved liquid-chromatographic method for determination of serum cortisol. *Clin Chem* 25:1293, 1979.
725. Gotelli GR, Wall JH, Kabra PM, Marton LJ: Fluorometric liquid-chromatographic determination of serum cortisol. *Clin Chem* 27:442, 1981.
726. Murphy BEP: Some studies of the protein-binding of steroids and their application to the routine micro and ultramicro measurement of various steroids in body fluids by competitive protein-binding radioassay. *J Clin Endocrinol Metab* 27:973, 1967.
727. Murphy BEP: Non-chromatographic radiotransinassay for cortisol: Application to human adult serum, umbilical cord serum and amniotic fluid. *J Clin Endocrinol Metab* 41:1050, 1975.
728. Porter CC, Silber RH: A quantitative color reaction for cortisone and related 17,21-dihydroxy-20-ketosteroids. *J Biol Chem* 185:201, 1950.
729. Nelson DH, Samuels LT: A method for the determination of 16-hydroxy-corticosteroids in blood: 17-Hydroxycorticosterone in the peripheral blood. *J Clin Endocrinol Metab* 12:519, 1952.
730. Mattingly D: A simple fluorimetric method for the estimation of free 11-hydroxycorticoids in human plasma. *J Clin Pathol* 15:374, 1962.
731. Nielsen E, Asfeldt VH: Studies on the specificity of fluorimetric determination of plasma corticosteroids ad modum de Moor and Steeno. *Scand J Clin Lab Invest* 20:185, 1967.
732. Dash RJ, England BG, Midgley AR, Niswender GD: A specific non-chromatographic radioimmunoassay for human plasma cortisol. *Steroids* 26:647, 1975.
733. Colburn WA: Radioimmunoassay for cortisol using antibodies against prednisolone conjugated at the 3-position. *J Clin Endocrinol Metab* 41:868, 1975.
734. Willig RP, Blunck W: Quantitation of plasma cortisol and other C21-steroids by radioimmunoassay, in Gupta D (ed): *Radioimmunoassay of Steroid Hormones*. Weinheim, Verlag-Chemie, Germany, 1975, p 135.
735. Newsome HH, Clements AS, Borum EA: The simultaneous assay of cortisol, corticosterone, 11-deoxycortisol and cortisone in human plasma. *J Clin Endocrinol Metab* 34:473, 1972.
736. Evans P, Peters J Dyas J, Walker R, Riad-Fahmy D, Hall R: Salivary cortisol levels in true and apparent hypercortisolism. *Clin Endocrinol (Oxf)* 20:709, 1984.
737. Tunn S, Mollmann H, Barth J, Derendorf H, Krieg M: Simultaneous measurement of cortisol in serum and saliva and different forms of cortisol administration. *Clin Chem* 38:1491, 1992.
738. Laudat MH, Cerdas S, Fournier C, Guiban D, Guilhaume B, Luton JP: Salivary cortisol measurement: A practical approach to assess pituitary-adrenal function. *J Clin Endocrinol Metab* 66:343, 1988.
739. Allolio B, Hoffmann J, Linton EA, Winkelmann W, Kusche M, Schulte HM: Diurnal salivary cortisol patterns during pregnancy and after delivery: Relationship to plasma corticotropin-releasing-hormone. *Clin Endocrinol (Oxf)* 33:279, 1990.
740. Krieger DT, Allen W, Rizzo F, Krieger HP: Characterization of the normal temporal pattern of plasma corticosteroid levels. *J Clin Endocrinol Metab* 32:266, 1971.
741. Gallagher TF, Yoshida K, Roffwarg HD, Fukushima D, Weitzman ED, Hellman L: ACTH and cortisol secretory patterns in man. *J Clin Endocrinol Metab* 36:1058, 1973.
742. DeLacerda L, Kowarski A, Migeon CJ: Integrated concentration and diurnal variation of plasma cortisol. *J Clin Endocrinol Metab* 36:227, 1973.
743. Silverberg A, Rizzo F, Krieger DT: Nyctohemeral periodicity of plasma 17-OHCS levels in elderly subjects. *J Clin Endocrinol Metab* 28:1661, 1968.
744. Jacobs HS, Nabarro JDN: Plasma 11-hydroxysteroid and growth hormone levels in acute medical illnesses. *Br Med J* 2:595, 1969.
745. Aron DC, Tyrrell JB, Fitzgerald PC, Findling JW, Forsham PH: Cushing's syndrome: Problems in diagnosis. *Medicine (Baltimore)* 160:25, 1981.
746. Rao KSJ, Srikantia SG, Gopalan C: Plasma cortisol levels in protein calorie malnutrition. *Arch Dis Child* 43:356, 1968.
747. Walsh BT, Katz JL, Levin J, Kream I, Fukushima DK, Hellman LD, Weiner H, Zumoff B: Adrenal activity in anorexia nervosa. *Psychosom Med* 40:499, 1978.
748. Wallace EZ, Rosman P, Toshav N, Sacerdote A, Balthazar A: Pituitary adrenocortical function in chronic renal failure: Studies of episodic secretion of cortisol and dexamethasone suppressibility. *J Clin Endocrinol Metab* 50:46, 1980.
749. Carr BR, Parker CR Jr, Maddin JD, MacDonald PC, Porter JC: Plasma levels of adrenocorticotropin and cortisol in women receiving oral contraceptive steroid treatment. *J Clin Endocrinol Metab* 49:346, 1979.
750. Abraham GE, Manlimos FS, Garza R: Radioimmunoassay of steroids, in Abraham GE (ed): *Handbook of Radioimmunoassay*. New York, Marcel Dekker, 1977, p 591.
751. Anderson DC, Hopper BR, Iasley BL, Yen SSC: A simple method for the assay of eight steroids in small volumes of plasma. *Steroids* 28:179, 1976.
752. Berson SA, Yalow RS: Radioimmunoassay of ACTH in plasma. *J Clin Invest* 47:2725, 1968.
753. Landon J, Greenwood FC: Homologous radioimmunoassay for plasma levels of corticotrophin in man. *Lancet* 1:273, 1968.
754. Orth DN: Adrenocorticotropic hormone and melanocyte stimulating hormone (ACTH and MSH), in Jaffe BM, Behrman HR (eds): *Methods of Hormone Radioimmunoassay*. New York, Academic, 1974, p 125.
755. Ruhmann-Wennhold A, Nelson DH: Adrenocorticotropic hormone, in Antoniades HN (ed): *Hormones in Human Blood*. Cambridge, MA, Harvard University Press, 1976, p 325.
756. Nicholson WE, Davis DR, Sherrell BJ, Orth DN: Rapid radioimmunoassay for corticotropin in unextracted human plasma. *Clin Chem* 30:259, 1984.
757. Hodgkinson SC, Allolio B, Landon J, Lowry PJ: Development of a non-extracted "two-site" immunoradiometric assay for corticotropin utilizing extreme amino- and carboxy-terminally directed antibodies. *Biochem J* 218:703, 1984.
758. White A, Smith H, Hoadley M, Dobson SH, Ratcliffe JG: Clinical evaluation of a two-site immunoradiometric assay for adrenocorticotrophin in unextracted human plasma using monoclonal antibodies. *Clin Endocrinol (Oxf)* 26:41, 1987.
759. Zahradnik R, Brennan G, Hutchison JS, Odell WD: Immunoradiometric assay of corticotropin with use of avidin-biotin separation. *Clin Chem* 35:804, 1989.
760. Raff H, Findling JW: A new immunoradiometric assay for corticotropin evaluated in normal subjects and patients with Cushing's syndrome. *Clin Chem* 35:596, 1989.
761. Findling JW: Clinical application of a new immunoradiometric assay for ACTH. *The Endocrinologist* 2:260, 1992.
762. Crapo L: Cushing's syndrome: A review of diagnostic tests. *Metabolism* 28:955, 1979.

763. Besser GM, Edwards CRW: Cushing's syndrome. *Clin Endocrinol Metab* 1:451, 1972.
764. Wolfsen AR, McIntyre HB, Odell WD: Adrenocorticotropin measurement by competitive binding receptor assay. *J Clin Endocrinol Metab* 34:684, 1972.
765. Daly JR, Fleisher MD, Chambers DJ, Bitensky L, Chayen J: Application of the cytochemical bioassay for corticotrophin to clinical and physiological studies in man. *Clin Endocrinol (Oxf)* 3:335, 1974.
766. Weidemann E, Saito T, Linfoot JA, Li C:Radioimmunoassay of human β-lipotropin in unextracted plasma. *J Clin Endocrinol Metab* 45:1108, 1977.
767. Jeffcoate WJ, Rees LH, Lowry PJ, Beser GM: A specific radioimmunoassay for human β-lipotropin. *J Clin Endocrinol Mebab* 47:160, 1978.
768. Krieger DT, Liotta AS, Suda T, Goodgold A, Condon E: Human plasma immunoreactive lipotropin and adrenocorticotropin in normal subjects and in patients with pituitary-adrenal disease. *J Clin Endocrinol Metab* 48:566, 1979.
769. Mullen PE, Jeffcoate WJ, Linsell C, Howard R, Rees LH: The circadian variation of immunoreactive lipotrophin and its relationship to ACTH and growth hormone in man. *Clin Endocrinol (Oxf)* 11:533, 1979.
770. Wardlow SL, Frantz AG: Measurement of β-endorphin in human plasma. *J Clin Endocrinol Metab* 48:176, 1979.
771. Wiedemann E, Saito T, Linfoot JA, Li CH: Specific radioimmunoassay of human β-endorphin in unextracted plasma. *J Clin Endocrinol Metab* 49:478, 1979.
772. Crosby SR, Stewart MF, Ratcliffe JG, White A: Direct measurement of the precursors of adrenocorticotropin in human plasma by two-site immunoradiometric assay. *J Clin Endocrinol Metab* 67:1272, 1988.
773. Beisel WR, Cos JJ, Horton R, Chao PY, Forsham PH: Physiology of urinary cortisol excretion. *J Clin Endocrinol Metab* 24:887, 1964.
774. Murphy BEP: Clinical evaluation of urinary cortisol determinations by competitive protein-binding radioassay. *J Clin Endocrinol Metab* 28:343, 1968.
775. Beardwell CG, Burke CW, Cope CL: Urinary free cortisol measured by competitive protein binding. *J Endocrinol* 42:79, 1968.
776. Nakamura J, Yakata M: Determination of urinary cortisol and 6β-hydroxycortisol by high performance liquid chromatography. *Clin Chim Acta* 149:215, 1985.
777. Contreras LN, Hane S, Tyrrell JB: Urinary cortisol in the assessment of pituitary-adrenal function: Utility of 24-hour and spot determinations. *J Clin Endocrinol Metab* 62:965, 1986.
778. Laudat MH, Billaud L, Thomopoulos P, Vera O, Yllia A, Luton JP: Evening urinary free corticoids: A screening test in Cushing's syndrome and incidentally discovered adrenal tumours. *Acta Endocrinol (Copenh)* 119:459, 1988.
779. Streeten DHP, Stevenson CT, Dalakos TG, Nicholas JJ, Dennick LG, Fellerman H: The diagnosis of hypercortisolism: Biochemical criteria differentiating patients from lean and obese normal subjects and from females on oral contraceptives. *J Clin Endocrinol Metab* 29:1191, 1969.
780. Burke CW: Hormones in urine: Uses and misuses. *J R Coll Physicians Lond* 8:335, 1974.
781. McCann VJ, Fulton TJ: Cortisol metabolism in chronic liver disease. *J Clin Endocrinol Metab* 40:1038, 1975.
782. Peterson RE: The influence of the thyroid on adrenal cortical function. *J Clin Invest* 37:736, 1958.
783. Brown H, Englert E, Wallack S: Metabolism of free and conjugated 17-hydroxycorticosteroids in subjects with thyroid disease. *J Clin Endocrinol Metab* 18:167, 1958.
784. Hellman K, Bradlow HL, Zumoff B, Gallagher TF: The influence of thyroid hormone on hydrocortisone production and metabolism. *J Clin Endocrinol* 21:1231, 1961.
785. Garib H, Munoz JM: Endocrine manifestations of diphenyl-hydantoin therapy. *Metabolism* 23:515, 1974.
786. Bledsoe T, Island DP, Ney RK, Liddle GW: An effect of o,p′-DDD in the extraadrenal metabolism of cortisol in man. *J Clin Endocrinol Metab* 24:1303, 1964.
787. Dillon RS: *Handbook of Endocrinology,* 2d ed. Philadelphia, Lea & Febiger, 1980.
788. Boruskek S, Gold JJ: Commonly used medications that interfere with routine endocrine laboratory procedures. *Clin Chem* 10:41, 1964.
789. Appleby JI, Gibson G, Normyberski JK, Stubbs RD: Indirect analysis of corticosteroids: I. The determination of 17-hydroxycorticosteroids. *Biochem J* 60:453, 1955.
790. Caro JF, Meikle AW, Check JH, Cohen SN: "Normal suppression" to dexamethasone in Cushing's disease: An expression of decreased metabolic clearance for dexamethasone. *J Clin Endocrinol Metab* 47:667, 1978.
791. Meikle AW: Dexamethasone suppression tests: Usefulness of simultaneous measurement of plasma cortisol and dexamethasone. *Clin Endocrinol (Oxf)* 16:401, 1982.
792. Liberman B, Wajchenberg BL, Tambascia MA, Mesquita CH: Periodic remission in Cushing's disease with paradoxical dexamethasone response: An expression of periodic hormonogenesis. *J Clin Endocrinol Metab* 43:913, 1976.
793. Liddle GW: Tests of pituitary adrenal suppressibility in the diagnosis of Cushing's syndrome. *J Clin Endocrinol Metab* 12:1539, 1960.
794. Eddy RL, Jones AL, Gilliland PF, Ibarra JD, Thompson JQ, McMurry IF: Cushing's syndrome: A prospective study of diagnostic methods. *Am J Med* 55:621, 1973.
795. Burke CW, Beardwell CG: Cushing's syndrome. An evaluation of the clinical usefulness of urinary free cortisol and other urinary steroid measurements in diagnosis. *Q J Med* 42:175, 1973.
796. Butler PWP, Besser GM: Pituitary-adrenal function in severe depressive illness. *Lancet* 1:1234, 1968.
797. Jubiz W, Meikle AW, Levinson RA, Mizutani S, West CD, Tyler FH: Effect of diphenylhydantoin on the metabolism of dexamethasone: Mechanism of the abnormal dexamethasone suppression in humans. *N Engl J Med* 283:11, 1970.
798. Ashcraft MW, Van Herle A, Vener SL, Geffner DL: Serum cortisol levels in Cushing's syndrome after low- and high-dose dexamethasone suppression. *Ann Intern Med* 97:21, 1982.
799. Cook DM, Kendall JW, Allen JP, Lagerquist LG: Nyctohemeral variation and suppressibility of plasma ACTH in various stages of Cushing's disease. *Clin Endocrinol (Oxf)* 5:303, 1976.
800. Tyrrell JB, Findling JW, Aron DC, Fitzgerald PA, Forsham PH: An overnight high-dose dexamethasone suppression test for rapid differential diagnosis of Cushing's syndrome. *Ann Intern Med* 104:180, 1986.
801. Nichols T, Nugent CA, Tyler FH: Steroid laboratory tests in the diagnosis of Cushing's syndrome. *Am J Med* 45:116, 1968.
802. Flack MR, Oldfield EH, Cutler GB Jr, Zweig MH, Malley JD, Chrousos GP, Loriaux L, Nieman LK: Urine free cortisol in the high-dose dexamethasone suppression test for the differential diagnosis of the Cushing syndrome. *Ann Intern Med* 116:211, 1992.
803. Chrousos GP, Schuermeyer TH, Doppman J, Oldfield EH, Schulte HM, Gold PW, Loriaux DL: Clinical applications of corticotropin-releasing factor. *Ann Intern Med* 102:344, 1985.
804. Chrousos GP, Schulte HM, Oldfield EH, Gold PW, Cutler GB Jr, Loriaux DL: The corticotropin releasing factor stimulation test: An aid in the evaluation of patients with Cushing's syndrome. *N Engl J Med* 310:622, 1984.
805. Lytras N, Grossman A, Perry L, Tomlin S, Wass JAH, Coy DH, Schally AV, Rees LH, et al: Corticotrophin releasing

factor: Responses in normal subjects and patients with disorders of the hypothalamus and pituitary. *Clin Endocrinol (Oxf)* 20:71, 1984.
806. Pieters GFFM, Hermus ARMM, Smals AGH, Bartelink AKM, Benraad TJ, Kloppenborg PWC: Responsiveness of the hypophyseal-adrenocortical axis to corticotropin-releasing factor in pituitary-dependent Cushing's disease. *J Clin Endocrinol Metab* 57:513, 1983.
807. Mezey E, Reisine TD, Brownstein MJ, Palkovits M, Axelrod J: β-Adrenergic mechanism of insulin induced adrenocorticotropin release from the anterior pituitary. *Science* 226:1085, 1984.
808. Wood JB, Frankland AW, James VHT, Landon J: A rapid test of adrenocortical function. *Lancet* 1:243, 1965.
809. Speckart PF, Nicoloff JT, Bethune JE: Screening for adrenocortical insufficiency with cosyntropin (synthetic ACTH). *Arch Intern Med* 128:761, 1971.
810. Grieg WR, Jasani MK, Boyle JA, Maxwell JD: Corticotrophin stimulation tests. *Mem Soc Endocrinol* 17:175, 1968.
811. May ME, Carey RM: Rapid adrenocorticotropic hormone test in practice. *Am J Med* 79:679, 1985.
812. Patel SR, Selby C, Jeffcoate WJ: The short Synacthen test in acute hospital admissions. *Clin Endocrinol (Oxf)* 35:259, 1991.
813. Dickstein G, Shechner C, Nicholson WE, Rosner I, Shen-Orr Z, Adawi F, Lahav M: Adrenocorticotropin stimulation test: Effects of basal cortisol level, time of day, and suggested new sensitive low dose test. *J Clin Endocrinol Metab* 72:773, 1991.
814. Hawkins JB, Burch WM: Rapid tests of adrenocortical function: Intravenous versus intramuscular administration of synthetic ACTH. *NC Med J* 50:306, 1989.
815. Nelson JC, Tindall DJ: A comparison of the adrenal responses to hypoglycemia, metyrapone and ACTH. *Am J Med Sci* 275:165, 1978.
816. Lindholm J, Kehlet H, Blickert-Toft M, Dinesen B, Rushede J: Reliability of the 30-minute ACTH test in assessing hypothalamic-pituitary-adrenal function. *J Clin Endocrinol Metab* 47:272, 1978.
817. Jasani MK, Boyle JA, Greig WR, Dalakos JG, Browning MCK, Thompson A, Buchanon WW: Corticosteroid-induced suppression of the hypothalamic-pituitary-adrenal axis: Observations on patients given oral corticosteroids for rheumatoid arthritis. *Q J Med* 36:261, 1967.
818. Jasani MK, Freeman PA, Boyle JA, Reid AM, Diver MJ, Buchanan WW: Studies of the rise in plasma 11-hydroxycorticosteroids (11-OHCS) in corticosteroid treated patients with rheumatoid arthritis during surgery: Correlations with the functional integrity of the hypothalamo-pituitary-adrenal axis. *Q J Med* 37:407, 1968.
819. Kehlet H, Binder C: Value of an ACTH test in assessing hypothalamic pituitary-adrenocortical function in glucocorticoid-treated patients. *Br Med J* 2:147, 1973.
820. Borst GC, Michenfelder HJ, O'Brian JT: Discordant cortisol response to exogenous ACTH and insulin-induced hypoglycemia in patients with pituitary disease. *N Engl J Med* 306:1462, 1982.
821. Landon J, Greenwood FC, Stamp TCB, Wynn V: The plasma sugar, free fatty acid, cortisol and growth hormone response to insulin, and the comparison of this procedure with other tests of pituitary and adrenal function: II. In patients with hypothalamic or pituitary dysfunction or anorexia nervosa. *J Clin Invest* 45:437, 1966.
822. Dluhy RG, Himathongkam T, Greenfield M: Rapid ACTH test with plasma aldosterone levels: Improved diagnostic discrimination. *Ann Intern Med* 80:693, 1974.
823. Spiger M, Jubiz W, Meikle AW, West CD, Tyler FH: Single-dose metyrapone test: Review of a four-year experience. *Arch Intern Med* 135:698, 1975.
824. Staub JS, Noelpp B, Girard J, Baumann JB, Graf S, Ratcliffe JG: The short metyrapone test: Comparison of the plasma ACTH response to metyrapone and insulin-induced hypoglycemia. *Clin Endocrinol (Oxf)* 10:595, 1979.
825. Orth DN: Corticotropin-releasing hormone in humans. *Endocr Rev* 13:164, 1992.
826. Malchoff CD, Orth DN, Abboud C, Carney JA, Pairolero PC, Carey RM: Ectopic ACTH syndrome caused by a bronchial carcinoid tumor responsive to dexamethasone, metyrapone and corticotropin-releasing factor. *Am J Med* 84:760, 1988.
827. Jacobs HS, Nabarro JDN: Tests of hypothalamic-pituitary-adrenal function in man. *Q J Med* 38:475, 1969.
828. Thorn GW: Adrenal cortical insufficiency, in Conn HF, Clohecy R, Conn RB (eds): *Current Diagnosis*. Philadelphia, Saunders, 1966, p 445.
829. Greenwood FC, Landon J, Stamp TCB: The plasma sugar, free fatty acid, cortisol, and growth hormone response to insulin: I. In control subjects. *J Clin Invest* 45:429, 1966.
830. Krieger DT, Glick SM: Growth hormone and cortisol responsiveness in Cushing's syndrome: Relation to a possible central nervous system etiology. *Am J Med* 52:25, 1972.
831. Donald RA: Plasma immunoreactive corticotrophin and cortisol response to insulin hypoglycemia in normal subjects and patients with pituitary disease. *J Clin Endocrinol Metab* 32:225, 1975.
832. Moll GW, Rosenfield RL: Testosterone binding and free plasma androgen concentrations under physiological conditions: Characterization by flow dialysis technique. *J Clin Endocrinol Metab* 49:730, 1979.
833. Vermeulen A, Ando S: Metabolic clearance rate and interconversion of androgens and the influence of the free androgen fraction. *J Clin Endocrinol Metab* 48:320, 1979.
834. Vermeulen A, Stoïca T, Verdonck K: The apparent free testosterone concentrations: An index of androgenicity. *J Clin Endocrinol Metab* 33:759, 1971.
835. Fisher RA, Anderson DC, Burke C: Simultaneous measurement of unbound testosterone and estradiol fractions in undiluted plasma at 37°C by steady-state gel filtration. *Steroids* 24:809, 1974.
836. Vermuelen A, Rubens R: Adrenal virilism, in James VHT (ed): *The Adrenal Gland*. New York, Raven, 1979, p 259.
837. Hammond GL, Nisker JA, Jones LA, Siiteri PK: Estimation of the percentage of free steroid in undiluted serum by centrifugal ultrafiltration-dialysis. *J Biol Chem* 255:5023, 1986.
838. Givens JR: Normal and abnormal androgen metabolism. *Clin Obstet Gynecol* 21:115, 1978.
839. Rosenfield RL: Studies of the relation of plasma androgen levels to androgen action in women. *J Steroid Biochem* 6:695, 1975.
840. Rosenfield RL: Plasma free androgen patterns in hirsute women and their diagnostic implications. *Am J Med* **66**: 417, 1979.
841. Anderson DC: The role of sex hormone binding globulin in health and disease, in James VHT, Serio M, Giusti G (eds): *The Endocrine Function of the Human Ovary*. London, Academic, 1976, p 141.
842. Horton R, Hawks D, Lobo R: 3α, 17β-Androstanediol glucuronide in plasma: A marker of androgen action in idiopathic hirsuitism. *J Clin Invest* 69:1203, 1982.
843. Nisula BC, Loriaux DL, Wilson YA: Solid phase method for measurement of the binding capacity of testosterone-estradiol binding globulin in human serum. *Steroids* 31:681, 1978.
844. Maroulis GB, Manlimos FS, Abraham GE: Comparison between urinary 17-ketosteroids and plasma androgens in hirsute patients. *Obstet Gynecol* 49:454, 1977.
845. Margraf HW, Weichselbaum TE: Laboratory procedures in diagnosis of adrenal cortical diseases, in Eisenstein AB (ed): *The Adrenal Cortex*. Boston, Little, Brown, 1967, p 405.

846. Abraham GE, Maroulis GB, Buster JE, Chang RJ, Marshall JR: Effect of dexamethasone on serum cortisol and androgen levels in hirsute patients. *Obstet Gynecol* 47:395, 1976.
847. Abraham GE, Chakmakjian ZH: Plasma steroids in hirsutism. *Obstet Gynecol* 44:171, 1974.
848. Paulson JD, Keller DW, Wiest WG, Warren JC: Free testosterone concentrations in serum: Elevations is the hallmark of hirsutism. *Am J Obstet Gynecol* 128:851, 1977.
849. New MI, del Balzo P, Crawford C, Speiser PW: The adrenal cortex in clinical pediatric endocrinology, in Kaplan SA (ed): *Endocrinology*. Philadelphia, Saunders, 1990, p 181.
850. Hindmarsh PC, Brook CGD: Single dose dexamethasone suppression test in children: Dose relationship to body size. *Clin Endocrinol (Oxf)* 23:67, 1985.
851. Speiser PW, Agdere L, Veshiba H, White PC, New MI: Aldosterone synthesis in patients with salt-wasting congenital adrenal hyperplasia (21-hydroxylase deficiency) and complete absence of adrenal 21-hydroxylase (P450c21). *N Engl J Med* 3221:145, 1991.
852. Miller DL: The congenital adrenal hyperplasias. *Endocrinol Metab Clin North Am* 20:721, 1991.
853. Miller DL: Genetics, diagnosis, and management of 21-hydroxylase deficiency. *J Clin Endocrinol Metab* 78:241, 1994.
854. Voutitainen R, Miller WL: Developmental expression of genes for the steroidogenic enzymes P450SCC (20, 22 desmolase), P450C17 (17α-hydroxylase/17, 20 lyase), and P450C21 (21-hydroxylase) in the human fetus. *J Clin Endocrinol Metab* 63:1145, 1986.
855. Grumbach MM, Conte FA: Disorders of sex differentiation, in Wilson JD, Foster DW (eds): *Williams' Textbook of Endocrinology,* 8th ed. Saunders, Philadelphia, 1992, p. 853.
856. Cara JF, Mashang TS, Bongiovanni AM, Marx BS: Elevated 17-hydroxyprogesterone and testosterone in a newborn with 3-beta-hydroxysteroid dehydrogenase deficiency. *N Engl J Med* 313:618, 1985.
857. Mulaikal RM, Migeon CJ, Rock JA: Fertility rates in female patients with congenital adrenal hyperplasia due to 21-hydroxylase deficiency. *N Engl J Med* 316:178, 1987.
858. Migeon CJ, Rosenwaks Z, Lee PA, Urban MD, Bias WB: The attenuated form of congenital adrenal hyperplasia as an allelic form of 21-hydroxylase deficiency. *J Clin Endocrinol Metab* 51:647, 1980.
859. Kohn B, Levine L, Pollack MS, Pang S, Lorenzen L, Levy D, Lerner AJ, Rondanini GF, et al: Late-onset steroid 21 hydroxylase deficiency: A variant of classical congenital adrenal hyperplasia. *J Clin Endocrinol Metab* 55:817, 1982.
860. Chrousos GP, Loriaux DL, Mann DL, Cutler GB Jr: Late-onset 21-hydroxylase deficiency mimicking idiopathic hirsutism or polycystic ovarian disease: An allelic variant of congenital virilizing adrenal hyperplasia with a milder enzymatic defect. *Ann Intern Med* 96:143, 1982.
861. Levine LS, Dupont B, Lorenzen F, Pang S, Pollack MS: et al: Genetic and hormonal characterization of the cryptic 21-hydroxylase deficiency. *J Clin Endocrinol Metab* 53:1193, 1981.
862. Fiet J, Gueux B, Gourmelen M, Kuttenn F, Vexiau P, Cuillin P, Pham-Huu-Trung M-T, Vilette J-M, et al: Comparison of basal and adreno-corticotropin-stimulated plasma 21-desoxycortisol and 17-hydroxyprogesterone values as biological markers of late-onset adrenal hyperplasia. *J Clin Endocrinol Metab* 66:659, 1988.
863. Pang S, Wallace MA, Hofman L, Thuline HC, Dorche C, Lyon ICT, Dobbind RH, Kling S, et al: Worldwide experience in newborn screening for classical congenital adrenal hyperplasia due to 21-hydroxylase deficiency. *Pediatrics* 81:866, 1988.
864. Speiser PW, Dupont BG, Rubinstein P, Piazza A, Kastelan A, New MI: High frequency of nonclassical steroid 21-hydroxylase deficiency. *Am J Hum Genet* 37:650, 1985.
865. Sherman SL, Aston CE, Morton NE, Speiser PW, New MI: A segregation and linkage study of classical and nonclassical 21-hydroxylase deficiency. *Am J Hum Genet* 42:830, 1988.
866. Dumic M, Brkljacic L, Speiser PW, Wood E, Crawford C, Plavsic V, Baniceviac M, Radmanovic S, et al: An update on the frequency of nonclassic deficiency of adrenal 21-hydroxylase in the Yugoslav population. *Acta Endocrinol (Copenh)* 122:703, 1990.
867. Kuttenn F, Couillin P, Girard F, Billaud L, Vincens M, Boucekkine C, Thalabard J-C, Maudelonde T, et al: Late-onset adrenal hyperplasia in hirsutism. *N Engl J Med* 313:224, 1985.
868. Chetkowski RJ, DeFazio J, Shamonki I, Judd HL, Chang RJ: The incidence of the late-onset congenital adrenal hyperplasia due to 21-hydroxylase deficiency among hirsute women. *J Clin Endocrinol Metab* 58:595, 1984.
869. Gourmelen M, Gueux B, Pham-Huu-Trung MT, Fiet J, Raux-Demay MC, Girard F: Detection of heterozygous carriers for 21-hydroxylase deficiency by plasma 21-deoxycortisol measurement. *Acta Endocrinol (Copenh)* 116:507, 1987.
870. Carroll MC, Campbell RD, Porter RR: Mapping of steroid 21-hydroxylase genes to complement component C4 genes in HLA, the major histocompatibility locus in man. *Proc Natl Acad Sci USA* 82:52, 1985.
871. White PC, Grossberger D, Onufer BJ, Chaplin DD, New MI, Dupont B, Strominger JL: Two genes encoding steroid 21-hydroxylase are located near the genes encoding the fourth component of the complement in man. *Proc Natl Acad Sci USA* 82:1089, 1985.
872. Chiou SH, Hu MC, Chung B-C: A missense mutation of Ile172 Asn or Arg356 Trp causes steroid 21-hydroxylase deficiency. *J Biol Chem* 265:3549, 1990.
873. Hood L, Campbell JH, Elgin SCR: The organization expression and evolution of antibody genes and other multigene families. *Annu Rev Genet* 9:305, 1975.
874. Liebhaber SA, Goossens M, Kan YW: Homology and concerted evolution of the α-1 and α-2 locus of human α-globin. *Nature* 290:26, 1981.
875. Miller WL, Eberhardt NL: Structure and evolution of the growth hormone gene family. *Endocr Rev* 4:97, 1983.
876. Amor M, Tosi M, Duponchel C, Steinmetz M, Meo T: Liver cDNA probes disclose two cytochrome P450 genes duplicated in tandem with the complement C4 loci of the mouse H-2S region. *Proc Natl Acad Sci USA* 82:4453, 1985.
877. Skow LE, Womack JE, Petresh JM, Miller WL: Synteny mapping of the genes for steroid 21-hydroxylase, alpha-A-crystallin, and class I bovine leukocyte antigen (BoLA) in cattle. *DNA* 7:143, 1988.
878. Chung B, Matteson KJ, Miller WL: Cloning and characterization of the bovine gene for steroid 21-hydroxylase (P450c21). *DNA* 4:211, 1985.
879. Parker KL, Chaplin DD, Wong M, Seidman JG, Smith JA, Schimmer BP: Expression of murine 21-hydroxylase in mouse adrenal glands and in transfected Y1 adrenocortical tumor cells. *Proc Natl Acad Sci USA* 82:7860, 1985.
880. Chaplin DD, Galbreath LG, Seidman JG, White PC, Parker KL: Nucleotide sequence analysis of murine 21-hydroxylase genes: Mutations affecting gene expression. *Proc Natl Acad Sci USA* 83:960, 1986.
881. Miller WL: Gene conversions, deletions, and polymorphisms in congenital adrenal hyperplasia. *Am J Hum Genet* 42:4, 1988.
882. Gitelman SE, Bristow J, Miller WL: Mechanism and consequences of the duplication of the human C4/P450c21/Gene X locus. *Mol Cell Biol* 12:12124, 1992.
883. Kay PH, Dawkins RL, Bowling AT, Bernoco D: Heterogeneity and linkage of equine C4 and steroid 21-hydroxylase genes. *J Immunogenet* 14:247, 1987.
884. Geffrotin C, Chardon P, DeAndres-Cara DF, Feil R, Re-

nard C, Vaiman M: The swine steroid 21-hydroxylase gene (CYP21): Cloning and mapping within the swine leukocyte antigen locus. *Anim Genet* 21:1, 1990.
885. Dupont B, Oberfield SE, Smithwick ER, Lee TD, Levine LS: Close genetic linkage between HLA and congenital adrenal hyperplasia (21-hydroxylase deficiency). *Lancet* 2:1309, 1977.
886. Dunham I, Sargent CA, Trowsdale J, Campbell RD: Molecular mapping of the human major histocompatibility complex by pulsed-field gel electrophoresis. *Proc Natl Acad Sci USA* 84:7237, 1987.
887. Spies T, Blanck G, Bresnarhan M, Sands J, Strominger JL: A new cluster of genes within the human major histocompatibility complex. *Science* 243:214, 1989.
888. Partanen J, Koskimies S, Sipila I, Lipsanen V: Major histocompatibility-complex gene markers and restriction fragment analysis of steroid 21-hydroxylase (CYP21) and complement C4 genes in classical adrenal hyperplasia patients in a single population. *Am J Hum Genet* 44:660, 1989.
889. Dupont B, Pollack MS, Levine LS, O'Neill GJ, Hawkins BR, New M: Congenital adrenal hyperplasia: Joint report from the eighth international histocompatibility workshop, in Terasaki PI (ed): *Histocompatibility Testing 1980*. Berlin, Springer-Verlag, 1981, p 693.
890. Fleischnick E, Awdeh ZL, Raum D, Granados J, Alosco SM, Crigler JR Jr, Gerald PS, Giles CM, et al: Extended MHC haplotypes in 21-hydroxylase deficiency congenital adrenal hyperplasia: Shared genotypes in unrelated patients. *Lancet* 1:152, 1983.
891. Holler W, Scholz S, Knorr D, Bidlingmaier F, Keller E, Ekkehard DA: Genetic differences between the salt-wasting, simple virilizing and nonclassical types of congenital adrenal hyperplasia. *J Clin Endocrinol Metab* 60:757, 1985.
892. Pollack MS, Levine LS, O'Neill GL: HLA linkage and B14, DR1, BfS haplotype association with the genes for late onset and cryptic 21-hydroxylase deficiency. *Am J Hum Genet* 33:540, 1981.
893. Speiser PW, New MI, White P: Molecular genetic analysis of nonclassical steroid 21-hydroxylase deficiency associated with HLA-B14DR1. *N Engl J Med* 319:19, 1988.
894. Morel Y, Andre J, Uring-Lambert B, Hauptman G, Betuel H, Tosi M, Forest MG, David M, et al: Rearrangements and point mutations of P450c21 genes are distinguished by five restriction endonuclease haplotypes identified by a new probing strategy in 57 families with congenital adrenal hyperplasia. *J Clin Invest* 83:527, 1989.
895. Rosenbloom NR, Smith DW: Varying expression for salt-losing in related patients with congenital adrenal hyperplasia. *Pediatrics* 38:215, 1966.
896. Stoner E, DiMartina J, Kuhnle U, Levine LS, Oberfield SE, New MI: Is salt-wasting in congenital adrenal hyperplasia genetic? *Clin Endocrinol (Oxf)* 24:9, 1986.
897. Morel Y, David M, Forest MG, Betuel H, Hauptman G, Andre J, Bertrand J, Miller WL: Gene conversions and rearrangements cause discordance between inheritance of forms of 21-hydroxylase deficiency and HLA types. *J Clin Endocrinol Metab* 68:592, 1989.
898. Sinnott PJ, Dyer PA, Price DA, Harris R, Strachan T: 21-Hydroxylase deficiency families with HLA identical affected and unaffected sibs. *J Med Genet* 26:10, 1989.
899. Carroll MC, Campbell RD, Bentley DR, Porter RR: A molecular map of the human major histocompatibility class III region lining complement genes C4, C2 and factor B. *Nature* 307:237, 1984.
900. Yu YC, Belt KT, Giles CM, Campbell RD, Porter RR: Structural basis of the polymorphism of the human complement components C4A and C4B: Gene size, reactivity and antigenicity. *EMBO J* 5:2873, 1986.
901. Levi-Strauss M, Carroll MC, Steinmetz M, Meo T: A previously undetected MHC gene with an unusual periodic structure. *Science* 240:201, 1988.
902. Speiser PW, White PC: Structure of the human RD gene: A highly conserved gene in the class III region of the major histocompatibility. *DNA* 8:745, 1989.
903. Sargent CA, Dunham I, Campbell RC: Identification of multiple HTF-island associated genes in the major histocompatibility complex class III region. *EMBO J* 8:2305, 1989.
904. Morel Y, Bristow J, Gitelman SE, Miller WL: Transcript encoded on the opposite strand of the human 21-hydroxylase/C4 locus. *Proc Natl Acad Sci USA* 86:6582, 1989.
905. Tokunaga K, Saueracker G, Kay PH, Christiansen FT, Anand R, Dawkins RL: Extensive deletions and insertions in different MHC supratypes detected by pulsed field gel electrophoresis. *J Exp Med* 168:933, 1988.
906. Collier S, Sinnott PJ, Dyer PA, Price DA, Harris R, Strachan T: Pulse field gel electrophoresis identifies a high degree of variability in the number of tandem 21-hydroxylase and complement C4 gene repeats in 21-hydroxylase deficiency haplotypes. *EMBO J* 8:1393, 1989.
907. Dunham I, Sargent CA, Dawkins RL, Campbell RD: Direct observation of the gene organization of the complement C4 and 21-hydroxylase loci by pulse field gel electrophoresis. *J Exp Med* 169:1989.
908. Partanen J, Kere J, Wessberg S, Koskimies S: Determination of deletion sizes in human C4 and CYP21 genes using pulsed field gel electrophoresis. *Genomics* 5:345, 1989.
909. Sinnott P, Collier S, Costigan C, Dyer PA, Harris R, Strachan T: Genetic by meiotic unequal crossover of a de novo deletion that contributes to steroid 21-hydroxylase deficiency. *Proc Natl Acad Sci USA* 87:2107, 1990.
910. Baltimore D: Gene conversion: Some implications for immunoglobulin genes. *Cell* 24:592, 1981.
911. Szostak JW, Orr-Weaver TL, Rothstein RJ: The double-stranded-break repair model for recombination. *Cell* 33:25, 1983.
912. Nicolas A, Treco D, Schultes NP, Szostak JW: An initiation site for meiotic gene conversion in the yeast *Saccharomyces cerevisiae*. *Nature* 338:35, 1989.
913. Fincham JRS, Oliver P: Initiation of recombination. *Nature* 338:14, 1989.
914. Donohoue PA, Van Dop C, McLean RH, White PC, Jospe N, Migeon CJ: Gene conversion in salt-losing congenital adrenal hyperplasia with absent complement C4B protein. *J Clin Endocrinol Metab* 62:995, 1986.
915. Higashi Y, Tanae A, Inoue H, Fujii-Kuriyama Y: Evidence for frequent gene conversions in the steroid 21-hydroxylase (P-450c21) gene: Implications for steroid 21-hydroxylase deficiency. *Am J Hum Genet* 42:17, 1988.
916. Harada F, Kimura A, Iwanaga T, Shimozawa K, Yata J, Sasazuki T: Gene conversion-like events cause steroid 21-hydroxylase deficiency in congenital adrenal hyperplasia. *Proc Natl Acad Sci USA* 84:8091, 1987
917. Jospe N, Donohoue PA, Van Dop C, McLean RH, Bias W, Migeon CJ: Prevalence of polymorphic 21-hydroxylase gene (CAH21B) mutations in salt-losing congenital adrenal hyperplasia. *Biochem Biophys Res Commun* 142:798, 1987.
918. Matteson KJ, Phillips JAI, Miller WL, Chung B, Orlando PJ, Frisch H, Ferrandez A, Burr IM: P450XXI (steroid 21-hydroxylase) gene deletions are not found in family studies of congenital adrenal hyperplasia. *Proc Natl Acad Sci USA* 84:5858, 1987.
919. White PC, Vitek B, Dupont B, New MI: Characterization of frequent deletions causing steroid 21-hydroxylase deficiency. *Proc Natl Acad Sci USA* 85:4436, 1988.
920. Amor M, Parker KL, Globerman H, New MI, White PC: Mutation in the CYP21B gene (Ile-172-Asn) causes steroid 21-hydroxylase deficiency. *Proc Natl Acad Sci USA* 85:1600, 1988.

921. Globerman H, Amor M, Parker PL, New MI, White PC: Nonsense mutation causing steroid 21-hydroxylase deficiency. *J Clin Invest* 82:139, 1988.
922. Higashi Y, Tanae A, Inoue Y, Fujii-Kuriyama HT: Aberrant splicing and missense mutations cause steroid 21-hydroxylase {P-450(C21)} deficiency in humans: Possible gene conversion products. *Proc Natl Acad Sci USA* 85:7486, 1988.
923. Hu MC, Chung B-C: Expression of human 21-hydroxylase (P450c21) in bacterial and mammalian cells—a system to characterize normal and mutant enzymes. *Mol Endocrinol* 4:893, 1990.
924. Urabe K, Kimura A, Harada F, Iwanaga T, Sasazuki T: Gene conversion in steroid 21-hydroxylase genes. *Am J Hum Genet* 46:1178, 1990.
925. Mornet E, Crété P, Kuttenn F, Raux-Demay MC, Boué J, White PC, Boué A: Distribution of deletions and seven point mutations on CYP21B genes in three clinical forms of steroid 21-hydroxylase deficiency. *Am J Hum Genet* 48:79, 1991.
926. Morel Y, Murena M, Forest MG, Nicolino M, David M: Frequency of the 8 known deleterious point mutations of the CYP21B gene in more than 100 families with 21-hydroxylase deficiency (CAH): Implications for prenatal diagnosis. *Abstracts of the 73rd Annual Meeting of the Endocrine Society*, 1991, 375.
927. Speiser PW, Dupont J, Zhu D, Serrat J, Buegeleisen M, Tusie-Luna M, Lesser M, New MI, et al: Disease expression and molecular genotype in congenital adrenal hyperplasia due to 21-hydroxylase deficiency. *J Clin Invest* 90:584, 1992.
928. Donohoue PA, Neto RS, Collins MM, Migeon CJ: Exon 7 Nco I restriction site within CYP21B (steroid 21-hydroxylase) is a normal polymorphism. *Mol Endocrinol* 4:1354, 1990.
929. Owerbach D, Crawford YM, Draznin MB: Direct analysis of CYP21B genes in 21-hydroxylase deficiency using polymerase chain reaction amplification. *Mol Endocrinol* 4:125, 1990.
930. Owerbach D, Ballard AL, Draznin MB: Salt-wasting congenital adrenal hyperplasia: Detection and characterization of mutations in the steroid 21-hydroxylase gene, CYP21, using the polymerase chain reaction. *J Clin Endocrinol Metab* 74:553, 1992.
931. Higashi Y, Hiromasa T, Tanae A, Miki T, Nakura J, Kondo T, Ohura T, Ogawa E, et al: Effects of individual mutations in the P450(c21) pseudogene on the P450(c21) activity and their distribution in the client genomes of congenital steroid 21-hydroxylase deficiency. *J Biochem* 109:638, 1991.
932. Picado-Leonard J, Miller WL: Homologous sequences in steroidogenic enzymes, steroid receptors and a steroid binding protein suggest a consensus steroid-binding sequence. *Mol Endocrinol* 2:1145, 1988.
933. Kitamura M, Buczko E, Dufau ML: Dissociation of hydroxylase and lyase activities by site-directed mutagenesis of the rat P450-17α. *Mol Endocrinol* 5:1373, 1991.
934. Wu DA, Chung B: Mutations of P450c21 at Cys^{428}, Val^{281}, or Ser^{268} result in complete, partial, or no loss of enzymatic activity. *J Clin Invest* 88:519, 1991.
935. Tusie-Luna M, Speiser PW, Dumic M, New MI, White PC: A mutation (Pro-30 to Leu) in CYP21 represents a potential nonclassic steroid 21-hydroxylase deficiency allele. *Mol Endocrinol* 5:685, 1991.
936. Morel Y: Personal communication. 1993.
937. Owerbach D, Sherman L, Ballard AL, Azziz R: Pro453 to Ser mutation in CYP21 is associated with nonclassic steroid 21-hydroxylase deficiency. *Mol Endocrinol* 6:1211, 1992.
938. Helmburg A, Tusie-Luna M, Tabarelli M, Kofler R, White PC: R339H and P453S: CYP21 mutations associated with nonclassic steroid 21-hydroxylase deficiency that are not apparent gene conversions. *Mol Endocrinol* 6:1318, 1992.
939. Monier S, VanLuc P, Kreibich G, Sabatini DD, Adesnik M: Signals for incorporation and orientation of cytochrome P450 in the endoplasmic reticulum membrane. *J Cell Biol* 107:457, 1988.
940. Hsu LC, Hu MC, Cheng HC, Lu JC, Chung B: The N-terminal hydrophobic domain of P450c21 is required for membrane insertion and enzyme stability. *J Biol Chem* 268:14682, 1993.
941. Forest MG, Bètuel H, Couillin P, Bouq A: Prenatal diagnosis of congenital adrenal hyperplasia (CAH) due to 21-hydroxylase deficiency by steroid analysis in the amniotic fluid of mid-pregnancy: Comparison with HLA typing in 17 pregnancies at risk for CAH. *Prenat Diagn* 1:197, 1981.
942. Forest MG, Bètuel H, David M: Prenatal treatment in congenital adrenal hyperplasia due to 21-hydroxylase deficiency: Update 88 of the French multicentric study. *Endocr Res* 15:277, 1989.
943. Pang S, Levine LS, Cederquist KK, Fuentes M, Riccari VM, Holcombe JH, Nitowski HM, Sachs G, et al: Amniotic fluid concentrations of Δ-5 and Δ-4 steroids in fetuses with congenital adrenal hyperplasia due to 21-hydroxylase deficiency and in anencephalic fetuses. *J Clin Endocrinol Metab* 51:223, 1980.
944. Pang S, Pollack MS, Loo M, Green O, Nussbaum R, Clayton G, Dupont B, New MI: Pitfalls of prenatal diagnosis of 21-hydroxylase deficiency congenital adrenal hyperplasia. *J Clin Endocrinol Metab* 61:89, 1985.
945. Hughes IA, Dyas J, Riad-Fahmy D, Laurence KM: Prenatal diagnosis of congenital adrenal hyperplasia: Reliability of amniotic fluid steroid analysis. *J Med Genet* 24:344, 1987.
946. Migeon CJ: Comments about the need for prenatal treatment of congenital adrenal hyperplasia due to 21-hydroxylase deficiency. *J Clin Endocrinol Metab* 70:836, 1990.
947. Pang S, Pollack MS, Marshall RN, Immken LD: Prenatal treatment of congenital adrenal hyperplasia due to 21-hydroxylase deficiency. *N Engl J Med* 322:111, 1990.
948. Speiser PW, Laforgia N, Kato K, Pareira J, Khan R, Yang SY, Whorwood C, White PC, et al:First trimester prenatal treatment and molecular genetic diagnosis of congenital adrenal hyperplasia (21-hydroxylase deficiency). *J Clin Endocrinol Metab* 70:838, 1990.
949. Lashansky G, Saenger P, Fishman K, Gautier T, Mayes D, Berg G, Di Martino Nardi J, Reiter E: Normative data for adrenal steroidogenesis in a healthy pediatric population: Age and sex related changes after adrenocorticotropin stimulation. *J Clin Endocrinol Met* 73:674, 1991.
950. New MI, Lorenzen F, Lerner AJ, Kohn B, Oberfield SE, Pollack MS, Dupont B, Stoner E, et al: Genotyping steroid 21 hydroxylase deficiency: Hormonal reference data. *J Clin Endocrinol Metab* 57:320, 1983.
951. Laue L, Cutler GB Jr: 21-Hydroxylase deficiency: Overview of treatment. *The Endocrinologist* 2:291, 1992.
952. Kenny FM, Preeyasombat C, Migeon CJ: Cortisol production rate: II Normal infants, children and adults. *Pediatrics* 37:34, 1966.
953. Kenny FM, Taylor FH, Richards C: Reference standards for cortisol production and 17-hydroxy corticosteroid excretion during growth: Variation in the pattern of excretion of radiolabeled cortisol metabolites. *Metabolism* 19:280, 1970.
954. Styne DM, Richards GE, Bell JJ, Conte FA, Morishima A, Kaplan SL, Grumbach MM: Growth patterns in congenital adrenal hyperplasia: Correlations of glucocorticoid therapy with stature, in Lee PA, Plotnick LP, Kowarski A, Migeon C (eds): *Congenital Adrenal Hyperplasia*. Baltimore, University Park Press, 1977, p 247.
955. Bongiovanni AM: The adrenogenital syndrome with deficiency of 3β-hydroxysteroid dehydrogenase. *J Clin Invest* 41:2086, 1962.

956. Rheaume E, Simard J, Morel Y, Mebarki F, Zachmann M, Forest MG, New MI, Labrie F: Congenital adrenal hyperplasia due to point mutations in the type II 3β-hydroxysteroid dehydrogenase gene. *Nature Genet* 1:239, 1992.
957. Simard J, Rheaume E, Sanchez R, Laflamme N, Heinrich U, Moshang T, New MI, Labrie F: Molecular basis of congenital adrenal hyperplasia due to 3β-hydroxysteroid dehydrogenase deficiency. *Mol Endocrinol* 7:716, 1993.
957a. Chang YT, Kappy MS, Iwamoto K, Wang J, Yang X, Pang S: Mutations in the type II 3β-hydroxysteroid dehydrogenase gene in a patient with classic salt-lasting 3β-hydroxysteroid dehydrogenase deficiency congenital adrenal hyperplasia. *Pediatr Res* 34:698, 1993.
958. Rosenfield RL, Rich BH, Wolfsdorf JI, Cassorla F, Parks JS, Bongiovanni AM, Wu CH, Shakleton CHL: Pubertal presentation of congenital 3β-hydroxysteroid dehydrogenase deficiency. *J Clin Endocrinol Metab* 51:345, 1980.
959. Pang S, Levine LS, Stoner E, Optiz JM, Pollack MS, Dupont B, New MI: Nonsalt-losing congenital adrenal hyperplasia due to 3β-hydroxysteroid dehydrogenase deficiency with normal glomerulosa function. *J Clin Endocrinol Metab* 56:808, 1983.
960. Pang S, Lerner AJ, Stoner E: Late onset adrenal 3β-hydroxysteroid dehydrogenase deficiency: I. A cause of hirsuitism in pubertal and post-pubertal women. *J Clin Endocrinol Metab* 60:428, 1985.
961. Yanase T, Simpson ER, Waterman MR: 17α-hydroxylase/17,20 lyase deficiency: From clinical investigation to molecular definition. *Endocr Rev* 12:91, 1991.
962. Scaroni C, Opocher G, Mantero F: Renin-angiotensin-aldosterone system: A long-term follow-up study in 17α-hydroxylase deficiency syndrome. *Hypertesion (Clin Exp Theory Pract)* A8:773, 1986.
963. Biglieri EG, Herron MA, Brust N: 17α-Hydroxylation deficiency in man. *J Clin Invest* 45:1946, 1966.
964. New MI: Male pseudohermaphroditism due to 17α-hydroxylase deficiency. *J Clin Invest* 49:1930, 1970.
965. Goldsmith O, Solomon DH, Horton R: Hypogonadism and mineralocorticoid excess: The 17-hydroxylase deficiency syndrome. *N Engl J Med* 277:673, 1976.
966. Zachmann M, Werder EA, Prader A: Two types of male pseudohermaphroditism due to 17,20 desmolase deficiency. *J Clin Endocrinol Metab* 55:487, 1982.
967. Biason A, Mantero F, Scaroni C, Simpson ER, Waterman MR: Deletion within the CYP17 gene together with insertion of foreign DNA is the cause of combined complete 17α-hydroxylase/17,20 lyase deficiency in an Italian patient. *Mol Endocrinol* 5:2037, 1991.
967a. Fardella CE, Hum DW, Homoki J, Miller WL: Point mutation of Arg440 to His in cytochrome P450c17 causes severe 17α-hydroxylase deficiency. *J. Clin Endocrinol Metab* 79:160, 1994.
968. Zachmann M, Tassinari D, Prader A: Clinical and biochemical variability of congenital adrenal hyperplasia due to 11β-hydroxylase deficiency. *J Clin Endocrinol Metab* 56:222, 1983.
969. Holcombe JH, Keenan BS, Nichols BL, Kirkland RT, Clayton GW: Neonatal salt loss in the hypertensive form of congenital adrenal hyperplasia. *Pediatrics* 65:777, 1980.
970. Sonino N, Levine LS, Vecscei P, New MI: Parallelism of 11β- and 18-hydroxylation demonstrated by urinary free hormones in man. *J Clin Endocrinol Metab* 51:557, 1980.
971. Helmberg A, Ausserer B, Kofler R: Frameshift by insertion of 2 basepairs in codon 394 of CYP11B1 causes congenital adrenal hyperplasia due to steroid 11β-hydroxylase deficiency. *J Clin Endocrinol Metab* 75:1278, 1992.
972. Curnow KM, Slutsker L, Vitek J, Cole T, Speiser PW, New MI, White PC, Pascoe L: Mutations in the CYP11B1 gene causing congenital adrenal hyperplasia and hypertension cluster in exons 6, 7, and 8. *Proc Natl Acad Sci USA* 90:4552, 1993.
973. Rosler A, White PC: Mutations in human 11β-hydroxylase genes: 11β-hydroxylase deficiency in Jews of Morocco and corticosterone methyl-oxidase II deficiency in Jews of Iran. *J Steroid Biochem Mol Biol* 45:99, 1993.
973a. Fardella CE, Hum DW, Miller WL: Gene conversion in exons 3 and 4 of the CYP11B2 gene encoding P450c11AS causes primary hypoaldosteronism (CMOII deficiency). Abstract of the 76th Annual Meeting of The Endocrine Society, Anaheim, CA, 1994.
974. Lifton RP, Dluhy RG, Powers M, Rich GM, Cook S, Ulick S, Lalovel JM: A chimaeric 11β-hydroxylase/aldosterone synthase gene causes glucocorticoid-remediable aldosteronism and human hypertension. *Nature* 355:262, 1992.
975. Pascoe L, Curnow KM, Slutsker L, Connell JMC, Speiser PW, New MI, White PC: Glucocorticoid-suppressible hyperaldosteronism results from hybrid genes created by unequal crossovers between CYP11B1 and CYP11B2. *Proc Natl Acad Sci USA* 89:8327, 1992.
976. Sandison AT: A form of lipidosis of the adrenal cortex in an infant. *Arch Dis Child* 30:538, 1955.
977. Prader A, Siebenmann RE: Nebennireninsuffizienz bei kongenitaler Lipoidhyperplasie der Nebennieren. *Helv Paediatr Acta* 12:569, 1957.
978. Kirkland RT, Kirkland JL, Johnson CM, Horning MG, Librik L, Clayton GW: Congenital lipoid adrenal hyperplasia in an eight-year-old phenotypic female. *J Clin Endocrinol Metab* 36:488, 1973.
979. Hauffa B, Miller WL, Grumbach MM, Conte FA, Kaplan SL: Congenital adrenal hyperplasia due to deficient cholesterol side-chain cleavage activity (20,22 desmolase) in a patient treated for 18 years. *Clin Endocrinol (Oxf)* 23:481, 1985.
980. Degenhart HJ, Visser HKA, Boon H, O'Doherty NJ: Evidence for deficient 20α-cholesterol-hydroxylase activity in adrenal tissue of a patient with lipoid adrenal hyperplasia. *Acta Endocrinol (Copenh)* 71:512, 1972.
981. Camacho AM, Kowarski A, Migeon CJ, Brough AJ: Congenital adrenal hyperplasia due to a deficiency of one of the enzymes involved in the biosynthesis of pregnenolone. *J Clin Endocrinol Metab* 28:153, 1968.
982. Koizumi S, Kyoya S, Miyawaki T, Kidani H, Funabashi T, Nakashima H, Nakanuma Y, Ohta G, et al: Cholesterol side-chain cleavage enzyme activity and cytochrome P450 content in adrenal mitochondria of a patient with congenital lipoid adrenal hyperplasia (Prader disease). *Clin Chim Acta* 77:301, 1977.
983. Lin D, Gitelman SE, Saenger PA, Miller WL: Normal genes for the cholesterol side-chain cleavage enzyme, P450scc in congenital lipoid adrenal hyperplasia. *J Clin Invest* 88:1955, 1991.
984. Björkhem I, Holmberg I, Oftebro H, Pedersen JI: Properties of a reconstituted vitamin D_3 25-hydroxylase from rat liver mitochondria. *J Biol Chem* 255:5244, 1980.
985. Wikvall K: Hydroxylations in biosynthesis of bile acids: Isolation of a cytochrome P-450 from rabbit liver mitochondria catalyzing 26-hydroxylation of C-27 steroids. *J Biol Chem* 259:3800, 1984.
986. Su P, Rennert H, Shayiq RM, Yamamoto R, Zheng Y, Addya S, Strauss JF III, Avadhani NG: A cDNA encoding a rat mitochondrial cytochrome P450 catalyzing both the 26-hydroxylations of cholesterol and the 25-hydroxylation of vitamin D_3: Gonadotropic regulation of the cognate mRNA in ovaries. *DNA Cell Biol* 9:657, 1990.
987. Shozu M, Akasofu K, Harada T, Kubota Y: A new cause of female pseudohermaphroditism: Placental aromatase deficiency. *J Clin Endocrinol Metab* 72:560, 1991.
988. Klonari Z, Miller WL, Fleischer A, Abram SC, Saenger P: Prenatal diagnosis of congenital lipoid adrenal hyperplasia (abstract). *Pediatr Res* 33(Suppl 5):S23, 1993.
989. Miller WL: The adrenal cortex, in Rudolph AM, Hoffman JIE, Rudolph CR (eds): *Rudolph's Pediatrics*, 19th ed. Norwalk, CT, Appleton & Lange, 1991, p 1584.
990. Yang X, Iwamoto K, Wang M, Artwohl J, Mason JI, Pang

S: Inherited congenital adrenal hyperplasia in the rabbit is caused by a deletion in the gene encoding cytochrome P450 cholesterol side-chain cleavage enzyme. *Endocrinology* 132:1977, 1993.

991. Irvine WJ, Barnes EW: Adrenocortical insufficiency. *Clin Endocrinol Metab* 1:549, 1972.
992. Doniach D, Cudworth AG, Khoury EL, Bottazzo GF: Autoimmunity and the HLA-system in endocrine disease, in O'Riordan JLH (ed): *Recent Advances in Endocrinology and Metabolism*. London, Churchill Livingstone, 1982.
993. Muir A, Maclaren NK: Autoimmune diseases of the adrenal glands, parathyroid glands, gonads, and hypothalamic-pituitary axis. *Endocrin Met Clin North Am* 20:619, 1991.
994. Leshin M: Southwestern internal medicine conference: Polyglandular autoimmune syndromes. *Am J Med Sci* 290:77, 1985.
995. Ahonen P, Myllarniemi S, Sipila I, Perheentupa J: Clinical variation of autoimmune polyendocrinopathy-candidiasis-ectodermal dystrophy (apeced) in a series of 68 patients. *N Engl J Med* 322:1829, 1990.
996. Kasperlik-Zaluska AA, Migdalska B, Czarnocka B, Drac-Kaniewska J, Niegowska E, Czech W: Association of Addison's disease with autoimmune disorders—a long-term observation of 180 patients. *Postgrad Med J* 67:984, 1991.
997. Neufeld M, Maclaren N, Blizzard R: Autoimmune polyglandular syndromes. *Pediatr Ann* 9:154, 1980.
998. Neufeld M, Maclaren NK, Blizzard RM: Two types of autoimmune Addison's disease associated with different polyglandular autoimmune (PGA) syndromes. *Medicine (Baltimore)* 60:355, 1981.
999. Trence DL, Morley JE, Handwerger BS: Polyglandular autoimmune syndromes. *Am J Med* 77:107, 1984.
1000. Nerup J: Addison's disease—a review of some clinical, pathological and immunological features. *Dan Med Bull* 21:201, 1974.
1001. Guttman PH: Addison's disease: A statistical analysis of 566 cases and a study of the pathology. *Arch Pathol* 10:742, 1930.
1002. Alvarez S, McCabe WR: Extrapulmonary tuberculosis revisited: A review of experience at Boston city and other hospitals. *Medicine (Baltimore)* 63:25, 1984.
1003. Dahlberg PJ, Goellner MH, Pehling GB: Adrenal insufficiency secondary to adrenal hemorrhage. Two case reports and a review of cases confirmed by computed tomography. *Arch Intern Med* 150:905, 1990.
1004. Rao RH, Vagnucci AH, Amico JA: Bilateral massive adrenal hemorrhage: Early recognition and treatment. *Ann Intern Med* 110:227, 1989.
1005. Rao RH, Vagnucci AH: The clinical profile and management of bilateral massive adrenal hemorrhage. *Adv Endocrinol Metab* 3:213, 1992.
1006. Xarli VP, Steele AA, Davis PJ, Buescher ES, Rios CN, Garcia-Bunuel R: Adrenal hemorrhage in the adult. *Medicine (Baltimore)* 57:211, 1978.
1007. Amador E: Adrenal hemorrhage during anticoagulant therapy. *Ann Intern Med* 63:559, 1965.
1008. Migeon CJ, Kenny FM, Hung W, Voorhess ML: Study of adrenal function in children with meningitis. *Pediatrics* 40:163, 1967.
1009. Margaretten W, Nakai H, Landing BH: Septicemic adrenal hemorrhage. *Am J Dis Child* 105:346, 1963.
1010. Guenthmer EE, Rabinowe SL, Van Niel A, Naftilian A, Dluhy R: Primary Addison's disease in a patient with the acquired immunodeficiency syndrome. *Ann Intern Med* 100:847, 1984.
1011. Stuart-Mason A, Mead TW, Lee JAH, Morris JN: Epidemiological and clinical picture of Addison's disease. *Lancet* 2:744, 1968.
1012. Nerup J: Addison's disease—clinical studies: A report of 108 cases. *Acta Endocrinol (Copenh)* 76:127, 1974.
1013. Maisey MN: Lessof MH: Addison's disease: A clinical study. *Guys Hosp Rep* 18:363, 1969.
1014. Wulffraat NM, Drexhage HA, Bottazzo GF, Wiersinga WM, Jeucken P, Van der Gaag R: Immunoglobulins of patients with idiopathic Addison's disease block the *in vitro* action of adrenocorticotropin. *J Clin Endocrinol Metab* 69:231, 1989.
1015. Krohn K, Uibo R, Aavik E, Peterson P, Savilahti K: Identification by molecular cloning of an autoantigen associated with Addison's disease as steroid 17α-hydroxylase. *Lancet* 339:770, 1992.
1016. Bednarek J, Furmaniak J, Wedlock N, Kiso Y, Baumann-Antczak A, Fowler S, Krishnan H, Craft JA, et al: Steroid 21-hydroxylase is a major autoantigen involved in adult onset autoimmune Addison's disease. *Fed Eur Biochem Soc* 309:51, 1992.
1017. Winqvist O, Karlsson FA, Kämpe O: 21-Hydroxylase, a major autoantigen in idiopathic Addison's disease. *Lancet* 339:1559, 1992.
1018. Enzymes as autoantigens (editorial). *Lancet* 339:779, 1992.
1019. Banga JP, McGregor AM: Enzymes as targets for autoantibodies in human autoimmune disease: Relevance to pathogenesis. *Autoimmunity* 9:177, 1991.
1020. Schmidt MB: Eine biglandulare erkrankung (nebennieren und Schilddruse) bei morbus Addisonii. *Verh Dtsch Ges Pathol* 212:1926.
1021. Turkington RW, Lebovitz HE: Extra-adrenal endocrine deficiencies in Addison's disease. *Am J Med* 43:499, 1967.
1022. Irvine WJ, Barnes EW: Addison's disease, ovarian failure and hypoparathyroidism. *Clin Endocrinol Metab* 4:379, 1975.
1023. Spinner MW, Blizzard RM, Childs B: Clinical and genetic heterogeneity in idiopathic Addison's disease and hypoparathyroidism. *J Clin Endocrinol Metab* 28:795, 1968.
1024. Chodosh LA, Daniels GH: Addison's disease. *The Endocrinologist* 16:102, 1993.
1025. Symington T: *Functional Pathology of the Human Adrenal Gland*. Edinburgh and London, Livingston, 1969.
1026. Glasgow BJ, Steinsapir KD, Anders K, Layfield LJ: Adrenal pathology in the acquired immune deficiency syndrome. *Am J Clin Pathol* 84:594, 1985.
1027. Vita JA, Silverberg SJ, Goland RS, Austin JHM, Knowlton AI: Clinical clues to the cause of Addison's disease. *Am J Med* 78:461, 1985.
1028. Buxi TBS, Vohra RB, Sujatha, Byotra SP, Mukherji S, Daniel M: CT in adrenal enlargement due to tuberculosis: A review of literature with five new cases. *Clin Imaging* 16:102, 1992.
1029. Sarosi GA, Voth DW, Dahl BA, Doto IL, Tosh FE: Disseminated histoplasmosis: Results of long-term follow-up. *Ann Intern Med* 75:511, 1971.
1030. Schonfeld AD, Jackson JA, Smith DJ, Hurley DL: Disseminated histoplasmosis with bilateral adrenal enlargement: Diagnosis by computed tomography-directed needle biopsy. *J Tex Med* 87:88, 1991.
1031. Wilson DA, Muchmore HG, Tisdal RG, Fahmy A, Pitha JV: Histoplasmosis of the adrenal glands studied by CT. *Radiology* 150:779, 1984.
1032. Washburn RG, Bennett JE: Reversal of adrenal glucocorticoid dysfunction in a patient with disseminated histoplasmosis. *Ann Intern Med* 110:86, 1989.
1033. Moreira AC, Martinez R, Castro M, Elias LLK: Adrenocortical dysfunction in paracoccidioidomycosis: Comparison between plasma β-lipotrophin/adrenocorticotrophin levels and adrenocortical tests. *Clin Endocrinol (Oxf)* 36:545, 1992.
1034. Chandler PT: Addison's disease secondary to North American blastomycosis. *South Med J* 70:863, 1977.
1035. Halvorsen RA Jr, Heaston DK, Johnston WW, Ashton PR, Burton GM: CT guided thin needle aspiration of adrenal blastomycosis. *J Comput Assist Tomogr* 6:389, 1982.

1036. Maloney PJ: Addison's disease due to chronic disseminated coccidioidomycosis. *Arch Intern Med* 90:869, 1952.
1037. Walker BF, Gunthel CJ, Bryan JA, Watts NB, Clark RV: Disseminated cryptococcosis in an apparently normal host presenting as primary adrenal insufficiency: Diagnosis by fine needle aspiration. *Am J Med* 86:715, 1989.
1038. Seidenwurm DJ, Elmer EB, Kaplan LM, Williams EK, Morris DG, Hoffman AR: Metastases to the adrenal glands and the development of Addison's disease. *Cancer* 54:552, 1984.
1039. Redman BG, Pazdur R, Zingas AP, Loredo R: Prospective evaluation of adrenal insufficiency in patients with adrenal metastasis. *Cancer* 60:103, 1987.
1040. Kung AWC, Pun KK, Lam K, Wang C, Leung CY: Addisonian crisis as presenting feature in malignancies. *Cancer* 65:177, 1990.
1041. Feinmann C, Gillett R, Irving MH: Hodgkin's disease presenting with hypoadrenalism. *Br Med J* 2:455, 1976.
1042. Gamelin E, Beldent V, Rousselet M, Rieux D, Rohmer V, Ifrah N, Boasson M, Bigorgne J: Non-Hodgkin's lymphoma presenting with primary adrenal insufficiency. *Cancer* 69:2333, 1992.
1043. Carey RW, Harris N, Kliman B: Addison's disease secondary to lymphomatous infiltration of the adrenal glands. *Cancer* 59:1087, 1987.
1044. Gruhn JG, Gould VE: The adrenal glands, in Kissane JM (ed): *Anderson's Pathology*. St. Louis, Mosby, 1990, vol 2, p 1586.
1045. Korobkin M, White EA, Kressel HY, Moss AA, Montagne J-P: Computed tomography in the diagnosis of adrenal disease. *AJR* 132:231, 1979.
1046. Danby P, Harris KPG, Williams B, Feehally J, Walls J: Adrenal dysfunction in patients with renal amyloid. *Q J Med* 76:915, 1990.
1047. Arik N, Tasdemir I, Karaaslan Y, Uasavul U, Turgan C, Caglar S: Subclinical adrenocortical insufficiency in renal amyloidosis. *Nephron* 56:246, 1990.
1048. Masharani U, Schambelan M: The endocrine complications of acquired immunodeficiency syndrome. *Adv Intern Med* 38:323, 1993.
1049. Bricaire F, Marche C: Adrenocortical lesions and AIDS. *Lancet* 1:881, 1988.
1050. Tapper ML, Rotterdam HZ, Lerner CW, Al Khafaji K, Seitzman PA: Adrenal necrosis in the acquired immunodeficiency syndrome. *Ann Intern Med* 100:239, 1984.
1051. Reichert CM, O'Leary TJ, Levens DL, et al: Autopsy pathology in AIDS. *Am J Pathol* 112:357, 1983.
1051a. Barboza A, Castro BA, Whalen M, Moore CCD, Harkin JS, Miller WL, Gonzales-Scarano F, Levy JA: Infection of cultured adrenal cells by different strains of HIV. *AIDS* 6:1437, 1992.
1052. Parker LN, Levin ER, Lifrak ER: Evidence for adrenocortical adaptation to severe illness. *J Clin Endocrinol Metab* 60:947, 1985.
1053. Norbiato G, Bevilacqua M, Vago T, Baldi G, Chebat E, Bertora P, Moroni M, Galli M, et al: Cortisol resistance in acquired immunodeficiency syndrome. *J Clin Endocrinol Metab* 74:608, 1992.
1054. Greendyke RM: Adrenal hemorrhage. *Am J Clin Pathol* 43:210, 1965.
1055. Siu SCB, Kitzman DW, Sheedy PF II, Northcutt RC: Adrenal insufficiency from bilateral adrenal hemorrhage. *Mayo Clin Proc* 65:664, 1990.
1056. Bosworth DC: Reversible adrenocortical insufficiency fulminant meningococcemia. *Arch Intern Med* 139:823, 1979.
1057. Feuerstein B, Streeten DHP: Recovery of adrenal function after failure resulting from traumatic bilateral adrenal hemorrhages. *Ann Intern Med* 115:785, 1991.
1058. Lia L, Haskin ME, Rose LI, Bemis CE: Diagnosis of bilateral adrenocortical hemorrhage by computed tomography. *Ann Intern Med* 97:720, 1982.
1059. Moser HW, Bergin A, Naidu S, Ladenson PW: Adrenoleukodystrophy. *Endocrinol Metab Clin North Am* 20:297, 1991.
1060. Rizzo WB: X-Linked adrenoleukodystrophy: A cause of primary adrenal insufficiency in males. *The Endocrinologist* 2:177, 1992.
1061. Sadeghi-Nejad A, Senior B: Adrenomyeloneuropathy presenting as Addison's disease in childhood. *N Engl J Med* 322:13, 1990.
1062. Wise JE, Matalon R, Morgan AM, McCabe ERB: Phenotypic features of patients with congenital adrenal hypoplasia and glycerol kinase deficiency. *Am J Dis Child* 141:744, 1987.
1063. Clark AJL, McLoughlin L, Grossman A: Familial glucocorticoid deficiency associated with point mutation in the adrenocorticotropin receptor. *Lancet* 341:461, 1993.
1064. Lanes R, Plotnick LP, Bynum TE, Lee PE, Casella JF, Fox CE, Kowarski AA, Migeon CJ: Glucocorticoid and partial mineralocorticoid deficiency associated with achalasia. *J Clin Endocrinol Metab* 50:268, 1980.
1065. Spark RF, Etzkorn JR: Absent aldosterone response to ACTH in familial glucocorticoid deficiency. *N Engl J Med* 297:917, 1977.
1066. Moshang T, Rosenfield RL, Bongiovanni AM, Parks JS, Amrhein JA: Familial glucocorticoid insufficiency. *J Pediatr* 82:821, 1973.
1067. Pombo M, Devesa J, Taborda A, Iglesias M, Garcia-Moreno F, Gaudiero GJ, Martinon JM, Castro-Gago M, et al: Glucocorticoid deficiency with achalasia of the cardia and lack of lacrimation. *Clin Endocrinol (Oxf)* 23:237, 1985.
1068. Stuckey BG, Mastaglia FL, Reed WD, Pullan PT: Glucocorticoid insufficiency, achalasia, alacrima with autonomic and motor neuropathy. *Ann Intern Med* 106:62, 1987.
1069. Thorn GW: *The Diagnosis and Treatment of Adrenal Insufficiency*. Springfield, IL, CC Thomas, 1951.
1070. Thorn GW, Koepf GF, Lewis RA, Olsen EF: Carbohydrate metabolism in Addison's disease. *J Clin Invest* 19:813, 1940.
1071. Cope CL: *Adrenal Steroids and Disease*. London, Pitman, 1972.
1072. Yamamoto T, Fukuyama J, Hasegawa K, Sugiura M: Isolated corticotropin deficiency in adults. *Arch Intern Med* 152:1705, 1992.
1073. Jensen MD, Handwerger BS, Scheithauer BW, Carpenter PC, Mirakian R, Banks PM: Lymphocytic hypophysitis with isolated corticotropin deficiency. *Ann Intern Med* 105:200, 1986.
1074. Sauter NP, Toni R, McLaughlin CD, Dyess EM, Kritzman J, Lechan RM: Isolated adrenocorticotropin deficiency associated with an autoantibody to a corticotroph antigen that is not adrenocorticotropin or other proopiomelanocortin-derived peptides. *J Clin Endocrinol Metab* 70:1391, 1989.
1075. Koide Y, Kimura S, Inoue S, Ikeda M, Uchida K, Ando J, Shimuzu A, Oda K, et al: Responsiveness of hypophyseal-adrenocortical axis to repetitive administration of synthetic ovine corticotropin-releasing hormone in patients with isolated adrenocorticotropin deficiency. *J Clin Endocrinol Metab* 63:329, 1986.
1076. Fukata J, Usui T, Tsukada T, Nakai Y, Koh T, Ishihara T, Tanaka I, Uchida K, et al: Effects of repetitive administration of corticotropin releasing hormone combined with lysine vasopressin on plasma adrenocorticotropin and cortisol levels in secondary adrenocortical insufficiency. *J Clin Endocrinol Metab* 71:1624, 1990.
1077. Major P, Kuchel O, Boucher R, Nowaczynski W, Genest J: Selective hypopituitarism with severe hyponatremia and secondary hyporeninism. *J Clin Endocrinol Metab* 46:15, 1978.
1078. Lieberman AH, Luetscher JA: Some effects of abnormali-

ties of pituitary, adrenal or thyroid function on excretion of aldosterone and the response to corticotropin or sodium deprivation. *J Clin Endocrinol Metab* 20:1004, 1960.
1079. May ME, Carey RM: Rapid adrenocorticotropic hormone test in practice. *Am J Med* 79:679, 1985.
1080. Borst GC, Michenfelder HJ, O'Brian JT: Discordant cortisol response to exogenous ACTH and insulin-induced hypoglycemia in patients with pituitary disease. *N Engl J Med* 306:1462, 1982.
1081. Besser GM, Cullen DR, Irvine WJ, Ratcliffe JG, Landon J: Immunoreactive corticotrophin levels in adrenocortical insufficiency. *Br Med J* 1:374, 1971.
1082. Fariss BL, Hane S, Shinsako J, Forsham PH: Comparison of absorption of cortisone acetate and hydrocortisone hemisuccinate. *J Clin Endocrinol Metab* 47:1137, 1978.
1083. Khalid BAK, Burke CW, Hurley DM, Funder JW, Stockigt JR: Steroid replacement in Addison's disease and in subjects adrenalectomized for Cushing's disease: Comparison of various glucocorticoids. *J Clin Endocrinol Metab* 55:551, 1982.
1084. Thompson DG, Stuart-Mason A, Goodwin FJ: Mineralocorticoid replacement in Addison's disease. *Clin Endocrinol (Oxf)* 10:499, 1979.
1085. Kyriazopoulou V, Parparousi O, Vagenakis A: Rifampicin induced adrenal crisis in addisonian patients receiving corticosteroid replacement therapy. *J Clin Endocrinol Metab* 59:1204, 1984.
1086. Feek CM, Ratacliffe JG, Setil J, Gray CE, Toft AD, Irvine WJ: Patterns of plasma cortisol and ACTH concentrations in patients with Addison's disease treated with conventional corticosteroid replacement. *Clin Endocrinol (Oxf)* 14:451, 1981.
1087. Scott RS, Donald RA, Espiner EA: Plasma ACTH and cortisol profiles in Addisonian patients receiving conventional substitution therapy. *Clin Endocrinol (Oxf)* 9:571, 1978.
1088. Nickelsen T, Schultz F, Demisch K: Studies on cortisol substitution therapy in patients with adrenal insufficiency. *Exp Clin Endocrinol* 82:35, 1983.
1089. Smith SJ, Markaandu ND, Banks RA, Dorrington Ward P, MacGregor GA, Bayliss J, Prentice MG, Wise P: Evidence that patients with Addison's disease are undertreated with fluorocortisone. *Lancet* 1:11, 1984.
1090. Oelkers W, Diederich S, Bahr V: Diagnosis and therapy surveillance in Addison's disease: Rapid adrenocorticotropin (ACTH) test and measurement of plasma ACTH, renin activity, and aldosterone. *J Clin Endocrinol Metab* 75:259, 1992.
1091. Plumpton FS, Besser GM, Cole PV: Corticosteroid treatment and surgery. II. The management of steroid cover. *Anaesthesia* 24:12, 1969.
1092. Hayes MA: Surgical treatment as complicated by prior adrenocortical steroid therapy. *Surgery* 40:945, 1956.
1093. Udelsman R, Ramp J, Gallucci WT, Gordon A, Lipford E, Norton JA, Loriaux DL, Chrousos GP: Adaptation during surgical stress: A reevaluation of the role of glucocorticoids. *J Clin Invest* 77:1377, 1986.
1094. Mulrow PJ: Aldosterone in hypertension and edema, in Bondy PK, Rosenberg LE (eds): *Metabolic Control and Disease*. Philadelphia, Saunders, 1979, p 1501.
1095. Sebastian A, Hernandez RE, Schambelan M: Disorders of renal handling of potassium, in Brenner BM, Rector FC Jr (eds): *The Kidney*. Philadelphia, Saunders, 1986, p 519.
1096. Schambelan M, Sebastian A: Hyporeninemic hypoaldosteronism. *Adv Intern Med* 24:385, 1979.
1097. Schambelan M, Sebastian A, Biglieri EG, Brust NL, Chang BC, Hirai J, Slater KL: Prevalence, pathogenesis, and functional significance of aldosterone deficiency in hyperkalemic patients with chronic renal insufficiency. *Kidney Int* 17:89, 1980.
1098. Phelps KR, Lieberman RL, Oh MS, Caroll HJ: Pathophysiology of the syndrome of hyporeninemic hypoaldosteronism. *Metabolism* 29:186, 1980.
1099. Tuck ML, Mayes DM: Mineralocorticoid biosynthesis in patients with hyporeninemic hypoaldosteronism. *J Clin Endocrinol Metab* 50:341, 1980.
1100. Williams GH: Hyporeninemic hypoaldosteronism. *N Engl J Med* 314:1041, 1986.
1101. Oster JR, Perez GO, Rosen MS: Hyporeninemic hypoaldosteronism after chronic sodium bicarbonate abuse. *Arch Intern Med* 136:1179, 1976.
1102. Obana K, Naruse M, Naruse K, et al: Synthetic rat atrial natriuretic factor inhibits *in vitro* and *in vivo* renin secretion in rats. *Endocrinology* 117:1282, 1985.
1103. Nadler JL, Lee FO, Hsueh W, Horton R: Evidence of prostacyclin deficiency in the syndrome of hyporeninemic hypoaldosteronism. *N Engl J Med* 314:1015, 1986.
1104. Sebastian A, Schambelan M: Amelioration of hyperchloremic acidosis with furosemide therapy in patients with chronic renal insufficiency and type 4 renal tubular acidosis. *Am J Nephrol* 4:287, 1984.
1105. Williams JAJ, Schambelan M, Biglieri EG, Carey RM: Acquired primary hypoaldosteronism due to an isolated zona glomerulosa defect. *N Engl J Med* 309:1623, 1983.
1106. Carey RM, Schambelan M, Biglieri EG, Bright GM: Primary hypoaldosteronism due to zona glomerulosa defect. *N Engl J Med* 310:1395, 1984.
1107. Stern N, Bech FWJ, Sowers JR, Tuck ML, Hsueh WA, Zipser R: Plasma corticosteroids in hyperreninemic hypoaldosteronism: Evidence for diffuse impairment of the zona glomerulosa. *J Clin Endocrinol Metab* 57:217, 1983.
1108. Zipser RD, Davenport MW, Martin KL, Tucck ML, Warner NF, Swinnery RR, Davis CL, Horton R: Hyperreninemic hypoaldosteronism in the critically ill: A new entity. *J Clin Endocrinol Metab* 53:867, 1981.
1109. Schambelan M, Sebastian A, Rector FC Jr: Mineralocorticoid-resistant renal hyperkalemia without salt wasting (type II pseudohypoaldosteronism): Role of increased renal chloride reabsorption. *Kidney Int* 19:716, 1981.
1110. Asa SL, Kalman K, Tindall GT, Barrow DL, Horvath E, Vecsei P: Cushing's disease associated with an intracellular gangliocytoma producing corticotrophin-releasing factor. *Ann Intern Med* 101:789, 1984.
1111. Carey RM, Varma SK, Drake CR, Thorner MO, Kovacs K, Rivier J, Vale W: Ectopic secretion of corticotropin-releasing factor as a cause of Cushing's syndrome. *N Engl J Med* 311:13, 1984.
1112. Belsky JL, Cuello B, Swanson LW, Simmons DM, Jarrett RM, Braza F: Cushing's syndrome due to ectopic production of corticotropin-releasing factor. *J Clin Endocrinol Metab* 60:496, 1985.
1113. Huff TA: Clinical syndromes related to disorders of adrenocococorticotrophic hormone, in Allen MB, Makesh VB (eds): *The Pituitary: A Current Review*. New York, Academic, 1977, p 153.
1114. Neville AM, O'Hare MJ: Aspects of structure, function and pathology, in James VHT (ed): *The Adrenal Gland*. New York, Raven, 1979, p 1.
1115. Plotz CM, Knowlton AI, Ragan C: The natural history of Cushing's syndrome. *Am J Med* 13:597, 1952.
1116. Mampalam TJ, Tyrrell JB, Wilson CB: Transsphenoidal microsurgery for Cushing disease: A report of 216 cases. *Ann Intern Med* 109:487, 1988.
1117. Findling JW, Aron DC, Tyrrell JB: Cushing's disease, in Imura H (ed): *The Pituitary Gland*. New York, Raven, 1985, p 441.
1118. Ratcliffe JG, Knight RA, Besser GM, Landon J, Stansfield AG: Tumor and plasma ACTH concentrations in patients with and without the ectopic ACTH syndrome. *Clin Endocrinol (Oxf)* 1:27, 1972.
1119. Azzopardi JG, Freeman E, Pook G: Endocrine and metabolic disorders in bronchial carcinoma. *Br Med J* 4:528, 1970.
1120. Gewirtz G, Yalow RS: Ectopic ACTH production in carcinoma of the lung. *J Clin Invest* 53:1022, 1974.
1121. Knight RA, Ratcliffe JG, Besser GM: Tumor ACTH con-

centrations in ectopic ACTH syndrome and in control tissues. *Proc R Soc Med* 64:1266, 1971.
1122. Bloomfield GA, Holdaway IM, Corrin B, Ratcliffe JG, Rees GM, Ellison M, Rees LH: Lung tumors and ACTH production. *Clin Endocrinol (Oxf)* 6:95, 1977.
1123. Neville AM, Symington T: The pathology of the adrenal gland in Cushing's syndrome. *J Pathol Bacteriol* 93:19, 1967.
1124. Hutter AM, Kayhoe DE: Adrenal cortical carcinoma: Clinical features of 138 patients. *Am J Med* 41:572, 1966.
1125. McArthur RG, Cloutier MD, Hayles AB, Sprague RG: Cushing's disease in children. *Mayo Clin Proc* 47:318, 1972.
1126. Jennings AS, Liddle GW, Orth DN: Results of treating childhood Cushing's disease with pituitary irradiation. *N Engl J Med* 297:958, 1977.
1127. Cassar J, Doyle FH, Mashiter K, Joplin GF: Treatment of Cushing's disease in juveniles with interstitial pituitary irradiation. *Clin Endocrinol (Oxf)* 11:313, 1979.
1128. Styne DM, Grumbach MM, Kaplan SL, Wilson CB, Conte FA: Treatment of Cushing's disease in childhood and adolescence by transsphenoidal microadenomectomy. *N Engl J Med* 310:889, 1984.
1129. Eisenhardt L, Thompson KW: A brief consideration of the present status of so-called pituitary basophilism. *Yale J Biol Med* 11:507, 1939.
1130. Robert F, Pelletier G, Hardy J: Pituitary adenomas in Cushing's disease. *Arch Pathol Lab Med* 102:448, 1978.
1131. Tyrrell JB, Brooks RM, Fitzgerald PA, Cofoid PB, Forsham PH, Wilson CW: Cushing's disease: Selective transsphenoidal resection of pituitary adenomas. *N Engl J Med* 298:753, 1978.
1132. Boggan JE, Tyrrell JB, Wilson CB: Transsphenoidal microsurgical management of Cushing's disease. *J Neurosurg* 59:195, 1983.
1133. Rovitt RL, Duane TD: Cushing's syndrome and pituitary tumors: Pathophysiology and ocular manifestations of ACTH-secreting pituitary adenomas. *Am J Med* 46:416, 1969.
1134. Kovacs K, Horvath E: Pathology of pituitary tumors. *Endocrinol Metab Clin* 16:529, 1987.
1135. Lloyd RV, Chandler WF, McKeever PE, Schteingart DE: The spectrum of ACTH-producing pituitary lesions. *Am J Surg Pathol* 10:618, 1986
1136. Grua JR, Nelson DH: ACTH-producing pituitary tumors. *Endocrinol Metab Clin North Am* 20:319, 1991.
1137. Suda T, Abe Y, Demura H, Demura R, Shizume K, Tamahashi N, Sasano N: ACTH, α-LPH and α-endorphin in pituitary adenomas of the patients with Cushing's disease: Activation of α-LPH conversion to α-endorphin. *J Clin Endocrinol Metab* 49:475, 1979.
1138. Suda T, Demura H, Demura R, Jibiki K, Tozawa F, Shizume K: Anterior pituitary hormones in plasma and pituitaries from patients with Cushing's disease. *J Clin Endocrinol Metab* 51:1048, 1980.
1139. Saeger W: Surgical pathology of the pituitary in Cushing's disease. *Pathol Res Pract* 187:613, 1991.
1140. Lüdecke D, Kautzky R, Saeger W, Schrader D: Selective removal of hypersecreting pituitary adenomas. *Acta Neurochir (Wien)* 35:27, 1976.
1141. Peillon F, Racador J, Oliver L, Vila-Porcile E: Microadenomas, structure and function, in Faglia G, Giovanelli MA, MacLeod RM (eds): *Microadenomas*. London, Academic, 1980, p 91.
1142. McKeever PE, Koppelman MC, Metcalf D, Quindlen E, Kornbluth PL, Strott CA, Howard R, Smith BH: Re-fractory Cushing's disease caused by multinodular ACTH cell hyperplasia. *J Neuropathol Exp Neurol* 41:490, 1982.
1143. Samuels MH: Cushing's syndrome associated with corticotroph hyperplasia. *The Endocrinologist* 3:242, 1993.
1144. Schnall AM, Kovacs K, Brodkey JS, Pearson OH: Pituitary Cushing's disease without adenoma. *Acta Endocrinol (Copenh)* 94:293, 1981.
1145. Taylor HC, Velasco ME, Brodkey JS: Remission of pituitary-dependent Cushing's disease after removal of nonneoplastic pituitary gland. *Arch Intern Med* 140:1366, 1980.
1146. Lamberts SWJ, DeLange SA, Stefanko SZ: Adrenocorticotropin secreting pituitary adenomas originate from the anterior or the intermediate lobe in Cushing's disease: Differences in the regulation of hormone secretion. *J Clin Endocrinol Metab* 54:286, 1982.
1147. McNicol AM, Teasdale GM, Beastal GH: A study of corticotroph adenomas in Cushing's disease: no evidence of intermediate lobe origin. *Clin Endocrinol (Oxf)* 24:715, 1986.
1148. Raffel C, Boggan JE, Eng LF, Davis RL, Wilson CW: Pituitary adenomas in Cushing's disease: Do they arise from the intermediate lobe? *Surg Neurol* 30:125, 1988.
1149. Neville AM, O'Hare MJ: Histopathology of the human adrenal cortex. *Clin Endocrinol Metab* 14:791, 1985.
1150. McNicol AM: The human adrenal gland: Aspects of structure, function and pathology, in James VHT (ed): *The Adrenal Gland*, 2d ed. New York, Raven, 1992.
1151. Anderson DC, Child DF, Sutcliffe CH, Buckley CH, Davies D, Longson D: Cushing's syndrome, nodular hyperplasia and virilizing carcinoma. *Clin Endocrinol (Oxf)* 9:1, 1978.
1152. Krieger DT, Amorosa L, Linick F: Cyproheptadine-induced remission of Cushing's disease. *N Engl J Med* 293:893, 1975.
1153. Krieger DT: Physiopathology of Cushing's disease. *Endocr Rev* 4:22, 1983.
1154. Hellman L, Weitzman ED, Roffwarg H, Fukushima DK, Yoshida K, Gallagher TF: Cortisol is secreted episodically in Cushing's syndrome. *J Clin Endocrinol Metab* 30:686, 1970.
1155. Sederberg-Olsen P, Binder C, Kehlet H, Neville AM, Nielsen LM: Episodic variation in plasma corticosteroids in subjects with Cushing's syndrome of differing etiology. *J Clin Endocrinol Metab* 36:906, 1973.
1156. Von Werder K, Smilo RP, Hane S, Forsham PH: Pituitary response to stress in Cushing's disease. *Acta Endocrinol (Copenh)* 67:127, 1971.
1157. Duick DS, Wahner HW: Thyroid axis in patients with Cushing's syndrome. *Arch Intern Med* 139:767, 1979.
1158. Smals AGH, Kloppenborg PWC, Benraad TJ: Plasma testosterone profiles in Cushing's syndrome. *J Clin Endocrinol Metab* 45:240, 1977.
1159. Fitzgerald PA, Aron DC, Findling JW, Brooks RM, Wilson CB, Tyrrell JB: Cushing's disease: Transient secondary adrenal insufficiency after selective removal of pituitary tumors. Evidence for a pituitary origin. *J Clin Endocrinol Metab* 54:413, 1982.
1160. Tyrrell JB: Cushing's disease. *Present Concepts Intern Med* 13:5, 1980.
1161. Gertz BJ, Contreras LN, McComb DJ, Kovacs K, Tyrrell JB, Dallman MF: Chronic administration of corticotropin-releasing factor increases pituitary corticotroph number. *Endocrinology* 120:381, 1987.
1162. Salassa RM, Laws ER Jr, Carpenter PC, Northcutt RC: Transsphenoidal removal of pituitary microadenoma in Cushing's disease. *Mayo Clin Proc* 53:24, 1978.
1163. Bigos ST, Somma M, Rasio E, Eastman RC, Lanthier A, Johnston NH, Hardy J: Cushing's disease: Management by transsphenoidal pituitary microsurgery. *J Clin Endocrinol Metab* 50:348, 1980.
1164. Schnall AM, Brodkey JS, Kaufman B, Pearson OH: Pituitary function after removal of pituitary microadenomas in Cushing's disease. *J Clin Endocrinol Metab* 47:410, 1978.
1165. Boyer RM, Witkin M, Carruth A, Ramsey J: Circadian cortisol rhythms in Cushing's disease. *J Clin Endocrinol Metab* 48:760, 1979.
1166. Doerr P, Pirke KM: Cortisol-induced suppression of plasma testosterone in normal adult males. *J Clin Endocrinol Metab* 43:622, 1976.
1167. Krieger DT, Gewirtz GP: Recovery of hypothalamic-pitu-

itary-adrenal function, growth hormone responsiveness, and sleep EEG pattern in a patient following removal of an adrenal cortical adenoma. *J Clin Endocrinol Metab* 38:1075, 1974.
1168. Jaquet P, Lissitzky JC, Boudouresque F, Guibout M, Goldstein E, Grisoli F, Oliver C: Peptides lipocorticotropes dans la maladie de Cushing: Etudes *in vitro, in vivo. 23rd International Symposium on Clinical Endocrinology*, Paris, 1980, p 54.
1169. Gillies G, Ratter S, Grossman A, Gaillard R, Lowry PJ, Besser GM, Rees LH: ACTH, LPH and β-endorphin secretion from perfused isolated human pituitary tumor cells *in vitro. Horm Res* 13:280, 1980.
1170. Lüdecke DK, Westphal M, Schabet M, Hollt V: *In vitro* secretion of ACTH beta-endorphin and beta-lipotropin in Cushing's disease and Nelson's syndrome. *Horm Res* 13:259, 1980.
1171. Lamberts SWJ, Klijn JGM, De Quijada M, Timmermans HAT, Uitterlinden P, De Jong FH, Birkenhager JC: The mechanism of the suppressive action of bromocryptine on adrenocorticotropin secretion in patients with Cushing's disease and Nelson's syndrome. *J Clin Endocrinol Metab* 51:307, 1980.
1172. Ishibashi M, Yamaji T: TRH stimulation and dopaminergic and antiserotonergic inhibition of ACTH release from cultured pituitary adenoma tissues of Nelson's syndrome. *Program of the VIth International Congress of Endocrinology*, Melbourne, 1980, p 407.
1173. Orth DN: Establishment of human malignant melanoma clonal cell lines that secrete ectopic adrenocorticotropin. *Nature (New Biol)* 242:26, 1973.
1174. Hashimoto K, Takahara J, Ogawa N, Yunoki S, Ofuji T, Arata A, Kanda S, Terada K: Adrenocorticotropin, β-lipotropin, β-endorphin and corticotropin-releasing factor-like activity in an adrenocorticotropin-producing nephroblastoma. *J Clin Endocrinol Metab* 50:461, 1980.
1175. Rees LH, Bloomfield GA, Gilkes JJH, Jeffcoate WJ, Besser GM: ACTH as a tumor marker. *Ann NY Acad Sci* 297:603, 1977.
1176. Allen RG, Orwell E, Kendall JW, Herbert E, Paxton H: The distribution of forms of adrenocorticotropin and β-endorphin in normal, tumorous, and autopsy human anterior pituitary tissue: Virtual absence of 13K adrenocorticotropin. *J Clin Endocrinol Metab* 51:376, 1980.
1177. Singer W, Kovacs K, Ryan N, Horvath E: Ectopic ACTH syndrome: Clinicopathological correlations. *J Clin Pathol* 31:591, 1978.
1178. Azzopardi JG, Williams ED: Pathology of nonendocrine tumors associated with Cushing's syndrome. *Cancer* 22:274, 1968.
1179. Liddle GW, Nicholson WE, Island DP, Orth DN, Abe K, Lowder SC: Clinical and laboratory studies of ectopic humoral syndromes. *Recent Prog Horm Res* 25:283, 1969.
1180. Luton J-P, Thieblot P, Valcke JC, Mahoudeau JA, Bicaire H: Reversible gonadotropin deficiency in male Cushing's disease. *J Clin Endocrinol Metab* 45:488, 1977.
1181. Friedman M, Marshall-Jones P, Ross EJ: Cushing's syndrome: Adrenocortical hyperactivity secondary to neoplasms arising outside the pituitary-adrenal system. *Q J Med* 35:193, 1966.
1182. Soffer LJ, Iannaccone A, Gabrilov JL: Cushing's syndrome: A study of fifty patients. *Am J Med* 30:129, 1961.
1183. Prunty FTG, Brooks RV, Dupre J, Gilmette TMD, Hutchinson JSM, McSwiney RR, Mills IH: Adrenocortical hyperfunction and potassium metabolism in patients with "non-endocrine" tumors and Cushing's syndrome. *J Clin Endocrinol Metab* 23:737, 1963.
1184. Taskinen M-R, Nikkila EA, Pelkonen R, Sane T: Plasma lipoproteins, lipolytic enzymes, and very low density lipoprotein triglyceride turnover in Cushing's syndrome. *J Clin Endocrinol Metab* 57:619, 1983.
1185. Findling JW, Tyrrell JB: Occult ectopic secretion of corticotropin. *Arch Intern Med* 146:929, 1986.
1186. Aron DC, Findling JW, Tyrrell JB, Fitzgerald PA, Brooks RM, Fisher FE, Forsham PH: Pituitary-ACTH dependency of nodular adrenal hyperplasia in Cushing's syndrome. *Am J Med* 71:302, 1981.
1187. Yamaji T, Ishibashi M, Sekihara H, Itabashi A, Yanaihara T: Serum dehydroepiandrosterone sulfate in Cushing's syndrome. *J Clin Endocrinol Metab* 59:1164, 1984.
1188. Aron DC, Findling JW, Tyrrell JB: Cushing's disease. *Endocrinol Metab Clin* 16:705, 1987.
1189. Meikle AW, Stanchfield JB, West CD, Tyler FH: Hydrocortisone suppression test for Cushing's syndrome. *Arch Intern Med* 134:1068, 1974.
1190. Bailey RE: Periodic hormonogenesis—a new phenomenon: Periodicity in function of a hormone-producing tumor in man. *J Clin Endocrinol Metab* 32:317, 1971.
1191. Blau N, Miller WE, Miller ER, Cervi-Skinner J: Spontaneous remission of Cushing's syndrome in a patient with an adrenal adenoma. *J Clin Endocrinol Metab* 40:659, 1975.
1192. Lamberts SWJ, Klijn JGM, DeJong FH, Birkenhäger JC: Hormone secretion in alcohol induced pseudo-Cushing's syndrome: Differential diagnosis with Cushing's disease. *JAMA* 242:1640, 1979.
1193. Gold PW, Loriaux DL, Roy A, Kling MA, Calabrese JR, Kellner CH, Nieman LK, Post RM, et al: Responses to corticotropin-releasing hormone in the hypercortisolism of depression and Cushing's disease. *N Engl J Med* 314:1329, 1986.
1194. Kaye TB, Crapo L: The Cushing syndrome: An update on diagnostic tests. *Ann Intern Med* 112:434, 1990.
1195. Orth DN: The old and the new in Cushing's syndrome. *N Engl J Med* 310:649, 1984.
1196. Fig LM, Gross MD, Shapiro B, Ehrmann DA, Freitas JE, Schteingart DE, Glazer GM, Francis RF: Adrenal localization in the adrenocorticotropic hormone-independent Cushing syndrome. *Ann Intern Med* 109:547, 1988.
1197. Perry RR, Nieman LK, Cutler GB Jr, Chrousos GP, Loriaux L, Doppman JL, Travis DT, Norton JA: Primary adrenal causes of Cushing's syndrome: Diagnosis and surgical management. *Ann Surg* 210:59, 1989.
1198. Carney JA, Young WF Jr: Primary pigmented nodular adrenocortical disease and its associated conditions. *The Endocrinologist* 2:6, 1992.
1199. Young WF, Carney JA: Cushing's syndrome: Primary pigmented nodular adrenal disease, in Mazzaferi EL (ed): *Advances in Endocrinology and Metabolism.* Mosby-Year Book, St. Louis, vol 3, p. 179. 1992
1200. Doppman JL, Travis WD, Nieman L, Miller DL, Crousos GP, Gomez MT, Cutler GB Jr, Loriaux DL, et al: Cushing syndrome due to primary pigmented nodular adrenocortical disease: Findings at CT and MR imaging. *Radiology* 172:415, 1989.
1201. Zeiger MA, Nieman LK, Cutler GB Jr, Chrousos GP, Doppman JL, Travis WD, Norton JA: Primary bilateral adrenocortical causes of Cushing's syndrome. *Surgery* 110:1106, 1991.
1202. Orloff DG, Cutler GB Jr: The spectrum of macronodular adrenal disease in Cushing's syndrome: Diagnosis and treatment, in Mazzaferi EL (ed): *Advances in Endocrinology and Metabolism.* Mosby-YearBook, St. Louis, 1992, vol 3 p. 199.
1203. Doppman JL, Miller DL, Dwyer AJ, Loughlin T, Nieman L, Cutler GB Jr, Chrousos GP, Oldfield E, et al: Macronodular adrenal hyperplasia in Cushing's disease. *Radiology* 166:347, 1988.
1204. Findlay JC, Sheeler LR, Engeland WC, Aron DC: Familial adrenocorticotropin-independent Cushing's syndrome with bilateral macronodular adrenal hyperplasia. *J Clin Endocrinol Metab* 76:189, 1993.
1205. DoppmanJL, Niemann LK, Travis WD, Miller DL, Cutler GB Jr, Chrousos GP, Norton JA: CT and MR imaging of

massive macronodular adrenocortical disease: A rare cause of autonomous primary hypercortisolism. *J Comput Assist Tomogr* 15:773, 1991.
1206. Malchoff CD, Rosa J, DeBold CR, Kozol RA, Ramsby GR, Page DL, Malchoff DM, Orth DN: Adrenocorticotropin-independent bilateral macronodular adrenal hyperplasia: An unusual cause of Cushing's syndrome. *J Clin Endocrinol Metab* 68:855, 1989.
1207. Trainer PJ, Grossman A: The diagnosis and differential diagnosis of Cushing's syndrome. *Clin Endocrinol (Oxf)* 34:317, 1991.
1208. Grossman AB, Howlett TA, Perry L, Coy DH, Savage MO, Lavender P, Rees LH, Bessier GM: CRF in the differential diagnosis of Cushing's syndrome: A comparison with the dexamethasone suppression test. *Clin Endocrinol (Oxf)* 29:167, 1988.
1209. Hermus AR, J PG, Benraad TJ, Pieters GF, Smals AG, Kloppenborg PW: The corticotropin-releasing-hormone test versus the high-dose dexamethasone test in the differential diagnosis of Cushing's syndrome. *Lancet* 2:540, 1986.
1210. Nieman LK, Chrousos GP, Oldfield EH, Avgerinos PC, Cutler GB Jr, Loriaux DL: The ovine corticotropin-releasing hormone stimulation test and the dexamethasone suppression test in the differential diagnosis of Cushing's syndrome. *Ann Intern Med* 105:862, 1986.
1211. Hermus AR, Pieters GF, Benraad TJ, Smals AG, Kloppenborg PW: The CRH test and the high-dose dexamethasone test in the differential diagnosis of Cushing's syndrome, in Casanueva FF, Dieguez C (eds): *Recent Advances in Basic and Clinical Neuroendocrinology*. New York, Elsevier, 1989, p 351.
1212. Oldfield EH, Doppman JL, Nieman LK, Chrousos GP, Miller DL, Katz DA, Cutler GB Jr, Loriaux DL: Petrosal sinus sampling with and without corticotropin-releasing hormone for the differential diagnosis of Cushing's syndrome. *N Engl J Med* 325:897, 1991.
1213. Doppman JL: The search for occult ectopic ACTH-producing tumors. *The Endocrinologist* 2:41, 1992.
1214. Doppman JL, Nieman L, Miller DL, Pass HI, Chang R, Cutler GB Jr, Schaaf M, Chrousos GP, et al: Ectopic adrenocorticotropic hormone syndrome: Localization studies in 28 patients. *Radiology* 172:115, 1989.
1215. Corrigan DF, Schaaf M, Whaley RA, Czerwinski CL, Earll JM: Selective venous sampling to differentiate ectopic ACTH secretion from pituitary Cushing's syndrome. *N Engl J Med* 296:861, 1971.
1216. Findling JW, Aron DC, Tyrrell JB, Shinsako JH, Fitzgerald PA, Norman D, Wilson CB, Forsham PH: Selective venous sampling for ACTH in Cushing's syndrome: Differentiation between Cushing's disease and the ectopic ACTH syndrome. *Ann Intern Med* 94:647, 1981.
1217. Howlett TA, Rees HL, Besser GM: Cushing's syndrome. *Clin Endocrinol Metab* 14:911, 1985.
1218. Manni A, Latshaw RF, Page R, Santen RJ: Simultaneous bilateral venous sampling for adrenocorticotropin in pituitary-dependent Cushing's disease: Evidence for lateralization of pituitary venous drainage. *J Clin Endocrinol Metab* 57:1070, 1983.
1219. Doppman JL, Oldfield E, Krudy AG, Chrousos GP, Schulte HM, Schaaf M, Loriaux DL: Petrosal sinus sampling for Cushing's syndrome: Anatomical and technical considerations. *Radiology* 150:99, 1984.
1220. Komanicky P, Spark RF, Melby JC: Treatment of Cushing's syndrome with trilostane (WIN 24,250), an inhibitor of adrenal steroid biosynthesis. *J Clin Endocrinol Metab* 47:1024, 1978.
1221. Sample WF, Sarti DA: Computed tomography and gray scale ultrasonography of the adrenal gland: A comparative study. *Radiology* 128:377, 1978.
1222. Thrall JH, Freitas JE, Beirwaltes WH: Adrenal scintigraphy. *Semin Nucl Med* 8:23, 1978.
1223. Orth DN, Liddle GW: Results of treatment in 108 patients with Cushing's syndrome. *N Engl J Med* 285:243, 1971.
1224. Kjellberg RN, Kliman B: Lifetime effectiveness—a system of therapy for pituitary adenomas, emphasizing Bragg peak proton hypophysectomy, in Linfoot JA (ed): *Recent Advances in the Diagnosis and Treatment of Pituitary Tumors*. New York, Raven, 1979, p 269.
1225. Linfoot JA: Heavy ion therapy: Alpha particle therapy of pituitary tumors, in Linfoot JA (ed): *Recent Advances in the Diagnosis and Treatment of Pituitary Tumors*. New York, Raven, 1979, p 245.
1226. Sheline GE: Role of conventional radiation therapy in the treatment of functional pituitary tumors, in Linfoot JA (ed): *Recent Advances in the Diagnosis and Treatment of Pituitary Tumors*. New York, Raven, 1979, p 289.
1227. Lamberts SWJ, DeJong FH, Birkenhager JC: Treatment of Cushing's disease by unilateral adrenalectomy followed by external pituitary irradiation, in Fahlbush R, von Werder K (eds): *Treatment of Pituitary Adenomas*. Stuttgart, Germany, Georg Thieme, 1978, p 339.
1228. Jeffcoate WJ, Rees LH, Tomlin S, Jones AE, Edwards CRW, Besser GM: Metyrapone in long-term management of Cushing's disease. *Br Med J* 2:215, 1977.
1229. Orth DN: Metyrapone is useful only as adjunctive therapy in Cushing's disease. *Ann Intern Med* 89:128, 1978.
1230. Burke CW, Doyle FH, Joplin GF, Arnot RN, MacErlean DP, Russell Fraser T: Cushing's disease: Treatment by pituitary implantation of radioactive gold or yttrium seeds. *Q J Med* 42:693, 1973.
1231. White MC, Doyle FH, Mashiter K, Joplin GF: Successful treatment of Cushing's disease using yttrium-90 rods. *Br Med J* 285:280, 1982.
1232. Welbourn RB, Montgomery DAD, Kennedy TL: The natural history of treated Cushing's syndrome. *Br J Surg* 58:1, 1971.
1233. Schteingart DE: Cushing's syndrome. *Endocrinol Metab Clin North Am* 18:311, 1989.
1234. Graber AL, New RL, Nicholson WE, Island DP, Liddle GW: Natural history of pituitary adrenal recovery following long term suppression with corticosteroids. *J Clin Endocrinol Metab* 25:11, 1965.
1235. Bertagna C, Orth DN: Clinical and laboratory findings and results of therapy in 58 patients with adrenocortical tumors admitted to a single medical center (1951 to 1978). *Am J Med* 71:855, 1981.
1236. Hutter AM, Kayhoe DE: Adrenocortical carcinoma: Results of treatment with o,p′DDD in 138 patients. *Am J Med* 41:581, 1966.
1237. Nelson DH, Meakin JW, Dealy JB, Matson DD, Emerson K, Thorn GW: ACTH-producing tumor of the pituitary gland. *N Engl J Med* 259:161, 1958.
1238. Moore TJ, Dluhy RG, Williams GH, Cain JP: Nelson's syndrome: Frequency, prognosis and effect of prior pituitary irradiation. *Ann Intern Med* 85:731, 1976.
1239. Barwich D, Bahner P: Pituitary tumors in adrenalectomized patients with Cushing's disease, in Fahlbush R, von Werder K (eds): *Treatment of Pituitary Adenomas*. Stuttgart, Germany, Georg Thieme, 1978, p 326.
1240. Weinstein M, Tyrrell JB, Newton TH: The sella turcica in Nelson's syndrome. *Radiology* 118:363, 1976.
1241. Findling JW, Tyrrell JB, Aron DC, Fitzgerald PA, Wilson CW, Forsham PH: Silent pituitary apoplexy: Subclinical infarction of an ACTH-producing adenoma. *J Clin Endocrinol Metab* 52:95, 1981.
1242. Stockigt JR: Mineralocorticoid excess, in James VHT (ed): *The Adrenal Gland*. New York, Raven, 1979, p 197.
1243. Ferris TF: Toxemia of pregnancy: A model of human hypertension. *Cardiovasc Med* 2:877, 1977.
1244. Gill JR: Bartter's syndrome. *Annu Rev Med* 31:405, 1980.

CHAPTER 13

Diseases of the Sympathochromaffin System

Philip E. Cryer

The sympathochromaffin system is a prototype neuroendocrine system.[1,2] Its major biologically active products—the catecholamines—serve as both neurotransmitters and hormones. The sympathochromaffin system includes two components: the sympathetic nervous system and the chromaffin tissues.[2] The major clusters of chromaffin cells that persist through postnatal life constitute the adrenal medullae. The catecholamines—epinephrine, norepinephrine, and dopamine—are neurotransmitters in the central nervous system (CNS). In the periphery, epinephrine serves as a hormone.[3] Although regulated epinephrine secretion from extraadrenal chromaffin cells occurs, biologically effective plasma epinephrine levels are derived only from the adrenal medullae, at least in adults.[2] Outside the CNS, norepinephrine functions primarily as a neurotransmitter of sympathetic postganglionic neurons;[4] it may also serve a hormonal function under some conditions. The physiologic function of dopamine outside the CNS is unclear, although it may also play a neurotransmitter role.

The sympathochromaffin system is a component of the autonomic nervous system (ANS).[5] The ANS consists of afferent, CNS, and efferent elements and is divided on autonomic grounds into parasympathetic and sympathetic divisions. Parasympathetic efferents include preganglionic and postganglionic neurons; the former arise from the brainstem and sacral spinal cord and synapse with the latter in ganglia which generally lie close to the innervated organs. Both preganglionic and postganglionic parasympathetic neurons release the neurotransmitter acetylcholine. Sympathetic efferents also include preganglionic and postganglionic neurons; the preganglionic neurons arise from the thoracolumbar spinal cord. Some sympathetic preganglionic neurons innervate chromaffin cells, including the adrenal medullae; the latter can be conceptualized as postganglionic neurons without axons.[3,6,7] The adrenal medullae release epinephrine, norepinephrine, or dopamine directly into the circulation. The remaining sympathetic preganglionic neurons synapse with postganglionic neurons in ganglia which are generally remote from the innervated organs (e.g., paravertebral ganglia). Like parasympathetic neurons, sympathetic preganglionic neurons release acetylcholine. A minority of sympathetic postganglionic neurons, such as those innervating sweat glands, also release acetylcholine. However, the vast majority of sympathetic postganglionic neurons release the neurotransmitter norepinephrine. In addition to catecholamines, components of the sympathochromaffin system contain a variety of peptides of potential but undefined biological importance.

The sympathochromaffin system is a rapid communication system. Its direct neural effects are virtually instantaneous, and its hormonal effects are detectable within minutes. The rapidity of the hormonal effects is comparable to that of pancreatic hormones such as insulin and glucagon but contrasts with the more gradual onset of action of pituitary hormones such as growth hormone, the adrenocortical and gonadal steroids, and, particularly, the thyroid hormones.

It has long been appreciated that the sympathochromaffin system is critically involved in cardiovascular homeostasis and that the catecholamines have prominent metabolic effects, but the precise physiologic roles of the catecholamines in human metabolic regulation have only begun to emerge. A better understanding of their physiology will provide further insight into the pathophysiologic roles of the catecholamines.

There are three established clinical disorders of sympathochromaffin function[3]: (1) hypertension and a variety of symptoms that result from excessive catecholamine release from a pheochromocytoma, a tumor of chromaffin cells, (2) postural (orthostatic) hypotension resulting from deficient sympathetic neural norepinephrine release in various forms of autonomic failure, and (3) hypoglycemia resulting from combined deficiencies of epinephrine and glucagon secretion.

SYMPATHOCHROMAFFIN PHYSIOLOGY

Biochemistry of the Catecholamines

Amines containing a 3,4-dihydroxyphenyl (catechol) nucleus are termed *catecholamines*. These include epinephrine (adrenaline), norepinephrine (noradrenaline), and dopamine. The conventions of catecholamine nomenclature and the structures of these catecholamines are shown in Fig. 13-1.

Catecholamine Biosynthesis

Catecholamines are synthesized from the amino acid tyrosine through the sequence tyrosine → dihydroxyphenylalanine (dopa) → dopamine → norepinephrine (NE) → epinephrine (E).[8] As shown in Fig. 13-2, some systems (e.g., most cells of the adrenal medullae) express all the necessary biosynthetic enzymes and produce epinephrine as their major product. Others, such as most sympathetic postganglionic neurons and some cells of the adrenal medullae, lack the final enzyme and release norepinephrine. Various CNS neurons release dopamine, norepinephrine, or epinephrine.

Tyrosine utilized in catecholamine biosynthesis is derived from the diet or formed from phenylalanine, in the presence of phenylalanine hydroxylase, in the liver (Fig. 13-2).[9,10]

The catecholamine biosynthetic sequence is illustrated in Fig. 13-3. The initial step—conversion of tyrosine to dopa—is catalyzed by tyrosine hydroxylase, the rate-limiting enzyme in catecholamine biosynthesis. Tyrosine hydroxylase (and phenylalanine and tryptophan hydroxylases) requires tetrahydrobiopterin as a cofactor. Tetrahydrobiopterin deficiency results in deficient catecholamine biosynthesis.[11] Tyrosine hydroxylase activity is product-inhibited. Accordingly, intracellular catecholamine depletion results in a rapid increase in enzyme activity and catecholamine biosynthesis. The activation of tyrosine hydroxylase involves phosphorylation of the enzyme;[12] both phosphorylation and activation are stimulated by acetylcholine, the preganglionic neurotransmitter. Further, prolonged sympathetic stimulation results in increased synthesis of tyrosine hydroxylase. Because of effective regulation of tyrosine hydroxylase, intracellular catecholamine stores are generally well maintained despite a marked variation in catecholamine release.

FIGURE 13-1 Conventions of catecholamine nomenclature.

HO- / HO- (positions 3, 4) ring (positions 1–6) –$CH(R_b)CH_2NHR_a$ (β, α)

	R_a	R_b
DOPAMINE	H	H
NOREPINEPHRINE	H	OH
EPINEPHRINE	CH_3	OH

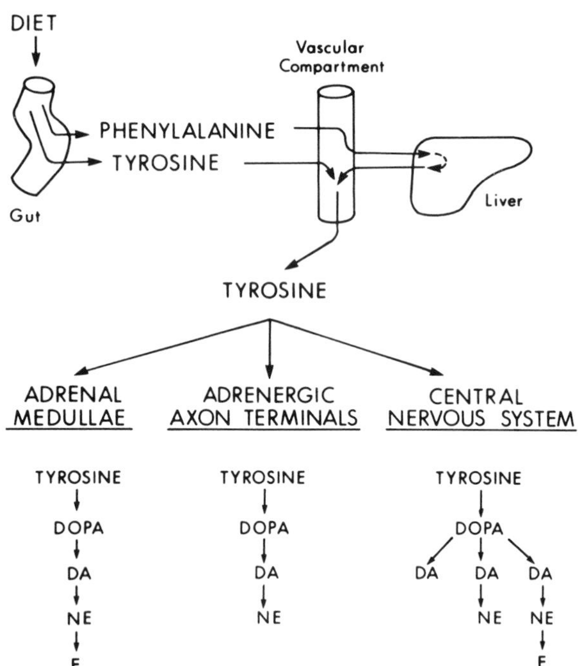

FIGURE 13-2 Sites of catecholamine biosynthesis from tyrosine and major end products in those sites.

In the presence of the relatively nonspecific enzyme aromatic L-amino acid decarboxylase, dopa is decarboxylated to form dopamine. As was noted earlier, subsequent enzymes are not expressed in some catecholamine-forming neurons in which dopamine is the final product.

In tissues containing dopamine β-hydroxylase, such as the adrenal medullae and sympathetic postganglionic neurons, dopamine is hydroxylated to form norepinephrine. Norepinephrine is the final product of most sympathetic postganglionic neurons.

In chromaffin tissues, such as the adrenal medullae, norepinephrine is methylated to form epinephrine in the presence of the enzyme phenylethanolamine *N*-methyl transferase (PNMT).[13] The methyl donor is *S*-adenosyl-L-methionine. PNMT is a glucocorticoid-inducible enzyme; this may explain the persistence of high activity of the enzyme in the adrenal medullae, which receive portal blood flow from the adrenal cortex. Indeed, histochemical studies suggest that norepinephrine-releasing adrenomedullary cells are located around medullary arteries, whereas epinephrine-releasing adrenomedullary cells appear to receive most of their blood supply from corticomedullary venous sinuses. Furthermore, the glucocorticoid receptor has been localized to epinephrine-producing adrenomedullary cells.[14] Inter-

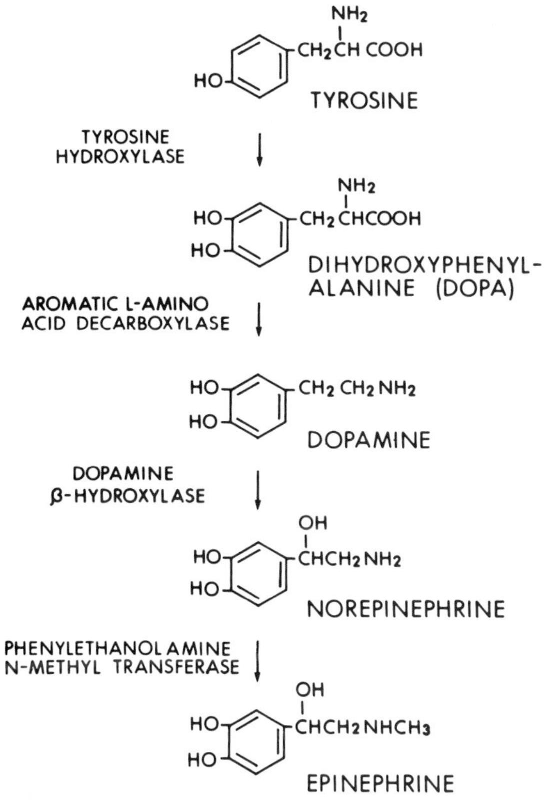

FIGURE 13-3 Catecholamine biosynthesis.

estingly, patients with secondary adrenocortical insufficiency (ACTH deficiency) have been reported to have reduced basal and postexercise plasma epinephrine concentrations.[15]

Catecholamine Degradation

The catecholamines are degraded by two principal intracellular enzyme systems, catechol-*O*-methyl transferase (COMT) and monoamine oxidase (MAO).[8] The major pathways of norepinephrine and epinephrine degradation are illustrated in Fig. 13-4.

In the presence of COMT and the methyl donor *S*-adenosyl-L-methionine, norepinephrine and epinephrine are converted to their respective *O*-methyl metabolites, normetanephrine (NMN) and metanephrine (MN). These metabolites can be converted, in the presence of MAO, to an aldehyde (3-methoxy-4-hydroxymandelaldehyde), which, in the presence of an aldehyde oxidase, is converted to 3-methoxy-4-hydroxymandelic acid, better known as vanillylmandelic acid (VMA). Alternatively, norepinephrine and epinephrine can be converted in the presence of MAO to 3,4-dihydroxymandelic acid. In the presence of COMT, the latter is also converted to VMA. Thus, VMA is a major end product of catecholamine degradation.

As indicated in Fig. 13-4, an alternative fate of the oxidative intermediate 3,4-dihydroxymandelaldehyde is *O*-methylation and conversion to 3-methoxy-4-hydroxyphenylglycol (MHPG). Although MHPG was formerly thought to be a marker for CNS norepinephrine metabolism, it is now known that it is formed from catecholamines in the periphery as well as in the CNS and that nearly half the MHPG formed is further converted to VMA. It has been estimated that the brain accounts for only 30 percent of total body production of MHPG.[16] Thus, although MHPG is produced by the human brain[17] and cerebrospinal fluid (CSF) MHPG can be used as an index of CNS norepinephrine metabolism if corrected for plasma MHPG,[18] neither urinary nor plasma MHPG can be considered a measure of CNS catecholamine metabolism.

The degradation of dopamine (not shown in Fig. 13-4) is similar to that outlined for norepinephrine and epinephrine except that the dopamine metabolites lack the hydroxyl group present on the β-carbon of norepinephrine and epinephrine metabolites. For example, dopamine is converted to 3-methoxytyramine via COMT and to 3-methoxy-4-hydroxyphenylacetic acid via MAO and COMT. Structurally, the latter compound, which is better known as homovanillic acid (HVA), corresponds to VMA except for the absence of the β-hydroxyl group.

COMT[19] is present in diverse body tissues, including the liver, kidneys, large intestine, and erythrocytes. It is involved in extraneuronal catecholamine degradation. MAO, which is also found in diverse tissues, plays an important role in intraneuronal catecholamine degradation. It exists in two forms—MAO A and MAO B—which are products of separate genes.[20]

Physiology of Adrenergic Axon Terminals and Chromaffin Cells

Organization of the Sympathochromaffin System

Afferent signals for sympathetic reflexes, which are derived primarily from the viscera, reach the CNS through a variety of visceral afferent nerves.[5] Central sympathetic connections include those in the spinal cord and medulla oblongata, where many sympathetic reflexes are mediated, and the hypothalamus, which is a principal site of autonomic integration. Efferent fibers from these central areas traverse the spinal cord and synapse, in the intermediolateral columns of the eighth cervical through the second or third lumbar cord segments, with cell bodies of sympathetic preganglionic neurons. The preganglionic axons leave the cord and synapse with sympathetic postganglionic neurons in the sympathetic ganglia. Preganglionic to postganglionic neurotransmission is cholinergic (mediated by acetylcholine). Neurotransmission from the axon terminals of sympathetic postganglionic neurons to effector cells is in the vast majority of instances adrenergic (mediated by norepinephrine).

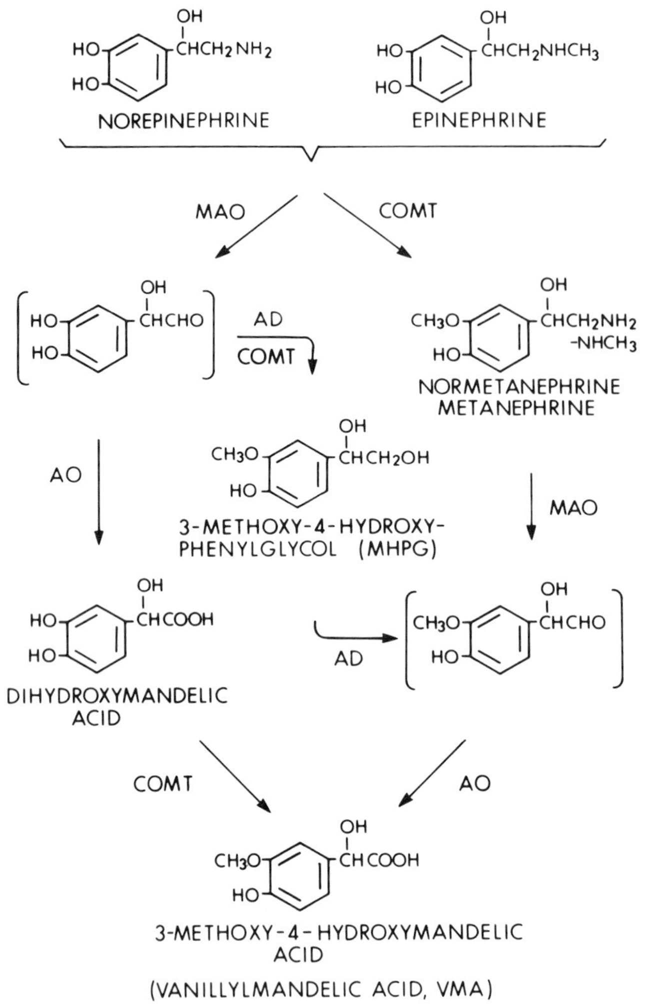

FIGURE 13-4 Catecholamine degradation. MAO = monoamine oxidase; COMT = catechol-*O*-methyl transferase; AD = alcohol dehydrogenase; AO = aldehyde oxidase.

The sympathetic ganglia include the paravertebral, prevertebral, and terminal ganglia. Postganglionic axons extend from the paravertebral ganglia to sympathetically innervated structures of the trunk and extremities via somatic nerves, to those of the head and neck (from the superior cervical ganglion), to the heart (from the cervical ganglia, stellate ganglia, and upper thoracic ganglia), and to the lungs and pulmonary vasculature (from the stellate ganglia and upper cervical ganglia). The major prevertebral sympathetic ganglia are the celiac (solar), aorticorenal, superior mesenteric, and inferior mesenteric ganglia. The greater splanchnic nerve carries preganglionic fibers to the adrenal medullae as well as the celiac ganglion. Sympathetic postganglionic axons from the celiac ganglion project to the liver, spleen, pancreas, stomach, small intestine, proximal colon, and kidneys. The kidneys also receive postganglionic fibers from the aorticorenal ganglion. Postganglionic fibers from the superior mesenteric ganglion extend to the distal colon, and those from the inferior mesenteric ganglion extend to the rectum, bladder, and external genitalia. Terminal sympathetic ganglia are found in the region of the bladder and rectum.

The anatomy of the sympathetic efferents facilitates progressive spreading of signals. A given preganglionic axon may traverse several vertebral ganglia before synapsing and may synapse with several postganglionic neurons. The long axons of the postganglionic neurons are highly branched and studded with thousands of axon terminals which release their neurotransmitter directly at their effector cells. This anatomic arrangement does not, of course, preclude regional organization of sympathetic firing.

Chromaffin cells are widely distributed and intimately associated with the sympathetic nervous system during fetal life. Most degenerate after birth; the major residual clusters of chromaffin cells constitute the adrenal medullae. However, extraadrenal chromaffin tissues adjacent to the aorta (paraganglia), in the carotid bodies, in the viscera, and within sympathetic ganglia persist in adults.[21] The physiologic function, if any, of these extraadrenal chromaffin cells is unknown.

Catecholamine Formation, Storage, and Release

The enzymes required for catecholamine biosynthesis are themselves synthesized in the cell bodies of chromaffin cells and postganglionic neurons. In the postganglionic neurons they are transported by axoplasmic flow to the axon terminals where the catecholamines are formed. Tyrosine is taken up from the circulation and, in the presence of the cytoplasmic enzymes tyrosine hydroxylase and aromatic L-amino acid decarboxylase, converted to dopa and then dopamine. Dopamine is transported into cytoplasmic vesicles (storage or secretion or chromaffin granules), where, in the presence of dopamine β-hydroxylase, it is converted to norepinephrine. In chromaffin cells containing PNMT (mainly in the adrenal medullae), which is located in the cytoplasm, norepinephrine must leave the granules to be converted to epinephrine, which is then reincorporated into granules. Norepinephrine and epinephrine are taken up from the cytoplasm into granules by an energy-dependent process.

The chromaffin granules of adrenomedullary cells have been studied extensively.[22] They concentrate catecholamines to high concentrations (approximately 0.5 mmol/L). This uptake into vesicles is a secondary transport coupled to and driven by a transmembrane proton electrochemical gradient generated by an inwardly directed proton pump adenosinetriphosphatase (ATPase) and mediated by a specific monamine transporter. This transporter has low specificity; it transports not only dopamine, norepinephrine, and epinephrine but also monamines not normally present in the adrenal medullae, including *m*-iodobenzylguanidine, which is used clinically to localize pheochromocytomas (see section on Diagnosis). It is antagonized by reserpine, which depletes catecholamines in vivo. It differs from the monamine uptake system that mediates uptake across the plasma membrane (see below) in that the monamine uptake system is antagonized by imipramine and guanethidine but not reserpine, is coupled to Na^+ and not to H^+ flux, and has other distinct pharmacologic properties. Despite lower catecholamine concentrations, uptake into vesicles into the axon terminals of sympathetic postganglionic neurons is thought to involve processes similar to those involved in uptake into vesicles in chromaffin cells.

The chromaffin cell vesicles contain catecholamines bound to ATP in association with specific proteins called chromogranins, forming a nondiffusible complex. Interestingly, chromogranin A has been found in a variety of peptide-producing tissues and tumors and may be a marker for peptide- as well as catecholamine-secreting cells.[23,24] Thus, chromogranins may be involved in storage mechanisms in a variety of granule-containing secretory cells. The adrenal medullae contain distinct epinephrine- and norepinephrine-containing cells that are distinguishable on the basis of differences in the electron microscopic appearance of the chromaffin granules as well as differences in biochemical composition.[25]

Catecholamine release into the extracellular fluid involves the release of the entire soluble contents of chromaffin granules (including catecholamines, dopamine β-hydroxylase, and chromogranins) through fusion and rupture of adjacent granule and plasma membranes. This release process is termed *exocytosis*. It normally results from an acetylcholine-stimulated influx of calcium from the extracellular fluid into the cytoplasm through a subset of voltage-dependent calcium channels.[26] It appears to involve cellular cytoskeletal elements and may be triggered by conformational changes in one or more fusion proteins.[27]

Norepinephrine storage and exocytotic release from axon terminals of sympathetic postganglionic neurons is similar to that of chromaffin cells, as was just described. Despite wide variations in norepinephrine release and some loss through intraneuronal oxidation (discussed below), the norepinephrine content of sympathetic axon terminals is normally well maintained. This is a result of regulated tyrosine hydroxylase activity and norepinephrine biosynthesis, as discussed above, and reuptake and storage of released norepinephrine, as discussed below. Because of release directly into the circulation rather than into a synaptic cleft, one might speculate that the adrenal medullae would less effectively recapture released catecholamines and therefore maintain their stores less effectively. Indeed, depletion of adrenomedullary catecholamines occurs in some experimental models of fasting hypoglycemia.[28]

Biological Inactivation of Catecholamines

A fundamental principle of neurotransmission is the existence of a mechanism or mechanisms capable of rapidly terminating the actions of a released neurotransmitter. At cholinergic junctions, for example, the action of released acetylcholine is terminated rapidly by degradation of the neurotransmitter by acetylcholinesterase. Biological inactivation of norepinephrine released from the adrenergic axon terminals of sympathetic postganglionic neurons is accomplished by (1) axonal reuptake, (2) local metabolism, and (3) escape into the circulation.

Axonal reuptake (uptake 1) is believed to be the major route of inactivation of released norepinephrine. Axonal reuptake is blocked by tricyclic antidepressants as well as by cocaine and guanethidine. Uptake 1 recognition sites have been measured with [^{3}H]desipramine and have been found to change in parallel with changes in norepinephrine content produced by MAO inhibition (increased norepinephrine) and reserpine treatment (decreased norepinephrine).[29] Through the reuptake process, norepinephrine is returned from the synaptic cleft to the axon terminal, where it can be stored in granules (approximately 75 percent) or metabolized via MAO. MAO is associated with mitochondria in axon terminals and is the major enzyme in the initial intraneuronal degradation of norepinephrine. In contrast, COMT is an extraneuronal enzyme. It is present in cells adjacent to the synaptic cleft and mediates the initial degradation of released norepinephrine after its uptake (uptake 2) into those cells. COMT is widely distributed. Thus, both oxidized metabolites and released catecholamines are rapidly *O*-methylated. Extraneuronal (and circulating) 3,4-dihydroxyphenylglycol (DHPG) is derived from norepinephrine metabolized intraneuronally (by MAO), while extraneuronal MHPG (Fig. 13-4) is derived from norepinephrine metabolized extraneuronally and from DHPG formed within sympathetic postganglionic neurons.[30]

From the foregoing, it is apparent that catecholamine metabolites in plasma and urine reflect not only local and systemic extraneuronal metabolism of released catecholamines but also metabolic degradation of catecholamines initiated within adrenergic axon terminals (or adrenomedullary cells). It has been estimated that only 25 percent of urinary norepinephrine metabolites are derived from the extraneuronal degradation of released norepinephrine.[31]

Catecholamines are cleared rapidly from the circulation; plasma half-times are 1 to 2 min. Clearance largely results from cellular uptake and metabolism. Only 2 to 3 percent of the norepinephrine that enters the circulation is excreted unchanged in the urine.[31] Catecholamine clearance sites are widespread. Removal by the liver, kidneys, and skeletal muscle, among other sites, has been demonstrated in humans.

In addition to cellular uptake and metabolism, catecholamines are conjugated, largely to the sulfate in humans, at least in part in the circulation.[32] The biological importance of conjugation is unclear, but it is a potentially important route of inactivation of circulating catecholamines. Plasma concentrations of conjugates are substantial. The concentrations of the corresponding sulfates exceed that of norepinephrine by about 50 percent and that of epinephrine about fourfold in the basal state. The ratio of the conjugated form to the unconjugated form of dopamine is so high that some have suggested that dopamine per se does not circulate in the basal state in humans. Amounts of conjugates also exceed those of catecholamines in the urine. At least during short-term physiologic adaptation, such as standing and exercise, changes in plasma catecholamine concentrations are not associated with corresponding changes in plasma concentrations of the conjugates.

Axonal reuptake and storage or metabolism and extraneuronal uptake and metabolism are the major processes that inactivate norepinephrine released from the axon terminals of sympathetic postganglionic neurons. Only a small fraction, estimated crudely to be about 10 percent, of released norepinephrine escapes from synaptic clefts into the circulation.[4]

Neurally stimulated norepinephrine release from adrenergic axon terminals may be modulated by several factors acting through receptors on the axon terminals.[33] These prejunctional receptors include adrenergic receptors (see below): Prejunctional α_2-adrenergic receptors mediate inhibition of norepinephrine release, whereas prejunctional β-adrenergic receptors mediate stimulation of norepinephrine release. An additional compound that facilitates release through prejunctional receptors is angiotensin II. Compounds that have been reported to diminish release include acetylcholine, prostaglandins, adenosine, histamine, serotonin, and opiates, as well as dopamine. The precise physiologic relevance of these factors has not been determined.

Mechanisms of Catecholamine Action

In order to produce biological actions, hormones and neurotransmitters must first interact with target cell receptors. It is the presence of specific receptors linked to intracellular effector mechanisms that makes a given cell a target cell for a given hormone or neurotransmitter. Whereas steroid and thyroid hormones bind to intracellular receptors, the initial cellular interaction of the catecholamines (as well as acetylcholine and the peptide hormones) is at the external surface of the cell with receptors in the plasma membrane. These concepts were discussed earlier (see Chap. 6).

Adrenergic receptors[34–42] are of two broad types: α- and β-adrenergic receptors (or adrenoceptors). Each is divided into subtypes that include α_1- and α_2-adrenergic receptors and β_1-, β_2-, and β_3-adrenergic receptors. Originally classified on the basis of the potency sequence of various agonists,[42] adrenergic receptor subtypes were studied extensively with ligand-binding techniques employing various antagonists and agonists. Representative agonists and antagonists are listed in Table 13-1. The genes that code for the four original subtypes (α_1, α_2, β_1, β_2) and for additional putative adrenergic receptors have been cloned,[34,41] permitting deduction of the amino acid sequences of the receptors, and chromosomal assignments have been made.[36] Among the recently discovered adrenergic receptors, the β_3-adrenergic receptor (which may be only one of the so-called variant β-adrenergic receptors) is of particular interest since it may mediate stimulation of metabolic rate among other actions of the catecholamines.[41]

Although the receptor subtype selectivity of some adrenergic receptor antagonists (Table 13-1) is high,

TABLE 13-1 Adrenergic Receptors

Type	Subtype	Agonist Potency Sequence	Agonists		Antagonists	
			Selective	Nonselective	Selective	Nonselective
Alpha	α_1	E>NE>ISP	Methoxamine Phenylephrine	Prazosin		
					Phenoxybenzamine Phentolamine	
				Epinephrine Norepinephrine		
	α_2	E>NE>ISP	Clonidine		Yohimbine	
Beta	β_1	ISP>E≅NE	Prenalterol (?)		Metoprolol Atenolol	
				Isoproterenol Epinephrine Norepinephrine		Propranolol Nadolol Timolol Oxprenolol Sotalol Alprenolol Pindolol
	β_2	ISP>E>NE	Terbutaline Salbutamol Soterenol		Butoxamine	
	β_3	ISP≅NE>E	Fenoterol BRL 37344 BRL 26830A	Isoproterenol Norepinephrine Epinephrine	None	Metoprolol ICI 118551 CGP 20712A

Note: E = epinephrine; NE = noepinephrine; ISP = isoproterenol.

it is important to recognize that subtype selectivity is not absolute. For example, although metoprolol is a relatively selective β_1-adrenergic receptor antagonist, it can produce β_2-adrenergic receptor antagonism if used in a large enough dose. In addition, it has been reported to antagonize β_3-adrenergic receptors in vitro.[41]

It is fundamental to recognize that the endogenous catecholamines norepinephrine and epinephrine are mixed agonists. They interact with both α- and β-adrenergic receptors. Thus, the response of a given tissue is largely a function of the types (and subtypes) of adrenergic receptors that populate that tissue. As shown in Table 13-1, there are, however, some differences between the two agonists. In general, epinephrine has a higher affinity for adrenergic receptors and exhibits greater potency in vivo as well as in vitro than does norepinephrine. Epinephrine has a particularly high affinity for β_2-adrenergic receptors relative to that of norepinephrine. Thus, β_2-mediated responses to epinephrine are more prominent than are those to norepinephrine. In contrast, norepinephrine has a higher affinity than epinephrine does for β_3-adrenergic receptors.[41]

Several adrenergic (and dopaminergic) receptors are linked, through guanine nucleotide regulatory (G) proteins, to adenylyl cyclase on the inner aspect of the plasma membrane of target cells.[34,35,41,43] Agonist occupancy of β-adrenergic receptors, through the action of a stimulatory G protein (G_s), increases adenylyl cyclase activity and, thus, levels of intracellular cyclic AMP. The latter, as well as the biochemical cascade that includes the protein kinase A activation that results from cyclic AMP elevation, mediates the cellular response. Agonist occupancy of α_2-adrenergic receptors, through the action of an inhibitory G protein (G_i), decreases adenylyl cyclase activity and, thus, intracellular cylic AMP levels. Agonist occupancy of D_1 receptors (see below) increases adenylyl cyclase activity, an effect that also involves a G protein. Although also G protein–linked, transmembrane signaling following agonist occupancy of α_1-adrenergic receptors differs. It generally involves the activation of phospholipase C and the generation of messengers including diacylglycerol (which activates protein kinase C) and inositol trisphosphate (which mobilizes intracellular calcium). There is, however, evidence of other subtypes of α_1-adrenergic receptors that open calcium channels and thus permit the influx of extracellular calcium into the cell.[39]

Adrenergic receptors are dynamic, not static, and are regulated by catecholamines.[37,38] The phenomenon of *desensitization*—a diminished cellular response over time despite the continued presence of the agonist—has been studied extensively.[38] Heterologous β-adrenergic receptor desensitization, which results in decreased adenylyl cyclase responsiveness to multiple agonists, is thought to involve phosphorylation of the receptor by protein kinase A (and perhaps by protein kinase C) and a functional alteration of G_s; phosphorylation of the catalytic subunit of adenylyl cyclase may also be involved. Homologous β-adrenergic receptor desensitization, which results in decreased adenylyl cyclase responsiveness only to the agonist that induced desensitization, is thought to involve, sequentially, functional uncoupling of the receptor from adenylyl cyclase, sequestration of the receptor away from the cell surface and into an intracellular compartment, and receptor down regulation. Down regulation—a decrease in the total number of receptors per cell—involves phosphorylation of the agonist-occupied receptor by a novel kinase named, initially, β-adrenergic receptor kinase (βARK). However, βARK may well be a more general adenylyl cyclase–coupled receptor kinase; it also phosphorylates, for example, the α_2- (but not the α_1-) adrenergic receptor.

In contrast to desensitization, little is known about the mechanisms of *hypersensitization*—an increased cellular response following a period of agonist deprivation. However, an increase in the numbers of adrenergic receptors has been reported in autonomic failure, as is discussed later in this chapter.

Hormones that are not adrenergic agonists, including thyroid hormones and steroids, also regulate adrenergic receptors.[44–46] For example, an excess of thyroid hormone results in increased β-adrenergic receptor densities in mononuclear leukocytes,[45] skeletal muscle, and fat.[46] Interestingly, this is not sufficient to enhance metabolic or hemodynamic sensitivity to epinephrine in vivo.[46]

Dopamine interacts with specific dopaminergic receptors.[40,47] These are of at least two subtypes: D-1 receptors linked to stimulation of adenylyl cyclase and D-2 receptors linked to inhibition of adenylyl cyclase or not linked to adenylyl cyclase. Dopamine is a full agonist at both D-1 and D-2 receptors. In contrast, apomorphine and the dopaminergic ergots such as bromocriptine are full agonists at D-2 receptors but only partial agonists at D-1 receptors. Phenothiazines and thioxanthenes are nonselective dopaminergic antagonists, whereas butyrophenones and related drugs (spiroperiodol, haloperidol, domperidone) are relatively selective D-2 receptor antagonists; substituted benzamides such as sulpiride are also D-2 antagonists.

Adrenergic receptors can be prejunctional (on axon terminals), postjunctional (on target cells adjacent to axon terminals), or extrajunctional (on noninnervated target cells). Prejunctional (presynaptic) α_2-adrenergic receptors on the axon terminals of sympathetic postganglionic neurons mediate suppression of norepinephrine release; their blockade, as with phentolamine, results in increased norepinephrine release. Prejunctional β-adrenergic receptors mediate facilitation of norepinephrine release. Postjunctional adrenergic receptors can be of the α_1 subtype (e.g., those which mediate arterial constriction), the α_2 subtype (e.g., those which mediate suppression of insulin secretion), the β_1 subtype (e.g., those which mediate an increase in heart rate), or, perhaps, the β_3 subtype (e.g. those which mediate an increase in the metabolic rate). Extrajunctional adrenergic receptors include those of the β_2 subtype (e.g., those which mediate lactate production and vasodilatation in skeletal muscle and those on lymphocytes) and those of the α_2 subtype (e.g., those which mediate platelet aggregation).

It has been postulated that there are physiologically distinct adrenergic receptors for neurally released norepinephrine and for circulating catecholamines such as epinephrine.[48–52] It has been observed that tissues with little sympathetic innervation, such as skeletal, uterine, and tracheal muscle, are more sensitive to epinephrine than to norepinephrine and are populated predominantly by β_2-adrenergic receptors. In contrast, tissues with rich sympathetic innervation, such as the heart and large intestine, tend to be more sensitive to norepinephrine and are populated predominantly by β_1-adrenergic receptors. Thus, it has been suggested that β_2-adrenergic receptors are extrajunctional and are the β-adrenergic receptors for the hormone epinephrine (β_H- or β_E-adrenergic receptors), whereas β_1-adrenergic receptors are postjunctional and are the β-adrenergic receptors for the neurotransmitter norepinephrine (β_T- or β_{NE}-adrenergic receptors). This notion is supported by the finding that neuronal catecholamine uptake inhibition potentiates β_1- but not β_2-adrenergic responses.[50] The findings that stimulated catecholamine release activates α_1- and β_1-adrenergic receptor processes at low doses of the releasing agent and α_2- and β_2-adrenergic receptor processes only at higher doses and that the latter is prevented by bilateral adrenalectomy[51] suggest a similar pattern for α-adrenergic receptors: α_2-adrenergic receptors are extrajunctional and are epinephrine receptors (α_H- or α_E-adrenergic receptors), and α_1-adrenergic receptors are postjunctional and norepinephrine receptors (α_T- or α_{NE}-adrenergic receptors). Nonetheless, it would seem too simplistic to consider all α_2- and β_2-adrenergic receptors to be hormone receptors, since prejunctional α_2- and β_2-adrenergic receptors are probably affected by released neurotransmitter.

Biological Effects of the Catecholamines

Catecholamines produce a variety of effects in vivo. The hemodynamic effects of the catecholamines—vasoconstriction (α), vasodilatation (β_2), and an increase in the rate and force of myocardial contraction (β_1)—are well known.[53] Norepinephrine causes generalized vasoconstriction and an increase in both systolic and diastolic blood pressure. The latter effect causes reflex (parasympathetic) limitation of the increase in heart rate and cardiac output that would otherwise be expected. Epinephrine causes vasoconstriction in many vascular beds (e.g., skin, kidney, mucosae) but vasodilatation (β_2) in others (e.g., skeletal muscle). It also increases hepatic blood flow. It causes substantial increments in heart rate and cardiac output. Systolic blood pressure increases. Diastolic blood pressure does not change at low doses but decreases with increasing plasma epinephrine concentrations that span the physiologic range.[54] Diastolic hypertension in patients with epinephrine-secreting tumors may reflect concomitant norepinephrine release; hypotension in such patients may reflect massive epinephrine release, although other tumor products may be responsible. Dopamine increases cardiac output, an effect mediated at least partially by β_1-adrenergic receptors; the increase may result from stimulation of norepinephrine release from adrenergic axon terminals.[53] Relatively small doses reduce mesenteric and renal vascular resistance but cause vasoconstriction in other vascular beds. Thus, systolic blood pressure rises more than does diastolic blood pressure.

Other effects of catecholamines include bronchodilation (β_2), mydriasis (α), decreased gastrointestinal motility (β_1), uterine contraction (α) and relaxation (β_2), and stimulation (α) and inhibition (β) of the release of mast cell mediators.

Catecholamines produce multiple metabolic effects through both direct and indirect actions. Indirect actions result from catecholamine-induced changes in the secretion of hormones that regulate metabolic processes. For example, catecholamines both suppress (α_2) and stimulate (β_2) insulin secretion; the suppressive effect generally predominates. They also stimulate glucagon (β), growth hormone (α), and renin (β_1) secretion under some conditions. Indeed, there is evidence of adrenergic modulation of the secretion of most hormones, although the physiologic relevance of this remains to be determined in most instances.

Direct metabolic actions of catecholamines include (1) stimulation of hepatic glucose production—both glycogenolysis and gluconeogenesis—and glucose release ($\beta_2 >> \alpha$ in humans) and limitation of extracentral nervous system glucose utilization (β_2),[4,54–61] (2) stimulation of glycogenolysis and glycolysis with increased lactate and pyruvate release from tissues such as muscle (β_2),[4,54,62] (3) stimulation of the release of some amino acids (e.g., alanine) from muscle (β),[63] (4) stimulation of lipolysis (β_1 and possibly β_3), with increased glycerol and fatty acid release, which predominates over the inhibition of lipolysis (α_2) in fat,[64] (5) stimulation of hepatic ketogenesis, largely secondary to lipolysis and increased fatty acid delivery to the liver,[65] (6) stimulation of shifts of potassium (β) and phosphate into cells, causing hypokalemia and hypophosphatemia,[66] and (7) stimulation of thermogenesis (possibly β_3).[67,68]

The mechanisms of the hyperglycemic effect of epinephrine are complex. They involve both indirect and direct actions of the hormone and both stimulation of glucose production and limitation of glucose utilization and are mediated through both β- and α-adrenergic receptors in humans.[54,55,56–62,69] These mechanisms are shown schematically in Fig. 13-5.

Limitation of insulin secretion is an important indirect hyperglycemic action of epinephrine.[61,69] α-Adrenergic blockade prevents this effect of epinephrine and reduces the glycemic response;[57] in contrast, α-adrenergic blockade has little effect on the glycemic response to epinephrine when changes in insulin (and glucagon or glucose) are prevented, i.e., when only the direct hyperglycemic action is examined.[58] By contrast, there is some insulin secretion, albeit limited, during sustained epinephrine elevations,[54,57] and this is physiologically important in that it normally limits the magnitude of the glycemic response to epinephrine.[61] Thus, patients with insulin-dependent diabetes mellitus, who are unable to release any insulin as the plasma glucose concentration rises, exhibit an enhanced glycemic response to epinephrine.[61] The role of epinephrine-stimulated glucagon secretion is less clear. Increments in plasma glucagon during epinephrine infusions have not been apparent in some studies[54,55,61] but have been observed in several studies in humans and dogs.[56,57,70] Although epinephrine-stimulated increments in glucose production clearly occur in the absence of glucagon release,[58] this does not exclude the possibility that glucagon normally mediates part of the hyperglycemic effect. However, using a somatostatin dose that suppressed glucagon secretion but not insulin secretion (as judged by peripheral insulin levels) in dogs, Gray et al. found no effect on the glycemic response to epinephrine and concluded that

FIGURE 13-5 Model of the mechanisms of catecholamine-induced increments in plasma glucose concentration in humans. (*From Rosen et al.*[60])

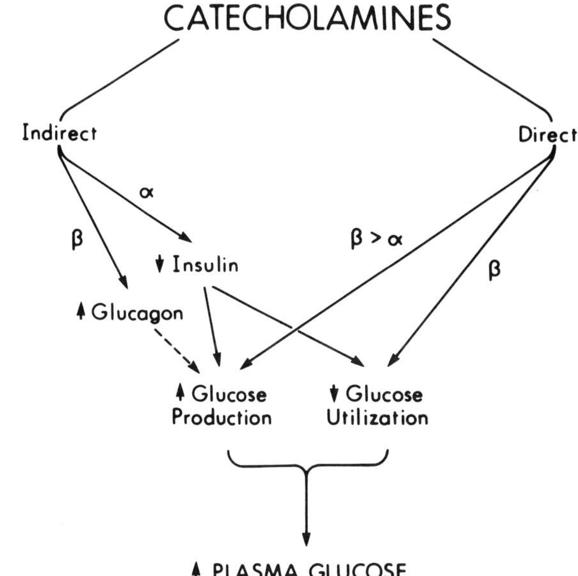

the effect of epinephrine on glucose production is normally independent of glucagon.[70]

The direct hyperglycemic actions of epinephrine involve both limitation of glucose utilization and stimulation of glucose production.[53,59] The first action is mediated through β-adrenergic mechanisms.[58,59] In humans, direct stimulation of hepatic glucose production is mediated predominantly through β-adrenergic mechanisms,[58] although direct α-adrenergic stimulation of glucose production can be demonstrated under some conditions.[60] However, there is also a large body of evidence indicating predominant (although not exclusive) α-adrenergic mediation in rats.[71]

The glucose concentration and kinetic responses to infused norepinephrine are similar to those during epinephrine infusion, although norepinephrine is less potent.[4,72] It is reasonable to assume that the mechanisms of the hyperglycemic effect of norepinephrine are fundamentally the same as those of epinephrine that were just discussed, although this has not been studied in detail.

Infusions of norepinephrine and epinephrine in doses that result in steady-state plasma norepinephrine and epinephrine concentrations that span the physiologic range have been used to estimate plasma concentration thresholds for the hemodynamic and metabolic effects of these catecholamines in normal humans.[4,54,55,67,69] Thresholds for the metabolic actions of epinephrine are listed in Table 13-2. Those for the cardiac chronotropic and systolic pressor effects of the hormone are also in the range of 410 to 680 pmol/L. It should be emphasized that these are estimates of *venous* plasma catecholamine threshold concentrations. Although they are relevant to comparisons with endogenous venous levels, they cannot be equated with biological thresholds because arterial epinephrine levels are commonly double the venous levels; venous norepinephrine concentrations tend to exceed arterial levels.[73]

It was estimated initially that plasma norepinephrine concentrations in excess of 9.0 nmol/L (~1500 pg/ml) are required to produce measurable hemodynamic and metabolic effects. At least with respect to the pressor effect, this estimate may be somewhat high. Subsequent studies have demonstrated diastolic pressor responses at venous plasma norepinephrine levels of about 6.0 nmol/L (~1000 pg/ml) or perhaps lower.[74,75] For example, Grimm et al. found that the mean extrapolated norepinephrine infusion rate that produced no change in mean arterial pressure in normal humans corresponded with plasma norepinephrine concentrations of about 4.7 nmol/L (~800 pg/ml); the rate required to produce a 20 mmHg increase in mean pressure corresponded to plasma norepinephrine concentrations of approximately 18.0 nmol/L (~3000 pg/ml).[74]

Integrated Physiology of the Sympathochromaffin System

Measurement of Catecholamines and Catecholamine Kinetics

The development of sensitive and precise methods for the measurement of catecholamines in plasma (as well as in urine and tissues) stimulated renewed interest in the study of human adrenergic physiology and pathophysiology.[76] Single-isotope-derivative (radioenzymatic) assays have become the reference methods, but high-pressure liquid chromatography (HPLC) using electrochemical detection is now used widely for measurements of catecholamines in plasma and urine.[77] Gas chromatography–mass spectroscopy (GC-MS) has also been used to measure catecholamines and their metabolites in plasma and urine.[78–80]

Venous plasma norepinephrine and epinephrine concentrations determined with a single-isotope-derivative assay in normal humans sampled in the supine and standing positions and during insulin-induced hypoglycemia are summarized in Table 13-3.

Spectrophotometric measurements of urinary catecholamine metabolites, such as MNs and VMA, continue to be used clinically. The clinically relevant analytic methods are discussed in more detail in Diagnostic Testing, below.

TABLE 13-2 Venous Plasma Epinephrine Threshold Concentrations for Metabolic Effects in Humans

Metabolic Process	Parameters Measured	Epinephrine Threshold pmol/L	Epinephrine Threshold pg/ml
Lipolytic effect	↑ Glycerol, ↑ nonesterified fatty acids, ↑ palmitate turnover	410–680	75–125
Thermogenic effect	↑ Resting metabolic rate	410–680	75–125
Glycemic effect	↑ Glucose, ↑ glucose production, ↓ glucose clearance	550–1100	100–200
Ketogenic effect	↑ β-Hydroxybutyrate	550–1100	100–200
Glycolytic effect	↑ Lactate	550–1100	100–200

TABLE 13-3 Venous Plasma Norepinephrine and Epinephrine Concentrations in Normal Humans

	Supine	Standing, 10 min	Hypoglycemia
No. of subjects	165	60	26
Norepinephrine, nmol/L (pg/ml)*			
Mean	1.30 (220)	3.13 (529)	2.92 (494)
Standard deviation	0.49 (83)	1.18 (199)	1.72 (291)
Range	0.38-3.37 (65-570)	1.38-6.15 (223-1040)	1.06-6.97 (179-1180)
Epinephrine, pmol/L (pg/ml)†			
Mean	160 (30)	270 (50)	5620 (1030)
Standard deviation	90 (17)	160 (29)	5840 (1070)
Range	<50-620 (<10-113)	70-810 (12-148)	560-24940 (103-4570)
Correlations (norepinephrine with epinephrine)			
Correlation coefficient (r)	0.115	0.080	0.829
P Value	n.s.	n.s.	<0.001

* To convert pg/ml to nmol/L, multiply by 0.005911.

† To convert pg/ml to pmol/L, multiply by 5.458.

n.s. = not significant.

There has been considerable interest in the application of newer analytic methods to estimations of catecholamine (particularly norepinephrine) kinetics. Since the plasma half-times of the catecholamines are short (1 to 2 min), steady-state plasma levels are achieved quickly during continuous catecholamine infusions. It is possible to estimate catecholamine clearance and plasma appearance rates from such infusions.[54,81] The metabolic clearance rate is the infusion rate divided by the difference between basal and steady-state plasma concentrations, and the plasma appearance rate is the product of the metabolic clearance rate and the basal plasma concentration. The calculated values are critically dependent on the sampling site. Because of arteriovenous differences,[73] epinephrine metabolic clearances calculated from venous samples are about twice those calculated from arterial samples;[81] norepinephrine clearances calculated from venous samples would be expected to be somewhat lower than those calculated from arterial samples. Furthermore, the calculations assume that endogenous catecholamine release does not change during infusions and that catecholamine flux into or out of the circulation is not altered by the infusion of biologically active catecholamines. Recent data support these assumptions, at least in the basal state (Marker JC, Cryer PE, and Clutter WE, unpublished observations).

An alternative approach is to calculate plasma appearance and plasma disappearance or clearance rates from infusions of trace amounts of radioactive catecholamines, specifically norepinephrine.[82–84] At steady state the clearance of norepinephrine is the infusion rate divided by the plasma concentration of labeled norepinephrine, and the plasma appearance rate is the infusion rate divided by the specific radioactivity of plasma norepinephrine. It should be emphasized that the plasma appearance rate is only a fraction (perhaps about 10 percent) of the rate of norepinephrine release, because released norepinephrine is largely dissipated locally, as was discussed earlier.[4] Esler et al. underscored this point by referring to the plasma appearance rate as the "spillover" rate.[82] Nonetheless, the plasma norepinephrine appearance rate should reflect the biologically relevant synaptic cleft concentration to the extent that norepinephrine is neurally derived. For the reasons discussed earlier, the sampling site affects the absolute calculated values. Venous sampling has been used extensively, but since both removal and release of norepinephrine occur in an extremity, arterial sampling has been advised.[84] Since there is norepinephrine extraction across the lungs, truly mixed venous (pulmonary arterial) sampling might be ideal,[84] but this is debatable. This technique assumes, reasonably, that both labeled and unlabeled norepinephrine are handled identically in the body and, more problematically, that recycling of labeled norepinephrine from sympathetic axon terminals back into the circulation is negligible.

Linares and colleagues[83] developed a compartmental model that includes a parameter considered to be the sympathetic neural norepinephrine release rate. This remains to be proved, but the model has gained empirical support.

Despite these methodologic reservations and others not discussed here, there is rather good agreement among the various methods used to calculate catecholamine kinetics.[85] Esler and colleagues reported basal plasma appearance rates of approximately 2.9 to 8.6 ng/kg per min for norepinephrine, 2.1 to 5.0 ng/kg per min for epinephrine, and 0.4 to 1.4 ng/kg per min for dopamine in adult humans.[82] Metabolic clearance rates are similar for the catecholamines, ranging from approximately 15 to 45 ml/kg per min.

In general, plasma norepinephrine concentrations correlate with plasma norepinephrine appearance rates rather than with norepinephrine metabolic clearance rates.[82,83,86] However, there are several cases in which altered clearance affects the plasma norepinephrine concentration.[82] For example, patients with a degenerative disorder of the sympathetic nervous system (see below) exhibit decreased norepinephrine clearance because the axon terminals of sympathetic postganglionic neurons are major sites of catecholamine removal, as was discussed earlier. Thus, plasma norepinephrine appearance rates are more clearly reduced than are plasma norepinephrine concentrations in such patients. Tricyclic antidepressant drugs, such as desipramine, also decrease norepinephrine clearance into nerve terminals and tend to elevate plasma levels. β-Adrenergic antagonists such as propranolol also reduce the clearance of catecholamines (both norepinephrine and epinephrine) from the circulation.[82,87] This has little effect on basal plasma catecholamine concentrations but results in markedly elevated levels when catecholamine release is stimulated. Reduced norepinephrine clearance in patients with cardiac failure has been reported.[88] Aging and reduced caloric intake have also been reported to decrease norepinephrine clearance.[82]

In a study of regional norepinephrine kinetics in humans, Esler and colleagues[82] found that the kidneys and skeletal muscle each contribute approximately 25 percent of norepinephrine appearance. The liver, gastrointestinal tract, heart, and skin contribute less than 10 percent each. They also found evidence of substantial norepinephrine release from the lungs and some from the CNS, although these sources are questionable.[82]

A different approach to the estimation of norepinephrine production rates is measurement of the quantities of norepinephrine metabolites excreted in the urine.[89,90] This method assumes that extraurinary losses are negligible, requires corrections for epinephrine-derived metabolites and adrenomedullary catecholamine production, and, if used to estimate peripheral norepinephrine production, requires corrections for CNS-derived metabolites.[89] It also includes norepinephrine that is degraded intraneuronally, a major fraction of total norepinephrine degradation.[31] Thus, the norepinephrine production rate calculated in this manner must be substantially greater than the norepinephrine release rate. Nonetheless, with this general approach it is possible to distinguish patients with degeneration of sympathetic postganglionic neurons as well as those with decreased central sympathetic outflow from normal subjects.[90]

Urinary norepinephrine and epinephrine excretion generally reflects circulating levels of these catecholamines. In contrast, dopamine in the urine is largely formed (from dopa) in the kidneys.[82] Therefore, urinary dopamine values are not a good index of circulating dopamine.

Patterns during Physiologic Adaptation

Human plasma norepinephrine and epinephrine concentrations under a variety of physiologic and pathophysiologic conditions are described in Figs. 13-6 and 13-7, respectively.[1] Note that plasma catecholamine levels vary markedly. For example, plasma norepinephrine concentrations increase two- to threefold when a subject stands. Plasma epinephrine concentrations increase up to 100-fold during hypoglycemia. The plasma levels of both catecholamines increase severalfold during vigorous exercise. Note also that plasma epinephrine concentrations commonly exceed their thresholds for the biological actions discussed earlier in this section. Plasma norepinephrine concentrations exceed their thresholds less commonly.

The sympathochromaffin system is known to be intimately involved in the maintenance of cardiovascular homeostasis during daily activities. For example, maintenance of blood pressure in the standing position requires an intact sympathetic neural reflex arc. Defects in this arc result in postural hypotension and syncope, as discussed later in this chapter. The roles of the sympathochromaffin system in metabolic regulation are only beginning to emerge. The importance of epinephrine, in concert with glucagon, in the prevention or correction of hypoglycemia is also discussed later in this chapter. It seems likely that epinephrine plays additional roles in the regulation of intermediary metabolism. Thus, the sympathochromaffin system can no longer be considered important only under conditions of "stress."

The Biological Roles of Epinephrine and Norepinephrine: Hormones and Neurotransmitters

The biological roles of epinephrine and norepinephrine outside of the CNS are shown schematically in Fig. 13-8. Epinephrine is a hormone of the adrenal medullae. Although regulated epinephrine secretion from extraadrenal chromaffin cells occurs, biologically effective plasma epinephrine levels are derived only from the adrenal medullae, at least in adults.[2] Thus, measurements of the plasma epinephrine concentration can be interpreted like those of other hormones—as measurements of a biologically active substance en route to its target cells and to metabolic degradation and elimination. Although it seems most reasonable to view peripheral epinephrine strictly as a hormone at the present time, it is conceivable that it also serves an autocrine, paracrine, or neurotransmitter function.

The interpretation of plasma norepinephrine measurements is less clear-cut. In the periphery, norepinephrine functions primarily as a neurotransmitter of sympathetic postganglionic neurons. Since its plasma concentrations exceed biological thresholds in some conditions, such as during vigorous ex-

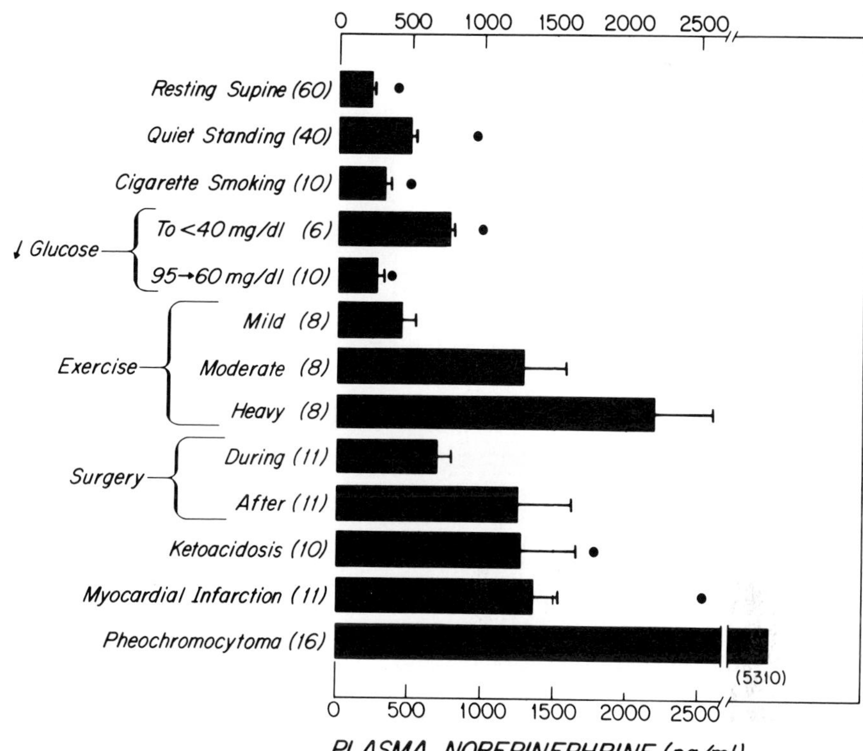

FIGURE 13-6 Mean (±SE) venous plasma norepinephrine concentrations in various physiologic and pathophysiologic states in humans. The numbers in parentheses indicate the number of subjects studied; solid circles represent the highest value observed. (*From Cryer.*[1])

ercise and in a variety of pathophysiologic states (Fig. 13-6), it may also serve a hormonal function under those conditions. Nonetheless, to the extent that norepinephrine is derived from sympathetic neurons, its neurotransmitter function must be considered primary.

Norepinephrine is released from the axon terminals of sympathetic postganglionic neurons in direct relation to postjunctional adrenergic receptors on effectors cells. Transport via the circulation is not required to explain its biological actions. As was discussed earlier, only a fraction, perhaps about 10 percent, of neurally released norepinephrine escapes into the circulation,[4,82] but it should reflect the biologically relevant synaptic cleft concentration of norepinephrine. Nonetheless, the plasma norepinephrine concentration is at best an index of sympathetic neural norepinephrine release.

There is considerable evidence (reviewed in Refs. 4, 91, and 92) that the plasma norepinephrine concentration is a valid index of sympathetic neuronal activity under common physiologic conditions. Under basal conditions in humans, the adrenal medullae have been estimated to produce only 2 to 8 percent of circulating norepinephrine;[89,93,94] bilaterally adrenalectomized humans have normal basal plasma norepinephrine concentrations and exhibit normal plasma norepinephrine increments in response to upright posture.[4] Further, plasma norepinephrine and epinephrine concentrations are not correlated in normal humans sampled in the supine resting state or after 10 min of standing (Table 13-3); these findings suggest different sources (and regulation) of norepinephrine and epinephrine release. Thus, the plasma norepinephrine concentration is a reasonable index of sympathetic neuronal activity in the basal site and during ordinary upright activity. It is not, however, an optimally sensitive measure of sympathetic neuronal activity. It is conceivable that directionally different changes in sympathetic activity in different target tissues could occur with no change in the plasma norepinephrine concentration.[91] It is clear that increments in sympathetic activity sufficient to produce measurable biological effects can be associated with small or even undetectable increments in plasma norepinephrine.[95,96] Finally, as was discussed earlier, altered norepinephrine clearance from the circulation can alter the impact of norepinephrine release on the plasma norepinephrine concentration.[82]

It cannot be assumed, however, that increments in plasma norepinephrine are derived from sympathetic neurons under all conditions. It has been estimated that the adrenal medullae contribute 30 to 45 percent of circulating norepinephrine in stressed animals,[92] and this contribution may be even greater during hypoglycemia. Studies in animals have consistently failed to demonstrate increased tissue (i.e., sympathetic neuronal) norepinephrine turnover during hypoglycemia despite increases in norepi-

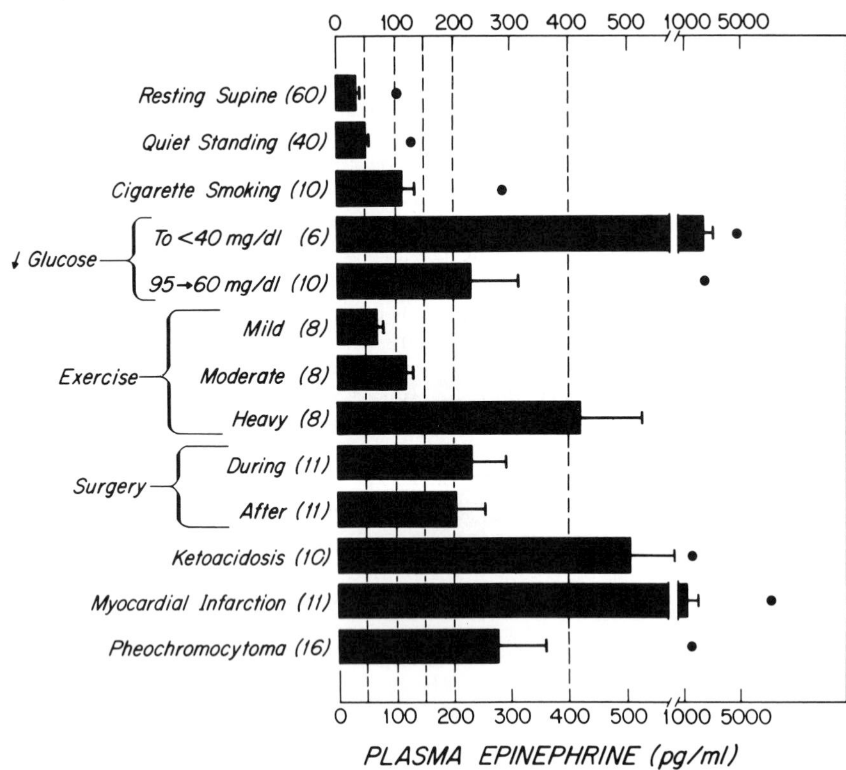

FIGURE 13-7 Mean (±SE) venous plasma epinephrine concentrations in various physiologic and pathophysiologic states in humans. The numbers in parentheses indicate the number of subjects studied; solid circles represent the highest value observed. (*From Cryer.*[1])

nephrine excretion;[28,97] such increases are prevented by adrenalectomy.[28] The capacity of the human adrenal medullae to release norepinephrine (along with large amounts of epinephrine) is well established.[93,94,98] Plasma norepinephrine and epinephrine concentrations are highly correlated during hypoglycemia in normal humans (Table 13-3), suggesting a predominant adrenomedullary source of the increases in norepinephrine. Further, in contrast to normal persons (Table 13-3), bilaterally adrenalectomized humans do not exhibit an increase in plasma norepinephrine during hypoglycemia.[2] Thus, the plasma norepinephrine response to hypoglycemia is derived predominantly from the adrenal medullae rather than from sympathetic neurons.[97] Clearly, the plasma norepinephrine concentration is not an index of sympathetic neuronal activity in this condition.

FIGURE 13-8 Schematic representation of the biological roles of epinephrine (E) and norepinephrine (NE) outside the CNS.

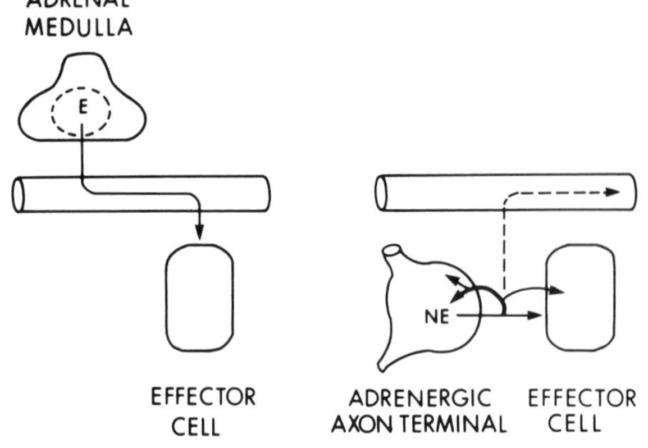

The origins of the increases in plasma norepinephrine (Fig. 13-6) that occur in other physiologic conditions such as exercise and in pathophysiologic states such as surgery, diabetic ketoacidosis, and acute myocardial infarction have not been established conclusively. However, since these states and conditions are often associated with substantial increases in plasma epinephrine (Fig. 13-7), the adrenal medullae probably contribute to the circulating norepinephrine pool. Thus, the plasma norepinephrine concentration is best viewed as an index of net sympathochromaffin activity under these conditions.

Despite the reservations just raised, the plasma norepinephrine concentration correlates remarkably well with muscle sympathetic nerve activity measured directly with microneurography in humans.[99,100]

SYMPATHOCHROMAFFIN PATHOPHYSIOLOGY

Pheochromocytoma

Pheochromocytomas are catecholamine-producing tumors of chromaffin cells that typically cause hypertension.[3,101,102] They are an uncommon cause of hypertension; approximately 1 in 1000 hypertensive patients harbors a pheochromocytoma.[103] However, for several reasons, it is important to detect a pheochromocytoma when it is present. First, hypertension due to a pheochromocytoma is often curable by means of surgical removal of the tumor. Second, patients with a pheochromocytoma are at risk for suffering a lethal hypertensive paroxysm. Third, there is an incidence, although probably only about 5 percent, of malignancy among pheochromocytomas, and early detection and removal can be expected to reduce the frequency of metastatic disease. Extraadrenal pheochromocytomas (paragangliomas) are more often malignant. Fourth, the presence of pheochromocytomas can be a clue to the presence of associated endocrine and nonendocrine familial disorders.

Pheochromocytomas are components of the multiple endocrine neoplasia (MEN) type 2a and type 2b syndromes.[104–106] These familial disorders are inherited as autosomal dominant traits. MEN 2a (Sipple's syndrome) includes medullary carcinoma of the thyroid, primary hyperparathyroidism, and pheochromocytoma. MEN 2b (sometimes called MEN 3) includes medullary carcinoma of the thyroid, multiple mucosal neuromas, and pheochromocytoma. It is fundamental to exclude pheochromocytoma before neck surgery in a member of such a family, since an unrecognized pheochromocytoma can result in a fatal hypertensive paroxysm during surgery. The gene for MEN 2a has been mapped to a region on chromosome 10. Restriction fragment length polymorphism analysis has been used to identify individuals at risk.[107] Familial pheochromocytoma also occurs as an isolated disorder, in neurofibromatosis, and in some kindreds with von Hippel-Lindau disease (including hemangioblastomas of the retinas, cerebellum, and other areas of the CNS). Pheochromocytomas occur in less than 1 percent of patients with neurofibromatosis but in up to 25 percent in some kindreds with von Hippel-Lindau disease.

Clinical manifestations of pheochromocytomas generally result from released catecholamines. They often contain a variety of peptides, including enkephalins,[108] somatostatin,[109] and calcitonin.[110] The clinical relevance of these, if any, is unknown. Pheochromocytomas can, however, be a source of clinically important ectopic hormone secretion.[111]

Origin and Distribution

Pheochromocytomas arise from chromaffin cells. These cells are widespread and generally are associated with sympathetic ganglia during fetal life. Postnatally, most chromaffin cells degenerate; the major residual clusters constitute the adrenal medullae. Thus, it is not surprising that approximately 90 percent of pheochromocytomas arise from the adrenal medullae. Extraadrenal pheochromocytomas have been found in sites ranging from the carotid body to the pelvic floor. However, the majority are associated with paravertebral sympathetic ganglia or the organ of Zuckerkandl near the aortic bifurcation in the abdomen, and most of the others are associated with ganglia in the posterior mediastinum. Multiple pheochromocytomas, including bilateral adrenomedullary tumors, occur in up to 10 percent of apparently sporadic cases.

Bilateral adrenomedullary pheochromocytomas with or without extraadrenal tumors are the rule in familial pheochromocytoma associated with multiple endocrine neoplasia.[105] Bilateral adrenomedullary hyperplasia, which is thought to be a precursor to pheochromocytoma, has been found in members of such families.[106] Some have reasoned that bilateral tumors are inevitable in a member of an affected family who is found to have a pheochromocytoma and have advocated bilateral adrenalectomy at the initial operation.[105] However, at least in some patients, decades may pass between the removal of one pheochromocytoma and the emergence of a clinically apparent contralateral pheochromocytoma. Thus, a more conservative approach coupled with careful, long-term follow-up seems reasonable.

Clinical Manifestations

The majority of pheochromocytomas release norepinephrine, and most also release epinephrine. Rarely, a pheochromocytoma releases epinephrine predominantly or even exclusively.[112,113] The clinical manifestations of pheochromocytomas are commonly due to the effects of released catecholamines, rarely to mass effects. There is marked variation in catecholamine release from a given pheochromocytoma and among different pheochromocytomas. Some pheochromocytomas have been discovered at autopsy or incidentally at surgery.[103] Whether these synthesized catecholamines which were degraded within the tumor and not released, released catecholamines at rates which did not produce plasma levels sufficient to cause biological effects or caused clinical manifestations that the physician failed to recognize during the patient's life is conjectural. However, retrospective analysis of patients whose pheochromocytomas were missed often yields suggestive symptoms or signs. In one series, more than half the patients with unrecognized pheochromocytomas had hypertension.[103] Clearly, the physician must have a high index of suspicion if this generally curable disease is to be diagnosed appropriately.

The common symptoms of pheochromocytoma are headache, palpitations, and diaphoresis.[102] Less common symptoms include abdominal or chest pain, gastrointestinal symptoms, weakness, and visual symptoms. The symptoms are typically paroxysmal and are associated with increases in blood pressure. During a paroxysm patients are commonly pale, soaked with perspiration, and markedly hypertensive. Tachycardia is not striking with common norepinephrine-releasing pheochromocytomas. The paroxysms often last only a few minutes but may persist for an hour or longer. Their frequency varies greatly.

Hypertension is sometimes truly intermittent; in many cases it is sustained but exhibits marked fluctuations, with peak values occurring during symptomatic episodes. In general, these paroxysmal clinical expressions can be explained by episodic catecholamine release; plasma catecholamine levels are higher during symptomatic hypertensive episodes than they are during asymptomatic, less hypertensive, or even normotensive intervals. The event that precipitates episodic catecholamine release is usually not identifiable. However, the relation between plasma catecholamine concentrations and blood pressure is not close.[114] This may reflect contrasting effects of norepinephrine and epinephrine but raises the possibility that hypertension in a patient with a pheochromocytoma is not exclusively the result of a direct effect of circulating norepinephrine on the cardiovascular system. Indeed, it has been suggested that hypertension may result from catecholamine release from an expanded sympathetic neuronal pool.[114] This would explain the relatively weak relation between blood pressure and the plasma norepinephrine concentration, the hypotensive response to clonidine without a decrease in plasma norepinephrine, and the occurrence of paroxysms that appear to be triggered by reflex mechanisms. However, this would require a coexistent abnormality of baroreflex regulation of sympathetic activity and conflicts with the concept of finely regulated norepinephrine stores in sympathetic neurons that was discussed earlier.

The metabolic features of pheochromocytoma include an increased metabolic rate (some patients complain of heat intolerance, weight loss, or both), limitation of insulin secretion, and an insulin-resistant state.[115] Glucose intolerance occurs, but overt diabetes is unusual and probably reflects a coexistent defect in insulin secretion, i.e., genetic diabetes mellitus.

The rare predominantly epinephrine-releasing pheochromocytomas can produce different paroxysms, including systolic hypertension, tachycardia, hypotension, noncardiac pulmonary edema, and cardiac arrhythmias.[112,113] Even with these clinical features attributable to massive overproduction of epinephrine, substantial overproduction of norepinephrine may also be present.[113]

Diagnosis

The diagnosis of pheochromocytoma is based on clinical suspicion and biochemical confirmation. Pheochromocytoma should be suspected in patients with paroxysmal symptoms; hypertension that is intermittent, unusually labile, or resistant to conventional therapy; or conditions known to be associated with pheochromocytoma. Persons with a history of familial pheochromocytoma or other components of MEN 2a or 2b should be evaluated thoroughly even if they are asymptomatic and normotensive. Radiographic studies should be used only to localize pheochromocytomas that are known or strongly suspected to be present on the basis of clinical and biochemical evidence. Nonfunctional adrenal masses are not infrequently found with modern imaging techniques (perhaps 2 to 4 percent of otherwise normal individuals). In the absence of other clinical clues, such lesions are rarely pheochromocytomas, although that diagnosis, as well as diagnoses of functioning adrenocortical tumors, must be considered once the lesion is detected. Members of MEN 2a or 2b families, particularly those known to have another component of the syndrome, are an exception to this general rule. In such patients an adrenal mass must be assumed to be a pheochromocytoma until proved otherwise.

Measurement of catecholamines, metanephrines, or VMA in 24-h urine collections is the traditional approach to the biochemical diagnosis of a pheochromocytoma.[116–118] Of the three, VMA determinations give a slightly higher frequency of false-negative findings. Nonetheless, the excretion of all three is substantially increased in most patients with a pheochromocytoma. For example, the urinary catecholamines were found to be more than twice the upper limit of normal in 90 percent of the patients in one large series.[116] These measurements provide somewhat different information. Catecholamine excretion (and perhaps that of metanephrines) provides an index of released catecholamines, whereas catecholamine degradation within the tumor also contributes to the excreted VMA.

With the development of sufficiently sensitive methods, specifically the single-isotope-derivative method that was discussed earlier and later HPLC methods, plasma catecholamine measurements have been effectively introduced into the diagnosis of pheochromocytoma.[3,119–121] After a direct comparison of plasma catecholamine measurements and 24-h urinary metanephrine and VMA measurements in the diagnosis of pheochromocytoma, Bravo and coworkers concluded that plasma catecholamine measurements were superior because there was less overlap in the data between affected and unaffected hypertensive patients.[121] Duncan and coworkers judged urinary norepinephrine values to be slightly superior to plasma norepinephrine values.[118] However, the two approaches yield somewhat different information. Urinary measurements provide an index of catecholamine release integrated over time. Thus, they may reflect intermittent plasma catecholamine elevations that could be missed by plasma measurements, which provide information relevant to a time frame of only a few minutes. The measurement of catecholamines in platelets is conceptually similar. Platelets take up and store circulating catecholamines. The platelet catecholamine content has been shown to be elevated in some pheochromocytoma patients whose plasma catecholamine concentrations were within the normal range.[122,123]

Our experience with plasma norepinephrine and epinephrine measurements in patients with proven pheochromocytomas is summarized in Fig. 13-9. As can be seen in the figure, most patients have markedly elevated values. Three points warrant emphasis, however. First, occasional patients with typical paroxysmal histories have normal plasma catecholamine concentrations when sampled during an asymptomatic, normotensive period. Second, some patients, commonly those investigated because of a family history of pheochromocytoma, have no symptoms or signs and have normal plasma catecholamine concentrations but are found to have pheochromocytomas. Measurement of epinephrine is particularly important in such patients.[106] These are not innocent tumors; lethal hypertensive paroxysms have occurred. Third, patients thought on clinical grounds to have predominantly epinephrine-secreting pheochromocytomas may also have substantial overproduction of norepinephrine.[113]

Strict attention to the details of sample collection, handling, and storage; to the sources of possible biological variation; and to the effects of drugs, as detailed below in Diagnostic Testing, is critical if diagnostic error is to be avoided in the biochemical assessment of patients with suspected pheochromocytomas. Patients should be studied in the drug-free state if possible.

When pheochromocytoma is suspected, samples for plasma norepinephrine and epinephrine should be obtained in the basal state, with the patient supine. Substantial elevations over reference values provide strong support for the diagnosis of a pheochromocytoma and are commonly found in affected patients. Samples are also obtained during symptomatic paroxysms. However, the interpretation of such values is more open to judgment, since reference values cannot be defined precisely; patients without pheochromocytomas may be expected to have somewhat elevated plasma norepinephrine and epinephrine levels during these symptomatic episodes. Thus, the biochemical diagnosis of pheochromocytoma is more convincing if plasma catecholamine levels are elevated in the basal state and rise further during symptomatic episodes.

It is useful to record the blood pressure and determine whether symptoms are present when plasma samples for catecholamine measurements are drawn from a patient suspected of having a pheochromocytoma. Normal plasma or urinary catecholamine values obtained when the patient is normotensive and free of symptoms do not exclude the presence of a pheochromocytoma. Theoretically, 24-h urinary catecholamine or metabolite measurements can detect intermittent catecholamine release missed by plasma sampling.

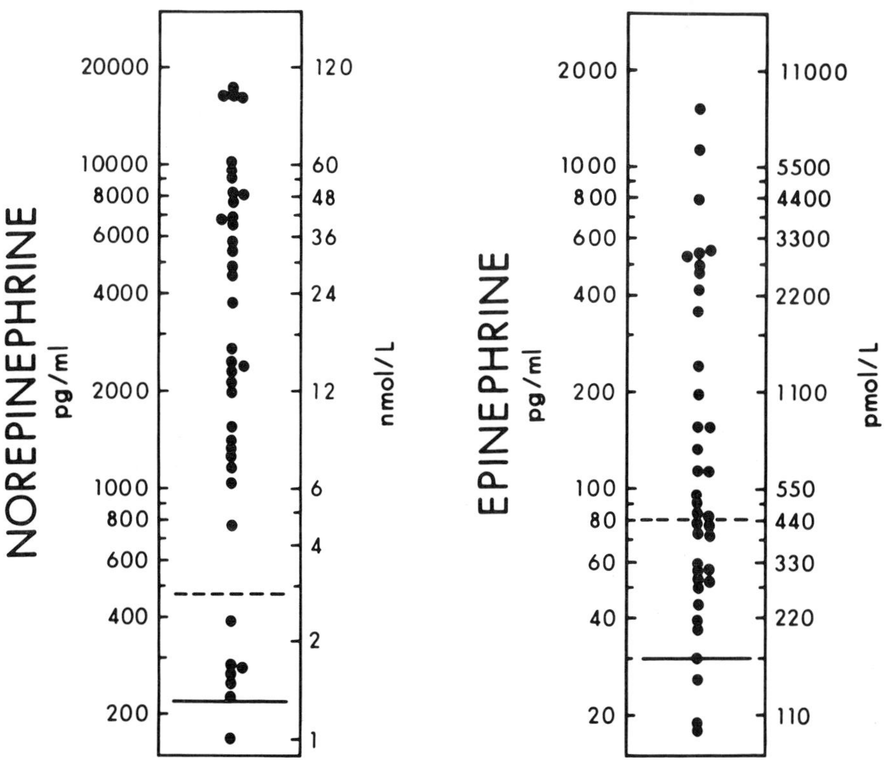

FIGURE 13-9 Plasma norepinephrine and epinephrine concentrations in the basal state (and supine position) in 38 patients with pheochromocytomas. Note the logarithmic scales. The interrupted horizontal lines are 3 SD above the mean (solid horizontal lines) of data from 165 normal humans.

Since substantial plasma norepinephrine elevations are required to produce hypertension in normal humans, as was discussed earlier, and since plasma epinephrine elevations within the physiologic range do not raise the diastolic blood pressure, it is reasonable to consider that normal or even minimally elevated plasma catecholamine levels measured when the patient is hypertensive constitute strong evidence against the diagnosis of pheochromocytoma. It could be argued, however, that this reasoning is flawed if hypertension results from excessive norepinephrine release from an expanded neuronal pool rather than being a direct result of elevated circulating norepinephrine, as was discussed earlier.

It should again be emphasized that most patients ultimately found to have pheochromocytomas have distinctly elevated plasma and urinary catecholamine levels. The considerations raised in the preceding paragraphs apply to the much less frequently encountered patients in whom the diagnosis is less clear-cut and to the problem of the degree of certainty of a negative conclusion. Obviously, one can never be absolutely certain that a given patient does not have a pheochromocytoma. As in many other areas of medicine, a clinical judgment based on probability must be made.

Blood pressure changes following the administration of pharmacologic agents, e.g., a precipitous fall in blood pressure after phentolamine in a hypertensive patient and an exaggerated rise in blood pressure after histamine, tyramine, or glucagon in a normotensive patient, were used in the past to test for pheochromocytoma. These tests are potentially dangerous, have unacceptably high false-positive and false-negative rates, and are not decisive. Consequently, they should not be used. Oral clonidine 0.3 mg has been reported to suppress plasma catecholamine levels in nonpheochromocytoma hypertensive patients but not in patients with a pheochromocytoma.[124] Thus, the clonidine suppression test has been suggested to separate essential hypertension patients with elevated basal plasma norepinephrine levels from patients with hypertension due to a pheochromocytoma. The utility of this test awaits further experience. False positives and negatives have been reported.[125] Further, clonidine commonly produces sedation and can produce hypotension (especially in patients treated with diuretics) or bradycardia (especially in patients treated with a β-adrenergic antagonist).

Plasma chromogranin A levels are also often elevated in patients with pheochromocytomas.[126]

After biochemical confirmation of a pheochromocytoma, anatomic localization is desirable. Pheochromocytomas are rarely palpable, although those associated with the carotid body may be. The rare mediastinal pheochromocytomas are usually but not invariably seen on chest radiographs. A history of paroxysms precipitated by micturition suggests strongly that the pheochromocytoma is in or adjacent to the urinary bladder. In the absence of this history, a mass seen on chest radiographs, or a palpable neck mass, the pheochromocytoma is probably in the abdomen.

Computed tomography (CT) can localize the majority of pheochromocytomas. Virtually all adrenomedullary tumors, about 90 percent of pheochromocytomas, are seen on CT scans. Magnetic resonance (MR) imaging appears to identify adrenomedullary tumors at least as well as CT and may identify extraadrenal pheochromocytomas more effectively.[127,128] Furthermore, MR often produces relatively distinct images—hyperintense T_2-weighted images—of pheochromocytomas.[127] Scintigraphy using [^{131}I]-*m*-iodobenzylguanidine (MIBG) has the advantage of measuring function rather than anatomy and permits scanning of the entire trunk. It appears to be superior to CT and perhaps MR in the localization of recurrent or metastatic pheochromocytoma[127] and to CT in the localization of extraadrenal tumors. In general, CT (and presumably MR) images and MIBG scans provide complementary information.[127,129,130] However, the availability of MIBG is limited, and the test is expensive, requires several days, and requires iodine administration to protect the thyroid gland. It is the author's practice to use MR imaging first and reserve MIBG scanning for difficult cases.

Screening

Since pheochromocytoma is a serious and generally treatable disease, it is tempting to suggest that all hypertensive patients should be screened for the presence of a pheochromocytoma, particularly since sensitive, noninvasive tests are available. However, given the high prevalence of hypertension in the population, the cost of screening would be appreciable. There are, of course, additional problems with screening. Screening tests require diagnostic sensitivity at the expense of specificity; false-negative tests are undesirable (since the diagnosis will be rejected), and some false-positive tests must therefore be accepted. The lower the prevalence of the disease sought in the population screened, the higher the number of false-positive tests. Clearly, the prevalence of pheochromocytoma is low (0.1 to 0.5 percent) in patients with hypertension.[131] Thus, screening results in a large number of false-positive tests. At the very least, these patients require repeat testing, increasing the cost. In some instances the test results can lead to more extensive diagnostic studies and perhaps unnecessary surgery, greatly increasing the monetary cost and making the human cost of screening inestimable. Thus, a high index of clinical suspicion is used to select patients in whom further testing is indicated for the diagnosis of pheochromocytoma.

Treatment

Most pheochromocytomas are benign and can be excised totally. Many believe that preoperative α-adrenergic blockade reduces surgical morbidity and mortality, although critical evidence is lacking.[102] The premises are that preoperative α-adrenergic blockade will permit reexpansion of intravascular volume, for which there is evidence,[116] and will reduce the frequency and severity of intraoperative pressor episodes. The long-acting, orally effective α-adrenergic antagonist phenoxybenzamine hydrochloride (Dibenzyline) is often used. Starting with 10 mg twice daily, the dose is increased over 7 to 10 days until the blood pressure is controlled and symptomatic paroxysms are prevented. Although total daily doses of 60 mg or more may be required, hypertension typically responds to phenoxybenzamine in patients with pheochromocytomas. The side effects include postural hypotension and occasionally the emergence of cardiac arrhythmias. The relatively selective α_1-adrenergic antagonist prazosin hydrochloride (Minipress) has also been used to prepare patients with pheochromocytomas for surgery.[102,132–139] Hypotensive responses to initial 1.0-mg oral doses of prazosin have been observed in patients with pheochromocytomas,[132–134] and an initial dose of 0.5 mg is recommended.[102] It has been suggested that prazosin may not be the preferred preoperative drug because of its inability to prevent perioperative pressor episodes.[134] However, these episodes can also occur in patients treated with phenoxybenzamine prior to surgery.

β-Adrenergic antagonists such as propranolol hydrochloride (Inderal) are generally not administered before surgery unless tachycardia or arrhythmias are or become a problem. It is generally recommended that a β-adrenergic antagonist be given only after effective α-adrenergic blockade has been established, because β-adrenergic blockade alone may result in an increase in blood pressure as a result of unopposed α-adrenergic stimulation. However, this does not occur invariably.[135] Pulmonary edema has been reported to follow the administration of propranolol to patients with pheochromocytomas.[136] Another alternative is the use of the tyrosine hydroxylase inhibitor α-methyl-L-tyrosine (Demser). However, intraoperative pressor episodes have also occurred after preparation with this drug.[137]

Pheochromocytoma surgery is high-risk surgery that requires a surgeon and an anesthesiologist who have experience with this disorder. Careful monitoring of the blood pressure and electrocardiogram is fundamental. Plasma catecholamine levels vary widely;[138] severe hypertension, arrhythmias, or both can occur during the induction of anesthesia, during manipulation of the tumor, or without obvious explanation. Pressor episodes can be treated with the rapid-acting α-adrenergic antagonist phentolamine (Regitine), among other drugs. Arrhythmias can be treated with a β-adrenergic antagonist or another antiarrhythmic agent. In view of the occurrence of multiple pheochromocytomas, including bilateral adrenomedullary ones, an anterior approach with a thorough exploration after the removal of a known intraabdominal tumor is most reasonable. Appropriate intraoperative fluid replacement is thought to reduce postoperative hypotension.[138]

Pheochromocytomas are occasionally first detected during pregnancy. Such patients have been treated to term with adrenergic antagonists, and the baby has been delivered by cesarean section, with removal of the tumor during the same operation.[139]

Given surgical and anesthesiologic experience and vigilance, the operative mortality is low, approximately 1 percent.[140] Reported surgical cure rates range from about two-thirds to 85 percent of patients. About 5 to 10 percent of patients initially thought to be cured suffer a recurrence.[140] Thus, lifelong follow-up is indicated. Probably because of postoperative stress, plasma and urinary catecholamine levels often remain elevated for about 1 week after surgery.[141] Therefore, thorough clinical and biochemical reassessment, which is fundamentally important, should be deferred until after discharge from the hospital. Persistent hypertension can be caused by a missed pheochromocytoma, a surgical complication resulting in renal ischemia,[142,143] or underlying essential hypertension. Surgery cannot be curative of malignant pheochromocytomas, since this diagnosis is based on the presence of metastases; histologic criteria are not reliable.

The biochemical effects of unresectable pheochromocytomas can be treated medically with adrenergic antagonists. A tyrosine hydroxylase inhibitor, α-methyl-L-tyrosine, has also been used effectively, although it can cause side effects, including postural hypotension and CNS dysfunction.[144]

Malignant pheochromocytomas are generally resistant to radiotherapy and chemotherapy.[145] Some success with streptozocin[145] and with a combination of cyclophosphamide, vincristine, and dacarbazine[146] has been reported. Beneficial effects of [^{131}I]-*m*-iodobenzylguanidine therapy have been noted in some patients, but there were no complete remissions.[147] The clinical course of patients with metastatic pheochromocytomas is quite variable: Some die within months; others live for more than two decades. The 5-year survival rate is about 45 percent.[140]

Other Sympathochromaffin Tumors

Pheochromocytomas are tumors of differentiated neural crest cells, the chromaffin cells. Tumors of more primitive cells and of cells differentiated toward neuronal elements also occur. These include neuroblastoma,[148] a common malignant tumor of infancy and early childhood which is responsible for 15 percent of cancer deaths in children, as well as generally benign tumors such as ganglioneuromas.

Neuroblastomas arise commonly in the adrenal medullae (40 percent) or paravertebral sympathetic ganglia in the abdomen (25 percent); mediastinal, pelvic, or cervical ganglia represent less common sites of origin.[148] These tumors synthesize catecholamines commonly but generally do not release sufficient quantities of biologically active catecholamines to produce clinical manifestations. Presumably, catecholamines are degraded within the tumors, since more than 90 percent of patients excrete excessive quantities of catecholamine metabolites such as HVA and VMA. Such measurements provide prognostic as well as diagnostic information: The duration of survival is correlated directly with the VMA/HVA ratio in patients with stage IV disease.[148] Measurements of catecholamine metabolites can also be used to follow the effects of therapy. Although mean plasma epinephrine, norepinephrine, and dopamine levels are increased in patients with neuroblastomas, there is considerable overlap with values from unaffected individuals.[149] In contrast, the majority of patients have elevated levels of plasma dihydroxyphenylalanine (dopa) and the enzyme aromatic L-amino acid decarboxylase.[149] These, as well as urinary VMA and HVA, appear to be useful markers for response to therapy and recurrence.

There have been notable advances in the treatment of neuroblastomas with surgery, radiation therapy, and chemotherapy.[148] A subset (about 10 percent) of patients with metastatic neuroblastomas, usually diagnosed at less than 1 year of age and with small primary tumors, is of particular interest because these patients exhibit a high spontaneous remission rate. More than 80 percent become long-term survivors with minimal or no therapy. Nonetheless, neuroblastoma is commonly a highly malignant tumor that requires aggressive therapy.

Generalized Autonomic Failure

Another established clinical disorder of sympathochromaffin function[3] is postural (orthostatic) hypotension resulting from deficient sympathetic neural norepinephrine release in various forms of autonomic failure. However, mechanisms other than autonomic failure more frequently cause postural hypotension.

Assumption of the upright position causes a sharp reduction in venous return (preload) to the heart because of pooling of an estimated 500 to 700 ml of blood in the distensible venous system in the lower extremities and abdomen. In the absence of compensatory mechanisms, this would result in a corresponding decrease in cardiac output, arterial pressure, and CNS perfusion; cerebrovascular autoregulation notwithstanding, syncope would result from the simple act of standing. Obviously, there are effective compensatory mechanisms. The primary, if not exclusive, compensatory mechanism is a baroreceptor-initiated, CNS-mediated sympathetic neural reflex that results in norepinephrine release from axon terminals within the tissues, which in turn results in a sharp increase in systemic vascular resistance (and limitation of the fall in venous return and cardiac output) and, thus, maintenance of blood pressure in the standing position. Postural activation of this sympathetic reflex is reflected in a rapid, approximately twofold rise in plasma norepinephrine concentrations,[150] as shown in Table 13-3 and Figure 13-10. Maximum levels are achieved within 5 min. Thus, measurement of the plasma norepinephrine response to standing provides a relatively simple means of assessing the integrity of this sympathetic reflex.

Postural Hypotension

Defective postural adaptation results in a decrement in blood pressure upon standing—postural (orthostatic) hypotension. Postural hypotension is a common clinical finding,[151] particularly in older persons.[152] Although a supine-to-standing decrement in systolic blood pressure of 30 mmHg is often used to define postural hypotension,[151] decrements of 20 mmHg have been found to be a significant risk

FIGURE 13-10 Mean (±SE) venous plasma norepinephrine concentrations measured in the supine (SU) and standing (ST) positions in posturally hypotensive patients with (1) severe sodium depletion (round symbols), (2) progressive autonomic failure (square symbols), or (3) diabetic adrenergic neuropathy (triangular symbols). The shaded areas encompass 1 SE around the mean for normal subjects.

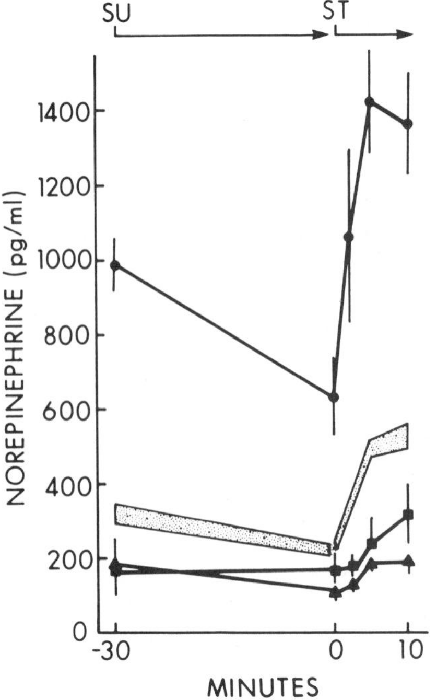

factor for falls and syncope and, in patients with diabetes mellitus, to be associated with an excess 5-year mortality rate.[152]

Upon standing, patients with postural hypotension note light-headedness, blurring or even loss of vision, and a profound weakness that may culminate in syncope. The symptoms clear rapidly if the patient lies down. Postural symptoms are commonly worse in the morning, after a meal, and after exercise.

Conceptually, postural hypotension can be caused by one or more of three general mechanisms: (1) absolute or relative intravascular volume contraction, (2) resistance to the cardiovascular actions of norepinephrine, and (3) an afferent, central, or efferent defect in the sympathetic neural reflex arc. Patients with postural hypotension due to intravascular volume contraction or resistance to the action of norepinephrine exhibit an exaggerated plasma norepinephrine response to standing.[153,154] They have hyperadrenergic postural hypotension. In contrast, patients with postural hypotension due to a defect in the sympathetic reflex arc have a blunted plasma norepinephrine response to standing.[155–157] They have hypoadrenergic postural hypotension. These patterns are shown in Fig. 13-10.

In a posturally hypotensive patient a supine-to-standing plasma norepinephrine increment of less than 140 pg/ml—the smallest increment we have observed in normal subjects—is indicative of hypoadrenergic postural hypotension. There is considerable scatter in the responses of normal subjects (Table 13-3). In a posturally hypotensive patient a maximum plasma norepinephrine concentration during standing of more than 1040 pg/ml—the highest value we have observed in normal subjects—is indicative of hyperadrenergic postural hypotension.

In practice, most patients with postural hypotension can be placed in the hyperadrenergic or hypoadrenergic categories on the basis of plasma norepinephrine measurements. Not infrequently, however, the plasma norepinephrine response overlaps the normal range. This may reflect the fact, discussed earlier, that plasma norepinephrine concentrations provide only an index of sympathetic activity, the scatter in the normal response, the presence of more than one mechanism of postural hypotension in a given patient, or a combination of these factors. One could reason that a normal norepinephrine response is inappropriately low and thus indicative of a hypoadrenergic component in a posturally hypotensive patient with intravascular volume contraction or resistance to norepinephrine. Obviously, this approach cannot be applied to all posturally hypotensive patients, since severely affected patients are unable to stand for any period of time.

The relative clinical utility of routine plasma norepinephrine measurements in posturally hypotensive patients who are able to stand remains to be determined; I belive these measurements are reasonable and have found them useful in individual patients. Typically, these are patients who are thought initially to have postural hypotension due to a defect in the sympathetic reflex arc, because of an associated disorder such as diabetes mellitus, or because of the absence of any other clinically apparent mechanism but are found to have a hyperadrenergic pattern caused by a potentially treatable abnormality.[154]

The heart rate and blood pressure should be recorded during supine and upright sampling for norepinephrine determinations. Although the heart rate response, which involves withdrawal of vagal tone as well as sympathetic stimulation, is not a sensitive measure for predicting the hypotensive mechanism, a marked supine-to-standing increase in the heart rate provides evidence against a defect in the sympathetic reflex arc. The forms of postural hypotension discussed here must, of course, be distinguished from bradycardic (vasovagal or vasodepressor) postural hypotension, which can occur in apparently normal persons and is generally not reproducible.

Mechanisms of Postural Hypotension

The mechanisms of hyperadrenergic postural hypotension are outlined in Table 13-4. Detailed discussion of these disorders is beyond the scope of this chapter. However, in the absence of drug administration, they most commonly result from intravascular volume contraction.[154,158,159] Clinically, they exhibit a spectrum ranging from postural symptoms without hypotension (the postural tachycardia syndrome), which can be disabling, to frank postural hypotension with recurrent syncope. This mechanism should be considered in all patients with postural symptoms and postural hypotension because it is commonly treatable. A given patient can have multiple hypotensive mechanisms, and correction of one can result in clinical improvement. For example, in a patient with relatively mild autonomic hypofunction, otherwise trivial sodium depletion can result in symptomatic postural hypotension that can be treated with sodium repletion.

TABLE 13-4 Mechanisms of Postural Hypotension

Hyperadrenergic (sympathicotonic) postural hypotension
Intravascular volume contraction (e.g., salt and water depletion, anemia)
Decreased vascular responsiveness to vasoconstrictors (e.g., vasodilator drugs, adrenocortical insufficiency, Bartter's syndrome)
Hypoadrenergic (asympathicotonic) postural hypotension-generalized autonomic failure
Primary
Secondary

Hypoadrenergic postural hypotension can result from afferent, central, or efferent lesions in the sympathetic neural arc. Diseases recognized to cause secondary hypoadrenergic postural hypotension produce lesions in the brain, spinal cord, or peripheral nerves.[160] These diseases are listed in Table 13-5. In the absence of such diseases, generalized autonomic failure is considered to be idiopathic or primary.

Primary autonomic failure can be divided into two clinical and pathophysiologic syndromes[151,160,161] (Table 13-5): progressive autonomic failure (idiopathic orthostatic hypotension; PAF) and progressive autonomic failure with parkinsonism or multiple system atrophy (PAF/MSA). Since the etiology, or etiologies, of these disorders is not known, it is not clear whether these are two separate diseases or portions of a spectrum of one disease. The fact that there is overlap in the pathologic findings, such as loss of neurons from the intermediolateral columns of the spinal cord, favors the latter interpretation and provides evidence against the simple designation of PAF as a primary peripheral neural disorder and of PAF/MSA as a primary central neural disorder.[160,161] Nonetheless, there are several clinical and pathophysiologic differences between the two syndromes.

Hypofunction of both the sympathetic and parasympathetic components of the ANS in the absence of other neurologic dysfunction characterizes PAF. Sympathetic hypofunction results in hypoadrenergic postural hypotension. In addition to reduced plasma norepinephrine responses to standing,[155–157,162] patients with PAF, but not those with PAF/MSA, exhibit reduced resting (supine) plasma norepinephrine concentrations.[155–157,161,163] Patients with PAF, but not those with PAF/MSA, also exhibit reduced plasma norepinephrine responses to stimulation of postganglionic neurons with edrophonium (an acetylcholinesterase inhibitor).[157,164] They also excrete smaller amounts of norepinephrine metabolites than do patients with PAF/MSA.[165] Collectively, these findings suggest more prominent damage to the norepinephrine-producing sympathetic postganglionic neurons in PAF than in PAF/MSA. Parasympathetic hypofunction can cause a variety of symptoms,[151,161,166] including those referable to genitourinary (urinary frequency, incontinence or retention, impotence), gastrointestinal (diarrhea, incontinence), and respiratory (sleep apnea, stridor) dysfunction, as well as hypohidrosis. Although typically slowly progressive, the course of PAF is variable.

TABLE 13-5 Classification of Generalized Autonomic Failure

- Primary autonomic failure
  - Progressive autonomic failure (idiopathic orthostatic hypotension, Bradbury-Eggleston syndrome)
  - Progressive autonomic failure with parkinsonism or multiple system atrophy (Shy-Drager syndrome)
- Secondary autonomic failure
  - Metabolic disorders: diabetes mellitus, alcoholism, amyloidosis, others (porphyria, Tangier disease, Fabry's disease)
  - Structural CNS disorders: trauma, tumors or vascular lesions of the brain or spinal cord
  - Paraneoplastic autonomic failure
  - Autoimmune disorders: acute and subacute dysautonomia, Guillian-Barre syndrome, pernicious anemia
  - CNS infections: syphilis, Chagas' disease
  - Others: hereditary sensory neuropathies, familial dysautonomia (Riley-Day syndrome)

Modified from Bannister.[160]

The clinical manifestations of autonomic hypofunction are similar in PAF and PAF/MSA. However, patients with PAF/MSA have additional neurologic disorders,[151,160,161,166] including extrapyramidal dysfunction that can resemble typical Parkinson's disease. In addition to striatonigral degeneration, olivopontocerebellar atrophy (with gait disturbance and truncal ataxia) and pyramidal dysfunction (with hyperreflexia and extensor plantar reflexes) can occur.[166] Somatic neuropathies are sometimes found.[161,166] However, intellectual function is generally preserved; dementia is not a feature of PAF/MSA. The course of PAF/MSA is progressive and debilitating. The disease is generally fatal. In one large series, death followed the onset of neurologic manifestations by an average of 4 to 5 years.[151]

Patients with primary autonomic failure have been found to have increased mononuclear leukocyte β_2-adrenergic receptor and platelet α_2-adrenergic receptor densities, probably representing receptor up regulation in response to decreased norepinephrine levels.[167] On the basis of increased cardiovascular sensitivity to agonists in vivo, receptor up regulation is thought to be a generalized phenomenon in such patients.

Rarely, hypoadrenergic postural hypotension occurs in the absence of other evidence of autonomic hypofunction. This has been attributed to dopamine β-hydroxylase deficiency resulting in deficient norepinephrine synthesis[168–170] and to a defect in norepinephrine release.[171]

As shown in Table 13-5, there are a variety of causes of secondary autonomic failure, of which diabetic autonomic neuropathy is the most common. Most of these causes result in chronic autonomic failure. However, acute autonomic neuropathy that often resolves completely also occurs.[172] It often occurs in young, previously healthy individuals, evolves over 1 to 3 weeks, and resolves over months, although recovery can be incomplete. Gastrointestinal symptoms (vomiting, abdominal pain, diarrhea) are common, but syncope and visual or urinary symptoms also occur.[172] The associations and known causes are listed in Table 13-6.

TABLE 13-6 Acute Autonomic Neuropathy

Primary (? autoimmune)
Associated with and perhaps secondary to
Antecedent viral syndrome, human immunodeficiency virus infection
Autoimmune disorders: systemic lupus erythematosus, ucerative colitis, thyroiditis
Malignancy
Secondary to
Porphyria
Botulism
Toxins: vincristine, rodenticide [pyriminil (Vacor)], podophyllin, others

Modified from Hart and Kanter.[172]

Treatment of Postural Hypotension

Treatment of a patient with postural hypotension[151,152,173] begins with a search for reversible pathogenic factors such as anemia, sodium depletion, or offending drugs. This is done even if the patient has autonomic failure, since treatment of such secondary factors can result in clinical improvement even though the basic neurologic disease cannot be corrected. For example, in a patient hospitalized for the management of Parkinson's disease who becomes further incapacitated by postural hypotension, discontinuation of a diet unnecessarily low in sodium, a diuretic, or both coupled with progressive ambulation will often resolve the orthostatic problem. In the absence of reversible factors, symptomatic therapy for postural hypotension is often required.

Mechanical measures are often recommended for patients with chronic postural hypotension.[151,152,173] These include sleeping with the head of the bed elevated and the use of elastic support garments that extend from the costal margin to the feet. The premise of the first is that it reduces fluid loss from the intravascular compartment during sleep, and that of the second is that external pressure reduces venous pooling when the patient stands.

The objective of drug therapy for patients with postural hypotension is to raise the blood pressure in the upright position to a level that prevents symptoms. One does not attempt to normalize the standing blood pressure, since supine hypertension is a predictable result. Indeed, an increase in the supine blood pressure is a concomitant of most effective therapies.

Administration of the mineralocorticoid fludrocortisone (9α-fluorohydrocortisone; Florinef) 0.1 to 0.3 mg or more daily is the mainstay of symptomatic treatment of chronic postural hypotension.[151,152,173] This potent sodium-retaining agent often increases the standing blood pressure and relieves symptoms. If it is not adequate in itself, most physicians then add other drugs. This drug increases plasma volume only transiently; in the long term it increases vascular resistance, perhaps by increasing vascular sensitivity to norepinephrine.[173,174] To the extent that the efficacy of fludrocortisone results from sodium retention, it would seem fundamental to ensure a liberal sodium intake, with sodium chloride tablets if necessary, and to document an initial positive sodium balance by means of serial measurements of body weight. Hypokalemia is a common complication and requires potassium supplementation. Cardiac failure is a potential but relatively uncommon complication. As with other therapies, supine hypertension occurs.[174] Administration of a β-adrenergic antagonist has been used to attempt to minimize this problem,[151] although it can precipitate cardiac failure.

Drugs with inconsistent efficacy in the treatment of chronic postural hypotension include MAO inhibitors (e.g., pargyline), cyclooxygenase inhibitors (e.g., indomethacin), dopaminergic agonists (e.g., metoclopramide), β-adrenergic antagonists (e.g., propranolol, pindolol), indirectly acting sympathomimetics (e.g., ephedrine, amphetamines, dietary tyramine), and directly acting vasoconstrictors (e.g., phenylephrine hydrochloride). Drugs that produce venous as well as arterial constriction include midodrine, the ergotamines, and clonidine. Midodrine, an α-adrenergic agonist, appears to be effective in some patients, specifically those with less severe impairment of autonomic reflexes.[175] Aside from one report involving ergotamine tartrate,[176] oral ergotamines have not been found to be effective, although parenteral dihydroergotamine has been reported to be effective. The α_2-adrenergic agonist clonidine has been shown to raise blood pressure in severely affected patients but to lower pressure in less severely affected patients; i.e., the blood pressure response was inversely related to the plasma norepinephrine level.[177] Clonidine lowers blood pressure in normal individuals by suppressing central sympathetic outflow, but it also has direct vasoconstrictive effects. Apparently the latter action predominates in patients with severe autonomic failure. The α_2-adrenergic antagonist yohimbine releases norepinephrine from adrenergic axon terminals and has been shown to raise blood pressure in some patients.[177] Finally, with respect to drug treatment, the somatostatin analogue octreotide has been reported to prevent postprandial hypotension in patients with PAF/MSA but not in those with PAF.[178]

Among other treatments, atrial pacing has been helpful in some but not all of these patients.[179] Finally, preliminary studies with a closed-loop computer-based system for blood pressure monitoring and controlled norepinephrine infusion have been reported.[180]

The preceding paragraphs have focused on supportive management of sympathetic hypofunction. Manifestations of parasympathetic hypofunction are common in patients with primary autonomic failure and are usually not treated. However, subcutaneous bethanechol chloride has been reported to improve tearing, salivation, sweating, and gastrointestinal and bladder functions.[181]

Hypoglycemia

The third established clinical disorder of sympathochromaffin function is symptomatic hypoglycemia resulting from combined, selective deficiencies of the epinephrine and glucagon secretory response to plasma glucose decrements. This has been well documented only in patients with insulin-dependent diabetes mellitus (IDDM).[182–184] However, because IDDM is a common disease and because deficient epinephrine and glucagon secretory responses to falling plasma glucose concentrations are common in these patients, iatrogenic hypoglycemia in IDDM is undoubtedly the most common clinical expression of abnormal sympathochromaffin function. As was mentioned in the preceding section, diabetic autonomic neuropathy[185] is the most common cause of generalized autonomic failure. However, that is not the subject of this section. Rather, a distinct form of hypoglycemia-associated autonomic failure that involves hypofunction of the adrenal medullae as well as the remainder of the autonomic nervous system and that is limited to the stimulus of falling plasma glucose levels and is associated with a high frequency of severe iatrogenic hypoglycemia in IDDM is described here.

Glucose is an obligate fuel for the brain under physiologic conditions. Even brief hypoglycemia can cause profound dysfunction of the brain, and prolonged severe hypoglycemia can cause brain death. Therefore, it is not surprising that mechanisms that effectively prevent or correct hypoglycemia have evolved. Indeed, because of the efficacy of these mechanisms, hypoglycemia is an uncommon clinical event except in persons who use drugs, such as insulin, that tend to lower the plasma glucose concentration.[184] Patients with IDDM must, of course, take insulin to survive.

Hypoglycemia is often the limiting factor in the management of IDDM.[183] Patients undergoing conventional therapy experience an average of one episode of symptomatic hypoglycemia per week; those undergoing intensive therapy experience an average of two such episodes per week. Ten percent of patients receiving conventional therapy and 25 percent of those receiving intensive therapy have at least one episode of severe, temporarily disabling hypoglycemia, often with seizure or coma, in a given year. Four percent of deaths of patients with IDDM have been attributed to hypoglycemia. In addition to recurrent physical morbidity and some mortality, hypoglycemia causes psychological morbidity. Many patients live in fear of hypoglycemia, and some feel guilty about that fear.

Although previously thought to be exclusively a result of imperfect insulin replacement in the setting of the variable carbohydrate intake and utilization that characterize daily life, it is now recognizedthat impaired defenses against plasma glucose decreases also play an important role in the pathogenesis of iatrogenic hypoglycemia in IDDM.[182–184]

Physiology of Glucose Counterregulation

The physiology of glucose counterregulation—the mechanisms that prevent or correct hypoglycemia—has been reviewed in detail[182–184] (see Chap. 21) and will only be summarized here. The prevention or correction of hypoglycemia involves both dissipation of insulin and activation of glucose counterregulatory (glucose-raising) systems. Whereas insulin is the dominant glucose-lowering factor, there are redundant glucose counterregulatory factors. There is also a hierarchy among the glucoregulatory factors.

Decreases in circulating insulin normally play an important role in defending against reductions in plasma glucose. However, glucose recovery from hypoglycemia can occur despite a degree of peripheral hyperinsulinemia and in the absence of decreases in portal insulin levels below baseline because of the efficacy of the counterregulatory systems.[186] Among the latter, glucagon plays a primary role (Fig. 13-11). Although it may be involved, epinephrine is not normally critical, but it compensates partially and becomes critical when glucagon secretion is deficient (Fig. 13-11). Hypoglycemia develops or progresses when both glucagon and epinephrine are deficient and insulin is present. Thus, these three hormones stand high in the hierarchy of glucoregulatory factors. Some of the studies leading to this conclusion are summarized in Fig. 13-11.

Growth hormone and cortisol are demonstrably involved in defending against prolonged, as opposed to short-term, hypoglycemia.[187–189] However, these hormones are not critical to the prevention of hypoglycemia, at least in adults, and are not critical to recovery from even prolonged hypoglycemia.[189] There is evidence consistent with the concept that glucose autoregulation (hepatic glucose production as an inverse function of the plasma glucose concentration independent of hormonal and neural regulatory factors) is operative in humans, although only during severe hypoglycemia.[190,191] Nonetheless, these factors stand low in the hierarchy of the redundant glucose counterregulatory factors, since hypoglycemia develops or progresses when both glucagon and epinephrine are deficient and insulin is present despite normal growth hormone and cortisol secretion and intact autoregulatory mechanisms. The same reasoning applies to the potential counterregulatory roles of other hormones, neurotransmitters, and substrates other than glucose.

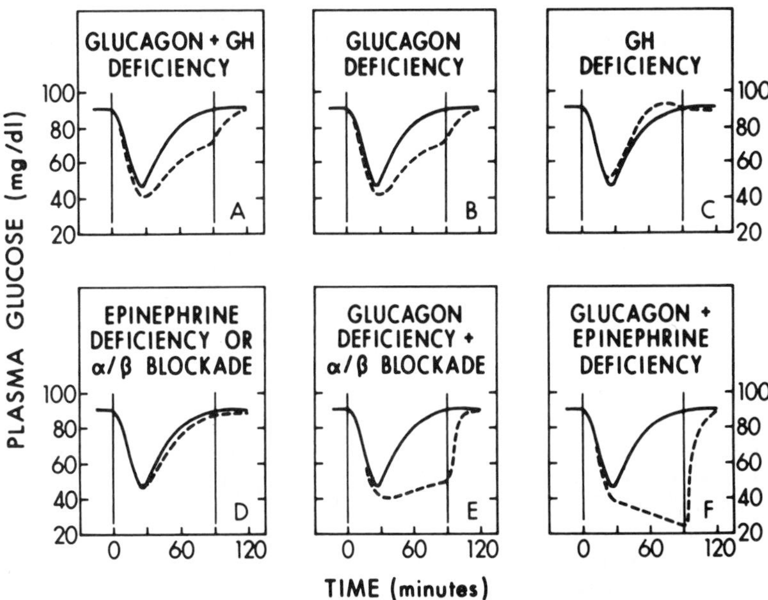

FIGURE 13-11 Plasma glucose curves following the intravenous injection of regular insulin at 0 min in human subjects during control studies (solid lines, same in all panels) and as modified (dashed lines) by (*A*) somatostatin infusion from 0 through 90 min (glucagon + GH deficiency); (*B*) somatostatin infusion with growth hormone replacement (glucagon deficiency); (*C*) somatostatin infusion with glucagon replacement (GH deficiency); (*D*) phentolamine plus propranolol infusion or studies in bilaterally adrenalectomized, glucocorticoid- and mineralocorticoid-replaced patients (α/β blockade or epinephrine deficiency); (*E*) somatostatin plus phentolamine and propranolol infusion (glucagon deficiency + α/β blockade); (*F*) somatostatin infusion in bilaterally adrenalectomized patients (glucagon + epinephrine deficiency). (*From Cryer.*[182])

Pathophysiology of Glucose Counterregulation in IDDM

There are three recognized hypoglycemia-associated clinical syndromes in patients with IDDM: defective glucose counterregulation, hypoglycemia unawareness, and elevated glycemic thresholds for the symptoms and activation of glucose counterregulatory systems during effective intensive therapy. Autonomic hypofunction distinct from diabetic autonomic neuropathy plays a central role in all three syndromes.

Deficient glucagon secretory responses to decreases in plasma glucose are the rule in IDDM.[183,184,192] This is an acquired defect, but it develops in the first few years of the disease. It is a selective defect in that glucagon secretory responses to other stimuli are generally normal. Its mechanism is unknown, although it is closely associated with absolute insulin deficiency. To the extent that they have deficient glucagon responses to hypoglycemia, patients with IDDM are largely dependent on epinephrine to prevent or correct hypoglycemia.[193] Thus, patients with established IDDM have altered glucose counterregulation, but this appears to be generally adequate, presumably because epinephrine compensates for deficient glucagon responses.

Many patients with IDDM, probably the majority of those with relatively long-standing disease, also develop deficient epinephrine secretory responses to decreases in plasma glucose.[183,184] The mechanism of this acquired defect, which also appears to be specific to the stimulus of hypoglycemia, is unknown. Pancreatic polypeptide responses to hypoglycemia are also reduced.[194] Nonetheless, as will be discussed below, the disorder is not linked closely with diabetic autonomic neuropathy.

Patients with combined deficiencies of glucagon and epinephrine responses to plasma glucose decrements have the syndrome of defective glucose counterregulation. Compared with patients with deficient glucagon but normal epinephrine responses, patients with the combined defect have been shown in prospective studies to have a 25-fold[195] or greater[196] increased risk for developing severe iatrogenic hypoglycemia, at least during intensive therapy.

Reduced sympathochromaffin responses to falling glucose levels can increase the frequency of severe hypoglycemia in patients with IDDM not only by impairing physiologic defenses against hypoglycemia, as just discussed, but also by impairing recognition of developing hypoglycemia. Indeed, reduced sympathochromaffin (sympathetic neural as well as adrenomedullary) responses to falling glucose levels are thought to underlie the clinical syndrome of hypoglycemia unawareness.[197,198] Affected patients no longer experience the neurogenic (autonomic) warning symptoms of developing hypoglycemia (e.g., palpitations, tremor, sweating) and therefore fail to act (e.g., eat) to prevent severe hypoglycemia. The result is recurrent episodes of neuroglycopenia.[199] Although the glycemic thresholds for the release of epinephrine, and probably pancreatic polypeptide, are high—i.e., at lower plasma glucose concentrations—hypoglycemia unawareness is not associated with diabetic autonomic neuropathy, as will be discussed below.

Glycemic thresholds for both symptoms and activation of glucose counterregulatory systems are also higher during intensive therapy that effectively lowers plasma glucose concentrations. Tightly controlled patients with IDDM require lower plasma glucose concentrations to elicit these responses.[200] Although this syndrome per se has not been shown to increase the frequency of severe iatrogenic hypoglycemia, it is reasonable to suspect that it does. Certainly the frequency of severe hypoglycemia is increased during intensive therapy.[201] Obviously, these elevated glycemic thresholds are not associated with diabetic autonomic neuropathy.

The syndromes of defective glucose counterregulation, hypoglycemia unawareness, and elevated glycemic thresholds during effective therapy have much in common. First, they segregate together.[202,203] Second, they are associated with a high frequency of iatrogenic hypoglycemia.[195,196,199,200] Third, they share several pathophysiologic features, including reduced adrenomedullary epinephrine responses to a given degree of hypoglycemia (i.e., high glycemic thresholds).[195,196,198,200,202,203] Thus, these are clinically, and perhaps at least in part pathogenetically, interrelated syndromes. Therefore, it is reasonable to group them as the syndromes of hypoglycemia-associated autonomic failure.

Hypoglycemia-associated autonomic failure (HAAF) is distinct from classical diabetic autonomic neuropathy (CDAN). First, HAAF and CDAN do not cosegregate.[195,198,199,202] Second, deficient autonomic responses are specific for hypoglycemia in HAAF but generalized in CDAN.[185] Third, whereas reduced adrenomedullary responses to a given degree of hypoglycemia constitute a central feature that is undoubtedly relevant to the pathogenesis of iatrogenic hypoglycemia in the setting of deficient glucagon responses in HAAF, epinephrine responses to hypoglycemia are reduced little if at all in CDAN.[185] Fourth, HAAF is associated with a high frequency of iatrogenic hypoglycemia, but there is no evidence that CDAN per se plays a role in the pathogenesis of hypoglycemia.[185] Fifth, for reasons discussed below, HAAF may be at least in part reversible[204] while CDAN is not.[185]

The pathogenesis of HAAF is not known, need not be the same in all three syndromes, and may be multifactorial in a given syndrome.[203]

In view of the finding that a single 2-h episode of afternoon hypoglycemia reduces the symptomatic and neuroendocrine (including adrenomedullary) responses (e.g., elevates the glycemic thresholds) to hypoglycemia the following morning in normal humans,[204] it is conceivable that recent antecedent hypoglycemia is one factor in the pathogenesis of the syndromes of HAAF. This hypothesis is illustrated in Fig. 13-12. Deficient glucagon responses to blood glucose decreases in the setting of imperfect insulin replacement would result in episodes of hypoglycemia. These episodes in turn would result in reduced symptomatic responses (i.e., decreased awareness) and a reduced adrenomedullary response (i.e., further compromised glucose counterregulation) to hypoglycemia, thus creating a vicious cycle. However,

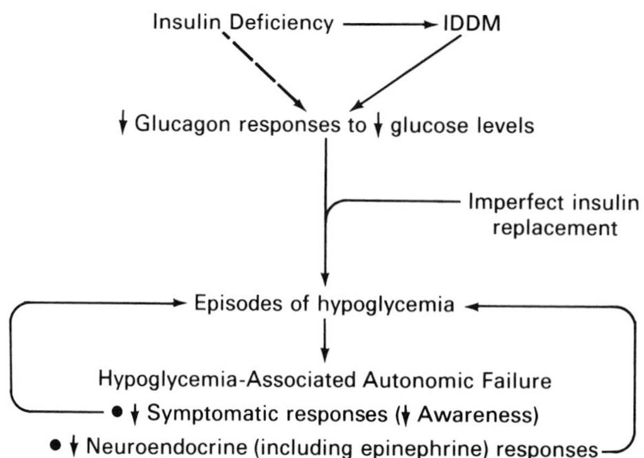

FIGURE 13-12 Proposed pathogenesis of hypoglycemia-associated autonomic failure.

it seems unlikely that this mechanism explains all the syndromes. For example, the syndrome of defective glucose counterregulation was defined in a group of patients with initially poorly controlled IDDM but was expressed clinically during subsequent intensive therapy.[195] Thus, it appears to be at least in part a fixed disorder that is not altered by improved glycemic control over time.

It is conceivable that administration of a β-adrenergic antagonist can produce HAAF. Compelling clinical evidence that this class of drugs increases the frequency or severity of clinical hypoglycemia in IDDM is lacking, but to the author's knowledge this issue has not been examined critically in the setting of intensive therapy in which hypoglycemia is particularly common. As was mentioned earlier, β-adrenergic antagonists impair recovery from experimental hypoglycemia in IDDM.[193] Furthermore, although β-adrenergic antagonism does not produce absolute unawareness of hypoglycemia, it shifts the glycemic thresholds for symptoms to lower plasma glucose concentrations.[205]

Clearly, pending the prevention or cure of IDDM, we need to learn to deliver insulin in a much more physiologic fashion or to prevent, correct, or compensate for compromised defenses against hypoglycemia if we are to achieve euglycemia safely in the majority of patients with IDDM. However, adherence to the principles of modern therapy—patient education and support, self blood glucose monitoring, flexible and more physiologic insulin regimens—coupled with prudent glycemic goals can minimize the frequency of severe hypoglycemia without compromising glycemic control completely.

The Sympathochromaffin System in Other Endocrine-Metabolic Disorders

Diabetes Mellitus

As has been emphasized throughout this chapter, diabetes mellitus can be involved in all three of the established clinical disorders of sympathochromaffin function. Although this probably occurs only in genetically susceptible individuals, pheochromocytoma can cause diabetes that resolves after the tumor is removed.[206] Furthermore, diabetic autonomic neuropathy[207] is the most common cause of generalized autonomic failure. Finally, selective autonomic hypofunction is a central feature of HAAF in IDDM, as was discussed in the preceding section.

Despite the "diabetogenic" glycemic, lipolytic, and ketogenic actions of the catecholamines, there is no compelling evidence that increased sympathochromaffin activity contributes to the metabolic abnormalities of diabetes mellitus in the long term.[208] It might, however, contribute to short-term abnormalities. For example, increased catecholamine levels might contribute to the perpetuation, if not the initiation, of diabetic ketoacidosis.[209,210] However, in patients with IDDM, β-adrenergic blockade was not found to delay the development of hyperglycemia and ketosis after insulin withdrawal.[211] Catecholamines are not involved in the pathogenesis of the dawn phenomenon (an increase in the nighttime-to-morning plasma glucose concentration or in the insulin dose required to maintain euglycemia in that time frame) in patients with diabetes.[212] Although increased catecholamine (along with cortisol and growth hormone) levels are demonstrably involved in the development of posthypoglycemic insulin resistance, the clinical relevance of the Somogyi phenomenon is open to serious question.[212–214] The conceptually attractive notion that catecholamines may mediate hyperglycemic responses to psychological stress has also not been supported convincingly.[215] Although these data do not exclude a role for catecholamines in short-term metabolic derangements in patients with diabetes, they do not support such a role.

Increased pressor sensitivity to norepinephrine in patients with diabetes has been reported.[216] This might contribute to the pathogenesis of hypertension. Alternatively, hypertension has been hypothetically attributed to metabolic insulin resistance, hyperinsulinemia, and increased sympathetic neural activity in the setting of obesity and NIDDM.[217] The ventricular fibrillation threshold has been found to be reduced, with a significantly greater decline in the threshold in response to epinephrine, in experimentally diabetic dogs.[218] This was prevented by β-adrenergic blockade and was associated with an increase in coronary sinus norepinephrine in diabetic, but not in nondiabetic, animals.

Obesity

Obesity can result from excessive caloric intake, deficient caloric expenditure, or both. Despite extensive study, clear-cut evidence that limited energy expenditure plays an important role has not been forthcoming.[219] However, it was observed that total energy expenditure at 3 months of age was approximately 20 percent lower in infants who became overweight, compared with those who did not, at 1 year of age.[220] An inverse relation between 24-h energy expenditure and subsequent weight gain in adults has also been reported.[221] Sympathochromaffin activity is one determinant of energy expenditure. Significant inverse relations between the percentage of body fat and plasma norepinephrine and epinephrine levels, as well as heart rate and beat-to-beat variation in heart rate, have been found.[222] These findings suggest but do not prove a mechanistic relation between decreased sympathochromaffin (and parasympathetic) activity and excessive body fat.

Thyroid Disorders

Several clinical manifestations of hyperthyroidism and hypothyroidism resemble the effects of increased and decreased catecholamine actions, respectively. Furthermore, β-adrenergic antagonists are often prescribed for symptomatic relief for patients with hyperthyroidism. However, if these manifestations reflect catecholamine actions, they must result from differences in sensitivity. Catecholamine production rates are increased in hypothyroidism and, if anything, decreased in hyperthyroidism.

Thyroid hormone excess increases β-adrenergic receptor densities in several tissues in humans.[46] Despite this, metabolic and hemodynamic sensitivity to epinephrine has been reported to be unaltered.[46] An apparent adaptive increase in insulin secretion is a plausible explanation for normal glycemic, glycogenolytic/glycolytic, lipolytic, and ketogenic sensitivity to epinephrine in the thyrotoxic state. The unaltered hemodynamic sensitivity to the hormone is not easily explained. Nonetheless, the data suggest that increased sensitivity to catecholamines may not mediate the clinical manifestations of thyrotoxicosis.

Idiopathic Edema

Idiopathic edema is a clinical syndrome characterized by seemingly excessive fluctuations in body weight, often in the premenstrual period, in women of childbearing age.[223] Morning to nighttime edema formation, which is indicative of sodium retention during upright activity, is the rule, and secondary aldosteronism has been observed. This syndrome has been reported to be associated with decreased urinary dopamine excretion,[223,224] leading to the postulate that decreased dopaminergic tone results in decreased sodium excretion through direct renal effects (dopamine, unlike norepinephrine, is natriuretic), decreased inhibition of aldosterone secretion, or both. Administration of the dopaminergic agonist bromocriptine has been reported to be beneficial.[225]

Bartter's Syndrome

Hypokalemia with urinary potassium wasting, elevated renin and aldosterone levels, and hyperplasia of the renal juxtaglomerular apparatus as well as the absence of hypertension and edema constitute Bartter's syndrome. Patients with Bartter's syndrome exhibit decreased pressor responses to infused norepinephrine and increased plasma[226] and urinary[227] norepinephrine values. Furthermore, the plasma norepinephrine response to standing is exaggerated, and some patients have postural hypotension. This is an example of hyperadrenergic postural hypotension caused by resistance of the vasculature to norepinephrine, as was discussed earlier in this chapter. The enhanced sympathetic activity in patients with Bartter's syndrome is therefore an appropriate compensatory response. Like many manifestations of this syndrome, it reverts toward or to normal during indomethacin administration.[226,227]

Pseudohypoparathyroidism

Albright's hereditary osteodystrophy (stocky short stature, brachydactyly, and subcutaneous calcification) is an autosomal dominant disorder associated with mutations that result in reduced production or activity of the alpha subunit of the stimulatory guanine nucleotide regulatory protein ($G_s\alpha$).[228,229] As was noted earlier, G_s links receptor occupancy with the activation of adenylyl cyclase for many agonists, including the catecholamines. Some individuals with the Albright's hereditary osteodystrophy phenotype and reduced $G_s\alpha$ have pseudohypoparathyroidism (type Ia)—the result of renal resistance to the actions of parathyroid hormone, in this instance including reduced cyclic AMP responses—but others have normal serum calcium and phosphate levels and no evidence of resistance to parathyroid hormone (pseudopseudohypoparathyroidism). Others with pseudohypoparathyroidism (type Ib) have normal G_s but reduced cyclic AMP responses, while a third group (type II) exhibits neither abnormality.[230]

Patients with pseudohypoparathyroidism (generally those with type Ia but apparently some with type Ib as well) can be shown to have evidence of reduced responsiveness to multiple hormones in addition to parathyroid hormone. These hormones include glucagon, catecholamines, thyroid stimulating hormone (TSH), and vasopressin. These are thought to reflect impaired G_s-mediated coupling of occupancy of the specific receptors, including β-adrenergic receptors,[231] to activation of adenylyl cyclase. However, despite reduced plasma cyclic AMP responses, the glycemic, blood pressure, and heart rate responses to a fixed dose of the β-adrenergic agonist isoproterenol[232] (and the glycemic response to a fixed dose of glucagon[233]) have been reported to be indistinguishable from those of unaffected individuals. Thus, the implications of these G_s abnormalities with respect to the function of the sympathochromaffin system are unclear.

Other Endocrine Disorders

Although catecholamines are involved in the regulation of the secretion of the vast majority of the hormones and a variety of hormones have been reported to affect adrenergic receptors,[44] clear-cut clinical expressions of disorders involving these interactions have not emerged.

As was mentioned earlier, because PNMT is a glucocorticoid-inducible enzyme, normal adrenomedullary epinephrine production probably is at least partially dependent on intact adrenocortical function. Reduced plasma epinephrine responses to exercise have been observed in patients with secondary adrenocortical insufficiency.[15]

DIAGNOSTIC TESTING

Measurement of Catecholamines and Their Metabolites

Measurements of catecholamines and of catecholamine metabolites are used clinically in the diagnosis of pheochromocytoma and other sympathochromaffin tumors. Measurement of the plasma norepinephrine response to standing (or tilting) can be used to define the mechanism of postural hypotension (hyperadrenergic vs. hypoadrenergic).

Determination of catecholamines, their metabolites, or both in urine, usually 24-h urine samples, have been used clinically for decades. Older fluorometric techniques[8] have been replaced by HPLC methods in the vast majority of clinical laboratories. Most HPLC methods employ electrochemical detection,[234] but other detection systems can be used.[235] These methods provide quantitative measurements of norepinephrine, epinephrine, and dopamine excretion. Normal urinary norepinephrine excretion is approximately 10 to 90 μ/24 h, while that of epinephrine is less than 15 μg/24 h. Urinary dopamine excretion, which is largely derived from the kidneys rather than the circulation, is generally in the range of 100 to 450 μg/24 h.

Although they were formerly determined by selective extraction and conversion to vanillin, as measured spectrophotometrically,[8] urinary MN and NMN (often reported as total metanephrines) and VMA can also be measured with HPLC methods.[234,235] Normal persons generally excrete less than 1.0 mg of total metanephrines and 7.0 mg of VMA per 24 h.

Single-isotope-derivative (radioenzymatic) methods, which are based on the conversion of the catecholamines to their respective tritiated *O*-methyl derivatives in the presence of *S*-adenosyl-L-methione containing a tritiated methyl group which is transferred to the catecholamines by the enzyme COMT, are the reference methods for measurements of catecholamines in plasma.[236,237] They provide the sensitivity, specificity, and precision needed for measurement of physiologic concentrations of epinephrine as well as norepinephrine in plasma. They can, of course, be used to measure catecholamines in urine (and tissue), but the high concentrations present in urine do not require a sensitive method.

However, isotope-derivative methods are technically demanding, time-consuming, and expensive. Most clinical laboratories now use HPLC methods to measure catecholamines, as well as precursors and metabolites, in plasma.[238–240] These methods are sufficiently sensitive to answer the clinical question, Are plasma catecholamine levels elevated above normal?

Representative venous plasma norepinephrine and epinephrine concentrations in normal individuals are listed in Table 13-3. Levels in various physiologic and pathophysiologic states are shown in Figs. 13-6, 13-7, 13-9, and 13-10.

Strict attention to the details of sample collection, handling, and storage; sources of possible biological variation; and the effects of drugs is critical if diagnostic error is to be avoided in the use of catecholamine measurements. This applies to both plasma and urinary catecholamine measurements but is perhaps more critical with plasma measurements.

Potential sources of error in the use of plasma catecholamine measurements are listed in Table 13-7. From a technical standpoint, it is important that the patient be in the supine position before and during sampling. Plasma norepinephrine and epinephrine concentrations double when a normal person stands, and the scatter in the values increases (Table 13-3). Although we have used a 30-min interval in the supine position, 10 to 15 min is probably sufficient. Because the stress of venipuncture elevates mean plasma catecholamine levels somewhat and increases the scatter in the values, some advocate sampling through a previously inserted indwelling intravenous needle or catheter.

Catecholamines are readily oxidized. They are most stable at low temperature, at low pH, and in the presence of an antioxidant. Furthermore, erythrocytes contain COMT. In whole blood catecholamines have been reported to degrade at a rate of approximately 30 percent per hour at room temperature,[236] although slower rates have also been reported.[241] Thus, blood samples for plasma catecholamine determinations should be drawn into iced tubes containing an anticoagulant and an antioxidant, and the plasma should be separated, preferably in a refrigerated centrifuge, promptly. Many laboratories, including ours, use the calcium chelating agent EGTA and the antioxidant reduced glutathione. 1,4-Dithiothreitol, but not metabisulfite or ascorbic acid, can be substituted for reduced glutathione. Once it is separated, the plasma should be frozen quickly. Catecholamines deteriorate at a rate of approximately 5 percent per month at −20°C. At −70°C they are stable for at least 1 year.[236] Finally, at the present time only single-isotope-derivative and HPLC methods are appropriate for the measurement of catecholamines in plasma.

Biological variation in plasma catecholamine concentrations can be substantial (Table 13-3 and Figs. 13-6 and 13-7). For example, plasma epineph-

TABLE 13-7 Potential Sources of Error in the Use of Plasma Catecholamine Measurements

1. Technical
   - *a.* Sampling: patient in supine position
   - *b.* Sample handling: iced, special tubes; prompt separation of plasma
   - *c.* Sample storage: −20°C (hours to days); −70°C (longer)
   - *d.* Analytic method: HPLC or radioenzymatic method
2. Biological variation: normally marked; increased catecholamine levels
   - *a.* Acute stress (physical or emotional)
   - *b.* Chronic illness
3. Drug-induced variation: increased catecholamine levels
   - *a.* Catecholamines and related compounds: methyldopa, dopa, isoproterenol, etc.
   - *b.* Increased catecholamine release
     - (1) Sympathomimetics: epinephrine, amphetamines, tyramine, etc.
     - (2) Vasodilators: nitrates/nitrites, hydralazine, minoxidil, methylxanthines, phenothiazines, calcium channel antagonists, etc.
     - (3) α-adrenergic antagonists: prazosin, phentolamine, phenoxybenzamine
     - (4) Diuretics (sodium depletion)
     - (5) Cigarette and marijuana smoking, caffeine ingestion
   - *c.* Decreased catecholamine clearance
     - (1) β-adrenergic antagonists: propranolol, etc.
     - (2) Others: cocaine, guanethidine, reserpine

rine concentrations increase as much as 100-fold during hypoglycemia. Smaller but substantial increments in norepinephrine and epinephrine levels occur during common activities. Thus, scrupulous attention to sampling conditions and reluctance to attach undue importance to single measurements are required if plasma catecholamine levels are to be interpreted correctly.

Elevated plasma catecholamine levels have been well documented during acute mental and physical stress. Stable elevations also occur in several chronic diseases, such as hypothyroidism, congestive cardiac failure, chronic pulmonary disease, and duodenal ulcer. Additional physiologic factors should be kept in mind. For example, plasma norepinephrine concentrations increase slightly with age.[242] Sodium depletion due to disease, diuretics, or dietary sodium restriction (less than 3.0 g per day) elevates resting plasma norepinephrine concentrations and increases the response to standing.[98,243]

Patients should be sampled in the drug-free state if possible. Drug-induced alterations are perhaps the most common cause of erroneous interpretation of plasma catecholamine determinations. Most antihypertensive drugs, other than clonidine, and many other drugs can elevate plasma and urinary catecholamines. Some of these mechanisms are summarized in Table 13-7. If the physician is compelled to treat hypertension before measuring catecholamines, clonidine is the drug of choice since it will not produce a false-positive result.

Urine samples for catecholamine determinations are commonly collected in refrigerated containers to which 15 ml of 6*N* HCl has been added, since catecholamines are more stable at low temperature and low pH. Urine samples for metanephrines and VMA need not be acidified, but the analytic methods are compatible with this form of collection if catecholamines are also to be measured. The collection of a complete 24-h urine specimen requires careful instruction of the patient and the nursing staff. The creatinine content should be measured in all specimens to detect major collection errors. Dietary restrictions are not necessary for specific measurements of urinary metanephrines and VMA.

Catecholamine and catecholamine metabolite excretion is subject to the same sources of biological variation as that apply to plasma catecholamine levels, as was discussed earlier. However, because these variations in catecholamine release are usually brief, their effect on 24-h excretion is relatively small and sampling conditions need not be controlled rigorously. Nonetheless, major stress should be avoided during these collections, as conditions known to produce stable elevations in plasma catecholamine levels will produce corresponding elevations in urinary catecholamine and metabolite excretion.

Drug-induced alterations are also common. All the drugs that elevate plasma catecholamine levels, as discussed earlier, can be expected to increase urinary catecholamine and metabolite values. Short-term administration of the mild analgesics acetylsalicylic acid, acetaminophen, and propoxyphene or of the sedative-tranquilizers diazepam, chlordiazepoxide, diphenhydramine, and phenobarbital does not alter catecholamine excretion.[244]

TABLE 13-8 Clinical Tests for Autonomic Hypofunction

Test	Normal	Borderline	Abnormal
Postural fall in blood pressure: fall in systolic blood pressure (mmHg) after 2 min standing	<11	11-29	>29
Heart rate variation: ratio of maximum to minimum heart rate (bpm) during deep breathing at 6 breaths per min	>15	11-14	<11
Heart rate response to standing: ratio of the R-R interval at approximately beat 30 to that at approximately beat 15 after initiation of standing (30:15 ratio)	>1.04	1.01-1.03	<1.01
Valsalva maneuver: ratio of longest R-R interval after to shortest R-R interval during the Valsalva maneuver (40 mmHg × 15 s) with an aneroid manometer or modified sphygmomanometer (Valsalva ratio)	>1.20	1.11-1.120	<1.11
Sustained handgrip: increase in diastolic blood pressure (mmHg) measured during 30% of maximal handgrip for up to 5 min with a handgrip dynamometer	>15	11-15	<11

From Ewing.[246]

Indirect Tests of Autonomic Function

Tests of cardiovascular reflexes are often used to assess autonomic function. Some relatively simple tests that can be used to document and to some extent quantitate autonomic failure[245–247] are described in Table 13-8. Measurement of blood pressure (and heart rate) in the supine and standing positions is the most widely used indirect clinical test of sympathetic function, as was discussed earlier in this chapter. Clearly, it is neither a sensitive nor a specific test of sympathetic function. Patients with other evidence of sympathochromaffin hypofunction may not have postural hypotension, and postural hypotension can result from mechanisms other than sympathetic hypofunction, as was discussed earlier. The utility of this maneuver is enhanced by the simultaneous measurement of the plasma norepinephrine response.

Among tests of parasympathetic function, measurements of the variation in heart rate associated with deep breathing is commonly used.[245–247] The normal variation is determined largely by vagal inputs; variation is decreased by parasympathetic hypofunction. A simple approach is to obtain an ECG recording during deep breathing at five to six cycles per minute in a resting subject.[245] R-R intervals are measured, and beat-to-beat variation is calculated as the difference between maximal and minimal heart rate and expressed as the mean of differences in five successive respirations. Values lower than 10 per minute are considered abnormal.

Acknowledgments The author is grateful for the efforts of his collaborators, whose names appear in the reference list, and for the support of U.S. Public Health Service grants AM 27085, RR 00036, and AM 20579. Particular thanks are due to Ms. Mary Kharibian for preparation of the manuscript.

REFERENCES

1. Cryer PE: Physiology and pathophysiology of the human sympathoadrenal neuroendocrine system. *N Engl J Med* 303:436, 1980.
2. Shah SD, Tse TF, Clutter WE, Cryer PE: The human sympathochromaffin system. *Am J Physiol* 247:E380, 1984.
3. Cryer PE: The adrenal medullae, in James VHT (ed): *The Adrenal Gland*, 2d ed. New York, Raven Press (in press).
4. Silverberg AB, Shah SD, Haymond MW, Cryer PE: Norepinephrine: Hormone and neurotransmitter in man. *Am J Physiol* 234:E252, 1978.
5. Mayer SE: Neurohumoral transmission and the autonomic nervous system, in Gilman AG, Goodman LS, Gilman A (eds): *The Pharmacological Basis of Therapeutics*. New York, Macmillan, 1980, pp 55–90.
6. Cryer PE: Decreased sympathochromaffin activity in IDDM. *Diabetes* 38:405, 1989.
7. Trifaró J-M: Cellular and molecular mechanisms in hormone and neurotransmitter secretion. *Can J Physiol Pharmacol* 68:1, 1990.
8. Nagatsu T: *Biochemistry of the Catecholamines*. Baltimore, University Park Press, 1973.
9. Clarke JTR, Bier DM: The conversion of phenylalanine to tyrosine in man: Direct measurement by continuous intravenous tracer infusions of L-[ring$^2H_5$]phenylalanine and L-[1-^{13}C]tyrosine in the postabsorptive state. *Metabolism* 31:999, 1982.
10. Fukami MH, Haavik J, Flatmark T: Phenylalanine as a substrate for tyrosine hydroxylase in bovine adrenal chromaffin cells. *Biochem J* 268:525, 1990.
11. McInnes RR, Kaufman S, Warsh JJ, Van Loon GR, Milstein S, Kapatos G, Soldin S, Walsh P, et al: Biopterin synthesis defect. *J Clin Invest* 73:458, 1984.
12. Haycock JW: Phosphorylation of tyrosine hydroxylase *in situ* at serine 8, 19, 31 and 40. *J Biol Chem* 265:11682, 1990.
13. Kaneda N, Ichinose H, Kobayashi K, Oka K, Kishi F, Nakazawa A, Kurosawa Y, Fujita K, Nagatsu T: Molecular cloning of cDNA and chromosomal assignment of the gene for human phenylethanolamine N-methyltransferase, the enzyme for epinephrine biosynthesis. *J Biol Chem* 263:7672, 1988.
14. Ceccatelli S, Dagerlind Å, Schalling M, Wikström A-C, Okret S, Gustafsson JÅ, Goldstein M, Hökfelt T: The glucocorticoid receptor in the adrenal gland is localized in the cytoplasm of adrenaline cells. *Acta Physiol Scand* 137:559, 1989.
15. Rudman D, Moffitt SD, Fernhoff PM, Blackston RD, Faraj BA: Epinephrine deficiency in hypocorticotropic hypopituitary children. *J Clin Endocrinol Metab* 53:722, 1981.
16. Blombery PA, Kopin IJ, Gordon EK, Markey SP, Ebert MH: Conversion of MHPG to vanillylmandelic acid. *Arch Gen Psychiatry* 37:1095, 1980.
17. Maas JW, Hattox SE, Greene NM, Landis DH: 3-Methoxy-4-hydroxyphenethyleneglycol production by human brain in vivo. *Science* 205:1025, 1979.
18. Kopin IJ, Gordon EK, Jimerson DC, Polinsky RJ: Relation between plasma and cerebrospinal fluid levels of 3-methoxy-4-hydroxphenylglycol. *Science* 219:73, 1983.
19. Axelrod J, Tomchick R: Enzymatic O-methylation of epinephrine and other catechols. *J Biol Chem* 233:702, 1958.
20. Shih JC: Molecular basis of human MAO A and B. *Neuropsychopharmacology* 4:1, 1991.
21. Coupland RE: *The Natural History of the Chromaffin Cell*. London, Longmans, 1965.
22. Johnson RG: Accumulation of biological amines into chromaffin granules: A model for hormone and neurotransmitter transport. *Physiol Rev* 68:232, 1988.
23. Takiyyudin MA, Cerrenka JH, Pandian MR, Stuenkel CA, Neumann HPH, O'Connor DT: Neuroendocrine sources of chromogranin-A in normal man: Clues from selective stimulation of endocrine glands. *J Clin Endocrinol Metab* 71:360, 1990.
24. Cryer PE, Wortsman J, Shah SD, Deftos LJ: Plasma chromogranin A as a marker of sympathochromaffin activity in humans. *Am J Physiol* 260:E243, 1991.
25. Kryvi H: Comparison of the ultrastructure of adrenaline and noradrenaline storage granules of bovine adrenal medulla. *Eur J Cell Biol* 20:76, 1979.
26. Miller RJ: Multiple calcium channels and neuronal function. *Science* 235:46, 1987.
27. Almers W: Exocytosis. *Annu Rev Physiol* 52:607, 1990.
28. Young JB, Landsberg L: Sympathoadrenal activity in fasting pregnant rats: Dissociation of adrenal medullary and sympathetic nervous system responses. *J Clin Invest* 64:109, 1979.
29. Lee C-M, Javitch JA, Snyder SH: Recognition sites for norepinephrine uptake: Regulation by neurotransmitter. *Science* 220:626, 1983.
30. Eisenhofer G, Goldstein DS, Ropchak TG, Nguyen HQ, Keiser HR, Kopin JJ: Source and physiological significance of plasma 3,4-dihydroxyphenylglycol and 3-methoxy-4-hydroxyphenylglycol. *J Auton Nerv Syst* 24:1, 1988.
31. Maas JW, Benensohn H, Landis HD: A kinetic study of the disposition of circulating norepinephrine in normal male subjects. *J Pharmacol Exp Ther* 174:381, 1970.
32. Wang P-C, Buu NT, Kuchel O, Genest J: Conjugation pat-

terns of endogenous plasma catecholamines in human and rat. *J Lab Clin Med* 101:141, 1983.
33. Starke K: Presynaptic α-autoreceptors. *Rev Physiol Biochem Pharmacol* 107:73, 1987.
34. Lefkowitz RJ, Caron MG: Adrenergic receptors. *J Biol Chem* 263:4993, 1988.
35. Levitski A: From epinephrine to cyclic AMP. *Science* 241:800, 1988.
36. Yang-Feng TL, Xue F, Zhong W, Cotecchia S, Frielle T, Caron MG, Lefkowitz RJ, Francke U: Chromosomal organization of adrenergic receptor genes. *Proc Natl Acad Sci USA* 87:1516, 1990.
37. Mahan LC, McKernan RM, Insel PA: Metabolism of alpha- and beta-adrenergic receptors in vitro and in vivo. *Ann Rev Pharmacol Toxicol* 27:215, 1987.
38. Benovic JL, Bouvier M, Caron MG, Lefkowitz RJ: Regulation of adenyl cyclase-coupled β-adrenergic receptors. *Annu Rev Cell Biol* 4:405, 1988.
39. Minneman KP: α_1-Adrenergic receptor subtypes, inositol phosphates, and sources of cell Ca^{2+}. *Pharmacol Rev* 40:87, 1988.
40. Todd RD, Khurana TS, Sajovic P, Stone KR, O'Malley KL: Cloning of ligand-specific cell lines via gene transfer: Identification of a D_2 dopamine receptor subtype. *Proc Natl Acad Sci USA* 86:10134, 1989.
41. Emorine LJ, Marullo S, Briend-Sutren M-M, Patey G, Tate K, Delavier-Klutchko C, Strosberg AD: Molecular characterization of the human β_3-adrenergic receptor. *Science* 245:1118, 1989.
42. Ahlquist RP: A study of adrenotropic receptors. *Am J Physiol* 153:586, 1948.
43. Hall A: The cellular functions of small GTP-binding proteins. *Science* 249:635, 1990.
44. Cryer PE: Adrenergic receptors in endocrine and metabolic diseases, in Insel PA (ed): *Adrenergic Receptors in Man*. New York, Marcel Dekker 1987, pp 285–301.
45. Ginsberg AM, Clutter WE, Shah SD, Cryer PE: Triiodothyronine induced thyrotoxicosis increases mononuclear leukocyte β-adrenergic receptor density in man. *J Clin Invest* 67:1785, 1981.
46. Liggett SB, Shah SD, Cryer PE: Increased fat and skeletal muscle β-adrenergic receptors but unaltered metabolic and hemodynamic sensitivity to epinephrine in vivo in experimental human thyrotoxicosis. *J Clin Invest* 83:803, 1989.
47. Creese I, Silbey DR, Hamblin MW, Leff SE: The classification of dopamine receptors. *Annu Rev Neurosci* 6:43, 1983.
48. Ariens EJ, Simonis AM: Receptors and receptor mechanisms, in Saxena PR, Forsyth RP (eds): *Beta-Adrenoceptor Blocking Agents*. Amsterdam, North-Holland, 1976, pp 3–27.
49. Ariens EJ: The classification of beta-adrenoceptors. *Trends Pharmacol Sci* 2:170, 1981.
50. Hawthorn MH, Broadley KJ: Evidence from use of neuronal uptake inhibition that β_1-adrenoceptors, but not β_2-adrenoceptors, are innervated. *J Pharm Pharmacol* 34:664, 1982.
51. Wilffert B, Timmermans PBMWM, van Zwieten PA: Extrasynaptic location of alpha-2 and noninnervated beta-2 adrenoceptors in the vascular system of the pithed normotensive rat. *J Pharmacol Exp Ther* 221:762, 1982.
52. Zukowska-Grojec Z, Bayorh MA, Kopin IJ: Effect of desipramine on the effects of α-adrenoceptor inhibitors on pressor responses and release of norepinephrine into plasma of pithed rats. *J Cardiovasc Pharmacol* 5:297, 1983.
53. Weiner N: Norepinephrine, epinephrine and the sympathochromimetic amines, in Gilman AG, Goodman LS, Gilman A (eds): *The Pharmacological Basis of Therapeutics*. New York, Macmillan, 1980, pp 138–175.
54. Clutter WE, Bier DM, Shah SD, Cryer PE: Epinephrine plasma metabolic clearance rates and physiologic thresholds for metabolic and hemodynamic actions in man. *J Clin Invest* 66:94, 1980.
55. Galster AD, Clutter WE, Cryer PE, Collins JA, Bier DM: Epinephrine plasma thresholds for lipolytic effects in man. *J Clin Invest* 67:1729, 1981.
56. Rizza RA, Haymond MW, Cryer PE, Gerich JE: Differential effects of physiological concentrations of epinephrine on glucose production and disposal in man. *Am J Physiol* 237:E356, 1979.
57. Rizza RA, Haymond MW, Miles JW, Verdonk CH, Cryer PE, Gerich JE: Effect of alpha-adrenergic stimulation and its blockade on glucose turnover in man. *Am J Physiol* 238:E467, 1980.
58. Rizza RA, Cryer PE, Haymond MW, Gerich JE: Adrenergic mechanisms for the effect of epinephrine on glucose production and clearance in man. *J Clin Invest* 65:682, 1980.
59. Deibert DC, DeFronzo RA: Epinephrine-induced insulin resistance in man. *J Clin Invest* 65:717, 1980.
60. Rosen SG, Clutter WE, Shah SD, Miller JP, Bier DM, Cryer PE: Direct, α-adrenergic stimulation of hepatic glucose production in postabsorptive human subjects. *Am J Physiol* 245:E616, 1983.
61. Berk MA, Clutter WE, Skor DS, Shah S, Cryer P: Enhanced glycemic responsiveness to epinephrine in insulin-dependent diabetes mellitus is the result of inability to secrete insulin. *J Clin Invest* 75:1842, 1985.
62. Chiasson J-L, Shikama H, Chu DTW, Exton JH: Inhibitory effect of epinephrine on insulin-stimulated glucose uptake by rat skeletal muscle. *J Clin Invest* 68:706, 1981.
63. Miles JM, Nissen S, Gerich JE, Haymond MW: Effects of epinephrine infusion on leucine and alanine kinetics in man. *Am J Physiol* 247:E166, 1984.
64. Fain JN, Garcia-Sainz JA: Adrenergic regulation of adipocyte metabolism. *J Lipid Res* 24:945, 1983.
65. Bahnsen M, Burrin JM, Johnston DG, Pernet A, Walker M, Alberti KGMM: Mechanisms of catecholamine effects on ketogenesis. *Am J Physiol* 247:E173, 1984.
66. Brown MJ, Brown DC, Murphy MB: Hypokalemia from $beta_2$-receptor stimulation by circulating epinephrine. *N Engl J Med* 309:1414, 1983.
67. Staten MA, Matthews DE, Cryer PE, Bier DM: Physiologic increments in epinephrine stimulate metabolic rate in humans. *Am J Physiol* 253:E322, 1987.
68. Staten MA, Matthews DE, Cryer PE, Bier DM: Epinephrine's effect on metabolic rate is independent of changes in insulin or glucagon. *Am J Physiol* 257:E185–E192, 1989.
69. Clutter WE, Rizza RA, Gerich JE, Cryer PE: Regulation of glucose metabolism by sympathochromaffin catecholamines. *Diabetes Metab Rev* 4:1, 1988.
70. Gray DE, Lickley HLA, Vranic M: Physiologic effects of epinephrine on glucose turnover and plasma free fatty acid concentrations mediated independently by glucagon. *Diabetes* 29:600, 1980.
71. Morgan NG, Blackmore PF, Exton JH: Age-related changes in the control of hepatic cyclic AMP levels by α_1- and β_2-adrenergic receptors in male rats. *J Biol Chem* 258:5103, 1983.
72. Sacca L, Morrone G, Cicala M, Corso G, Ungaro B: Influence of epinephrine, norepinephrine and isoproterenol on glucose homeostasis in normal man. *J Clin Endocrinol Metab* 50:680, 1980.
73. Halter JB, Pflug AE, Tolas AG: Arterial-venous differences of plasma catecholamines in man. *Metabolism* 29:9, 1980.
74. Grimm M, Weidmann P, Keusch G, Meier A, Gluck Z: Norepinephrine clearance and pressor effect in normal and hypertensive man. *Klin Wochenschr* 58:1175, 1980.
75. Izzo J Jr: Cardiovascular hormonal effects of circulating norepinephrine. *Hypertension* 5:787, 1983.
76. Cryer PE: Catecholamines and metabolism. *Am J Physiol* 247:E1, 1984.
77. Hjemdahl P: Catecholamine measurements by high performance liquid chromatography. *Am J Physiol* 247:E13, 1984.
78. Wang M-T, Imai K, Yoshioka M, Tamura Z: Gas-liquid chromatographic and mass fragmentographic determination of

catecholamines in human plasma. *Clin Chim Acta* 63:13, 1975.
79. Wang M-T, Yoshioka M, Imai K, Tamura Z: Gas-liquid chromatographic and mass fragmentographic determination of 3-O-methylated catecholamines in human plasma. *Clin Chim Acta* 63:21, 1975.
80. Elshisak MA, Polinsky RJ, Ebert MH, Kopin IJ: Kinetics of homovanillic acid and determination of its production rate in humans. *J Neurochem* 38:380, 1982.
81. Best JC, Halter JB: Release and clearance rates of epinephrine in man: Importance of arterial measurements. *J Clin Endocrinol Metab* 55:263, 1982.
82. Esler M, Jennings G, Lambert G, Meredith I, Horne M, Eisenhofer G: Overflow of catecholamine neurotransmitters to the circulation: Source, fate and functions. *Physiol Rev* 70:963, 1990.
83. Linares OA, Jaquez JA, Zech LA, Smith MJ, Sanfield JA, Morrow LA, Rosen SG, Halter JB: Norepinephrine metabolism in humans: Kinetic analysis and model. *J Clin Invest* 80:1332, 1987.
84. Christensen NJ, Hilsted J, Hegedus L, Madsbad S: Effects of surgical stress and insulin on cardiovascular function and norepinephrine kinetics. *Am J Physiol* 247:E29, 1984.
85. Cryer PE: Diseases of the sympathochromaffin system, in Felig P, Baxter J, Broadus A, Frohman L (eds): *Endocrinology and Metabolism*, 2d ed. New York, McGraw-Hill, 1987, pp 651–692.
86. Goldstein DS, Horwitz D, Keiser HR, Polinsky RJ, Koprin IJ: Plasma l-[^{3}H]norepinephrine, d-[^{14}C]norepinephrine and d,l-[^{3}H]isoproterenol kinetics in essential hypertension. *J Clin Invest* 72:1748, 1983.
87. Cryer PE, Rizza RA, Haymond MW, Gerich JE: Epinephrine and norepinephrine are cleared through β-adrenergic, but not α-adrenergic, mechanisms in man. *Metabolism* 29:1114, 1980.
88. Ghione S, Palombo C, Pellegrini M, Fommei E, Pilo A, Donato L: The kinetics of plasma noradrenaline in normal and hypertensive subjects. *Clin Sci* 55:89S, 1978.
89. Hoeldtke RD, Cilmi KM, Reichard GA Jr, Boden G, Owen OE: Assessment of norepinephrine secretion and production. *J Lab Clin Med* 101:772, 1983.
90. Kopin IJ, Polinsky RJ, Oliver JA, Oddershede IR, Ebert MH: Urinary catecholamine metabolites distinguish different types of sympathetic neural dysfunction in patients with orthostatic hypotension. *J Clin Endocrinol Metab* 57:632, 1983.
91. Folkow B, DiBona GF, Hjemdahl P, Toren PH, Wallin BG: Measurements of plasma norepinephrine concentrations in human primary hypertension. *Hypertension* 5:399, 1983.
92. Goldstein DS, McCarty R, Polinsky RJ, Kopin IJ: Relationship between plasma norepinephrine and sympathetic neural activity. *Hypertension* 5:552, 1983.
93. Brown MJ, Jenner DA, Allison DJ, Dollery CT: Variations in individual organ release of noradrenaline measured by an improved radioenzymatic technique: Limitations of peripheral venous measurements in the assessment of sympathetic nervous activity. *Clin Sci* 61:585, 1981.
94. Planz G: Adrenaline and noradrenaline concentration in blood of suprarenal and renal vein of man with normal blood pressure and with essential hypertension. *Klin Wochenschr* 56:1109, 1978.
95. Cryer PE, Haymond MW, Santiago JV, Shah SD: Norepinephrine and epinephrine release and adrenergic mediation of smoking-associated hemodynamic and metabolic events. *N Engl J Med* 295:573, 1976.
96. Mancia G, Ferrari A, Gregorini L, Leonetti G, Parati G, Picotti GB, Ravazzani C, Zanchetti A: Plasma catecholamines do not invariably reflect sympathetically induced changes in blood pressure in man. *Clin Sci* 65:227, 1983.
97. Young JB, Rose RM, Landsberg L: Dissociation of sympathetic nervous system and adrenal medullary responses. *Am J Physiol* 247:E35, 1984.
98. Cryer PE: Isotope derivative measurements of plasma norepinephrine and epinephrine in man. *Diabetes* 25:1071, 1976.
99. Wallin GB: Peripheral sympathetic neural activity in conscious humans. *Annu Rev Physiol* 50:565, 1988.
100. Rea RF, Eckberg DL, Fritsch JM, Goldstein DS: Relation of plasma norepinephrine and sympathetic traffic during hypotension in humans. *Am J Physiol* 258:R982, 1990.
101. Cryer PE: Pheochromocytoma. *West J Med* (in press).
102. Manger WM, Gifford RW Jr: Hypertension secondary to pheochromocytoma. *Bull NY Acad Med* 58:139, 1982.
103. Sutton MGS, Sheps SG, Lie JT: Prevalence of clinically unsuspected pheochromocytoma: Review of a 50-year autopsy series. *Mayo Clin Proc* 56:354, 1981.
104. Steiner AL, Goodman AD, Powers SR: Study of a kindred with pheochromocytoma, medullary thyroid carcinoma, hyperparathyroidism and Cushing's disease: Multiple endocrine neoplasia, type 2. *Medicine (Baltimore)* 47:371, 1968.
105. Lips KJM, Veer JVDS, Struyvenberg A, Alleman A, Leo JR, Wittebol P, Minder WH, Kooiker CJ, et al: Bilateral occurrence of pheochromocytoma in patients with the multiple endocrine neoplasia syndrome type 2a (Sipple's syndrome). *Am J Med* 70:1051, 1981.
106. DeLellis RA, Wolfe HJ, Gagel RF, Feldman ZT, Miller HH, Gang DL, Reichlin S: Adrenal medullary hyperplasia. *Am J Physiol* 83:177, 1976.
107. Sobol H, Narod SA, Nakamura Y, Boneu A, Calmettes C, Chadenas D, Charpentier G, Chatal JF, et al: Screening for multiple endocrine neoplasia type 2a with DNA polymorphism analysis. *N Engl J Med* 321:996, 1989.
108. Yoshimasa T, Nakao K, Li S, Ikeda Y, Suda M, Sakamoto M, Imura H: Plasma methionine-enkephalin and leucine-enkephalin in normal subjects and patients with pheochromocytoma. *J Clin Endocrinol Metab* 57:706, 1983.
109. Berelowitz M, Szabo M, Barowsky HW, Arbel ER, Frohman LA: Somatostatin-like immunoactivity and biological activity is present in a human pheochromocytoma. *J Clin Endocrinol Metab* 56:134, 1983.
110. Weinstein RS, Ide LF: Immunoreactive calcitonin in pheochromocytomas. *Proc Soc Exp Biol Med* 165:215, 1980.
111. Spark RF, Connolly PB, Gluckin DS, White R, Sacks B, Landsberg L: ACTH secretion from a functioning pheochromocytoma. *N Engl J Med* 301:416, 1979.
112. Page LB, Raker JW, Beberich FR: Pheochromocytoma with predominant epinephrine secretion. *Am J Med* 47:648, 1969.
113. Aronoff SL, Passamani E, Borowsky BA, Weiss AN, Roberts R, Cryer PE: Norepinephrine and epinephrine secretion from a clinically epinephrine-secreting pheochromocytoma. *Am J Med* 69:321, 1980.
114. Bravo EL, Tarazi RC, Fouad FM, Textor SC, Gifford RW Jr, Vidt DG: Blood pressure regulation in pheochromocytoma. *Hypertension* 4(Suppl 2):193, 1982.
115. Turnbull DM, Johnston DG, Alberti KGMM, Hall R: Hormonal and metabolic studies in a patient with a pheochromocytoma. *J Clin Endocrinol Metab* 51:930, 1980.
116. Sjoerdsma A, Engelman K, Waldmann TA, Cooperman LH, Hammond WG: Pheochromocytoma: Current concepts of diagnosis and treatment. *Ann Intern Med* 65:1302, 1966.
117. Sheps SG, Jiang NS, Klee GG, van Heerden JA: Recent developments in the diagnosis and treatment of pheochromocytoma. *Mayo Clinic Proc* 65:88, 1990.
118. Duncan MW, Compton P, Lazarus L, Smythe GA: Measurement of norepinephrine and 3,4-dihydroxyphenylglycol in urine and plasma for the diagnosis of pheochromocytoma. *N Engl J Med* 319:136, 1988.
119. Engelman K, Portnoy B, Sjoerdsma A: Plasma catecholamine concentrations in patients with hypertension. *Circ Res* 26(Suppl 1):141, 1970.
120. Geffen LB, Rush RA, Louis WJ, Doyle AE: Plasma catecholamine and dopamine β-hydroxylase amounts in phaeochromocytoma. *Clin Sci* 44:421, 1973.

121. Bravo EL, Tarazi RC, Gifford RW Jr, Stewart BH: Circulating and urinary catecholamines in pheochromocytoma. *N Engl J Med* 301:682, 1979.
122. Feldman JM, Klatt C: Elevated platelet norepinephrine concentration in patients with pheochromocytomas. *Clin Chim Acta* 117:279, 1981.
123. Zweifler AJ, Julius S: Increased platelet catecholamine content in pheochromocytoma. *N Engl J Med* 306:890, 1982.
124. Bravo EL, Tarazi RC, Fouad FM, Vidt DG, Gifford GW Jr: Clonidine suppression test: A useful aid in the diagnosis of pheochromocytoma. *N Engl J Med* 305:623, 1981.
125. Taylor HC, Mayes D, Anton AH: Clonidine suppression test for pheochromocytoma: Examples of misleading results. *J Clin Endocrinol Metab* 63:238, 1986.
126. Hsiao RJ, Parmer RJ, Takiyyudin MA, O'Connor DT: Chromogranin A storage and secretion: Sensitivity and specificity for the diagnosis of pheochromocytoma. *Medicine (Baltimore)* 70:33, 1991.
127. Quint LE, Glazer GM, Francis IR, Shapiro B, Chenevert TL: Pheochromocytoma and paraganglioma: Comparison of MR imaging with CT and I-131 MIBG scintigraphy. *Radiology* 165:89, 1987.
128. Schmedtje JF Jr, Sax S, Pool JL, Goldfarb RA, Nelson EB: Localization of ectopic pheochromocytomas by magnetic resonance imaging. *Am J Med* 83:770, 1987.
129. Shapiro B, Copp JE, Sisson JC, Eyre PL, Wallis J, Bierwaltes WH: Iodine-131 metaiodobenzylguanidine for the locating of suspected pheochromocytomas: Experience in 400 cases. *J Nucl Med* 26:576, 1985.
130. Chatal JR, Charbonel B: Comparison of iodobenzylguanidine imaging with computed tomography in locating pheochromocytoma. *J Clin Endocrinol Metab* 61:769, 1985.
131. Mellicow MM: One hundred cases of pheochromocytoma (107 tumors) at the Columbia-Presbyterian Medical Center. *Cancer* 40:1907–1977.
132. Cubbeddu LX, Zarate NA, Rosales CB, Zshaeck DW: Prazosin and propranolol in preoperative management of pheochromocytoma. *Clin Pharmacol Ther* 32:156, 1982.
133. Glass AR, Ballou R: Pheochromocytoma, prazosin and hypotension. *Ann Intern Med* 97:455, 1982.
134. Nicholson JP Jr, Vaugh ED Jr, Pickering TG, Resnick LM, Artusio J, Kleinert HD, Lopez-Overjero JA, Laragh JH: Pheochromocytoma and prazosin. *Ann Intern Med* 99:477, 1983.
135. Plouin P-F, Menard J, Corvol P: Noradrenaline producing pheochromocytomas with absent pressor response to beta-blockade. *Br Heart J* 42:359, 1979.
136. Wark JD, Larkins RG: Pulmonary edema after propranolol therapy in two cases of phaeochromocytoma. *Br Med J* 1:1395, 1978.
137. Ram CVS, Meese R, Hill SC: Failure of α-methyltyrosine to prevent hypertensive crisis in pheochromocytoma. *Arch Intern Med* 145:2114, 1985.
138. Feldman JM, Blalock JA, Fagraeus L, Miller JN, Farrell RE, Wells SA Jr: Alterations in plasma norepinephrine concentration during surgical resection of pheochromocytoma. *Ann Surg* 188:758, 1978.
139. Leak D, Carroll JJ, Robinson DC, Ashworth EJ: Management of pheochromocytoma during pregnancy. *Can Med Assoc J* 116:371, 1977.
140. Sheps SG, Jiang N-S, Klee GG, van Heerden JA: Recent developments in the diagnosis and treatment of pheochromocytoma. *Mayo Clin Proc* 65:88, 1990.
141. Hengstmann JH, Dengler HJ: Evidence for extratumoral storage of catecholamines in pheochromocytoma patients. *Acta Endocrinol (Copenh)* 87:589, 1978.
142. Hammerman M, Levitt R, Clutter WE, Meltzer V, Bobzein B: Persistent hypertension after resection of a pheochromocytoma. *Am J Med* 73:97, 1982.
143. Castle CH: Iatrogenic renal hypertension: Two unusual complications of surgery for familial pheochromocytoma. *JAMA* 225:1085, 1973.
144. Jones NF, Walker G, Ruthven CRJ, Sandler M: α-Methyl-p-tyrosine in the management of phaeochromocytoma. *Lancet* ii:1105, 1968.
145. Feldman JM: Treatment of metastic pheochromocytoma with streptozotocin. *Arch Intern Med* 143:1799, 1983.
146. Averbuch SD, Steakley CS, Young RC, Gelman EP, Goldstein DS, Stull R, Keiser HR: Malignant pheochromocytoma: Effective treatment with a combination of cyclophosphamide, vincristine and decarbazine. *Ann Intern Med* 109:267, 1988.
147. Krempf M, Lumbroso J, Mornex R, Brendel AJ, Wemeau JL, Delisle MJ, Aubert B, Carpentier P, et al: Use of m-[^{131}I]iodobenzylguanidine in the treatment of malignant pheochromocytoma. *J Clin Endocrinol Metab* 72:455, 1991.
148. Seeger RC, Siegel SE, Sidell N: Neuroblastoma: Clinical perspectives, monoclonal antibodies and retinoic acid. *Ann Intern Med* 97:873, 1982.
149. Boomsma F, Ausema L, Hakvoort-Cammel FGA, Oosterom R, Man in't Veld AJ, Krenning EP, Hahlen K, Schalekamp MADH: Combined measurements of plasma aromatic L-amino acid decarboxylase and DOPA as tumor markers in diagnosis and follow-up of neuroblastoma. *Eur J Cancer Clin Oncol* 25:1045, 1989.
150. Cryer PE, Santiago JV, Shah SD: Measurement of norepinephrine and epinephrine in small volumes of human plasma by a single isotope derivative method: Response to the upright posture. *J Clin Endocrinol Metab* 39:1025, 1974.
151. Thomas JE, Schirger A, Fealey RD, Sheps SG: Orthostatic hypotension. *Mayo Clin Proc* 56:117, 1981.
152. Lipsitz LA: Orthostatic hypotension in the elderly. *N Engl J Med* 321:952, 1989.
153. Cryer PE: Silverberg AB, Santiago JV, Shah SD: Plasma catecholamines in diabetes: The syndromes of hypoadrenergic and hyperadrenergic postural hypotension. *Am J Med* 64:407, 1978.
154. Tohmeh JF, Shah SD, Cryer PE: The pathogenesis of hyperadrenergic postural hypotension in patient with diabetes. *Am J Med* 67:772, 1979.
155. Cryer PE, Weiss S: Reduced plasma norepinephrine response to standing in autonomic dysfunction. *Arch Neurol* 33:275, 1976.
156. Ziegler MG, Lake CR, Kopin IJ: The sympathetic nervous system defect in primary orthostatic hypotension. *N Engl J Med* 296:293, 1977.
157. Leveston SA, Shah SD, Cryer PE: Cholinergic stimulation of norepinephrine release in man: Evidence of a sympathetic postganglionic axonal lesion in diabetic adrenergic neuropathy. *J Clin Invest* 64:374, 1979.
158. Fouad FM, Tadena-Thoma L, Bravo EL, Tarazi RC: Idiopathic hypovolemia. *Ann Intern Med* 104:298, 1986.
159. Streeten DHP: Pathogenesis of hyperadrenergic orthostatic hypotension. *J Clin Invest* 86:1582, 1990.
160. Bannister R: Introduction and classification, in Bannister R (ed): *Autonomic Failure*. New York, Oxford University Press, 1983, p 1.
161. Cohen J, Low P, Fealey R, Sheps S, Jiang N-S: Somatic and autonomic function in progressive autonomic failure and multiple system atrophy. *Ann Neurol* 22:692, 1987.
162. Sever PS: Plasma noradrenaline in autonomic failure, in Bannister R (ed): *Autonomic Failure*. New York, Oxford University Press, 1983, p 155.
163. Goldstein DS, Polinsky RJ, Garty M, Robertson D, Brown RT, Biaggioni I, Stull R, Kopin IJ: Patterns of plasma levels of catechols in neurogenic orthostatic hypotension. *Ann Neurol* 26:558, 1989.
164. Gemmill JD, Venables GS, Ewing DJ: Noradrenaline response to edrophonium in primary autonomic failure: Distinction between central and peripheral damage. *Lancet* i:1018, 1988.
165. Kopin IJ, Polinsky RJ, Oliver JA, Oddershede IR, Ebert MH: Urinary catecholamine metabolites distinguish different

types of sympathetic neuronal dysfunction in patients with orthostatic hypotension. *J Clin Endocrinol Metab* 57:632, 1983.

166. Bannister R: Clinical features of progressive autonomic failure, in Bannister R (ed): *Autonomic Failure*. New York, Oxford University Press, 1983, p 67.
167. Davies B: Adrenergic receptors in autonomic failure, in Bannister R (ed): *Autonomic Failure*. New York, Oxford University Press, 1983, p 174.
168. Robertson D, Goldberg MR, Onrot J, Hollister AS, Wiley R, Thompson JG Jr, Robertson RM: Isolated failure of autonomic noradrenergic neurotransmission. *N Engl J Med* 314:1494, 1986.
169. Biaggioni I, Robertson D: Endogenous restoration of noradrenaline by precursor therapy in dopamine-beta-hydroxylase deficiency. *Lancet* 2:1170, 1987.
170. Man in't Veld AJ, Boomsma F, van den Meiracker AH, Schalekamp MADH: Effect of an unnatural noradrenaline precursor on sympathetic control and orthostatic hypotension in dopamine-beta-hydroxylase deficiency. *Lancet* ii:1172, 1987.
171. Nanda RN, Boyle FC, Gillespie JS, Johnson RH, Keogh HJ: Idiopathic orthostatic hypotension from failure of noradrenaline release in a patient with vasomotor innervation. *J Neurol Neurosurg Psychiatry* 40:11, 1977.
172. Hart RG, Kanter MC: Acute autonomic neuropathy. *Arch Intern Med* 150:2373, 1990.
173. Bannister R: Treatment of progressive autonomic failure, in Bannister R (ed): *Autonomic Failure*. New York, Oxford University Press, 1983, p 316.
174. Chobanian AV, Volicer L, Tifft CCP, Gavras H, Liang C-S, Faxon D: Mineralocorticoid-induced hypertension in patients with orthostatic hypotension. *N Engl J Med* 301:68, 1979.
175. Kauffmann H, Brannan T, Krakoff L, Yahr MD, Mandelli J: Treatment of orthostatic hypotension due to autonomic failure with a peripheral alpha-adrenergic agonist (midodrine). *Neurology* 38:951, 1988.
176. Chobanian AV, Tifft CP, Faxon DP, Creager MA, Sackel H: Treatment of chronic orthostatic hypotension with ergotamine. *Circulation* 67:602, 1983.
177. Robertson D, Goldberg MR, Tung C-S, Hollister AS, Robertson RM: Use of $alpha_2$ adrenoreceptor agonists and antagonists in the functional assessment of the sympathetic nervous system. *J Clin Invest* 78:576, 1986.
178. Hoeldtke RD, Dworkin GE, Gaspar SR, Israel BC, Boden G: Effect of the somatostatin analogue SMS-201-995 on the adrenergic response to glucose ingestion in patients with postprandial hypotension. *Am J Med* 86:673, 1989.
179. Kristinsson A: Programmed atrial pacing for orthostatic hypotension. *Acta Med Scand* 214:79, 1983.
180. Polinsky RJ, Samaras GM, Kopin IJ: Sympathetic neural prothesis for managing orthostatic hypotension. *Lancet* i:901, 1983.
181. Khurama RK, Nelson E, Azzarelli B, Garcia JH: Shy-Drager syndrome: Diagnosis and treatment of cholinergic dysfunction. *Neurology* 30:805, 1980.
182. Cryer PE: Glucose counterregulation in man. *Diabetes* 30:261, 1981.
183. Cryer PE, Gerich JE: Hypoglycemia in insulin dependent diabetes mellitus, in Rifkin H, Porte D (eds): *Ellenberg and Rifkin's Diabetes Mellitus, Theory and Practice*, 4th ed. New York, Elsevier, 1990, p 526.
184. Cryer PE: Glucose homeostasis and hypoglycemia, in Wilson JD, Foster DW (eds): *Williams Textbook of Endocrinology*, 8th ed. Philadelphia, Saunders 1992, p 1223.
185. Hilsted J, Madsbad S, Krarup T, Sestoft L, Christensen NJ, Tronier B, Galbo H: Hormonal, metabolic and cardiovascular responses to hypoglycemia in diabetic autonomic neuropathy. *Diabetes* 30:626, 1981.
186. Heller SR, Cryer PE: Hypoinsulinemia is not critical to glucose recovery from hypoglycemia in humans. *Am J Physiol* 261:E41, 1991.
187. DeFeo P, Periello G, Torlone E, Ventura MM, Santeusanio F, Brunetti P, Gerich JE, Bolli GB: Demonstration of a role for growth hormone in glucose counterregulation. *Am J Physiol* 256:E835, 1989.
188. DeFeo P, Periello G, Torlone E, Venture MM, Fanelli C, Santeusanio F, Brunetti P, Gerich JE, Bolli GB: Contribution of cortisol to glucose counterregulation in humans. *Am J Physiol* 257:E35, 1989.
189. Boyle PJ, Cryer PE: Growth hormone, cortisol, or both are involved in defense against, but are not critical to recovery from, prolonged hypoglycemia in humans. *Am J Physiol* 260:E395–E402, 1991.
190. Bolli G, DeFeo P, Perriello G, DeCosmo S, Ventura M, Campbell P, Brunetti P, Gerich J: Role of hepatic autoregulation in defense against hypoglycemia in humans. *J Clin Invest* 75:1623, 1985.
191. Hansen I, Firth R, Haymond M, Cryer P, Rizza R: The role of autoregulation of hepatic glucose production in man. *Diabetes* 35:186, 1986.
192. Gerich J, Langlois M, Noacco C, Karam J, Forsham P: Lack of glucagon response to hypoglycemia in diabetes: Evidence for an intrinsic pancreatic alpha-cell defect. *Science* 182:171, 1973.
193. Popp DA, Shah SD, Cryer PE: The role of epinephrine-mediated β-adrenergic mechanisms in hypoglycemic glucose counterregulation and posthypoglycemic hyperglycemia in insulin dependent diabetes mellitus. *J Clin Invest* 69:315, 1982.
194. White NH, Gingerich R, Levandoski L, Cryer P, Santiago J: Plasma pancreatic polypeptide response to insulin induced hypoglycemia as a marker for defective glucose counterregulation in insulin-dependent diabetes mellitus. *Diabetes* 34:870, 1985.
195. White NH, Skor DA, Cryer PE, Bier DM, Levandoski L, Santiago JV: Identification of type 1 diabetic patients at increased risk for hypoglycemia during intensive therapy. *N Engl J Med* 308:485, 1983.
196. Bolli GB, DeFeo P, DeCosmo S, Periello G, Ventura MM, Massi-Bendetti M, Santeusanio F, Gerich J, Brunetti P: A reliable and reproducible test for adequate glucose counterregulation in type 1 diabetes mellitus. *Diabetes* 33:732, 1984.
197. Cryer PE, Binder C, Bolli GB, Cherrington AD, Gale EAM, Gerich JE, Sherwin RS: Hypoglycemia in insulin dependent diabetes mellitus. *Diabetes* 33:1193, 1989.
198. Heller SR, Herbert M, Macdonald IA, Tattersall RB: Influence of sympathetic nervous system on hypoglycaemic warning symptoms. *Lancet* ii:359, 1987.
199. Hepburn DA, Patrick AW, Eadington DW, Ewing DJ, Frier BM: Unawareness of hypoglycemia in insulin treated diabetes patients: Prevalence and relation to autonomic neuropathy. *Diabetic Med* 7:711, 1990.
200. Amiel SA, Sherwin RS, Simonson DC, Tamborlane WV: Effect of intensive insulin therapy on glycemic thresholds for counterregulatory hormone release. *Diabetes* 37:901, 1988.
201. Diabetes Control and Complications Trial: Results of feasibility study. *Diabetes Care* 10:1, 1987.
202. Ryder REJ, Owens DR, Hayes TM, Ghatei MA, Bloom SR: Unawareness of hypoglycaemia and inadequate hypoglcaemic counterregulation: No causal relation with diabetic autonomic neuropathy. *Br Med J* 301:783, 1990.
203. Clarke WL, Gonder-Frederick LA, Richards FE, Cryer PE: Multifactorial origin of hypoglycemic symptom unawareness in insulin dependent diabetes mellitus. *Diabetes* 40:680, 1991.
204. Heller SR, Cryer PE: Reduced neuroendocrine and symptomatic responses to subsequent hypoglycemia after one episode of hypoglycemia in normal humans. *Diabetes* 40:223, 1991.
205. Hirsch IB, Boyle PJ, Craft S, Cryer PE: β-adrenergic blockade shifts glycemic thresholds for symptoms to lower plasma glucose concentrations in insulin dependent diabetes mellitus. *Diabetes* 40:1177, 1991.

206. Stenström G, Sjöström L, Smith U: Diabetes mellitus in pheochromocytoma. *Acta Endocrinol (Copenh)* 106:511, 1984.
207. Hilsted J: Pathophysiology in diabetic autonomic neuropathy: Cardiovascular, hormonal and metabolic studies. *Diabetes* 31:730, 1982.
208. Cryer PE: Decreased sympathochromaffin activity in IDDM. *Diabetes* 38:405, 1989.
209. Alberti KGMM, Christensen NJ, Iversen J, Orskov H: Role of glucagon and other hormones in development of diabetic ketoacidosis. *Lancet* i:1307, 1975.
210. Schade DS, Eaton RP: Pathogenesis of diabetic ketoacidosis: A reappraisal. *Diabetes Care* 2:296, 1979.
211. Beylot M, Sautot G, Dechaud H, Cohen R, Riou JP, Serrusclat P, Mornex R: Lack of β-adrenergic role for catecholamines in the development of hyperglycemia and ketonemia following acute insulin withdrawal in type 1 diabetic patients. *Diabete Metab* 11:111, 1985.
212. Cryer PE: Morning hyperglycemia in insulin dependent diabetes mellitus: Insulin lack versus the dawn and Somogyi phenomena, in Mazzaferri EL (ed): *Advances in Endocrinology and Metabolism*. Chicago, Year Book, 1990, p 231.
213. Tordjman KM, Havlin CE, Levandoski L, White NH, Santiago JV, Cryer PE: Failure of nocturnal hypoglycemia to cause fasting hyperglycemia in patients with insulin dependent diabetes mellitus. *N Engl J Med* 317:1552, 1987.
214. Hirsch IB, Smith LB, Havlin CE, Shah SD, Clutter WE, Cryer PE: Failure of nocturnal hypoglycemia to cause daytime hyperglycemia in patients with insulin dependent diabetes mellitus. *Diabetes Care* 13:133, 1990.
215. Kemmer FW, Bisping R, Steingrüber HJ, Baar H, Hardtmann F, Schlaghecke R, Berger M: Psychological stress and metabolic control in patients with type I diabetes mellitus. *N Engl J Med* 314:1078, 1986.
216. Berretta-Piccoli C, Weidman P: Exaggerated pressor responses to norepinephrine in nonazotemic diabetes mellitus. *Am J Med* 71:829, 1981.
217. Daly PA, Landsberg L: Hyptertension in obesity and NIDDM. *Diabetes Care* 14:240, 1991.
218. Fusilli L, Lyons M, Patel B, Torres R, Hernandez F, Regan T: Ventricular vulnerability in diabetes and myocardial norepinephrine release. *Am J Med Sci* 298:207, 1989.
219. Jéquier E, Schutz Y: Energy expenditure in obesity and diabetes. *Diabetes Metab Rev* 4:583, 1988.
220. Roberts SB, Savage J, Coward WA, Chew B, Lucas A: Energy expenditure and intake in infants born to lean and overweight mothers. *N Engl J Med* 318:461, 1988.
221. Ravussin E, Lillioja S, Knowler WC, Christin L, Freymond D, Abbott WGH, Boyce V, Howard BV, Bogardus C: Reduced rate of energy expenditure as a risk factor for body-weight gain. *N Engl J Med* 318:467, 1988.
222. Peterson HR, Rothschild M, Weinberg CR, Fell RD, McLeish KR, Pfeifer MA: Body fat and the activity of the autonomic nervous system. *N Engl J Med* 318:1077, 1988.
223. Kuchel O, Cuche JL, Hamet P, Buu NT, Nowaczynski W, Boucher R, Genest J: Idiopathic edema: New pathogenic and therapeutic aspects. *Mod Med Can* 31:619, 1976.
224. Kuchel O, Cuche JL, Buu NT, Guthrie GP, Unger T, Nowaczynski W, Boucher R, Genest J: Catecholamine excretion in "idiopathic" edema: Decreased dopamine excretion, a pathogenic factor? *J Clin Endocrinol Metab* 44:639, 1977.
225. Sowers J, Catania R, Paris J, Tuck M: Effects of bromocriptine on renin, aldosterone and prolactin responses to posture and metoclopramide in idiopathic edema: Possible therapeutic approach. *J Clin Endocrinol Metab* 54:510, 1982.
226. Silverberg AB, Mennes PA, Cryer PE: Resistance to endogenous norepinephrine in Bartter's syndrome. *Am J Med* 64:231, 1978.
227. Gullner HG, Gill JR Jr, Bartter FC, Lake CR, Lakatua DJ: Correction of increased sympathoadrenal activity in Bartter's syndrome by inhibition of prostaglandin synthesis. *J Clin Endocrinol Metab* 50:857, 1980.
228. Levine MA, Ahn TG, Klupt SF, Kaufman KD, Smallwood PM, Bourne HR, Sullivan KA, Van Dop C: Genetic deficiency of the α subunit of the guanine nucleotide-binding protein G_s as the molecular basis for Albright hereditary osteodystrophy. *Proc Natl Acad Sci USA* 85:617, 1988.
229. Pattern JL, Johns DR, Valle D, Eil C, Gruppuso PA, Steele G, Smallwood PM, Levine MA: Mutation in the gene encoding the stimulatory G protein of adenylate cyclase in Albright's hereditary osteodystrophy. *N Engl J Med* 322:1412, 1990.
230. Kerr D, Hosking DJ: Pseudohypoparathyroidism: Clinical expression of PTH resistance. *Q J Med* 65:889, 1987.
231. Heinsimer JA, Davies AO, Downs RW, Levine MA, Spiegel AM, Drezner MK, DeLean A, Wreggett KA, et al: Impaired formation of β-adrenergic receptor-nucleotide regulatory protein complexes in pseudohypoparathyroidism. *J Clin Invest* 73:1335, 1984.
232. Carlson HE, Brickman AS: Blunted plasma cyclic adenosine monophosphate response to isoproterenol in pseudohypoparathyroidism. *J Clin Endocrinol Metab* 56:1323, 1983.
233. Brickman AS, Carlson HE, Levin SR: Responses to glucagon infusion in pseudohypoparathyroidism. *J Clin Endocrinol Metab* 63:1354, 1986.
234. Parker NC, Levtzow CB, Wright PW, Woodard LL, Chapman JF: Uniform chromatographic conditions for quantifying urinary catecholamines, metanephrines, vanillylmandelic acid, 5-hydroxyindoleacetic acid by liquid chromatography with electrochemical detection. *Clin Chem* 32:1473, 1986.
235. Moleman P, van Dijk J: Determination of urinary norepinephrine and epinephrine by liquid chromotography with fluorescence detection and pre-column devirilization. *Clin Chem* 36:732, 1990.
236. Johnson GA, Kupiecki RM, Baker CH: Single isotope derivative (radioenzymatic) methods in the measurement of catecholamines. *Metabolism* 29(Suppl 1):1106, 1980.
237. Shah SD, Clutter WE, Cryer PE: External and internal standards in the single isotope derivative (radioenzymatic) measurement of plasma norepinephrine and epinephrine in normal humans and persons with diabetes mellitus or chronic renal failure. *J Lab Clin Med* 106:624, 1985.
238. Hjemdahl P: Catecholamine measurements in plasma by high performance liquid chromatography with electrochemical detection. *Methods Enzymol* 142:521, 1987.
239. Bouloux P, Perrett D, Besser GM: Methodological considerations in the determination of plasma catecholamines by high performance liquid chromatography with electrochemical detection. *Ann Clin Biochem* 22:194, 1985.
240. Eisenhofer G, Goldstein DS, Stull R, Keiser HR, Sunderland T, Murphy DL, Kopin IJ: Simultaneous liquid-chromatographic determination of 3,4-dihydroxyphenylglycol, catecholamines and 3,4-dihydroxyphenylalanine in plasma, and their responses to inhibition of monoamine oxidase. *Clin Chem* 32:2030, 1986.
241. Weir TB, Smith CCT, Round JM, Betteridge DJ: Stability of catecholamines in whole blood, plasma and platelets. *Clin Chem* 32:882, 1986.
242. Christensen NJ: Sympathetic nervous activity and age. *Eur J Clin Invest* 12:91, 1982.
243. Romoff MS, Keusch G, Campese VM, Wang M-S, Friedler RM, Weidman P, Massry SG: Effect of sodium intake on plasma catecholamines in normal subjects. *J Clin Endocrinol Metab* 48:26, 1978.
244. Cryer PE, Sode J: Drug interference with measurement of adrenal hormones in urine: Common analgesics and tranquilizer-sedatives. *Ann Intern Med* 75:697, 1971.
245. Hilsted J, Jensen SB: A simple test for autonomic neuropathy in juvenile diabetics. *Acta Med Scand* 205:385, 1979.
246. Ewing DJ: Practical bedside investigation of diabetic autonomic failure, in Bannister R (ed): *Autonomic Failure*. New York, Oxford University Press, 1983, p 371.
247. Johnson RH: Clinical assessment of sympathetic function in man. *Methods Find Exp Clin Pharmacol* 6:187, 1984.-

CHAPTER 14

The Endocrinology of Hypertension

John D. Baxter
Dorothee Perloff
Willa Hsueh
Edward G. Biglieri

Hypertension is defined as an inappropriate elevation of arterial pressure and affects 20 percent of the adult population in the United States.[1,2] This disorder is a major risk factor for the development of atherosclerosis (with resultant strokes, myocardial infarctions, and other problems), renal failure, and left ventricular hypertrophy.[1–3] Table 14-1 provides current recommendations for defining hypertension by the level of the blood pressure.[1,2]

Blood pressure levels sufficient for the perfusion of vital organs are controlled by interactions of multiple, complex, delicately balanced, and counterbalanced systems which facilitate adjustments to physiologic and pathologic changes in activity, posture, and volume status. Hormones, acting as endocrine, autocrine, and/or paracrine factors (see Chap. 1) play key roles in this control. These hormones are produced in multiple tissues, including the kidneys, liver, adrenals, heart, vasculature, peripheral nerves, and brain. They display diverse mechanisms of actions and interactions. These actions are further modified by the major anions and cations, the nervous system, and other factors.

Hypertension has traditionally been separated into "essential" ("primary") and "secondary" forms. The majority of these patients have essential hypertension in which the underlying mechanisms for elevated blood pressure are understood incompletely (but are being rapidly unraveled). A minority of patients have secondary hypertension with an identifiable cause for the elevated blood pressure. The common types of secondary hypertension are listed in Table 14-2.

The etiology of essential hypertension is heterogeneous and involves multiple genetic and environmental factors. This heterogeneity is reflected by the fact that any one type of drug is fully effective only in 30 to 50 percent of patients at best[4,5] and by highly variable individual patient responses. Various factors influence renal mechanisms, the release of pressor and depressor substances, and transmembrane transport of ions such as Na^+ and Ca^{2+}. Much of the information about the mechanisms involved in essential hypertension is derived from observations of patients with both essential and secondary hypertension, experimentally produced hypertension in animals, and strains of animals that develop hypertension spontaneously. These studies have led to the realization that abnormalities in levels of and responses to hormones play a dominant role in essential hypertension. Thus, whereas a comprehensive discussion of all the clinical aspects of essential hypertension is beyond the scope of this chapter, a discussion of the overall involvement of hormones in hypertension is warranted.

The exact prevalence of secondary forms of hypertension is not known. Many researchers feel that the incidence of these forms is lower than originally was thought. This view is partly due to the fact that many reports originate from referral centers where the patient population is preselected.[6,7] For example, the incidence of renovascular hypertension has recently been estimated to be around 0.5 percent in the general hypertensive population.[8] This is possibly the most common known form of treatable secondary hypertension, and this estimate is lower than previous values in the 5 percent range.[8–11]

By contrast, the prevalence of secondary forms of hypertension may actually be greater than is currently thought. Current estimates are based on diagnostic criteria that direct the physician to specific remedies, such as revascularization procedures with renovascular hypertension and adrenalectomy with primary aldosteronism. These estimates do not exclude the possibility that many patients with milder forms of a given disorder are misdiagnosed as having essential hypertension. This point is clearly evident from analysis of a rare form of primary aldosteronism, glucocorticoid-remediable aldosteronism (see Primary Aldosteronism below). This disorder can

TABLE 14-1 Classification of Blood Pressure Levels*

	Pressure, mmHg			
	JNC V*		WHO†	
Classification†	Systolic	Diastolic	Systolic	Diastolic
Normal	<130	<85	<140	<90
High normal	130–139	85–89		
Borderline			140–160	90–95
Hypertension				
Mild (stage 1)	140–159	90–99	140–180	90–105
Moderate (stage 2)	160–179	100–109		
Moderate and severe			180	>105
Severe (stage 3)	180–209	110–119		
Very severe (stage 4)	≥210	≥120		

* Data from the Joint National Committee on Detection, Evaluation, and Treatment of High Blood Pressure (JNC V).[1] Classification is for adults age 18 years and older. When the pressures are in more than one category, the higher category should be used.

† Data from the World Health Organization (WHO) International Society of Hypertension Meeting.[2] The subgroup with isolated systolic hypertension defined by the WHO is not included.

now be diagnosed at a very early stage; this had led to the recognition that most patients with the disorder do not have hypokalemia. Hypokalemia has been used over the years as the initial screening procedure to detect primary aldosteronism. Thus, most patients with this form of primary aldosteronism were not diagnosed properly in the past. It is likely that most patients with other causes of primary aldosteronism have also been diagnosed as having essential hypertension or are diagnosed only at a late stage in the progression of the disorder. Similar arguments could be made for other secondary forms of hypertension.

It is important to identify patients with secondary hypertension from among the large population of hypertensive individuals. If the primary cause for the hypertension can be corrected, the progressive complications of hypertension and the need for lifelong drug therapy in these patients often can be reduced. There is also evidence that correcting secondary hypertension earlier in life is associated in the long term with better correction of the hypertension.[12] Thus, a careful search for a curable cause of hypertension is justified in all patients with significant and sustained hypertension.

Secondary forms of hypertension are commonly the subject of referral to an endocrinologist. The pathogenesis of these disorders and the clinical approach to them are discussed in this chapter. Here, we focus on mechanisms, diagnosis, and management of hypertension due to excessive levels of steroids, such as mineralocorticoids, and on activation of the renin-angiotensin-aldosterone system (RAS) in patients with renovascular hypertension. Hypertension due to pheochromocytoma is discussed in Chap. 13. Outside the scope of this chapter are certain forms of hypertension that are influenced by the endocrine system, including renal parenchymal disease, pregnancy, and disorders in which the pathogenesis is poorly understood. In addition, the central nervous system (CNS) plays a critical role in regulating the blood pressure; a discussion of the role of the CNS in hypertension is beyond the scope of this chapter.

The physician should also be aware that the hypertension in any patient may have more than one etiology. For example, primary aldosteronism and pheochromocytoma[13] and primary aldosteronism and renovascular hypertension[14] can occur in the same patient. Hypertension in pregnancy may be the warning for the subsequent development of another form of hypertension. Commonly, patients with currently understood secondary forms of hypertension also have a form of essential hypertension that blunts the response of definitive treatment and results in a need for long-term treatment. However, this should not discourage the physician from looking for secondary causes of the hypertension, because the removal of these causes will reduce the need for medications.

GENERAL FEATURES OF HYPERTENSION

Some general features of hypertension relevant to endocrine hypertension are reviewed briefly below.

Epidemiology

As many as 50 million Americans have elevated blood pressure.[1,2] The prevalence of hypertension increases with age, is greater for blacks than for whites, is greater in less educated than more educated people of both races, is greater for men than for women in young adulthood and early middle age, and is greater for women than men after that age.[1]

TABLE 14-2 Types of Hypertension

- Essential, primary or idiopathic (multiple causes)
- Systolic hypertension
  - Aortic valvular insufficiency
  - Arteriovenous fistula, patent ductus arteriosus
  - Hyperthyroidism
  - Paget disease of bone
  - Beriberi heart disease
  - Hyperkinetic circulation
  - Complete heart block
  - Rigidity of aorta and great vessels due to atherosclerosis
- Renal
  - Parenchymal disease: glomerulonephritis, pyelonephritis, interstitial nephritis, radiation nephritis; polycystic disease; connective tissue diseases; trauma
  - Obstructive uropathies; hydronephrosis
  - Renovascular; renal arterial stenosis; extrarenal-induced renal ischemia (e.g., vasculitis, coarctation of the aorta); vasculitis
  - Primary sodium retention
    - (Liddle's and Gordon's syndromes)
- Endocrine
  - Acromegaly
  - Adrenal cortical hormones
    - Apparent mineralocorticoid excess
    - Congenital adrenal hyperplasia
    - Cushing's syndrome
    - Deoxycorticosterone-producing tumors
    - Glucocorticoid resistance
    - Primary aldosteronism
  - Catecholamine-producing tumors
    - Glioma
    - Neurofibroma
    - Pheochromocytoma
  - Hyperparathyroidism
  - Hyperthyroidism
  - Hypothyroidism
  - Renin-producing tumors
- Exogenous
  - Alcohol abuse
  - Cyclosporine
  - Erythropoietin therapy
  - Estrogen/oral contraceptives
  - Excessive salt intake
  - Glucocorticoids
  - Mineralocorticoids: licorice, carbenoxolone
  - Sympathomimetics
  - Tyramine-containing foods and monoamine oxidase inhibitors
  - Thyroid hormone
- Coarctation of the aorta
- Hypertensive diseases of pregnancy
- Neurogenic
  - Acute lead poisoning
  - Acute porphyria
  - Familial dysautonomia
  - Increased intracranial pressure
    - Respiratory acidosis (CO_2 retention): lung or CNS disease (polio)
    - Encephalitis
    - Brain tumor
  - Psychogenic
  - Spinal cord damage
- Miscellaneous
  - Polycythemia
  - Burns (extensive)

Hypertension is a major risk factor for premature death and morbidity from cardiovascular disease and renal failure.[1–3,15–19] Cardiovascular morbidity and mortality increase with higher levels of the systolic and/or diastolic blood pressure, even at levels not considered hypertensive (Fig. 14-1).[1–3,15,17,20,21] For example, men with initial blood pressures of 152/95 and 162/85 mmHg had nearly twice and three times, respectively, the mortality rate within the first 10 years of follow-up of those with a blood pressure below 132/85 mmHg at entry.[22] The age-adjusted average annual incidence of coronary artery disease events can be three times as great in women with blood pressures >160/94 mmHg than in those with pressures <140/90 mmHg.[23] Although there is no dividing line between normotensive and hypertensive, it is estimated that optimal blood pressure with respect to cardiovascular risk is <120 mmHg systolic and <80 mmHg diastolic.[1] Mild hypertension (stage 1) is the most common form of hypertension and because of this is responsible for most of the excess morbidity, disability, and mortality attributed to hypertension.[1] Other risk factors, cigarette smoking, hyperlipidemia, glucose intolerance, and male sex amplify the risk.[1,17]

Treatment of hypertension can have a significant influence on the clinical outcome. The most impressive data are associated with malignant or accelerated hypertension, in which the reduction of mortality by drug therapy is marked.[1,24,25] Similarly, the data are impressive in terms of preventing the development of stroke.[1,16,25] Protection for coronary events and regression of left ventricular hypertrophy have also been demonstrated.[1–3,17,18] Since the prevalence of heart attacks is greater than that of strokes, the absolute reduction in coronary events due to treatment of hypertension is about half that for strokes.[3] It was recently concluded that a reduction by as little as 5 to 6 mmHg in diastolic blood pressure and of 10 mmHg in systolic pressure can reduce stroke risk by about a third and the risk for coronary events by about a sixth.[2,3] It has also been suggested that the benefits of hypertensive therapy have probably been underestimated in most of the randomized trials because of crossover of patients from placebo to active treatment, preferential inclusion of low-risk patients in trials, and the short-term duration.[2] Therapy has also been shown to slow the progression of loss of renal function significantly.[19,26]

FIGURE 14-1 Annual incidence of cardiovascular disease among the Framingham group over an 18-year follow-up based on systolic blood pressure at the onset of the study. The upper and lower curves are for men and women, respectively. *(From Kaplan,[20] as drawn from data of Kannel and Sorlie.[21])*

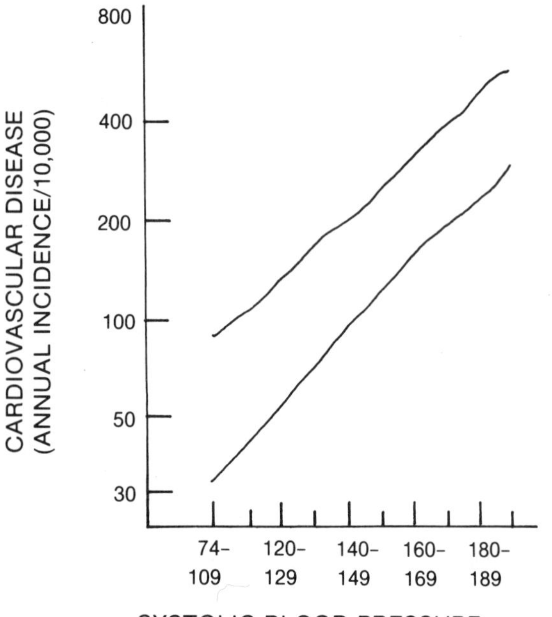

Genetic and Environmental Influences

The development of essential hypertension depends on the interaction of both genetic and environmental influences. The familial correlations for blood pressure range from 0.14 to 0.34 between parents and offspring and adult siblings to 0.75 with identical twins, and a positive family history is a good predictor of the development of hypertension.[19,27] The inherited nature of the disorder is also reflected by the differences in its prevalence in men and women and in blacks and whites, as discussed above.[1] Relatives of hypertensives have significantly higher mean blood pressure levels at all ages than do those of normotensives.[19,27] The distribution of blood pressure in the general population is unimodal rather than bimodal, suggesting that the etiology of the elevated blood pressure is polygenic or multifactorial.[19]

Known biochemical markers of hypertension relate to hormones or hormone-related systems. Prominent among these are abnormal ion fluxes in red blood cells, with the best correlations having been established between certain subgroups of hypertensives and the Na^+-Li^+ countertransport and possibly others (see the sections on sodium and ion transport).[27] Second, there is a correlation between an inherited tendency toward high urinary kallikrein excretion and a decreased likelihood of developing hypertension.[28] This correlation is one of the strongest major genetic factors identified as being associated with essential hypertension, although it is not known whether this phenomenon reflects a primary or a secondary event.[28] Genetic influences on the renin-angiotensin-aldosterone system are discussed later in this chapter. The restriction fragment length polymorphism (RFLP) in the angiotensinogen gene is the only genetic correlation that has been linked to human hypertension.[29] In animals, several genes have been linked to elevated blood pressure.[30–33] Other factors associated with increased blood pressure include obesity, increased sodium chloride intake, decreased potassium and magnesium intake, psychosocial stress, and alcohol consumption.[1,2,17,34] The development of hypertension in genetically predisposed individuals is accelerated when they are exposed to other influences that elevate the blood pressure.

Regulation of Blood Pressure

Mean arterial pressure is a function of cardiac output, systemic blood flow, and resistance to flow in the perfused organs.[35–37] These functions are regulated by hormones, neurotransmitters, and local factors and are affected by structural and functional abnormalities in the heart and vasculature that occur with chronic hypertension. Derangements in any or several of these functions can lead to hypertension, although in the long term, the increased vascular resistance is primarily responsible for the elevated blood pressure in most patients with essential and secondary hypertension. The hemodynamic derangements in hypertension vary with the etiology, duration, and severity of the disorder. In general, in patients with borderline hypertension,[35–41] cardiac output, stroke volume, and heart rate are relatively high and total peripheral resistance is normal. However, peripheral resistance is inappropriate for the elevated level of cardiac output and is abnormal during exercise. The plasma volume is typically normal or slightly decreased with attenuation of the microcirculation. Cardiac and renal function are normal, but myocardial contractility is increased and arterial compliance, coronary reserve, and renal blood flow are decreased. With exercise, cardiac output decreases and stroke volume does not increase sufficiently, while cardiac index and heart rate are elevated.

Patients with established or long-standing hypertension[35–42] and older hypertensives characteristically have an increase in total peripheral resistance that is attributable both to structural changes in the resistance vessels and to the influence of vasoactive mediators. Cardiac output and cardiac index are normal or decreased, and myocardial contractility is normal to increased. However, early left ventricular filling is delayed, left ventricular compliance is decreased, and left ventricular mass is increased. Renal blood flow is normal to decreased.

Complications of Hypertension

Hypertension is a chronic disease which normally evolves over the course of 20 to 30 years. Most patients remain asymptomatic until target organ damage is well advanced. The major complications of hypertension result from its acceleration of atherosclerosis in large elastic arteries and medium-sized muscular arteries such as the carotid, coronary, cerebral, mesenteric, aortoiliac, and renal arteries.[15,18,43–45] This is associated with early alterations in endothelial cell function and is followed by changes in vascular smooth muscle cell remodeling processes. Atherosclerosis accelerated by hypertension in turn leads to the development of thrombotic brain infarction; occlusive coronary artery disease; thromboembolic occlusive disease in the aortoiliac, mesenteric, and peripheral arteries; and aneurysm formation. Atherosclerosis also causes stiffening, decreased elasticity, and tortuosity in medium size and large arteries. This leads to altered pressure and flow relationship and further raises systolic pressure. The incidence of these events is compounded by the association of additional risk factors for atherosclerosis such as advancing age, male sex, cigarette smoking, hyperlipidemia, and glucose intolerance.[1,17,34]

Changes in the heart are due both to atherosclerosis and to left ventricular hypertrophy.[1–3,18] The left ventricle hypertrophies by increasing wall thickness. This maintains normal wall tension, compensates for the increased afterload, and maintains normal systolic cardiac performance. However, even mild left ventricular enlargement impairs diastolic function.[42] Left ventricular hypertrophy is an independent atherosclerotic risk factor and is a predictor of a poor prognosis among untreated patients with hypertension.[15,18] Ultimately, left ventricular systolic function can become impaired sufficiently to lead to heart failure. In the absence of coronary artery disease, this complication has become rare since the advent of antihypertensive medication, but it was previously a major cause of death.

In chronic hypertension, structural alterations occur in the microvascular circulation.[1,41,46,47] These alterations consist of increased thickness of the resistance arterioles as a result of hypertrophy and hyperplasia of smooth muscle cells and osmotic trapping of water. These changes reduce the size of the arterial lumen and increase the resistance to flow. There is also a reduction in the number of arterioles. Hypertension also accelerates the rate of endothelial cell turnover. These changes may play a role in the increased lipid transport and accumulation in the vessels of hypertensive patients.

In the cerebral circulation, chronic hypertension accelerates the development of atherosclerosis and aneurysm formation in the larger arteries and of specific degenerative changes in the small arteries.[16–18,25,45] These abnormalities can lead to ischemic infarcts of the brain, transient ischemic attacks, intracerebral hemmorhage, and dementia. Retinal changes reflect similar processes and eventual cerebral edema manifested as papilledema. In hypertensive encephalopathy, the extreme and rapid rise of blood pressure exceeds the ability of the cerebral vasculature to adapt (autoregulate), and there is segmental overdistension alternating with areas of vasoconstriction of cerebral arterioles. This can lead to cerebral edema, hemorrhage, and herniation unless the blood pressure is reduced rapidly.

There are progressive changes in the kidneys during the course of hypertension. Renal blood flow is reduced early in many patients, with preservation of the glomerular filtration rate, resulting in an increased filtration fraction.[48–50] A hallmark of the disorder is afferent arteriolar narrowing.[51] There can also be impressive heterogeneity in this response.[51] Nephrosclerosis is common in the kidneys of hypertensives.[48] As described in the section on renovascular hypertension, atherosclerosis in the larger arteries can also contribute to renal damage, leading to renal failure.[52,53] There can be microalbuminuria.[54] As described in the section on the renin-angiotensin system, plasma prorenin levels can be increased. An increase in serum uric acid levels reflects increased intrarenal vascular resistance and decreased glomerular filtration.[55] In the era before effective drug therapy was available, about 40 percent of hypertensives developed proteinuria and about 20 percent developed nitrogen retention.[56] Renal failure can be progressive in a poorly treated patient. An elevated serum creatinine remains a very potent independent risk factor for mortality.[57] It can develop rapidly with malignant hypertension and exacerbate the condition. Renal failure was the cause of death in up to 60 percent of patients before effective drug therapy was available,[24] and among blacks hypertension is still a major cause of renal failure. Overall, as many as 20 percent of chronic dialysis patients may have hypertension as the primary cause of their renal failure.[19]

HORMONAL MODIFIERS OF BLOOD PRESSURE

Many hormone-regulated processes affect blood pressure. Abnormalities in the release of and/or responsiveness to hormones are important in essential and secondary hypertension. In the latter, the abnormalities are typically more obvious, where systems such as the renin-angiotensin-aldosterone axis and catecholamines are involved. Other interrelations of hormonal and effector systems and hypertension, such as with insulin and obesity and Ca^{2+} and Na^{+} ion transporters, have been studied intensively but are inadequately understood. The role of some systems, such as those involving the endothelins and endothelial-derived releasing factors, are just beginning to be understood. There are poorly characterized factors such as the putative hypertensinogenic factor from the parathyroid gland. A number of these factors are discussed below in relation to essential and secondary forms of hypertension and their effects on blood pressure.

The Renin-Angiotensin System

The renin-angiotensin system (Figs. 14-2 and 14-3) is important in adaptive blood pressure responses and is involved in essential and secondary forms of hypertension. The effector substance of this system is angiotensin II, an octapeptide. A glycoprotein enzyme, renin, acts on angiotensinogen, an α_2-globulin substrate made in the liver, to form the decapeptide angiotensin I, the precursor to angiotensin II. The two carboxyl-terminal amino acids of angiotensin I are then cleaved in vascular beds by converting enzyme to form angiotensin II. Proteases in the circulation inactivate angiotensin II. Its activity is mediated by two angiotensin receptor subtypes: AT_1 and AT_2.

Components of the Renin-Angiotensin System

Renin and Prorenin

Renin occurs in two major forms at low concentrations in blood.[58–63] The active form of this aspartyl protease[58–61] has a molecular weight of about 40,000.[63] Prorenin, the precursor of renin, has a small amount of renin activity and a molecular weight of 47,000 and can be acid- or protease-activated. Prorenin constitutes most of the renin proteins in the normal circulation.[62,64–66]

A single human renin gene[67–69] located on chromosome 1[70] encodes for the 406 amino acids of preprorenin.[71] A 20-amino acid signal peptide is cleaved from preprorenin as it enters the rough endoplasmic reticulum to form prorenin.[72] Prorenin is then glycosylated and transported to the Golgi.[72] Renin in the circulation is variably glycosylated and exists as four to five isoenzymes with differing isoelectric points.[63] At the trans-Golgi, about half the prorenin is constitutively secreted without proteolytic processing and the other half is sorted to secretory granules, where prorenin is processed to renin by cleavage of the 46-amino acid prosegment.[72] Less than 5 percent of the prorenin is sorted to lysosomes, where it is metabolized.[73] Cathepsin B in juxtaglomerular cell granules probably cleaves human prorenin to renin.[72,74] Constitutive secretion of prorenin is nonregulated and operates continuously, while release of renin stored in secretory granules is regulated, for example, by cAMP.[72,75,76]

Renal and Extrarenal Sources of Renin Circulating active renin arises almost exclusively from the kidney, whereas most plasma prorenin comes from extrarenal sources. After nephrectomy, plasma renin activity (PRA) and protein and angiotensin II concentrations drop to levels about6 percent of normal.[65] The prorenin levels are decreased by only around 35 to 55 percent, depending on the assay.[65,77] These data also indicate that plasma angiotensin II

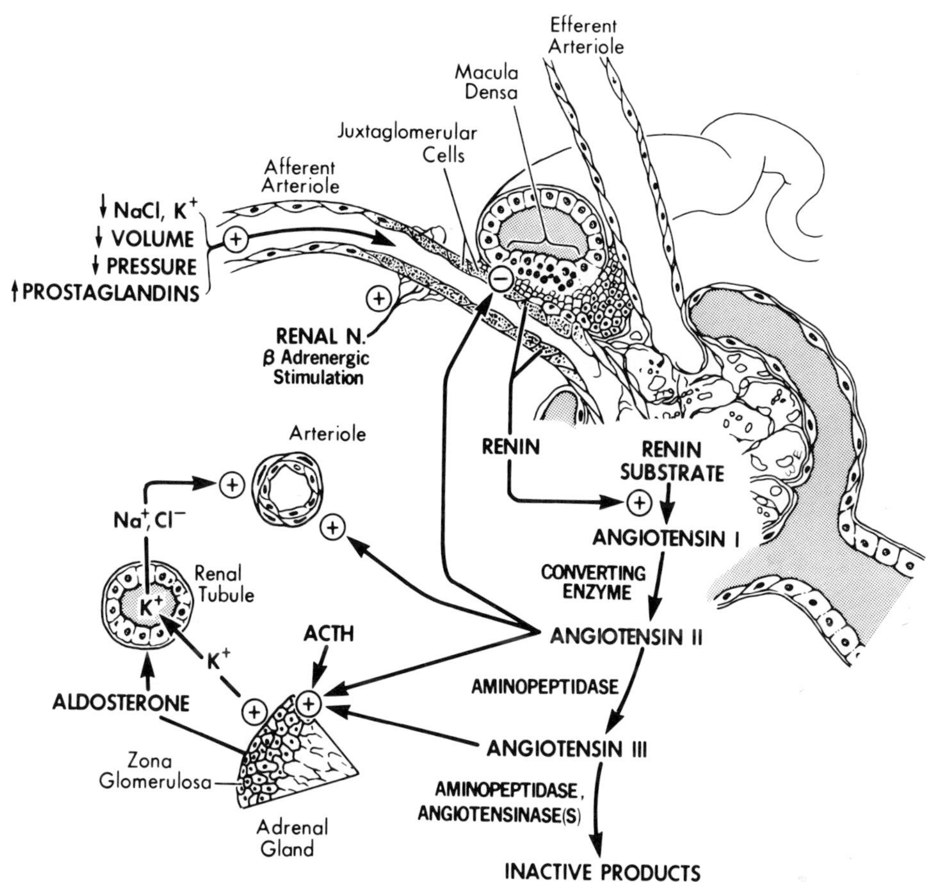

FIGURE 14-2 The renin-angiotensin system. Plus and minus signs indicate stimulation and inhibition, respectively. Only the major influences on the system are shown.

levels are mostly dependent on renin of renal origin, although there can be a small contribution by extrarenally produced renin and/or prorenin. Evidence for extrarenal production of prorenin and renin is supported by other studies in humans and animals that have demonstrated prorenin, renin, and/or renin mRNA in pituitary, brain, vascular endothelial and smooth muscle tissue, adrenal gland, chorion, decidua, pituitary, testes, ovary, and other tissues.[77–86a]

The finding that most extrarenal prorenin is not processed to active renin has led to speculation that prorenin may be active locally (Figs. 14-4 and 14-5). Prorenin has a small amount of renin activity and might also be activated locally through means that do not remove its prosegment.[72,87,88] Prorenin could also be activated locally by removal of its prosegment in the tissue; this probably occurs in the adrenal.[86] Prorenin could also have activity in addition to its angiotensinogen-cleaving function.[87]

In animals, injected renin can be taken up by the vasculature, and levels of vascular renin generally parallel those in the plasma.[84] Infused prorenin in monkeys is mostly taken up by the kidneys and liver, where it is probably degraded; very little active renin enters the circulation.[89] A small amount of this prorenin may be taken up by other tissues; this uptake could account for angiotensin I–generating activity in the extremities.[89] As shown in Fig. 14-4[86a,90], isoproterenol infusion increases renin release from the extremities. The fact that this release is increased in patients with renovascular hypertension and is decreased in patients with primary aldosteronism suggests that the renin is of renal origin.[82] Elements of the expressions of the renin-angiotensin system are in the vasculature, as shown in Fig. 14-5.[90]

Nonrenin Reninlike Enzymes Several nonrenin proteolytic enzymes can generate angiotensin I or angiotensin II from renin substrate.[83,91,92] For example, tonin can act on angiotensinogen, tetradecapeptide renin substrate, and angiotensin I to form angiotensin II.[93] Tonin does not modify blood pressure when injected into rats but has a pressor effect in nephrectomized animals. Cathepsins other than cathepsin B can generate an-

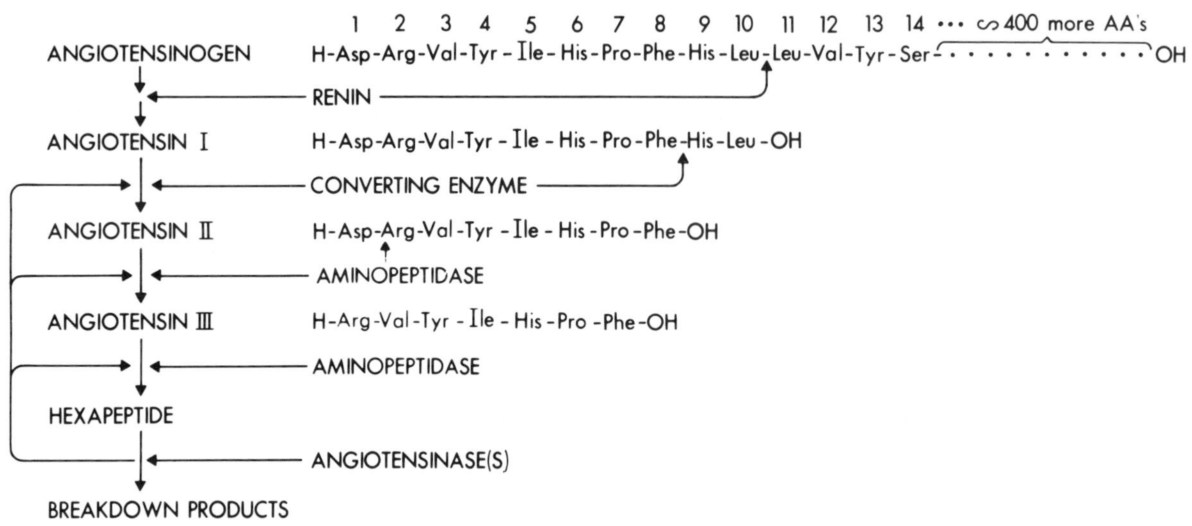

FIGURE 14-3 Formation and metabolism of angiotensins. *(Modified from Boucher et al.[57a])*

giotensins I and II and are found in several tissues.[94,95] However, their angiotensin I or II–generating activity at physiologic pH is very low. The importance of these enzymes in blood pressure regulation is unknown.

Regulation of Renal Renin Renin is rate-limiting for the cascade of events that generate angiotensin II. Renal renin is synthesized in the juxtaglomerular cells of the afferent renal arteriole (Fig. 14-2) and is stored as rhomboid-appearing granules.[96,97] It is released into both the bloodstream and the renal lymphatics in response to stimuli (Fig. 14-2).[72,95–110] Some of these stimuli are discussed in later sections on these individual hormones. These stimuli act mostly through (1) renal baroreceptors, (2) adrenergic receptors, and (3) circulating factors such as ions and hormones. Renin release is stimulated by lowering the blood pressure, changing from supine to erect posture, salt depletion, β-adrenergic or CNS stimulation, vasodilating prostaglandins and hormones, opiate peptides, kallikrein, calcitonin, calcitonin gene-related peptide (CGRP), growth factors and a high-protein diet. Renin release is inhibited by increases in blood pressure, assumption of the supine posture, salt loading, angiotensin II, vasopressin, inhibitors of prostaglandin biosynthesis, potassium, calcium, endothelin, endothelium-derived releasing factor (EDRF), adenosine, and atrial natriuretic peptide (ANP). It is also inhibited by certain antihypertensive drugs, including β-adrenergic blockers, α-methyldopa,[111] and clonidine.[112] The importance of only some of these factors is well understood.

Renin is inactivated by proteolytic enzymes in the liver, kidney, and plasma or is excreted by the kidney and in the bile. Its half-life in plasma is 10 to 20 min.[89,90]

The macula densa is a specialized segment of the distal nephron where the distal tubule contacts the afferent arteriole before it enters the glomerulus (Fig. 14-2). The macula densa has an intimate anatomic relation to the juxtaglomerular apparatus and inhibits renin release.[72,76,96,107,113–115] This inhibitory influence is inversely proportional to the renal tubular fluid NaCl concentration and may be due to release from macula densa cells of adenosine that acts through juxtaglomerular cell α_1-adenosine receptors.[76,110,114,116] The macula densa detects renal tubular fluid sodium[96,99,115] or its associated chloride concentration.[117] The concentration of NaCl may be more important than the flux.[115] NaCl may stimulate adenosine release by blocking $Na^+,K^+,2K^+$-cotransporter activity.[115] Whatever the mechanism, factors that reduce volume and/or lower the plasma [NaCl], such as dehydration or a loss of fluid or blood, stimulate renin release. The relation between plasma renin activity and sodium intake as reflected by the urinary sodium excretion is shown in Fig. 14-6.[118]

Renal baroreceptors stimulate renin release in response to decreased renal perfusion pressure.[97,99,107] Apparently, changes are more important than the absolute perfusion pressure, because they can influence renin release in the presence of renal arteriolar constriction or dilation. These receptors can function independently of innervation and of the influences of NaCl delivery to the macula densa. They probably regulate renin release in response to fluid loss and decreased blood pressure.

Renal sympathetic nerves that terminate in the juxtaglomerular cells and in smooth muscle cells of

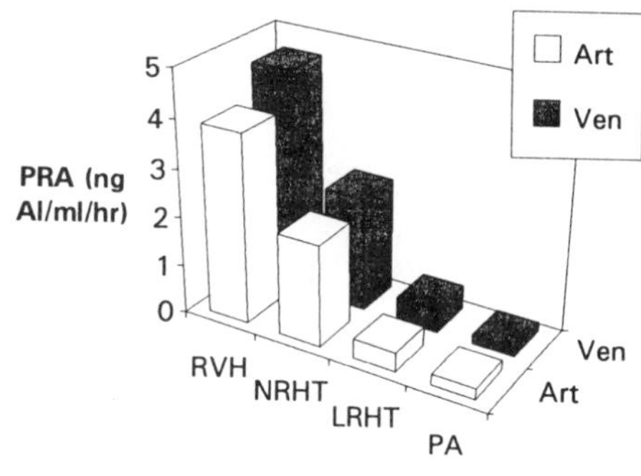

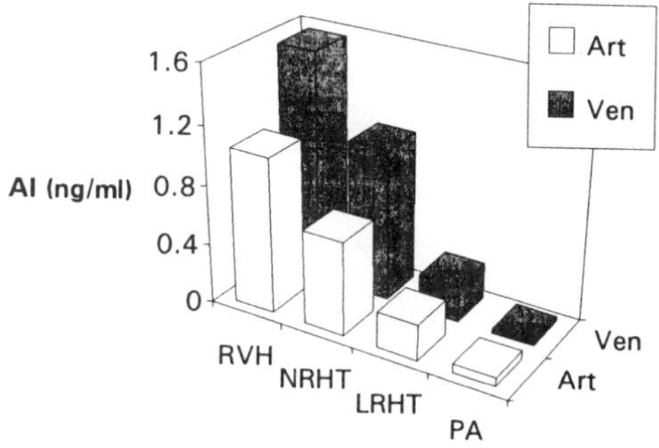

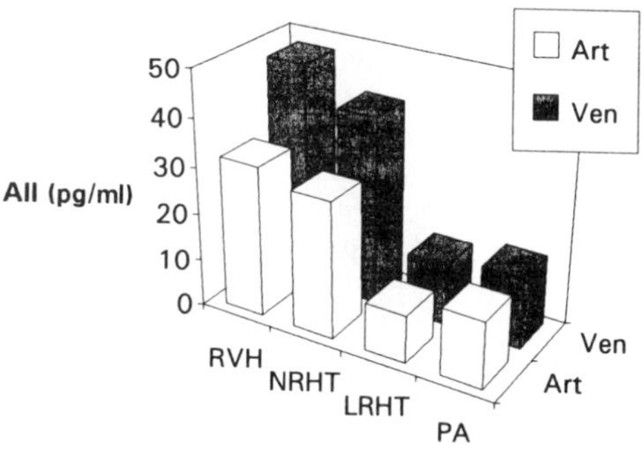

FIGURE 14-4 Release of renin (expressed as PRA), angiotensin I (AI), and angiotension II (AII) from the forearm in response to isoproterenol. Note the higher venous than arterial levels, indicating release from the forearm. *(Drawn from data taken from Taddei et al.*[86a]*)*

renal afferent arterioles secrete norepinephrine and stimulate renin release.[97,99,104] These nerves mediate CNS stimuli and responses to posture, changes in blood pressure, and salt depletion. They can act independently of baroreceptors and salt influences on the macula densa. The activity of these nerves is stimulated primarily by low-pressure cardiopulmonary venous receptors; an independent role for arterial baroreceptors has not been established, although effects through baroreceptors in concert with those through low-pressure receptors probably operate.[119]

β-Adrenergic receptors mediate catecholamine influences on renin release.[97,99,104] Thus, the effects of norepinephrine released by the sympathetic nerves are abolished by β- but not α-adrenergic blockers in most studies. Some of the efficacy of β-adrenergic blockers in treating essential hypertension may be due to blocking of renin release.[120] β-Adrenergic stimulation of renin release is independent of the vasoconstrictor effects of catecholamines that affect the renal glomerular filtration rate and filtered sodium load. Conversely, the effects of NaCl and other influences on renin release can occur independently of β-adrenergic receptors.

Angiotensin II is a potent inhibitor of renin release.[96–99,121] This occurs under all conditions of sodium intake. Thus, inhibition of converting enzyme stimulates renin release even when it does not decrease blood pressure. This negative feedback inhibition appears to be calcium-dependent. Calcium-channel blockers thus enhance renin release.[122] However, these blockers also inhibit the release of aldosterone (whose production is stimulated by intracellular Ca^{2+}) and thus uncouple renin-aldosterone responses. Ca^{2+}-mediated inhibition of renin release may be mediated in part by nitric oxide.[98] Renal prostaglandins are important mediators of renal renin release and may mediate baroreceptor and macula densa signals to release renin.[99,123–129] Administration of either the prostaglandin precursor arachidonic acid or various prostaglandins increases renin secretion. The vasodilator prostacyclin (PGI_2) is the major prostaglandin produced in the human renal cortex.[123] PGI_2 stimulates renin secretion.[125] This influence is independent of changes in renal hemodynamics or the sympathetic nervous system.[126] Inhibition of prostaglandin synthesis, for example, with indomethacin, reduces renin production, decreases plasma renin levels, and can induce hyporeninemic hypoaldosteronism in some patients with renal disease (see Chap. 12).[130] Arachidonic acid precursors can form lipoxygenase products that impair renin release.[127] In patients with hyporeninemic hypoaldosteronism, renal prostacyclin production is low, while lipoxygenase products are increased.[131]

Renin release is affected by several growth factors and cytokines.[100,101,132] Tumor necrosis factor (TNF) and interleukin 1 (IL-1) stimulate renin release from rat cortical slices and suppress aldosterone secretion.[132] These changes have been implicated in hyperreninemic hyperaldosteronism with severe illness.[100] Transforming growth factor β (TGF-β) stimulates renin at a concentration of $10^{-12}M$, but enhances the angiotensin II suppressive effect at $10^{-10}M$. TGF-β levels are increased in the streptozotocin diabetic rat kidney[101] and may contribute to renin suppression in this model.

The quantitative contributions of the nervous and vascular systems, the macula densa, and other factors to the regulation of the renin release have not been fully delineated.[97,104] It appears that each can act independently and that when one system is

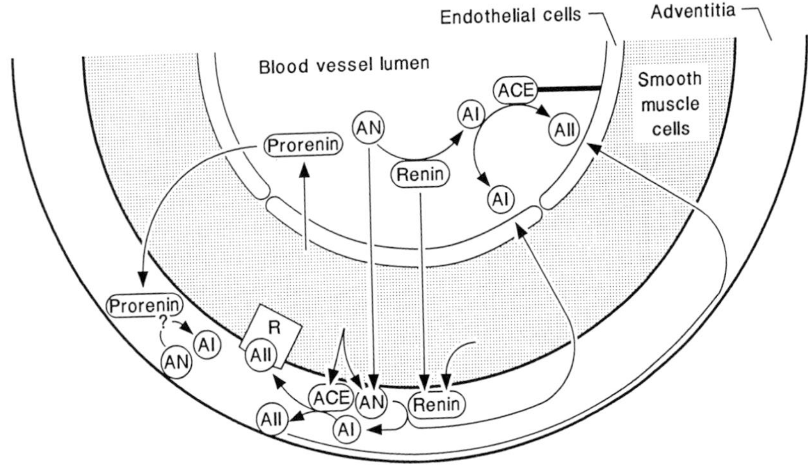

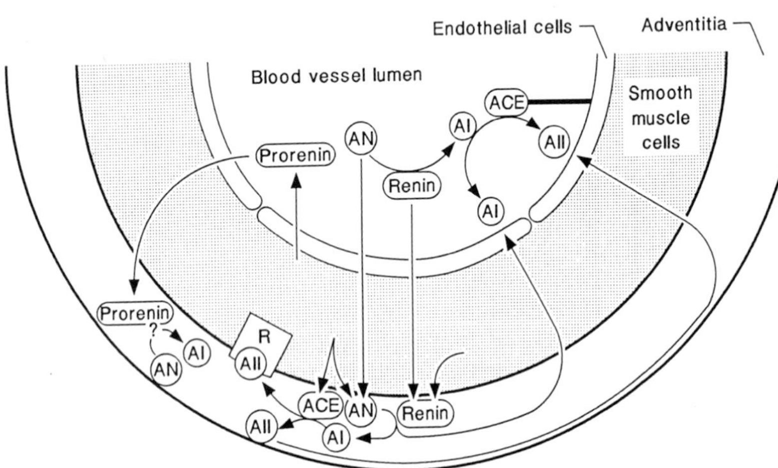

FIGURE 14-5 Circulating and tissue renin-angiotensin systems. The generation of angiotensins I (AI) and II (AII) both in the circulation and in peripheral tissues. Renin, prorenin, and angiotensinogen (An) are present in the circulation or in tissues. Tissue renin, prorenin, and angiotensinogen are derived from the circulation or from local synthesis. The question mark indicates that the role of prorenin in angiotensin I generation in tissues is not established. Angiotensin-coverting enzyme (ACE) is produced locally and is present either on the vascular endothelium, where it can generate angiotensin II in the circulation, or in the tissues.

blocked (e.g., the kidney denervated and the vascular receptors blocked by papaverine), the other systems are capable of appreciable compensation.

Acute stimulation results in the release of almost exclusively renin with either little effect on or a decrease in prorenin.[64,66] By contrast, with chronic stimulation, there is a parallel increase in both renin and prorenin.[66] During periods of relative suppression, more prorenin than renin is released, although as described above, some of the prorenin may be derived from extrarenal sources. Nevertheless, certain stimuli probably result in a preferential processing of prorenin to renin or preferential release of renin as a result of increased shuttling of newly synthesized protein to secretory granules where the conversion of prorenin to renin occurs. It is not known whether the processing is specifically regulated. Prostaglandins may regulate prorenin to renin conversion.[133] The idea that there is control of the processing of prorenin to renin is also suggested by the finding in diabetic nephropathy of an increase in prorenin but not renin levels.[134,135] These observations could also imply that tissue damage may impair the conversion pathways; however, it is not known whether the increased prorenin in diabetic nephropathy comes from renal or extrarenal sources.[134,135]

Certain stimuli affect not only renin release and synthesis but also the number of cells that produce renin. Prolonged stimulation by salt deprivation increases the cellular content of both renin and its mRNA in the rat.[136] However, the major influence of removal of the negative effect of angiotensin II (e.g., by converting enzyme inhibitor treatment of rats) is to recruit more cells that release renin.[103]

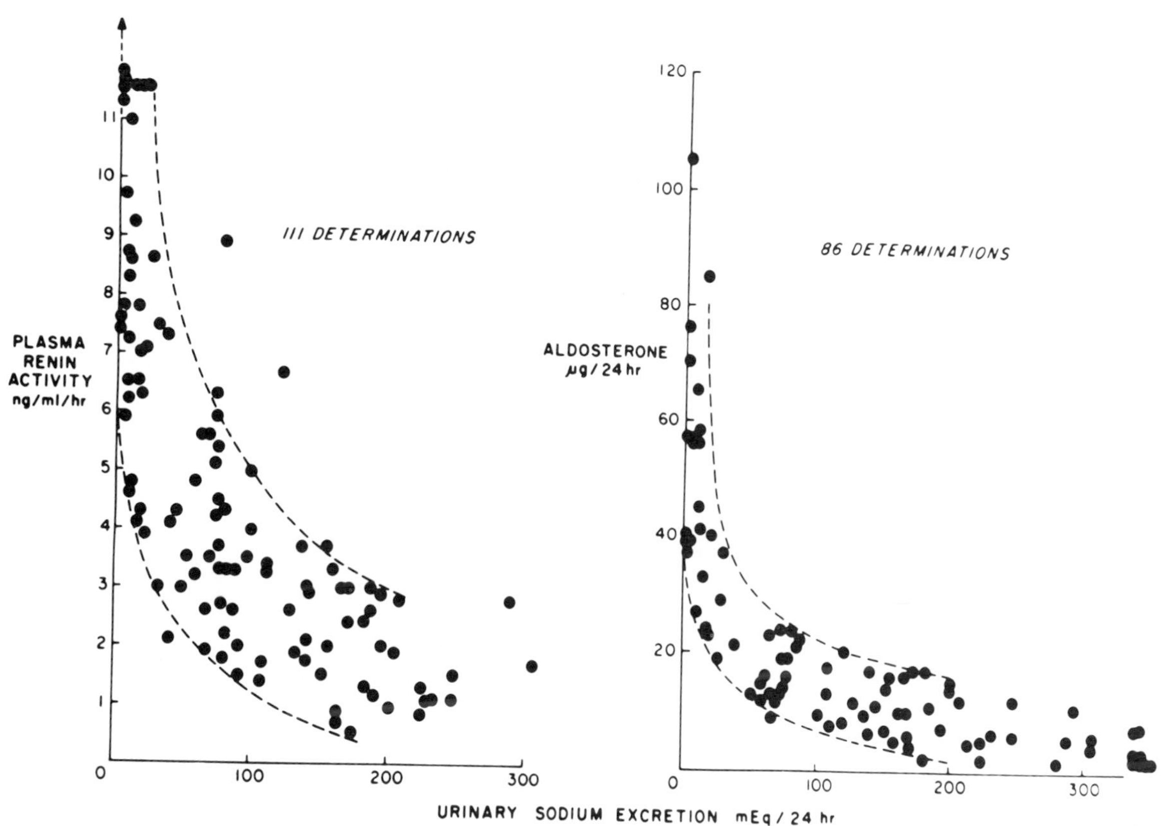

FIGURE 14-6 Relation of 4-h plasma renin activity (PRA, upright posture, *left*) or 24-h urinary aldosterone levels (*right*) to the daily rate of sodium excretion in 52 normal subjects with 111 determinations. *(From Brunner et al.*[118]*)*

Renin Inhibitors Several compounds have been developed that can specifically inhibit renin enzyme activity.[137,138] Their long-term therapeutic effectiveness has not been established.

Angiotensinogen (Renin Substrate)

Angiotensinogen is a glycoprotein synthesized predominantly in the liver, with a molecular weight of 55,000 to 100,000 that varies according to the carbohydrate content of the protein (Fig. 14-3).[90] Several molecular-weight forms are present in the circulation, and higher-molecular-weight forms are synthesized in greater quantities during pregnancy or oral contraceptive administration.[139] The protein is also synthesized at lower levels in a variety of extrahepatic tissues, including kidney (primarily the proximal convoluted tubule), brain, adrenal, aorta, heart, testis, and perivascular fat.[139–141] Release of angiotensinogen from the liver is constitutive, and regulators of angiotensinogen levels affect the synthesis of the protein. Circulating angiotensinogen levels are increased by angiotensin II, estrogens, glucocorticoids, thyroid hormone, and inflammatory mediators.[139,142,143] Angiotensinogen production is decreased by glucagon and certain prostaglandins[142] and in untreated Addison's disease.[139]

Under most circumstances, angiotensinogen appears to circulate at concentrations that do not greatly exceed the K_m for renin, that is, around 1.15 *M*, using pure human renin substrate.[61] This implies that variations in angiotensinogen levels influence the amount of angiotensin I that is generated. However, the extent to which circulating angiotensinogen is limiting for angiotensin I production in the circulation has not been resolved.[139] The finding of an RFLP in the angiotensinogen gene that correlates with hypertension,[29] as discussed in the section on the role of the renin-angiotensin system in hypertension below, could imply that the levels of expression of the gene in the liver or extrahepatic tissues is an important determinant of ultimate angiotensin II generation.

Angiotensin-Converting Enzyme

Expression and Actions Angiotensin-converting enzyme (ACE) is a zinc-containing glycoprotein found in lung, plasma, brush borders of the proximal renal tubule, endothelium of vascular beds, heart, brain, and testis (Figs. 14-3 and 14-4).[144,145] A single gene encodes for ACE, but alternative transcription start sites generate differences in size between pulmonary and testicular ACE.[146] The enzyme is mostly membrane-bound, although there is a soluble form.[145] This enzyme removes two carboxyl-terminal amino acids from a number of peptide substrates. Its two most important actions are the inactivation of bradykinin and the conversion of angiotensin I to angiotensin II (Figs. 14-3 and 14-5). It can also have actions on other proteins.[145,147]

Converting enzymes have an enormous capacity for generating angiotensin II. Thus, even though in certain diseases (e.g., pulmonary disease) there can be a decrease in the plasma levels of converting enzyme, this does not noticeably affect angiotensin II generation.[148] Converting enzyme levels are increased in patients with essential and renovascular hypertension, by diuretic therapy, in some patients with diabetes mellitus,[149] and in hyperthyroidism.[150,151] The activity of the enzyme is increased by glucocorticoids (see Chap. 12) and in rat heart after aortic banding.[152] An RFLP in the converting enzyme gene has been linked to the development of diabetic nephropathy.[153]

Converting Enzyme Inhibitors A number of converting enzyme inhibitors are now available. They have great clinical utility for treating hypertension and heart failure, promoting remodeling after myocardial infarction, and preventing renal failure.[51,154–161] They are also useful for the diagnosis and treatment of renin-dependent hypertension[51,156,162–164] (see also the sections on the role of the renin-angiotensin system in hypertension and on renovascular hypertension, below). Activation of the renin-angiotensin system plays a pathophysiologic role in the development of congestive heart failure, and converting enzyme inhibitors improve hemodynamics and decrease mortality in this condition. Converting enzyme inhibition can also lessen mortality and prevent the development of severe heart failure after myocardial infarction, suggesting that angiotensin II plays a role in cardiac remodeling. Another potential use of converting enzyme inhibitors is in diabetic and other forms of nephropathy, where these drugs can decrease proteinuria.[158,160] Captopril was demonstrated to decrease mortality and the progression of renal disease in more than 400 type I diabetic patients.[158]

Interpretation of the actions of converting enzyme inhibitors must be made in light of the fact that the enzyme can also degrade bradykinin and other proteins.[141,147,148,155,165–168] This bradykinin-metabolizing activity has been termed kininase II or peptidyldipeptide hydroxylase. Bradykinin is also inactivated by another enzyme, kininase I (carboxypeptidase N).[169] Inhibitors of converting enzyme can increase bradykinin concentrations.[165,166] However, captopril treatment of patients with essential hypertension does not consistently increase plasma bradykinin concentrations.[166] An argument for a role for increased bradykinin production in the effectiveness of converting enzyme therapy is that administration of a bradykinin antagonist can attenuate the effects of these inhibitors.[166a]

Angiotensins I, II, and III

Production Although a significant amount of angiotensin I is produced in the circulation, more than half of it occurs in tissues (Figs. 14-4 and 14-5).[65,82,92] Most of this angiotensin I generation appears to be due to renin of renal origin that has been taken up by these tissues, since plasma angiotensin II levels are very low in anephric individuals[65] (also discussed in the section on renin). Conversely, most of the plasma angiotensin II appears to be derived in the circulation as a result of tissue-bound converting enzyme (Figs. 14-3 and 14-4).[170]

Actions Angiotensin I is not known to have physiologically important actions, although it can, at very large doses, stimulate the adrenal medulla to produce catecholamines and the CNS to increase blood pressure and induce thirst.[78,171,172]

Angiotensin II has effects on the cardiovascular system and other systems. The actions of angiotensin II in inhibiting renin release are discussed in the preceding section (Fig. 14-2).[95,121] Angiotensin II actions as one of the most potent stimulators of aldosterone production by the adrenal zona glomerulosa are described in Chap. 12. Angiotensin II also stimulates the production of its substrate, angiotensinogen.[142]

Angiotensin II has potent vasoconstrictor activity and can elevate the blood pressure through direct action on arterioles.[78,121] These blood pressure–elevating effects may be amplified by angiotensin II actions in the CNS, kidney, and other vasoactive substances.[78,121] Angiotensin II stimulates sympathetic nervous system activity through actions on muscle sympathetic nerve activity, adrenergic nerve endings, sympathetic ganglia, and the CNS.[173] Angiotensin II acts within a few seconds, and the duration of action is a few minutes.

Angiotensin II induces a coordinated set of responses in the kidney that affect blood flow, glomerular function, and ion and solute transport. These effects are also modified by angiotensin II–mediated aldosterone release. Angiotensin II decreases renal blood flow and the glomerular filtration rate.[78,121,172,174,175] There is renal vasoconstriction with greater effects on efferent than afferent glomerular arterioles.[121,174–176] These influences modify glomerular filtration and sodium balance. The effects on glomerular blood flow are especially important when renal function is compromised. In this case, angiotensin II maintains the glomerular filtration rate; loss of this effect explains why converting enzyme inhibitors sometimes lead to a decrease in renal function[159,177] (see the section on renovascular hypertension). Angiotensin II increases the activity of the Na^+-H^+ antiporter that enhances Na^+ and Cl^-reabsorption in the proximal convoluted tubule.[176] Na^+ retention can be further increased by angiotensin II–induced vasoconstriction in the medullary circulation and in the cortical collecting tubules secondary to aldosterone actions.[176] Some renal effects of angiotensin II may be mediated through changes in the kallikrein and prostaglandin systems, endothelial-derived releasing factors, and norepinephrine release.[78,121,166a,172,174,175]

Whereas administration of angiotensin II to a nonhypertensive normal subject results in sodium retention, natriuresis is observed in a subset of patients with hypertension.[78,172,178] These different effects are probably due to the fact that in the hypertensive patients, substantial influences of endogenous angiotensin II on the kidney are operative and pressor and other actions of the peptide stimulate the natriuresis.[178] This group (nonmodulators) apparently forms a large proportion of the salt-sensitive hypertensive population and is discussed below under the role of the renin-angiotensin system in hypertension.

There are a number of other effects of angiotensin II.[78,121,141,179] In the heart, angiotensin II can affect coronary blood flow, induce positive ionotropic effects, stimulate the development of cardiac hypertrophy, increase intracellular Ca^{2+}, and influence ion channel responses.[121,166a] In the brain, angiotensin II stimulates dipsogenic behavior, elevates blood pressure, and stimulates the release of vasopressin, corticotropin (ACTH), prolactin, oxytocin, and luteinizing hormone (LH).[78,121,179] Angiotensin II stimulates a "resetting" of the baroreceptor reflex,[121] absorption of salt and water across extrarenal epithelial tissues such as jejunum and colon,[78] uterine smooth muscle contraction, blood coagulation, erythropoietin production, and catecholamine production from nerve endings and the adrenal medulla. Angiotensin II can stimulate insulin-mediated glucose uptake, inhibit glucagon effects on the liver, and decrease plasma fatty acid and elevate plasma lactate levels; some of these effects may be secondary to the vasoconstrictor actions of the peptide.

Important actions of angiotensin II include promoting the growth of vascular smooth muscle cells, renal mesangial cells, and cardiac fibroblasts.[121,180–187] In cultured vascular smooth muscle cells, angiotensin II induces hypertrophy but not proliferation and increases the levels of platelet-derived growth factor (PDGF)-A chain, c-fos, c-myc, TFG-β mRNAs. Whereas PDGF may stimulate the growth of these cells, TGF-β inhibits their growth and thus the proliferative response to PDGF, resulting in hypertrophy. Angiotensin II can induce hyperplasia in human fetal mesangial cells and in vascular smooth muscle cells from the spontaneously hypertensive rat (SHR). Thus, angiotensin II may enhance growth by altering the balance of autocrine growth factors and growth inhibitors in smooth muscle cells. The actions of angiotensin II in inducing proliferation and collagen production in cardiac fibroblasts may contribute to its role in hypertrophic and remodeling processes in the heart.[182,183,188]

Circulation and Metabolism The concentrations of angiotensin II in plasma vary between 5 and 100 p*M*.[48,65,82,91] Tissue levels of angiotensin II are probably higher, in the nanomolar range. Physiologic stimuli may increase the plasma concentrations 10- to 25-fold. Angiotensin II may circulate partly bound by plasma proteins. It has a half-life of a very few minutes in plasma; 50 percent or more of the activity disappears in a single passage through the vascular beds.

There are other angiotensin products whose roles have not been clarified. The heptapeptide angiotensin III has activity that differs from that of angiotensin II quantitatively.[171] The plasma concentrations of angiotensin III are perhaps only 20 percent of those of angiotensin II, and the former is even more susceptible to proteolytic degradation than is angiotensin II. The brain can produce angiotensin-(1–7) and other angiotensin peptides that have actions that partly resemble and partly differ from those of angiotensin II.[83,193]

Mechanisms of Action Angiotensin binds to specific receptors on the cell membrane (see Chaps. 5 and 12). Two types of angiotensin II receptors have been identified.[194–196] The AT_1 receptor defined by binding to the angiotensin II antagonist losartan (Dup 753) has been identified in vasculature, kidney, adrenal, and heart and probably mediates the cardiovascular and renal effects of angiotensin II.[121,197] The AT_2 receptor is defined by its binding to PD123177; the function of this receptor is unknown, although it is present in fetal tissue, suggesting a role in growth and development.[121,198] In the adult, AT_2 receptors have been found in brain, heart, uterus, and adrenal medulla.[121,199,200] Both receptor types have seven transmembrane-spanning domains.[191–196,201,202] The AT_1 receptor is G protein–linked.[194–196] The AT_2 receptor apparently can inhibit protein tyrosine phosphatase activity.[201]

Immediate post-angiotensin II–receptor binding events involve effects on phospholipids, with increased intracellular levels of inositol 1,4,5-triphosphate (IP_3) and mobilization of intracellular Ca^{2+} (see Chaps. 5 and 12), which occur in all angiotensin II–responsive tissues.[121,203,204] Many angiotensin II–

receptor interactions may be negatively coupled to adenylyl cyclase.[121,176] Mechanisms for angiotensin II stimulation of aldosterone release are described in Chap. 12. The initial events in the vasculature are mostly similar; angiotensin II-induced increases in intracellular Ca^{2+} mobilization initiate the formation of Ca^{2+} calmodulin complexes, activation of myosin light-chain kinase phosphorylation of myosin light chain, and ultimately actin-myosin interaction and contraction.[121] Effects on prostaglandins and lipoxygenase production may also contribute, although the precise role of these systems has not been elucidated.[205]

Regulation of Responsiveness to Angiotensin Cellular sensitivity to angiotensin II can vary in physiologic circumstances and disease states. Such variations occur partly through influences on cellular receptor levels (see Chap. 5).[206,207] In the rat, angiotensin II increases the concentration of adrenal receptors (an exception to the general case with polypeptide hormones) and decreases the concentration of uterine, vascular, and cardiac fibroblast receptors.[206] Prolonged infusion of angiotensin II increases the sensitivity of the adrenal gland to the hormone. However, in some circumstances in which plasma angiotensin concentrations are chronically low (e.g., in low-renin essential hypertension, discussed below), the sensitivity of the adrenal gland to angiotensin II is increased. Hyperkalemia and decreased sodium increase and hypokalemia and increased sodium decrease the adrenal content of angiotensin receptors.[206] The affinity of these receptors for angiotensin II can also be increased transiently by sodium restriction.[206] As discussed below in the section on the role of the renin-angiotensin system in essential hypertension, there is blunted renal responsiveness to angiotensin II in a common form of salt-sensitive essential hypertension.

Angiotensin II Receptor Antagonists As was described above, these antagonists have been useful in defining the subclasses of angiotensin receptors. They are also being examined for effectiveness in treating hypertension and other conditions.[208,209]

Participation of Renal versus Extrarenal Renin-Angiotensin Systems

As noted above, there is extensive expression of components of the renin-angiotensin system[77–85, 210] and angiotensin I and probably angiotensin II can be produced outside the circulation (Figs. 14-4 and 14-5).[65,82,92] The relative contributions of the renal and extrarenal systems to blood pressure control are currently being unraveled.

There are several arguments for the importance of extrarenal renin-angiotensin systems. One is that there are poor correlations between the effects of converting enzyme inhibitors on the blood pressure and plasma renin levels[84,166a] and poor kinetic correlations between the effects of blockade of the circulating system and blood pressure effects.[84] Administration of ACE inhibitors into the brains of SHRs lowers blood pressure without inhibiting the peripheral renin-angiotensin system.[166a] Transgenic rats that overexpress the renin gene in multiple extrarenal tissues have profound angiotensin II–dependent hypertension, slightly depressed plasma renin and angiotensin II levels, and suppressed renal renin gene expression.[166a,211–213] These animals are discussed below under the role of the renin-angiotensin system in experimental hypertension.

The RFLP analyses described in the preceding section on angiotensinogen could imply that the level of extrarenal expression of the gene for this protein is an independent risk factor for hypertension. Changes in hepatic expression of the gene that affect plasma angiotensinogen levels may be compensated for by angiotensin II–induced feedback influences on renin release. Thus, the important differences in angiotensinogen expression may occur at extrahepatic sites that are not subjected to the feedback control. However, studies of the effects of converting enzyme inhibitors and angiotensin II antagonists in anephric individuals and animal models have not provided clear indications that inhibition of any kidney-independent renin-angiotensin system has significant effects on blood pressure.[65,214]

It is unresolved how extrarenal renin-angiotensin systems work. The various components are not all expressed in all the tissues, and the levels of expression are disputed.[215,216] Substrates (angiotensinogen and angiotensin I) may need to be delivered to the sites (Fig. 14-5), and perhaps the systems generate peptides other than angiotensin II (discussed above). As discussed in the preceding section on renin, in most cases the renin expressed is prorenin, although this protein has low renin activity and can be activated by means other than proteolysis of the prosegment. Infusion of prorenin results in very weak vasodilatory effects, leading to the hypothesis that it may act in this way in local areas.[51]

Maintenance of Blood Pressure

Information about the physiologic role of angiotensin II in blood pressure control has been provided by the development of angiotensin antagonists and converting enzyme and renin inhibitors. In sodium-replete normotensive individuals, blockade of the renin-angiotensin system does not reduce blood pressure, even with changes in posture, but it does induce a significant fall in blood pressure in volume-depleted (salt-deprived, etc.) normotensive individuals.[217,218] The failure to reduce the blood pressure in the salt-replete state probably reflects the fact that mechanisms that compensate for the angiotensin II deficiency can normalize the blood pressure under these conditions.

Role of the Renin-Angiotensin System in Hypertension

Experimental Hypertension

Studies with animal models have elucidated how the renin-angiotensin system can cause hypertension.[219–221] The two-kidney one-clip model resembles the acute stages of renovascular hypertension in humans. Plasma renin activity and blood pressure increase after the renal artery is clamped. Sodium balance is positive in the early stages and returns to normal or becomes negative in the chronic phase. The sodium balance is inversely related to the degree of hypertension. Inhibition of renin, converting enzyme, or angiotensin II action lowers blood pressure in animals with two-kidney Goldblatt hypertension.[128] Thus, in the two-kidney model, increased renin activity not only initiates but maintains the hypertension. However, with longer periods of time (e.g., 2 to 4 months), the hypertension becomes non-angiotensin II–dependent and more volume-dependent.[128,222] This appears to be due to a hypertension-induced decrease in the ability of the contralateral kidney to excrete salt. At this stage, the two-kidney preparation resembles the one-kidney preparation described below.

A different sequence of events occurs in the one-kidney Goldblatt model.[128,222,223] There is a prompt increase in arterial blood pressure and an increase in plasma renin activity. During the chronic phase, hypertension persists and there is sodium retention. The sodium retention depresses renin release, and plasma renin levels return to the normal range but are slightly elevated compared with those in control nonclipped rats. The use of an angiotensin antagonist or a converting enzyme inhibitor can prevent the occurrence of hypertension early after the experimental lesion is produced, but neither is persistently effective. However, blood pressure can be reduced by inhibiting angiotensin II action if the rats are first given a low-sodium diet. The hypertension can be reversed in the chronic phase by removal of the renal artery constriction, and this is accompanied by a negative sodium balance that correlates with the drop in blood pressure. Although the increase in renin activity is the primary initiating event, other factors (most likely the solution retention) participate more in the maintenance of the hypertension. This model may be useful for understanding chronic renovascular hypertension in humans. The hypertension in this state can become volume-dependent, possibly as a result of chronic hypertensive changes in the nonstenotic kidney. The hypertension during this phase in humans is not responsive to correction of the stenosis.

Two transgenic animal models illustrate differences in the ways in which the renin-angiotensin system can generate hypertension. In a chimeric mouse model, hypertension results from the hypersecretion of human renin and angiotensinogen in the circulation.[211] Transgenic rats that overexpress the mouse renin gene in multiple tissues were discussed above. These animals have fulminant angiotensin II–dependent hypertension[212,213] with low levels of plasma renin activity, circulating angiotensin II, and kidney renin mRNA and high levels of plasma prorenin, adrenal renin, and plasma aldosterone. In these animals, the mouse renin gene is expressed primarily in the rat adrenal, which hypersecretes prorenin and mineralocorticoids. Adrenal-derived renin is thought to mediate the hypertension, which is lowered by treatment with converting enzyme inhibitors. This model demonstrates the role of a tissue renin angiotensin system, i.e., the adrenal, in the development and maintenance of hypertension.

Renin-Secreting Tumors

As described in the section on renovascular hypertension, there are rare renin-secreting tumors (Fig. 14-7).[224,225] These tumors result in severe hypertension, hypokalemia, hyperreninemia, and markedly elevated prorenin levels.

Human Renovascular Hypertension

In human renovascular hypertension, renal ischemia and hypoperfusion resulting from renal artery lesions lead to excessive renin release, with consequences similar to those in animals.[128] The overall results depend on the severity of the lesions and the functional capacity of both the contralateral kidney and the involved kidney. Functional capacity depends on both the extent of preceding renal impairment and hypertension-induced changes.[226] Plasma renin levels can be high, normal, or even low normal and are determined by the degree of stimulus induced by the ischemic kidney and the extent to which subsequent sodium retention suppresses renin levels. Sodium retention is greatly affected by the functional capacity of the kidneys. Thus, when human renovascular hypertension occurs in the absence of a severe impairment in renal function, the hemodynamic and hormonal profile resembles more that of the two-kidney model, whereas with major impairment in renal function, there can be sodium dependency of the hypertension similar to that which occurs with the one-kidney model. This heterogeneity of clinical presentation accounts for some of the problems in the diagnosis and management of renovascular hypertension.

Other Forms of Secondary Hypertension

Given the large number of factors that influence the renin-angiotension system or are influenced by this system, it is expected that abnormalities in it participate in other forms of hypertension. These are

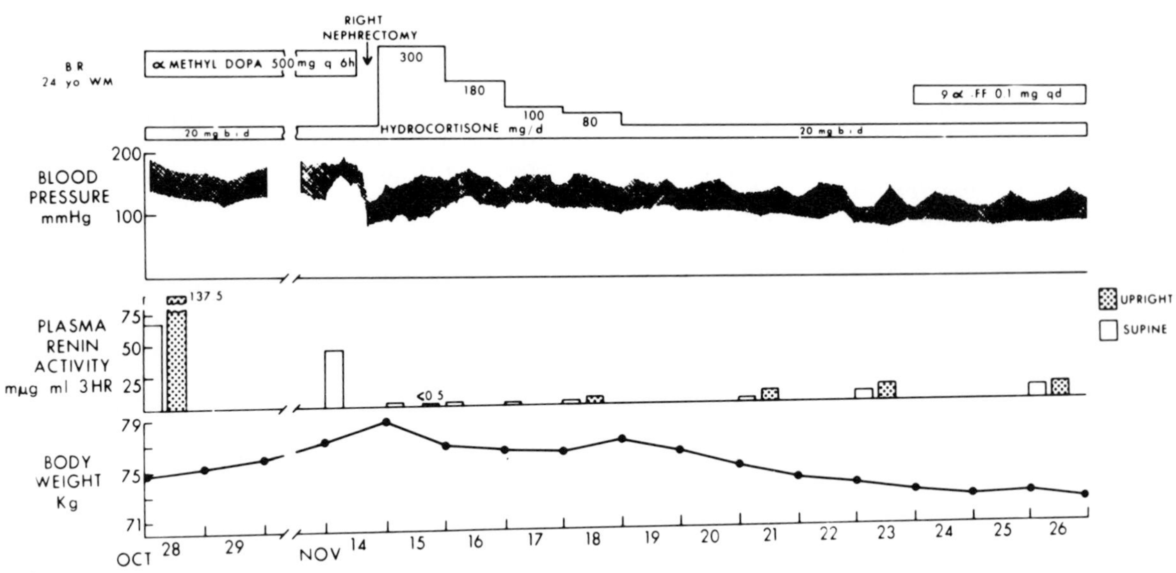

FIGURE 14-7 Preoperative and postoperative measurements of blood pressure, plasma renin activity (PRA), and body weight in a patient with a renin-secreting tumor (previous surgery was subtotal adrenalectomy). Note the prompt fall in blood pressure and PRA after right nephrectomy. Normal PRA was seen on the ninth prospective day. Adrenal hormone replacement was required because of reduced adrenal mass from previous surgery. *(From Schambelan et al.[224])*

discussed in the sections on individual hormonal modifiers of blood pressure.

Accelerated Hypertension

Accelerated hypertension is characterized by marked elevation of blood pressure, decreased renal function, and severe retinopathy. Renin levels are usually extremely high and result in secondary aldosteronism.[227,228] Activation of the renin system in these patients is due predominatly to altered renal hemodynamics that result in ischemia. This activation enhances further the vasoconstriction and arterial hypertension. Patients with chronic renal failure are particularly susceptible to this form of hypertension, and an increased blood volume usually aggravates the condition. This renin-dependent form of accelerated hypertension occurs in a small subgroup of hypertensive patients and is an acute disorder that requires immediate treatment.

Genetic Linkage

Polymorphisms of genes that express components of the renin-angiotensin system have been linked to human and animal forms of hypertension. Variants of the angiotensinogen gene have been linked to hypertension in over 400 families with essential hypertension.[29] The ACE and renin genes have not been linked to hypertension.[229,230] However, RFLPs of the rat renin gene are linked to hypertension in the Dahl salt-sensitive model and in the SHR,[30,32] and polymorphisms in the ACE gene have been linked to blood pressure in the stroke-prone SHR.[31,33] Associations have been identified between polymorphisms in the ACE gene and increased risks of myocardial infarction[231] and diabetic nephropathy.[153] It is not known whether variants in the AT_1 receptor gene are related to hypertension.

Essential Hypertension

Several lines of evidence document participation of the renin-angiotensin system in the pathogenesis of essential hypertension. Genetic evidence for this was cited in the preceding section.

The heterogeneity of essential hypertension is reflected to a major event by variations in components of the renin-angiotensin system. As shown in Figs. 14-6 and 14-8, plasma renin levels show considerable variation as a function of urinary sodium excretion in patients with essential hypertension (a reflection of sodium intake) in comparison to normal subjects. This type of comparison has been the basis for classifying patients as having low-, normal-, or high-renin essential hypertension.

Blockade of the Renin-Angiotensin System in Essential Hypertension The therapeutic effectiveness of converting enzyme inhibitors provides strong evidence for participation of the renin-angiotensin system in essential hypertension.[51,154–162,166a,232] Con-

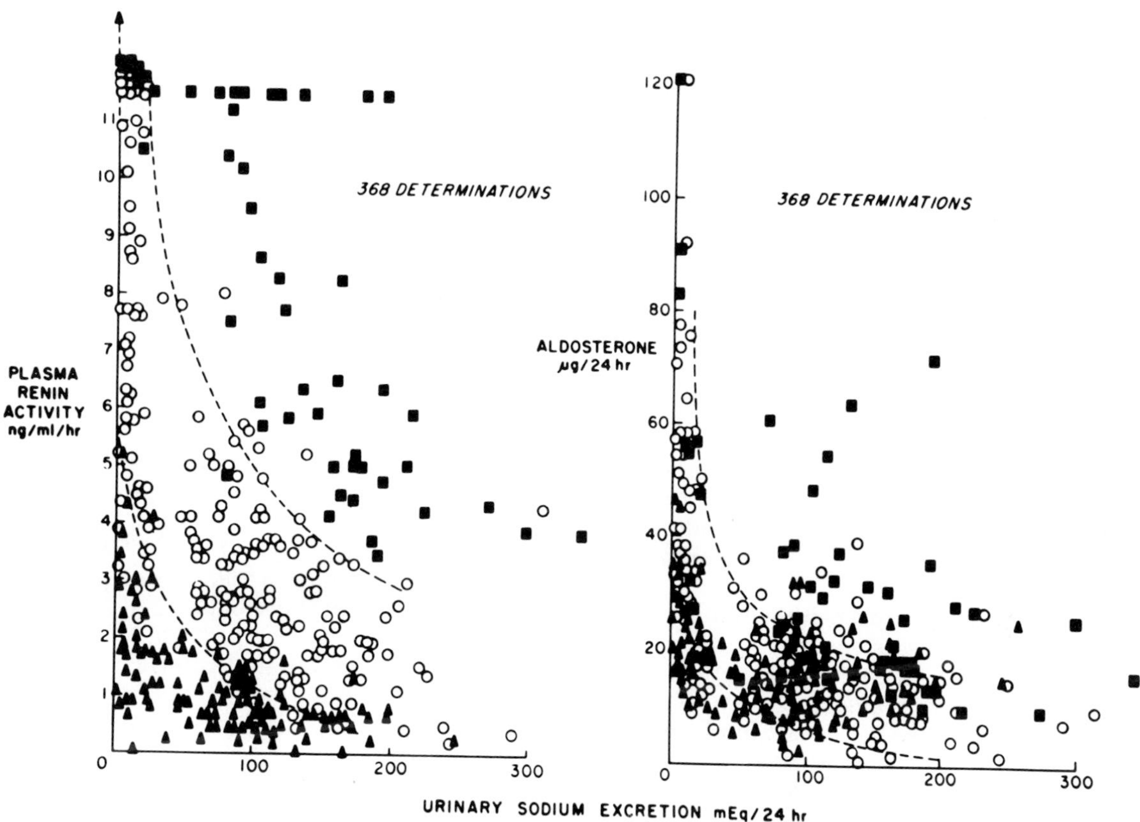

FIGURE 14-8 Plasma renin activity measured at noon after 4 h upright (*left*) and corresponding daily urinary aldosterone excretion (*right*) plotted against the concurrent daily rate of sodium excretion in 219 patients with essential hypertension. Plasma renin activity levels are indicated by triangles for low, open circles for normal, and squares for high activity. Values for 52 normal individuals are represented by the dotted line. In some cases, individual points fall outside the indicated classification. This is due to the fact that repeated samples in these patients mostly fall into another category. *(From Brunner et al.[118])*

verting enzyme inhibitors are as effective as other forms of therapy in the general hypertensive population[232] and, as described below, are especially effective in subsets of patients. Blockade of the renin-angiotensin system probably has additional usefulness in hypertensive patients for inhibiting vascular proliferative and other responses.[51,82,159—162]

As discussed above, the effects of converting enzyme inhibitors should be interpreted in light of the knowledge that some actions of these drugs may increase bradykinin levels.[153,166a,168] However, the effectiveness of these inhibitors appears to be generally similar to that of the renin inhibitors[137,138] and angiotensin receptor antagonists.[208,209] There is also some correlation between the effectiveness of the converting enzyme inhibitors for treating essential hypertension and levels of plasma renin activity.[51,80,156,219] Patients with normal or high levels of plasma renin tend also to respond better to β-adrenergic blocking agents.[156] Conversely, patients with lower renin levels tend to respond better to diuretic therapy, calcium-channel blockers, and α-adrenergic blockers.[156]

Normal and High-Renin Essential Hypertension The presence of normal or high plasma renin levels in essential hypertension could be taken as an abnormality, since the expected response to an elevation of blood pressure would be to suppress the plasma renin activity. "Abnormally normal" or elevated plasma renin levels have been attributed to a primary renal abnormality with heterogeneity of the nephrons.[51] In this abnormality, some nephrons are proposed to oversecrete renin because of vasospasm, whereas in others, there is more dilatation with glomerular hyperfiltration.[51] Renal biopsy data showing heterogeneity in afferent arteriolar narrowing support this model.[51] In essence, these patients are proposed to have a micro form of renovascular hypertension. Variations on this theme could also explain some of the wide differences in plasma renin

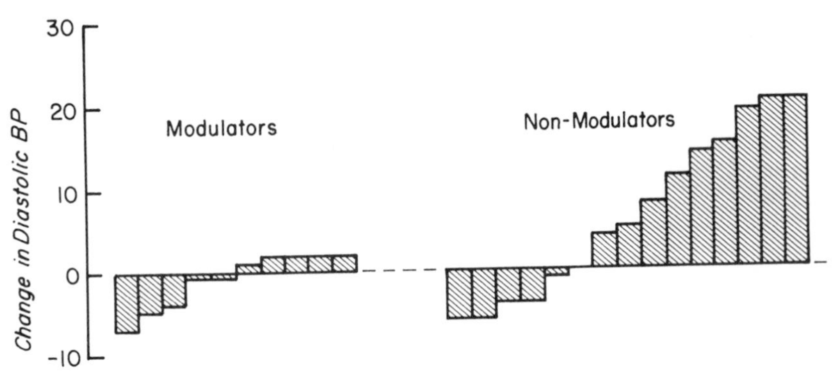

FIGURE 14-9 Frequency distribution of increment in diastolic blood pressure after 5 days of high sodium intake in 25 hypertensive subjects. The hypertensive subjects have been divided into modulators ($n = 10$) and nonmodulators ($n = 15$) according to their renal vascular response to angiotensin II. A significant pressor response (>10 mmHg) with sodium loading occurred only in the nonmodulating group. The difference in the blood pressure response in the two groups was highly significant ($p < 0.004$) *(From Redgrave et al.[241])*

levels in essential hypertension. As will be discussed later, activity of the adrenergic nervous system is enhanced in essential hypertension; this would stimulate renin release and contribute to inappropriate levels of plasma renin.[233]

There is significant heterogeneity within the normal-renin subgroup of essential hypertension, and many of the differences probably are determined by factors other than the renin-angiotensin system. One differentiating influence is that of salt intake on the blood pressure, with subdivision of patients into salt-sensitive and salt-resistant (see the section on sodium chloride).

Salt-sensitive patients can be separated further into modulating and nonmodulating essential hypertension as reflected by certain abnormalities of the renin-angiotensin-aldosterone axis (Fig. 14-9).[234–241] Unlike the case with normotensives and modulating hypertensive patients, in response to salt loading, nonmodulating patients display a failure of renal blood flow to increase, leading to a reduced ability to excrete a salt load; reduced responsiveness of renin and aldosterone release (also in response to angiotensin II); and impaired responsiveness of ANP release. The plasma aldosterone levels in nonmodulating patients tend to be lower than those in other patients. This results in a normal to high plasma renin level. The sodium sensitivity of their blood pressures appears to arise from the sodium-dependent changes in renal blood flow mediated by endogenous angiotensin II. The abnormalities in the nonmodulators are corrected by the administration of converting enzyme inhibitors or calcium-channel blocking agents. These classes of drugs therefore constitute a specific form of therapy in these patients. As in other salt-sensitive hypertensives, nonmodulators typically have a strong family history for hypertension. They also tend to have an increase in erythrocyte Na^+-Li^+ countertransport (also discussed in the section on sodium transport and blood pressure). It has been argued that this may be the most common form of hypertension. Although at present the classification of modulators vs. nonomodulators is cumbersome and restricted to research uses, ultimately drug therapy may be tailored to this type of evaluation.

Low-Renin Essential Hypertension The low-renin subgroup (Fig. 14-8) includes approximately 5 to 15 percent of patients with essential hypertension, depending on the study group.[51,238,239] The condition is more common in blacks and may be present in up to 50 percent of elderly patients.[51,156,242] These patients have salt-sensitive hypertension, a tendency toward sodium retention, blunted catecholamine responses to provocative stimuli, abnormal sensitivity to angiotensin II, and possible ion transport abnormalities.[50,51,156,235,237–239]

The existence of low plasma renin activity in essential hypertension could reflect an attempt by the body to adapt to the hypertension. The idea that low plasma renin levels reflect in part adaptive responses is supported by findings of an inverse correlation between blood pressure and plasma renin activity in hypertensive and normotensive persons[50,51, 156,166a] and the fact that borderline hypertensive patients have greater variations in plasma renin levels than do age-matched normotensive control subjects.[243] In the normotensive offspring of hypertensive parents, there tend to be lower levels of plasma renin activity and aldosterone, with increased renal vasoconstriction, compared to the offspring of normotensive parents.[50]

Although patients with low-renin essential hypertension show reduced blood pressure–lowering responses to converting enzyme inhibition compared to normal-renin and high-renin hypertensives,[51,141, 156,219] these patients do respond to some extent. The responses observed in low-renin patients may be due to the fact that they are more sensitive to the low levels of circulating angiotensin II that are present than are normal-renin hypertensives (also discussed below).[219,238,239] Alternatively, the responses could reflect participation of extrarenal renin-angiotensin systems in the hypertension[141] (discussed above).

The abnormal sensitivity to angiotension II in patients with low-renin essential hypertension is observed in both the adrenal and the kidneys.[235,237–239] In normal subjects, the response of the adrenal glomerulosa to angiotensin II varies with the level of sodium intake; sodium restriction enhances the re-

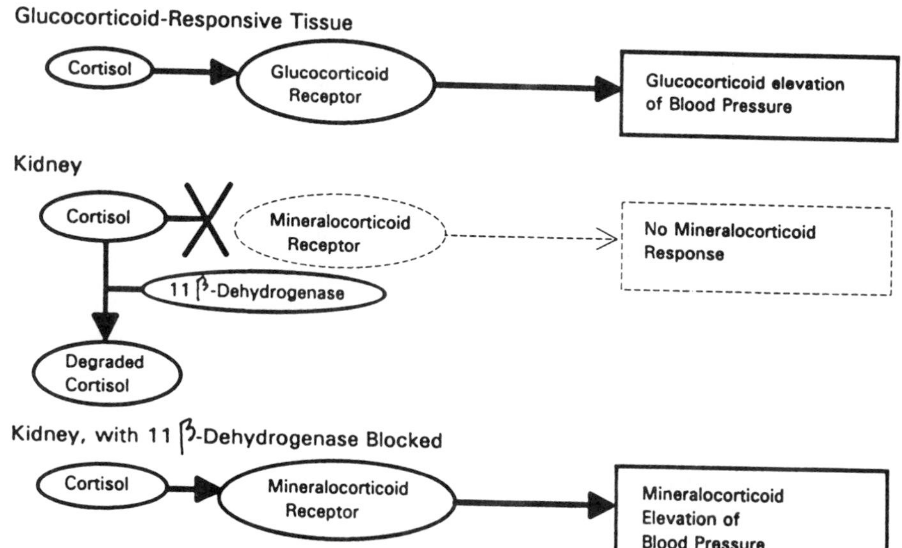

FIGURE 14-10 Actions of glucocorticoids and mineralocorticoids on the blood pressure. Glucocorticoids can elevate the blood pressure by binding to the glucocorticoid receptor. Cortisol exhibits major actions through the mineralocorticoid receptors in the kidney when its degradation is blocked. 11β-Dehydrogenase = 11β-hydroxysteroid dehydrogenase.

sponse,[235,237] while a high sodium intake enhances the renal blood flow response.[237] In patients with low-renin essential hypertension, the normally reduced response of aldosterone release to angiotensin II on the high-salt diet do not occur, and these individuals release angiotensin II that induces an inappropriately enhanced aldosterone release.[235,237–239] This leads to lower plasma renin levels and a tendency toward sodium retention.[237,237]

The putative ion-transport abnormalities in low-renin patients involve either a Ca^{2+} leak or impaired cell membrane Ca^{2+} pumping activity.[51,244,245] The effect of the abnormality is to elevate intracellular [Ca^{2+}] and lower serum [Ca^{2+}] levels and to enhance blood pressure responses to calcium-channel blockers and dietary calcium supplementation[51,246,247] (see also the section on Ca^{2+} and hypertension). Such a defect could simultaneously affect the blood pressure and the adrenal glomerulosa response to angiotensin II.

Patients with low-renin essential hypertension do not have hypokalemia and elevated plasma and/or urinary aldosterone levels and thus differ from those with primary aldosteronism and hypokalemia, as described in the section on primary aldosteronism. However, there may be only a quantitative distinction between low-renin essential hypertension and primary aldosteronism with hyperplasia. The normal plasma aldosterone levels in patients with low-renin essential hypertension are high relative to the suppressed plasma renin levels. Thus, these patients have high plasma aldosterone/renin ratios. Their inappropriately high aldosterone levels are due to enhanced adrenal sensitivity to angiotensin II, and abnormality also present in primary aldosteronism with hyperplasia. Aldosterone and plasma renin responses to posture and other stimuli in patients with low-renin essential hypertension also resemble primary aldosteronism with hyperplasia. In fact, some patients with low-renin essential hypertension do have primary aldosteronism, since many patients with the latter disorder can have normal plasma aldosterone levels and be normokalemic. However, the proportion of low-renin hypertensive patients with occult primary aldosteronism has not been determined.

Role of the Renin-Angiotensin System in Complications of Atherosclerosis

Angiotensin II is a growth factor and might promote atherosclerosis, and its vasoconstrictor actions might promote thrombotic events.[51,248,249] Angiotensin II also stimulates other functions related to atherosclerosis, such as circulating levels of plasminogen activator inhibitor–1.[248] Other evidence cited in support of a relation between renin and thrombotic complications includes data from stroke-prone hypertensive rats and renin-producing tumors, in which there are high plasma renin levels and significant vascular damage.[51] However, epidemiologic data are conflicting in terms of the relation between the renin status and the development of heart attack and stroke.[51,249,250]

Mineralocorticoids

Adrenal glucocorticoids and mineralocorticoids have been implicated in hypertension (Fig. 14-10). *Glucocorticoid* and *mineralocorticoid* are described in Chap. 12. An excess of mineralocorticoid activity can cause hypertension, and aldosterone, deoxycorticosterone (DOC), and cortisol can all lead to a mineralocorticoid excess state. Glucocorticoids can also elevate the blood pressure through mineralocorticoid receptor–independent mechanisms, as discussed in the following section. Other adrenal steroids may be capable of elevating blood pressure, but it is not known whether they contribute to human disease.

The identification of aldosterone as a mineralocorticoid that can cause hypertension was made in 1955 by Conn, who described primary aldosteronism.[251] In 1956, Eberlein and Bongiovanni identified the tetrahydro metabolite of DOC in patients with 11β-hydroxylase deficiency.[252] Further evidence that DOC excess can lead to hypertension was reported in 1966 with the discovery of the 17α-hydroxylase syndrome.[253]

Steroids with Mineralocorticoid Activity

Aldosterone

Aldosterone is the major mineralocorticoid in humans (Chap. 12). Regulation of synthesis and release and states of deficiency and secondary excess of aldosterone are discussed in Chap. 12. The hormone is released in response to posture or fluid loss to conserve sodium and to potassium intake to protect against hyperkalemia. In contrast to cortisol, aldosterone probably is not critical for maintenance of blood pressure in the sodium-replete state under normal circumstances. However, in children with mineralocorticoid deficiency and in salt-deprived adults the sodium-retaining actions of the steroid can be critical for maintaining blood pressure. Administration of mineralocorticoids without concomitant glucocorticoid replacement does not ameloriate the hypotension in Addison's disease.

Aldosterone excess can result from primary aldosteronism (see the section on primary aldosteronism) or from secondary causes (see Chap. 12). Whereas hypersecretion of aldosterone in primary aldosteronism results in hypertension, the steroid usually does not cause hypertension in most cases of secondary aldosterone excess, such as cirrhosis and heart failure. In those states, elevations of the steroid occur in response to a perceived decrease in intravascular volume. Aldosterone excess can also occur with renin-producing tumors, renovascular hypertension, high-renin essential hypertension, and accelerated hypertension, and in these cases it aggravates the hypertension (see the discussion on the role of the renin-angiotensin system in hypertension). The potential role of aldosterone in essential hypertension is discussed below.

Mineralocorticoid Actions of Cortisol and Other Steroids with Glucocorticoid Activity

Cortisol and other steroids with glucocorticoid activity can act as mineralocorticoids by binding to the mineralocorticoid receptor (Fig. 14-10) (Chap. 12).[254–257] The affinity of cortisol for the mineralocorticoid receptor is about 10 percent that of aldosterone (Chap. 12). Cortisol circulates at approximately 1000-fold higher total concentrations than does aldosterone. Thus, at levels in the normal range, cortisol would ordinarily be expected to occupy the mineralocorticoid receptor instead of aldosterone and to cause a mineralocorticoid-excess state. However, at least two mechanisms prevent this from happening in the kidney (see also Chap. 12).[254–257]

First, cortisol is about 92 percent bound to plasma proteins, whereas only about 50 percent of the aldosterone is so bound (Chap. 12). Thus, the free concentrations of cortisol are only about 200-fold those of aldosterone, and the effective concentration would be only about 20-fold higher based on the relative receptor-binding affinities of the two steroids. Cortisol access to the mineralocorticoid receptor in the kidney also may be blunted by sequestering of the steroid by renal intracellular cortisol-binding proteins.

Second, renal 11β-hydroxysteroid dehydrogenase degrades cortisol to the inactive metabolite cortisone by converting the 11β-OH group of cortisol (and other steroids) to a keto group[254–257] (Fig. 14-10) (Chap. 12). The hemiacetyl group of aldosterone, which links its 11- and 19-positions, prevents the enzyme from degrading aldosterone. In some tissues, such as brain, this enzyme is not as active, and cortisol can have greater actions through the mineralocorticoid receptors.

Thus, cortisol and other glucocorticoids can apparently elicit potent mineralocorticoid activities only when they are present in sufficient excess to overwhelm 11β-hydroxysteroid dehydrogenase or when this enzyme is blocked. The former mechanism may occur in patients with severe Cushing's syndrome, in the syndrome of primary glucocorticoid resistance, or with glucocorticoid antagonist treatment when the body produces large quantities of cortisol to overcome the resistance to glucocorticoid suppression of ACTH (see the section on other low-renin hypertension syndromes below).[258–260] However, the mineralocorticoid excess could also be due to DOC, which is usually produced in excess in these states (see the section on other low-renin hypertension syndromes).

Defective function of 11β-hydroxysteroid dehydrogenase resulting in a cortisol-induced mineralocorticoid-excess state is observed after ingestion of licorice or carbenoxolone which blocks the enzyme, or in a rare syndrome of apparent mineralocorticoid excess in which the defect has not been defined.[255–257,261–264] These syndromes are discussed in the section on low-renin hypertension.

Changes in the inactivation of cortisol to cortisone have been proposed to be potentially important in other settings. An increase in the ratio of plasma cortisol to cortisone has been reported in patients with renal impairment, leading to the suggestion that defective renal 11β-hydroxysteroid dehydrogenase activity might cause renal cortisol excess and contribute to hypertension in this state.[265] It has been proposed that glucocorticoid excess is responsible for the hypertension associated with low birthweight.[266] There are correlations in animals between excess fetal glucocorticoid exposure and hypertension,[266] and in humans between hypertension in the fetus and low placental 11β-hydroxysteroid dehydrogenase activity.[266] Finally, it has been speculated that the subtle abnormalities in the metabolism of cortisol to cortisone could contribute to elevated blood pressure in other patients with essential hypertension.[256]

Deoxycorticosterone

DOC is as potent as aldosterone in eliciting mineralocorticoid responses, but its free concentrations in plasma are normally too low to contribute substantially to plasma mineralocorticoid activity (Chap. 12). Exogenous DOC can lead to hypertension in animal models of hypertension and in humans.[267–270] Secretion of DOC is predominantly under ACTH control (Chap. 12). States in which DOC produces mineralocorticoid-excess hypertension are described in the section on deoxycorticosterone-excess hypertension. These states occur with adrenal enzymatic defects, in some patients with Cushing's syndrome, and in rare patients with predominantly DOC-secreting tumors (Chap. 12).

19-Nor-Deoxycorticosterone (19-Nor-DOC)

19-Nor-DOC is produced in the adrenals, the kidney, and aldosterone-producing adenomas from precursors synthesized in the adrenal and has mineralocorticoid activity equivalent to that of aldosterone.[267,271] Its adrenal production is regulated by ACTH.[271] It has not been detected in normal plasma.[271] Elevated levels of urinary 19-nor-DOC have been found in three rat models of hypertension[267] and in the plasma of patients with aldosterone-producing adenomas.[271] Thus, this steroid is a candidate for contributing to mineralocorticoid action in primary aldosteronism, although its importance is unknown.

Other Steroids

Several other steroids have mineralocorticoid activity, including 18-hydroxydeoxycorticosterone (10-OH-DOC), 18-hydroxycorticosterone (18-OHB), 19-nor-DOC, 10-oxo-cortisol, 18-OH-cortisol, and 18-deoxy-19-noraldosterone. 18-OH-DOC, 18-OHB, 18-oxo-cortisol, and 18-OH-cortisol have weak mineralocorticoid activity. 18-OH-DOC production is predominantly under ACTH control (Chap. 12), and its levels are elevated in ACTH-excess states.[267] Given the weak activities and low levels of 10-OH-DOC and 18-OHB, these steroids are unlikely to contribute to known mineralocorticoid-excess states.[272] 18-Deoxy-19-noraldosterone has potent mineralocorticoid antagonist activity and is made in normal and adenomatous adrenal tissue,[273] and the aldosterone metabolites dihydroaldosterone and tetrahydroaldosterone can elevate the blood pressure in rats;[274] however, the importance of these steroids is not documented.

Mechanisms of Mineralocorticoid Elevation of Blood Pressure

Mineralocorticoids regulate ion transport in secretory tissues, such as sweat glands, salivary glands, kidney, and intestinal tract, and possibly in arterial walls (see Chap. 12). These actions promote Na^+ reabsorption and secretion of K^+ and H^+.[275,276] The effects of mineralocorticoids on the kidney are the greatest quantitatively.

Mineralocorticoid excess leads to sodium retention, increased extracellular fluid volume, and increased total body sodium content. The changes are reflected by normal or elevated serum sodium ion concentrations and a reduced hematocrit.[277] The increased extracellular fluid volume suppresses plasma renin levels and abolishes the usual parallel relations between renin and aldosterone.[278]

Sodium and fluid overload are essential for the initiation of mineralocorticoid hypertension,[279] although this may not be the sole mechanism.[280,281] Continued sodium retention increases the intracellular sodium content in tissues.[282] Excess intracellular Na^+ increases intracellular $[Ca^{2+}]$, which enhances vascular reactivity (see the section on Ca^{2+} and hypertension below). These changes can further elevate the blood pressure. However, in some studies, intracellular $[Ca^{2+}]$ was not found to be elevated in the platelets of patients with primary aldosteronism.[283]

Mineralocorticoid excess also leads to a depletion of potassium and magnesium. Potassium depletion results in hypokalemia, alkalosis and increased ammonia production,[284] decreased carbohydrate tolerance, and resistance to vasopressin (nephrogenic diabetes insipidus). Depletion of K^+ also causes diminished adrenergic nervous system activity, decreased catecholamine levels, abnormalities in baroreceptor functions, and postural falls in blood pressure without reflex tachycardia.[276,285] Baroreceptor function may also be more directly affected by aldosterone.[286] These influences enhance blood pressure dependency on intravascular volume and decrease dependency on the nervous system. Hypokalemia also creates a special problem with diuretic therapy in these patients; such therapy can precipitously lower both the blood pressure and serum K^+ concentrations to dangerously low levels. Severe hypokalemia can also lead to renal damage with scarring and the development of renal cysts.[287] The hypomagnesemia increases vascular activity (see also the section on magnesium) and perpetuates the hypertension.

Direct actions of aldosterone on other organ systems, such as the vasculature and the CNS, may also contribute to the production of hypertension, but the role of these influences is not known. For example, in rats, injection of either aldosterone or glycyrrhetinic acid (which blocks the conversion of cortisol to cortisone) into the CNS causes hypertension.[288] Mineralocorticoids can increase ouabain-sensitive Na^+-K^+-ATPase activity.[289]

Some time (e.g., weeks to months) is required for mineralocorticoid hypertension to develop. Short-term administration of large amounts of mineralocorticoids to normotensive subjects has modest effects on blood pressure, even though the mineralocorticoid promotes sodium retention.[290–293] The time course of the development of mineralocorticoid hypertension can be observed after withdrawal of spironolactone therapy in patients with primary aldosteronism whose blood pressures have been normalized with the drug.[282,292] When this antimineralocorticoid therapy is withdrawn, these patients begin to retain sodium and gain weight until the usual mineralocorticoid "escape" occurs, and they develop progressive renal potassium wasting. Their blood pressures increase only gradually over a period of weeks. The hypertension is sodium- and volume-dependent, but sodium restriction does not prevent it.[282] Thus, more slowly developing events in the arteriole, such as intracellular changes in ionic concentrations or other effects on vascular reactivity, also must take place to produce the sustained elevated blood pressure of long-term mineralocorticoid administration.

With the development of sustained hypertension, as with all forms of hypertension, the body apparently attempts to compensate by decreasing the plasma volume. Thus, even though the increased level of exchangeable sodium and extracellular fluid volume persists, patients with long-established hypertension can have normal blood volumes.[282] Under these circumstances, the hypertension may be due to a large extent to the increased peripheral vascular resistance with normal cardiac output.[280–282] Nevertheless, even in this circumstance, continued mineralocorticoid actions contribute to the hypertensive state: Removal of an adenoma or treatment of hyperplasia with mineralocorticoid antagonists can ameliorate the hypertension. Rarely, the hypertension can progress to a malignant phase and stimulate the kidney to relase renin, resulting in a "high-renin" primary aldosteronism state.[294]

A number of other changes are observed in mineralocorticoid-excess states. Some of these changes may be secondary to the hypertension, and in most cases their participation in the development of the hypertension has not been established. There can be an impairment of endothelium-dependent vasodilation.[295] Unlike the case with essential hypertension, this is not blunted by blocking prostaglandin synthesis.[295] The decreased adrenergic system activity discussed above also may be influenced by increases in plasma ANP.[296] By contrast, in deoxycorticosterone acetate (DOCA)-salt hypertensive animals, there is a secondary increase in vasopressin and plasma catecholamines.[297,298] There is also increased endothelin-1 in the blood vessels of these rats, which could contribute to the increased blood pressure.[299]

Mineralocorticoid excess also may have direct effects on organs. It can induce fibrosis in the myocardium and other tissues in excess of that expected from the hypertension alone; this can affect myocardial stiffness, cardiac hypertrophy, and cardiac arrhythmias.[300,301]

Mineralocorticoids and Essential Hypertension

It is not known whether mineralocorticoid action contributes to essential hypertension. As dissussed in the section on primary aldosteronism, the answer to this question is complicated by the fact that primary aldosteronism may be more common than previously suspected in patients currently thought to have essential hypertension. The relations between low-renin essential hypertension and primary aldosteronism were discussed in the section on low-renin essential hypertension.

As discussed above in the section on the role of the renin-agiotensin system in hypertension, aldosterone levels tend to be normal to low in patients with essential hypertension with normal or suppressed renin levels, and these patients do not have other stigmata of mineralocorticoid excess, such as hypokalemia. However, mineralocorticoid excess can elevate the blood pressure in the absence of frank stigmata of mineralocorticoid excess (see section on glucocorticoid-remediable aldosteronism).[302–304] Therefore, normal aldosterone levels in many patients with essential hypertension may be inappropriate and contribute to blood pressure elevation.

Participation of mineralocorticoid activity in essential hypertension is suggested by studies with spironolactone. This drug reduces both systolic and diastolic blood pressure in patients with essential hypertension.[305,306] Further, the overall effects in patients over 50 years of age were comparable to those of a converting enzyme inhibitor.[306] However, it is difficult to intrepret the results of treatment with spironolactone. First, this antimineralocorticoid has significant side effects (largely gynecomastia in men and menstrual irregularities in women) (see the section on primary aldosteronism)[305] that limit the dose that can be given. Second, spironolactone may have other mechanisms of action, for example, to block actions of endogenous Na^+-K^+-ATPase inhibitors.[307]

Glucocorticoids

The natural glucocorticoid cortisol and the synthetic steroids used in glucocorticoid therapy can elevate the blood pressure through their actions as glucocorticoids. These effects are independent of any mineralocorticoid activities of these steroids (Fig. 14-10). Circumstances in which cortisol can cause mineralocorticoid-excess hypertension through mineralocorticoid-receptor interactions are discussed above and in the section on the other low-renin hypertension syndromes. The importance of glucocorticoids in maintaining normal blood pressure is demonstrated by the hypotension that occurs in adrenal insufficiency; this is correctable with glucocorticoid but not mineralocorticoid replacement (see Chap. 12).

Clinical features of hypertension in patients with spontaneous and iatrogenic Cushing's syndrome are described in the section on Cushing's syndrome. Most patients with spontaneous Cushing's syndrome have hypertension (see also Chap. 12) without the sitgmata of frank mineralocorticoid excess.[268,308–311] It is thought that the glucocorticoid actions of cortisol in this condition is predominantly responsible for the hypertension.

Additional evidence for blood pressure–elevating actions of glucocorticoids is derived from studies of responses to administered steroids. Synthetic glucocorticoids such as prednisolone, methylprednisolone, triamcinolone, and dexamethasone have much lower relative mineralocorticoid activity than does cortisol (see Chaps. 12 and 15) but can all increase the blood pressure. However, in short-term experiments, the effects are modest.[312] Estimates of the incidence of hypertension in patients treated with glucocorticoids have ranged from 17 to 69 percent.[302,311,314–317] The lower range of these values is not very different from the incidence of hypertension in the general population of around 20 percent.[1,2] Since hypertension in spontaneous Cushing's syndrome may be aggravated by mineralocorticoid actions of the cortisol excess, the overall influences of glucocorticoids in causing hypertension may be modest.

Hypertension can also be induced in animals by administering glucocorticoids.[316,318–320] Dexamethasone-induced increases in blood pressure in these animals can be blocked by glucocorticoid but not mineralocorticoid antagonists, suggesting a role for the glucocorticoid receptor in mediating the blood pressure elevations (see Chap. 12).[318] Glucocorticoid action is also required for full expression of hypertension in the SHR.[320]

Blood pressure–elevating effects of glucocorticoids could be explained by a number of mechanisms (see Chap. 12). Candidate actions include glucocorticoid-mediated increases in plasma angiotensinogen[311] and prorenin levels.[312] These actions may partly explain why plasma renin levels are not suppressed in Cushing's syndrome.[311] Hypertension in patients with spontaneous Cushing's syndrome and high or normal plasma renin activity does respond well to converting enzyme inhibition.[267,311] Other actions to reduce the production of prostaglandins or components of the kallikrein-kinin system[311] (see Chap. 12), to enhance the sensitivity to pressor substances such as epinephrine and angiotensin II,[321] or on endothelial and smooth muscle cells and the heart also may contribute. Glucocorticoids can induce phenylethanolamine *N*-methyltransferase and in this way could increase epinephrine production; inhibitors of the enzyme can ameloriate glucocorticoid hypertension in rats.[322] Glucocorticoid-induced hypertension in these animals is blocked by lesions in the anterioventral third ventricle, implying steroid actions through the CNS.[319] Experimental cortisol-induced hypertension[311,323] is associated with increased cardiac output and forearm vascular responsiveness to norepinephrine, decreased total peripheral resistance, and no change in sympathetic tone. Blocking the increase in cardiac output with an α-adrenergic antagonist does not block the blood pressure rise.[311,323] There can be cortisol-induced Na^+ retention (that is mineralocorticoid- and possibly glucocorticoid receptor–independent),[324] and glucocorticoids can increase Na^+ influx into vascular smooth muscle cells.[325] It is possible that a combination of these influences is operative (Chap. 12).[326]

The question of whether variations in either the levels or the responsiveness of glucocorticoids could contribute to essential hypertension has also been considered. Offspring of parents with high blood pressures whose personal blood pressures were higher had higher plasma cortisol and angiotensinogen levels (mean, 14.0 μg/dl) than did those with lower personal blood pressures (9.6 μg/dl).[327] The offspring with higher blood pressures also had a greater likelihood of having a certain glucocorticoid receptor genotype.[327] Spontaneously hypertensive rats also have higher plasma corticosterone levels than do comparable Wistar-Kyoto (WKY) rats.[266] Further work will be required to assess the significance of these observations. The idea that glucocorticoid exposure to the fetus can contribute to hypertension is discussed above in the section on mineralocorticoids.

Corticotropin (ACTH)

Hypertension in spontaneous ACTH-excess states is described in the section on Cushing's syndrome. Hypertension can also be induced by ACTH treatment.[317,328] The increase in cortisol (corticosterone in the rat) is thought to be primarily responsible for the elevations in blood pressure, and the hypertension can be observed in the absence of suppressed plasma renin and hypokalemia. Nevertheless, DOC production is increased by ACTH treatment and could contribute to the blood pressure elevations. Other adrenal-derived steroids have also been proposed to participate in ACTH-induced elevations of blood pressure in sheep, but a role for these steroids in humans has not been established. Finally, the adrenal is a major source for the ouabain-like factor that may have blood pressure–elevating actions (discussed in a subsequent section), and the levels of this factor are increased with ACTH induction of hypertension in rats.[328]

Estrogens, Progestins, and Androgens

Men have higher blood pressures than women at younger ages, with a crossover in which women have higher pressures in the fourth to sixth decades.[1] There are no known sex differences in children. These studies raise the issue of the role of sex steroids in hypertension.

Little is known regarding the role of testosterone in hypertension in humans. In spontaneously hypertensive rats, genetic studies have linked the Y chromosome to hypertension.[329] Castration results in a lower blood pressure. Androgen-resistant animals have lower blood pressures than controls but have higher levels than females. Thus, both androgen action and other factors could be contributory.

Most women receiving oral contraceptives experience a small but detectable increase in blood pressure within the normal range.[1] A few women also experience blood pressure rises when estrogen replacement is initiated.[1] Hypertension is more common in women who have taken contraceptives for several years, and this incidence increases with the duration of use.[1] The mechanisms are not clear.[1] Estrogens can have vasodilatory actions in pregnancy and other conditions; these actions are probably due to estrogen-mediated effects on prostacyclin synthesis.[330,331] Estrogens can also increase the levels of angiotensinogen[139] and nitric oxide synthetase.[332,333] Progestin-only preparations are not known to cause hypertension.[330]

Thyroid Hormone

There are abnormalities in blood pressure in both hyperthyroidism and hypothyroidism. In hyperthyroidism, diastolic pressure may be decreased but systolic pressure is typically either increased or normal.[334–336] Hypothyroidism has been associated with diastolic hypertension.

Systolic hypertension with hyperthyroidism is due to increased cardiac stroke volume, whereas the decreased diastolic pressure is due to peripheral vasodilation. The increased cardiac stroke volume is probably due to direct thyroid hormone actions on the heart. Thyroid hormone excess can enhance cardiac β-adrenergic responsivenes and probably has other direct effects on tension development and shortening velocity.[334] Mechanisms for decreased diastolic pressure in hyperthyroidism are less well understood; increases in metabolism or Na^+-K^+-ATPase[336] may enhance vasodilator mechanisms in peripheral tissues.

The incidence of hypertension in patients with hypothyroidism has been difficult to document. In a survey of 688 consecutive hypertensive outpatients,[337] 3.6 percent were found to be hypothyroid. The blood pressures decreased in these patients with replacement thyroid hormone, suggesting a cause-and-effect relation. These data suggest that hypothyroidism may be one of the most common causes of secondary hypertension. Conversely, when the incidence of hypertension in patients with hypothyroidism is compared with that in the general population, an increased incidence is not evident.[336]

Changes with hypothyroidism are the converse of those with hyperthyroidism.There is increased vasoconstriction and decreased stroke volume. Patients with hypothyroidism also tend to have decreased plasma renin activity and angiotensinogen levels[334,337] and increased arginine vasopressin (AVP) levels. The significance of these changes is not known.

Vasopressin

AVP has potent vasoconstrictor properties in addition to its actions on the kidney to regulate water balance (Chap. 8). AVP is thought to regulate blood pressure mainly when other systems are suppressed.[338,339] The peptide interacts with three classes of receptors; V_{1a} and V_{1b} are linked to phospholipase C activation and calcium mobilization, and V_2 is linked to adenylyl cyclase activation (see Chap. 8). V_{1a} receptors probably mediate the effects of AVP on blood pressure. The use of vasopressin antagonists suggests that AVP elicits vasopressor activity in patients with severe accelerated hypertension and with diabetes with impaired sympathetic nervous system activity, when the activities of the sympathetic nervous or renin-angiotensin systems are blocked, and with salt loading. AVP has not been implicated in most forms of essential hypertension. However, it is not known whether AVP is active in other states, for example those in which there is modest impairment of sympathetic nervous system activity. AVP receptor blockade can decrease the blood pressure in the upright posture, implying a role for AVP in the maintenance of orthostatic blood pressure.[338] These effects were more prominent in elderly and black than in young and white patients.[338] Increased vasopressin may also play a role in DOCA-salt hypertension in which AVP levels are increased and the blood pressure can be reduced by means of the administration of antisera to vasopressin.[297]

Erythropoietin

Erythropoietin is used extensively to treat anemia of chronic renal disease.[340,341] Hypertension is the major complication with erythropoietin therapy. Mechanisms for these actions are not understood; candidates include increases in blood cell volumes and viscosity, diminished hypoxic vasodilation, and direct vasopressor effects. The effects on blood cell volume appear to be a minor contributor in short-term experiments. Vasoconstrictor effects tend to be observed only at high hormone concentrations. Erythropoietin may stimulate renal production of angiotensin II; the administration of erythropoietin to rats decreases sodium excretion with no change in glomerular filtration rate. These effects are blocked by captopril. It is not known whether endogenous erythropoietin is involved in blood pressure control; however, erythropoietin levels are increased with a high-salt diet.

Growth Hormone

Patients with acromegaly usually have hypertension (Chap. 8), and growth hormone–deficient adults treated with growth hormone can develop hypertension and fluid retention.[342] Growth hormone–deficient children treated with growth hormone generally do not develop hypertension but can have transient blood pressure elevation and some fluid retention.[343] The mechanisms are unknown. Growth hormone excess causes insulin resistance, but the transient blood pressure–elevating actions of growth hormone in children precede insulin resistance.[343] Growth hormone treatment has also been reported to increase the activity of the renin-angiotensin-aldosterone axis in adults,[342] but this has not been observed in children.[343] There is no evidence implicating growth hormone in the pathogenesis of essential hypertension.

Calcitonin Gene–Related Peptide

Calcitonin gene–related peptide (CGRP) has potent vasodilator actions and can lower blood pressure in humans and animals.[245,344,345] CGRP is produced in the CNS and in peripheral nerves in the vascular wall, and its receptors are widely distributed in the CNS and the cardiovascular system. The peptide can also increase urinary volume and sodium excretion, inhibit angiotensin II–mediated contraction of renal mesangial cells, and increase renal blood flow and glomerular filtration. Thus, it could be an important component of the vasodilatory system. Little is known about its potential function in hypertension. Measurements of the blood levels of the peptide, which may not reflect the hormone's autocrine or paracrine functions, have shown conflicting results, with elevations or depressions of the levels in essential hypertension, for example. CGRP levels have been reported to increase with calcium supplementation and lowering of the blood pressure in patients with essential hypertension, leading to speculation that the peptide could be involved in the hypotensive effects of calcium supplementation.[345]

Calcium-Regulating Hormones

The primary calcium-regulating hormones affect the blood pressure. These include parathyroid hormone (PTH), 1,25$(OH)_2$ vitamin D_3, and parathyroid gland hypotensive factor. A case can be made for a role for each of these factors in Ca^{2+} mediated influences on the blood pressure (see the section on Ca^{2+} and hypertension). However, these roles are undefined. Calcitonin has been reported to have blood pressure–lowering actions, but these effects are modest.[345]

Parathyroid Hormone and Parathyroid Hormone–Related Peptide

PTH and parathyroid hormone–related protein PTH-rp, can induce hypotension.[245,346,347] They relax vascular tissues by blocking voltage gated channels and reducing intracellular Ca^{2+} concentrations.[347] PTH may increase renin release[348] and potentiate the pressor effects of hypercalcemia.[349] Angiotensin II can increase PTH release; this may occur when angiotensin II levels increase in response to decreases in serum Ca^{2+}. Hypertension is commonly observed in primary hyperparathyroidism,[350] although this may be due to other hormones, such as parathyroid hypertensive factor (see below). Low-calcium diets that elevate PTH levels decrease the blood pressure–lowering effects of PTH.[245]

Vitamin D

Vitamin D is thought to act on the vasculature, but its role is poorly defined. 1,25$(OH)_2$ Vitamin D_3 increases vascular responses in mesenteric arteries,[351] increases blood pressure in Wistar rats,[351] modulates vascular cell growth,[351] and may have vasoconstrictor activities.[345] Administration of 1-α-$(OH)D_3$ has been reported to abolish calcium-induced decreases in blood pressure.[345] Conversely, vitamin D administration lowers the blood pressure in patients with primary hyperparathyroidism.[347]

Parathyroid Gland Hypertensinogenic Factor

A parathyroid gland hypertensinogenic factor has been proposed.[346,352,353] This factor may be released in response to salt ingestion, and its levels are increased in the plasma of patients with low renin and salt-sensitive hypertension, in spontaneously hypertensive DOCA-salt treated and Dahl-S rats and with low calcium intakes, but not in two-kidney, one-clip hypertensive rats. Parathyroid glands from spontaneously hypertensive rats transplanted to normotensive Sprague-Dawley or Wistar-Kyoto rats elevate the recipients' blood pressures and release the factor in the serum.[346] This factor could explain the influence of Ca^{2+} on blood pressure and demonstrate how both calcium antagonists and dietary calcium often reduce mean arterial pressure in the same patients.[346]

Endothelin

The vascular endothelium produces both vasoconstrictor and vasodilator substances. The vasoconstrictor substances include the endothelins[354–356] and PDGF; the vasodilator substances are discussed below.

The endothelins are a family of three peptides with extremely potent and sustained vasoconstrictor and vasopressor actions.[354–356] Infused endothelin induces transient vasodilation, followed by a profound and long-lasting increase in blood pressure. These peptides also potentiate the actions of vasopressors such as catecholamines, stimulate sympathetic tone, and induce the release of vasopressin and epinephrine. They also have proliferative effects on vascular smooth muscle and renal mesangial cells. Their actions can be inhibited by cGMP produced in response to vasodilators such as nitrous oxide and ANP.

Endothelin-1 predominates in the vascular endothelium and is generated from proendothelin-1 through the actions of a unique neutral metalloprotease, "endothelin-converting enzyme."[354–356] Certain vasoconstrictor substances, angiotensin II, catecholamines and vasopressin, and ouabain-like factors can increase endothelin production, and their actions may be mediated in part through endothelin. Endothelin appears to act predominantly paracrine, and its release is mainly abluminal.

There are at least two distinct endothelin receptor subtypes.[354,355] The ET_A receptor is preferentially activated by endothelin-1, highly expressed in vascular smooth muscle, and the major receptor subtype that causes vasoconstriction. Binding of endothelin with this receptor activates phosphoinositide hydrolysis and/or calcium channels. The ET_B receptor is activated equally by all three endothelin subtypes and is present on the luminal surface of endothelial cells, where it mediates release of endothelium-dependent vasodilator substances. It is also present in smooth muscle in some tissues where it participates in vasoconstrictor actions. The existence of the ET_C subtype remains controversial. Specific endothelin receptor antagonists can inhibit pressure responses to the peptide.

The potential of endothelin to cause hypertension is suggested by the rare occurrence of hemangioendotheliomas. These tumors release large amounts of endothelin into the circulation, and patients with these tumors have profound hypertension.[356] Removal of the tumor ameloriates the hypertension and lowers plasma endothelin levels.

A role for endothelin in essential hypertension has not been established. Plasma concentrations of endothelin may be a poor reflection of endothelin-1 activity, given the probable paracrine/autocrine activities of the peptide. Nevertheless, most studies suggest that circulating levels of endothelin are not increased or modestly increased in patients with essential hypertension.[354,355]

However, the data suggest that endothelin does play a role in malignant hypertension, other specialized circumstances, and certain animal models.[354,355] Plasma concentrations of endothelin are elevated[354,355] in conditions associated with vasoconstriction, such as heart failure, pulmonary hypertension, vasospastic disorders (Raynaud's disease, Prinzmetal's angina), and myocardial infarction. Increased tissue concentrations of and/or binding sites for endothelin-1 have been found in sustained cerebral vasospasm after subarachnoid hemmorhage. Circulating endothelin levels can be elevated with renal failure, atherosclerosis, severe hypertension and end organ complications, and disseminated intravascular coagulation.[354,356] Endothelin-converting enzyme inhibitors and receptor antagonists decrease hypertension in spontaneously hypertensive and DOCA-sensitive salt-treated rats.[354,355] An ET_A-specific antagonist ameloriated renal dysfunction and structural changes in a rat model of renal failure, and the stroke-prone SHR but not in the normal SHR.[340] Thus, endothelin may be more important in more malignant forms of hypertension.

Studies of endothelin have been complicated by the observation that vascular responsiveness to the peptide varies in different parts of the body.[345] For example, reduced sensitivity has been reported in the aorta and mesenteric arteries of spontaneously hypertensive, DOCA-salt-sensitive, and two-kidney, one-clip renovascular hypertensive rats and in hypertensive humans. This could reflect endothelin-induced down regulation of endothelin responsiveness. Conversely, enhanced responses to endothelin have been reported in the renal arteries of spontaneously hypertensive rats, and enhanced release of the peptide has been reported in the mesenteric arteries of spontaneously hypertensive and salt-sensitive Dahl rats.

Cyclosporin-induced hypertension may be mediated in part through endothelin release.[354] Cyclosporin A increases plasma levels of endothelin and increases endothelin release from cells in culture. Endothelin receptor antagonists protect against cyclosporin toxicity in the rat renal circulation.

Nitric Oxide (Endothelium-Derived Releasing Factor)

The endothelium is important for vasodilator responses and is necessary for the vasodilator actions of bradykinin and acetylcholine. The endothelium releases relaxing factors, termed endothelium-derived relaxing factors (EDRFs). The major EDRF appears to be nitric oxide (NO), a water-soluble gas. EDRF is responsible for the vasodilator tone that is essential for the regulation of blood pressure[98,332,333] (Fig. 14-11). The molecule also regulates a number of other diverse functions, including neurotransmitter,

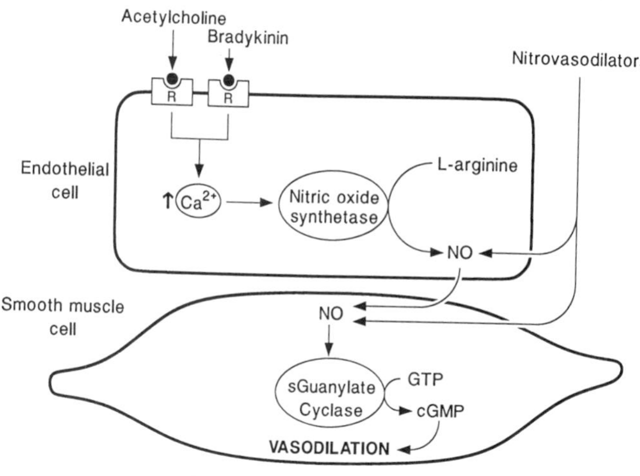

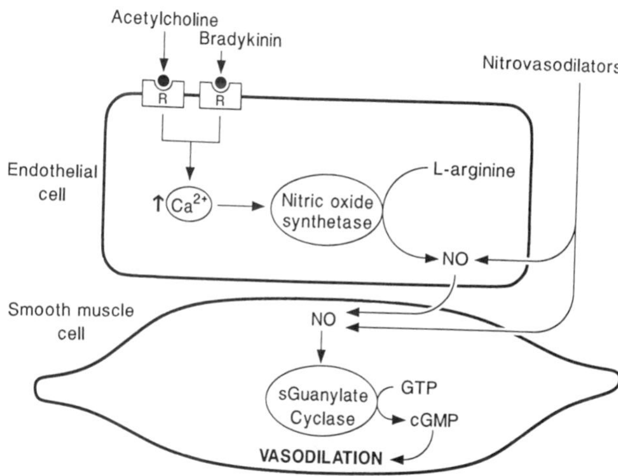

FIGURE 14-11 Synthesis and actions of nitric oxide (NO). s = soluble. The arrow next to the Ca^{2+} indicates that bradykinin and acetylcholine increase intracellular Ca^{2+}. Cytokines can induce Ca^{2+}-independent NO synthetase, and this can be blocked by glucocorticoids (not shown). *(From Moncada and Higgs.[332])*

platelet aggregation, gastrointestinal, genitourinary, respiratory, inflammatory, and immunologic processes,[332] as well as renin release[98] and cardiac hypertrophy.[99] Endogenously produced NO appears to act predominantly in a paracrine or autocrine manner.

All known NO actions are mediated by the activation of soluble guanylate cyclase. NO binds directly to a heme prosthetic group of this enzyme. Actions of the cGMP formed directly induce vasorelaxation and inhibit the production of other vasoconstrictor substances, such as endothelin.[357]

Nitric oxide is produced by nitric oxide synthetases from L-arginine.[155,332,333] There are at least three different enzymes. A major form of the enzyme is constitutive, and its activity is dependent on calcium and calmodulin. This enzyme is activated by acetylcholine and bradykinin, which increase intracellular Ca^{2+}. Other forms are inducible, for example, with cytokines; this induction can be blocked by glucocorticoids. Estrogens induce nitric oxide synthetase in some cases. Most of the NO is released from the vascular endothelium, although there can be some release from nonadrenergic, noncholinergic terminals. The actions of nitric oxide are mimicked by compounds such as nitroglycerin and sodium nitroprusside, which are converted to nitric oxide.

Competitive inhibitors of nitric oxide synthetase, such as N^G-monomethyl-L-arginine, have been useful for studying the role of NO in blood pressure control. These inhibitors are potent vasoconstrictors and can produce decreased forearm blood flow responses in patients with essential hypertension.[333,358] Inhibition of nitric oxide synthetase in animals induces hypertension and glomerular damage,[333,359,360] exacerbates the development of cardiac hypertrophy,[361] and attenuates pressure-induced natriuresis.[362] Hypertension induced by blockade of the enzyme in Wistar rats was prevented by an angiotensin II receptor antagonist but not by sodium restriction.[363]

Endothelium-dependent relaxation may be involved in various forms of hypertension.[155,332,333,358–369] Acetylcholine activates NO synthetase and is a probe for endothelium-dependent relaxation. Several groups have reported that the vasodilator response to acetylcholine is decreased in patients with essential hypertension,[332,364,367–369] although these findings have been disputed.[370] These defects have not been reversed with hypertensive therapy. This finding suggests that in essential hypertension there is defective EDRF action and that the defect, if it exists, either is primary or becomes long-standing with time.[368]

The putative defect in hypertension appears to reside in the ability to synthetize NO rather than respond to it.[369] This is suggested by the lack of differences in response to nitroprusside between normotensive and hypertensive subjects.[344]

Studies addressing whether there is a defect in the availability of the NO precursor, arginine, in essential hypertension have yielded conflicting results. In support of such a defect, arginine infusion decreased the blood pressure in normal subjects and patients with essential hypertension.[332,365] However, in other studies, intraarterial administration of L-arginine failed to augment the forearm vascular response to acetylcholine in patients with essential hypertension but did so in normal subjects.[367]

Reduced vasodilation in response to activators of nitric oxide synthetase can occur as a secondary phenomenon. This is observed in primary aldosteronism and renovascular hypertension.[369] However, patients with essential hypertension differed from

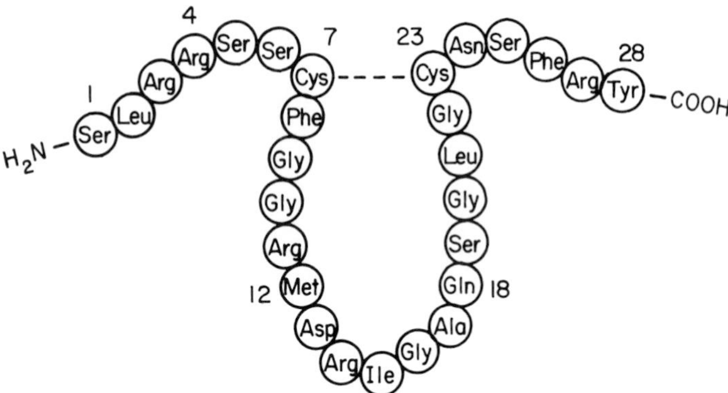

FIGURE 14-12 Structure of human atrial natriuretic peptide. *(Data from Schwartz et al.*[372] *and Greenberg et al.*[373]*)*

those with primary aldosteronism or renovascular hypertension in that a cyclooxygenase inhibitor increased the vasodilatory effect of acetylcholine only in the essential hypertensives. This result implies that eicosanoid-dependent vasoconstrictor mechanisms may blunt endothelium-dependent vasodilation in essential hypertension.[369]

Overall, the data suggests that the cardiovascular system is in a state of active vasodilation but that there is defective NO action in certain forms of hypertension. However, it remains to be clarified whether the abnormalities are primary or secondary and how they are generated.

Impairment in endothelium-dependent vasorelaxation also occurs in hypertensive animals. For example, in hypertensive rats, blockade of NO synthetase produces smaller increases in arterial pressure,[366] and there are blunted vasodilator responses to acetylcholine[369] compared to control rats. Arginine administration prevents the development of hypertension in several types of animal models[332,363,365] but not in DOCA-salt hypertension,[366] implying differences in the mechanisms for the attenuation.

Endothelium-Derived Hyperpolarizing Factor (EDHF)

Endothelium-derived hyperpolarizing factor (EDHF) is a vasodilator that is distinct from NO.[371] Its existence can explain endothelium-dependent vasorelaxation that is resistant to inhibition of nitric oxide synthetase and cyclooxygenase. It contributes to endothelium-dependent vasorelaxation by opening K^+ channels in the vascular smooth muscle. It can be induced by bradykinin. The identity of EDHF and its role in hypertension are unknown.

Atrial Natriuretic Peptides

Atrial natriuretic peptides constitute a family of hormones that oppose influences that elevate the blood pressure and promote sodium retention (Figs. 14-12 and 14-13).[372,373] Thus, they guard against excessive increases in blood pressure and fluid volume. However, the actions of these peptides are extensive and complex. deBold[374] first demonstrated that atrial extracts possess vasodilatory and natriuretic activity. It was known even earlier that the cardiac atrium contains secretory granules[374,375] and that atrial distension causes diuresis, bradycardia, hypotension, and a release of the granules.[374,375] This work led to the characterization of the atrial natriuretic peptides and to the recognition that the heart is a major endocrine organ (Figs. 14-12 and 14-13).[374–376]

Production and Forms

Natriuretic peptides are encoded by at least three genes. These genes encode ANP, brain natriuretic peptide (BNP), and C-type natriuretic peptide (CNP).

ANP is a 28-amino acid peptide (Fig. 14-12) that is derived from the carboxy terminus of a 126-amino acid precursor protein (pro-ANP) that is stored in the heart.[374–380] ANP is cleaved from pro-ANP with release of the storage vesicles and secretion of ANP.[374,376–378] The major sites of ANP production are the cardiac atria.[374,375,378] The right atrium produces more ANP than does the left.[374,375] ANP is produced in much lower quantities in the ventricles and in other tissues, where the peptide probably exerts autocrine or paracrine actions.[381] These include lung, aortic arch, CNS, and pituitary.[381,382]

Urodilan contains 32 amino acids that are derived from the carboxy terminus of pro-ANP.[378,383] It is produced in the kidney and has not been detected in other tissues or in the circulation.[378] It is resistant to endopeptidase and is more stable than ANP and may be more effective than ANP in the kidney.[378]

BNP contains 32 amino acids and is cleaved from the carboxy terminus of a 108-amino acid precursor protein.[384–386] BNP was originally discovered in the brain, but the major source of the peptide are the cardiac ventricles.[385,386] BNP has a high homology to ANP.[384]

CNP is a 22-amino acid peptide derived from the carboxy terminus of a larger precursor protein.[378,385]

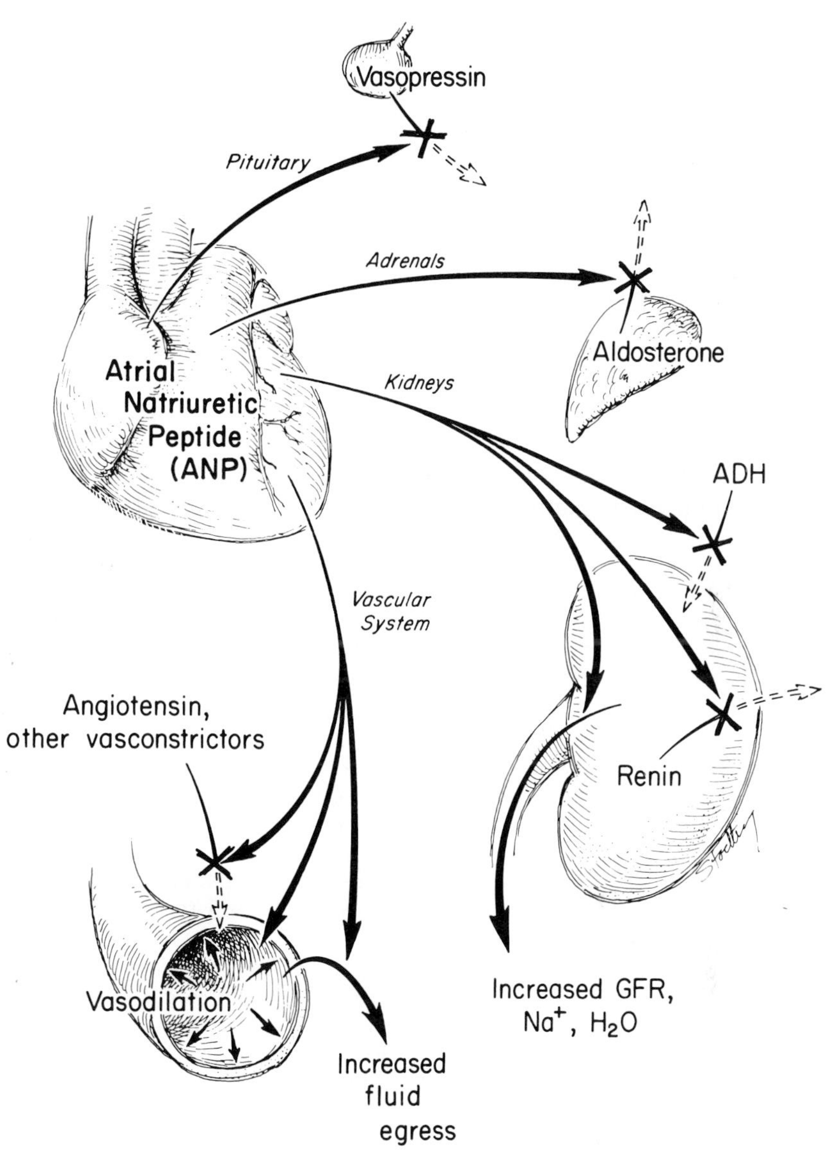

FIGURE 14-13 Actions of ANP.

It is produced predominantly in the CNS, where it acts as a neuropeptide.[378] It has also been found in the kidney and in vascular endothelial cells.[378,380]

Regulation of Release

Regulation of the release of the three types of peptides differs. The major control of ANP release is through stretch influences on the atria.[374–377,382,387] By contrast, BNP release is thought to be mostly constitutive but is also increased with left ventricular hypertrophy and in heart failure.[386,388] Little is known about the regulation of CNP.

Stretch influences that increase ANP release occur through stimuli such as vasopressors, volume increases, postural changes, tachycardia, and mineralocorticoid treatment.[374–377,382,387,389] ANP release also may be increased by glucocorticoid and thyroid hormones.[390] Synthesis of the peptide is also increased in the ventricles in myocardial adaptations such as heart failure and cardiac hypertrophy, along with other proteins, including embryonic contractile protein isoforms (myosin light chain-2, α-myosin heavy chain, and skeletal α-actin).[390a]

ANP has a half-life in the circulation of only a few minutes.[374] The peptide is eliminated through three routes.[386,391,392] First, there is loss by renal glomerular filtration. Second, elimination through the C-type "clearance" receptors (see below) is the most important quantitatively. Third, ANP is cleaved at a Cys-Phe bond within its 17-member ring by a neutral endopeptidase 24.11 (NEP). This enzyme also cleaves insulin, kinins, and other peptides and is widely distributed in the body.[386,391,392] BNP is cleared more slowly than is ANP and has a plasma half-life of around 19 mins.[379,388]

Radioimmunoassays yield normal plasma levels of ANP to 6 to 8 p*M*, of BNP of around 4 to 6 p*M*, and no detectable CNP.[378–380,393] Levels of ANP and BNP are increased with age, essential hypertension, primary aldosteronism, pheochromocytoma, renal failure, and heart failure.[379,384,393–395] ANP levels are elevated with paroxysmal atrial arrhythmias.[374–376] BNP levels are not affected by acute atrial or ventricular pacing.[379] BNP plasma levels are elevated in left ventricular hypertrophy.[384,386]

Actions

The actions of ANP and BNP are similar.[386,388] These actions are natriuretic, diuretic, and vasorelaxant and tend to oppose the effects of other sodium- and water-retaining and pressor stimuli (Fig. 14-13).

In the kidney, ANP increases the glomerular filtration rate (GFR) and the renal excretion of water and sodium, chloride, magnesium, calcium, and phosphate ions.[377,385,394,396–398] ANP has either no effect or a modest effect on potassium and hydrogen ion excretion. The effects of ANP on sodium and water excretion are due to direct actions on renal tubules, although these are enhanced by its effects on the GFR.[394,398] ANP inhibits water and Na^+ reabsorption in the inner medullary and cortical collecting ducts, blocks AVP actions, and decreases Cl^-reabsorption in the juxtamedullary loop of Henele.[398] The increase in GFR is due to afferent glomerular arteriolar dilatation, efferent arteriolar constriction, and possibly other effects on glomerular cells. The hormone modifies intrarenal hemodynamics by increasing blood flow through the middle and outer cortices, medulla, and papilla.[376,377,397] Effects on total renal blood flow are variable; ANP can block renal artery vasoconstriction in response to other agents[377,399] but increases renal plasma flow in patients with essential hypertension.[394]

ANP blunts the release of several classes of hormones, including renin, AVP, aldosterone, and catecholamines.[374–377,385,392,396,399–402] Effects on renin release blunt increases in response to a variety of stimuli and lower plasma renin levels. The effects are more prominent when there is excessive renin production, as with renovascular hypertension. These effects could be due to increased delivery of NaCl to the macula densa, renal vasodilation, or direct effects on juxtaglomerular cells.

The effects on aldosterone are observed under basal conditions and in response to angiotensin II, K^+, cAMP, prostaglandins, or ACTH. ANP does not affect cortisol release. These actions are independent of effects on renin and involve early steps in steroid biosynthesis.

ANP has additional actions, independent of its effects on fluid balance, that can lower blood pressure.[375,377,392,394,403–406] These actions promote vasodilation, decrease thirst, and induce shifts from the intravascular to the interstitial spaces. The vasodilatory actions of ANP are direct and can also oppose the actions of other vasoconstrictors. ANP also blunts baroreceptor responses; this effect favors bradycardia and opposes increases in heart rate. These actions are relatively selective in their effects on specific vascular beds.

ANP has growth-inhibitory properties and blocks the actions of other growth factors in several tissues, including the adrenal glomerulosa, vascular smooth muscle, and renal glomerular mesangial cells.[407,408]

Molecular Mechanisms of Action

Three different receptors mediate ANP action.[378,383,385,392,398,407–409] Two of these are membrane-bound guanylate cyclases. The ANP-A (ANP-$R_{GC(A)}$) guanylate cyclase–linked receptor binds ANP≥ BNP>>CNP. The ANP-B (ANP-$R_{GC(B)}$, also called the CNP receptor) guanylate cyclase–linked receptor binds CNP>ANP≥BNP. The third receptor, the ANP-C receptor (ANP-R_c), was formerly called the clearance receptor. This receptor serves to degrade ANP and is also linked to inhibition of adenylyl cyclase and phosphoinositide hydrolysis. The ANP-C receptor has less specificity for binding various ANP compounds and can bind truncated versions of ANP. It binds ANP>CNP>BNP.

Mechanisms by which the cGMP generated in response to ANP affects various responses are being unraveled.[409] ANP-stimulated cGMP inhibits hormone secretion in the pituitary by increasing membrane conductance to potassium by activating large-conductance calcium- and voltage-activated potassium channels through protein dephosphorylation. cGMP activates a kinase that activates protein phosphatase 2A, which regulates these channels. By simultaneously inhibiting calcium channels and activating potassium channels, ANP could profoundly reduce electrical excitability.

The specific effects mediate by each of the receptors are being deciphered.[378,380,392,401,402,408] All three receptor forms are widely distributed, but there are differences in their relative expression in various tissues. For example, ANPR-A is preferentially expressed in endothelial cells.[380] The ANP-C receptor accounts for over 90 percent of the total ANP receptors in most cell types. Nevertheless, most effects appear to be mediated through the other guanylyl cyclase–linked receptors, for example, those in the kidney, and through aldosterone release in the adrenal. However, other actions, such as suppression of sympathetic neurotransmission, occur independently of guanylyl cyclase activation.

Role in Hypertension and Heart Failure

The elevations of ANP and BNP in essential hypertension and heart failure discussed above imply that these hormones counteract elevations of blood pressure and fluid overload in these conditions.[384,394,395,400,410] There is blunted responsiveness to ANP in heart failure. It has been reported that there is impaired release of ANP in patients with salt-sensitive essential hypertension.[411] It is not known whether there are any primary abnormalities in ANP in hypertension. Effects of infused ANP on systemic hemodynamics are more, not less, pronounced in patients with essential hypertension.[394]

Therapeutic Uses of ANP

ANP, BNP, urodilatin, and analogues and inhibitors of neutral endopeptidase show promise for their usefulness in treating hypertension, renal failure, heart failure, and other indications.[383,386,387,391,392,394,400,412–414] The short half-life of ANP has limited its effectiveness as a therapeutic agent. BNP may be more effective. The neutral endopeptidase inhibitors can be given orally. Even though the neutral endopeptidase is responsible for a minority of ANP clearance, administration of inhibitors of it elevate plasma levels of ANP (but suppress BNP levels), lower blood pressure, and induce natriuresis.

Catecholamines and the Autonomic Nervous System

Catecholamines, the autonomic nervous system, and the CNS are involved in multiple aspects of blood pressure control and essential hypertension. The synthesis, actions, and molecular actions of catecholamines are described in Chaps. 4, 5, and 13. Hypertension due to catecholamine-producing tumors is addressed in Chap. 13. Many aspects of catecholamines relevant to blood pressure control are described in other sections of this chapter. The role of beta-adrenergic activation in regulation of renin release and that of angiotensin II in stimulating adrenergic activity are described above in the section on the renin-angiotensin system. The role of adrenergic mechanisms in obesity, insulin resistance and salt-sensitivity of blood pressure responses, stimulation by insulin and food intake of central adrenergic activity, and use of drugs that affect sympathetic nervous system activity are described below in the section on obesity, insulin, and insulin resistance in hypertension. The role of the sympathetic nervous system in hypertension is also reflected by the usefulness of drugs that affect adrenergic activity in treating essential hypertension.[120,233] Although an extensive analysis of the role of the autonomic nervous system in blood pressure control is beyond the scope of this chapter, certain comments may be useful.

Several aspects of the release of and the responsiveness to catecholamines may be inappropriate in certain subgroups of individuals with essential hypertension.[19,27,120,233,415] Studies of plasma levels of catecholamines are complicated by the fact that norepinephrine levels are determined by spillover of the catecholamine into the blood, which reflects a small proportion of its release; differences could reflect either production or elimination, and there are regional differences in activity in various states.[120,233]

Nevertheless, the sympathetic nervous system appears overall to be overactive in essential hypertension.[120,233] Plasma norepinephrine levels are higher in young patients with essential hypertension than in control subjects.[120,223] Plasma norepinephrine levels increase with age.[120,233] These increases are greater in normotensives than in hypertensives, so that differences in plasma norepinephrine levels are blunted with advancing age. This may explain some of the controversy regarding differences between normotensives and hypertensives.[27,120,233] There is also enhanced regional release of norepinephrine in essential hypertension that is selective for the heart and kidneys.[120,233,415] It has been proposed that as hypertension progresses, there is a transition from hyperkinetic, sympathetic nervous system–dependent hypertension to a state of increased vascular resistance with normal sympathetic nervous system activity.[120] Plasma epinephrine levels are usually normal or elevated in essential hypertension.[120] Dopamine exerts natriuretic actions in and is produced in the kidneys.[233] Plasma levels of conjugated dopamine appear to be elevated, but urinary free dopamine is depressed in essential hypertension.[120,233] Decreased dopamine levels or responses could result in impaired sodium excretion.[233] Abnormal dopamine-receptor coupling has been linked to the hypertension in the Okomato-Aoki SHR.[416]

Neuropeptide Y is a 36-amino acid peptide that is coreleased with norepinephrine and epinephrine, has vasoconstrictor activities, and can inhibit norepinephrine release.[417] This peptide is found in brain, adrenal medulla, and peripheral nerves.[417] It has been proposed to be involved in blood pressure control, but there is insufficient evidence to determine its role. A neuropeptide Y locus on chromosome 4 of the SHR cosegregates with blood pressure.[418]

There is also evidence for enhanced pressor sensitivity to catecholamines in essential hypertension.[120,233] β-adrenergic blockers and other sympatholytic agonists produce greater depressor responses in essential hypertensive than in normotensive subjects.[120] Blood pressure responses to these agents are correlated with plasma norepinephrine levels.[120] This enhanced responsiveness in the fact of excessive norepinephrine production differs from the usual case of negative regulation of adrenergic responsiveness by catecholamines (see Chap. 5). Firing rates of sympathetic nerves are increased in young patients with essential hypertension and are normal to increased in essential hypertension in general.[120,233] There is a blunting in some essential hypertensives of baroreceptor-mediated heart rate slowing and reduced sympathetic nervous system activity in response to blood pressure increases.[19] Efferent renal nerve sympathetic nerve activity is elevated in essential hypertension and in several animal models of hypertension.[415] This enhanced renal activity is influenced by dietary sodium and environmental stress, tends to be inherited, and influences renal sodium handling and renin release.[415]

The reasons for enhanced sympathetic nervous system activity in many patients with essential hypertension are not fully understood. However, since enhanced activity is common in the general hypertensive population, it may reflect the common abnormalities discussed in other sections. These include (1) stimulation of sympathetic nervous system activity by insulin, food intake, and obesity and possible associated ion transport defects; (2) defective salt-induced decreases in adrenergic nervous system activity in salt-sensitive essential hypertension; and (3) inappropriate angiotensin II activity that might stimulate adrenergic activity in some salt-sensitive hypertensives (modulators). Other factors that have been proposed include a sedentary lifestyle, stress and behavorial factors, and primary CNS defects.[233] There have also been extensive studies of various adrenergic receptors in humans and in animal models of hypertension.[419] A number of changes have been found that are mostly secondary. However, there is evidence linking the α_{2A}-adrenoreceptor in genetic hypertension of the SHR.[419] It has been speculated that there may be primary abnormalities in this receptor for some humans with essential hypertension.[419]

Prostaglandins and Other Eicosanoids

Prostaglandins and other eicosanoids are not known to act as hormones but play extensive roles in the regulation of processes related to blood pressure control as autocrine and paracrine factors. These actions affect the release of renin and other hormones, renal functions, and systemic resistance vessels.[420]

Eicosanoids have received intensive study in terms of their roles in essential hypertension and other forms of hypertension.[420] There are discussions about these agents in several parts of this chapter, including the sections on the renin-angiotensin system; kallikreins and kinins; endothelial-derived releasing factors; ions, hormones, and blood pressure; obesity, insulin, and insulin resistance; mineralocorticoids; and glucocorticoids. Thus, whereas an extensive discussion of their actions is outside the focus of this chapter, some general comments are warranted.

Evidence for a role of prostaglandins in essential hypertension has been obtained through the observation that inhibitors of cyclooxygenase blunt the response to hypertensive therapy.[421] These inhibitors can also selectively elevate blood pressure and decrease urinary Na^+ excretion in salt-sensitive hypertensives.[421] In this case, sodium sensitivity, rather than the renin status, appears to be the better indicator of a hypotensive response. Blood pressure is lowered by dietary omega-3 polyunsaturated fatty acids that increase vasodilatory prostaglandin biosynthesis. Salt sensitivity in the SHR is accelerated by cicletanine which stimulates prostaglandin production; this may work through prostaglandin-induced renal hemodynamic changes.[422]

Thromboxane A_2 has potent vasoconstrictor actions, and prostaglandin I_2 has vasodilator and natriuretic actions.[420,421] These molecules are produced in endothelial cells. Abnormalities in thromboxane metabolites have been reported to precede hypertension in Dahl salt-sensitive rats.[421] Overall, imbalances in the production of and responsiveness of these molecules are observed in subsets of patients with essential hypertension.[421] Vasoconstrictor eicosanoids are thought to contribute to the elevated blood pressure in pregnancy-induced hypertension and renovascular hypertension.[423] The generation of vasodilator prostaglandins may be reduced in these situations.[423] However, blockade of thromboxane A_2 synthesis and action, which results in a significant imbalance of thromboxane A_2 and prostaglandin I_2, does not affect blood pressure in humans with essential hypertension.[420]

Kallikreins and Kinins

Kinins, including bradykinin, are released from kininogen by proteolytic actions of kallikrein and have potent vasodilatory actions; these actions are due mainly to stimulation of the release of prostaglandins, NO, and other endothelium-derived vasodilators.[424,425] Kinins also stimulate the release of renin, catecholamines, and vasopressin.[426] These substances act mostly in an autocrine or paracrine mode and circulate at very low concentrations.[424] Kallikrein is produced in and released from both kidney and blood vessels.[424] Transgenic animals that overexpress the kallikrein gene have hypotension.[427] Chronic kinin receptor blockade induces hypertension in DOCA-treated rats, implying that kinins blunt mineralocorticoid-induced increases in blood pressure in these animals.[428,429] Shorter-term experiments give depressor followed by pressor responses; the latter responses are probably due to induced release of vasopressor substances.[426]

Arterial kallikrein is decreased in essential hypertension, particularly salt-sensitive hypertension, and renovascular hypertension.[421,424,430] Kallikrein excretion is also lower in black than in white patients with essential hypertension.[411] Kallikrein appears to be induced by mineralocorticoids in both the vasculature and kidneys.[421,424,430] Additional interest in the generation of bradykinin derives from the fact that converting enzyme inactivates bradykinin breakdown and that treatment with converting enzyme inhibitors elevates bradykinin production and may utilize this mechanism for part of its blood pressure–lowering actions.[155,166a,168] In SHRs, a bradykinin antagonist attenuated the effects of a converting enzyme inhibitor, but did not block the actions of an angiotensin receptor antagonist.[155]

There is interest in the role of kallikreins in the kidney. Lower urinary kallikrein levels have been found in patients with essential hypertension (discussed in the section on genetic and environmental influences above),[28,431] although in some studies this association was detected only in individuals with mild renal insufficiency.[431] It has been proposed that this lower excretion of kallikrein is determined by a major, albeit unidentified, gene that increases the risk for hypertension in up to 30 percent of the population.[19] The gene effect, assessed by detection of lower urinary kallikrein levels, is also associated with a positive family history of hypertension, stroke, and coronary artery disease.[19] In hypertensive rats, there is also cosegregation of a kallikrein gene polymorphism with hypertension.[432]

The role of potassium in blood pressure control is discussed later in this chapter. Increased dietary potassium increases urinary kallikrein excretion; this effect appears to be blunted in individuals who are homozygous for either low or high urinary kallikrein excretion but not in heterozygotes.[19] The effects of potassium in this setting may be due to influences on adrenal aldosterone release, with secondary effects on kallikrein.[19] Thus, potassium may have blood pressure–lowering actions through influences on kallikrein. Such variations in responsiveness to dietary potassium may also explain the inconsistencies in blood pressure responses to potassium supplementation discussed in the section on potassium below.

Ions, Hormones, and Blood Pressure

Sodium Chloride

Sodium chloride controls intravascular volume, and many hormones that regulate blood pressure affect salt dynamics. Blood pressure rises with age in societies with a high salt-intake. This is not seen in populations with little access to salt; however, the blood pressures of these individuals rise when they migrate to places where salt intake is high.[244] Potassium intake is high in societies where salt intake is low. Potassium has blood pressure–lowering effects (see below), and decreased potassium intake increases the salt sensitivity of blood pressure.[352] However, changes in potassium do not appear to account for most of the relation between blood pressure and salt intake.[34,244,433] Further, increased salt intake increases blood pressure in many individuals with essential hypertension, several forms of secondary hypertension (discussed below), and several forms of experimental hypertension.[34,411,422]

A role for sodium in the pathogenesis of hypertension is further suggested by blood pressure–lowering influences of decreased sodium intake and the use of diuretics (Figs. 14-14 and 14-15).[433,434] A marked reduction of salt intake can lower blood pressure in many patients with hypertension.[34,244,352,435] Reducing salt intake can blunt blood pressure rises with age in adolescents.[436] Moderate salt restriction probably has some blood pressure–lowering effectiveness (Fig. 14-14).[241,435] Overall efforts to reduce blood pressure with dietary salt reductions in patients with essential hypertension have produced only modest results[34,244,437,438] and are effective in only a subset of patients.[439,440] Many investigators feel that weight reduction is more easily achievable than modification of dietary sodium and potassium.[34,441] Short-term salt restriction can also have adverse effects on serum lipids.[442] However, salt restriction in the general population may take on greater importance in countries such as Japan, where there is a higher incidence of stroke relative to coronary disease.[34] Further, the effectiveness of diuretic agents in lowering blood pressure in hypertensive patients is mainly sodium-dependent.[443]

The minor influence of modest reductions in salt intake on blood pressure in the general hypertensive population is due in part to individual variations in sensitivity to the effects of salt on blood pressure.[178,244,246,411,444,446] Patients with essential hypertension can be subdivided into salt-sensitive and salt-resistant according to the influence of salt on their blood pressures. The distinctions are arbitrary, since there is a spectrum of sensitivities rather than a bimodal distribution, and there are substantial differences in the criteria used for standardization. However, when standardized, the effects of increased salt intake on blood pressure are reproducible in individual subjects. The prevalence of salt sensitivity varies from 15 to 60 percent depending on the means of classification and patient selection criteria.[178,244,411,446]

Salt sensitivity in essential hypertension occurs more frequently in people who are older and have positive family histories for hypertension.[445] Salt sensitivity in normotensives is a predictor of the subsequent development of hypertension.[444,445] This is evidenced by twin studies, relations to a positive family history of hypertension, the haptoglobin 1-1 phenotype, and certain leukocyte antigens.[444,445] Salt-sensitive normotensives display increased pressor responses to norepinephrine and angiotensin II, increased forearm vascular resistance, and suppressed plasma renin activity.[444] Salt sensitivity in secondary hypertension is observed with primary aldosteronism, renovascular hypertension, acromegaly, renal parenchymal disease, and bilateral renal artery stenosis.[178]

As discussed in the section on the renin-angiotensin system, the responsiveness of renal renin release to various measures and to angiotensin II differs in various patients with essential hypertension, suggesting that these traits identify discrete subgroups.[51,235,237–240,438] Patients with essential hypertension and low plasma renin levels tend to be salt-sensitive and sodium-retaining, whereas those with essential hypertension and high plasma renin levels tend to be salt-resistant. Essential hypertension patients with normal plasma renin levels can be salt-resistant or salt-sensitive. Patients with normal-renin essential hypertension can be divided into modulators and the more common nonmodulators; the latter have more angiotensin II–dependent hypertension and defective renal responses to a sodium load (Fig. 14-9).

Several mechanisms probably contribute to salt actions to elevate the blood pressure. The possibility that there are abnormalities in the actions of prostaglandins in salt-sensitive hypertension is discussed in the section on prostaglandins and other eicosanoids. Na^+ retention increases extracellular volume, urinary calcium and potassium excretion,[244] and the release of ANP (discussed above) and ouabain-like natriuretic factors (discussed below).[244,411] Increases in the ouabain-like factor would increase the salt-induced blood pressure elevations (discussed below). Reduced release of ANP in salt-sensitive essential hypertension was mentioned in the section on ANP.[411] This would blunt the ability of this peptide to lower blood pressure in response to salt loading.[411] The influence of increased extracellular volume is prominent in certain forms of secondary hypertension, such as with renal parenchymal disease, bilateral renal artery stenosis, and primary aldosteronism. The mechanisms by which calcium and potassium deficiency can increase blood pressure are discussed below.

FIGURE 14-14 Fall in supine systolic blood pressure with sodium restriction plotted against pretreatment supine systolic blood pressure. The data were obtained from multiple studies. *(Reviewed in and redrawn from MacGregor.[433])*

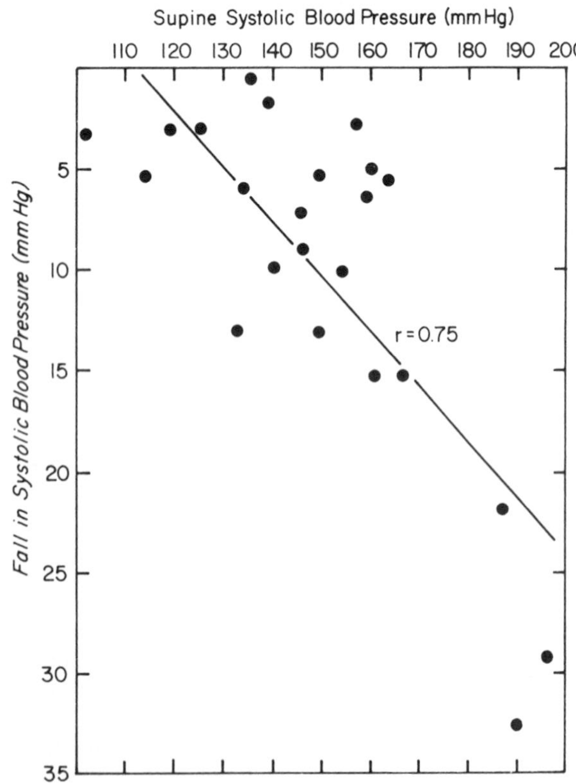

The possibility that there are abnormalities in components of the membrane handling of Na^+ or Ca^{2+} in salt-sensitive essential hypertension are discussed below. Intracellular Na^+ is elevated in individuals with low- and normal-renin essential hypertension (discussed earlier).[247,411] Intracellular Na^+ was higher and rose higher with salt intake in salt-sensitive essential hypertensives.[247,411] Na^+ can also affect Ca^{2+}, as described below. Increased intracellular $[Ca^{2+}]$ has been reported in salt-sensitive but not in salt-resistant subjects after sodium loading.[446] Salt sensitivity in hypertensives is significantly correlated with plasma ionized and total $[Ca^{2+}]$.[447]

Essential hypertension associated with hyperinsulinemia, insulin resistance and obesity (discussed in a following section) is generally salt-sensitive.[411,444,448,449] Insulin actions to stimulate renal sodium reabsorption and increase intracellular $[Na^+]$[449] and to stimulate sympathetic nervous system activity, as discussed below, could contribute to sodium sensitivity in hypertension. However, it has not been established whether insulin is responsible for the salt sensitivity or whether this is an associated defect.

Sodium retention in essential hypertension may depend on increased sympathetic nervous system activity.[244,411,415,445,450] Plasma norepinephrine levels decrease with high sodium intake in normal subjects and individuals with salt-resistant hypertension; this response is blunted in salt-sensitive hypertensive patients. With time, there may even be a salt-induced increase in sympathetic nervous system activity in salt-sensitive subjects. Salt-sensitive patients also tend to display greater basal and postural increments in plasma norepinephrine concentrations. Patients with salt-sensitive essential hypertension also display decreased urinary dopamine responses to salt loading; reduced levels of this natriuretic factor could enhance sodium retention. Central mechanisms have been suggested to explain salt sensitivity in SHR, in which a high salt intake increases norepinephrine levels in hypothalamic nuclei implicated in cardiovascular regulation and in

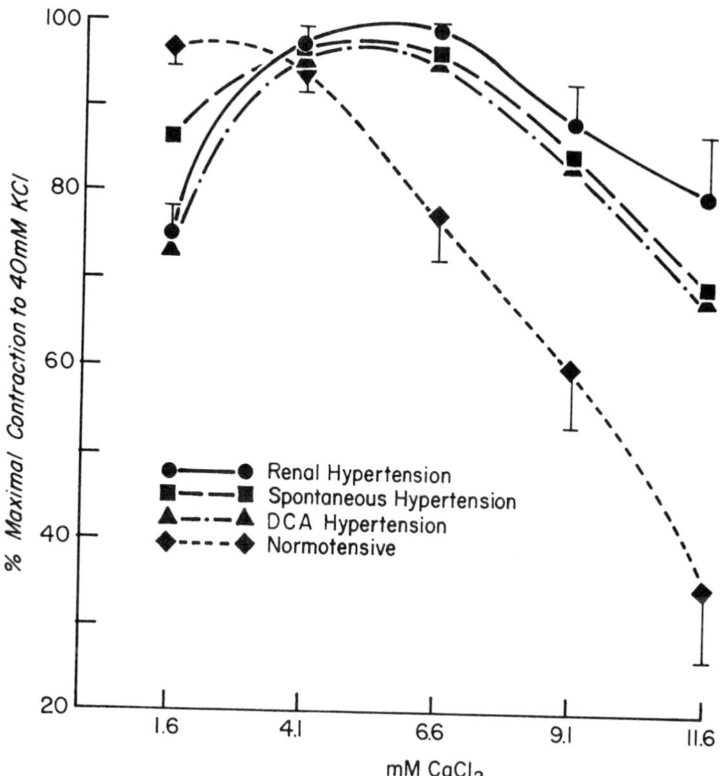

FIGURE 14-15 Normalized (see text) average of responses of aortic strips from normotensive, spontaneously hypertensive, renal hypertensive, and deoxycorticosterone hypertensive (DCA Hypertension) rats to 40 m*M* KC1 at various calcium concentrations. The greatest response of strips (eight or nine from each group) from the normotensive rats was at 1.6 m*M* Ca^{2+}, from the spontaneously hypertensive rats was at 4.1 m*M*, and from the DCA and renal hypertensive rats was at 6.6 m*M*. Brackets indicate standard errors, and an asterisk indicates a significant difference from the normotensive value at $p < 0.05$. *(From Holloway and Bohr.[434])*

Dahl salt-sensitive rats in which lesions in specific brain regions eliminate salt sensitivity.[451] Salt-sensitive hypertensives also have increased vascular responses to norepinephrine.[411] Rats also can be induced to develop salt-sensitive hypertension by α-adrenergic blockade.[452]

The majority of salt-sensitive patients with hypertension tend to have the nonmodulating phenotype discussed in the section on the renin-angiotensin system. This phenotype is associated with abnormal angiotensin II responses; it is not known whether these responses reflect a primary abnormality or are associated with another abnormality that is responsible for the salt sensitivity. These modulators also tend to have abnormal sympathetic nervous system activity.[239] The cause-and-effect relations between these overlapping characteristics have not been defined.

Chloride

Studies of salt and hypertension have focused primarily on sodium; the role of Cl^- has received less attention and is unclear.[244] In both humans and animals, there is little influence of selective loading of Na^+ without Cl^- on blood pressure.[244,453,454] NaCl leads to more fluid retention than $NaHCO_3$ or sodium citrate and to greater urinary calcium excretion than does sodium citrate. Conversely, selective Cl^- loading has not consistently elevated blood pressure in humans but has done so in some animal hypertension models.[244] Thus, both Na^+ and Cl^- may be required for the optimal blood pressure–elevating influences of salt.

Potassium

Oral potassium supplementation can lower the blood pressure in humans and animals.[34,244,436,440,455–458] A negative correlation has been reported between serum potassium concentrations and prevalence of hypertension in several populations. Potassium depletion increases blood pressure of patients with essential hypertension. Reduced potassium intake might contribute to higher prevalence of hypertension in blacks compared with whites in some areas. However, effects of sodium restriction and potassium supplementation have not been shown to be additive.

Several mechanisms have been proposed to explain the blood pressure lowering–actions of potassium. Earlier reports that high potassium intakes affect autonomic nervous system activity and plasma norepinephrine levels have not been confirmed[458] Potassium can decrease plasma renin activity in humans[458] and rats[459] and can inhibit proximal tubular sodium reabsorption in the rat.[460] Elevated serum K^+ increases urinary Na^+ and decreases Ca^{2+} loss.[458] Potassium increases endothelium-dependent vasodilation and enhances EDRF action in patients with essential hypertension[457] and in hypertensive Dahl salt-sensitive rats[455] but not in normotensive controls.[457] K^+ increases EDRF release in cultured cells.[455]

Potassium supplementation has not been recommended as a general measure for treating essential hypertension.[440] However, diuretic-induced hypokalemia increases the risk of cardiac arrhythmias,[461] so that potassium supplementation or the use of a potassium-sparing agent is indicated if the serum potassium concentration falls with diuretic administration. Further, a recent study does indicate that decreasing dietary potassium intake from natural foods is a feasible way to reduce antihypertensive drug treatment.[458]

Calcium Ion and Calcium Regulatory Hormones

Actions and Regulation of Ca^{2+}

Intracellular [Ca^{2+}] dictates contractile tone in the vascular smooth muscle that regulates the blood pressure and mediates the release and actions of hormones, neurotransmitters, and other effectors that regulate blood pressure (Chaps. 4 and 5). The participation of calcium in hypertension is illustrated by the utility of calcium-channel blockers in treating essential and other forms of hypertension.[462] There is interest in the relations between serum calcium levels, dietary calcium intake, and blood pressure.

Extracellular Ca^{2+} affects vascular smooth and cardiac muscle contractility through its influences on intracellular Ca^{2+}. Calcium binds to calmodulin and increases Ca^{2+}-ATPase activity that lowers intracellular [Ca^{2+}] levels.[245] The relation of extracellular [Ca^{2+}] and vascular smooth muscle contraction is parabolic in isolated rat aortic strips, with increasing contractility at lower concentrations up to a certain level, at which point relaxation occurs with further increases in [Ca^{2+}] (Fig. 14-15). These dichotomous effects of calcium on vascular reactivity may contribute to the effects of calcium on blood pressure.

The endothelium and the automatic nerves are major determinants of [Ca^{2+}] in arteries.[463] As discussed in the section on EDRF, the endothelium exerts inhibitory influences mediated by voltage-dependent Ca^{2+} channels.[463] Smooth muscle potassium channels and Na^+-K^+-ATPase hyperpolarize the membrane potential, counter the effects of voltage-dependent calcium channels, and inhibit contraction.[463]

Role of Ca^{2+} in Hypertension

Studies of the role of Ca^{2+} in hypertension have focused on levels of extracellular and/or intracellular Ca^{2+}, effects of Ca^{2+} channel blockade and Ca^{2+}-regulating hormones, influences of dietary calcium, and Ca^{2+} transport abnormalities.

Although hypercalcemia can acutely elevate blood pressure, increased dietary calcium intake is more related to lower blood pressure levels in a subset of individuals with essential hypertension.[20,245,345,352,464] Calcium supplementation is more effective for blood pressure lowering in patients who are older, have low-renin hypertension, are black, or are salt-sensitive. The blood pressure–lowering actions of calcium appear to be more evident in subjects who previously had a low dietary intake of calcium and who may have a relative or absolute deficiency of calcium. Calcium supplementation has been reported to reduce hypertension in the general population when the calcium intake is above 800 mg/day compared to below 400 mg/day.[352] However, most do not recommend the administration of oral calcium as a general treatment for hypertension.

Other abnormalities in Ca^{2+} and related factors are correlated with essential hypertension. A profile of extracellular Ca^{2+} deficiency and elevated intracellular [Ca^{2+}] was discussed in the section on low-renin essential hypertension below. By contrast, patients with high-renin or salt-insensitive essential hypertension have higher serum levels of ionized calcium and lower PTH concentrations.[352] Calcium-channel blockers lower intracellular Ca^{2+} levels.[352,465] Calcium-channel blockers are particularly effective in lowering blood pressure in patients with salt-sensitive or low-renin hypertension and are less effective in high-renin and salt-resistant essential hypertension.[352] This is consistent with the formulation that increased intracellular Ca^{2+} participates significantly in the pathogenesis of low-renin essential hypertension.

However, elements of a profile with increased intracellular Ca^{2+} are observed in patients with essential hypertension not selected by their renin status and in the children of hypertensive parents. This profile includes elevations of PTH, slight elevations of urine and intracellular Ca^{2+}, and slightly reduced mean serum Ca^{2+}, Mg^{2+}, and PO^{4-2} concentrations, as well as renal excretion of PO_{4-2} and Mg^{2+}.[464–467] There are conflicting reports on changes in vitamin D (1,25D3) levels.[351,464–467] Patients with primary aldosteronism and renovascular hypertension do not have increased intracellular [Ca^{2+}].[283] Increased intracellular Ca^{2+} is also related to other abnormalities seen in essential hypertension, including the level of blood pressure, cardiac left ventricular mass index, obesity, oral glucose loading, hyperinsulinemia, and insulin resistance.[245,465,468,469]

The reasons for these abnormalities are not understood. Extracellular Ca^{2+} does not always reflect intracellular concentrations of the ion, and it has seemed paradoxic why a decreased extracellular Ca^{2+} would be associated with an increased intracellular Ca^{2+}.[245] Proposed possibilities are listed in Table 14-3.[245] However, none of these have been established as primary mechanisms. Confounding these considerations is the fact that changes in Ca^{2+} also affect the levels of and/or the actions of most hormones that regulate blood pressure (discussed in other sections and in Chaps. 4 and 5). Most investigators feel that the primary abnormality leads to aberrant transmembrane calcium transport, with increased intracellular Ca^{2+} in the vascular smooth muscle, and lower extracellular Ca^{2+} levels in hypertensive patients.

A common defect in ion handling might link the multiple associations of insulin resistance, salt sensitivity, and ion abnormalities.[465] Increased uptake of Ca^{2+} would cause increased release of insulin with hyperinsulinemia, insulin resistance, increased proximal sodium reabsorption, increased urinary calcium excretion, vasoconstriction, increased cardiac contractility, and a tendency to left ventricular hypertrophy. However, not all these abnormalities are observed in all hypertensive patients, and this could imply that there is more than one type of defect.

Magnesium

Indications that magnesium plays a role in hypertension come from observations of hypomagnesemia in several hypertensive populations.[470,471] The administration of magnesium salts can lower blood pressure, particularly in pregnancy-induced hypertension.[472] Long-term administration of lower doses of magnesium salts has decreased requirements for antihypertensive drugs.[473] Diuretics used to treat hypertension enhance urinary magnesium loss. Magnesium supplementation in hypertensive patients on thiazide diuretics decreases both the blood pressure and the risk of developing an arrythmia.[461,474]

Intracellular Mg^{2+} levels can affect vascular tone; lowering the Mg^{2+} content of blood vessels induces contractile responses, potentiates the actions of vasoconstrictors such as angiotensin II and norepinephrine, decreases the production of the vasodilator prostaglandin I_2, and enhances aldosterone synthesis.[475,476] Mg^{2+} affects vascular smooth muscle by regulating the intracellular Ca^{2+} and Na^+ content of smooth muscle cells. Lowering extracellular $[Mg^{2+}]$ impairs Na^+-Ca^{2+} exchange, and increases intracellular free $[Ca^{2+}]$ and $[Na^{2+}]$ in blood vessels.[247,475–477] The tendency to have reduced serum and intracellular $[Mg^{2+}]$ and excretion of Mg^{2+} in essential hypertension was discussed in the preceding section.[464–466]

Ion Transport and Blood Pressure

Ion transport and blood pressure are intimately linked. Transmembrane proteins in the cell membrane mediate ion transport. These include ion channels (Na^+ channel), carriers and exchangers [Na^+-independent Cl^--HCO_3^- anion exchanger, Na^+-H^+ exchanger, Na^+-Na^+ countertransport (Na+Li+ countertransport)], cotransporters (Na^+-glucose cotransporter, Na^+-K^+-$2Cl^-$ cotransport), and pumps (Na^+, K^+-ATPase, Ca^{2+}-ATPase, H^+-ATPase).[478–480] Transport processes control intracellular $[Ca^{2+}]$, which in turn regulates processes such as smooth and cardiac muscular contraction, release of hormones, and cellular sensitivity to vasoactive substances and hormones. These processes also regulate salt balance. Their activities are affected by hormones and genetic influences. The fact that there are potential abnormalities in the transport of Na^+ and Ca^{2+} in essential hypertension is discussed in the preceding sections.

A number of methodologic problems affect the assessment of ion transport. For example, vascular tone is dependent on the ion concentrations in smooth muscle, and it is difficult to obtain in vivo measurements of this tissue. Instead, investigators have utilized other cells in which measurements can be made. These include peripheral blood erythrocytes and leukocytes, each of which have advantages and drawbacks.

Na^+, K^+-ATPase

Na^+, K^+-ATPase couples ATP hydrolysis to extrusion of Na^+ out of the cell and K^+ transport into the cell. It is the major element responsible for intracellular-extracellular and electrochemical gradients of Na^+ and K^+ and for membrane polarization. These ATPases contain several different subunits. Ordinarily, activity of the ATPase is greater with higher intracellular Na^+ and extracellular K^+ concentrations. Increased pumping hyperpolarizes the membrane, and decreased pumping depolarizes it.

The role of ATPase in hypertension has been studied mainly in terms of circulating factors that affect pump activity (discussed in the section on ouabain-like factors below). Reduced Na^+, K^+-ATPase activity found during salt loading in salt-sensitive but not salt-insensitive individuals could be due to enhanced release of these factors and could contribute to blood pressure elevations, as described below.[446] In addition, erythrocyte pump activity has been found to be lower and intracellular Na^+ concentrations to be higher in normotensive blacks than in whites and in men than in women; it has been suggested that this could contribute to the higher prevalence of hypertension in blacks and men vs. whites and women.[411,481]

TABLE 14-3 Potential Mechanisms of Dietary Calcium-Induced Influences on Blood Pressure

↑ Membrane stabilization
↑ Na^+-K^+-ATPase
↑ Ca^{2+}-ATPase
Changes in Ca^{2+} regulating hormones: PTH, 1,25$(OH)_2$ vitamin D_3, calcitonin, parathyroid hypertensive factor, etc.
Changes in release of other hormones in response to Ca^{2+}: ANP, renin, CGRP, etc.
↓ Sympathetic activity
↑ Natriuresis

Reviewed in Resnick et al.[246]

Na^+-K^+-Cl^- Cotransport

This facilitated diffusion mechanism allows sodium and potassium ions to enter or leave cells, depending on their concentrations.[411,446,482] Na^+-K^+-Cl^- cotransport activity can be inhibited by furosemide, and regulated by vasoactive substances.[482] The physiologic role of the system is uncertain, but it probably supports Na^+ extrusion when intracellular Na^+ levels are high. Enhanced Na^+-K^+-Cl^- cotransport activity might increase renal tubular Na^+ reabsorption[482] and intracellular $[Na^+]$ in hypertension during high salt intake.[446] The existence of abnormalities in this transporter in hypertension is controversial.[411] However, it has been reported that red blood cell Na^+-K^+-Cl^- cotransport activity increases with increased salt in hypertensive but not normotensive patients[446] and is higher in patients with low-renin essential hypertension,[482] possibly secondary to a primary salt-loaded state in this condition. However, blacks with low-renin hypertension have low levels of the transporter, indicating that the renin status is not the only determinant of its activity.[482] Thus, dysregulation of this transporter may contribute to the salt sensitivity of essential hypertension.[411]

Na^+-Na^+ Countertransport (Na^+-Li^+ Countertransport)

Na^+-Li^+ countertransport exchanges Na^+ for Na^+ by passive facilitated diffusion. Li^+ can substitute for Na^+. The activity of this element is studied by measuring Li^+ efflux from Li^+ loaded cells; it is thus usually called the Na^+-Li^+ countertransport.[483] This system is inhibited by furosemide plus phloretin or by phloretin alone.[480] This system may be the same one that mediates Na^+-H^+ antiport activity, as discussed below.[411] However, the activities of the two systems assayed under various conditions differ.

Na^+-Li^+ countertransport activity is influenced by a number of factors, including hypertension.[446,480,484,485] Insulin increases,[486] and physical training decreases[487] its activity. Na^+-Li^+ countertransport activity is higher in hypertensive whites but not blacks.[483,485,486,488] It is higher in normotensive whites than in blacks.[486] Although there a lack of general agreement,[489] the activity of this transporter has been correlated with subsequent development of hypertension and a family history of hypertension.[488,490] Na^+-Li^+ countertransport activity has also been correlated directly with waist/hip ratio and a higher risk for developing renal and cardiovascular complications of hypertension.[488,490] and has been negatively correlated with high-density lipoprotein (HDL) cholesterol.[489] Some researchers have concluded that Na^+-Li^+ countertransport suggests a cardiovascular risk more than a hypertension risk.[489] Na^+-Li^+ countertransport activity is higher in insulin-resistant blacks and whites.[485,486,488] In diabetic patients, activity is higher with insulin resistance than with normal insulin sensitivity, lipid abnormalities, left ventricular hypertrophy, and an increased risk for developing nephropathy.[485,491] In diabetic patients, an inverse correlation has been found between abnormalities in Na^+-Li^+ countertransport and endothelium-dependent vascular relaxation.[485] Thus, the subgroup of people with hypertension, insulin resistance, and salt sensitivity appear to have the abnormality,[446,485] although one group found a lack of correlation between elevations of this transporter and insulin resistance in the normotensive offspring of hypertensive parents.[492]

The role of the system in physiology and hypertension is not known. It is thought that the exchange of Na^+ for Na^+ cannot lead to net Na^+ transport. Thus, some researchers have regarded the system as an epiphenomenon that may not play a role in hypertension. It has been suggested that elevations of the Na^+-Li^+ countertransporter in essential hypertension result in a rate of cellular sodium efflux that exceeds that of the influx that would increase extracellular fluid volume.[483]

As was mentioned above, it has also been speculated that the Na^+-Li^+ countertransporter participates in Na^+-H^+ exchange in the proximal renal tube.[411,480] If this were true, increased erythrocyte countertransport would increase proximal tubular Na^+-H^+ exchange and sodium reabsorption. This would decrease the renal capacity to excrete sodium.[27,493] In support of this notion, Li^+ clearance as a potential reflection of renal Na^+-Li^+ countertransport activity was decreased in subjects with essential hypertension.[494] This hypothesis could explain the limitations in proximal tubular sodium responses reported in salt-sensitive human hypertension.

Regulation of Intracellular pH

Alterations in intracellular pH have been proposed to contribute to vasoconstriction and vascular hypertrophy in hypertension.[247,495] Although studies of intracellular pH have produced variable results and have been hindered by methodologic issues, erythrocyte pH appears to be lower in hypertensives.[247,495] Intracellular pH is regulated by the Na^+-H^+ exchanger and the Na^+-independent $C1^-$-HCO_3^- anion exchanger.[495] The mechanisms by which pH affects blood pressure have not been clarified.

Na^+-H^+ Exchanger (Na^+-H^+ Antiport) Na^+-H^+ exchangers move Na^+ into and H^+ out of the cell, utilizing the Na^+ gradient across the cell membrane.[478,496,497] Na^+-H^+ exchange could affect blood pressure by increasing renal Na^+ reabsorption.[486,498] In vascular smooth muscle cells, increased Na^+-H^+ exchange could increase intracellular Ca^{2+} through inhibition of sarcolemmal Na^+-Ca^{2+} exchange.[499] It is inhibited by amiloride.[411] These exchangers are members of a gene family with different isoforms referred to as NHE-1 to NHE-4.[497,500]

An enhancement of Na^+-H^+ exchange is frequently observed in black and white persons with essential hypertension.[411,486,495,496] and is measureable in both blood cells and skeletal muscle.[496] Increased activity is found only in a subgroup of patients with high blood pressure, is not tightly correlated to the severity or duration of the hypertension, persists over time, and is not affected by treatment.[496] In blacks, the activity is higher in hypertensive insulin-resistant subjects than in normotensive insulin-resistant or hypertensive insulin-sensitive subjects.[486] Elevated Na^+-H^+ exchange in blacks is usually associated with normal Na^+-Li^+ countertransport activity.[486] In normotensives, activity is higher in whites than in blacks.[486] Whites with elevated Na^+-Li^+ countertransport activity tend to have normal Na^+-H^+ exchange activity.[486]

Increased Na^+-H^+ exchange, a decreased maximal rate for Na^+-K^+-Cl^--cotransport, and no differences in Na^+-Li^+ countertransport are correlated with left ventricular hypertrophy in patients with essential hypertension; these changes could increase intracellular Na^+ content as a result of increased Na^+ influx and enhanced H^+ efflux and could be involved in the pathogenesis of the hypertrophy.[499]

Increased Na^+-H^+ exchange activity has been found to persist in lymphocytes immortalized from hypertensive patients, implying a cellular defect.[497] These lymphocytes also were found to proliferate more rapidly than control cells, an observation that would be relevant to hypertension if the defect were also present in vascular smooth muscle and/or cardiac cells.

Na^+-Independent Cl^--HCO_3^- Anion Exchanger The Na^+-independent Cl^--HCO_3^--anion exchanger ordinarily results in a net efflux of HCO_3^- as a result of the usual inward gradient of Cl^- in excess of HCO_3^-[495] that acts as a cell-acidifying mechanism.[495] Levels of this transporter have been reported to be elevated in a subset of patients with essential hypertension.[495] This abnormality was not found in normotensive family members of the hypertensive individuals.[495] The abnormality (but not that in Na^+-H^+ exchange) was correlated with diminished intracellular pH.[495]

Ouabain-like Factors

Ouabain directly inhibits Na^+, K^+-ATPase.[415,446,501–506] Ouabain analogues such as digoxin are used to treat heart failure and cardiac arrythmias. Low concentrations of ouabain result in modest rises in intracellular Na^+ and declines in membrane potential.[503] This may lead to a secondary increase in cytosolic $[Ca^{2+}]$ and Ca^{2+} stores in intracellular organelles mediated by increased Na^+-Ca^{2+}-exchange. Increased intracellular $[Ca^{2+}]$ would enhance vascular tone, secretory processes, and Ca^{2+} availability for mobilization when cells are activated.[503] Thus, endogenous ouabain could influence blood pressure control in several ways (Fig. 14-16).[503]

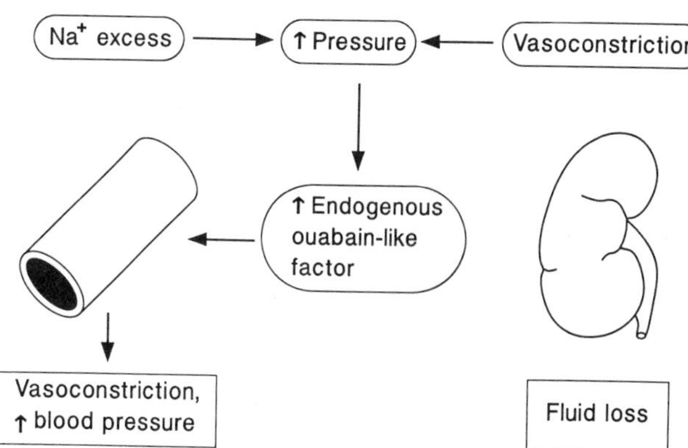

FIGURE 14-16 Release and actions of endogenous ouabain-like factors.

Early studies in salt-sensitive rats suggested that increased salt intake stimulates release from the kidneys of a factor that elevates blood pressure.[446] This factor inhibited Na^+-K^+-ATPase, which normally promotes renal sodium and water excretion. Levels of this inhibitor increased enough also to affect vascular Na^+, K^+-ATPase in individuals who had defective renal Na^+ excretory capacity or in whom Na^+ intake exceeded renal excretory capacity. This influence would increase cytosolic $[Ca^{2+}]$ and promote vasoconstriction, as described above.[446]

This class of inhibitors are assessed by their capacity to inhibit the sodium pump in intact cells, compete with ouabain for binding to the ATPase, inhibit ATPase activity, or react to antiserum to digoxin.[415,446,505] For studies of cells of individual subjects, data using white blood cells are the most convincing.[446]

These studies indicate that ouabain-like factors are present in human plasma and tissues. Although chemical characterization of these factors has been elusive, it appears that ouabain itself is present in human tissues and plasma.[446,504–507] However, there is also evidence for ouabain-like factors with different properties and indications that their regulation differs from that of ouabain.[507] Endogenous ouabain-like activity is found in the CNS, especially the hypothalamus, and in the adrenals, hearts, and plasma.[503,504,507]

Ouabain blocks sodium reabsorption by the kidney and increases blood pressure and myocardial contractility.[484] There has been confusion regarding the activities of endogenous ouabain, based on whether plasma levels of the glycoside reach levels high enough to be active and on clinical observations that treatment of patients with digoxin preparations is not ordinarily associated with hypertension.[507,508] However, chronic ouabain-induced increases in blood pressure have been demonstrated by administering the compound to rats with normal kidneys or reduced renal masses.[501] The treatment increased tissue but not plasma ouabain levels significantly;[501] this may imply that plasma levels do not reflect the activity of the factors. In humans, acute administration of ouabain can increase calf vascular resistance and reduce blood flow without affecting blood pressure.[509] Canrenoate (the active metabolite of spironolactone) may also have ouabain-like antagonist activity and can attenuate these effects and lower blood pressure.[509]

Ouabain-like activity is increased with volume expansion in a number of tissues.[504,507] There are salt-induced increases in this activity; these are greater in SHRs than in control rats.[504] The increases occur earlier in the hypothalamus and pituitary than in peripheral tissues and plasma.[504] In these rats, adrenalectomy (with replacement aldosterone and corticosterone) blunts the development of hypertension and has little effect on or diminishes circulating and central ouabain-like activity but does not prevent the 50 to 90 percent increases in plasma, hypothalamic, and pituitary ouabain-like activity caused by a high sodium intake.[502] In humans, with elevated ouabain activities, there was no significant increase in ouabain levels in the effluent from the adrenal veins, and plasma levels of ouabain were in the normal range after adrenalectomy.[505] These data suggest that the major source of both central and peripheral activity is the CNS.[502]

Increased plasma ouabain-like activity has been reported in a number of states associated with hypertension and/or fluid overload. These include ACTH-induced hypertension, renal insufficiency, cirrhosis, pregnancy-induced hypertension, essential hypertension, relation to patients with essential hypertension, low-renin hypertension, primary aldosteronism, acromegaly, and pheochromocytoma.[328,395,446,501,507] Levels of the factor have been correlated with the salt sensitivity of the blood pressure.[446] An ouabain-producing adrenal tumor associated with hypertension has been reported.[510]

Actions of these factors to elevate blood pressure, promote natriuresis, and stimulate cardiac contractiliy could allow them to form part of the body's defense against fluid overload at the expense of elevating blood pressure. Their actions contrast with those of ANP (see above), which does not elevate blood pressure. However, their overall roles remain to be elucidated. The use of infused antiserum to ouabain have yielded conflicting results, although in some cases these antisera did decrease blood pressure.[507]

Elevations of the levels of these compounds in tissues and plasma in various hypertensive states could contribute to the blood pressure elevations.[446,501,507] It is not known in these situations whether the elevations are primary or secondary, although in some cases they are likely to be secondary.

Obesity, Insulin, and Insulin Resistance in Hypertension

There are strong associations between essential hypertension, insulin resistance, hyperinsulinemia, and obesity.[466,511,512a,512b] There is a high incidence of hypertension in diabetes.[511,513,514] Hypertension, insulin resistance, and hyperinsulinemia are further linked to glucose intolerance, hypertriglyceridemia with elevated very low density lipoprotein (VLDL) levels and VLDL cholesterol, low levels of HDL cholesterol and other abnormalities; this constellation of aberrations has been termed syndrome X[514–517] or the insulin resistance syndrome.[515] However, all these abnormalities are not consistently present in all patients; thus, several different defects may dictate the spectrum of features that are observed. The insulin resistance syndrome abnormalities are associated with aberrations in ions, ion transporters, and other functions related to blood pressure control. In spite of intense study, the primary defects and cause-and-effect relations of many aspects of these associations are poorly understood.

Correlations between Hypertension, Insulin Resistance, Hyperinsulinemia, and Obesity

The incidence of hypertension in obese individuals is about 50 percent and about 50 percent of hypertensives are obese.[511,512] The term *obesity* denotes an increase in adipose tissue mass and generally refers to a body weight of >120 percent of the ideal.[518] Hypertension is twice as prevalent in overweight adolescents and young adults.[511] The association between obesity and hypertension exists in populations (e.g., blacks and whites in the United States) that differ in the prevalence of the two disorders, although this is not true for all groups, Pima Indians and Mexican Americans, for example. The association between obesity and hypertension appears to weaken with advancing age. Body fat distribution is also related to the risk of developing hypertension; increased abdominal fat with a high waist-to-hip ratio is associated with high blood pressure and insulin resistance.[512] The correlation is even greater in subjects with increased visceral fat as measured by CT scanning.[518a] There are also correlations between hypertension and obesity in diabetic patients.[513]

In addition to obesity, both hyperinsulinemia and insulin resistance have been identified as independent risk factors for predicting the development of hypertension.[247,486,511,512,519] Insulin resistance is a defect in insulin-mediated glucose uptake. This defect is generally associated with a resultant increase in pancreatic insulin secretion. Insulin resistance is better correlated with hypertension in Caucasian populations. Insulin resistance is the common feature shared by obesity, diabetes, and hypertension.[511,520] Insulin resistance is correlated with essential hypertension even in thin patients,[466,511,518,521–524] is greater in obese hypertensives than in obese normotensives,[520] and is present in the offspring of hypertensives before the development of either obesity or hypertension.[492,516,525] Insulin resistance and hypertension are also correlated in Chinese Americans and in normal or low-weight Mexican Americans.[515] The issue is unclear in black populations.[525a,525b]

Insulin resistance and hyperinsulinemia are not a consequence of hypertension. For example, patients with hyperaldosteronism or renovascular hypertension have higher sensitivity to insulin than do those with essential hypertension.[526] Hypertension does not alter the suppressive effects of insulin on hepatic glucose production in obese or type II diabetic subjects.[527] Hyperinsulinemia in hypertensive subjects does not change with blood pressure control.[528]

There is evidence in clinical studies that insulin resistance and hyperinsulinemia are antecedents to hypertension. These derangements were found to predict the development of hypertension in normal weight individuals in an 8-year prospective study of Mexican Americans[515] and to be present in (1) normotensive children of hypertensive but normotensive patients,[528a] (2) borderline hypertensive subjects in the Tecumseh study,[528b] and (3) borderline hypertensive, but not normotensive African-American adolescents.[528c]

However, the association between hypertension and insulin resistance and/or hyperinsulinemia is not universal.[517,520,529] Some studies have failed to show a correlation between hyperinsulinemia and hypertension in obese subjects.[511] There are a number of patients with type II diabetes mellitus and marked insulin resistance who do not have hypertension.[527] More than 40 percent of hypertensives have normal insulin-stimulated whole-body glucose uptake.[511,530] In Pima Indians and Mexican Americans in the United States and some other groups, hypertension is uncommon but insulin resistance is common.[517,520,531] Finally, some states with clear hyperinsulinemia, for example, insulinomas, do not regularly lead to hypertension.[466]

Insulin resistance is induced with glucororticoid or growth hormone excess. Both of these states are associated with hypertension, and insulin resistance has been correlated with hypertension in acromegaly.[532] However, except for this association, there is no evidence that the hypertension in these states is caused by the insulin resistance (also see the section on growth hormone).[343,533] For example, in glucocorticoid hypertension, octreotide lowered plasma insulin concentrations but did not modify the blood pressure.[533] The effects of growth hormone on blood pressure can occur independently of changes in insulin resistance.[343]

Insulin resistance and hyperinsulinemia are also seen in SHRs,[511] salt-sensitive and salt-resistant hypertensive Dahl rats,[521] and genetically obese hypertensive Zucker rats.[511] However, some SHRs are more sensitive than resistant to insulin.[511] Rats with renovascular hypertension are not insulin-resistant or hyperinsulinemic.[533a]

Hypertension can be improved by correcting insulin resistance.[511] Weight loss lowers blood pressure; this is associated with decreased insulin resistance and is independent of simple energy restriction[534] or salt intake.[520] Exercise programs can reduce blood pressure; the greatest reductions occur in individuals with the greatest fall in plasma insulin levels (a reflection of insulin sensitivity).[511] Some antihypertensive agents, converting enzyme inhibitors,[535,536] and alpha-adrenergic blockers[523,536] can improve glucose tolerance,[535] although improved insulin sensitivity has not been linked to the antihypertensive effects of these drugs.

Hypertension and insulin resistance are correlated with higher concentrations of triglyceride and VLDL, lower levels of HDL, smaller low-density lipoprotein (LDL) particles, and higher serum uric acid and plasminogen activator inhibitor-I concentrations.[514,517,537] The LDL subclass patterns are correlated with an increased risk of developing coronary heart disease because of the greater oxidation of the apo B moiety on this particle, [537] and are influenced by a gene located near the LDL and insulin receptor genes.[537,538] Thus, it is conceivable that this allele predisposes to insulin resistance.[537]

Hypertension and Diabetes Mellitus

About 2.5 million to 3 million Americans have both diabetes and hypertension.[513] The prevalence of hypertension in type I diabetes mellitus and probably type II diabetes mellitus is about twofold that in the nondiabetic population.[513] Around 30 to 40 percent of patients with type II diabetes mellitus are hypertensive when the diagnosis is made.[513] By the fifth decade of life, 85 percent of all diabetic individuals (most of whom have type II diabetes) are estimated to be hypertensive and obese.[511] The prevalence of the hypertension in type II diabetes increases markedly once proteinuria first develops.[513] The presence of hypertension increases both morbidity and mortality in diabetic patients and accelerates the course of diabetes nephropathy.[513] Hypertension has been implicated in 44 percent of deaths coded to diabetes, and diabetes has been attributed to around 10 percent of deaths caused by hypertension.[513] An absence of hypertension is the usual finding in long-term survivors of diabetes.[513]

Insulin resistance is common in both type I and type II diabetes mellitus and is more prominent with type II diabetes. This resistance may participate in the pathogenesis of hypertension in these patients. However, the degree of insulin resistance in patients with type II diabetes mellitus has not been correlated with the presence of hypertension.[527] The in-

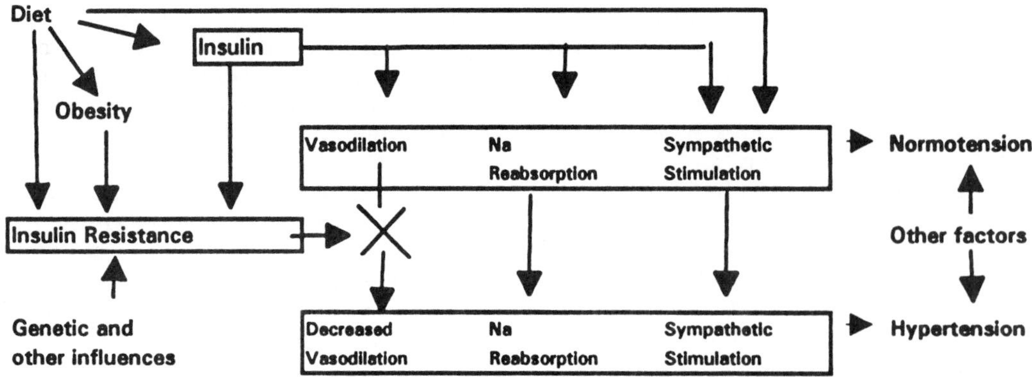

FIGURE 14-17 Representation of the development of insulin resistance and the influence of insulin and insulin resistance on blood pressure.

creased blood pressure in these patients is also in part independent of body weight.[513]

Multiple factors, in addition to insulin resistance, can contribute to hypertension in diabetes. Hypertension with type I diabetes mellitus is predominantly related to nephropathy.[513] Nephropathy also accelerates the development of hypertension in type II diabetes mellitus.[513] Diabetic patients tend to have decreased baroreceptor reflex sensitivity, increased exchangeable sodium with an impaired ability to excrete an intravenous saline load, increased peripheral vascular resistance, and enhanced vascular smooth muscle contractility responses to various agonists.[513]

Glucose intolerance itself, independent of obesity, may also exacerbate the hypertension.[511] Hyperglycemia with glomerular hyperfiltration of glucose can stimulate proximal tubular glucose-Na^+ cotransport, elevate Na^+, K^+-ATPase activity in an insulin-independent manner,[513] and promote vascular structural changes, including overexpression of fibronectin and collagen, endothelial dysfunction, accumulation of glycosylation products, and others.[513]

Effects of Insulin on Blood Pressure

Insulin has little or no effect on blood pressure in short-term experiments.[466,539,540] This has been demonstrated in both normotensive, borderline hypertensive, and in obese, insulin-resistant hypertensive individuals. Hypotension can be a complication of insulin treatment in diabetic patients with neuropathy.[541]

Studies of blockade of insulin release or modulation of responsiveness to insulin suggest an effect of hyperinsulinemia on blood pressure.[466,524] However, these experiments should be interpreted with caution, since other actions of the drugs might explain the results. Nevertheless, treatment with the somatostatin analogue octreotide decreased both plasma insulin levels and hypertension in obese hypertensive, hyperinsulinemic humans but not in normoinsulinemic, hypertensive humans[466] and enhanced natriuretic responses to a sodium load in lean, non-insulin-resistant hypertensive and normal subjects.[524] Metformin, which may increase insulin sensitivity, decreased blood pressure in insulin-resistant hypertensive men.[466]

Experiments with various animal models also suggest that insulin can influence blood pressure under some circumstances.[466,511,517,542] Most dog studies have not shown blood pressure–elevating actions of insulin,[466] although chronic insulin infusion has resulted in hypertension in some studies[511] and weight gain was associated with increased blood pressure and plasma insulin levels in a dog model of obesity hypertension.[511] In several rat model systems, there is insulin resistance and hypertension.[511] Insulin can increase blood pressure[543a,541b] and sodium retention, and a high-fructose diet can lead to insulin resistance and hypertension.[511,542] In female but not male stroke-prone hypertensive rats, glyburide, which stimulates insulin release and increases sensitivity to insulin, increases blood pressure, insulin release, and vascular responsiveness.[543]

As described below, insulin has actions that can either elevate or lower the blood pressure. It is thought that insulin usually does not increase the blood pressure, because influences on sympathetic nervous system activity and on sodium retention that might elevate the blood pressure are counterbalanced by vasodilatory actions in the periphery.

Actions of Insulin that Influence Blood Pressure

Insulin has a number of actions that may influence blood pressure either positively or negatively (Fig. 14-17).[466,520,541] Among these, vasodilator actions on peripheral blood vessels tend to lower blood pressure and influences on renal sodium handling and sympathetic activity tend to elevate blood pressure. The actions are also associated with effects on intracellular ion handling that may contribute to these processes.

Actions on Blood Vessels

Insulin and IGF have direct vascular action, which appear to be endothelial-mediated and depends on the geographic location of the vessel.[541a,543a] In intact mesenteric artery, insulin enhances vasoconstrictor effects through the stimulation of an endothelial-dependent cyclooxygenase product. In contrast, in rat aortic ring, insulin opposes vasoconstrictor effects by stimulating endothelial nitric oxide production. Thus, the overall effect of insulin on blood pressure may be a balance between vasoconstrictor and vasodilator responses, which may be altered in the setting of obesity, diabetes, etc. In normal subjects insulin increases vasodilation of skeletal muscle beds.[466,520] Insulin mediated glucose uptake is enhanced in the presence of vasodilation.[543b] Insulin can increase skeletal muscle blood flow,[544,545] decrease forearm vascular resistance, and attenuate responses to various vasoconstrictors.[546] These actions are selective for certain vascular beds. They are blunted in obesity and in type II diabetes mellitus.[545,546a] Blood vessels from insulin-deficient or insulin-resistant/hyperinsulinemic rats exhibit enhanced pressor responses to vasoconstrictor substances.[247] Exogenous insulin restores normal vascular responsiveness and blunts the vasoconstrictor effects of catecholamines; higher concentrations are required for these effects in obese and insulin-resistant hypertensive rats (SHRs).[247] Insulin actions on skeletal muscle blood flow can occur independently of hypoglycemia,[544,545] are not secondary to insulin stimulation of glucose uptake, and probably contribute to insulin-stimulated glucose update.[547]

Multiple, possibly interrrelated mechanisms may contribute to the influences in the intact animal; their relative contributions have not been established. Evidence for involvement of adrenergic mechanisms is suggested by the finding that the vasodilator effects of insulin can be blunted by treatment with beta-adrenergic blockers.[466] The effects on ion transport and intracellular [Ca^{2+}], pH and [Mg^{2+}], and ion responses to various stimuli discussed below are probably important. There can be metabolic vasodilation secondary to increased skeletal muscle oxygen consumption.[466] The vasodilatory effects of insulin can be mimicked by cGMP analogues, and inhibition of arginine-derived NO generation blocks insulin's effects on IP_3-sensitive Ca^{2+} release.[541]

Renal

Insulin increases renal sodium reabsorption and can cause sodium retention.[466,511,520,548,549] The major mechanism for this effect appears to involve insulin stimulation of sodium reabsorption in the loop of Henle.[548] The sodium-retaining actions of insulin may be enhanced through indirect stimulatory influences on sympathetic nervous system activity and on angiotensin II–mediated aldosterone secretion.[511,550] The effects of insulin on sodium retention can occur indpendently of insulin-induced hypokalemia, stimulation of angiotensin II production, or decreases in prostaglandin production and of changes in the GFR.[548,551] They can be blocked by calcium-channel blockers,[548] in vasopressin deficient animals,[548] and by ANP.[552] These results suggest that the renal effects of insulin may be blunted in a number of circumstances.[552] Insulin can affect glomerular hemodynamics by increasing glomerular efferent arteriolar vasodilation and afferent arteriole vasoconstriction[551] and can increase renal plasma flow at high concentrations.[540]

Sympathetic

Insulin can increase noradrenergic sympathetic activity, plasma norepinephrine levels, urinary norepinephrine, and norepinephrine turnover.[120,466,511,512,547] Insulin actions in the CNS probably elicit these responses. There is regional nonuniformity in the stimulation. Thus, insulin increases lumbar but not renal or adrenal activity in rats and increases medial hypothalamic and muscle but not skin activity in humans. Some sympathetic effects could be secondary to baroreceptor reflex responses. The effects of insulin occur in the absence of hypoglycemia (which suppresses the sympathetic nervous system and stimulated adrenal epinephrine release) and are independent of insulin stimulation of carbohydrate metabolism.

Vascular Structure

Insulin is a growth factor and can stimulate smooth muscle and fibroblast proliferation in cell culture and the uptake and esterification of lipoprotein by smooth muscle cells.[511,513,553] These actions could accelerate the development of secondary changes in hypertension and atherosclerosis.[513]

Effects on Ions

Insulin regulates cation transport activity[513] and has other effects on ions and ion channels that may influence blood pressure. Insulin stimulates Na^+, K^+-ATPase and Ca^{2+}, Mg^{2+}-ATPase activities; these actions decrease Ca^{2+} influx and block Ca^{2+} currents and Ca^{2+} action potentials.[511,513,548,553–555] Insulin effects on Ca^{2+} are observed in vascular smooth muscle, where the peptide promotes vasodilation, inhibits K^+ and vasopressor-induced contractions, attenuates agonist-induced intracellular Ca^{2+} transients,[554] and decreases inositol trisphosphate–releasable Ca^{2+}.[513,541,553,556] Insulin increases the activity of the Na^+-Li^+ countertransport;[486,511] Na^+-Li^+ countertransport activity decreases with weight loss.[557] Insulin may affect Na^+-K^+ cotransport.[511] The significance of these changes is not understood.

Insulin can increase Na^+-phosphate cotransport and Na^+-H^+ antiport activity.[486,513,548,553] Enhanced

Na^+-H^+ exchange might increase intracellular Ca^{2+} and vascular contractility and increase intracellular alkalinization, which stimulates protein synthesis and cell proliferation; both of these influences would promote hypertension.[513] Insulin-mediated Na^+-H^+ exchange could also increase renal Na^+ reabsorption.[486]

Insulin Resistance and Actions in Essential Hypertension

Interpretation of the actions of insulin in hypertension is complicated by coexisting influences (Fig. 14-17). There is both insulin resistance and hyperinsulinemia. The insulin resistance is selective. Thus, abnormalities can be due to either excessive insulin action or insulinopenia. Concomitant insulin-mediated influences on glucose uptake, obesity, and food intake influence ion transport, sympathetic nervous system activity, and other parameters. Finally, the patient population is heterogeneous.

Insulin resistance in hypertension and obesity is selective for skeletal muscle. In this tissue, there are blunted insulin effects on vasodilation and increased skeletal muscle blood flow and glucose update.[466,544,545,537] Skeletal muscle resistance to insulin also contributes to a decrease in the ability of insulin to dispose of glucose. Resistance to glucose uptake is not found in the liver. Resistance to insulin-mediated increases in skeletal muscle blood flow and glucose uptake are proportional to basal blood pressure and occur independently of age or body fat content.[466,544] However, they can also be correlated with body mass index.[558] Hypertensive rats can also have selective insulin resistance[511] and augmented adrenal sympathetic nerve responses to insulin compared with normotensive strains.[466,559] Rats made insulin-resistant with fructose also have exaggerated pressor and sympathetic responses to insulin.[466]

By contrast, there is less resistance to insulin actions on the sympathetic nervous system and kidneys.[444,466,511,524,544,545,549] This selective resistance potentially leads to excessive sympathetic nervous system activity, an enhanced tendency to sodium retention, and a greater tendency to develop hypertension. The contribution of insulin to activation of the autonomic nervous system and that of renal sodium retention to insulin-resistant states has not been accurately defined. The contributions of autonomic nervous system activity and renal salt retention to the hypertension in these states are also not known. However, with insulin resistance and hyperinsulinemia, there is excessive sympathetic nervous system activity and salt sensitivity of the blood pressure. The correlations between enhanced sympathetic nervous system activity and hypertension in general are discussed in the section on catecholamines and the autonomic nervous system above.

Many studies of sympathetic nervous system activity have focused on obesity.[120,512] Plasma norepinephrine levels and sympathetic nervous system activity have been reported to be low, normal, or high in obesity.[120] Plasma epinephrine levels are normal.[120,512] It has been proposed that autonomic deficiency may cause obesity.[120] However, overall there appears to be increased sympathetic nervous system activity with insulin resistance, obesity, and hypertension.[120,512] There is a positive correlation between plasma norepinephrine levels and the abdominal form of obesity, the phenotype associated with hypertension and insulin resistance.[512] There are accentuated plasma norepinephrine responses to postural and other stimuli and to glucose ingestion in obesity.[120] Obese and salt-sensitive hypertensive subjects also have enhanced sympathetic activity.[120] Urinary norepinephrine levels are highest in those with the highest fasting levels of insulin and glucose.[512] Both insulin and food intake can stimulate the sympathetic nervous system in obesity.[120,512] The overall weight probably contributes as well.[120]

Insulin resistance is strongly correlated in obese and nonobese hypertensives with enhanced sodium sensitivity of blood pressure.[444,448,511] Plasma insulin levels correlate with salt-induced changes in blood pressure in obese subjects. Improvement of insulin sensitivity by means of weight reduction reduces salt sensitivity. A hyperinsulinemic response to oral glucose occurs in normotensive salt-sensitive men.[444] The blood pressure of obese adolesents is more dependent on salt than is that of nonobese adolesents; this sodium sensitivity is attenuated with weight loss.[448,511] Hypertension with weight gain in the dog occurs only if adequate salt is present in the diet.[511] Further, in contrast to previous reports, sodium restriction probably does not affect insulin sensitivity.[444] However, plasma insulin levels were similar in salt-sensitive vs. salt-resistant hypertensives,[560] this could imply that insulin does not induce salt sensitivity in all individuals. However, the salt-retaining actions of insulin can be demonstrated in hypertensives.[549]

Weight loss has a hypotensive effect.[120,512] Overall, this is correlated with decreases in plasma norepinephrine levels.[120] However, there is some decrease in blood pressure before plasma norepinephrine levels fall, and this may be mediated in part by changes in sodium balance caused by decreases in plasma insulin levels and salt intake.[120] Dopamine levels may increase during caloric restriction, and this may enhance natriuresis.[120]

Thus, it is hypothesized that in insulin-resistant states hyperinsulinemia stimulates the sympathetic nervous system activity and renal sodium retention and that these actions elevate blood pressure (Fig. 14-17). These effects are ordinarily counterbalanced by the peripheral vasodilator actions of insulin, but selective resistance to this effect in insulin-resistant states leaves the renal and sympathetic nervous system actions unopposed. This formulation could imply that the administration of more insulin might overcome the resistance and lower the blood pressure; this idea would be consistent with the finding that hypertension generally does not occur with insulinomas, where the insulin excess would overcome insulin resistance. This formulation is also consistent with other findings, for example, that blood pressure responses to angiotensin II are blunted during maximal hyperinsulinemia but not at lower concentrations of insulin.[540]

Ion Transport Abnormalities in Insulin Resistance

Changes in intracellular ions (Ca^{2+}, Mg^{2+}, and pH) and transport processes occur with insulin resistance, obesity, insulin action, glucose uptake, and diabetes.[247] It is not understood which of these influences are primary vs. secondary, and their overall role in hypertension is undefined.

Elevated intracellular [Ca^{2+}] and depressed intracellular [Mg^{2+}] and pH values are correlated with hypertension in insulin-resistant and obese individuals.[247] Patients with type II diabetes mellitus also tend to have higher intracellular Ca^{2+} irrespective of hypertension, but even in these patients, there is a correlation between hypertension and higher intracellular Ca^{2+} levels and lower intracellular [Mg^{2+}] and pH levels.[247,475] pH and Mg^{2+} differences between hypertensive and normotensive diabetic patients are similar to those in nondiabetics.[247,475] These changes in essential hypertension tend to normalize with correction of the hypertension.[247] There is also increased cytosolic free [Ca^{2+}] with insulin resistance in cells in culture.[247,513,518]

The effects of glucose ingestion are the opposite of those of insulin and may blunt those of insulin. Glucose increases intracellular pH, Na^+, and Ca^{2+} levels and decreases Mg^{2+} levels.[246,247,556] These influences are blunted in essential hypertension, obesity, and type II diabetes mellitus,[246,247,556] implying that the ion transport abnormalities present in essential hypertension also affect the influences of glucose.

The higher levels of intracellular Ca^{2+} in insulin-resistant states could contribute to a number of abnormalities associated with hypertension, obesity, and type II diabetes mellitus.[246,247] Increased intracellular Ca^{2+} in vascular smooth muscle could increase the blood pressure directly through vasoconstriction and indirectly by enhancing responses to vasoconstrictor agents and stimulating vascular smooth muscle proliferation.[247,513] Increased intracellular Ca^{2+} could also lead to resistance to insulin release in pancreatic beta-cells, suppression of renal renin release, and enhanced release of vasoactive substances.[247] It could also stimulate platelet aggregation and enhance endothelial cell release of protective glycosaminoglycans and heparin.[247] The decreased Mg^{2+} may further increase the intracellular Ca^{2+} and hypertension and also amplify insulin resistance.[475]

Changes in ion transporters in insulin-resistant states include diminished Na^+, K^+-ATPase and Ca^{2+}-ATPase activities.[553] These influences could participate in increasing intracellular Ca^{2+} levels. Na^+-Li^+ countertransport activity is higher in insulin-resistant blacks and whites and in white hypertensives with insulin resistance[486] but is not correlated with hyperinsulinemia in offspring of hypertensive parents.[492] Na^+-Li^+ countertransport activity decreases with exercise but not with weight reduction.[487] In blacks, Na^+-H^+ exchange is higher in hypertensive insulin-resistant subjects than in normotensive insulin-resistant or hypertensive insulin-sensitive subjects.[486] The insulin-resistant Zucker rat has decreased membrane Ca^{2+}-ATPase activity and increased intracellular Ca^{2+} levels, implying that insulinopenia may elevate the blood pressure.[555]

Thus, it is attractive to postulate a defect in ion transport to explain the insulin resistance syndrome or aspects of it. However, it is unkown whether one of the processes described above or an influence that affects them is involved. Further, since there is a spectrum of abnormalities that includes hypertension, insulin resistance, obesity, type II diabetes mellitus, and other aberrations, it appears likely that there is more than one primary abnormality.

Therapeutic Implications

As the insulin resistance syndrome becomes better understood, there may be increasing discussion on prevention and treatment. Hypertension in individuals with insulin resistance, obesity, or type II diabetes mellitus responds especially well to caloric restriction.[120,511–513,528] Even small reductions in weight can have a significant effect on blood pressure. The blood pressure and insulin resistance also respond favorably to exercise.[511] Salt restriction is helpful when there is moderate caloric restriction but is less beneficial with very low calorie diets.[528]

Antihypertensive agents that enhance sodium excretion and reduce sympathetic nervous system activity would seem to be ideal in these patients.[120] However, most antihypertensive agents affect the sympathetic nervous system in some way, and the resultant effects are somewhat complex. For example, diuretic agents lower blood pressure by reducing intravascular volume and cardiac output, but these changes also activate sympathetic nervous system activity. β, α-adrenergic blockers have varied effects on different components of the sympathetic nervous system; whereas the β-blockers enhance insulin resistance. α-blockers improve it.[120] Centrally acting antihypertensive agents such as clonidine, methyldopa, and guanabenz inhibit sympathetic outflow and may be especially useful in this population. Calcium-channel blockers have had modest and mixed effects on sympathetic nervous system activity, but may influence some of the ion abnormalities in the syndrome and have had a high rate of efficacy in obese hypertensives.[120] Converting enzyme inhibitors are also useful, since they block angiotensin II actions on sympathetic nervous system activity (as discussed earlier) and have favorable effects on glucose control and the kidney in diabetes.[120] There will also be interest in utilizing drugs that improve the sensitivity to insulin action and result in weight reduction through a variety of mechanisms.

EVALUATION OF THE HYPERTENSIVE PATIENT

Evaluation of a hypertensive patient should provide sufficient information to (1) confirm the presence and level of persistent inappropriately elevated blood pressure, (2) assess the presence and severity of secondary target organ involvement of the heart, brain, kidneys, and vasculature, (3) identify clues for secondary forms of hypertension which would lead to more extensive evaluation, (4) identify coexistent medical illnesses and other treatable risk factors for accelerated atherosclerosis, (5) determine the urgency and basis for the selection of specific antihypertensive therapy, and (6) assess previous therapy for hypertension and responses to or side effects from such therapy. This evaluation can be obtained from a careful medical history, physical examination, and selected screening laboratory studies as outlined elsewhere.[1,2,4] The evaluation should also allow the physician to decide whether a further work-up should be performed to look for a secondary form of hypertension. Features from the history and physical examination that suggest secondary hypertension are provided in Tables 14-4 and 14-5.

Clinical History

The clinical history should provide (1) information on timing of the onset and known duration of hypertension, (2) the family history, including the presence of hypertension and its complications or premature arteriosclerosis in close relatives, (3) evidence of target organ involvement manifested as symptoms or clinical episodes of ischemic cerebral, cardiac, or peripheral vascular disease or renal disease, (4) clues such as symptoms or events suggesting secondary hypertension, such as congenital, acquired, or iatrogenic endocrine diseases (Table 14-4), (5) history of coexistent systemic diseases that could influence management, such as asthma, gout, diabetes mellitus, arthritis, and thyroid disease, (6) use of substances that have the potential to raise the blood pressure, such as glucocorticoids, erythropoietin, nonsteroidal anti-inflammatory agents, estrogens, over-the-counter nasal decongestants, licorice, or recreational drugs (cocaine, tobacco, and alcohol), and (7) dietary habits (sodium, potassium, calories, and fat intake).

Secondary hypertension is suggested when the hypertension occurs in younger (<20 years of age) or older (>60 years of age) patients, when blood pressure responds very poorly to drug therapy, with accelerated or malignant hypertension, in well-controlled patients whose hypertension becomes worse, and with sudden onset of hypertension. The diagnosis of essential hypertension is made by exclusion.

Physical Examination

Physical examination should begin with careful measurement of the blood pressure, since the level of the pressure determines the diagnosis of hypertension, predicts the long-term prognosis, justifies a search for secondary hypertension, and becomes the

TABLE 14-4 Features on History Suggestive of Secondary Hypertension

No family history of hypertension
Very strong family history, particularly of severe hypertension, hypertension at an early age, or a disorder such as renal disease that is associated with hypertension
Abrupt onset of hypertension
Onset of hypertension before age 20 or after age 60
Sudden acceleration of previously existing hypertension or development of malignant hypertension de novo
Rapid deterioration of renal function despite well-controlled hypertension or after treatment with converting enzyme inhibitors
Unresponsiveness to standard antihypertensive therapy (other than converting enzyme inhibitor therapy)
Rapid development of hypokalemia with standard doses of diuretics
History of renal trauma, flank pain, and hematuria, suggesting renal infarction
Sudden onset of hypertension in a patient with systemic emboli or vasculitis
Development of hypertension in association with lower-extremity ischemia, calf or buttock claudication, and erectile incompetence, abdominal angina, or aortic aneurysm
Nocturnal polyuria
Periodic paralysis or muscle weakness
Weight loss or gain; change in fat distribution
Change in menses
Change in appearance (e.g., with Cushing's syndrome, acromegaly)
Headaches
Palpitations
Tremulousness
Symptoms of postural hypotension
Skin changes (acne, excessive bruising, pigmentation, dry skin)
Muscle weakness
Edema
Excessive sweating

basis for initiating therapy. Recommendations for the indirect measurement of blood pressure with a sphygmomanometer, using the Korotkoff sounds, have been recently updated by a task force of the American Heart Association.[560a] For accurate measurements, the equipment must be properly calibrated, the width and length of the cuff and inflation bladder should be appropriate for the circumference of the arm, the subject should be comfortably positioned with the arm in which the measurement is made at the level of the heart, and the observer should be seated to minimize distraction.[1] The disappearance of sound (phase V) should be used for the diastolic measurement. However, in children and patients with high cardiac output, such as in hyperthyroidism, aortic insufficiency, pregnancy, and after exercise, phase IV, or muffling of the Korotkoff sounds, is a more accurate reflection of the diastolic pressure.[561]

To establish the diagnosis of hypertension, multiple blood pressure determination should be made. Elevated readings should be confirmed on at least two subsequent visits during one to several weeks unless hypertension is very severe (Table 14-1), in which case more immediate treatment is indicated. Normal fluctuations in blood pressure levels resulting from diurnal variations, effects of ambient temperature, activity, hospitalization, emotional factors, and so on, must be appreciated.[1,562,563] In some patients, home blood pressure recordings or automated 24-h recordings are needed to define whether the blood pressure is elevated persistently or only in the physician's office. Target organ damage is correlated better with out of office than with office pressure readings.[1] Average levels of diastolic blood pressure of >90 mmHg or of systolic of over 140 mmHg are required for the diagnosis of hypertension (Table 14-1).[1] Blood pressure should also be measured in supine, erect, and sitting positions. A marked postural fall in blood pressure (e.g., >10 mmHg systolic) suggests volume depletion, blunted baroreceptor reflexes, or peripheral neuropathy.[561]

The remainder of the general physical examination should include careful inspection of the skin, head, and neck, including the optic fundi; detailed cardiovascular examination with palpation and auscultation of the major vessels; determination of cardiac size, rhythm, and the presence of murmurs; examination of the chest, abdomen, and extremities; and a screening neurologic examination. Features on physical examination that suggest the presence of secondary hypertension are listed in Table 14-5.

TABLE 14-5 Findings on Physical Examination Suggestive of Secondary Hypertension

Malignant hypertension, grade III or IV Keith Wagener retinopathy
Widespread occlusive vascular disease in the carotid, aortoiliac, or femoral arteries manifested by decreased pulses or bruits
Epigastric or flank bruit with both systolic and diastolic components
Abdominal aortic aneurysm
Positive Chvostek's or Trousseau's sign, suggesting alkalosis
Impaired autonomic reflexes; postural hypotension
Central obesity with thinning of the extremities, hirsutism, etc., suggesting Cushing's syndrome
Tremor, weight loss, etc., suggesting thyrotoxicosis
Hypertension in the upper extremities only or radiofemoral pulse disparity (suggesting coarctation)
Skin: striae, acne, sweating, café au lait spots and neurofibromas
Mumurs: interscapular late systolic murmur (coarctation of the aorta)
Radiofemoral pulse delay (coarctation of the aorta)
Abnormal fat distribution
Muscle wasting
Postural hypotension with and without reflex tachycardia
Wide swings in blood pressure levels
Abdominal or flank masses (polycystic kidneys)
Tachycardia, tremor, orthostatic hypotension, sweating, and pallor (pheochromocytoma)

Laboratory Tests

Laboratory tests are used to obtain clues about secondary forms of hypertension and assess end organ damage and associated risk factors. Some general tests should be performed in all hypertensive patients, as outlined below. More specialized tests should be performed as described in the section that follows the discussion of general tests. Except for the plasma renin determination, the specialized tests described in this chapter are intended to evaluate the renovascular hypertension or mineralocorticoid-excess states; these tests are described in the sections dealing with those disorders.

General Tests

General tests that should be performed in all hypertensive patients are listed in Table 14-6.[564,565] Additional studies such as chest x-ray, echocardiogram, and treadmill exercise test should be performed if additional cardiac evaluation is suggested by the clinical findings. There is growing interest in determining the plasma aldosterone/renin ratios (see the section on primary aldosteronism). Table 14-6 lists common laboratory tests.

Specific Tests

Specialized tests for the evaluation of specific secondary forms of hypertension are performed in general when indicated by information from the history, physical examination, or routine laboratory testing, as described above and in sections on specific secondary forms of hypertension below. The decision to perform additional tests should be made with the under-

TABLE 14-6 Laboratory Evaluation of the Hypertensive Patient*

Complete blood count
Urinalysis
Serum creatinine, uric acid, and electrolytes
Blood urea nitrogen
Fasting blood glucose
Fasting serum LDL and HDL cholesterol and triglycerides
Electrocardiogram

* General tests that should be performed in all hypertensive patients.

standing that many of these tests are imprecise. Their use for screening general hypertensive populations can result in a large number of false-positive test results, and an excessive number of unfruitful follow-up evaluations.

The usefulness of these tests is frequently described in terms of their sensitivity and specificity. *Sensitivity* refers to the percentage of the time the test will detect the abnormality when it is present. *Specificity* refers to the percentage of the time the disorder will be present when the test is abnormal. The utility of a test with a 90 percent sensitivity and specificity is shown in Table 14-7. For a disorder with a prevalence of 1 percent and a test with a sensitivity of 90 percent, there would be 10 false positives and one correct positive in a screening of 100 patients. This number of false positives is ordinarily unacceptable for further extensive analysis. However, if clinical assessment could identify patients with a 50 percent probability of having the disorder, screening 100 patients would yield 45 correct and only 5 false positives. This analysis illustrates the need for preselecting patients to be screened when only tests with lower sensitivities are available.

Plasma Renin Activity

PRA is measured to assess renovascular hypertension and low-renin states and has been recommended as a general screening procedure to indicate the type of hypertensive medication to be used.[156] PRA can be measured under basal conditions or after stimulatory maneuvers. It is sometimes measured in samples taken from the renal veins.

PRA is measured by its ability to generate angiotensin I from the substrate angiotensinogen.[66,214,566–570] In vivo, this reaction occurs in the circulation, within blood vessel walls, and probably within some tissues. PRA is determined by incubation of plasma at 37°C followed by radioimmunoassay (RIA) of the generated angiotensin I.[66,569–571] Thus, plasma samples for renin determination must be processed quickly on collection (usually in tubes containing EDTA) and stored frozen at temperatures <20°C until assay. Prolonged storage of plasma at temperatures just below freezing can result in a slow activation of prorenin that can invalidate the results. The incubation pH is critical. A pH around 5.7 is used by some laboratories because it is the optimum pH for the reaction between human renin and human angiotensinogen. Conversely, a neutral pH is used by others to mimic in vivo conditions and eliminate the effects of plasma proteases which may have reninlike activity. Generation of angiotensin I at neutrality generally gives lower PRA values than generation at pH 5.7. The reactions should include angiotensinase inhibitors; the choice depends on the incubation pH. PRA is usually expressed as nanograms of angiotensin I generated per milliliter per hour and is dependent on linear angiotensin I generation with time.

There is also a direct RIA for renin.[567] The values obtained with it in general correlate with the PRA values.[567]

In human plasma, the reaction between renin and angiotensinogen occurs at substrate concentrations near the K_m for renin, so that the reaction rate is proportional to concentrations of both renin and substrate. Ordinarily, the plasma renin substrate concentration is quite constant. However, in some clinical conditions it may be altered, leading to a change in the measured rate of angiotensin I generation. During estrogen administration and pregnancy and in patients with glucocorticoid excess, renin substrate concentration is increased, leading to elevated PRA.[139] Renin substrate concentration is reduced in liver disease and in states of glucocorticoid deficiency.[139]

TABLE 14-7 Tests for Sensitivity and Specificity: Analysis of Hypothetical Population of 100 Patients Using a Test with 90% Specificity and Sensitivity

	Screening					
Test Population Prevalence, %	False Positives		Correct Positives		Missed Diagnoses	
	Number	Percent	Number	Percent	Number	Percent
1	10	9.9	1	0.9	0	0.1
5	10	9.5	5	4.5	1	0.5
20	8	8	18	18	2	2
50	5	5	45	45	5	5
80	2	2	72	72	8	8

Plasma renin concentration (PRC) is measured by generating angiotensin I in the presence of excess substrate so that the reaction between renin and angiotensinogen is not limited by the concentration of angiotensinogen (i.e., is zero-order). Except in situations where the human substrate concentration is altered, PRA and PRC are directly proportional. PRC measurements are not generally performed but can be useful in situations where angiotensinogen concentration is altered or to better define a low-renin state such as primary aldosteronism.

Plasma prorenin concentrations can also be measured by assaying PRC before and after acid or protease treatment of plasma to activate prorenin to renin.[62,72] Some patients with diabetes mellitus, patients with renin-secreting tumors, and pregnant women have elevated plasma levels of prorenin (5 to 10 times normal).[72]

PRA levels fluctuate spontaneously.[4,51,63,66,87,97,104,122,135,153,156,214,250] They are influenced by sex, race, age, sodium balance, position, activity, severity of hypertension, concurrent medication such as birth control pills and antihypertensive drugs, and illnesses such as diabetes mellitus, congestive heart failure, and cirrhosis (see above).[4,51,63,66,87,97,104,122,135,153,156,214,250]

Several protocols have been proposed to standardize the measurement of PRA. They include normal and low-sodium diet, pretreatment with a diuretic, and measurement of PRA after overnight recumbency before the patient arises; others measure PRA after the patient has been ambulatory and upright for 4 h. Hence, "normal" values differ from laboratory to laboratory and under different circumstances.

PRA values (Table 14-8)[4,51,63,66,87,97,104,122,135,153,156,214,250,291] can be more easily interpreted by comparing them with concurrent 24-h urinary sodium excretion rates after several days with a stable sodium intake and without antihypertensive medications for at least 2 weeks (Figs. 14-6 and 14-8).[4,156] If renal, endocrine, and cardiac functions are normal, the sodium excretion rate is a convenient marker for extracellular fluid volume. Sodium excretion and extracellular fluid volume normally are inversely related to PRA and plasma aldosterone levels. The sodium/creatinine concentration ratio in a specimen of urine collected at the same time as the blood for PRA can also be used as a marker of volume status. PRA falls with age, and normal subjects above 55 years of age have PRA values that range up to 50 percent less than in younger subjects. Patients with diabetes mellitus with and without renal failure may have lower PRA levels.

In hypertensive patients, PRA levels are low in primary aldosteronism and other mineralocorticoid-excess states (see the sections on primary aldosteronism and other mineralocorticoid-excess states). They can also be low in low-renin essential hypertension and in renal disease.[50,51,141,156,219] PRA can also be low with excessive salt loading.

To diagnose a low-renin state, PRA can be measured before and after stimulation of the renin system. Stimulatory maneuvers include provision of a low-sodium diet, standing (1 to 4 h), intravenous (IV) administration of furosemide (40 to 60 mg), and oral captopril. These maneuvers are described in the section on primary aldosteronism.

In hypertensive patients, PRA values are elevated in some patients with essential hypertension, renovascular hypertension, accelerated hypertension, renin-secreting tumors, and diuretic therapy.[225,572–575] In states not associated with hypertension, they can be high with dehydration, blood loss, and diuretic therapy. In patients with renin-secreting tumors, plasma prorenin levels are also markedly elevated.[225,572] In patients with unexplained hyperkalemia, a PRA determination is necessary in the diagnosis of hyporeninemic hypoaldosteronism (see Chap. 12).

Increased PRA in renovascular hypertension is seen in 50 to 80 percent of patients subsequently improved by angioplasty.[8,573,575] Since discontinuation of medication is not possible in patients with severe hypertension, depending on the standards for the particular laboratory, up to 20 percent of patients with proven renovascular hypertension can have normal to low PRA and approximately 15 percent of patients with essential hypertension can have elevated PRA. Thus, random determination of PRA per se has limited use in screening for renovascular hypertension.[573–575] Further, in chronic renovascular hypertension, especially if both renal arteries are stenotic, extracellular fluid volume can increase and PRA can be suppressed.

Measurement of PRA after the administration of a converting enzyme inhibitor may be helpful in differentiating patients with high-renin essential hypertension from those with renovascular hypertension[572] (see the sections on the evaluation of renovascular hypertension).

RENOVASCULAR HYPERTENSION

Clarification of the pathogenesis of renovascular hypertension has increased our understanding of the role of the kidney and the renin-angiotensin system in the regulation of blood pressure. By the late 1890s, investigators recognized the relations between hypertension and cardiac and renal disease and produced experimental hypertension by injecting renal extracts into rabbits.[576,577] There followed pioneering work by Goldblatt and coworkers in 1934,[578] who produced hypertension in the dog by constricting the renal artery, and subsequent observations by Page and associates and Braun-Menendez and coworkers describing the renin-angiontensin system.[579,580] This set the stage for later work that demonstrated the origin of renin,[581] identified angiotensin II[582] and aldosterone,[583] and defined the relations between aldosterone, renin, angiotensin II, the kidney, sodium and potassium, and hypertension in humans.[584–586]

Subsequent developments have led to improved tests for the diagnosis and treatment of renovascular hypertension, the most common known form of "curable" hypertension in adults, infants, and children. The value of revascularization for improving renal function is increasingly recognized, since even older patients with extensive atherosclerotic disease can be treated successfully. Although the utility of current diagnostic tests is limited in terms of sensitivity and specificity, the benefits gained from searching for and treating renovascular hypertension are generally recognized. The pathogenesis of renovascular hypertension is discussed in the section on the renin-angiotensin system. Clinical aspects of renovascular hypertension are described below.

The precise incidence of renovascular hypertension is not clear.[8–11] As was stated earlier, some estimate an incidence of only 0.5 percent among unselected hypertensives,[8] a value considerably lower than previous estimates in the 5 percent range.[8–11] However, in certain groups of patients, such as those with accelerated or malignant hypertension, children under age 10, those developing hypertension after age 50, diabetic patients, and patients with peripheral vascular disease, the prevalence of renovascular hypertension is higher.[8–11] For example, renal artery stenosis of 50 percent or more was observed in 45 percent of patients presenting with intermittent claudication or lower limb ischemic ulceration.[11] Autopsy studies indicate that the prevalence of renal artery stenosis is high, although the functional significance of these lesions cannot be assessed.[587,588] In a study of subjects older than 50 years, stenosis of more than 50 percent was seen in 53 percent of subjects whose diastolic blood pressures were more than 100 mmHg and in 22.5 percent of subjects whose diastolic blood pressures were less than 100 mmHg.[588,589]

TABLE 14-8 Normal Peripheral Plasma Renin Activity Values*

	Incubation pH	
	5.5	7.5
Supine 1 h	1–3	0–0.7
Standing 1 h	3–6	0.7–3.5
Sodium-restricted diet and standing	5–10	3.7–7.0

* Values in ng/ml per hour for subjects on a normal sodium intake of ~110 mEq/24 h. Low-salt diet and furosemide increase PRA twofold to threefold; captopril increases PRA threefold to fivefold. Data from Oparil.[569]

Not included in these estimates are situations in which smaller segmental artery lesions could be inducing excessive renin release, especially with multiple lesions. It would be difficult to diagnose these situations with current methods. As discussed in the section on the role of the renin-angiotensin system in hypertension, it has been proposed that the kidneys of many patients with normal- and high-renin essential hypertension have regions of relative ischemia that hypersecrete renin.[51] By this formulation, there could be a continuum from the relatively large artery lesions causing renovascular hypertension that can be treated by revascularization procedures to smaller lesions that may be driving the hypertension but are less accessible to revascularization corrective approaches.

The pathophysiology of both experimental and human renovascular hypertension is described in the section on the role of the renin-angiotensin system in hypertension above. Human renovascular hypertension resembles the early phase of the two-kidney, one-clip Goldblatt animal model discussed in that section in that the kidney with decreased blood flow secretes increased amounts of renin and the opposite, nonischemic kidney is suppressed and secretes less renin.[128] However, in patients with long-standing renovascular hypertension, the pattern is more like the one-kidney, one-clip animal model and resistance to converting enzyme blockade occurs unless the animal is sodium-depleted.

Pathology of Renovascular Hypertension

The most common causes of renovascular hypertension are atherosclerosis (Fig. 14-18) and fibromuscular dysplasia (Fig. 14-19); other causes (Table 14-9) are much less frequent.[163,590–603]

Atherosclerosis

Atherosclerotic renal artery lesions resemble those in other muscular arteries (Fig. 14-19).[10,11,163,587,599] The atheromatous intimal plaque may be focal or extensive, eccentric or concentric; it may be complicated by adherent platelet clumps and hemorrhage, resulting in occlusion or dissection. Emboli from ulcerating plaques to distal vessels may also occur. Atherosclerotic lesions may be unilateral but are frequently bilateral and are associated with plaques in the abdominal aorta. These lesions are characteristically located at the orifice of or in the initial one-third of the renal arteries. They occur predominantly in older male patients and in those with atherosclerosis in other arteries and with risk factors for atherosclerosis, such as hypertension, diabetes mellitus, hyperlipidemia, and cigarette smoking.[10,163,604] Atherosclerotic plaques in the renal arteries may also develop as a complication in pa-

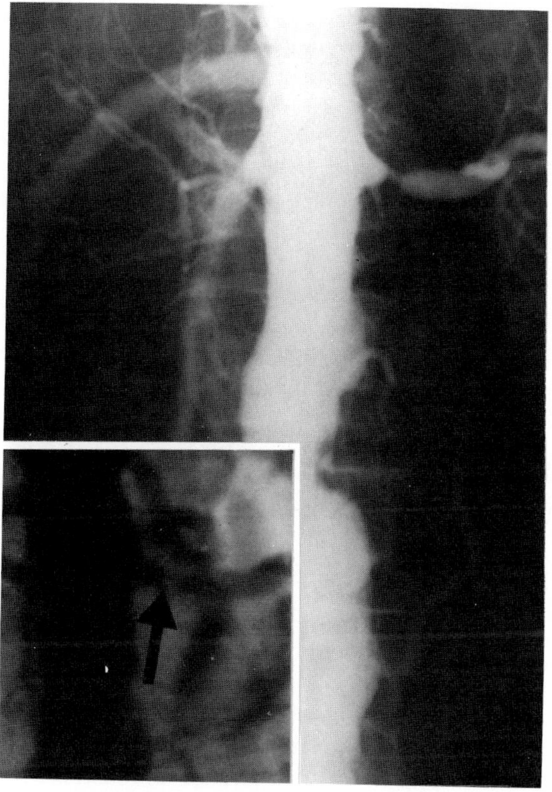

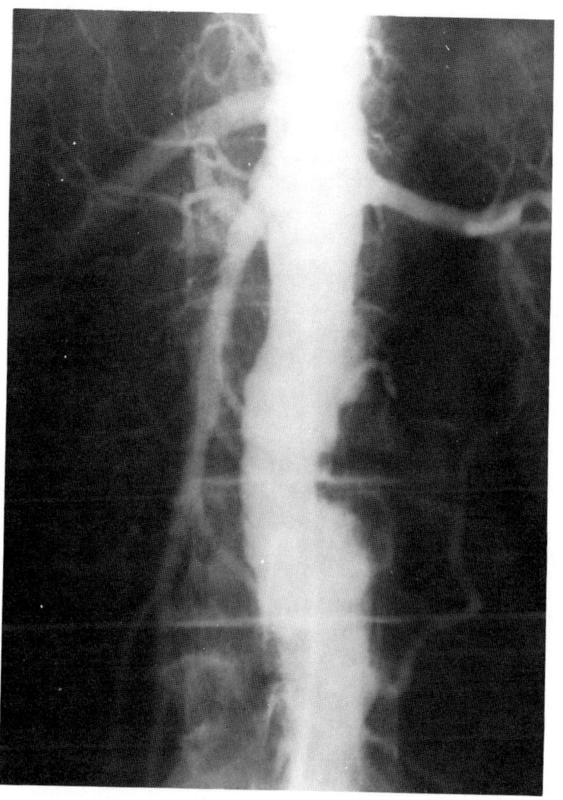

FIGURE 14-18 Renal arteriogram before (*left*) and after (*right*) balloon catheter percutaneous and transluminal angioplasty (PTLA). The insert in the left photograph shows the IV digital subtraction angiogram of the same lesion.

tients with preexisting hypertension and can lead to an abrupt decrease in renal function or acceleration of the hypertension. Conversely, incidental plaques have been observed at autopsy in the arteries of older normotensive patients.[587,605]

Fibromuscular Dysplasia

These nonatheromatous lesions (Fig. 14-19)[590,591,593] are subgrouped on the basis of (1) location of the predominant histopathology in the arterial wall (intimal, medial, perimedial, or subadventitial), (2) degree of destruction of the elastica interna and externa, and (3) predominant cell type. This subgrouping helps define differences in the angiographic appearance, natural history, and prevalence of the lesions. The cause of these lesions is not understood.

Intimal Fibroplasia

Intimal fibroplasia, which is present in 5 to 10 percent of patients with fibrodysplastic lesions, is characterized by the accumulation of irregularly arranged mesenchymal cells within subendothelial fibrous connective tissue, resulting in long, irregular but smooth focal tubular stenoses. These lesions are common in infants and children, occur with equal frequency in both sexes, may be associated with arteritis of the aorta and medial lesions, occasionally result from intimal trauma, can be complicated by dissection, and may be unilateral or bilateral.[590,592,597,606–608] In children, the elastica interna is reduplicated and there is often medial disorganization. Only intimal collagen accumulation is seen in the adult.

Medial Fibromuscular Dysplasia

Medial fibromuscular dysplasia is subdivided into medial and perimedial fibroplasia and medial hyperplasia.

Medial Fibroplasia (Fibromuscular Hyperplasia) This condition accounts for about 85 percent of patients with fibrodysplastic lesions and occurs predominantly in women age 25 to 50 years. The lesions consist of multifocal stenoses resulting from thick fibrous ridges and circumferential rings of collagen replacing muscle, alternating with arterial wall thinning and aneurysm formation with loss of normal medial and internal elastica. This results in the typical "string of beads" appearance on the arteriogram.[609,610] The lesion is often bilateral, occurs in the middle and distal thirds of the renal artery, and may

TABLE 14-9 Anatomic Causes of Renal Artery Obstruction

Atherosclerosis
Fibromuscular dysplasia
Arterial emboli
Aortic dissection or isolated renal artery dissection
Extrarenal compression by tumor, neurofibroma, retroperitoneal fibrosis, perirenal or subcapsular hematoma, or scarring
Arteriovenous malformation, fistula, hemangioma
Hypoplasia of suprarenal abdominal aorta
Renal artery aneurysm; intra- or extrarenal
Generalized arteritis, aortitis syndromes: Takayasu's disease
Stenosis in the artery supplying a transplanted kidney

extend into the intrarenal branches. These lesions can progress but rarely dissect or thrombose.

Medial Hyperplasia This form occurs in 1 to 2 percent of patients. It is characterized by a hyperplasia of muscular and fibrous tissue cells in the media, resulting in smooth focal stenoses on the arteriogram. This process may involve the main renal artery or its branches, occurs with equal frequency in men and women, is usually progressive, and is frequently complicated by dissection.[590,611]

Perimedial Fibroplasia This type, also referred to as subadventitial fibroplasia, is intermediate in frequency between the two varieties discussed above and is characterized by intense fibroplasia of the outer half of the media, forming a stenotic collar of collagen, variably enveloping the artery and replacing the elastica externa with fibrous tissue. The resulting appearance of the vessel is one of intermittent irregularities with small beads or "accordion pleating" but no true aneurysm formation.[590,591]

Medial Dissection Medial dissection occurs in 5 to 10 percent of fibrodysplastic lesions. It can be isolated or associated with the lesions described above, especially medial hyperplasia.[590,591]

Periarterial Hyperplasia

Periarterial hyperplasia is characterized by excessive collagen formation in the periarterial adventitia. It is rare and may be a variant of retroperitoneal fibrosis. Its natural history is not well described.[590,591]

Takayasu's Arteritis

Takayasu's arteritis is a rare cause of renovascular hypertension in the western nations but is a common cause in Asian and African populations.[598] It has been reported to account for 61 percent of patients with renovascular hypertension in India.[598]

Other Causes of Renovascular Hypertension

There are several less frequent causes of renovascular hypertension. Renal artery thrombosis may occur in situ or result from arterial emboli, occasionally in showers, from a variety of sources (vegetations from endocarditis, mural thrombi, cardiac tumors, paradoxic venous thromboemboli via a patent foramen ovale or atrial septal defect, and ulcerating aortic atherosclerotic plaques).[10,11,587,599,605,607,612] Rarer causes include aortic dissection,[613] renal artery aneurysm,[614] vasculitis,[615–618] and mechanical

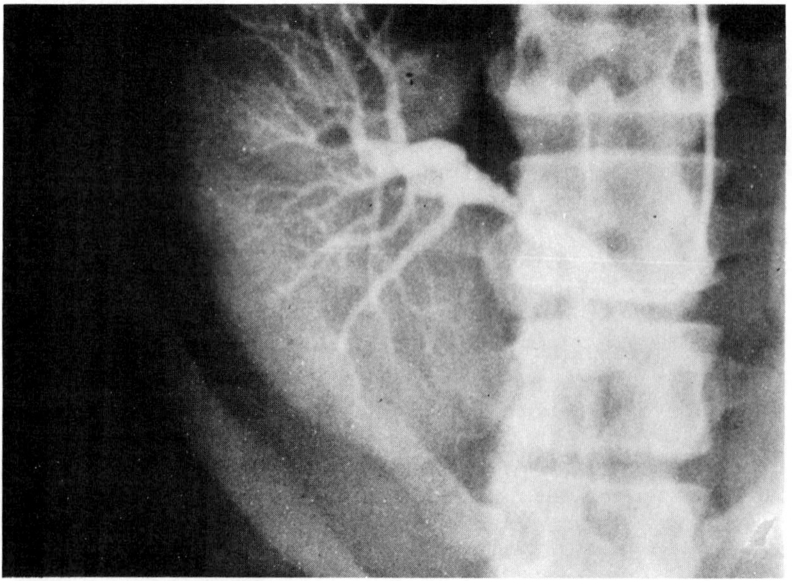

FIGURE 14-19 Renovascular hypertension resulting from fibromuscular disease. Note the "corkscrew" constriction with poststenotic dilatation.

compression of the artery due to retroperitoneal fibrosis (idiopathic or caused by drugs such as methylsergide maleate or infection),[619,620] neurofibromas, or other mass lesions.[621,622] Stenosis in the artery supplying a transplanted kidney accounts for 5 to 15 percent of posttransplant hypertension and therefore must be considered in this group of patients.[8,623]

Renin-Secreting Tumors

Hypertension results from excessive renin secretion with various types of rare renal and extrarenal tumors (Fig. 14-7).[225,624–626] Most of these tumors are small benign encapsulated hemangiopericytomas or hamartomas composed of juxtaglomerular cells, but renin-secreting adenocarcinomas of the pancreas, lung, and ovaries and Wilms' tumors have been reported. These tumors tend to produce a relatively high proportion of prorenin relative to renin; some produce only protein with minimal sequelae. Patients with pheochromocytomas can sometimes have hyperreninemia secondary to the catecholamine excess, and this can lead to a misdiagnosis of the tumor. Renin-producing tumors usually are not associated with markedly elevated catecholamine levels.

The diagnosis should be suspected in a patient whose hypertension is severe or responds poorly to therapy and in whom evaluation reveals hyperreninemia, hyperaldosteronism, and no arterial lesion on arteriography. Patients with renin-secreting renal adenomas often present with malignant or accelerated hypertension, severe headaches and papilledema, and symptoms of hyperaldosteronsim, polyuria, thirst, muscle cramps, weakness, and hypokalemic alkalosis. Occasional patients have only mild hypertension without obvious clues. Patients with renal or extrarenal renin-secreting carcinomas may have lesser degrees of hypertension, and their symptoms are due directly to the mechanical effects of the tumor. Abdominal CT scanning or MRI can be helpful in localizing the tumor.

Treatment consists of local excision, segmental resection, or rarely nephrectomy. This usually results in a "cure" of the hypertension. If surgical resection is not possible, converting enzyme inhibition can effectively control the hypertension.

Natural History of Renal Artery Lesions

Information regarding the natural history of stenotic renal arterial lesions is derived from serial angiographic studies and autopsies.[163,587,627,628] These studies may overestimate the rate of progression, since only patients with changes in the anatomic lesion and worsening of renal function of hypertension are likely to be restudied.

All investigators report progression of atherosclerotic lesions in terms of increased narrowing, extent of narrowing, and number of vessels involved;[163,627,628] 10 to 17 percent of patients will occlude within 2 to 3 years, and 40 percent of unilateral stenoses will proceed to contralateral involvement within a year.[163] There can also be thrombosis, hemorrhage into the plaque, embolization, or dissection.[628] The likelihood of progression to occlusion is related directly to the degree of stenosis.

Fibromuscular dysplastic lesions have variable rates of progression because of heterogeneous pathologic processes that are involved. For example, in one study, progression was found in 33 percent of patients with medial fibroplasia after a mean interval of 45 months, but there was no progression to occlusion.[628] Only 2 of 66 patients had a rise in the serum creatinine level, while kidney size decreased in 10 percent and blood pressure control became inadequate in 15 percent. Progression tends to be slower in patients over age 40.[627] In medial hyperplasia, reports of the incidence of dissection vary.[610,627] Progression to renal infarction can rarely occur,[611] especially with perimedial fibrosis or intimal fibroplasia. In intimal fibroplasia, dissection is frequent and there is progression in most patients.[629] Perimedial fibroplasia can progress to severe stenosis.[593]

Aneurysms can rupture, thrombose, or expand with further compression of the surrounding vasculature.[614] Patients with aortic dissection may have a second, more devastating dissection, with a further decrease in renal blood flow. Arteritis such as Takayasu's often progresses but may be arrested unpredictably.[630]

Progressive stenosis leads to increasing renal ischemia and progressive renal destruction (ischemic nephropathy) and deterioriation in renal function, especially when the lesions are bilateral.[52,53] Hypertension in these patients tends to be more resistant to therapy. In one survey, ischemic nephropathy was present in about 33 percent of patients who were treated for renovascular occlusive disease.[52,53] Revascularization can decrease progression of these lesions.

Clinical Characteristics of Patients with Renovascular Hypertension

Certain clinical features help differentiate patients with essential hypertension from those with renovascular hypertension.[8,9,573–575,631–634] These features are included in the more general lists in Tables 14-4 and 14-5. Some of those most relevant to renovascular hypertension are listed in Table 14-10. These elements relate to the severity of the blood pressure elevation; the onset, progression, and responsiveness to therapy of the hypertension; and evidence for atherosclerotic disease in the kidneys or elsewhere.

Patients who are ultimately evaluated tend to have more severe and inappropriate hypertension that is difficult to control on standard medications or have established hypertension with blood pressures that have increased significantly. There is an enhanced likelihood of finding renovascular hypertension if there is malignant hypertension. Patients with renovascular hypertension may develop hypertension abruptly rather than gradually before age 20 or after age 50. Hypertension in infancy or childhood and de novo onset of hypertension in older patients are especially suggestive.

Patients often give a history of poor responses to most medical therapy for hypertension but may have experienced an excellent response to converting enzyme inhibitor therapy. In patients with bilateral disease, blood pressure reduction with β-adrenergic antagonists or converting enzyme inhibitors can result in a deterioration in renal function[159,163,177] that can be a clue to the presence of stenosis.

Patients with renovascular hypertension often give no family history of hypertension. It has traditionally been felt that renovascular hypertension is rare among blacks, but this is disputed in a recent study.[635] In the Cooperative Study on Renovascular Hypertension, which included 2442 patients from 15 medical centers, blacks represented 30 percent of all patients studied but only 8 percent of those with renovascular hypertension.[631]

The likelihood of the presence of the disorder is increased if there is evidence for other manifestations of atherosclerotic disease, especially aortico-iliac disease, or deterioration of renal function. Patients may give a history of flank pain or trauma, hematuria, or a source of systemic emboli. Older patients may have symptoms of occlusive atherosclerotic vascular disease in other organ systems.

On physical examination,[8,9,574,634,636–638] patients with renovascular hypertension are more likely to have accelerated or malignant hypertension, with advanced hypertensive changes in the optic fundi. A bruit is often heard in the epigastrium or over the abdominal aorta. In various series, an abdominal and/or flank bruit has been heard six to nine times as often in patients with renovascular hypertension as in patients with essential hypertension. The presence of occlusive aortoiliac disease or aortic aneurysm enhances the probability of atherosclerotic renal artery involvement.

The only routine laboratory clues to renovascular hypertension are hypokalemic alkalosis (caused by secondary hyperaldosteronism), proteinuria, and impaired renal function in patients with bilateral disease.[8,9,574,634,636–638] Atheroembolic disease is commonly associated with eosinophilia and eosinophiluria detected by Wright's stain.

Initiating the Evaluation for Renovascular Hypertension

A blanket approach of performing specific tests in search of renovascular hypertension in all hypertensive patients would have a low yield and a high overall cost. Thus, most researchers agree that patients should not be evaluated if they have borderline, mild, or moderate hypertension and no specific clinical clues. It is estimated that only 0.2 percent of hypertensives have renovascular hypertension in the absence of suggestive clinical clues.[8]

More extensive testing for renovascular hypertension should be initiated only if revascularization will be attempted after the diagnosis is made. Medical and revascularization treatments are discussed in more detail in the section on therapy below. In general practice and areas remote from major medical centers, many physicians initiate standard antihypertensive therapy and pursue the possibility of renovascular hypertension only if standard treatment fails, hypertension accelerates, or renal function deteriorates. The use of β-adrenergic blocking agents and converting enzyme inhibitors allows many patients with renovascular hypertension to be treated effectively; blood pressure can be reduced to normal and renal function may not deteriorate for many years, especially in patients with unilateral disease. However, this approach sentences many patients with curable disease to a life of drug therapy instead of a possible "cure." In addition, medical therapy does not offer the same level of protection against the development of ischemic nephropathy as does a revascularization procedure.[52,53] Percutaneous transluminal angioplasty can be performed safely even in elderly, seriously ill patients. As skill with this techniques has become more widespread, complication rates from this procedure are decreasing and success rates are improving. Even if stenosis recurs, repeat angioplasty is possible. Thus, the trend is increasingly to perform revascularization if a diagnosis of renovascular hypertension is made.[574,601–603,639–641]

If revascularization will be performed after renovascular hypertension is diagnosed, the decision to initiate more definite testing should be based on finding clues as outlined above and in Table 14-10. These clues can be found by history, physical exami-

TABLE 14-10 Clues to the Presence of Renovascular Hypertension

Onset at age <20 or >60
Recent onset of hypertension
Accelerated/malignant hypertension
Abdominal bruit
Worsening of previously well controlled hypertension
Deterioriating renal function
Hypertension refractory to an appropriate three-drug regimen
Acute impairment in renal function with converting enzyme inhibitor therapy
Severe retinopathy
Unilateral small kidney
Known occlusive disease in another vascular bed

nation, or laboratory testing.[4,8,9,573,574,642] It has been estimated that 5 to 15 percent of patients with suggestive clinical clues and 30 percent of patients with accelerated hypertension have renovascular hypertension.[8] Some groups feel that this diagnosis should be pursued in any patient in whom there is significant and sustained hypertension.[4] The diagnosis should probably be pursued in all patients with severe hypertension with either progressive renal insufficiency or refractoriness to aggressive treatment, particularly patients with a history of smoking or evidence of peripheral vascular disease. It should be pursued in all patients with accelerated or malignant hypertension with grade III or IV changes in the optic fundi and in patients with moderate to severe hypertension with incidentally detected asymmetry of renal size. However, clinical judgment is the ultimate determinant in the decision to evaluate a given patient.

Specific Diagnostic Studies for Renovascular Hypertension

There is no gold standard diagnostic test for renovascular hypertension. The diagnosis requires the demonstration of both an occlusive arterial lesion and activation of the renin-angiotensin-alderosterone system.

The definitive diagnosis is made only in retrospect, when correction of a renal arterial lesion by revascularization or nephrectomy results in sustained reduction of blood pressure levels. However, a lack of fall in blood pressure after relief of the obstruction does not exclude the possibility that renal artery stenosis was previously responsible for elevating the blood pressure, since other mechanisms, such as a deterioration in renal function, could maintain hypertension that was initiated by renal ischemia. The response to therapy is also determined by the adequacy of the revascularization, the duration of the hypertension, and the presence of associated nephrosclerosis.

The lack of a definitive standard for the diagnosis of renovascular hypertension and the varying prevalence of the disease in different populations limit the diagnostic accuracy of currently available tests. The prevalence of bilateral renal artery stenosis further confounds the diagnostic accuracy of tests such as renal isotope scintigraphy, intravenous urography, and reval vein PRA determinations that depend on demonstrating a difference between the "ischemic" kidney and the normal kidney. Furthermore, in bilateral renal artery stenosis which has resulted in renal functional impairment, renin levels may be suppressed and tests that depend on demonstration of activation of the renin-angiotensin system may be negative.

The only method for visualizing the arterial lesion is arteriography. However, the presence of an anatomic lesion does not prove functional obstruction to renal blood flow, since major arterial stenoses can occur in patients without hypertension.[573] Since renal arteriography is invasive with a definite risk and expense, various screening tests are used to preselect patients in whom arteriography is likely to reveal a functionally important lesion.

Screening and predictive tests assess the relative function of the two kidneys and activation of the renin-angiotensin-aldosterone mechanism. The relative function of the kidneys with either unilateral or bilateral ischemic lesions can be assessed by the isotope renogram after captopril administration. Activation of the renin-angiotensin system can be detected more directly by finding an elevated PRA level either in the periphery or selectively in the renal veins under basal conditions or after captopril administration. These tests are relatively sensitive and specific when performed carefully in preselected patients.

Determination of Plasma Renin Activity

Measurement of PRA levels is described in the section on laboratory testing. Measurements should be made under standardized conditions, such as by comparing the PRA to the 24-h urinary sodium determination. It is emphasized in the section on laboratory testing that PRA can be elevated in essential hypertension and that PRA levels vary in a number of circumstances, such as with changes in sodium intake, posture, antihypertensive therapy, and the use of other drugs. Thus, there are patients with increased PRA who do not have renovascular hypertension and patients who can benefit from revascularization whose PRA levels are not elevated (Fig. 14-20).[643] About 16 percent of patients with essential hypertension have an elevated renin level, and only 50 to 80 percent of patients with renovascular hypertension have elevated plasma renin levels.[8,118]

There are also patients with long-standing renovascular hypertension in whom the activation of secondary mechanisms results in suppression of PRA levels. For example, the development of nephrosclerosis and renal failure can sustain hypertension independently of the initiating renal arterial ischemia and can result in renal sodium retention, volume increase, and secondary suppression of renin levels.[644] Under these circumstances, measurement of renin levels can give misleading results.

For these reasons, there has been less use of basal PRA determinations for assessing the presence of renovascular hypertension and investigators have relied increasingly on the changes in PRA in response to captopril, described below, assayed in samples from either peripheral blood (captopril test) or the renal veins (differential renal vein renin determinations). Both tests require standardization and this has limited their use in centers where the standardization has not been performed.

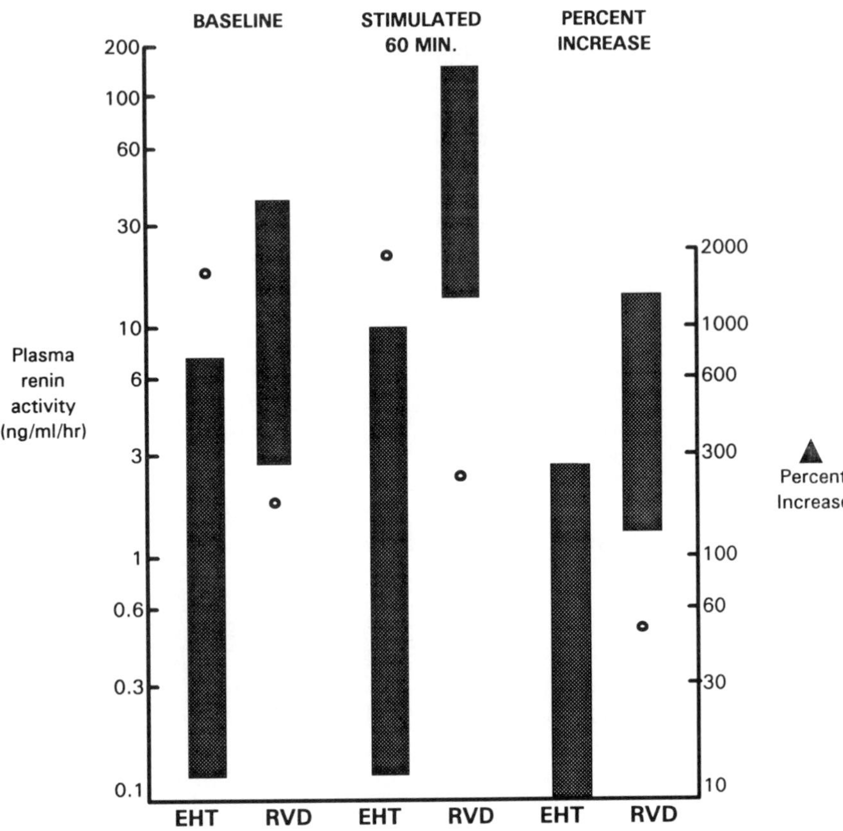

FIGURE 14-20 Captopril test for the evaluation of renovascular hypertension. The figure shows baseline and postcaptopril (60 min) values (shown as actual values, stimulated, or % increase) for patients with essential hypertension (EHT) and renovascular hypertension (RVD). Note the decreased overlap after captopril. The shaded areas indicate the location of most of the data points, with rare exceptions indicated as separate points. *(Data redrawn from Müller et al.[643])*

Blockade of the Renin-Angiotensin System (Captopril Tests)

The captopril test has been used to screen for both renovascular hypertension and primary aldosteronism (Fig. 14-20). However, the protocols used differ for the two indications. The test for renovascular hypertension[4,8,156,573,575,642,643,645–648] relies on the effect of the converting enzyme inhibitor on PRA, whereas that for primary aldosteronism relies on the influence of the blockade on plasma aldosterone (described in the section on primary aldosteronism).

In screening for renovascular hypertension, oral administration of captopril usually reduces blood pressure in 10 to 15 min with a peak fall at 90 min, and the magnitude of blood pressure reduction is proportional to PRA. In patients with correctable renovascular hypertension and high PRA, converting enzyme inhibition not only lowers blood pressure but produces a reactive hyperreninemia resulting from blockade of the negative feedback exerted by intrarenal angiotensin II. This reactive hyperreninemia is less pronounced in patients with essential hypertension.

The protocol for the captropil test[4,156,643] is as follows: Antihypertensive medications are withheld for 2 weeks if possible, especially diuretics, converting enzyme inhibitors, and nonsteroidal anti-inflammatory agents. The results are affected only marginally when patients are continued on other medications, other than those which block the renin-angiotensin system.[642,643] The patient is maintained on a normal or high-sodium diet, and a baseline 24-h urinary sodium excretion is measured. The patient is seated for at least 30 min, and blood pressure measurements are taken at 20, 25, and 30 min and averaged for a baseline. After a baseline blood sample is drawn for PRA determination, a crushed 25-mg tablet of captopril dissolved in 10 ml of water is administered orally. Earlier tests used 50 mg of captopril, but this dose has been reduced because of occasional episodes of hypotension.[4,642,643] Blood pressure is measured at 15, 30, 45, 50, 55, and 60 min after captopril ingestion; at 60 min, another blood sample is drawn for PRA determination (stimulated PRA).

The criteria for a positive test vary. Recent criteria of Müller and Laragh[4,643] are (1) stimulated PRA of 12 μg/ml per hour, (2) an absolute increase of plasma renin activity over the baseline level of 10 μg/liter per hour, (3) a 150 percent increase in plasma renin activity or a 400 percent increase if the baseline plasma renin activity is <3 μg/liter per hour. Since absolute values for PRA differ in various laboratories, these criteria may have to be modified depending on the individual techniques and laboratory normal values.

In the hands of well-equipped dedicated research

laboratories that handle large volumes of samples, both the sensitivity and the specificity of the captopril test have been reported to be as high as 95 percent.[4,643] For example, in one series, these criteria identified retrospectively all 56 patients with proven renovascular disease among 200 hypertensive patients with normal renal function. False-positive responses occurred in only 2 of 112 patients with essential hypertension and in 6 with secondary hypertension from other causes. The test was not as specific or sensitive in patients with renal insufficiency.

Other clinical variables that can influence the predictive accuracy of the test include variable sodium intake, use of antihypertensive drugs, and bilateral renal artery stenosis, which can result in renin suppression. Although the captopril-induced decrease in blood pressure was greater in patients with renovascular hypertension than in those with essential hypertension, there was a significant overlap in the responses between the two groups. Other investigators have reported less favorable results, with sensitivities as low as 39 percent and specificities in the range of 76 to 82 percent, respectively.[642, 646–649] This test is cumbersome and time-consuming. Nevertheless, when properly standardized, the captopril test is an excellent outpatient screening test for renovascular hypertension.

Differential Renal Vein Renin Determinations

Measurement of PRA in both renal veins has been used to establish whether a lesion in the renal artery is causing hypertension and to predict the outcome of revascularization.[9,574,575,650] The technique had fallen into disfavor in some centers because of its invasiveness and problems with sampling (especially branch lesions). The test is less useful in patients with bilateral disease. It also can be affected by a high sodium intake or β-adrenergic blocking agents that suppress renin release.

Enthusiasm for the procedure increased with the addition of captopril administration before the sampling, since the inhibitor preferentially stimulates renin release from the ischemic kidney.[9,574,575,650] The improvement with captopril is especially true for bilateral disease, in which the converting enzyme inhibitor enhances renin release from both kidneys.[650]

The technique is performed as follows. Blood for PRA is collected from the vena cava upstream from the renal veins as an index of peripheral PRA and in both renal veins 30 min after the oral administration of 25 mg of captopril. Two types of abnormalities suggest renovascular hypertension: (1) unilateral hypersecretion with an ischemic/peripheral PRA ratio of 2.0 with contralateral suppression where the contralateral/peripheral PRA ratio is <1.25 and (2) bilateral hypersecretion with a ratio from one renal vein of >2.0 and a ratio from the contralateral side of >1.25. With these criteria, the sensitivity and specificity for unilateral stenosis were found to be 61 percent and 96 percent, respectively, and for bilateral stenosis to be 96 percent and 92 percent, respectively.[650] These criteria differ from the lateralizing ratios of 1.5 or above used in the past.[650] Whereas abnormal results are highly suggestive of renovascular hypertension, a negative test does not exclude a curable lesion.

Radioisotope Renography (Scintigraphy)

Isotope renography, especially when augmented by pretreatment with captopril, is widely used for the evaluation of patients suspected of having renal artery stenosis (Figs. 14-21 and 14-22).[8,573–575,642,651–654] The procedure is relatively noninvasive and safe in patients with impaired renal function, and the dose of tracer isotope is minimal. Both bilateral and unilateral lesions can be recognized. The test is useful for a screening test for renovascular hypertension in selected patients but is not appropriate for screening of the general hypertensive population. It is useful for assessing the functional hemodynamic significance of a lesion seen on arteriography and for predicting the outcome from revascularization. It is also useful in the postoperative evaluation of renal blood

FIGURE 14-21 Schematic representation of normal and abnormal isotope renograms as outlined by the consensus committee.[654] The curve shows the three phases in normal subjects and abnormal curves of varying degrees graded as suggested by the committee. Grade 1 is borderline and is not considered abnormal if obtained after captopril treatment. However, if obtained without captopril treatment, this curve may shift to grade 2 or grade 3, which are considered to suggest renovascular hypertension. *(Redrawn from Nally et al.[654])*

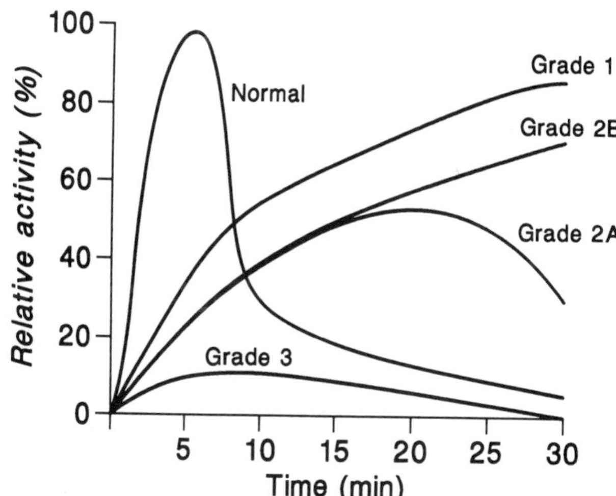

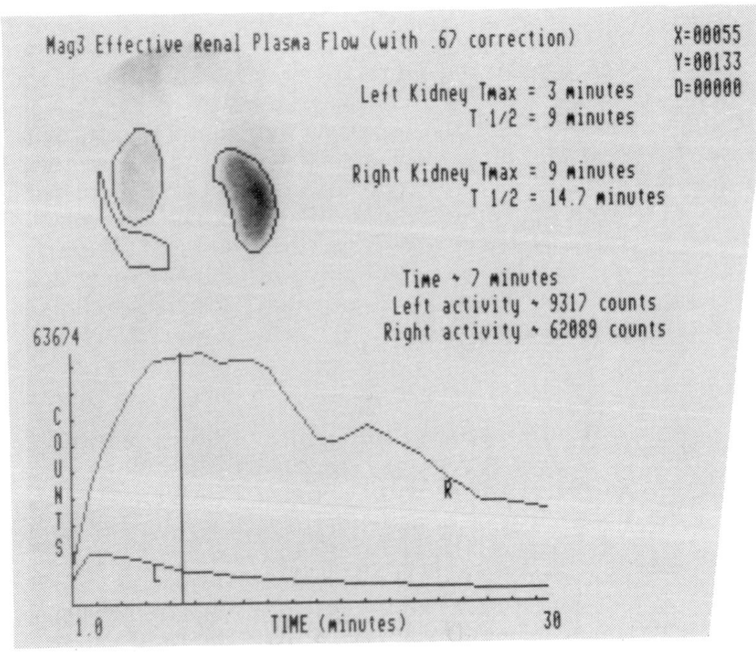

FIGURE 14-22 Captopril isotope renogram using Mag3 in a patient with renovascular hypertension. Shown at the bottom is the time curve of uptake that indicates marked differences between the right (R) and left (L) kidneys. However, the scan at the top shows good perfusion of the left kidney, suggesting that there is good cortical function and that the patient would benefit from a revascularization procedure.

flow and function after revascularization and in patients with renal transplants.

The test requires no patient preparation and takes 1 to 2 h to perform. It is not necessary to discontinue antihypertensive medications. Before the test, the patient is hydrated orally (10 ml water per kilogram), and captopril, when used, is given orally (25 to 50 mg) or 50 μg/kg of enalapriat can be given IV. The isotope-labeled tracer is injected IV 1 h after the oral or 15 min after the IV converting enzyme inhibitor. Static and dynamic scintigraphic images are then obtained using a scintillation camera and are anlayzed by computer. The rate of accumulation and disappearance or clearance of the radiolabeled tracer provides information on renal morphology, blood flow, flow characteristics, excretory function, and GFR for each kidney individually.

The currently preferred radionuclide is ^{99m}Tc-mercuraptoacetyltriglycine (Mag$_3$).[573,574,642,655] Mag$_3$ is extracted by the proximal renal tubule. Although expensive compared with other radionuclides, it provides better images, more accurate counts and quantitation with a shorter scan time, and less radiation exposure, especially in patients with impaired renal function. Other radionuclides contain [^{123}I]hippuran [sodium [^{123}I]orthoiodohippurate (OIH)] and ^{99m}Tc [such as ^{99m}Tc diethylenetriamine pentaacetic acid (DPTA)].[573,574,642,655] [^{123}I]Iodohippurate has replaced [^{131}I]iodohippurate because of the lower radiation dose.[656] ^{99m}Tc-DTPA excreted by glomerular filtration is a marker for GFR and should be avoided in patients with impaired renal function.[656] OIH is excreted by glomerular filtration plus renal tubular secretion and is a marker for renal plasma flow.

Scintigraphic images may be visually analyzed for renal perfusion, kidney size and excretory capacity, and differences between the two kidneys (Figs. 14-21 and 14-22). The time activity curves are analyzed according to effects on the upslope, time to peak accumulation, and clearance. Renal artery stenosis (reduced renal blood flow) prolongs the upslope and time to peak accumulation, reduces the absolute peak, and delays clearance of the radionuclide. Figure 14-21 shows a schematic representation of the range of abnormalities that can be observed. Figure 14-22 shows an abnormal scintigram. Confusing results are seen in patients with low urinary flow rates, renal parenchymal disease, and pelvoureteral obstruction. The scintigram is considered abnormal if any of the following are noted[642]: a delay in peak perfusion of one kidney longer than 5 s compared with the contralateral side, an absolute difference in GFR (right vs. left kidney) of more than 10 percent 2 to 3 min after the injection of the tracer, or a delay in excretion of more than 5 min compared with the contralateral kidney.

Without the use of captopril, the sensitivity and specificity of this procedure for detecting functional renovascular lesions have been in the range of 75 to 85 percent.[8] However, with captopril, sensitivities and specificities in the range of 91 to 94 percent and 93 to 97 percent, respectively, have been reported in patients with unilateral renal artery stenosis.[642] Even in patients with bilateral renal artery stenosis, the test can identify the more severely involved kidney, and with quantitative methods a reduction in peak concentration in both kidneys can be identified.

Some advocate that the test be repeated without

captopril if it is abnormal with captopril[642] to determine if the renal ischemia revealed by the captopril is reversible (captopril causes an increase in Mag_3 cortical retention in renovascular hypertension).[574] However, others believe that this procedure adds insufficient data to warrant its cost.[8]

Renal Arteriography

Renal arteriography[573–575,642] is the definitive technique for visualizing the renal arteries and to determine the presence, location, etiology, extent, and degree of obstruction (Figs. 14-19 and 14-20). This technique utilizes a percutaneous femoral catheter, multiple injections of contrast material, and multiple views obtained with the patient in various positions and respiratory phases. Recent improvements in methodology and new contrast media have reduced markedly the complications that were observed in the past. The reduction of complications is also correlated with the total experience of the arteriographer.[8,655–658] The complication rate appears to be much lower than that for cardiac angiography, in which current estimates of the fatality rate are around 0.03 percent and the total rate of complications, both major and minor, is less than 2 percent.[658]

Renal arteriography allows visualization of the renal artery orifices and the "unfolding" of tortuous overlapping vessels, the primary branches of the renal arteries, and intrarenal vessels.[573–575,642] It can help determine the presence, degree, and pathologic etiology of the obstruction and the presence of collateral circulation, poststenotic dilatation, accessory renal arteries, arterial aneurysms, and vascular malformations. To assess the degree and extent of arterial narrowing, it may be necessary to obtain multiple views of the artery from different angles. Since the renal artery orifices do not arise from the aorta in the same plane, multiple views are often needed to visualize orifice lesions, as is the case in patients with fibromuscular disease and septate lesions, in whom the degree of stenosis is also difficult to estimate.

Supplementation of digital subtraction methodology [digital subtraction angiography (DSA)] for intraarterial angiography is now generally used.[575,659–661] DSA involves computer subtraction of the precontrast from postcontrast images, thus canceling out overlying bone, gas, and soft tissue shadows.[659–661] Intraarterial DSA provides better detail of small vessels, requires less imaging time and thus minimizes motion artifacts, and requires only a fraction of the usual dose of contrast agent.[661] Since the image can be displayed rapidly, less time is required for the procedure, and fewer injections are required for assessment of the lesion. The use of smaller catheters has permitted the safe use of this technique in outpatients with little patient discomfort. However, despite the increased contrast resolution of DSA, the technique provides decreased spatial resolution compared with conventional arteriography.[661] Intraarterial DSA has routinely replaced conventional arteriography in centers where the equipment is available.

The degree of obstruction, measured as the percentage of reduction in luminal diameter, and/or the finding of collateral blood flow around a stenotic renal artery[662] have been used to assess the functional significance of a lesion and to predict the response to revascularization. For example, if the artery is narrowed by more than 70 percent, it is probable that the lesion is the cause of the hypertension and that the renin-angiotensin-aldosterone system is activated.[573–575,641]

However, the presence of a stenotic lesion does not necessarily mean that the lesion is causing enough ischemia to activate the renin-angiotensin system, and narrowing of the renal artery lumen by up to 50 percent is common in older patients with generalized atherosclerosis and may occur incidentally in normotensive individuals.[573–575] In autopsy series, approximately 30 percent of patients with a 50 percent stenosis were normotensive.[587] Furthermore, in early series when surgery was based solely on the appearance of the arterial lesion, not all patients with arterial lesions benefited from surgery. Therefore, it is preferred to document the physiologic significance of the renal artery stenosis with other techniques before corrective surgical revascularization is undertaken.

Other Methods

Several other tests are not in standard use for diagnosing renovascular hypertension. Tests described below that may come into more general use include duplex Doppler ultrasonography, and computed tomography (CT) scanning and MRI. Tests that are no longer used include the divided (or split) renal function test (Howard-Stamey), which necessitated bilateral ureteral catheterization and bilateral renal biopsy, and the saralasin infusion test, a forerunner of the captopril test.[8,573] The intravenous urogram [intravenous pyelogram (IVP)], although the standard screening test in the past, with a sensitivity of 75 percent and a specificity of 86 percent, is no longer used for screening for renovascular hypertension, although it remains useful for defining renal anatomy.[663]

Duplex Doppler Ultrasonography

Duplex Doppler ultrasonography is a noninvasive technique for evaluating flow in renal arteries that does not require the injection of a contrast agent.[2,573,575,642,664–668] The technique involves the combination of imaging of the renal arteries with ultrasound and Doppler techniques to measure the velocity of flow in the renal artery and aorta. Renal artery stenosis is suspected from altered flow velocity, acceleration time, and peak frequency or evidence of turbulence. The technique is difficult, time-consuming, and operator-dependent. Assessment of renal artery flow can be hindered by large amounts of bowel gas or peristaltic activity. Even in experienced hands, only 85 percent of studies are technically successful.[642] Sensitivities and specificities of around 85 percent and 95 percent have been reported by a few centers,[2,665] but the test has not found widespread use.[666–668]

Intravenous Digital Subtraction Angiography

Intravenous angiography using computerized digital subtraction techniques, as described above for arteriography is a simple, less invasive procedure for visualizing the renal arteries, especially in children.[8,574,575,634] Although there are advocates for the procedure,[8,574,575,634] the technique is not widely used because a large volume of contrast agent is required to visualize the arteries from an IV injection. This is poorly tolerated by older patients with impaired renal function, and the studies are technically unsatisfactory in the hands of many investigators. The images are commonly inadequate for visualizing the entire renal vasculature, and multiple injections with oblique or angled views are not possible.[8,574,669]

Computed Tomography Scanning and Magnetic Resonance Imaging

CT scanning and MRI are being evaluated as noninvasive means for detecting flow in renal arteries.[8] Both methods have shown encouraging preliminary results, but further evaluation will be required before they can be generally recommended.[8,670]

Selection and Sequencing of Diagnostic Tests

Once the decision has been made to pursue the diagnosis of renovascular hypertension (discussed above), the physician must decide which of the various tests are most appropriate. Various protocols have been suggested.[4,8,9,573,574,642,671–673] Figure 14-23 shows possible algorithms. Sequencing of tests by most investigators depends on the degree of clinical suspicion.

If renovascular hypertension is strongly suspected, many proceed directly to renal arteriography. If a lesion is found, its functional significance can then be assessed by using renal vein renin determinations or isotope renography. This should be done especially when surgery is planned as a possible treatment. However, many experts proceed directly to angioplasty if there is strong evidence by arteriography for a significant lesion. Lesions that might be treated by angioplasty at the time of arteriography include those where there is 70 percent or more occlusion and occasionally those with less occlusion when the angiogram shows significant poststenotic dilatation, evidence for collateral circulation into the region distal to the obstruction, or a significant reduction in renal size.

In patients in whom there is a moderate level of suspicion of renovascular hypertension, the captopril test or isotope renogram is recommended as the initial test. If these tests are positive, the arteriography should be performed, followed by renal vein renin determinations, if indicated.

Therapy for Renovascular Hypertension

Medical Therapy

Medical therapy for renovascular hypertension is something of an anachronism, since the diagnosis should be pursued only if there is hope of finding a treatable lesion or because medical therapy for the hypertension has been unsuccessful. Considerations in deciding to pursue the diagnosis instead of treating patients medically are discussed above. Medical therapy is used to treat patients in whom a definitive diagnosis is not pursued and before and after revascularization procedures. Continued medical supervision is required even for patients who have had revascularization procedures, since cure from surgery may not be permanent, both atherosclerotic and fibromuscular lesions progress, and many patients have underlying essential hypertension.

Medical therapy was previously more important in terms of its lower immediate mortality and morbidity. This was especially true for older patients in whom there was widespread arteriosclerotic disease, more end organ damage, a longer duration of hypertension, and a greater risk for operative complications.[674–676] Before the general availability of transluminal angioplasty but in the era of potent antihypertensive drugs, there was considerable controversy regarding surgical vs. medical therapy.[677–679] Although atherosclerotic lesions are more likely to progress to renal failure on medical therapy, these patients also have a higher operative mortality and morbidity and a higher incidence of recurring hypertension. Conversely, whereas fibromuscular lesions are less likely to progress on medical therapy, patients with these lesions tend to be younger and respond well to surgery. Published earlier series[628,674,676,680] suggested that surgical approaches were preferable, since about 25 percent of medically treated patients developed cardiovascular complications within two years and after 7 years 42 percent had a significant decline in renal function despite adequate blood pressure control. Overall mortality after 1 to 14 years was 16 percent for surgically treated and 40 percent for medically treated patients. Unfortunately, many of the early data are difficult to interpret because converting enzyme inhibitors were not available, trials were not random-

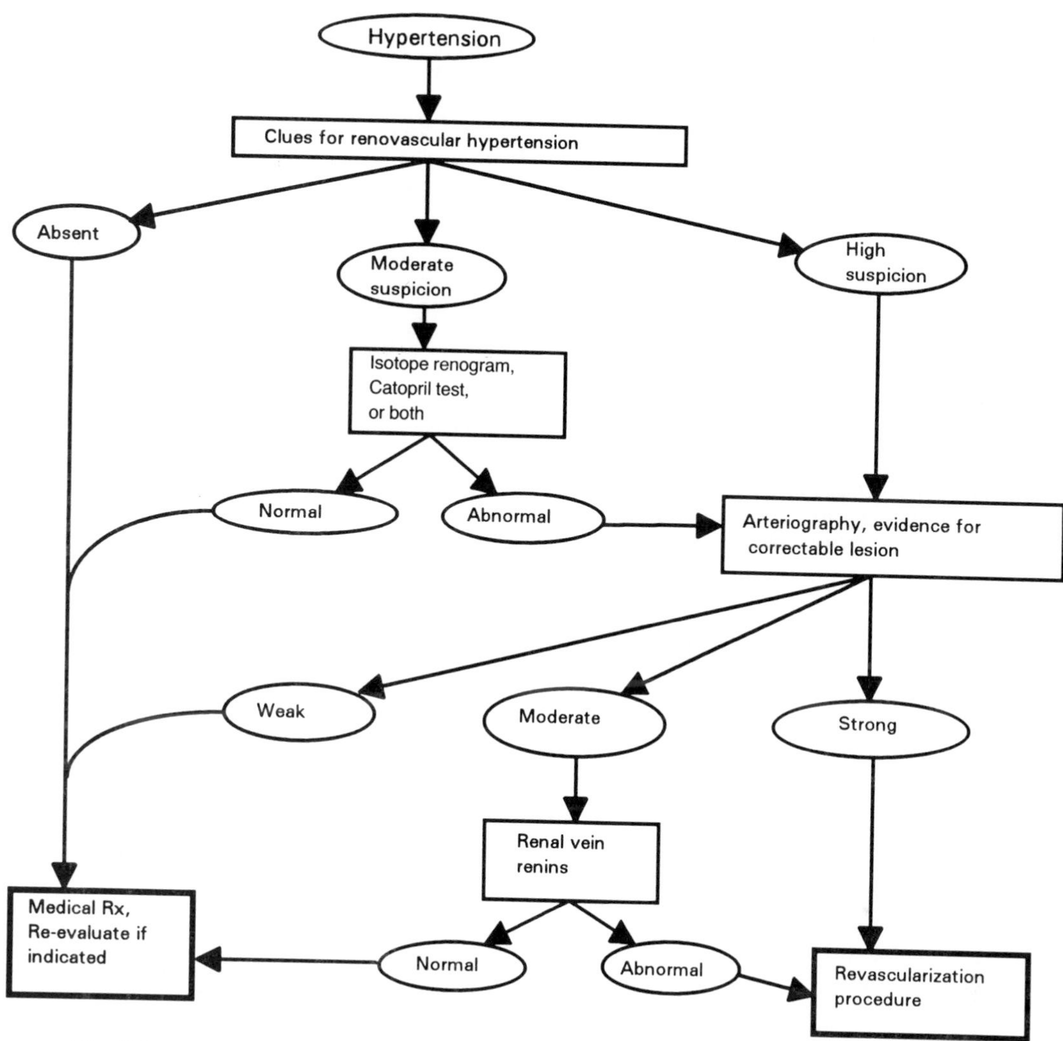

FIGURE 14-23 Algorithm for evaluating renovascular hypertension. Considerations are discussed in the text.

ized, and a higher proportion of older patients with more progressive disease were allocated to medical therapy.

Therapy for renovascular hypertension that blocks the renin-angiotensin system offers the specific advantage that it is directed at the cause of the hypertension.[162,164] Converting enzyme inhibitors are the only agents available today that can block this system, although angiotensin II receptor antagonists may be available in the future (see the section on the renin-angiotensin system above). Calcium-channel blockers and β-adrenergic antagonists are also effective for treating these patients.[681]

The major problem with converting enzyme inhibitor therapy (and β-adrenergic blocking agents) is that it can cause renal failure in patients with bilateral renovascular disease or a stenotic artery to a solitary kidney.[53,159,177,682,683] In a series of patients who presented with renal failure, over 50 percent had been on ACE inhibitors when renal failure developed.[163] Converting enzyme inhibitor therapy for renovascular hypertension can rarely precipitate renal artery thrombosis.[163,684]

Converting enzyme inhibitors reduce renal function in these situations by blocking angiotensin II actions that preserve renal function (see also the section on the renin-angiotensin system). When there is decreased blood flow to a compromised kidney with decreased afferent glomerular arterial pressure, angiotensin II preserves glomerular filtration by constricting the glomerular efferent arterioles. In this circumstance, converting enzyme inhibitor treatment can lower intrarenal efferent arteriolar resistance to such a degree that the GFR is reduced. Other factors can contribute to impaired renal function with converting enzyme inhibitor therapy. These include decreased arterial pressure, concurrent diuretic therapy, and other hemodynamic factors that maintain glomerular filtration. There can also be decreased renal function following β-adrenergic blocking agent therapy; this results both from a reduction in renin release and from decreased cardiac output and hence renal blood flow.[682]

Nevertheless, converting enzyme inhibitors are effective for treating renovascular hypertension, and their use is encouraged provided that renal function is carefully monitored. If renal function deteriorates with this therapy, revascularization therapy should be attempted.[685] In 269 patients with renovascular hypertension, captopril treatment produced complete control of blood pressure in 74 percent and partial control in an additional 8 percent.[164] The response to converting enzyme inhibitor therapy also predicts the response to revascularization.[686]

If revascularization is planned, patients should be treated medically, with special attention paid to maintaining normal potassium levels, until the morning of the procedure. Intra- and postoperative hypertension can best be managed with oral nifedipine or intravenous labetalol. Intravenous furosemide can be added on the third or fourth postoperative day when "third space" fluid mobilization occurs. Many patients, especially those with fibrodysplastic lesions, become normotensive after surgery or angioplasty and require no further medical therapy. Patients with atherosclerotic lesions are slower to return to normal levels.[163,602,608,687]

Revascularization Approaches to Renovascular Hypertension

The only method for relieving an anatomic obstruction to renal blood flow is mechanical. Revascularization of the afflicted renal artery can be accomplished by transluminal balloon angioplasty or surgically by resection, endarterectomy, bypass of the lesion, or replacement of the affected artery with endogenous or exogenous materials. Revascularization offers the chance for a definitive cure of the hypertension, preservation of renal function, and obviation of continued medical therapy.

Revascularization should relieve the cause of the hypertension. However, in some cases preexisting essential hypertension has accelerated the development of atherosclerotic renovascular hypertension. Although revascularization does not "cure" the hypertension in these patients, it results in reversal of superimposed accelerated hypertension, increases the ease with which blood pressure can be controlled medically, and preserves renal function.

A successful outcome from revascularization is predicted by the tests described earlier and by certain clinical features, including fibromuscular dysplastic lesions, young age, short duration of function.[8,9,52,53,164,574,575,601,602,687] A successful outcome from revascularization is less likely in older patients with atherosclerotic lesions and in patients with impaired renal function, inadequate operative repair, residual intrarenal arterial disease such as nephrosclerosis, and coexistence of essential hypertension predating the development of renovascular hypertension.

Revascularization is especially important for patients with impaired renal function, since renal function continues to deteriorate when there is no correction of the ischemia.[52,603] Revascularization can preserve renal function, delay progressive deterioriation, and occasionally reverse the process.[52,603] Nephrectomy is indicated only if renal infarction or atrophy has occurred and revascularization is technically not feasible, since preserving functioning renal tissue is of prime importance.

The two approaches to revascularization, surgery and balloon catheter percutaneous transluminal angioplasty (PTLA), and the results of treatment are described below.[574,601–603,608,639–641,688–690] PTLA has become more widely used even in high-risk patients because of the relative ease of the procedure and the lack of a need for hospitalization. However, as summarized below, it is not clear whether this approach gives better long term-results than surgery. With both approaches, the techniques for the procedures and for postprocedure management are improving. Thus, published data on complications may be overestimates that reflect results when the expertise was lower than it is currently.

The high perioperative mortality with revascularization reported in older series, especially in debilitated patients with atherosclerotic lesions, bilateral lesions, and associated aortoiliac surgery, was largely due to associated coronary and cerebrovascular disease. Morbidity in these patients was due to postoperative myocardial infarction, congestive heart failure and cerebrovascular accidents, hemorrhage, hypotension, and acute renal tubular necrosis. It is the general policy now to perform cartoid endarterectomy and coronary artery bypass grafting when indicated before undertaking renal and aortoiliac revascularization, thus decreasing the operative mortality and morbidity.

Surgical Techniques

A variety of surgical techniques are available, some of which are described below. The results using these techniques are detailed in the section on results of revascularization procedures below. Segmental resection of a focal stenosis in a main renal artery with end-to-end reanastomosis of the artery has been supplanted by newer modalities.

Endarterectomy

Endarterectomy,[691,692] preferably transaortic, is an effective technique for the removal of atherosclerotic plaques in the aorta or at the orifices of the renal arteries. For more distal lesions, direct incision and endarterectomy are rarely performed, since bypass techniques are preferable.

Bypass Techniques

Various bypass techniques can be employed if resection of a lesion is not possible.[53,687,690–692] Earlier experience using the splenic artery as a bypass to the left renal artery led to the use of other vessels, such as the saphenous veins or the hypogastric artery, for bypass grafts.[53,690] This is especially important for patients with renal insufficiency in whom transluminal angioplasty has been less successful. Synthetic Dacron grafts have also been employed, especially in patients in whom associated aortic aneurysm or extensive aortoiliac disease precludes the use of native vessels and necessitates additional reconstructive grafting and bypassing. In patients with bilateral lesions, bypass grafting is usually carried out as a one-stage procedure. Simultaneous aortic reconstruction is required in some patients with severe disease.

Microsurgical Techniques

Revascularization by microsurgical techniques and autotransplantation is employed particularly for segmental disease, distal fibrodysplastic lesions which extend into the primary branches of the renal arteries, small intrarenal aneurysms, pediatric cases, and situations in which "bench surgery" is necessary for the repair of extensive lesions.[53,691–693]

Nephrectomy

Nephrectomy is now performed only if the kidney is atrophied and nonfunctioning or is nearly totally infarcted but still produces renin. Although nephrectomy was formerly used when the arterial lesion was inoperable or irreparable, the removal of potentially functioning renal tissue is now avoided if at all possible.[687] Even in patients with occlusion of a renal artery, if collateral circulation maintains some renal perfusion, revascularization with restoration of blood flow is possible and should be attempted.[694] In patients with malignant hypertension, removal of a small ischemic kidney which is nevertheless "protected" from the impact of the markedly elevated blood pressure can actually result in progressive renal failure, since the remaining kidney, which bears the brunt of the elevated pressure, develops rapidly progressive nephrosclerosis.[695]

Transluminal Angioplasty

PTLA was applied at first in the peripheral vasculature and then in coronary arteries and is now widely used to dilate renal arteries (Fig. 14-18).[601–603,608,653,692,696,697] Despite earlier concerns, PTLA has become the first-line procedure for patients with renal artery stenosis in many centers unless they have indications that exclude its use.[574,601–603,641,697–699] PTLA also has the advantage, mentioned above, that it can be performed at the time of renal arteriography without exposing the patient to an additional procedure.[642]

For PTLA, a polyethylene double-lumen cathether is introduced percutaneously over a guide wire and is maneuvered to locate the inflatable portion of the cathether at the site of the stenosis. The balloon is then inflated for about 10 s and then deflated. This process can be repeated several times until a satisfactory result is demonstrated on angiography. Fibromuscular lesions can be "stretched" or dilated, and atherosclerotic plaques can be fragmented, remodeled, and compressed or flattened against and into the vessel wall, thus enlarging the arterial lumen. Pressure gradients can be measured across the lesion before and after the procedure. The cathether is then withdrawn, and prolonged pressure is applied at the femoral artery puncture site. It is important to use a balloon size that will produce slight overdistension of the renal artery during dilation; otherwise, stenosis is likely to recur. A good initial cosmetic appearance after angioplasty is a predictor of long-term patency.

Immediately after the procedure, the arteriogram shows roughening and fuzziness at the site of the lesion, suggesting that there is intimal abrasion and injury, perhaps with rupture of the fibrous cap of the plaque in atherosclerotic lesions.[696] Hence, anticoagulation with heparin and antiplatelet drugs during and for a short time after the procedure is generally recommended.

Angioplasty is a relatively low-risk procedure done under local anesthesia. The blood pressure usually falls promptly. In experienced hands, complications with this technique occur in 5 to 20 percent of patients.[574,588,601–603,641,692,696] Mortality has been reported to be in the range of 6 to 7 percent in series that include high-risk elderly patients.[588] However, in some series the mortality was much lower,[588] and this is also the experience of the authors. Complications are of three types. (1) Problems at the arterial puncture site include occlusion, bleeding, and pseudoaneurysm in about 1 percent of patients. There is distal embolization in less than 1 percent of patients. (2) Problems at the intervention site include trauma to the renal artery, resulting in occlusion, perforation, intimal dissection, or raising of a subintimal flap; arterial thrombosis and acute renal infarction; arterial spasm; hemorrhage and balloon rupture,[636,696] sometimes[696] requiring surgical bypass or nephrectomy. These complications occur in about 2 percent of cases. (3) General problems include myocardial infarction in <1 percent of patients, transient or chronic renal failure in <2 percent and blood loss. Major cholesterol embolization is a rare complication.[700] The load of contrast medium can lead to further deterioration of renal function in patients with impaired renal function.[661] Emergency surgery for arterial tear or balloon rupture or impaction is rarely necessary, but facilities and staff should be available for such an eventuality, especially in high-risk patients.

Problems may also be encountered passing the

catheter through tortuous femoral arteries.[601–603,641,661,697–699] The axillary approach is associated with an increased number of complications, such as hematoma and brachial plexus injury. The most common reason for failure is inability to pass the guide wire across the stenosis in a lesion that is too tight, especially in an arteriosclerotic lesion, or multiple lesions in a tortuous artery.

Patients likely to respond well to angioplasty include those with fibromuscular dysplastic lesions which do not involve the primary branches and are not associated with aneurysms.[574,601–603,641,692,697,698] Atherosclerotic plaques can also be successfully fragmented and flattened unless they are heavily calcified or contiguous with a larger intraaortic periorifice plaque. Transluminal angioplasty can be used in children and in stenoses in the arteries to transplanted kidneys.

PTLA should not be performed on fibromuscular lesions with aneurysmal dilatation, since they are more likely to rupture if treated in this way. In addition, atherosclerotic lesions that extend into the aorta are not effectively treated by PTLA and should be treated surgically.

Results of Revascularization Procedures

Information about surgical results is more widely available than are results from angioplasty. Results from 1960 to 1980[701,702] for patients with atherosclerosis and fibromuscular dysplasia resulted in surgical cures for 39 to 64 percent, improvement in 29 to 42 percent, failure in 11 to 35 percent, and operative mortality in 1.6 to 5.4 percent. Subsequent improvements in patient selection, surgical techniques, and perioperative management led to even better results. With fibrodysplastic lesions about 70 to 95 percent were cured or improved, with operative mortality approaching zero, while benefit with atherosclerotic lesions occurred in 55 to 80 percent, with operative mortality ranging from 0 to 10 percent.[703–707] Particularly dramatic results were reported in children with renovascular hypertension.[708] However, even older (>65 years of age) patients had marked benefit from revascularization.[53,687,690,709] Revascularization improved renal function in 34 to 56 percent of patients.[687,710]

Long-term results are also excellent. In patients with an initial successful surgical result followed for a number of years, about one-third of patients with atherosclerotic disease and two-thirds with fibrodysplastic lesions have normal blood pressures.[711,712] Among the remainder, most have hypertension caused by progression or recurrence of renovascular lesions and many develop essential hypertension. Many patients with recurring or progressive disease can be re-revascularized.[713] In any case, continued regular follow-up of patients after surgery is important.

Even though surgery is now being performed on patients with more severe disease, the overall results are favorable.[588,687,690] A recent review of the published literature summarized the overall surgical mortality at 6 percent.[588] However, in two very recent series in which a variety of surgical techniques were used, operative deaths were in the range of 1 to 3 percent. In one series, hypertension was considered cured in 21 percent and improved in 70 percent of patients, and 1.4 percent of patients had an occlusion of the renal artery within the first 30 days after surgery.[687] Improvement of renal function was recently summarized at 55 percent, with 31 percent of patients having stable renal function and 14 percent showing deterioration.[588]

The results of transluminal angioplasty are encouraging, and there is overall agreement in a number of studies.[574,588,601–603,639–641] The results are somewhat better with fibrodysplastic than with atherosclerotic lesions.[601,602] Initial success rates are around 79 to 100 percent. The hypertension is cured in 13 to 40 percent of patients and improved in 50 to 70 percent. In one series of patients with fibromuscular disease, the mean systolic and diastolic blood pressure decreases were 52 and 35 mmHg, respectively.[603] Reported series show marked differences in rates of improvement of renal function.[588,603] Overall, there appears to be improvement in around 50 percent of patients.[588]

Restenosis occurs in about 20 to 25 percent of atheromatous[602] and 8 percent of fibrodysplastic lesions.[603] This can occur early, usually as a result of elastic recoil of an incompletely dilated artery, and later, usually because of neointimal hyperplasia.[602] Anticoagulation therapy has not reduced the rate of restenosis.[602]

PRIMARY ALDOSTERONISM

Primary aldosteronism (primary hyperaldosteronism) is the most frequent type of hypertension caused by the adrenal gland.[714] This syndrome, which was described by Conn and Heinerman in 1955,[251,715] is defined as a condition in which there is increased and inappropriate production of aldosterone by the adrenal zona glomerulosa, leading to a mineralocorticoid excess state (Fig. 14-24). This is accompanied by suppression of PRA, elevation of blood pressure, and ultimately hypokalemia. Cortisol production is usually normal. Primary aldosteronism is only one cause of low-renin hypertension, but it is the most common form for which there is an agreed on specific "cure." Other forms of hypertension associated with low renin activity and/or low potassium levels are listed in Table 14-11 and are discussed below.

Occurrence and Classification

The exact prevalence of primary aldosteronism among hypertensive patients has not been precisely

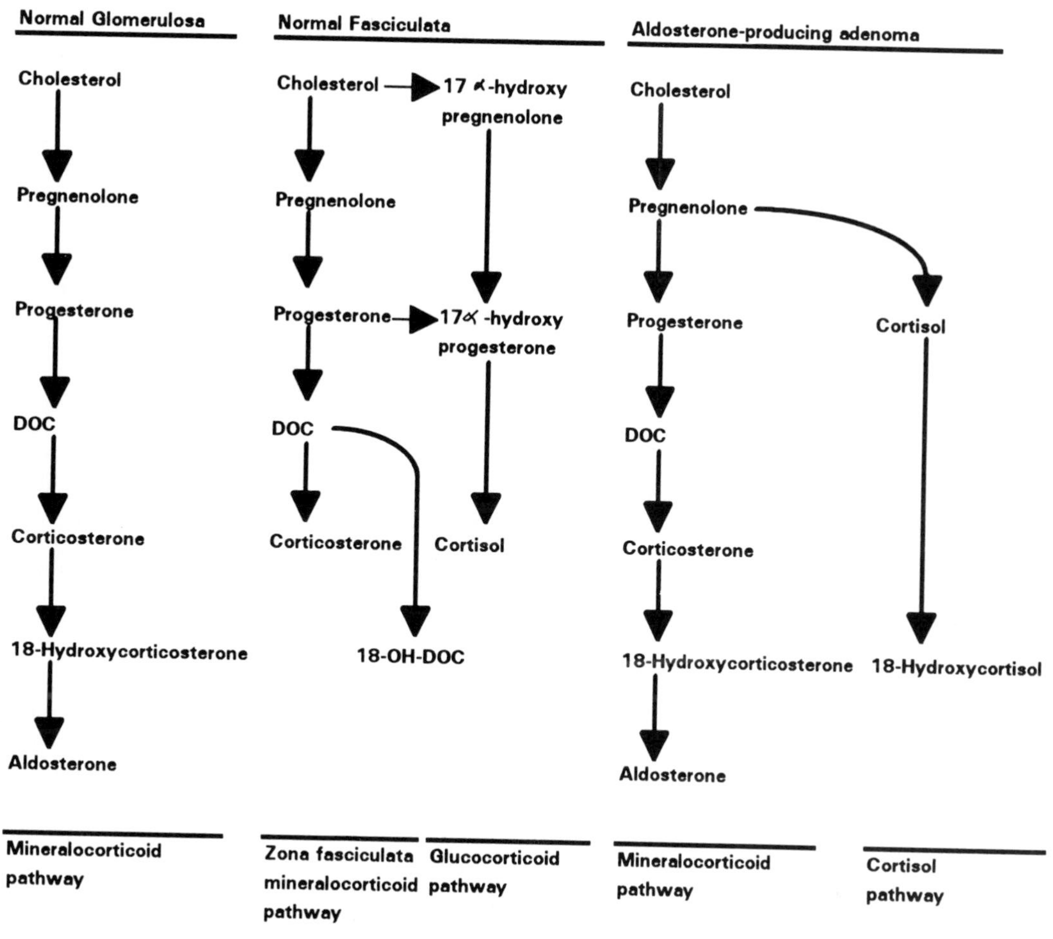

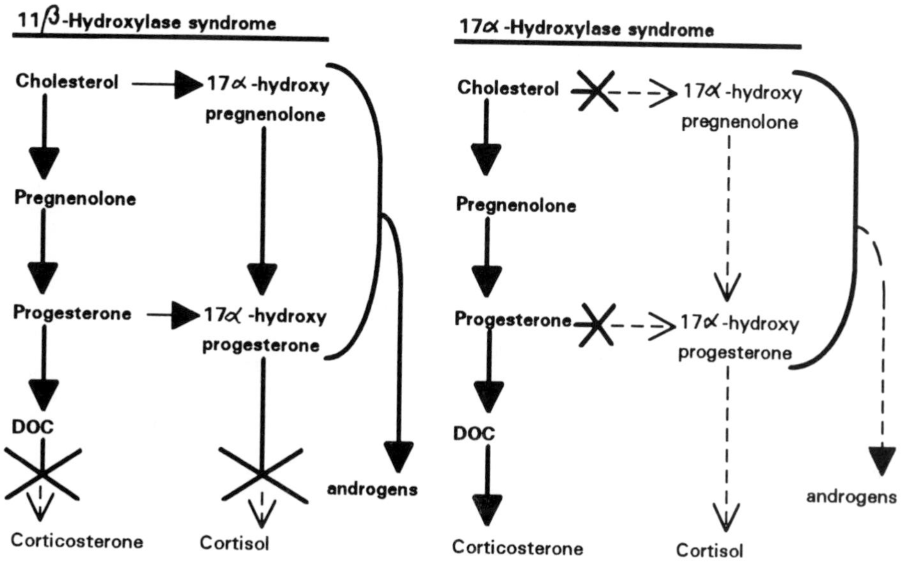

FIGURE 14-24 Pathways of steriod synthesis in the normal adrenal, aldosterone-producing adenomas, and the 11β- and 17α-hydroxylase syndromes. Only those pathways that are major or emphasized are indicated.

TABLE 14-11 Differential Diagnosis of Hypertension with Hypokalemia

Low plasma renin activity
- Primary aldosteronism
  - Adrenal adenomas
    - Aldosterone-producing (APA)
    - Responsive (AP-RA)
  - Adrenal hyperplasia
    - Idiopathic (IHA)
    - Primary (PAH)
    - Glucocorticoid-remediable (GSA)
  - Adrenal carcinomas
- Deoxycorticosterone-excess states
  - 11β-Hydroxylase deficiency
  - 17α-Hydroxylase deficiency
  - Adrenal adenomas
  - Adrenal carcinomas
  - Spontaneous Cushing's syndrome (usually with ectopic ACTH production)
  - ACTH therapy
  - Primary cortisol resistance
- Iatrogenic
  - Mineralocorticoid ingestion
  - Licorice ingestion
  - Glucocorticoid antagonist therapy
- Liddle's syndrome

Normal or elevated plasma renin activity
- Renovascular hypertension
- Pheochromocytoma
- Renin-producing tumors
- Essential or other forms of hypertension treated with diuretics

defined. It was originally predicted that up to 20 percent of unselected hypertensive patients have this disorder,[304,714–716] and it was subsequently thought that the incidence is very low. Current estimates range from less than 0.5 percent to as high as 12 percent of hypertensive patients.[13,302,303,307,425,717,718] These differences are due to controversy over diagnosing milder forms of the disorder. In series with lower incidence rates, hypokalemia has been a requirement for making the diagnosis. However, there are normokalemic patients with the disorder, as noted by Conn and associates.[304] In fact, as discussed in the section on glucocorticoid-remediable aldosteronism below, a large number of patients with primary aldosteronism are probably normokalemic, albeit with milder forms of the disorder. Therefore, the incidence of the disorder is higher than has been reflected in most previous estimates. In series where the incidence of primary aldosteronism has been reported to be higher, many patients did not have hypokalemia. However, there remains a dispute about whether some of these patients have low-renin essential hypertension.

There is general agreement that the prevalence of primary aldosteronism with frank mineralocorticoid excess and with hypokalemia and suppressed PRA is less common than renovascular hypertension but more common than pheochromocytoma; this form of primary aldosteronism probably occurs in less than 0.5 percent of patients with hypertension. Primary aldosteronism occurs in all age groups but has its peak incidence during the third and fourth decades. This coincides with the peak decades of recognition of essential hypertension.

There are three principal pathologic types (Table 14-12).[13,302–304,719–727] These are (1) unilateral benign adrenocortical adenoma (Figs. 14-25 and 14-26), further subclassified into two subtypes, autonomously functioning or unresponsive [aldosterone-producing adenoma (APA)] and responsive [aldosterone-producing/renin responsive adenoma (AP-RA)], (2) adrenocortical hyperplasia that is also subclassified into either nonautonomous [idiopathic hyperaldosteronism (IHA)] or autonomous [primary adrenal hyperplasia (PAH)] forms, and (3) adrenocortical carcinoma (rare). A third rare form of hyperplasia is glucocorticoid-responsive [glucocorticoid-remediable hyperaldosteronism (GSA)] with a well-defined autosomal dominant genetic defect.

Table 14-12 also shows the relative incidence of the disorders in patients with hypokalemia.[719] These data are in general agreement with those of others.[13,303,307,714,717,728,729] About 60 percent of patients have an adenoma, and about 5 percent of these are the responsive variant (AP-RA). Among those with hyperplasia, about 90 percent have IHA and 10 percent have PAH. Most large series indicate a greater incidence of adenoma in women (about 70 percent), but the prevalence of hyperplastic disorders is equally divided between the sexes. The relative prevalence of hyperplasia vs. adenoma is similar in series in which the overall incidence of the disorder is higher,[302,729a] but in these series a higher proportion of the adenomas are of the responsive form (AP-RA). This higher prevalence of the responsive variety in

TABLE 14-12 Syndrome of Primary Aldosteronism and Incidence of Various Forms of the Disorders

Etiology	Number	%
Adenoma		
Aldosterone-producing adenoma (APA)	88	57
Aldosterone-producing/renin-responsive adenoma (AP-RA)	4	3
Hyperplasia		
Idiopathic hyperaldosteronism (IHA)	54	35
Primary adrenal hyperplasia (PAH)	8	5
Glucocorticoid-remediable	0	<1
Carcinoma	0	<1
Total	154	100

Data from Irony et al.[719]

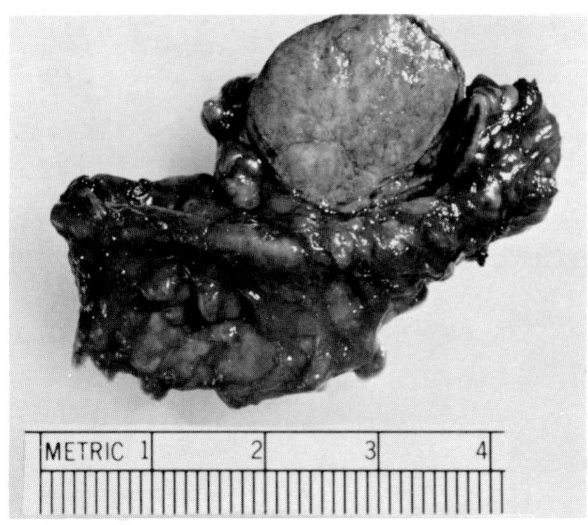

FIGURE 14-25 Aldosterone-producing adenoma. Note lack of suppression in the contiguous adrenal gland.

milder cases might imply that autonomy (discussed below) is more common with severe disease.

Autonomous vs. Nonautonomous Primary Aldosteronism

Classification of aldosterone release in primary aldosteronism as either "autonomous" (nonresponsive) or "nonautonomous" (responsive) is important in considering therapy.[13,307,425,719–727] With autonomous forms of the disorder, aldosterone release does not respond to the usual suppressive maneuvers, such as salt loading and mineralocorticoid administration (Table 14-13 and Figs. 14-27 through 14-29)[278,723] or to stimulatory maneuvers such as upright posture, salt deprivation, and diuretic or angiotensin II administration. However, this release is not truly autonomous in that it does increase in response to ACTH and K^+. Conversely, release in the responsive varieties responds to the suppressive and stimulatory maneuvers described above (Table 14-13 and Figs. 14-27, 14-29, and 14-30). All these subsets retain their characteristics, with no clear progression from hyperplasia to adenoma. Patients with unilateral adenoma and autonomous hyperplasia have excellent results from unilateral or bilateral adrenalectomy, respectively. Those with IHA do not respond as well to surgery.[254,730,731]

Adenoma

Most adenomas are autonomous (APA), as described above. However, small tumors and rarely larger tumors can be nonautonomous (AP-RA), with a pattern of responsiveness that resembles idiopathic hyperplasia.[302,727,729a,919] Adenomas typically are slow growing and well demarcated.[13,278,714,732] Solitary adenomas causing the disease are the rule (Figs. 14-25 and 14-26), although bilateral adenomas rarely occur. There are also rare ovarian adenomas that hypersecrete aldosterone and cause the syndrome.[733] In contrast to many types of endocrine tumors, most aldosterone-producing tumors do not have a familial basis. However, familial aldosterone-producing adenomas have been reported.[302,734] Adrenal aldosterone-producing adenomas can vary in size, but it is common for adenomas less than 1 cm in diameter to cause disease. This small size is difficult to identify by CT scanning of the adrenals and poses a diagnostic problem. The ipsilateral or contralateral glands of patients with either small or dominant adenomas frequently have additional small adenomas.

FIGURE 14-26 Coaxial computed tomography of (*A*) hyperplasia and (*B*) an adrenal adenoma in patients with primary aldosteronism.

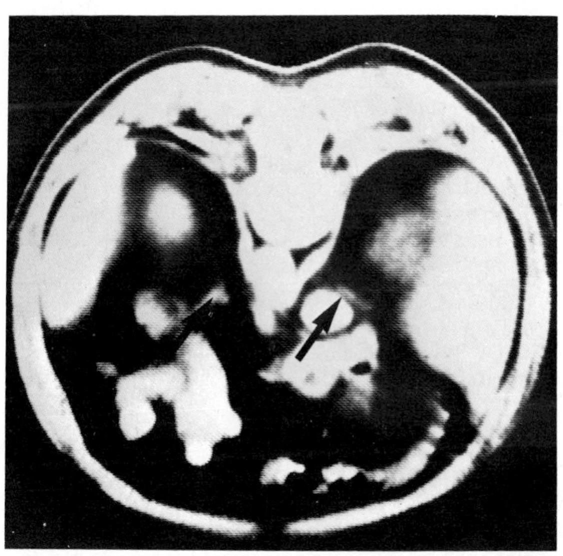

A

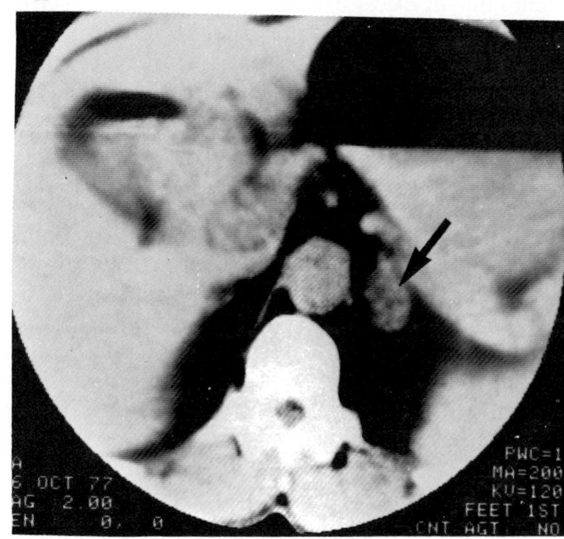

B

TABLE 14-13 Common Biochemical Parameters and Blood Pressure Responses in Low-Renin Hypertension

	Syndrome of primary aldosteronism					Congenital adrenal hyperplasia	
	Aldosterone-producing adenoma		Adrenal hyperplasia				
	APA	AP-RA	Idiopathic	Primary adrenal hyperplasia	Glucocorticoid-remediable	11α-Hydroxylase deficiency	17α-Hydroxylase deficiency
PAC after overnight recumbency	>20 ng/dl	<20 ng/dl	<20 ng/dl	V	V	↓	↓
PAC after 2 to 4 h upright	↓	↑	↑	↓	V		
Cortisol	N	N	N	N	N	N to ↓	↓
Corticosterone	N	N	N	N	N	N to ↓	↑
DOC	Occ ↑	N	N	N	N	↑	↑
18-OHB		N to slight ↑	N to slight ↑	↑	±	↓	↑
18-OHDOC	Occ ↑	N	N	N to slight ↑	N	↓	↑
18-OHF	↑	N	N	↑ N	↑↑	—	—
PRA	↓↓	↓	↓	↓	↓	↓	↓↓
PAC after DOCA maneuver or fludrocortisone	0	—	0	0	±	±	±
Blood pressure response to spironolactone	+	—	0	+	±	±	±
Blood pressure response to dexamethasone	0	0	0	0	+	+	+

Note: PAC = plasma aldosterone concentration; DOC = plasma deoxycorticosterone concentration; 18-OHB = plasma 18-hydroxycorticosterone concentration; 18-OHDOC = plasma 18-hydroxydeoxycorticosterone concentration; 18-OHF = plasma 18-hydroxycortisol concentration; PRA = plasma renin activity; N = normal; V = variable; ± = not established; ↑ = increased; ↓ = decreased; ↓↓ = markedly suppressed; 0 = no change; + = response; occ = occasionally.

The significance of these adenomas is currently unclear, since recurrence of primary aldosteronism in patients who have had successful resection of a functioning adenoma is rare. CT and MRI studies reveal an incidence of adrenal masses of 1 to 10 percent in patients studied for reasons other than adrenal disease, and autopsy studies document microscopic and macroscopic adrenal nodules in 2 to 9 percent of patients without premortem evidence of adrenal dysfunction.[735]

The characteristic adenoma (Figs. 14-25 and 14-26) is readily identified by its golden yellow color. In addition, small satellite adenomas are often found, and distinction from micro- or macronodular hyperplasia can be difficult. In these patients, the contiguous adrenal gland can show hyperplasia of the glomerulosa or micro- or macronodular hyperplasia throughout the gland. Often this pathology is also present in the contralateral adrenal gland but is not associated with aldosterone abnormalities after removal of the primary adenoma. The adenoma is composed of cell types resembling those of all three zones of the adrenal gland, including hybrid cells resembling zonae glomerulosa and fasciculata cells. These hybrid cells in monolayer cultures can produce aldosterone, corticosterone, and cortisol.

The cells of unresponsive adenomas tend to have a higher proportion of fasciculata-like cells and to produce more cortisol than does the usual adrenal glomerulosa (Fig. 14-24).[13,719,721,736,737] This is also reflected by increased production of certain cortisol metabolites, such as 18-hydroxycortisol (discussed below). The cortisol production is responsive to ACTH.[738] These abnormalities may reflect overall lack of differentiation in the tumors.

The nature of the defect causing tumors has not been defined, although karyotypic abnormalities in the tumors have been reported.[739] The adrenal and other endocrine glands (thyroid and pituitary), unlike most body organs, have developed to become hyperplastic in response to physiologic stimuli. Thus, it is not surprising that abnormalities in growth are common. It is noteworthy that like many endocrine tumors, adenoma is the rule and carcinomas are rare.

Whereas the clinical features of adenoma vs. hyperplasia remain constant, the two disorders may reflect a spectrum of adrenal abnormalities rather

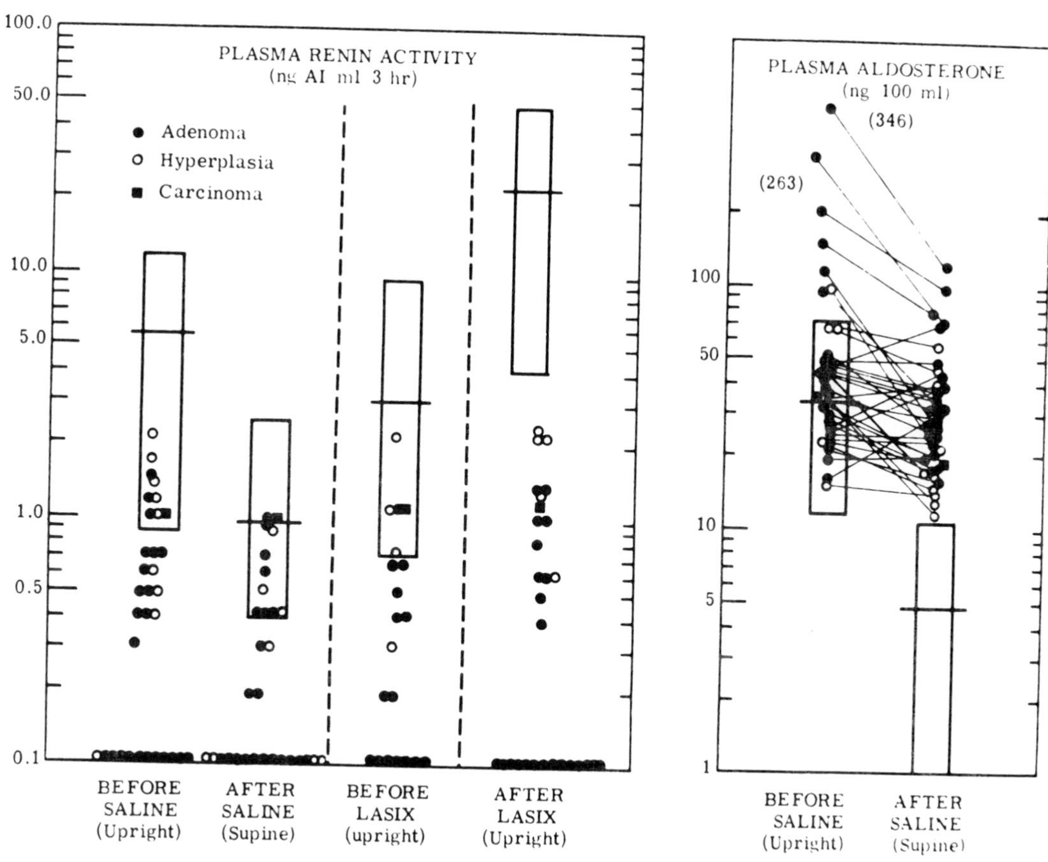

FIGURE 14-27 Responses of plasma renin activity (*left*) and plasma aldosterone concentration (*right*) to suppressive and stimulating maneuvers. Scales are logarithmic to accommodate the range of values. Normal values (114 subjects) are represented as mean (bars) ± 95 percent confidence limits (boxes). Values for patients with primary aldosteronism are indicated by symbols (see key); connecting lines for plasma aldosterone concentration represent values for a given patient. A1=angiotensin 1. *(From Weinberger et al.[278])*

than two distinct entities. This is suggested by the features noted above: (1) both adenomas and hyperplasias can be either responsive or unresponsive to stimulatory maneuvers, (2) adenomatous and hyperplastic abnormalities are commonly observed in the same patient, and (3) hyperplasia can be more diffuse or macro- or micronodular. The overall pattern is reminiscent of the thyroid gland, which can have isolated nodules or diffuse or nodular goiter (see Chap. 11). Nevertheless, it remains more convenient to discuss adenoma and hyperplasia as separate entities, since it allows a distinction between the extremes and the clinical management.

Hyperplasia

Hyperplasias resulting in primary aldosteronism involve the glomerulosa portions of the adrenals. With the idiopathic variety, hyperplasia is usually bilateral (Fig. 14-26), and micro- and macronodular forms of hyperplasia occur. The nodules of the hyperplastic adrenal gland are composed of a mixture of cells, and more of them resemble glomerulosa cells than is the case with unresponsive aldosterone-producing adenomas.[736] However, there can be unilateral hyperplasia with aldosterone hypersecretion by only one adrenal gland as examined by adrenal vein sampling; this can lead to the misinterpretation of a tumor.[721]

The nature of the defect causing hyperplasias has not been defined, with the exception of glucocorticoid-suppressible primary aldosteronism. The considerations mentioned with respect to hyperplasias and adenomas in endocrine glands in general in the preceding section also apply to hyperplasias. As discussed below, the hypertension in patients with hyperplasia does not respond as well to adrenalectomy as does that in patients with adenomas. This could imply that the primary defect is one that both causes hypertension and stimulates the adrenal glomerulosa to hypersecrete aldosterone. As discussed below, aldosterone release in these patients is hypersensitive to angiotensin II. This observation raises the

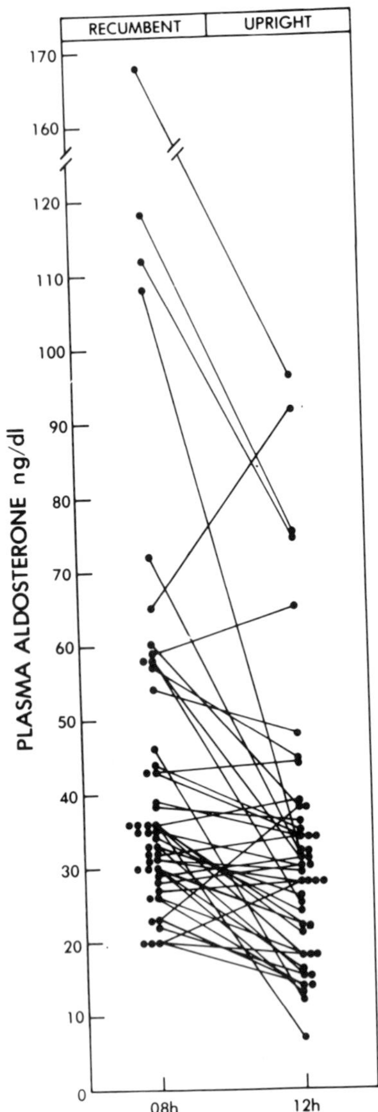

FIGURE 14-28 Effect of 4 h in the upright position after overnight recumbency in 47 patients with proven aldosterone-producing adenoma while on a sodium intake of 120 mEq. Note: At 8 A.M. plasma aldosterone concentrations are above 20 ng/dl.

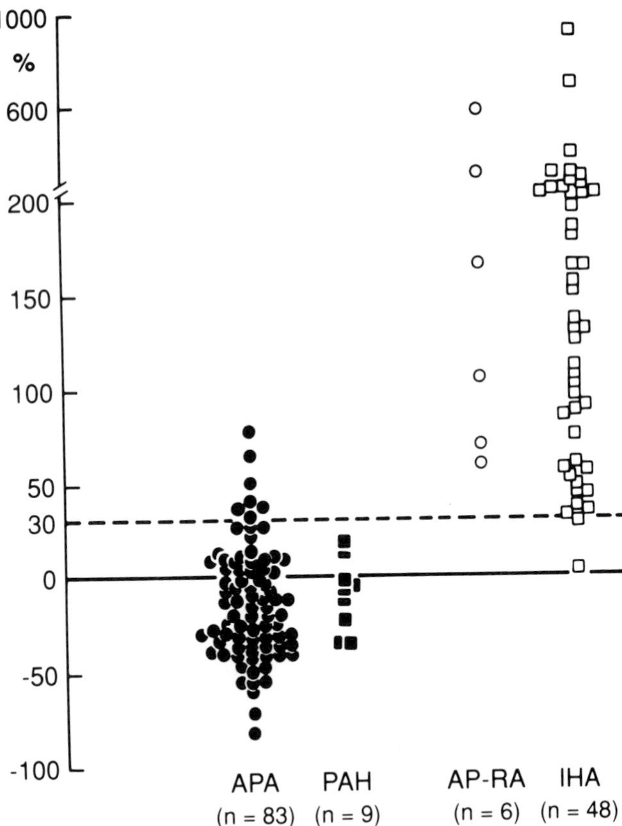

FIGURE 14-29 Individual plasma aldosterone responses to postural stimulation (described in the text) expressed as percentage changes from baseline lying values in patients with various forms of primary aldosteronism. Whenever the plasma cortisol increased during the study period, the percentage increase in plasma cortisol was subtracted from the percentage change in plasma aldosterone. Abbreviations are as described in the text. The dotted line at 30 percent shows the upper limits from normal subjects. *(Reprinted from Fontes et al.[723])*

question whether a more generalized sensitivity to angiotensin II accounts for the disorder. An argument against this notion is that the hypertension in these patients responds only modestly to treatment with ACE inhibitors.[729]

Idiopathic Hyperaldosteronism

Patients with IHA and adrenal hyperplasia by definition have nonautonomous primary aldosteronism.[242,254,303,425,719,721–726,740,741] Thus, although PRA is markedly suppressed, it responds slightly but significantly to postural or other stimuli, and small increases in PRA result in substantial increases in aldosterone production (Table 14-13 and Figs. 14-27, 14-29, and 14-30). This reflects a hypersensitivity of the hyperplastic adrenal gland to the low quantities of angiotensin II generated by the low renin levels. Conversely, in contrast to most patients with adenomas, aldosterone release can be suppressed in most patients with hyperplasia by maneuvers such as sodium loading and mineralocorticoid treatment.

In patients diagnosed in most centers, the aldosterone excess and the tendency to hypokalemia in general are not as severe in patients with IHA as they are in those with adenoma.[242,254,303,719,721–726] The production of other steroids in the aldosterone biosynthetic pathway (DOC, corticosterone, and 18-OHB) is also not as increased as in adenoma; measurement of plasma levels of various steriods has proved to be useful in differentiating adenoma from hyperplasia (Table 14-13; also see below).

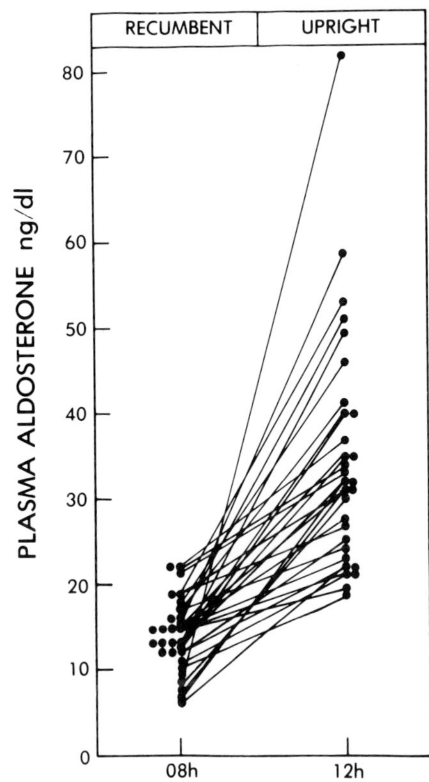

FIGURE 14-30 Effect of 4 h in the upright position after overnight recumbency in 31 patients on a sodium intake of 120 mEq who have primary aldosteronism caused by adrenal hyperplasia.

Primary Arenal Hyperplasia

Aldosterone release in patients with primary adrenal hyperplasia (PAH) is autonomous and resembles that of most larger adenomas.[719,725,726] It can be speculated that this condition represents an early phase of adenoma. The adrenal glands of these patients are nodular and often have a dominant nodule. Patients with adenomas also tend to have such nodularity in both the contiguous and the contralateral adrenal glands. However, the hyperplasia is usually bilateral. The blood pressures and hypokalemia in these patients respond to surgical reduction in adrenal mass.

Glucocorticoid-Remediable Hyperaldosteronism

Glucocorticoid-remediable aldosteronism [glucocorticoid-suppressible aldosteronism (GSA)] is a form of hyperplasia in which the hypertension and hypokalemia ordinarily can be ameliorated by treatment with dexamethasone. This is a mostly familial disorder with an autosomal dominant pattern of inheritance for which the genetic defect for many cases has been defined.[254,728,742–745] It is probably a rare disease, since in our experience (unpublished) and that of others[302] dexamethasone testing of patients with primary aldosteronism only rarely detects its presence. However, the true prevalence of the disorder is much greater than was previously thought, since most patients with the syndrome and hypertension have normal serum potassium levels (Table 14-14), and were probably diagnosed previously as having essential hypertension.[744]

Moderately low doses of glucocorticoids (0.5 to 2 mg of dexamethasone daily) usually reverse the biochemical abnormalities and ultimately reduce the blood pressure in GSA. Dexamethasone treatment also lowers plasma aldosterone concentrations into the normal range in patients with the more common types of hyperplasia (IHA) and even those with an adenoma, but these effects are transient and plasma aldosterone concentrations return to elevated levels after 24 to 48 h.[746] However, in patients with GSA, normalization of plasma aldosterone concentrations, the other biochemical abnormalities, and the hypertension persist with continued therapy, although eventually the disorder can become dexamethasone-insensitive.[747]

The mechanism for the defect in the cases studied appears to involve a gene duplication with unequal crossing over between the two homologous genes that encode aldosterone synthetase [also termed CYP11B2, corticosterone methyloxidase type II, p450aldo, p450cmo, p450c18, p450XIB2, and steriod 18-hydroxylase (see Chap. 12)] and steriod 11β-hydroxylase [also termed CYP11B1, p450c11, and p450XIB1 (Fig. 14-31)]. The crossing over occurs between intron 2 and exon 4 of the two genes.[728,742,743] The result is that the coding sequences of aldosterone synthetase are under control of the promoter for the 11β-hydroxylase gene. Since 11β-hydroxylase is expressed in the zona fasciculata under the control of ACTH, the mutated gene and consequently the production of aldosterone are placed under the control of ACTH. The zona fasciculata aldosterone production in this case is excessive and is not suppressed by the usual feedback mechanisms. Other 18-hydroxylation products of steroids made in the zona fasciculata—18-OH-cortisol and 18-oxocortisol—are also produced in excess. Thus, the dramatic response to dexamethasone in the syndrome is due to suppression of ACTH and subsequently of the synthesis of these steroids.[254,744,745]

There is a high prevalence of hypertension in afflicted members, and these individuals have elevated blood pressures relative to unafflicted members even before they develop frank hypertension. In the family described in Table 14-14, all afflicted members had developed hypertension by 20 years of age. In this and other families, there is a very high incidence of early mortality from strokes.[744] As shown in Table 14-14, serum potassium and aldosterone values cannot ordinarily be used to diagnose the syndrome.

TABLE 14-14 Clinical Features of Glucocorticoid-Remediable Aldosteronism

Feature	Afflicted		Nonafflicted
Blood			
Potassium (mmol/L)	4.3	(3.7–5.0)	4.3 ± 0.4
PRA (ng/L s)	0.14	(0.11–2.06)	0.92 ± 0.41
Aldosterone (pmol/L)	597	(55–1220)	314 ± 170
Urine			
K^+ (mmol/day)	37	(10–77*)	51 ± 20
THAldo (nmol/day)	125	(41–242*)	74 ± 39
TH18-oxoF (nmol/day)	1683	(297–5168*)	84 ± 46
18-OHF (nmol/day)	393	(120–888*)	12 ± 7
TH18-oxoF/THAldo	3.0	(2.0–4.1)	0.19 ± 0.09

Results are an analysis of a single family, and the comparisons are between afflicted and nonafflicted family members. Shown are mean values, with the range in parentheses for the afflicted members and ± SD for the nonafflicted members. Abbreviations: THAldo = tetrahydroaldosterone; TH18-oxoF = tetrahydro-18-oxocortisol; 10-oxoF = 18-oxo-cortisol.

* Some values are per liter rather than per day.

Source: Rich et al.[744]

These findings are the strongest indication that primary aldosteronism may exist commonly in the absence of hypokalemia. If the history of the development of hypertension and biochemical abnormalities could be extended to other causes of primary aldosteronism, it would be concluded that those patients with hypokalemia account for a small percentage of the total patients with primary aldosteronism. By this formulation, hypokalemia would be only a manifestation of the syndrome in its more severe form. This issue needs to be resolved. The analysis, if correct, implies that a substantial percentage of patients with essential hypertension, perhaps many or most of those with low-renin essential hypertension, actually have mild primary aldosteronism.

Overproduction of 18-hydroxycortisol and 18-oxocortisol is even greater than that in primary aldosteronism (discussed below) and can be used to diagnose the condition (Table 14-14).[744] The ratio of 18-oxocortisol to tetrahydroaldosterone proves to be a

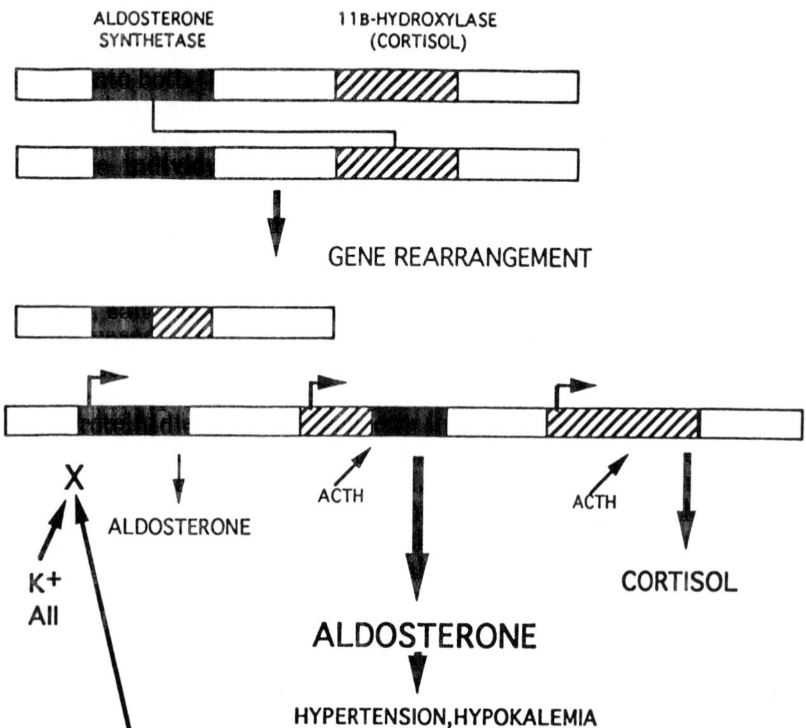

FIGURE 14-31 Schematic representation of the genetic defect in glucocorticoid-remediable primary aldosteronism.[728,742,743] The gene sequences for aldosterone synthetase CYP11β2 are shown in black, and those for 11β-hydroxylase (CYP11β1) are shown hatched. The rearrangement leaves three functional genes on one chromosome and one nonfunctional gene on the other chromosome. Note that in the hybrid gene containing the upstream portion of 11β-hydroxylase and the downstream portion of aldosterone synthetase, the coding sequences of aldosterone synthetase (and thus aldosterone synthesis) are under the control of the same influences (ACTH, etc.) that regulate cortisol release.

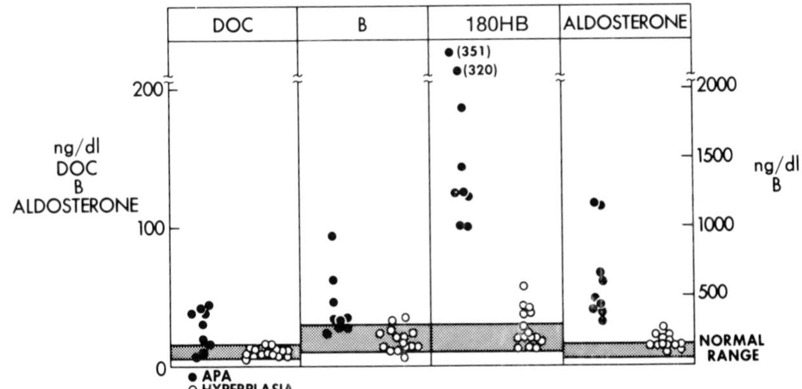

FIGURE 14-32 8 A.M. values (after overnight recumbency) of concentration of the steroids of the mineralocorticoid pathway [deoxycorticosterone (DOC), corticosterone (B), 18-hydroxycorticosterone (18-OHB), and aldosterone] in patients with primary aldosteronism caused by an adenoma (APA) and hyperplasia.

useful index, as shown in Table 14-14. This ratio does not show any overlap in nonafflicted individuals, and even in primary aldosteronism, the ratio usually does not exceed 1. Thus, this test is excellent for diagnosing the syndrome and has supplanted the previous laborious method of testing the patient's blood pressure response to dexamethasone.[744]

Carcinoma

Adrenal carcinomas resulting in primary aldosteronism are extremely rare. Adrenal carcinomas in general exhibit a varied pattern of steroid production, and there is no typical pattern (see Chap. 12). Although many of these tumors probably produce some aldosterone, production of this steroid in excess is rare. When aldosterone is produced in excess, it is almost always accompanied by production of other steroids, including DOC, corticosterone, cortisol, and aldosterone.[748] The survival rate seems to be prolonged slightly in cases where there is excessive production only by the mineralocorticoid pathway, probably reflecting a more differentiated tumor. Most patients with adrenal carcinomas are first seen because of general symptoms related to the tumor or tumor mass or because of excess androgens or glucocorticoids (see Chap. 12). Plasma concentrations of mineralocorticoid hormone can be extremely high with these carcinomas, and profound hypokalemia is common. For instance, the finding of a plasma aldosterone concentration over 100 ng/dl should raise a strong suspicion of malignancy. Furthermore, steroid production does not respond to stimuli such as postural changes, ACTH, and salt loading (Fig. 14-27). Changes in the clinical course are usually identifiable by sudden or gradual increases in aldosterone production and the appearance of increasing amounts of other adrenal steroids. Adrenal carcinomas causing primary aldosteronism usually do not concentrate iodocholesterol. This may be due to the fact that these tumors are usually large, i.e., >6 cm, and the iodocholesterol may be too diffuse within the tumor to be adequately visualized. CT and IVP may be adequate for locating the tumor.

Pathophysiology

The intensified synthesis of aldosterone in primary aldosteronism is reflected by activation of the entire aldosterone biosynthetic pathway. Increased quantities of steroids such as DOC, corticosterone, and 18-OHB, which are precursors to aldosterone, are released into the circulation (Figs. 14-24 and 14-32).

The mechanisms of the development of hypertension in mineralocorticoid-excess states are described in the section on mineralocorticoids above. As noted, the hypertension is due primarily to sodium retention, but it may be exacerbated by concomitant depletion of potassium and magnesium and other effects of the mineralocorticoids. It was also noted that some time is required for mineralocorticoid-induced hypertension to develop. This fact, plus the usual slow progression of tumor or hyperplasia causing primary aldosteronism, indicates a slowly developing process.

Primary aldosteronism is also likely to develop more rapidly in patients with underlying essential hypertension. The data with glucocorticoid-remediable aldosteronism, discussed above, suggest that hypertension does not develop in all patients with primary aldosteronism. Another indication of this and/or the overall slow development of the syndrome is that women with primary aldosteronism commonly give a history of transient hypertension during pregnancy.[749] Short-term administration of large amounts of DOCA to normal subjects rarely causes hypertension, even though the treatment results in sodium retention, whereas DOCA administration to borderline hypertensives made normotensive with hospitalization readily induces hypertension.[731] When DOCA is administered to patients with sustained essential hypertension or primary aldosteronism, there is little or no acute or chronic sodium retention or change in the blood pressure, indicating that they are already in an escape state.[731] This probably reflects the body's efforts to adapt to the hypertension from any of a number of causes by secreting salt maximally.[731] As stated in the discussion of hyperplasias, the response to adrenalectomy in patients with hyperplasia has suggested that there may be a disorder in addition to the mineralocorticoid excess that promotes the hypertension.

History and Physical Findings

Patients usually present because elevated blood pressure was detected on routine screening, and the medical history usually does not reveal any characteristic symptoms. In the past, many patients were detected because of symptoms of hypokalemia, but this disease is now recognized earlier, and thus the incidence of nonspecific symptoms or extreme abnormalities resulting from potassium depletion has decreased. Potassium depletion can produce the nonspecific complaints of tiredness, loss of stamina, weakness, nocturia, lassitude, and headache. With more severe depletion, there can be alkalosis, increased thirst, polyuria, paresthesias, and even flaccid paralysis. Severe potassium depletion can also precipitate cardiac arrhythmias, including ventricular tachycardia, with related symptoms of palpitations or shortness of breath.

Excessive production of mineralocorticoids also produces no characteristic physical findings. Retinopathy is mild, and hemorrhages are rarely, if ever, present. Postural falls in blood pressure without reflex tachycardia are observed in severely potassium-depleted patients. Although the extracellular fluid volume is increased, clinical edema is practically never seen. A positive Trousseau's or Chvostek's sign can rarely occur when alkalosis accompanies severe potassium depletion. The heart is usually enlarged only mildly if at all, and electrocardiographic changes are usually those of modest left ventricular hypertrophy and/or potassium depletion, although arrhythmias also may be seen. In the authors' experience, the incidence of cerebrovascular disease in these patients is much lower than in other forms of hypertension, although it is unexplained why this experience differs from that with GSA discussed above.

Hypertension

Blood pressure in patients with primary aldosteronism can range from normal (see the discussion above) to severe hypertensive levels; levels up to 250/160 mmHg have been reported.[714] The mean blood pressure in 136 patients reported by the unit in Glasgow was 205/123 ± 21/18 (SE) mmHg, and the means for the adenoma and hyperplasia groups did not differ significantly.[714] However, these data probably represent more severely affected patients. Accelerated (malignant) hypertension is extremely rare in patients with primary aldosteronism, even though renal biopsies may occasionally show some fibrinoid necrosis typical of accelerated disease. Before primary aldosteronism was recognized and appropriately treated, long-standing hypertension resulted in the expected consequences: congestive heart failure, stroke, and repeated episodes of pyelonephritis and consequent renal failure. These complications still occur in older patients.

Diagnostic Procedures

Initial Studies

The traditional hallmarks of this disease are hypertension with hypokalemia, suppression of the renin-angiotensin system, and increased aldosterone production in the presence of normal cortisol production. The rationale discussed above that many patients with primary aldosteronism may not have hypokalemia has led to a reconsideration of the overall approach to evaluation and to a current lack of consensus about how to pursue the diagnosis.

There is general agreement, however, that the initial determination of the presence or absence of hypokalemia is a critical screening procedure (Fig. 14-33).[13,242,303,307,425,719–727,750] This should be carried out for all hypertensive persons and should be assessed under conditions of adequate sodium intake (described below) so that significant hypokalemia is not missed. The detection of hypokalemia requires further investigation.

There is no general agreement regarding the evaluation of patients with normokalemic primary aldosteronism.[13,242,303,307,425,719–727,750] There are several arguments in favor of searching for these patients. First, a surgically correctable lesion may be found in some cases. Second, knowledge of the diagnosis is useful even if a tumor is not obvious or a surgical approach is not anticipated. This knowledge can alert the physician to conduct careful follow-up and pursue surgery if indicated at a later date and may influence the hypertensive medications that will be used. For example, these patients respond well to spironolactone and triamterene. They respond moderately well to calcium-channel blockers. Although they have sodium-dependent hypertension and respond to thiazide diuretics, they also have an enhanced probability of developing serious hypokalemia on these diuretics and should be followed carefully when these medications are used. An argument against searching for normokalemic primary aldosteronism is that we do not yet know the utility of surgery in these milder cases. Surgery may not yield as good a response in milder cases. Most of these patients would previously have been labeled as having low-renin essential hypertension. As discussed in the section on the role of the renin-angiotensin system in hypertension, the merits of renin profiling for patients with essential hypertension have been debated for years with no clear consensus.

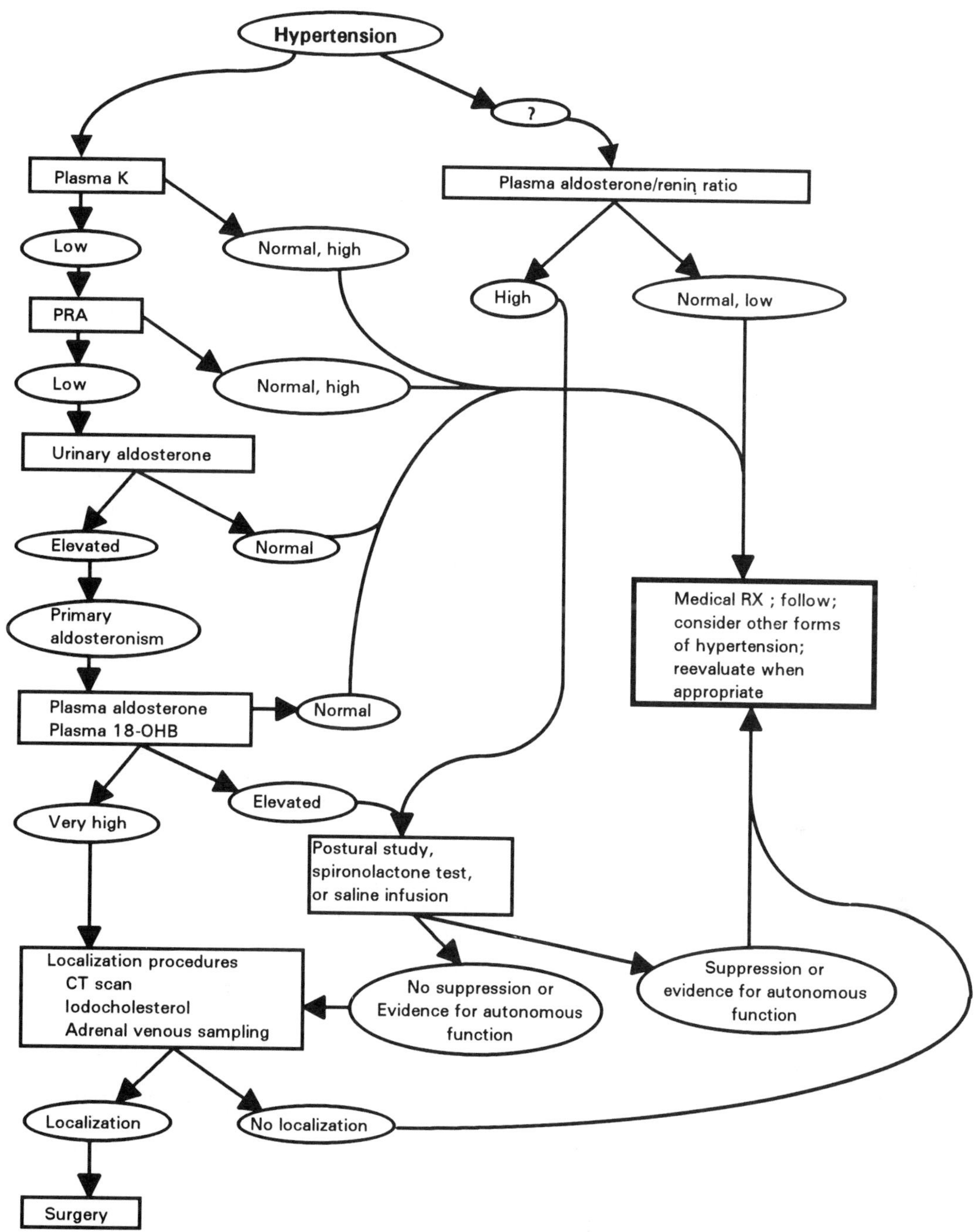

FIGURE 14-33 Algorithm for evaluation of primary aldosteronism.

Thus, more studies will be required to resolve these important issues before firm recommendations can be made. Nevertheless, because of the increasing use of the plasma aldosterone/renin ratio (discussed below), this test as a screening test is included as an option in the algorithm in Fig.14-33.

Hypokalemia

In assessing hypokalemia, care must be taken to control the sodium intake or balance in the patient before serum electrolyte levels are measured; serum potassium concentration and 24-h urinary excretion of potassium are closely related to and determined to a great extent by sodium chloride intake in these patients.[13,242,303,307,425,719–727,750] A low-sodium diet can correct major potassium abnormalities by retarding potassium secretion in the distal tubule as the amount of sodium ion available for reabsorption and exchange is reduced. In the presence of normal renal function and aldosterone excess, salt loading

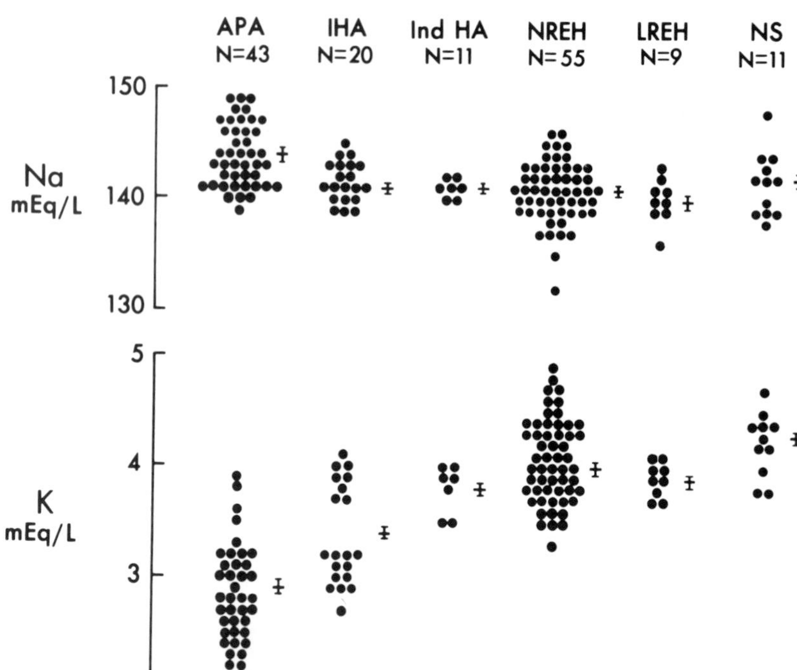

FIGURE 14-34 Serum sodium and potassium concentrations on a 120-mEq sodium intake in patients with an aldosterone-producing adenoma (APA), idiopathic hyperaldosteronism (IHA), indeterminate hyperaldosteronism (Ind HA; this category is no longer used), normal-renin essential hypertension (NREH), low-renin essential hypertension (LREH), and normal subjects (NS). High-salt challenge was not performed.

should effectively unmask hypokalemia as a manifestation of potassium depletion. On sodium intakes greater than 120 mEq per day, hypokalemia will be apparent in potassium-depleted patients by the fourth day (Fig. 14-34).

Excessive renal potassium secretion should also be demonstrable under these conditions. Thus, a urinary potassium excretion of >50 mEq per 24 h is inappropriate in the presence of hypokalemia.

In the United States, Japan, and Europe, among other areas, the average person consumes over 110 to 120 mEq of sodium per day, enough to allow hypokalemia to be manifest. Thus, in practice, if such a dietary history is obtained and the serum potassium concentrations are normal on three occasions, a further work-up for hypokalemia probably is not indicated.

Previous diuretic therapy always poses a problem in interpreting serum potassium concentrations and is the most common cause of hypokalemia in patients with hypertension. The patient should be off diuretics for at least 3 weeks. Normal dietary intake of potassium will restore depleted potassium levels that are not related to primary aldosteronism. Potassium excretion may decrease immediately after the cessation of diuretic treatment in the absence of primary aldosteronism. Sudden falls in serum potassium concentration when hypertensive patients are placed on diuretics, especially when the changes are marked with paralysis or profound weakness, suggest that primary aldosteronism is present.

There are a number of other causes of hypokalemia in patients with hypertension (Table 14-11). These include excessive gastrointestinal loss due to vomiting or diarrhea, other mineralocorticoid excess or "mineralocorticoid-excess-like" syndromes (discussed later), starvation, insulin and glucose therapy, metabolic alkalosis, renal disease, renovascular hypertension, and accelerated hypertension. These causes can be ruled out with the tests described below.

Plasma Renin Activity

If hypokalemia is documented or if there are other indications that further evaluations are necessary, the PRA should be measured (Fig. 14-27).[13,242,303,307,425,719–727,750] Methods for measurement of PRA are described in the section on laboratory testing.

The PRA can be a random measurement in the unstimulated state because in patients with primary aldosteronism, the increase in extracellular fluid volume results in continuous PRA suppression. Factors such as posture, eating, exercise, salt intake, and to some extent diuretic therapy tend to have a minimal influence on suppressed PRA in patients with this disorder. Thus, if PRA is normal or high in a patient who has been off diuretic therapy for 3 weeks, it is unlikely that primary aldosteronism is present. If the random PRA is suppressed in this setting, no assessment is required in a stimulated state. If the random PRA is marginally suppressed and hypokalemia and aldosterone excess are present, further evaluations along the lines discussed below are indicated.

Urinary Aldosterone

Aldosterone production can best be assessed by measuring aldosterone excretion over a 24-h period. This test is recommended as a better screening test for aldosterone hypersecretion than measurement of plasma aldosterone levels and should be performed in all patients with hypokalemia and suppressed PRA (Fig. 14-33).[13,242,303,307,425,719–727,750,751] The urinary measurement provides a reflection of the integrated aldosterone secretion over the 24-h period. As with cortisol (Chap. 12), aldosterone is released in a pulsatile fashion from the adrenal, and its release from the gland can vary enormously in response to posture, other stimuli, and circadian influences directed mostly by ACTH (Chap. 12).

Ordinarily, the concentration of the urinary 18-glucuronide metabolite of aldosterone is measured. For this procedure, urine is collected at around pH 5 in the presence of a preservative to prevent bacterial growth. The urine is treated with acid to convert the 18-glucuronide metabolite of aldosterone to free aldosterone, which is then measured by RIA. The 18-glucuronidation occurs predominantly in the kidney and accounts for about 15 percent of total aldosterone production. Less commonly, the urinary tetrahydroaldosterone concentration is measured.

Both plasma and urinary aldosterone measurements should be performed while the patient is on a high-salt intake (>120 mEq per day for at least 4 days) and after being recumbent overnight (at least 6 h). This is crucial, because a diminution of salt intake in patients with essential hypertension normally increases the plasma aldosterone level and aldosterone production. In patients who have recently received diuretic therapy, both renin and aldosterone values may remain elevated until the extracellular fluid volume increases and sodium repletion has occurred.

The production of aldosterone is influenced by the potassium balance; it decreases with progressive hypokalemia (see Chap. 21). Such depletion may reduce both aldosterone production and plasma levels into the normal or even below-normal range.[752] Thus, normal values in the presence of hypokalemia in these patients are really abnormal.

Typical normal urinary aldosterone excretion values range from 4 to 17 μg/24 h. In one series, there were mean values of 37.6 ± 3.1 μg/24 h for adenoma and 22.5 ± 1.5 μg/24 h for hyperplasia.[753]

The sensitivity may be further improved with the use of nomograms to correct for age and sodium intake, although these have not come into standard practice and proper normalization for this has been done in only a few centers.

Some researchers advocate measurement of 24-h urinary aldosterone after salt loading.[750] For this, 25 ml/kg of physiologic saline is administered over 4 h for 3 days; 24-h urinary aldosterone levels over 140 μg/24 h after the loading are taken as evidence for aldosterone overproduction.[750] The reported sensitivity and specificity of this test for detecting patients with primary aldosteronism are 96 percent and 93 percent, respectively.[750]

Plasma Aldosterone

Measurement of plasma aldosterone concentrations can be useful in diagnosing primary aldosteronism when levels of the steroid are very high and are more useful than urinary measurements for discriminating between adenoma and hyperplasia when a mineralocorticoid-excess state is already documented (compare Figs. 14-27, 14-28, 14-30, and 14-32).[13,242,303,307,425,719–727,750] Plasma aldosterone measurements can also be helpful in screening for primary aldosteronism when they are evaluated in conjunction with the PRA measurements (see the section on aldosterone/renin ratios below).

Conditions under which blood samples are obtained are critical in yielding diagnostic information and are similar to those for which urinary determinations are made, as described in the preceding section. Plasma aldosterone concentration can be measured in either heparinized or EDTA-treated blood. The steroid is extracted from the blood, isolated by high-performance liquid chromatography (HPLC), and assayed by RIA.[741] Plasma direct assays are also available.

In normal subjects, plasma aldosterone concentrations at 8 A.M. after overnight recumbency range from 4 to 12 ng/dl.[753] In patients with an adenoma and hypokalemia, they are almost always >20 ng/dl and may reach very high levels (Figs. 14-27 and 14-28). In patients with hyperplasia, they are commonly <20 ng/dl but can be higher;[753,754] in a group of 31 patients with hyperplasia, the mean value was 13 ± 1.2 (standard error of the mean) ng/dl (Figs. 14-30 and 14-32). Many values were in the normal range. Thus, many patients with primary aldosteronism have random plasma aldosterone levels that are in the normal range, and such determinations thus can be misleading, especially in milder cases.

Thus, the use of random plasma aldosterone determinations for making the initial diagnosis is discouraged. In principle, multiple measurements of the plasma aldosterone levels with calculation of production rates would also be acceptable, but this is not practical in a general clinical setting.

Plasma Aldosterone/Renin Ratio

Determination of the ratio of random plasma aldosterone to renin activity has been utilized as a more sensitive index for detecting primary aldosteronism (Fig. 14-35).[13,303,717,729a,755] This ratio is usually elevated in patients with primary aldosteronism with either an adenoma or hyperplasia but shows

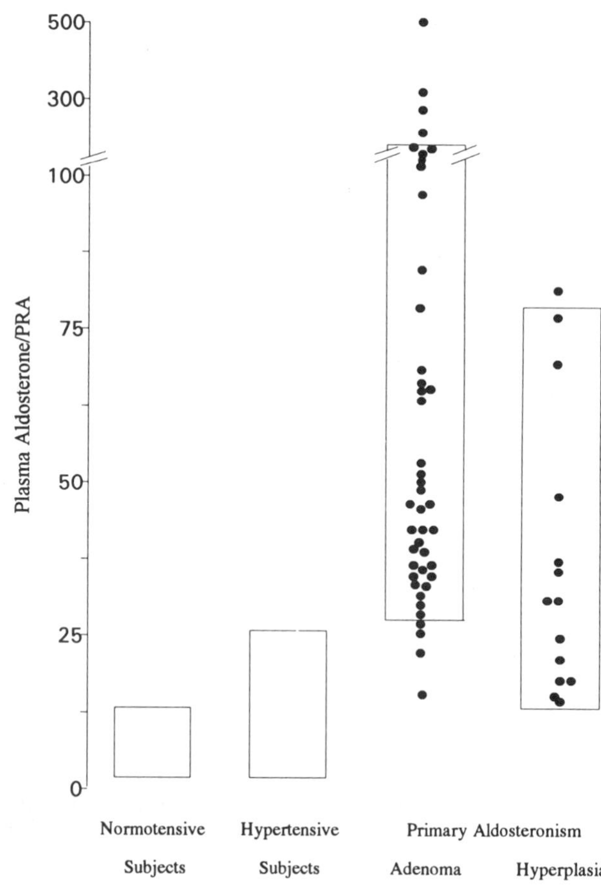

FIGURE 14-35 Use of the plasma aldosterone/PRA ratio for the diagnosis of primary aldosteronism. Shown are values for normotensive and hypertensive subjects and for primary aldosteronism caused by either adenoma or hyperplasia. The 90 percent confidence limits are shown with the boxes. n = number of subjects. *(Redrawn from Weinberger and Fineberf.[755])*

some overlap with patients with essential hypertension (Fig. 14-35). Normal values vary in different centers and are expressed in different units. For example, in one center, the ratio is abnormal if it is >30 when the aldosterone is expressed in ng/100 ml and the renin is expressed in ng/ml per h.[729a] This method has the advantage of detecting normokalemic patients with primary aldosteronism. False-positive values are seen predominantly in patients with renal impairment and sometimes in patients with the syndrome of inappropriate antidiuretic hormone. The ratios are similar if the blood samples are taken after subjects are upright or recumbent and with varied salt intakes and are not abnormal in patients with secondary hyperaldosteronism as, for example, with chronic diuretic therapy. However, they can be suppressed acutely with furosemide administration.

Plasma Aldosterone Response to Captopril (Captopril Test)

For this test, captopril is administered to block angiotensin II production and any effect on aldosterone release.[4,643,721,756,756a] PRA is markedly suppressed with APA, moderately suppressed with hyperplasia, and not suppressed with normal-renin essential hypertension; thus, after captopril, plasma aldosterone levels show no change in patients with an adenoma, shows some change with hyperplasia, and show greater changes in patients with normal-renin essential hypertension. There is also some effect of captopril on the blood pressure with IHA, but none with APA.[756a] Thus, the test may be useful for both detecting primary aldosteronism and differentiating between the subtypes.[756a] One protocol is to administer 50 mg of captopril orally at 9 A.M. after fasting from midnight and take blood samples before and 90 min after the administration.[756a] A normal response for this group is a decrease in plasma aldosterone of >20 percent.[756a] Others utilize the ratio of plasma aldosterone to renin with a slightly different protocol.[756] In two series, the ranges were: sensitivity, 88 to 100 percent; specificity, 53 to 83 percent; and a predictive value of 72 to 82 percent.[756,756a] PRA also remains suppressed by the test.[756a] These values are improved when the results of this test and the postural test (described below) are considered together.[425] Overall, whereas the test has some value, it may not be superior to the other measurements described.[756]

Other Blood Test Values

In initial screening, scrutiny of the serum or plasma concentrations of sodium (Fig. 14-34) and bicarbonate and of the hematocrit also yields clues about the presence or absence of a mineralocorticoid-excess state. Carbohydrate intolerance and failure of urinary osmolality or specific gravity to increase are additional manifestations of potassium depletion. In the absence of previous diuretic therapy, serum Na^+ concentrations <139 mEq/liter are rare in primary aldosteronism, but they are common with diuretic therapy (Fig. 14-34). The hematocrit can be reduced by increased extracellular fluid and plasma volume from sodium retention. Thus, a high serum sodium concentration in the presence of a reduced hematocrit provides presumptive evidence of a mineralocorticoid-excess state (Fig. 14-34).

Further Tests in Borderline Cases

During normal sodium intake, a suppressed renin level and high urinary or plasma aldosterone levels in the presence of hypertension and hypokalemia confirm the diagnosis of primary aldosteronism. However, suppression tests of aldosterone to demonstrate autonomy of production in primary aldosteronism are required in a number of circumstances. These tests are used when aldosterone/renin ratios are used for screening, patients have normokalemia, and urinary levels of aldosterone are normal and the diagnosis is still questioned. The tests include (1) a high-sodium diet (300 mEq per day for 5 days), (2) fludrocortisone acetate or DOCA administration (see below), or (3) 2 liters of saline IV over 4 h (discussed below).[716,757,758] In normal subjects, these maneuvers decrease the plasma aldosterone concentration to <5 ng/dl, while in patients with hyperaldosteronism, the concentration is not reduced to less than 10 mg/dl. In patients with primary aldosteronism, serum potassium levels and blood pressure must be monitored carefully during these maneuvers, as the hypokalemia in hypertension is extremely sensitive to sodium loading.

Fludrocortisone or DOCA Administration

The administration of fludrocortisone or DOCA in the hospital is another means of provoking volume expansion to provide evidence for nonsuppressibility of aldosterone production.[721,727,729a,745] It may be particularly useful for identifying patients with milder forms of primary aldosteronism. The technique is inconvenient and has the serious risk of provoking hypokalemia. Therefore, patients must be followed extremely carefully. For this reason, this test is not recommended in the general setting and probably should be reserved for specialized centers.

Localization Procedures

If the urinary excretion of aldosterone is elevated in the face of suppressed PRA and documented renal potassium wasting, the diagnosis of primary aldosteronism is confirmed. If the plasma aldosterone and/or plasma 18-hydroxycorticosterone levels are in a range suggestive of an APA (e.g., >20 ng/dl or >100 ng/dl, respectively, it is reasonable to proceed with localization procedures to detect the probable adenoma (Fig. 14-33). The next procedure is a CT scan of the adrenal glands. This presence of a tumor confirms an APA. If no tumor is identified, other diagnostic maneuvers can be applied to identify the surgically correctable form of adrenal hyperplasia (PAH) from the noncorrectable form (IHA). These maneuvers include other localization studies such as ^{131}I-cholesterol scanning and adrenal vein catheterization and bilateral sampling,[759–761] biochemical studies, and provocative tests.

Computed Tomographic Scanning and Magnetic Resonance Imaging

Traditionally, CT scanning has provided better localization of adrenal tumors causing Cushing's syndrome (Chap. 12) or pheochromocytomas (Chap. 13) than of aldosteronomas, which tend to be smaller than the other tumors. Many aldosteronomas are 1 cm or less in diameter. Nevertheless, CT scanning is currently the standard diagnostic approach for differentiating adenoma from hyperplasia (Figs. 14-26 and 14-33). CT scanning can be used to identify the larger aldosteronomas.[13,729,750,756a,759,761–763] In a study of 23 patients with adenoma and primary aldosteronism, CT scan was 70 percent accurate in localizing the adenoma. All nodules ≥1.5 cm in diameter were recognized, and 50 percent of nodules 1.0 to 1.4 cm in diameter were identified.[750,759] High-resolution CT scanning has improved the sensitivity of the technique, especially for lesions as small as 0.5 cm in diameter. The authors' experience is in agreement with that of others[756a] and suggests that CT scanning should locate the adenoma 80 to 95 percent of the time in patients with such tumors in the presence of hypertension, hypokalemia, and suppressed plasma renin. In comparison, bilateral adrenal venous sampling (discussed below) accurately located the tumor in 22 of 23 patients; in one patient with an adenoma diagnosed by CT scan, venous sampling was insufficient.

However, detection of small adenomas can be especially difficult if the adenoma is totally surrounded by normal adrenal tissue so that the tumor produces no defect in the center of the gland. It can also be difficult in patients who lack sufficient retroperitoneal fat, which is necessary to delineate adrenal anatomy. In addition, nonfunctioning adenomas can be present in the gland contralateral to the one that hypersecretes aldosterone.

MRI can also be used to identify aldosteronomas. In our experience, this method does not offer any advantages over CT scanning. However, it has been claimed that MRI has higher sensitivity, although lower specificity than CT scanning and should be used initially.[764]

Bilateral Adrenal Vein Catheterization

Bilateral adrenal vein catheterization with sampling for plasma aldosterone and cortisol can be used to localize the site of aldosterone hypersecretion.[13,729,750,759,760,762,765] The authors ordinarily reserve this method for patients with an adenoma that is not identifiable by CT scan and in the few patients in whom biochemical studies have not clearly differentiated an adenoma from hyperplasia. However, this technique is used more frequently in some centers.[13,762,765] Samples from the caudal inferior vena cava are also obtained. A higher cortisol concentration in the adrenal vein than in the caudal vena cava helps document the fact that the catheter is in or near the adrenal vein. Failure to catheterize the right adrenal vein is especially apt to happen because of visualization difficulties. A major increase in the concentration of aldosterone in one adrenal vein relative to that in the caudal vena cava or the contralateral adrenal vein indicates a unilateral source of the excess aldosterone. If the biochemical evidence strongly suggests a tumor, catheterization of only the left adrenal vein may yield sufficient information; that is, if there is a considerable increase in the plasma aldosterone concentration between peripheral and left adrenal venous blood samples, the adenoma is most likely in the left adrenal gland. In contrast, if the plasma aldosterone concentration in the left adrenal vein is similar to that in the periphery, it can be inferred that aldosterone production by the left adrenal gland is markedly suppressed and that the adenoma is in the right adrenal gland. Simultaneous ACTH infusions can be used to block possible episodic ACTH secretion in patients with tumors,[278] although this has not been found to be necessary. Bilateral adrenal vein catheterization has been shown to have a predictive value as high as 96 percent.[307,425,729,759,765] Thus, with technical proficiency and familiarity with adrenal vein sampling, which are essential, this is a valuable diagnostic tool. Adrenal venography was previously used to locate the tumor but is a potentially traumatic procedure and is rarely performed today.

Iodocholesterol Scanning Technique

Cholesterol and radiolabeled derivatives concentrate in steroid-synthesizing tissues; thus, uptake of radiolabeled iodocholesterol or selenomethylcholesterol can provide some indication of unilateral versus bilateral hyperfunction or normal function.[304,425,750,756a,761,766] This technique is rarely used in our institutions because of the availability of other methods. For this technique, the patient is scanned for several days after IV administration of the radiolabeled cholesterol. Dexamethasone is administered to suppress zonae fasciculata and reticularis uptake of radioactivity. For scanning with radiolabeled iodine, Lugol's solution is given to avoid thyroid uptake of radioiodine. The diagnostic accuracy for localization of aldosteronomas of this technique has been reported to be 70 to 90 percent.[304,425,756,766]

Biochemical Determination of the Subtypes of Primary Aldosteronism

In the absence of a demonstrable tumor, a series of other diagnostic maneuvers are helpful in separating occult tumors and PAH from IHA (Table 14-13).[13,242,303,307,719–727,750,756a,766] These maneuvers have utilized (1) differences in responsiveness of the various forms to various stimuli, (2) differences in the patterns of release of precursor steroids, including 18-OH-corticosterone and 18-hydroxycortisol, and (3) the fact that in general, patients with adenomas have higher levels of aldosterone and other steroids and more hypokalemia. The distinctions in the following discussions have been established for primary aldosteronism with hypokalemia; they may change for milder cases of the disorder.

Aldosterone

In general, patients with APA have higher aldosterone secretion and more suppression of PRA than those with IHA (Figs. 14-27, 14-28, and 14-30).[13,242,303,307,719–727,750,756a]

Precursor Steroids

The precursors of aldosterone in the zona glomerulosa [DOC, corticosterone, and 18-hydroxycorticosterone (18-OHB)], while similar to those in the 17-deoxy pathway in the zona fasciculata, do not ordinarily contribute to the peripheral plasma levels of these steroids (Figs. 14-24 and 14-32 and Table 14-13). Thus, overactivity of the zona glomerulosa pathways is suggested when these precursors are elevated in the presence of normal cortisol (produced in the zona fasciculata). Among all the precursor steroids, 18-OHB is elevated to a greater extent than are other precursors in APA and is clearly greater than in IHA, although there can be some overlap with the normals when they are sampled at 8 A.M. after overnight recumbency (Fig. 14-32 and Table 14-13).[729,750,756a,767,768] This separation of 18-OHB levels is due in part to the fact that potassium depletion can influence aldosterone production by retarding the final conversion of 18-OHB by dehydrogenation to aldosterone. Plasma DOC and corticosterone levels can be slightly elevated at 8 A.M. in patients with hyperplasia. Nevertheless, differences in 18-OHB levels between adenoma and hyperplasia patients are greater than for the other precursor steroids. In patients with PAH, DOC, corticosterone, and 18-OHB are likely to be elevated as they are in APA.

Postural Test

The pathologic cause of primary aldosteronism can be inferred by examining the circadian rhythm of aldosterone production.[460,721,723,724,769] Under normal circumstances, the plasma aldosterone level shows an early morning peak that is associated with increased ACTH release at that time, followed by a decline in the early morning hours. If the subject remains supine, this is the only peak seen. However, the plasma aldosterone level shows a second peak when upright posture is assumed, ordinarily between 8 A.M. and noon (see also Chap. 12). Plasma aldosterone levels show the early ACTH-induced peak in patients with both autonomous and nonautonomous primary aldosteronism. However, the autonomous and nonautonomous forms differ in their patterns in response to posture.

In patients with autonomous aldosterone production (APA and PAH), plasma aldosterone concentrations generally show no significant change or decrease in response to assumption of the upright posture; after 2 to 4 h in the upright position, the plasma aldosterone concentration falls in 90 percent of these patients (Figs. 14-28 and 14-29). Even in those (<10 percent) who show a slight increase, the overnight recumbent value is >20 ng/dl and the increases are less than in normal subjects, that is, less than a doubling of the level. This general lack of a posture-induced increase in aldosterone levels in patients with adenoma and PAH is due to the profound suppression of the renin-angiotensin system and the consequent insensitivity to posture induced by the aldosterone excess. The fall or downward drift of plasma aldosterone levels in these patients between 8 A.M. and noon may reflect the diminishing influence of ACTH resulting from its circadian rhythm.

By contrast, in patients with nonautonomous primary aldosteronism (IHA and AP-RA), plasma aldosterone concentrations almost always increase after 2 to 4 h in the erect posture (Figs. 14-29 and 14-30).[723,724] In these patients, the increase in plasma aldosterone levels is due in part to the increased sensitivity of the hyperplastic gland to minute but definite posture-induced changes in renin release (Figs. 14-29 and 14-30).[746]

To performed the test, patients are maintained on a normal sodium diet (120 mEq of Na^+ per day and 50 to 80 mEq of K^+ per day) and medications are discontinued for at least 3 weeks before the test.[723] After overnight recumbency and fasting, a blood sample is drawn in the morning (8 A.M.) and again after 2 to 4 h in the upright position during quiet ambulation. Whereas 4 h in the upright posture was used in the past, 2 h is now considered sufficient.

The diagnostic accuracy of the test is improved by simultaneous measurement of plasma cortisol levels in the recumbent and upright positions (Fig. 14-29). Changes in plasma cortisol levels reflect variations in ACTH-induced contributions to plasma aldosterone levels during the test (Chap. 12). This correction for the ACTH influence is made by subtracting the percentage increase in cortisol from the percentage change in plasma aldosterone.

A corrected increase in plasma aldosterone of less than 30 percent has a positive predictive value of 98 percent for autonomous primary aldosteronism, including APA and PAH.[723,724] The predictive value would be 87 percent for adrenal adenoma alone, but this is probably not as valid an index, since patients with primary adrenal hyperplasia respond to surgery.[723,724] This high predictive value resides in the fact that almost all patients with APA and all with PAH had values <30 percent, whereas only two patients with IHA had values of <30 percent. Thus, if the response is <30 percent, an excellent response to surgery should be anticipated. The major problem with the test is that about 10 percent of patients with adenoma, who would probably respond to surgery, have values >30 percent and will be missed.

Lower success rates with this test were reported when different methods of patient preparation were employed or when the results were not normalized to changes in plasma cortisol.[278,720,729,770] Equivocal responses can be evaluated further by more frequent sampling during a 24-h period, which will yield a discriminating pattern, or by the other studies described below. In interpreting the results, however, it must be remembered that physiologic stimuli such as posture and exercise can increase the plasma aldosterone concentration to quite high levels in normal subjects.

Saline Infusion Test

The saline infusion test shows promise for differentiating autonomous from nonautonomous primary aldosteronism.[723,755,771] Patients on a balanced diet containing 120 mEq of sodium receive 1250 ml of isotonic saline IV between 8 A.M. and 10 A.M. after overnight recumbency. Plasma samples are obtained immediately before and after the infusion, and the 18-OHB/cortisol or aldosterone/cortisol ratio is measured. This ratio increases in patients with an aldosterone-producing adenoma but remains unchanged or decreases in patients with hyperplasia. The ratio increases in primary aldosteronism with adenoma because of the greater effect over the time of study of diminishing ACTH on cortisol release from the normal adrenal compared with 18-OHB or aldosterone release from the adenoma. The infusion has little influence on this ratio in APA and PAH, since the PRA is suppressed and the tumor or autonomous hyperplastic gland is not under the control of angiotensin II. By contrast, the infusion decreases the release of 18-OHB or aldosterone by nonautonomous hyperplastic tissue and/or AP-RA that are in part under angiotensin II control, so that the 18-OHB/cortisol and/or aldosterone/cortisol ratios will not increase. The aldosterone/cortisol and 18-OHB/cortisol ratios are greater than 3 in patients with adenoma or primary hyperplasia, whereas with IHA or AP-RA the ratios are <3 because of the sensitivity of renin release in these states.

Response to Spironolactone

Spironolactone is a competitive antagonist for the mineralocorticoid receptor. In doses of 200 to 400 mg/dl, it corrects the hypertension and hypokalemia in patients with PAH and APA but not in those with IHA. Autonomous lesions (APA and PAH) do not increase aldosterone production in response to the inhibitor.[722] This is in marked contrast to patients with IHA, in whom aldosterone increases occur with the restoration of plasma potassium and PRA to normal.[722]

18-Hydroxycortisol

Measurement of the naturally occurring steroids 18-oxo-cortisol (18-oxoF) and 18-OH-cortisol (18-OHF) may have utility in differentiating adenomas from hyperplasias, although these tests are not generally available. 18-oxoF and 18-OHF are produced by aldosterone synthetase (CYP11B2) from cortisol; they are generally produced in higher quantities with APA and PAH but not in IHA and AP-RA.[714,738,768,772] Table 14-15 shows data from two series; the use of the criterion of urinary 18-OHF levels of >100 μg/day or of a ratio of 18-OHF/total cortisol metabolites would have detected all but one patient

TABLE 14-15 Urinary 18-Hydroxycortisol Metabolites in Primary Aldosteronism

	18-OHF/TCM (>0.022)*		18-OHF (>100 μg/d)	
	%	Number	%	Number
Normals	0	0/18	0	0/17
APA	100	6/6	92	11/12
IHA	0	0/6	0	0/20
AP-RA	0	0/2	0	0/2
PAH	67	2/3	—	—

* Ratio of urinary 18OHF to total cortisol metabolites.

Source: Hamlet et al.[738] and Ulick et al.[772]

with APA and would have included two of three patients with surgically correctable PAH. Patients with AP-RA tend to have lower levels and would not be detected. The mechanisms for the increased production of these steroids may be due to the fact that cortisol synthesis is increased in the adenomas relative to the normal or hyperplastic adrenal glomerulosa and that this provides increased substrate for the reaction (Fig. 14-24) (discussed above).

Treatment

The decision to use surgical treatment depends for the most part on the precision of diagnosis.[13,242,719,721,722,724–727,731,750] In general, IHA should be treated medically and APA, AP-RA, and PAH respond to surgery but can be treated medically.

Adenoma

In patients with an aldosterone-producing adenoma [both autonomous aldosterone-producing adenomas (APAs) and AP-RA] without a contraindication for surgical intervention, unilateral adrenalectomy is recommended.

Standard surgical approaches are still used in most centers. The transperitoneal surgical approach has been employed for many years with good success.[732] However, with lateralization techniques, the unilateral posterior approach has been employed with considerably less postoperative morbidity. Unilateral adrenalectomy is generally performed. If the tumor is identified at surgery, exploration of the contralateral adrenal gland is not indicated. Less invasive laparoscopic techniques are also beginning to be employed with increasing frequency. Although it is too soon to know how effective these techniques will be, early reports are optimistic that this will reduce the overall morbidity in removing these tumors.[773,774]

Neither the duration of hypertension nor the severity of the hypertension is a predictor of a response.[750] Many patients require additional antihypertensive therapy.[750] This may be due largely to the fact that many of these patients have underlying essential hypertension. By contrast, the blood pressure response to spironolactone before surgery provides a surprisingly close approximation of the actual response to surgery, although greater reductions often occur postoperatively, presumably because of a greater reduction of extracellular fluid volume. Table 14-16 shows the responses of patients with adenoma to adrenalectomy. As noted, in these series, there were significant lowerings of both systolic and diastolic blood pressures but not normalization in all cases.[730,731] The overall surgical cure rate of hypertension associated with an adenoma is

TABLE 14-16 Effect of Adrenalectomy on Blood Pressure in Patients with Primary Aldosteronism with Adenoma or Hyperplasia

		Systolic			Diastolic			
Disorder	Series	Before	After	Change	Before	After	Change	Follow, months
Adenoma	Baer et. al.*	179	135	44	113	87	33	2–108
	Biglieri et. al.†	195	155	40	120	100	20	6
Hyperplasia								
Bilateral Adx.	Baer et. al.	185	157	28	130	112	18	8–48
	Biglieri et. al.	175	160	15	115	110	5	6
Subtotal Adx.	Baer et. al.	172	165	7	112	109	3	1–48
	Biglieri et. al.	215	185	30	125	105	20	6

* Data taken from Baer et al.[730] One patient was reported to have a "normal" blood pressure after surgery and was assigned a pressure of 120/80 mmHg for the calculation.

† Data taken from Biglieri et al.[731]

>50 percent in several series, with reduction of hypertension in another 25 percent.[27,729–731,775,776] Normalization of blood pressure in 60 to 70 percent has been reported, and the hypertension decreased in all other patients. The authors' more recent experience is that with APA, the cure rate approaches 85 percent, with significant improvement in the control of the hypertension in the remaining patients. The authors have also not noted a recurrence in tumors after surgery in any of our patients with follow-up periods up to 25 years.

Given that an additional cause for the hypertension, such as one of the causes of essential hypertension probably is present in many cases, it should not be surprising that in many cases hypertension, but not primary aldosteronism, can recur many years after surgery[731,756a,776] and usually requires antihypertensive drugs. In fact, the best predictor of the recurrence of hypertension after treatment is the presence of a positive family history of hypertension.[776] Thus, the blood pressure should be followed forever after surgical removal of an adenoma. Similar to the experience of patients with PAH, subtotal adrenalectomy produced sustained normalization of aldosterone production and correction of hypertension and hypokalemia in patients with PAH.

Preoperative treatment with 200 to 400 mg of spironolactone daily is recommended. This should be continued until the blood pressure and serum potassium concentration are normalized. This drug is particularly beneficial because of its unique mechanism of action as an antagonist that blocks steroid binding by the mineralocorticoid receptor. These high doses normalize blood pressure, reduce the expanded sodium spaces, restore normal serum potassium concentration, and promote potassium retention in 1 to 3 months. Once normalization of blood pressure and the serum potassium level has occurred, the dose can be reduced gradually to maintenance, approximately 100 to 150 mg of spironolactone per day. During the initial treatment period, further confirmation of the diagnosis can be obtained by demonstrating that PRA has not increased and aldosterone production has not been altered during the first few days. Spironolactone therapy also has the desirable effect of usually activating (after 1 or 2 months) the suppressed renin-angiotensin system.[777,778] This will stimulate the suppressed zona glomerulosa of the nonadenomatous adrenal gland so that postoperative aldosteronism with hyperkalemia is rare. Treatment will also permit reversal, to some extent, of some of the target organ changes that have been produced by the hypertensive and hypokalemic states.

The side effects of spironolactone stem largely from its antiandrogenic capabilities.[425] Spironolactone can impair testosterone production and act as an androgen antagonist.[779] Thus, loss of libido and gynecomastia can occur in up to 80 and 40 percent, respectively, of male patients persistently ingesting spironolactone. Menstrual irregularities occur in women. Rash and epigastric discomfort occur rarely.

Interestingly, spironolactone bodies appear in the adrenal cortex during the first 4 to 5 weeks of therapy and then disappear. These intercellular whorls, several microns in size, are seen in the glomerulosa on histologic examination. Their function and mechanisms of appearance are unknown, but they often appear in relation to transient decreases in aldosterone production, which may result from interruption by the drug of the late steps of aldosterone synthesis[715] (see also Chap. 12).

Amiloride (a diuretic that retards potassium secretion and sodium entry), up to 20 to 40 mg per day, has been used instead of spironolactone and has effected similar reductions in blood pressure and correction of hypokalemia.[729,780]

In patients whose blood pressures do not normalize with spironolactone or triamterene, calcium-channel blockers and diuretics can be effective.[750,754,781] Nadler and associates reported that nifedipine decreased blood pressure and plasma aldosterone levels in five patients with adenoma and five patients with hyperplasia.[754] After 4 weeks of nifedipine administration (20 mg sublingually tid), four patients with hyperplasia and two with adenoma had decreases in plasma aldosterone levels and normalization of blood pressure and serum potassium levels. The addition of spironolactone with nifedipine led to supranormal elevations of serum potassium levels; this suggests that combinations of antialdosterone agents should be used with caution. In another study, nifedipine was found not to be as effective as spironolactone, and so further evaluation of the effects of calcium-channel blockers is necessary.[781] After surgery, the blood pressure needs careful monitoring. As stated, some patients will require blood pressure–lowering medications. In addition, some patients can become symptomatically hypotensive after surgery, and hypotension can last at least 2 years.[782] This may be due in part to secondary suppression of the remaining adrenal gland with decreased aldosterone production.[782] Interestingly, plasma cortisol levels were also lower in this group.[782]

If there are contraindications for or if the patient refuses surgery, long-term treatment with spironolactone can be effective. The initial dose of 200 to 400 mg of spironolactone per day must be continued for 4 to 6 weeks before the full effect on blood pressure is realized. With prolonged treatment, aldosterone production increases, probably because of modest activation of the renin-angiotensin system by potassium replenishment and diminution of expanded sodium and fluid volume. The authors have had patients with adenomas who have been treated successfully with spironolactone for over 10 years. Patients who do not respond to spironolactone with normalization of blood pressure are likely to have other causes for their hypertension (i.e., background essential hypertension).

Primary Adrenal Hyperplasia

The small subset of patients with primary adrenal hyperplasia respond favorably to a reduction in adrenal mass.[719,725,726] In these patients, unilateral adrenalectomy, usually of the left adrenal gland, is sufficient to produce a sustained cure or amelioriation of the hypertension. In the authors' experience with eight patients treated in this way, there has been no recurrence of primary aldosteronism after follow-up for up to 12 years.

Idiopathic Hyperplasia

Medical therapy is recommended for patients with hyperplasia. The response to surgery in these patients is shown in Table 14-16.[730,731] Surgery reduced both systolic and diastolic blood pressures in some patients, but overall the responses to subtotal adrenalectomy were modest; those to bilateral adrenalectomy were better but were less than in patients with adenoma. Subtotal adrenalectomy will also correct the hypokalemia in these patients.[228,730–732,750,762,780,783,784] Primary aldosteronism also tends to recur with subtotal adrenalectomy. Thus, because of the modest responses to surgery, this is not recommended for patients with hyperplasia.

In patients with idiopathic hyperplasia, large doses of spironolactone alone are useful for treating the hypokalemia, but the drug alone is usually ineffective in controlling the hypertension. Thus, other antihypertensive measures must be added to normalize blood pressure. Calcium-channel blockers are useful for treatment of these patients, although they are not effective in all patients, and additional drugs are commonly required.[4,156,750,781] These patients also respond to thiazide diuretics, but spironolactone should be given concomitantly and the serum potassium levels should be monitored.[750]

Glucocorticoid-Remediable Aldosteronism

In patients with glucocorticoid-remediable aldosteronism, a replacement dose of 0.5 to 2 mg of dexamethasone per day frequently normalizes blood pressure and hypokalemia in 3 to 4 weeks; prolonged treatment with 1 to 2 mg per day is necessary to maintain normal blood pressure and potassium concentration.[744,745] However, cushingoid side effects should be avoided and have been a problem with treatment. The blood pressure, as well as hypokalemia, if present, also responds to antimineralocorticoid therapy, and these patients also respond well to calcium-channel blockers. Many patients require additional hypertensive therapy either initially or later; this is not surprising, since many of those with frank hypertension probably have an additional defect causing essential hypertension.

Carcinoma

When identified, carcinomas are usually large and the prognosis is extremely grim, with a life expectancy of less than 6 months. The palliative measure of reduction of adrenal mass can modify the hypertension and the other effects of aldosterone excess to some extent. Also, chemotherapeutic agents such as aminoglutethimide, ketoconazole, and mitotane can help reduce the effects of steroid excess, although they are only rarely curative.

OTHER LOW-RENIN HYPERTENSION SYNDROMES

Known causes of low-renin hypertension that are not attributable to aldosterone are listed in Table 14-11. Hypertension can be due to excessive DOC, cortisol, or other unknown factors. Low-renin essential hypertension was discussed in the section on the renin-angiotensin system above.

Deoxycorticosterone-Excess Hypertension

DOC excess plays a role in several forms of hypertension. DOC is measured by RIA, and in normal subjects, circulating levels (4 to 12 ng/dl) probably contribute negligibly to the mineralocorticoid activity of plasma. Circulating levels of DOC can be 10 times normal in certain syndromes, and these levels can contribute to the mineralocorticoid excess. This occurs in syndromes of defective 11β- or 17α-hydroxylation of steroids (Chap. 12). It occurs with rare tumors that produce DOC in excess. These syndromes are discussed below (see also Chap. 12). DOC excess participates in hypertension in certain cases of Cushing's syndrome (particularly with ectopic ACTH production), adrenal adenoma, and adrenal carcinoma, this role is discussed in the section on Cushing's syndrome below.

Congenital Adrenal Hyperplasia

Two forms of congenital adrenal hyperplasia, the 11β-hydroxylase ($P450_{c11}$ and 17α-hydroxylase ($P450_{c17}$ deficiencies, are associated with hypertension (Fig. 14-24 and Table 14-13). The molecular biology and other aspects of these disorders are discussed in Chap. 12. These disorders are rare in individuals of European ancestry, but 11β-hydroxylation deficiency accounts for about 15 percent of cases of congenital adrenal hyperplasia in Moslem and Jewish Middle Eastern populations (see Chap. 12). These syndromes usually can be readily identified. Salient features of these disorders are listed in

Table 14-13, and the site of the defect is depicted in Fig. 14-24.

11β-Hydroxylase deficiency is usually recognized in infants and children because of virilization and the frequent presence of both hypertension and hypokalemia. Although growth is accelerated, the ultimate height achieved by these patients tends to be abnormally low. Plasma levels of 17α-hydroxyprogesterone and its urinary metabolite pregnanetriol and urinary levels of 17-ketosteroids are increased, similar to the case with the simple virilizing form of congenital adrenal hyperplasia, 21α-hydroxylase deficiency (see Chap. 12). The defect is usually partial, so that some cortisol is produced, but it does not increase with further stimulation by ACTH. The level of cortisol finally attained is due in part to the increased ACTH production in the presence of cortisol deficiency. Blood levels and production rates of cortisol are usually within normal limits or slightly decreased.[785] A partial defect of 11β-hydroxylation with increased ACTH levels results in increased production and blood levels of DOC, 11-deoxycortisol, and androgens.[786] Hypertension, hypokalemia, and suppression of PRA can result from excessive production of DOC. Suppressed PRA results in reduced or normal plasma levels of aldosterone.[787]

The 17α-hydroxylase deficiency syndrome is usually recognized at the time of puberty in young adults by the presence of hypertension, hypokalemia, and primary amenorrhea in the female or pseudohermaphroditism in the male (Chap. 12).[788,789] These features become more evident at this time because of the increased steroid production associated with puberty. In contrast to 11β-hydroxylation deficiency, there is no virilization or restricted growth. Patients often present with eunuchoid proportions and appearance. The levels of 17β-hydroxyprogesterone and pregnanetriol are low and are almost diagnostic. The block in this syndrome results in compensatory ACTH hypersecretion, with increased production of corticosterone and DOC. The corticosterone provides glucocorticoid activity, and both DOC and corticosterone lead to a mineralocorticoid-excess state with suppressed PRA, hypokalemia, and suppressed aldosterone production.

Treatment of both the 11β-hydroxylase and the 17α-hydroxylase deficiency syndromes is similar to that of other non-salt-losing forms of congenital adrenal hyperplasia (see Chap. 12). The administration of small doses of glucocorticoids such as dexamethasone restores blood pressure to normal levels, corrects potassium depletion, and reduces excessive DOC and corticosterone production in the 17α-hydroxylase deficiency syndrome and reduces DOC and 11-deoxycortisol production in the 11β-hydroxylase deficiency syndrome. Prompt natriuresis usually occurs when treatment is started. In the 17α-hydroxylase deficiency syndrome, restoration of normal levels of DOC results in a return of PRA and aldosterone concentration to normal values. In patients with extremely low cortisol production, care should be exercised during the early treatment period; a delay in the return of the suppressed renin-aldosterone system toward normal can result in a hypovolemic crisis after the initial natriuresis and diuresis. It may take up to several years before the aldosterone and renin systems become normalized. The amount of glucocorticoid administered must be carefully monitored to avoid the induction of Cushing's syndrome. Cushingoid changes have been effected with as little as 0.125 mg of dexamethasone per day; often a very small dose must be given intermittently.

Deoxycorticosterone-Producing Adrenocortical Adenoma

Most tumors that hypersecrete DOC are found in association with the ectopic ACTH syndrome and adrenocortical carcinomas (see Chap. 12; also discussed below). However, a few patients have been described with hypertension and hypokalemia associated with DOC excess, suppressed PRA, and low-normal plasma aldosterone and cortisol concentrations.[790,791] In one tumor, a unique pattern of steroid production after surgical removal of the tumor was observed in which there was a relatively prolonged and selective suppression of 17-deoxy steroids (including DOC) with normal cortisol production, implying the existence of a factor that selectively regulates this pathway.[791]

Iatrogenic Syndromes

There are several circumstances in which iatrogenic mineralocorticoid-excess hypertension can occur. These include ingestion of large quantities of licorice,[261,262] use of chewing tobacco,[792] administration of carbenoxolone for gastric ulcer,[255–257] administration of moderate doses of fludrocortisone for postural hypotension,[793] and use of mineralocorticoid-containing nasal sprays.[290,311] For all these syndromes, the diagnosis depends on uncovering a history of ingestion of the offending substance in a patient with hypertension, hypokalemia, suppressed PRA, low aldosterone concentration, and no excess of other steroids. The metabolic abnormalities become normal several weeks after discontinuance of the agent. Such a normalization also helps confirm the diagnosis.

Licorice Ingestion

Persons who ingest large quantities (e.g., 1 lb per week) of certain types of licorice can develop mineralocorticoid-excess hypertension.[261,262,264] The types of licorice that produce the syndrome contain glycyrrhizic acid and its hydrolytic product, glycyrrhetinic acid, the major active principal.[261,262] Glycyrrhizic acid inhibits 11β-hydroxysteroid dehydrogenase activity[255–257,261,262] and thus blocks renal conversion of cortisol to cortisone (see Chap. 12). This results in exposure of renal mineralocorticoid receptors to cortisol, which binds to these receptors and produces a mineralocorticoid-excess state with hypertension, hypokalemia, suppressed PRA, and low plasma and urinary levels of aldosterone. The activity of 11β-hydroxysteroid dehydrogenase and cortisol as a mineralocorticoid are also discussed in the section on mineralocorticoids. Patients with this disorder have a prolonged plasma half-life of cortisol, increased urinary excretion of cortisol, and decreased urinary ratios of cortisone to cortisol metabolites.[262] After withdrawal of the licorice, the pattern of steroid metabolism can return to normal in about 2 weeks as the licorice metabolites are cleared, but it can take months for the renin-angiotensin-aldosterone axis to normalize.[262]

Carbenoxolone Ingestion

Carbenoxolone has been used for the treatment of gastric and peptic ulcers, mostly in Europe. Its use has declined in recent years because of the effectiveness of newer pharmaceuticals. The ingestion of this material produces a mineralocorticoid-excess-like syndrome with hypertension, hypokalemia, and suppressed renin with low levels of aldosterone.[255,256] Carbenoxolone has been found to inhibit 11β-hydroxysteroid dehydrogenase and may cause hypertension by means similar to those described above for licorice ingestion, although other mechanisms have been suggested.[255–257]

Steroid Ingestion

Mineralocorticoid hypertension with hypokalemia and suppressed PRA caused by steroid ingestion is uncommon because compounds with predominant mineralocorticoid activity are not often used except for replacement therapy. However, fludrocortisone sometimes is used to treat postural hypotension, and this can lead to moderate hypertension (particularly in the supine state), hypokalemia, and a suppressed plasma renin level. Mineralocorticoid-excess hypertension has been reported in several patients in Italy who were using a steroid-containing nasal spray (Biorinil) for allergic rhinitis.[311] The active component of the spray was found to be fluprednisolone, which was shown to have potent mineralocorticoid activity.

Syndrome of Apparent Mineralocorticoid Excess

This is a rare syndrome that has been observed mostly in children and in one adult with low-renin hypokalemic hypertension.[256,257,261,263,311,794,795] Children have usually presented with failure to thrive, short stature, and thirst, polyuria, and polydipsia secondary to nephrogenic diabetes insipidus induced by the hypokalemia. The disorder can be familial, and in one situation where three patients were siblings, the mother had mild low-renin hypertension, hypokalemia, and a prolonged cortisol half-life.[256,264] Plasma aldosterone concentrations are low, and plasma cortisol concentrations are normal to low. The low PRA levels, hypokalemia, and hypertension responded to the mineralocorticoid antagonist spironolactone but not to a glucocorticoid antagonist, suggesting that the abnormalities were due to mineralocorticoid excess.[263] The hypertension can be aggravated by the administration of ACTH. This suggests that the steroids involved come from the cortisol producing adrenal fasciculata-reticularis. The patterns of steroid metabolism resemble those described above with licorice ingestion, with a delayed clearance of cortisol, increased urinary cortisol, and increased ratios of urinary cortisone to cortisol metabolites.[262] The data suggest that there is decreased 11β-hydroxysteroid dehydrogenase activity with excessive access of cortisol to the mineralocorticoid receptor and a cortisol-driven mineralocorticoid-excess state in these patients.[794,795] However, there are some differences in the patterns of steroid metabolism in apparent mineralocorticoid excess vs. licorice ingestion that could imply that there are differences between the two syndromes. In contrast to licorice ingestion, in the syndrome of apparent mineralocorticoid excess, there is an increase in cortisol 5α-reductase relative to 5α-reductase activity and reduced activity of metabolites of the A ring of the steroid, resulting in a high level of relative excretion of conjugated cortisol metabolites.[255,256,262–264,794,795] The mechanisms for the decreased enzyme activity in the syndrome of apparent mineralocorticoid excess have not been elucidated, and efforts to find a mutation in the gene for this enzyme have been unsuccessful. Although this volume-dependent hypertension often can be treated with spironolactone and dexamethasone in addition to agents such as calcium-channel blockers, the disease can also be fatal and can respond poorly to therapy.

Spironolactone-Unresponsive Subgroup (Liddle's Syndrome)

This is a rare disorder originally described by Liddle and associates[796] in which patients present with hypertension, hypokalemia (usually), suppressed plasma renin levels, and low aldosterone levels. In the families studied, it is inherited as an autosomal dominant disorder with variable penetrance.[796] Potassium depletion and low serum levels of potassium are not corrected by the administration of the antimineralocorticoid spironolactone or a low-sodium diet but are ameliorated by triamterene or amiloride, diuretics that block renal sodium reabsorption and potassium excretion by mineralocorticoid receptor–independent mechanisms.[796] The syndrome is also ameliorated by renal transplantation. The syndrome is thought to be caused by a primary defect in the distal nephron[796] that also may be more generalized, since erythrocyte sodium is enhanced in these patients.[795,796]

Primary or Secondary Glucocorticoid Resistance

Glucocorticoid resistance can occur as a primary genetic defect, or can be induced by treatment with a glucocorticoid antagonist.[258–260] The genetic defects studied are in the glucocorticoid receptor and result in a lowered affinity. To compensate for the defect, the body produces more ACTH, with consequent increases in the release of cortisol, DOC, and adrenal androgens. Thus, in women, the disorder can present with acne, hirsutism, and menstrual irregularities. In its severe form, the cortisol and DOC excess cause a mineralocorticoid-excess syndrome, with hypokalemia, hypertension, suppressed plasma renin levels, and low plasma and urinary aldosterone levels. The relative contributions of DOC and cortisol to the mineralocorticoid excess have not been established.

CUSHING'S SYNDROME

Most patients with spontaneous Cushing's syndrome have hypertension (see Chap. 12).[268,308,311] Hypertension is present in 17 to 70 percent of patients treated with glucocorticoids for other conditions (see Chap. 15).[308,311,316,317] The incidence of hypertension in spontaneous Cushing's syndrome is highest in patients with ectopic ACTH-producing tumors and adrenal carcinomas.[311] Hypertension is present in around 70 percent of patients with Cushing's disease (pituitary ACTH hypersecretion; see Chap. 12) and cortisol-producing adrenal adenomas.

In patients with Cushing's disease (pituitary ACTH hypersecretion), cortisol production is increased but aldosterone and corticosterone excretion and secretion are usually normal.[268,269,308] In some cases, urinary aldosterone excretion is low; rarely, it may be increased.[269] The lack of an increase in aldosterone levels is expected, because stimulatory influences of ACTH on aldosterone production are transient, and with prolonged exposure, ACTH may inhibit aldosterone production. Plasma DOC concentrations are usually normal[269] or increased modestly. In patients with ectopic ACTH syndrome, overall production of cortisol and other steroids, including DOC, can be much higher. Adrenal malignancies can result in a variety of patterns of steroid production; elevated levels of DOC, corticosterone, and aldosterone occur in some patients, whereas levels of cortisol and 11β-deoxycortisol are elevated in others.

Clear evidence for mineralocorticoid excess with hypokalemia and suppressed PRA is absent in 60 to 90 percent of patients with Cushing's disease, many patients with cortisol-producing adrenal adenomas, and patients who develop hypertension on glucocorticoid therapy.[311] However, in one study, PRA values measured with the patient upright were low in 9 of 16 patients with Cushing's disease, even though the mean PRA for the group was normal and only 3 patients had plasma potassium concentration values of <3.5 mEq/liter.[309] Conversely, PRA is high in some cases.[267]

Frank mineralocorticoid excess with hypokalemia and suppressed PRA is observed more commonly in severe cases of Cushing's disease, with ectopic ACTH production, or with adrenal adenoma or carcinoma.[268,311] In these cases, plasma cortisol concentrations may be higher than in most patients with Cushing's disease and may contribute to a mineralocorticoid-excess state. However, DOC levels can be very high (i.e., >75 ng/dl) in these cases and may be the major contributor to the mineralocorticoid-excess state. There may also be increased production of corticosterone and other steroids that could contribute mineralocorticoid activity, but the role of these steroids is not established.[268] Thus, the hypertension in these patients could be due to both mineralocorticoid and glucocorticoid excess.

However, mineralocorticoid excess may not account for the hypertension in the majority of patients with spontaneous Cushing's syndrome who have normal serum potassium and PRA levels. The mechanisms for the hypertension in these patients is discussed in the sections on glucocorticoids and ACTH and hypertension above. The glucocorticoid excess is likely to be the major factor, but other steroids and factors, such as the ouabain-related factor, have been considered. Hypertension in these cases is responsive to treatment with antiglucocorticoids, but it does not respond to treatment with the antimineralocorticoid spironolactone and is not salt-responsive.[311,797,798]

Cure or improvement of hypertension usually follows successful treatment of Cushing's syndrome and remission of other stigmata of the syndrome. However, this is not the case in about a third of the patients, and this could reflect underlying essential hypertension.

REFERENCES

1. Fifth Report of the Joint National Committee on High Blood Pressure. *Arch Intern Med* 153:154, 1993.
2. 1993 Guidelines for the management of mild hypertension: Memorandum from a World Health Organization/International Society of Hypertension Meeting. *Hypertension* 22:392, 1993.
3. Collins R, Peto R, MacMahon S, et al: Blood pressure, stroke, and coronary heart disease: II. Short term reduction

in blood pressure: Overview of randomized drug trials in their epidemiological context. *Lancet* 335:827, 1990.

4. Müeller F, and Laragh J: Clinical evaluation and differential diagnosis of the individual hypertensive patient. *Clin Chem* 37:1868, 1991.
5. Ménard J: Improving hypertension treatment: Where should we put our efforts: new drugs, new concepts or new management. *Am J Hypertens* 5:252, 1992.
6. Berglund G, Andersson O, Wilhelmsen L: Prevalence of primary and secondary hypertension: Studies in a random population sample. *Br Med J* 2:554, 1976.
7. Bech K, Hilden T: The frequency of secondary hypertension. *Acta Med Scand* 197:65, 1975.
8. Mann S, Pickering T: Detection of renovascular hypertension. *Ann Intern Med* 117:845, 1992.
9. Detection, evaluation, and treatment of renovascular hypertension: Final Report. Working Group on Renovascular Hypertension. *Arch Intern Med* 147:820, 1987.
10. Swartbol P, Thorvinger B, Pärsson H, et al: Renal artery stenosis in patients with peripheral vascular disease and its correlation to hypertension. *Int Angiol* 11:195, 1992.
11. Missouris C, Buchenham T, Cappuccio F, et al: Renal artery stenosis: A common and important problem in patients with peripheral vascular disease. *Am J Med* 96:10, 1994.
12. Streetan D, Anderson GI, Wagner S: Effect of age on response of secondary hypertension to specific treatment. *Am J Hypertens* 3:360,1990.
13. Gordon R: Primary aldosteronism: A new understanding. *Med J Aust* 158:729, 1993.
14. Stokes G, Monaghan J, Roche J, et al: Concurrence of primary aldosteronism and renal artery stenosis. *Clin Exp Pharmacol Physiol* 19:300, 1992.
15. Stokes J, Kannel W, Wolff P, et al: Blood pressure as a risk factor for cardiovascular disease: The Framingham study—30 years of follow-up. *Hypertension* 13:I–13, 1989.
16. Kannel W: The clinical heterogenity of hypertension. *Am J Hypertens* 4:283, 1991.
17. Agabiti E, Muiesan M, Muiesan G: Regression of structural alterations in hypertension. *Am J Hypertens* 2:70, 1989.
18. Russel R: Pathological changes in small cerebral arteries causing occlusion and hemorrhage. *J Cardiovasc Pharmacol* 6:S691, 1984.
19. Havlik R: Predictors of hypertension, population studies. *Am J Hypertens* 4:586, 1991.
20. Kaplan NM: *Clinical Hypertension*. Baltimore, Williams & Wilkins, 1978.
21. Kannel WB, Sorlie P: Hypertension in Framingham, in *Epidemiology and Control of Hypertension*. New York, Stratton, 1975, p. 553.
22. *Build and Blood Pressure Study*, Chicago, Society of Actuaries, Vol 1, 1959.
23. Castelli WP: Epidemiology of coronary heart disease: The Framingham study. *Am J Med* 76:4, 1984.
24. Harrington, M, Kincaid-Smith P, McMichael J: Results of treatment in malignant hypertension: A seven-year experience in 94 cases. *Br Med J* 2:969, 1959.
25. Doyle A: A review of the short-term benefits of antihypertensive treatment with emphasis on stroke. *Am J Hypertens* 6:6, 1993.
26. Klahr S, Levey A, Beck G, et al: The effects of dietary protein restriction and blood-pressure control on the progression of chronic renal disease. *N Engl J Med* 330:877, 1994.
27. Muldoon M, Terrell D, Bunker C, et al: Family history studies in hypertension research. *Am J Hypertens* 6:76, 1993.
28. Berry T, Hasstedt S, Hunt S, et al: A gene for high urinary kallikrein may protect against hypertension in Utah kindreds. *Hypertension* 13:3, 1989.
29. Jeunemaltre X, Soubrier F, Kotekevstev W, et al: Molecular basis of human hypertension: Role of angiotensinogen. *Cell* 71:169, 1992.
30. Rapp J, Wang S, Dene H: A genetic polymorphism in the renin gene of dahl rats cosegregates with blood pressure. *Science* 243:542, 1989.
31. Kilbert P, Lindpainter K, Lincoln J, et al: Chromosomal mapping of two genetic loci associated with blood pressure regulation in hereditary hypertensive rats. *Nature* 353:521, 1991.
32. Kurk T, Simonet L, Kabra P, et al: Cosegregation of the renin allele of the spontaneously hypertensive rat with an increase in blood pressure. *J Clin Invest* 85:1328, 1990.
33. Jacob H, Lindpainter K, Lincoln S, et al: Genetic mapping of a gene causing hypertension in the stroke prone spontaneously hypertensive rat. *Cell* 67:213, 1992.
34. Beilin L: Dietary salt and risk factors for cardiovascular disease. *Kidney Int* 37:S90, 1992.
35. Conway J: Hemodynamic aspects of essential hypertension. *Physiol Rev* 64:617, 1984.
36. Pickering T: Pathophysiology of systemic hypertension. *Am J Cardiol* 58:12, 1986.
37. Lund-Johansen P, Omvik P: Hemodynamic patterns of untreated hypertensive disease, in Laragh J, Brenner B (eds): *Hypertension: Pathophysiology, Diagnosis and Management*. New York, Raven, 1990, p 305.
38. Folkow B: Physiological aspects of primary hypertension. *Physiol Rev* 62:347, 1982.
39. Webb RC, Bohr DF: Recent advances in the pathogenesis of hypertension: Consideration of structural, functional, and metabolic vascular abnormalities resulting in elevated arterial resistance. *Am Heart J* 102:251, 1981.
40. Ventura H, Messerli FH, Oigman W, et al: Impaired systemic arterial compliance in borderline hypertension. *Am Heart J* 108:132, 1984.
41. Sullivan JM, Prewitt RL, Josephs JA: Attenuation of the microcirculation in young patients with high-output borderline hypertension. *Hypertension* 5:844, 1983.
42. Frohlich ED: Physiologic considerations in left ventricular hypertrophy. *Am J Med* 75:12, 1983.
43. Chobanian AV, Brecher PL, Haudenschild CC: Effects of hypertension and antihypertensive therapy on atherosclerosis: State of the art lecture. *Hypertension* 8 (Suppl 1):15, 1986.
44. Ross R: The pathogenesis of atherosclerosis: An update. *N Engl J Med* 314:488, 1986.
45. Phillips S, Whisnant J: Hypertension and the brain. *Arch Intern Med* 152:938, 1992.
46. Schalekamp MADH, Man in't Veld AJ, Wenting GJ: The second Sir George Pickering Memorial Lecture: What regulates whole body autoregulation? Clinical observations. *J Hypertens* 3:97, 1985.
47. Schwartz SM: Smooth muscle proliferation in hypertension. *Hypertension* 6 (Suppl 1):56, 1984.
48. Lindeman RD, Tobin JD, Shock NW: Association between hypertension and the rate of decline of renal function. *Kidney Intl* 26:861, 1984.
49. Ledingham JGC: Early assessment of organ involvement in hypertension: *J Hypertens* 3 (Suppl 2):S33, 1985.
50. van Hooft I, Grobbee D, Derkx F, et al: Renal hemodynamics and the renin-angiotensin-aldosterone system in normotensive subjects with hypertensive and normotensive parents. *N Engl J Med* 324:1305, 1994.
51. Laragh J: The renin system and four lines of hypertension research: Nephron heterogeneity, the calcium connection, the prorenin vasodilator limb, and plasma renin and heart attack. *Hypertension* 20:267,1992.
52. Dean R, Tribble R, Kansen K, et al: Evolution of renal insufficiency in ischemic nephropathy. *Ann Surg* 213:446, 1991.
53. Hallet JJ, Schriger A, Bower T, et al: The current role of surgical revascularization for combined renovascular and renal insufficiency. *Int Angiol* 11:64, 1992.
54. Bianchi S, Bigazzi R, Baldari G, et al: Microalbuminuria in patients with essential hypertension: Effects of an an-

giotension converting enzyme inhibitor and of a calcium channel blocker. *Am J Hypertens* 4:291, 1991.

55. Messerli FH, Frohlich ED, Dreslinski GR, et al: Serum uric acid in essential hypertension: An indication of renal vascular involvement. *Ann Intern Med* 93:817, 1980.
56. Perera GA: Hypertensive vascular disease: Description and natural history. *J Chronic Dis* 1:33, 1955.
57. Schulman N, Ford C, Hall W, et al: Prognostic value of serum creatinine and effect of treatment of hypertension on renal function. Results from the hypertension detection and follow-up program. *Hypertension* 13:I80, 1989.

57a. Boucher R, Rojo-Ortega JM, Genest J: Description of renin-angiotensin system and methods of measurement, in Genest J, Koiw E, Kuchel O (eds): *Hypertension: Physiopathology and Treatment.* New York, McGraw-Hill, 1977, pp 140–155.

58. Yokosawa H, Holladay LA, Inagami T, et al: Human renal renin: Complete purification and characterization. *J Biol Chem* 265:3498, 1980.
59. Slater EE, Strout HV: Pure human renin: Identification and characterization of two molecular weight forms. *J Biol Chem* 256:8164, 1981.
60. Galen FX, Devaux J, Guyenne TT, et al: Multiple forms of human renin, purification and characterization. *J Biol Chem* 254:4848, 1981.
61. Do YS, Shinagawa T, Tam H, et al: Characterization of pure human renal renin: Evidence for its subunit structure. *J Biol Chem* 1986:1986.
62. Sealey JE, Atlas SA, Laragh JH: Prorenin and other large molecular weight forms of renin. *Endocr Rev* 1:365, 1980.
63. Opsahl J, Abraham P, Katz S: Acute stimulation of renin secretion changes the multiple form profile of active plasma renin. *Am H Hypertens* 4:126, 1991.
64. Goldstone R, Horton R, Carlson EJ, et al: Reciprocal changes in active and inactive renin after converting enzyme inhibition in normal man. *J Clin Endocrinol Metab* 56:264, 1983.
65. Campbell D, Kladis A, Skinner S, et al: Characterization of angiotensin peptides in plasma of anephric man. *J Hypertens* 9:265, 1991.
66. Toffelmire E, Slater K, Corvol P, et al: Response of plasma prorenin and active renin to chronic and acute alteration of renin secretion in normal humans. *J Clin Invest* 83:679, 1989.
67. Hobart PM, Fogliano M, O'Connor BA, et al: Human renin gene: Structure and sequence analysis. *Proc Natl Acad Sci USA* 81:5026, 1984.
68. Hardman JA, Hort YJ, Catanzaro DF, et al: Primary structure of the human renin gene. *DNA* 3:457, 1984.
69. Miyazaki H, Fukamizu A, Hirose S, et al: Structure of the human renin gene. *Proc Natl Acad Sci USA* 81:5999, 1984.
70. Soubrier F, Panthier JT, Corvol P, et al: Molecular cloning and nucleotide sequence of a human renin cDNA fragment. *Nucleic Acids Res* 20:7181, 1983.
71. Imai T, Miyazaki H, Hirose S, et al: Cloning and sequence analysis of cDNA for human renin precursor. *Proc Natl Acad Sci USA* 80:7405, 1983.
72. Hsueh W, Baxter J: Human prorenin. *Hypertension* 17:469, 1991.
73. Faust P, Chirgwin J, Kornfield S: Renin, a secretory-glycoprotein, acquires phosphomannosyl residues. *J Biol Chem* 105:1947, 1987.
74. Wang P-H, Do Y, Macauley L, et al: Identification of renal cathepsin B as a human prorenin processing enzyme. *J Biol Chem* 266:12633, 1991.
75. Fritz L, Hadar M, Arfsten A, et al: Human renin is correctly processed and targeted to the regulated secretory pathway in mouse pituitary AtT-20 cells. *J Biol Chem* 262:12409, 1987.
76. Pratt R, Flynn J, Hobart P, et al: Different secretory pathways of renin from mouse cells transfected with the human renin gene. *J Biol Chem* 263:3137, 1987.
77. Campbell D: Extrarenal renin and blood pressure regulation: An alternative viewpoint. *Am J Hypertens* 2:266, 1989.
78. Re RN: Cellular biology of the renin-angiotensin systems. *Arch Intern Med* 144:2037, 1984.
79. Deschepper CF, Mellon SH, Cumin F, et al: Analysis by immunocytochemistry and in situ hybridization of renin and its mRNA in kidney, testis, adrenal, and pituitary of the rat. *Proc Natl Acad Sci USA* 83:7552, 1986.
80. Lee M, Paul M, Böhm M, et al: Effects of angiotensin-converting enzyme inhibitors on tissue renin-angiotensin systems. *Am J Cardiol* 70:12, 1992.
81. Lou Y, Smith D, Robinson B, et al: Renin gene expression in various tissues determined by single-step polymerase chain reaction. *Clin Exp Pharmacol Physiol* 18:357, 1991.
82. Lee MA, Böhm M, Paul M, et al: Tissue renin-angiotensin systems: Their role in cardiovascular disease. *Circulation* 87:IV7, 1993.
83. Ferrario C, Barnes K, Block C, et al: Pathways of angiotensin formation and function in the brain. *Hypertension* 15(Suppl 1):I–13, 1990.
84. Lever A: Endocrine, paracrine, or part-paracrine control of blood pressure. *Am J Hypertens* 2:276, 1989.
85. Danser A, van den Dorper M, Deinum J, et al: Renin, prorenin and immunoreactive renin in vitreous fluid from eyes with and without diabetic retinopathy. *J Clin Endocrinol Metab* 68:160, 1989.
86. Yamahuchi T, Franco-Saenz R, Mulrow P: Effect of angiotensin II on renin production by rat adrenal glomerulosa cells in culture. *Hypertension* 19:263, 1992.

86a. Taddei S, Favilla S, Duranti P, et al: Vascular renin-angiotension system and neurotransmission in hypertensive persons. *Hypertension* 18:266, 1991.

87. Sealey J, von Lutterotti N, Rubattu S, et al: The greater renin system: Its prorenin-directed vasodilator limb: Relevance to diabetes mellitus, pregnancy, and hypertension. *Am J Hypertens* 4:972, 1991.
88. Heinrikson R, Hui J, Zürcher-Neely H, et al: A structural model to explain the partial catalytic activity of human prorenin. *Am J Hypertens* 2:367, 1989.
89. Kim S, Hosoi M, Ikemoto F, et al: Conversion to renin of exogenously administered recombinant human prorenin in liver and kidney of monkeys. *Am J Physiol* 285:E-151, 1990.
90. Boucher R, Rojo-Ortega JM, Genest J: Description of renin angiotensin system and methods of measurement, in Genest J, Koiw E, Kuchel O (eds): *Hypertension: Physiopathology and Treatment.* New York, McGraw-Hill, 1977, p 140.
91. Rosenthal J, Thurnreiter M, Plaschke M, et al: Reninlike enzymes in human vasculature. *Hypertension* 15:848, 1990.
92. Admiraal P, Derkx F, Danser A, et al: Metabolism and production of angiotensin I in different vascular beds in subjects with hypertension. *Hypertension* 15:44, 1990.
93. Ikeda M, Sasaguri M, Maruta H, et al: Formation of angiotensin II by tonin-inhibitor complex. *Hypertension* 11:63, 1988.
94. Wintroub B, Klickstein LD, Watt KWK: A human neutrophil dependent pathway for generation of angiotensin II. *J Clin Invest* 68:484, 1981.
95. Taugner R, Yokota S, Buhrle CP, et al: Cathepsin D coexists with renin in the secretory granules of juxtaglomerular epithelioid cells. *Histochemistry* 84:19, 1986.
96. Davis JO, Freeman RH: Mechanisms regulating renin release. *Physiol Rev* 56:1, 1976.
97. Hachenthal E, Ganten P, Taugner R: Morphology, physiology and molecular biology of renin secretion. *Physiol Rev* 70:1067, 1990.
98. Beierwaltes W: Nitric oxide participates in calcium-mediated regulation of renin release. *Hypertension* 23(Suppl 1):I–40, 1994.

99. Chuchill P: Second messengers in renin secretion. *Am J Physiol* 245:F175, 1985.
100. Zipser R, Davenport M, Martin K, et al: Hyperreninemic hypoaldosteronism in the critically ill: A new entity. *J Clin Endocrinol Metab* 53:867, 1981.
101. Yamamoto T, Nakamura T, Noble N, et al: Expression of transforming growth factor β is elevated in human and experimental diabetic nephropathy. *Proc Natl Acad Sci USA* 90:1814, 1993.
102. Rosenberg M, Chmlelewski D, Hostetter T: Effect of dietary protein on rat renin and angiotensinogen gene expression. *J Clin Invest* 85:1144, 1990.
103. Geary K, Hunt M, Peach M, et al: Effects of angiotensin converting enzyme inhibition, sodium depletion, calcium, isoproterenol, and angiotensin II on renin secretion by individual renocortical cells. *Endocrinology* 131:1588, 1992.
104. Stella GR, Zanchetti A: Neural control of renin release. *Am J Hypertens* 2:7, 1989.
105. Kurtz A, Kaissling B, Busse R, et al: Endothelial cells modulate renin secretion from isolated mouse juxtaglomerular cells. *J Clin Invest* 88:1147, 1991.
106. Kurtz A, Muff R, Born W, et al: Calcitonin gene-related peptide is a stimulator of renin secretion. *J Clin Invest* 82:538, 1988.
107. Martinez-Maldonada M, Gely R, Tapia E, et al: Role of macula densa in diuretic-induced renin release. *Hypertension* 16:261, 1990.
108. Beierwaltes W, Carretero O: Non-prostanoid endothelium-derived factors inhibit renin release. *Hypertension* 19 (Suppl II):II–68, 1992.
109. Resnick L, Churchill M, Churchill P, et al: Effects of calcitonin calcitonin analogues, and calcitonin gene-related peptide on basal in vitro renin secretion. *Am J Hypertens* 2:453, 1989.
110. Taddei S, Arzilli F, Arrighi P, et al: Dipyridamole decreases circulating renin-angiotensin system activity in hypertensive patients. *Am J Hypertens* 5:29, 1992.
111. Weidmann P, Hirsch D, Maxwell MH, et al: Plasma renin and blood pressure during treatment with methyldopa. *Am J Cardiol* 34:671, 1974.
112. Niarchos AP, Baer L, Radichevich I: Role of renin and aldosterone suppression in the antihypertensive mechanism of clonidine. *Am J Med* 65:614, 1978.
113. Itoh S: Role of the macula densa in renin release. *Hypertension* 7(Suppl 1):49, 1985.
114. Itoh S, Carretero OA, Murray RD: Possible role of adenosine in the macula densa mechanism of renin release in rabbits. *J Clin Invest* 76:1412, 1985.
115. Briggs J, Lorenz J, Weihprecht H, et al: Macula densa control of renin secretion. *Renal Physiol Biochem* 14:164, 1991.
116. Briggs J, Skatt O: Direct demonstration of macular densa-mediated renin secretion. *Science* 237:1618, 1987.
117. Kotchen TA, Galla JH, Luke RG: Contribution of chloride to the inhibition of plasma renin by sodium chloride in the rat. *Kidney Int* 13:201, 1978.
118. Brunner HR, Laragh JH, Baer L, et al: Essential hypertension: Renin and aldosterone, heart attack and stroke. *N Engl J Med* 286:441, 1972.
119. Egan BM, Julius S, Cottier C, et al: Role of cardiovascular receptors on the neural regulation of renin release in normal men. *Hypertension* 5:779, 1983.
120. Tuck M: Obesity, the sympathetic nervous system, and essential hypertension. *Hypertension* 19:I–67, 1992.
121. Timmermans P, Benfield P, Chiu A, et al: Angiotensin II receptors and functional correlates. *Am J Hypertens* 5:221, 1992.
122. Kotchen T, Guthrie G: Effects of calcium on renin and aldosterone. *Am J Cardiol* 62:41, 1988.
123. Gerber JG, Olson RD, Nies AS: Interrelationship between prostaglandins and renin release. *Kidney Int* 19:816, 1981.
124. Oates J, Whorton AR, Gerkens JF, et al: The participation of prostaglandins in the control of renin release. *Fed Proc* 38:72, 1979.
125. Whorton AR, Misono K, Hollifield J, et al: Prostaglandins and renin release: I. Stimulation of renin release from rabbit renal cortical slices by PGI2. *Prostaglandins* 14:1095, 1977.
126. Patrono C, Pugliese F, Ciabattoni G, et al: Evidence for a direct stimulatory effect of prostacyclin on renin release in man. *J Clin Invest* 69:231, 1982.
127. Antonipillal I: 12-Lipoxygenase products are potent inhibitors of prostacyclin-induced renin release. *Proc Soc Exp Biol Med* 194:224, 1990.
128. Martinez-Maldonado M: Pathophysiology of renovascular hypertension. *Hypertension* 17:707, 1991.
129. Imanishi M, Kawamura M, Akabane S, et al: Aspirin lowers blood pressure in patients with renovascular hypertension. *Hypertension* 14:461, 1989.
130. Tan SY, Shapiro R, Franco R, et al: Indomethacin induced prostaglandin inhibition with hyperkalemia: A reversible cause of hyporeninemic hypoaldosteronism. *Ann Intern Med* 90:783, 1979.
131. Antonipillal I, Jost-Vu A, Horton R, et al: Altered production of 12-lipoxygenase product, 12-hydroxyeicosatetraenoic acid in diabetes. International Conference on Prostaglandins and Related Compounds. Montreal, Canada, 1992.
132. Antonipillal I, Wang Y, Horton R: Tumor necrosis factor and interleukin-1 may regulate renin secretion. *Endocrinology* 126:273, 1990.
133. Hsueh WA, Goldstone R, Carlson EJ, et al: Evidence that the beta-adrenergic system and prostaglandins stimulate renin release through different mechanisms. *J Clin Endocrinol Metab* 61:399, 1985.
134. Leutscher JA, Kraemer FB, Wilson DM, et al: Increased plasma inactive renin in diabetes mellitus. *N Engl J Med* 312:1412, 1985.
135. Wilson D, Leutscher J: Plasma prorenin activity and complications in children with insulin-dependent diabetes mellitus. *N Engl J Med* 323:1101, 1990.
136. Nakamura N, Soubrier F, Menard J, et al: Nonproportional changes in plasma renin concentration, renal renin content, and rat renin messenger RNA. *Hypertension* 7:855, 1986.
137. Kobrin I, Viskoper RJ, Laszt A, et al: Effects of an orally active renin inhibitor, Ro 42–5892, in patients with essential hypertension. *Am J Hypertens* 6:349, 1993.
138. Kleinert HD, Stein HH, Boyd S, et al: Discovery of a well-absorbed, efficacious renin inhibitor, A-74273. *Hypertension* 20:768, 1992.
139. Lynd K, Peach M: Molecular biology of angiotensinogen. *Hypertension* 17:263, 1991.
140. Campbell DJ, Habener JF: Angiotensin gene is expressed and differentially regulated in multiple tissues of the rat. *J Clin Invest* 78:31, 1986.
141. Lee M, Paul M, Böhm M, Ganten D: Effects of angiotensin-converting enzyme inhibitors on tissue renin-angiotensin systems. *Am J Cardiol* 70:12, 1992.
142. Klett C, Bader M, Ganten D, et al: Mechanism by which angiotensin II stabilizes messenger RNA for angiotensinogen. *Hypertension* 23(Suppl I):I–120, 1994.
143. Bouhnik J, Galen FX, Clauser E, et al: The renin-angiotensin system in thyroidectomized rats. *Endocrinology* 108:647, 1981.
144. Strittmatter SM, Thiele EA, DeSouza EB, et al: Angiotensin-converting enzyme in the testis and epididymis: Differential development and pituitary regulation of isozymes. *Endocrinology* 117:1374, 1985.
145. Erdos EG, Skidgel RA: The unusual substrate specificity and the distribution of human angiotensin I converting enzyme. *Hypertension* 8(Suppl 1):1, 1986.
146. Kumar R, Thekkumkara T, and Sen G: The mRNA's encoding the two angiotensin-converting isozymes are tran-

scribed from the same gene by a tissue-specific choice of alternative transcription initiation sites. *J Biol Chem* 266:2854, 1991.
147. Skidgel RA, Erdos EG: Novel activity of human angiotensin I converting enzyme: Release of the NH2- and COOH-terminal tripeptides from the luteinizing hormone-releasing hormone. *Proc Natl Acad Sci USA* 82:1025, 1985.
148. Fantone JC, Schrier D, Weingarten B: Inhibition of vascular permeability changes in rats by captopril. *J Clin Invest* 69:1207, 1982.
149. Liberman J, Sastri A: Serum angiotensin-converting enzyme: Elevations in diabetes mellitus. *Ann Intern Med* 93:825, 1980.
150. Niarchos AP, Resnick LM, Weinstein DL, et al: Angiotensin I converting enzyme activity in hypertension: Relationship to blood pressure, renin-sodium profiles, and antihypertensive therapy. *Am J Med* 79:435, 1985.
151. Silverstein E, Schussler GC, Friedland J: Elevated serum angiotensin-converting enzyme in hyperthyroidism. *Am J Med* 75:233, 1983.
152. Schunkert H, Dzau V, Tang S, et al: Increased rat cardiac angiotensin converting enzyme activity and mRNA expression in pressure overload left ventricular hypertrophy: Effects of coronary resistance, contractility and relaxation. *J Clin Invest* 86:1913, 1990.
153. Doria A, Warram J, Krolewski A: Genetic predisposition to diabetic nephropathy: Evidence for a role of the angiotensin I-converting enzyme gene. *Diabetes* 43:690, 1994.
154. Helgeland A, Strömmen R, Hagelund CH, et al: Enalapril, atenolol and hydrochlorothiazide in mild to moderate hypertension: A comparative multicentre study in general practice in Norway. *Lancet* 1:872, 1986.
155. Cachofeiro V, Sakakibara T, Nasjletti A: Kinins, nitric oxide, and the hypotensive effect of captopril and ramiprilat in hypertension. *Hypertension* 19:138, 1992.
156. Laragh J: Issues, goals, and guidelines in selecting first-line drug therapy for hypertension. *Hypertension* 13(Suppl I):I–103, 1989.
157. Pfeifer M, Braunwald E, Moye L, et al. Effect of captopril on morbidity and mortality in patients with left ventricular dysfunction after myocardial infarction. *N Engl J Med* 327:669, 1992.
158. Lewis EJ, Hunsicker LG, Bain RP, Rodhe RD: The effect of angiotensin-converting-enzyme inhibition on diabetic nephropathy: The Collaborative Study Group. *N Engl J Med* 329:1456, 1993.
159. Hollenberg N: Renal perfusion and function: The implication of converting enzyme inhibition. *Am J Med* 84:9, 1988.
160. Kamper AL, Strandgaard S, Leyssac PP: Effect of enalapril on the progression of chronic renal failure: A randomized controlled trial. *Am J Hypertens* 5:423, 1992.
161. Albaladejo P, Bouaziz H, Duriez M, et al: Angiotensin converting enzyme inhibition prevents the increase in aortic collagen in rats. *Hypertension* 23:74, 1994.
162. Todd PA, Heel RC: Enalapril: A review of its pharmacodynamic and pharmacokinetic properties, and therapeutic use in hypertension and congestive heart failure. *Drugs* 3:198, 1986.
163. Stansby G, Hamilton G: Atherosclerotic renal artery stenosis. *Br J Hosp Med* 49:388, 1993.
164. Hollenberg NK: Medical therapy for renovascular hypertension: A review. *Am J Hypertens* 1:338, 1988.
165. Mersey JH, Williams HG, Hollenberg NK, et al: Relationship between aldosterone and bradykinin. *Circ Res* 40(Suppl 1):84, 1977.
166. Williams GH, Hollenberg NK: Accentuated vascular and endocrine response to SQ 20881 in hypertension. *N Engl J Med* 297:184, 1977.
166a. Sambhi M: Long-term safety and protective benefits of angiotensin-converting enzyme inhibitors for hypertension: Do we need more clinical trials? *West J Med* 158:286, 1993.
167. Johnston CJ, Miller JA, McGrath BP, et al: Long-term effects of captopril (SQ 14225) on blood pressure and hormone levels in essential hypertension. *Lancet* 2:493, 1979.
168. Campbell D, Kladis A, Duncan AM: Effects of converting enzyme inhibitors on angiotensin and bradykinin peptides. *Hypertension*23:439, 1994.
169. Oparil S: Angiotensin I converting enzyme inhibitors and analogues of angiotensin II, in Genest J, Kuchel O, Hamet P, Cantin M (eds): *Hypertension*. New York, McGraw-Hill, 1983, p 250.
170. Admiraal PJ, Danser AH, Jong MS, et al: Regional angiotensin II production in essential hypertension and renal artery stenosis. *Hypertension* 21:173, 1993.
171. Goodfriend TL: Angiotensin receptors and specific functions of angiotensins I, II and III, in Genest J, Kuchel O, Hamet P, Cantin M (eds): *Hypertension*. New York, McGraw-Hill, 1983, p 271.
172. Levens NR, Freedlender AE, Peace NJ, et al: Control of renal function by intrarenal angiotensin II. *Endocrinology* 112:43, 1983.
173. Matsukawa T, Mano T, Gotoh E, et al: Elevated sympathetic nerve activity in patients with accelerated essential hypertension. *J Clin Invest* 92:25, 1993.
174. Carmines P, Inscho E: Renal arteriolar angiotensin responses during varied adenosine receptor activation. *Hypertension* 23(Suppl 1):I–114, 1994.
175. Carmines P, Flemming J: Control of the renal microvasculature by vasoactive peptides. *FASEB J* 4:3300, 1990.
176. Cogan M: Angiotensin II: A powerful controller of sodium transport in the early proximal tubule. *Hypertension* 15:451, 1990.
177. Crysant SG, Dunn M, Marples D, et al: Severe reversible azotemia from captopril therapy: Report of three cases and review of the literature. *Arch Intern Med* 143:437, 1983.
178. Hollenberg NK, Williams GH: Sodium-sensitive hypertension: Implications of pathogenesis for therapy. *Am J Hypertens* 2:809, 1989.
179. Saaveda J: Brain and pituitary angiotensin. *Endocr Rev* 13:329, 1992.
180. Anderson P, Do Y, Hsueh W: Angiotensin II causes mesangial cell hypertrophy. *Hypertension* 21:29, 1993.
181. Gelsterfer A, Peach M, Owens G: Angiotensin II induces hypertrophy, not hyperplasia, of cultured rat aortic smooth muscle cells. *Circ Res* 62:749, 1988.
182. Schorb W, Booz G, Dostal D, et al: Angiotensin II is mitogenic in neonatal rat cardiac fibroblasts. *Circ Res* 72:1245, 1993.
183. Iwami K, Do Y, Hsueh W: Intracardiac distribution of angiotensin II, AT1 receptors (abstract). Council for High Blood Pressure Research. San Francisco, 1993, American Heart Association.
184. Gibbons G, Pratt R, Dzau V: Vascular smooth muscle cell hypertrophy vs. hyperplasia: Autocrine transforming growth factor-13 expression determines growth response to angiotensin II. *J Clin Invest* 90:456, 1992.
185. Naftilan A, Pran R, Dzau V: Induction of platelet-derived growth factor A-chain and c-mycogene expressions by angiotensin II in cultured rat vascular smooth muscle cells. *J Clin Invest* 83:1419, 1989.
186. Stouffer G, Owens G: Angiotensin II-induced mitogenesis of spontaneously hypertensive rat-derived cultured smooth muscle cells is dependent on autocrine production of transforming growth factor-13. *Circ Res* 70:820, 1992.
187. Ray P, Aguilera G, Kipp J, et al: Angiotensin II receptor-mediated proliferation of cultured human fetal mesangial cells. *Kidney Int* 40:764, 1991.
188. Kim N, Villareal F, Dillman W, et al: Distribution of angiotensin II receptors on rat cardiac fibroblasts and myocytes (abstract). Inter-American Society of Hypertension, La Jolla, CA, 1993.
189. Block CH, Santos RAS, Brosnihan KB, Ferrario CM: Immunocytochemical localization of angiotensin-(1–7) in the rat forebrain. *Peptides* 9:1395, 1988.

190. Campagnole-Santos ML, Diz DI, Santos RAS, Khosla MC, Brosnihan KB, Ferrario CM: Cardiovascular effects of angiotensin-(1–7) injected in the dorsal medulla of rats. *Am J Physiol* 257:H324, 1989.
191. Kohara K, Brosnihan KB, Chappell MC, Khosla MC, Ferrario CM: Angiotensin-(1–7): A member of circulating angiotensin peptides. *Hypertension* 17:131, 1991.
192. Lawrence AC, Evin G, Kladis A, Campbell DJ: An alternative strategy for the radioimmunoassay of angiotensin peptides using amino-termination-directed antisera: Measurement of eight angiotensin peptides in human plasma. *Hypertension* 8:715, 1990.
193. Welches W, Santos R, Chappell M, et al: Evidence that prolyl endopeptidase participates in the processing of brain angiotensin. *J Hypertens* 9:631, 1991.
194. Chiu A, Herblin W, McCall D, et al: Identification of angiotensin II receptor subtypes. *Biochem Biophys Res Commun* 265:196, 1989.
195. Murphy T, Alexander R, Griendling K, et al: Isolation of a cDNA encoding the vascular type-1 angiotensin II receptor. *Nature* 351:233, 1991.
196. Sasaki K, Yamamono Y, Bardham S, et al: Cloning and expression of a complementary DNA encoding a bovine adrenal angiotensin II type-1 receptor. *Nature* 351:230, 1991.
197. Bernstein K, Alexander R: Counterpoint: Molecular analysis of the angiotensin II receptor. *Endocr Rev* 13:381, 1992.
198. Grady E, Sechl L, Griffin C, et al: Expression of AT2 receptors in the developing rat fetus. *J Clin Invest* 88:921, 1991.
199. Sechi L, Griffin C, Grady E, et al: Characterization of angiotensin II receptor subtypes in rat heart. *Circ Res* 71:1482, 1992.
200. Millan M, Jacobowitz D, Aguilera G, et al: Differential distribution of AT1, and AT2 angiotensin II receptor subtypes in the rat brain during development. *Proc Natl Acad Sci USA* 88:11440, 1991.
201. Kambayashi Y, Bardham S, Takahashi K, et al: Molecular cloning of a noval angiotensin II receptor, type 1. *J Biol Chem* 268:24543, 1993.
202. Mukoyama M, Nakajuma M, Horiuchi M, et al: Expression cloning of type 2 angiotensin II receptor reveals a unique class of seven-transmembrane receptors. *J Biol Chem* 268:24539, 1993.
203. Ambroz C, Catt K: Angiotensin II receptor-mediated calcium influx in bovine adrenal glomerulosa cells. *Endocrinology* 131:408, 1992.
204. Barrett P, Bollag W, Isales C, et al: Role of calcium in angiotensin II-mediated aldosterone secretion. *Endocr Rev* 10:496, 1989.
205. Diz DI, Bear PG, Nasjletti A: Angiotensin II-induced hypertension in the rat: Effects on the plasma concentration, renal excretion, and tissue release of prostaglandins. *J Clin Invest* 72:466,1983.
206. Catt KJ, Harwood JP, Aquilera G, et al: Hormonal regulation of peptide receptors and target cell responses. *Nature* 280:109, 1979.
207. Lehoux JG, Bird I, Rainey W, et al: Both low sodium and high potassium intake increase the level of adrenal angiotensin-II receptor type 1, but not that of adrenocorticotropin receptor. *Endocrinology* 134:776, 1994.
208. Weber MA: Clinical experience with the angiotensin II receptor antagonist losartan: A preliminary report. *Am J Hypertens* 5:247, 1992.
209. Brunner HR, Christen Y, Munafo A, et al: Clinical experience with antiotensin II receptor antagonists. *Am J Hypertens* 5:243, 1992.
210. Hsueh WA, Do YS, Shinagawa T, et al: Biochemical similarity of expressed human prorenin and native inactive renin. *Hypertension* 8(Suppl II):78, 1986.
211. Fukamizu A, Sugimura K, Takimoto E, et al: Chimeric renin-angiotensin system demonstrates sustained increase in blood pressure of transgenic mice carrying both human renin and human angiotensinogen genes. *J Biol Chem* 268:11617, 1993.
212. Mullins J, Peters J, Ganten D: Fulminant hypertension in transgenic rats harbouring the mouse Ren-2 gene. *Nature* 344:541, 1990.
213. Mullins JJ, Mullins LJ: Transgenes, hypotheses, and hypertension. *Hypertension* 23:428, 1994.
214. Inagami T, Murakami T, Higuchi K, et al: Roles of renal and vascular renin in spontaneous hypertension and switching of the mechanism upon nephrectomy. *Am J Hypertens* 4:15, 1991.
215. Dzau VJ, Re R: Tissue angiotensin system in cardiovascular medicine: A paradigm shift? *Circulation* 89:493, 1994.
216. Von Lutteroi N, Catanzaro DF, Sealey JE, et al: Renin is not synthesized by cardiac and extrarenal tissues: A review of experimental evidence. *Circulation* 89:458, 1994.
217. Haber E, Sancho J, Re R, et al: The role of the renin-angiotensin-aldosterone system in the cardiovascular homeostasis in normal man. *Clin Sci Mol Med* 48(Suppl 2):49, 1975
218. Noth RH, Tan SY, Mulrow PJ: Effects of angiotensin II blockade by saralasin in normal man. *J Clin Endocrinol Metab* 45:10, 1977
219. Gavras H, Ribeiro AB, Gavras I, et al: Reciprocal relation between renin dependency and sodium dependency in essential hypertension. *N Engl J Med* 295:1278, 1976
220. Miller EDJ, Samuels AI, Haber E, et al: Inhibition of angiotensin conversion and prevention of renal hypertension. *Am J Physiol* 228:448, 1975.
221. Carretero OA, Romero JC: Production and characteristics of experimental hypertension in animals, in Genest J, Koiw E, Kuchel O (eds): *Hypertension: Physiopathology and Treatment.* New York, McGraw-Hill, 1977, p 485.
222. Waeber B, Gavras I, Brunner HR, et al: Safety and efficacy of chronic therapy with captopril in hypertensive patients: An update. *J Clin Pharmacol* 21:508, 1981.
223. Akahoshi M, Carretero O: Body fluid volume and angiotensin II in maintenance of one-kidney, one clip hypertension. *Hypertension* 14:269,1989.
224. Schambelan M, Howes ELJ, Stockigt JR, et al: Role of renin and aldosterone in hypertension due to a renin-secreting tumor. *Am J Med* 55:86, 1973.
225. Anderson P, Macaulay L, Do Y, et al: Insights into hypertension and ovarian renin production. *Medicine (Baltimore)* 68:257, 1990.
226. London G, Safr M: Renal hemodynamics in patients with sustained essential hypertension and in patients with unilateral stenosis of the renal artery. *Am J Hypertens* 2:244, 1989.
227. Brown JJ, Davies DL, Lever AF, et al: Variations in plasma renin concentration in several physiological and pathological states. *Can Med Assoc J* 90:201, 1964.
228. McAllister RGJ, Van Way CWI, Dayani K, et al: Malignant hypertension: Effect of therapy on renin and aldosterone. *Circ Res* 8(Suppl 2):160, 1971.
229. Harrap S, Davidson H, Connor J, et al: The angiotensin I converting enzyme gene and predisposition to high blood pressure. *Hypertension* 21:455, 1993.
230. Soubrier F, Jeunemaitre X, Rigat B, et al: Similar frequencies of renin gene restriction fragment length polymorphisms in hypertensive and normotensive subjects. *Hypertension* 16:712, 1990.
231. Cambien F, Poirier O, Lacerf L, et al: Deletion polymorphism in the gene for angiotensin-converting enzyme is a potent risk factor for myocardial infarction. *Nature* 359:641, 1992.
232. Materson B, Domenic J, Reda M, et al: Single drug therapy for hypertension in men. *N Engl J Med* 328:914, 1993.
233. Esler MD: Catecholamines and essential hypertension. *Baillieres Clinic Endrocrinol Metab* 7:415, 1993.
234. Luparini R, Ferri C, Santucci A, et al: Atrial natriuretic peptide in non-modulating essential hypertension. *Hypertension* 21:803, 1993.

235. Williams G, Dluhy R, Lifton R, et al: Non-modulation as an intermediate phenotype in essential hypertension. *Hypertension* 20:788, 1992.
236. Grant F, Mandel S, Brown E, et al: Interrelationship between the renin-angiotensin-aldosterone and calcium homeostatic systems. *J Clin Endocrinol Metab* 75:988, 1992.
237. Williams G, Moore T, Hollenberg K: Dysregulation of aldosterone secretion and its relationship to the pathogenesis of essential hypertension. *Endocrinol Metab Clin North Am* 20:423, 1991.
238. Williams G, Hollenberg N: Functional derangements in the regulation of aldosterone secretion in hypertension. *Hypertension* 5(Suppl III):143, 1991.
239. Conlin PR, Braley LM, Menachery AI, et al: Abnormal norepinephrine and aldosterone responses to upright posture in nonmodulating hypertension. *J Clin Endocrinol Metab* 75:1017, 1992.
240. Williams G, Hollenberg N: Non-modulating hypertension: A subset of sodium-sensitive hypertension. *Hypertension* 17:I–81, 1991.
241. Redgrave J, Rabinowe S, Hollenberg NK, et al: Correction of abnormal renal blood flow response to angiotensin II by converting enzyme inhibition in essential hypertensives. *J Clin Invest* 75:1285, 1985.
242. Drury P: Disorders of mineralocorticoid activity. *J Clin Endocrinol Metab* 14:175, 1985.
243. Kotchen TA, Guthrie GPJ, Cottrill CM, et al: Low renin-aldosterone in "prehypertensive" young adults. *J Clin Endocrinol Metab* 54:808, 1982.
244. Muntzel M, Drueke T: A comprehensive review of the salt and blood pressure relationships. *Am J Hypertens* 5:1, 1992.
245. Hatton D, McCarron D: Dietary calcium and blood pressure in experimental models of hypertension: A review. *Hypertension* 23:513, 1994.
246. Resnick L, Barbagallo M, Gupta R, et al: Ionic basis of hypertension in diabetes mellitus. *Am J Hypertens* 6:413, 1993.
247. Resnick L: Ionic basis of hypertension, insulin resistance, vascular disease, and related disorder. *Am J Hypertens* 6:123, 1993.
248. Ridker P, Gaboury C, Conlin P, et al: Stimulation of plasminogen activator inhibitor in vivo by infusion of angiotensin II: Evidence of a potential interaction between the renin-angiotensin system and fibrinolytic function. *Circulation* 87:1969, 1993.
249. Alderman M, Madhavan S, Ooi W, et al: Association of the renin-sodium profile with the risk of myocardial infarction in patients with hypertension. *N Engl J Med* 324:1098, 1991.
250. Meade T, Cooper J, Peart W: Plasma renin activity and ischemic heart disease. *N Engl J Med* 329:616, 1993.
251. Conn JW: Presidential address: Primary aldosteronism: A new clinical syndrome. *J Lab Clin Med* 45:3, 1955.
252. Eberlein WB, Bongiovanni AM: Plasma and urinary corticosteroids in the hypertensive form of congenital adrenal hyperplasia. *J Biol Chem* 223:85, 1956.
253. Biglieri EG, Herron MA, Brust N: 17α-Hydroxylation deficiency in man. *J Clin Invest* 45:1946, 1966.
254. Ulick S: Evidence for defective functional zonation of adrenal hyperplasia syndromes in man, in Mantero F, Biglieri E, Funder J, Scoggins B (eds): *The Adrenal Gland and Hypertension*. New York, Raven Press, 1985, p 357.
255. Monder C: Corticosteroids, kidneys, sweet roots and dirty drugs. *Mol Cell Endocrinol* 78:C95, 1991.
256. Stewart P and Edwards C: The cortisol-cortisone shuttle and hypertension. *J Steroid Biochem Mol Biol* 40:501, 1991.
257. Monder C, and White P: 11β-Hydroxysteroid dehydrogenase. *Vitam Horm* 47:187, 1993.
258. Lamberts S, Koper J, Biemond P, et al: Cortisol receptor resistance: The variability of its clinical presentation and response to treatment. *J Clin Endocrinol Metab* 74:313, 1992.
259. Lamberts S, Koper J, Biemond P, et al: Familial and iatrogenic cortisol receptor resistance. *Cancer Res* (Suppl): 49:2217, 1989.
260. Malchoff CD, Javier EC, Malchoff DM, et al: Primary cortisol resistance presenting as sexual precocity. *J Clin Endocrinol Metab* 70:503, 1990.
261. Edwards C: Lessons from licorice. *N Engl J Med* 325:1242, 1991.
262. Farese RJ, Biglieri E, Schakleton C, et al: Licorice-induced hypertension. *N Engl J Med* 325:1223, 1991.
263. Speiser P, Riddick L, Martin K, et al: Investigation of the mechanism of hypertension in apparent mineralocorticoid excess. *Metab Clin Exp* 42:843, 1993.
264. Shackelton C, Rodriguez J, Arteaga G, et al: Congenital 11β-hydroxysteroid dehydrogenase deficiency associated with juvenile hypertension: Corticosteroid metabolite profiles of four patients and their families. *Clin Endocrinol (Oxf)* 22:701, 1985.
265. Whitworth J, Brown M: Hypertension and the kidney. *Kidney Int* 44(Suppl 42):S52, 1993.
266. Edwards C, Benediktsson R, Lindsay R, et al: Hypothesis: Dysfunction of placental glucocorticoid barrier: Link between fetal environment and adult hypertension? *Lancet* 341:355, 1993.
267. Griffing GT, Melby JC: Adrenocortical factors in hypertension. *J Clin Pharmacol* 25:218, 1985.
268. Krakoff L, Nicolis G, Amsel B: Pathogenesis of hypertension in Cushing's syndrome. *Am J Med* 58:216, 1975.
269. Cassar J, Loizou S, Kely WF, et al: Deoxycorticosterone and aldosterone excretion in Cushing's syndrome. *Metabolism* 29:115, 1980.
270. Hogan MJ, Schambelan M, Biglieri EG: Concurrent hypercortisolism and hypermineralocorticoidism. *Am J Med* 62:777, 1977.
271. Azar S, Melby J: 19-Nor-deoxycorticosterone production from aldosterone-producing adenomas. *Hypertension* 19: 362, 1992.
272. Baxter JD, Schambelan M, Matulich D, et al: Aldosterone receptors and the evaluation of plasma mineralocorticoid activity in normal and hypertensive states. *J Clin Invest* 58:579, 1976.
273. Takeda Y, Iki K, Takeda R: Formation of 18-deoxy-19-noraldosterone by a human aldosterone-producing adenoma. *Steroids* 58:282, 1993.
274. Gorsline J, Harnik M, Tresco PA, et al: Hypertensinogenic activities of ring A-reduced metabolites of aldosterone. *Hypertension* 8(Suppl 1):187, 1986.
275. Pelletier M, Ludens JH, Fanestil DD: The role of aldosterone in active sodium transport. *Arch Intern Med* 129:248, 1972.
276. Mion DJ, Rea R, Anderson E, et al: Effects of fludrocortisone on sympathetic nerve activity in humans. *Hypertension* 23:123, 1994.
277. Biglieri EG, Forsham PH: Studies on expanded extracellular fluid and responses to various stimuli in primary aldosteronism. *Am J Med* 30:564, 1961.
278. Weinberger MH, Grim CE, Hollifield JW, et al: Primary aldosteronism: Diagnosis, localization, and treatment. *Ann Intern Med* 90:386, 1979.
279. Slaton PE, Biglieri EG: Hypertension and hyperaldosteronism renal artery stenosis: Serial observations on 54 patients treated medically. *Clin Pharmacol Ther* 6:700, 1965.
280. Bravo EL, Dustan HP, Tarazi RC: Spironolactone as a nonspecific treatment for primary aldosteronism. *Circulation* 48:491, 1973.
281. Tarazi RC, Ibrahim MM, Bravo EL, et al: Hemodynamic characteristics of primary aldosteronism. *N Engl J Med* 289:1330, 1973.
282. Went GJ, MarintVeld AJ, Verhoeven RP, et al: Volume-pressure relationships during development of mineralocorticoid hypertension in man. *Circ Res* 40(Suppl 1):163, 1977.
283. Oh-hashi S, Takata M, Ueno H, et al: Cytosolic free calcium

concentration in platelets in patients with renovascular hypertension and primary aldosteronism. *J Human Hypertens* 6:71, 1992.

284. Tannen RL: Potassium handling by the kidney, in Tannen RL, Massry S, Glassock RJ (eds): *Textbook of Nephrology*. Baltimore, Williams & Wilkins, 1983, p 3.
285. Miyajima E, Yamada Y, Yoshida Y, et al: Muscle sympathetic nerve activity in renovascular hypertension and primary aldosteronism. *Hypertension* 17:1057, 1991.
286. Wang W, McClain J, Zucker I: Aldosterone reduces baroreceptor discharge in the dog. *Hypertension* 19:270, 1992.
287. Torres, Young WJ, Offord KP, et al: Association of hypokalemia, aldosteronism, and renal cysts. *N Engl J Med* 322:345, 1990.
288. Gomez-Sanchez E: Intracerebroventricular infusion of aldosterone induces hypertension in rats. *Endocrinology* 118:819, 1986.
289. Smith J, Wade M, Fineberg N, et al: Sodium transport parameters in erythrocytes of patients with primary aldosteronism. *Hypertension* 11:141, 1988.
290. Funder JW, Adam WR, Mantero F, et al: The etiology of a syndrome of factitious mineralocorticoid excess: A steroid-containing nasal spray. *J Clin Endocrinol Metab* 49:842, 1979.
291. August JT, Nelson DH, Thorn GW: Response of normal subjects to large amounts of aldosterone. *J Clin Invest* 37:1549, 1958.
292. Schalekamp M, Wenting G, Man A: Pathogenesis of mineralocorticoid hypertension. *Clin Endocrinol Metab* 10:397, 1981.
293. Whitworth J, Saines D, Thatcher R: Differential blood pressure and metabolic effects of 9α-fluorocortisol in man. *Clin Exp Pharmacol Physiol* 10:351, 1983.
294. Idewhi M, Kishikawa K, Kinoshita A, et al: High-renin malignant hypertension secondary to an aldosterone-producing adenoma. *Nephron* 54:259, 1990.
295. Taddi S, Virdis A, Mattei P, et al: Vasodilation to acetylcholine in primary and secondary forms of human hypertension. *Hypertension* 21:929, 1993.
296. O'Neil RG, Helman SI: Transport characteristics of renal collecting tubules: Influences of DOCA and diet. *Am J Physiol* 233:F544, 1977.
297. Trinder D, Phillips P, Rievanis J, et al: Regulation of vasopressin receptors in deoxycorticosterone acetate-salt hypertension. *Hypertension* 20:569, 1992.
298. Nakata T, Takeda K, Itho H, et al: Paraventricular nucleus lesions attenuate the development of hypertension in DOCA/salt-treated rats. *Am J Hypertens* 2:625, 1989.
299. Lavriviere R, Day R, Schiffrin E: Increased expression of endothelin-1 gene in blood vessels of deoxycorticosterone acetate-salt hypertensive rats. *Hypertension* 21:916, 1993.
300. Brills C, Matsubara L, Wever K: Anti-aldosterone treatment and the prevention of myocardial fibrosis in primary and secondary hyperaldosteronism. *J Mol Cell Cardiol* 25:563, 1993.
301. Campbell S, Janicki J, Matsubara B, et al: Myocardial fibrosis in the rat with mineralocorticoid excess: Prevention of scarring by amiloride. *Am J Hypertens* 6:487, 1993.
302. Gordon R, Klemm D, Tunny T, et al: Primary aldosteronism with a genetic basis. *Lancet* 340:159, 1992.
303. McKenna T, Sequeira S, Hefferman A, et al: Diagnosis under random conditions of all disorders of the renin-angiotensin-aldosterone axis, including primary aldosteronism. *J Clin Endocrinol Metab* 73:952, 1991.
304. Conn J, Tovner D, Nesbit R: Normokalemic primary aldosteronism: A detectable cause of curable "essential hypertension." *JAMA* 193:200, 1965.
305. Xavier J, Chatellier G, Kreft-Jais C, et al: Efficacy and tolerance of spironolactone in essential hypertension. *Am J Cardiol* 60:820, 1987.
306. Plouin P-F, Battaglia C, Athene-Gelas F, et al: Are angiotensin converting enzyme inhibition and aldosterone antagonism equivalent in hypertensive patients over fifty. *Am J Hypertens* 4:356, 1991.
307. Semplicini A, Buzzaccarini F, Ceoletto G, et al: Effects of canrenoate on red cell sodium transport and calf flow in essential hypertension. *Am J Hypertens* 6:295,1993.
308. Gomez-Sanchez CE: Cushing's syndrome and hypertension. *Hypertension* 8:258, 1986.
309. Mantero F, Armanini D, Boscaro M: Plasma renin activity and urinary aldosterone in Cushing's syndrome. *Horm Metab Res* 10:65, 1978.
310. Cristy NP: Cushing's syndrome: The natural disease, in Christy NP (ed): *The Human Adrenal Cortex*. New York, Harper & Row, 1971, p 359.
311. Mantero F, Boscardo M: Glucocorticoid-dependent hypertension. *J Steroid Biochem Mol Biol* 43:409, 1992.
312. Whitworth J, Gordon D, Andrew J, et al: The hypertensive effect of synthetic glucocorticoids in man: Role of sodium and volume. *J Hypertens* 7:537, 1989.
313. Siegel RR, Luke RG, Hellebusch AA: Reduction of toxicity of corticosteroid therapy after renal transplantation. *Am J Med* 53:159, 1972.
314. Reed WP, Lucas ZJ, Cohn R: Alternate day prednisone therapy after renal transplantation. *Lancet* 1:747, 1970.
315. Soyka L: Treatment of the nephrotic syndrome in childhood. *Am J Dis Child* 113:693, 1967.
316. Thomas TPL: The complications of systemic corticosteroid therapy in the elderly. *Gerontology* 30:60, 1984.
317. Whitworth J: Adrenocorticotropin and steroid-induced hypertension in humans. *Kidney Int* 41 (Suppl 37):S34, 1992.
318. Grunfeld J, Eloy L, Moura A, et al: Effects of antiglucocorticoids on glucocorticoid hypertension in the rat. *Hypertension* 7:292, 1985.
319. Marson O, Ribeiro A, Tufik S, et al: Role of the anteroventral third ventricle region and the renin angiotensin system in methylprednisolone hypertension. *Hypertension* 3(Suppl II):II–142, 1981.
320. Yagil Y, Levin M, Krakogg L: Effect of glucocorticoid deficiency on arterial pressure in conscious spontaneously hypertensive rats. *Am J Hypertens* 2:99, 1989.
321. Sato A, Suzuki H, Murakami M, et al: Glucocorticoid increases angiotensin II type 1 receptor and its gene expression. *Hypertension* 23:25, 1994.
322. Kennedy B, Elayan H, Ziegler M: Glucocorticoid hypertension and nonadrenal phenylethanolmine N-methyltransferase. *Hypertension* 21:415, 1993.
323. Pirpiris M, Yeung S, Dewar E, et al: Hydrocortisone-induced hypertension in man: The role of cardiac output. *Am J Hypertens* 6:287, 1993.
324. Montrella-Waybill M, Clore J, Schoolwerth A, et al: Evidence that high dose cortisol-induced Na^+ retention in man is not mediated by the mineralocorticoid receptor. *J Clin Endocrinol Metab* 72:1060, 1991
325. Kornel L, Manisundaram B, Nelson W: Glucocorticoids regulate Na^+ transport in vascular smooth muscle through the glucocorticoid receptor-mediated mechanism. *Am J Hypertens* 6:736, 1993.
326. Saruta T, Suzuki H, Handa M, et al: Multiple factors contribute to the pathogenesis of hypertension in Cushing's syndrome. *J Clin Endocrinol Metab* 62:275,1986.
327. Watt G, Harrap S, Foy C, et al: Abnormalities of glucocorticoid metabolism and the renin-angiotensin system: A four-corners approach to the identification of genetic determinants of blood pressure. *J Hypertens* 10:473, 1992.
328. Liu M, Wong KS, Martin A, et al: Adrenocorticotropin-induced hypertension in rats: Role of progesterone and digoxin-like substances. *Am J Hypertens* 7:59, 1994.
329. Ely D, Salisbury R, Hadi D, et al: Androgen receptor and the testes influence hypertension in a hybrid rat model. *Hypertension* 17:1104, 1991.
330. Sondheimer S: Update on the metabolic effects of steroidal contraceptives. *Endocrinol Metab Clin North Am* 20:911, 1991.

331. Radwanska E: The role of reproductive hormones in vascular disease and hypertension. *Steroids* 58:605, 1993.
332. Moncada S, and Higgs A: The L-arginine-nitric oxide pathway. *N Engl J Med* 329:2002, 1993.
333. Moncada S: The L-arginine-nitric oxide pathway. *Acta Physiol Scand* 145:201, 1992.
334. Polikar R, Burger AG, Scherrer U, et al: The thryoid and the heart. *Circulation* 87:1435, 1993.
335. Streeten D, Anderson G, Howland T, et al: Effects of thyroid function on blood pressure: Recognition of hypothyroid hypertension. *Hypertension* 11:78, 1988.
336. Klein I: Thyroid hormone and blood pressure regulation, in Laragh J, Brenner B (eds): *Hypertension: Pathophysiology, diagnosis, and management.* New York, Raven Press, 1990, p 1661.
337. Bing R, Briggs R, Burden A, et al: Reversible hypertension and hypothyroidism. *Clin Endocrinal (Oxf)* 13:339, 1980.
338. De Paula R, Plavnik F, Rodrigues C, et al: Contribution of vasopressin to orthostatic blood pressure maintenance in essential hypertension. *Am J Hypertens* 6:794, 1993.
339. Laszlo F, Laszlo F, De Wood D: Pharmacology and clinical perspectives of vasopressin antagonists. *Pharmacol Rev* 4:73, 1991.
340. Brier M, Bunke C, Lathon P, et al: Erythropoietin-induced antinatriuresis mediated by angiotensin II in perfused kidneys. *J Am Soc Nephrol* 3:1583, 1993.
341. Naomi S, Umeda T, Iwaoka T, et al: Endogenous erythropoietin and salt sensitivity of blood pressure in patients with essential hypertension. *Am J Hypertens* 6:15, 1993.
342. Cuneo R, Salomon F, Wilmshurst P, et al: Cardiovascular effects of growth hormone treatment in growth-hormone-deficient adults: Stimulation of the renin-aldosterone system.*Clin Sci* 81:587, 1991.
343. Barton J, Hindmarshi P, Preece M, et al: Blood pressure and the renin-angiotensin-aldosterone system in children receiving recombinant growth hormone. *J Clin Endocrinol* 38:245, 1993.
344. Masuda A, Kazuaki S, Mori Y, et al: Plasma calcitonin gene-related peptide levels in patients with various hypertensive diseases. *J Hyperten* 10:1499, 1992.
345. Wimalawansa S: Antihypertensive effects of oral calcium supplementation may be mediated through the potent vasodilator CGRP. *Am J Hypertens* 6:996, 1993.
346. Benishin C, Labedz T, Guo D, et al: Identification and purification of parathyroid hypertensive factor from organ culture of parathyroid glands from spontaneously hypertensive rats. *Am J Hypertens* 6:134, 1993.
347. Pirola C, Wang H, Kamyar A, et al: Angiotension II regulates parathyroid hormone-related protein expression in cultured rat aortic smooth muscle cells through transcriptional and post-transcriptional mechanisms. *J Biol Chem* 268: 1987, 1993.
348. Grant FD, Mandel SJ, Brown EM, et al: Interrelationships between the renin-angiotensin-aldosterone and calcium homeostatic systems. *J Clin Endocrinol Metab* 75:988, 1992.
349. Campese V: Calcium, parathyroid hormone and blood pressure. *Am J Hypertens* 2:34, 1989.
350. Lind L, Wengle B, Wide L, et al: Hypertension in primary hyperparathyroidism—reduction of blood pressure by long-term treatment with vitamin D (Alphacalcidol): A double-blind placebo-controlled study. *Am J Hypertens* 1:397, 1988.
351. Bukoski R, Xue H: On the vascular inotropic action of 1,25-(OH)2 vitamin D3. *Am J Hypertens* 6:388, 1993.
352. Sowers J, Zemel M, Zemel P, et al: Calcium metabolism and dietary calcium in salt sensitive hypertension. *Am J Hypertens* 4:557, 1991.
353. Lewanczuk R, Pang P: Parathyroid hypertensive factor is present in DOCA-salt but not two-kidney-one-clip hypertensive rats. *Am J Hypertens* 4:802, 1991.
354. Lüscher T, Sco B, Bühler F: Potential role of endothelin in hypertension: Controversy on endothelin in hypertension. *Hypertension* 21:752, 1993.
355. Vanhoutte P: Is endothelin involved in the pathogenesis of hypertension. *Hypertension* 21:747, 1993.
356. Yokokawa K, Tahara H, Kohno M, et al. Hypertension associated with endothelin-secreting malignant hemangioendothelinoma. *Ann Intern Med* 114:213, 1991.
357. Kourembanas S, McQuillan L, Leung G, et al. Nitric oxide regulates the expression of vasoconstrictors and growth factors by vascular endothelium under both normoxia and hypoxia. *J Clin Invest* 92:99, 1993.
358. Calver A, Collier J, Moncada S, et al: Effect of local intra-arterial N^G-monomethyl-L-arginine in patients with hypertension: The nitric oxide dilator mechanism appears abnormal. *J Hypertension* 10:1025, 1992.
359. Salazar F, Alberola A, Pinila J, et al: Salt-induced increase in arterial pressure during nitric oxide synthesis inhibition. *Hypertension* 22:49, 1993.
360. Baylis C, Mitruka B, Deng A: Chronic blockade of nitric oxide synthesis in the rat produces systemic hypertension and glomerular damage. *J Clin Invest* 90:278, 1992.
361. Arnal J-F, Armrani A-I, Chatellier G, et al: Cardiac weight in hypertension induced by nitric oxide synthetase blockade. *Hypertension* 22:380,1993.
362. Ikenaga H, Suzuki H, Ishii N, et al: Role of NO on pressure-natriuresis in Wistar-Kyoto and spontaneously hypertensive rats. *Kidney Int* 43:205, 1993.
363. Jover B, Herizi A, Ventre F, et al: Sodium and angiotensin in hypertension induced by long-term nitric oxide blockade. *Hypertension* 21:944, 1993.
364. Panza J, Quyyuma A, Brush JJ, et al: Abnormal endothelium-dependent vascular relaxation in patients with essential hypertension. *N Engl J Med* 323:22, 1990.
365. Petros A, Hewletyt A, Bogle R, et al: L-arginine-induced hypotension. *Lancet* 337:1044, 1991.
366. Kirchner K, Scanlon PJ, Dzielak D, et al: Endothelium derived relaxing factor responses in DOCA-salt hypertensive rats. *Am J Physiol* 265:R568, 1993.
367. Panza J, Casino P, Badar D, et al: Effect of increased availability of endothelium-derived nitric oxide precursor on endothelium-dependent vascular relaxation in normal subjects and in patients with essential hypertension. *Circulation* 87:1475, 1993.
368. Panza J, Quyyumi A, Callahan T, et al: Effect of antihypertensive treatment on endothelium-dependent vascular relaxation in patients with essential hypertension. *J Am Coll Cardiol* 12:1145, 1993.
369. Taddei S, Virdis A, Mattei P, et al: Vasodilation to acetylcholine in primary and secondary forms of human hypertension. *Hypertension* 21:929, 1993.
370. Cockcroft J, Chowienczyk P, Benjamin N, et al: Preserved endothelium-dependent vasodilatation in patients with essential hypertension. *N Engl J Med* 330:1036, 1994.
371. Nakashima M, Mombouli J-V, Taylor A, et al: Endothelium-dependent hyperpolarization caused by bradykinin in human coronary arteries. *J Clin Invest* 92:2867, 1993.
372. Schwartz D, Geller DM, Manning PT, et al: Ser-Leu-Arg-Arg-atriopeptin III: The major circulating form of atrial peptide. *Science* 229:397, 1985.
373. Greenberg BD, Bencen GH, Seilhamer JJ, et al: Nucleotide sequence of the gene encoding human atrial natriuretic factor precursor. *Nature* 312:656, 1984.
374. De Bold AJ: Atrial natriuretic factor: A hormone produced by the heart. *Science* 230:767, 1985.
375. Cantin M, Genest J: The heart as an endocrine gland. *Sci Am* 254:76, 1986.
376. Needleman P, Greenwald JE: Atriopeptin: A cardiac hormone intimately involved in fluid, electrolyte, and blood-pressure homeostasis. *N Engl J Med* 314:828, 1986.
377. Ballermann BJ, Brenner BM: Biologically active atrial peptides. *J Clin Invest* 76:2041, 1985.
378. Jamison R, Canaan-Kuhl S, Pratt R: The natriuretic peptides and their receptors. *Am J Kidney Dis* 20:519, 1992.

379. Naruse M, Takeyama Y, Tanabe A, et al: Atrial and brain natriuretic peptides in cardiovascular diseases. *Hypertension* 23:I231, 1994.
380. Wei C-M, Heublein D, Perrella M, et al: Natriuretic peptide system in human heart failure. *Circulation* 88:1004, 1993.
381. Gardner DG, Deschepper CF, Ganong WF, et al: Extraatrial expression of the gene for atrial natriuretic factor. *Proc Natl Acad Sci USA* 83:6697, 1986.
382. Chen Y-F, Elton T, Oparil S: Quantitation of hypothalamic atrial natriuretic peptide messenger RNA in hypertensive rats. *Hypertension* 19:296, 1992.
383. Hummel M, Kuhn M, Bub A, et al: Urodilatin, a new therapy to prevent kidney failure after heart transplantation. *J Heart Transplant* 12:209, 1993.
384. Kohno M, Horio T, Yokokawa K, et al: Brain natriuretic peptide as a cardiac hormone in essential hypertension. *Am J Med* 92:29, 1992.
385. Suga S-I, Nakao K, Hosoda K, et al: Receptor selectivity of natriuretic peptide family: Atrial natriuretic peptide, brain natriuretic peptide, and c-type natriuretic peptide. *Endocrinology* 130:229, 1992.
386. Richards A, Crozier I, Espiner E, et al: Plasma brain natriuretic peptide and endopeptidase 24.11 inhibition in hypertension. *Hypertension* 22:231, 1993.
387. Hoffman A, Grossman E, Keiser H: Increased plasma levels and blunted effects of brain natriuretic peptide in rats with congestive heart failure. *Am J Hypertension* 4:597, 1991.
388. Richards A, Crozier I, Holmes S, et al: Brain natriuretic peptide: Natriuretic and endocrine effects in essential hypertension. *J Hypertens* 11:163, 1993.
389. Metzler CH, Gardner DG, Keil LC, et al: Increased synthesis and release of atrial peptide during mineralocorticoid escape in conscious dogs. *Am J Physiol* 252:R188, 1987.
390. Gardner DG, Hane S, Trachewsky D, et al: Atrial natriuretic peptide mRNA is regulated by glucocorticoids in vivo. *Biochem Biophys Res Commun* 139:1047, 1986.
390a. McDonough P, Glembotski C: Induction of atrial natriuretic factor and myosin light chain-2 gene expression in cultured ventricular myocytes by electrical stimulation of contraction. *J Biol Chem* 267:11665, 1992.
391. Watkins R, Vemulapalli S, Chiu P, et al: Atrial natriuretic factor potentiating and hemodynamic effects of SCH 42495, a new, neutral metalloendopeptidase inhibitor. *Am J Hypertens* 6:357, 1993.
392. Wilkins M, Needleman P: Effect of pharmacological manipulation of endogenous atriopeptin activity on renal function. *Am J Physiol* 262:F161, 1992.
393. Yandle T, Richards A, Gilbert A, et al: Assay of brain natriuretic peptide (BNP) in human plasma: Evidence for high molecular weight BNP as a major plasma component in heart failure. *J Clin Endocrinol Metab* 76:832, 1993.
394. Predel H-G, Schulte-vels O, Glanzer K, et al: Atrial natriuretic peptide in patients with essential hypertension: Hemodynamic, renal, and hormonal responses. *Am J Hypertens* 4:871, 1991.
395. Musca A, Cammarella I, Ferri C, et al: Natriuretic hormones in young hypertensives and in young normotensives with or without a family history of hypertension. *Am J Hypertens* 5:592, 1992.
396. Atlas SA: Atrial natriuretic factor: A new hormone of cardiac origin. *Rec Prog Horm Res* 42:207, 1986.
397. Maack T, Camargo MJF, Kleinert HD, et al: Atrial natriuretic factor: Structure and functional properties. *Kidney Int* 27:607, 1985.
398. Nonoguchi H, Tomita K, Marumo F: Effects of atrial natriuretic peptide and vasopressin on chloride transport in long- and short-looped medullary thick ascending limbs. *J Clin Invest* 90:349, 1992.
399. Arendt RM, Gerbes AL, Ritter D, et al: Plasma-ANF in various disease states. Congress on Biologically Active Atrial Peptides. New York, Raven, 1986.
400. Hollister A, Inagami T: Atrial natriuretic factor and hypertension, a review and metaanalysis. *Am J Hypertens* 4:2, 1991.
401. Trachte G, Drewett J: C-type natriuretic peptide neuromodulates independently of guanylyl cyclase activation. *Hypertension* 23:38, 1993.
402. Bahr V, Sander-Bahr C, Ardevol R, et al: Effects of atrial natriuretic factor on the renin-aldosterone system: *In vivo* and *in vitro* studies. *J Steroid Biochem* 45:173, 1993.
403. Winquist RJ, Faison EP, Nutt RF: Vasodilator profile of synthetic atrial natriuretic factor. *Eur J Pharmacol* 102:168, 1984.
404. Cody RJ, Kubo SH, Atlas SA, et al: Atrial natriuretic factor in heart failure: Endogenous activity and response to exogenous administration. *Congress on Biologically Active Atrial Peptides*. New York, Raven Press, 1986.
405. Antunes-Rodrigues J, McCann SM, Rogers LC, et al: Atrial natriuretic factor inhibits dehydration and angiotensin II induced water intake in the conscious, unrestrained rat. *Proc Natl Acad Sci USA* 82:8720, 1985.
406. Volpe M: Atrial natriuretic peptide and the baroreflex control of circulation. *Am J Hypertens* 5:488, 1992.
407. Appel R: Growth-regulatory properties of atrial natriuretic factor. *Am J Physiol* 262:F911, 1992.
408. Levin E: Natriuretic peptide c-receptor: More than a clearance receptor. *Am J Physiol* 264:E483, 1993.
409. White R, Lee A, Shcherbatko A, et al: Potassium channel stimulation by natriuretic peptides through cGMP-dependent dephosphorylation. *Nature* 361:263, 1993.
410. Awazu M, Ichikawa I: Biological significance of atrial natriuretic peptide in the kidney. *Nephron* 63:1, 1993.
411. Campese VM: Salt sensitivity in hypertension. *Hypertension* 23:531, 1994.
412. Watkins R, Vemulapalli S, Chiu P, et al: Atrial natriuretic factor potentiating and hemodynamic effects of SCH 42495, a new neutral metalloendopeptidase inhibitor. *Am J Hypertens* 6:357, 1993.
413. Wazna J, Shenker Y: Atrial natriuretic peptide—alive and well? *Am J Hypertens* 5:336, 1992.
414. Giles T, Quiroz A, Roffidal L, et al: Prolonged hemodynamic benefits from a high-dose bolus injection of human atrial natriuretic factor in congestive heart failure. *Clin Pharmacol Ther* 50:557, 1991.
415. DiBona G: Sympathetic neural control of the kidney in hypertension. *Hypertension* 19:I28, 1992.
416. Ohbu K, Hendley ED, Yamaguchi I, et al: Renal dopamine-1 receptors in hypertensive inbred rat strains with and without hyperactivity. *Hypertension* 21:485, 1993.
417. Waeber B, Aubert J-F, Corder R, et al: Cardiovascular effects of neuropeptide Y. *Am J Hypertens* 1:193, 1988.
418. Katsuya T, Higaki, J, Zhao Y, et al: A neuropeptide Y locus on chromosome 4 cosegregates with blood pressure in the spontaneously hypertensive rat. *Biochem Biophys Res Commun* 192:261, 1993.
419. Michel MC, Philipp T, Brodde O-E: α- and β-Adrenoceptors in hypertension: Molecular biology and pharmacological studies. *Pharmacol Toxicol* 70:sl, 1992.
420. Ritter J, Barrow S, Doktor H, et al: Thromboxane A_2 receptor antagonism and synthetase inhibition in essential hypertension. *Hypertension* 22:197, 1993.
421. Ferri C, Bellini C, Piccoli A, et al: Enhanced blood pressure response to cyclooxygenase inhibition in salt-sensitive human essential hypertension. *Hypertension* 21:875, 1993.
422. Ando K, Ono A, Sato Y, et al: Involvement of prostaglandins and renal haemodynamics in salt-sensitivity of young spontaneously hypertensive rats. *Hypertension* 11:373, 1993.
423. Schror K: Prostoglandin-mediated actions of the renin-angiotensin system. *Arzneimittelforschung* 43:236, 1993.
424. Nolly H, Carretero O, Lama M, et al: Vascular kallikrein in deoxycorticosterone acetate-salt hypertensive rats. *Hypertension* 23(Suppl I):I–85, 1994.
425. Carretero OA, Scicli AG: Kinins, paracrine hormones, in the regulation of blood flow, renal function, and blood pres-

sure, in Laragh JH, Brenner BM, Kaplan NM (eds): *Endocrine Mechanisms in Hypertension: Perspectives in Hypertension*. New York, Raven Press, 1989, vol 2, p 219.
426. Carbonell L, Carretero O, Madeddu P, et al: Effects of a kinin antagonist on mean blood pressure. *Hypertension* 11:I–84, 1988.
427. Wang J, Xiong W, Yang Z, et al: Human tissue kallikrein induces hypotension in transgenic mice. *Hypertension* 23:236, 1994.
428. Madeddu P, Parpaglia P, Demontis M, et al: Chronic kinin receptor blockade induces hypertension in deoxycorticosterone-treated rats. *Br J Pharmacol* 108:651, 1993.
429. Madeddu P, Parpaglia P, Demontis M, et al: Bradykinin B_2-receptor blockade facilitates deoxycorticosterone-salt hypertension. *Hypertension* 21:980, 1993.
430. Carratero O, Scicli A: Local hormone factors (intracrine, autocrine and paracrine). *Hypertension* 18:I-58, 1991.
431. Hunt S, Hasstedt S, Wu L, et al: A gene-environment interaction between inferred kallikrein genotype and potassium. *Hypertension* 22:161, 1993.
432. Li F, Joshua J: Decreased arteriolar endothelium-derived relaxing factor production during the development of genetic hypertension. *Clin Exp Hypertens* 15:511, 1993.
433. MacGregor GA: Sodium is more important than calcium in essential hypertension. *Hypertension* 7:628, 1985.
434. Holloway ET, Bohr DF: Reactivity of vascular smooth muscle in hypertensive rats. *Circ Res* 33:678, 1973.
435. Nicholls MG: Reduction of dietary sodium in western society: Benefit or risk? *Hypertension* 6:795, 1984.
436. Sinaiko A, Gomez-Martin O, Prineas R: Effect of low sodium diet or potassium supplementation on adolescent blood pressure. *Hypertension* 21:989, 1993.
437. Kumanyika SK, Hebert PR, Cutler JA, et al: Feasibility and efficacy of sodium reduction in the trials of hypertension prevention, phase I: Trials of Hypertension Prevention Collaboration Research Group. *Hypertension* 22:502, 1993.
438. Intersalt Cooperative Research Group I: An international study of electrolyte excretion and blood pressure: Results for 24 hour urinary sodium and potassium excretion. *Br Med J* 297:319, 1988.
439. Fotherby MD, Potter JF: Effects of moderate sodium restriction on clinic and twenty-four-hour ambulatory blood pressure in elderly hypertensive subjects. *J Hypertens* 11:657, 1993.
440. Stein P, Black H: The role of diet in the genesis and treatment of hypertension. *Med Clin North Am* 77:831, 1993.
441. Wylie-Rosett J, Wassertheil-Smoller S, Blaufox M, et al: Trial of antihypertensive intervention and management: Greater efficacy with weight reduction than with a sodium-potassium intervention. *J Am Diet Assoc* 93:408, 1993.
442. Del Rio A, Rodriguez-Villamil JL: Metabolic effects of strict salt restriction in essential hypertensive patient. *J Intern Med* 233:409, 1993.
443. Winer BH: The antihypertensive actions of benzothiadiazines. *Circulation* 23:211, 1961.
444. Sharma A, Schorr U, Distler A: Insulin resistance in young salt-sensitive normotensive subjects. *Hypertension* 21:273, 1993.
445. Overlack A, Ruppert M, Kollock R, et al: Divergent hemodynamic and hormonal responses to varying salt intake in normotensive subjects. *Hypertension* 22:331, 1993.
446. Weder A: Membrane sodium transport and salt sensitivity of blood pressure. *Hypertension* 17:I74, 1991.
447. Lind L, Lithell H, Gustafasson I, et al: Calcium metabolism and sodium sensitivity in hypertensive subjects. *J Hum Hypertens* 7:53, 1993.
448. Rocchini AP: Cardiovascular regulation in obesity-induced hypertension. *Hypertension* 19:I56, 1992.
449. Barbagallo M, Gupta R, Resnick L: Independent effects of hyperinsulinemia and hyperglycemia on intracellular sodium in normal human red cells. *Am J Hypertens* 6:264, 1993.
450. Campese VM, Romoff MS, Levitan D, et al: Abnormal relationship between sodium intake and sympathetic nervous system activity in salt-sensitive patients with essential hypertension. *Kidney Int* 21:371, 1982.
451. Tobian L: Salt and hypertension. *Am J Nephrol* 3:80, 1983.
452. Osborn J, Provo B, Montana J, et al: Salt-sensitive hypertension caused by long-term (alpha)-adrenergic blockade in the rat. *Hypertension* 21:995, 1993.
453. Passmore JC, Whitescarver SA, Ott CE, et al: Importance of chloride for deoxycorticosterone acetate-salt hypertension in the rat. *Hypertension* 7:1115, 1985.
454. Kurtz TWJ, Morris RCJ: Dietary chloride as a determinant of sodium-dependent hypertension. *Science* 22:1139, 1983.
455. Sudhir K, Kurtz TW, Yock PG, et al: Potassium preserves endothelial function and enhances aortic compliance in Dahl rats. *Hypertension* 22:315, 1993.
456. Krishna G, Kapoor S: Potassium depletion exacerbates essential hypertension. *Ann Intern Med* 115:77, 1991.
457. Taddel S, Mattei P, Virdis A, et al: Effect of potassium on vasodilation to acetylcholine in essential hypertension. *Hypertension* 23:485, 1994.
458. Siani A, Strazzullo P, Giacco A, et al: Increasing the dietary potassium intake reduces the need for antihypertensive medication. *Ann Intern Med* 115:753, 1991.
459. Susuki H, Kondo K, Saruta T: Effect of potassium chloride on the blood pressure in two-kidney, one clip Goldblatt hypertensive rats. *Hypertension* 3:566, 1981.
460. Brandis M, Keyes J, Windhager EE: Potassium-induced inhibition of proximal tubular fluid reabsorption in rats. *Am J Physiol* 222:421, 1972.
461. Helfant RH: Hypokalemia and arrhythmias. *Am J Med* 80(Suppl 4A):13, 1986.
462. Oparil S, Calhoun A: The calcium antagonists in the 1990's. *Am J Hypertens* 4:396, 1991.
463. Cohen R: Pathways controlling healthy and diseases arterial smooth muscle. *Am J Cardiol* 72:39, 1993.
464. Van Hooft IM, Grobbee DE, Frölich M, et al: Alterations in calcium metabolism in young people at risk for primary hypertension. *Hypertension* 21:267, 1993.
465. Resnick L: Cellular calcium and magnesium metabolism in the pathophysiology and treatment of hypertension and related metabolic disorders. *Am J Med* 93:2, 1992.
466. Anderson E, Mark A: The vasodilator action of insulin: Implications for the insulin hypothesis of hypertension. *Hypertension* 21:136, 1993.
467. Papagalanis N, Kourti A, Tolis A, et al: Effect of intravenous calcium infusion on indices of activity of the parathyroid glands and on urinary calcium and sodium excretion in normotensive and hypertensive subjects. *Am J Hypertens* 6:59, 1993.
468. Byyny R, LoVerde M, Lloyd S, et al: Cytosolic calcium and insulin resistence in elderly patients with essential hypertension. *Am J Hypertens* 5:459, 1992.
469. Brickman A, Nyby M, von Hungen K, et al: Parathyroid hormone, platelet calcium, and blood pressure in normotensive subjects. *Hypertension* 18:176, 1991.
470. Whelton PK, Klag MJ: Magnesium and blood pressure: Review of the epidemiologic and clinical trial experience. *Am J Cardiol* 63:26, 1989.
471. Joffreys MR, Reed DM, Yano K: Relationship of magnesium intake and other dietary factors to blood pressure: The Honolulu heart study. *Am J Clin Nutr* 45:469, 1987.
472. Pritchard JA: The use of magnesium ion in the management of eclamptogenic toxeimas. *Surg Gynecol Obstet* 100:131, 1955.
473. Dyckner I: Wester PO: Effect of magensium on blood pressure. *Br Med J* 286:1847, 1983.
474. Holliheld JW: Thiazide treatment of hypertension: Effects of thiazide diuretics on serum, potassium magnesium, and ventricularectopy. *Am J Med* 80:8, 1986.
475. Nadler J, Buchanan T, Natarajan R, et al: Magnesium deficiency produces insulin resistance and increased thromboxane synthesis. *Hypertension* 21:1024, 1993.

476. Altura BM, Altura BT, Gebrewold A: Magnesium deficiency and hypertension: Correlation between magnesium-deficient diets and microcirculatory changes in situ. *Science* 223:1315, 1984.
477. Altura BM, Altura BT: Magnesium ions and contraction of vascular smooth muscles: Relationships to some vascular diseases. *Fed Proc* 40:2672, 1981.
478. Stokes J: Principles of epithelial transport, in (ed): *Dynamics of Body Water and Electrolyte Distribution and Transport.* 1990, p 21.
479. Aalkjaer C, Parvin SD, Bing RF, et al: Cell membrane sodium transport: A correlation between human resistance vessels and leucocytes. *Lancet* 1:649, 1986.
480. Hilton PJ: Cellular sodium transport in essential hypertension. *N Engl J Med* 314:222, 1986.
481. Lasker N, Hopp L, Grossman S, et al: Race and sex differences in erythrocyte Na+, K+, and Na+-K+-adenosine triphosphatase. *J Clin Invest* 75:1813, 1985.
482. Cacciafesta M, Ferri C, Carlomagno A, et al: Erythrocyte Na-K-Cl cotransport activity in low renin essential hypertensive patients: A ^{23}Na nuclear magnetic resonance study. *Am J Hypertens* 7:151, 1994.
483. Brearley CJ, Wood AJ, Aronson JK, et al: Evidence for an altered mode of action of the sodium-lithium countertransporter in vivo in patients with untreated essential hypertension. *Hypertension* 11:147, 1993.
484. Haddy FJ: Abnormalities of membrane transport in hypertension. *Hypertension* 5:66, 1983.
485. Doria A, Fioretto P, Avogaro A, et al: Insulin resistance is associated with high sodium-lithium countertransport in essential hypertension. *Insulin Resist Hypertens* 261:E684, 1991.
486. Canessa M, Falkner B, Hulman S: Red blood cell sodium-proton exchange in hypertensive blacks with insulin-resistant glucose disposal. *Hypertension* 22:204, 1993.
487. Wolpert H, Steen S, Istfan N, et al: Disparate effects of weight loss on insulin sensitivity and erythrocyte sodium-lithium countertransport activity. *Am J Hypertens* 5:754, 1992.
488. Mangili R, Zerbini G, Barlassina C, et al: Sodium-lithium countertransport and triglycerides in diabetic nephropathy. *Int Soc Nephrol* 127, 1993.
489. Krzesinski JM, Saint-Remy A, Du F, et al: Red blood cell Na-Li countertransport, hypertensive heredity, and cardiovascular risk in young adults. *Hypertension* 6:314, 1993.
490. Rebbect TR, Turner ST, Sing FC: Sodium-lithium countertransport genotype and the probability of hypertension in adults. *Hypertension* 22:560, 1993.
491. Lopes De Faria J, Jones S, Macdonald F, et al: Sodium-lithium countertransport activity and insulin resistance in normotensive IDDM patients. *Diabetes* 41:610, 1992.
492. Grunfeld B, Balzareti M, Romo M, et al: Hyperinsulinemia in normotensive offspring of hypertensive parents. *Hypertension* 23:I12, 1994.
493. Lifton R, Hunt S, Williams R, et al: Exclusion of the Na^+-H^+ antiporter as a candidate gene in human essential hypertension. *Hypertension* 17:8, 1991.
494. Weber AB: Red-cell lithium-sodium countertransport and renal lithium clearance in hypertension. *N Engl J Med* 314:198, 1986.
495. Alonsa A, Arrazola A, Garciandia A, et al: Erythrocyte anion exchanger activity and intracellular pH in essential hypertension. *Hypertension* 22:348, 1993.
496. Rosskopf D, Dusing R, Siffert W: Membrane sodium-proton exchange and primary hypertension. *Hypertension* 21:607, 1993.
497. Rosskopf D, Frömter E, Aiffert W: Hypertensive sodium-proton exchanger phenotype persists in immortalized lymphocytes from essential hypertensive patients. *J Clin Invest* 92:2553, 1993.
498. Mahnensmith RL, Aronson PS: The plasma membrance sodium-hydrogen exchanger and its role in physiological and pathophysiological processes. *Circ Res* 56:773, 1985.
499. Sierra A, Coca A, Pare CJ, et al: Erythrocyte ion fluxes in essential hypertensive patients with left ventricular hypertrophy. *Hypertension* 1628, 1993.
500. Wakabayashi S, Sarder C, Fafournoux P, et al: Structure function of the growth factor activatable Na^+/H^+ exchanger (NHE1). *Rev Physiol Biochem Pharmacol* 119:157, 1992.
501. Yuan CM, Manunta P, Hamlyn JM, et al: Long-term ouabain adminstration produces hypertension in rats. *Int J Clin Pharmacol Ther Toxicol* 31:89, 1993.
502. Leenen FHH, Harmsen E, Yu H, et al: Dietary sodium stimulates ouabainlike activity in adrenalectomized spontaneously hypertensive rats. *Am J Physiol* 265:H421, 1993.
503. Blaustein M: Physiological effects of endogenous ouabain: Control of intracellular Ca^{2+} stores and cell responsiveness. *Am J Physiol* 264:C1367, 1993.
504. Leenen F, Harmsen E, Yu H, et al: Effects of dietary sodium on central and peripheral ouabain-like activity in spontaneously hypertensive rats. Am J Physiol 264:H2051, 1993.
505. Naruse K, Naruse M, Tanabe A, et al: Does plasma immunoreactive ouabain originate from the adrenal gland? *Hypertension* 23:I102, 1994
506. Hamlyn JM, Blaustein MP, Bova S, et al: Identification and characterization of an ouabain-like compound from human plasma. *Proc Natl Acad Sci USA* 88:6259, 1991.
507. Schoner W: Endogenous digitalis-llke factors. *Clin Exp Hypertens* 14:767, 1992.
508. Tibblin G: High blood pressure in men aged 50: A population study of men born in 1913. *Acta Med Scand [Suppl]* 470:1, 1967.
509. Semplicini A, Buzzaccarini F, Ceolotto G, et al: Effects of canrenoate on red cell sodium transport and calf flow in essential hypertension. *Hypertension* 6:295, 1993.
510. Manunta P, Evans G, Hamilton BP, et al: A new syndrome with elevated plasma ouabain and hypertension secondary to an adrenocortical tumor. *J Hypertens* 10:S27, 1992.
511. Rocchini A: Insulin resistance and blood pressure regulation in obese and nonobese subjects. *Hypertension* 17:837, 1991.
512. Landsberg L: Hyperinsulinemia: Possible role in obesity-induced hypertension. *Hypertension* 19:61, 1992.
512a. Hsueh WA, Buchanan TA: Obesity and hypertension. *Endocr Hyper* 23:405, 1994.
512b. Hsueh WA: Insulin resistance in essential hypertension, *Yearbook of Nephrology.*
513. Epstein M, Sowers J: Diabetes mellitus and hypertension. *Hypertension* 19:403, 1992.
514. Reaven G: Role of insulin resistance in human disease (syndrome X): An expanded definition. *Annu Rev Med* 44:121, 1993.
515. Stern M, Morales P, Haffner S, et al: Hyperdynamic circulation and the insulin resistance syndrome ("syndrome X"). *Hypertension* 20:802, 1992.
516. Facchini F, Chen I, Clinkingbeard C, et al: Insulin resistance, hyperinsulinemia, and dyslipidemia in nonobese individuals with a family history of hypertension. *Am J Hypertens* 5:694,1992.
517. Jarrett R: In defense of insulin: A critique of syndrome X. *Lancet* 340:469, 1992.
518. Caro J: Insulin resistance in obese and nonobese man. *J Clin Endrocinol Metab* 73:691, 1991.
518a Brunzell, JD: Personal correspondence.
519. Lissner L, Bengtsson C, Lapidus L, et al: Fasting insulin in relation to subsequent blood pressure changes and hypertension in women. *Hypertension* 20:797, 1992.
520. Hall J, Brands M, Hildebrandt D, et al: Obesity-associated hypertension. *Hypertension* 19:45, 1992.
521. Ferrannini E: Metabolic abnormalities of hypertension: A lesson in complexities. *Hypertension* 18:636, 1991.
522. Kautzky-Willer A, Pacini G, Weissel M, et al: Elevated hepatic insulin extraction in essential hypertension. *Hypertension* 21:646, 1993.
523. Suzuki M, Hirose J, Asakura Y, et al: Insulin insensitivity

in nonobese, nondiabetic essential hypertension and its improvement by an α1-blocker (Bunazosin). *Am J Hypertens* 5:689, 1992.

524. Ferri C, De Mattia G, Bellini C, et al: Octreotide, a somatostatin analog, reduces insulin secretion and increases renal Na excretion in lean essential hypertensive patients. *Am J Hypertens* 6:276, 1993.
525. Allemann Y, Horber F, Colombo M, et al: Insulin sensitivity and body fat distribution in normotensive offspring of hypertensive patients. *Lancet* 341:327, 1993.
525a. Saad MF, Lillioja S, Nyomba BL, et al.: Racial differences in the relation between blood pressure and insulin resistance. *N Engl J Med* 324:733, 1991.
525b. Saad MF, Howard G, Rewers M, et al.:. Insulin resistance but not Insulinemia is associated with hypertension: The insulin resistance atherosclerosis study. *Circulation* 89:934, 1994.
526. Shamiss A, Carroll J, Rosenthal T: Insulin resistance in secondary hypertension. *Am J Hypertens* 5:26, 1992.
527. Bonora E, Bonadona R, Del Prat S, et al: In vivo glucose metabolism in obese and type II diabetic subjects with or without hypertension. *Diabetes* 42:764, 1993.
528. Nilsson P, Lindholm L, Scherstein B: Hyperinsulinemia and other metabolic disturbances in well controlled hypertensive men and women: An epidemiological study of the Dalby population. *J Hypertens* 8:953, 1990.
528a. Ferrari P, Weidmann P, Shaw S, et al: Altered insulin sensitivity, hyperinsulinemia, and dyslipidemia in individuals with a hypertensive parent. *Am J Med* 91:589, 1991.
528b. Julius S, Jamerson K, Mejiia A, et al: The association of borderline hypertension with target organ changes and higher coronary risk. Techumseh Blood Pressure Study. *JAMA* 264:354, 1990.
529. Dowse G, Collins V, Alberti K, et al: Insulin and blood pressure levels are not independently related in Mauritians of Asian Indian, Creole or Chinese origin. *J Hypertens* 11:297, 1993.
530. Hypertension Detection and Follow-up Program Cooperative Group: Five-year findings of the hypertension detection and follow up program: I. Reduction in mortality of persons with high blood pressure, including mild hypertension. *JAMA* 242:2562, 1979.
531. Ferrannini E, Haffner SM, Stern MP: Essential hypertension: An insulin-resistance state. *J Cardiovasc Pharmacol* 15:s18, 1990.
532. Ikeda T, Terasawa H, Ishimura H, et al: Correlation between blood pressure and plasma insulin in acromegaly. *J Intern Med* 234:61, 1993.
533. Whitworth J: Studies on the mechanisms of glucocorticoid hypertension in humans. *Blood Pressure* 3:24, 1994.
533a. Buchanan TA, Sipos GF, Gadalah S, et al.: Glucose tolerance and insulin action in rat with renovascular hypertension. *Hypertension* 18:341, 1991.
534. Weinsier R, James D, Darnell B, et al: Obesity-related hypertension: Evaluation of the separate effects of energy restriction and weight reduction on hemodynamic and neuroendocrine status. *Am JMed* 90:460, 1991.
535. Santoro D, Natali A, Palombo C, et al: Effects of chronic angiotensin coverting enzyme inhibition on glucose tolerance and insulin sensitivity in essential hypertension. *Hypertension* 20:181, 1992.
536. Kaplan N: Effects of antihypertensive therapy on insulin resistance. *Hypertension* 19:116, 1992.
537. Reaven G, Chen Y, Jeppesen J, et al: Insulin resistance and hyperinsulinemia in individuals with small, dense, low density lipoprotein particles. *J Clin Invest* 92:141, 1993.
538. Nishina P, Johnson J, Naggert J, et al: Linkage of atherogenic lipoprotein phenotype to the low density lipoprotein receptor locus on the short arm of chromosome 19. *Proc Natl Acad Sci USA* 89:708, 1992.
539. Anderson E, Balon T, Hoffman R, et al: Insulin increases sympathetic activity but not blood pressure in borderline hypertensive humans. *Hypertension* 19:621, 1992.
540. Buchanan T, Thawani H, Kades J, et al: Angiotensin II increases glucose utilization during acute hyperinsulinemia via a hemodynamic mechanism. *J Clin Invest* 92:720, 1993.
541. Saito F, Hori M, Fittingoff M, et al: Insulin attenuates agonist-mediated calcium mobilization in cultured rat vascular smooth muscle cell. *J Clin Invest* 92:1161, 1993.
541a. Meehan WP, Buchanan TA, Hsueh W: Chronic insulin administration elevates blood pressure in rats. *Hypertension* 23:1012, 1994.
541b. Hall JE, Coleman TG, Mizelle HL, Smith MJ: Chronic hyperinsulinemia and blood pressure regulation. *Am J Physiol* 258:F722, 1990.
542. Tomiyama H, Kushiro T, Abeta H, et al: Blood pressure response to hyperinsulinemia in salt-sensitive and salt-resistant rats. *Hypertension* 20:596, 1992.
543. Peuler JD, Johnson BAB, Phare SM, et al: Sex-specific effects of an insulin secretagogue in stroke-prone hypertensive rats. *Hypertension* 22:214, 1993.
543a. Wu H-y, Jeng YY, Yue C-j, et al.: Endothelial-dependent vascular effects of insulin and insulin-like growth factor I in the perfused rat mesenteric artery and aortic ring. *Diabetes* 43:1994.
543b. Buchanan TA, Thawani H, Kades W, et al.: Angiotensin II increases glucose utilization during acute hyperinsulinemia via a hemodynamic mechanism. *J Clin Invest* 92:720, 1993.
544. Baron A, Brechtel-Hook G, Johnson A, et al: Skeletal muscle blood flow. *Hypertension* 21:129, 1993.
545. Baron A, Brechtel G: Insulin differentially regulares systemic and skeletal muscle vascular resistance. *Am J Physiol* 265:E61, 1993.
546. Sakai K, Imaizumi T, Masaki H, et al: Intra-arterial infusion of insulin attenuates vasoreactivity in human forearm. *Hypertension* 22:67, 1993.
546a. Laakso M, Edelman SV, Brechtel G, Baron AD: Decreased effect of insulin to stimulate skeletal muscle blood flow in obese man: A novel mechanism for insulin resistance. *J Clin Invest* 85:1844, 1990.
547. Vollenweider P, Tappy L, Randin D, et al: Differential effects of hyperinsulinemia and carbohydrate metabolism on sympathetic nerve activity and muscle blood flow in humans. *I Clin Invest* 92:147, 1993.
548. Gupta A, Clark R, Kirchner K: Effects on insulin on renal sodium excretion. *Hypertension* 19:I78, 1992.
549. Shimamoto K, Kirata A, Masatada F, et al: Insulin sensitivity and the effects of insulin on renal sodium handling and pressor systems in essential hypertensive patients. *Hypertension* 23:I29, 1994.
550. Goodfriend T, Ball D, Elliott M, et al: Fatty acids may regulate aldosterone secretion and mediate some of insulin's effects on blood pressure. *Prostaglandins Leukotrienes Essential Fatty Acids* 48:43, 1993.
551. Juncos L, Ito S: Disparate effects of insulin on isolated rabbit afferent and efferent arterioles. *J Clin Invest* 92:1981, 1993.
552. Miller J. Abouchacra S, Zimman B, et al: Atrial natriuretic factor counteracts sodium-retaining action of insulin in normal men. *Am J Physiol* 265:R584, 1993.
553. Standley P, Bakir M, Sowers J: Vascular insulin abnormalities, hypertension. *Am J Kidney Dis* 21:1993.
554. Kahn A, Seidel C, Allen J, et al: Insulin reduces contraction and intracellular calcium concentration in vascular muscle. *Hypertension* 22:735,1993.
555. Sowers J, Khoury S, Standley P, et al: Mechanisms of hypertension in diabetes. *Am J Med* 4:177, 1991.
556. Sowers J, Standley P, Jacober S, et al: Postpartum abnormalities of carbohydrate and cellular calcium metabolism in pregnancy induced hypertension. *Am J Hypertens* 6:302, 1993.
557. Bunker C, Wing R, Becker D, et al: Sodium-lithium countertransport activity is decreased after weight loss in healthy obese men. *Metabolism* 42:1052, 1993.

558. Feldman R, Bierbrier G: Insulin-mediated vasodilation: Impairment with increased blood pressure and body mass. *Lancet* 342:707, 1993.
559. Gavras H, Hatzinikolaou P, North WG, Bresnahan M, Gavras I: Interaction of the sympathetic nervous system with vasopressin and renin in the maintenance of blood pressure. *Hypertension* 4:400, 1982.
560. Egan BM, Stepniakowski K, Nazzaro P: Insulin levels are similar in obese salt-sensitive and salt-resistant hypertensive subjects. *Hypertension* 23:I1, 1994.
560a. Perloff, D, Grim C, Flack J, Frohlich ED, Hill M, McDonald M, Morgenstern BZ, Writing Group: Human blood pressure determination by sphygmomanometry: Special Report. *Circulation* 88:2460, 1993.
561. Kirkendall WM, Feinleib M, Freis ED, et al: Recommendations for human blood pressure determination by sphygmomanometers. *Circulation* 62:1145, 1980.
562. Hossmann V, Fitzgerald GA, Dollery CT: Influence of hospitalization and placebo therapy on blood pressure and sympathetic function in essential hypertension. *Hypertension* 3:113, 1981.
563. Pickering TG, Harshfield GA, Devereux RB, et al: What is the role of ambulatory blood pressure monitoring in the management of hypertensive patients? *Hypertension* 7:171, 1985.
564. Levy D, Labib SB, Anderson KM, Christiansen JC, Kannel WB, Castelli WP. Determinants of sensitivity and specificity of electrocardiographic criteria for left ventricular hypertrophy. *Circulation* 81(3):815, 1990.
565. Devereux R, Alonso D, Lutas E, et al: Echocardiographic assessment of left ventricular hypertrophy: Comparison to necropsy findings. *Am J Cardiol* 57:45, 1986.
566. Campbell D, Kladis S: Simultaneous radioimmunoassay of six angiotensin peptides in arterial and venous plasma of man. *J Hypertens* 8:165, 1990.
567. Thatcher R, Whitworth J, Casley D, et al: A two-site monoclonal immunoradiometric assay for total renin protein: Comparison with an established enzyme kinetic assay. *Clin Exp Pharmacol Physiol* 15:285, 1988.
568. Galen FX, Guyenne TT, Devaux C, et al: Direct radioimmunoassay of human renin. *J Clin Endocrinol Metab* 48:1041, 1979.
569. Oparil S: Theoretical approaches to estimation of plasma renin activity: A review and some original observations. *Clin Chem* 22:583, 1976.
570. Bennett CM, Hsueh WA: Measurement of renin and interpretations of plasma renin activity, in Massry SG, Glassack RJ (eds): *Textbook of Nephrology*. Baltimore, Williams & Wilkins, 1983, p 1125.
571. Pickering TG, Sos TA, Vaughn EDJ, et al: Predictive value and changes of renin secretion in patients undergoing successful renal angioplasty. *Am J Med* 76:398, 1984.
572. Ruddy MC, Atlas SA, Salerno FG: Hypertension associated with a renin-secreting adenocarcinoma of the pancreas. *N Engl J Med* 307:993, 1982.
573. Davidson R, Wilcox C: Newer tests for the diagnosis of renovascular disease. *Renovasc Dis* 268:3353, 1992.
574. Dunnick N, Sfakianakis G: Screening for renovascular hypertension. *Radiol Clin North Am* 29:497, 1991.
575. Distler A, Spics K-P: Diagnostic procedure in renovascular hypertension. *Clin Nephrol* 36:174, 1991.
576. Mahomed F: Chronic Bright's disease without albuminuria. *Guys Hosp Rep* 25:295, 1881.
577. Tigerstedt R, Bergman G: Niere and Kreislauf. *Scand Arch Physiol* 8:223, 1898.
578. Goldblatt H, Lynch J, Hanzal RF, et al: Studies on experimental hypertension: I. The production of persistent elevation of systolic blood pressure by means of renal ischemia. *J Exp Med* 59:347, 1934.
579. Page IH: On the nature of the pressor action of renin. *J Exp Med* 70:521, 1939.
580. Braun-Menendez E, Fasciolo JC, Leloir LF, et al: La substance hypertensive extraite du sang des reins ischemies. *C R Soc Biol* 133:731, 1940.
581. Goormaghtigh N: Facts in favor of an endocrine function of the renal arterioles. *J Pathol* 57:393, 1945.
582. Bumpus FM, Schwartz H, Page IH: Synthesis and pharmacology of the octapeptide angiotensin. *Science* 125:886, 1957
583. Deming QB, Luetscher JA: Bioassay of desoxycorticosterone like material in urine. *Proc Soc Exp Biol Med* 73:171, 1950.
584. Goldblatt H: Studies on experimental hypertension: V. The pathogenesis of experimental hypertension due to renal ischemia. *Ann Intern Med* 11:69, 1937.
585. Laragh JH: The role of aldosterone in man: Evidence for regulation of electrolyte balance and arterial pressure by renal-adrenal system which may be involved in malignant hypertension. *JAMA* 174:293, 1960.
586. Bumpus FM, Khosla MC: Pathogenetic factors involved in renovascular hypertension-state of the art. *Mayo Clin Proc* 52:417, 1977.
587. Sawicki P, Kaiser S, Heinemann L, et al: Prevalence of renal artery stenosis in diabetes mellitus—an autopsy study. *J Intern Med* 229:489, 1991.
588. Rimmer JM, Gennari FJ: Atherosclerotic renovascular disease and progressive renal failure. *Ann Intern Med* 118: 712, 1993.
589. Rudnick MR, Goldfarb S, Ludbrook P, et al: Nephrotoxicity following cardiac angiography: A double-blind multicenter trial of ionic and nonionic contrast media in 1194 patients. *J Am Soc Nephrol* 2:688, 1991.
590. Harrison EG Jr, McCormack LJ: Pathologic classification of renal arterial disease in renovascular hypertension. *Mayo Clin Proc* 46:161, 1971.
591. Stanley JC, Gewartz BL, Boue EL, et al: Arterial fibrodysplasia: Histopathologic character and current etiologic concepts. *Arch Surg* 110:561, 1975.
592. McCormack LJ, Poutasse EF, Meaney TF, et al: A pathologic-arteriographic correlation of renal arterial disease. *Am Heart J* 72:188, 1966.
593. Kincaid OW, David GD, Hallermann FJ, et al: Fibromuscular dysplasia of the renal arteries—arteriographic features, classification and observation on natural history of the disease. *AJR* 104:271,1968.
594. Wylie EJ, Wellington JS: Hypertension caused by fibromuscular hyperplasia of the renal arteries. *Am J Surg* 100:183, 1960.
595. Wylie EJ, Binkley FM, Palubinskas AJ: Extrarenal fibromuscular hyperplasia. *Am J Surg* 112:149, 1966.
596. Keim HJ, Johnson PM, Vaughan ED, et al: Computer-assisted static/dynamic renal imaging: A screening test for renovascular hypertension? *J Nucl Med* 20:11, 1979.
597. Makker SP, Moorthy B: Fibromuscular dysplasia of renal arteries: An important cause of renovascular hypertension in children. *J Pediatr* 95:940, 1979.
598. Chugh K, Jain S, Sakhuja V, et al: Renovascular hypertension due to Takayasu's arteritis among Indian patients. *Q J Med* 85:833, 1992.
599. Vidt D, Eisele G, Gephardt G, et al: Atheroembolic renal disease: Association with renal arterial stenosis. *Cleve J Med* 56:407, 1989.
600. Sang C, Whelton P, Hamper U, et al: Etiologic factors in renovascular fibromuscular dysplasia. *Hypertension* 14: 472, 1989.
601. Martinez-Amenós A, Rama H, Sarrias X, et al: Percutaneous transluminal angioplasty in the treatment of renovascular hypertension. *J Hum Hypertens* 5:97, 1991.
602. Sos T: Angioplasty for the treatment of azotemia and renovascular hypertension in atherosclerotic renal artery disease. *Circulation* 83:I162, 1991.
603. Tegtmeyer C, Selby J, Hartwell G, et al: Results and complication of angioplasty in fibromuscular disease. *Circulation* 83:I-155, 1991.
604. Poutasse EF, Dustan HP: Arteriosclerosis and renal hyper-

tension: Indications for aortography in hypertensive patients and results of surgical treatment of obstructive lesions of renal artery. *JAMA* 165:1521, 1957.
605. Perloff D, Sokolow M, Wylie E, et al: Renal vascular hypertension: Further experiences. *Am Heart J* 74:614, 1967.
606. Schmidt DM, Rambo ON: Segmental intimal hyperplasia of the abdominal aorta and renal arteries producing hypertension in an infant. *Am J Clin Pathol* 44:546, 1965.
607. Sharma BK, Sagar S, Chugh KS, et al: Spectrum of renovascular hypertension in the young in north India: A hospital based study on occurrence and clinical features. *Angiology* 36:370, 1985.
608. McAllister M, Thompson W III, Pabian C: Percutaneous angioplasty for renovascular hypertension due to fibromuscular dysplasia. *Am Fam Physician* 46:1225, 1992.
609. Palubinskas AJ, Wylie EJ: Roentgen diagnosis of fibromuscular hyperplasia of the renal arteries. *Radiology* 76:634, 1961.
610. Ekelund L, Gerlock J, Molin J, et al: Roentgenologic appearance of fibromuscular dysplasia. *Acta Radiol* 19:433, 1978.
611. Goncharenko V, Gerlock AJJ, Shaff MI, et al: Progression of renal artery fibromuscular dysplasia in 42 patients as seen on angiography. *Radiology* 139:45, 1981.
612. Golbus SM, Swerdlin AR, Mitas JA, et al: Renal artery thrombosis in a young woman taking oral contraceptives. *Ann Intern Med* 90:989,1979.
613. Slater EE and DeSanctis RW: Disease of the aorta, in E B (ed): *Heart Disease*. Philadephia, Saunders, 1980, p 1548.
614. Smith JN, Hinman FJ: Intrarenal arterial aneurysms. *J Urol* 97:990, 1967.
615. Shelhamer JH, Volkman DJ, Parillo J, et al: Takayasu's arteritis and its therapy. *Ann Intern Med* 103:121, 1985.
616. Lagneau P, Michel JB: Renovascular hypertension and Takayasu's disease. *J Urol* 134:876, 1985.
617. Scully RE, Mark EJ, McNeely BU: Weekly clinicopathological exercises: Case 36-1985. *N Engl J Med* 313:622, 1985.
618. Duffy J, Lidsky MD, Sharp JT, et al: Polyarthritis, polyarteritis and hepatitis B. *Medicine (Baltimore)* 55:19, 1976.
619. Silver D, Clements JB: Renovascular hypertension from renal artery compression by congenital bands. *Ann Surg* 183:161, 1976.
620. Patel SR, Mooppan MM, Kim H: Subcapsular urinoma: Unusual form of page kidney in newborn. *Urology* 23:585, 1984.
621. Halpern M, Currarino G: Vascular lesions causing hypertension in neurofibromatosis. *N Engl J Med* 273:248, 1965.
622. Flynn MP, Buchanan JP: Neurofibromatosis, hypertension, and renal artery aneurysms. *South Med J* 73:618, 1980.
623. Erley C, Duda S, Wakat JP, et al: Noninvasive procedures for diagnosis of renovascular hypertension in renal transplant recipients—a prospective analysis. *Transplantation* 54:863, 1992.
624. Scully RE, Mark EJ, McNeely BN: Weekly clinicopathological exercises: Case 51-1985. *N Engl J. Med* 313:1594, 1985.
625. Sheth KJ, Tang TT, Blaedel ME, et al: Polydipsia, polyuria and hypertension associated with renin-secreting Wilms tumor. *J Pediatr* 92:921, 1978.
626. Aurell M, Rudin A, Tisell LE, et al: Captopril effect on hypertension in patient with renin-producing tumour. *Lancet* 2:149, 1979.
627. Meaney TF, Dustan HP, McCormack LJ: Natural history of renal arterial disease. *Radiology* 91:881, 1968.
628. Schreiber MJ, Pohl MA, Novick AC: The natural history of atherosclerotic and fibrous renal artery disease. *Urol Clin North Am* 11:383, 1984.
629. Stewart BH, Dustan HP, Kiser WS, et al: Correlation of angiography and natural history in evaluation of patients with renovascular hypertension. *J Urol* 104:231, 1970.
630. Ishikawa K: Natural history and classification of occlusive thromboaortopathy (Takayasu's disease). *Circulation* 57: 27, 1978.
631. Simon N, Franklin SS, Bleifer KH, et al: Cooperative Study of Renovascular Hypertension: Clinical characteristics of renovascular hypertension. *JAMA* 220:1209, 1972.
632. Londe S: Causes of hypertension in the young. *Pediatr Clin North Am* 25:55, 1978.
633. Keith TA: Renovascular hypertension in black patients. *Hypertension* 4:438, 1982.
634. Vidt D: The diagnosis of renovascular hypertension: A clinician's viewpoint. *Am J Hypertens* 4:663, 1991.
635. Svetkey LP, Kadir S, Dunnick NR, et al: Similar prevelance of renovascular hypertension in selected blacks and whites. *Hypertension* 17:678, 1991.
636. Davis BA, Crook JE, Vestal RE, et al: Prevalence of renovascular hypertension in patients with grade III or IV hypertensive retinopathy. *N Engl J Med* 301:1273, 1979.
637. Perloff D, Sokolow M, Wylie EJ, et al: Hypertension secondary to renal artery occlusive disease. *Circulation* 24:1286, 1961.
638. Foster JH, Pettinger WA, Oates JA, et al: Malignant hypertension secondary to renal artery stenosis in children. *Ann Surg* 164:700, 1966.
639. Martin LG, Casarella WJ, Alspaugh JP, et al: Renal artery angioplasty: Increased technical success and decreased complications in the second 100 patients. *Radiology* 159:631, 1986.
640. Freiman DB: Transluminal angioplasty of the renal arteries. *Urol Clin North Am* 12:737, 1985.
641. Klinge J, Mali W, Puijaert C, et al: Percutaneous transluminal renal angioplasty. *Radiology* 171:501, 1989.
642. Elliott W, Martin W, Murphy M. Comparison of two noninvasive screening tests for renovascular hypertension. *Arch Intern Med* 153:755, 1993.
643. Müller FB, Sealey JE, Case DB, et al: The captopril test for identifying renovascular disease in hypertension patients. *Ann J Med* 80:633, 1986.
644. Kashgarian M: Pathology of small blood vessel disease in hypertension. *Am J Kidney Dis* 5:A104, 1985.
645. Vaughn EDJ: Renovascular hypertension. *Kidney Int* 27:811, 1985.
646. Kutkuhn B, Godehardt E, Kunert J, et al: Validity of the captopril test for identifying correctable unilateral renovascular hypertension. *Clin Exp Hypertens [A]* 13:143, 1991.
647. Hamed R, Balfe J, Ellis G: Use of the captopril test to assess renin responsiveness in children with hypertension and renal disease. *Child Nephrol Urol* 11:10, 1991.
648. Kaplan N: The captopril challenge for renovascular hypertension. *Am J Hypertens* 3:588, 1990.
649. Postma C, van der Steen P, Hoefnagels W, et al: The captopril test in the detection of renovascular disease in hypertensive patients. *Arch Intern Med* 150:625, 1990.
650. Simon G, Coleman C: Captopril-stimulated renal vein renin measurements in the diagnosis of atherosclerotic renovascular hypertension. *Am J Hypertens* 7:1, 1994.
651. Fommei E, Bellina CR, Carmellini M, et al: High sensitivity of a computerized radioisotopic method to evaluate unilateral renal blood flow reduction by firstpass analysis and static imaging with 99mTc-glucoheptonate. *J Nucl Med Allied Sci* 27:303, 1983.
652. Lamki L, Spence JD, MacDonald AC, et al: Differential glomerular filtration rate in diagnosis of renovascular hypertension and follow-up of balloon angioplasty. *Clin Nucl Med* 11:188, 1986.
653. Geyskes G, de Bruyn J: Captopril renography and the effect of percutaneous transluminal angioplasty on blood pressure in 94 patients with renal artery stenosis. *Am J Hypertens* 4:685, 1991.
654. Nally JJ, Chen C, Fine E, et al: Diagnostic criteria of renovascular hypertension with captopril renography. *Am J Hypertens* 4:749, 1991.
655. Chervu LR, Blaufox MD: Renal radiopharmaceuticals—an update. *Semin Nucl Med* 12:224, 1982.
656. Blaufox R, Dubovsky E, Hilson A, et al: Report on the work-

ing party group on determining the radionuclide of choice. *Am J Hypertens* 4:747, 1991.

657. Hessel SJ: Complications of angiography and other catheter procedures, in Abrams HL (ed): *Angiography*. Boston, Little Brown, 1983, p 1041.
658. Steinberg E, Moore R. Powe N, et al: Safety and cost-effectiveness of high-osmolality as compared with low-osmolality contrast materials in patients undergoing cardiac angiography. *N Engl J Med* 326:425, 1992.
659. Hillman BJ, Ovitt TW, Nudelman S, et al: Digital video subtraction angiography of renal vascular abnormalities. *Radiology* 139:277, 1981.
660. Buonocore E, Meaney TF, Borkowski GP, et al: Digital subtraction angiography of the abdominal aorta and renal arteries. *Radiology*, 139:281, 1981.
661. Kerlan RKJ, Pogany AC, Burke DR, et al: Recognition and management of renovascular hypertension (clinical conference). *AJR* 45:119, 1985.
662. Bookstein J, Walter JF, Stanley JC, et al: Pharmacoangiographic manipulation of renal collateral blood flow. *Circulation* 54:328, 1976.
663. Cameron H, Close C, Yeo W, et al: Investigation of selected patients with hypertension by the rapid-sequence intravenous urogram. *Lancet* 339:658, 1992.
664. Kohler TR, Zierler RE, Martin RL, et al: Noninvasive diagnosis of renal artery stenosis by ultrasonic duplex scanning. *J Vasc Surg* 4:450, 1986.
665. Bardelli M, Jensen G, Volknamm R, et al: Non-invasive ultrasound assessment of renal artery stenosis by means of the Gosling pulsatility index. *J Hypertens* 10:985, 1992.
666. Postma C, van Aalen J, de Boo T, et al: Doppler ultrasound scanning in the detection of renal artery stenosis in hypertensive patients. *Br J Radiol* 65:857, 1992.
667. Edwards J, Zaccardi M, Strandness D: A preliminary study of the role of duplex scanning in defining the adequacy of treatment of patients with renal artery fibromuscular dysplasia. *J Vasc Surg* 15:604, 1992.
668. Miralles M, Santiso A, Gimenez A, et al: Renal duplex scanning: Correlation with angiography and isotopic renography. *Eur J Vasc Surg* 7:188, 1993.
669. Hillman BJ: Digital radiology of the kidney. *Radiol Clin North Am* 23:211, 1985.
670. Galanski M, Prokop M, Chavan A, et al: Renal arterial stenoses: Spiral CT angiography. *Radiology* 189:185, 1993.
671. Dzau VJ, Gibbons GH, Levine DC: Renovascular hypertension: An update on pathophysiology diagnosis and treatment. *Am J Nephrol* 3:172, 1983.
672. Grim CE, Luft FC, Weinberger MH, et al: Sensitivity and specificity of screening tests for renal vascular hypertension. *Ann Intern Med* 91:617, 1979.
673. Thornbury JR, Stanley JC, Fryback DG: Optimizing workup of adult hypertensive patients for renal artery stenosis. *Radiol Clin North Am* 22:333, 1984.
674. Hunt JC, Strong CG: Renovascular hypertension: Mechanisms natural history and treatment. *Am J Cardiol* 32:563, 1973.
675. Gifford RW Jr: Epidemiology and clinical manifestations of renovascular hypertension, in Stanley JC, Ernst CN, Fry WJ (eds): *Renovascular Hypertension*. Philadelphia, Saunders, 1984, p 77.
676. Whelton PK, Harris AP, Russell RP, et al: Renovascular hypertension: Results of medical and surgical therapy. *Johns Hopkins Med J* 149:213, 1981.
677. Vidt DG: Advances in the medical management of renovascular hypertension. *Urol Clin North Am* 11:417, 1984.
678. Breslin DJ, Swinton NW: Renovascular hypertension: Surgical versus medical therapeutic consideration. *Med Clin North Am* 63:397, 1979.
679. Schreiber MJ, Novick AC: Medical versus surgical management of renovascular hypertension. *Cardiovasc Clin* 2:93, 1982.
680. Dean RH, Kieffer RW, Smith BM, et al: Renovascular hypertension: Anatomic and renal functional changes during drug therapy. *Arch Surg* 116:1408, 1981.
681. Rosenthal T: Drug therapy of renovascular hypertension. *Drugs* 45:895, 1993.
682. Epstein M, Oster JR: Beta blockers and renal function: A reappraisal. *J Clin Hypertens* 1:85, 1985.
683. Mimran A, Ribstein J, Ducailar G: Converting enzyme inhibitors and renal function in essential and renovascular hypertension. *Am J Hypertens* 4:7, 1991.
684. Hannedouch T, Godin M, Fries D, et al: Acute renal thrombosis induced by angiotensin-converting enzyme inhibitors in patients with renovascular hypertension. *Nephron* 578: 230, 1991.
685. Staessen J, Bulpitt CJ, Fagard R, et al: Long-term converting enzyme inhibition versus surgical treatment in hypertensive patients with renovascular disease. *Neth J Med* 27: 161, 1984.
686. Staessen J, Bulpitt C, Fagard R, et al: Long-term converting-enzyme inhibition as a guide to surgical curability of hypertension associated with renovascular disease. *Am J Cardiol* 51:1317, 1983.
687. Hansen K, Starr S, Sands R, et al: Contemporary surgical management of renovascular disease. *J Vasc Surg* 16:319, 1992.
688. Horvath JS, Tiller DJ: Indications for renal artery surgery: A review. *J R Soc Med* 77:221, 1984.
689. Novick AC, Straffon RA, Stewart BH, et al: Diminished operative morbidity and mortality in renal revascularization. *JAMA* 246:749, 1981.
690. Messina L, Zelenock G, Yao K, et al: Renal vascularization for recurrent pulmonary edema in patients with poorly controlled hypertension and renal insufficiency: A distinct subgroup of patients with arteriosclerotic renal artery occlusive disease. *J Vasc Surg* 15:73, 1992.
691. Van Bockel J, van den Acker P, Chang P, et al: Extracorporeal renal artery reconstruction for renovascular hypertension. *J Vasc Surg* 13:101, 1991.
692. Novick AC: Management of renovascular disease: A surgical perspective. *Circulation* 83(Suppl I):I167, 1991.
693. Sinaiko A, Najarian J, Michael AF, et al: Renal autotransplantation in the treatment of bilateral renal artery stenosis: Relief of hypertension in an 8-year-old boy. *J Pediatr* 83:409, 1973.
694. Vogt PA, Pairolero PC, Hollier LH, et al: The occluded renal artery: Durability of revascularization. *J Vasc Surg* 2:125, 1985.
695. Bauer H, Forbes GL: Unilateral renal artery obstruction associated with malignant nephrosclerosis confined to the opposite kidney. *Am Heart J* 44:634, 1952.
696. Ring EJ, McLean GK: *Interventional Radiology: Principles and Techniques*. Boston, Little, Brown, 1981.
697. Sos TA, Pickering TG, Sniderman K, et al: Percutaneous transluminal renal angioplasty in renovascular hypertension due to atheroma or fibromuscular dysplasia. *N Engl J Med* 309:274, 1983.
698. Tegtmeyer CJ, Elson J, Glass TA, et al: Percutaneous transluminal angioplasty: The treatment for choice for renovascular hypertension due to fibromuscular dysplasia. *Radiology* 143:631, 1982.
699. Slater EE: Renal artery angioplasty versus surgery: A hypertensionologist's dilemma. *AJR* 135:1085, 1980.
700. Koga T, Okuda S, Takishita S, et al: Renal failure due to cholestrol embolization following percutaneous transluminal renal angioplasty. *Jpn J Med* 30:35, 1991.
701. Stanley JC, Graham LM: Renal artery fibrodysplasia and renovascular hypertension, in Rutherford RB (ed): *Vascular Surgery*. Philadelphia, Saunders, 1984, p 1145.
702. Fry WJ: Treatment of renovascular hypertension. *Adv Surg* 19:51, 1986.
703. Novick AC, Straffon RA: Surgical treatment of renovascular hypertension. *Urol Surv* 30:61, 1980.
704. Sheps SG, Colville DS: Occlusive renovsacular disease. *Cardiovasc Clin* 13:219, 1983.

705. Morin J, Hutchinson T, Lisbona R: Long-term prognosis of surgical treatment of renovascular hypertension: A fifteen-year experience. *J Vasc Surg* 3:545, 1986.
706. Jordan ML, Novick AC, Cunningham RL: The role of renal autotransplantation in pediatric and young adult patients with renal artery disease. *J Vasc Surg* 2:385, 1985.
707. Fowl RJ, Hollier LH, Bernatz PE, et al: Repeat vascularization versus nephrectomy in the treatment of recurrent renovascular hypertension. *Surg Gynecol Obstet* 162:37, 1986.
708. Stanley JC: Renal vascular disease and renovascular hypertension in children. *Urol Clin North Am* 11:451, 1984.
709. Dean RH, Krueger TC, Whiteneck JM, et al: Operative management of renovascular hypertension: Results after 15–23 years follow-up. *J Vasc Surg* 1:234, 1984.
710. Dean RH, Englund R, Dupont WD, et al: Retrieval of renal function by revascularization: Study of preoperative outcome predictors. *Ann Surg* 202:367, 1985.
711. Bardram L, Helgstrand U, Bentzen MH, et al: Late results after surgical treatment of renovascular hypertension: A follow-up study of 122 patients 2–18 years after surgery. *Ann Surg* 201:219, 1985.
712. Starr DS, Lawrie GM, Morris GCJ: Surgical treatment of renovascular hypertension: Long-term follow-up of 216 patients up to 20 years. *Arch Surg* 115:494, 1980.
713. Stanley JC, Whitehouse WMJ, Zelenock GB, et al: Reoperation for complications of renal artery reconstructive surgery undertaken for treatment of renovascular hypertension. *J Vasc Surg* 2:133,1985.
714. Ferriss JB, Beevers DG, Brown JJ, et al: Low-renin (primary) hyperaldosteronism. *Am Heart J* 95:641, 1978.
715. Conn JW, Hinerman DL: Spironolactone-induced inhibitions of aldosterone biosynthesis in primary aldosteronism: Morphological and functional studies. *Metabolism* 26:1293, 1971.
716. Streeten DHP, Tomycz N, Anderson GHJ: Reliability of screening methods for primary aldosteronism. *Am J Med* 67:412, 1979.
717. Hiramatsu K, Yamada T, Yukumura Y, et al: A screening test to identify aldosterone-producing adenoma by measuring plasma renin activity. *Arch Intern Med* 141:1589, 1981.
718. Gordon R, Stowasser M, Tunny T, et al: High incidence of primary aldosteronism in 199 patients referred with hypertension. High Blood Pressure Research Council of Australia, Australia, 1993, *Clin Experi. Pharmacol Physiol,* 21: 315, 1994.
719. Irony I, Kater C, Biglieri E, et al: Correctable subsets of primary aldosteronism: Primary adrenal hyperplasia and renin responsive adenoma. *Am J Hypertens* 3:576, 1990.
720. Nomura K, Toraya S, Horiba N, et al: Plasma aldosterone response to upright posture and angiotensin II infusion in aldosterone-producing adenoma. *J Clin Endocrinol Metab* 75:323, 1992.
721. Noth R, Biglieri E: Primary aldosteronism. *Med Clin North Am* 72:1117, 1988.
722. Biglieri E, Irony I, Kater C: Identification and implications of new types of mineralocorticoid hypertension. *J Steroid Biochem* 32:199, 1989.
723. Fontes R, Kater C, Biglieri E, et al: Reassessment of the predictive value of the posture test in primary aldosteronism. *Am J Hypertens* 4:786, 1991.
724. Ganguly A, Melada G, Leutscher J, et al: Control of plasma aldosterone in primary aldosteronism: Distinction between adenoma and hyperplasia. *J Clin Endocrinol Metab* 37:765, 1973.
725. Kater CE, Biglieri EG, Rost CR, Schambelan M, Hirai J, Chang BCF, Brust N: The constant plasma 18-hydroxycorticosterone to aldosterone ratio: An expression of the efficacy of corticosterone methyloxidase type II activity in disorders with variable aldosterone production. *J Clin Endocrinol Metab* 60:225, 1985.
726. Banks W, Kastin A, Ruiz A, et al: Primary adrenal hyperplasia: A new subset of primary aldosteronism. *J Clin Endocrinol Metab* 58:783, 1984.
727. Gordon R, Gomez-Sanchez C, Hamlet S, et al: Angiotensin responsive aldosterone producing adenoma masquerades as idiopathic hyperaldosteronism or low-renin essential hypertension. *J Hypertens* 5(Suppl 5):S103, 1987.
728. Lifton R, Dluhy R, Power M, et al: A chimeric 11-hydroxylase/aldosterone synthetase gene causes glucocorticoid-remediable aldosteronism and human hypertension. *Nature* 355:262, 1992.
729. Melby JC: Primary aldosteronism. *Kidney Int* 26:769, 1984.
729a. Gordon R, Ziesak M, Tunny T, et al: Evidence that primary aldesteronism may not be uncommon: 12% incidence among antihypertensive drug trial volunteers. *Clin Exp Pharm Physiol* 20:296, 1993.
730. Baer L, Sommers SC, Krakoff LR, et al: Pseudoprimary aldosteronism: An entity distinct from true aldosteronism. *Circ Res* 26/27(Suppl 1):203, 1970.
731. Biglieri E, Schambelan M, Slanton P, et al: The intercurrent hypertension of primary aldosteronism. *Circ Res* 20/21:I-195, 1970.
732. Hunt TK, Schambelan M, Biglieri EG: Selection of patients and operative approach in primary aldosteronism. *Ann Surg* 182:353, 1975.
733. Kulkarni J, Nistry R, Kamat M, et al: Autonomous aldosterone-secreting ovarian tumor. *Gynecol Oncol* 37:284, 1990.
734. Stowasser M, Gordon R, Tunny T, et al: Familiar hyper aldosteronism type II: Five families with a new variety of primary aldosteronism. *Clin Exp Pharmacol Physiol* 19(5):319, 1992.
735. Gross M, Shapiro B: Clinical review 50: Clinically silent adrenal masses. *J Clin Endocrinol Metab* 77:885, 1993.
736. Tunny T, Gordon R, Klemm S, et al: Histological and biochemical distinctiveness of atypical aldosterone-producing adenomas responsive to upright posture and angiotensin. *Clin Endocrinol (Oxf)* 34:363, 1991.
737. Stowasser M, Tunny T, Klemm S, et al: Cortisol production by aldosterone-producing adenomas *in vitro*. *Clin Exp Pharmacol Physiol* 20:292, 1993.
738. Hamlet S, Gordon R, Gomez-Sanchez C, et al: Adrenal transitional zone steroids, 18-oxo and 18-hydroxycortisol, useful in the diagnosis of primary aldosteronism, are ACTH-dependent. *Clin Exp Pharmacol Physiol* 15:317, 1988.
739. Gordon R, Stowasser M, Martin N, et al: Karyotypic abnormalities in benign adrenocortical tumors producing aldosterone. *Cancer Genet Cytogenet* 68:78, 1993.
740. Stockigt JR, Collins RD, Biglieri EG: Determination of plasma renin concentration by angiotensin immunoassay: Diagnostic import of precise measurement of subnormal renin in hyperaldosteronism. *Circ Res* 28/29(Suppl 2):175, 1971.
741. Cain JP, Tuck ML, Williams GH, et al: The regulation of aldosterone secretion in primary aldosteronism. *Am J Med* 53:627, 1972.
742. Pascoe L, Curnow K, Slutsker L, et al: Glucocorticoid-suppressible hyperaldosteronism results from hybrid genes created by unequal crossovers between Cyp11B1 and CYP11B2. *Proc Natl Acad Sci USA* 89:8327, 1992.
743. Miyahara K. Kawamoto T, Mitsuuchi Y, et al: The chimeric gene linked to glucocorticoid suppressible hyperaldosteronism encodes a fused P-450 protein possessing aldosterone synthetase activity. *Biochem Biophys Res Commun* 189:885, 1992.
744. Rich G, Ulick S, Cook S, et al: Glucocorticoid-remediable aldosteronism in a large kindred: Clinical spectrum and diagnosis using a characteristic biochemical phenotype. *Ann Intern Med* 116:813, 1992.
745. Gomez-Sanchez C, Gill J, Ganguly A, et al: Glucocorticoid-suppressible aldosteronism: A disorder of the transitional zone. *J Clin Endocrinol Metab* 67:444, 1988.
746. Schambelan M, Brust NL, Chang BCF, et al: Circadian rhythm and effect of posture on plasma aldosterone concentration in primary aldosteronism. *J Clin Endocrinol Metab* 43:115, 1976.

747. Stockight J, Scoggins B: Long term evolution of glucocorticoid-suppressible hyperaldosteronism. *J Clin Endocrinol Metab* 64:22, 1987.
748. Biglieri EG, Slaton PE, Schambelan M, et al: Hypermineralocorticism. *Am J Med* 45:170, 1968.
749. Gordon R, Tunny T: Aldosterone-producing-adenoma (A-P-A): Effect of pregnancy. *Clin Exp Hypertens [A]* 4:1685, 1982.
750. Bravo E: Primary aldosteronism: New approaches to diagnosis and management. *Cleve Clin J Med* 60:379, 1993.
751. Biglieri EG, Stockigt JR, Schambelan M: Adrenal mineralocorticoids causing hypertension. *Am J Med* 52:623, 1972.
752. Himathongkam T, Dluhy RG, Williams GH: Potassium-aldosterone-renin interrelationships. *J Clin Endocrinol Metab* 41:115, 1976.
753. Biglieri EG: Effect of posture on plasma concentrations of aldosterone in hypertension and primary hyperaldosteronism. *Nephron* 23:112, 1979.
754. Nadler JL, Hsueh W, Horton R: Therapeutic effect of calcium channel blockade in primary aldosteronism. *J Clin Endocrinol Metab* 60:1896, 1985.
755. Weinberger M, Fineberf N: The diagnosis of primary aldosteronism and separation of two major subtypes. *Arch Intern Med* 153:2125, 1993.
756. Hambling C, Jung R, Gunn A, et al: Re-evaluation of the captopril test for the diagnosis of primary aldosteronism. *Clin Endocrinol (Oxf)* 36:499, 1992.
756a. Opocher G, Rocco S, Carpene G, et al: Different diagnosis in primary aldosteronism. *J Steroid Biochem* 45:49, 1993.
757. Horton R: Stimulation and suppression of aldosterone in plasma of normal man and in primary aldosteronism. *J Clin Invest* 48:1230, 1969.
758. Kem DC, Weinberger MH, Mayes DM, et al: Saline suppression of plasma aldosterone in hypertension. *Arch Intern Med* 128:380, 1971.
759. Scoggins BA, Odie CJ, Hare WSC, et al: Preopreative lateralization of aldosterone producing tumors in primary aldosteronism. *Ann Intern Med* 76:891, 1972.
760. Horton R, Frinck E: Diagnosis and localization in primary aldosteronism. *Ann Intern Med* 76:885, 1972.
761. Geisinger MA, Zelch MG, Bravo EL, et al: Primary hyperaldosteronism: Comparison of CT, adrenal venography, and venous sampling. *AJR* 141:299, 1983.
762. Bleason P, Weinberger M, Pratt J, et al: Evaluation of diagnostic tests in the differential diagnosis of primary aldosteronism. *J Urol* 150:1365, 1993.
763. Dunnick N, Leight GJ, Roubidoux M, et al: CT in the diagnosis of primary aldosteronism: Sensitivity in 29 patients. *AJR* 160:321, 1993.
764. Rossi G-P, Chiesura-Corona M, Tregnaghi A, et al: Imaging of aldosterone-secreting adenomas: A prospective comparison of computed tomography and magnetic resonance imaging in 27 patients with suspected primary aldosteronism. *J Hum Hypertens* 7:357, 1993.
765. Doppman J, Gill J, Miller D, et al: Distinction between hyperaldosteronism due to bilateral hyperplasia and unilateral aldosteronoma: Reliability of CT. *Radiology* 184:677, 1992.
766. Kazeroomi E, Sisson J, Shapiro B, et al: Diagnostic accuracy and pitfalls of $[^{131}I]6\beta$-iodomethyl-19-norcholesterol (NP59) imaging. *J Nucl Med* 31:526, 1990.
767. Connell M, Fraser R: Adrenal corticosteroid synthesis and hypertension. *J Hypertens* 9:97, 1991.
768. Takeda Y, Miyamori I, Iki K, et al: Urinary excretion of 19-noraldosterone, 18, 19-dihydrocorticosterone and 18-hydroxy-19-norcorticosterone in patients with aldosterone-producing adenoma or idiopathic hyperaldosteronism. *Acta Endocrinol (Copenh)* 126:484, 1992.
769. Gordon R, Stowasser M, Tunny T, et al: Clinical and pathological diversity of primary aldosteronism, including a new familial variety. *Clin Exp Pharmacol Physiol* 18:283, 1991.
770. Vetter H, Siebenschein R, Studer A, et al: Primary aldosteronism: Inability to differentiate unilateral from bilateral adrenal lesions by various routine clinical and laboratory data and by peripheral plasma aldosterone. *Acta Endocrinol (Copenh)* 89:710, 1978.
771. Arteage E, Klein R, Biglieri EG: Use of the saline infusion test to diagnose the cause of primary aldosteronism. *Am J Med* 79:722, 1985.
772. Ulick S, Blumenfeld J, Atlas S, et al: The unique steroidogenesis of the aldosteronoma in the differential diagnosis of primary aldosteronism. *J Clin Endocrinol Metab* 76:873, 1993.
773. Higashihara E, Tanaka Y, Horie S, et al: Laproscopic adrenalectomy: The initial three cases. *J Urol* 149:973, 1993.
774. Sardi A, McKinnon W: Laproscopic adrenalectomy for primary aldosteronism. *JAMA* 269:989, 1993.
775. Franco-Saenz R, Mulrow PJ, Kin K: Idiopathic aldosteronism: A possible disease of the intermediate lobe of the pituitary. *JAMA* 251:2555, 1984.
776. Itoh N, Kumamoto Y, Akagashi K, et al: Study of the predictive factors of postoperative blood pressure in cases with primary aldosteronism. *Nippon Naibunpi Gakkai Zasshi* 67:1211, 1991.
777. Morimoto S, Takeda R, Murakami M: Does prolonged treatment with large doses of spironolactone hasten recovery of juxtaglomerular adrenal suppression in primary aldosteronism? *J Clin Endocrinol Metab* 31:659, 1970.
778. Ganguly A, Zager PG, Luetscher JA: Primary aldosteronism due to unilateral hyperplasia. *J Clin Endocrinol Metab* 51:1190, 1980.
779. Horton R, Hsueh WA: Treatment of hyperaldosteronism, in Krieger D, Barden CW (eds): *Current Therapy in Endocrinology*. Philadelphia, Mosby, 1983, p 127.
780. Ferriss JB, Bleevers DG, Boddy K, et al: The treatment of low-renin ("primary") hyperaldosteronism. *Am Heart J* 96: 97, 1978.
781. Bravo EL, Fouad FM, Tarazi RC: Calcium channel blockade with nifedipine in primary aldosteronism. *Hypertension* 8(Suppl 1):1191, 1986.
782. Gordon R, Hawkins P, Hamlet S, et al: Reduced adrenal secretory mass after unilateral adrenalectomy for aldosterone-producing adenoma may explain unexpected incidence of hypotension. *J Hypertens* 7:S210, 1989.
783. George JM, Wright L, Bell NH, et al: The syndrome of primary aldosteronism. *Am J Med* 48:343, 1970.
784. Grim CE, Weinberger MH, Kanand S: Familial dexamethasone-suppressible normokalemic hyperaldosteronism, in New MI, Levine LS (eds): *Juvenile Hypertension*. New York, Raven Press, 1977, p 109.
785. New MI, Seaman MP: Secretion rates of cortisol and aldosterone precursors in various forms of congenital adrenal hyperplasia. *J Clin Endocrinol Metab* 30:361, 1970.
786. Bongiovanni AM, Root AW: The adrenogenital syndrome. *N Engl J Med* 268:1283, 1963.
787. Levine LS, Rauh W, Gottesdiener K, et al: New studies of the β-hydroxylase and 18-hydroxylase enzymes in the hypertensive form of congenital adrenal hyperplasia. *J Clin Endocrinol Metab* 50:258, 1980.
788. New MI: Male pseudohermaphroditism due to 17α-hydroxylase deficiency. *J Clin Invest* 49:1930, 1970.
789. Biglieri EG, Mantero F: The characteristics, course and implications of the 17 hydroxylation deficiency in man, in Finkelstein Jungblut P, Klopper A, Conti C (eds): *Research on Steriods*. Rome, Societa Editrice Universo, 1973, vol 5, p 385.
790. Kondo K, Saruta T, Saito I, et al: Benign desoxycorticosterone-producing adrenal tumor. *JAMA* 236:1042, 1976.
791. Irony I, Biglieri E, Perloff D, et al: Pathophysiology of deoxycorticosterone-secreting adrenal tumors. *J Clin Endocrinol Metab* 65:836, 1987.
792. Blachley JD, Knochel JP: Tobacco chewer's hypokalemia licorice revisited. *N Engl J. Med* 302:784, 1980.
793. Chobanian AV, Volicer L. Tifft CP, et al: Mineralocorticoid-

induced hypertension in patients with orthostatic hypotension. *N Engl J Med* 301:68, 1979.
794. Ulick S, Levine LS, Gunczler P, et al: A syndrome of apparent mineralocorticoid excess associated with defects in the peripheral metabolism of cortisol. *J Clin Endocrinol Metab* 49:757, 1979.
795. Oberfield SE, Levine LS, Carey RM, et al: Metabolic and blood pressure responses to hydocortisone in the syndrome of apparent mineralocorticoid excess. *J Clin Endocrinol Metab* 56:332, 1983.
796. Botero-Veltz M, Curtis J, Warnock D: Brief report: Liddle's syndrome revisited—a disorder of sodium reabsorption in the distal tubule. *N Engl J Med* 330:178, 1994.
797. Chrousos G, Laue L, Mioeman L, et al: Gulcocorticoids and glucocorticoid antagonists: Lessons from RU 486. *Kidney Int* 34(Suppl 26):S18, 1988.
798. Whitworth J: Mechanisms of glucocorticoid-induced hypertension. *Kidney Int* 31:1213, 1987.

CHAPTER 15

Glucocorticoid Therapy

J. Blake Tyrrell

Glucocorticoids are among the most commonly used drugs. They are employed to treat a number of medical problems, varying from self-limited processes such as poison ivy, poison oak, and other hypersensitivity reactions to life-threatening problems such as leukemia. A partial list of these conditions is shown in Table 15-1.[1] Christy estimated in 1971[2] that 5 million persons in the United States receive some form of steroids (Fig. 15-1) annually in therapy. The overall use has, if anything, increased with the expanding population. Because of such extensive use and the numerous conditions for which steroids are given, glucocorticoid-treated patients are encountered in all medical and surgical specialties.

Although glucocorticoids have many beneficial influences, their use is frequently accompanied by deleterious side effects. Physicians must be aware of these effects and must exercise judgment in the decision to use steroids in the first place. It is also important to be aware of methods for reducing the total dosage by manipulating the timing and route of administration while maximizing adjunctive measures. This allows maximum therapeutic benefit while minimizing adverse effects. Many of the sequelae of long-term glucocorticoid therapy are similar to those of the diseases for which steroids are given (weakness, bruising, etc.). Thus, clinicians must also know the features that can be helpful in differentiating the cause of such disturbances in glucocorticoid-treated patients.

Many endocrinologists encounter steroid-treated patients less commonly than do other specialists (e.g., nephrologists, rheumatologists, dermatologists), yet the endocrinologist commonly is asked to evaluate whether clinical stigmata are due to the steroid or to another process and to give advice on therapy or its withdrawal. An endocrinologist is also asked to evaluate the hypothalamic-pituitary-adrenal axis, which may be suppressed in glucocorticoid-treated patients, and to give advice on patient management in such situations.

Over the past 20 years, much has been learned about the pharmacokinetics of glucocorticoids and the mechanisms by which these steroids elicit their diverse effects (Chap. 12). This knowledge, although incomplete, is helping physician's formulate more rational approaches to steroid therapy. This may increase the scope of steroid use in therapy and diminish the deleterious effects.

In this chapter, the pharmacology of the glucocorticoids is reviewed with the hope of providing a rational basis for the use of these steroids in therapy. For the most part, specific clinical indications for glucocorticoid administration are avoided, as they require discussions of the particular diseases that are found in the literature about them.

PHYSIOLOGIC AND PHARMACOLOGIC ACTIONS OF GLUCOCORTICOIDS IN RELATION TO STEROID THERAPY

Therapeutic Influences

The diverse actions of the glucocorticoids and the manifestations of excessive concentrations are detailed in Chap. 12. Several different types of these actions are exploited in glucocorticoid therapy.

In most circumstances, the anti-inflammatory and/or immunosuppressive actions of the glucocorticoids are responsible for the therapeutic response. As detailed in Chap. 12, glucocorticoids can affect nearly every component involved in the inflammatory and immunologic response, although in humans some components are more sensitive than others (e.g., cell-mediated more than humoral responses) (for a review, see Refs. 3 and 4). It is less clear which particular responses account for the beneficial therapeutic influences. For instance, the anti-inflammatory actions are clearly important when steroids are given topically for inflammatory conditions. Thus, certain skin diseases benefit from glucocorticoid therapy because the inflammatory response to the offending agent is excessive. In other cases (e.g., lupus erythematosus, other collagen vascular disorders, transplant rejection, and the nephrotic syndrome), it is not clear whether immunosuppressive or anti-inflammatory actions are more important. In general, glucocorticoid therapy for conditions of ex-

TABLE 15-1 Selected Clinical Conditions for Which Glucocorticoids Are Used

Addison's disease: replacement therapy	Eye diseases
Adrenal hyperplasia due to enzymatic defects (e.g., 11β-, 17α-, and 21-hydroxylase syndromes)	Acute uveitis
Allergic diseases	Allergic conjunctivitis
Angioneurotic edema	Choroiditis
Bee stings	Optic neuritis
Contact dermatitis	Gastrointestinal diseases
Drug reactions	Inflammatory bowel disease
Hay fever	Nontropical sprue
Serum sickness	Regional enteritis
Urticaria	Subacute hepatic necrosis
Arthritis, bursitis, and tenosynovitis; inflammatory complications of a variety of types of arthritis	Ulcerative colitis
Blood dyscrasias	Hypercalcemia (e.g., due to sarcoidosis; most hypercalcemias not responsive)
Acquired hemolytic anemia	Infections (occasionally helpful to suppress excessive inflammation)
Allergic purpura	Malignant exophthalmos
Autoimmune hemolytic anemia	Neurologic diseases
Idiopathic thrombocytopenic purpura	Pulmonary diseases
Lymphoblastic leukemia	Aspiration pneumonia
Multiple myeloma	Bronchial asthma
Collagen vascular disorders	Infant respiratory distress syndrome
Giant cell arteritis	Sarcoidosis
Lupus erythematosus	Renal diseases: certain nephrotic syndromes
Mixed connective tissue syndromes	Skin conditions
Polymyositis	Atopic dermatitis
Polymyalgia rheumatic	Dermatoses
Rheumatoid arthritis	Lichen simplex chronicus (localized neurodermatitis)
Temporal arteritis	Mycosis fungoides
	Pemphigus
	Seborrheic dermatitis
	Xerosis
	Transplantation: prevention of rejection

* This table is not meant to be comprehensive, nor are steroids always indicated for the condition listed.

Source: Baxter and Rousseau.[1]

cessive inflammatory and/or immunologic activity does not cure the primary condition but instead ameliorates its manifestations. Sometimes this "buys time" for the body's natural defenses to cure the problem or for more definitive therapy to work. Unfortunately, in many of the chronic problems for which glucocorticoids are used, the primary process is not curable by currently known measures and the manifestations return after the withdrawal of steroid therapy. As a result, in spite of symptomatic improvement, steroid therapy has no effect on the long-term prognosis or even worsens it.

When steroids are used to treat certain lymphoid cell malignancies, they act by killing or inhibiting the functions of lymphoid cells that mediate the response.[5,6] The different subpopulations of lymphoid cells vary markedly in their sensitivity to glucocorticoids (Chap. 12), and in humans under normal conditions (in contrast to certain animal species), glucocorticoids exhibit minimal lymphoid cell killing.[6] Thus, many leukemias are steroid-resistant. Acute lymphoblastic leukemia of childhood is the most commonly occurring steroid-sensitive leukemia, yet even this disease has a tendency to become steroid-resistant (see below).[5,6]

Whereas most malignancies are steroid-resistant, one occasionally observes patients with ordinarily steroid-resistant malignancies who respond to glucocorticoids. For instance, in a study of the preleukemic syndrome (hemopoietic dysplasia), 3 of 34 patients responded favorably to glucocorticoids.[7]

The actions of glucocorticoids on cell growth may also explain how these steroids inhibit solid tumors such as carcinomas of the breast and juvenile hemangiomas.[8]

In certain circumstances, glucocorticoid therapy is used not to affect the primary process but to ameliorate associated problems. For example, steroids are used to treat the hemolytic anemia that occurs in association with chronic granulocytic leukemia in

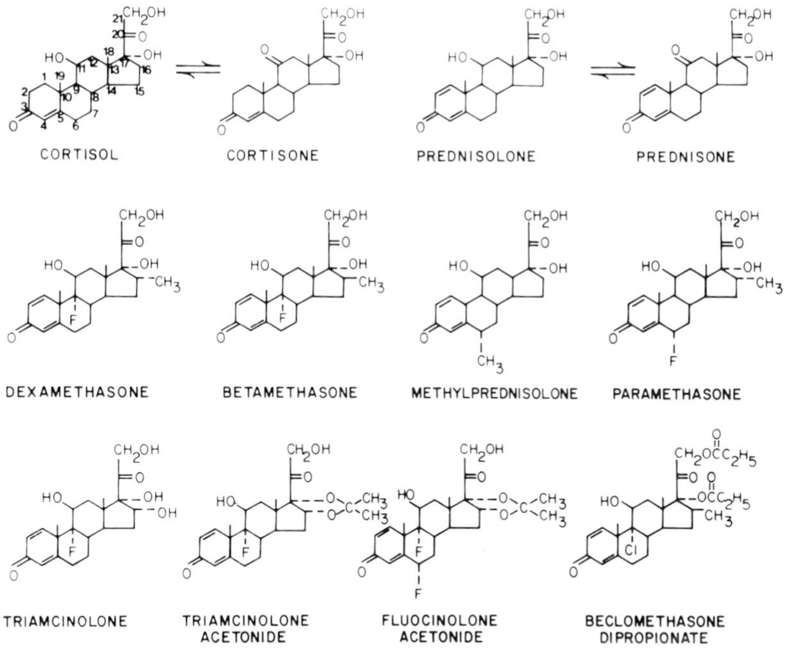

CORTISOL ⇌ CORTISONE PREDNISOLONE ⇌ PREDNISONE

DEXAMETHASONE BETAMETHASONE METHYLPREDNISOLONE PARAMETHASONE

TRIAMCINOLONE TRIAMCINOLONE ACETONIDE FLUOCINOLONE ACETONIDE BECLOMETHASONE DIPROPIONATE

FIGURE 15-1 Structures of some steroids commonly used for glucocorticoid therapy. The numbers of the carbon atoms are shown for cortisol (upper left). Arrows indicate the interconvertibility of cortisol and cortisone and of prednisolone and prednisone. Dotted lines indicate side groups in the α position; solid lines indicate steroids in the β position (see also Chap. 12).

adults[9] and to treat the hypercalcemias associated with malignancy or sarcoidosis (Chaps. 12 and 23).

Glucocorticoids are commonly used to treat patients with severe or moderately severe asthma (Fig. 15-2)[10–14] and some patients with chronic obstructive pulmonary disease.[15,16] Pulmonary function in asthma can improve after steroid administration, although several hours must pass for this to occur.[10,17] The improvement is due to one or a combination of several effects. First, the steroid may directly promote bronchodilation by sensitizing the bronchioles to β-adrenergic agonists (Chap. 12).[10,18] Second, glucocorticoids may also inhibit the production of bronchoconstrictor substances, such as leukotrienes, other eicosanoids (Chap. 12), and histamine,[11] generated by immunologic mechanisms. The suppression of phospholipase A_2 activity by glucocorticoids may be of critical importance in this respect (Chap. 12). Third, the steroid may suppress inflammatory responses in the lung and thus improve pulmonary function.[12]

FIGURE 15-2 Effect of hydrocortisone hemisuccinate (4 mg per kilogram of body weight, followed in some cases by 3 mg per kilogram of body weight at 3-h intervals and in other cases by a continuous intravenous infusion at 3 mg per kilogram of body weight every 6 h) and of cosyntropin depot (1 mg IM) on pulmonary function (FEV_1 and FVC) in acute asthma. *(From Collins et al.*[10]*)*

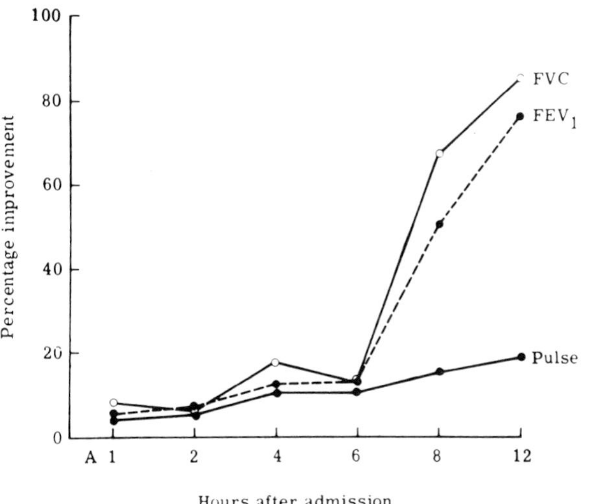

There are several examples of steroid actions not primarily directed at inflammatory or immunologic responses. For instance, in sarcoidosis, the steroid ameliorates the hypercalcemia by inhibiting the conversion of 25-hydroxycholecalciferol to 1α,25-dihydroxycholecalciferol (Chap. 23).[19] Glucocorticoids are used to decrease brain edema in some patients with brain tumors, meningitis, and other conditions[20–22] and are also beneficial in conditions such as acute mountain sickness (which is believed to be due to cerebral edema unassociated with inflammation).[23] The effectiveness of glucocorticoids in reducing damage resulting from spinal cord injury is probably not mediated by suppression of inflammation. The antiemetic actions of the steroids are sometimes useful in cancer chemotherapy.[24]

Adverse Influences

Glucocorticoids have a number of adverse influences that lead to Cushing's syndrome and limit their usefulness in therapy. These problems are discussed in

Chap. 12 and below. The actions on immunologic and inflammatory responses play a dominant role in generating these adverse effects because they increase the incidence and severity of infections.[25–28] However, the actions on carbohydrate metabolism, fibroblasts, bone, and other tissues are much more prominent in the pathogenesis of iatrogenic Cushing's syndrome than are the therapeutically beneficial responses.

MOLECULAR MECHANISMS FOR GLUCOCORTICOID-MEDIATED THERAPEUTIC INFLUENCES

Most physiologic and pharmacologic actions of glucocorticoids are mediated through intracellular receptors, termed "glucocorticoid receptors" that bind the steroid, associate with the nucleus, and then affect transcription of specific genes (for a review see Refs. 3 and 12 and Chaps. 5 and 12). The relative potency of steroids in eliciting therapeutic responses correlates with receptor-binding activities. The receptors are widely distributed and are generally present in the relevant target tissues thought to be involved in both therapeutic and deleterious glucocorticoid responses. Further, with lymphoblastic leukemia cells, as discussed above and in Chap. 12, loss of the glucocorticoid receptor is associated with unresponsiveness to glucocorticoids.[5] The existence of similar receptors in many different tissues explains how glucocorticoids can influence all these tissues.[29] The responses differ in the various tissues (e.g., killing in lymphoid cells and glucoconeogenesis in liver) because of postreceptor cellular differentiation (Chap. 12). The fact that the receptors are similar in different glucocorticoid-responsive tissues probably explains the failure of the pharmaceutical industry to find a steroid that when administered systemically has one type of beneficial therapeutic response (e.g., an immunosuppressive one) but does not have other deleterious ones (e.g., induction of osteoporosis); the compounds may bind to all the receptors and mediate all the responses. Thus, caution should be exercised in interpreting differential effects of various glucocorticoids as being due to qualitatively different actions, rather than to factors such as potency and duration of action.

As discussed in Chaps. 5, 12 and 14, some glucocorticoid actions are mediated through "mineralocorticoid receptors." These receptors are present in several different tissues in addition to the kidneys, and they regulate transcription in a manner analogous to the glucocorticoid receptors (Chaps. 5 and 12). Mineralocorticoid receptors regulate renal sodium and potassium transport, mostly in response to aldosterone. Cortisol and other steroids with glucocorticoid activity bind tightly to the mineralocorticoid receptors (Table 15-2). However, in the kidney, many of these steroids are prevented from acting through mineralocorticoid receptors due to local degradation. This degradation does not occur in some other tissues with mineralocorticoid receptors. Thus, some actions of glucocorticoids used in therapy could be mediated through nonrenal mineralocorticoid receptors, e.g., the feedback inhibition of ACTH release by glucocorticoids (Chap. 12). However, it is not known whether other therapeutic or deleterious actions of glucocorticoids are mediated through these receptors.

The sodium-retaining actions of various steroids mediated through mineralocorticoid receptors affect the selection of the steroid to be used in therapy. This selection is dictated by both the affinities of these steroids for the mineralocorticoid receptor (Table 15-2) and the stability of the steroids to metabolic degradation. The overall weaker mineralocorticoid activities of steroids such as prednisone, prednisolone, dexamethasone, and betamethasone (Chap. 12) constitute one reason why these steroids are ordinarily used in preference to cortisol.

Glucocorticoid responses usually require hours to days to be observed. These kinetics are consistent with a requirement for influences on macromolecular synthesis mediated through nuclear receptors.[29] Nevertheless, in some cases glucocorticoids act by mechanisms that do not involve transcription [e.g., fast feedback of adrenocorticotropic hormone (ACTH) release; see Chap. 12]. The receptors that mediate this effect are not known.

TABLE 15-2 Affinities of Some Steroids for Human Glucocorticoid Receptors and Relative Mineralocorticoid-Glucocorticoid Receptor Affinities

Steroid	Affinity for Glucocorticoid receptor*	Mineralocorticoid/ Glucocorticoid Receptor Affinity Ratio*
Cortisol	1.0	1.0
Fludrocortisone	3.5	11.6
Triamcinolone acetonide	1.9	
Prednisolone	2.1	0.9
Betamethasone	5.4	0.8
Dexamethasone	7.1	0.2
Fluocinolone acetonide	11.4	

* Relative to cortisol.

Source: Data for human receptor binding from Ballard PL, Carter JP, Graham BS, Baxter JD: A radioreceptor assay for evaluation of the plasma glucocorticoid activity of natural and synthetic steroids in man. *J Clin Endocrinol Metab* 41:290, 1975. Data for the ratio of affinities using rat mineralocorticoid receptors and human glucocorticoid receptors for unpublished data of Lan NC, Matulich DT, and Baxter JD.

KINETIC CONSIDERATIONS

The actions of glucocorticoids through their specific receptors and the subsequent modulation of DNA transcription require some time before a response is observed (Chap. 12). Similarly, in terminating the response, some time is required for the steroid to leave the circulation. When this occurs, dissociation of the steroid from the receptor occurs within a few minutes,[29] resulting in the termination of further steroid action. However, some time is required for the levels of the induced mRNAs and their protein products to return to baseline before the response is terminated.[30] Further, the response may be even more prolonged because the steroid might have induced other factors that affect transcription; thus, a stimulation of transcription may occur for some time after removal of the steroid because of the period required for the concentrations of these factors to decrease to basal levels. The time required for induced mRNAs and proteins to return to basal levels depends on their rates of turnover.[30] These rates vary for different mRNAs. The rates of protein and mRNA turnover also affect the kinetics of induction (for a discussion, see Ref. 30 and Chap. 12); for steroid-regulated mRNAs and proteins that turn over with a long half-life, a longer time is required for the response to reach a maximum (and to terminate) than is the case with the more rapidly turning over macromolecules. Thus, there may be considerable variation in the time required for the onset and disappearance of various glucocorticoid responses; these variations form the basis for alternate-day steroid therapy (discussed below) and emphasize that the kinetics of each response must be determined independently in order to develop the most rational approach to glucocorticoid therapy.

MANIFESTATIONS OF IATROGENIC CUSHING'S SYNDROME

Comparisons with Spontaneous Cushing's Syndrome

The clinical features of iatrogenic Cushing's syndrome are similar to those of spontaneous Cushing's syndrome with several exceptions (Chap. 12). In fact, since many patients receive very high doses over prolonged periods, the symptoms and signs are commonly more prominent than is the case with spontaneous Cushing's syndrome. Thus, there can be weight gain with redistribution of fat to the truncal areas, "moon face," plethora, "buffalo hump," thin skin, easy bruising, osteoporosis, avascular necrosis, striae, poor wound healing, increased incidence of infections, psychiatric problems, myopathy and muscular weakness, decreased carbohydrate tolerance, negative nitrogen balance, renal calculi, and other stigmata. An extensive analysis of these and other factors and of the pathophysiology is provided in Chap. 12.

The major differences between iatrogenic and spontaneous Cushing's syndrome (unless ACTH therapy is used) relate to the presence of androgens and mineralocorticoids, Since adrenal androgen excess is not present in the iatrogenic syndrome, the hirsutism and other virilizing features are not observed. However, glucocorticoid-treated individuals develop an increase in fine lanugo hair on the face and elsewhere.[31] Steroids with less mineralocorticoid potency (relative to their glucocorticoid potency) than cortisol are ordinarily used for steroid therapy (Table 15-2). Further, steroids with mineralocorticoid potency, such as 11-deoxycorticosterone (DOC), are sometimes present in excess in spontaneous Cushing's syndrome (Chaps. 12 and 14). Thus, the features of mineralocorticoid excess—hypertension and hypokalemia (Chap. 14)—are much less common in the iatrogenic syndrome. However, in iatrogenic Cushing's syndrome there is an increased frequency of hypertension (Chaps. 12 and 14), and fluid retention can be exaggerated in patients with congestive heart failure (Chap. 12).

Whereas steroid-treated patients can become euphoric or depressed, it appears that euphoria is more common in iatrogenic than in spontaneous Cushing's syndrome. In some individuals, this may be due to improvement in the disease for which steroids were given; however, others develop euphoria without any detectable beneficial effect on the primary disease.[2,21,32]

It has been reported that several other features are unique to iatrogenic Cushing's syndrome.[2,33] Some of these features are uncommon; they include benign intracranial hypertension, pancreatitis, and vasculitis. Although it has been reported that an increased incidence of glaucoma and avascular necrosis of bone (discussed below) is unique to the iatrogenic syndrome,[2,34] glaucoma has been reported[35] and some authors have observed avascular necrosis of bone in the spontaneous syndrome. Whereas this deposition of fat in various body areas in Cushing's syndrome is well known, excessive deposition of fat around the spinal cord has been reported rarely in iatrogenic Cushing's syndrome.[36,37]

Ocular Changes

Posterior subcapsular cataracts occur commonly in both pediatric and adult steroid-treated individuals (Chap. 12), especially with prolonged treatment.[38–42] As discussed in Chap. 12, there is some evidence that steroid-induced cataract may be a result of the formation of covalent complexes between the steroids and lens proteins.[43]

Steroid-induced increases in intraocular pressure with subsequent development of glaucoma occur in a subset of patients who are susceptible to this action.[38,39] There are a significant number of these individuals,[38] and all glucocorticoid-treated patients should be monitored for changes in intraocular pressure.

Avascular Necrosis of Bone

Avascular or ischemic necrosis of bone has been reported in up to 50 percent of patients in some series and is apparently related more to the dose than to the duration of therapy.[44,45] It is also more prevalent in patients with vasculitis and Raynaud's phenomenon, although it also occurs frequently with steroid therapy in other conditions, such as in transplant recipients.[44–46] It has been proposed that this complication is due to steroid-induced enlargement of intramedullary lipocytes, with resulting pressure on the bone leading to ischemia.[44–46]

Osteoporosis

Osteoporosis is one of the major limitations of long-term glucocorticoid therapy (see also Chap. 24).[2,47,48] The precise prevalence is difficult to determine, but most patients on chronic therapy develop decreased bone density when studied by sophisticated methods.[49,50] In a study of patients with rheumatoid arthritis who were given prednisone in a mean daily dose of 7.5 mg/day for 20 weeks, bone density of the lumbar spine decreased by 8% and this was partially reversible after discontinuation of the steroid.[49] In another study, about two-thirds of patients receiving chronic glucocorticoid therapy were classified as having osteoporosis.[50] In addition, many of these patients develop fractures. In a study of asthmatic patients who received steroids for at least a year, 11 percent developed fractures, compared with none of the control patients; in a prospective study, 8 of 19 patients and none of 11 control patients had fractures.[51] The long-term steroid-treated patients also had decreased trabecular but not cortical bone density, as measured by photon absorptiometry (Fig. 15-3).[51] Further, alternate-day steroid therapy (see below) did not protect them against osteoporosis.[52]

The pattern of bone loss due to glucocorticoids is similar to that seen with primary hyperparathyroidism but differs from that observed in idiopathic osteoporosis (Fig. 15-4) (see also Chap. 24). The osteoporosis is most prominent in trabecular bone, with less dramatic changes in the more slowly turning over cortical bone.[48–52] Thus, the most pronounced bone loss occurs in the axial skeleton, such as the ribs and vertebrae, rather than in the long bones. Steroid-induced bone loss is more profound in patients with previously reduced bone mineral, such as postmenopausal or oophorectomized women; alcoholics in whom endogenous hypercortisolism may already be contributing to bone loss[53]; patients with bowel disease and decreased calcium absorption; and those with liver or renal disease and impaired vitamin D metabolism (Chap. 24). Children are also susceptible to steroid-induced osteopenia, presumably because of their lower bone mass and higher initial bone turnover.[47,54] The mechanisms of corticosteroid-induced bone loss are discussed in Chap. 12.

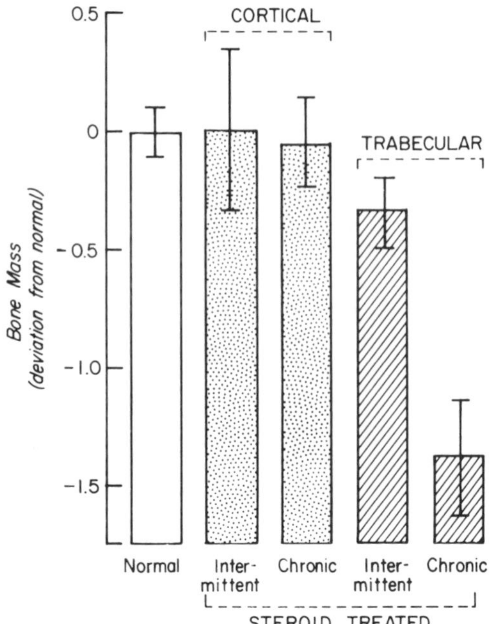

FIGURE 15-3 Trabecular and cortical bone mass in control and glucocorticoid-treated asthmatic patients. Bone mass was measured by single-photon absorption and was calculated by dividing the bone mineral content by bone width. Trabecular mass was taken from a metaphyseal site 2 cm proximal to the distal end of the ulnar styloid process, which contains a large proportion of trabecular bone. Cortical mass was taken from a diaphyseal site one-third the distance from the distal to the proximal end of the ulna, which is composed primarily of cortical bone. The bone mass is expressed as a fraction of the standard deviation of the mean of the normal value for the patient's sex and decade of age (*z* score). "Intermittent" refers to patients who had received intermittent courses of steroids but who did not require constant treatment for as long as a year. "Chronic" refers to patients who received daily or alternate-day corticosteroids for 1 year or more or at least eight short courses for 10 days or less of high-dose steroids for as long as a year. (*Data taken from Adinoff and Hollister.*[51])

Prevention and treatment of glucocorticoid osteopenia have been unsatisfactory and controversial.[55–58] However, several promising studies have been reported and hold promise for future long-term regimens. Bone density studies should be performed before the initiation of glucocorticoid therapy if long-term or high-dose treatment is being contemplated or if the patient has other risk factors for osteoporosis. In addition, every effort should be directed toward minimizing the dose and the duration of ther-

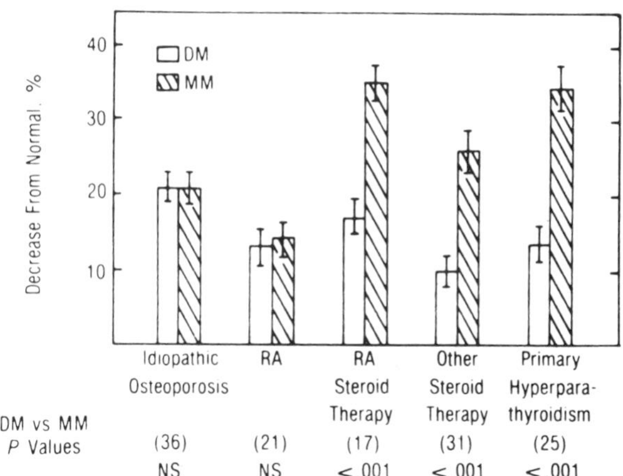

FIGURE 15-4 Decrease in bone mass (percent decrease from normal) estimated by photon absorption measurements of bone mass in the midshaft diaphyseal site (DM) and the distal metaphyseal site (MM) in patients with idiopathic osteoporosis, rheumatoid arthritis (RA) that was not treated or was treated with glucocorticoids, and primary hyperparathyroidism. Vertical bars indicate mean percent decrease from normal for age and sex (±SEM). Number of patients studied is indicated in parentheses. (*From Hahn.*[54])

apy, and if possible, topical or inhaled corticosteroids should be used in conjunction with other ancillary therapies.

Dietary calcium intake should be supplemented to a total intake of 1200 to 1500 mg of elemental calcium per day, and vitamin D should be given in a minimum dose of 400 U/day. Appropriate replacement therapy for decreased gonadal function also retards bone loss, and serial assessment of gonadal function should be undertaken since glucocorticoids in excess suppress gonadotropin secretion and gonadal function (Chap. 12).

Treatment with pharmacologic doses of vitamin D and its active metabolites can restore intestinal calcium absorption and suppress the secondary hyperparathyroidism. The doses used have been ergocalciferol 50,000 U three times weekly,[59] calcifidiol (25-hydroxyvitamin D) 40 μg/day,[58,59] and calcitriol (1, 25-dihydroxyvitamin D) 0.5 to 1.0 μg/day.[60] The risks of this therapy include hypercalcemia (especially with calcitriol) and hypercalcuria, which can occur with all forms of vitamin D and is correctable with thiazide diuretics.[52,58–60]

In addition, antiresorptive agents such as calcitonin and biphosphonates may be useful. Salmon calcitonin given either by injection or intranasally was useful in both the prevention and the treatment of glucocorticoid oseteopenia.[61] The bisphosphonates etidronate and pamidronate have also been reported to prevent bone loss in steroid-treated patients.[62,63]

Finally, fluoride salts have been used to increase bone formation in glucocorticoid-treated patients.[58,64] However, long-term efficacy has not been established.

In summary, promising data are emerging which suggest that glucocorticoid-induced osteopenia may be prevented, at least in part. However, longer-term controlled studies will be required to determine appropriate treatment regimens.

Infections

Infections are a major problem with long-term glucocorticoid therapy (Chap. 12).[2,26–28,65–67] Several types of infections can occur (Chap. 12), including bacterial, viral, fungal, and parasitic; gram-negative and fungal infections appear to be particularly prevalent.[2,26–28,66] Except in specific situations (e.g., reactivation of quiescent tuberculosis, abscesses, osteomyelitis), it is not possible to predict the organism that will cause a complicating infection,[26] and opportunistic organisms can be responsible.[66] Hepatitis B virus poses a special concern because steroids are used to treat chronic active hepatitis[68] but can be harmful when this form of hepatitis is associated with hepatitis B surface antigen positivity.[69,70] Because glucocorticoids decrease the inflammatory response, it may be particularly difficult to detect and diagnose infections in glucocorticoid-treated individuals. The incidence, severity, and frequency of serious infections increase with both the dose and duration of steroid therapy.[67,71] Infectious complications may be decreased when alternate-day steroid therapy is used.[71] The mechanisms of glucocorticoid-mediated decreased host defense against infection are discussed in Chap. 12.

The probable increase in the incidence and severity of tuberculosis in steroid-treated patients with systemic disease has been of particular concern.[26,72] Diagnosis may be difficult in the presence of the systemic disease for which the steroid is administered, and in addition, the tuberculin response may be suppressed by glucocorticoids. However, reactivation of tuberculosis does not appear to occur with increased frequency in patients on long-term steroid therapy.[72] Thus, patients receiving glucocorticoids who are tuberculin-positive do not require antituberculosis therapy unless active disease is present.

Myopathy

Myopathy is a common manifestation of prolonged steroid therapy (Chap. 12).[2,33,73] The onset is usually gradual and often requires weeks or months to develop. It first affects the proximal muscles, although distal muscles can also be involved and muscle atrophy may be profound with prolonged high-dose therapy. Levels of serum enzymes [glutamic oxaloacetic transaminase (SGOT), creatine phosphokinase, and aldolase] are normal in glucocorticoid-induced myopathy, although they may be elevated in myopathy resulting from hypokalemia, polymyositis, or other causes.[73] However, creatine excretion is increased with glucocorticoid-induced and other myopathies, and its measurement can be useful. Muscle biopsy has not been shown to be helpful. Changes in muscle may also be monitored with the use of CT and isokinetic dynamic testing.[74] A study has suggested that glucocorticoid-induced muscle wasting can be reversed by physical training.[74] Thus, steroid-treated patients should exercise when possible.

Atherosclerosis

Atherosclerosis has not traditionally been considered a complication of glucocorticoid therapy. However, a body of retrospectively obtained data suggests that atherosclerosis is more prevalent in glucocortisol-treated individuals,[75] and in one study prednisone was found to be an independent risk factor for coronary artery disease.[76] In addition, patients with spontaneous Cushing's syndrome have an increased mortality from atherosclerotic disease.[77] Whether these atherogenic effects are due to a specific glucocorticoid effect or to the secondary effects of hypertension or hyperglycemia is unknown. Thus, the potential for increasing the rate of progression of atherosclerosis should be considered in the overall decision to administer glucocorticoids on a long-term basis.

Dose and Time Dependency and Reversibility

The manifestations of iatrogenic Cushing's syndrome are generally dose- and time-dependent, although the time required to develop particular features varies considerably. Further, some complications also occur less frequently with alternate-day therapy (see below). Increased appetite and euphoria can be observed within hours, whereas days to weeks are ordinarily required for the development of a cushingoid appearance. Effects on carbohydrate metabolism can occur within hours, although they become more pronounced with time (Chap. 12). The time required to develop an increased susceptibility to infections is not known, although it is likely that this happens within hours, since influences on leukocytes and other factors involved in inflammatory and immunologic responses occur by this time (Chap. 12). The development of frank osteoporosis[54–57,78] usually occurs after weeks or months of therapy, although occasional patients have experienced the onset of muscular weakness after a few days.[73] Psychiatric problems may develop soon after the institution of therapy or may develop later.[2,22,79–81] Other, rarer stigmata caused by glucocorticoid excess usually develop after weeks of therapy, although their appearance is unpredictable.

Most of the manifestations of glucocorticoid excess are reversible. Thus, within weeks to several months after the discontinuation of therapy, weight and fat distribution can return to normal, the skin changes and cushingoid appearance disappear, and muscular strength returns. The immunosuppressive and metabolic effects (e.g., on carbohydrate tolerance) return to normal within hours to days after the discontinuation of therapy. Unfortunately, the osteoporosis is not reversible with current therapy, even though further steroid-mediated bone destruction ceases.

DIAGNOSIS OF IATROGENIC CUSHING'S SYNDROME

The diagnosis of iatrogenic Cushing's syndrome is usually obvious from the clinical manifestations, the history of steroid therapy, and the finding of suppression of the hypothalamic-pituitary-adrenal axis (see below and Chap. 12). Thus, plasma cortisol and ACTH levels are low, and the rapid ACTH stimulation test result is subnormal.

DETERMINANTS OF GLUCOCORTICOID POTENCY

The potency of a steroid depends on its absorption ("bioavailability"), distribution, rate of metabolic clearance, concentration at sites of action, affinity for the glucocorticoid receptors, and ability to act as an agonist once it is bound (Chap. 12). It is important to consider each of these factors in using steroids for therapy.

Bioavailability

Most glucocorticoids are readily absorbed after oral administration. The estimates of fractional cortisol absorption expressed as bioavailability range from 0.45 to 0.8 (45 to 80 percent).[82] The absolute bioavailability of prednisolone from all forms of oral prednisone ranges from 77 to 99 percent.[82] Although glucocorticoid uptake is not impaired in most patients with intrinsic intestinal disease,[82] this can occur rarely, usually in association with severe disease.[83] Food intake does not have an appreciable effect on uptake.[82] Uptake is generally not impaired in renal or pulmonary disease.[82] Rare patients have decreased absorption of oral glucocorticoids in the absence of obvious bowel disease.

In the case of intramuscular (IM) injections, the uptake of steroids can vary markedly, depending on the preparation. For instance, triamcinolone acetonide is absorbed very slowly by the intramuscular route, and so the effect of a single injection may last for several weeks (see also Intrarticular Preparations, below).[84] Intramuscular injections of cortisone acetate do not reproducibly yield adequate blood levels of cortisol in the first 4 to 6 h after injection (Chap. 12),[85,86] although ultimately the steroid is absorbed. However, when more soluble derivatives of cortisol (e.g., hydrocortisone hemisuccinate) are injected IM, maximal cortisol levels are attained within an hour.[85,86] Thus, a physician must be aware of the properties of each preparation when the IM route is anticipated.

Inhaled glucocorticoids are highly effective in the treatment of asthma. Current preparations include beclomethasone dipropionate, triamcinolone acetonide, budesonide, and flunisolide. Their efficacy and systemic side effects vary with the method of administration and the dosage form.[12] Current types of inhaled steroid administration include metered-dose inhalers, large-volume spacer attachments, dry powder inhalers, and nebulizers. For current use, a metered-dose inhaler with a large-volume attachment is preferred since this method reduces the amount of the steroid deposited in the oropharynx and then swallowed and absorbed systemically. This method maximizes the dose delivered to the intrapulmonary airways while minimizing the total systemic dose.[12] When a steroid is inhaled, peak plasma concentrations are achieved within an hour and plasma half-life is about 2 h.[12]

Compounds topically administered to the skin must penetrate the keratin layer of the stratum corneum to reach the squamous cell layer of the epidermis; high lipid solubility favors such penetration. For instance, the more lipophilic triamcinolone acetonide is 10 times as active as triamcinolone topically but is only equiactive systemically.[87–89] However, both compounds are more active than cortisol, which penetrates very poorly. By contrast, hydrocortisone butyrate appears to have an activity similar to that of triamcinolone acetonide.[88] Nevertheless, only a small fraction of the topically applied steroid is actually absorbed.[88,89] With cortisol, only 1 percent is so taken up; the remainder rubs off, exfoliates with the stratum corneum, or washes off. Percutaneous penetration of glucocorticoids can vary in different anatomic regions. For instance, uptake by the scrotum and forehead is about 42 and 6 times, respectively, that of the forearm.[88] Absorption is enhanced when skin is damaged and when occlusive dressings are applied, particularly to open areas.[88] Uptake is affected by the vehicle; for example, ointment bases are taken up better than are creams and lotions.[88,89]

Uptake of steroids applied topically to the eyes presents a special problem in that they must penetrate both the corneal epithelium, which is hydrophobic, and the corneal stroma, which is hydrophilic.[38,39] For this reason, acetate steroid derivatives have been shown to be the most effective.[38,39] They are applied as aqueous suspensions and are most effective when applied frequently.[38,39]

Uptake in specific tissues after systemic administration can also vary. For example, in lung, the uptake of cortisol and methylprednisolone is greater than that of prednisone.[90] Dexamethasone is sometimes given to mothers at risk for premature delivery to prevent respiratory distress syndrome in the newborn.[91] In this case, the blood levels attained in the fetus are only a fraction of those reached in the mother.[91,92] Although this may be due in part to decreased uptake, there is enhanced metabolism of the drug as well.[92]

Distribution

The effect of distribution on steroid dynamics is discussed in Chap. 12; corticosteroid-binding globulin (CBG), other plasma proteins, and the peripheral tissues sequester administered steroids to a variable extent. For steroids that bind to CBG, variations in the protein affect the rate of metabolic clearance. The presence of the protein also changes the rate of clearance of prednisolone after prednisone administration; this is more rapid shortly after the dose is given than it is later[82] because at the early time the plasma prednisolone level exceeds the CBG binding capacity and more of the steroid is available for metabolic degradation or excretion. With prednisolone, it has also been reported that individual patient differences in the volume of distribution may explain in part why certain patients are more prone to develop cushingoid side effects,[31] and it has been reported that patients with low serum albumin concentrations are more likely to develop cushingoid side effects.[93] This might affect the volume of distribution (although this was not measured), and other associated factors (e.g., the severity of the illness) also might contribute. Dexamethasone has only about sevenfold greater intrinsic activity than cortisol (Table 15-2) but was found in vivo to have 17 times the potency of cortisol when the data were extrapolated to zero time to eliminate any influence of clearance.[94] This greater activity may be due in part to enhanced availability of this steroid relative to cortisol because of less plasma binding.

Metabolism and Clearance

Metabolic pathways convert inactive compounds to active forms and vice versa. Although most glucocorticoids are active without metabolic alteration, two commonly used compounds—prednisone and cortisone—are themselves antagonists, although their affinities for the glucocorticoid receptor (see Chap. 12) are so low[95] that these compounds are effectively inactive. These 11-ketosteroids are, however, rapidly converted, mostly by the liver, to the 11-hydroxyl

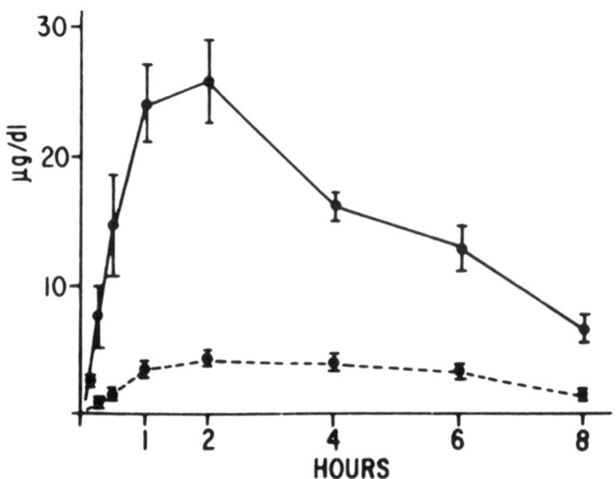

FIGURE 15-5 Plasma concentrations of prednisone (– – –) and prednisolone (——) after oral administration of 10 mg of prednisone. (*From Meikle et al.*[96])

forms—prednisolone and cortisol—which have full agonist activity (Chap. 12). Ordinarily this conversion proceeds readily (Fig. 15-5); in the study shown in the figure, the concentration of prednisolone was 10 times that of prednisone even in the first 30 min after a 10-mg oral dose of prednisone.[96] However, inadequate 11-hydroxylation could explain certain clinical findings, such as the fact that cortisone, which can penetrate human skin, does not exhibit glucocorticoid activity when applied topically[88] or injected into joints[97] and the fact that cortisone acetate injections are sometimes ineffective in the first few hours after injection[85,86] (see above and Chap. 12). In liver disease, the conversion of cortisone to cortisol is rarely affected, although the conversion of prednisone to prednisolone can be impaired.[82] For this reason, it is generally recommended that prednisolone rather than prednisone be used in patients with liver disease.[65,82] Other than with the 11-keto-steroids, there is only a small role for metabolic conversion in the formation of more active steroids; instead, the rate of inactivation is an important determinant of biological potency. The plasma half-life is commonly used as an index of the rate of clearance of corticosteroids; this parameter has some utility. However, since both the distribution and the clearance can vary differentially for various steroids and in states where these parameters change, the use of half-life alone can sometimes be misleading and can underestimate true differences in clearance.[82]

The rates of clearance of the steroids used in therapy show considerable variation (Table 15-3), and the decreased clearance of many of the commonly used steroids (prednisone, dexamethasone, etc.) relative to cortisol is one of the most important factors explaining their enhanced potency.[82,94,98–102] To a large extent, it is the modification of the steroid molecule around the A ring and the AB ring angle that accounts for the delayed clearance, as these modifications decrease the ability of the liver to reduce the ring (Chap. 12). In these cases, the 6-methylation and 21-conjugation pathways become more important.

There also appear to be some variations in the rates of clearance of the steroids in different individuals.[103] For example, in one study the half-life for prednisolone clearance in nine subjects ranged from 134 to 342 min.[83] In another study, 11 of 54 patients had accelerated clearance of methylprednisolone.[104] Although it has been reported that the plasma clearance of prednisolone is lower in steroid-treated patients who develop cushingoid side effects than in those who do not (Fig. 15-5),[31,105] this was not confirmed in a later study.[106] However, in the latter case, in the cushingoid steroid-treated patients the affinity of prednisolone for CBG was increased and plasma cortisol levels while on the steroid were higher.[106] This may imply that the hypothalamic-pituitary-adrenal axis is more resistant to suppression in cushingoid patients so that higher endogenous cortisol levels contribute to the development of side effects.

As outlined in Chap. 12, drugs and disease states can affect the clearance of administered glucocorticoids. There is impaired steroid clearance in liver disease.[82] In renal diseases, some researchers have reported that the pharmacokinetics of steroids are unchanged.[82] However, a later report suggests that the clearance and half-life of prednisolone are decreased but that those of dexamethasone are increased in renal disease.[107] Drugs such as phenytoin (diphenylhydantoin), phenobarbital, and rifampin can increase the rate of steroid clearance by inducing hepatic metabolizing enzymes.[82]

Estrogen-containing oral contraceptives and estrogen therapy in general result in decreased clearance of administered steroids.[82,108] Nonsteroidal anti-inflammatory agents may increase steroid availability, although this has not been rigorously studied.[82] It appears that the use of antacids or cimetidine does not appreciably affect steroid pharmacokinetics.[82] In general, clearance is similar in children and adults but may decrease slightly with advancing age.[82] As mentioned above, the metabolic clearance of dexamethasone in the fetus appears to be markedly enhanced relative to clearance in the mother.[94]

Concentration at Sites of Action

The potency of compounds with agonist activity, including all the major steroids used for glucocorticoid therapy (see the earlier discussions regarding the exceptions with cortisone and prednisone), is directly related to affinity for glucocorticoid receptors

TABLE 15-3 Plasma Half-Life and Glucocorticoid and Mineralocorticoid Potencies of Some Commonly Used Glucocorticoid Preparations

Steroid	Half time, min	Ref.	Relative Potency: Glucocorticoid	Relative Potency: Mineralocorticoid	Ref.
Cortisol	80–120	82	1.0	1.0	100–102
Cortisone			0.8	0.8	100–102
Prednisone	200–210	98	3.5–4.0		100, 101
			1.05–5.2		94
Prednisolone	120–300	82	4.0	0.8	100
Methylprednisolone	120–180	82	5.0	0.5	100
Triamcinolone			5.0	0	100
Dexamethasone	150–270	82	30.0	~0	100
			17–154		94
Betamethasone	130–330	82	25–30	~0	100

(see Chap. 12 and Table 15-2). Thus, once the steroid has been delivered to the target tissue, affinity is the overwhelming determinant of activity. For instance, dexamethasone and prednisolone have, respectively, about eight and two times the affinity of cortisol for the receptors.[95] Initially, this is a major determinant of the relative differences in their potencies.

Agonist Activity

Most of the steroids that are used in glucocorticoid therapy are full agonists (Chap. 12). The major exceptions are the steroids with an 11-keto group, prednisone and cortisone (discussed above), which are rapidly converted in vivo to the agonists prednisolone and cortisol.

Overall Estimation of Glucocorticoid Potency

Because the relative potencies of steroids vary even with the time after administration, it is an oversimplification to consider only a single set of potency ratios. Thus, whereas dexamethasone and prednisone were found to be, respectively, 154 and 5.2 times as potent as cortisol when examined at 14 h, they were only 17 and 1.05 times as potent when the data were extrapolated to zero time.[94] Because other responses have different kinetics, it is likely that the changes in relative potency with time will also differ, depending on the particular response. For all these reasons, the safest way to develop clinical protocols would be to standardize each drug for each disease, adjust the dose for each patient (see below), and exercise caution when switching steroids.

Over the years, a number of estimates of relative potency have been made (Table 15-3). In spite of the inherent problems, the relative potency values serve as a rough index of relative activity; these relative activities are generally similar for various responses in a number of different tissues in animals and humans (Chap. 4).[29,94] The data have been obtained from a variety of assays, including those which quantify glycogen deposition (Chap. 12), lymphocyte killing (Chap. 12), and clinical responses (e.g., antiarthritic).[33]

Variations in Sensitivity to Glucocorticoids: Glucocorticoid Resistance

Variations in intrinsic sensitivity to glucocorticoids are discussed in Chap. 12 and reviewed in Ref. 109. It is clear that marked and generalized hyposensitivity is rare; when this occurs, a mineralocorticoid excess syndrome occurs (Chap. 14). Similarly, there is no evidence for a syndrome of primary increased sensitivity to glucocorticoids. Nevertheless, there are known situations in which the steroid dosage must be altered because of individual differences (discussed under Metabolism and Clearance, above) or therapy with other drugs (e.g., phenytoin or barbiturates) that increase the hepatic metabolism of glucocorticoids (Chap. 12). However, it is possible that there are also variations in intrinsic sensitivity between individuals and between various tissues in an individual. Individual differences in the steroid's ability to suppress the hypothalamic-pituitary-adrenal axis could explain the higher cortisol levels in the cushingoid patients in the study of Benet and associates.[106] If this is the case, it is likely that the lowered sensitivity of the axis in certain individuals is also selective for the tissues involved in axis suppression, since the presence in these individuals of effects of the steroid sufficient to produce Cushing's syndrome indicates that other target tissues are sensitive to glucocorticoids. Individual differences could also explain why only subpopulations of patients with certain diseases respond to glucocorticoid therapy; the study quoted under Therapeutic Influences, above, of patients with the preleukemic syndrome[7] underscores this point.

The concentrations of glucocorticoid receptors, unlike those of receptors for other classes of hormones, such as the polypeptide and catecholamine hormones, are not extensively regulated; however, they can be regulated to some extent, and other factors have a pronounced effect on cellular sensitivity to glucocorticoids (Chap. 12). Although the clinical importance of these phenomena is not known, they could affect the sensitivity of selected target tissues to glucocorticoids and be of therapeutic relevance. It is possible that studies of these influences may yield information that will facilitate the design of protocols to enhance specifically the effectiveness of glucocorticoids on certain tissues while minimizing that on other tissues.

In the treatment of lymphoid leukemias, patients who initially respond can become resistant to the steroid.[6] This appears to be due to a mutation in the gene for the receptor and the selection of a population of cells that have functionally defective receptors that cannot respond to the steroid (Fig. 15-6).

GLUCOCORTICOID PREPARATIONS

Steroids with Glucocorticoid Activity Available for Therapy

A great number of steroids with glucocorticoid potency are available. The structures of some of the more commonly used synthetic glucocorticoid preparations are shown in Fig. 15-1. The modifications that enhance activity are discussed above and in Chap. 12. The steroids may be given orally, parenterally, topically, intraarticularly, or as aerosols. The advantage of topical, intraarticular, or aerosol therapy is that certain areas (skin, joints, and the bronchial tree) can be exposed to high concentrations of glucocorticoids while systemic exposure and side effects are minimized.

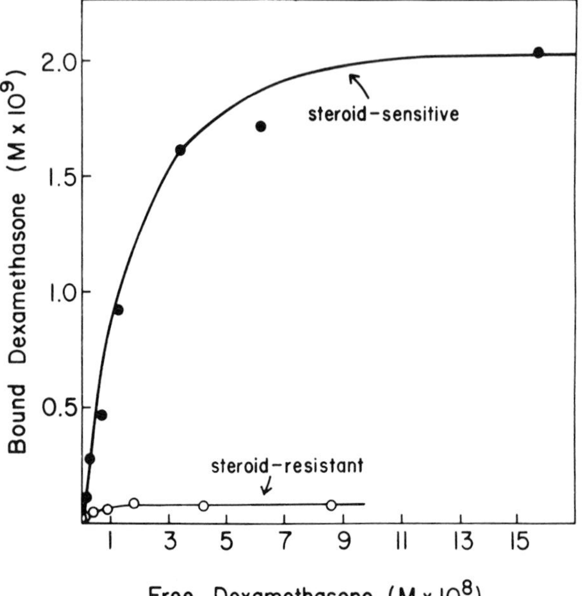

FIGURE 15-6 Binding of radioactive dexamethasone to receptors from glucocorticoid-sensitive lymphoma cells and to glucocorticoid-resistant cells selected by growing steroid-sensitive cells in the presence of dexamethasone. [*From Rosenau W, Baxter JD, Rousseau GG, Tomkins GM: Mechanism of resistance to steroids: Glucocorticoid receptor defect in lymphoma cells. Nature (New Biol) 237:20, 1972.*]

Orally and Parenterally Active Preparations

In general, with oral administration, the unmodified steroid is given, since for the commonly used steroids (e.g., prednisone, prednisolone, dexamethasone, cortisol), substitutions (21-phosphate, etc.) are not needed for absorption (see Bioavailability, above).

Parenteral administration is indicated in the immediate treatment of addisonian patients in crisis (Chap. 12) and patients who cannot take oral medications. There appears to be no acute danger in giving moderate doses (1 g or less) intravenously (IV), although in general the oral route is effective. The preparations used intravenously are ordinarily compounds with C-21 substitutions to enhance solubility (Table 15-4). Intramuscular administration is described in the preceding section.

The four major considerations in selecting the particular steroid to be used are experience with prescribing it for the disease in question, duration of action, the possible need to avoid concomitant mineralocorticoid activity, and cost. Whereas in principle all the various glucocorticoids should be effective when given in equivalent doses, caution should be exercised in substituting them because the relative potencies have not been established as clearly as has generally been assumed (see above and Chap. 12). Thus, in general, it is best to use preparations that have been shown to be effective for a particular condition. For instance, if a physician were treating an asthmatic crisis and wanted to administer the equivalent of 100 mg of cortisol, the prednisolone equivalent over the first few hours would be around 50 to 95 mg rather than the usually considered value of 20 to 25 mg (Table 15-2).[94] Whereas in the acute treatment of primary adrenocortical insufficiency cortisol is preferred because of its relatively greater mineralocorticoid activity, in other circumstances it is generally preferable to avoid sodium-retaining actions by giving a steroid with less mineralocorticoid activity. Duration of action is particularly relevant for alternate-day steroid therapy (discussed below). Finally, physicians should be aware that the various steroid preparations vary considerably in cost, and when possible, less expensive preparations should be used.

Intraarticular Preparations

Glucocorticoids can be injected into joints for the relief of inflammation.[33,97,110] Although these measures are usually for supplemental and temporary ther-

TABLE 15-4 Some Parenteral and Topical Glucocorticoid Preparations

Intravenous	Intraarticular
Hydrdocortisone phosphate	Hydrocortisone acetate
Hydrocortisone hemisuccinate	Prednisolone tebutate
Prednisolone phosphate	Triamcinolone hexacetonide
Dexamethasone phosphate	Betamethasone acetate phosphate
Methylprednisolone hemisuccinate	Methylprednisolone acetate
Topical	
Lowest potency	Low potency
0.25–0.5% cortisol	0.01% fluocinolone acetonide
0.04–0.1% dexamethasone	0.01% betamethasone valerate
0.5% prednisolone	0.025% fluorometholone
0.2% betamethasone	0.025% triamcinolone acetonide
Intermediate potency	High potency
0.1% betamethasone valerate	0.05% betamethasone dipropionate
0.025% halcinolone	0.5% triamcinolone acetonide
0.1% triamcinolone acetonide	0.2% fluocinolone acetonide
0.025% fluocinolone acetonide	0.1% halcinonide

Source: Data on topical preparations from Robertson and Maibach.[88]

apy, they can provide dramatic symptomatic relief. In general, the preparations are relatively insoluble and form microcrystals. Substitution with a *tert*-butylacetate or a hexacetonide group has proved to be particularly effective in this respect (Table 15-4).[33,97,110] These properties retard systemic absorption, promote retention within the joint space, and lead to a longer period of clinical effect; a single injection of such a preparation can last for weeks.[97] As stated earlier, preparations containing cortisone are not effective.[33,97,110]

When intraarticular preparations are used, generalized problems caused by glucocorticoid excess, including suppression of the hypothalamic-pituitary-adrenal axis, are uncommon.[97] Intraarticular steroid administration is not, however, without risk. It is important to adhere to scrupulous aseptic technique and avoid injection into potentially infected joints, as steroids can worsen the course of such infections. Nevertheless, infections in the joint or needle tract occur infrequently in spite of strict aseptic techniques.[33] Other problems with intraarticular steroids include the infrequent occurrence of synovitis, induced presumably by the steroid-containing crystals; occasional damage to the cartilage, supporting ligaments, and surrounding bone; partial absorption of bony margins; and cutaneous atrophy at the site of injection.[33,97,110] The last condition can be minimized by avoiding overdistension of the synovial cavity and leakage along the needle track.[97]

Topical Preparations

The use of topical glucocorticoid preparations constitutes the major advance in the pharmacology of dermatology.[88,89] Some of the factors involved in topical uptake of glucocorticoids are discussed above under Determinants of Glucocorticoid Potency. Thus, many of the cortisol analogues are much more effective than cortisol itself. Some of the commonly used steroids are listed in Table 15-4. These steroids come in ointment, cream, lotion, or aerosol vehicles and in varying strengths. The ointment bases tend to give better activity than do cream or lotion vehicles but also tend to be less acceptable cosmetically to the patient in spite of the fact that they are more soothing to dry skin.[88,89] However, hairy areas are best treated with lotions or aerosol vehicles.[88] The availability of several strengths helps a physician provide the needed dosage while minimizing excess dosage. For most indications, high-potency steroid preparations are unnecessary; they carry a higher risk of local side effects (see below) and are used primarily on areas of skin that have been thickened by disease.[88,89] Although topical steroid preparations are commonly given without occlusion, they can be used (e.g., with plastic wrap, sometimes intermittently,[88] or with wet dressings[89]) to enhance penetration.[88,89] Single daily applications of an ointment are probably as effective as three daily applications.[88,89] In general, topical steroid use on ulcerated skin should be avoided. Except for circumstances under which there is markedly increased absorption, systemic toxicity, including suppression of the hypothalamic-pituitary-adrenal axis, is uncommon, although the possibility that it may develop must be kept in mind.[88] Other complications of topical therapy include exacerbation of an infection when steroids are given inappropriately, localized striae (usually in areas of increased uptake such as the groin), rosacea-like eruptions, pustules (steroid acne), and, rarely, an allergic contact dermatitis from the steroids themselves.[88]

Inhaled Corticosteroids

Corticosteroid aerosols are effective in the treatment of asthma.[12,40,111,112] Beclomethasone dipropionate, trimacinolone acetonide, budesonide, flunisolide, and betamethasone valerate are the most commonly used preparations.[12,40,111,112] These preparations are preferable to other steroids because they are not absorbed as well systematically as many other steroids, such as cortisol.[40] Inhalers that deliver higher doses of up to 250 μg of beclomethasone dipropionate per puff have been shown to have significant efficacy.[112] In general, aerosols are used for maintenance therapy for asthma and are substituted for oral or parenteral steroids after they have induced a good response.[40] In some cases, delivery of the steroid to the lower bronchial tissue is enhanced by prior administration of a bronchodilator such as albuterol.[111] Delivery can be difficult during heavy sputum production. Although it is clear that steroids given in this way improve the ratio of therapeutic to toxic effects, this form of therapy is not without problems.[113] First, there is an increased incidence of fungal infections of the upper respiratory tract, including candidiasis of the pharynx.[113] Second, patients can experience dysphonia, which may be a steroid-induced myopathy of the phonatory muscle.[113] Although suppression of the hypothalamic-pituitary-adrenal axis with corticosteroid aerosol therapy[12,40] can occur, it is overall much less severe than suppression with the same dose given systemically; this can be minimized further in asthmatic patients by holding the aerosol canister outside the mouth, using the inhaler before meals, rinsing the mouth and throat after inhalation, and using a spacer or holding chamber into which the medication is delivered.[12,40] The extent to which aerosols produce atrophy of the pharynx and airways has not been determined.[40]

ACTH

ACTH can be given instead of a glucocorticoid, and such preparations are occasionally used. Cosyntropin ($ACTH_{1-24}$; see Chap. 12) is not commonly used because of its short duration of action (unless continuous intravenous ACTH is given); instead, repository ACTH preparations are available for IM injection.[34] When given in this way, the peptide is released slowly and daily injections can be used to provide therapeutically effective steroid levels. These injections vary in composition and can include zinc or gelatin (the zinc preparations have a greater duration of action); 15 to 40 U of ACTH given in this way is roughly equivalent to 37.5 to 100 mg of cortisol.[34] However, a problem in comparing the efficacy of ACTH and glucocorticoids involves determining the equivalency of doses.[34]

ACTH stimulates the production of cortisol, adrenal androgens, and other steroids. Thus, the observed effects are due not only to cortisol but also to the other steroids and resemble spontaneous Cushing's syndrome, in which acne and hirsutism in females can be prominent.[99] Also, patients receiving ACTH appear to have a greater prevalence of hypertension than do those receiving synthetic steroids.[34] This may be due to the greater mineralocorticoid activity of cortisol compared with the other, more commonly used synthetic glucocorticoid preparations and to increased secretion of deoxycorticosterone (Chap. 14). Further, ACTH itself can cause pigmentation.[34]

ACTH produces less suppression of the hypothalamic-pituitary-adrenal axis than do glucocorticoids. In almost all ACTH-treated patients, the responses to provocative testing with insulin-induced hypoglycemia are normal or only slighty impaired.[34] For instance, Daly and associates found a diminished plasma ACTH response but a normal cortisol response to insulin hypoglycemia testing.[114] These data suggest that ACTH therapy does suppress the axis to some extent but that the adrenal, when stimulated by the therapy, can respond to lower ACTH concentrations.[34] However, some patients on prolonged ACTH therapy show suppression of the hypothalamic-pituitary-adrenal axis.[115] The decreased frequency of suppression of the axis by ACTH compared with the frequency of suppression by glucocorticoids probably reflects differences in the maximal plasma glucocorticoid level attained and the duration of the effect. ACTH gel (20 to 40 U) given once daily results in only a moderate increase in plasma cortisol levels (maximum approximately 40 to 50 μg/dl), and these levels return to normal by approximately 16 h.[115] Thus, the effect of daily ACTH injections appears to be roughly comparable to that of a single morning dose of a short-acting glucocorticoid.[34] If ACTH were given twice daily, the degree of suppression of the axis might approximate that seen with glucocorticoids given in multiple doses. The fact that glucocorticoid concentrations are only moderately elevated and are not sustained over 24 h by once-daily ACTH therapy[115] may also explain the observation that ACTH causes less suppression of linear growth in children than does daily glucocorticoid therapy.[34]

The disadvantages of ACTH therapy are the necessity for daily injection and the side effects of androgen excess and hypertension.[34] Since there is no clear advantage over oral glucocorticoids, ACTH in doses which achieve similar plasma glucocorticoid concentration is not commonly used for prolonged therapy.[116]

SOME GENERAL PRINCIPLES

Selection of Patients

The decision to use glucocorticoids implies that the benefits will outweigh the serious side effects. Thus, it should be clear that there is a reasonable chance that the patient will respond.

Need for Empirical Data

If there are no data to suggest that a given condition will respond to glucocorticoids, their use for that condition constitutes experimentation. Clearly, the decision to use corticosteroids should be based on verification that the drugs are effective.

Short-Term Versus Long-Term

The major complications of glucocorticoid therapy are ones that require a considerable time to develop (see above). Thus, in general, the use of steroids over a short period of time is not associated with major risk.[117] If steroids will significantly benefit a patient and need be given for only a few days, they should not be withheld. For instance, severe poison oak or poison ivy or an allergic skin reaction that is not responsive to topical steroids is an indication for a short course of systemic steroids. However, short courses of glucocorticoids may induce hyperglycemia in susceptible individuals and can rarely precipitate avascular necrosis.[44,45]

The decision to initiate steroid therapy when it may involve treatment for a longer period is a more serious one. For instance, with asthma, once steroid therapy is started, it may be necessary to continue the drug for months to years. Clearly, the seriousness of the primary disease commonly mandates this, but the physician must be aware of the consequences of such long-term therapy.

Testing the Sensitivity

With many conditions (e.g., acute lymphoblastic leukemia of childhood[5] and suppression of transplant rejection[118]), most patients respond to glucocorticoids, whereas with other conditions only a subgroup of patients with the disease will respond. In the latter case, it is sometimes possible to identify the patients who will respond. For instance, asthmatic patients with less fixed airway obstruction respond better than do those with a greater complement of this.[113] Thus, documentation of such factors may assist in the selection of patients who can benefit from therapy. The identification of steroid-responsive patients also may be achieved by in vitro testing. This appears to be the case with the preleukemic syndrome mentioned under Therapeutic Influences, above. In this study, bone marrow cells of 34 patients were tested in vitro; the cells of 5 patients responsed to the steroid, and 3 of these patients responded to glucocorticoid therapy.[7] In acute lymphoblastic leukemia and several other hematologic malignancies, there is a good correlation between the concentration of glucocorticoid receptors measured in the malignant cells in vitro and the responsiveness of the disease to glucocorticoid therapy.[5] In a study of T lymphocyte–mediated granulopoietic failure, prednisone-responsive patients could be identified by in vitro testing of the ability of the steroid to stimulate clonal growth of bone marrow cells.[119] It is hoped that approaches such as these will be applied to other conditions to increase the ability to detect glucocorticoid-sensitive patients.

Dose-Response Considerations

The recommended doses of glucocorticoids used in therapy are based on empirical observations; this approach is reasonable and is probably safest. As more is learned about glucocorticoid action, it will be possible to predict which doses will be required. This may facilitate the development of therapeutic trials and help optimize the dosage in order to minimize toxicity while maximizing therapeutic responses.

The application of current information about glucocorticoid receptors illustrates this point. For responses that are mediated by the receptors, doses resulting in steroid levels far in excess of those necessary to saturate the receptors will not provide greater short-term benefit than will those minimally required to do this. Such "excess" doses may, however, produce a greater effect, since higher levels of the steroid will be present longer.

As emphasized in Chap. 12, there is in general a close correlation between the relative saturation of the hormone by the receptor and the relative magnitude of the hormone response. In such cases, the effectiveness of a steroid can be calculated from its affinity for the receptor and the free concentrations of the steroid with time. However, in vitro there appear to be circumstances[109] in which the steroid achieves a maximal response at concentrations lower than those required to fully saturate the receptors. Knowledge of whether this ever occurs in therapeutic situations would be particularly important, since lower than usual steroid concentrations might be used and would have fewer undesirable side effects.

With human systems, precise data on the doses of steroids required to occupy the receptors have not been collected; however, from the known binding constants, free steroid levels, and so on, it can be calculated that oral doses of 7.5 and 15 mg of prednisolone would result in blood levels 8 h after the dose that would bind the receptors to 42 and 63 percent, respectively, of saturation. Much higher doses (e.g., 100 mg or more) would be required to result in nearly complete receptor saturation for long periods. Thus, a dose this large given several times a day should stimulate nearly maximal receptor-mediated responses.

There are situations, such as acute renal transplant rejection,[118] gram-negative sepsis with shock,[20,120–122] tumors of the central nervous system,[21] and certain immune-mediated hematologic dyscrasias,[123] in which the use of even larger doses of glucocorticoids has been recommended. Subsequent studies of renal transplant rejection have indicated that such large doses actually decrease survival,[118] and for this indication the trend has been toward the use of progressively lower steroid doses.[124] Studies in baboons show clear beneficial effects of high-dose glucocorticoids given early in the course of bacteria-induced shock.[125] Dexamethasone at doses of 3 to 5 mg per kilogram of body weight per day has been shown to be beneficial in patients with suspected typhoid fever who are delirious, obtunded, stuporous, comatose, or in shock.[126] A single bolus of 30 mg per kilogram of body weight of methylprednisolone sodium succinate or 6 mg per kilogram of body weight of dexamethasone sodium phosphate was associated with a reversal of shock during the first 24 h in 27 percent of patients with septic shock, versus none of the nonsteroid-treated patients and was found to reduce mortality early in the hospital course, although improvement in mortality was not evident on a long-term basis.[122] These workers suggested that this improved short-term survival and the reversal of shock may be beneficial in that they may allow the physician to buy time for the institution of other measures.[122] Overall, it appears that glucocorticoids must be given early to be beneficial. It has not been demonstrated in these circumstances whether smaller doses of corticosteroids would be equally effective. Based on the preceding considerations, these very large doses might not be expected to produce a greater effect than do the large doses if the therapeutic influences are glucocorticoid receptor–mediated, and they might have other undesirable side effects. However, some argue that receptor-independent mechanisms, such as those resulting from membrane effects secondary to the lipid properties of the steroids, are operative in these conditions.[5,123]

The Use of Adjunctive Therapy

In the majority of conditions for which glucocorticoids are used, there are either alternative or adjunctive therapeutic modalities; these modalities must be considered and if possible used before beginning steroid therapy, since their use may be associated with a lower incidence of complications. Further, if the patient's condition can be adequately controlled by such methods, glucocorticoid therapy may not be indicated. Conversely, failure to respond to maximal utilization of conventional treatment may be an indication for the use of glucocorticoids in certain conditions.

If glucocorticoid therapy is used, adjunctive therapy should in most cases be continued, as it may be beneficial, improve the overall response to therapy, and allow the use of lower steroid doses. For instance, in rheumatoid arthritis, the use of physical therapy, braces, salicylates, and other nonsteroidal anti-inflammatory agents may obviate the need for steroids or provide additional benefit. In asthma, other bronchodilators, such as beta-adrenergic agents, are used in conjunction with steroids. Immunosuppressants in addition to a glucocorticoid may be helpful in the treatment of nephritis[127] or the prevention of renal transplant rejection.[118] Other chemotherapeutic agents can be helpful in malignancies or in conditions such as amyloidosis.[128]

Specific Measures to Reduce Side Effects

There is a growing awareness that certain specific measures may reduce side effects. The potential use of measures to reduce osteoporosis and myopathy and of insulin to control diabetes is discussed elsewhere in this chapter. An increased protein intake can reduce steroid-induced nitrogen wasting.[129] Vitamin A may decrease the steroid effect of impaired wound healing.[130]

Cognizance of Objective Criteria

In evaluating the response to steroid therapy, objective criteria should be used whenever possible since glucocorticoids can induce a sense of well-being[2,21,32,79–81] that is not necessarily accompanied by improvement in the primary disease for which the steroids are being administered. Conversely, patients on long-term therapy frequently develop symptoms of steroid withdrawal when the dose is lowered (see below), and these symptoms may be misinterpreted as an exacerbation of the primary disease. For example, arthralgias and myalgias are common during steroid withdrawal and do not necessarily indicate increased activity of rheumatoid arthritis. Similarly, lowering the steroid dose in patients with inflammatory bowel disease may provoke anorexia and nausea which may not be due to an exacerbation of the gastrointestinal disorder. Thus, subjective changes may be misleading and may lead to inappropriate alterations in dosage. Although many of the disorders for which steroids are used have no clearly identifiable chemical criteria which can be used to quantify maximal benefit or improvement, objective criteria should be used when possible. Such criteria include pulmonary function studies or blood and sputum eosinophil determinations in patients with asthma,[131] gallium lung scanning or assay of the activity of serum angiotensin converting enzyme in sarcoidosis,[132] evaluation of serum complement levels in patients with lupus erythematosus, determination of serum Ca^{2+} concentrations in patients with hypercalcemia and sarcoidosis, serial creatinine clearance measurements in patients treated for renal transplant rejection, and evidence of true joint inflammation in patients with arthritis.

The Circadian Rhythm

When moderate doses of glucocorticoids are given for a short time (e.g., a few days or less), the circadian rhythm of endogenous steorid production (Chap. 12) is ignored; the transient suppression of the hypothalamic-pituitary-adrenal axis in this setting is not a problem. When it is necessary to give moderate to large doses of steroids on a daily basis for a longer period, suppression of the axis is unavoidable and must be considered and dealt with as described below (see Withdrawal of Glucocorticoids and Suppression of the Hypothalamic-Pituitary-Adrenal Axis).

However, there are other circumstances in which it is important to tailor glucocorticoid therapy to the circadian rhythm; this is the case with alternate-day therapy (discussed below), with replacement therapy in a patient whose hypothalamic-pituitary-adrenal axis is suppressed (discussed below), and sometimes when low doses of steroids are required. In the latter situation, a patient with lupus arthritis or asthma refractory to other therapy may sometimes respond to low doses of glucocorticoids (e.g., 5 mg or less of prednisone per day). If these doses are given in the evening, there will be suppression of the rise in plasma ACTH concentration and therefore in the cortisol level. In this case, the total additional effect will be minor, since the suppression of endogenous cortisol production will offset the effect of the steroid administered. However, if the steroid is given in the morning, when ACTH levels spontaneously fall, the net effect can be additive, with a minimal influence on the body's normal rhythm of steroid secretion.

Adjusting the Dose

Once glucocorticoid therapy has been instituted, it is important to monitor the dose carefully. The major endpoint is clinical response; side effects can be minimized by decreasing the dose when the patient is responding. Alternatively, it may be necessary to increase the dose when the patient is not responding, and the literature regarding that condition suggests that higher doses may be more effective.

The factors that lead to variations in response were discussed earlier. Because variations exist in metabolism and distribution, absorption, and possibly even intrinsic sensitivity, it should be obvious that adherence to a fixed drug protocol is not ideal, although in certain situations this may be necessary because other information is not available.

It is hoped that plasma measurements of the glucocorticoids used in therapy will be used more in the future to minimize variations resulting from uptake, metabolism, and distribution. In this way, patients in whom higher drug levels develop could have their doses lowered sooner, minimizing cushingoid side effects. Conversely, patients in whom adequate blood levels are not attained could receive an increased dose (and possible improvement) sooner.

ALTERNATE-DAY THERAPY

Alternate-day therapy emerged after it was found that if a single dose of glucocorticoid was given once in the morning on alternate days, certain adverse effects of the steroid could be minimized while a therapeutically beneficial response could still be obtained.[34,40,116,133,134] Conditions in which alternate-day glucocorticoid therapy has been effective include certain nephrotic syndromes (particularly in children), renal transplantation rejection and other renal diseases, ulcerative colitis, rheumatoid arthritis and some other arthritic disorders, rheumatic fever, myasthenia gravis, muscular dystrophy, sarcoidosis, alopecia areata, chronic dermatoses, asthma, and pemphigus vulgaris.[34,40,72,116,135,136] However, alternate-day therapy has been shown not to be effective in giant cell arteritis.[137] Thus, before the use of alternate-day steroid therapy is contemplated, the specific literature about each condition should be examined.

Based on studies in which the same dose of steroid was given once in the morning on alternate days rather than over a 48 h period, a number of glucocorticoid side effects are decreased.[34,40,116,134] These side effects include suppression of the hypothalamic-pituitary-adrenal axis, growth inhibition in children, cushingoid facies, abnormal fat deposition, obesity, excessive appetite, striae, easy bruisability, carbohydrate intolerance, infections, myopathy, and other features. The decrease in growth inhibition constitutes a major advantage of alternate-day glucocorticoid therapy in the pediatric group.[34,40,116,138]

The effect of alternate-day steroid therapy on the hypothalamic-pituitary-adrenal axis has been studied by ACTH stimulation, metyrapone testing, insulin hypoglycemia testing, and corticotropin releasing hormone (CRH) stimulation.[34,136,139,140] These studies show less suppression than with equivalent divided doses given on a daily basis, and in one study there was recovery of a suppressed axis when children were switched from daily to alternate-day therapy.[136] However, some suppression of the hypothalamic-pituitary-adrenal axis does occur with alternate-day therapy.[34,136,139–141] For example, in a study of patients receiving 5 to 60 mg of prednisone on alternate days, the response to CRH was markedly suppressed on the day of treatment and was mildly blunted on the day off treatment.[140] However, the cortisol response to ACTH was normal in all cases, including that enough ACTH was secreted to maintain normal adrenal function.[140]

The precise mechanisms of the effectiveness of alternate-day therapy are not known. However, when various responses to glucocorticoids are examined, some persist on the "off steroid" day of alternate-day therapy, whereas other influences are present only during the "on" day. For instance, Fauci and Dale[142] found that glucocorticoid-induced lymphocytopenia and monocytopenia returned to normal by 8 A.M. on the day off prednisone, yet at this time there was evidence that the steroid was suppressing disease activity. Considerations such as these underscore a general problem that must be faced with glucocorticoid therapy: The dose response and the kinetics of each particular beneficial and deleterious effect must be known. It might then be possible to optimize even more precisely the dose and the interval between doses. However, other dosage intervals have been tried and have not been found to be superior.[34,133,143]

If alternate-day therapy is used, one of the short-acting glucocorticoids should be administered (Table 15-5).[34,133–135,143] These include prednisone, prednisolone, methylprednisolone, cortisol, and cortisone, which are cleared more rapidly from the plasma (Table 15-3). The optimal alternate-day therapy requires that the steroid be administered in the morning (preferably before breakfast) as a single dose.[34,133,135] If the steroid is given in divided doses, the effect of the later doses may persist into the alternate day. Avoidance of late afternoon and evening doses is especially important in terms of minimizing suppression of the hypothalamic-pituitary adrenal axis (discussed below), and with the short-acting steroid, morning-only administration allows the steroid to be cleared from the circulation before the nocturnal increase in ACTH release. Steroids such as dexamethasone, betamethasone, triamcinolone, triamcinolone acetonide, and fluocinolone acetonide are cleared more slowly, are longer-acting, and should not be used for alternate-day therapy.[34,133,135]

Alternate-day therapy is best used for prolonged[136] therapy and is not in general indicated for initial treatment, especially when glucocorticoids are used for acute problems (Tables 15-1 and 15-5).[34,133,135,136] Thus, most people experienced in the use of steroids recommend that even for chronic diseases, daily therapy should be used initially. In fact, if only short-term treatment is anticipated, alternate-day therapy may not be necessary. Thus, in instituting steroid therapy, the glucocorticoid is given on a daily (or more frequent) basis and then, once there is amelioration or control, the patient is switched to alternate-day therapy. The change to alternate-day therapy should be made as soon as possible (within several weeks) after beginning steroid therapy and before there is major suppression of the hypothalamic-pituitary-adrenal axis, as the change is more difficult if the axis is suppressed.

In patients in whom the axis is not suppressed, the change can be made abruptly. In changing to alternate-day therapy, it is generally best not to reduce the total dose of steroid given.[34,133–135] In fact, sometimes it may be advantageous to increase the total dose. Thus, the overall dosage for two days used with daily therapy can be administered as a single dose on the mornings of alternate days. Then the overall dose can be reduced as indicated by the condition of the problem for which the steroid was given.

Patients on long-term daily multiple-dose therapy in whom the axis is suppressed frequently have manifestations of adrenal insufficiency and steroid withdrawal (discussed below) on the off day when switched abruptly to alternate-day therapy.[34,133–135] In these patients, the change can be made slowly; it may first require gradual reduction in the total dose, then a change to single daily doses, and finally a switch to alternate-day therapy. This can be done by gradually reducing (e.g., by 5 mg every 4 to 5 days) the steroid dose on alternate days and adding this dose to the one given on the other days until the transition is achieved. In making this transition, the physician should be concerned not only with an exacerbation of the primary disease but also with the problem of a lack of well-being while the patient is off the steroid. This can be due to symptoms of adrenal insufficiency in cases where the hypothalamic-pituitary adrenal axis is suppressed, to a lack of the general euphoric influences of the steroid independent of the primary disease, or to the primary disease. Thus, the patient is likely to complain on the off day. The physician and patient must be committed to alternate-day therapy once the decision to use it has been made, and in a patient who has symptoms on the off day, special attention must be given to objective criteria and to whether the therapy is ineffective or effective and whether the complaints are due to the other factors discussed above. However, during this time, if there is a documented flare-up of the primary disease, it may be necessary to switch to daily therapy for a short time, and several attempts at conversion to alternate-day therapy may be required. In switching to alternate-day therapy, the physician should be especially aware of the use of adjunctive modalities (see above) that may minimize symptoms.

TABLE 15-5 Recommendations Regarding Alternate-Day Glucocorticoid Therapy

1. Use a short-acting glucocorticoid.
2. Avoid in acute situations or if only short-term therapy (e.g., <3 weeks) is anticipated.
3. Inform patient fully of the advantages, then be diligent.
4. Give special attention if there is already suppression of the hypothalamic-pituitary-adrenal axis.
5. Maximize adjuctive therapy, particularly on the "off" day.
6. Check the literature: may not be effective for certain diseases

SPECIAL SITUATIONS

Pregnancy

There has been concern that the use of glucocorticoids in pregnancy may increase the incidence of fetal deaths or congenital abnormalities.[33,65,144–146] Indeed, glucocorticoid-treated pregnant animals have an increased incidence of abortions, placental insufficiency, and congenital malformations, including cleft palate, in their offspring.[33,65,144,145] Despite these valid concerns, there are circumstances in which pregnant patients with life-threatening conditions such as asthma and systemic lupus erythematosus may require steroid therapy. Fortunately, the overall experience with glucocorticoids in pregnancy has not been as bad as expected.[33,65,144,145] For instance, during 70 pregnancies in 55 asthmatic patients, there were 71 live births, only 1 spontaneous abortion, and possibly a slight increase in premature births.[144] Furthere, there were no fetal, maternal, or neonatal deaths, and the incidence of toxemia, uterine hemorrhage, and congenital malformations was not increased. In a series of 260 pregnancies (reviewed in Ref. 33), seven full-term infants had disorders. One had apparent adrenocortical failure for 3 days, and there were two cases of cleft palate. Cleft palate has also been noted in a few instances in which steroids were used at the time of conception and were continued for significant periods thereafter.[33] However, cleft palate was not observed in two other series of 46 mothers who were on steroids during and after conception.[33] Thus, glucocorticoids should not be used indiscriminately during pregnancy and should be avoided especially in the first trimester. However, they should not be withheld in conditions where a steroid may ameliorate life-threatening disease.

When glucocorticoids are required in pregnant individuals, it is best to use cortisol or prednisolone since they are short-acting and are changed to their inactive 11-keto forms, cortisone and prednisone, by the placenta and thus minimize the exposure of the fetus (see Chap. 12). Steroids such as dexamethasone and betamethasone cross the placenta unchanged and thus should not be used during pregnancy (Chap. 12).

Prednisone and prednisolone administration are not contraindicated in breast-feeding women even though small amounts are excreted in breast milk.[147–149] In general, higher doses such as >20 mg/day of prednisone should be avoided.

The use of steroid aerosols in pregnancy appears to be safe when recommended doses are used.[145]

Diabetes

Glucocorticoids alter carbohydrate metabolism by increasing gluconeogenesis and antagonizing the peripheral uptake of glucose. However, in glucocorticoid-treated patients without subclinical or overt diabetes, significant clinical problems with hyperglycemia are unusual (Chap. 12). Thus, in most patients, fasting blood sugar levels are usually normal or only mildly elevated, although glucose tolerance may be impaired. However, in patients with subclinical or overt diabetes, steroid therapy may provoke or worsen hyperglycemia. Steroid therapy is not contraindicated in such patients, although oral hypoglycemic agents, insulin therapy, or an increase in the insulin dose may be required. In the rare patient with insulin resistance ascribable to the development of anti-insulin antibodies, glucocorticoids may be beneficial and may reduce the insulin requirement by suppressing the immune response.[33]

Surgery

It is generally recommended that patients on prolonged high-dose glucocorticoids receive additional steroid coverage for the stress of surgery (discussed below and in Chap. 12). Patients with iatrogenic Cushing's syndrome also have an increased risk of developing serious postoperative complications. Local problems include poor healing, wound infections, and occasionally dehiscence of the incision; hematomas and abscesses may occur with abdominal or thoracic surgery. The courses of these patients may also be complicated by systemic infection. Thus, morbidity is increased and recovery is prolonged; if time allows, elective surgery should be deferred and the steroid dose should be decreased.

Psychiatry

Changes in mood and psychological state occur frequently in glucocorticoid-treated patients, and although many patients initially note a feeling of mental well-being, depression and several types of psychosis may also occur.[2,21,32,79–81] The type of disorder that may occur is not predictable by the patient's pretherapy condition, but it is ordinarily reversible after the discontinuation of therapy. Previous psychiatric disorders are in general not a contraindication to steroid therapy.

Peptic Ulcer

The relationship between glucocorticoid therapy and peptic ulcer disease is reviewed in Chap. 12. Recent studies have demonstrated a twofold increased risk of peptic ulcer in glucocorticoid-treated individuals.[150,151] However, this risk was present only in patients who were concomitantly receiving nonsteroidal antiinflammatory drugs (NSAIDs),[151] and in this study patients who used both drugs concurrently had a 15-fold estimated increased risk of peptic ulcer.[151] This study also suggested that among NSAID users, both the dose and the duration of glucocorticoid therapy were associated with increased risk.[151] Thus, caution should be observed in prescribing these drugs together, and when this is done, patients should be informed of the risk of peptic ulcer disease.

Pediatrics

In children, glucocorticoid therapy has the major additional disadvantage of causing growth failure (for a review, see Ref. 12 and Chap. 12). There tends to be a growth spurt after discontinuation of the steroid, since it also inhibits bone maturation (Chap. 12); however, chronic therapy leads to permanent growth retardation.[12] Nevertheless, alternate-day therapy in children results in a less inhibitory effect on growth (see above) and decreased cushingoid effects in general.[40] In addition, inhaled steroids do not inhibit growth in childhood asthma.[12]

Kaposi's Sarcoma

Kaposi's sarcoma occurs with an increased prevalence in patients who receive immunosuppressive therapy or have the acquired immune deficiency syndrome (AIDS).[152] There are several case reports of regression of their tumors in association with discontinuation of treatment with glucocorticoids.[152] Thus, glucocorticoids should be used with caution in such patients, and their use should be avoided in patients who are at a greater risk for developing Kaposi's sarcoma.

WITHDRAWAL OF GLUCOCORTICOIDS AND SUPPRESSION OF THE HYPOTHALAMIC-PITUITARY-ADRENAL AXIS

As was mentioned above, spontaneous Cushing's syndrome or glucocorticoid therapy can result in suppression of the hypothalamic-pituitary-adrenal axis. However, such suppression is most frequently encountered in glucocorticoid therapy because of the large number of patients receiving these steroids and must be considered in all patients who will discontinue or have discontinued glucocorticoid therapy.

Kinetics and Dosage Required for Suppression

Glucocorticoid suppression of the hypothalamic-pituitary-adrenal axis is discussed in Chap. 12. Even a single dose of a glucocorticoid can for some hours prevent a response of the axis to a major insult such as surgery. However, with short exposure, i.e., one or two doses, the axis recovers rapidly and the suppression occurs for the most part while the glucocorticoid is present in the circulation.[153] Thus, after short-term glucocorticoid therapy, suppression of the hypothalamic-pituitary-adrenal axis is rarely pronounced for more than a few hours. With more prolonged therapy, suppression increases with both duration and total dose. When glucocorticoids are administered for a period of days, there may be both suppression of basal cortisol levels (Fig. 15-7), if doses are sufficiently high and decreased responsiveness of both the hypothalamic-pituitary-adrenal axis and the adrenal to stimulation.[153] Thus, in one study (Fig. 15-8), the administration of 50 mg of prednisone per day for 5 days resulted in decreased responsiveness to both insulin-induced hypoglycemia and exogenous ACTH 2 days after discontinuation of the steroid, but responses returned to normal at 5 days.[153] In another study, asthmatic children who were given high-dose prednisone (up to 2 mg/kg per day) for 5 days had normal responses to insulin hypoglycemia 10 days after discontinuing the drug.[154] In addition, the administration of high-dose steroids for as long as a month does not seriously impair the hypothalamic-pituitary-adrenal axis. Children with leukemia who were given high-dose prednisone (2 mg/kg per day) for 1 month had normal basal plasma

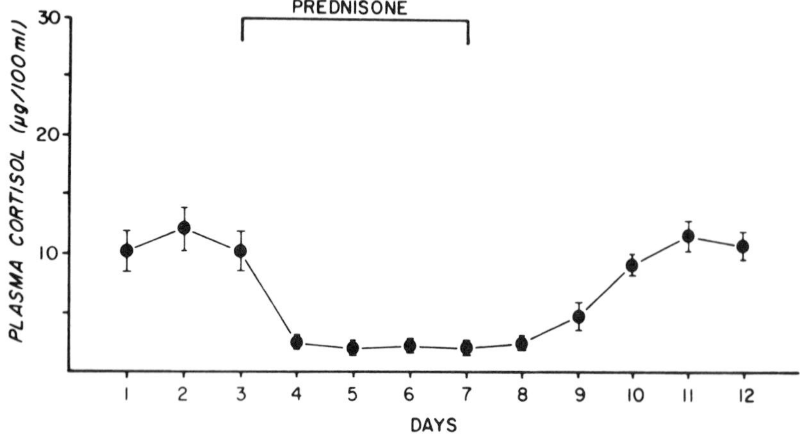

FIGURE 15-7 Fasting plasma cortisol levels (mean ± SEM) in 10 subjects before, during, and after the oral administration of prednisone, 25 mg twice daily on days 3 to 7. (*From Streck and Lockwood.*[153])

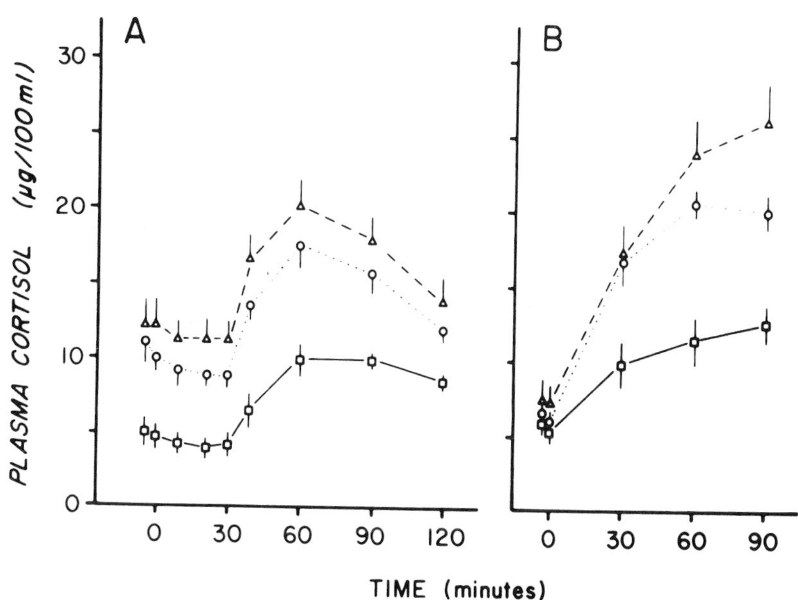

FIGURE 15-8 Plasma cortisol response (mean ± SEM) to insulin-induced hypoglycemia (*A*) and synthetic ACTH (*B*) in 10 subjects before (△) and at 2 days (○) and 5 days (□) after oral prednisone, 25 mg twice daily for 5 days. (*From Streck and Lockwood.*[153])

cortisol 9 days after discontinuation, and this group of patients had normal clinical and plasma cortisol responses to intercurrent stress in the 3 months after prednisone was discontinued.[155] With lower doses, there may be suppression of basal secretion but normal responsiveness of the axis to stimulation even when the steroid is given for a more prolonged period.[156] Finally, with long-term therapy, particularly in high doses, there is profound and prolonged suppression of the axis and absent responsiveness to major stimuli (Fig. 15-9).[156,157]

The degree of pituitary-adrenal suppression also depends on the timing of the dose and the steroid preparation used.[158] As discussed under Alternate-Day Therapy, above, longer-acting steroids such as dexamethasone result in greater suppression than do short-acting ones such as cortisol, prednisolone, and prednisone, since they are present in the circulation for a longer period.[94,103] Suppression is also greater if glucocorticoids are administered in the evening or at night rather than in the morning, since this results in maximal suppression of the normal early morning circadian rise in ACTH.[159] This timing of steroid administration is essential to the success of alternate-day therapy (see above).[139] Also discussed previously was the fact that therapy with ACTH, if given once daily, causes less suppression than does therapy with oral corticosteroids.[114,115]

Kinetics of Return to Normal Axis Function

The kinetics of the return of the hypothalamic-pituitary-adrenal axis are also time- and dose-dependent. Recovery of the axis may require hours to months.[153,156,157] Thus, as mentioned above, hypothalamic-pituitary-adrenal responsiveness remains normal after single doses and returns to normal within several days after short courses of glucocorticoids (Fig. 15-8).[153–155] When moderate doses of glucocorticoids have been continued for months to

FIGURE 15-9 Plasma cortisol response (shown as the increment) after insulin hypoglycemia testing in control subjects and patients on various doses of glucocorticoids for various times. A dashed line connects median values, the solid line shows the median value for the control subjects, and the horizontal dashed lines show the upper and lower values for the control subjects. For the steroid-treated patients, open circles indicate that the test was performed while the patient was on steroids, and closed circles indicate that the test was performed 48 h after discontinuing therapy. (*Based on data from Livanou et al.*[156])

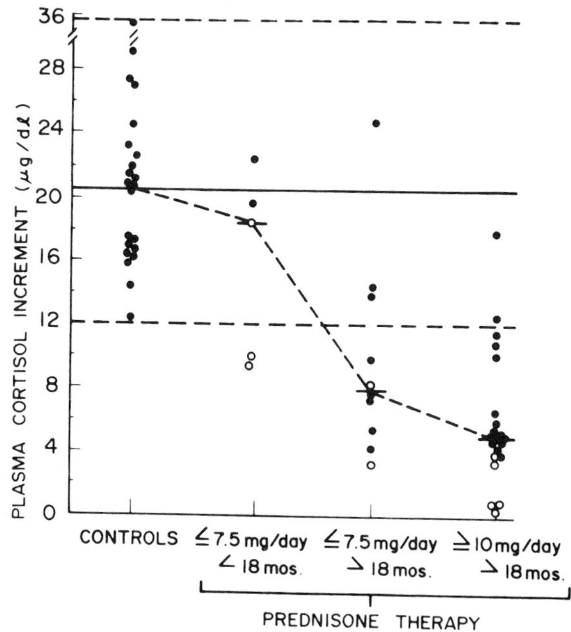

years, recovery is prolonged in general, although considerable individual variability is present (Fig. 15-10).[156] Recovery of both basal cortisol secretion and stress responsiveness is more rapid in patients who have received lower glucocorticoid doses (7.5 mg or less of prednisone per day) and those in whom therapy was of shorter duration.[156] Basal plasma cortisol levels return to normal first, usually within 1 month of the cessation of therapy, but months may be required before the response to insulin-induced hypoglycemia returns to normal (Fig. 15-10).[156]

The kinetics of the return of the axis in patients exposed to higher glucocorticoid concentrations for more prolonged periods, i.e., 1 to 10 years, are shown in Fig. 15-11.[157] In the first month after withdrawal of glucocorticoid excess, both plasma cortisol and ACTH levels were subnormal. During the next several months, plasma ACTH levels increased to supranormal in most of these patients. Despite this, cortisol levels remained low and were subnormally responsive to stimulation with exogenous ACTH, indicating persisting adrenal atrophy.[157] However, at 5 to 9 months the plasma cortisol levels gradually increased into the normal range because of the trophic influence of ACTH, and in this study normal concentrations of plasma cortisol and ACTH were attained in all patients more than 9 months after glucocorticoid withdrawal.[157] Although suppression after more than a year is rare, the author has followed one patient with a successfully resected cortisol-producing adrenal adenoma whose axis has remained suppression for 2.5 years in spite of otherwise normal pituitary function. Thus, the return of normal axis function requires sequential recovery of the hypothalamus, pituitary, and adrenal. The recovery of pituitary ACTH secretion is the primary and limiting determinant for recovery; with recovery, ACTH levels gradually rise and stimulate the adrenal. However, they generally need to become elevated before adequate adrenal stimulation occurs with reversal of the adrenal atrophy. As plasma cortisol levels reach the normal range, the feedback inhibition by hydrocortisone begins to suppress ACTH production; as this happens, this axis returns to normal.

As mentioned in Chap. 12, administration of ACTH for 3 to 5 days can increase the responsiveness of the adrenal gland to normal or nearly normal.[156–161] It might therefore seem desirable to administer ACTH to restore such responsiveness to the adrenal. However, the limiting factor in the return of the axis is the ability of the pituitary to release ACTH. Thus, if ACTH is administered, the subsequent increase in steroid production may impair the return of the pituitary to normal.[160] Further, once ACTH is withdrawn, it is still necessary to wait until the pituitary returns to normal function[160] before it can be predicted with confidence that the patient will respond to an insult requiring increased cortisol production. Thus, there is no evidence that ACTH hastens

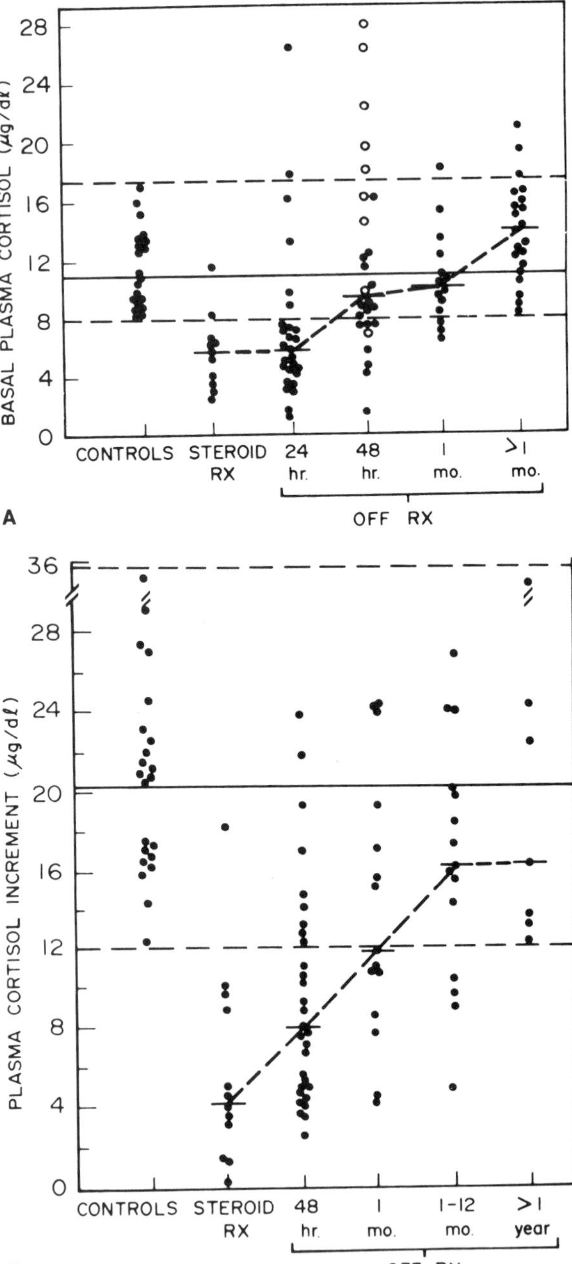

FIGURE 15-10 (*A*) Basal plasma cortisol levels in control subjects, patients on glucocorticoid therapy, and patients in whom glucocorticoid therapy had been withdrawn ("off Rx") for the indicated times. For the period 48 h after steroid withdrawal, open circles indicate the patients who had been on 7.5 mg of prednisone or less and closed circles indicate patients who had been on 10 mg of prednisone or more. (*B*) Plasma cortisol response to insulin-induced hypoglycemia testing in control subjects and patients on glucocorticoid therapy and after withdrawal of therapy for the indicated times. For both panels, heavy dashed lines connect median values. The solid line indicates the median value for the controls, and the lighter dashed line shows the upper and lower values for the control subjects. (*Based on data from Livanou et al.*[156])

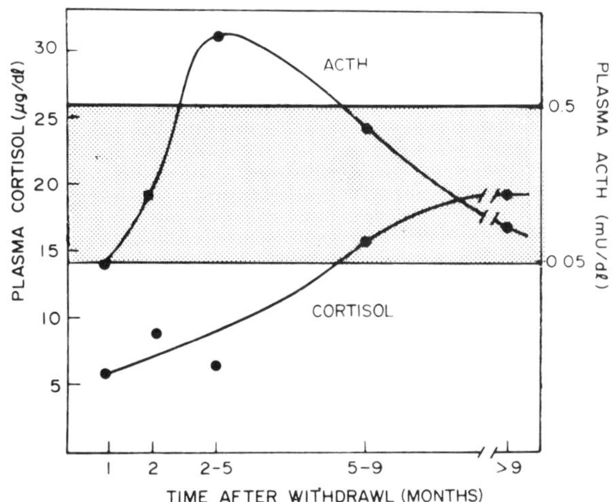

FIGURE 15-11 Median plasma cortisol and ACTH levels (at 6 A.M.) in patients after withdrawal of glucorticoids. The shaded area indicates the range of values for control subjects. The data were obtained from eight patients with spontaneous Cushing's syndrome after removal of an adrenal tumor and from six patients on high-dose glucocorticoid therapy for 1 to 10 years. Glucocorticoids were not abruptly withdrawn in these patients but instead were tapered over periods of 1 to 4 weeks. The time after withdrawal indicates the period following complete cessation of therapy. (*Based on data from Graber et al.*[157])

recovery of the axis[158,160,161] when given either as a single course or intermittently for months, and ACTH administration is therefore not recommended.

Steroid Withdrawal Syndromes

The response to withdrawal of steroids can vary. First, the primary disease may remain in remission, and the patient may be asymptomatic. Second, there may be a recurrence or worsening of the disease, and the patient may or may not experience other symptoms of withdrawal. Third, the patient may experience symptoms caused by adrenal insufficiency. Fourth, the patient may experience symptoms similar to those of adrenal insufficiency yet have no biochemical evidence of deficient adrenal secretion ("steroid withdrawal syndrome").[162,163] Perhaps a subclass within the last category is the case in which there is a general lack of well-being without other symptoms of adrenal insufficiency.

In the first case, in which there are no symptoms and the disease for which steroids were given is quiescent, has improved, or has resolved, it is necessary only to follow the disease and the potential for a suppressed axis. Many patients can have a suppressed hypothalamic-pituitary-adrenal axis without symptoms of adrenal insufficiency, and if these patients are exposed to stress (see Chap. 12), they can develop acute adrenal insufficiency. Thus, all the precautions outlined below for the withdrawal procedures should be taken.

In the second case, where there is exacerbation of the primary disease, it may be necessary to reinstitute glucocorticoid therapy. Of course, there are times when this is not warranted. For instance, in acute lymphocytic leukemia of childhood, the development of glucocorticoid resistance precludes further glucocorticoid therapy. In other cases, serious complications of glucocorticoid therapy (e.g., compression fractures and severe osteoporosis) may be present to such an extent that further steroid administration may be more damaging than relief of the primary condition. In cases where therapy is not reinstituted, the precautions relative to hypothalamic-pituitary-adrenal axis suppression must be followed.

The symptoms of adrenal insufficiency that occur with a suppressed hypothalamic-pituitary-adrenal axis are similar to those of secondary adrenal insufficiency discussed in Chap. 12. Thus, the adrenal glomerulosa, with its electrolyte-regulating properties, is almost always intact, so that dehydration, hypotension, hyponatremia, and hyperkalemia are uncommon (see Chap. 12).

The steroid withdrawal syndrome is characterized by symptoms similar or identical to those of adrenocortical insufficiency in a patient who is receiving physiologic doses of glucocorticoids or has a normally responsive hypothalamic-pituitary-adrenal axis.[162,163] The syndrome occurs in patients in whom exogenous glucocorticoid doses are either reduced or withdrawn. Thus, patients may develop the syndrome even though they continue to receive "physiologic" or even supraphysiologic doses of glucocorticoids. The most prominent clinical features are lethargy, malaise, anorexia, nausea, arthralgias, myalgias, weight loss, desquamation of the skin, headache, and fever.[163] Vomiting is less common; postural hypotension may occur occasionally.[163] These symptoms are variable and may be transient.[163] For example, the reduction of the steroid dosage may be accompanied by mild to moderate symptoms that resolve within several days and permit continuation of the lower dose. However, in other patients, the symptoms may be severe and disabling; the persistence of severe symptoms for more than several days is an indication to reinstitute glucocorticoids in small doses (e.g., 10 to 20 mg of cortisol) or to increase the steroid dose to its former level and then to taper it by smaller decrements over a more prolonged period.

The mechanisms of the steroid withdrawal syndrome are unknown: however, there are two potential explanations. First, it is possible that the transition from higher to lower doses of glucocorticoids, even when the lower dose is "normal," causes the same type of subjective findings as those observed in adrenal insufficiency. Second, it is possible that these patients have a relative state of glucocorticoid resistance that renders them effectively hypoadrenal. However, there is no evidence that this group is in danger of developing acute adrenal insufficiency, suggesting that any resistance, if present, is not severe or complete enough to prevent certain responses to stress.

Evaluation of Axis Function

The same considerations discussed in Chap. 12 for evaluation of adrenal insufficiency apply in evaluating suppression of the hypothalamic-pituitary-adrenal axis. First, a normal random cortisol determination does not exclude significant suppression; however, a random plasma cortisol of 20 μg/dl or greater excludes adrenal insufficiency in virtually all circumstances. Conversely, a subnormal random cortisol level may occur during episodic cortisol secretion and thus does not prove suppression of the axis. If the plasma cortisol concentration is low or low normal during an obvious acute stress (e.g., during shock), significant suppression is likely. However, stimulation tests of the axis are usually required for verification.

The tests used to assess the integrity of the axis are discussed in Chap. 12. Among them, the rapid ACTH stimulation, metyrapone, and insulin-induced hypoglycemia tests are most frequently used. The rapid ACTH stimulation test is more commonly used because of its ease; it is a simple and safe outpatient procedure. If the cortisol response is subnormal, this test confirms suppression of the axis, since deficient cortisol responsiveness indicates adrenal atrophy secondary to ACTH deficiency. However, a normal response to this test does not necessarily predict normal pituitary responsiveness to stress (see Chap. 12), and in this circumstance more definitive information is obtained with metyrapone or insulin-induced hypoglycemia. Thus, in usual circumstances, a normal response to the rapid ACTH test is sufficient to preclude the necessity of daily maintenance therapy. However, if stress such as elective surgery is anticipated, further testing should be carried out or the patient should receive glucocorticoid coverage (Chap. 12).

Withdrawal Protocols and Indications for Steroid Coverage

When the status of the disease being treated permits withdrawal of glucocorticoids, both the patient and the physician must be fully aware of the tedious nature and potential difficulty of the process. The patient should be informed of the symptoms of steroid withdrawal; this knowledge may allow differentiation of these symptoms for those caused by worsening of the disease. The patient should also be aware of the potential time required for the return to normal of the axis.

Patients who have undergone only short courses of steroid therapy usually do not have great difficulty during steroid withdrawal, but patients on high-dose long-term therapy may require close monitoring for as long as a year before pituitary-adrenal function returns to normal. In assessing these patients, the physician must assess the underlying disease and the potential symptoms of steroid withdrawal and in addition must serially assess the hypothalamic-pituitary-adrenal-axis.[158]

In patients who have been on long-term glucocorticoid therapy, it is usually necessary to reduce the total dosage more gradually toward physiologic levels, since abrupt changes may precipitate exacerbation of the underlying disease and steroid withdrawal symptoms. For instance, the glucocorticoid dose may be reduced by 2.5 to 5.0 mg of prednisone (or its equivalent) per week. As the dose is being reduced, an attempt should also be made to administer the dose either once daily in the morning or on alternate days to give the hypothalamic-pituitary-adrenal axis a better chance to recover (see above). The dose may have to be increased if there is worsening of the underlying disease or if severe symptoms of steroid withdrawal develop. Acute flare-ups or unrelated acute illness should be managed by means of short-term administration of high-dose steroids, with a return to the previous dosage as soon as the clinical situation permits. During this period, adjunctive therapy (see above) should also be continued or increased, as this will assist in the control of the primary disorder.

When the total steroid dosage has been tapered to the equivalent of 20 to 30 mg of cortisol or 5 mg of prednisone given as a single morning dose, the function of the hypothalamic-pituitary-adrenal axis should be assessed. The simplest method is to measure basal morning cortisol levels before the daily glucocorticoid dose at 1- to 2-month intervals. When basal cortisol levels are normal (>10 μg/dl), therapy may be withdrawn, since this indicates normal basal steroid section. Additionally, at this point serial assessment of the axis may be begun, also at 1- to 2-month intervals. Persisting subnormal responses to the rapid ACTH stimulation test indicate continuing suppression of the axis (Chap. 12). When normal responsiveness to ACTH occurs, the axis can be presumed to be normal in most patients; confirmation can be readily obtained by demonstrating a normal response to the overnight metyrapone test (Chap. 12). If the responses to both rapid ACTH stimulation and metyrapone tests are normal, the return of the normal function of the hypothalamic-pituitary-adrenal axis is demonstrated.

Supplementation with high doses of glucocorticoids may be required at any point in the withdrawal process for acute illness or elective surgery. In these circumstances, increased steroid doses should be administered to patients who have (1) a continuing requirement for glucocorticoid therapy, (2) subnormal basal cortisol levels, (3) subnormal responsiveness to the rapid ACTH stimulation test, or (4) a subnormal response to metyrapone testing. A patient who presents with an acute illness and for whom no previous data are available should empirically be covered with steroids, which may be withdrawn rapidly as the acute stress resolves. Similarly, patients undergoing surgery who have a history of prior glucocorticoid therapy may require additional steroid coverage. In these patients, a normal response to metyrapone indicates normal function of the axis, and glucocorticoid therapy is not required. If time does not allow an assessment of hypothalamic-pituitary-adrenal axis function, steroid coverage should be given during surgery and the postoperative period. The doses and ancillary procedures for the treatment of acute illness and steroid coverage for surgery in these patients with secondary adrenocortical insufficiency caused by glucocorticoid suppression are detailed in Chap. 12.

REFERENCES

1. Baxter JD, Rousseau GG: Glucocorticoid hormone action: An overview, in Baxter JD, Rouseau GG (eds): *Glucocorticoid Hormone Action.* New York, Springer-Verlag, 1979, p. 1.
2. Christy NP: Iatrogenic Cushing's syndrome, in Christy NP (ed): *The Human Adrenal Cortex.* New York, Harper & Row, 1971, p 395.
3. Boumpas DM: Glucocorticoid therapy for immune-mediated diseases: Basic and clinical correlates. *Ann Intern Med* 119:1198, 1993.
4. Schleimer R, Claman H, Oronsky A (eds): *Anti-Inflammatory Steroid Action: Basic and Clinical Aspects.* San Diego, Academic, 1989.
5. Lippman ME: Steroids in malignant diseases: Progress in patient selection. *Hosp Pract* 19:93, 1984.
6. Cohen J: Lymphocyte death induced by glucocorticoids, in Schleimer R, Claman H, Ornonsky A (eds): *Anti-Inflammatory Steroid Action: Basic and Clinical Aspects.* San Diego, Academic, 1989, p 110.
7. Bagby GC, Gabourel JD, Linman JW: Glucocorticoid therapy in the preleukemic syndrome (hemopoietic dysplasia). *Ann Intern Med* 92:55, 1980.
8. Brennan MJ: Corticosteroids in the treatment of solid tumors, in Azarnoff DL (ed): *Steroid Therapy.* Philadelphia, Saunders, 1975, p 134.
9. Atkinson JP, Frank MN: Glucocorticoids in the treatment of hemolytic disorders, in Azarnoff DL (ed): *Steroid Therapy.* Philadelphia, Saunders, 1975, p. 49.
10. Collins JV, Clark TJH, Brown D, Townsend J: The use of corticosteroids in the treatment of acute asthma. *Q J Med* 44:259, 1975.
11. Bruce C, Weatherstone R, Seaton A, Taylor WH: Histamine levels in plasma, blood and urine in severe asthma and the effect of corticosteroid treatment. *Thorax* 31:724, 1976.
12. Barnes P, Pedersen S: Efficacy and safety of inhaled corticosteroids in asthma. *Am Rev Respir Dis* 148:S1, 1993.
13. Szefler S: Glucocorticoid therapy for asthma: Clinical pharmacology. *J Allergy Clin Immunol* 88:147, 1991.
14. Corrigan C: Mechanism of glucocorticoid action in asthma: Too little, too late. *Clin Exp Allergy* 22:315, 1992.
15. Mitchell DM, Gilfeh P, Rehahn M, Diamond AH, Collins JV: Effects of prednisolone in chronic airflow limitation. *Lancet* 2:193, 1984.
16. Mendella LA, Manfreda J, Warren CPW, Anthonisen NR: Steroid response in stable chronic obstructive pulmonary disease. *Ann Intern Med* 96:17, 1982.
17. Fanta FH, Rossing TH, McFadden ER Jr: Glucocorticoids in acute asthma: A critical controlled trial. *Am J Med* 74:845, 1983.
18. Collins JV, Jones D: Corticosteroid mechanisms and therapeutic schedules, in Weiss EB (ed): *Status Asthmaticus.* Baltimore, University Park Press, 1978, p 235.
19. Frame B, Parfitt AM: Corticosteroid-responsive hypercalcemia with elevated serum 1-alpha,25-dihydroxyvitamin D. *Ann Intern Med* 93:449, 1980.
20. Tauber MG, Khayam-Bashi H, Sande MA: Effects of ampicillin and corticosteroids on brain water content, cerebral spinal fluid pressure and lactate in experimental pneumococcal meningitis. *J Infect Dis* 151:528, 1985.
21. Ellison GW: Corticosteroids in neurological disease. *Hosp Pract* 19:105, 1984.
22. Fishman RA: Steroids in the treatment of brain edema. *N Engl J Med* 306:359, 1982.
23. Johnson TS, Rock PB, Fulco CS, Trad LA, Spark RF, Maher JT: Prevention of acute mountain sickness by dexamethasone. *N Engl J Med* 310:683, 1984.
24. Markman M, Sheidler V, Ettinger DS, Quaskey SA, Mellits ED: Antiemetic efficacy of dexamethasone: Randomized, double-blind, crossover study with prochlorperazine in patients receiving cancer chemotherapy. *N Engl J Med* 9:549, 1984.
25. Baxter JD: Glucocorticoid hormone action, in Gill GN (ed): *Pharmacology of Adrenal Cortical Hormones.* Oxford, UK, Pergamon, 1979, p 67.
26. Dale DC, Petersdorf RG: Corticosteroids and infectious diseases, in Azarnoff DL (ed): *Steroid Therapy.* Philadelphia, Saunders, 1975, p 209.
27. Kass EH, Finland M: Corticosteroids and infections. *Adv Intern Med* 9:45, 1958.
28. Parrillo JE, Fauci AS: Mechanisms of glucocorticoid action on immune processes. *Annu Rev Pharmacol Toxicol* 19:179, 1979.
29. Rousseau GG, Baxter JD: Glucocorticoid receptors, in Baxter JD, Rousseau GG (ed): *Glucocorticoid Hormone Action.* New York, Springer-Verlag, 1979, p. 49.
30. Baxter JD, MacLeod KM: The molecular basis for hormone action, in Bondy PK, Rosenberg LE (ed): *Metabolic Control and Disease.* Philadelphia, Saunders, 1979, p 104.
31. Gambertoglio JG, Vincenti F, Feduska NJ, Birnbaum J, Salvatierra O, Amend WJC Jr; Prednisolone disposition in cushingoid and noncushingoid kidney transplant patients. *J Clin Endocrinol Metab* 51:561, 1980.
32. Thorn GW, Jenkins D, Laidlow JC, Goetz FC, Dingman JF, Arons WL, Streeten DHP, McCraken BH: Medical progress: Pharmacological aspects of adrenocortical steroids and ACTH in man. *N Engl J Med* 248:232, 1953.
33. Cope CL: *Adrenal Steroids and Disease,* London, Pittman Medical, 1977.
34. Axelrod L: Glucocorticoid therapy. *Medicine* Baltimore 55:39, 1976.
35. Bayer JM, Neuner H-P: Cushing-Syndrom und erhöhter Augeninnedruck. *Dtsch Med Wochenschr* 40:1791, 1967.
36. George WE Jr, Wilmot M, Greenhouse A, Hammeke M: Medical management of steroid-induced epidural lipomatosis. *N Engl J Med* 308:316, 1983.
37. Russell N, Belanger G, Benoit B, Latter D, Finestone D, Armstrong G: Spinal epidural lipomatosis: A complication of glucocorticoid therapy. *J Can Sci Neurol* 11:383, 1984.
38. Polansky JR, Weinreb RN: Anti-inflammatory agents: Steroids as anti-inflammatory agents, in Sears ML (ed): *Handbook of Experimental Pharmacology.* Heidelberg, Springer-Verlag, 1984, vol 69, p 459.
39. Roberts AM, Leibowtiz HM: Corticosteroid therapy of ophthalmologic diseases. *Hosp Pract* 19:181, 1984.
40. Ellis EF: Corticosteroid regimens in pediatric practice. *Hosp Pract* 19:143, 1984.
41. Brocklebank JT, Harcourt RB, Meadow SR: Corticosteroid induced cataracts in idiopathic nephrotic syndrome. *Arch Dis Child* 53:30, 1982.

42. Toogood J, Markov A, Baskerville J, Dyson C: Association of ocular cataracts with inhaled and oral steroid therapy during long term treatment for asthma. *J Allergy Clin Immunol* 91:571, 1993.
43. Manabe S, Bucala R, Cerami A: Nonenzymatic addition of glucocorticoids to lens proteins in steroid-induced cataracts. *J Clin Invest* 74:1803, 1984.
44. Mankin H: Nontraumatic necrosis of bone (osteonecrosis). *N Engl J Med* 326:1473, 1992.
45. Zizic T: Osteonecrosis. *Curr Opin Rheumatol* 3:481, 1991.
46. Zizic TM, Marcoux C, Hungerford DS, Dansereau J-V, Stevens MB: Corticosteroid therapy associated with ischemic necrosis of bone in systemic lupus erythematosis. *Am J Med* 79:596, 1985.
47. Chesney RW, Mayess RB, Rose P, Jax DK: Effect of prednisone on growth and bone mineral content in childhood glomerular disease. *Am J Dis Child* 132:768, 1978.
48. Baylink DJ: Glucocorticoid-induced osteoporosis. *N Engl J Med* 309:306, 1983.
49. Laan R, van Riel P, van de Putte L, van Erning L, van't Hof M, Lemmens J: Low-dose prednisone induces rapid reversible axial bone loss in patients with rheumatoid arthritis. *Ann Intern Med* 119:963, 1993.
50. Reid I, Evans M, Stapleton J: Lateral spine densitometry is a more sensitive indicator of glucocorticoid-induced bone loss. *J Bone Mineral Res* 7:1221, 1992.
51. Adinoff AD, Hollister JR: Steroid-induced fractures and bone loss in patients with asthma. *N Engl J Med* 309:265, 1983.
52. Gluck OS, Murphy WA, Hahn TJ, Hahn B: Bone loss in adults receiving alternate day glucocorticoid therapy. A comparison with daily therapy. *Arthritis Rheum* 24:892, 1981.
53. Spencer H, Rubio N, Rubio E, Indreika M, Seitam A: Chronic alcoholism: Frequently overlooked cause of osteoporosis in men. *Am J Med* 80:393, 1986.
54. Hahn TJ; Corticosteroid-induced osteopenia. *Arch Intern Med* 138:882, 1978.
55. Lukert B, Raisz L: Glucocorticoid-induced osteoporosis: Pathogenesis and management. *Ann Intern Med* 112:352, 1990.
56. Hodgson S: Corticosteroid-induced osteoporosis. *Endocrinol Metab Clin North Am* 19:95, 1990.
57. Libanati C, Baylink D: Prevention and treatment of glucocorticoid-induced osteoporosis. *Chest* 102:1426, 1992.
58. Meunier P: Is steroid-induced osteoporosis preventable? *N Engl J Med* 328:1781, 1993.
59. Hahn T, Halstead L, Teitelbaum S, Hahn B: Altered mineral metabolism in glucocorticoid-induced osteopenia: Effect of 25-hydroxyvitamin D administration. *J Clin Invest* 64:655, 1979.
60. Sambrook P, Birmingham J, Kelly P, Kempler S, Nguyen T, Pocock N, Eisman J: Prevention of corticosteroid osteoporosis. *N Engl J Med* 328:1747, 1993.
61. Ringe J-D, Welzel D: Salmon calcitonin in the therapy of corticoid-induced osteoporosis. *Eur J Clin Pharmacol* 33:35, 1987.
62. Reid I, King A, Alexander C, Ibbertson H: Prevention of steroid-induced osteoporosis with (3-amino-1-hydroxypropylidene)-1, 1-bisphonsphonate (APD). *Lancet* 1:143, 1988.
63. Mulder H, Shelder H: Effect of cyclical etidronate regimen on prophylaxis of bone loss of glucocorticoid therapy in postmenopausal women. *Bone Miner* 17:168, 1992.
64. Greenwald M, Brandli D, Spector S, Silverman S, Golde G: Corticosteroid-induced osteoporosis: Effects of a treatment with slow-release sodium fluoride. *Osteoporosis Int* 2:303, 1992.
65. Claman HN: Glucocorticosteroids: II. The clinical responses. *Hosp Pract* 18:143, 1983.
66. Graham BS, Tucker WS Jr: Opportunistic infections in endogenous Cushing's syndrome. *Ann Intern Med* 101:334, 1984.
67. Sheagren J: Glucocorticoid action: Infectious diseases, in Schleimer R, Claman H, Oronsky A (eds): *Anti-Inflammatory Steroid Action: Basic and Clinical Aspects*. San Diego, Academic, 1989, p 525.
68. Czaja AJ, Ludwig J, Baggenstoss AH, Wolff A: Corticosteroid-treated chronic active hepatitis in remission: Uncertain prognosis of chronic persistent hepatitis. *N Engl J Med* 304:5, 1981.
69. Lam KC, Lai CL, Ng RP, Trepo C, Wu PC: Deleterious effect of prednisolone in HBsAg-positive chronic active hepatitis. *N Engl J Med* 304:380, 1981.
70. Hoofnagle JH, Davis GL, Pappas C, Hanson RG, Peters M, Avigan MI, Waggoner JG, Jones EA, Seeff LB: A short course of prednisolone in chronic type B hepatitis: Report of a randomized, double-blind, placebo-controlled trial. *Ann Intern Med* 104:12, 1986.
71. Tuberculosis in corticosteroid-treated asthmatics (editorial). *Br Med J* 2:266, 1976.
72. Fauci AS, Dale DC, Balow JE: Glucocorticosteroid therapy: Mechanisms of action and clinical considerations. *Ann Intern Med* 84:304, 1976.
73. Askari A, Vignos PJ, Moskowitz RW: Steroid myopathy in connective tissue disease. *Am J Med* 61:485, 1976.
74. Horker FF, Scheidegger JR, Grunig BE, Frey FJ: Evidence that prednisone-induced myopathy is reversed by physical training. *J Clin Endocrinol Metab* 61:83, 1985.
75. Nashel DJ: Is atherosclerosis a complication of long-term corticosteroid treatment? *Am J Med* 80:925, 1986.
76. Petri M, Perez-Gutthann S, Spence D, Hochberg M: Risk factors for coronary artery disease in patients with systemic lupus erythematosus. *Am J Med* 93:513, 1992.
77. Plotz C, Knowlton A, Ragan C: The natural history of Cushing's syndrome. *Am J Med* 13:597, 1952.
78. Gordan GS: Drug treatment of the osteoporoses. *Annu Rev Pharmacol Toxicol* 18:253, 1978.
79. Litz T, Carter JD, Lewis BI, Suvratt C: Effects of ACTH and cortisone on mood and mentation. *Psychosom Med* 14:363, 1952.
80. Woodbury DM: Relation between the adrenal cortex and the central nervous system. *Pharmacol Rev* 10:275, 1958.
81. Gookler P, Schein J: Psychic effects of ACTH and cortisone. *Psychosom Med* 15:589, 1953.
82. Gustavson LE, Benet LZ: Pharmacokinetics of natural and synthetic glucocorticoids, in Anderson DC, Winter JSD (eds): *The Actual Cortex* Cornwall, UK, Butterworth, 1985, p 235.
83. Hsueh WA, Pay-Guevara A, Bledsoe T: Studies comparing the clearance rate of 11β,17,21-trihydroxypreg-1,4-diene-3,20-dione (prednisolone) after oral 17,21-dihydroxypreg-1,4-diene-3,11,20-trione and intravenous prednisolone. *J Clin Endocrinol Metab* 48:748, 1959.
84. Melby JC: Clinical pharmacology of adrenal steroids, in Thorn GW (ed): *Steroid Therapy*. Kalamazoo, MI, Medcom, 1974, p 16.
85. Fariss BL, Hane S, Shinsako J, Forsham PH: Comparison of absorption of cortisone acetate and hydrocortisone hemisuccinate. *J Clin Endocrinol Metab* 47:1137, 1978.
86. Plumpton FS, Besser GM, Cole PV: Corticosteroid treatment and surgery: II. The management of steroid cover. *Anaesthesia* 24:12, 1969.
87. Wolff ME: Structure-activity relationships in glucocorticoids, in Baxter JD, Rousseau GG (eds): *Glucocorticoid Hormone Action*. New York, Springer-Verlag, 1979, p 97.
88. Robertson DB, Maibach HI: Topical corticosteroids. *Hosp Formulary* 16:1130, 1981.
89. Weston WL: Topical corticosteroids in dermatologic disorders. *Hosp Pract* 19:159, 1984.
90. Braude AC, Rebuck AS: Prednisone and methylprednisolone disposition in the lung. *Lancet* 2:995, 1983.
91. Collaborative Group on Antenatal Steroid Therapy: Effect of antenatal dexamethasone administration on the prevention of respiratory distress syndrome. *Am J Obstet Gynecol* 141:276, 1981.
92. Kream J, Mulay S, Fukushima DK, Solomon S: Determination of plasma dexamethasone in the mother and the new-

born after administration of the hormone in a clinical trial. *J Clin Endocrinol Metab* 56:127, 1983.
93. Lewis GP, Jusko WJ, Burke CW, Graves L: Prednisone side effects and serum protein levels. *Lancet* 2:778, 1971.
94. Meikle AW, Tyler FH: Potency and duration of action of glucocorticoids: Effects of hydrocortisone, prednisone and dexamethasone on human pituitary-adrenal function. *Am J Med* 63:200, 1977.
95. Ballard PL, Carter JP, Graham BS, Baxter JD: A radioreceptor assay for evaluation of the plasma glucocorticoid activity of natural and synthetic steroids in man. *J. Clin Endocrinol Metab* 41:290, 1975.
96. Meikle AW, Weed JA, Tyler FH: Kinetics and interconversion of prednisolone and prednisone studied with new radioimmunoassays. *J Clin Endocrinol Metab* 41:717, 1975.
97. Gifford RH: Corticosteroid therapy for rheumatoid arthritis, in Azarnoff DL (ed): *Steroid Therapy*. Philadelphia, Saunders, 1975, p 78.
98. Rose JQ, Yurchak AM, Jusko WJ: Dose dependent pharmacokinetics of prednisone and prednisolone in man. *J Pharmacokinet Biopharm* 9:389, 1981.
99. Bondy PK: The adrenal cortex, in Bondy PK, Rosenberg LE (eds): *Metabolic Control and Disease*. Philadelphia, Saunders, 1979, p 1427.
100. Haynes RC Jr, Murad F: Adrenocorticotropic hormone; adrenocortical steroids and their synthetic analogs: Inhibitors of adrenocortical steroid biosynthesis, in Gilman AG, Goodman LS, Rall TW, Murad F (eds): *The Pharmacological Basis of Therapeutics*. New York, Macmillan, 1985, p 1459.
101. Dluhy RG, Newmark SR, Lauler DP, Thorn GW: Pharmacology and chemistry of adrenal glucocorticoids, in Azarnoff DL (ed): *Steroid Therapy*. Philadelphia, Saunders, 1975, p 1.
102. Brooks RV: Biosynthesis of adrenocortical steroids, in James VHT (ed): *The Adrenal Gland*. New York, Raven, 1979, p 67.
103. Meikle AW, Clarke DH, Tyler FH: Cushing's syndrome from low doses of dexamethasone. *JAMA* 235:1592, 1976.
104. Hill M, Szefler S, Ball B, Bartoszek M, Brenner A: Monitoring glucocorticoid therapy: A pharmacokinetic approach. *Clin Pharmacol Ther* 48:390, 1990.
105. Kozower M, Veatch L, Kaplan MM: Decreased clearance of prednisone, a factor in the development of corticosteroid side effects. *J Clin Endocrinol Metab* 38:407, 1974.
106. Benet LZ, Frey FJ, Amend JC Jr, Lozada F, Frey BM: Endogenous and exogenous glucocorticoids in cushingoid patients. *Drug Intell Clin Pharm* 16:863, 1982.
107. Kawai S, Ichikawa Y, Homma M: Differences in metabolic properties among cortisol, prednisolone, and dexamethasone in liver and renal diseases: Accelerated metabolism of dexamethasone in renal failure. *J Clin Endocrinol Metab* 60:848, 1985
108. Boekenoogen SJ, Szefler SJ, Jusko WJ: Prednisolone disposition and protein binding in oral contraceptive users. *J. Clin Endocrinol Metab* 56:702, 1983.
109. Harris AW, Baxter JD: Variations in cellular sensitivity to glucocorticoids: Observations and mechanisms, in Baxter JD, Rousseau GG (eds): *Glucocorticoid Hormone Action*. New York, Springer-Verlag, 1979, p 423.
110. Intra-articular steroids (editorial). *Lancet* 1:38, 1984.
111. Clark RA, Anderson PB: Combined therapy with salbutamol and beclomethasone inhalers in chronic asthma. *Lancet* 2:70, 1978.
112. High dose corticosteroid inhalers for asthma (editorial). *Lancet* 2:23, 1984.
113. McAllen MK, Kochanowski SJ, Shaw KM: Steroid aerosols in asthma: An assessment of betamethasone valerate and a twelve month study of patients on maintenance treatment. *Br Med J* 1:171, 1974.
114. Daly JR, Fletcher MR, Glass D, Chambers DJ, Bitensky L, Chayen L: Comparison of effects of long term corticotrophin and corticosteroid treatment on responses of plasma growth hormone, ACTH and corticosteroid to hypoglycemia. *Br Med J* 2:521, 1974.
115. Bacon PA, Daly JR, Myles AB, Savage O: Hypothalamo-pituitary-adrenal function in patients on long-term adrenocorticotrophin therapy. *Ann Rheum Dis* 27:7, 1968.
116. Axelrod L: Glucocorticoids, in Kelly W, Harris E, Ruddy S, Sledge C (eds): *Textbook of Rheumatology*. Philadelphia, Saunders, 1989, 845.
117. Chrousos G, Kattah J, Beck R, Cleary P, Group ONS: Side effects of glucocorticoid treatment: Experience of the optic neuritis treatment trial. *JAMA* 269:2110, 1993.
118. Vincenti F, Amend W, Feduska NJ, Duca RM, Salvatierra JRO: Improved outcome following renal transplantation with reduction in the immunosuppression therapy for rejection episodes. *Am J Med* 69:107, 1980.
119. Bagby GC Jr, Lawrence HJ, Neerhout RC: T-Lymphocyte-mediated granulopoietic failure: *In vitro* identification of prednisone-responsive patients. *N Engl J Med* 309:1073, 1983.
120. Schumer W: Steroids in the treatment of clinical septic shock. *Ann Surg* 184:333, 1976.
121. Sheagren JN: Septic shock and corticosteroids. *N Engl J Med* 305:456, 1981.
122. Sprung CL, Panagiota V, Caralis MD, Marcial RTT, Pierce M, Gelbard MA, Long WM, Duncan RC, et al: The effects of high dose corticosteroids in patients with septic shock. *N Engl J Med* 311:1137, 1984.
123. Jacob HS: Pulse steroids in hematologic diseases. *Hosp Pract* 20:87, 1985.
124. Morris PJ, Chan L, French ME, Ting A: Low dose oral prednisolone in renal transplantation. *Lancet* 1:525, 1982.
125. Hinshaw LB, Archer LT, Beller-Todd BK, Coalson JJ, Flournoy DJ, Passey R, Benjamin B, White GL: Survival of primates in LD_{100} septic shock following steroid/antibiotic therapy. *J. Surg Res* 28:151, 1980.
126. Hoffman SL, Punjabi NH, Kumala S, Moechtar A, Pulungsih SP, Rivai AR, Rockhill RC, Woodward TE, Loedin AA: Reduction of mortality in chloramphenicol-treated severe typhoid fever by high-dose dexamethasone. *N Engl J Med* 310:82, 1984.
127. Felson DT, Anderson J: Evidence for the superiority of immunosuppressive drugs and prednisone over prednisone alone in lupus nephritis. *N Engl J Med* 311:1528, 1984.
128. Kyle RA, Greipp PR, Garton JP, Gertz MA: Primary systemic amyloidosis: Comparison of melphalan/prednisone versus colchicine. *Am J Med* 79:708, 1985.
129. Cogan MG, Sargent JA, Yarbrough SG, Vincenti F, Amend WJ Jr: Prevention of prednisone-induced negative nitrogen balance: Effect of dietary modification on urea generation rate in hemodialyzed patients receiving high dose glucocorticoids. *Ann Intern Med* 95:158, 1981.
130. Hunt TK, Ehrlich HP, Garcia JA, Dunphy JE: Effect of vitamin A on reversing the inhibitory effect of cortisone on healing of open wounds in animals and man. *Ann Surg* 170:633, 1969.
131. Baigelman W, Chodosh S, Pizzuto D, Cupples LA: Sputum and blood eosinophils during corticosteroid treatment of acute exacerbations of asthma. *Am J Med* 75:929, 1983.
132. Lawrence EC, Teague RB, Gottlieb MS, Jhingran SG, Liberman J: Serial changes in markers of disease activity with corticosteroid treatment in sarcoidosis. *Am J Med* 74:747, 1983.
133. Harter JG, Reddy WJ, Thorn GW: Studies on an intermittent corticosteroid dosage regimen. *N Engl J Med* 269:591, 1963.
134. Fauci AS: Corticosteroids in autoimmune disease. *Hosp Pract* 18:99, 1983.
135. Fauci AS: Alternate-day corticosteroid therapy. *Am J Med* 64:729, 1978.
136. Fleisher DS, Pellecchier P: Pituitary-adrenal responsiveness after corticosteroid therapy in children with nephrosis. *J. Pediatr* 70:54, 1967.
137. Hunder GG, Sheps SG, Allen GL, Joyce JW: Daily and alternate day corticosteroid regimens in treatment of giant cell

arteritis: Comparison in a prospective study. *Ann Intern Med* 82:613, 1975.
138. Foote KD, Brocklebank JT, Meadow SR: Height attainment in children with steroid-responsive nephrotic syndrome. *Lancet* 2:917, 1985.
139. Ackerman GL, Nolan CM: Adrenocortical responsiveness after alternate-day corticosteroid therapy. *N Engl J Med* 278:405, 1968.
140. Schurmeyer TH, Tsokos GC, Avgerinos PC, Balow JE, D'Agata R, Loriaux DL, Chrousos GP: Pituitary-adrenal responsiveness to corticotropin-releasing hormone in patients receiving chronic, alternate day glucocorticoid therapy. *J Clin Endocrinol Metab* 61:22, 1985.
141. Wyatt R, Waschek J, Weinberger M, Sherman B: Effects of inhaled beclomethasone dipropionate and alternate day prednisone on pituitary-adrenal function in children with chronic asthma. *N Engl J Med* 299:1387, 1978.
142. Fauci AS, Dale DC: Alternate day prednisone therapy and human lymphocyte subpopulations. *J Clin Invest* 55:22, 1975.
143. Harter JG: Alternate day therapy, in Thorn GW (ed): *Steroid Therapy*. Kalamazoo, MI, Medcom, 1974, p 42.
144. Schatz M, Patterson R, Zeit S, O'Rourke J, Melam H: Corticosteroid therapy for the pregnant asthmatic patient. *JAMA* 233:804, 1975.
145. Greenberger PA, Patterson R: Beclomethasone dipropionate for severe asthma during pregnancy. *Ann Intern Med* 98:478, 1983.
146. Rayburn W: Glucocorticoid therapy for rheumatic diseases: maternal, fetal, and breast-feeding considerations. *Am J Reprod Immunol Microbiol* 28:138, 1992.
147. Committee on Drugs AAoP: The transfer of drugs and other chemicals into human breask milk. *Pediatrics* 84:924, 1989.
148. Katz F, Duncan B: Entry of prednisone into human milk. *N Engl J Med* 293:1154, 1975.
149. Ost L, Wettrell G, Bjorkhem I, Rane A: Prednisolone excretion in human milk. *J Pediatr* 106:1008, 1985.
150. Messer J, Reitman D, Sacko H, Smith H, Chalmer T: Association of adrenocorticosteroid therapy and peptic ulcer disease. *N Engl J Med* 309:21, 1983.
151. Piper J, Ray W, Daugherty J, Griffin M: Corticosteroid use and peptic ulcer disease: Role of nonsteroidal anti-inflammatory drugs. *Ann Intern Med* 114:735, 1991.
152. Real FX, Krown SE, Koziner B: Steroid-related development of Kaposi's sarcoma in a homosexual man with Burkitt's lymphoma. *Am J Med* 30:119, 1986.
153. Streck WF, Lockwood DH: Pituitary adrenal recovery following short-term suppression with corticosteroids. *Am J Med* 66:910, 1979.
154. Zora J, Zimmerman D, Carey T, O'Connell E, Yunginger J: Hypothalamic-pituitary-adrenal axis suppression after short-term, high-dose glucocorticoid therapy in children with asthma. *J Allergy Clin Immunol* 77:9, 1986.
155. Lightner E, Johnson H, Corrigan J: Rapid adrenocortical recovery after short-term glucocorticoid therapy. *Am J Dis Child* 135:790, 1981.
156. Livanou T, Ferriman D, James VHT: Recovery of hypothalamo-pituitary-adrenal function after corticosteroid therapy. *Lancet* 2:856, 1967.
157. Graber AL, Ney RL, Nicholson WE, Island DP, Liddle GW: Natural history of pituitary-adrenal recovery following long-term suppression with corticosteroids. *J Clin Endocrinol Metab* 25:11, 1965.
158. Byyny RL: Withdrawal from glucocorticoid therapy. *N Engl J Med* 295:30, 1976.
159. Nichols T, Nugent CA, Tyler FH: Diurnal variation in suppression of adrenal function by glucocorticoids. *J Clin Endocrinol Metab* 25:343, 1965.
160. Donald RA, Espiner EA: The plasma cortisol and corticotropin response to hypoglycemia following adrenal steroid and ACTH administration. *J Clin Endocrinol Metab* 41:1, 1975.
161. Steroid therapy and the adrenals (editorial). *Lancet* 2:537, 1975.
162. Dixon RB, Christy NP: On the various forms of corticosteroid withdrawal syndrome. *Am J Med* 68:224, 1980.
163. Amatruda TT, Hurst MM, D'Esopo ND: Certain endocrine and metabolic facets of the steroid withdrawal syndrome. *J Clin Endocrinol Metab* 25:1207, 1965. 6

PART V

Gonadal Disease

CHAPTER 16

The Testis

Richard J. Santen

The human testis has two separate functions: secretion of androgens and excretion of mature spermatozoa. Although the functional anatomy and physiologic control of these two processes are interrelated, this chapter approaches androgen secretion and germinal cell maturation separately. This strategy minimizes the complexity of this system and reduces physiologic principles to their functional components. The important integrative interactions between the two testicular elements are addressed after full discussion of the discrete systems.

ANATOMY

Central Nervous System and Hypothalamic-Pituitary Axis

Major regulatory centers for the control of testicular function are highly concentrated within the hypothalamus.[1] Reference landmarks that delineate the critical areas include the optic chiasma anteriorly, the mammillary body posteriorly, and the infundibulum (Latin for "funnel") inferiorly (Fig. 16-1*A*). Most important is a small triangular area within these boundaries called the *medial basal hypothalamus,* which contains a dense aggregation of structures that are involved in the integrated control of testicular function. The major regulatory systems present include the peptidergic neurons (i.e., gonadotropin releasing hormone and opiate systems), the aminergic systems (i.e., dopamine, norepinephrine, serotonin), and the steroid receptor–containing neurons.

Peptidergic and Aminergic Systems

The greatest concentrations of neurons containing the peptide gonadotropin releasing hormone (GnRH) are found in two general regions: the anterior hypothalamic nuclear groups and the medial basal hypothalamus. The anterior region contains the suprachiasmatic and preoptic nuclei, the retrochiasmatic areas, and the organum vasculosum of the lamina terminalis (OVLT). In the medial basal hypothalamus are the arcuate nucleus and the median eminence.[2–4] Axons from cell bodies in the anterior hypothalamus and medial basal hypothalamus terminate on the "neurohemal" contact zone (see below), which lies in the external portion as well as the internal portion of the median eminence. Here GnRH is secreted into the pituitary portal capillaries for transport into the anterior pituitary.

The other peptidergic system of neurons contains the endogenous opiates.[5] The medial basal hypothalamus is rich in opiate receptors and contains measurable quantities of the enkephalins. The presence of endogenous opiates and their receptors in regions that are known to control gonadotropin secretion provides a neuroanatomic basis for physiologic observations that the opiates can modulate the secretion of luteinizing hormone (LH).[6] Also concentrated in the medial basal hypothalamus are aminergic neurons containing serotonin, norepinephrine, and dopamine (Fig. 16-1*C*). These axons represent the final termination of pathways that carry both stimulatory and inhibitory neural afferent systems into the hypothalamus.[1,2] Axons from this system terminate directly on portal capillaries in the median eminence, allowing direct access of dopamine to the portal system.

Steroid Receptor Neurons

Steroid binding is most dense in the region along the third ventricle extending from the suprachiasmatic area to the caudal part of the arcuate nucleus. In the most intensely labeled areas, 4000 to 5000 molecules of estradiol are bound per neuron. Concentrations of androgen receptors are much lower than concentrations of estrogen receptors in these areas.[7–9] The receptors for both of these sex steroids are present in areas which largely overlap those of GnRH-containing neurons; this finding suggests that a functional interaction takes place between peptidergic and sex steroid–binding neurons.

Portal Venous System

The superior hypophyseal arteries deliver arterial blood into the median eminence, where a capillary bed forms within a highly complex network of neurons. The axons here terminate directly onto the walls of capillaries (Fig. 16-2), allowing transport of

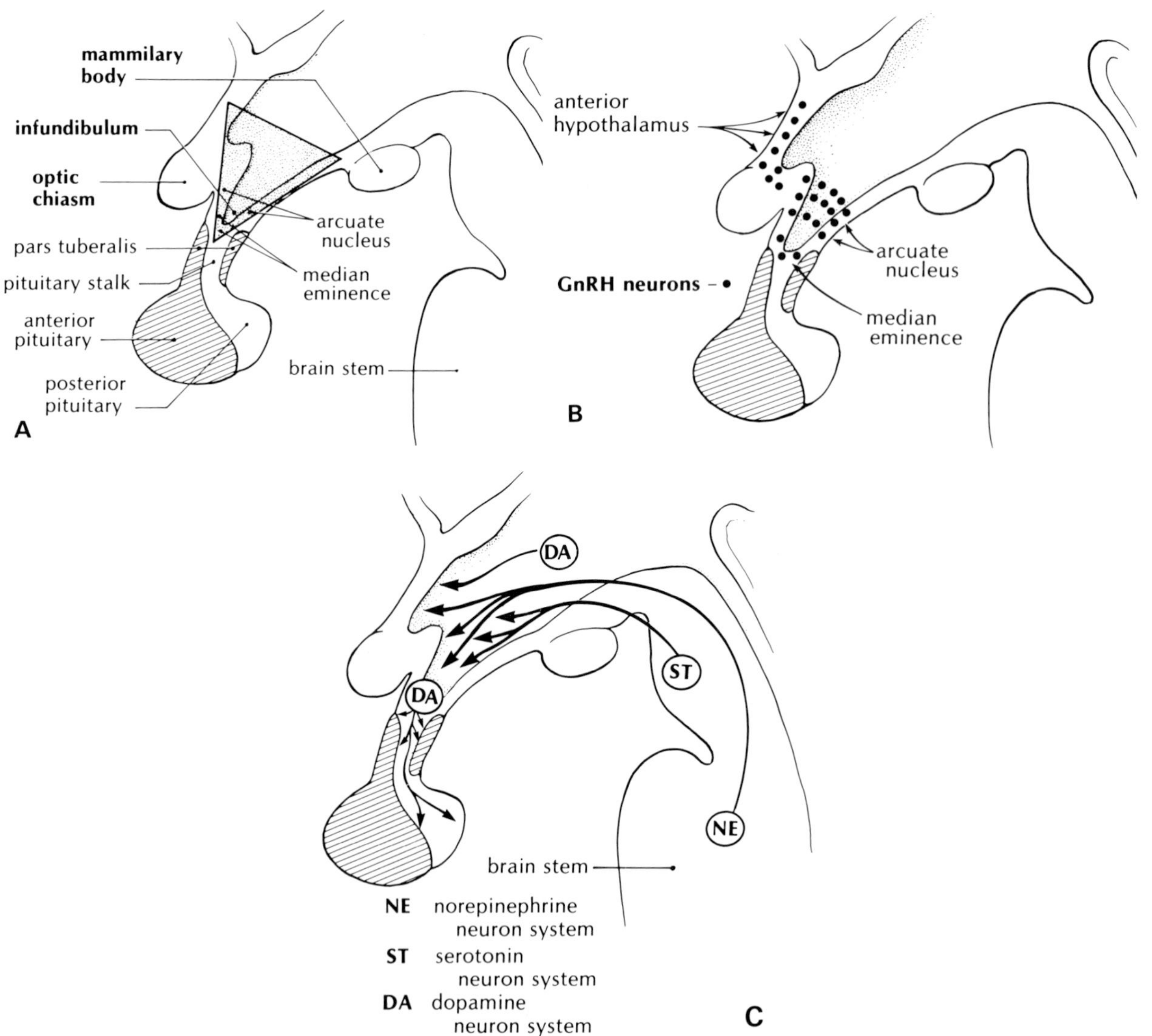

FIGURE 16-1 *(A)* Diagrammatic representation of the brainstem, hypothalamus, and pituitary with important anatomic landmarks labeled. The shaded triangular area indicates the region of the medial basal hypothalamus, a critical regulatory center. *(B)* Location of the major GnRH neuron cell bodies. *(C)* Diagrammatic representation of the aminergic neuronal systems. The superior dopamine system is called the *incertohypothalamic,* and the inferior system is called the *tuberohypophyseal.* The serotonin pathway is called the *raphe* serotonin neuron system. The norepinephrine system arises from lateral tegmental cell groups in the caudal medulla, midpons, and rostral pons. (*Adapted from Moore.*[1])

GnRH and other substances from neurons into the vascular channels (Fig. 16-2).[10] These capillaries form portal veins, which descend down the pituitary stalk to re-form in a capillary bed in the anterior pituitary.

Anterior Pituitary

Interspersed among the multiple anterior pituitary cell types are the *gonadotrophs,* cells containing both LH and follicle stimulating hormone (FSH) and receptors for GnRH. Morphometric analyses indicate that most of these cells produce LH and FSH conjointly, and that only a few contain LH or FSH exclusively.[11]

Testes

The testes are paired organs measuring approximately 5 by 3 cm and containing a volume of 20 to 30 ml. They hang in the scrotum in an environment with a temperature 2.2°C lower than that in the abdomen. The *cremasteric* muscle allows retraction of the testes closer to the areas of core body temperature, a mechanism for keeping testicular tempera-

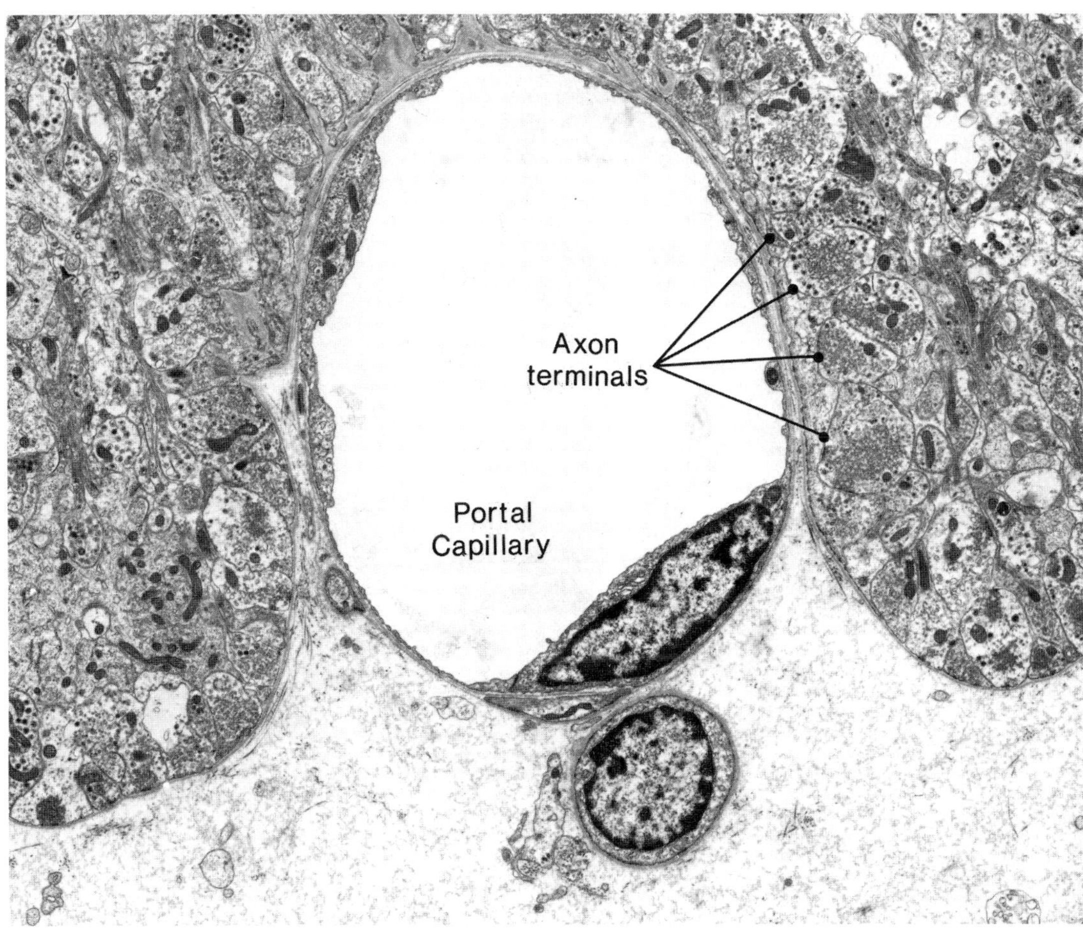

FIGURE 16-2 Electron micrograph of the neurohemal contact zone. A single portal capillary is surrounded by numerous axon terminals, only four of which are labeled. (*From Page and Dovey-Hartman.*[651])

ture relatively constant. Arterial blood to the testis is supplied by the internal spermatic, cremasteric, and vas deferential arteries. Beneath the tunica albuginea in the testis, the main branches of the testicular artery are variably located but are likely to be present over the medial, anterior, and lateral surfaces of the lower pole.[12] Venous blood drains into the pampiniform plexus and then into the internal spermatic veins. On the right, the internal spermatic vein enters the inferior vena cava; on the left, it drains into the renal vein. The close apposition of testicular arteries with the pampiniform plexus forms a functional countercurrent heat exchange mechanism and helps maintain testicular temperature. The anterior and lateral portions of the testes are covered by the *tunica vaginalis*. Beneath this, the entire testis is surrounded by the *tunica albuginea,* from which fibrous septa pass into the parenchyma and divide the testis into lobules.

The testis can be considered as two functional regions (Fig. 16-3*A* and *B*): the interstitial cell compartment with its androgen-secreting *Leydig* cells and the seminiferous tubular compartment, which contains *germinal* and *Sertoli* cells. Each serves a distinct function and thus is considered separately here.

Interstitial Cell Compartment

The Leydig, or interstitial, cells of the testis are highly specialized, with the typical appearance of highly active steroid-secreting tissue. In the adult male, the paired testes contain 432 ($\pm$ 45) $\times 10^6$ Leydig cells.[13] On light microscopy, these cells are polygonal, measure 10 to 25 μm in diameter, and represent approximately 5 percent of the total testicular volume (Fig. 16-3*A*). They contain lipid droplets, the ratios of cytoplasm to nucleus are large, and nucleoli are prominent. These cells are contiguous to capillaries; they deliver the secreted steroids into the testicular veins and, less so, into the lymphatics that drain the interstitial cell compartment. Clusters of Leydig cells are interspersed in the spaces adjacent to the seminiferous tubules. On electron microscopy (Fig. 16-4), Leydig cell cytoplasm contains large

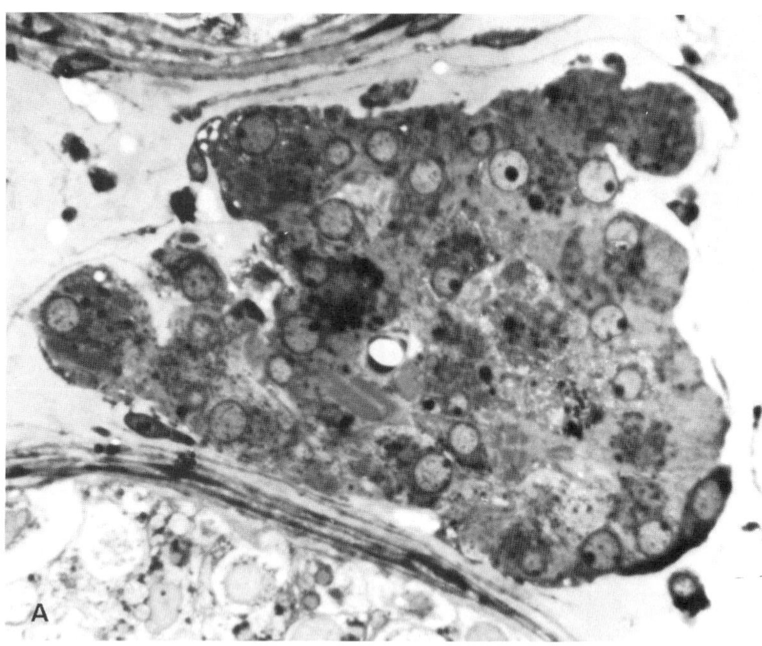

FIGURE 16-3 *(A)* Light microscopic appearance of Leydig cells from a human testis. *(B)* Light microscopic appearance of a seminiferous tubule from a human testis. *(Courtesy of Dr. Hugh F. English.)*

amounts of smooth endoplasmic reticulum, a morphologic structure characteristically abundant in steroid-producing cells, as well as numerous lipid droplets and mitochondria. Crystalloids of Reinke, a structure of unknown function unique to the Leydig cell, may also be seen.

Seminiferous Tubular Compartment

Individual seminiferous tubules are tightly coiled and measure approximately 0.12 to 0.30 mm in diameter and up to 70 cm in length. These structures provide a continuous pathway for the delivery of sperm from the testes to the rete testis, caput epididymis, and vas deferens. The seminiferous tubule is lined by a basal laminar layer and by myoid cells which give it the ability to propel fluids within the lumen (Fig. 16-5). Immature stem cells called *spermatogonia* lie along the basal lamina, interspersed between Sertoli or supporting cells. Lateral projections of Sertoli cell cytoplasm envelop the spermatogonia, sealing them off from the remainder of the tubular contents and creating the basal or outer compartment (Fig. 16-5). Unimpeded diffusion across the basal lamina allows the spermatogonia free access to substances in interstitial tissues. The Sertoli cells also project their cytoplasm upward toward the seminiferous tubular lumen. Specialized tight junctions between them form a blood-testis barrier and divide the tubule into the outer, or basal, compartment and the inner, or adluminal, compartment (Fig. 16-5). The inner segment contains the spermatocytes and spermatids, which rest within evaginations of Sertoli cell cytoplasm. Physiologic studies have demonstrated that diffusion of dyes, steroids, proteins, and ions into the inner compartment is impeded and have confirmed the functional significance of the blood-testis barrier.[14]

Sertoli Cells

The Sertoli cells are basically columnar in form (Fig. 16-5). Their structural arrangement surrounding germinal cells, in conjunction with the anatomic distinction of the compartment formed by the blood-testis barrier, allows an intimate interaction between Sertoli cells and germ cells. By surrounding each cell type, Sertoli cell cytoplasm provides a controlled microenvironment and creates an immunologically protected space. Morphologically, Sertoli cells have a basally placed nucleolus. On electron microscopy, the cytoplasm contains mitochondria, rough endoplasmic reticulum along the basal region, widely dispersed smooth endoplasmic reticulum, lysosomes, and numerous microtubular elements.

Germinal Epithelia

The human testis manufactures 123 ($\pm$ 18) $\times 10^6$ sperm daily.[15] This requires a process of cellular replication with provision for a pool of undifferentiated cells held in reserve as well as a pool committed to full differentiation. The spermatogonia serve as the pool of undifferentiated cells (Fig. 16-6). The majority undergo continuous mitotic division in a manner analogous to that of other somatic cells; in this way they provide a renewal pathway for stem cells.[16] These cells remain in the outer compartment. A minority become committed to further differentiation and undergo meiosis, a process unique to germinal cell tissue. After meiotic division, these cells ultimately form mature spermatozoa; the series of maturing cells is detailed in Fig. 16-7. This process of

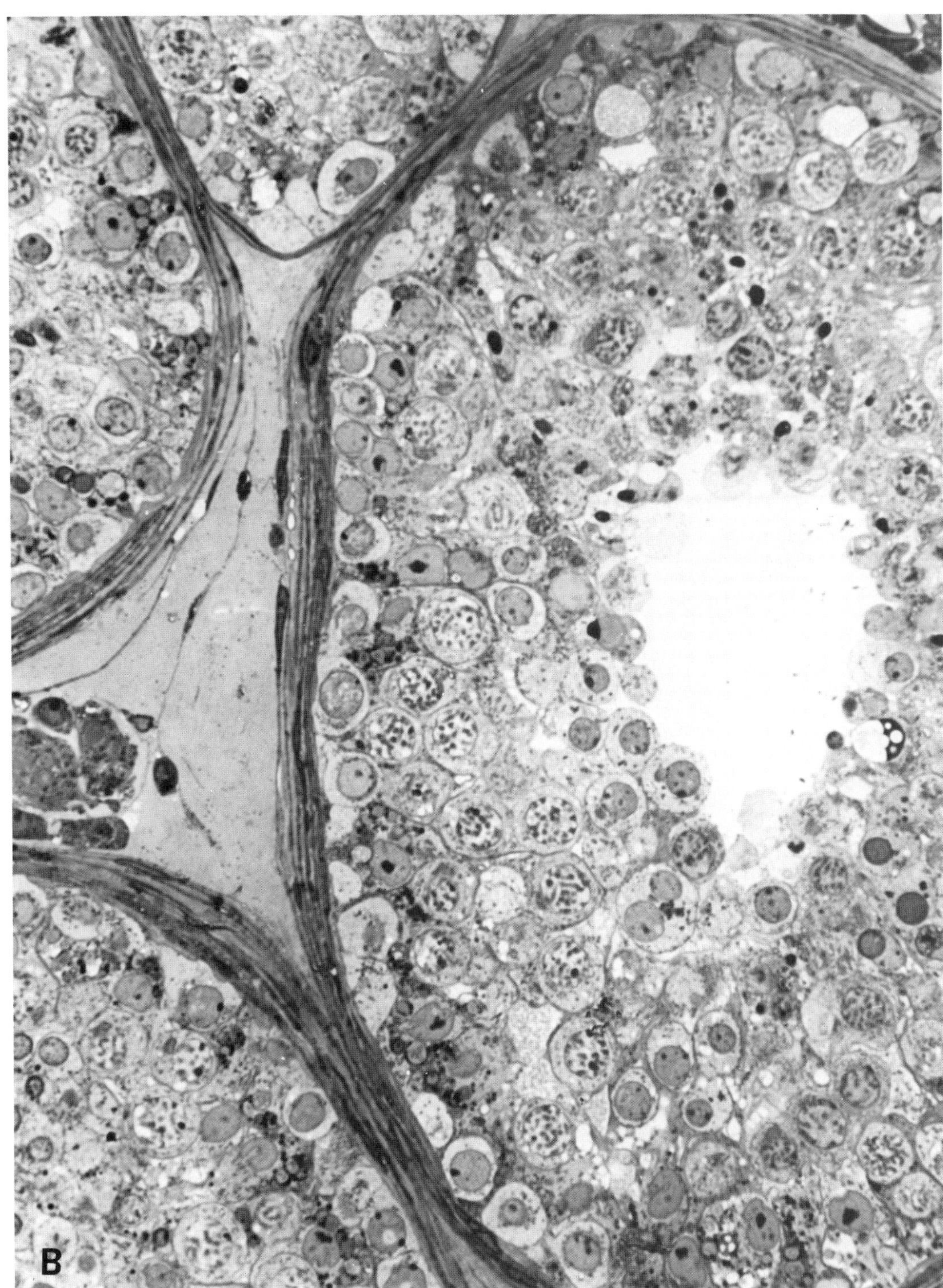

FIGURE 16-3 *(Continued)*

differentiation of cells takes place in the inner or adluminal, compartment.

In the process of meiosis, a new complement of DNA is synthesized to replicate each of the 46 chromosomes. In this way, chromosomes with twice the normal amount of DNA per chromosome are formed. Newly synthesized chromatin material progressively condenses. Each chromatid separates along its length, except at the common centromere (Fig. 16-8). During this process, crossing over between contiguous chromosomes can take place. This mechanism allows the formation of new combinations of maternal and paternal genetic material and explains the numerous translocations observed in banding stud-

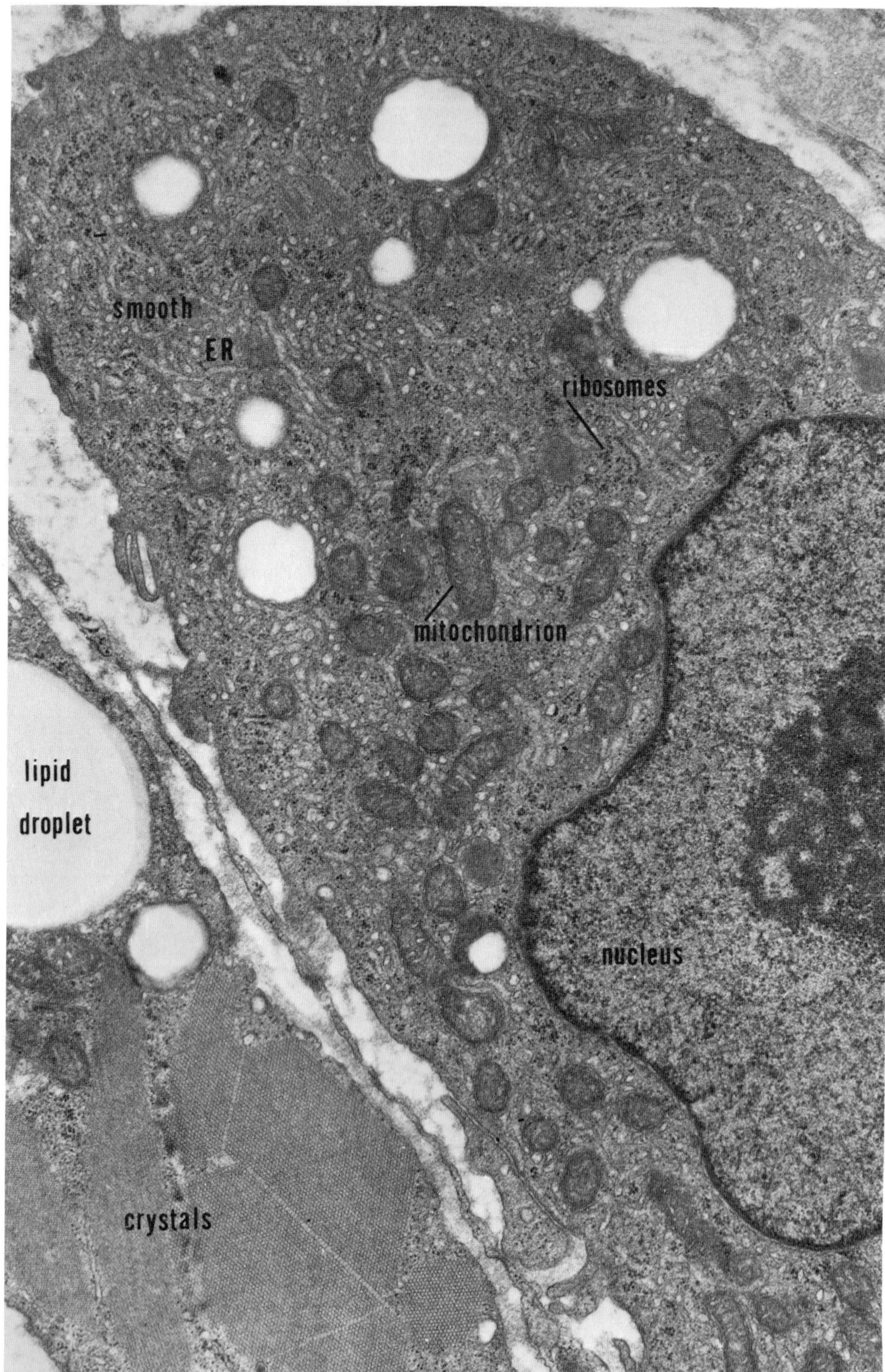

FIGURE 16-4 Electron micrograph of a Leydig cell from a human testis. Crystals refer to crystalloids of Reinke (see text). (*From Christensen.*[652])

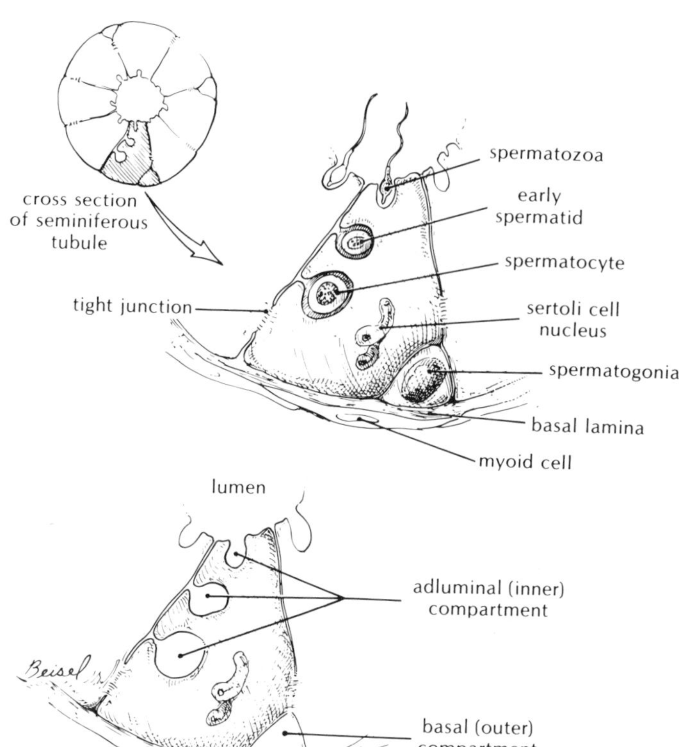

FIGURE 16-5 *(Top)* Diagrammatic representation of a seminiferous tubule to illustrate the relation between the lining membrane structures (i.e., basal lamina and myoid cells), Sertoli cell cytoplasm, and germinal epithelial cells. *(Bottom)* As above, with deletion of germinal cells. The basal or outer compartment lies outside the tight-junction barrier formed by the Sertoli cells, whereas the adluminal compartment lies within it.

ies during karyotype analysis. After DNA synthesis, the first meiotic division takes place. Rather than splitting into daughter cells with 46 single chromosomes, the first meiotic division involves reduction into daughter cells with 23 chromosome pairs per cell. The *primary spermatocytes* formed by this meiotic division then quickly undergo a second meiotic division to produce daughter cells with 23 single chromosomes, each with a normal amount of DNA. These *secondary spermatocytes* then mature further to spermatozoa, a process called *spermiogenesis,* and develop the cellular machinery necessary for motility. The sperm tail, a structure capable of generating linear, wavelike motion, is required for cellular propulsion (Figs. 16-9 and 16-10). Called a *cilium,* this highly conserved structure[17] contains nine pairs of microtubules surrounding an additional central pair, the so-called 9 + 9 + 2 configuration (Fig. 16-10).[17] Pieces of electron-dense material, the *dynein* (outer and inner) arms, are connected to the outer pairs of tubules. Moderate variability in the presence of individual features occurs in a population of normal sperm.[17] Reconstructed models (Fig. 16-10) reveal a series of linear tubules which can slide against one another to generate wave motion. Called the *sliding microtubule hypothesis,* this mechanism is invoked to explain the motility of all cilia or flagella.

Spermatogenesis in many lower species is synchronous throughout the four quadrants of each seminiferous tubule and is easy to assess quantitatively. In humans, spermatogenesis is asynchronous between various quadrants. Although difficult to recognize morphologically, six separate stages of spermatogenic maturation are present. A complete cycle through six stages takes 16 days; 4.5 cycles (74 ± 5 days) are required for full spermatogenesis (Fig. 16-11).[18]

After the process of spermiogenesis is complete, the spermatozoa are released into the tubular lumen and carried by passive fluid flow to the rete testes, ductuli efferentes, and into the epididymis. In the caput epididymis, the sperm first become[19] actively motile, a process which requires exposure of the epididymal cells to androgen. Further spermatozoal maturation occurs during passage through the corpus epididymis and cauda epididymis. The average time for transit of sperm through the excurrent duct system is 12 days. After ejaculation, these spermatozoa acquire fertilization potential through a process called *capacitation,* which takes place after entry into the female reproductive tract.[20] The fate of those not ejaculated is unclear; macrophage ingestion, local resorption, and passage into the urine are likely possibilities.[15]

PHYSIOLOGY

Hypothalamic-Pituitary-Leydig Cell Axis

Overview

An integrated, highly complex system regulates the level of circulating androgens within a relatively

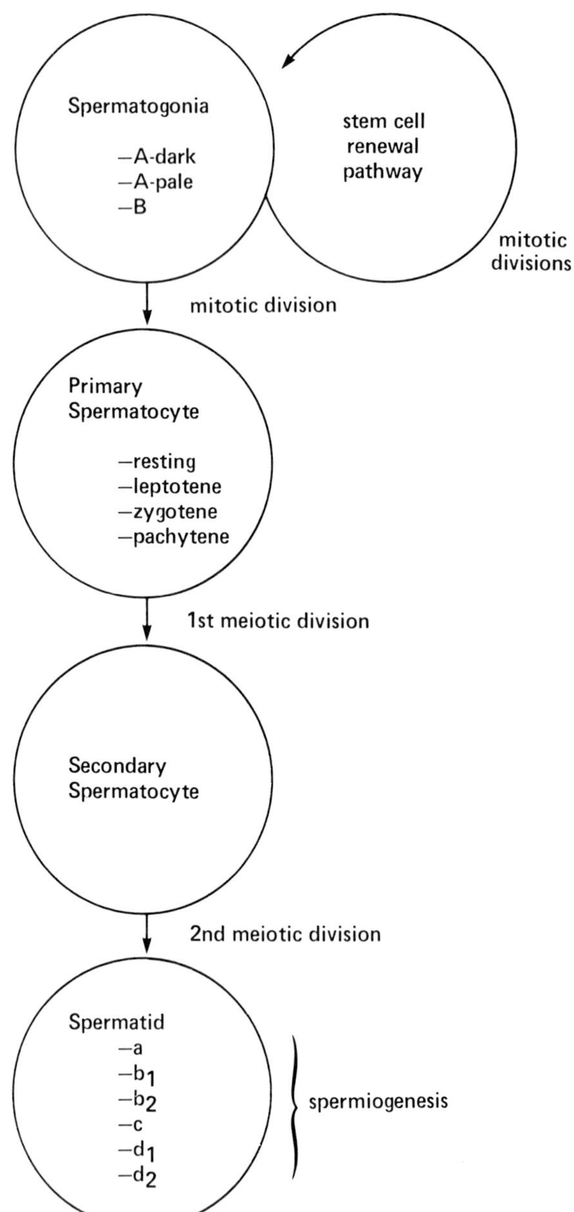

FIGURE 16-6 Diagrammatic representation of the stem cell renewal pathway and the differentiation pathway of the germinal cells. Specific cell types are listed for each major grouping.

narrow range in humans. The hypothalamus plays a major regulatory role through the release of GnRH, a decapeptide that controls both LH and FSH secretion. The pituitary secretes LH, which in turn binds to Leydig cell receptors in the testes and stimulates androgen production. Superimposed upon this hypothalamic-pituitary-testicular regulatory axis are neuronal pathways imparting input from higher central nervous system (CNS) centers.

Hypothalamus

Afferent Neural Input

The primary center for tonic control of gonadotropin regulation is located in the medial basal hypothalamus, primarily in the arcuate nucleus. Hormonal feedback exerted directly at this site and neural modulation from axons arising within or beyond the hypothalamus regulate GnRH secretion. The identities of the specific neuronal pathways involved and of the specific neurotransmitters modulating these effects are controversial. Current evidence suggests that catecholaminergic pathways using norepinephrine as a neurotransmitter (Fig. 16-1*C*) stimulate the release of GnRH.[2] Dopaminergic pathways are inhibitory in nature under certain experimental conditions and stimulatory under others,[2,21,22] whereas serotonergic neuronal systems generally appear to be inhibitory.[23,24] An integrated view of these regulatory pathways in humans, however, has not yet emerged.

Inhibitory neuronal pathways, particularly those modulated by endogenous opiates, have recently been a major topic of interest.[25] Exogenous opiates suppress LH secretion under certain conditions, and opiate antagonists increase LH output.[26,27] A reduction in the tone of the opiate system may be associated with the rises in gonadotropin concentrations which occur at puberty.[28] Another potential inhibitory pathway involves neural control of melatonin secretion by the pineal. This pathway appears to be important in the seasonal regression of reproductive activity in certain animal species but is of uncertain import in primates.[29]

Hypothalamic Pulse Generator

The release of GnRH is controlled by peptidergic neurons whose axons are highly concentrated in the arcuate (Fig. 16-1*A–C*) nucleus and the median eminence. A characteristic property of neuronal function is an intrinsic periodicity of firing with variable amplitude and frequency modulation. The pattern of release of GnRH into the pituitary portal capillaries reflects the nature of its neuronal control. GnRH is secreted in a series of pulses with variable amplitude and frequency.[30] The pituitary responds to this releasing hormone with pulsatile secretion of LH and, to a lesser extent, FSH into the peripheral circulation (Fig. 16-12).[31] Simultaneous measurement of portal GnRH and peripheral plasma LH concentrations reveals an excellent concordance.[30,32] Inference from a variety of observations regarding pulsatile LH secretion has led to the concept of a hypothalamic "pulse generator" (Fig. 16–13).[30,32] The neurons responsible for pulse generation reside in the medial basal hypothalamus. Episodic neuronal firing in this area precedes each LH pulse by 2 to 5 min.[33] Highly selective radio wave lesions produced in the arcuate nucleus in the rhesus monkey

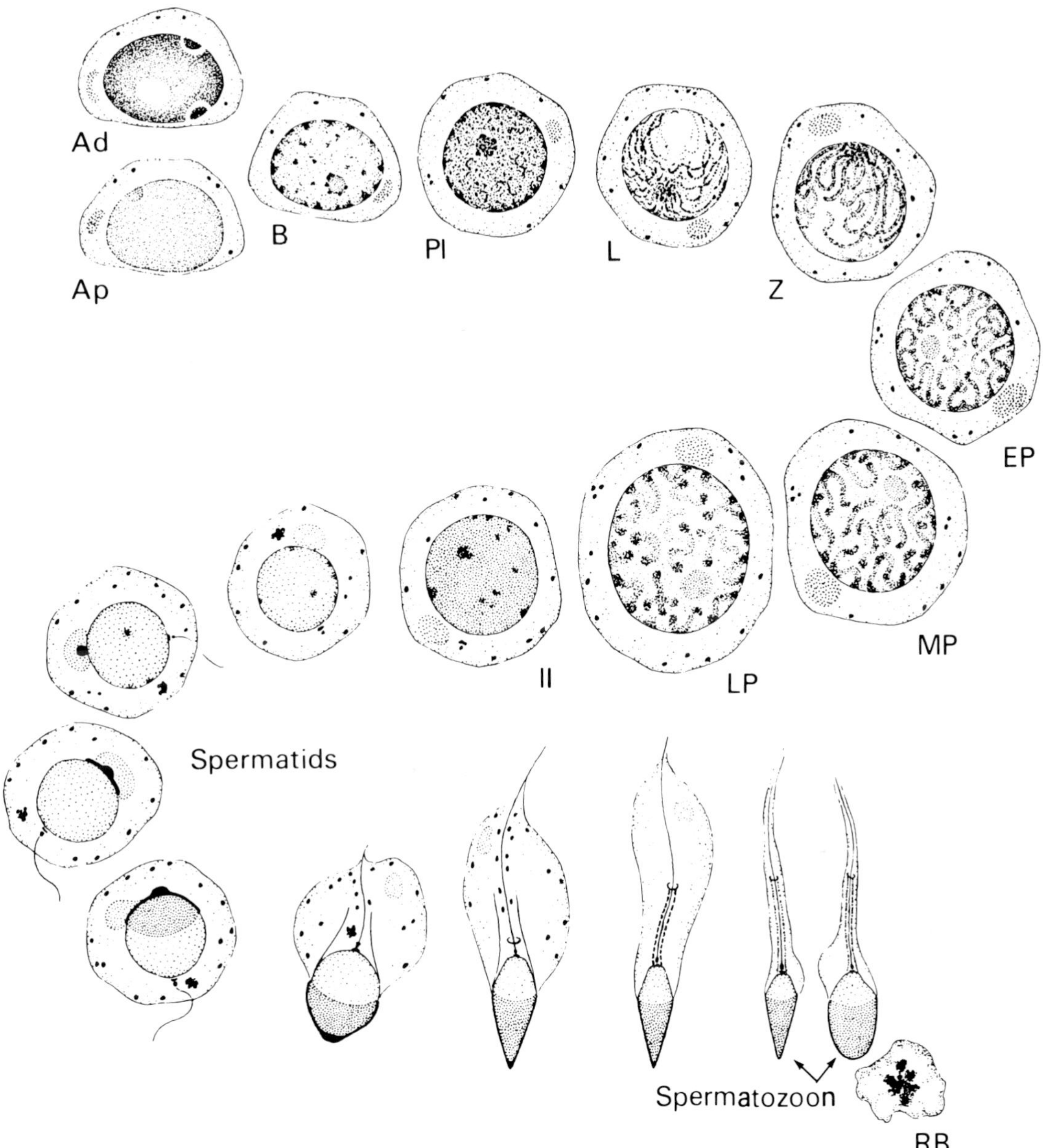

FIGURE 16-7 Appearance of the various germinal cell types in men. Ad = dark type A spermatogonium; Ap = pale type A spermatogonium; B = type B spermatogonium; Pl = preleptotene spermatocyte; L = leptotene spermatocyte; Z = zygotene spermatocyte; P = pachytene spermatocyte; II = secondary spermatocyte; Sa, Sb_1, Sb_2, Sc, Sd_1, Sd_2 = spermatids at different stages of spermatogenesis; RB=residual body. (*From Clermont.*[18])

completely abolish pulsatile LH release,[34,35] and electrical stimulation of this area induces pulses.[36] Generation of GnRH pulses may involve the glutamate receptor as *N*-methyl-D-L-aspartic acid (NMA); a neuroexcitatory amino acid elicits LH pulses; and AP5, a selective antagonist, abolishes LH pulses in vivo.[37,38] Sex steroid, catecholamine, and opiate agonists and antagonists, and the 29-amino acid galanin can alter the amplitude and frequency of LH pulses, presumably through interactions with the neuronal pulse generator.[2,26,27,31,39–41]

The concentration of GnRH in the portal capillary system has not been directly measured in men but has been estimated indirectly to range from 30 to 300 pg/ml.[42] These levels are higher than the amounts found by direct measurements in sheep, 10 to 30 pg/ml.[30] Little GnRH accumulates in peripheral plasma because of the rapid rate of metabolism

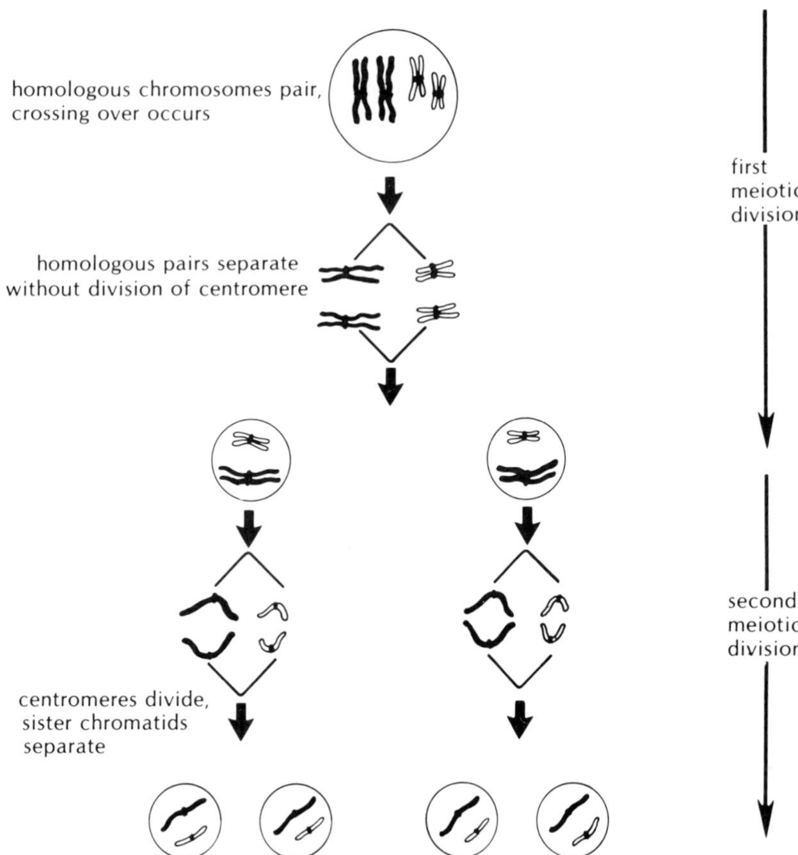

FIGURE 16-8 Diagrammatic representation of meiosis. *(Adapted from Flickinger et al.[653])*

of this releasing hormone.[42] A total of 802 ± 74 liters of plasma is cleared per day per square meter of body surface. Consequently, radioimmunoassay (RIA) methods for the measurement of peripheral plasma levels of GnRH are insufficiently sensitive for routine clinical assessment. GnRH, as well as immunologically detectable cleavage products, is concentrated in the urine. Measurements in this biological fluid correlate with LH and FSH secretion in adult men and increase appropriately during puberty in parallel with the plasma gonadotropins.[38]

Hypothalamic Behavioral Centers

The hypothalamus may play a role in the behavioral patterning induced by sex steroids. These actions can be divided into two types: those which exert organizational or permanent effects and those which are "activational" or transient.

Organizational Effects Based on extensive studies in the rodent and several other species, the organizational effects are believed to correlate with sex steroid receptor–mediated structural changes in the hypothalamus. In the rat, the dimorphic nucleus undergoes characteristic structural changes upon androgen administration.[43] Definable behavioral functions such as male-related singing behavior in the songbird and male lordosis patterns in the rat can be correlated with characteristic hypothalamic histologic patterns.[44] Prenatal exposure to androgens imprints later patterns of gonadotropin regulatory control in the guinea pig, sheep, hamster, mouse, and rat.[44] In the rat, perinatal exposure to androgens influences aggressiveness and other definable behavioral parameters.[44]

The relevance of these structural studies in animals to an understanding of the behavioral effects of androgens in men has not been established. In a number of clinical disorders, exposure of the brain to androgen in the prenatal period is altered. Males with androgen-resistant syndromes or 5α-reductase deficiency lack appropriate prenatal androgen exposure; females with congenital adrenal hyperplasia and those exposed to steroids prenatally are subject to increased androgenic effects. These disorders would be expected to provide insight into the relative importance of prenatal androgen exposure versus postnatal socialization on patterns of sexual behavior. However, no clear conclusions have emerged from observations of these disorders. It should be noted that little support has been provided for the concept of organizational imprinting of the brain by

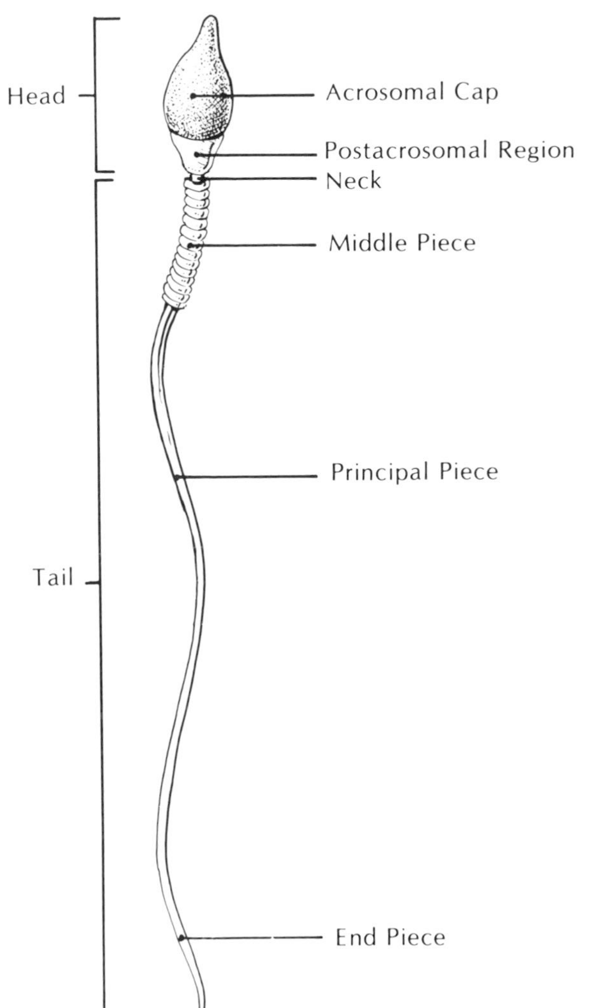

FIGURE 16-9 Drawing of human sperm. (*Adapted from Fawcett.*[654])

prenatal exposure to androgens in humans.[44] Further evidence against androgen imprinting comes from observations in men who were castrated after prenatal androgen exposure.[45] The administration of estrogen in an appropriate dose causes a stimulatory release of LH in these subjects. In rodents and many other species, by contrast, prenatal androgenic imprinting of the hypothalamus prevents such a stimulatory response.[44]

Activational Effects Specific behavior effects of androgens in adult men are observable but appear to be of the activational or transient type. The exact site which induces these actions is not known. Androgen deprivation reduces the frequency of nocturnal as well as spontaneous daytime erections; androgen replacement rapidly returns these functions to normal. Androgens also appear to influence *libido,* the behavioral activity which includes cognitive events leading to engagement in sexual activity.[46] The role of androgens in aggressive behavior remains unclear, since the effect of social learning confounds interpretation. While hypothalamic, cortical, or other CNS sites could mediate the actions of androgens, no data are available to localize these functions in men.

Pituitary

The dominant factor controlling gonadotropin release by the pituitary is exposure to GnRH. This hormone binds to specific receptors on cells which synthesize and release both LH and FSH.[47] Binding of hormone to the GnRH receptor translocates uniformly distributed receptor units into patches, stimulates the mobilization of ionized calcium within the cell, and induces the release of LH.[47] This coupling-activation sequence depends on calcium binding to the calcium-binding protein calmodulin for maximal function and may involve protein kinase C activation and diacylglycerol.[47,48] Calcium channel blockers and calcium ionophores exert profound influences on this process.

In response to a discrete GnRH bolus, the pituitary promptly releases LH into the peripheral circulation. With exposure to constantly infused GnRH for 2 to 4 h, a bimodal pattern of LH release becomes apparent.[49] After the initial burst of LH secretion over a 30-min period, the levels of this gonadotropin decline, only to increase slowly again over the next 4 h. This secretory pattern has been attributed to the presence of two functional pools of LH within the pituitary. Whether these pools represent molecular processing, compartmentalization of storage granules, or previously and newly synthesized hormone has not been established. Exposure of the pituitary to two successive discrete boluses of GnRH separated by 1 to 2 h enhances the response to the second dose.[50] Termed the *self-priming effect,* this phenomenon may reflect the same functional alterations observed during constant infusion but could also represent separate mechanistic changes.

LH is a glycoprotein with a molecular weight of 28,000 which is composed of two separate subunits. The α subunit contains 92 amino acids and is identical to the α subunits of thyroid stimulating hormone (TSH), FSH, and human chorionic gonadotropin (hCG); the β subunit contains 115 amino acids and is specific to LH. While the β subunit of hCG shares homology with the 115 amino acids of β-LH, β-hCG contains an additional 30 amino acids beyond the β-LH peptide sequence.[51] The gonadotrophs independently synthesize both the α and β subunits of LH from separate gene sequences and separate mRNA. The rate of synthesis of the mRNAs from each subunit can be regulated differentially.[52] After transcription and translation are completed, these subunits join to form the native LH molecule. During additional processing, a variable amount of carbohydrate is inserted into the molecule, resulting in a high degree of microheterogeneity. A family of LH

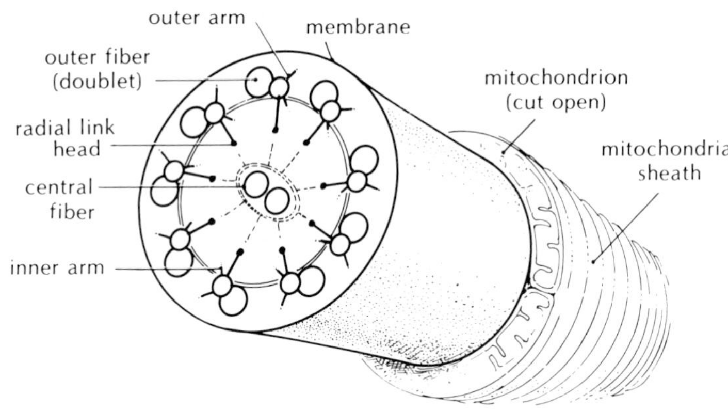

FIGURE 16-10 Drawing of cross section of midpiece of sperm and diagrammatic representation of its microtubules. Dynein represents outer and inner arms. Outer dense fibers not shown. (*Adapted from Fawcett.*[654])

molecules with various isoelectric points can be demonstrated with isoelectric focusing techniques.[53] The amount of carbohydrate contained in the LH molecule after secretion is physiologically important, since this determines its rate of metabolic clearance in plasma and its degree of inherent physiologic potency. A reduction in the carbohydrate content of LH enhances its rate of clearance and reduces its biological potency when tested by in vivo bioassay techniques.[53]

As a result of variable carbohydrate content, qualitative differences exist in the molecular structure of circulating LH under various clinical circumstances. One potential marker for such qualitative change is the ratio of biological to immunologic activity of circulating LH (B/I ratio). Techniques recently

FIGURE 16-11 Germ cell association (stages I to VI), including each cycle of spermatogenesis. (This illustration appeared originally in the first edition of *Endocrinology* in 1981. It is reproduced here by courtesy of Dr. Philip Troen.)

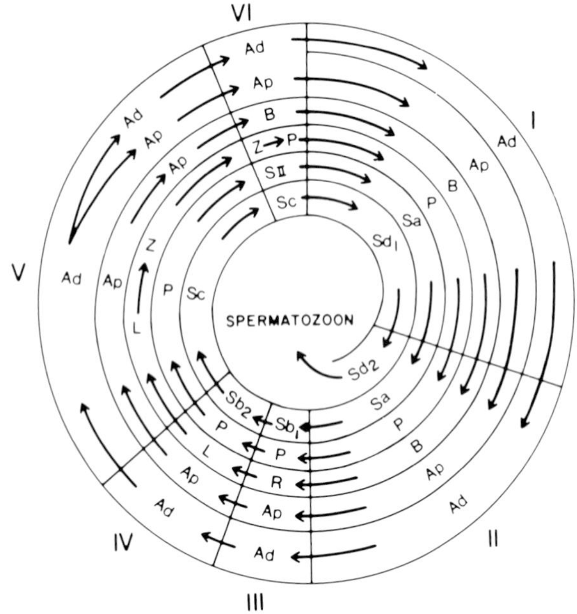

made available allow the measurement of LH and FSH bioactivity.[53,54] Testosterone production from isolated rat or mouse Leydig cells exposed to LH in vitro serves as the biological endpoint for LH measurements.[53,55] Estradiol production from Sertoli cells exposed to FSH serves as the endpoint for FSH bioactivity.[56] These techniques are highly sensitive. Most bioassays detect a greater amount of gonadotropin than do immunoassays, and B/I ratios are usually greater than unity.[53] Controversy regarding the use of B/I ratios exists since assay conditions, gonadotropin standards, the species used for Leydig cell harvest, and physiologic circumstances[57–60] can alter the results. Changes in B/I ratios occur with aging, pubertal maturation, androgen deprivation, GnRH agonists, GnRH antagonists, and estrogen administration.[53,54,58,61–63] These changes have been interpreted to reflect alterations in the physicochemical properties of secreted LH under these circumstances. However, much of the prior data documenting B/I ratio changes may be artifactual and may reflect a lack of sensitivity of the available RIAs.[60,64,65] The availability of highly sensitive two-site fluorescent or chemiluminescent assays eliminates this measurement artifact. Consequently, previously published studies which used insensitive LH assays must be interpreted with caution and additional data must be collected to establish the extent and biological relevance of alterations in the B/I ratio. In spite of these major questions regarding changes in the B/I ratio, the concept of secretion of LH molecules with altered carbohydrate content and bioactivity remains valid. Isoelectric focusing studies clearly demonstrate LH species with varying changes and biological activity. Physiologic manipulations alter the proportion of the basic or acidic LH molecules secreted.[53]

The gonadotroph is ordinarily exposed to intermittent pulses of GnRH which occur at intervals of 90 to 120 min.[30–32] This periodicity of exposure appears to be necessary for the preservation of normal secretory function. Paradoxically, exposure of the pituitary to constant amounts of GnRH for periods of

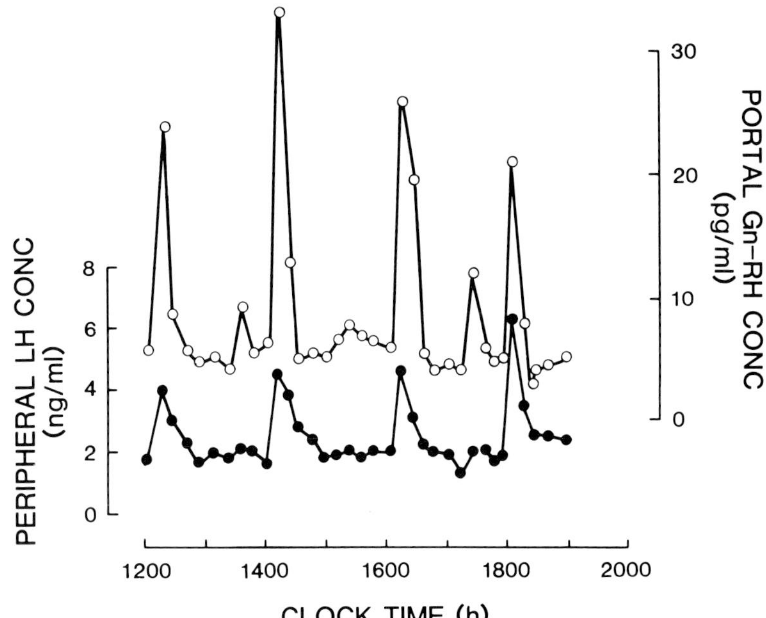

FIGURE 16-12 Simultaneous measurement of concentrations of GnRH in pituitary portal plasma and LH in peripheral plasma of the sheep. Open circles = GnRH; closed circles = LH. *(Adapted from Clarke and Cummins.*[30]*)*

24 to 48 h suppresses LH production.[66] For this reason, potent synthetic analogues of GnRH which are resistant to metabolic cleavage and bind to the GnRH receptor with higher than normal affinity produce a paradoxic inhibition of gonadotropin release on long-term administration.[67]

Episodic exposure of the pituitary to GnRH results in LH and α subunit LH pulses with quantifiable amplitude and frequency.[31,68,69] Several computer programs based on setting thresholds to detect pulses allow precise estimation of pulse frequency and amplitude.[31,70–74] Additional computer programs utilize the rate of hormone disappearance as well as pulse detection for analysis. Called "deconvolution techniques," these methods allow calculation of the frequency, duration, and amplitude of secretory episodes; the half-life of disappearance of secreted hormones; the instantaneous secretion rate of hormone during discrete pulses; and integrated endogenous production rates.[74–76] Data from this methodology suggest that pituitary LH secretion ceases completely during intervals between pulses. In men, pulse frequency averages 12 to 14 pulses/24 h. Pulse amplitude ranges from 20 to 400 percent between nadir and peak, with an average change of 70 percent.

FIGURE 16-13 Diagrammatic representation of the GnRH pulse generator. Triangle = medial basal hypothalamus (see Fig. 16-1*A*); oval = pituitary. Pulsatile release of GnRH results in pulsatile LH release with measurable amplitude and frequency.

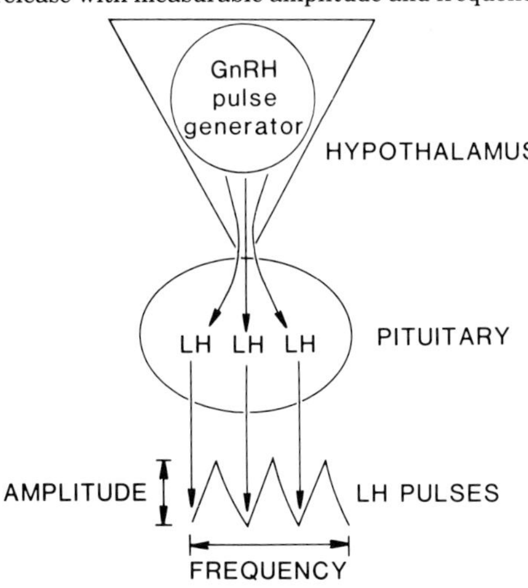

After release into the peripheral circulation, LH is cleared by the kidney, liver, and gonads and from other sites. The metabolic clearance rate of LH, as determined by constant infusion of exogenous gonadotropin, is in the range of 34 ± 3 ml/min for immunoactive LH[76–78] and 26 ± 3 ml/min for bioactive LH. Using the radiolabeled LH method, values are slightly higher at 44 ± 8 ml/min.[78] The value determined for the daily production rate depends on which assay is used to measure plasma LH concentration. Estimates include production rates of 600 IU/24 h for immunoactive LH and 1900 IU/24 h for bioactive LH.[77] These estimates generally correlate with the amounts of exogenous human LH necessary to maintain normal testosterone levels in patients with isolated gonadotropin deficiency.

Measurements of LH can be made in urine or plasma and by RIA or bioassay. Only a small fraction of LH is excreted intact into the urine; levels detected by immunoassay range from 12 to 60 IU/24 h.[78,79] Plasma LH concentration can be measured by standard RIA or by highly sensitive immunologic assays which utilize two antibodies to recognize separate epitopes of the molecule. These newer methods correlate well with highly sensitive bioassays.[80] These bioassays involve the stimulation of testosterone in vitro by Leydig cells isolated from rats or mice.[53,55] Normal ranges for bioactive LH vary widely, depending on the species of Leydig cell and the standard utilized, but generally are 3.0 to 10 times higher than immunologic measurements. The degree of carbohydrate content, the tertiary structure, and other minor molecular modifications appear to affect LH biological activity to a greater extent than immunologic recognition.[53,60]

Testis

In the testes, the Leydig or interstitial cells contain membrane receptors which bind LH with high affinity. The LH receptor is a member of the G-protein-coupled superfamily, which also includes rhodopsin, β-adrenergic, angiotensin, muscarinic, substance K, α-adrenergic, serotonin, dopamine, TSH, and FSH receptors, among others.[79] The LH receptor contains an extracellular domain of approximately 340 amino acids and a 330-amino acid residue C-terminal region containing seven transmembrane spanning elements.[80,81] The extracellular domain binds LH with high affinity and is relatively unique structurally. The transmembrane portion displays sequence similarity with all members of the G-protein-coupled receptor genes.[81–83]

The interaction of LH with its receptor initiates a cascade of events similar to those for other polypeptide hormones with their respective receptors. This sequence consists of receptor binding, aggregation of receptor proteins in the cell membrane, the appearance of membrane pitting, binding of GTP (guanosine triphosphate) to the alpha subunit of the G-protein, activation of adenylate cyclase, the generation of cyclic AMP, binding to the regulatory subunit of cAMP-dependent protein kinase A, release of the cAMP-dependent catalytic subunit, and phosphorylation of one or more protein substrates in the Leydig cell[76,84] (see Chap. 4). These events induce an increase in Leydig cell steroidogenesis and ultimately lead to an increase in testosterone production.[85] Only a small fraction of receptors must be occupied by hormone for testosterone stimulation to be maximal.[86] The unoccupied or "spare receptors," a commonly observed phenomenon in many tissues, may relate to a large subpopulation of Leydig cells characterized by low density on centrifugation. These "low-density" cells have LH receptors but little steroidogenic responsiveness. "High-density" Leydig cells respond in a more sensitive fashion and do not appear to have "spare receptors."[87]

Exposure to high concentrations of LH over several hours reduces receptor content, a process of suppression generally termed *down regulation*. The synthesis of new receptors is inhibited via cAMP-mediated processes.[88] Increased receptor internalization and lysosomal degradation also occur. Reduced LH levels induce higher receptor concentrations (up regulation), a process which is prevented by the addition of protein synthesis inhibitors.[88]

Extensive in vitro studies of rodent testis tissue have demonstrated that the biological consequences of receptor suppression involve the inhibition of C_{17-20}-lyase and 17α-hydroxylase activities, both distal steps in the androgen biosynthetic pathway. These actions may be partially related to an associated increase in estradiol induced by the aromatase-stimulating effect of LH.[85,89] The biological relevance of the estrogen inhibitory hypothesis is supported by the observation that estrogen-producing Leydig cell tumors are associated with precursor steroid patterns compatible with C_{17-20}-lyase inhibition.[90]

Experiments in men given hCG also suggest the potential physiologic relevance of LH receptor suppression in patients. For example, increments in 17α-hydroxyprogesterone concentration greater than those of testosterone concentration, reflecting the C_{17-20}-lyase block, are observed for 1 to 2 days after exposure to high doses of hCG. The disproportionate rise in 17α-hydroxyprogesterone concentration correlates with increments in plasma estradiol concentration. Lower doses of hCG given more frequently cause exaggerated rises in neither 17α-hydroxyprogesterone nor estradiol concentrations.[91,92]

Receptor down regulation could explain why men with very high circulating levels of hCG due to choriocarcinoma secrete reduced instead of increased amounts of testosterone. However, other studies call into question the general relevance of receptor down regulation in men. When physiologic amounts of hCG or LH are administered to men for long periods, Leydig cell responsiveness is not substantially altered.[93] Comparison of pulsatile and continuous LH administration in rodents reveals equal testosterone secretion with both modes of administration. Further correlation between in vitro studies using animal tissue and in vivo studies in humans is thus necessary to determine the significance of receptor down regulation in the regulation of intratesticular steroidogenic events.

Factors other than LH may modulate Leydig cell responsiveness (Fig. 16-14).[94–98] Growth hormone (GH) appears to enhance hCG-induced testosterone secretion in GH-deficient subjects.[98] FSH given to men with isolated gonadotropin deficiency during long-term hCG treatment increases testosterone levels twofold.[99] Other peptide hormones may also exert either an inhibitory or a stimulatory effect. For example, GnRH, arginine vasopressin, oxytocin, transforming growth factor β (TGFβ), activin, and β-endorphin can inhibit testosterone biosynthesis in isolated Leydig cells in a dose-dependent fashion, whereas inhibin reverses the effects of activin.[94,96,100–102] At least some of these substances, such as β-endorphin

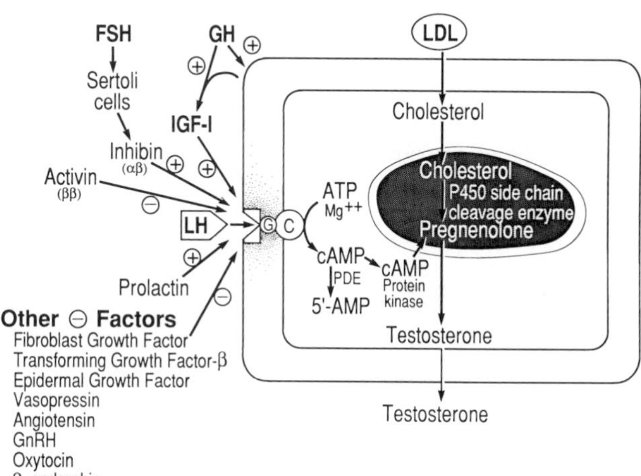

FIGURE 16-14 Schematic diagram of the effects of various peptides on the responses of the testis to LH. *(Figure obtained from Dr. Tu Lin, University of South Carolina, Columbia, South Carolina.)*

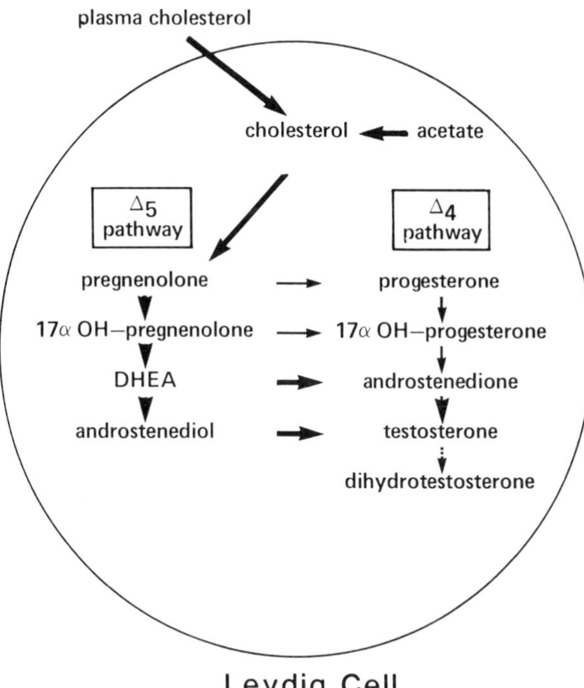

FIGURE 16-15 Diagrammatic representation of the androgen synthetic pathway in the Leydig cells of the testis. Preferred pathways are shown by heavy arrows. Only small amounts of dihydrotestosterone are synthesized from testosterone within the Leydig cell.

and oxytocin,[103] can be synthesized directly in the testes as shown by RNA hybridization. Other peptides, such as the tachykinins, somatostatin, and pro-renin, are present in the testes but have no assigned role.[104–106] In this rapidly advancing area, additional information is required before apparently conflicting reports can be resolved.[101] However, it is apparent that much variation between species exists. For example, while receptors for GnRH can be demonstrated to exist in the testes of the rat, such is not the case in men, mice, and monkeys.[107] Therefore, a clear understanding of the importance of these substances (called gonadocrinins) awaits further detailed studies in men.

Upon exposure to LH, the Leydig cells increase their rate of testosterone production by increasing pregnenolone synthesis. The substrate for this steroidogenic process can come from either de novo synthesis of cholesterol from acetate in the Leydig cells or tissue uptake of plasma cholesterol (Fig. 16-15)[108] via low-density lipoprotein (LDL) receptors. Androgen biosynthesis in the human testis preferentially proceeds via the Δ^5 pathway from pregnenolone to dehydroepiandrosterone (DHEA) and androstenediol before entering the Δ^4 pathway as *androstenedione* (and testosterone). Androgen precursors and products can be converted to steroid sulfates for storage in the testis. Enzymatic cleavage to the free steroids then precedes release into the circulation. The physiologic significance of this *sulfate storage shunt* remains controversial.[109]

The major androgen secreted by the testes is testosterone; approximately 7000 μg per day enters the peripheral circulation. Using calculations from spermatic vein–peripheral vein gradients, the testes are also found to secrete significant amounts (Fig. 16-16) of 17α-hydroxyprogesterone, androstenedione, and pregnenolone but relatively little dihydrotestosterone (DHT) (i.e., 69 μg/24 h) and even smaller amounts of estradiol (10 μg/24 h).[110]

Testosterone is secreted into the peripheral plasma via the spermatic veins in a pulsatile manner. While LH and testosterone pulses would be expected to be in concord, they appear to be poorly correlated in men.[111] Two factors probably explain this finding. First, testosterone is largely protein-bound in peripheral plasma.[112] The small fraction of newly secreted testosterone enters a large pool of bound testosterone, and pulses are masked by this dilution factor. Supporting this concept is the fact that an excellent concordance between testosterone and LH pulses is observed in animal species that lack testosterone-binding proteins. Second, the response of the human testis to LH is relatively sluggish.[111] Although small rises in testosterone concentrations occur within 2 to 4 h after LH or hCG is administered, peak increases are not observed until 24 to 72 h later.[91] For these reasons, the variation in testosterone levels due to pulsatile secretion is only 25 percent; in comparison, LH concentrations vary by 65 percent[31,113] as a reflection of episodic secretion.

A diurnal rhythm of testosterone level, with a peak at 4 to 8 A.M. and a nadir concentration at 4 to 8 P.M., occurs in younger men and less so in elderly

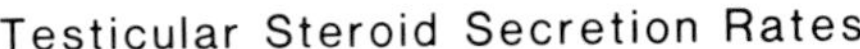

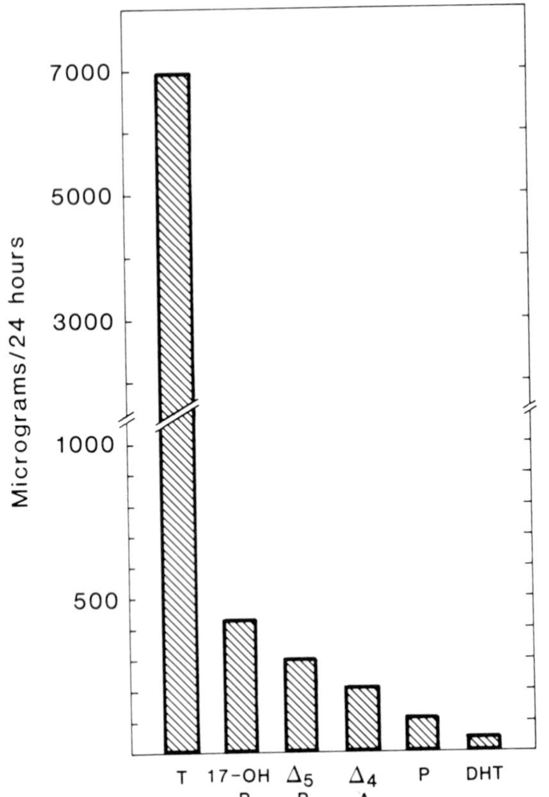

FIGURE 16-16 Testicular secretion rates of various androgens. T = testosterone; 17-OHP = 17α-hydroxyprogesterone; Δ^5P = pregnenolone; Δ^4A = androstenedione; P = progesterone; DHT = dihydrotestosterone. Secretion rates (SR) calculated from the arteriovenous (av) differences across the testis as measured by Hammond et al.[110] Calculations based on assumptions used by Kirchner et al.[655] for adrenal secretion rates, represented by the formula

$$\text{Secretion rate (SR)} = \frac{\text{Assumed testosterone SR}}{\text{testosterone av difference} \times \text{av difference of steroid in question}}$$

Testosterone SR assumed to be 7000 μg/day.

men.[111,114] The overall excursion from nadir to peak levels ranges from 20 to 30 percent. This rhythm is not associated with diurnal increments in LH. Its cause is unknown, but it may be related to nocturnal prolactin increments,[115] changes in the testosterone metabolic clearance rate, altered sensitivity of the testis to LH, or other factors.

The adrenal provides an additional source of testosterone. Direct measurements of testosterone concentration in adrenal venous plasma indicate that approximately 200 μg per day of testosterone arises from this source.[116] The peripheral conversion of androstenedione, which is secreted by the adrenal and converted into testosterone, accounts for another 200 to 300 μg. Therefore, adrenal sources provide approximately 5 percent of the total testosterone produced (i.e., 400 to 600 μg per day).[116]

A small percentage of testosterone (approximately 2 percent) circulates in a free state in plasma, whereas the remainder is bound either to testosterone-estrogen–binding globulin (TeBG) or to albumin (Fig. 16-17).[112] The affinity of TeBG for testosterone (1.6×10^{-9} M) is several orders of magnitude higher than that of albumin ($4 \times 10^{-4}M$).[117] Only TeBG binds testosterone with sufficiently high affinity to retard its entry into tissues. Vermeulen et al. initially demonstrated an excellent correlation between the levels of non-TeBG-bound testosterone and the rate of its metabolic clearance, a variable reflecting tissue entry.[118] Perturbation of the amount of TeBG present or drug saturation of its functional binding capacity alters the degree of tissue entry in a predictable fashion. However, a high degree of complexity is present to control tissue delivery. Experimental studies and mathematical modeling have identified the major factors that affect the retardation of tissue entry by plasma protein binders. These factors include the rate of plasma flow to a specific organ, the dissociation of hormone from plasma-binding proteins, the influx rate of free hormone to that tissue, and the rate of intracellular elimination of hormone.[112,117,119] Taking these factors into account, TeBG-bound but not albumin-bound testosterone is retarded from entry into certain tissues whereas TeBG-bound steroid can enter other tissues.[118,120]

Several clinicopathologic events alter the absolute levels of TeBG in plasma (Fig. 16-17). Reduced TeBG levels occur in association with obesity, acromegaly, hyperprolactinemia, hypothyroidism, and glycocorticoid ingestion. Increased levels accompany aging; hyperthyroidism; ingestion of birth control pills, tamoxifen, or phenytoin; cirrhosis; hypogonadism; and pregnancy.[121] Estrogens stimulate, and androgens inhibit, its biosynthesis. Several drugs can alter the functional binding of TeBG. The most commonly observed effects occur with spironolactone and its metabolites; fluoxymesterone, danazol, 17-methyltestosterone, megestrol acetate, and a large group of natural and synthetic steroids also produce this effect.[117,122,123] Measurement of non-TeBG-bound testosterone provides a better indication of physiologically available testosterone than do total testosterone levels when conditions of altered TeBG concentrations or functional binding exist (Fig. 16-18).

TeBG is a homodimeric glycoprotein, composed of two 50-kDa subunits, which is synthesized in the liver.[124,125] A single gene on chromosome 17 containing 8 exons codes for both TeBG and the testicular analogue, androgen-binding protein (ABP). Tissue-specific variations in the start of transcription and/or modification of a common primary transcript or its translation products account for the differences between TeBG and ABP. Receptors for TeBG on cell

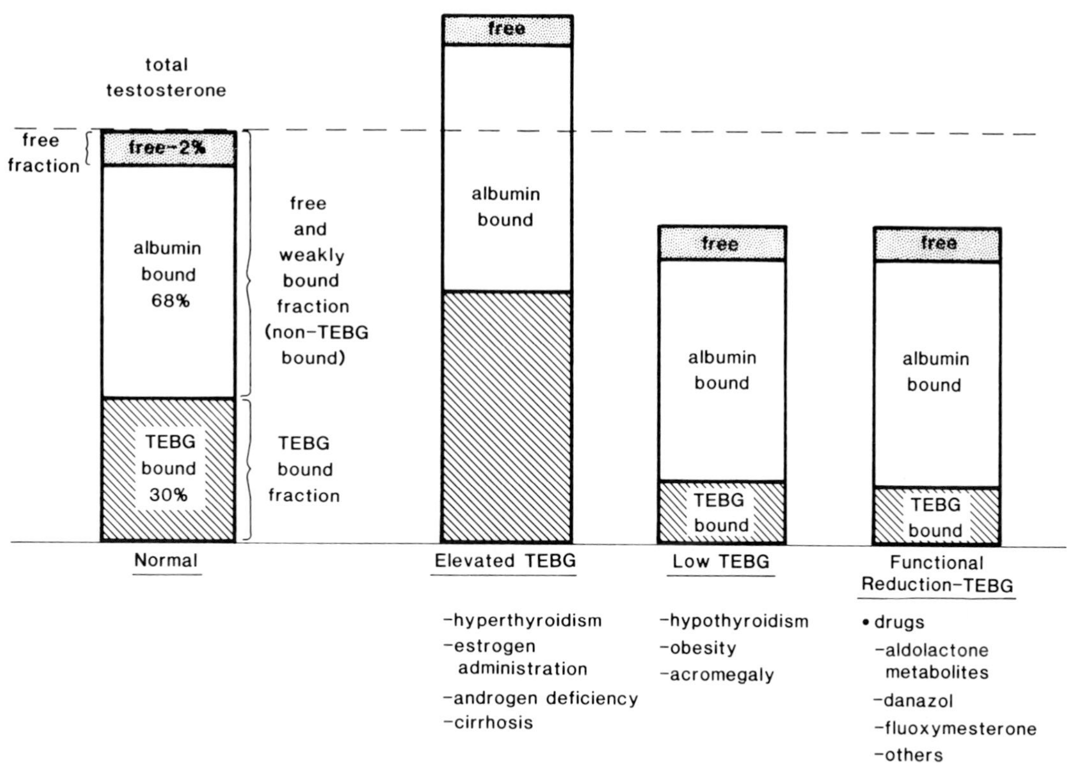

FIGURE 16-17 Fractions of bound, weakly bound, and free testosterone in normal men and in men with disorders producing high or low levels of testosterone-estrogen–binding globulin (TeBG).

membranes and a role for TeBG in cAMP generation in target tissues has been postulated.[126] RIAs are now available for the specific measurement of the mass of TeBG in plasma.[127] Other methods for quantitating the level of this protein involve saturation analysis after purification on lectin or ion-exchange columns, quantitative polyacrylamide gel or agar gel electrophoresis, or precipitation with ammonium sulfate. For routine clinical purposes, the percentage of non-TeBG-bound androgen can be determined under equilibrium conditions using dialysis against an albumin buffer or precipitation with ammonium sulfate.[117,122,128]

FIGURE 16-18 Correlation between non-TeBG-bound testosterone determined by the ammonium sulfate precipitation technique and bioavailable testosterone measured by the Oldendorf method. *(From Manni et al.*[128]*)*

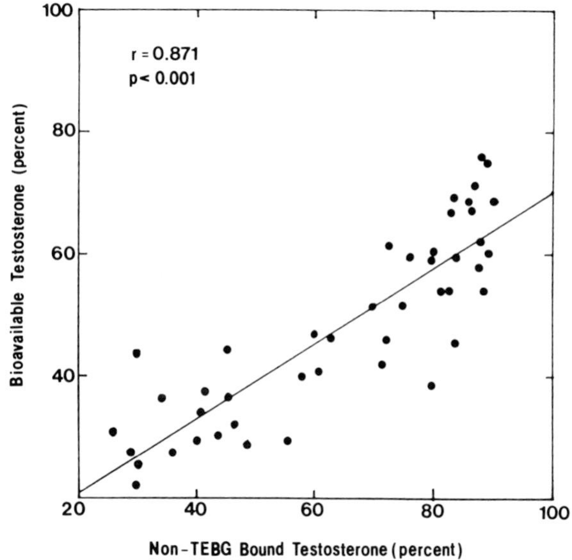

The optimal clinical method for measuring the amount of testosterone free to enter tissue remains controversial. Because recent evidence indicates that non-TeBG-bound testosterone is the functionally free fraction (see above), the measurement of this fraction is preferred for assessing testosterone levels. Such "free and weakly bound" testosterone measurements assess the albumin-bound as well as free fractions and correlate well with most clinical indexes of androgenicity. Measurement of the free fraction using methods that do not detect albumin binding also correlate better with clinical findings than does an assay of total testosterone. However, the partition between albumin-bound and free testosterone is occasionally observed to be altered; this could confound the interpretation of free testosterone measurements.[129]

The peripheral metabolism of secreted testosterone involves a series of enzymatic steps which can either activate or degrade the hormone. Two activation pathways exist by which testosterone serves as a prohormone and undergoes conversion to more potent metabolites. First, testosterone can be converted to estradiol, a compound with 200-fold greater gonadotropin-suppressive potency per unit mass than testosterone. The enzyme *aromatase,* which converts testosterone to estradiol, is present in fatty tissue, liver, muscle, hair follicles, Leydig and Sertoli cells, and specific sites in the brain. Approximately 0.4 percent of the 7000 μg of testosterone produced daily is converted to estradiol outside the testes.[130] The 30 μg of estradiol produced in this manner and the 10 μg secreted directly by the testes[131] account for most of the 40 to 50 μg of estradiol made daily in males. The remainder arises from the peripheral aromatization of androstenedione to estrone and its subsequent reduction to estradiol.

Testosterone can also be converted to DHT, an androgen with 2.5 times greater potency than testosterone. This reaction is catalyzed by 5α-reductase, an enzyme present in the prostate, seminal vesicles, sebaceous glands, kidney, skin, brain, and other tissues.[132] Genes for two forms of the enzyme have now been cloned.[133] Of the approximately 200 to 300 μg of DHT produced daily, the majority arises from peripherally converted testosterone; less than half is secreted by the testes.[110] In a study of men with congenital deficiency of 5α-reductase, DHT was inferred to be necessary for the mediation of androgenic effects on beard growth and prostatic hypertrophy.[134] Stimulatory effects on muscle and sexual potency do not appear to require reduction at the 5α position. The requirement for 5α reduction of testosterone for germ cell maturation is controversial. Inhibitors of 5α-reductase activity are being developed for potential exploration of these specific effects.[135]

Degradative androgen metabolism takes place in the liver (50 to 70 percent) as well as in peripheral tissues (30 to 50 percent). Nearly 50 percent of testosterone in the plasma is taken up by the liver during one pass through this organ (Figs. 16-19 and 16-20). Testosterone is then converted to the inactive metabolites androsterone and etiocholanolone, both 17-ketosteroids, and to DHT and 3α-androstanediol. These compounds can then be converted to their glucuronide or sulfate derivatives for reentry into plasma and excretion in urine. Genetic and nongenetic factors can alter the rate of these androgen transformations.[136]

Biosynthetic activation of androgens can be hormonally regulated at specific target organ sites.[137,138] For example, 5α-reductase is under androgenic control in skin. In conditions of androgen deficiency, such as hypogonadism in men, the levels of activity of this enzyme are reduced. Androgen administration increases the activity of 5α-reductase in these men.

Local degradative inactivation occurs in target organ sites as well but is not clearly androgen-regulated. DHT is reversibly converted to 3α-androstanediol and then to 3α-androstanediol glucuronide. Each of these compounds can reenter plasma and ultimately be excreted in the urine.[139] Mauvais-Jarvis et al. first pointed out the significance of the local skin metabolic pathway for androgens.[139] They demonstrated that the quantity of urinary 3α-androstanediol glucuronide reflects not only the amount of androgen initially secreted into the plasma but also the rate of its metabolism in target tissues. Local metabolism of androgens in the skin increases in states of androgen excess; skin metabolism of androgens correlates with the results of 3α-androstanediol glucuronide measurements in urine. Horton et al.[140] and others[141,142] later extended these observations by demonstrating a marked elevation of 3α-androstanediol glucuronide concentration in plasma in states of androgen excess. The extent of acne and body hair in men correlates with plasma levels of 3α-androstanediol glucuronide.[143]

Testosterone induces its hormonal effects through a sequence of events which are analogous to those initiated by other steroid hormones. Either directly in tissues such as the testis or after metabolic activation to DHT, testosterone binds to a specific receptor.[144] The human androgen receptor is a 919-amino acid protein which is a member of the steroid receptor superfamily. It has 82 percent homology with the progesterone receptor, 79 percent with the mineralocorticoid receptor, and 79 percent with the glucocorticoid receptor. The androgen receptor binds DHT with 1.2 times greater affinity than it binds testosterone.[145] A nuclear targeting signal is present on the receptor which allows ligand-bound receptor to be transported to the nucleus. There, binding to an androgen-responsive element (ARE) on a segment of DNA initiates transcriptional activation.[146,147] The affinity of binding to specific nuclear structures varies. Certain nuclear receptor fractions elute under conditions of low salt concentration and others elute under high salt concentration. An additional fraction is highly resistant to extraction. Evidence is accumulating to suggest that only a small fraction of all nuclear androgen receptors mediate androgen effects.[148] This fraction binds preferentially to the nuclear matrix, the DNA cytoskeleton which forms a supporting infrastructure in the nucleus.[148]

Receptor binding to nuclear DNA initiates a sequence of events which involves the activation of RNA polymerases I and II, the initiation of protein synthesis, and the induction of androgenic effects. Two general categories of androgenic actions on the body occur: those which are called anabolic effects and those which are more properly androgenic.[149] Assays that are more responsive to the anabolic effects of steroids (such as mass assessment of the levator ani muscle in the rat) or to the androgenic effects (e.g., ventral prostate weight) have been developed in animals. Structural manipulations of the synthetic androgens can produce substances which are relatively more anabolic than androgenic and

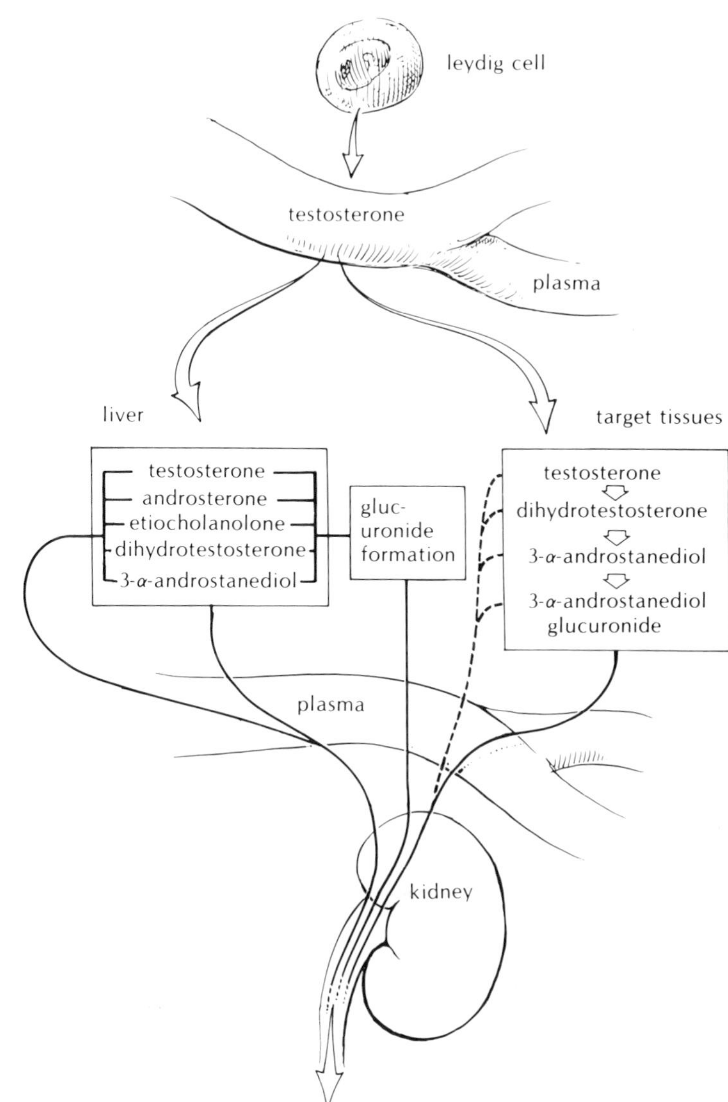

FIGURE 16-19 Diagrammatic representation of the metabolism of testosterone. After secretion by the Leydig cell, testosterone travels through the plasma to the liver or target tissues. After metabolism and conjugation, products are excreted into the urine.

vice versa. The exact molecular basis for determining whether actions will be androgenic or anabolic is uncertain.[149] Recent experiments, however, suggest that substitutions of the androgen molecule at the 7th carbon position prevent 5α redution and render the actions more anabolic than androgenic.[150] The specific actions of androgens at various times in life are listed in Table 16-1. Anabolic and androgenic actions are not differentiated in the table because of the uncertainty in distinguishing these effects on a mechanistic basis.

Feedback Interaction

Overview

Complementary and redundant servomechanisms are present to control LH secretion precisely in men. Two steroids—testosterone and estradiol—independently control LH secretion at two separate anatomic sites: the hypothalamus and pituitary (Fig. 16-21).[40] Negative feedback—the primary mechanism of this control—consists of two phases: the *suppressive* and *recovery* phases.[151] During the suppressive phase, an elevation of sex steroid concentrations causes a reduction in LH secretion (Fig. 16-22) and in pituitary mRNA levels for the LH subunits.[152] Later, during the recovery phase, LH concentration returns to basal levels upon the lowering of concentrations of sex steroids. Negative feedback effects can be mediated either by an alteration in the frequency or by modulation of the amplitude of LH pulses. Another mechanism—positive feedback—allows estradiol but not testosterone to stimulate LH under precisely defined conditions.[45]

Testosterone exerts negative feedback effects through interaction with androgen receptors or after aromatization to estradiol. Several lines of evidence support the independent actions of testosterone as an androgen on LH secretion.[40,41,153–155] Nonaromatizable androgens such as DHT and fluoxymesterone

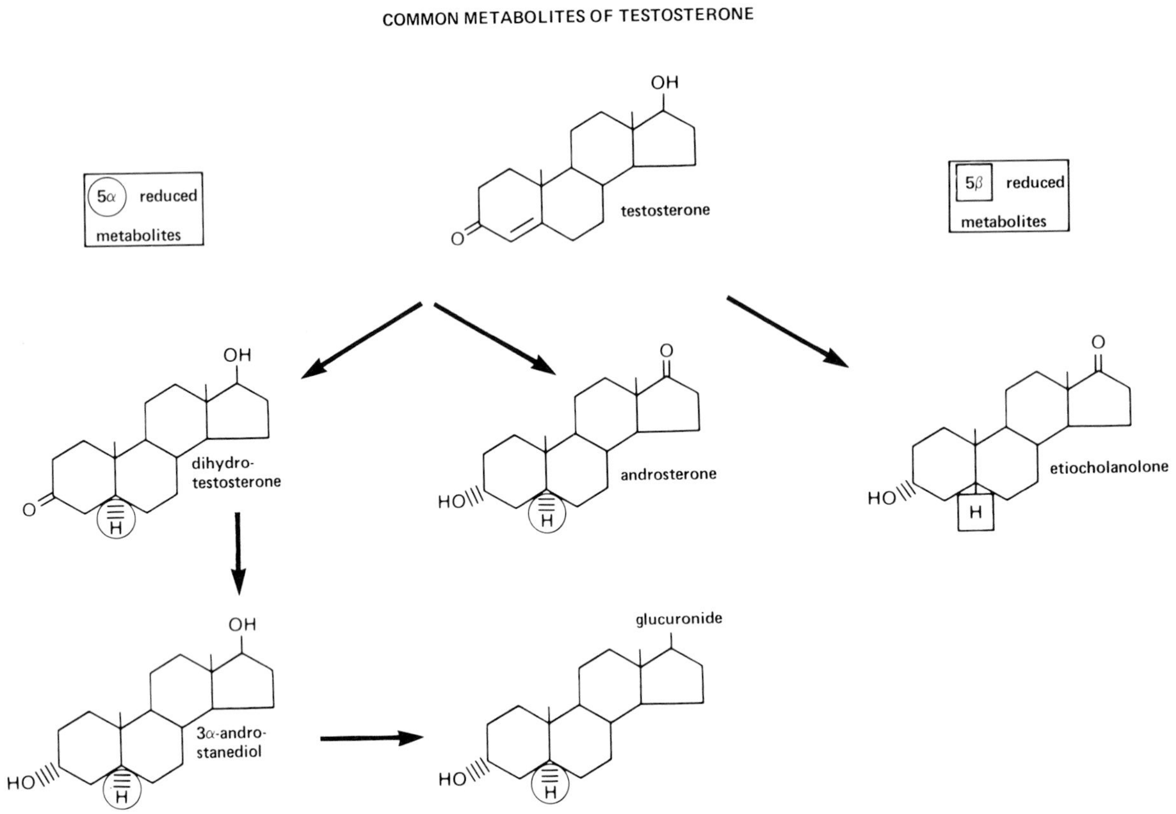

COMMON METABOLITES OF TESTOSTERONE

5α reduced metabolites

testosterone

5β reduced metabolites

dihydrotestosterone

androsterone

etiocholanolone

3α-androstanediol

glucuronide

FIGURE 16-20 Structures of the testosterone metabolites.

inhibit LH. The antiandrogen flutamide increases LH levels.[156] When administered with an aromatase inhibitor such as testolactone, testosterone suppresses LH release without a concomitant increase in estradiol concentration.[153] Androgens and estrogens produce differential effects on the frequency of pulsatile LH secretion as well as on its amplitude. Finally, hypogonadal men are relatively resistant to the LH-suppressive effects of androgens but not those of estrogens.[155] However, the amount of estradiol aromatized daily from secreted testosterone can also inhibit LH. Based on these data, current opinion considers that two negative feedback systems, one mediated by androgens and the other by estrogens, operate independently (Fig. 16-21). Both systems exert rapid effects on LH secretion within 3 to 6 h (Fig. 16-22).[41]

Androgen Negative Feedback

Testosterone reduces the amount of GnRH released from hypothalamic tissue in vitro and the amount secreted into the pituitary portal circulation in vivo.[32,157,158] When given for a short period of time (6 h to 4 days) testosterone inhibits LH exclusively through hypothalamic effects. This conclusion is inferred from the observation that the LH response to exogenous GnRH is not blunted during periods of androgen-induced LH suppression.[40,41,159] The mechanism of LH inhibition is through a specific effect on the frequency modulation of the pulse generator. Testosterone reduces GnRH pulse frequency from 1/100 min to 1/200 min on average in adult men.[40,41,159] This effect also has been observed in pubertal subjects.[160] Both testosterone and androgens incapable of conversion to estrogens such as DHT or fluoxymesterone lower pulse frequency.[159,161] The potent antiandrogen flutamide exerts opposite effects to increase LH frequency.[156] The negative feedback effect of androgens appears to be mediated through an opiatergic system.[161] The inhibitory effects of testosterone can be blocked by μ-opiate receptor antagonists, and these agents can stimulate LH and testosterone levels.[26] Opiate agonists are known to inhibit LH release,[162] and in primates, androgens increase the mRNA for pro-opiomelanocortin (POMC); this mRNA is translated into the precursor of β-endorphin, a potent endogenous opiate.[163]

Whether androgens play an inhibitory role at the pituitary level through androgen receptors in men is less certain. Androgen receptors are present in the pituitary of many species,[7] and DHT lowers LH secretion and content when it is directly implanted into the rodent pituitary.[164] Cultured pituitary cells respond to DHT by decreasing the amount of LH released in response to GnRH.[165] In contrast to these suggestive studies, more direct observation in male

TABLE 16-1 Clinical Actions of Androgen

In utero
- External genitalia development
- Wolffian duct development

Prepubertal
- Possible male behavioral effects

Pubertal
- External genitalia
  - Penis and scrotum increase in size and become pigmented
  - Rugal folds appear in scrotal skin
- Hair growth
  - Mustache and beard develop; scalp line undergoes recession
  - Pubic hair develops
  - Axillary, body, extremity, and perianal hair appears
- Linear growth
  - Pubertal growth spurt
  - Androgens interact with growth hormone to increase somatomedin C levels
- Accessory sex organs
  - Prostate and seminal vesicles enlarge, and secretion begins
- Voice
  - The pitch is lowered because of enlargement of larynx and thickening of vocal cords
- Psyche
  - More aggressive attitudes are manifest
  - Sexual potential develops
- Muscle mass
  - Muscle bulk increases
  - Positive nitrogen balance is demonstrable

Adult
- Hair growth
  - Androgenic patterns are maintained
  - Male baldness may be initiated
- Psyche
  - Behavioral attitudes and sexual potency are maintained
- Bone
  - Bone loss and osteoporosis are prevented
- Spermatogenesis
  - Interaction with FSH to modulate Sertoli cell function and stimulate spermatogenesis
- Hematopoiesis
  - Erythropoietin-stimulated
  - Direct marrow effect on erythropoiesis

Source: Adapted from Bardin and Paulsen.[282]

monkeys suggests that the direct pituitary effects of androgens play only a minor role. Lesions made by radio-frequency waves are used to ablate the hypothalamic pulse generator in these animals; GnRH is then administered to reestablish these pulses artificially. Completely normal patterns of LH secretion persist in these animals in response to acute androgen depletion or repletion. Only during chronic androgen deprivation are minor effects on LH observed.[35] Similar effects occur in GnRH-deficient patients who receive GnRH pulses. Although testosterone inhibits LH secretion under these circum-

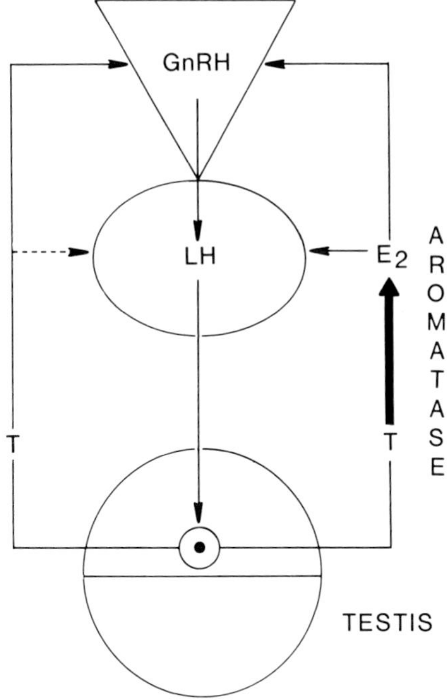

FIGURE 16-21 Diagrammatic representation of the hypothalamus (triangle), pituitary (oval), and testis (circle) with its Leydig cell depicted. T = testosterone; E = estradiol. Dotted line indicates questionable effect.

stances, this effect can be blocked by aromatase inhibitors and is mediated by estradiol.[166,167] Taken together, these observations suggest that androgens, acting through the androgen receptor, play a major inhibitory role at the hypothalamic level and a minor role at the pituitary.

Testosterone could act on the hypothalamus by binding to androgen receptors directly or by undergoing 5α reduction to DHT before receptor binding; no direct data are available to clearly establish which pathway predominates. 5α-Reductase exists in the hypothalami of several species.[133] Men with 5α-reductase deficiency exhibit slightly higher mean levels of LH and testosterone concentration than do their unaffected siblings.[134] By contrast, 5α reductase inhibitors lower DHT levels but do not increase LH levels in normal men.[135] Taken together, these observations suggest only a minor role for DHT in the physiologic regulation of LH.[135]

Estrogen Negative Feedback

In contrast to testosterone, the earliest effect of estradiol is mediated by a direct pituitary action. Within 3 to 6 h of estradiol administration, mean LH levels fall by 20 to 30 percent (Fig. 16-22), as do responses to exogenous GnRH.[40,41] This direct pituitary effect induces a 30 percent diminution in the amplitude of spontaneous LH pulses. Direct measurements of GnRH level in portal plasma in sheep further substantiate the direct pituitary effects of

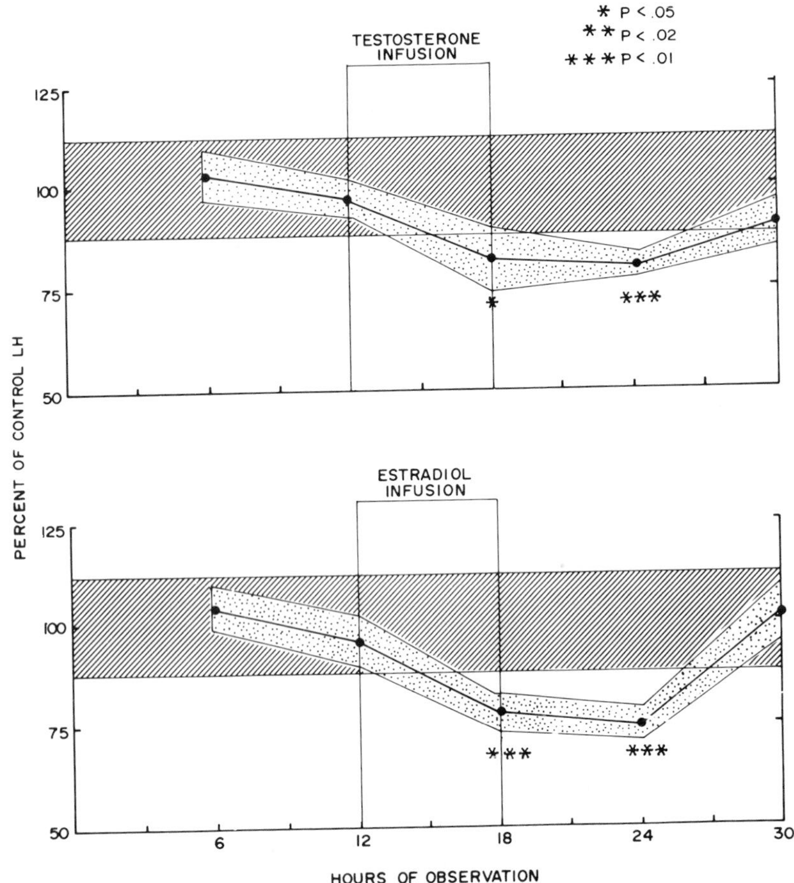

FIGURE 16-22 Effect of testosterone and estradiol infusions on mean LH concentration. Six-hour mean LH levels represented by solid circles; standard error of the mean represented by shaded area. With this method (6-h mean LH concentration), changes of >12 percent (cross-hatched area) are significant. (*From Santen.*[41])

brief administrations of estradiol.[168] During more prolonged infusions (e.g., 4 days), GnRH responsiveness returns to normal levels, indicating that the direct pituitary effect is transient.[169] This is not surprising, since a variety of observations suggest that the pituitary responds to estrogen in a biphasic fashion.[170] When briefly exposed to estradiol, the pituitary initially responds to exogenous GnRH with a blunted LH release; this is followed by enhancement of LH release. While such an effect has not been tested directly in men, measurements of LH responses to GnRH during estradiol infusion suggest that a similar biphasic pattern occurs.[41,169,170]

Several studies imply that estrogens act on a hypothalamic site in addition to affecting the pituitary directly. Receptors exist for estradiol in the hypothalamus as well as in the pituitary.[8] Estrogens inhibit the release of GnRH from neurons and increase the tissue concentrations of this neuropeptide in the hypothalamus.[157,158] Neurons in the medial basal hypothalamus alter their firing rates upon exposure to estradiol.[171] Clinical observations also suggest that estradiol has a hypothalamic effect. In men, the administration of an antiestrogen such as clomiphene stimulates LH secretion and pulse amplitude without enhancing the responsiveness to exogenous GnRH.[172,173] By the fourth day of intravenous (IV) infusion of physiologic amounts of estradiol, mean LH levels are suppressed but responsiveness to exogenous GnRH is not.[169]

The estradiol which acts at the hypothalamic level could be synthesized locally from androgen precursors or could be delivered to the hypothalamus from plasma. Aromatase, the enzyme which catalyzes the conversion of testosterone to estradiol, is present in the hypothalamus.[174] Aromatase is localized to certain hypothalamic nuclei; in the medial preoptic nucleus, for example, levels of aromatase are 10-fold higher than they are in the arcuate nucleus. This localization suggests that local estrogen production at these sites may play an important role.[175] Experiments with aromatase inhibitors in dogs are most compatible with the hypothesis that local estradiol synthesis in the hypothalamus is required for LH feedback.[176] Taken together, these data imply that there are major negative feedback effects of the estrogens at both the hypothalamic and pituitary levels.

Estrogen Positive Feedback

In women, the administration of estrogens in an appropriate dose and for an appropriate duration can transiently stimulate LH release after an initial inhibitory phase.[177] This positive feedback phenomenon is responsible for the abrupt midcycle rise in LH concentration which causes ovulation. An estrogen dose equivalent to 50 to 100 μg of estradiol daily for 4 to 7 days is required to stimulate LH through positive feedback. Androgens blunt or abolish the positive feedback response to estrogens. For this reason, castrated or hypogonadal men respond to estrogen with clearly defined positive feedback responses.[45] In contrast, men with normal circulating testosterone levels exhibit inconsistent and only modest increases in LH concentration.[178]

Hypothalamic-Pituitary-Germ Cell Axis

Overview

In addition to their role in androgen secretion, the testes produce sperm and emit them via an excretory ductal system. Germinal cell function is controlled by FSH as well as by intratesticular androgens; the separate determinants of FSH secretion are emphasized in this section. The pituitary releases FSH, which stimulates the Sertoli cells of the testis to initiate the secretion of a number of regulatory proteins. One of these proteins—*inhibin*—enters plasma and exerts negative feedback effects on FSH secretion by the pituitary (Fig. 16-23).

Hypothalamus

GnRH stimulates FSH as well as LH release by the pituitary. The existence of a separate FSH-releasing factor has been suggested by electrostimulative and biochemical studies in rodents.[179] However, the discordance between FSH and LH levels observed in a variety of clinical conditions can be explained without postulating that a separate FSH-releasing factor exists. Based on a variety of data, current opinion favors GnRH as the single physiologic releasing factor for FSH.

FIGURE 16-23 Control of FSH secretion. Diagrammatic representation of feedback relation between the hypothalamus (triangle), pituitary (oval), and testis (circle) with its Sertoli germ cell unit.

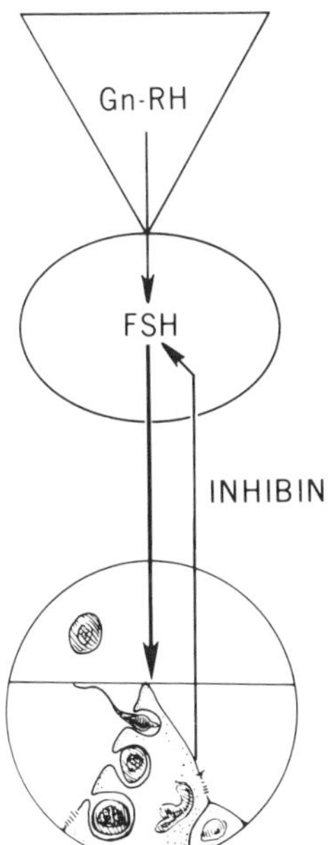

Pituitary

One pituitary cell, the gonadotroph, releases FSH as well as LH upon exposure to GnRH. FSH is a glycoprotein with a unique β subunit and an α subunit identical to α-LH.[180] Posttranslational processing alters several properties of this molecule in a fashion analogous to the processing of LH. The amount of carbohydrate introduced into its structure alters its intrinsic biological activity, the rapidity of its clearance from the peripheral circulation, and its ability to be recognized by RIA. The androgen depletion state associated with long-standing hypogonadism, readministration of androgens, or therapy with estrogens can modulate the degree of posttranscriptional processing by the pituitary. Circulating FSH molecules are modified as a result so that they exert altered effects on gonadal stimulation. Under other circumstances, such as the administration of GnRH antagonist analogues, FSH molecules with FSH antagonistic activity can be secreted.[181] This process provides a potentially important regulatory step in controlling the male reproductive process.

Under a variety of circumstances, the amount of FSH released in proportion to LH increases. Mechanisms for controlling the specific modulation of the amount of FSH released must therefore exist. As theorized by Franchimont et al., the gonadotroph releases FSH preferentially when exposed to minimal amounts of GnRH.[182,183] For example, fetal pituitary cultures secrete a predominance of FSH in the absence of GnRH in vitro.[184] FSH secretion predominates in a variety of clinical conditions characterized by reduced GnRH secretion, such as early puberty, hypothalamic amenorrhea, anorexia nervosa, and hyperprolactinemia.[185]

The frequency of GnRH pulses can also alter the amount of FSH secreted relative to LH.[186] Administration of the same total dose of GnRH but in pulses every 3 h rather than every hour caused a twofold rise in FSH level without altering LH levels in men with isolated gonadotropin deficiency.[186] The generation of low-frequency GnRH pulses in monkeys also produces higher FSH than LH plasma levels.[187] High-frequency GnRH pulses, by contrast, decrease the FSH/LH ratio. The disparity between FSH and LH responses to frequency modulation is dampened by increasing amounts of circulating testosterone.[166,167]

The exposure of the pituitary to inhibin also alters the proportion of FSH and LH released in response to GnRH.[182] In culture, pituitary cells exhibit a dose-dependent decrease in FSH but not LH released in response to purified inhibin preparations.

After release into the circulation, FSH is cleared by the liver, kidneys, and other sites. Metabolic clearance rates (MCR) of 14 ml/min are found in premenopausal women, and 4 to 12 ml/min in men.[188–190] FSH production rates calculated from this MCR and mean plasma levels of 10 to 20 mIU/ml equal 140 to 280 IU per day in men. Approximately 5 percent of secreted FSH appears in the urine as immunologically detectable hormone (5 to 20 IU per day).[79] The remainder is degraded in the liver and kidneys and at other sites. The half-life of FSH in plasma is markedly prolonged compared to that of LH. The first-phase half-life has been reported to be 1.7 h in one study and 3.9 h in another,[188] whereas the second-phase half-life was 8.3 and 70.4 h.[191] Because the half-life of FSH is longer than that of LH in plasma, pulsatile FSH secretion is difficult to discern. With each secretory pulse, a small amount of newly released FSH enters a large, slowly turning over pool of plasma FSH.[180] In contrast, newly secreted LH is added to a small, rapidly turning over pool. Based on these phenomena, LH pulses are readily apparent, whereas FSH pulses are less obvious.[192] However, with the appropriate methodology, pulsatile FSH secretion can be easily documented.[192,193] As would be predicted, the concordance of FSH and LH pulses increases as LH pulse amplitude (and the amount of GnRH released) increases.[31,193]

Testis

FSH binds to specific receptors located in the Sertoli cell.[194] The typical sequence of receptor binding, adenylate cyclase activation, stimulation of cyclic AMP, binding to the regulatory subunit, activation of the catalytic subunit, and protein phosphorylation occurs as for the other polypeptide hormones. FSH induces increased synthesis and secretion of several Sertoli cell proteins, including inhibin, transferrin, and ABP. The best characterized is ABP, the intratesticular analogue of the plasma protein TeBG, with which it shares many amino acid homologies.[125,195,196] In the rodent, ABP is a dimeric glycoprotein of known amino acid sequence[197] containing H and L monomers of molecular weights 45,000 and 41,000, respectively. Human ABP is similar, with monomers called *form 1,* which does not bind to concanavalin A, and *form 2,* a glycopeptide which does. Extensive physiologic studies in rodents indicate that ABP synthesis is controlled by both FSH and testosterone.[125] ABP requires FSH for initial synthesis, but ABP levels can be maintained by high androgen concentrations after induction.

ABP is secreted into the seminiferous tubular lumen and travels by fluid flow to the epididymis, where it is actively concentrated.[198] ABP has been suggested to play a physiologic role in maintaining high local testosterone concentrations in the seminiferous tubular compartment and epididymis, but this hypothesis has not been substantiated. In the rodent, ABP is also secreted into the peripheral plasma,[199] but this has not been demonstrated in men.[197]

Inhibin is another well-studied Sertoli cell protein. Its activity is currently detected by bioassay[182] or specific RIA.[200] Many other proteins, some of which are identical to serum proteins and others of which are not,[125] are also secreted by the Sertoli cells. Two of these—somatomedin C and interleukin 1—serve as mitogens in other tissues and could exert similar effects on seminiferous tubule cells.[201,202] The responsiveness of most of these additional proteins to FSH is under study. Only aromatase, however, is known to be FSH-responsive.

The Sertoli cells serve a number of physiologic functions in the germinal cell compartment. These include maintenance of the blood-testis barrier, provision of potassium- and bicarbonate-rich tubular fluid in the seminiferous tubules, phagocytosis of damaged germ cells, regulation of germ cell maturation, conversion of androgen precursors to estrogens by the action of aromatase, and the production of specific proteins for secretion into the seminiferous tubule lumen and blood.[125]

Control of the process of spermatogenesis is not completely understood at present.[203] Data from studies in animals suggest that FSH is required to *initiate* spermatogenesis and that testosterone in high intratesticular concentrations can *maintain* this process.[16] By stimulating Leydig cells, LH produces high intratesticular testosterone levels. Testosterone or, alternatively, DHT then acts on the spermatogonia and primary spermatocytes to complete the meiotic divisions. FSH facilitates maturation of spermatids to spermatozoa during the process of spermiogenesis and may also enhance the rate of initial spermatogonial maturation.[204] After the initiation of full spermatogenesis by this means, testosterone alone, if given in amounts sufficient to maintain high intratesticular concentrations, can maintain this process. For example, after hypophysectomy in male monkeys and rats, prolonged administration of testosterone at a high dose can maintain spermatogenesis.[205] The effects of testosterone are probably mediated by direct actions on peritubular myoid cells and Sertoli cells, and indirect actions are exerted on the germinal epithelium. Androgen receptors are present only on Sertoli and peritubular cell elements but not on the germinal cell elements themselves.[206,207]

After the process of spermiogenesis is complete, spermatozoa enter the seminiferous tubular lumen and the caput epididymis. Motility is acquired during their passage through the epididymis.[19,208] A variety of factors have been identified as possible physiologic regulators of sperm motility, including calcium ions,[209,210] cyclic AMP,[211,212] catecholamines,[213] a protein motility factor,[214] and protein carboxymethylase.[215] The exact manner in which these diverse factors coordinately regulate motility has yet to be established. Spermatozoa that are present in the fresh ejaculate are not capable of fertilization despite their rapid motility. A further change occurs in the female reproductive tract, in which the ability to fertilize is acquired through a process called *capacitation.*[216]

The way in which this proposed sequence relates to human physiology is problematic. The congenitally hypogonadotropic male serves as a model for studying the initiation of spermatogenesis in patients. The administration of hCG, an LH-like material, stimulates germ cell maturation to the spermatid level but does not lead to the production of mature spermatozoa. FSH is necessary to complete the process of spermiogenesis and allow the exit of normal amounts of spermatozoa into the ejaculate.[99,217,218] These observations are consistent with theories that have been proposed to explain the initiation of spermatogenesis in animals.

An interesting experimental paradigm has been used to directly determine the requirement for the *maintenance* of spermatogenesis in men.[219] Volunteers receive high doses of exogenous testosterone, which inhibits the production of LH and FSH while it is being administered but does not produce normal intratesticular testosterone levels. Separate replacement of exogenous LH or FSH allows quantitative assessment of the effects of these individual gonadotropins on the maintenance of spermatogenesis. With physiologic replacement amounts of pure LH, spermatogenesis is rapidly restored, although not to quantitatively normal levels. This presumably occurs through the induction of high intratesticular levels of testosterone. FSH alone also restores spermatogenesis under these conditions, but not to normal levels.[220] Thus, the maintenance of quantitatively normal spermatogenesis requires both gonadotropins. It should be noted that exogenous testosterone replacement in gonadotropin-deficient patients usually does not support spermatogenesis, since high intratesticular concentrations are not maintained as with exogenous LH or hCG.

Feedback Control of FSH Release

A specific feedback interaction between the germ cell compartment of the testis and FSH was first suggested by the observation of isolated FSH elevations in patients with syndromes of germ cell failure. Irradiation of the testis in animals and men[221] induces germ cell arrest and FSH increments without altering LH and testosterone levels. Oligospermic males frequently exhibit monotrophic FSH increments.[222] These observations initially suggested that the germinal cell compartment, specifically the Sertoli cells, secretes a substance which inhibits FSH into the peripheral plasma. Such a factor has been identified in extensive studies and is called inhibin.[223] It has been purified and sequenced by analysis of its complementary DNA. Inhibin consists of a 31-kDa heterodimeric protein with α and β subunits connected by a disulfide bridge. Two alternate β subunits called β_A and β_B combine with the α subunit to form inhibins β_A and β_B. Homodimers and heterodimers of the β subunit also form and are called activin A (B_A-B_B) and activin AB (B_B-B_B). These peptides stimulate FSH at concentrations (0.4 to 1.0 ng/ml) 10-fold less than those required for GnRH to exert similar effects. Inhibin and activin are part of a family of peptides which also includes TGF_β; müllerian inhibitory substance, a Sertoli cell glycoprotein that causes regression of müllerian ducts in male fetuses; the decapentapalegic gene complex in *Drosophila;* and the VG gene in *Xenopus.*

The relative roles of activin and inhibin in the feedback regulation of FSH are incompletely understood. A current hypothesis postulates a negative feedback loop by which FSH stimulates the secretion of inhibin by the Sertoli cell and inhibin in turn reduces the secretion of FSH. Data in men demonstrate that FSH increases the production of inhibin, and LH can also exert this effect.[224] The biological role of inhibin in the negative feedback loop to reduce FSH secretion is controversial. The most convincing evidence regarding an FSH-inhibin feedback loop consists of observations demonstrating an inverse relation between plasma FSH and inhibin levels in ewes and in male rats.[225] Further support comes from the observation that anti-inhibin antibodies increase FSH levels in monkeys.[226] One study also found a negative correlation between FSH and inhibin in normal men and in men receiving chemotherapy, as would be expected if such a feedback loop were operative.[227,228] In contrast, no inverse correlation between inhibin and FSH was observed in oligospermic men.[229,230] A biological role for inhibin in FSH regulation in men thus remains an open question.

Both activin and inhibin share homology with many growth factors and are present in many tissues in the body, such as brain, spleen, adrenal, pituitary, kidney, and bone marrow.[223,230] Recent data suggest that these peptides exert local regulatory effects in many tissues in addition to the testes. Activin, for example, exerts a mitogenic effect on thymocytes and 3T3 cells, a stimulatory effect on erythroid precursors,[231] and a potential regulatory role during embryogenesis, including the induction of CNS differentiation, mesodermal development, and axial patterning.[231–233] Its role in the basal secretion of FSH is suggested by in vitro experiments[231–233] but remains to be established by in vivo observations.

Several other factors which inhibit FSH secretion in vitro have also been purified, including two distinct seminal plasma proteins (α and β inhibins),[230] which have no homology with inhibin or activin, and follistatin, another FSH inhibitory protein. Follistatin also functions as an inhibin-binding protein.[234] These peptides are under study to determine their biological roles.

Interactions between the LH-Leydig Cell and FSH-Germ Cell Axes

Hypothalamus and Pituitary

Since GnRH stimulates the release of LH as well as FSH, the regulation of GnRH affects both the Leydig cell and germ cell axes of the testis (Fig. 16-24). Through the inhibition of GnRH release, testosterone and estradiol exert negative feedback effects on FSH as well as on LH at the hypothalamic level.[40] The differential effects of these sex steroids directly at the pituitary level have not been clearly delineated. Reports on the effect of testosterone are conflicting: In some studies LH secretion is suppressed to a greater extent with testosterone than is FSH, whereas the converse is observed in other studies.[185] A similar lack of agreement exists regarding the differential effects of estradiol on LH and FSH secretion at the pituitary level. Present data, then, indicate that there are multiple interactions between control of the LH-Leydig cell axis and control of the germ cell-FSH axis.

Testis

The germ cell and Leydig cell compartments are contiguous anatomically in order to facilitate local interactions between separate biological functions, namely, testosterone production and the manufacture and release of germ cells (Fig. 16-25). The Leydig cells maintain 100-fold higher testosterone concentrations locally in the testes than in peripheral plasma.[235] This facilitates concentration-dependent diffusion through the limiting blood–Sertoli cell barrier. As was noted above, testosterone interacts with FSH to maintain ABP synthesis in Sertoli cells.[125] While FSH is required to initiate ABP synthesis, large amounts of testosterone can maintain this process, at least in the rodent.[236] The effects of androgen on germinal cell epithelium are indirect, since androgen receptors are present in Sertoli and peritubular cells but not in germinal epithelium.[206,207] Whether DHT or testosterone itself is the primary mediator of androgenic action here remains a matter of controversy. Leydig cells also secrete prodynorphin, renin, oxytocin, β-endorphin, α-melanocyte stimulating hormone (α-MSH), and ACTH, which may also regulate Sertoli cell function, although this requires further study.[94]

Peritubular myoid cells also respond to androgen by producing a factor or factors which reduce aromatase activity in the Sertoli cell.[237] These factors, called P-mod-S, also modulate the secretion by the Sertoli cell of proteins such as transferrin and androgen-binding protein.[94] Growth factors such as TGF_α and TGF_β, insulin-like growth factor-1 (IGF-1) and insulin-like growth factor binding proteins[238] may also regulate Sertoli cell function after synthesis and secretion by peritubular cells.[94]

FIGURE 16-24 Integrated control of LH and FSH secretion involving both the Leydig cell and Sertoli cell compartments of the testis. T=testosterone; E_2=estradiol.

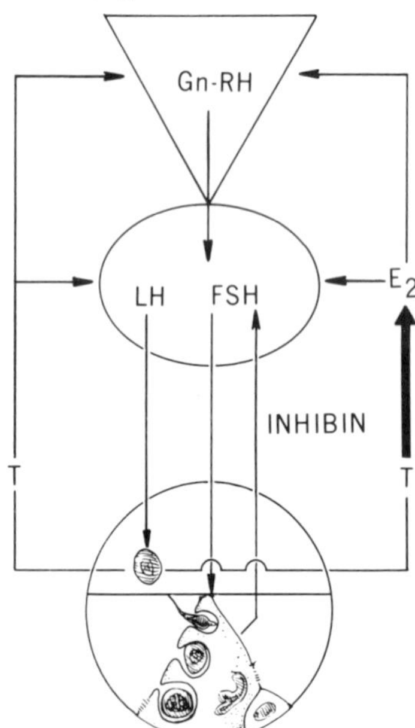

FIGURE 16-25 Diagrammatic representation of the relation between the seminiferous tubular compartment of the testis and the Leydig cells. Testosterone crosses into the seminiferous tubular compartment, where it stimulates spermatogenesis as well as synthesis of androgen-binding protein (ABP).

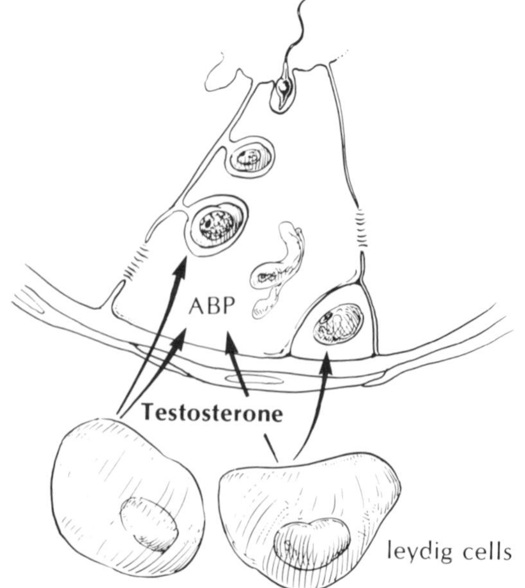

The Sertoli cells can also influence Leydig cell function through local regulatory mechanisms. Growth factors, inhibin, activin, and aromatase may all play a regulatory role.[94] Within the Sertoli cell, sufficient aromatase is present to convert testosterone to estradiol. This enzyme and, thus, local estradiol synthesis are under the control of FSH.[125] Receptors for estradiol are present in the Leydig cell. A current hypothesis suggests that estradiol of Sertoli cell origin diffuses back into the Leydig cells, where it inhibits 17α-hydroxylase and $C_{17\text{-}20}$-lyase and modulates local testosterone production.[91,92] Leydig cell aromatase may contribute to this process.[239] Not all investigators agree with the estradiol inhibition hypothesis. They base their conclusions on the observation that hypogonadotropic patients who are given hCG for 4 to 6 months have persistent fourfold increases in estradiol concentration but no alteration in testosterone biosynthesis.[93]

Prolactin Effects on Male Reproduction

The secretion of prolactin in physiologic amounts is required in animals for the maintenance of testosterone biosynthesis.[240] In men, prolactin may also influence the degree of tissue sensitivity to androgens by increasing androgen binding in reproductive tissues.[241] Pharmacologic amounts of prolactin, in contrast, exert an inhibitory effect on testosterone synthesis in both men and animals. These actions are mediated primarily at the hypothalamic level. Prolactin appears to inhibit GnRH release by influencing hypothalamic aminergic function.[24] Consequently, LH secretion is reduced and testosterone levels fall. In the clinic, men with prolactin-secreting adenomas are found to have a reduction in pulsatile LH release[242] and low testosterone levels.[243,244] A direct testicular action of prolactin, while possible, is difficult to demonstrate in men. Prolactin receptors are present in the testes of several species and may also exist in men.[240,245] However, testosterone responses to hCG are completely normal in men with elevated prolactin levels. This is observed whether the prolactin increments are induced by pharmacologic means or by functioning tumors.[246,247]

Another important effect of prolactin is a reduction in 5α-reductase activity in peripheral tissues.[248] This results in a lower ratio of DHT to testosterone in plasma both in the unstimulated state and during hCG stimulation.[247,249] Diminished androgenic effects at the tissue level would be expected but have not been clearly demonstrated. Hyperprolactinemic men frequently complain of impotence. This symptom does not respond to testosterone administration until prolactin levels are normalized.[250,251] Whether this observation can be explained on the basis of the 5α-reductase-inhibitory effects of prolactin or other mechanisms is unknown.

CLINICAL EVALUATION OF THE HYPOTHALAMIC-PITUITARY-TESTICULAR AXIS

Assessment of patients is based on an understanding of the normal actions of androgens in utero, during puberty, and in adult men (Table 16-1). Patients with congenital hypogonadism present with sexual infantilism and retarded growth for age. The history and physical examination focus on external genitalia, hair growth, linear growth, accessory sex organs, voice, psyche, and muscle mass. Acquired hypogonadism results in a loss of maintenance of normal androgen-mediated effects (Table 16-1). Evaluation in these men is directed toward patterns of hair growth, testis size, sexual potential, behavioral patterns, maintenance of bone density, spermatogenesis, and normal hematopoiesis.

Assessment of Hormonal Status

Basal Levels

GnRH circulates in plasma in concentrations too low for practical measurement.[252] Plasma LH and FSH may be quantitated by several methods, but three potential problems may confound interpretation: pulsatile secretion, assay sensitivity, and secretion of heterogeneous gonadotropin molecules. *Pulsatile secretion* introduces errors in estimates of integrated gonadotropin levels when single samples are obtained. Estimates from single samples may differ from integrated concentrations by approximately ± 60 percent for LH and ± 20 percent for FSH.[31] Most standard RIAs have limits of *sensitivity* close to those representing the lower range of normal values. However, two-site radioimmunometric, time-resolved fluorometric, or chemiluminescent assays are characterized by a marked enhancement in sensitivity. Values can be reliably detected in plasma in most subjects with the exception of prepubertal and severely hypogonadotropic subjects.[60] Gonadotropin molecules with hetereogeneous properties due to altered carbohydrate content are secreted. These molecules may vary in biological potency. In general, the two-site radioimmunometric and other highly sensitive immunoassay methods detect levels of gonadotropin which correlate with in vitro bioassay results, whereas standard RIAs may not. For this reason, ratios of bioassayable to immunoassayable LH (B/I ratios) vary substantially in patients with androgen deficiency, aging, or illness[53,55,57,58,253,254] when standard RIAs are used. These ratios, however, are relatively constant when newer, highly sensitive assays are employed.[64,65]

A practical recommendation for gonadotropin assessment, based on cost and precision, includes the following algorithm. Initially, measure LH and FSH in a single plasma sample, using a highly sensitive assay. Markedly elevated or clearly low values can usually be interpreted without further measurements. However, if the initial value is borderline high, confirm by repeat measurements in a pool of four samples taken at 20-min intervals or in a precisely timed 3-h urine (Fig. 16-26). Both methods integrate fluctuations from pulsatile secretion.[114,255,256] If the initial value is borderline low, confirm by measurements in a 3-h urine prepared with a concentrating step[255,256] or in a pool of four plasma samples.

Measurement of gonadal steroid levels for clinical purposes presents fewer inherent problems than do gonadotropin determinations. Assay sensitivity can be easily enhanced when necessary by extracting larger volumes of plasma before an RIA. The lower amplitude of secretory pulses attenuates the error introduced by single-sample measurements to approximately half that for LH determinations.[111,114] Single samples are usually adequate for clinical assessment of testosterone and DHT levels. Testosterone levels, but not LH and FSH concentrations, vary diurnally; peak concentrations occur between 4 and 8 A.M., and nadir levels occur between 4 and 8 P.M.[257] Normal ranges should be established using early-morning samples, and attempts should be made to collect patient samples at the same time of day. When abnormal values for total testosterone concentration are detected, attention should be directed toward the possibility of TeBG abnormalities (Fig. 16-17), and free and weakly bound (i.e., non-TeBG-bound) or free testosterone levels should be specifically determined.[129] Certain clinical circumstances warrant the measurement of adrenal androgens. Determination of 17-ketosteroid levels has been superseded by measurements of plasma DHEA sulfate concentration for this purpose.

Inhibin RIAs are currently available as a research tool to assess Sertoli cell function[258] but are limited by lack of specificity. The free α subunit of inhibin and the intact inhibin molecule are measured by current assays.[259] Routine clinical use awaits further characterization of levels in pathologic states.[228,229,260,261]

Dynamic Tests

Interruption of the estrogen negative feedback axis with clomiphene citrate (Figs. 16-27 and 16-28) stimulates the release of LH and FSH and, secondarily, the release of testosterone and estradiol.[262] Clomiphene is a potent estrogen antagonist (and weak agonist) which exerts antiestrogenic effects predominantly at the hypothalamic level. In men, the administration of 100 mg daily for 7 days can be used as a provocative test to evaluate the entire hypothalamic-pituitary axis (Fig. 16-28). A 100 percent rise in LH and a 50 percent rise in FSH concentrations represent mean normal increments observed

FIGURE 16-26 Correlation of LH levels *(left)* in matched samples of blood and urine; similar correlations of FSH levels *(right)*. Arrows indicate samples that fall below (<) or above (>) assay sensitivity. Results indicate that either blood or timed 3-h urine samples may be used to assay basal gonadotropin levels. *(From Kulin et al.*[255] *and Santen and Kulin.*[256]*)*

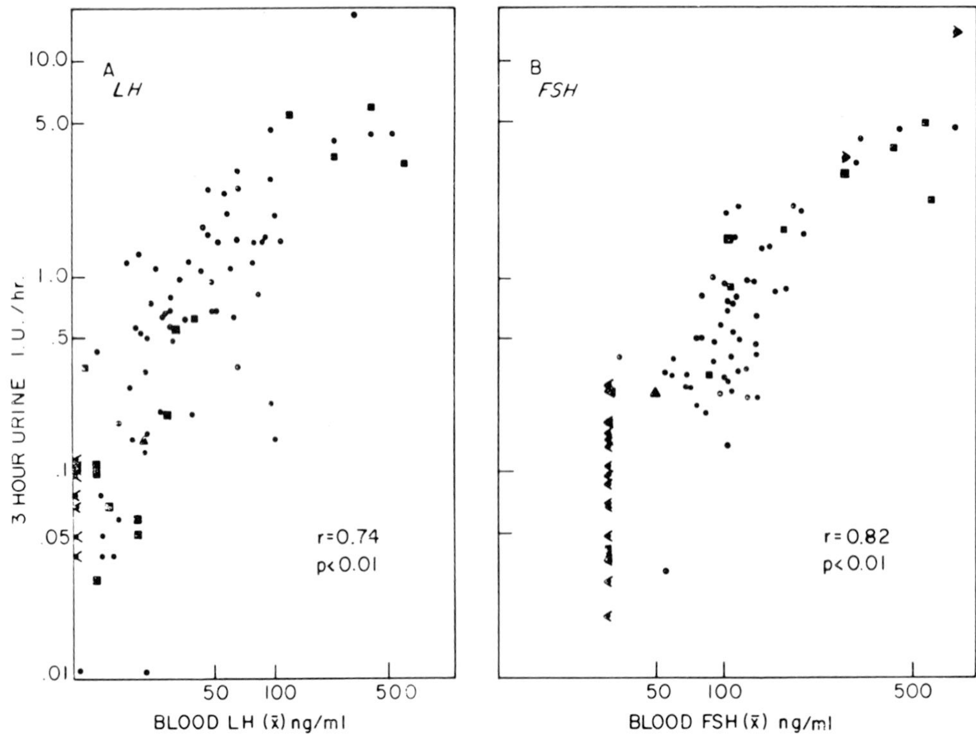

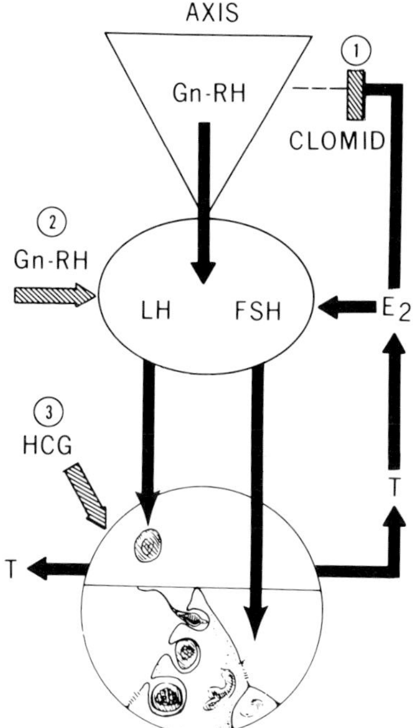

FIGURE 16-27 Diagrammatic representation of sites of action of stimulation tests of the testis: (1) clomiphene citrate; (2) GnRH; (3) hCG. Triangle = hypothalamus; oval = pituitary; circle = Leydig and germ cell compartments of the testis.

with this test and indicate an intact hypothalamic-pituitary axis. When clomiphene is given over a 6-week period, the LH concentration increases further by 200 to 700 percent, and FSH by 70 to 360 percent, reaching a plateau at approximately 1 month. Interruption of the androgen negative feedback axis with ketoconazole has also been proposed as a possible provocative test for LH and FSH secretion, but comprehensive clinical data are not available.[263]

The GnRH test evaluates the functional capacity of the gonadotrophs to release LH and FSH (Figs. 16-27 and 16-28). Two factors influence this response: the number of gonadotrophs present and the priming of these cells by prior exposure to endogenous GnRH secretion. If the gonadotrophs are not primed, the response to a single bolus of GnRH is limited. For this reason, use of the GnRH test to distinguish between hypothalamic and pituitary causes of reduced gonadotropin secretion is problematic. Operationally, the test consists of the administration of 25 μg of GnRH as a single bolus with a measurement of plasma LH before and three to six measurements after the injection over a 3-h period. Collection of timed 3-h urine samples before and after injection is a method particularly suitable for patients with low basal gonadotropin levels.[80] No general agreement exists on whether the results are best interpreted with respect to peak response, area under the response curve, absolute changes in gonadotropin level, or percent response. As a general guideline, a doubling of LH and a 50 percent increase in FSH concentrations represent minimally normal results (Table 16-2).

Direct provocative testing of the testes requires the administration of hCG and the assessment of plasma testosterone increments at various time intervals (Figs. 16-27 and 16-28). Traditional test procedures use multiple injections on a daily basis; however, more recent data indicate that one injection of 1500 to 4000 IU intramuscularly (IM) is a sufficient stimulus.[264] Plasma testosterone is then measured before and 5 days after hCG injections. Normal responses vary from a doubling of the initial testosterone level in adult patients to a rise greater than 150 ng/100 ml in prepubertal subjects (Table 16-2). Alternatively, in prepubertal boys, a longer protocol can be used during which testosterone reaches the adult male range after 16 days of stimulation.[265]

Biological Effects of Sex Steroids on Target Organs

Structural changes of the epiphyseal growth centers in the wrist and hands occur in response to changes in testosterone levels during pubertal maturation. X-rays of these structures allow the determination of bone age and provide functional information reflecting prior exposure of these structures to hormonal stimulation. In pubertal and prepubertal subjects, bone age correlates with the degree of pubertal maturation of the hypothalamus, provided that GH and thyroxine levels are normal. In adult men, androgens act to maintain bone mass; hypogonadism is associated with reductions in quantitatively assessed bone density.[266–268]

Genetic Tests

Several disorders of testicular function are associated with chromosomal abnormalities, particularly of the heterotopic sex chromatin. A number of methods are available to detect chromosomal abnormalities. When two X chromosomes are present, one of them condenses to form a Barr body, a dark-staining inclusion along the nuclear membrane of the cell. Examination of a buccal smear can therefore be used to detect an extra X chromosome in a male. Karyotype analysis of blood lymphocytes, skin fibroblasts, or gonadal tissues provides more definitive information. Special banding stains allow the identification of individual chromosomes and portions of them. Special fluorescent stains are available which can identify the Y chromosomes in cells from buccal smears, metaphase plates, or meiotic spreads of gonadal tissue. Recently, the DNA sequences of the gene on the Y chromosome which control testicular

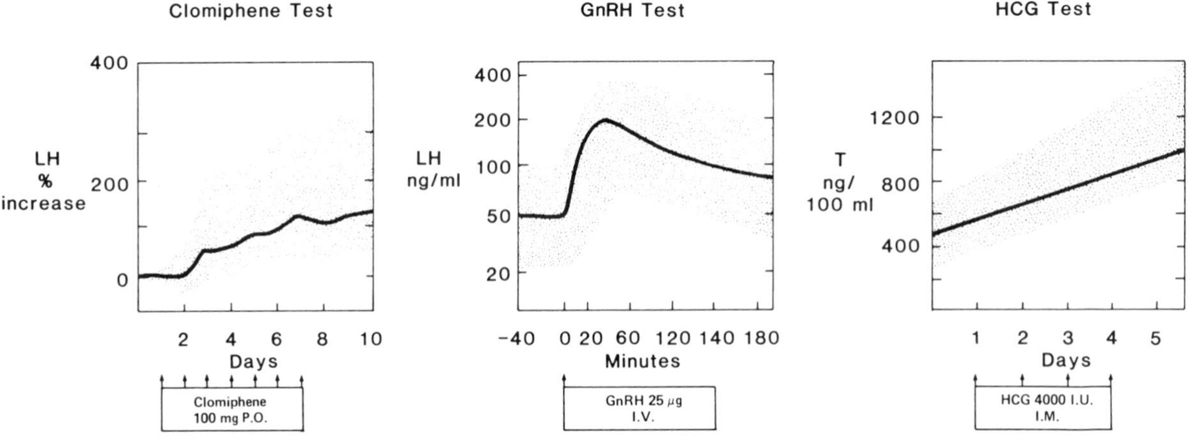

FIGURE 16-28 Mean (solid lines) and ranges (shaded areas) of LH and testosterone concentration increments during clomiphene, GnRH, and hCG stimulation tests. *(Data from Refs. 41, 172, 256, 262, 656, 657.)*

development (SRY gene) were determined.[269] cDNA probes are now available to identify this region and can be used to determine the presence of this portion of the Y chromosome. The use of polymerase chain reaction methodology enhances sensitivity and is practically applicable.[270]

TABLE 16-2 Normal Basal and Stimulated Hormone Levels

		Stimulated Mean % Increase*		
	Basal	Clomiphene	GnRH	hCG
Plasma concentration†				
LH	4–20 mIU/ml	100 (30–400)	450 (50–1200)	
FSH	4–20 mIU/ml	50 (20–200)	70 (9–176)	
Testosterone	300–1200 ng/100 ml	25 (0–65)	0	100 (50–200)
Urine excretion rate				
LH	500–2500 mIU/h	100 (0–200)	100 (15–200)	
FSH	200–3300 mIU/h	100 (20–180)	63 (30–100)	

* Range of percent increase in parenthesis.

† Normal ranges in laboratories that do not use external control standards vary.

Test protocols (see Fig. 16-28): Clomiphene: 100 mg clomiphene citrate daily by mouth for 7 days; draw blood sample or collect timed 3-h urine samples before and on day 8; GnRH, plasma: 25 μg GnRH IV with collection of blood before and 30, 60, 90, and 120 min later; GnRH, urine: 100 μg GnRH IV with collection of timed 3-h urine samples before and after injection; hCG: 5000 IU hCG IM daily for 4 days; draw blood samples before and on day 5.

Structural and Functional Assessment

Pituitary and Hypothalamus

Magnetic resonance imaging (MRI) scans with contrast enhancement have replaced skull x-rays and tomograms as methods for delineating anatomic structures. Computed tomography (CT) scans provide inferior delineation of pituitary lesions but can be used to evaluate bony changes contiguous with the pituitary. Digital subtraction angiography allows precise definition of vascular relations among the pituitary, the hypothalamus, and the surrounding structures but is now used only in patients who require pituitary surgery. Histologic assessment of the pituitary is useful when a functioning tumor is present and immunohistochemistry is desired to delineate the various cell types present.

Testis and Surrounding Structures

Physical examination provides information regarding the anatomy of the epididymis, vas deferens, and testes. Testis size is assessed by means of simple measurement of the longitudinal and horizontal axes or comparison with a series of ellipsoids of increasing volume (Table 16-3), using an apparatus called a Prader orchidometer.[271] This technique correlates precisely with objective ultrasonic measurements.[272] Special techniques of testicular examination must be used under certain circumstances. In boys with pseudocryptorchism or retractile testes, the gonads may be palpated only when the patient exits from a warm bath or assumes a squatting position. Dilatation of veins in the scrotum, a condition called *varicocele,* may be detected only when the patient is upright and performing a Valsalva maneuver.

Special diagnostic tools are available to provide further anatomic information.[273] Pelvic ultrasound can help locate intraabdominal testicular structures in older boys and adults or identify occult testicular

TABLE 16-3 Assessment of Testicular Size

Method	Prepubertal	Pubertal	Adult
Orchidometer*	1-6	8-15	20-30†
Ruler measurement‡			
Length	1.6-2.9	3.1-4.0	4.1-5.5
Width	1.0-1.8	2.0-2.5	2.7-3.2

* Measured in milliliters.

† 24 ± 4 SD ml; $n = 44$.

‡ Measured in centimeters.

Source: Adapted from Sherins and Howards.[271]

tumors.[274] Spermatic venography detects and delineates the location of cryptorchid testes.[275] Laparoscopy allows visualization of the vas deferens and testicular structures.[276] The presence of varicocele can be demonstrated by a venogram with dye injected into the testicular vein. The vas deferens may be cannulated during surgery and injected with dye (called an *operative vasogram*) to establish patency of the epididymis and vas deferens.

Testis biopsy permits the determination of the number of germ cells of each cell type and the degree of hyalinization of the seminiferous tubules.[277] Precise quantitation of germ cell parameters is time-consuming and difficult. Special competence in processing (e.g., use of Cleland's or Buin's fixative rather than Formalin) and quantifying is required. A well-studied technique[277] expresses the number of germ cells as a function of the number of Sertoli cells and evaluates the degree of cellular maturation, amounts of peritubular hyalinization, and the degree of tubular sclerosis (Table 16-4).

Before the availability of plasma FSH assays, testis biopsy provided the only information regarding the degree of functional impairment of the spermatogenic process. Currently, plasma FSH measurements are also used to assess the amount of testicular damage, as FSH concentration rises with increasing testicular destruction.[222] For this reason, testis biopsy is now used less commonly. However,

TABLE 16-4 Abundances of Germinal Cell Components Quantified on Testicular Biopsy*

Cell type	Number/ Sertoli cell	Range
Spermatogonia	1.77	1.05-2.83
Preleptotene	0.25	0.06-0.44
Leptotene	0.22	0.08-0.38
Zygotene + pachytene	1.96	1.03-2.86
Sa + Sb spermatids	3.05	1.59-4.87
Sc + Sd spermatids	2.14	1.44-3.63

* Cellular abundance is expressed as the number of cells per Sertoli cell in cross sections of seminiferous tubules. Other methods are more practical but are considered less precise.

Source: Data adapted from Skakkebaek and Heller.[662]

this procedure may be helpful in distinguishing obstructive azoospermia from idiopathic azoospermia with peritubular hyalinization. With obstruction of the excurrent duct system, normal spermatogenesis is found on biopsy; with idiopathic azoospermia, severe tubular sclerosis and peritubular hyalinization are observed. FSH determination also distinguishes these two groups of patients since those with obstruction exhibit normal FSH levels while those with hyalinization have high titers.[222,278] The clinician should be aware that testis biopsy causes a transient but reversible reduction in sperm count.[279]

Seminal fluid analysis provides information regarding the production of sperm by the testes and patency of the excurrent duct system. Standardized collection involves abstinence from ejaculation for 3 or more days, submission of the specimen by masturbation into a clean and dry wide-mouthed container, and completion of sperm counting and other analyses within 2 h of collection. The presence of fructose indicates patency of the excurrent duct system from the seminal vesicles distally into the urethra. Quantitative analysis of several sperm parameters provides information about the process of spermatogenesis. Computerized video analytic procedures are available for these analyses, but careful standardization is required.[280] The sperm count in multiple specimens from the same subject usually varies by an average of 75 percent but may vary more extremely.[281] For example, counts in samples from normal volunteers ranged from 5×10^6/ml to 200×10^6/ml in the same individuals over a 2- to 3-year period.[282] Some of the variability may be seasonal and related to the summer climate.[283] Independently assessed variables such as total sperm count, sperm concentration, percent motility, and percent normal forms covary in the same individual.[284] For example, specimens with decreased sperm counts commonly contain spermatozoa with decreased motility and decreased percent normal forms. Under some circumstances, however, specimens with counts as low as 5×10^6/ml can be normal with respect to motility and morphology and consequently may have high fertilization potential. For these reasons, only general ranges describing relative normality can be given (Table 16-5). It is recommended that a minimum of three samples collected over a 3-month period be obtained. The variability observed in single

TABLE 16-5 Normal Values for Semen Analysis

Parameter	Normal Value
Sperm concentration	$>20 \times 10^6$/ml
Total sperm in ejaculate	$>50 \times 10^6$
Semen volume	>1 ml
Percent motile	>60

Source: Based on data from four studies.[663-666]

samples can be minimized by averaging the results from these separate collections.

The functional capability of sperm to fertilize can be examined in vitro with the zona free hamster oocyte penetration test and the hypo-osmotic swelling test. These assays add independent information to that gained from an analysis of semen volumes, sperm count, percent sperm motility, and percent normal spermatozoa. However, a recent study[284] found that the overall prediction of fertility increased only from 70 to 78 percent when these two functional tests were added to the routine semen parameters. For this reason and because of difficulties in standardization, these functional tests have not been widely applied.

AGE-DEPENDENT PHYSIOLOGIC CHANGES IN TESTICULAR FUNCTION

Prepuberty

During the first 2 months of fetal life, hCG of placental origin stimulates testosterone secretion by the testes. Testosterone induces wolffian duct development directly; its metabolite, DHT, mediates male differentiation of the external genitalia. During the last third of gestation, pituitary LH supplants the effects of hCG in the stimulation of testosterone. Pituitary gonadotropin secretion is needed to achieve normal penis size and induce testicular descent.[285] Consequently, congenital LH deficiency is associated with microphallus, a high incidence of cryptorchidism, and subtle abnormalities in the morphologic appearance of Leydig cells.

During the first 2 months of life, LH and testosterone levels approach the levels which occur in adult life.[286] A Sertoli cell protein, müllerian inhibitory substance, increases at the same time period and then declines gradually during the prepubertal period.[287,288] After this brief interval, the hypothalamic-pituitary-testicular axis becomes quiescent during childhood and LH and testosterone levels remain low (<1 mIU/ml and <20 ng/100 ml, respectively). Testicular size is stable until age 6 and then gradually increases in proportion to somatic growth (Fig. 16-29). With ultrasensitive gonadotropin assays, LH pulses of low amplitude and frequency can be demonstrated in the prepubertal period.[289–291] One to 2 years before puberty, the frequency increases and nocturnal pulses increase.[289]

Puberty

The pubertal process begins on average at age 11 in boys (95 percent confidence limits, 9.0 to 13.0). The first physical evidence of puberty is testicular enlargement with an increase to >2.9 cm on the long axis or 6 ml in volume. Once the process begins, pubertal testosterone increments occur relatively rapidly over a 10- to 12-month period and reach levels 20-fold greater than those observed in the prepubertal period (Fig. 16-30).

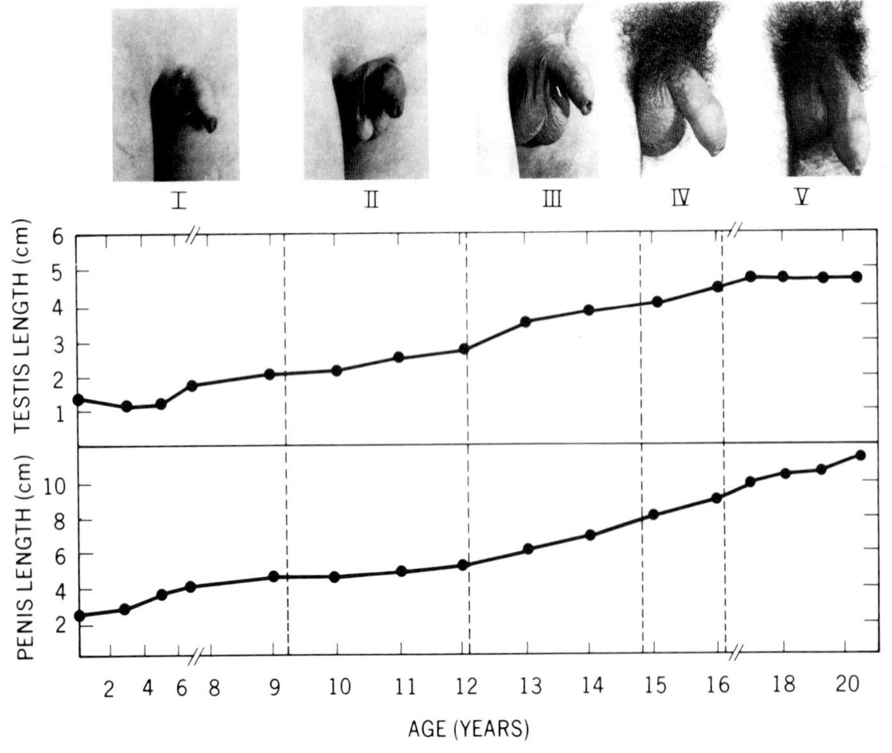

FIGURE 16-29 Genital changes during puberty. I to V represent the pubertal stages of Marshall and Tanner.[658] (*From Faiman and Winter.*[659])

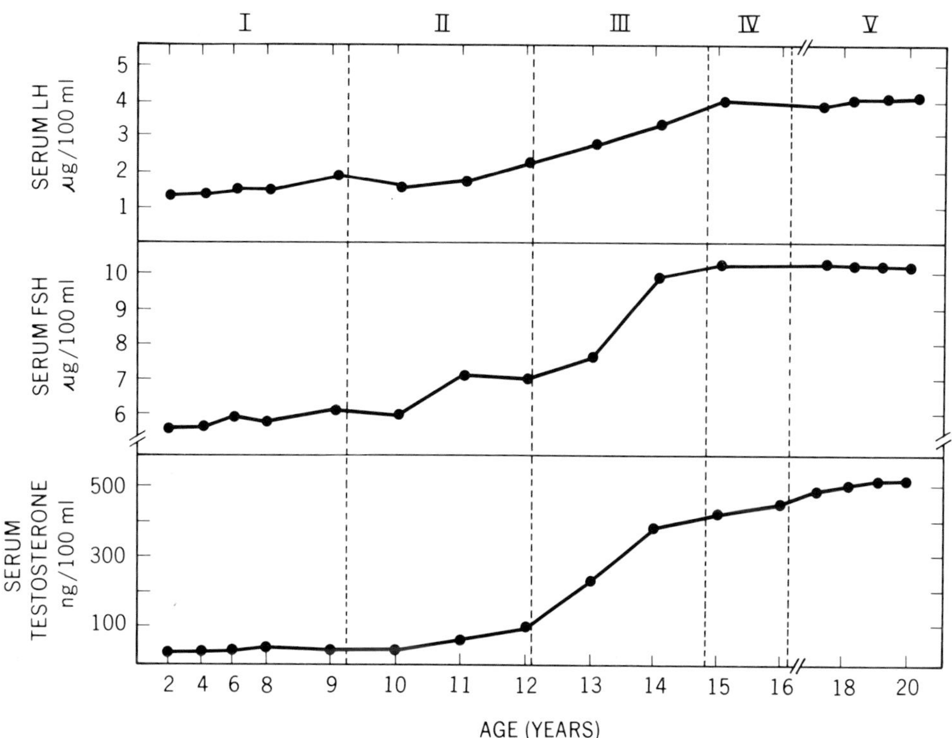

FIGURE 16-30 Hormonal changes during puberty.

During puberty, the major testosterone increase occurs during sleep, when simultaneous nocturnal LH and testosterone secretory pulses are observed (Fig. 16-31).[292] With progression into late puberty, the nocturnal LH increment ceases but the diurnal testosterone rhythm persists.

Two mechanisms have been proposed to mediate the initiation of puberty: (1) altered negative feedback sensitivity of the hypothalamus and pituitary (the gonadostat theory) and (2) an altered balance between the stimulatory and inhibitory neuronal pathways in the CNS which control gonadotropin secretion.[293] Until recently, the gonadostat theory was considered an adequate explanation for the onset of puberty. However, increments in LH and FSH concentrations are now known to occur in castrated animals and in patients with gonadal dysgenesis at the time of puberty, even though sex steroid levels are negligible and invariant.[293,294] These data suggest that CNS events are primary and that the pubertal process is mediated by the development of an organized pattern of neuronal activity that results in pulsatile GnRH and LH secretion. The limiting event in pubertal maturation is not a deficiency of GnRH, since GnRH and LH pulses can be initiated by the administration of *N*-methyl-D-L-aspartate acid, a tripeptide which binds to the glutamic acid receptor in the hypothalamus and stimulates GnRH.[37,38] An organized pattern of hypothalamic neuronal firing might require an alteration in the balance of stimulatory and inhibitory pathways entering the hypothalamus from higher centers. Brain lesion experiments designed to test this hypothesis are capable of inducing puberty, supporting the possibility that such CNS mechanisms are primary. Nonetheless, decreased negative feedback sensitivity to sex steroids also occurs during puberty and may contribute to the marked increases in gonadotropin levels observed during this process.[295–297]

CLINICAL DISORDERS

Introduction

Physicians require a logical framework to treat patients with complaints that can be traced to reproductive dysfunction. A useful classification scheme on which to initiate a rational evaluation is based on the functional status of gonadotropin secretion; it delineates hypogonadotropic, hypergonadotropic, and eugonadotropic syndromes. With this conceptual framework, Leydig cell and germinal cell dysfunction, considered separately, can be placed in one of these three categories.

Hypogonadotropic Syndromes

Hypogonadotropic syndromes are classified in Table 16-6 and depicted in Fig. 16-32.

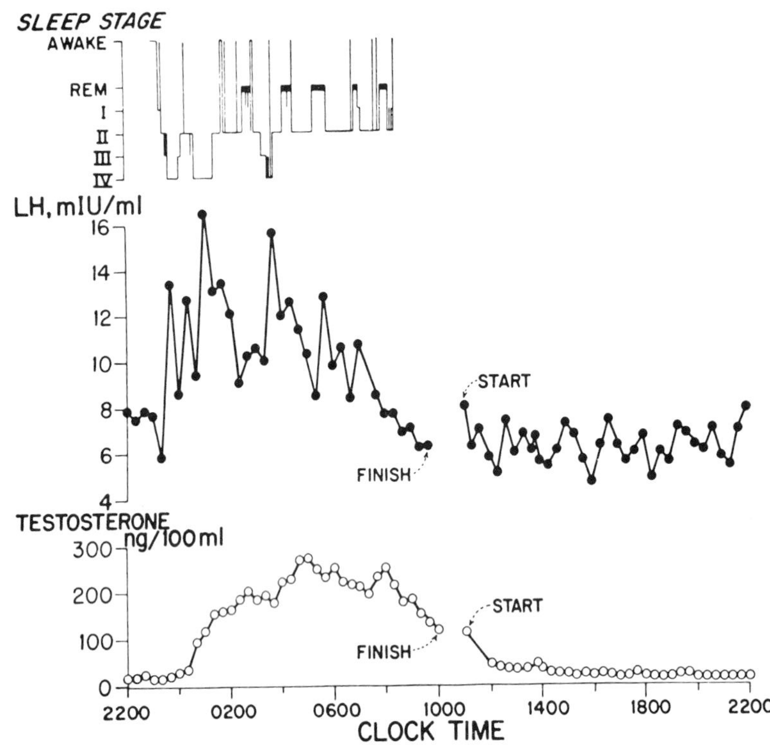

FIGURE 16-31 Levels of LH and testosterone concentration during sleep in a pubertal boy. (*From Boyar et al.*[292])

Organic Causes

Multiple Trophic Hormone Deficiency

Prepubertal patients with multiple trophic hormone deficiencies (hypopituitarism) commonly present with severe growth retardation, whereas older boys present with delayed adolescence. Adults come to medical attention because of impotence, headaches, or visual disturbance. Lethargy or symptoms of hypoglycemia may be present, suggesting deficient secretion of TSH or ACTH and growth hormone. The patient may complain of progressive headache, visual disturbances, or symptoms of diabetes insipidus caused by a pituitary tumor. Idiopathic hypopituitarism is the most common cause of multiple pituitary hormone deficiencies in early childhood and early adolescence. Pituitary tumors are common in adult patients. Specific etiologies include craniopharyngioma and other suprasellar lesions, such as pinealoma, dysgerminoma, and glial tumors. Autoimmune or necrotizing hypophysitis frequently causes deficiencies of multiple pituitary hormones.[298] A number of miscellaneous disorders which are recognizable by their extrapituitary manifestations may also cause hypogonadotropism (Table 16-6). These include histiocytosis X, tuberculosis, sarcoidosis, and certain collagen vascular diseases with CNS vasculitis. Pituitary irradiation for nasopharyngeal carcinoma or other disorders may also result in gonadotropin deficiency many years later.[299,300]

LH, FSH, and testosterone concentrations are low in patients with these etiologies; release of these hormones in response to clomiphene is blunted or absent. GnRH produces a variable release of LH and FSH, depending on the degree of pituitary gonadotropin reserve and preexposure to endogenous GnRH from the hypothalamus. Elevated lipid levels and decreased bone density are observed as a reflection of long-standing androgen deficiency.[266–268,301]

Hyperprolactinemia

Elevations of serum prolactin may result in hypogonadism through a variety of direct and indirect mechanisms. Prolactin acts directly on the hypothalamus to alter aminergic function and thus inhibit GnRH release.[302] This results in a reduction in gonadotropin and testosterone secretion. Prolactin also reduces the concentration of 5α-reductase in androgen-dependent tissues.[248] A disproportionate reduction in DHT as opposed to testosterone levels may then occur.[247,249] A direct antagonistic effect of prolactin on the testes has been suggested[303] but is probably not functionally important, since testosterone responses to hCG are normal in hyperprolactinemia that results from a variety of drug-induced or organic causes.[246,247] Hyperprolactinemia may also be associated with hypogonadism through indirect mechanisms. Prolactin-producing tumors can reach sufficient size to displace or destroy functional gonadotrophs in the pituitary. Under these circumstances, LH, FSH, and testosterone levels are re-

TABLE 16-6 Classification of Hypogonadotropic Hypogonadism

Organic causes
- Multiple trophic hormone deficiencies (hypopituitarism)
  - Idiopathic
  - Secondary to tumor of pituitary or adjacent structures
- Miscellaneous causes
  - Histiocytosis X
  - Tuberculosis
  - Sarcoidosis
  - Collagen vascular diseases
  - Hypophysitis
  - Sequela of pituitary irradiation
- Secondary to hyperprolactinemia
- Isolated gonadotropin deficiency
  - Hypogonadotropic eunuchoidism (Kallmann's syndrome)
    - Complete
    - Partial (predominant LH deficiency, "fertile eunuch syndrome")
    - Variant form (isolated FSH deficiency)
  - Specific genetic syndromes
    - Prader-Labhart-Willi
    - Laurence-Moon
    - Bardet-Biedl
    - Möbius
    - Other rarer disorders
- Acute and chronic illness
  - Chronic illnesses
  - Emotional disorders
  - AIDS
  - Obesity
  - Drugs
  - Liver disease (one subgroup)
  - Renal disease (one component)
  - Hemochromatosis
  - Spinal cord damage
- Glucocorticoids

Functional causes
- Physiologic delayed puberty

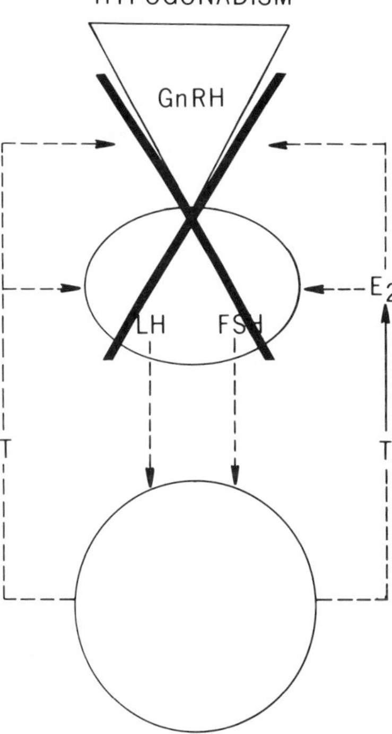

FIGURE 16-32 Diagrammatic representation of hypogonadotropic hypogonadism. Triangle = hypothalamus; oval = pituitary; circle = testis; T = testosterone; E_2 = estradiol.

duced as a result of an insufficient number of gonadotropin-producing cells. Alternatively, a prolactinoma extending superiorly may compress the pituitary venous system and functionally disconnect the hypothalamus from the pituitary. Under these circumstances, the gonadotrophs are exposed to insufficient amounts of GnRH to maintain adequate secretion.

Elevations of prolactin in patients result from secretory tumors of the pituitary (prolactinomas) and from functional causes. With small prolactinomas, the major clinical manifestations are delayed puberty[304] in children and hypogonadism in adults.[250] Impotence resulting from androgen deficiency or possibly from the direct effects of elevated prolactin on erectile function is nearly always present in adult men. With large prolactinomas, symptoms related to growing tumor mass such as headache, visual field abnormalities, and functional hypopituitarism predominate. Notably, most men with prolactinomas are found to have large lesions on presentation.[250] While this finding could reflect rapid tumor growth rates, it more likely indicates delayed clinical ascertainment. Patients with this problem present late to the physician. With careful history taking, they frequently relate a long history of impotence but a reluctance to seek medical evaluation for this complaint.

The functional causes of hyperprolactinemia are either idiopathic or drug-induced secondary to centrally acting pharmacologic agents. Drugs such as the phenothiazines commonly lower LH and testosterone levels in association with prolactin increments.[305] Antihypertensive medications with alpha-adrenergic or beta-adrenergic or dopamine-blocking properties also produce this syndrome. The reduction of androgen secretion in association with functional hyperprolactinemia results predominantly from inhibition of GnRH and gonadotropin secretion. Pulsatile administration of GnRH in men with prolactin excess restores normal secretion of both LH and testosterone.[306]

Among men presenting with impotence, 5 percent are found to have elevated prolactin levels. Nearly half of these elevations are idiopathic, whereas prolactinoma (10 percent), drugs (30 percent), and chronic renal failure (6 percent) account for the remainder.[307] A small group of men with oligospermia and unexplained hyperprolactinemia have also been reported.[308] A direct effect of prolactin on spermatogenesis in these patients, while possible, is unsupported by convincing evidence.

Evaluation of hypogonadism in men with hyperprolactinemia is directed toward identification of the cause or causes of prolactin excess. An MRI scan with gadolinium contrast provides a sensitive tool for identifying pituitary lesions. When a tumor is present, functional assessment (i.e., GnRH or clomiphene testing) to determine the mechanism causing gonadotropin deficiency is possible but not usually relevant clinically.

Treatment when a tumor is present consists of bromocriptine or pergolide[309] therapy alone or in combination with surgery. Testosterone levels rise slowly over a period of 1 year upon the administration of bromocriptine[309] and usually return toward but not into the normal range. Exogenous testosterone administration may be necessary, but caution is advised since tumor stimulation secondary to increased aromatization of testosterone to estradiol has occasionally been observed.[310] Correction of androgen deficiency alone is usually insufficient to relieve the symptoms of impotence; reduction of prolactin concentration is also necessary. This observation, which suggests that prolactin plays a direct role in the erectile process, remains to be explained in rigorous physiologic studies.

Hyperprolactinemia of a functional nature is usually diagnosed by identifying the drugs causing this condition. Treatment consists of withholding the offending agent or substituting other drugs, if possible.

Isolated Gonadotropin Deficiency

Gonadotropin deficiency without the loss of other anterior pituitary hormones results from a number of different genetic disorders. Patients with these conditions present with sexual infantilism or incomplete sexual development.[311] The specific diagnosis may be made easily if a family history is elicited or if characteristic physical findings are demonstrated. The specific disorders and their associated anomalies are discussed below.

Kallmann's Syndrome *Hypogonadotropic eunuchoidism,* or *Kallmann's syndrome,* is the most common cause of isolated gonadotropin deficiency; it is inherited either as an autosomal dominant syndrome with relative sex limitation to males[312,313] or by X-linked autosomal recessive inheritance in other kindreds.[314] While karyotypic abnormalities are described, including Xp deletions, the majority of patients have normal 46XY patterns.[315–317] This disorder results from a reduction in the secretion of GnRH by the hypothalamus. A recent study demonstrated that GnRH neurons originate in olfactory tissue in early fetal life and then migrate into the hypothalamus (Fig. 16-33).[318] The olfactory bulb and tracts are absent in many patients with Kallmann's syndrome, as seen at autopsy or on MRI scans (Fig. 16-34).[319] Consequently, the deficiency in GnRH may reflect an embryologic absence of the anlage for GnRH neurons.[318]

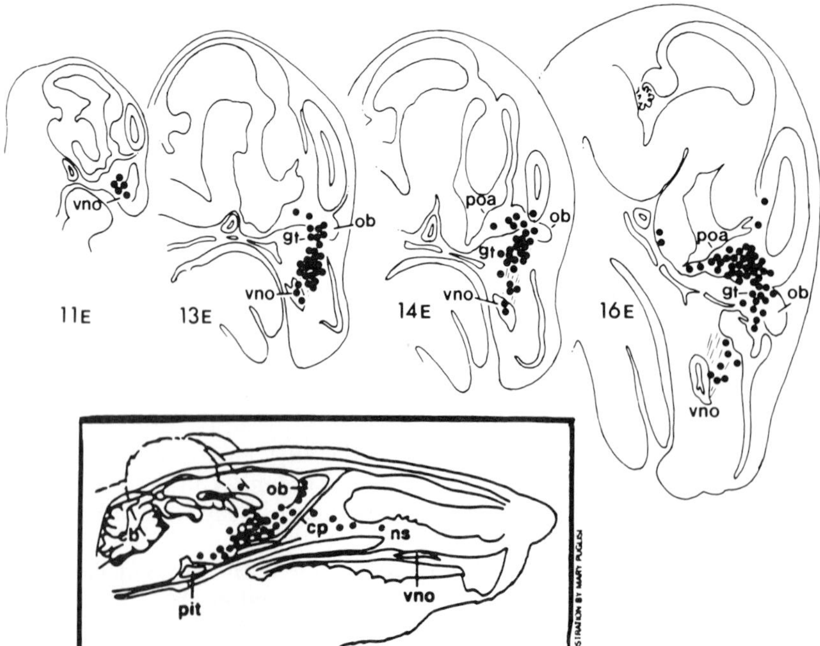

FIGURE 16-33 Migration of gonadotropin releasing hormone (GnRH) cells from the olfactory pit to the brain begins at about 11.5 days after conception in the mouse. (*11E*) Most cells are still close to the vomeronasal organ (vno) at embryonic day 11 to 11.5. (*13E*) By 13 days, the number of GnRH neurons has increased and the first cells are crossing into the brain near the olfactory bulb (ob). (*14E*) By 14 days, GnRH neurons have begun to arch back through the forebrain to the preoptic area (poa). Migration is largely complete 15 to 16.5 days after conception (*16E*). CTX = cerebral cortex; TG = ganglion terminale. (*Adapted from Schwanzel-Fukada and Pfaff.*[660])

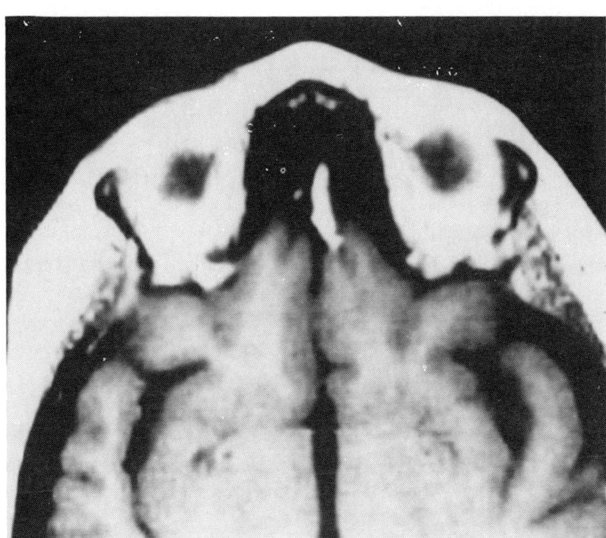

FIGURE 16-34 Five-mm T_1-weighted axial image by MRI demonstrating hypoplastic olfactory gyri. (*Reprinted from Brackett et al.*[359])

Abnormalities observed in Kallmann's syndrome (Fig. 16-35) include hyposmia or anosmia, cryptorchidism, cleft lip or cleft palate, and congenital deafness in addition to hypogonadism.[312,314] A recent study also detected mirror movements, eye movement abnormalities, cerebellar dysfunction, pes cavus deformity of feet, and café-au-lait macules in a substantial fraction of patients with Kallmann's syndrome.[320] No pathophysiologic distinction can be made between subjects with a familial pattern of gonadotrophin deficiency and sporadic or nonfamilial forms.[321] It is probably best to consider the familial and sporadic types of isolated gonadotrophin deficiency as a group, even though several discrete disorders may be represented.

The degree of gonadotropin deficiency in patients with Kallmann's syndrome may vary. In the complete form, both FSH and LH levels are low and no evidence of sexual maturation is apparent. With partial deficits, incomplete sexual development results. With partial GnRH deficiency, FSH secretion predominates and germinal cell maturation of the testis proceeds even to late spermatid or spermatozoa formation. These patients have been referred to as "fertile eunuchs," since spermatozoa may be present on testicular biopsy or in the ejaculate,[262] but few of these patients are actually fertile. On clinical examination, the presence of gynecomastia is more frequent in these subjects than in those with complete gonadotropin deficiency. The fertile eunuch syndrome is considered a variant of hypogonadotropic eunuchoidism, since anosmia and other anomalies of the genetic disorder may be present. Another variant, isolated FSH deficiency, has been described.[322] However, even in a well-documented recent case, the exact nature of the defect was unclear.

A large degree of heterogeneity of gonadotropin deficiency exists in patients with Kallmann's syndrome. For this reason, plasma LH and FSH levels in these patients may overlap the normal range, particularly if less sensitive RIAs are used to measure them. The degree of heterogeneity is best demonstrated with highly sensitive assays, such as two-site radiometric plasma assays and assays of urinary concentrates.[60,64] In a group of 16 subjects with this disorder (Fig. 16-36), basal urinary FSH excretion ranged from 10 to 500 mIU/h (a 50-fold variation), whereas LH excretion varied from 10 to 700 mIU/h. Plasma testosterone concentration was as low as 5 ng/100 ml and as high as 60 ng/100 ml.[323]

Heterogeneity in the amplitude and frequency of spontaneous LH pulses has also been observed.[324] Spratt et al. demonstrated a spectrum of patterns of pulsatile LH secretion, ranging from absent LH pulses or only minimal pulses to pulses of normal amplitude but diminished frequency (Fig. 16-37).[324,325] Subjects with infrequent pulses could be returned to normal testicular function by the administration of GnRH episodically at a frequency comparable to that in normal individuals. Surprisingly, a few of these patients (approximately 5 percent) maintained normal function even after the cessation of GnRH therapy, perhaps as a result of pituitary priming or further hypothalamic maturation.[326]

The severity of the gonadotropin secretory defect may have practical significance in regard to therapy. Subjects with relative preservation of FSH may respond with normal spermatogenesis to treatment with hCG alone.[327] Presumably, a sufficient amount of FSH is present to initiate and complete normal spermatogenesis after intratesticular testosterone levels are normalized by the effects of exogenous LH or hCG. Rowe et al. reported that two subjects with incomplete gonadotropin deficiency developed normal spermatogenesis with testosterone treatment alone,[328] but this phenomenon is probably uncommon.

The major problem in diagnosing isolated gonadotropin deficiency is differentiating patients with an organic defect from those with physiologic delayed puberty. Demonstration of the nongonadal clinical abnormalities associated with hypogonadotropic eunuchoidism (e.g., anosmia, cleft lip) provides the best means of confirming the diagnosis of Kallmann's syndrome.[312,314] Approximately 80 percent of boys with hypogonadotropic hypogonadism exhibit either anosmia or hyposmia; therefore, this clinical finding is useful.[312] Precise determination of the olfactory threshold may be accomplished using a scratch, sniff, and smell test developed by Doty et al.[329] If no associated congenital abnormalities are present, serial measurements of LH and FSH concentrations over a period of several months strongly

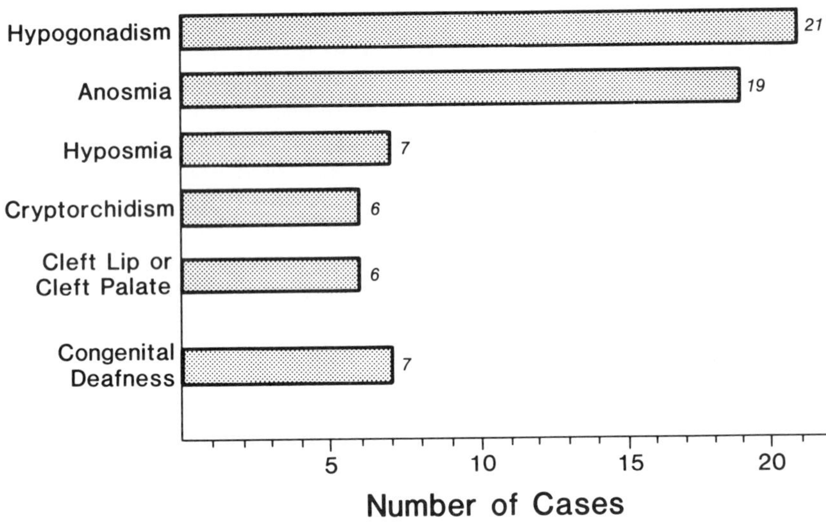

FIGURE 16-35 Frequency of anomalies in patients with Kallmann's syndrome. (*From Santen and Paulsen.*[312])

suggest physiologic delayed puberty if progressive increments in the levels of these hormones are observed (Fig. 16-38). However, it may be necessary to wait until the patient is older than 18 to 20 years of age, when most boys with a physiologic delay will have undergone pubertal changes, to be certain about permanent hypogonadotropism. It should be kept in mind, however, that some patients undergo spontaneous puberty even after age 20.[330]

It was originally thought that the gonadotropin response to GnRH might allow earlier differentiation between subjects with physiologic delay of puberty and those with isolated gonadotropin deficiency. However, variable increments in LH and FSH concentrations have been observed after single injections of GnRH and after 4-h infusions[331–333] in patients with hypogonadotropic eunuchoidism, particularly in those with the incomplete forms (Fig. 16-39). Patients with physiologic delayed puberty, by contrast, may exhibit diminished responses to GnRH before the onset of testicular enlargement. When sexual maturation has progressed, as reflected by testicular enlargement, the LH concentration increments after GnRH stimulation may become normal. These considerations limit the clinical utility of GnRH infusions or prolonged administration as a diagnostic test to distinguish organic from physiologic delay of puberty.

Stimulation of the hypothalamic-pituitary axis with clomiphene has also been suggested as a means of differentiating organic from physiologic disorders of sexual maturation. However, both boys with delayed puberty and those with hypogonadotropic eunuchoidism respond to clomiphene similarly, with a paradoxic suppression of LH and FSH concentrations.[262,334] The fall in gonadotropin levels reflects their sensitivity to the minimally estrogenic properties of clomiphene. Other proposed tests involve stimulation of prolactin release with thyrotropin releasing hormone (TRH), metoclopramide, or chlorpromazine.[335] However, recent data from these tests suggest marked variability among patients and an overlap in the response observed between boys with physiologically delayed puberty[321,335,336] and those with organic forms of gonadotropin deficiency. Heterogeneity in the degree of gonadotropin deficiency is the major problem in the diagnosis of hypogonadotropic hypogonadism. The sensitivity of plasma and urinary gonadotropin assays is another problem. With the use of highly sensitive immunoassays, most patients with hypogonadotropic hypogonadism have lower basal and post-GnRH gonadotropin levels than do patients with constitutional delay.[337] The use of a long-acting GnRH agonist in conjunction with sensitive RIAs also provides a more discriminative provocative stimulation test.[337] Nonetheless, none of these methods is likely to provide complete discrimination because of the overlap in the amount of gonadotropin secretion between patients with constitutional delay and those with hypogonadotropic hypogonadism.

Clinical observations suggest that certain patients with hypogonadotropic eunuchoidism may have Leydig cells that are relatively unresponsive to hCG[338] or to GnRH-induced LH increments.[339] This concept has been controversial, since the majority of patients in other series achieved normal testosterone levels when sufficient amounts of hCG were given for 6 to 8 weeks.[340] The associated Leydig cell defect may be limited to patients with bilateral cryptorchidism[341] or to subjects with more severe intrauterine GnRH deficiency.[339]

Evaluation of patients with isolated gonadotropin deficiency requires a careful family history to identify other affected family members, many of whom may have hyposmia or anosmia without reproductive dysfunction.[323] Quantitative estimation of olfactory threshold or an MRI scan (Fig. 16-34) can

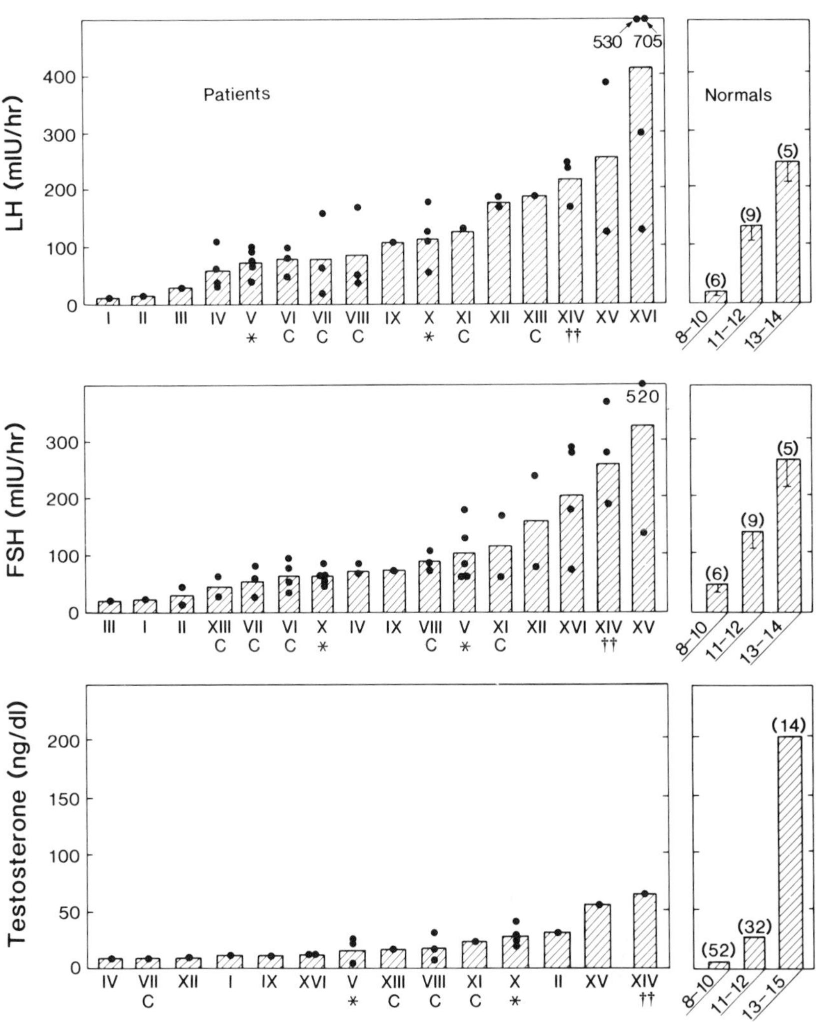

FIGURE 16-36 *(Top)* Levels of urinary LH were ranked according to increased concentration in subjects 1 to 16 with hypogonadotropic hypogonadism. Circles represent separate determinations; height of bar indicates mean level. For comparison *(middle, bottom)*, levels of urinary FSH and plasma testosterone are shown. * = testis size, 2.0 to 2.5 cm on the long axis, all others less than 2.0 cm; C = unilateral cryptorchism. Normal ranges and number of individuals in normal range (in parentheses) shown on right panels for comparison. *(From Santen and Kulin.*[323]*)*

identify 80 percent of subjects with this disorder. Measurements of LH, FSH, and testosterone concentrations define the degree of deficit. Additional evaluation includes the demonstration of normal GH and thyroid function and the exclusion of hyperprolactinemia and sellar or parasellar mass lesions. An assay of the DHEA sulfate level as an indicator of adrenarche is useful in patients with Kallmann's syndrome. It should be recalled that gonadarche and adrenarche reflect two separate physiologic processes which can be dissociated clinically. Adrenarche, as reflected by DHEA sulfate levels, is normal for age in Kallmann's syndrome. Delayed adrenarche with low DHEA sulfate levels is found with physiologic delayed puberty or organic lesions of the pituitary.[342]

Specific Genetic Syndromes with Predominant Hypogonadotropism *Prader-Labhart-Willi Syndrome* This syndrome[343,344] is an inherited disorder that causes hypogonadism (Table 16-7). Boys with this disorder may have hypotonia (especially in infancy), obesity, mental retardation, short stature, and adult-onset diabetes mellitus. The mnemonic HHHO syndrome (hypomentia, hypotonia, hypogonadism, obesity) has been applied in these cases. Other distinguishing features that are often present include acromicria, micrognathia, strabismus, fishlike or Cupid's-bow mouth, clinodactylism, and an absence of auricular cartilage. The degree of hypogonadotropism in this disorder is variable, ranging from partial to severe. Paradoxically, some patients with hypergonadotropic hypogonadism or diminished responsiveness to hCG have been recognized.[344] The diagnosis is made by identifying the clinical stigmata of this syndrome and documenting the presence of reduced LH and FSH levels in blood or urine. A karyotypic analysis of peripheral blood lymphocytes may also be helpful. A defect in chromosome 15 has been described in approximately half the cases.[345,346] It should be noted that a few older subjects with this disorder have responded to clomiphene citrate with reversal of hy-

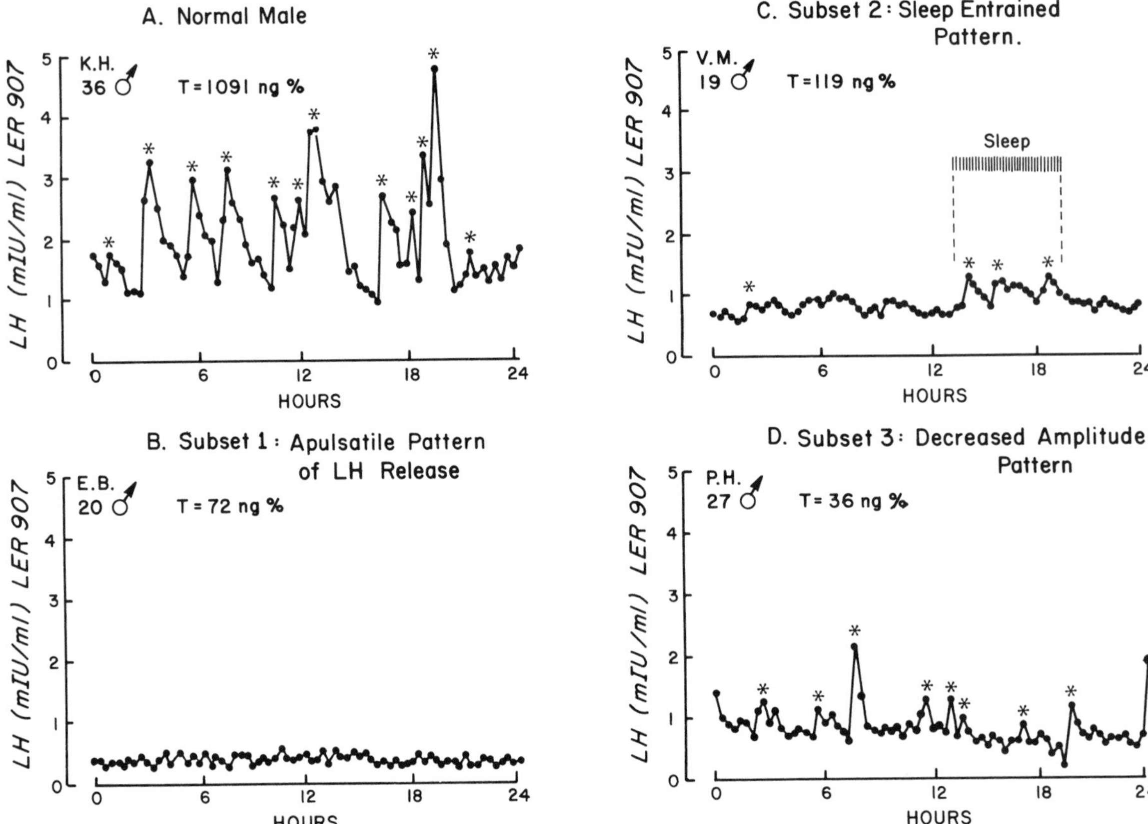

FIGURE 16-37 Patterns of endogenous LH secretion in idiopathic hypogonadotropic hypogonadal men. *(A)*: LH values determined every 20 min for 24 h in a normal male displaying discrete LH pulsations occurring about every 2 h and resulting in a normal plasma testosterone concentration. *(B)* LH determinations in a male with idiopathic hypogonadotropic hypogonadism displaying no detectable LH pulsations and a prepubertal testosterone level. *(C)* Sleep LH entrained pulsations have decreased amplitude associated with prepubertal testosterone levels in an 18-year-old idiopathic hypogonadotropic hypogonadal male. *(D)* LH pulsations of decreased amplitude occurring throughout sleep and wake periods in a 27-year-old idiopathic hypogonadotropic hypogonadal male. *(From Spratt DI, Hoffman AR, Crowley WF Jr: Hypogonadotropic hypogonadism and its treatment, in Santen and Swerdloff.*[661]*)*

pogonadotropism and the onset of spontaneous puberty.[347] The pathogenic mechanism for this response has not been fully explained.

Laurence-Moon and Bardet-Biedl Syndromes Hypogonadism in association with retinitis pigmentosa, obesity, mental retardation, and polydactyly has commonly been termed the Laurence-Moon-Biedl syndrome.[348] Recent reviews distinguish two distinct entities: the Laurence-Moon and Bardet-Biedl syndromes (Table 16-7).[349,350] Distinguishing features include the presence of spastic paraplegia and rarity of polydactyly in the Laurence-Moon syndrome and the presence of polydactyly or other dysmorphic extremity features and renal disease in the Bardet-Biedl syndrome.

Most studies of endocrine function have not distinguished these two syndromes and describe abnormalities in groups of patients that include both entities. Early reports suggested that hypogonadism occurs in 80 percent of boys with Laurence-Moon-Biedl syndrome. However, more than half of these patients were <15 years of age at diagnosis; examination of older boys revealed only a 50 percent prevalence of hypogonadism.[351] This finding suggests that delayed adolescence is a common feature of this syndrome. In prepubertal boys, microphallus, hypospadias, and undescended testes are common. The major manifestations of this syndrome are apparent early in life. Retinal degeneration occurs between 4 and 10 years of age, and obesity begins somewhat earlier.[351] Many reports attribute the hypogonadism to a hypothalamic-pituitary disorder.[348,352,353] Other studies have identified patients with hypergonadotropic hypogonadism.[354,355] A recent family study of eight males with the Bardet-Biedl syndrome identified seven with small testes and genitalia and two with low serum testosterone.[349] These two subjects

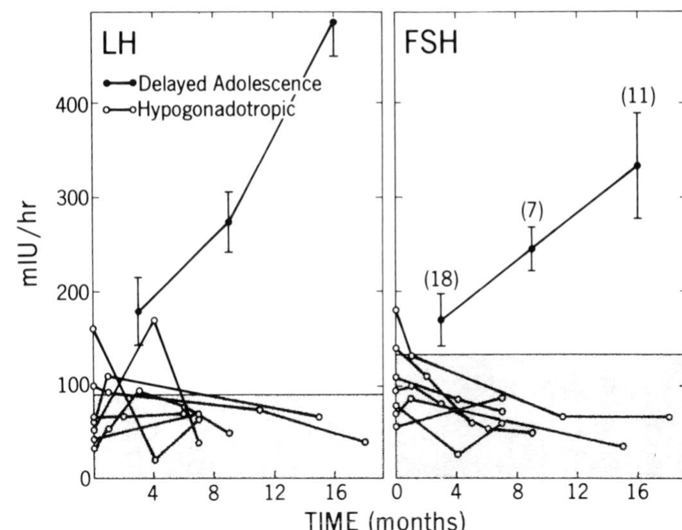

FIGURE 16-38 Sequential gonadotropin changes in 10 boys with constitutionally delayed adolescence and in 7 patients with hypogonadotropic hypogonadism followed over a period of 6 to 28 months. Shaded areas indicate normal prepubertal male ranges. (*From Kulin and Santen.*[578])

had low to normal LH levels and an exaggerated response to GnRH. Although interpreted differently,[349] these findings suggest an incomplete form of hypogonadotropic hypogonadism. Thus, both hypo- and hypergonadotropic forms of these syndromes probably exist.

Other Syndromes Hypogonadotropic hypogonadism may also be associated with the multiple lentigines syndrome,[356] congenital ichthyosis,[357] Rud's syndrome,[357] cerebellar ataxia,[358] and Möbius' syndrome.[359] The diagnosis of these disorders is made by recognizing the characteristic congenital anomalies (Table 16-7). A wide variety of other inherited disorders are also associated with hypo- or hypergonadotropic hypogonadism. The list is encyclopedic, and the associated features cannot be systematically recalled by most clinicians. The approach suggested is to consult the compendium of genetic disorders written by Rimoin and Schimke[360] when unusual congenital malformations are noted in a patient with hypogonadism.

A unifying feature in most of these congenital syndromes as well as in Kallmann's syndrome may be a disruption of neural afferent input into the hypothalamus (Fig. 16-40). The input necessary to maintain normal release of GnRH may be deficient and, as a consequence, hypogonadotropism will result. Although hypothetical, this possibility would explain the coexistence of multiple defects in CNS function found in these various syndromes and the presence of gonadotropin deficiency.

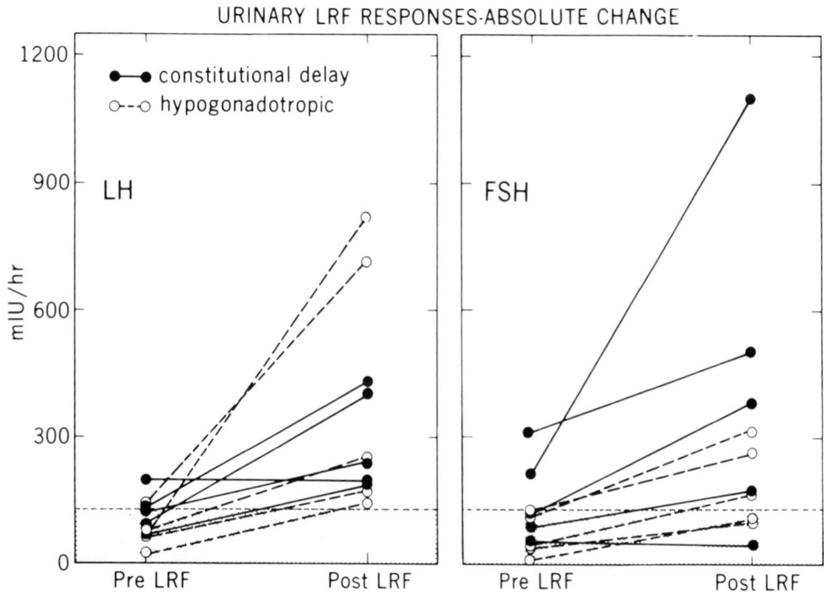

FIGURE 16-39 Response to GnRH in five males with constitutionally delayed adolescence and five with hypogonadotropic hypogonadism. LH and FSH concentrations were determined in urine specimens collected over a 3-h period before and after the subcutaneous administration of 100 μg GnRH. Shaded areas represent normal prepubertal male levels. (*From Kulin and Santen.*[578])

TABLE 16-7 Clinical Features of Common Genetic Hypogonadotropic Hypogonadal Syndromes

Prader-Labhart-Willi	Lawrence-Moon	Bardet-Biedl	Rud's	Hypogonatropism/ Ataxia	Möbius'	Multiple Lentigenes
Hypomentia	Hypogonadism*	Hypogonadism*	Mental retardation	Cerebellar ataxia	Multiple cranial nerve abnormalities	Multiple lentigenes
Hypotonia	Mental retardation Ataxia Nystagmus	Dysmorphic extremities, (polydactyly, syndactyly, or bradydactyly)	Epilepsy	Pes cavus	Anosmia	Cardiac defects, hypertelorism Short stature Deafness
Short stature	Pigmentary retinopathy	Retinal dystrophy	Congenital ichthyosis	Spina bifida	Mental retardation	Delayed or no puberty
Cupid's-bow mouth	Spastic paraplegia	Renal disease Obesity				Genital and urologic defects
Diabetes mellitus Hypogonadism* Obesity	Obesity Short stature Nystagmus					

* Hypergonadotropic types also have been described.

Chronic Illnesses

Systemic illness of sufficient severity may cause hypogonadism in an adult.[361] Malnutrition is a factor in some instances.[362] Studies in male primates suggest that there is a defect in GnRH release at the level of the hypothalamic pulse generator during restricted food intake.[363] Intestinal disease which produces weight loss or frank malabsorption may be associated with hypogonadotropic hypogonadism. Adolescents are particularly sensitive to the gonadotropin-suppressing effects of systemic illness and weight loss. Recurrent infections, repeated hospitalizations, severe burns,[364] and neoplastic disease may also cause poor growth and delayed pubertal progression.[365] Major head injuries, septic shock, and sleep apnea syndrome are also associated with hypogonadotropic hypogonadism.[366–369]

Another group of patients present with impotence and have low testosterone but normal LH levels. These men frequently take multiple medications and have a variety of underlying medical conditions. Normal responses to clomiphene suggest that the problem is functional and may be related to chronic illness.[370]

Emotional Disorders Adult men with anorexia nervosa present with gonadotropin deficiency and hypogonadism in association with weight loss. In adolescents, psychiatric illness or emotional stress may cause an inhibition of gonadotropin secretion or delay the pubertal process. In children, severe psychiatric illness as a cause of delayed puberty is usually not difficult to diagnose. Milder forms of psychological problems, however, may be confirmed only by excluding the presence of organic disease. One variant of this condition appears to be a fear of becoming obese.[371]

A unifying pathophysiologic mechanism for hypogonadotropic hypogonadism in these disorders may relate to the effects of stress. Corticotropin releasing hormone (CRH) levels[372] increase in response to stress. CRH in turn stimulates β-endorphin levels, which then directly inhibit the release of GnRH. The administration of opiate antagonists to experimentally stressed primates reverses the inhibition of stress-induced gonadotropin secretion.[373] These observations suggest that various systemic illnesses induce stress, which in turn produces increased CRH levels, increased endogenous opiate secretion, and decreased GnRH release.[374] Hypogonadotropic hypogonadism then occurs as a result.

AIDS Low testosterone levels occur in men with AIDS and the AIDS-related complex. In one study, measurement of LH levels indicated hypogonadotropism as the cause of androgen deficiency in 75 percent of these men.[375] Adequate responses to GnRH suggested a lack of involvement of the pituitary, which can be secondarily involved by infectious processes in patients with AIDS.[376] The mechanism for low androgen levels is controversial, however, since other investigators detected primarily hypergonadotropic hypogonadism.[377]

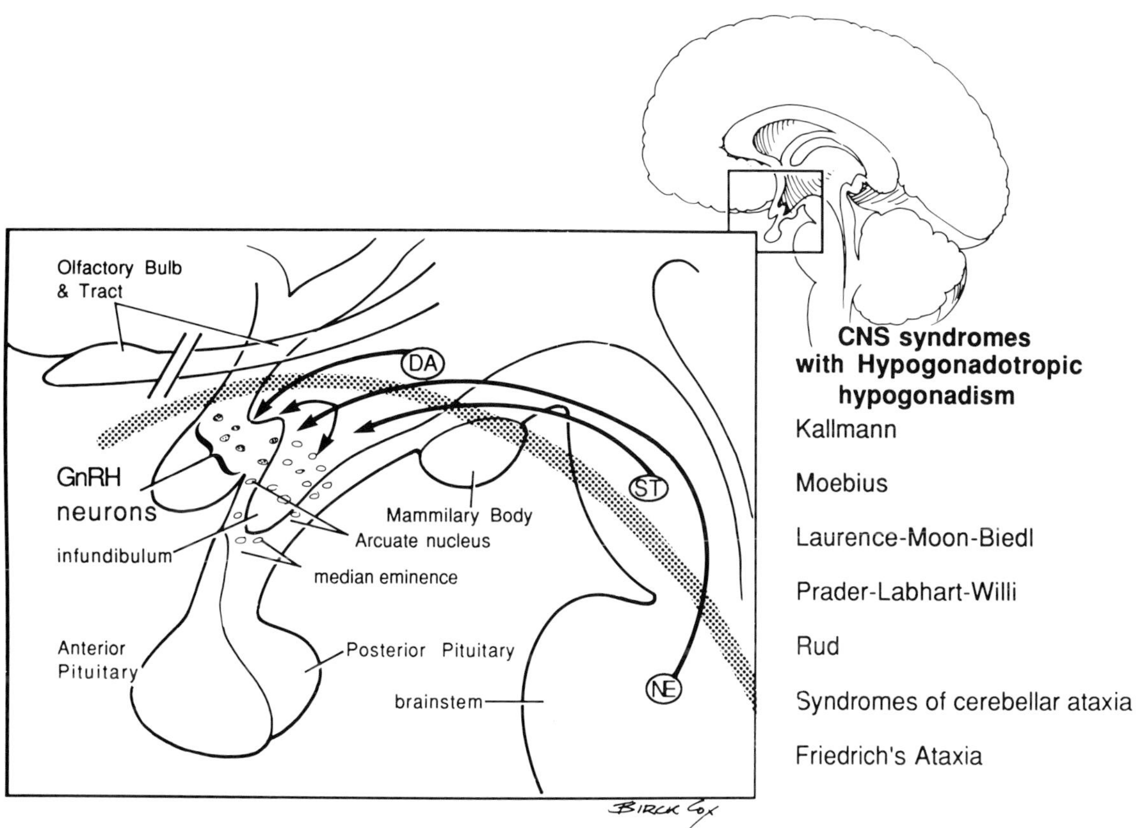

FIGURE 16-40 The disruption of neural afferent input into the hypothalamus in patients with a variety of central nervous system (CNS) syndromes associated with hypogonadotropic hypogonadism. The hypothesis illustrated could explain the association of multiple CNS abnormalities with hypogonadotropic hypogonadism. Congenital defects disrupt the neural pathways into the hypothalamus; in the case of Kallmann's syndrome, the neurons migrating into the hypothalamus are absent (see text). GnRH = gonadotropin releasing hormone; DA = dopamine; NE = norepinephrine; ST = serotonin. (*From Brackett et al.*[359])

Obesity Massive obesity is associated with low testosterone levels and low to low normal LH levels. Reductions in sex hormone–binding globulin (SHBG) (Fig. 16-17) levels are partially responsible for the lowering of total testosterone, but free or weakly bound testosterone levels are low as well. Increased aromatization of testosterone to estradiol is present, but the testosterone levels can be returned to normal with weight loss of insufficient degree to lower estradiol levels. Consequently, aromatization of testosterone to estradiol is not the only factor involved in diminished gonadotropin secretion.[378]

Drugs Narcotic analgesics reduce the secretion of LH and testosterone, resulting in hypogonadotropic hypogonadism of the reversible type. Men who abuse narcotics often develop symptoms of impotence.[379]

Liver Disease Hypogonadism, gynecomastia, and testicular atrophy are commonly observed in men with hepatic cirrhosis.[380] The reduction in testosterone correlates with the severity of liver disease.[381] One of several different mechanisms may be responsible for these findings. Men with both hypo- and hypergonadotropic subtypes of hypogonadism are encountered. In the hypogonadotropic subgroup, LH and FSH levels may be suppressed because of associated malnutrition or enhanced aromatization of testosterone to estradiol and increased estrogen negative feedback.[380] The hypergonadotropic group has a form of primary gonadal disease characterized by high LH levels and a diminished testosterone response to exogenous hCG. The direct inhibiting effects of alcohol on testicular steroidogenesis[382] may partially explain this abnormality. Additional effects of alcohol on the liver which increase the MCR of testosterone may also lower circulating androgen concentrations.

Renal Disease Chronic renal failure is associated with hypogonadism and hyperprolactinemia.[383] Impotence, related partially to the low androgen levels and partially to associated neuropathy and vascular disease, is a common complaint. The pathophysiology of the hypogonadism is complex. A reduced metabolic clearance rate of LH leads to an increased plasma LH concentration in patients with a marked reduction in renal function. A component of primary testicular failure leads to an increase in the LH production rate in approximately 20 percent of men. However, the major defect involves hypothalamic dysfunction, which results in relative hypogonadotropism. Administration of the antiestrogen clomiphene citrate stimulates the return of gonadotropin and testosterone secretion to normal in these patients, suggesting that an abnormality of the negative feedback set point exists.[383]

Hemochromatosis Hemochromatosis of both primary and secondary (i.e., β-thalassemia with transfusion-induced iron overload) origin involves the pituitary, and iron can be demonstrated there by MRI scan.[384] Gonadotropin deficiency and hypogonadism are commonly present. Impotence usually precedes the diagnosis of hemochromatosis. The symptoms are exacerbated in the presence of diabetes, but cirrhosis does not contribute to the symptoms.[385,386] Although primary testicular involvement may also be present, the pituitary defect appears to predominate. Marked iron deposition in the pituitary leads to functional impairment of the gonadotrophs. Some but not all of these patients experience improved gonadal function after prolonged therapy with phlebotomy.[387,388]

Spinal Cord Damage Injury to the spinal cord induces a variable reduction in testosterone production, resulting in impotence and hypospermatogenesis in more than half of these patients.[389]

Hypophysitis Lymphocytic hypophysitis causes isolated gonadotropin deficiency and fractional panhypopituitarism. This rare disorder occurs predominantly in women and is associated with autoantibodies to multiple endocrine organs, particularly the thyroid.[390,391]

Glucocorticoids Cushing's syndrome and glucocorticoid administration are associated with reduced testosterone levels. Both central and direct gonadal effects of glucocorticoids are involved.[392]

Exercise Serum testosterone levels increase after acute forms of strenuous exercise but decrease with prolonged activity.[393] Although gonadotropin levels are not significantly altered, both hypothalamic and testicular mechanisms for the low testosterone levels have been invoked.[394] There have been only anecdotal reports of diminished libido, and no systematic studies have shed light on the presence, degree, or severity of hypogonadal symptoms which may occur as a result of prolonged strenuous activity.[395] (see Chap. 33).

Physiologic Delayed Puberty (Constitutional Delay)

Physiologic delayed puberty is a common disorder which often appears to be familial but may occur sporadically.[396] From an early age, boys with this disorder lag 1 to 3 years behind their peers in growth and bone age; they may fall as low as the first percentile on growth charts. Puberty is usually initiated between ages 14 and 18 but may be delayed to ages 20 to 24 in rare instances. The diagnosis is suspected in a short, adolescent boy with no significant testicular enlargement by age 14 whose father, brothers, or cousins initiated puberty between the ages of 14 and 18. In some instances, no family history can be elicited. The absence of hyposmia, anosmia, cryptorchidism, or other congenital anomalies supports the diagnosis of physiologic delay. Retardation in bone age and/or height to more than 3.5 SD below the mean raises the possibility that there is an organic cause of delayed puberty. Additionally, clinical evidence of GH, thyroxine, or cortisol deficiency by history or physical examination points to organic rather than physiologic causes of delayed sexual maturation.

The major problem in diagnosis is the differentiation of boys with physiologic delayed puberty from those with complete or incomplete forms of hypogonadotropic eunuchoidism. Since it is inappropriate to withhold treatment until late in the teenage period in patients with organic hypogonadotropic hypogonadism, efforts have been made to develop functional tests to identify patients who will ultimately undergo spontaneous sexual development. No definitive methods to make this distinction currently exist (see Kallmann's Syndrome, above). Progressive increments in gonadotropin titers over a period of months point to physiologic delayed adolescence rather than to organic hypogonadotropic hypogonadism (Fig. 16-38). A clearly pubertal response to a single bolus of GnRH, GnRH infusions, or long-acting GnRH favors physiologic delay, although caution must be advised in drawing definitive conclusions from these tests.

Hypergonadotropic Hypogonadism

Overview

Primary disorders of testicular function result in incomplete sexual maturation and hypogonadism (Table 16-8 and Fig. 16-41). Demonstration of hypergonadotropism allows this group of patients to be differentiated from those with hypothalamic-pituitary disorders in whom gonadotropin secretion is diminished. The clinical presentation differs depending on the patient's age. In boys, the defect in testosterone secretion is often partial; androgen-related somatic changes occur at puberty but are incomplete. Testicular growth is diminished because of the dysgenetic nature of the gonad. The gynecomastia which frequently develops during puberty is more

TABLE 16-8 Classification of Hypergonadotropic Hypogonadism

- Gonadal defects
  - Genetic
    - Klinefelter's syndrome
    - Myotonic dystrophy
    - Webbed neck, ptosis (etc.)
    - XYY syndrome
    - Down syndrome
    - Miscellaneous
  - Anatomic
    - Functional prepubertal castrate
  - Gonadal toxin-induced
    - Drugs
    - Ionizing radiation
  - Enzymatic
    - 17α-hydroxylase deficiency
    - 17-ketoreductase deficiency
    - $C_{17\text{-}20}$-lyase
  - Viral
    - Mumps orchitis
  - Diabetes mellitus
  - Gerontologic
    - Male climacteric
- Hormone resistance
  - Androgen insensitivity
  - Luteinizing hormone resistance

severe than that observed in normal boys. In adults, testicular failure produces impotence as an early symptom; loss of secondary sex characteristics occurs later, often taking 5 to 10 years to develop.

Genetic Disorders

Klinefelter's Syndrome

Klinefelter's syndrome, the most common disorder causing male hypogonadism, is defined as a type of testicular dysgenesis characterized by the presence of one or more supernumerary X chromosomes (Table 16-9). Classic and variant forms have been described. The classic (XXY) form occurs in approximately 1 in 500 males (0.21 percent of infants and 0.15 to 0.24 percent of adults).[282,397] This disorder is highly suspect in an adult with firm testes <2.0 cm in length who has clinical signs of androgen deficiency of variable degree. Gynecomastia occurs in 85 percent of these patients. The arm span is usually >2 cm longer than the patient's height, and the floor-to-pubis length is usually 2 cm greater than the distance from the pubis to the crown of the head. These disproportionate body measurements are called *eunuchoidal proportions.* It is a common misconception that short stature is associated with Klinefelter's syndrome; in general, these patients are of normal stature or are taller than normal. Large prospective surveys show that mean intelligence test scores and educational levels achieved are lower in men with Klinefelter's syndrome than in controls of a similar age.[398] A slightly increased proportion of patients with Klinefelter's syndrome may have frankly subnormal intelligence[399]; however, case selection methods may bias these results toward identification of a greater number of patients of subnormal intelligence than occurs among the general population. Personality disorders are reported to occur more commonly in men with Klinefelter's syndrome than in the normal population. This finding could be ascribed to the problems encountered in adjusting to androgen deficiency and an altered physical habitus or could occur as a primary manifestation of the genetic process.

Patients with this disorder are most commonly detected on routine physical examination on the basis of small testes. Additional cases are discovered among patients with azoospermia (i.e., complete lack of spermatozoa) presenting to infertility clinics. Klinefelter's syndrome patients usually do not seek medical attention because of the signs or symptoms of androgen deficiency, even though these features are commonly present. For this reason, the large majority of patients with this common syndrome escape diagnosis.

The testes of pubertal boys with Klinefelter's syndrome are smaller than normal. By adulthood, nearly all patients with classic Klinefelter's syndrome have lost their total complement of germinal cells in the testes. As a consequence, their testes remain small and their semen contains no spermatozoa, a condition called azoospermia. The exact mechanisms responsible for the testicular dysfunction are inferred from observations in animals. The presence of an extra X chromosome commits the germ cells to a shortened life span. In a variety of animal species as well as in humans, a normal complement of primordial germ cells is present in the fetal testes of XXY males, but these cells degenerate at an accelerated rate during childhood.[400]

FIGURE 16-41 Diagrammatic representation of hypergonadotropic hypogonadism. Triangle = hypothalamus; oval = pituitary; circle = testis; T = testosterone; E_2 = estradiol.

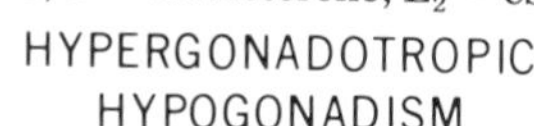

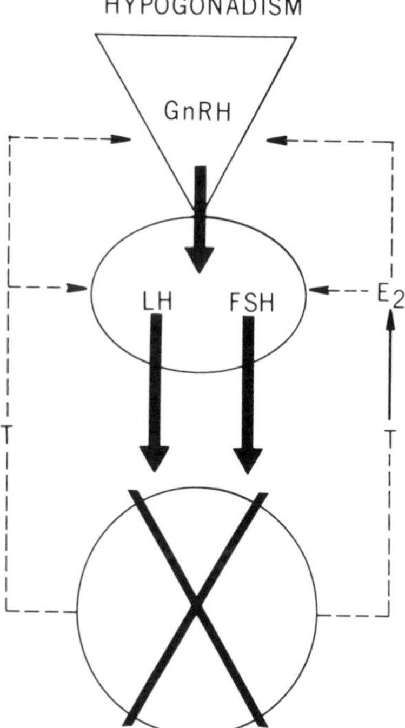

TABLE 16-9 Features of Klinefelter's Syndrome

		Variant Forms*		
Parameter	Classic form (XXY)	XX	Mosaic Forms*	Poly X + Y
Incidence	1/500	1/9000	Unknown	Unknown
Clinical features	Testes <2 cm and firm Eunuchoidal proportions Gynecomastia Personality disorder Androgen deficiency of variable degree	Shorter in stature Hypospadias	Testes may be normal-sized	Increased incidence of cryptorchism Radioulnar synostosis
Laboratory determinations	LH elevated FSH extremely elevated Testosterone lowered (in 50%)			
Karyotype	Barr body present 47,XXY	46,XX	XXY/XY; XXY/XX	XXXY, XXXXY, XXXXXY
Spermatogenesis	Azoospermia		Impairment less severe	
Testis biopsy	Hyalinized tubules Relative Leydig cell hyperplasia		Less severe damage	

* Only divergent features are listed.

Source: Adapted from Bardin and Paulsen.[282]

The exact mechanism that causes the androgen deficiency in Klinefelter's syndrome is unknown, and the degree of Leydig cell dysfunction is variable. Mean testosterone concentrations in patients with Klinefelter's syndrome as a group are approximately half those in normal men (300 ng/100 ml vs. 600 ng/100 ml). However, 43 percent of men in one series had total testosterone levels in the normal (albeit low normal) range.[401] Plasma estradiol concentration, by contrast, was twofold higher in patients than in control subjects (30 vs. 15 pg/ml).[401] This results from an increased fraction of testosterone converted into estradiol in peripheral tissues (0.60 percent in Klinefelter's syndrome vs. 0.38 percent in normal men).[401] In response to an elevated estradiol concentration, the plasma TeBG level increases and the fraction of non-TeBG-bound testosterone is reduced. Consequently, some patients with normal total testosterone levels exhibit low free and weakly bound testosterone concentrations.

Variant forms of Klinefelter's syndrome include individuals with a 46,XX karyotype, those with mosaic forms, and those with the poly X (XXX, XXXX, and XXXXX) + Y varieties (Table 16-9). The XX subtype (the "sex reversal syndrome") occurs in 1 in 9000 men; it mimics the XXY variety in most respects. XX individuals, however, are shorter (168 ± 0.77 cm) and have a 9 percent incidence of hypospadias.[402] The testis determining factor gene (SRY), which is present in normal males on the Y chromosome, can uniformly be demonstrated to be on the X chromosome in such patients by means of DNA hybridization testing.[269,403]

Patients with mosaic forms of Klinefelter's syndrome exhibit variable cytogenetic findings. Mosaicism may be present in cell lines from all tissues.[282] Supernumerary X cell lines may also exist exclusively in testicular tissue. Testicular biopsy with karyotyping of the testicular fibroblasts is required to diagnose such patients. Variable degrees of spermatogenesis and, occasionally, normal-sized testes may be present in some of these individuals; fertility is possible. Such individuals usually undergo a progressive loss of spermatogenesis, Leydig cell function, and testicular size if followed over time. In the poly X + Y variant of Klinefelter's syndrome, the incidence of cryptorchidism is increased, severe deficits in intellectual function occur, and radioulnar synostosis is found.[282]

The diagnosis of Klinefelter's syndrome of any type is presumed when buccal smear analysis reveals Barr bodies in a phenotypic male. Confirmation requires karyotype analysis of blood lymphocytes (commonly) or of fibroblasts grown from testicular biopsy specimens (rarely). Elevation of the plasma FSH concentration always occurs, and LH elevation nearly always occurs. The response to exogenous hCG is blunted, indicating that testicular reserve function is decreased.

Testis biopsy reveals peritubular hyalinization, tubular sclerosis, and adenomatous hyperplasia of Leydig cells. The hyperplastic appearance of the

Leydig cells is deceiving; it reflects the marked reduction in seminiferous tubular mass with relative preservation of interstitial tissue. In actuality, quantitative morphometric studies reveal a reduced Leydig cell volume.

Treatment consists of counseling regarding the presence of infertility and provision of androgen replacement therapy when the clinical circumstances warrant. Individuals with testosterone levels in the low normal range in the face of high LH levels should receive a therapeutic trial of androgen replacement, even though they may not complain of androgen deficiency symptoms. Many of these individuals improve in well-being and sexual potency during such therapy. These patients may be considered analogous to subjects with high TSH levels but normal serum thyroxine concentrations ("compensated hypothyroidism").

Myotonic Dystrophy

Myotonic dystrophy is a familial disorder characterized by cataracts, baldness, muscle weakness, and hypogonadism in 80 percent of affected males. The testes are small and soft as a result of partial to complete germinal cell destruction. Leydig cell morphology appears normal, but function is compromised and maintained only by the secretion of high levels of LH. The testosterone concentration ranges from moderately reduced to low normal. Clinical signs of androgen deficiency vary and correlate with the level of plasma testosterone. FSH concentration was found to be increased in all 32 patients studied by Harper et al.[404] Testicular biopsy revealed a range from complete tubular sclerosis and peritubular hyalinization to moderate derangement of spermatogenesis.[405] No treatment exists for the infertility; androgen replacement is available for patients with low testosterone levels.

Syndrome of Webbed Neck, Ptosis, Hypogonadism, Congenital Heart Disease, and Short Stature (Noonan's Syndrome, Male Turner's Syndrome)

The clinical association of diminished testicular function and the phenotypic stigmata of Turner's syndrome was once classified as the male Turner's syndrome.[406] Clinical findings in these patients may include facies typical of Turner's syndrome in girls: a webbed neck, short stature, low-set ears, ptosis, a shieldlike chest, cryptorchidism, diminished spermatogenesis, decreased Leydig cell function, cubitus valgus, and cardiovascular anomalies (especially pulmonary stenosis).[406,407] Mental retardation, low hairline, a small penis, and lymphedema of the hands and feet, particularly at birth, may also be present.

The diagnosis is limited to patients with four or more cardinal features of the syndrome and a normal chromosomal constitution. The term *male Turner's syndrome* has been discouraged because >95 percent of patients with the cardinal features of this syndrome have a normal karyotype.[407] Gonadotropin levels may be elevated, reflecting a reduction in germ cell or Leydig cell function. Sterility and cryptorchidism are common. Testis biopsy reveals only Sertoli cells in the seminiferous tubules of some patients and a moderate reduction in germ cells in others. Treatment consists of androgen replacement when testosterone levels are low. Orchidopexy is required for cryptorchidism.

XYY Syndrome

Patients with this disorder have been identified with higher frequency among men with tall stature and severe nodular cystic acne. The prevalence is common; 0.1 to 0.2 percent of live male newborns are found to have this abnormality.[397,408] In adults, the disorder has been identified primarily in prisoners and mental hospital patients. Early studies recorded aggressive tendencies in affected individuals and suggested a behavioral effect of the extra Y chromosome. More recent observations suggest that the mean intelligence and educational level achieved in these patients are lower than in normal controls of the same age.[398] These individuals have a high incidence of convictions for criminal behavior (45 percent) compared to a control group (9.3 percent) in one study.[398] However, the criminal behavior appears to relate more to the diminished intellectual function and its concomitant male adjustment patterns than to aggressive behavior imparted by the extra Y chromosome.

Endocrine studies reveal normal LH, FSH, and testosterone levels in the majority of these patients and elevated gonadotropin titers in the minority.[409,410] Numerous case reports of patients with an XYY karyotype with defective sperm production or Leydig cell function have appeared. The actual frequency of these abnormalities among all patients with this karyotype is unknown. The significance of an XYY karyotype in an otherwise normal boy is unclear, and caution is advised with respect to alarming the patient or his parents if the diagnosis is made fortuitously on the basis of routine screening.

Down's Syndrome

A mild degree of testicular dysfunction occurs in patients with Down's syndrome. LH levels are elevated even though Leydig cells appear normal on testicular biopsy.[411] A moderate to severe reduction in all germ cell types, germ cell arrest, and Sertoli cell only patterns can be seen. Peritubular hyalinization is not prominent. FSH levels may be normal or elevated. The degree of reduction of testicular size or body hair in reported series has been variable.

Miscellaneous Genetic Disorders

A variety of clinical syndromes identified on the basis of their specific nontesticular features involve testicular dysfunction. Sickle cell disease is associated with low testosterone levels in conjunction with high LH and FSH concentrations and a reduced response to exogenous GnRH.[412] Certain autoimmune disorders are associated with testicular failure and other endocrine deficiency states.[413] The reader is referred to the compendium of syndromes by Rimoin and Schimke[360] for the identification of several additional disorders which occur rarely.

Functional Prepubertal Castrate Syndrome (Anorchia)

Individuals with the functional prepubertal castrate syndrome[414] present with signs and symptoms of severe androgen deficiency and lack anatomically demonstrable or functioning testes. The appearance of the external genitalia is normal, with the exception of an empty scrotum. Since testosterone is required for development of the external genitalia during the critical fetal period of 8 to 14 weeks, it is assumed that testes were present at the time of fetal development; testicular degeneration must have occurred at a later time. Bilateral testicular torsion may explain the loss of testes in most patients with this disorder, but proof is usually lacking. Regardless of etiology, this disorder has been called a variety of names, including the syndrome of "vanishing testes," anorchia, and functional prepubertal castrate syndrome. This disorder may be partial, resulting from incomplete interference with the vascular supply to the testes. This occurs on occasion during bilateral hernia repair or the performance of bilateral orchidopexy. Affected individuals may retain some degree of testicular tissue and the ability to secrete testosterone.

Patients with complete anorchia present either with suspected bilateral cryptorchism before puberty or with sexual infantilism in the teenage or adult years. Palpation of the scrotum reveals the vas deferens or small masses of tissue consisting of wolffian duct remnants. With gonadotropin assays, elevated levels for age may be documented even in childhood.[415] In the pubertal years, the levels of LH and FSH increase and ultimately reach adult castrate levels in patients with anorchia. The finding of normal gonadotropin levels in a pubertal or adult patient suspected of having anorchia would exclude this condition and prompt a search for cryptorchid testes. Alternatively, levels of LH and FSH in the castrate (high) range, in conjunction with very low testosterone, strongly suggest anorchia.

The differential diagnosis between bilateral cryptorchism and anorchia can usually be made at any age by employing the hCG test.[416] After 2 weeks of administration of 1000 to 2000 IU of hCG three times per week, patients with functioning testes generally attain adult male testosterone levels, whereas those without testes exhibit no increase in testosterone concentration. Cryptorchid testes often descend during this regimen. Exceptions to the expected responses to hCG exist, since patients with isolated gonadotropin deficiency and bilateral cryptorchism exhibit no rise in testosterone concentration during up to 6 weeks of hCG therapy. The hCG test may be omitted if gonadotropin levels are very high under basal conditions and testosterone concentrations are nonetheless very low. Abdominal exploration may be avoided in anorchic patients if gonadotropin levels are high, provided that a prepubertal testosterone level is demonstrated and/or a response to hCG is absent. When intermediate responses are found, surgical exploration may still be indicated. Experience with laparoscopy indicates that this technique is useful.[273] When a blind-ending vas deferens and vascular structures are clearly seen, laparotomy may also be avoided.

Gonadal Toxins

Cytotoxic drugs used as treatment for the nephrotic syndrome or neoplastic diseases commonly produce testicular damage.[261,417,418] The alkylating agents and procarbazine are particularly common offenders. Nearly 100 percent of patients receiving MOPP chemotherapy (mechlorethamine, vincristine, procarbazine, and prednisone) develop azoospermia. Dactinomycin, vincristine, and vinblastine appear not to affect spermatogenesis regardless of dose, whereas agents such as cisplatin produce intermediate effects. At times, chemotherapeutic regimens can be based on the degree of gonadal toxicity. For example, for Hodgkin's disease, ABVD (doxorubicin, bleomycin, vinblastine, and dacarbazine) produces azoospermia in only 35 percent of patients whereas an equally efficacious regimen such as MOPP produces azoospermia in 100 percent of subjects.

Radiation therapy that includes the gonads also results in testicular failure.[419] Damage occurs in prepubertal as well as pubertal and adult men receiving cytotoxic chemotherapy.[228,261,420,421] Damage is dependent on the dose and the duration of therapy.[418] Spermatogenic elements are more sensitive than Leydig cells to radiation therapy and radiomimetic drugs. Consequently, each of these cytotoxic agents may compromise spermatogenesis to a greater extent than androgen production, and monotrophic FSH rises may be observed. Radiation doses as low as 15 rad transiently compromise the pool of spermatogonial cells, and 600 rad permanently destroys germinal elements.[422,423] Permanent Leydig cell dysfunction occurs with doses of 2000 to 3000 rad, as in the treatment of lymphoblastic leukemia with testicular involvement. Subtle defects in LH secretion occur in patients receiving chemotherapeutic agents[424] as well. Various regimens designed to induce protection of the testes during chemotherapy have been attempted, but the results have generally been disappointing.

When potential fertility is discussed with patients who are about to undergo cytotoxic therapy, the possibility of banking sperm requires exploration. It should be recognized, however, that studies have revealed a high incidence of hypogonadism prior to the initiation of therapy in groups of patients with malignant disorders.[425] Defects in both pituitary and gonadal function are encountered which explain the reduction in testosterone levels.

Environmental toxins or habitually abused agents which adversely affect Leydig cell function or spermatogenesis have been insufficiently investigated. Under experimental conditions, marijuana causes a reduction in sperm count and motility[426]; the frequency and severity of the abnormalities produced under uncontrolled conditions are currently unknown. Alcohol also exerts a direct effect on testicular steroidogenesis and may contribute to testicular dysfunction.[382] Industrial hydrocarbon exposure, particularly to polychlorinated insecticides and dibromochloropropane, has been associated with a reduction in sperm count.[427] The clinician should be alert to and suspicious of other possible toxins which have not yet been identified.

Enzyme Defects

Several defects in steroidogenic enzymes result in deficient testosterone production and reflex elevations in gonadotropin production (see Chap. 12). Two of these defects—cholesterol side-chain cleavage and 3β-ol-dehydrogenase, Δ_4, Δ_5-isomerase—profoundly affect cortisol and aldosterone biosynthesis, and patients usually present with the signs and symptoms of classical adrenal insufficiency. Defects in 17-ketoreductase, $C_{17\text{-}20}$ lyase, and 17α-hydroxylase, however, usually cause symptoms of androgen deficiency with elevated gonadotropin secretion.[428–430]

Genetic males with complete 17α-hydroxylase, $C_{17\text{-}20}$lyase and 17-ketosteroid reductase deficiencies[431,432] present as phenotypic females with partial virilization at puberty. However, incomplete defects may result in androgenized males with hypospadias, gynecomastia, and lack of full pubertal development. In the 17α-hydroxylase defect, hypertension and hypokalemia are present because of increased adrenal mineralocorticoid production. Definitive diagnosis is made by demonstrating elevated levels of precursor steroids (progesterone in the 17α-hydroxylase defect, androstenedione in the 17-ketoreductase defect, and 17α-hydroxyprogesterone in the $C_{17\text{-}20}$ lyase defect).

Mumps Orchitis

In 15 to 25 percent of pubertal or postpubertal subjects, mumps involves the testes and produces a highly painful inflammatory disorder. Cytoplasmic swelling of interstitial and germ cells progresses to complete germ cell sloughing. After the acute illness subsides, the germ cells gradually degenerate over a period of several years and Leydig cell dysfunction develops. In later years, patients present with symptoms of androgen deficiency or infertility and relate a history of painful orchitis.[433] Gynecomastia and testicular atrophy may be present, along with clinical evidence of androgen deficiency. Evaluation reveals low testosterone levels, low sperm counts, and high serum or urine LH and FSH concentrations. Testis biopsy specimens appear similar to those seen in patients with Klinefelter's syndrome, with seminiferous tubular hyalinization and relative Leydig cell hyperplasia. The diagnosis is made in a patient with a clinical picture suggesting Klinefelter's syndrome but with a normal blood cell karyotype and a history of mumps with painful testes. The disorder is treated with androgen replacement. This entity will probably be seen much less frequently in the future as a result of the advent of the mumps vaccine.

Diabetes Mellitus

Impotence occurs in 50 percent of diabetic men[434] and may reflect neurologic, vascular, psychologic, drug-induced, or endocrine etiologies. The possibility that primary gonadal failure may explain impotence in a subset of diabetic patients is controversial. Conflicting reports indicate normal or low serum testosterone[435,436] and variable gonadotropin concentrations in these patients.[434–436] A recent study[434,436] separated diabetic patients with impotence into psychogenic and organic subgroups based on nocturnal penile tumescence testing. In the organic impotence subgroup, extensive evaluation revealed convincing evidence of gonadal dysfunction. Specifically, free testosterone concentrations were low and urinary and integrated plasma LH levels were high compared with control subjects and diabetic men with psychogenic impotence.[434,437] Androgen replacement in the group with organic impotence without vascular disease improved nocturnal penile tumescence testing, and symptoms of impotence improved.[434]

Male Climacteric

Clinical, histopathologic, and hormonal studies indicate that gonadal function declines gradually as a function of age in men.[438] This defect exists primarily at the level of the testes. Clinical observations include a gradual reduction in total, free, or bioavailable testosterone; increases in the levels of LH and FSH measured by RIA; and blunted testosterone responses to hCG.[439] Inhibin levels[260] are lower in elderly men than in young men as a reflection of reduced Sertoli cell function. Histologic studies reveal an age-related decline in Leydig cells[440] as well as Sertoli cells,[441] and sperm production diminishes.[442] Symptoms of decreased sexual function may correlate with these changes.[443] Subsets of very healthy men exhibit lesser degrees of these abnormalities,[439,444,445] suggesting that an age-related increase in chronic illness may contribute to the observed gonadal dysfunction.[58]

While a primary testicular defect predominates, hypothalamic and pituitary abnormalities with aging have been suggested but are controversial. These abnormalities include loss of the diurnal pattern of testosterone secretion,[446] altered ratios of biological to immunologic LH and FSH in some[58,253,254] but not all studies,[447,448] inconsistent reports of altered LH pulse frequency,[449,450] and alterations of opiate tone[450] and androgen negative feedback.[451,452]

When there is evidence of primary gonadal failure in an older man with symptoms of impotence, replacement of testosterone is a reasonable consideration, and preliminary trials support the benefit of this approach.[453] This therapeutic option must be weighed against the possibility of adversely affecting prostatic size and uroflow dynamics. Further study is required for the development of clear guidelines regarding the evaluation and treatment of such patients.

Hormone Resistance

Androgen Insensitivity

A genetic male with complete insensitivity to androgens presents as a phenotypic female with primary amenorrhea and breast development, the so-called testicular feminization syndrome.[454] As a manifestation of androgen resistance, these individuals lack facial, axillary, and pubic hair and have female external genitalia. The distal two-thirds of the vagina is well developed, but the proximal one-third, the uterus, and the fallopian tubes are absent. Testosterone, estradiol, and LH levels are high, whereas FSH is normal. Testis biopsy reveals immature germ cells because of the insensitivity to androgen. The Leydig cells are hyperplastic as a result of the elevated LH levels, and adenomatous clumps may be observed. The androgen resistance may be due to a complete lack of androgen receptors, a diminution of receptor number,[455] or a defect in receptor function or to postreceptor defects. Highly sensitive techniques for detecting gene deletions or point mutations allow precise identification of the defects present (Fig. 16-42). Most commonly, point mutations of the androgen receptor occur. These mutations can result in the synthesis of androgen receptors with reduced affinity for androgen, premature termination of transcription of the androgen receptor mRNA, or derangements of splicing of the mRNA sequences. Less commonly,[456] whole exons are deleted and the androgen receptor mRNA is markedly truncated. Each of these mutations produces androgen receptors with a reduced or absent capacity to mediate androgenic effects.[457–463]

Incomplete insensitivity to androgens produces a clinical spectrum ranging from features of severe undervirilization to normally virilized men with infertility or even fertile men with minimal underviriliza-

FIGURE 16-42 Diagrammatic representation of recently described genetic mutations associated with androgen insensitivity. Gene deletions, sites of point mutations, and locations of amino acid changes indicated. See text for references.

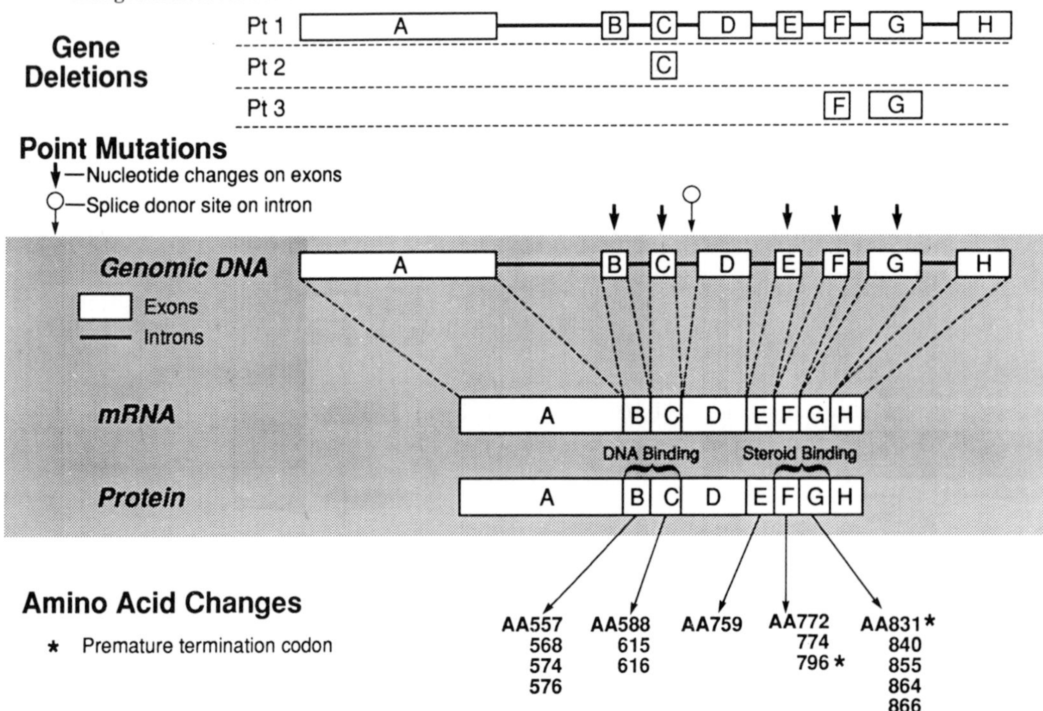

tion.[464–466] These patients experience pubertal onset at an appropriate age but usually fail to androgenize completely. Gynecomastia, hypospadias,[467,468] a bifid scrotum, and cryptorchidism are common. The disorder in these patients encompasses entities previously called the syndromes of Rosewater, Dreyfus, Lubs, and Reifenstein. LH levels are usually elevated, reflecting resistance to androgens at the hypothalamic-pituitary level. FSH levels are usually normal.

Testicular biopsy reveals a variable picture. Complete tubular sclerosis and peritubular hyalinization constitute one extreme, and immature germ cells without sclerosis make up the other. Diagnosis requires[464] the demonstration of quantitative or qualitative abnormalities of the androgen receptor. Lack of suppression of SHBG levels with the anabolic androgen stanozolol may provide a screening method to identify patients for definitive receptor measurements,[469] but this test requires wider confirmation. Treatment with high-dose androgen therapy in postpubertal patients produces limited results. However, encouraging beneficial effects were observed in one prepubertal patient with an androgen receptor defect characterized by a rapid dissociation rate of androgen from its receptor.[464]

Partial androgen resistance may represent a common cause of oligo- or azoospermia in patients who present with infertility.[470] Clinically, these men exhibit minimal evidence of undervirilization and normal levels of LH and testosterone. LH/testosterone product indexes (i.e., LH times testosterone) were initially found to be elevated,[471] but later studies have not confirmed this observation.[470,472] The frequency of this disorder in azoospermic patients is a matter of controversy, with a prevalence of 12.5 to 40 percent in two series and no cases found in two other series.[470,472–474]

Another type of partial androgen resistance results from a deficiency of the enzyme 5α-reductase, which converts testosterone to dihydrotestosterone.[475] These patients exhibit a characteristic form of male pseudohermaphroditism, originally termed pseudovaginal perineoscrotal hypospadias, and are usually raised as females. Their excretory duct system, including epididymides, vas deferentiae, seminal vesicles, and ejaculatory ducts, are normal male in type, but the ejaculatory ducts terminate in a vagina and the external genitalia are ambiguous. At puberty, partial virilization with penile growth and an increase in muscle mass ensue. Facial hair, acne, and frontal balding are lacking. In primitive cultures, these individuals take on a male role at puberty. Spermatogenesis is usually impaired either as a result of 5α-reductase deficiency and subsequent reduction of testicular dihydrotestosterone levels or as a consequence of the cryptorchid position of the testes.[476]

LH Resistance

LH resistance was first described in the rodent. The predicted findings of elevated LH and low testosterone concentration and unstimulated testes were found.[477] Patients with this disorder have similar hormonal changes in addition to sexual immaturity.[478] Secretion of an immunologically recognizable but biologically inactive LH molecule exactly mimics this syndrome.[479] Measurement of LH concentration by bioassay as well as by RIA is required to identify the latter disorder.

Treatment of Hypogonadism

Approaches to treatment differ depending on the clinical circumstances and the desire of the patient (Table 16-10).

Delayed Adolescence

Major psychologic effects may result from a delay in adolescent sexual development. Precise differentiation of physiologically delayed adolescence from isolated gonadotropin deficiency is not usually possible in boys of pubertal age. These considerations favor treatment empirically in patients over 14 years of age when clinical circumstances, specifically the psychological needs of the patient, warrant. The usual goal of therapy is to initiate androgenic effects with intermittent subreplacement doses of testosterone (i.e., maintenance of testosterone at levels of 100 to 300 ng/100 ml) while observing for spontaneous maturational changes during periods off medication. Two therapeutic modalities—hCG and synthetic androgen replacement—are available. hCG is efficacious in hypogonadotropic syndromes when Leydig cell responsiveness is adequate. A dose of 1500 IU once to twice weekly stimulates testosterone to levels between 100 and 300 ng/100 ml.[480] This regimen is expensive and requires frequent injections. Its only advantage over replacement testosterone is the direct stimulation of testis size. Consequently, hCG is infrequently used as a long-term treatment modality.

Injectable esters such as testosterone enanthate and testosterone cypionate provide sustained blood levels of testosterone over a 1- to 2-week period. To initiate pubertal changes, 50 to 100 mg is administered intramuscularly every 3 to 4 weeks for 3 to 4 months with cessation for an equal period. The goal is to promote secondary sex characteristics and normal linear growth. Evidence of spontaneous pubertal development such as testicular enlargement and spontaneous increments of gonadotropins and testosterone should be sought during the 3 to 4 months off therapy. The onset of pubertal progression under these circumstances is thought by some to reflect a maturing effect of exogenous testosterone on the hypothalamic-pituitary axis. If no significant progression is noted, several intermittent courses of low-

TABLE 16-10 Treatment of Hypogonadism

Group	Goal of Treatment	Treatment Modality	Dosage
Delayed adolescence	Short-term maintenance of plasma testosterone at 100-300 ng/dl	hCG	1500 IU IM 1-2 times/wk
		Testosterone enanthate or cypionate	50-100 mg IM q 3-4 wk
Adult hypogonadotropic hypogonadism	Long-term maintenance of testosterone levels at 300-1200 ng/dl	GnRH*	5-30 μg SC q 2 h
		hCG	1000-4000 IU IM 1-3 times/wk
		Testosterone enanthate or cypionate	300 mg q 14-21 days 200 mg q 10-17 days 100 mg q 5-10 days
Adult hypergonadotropic hypogonadism	Long-term maintenance of testosterone levels at 300-1200 ng/dl	Testosterone enanthate or cypionate	300 mg q 14-21 days 200 mg q 10-17 days 100 mg q 5-10 days
	Subreplacement doses of androgen	Fluoxymesterone	5-10 mg PO daily
		Methyltestosterone	25 mg daily by linguet
		Testosterone undecanoate†	200 mg PO 4 times daily

* Experimental, requires programmed pump.

† Not available in United States.

dose testosterone can be administered until spontaneous puberty is initiated or the need for long-term exogenous therapy is confirmed. When the doses are kept small, this regimen does not have a harmful effect on the potential for full somatic growth or subsequent testicular function.

Hypergonadotropic Hypogonadism

Direct replacement of androgen provides the only effective therapy in adults with hypergonadotropic hypogonadism and can also be used in hypogonadotropic patients who do not immediately want to father children.[481] The goal of therapy is to maintain the plasma testosterone concentration in the range of 300 to 1200 ng/100 ml. After a sufficient time, full secondary sex characteristics and sexual potency are attained. Testicular enlargement, an effect observed only with gonadotropin therapy, does not occur. Injectable testosterone esters are required for full androgen maintenance. Pharmacologic studies have fully characterized the profiles of dose response over time for the available agents (Fig. 16-43).[482] Higher doses produce more prolonged effects at the expense of higher peak levels.[481,482] As the toxic effects of pharmacologic plasma concentrations of testosterone are quite rare, higher doses are usually chosen to prolong the effect. Suggested regimens include 300 mg testosterone enanthate or testosterone 17β-cypionate every 14 to 21 days IM, 200 mg every 10 to 17 days, or 100 mg every 5 to 10 days. Measurement of the plasma testosterone concentration at the nadir, just before the next injection, allows empirical adjustment of the dose. Levels of testosterone below 250 ng/100 ml during therapy can often be perceived by patients as causing impaired sexual potency or reduced endurance during physical activity.

Side effects or toxicity caused by testosterone replacement are uncommon. However, an increased hematocrit due to bone marrow stimulation,[483] acne, sleep apnea syndrome,[484] gynecomastia as a result of aromatization of testosterone to estradiol, and prostatic hypertrophy in the elderly are physiologic consequences of this therapeutic approach. Rarely, hepatic tumors occur in patients who receive pharmacologic levels of androgen.[485] Only anecdotal reports have associated androgen therapy with prostatic carcinoma, and systematic data regarding this association are required.[486,487] Nonaromatizable an-

FIGURE 16-43 Testosterone and estradiol levels in hypogonadal subjects after a single dose of testosterone enanthate. (*Adapted from Sokol et al.*[482])

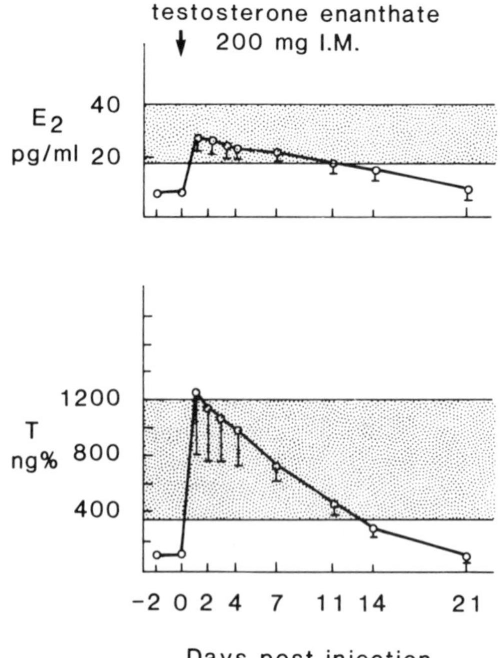

drogens (anabolic steroids) increase LDL and decrease high-density lipoprotein (HDL) cholesterol levels and potentially could increase the risk of developing cardiovascular disease. With aromatizable androgens (e.g., testosterone), these effects are offset by the concomitant increase in estrogen levels.[488] Recognition of these problems and clinical monitoring allow prompt recognition and a change of therapy when warranted.

The available oral androgens are insufficiently potent for full androgen replacement at doses compatible with reasonable safety; they are useful, however, for achieving anabolic effects in selected patients. Either fluoxymesterone or methyltestosterone can be used. Testosterone undecanoate, another orally absorbable androgen ester, is not available for use in the United States[481] but is sufficiently potent for full androgen replacement. Patients should be monitored for the development of cholestatic jaundice with liver function tests when they receive fluoxymesterone or methyltestosterone.

Transdermal patches containing testosterone provide another effective means of maintaining plasma testosterone levels between 300 and 1200 ng/100 ml (Fig. 16-44). Well tolerated and preferred to injections by many patients, this delivery system is undergoing review by the U.S. Food and Drug Administration for potential approval.[489] Testosterone microsphere pellets and long-acting analogues are also undergoing development as approved means of maintaining stable testosterone levels during replacement therapy.[490,491]

FIGURE 16-44 Mean (±SEM) serum testosterone concentrations in five hypogonadal men before and during long-term therapy with transdermal testosterone. (*From Ahmed et al.*[489])

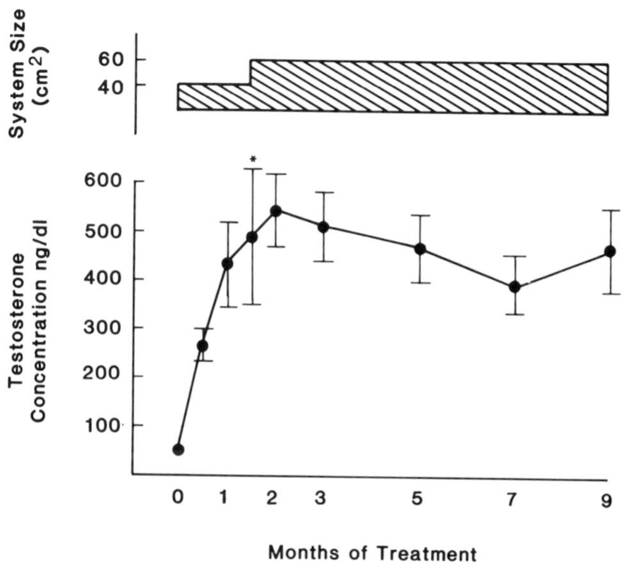

Adult Hypogonadotropic Hypogonadism

Treatment goals in patients with adult hypogonadotropic hypogonadism include (1) maintenance of androgen levels in the normal adult male range (i.e., 300 to 1200 ng/100 ml) to allow full virilization and maintenance of normal bone density[492] and (2) stimulation of spermatogenesis to allow fertility.

Maintenance of Androgen Levels

Therapy with exogenous testosterone is usually chosen to allow virilization, since this approach requires less frequent injections and is less costly than hCG. Exogenous androgen administration does not compromise the potential for later fertility. The approach is identical to that used in patients with hypergonadotropic hypogonadism.

hCG administration provides another means of maintaining normal adult male androgen levels (Fig. 16-45). A dose of 1000 to 4000 IU is given intramuscularly two to three times per week. The exact dose is established empirically in individual patients by measuring plasma testosterone concentrations. Testicular enlargement can be achieved, but the testes seldom exceed 3.5 cm in length in response to hCG alone. This approach is expensive, requires frequent injections, and has no advantage over direct androgen replacement therapy unless fertility is an immediate goal.

Stimulation of Spermatogenesis

Two approaches are available: the use of hCG/hMG and treatment with pulsatile GnRH.

hCG/hMG This method administers exogenous LH-like material in the form of hCG initially, followed by the coadministration of FSH [in the form of human menopausal gonadotropin (hMG)] if necessary. Patients with adult-onset (acquired) hypogonadotropism and incomplete forms of gonadotropin deficiency frequently achieve normal spermatogenesis when given 1000 to 4000 IU of hCG alone over a period of 1 to 2 years. The response to monotherapy is predicted by the presence of testes which exceed prepubertal size before therapy is initiated.[218] Other patients require the addition of 75 to 150 IU of Pergonal (hMG) three times weekly for 1 to 2 years. Pergonal is started after testosterone levels have been normalized in response to hCG for at least 6 months. On average, sperm appear in the ejaculate after 18 months, and maximal sperm counts are observed after approximately 2 years of therapy. Even though quantitatively normal spermatogenesis is not achieved, more than half of these patients are successful in impregnating their partners.[218,327] After full stimulation of spermatogenesis with hCG/hMG, maintenance of sperm production is often possible with hCG administration alone. Antibodies to hCG occasionally develop but rarely present a clinical problem.

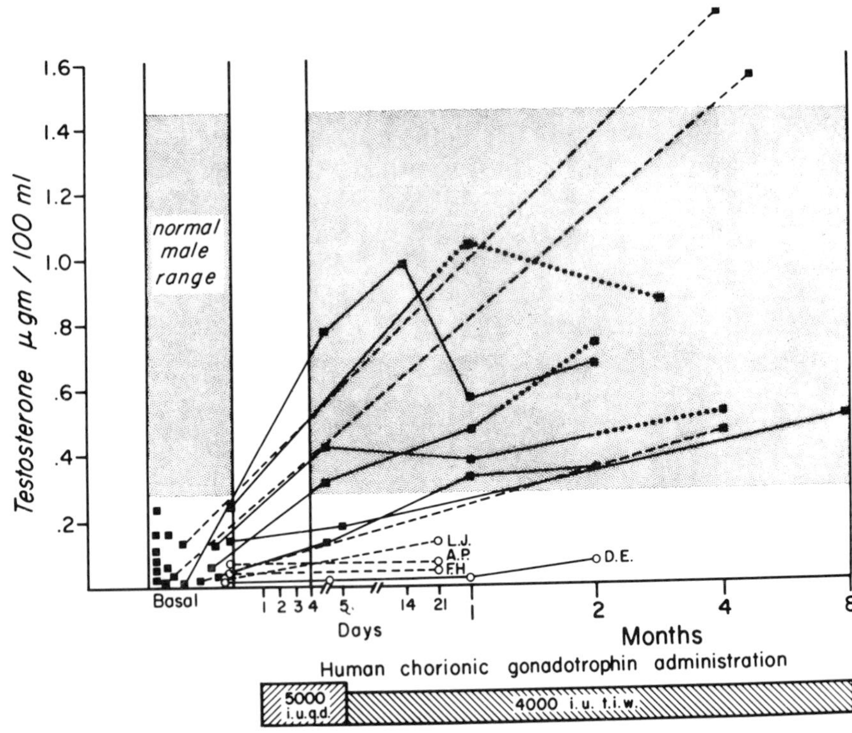

FIGURE 16-45 Basal and stimulated levels of serum testosterone concentration in men with hypogonadotropic hypogonadism. Open circles refer to men with bilateral cryptorchism. Broken lines refer to patients not studied with 4-day hCG stimulation. Dotted lines refer to nonconsecutive observations of serum testosterone concentration. (*From Santen and Paulsen.*[656])

Pulsatile GnRH Therapy. On theoretical grounds, it was predicted that pulsatile GnRH treatment might provide more physiologic normalization of LH and FSH levels in patients with GnRH deficiency (Kallmann's syndrome). In initial trials, patients received 5 to 30 µg of GnRH subcutaneously every 2 h by programmed pump for 2 years or longer. Sperm production occurred, and the patients were often able to impregnate their partners. Direct comparisons of GnRH and hCG/hMG regimens in both randomized and crossover designs revealed that larger testis size was achieved during the GnRH treatment, but no significantly greater sperm concentrations.[493,494] Since GnRH therapy by pulsatile pump is more difficult for the patient to tolerate, the authors prefer to use hCG/hMG until more data on the use of GnRH are available.

GERMINAL CELL FAILURE

Overview

Men with germinal cell failure usually seek medical attention for evaluation of infertility. If it is defined as a lack of conception for 1 year of adequate, unprotected intercourse, infertility occurs in 10 percent of marriages. In 30 to 50 percent of cases, the male partner in an infertile marriage is found to have oligospermia or azoospermia. Appropriate calculations from these data indicate that the prevalence of germinal cell dysfunction in men approaches 3 to 5 percent. Thus, on a statistical basis, hypospermatogenesis constitutes one of the most common clinical disorders involving the reproductive system.

The initial evaluation of an infertile male involves documentation of low sperm counts with at least three semen analyses at monthly intervals. Specimens are obtained after 3 days of abstinence from intercourse. If counts are consistently below 20×10^6 ml or 50×10^6 total, germinal cell dysfunction is highly suspected. A work-up should then be initiated to identify possible causes (Table 16-11). Disorders of germinal cell function can be classified as hypogonadotropic, hypergonadotropic, and eugonadotropic in type. The hypogonadotropic forms produce a clinical picture of Leydig cell dysfunction as well as germinal cell failure; they can be classified under the hypogonadotropic syndromes discussed above. In contrast, germinal cell failure of the hypergonadotropic and eugonadotropic types produces only subclinical Leydig cell dysfunction and is generally recognized clinically because of infertility rather than testosterone deficiency.

Hypergonadotropic Syndromes

When germinal cell mass or Sertoli cell function is sufficiently reduced, plasma or urinary FSH levels increase, often without a concomitant rise in the LH concentration (Fig. 16-46). Most but not all studies demonstrate similar increases in FSH levels with in vitro bioassays and with immunoassays.[495–497] Detailed clinical observations demonstrate an inverse

TABLE 16-11 Relative Frequency of Etiologies and Histologic Findings in Infertile Men

Causes, %		Histologic Findings, %	
Idiopathic	33	Hypospermatogenesis	61
Varicocele	25	Maturation arrest	15
Undescended testes (surgically corrected or uncorrected)	7	Sertoli cell only	13
Excurrent duct obstruction	4.8	Normal appearance	8
Mumps orchitis	3.3	Hyalinized tubules	2
Hypogonadotropism	2.3	Immature testis	1
Klinefelter's syndrome	1.9		
Miscellaneous	23		

Source: Data from Baker HWG, Burger HG, deKretser DM, Hudson B: Relative incidence of etiologic disorders in male infertility, in Santen and Swerdloff[661]; Tyler ET, Singher HO: Male infertility—status of treatment, prevention, and current research. *JAMA* 160:91, 1956; Dubin L, Amelar RD: Etiologic factors in 1294 consecutive cases of male infertility. *Fertil Steril* 22:469, 1971; Greenberg SH, Lipshultz LI, Wein AJ: Experience with 425 subfertile male patients. *J Urol* 119:507, 1978; and Abyholm T: Azoospermia and oligozoospermia etiology and clinical findings. *Arch Androl* 10:57, 1983.

correlation between the remaining germinal cell mass and the level of circulating FSH.[222] An exact relation between FSH secretion and the absence of a specific germinal cell type is not found. Several lines of evidence suggest that FSH secretion may correlate directly with Sertoli cell function and only indirectly with germinal cell maturation.[222,498] Regardless of the exact relations, the degree of elevation of FSH concentration in plasma can be used as an index of the severity of germinal cell dysfunction.[222] An exaggerated release of FSH in response to GnRH appears to uncover lesser degrees of germinal cell failure.[499] Several specific disorders produce monotropic FSH elevation or disproportionate FSH/LH ratios in association with germinal cell failure.[499,500]

The mechanistic basis for monotropic FSH elevations is unclear. At least four possibilities exist: (1) the effect of a specific FSH releasing hormone, (2) a deficiency of inhibin, (3) reduced frequency of GnRH pulses,[501] and (4) differential sensitivity of FSH and LH to sex steroid feedback. With respect to the first two possibilities, a specific FSH-releasing hormone has not been identified and a lack of negative correlation of inhibin with FSH has been recently shown.[229] Reduced GnRH pulse frequency remains a possible explanation, but careful study of a large number of oligospermic men revealed a normal or increased frequency of gonadotropin pulses.[502] Differential sensitivity to sex steroids has gained experimental support as well. Castrate rats respond to slight reductions in testosterone concentrations with monotropic increments in FSH.[503] Men with monotropic FSH increments frequently have slightly reduced testosterone secretion.[504] From this analysis, it is clear that further studies are required to delineate the mechanism or mechanisms for monotropic FSH increments.

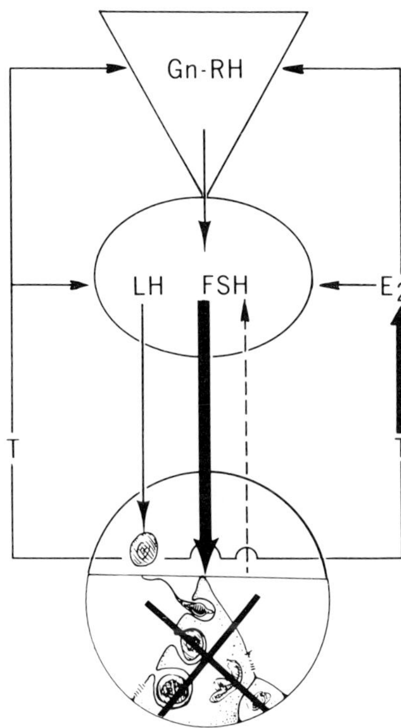

FIGURE 16-46 Diagrammatic representation of monotrophic FSH increments in patients with seminiferous tubular failure. Triangle = hypothalamus; oval = pituitary; circle = testis with Leydig cell and Sertoli cell compartments represented; T = testosterone; E_2 = estradiol.

Sertoli-Cell-Only Syndrome

The Sertoli-cell-only syndrome is a disorder diagnosed by means of testicular biopsy and characterized by azoospermia, elevated FSH, and absence of germinal cells on testicular biopsy. Clinical examination reveals normal pubic and axillary hair but small, soft testes averaging 2 to 4 cm on their long axes (volume 10 to 20 ml). Half of these patients exhibit subclinical Leydig cell dysfunction, characterized by elevated LH with a normal or slightly reduced testosterone concentration and a blunted response to hCG.[499] Analysis of testicular biopsy specimens reveals that the seminiferous tubules are slightly reduced in diameter, contain only Sertoli cells, and are not sclerotic in appearance. No peritubular hyalinization is present. The Sertoli and Leydig cells appear normal on light microscopy, but on electron microscopy they contain minor abnormalities.[505] Normal seminiferous tubules with full germinal cell maturation are occasionally seen, but the majority are completely depleted of germinal elements. A definitive diagnosis requires a testicular biopsy and the demonstration of markedly depleted germinal cells. The etiology of this syndrome is unknown, and multiple causes are possible.

Idiopathic Seminiferous Tubular Failure with Hyalinization

In a major subgroup of men with oligospermia or azoospermia, no specific cause is found but FSH concentrations are elevated.[222] These men appear to have testicular hyperthermia, whereas those with normal FSH levels as a group do not.[506] It is not known whether the hyperthermia is a cause or a result of the oligospermia. Testis biopsies reveal hyalinization of the peritubular elements in conjunction with variable degrees of germinal cell loss. Testis size may be reduced to below adult normal limits of 4.0 cm on the long axis or 20 ml. Because serum FSH levels generally correlate with the degree of hyalinization and testicular damage, a biopsy is usually not performed to establish this diagnosis.

Eugonadotropic Germinal Cell Failure

Idiopathic Germinal Cell Failure

Oligospermia or azoospermia of unknown cause may be less severe and may be associated with normal basal FSH levels. Two subtypes have been described: arrest of germinal cell maturation at a specific step and generalized hypospermatogenesis that affects all germinal cell elements (Table 16-11). Clinical examination reveals no abnormality; testis size is usually normal. On testis biopsy, only minimal peritubular hyalinization or normal peritubular elements are present. Subclinical hypergonadotropism can be uncovered in approximately 30 percent of these patients by the demonstration of exaggerated FSH (and often LH) increments after the administration of exogenous GnRH.[500] Prolactin levels are elevated in 5 percent of oligospermic patients, but the pathophysiologic significance of this is unclear.[308]

Numerous treatments for patients with germinal cell failure, particularly the eugonadotropic subgroup, have been proposed, including (1) induction of rebound from testosterone or anabolic androgen-induced azoospermia, (2) administration of exogenous gonadotropins or gonadotropin-releasing factors, (3) use of clomiphene citrate or tamoxifen to stimulate endogenous gonadotropin secretion, (4) administration of low doses of mesterolone, an oral synthetic androgen, and (5) use of an aromatase inhibitor such as testolactone.[507–512] A general review of the available data reveals that sperm count increases in 20 to 40 percent of these patients in association with each of these treatments.[507–512] Baker suggested that these increments merely represent regression to the mean in men selected on the basis of a limited number of sperm counts.[512] Increased sperm counts in men receiving a placebo in one study supported his conclusion.[513] Few controlled randomized trials using a placebo have been conducted, and no study has conclusively established the benefit of these treatments.[510,513,514] Strictly controlled studies of extensively characterized patients will be required to establish that any of the currently available treatment modalities has a role in reversing the spermatogenic deficiency.

Varicocele

Incompetence of the left testicular vein or, less commonly, the right results in the formation of dilated veins in the scrotum, a condition called *varicocele*. Detection of varicocele clinically requires examination of a standing patient during the Valsalva maneuver. Subclinical varicocele is suggested by thermography and confirmed by retrograde testicular vein venography,[515] but the significance of this finding remains controversial.

A series of clinical observations suggest an etiologic association between varicocele and infertility.[516] Varicoceles can be palpated in approximately 40 percent of men with oligo- or azoospermia[517] and 8 to 23 percent of normal men.[518,519] Sperm motility is often reduced, and a stress pattern of sperm morphology with increased numbers of immature or tapered forms is commonly found.[520] These abnormalities, however, occur no more frequently than they do in other men with infertility.[521] Sperm from patients with varicocele penetrate into denuded ova from hamsters as a test of sperm function less well than do normal sperm.[522]

High venous ligation of the testicular veins in the inguinal canal is the standard treatment for varicocele.[515,517] Venous occlusion can also be induced by the injection of thrombogenic agents through a venous catheter.[515] The clinician should be aware that 10 percent of varicoceles recur after surgery and can be detected on careful repeat examination.[515] The majority of reports indicate a pregnancy rate in operated patients of approximately 30 percent, compared with 16 percent in control patients receiving either medical treatment or no therapy.[516] Because the mechanism of induction of oligospermia is unknown and prospective controlled trials of therapy have not been completed, some investigators question the etiologic association of varicocele with infertility and the efficacy of surgical therapy.[523] Recent data for and against this conclusion have been presented.[523–526] Until a definitive answer is obtained from controlled studies (one is currently ongoing), the question of the efficacy of varicocele repair will remain open. However, the majority of studies indicate an improved rate of fertility of approximately 20 percent in men undergoing correction. Based on this finding, an informed patient can rationally choose varicocele repair.

No clearly defined criteria allow a prediction of

responders to corrective surgery. Carefully conducted studies suggest that patients with subclinical Leydig cell dysfunction, as detected by exaggerated LH and FSH responses to GnRH infusion, may be more likely to respond to varicocele repair.[527,528] Azoospermic patients are unlikely to benefit from this procedure.

Varicoceles occur in approximately 15 percent of adolescent boys.[519] Progressive testicular atrophy has been observed in some of these subjects.[529] An increase in the volume of the affected testis follows varicocele repair in the majority of patients with an ipsilateral testis smaller than the contralateral one.[530] Histologic abnormalities in the testis on the side of the varicocele have been demonstrated.[531] These findings raise questions about the management of adolescent patients with varicocele.[532] Many researchers advocate varicocele repair for patients with large varicoceles and progressive atrophy of the ipsilateral testis.[530] An operation for oligospermia is generally not performed, because systematic collection of prospective data based on semen analyses is not practical. Adolescents with varicocele should probably be followed with a physical examination every 6 months, and an attempt should be made to obtain a baseline semen analysis. Growth failure of the testis ipsilateral to the varicocele is an indication for varicocele ligation.

Ductal Obstruction

Nearly 40 percent of patients with azoospermia are found to have ductal obstruction. Inflammatory, iatrogenic, or congenital defects of the vas deferens or epididymis are the most common causes. These patients have normal FSH levels and testis size and are diagnosed by demonstrating normal spermatogenesis on testicular biopsy and obstructed ducts on vasographic study. An algorithm for the evaluation of azoospermic patients recommends testicular biopsy only for those with normal testes and vas deferentiae on physical examination and normal FSH levels.[533]

Congenital Adrenal Hyperplasia

Elevated adrenal androgens suppress the production of LH and FSH in men with congenital adrenal hyperplasia (CAH). The majority of these patients have normal spermatogenesis.[534] Some, particularly those with adrenal rest tumors in the testes, exhibit oligospermia. Treatment with exogenous glucocorticoids reverses the oligospermia and reduces the size of testicular masses in such patients.[535–538]

Heat

Exposure to heat reproducibly reduces sperm production temporarily in a number of animal species. While this effect has been incompletely documented in men, studies suggest that the heat encountered in a sauna may be sufficient to reduce sperm production temporarily.[539]

Infections

In the majority of patients with eugonadotropic seminiferous tubular failure, no cause can be identified. A thorough search for infectious agents has identified a variety of organisms in the seminal fluid of men with oligospermia or decreased sperm motility.[540] Mycoplasma infection, particularly by *Ureaplasma urealyticum,* has been suggested as a causative agent in infertility, but this conclusion remains controversial.[541] *U. urealyticum* was found in 26 percent of 100 infertile men compared with 13 percent of 30 fertile men in one study. *Escherichia coli* has been implicated in other studies. No characteristic features are apparent by history or physical examination in these men. The presence of an excess number of leukocytes in the seminal fluid suggests the possibility of infection. A cause-and-effect relation between the documented infection and the associated infertility has not been established. However, most large infertility clinics routinely treat patients with antibiotics such as doxycycline when infection is suspected on the basis of the presence of pus cells on several seminal fluid examinations or positive cultures.

Sinopulmonary-Infertility Syndrome

In a number of recently described disorders, a correlation between infertility and recurrent sinopulmonary infections is apparent (Table 16-12).[542] Although no single mechanism explains this association, the characterization of these disorders as a group is useful for the clinician. In the *immotile cilia syndrome,* sperm motility and ciliary function in the respiratory tract are defective because of abnormal flagellar function.[543] One subtype of this syndrome is identified by electron microscopic study. It consists of the absence of dynein arms on the sperm tail and respiratory cilia. Partial deletions of the dynein arms may also exist but are difficult to detect because of considerable variability in the appearance of normal sperm tails on electron microscopy. A deficiency of protein carboxymethylase, an enzyme required for motility,[544] has been demonstrated in the sperm of patients with necrospermia.

Cystic fibrosis is characterized by congenital malformation of the vas deferens with azoospermia and tenacious bronchopulmonary secretions. Young's syndrome, by contrast, is associated with inspissated secretions in the vas deferens in association with azoospermia. Both disorders produce recurrent respiratory infections; the infections are severe in cystic fibrosis and mild in Young's syndrome.[542,545]

Genetic Syndromes

Surveys of karyotype analyses or of meiotic chromosomes in men with infertility document the fre-

TABLE 16-12 **Clinical Features of the Sinopulmonary-Infertility Syndrome**

Syndrome	Sinopulmonary infection	Sperm and cilia ultrastructure	Vas and epididymis	Sperm analysis	Pancreatic function	Sweat test
Immotile cilia syndrome	Present	Abnormal*	Normal sperm	Immotile	Normal	Normal
Cystic fibrosis	Present	Normal	Malformation†	Azoospermia	Abnormal	Abnormal
Young's syndrome	Present	Normal	Obstruction by inspissated secretions	Azoospermia	Normal	Normal

* Biochemical variants with enzymatic defects may also exist.

† Rare cases with intact vas and epididymides and fertility have been reported.

Source: Adapted from Handelsman et al.[542]

quency of genetic disorders.[546] Fifteen percent of men with azoospermia are found to have various genetic abnormalities, including XXY and XYY karyotypes, reciprocal autosomal and robertsonian translocations, and a variety of other abnormalities.[546] The frequency of these disorders in oligospermic men with sperm counts of 1 to 20 $\times$ 10^6/ml was 1.65 percent. In 2372 infertile men screened by Chandley, 24 had an XXY karyotype, 10 had reciprocal autosomal translocations, 5 were of the XYY karyotype, 4 had robertsonian translocations, and 8 had miscellaneous abnormalities on somatic karyotype analysis.[546]

Autoimmunity

Infertility and oligospermia occur in association with certain autoimmune disorders, such as Addison's disease and the familial autoimmune endocrine deficiency syndrome.[413] The presence of autoantibodies against the testis has been demonstrated in these subjects as well as in other patients with oligo- or azoospermia.[547] Indirect quantitative RIA detects antisperm antibodies on spermatozoa, in seminal plasma, and in the sera of men with oligospermia with greater frequency than it does in the normal population.[548] Anecdotal reports of successful immunosuppression with glucocorticoids in these patients have been published,[548] but a single randomized trial showed no benefit.[549] The exact etiologic relation between antibody formation and infertility is poorly understood.

Approach to the Diagnosis of the Infertile Male

After documentation of oligo- or azoospermia with three appropriate semen analyses, a carefully directed history should be attained.[550] A decrease in libido and potency, energy, and shaving frequency and a loss of body hair are consistent with hypogonadism. Retrograde ejaculation with spermaturia is suggested if patients void cloudy urine after intercourse. A history of testicular maldescent or trauma, prior genitourinary or hernia surgery, a past history of genitourinary infection, and a history of pain or swelling of the testes should be elicited. Systemic illnesses such as recent febrile episodes, renal disease, and inflammatory bowel disease can impair fertility. A history of recurrent respiratory illnesses is associated with Young's syndrome and obstructive azoospermia. Since in utero exposure to diethylstilbestrol may be associated with infertility in males, information regarding this risk factor should be obtained.[551] Medications and drugs can affect germ cell function. Examples include marijuana and anabolic steroids. Marijuana has been shown to damage germ cells, usually in a dose-dependent fashion, while anabolic steroids cause hypogonadotropic hypogonadism and may have a direct effect on the testes as well. Chemotherapeutic agents, primarily alkylating agents, can cause selective germ cell damage. Excessive alcohol intake can also adversely affect hypothalamic, pituitary, and gonadal function.

Physical examination requires an overall assessment of the patient's degree of virilization, body proportions, musculature, and hair distribution. Examination of the scrotal veins during a Valsalva maneuver is required to exclude a minimal varicocele. Examination of the genitourinary system should include accurate measurement of testicular volume (using a ruler, an orchidometer, or ultrasound examination) and palpation of the epididymis, checking specifically for tenderness (infection) and fullness (obstruction). Necessary laboratory data include measurements of LH, FSH, testosterone, and prolactin concentrations. Seminal fluid should be cultured if pus cells are detected on semen analysis or if excurrent duct infection is apparent. Examination of urine voided after intercourse allows documentation of retrograde ejaculation.[552] Testicular biopsy may be requested in subjects with normal FSH levels, normal testicular size, and a palpable vas deferens on physical examination. This procedure is now less commonly performed but is useful in identifying patients who are likely to have ductal obstruction. Special techniques such as assessment of hamster egg penetration or antisperm antibodies are available only to certain investigative groups but may be useful under certain circumstances. It should be emphasized that the female partner of an oligospermic male requires complete evaluation as well. Reproductive abnormalities commonly exist in both partners.

The clinician should keep in mind the relative prevalence of different etiologic disorders in infertile men. Five series which involved 3478 men[278] revealed the following frequencies of etiologies: idiopathic, 33 percent; varicocele, 25 percent; undescended testes, 7 percent; excurrent duct obstruction, 4.8 percent; mumps orchitis, 3.3 percent; hypogonadotropism, 2.3 percent; and Klinefelter's syndrome, 1.9 percent. A large category of miscellaneous etiologies remains. In another series of 280 men, testicular biopsy revealed hypospermatogenesis in 61 percent, maturation arrest in 15 percent, Sertoli-cell-only syndrome in 13 percent, normal appearance in 8 percent, hyalinized tubules in 2 percent, and immature testes in 1 percent[278] (Table 16-11).

DISORDERS ASSOCIATED WITH NONPHYSIOLOGIC SECRETION OF GONADOTROPINS

Gonadotropin-Producing Tumors

Functioning tumors of the pituitary are usually recognized because of clinical signs of hormone excess, such as acromegaly or Cushing's syndrome. Gonadotropin-producing tumors result in no distinctive clinical features. In the last several years, a group of men with large pituitary tumors and elevated FSH levels were detected during routine preoperative screening. Immunohistochemical staining of the tumor cells and demonstration of gonadotropin secretion in cell culture definitively established that these were functioning tumors.[553] One series reported elevated FSH levels in 12 of 50 men with untreated pituitary adenomas, suggesting that this tumor is not rare.[554] Clinically, the majority of these patients are men, tumors are large, and FSH concentrations correlate with tumor size. Diagnosis in postmenopausal women is difficult because both gonadotropin-producing tumors and the postmenopausal state are associated with increased FSH levels. Stimulation of the free α subunit with TRH has been proposed as a means of identifying these tumors in women.[555]

These tumors most commonly secrete FSH but may produce both LH and FSH and/or the free α and β subunits.[556,557] The production of LH alone is unusual.[558] Men with gonadotropin-producing tumors often complain of impotence and have low testosterone levels. Physiologically, these tumors are variably autonomous and are incompletely suppressed during testosterone administration.[558–560] Clomiphene citrate given as a provocative stimulatory test produces a blunted response.[559] Acute administration of GnRH causes stimulation of LH, FSH and α subunit levels in the majority of patients. Chronic administration of GnRH agonist analogues in an attempt to suppress LH and FSH is usually not effective, although gonadotropin inhibition occasionally is observed.[561] GnRH antagonist analogues do routinely suppress FSH levels[562] in short-term studies, but observation has been too short to evaluate for a reduction in tumor size. Both dopamine and bromocriptine can lower gonadotropin levels in these patients, but tumor regression is minimal.[563] Somatostatin lowered LH in one patient with an LH-producing tumor,[564] but extensive experience with this analogue is not available.

Clinically, the majority of FSH-producing tumors arise de novo, while the minority occur in the setting of long-standing testicular failure.[559,565] Because there are no detrimental effects from excess secretion of FSH, treatment includes standard surgery and radiotherapy to control mass lesion effects and testosterone replacement for the symptoms of androgen deficiency.

Precocious Puberty

Sexual precocity in boys is defined as the appearance of the physical signs of puberty before age 9. "True" precocious puberty encompasses a group of disorders characterized by premature activation of the hypothalamic-pituitary-gonadotropic axis. Two forms occur: the cerebral and idiopathic types. The specific causes are listed in Table 16-13. Hamartomas are of special interest since they contain a large amount of GnRH, have the electron microscopic characteristics of neurosecretory tissue, and may be considered GnRH-producing neoplasms.[566]

The idiopathic type includes cases of sexual precocity in which careful investigation reveals no CNS or gonadal lesion. An equal frequency of cerebral and idiopathic varieties of true precocious puberty occurs in boys. The availability of CT and MRI scans, however, will probably increase the number of patients in whom specific CNS lesions are found.

True sexual precocity begins at any age after birth and progresses in a normal, albeit premature sequence. The clinical hallmark in boys is testicular enlargement, a sign which reflects increased circulating gonadotropin concentrations. Treatment with large amounts of GnRH agonist analogues, particularly of the long-acting type, paradoxically suppresses LH secretion and provides effective therapy for these patients. The effects of these agents are rapidly reversible upon discontinuation of therapy.[567–569]

TABLE 16-13 Classification of Sexual Precocity

True or central precocity
- Idiopathic
- CNS tumors
  - Hypothalamic hamartoma (ectopic GnRH pulse generator)
  - Other tumors, e.g., optic glioma, hypothalamic astrocytoma
  - Other CNS disorders: developmental abnormalities, arachnoid cyst, infections, vascular, head trauma, cranial irradiation
  - True precocious puberty after late treatment of congenital virilizing adrenal hyperplasia or other previous chronic exposure to sex steroids

Pseudo precocious puberty
- Gonadotropin-producing tumors
  - hCG-secreting CNS tumors (e.g., chorioepithelioma, germinoma, teratoma)
  - LH-secreting pituitary adenoma
  - hCG-secreting tumors outside the CNS (hepatoma, teratoma, choriocarcinoma)
- Increased androgen secretion by adrenal or testis
  - Congenital adrenal hyperplasia
  - Primary cortisol resistance
  - Virilizing adrenal neoplasm
  - Leydig cell adenoma
  - Testis toxicosis syndrome
- Hypothyroidism
- Exogenous androgen administration

Source: Adapted from Kaplan and Grumbach.[569]

Pseudo precocious puberty occurs as a result of a primary excess in androgen secretion, independent of gonadotropic control. Congenital adrenal hyperplasia is the most common cause,[570] followed by virilizing adrenal and testicular tumors (Table 16-13). Forms of the McCune-Albright syndrome with pseudo precocious puberty, in addition to forms with true precocious puberty, have been described.[571] Recently, a type of testicular hyperplasia occurring independently of gonadotropin secretion, termed the *testis toxicosis syndrome,* has been described in several families.[572] Boys with this disorder have high testosterone levels but low gonadotropin levels. A circulating Leydig cell stimulatory factor which is not LH or hCG has been demonstrated in the blood of these patients.[572]

Treatment of pseudoprecocious puberty consists of adrenal suppression with cortisol for congenital adrenal hyperplasia and excision of virilizing tumors if present. *Testis toxicosis syndrome* can be treated with ketoconazole,[573] an inhibitor of adrenal and testicular steroidogenesis; testolactone, an aromatase inhibitor; and spironolactone, an antiandrogen.[569] Each of these approaches decreases the rate of skeletal maturation and height velocity.

CRYPTORCHISM

Pathophysiology

Cryptorchism is present when the testis does not occupy a scrotal position. In the clinical assessment of these patients, two functional types of cryptorchism exist which should be considered separately. True cryptorchism requires that the testis reside outside the scrotum permanently. *Pseudocryptorchism* or *retractile testis* is present if the gonad at times occupies a scrotal position and at other times retracts into the inguinal canal. Compensatory hypertrophy of the contralateral scrotal testis is often observed in association with true cryptorchism.

The embryologic causes of true cryptorchism are incompletely understood. One view states that the primary defect is in the testis itself. Histologic studies demonstrate that severely atrophic or dysgenetic testes may be the cause of cryptorchism in some cases. However, examination of a large number of cryptorchid testes biopsied during orchiopexy reveals that the majority of these gonads are not severely dysgenetic. The latter observation has led to the position that factors other than testicular atrophy are operative in most instances. Possible contributing causes include inadequate length of the spermatic vessels or vas deferens, insufficient size of the inguinal canal or superficial inguinal ring, and insufficient abdominal pressure to push the testes through the inguinal ring.

Another explanation—partial gonadotropin deficiency—has gained support from several recent observations. The basal LH level is low and the response to GnRH is blunted in some but not all boys with cryptorchism. Perhaps as a reflection of decreased testicular priming, increments in testosterone concentration after hCG administration are diminished in some patients. It should be noted, however, that not all investigators have confirmed these hormonal abnormalities.[574] The postulated basis for cryptorchism is that LH, in addition to maternal hCG, may be involved in the process of testicular descent during fetal life. The *gubernaculum* (Latin for "helmsman") of the testis, which pulls the testis into the scrotum, is an androgen-dependent tissue.[575] Lack of LH late in gestation might lower the testosterone concentration to a level supported only by residual hCG secretion. Consequently, gubernacular function might be insufficient to guide the testis into the scrotum. Two clinical observations support this hypothesis. First, patients with isolated gonadotropin deficiency or absent pituitaries (anencephalic patients) have a high incidence of cryptorchism. Second, treatment of cryptorchid boys with exogenous GnRH to increase their LH levels induces testicular descent.[576]

Whatever the mechanism, the descent of the testis through its normal pathway may be arrested at an abdominal, inguinal, or high scrotal position (Fig. 16-47). A patent processus vaginalis often accompanies true cryptorchism. This evagination may extend considerably farther down the scrotum than the testis and predispose to inguinal hernia, which may be associated with cryptorchism in 50 to 80 percent of cases. In certain instances, the testis may migrate through an abnormal or ectopic pathway and occupy a pubic, femoral, peritoneal, or superficial inguinal position (Fig. 16-47). When this occurs, the testis is contained in the superficial inguinal pouch, a recessed line lateral to the superficial inguinal ring. Although it has been suggested that ectopic testes result from etiologic factors that differ from those leading to inguinal cryptorchid testes, the coexistence of both ectopic and inguinal testes in patients with bilateral cryptorchism suggests that similar causes are operative in both types.

Unilateral cryptorchism is a condition which occurs in 2 to 5 percent of newborn males. The incidence decreases to approximately 0.8 percent after the first 3 months of life. Based on older studies, it was held that cryptorchid testes spontaneously enter the scrotum in late childhood or during early puberty. However, these studies failed to distinguish between retractile and truly cryptorchid testes. The natural history of pseudocryptorchid testes is that they occupy the scrotum for greater periods of time as the boy approaches puberty. Because of increasing gonadal size and a diminished cremasteric reflex, they eventually reside permanently in the scrotum. No increased risk of infertility or testicular tumor has been observed during long-term follow-up of patients with pseudocryptorchid testes.[577] By contrast, truly cryptorchid testes never reach a normal scrotal position even though they may descend somewhat as the boy approaches puberty.

Bilateral cryptorchism occurs much less commonly than does unilateral involvement. When present, this condition is more likely to be associated with a dysgenetic or defective testis than is unilateral cryptorchism. A primary cause of hypogonadism may be present; this should be suspected in patients with bilateral cryptorchism and androgen deficiency. Specific causes include isolated gonadotropin deficiency, idiopathic hypopituitarism, Prader-Labhart-Willi syndrome, Laurence-Moon syndrome, Bardet-Biedl syndrome, poly X + Y Klinefelter's syndrome (but not classic XXY Klinefelter's), and various rarer syndromes.[360] Cryptorchism is also common in patients with cerebral palsy and occurs in 40 percent of patients with mental retardation.[578]

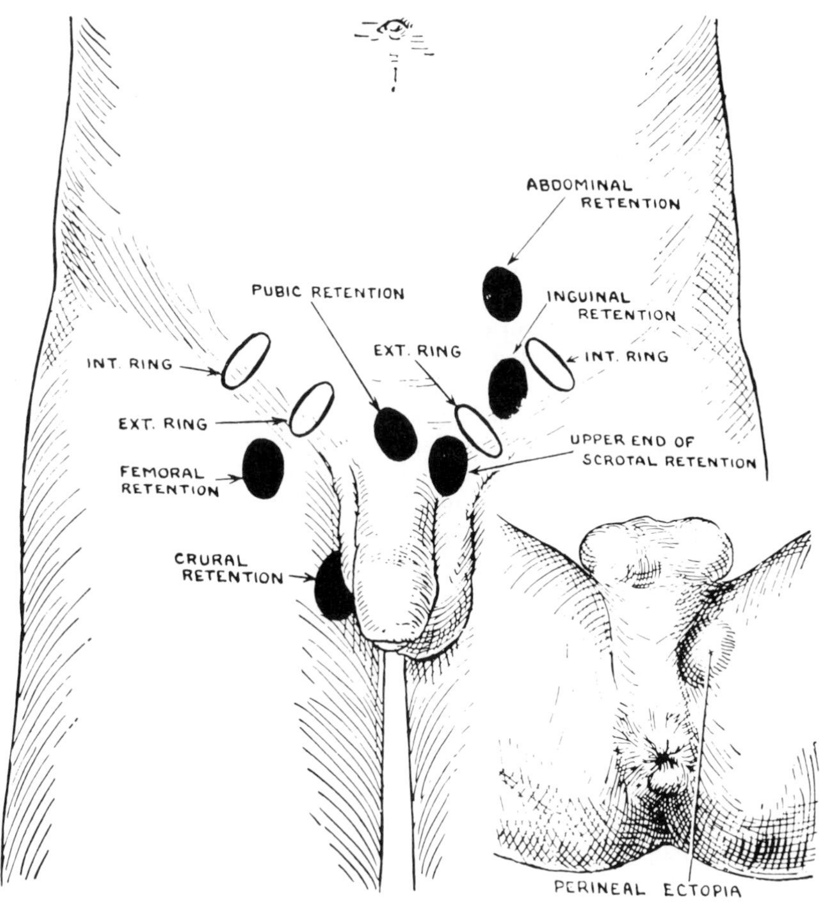

FIGURE 16-47 Sites of maldescent of the testes. [*From Santen RJ and Kulin HE, The male reproductive system, in Kelley VC (ed): Practice of Pediatrics. Philadelphia, Harper & Row, 1976.*]

The evaluation of unilateral cryptorchism requires that a pseudocryptorchid or retractile testis be differentiated from a truly cryptorchid one. This involves repeated physical examinations using special techniques. For example, the squatting position often causes retractile testes to descend spontaneously because of increased intraabdominal pressure. Examination after a warm bath may also reveal a scrotal testis when it had previously occupied an inguinal position. The parents can be instructed to examine the child at home after a bath to uncover this phenomenon.

Rationale for Treatment

Considerations regarding treatment are based on the known effects of cryptorchism on testicular function. It was initially recognized that the undescended testis is always smaller than the contralateral descended one and that the undescended testis appears somewhat atrophic on histologic examination. In patients less than 7 years of age, the volume of the unilaterally cryptorchid testis is only 64 percent of normal.[579] Recent evidence from experimental studies in rats and clinical studies in men suggests that the cryptorchid position itself is detrimental and is the primary cause of the testicular damage. For example, surgically induced cryptorchism in rats produces a progressive diminution of germ cell maturation and ultimately leads to tubular atrophy. In response to the loss of germ cells, the serum FSH concentration rises. In these animals, LH concentration also rises as a reflection of damage to Leydig cells. It is likely that germ cell destruction results at least in part from an increase in testis temperature which is produced by the intraabdominal position. Similar disruption of germ cells can be produced in rats by warming the testes by means of immersion in warm water to the temperature of the abdomen. In men, transient elevations of testicular temperature also may inhibit spermatogenesis.

Further evidence that the cryptorchid position is detrimental to germ cell maturation has been obtained in longitudinal studies. Mengel et al.[580] and Waaler[579] studied the histologic appearance of cryptorchid testes in boys of increasing age and compared them with the subjects' contralateral normal testes. For precise characterization, they accurately counted the germ cells and measured the diameter of the seminiferous tubule. It was clear that the cryptorchid testis becomes progressively more atrophic compared with the age-matched normal testis. From these observations, they concluded that the cryptorchid position itself produces progressive testicular damage. Additional studies have shown that the contralateral scrotal testis may also undergo progressive damage in boys with unilateral cryptorchism. Although this phenomenon can be produced experimentally in dogs, the mechanism is unknown.

An important practical question is whether cryptorchid testes brought into the scrotum recover function as a result of the altered position of the testis. The available data suggest that some improvement in the histologic appearance of cryptorchid testes may be expected if the operation is performed before the onset of puberty. The functional capacity for sperm production may be improved as well. Studies of patients with bilateral cryptorchism reveal that the fertility rate may be as high as 70 to 80 percent in subjects operated on before age 10. Without an operation, such individuals are rarely fertile. Even though improvement in function occurs after orchiopexy, some degree of functional impairment persists after surgery. In one elegantly conceived study, unilateral vasectomy on the contralateral side allowed the study of the function of the once-cryptorchid testis. Sperm were detected in only 4 of 12 men.[581] Follow-up studies have revealed elevations of FSH and, on occasion, LH concentrations in boys operated on for bilateral cryptorchism. It is encouraging to note that serum gonadotropin levels remained normal in boys with unilateral cryptorchism who were treated with surgical intervention.

David et al.[582] extensively reviewed the available literature regarding sperm counts in men who had previously undergone unilateral or bilateral orchiopexy. Fifty-two percent of 296 men with bilateral orchiopexy and 21 percent of 247 with unilateral orchiopexy exhibited azoospermia on later semen analysis. Similarly, spermatogenesis was adequate in only 13 percent and 30 percent, respectively. Unfortunately, the age at which these patients underwent surgery did not correlate with the degree of germ cell abnormalities found.

Another consideration regarding treatment is the malignant potential of a cryptorchid testis. It has been stated that a cryptorchid testis has a 20-fold greater chance of becoming malignant than a scrotal one if it resides in the inguinal canal and a 50-fold greater risk if it is intraabdominal. Testicular tumors are rare, however, occurring in only 1 to 2 in 100,000 males. Thus, the prevalence of malignancy in cryptorchid testes should approximate only 20 to 100 per 100,000. However, over a 60-year lifetime, the incidence may be as high as 6000 per 100,000 (6 percent). One study found a prevalence of malignancy of 8 percent,[583] predominantly carcinoma in situ, in prospectively biopsied cryptorchid testes.

Even when brought into the scrotum, a cryptorchid testis retains its malignant potential.[584] It has been argued that early detection of a testicular tumor is easier if the testis resides in the scrotum rather than in the inguinal canal. This rationale for treating by orchiopexy is not totally convincing; several investigators now recommend orchiectomy for unilaterally cryptorchid testes in older boys or when the testis is small or dysgenetic.

Treatment

A current recommendation regarding the treatment of boys is that orchiopexy be carried out if testicular descent is not observed after hCG therapy.[584] Medical treatment with hCG produces varying results, depending on the group studied. When pseudocryptorchism was carefully excluded, 24 percent of patients with unilateral cryptorchism aged 2 to 5 responded with testicular descent in one study.[585] In a randomized trial, only 4 out of 33 boys experienced testicular descent with either hCG or GnRH.[586]

As a matter of clinical practice, it is reasonable to administer a trial course of hCG, 1000 to 4000 IU three times weekly for 6 weeks, to avoid unnecessary surgery in boys proved to have true cryptorchism on repeated examination.[587] GnRH represents an alternative therapy. Subjects who do not respond to hCG (or GnRH) should undergo orchiopexy and correction of the associated hernia if one is present.[587] The appropriate age for performing the orchiopexy is controversial. Some experts recommend the procedure between ages 6 months and 18 months to allow preservation of spermatogenesis.[584] Others find no evidence favoring early operation[588,589] and suggest a delay until just before puberty.

GYNECOMASTIA

Overview

In prepubertal boys, as in girls, parenchymal and stromal cells with a potential for full breast development are present beneath the nipples. Experimental and clinical studies indicate that both stimulatory and inhibitory hormones control the growth and differentiation of these tissues (Fig. 16-48). Estradiol stimulates the cellular growth and proliferation of parenchymal epithelium to form ductal elements. Prolactin primarily acts on differentiated breast acini to stimulate the synthesis of milk protein. In tissue culture, mammary cells require the presence of GH, insulin, and cortisol as permissive factors for growth, but specific effects on differentiated function are not clearly defined. Testosterone exerts a generalized inhibitory action on breast tissue growth and differentiation, perhaps through a specific antiestrogenic action.[590] Also, certain regulatory hormones modulate systemic hormonal effects, which in turn influence breast growth and differentiation. Thyroxine increases the levels of TeBG and serum estradiol concentration and thus exerts indirect effects on the breast. Both cortisol and prolactin lower circulating testosterone levels through hypothalamic and testicular effects. Thus, they diminish inhibitory influences on the breast.

The application of these physiologic principles allows gynecomastia to be considered on a pathophysiologic basis. A disordered balance between secretion of stimulatory hormones and that of inhibitory hormones underlies the development of the pathologic forms of gynecomastia in men. Gynecomastia may also occur as a normal physiologic process at various stages of life. Major emphasis has been placed on the balance between estradiol, the major facilitative hormone, and testosterone as an inhibitor in both the physiologic and pathologic types.

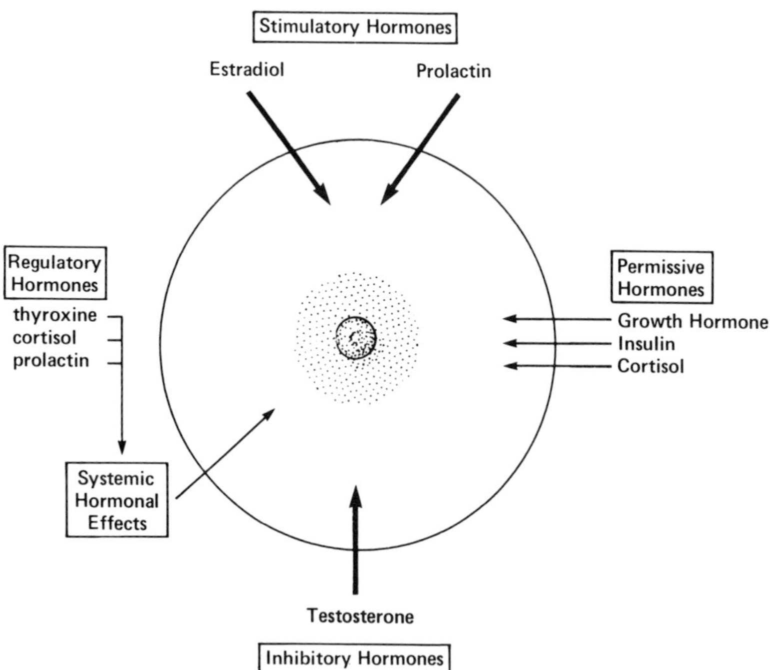

FIGURE 16-48 Diagrammatic representation of the hormones which affect breast tissue.

Physiologic Forms of Gynecomastia

Pubertal Gynecomastia

Beginning at age 11, approximately 30 percent of boys develop detectable gynecomastia (i.e., glandular tissue >0.5 cm in diameter); by age 14, gynecomastia is detectable in 65 percent.[591] Surprisingly, unilateral gynecomastia is common, occurring on the left in 19 percent, the right in 26 percent, and bilaterally in 55 percent of those with palpable breast tissue.[592] Gynecomastia resolves spontaneously in the majority after 1 year. Hormonal alterations in boys with gynecomastia are not consistently found and are variably reported as low free testosterone, increased estradiol, elevated estradiol/testosterone ratio, and increased TeBG levels.[592–597]

Adult Gynecomastia

Four studies[598–601] found that gynecomastia was present in hospitalized adults with high prevalence; patients and physicians, however, were found to have minimal awareness of the existence of the condition. Thirty-three percent of men in their mid-20s and 57 percent between ages 45 and 59 had palpable breast tissue which exceeded 2 cm in diameter. These findings do not appear to represent pseudogynecomastia as a result of fat deposition beneath the nipple. Autopsy confirmed the physical findings in 60 consecutive cases in one study[601] and independently detected gynecomastia in another. For example, in Williams's study,[602] 50 percent of the men had gynecomastia, 31 percent with stromal and 9 percent with glandular predominance at autopsy.

In 83 percent of hospitalized men with gynecomastia, the diameter of breast tissue was 5 cm or less.[601] The etiology of this form of physiologic gynecomastia is not clear but is thought to reflect increased aromatase activity in adipose tissue. Aromatase activity increases as a function of body fat. In support of this theory, the diameter of breast tissue correlated significantly ($r = 0.52$) with body mass index in a group of 214 well-studied men.[601]

Pathologic Forms of Gynecomastia

In adolescence, a group of boys develop an exaggerated form of gynecomastia with breast development to Tanner stages III (>4 cm of glandular breast tissue), IV (nearly adult female), or V (normal adult female). This condition, called *persistent pubertal macromastia,* is not associated with specific endocrine disorders or recognized hormonal or receptor abnormalities.[603] Tumors of the testis or adrenal and exogenous sources of estrogen are rare causes of gynecomastia in prepubertal or pubertal boys.

Etiologies of the pathologic forms of gynecomastia in adults are multiple, but the physiologic variety is common. Consequently, the clinician must be concerned only when there is breast tenderness, a progressive increase in breast size, or enlargement beyond the physiologic range (2 to 5 cm). A logical approach to the differential diagnosis can then be based on known physiology (Table 16-14). An excess of breast-stimulatory hormones, a deficiency of inhibitory ones, a stimulatory-inhibitory imbalance, or abnormalities of the regulatory hormones cause gynecomastia in the majority of patients. The remainder of cases remain largely idiopathic or of uncertain cause.

The differential diagnosis of gynecomastia is extensive and difficult to remember because of the variety of causes. Two approaches are useful for the clinician: consideration of the various disorders on a pathophysiologic basis (Table 16-14) and practical attention to the most frequent causes of this condition (Fig. 16-49). With the first approach, the etiologies of gynecomastia are considered with respect to each specific hormone. Certain disorders, such as adrenal tumors, are associated with clear elevations of plasma estradiol secretion. Other conditions are characterized by increased conversion of androgens to estrogens in glandular and nonglandular tissues. The enzyme responsible for this conversion—aromatase—is present in fat, muscle, and liver as well as in breast tissue. Obesity, liver disease, and rare genetic disorders are associated with increased aromatase activity and gynecomastia.[604] Aromatase may also be increased in pubic skin fibroblasts,[605] testis tissue,[606] and testicular tumors.[274] In addition, the gynecomastia associated with early puberty and the administration of aromatizable androgens to hypogonadal men may be related to excess aromatase activity.[607]

Prolactin secretion is modulated by central aminergic neuronal pathways, particularly of the dopaminergic variety. A wide range of drugs with catecholamine-antagonizing or depleting actions can stimulate prolactin release. Either through direct effects on the breast or through a regulatory alteration of gonadotropin and testosterone secretion, these drugs can cause gynecomastia.

Drugs which inhibit the biosynthesis or action of androgens may be associated with gynecomastia. Syndromes of androgen resistance represent experiments of nature in which a deficiency of androgen action causes gynecomastia. Among the most common examples of androgen antagonistic drugs are spironolactone, flutamide, and cimetidine.[599,608] Drugs with estrogenic effects such as digitoxin also cause gynecomastia.

The hypergonadotropic syndromes as a group are associated with relative deficiency of androgen secretion. The compensatory increase in LH and FSH secretion appears to induce a relative rise in estradiol concentration. The resulting imbalance between estrogen and androgen commonly produces gynecomastia. Klinefelter's syndrome, with an 85 percent prevalence of gynecomastia, is typical of this condition, but

TABLE 16-14 Causes of Gynecomastia

Stimulatory hormone excess
  Estradiol
    Adrenal or testicular tumors
    Drug therapy with
      Estrogens
      Estrogen analogues: *digitoxin**
      Estrogen precursors: aromatizable androgens
        Testosterone enanthate
        Testosterone propionate
  Increased peripheral aromatase activity due to
    Heredity
    Obesity
  Prolactin
    Pituitary tumor
    Drug therapy with
      Catecholamine antagonists or depleters
        Sulpiride *Phenothiazines*
        Metoclopropamide *Reserpine*
        Domperidone *Tricyclic antidepressants*
        Methyldopa
    Hypothyroidism
Inhibitory hormone deficiency
  Androgen resistance
    Complete testicular feminization
    Partial: Reifenstein, Lubbs, Rosewater, and Dreyfus syndromes
  Androgen antagonist drugs
    Spironolactone *Progestagens*
    Cimetidine *Flutamide*
    Marijuana
Stimulatory-inhibitory hormone imbalance
  Hypergonadotropic syndromes
    Primary gonadal diseases
    Cytotoxic drug-induced hypogonadism from
      Busulfan *Nitrosourea*
      Vincristine *Combination chemotherapy*
    Tumor-related: hCG-producing tumors (testis, lung, GI tract, etc.)
    hCG administration
  Hypogonadotropic syndromes
    Isolated gonadotropin deficiency, particularly "fertile eunuch syndrome"
    Panhypopituitarism
  System illnesses
    Severe liver disease
    Renal disease
Miscellaneous endocrine causes
  Hyperthyroidism
  Acromegaly
  Cushing's syndrome
Local trauma
  Hip spica cast
  Chest injury
Primary breast tumor
Uncertain causes
  Refeeding
  Other chronic illnesses
    Pulmonary tuberculosis
    Diabetes mellitus
  Persistent pubertal macromastia
  Idiopathic

* Drugs are listed in *italics*.

other genetic disorders and drugs can produce similar findings. Less well explained is the estrogen-androgen imbalance associated with hypopituitarism and systemic illness such as renal disease.

The rapid onset of gynecomastia in an adult patient should elicit suspicion of an underlying neoplastic disease. Lung, gastrointestinal (GI), and testis tumors produce hCG, which stimulates estradiol out of proportion to testosterone and causes gynecomastia. Other endocrine disorders produce gynecomastia through the secretion of hormones which indirectly influence breast growth. For example, hyperthyroidism appears to increase estradiol levels[609] and cortisol excess inhibits testosterone production. Prolactin excess may cause gynecomastia by this mechanism as well, since it reduces testosterone secretion.

Local chest trauma is associated with gynecomastia, probably related to local stimulation of breast tissue or afferent neurologic influences. Breast neoplasms characteristically are asymmetric. A hard nodule is palpable on examination. Breast carcinoma is rare in males and is not usually confused with gynecomastia.

The remaining causes of gynecomastia are uncertain. One form associated with refeeding was first recognized when prisoners of war in World War II were renourished after a period of starvation. A similar situation pertains when patients with chronic illnesses recover and regain weight. The gynecomastia associated with tuberculosis or diabetes mellitus may be similarly related to regain of weight.[599] An idiopathic category is also seen in which extensive evaluation reveals no definite cause.

For the clinician, knowledge of the frequency of these disorders provides information of practical use. To the general internist, the most frequent causes of gynecomastia are (1) the combination of systemic illness and use of drugs known to cause gynecomastia, (2) the use of drugs alone, and (3) regain of weight after a severe nutritional insult (refeeding gynecomastia) (Fig. 16-49). Liver disease is also commonly associated with gynecomastia, but the frequency of this finding in men with cirrhosis compared with other hospitalized patients has recently been questioned.[610] Patients with various disorders of hormone excess or gonadal insufficiency are referred to the endocrinologist. Endocrinologists are also asked to evaluate many patients in whom no etiology is diagnosed.

Evaluation

The clinician must decide when to evaluate men with gynecomastia, a condition found in approximately 50 percent of hospitalized men. Clear indications for evaluation include breast tenderness, rapid enlargement, and eccentric or hard irregular masses and lesions >5 cm. Asymptomatic stable gynecomastia

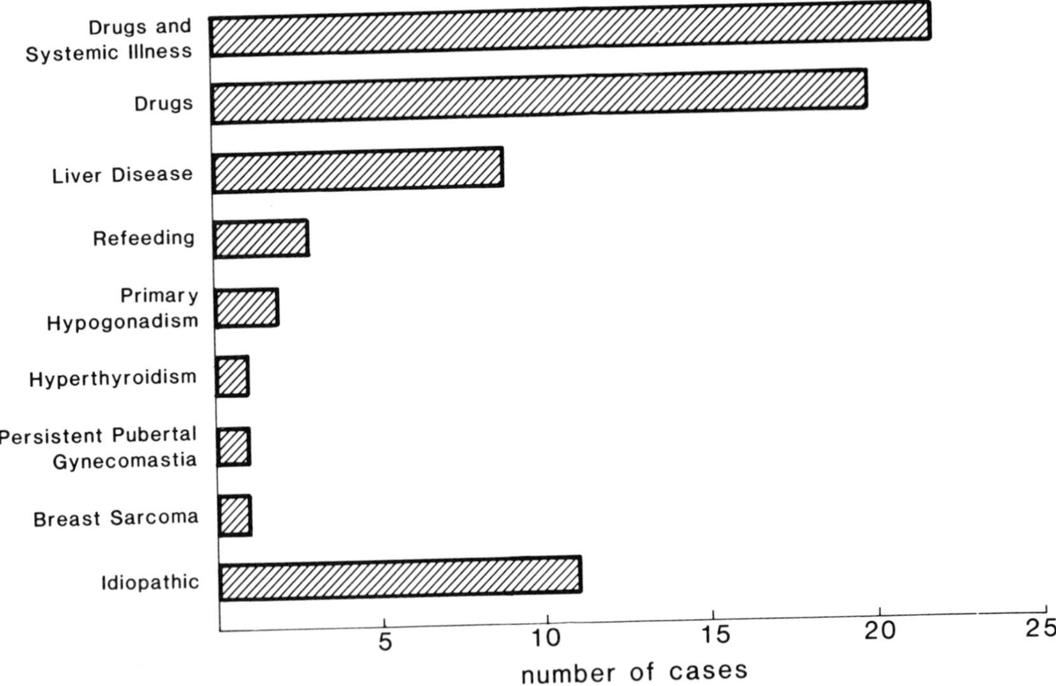

FIGURE 16-49 Frequency of etiologies of gynecomastia in men hospitalized at a Veterans Administration hospital. The "drugs and systemic illness" category included patients with male climacteric, cirrhosis, hepatitis, hyperthyroidism, refeeding syndrome, and primary hypogonadism. The "drugs" category included α-methyldopa, phenothiazines, amitriptyline, imipramine, spironolactone, isoniazid, testosterone, narcotics, estradiol, amphetamines, and reserpine. (*From Carlson.*[599])

<5 cm in diameter, particularly in obese patients, probably requires only a careful history and physical examination for evaluation. In lean subjects, gynecomastia with a breast diameter of 2 to 5 cm should probably be evaluated more extensively.

After deciding that it is warranted, an evaluation should be initiated, including in all patients (1) a careful drug history, (2) identification of the presence of systemic renal, hepatic, cardiac, or pulmonary disease and particularly previous malnutrition due to other disorders, (3) detection of obvious signs and symptoms of underlying malignancy, especially testicular, and (4) detection of clinically evident syndromes of estradiol, prolactin, GH, cortisol, or thyroxine excess or androgen deficiency.

If the initial evaluation is unrevealing, screening tests to exclude the presence of a neoplasm, including measurement of β-hCG as a tumor marker and a chest x-ray to rule out pulmonary carcinoma, should be performed on all patients. Clinical judgement then dictates whether additional studies such as thyroxine, prolactin, LH, FSH, estradiol, testosterone, and DHEA sulfate concentrations should be obtained. After this evaluation, many patients, particularly those referred to an endocrinologist, remain in the idiopathic category.

Treatment

Specific therapy for treatable disease should be used when feasible, and offending drugs should be discontinued. Reduction mammoplasty is required under certain clinical circumstances. Persistent pubertal macromastia resistant to medical therapy requires surgical excision.[603] Reduction mammoplasty occasionally is necessary in men with painful or cosmetically disabling lesions. A highly experienced surgeon should be asked to perform this procedure because of the precise sculpturing necessary to produce the desired cosmetic effects. Boys with pubertal gynecomastia can generally be reassured that regression usually occurs after 1 year and at most after 3 years.[591,592] Medical therapy has been considered when gynecomastia is severe or of prolonged duration. The use of antiestrogens to block estrogen action, stimulate testosterone secretion, and alter the estrogen-androgen balance has been evaluated. Improvement has been seen in some but not all patients.[611,612] The administration of nonaromatizable androgens, such as DHT, which lower estradiol concentration and increase androgen levels is associated with an improvement in gynecomastia.[613,614] The aromatase inhibitor testolactone has also been used to suppress estradiol but not androgen levels.[615] While each of these medications can be considered, the results are generally disappointing. Surgical therapy with reduction mammoplasty is usually required for a successful outcome, and this approach is offered without a prior trial of medical therapy.

IMPOTENCE

Impotence is defined as the inability to achieve or sustain an erection for a sufficient duration to have coitus. Disorders of libido or orgasmic potential should be distinguished from impotence. The frequency of impotence increases with age such that 1.9 percent of men at age 40 and 25 percent of men at age 65 experience this symptom.[616] The causes of impotence can be divided into five general categories: psychogenic, vascular, neuropathic, endocrinologic, and drug-related.

Psychogenic impotence is the most common type and the primary one in approximately 90 percent of individuals who present with this complaint for the first time. Patients with psychogenic impotence often recount alternating periods of normal potency and impotence. Suggestive historical features include a history of premature ejaculation or stress-related premature detumescence, abrupt onset of impotence after heavy alcohol ingestion, and maintenance of normal libido but loss of potency. Characteristically, physiologic control of the erectile process remains intact; these individuals continue to experience morning and sleep-related erections and retain the ability to masturbate.

Impotence of vascular insufficiency is often associated with symptoms of intermittent claudication, angina, or transient ischemic attacks of the anterior or posterior cerebral circulation. Historical features suggesting *neuropathic impotence* include stocking-glove paresthesias, symptoms of autonomic insufficiency, and a history of diabetes mellitus or renal disease. *Endocrine-related impotence* causes decreased libido as well as potency, loss of morning erections, inability to masturbate, and, after a prolonged period, loss of secondary sex characteristics. *Drug-related impotence* is obvious, provided that the physician considers the diagnosis.

The physical examination is directed toward careful assessment of secondary sex characteristics and testicular size. The neurologic examination should include sensory testing of the penis and perineum and an evaluation of the bulbocavernous reflex. The vascular examination involves assessment of the arteries in the penis and lower extremities. Detection of normal prolactin and free testosterone concentrations in the morning (to eliminate diurnal variability) practically excludes an endocrinologic cause. The major clinical problem, then, is to distinguish between organic and psychogenic impotence. Quantitative assessment of nocturnal penile tumescence and correlation with EEG sleep stages are the best methods for assessing nocturnal erections. The snap gauge band provides a home screening device, and the Rigiscan provides a more quantitative instrument for home detection of nocturnal erections.[617,618] Documentation of a low testosterone concentration in the morning favors the diagnosis of endocrine-related impotence. A specific endocrinologic etiology should then be sought among the various causes of hypo- and hypergonadotropic hypogonadism described in this chapter.

A recent report described a group of impotent men with low testosterone concentration and secretion of normal amounts of immunologically detectable but reduced bioactive LH in association with mild reductions in plasma testosterone.[619] The altered ratio of biological to immunologically detectable LH was ascribed to pulsatile GnRH secretion of lower than normal amplitude. Further studies of these patients are required to establish physicochemical alterations of the LH molecule.[620]

Treatment of impotence related to androgen deficiency involves the administration of adequate amounts of testosterone. Objective measures of erectile function improve in hypogonadal men who receive this therapy.[621] Testosterone enanthate, 200 mg every 2 weeks, can be given as a therapeutic trial. As confirmation of a physiologic rather than a placebo response, the physician can substitute a sterile vehicle for 1-month periods with 1-month androgen replacement therapy interspersed.

Treatment of impotence related to prolactin excess first requires that the specific etiology of hyperprolactinemia be evaluated. Prolactin levels should then be lowered with bromocriptine before androgen therapy is initiated. As emphasized above, impotence often persists when prolactin levels are elevated even if the testosterone deficiency is corrected.

Approaches to the diagnosis and therapy of impotence of a nonendocrine nature requires extensive laboratory and clinical support. A full discussion is beyond the scope of this chapter. Several reviews provide comprehensive information on this topic.[616,622–624]

MALE CONTRACEPTION

Investigative groups are actively pursuing the development of a practical male contraceptive. Suppression of LH and FSH release with weekly or biweekly injections of testosterone enanthate reduces spermatogenesis but does not produce azoospermia in all men.[625,626] In the subgroup achieving azoospermia, the fertility rate is quite low when observed prospectively.[625] However, 20 to 40 percent of men do not achieve azoospermia with these regimens, and trials are being initiated to determine the fertility of those with reduced sperm production. The basis for these trials is that sperm function may be reduced sufficiently in these oligospermic men to render them infertile. Combinations of injectable testosterone with impeded androgens such as danazole, progestins such as medroxyprogesterone acetate, or antiandrogens such as cyproterone are also incompletely effective. A direct inhibitor of spermatogenesis—gossypol—produces azoospermia without androgen deficiency but has been abandoned because it is too toxic. Another approach combines injectable testosterone with agonist analogues of GnRH which paradoxically inhibit LH and FSH release. While azoospermia can be achieved in some men, uniform and complete reduction of spermatogenesis may not be possible.[627] The most recent approach utilizes GnRH antagonists followed 2 weeks later by injectable androgen supplementation. Azoospermia occurred in the majority of the small number of subjects observed in two trials.[628,629] Further studies with these regimens are being pursued.

Several years will be required for the development of safe, practical, acceptable pharmacologic contraception for men. In the meantime, vasectomy and the use of condoms are generally applicable methods. Immunologic abnormalities detected in the monkey as a complication of vasectomy and accelerated coronary artery disease[630] have not been demonstrated in human patients, although further surveillance will be required.

TESTICULAR TUMORS

Testicular neoplasms represent 1 percent of all malignant tumors in men. They are 20-fold to 50-fold more common in cryptorchid or once-cryptorchid testes. Four predominant types of germ cell malignancies affect the testis: seminomas, embryonal cell carcinomas, teratomas, and choriocarcinomas. Fourteen possible combinations of these basic types, called *compound tumors,* are observed. Two tumor markers, β-hCG and alpha-fetoprotein, provide useful information regarding the prognosis at the time of initial evaluation and permit detection of early recurrence during follow-up observation. While seminoma has always been a highly curable tumor, major advances in chemotherapy for the other germinal cell tumors have markedly improved the prognosis in these patients. The reader is referred to reviews for a full discussion of the diagnosis, surgery, and chemotherapeutic regimens for the treatment of these neoplasms.[631–634]

Recent studies have identified an early form of testicular carcinoma in situ. This lesion was first recognized in 6 of 555 testes examined during studies of infertile men.[635] Within 1.3 to 4.5 years, four of these men developed invasive carcinoma. Krabbe and coworkers then recalled 180 men with corrected cryptorchism; 50 agreed to undergo biopsy of the testes. Eight percent were found to have carcinoma in situ on biopsy.[583] This preliminary observation suggests that testicular cancer may be identified early.

Nongerminal cell tumors of the testis are rare; they are diagnosed because of their steroid hormone–secreting nature. Sertoli or Leydig cell tumors may produce estrogens or androgens; they are generally benign.[90,636] Patients with these tumors develop gynecomastia or pseudo precocious puberty. In those with gynecomastia, basal estradiol levels may be elevated and estradiol responses to hCG may be prolonged. This latter finding, which initially was proposed as a method to detect testicular tumors, is nonspecific and has been seen in other patients with gynecomastia.[637]

One type of Sertoli cell tumor occurs in patients with familial Peutz-Jeghers syndrome. In this condition, enhanced estrogen synthesis occurs as a direct result of very high tumor levels of aromatase, even in the absence of elevated testosterone substrate.[274] Adrenal rest tumors occur in boys with incompletely treated congenital adrenal hyperplasia.[638] Tumor regression in these patients is observed after adequate suppression of ACTH with exogenous hydrocortisone. Gonadal, stromal, and compound tumors of nongerminal cell origin may also be encountered. A recent advance is the use of testicular ultrasound to detect occult testicular tumors even before they are palpable on physical examination.[639]

ANDROGEN-DEPENDENT NEOPLASIA

One hundred twenty-two thousand new cases of prostate cancer are diagnosed in the United States yearly. A clinical staging system has been developed and is widely applied to this disease.[640] Treatment decisions are based on prior studies with patients in each of these stages.[640a] Current recommendations advise that only patients with stage D_2 (metastatic) disease and preferably those who are symptomatic be started on endocrine therapy. This recommendation is based on the fact that hormonal therapies have not been shown to cure prostate cancer or prolong patient survival. Although a preliminary report from the Mayo Clinic suggested an improved chance of survival from endocrine therapy in stage D_1 disease, confirmation is required since an imbalance in prognostic factors such as tumor ploidy might explain this finding.[641]

Choices of endocrine therapy at present include surgical orchiectomy, estrogen treatment, the use of GnRH analogues, inhibition of androgen biosynthesis, combination of low-dose estrogen with progestin, and combinations of agents which eliminate the effects of both testicular and adrenal androgens (complete androgen blockade) (Fig. 16-50). A number of

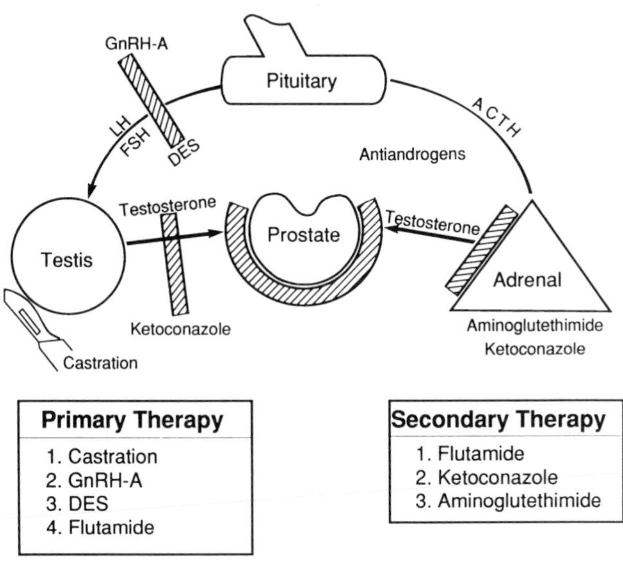

FIGURE 16-50 Diagrammatic representation of various types of primary and secondary hormonal therapies for prostate cancer. Complete androgen blockade involves measures designed to block the synthesis or action of androgens and androgen precursors made by the testes and adrenals.

considerations favor the use of orchiectomy as the method of first choice for reducing androgen levels. No therapy has been shown to be clearly superior to orchiectomy in relieving symptoms or providing a durable progression-free interval. Problems with accelerated cardiovascular disease have not been encountered as with estrogen therapy. The reduction in androgen levels takes place within hours of the removal of the testes. Patient compliance is not an issue. The incidence of impotence and loss of libido is the same as with other therapies. The lowering of androgen levels continues no matter what later therapy is chosen.

A number of patients refuse orchiectomy and prefer medical therapy. Prior to studies with the GnRH superagonist analogues, estrogen was the preferred form of "medical castration." The rationale is to inhibit LH release by the pituitary and thereby lower plasma androgens to castrate levels. However, in a series of studies, excessive estrogen doses accelerated cardiovascular death rates while insufficient amounts did not completely suppress testosterone levels.[640] These data suggest that it may not be possible to suppress testicular androgens completely without enhancing the risk of cardiovascular death. Estrogens also may produce gynecomastia, fluid retention and congestive heart failure, thrombophlebitis, and nausea. These problems with estrogen provided an impetus for the development of GnRH superagonist analogues (GnRH-A) as a means of suppressing androgen. The GnRH-A paradoxically inhibit LH secretion by the pituitary and thus suppress testicular testosterone production to castrate levels (approximately 20 ng/dl). No escape from inhibition occurs during the 5 years of continuous treatment,[642] and efficacy is equal to that of surgical orchiectomy.

All the GnRH-A transiently stimulate LH threefold to fourfold and testosterone twofold for 1 to 2 weeks immediately upon the initiation of therapy. Thereafter, LH levels are profoundly suppressed. The transient increase in testosterone can be associated with worsening of bone pain or other cancer-related symptoms in up to 10 percent of patients and with an objective tumor "flare" in approximately 3 percent. However, no cardiovascular or other toxic effects have been associated with GnRH-A use. Randomized, controlled trials of GnRH-A in adequate dosage vs. orchiectomy or diethylstilbestrol (DES) have demonstrated similar rates and durations of response with each of these treatments. These considerations favor the use of the GnRH-A over the use of estrogens to produce medical castration. With the availability of once-monthly biodegradable preparations of GnRH-A, this approach should supplant estrogen therapy and possibly orchiectomy in the future.

One problem remains with the GnRH agonists: the initial disease flare phenomenon. While rare, severe complications such as tumor-induced spinal cord compression have been reported to occur. For this reason, coadministration of an antiandrogen such as flutamide, an androgen biosynthesis inhibitor such as ketoconazole, or an estrogen (DES) for 1 week before and 2 to 3 weeks after the initiation of GnRH-A is advisable, particularly in patients with a large tumor burden.

Other medical approaches, such as the antiandrogens flutamide and cyproterone acetate, the androgen biosynthesis inhibitor ketoconazole, and low-dose estrogen plus antiandrogen, are efficacious therapies for prostate cancer.[643–646] However, the various side effects of these agents and a lack of comparable data from controlled trials relegate their use to second-line treatment.

Secondary Endocrine Treatments

Initial responses to hormonal treatment in men with prostate cancer persist for a median duration of 12 to 18 months. After relapse, several means of further reducing hormone secretion remain. However, the use of secondary maneuvers is controversial. The dispute rests on two issues: the degree of production of androgens or preandrogens by the adrenal and the persistence of hormonally dependent cells in the tumor after orchiectomy. Direct venous catheterization studies indicate that the production of androgens by the adrenals accounts for 5 percent of the total androgen pool in adult men.[644] One-twelfth of the DHT in prostatic tissue originates from adrenal androgen precursors.[643] Evidence for the existence of an androgen-dependent subpopulation of cells that persists after surgical orchiectomy is provided by two observations. First, objective responses to surgical adrenalectomy or medical adrenalectomy with aminoglutethimide occur in 10 to 20 percent of castrate men with prostate cancer.[645,646] Second, early studies of androgen administration in such patients, a maneuver analogous to DES administration to breast cancer patients, results in increased bone pain or objective disease progression in nearly three-quarters of patients. Practical clinical considerations have tempered enthusiasm for secondary endocrine therapy for prostate cancer. Responses consist predominantly of stabilization of disease or relief of bone pain, whereas fewer men experience objective tumor regression. In contrast to the situation in breast cancer, receptor determinations have not been studied as a potential means of identifying patients who will respond objectively. The average duration of benefit is short, with a median of only 6 months.

Nonetheless, nontoxic medical treatments to inhibit androgen biosynthesis or antagonize androgen action as secondary therapy for prostate cancer are probably warranted in selected patients. The adrenal steroidogenesis inhibitor aminoglutethimide, in combination with hydrocortisone, produces objective tumor regression in 10 to 20 percent of patients and disease stabilization in 25 percent of the others.[645,646] Responders survive approximately 12 months longer than do nonresponders. This therapy is associated with a transient skin rash and persistent lethargy but can produce impressive relief of bone pain. The antiandrogen flutamide produced similar responses, with a 15.8 percent rate of objective regression and 18.7 percent stabilization in 209 patients.[647] Other than mild nausea and diarrhea, this agent causes few side effects. Ketoconazole, an inhibitor of $C_{17\text{-}20}$ lyase, also blocks adrenal androgens and produces secondary responses. The side effects of this agent (nausea and occasional hepatotoxicity) make it less desirable than flutamide or aminoglutethimide. Based on this analysis, flutamide is the preferred secondary endocrine treatment for prostate cancer.

Proper selection of appropriate patients for secondary therapy is important. Men with a prolonged response to the first endocrine therapy or with a relatively indolent course are the best candidates. The physician must balance the benefits of relatively nontoxic endocrine therapy against the more toxic and not necessarily more effective chemotherapy. It should be emphasized that radiation therapy to painful bony lesions should be utilized liberally at the same time hormonal therapy is being used.

Complete Androgen Blockade

A new strategy for the endocrine treatment of prostate cancer—complete androgen blockade—has been proposed.[648] The rationale for this approach is based on the concept that the adrenal contributes 5 percent to the total androgen pool and that this amount of androgen supports the viability of a fraction of hormone-dependent cells. Ablation of adrenal as well as testicular androgens initially rather than sequentially might then produce more efficacious results in patients. Based on this rationale, men with stage D (metastatic) disease have been treated primarily with a combination of either orchiectomy or a GnRH superagonist analogue to eliminate testicular androgens and a nonsteroidal antiandrogen (either flutamide or anandron) to block adrenal androgen action.

This approach has been highly controversial, particularly since initial reports involving nonrandomized trials suggested highly favorable results.[648] Data from a wide variety of randomized trials are becoming available.[643] The majority indicate no prolongation of disease-free or overall survival with complete androgen blockade.[643,649] However, an ongoing, large, well-designed multicenter trial in the United States is allowing this controversial issue to be placed in a more focused perspective. At present, 617 patients have been entered into this study (National Institutes of Health–sponsored Southwestern Oncology Group/Eastern Cooperative Oncology Intergroup Study), and 603 patients are evaluable. The combination of Leuprolide (a GnRH-A) and a placebo is being compared with GnRH-A plus flutamide as an initial treatment in stage D_2 patients.[649,650] Only a modest benefit results from the concomitant use of antiandrogen. For example, the median time to progression was 16.9 months for men receiving GnRH-A plus flutamide vs. 13.9 months for men receiving GnRH-A plus placebo. Median survival was prolonged to 35.9 months vs. 28.3 months. These data suggest that adrenal androgens provide a real but minimal stimulus to prostate tumor growth under these circumstances. Another interpretation is that only a subset of men benefit from complete androgen blockade. To address this issue, the Intergroup study (SWOG-ECOG) performed a post hoc subset analysis.[649,650] Eighty-two patients with minimal disease were identified. The criteria for minimal disease included disease limited to retroperitoneal nodes and/or the axial but not appendicular skeleton. The 41 patients in the placebo group had a median survival of 39.6 months, whereas those in the flutamide group have not yet reached the median survival duration at the 50-month follow-up. It appears that this subgroup may achieve an important benefit from complete androgen blockade.

Several issues regarding complete androgen blockade remain to be resolved. First, the results in stage D_2 patients with minimal disease require confirmation in additional studies with patients in this category randomized prospectively to each treatment group. Second, the superiority of complete androgen blockade to sequential use of castration (or GnRH-A) followed by adrenal blockade should be confirmed in additional studies. Third, the intergroup study should be supported by additional trials, preferably comparing castration alone with castration plus antiandrogens, before definitive conclusions regarding complete androgen blockade can be made.

A conservative assessment suggests that complete androgen blockade offers some advantage over standard approaches, particularly in the subset of patients with minimal disease (i.e., retroperitoneal nodes and/or axial skeletal metastases). While additional studies are being completed, the approach of complete androgen blockade could be offered to patients after a full discussion of the currently known risks and benefits.

REFERENCES

1. Moore RY: Neuroendocrine regulation of reproduction, in Yen SSC, Jaffe RB (eds): *Reproductive Endocrinology*. Philadelphia, Saunders, 1986, p 13.
2. Barraclough CA, Wise PM: The role of catecholamines in the regulation of pituitary luteinizing hormone and follicle-stimulating hormone secretion. *Endocr Rev* 3:91, 1982.
3. Merchenthaler I, Kovacs G, Lovasz G, Setalo G: The preoptico-infundibular LH-RH tract of the rat. *Brain Res* 198:63, 1980.
4. Halasz B, Kiss J, Molnar J: Regulation of the gonadotropin-releasing hormone (GnRH) neuronal system: Morphological aspects. *J Steroid Biochem* 33:663, 1989.
5. Morley JE: The endocrinology of the opiates and opioid peptides. *Metabolism* 30:195, 1981.
6. Ferin M, van Vugt D, Wardlaw S: The hypothalamic control of the menstrual cycle and the role of endogenous opioid peptides. *Recent Prog Horm Res* 40:441, 1984.
7. Sheridan PJ: Androgen receptors in the brain: What are we measuring? *Endocr Rev* 4:171, 1983.
8. McEwen BS, Davis PG, Parsons B, Pfaff DW: The brain as a target for steroid hormone action. *Annu Rev Neurosci* 2:65, 1979.
9. Sar M, Stumpf WE: Central noradrenergic neurones concentrate ^{3}H-oestradiol. *Nature* 289:500, 1981.
10. Page RB: Pituitary blood flow: A review. *Am J Physiol* 243:E427, 1982.
11. Phifer RF, Midgley AR, Spicer SS: Immunohistologic and histologic evidence that follicle-stimulating hormone and luteinizing hormone are present in the same cell type in the human pars distalis. *J Clin Endocrinol Metab* 36:125, 1973.
12. Jarow JP: Intratesticular arterial anatomy. *J Androl* 11:255, 1990.
13. Neaves WB, Johnson L: Age-related change in numbers of other interstitial cells in the human testis: Evidence bearing on the fate of Leydig cells lost with increasing age. 17th Annual Meeting of the Society for the Study of Reproduction, Laramie, Wyoming, Abstr 100, 1984.
14. Waites GMH, Gladwell RT: Physiological significance of fluid secretion in the testis and blood-testis barrier. *Physiol Rev* 62:624, 1982.
15. Amann RP, Howards SS: Daily spermatozoal production and epididymal spermatozoal reserves of the human male. *J Urol* 124:211, 1980.
16. Parvinen M: Regulation of the seminiferous epithelium. *Endocr Rev* 3:404, 1982.
17. Wilton LJ, Teichtahl H, Temple-Smith PD, de Kretser DM: Structural heterogeneity of the axonemes of respiratory cilia and sperm flagella in normal men. *J Clin Invest* 75:825, 1985.
18. Heller CG, Clermont Y: Kinetics of the germinal epithelium in man. *Recent Prog Horm Res* 20:545, 1964.
19. Bedford JM: Maturation, transport, and fate of spermatozoa in the epididymis, in Hamilton DW, Greep RO (eds): *Handbook of Physiology: Endocrinology*. Baltimore, Williams & Wilkins, 1975, vol 5, p 303.
20. Chang MC: The meaning of sperm capacitation: A historical perspective *J Androl* 5:45, 1984.
21. Kaufman J-M, Kesner JS, Wilson RC, Knobil E: Electrophysiological manifestation of luteinizing hormone-releasing hormone pulse generator activity in the rhesus monkey: Influence of α-adrenergic and dopaminergic blocking agents. *Endocrinology* 116:1327, 1985.
22. Rasmussen DD, Liu JH, Wolf PL, Yen SSC: Gonadotropin-releasing hormone neurosecretion in the human hypothalamus: *In vitro* regulation by dopamine. *J Clin Endocrinol Metab* 62:479, 1986.
23. Fraschini J: Role of indoleamines in the control of the secretion of pituitary gonadotropins, in Martini L, Meites J (eds); *Neurochemical Aspects of Hypothalamic Function*. New York, Academic, 1971, p 141.
24. Pontiroli AE, Alberetto M, Pellicciotta G, de Castro e Silva E, De Pasqua A, Girardi AM, Pozza G: Interaction of dopaminergic and anti-serotoninergic drugs in the control of prolactin and LH release in normal women. *Acta Endocrinol (Copenh)* 93:271, 1980.
25. Martini L, Dondi D, Limonta P, Maggi R, Piva F: Modulation by sex steroids of brain opioid receptors: Implications for the control of gonadotropins and prolactin secretion. *J Steroid Biochem* 33:673–681, 1989.
26. Ellingboe J, Veldhuis JD, Mendelson JH, Kuehnle JC, Mello NK: Effect of endogenous opioid blockade on the amplitude and frequency of pulsatile luteinizing hormone secretion in normal men. *J Clin Endocrinol Metab* 54:854, 1982.
27. Veldhuis JD, Rogol AD, Williams FA, Johnson ML: Do α-adrenergic mechanisms regulate spontaneous or opiate-modulated pulsatile luteinizing hormone secretion in man? *J Clin Endocrinol Metab* 57:1292, 1983.
28. Blank MS, Panerai AE, Firesen HG: Opioid peptides modulate luteinizing hormone secretion during sexual maturation. *Science* 203:1129, 1979.
29. Plant TM, Zorub DS: Pinealectomy in agonadal infantile male rhesus monkeys *(Macaca mulatta)* does not interrupt initiation of the prepubertal hiatus in gonadotropin secretion. *Endocrinology* 118:227, 1986.
30. Clarke IJ, Cummins JT: The temporal relationship between gonadotropin releasing hormone (GnRH) and luteinizing hormone (LH) secretion in ovariectomized ewes. *Endocrinology* 111:1737, 1982.
31. Santen RJ, Bardin CW: Episodic luteinizing hormone secretion in man: Pulse analysis, clinical interpretation, physiologic mechanisms. *J Clin Invest* 52:2617, 1973.
32. Jackson GL, Kuehl D, Rhim TJ: Testosterone inhibits gonadotropin-releasing hormone pulse frequency in the male sheep. *Biol Reprod* 45:188–194, 1991.
33. Wilson RC, Knobil E: Central electrophysiologic correlates of pulsatile luteinizing hormone secretion in the rhesus monkey. 7th International Congress on Endocrinology, Quebec, Canada, Abstr S204, 1984.
34. Plant TM, Krey LC, Moossy J, McCormack JT, Hess DL, Knobil E: The arcuate nucleus and the control of gonadotropin and prolactin secretion in the female rhesus monkey *(Macaca mulatta)*. *Endocrinology* 102:52, 1978.

35. Plant TM, Dubey AK: Evidence from the rhesus monkey (*Macaca mulatta*) for the view that negative feedback control of LH secretion by the testis is mediated by a deceleration of hypothalamic gonadotropin-releasing hormone pulse frequency. *Endocrinology* 115:2145, 1984.
36. Claypool LE, Watanabe G, Terasawa E: Effects of electrical stimulation of the medial basal hypothalamus on the *in vivo* release of luteinizing hormone-releasing hormone in the prepubertal and peripubertal female monkey. *Endocrinology* 127:3014, 1990.
37. Gay VL, Plant TM: *N*-Methyl-D,L-aspartate (NMA) elicits hypothalamic GnRH release in prepubertal male rhesus monkeys (*Macaca mulatta*). *Endocrinology* 120: 2289, 1987.
38. Bourguignon J-P, Gerard A, Mathieu J, Simons J, Franchimont P: Pulsatile release of gonadotropin-releasing hormone from hypothalamic explants is restrained by blockade of *N*-methyl-D,L-aspartate receptors. *Endocrinology* 125: 1090, 1989.
39. Lopez FJ, Negro-Vilar A: Galanin stimulates luteinizing hormone-releasing hormone secretion from arcuate nucleus-median eminence fragments *in vitro:* Involvement of an α-adrenergic mechanism. *Endocrinology* 127:2431, 1990.
40. Santen RJ: Independent control of luteinizing hormone secretion by testosterone and estradiol in males, in Fotherby K, Pal SB (eds): *Hormones in Normal and Abnormal Human Tissues*. Berlin and New York, Walter de Gruyter, 1981, p 459.
41. Santen RJ: Is aromatization of testosterone to estradiol required for inhibition of LH secretion in men? *J Clin Invest* 56:1555, 1975.
42. Huseman CA, Kelch RP: Gonadotropin responses and metabolism of synthetic gonadotropin-releasing hormone (GnRH) during constant infusion of GnRH in men and boys with delayed adolescence. *J Clin Endocrinol Metab* 47: 1325, 1978.
43. Gorski RA, Harlan RE, Jacobson CD, Shryne JE, Southam AM: Evidence for the existence of a sexually dimorphic nucleus in the preoptic area of the rat. *J Comp Neurol* 193:529, 1980.
44. Pardridge WM, Gorski RA, Lippe BM, Green R: Androgens and sexual behavior. *Ann Intern Med* 96:488, 1982.
45. Barbarino A, de Marinis L: Estrogen induction of luteinizing hormone release in castrated adult human males. *J Clin Endocrinol Metab* 51:280, 1980.
46. Kwan M, Greenleaf WJ, Mann J, Crapo L, Davidson JM: The nature of androgen action on male sexuality: A combined laboratory-self-report study on hypogonadal men. *J Clin Endocrinol Metab* 57:557, 1983.
47. Conn PM: The molecular basis of gonadotropin releasing hormone action. *Endocr Rev* 7:3, 1986.
48. Conn PM: Receptor and post receptor actions of GnRH. Proceedings of the 73rd Annual Meeting of the Endocrine Society, Washington, D.C., 1991, p 13.
49. Bremner WJ, Findlay JK, Cumming IA, Hudson B, de Kretser DM: Pituitary-testicular responses in rams to prolonged infusions of luteinizing hormone-releasing hormone (LHRH). *Biol Reprod* 15:141, 1976.
50. Evans WS, Uskavitch DR, Kaiser DL, Hellmann P, Borges JLC, Thorner MO: The self-priming effect of gonadotropin-releasing hormone on luteinizing hormone release: Observations using rat anterior pituitary fragments and dispersed cells continuously perifused in parallel. *Endocrinology* 114:861, 1984.
51. Odell WD: LH, in Degroot LJ, Cahill GF, Odell WD, Martini L, Potts JT, Nelson DH, Steinberger E, Winegrad AI (eds): *Endocrinology*. New York, Grune & Stratton, 1979, vol 1, p 151.
52. Dalkin AC, Haisenleder DJ, Ortolano GA, Ellis TR, Marshall JC: The frequency of gonadotropin-releasing-hormone stimulation differentially regulates gonadotropin subunit messenger ribonucleic acid expression. *Endocrinology* 125:917, 1989.
53. Wilson CA, Leigh AJ, Chapman AJ: Gonadotrophin glycosylation and function. *J Endocrinol* 125:3, 1990.
54. Dahl KD, Stone MP: FSH isoforms, radioimmunoassays, bioassays, and their significance. *J Androl* 13:11–22, 1992.
55. Dufau ML, Veldhuis JD: Pathophysiological relationships between the biological and immunological activities of luteinizing hormone. *Bailleres Clin Endocrinol Metab* 1: 153, 1987.
56. Jia X-C, Kessel B, Yen SSC, Tucker EM, Hsueh AJW: Serum bioactive follicle-stimulating hormone during the human menstrual cycle in hyper- and hypogonadotropic states: Application of a sensitive granulosa cell aromatase bioassay. *J Clin Endocrinol Metab* 62:1243, 1986.
57. Tsatsoulis A, Shalet SM, Robertson WR: Changes in the qualitative and quantitative secretion of luteinizing hormone (LH) following orchidectomy in man. *Clin Endocrinol (Oxf)* 29:189, 1988.
58. Warner BA, Dufau ML, Santen RJ: Effects of aging and illness on the pituitary testicular axis in men: Qualitative as well as quantitative changes in luteinizing hormone. *J Clin Endocrinol Metab* 60:263, 1985.
59. Burstein S, Schaff-Blass E, Blass J, Rosenfield RL: The changing ratio of bioactive to immunoreactive luteinizing hormone (LH) through puberty principally reflects changing LH radioimmunoassay dose-response characteristics. *J Clin Endocrinol Metab* 61:508, 1985.
60. Rosenfield RL, Helke J: Is an immunoassay available for the measurement of bioactive LH in serum? *J Androl* 13:1–10, 1992.
61. Rich BH, Rosenfield RL, Moll GW Jr, Lucky AW, Roche-Bender N, Fang V: Bioactive luteinizing hormone pituitary reserves during normal and abnormal male puberty. *J Clin Endocrinol Metab* 55:140, 1982.
62. Reiter EO, Beitins IZ, Ostrea T, Gutai JP: Bioassayable luteinizing hormone during childhood and adolescence and in patients with delayed pubertal development. *J Clin Endocrinol Metab* 54:155, 1982.
63. Torresani T, Schuster E, Illig R: Bioactivity of plasma luteinizing hormone in infants and young children. *Acta Endocrinol (Copenh)* 103:326, 1983.
64. Jaakkola T, Ding Y-Q, Kellokumpu-Lehtinen P, Valavaara R, Martikainen H, Tapanainen J, Ronnberg L, Huhtaniemi I: The ratios of serum bioactive/immunoreactive luteinizing hormone and follicle-stimulating hormone in various clinical conditions with increased and decreased gonadotropin secretion: Reevaluation by a highly sensitive immunometric assay. *J Clin Endocrinol Metab* 70:1496, 1990.
65. Chappel S: Biological to immunological ratios: Reevaluation of a concept. *J Clin Endocrinol Metab* 70:1494-1495, 1990.
66. Nakai Y, Plant TM, Hess DL, Keogh EJ, Knobil E: On the sites of the negative and positive feedback actions of estradiol in the control of gonadotropin secretion in the rhesus monkey. *Endocrinology* 102:1008, 1978.
67. Corbin A, Bex FJ: Inhibition of male reproductive processes with an LH-RH agonist, in Cunningham GR, Schill W-B, Hafez ESE (eds): *Regulation of Male Fertility*. Hague, Boston, and London, Martinus Nijhoff, 1980, p 55.
68. Whitcomb RW, O'Dea LSL, Finkelstein JS, Heavern DM, Crowley WF Jr: Utility of free α-subunit as an alternative neuroendocrine marker of gonadotropin-releasing hormone (GnRH) stimulation of the gonadotroph in the human: Evidence from normal and GnRH-deficient men. *J Clin Endocrinol Metab* 70:1654, 1990.
69. Winters SJ, Troen P: Pulsatile secretion of immunoreactive alpha-subunit secretion in man. *J Clin Endocrinol Metab* 60:344, 1985.
70. Clifton DK, Steiner RA: Cycle detection: A technique for estimating the frequency and amplitude of episodic fluctu-

ations in blood hormone and substrate concentrations. *Endocrinology* 112:1057, 1983.
71. Merriam GR, Wachter KW: Algorithms for the study of episodic hormone secretion. *Am J Physiol* 243:E310, 1982.
72. Van Cauter E: Estimating false-positive and false-negative errors in analyses of hormonal pulsatility. *Am J Physiol* 254:E786, 1988.
73. Guardabasso V, DeNicolao G, Rocchett M, Rodbard D: Evaluation of pulse-detection algorithms by computer simulation of hormone secretion. *Am J Physiol* 255:E775, 1988.
74. Urban RJ, Johnson ML, Veldhuis JD: Biophysical modeling of the sensitivity and positive accuracy of detecting episodic endocrine signals. *Am J Physiol* 257:E88, 1989.
75. Veldhuis JD, Johnson ML: A novel general biophysical model for simulating episodic endocrine gland signaling. *Am J Physiol* 255:E749, 1988.
76. Veldhuis J: The hypothalamic-pituitary-testicular axis, in Yen SSC, Jaffe RB (eds): *Reproductive Endocrinology*. Philadelphia, Saunders, 1991, p 409.
77. Veldhuis JD, Fraioli F, Rogol AD, Dufau ML: Metabolic clearance of biologically active luteinizing hormone in man. *J Clin Invest* 77:1122, 1986.
78. Pepperell RJ, de Kretser DM, Burger HG: Studies on the metabolic clearance rate and production rate of human luteinizing hormone and on the initial half-time of its subunits in man. *J Clin Invest* 56:118, 1975.
79. Kulin HE, Santner SJ, Santen RJ, Murray FT, Hammond JM: The use of urinary gonadotropin measurements to evaluate LRH responsiveness in hypogonadotropic states, in Berling CG, Wentz A (eds): *The LH-Releasing Hormone*. New York, Masson, 1980, p 75.
80. Koo YB, Ji I, Slaughter RG, Ji TH: Structure of the luteinizing hormone receptor gene and multiple exons of the coding sequence. *Endocrinology* 128:2297–2308, 1991.
81. McFarland KC, Sprengel R, Phillips HS, Kohler M, Rosemblit N, Nikolics K, Segaloff DL, Seeburg PH: Lutropin-choriogonadotropin receptor: An unusual member of the G protein-coupled receptor family. *Science* 245:494–499, 1989.
82. Wang H, Ascoli M, Segaloff DL: Multiple luteinizing hormone/chorionic gonadotropin receptor messenger ribonucleic acid transcripts. *Endocrinology* 129:133–138, 1991.
83. Ji I, Ji TH: Exons 1-10 of the rat LH receptor encode a high affinity hormone binding site and exon 11 encodes G-protein modulation and a potential second hormone binding site. *Endocrinology* 128:2648–2650, 1991.
84. Podesta EJ, Dufau ML, Solano AR, Catt KJ: Hormonal activation of protein kinase in isolated Leydig cells: Electrophoretic analysis of cyclic AMP receptors. *J Biol Chem* 253:8994, 1978.
85. Nozu K, Dehejia A, Zawistowich L, Catt KJ, Dufau ML: Gonadotropin-induced receptor regulation and steroidogenic lesions in cultured Leydig cells: Induction of specific protein synthesis by chorionic gonadotropin and estradiol. *J Biol Chem* 256:12875, 1981.
86. Catt KJ, Dufau ML: Spare gonadotropin receptors in rat testis. *Nature New Biol* 244:219, 1973.
87. Browne ES, Bhalla VK: Does gonadotropin receptor complex have an amplifying role in cAMP/testosterone production in Leydig cells? *J Androl* 12:132, 1991.
88. Schwall RH, Erickson GF: Inhibition of synthesis of luteinizing hormone (LH) receptors by a down-regulating dose of LH. *Endocrinology* 114:1114, 1984.
89. Tsai-Morris C-H, Aquilano DR, Dufau ML: Gonadotropic regulation of aromatase activity in the adult rat testis. *Endocrinology* 116:31, 1985.
90. Bercovici JP, Nahoul K, Tater D, Charles JF, Scholler R: Hormonal profile of Leydig cell tumors with gynecomastia. *J Clin Endocrinol Metab* 59:625, 1984.
91. Forest MG, Lecoq A, Saez JM: Kinetics of human chorionic gonadotropin-induced steroidogenic response of the human testis: II. Plasma 17α-hydroxyprogesterone, Δ^4-androstenedione, estrone, and 17-β-estradiol: Evidence for the action of human chorionic gonadotropin on intermediate enzymes implicated in steroid biosynthesis. *J Clin Endocrinol Metab* 49:284, 1979.
92. Smals AGH, Pieters GFFM, Boers GHJ, Raemakers JMM, Hermus ARMM, Benraad ThJ, Kloppenborg PWC: Differential effect of single high dose and divided small dose administration of human chorionic gonadotropin on Leydig cell steroidogenic desensitization. *J Clin Endocrinol Metab* 58:327, 1984.
93. Matsumoto AM, Paulsen CA, Hopper BR, Rebar RW, Bremner WJ: Human chorionic gonadotropin and testicular function: Stimulation of testosterone, testosterone precursors and sperm production despite high estradiol levels. *J Clin Endocrinol Metab* 56:720, 1983.
94. Skinner MK: Cell-cell interactions in the testis. *Endoc Rev* 12:45, 1991.
95. Sordoillet C, Chauvin MA, DePeretti E, Morera AM, Benahmed M: Epidermal growth factor directly stimulates steroidogenesis in primary cultures of porcine Leydig cells: Actions and sites of action. *Endocrinology* 128:2160, 1991.
96. Lin T, Calkins JH, Morris PL, Vale W, Bardin CW: Regulation of Leydig cell function in primary culture by inhibin and activin. *Endocrinology* 125:2134, 1989.
97. Foresta C, Mioni R, Miotto D, DeCarlo E, Facchin F, Varotto A: Stimulatory effects of α-hANP on testosterone secretion in man. *J Clin Endocrinol Metab* 72:392–395, 1991.
98. Kulin HE, Samojlik E, Santen R, Santner S: The effect of growth hormone on the Leydig cell response to chorionic gonadotrophin in boys with hypopituitarism. *Clin Endocrinol (Oxf)* 15:463, 1981.
99. Sherins RJ, Winters SJ, Wachslicht H: Studies of the role of HCG and low dose FSH in initiating spermatogenesis in hypogonadotropic men. *Proceedings of the 59th Annual Meeting of the Endocrine Society,* Chicago, IL, Abstr 312, 1977.
100. Sharpe RM: Intratesticular factors controlling testicular function. *Biol Reprod* 30:29, 1984.
101. Tahri-Joutei A, Pointis G: Developmental changes in arginine vasopressin receptors and testosterone stimulation in Leydig cells. *Endocrinology* 125:605, 1989.
102. Bebakar WMW, Honour JW, Foster D, Liu YL, Jacobs HS: Regulation of testicular function by insulin and transforming growth factor-β. *Steroids* 55:266, 1990.
103. Ang H-L, Ungefroren H, DeBree F, Foo N-C, Carter D, Burbach JP, Ivell R, Murphy D: Testicular oxytocin gene expression in seminiferous tubules of cattle and transgenic mice. *Endocrinology* 128:2110, 1991.
104. Sasaki A, Yoshinaga K: Immunoreactive somatostatin in male reproductive system in humans. *J Clin Endocrinol Metab* 68:996, 1989.
105. Sealey JE, Goldstein M, Pitarresi T, Kudlak TT, Glorioso N, Fiamengo SA, Laragh JH: Prorenin secretion from human testis: No evidence for secretion of active renin or angiotensinogen. *J Clin Endocrinol Metab* 66:974, 1988.
106. Chiwakata C, Brackmann B, Hunt N, Davidoff M, Schulze W, Ivell R: Tachykinin (substance-P) gene expression in Leydig cells of the human and mouse testis. *Endocrinology* 128:2441, 1991.
107. Clayton RN, Catt KJ: Gonadotropin-releasing hormone receptors: Characterization, physiological regulation, and relationship to reproductive function. *Endocr Rev* 2:186, 1981.
108. Hou JW, Collins DC, Schleicher RL: Sources of cholesterol for testosterone biosynthesis in murine Leydig cells. *Endocrinology* 127:2047, 1990.
109. Ruokonen AO, Vihko RK: Quantitative changes of endogenous unconjugated and sulfated steroids in human testis in relation to synthesis of testosterone *in vitro*. *J Androl* 4:104, 1983.

110. Hammond GL, Ruokonen A, Kontturi M, Koskela E, Vihko R: The simultaneous radioimmunoassay of seven steroids in human spermatic and peripheral venous blood. *J Clin Endocrinol Metab* 45:16, 1977.
111. Baker HWG, Santen RJ, Burger HG, de Kretser DM, Hudson B, Pepperell RJ, Bardin CW: Rhythms in the secretion of gonadotropins and gonadal steroids. *J Steroid Biochem* 6:793, 1975.
112. Pardridge WM: Transport of protein-bound hormones into tissues *in vivo*. *Endocr Rev* 2:103, 1981.
113. Goldzieher JW, Dozier TS, Smith KD, Steinberger E: Improving the diagnostic reliability of rapidly fluctuating plasma hormone levels by optimized multiple-sampling techniques. *J Clin Endocrinol Metab* 43:824, 1976.
114. Tenover JS, Matsumoto AM, Clifton DK, Bremner WJ: Age-related alterations in the circadian rhythms of pulsatile luteinizing hormone and testosterone secretion in healthy men. *J Gerontol* 43:M163, 1988.
115. Rubin RT, Poland RE, Tower BB: Prolactin-related testosterone secretion in normal adult men. *J Clin Endocrinol Metab* 42:112, 1976.
116. Sanford EJ, Paulson DF, Rohner TJ Jr, Drago JR, Santen RJ, Bardin CW: The effects of castration on adrenal testosterone secretion in men with prostatic carcinoma. *J Urol* 118:1019, 1977.
117. Dunn JF, Nisula BC, Rodbard D: Transport of steroid hormones: Binding of 21 endogenous steroids to both testosterone-binding globulin and corticosteroid-binding globulin in human plasma. *J Clin Endocrinol Metab* 53:58, 1981.
118. Vermeulen A, Verdonck L, Van der Straeten M, Orie N: Capacity of the testosterone binding globulin in human plasma and influence of specific binding of testosterone on its metabolic clearance rate. *J Clin Endocrinol Metab* 29:1470, 1969.
119. Mendel CM: The free hormone hypothesis: Distinction from the free hormone transport hypothesis. *J Androl* 13:107–116, 1992.
120. Hobbs CJ, Jones RE, Plymate SR: The effect of sex hormone binding globulin (SHBG) on testosterone transport into the cerebrospinal fluid. *J Steroid Biochem Mol Biol* 42:629, 1992.
121. Rosner W: The functions of corticosteroid-binding globulin and sex hormone-binding globulin: Recent advances. *Endocr Rev* 11:80-91, 1990.
122. Pugeat MM, Dunn JF, Nisula BC: Transport of steroid hormones: Interaction of 70 drugs with testosterone-binding globulin and corticosteroid-binding globulin in human plasma. *J Clin Endocrinol Metab* 53:69, 1981.
123. Cunningham SK, Loughlin T, Culliton M, McKenna TJ: Plasma sex hormone-binding globulin levels decrease during the second decade of life irrespective of pubertal status. *J Clin Endocrinol Metab* 58:915, 1984.
124. Hammond GL, Pallesen M: Molecular biology of androgen transport proteins. *J Androl* (submitted for publication).
125. Musto NA, Cheng CY, Gunsalus GL, Escobar N, Bardin CW: The use of androgen binding protein and other Sertoli cell products to monitor seminiferous tubular physiology and pathophysiology, in Santen RJ, Swerdloff RS (eds): *Male Sexual Dysfunction: Diagnosis and Management of Hypogonadism, Infertility and Impotence*. New York, Marcel Dekker, 1985.
126. Rosner W, Hryb DJ, Khan MS, Nakhla AM, Romas NA: Sex hormone-binding globulin-binding to cell membranes and generation of a second messenger. *J Androl* 13:101–106, 1992.
127. Cheng CY, Bardin CW, Musto NA, Gunsalus GL, Cheng SL, Ganguly M: Radioimmunoassay of testosterone-estradiol-binding globulin in humans: A reassessment of normal values. *J Clin Endocrinol Metab* 56:68, 1983.
128. Manni A, Pardridge WM, Cefalu W, Nisula BC, Bardin CW, Santner SJ, Santen RJ: Bioavailability of albumin-bound testosterone. *J Clin Endocrinol Metab* 61:705, 1985.
129. Demisch K, Nickelsen T: Distribution of testosterone in plasma proteins during replacement therapy with testosterone enanthate in patients suffering from hypogonadism. *Andrologia* 15:536, 1983.
130. Longcope C, Sato K, McKay C, Horton R: Aromatization by splanchnic tissue in men. *J Clin Endocrinol Metab* 58:1089, 1984.
131. Weinstein RL, Kelch RP, Jenner MR, Kaplan SL, Grumbach MM: Secretion of unconjugated androgens and estrogens by the normal and abnormal human testis before and after human chorionic gonadotropin. *J Clin Invest* 53:1, 1974.
132. Martini L: The 5α-reduction of testosterone in the neuroendocrine structures: Biochemical and physiological implications. *Endocr Rev* 3:1, 1982.
133. Jenkins EP, Andersson S, Imperato-McGinley J, Wilson JD, Russell DW: Genetic and pharmacological evidence for more than one human steroid 5α-reductase. *J Clin Invest* 89:293–300, 1992.
134. Peterson RE, Imperato-McGinley J, Gautier T, Sturla E: Male pseudohermaphroditism due to steroid 5α-reductase deficiency. *Am J Med* 62:170, 1977.
135. The MK-906 (Finasteride) Study Group: One-year experience in the treatment of benign prostatic hyperplasia with finasteride. *J Androl* 12:372–375, 1991.
136. Meikle AW, Stringham JD, Bishop DT, West DW: Quantitating genetic and nongenetic factors influencing androgen production and clearance rates in men. *J Clin Endocrinol Metab* 67:104–109, 1988.
137. Mowszowicz I, Melanitou E, Kirchhoffer M-O, Mauvais-Jarvis P: Dihydrotestosterone stimulates 5α-reductase activity in pubic skin fibroblasts. *J Clin Endocrinol Metab* 56:320, 1983.
138. Goos CMAA, Wirtz P, Vermorken AJM, Mauvais-Jarvis P: Androgenic effect of testosterone and some of its metabolites in relation to their biotransformation in the skin. *Br J Dermatol* 107:549, 1982.
139. Mauvais-Jarvis P, Kuttenn F, Mowszowicz I (eds): *Hirsutism*. New York, Springer-Verlag, 1981.
140. Horton R, Hawks D, Lobo R: 3α, 17β-androstanediol glucuronide in plasma: A marker of androgen action in idiopathic hirsutism. *J Clin Invest* 69:1203, 1982.
141. Lookingbill DP, Horton R, Demers LM, Egan N, Marks JG Jr, Santen RJ: Tissue production of androgens in women with acne. *J Am Acad Dermatol* 12:481, 1985.
142. Samojlik E, Kirschner MA, Silber D, Schneider G, Ertel NH: Elevated production and metabolic clearance rates of androgens in morbidly obese women. *J Clin Endocrinol Metab* 59:949, 1984.
143. Lookingbill DP, Demers LM, Wang C, Leung A, Rittmaster RS, Santen RJ: Clinical and biochemical parameters of androgen action in normal healthy Caucasian versus Chinese subjects. *J Clin Endocrinol Metab* 72:1242, 1991.
144. Chan L, O'Malley BW: Mechanism of action of the sex steroid hormones. *N Engl J Med* 294:1322, 1976.
145. Chang CH, Rowley DR, Tindall DJ: Purification and characterization of the androgen receptor from rat ventral prostate. *Biochemistry* 22:6170, 1983.
146. Lubahn DB, Tan J-A, Quarmby VE, Sar M, Joseph DR, French FS, Wilson EM: Structural analysis of the human and rat androgen receptors and expression in male reproductive tract tissues. *Ann NY Acad Sci* 564:48-56, 1989.
147. Simental JA, Sar M, Lane MV, French FS, Wilson EM: Transcriptional activation and nuclear targeting signals of the human androgen receptor. *J Biol Chem* 266:510, 1991.
148. Barrack ER: The nuclear matrix of the prostate contains acceptor sites for androgen receptors. *Endocrinology* 113: 430, 1983.
149. Saartok T, Dahlberg E, Gustafsson J-A: Relative binding affinity of anabolic-androgenic steroids: Comparison of the binding to the androgen receptors in skeletal muscle and in

prostate, as well as to sex hormone-binding globulin. *Endocrinology* 114:2100, 1984.
150. Kumar N, Didolkar AK, Sundaram K: Biological activity of 7α-methyl-19-nortestosterone (7MENT) in castrated rats. 73rd Annual Meeting of the Endocrine Society, Washington, D.C., Abstr. 1394, 1991.
151. Santen RJ, Friend JN, Trojanowski D, Davis B, Samojlik E, Bardin CW: Prolonged negative feedback suppression after estradiol administration: Proposed mechanism of eugonadal secondary amenorrhea. *J Clin Endocrinol Metab* 47:1220, 1978.
152. Gharib SD, Bowers SM, Need LR, Chin WW: Regulation of rat luteinizing hormone subunit messenger ribonucleic acids by gonadal steroid hormones. *J Clin Invest* 77:582, 1986.
153. Marynick SP, Loriaux DL, Sherins RJ, Pita JC Jr, Lipsett MB: Evidence that testosterone can suppress pituitary gonadotropin secretion independently of peripheral aromatization. *J Clin Endocrinol Metab* 49:396, 1979.
154. Kuhn JM, Rieu M, Laudat MH, Forest MG, Pugeat M, Bricaire H, Luton JP: Effects of 10 days administration of percutaneous dihydrotestosterone on the pituitary-testicular axis in normal men. *J Clin Endocrinol Metab* 58:231, 1984.
155. Winters SJ, Sherins RJ, Loriaux DL: Studies on the role of sex steroids in the feedback control of gonadotropin concentrations in men: III. Androgen resistance in primary gonadal failure. *J Clin Endocrinol Metab* 48:553, 1979.
156. Urban RJ, Davis MR, Rogol AD, Johnson ML, Veldhuis JD: Acute androgen receptor blockade increases luteinizing hormone secretory activity in men. *J Clin Endocrinol Metab* 67:1149, 1988.
157. Gross DS: Effect of castration and steroid replacement on immunoreactive gonadotropin-releasing hormone in the hypothalamus and preoptic area. *Endocrinology* 106:1442, 1980.
158. Rudenstein RS, Bigdeli H, McDonald MH, Snyder PJ: Administration of gonadal steroids to the castrated male rat prevents a decrease in the release of gonadotropin-releasing hormone from the incubated hypothalamus. *J Clin Invest* 63:262, 1979.
159. Loriaux DL, Vigersky RA, Marynick SP, Janick JJ, Sherins RJ: Androgen and estrogen effects in the regulation of LH in man, in Troen P, Nankin HR (eds): *The Testis in Normal and Infertile Men*. New York, Raven, 1977, p 213.
160. Foster CM, Hassing JM, Mendes TM, Hale PM, Padmanabhan V, Hopwood NJ, Beitins IZ, Marshall JC, Kelch RP: Testosterone infusion reduces nocturnal luteinizing hormone pulse frequency in pubertal boys. *J Clin Endocrinol Metab* 69:1213, 1989.
161. Veldhuis JD, Rogol AD, Samojlik E, Ertel NH: Role of endogenous opiates in the expression of negative feedback actions of androgen and estrogen on pulsatile properties of luteinizing hormone secretion in man. *J Clin Invest* 74:47, 1984.
162. Ieiri T, Chen HT, Campbell GA, Meites J: Effects of naloxone and morphine on the proestrous surge of prolactin and gonadotropins in the rat. *Endocrinology* 106:1568, 1980.
163. Adams LA, Vician L, Clifton DK, Steiner RA: Testosterone regulates proopiomelanocortin gene expression in the primate brain. *Endocrinology* 128:1881, 1991.
164. Kingsley TR, Bogdanove EM: Direct feedback of androgens: Localized effects of intrapituitary implants of androgens on gonadotrophic cells and hormone stores. *Endocrinology* 93:1398, 1973.
165. Leveque NW, Grotjan HE Jr: Testosterone inhibition of LRH-induced luteinizing hormone release by cultures of rat anterior pituitary cells: Effect of inhibitors of steroid 5α-reductase. *Acta Endocrinol (Copenh)* 100:196, 1982.
166. Finkelstein JS, Whitcomb RW, O'Dea LSL, Longcope C, Schoenfeld DA, Crowley WF: Sex steroid control of gonadotropin secretion in the human male: I. Effects of testosterone administration in normal and gonadotropin-releasing hormone-deficient men. *J Clin Endocrinol Metab* 73:609–620, 1991.
167. Bagatell CJ, Bremner WJ: Estradiol, but not dihydrotestosterone, mediates the direct pituitary suppression of gonadotropin secretion induced by testosterone administration to men. Proceedings of the 73rd Annual Meeting of the Endocrine Society, Washington, D.C., Abstr 857, 1991.
168. Clarke IJ: The relationships between GnRH and LH secretion, in Labrie F, Proulx L (eds): *Endocrinology*. Amsterdam, Excerpta Medica, 1984, pp 366–369.
169. Winters SJ, Janick JJ, Loriaux DL, Sherins RJ: Studies on the role of sex steroids in the feedback control of gonadotropin concentrations in men: II. Use of the estrogen antagonist, clomiphene citrate. *J Clin Endocrinol Metab* 48:222, 1979.
170. Frawley LS, Neill JD: Biphasic effects of estrogen on gonadotropin-releasing hormone-induced luteinizing hormone release in monolayer cultures of rat and monkey pituitary cells. *Endocrinology* 114:659, 1984.
171. Pfaff DW, McEwen BS: Actions of estrogens and progestins on nerve cells. *Science* 219:808, 1983.
172. Santen RJ, Ruby EB: Enhanced frequency and magnitude of episodic luteinizing hormone-releasing hormone discharge as a hypothalamic mechanism for increased luteinizing hormone secretion. *J Clin Endocrinol Metab* 48:315, 1979.
173. Winters SJ, Troen P: Evidence for a role of endogenous estrogen in the hypothalamic control of gonadotropin secretion in men. *J Clin Endocrinol Metab* 61:842, 1985.
174. Naftolin F, Ryan KJ, Davies IJ, Reddy VV, Flores F, Petro Z, Kuhn M, White RJ, et al: The formation of estrogens by central neuroendocrine tissues. *Recent Prog Horm Res* 31: 295, 1975.
175. Roselli CE, Resko JA: Androgens regulate brain aromatase activity in adult male rats through a receptor mechanism. *Endocrinology* 114:1, 1984.
176. Worgul TJ, Santen RJ, Samojlik E, Irwin G, Falvo RE: Evidence that brain aromatization regulates LH secretion in the male dog. *Am J Physiol* 241:E246, 1981.
177. Keye WR Jr, Jaffe RB: Strength-duration characteristics of estrogen effects on gonadotropin response to gonadotropin-releasing hormone in women: I. Effects of varying duration of estradiol administration. *J Clin Endocrinol Metab* 41:1003, 1975.
178. Kulin HE, Reiter EO: Gonadotropin and testosterone measurements after estrogen administration to adult men, prepubertal and pubertal boys, and men with hypogonadotropism: Evidence for maturation of positive feedback in the male. *Pediatr Res* 10:46, 1976.
179. Bowers CY, Currie BL, Johansson NG, Folkers K: Biological evidence that separate hypothalamic hormones release the follicle stimulating and luteinizing hormones. *Biochem Biophys Res Commun* 50:20, 1973.
180. Chappel SC, Ulloa-Aguirre A, Coutifaris C: Biosynthesis and secretion of follicle-stimulating hormone. *Endocr Rev* 4:179, 1983.
181. Dahl KD, Bicsak TA, Hsueh AJW: Naturally occurring antihormones: Secretion of FSH antagonists by women treated with a GnRH analog. *Science* 239:72, 1988.
182. Franchimont P, Demoulin A, Bourguignon JP, Santen R: Role of inhibin in the regulation of gonadotrophin secretion in the male, in Job, J.-C. (ed): *Pediatric and Adolescent Endocrinology: Cryptorchidism: Diagnosis and Treatment*. Basel, Karger, 1979, vol 6, p 47.
183. Kitahara S, Winters SJ, Attardi B, Oshima H, Troen P: Effects of castration on luteinizing hormone and follicle-stimulating hormone secretion by pituitary cells from male rats. *Endocrinology* 126:2642, 1990.
184. Pasteels JL, Sheridan R, Gaspar S, Franchimont P: Syn-

thesis and release of gonadotrophins and their subunits by long term organ cultures of human foetal hypophyses. *Mol Cell Endocrinol* 9:1, 1977.

185. Franchimont P, Demoulin A, Bourguignon JP: Regulation of gonadotropin secretion, in Santen RJ, Swerdloff RS (eds): *Male Sexual Dysfunction: Diagnosis and Management of Hypogonadism, Infertility and Impotence.* New York, Marcel Dekker, 1986, pp 101–126.
186. Gross KM, Matsumoto AM, Berger RE, Bremner WJ: Increased frequency of pulsatile luteinizing hormone-releasing hormone administration selectively decreases follicle-stimulating hormone levels in men with idiopathic azoospermia. *Fertil Steril* 45:392, 1986.
187. Wildt L, Hausler A, Marshall G, Hutchison JS, Plant TM, Belchetz PE, Knobil E: Frequency and amplitude of gonadotropin-releasing hormone stimulation and gonadotropin secretion in the rhesus monkey. *Endocrinology* 109:376, 1981.
188. Urban RJ, Padmanabhan V, Beitins I, Veldhuis JD: Metabolic clearance of human follicle-stimulating hormone assessed by radioimmunoassay, immunoradiometric assay, and *in vitro* sertoli cell bioassay. *J Clin Endocrinol Metab* 73:818–823, 1991.
189. Coble YD Jr, Kohler PO, Cargille CM, Ross GT: Production rates and metabolic clearance rates of human follicle-stimulating hormone in premenopausal and postmenopausal women. *J Clin Invest* 48:359, 1969.
190. Amin HK, Hunter WM: Human pituitary follicle-stimulating hormone: Distribution, plasma clearance and urinary excretion as determined by radioimmunoassay. *J Endocrinol* 48:307, 1970.
191. Yen SSC, Llerena LA, Pearson OH, Littell AS: Disappearance rates of endogenous follicle-stimulating hormone in serum following surgical hypophysectomy in man. *J Clin Endocrinol Metab* 30:325, 1970.
192. Urban RJ, Johnson ML, Veldhuis JD: In vivo biological validation and biophysical modeling of the sensitivity and positive accuracy of endocrine peak detection: II. The follicle-stimulating hormone pulse signal. *Endocrinology* 128:2008, 1991.
193. Veldhuis JD, Iranmanesh A, Clarke I, Kaiser DL, Johnson ML: Random and non-random coincidence between LH peaks and FSH, alpha subunit, prolactin, and GnRH pulsations. *J Neuroendocrinol* 1:1, 1989.
194. Lipshultz LI, Murthy L, Tindall DJ: Characterization of human Sertoli cells *in vitro*. *J Clin Endocrinol Metab* 55:228, 1982.
195. Petra PH, Titani K, Walsh K: Purification and chemical characterization of SBP, the sex steroid binding protein of plasma. *First International Symposium on Binding Proteins: Steroid Hormones.* Lyons, France, 1986, p 1.
196. Cheng CY, Frick J, Gunsalus GL, Musto NA, Bardin CW: Human testicular androgen-binding protein shares immunodeterminants with serum testosterone-estradiol-binding globulin. *Endocrinology* 114:1395, 1984.
197. Joseph DR, Hall SH, French FS: Rat androgen binding protein: Structure of the gene, mRNA and protein. *First International Symposium on Binding Proteins: Steroid Hormones.* Lyons, France, 1986, p 1.
198. Becker RR, Gunsalus GL, Musto NA, Bardin CW: The epididymis contributes minimally to serum androgen-binding protein in the rat: A whole body kinetic study. *Endocrinology* 114:2354, 1984.
199. Gunsalus GL, Musto NA, Bardin CW: Immunoassay of androgen binding protein in blood: A new approach for study of the seminiferous tubule. *Science* 200:65, 1978.
200. Robertson DM, Tsonis CG, McLachlan RI, Handelsman DJ, Leask R, Baird DT, McNeilly AS, Hayward S, et al: Comparison of inhibin immunological and *in vitro* biological activities in human serum. *J Clin Endocrinol Metab* 67:438, 1988.
201. Khan SA, Soder O, Syed V, Ritzen M: Secretion of interleukin-1 by the rat testis. *Fourth International Workshop on Molecular and Cellular Endocrinology of the Testis.* Capri, Italy, 1986, p 91.
202. Benahmed M, Morera AM, Chauvin DC, Peretti E: Is somatomedin C a mediating factor between Sertoli and Leydig cells? Fourth International Workshop on Molecular and Cellular Endocrinology of the Testis. Capri, Italy, 1986, p 55.
203. Sharpe RM: Follicle-stimulating hormone and spermatogenesis in the adult male. *J Endocrinol* 121:405–407, 1989.
204. Van Alphen MMA, Van de Kant HJG, De Rooij DG: Follicle-stimulating hormone stimulates spermatogenesis in the adult monkey. *Endocrinology* 123:1449–1455, 1988.
205. Marshall GR, Wickings EJ, Ludecke DK, Nieschlag E: Stimulation of spermatogenesis in stalk-sectioned rhesus monkeys by testosterone alone. *J Clin Endocrinol Metab* 57:152, 1983.
206. Sar M, Lubahn DB, French FS, Wilson EM: Immunohistochemical localization of the androgen receptor in rat and human tissues. *Endocrinology* 127:3180, 1990.
207. Takeda H, Chodak G, Mutchnik S, Nakamoto T, Chang C: Immunohistochemical localization of androgen receptors with mono- and polyclonal antibodies to androgen receptor. *J Endocrinol* 126:17, 1990.
208. Orgebin-Crist MCV, Danzo BJ, Davies J: Endocrine control of the development and maintenance of sperm fertilizing ability in the epididymis, in Greep RO, Astwood EB (eds): *Handbook of Physiology,* Sect. 7, Vol. V, Baltimore, Williams & Wilkins, 1975, pp 319–338.
209. Schmidt JA, Eckert R: Calcium couples flagellar reversal to photostimulation in *Chlamydomonas reinhardtii. Nature* 262:713, 1976.
210. Gibbons BH, Gibbons IR: Calcium induced quiescence in reactivated sea urchin sperm. *J Cell Biol* 84:13, 1980.
211. Garbers DL, Lust WD, First NL, Lardy HA: Effects of phosphodiesterase inhibitors and cyclic nucleotides on sperm respiration and motility. *Biochemistry* 10:1825, 1971.
212. Mohri H, Yanagimashi R: Characteristics of motor apparatus in testicular epididymal and ejaculated spermatozoa. *Exp Cell Res* 127:191, 1980.
213. Bavister BD, Chen AF, Fu PC: Catecholamine requirement for hamster sperm motility *in vitro*. *J Reprod Fertil* 56:507, 1979.
214. Acott TS, Hoskins DD: Bovine sperm forward motility protein: Partial purification and characterization. *J Biol Chem* 253:6744, 1978.
215. Bouchard P, Gagnon C, Phillips DM, Bardin CW: The localization of protein carboxylmethylase in sperm tails. *J Cell Biol* 86:417, 1980.
216. Austin CR: *Fertilization.* Englewood Cliffs, NJ, Prentice-Hall, 1965.
217. Paulsen CA, Espeland DH, Michals EL: Effects of hCG, hMG, hLH and hGH administration on testicular function, in Rosemberg E, Paulsen CA (eds): *The Human Testis.* New York, Plenum, 1970, p 47.
218. Burris AS, Rodbard HW, Winters SJ, Sherins RJ: Gonadotropin therapy in men with isolated hypogonadotropic hypogonadism: The response to human chorionic gonadotropin is predicted by initial testicular size. *J Clin Endocrinol Metab* 66:1144, 1988.
219. Matsumoto AM, Paulsen CA, Bremner WJ: Stimulation of sperm production by human luteinizing hormone in gonadotropin-suppressed normal men. *J Clin Endocrinol Metab* 59:882, 1984.
220. Matsumoto AM, Karpas AE, Paulsen CA, Bremner WJ: Reinitiation of sperm production in gonadotropin-suppressed normal men by administration of follicle-stimulating hormone. *J Clin Invest* 72:1005, 1983.
221. Clifton DK, Bremner WJ: The effect of testicular-irradiation on spermatogenesis in man. *J Androl* 4:387, 1983.

222. De Kretser DM, Burger HG, Fortune D, Hudson B, Long AR, Paulsen CA, Taft HP: Hormonal, histological and chromosomal studies in adult males with testicular disorders. *J Clin Endocrinol Metab* 35:392, 1972.
223. De Kretser DM, Robertson DM: The isolation and physiology of inhibin and related proteins. *Biol Reprod* 40:33–47, 1989.
224. McLachlan RI, Matsumoto AM, Burger HG, deKretser DM, Bremner WJ: Relative roles of follicle-stimulating hormone and luteinizing hormone in the control of inhibin secretion in normal men. *J Clin Invest* 82:880, 1988.
225. Ackland JF, Schwartz NB: Developmental changes in inhibin and FSH in female and male rats. Proceedings of the 73rd Annual Meeting of the Endocrine Society, Washington, D.C., Abstr. 1085, 1991.
226. Medhamurthy R, Culler MD, Gay VL, Negro-Vilar A, Plant TM: Evidence that inhibin plays a major role in the regulation of follicle-stimulating hormone secretion in the fully adult male rhesus monkey *(Macaca mulatta). Endocrinology* 129:389–395, 1991.
227. Nagao RR, Plymate SR, Berger RE, Perin EB, Paulsen CA: Comparison of gonadal function between fertile and infertile men with varicoceles. *Fertil Steril* 46:930–933, 1986.
228. Tsatsoulis A, Shalet SM, Robertson WR, Morris ID, Burger HG, de Kretser DM: Plasma inhibin levels in men with chemotherapy-induced severe damage to the seminiferous epithelium. *Clin Endocrinol (Oxf)* 29:659, 1988.
229. De Kretser DM, McLachlan RI, Robertson DM, Burger HG: Serum inhibin levels in normal men and men with testicular disorders. *J Endocrinol* 120:517, 1989.
230. McLachlan RI, Robertson DM, deKretser DM, Burger HG: Advances in the physiology of inhibin and inhibin-related peptides. *Clin Endocrinol (Oxf)* 29:77, 1988.
231. Vale W, Corrigan A, Bilezikjian L, Vaughan J, Roberts V, Carroll R, Chin W, Schwall R, et al: Roles of activin in the anterior pituitary. Proceedings of the 73rd Annual Meeting of the Endocrine Society, Washington, D.C., Abstr 5C, 1991.
232. Thomsen G, Woolf T, Whitman M, Sokol S, Ziv T, Shomoni Y, Bril A, Mitrani E, Melton D: Activin's role in vertebrate embryogenesis. Proceedings of the 73rd Annual Meeting of the Endocrine Society, Washington, D.C., Abstr 5C, 1991.
233. Yu J: Roles of activin in the regulation of human erythropoiesis. Proceedings of the 73rd Annual Meeting of the Endocrine Society, Washington, D.C., Abstr 5C, 1991.
234. Shimonaka M, Inouye S, Shimasaki S, Ling N: Follistatin binds to both activin and inhibin through the common beta-subunit. *Endocrinology* 128:3313–3315, 1991.
235. Takahashi J, Higashi Y, LaNasa JA, Winters SJ, Oshima H, Troen P: Studies of the human testis: XVII. Gonadotropin regulation of intratesticular testosterone and estradiol in infertile men. *J Clin Endocrinol Metab* 55:1073, 1982.
236. Hansson V, Ritzen EM, French FS, Nayfeh SN: Androgen transport and receptor mechanisms in testis and epididymis, in Hamilton DW, Greep RO (eds): *Handbook of Physiology: Endocrinology.* Baltimore, Williams & Wilkins, 1975, vol 5, p 173.
237. Verhoeven G, Cailleau J: Testicular peritubular cells secrete a protein under androgen control that inhibits induction of aromatase activity in Sertoli cells. *Endocrinology* 123:2100, 1988.
238. Smith EP, Dickson BA, Chernausek SD: Insulin-like growth factor binding protein-3 secretion from cultured rat Sertoli cells: Dual regulation by follicle stimulating hormone and insulin-like growth factor-I. *Endocrinology* 127:2744, 1990.
239. Dufau ML, Nozu K, Dehejia A, Garcia Vela A, Solano AR, Fraioli F, Catt KJ: Biological activity and target cell actions of luteinizing hormone, in Motta M, Zonisi M, Piva F (eds): *Serono Symposium, Pituitary Hormones and Related Peptides.* New York, Academic, 1982, pp 118–119.
240. Klemcke HG, Bartke A, Borer KT: Regulation of testicular prolactin and luteinizing hormone receptors in golden hamsters. *Endocrinology* 114:594, 1984.
241. Baranao JLS, Tesone M, Oliveira-Filho RM, Chiauzzi VA, Calvo JC, Charreau EH, Calandra RS: Effects of prolactin on prostate androgen receptors in male rats. *J Androl* 3:281, 1982.
242. Winters SJ, Troen P: Altered pulsatile secretion of luteinizing hormone in hypogonadal men with hyperprolactinemia. *Clin Endocrinol (Oxf)* 21:257, 1982.
243. Thorner MO, Edwards CRW, Hanker JP, Abraham G, Besser GM: Prolactin and gonadotropin interaction in the male, in Troen P and Nankin H (eds): *The Testis in Normal and Infertile Men.* New York, Raven, 1977, p 351.
244. Beumont PJV, Corker C, Friesen HG, Kolakowska T, Mandelbrote BM, Marshall J, Murray MA, Wiles DH: The effect of phenothiazines on endocrine function: II. Effects in men and postmenopausal women. *Br J Psychiatry* 124:420, 1974.
245. Wahlstrom T, Huhtaniemi I, Hovatta O, Seppala M: Localization of luteinizing hormone, follicle-stimulating hormone, prolactin and their receptors in human and rat testis using immunohistochemistry and radioreceptor assay. *J Clin Endocrinol Metab* 57:825, 1983.
246. Martikainen H, Vihko R: hCG-stimulation of testicular steroidogenesis during induced hyper- and hypoprolactinaemia in man. *Clin Endocrinol (Oxf)* 16:227, 1982.
247. Bernini GP, Gasperi M, Franchi F, Luisi M: Effects of sulpiride induced hyperprolactinemia on testosterone secretion and metabolism before and after hCG in normal men. *J Endocrinol Invest* 6:287, 1983.
248. Magrini G, Pellaton M, Felber JP: Prolactin induced modifications of testosterone metabolism in man. *Acta Endocrinol [Supp] (Copenh)* 212:143, 1977.
249. Magrini G, Ebiner JR, Burckhardt P, Felber JP: Study on the relationship between plasma prolactin levels and androgen metabolism in man. *J Clin Endocrinol Metab* 43:944, 1976.
250. Carter JN, Tyson JE, Tolis G, Van Vliet S, Faiman C, Friesen HG: Prolactin-secreting tumors and hypogonadism in 22 men. *N Engl J Med* 299:847, 1978.
251. Evans WS, Cronin MJ, Thorner MO: Hypogonadism in hyperprolactinemia: Proposed mechanisms, in Ganong WJ, Martin L (eds): *Frontiers in Neuroendocrinology.* New York, Raven, 1982, vol 7, pp 77–122.
252. Bourguignon JP, Hoyoux C, Reuter A, Franchimont P, Leinartz-Dourcy C, Vrinats-Geraert Y: Urinary excretion of immunoreactive luteinizing hormone-releasing hormone-like material and gonadotropins at different stages of life. *J Clin Endocrinol Metab* 48:78, 1979.
253. Tenover JS, Dahl KD, Hsueh AJW, Lim P, Matsumoto AM, Bremner WJ: Serum bioactive and immunoreactive follicle-stimulating hormone levels and the response to clomiphene in healthy young and elderly men. *J Clin Endocrinol Metab* 64:1103, 1987.
254. Marrama P, Montanini V, Celani MF, Carani C, Cioni K, Bazzani M, Cavani D, Baraghini GF: Decrease in luteinizing hormone biological activity/immunoreactivity ratio in elderly men. *Maturitas* 5:223, 1984.
255. Kulin HE, Bell PM, Santen RJ, Ferber AJ: Integration of pulsatile gonadotropin secretion by timed urinary measurements: An accurate and sensitive 3-hour test. *J Clin Endocrinol Metab* 40:783, 1975.
256. Santen RJ, Kulin HE: Evaluation of gonadotropins in man, in Hafez ESE (ed): *Techniques of Human Andrology.* Amsterdam, Elsevier, North-Holland, 1977, p 251.
257. Nieschlag E: Circadian rhythm of plasma testosterone, in Aschoff J, Ceresa F, Halberg F (eds): *Chronobiological Aspects of Endocrinology.* Schattauer, Verlag, Stuttgart, and New York, 1977, p 117.
258. Robertson DM, Tsonis CG, McLachlan RI, Handelsman DJ, Leask R, Baird DT, McNeilly AS, Hayward S, et al: Com-

parison of inhibin immunological and *in vitro* biological activities in human serum. *J Clin Endocrinol Metab* 67:438, 1988.
259. Schneyer AL, Mason AJ, Burton LE, Ziegner JR, Crowley WF Jr: Immunoreactive inhibin α-subunit in human serum: Implications for radioimmunoassay. *J Clin Endocrinol Metab* 70:1208, 1990.
260. Tenover JS, McLachlan RI, Dahl KD, Burger HG, de Kretser DM, Bremner WJ: Decreased serum inhibin levels in normal elderly men: Evidence for a decline in Sertoli cell function with aging. *J Clin Endocrinol Metab* 67:455, 1988.
261. Quigley C, Cowell C, Jimenez M, Burger H, Kirk J, Bergin M, Stevens M, Simpson J, Silink M: Normal or early development of puberty despite gonadal damage in children treated for acute lymphoblastic leukemia. *N Engl J Med* 321:143, 1989.
262. Santen RJ, Leonard JM, Sherins RJ, Gandy HM, Paulsen CA: Short- and long-term effects of clomiphene citrate on the pituitary-testicular axis. *J Clin Endocrinol Metab* 33:970, 1971.
263. Glass AR: Ketoconazole-induced stimulation of gonadotropin output in men: Basis for a potential test of gonadotropin reserve. *J Clin Endocrinol Metab* 63:1121, 1986.
264. Forest MG: How should we perform the human chorionic gonadotrophin (hCG) stimulation test? *Int J Androl* 6:1, 1983.
265. Saez JM, Bertrand J: Studies on testicular function in children: Plasma concentrations of testosterone, dehydroepiandrosterone and its sulfate before and after stimulation with human chorionic gonadotropins. *Steroids* 12:749, 1968.
266. Stepan JJ, Lachman M, Zverina J, Pacovsky V, Baylink DJ: Castrated men exhibit bone loss: Effect of calcitonin treatment on biochemical indices of bone remodeling. *J Clin Endocrinol Metab* 69:523, 1989.
267. Jackson JA, Kleerekoper M, Parfitt AM, Rao DS, Villanueva AR, Frame B: Bone histomorphometry in hypogonadal and eugonadal men with spinal osteoporosis. *J Clin Endocrinol Metab* 65:53, 1987.
268. Finkelstein JS, Klibanski A, Neer RM, Greenspan SL, Rosenthal DI, Crowley WF Jr: Osteoporosis in men with idiopathic hypogonadotropic hypogonadism. *Ann Intern Med* 106:354, 1987.
269. Koopman P, Munsterberg A, Capel B, Vivian N, Lovell-Badge A: Expression of a candidate sex-determining gene during mouse testis differentiation. *Nature* 348:450–452, 1990.
270. Ebensperger C, Studer R, Epplen JT: Specific amplification of the ZFY gene to screen sex in man. *Hum Genet* 82:289, 1989.
271. Sherins RJ, Howards SS: Male infertility, in Harrison JH, Gittes RF, Perlmutter AD, Stamey TA, Walsh PC (eds): *Campbell's Urology,* 4th ed. Philadelphia, Saunders, 1978, vol 1, p 715.
272. Behre HM, Nashan D, Nieschlag E: Objective measurement of testicular volume by ultrasonography: Evaluation of the technique and comparison with orchidometer estimates. *Int J Androl* 12:395, 1989.
273. Lowe DH, Brock WA, Kaplan GW: Laparoscopy for localization of nonpalpable testes. *J Urol* 131:728, 1984.
274. Coen P, Kulin H, Ballantine T, Zaino R, Frauenhoffer E, Boal D, Inkster S, Brodie A, Santen RJ: An aromatase-producing sex-cord tumor resulting in prepubertal gynecomastia. *N Engl J Med* 324:317–322, 1991.
275. Weiss RM, Glickman MG, Lytton B: Clinical implications of gonadal venography in the management of the non-palpable undescended testis. *J Urol* 121:745, 1979.
276. Naslund MJ, Gearhart JP, Jeffs RD: Laparoscopy: Its selected use in patients with unilateral nonpalpable testis after human chorionic gonadotropin stimulation. *J Urol* 142:108–110, 1989.
277. Muller J, Skakkebaek NE: Quantitative assessment of the seminiferous epithelium in male infertility, in Santen RJ, Swerdloff RS (eds): *Male Reproductive Dysfunction: Diagnosis and Management of Hypogonadism, Infertility and Impotence.* New York, Marcel Dekker, 1986, pp 321–340.
278. Baker HWG, Burger HG, de Kretser DM, Hudson B: Relative incidence of etiologic disorders in male infertility, in Santen RJ, Swerdloff RS (eds): *Male Reproductive Dysfunction: Diagnosis and Management of Hypogonadism, Infertility and Impotence.* New York, Marcel Dekker, 1986, pp 341–372.
279. Gordon DL, Barr AB, Herrigel FE, Paulsen CA: Testicular biopsy in man: Effect upon sperm concentration. *Fertil Steril* 16:522, 1965.
280. Vantman D, Koukoulis G, Dennison L, Zinaman M, Sherins RJ: Computer-assisted semen analysis: Evaluation of method and assessment of the influence of sperm concentration on linear velocity determination. *Fertil Steril* 49:510, 1988.
281. Schwartz D, Laplanche A, Jouannet P, David G: Within subject variability of human semen in regard to sperm count, volume, total number of spermatozoa and length of abstinence. *J Reprod Fertil* 57:391, 1979.
282. Bardin CW, Paulsen CA: The testes, in Williams RD (ed): *Textbook of Endocrinology,* 6th ed. Philadelphia, Saunders, 1981, p 293.
283. Levine RJ, Mathew RM, Chenault CB, Brown MH, Hurtt ME, Bentley KS, Mohr KL, Working PK: Differences in the quality of semen in outdoor workers during summer and winter. *N Engl J Med* 323:12–16, 1990.
284. Wang C, Chan SYW, Ng M, So WWK, Tsoi W-L, Lo T, Leung A: Diagnostic value of sperm function tests and routine semen analyses in fertile and infertile men. *J Androl* 9:384, 1988.
285. George FW, Catt KJ, Wilson JD: Regulation of the onset of steroid hormone synthesis in fetal gonads, in Hamilton TH, Clark JH, Sadler WA (eds): *Ontogeny of Receptors and Reproductive Hormone Action.* New York, Raven, 1979, p 411.
286. Winter JSD, Hughes IA, Reyes FI, Faiman C: Pituitary-gonadal relations in infancy: II. Patterns of serum gonadal steroid concentrations in man from birth to two years of age. *J Clin Endocrinol Metab* 42:679, 1976.
287. Baker ML, Metcalfe SA, Hutson JM: Serum levels of Mullerian inhibiting substance in boys from birth to 18 years, as determined by enzyme immunoassay. *J Clin Endocrinol Metab* 70:11–15, 1990.
288. Josso N, Legeai L, Forest MG, Chaussain J-L, Brauner R: An enzyme linked immunoassay for anti-Mullerian hormone: A new tool for the evaluation of testicular function in infants and children. *J Clin Endocrinol Metab* 70:23–27, 1990.
289. Wu FCW, Butler GE, Kelnar CJH, Sellar RE: Patterns of pulsatile luteinizing hormone secretion before and during the onset of puberty in boys: A study using an immunoradiometric assay. *J Clin Endocrinol Metab* 70:629–637, 1990.
290. Dunkel L, Alfthan H, Stenman U-H, Tapanainen P, Perheentupa J: Pulsatile secretion of LH and FSH in prepubertal and early pubertal boys revealed by ultrasensitive time-resolved immunofluorometric assays. *Pediatr Res* 27:215–219, 1990.
291. Dunkel L, Alfthan H, Stenman U-H, Perheentupa J: Gonadal control of pulsatile secretion of luteinizing hormone and follicle-stimulating hormone in prepubertal boys evaluated by ultrasensitive time-resolved immunofluorometric assays. *J Clin Endocrinol Metab* 70:107–114, 1990.
292. Boyar RM, Rosenfeld RS, Kapen S, Finkelstein JW, Roffwarg HP, Weitzman ED, Hellman L: Human puberty: Simultaneous augmented secretion of luteinizing hormone and testosterone during sleep. *J Clin Invest* 54:609, 1974.
293. Ojeda SR, Andrews WW, Advis JP, White SS: Recent advances in the endocrinology of puberty. *Endocr Rev* 1:228, 1980.
294. Conte FA, Grumbach MM, Kaplan SL, Reiter EO: Correla-

tion of luteinizing hormone-releasing factor-induced luteinizing hormone and follicle-stimulating hormone release from infancy to 19 years with the changing pattern of gonadotropin secretion in agonadal patients: Relation to the restraint of puberty. *J Clin Endocrinol Metab* 50:163, 1980.
295. Garibaldi LR, Picco P, Magier S, Chevli R, Aceto T Jr: Serum luteinizing hormone concentrations, as measured by a sensitive immunoradiometric assay, in children with normal, precocious or delayed pubertal development. *J Clin Endocrinol Metab* 72:888–898, 1991.
296. Lucky AW, Rich BH, Rosenfield RL, Fang VS, Roche-Bender N: LH bioactivity increases more than immunoreactivity during puberty. *J Pediatr* 97:205–213, 1980.
297. Haavisto AM, Dunkel L, Pettersson K, Huhtaniemi I: LH measurements by *in vitro* bioassay and a highly sensitive immunofluorometric assay improve the distinction between boys with constitutional delay of puberty and hypogonadotropic hypogonadism. *Pediatr Res* 27:211–214, 1990.
298. Ahmed SR, Aiello DP, Page R, Hopper K, Towfighi J, Santen RJ: Necrotizing infundibulo-hypophysitis: A new syndrome of diabetes insipidus and hypopituitarism. *Clin Endocrinol* 1992 (submitted for publication).
299. Lam KSL, Tse VKC, Wang C, Yeung RTT, Ma JTC, Ho JHC: Early effects of cranial irradiation on hypothalamic-pituitary function. *J Clin Endocrinol Metab* 64:418, 1987.
300. Rappaport R, Brauner R, Czernichow P, Thiband E, Renier D, Zucker JM, Lemerle J: Effect of hypothalamic and pituitary irradiation on puberty development in children with cranial tumours. *J Clin Endocrinol Metab* 54:1164, 1982.
301. Oppenheim DS, Greenspan SL, Zervas NT, Schoenfeld DA, Klibanski A: Elevated serum lipids in hypogonadal men with and without hyperprolactinemia. *Ann Intern Med* 111:288, 1989.
302. Thorner MO, Evans WS, MacLeod RM, Nunley WC Jr, Rogol AD, Morris JL, Besser GM: Hyperprolactinemia: Current concepts of management including medical therapy with bromocriptine, in Goldstein M, Calne DB, Lieberman A, Thorner MO (eds): *Ergot Compounds and Brain Function: Neuroendocrine and Neuropsychiatric Aspects.* New York, Raven, 1980, p 165.
303. Fung MC, Wah GC, Odell WD: Effects of prolactin on luteinizing hormone-stimulated testosterone secretion in isolated perfused rat testis. *J Androl* 10:37, 1989.
304. Patton ML, Woolf PD: Hyperprolactinemia and delayed puberty: A report of three cases and their response to therapy. *Pediatrics* 71:572, 1983.
305. Bixler EO, Santen RJ, Kales A, Soldatos CR, Scharf MB: Inverse effects of thioridazine (Mellaril) on serum prolactin and testosterone concentrations in normal men, in Troen P, Nankin HR (eds): *The Testis in Normal and Infertile Men,* New York, Raven, 1977, p 403.
306. Bouchard P, Lagoguey M, Brailly S, Schaison G: Gonadotropin-releasing hormone pulsatile administration restores luteinizing hormone pulsatility and normal testosterone levels in males with hyperprolactinemia. *J Clin Endocrinol Metab* 60:258, 1985.
307. Leonard MP, Nickel CJ, Morales A: Hyperprolactinemia and impotence: Why, when and how to investigate. *J Urol* 142:992, 1989.
308. Rjosk HK, Schill WB: Serum prolactin in male infertility. *Andrologia* 11:297, 1979.
309. Vance ML, Evans WS, Thorner MO: Bromocriptine. *Ann Intern Med* 100:78, 1984.
310. Prior JC, Cox TA, Fairholm D, Kostashuk E, Nugent R: Testosterone-related exacerbation of a prolactin-producing macroadenoma: Possible role for estrogen. *J Clin Endocrinol Metab* 64:391, 1987.
311. Spitz IM, Diamant Y, Rosen E, Bell J, David MB, Polishuk W, Rabinowitz D: Isolated gonadotropin deficiency. *N Engl J Med* 290:10, 1974.
312. Santen RJ, Paulsen CA: Hypogonadotropic eunuchoidism: I. Clinical study of the mode of inheritance. *J Clin Endocrinol Metab* 36:47, 1973.
313. Dean JCS, Johnston AW, Klopper AI: Isolated hypogonadotrophic hypogonadism: A family with autosomal dominant inheritance. *Clin Endocrinol (Oxf)* 32:341, 1990.
314. Lieblich JM, Rogol AD, White BJ, Rosen SW: Syndrome of anosmia with hypogonadotropic hypogonadism (Kallmann syndrome): Clinical and laboratory studies in 23 cases. *Am J Med* 73:506, 1982.
315. White BJ, Rogol AD, Brown KS, Lieblich JM, Rosen SW: The syndrome of anosmia with hypogonadotropic hypogonadism: A genetic study of 18 new families and a review. *Am J Med Genet* 15:417, 1983.
316. Bick D, Sneed M, Yen PH, McGill J, Schorderet D, Hejtmancik JF, Ballabio A, Campbell L, et al: Mapping chondrodysplasia punctata ichthyosis, Kallmann syndrome and DNA markers in male patients with Xp chromosome deletions. *Cytogenet Cell Genet* (in press).
317. Nakayama Y, Wondisford FE, Lash RW, Bale AE, Weintraub BD, Cutler GB Jr, Radovick S: Analysis of gonadotropin-releasing hormone gene structure in families with familial central precocious puberty and idiopathic hypogonadotropic hypogonadism. *J Clin Endocrinol Metab* 70:1233, 1990.
318. Schwanzel-Fukuda M, Pfaff DW: Origin of luteinizing hormone-releasing hormone neurons. *Nature* 338:161, 1989.
319. Klingmuller D, Dewes W, Krahe T, Brecht G, Schweikert HU: Magnetic resonance imaging of the brain in patients with anosmia and hypothalamic hypogonadism (Kallmann's Syndrome). *J Clin Endocrinol Metab* 65:581, 1987.
320. Schwankhaus JD, Currie J, Jaffe MJ, Rose SR, Sherins RJ: Neurologic findings in men with isolated hypogonadotropic hypogonadism. *Neurology* 39:223, 1989.
321. Yeh J, Rebar RW, Liu JH, Yen SSC: Pituitary function in isolated gonadotrophin deficiency. *Clin Endocrinol (Oxf)* 31:375, 1989.
322. Mozaffarian GA, Higley M, Paulsen CA: Clinical studies in an adult male patient with "isolated follicle stimulating hormone (FSH) deficiency." *J Androl* 4:393, 1983.
323. Santen RJ, Kulin HE: Evaluation of delayed puberty and hypogonadotropism, in Santen RJ, Swerdloff RS (eds): *Male Reproductive Dysfunction: Diagnosis and Management of Hypogonadism, Infertility and Impotence.* New York, Marcel Dekker, 1986, pp 145–190.
324. Spratt DI, Hoffman AR, Crowley WF Jr: Hypogonadotropic hypogonadism and its treatment, in Santen RJ, Swerdloff RS (eds): *Male Reproductive Dysfunction: Diagnosis and Management of Hypogonadism, Infertility and Impotence.* New York, Marcel Dekker, 1986, p 227.
325. Spratt DI, Carr DB, Merriam GR, Scully RE, Rao PN, Crowley WF Jr: The spectrum of abnormal patterns of gonadotropin-releasing hormone secretion in men with idiopathic hypogonadotropic hypogonadism: Clinical and laboratory correlations. *J Clin Endocrinol Metab* 64:283, 1987.
326. Finkelstein JS, Spratt DI, O'Dea LStL, Whitcomb RW, Klibanski A, Schoenfeld DA, Crowley WF Jr: Pulsatile gonadotropin secretion after discontinuation of long term gonadotropin-releasing hormone (GnRH) administration in a subset of GnRH-deficient men. *J Clin Endocrinol Metab* 69:377, 1989.
327. Finkel DM, Phillips JL, Snyder PJ: Stimulation of spermatogenesis by gonadotropins in men with hypogonadotropic hypogonadism. *N Engl J Med* 313:651, 1985.
328. Rowe RC, Schroeder ML, Faiman C: Testosterone-induced fertility in a patient with previously untreated Kallmann's syndrome. *Fertil Steril* 40:400, 1983.
329. Doty RL, Shaman P, Dann M: Development of the University of Pennsylvania smell identification test: A standardized microencapsulated test of olfactory function. *Physiol Behav* 32:489, 1984.
330. Bauman A: Markedly delayed puberty or Kallmann's syndrome variant. *J Androl* 7:224–227, 1986.

331. Partsch C-J, Hermanussen M, Sippell WG: Differentiation of male hypogonadotropic hypogonadism and constitutional delay of puberty by pulsatile administration of gonadotropin releasing hormone. *J Clin Endocrinol Metab* 60:1196, 1985.
332. De Lange WE, Sluiter WJ, Snoep MC, Doorenbos H: The assessment of hypothalamic pituitary maturation during puberty with combined clomiphene citrate/GnRH test in boys. *J Endocrinol Invest* 7:611, 1984.
333. Barkan AL, Reame NE, Kelch RP, Marshall JC: Idiopathic hypogonadotropic hypogonadism in men: Dependence of the hormone responses to gonadotropin-releasing hormone (GnRH) on the magnitude of the endogenous GnRH secretory defect. *J Clin Endocrinol Metab* 61:1118, 1985.
334. Sizonenko PC: Endocrine laboratory findings in pubertal disturbances. *J Clin Endocrinol Metab* 4:173, 1975.
335. Moshang T Jr, Marx BS, Cara JF, Snyder PJ: The prolactin response to thyrotropin-releasing hormone does not distinguish teenaged males with hypogonadotropic hypogonadism from those with constitutional delay of growth and development. *J Clin Endocrinol Metab* 61:1211, 1985.
336. Cristiano AM, Munabi A, Sabbagh HE, Cassorla F, Sherins RJ: Prolactin response to metoclopramide does not distinguish patients with hypogonadotrophic hypogonadism from delayed puberty. *Clin Endocrinol (Oxf)* 28:75, 1988.
337. Ehrmann DA, Rosenfield RL, Cuttler L, Burstein S, Cara JF, Levitsky LL: A new test of combined pituitary-testicular function using the gonadotropin-releasing hormone agonist nafarelin in the differentiation of gonadotropin deficiency from delayed puberty: Pilot studies. *J Clin Endocrinol Metab* 69:963, 1989.
338. Bardin CW, Ross GT, Rifkind AB, Cargille CM, Lipsett MB: Studies of the pituitary-Leydig cell axis in young men with hypogonadotropic hypogonadism and hyposmia: Comparison with normal men, prepuberal boys, and hypopituitary patients. *J Clin Invest* 48:2046, 1969.
339. Sheckter CB, McLachlan RI, Tenover JS, Matsumoto AM, Burger HG, de Kretser DM, Bremner WJ: Stimulation of serum inhibin concentrations by gonadotropin-releasing hormone in men with idiopathic hypogonadotropic hypogonadism. *J Clin Endocrinol Metab* 67:1221, 1988.
340. Weinstein RL, Reitz RE: Pituitary-testicular responsiveness in male hypogonadotropic hypogonadism. *J Clin Invest* 53:408, 1974.
341. Santen RJ, Kulin HE: Hypogonadotropic hypogonadism and delayed puberty, in Burger H, de Kretser D (eds): *The Testis*. New York, Raven Press, 1981, p 329.
342. Counts DR, Pescovitz OH, Barnes KM, Hench KD, Chrousos GP, Sherins RJ, Comite F, Loriaux DL, Cutler GB Jr: Dissociation of adrenarche and gonadarche in precocious puberty and in isolated hypogonadotropic hypogonadism. *J Clin Endocrinol Metab* 64:1174, 1987.
343. Tolis G, Lewis W, Verdy M, Friesen HG, Solomon S, Pagalis G, Pavlatos F, Fessas PH, Rochefort JG: Anterior pituitary function in the Prader-Labhart-Willi (PLW) syndrome. *J Clin Endocrinol Metab* 39:1061, 1974.
344. Jeffcoate WJ, Laurence BM, Edwards CRW, Besser GM: Endocrine function in the Prader-Willi syndrome. *Clin Endocrinol (Oxf)* 12:81, 1980.
345. Pauli RM, Meisner LF, Szmanda RJ: Expanded Prader-Willi syndrome in a boy with an unusual 15q chromosome deletion. *Am J Dis Child* 137:1087, 1983.
346. Ledbetter DH, Mascarello JI, Riccardi VM, Harper VD, Hirhart SD, Strobel RJ: Chromosome 15 abnormalities and the Prader-Willi syndrome: A follow-up report of 40 cases. *Am J Hum Genet* 34:278, 1982.
347. Hamilton CR Jr, Scully RE, Kliman B: Hypogonadotropism in Prader-Willi syndrome. *Am J Med* 52:322, 1972.
348. Perez-Palacios G, Uribe M, Scaglia H, Lisker R, Pasapera A, Maillard M, Medina M: Pituitary and gonadal function in patients with the Laurence-Moon-Biedl syndrome. *Acta Endocrinol (Copenh)* 84:191, 1977.
349. Green JS, Parfrey PS, Harnett JD, Farid NR, Cramer BC, Johnson G, Heath O, McManamon PJ, et al: The cardinal manifestations of Bardet-Biedl syndrome, a form of Laurence-Moon-Biedl syndrome. *N Engl J Med* 321:1002, 1989.
350. Schachat AP, Maumenee IH: Bardet-Biedl syndrome and related disorders. *Arch Opthalmol* 100:285, 1982.
351. Dekaban NS, Parks JS, Ross GT: Laurence-Moon syndrome: Evaluation of endocrinological function and phenotypic concordance and report of cases. *Med Ann DC* 41:687, 1972.
352. Klein D, Amman F: The syndrome of Laurence-Moon-Bardet-Biedl and allied diseases in Switzerland. *J Neurol Sci* 9:479, 1969.
353. Lee CSN, Butler HG: The Laurence-Moon syndrome: Association with hypogonadotropic-hypogonadism and sex chromosome aneuploidy. *Arch Intern Med* 116:598, 1965.
354. Toledo SP, Medeiros-Neto GA, Knobel M, Mattar E: Evaluation of the hypothalamic-pituitary gonadal function in the Bardet-Biedl syndrome metabolism. *Metabolism* 26:1277, 1977.
355. Leroith D, Farkash Y, Bar-Ziev J, Spitz IM: Hypothalamic-pituitary function in the Bardet-Biedl syndrome. *Isr J Med Sci* 16:514, 1980.
356. Gorlin RJ, Anderson RC, Blaw M: Multiple lentigenes syndrome. *Am J Dis Child* 117:652, 1969.
357. Bardin CW: Hypogonadotropic hypogonadism in patients with multiple congenital defects, in Bergsma D (ed): *Birth Defects*, Baltimore, Williams & Wilkins, 1971, vol. 7, p 175.
358. Volpe R, Metzler WS, Johnston MW: Familial hypogonadotropic eunuchoidism with cerebellar ataxia. *J Clin Endocrinol Metab* 23:107, 1963.
359. Brackett E, Demers L, Mamourian AC, Ellenberger C Jr, Santen RJ: Moebius syndrome in association with hypogonadotropic hypogonadism: Case report. *J Endocrinol Invest*, 1992 (in press).
360. Rimoin DL, Schimke RN: The gonads, in Rimoin DL, Schimke RN (eds): *Genetic Disorders of the Endocrine Glands*. St. Louis, Mosby, 1971, pp 258–356.
361. Woolf PD, Hamill RW, McDonald JV, Lee LA, Kelly M: Transient hypogonadotropic hypogonadism caused by critical illness. *J Clin Endocrinol Metab* 60:444, 1985.
362. Hoffer LJ, Beitins IZ, Kyung N-H, Bistrian BR: Effects of severe dietary restriction on male reproductive hormones. *J Clin Endocrinol Metab* 62:288, 1986.
363. Dubey AK, Cameron JL, Steiner RA, Plant TM: Inhibition of gonadotropin secretion in castrated male rhesus monkeys (*Macaca mulatta*) induced by dietary restriction: Analogy with the prepubertal hiatus of gonadotropin release. *Endocrinology* 118:518, 1986.
364. Vogel AV, Peake GT, Rada RT: Pituitary-testicular axis dysfunction in burned men. *J Clin Endocrinol Metab* 60:658, 1985.
365. Blackman MR, Weintraub BD, Rosen SW, Harman SM: Comparison of the effects of lung cancer, benign lung disease, and normal aging on pituitary-gonadal function in men. *J Clin Endocrinol Metab* 66:88–95, 1988.
366. Christeff N, Benassayag C, Carli-Vielle C, Carli A, Nunez EA: Elevated oestrogen and reduced testosterone levels in the serum of male septic shock patients. *J Steroid Biochem* 29:435, 1988.
367. Santamaria JD, Prior JC, Fleetham JA: Reversible reproductive dysfunction in men with obstructive sleep apnoea. *Clin Endocrinol (Oxf)* 28:461, 1988.
368. Wortsman J, Eagleton LE, Rosner W, Dufau ML: Mechanism for the hypotestosteronemia of the sleep apnea syndrome. *Am J Med Sci* 293:221, 1987.
369. Clark JDA, Raggatt PR, Edwards OM: Hypothalamic hypogonadism following major head injury. *Clin Endocrinol (Oxf)* 29:153, 1988.
370. Glass AR: Pituitary-testicular reserve in men with low serum testosterone and normal serum luteinizing hormone. *J Androl* 9:224, 1988.

371. Pugliese MT, Lifshitz F, Grad G, Fort P, Marks-Katz M: Fear of obesity: A cause of short stature and delayed puberty. *N Engl J Med* 309:513, 1983.
372. Taylor AL, Fishman LM: Corticotropin-releasing hormone. *N Engl J Med* 319:213, 1988.
373. Sapolsky RM, Krey LC: Stress-induced suppression of luteinizing hormone concentrations in wild baboons: Role of opiates. *J Clin Endocrinol Metab* 66:722, 1988.
374. Barbarino A, de Marinis L, Tofani A, Casa SD, D'Amico C, Mancini A, Corsello SM, Sciuto R, Barini A: Corticotropin-releasing hormone inhibition of gonadotropin release and the effect of opioid blockade. *J Clin Endocrinol Metab* 68:523, 1989.
375. Dobs AS, Dempsey MA, Ladenson PW, Polk BF: Endocrine disorders in men infected with human immunodeficiency virus. *Am J Med* 84:611, 1988.
376. Milligan SA, Katz MS, Craven PC, Strandberg DA, Russel IJ, Becker RA: Toxoplasmosis presenting as panhypopituitarism in a patient with the acquired immune deficiency syndrome. *Am J Med* 77:760, 1984.
377. Croxson TS, Chapman WE, Miller LK, Levit CD, Senie R, Zumoff B: Changes in the hypothalamic-pituitary-gonadal axis in human immunodeficiency virus-infected homosexual men. *J Clin Endocrinol Metab* 68:317, 1989.
378. Strain GW, Zumoff B, Miller LK, Rosner W, Levit C, Kalin M, Hershcopf RJ, Rosenfeld RS: Effect of massive weight loss on hypothalamic-pituitary-gonadal function in obese men. *J Clin Endocrinol Metab* 66:1019, 1988.
379. Azizi F, Vagenakis AG, Longcope C, Ingbar SH, Braverman LE: Decreased serum testosterone concentration in male heroin and methadone addicts. *Steroids* 22:467, 1973.
380. Baker HWG, Burger HG, de Kretser DM, Dulmanis A, Hudson B, O'Connor S, Paulsen CA, Purcell N, et al: A study of the endocrine manifestations of hepatic cirrhosis. *Q J Med* 45:145, 1976.
381. De Besi L, Zucchetta P, Zotti S, Mastrogiacomo I: Sex hormones and sex hormone binding globulin in males with compensated and decompensated cirrhosis of the liver. *Acta Endocrinol (Copenh)* 120:271, 1989.
382. Van Thiehl DH, Lester R: Alcoholism: Its effect on hypothalamic pituitary gonadal function. *Gastroenterology* 71:318, 1976.
383. Emmanouel DS, Lindheimer MD, Katz AI: Pathogenesis of endocrine abnormalities in uremia. *Endocr Rev* 1:28, 1980.
384. Balducci R, Toscano V, Finocchi G, Municchi G, Mangiantini A, Boscherini B: Effect of hCG or hCG + FSH treatments in young thalassemic patients with hypogonadotropic hypogonadism. *J Endocrinol Invest* 13:1–7, 1990.
385. Cundy T, Bomford A, Butler J, Wheeler M, Williams R: Hypogonadism and sexual dysfunction in hemochromatosis: The effects of cirrhosis and diabetes. *J Clin Endocrinol Metab* 69:110, 1989.
386. Kley HK, Niederau C, Stremmel W, Lax R, Strohmeyer G, Kruskemper HL: Conversion of androgens to estrogens in idiopathic hemochromatosis: Comparison with alcoholic liver cirrhosis. *J Clin Endocrinol Metab* 61:1, 1985.
387. Siemons LJ, Mahler CH: Hypogonadotropic hypogonadism in hemochromatosis: Recovery of reproductive function after iron depletion. *J Clin Endocrinol Metab* 65:585, 1987.
388. Wang C, Tso SC, Todd D: Hypogonadotropic hypogonadism in severe β-thalassemia: Effect of chelation and pulsatile gonadotropin-releasing hormone therapy. *J Clin Endocrinol Metab* 68:511, 1989.
389. Claus-Walker J, Scurry M, Carter RE, Campos RJ: Steady state hormonal secretion in traumatic quadriplegia. *J Clin Endocrinol Metab* 44:530, 1977.
390. Barkan AL, Kelch RP Jr, Marshall JC: Isolated gonadotrope failure in the polyglandular autoimmune syndrome. *N Engl J Med* 312:1535, 1985.
391. Guay AT, Agnello V, Tronic BC, Gresham DG, Freidberg SR: Lymphocytic hypophysitis in a man. *J Clin Endocrinol Metab* 64:631, 1987.
392. MacAdams MR, White RH, Chipps BE: Reduction of serum testosterone levels during chronic glucocorticoid therapy. *Ann Intern Med* 104:648, 1986.
393. Wheeler GD, Singh M, Pierce WD, Epling WF, Cumming DC: Endurance training decreases serum testosterone levels in men without change in luteinizing hormone pulsatile release. *J Clin Endocrinol Metab* 72:422–425, 1991.
394. Kujala UM, Alen M, Huhtaniemi IT: Gonadotrophin-releasing hormone and human chorionic gonadotrophin tests reveal that both hypothalamic and testicular endocrine functions are suppressed during acute prolonged physical exercise. *Clin Endocrinol (Oxf)* 33:219, 1990.
395. Howlett TA: Hormonal responses to exercise and training: A short review. *Clin Endocrinol (Oxf)* 26:723, 1987.
396. Rosenfield RL: Diagnosis and management of delayed puberty. *J Clin Endocrinol Metab* 70:559–562, 1990.
397. Philip J, Lundsteen C, Owen D: The frequency of chromosome aberrations in tall men with special reference to 47,XYY and 47,XXY. *Am J Hum Genet* 28:404, 1976.
398. Witkin HA, Mednick SA, Schulsinger F, Bakkestrom E, Christiansen KO, Goodenough DR, Hirschhorn K, Lundsteen C, et al: Criminality in XYY and XXY men. *Science* 193:547, 1976.
399. Raboch J, Sipova I: The mental level in 47 cases of true Klinefelter's syndrome. *Acta Endocrinol (Copenh)* 36:404, 1961.
400. Ferguson-Smith MA: The prepubertal testicular lesion in chromatin-positive Klinefelter's syndrome (primary microorchidism) as seen in mentally handicapped children. *Lancet* 1:219, 1959.
401. Wang C, Baker HWG, Burger HG, de Kretser DM, Hudson B: Hormonal studies in Klinefelter's syndrome. *Clin Endocrinol (Oxf)* 4:399, 1975.
402. De la Chappelle A: Analytic review: Nature and origin of males with XX sex chromosomes. *Am J Hum Genet* 24:71, 1972.
403. Page DC, Mosher R, Simpson EM, Fisher EMC, Mardon G, Polack J, McGillivray B, de la Chapelle A, Brown LG: The sex determining region of the human Y chromosome encodes a finger protein. *Cell* 51:1091, 1987.
404. Harper P, Penny R, Foley TP Jr, Migeon CJ, Blizzard RM: Gonadal function in males with myotonic dystrophy. *J Clin Endocrinol Metab* 35:852, 1972.
405. Drucker WD, Blanc WA, Rowland LP, Grumbach MM, Christy NP: The testis in myotonic muscular dystrophy: A clinical and pathologic study with a comparison with the Klinefelter syndrome. *J Clin Endocrinol Metab* 23:59, 1963.
406. Chaves-Carballo E, Hayles AB: Ullrich-Turner syndrome in the male: Review of the literature and report of a case with lymphocytic (Hashimoto's) thyroiditis. *Mayo Clin Proc* 41:843, 1966.
407. Grumbach MM, Conte FA: Disorders of sexual differentiation, in Wilson JD, Foster DW (eds): *Textbook of Endocrinology*, 7th ed. Philadelphia, Saunders, 1985, p 312.
408. Friedrich V, Nielson J: Chromosome studies in 5,049 consecutive newborn children. *Clin Genet* 4:333, 1973.
409. Santen RJ, de Kretser DM, Paulsen CA, Vorhees J: Gonadotrophins and testosterone in the XYY syndrome. *Lancet* 2:371, 1970.
410. Schiavi RC, Owen D, Fogel M, White D, Szechter R: Pituitary-gonadal function in XYY and XXY men identified in a population survey. *Clin Endocrinol (Oxf)* 9:233, 1978.
411. Swersie S, Hueckel J, Hudson B, Paulsen CA: Endocrine, histologic and genetic features of the hypogonadism in patients with Down's syndrome. 53d Annual Meeting of the Endocrine Society, San Francisco, Abstr 440, 1971.
412. Abbasi AA, Prasad AS, Ortega J, Congco E, Oberleas D: Gonadal function abnormalities in sickle cell anemia: Studies in adult male patients. *Ann Intern Med* 85:601, 1976.
413. Elder M, Maclaren N, Riley W: Gonadal autoantibodies in patients with hypogonadism and/or Addison's disease. *J Clin Endocrinol Metab* 52:1137, 1981.

414. Aynsley-Green A, Zachmann M, Illig R, Rampini S, Prader A: Congenital bilateral anorchia in childhood: A clinical, endocrine and therapeutic evaluation of twenty-one cases. *Clin Endocrinol (Oxf)* 5:381, 1976.
415. Winter JSD, Faiman C: Serum gonadotropin concentrations in agonadal children and adults. *J Clin Endocrinol Metab* 35:561, 1972.
416. Levine LS, New MI: Preoperative detection of hidden testes. *Am J Dis Child* 121:176, 1971.
417. Schilsky RL, Lewis BJ, Sherins RJ, Young RC: Gonadal dysfunction in patients receiving chemotherapy for cancer. *Ann Intern Med* 93:109, 1980.
418. Da Cunha MF, Meistrich ML, Fuller LM, Cundiff JH, Hagemeister FB, Velasquez WS, McLaughlin P, Riggs SA, et al: Recovery of spermatogenesis after treatment for Hodgkin's disease: Limiting dose of MOPP chemotherapy. *J Clin Oncol* 2:571, 1984.
419. Brauner R, Czernichow P, Cramer P, Schaison G, Rappaport R: Leydig-cell function in children after direct testicular irradiation for acute lymphoblastic leukemia. *N Engl J Med* 309:25, 1983.
420. Aubier F, Flamant F, Brauner R, Caillaud JM, Chaussain JM, Lemerle J: Male gonadal function after chemotherapy for solid tumors in childhood. *J Clin Oncol* 7:304, 1989.
421. Schilsky RL: Male fertility following cancer chemotherapy. *J Clin Oncol* 7:295, 1989.
422. Paulsen CA: The study of radiation effects of the human testis: Including histologic, chromosomal and hormonal aspects. *Final Progress Report AEC Contract AT(45-1)-2225,* Task agreement 6, RLO-2225-2, 1973.
423. Ash P: The influence of radiation on fertility in man. *Br J Radiol* 53:271, 1980.
424. Talbot JA, Shalet SM, Tsatsoulis A, Grabinski M, Robertson WR: Luteinizing hormone pulsatility in men with damage to the germinal epithelium. *Int J Androl* 13:223, 1990.
425. Chlebowski RT, Heber D: Hypogonadism in male patients with metastatic cancer prior to chemotherapy. *Cancer Res* 42:2495, 1982.
426. Hembree WC III, Nahas GG, Zeidenberg P, Huang HFS: Changes in human spermatoza associated with high dose marihuana smoking, in Nahas GG, Paton WDM (eds): *Marihuana: Biological Effects.* New York, Pergamon, 1979, p 429.
427. Lantz GD, Cunningham GR, Huckins C, Lipshultz LI: Recovery from severe oligospermia after exposure to dibromochloropropane (DBCP). *Fertil Steril* 35:46, 1981.
428. Imperato-McGinley J, Akgun S, Ertel NH, Sayli B, Shackleton C: The coexistence of male pseudohermaphrodites with 17-ketosteroid reductase deficiency and 5α-reductase deficiency within a Turkish kindred. *Clin Endocrinol (Oxf)* 27:135, 1987.
429. Wilson SC, Hodgins MB, Scott JS: Incomplete masculinization due to a deficiency of 17β-hydroxysteroid dehydrogenase: Comparison of prepubertal and peripubertal siblings. *Clin Endocrinol (Oxf)* 26:459, 1987.
430. Eckstein B, Cohen S, Farkas A, Rosler A: The nature of the defect in familial male pseudohermaphroditism in Arabs of Gaza. *J Clin Endocrinol Metab* 68:477, 1989.
431. Kershnar AK, Borut D, Kogut MD, Biglieri EG, Schambelan M: Studies in a phenotypic female with 17-alpha-hydroxylase deficiency. *J Pediatr* 89:395, 1976.
432. Imperato-McGinley J, Peterson RE, Stoller R, Goodwin WE: Male pseudohermaphroditism secondary to 17β-hydroxysteroid dehydrogenase deficiency: Gender role change with puberty. *J Clin Endocrinol Metab* 49:391, 1979.
433. Ballew JW, Masters WH: Mumps, a cause of infertility: I. Present consideration. *Fertil Steril* 5:536, 1954.
434. Murray FT, Wyss HU, Thomas RG, Spevack M, Glaros AG: Gonadal dysfunction in diabetic men with organic impotence. *J Clin Endocrinol Metab* 65:127, 1987.
435. McCulloch DK, Campbell IW, Wu FC, Prescott RJ, Clarke BE: The prevalence of diabetic impotence. *Diabetologia* 18:279, 1980.
436. Murray FT, Cameron DF, Vogel RB, Thomas RG, Wyss HU, Zauner CW: The pituitary-testicular axis at rest and during moderate exercise in males with diabetes mellitus and normal sexual function. *J Androl* 9:197, 1988.
437. Murray FT, Rountree J, Sciadini M, Wyss HU, Thomas RG: Alterations in the pulsatile properties of luteinizing hormone (LH) in diabetic men with organic impotence. American Society Andrology, 14th Annual Meeting, Abstr 2, April 13–16, 1989.
438. Veremeulen A: Androgens in the aging male. *J Clin Endocrinol Metab* 73:221–250, 1991.
439. Harman SM, Tsitouras PD: Reproductive hormones in aging men: I. Measurement of sex steroids, basal luteinizing hormone, and Leydig cell response to human chorionic gonadotropin. *J Clin Endocrinol Metab* 51:35, 1980.
440. Kaler LW, Neaves WB: Attrition of the human Leydig cell population with advancing age. *Anat Rec* 192:513, 1978.
441. Johnson L, Zane RS, Petty CS, Neaves WB: Quantification of the human Sertoli cell population: Its distribution, relation to germ cell numbers, and age-related decline. *Biol Reprod* 31:785, 1984.
442. Johnson L, Petty CS, Neaves WB: Influence of age on sperm production and testicular weights in men. *J Reprod Fertil* 70:211, 1984.
443. Davidson JM, Chen JJ, Crapo L, Gray GD, Greenleaf WJ, Catania JA: Hormonal changes and sexual function in aging men. *J Clin Endocrinol Metab* 57:71, 1983.
444. Paniagua R, Martin A, Nistal M, Amat P: Testicular involution in elderly men: Comparison of histologic quantitative studies with hormone patterns. *Fertil Steril* 47:671, 1987.
445. Tsitouras PD, Martin CE, Harman SM: Relationship of serum testosterone to sexual activity in healthy elderly men. *J Gerontol* 37:288, 1982.
446. Plymate SR, Tenover JS, Bremner WJ: Circadian variation in testosterone, sex hormone-binding globulin, and calculated non-sex hormone-binding globulin bound testosterone in healthy young and elderly men. *J Androl* 10:366, 1989.
447. Carani C, Celani MF, Zini D, Baldini A, Della Casa L, Marrama P: Changes in the bioactivity to immunoreactivity ratio of circulating luteinizing hormone in impotent men treated with testosterone undecanoate. *Acta Endocrinol (Copenh)* 120:284, 1989.
448. Tenover JS, Matsumoto AM, Plymate SR, Bremner WJ: The effects of aging in normal men on bioavailable testosterone and luteinizing hormone secretion: Response to clomiphene citrate. *J Clin Endocrinol Metab* 65:1118, 1987.
449. Deslypere JP, Kaufman JM, Vermeulen T, Vogelaers D, Vandalem JL, Vermeulen A: Influence of age on pulsatile luteinizing hormone release and responsiveness of the gonadotrophs to sex hormone feedback in men. *J Clin Endocrinol Metab* 64:68, 1987.
450. Vermeulen A, Deslypere JP, Kaufman JM: Influence of anti-opioids on luteinizing hormone pulsatility in aging men. *J Clin Endocrinol Metab* 68:68, 1989.
451. Deslypere JP, Vermeulen A: Leydig cell function in normal men: Effect of age, life style, residence, diet and activity. *J Clin Endocrinol Metab* 59:955, 1984.
452. Winters S, Shawns R, Troen P: The gonadotropin suppressive activity of androgens is increased in elderly men. *Metabolism* 33:1052, 1984.
453. Korenman SG, Morley JE, Mooradian AD, Davis SS, Kaiser FE, Silver AJ, Viosca SP, Garza D: Secondary hypogonadism in older men: Its relation to impotence. *J Clin Endocrinol Metab* 71:963–969, 1990.
454. Migeon CJ, Brown TR, Fichman KR: Androgen insensitivity syndrome, in Josso N (ed): *Pediatric and Adolescent Endocrinology: The Intersex Child.* Basel, Karger, 1981, vol 8, p 171.

455. Grino PB, Griffin JE, Wilson JD: Androgen resistance due to decreased amounts of androgen receptor: A reinvestigation. *J Steroid Biochem* 35:647, 1990.
456. DiLauro SL, Behzadian A, Tho SPT, McDonough PG: Probing genomic deoxyribonucleic acid for gene rearrangement in 14 patients with androgen insensitivity syndrome. *Fertil Steril* 55:481, 1991.
457. Marcelli M, Tilley WD, Wilson CM, Griffin JE, Wilson JD, McPhaul MJ: Definition of the human androgen receptor gene structure permits the identification of mutations that cause androgen resistance: Premature termination of the receptor protein at amino acid residue 588 causes complete androgen resistance. *Mol Cell Endocrinol* 4:1105, 1990.
458. French FS, Lubahn DB, Brown TR, Simental JA, Quigley CA, Yarbrough WG, Tan J-A, Sar M, et al: Molecular basis of androgen insensitivity. *Recent Prog Horm Res* 46:1, 1990.
459. Ris-Stalpers C, Kuiper GGJM, Faber PW, Schweikert HU, van Rooij HCJ, Zegers ND, Hodgins MB, Degenhart HJ, et al: Aberrant splicing of androgen receptor mRNA results in synthesis of a nonfunctional receptor protein in a patient with androgen insensitivity. *Proc Natl Acad Sci USA* 87:7866, 1990.
460. Lubahn DB, Brown TR, Simental JA, Higgs HN, Migeon CJ, Wilson EM, French FS: Sequence of the intron/exon junctions of the coding region of the human androgen receptor gene and identification of a point mutation in a family with complete androgen insensitivity. *Proc Natl Acad Sci USA* 86:9534, 1989.
461. Brown TR, Lubahn DB, Wilson EM, Joseph DR, French FW, Migeon CJ: Deletion of the steroid-binding domain of the human androgen receptor gene in one family with complete androgen insensitivity syndrome: Evidence for further genetic heterogeneity in this syndrome. *Proc Natl Acad Sci USA* 85:8151–8155, 1988.
462. Marcelli M, Tilley WD, Wilson CM, Wilson JD, Griffin JE, McPhaul MJ: A single nucleotide substitution introduces a premature termination codon into the androgen receptor gene of a patient with receptor-negative androgen resistance. *J Clin Invest* 85:1522, 1990.
463. Griffin JE, Wilson JD: The androgen resistance syndromes: 5α-reductase deficiency, testicular feminization, and related disorders, in Scriver CR, Beaudet AL, Sly WS, Valle D (eds): *The Metabolic Basis of Inherited Disease,* 6th ed. New York, McGraw-Hill, 1989, pp 1919–1944.
464. Grino PB, Isidro-Gutierrez RF, Griffin JE, Wilson JD: Androgen resistance associated with a qualitative abnormality of the androgen receptor and responsive to high dose androgen therapy. *J Clin Endocrinol Metab* 68:578, 1989.
465. Grino PB, Griffin JE, Cushard WG Jr, Wilson JD: A mutation of the androgen receptor associated with partial androgen resistance, familial gynecomastia, and fertility. *J Clin Endocrinol Metab* 66:754, 1988.
466. Hughes JA, Evans BAJ, Ismail R, Matthews J: Complete androgen insensitivity syndrome characterized by increased concentration of a normal androgen receptor in genital skin fibroblasts. *J Clin Endocrinol Metab* 63:309, 1986.
467. Schweikert H-U, Schluter M, Romalo G: Intracellular and nuclear binding of [^{3}H]dihydrotestosterone in cultured genital skin fibroblasts of patients with severe hypospadias. *J Clin Invest* 83:662, 1989.
468. Guerami A, Griffin JE, Kovacs WJ, Grino PB, MacDonald PC, Wilson JD: Estrogen and androgen production rates in two brothers with Reifenstein syndrome. *J Clin Endocrinol Metab* 71:247, 1990.
469. Sinnecker G, Kohler S: Sex hormone-binding globulin response to the anabolic steroid stanozolol: Evidence for its suitability as a biological androgen sensitivity test. *J Clin Endocrinol Metab* 68:1195, 1989.
470. Bouchard P, Wright F, Portois MC, Couzinet B, Schaison G, Mowszowicz I: Androgen insensitivity in oligospermic men: A reappraisal. *J Clin Endocrinol Metab* 63:1242, 1986.
471. Aiman J, Griffin JE, Gazak JM, Wilson JD, MacDonald PC: Androgen insensitivity as a cause of infertility in otherwise normal men. *N Engl J Med* 300:223, 1979.
472. Aiman J, Griffin JE: The frequency of androgen receptor deficiency in infertile men. *J Clin Endocrinol Metab* 54:725, 1982.
473. Migeon CJ, Brown TR, Lanes R, Palacios A, Amrhein JA, Schoen EJ: A clinical syndrome of mild androgen insensitivity. *J Clin Endocrinol Metab* 59:672, 1984.
474. Eil C, Gamblin GT, Hodge JW, Clark RV, Sherins RJ: Whole cell and nuclear androgen uptake in skin fibroblasts from infertile men. *J Androl* 6:365, 1985.
475. Wilson JD, Griffin JE, George FW, Leshin M: The role of gonadal steroids in sexual differentiation. *Recent Prog Horm Res* 37:1, 1981.
476. Johnson L, George FW, Neaves WB, Rosenthal IM, Christensen RA, Decristoforo A, Schweikert HU, Sauer MV, et al: Characterization of the testicular abnormality in 5α-reductase deficiency. *J Clin Endocrinol Metab* 63:1091, 1986.
477. Bardin CW, Bullock LP, Sherins RJ, Mowszowicz I, Blackburn WR: Androgen metabolism and mechanism of action in male pseudohermaphroditism: II. A study of testicular feminization. *Recent Prog Horm Res* 29:65, 1973.
478. David R, Yoon DJ, Landin L, Lew L, Sklar C, Schinella R, Golimbu M: A syndrome of gonadotropin resistance possibly due to a luteinizing hormone receptor defect. *J Clin Endocrinol Metab* 59:156, 1984.
479. Jameson JL, Arnold A: Recombinant DNA strategies for determining the molecular basis of endocrine disorders. *J Clin Endocrinol Metab* 70:301, 1990.
480. Balducci R, Toscano V, Casilli D, Maroder M, Sciarra F, Boscherini B: Testicular responsiveness following chronic administration of hCG (1500 IU every six days) in untreated hypogonadotropic hypogonadism. *Horm Metabol Res* 19:216, 1987.
481. Snyder PJ: Clinical use of androgens. *Ann Rev Med* 35:207, 1984.
482. Sokol RZ, Palacios A, Campfield LA, Saul C, Swerdloff RS: Comparison of the kinetics of injectable testosterone in eugonadal and hypogonadal men. *Fertil Steril* 37:425, 1982.
483. Palacios A, Campfield LA, McClure RD, Steiner B, Swerdloff RS: Effect of testosterone enanthate on hematopoiesis in normal men. *Fertil Steril* 40:100, 1983.
484. Sandblom RE, Matsumoto AM, Schoene RB, Lee KA, Giblin EC, Bremner WJ, Pierson DJ: Obstructive sleep apnea syndrome induced by testosterone administration. *N Engl J Med* 308:508, 1983.
485. Boyer JL, Preisig R, Zbinden G, de Kretser DM, Wang C, Paulsen CA: Guidelines for assessment of potential hepatotoxic effects of synthetic androgens, anabolic agents and progestagens in their use in males as antifertility agents. *Contraception* 13:461, 1976.
486. Jackson JA, Waxman J, Spiekerman M: Prostatic complications of testosterone replacement therapy. *Arch Intern Med* 149:2365, 1989.
487. Bardin CW, Swerdloff RS, Santen RJ: Androgens: Risk and benefits. *J Clin Endocrinol Metab* 73:4, 1991.
488. Friedl KE, Hannan CJ, Jones RE, Plymate SR: High-density lipoprotein cholesterol is not decreased if an aromatizable androgen is administered. *Metabolism* 39:69–74, 1990.
489. Ahmed SR, Boucher AE, Manni A, Santen RJ, Bartholomew M, Demers LM: Transdermal testosterone therapy in the treatment of male hypogonadism. *J Clin Endocrinol Metab* 66:546, 1988.
490. Burris AS, Ewing LL, Sherins RJ: Initial trial of slow-release testosterone microspheres in hypogonadal men. *Fertil Steril* 50:493, 1988.
491. Handelsman DJ, Conway AJ, Boylan LM: Pharmacokinet-

ics and pharmacodynamics of testosterone pellets in man. *J Clin Endocrinol Metab* 70:216, 1990.

492. Finkelstein JS, Klibanski A, Neer RM, Doppelt SH, Rosenthal DI, Segre GV, Crowley WF Jr: Increases in bone density during treatment of men with idiopathic hypogonadotropic hypogonadism. *J Clin Endocrinol Metab* 69:776, 1989.
493. Liu L, Banks SM, Barnes KM, Sherins RJ: Two-year comparison of testicular responses to pulsatile gonadotropin-releasing hormone and exogenous gonadotropins from the inception of therapy in men with isolated hypogonadotropic hypogonadism. *J Clin Endocrinol Metab* 67:1140, 1988.
494. Liu L, Chaudhari N, Corle D, Sherins RJ: Comparison of pulsatile subcutaneous gonadotropin-releasing hormone and exogenous gonadotropins in the treatment of men with isolated hypogonadotropic hypogonadism. *Fertil Steril* 49: 302, 1988.
495. Jockenhovel F, Khan SA, Nieschlag E: Diagnostic value of bioactive FSH in male infertility. *Acta Endocrinol (Copenh)* 121:802, 1989.
496. Fauser BCJM, Bogers JW, Hop WCJ, De Jong FH: Bioactive and immunoreactive FSH in serum of normal and oligospermic men. *Clin Endocrinol (Oxf)* 32:433, 1990.
497. Wang C, Dahl KD, Leung A, Chan SYW, Hsueh AJW: Serum bioactive follicle-stimulating hormone in men with idiopathic azoospermia and oligospermia. *J Clin Endocrinol Metab* 65:629, 1987.
498. Franchimont P, Demoulin A, Bourguignon JP, Santen R: Role of inhibin in the regulation of gonadotrophin secretion in the male, in Job J-C (ed): *Pediatric and Adolescent Endocrinology: Cryptorchidism, Diagnosis and Treatment.* Basel, Karger, 1979, vol 6, p 47.
499. Bain J, Moskowitz JP, Clapp JJ: LH and FSH response to gonadotropin releasing hormone (GnRH) in normospermic, oligospermic and azoospermic men. *Arch Androl* 1:147, 1978.
500. Wu FCW, Edmond P, Raab G, Hunter WM: Endocrine assessment of the subfertile male. *Clin Endocrinol (Oxf)* 14:493, 1981.
501. Gross KM, Matsumoto AM, Bremner WJ: Differential control of luteinizing hormone and follicle-stimulating hormone secretion by luteinizing hormone-releasing hormone pulse frequency in man. *J Clin Endocrinol Metab* 64:675, 1987.
502. Wu FCW, Taylor PL, Sellar RE: LHRH pulse frequency in normal and infertile men. *J Endocrinol* 123:149, 1989.
503. Decker MH, Loriaux DL, Cutler GB: A seminiferous tubular factor is not obligatory for regulation of plasma follicle-stimulating hormone in the rat. *Endocrinology* 108:1035, 1981.
504. Giagulli VA, Vermeulen A: Leydig cell function in infertile men with idiopathic oligospermic infertility. *J Clin Endocrinol Metab* 66:62, 1988.
505. Chemes HE, Dym M, Fawcett DW, Jayadpour N, Sherins RJ: Pathophysiological observations of Sertoli cells in patients with germinal aplasia or severe germ cell depletion. *Biol Reprod* 17:108, 1977.
506. Mieusset R, Bujan L, Plantavid M, Grandjean H: Increased levels of serum follicle-stimulating hormone and luteinizing hormone associated with intrinsic testicular hyperthermia in oligospermic infertile men. *J Clin Endocrinol Metab* 68:419, 1989.
507. Clark RV, Sherins RJ: Treatment of men with idiopathic oligozoospermic infertility using the aromatase inhibitor, testolactone: Results of a double-blinded, randomized, placebo-controlled trial with crossover. *J Androl* 10:240, 1989.
508. Bals-Pratsch M, Knuth UA, Honigl W, Klein HM, Bergmann M, Nieschlag E: Pulsatile GnRH-therapy in oligozoospermic men does not improve seminal parameters despite decreased FSH levels. *Clin Endocrinol* 30:549, 1989.
509. Knuth UA, Honigl W, Bals-Pratsch M, Schleicher G, Nieschlag E: Treatment of severe oligospermia with human chorionic gonadotropin/human menopausal gonadotropin: A placebo-controlled, double-blind trial. *J Clin Endocrinol Metab* 65:1081, 1987.
510. AinMelk Y, Belisle S, Carmel M, Jean-Pierre T: Tamoxifen citrate therapy in male infertility. *Fertil Steril* 48:113, 1987.
511. Sokol RZ, Swerdloff RS: Male infertility: Diagnosis and medical management, in Aiman J (ed): *Infertility: Diagnosis and Management,* New York, Springer-Verlag, 1984, p 185.
512. Baker HWG: Development of clinical trials in male infertility research, in Serio M (ed): *Perspectives in Andrology.* New York, Raven, 1989, vol 53, p 307.
513. World Health Organization Task Force on the Diagnosis and Treatment of Infertility: Mesterolone and idiopathic male infertility: A double-blind study. *Int J Androl* 12:254, 1989.
514. Sokol RZ, Steiner BS, Bustillo M, Petersen G, Swerdloff RS: A controlled comparison of the efficacy of clomiphene citrate in male infertility. *Fertil Steril* 49:865, 1988.
515. Comhaire FH: Evaluation and treatment of varicocele, in Santen RJ, Swerdloff RS (eds): *Male Reproductive Dysfunction: Diagnosis and Management of Hypogonadism, Infertility and Impotence.* New York, Marcel Dekker, 1986, pp 387–406.
516. Pryor JL, Howards SS: Varicocele. *Urol Clin North Am* 14:499–513, 1987.
517. Dubin L, Amelar RD: Varicocelectomy: 986 cases in a twelve-year study. *Urology* 10:446, 1977.
518. Kursh ED: What is the incidence of varicocele in a fertile population? *Fertil Steril* 48:510–511, 1987.
519. Steeno O, Knops J, Declerck L, Adernoelja A, VanDeVoorde H: Prevention of fertility disorders by detection and treatment of varicocele at school and college age. *Andrologia* 8:47, 1971.
520. MacLeod J: Further observations on the role of varicocele in human male infertility. *Fertil Steril* 20:545, 1969.
521. Ayodeji O, Baker HWG: Is there a specific abnormality of sperm morphology in men with varicoceles? *Fertil Steril* 45:839–842, 1986.
522. Plymate SR, Nagao RR, Muller CH, Paulsen CA: The use of sperm penetration assay in evaluation of men with varicocele. *Fertil Steril* 47:680–683, 1987.
523. Clark RV, Sherins RJ: Male infertility, in Becker KL (ed): *Principles and Practice of Endocrinology and Metabolism.* Philadelphia, Lippincott, 1990, pp 985–991.
524. Baker HWG, Burger HG, de Kretser DM, Hudson B, Rennie GC, Straffon WGE: Testicular vein ligation and fertility in men with varicoceles. *Br Med J* 291:1678–1680, 1985.
525. Vermeulen A, Vandeweghe M: Improved fertility after varicocele correction: Fact or fiction? *Fertil Steril* 42:249–256, 1984.
526. Okuyama A, Fujisue H, Doi MY, Takeyama M, Nakamura M, Namiki M, Fujioka H, Matsuda M: Surgical repair of varicocele: Effective treatment from subfertile men in a controlled study. *Eur Urol* 14:298–300, 1988.
527. Hudson RW: The endocrinology of varicoceles. *Fertil Steril* 49:199–208, 1988.
528. Bickel A, Dickstein G: Factors predicting the outcome of varicocele repair for subfertility: The value of the luteinizing hormone-releasing hormone test. *J Urol* 142:1230–1234, 1989.
529. Lipshultz Ll, Corriere JN Jr: Progressive testicular atrophy in the varicocele patient. *J Urol* 117:175–176, 1977.
530. Kass EJ, Belman AB: Reversal of testicular growth failure by varicocele ligation. *J Urol* 137:475–476, 1987.
531. Kass EJ, Chandra RS, Belman AB: Testicular histology in the adolescent with a varicocele. *Pediatrics* 79:996–998, 1987.
532. Lyon RP, Marshall S, Scott MP: Varicocele in childhood and adolescence: Implication in adulthood infertility? *Urology* XIX:641–644, 1982.

533. Jarow JP, Espeland MA, Lipshultz LI: Evaluation of the azoospermic patient. *J Urol* 142:62, 1989.
534. Urban MD, Lee PA, Migeon CJ: Adult height and fertility in men with congenital virilizing adrenal hyperplasia. *N Engl J Med* 299:1392, 1978.
535. Bonaccorsi AC, Adler I, Figueiredo JG: Male infertility due to congenital adrenal hyperplasia: Testicular biopsy findings, hormonal evaluation, and therapeutic results in three patients. *Fertil Steril* 47:664, 1987.
536. Radfar N, Bartter FC, Easley R, Kolins J, Javadpour N, Sherins RJ: Evidence for endogenous LH suppression in a man with bilateral testicular tumors and congenital adrenal hyperplasia. *J Clin Endocrinol Metab* 45:1194, 1977.
537. Cutfield RG, Bateman JM, Odell WE: Infertility caused by bilateral testicular masses secondary to congenital adrenal hyperplasia (21-hydroxylase deficiency). *Fertil Steril* 40:809, 1983.
538. Uehling DT: Adrenal rest tumors of the testis: A case report of fertility following treatment. *Fertil Steril* 29:583, 1978.
539. Brown-Woodman PDC, Post EJ, Gass GC, White IG: The effect of a single sauna exposure on spermatozoa. *Arch Androl* 12:9, 1984.
540. Berger RE, Holmes KK: Infection and male infertility, in Santen RJ, Swerdloff RS (eds): *Male Reproductive Dysfunction: Diagnosis and Management of Hypogonadism, Infertility and Impotence.* New York, Marcel Dekker, 1986, p 407.
541. Gump DW, Gibson M, Ashikaga T: Lack of association between genital mycoplasmas and infertility. *N Engl J Med* 310:937, 1984.
542. Handelsman DJ, Conway AJ, Boylan LM, Turtle JR: Young's syndrome: Obstructive azoospermia and chronic sinopulmonary infections. *N Engl J Med* 310:3, 1984.
543. Afzelius BA: "Immotile-cilia" syndrome and ciliary abnormalities induced by infection and injury. *Am Rev Respir Dis* 124:107, 1981.
544. Gagnon C, Sherins RJ, Phillips DM, Bardin CW: Deficiency of protein-carboxyl methylase in immotile spermatozoa of infertile men. *N Engl J Med* 306:821, 1982.
545. Wang C, So SY, Wong KK, So WWK, Chan SYW: Chronic sinopulmonary disease in Chinese patients with obstructive azoospermia. *J Androl* 8:225, 1987.
546. Chandley AC: Assessment of blood karyotypes and germinal cell meiosis in the evaluation of male infertility, in Santen RJ, Swerdloff RS (eds): *Male Reproductive Dysfunction: Diagnosis and Management of Hypogonadism, Infertility and Impotence.* New York, Marcel Dekker, 1986, p 457.
547. Rabin BS, Nankin HR, Troen P: Immunologic studies of patients with idiopathic oligospermia, in Troen P, Troen HR (eds): *The Testis in Normal and Infertile Man.* New York, Raven Press, 1977, p 435.
548. Haas GG Jr: Evaluation of sperm antibodies and autoimmunity in the infertile male, in Santen RJ, Swerdloff RS (eds): *Male Reproductive Dysfunction: Diagnosis and Management of Hypogonadism, Infertility and Impotence.* New York, Marcel Dekker, 1986, p 439.
549. Haas GG Jr, Manganiello P: A double-blind, placebo-controlled study of the use of methylprednisolone in infertile men with sperm-associated immunoglobulins. *Fertil Steril* 47:295, 1987.
550. Whitcomb RW: The approach to the oligo/azoospermic male. *The Endocrinologist* 1:125–130, 1991.
551. Stenchever MA, Williamson RA, Leonard J, Karp LE, Ley B, Shy K, Smith D: Possible relationship between *in utero* diethylstilbestrol exposure and male fertility. *Am J Obstet Gynecol* 140:186, 1981.
552. Shangold GA, Cantor B, Schreiber JR: Treatment of infertility due to retrograde ejaculation: A simple, cost-effective method. *Fertil Steril* 54:175–177, 1990.
553. Snyder PJ, Bashey HM, Phillips JL, Gennarelli TA: Comparison of hormonal secretory behavior of gonadotroph cell adenomas *in vivo* and in culture. *J Clin Endocrinol Metab* 61:1061, 1985.
554. Snyder PJ, Bigdeli H, Gardner DF, Mihailovic V, Rudenstein RS, Sterling FH, Utiger RD: Gonadal function in fifty men with untreated pituitary adenomas. *J Clin Endocrinol Metab* 48:309, 1979.
555. Daneshdoost L, Gennarelli TA, Bashey HM, Savino PJ, Sergott RC, Bosley TM, Synder PJ: Recognition of gonadotroph adenomas in women. *N Engl J Med* 324:589–594, 1991.
556. Ishibashi M, Yamaji T, Takaku F, Teramoto A, Fukushima T: Secretion of glycoprotein hormone α-subunit by pituitary tumors. *J Clin Endocrinol Metab* 64:1187, 1987.
557. Yamada S, Asa SL, Kovacs K, Muller P, Smyth HS: Analysis of hormone secretion by clinically nonfunctioning human pituitary adenomas using the reverse hemolytic plaque assay. *J Clin Endocrinol Metab* 68:73, 1989.
558. Klibanski A, Deutsch PJ, Jameson JL, Ridgway EC, Crowley WF, Hsu DW, Habener JF, Black PMcL: Luteinizing hormone-secreting pituitary tumor: Biosynthetic characterization and clinical studies. *J Clin Endocrinol Metab* 64:536, 1987.
559. Friend JN, Judge DM, Sherman BM, Santen RJ: FSH-secreting pituitary adenomas: Stimulation and suppression studies in two patients. *J Clin Endocrinol Metab* 43:650, 1976.
560. Demura R, Jibiki K, Kubo O, Odagiri E, Demura H, Kitamura K, Shizume K: The significance of α-subunit as a tumor marker for gonadotropin-producing pituitary adenomas. *J Clin Endocrinol Metab* 63:564, 1986.
561. Klibanski A, Jameson JL, Biller BMK, Crowley WF Jr, Zervas NT, Rivier J, Vale WW, Bikkal H: Gonadotropin and α-subunit responses to chronic gonadotropin-releasing hormone analog administration in patients with glycoprotein hormone-secreting pituitary tumors. *J Clin Endocrinol Metab* 68:81, 1989.
562. Daneshdoost L, Pavlou SN, Molitch ME, Gennarelli TA, Savino PJ, Sergott RC, Bosley TM, River JE, et al: Inhibition of follicle-stimulating hormone secretion from gonadotroph adenomas by repetitive administration of a gonadotropin-releasing hormone antagonist. *J Clin Endocrinol Metab* 71:92, 1990.
563. Lamberts SWJ, Verleun T, Oosterom R, Hofland L, van Ginkel LA, Loeber JG, van Vroonhoven CCJ, Stefanko SZ, de Jong FH: The effects of bromocriptine, thyrotropin-releasing hormone, and gonadotropin-releasing hormone on hormone secretion by gonadotropin-secreting pituitary adenomas *in vivo* and *in vitro*. *J Clin Endocrinol Metab* 64:524, 1987.
564. Vos P, Croughs RJM, Thijssen JHH, van't Verlaat JW, van Ginkel LA: Response of luteinizing hormone secreting pituitary adenoma to a long-acting somatostatin analogue. *Acta Endocrinol (Copenh)* 118:587, 1988.
565. Kwekkeboom DJ, de Jong FH, Lamberts SWJ: Gonadotropin release by clinically nonfunctioning and gonadotroph pituitary adenomas *in vivo* and *in vitro:* Relation to sex and effects of thyrotropin-releasing hormone, gonadotropin-releasing hormone, and bromocriptine. *J Clin Endocrinol Metab* 68:1128, 1989.
566. Judge DM, Kulin HE, Page R, Santen R, Trapukdi S: Hypothalamic hamartoma: A source of luteinizing-hormone-releasing factor in precocious puberty. *N Engl J Med* 296:7, 1977.
567. Manasco PK, Pescovitz OH, Feuillan PP, Hench KD, Barnes KM, Jones J, Hill SC, Loriaux DL, Cutler GB Jr: Resumption of puberty after long term luteinizing hormone-releasing hormone agonist treatment of central precocious puberty. *J Clin Endocrinol Metab* 67:368, 1988.
568. Kappy M, Stuart T, Perelman A, Clemons R: Suppression of gonadotropin secretion by a long-acting gonadotropin-releasing hormone analog (Leuprolide acetate, Lupron depot)

in children with precocious puberty. *J Clin Endocrinol Metab* 69:1087–1089, 1989.

569. Kaplan SL, Grumbach MM: Clinical Review 14: Pathophysiology and treatment of sexual precocity. *J Clin Endocrinol Metab* 71:785–789, 1990.
570. Pescovitz OH, Comite F, Cassorla F, Dwyer AJ, Poth MA, Sperling MA, Hench K, McNemar A, et al: True precocious puberty complicating congenital adrenal hyperplasia: Treatment with a luteinizing hormone-releasing hormone analog. *J Clin Endocrinol Metab* 58:857, 1984.
571. Foster CM, Ross JL, Shawker T, Pescovitz OH, Loriaux DL, Cutler GB Jr, Comite F: Absence of pubertal gonadotropin secretion in girls with McCune-Albright syndrome. *J Clin Endocrinol Metab* 58:1161, 1984.
572. Manasco PK, Girton ME, Diggs RL, Doppman JL, Feuillan PP, Barnes KM, Cutler GB Jr, Loriaux DL, Albertson BD: A novel testis-stimulating factor in familial male precocious puberty. *N Engl J Med* 324:227–231, 1991.
573. Holland FJ, Kirsch SE, Selby R. Gonadotropin-independent precocious puberty ("Testotoxicosis"): Influence of maturational status on response to ketoconazole. *J Clin Endocrinol Metab* 64:328–333, 1987.
574. De Muinck Keizer-Schrama SMPF, Hazebroek FWJ, Drop SLS, Degenhart HJ, Molenaar JC, Visser HKA: Hormonal evaluation of boys born with undescended testes during their first year of life. *J Clin Endocrinol Metab* 66:159–164, 1988.
575. Elder JS, Issacs JT, Walsh PC: Androgenic sensitivity of the gubernaculum testis: Evidence for hormonal/mechanical interactions in testicular descent. *J Urol* 127:170, 1982.
576. Illig R, Torresani T, Bucher H, Zachmann M, Prader A: Effect of intranasal LHRH therapy on plasma LH, FSH and testosterone and relation to clinical results in prepubertal boys with cryptorchidism. *Clin Endocrinol (Oxf)* 12:91, 1980.
577. Puri P, Nixon HH: Bilateral retractile testes—subsequent effects on fertility. *J Pediatr Surg* 12:563, 1977.
578. Kulin HE, Santen RJ: Normal and aberrant pubertal development in man, in Vaitukaitis JL (ed): *Current Endocrinology: Clinical Reproductive Neuroendocrinology*. New York, Elsevier, 1982, p 19.
579. Waaler PE: Morphometric studies in undescended testes, in Job JC (ed): *Cryptorchidism*. Basel and New York, Karger, 1979, p 27.
580. Mengel W, Heinz HA, Sippe WG, Hecker WC: Studies on cryptorchidism: A comparison of histologic findings in the germinative epithelium before and after the second year of life. *J Pediatr Surg* 9:445, 1974.
581. Alpert PF, Klein RS: Spermatogenesis in the unilateral cryptorchid testis after orchiopexy. *J Urol* 129:301, 1983.
582. David G, Bisson JP, Martin-Boyce A, Feneux D: Sperm characteristics and fertility in previously cryptorchid adults, in Job JC (ed): *Cryptorchidism*. Basel and New York, Karger, 1979, p 187.
583. Krabbe S, Skakkebaek NE, Berthelson JG, Eyben FV, Volsted P, Mauritzen K, Eldrup J, Nielsen AH: High incidence of undetected neoplasia in maldescended testes. *Lancet* 1:999, 1979.
584. King LR: Optimal treatment of children with undescended testes. *J Urol* 131:734, 1984.
585. Ehrlich RM, Dougherty LJ, Tomashefsky P, Lattimer JK: Effect of gonadotropin in cryptorchidism. *J Urol* 102:793, 1969.
586. Rajfer J, Handelsman DJ, Swerdloff RS, Hurwitz R, Kaplan H, Vandergast T, Ehrlich RM: Hormonal therapy of cryptorchidism: A randomized, double-blind study comparing human chorionic gonadotropin and gonadotropin-releasing hormone. *N Engl J Med* 314:466, 1986.
587. Colodny AH: Undescended testes—is surgery necessary? *N Engl J Med* 314:510, 1986.
588. Chilvers C, Dudley NE, Gough MH, Jackson MB, Pike MC: Undescended testis: The effect of treatment on subsequent risk of subfertility and malignancy. *J Pediatr Surg* 21:691, 1986.
589. Thorup J, Kvist N, Larsen P, Tygstrup I, Mauritzen K: Clinical results of early and late operative correction of undescended testes. *Br J Urol* 56:322–325, 1984.
590. Wilson JD, Aiman J, MacDonald PC: The pathogenesis of gynecomastia, in Stollerman GH (ed): *Advances in Internal Medicine*. Chicago, Yearbook, 1980, vol 25, pp 1–32.
591. Nydick M, Bustos J, Dale JH Jr, Rawson RW: Gynecomastia in adolescent boys. *JAMA* 178:449, 1961.
592. Biro FM, Lucky AW, Huster GA, Morrison JA: Hormonal studies and physical maturation in adolescent gynecomastia. *J Pediatr* 116:450–455, 1990.
593. Lee PA: The relationship of concentrations of serum hormones to pubertal gynecomastia. *J Pediatr* 86:212–215, 1975.
594. La Franchi SH, Parlow AF, Luppe BM, Coytupa J, Kaplan SA: Pubertal gynecomastia and transient elevation of serum estradiol level. *Am J Dis Child* 129:927–931, 1975.
595. Knorr D, Bidlingmaier F: Gynecomastia in male adolescents. *J Clin Endocrinol Metab* 4:157–171, 1975.
596. Large DM, Anderson DC: Twenty-four hour profiles of circulating androgens and estrogens in male puberty with and without gynecomastia. *Clin Endocrinol (Oxf)* 11:505–521, 1979.
597. Moore DC. Schlaepfor LV, Paunier L, Sizonenko PC: Hormonal changes during puberty: V. Transient pubertal gynecomastia: Abnormal androgen-estrogen ratios. *J Clin Endocrinol Metab* 58:492–499, 1984.
598. Nuttal FQ: Gynecomastia as a physical finding in normal men. *J Clin Endocrinol Metab* 48:338, 1979.
599. Carlson HE: Current concepts: Gynecomastia. *N Engl J Med* 303:795, 1980.
600. Ley SB, Mozaffarian GA, Leonard JM, Higley M, Paulsen CA: Palpable breast tissue versus gynecomastia as a normal physical finding. *Clin Res* 28:24A, 1980.
601. Niewoehner CB, Nuttal FQ: Gynecomastia in a hospitalized male population. *Am J Med* 77:633–638, 1984.
602. Williams MJ: Gynecomastia: Its incidence, recognition and host characterization in 447 autopsy cases. *Am J Med* 34:103, 1963.
603. Eil C, Lippman ME, de Moss EV, Loriaux DL: Androgen receptor characteristics in skin fibroblasts from men with pubertal macromastia. *Clin Endocrinol (Oxf)* 19:223, 1983.
604. Berkovitz GD, Guerami A, Brown TR, MacDonald PC, Migeon CJ: Familial gynecomastia with increased extraglandular aromatization of plasma $carbon_{19}$-steroids. *J Clin Invest* 75:1763–1769, 1985.
605. Bulard J, Mowszowicz I, Schaison G: Increased aromatase activity in pubic skin fibroblasts from patients with isolated gynecomastia. *J Clin Endocrinol Metab* 64:618–623, 1987.
606. Elias AN, Valenta LJ, Domurat ES: Male hypogonadism due to nontumorous hyperestrogenism. *J Androl* 11:485–490, 1990.
607. Siiteri PK, MacDonald PC: Role of extraglandular estrogen in human endocrinology, in Greep RO, Astwood EB (eds): *Handbook of Physiology*. Baltimore, Waverly, 1973, vol 2, p 615.
608. Jensen RT, Collen MJ, Pandol SJ, Allende HD, Raufman JP, Bissonnette BM, Duncan WC, Durgin PL, et al: Cimetidine-induced impotence and breast changes in patients with gastric hypersecretory states. *N Engl J Med* 308:883, 1983.
609. Chopra IJ, Abraham GE, Chopra U, Solomon DH, Odell WD: Alterations in circulating estradiol-17β in male patients with Grave's disease. *N Engl J Med* 286:124, 1972.
610. Cavanaugh J, Niewoehner CB, Nuttall FQ: Gynecomastia and cirrhosis of the liver. *Arch Intern Med* 150:563–565, 1990.
611. Plourde PV, Kulin HE, Santner SJ: Clomiphene in the

treatment of adolescent gynecomastia. *Am J Dis Child* 137:1080, 1983.
612. Parker LN, Gray DR, Lai MK, Levin ER: Treatment of gynecomastia with tamoxifen: A double-blind crossover study. *Metabolism* 35:705–708, 1986.
613. Kuhn JM, Laudat MH, Roca R, Dugue MA, Luton JP, Bricaire H: Gynecomasties: Effect du traitement prolongé par la dihydrotestosterone par voie per-cutanée. *Press Med* 12:21, 1983.
614. Eberle AJ, Sparrow JT, Keenan BS: Treatment of persistent pubertal gynecomastia with dihydrotestosterone heptanoate. *J Pediatr* 109:144–149, 1986.
615. Zachmann M, Eiholzer U, Muritano M, Werder EA, Manella B: Treatment of pubertal gynecomastia with testolactone. *Acta Endocrinol [suppl] (Copenh)* 279:218–226, 1986.
616. Krane RJ, Goldstein I, De Tejada IS: Impotence. *N Engl J Med* 321:1648, 1989.
617. Morales A, Condra M, Reid K: The role of nocturnal penile tumescence monitoring in the diagnosis of impotence: A review. *J Urol* 143:441–446, 1990.
618. Burris AS, Banks SM, Sherins RJ: Quantitative assessment of nocturnal penile tumescence and rigidity in normal men using a home monitor. *J Androl* 10:492–497, 1989.
619. Fabbri A, Jannini EA, Ulisse S, Gnessi L, Moretti C, Frajese G, Isidori A: Low serum bioactive luteinizing hormone in nonorganic male impotence: Possible relationship with altered gonadotropin-releasing hormone pulsatility. *J Clin Endocrinol Metab* 67:867, 1988.
620. Plourde PV, Dufau ML, Plourde N, Santen RJ: Impotence associated with low biological to immunological ratio of luteinizing hormone in a man with a pituitary stone. *J Clin Endocrinol Metab* 60:797, 1985.
621. Cunningham GR, Hirshkowitz M, Korenman SG, Karacan I: Testosterone replacement therapy and sleep-related erections in hypogonadal men. *J Clin Endocrinol Metab* 70:792–797, 1990.
622. Karacan I, Moore CA: Objective methods of differentiation between organic and psychogenic impotence, in Santen RJ, Swerdloff RS (eds): *Male Reproductive Dysfunction: Diagnosis and Management of Hypogonadism, Infertility and Impotence*. New York, Marcel Dekker, 1986, p 545.
623. Spark RF, White RA, Connolly PB: Impotence is not always psychogenic: Newer insights into hypothalamic-pituitary-gonadal dysfunction. *JAMA* 243:750, 1980.
624. Hampson JL: Evaluation and treatment of psychogenic male erectile dysfunctions, in Santen RJ, Swerdloff RS (eds): *Male Reproductive Dysfunction: Diagnosis and Management of Hypogonadism, Infertility and Impotence*. New York, Marcel Dekker, 1986, p 521.
625. World Health Organization Task Force on Methods for the Regulation of Male Fertility: Contraceptive efficacy of testosterone-induced azoospermia in normal men. *Lancet* 336:955–959, 1990.
626. Matsumoto AM: Effects of chronic testosterone administration in normal men: Safety and efficacy of high dosage testosterone and parallel dose-dependent suppression of luteinizing hormone, follicle-stimulating hormone, and sperm production. *J Clin Endocrinol Metab* 70:282–287, 1990.
627. Rabin D, Evans RM, Alexander AN, Doelle GC, River J, Vale W, Liddle GW: Heterogeneity of sperm density profiles following 20-week therapy with high-dose LHRH analog plus testosterone. *J Androl* 5:176, 1984.
628. Pavlou SN: GnRH antagonists in men. 73rd Annual Meeting of the Endocrine Society, Washington, D.C., Session 15A, 1991, p 21.
629. Tom L, Salameh W, Bhasin S, Steiner B, Peterson M, Swerdloff RS: Male contraception: Achievement of reversible azoospermia by combined gonadotropin releasing hormone antagonist and testosterone enanthate regimen. 73rd Annual Meeting of the Endocrine Society, Washington, D.C., Abstr. 1154, 1991, p. 319.
630. Alexander NJ, Clarkson TB: Vasectomy increases the severity of diet-induced atherosclerosis in *Macaca fascicularis. Science* 201:538, 1978.
631. Hesketh PJ, Krane RJ. Prognostic assessment in nonseminomatous testicular cancer: Implications for therapy. *J Urol* 144:1–9, 1990.
632. Einhorn LH: Testicular cancer as a model for a curable neoplasm: The Richard and Linda Rosenthal Foundation Award Lecture. *Cancer Res* 41:3275, 1981.
633. DeWys WD, Muggia FM: Staging of testicular cancer. *Cancer Treat Rep* 63:1675, 1980.
634. Vugrin D, Herr HW, Whitmore WR Jr, Sogani PC, Golbey RB: VAB-6 combination chemotherapy in disseminated cancer of testis. *Ann Intern Med* 95:59, 1981.
635. Skakkebaek NE: Carcinoma-in-situ of the testis: Frequency and relationship to invasive germ cell tumors in infertile men. *Histopathology* 2:157, 1978.
636. Roth LM, Anderson MC, Govan ADT, Langley FA, Gowing NFC, Woodcock AS: Sertoli-Leydig cell tumors: A clinicopathologic study of 34 cases. *Cancer* 48:187, 1981.
637. Kuhn JM, Reznik Y, Mahoudeau JA, Courtois H, Lefebvre H, Wolf LM, Luton JP: hCG test in gynaecomastia: Further study. *Clin Endocrinol (Oxf)* 31:581–590, 1989.
638. Clark RV, Albertson BD, Munabi A, Cassorla F, Aguilera G, Warren DW, Sherins RJ, Loriaux DL: Steroidogenic enzyme activities, morphology, and receptor studies of a testicular adrenal rest in a patient with congenital adrenal hyperplasia. *J Clin Endocrinol Metab* 70:1408–1413, 1990.
639. Kuhn JM, Mahoudeau JA, Billaud L, Joly J, Rieu M, Gancel A, Archambeaud-Mouveroux F, Steg A, Luton JP: Evaluation of diagnostic criteria for Leydig cell tumours in adult men revealed by gynaecomastia. *Clin Endocrinol (Oxf)* 26:407–416, 1987.
640. Santen RJ: Endocrine aspects of prostate cancer, in Becker KL (ed): *Principles and Practice of Endocrinology and Metabolism,* Philadelphia, Lippincott, 1990, pp 1656–1663.
640a. Byar DP, Corle DK: Hormone therapy for prostate cancer: Results of the Veteran's Administration Cooperative Urological Research Group Studies. *NCI Monographs* 7:165–170, 1988.
641. Zincke H: The role of pathologic variables and hormonal treatment after radical prostatectomy for stage D1 disease. Oncology 5:129–140, 1991.
642. Santen RJ, Demers LM, Max DT, Smith J, Stein BS, Glode LM: Long term effects of administration of a gonadotropin-releasing hormone superagonist analog in men with prostatic carcinoma. *J Clin Endocrinol Metab* 58:397–400, 1984.
643. Geller J: Overview of enzyme inhibitors and anti-androgens in prostatic cancer. *J Androl* 12:364–370, 1991.
644. Sanford EJ, Paulson DF, Rohner TJ, Drago JR, Santen RJ, Bardin CW: The effects of castration on adrenal testosterone secretion in men with prostatic carcinoma. *J Urol* 118:1019–1021, 1977.
645. Crawford ED: Aminoglutethimide in metastatic carcinoma of the prostate. *Prog Clin Biol Res* 243A:283, 1987.
646. Harnett PR, Raghavan D, Caterson I, Pearson B, Watt H, Teriana N, Coates A, Coorey G: Aminoglutethimide in advanced prostate carcinoma. *Br J Urol* 59:323–327, 1987.
647. Labrie F, Dupont A, Giguere M, Borsanyi JP, Lacourciere Y, Monfette G, Emond J, Bergeron N: Important benefits of combination therapy with flutamide in patients relapsing after castration. *Br J Urol* 61:341–346, 1988.
648. Labrie F, Dupont A, Belanger A: Complete androgen blockade for the treatment of prostate cancer, in DeVita VT, Hellman D, Rosenberg SA (eds): *Important Advances in Oncology,* Philadelphia, Lippincott, 1985, pp 103–210.
649. Crawford ED, Nabors W: Hormone therapy of advanced prostate cancer: Where we stand today. *Oncology* 5:21–30, 1991.
650. Crawford ED, Eisenberger MA, McLeod DG, Spaulding JT, Benson R, Dorr FA, Blumenstein BA, Davis MA, Goodman

PJ: A controlled trial of leuprolide with and without flutamide in prostatic carcinoma. *N Engl J Med* 321(7):419–424, 1989.

651. Page RB, Dovey-Hartman BJ: Neurohemal contact in the internal zone of the rabbit median eminence. *J Comp Neurol* 226:274, 1984.
652. Christensen AK: Leydig cells, in Hamilton DW, Greep RO (eds): *Handbook of Physiology: Endocrinology*. Baltimore, Williams & Wilkins, 1975, vol 5, p 57.
653. Flickinger CJ, Brown JC, Kutchai HC, Ogilvie JW: *Medical Cell Biology*. Philadelphia, Saunders, 1979.
654. Fawcett DW: The mammalian spermatozoon. *Dev Biol* 44:394, 1975.
655. Kirschner MA, Zucker R, Jespersen D: Idiopathic hirsutism—an ovarian abnormality. *N Engl J Med* 294:637, 1976.
656. Santen RJ, Paulsen CA: Hypogonadotropic eunuchoidism: II. Gonadal responsiveness to exogenous gonadotropins. *J Clin Endocrinol Metab* 36:55, 1973.
657. Santen RJ: Independent effects of testosterone and estradiol on the secretion of gonadotropins in man, in Troen P, Nankin HR (eds): *The Testis in Normal and Infertile Men*. New York, Raven, 1977, p 197.
658. Marshall WA, Tanner JM: Variations in the pattern of pubertal changes in boys. *Arch Dis Child* 45:13, 1970.
659. Faiman C, Winter JSD: Gonadotropins and sex hormone patterns in puberty, in Grumbach MM, Grave GD, Mayer EF (eds): *The Control of the Onset of Puberty*. New York, Wiley, 1974, p 32.
660. Schwanzel-Fukada M, Pfaff DW: Origin of luteinizing hormone releasing hormone neurons. *Nature* 338:162, 1989.
661. Santen RJ, Swerdloff RS (eds): *Male Reproductive Dysfunction: Diagnosis and Management of Hypogonadism, Infertility and Impotence*. New York, Marcel Dekker, 1986.
662. Skakkebaek NE, Heller CG: Quantification of human seminiferous epithelium: I. Histological studies in twenty-one fertile men with normal chromosome complements. *J Reprod Fertil* 32:379, 1973.
663. MacLeod J, Gold RZ: The male factor in fertility and infertility: II. Spermatozoon counts in 1000 men of known fertility and in 1000 cases of infertile marriage. *J Urol* 66:436, 1951.
664. Naghma-E-Rehan, Sobrero AJ, Fertig JW: The semen of fertile men: Statistical analysis of 1300 men. *Fertil Steril* 26:492, 1975.
665. Nelson CMK, Bunge RG: Semen analysis: Evidence for changing parameters of male fertility potential. *Fertil Steril* 25:503, 1974.
666. Smith KD, Steinberger E: What is oligospeermia? in Troen P, Nankin HR (eds): *The Testis in Normal and Infertile Men*. New York, Raven, 1977, p 489.-

CHAPTER 17

The Ovary: Basic Principles and Concepts

A. PHYSIOLOGY*

Gregory F. Erickson

ANATOMY

Morphology

The mature human ovaries are oval-shaped bodies that each measure 2.5 to 5.0 cm in length, 1.5 to 3 cm in width, and 0.6 to 1.5 cm in thickness. The medial edge of the ovary is attached by the mesovarium to the broad ligament, which extends from the uterus laterally to the wall of the pelvic cavity. The surface of the ovary is a layer of cuboidal cells resting on a basement membrane. This layer, termed the *germinal* or *serous* epithelium, is continuous with the peritoneum. Underlying the serous epithelium is a layer of dense connective tissue termed the *tunica albuginea*.

The ovary is organized into two principal parts: a central zone called the *medulla*, which is surrounded by a particularly prominent peripheral zone called the *cortex* (Fig. 17A-1). A characteristic feature of the cortex is the presence of follicles containing the female gametes or *oocytes*. The number and size of the follicles vary depending on the age and reproductive state of the female. The existence of follicles of different sizes reflects internal changes associated with their growth and development. At the end of the follicular phase, the follicle that reaches maturity secretes its ovum into the peritoneal cavity (Fig. 17A-1). After ovulation, the wall of the follicle develops into a *corpus luteum* (Fig. 17A-1). If implantation does not occur, the corpus luteum deteriorates and eventually becomes a nodule of dense connective tissue called the *corpus albicans*. Another class of cells in the cortex is the steroidogenic cells termed *interstitial* cells. These cells are found in nests or cords and are present throughout the life of the female. At the medial border of the cortex is a mass of loose connective tissue, the *medulla*. This tissue contains a network of convoluted blood vessels and associated nerves which pass through the connective tissue toward the cortex.

Blood Vessels

The arterial supply to the ovary originates from two principal sources: One, the ovarian artery, arises from the abdominal aorta; the other is derived from the uterine artery.[1] These two vessels, which enter the mesovarium from opposite directions, form an anastomotic trunk and become a common vessel called the *ramus ovaricus* artery. At frequent intervals this artery gives rise to a series of primary branches which enter the hilum like teeth on a rake (Fig. 17A-2). In the hilum, numerous secondary and tertiary branches are given off to supply the medulla.

A characteristic feature of the secondary and tertiary arteries in the hilum and medulla is that they exhibit extensive spiraling.[1] The spiraling is in a counterclockwise direction with a gradually diminishing diameter (Fig. 17A-2). The degree of spiraling in the ovarian arteries undergoes dramatic changes during aging. In the fetal ovary, there is little or no spiraling of the ovarian arteries; however, in the neonatal period, extensive spiraling and profuse branching of these arteries occur. The spiral ovarian arteries are most highly developed in sexually mature women and remain prominent throughout the reproductive years. During the menopause, the spiral ovarian arteries diminish in number until finally only the main branches of the ovarian artery exist in the hilus.

What is the importance of spiral arteries in the ovary? Evidence suggests that the number and distribution of ovarian spiral arteries are influenced by local changes in ovarian sex hormones,[1] in a manner not unlike that reported for spiral arteries in the uterus. During growth and development of the dominant follicle and the corpus luteum tremendous in-

* This work was supported in part by National Institutes of Child Health and Human Development Research Center Grant HD-12303.

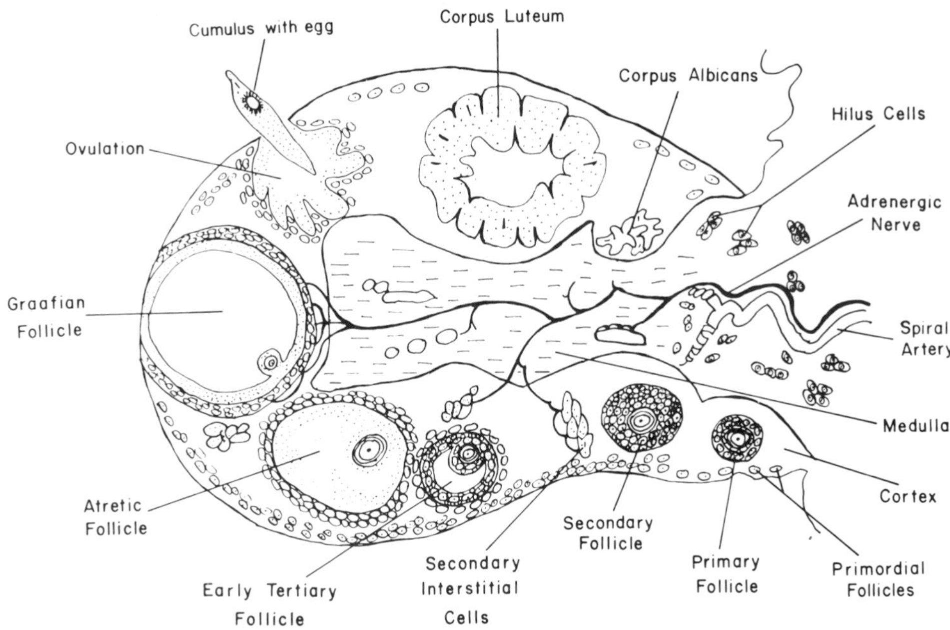

FIGURE 17A-1 Diagram summarizing the architecture of the human ovary during the reproductive years. The follicles, corpora lutea, and interstitial cells are located in the outer cortex, while the hilus cells, autonomic nerves, and spiral arteries are found in the medulla.

creases occur in the vascular bed which supplies these two organs; such increases are associated with the induction of a high order of spiraling of the arteries that serve the organs. Thus, it seems that when the dominant follicle is selected, local control mechanisms are initiated which increase the arterial supply and the degree of vessel spiraling. Although the nature of the inductive influences remains unknown, one such factor might be estrogen.[1] The physiologic significance of this phenomenon would be the adaptation of the vasculature to accommodate differential ovarian growth, which occurs during the

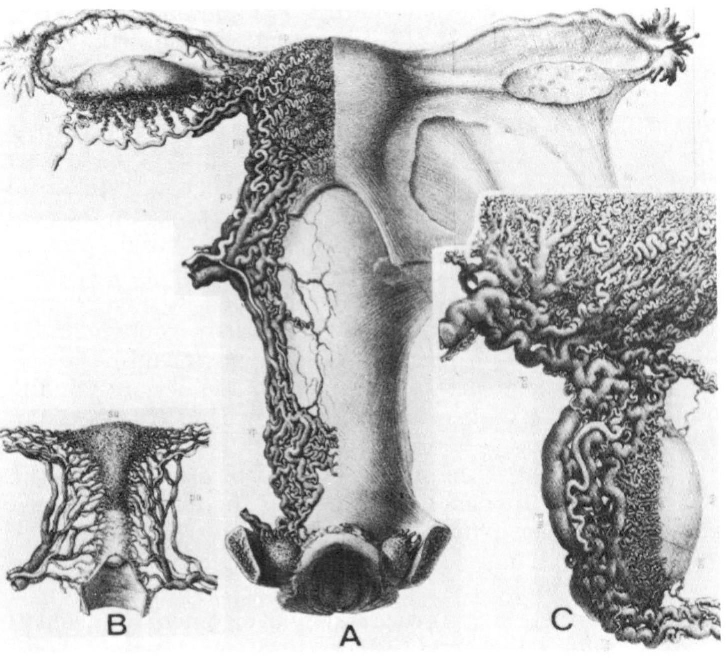

FIGURE 17A-2 Demonstration of extensive spiraling of arteries and veins in the genital tract of an adult woman. (*A*) Ovaries, fallopian tubes, uterus. (*B*) Details of uterus. (*C*) Details of ovary (note anastomoses of ovarian and uterine arteries). *(From Calza L: Arch Physiol Reils 7:341, 1807.)*

menstrual cycle. A physiologic sequela of the increased spiraling could be to provide a mechanism for regulating blood pressure within the ovary.[1]

Certainly the ovary contains within itself the capacity for vascular adaptation. In this sense, it seems possible that disturbed vascular activities may be etiologic factors in pathologic ovarian endocrine functions.

Innervation

Coursing through the human ovary is an extensive network of sympathetic and parasympathetic nerves reflecting both pre- and postganglionic fibers.[2] The preganglionic sympathetic fibers originate from cell bodies in the intermediolateral horn of the spinal cord at the 10th and 11th thoracic segments, and postganglionic sympathetic fibers originate from the ovarian and celiac plexuses. These nerves travel along the ovarian artery and enter the ovary at the hilus. The parasympathetic system consists of two main parts. One is derived from the vagus nerve and enters the hilum via the ovarian plexus. The other represents preganglionic parasympathetic fibers from the third and fourth sacral nerves, which are derived from the inferior hypogastric nerve. Thus, ovarian cells are capable of interacting with both adrenergic and cholinergic nerves.

The target tissues for adrenergic[3,4] and cholinergic fibers are in the cortex and medulla and include the smooth muscle cells of large arteries and veins and the smooth muscle cells in the outermost layer of the follicle, the theca externa (Fig. 17A-1). In the past few years considerable evidence has shown that ovarian cells respond to specific neurochemical transmitters with changes in steroidogenesis. The best examples come from studies in which catecholamine stimulated corpus luteum function and granulosa cell activity.[5,6] However, the physiologic significance of these studies remains unclear because neither the corpora lutea nor the granulosa cells are innervated.[7]

Ultrastructural studies in laboratory animals have clearly demonstrated that naked sympathetic adrenergic axons end directly on steroidogenic interstitial cells.[8] The innervation between these cells is not a typical synapse but rather a "buton de passage" type that is often seen between adrenergic terminals and glandular cells.[8] The importance of nerves in regulating ovarian functions is an important issue, which is discussed below.

HISTOLOGY

Ovarian Follicles

In the mammalian ovary, all follicles are embedded in the loose connective tissue of the cortex, medial to the tunica albuginea. Each follicle exhibits a specialized cytologic character which is related to the steps in its development. In a broad sense, there are two major classes of follicles: nongrowing and growing. The nongrowing follicles, which are referred to as *primordial* follicles, constitute 90 to 95 percent of the ovarian follicles throughout most of the life of the female. Once a primordial follicle has been recruited to initiate growth, its size, orientation, and relative position in the ovary change dramatically. Morphologically, the growing follicles can be divided into five classes: primary, secondary, tertiary, graafian, and atretic (Fig. 17A-3). It has been established in animal models that a recruited primordial follicle undergoes self-differentiation into the primary, secondary, and early tertiary stages in the absence of the pituitary.[9] Therefore, the mechanisms controlling differentiation of preantral follicle development are under intraovarian regulation. By contrast, when a growing follicle reaches the early tertiary stage (Fig. 17A-3), its survival and continued development depend on follicle stimulating hormone (FSH) and luteinizing hormone (LH).[10]

Preantral Follicles

Primordial Follicle

The primordial follicles represent a pool of nongrowing follicles from which all dominant preovulatory follicles are selected. In this sense, primordial follicles are the fundamental reproductive units of the ovary. Morphologically, each primordial follicle is composed of an outer single layer of squamous epithelial cells that are termed granulosa or follicle cells and a small (approximately 15 μm in diameter) immature oocyte arrested in the dictyotene stage of meiosis; both the granulosa and the oocyte are enveloped by a thin, delicate membrane called the *basal lamina* (Fig. 17A-4B). Because of the basal lamina, the granulosa and the oocyte exist in a microenvironment in which direct contact with other cells does not occur. Although small capillaries are occasionally observed in proximity to primordial follicles, these follicles do not have an independent blood supply.

Developmentally, the primordial follicles are formed in the cortical cords of the fetal ovaries between the sixth and ninth months of gestation (Fig. 17A-4A).[11] During this period the oocytes are stimulated to initiate meiosis in an asynchronous manner. Since the oocytes in the primordial follicles have entered meiotic prophase, all oocytes that are capable of participating in reproduction during a woman's life are formed at birth.[12] Soon after primordial follicle formation, some are recruited or activated to initiate growth.[13] As successive recruitments proceed, the size of the pool of primordial follicles becomes small.[14] Between the times of birth and menarche[12] the number of primordial follicles (and thus oocytes) decreases from several million to several hundred

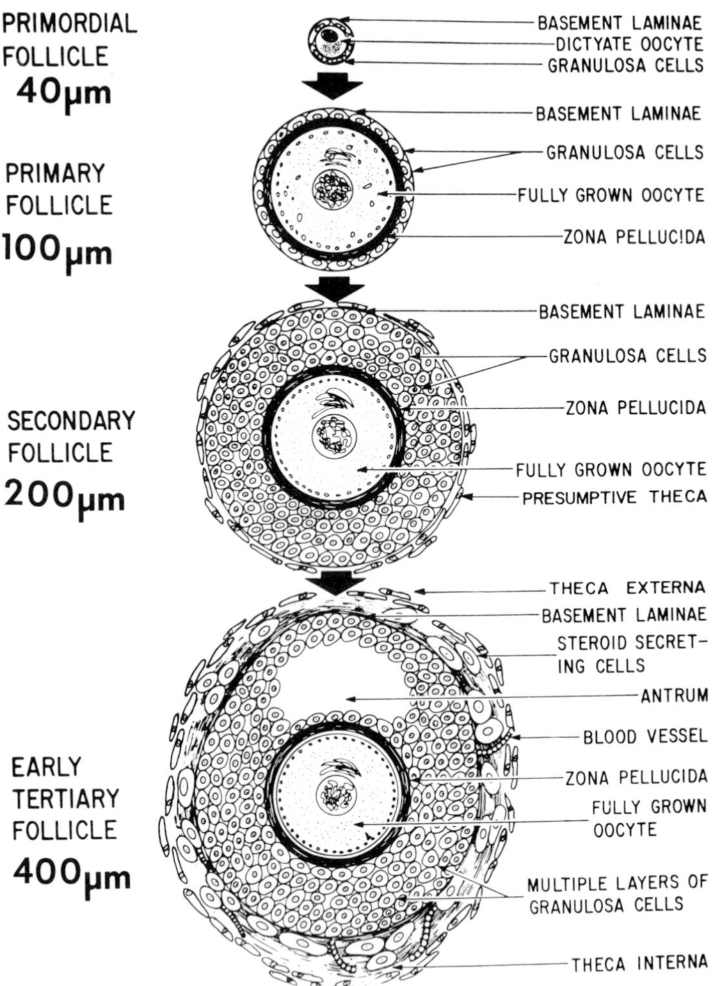

FIGURE 17A-3 Schematic drawing of the stages of preantral folliculogenesis. Note that the oocyte completes its growth very early in folliculogenesis, at the secondary stage. The average size of the follicles is indicated in micrometers. According to the work of Gougeon[156] it takes about 300 days for a recruited primordial follicle to grow to the early tertiary stage.

thousand (Fig. 17A-5). As a woman ages, the number of primordial follicles continues to decline until at menopause they are difficult to find (Fig. 17A-6).

Primary Follicle

A *primary follicle* is defined as one which contains a growing oocyte surrounded by a single layer of granulosa cells which is becoming cuboidal or low-columnar in shape (Fig. 17A-3). During primary follicular growth, both the granulosa and the oocyte undergo striking changes. The first indication of primary follicle development (recruitment) is that individual granulosa cells begin to become round and appear cuboidal rather than squamous in shape; at about this time, the oocyte begins to change, primarily by increasing in size. As oocyte growth progresses, small patches of glycoprotein material begin to form between the granulosa cells juxtaposed to the oolemma; this material eventually covers the entire egg and is termed the *zona pellucida*. At the later primary stage, the oocyte is nearly fully grown (100 µm in diameter) and is completely enveloped by a thin zona pellucida, a single layer of cuboidal granulosa cells, and a basal lamina (Fig. 17A-3).

Secondary Follicle

During the stages of secondary follicle development, the granulosa cells proliferate and the oocyte completes its growth. By the end of the secondary stage, the follicle is organized into a multilayered structure which is strikingly symmetrical. In the center is a full-grown oocyte (120 µm in diameter) covered by a thick zona pellucida, four to eight layers of stratified low-columnar granulosa cells, and a basal lamina (Fig. 17A-7).

During the course of secondary follicle development, several important morphologic events occur. One critical event involves the acquisition of cells of the prospective theca. When a secondary follicle acquires two to three layers of granulosa cells, a signal is generated which causes a stream of mesenchymal cells to migrate to the outer surface of the follicle.[9,15] The precise origin of these cells and the pathway they take remain unknown, but there is evidence in

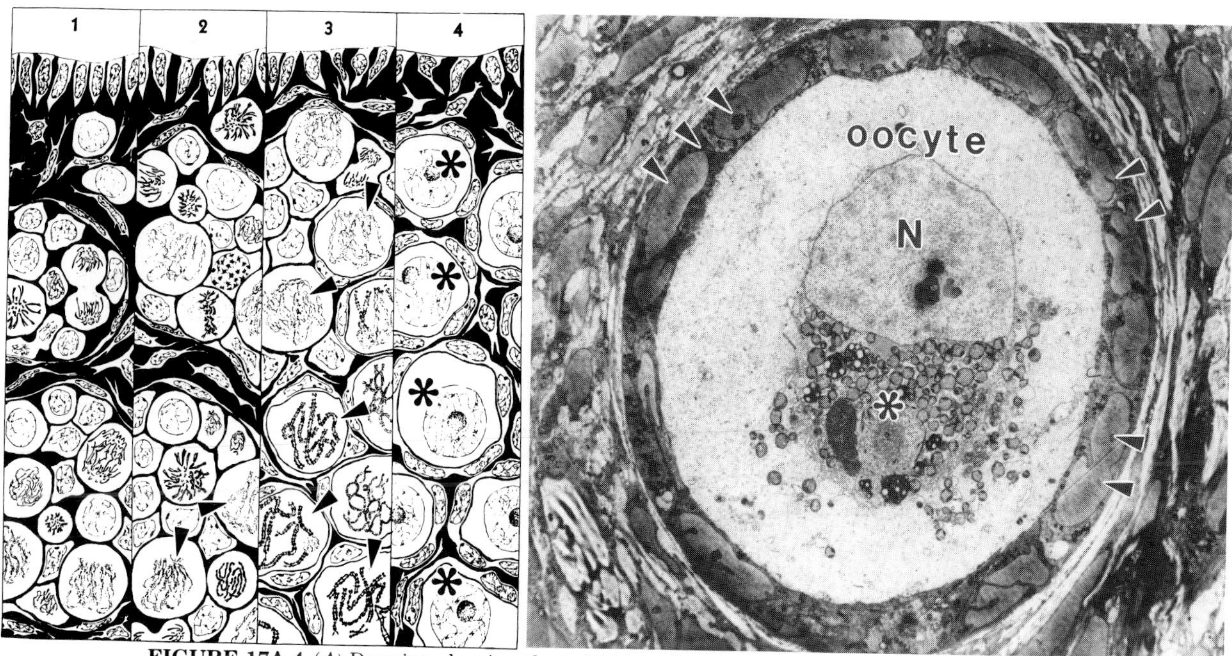

FIGURE 17A-4 *(A)* Drawing showing the initiation of meiosis in the cortex of the human fetal ovary, leading to the formation of the pool of primordial follicles. At 3 months (1), most of the oogonia are dividing mitotically. At 4 months (2), some oocytes deep within the cortical cords enter meiosis (arrowheads). At 7 months (3), the cords are no longer distinct and all germ cells are in meiotic prophase I. At 9 months (4), the oocytes become associated with pregranulosa cells and appear as primordial follicles (asterisks). *(From Ohno et al.,[11] by permission of S. Karger.)* *(B)* Electron micrograph of human primordial follicle. Granulosa cells (arrowheads), oocyte nucleus (N), and Balbiani body (asterisk) are shown.

the rodent that they arise from stromal fibroblasts outside the immediate vicinity of the secondary follicle.[16] After the mesenchymal cells reach the basal lamina, they align themselves in parallel and form a radial arrangement of highly elongated, fibroblast-like cells around the entire follicle (Fig. 17A-7). This newly acquired connective tissue layer of the secondary follicle ultimately gives rise to both the theca interna and the theca externa. Thus, it is apparent that when a follicle reaches the secondary stage, it has acquired a presumptive theca (Fig. 17A-7).

Another critical event which occurs during secondary follicle growth is the acquisition of an independent blood supply. At the secondary stage, a follicle is supplied by one or two arterioles which terminate in a wreathlike network of capillaries.[1] In a broad sense, the investing vessels form two sets of capillaries which are interconnected: an inner wreath of capillaries in the theca interna, which is supplied by branches from an outer wreath of capillaries in the theca externa. Characteristically, the capillaries of the inner wreath become closely associated with the basal lamina; however, they never penetrate beyond this membrane, and thus the granulosa and egg are avascular. The inner capillary wreath is drained by small venules which connect in

FIGURE 17A-5 Changes in the total number of germ cells in the human ovaries during aging. At early to midgestation the number of germ cells increases to almost 7×10^6. Shortly thereafter the number declines rapidly to about 2×10^6 at birth. The number continues to decline until no oocytes are detected at 50 years of age. *(From Baker and Sum, by permission.)*

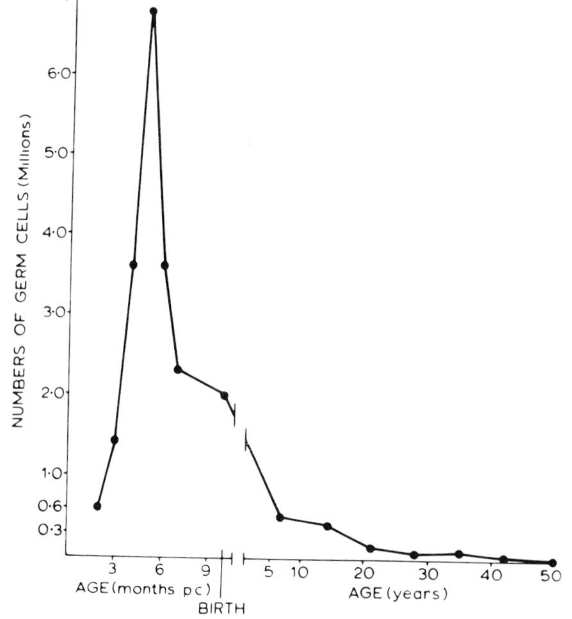

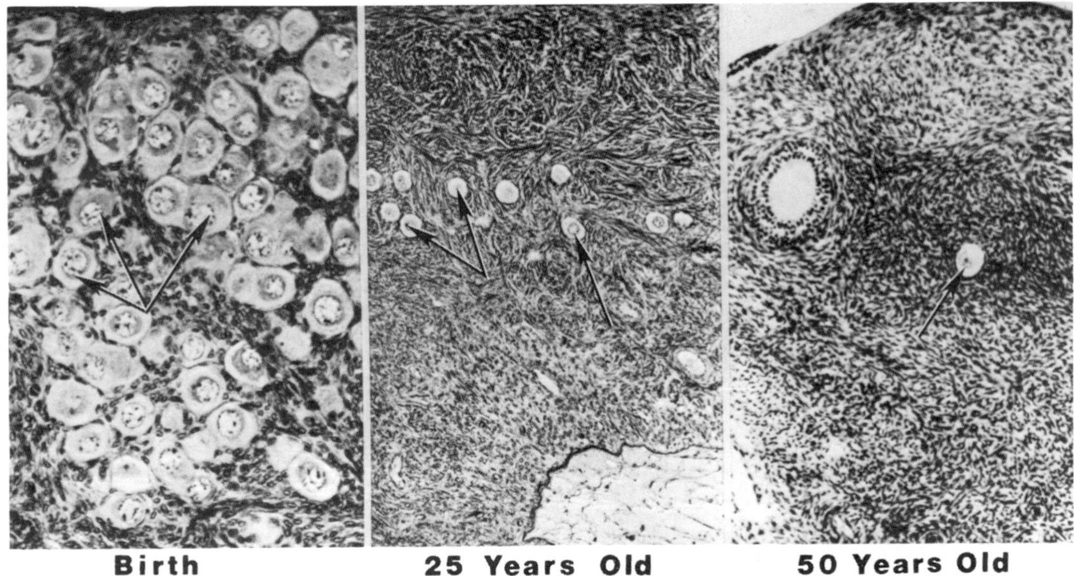

FIGURE 17A-6 Photomicrographs of sections through the cortex of human ovaries at different periods in life, showing the progressive decrease in the number of primordial follicles (arrows).

the theca externa into larger venules, which in turn enter the ovarian veins.[1]

Another interesting morphologic feature which appears in the secondary follicle is the formation of Call-Exner bodies among the granulosa cells (Fig. 17A-7). These bodies have been characterized ultrastructurally (Fig. 17A-8), but nothing is known about the manner in which they form or their physiologic importance. They may play a role in regulating granulosa differentiation by providing novel substrate-to-cell interactions.

Tertiary Follicle

The primary characteristic of a tertiary follicle is the presence of a small antrum. Antrum formation occurs when a follicle reaches approximately 400 μm in diameter.[10] The process of antrum formation in its earliest phase is termed *cavitation* (Fig. 17A-3). This

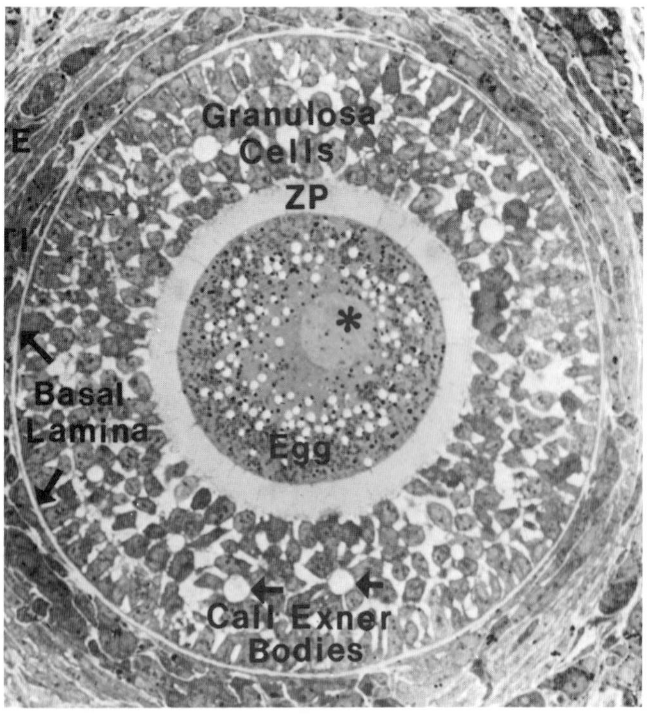

FIGURE 17A-7 Photomicrograph of a section through a preantral secondary follicle. The dictyotene oocyte contains a large germinal vesicle (asterisk) and a zona pellucida (ZP). The egg is surrounded by five layers of granulosa cells, which in turn are enclosed by a basal lamina. The presumptive cells of the theca interna (TI) and theca externa (TE) have become associated with the follicle. *(Courtesy of Dr. Everett Anderson, by permission of Saunders.)*

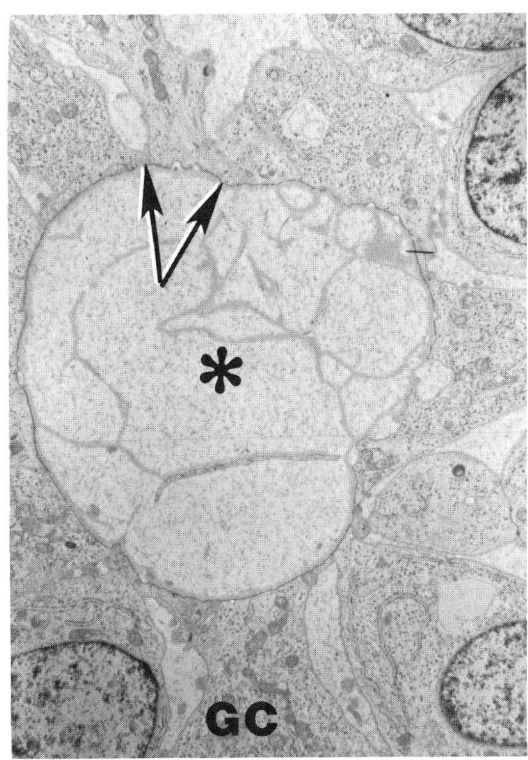

FIGURE 17A-8 Electron micrograph of a Call-Exner body. It consists of a distinct basal lamina (arrow) to which membrana granulosa cells (GC) are attached and a cavity (asterisk) with excess basal lamina material and a flocculant protein-like material. The question of its function remains unanswered.

event is characterized by the uptake or accumulation of fluid between the granulosa cells and, therefore, the formation of a small internal cavity at one pole of the oocyte. Histologic evidence indicates that the site of initiation of antrum formation is controlled in a highly specific manner (Fig. 17A-9). Although the underlying mechanism for cavitation is unknown, it occurs in the absence of the pituitary and thus seems to result from a developmental program within the follicle itself.[10] As a result of cavitation, the follicle acquires an inherent polarity and internal organization which remain throughout the rest of folliculogenesis.

Concurrent with the initiation of antrum formation, numerous histologic changes occur in both the theca interna and the granulosa cells. In the case of the theca interna,[15] subpopulations of stromal fibroblasts begin to be transformed into large epithelial cells termed *theca interstitial cells* (Fig. 17A-3). Eventually, the theca cells become highly differentiated steroidogenic cells which synthesize and secrete androgens in response to LH stimulation.[15]

At cavitation, there is a particularly dramatic increase in the size and number of gap junctions (Fig. 17A-10)[16,17] in the granulosa. The gap junction, or *nexus*, is a membrane specialization composed of a protein called *connexin*. Studies of the permeability of this cell-to-cell membrane channel have indicated that molecules with a molecular mass up to 1800 daltons can pass from one cell to another.[18] Gap junctions also develop between the oocyte and presumptive corona radiata granulosa cells. It appears from work in animals that this communication begins in the primary follicle and reaches a maximum at cavitation.[19] Gap junctions have also been found between differentiating theca interstitial cells at cavitation.[20] The concept which emerges is that, as a result of gap junctions, the entire follicle has the potential to undergo a synchronized pattern of activities, either positive or negative, in response to hormone stimulation.

Antral Follicles

Graafian Follicle

In response to FSH and LH brought to the follicle by the inner and outer capillary wreaths, the tertiary follicle increases tremendously in size.[10] If a developing human tertiary follicle is selected to ovulate, it may grow 75-fold, increasing from 0.4 mm to 30 mm in diameter; the growth of the graafian follicle is accomplished by granulosa and theca proliferation and follicular fluid accumulation in the antrum.[21] Contrary to preantral follicles, this change in size and differentiation is not under autonomous control but is dependent on FSH and LH.[10]

As seen in Fig. 17A-11, the graafian follicle is a highly structured mass of precisely positioned cells. Granulosa cells develop as pseudostratified epithelium and are limited peripherally by a basal lamina. By virtue of this architecture, the granulosa cells (and the egg) develop within the microenvironment of the follicular fluid. In the graafian follicle, both the number and the size of the gap junctions between the granulosa cells increase, suggesting that the levels of electric and metabolic coupling in this tissue become amplified during folliculogenesis.

During graafian follicle development the granulosa cells become different from one another with respect to polarity and relative position within the whole follicle (Fig. 17A-11). An important concept states that granulosa cells are a complex tissue containing several subgroups of different cell populations: the corona radiata cells, which make cell-to-cell contact with the egg and the zona pellucida; the cumulus cells, which make cell-to-cell contact with both the corona and membrana granulosa cells; and the membrana cells, which make direct contact with the basal lamina and Call-Exner bodies (Fig. 17A-11). This has led to the concept of heterogeneity in granulosa cell organization and function. An interesting and basic question (considered below) is to what extent the relative position of a granulosa cell or a group of granulosa cells within the follicle can determine the direction in which that cell differentiates.

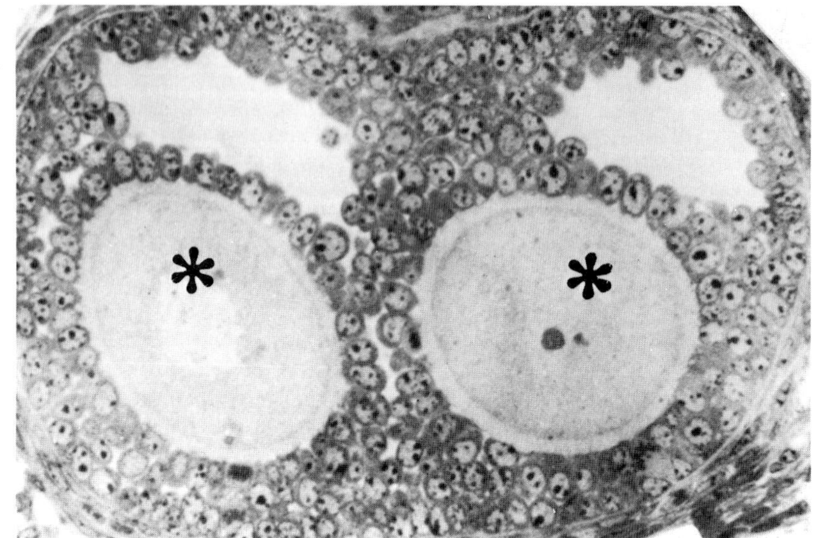

FIGURE 17A-9 Photomicrograph of a polyovular follicle at the early tertiary stage, showing the sites of cavitation or early antrum formation (clear spaces) just above oocytes (asterisk). This event, which is under intraovarian control, seems to arise in a specific synchronized manner and establishes the polarity of the follicle. *[From Zamboni, L: Comparative studies on the ultrastructure of mammalian oocytes. In* Oogenesis. *(Biggers JD and Schultz AW (eds). University Park Press, Baltimore, MD, pp 5–46, 1972.]*

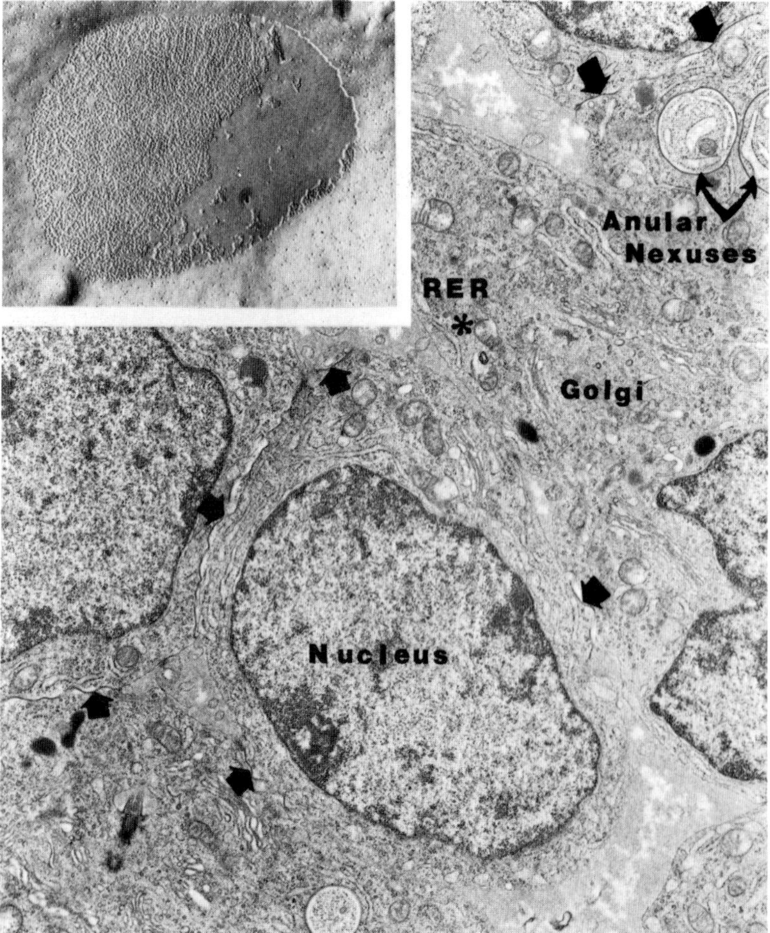

FIGURE 17A-10 Electron micrograph showing extensive gap junctional contacts (arrows) between granulosa cells of a healthy graafian follicle. *(Inset)* Replica of a granulosa cell fracture showing the hexagonally ordered particles of the gap junction. *(Courtesy of Dr. David Albertini.)*

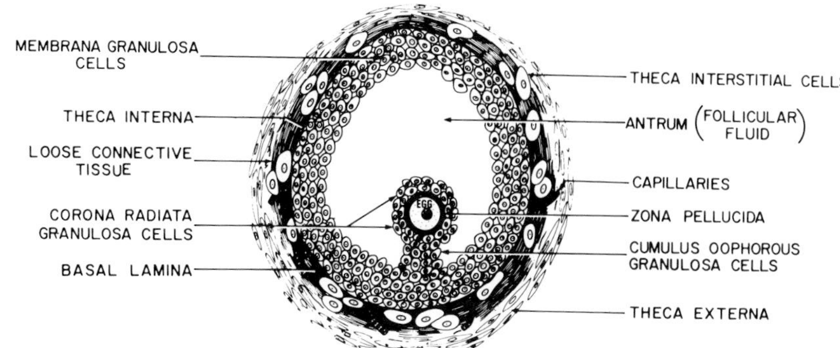

FIGURE 17A-11 Diagrammatic representation of the histology of a section through a dominant preovulatory graafian follicle. *(Revised from Erickson,[64] by permission by Elsevier Scientific.)*

Throughout graafian follicle development, the morphologic characteristics of the theca that are established at cavitation remain. Highly differentiated theca interstitial cells progressively accumulate until there are eventually five to eight layers of these cells in a dominant preovulatory follicle (Fig. 17A-11). The production of theca interstitial cells results, through mitotic division of cells in the theca interna.[21]

Electron microscopic studies of the theca externa of graafian follicles reveal the presence of smooth muscle cells[22] which contain actin and myosin.[23] The contractile cells in the theca externa (Figs. 17A-1 and 17A-11) are innervated by both sympathetic and parasympathetic nerves,[2] and the influence of the associated nerves presumably determines the extent to which the theca externa cells contract. Several lines of evidence point to a role of these cells in ovulation. This issue is addressed below.

Atretic Follicles

Once a primordial follicle is recruited to initiate growth, it either develops into a dominant preovulatory follicle or degenerates by a process termed *atresia*.[24] Atresia results in the selective death and clearance of the oocyte and granulosa, but the surrounding theca cells undergo extensive hypertrophy and eventually become interstitial gland cells, remaining permanently in the ovarian cortex.[15]

Differentiating between healthy and atretic follicles is difficult. Most researchers contend that a healthy follicle is completely free of degenerative necrotic changes; thus, any follicle which exhibits signs of cell death, regardless of how slight, would be atretic.

Based on studies in animal models, there seems to be two types of atresia: *type A* atresia, in which primary changes occur in the oocyte, and *type B* atresia, in which there are primary changes in granulosa cells.[25] Type A atresia is most common in preantral follicles, whereas type B atresia is most common in graafian follicles. During the course of both types of atresia, three major successive changes have been identified morphologically: the primary, secondary, and tertiary stages.

In the primary stage of type B atresia (in graafian follicles), necrotic changes first appear in some granulosa cells bordering the antrum (Fig. 17A-12).[26] In time, the margin of necrosis expands until all granulosa cells along the antrum are pyknotic. At the secondary stage, major zones of necrosis develop in the membrana granulosa cells. As necrosis continues,

FIGURE 17A-12 Photomicrograph of type B atresia in a graafian follicle. Note that large clumps of granulosa cells (open arrowhead) have detached from the basal lamina and that many appear pyknotic. By contrast, the dictyate egg appears healthy. The theca interstitial cells exhibit marked hypertrophy (arrows) and are surrounded by a thin theca interna (arrowheads).

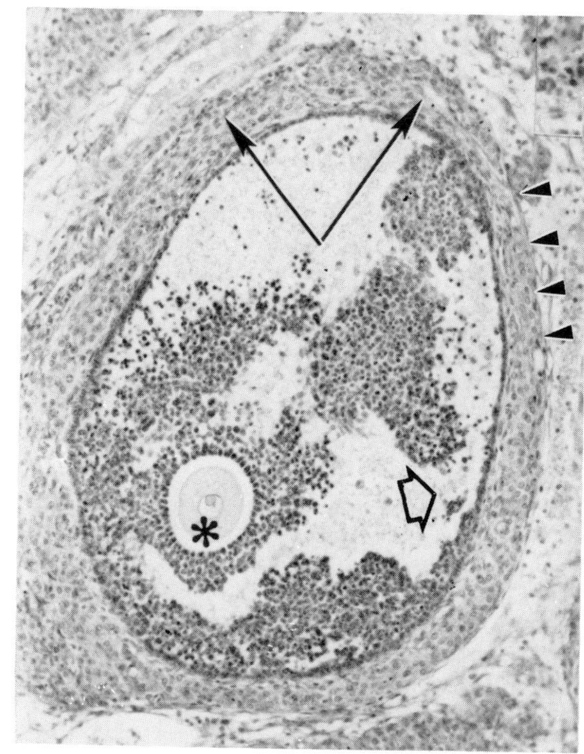

large numbers of granulosa cells undergo autophagy and their nuclei begin to fuse, forming so-called atretic bodies.[26] Atretic bodies usually have a diameter of about 15 μm but occasionally reach 400 μm in size and may contain DNA equivalent to 500,000 pyknotic granulosa nuclei.[27] It seems that some membrana granulosa cells become phagocytic cells which engulf membrane, lipid bodies, mitochondria, chromatin, and gap junctions. Directly next to the granulosa cells that are extruding their cytoplasmic and nuclear contents, there are granulosa cells which appear healthy and show mitotic activity. In this light, cumulus cells show little or no sign of necrosis during secondary atresia and thus seem to occupy a privileged position in comparison with membrana granulosa cells in the atretic process.[26] At the tertiary stage, the entire membrana granulosa is necrotic and large parts of it are often seen lying free in the antrum (Fig. 17A-12). During these late stages of atresia, intense necrosis begins appearing in the cumulus cells and the first signs of oocyte degeneration are detected. In some cases, the cumulus breaks up and the oocyte, surrounded only by corona radiata, is set free within the antral cavity. Finally, there is the complete clearance of the granulosa and oocyte; the follicle collapses. With the collapse of the follicle, the theca interstitial cells hypertrophy and become the secondary interstitial gland cells.[15]

The route taken in type A atresia (in preantral follicles) is completely different from that in the type B pattern. An early morphologic event seen in type A atresia involves the oocyte rather than the granulosa cells.[25–27] In the early phases of type A atresia the oocyte initiates meiotic maturation and begins to exhibit maturation spindles and polar bodies. In some instances, the activated oocytes in preantral follicles undergo pseudo cleavage or fragmentation into embryoid bodies.[28] Such activated eggs may be the source of ovarian teratomas. Subsequently, necrotic zones and atretic bodies develop in surrounding granulosa cells. This is followed by autophagy and removal of all granulosa and oocyte material from the preantral follicle. The basal lamina becomes hyalinized and the theca interna hypertrophies, after which the unit becomes part of the secondary interstitial gland cells.[15]

Ovarian Interstitial Cells

A characteristic feature of the human ovary is the presence of several different types of interstitial cells which can synthesize and secrete androgens. These cells are found in the stroma of both the cortex and the medulla (Fig. 17A-1). Over the years, considerable attention has been paid to the development of these cells, and as a result, the life cycle of the ovarian interstitial cell type has been well worked out. In all cases, the cells which eventually give rise to interstitial cells are derived from mesenchymal cells in the ovarian stroma.[15] In the human, there are four major classes of ovarian interstitial cells: (1) primary, (2) theca interstitial, (3) secondary interstitial, and (4) hilus cells. Because ovarian interstitial cells produce androgens, they are central in regulating a number of fundamental reproductive processes and therefore are of enormous physiologic importance.[15]

Primary Interstitial Cells

The first interstitial cells to develop in the ovary are termed primary interstitial cells. In the human, primary interstitial cells are first distinguished at 12 weeks gestation in the fetal ovary; they remain visible there until about the 20th week.[29] During their presence in the fetal ovary, the primary interstitial cells are juxtaposed to the basal lamina of the ovarian cortical cords which contain the oogonia and oocytes (Fig. 17A-13).

The ultrastructural properties of primary interstitial cells are consistent with those of active, steroid-secreting cells. It is interesting that these cells bear a striking resemblance to the Leydig cells in the human fetal testis.[29] If their ultrastructure is considered, it is suggested that primary interstitial cells are producing steroids, perhaps androgens, at high rates. This point is considered below.

Theca Interstitial Cells

The most widely studied class of ovarian interstitial cells is the theca interstitial cells.[15] Such cells are present in the theca interna of all tertiary follicles (Figs. 17A-3 and 17A-11). In the human, theca interstitial cells are the site of follicular androgen, most notably androstenedione, synthesis.[15,30–32]

As was pointed out earlier, presumptive theca interstitial cells first develop when a follicle reaches the secondary stage (Figs. 17A-3 and 17A-7). At this point, some mesenchymal cells undergo significant change and become directed along a path of theca interstitial cell differentiation. This developmental shift involves the acquisition of two constitutive molecules characteristic of a theca interstitial cell:[15,33] LH receptor and the 3β-hydroxysteroid dehydrogenase (3β-HSD)-$\Delta^{4,5}$-isomerase enzyme. The stimulus which causes some mesenchymal cells to undergo this change is unknown, but it appears to be directed by local information emanating from the secondary follicle itself and is independent of the pituitary. In this sense, it appears the acquisition of LH receptors and 3β-HSD in theca cells is determined by a basic clock mechanism operating within the secondary follicle. The remaining mesenchymal cells are thought to be pluripotent stem cells that can divide to produce other theca interstitial cells or differentiate into loose connective tissue as the follicle grows.[15]

The consequence of the transformation from a mesenchymal to a theca interstitial cell is evident. With the acquisition of LH receptors, theca interstitial cells are committed to respond to plasma LH,

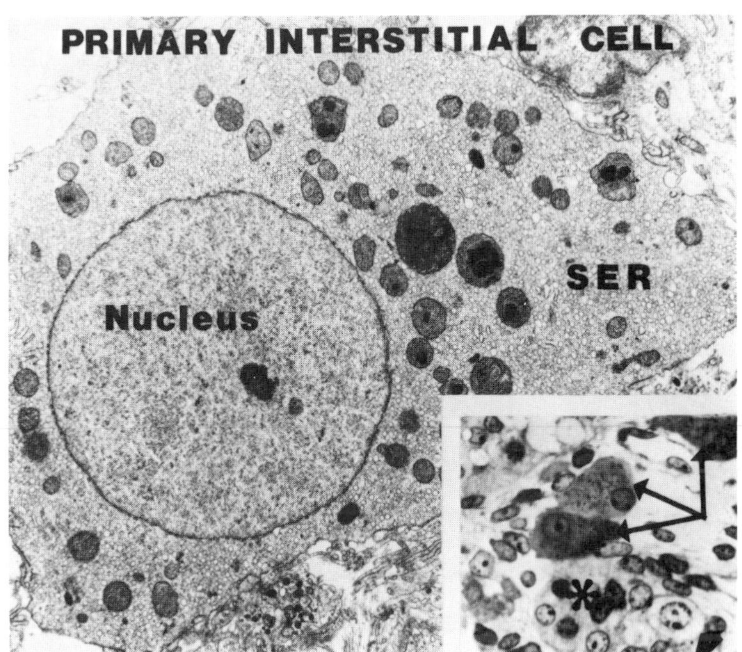

FIGURE 17A-13 Electron micrograph of primary interstitial cells in the human fetal ovary at 15 weeks gestation. Such ovarian cells strongly resemble steroidogenically active Leydig cells. *Inset* shows the intimate relation between primary interstitial cells (arrows) and oogonia (arrowhead) in the cortical cords (asterisk). *(From Ref. 29, courtesy of Dr. B. Gondos, by permission of Williams & Wilkins.)*

which is brought to the follicle by the inner capillary wreath. When a follicle reaches the early tertiary stage, the presumptive theca interstitial cells respond to LH by undergoing a major shape change from an elongated fibroblast to an epithelial cell.[15] Once the shape change is initiated (Fig. 17A-3), the cells begin to develop properties that are not found in the precursor stem cells. With increasing periods of time, theca interstitial cells increase markedly in size to 15 to 20 μm in diameter and acquire the fine structure typical of active steroid-synthesizing cells (Fig. 17A-14). This step is particularly striking and is characterized by the increased use of cytoplasmic organelles for de novo androgen biosynthesis. As folliculogenesis proceeds, the number of terminally differentiated theca interstitial cells increases as a result of mitosis.[21] Within the theca interna of developing follicles are transitional cells whose ultrastructure reflects intermediate stages between the ultrastructure of unspecialized mesenchymal cells and that of fully differentiated steroidogenic cells, providing support for the concept of a theca interstitial stem cell.

A characteristic feature of the human theca interna is the presence of what seem to be subpopulations of differentiated theca interstitial cells (Fig. 17A-14). Electron micrographs show that the two main types (dark and light cells) both have the ultrastructure of active steroidogenic cells. Even though data are lacking, the demonstration of cytologic heterogeneity raises the possibility that within a follicle there are theca interstitial cells with differing endocrine capabilities and responsiveness.[15] Whether these cells secrete different classes of steroids or are regulated independently is an intriguing and unanswered question.

Secondary Interstitial Cells

During the process of atresia, the granulosa and the egg degenerate; however, the theca interstitial cells[15] of atretic follicles undergo a striking hypertrophy (Fig. 17A-12) and survive as cords or clusters of large epithelial cells called *secondary interstitial cells*.[15,34,35] In this sense, secondary interstitial cells are direct descendants of theca interstitial cells of atretic follicles. Thus, theca interstitial cells never die but are actually accumulated in the ovary. In humans, secondary interstitial cells maintain their specialized ultrastructure characteristic of active steroidogenic cells (Fig. 17A-15) and continue responding to LH with increased androstenedione production.[21] This indicates that the secondary interstitial cells continue to exhibit properties of their precursors, the theca interstitial cells, throughout the life of the female.

There is, however, one very important property that these two cell types do not have in common: Secondary, but not theca, interstitial cells are innervated.[15] As was mentioned earlier, secondary interstitial cells are unique in that they seem to be innervated by sympathetic nerves. Evidence in rodents strongly suggests the existence of point-to-point communication between neurons in the brain and the ovarian steroidogenic cells.[36] Stimulation of selected hypothalamic nuclei in hypophysectomized and adrenalectomized rats stimulates or inhibits estrogen and progesterone synthesis, depending on which nucleus is stimulated.[36] It seems, therefore,

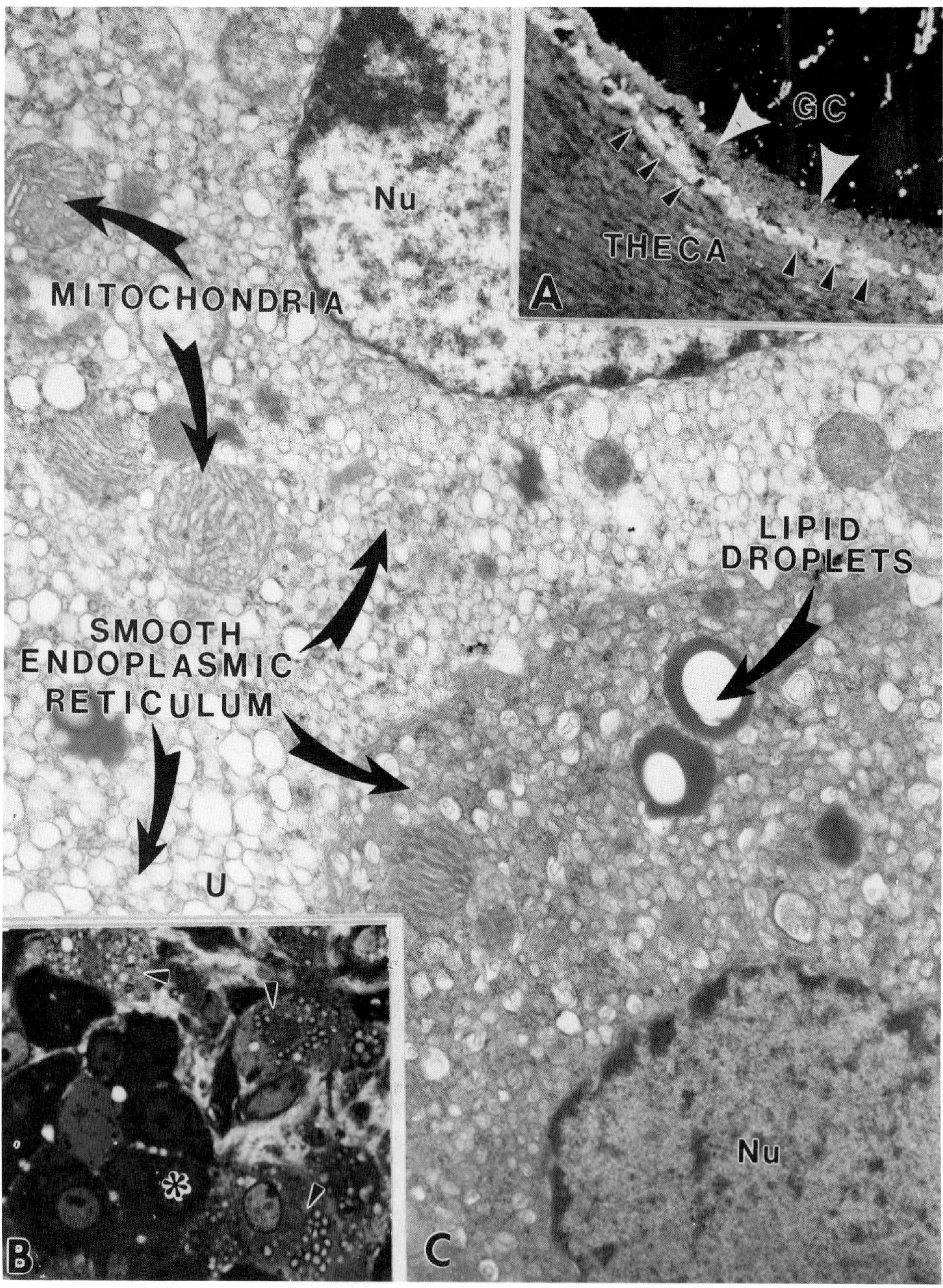

FIGURE 17A-14 Histology of human theca interstitial cells. (*A*) Localization of $P450_{17\alpha}$ in theca cells. $P450_{17\alpha}$ was detected by immunocytochemistry. Note that $P450_{17\alpha}$ is not detected in the granulosa (GC). (*B*) Photomicrograph of theca interna showing the two populations of differentiated theca interstitial cells: dark ones (asterisk) and light ones (arrowheads). (*C*) Electron micrograph of the dark and light cells. Note that both contain mitochondria with tubular cristae (the site of $P450_{ssc}$) and lipid droplets (site of cholesterol ester storage).

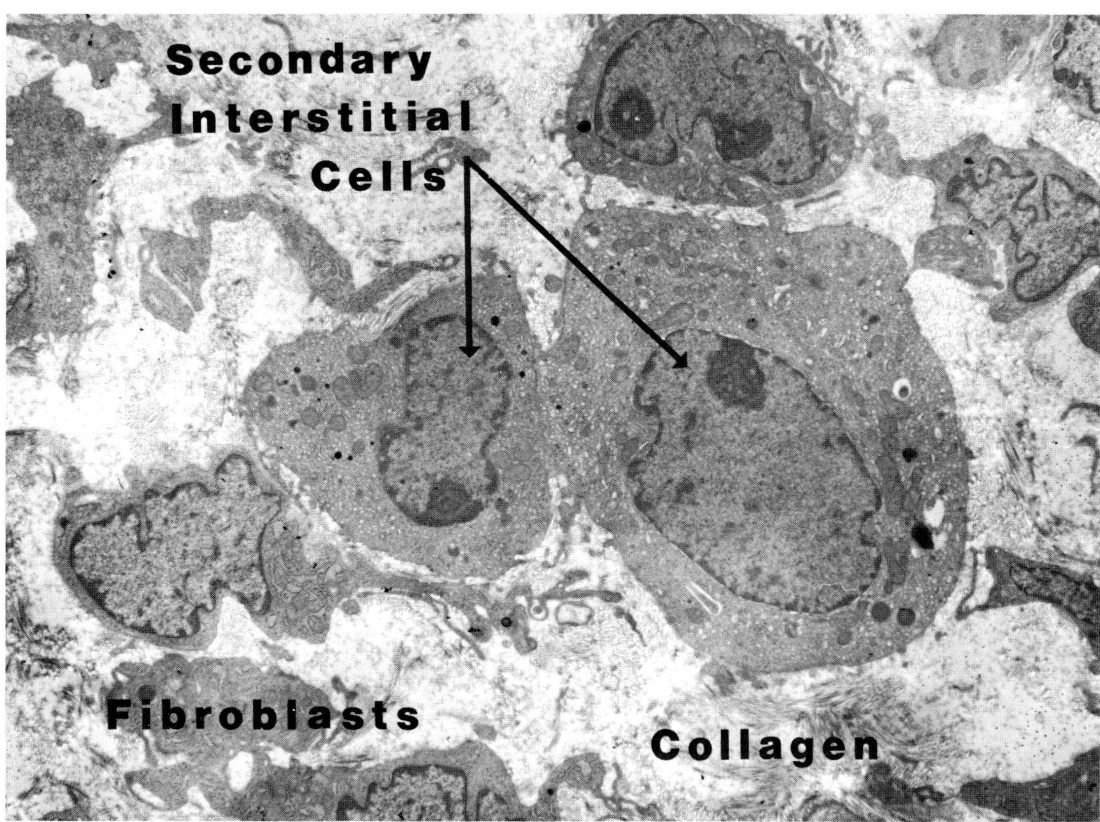

FIGURE 17A-15 Electron micrograph of a cluster of secondary interstitial cells found in the connective tissue of the cortex of a normal human ovary. Their fine structure is typical of active steroidogenic cells in that they have smooth endoplasmic reticulum, lipid droplets, and mitochondria with tubular cristae. During the life of a woman, they remain as hormone-responsive androgen-producing cells.

that precise information from the brain can be transmitted directly to the ovaries via the secondary interstitial cells. In this regard, direct evidence in the rat that catecholamines can stimulate structural and functional changes in secondary interstitial cells has been reported.[37] Thus, the concept which is emerging is that catecholamines pass across a synapse bind to receptors and thus regulate androgen activity in the secondary interstitial cell.

Hilus Cells

Along the length of the ovarian hilus are clusters of large (15 to 25 μm in diameter) steroidogenic cells called *hilus cells* (Fig. 17A-1). These are highly unusual cells because all aspects of their structure and function are identical to those of differentiated testicular Leydig cells.[38,39] The hilus and Leydig cells cannot be distinguished on morphologic criteria (Fig. 17A-16): Both contain a unique hexagonal array of crystal lattice termed *crystalloids of Reinke*.[40,41] The nature and importance of these crystalloids are unknown; however, they may be albuminlike material which provide a reservoir of binding sites for testosterone molecules. It has been established that hilus cells (like Leydig cells) synthesize and secrete testosterone in response to LH stimulation.[42–44] In this context, ovarian tumors of the hilus cell cause virilization. For all intents and purposes, a hilus cell is an ovarian Leydig cell.

What are the endocrine controls and physical importance of ovarian hilus cells? One intriguing feature is the intimate association of hilus cells with nonmyelinated sympathetic nerve fibers (Fig. 17A-1)[39] and the ovarian spiral arteries.[1] Perhaps interactions occur between hilus cells and the nerves and blood vessels which directly or indirectly alter ovarian function. In this light, since testosterone induces atresia, hilus cells may have an impact on the decision-making processes in follicular growth and development. It has been proposed that hilus cells may be a source of testosterone needed for increased striated muscle activities in women during exercise.[45]

Corpora Lutea

After ovulation of the egg-cumulus complex, the follicle undergoes a series of histologic changes that result in the formation of a corpus luteum.[46] Cells that

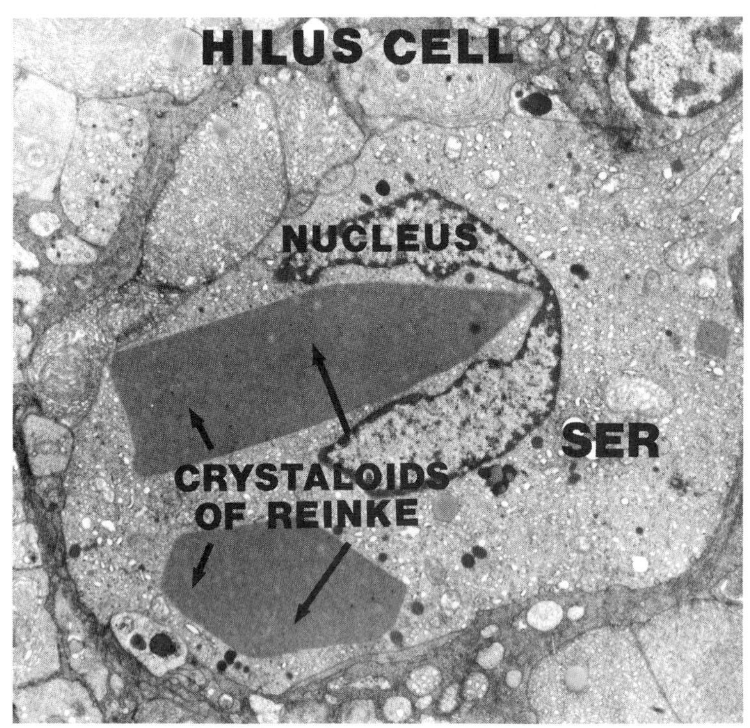

FIGURE 17A-16 Electron micrograph of a hilus cell, showing both abundant smooth endoplasmic reticulum (SER) and numerous large crystalloids of Reinke. *(Courtesy of Dr. Norbert Schnoy, by permission of Springer-Verlag.)*

make up the corpus luteum are contributed by the membrana granulosa, theca interna, and theca externa. Morphologically, a corpus luteum is roughly equivalent to a graafian follicle (Fig. 17A-17; compare with Fig. 17A-11). In the center, where the antrum and liquor folliculi are located, is a fibrin clot in which there has been an invasion of loose connective tissue and blood cells (angiogenesis). At ovulation, the wall of the graafian follicle undergoes extensive hypertrophy (Fig. 17A-17).

During luteinization, the membrana granulosa cells undergo tremendous changes and attain a large size of 35 to 60 μm in diameter.[47] Such cells are termed *granulosa-lutein* cells. Perhaps the most dramatic event that occurs in the newly forming granulosa-lutein cell is its transformation from a protein secretory-like cell into a highly differentiated steroidogenic cell. In the cytoplasm prominent regions of smooth endoplasmic reticulum develop, the mitochondria develop tubular cristae, and large clusters of lipid droplets containing cholesterol esters accumulate (Fig. 17A-18). Granulosa-lutein cells contain substantial quantities of rough endoplasmic reticulum, indicating that these cells also have protein-synthesizing activity (Fig. 17A-18). These cells have a series of long microvilli which can measure 2 μm or more in length projecting from their apical surface.[47] In rodents, these microvilli have been shown to contain the functional LH receptors, suggesting that they may play important endocrine roles.[48]

During luteinization, the theca interstitial cells become incorporated into the corpus luteum and are termed *theca lutein* cells. Theca lutein cells can be distinguished from granulosa-lutein cells (Fig. 17A-19) because they are typically smaller (15 μm in diameter) and stain more darkly.[47,49,50] Ultrastructurally, they appear as active steroid-producing cells, but they also contain stacks of rough endoplasmic reticulum, suggesting that they may also synthesize protein hormones.[47] Like the theca interna, the theca lutein tissue contains cells with differing degrees of density (light, dark, intermediate) (Fig. 17A-19), suggesting that there may be subpopulations of theca lutein cells.[47] Scattered throughout the corpus luteum are many macrophages,[49] the so-called K cells (Fig. 17A-19). Finally, as with the follicle, the entire corpus luteum is surrounded by a theca externa.

If fertilization and implantation do not occur, the corpus luteum undergoes degeneration. This process, which is termed *luteolysis*, becomes apparent 8 days after ovulation.[50] The first histologic indication of luteolysis is shrinkage of the granulosa-lutein cells. This is characterized by specific decreases in the amount of endoplasmic reticulum and general decreases in the amount of cytoplasmic matrix.[50] Initially the regression seems to be selective for granulosa-lutein cells as theca lutein cells actually become more prominent.[50] At this time, the theca layer is formed of tightly packed theca-lutein cells which contain profuse amounts of smooth endoplasmic reticulum and large mitochondria with tubular cristae. In this sense, luteolysis seems to be associated with hyperstimulation of the theca lutein cells. This is

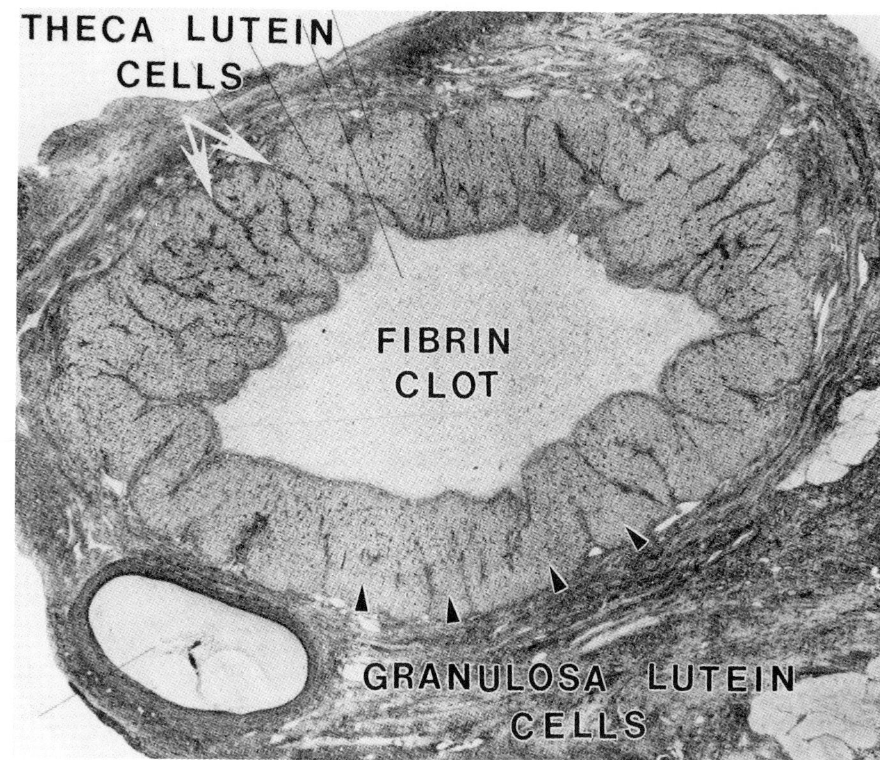

FIGURE 17A-17 Photomicrograph of a section of a human corpus luteum, showing the fibrin clot in the antrum and the collapsed follicle wall composed of granulosa and theca lutein cells. *(Revised from Bloom and Fawcett,[51] by permission of WB Saunders.)*

followed by the development of large zones of autophagy and necrosis. When the glandular corpus luteum disintegrates, all that is left is a nodule of dense connective tissue called the *corpus albicans*.

BIOGENESIS OF OVARIAN HORMONES

Steroids

In a broad sense, the adult human ovaries secrete three major types of biologically active steroid hormones: progesterone, androstenedione, and estradiol. The ability to produce these steroids depends on the presence of a special collection of enzymes termed *mixed-function oxidases* (Fig. 17A-20). These enzymes are involved in a variety of oxidation-reduction reactions and require an NADPH-generating system and an oxygen transport system involving cytochrome P450. Recently, researchers have isolated, cloned, and sequenced the genes which encode the human cytochrome P450 enzymes responsible for ovarian steroidogenesis.[51] Therefore, it is now possible to study physiologic and pathologic aspects of their expression at the molecular level. Ultimately, this work could lead to a new understanding of the role of these key regulatory enzymes in both health and disease.

An important concept in ovarian physiology is that steroidogenic enzymes are distributed throughout the endocrine compartments in a highly specialized manner. The basis for this process of specification is the selective transcription of genes which code for specific steroid-metabolizing enzymes. By virtue of differential gene activities, the various steroidogenic cells in the ovary respond to effectors with increases and/or decreases in selective classes of steroid hormones. Consequently, luteal cells secrete primarily C_{21} progestins and interstitial cells preferentially produce C_{19} androgens. Importantly, the capacity to produce C_{18} estrogens de novo does not exist in any one cell type. Rather, ovarian aromatase enzymes are selectively expressed in the granulosa and granulosa-lutein cells.

Cholesterol Substrate

All steroids are derived from cholesterol. Normally, three systems operate to provide a steroidogenic cell with cholesterol: (1) de novo synthesis from acetate, (2) mobilization from intracellular lipid droplets, (3) liberation from low-density lipoprotein (LDL). Under normal physiologic conditions, the de novo synthesis of cholesterol provides little substrate for steroid hormone production by the ovary. Similarly, the storage pool of cholesterol esters in the lipid droplets is not a primary source of cholesterol under normal conditions.[52] The most important source of cholesterol used for steroid biosynthesis is the cholesterol liberated from LDL.[53] As can be seen in Fig. 17A-21, the process begins with the

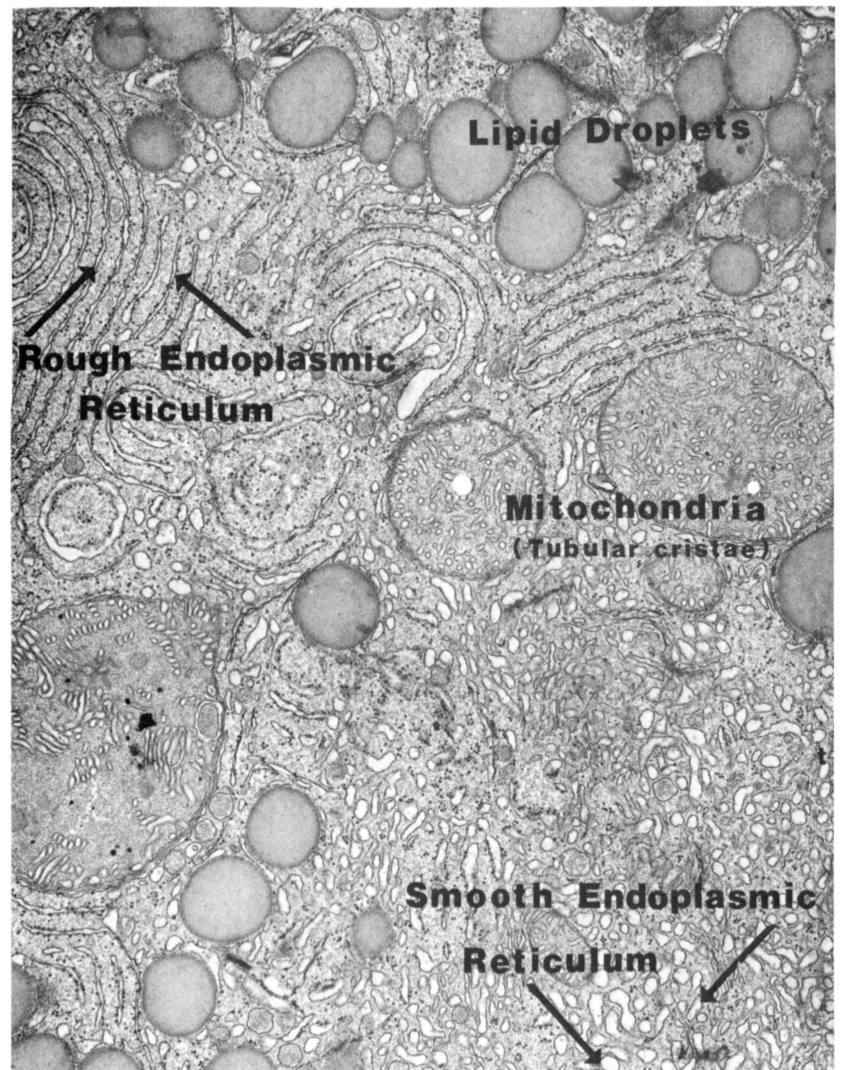

FIGURE 17A-18 Electron micrograph of a section through a human granulosa cell, showing both protein-synthesizing [rough endoplasmic reticulum (ER)] and steroid-synthesizing (smooth ER) potential. The smooth ER is the site of $P450_{AROM}$. Note the prominent tubular cristae (the site of $P450_{scc}$) in the mitochondria and the large number of lipid droplets containing stored cholesterol esters. *(Courtesy of Dr. Tom Crisp, by permission of CV Mosby.)*

binding of LDL to a high-affinity receptor site and the subsequent internalization of the receptor-LDL particle in the form of a coated or endocytic vesicle.[54,55] This is followed by the delivery of the endocytic vesicle to a lysosome, where the LDL particle is hydrolyzed to amino acids by proteinases and the cholesterol esters are cleaved by an acid lipase to generate free cholesterol, which leaves the lysosome for use in cellular reactions.[55]

The cholesterol which is liberated from LDL initiates a set of three feedback control mechanisms within the steroidogenic cell (Fig. 17A-21). First, liberated cholesterol turns off de novo cholesterol synthesis from acetate by inhibiting 3-hydroxy-3-methyl-glutaryl coenzyme A reductase, which is the rate-controlling enzyme in cholesterol biosynthesis. Second, the LDL-derived cholesterol stimulates the enzyme acyl CoA:cholesterol acyltransferase, which reesterifies excess cholesterol and stores it as cholesterol ester lipid droplets. Third, the incoming cholesterol inhibits the synthesis of new LDL receptors, preventing the entry of LDL and the overaccumulation of cholesterol.

Intracellular Cholesterol Transport

The rate-limiting step in the conversion of cholesterol to steroid hormones is the transfer of the liberated cholesterol into the mitochondrion, where the cholesterol side-chain cleavage enzyme ($P450_{scc}$) is located.[56] It has been proposed that this process involves activation of the cytoskeletal systems (microfilaments and microtubules) by a cyclic AMP (cAMP)-protein A kinase–dependent mechanism.[53] As a consequence of this putative transport system, free cholesterol accumulates in the outer membrane of the mitochondrion (Fig. 17A-21). Here, movement from the outer into the inner mitochondrial membrane, where the cholesterol side-chain cleavage enzyme is located, depends on a labile protein.[56]

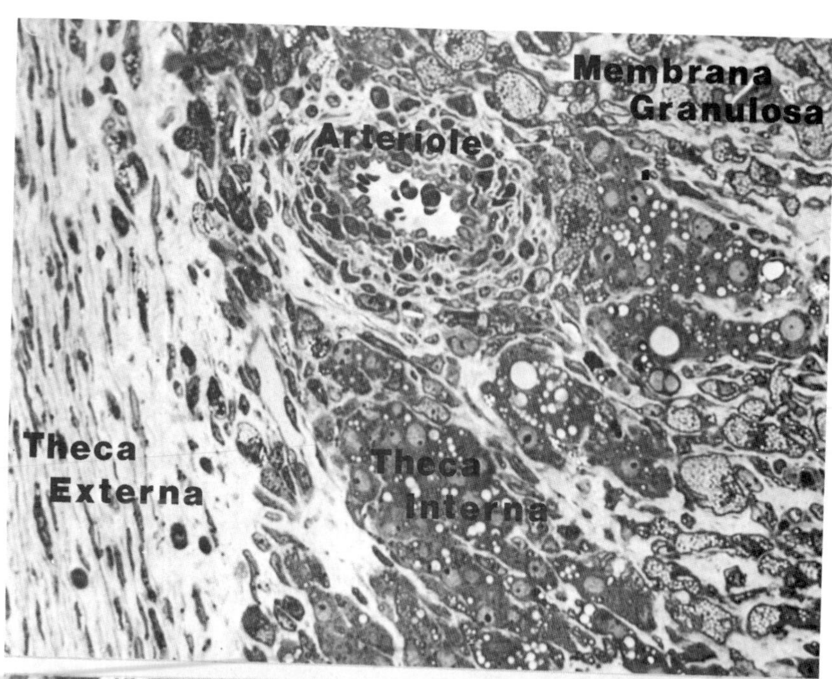

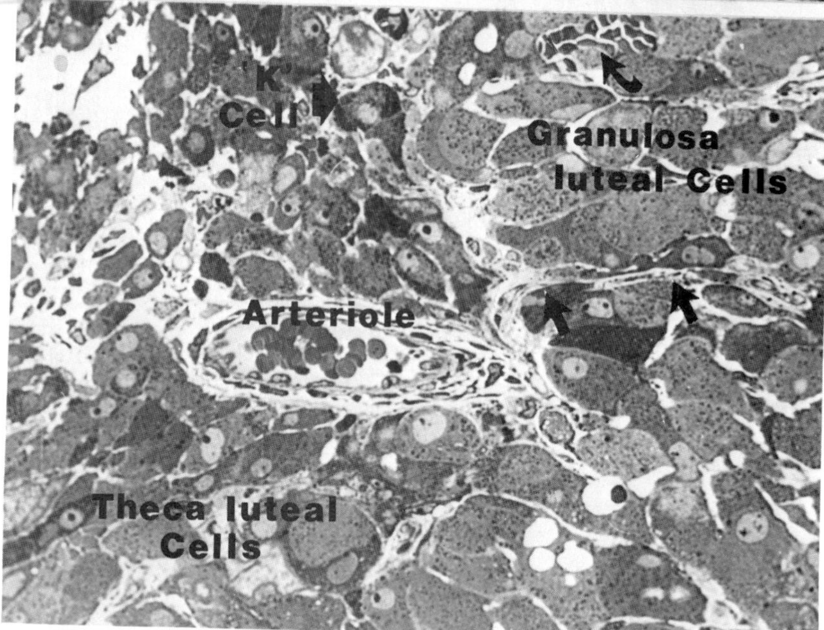

FIGURE 17A-19 Photomicrographs of a section through a human corpus luteum. *(Top)* The three main parts—theca externa, theca lutein, and granulosa lutein—are readily distinguished from one another. *(Bottom)* Larger pale granulosa-lutein cells readily distinguished from smaller (light and dark) theca lutein cells. Note intimate relation between the K cell (macrophage) and luteal cells. *(Courtesy of Dr. Tom Crisp, by permission of CV Mosby.)*

Cholesterol Side-Chain Cleavage

The enzyme which is responsible for converting free cholesterol to pregnenolone (the initial step in steroidogenesis) is located at the inner mitochondrial membrane (Fig. 17A-22). In this enzyme complex, cytochrome $P450_{scc}$ is a terminal oxidase of the mitochondrial electron transport system, which consists of a flavoprotein and an iron-sulfur protein which transports electrons from NADPH to O_2.[56,57] The consequence of the side-chain cleavage is the transformation of C_{27} cholesterol to C_{21} pregnenolone and a 6-carbon fragment called *isocaproic acid*.

FIGURE 17A-20 The cytochrome P450e play a critical role in the ovarian metabolism of steroid hormones. They are involved in the stepwise removal of carbon atoms from the C_{27} skeleton of cholesterol.

$$C_{27} \xrightarrow{P450_{scc}} C_{21} \xrightarrow{P450_{17\alpha}} C_{19} \xrightarrow{P450_{AROM}} C_{18}$$

CHOLESTEROL PROGESTINS ANDROGENS ESTROGENS

Metabolism of Steroid Hormones

Pregnenolone is the precursor to all steroid hormones. Once formed, pregnenolone is rapidly converted to the biologically active hormone progesterone

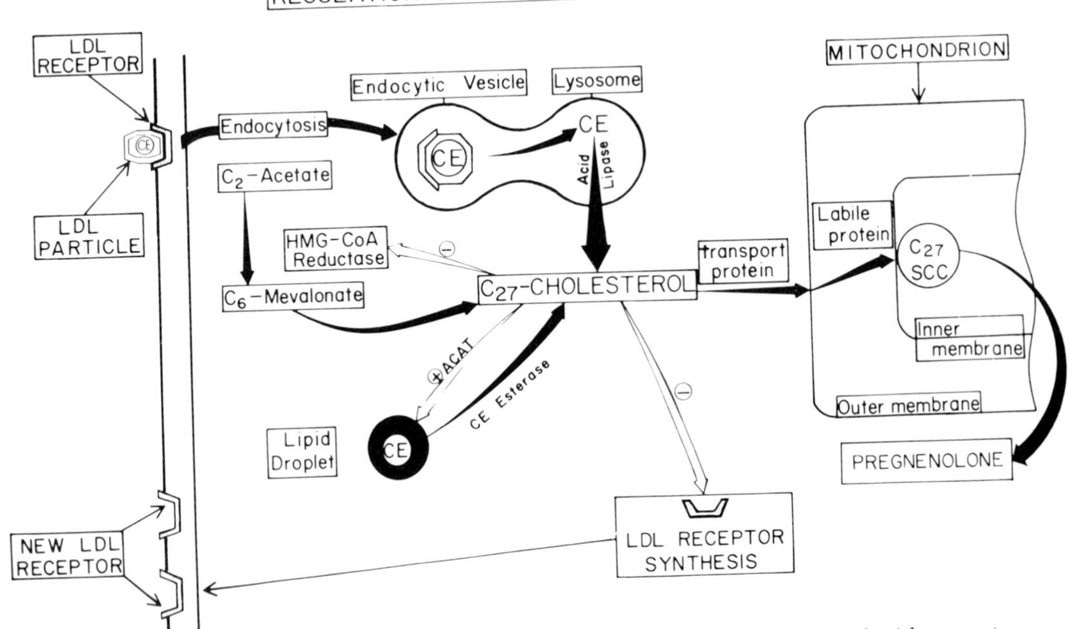

FIGURE 17A-21 Diagram showing the ovarian cellular responses to cholesterol with respect to steroidogenesis.

through the action of Δ^5-3β-ol dehydrogenase–$\Delta^{4,5}$-isomerase.[58] This enzyme is located within the outer mitochondrial membrane and in the smooth endoplasmic reticulum of steroid-secreting cells.[59] The main pathway of steroid synthesis in the human ovary is the Δ^4 pathway, which involves the conversion of progesterone to various C_{19} and C_{18} steroids. The cytochrome P450 ($P450_{scc}$, $P450_{17\alpha}$, and P450 aromatase) enzymes in the Δ^4 pathway are involved principally with the stepwise removal of carbon atoms from the C_{21} skeleton of progesterone (Fig. 17A-20). The formation of C_{19} androgens involves the enzyme $P450_{17\alpha}$, which contains both 17α-hydroxylase and 17,20-lyase activities.[51] The $P450_{17\alpha}$ is located in the smooth endoplasmic reticulum and is responsible for cleavage of the side chain of progesterone to yield Δ^4-androstenedione (Fig. 17A-20). In the ovary, the $P450_{17\alpha}$ is selectively found in the interstitial cells, including the theca lutein cells (Fig. 17A-14). Importantly, granulosa cells do not contain these en-

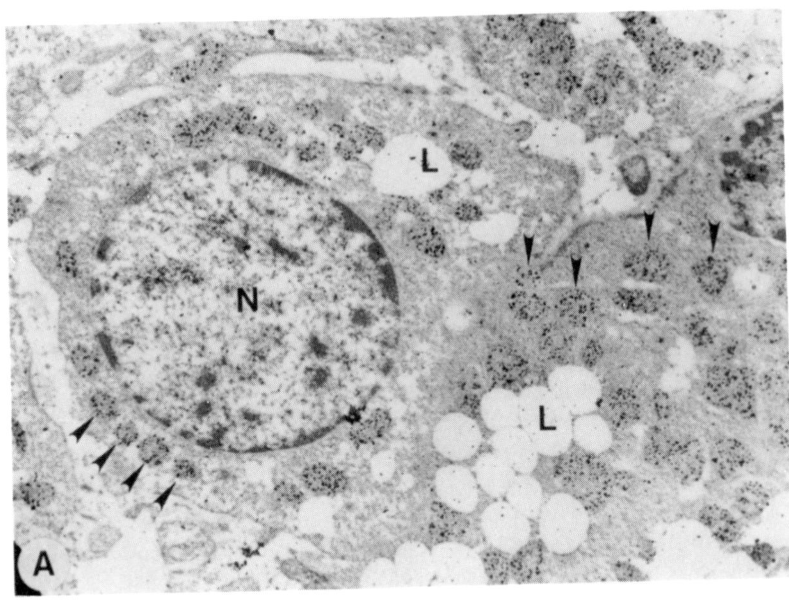

FIGURE 17A-22 Localization of $P450_{scc}$ in mitochondria by staining with immunogold. Colloidal gold particles are specifically located in the mitochondria (arrowheads). N-nucleus; L-lipid droplets. *(Courtesy of Dr. Yosi Orly.)*

zymes and therefore are unable to convert progesterone to androstenedione (Fig. 17A-14).

The degree to which androstenedione is further metabolized depends on the ovarian cell type. The hilus cells, for example, contain the enzyme 17β-hydroxysteroid dehydrogenase, which converts androstenedione to testosterone.[42] This enzyme is also present in rat granulosa cells,[60] where it converts androstenedione to testosterone and estrone to estradiol. In the ovary, one of the most important steps in androstenedione metabolism is its conversion to estrogen via a 19-hydroxylase-aromatase enzyme complex, P450 aromatase (Fig. 17A-20). This enzyme, which holds the key to much that is characteristic of the female, is primarily found in the granulosa cells.[61] The presence of the aromatase leads to the removal of the angular carbon between rings A and B, followed by the aromatization of the A ring of the C_{18} steroid. Finally, the interstitial cells contain a 5α-reductase (NADPH: Δ^4-3-ketosteroid-5α-reductase), which can convert ring A metabolites to 5α-reduced steroids.[62] The 5α-reductase is potentially an important enzyme because (1) the 5α-reduced steroids [such as dihydrotestosterone (DHT)] are extremely potent androgens and because (2) they are competitive inhibitors of the aromatase.[63] Thus, they may play a role in inhibiting estradiol production.

Gonadotropin Control

The control mechanisms governing de novo steroid synthesis in the ovary are almost exclusively regulated by LH and human chorionic gonadotropin (hCG). The ability of LH to stimulate de novo steroidogenesis involves both acute and long-acting mechanisms. The acute effects of LH occur within minutes and involve a G-protein-linked receptor-signaling, A-kinase mechanism followed by phosphorylation of regulatory proteins. The rate-determining step in ovarian steroid biosynthesis is the conversion of cholesterol to pregnenolone by $P450_{scc}$.[56] LH, through its second message, cAMP, causes dramatic and rapid increases in the capacity of $P450_{scc}$ to convert cholesterol to pregnenolone. The underlying control mechanism involves LH-induced increases in the amount of cholesterol which is specifically bound to $P450_{scc}$.[56] The mechanism remains a mystery but seems to involve LH-dependent increases in the amount or activity of the "labile protein" (Fig. 17A-21). Thus, the basis of the immediate effect of LH on steroidogenesis seems to be a rapid delivery of cholesterol to $P450_{scc}$.

The long-term effect of LH on steroidogenesis involves the expression of the genes which encode steroid-metabolizing enzymes.[57] Specifically, LH stimulates the synthesis of $P450_{scc}$, 3β-HSD, and $P450_{17\alpha}$. Consequently, the long-term control of steroidogenesis by LH occurs at a rate which is governed by the rate of the synthesis of new enzyme molecules. Although the relation between FSH and de novo steroidogenesis is minimal, FSH plays a central role in regulating ovarian steroid formation by virtue of its control of the activities of ovarian P450 aromatase and 17β-HSD.[61,63–65] In this sense, FSH is most important in controlling immediate and long-term estrogen responses in the ovary.

OVARIAN CYTODIFFERENTIATION: UNDERLYING CONTROL MECHANISMS

The changing morphologic pattern of the developing follicle and corpus luteum is accompanied by dramatic biochemical changes that reflect continuing processes of cellular differentiation. The underlying basis for this differentiation is the acquisition of specific cell surface and intracellular receptors which provide cells with the ability to respond in a specific way to various ligands, such as the hormones (amino acid derivatives, peptides, and steroid derivatives) and the growth factors. The development of the receptors occurs in a highly predictable pattern and involves both intraovarian and extraovarian mechanisms. In essence, the continued transformation of cells from the undifferentiated state to the fully differentiated state is the underlying principle of ovarian physiology.[64]

The Granulosa Cell

Cytodifferentiation

The differentiation of a granulosa cell begins in the primordial follicle when it is recruited to initiate growth. After being committed to the granulosa pathway, these morphologically unspecialized cells start to proliferate and produce new cells whose subsequent differentiation is under hormonal control. Granulosa cytodifferentiation can thus be divided into four levels which parallel follicular morphology (Fig. 17A-3).

First Level

Only when a primordial follicle is recruited does granulosa cytodifferentiation begin. After changing from a squamous to a cuboidal shape, the granulosa cells are shifted into mitosis. This transition is accompanied by the acquisition of FSH receptors in the plasma membrane.[66] Therefore, the first step in granulosa differentiation occurs in primary follicles and involves FSH receptor induction. The basis of FSH receptor induction is obscure but seems to involve intraovarian control mechanisms. In the rat, binding studies indicate that when the follicle reaches the secondary stage, the granulosa cell has approximately 1500 specific high-affinity FSH receptors and that this number remains constant in the granulosa cells throughout the remainder of follicle development.[67] It can be concluded, therefore, that the first level of granulosa cytodifferentiation involves a shape change from squamous to cuboidal which then results in mitosis and the induction of a maximum number of FSH receptors.

Second Level

When a rat follicle reaches the secondary or early tertiary stage, the granulosa cells reach a second level of differentiation. The second transition is accompanied by the acquisition of intracellular receptors for estradiol, progesterone, testosterone, and glucocorticoids.[64] The factor responsible for inducing these important changes is unknown but seems to be regulated by intraovarian processes. In the rat, this differentiative change is fundamental because the granulosa cells (and thus the follicle) are now competent to react in a specific way to a set of very potent determinative stimuli which can modulate folliculogenesis in a positive or negative manner.

Surprisingly, the concept of steroid receptors in the human ovary has not been addressed; there is no evidence for the existence of any class of steroid receptors in the human ovary. On the basis of immunocytochemical studies in the monkey ovary, it seems that there is no estrogen receptor in any developing follicle.[68] Accordingly, the concept of autocrine control of granulosa cell differentiation by estradiol in humans is open to question.

Third Level

Up to this point, granulosa cytodifferentiation occurs independently of the pituitary. This is not the case for its subsequent differentiation, which is completely dependent on pituitary FSH. FSH, which is brought to a tertiary follicle by capillaries in the theca interna, crosses the basal lamina, where it binds to the G-protein-linked FSH receptor in the granulosa and stimulates adenylate cyclase. This causes an increase in cAMP which binds to the cAMP-dependent protein A kinases and causes phosphorylation of regulatory proteins. In this context, estrogen plays a permissive role in FSH action by facilitating FSH-stimulated cAMP formation in rat granulosa cells. This action of estrogen is particularly important in the rat because it increases the sensitivity of the granulosa cell to FSH, which is known to be present in relatively low concentrations in follicular fluid. However, as was discussed above, there may not be estrogen receptor in the human ovary.[68] Therefore, this autocrine concept may not apply to the human folliculogenesis.

The critical role of FSH in granulosa cytodifferentiation is illustrated by the number of specialized functions which are dependent on FSH stimulation. One of the primary consequences of FSH action is the activation of proliferative cell cycles which lead to increased numbers of granulosa cells.[69,70] The growth of a tertiary follicle to the preantral stage (Fig. 17A-22) is associated with an increase in the number of granulosa cells from about 1×10^4 to over 50×10^6 cells.[69,70] It is clear that FSH is responsible for the stimulation of mitosis in human granulosa cells.[71] Whether this effect is direct or is controlled indirectly by the production of regulatory molecules such as growth factors is unknown. Two growth factors—basic fibroblast growth factor (bFGF) and epidermal growth factor (EGF)—have been observed to stimulate mitosis in human granulosa cells in vitro.[72] Based on such evidence, one explanation for the FSH stimulation of mitosis is that it results from the local production of EGF and/or bFGF.

FSH interaction also causes the granulosa cells to develop increasing amounts of $P450_{AROM}$.[63,64] This regulatory process is fundamentally important in the maintenance of the estrogen-synthetic activities of the follicle and thus the homeostatic activities of the female. It appears that FSH stimulation of its G-protein-linked receptor activates the adenylate cyclase–cAMP–A kinase cascade. This results in the phosphorylation of key regulatory peptides, leading to the activation of the transcription of the gene encoding $P450_{AROM}$.[61,73] This positive regulatory effect of FSH on $P450_{AROM}$ activity increases progressively as a function of both follicle growth and the stage in the follicular phase of the menstrual cycle.[63,65]

Fourth Level

In the fourth level, the granulosa cells in the dominant follicle develop LH receptors in their plasma membranes.[64] Recent in vitro experiments with monkey granulosa cells have shown that FSH regulates the induction of LH receptors.[74] The LH receptors are members of the G-protein-linked receptor family which can stimulate the effector adenylate cyclase.[75] It is significant that when granulosa cells develop LH receptors, they become competent to respond to the LH that enters the follicular fluid during the late follicular phase.[76] Thus, it is possible that LH in the dominant follicle becomes a primary regulator of granulosa cell differentiation during the period when FSH levels in the blood are declining.

It is clear from this discussion that FSH plays a fundamental role in controlling the differentiation processes that occur in granulosa cells during the growth and development of a primary follicle to the preovulatory stage. In this regard, it should be noted that once granulosa cytodifferentiation has been initiated by FSH, the cells become completely dependent on FSH for their survival. In this context, FSH withdrawal results in the loss of all available receptors and aromatase enzymes, followed by cell death by atresia. Therefore, FSH is critical for the life of any granulosa cell that it has activated.

Granulosa Heterogeneity

In developing animal graafian follicles, it appears that every granulosa cell contains FSH receptors.[77] Surprisingly, however, groups of differentiating granulosa cells respond to FSH differently.[64] For example, when challenged by FSH in vivo or in vitro, the LH receptor and aromatase enzymes are selectively induced in the membrana granulosa cells.[64] These data argue strongly that the granulosa cells are not a simple equipotent tissue, even though they all presumably have FSH receptors. In this view, it seems certain that the position of the granulosa cell within the follicle determines which way it will differentiate in response to FSH stimulation. How the relative position within the granulosa cell mass determines the direction of its differentiation is unknown, but this process probably involves the microenvironment of the follicular fluid as well as cell contacts with the basal lamina, oocyte, and/or other granulosa cells.[64] It had been proposed that granulosa cells are really a complex tissue containing several subgroups of functionally different cells. It is noteworthy that evidence is emerging which indicates heterogeneity in human granulosa cells in graafian follicles.[78]

The Interstitial Cells

Androgens produced by interstitial cells are involved in both constructive and destructive processes in the ovary.[15] Follicular estradiol formation is causally linked to androgens produced by interstitial cells (Fig. 17A-20). This contrasts with other evidence that androgens arising from interstitial cells can induce necrosis and destruction of granulosa cells and ova through atresia.[15] Therefore, androgens derived from interstitial cells are important in both follicle selection and atresia. Consequently, changes in interstitial androgen production affect the direction of folliculogenesis and thus may have important consequences for the reproductive state of the female.

The most important stimulating force in interstitial androgen production is LH.[15] All interstitial cells are competent to react to LH (or hCG) by way of G-protein-linked LH receptors in the plasma membrane.[33] When LH binds to its receptor, there is an allosteric change which causes the LH-receptor complex to interact with G-proteins. This results in the release of the G-stimulatory protein, which then activates adenylate cyclase, which converts ATP to the second messenger, cAMP; the cAMP binds to the regulatory subunit of A kinase, which then allows the catalytic subunits of protein kinase A to phosphorylate the serine and threonine residues of regulatory proteins.[79] This cascade then results in the transcription of genes which encode the steroidogenic enzymes, $P450_{scc}$ and $P450_{17\alpha}$.[80] In this regard, theca interstitial cells in preantral follicles express $P450_{scc}$ but not $P450_{17\alpha}$. This indicates that during the first stages of differentiation, the theca cells are primarily progesterone-producing cells (Fig. 17A-23). The failure of theca interstitial cells to produce androgens during early folliculogenesis could ensure that none of the developing preantral follicles dies by atresia. Once antrum formation occurs, an unknown mechanism causes the expression of the $P450_{17\alpha}$ in the theca cells, thus switching them into androgen-producing cell (Fig. 17A-23). The development of $P450_{17\alpha}$ ensures that aromatase substrate is produced by the cohort of graafian follicles. Interestingly, after the surge of LH at midcycle, the theca cells once again lose $P450_{17\alpha}$ and become primarily a progestin-producing tissue during ovulation (Fig. 17A-23). Then, as the process of luteinization occurs, the theca interstitial cells (now called theca lutein cells) reexpress $P450_{17\alpha}$ activity and once again produce C_{19} androgens (Fig. 17A-23). Thus, the concept that differentiating theca interstitial cells switch back and forth between progesterone- and androgen-producing cells during their life cycle is clearly established.[81] We will return to the physiologic significance of this concept later.

The Corpus Luteum

Corpus luteum differentiation is typically divided into two periods. It begins in response to the preovulatory surge of gonadotropins by the process called luteinization. After maximal differentiated function is reached at the end of 1 week (day 21 to day 22 of the cycle), the corpus luteum normally undergoes

FIGURE 17A-23 Diagram of the steroidogenic changes in the human theca interstitial cells throughout their life cycle.

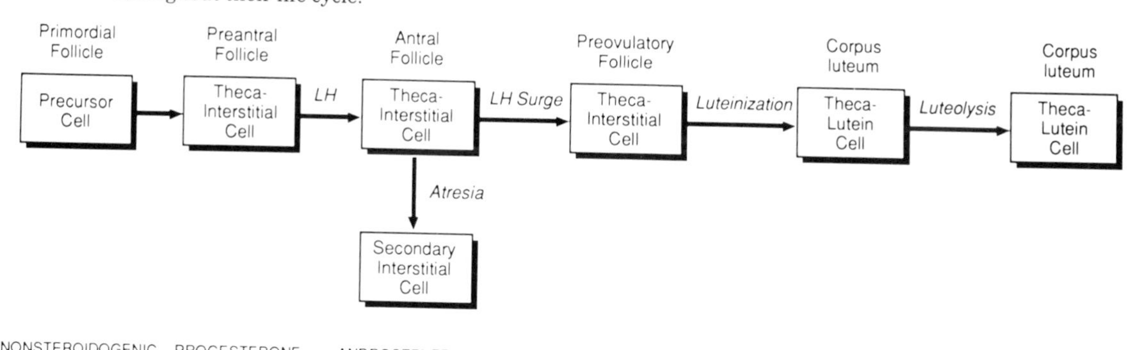

degeneration by the process of luteolysis. What are the primary events leading to luteinization and luteolysis?

Luteinization

Much of what is known about the control of the human corpus luteum has come from studies of hormone levels in peripheral and ovarian venous blood and follicular fluid.[82–87] Collectively, the evidence indicates that luteal differentiation is associated with a biphasic secretion of ovarian regulatory steroids, namely, progesterone, 17α-hydroxyprogesterone, androstenedione, and estradiol. This conclusion has been corroborated by in vitro experiments with isolated corpus luteum tissue.[88,89] The concept which emerges is that the biphasic production of a steroid in the corpus luteum is causally connected with biphasic changes of activities of the regulatory steroidogenic enzymes in the Δ^4 pathway, namely, $P450_{scc}$, 3β-SDH, $P450_{17\alpha}$, and $P450_{AROM}$.

What agents are responsible for biphasic changes in corpus luteum steroidogenic enzymes? The fundamental regulator in promoting and maintaining the life of a corpus luteum is LH. LH is the inducer of luteinization, and low levels of LH are critical for maintaining active luteal tissue during the early and midluteal phases.[90] Importantly, hCG produced by the blastocyst can prevent luteolysis and promote further increases in corpus luteum activity; however, this effect is only temporary.[90] The conclusion can therefore be reached that induction and maintenance of the differentiated state of the corpus luteum are controlled directly by LH/hCG, but other regulatory molecules must also be involved.

Considering the fact that LH/hCG action is mediated by receptors, the question of the factors involved in changes in the corpus luteum becomes intimately connected with how the LH receptor is controlled by luteal cells. LH receptors in developing human corpora lutea undergo a predictable pattern of activity. As ovulation approaches, a striking decrease in the LH receptor number occurs in granulosa cells, while during the early luteal phase, the LH receptor number increases sharply, reaching a nearly-maximal level in the midluteal phase, where it remains until the end of the cycle.[91–93] It thus can be concluded that the LH receptor is first desensitized and down regulated and then reinduced during the process of luteinization.[94–97]

Since reinduction of LH receptor renders the corpus luteum sensitive to hCG secreted by the implanting blastocyst, an important question is how the LH receptor is reinduced in luteal cells. In vitro studies with human granulosa luteal cells have shown that the recovery of LH/hCG sensitivity is due to the reinduction of functional LH/hCG receptors in the plasma membrane; significantly, this process is regulated by LH itself.[98] This is an important question clinically because foremost among the characteristics of luteal-phase defects in women is the inability of the corpus luteum to respond appropriately to LH/hCG. This defect may be caused by inappropriate formation of new LH/hCG receptors.[99–101]

The physiologic importance of LH/hCG in regulating progesterone secretion by the human corpus luteum has been clearly established. FSH itself does not stimulate progesterone biosynthesis during luteinization in women. In vitro[102,103] and in vivo[104] studies have demonstrated that progesterone levels are not increased in response to purified FSH during the early, middle, or late luteal phase of the menstrual cycle. The concept which emerges is that FSH, unlike LH/hCG, does not play a physiologic role in controlling progesterone production by the human corpus luteum. Importantly, however, FSH has a high capacity for stimulating estradiol formation by human copora luteal cells in vivo[104] and in vitro.[105] Hence, the physiologic actions of FSH in luteinization seem to promote estradiol rather than progesterone synthesis. It is interesting that LH/hCG can also stimulate estradiol production.[105] Therefore, by comparison to FSH, the LH/hCG signaling pathway in human granulosa-lutein cells is capable of stimulating both estradiol and progesterone synthesis.

Luteolysis

At the time of luteolysis, a cell death mechanism is initiated which leads to the destruction of the corpus luteum approximately 5 to 7 days later. Once this mechanism has been initiated, there is a sharp decrease in progesterone production, an event which is unfavorable to pregnancy. What is the mechanism of luteolysis? The answer to this fundamental question is uncertain, but evidence suggests that aromatase activity may be particularly important. Aromatase activity in the corpus luteum increases prior to luteolysis, and the concentration of estrogen in the corpus luteum reaches a peak at that time.[92,106,107] Can the two processes—a decrease in progesterone production and an increase in aromatase activity, be causally linked in luteolysis? In women, injection of estrogen directly into the ovary causes an early onset of menstrual bleeding.[108] Furthermore, treatment with exogenous estrogen inhibits progesterone production by human corpus luteum cells in vitro.[109,110] The site of estrogen action seems to be directly at the level of Δ^4-3β-HDH-$\Delta^{4,5}$-isomerase.[111] Consequently, the conclusion may be drawn that estradiol is an important luteolytic agent in humans.

With this concept in mind, a very important question in the differentiation of the corpus luteum concerns the underlying mechanisms for controlling estrogen biosynthesis. The mechanism that controls estrogen formation could act directly at the $P450_{AROM}$ and/or at the level of androgen substrate production. As was noted above, LH/hCG can increase estrogen and progesterone secretion in human corpora lutea while FSH selectively stimulates estrogen but not progesterone production.[102–105] The picture that emerges is that FSH and LH may be responsible for progressive increases in corpora lutea aromatase activity and progesterone levels, respectively, during the differentiation of the corpus luteum in the early to midluteal phases.

In this context, clomiphene acts directly on the human placenta to decrease progesterone production while increasing 17-hydroxyprogesterone, androstenedione, and estradiol production.[112] How clomiphene exerts this action is unknown, but clomiphene can increase the aromatization of testosterone to estradiol. With respect to luteolysis, the induction of aromatase activity by clomiphene may result in increased concentrations of cellular estrogen, which then enters into the process of luteolysis. This scenario could have important implications for the way in which clomiphene induces luteal defects in women.

To what extent is luteal cytodifferentiation determined by interactions with modulators? It seems clear that LH, FSH, and hCG are the principal positive regulators of corpus luteum differentiation. Several putative hormone modulators of human corpus luteum function have been identified, including prolactin, gonadotropin releasing hormone (GnRH), $PGF_{2\alpha}$, estradiol, and oxytocin.

In human granulosa cells which are undergoing luteinization in vitro, prolactin can inhibit LH/FSH-stimulated progesterone production[113] and prolactin inhibits basal and gonadotropin-stimulated progesterone and estrogen secretion by human ovaries in vitro. By contrast, experiments with human corpus luteum cells have failed to find consistent direct effects of prolactin on hCG-stimulated progesterone production, although prolactin was found to modulate hCG-stimulated estrogen formation.[114] Despite great clinical interest, the consequences of prolactin action on the human corpus luteum remain unsolved.

As with prolactin, a direct effect of GnRH on human ovarian cells is equivocal. Evidence suggests that human corpora lutea do not have high-affinity GnRH receptors[115] and that GnRH does not influence steroidogenesis by human corpus luteum cells in vitro. It was reported that GnRH inhibits granulosa luteinization in culture,[117] but this was not subsequently confirmed.[118] The question of whether GnRH can modulate the differentiation of human corpus luteum cells is still controversial. It is notable that a GnRH-like molecule has been found in the human ovary, raising the possibility that this protein mediates antigonadotropic responses during the luteal phase of the menstrual cycle.[119]

In some animals $PGF_{2\alpha}$ directly inhibits progesterone production by the corpus luteum and therefore has been termed a physiologic luteolysin. In human corpora lutea, $PGF_{2\alpha}$ receptors have been reported[120] and luteal cells have the synthetic capability of producing PGs.[121,122] Again, despite considerable clinical interest, definitive evidence that $PGF_{2\alpha}$ is a physiologic modulator in human luteal cytodifferentiation is lacking.[123]

As was stated earlier, there is evidence that estradiol and oxytocin act directly on human corpus luteum cells to block LH/hCG activation of progesterone synthesis. Thus, the concept is emerging that the differentiation of the human corpus luteum (like that of the granulosa and interstitial cells) is controlled by multiple hormone responses, some of which are themselves the products of the corpus luteum.

The Oocyte

Primordial Germ Cells

The eggs within the ovary are derived from primordial germ cells (PGCs). These cells, which are set aside very early in embryonic development, arise in the yolk sac endoderm, far from the eventual site of gonad formation. In humans, PGCs can be selectively identified histochemically by virtue of an alkaline phosphatase which is located in their plasma membrane.[124] It is known that from their location in the hindgut they migrate through the dorsal mesentery and into the gonadal ridges; PGCs migrate to the gonad by ameboid movement, presumably via chemotaxis.[125]

When PGCs enter the female genital ridge, they migrate toward the germinal epithelium and are incorporated into cortical cords.[125] Coincident with the colonization of the gonad by PGCs, epithelial cells from mesonephric tubules migrate into the genital area, where they probably become the granulosa and interstitial cells.[126] The conclusion, therefore, is that all the cellular components of the follicle (oocyte, granulosa, theca) originate outside the gonad itself.[126,127]

Oogonia

In the PGCs, only one X chromosome in an XX female is expressed; however, once PGCs enter the presumptive ovary, both X chromosomes are expressed and the germ cells are now called *oogonia*.[128] Subsequently, oogonia initiate an active phase of proliferation, and their number increases tremendously. As the oogonia proliferate, there are dramatic increases in the activity of enzymes which are encoded by genes on the X chromosome. The importance of the expression of twice the gene product in developing female germ cells is emphasized by the fact that XO genetic females exhibit oocyte depletion and sterility.[129] The oogonium is unique in that it is the only cell in which both X chromosomes are active.

As mitosis proceeds and cortical cord growth continues, the dividing oogonia fail to complete cytokinesis. Consequently, subpopulations of oogonia remain joined together by intercellular bridges,[130] and their differentiation then proceeds synchronously in a way resembling germ cell differentiation in the testis.

Oocytes

Beginning at 12 weeks gestation,[11] some of the connected oogonia (those in the deepest regions of the cortical cords nearest the medullary tissue) initiate meiosis (Fig. 17A-4). There is evidence that the mesonephric system is important in triggering the initiation of meiosis in the oocytes and their subsequent incorporation into primordial follicles.[131] In response to the putative meiosis-inducing substance, subgroups of oogonia initiate meiotic DNA synthesis and begin to proceed through leptotene, zygotene, pachytene, and diplotene stages of meiotic prophase (Fig. 17A-4). At the diplotene, the paired homologous chromosomes become less condensed and the oocyte enters a protracted interphase-like stage called the *dictyotene*. It is at this time that the oocytes become incorporated into primordial follicles (Fig. 17A-4).[11] At its shortest, an oocyte will remain in this arrested state for about 12 years (until puberty); at its longest, it can last about 50 years (until the menopause).

Oocyte Growth

To understand oogenesis, two interrelated processes must be considered: oocyte growth and completion of meiosis. Oocyte growth is associated with the accumulation and storage of nutritional and informational materials, some of which are critical to the development of the preimplantation blastocyst. During growth the human oocyte increases in diameter from 20 μm to 120 μm. The basis for growth resides in the active transcription of stable messenger RNA, ribosomal RNA, transfer RNA, and heterogeneous RNA by lampbrush chromosomes of the oocyte.[132,133] A fundamental concept is that the growth of the follicle relative to that of the oocyte can be divided into two distinct phases: Initially, oocyte and follicle diameter are positively and linearly correlated until the follicle reaches the early tertiary stage (cavitation); after that, the oocyte ceases to grow while follicular growth continues (Fig. 17A-24).

The presence of granulosa cells is an absolute requirement for mouse oocyte growth.[134,135] As growth progresses, the oocyte is closely surrounded by corona radiata granulosa cells which interact directly with the oocyte via gap junctions and desmosomes.[136] As a result of this metabolic coupling, the oocyte can capitalize on unique nutritional and/or regulatory capacities of granulosa cells. Results obtained with animal species indicate that 85 percent of the metabolites present in follicle-enclosed oocytes are originally taken up by the granulosa cell and then transferred into the oocyte through the gap junctions.[137,138] The concept which emerges is that the obligatory role of granulosa cells in oocyte growth involves special gap junctional contacts which are responsible for the transfer of fundamental nutrients into the oocyte.

During oocyte growth, the zona pellucida is formed. The zona pellucida is a relatively thick, translucent acellular coat which surrounds the oolemma of the fully grown oocyte. The zona pellucida plays an important role in a number of vital biological functions:[139,140] (1) It contains species-specific receptors for capacitated sperm, (2) it provides a block to polyspermy, and (3) it is critical in allowing the embryo to move freely through the fallopian tube into the uterus.

It is apparent that the proteins in the zona pellucida are synthesized and secreted by the growing oocytes.[139,140] The morphologic basis for this event involves multiple replications of the Golgi apparatus and their subsequent migration to the periphery of the oocyte, just beneath the oolemma. The zona pellucida contains three glycoproteins, designated ZP-1 (molecular weight of 200,000), ZP-2 (molecular weight of 120,000), and ZP-3 (molecular weight of 83,000).[139,140] The physiologic significance of the zona pellucida proteins produced by the egg is em-

FIGURE 17A-24 Regression lines showing the relation between the sizes of the oocyte and follicle in the human ovary. *(From Green and Zuckerman,[199] by permission of Cambridge University Press.)*

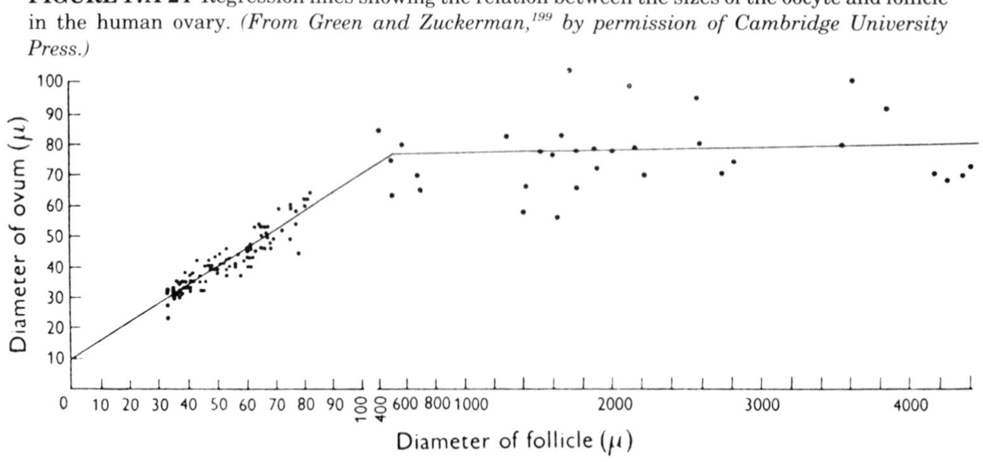

phasized by the fact that they contain the species-specific sperm receptor and initiate the acrosome reaction. The ZP-3 molecule is responsible for these two critical events.[139,140] Clinically, there is growing evidence that infertility in some women may be caused by the presence of circulating antibodies to the ZP-3 protein which block the binding of the sperm to its ZP-3 receptor on the zona pellucida.[141] In this regard, ongoing research is headed toward using ZP-3 as an antigen to develop novel immunologic approaches to contraception.[142,143]

Meiotic Maturation The capacity to resume meiosis is acquired at a specific stage in oocyte growth and differentiation; the ability to complete meiotic maturation is acquired subsequently. Meiotic maturation or resumption of meiosis (Fig. 17A-25) is a process characterized by (1) the dissolution of the nuclear or germinal vesicle membrane, (2) the condensation of dictyotene chromatin into discrete bivalents, (3) the separation of homologous chromosomes, (4) the release of a first polar body, and (5) the arrest of the meiotic process at metaphase II. The completion of meiosis and the release of the second polar body are triggered by fertilization or parthenogenetic activation.

During follicle development, the oocyte acquires the capacity to resume meiosis at the stage of early antrum formation (small graafian follicles 3 to 4 mm in diameter).[144] The acquisition of the capacity for meiotic maturation seems to be a two-step process.[145] First, the oocyte acquires the capacity to undergo germinal vesicle breakdown and progress to metaphase I; second, it acquires the capacity to complete the first reductional division and release the first polar body. The mechanisms responsible for the acquisition of meiotic potential are unknown, but they seem to be under intraovarian control. In this connection, it is interesting that isolated mice oocytes which have been allowed to complete their growth in vitro undergo meiotic maturation spontaneously; such eggs can be fertilized in the dish and then give rise to live young when transferred into foster mothers.[146]

Although the oocyte is capable of resuming meiosis early in follicle development, it is kept from doing so by an inhibitory influence. Under normal physiologic conditions, the resumption of meiotic maturation is a highly selective process that occurs only in oocytes which are in dominant preovulatory follicles. There is little doubt that the resumption of meiosis in such oocytes occurs as a result of the preovulatory

FIGURE 17A-25 Photomicrographs showing the process of meiotic maturation or resumption of meiosis induced by preovulatory surge of LH. (*A*) Germinal vesicle stage of primary (4N) oocyte; (*B*) germinal vesicle breakdown followed by condensation of chromosomes into bivalents; (*C, D*) release of first polar body and arrest of meiotic process at metaphase II of the secondary (2N) oocyte.

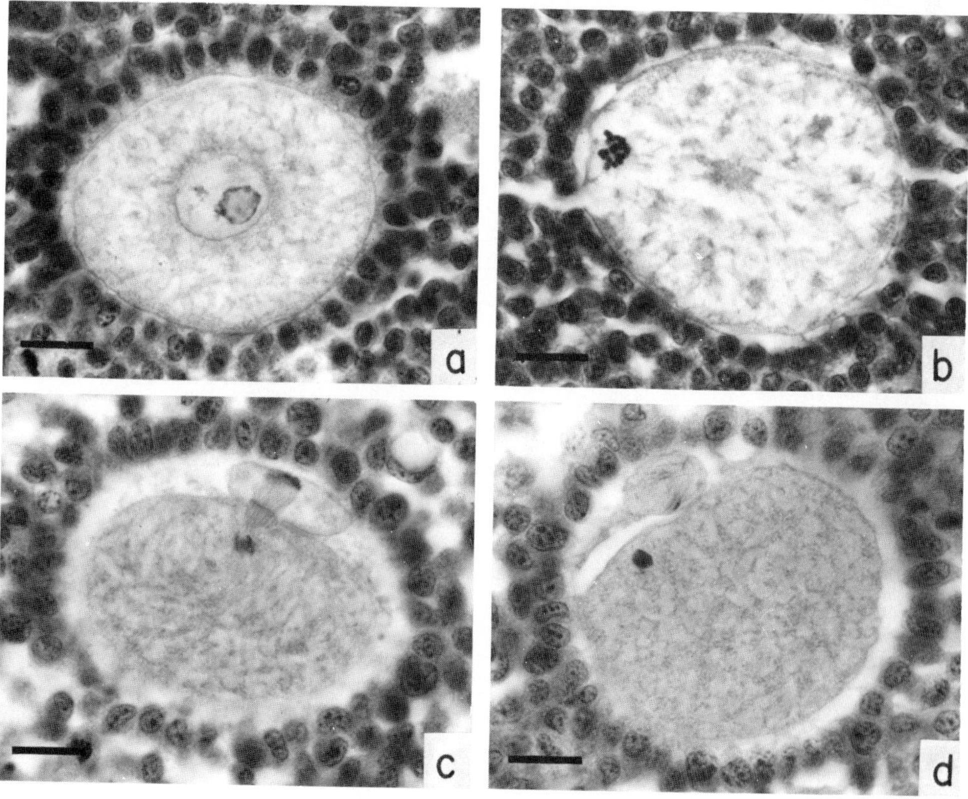

surge of LH.[147] Interestingly, studies in rodents have demonstrated that EGF[148] and GnRH[149] can induce meiotic maturation. Therefore, the possibility exists that other regulatory molecules play a role in this important process. Based on a large body of data, it is evident that fully grown oocytes from any tertiary or graafian follicle undergo meiotic maturation spontaneously when the oocyte is placed in tissue culture. Collectively, these observations have led to the hypothesis that there is an inhibiting substance which blocks meiotic maturation in the follicle and that high levels of LH can override the inhibitory influence.

Evidence suggests that granulosa cells supply to the ovum a substance which blocks meiotic maturation.[150] This substance, termed *oocyte meiotic inhibitor* (OMI), is putatively a protein. What is the underlying mechanism by which LH and OMI regulate meiotic maturation? In this concept it is proposed that the membrana granulosa cells secrete OMI into the follicular fluid in response to gonadotropin stimulation. Evidence indicates that OMI does not act directly on the oocyte but exerts its inhibitory influence indirectly through interactions with the cumulus and the corona radiata granulosa cells.[150] It has been proposed that OMI acts as a signal to these cells to stimulate cAMP, which subsequently diffuses through gap junctions into the oocyte, where it suppresses meiotic maturation.[150] When the preovulatory surge of LH occurs, the membrana granulosa becomes desensitized and stops producing OMI. Ultimately, this response leads to decreases in oocyte cAMP levels, followed by a release of intracellular calcium stores and germinal vesicle breakdown (Fig. 17A-26).[151] An important question concerns the nature of the OMI molecule, which remains unknown. However, there is evidence that it may be the glycoprotein hormone müllerian inhibiting substance (MIS)[152] or perhaps the glycoprotein hormone inhibin.[153] However, more work is necessary to prove the nature of physiologic OMI.

An important aspect of this concept concerns the role of steroids in the initiation of meiosis. The best results to date have been obtained in animal species. High concentrations of estradiol are essential for normal cytoplasmic maturation of the oocyte. If there is inadequate estrogen support, meiotic maturation results in abnormalities in fertilization, delayed cleavage, and almost total failure of the embryo to undergo blastocyst formation.[154] The conclusion is that high levels of estradiol in follicular fluid facilitate the complete differentiation of the egg in vivo and in vitro. The mechanism for this is unknown.

FOLLICLE DEVELOPMENT: CONTROL MECHANISMS

Recruitment

Recruitment is the process in which a primordial follicle is stimulated to leave the pool of nongrowing follicles and initiate development. In humans, recruitment begins in the embryo when primordial follicles are first formed and ends at the menopause when the pool of primordial follicles is depleted.[11,12]

What mechanisms are responsible for recruitment? It is well established that the first transition to the recruited state is accompanied by the transformation of the granulosa cells from a squamous to a cuboidal shape.[155] Thus, the activation in the granulosa must be considered a major event in recruitment. As granulosa cells become round, they acquire the capability to incorporate [^{3}H]thymidine and begin to divide, albeit very slowly.[156] When ≥ 90 per-

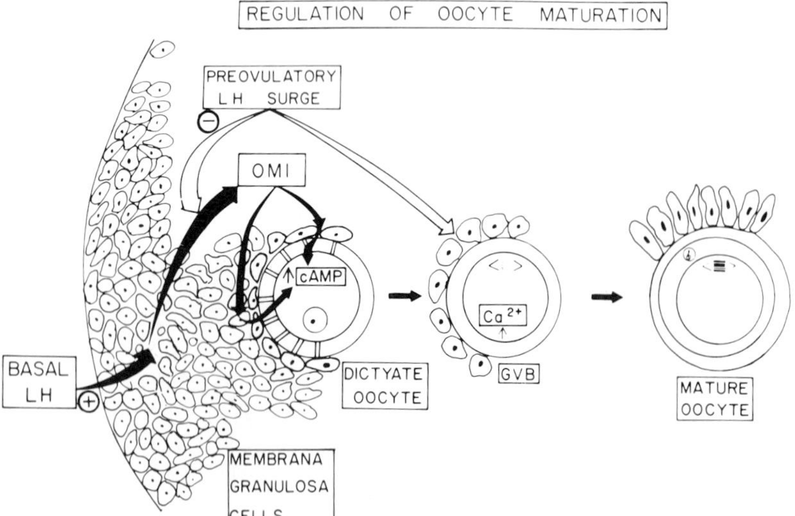

FIGURE 17A-26 Diagram of current concept of control of meiotic maturation.

cent of the granulosa cells are cuboidal, there occurs a dramatic activation in rodent oocyte RNA synthesis which results in rapid growth of the cytoplasm and the germinal vesicle.[132,133] Since changes in the synthetic activity of the oocyte arise after prior changes in the granulosa cells, it would seem that the granulosa either responds to or generates a signal that triggers the primordial follicle to follow the pathway of recruitment.

Although the whole process is poorly understood, some information about the nature of the cues for recruitment does exist in animal models. First, the ovaries are endowed with a message capable of initiating recruitment. It has long been recognized that recruitment (including oocyte growth and granulosa proliferation) does not depend on extragonadal hormones such as FSH and LH.[9] The cellular source or chemical nature of recruitment inducers is unknown.

An important concept in laboratory animals is that the process of recruitment can be modulated. Normally, the number of primordial follicles recruited is not constant but varies with age.[157] The greatest growth activity occurs early in life, after which the number of recruited follicles decreases progressively with advancing age.[158] This would indicate that the normal inducers of recruitment are somehow regulated by the actual size of the pool of primordial follicles. In this context, there is a marked reduction (by 30 percent) in the number of follicles recruited during pregnancy compared to the number during the cycle.[159] This suggests that the conditions leading to recruitment may be modulated by hormones. It is clear that the presence of testosterone severely reduces the number of primordial follicles and thus influences the recruitment process.[160] On the basis of these experiments, it has been proposed that recruitment is regulated by intraovarian androgens produced by the interstitial cells. Other experiments of a more complicated nature indicate that recruitment can also be modulated (i.e., attenuated) by the thymus gland,[161] food intake or starvation,[162] and opioid peptides.[163] No modulator has yet been found which can stimulate or amplify the process of recruitment. Finally, next to nothing is known about the recruitment process in humans.

Atresia

Of the estimated 2 million primary oocytes present in the female at birth (Fig. 17A-5), only about 400 are destined to leave the ovary through ovulation. Thus, 99.9 percent of the eggs are destroyed by the process of atresia. There are two classes of atresia (see Ovarian Follicles, above): type A, which occurs in preantral follicles, and type B, which occurs in antral or graafian follicles.[15] Despite the fact that atresia embraces so much that is central to ovarian function, almost nothing is known about the nature of the atretic signal or the steps in the atretic process in humans.

Selection

One of the most profound questions for ovarian physiologists has been how the dominant preovulatory follicle is selected from a cohort of developing follicles. An important insight into the mechanism was obtained when it was found that this basic process requires both LH and FSH as well as both granulosa and theca interstitial cells. This has led to a fundamental principle in ovarian physiology, called the two-cell-two-gonadotropin principle of follicular estrogen biosynthesis (Fig. 17A-27). When LH binds to the LH receptor in the theca interstitial cells of developing antral follicles, the hormone-receptor complex interacts with a guanine nucleotide-binding protein (G-protein) that mediates signal transduction.[164] The α-G stimulatory (α-G_s) binds GTP and stimulates the effector adenyl cyclase. The cyclic AMP–protein kinase A pathway then increases the activity of two steroidogenic enzymes, $P450_{scc}$ and $P450_{17\alpha}$, resulting in an increase in androgen biosynthesis. The androstenedione diffuses across the basal lamina into the follicular fluid and then enters the granulosa cells, where it is metabolized to estradiol by $P450_{AROM}$ induced by the interaction of FSH with its G-protein-linked receptor (Fig. 17A-27). The newly synthesized estrogen is released into the follicular fluid and the peripheral circulation, where it leads to the formation of a permissive estrogenic environment. The presence and maintenance of this process constitute the basis of follicle selection.

What is the primary event leading to sustained follicular estrogen biosynthesis? Much of what is known has come from studies by McNatty and coworkers conducted on the microenvironment of developing follicles in normal women during the follicular phase of the menstrual cycle.[21] Some relevant data are illustrated in Table 17A-1. In regard to the gonadotropins, it is evident that plasma FSH enters follicular fluid early on day 1 of the cycle, after which its concentration increases progressively with follicular growth. This finding is important because it strongly suggests that a selected follicle has the ability to sequester FSH against the declining FSH levels in the peripheral plasma. Interestingly, the situation is not the same for other gonadotropins. Table 17A-1 shows that the patterns of LH and prolactin concentrations in follicular fluid differ from each other and from that of FSH. This type of finding has implications for the way in which selection occurs because it demonstrates that a mechanism is operating at the level of the follicle both to inhibit and to stimulate the entry of potent regulatory molecules into the microenvironment of the follicular fluid. The nature of this mechanism is totally obscure.

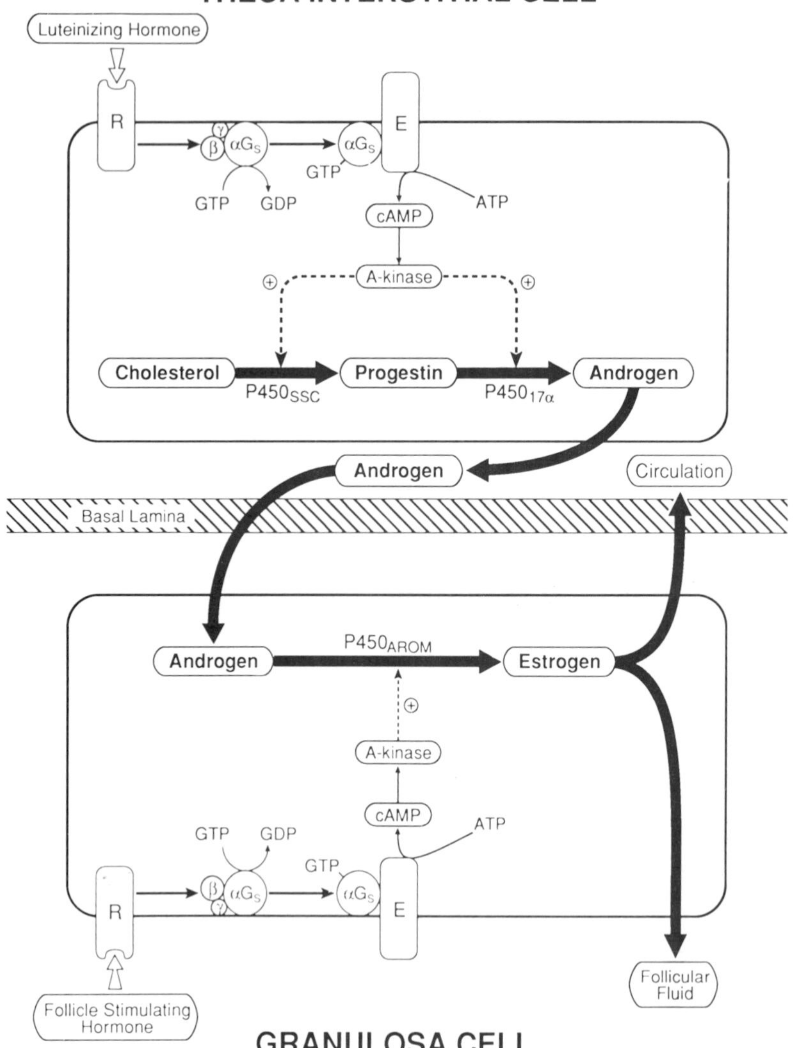

FIGURE 17A-27 Diagram illustrating the two-cell, two-gonadotropin concept of follicle estrogen biosynthesis.

Studies of human follicular fluid indicate that the major proteins are plasma proteins and that both total protein and protein composition are basically the same in follicular fluid and serum. The relative proportions, however, of proteins in follicular fluid are strikingly different from those in plasma.[165] As a rule, the ability of a protein to enter follicular fluid is inversely proportional to its molecular weight. This has led to the concept that the follicle (most likely the basal lamina) filters thecal blood in a sievelike manner so that it blocks 50 percent of the proteins with a molecular weight of 250,000 and is impermeable to proteins with a molecular weight above 850,000. In this light, it could be argued that the gonadotropins,

TABLE 17A-1 Microenvironment of Healthy Human Follicles

Day of Cycle	Follicle Size, mm	Volume of Follicular Fluid, µl	Hormone Concentration, mIU or ng/ml						
			FSH	LH	PRL	Δ4	E_2	P	DHT
1	4	30	2.5	ND	60	800	100	ND	100
4	7	150	2.5	ND	40	800	500	100	100
7	12	500	3.6	2.8	20	800	1000	300	100
12	20	6500	3.6	6	5	800	2000	2000	100

Note: Data based on the work of McNatty et al.[21]

PRL = prolactin; Δ4 = androstenedione; E_2 = estradiol; P = progesterone; DHT = dihydrotestosterone; ND = nondetectable.

which are relatively small molecules, should have no difficulty penetrating the blood-follicle barrier. It is apparent (Table 17A-1) that these molecules are not freely diffusible; thus, some mechanism must exist to account for their passage into and out of the follicles. The basis for this control is unknown, but this mechanism seems to be central to the selection process.

To what extent is the estrogen potential of a follicle attributable to androgen substrate? It has been shown that aromatase substrate (androstenedione) in all follicles attains a maximum concentration of about 10^{-6} to 10^{-5} M at day 1 of the menstrual cycle (Table 17A-1). Despite these very high levels of aromatase substrate, the concentration of estradiol in the follicular fluid of all developing follicles is low during the first 7 days of the follicular phase. At the midfollicular phase, however, there occurs a rather sharp increase in estradiol concentration, which reaches levels of about 1 to 2 μg/ml. Since androstenedione levels are so high, it can be concluded that the dramatic increases in follicle estradiol production that accompany selection are not causally related to the level of aromatase substrate. Rather, the underlying basis for the estrogen switch must depend on the induction or activation of follicular aromatase enzyme. An important sidelight is that the aromatase inhibitor DHT does not appear to be an important factor in regulating follicular estrogen production because DHT (at a concentration found in follicular fluid; Table 17A-1) does not suppress aromatization of androstenedione by the human follicle.[166] This indicates that the aromatase inhibitors do not play a role in the selection process.

The study of atretic follicles has been very valuable in understanding selection. One of the most characteristic features of the atretic or nondominant follicle is the absence of FSH in the follicular fluid (Fig. 17A-28). Given the evidence that FSH is the primary stimulus for the induction of aromatase enzymes in granulosa cells, the conclusion can be drawn that the very essence of atresia in graafian follicles is the failure to sequester or concentrate FSH in the follicular fluid. Accordingly, dramatic decreases in follicular fluid estradiol concentration occur, and the follicle dies. It follows, therefore, that the mechanism controlling the selection of a dominant preovulatory follicle certainly involves the continued ability to selectively increase the concentration of FSH in the microenvironment. Physiologi-

FIGURE 17A-28 Photomicrographs showing basic differences between the microenvironments of dominant and nondominant follicles at the midfollicular phase of the menstrual cycle. *(From Erickson and Yen,[167] by permission of Thieme-Stratton.)*

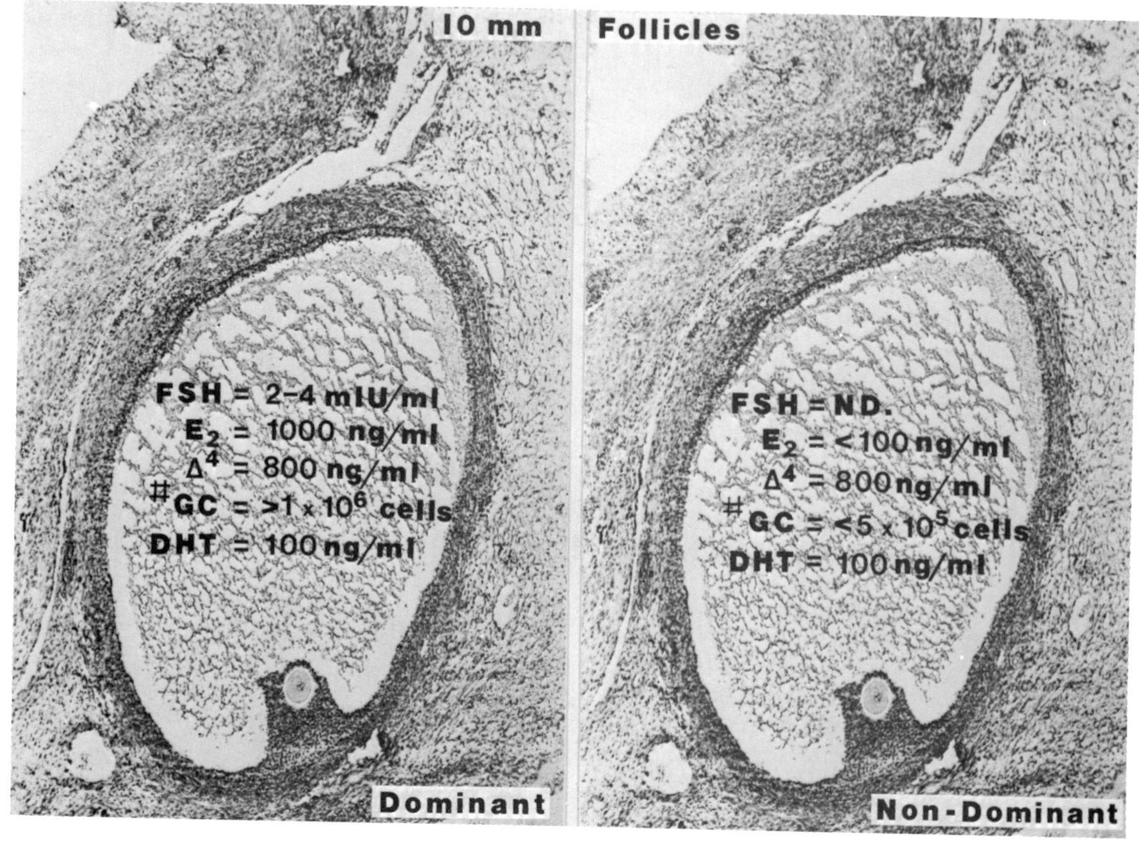

cally, this would mean more aromatase enzyme and more estradiol, both of which would shift a follicle along the path of selection as opposed to atresia.

Inasmuch as the follicle contains two major populations of endocrine cells—the granulosa cells and theca interstitial cells—each with differing hormonal sensitivities and steroidogenic capacities, the question arises whether modulators are involved in the selection process. To become a dominant preovulatory follicle, the theca and the granulosa must complete all the steps in the selection process; interruption of the maturation sequence at any step in the process could potentially prevent selection and result in atresia. As was pointed out earlier, many hormones and factors can alter follicular estrogen biosynthesis and thus influence the process of follicular maturation and selection. In physiologic terms, it is interesting that high concentrations of prolactin in human follicular fluid are associated with low estradiol levels.[168] This suggests that the continued entry of prolactin into the follicle may lead to suppression of the physiologic changes underlying estrogen biosynthesis (Table 17A-1). Considering what is known about the control of granulosa and interstitial cell differentiation, the implications for estrogen synthetic potential and therefore selection are obvious (Fig. 17A-28).

Ovulation

The expulsion of a mature oocyte from the ovary involves the release of hydrolytic enzymes in selected regions of the preovulatory follicle and a squeezing process in the basal region of the follicle wall (Fig. 17A-29). It follows, therefore, that questions concerning the phenomenon of ovulation center on the generation of proteolytic activity and contractile mechanisms in the theca externa.

There are seven cellular and extracellular components which together serve as a barrier to prevent the escape of the oocyte from the preovulatory follicle. Beginning at the surface of the ovary and moving inward, these components include (1) the surface or germinal epithelium, (2) the basement membrane, (3) the dense connective tissue of the tunica albuginea, (4) the theca externa, (5) the theca interna, (6) the basal lamina of the follicle, and (7) the membrana granulosa cells. It is evident that if an oocyte-cumulus complex is to exit from its follicle, this organized network of cells and extracellular material must be broken down.

One important aspect of the destructive mechanism is that it occurs in a highly localized area called the *stigma* (Fig. 17A-29). How do the cells in the presumptive stigma become activated to fulfill this fundamental degradative process? Morphologic and biochemical studies have shown that during the ovulatory period surface epithelial cells in the presumptive stigma become filled with large lysosome-like

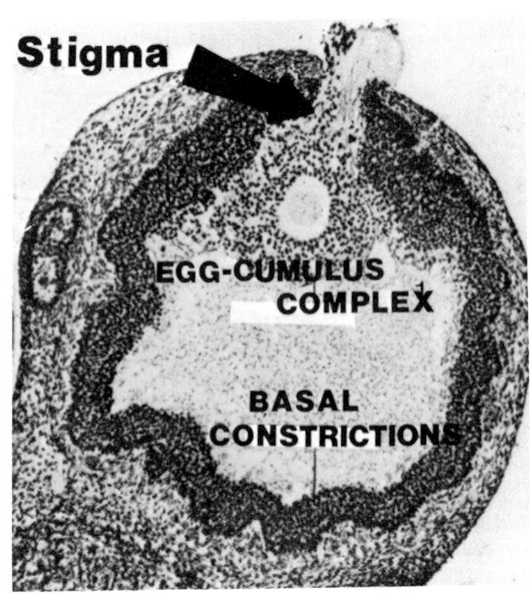

FIGURE 17A-29 Photomicrograph through a preovulatory follicle during ovulation. Note the selective destruction of tissue in the stigma and the constrictions of the basal follicular wall. *(From Hartman and Leathem,[169] by permission of Pergamon.)*

inclusions.[170] With increasing periods of time, the lysosome-like inclusions fuse with the plasma membrane and release their contents toward the tunica albuginea. This is accompanied by the progressive destruction of the basement membrane. This situation continues to progress medially, causing disruptive changes in the theca layers. It appears, therefore, that the steps leading to the formation of the stigma are initiated in a specialized population of surface epithelial cells and involve the formation and subsequent release of large amounts of hydrolytic enzymes. The question that must be analyzed is how this event occurs.

It is well established that the most important stimulating force in ovulation is LH. Although the basic mechanisms involved in LH-induced ovulation are unclear, some insights have been generated from studies carried out primarily in laboratory animals. First, the LH surge starts the preovulatory follicle on the path of progesterone production. An interesting observation in animals hypophysectomized during the preovulatory LH rise is that treatment with exogenous progesterone completely restores ovulation.[171] Consequently, it appears that progesterone plays a physiologic role in the ovulation process and may be a mediator of LH action.

Results from an extensive variety of animal studies indicate that the mechanisms underlying ovulation involve the generation of PGs by the preovulatory follicle.[172,173] Following the preovulatory surge of LH and the stimulation of progesterone production, marked increases in the synthesis of PGE and PGF occur. If an LH-stimulated preovulatory follicle is injected with indomethacin or antiprostaglandin serum, ovulation is completely blocked.[174] The conclusion that emerges is that LH-stimulated PG production is an obligatory trigger eliciting ovulation. Interestingly, morphologic studies of indomethacin-treated ovaries suggest that the prostaglandins are involved in the steps by which the stigma is formed.[175] It appears, therefore, that the underlying mechanisms of LH-induced ovulation involve the following scenario: The elevated level of progesterone serves to activate PG production, which then promotes the release of hydrolytic enzymes by a subpopulation of surface epithelial cells, which then cause stigma formation (Fig. 17A-30).

Another highly active protease that is involved in ovulation is plasmin.[176] The follicular fluid of a preovulatory follicle contains the plasmin precursor *plasminogen* at the same levels that are found in serum. The granulosa cells in a preovulatory follicle are selectively stimulated by very low levels of FSH to release the protein plasminogen activator.[177] This regulatory molecule then converts plasminogen to the active protease plasmin. Once the process is initiated, holes are formed in the basal lamina and there is a general weakening of the follicular wall, presumably caused by the proteolytic action of plasmin.[178] Questions concerning the physiologic importance of the plasminogen activator in ovulation are unanswered, but the concept is intriguing and raises the possibility that FSH, like LH, plays a basic role in ovulation, perhaps by causing destructive changes in the follicular basal lamina.

As was discussed above, the meiotically competent oocyte in the dominant follicle is inhibited from resuming meiosis by an OMI substance. However, under normal physiologic conditions, the high levels of LH at midcycle are capable of overriding the inhibitory influence of OMI. Consequently, meiosis resumes and the oocyte reaches the second meiotic metaphase or first polar body stage (Fig. 17A-30). Meiotic maturation is again arrested, and the egg awaits fertilization. The process of meiotic maturation occurs only in the oocyte of the dominant preovulatory follicle and results from specific stimulation by the high levels of LH reached at midcycle.

During the ovulatory sequence, the cumulus granulosa cells undergo a series of structural and functional changes termed *mucification* or *expansion* (Fig. 17A-30). In response to the preovulatory surge of gonadotropins, the granulosa cells in the cumulus secrete a hyaluronidase-sensitive mucous substance. This results in the dispersal of the cumulus cells and causes the egg-cumulus complex to expand tremendously.[179] The specific stimulus for mucification is believed to be FSH. The functional significance of mucification is thought to involve the pickup and transport of the egg-cumulus complex in the fallopian tube.

To what extent are contractile mechanisms involved in ovulation? It has been established that cells with the ultrastructure of smooth muscle cells are found only in the basal hemisphere of the follicle and that these cells contract before follicle rupture.[180] A number of experiments have been done

FIGURE 17A-30 Diagram illustrating the mechanisms by which the preovulatory surges of FSH and LH cause the ovulation of a fertilizable egg at midcycle.

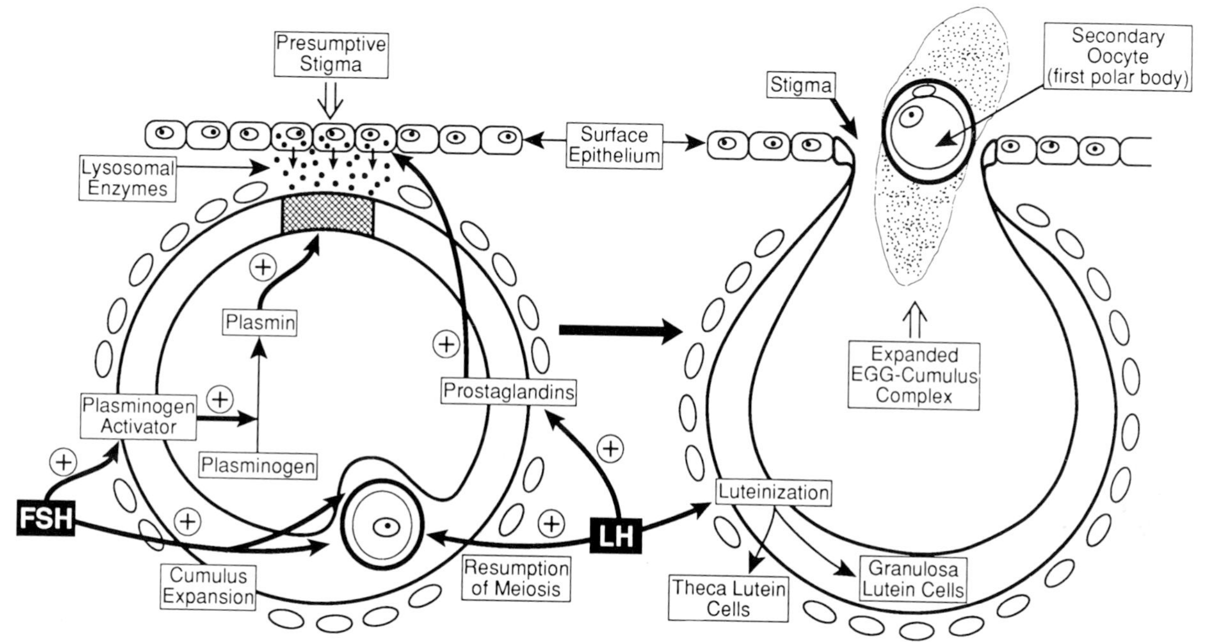

with human ovarian follicles with regard to the contractile effects of various hormones. The conclusion which emerges is that the smooth muscle cells in the theca externa have beta-adrenergic receptors for norepinephrine and muscarinic receptors for acetylcholine, both of which, when activated by ligand, will stimulate follicle contraction.[181] Since smooth muscle cells in the theca externa are innervated by sympathetic and parasympathetic nerves, it seems certain that autonomic nerves are involved in the contractile mechanisms which occur prior to ovulation. Importantly, direct analysis of intrafollicular pressure during ovulation has ruled out a buildup of intrafollicular pressure in the ovulatory process.[182] These results suggest that contractile mechanisms do not play a direct role in follicular rupture. However, based on morphologic studies, there is little doubt that contractile mechanisms occur prior to ovulation and play an important role in the collapse of the follicle and the actual expulsion of the cumulus-egg complex onto the surface of the ovary.

PHYSIOLOGIC CORRELATES OF OVARIAN ACTIVITY WITH AGING

The Fetal Period

To what extent is the human fetal ovary steroidogenically active? It was pointed out earlier that fetal ovaries at 12 to 20 weeks gestation contain a population of differentiated primary interstitial cells (Fig. 17A-13). Analysis of steroid metabolism has led to the concept that the human fetal ovaries do not have the ability to synthesize steroids de novo, presumably because they are unable to metabolize cholesterol to pregnenolone.[183] Furthermore, if human fetal ovaries are incubated with either exogenous pregnenolone or progesterone, there is little or no metabolism to steroid hormones.[184,185]

By contrast, when fetal ovary cells at 12 weeks gestation are incubated with pregnenolone sulfate, it is metabolized to pregnenolone, 17α-hydroxypregnenolone, dehydroepiandrosterone, and androstenedione but not to estrogen or testosterone.[186] This finding indicates that the fetal ovaries at 12 weeks gestation contain a very active sulfatase (three to seven times more active than in the fetal adrenal), as well as key steroidogenic enzymes in the Δ^5 pathway.[186] As development proceeds, there is a progressive decline in the steroidogenic enzymes such that by 17 weeks, the ability of the fetal ovary to metabolize pregnenolone sulfate to C_{19} steroids is very low.[186] It follows from these types of experiments that cells in human fetal ovaries can effectively use pregnenolone sulfate to produce biologically active androgens. The physiologic implications of this work lie in the fact that pregnenolone sulfate is present in very high concentrations in the fetal circulation.[187] Taken together, these observations support the concept that during their short existence (between 12 and 20 weeks of gestation), the primary interstitial cells are actively engaged in the production of biologically active androgens, using as substrate the steroid sulfates present in the fetal circulation. The physiologic significance of the androgens produced by the fetal ovaries is unknown. Importantly, LH, FSH, and hCG do not stimulate steroid metabolism by fetal ovarian cells in vitro,[188] suggesting that their activity is independent of gonadotropin control.

By 26 weeks gestation, the fetal ovaries contain a population of graafian follicles that have well-developed thecae internae.[189] During the remainder of gestation, the frequency and size of graafian follicles increase; the largest diameter reached is about 5 mm at 28 weeks. No follicles progress beyond this size, and all are destroyed by atresia. Nothing is known about the steroidogenic potential of the human fetal ovaries during this latter period, but the presence of well-developed theca interstitial cells implies they are active in androgen formation.

Premenarche

Typically, the normal ovary in childhood is a dynamic organ which is undergoing constant internal changes associated with recruitment, follicular growth, and atresia.[190–192] A characteristic feature of the human ovary from birth until menarche is the presence of large numbers of graafian follicles which measure between 1 and 6 mm in diameter (Fig. 17A-31). Generally, these follicles contain three to five layers of granulosa cells, a fully grown oocyte, and a thickened theca interna with apparently highly differentiated theca interstitial cells (Fig. 17A-31). In this sense, the infant and prepubertal ovary is morphologically indistinguishable from that of a woman with polycystic ovary syndrome (PCO). Although evidence is lacking, the premenarcheal ovaries (like those in PCO) may be actively engaged in androgen biosynthesis. Under normal circumstances, these follicles in the premenarcheal ovary grow to the graafian state, but all of them undergo atresia.[192] Thus, as in PCO, the regulatory mechanisms of selection are not operative in the prepubertal ovary.

Menarche

When a child reaches 6 years of age, some follicles begin to grow and develop beyond the 5- and 6-mm stage.[193] This situation is accompanied by progressive increases in the levels of estrogen in plasma (Fig. 17A-32).[194] At the same time, steady increases in FSH and LH concentrations in the peripheral plasma occur. Importantly, at about age 10, the concentration of FSH is greater than that of LH, similar to the situation in the early follicular phase of the menstrual cycle.[194] The underlying mechanism that

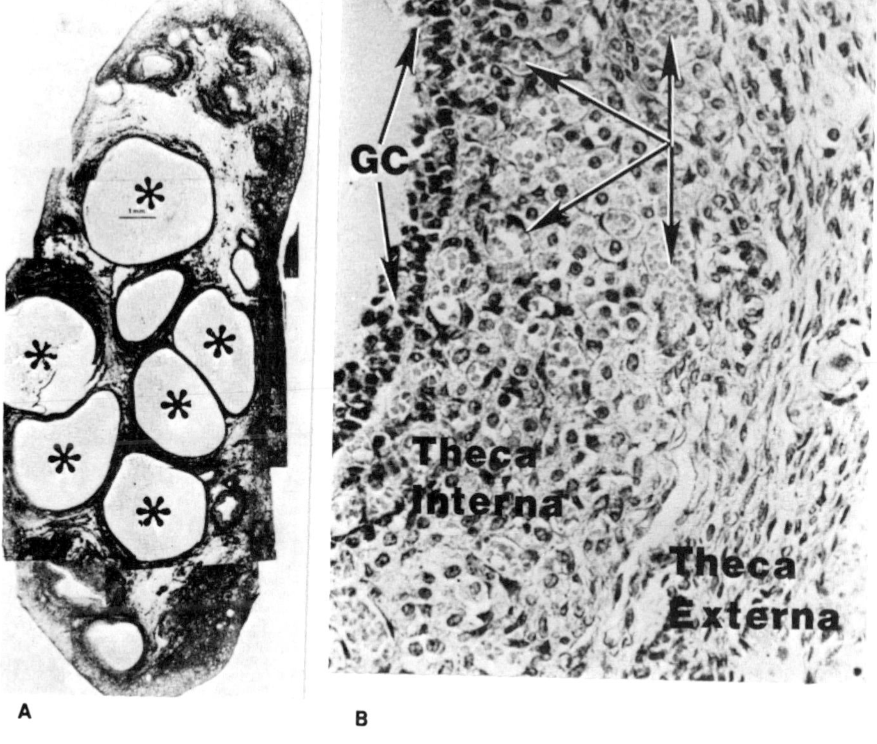

FIGURE 17A-31 Photomicrographs of actively growing human ovary at 7½ years of age. (*A*) Ovaries are polycystic-like with large numbers of graafian follicles (asterisk) measuring 2 to 6 mm in diameter. (*B*) Higher magnification of follicle shows paucity of granulosa cells (GC) and well-developed theca interna with five to seven layers of highly differentiated theca interstitial cells and numerous large capillaries (arrows). *(From Peters et al,[191] by permission.)*

controls the onset of follicular estrogen synthesis certainly involves the stimulatory effect of LH and FSH, in particular the FSH induction of $P450_{AROM}$ activity in the granulosa cells. As a result of this scenario, the prepubertal ovaries show a progressive increase in the capacity for estrogen production and follicular growth, a process which continues until the events responsible for the initiation of selection occur. After commitment to a dominant follicle occurs, the ovulatory process is initiated and the follicle becomes a corpus luteum. At this time menarche occurs; the basis for the commitment toward menarche certainly involves a steady increase in the FSH level, which, when high enough in the follicular fluid, drives granulosa cells in ovarian follicles to produce an appropriate estrogenic environment suitable for initiating the selection process.

Currently, there is great interest in the concept that insulin-like growth factor I (IGF-I) acts synergistically with FSH and LH to control the level of androgen and estrogen expression by prepubertal and pubertal ovaries. The basis for this interest is twofold. First, IGF-I levels in the blood of females increase dramatically during normal puberty.[195]

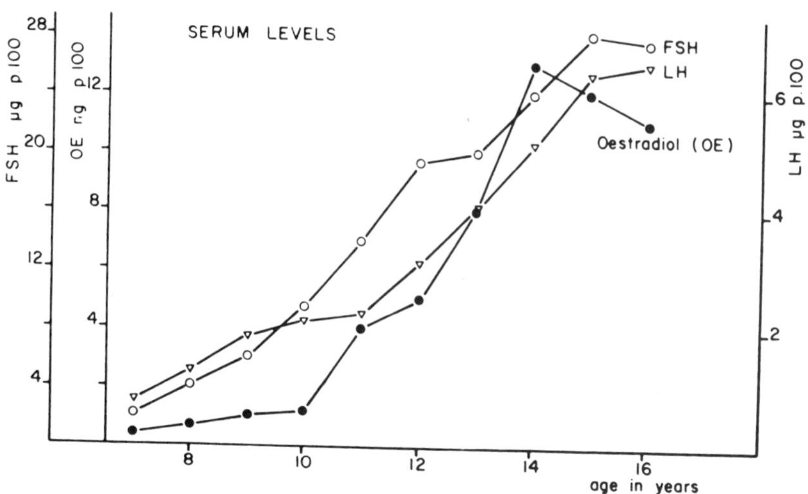

FIGURE 17A-32 Serum concentration of FSH, LH, and estradiol in girls of different ages. *(From Peters,[198] by permission of Gauthier Villars.)*

Second, specific synergistic interactions between IGF-I and the gonadotropins have been observed in human granulosa and theca cells in vitro.[196,197] Thus, IGF-I is a candidate for controlling the increase in ovarian estradiol expression that accompanies menarche in women.

Postmenarche: The Normal Menstrual Cycle

The menstrual cycle is accompanied by the sequence of recruitment, selection, ovulation, luteinization, and luteolysis. The underlying mechanisms responsible for these individual processes have already been described.

Typically, the menstrual cycle is divided into two major periods (Fig. 17A-33): the follicular phase (days 1 to 14) and the luteal phase (days 15 to 28); these major events are divided by ovulation, which occurs early on day 15. If the length of the normal menstrual cycle changes (becoming either shorter or longer), the shift occurs in the length of the follicular phase; normally, the programming of the corpus luteum is highly constant at 14 days.

As the name implies, the follicular phase concerns the evolution and development of a preovulatory follicle. In women, folliculogenesis is a very long process.[155,156] The dominant preovulatory follicle in any given cycle originates from a cohort of primordial follicles that were recruited into the pool of growing follicles about 1 year earlier (Fig. 17A-34). The very early stages of folliculogenesis take the most time to complete. A primordial follicle that has been recruited to grow takes approximately 9 months to reach the secondary follicle stage (Figs. 17A-34 and 17A-35). These follicles then develop an antrum and grow into a cohort of small graafian follicles, each measuring about 2 mm in diameter. It takes about 65 days to complete this growth phase (Fig. 17A-34).

Selection is the next step in this long sequence of events. The decision to select the dominant follicle is made at the end of the luteal phase of the preceding cycle. At this time, each ovary contains a cohort of small, rapidly growing graafian follicles (2 to 5 mm in diameter); it is from this pool that the follicle destined to ovulate in the next cycle is selected (Figs. 17A-34 and 17A-36). Initially, the chosen follicle is visibly defined only by its size, but after it reaches 6 to 8 mm in diameter in the early follicular phase, the mitotic activities in the granulosa and theca cells increase considerably. This sustained capacity for rapid growth and cell division constitutes the difference between the dominant and nondominant follicles. The consequence of the loss of growth potential in nondominant follicles is death by atresia (Fig. 17A-34).

FIGURE 17A-33 Diagrammatic illustration of endocrine events in the human menstrual cycle. The *inset* (lower left) indicates differences in levels of steroids in ovarian venous effluent between ovaries with (active) and without (inactive) the selected follicle. *(Revised from Erickson and Yen,[167] by permission of Thieme-Stratton.)*

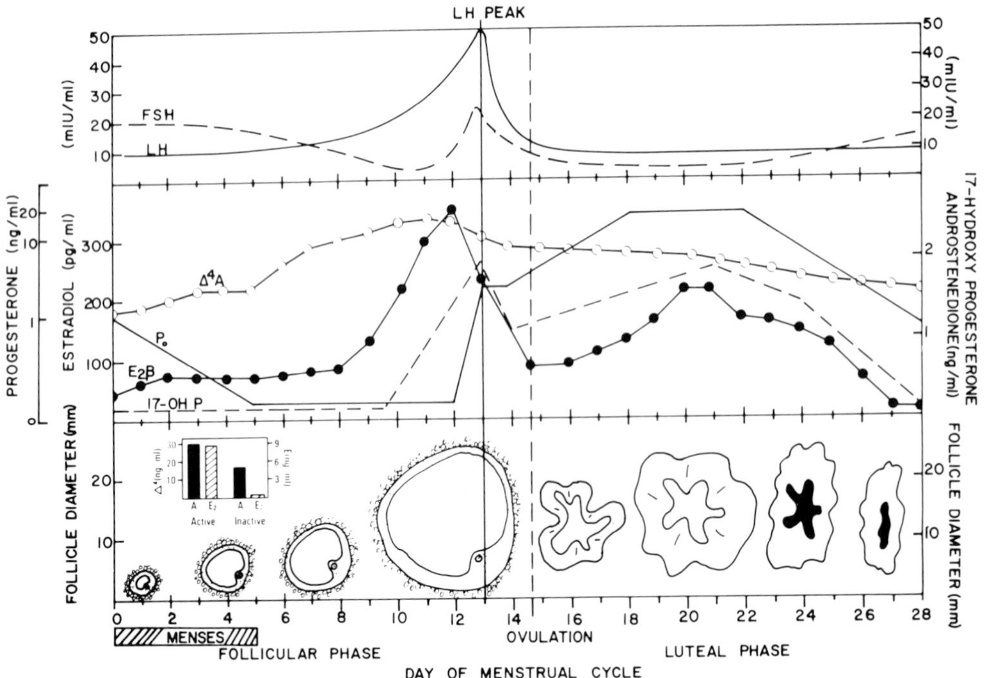

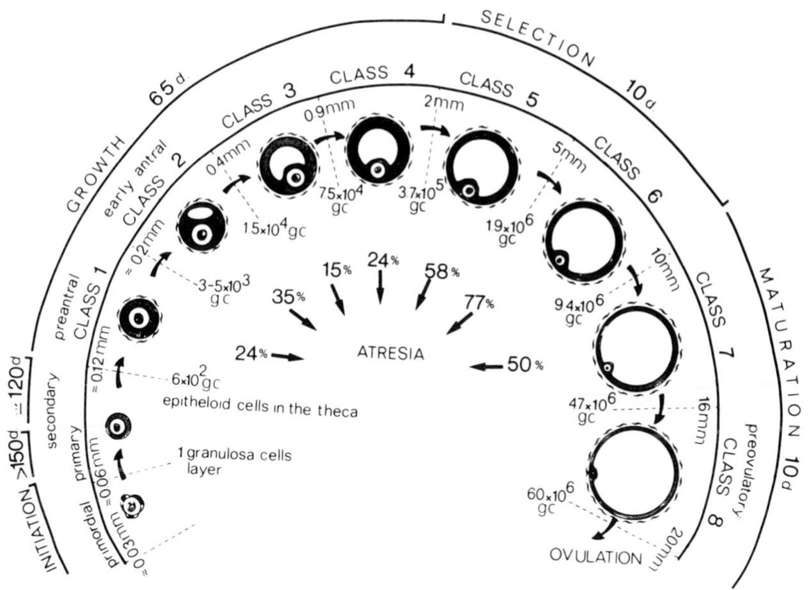

FIGURE 17A-34 The temporal pattern of folliculogenesis in normal human ovaries. The rates (in days) and stages (classes 1 through 8) of folliculogenesis and the levels of atresia (%) in the eight follicle classes are shown. The number of granulosa cells (gc) and the diameters of corresponding follicles are indicated. *(From Gougeon,[156] by permission of Oxford University Press.)*

The first question to consider is how a graafian follicle is selected in the follicular phase. As was discussed earlier, the selective influences involve FSH and estrogen. As illustrated in Fig. 17A-33, FSH is the predominant gonadotropin in the peripheral circulation when the dominant follicle is selected. The importance of elevated FSH concentrations in selection is best revealed by studies employing estradiol implants.[200] When the FSH rise is blocked by estradiol, the selected follicle is rendered inactive and the follicular phase is substantially lengthened. In conjunction with the previous discussion, the basis for this process is that the chosen follicle sequesters plasma FSH which stimulates DNA synthesis and the induction of $P450_{AROM}$ activity in the granulosa cells, followed by dramatic increases in both granulosa cell number and follicular estrogen production (Table 17A-1). As a result of the selectivity of the FSH response, plasma estradiol levels begin to increase gradually between days 1 and 7, followed by a rapid and sharp increase of estrogen concentration, reaching peak values of about 300

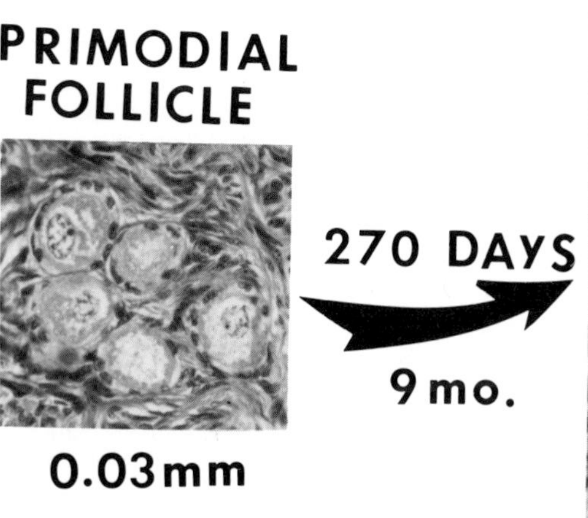

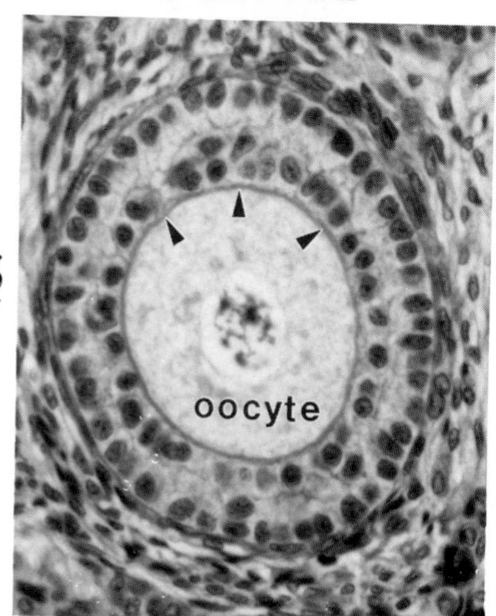

FIGURE 17A-35 Time required for a recruited primordial follicle (0.03 mm in diameter) to grow and develop into a secondary follicle (0.12 mm in diameter) in the human ovary. During the 9-month period, the oocyte completes its growth and becomes surrounded by a zona pellucida (arrowheads), and the granulosa divide slowly, increasing in number from about 7 in the primordial follicle to a total of 700 in the secondary follicle.

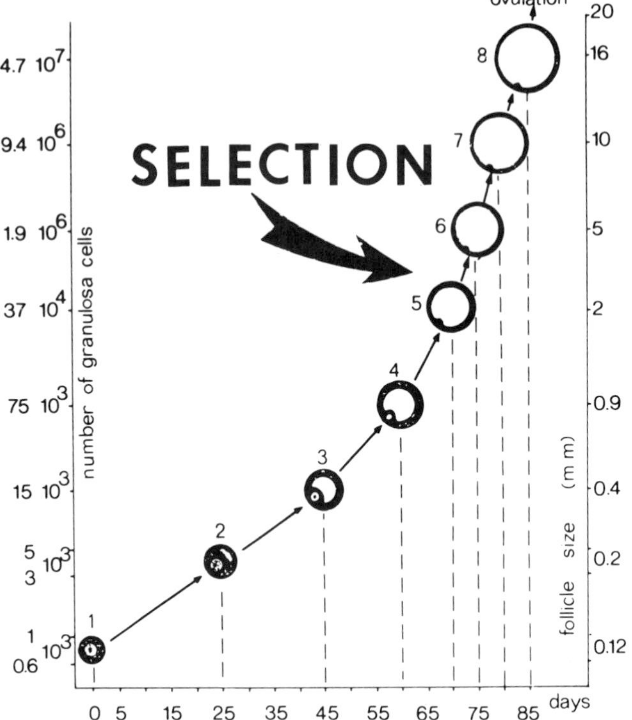

FIGURE 17A-36 In the human ovary, the dominant follicle is selected from a cohort of rapidly growing small graafian follicles (2 to 5 mm in diameter) at about the beginning of the follicular phase of the menstrual cycle. *(Modified from Gougeon[156] by permission of Oxford University Press.)*

pg/ml on day 12, when the dominant follicle reaches about 20 mm in diameter (Fig. 17A-33).

Unlike FSH, LH levels remain low and uniform during the early to midfollicular phase (Fig. 17A-33). Even though the LH concentration is low, it is evident from the androstenedione levels that LH stimulates theca interstitial cells to secrete large amounts of the aromatase substrate and that the amount formed is the same in both ovaries (Fig. 17A-33, *inset*). In contrast to estradiol, the concentration of androstenedione (1 to 2 ng/ml) in the peripheral plasma (and ovarian venous effluent) remains relatively constant throughout the menstrual cycle. This is supported by the fact that the concentration of follicular fluid androstenedione is maximal on day 1 of the cycle (Table 17A-1). Thus, the conclusion can be drawn that LH-stimulated androgen production in the follicular phase is sufficient to ensure that the levels of aromatase substrate are nearly maximal throughout the development of the selected follicle to the preovulatory stage.

Once the estradiol levels rise, the gonadotropins (LH and FSH) undergo a predictable pattern of activity characteristic of negative and positive feedback, respectively (Fig. 17A-33). When LH reaches a concentration of about 30 to 40 mIU/ml on day 12 of the cycle, a signal is triggered in the preovulatory follicle which results in the cessation of estradiol production. The mechanism underlying this change involves a selective inhibition of the $P450_{17\alpha}$ enzyme in the theca interstitial cells.[201] Consequently, the selected follicle stops producing androstenedione (and therefore estradiol) and begins to secrete increased amounts of progestin. The physiologic mechanism by which the $P450_{17\alpha}$ is suppressed might involve a local negative feedback action of estradiol directly on the theca interstitial cells.[202,203] Altogether, the increases in the plasma progestin (17-hydroxyprogesterone) level during the late follicular phase seem to be a consequence of steroidogenic changes within the affected preovulatory follicle.

In response to the peak levels of LH and FSH which occur on day 13, the process of ovulation is initiated in the dominant follicle and an egg-cumulus complex is released 36 to 38 h later.[204] As a consequence of breaks in the basal lamina caused by plasmin activity, LDL enters the granulosa cell microenvironment for the first time[205] and causes rapid increases in progesterone production by a mechanism that was discussed earlier. Considering the low levels of LH and FSH in the luteal phase (Fig. 17A-33), it is believed that LDL is the principal force stimulating progesterone production in the corpus luteum.[205] Normally, the plasma progesterone concentration reaches maximum levels of 10 to 20 ng/ml on day 19 (the consequence of luteinization) and remains elevated until day 22, when it declines sharply, reaching levels of about 0.8 ng/ml on the first day of menses (the consequence of luteolysis).

It is evident that as the corpus luteum differentiates, estrogen production is reinitiated and the corpus luteum begins progressively increasing estradiol secretion, reaching peak levels on days 21 to 22 of the luteal phase. Afterward, a sharp decline in estradiol concentration occurs, reaching levels of about 40 pg/ml at the end of the luteal phase (Fig. 17A-33). Importantly, as estradiol levels decline in the late luteal phase, the plasma FSH level begins to rise. Undoubtedly, this event is physiologically coupled with the selection of the dominant follicle which will generate the next menstrual cycle.

Menopause

The basis for the menopause is the depletion of the pool of primordial follicles (Fig. 17A-6). Consequently, the processes of recruitment and selection no longer occur, and the ovary loses its ability to synthesize and secrete estradiol and progesterone. Therefore, the menstrual cycle ceases.

Although all the aspects of folliculogenesis cease, the postmenopausal ovaries are active steroidogenically. As was discussed earlier, the theca interstitial cells of atretic follicles hypertrophy and subsequently accumulate in the ovarian stroma as the secondary interstitial cells. Thus, with increasing age, the number of secondary interstitial cells increases in human ovaries. It is obvious from the previous discussion that these cells, together with the hilar cells, respond to LH with increased synthesis of androstenedione and testosterone. During the menopause, plasma LH levels are elevated, and therefore the interstitial cells in the postmenopausal ovaries are active secretors of C_{19} androgens, but not of C_{18} estrogens.[206,207] As might be expected, the androgenic capacity of the postmenopausal ovaries is greater than that found in the ovaries of normal, nonhirsute women.

Altogether, it can be concluded that secondary interstitial and hilar cells in postmenopausal ovaries retain their full capacity for androgen biosynthesis and are constantly activated by the high levels of circulating LH in the peripheral plasma. The absence of estradiol production by the postmenopausal ovary certainly is causally connected with the absence of follicular granulosa cells.

THE CONCEPT OF OVARIAN GROWTH FACTORS

It is clear that FSH and LH play an essential role in the physiologic mechanisms of follicle section. However, only a single follicle is selected during each menstrual cycle, despite the fact that the concentrations of LH and FSH are identical in the blood perfusing both ovaries. To explain the variance in behavior between the two ovaries and among the follicles themselves, it is necessary to invoke the existence of local intraovarian/intrafollicular regulatory elements.

Historically, this concept evolved when Gospodarowitz and Bialecki[72] discovered that a number of potent growth factors act directly on human granulosa cells to stimulate mitosis. This finding was of considerable interest because it implied that folliculogenesis may be regulated by regulatory elements other than FSH and LH. As researchers began to look more closely at the issue, two significant discoveries were made using animal models. First, the theca and granulosa cells were found to actually synthesize and secrete growth factors and their binding proteins. Second, these growth factors can act directly on all follicle cells (theca, granulosa, and oocyte) to regulate their activities independently of proliferation.[72,208–222] Such discoveries have led to the novel theory that growth and development of follicles are influenced by interactions with growth factors via autocrine and paracrine mechanisms which serve to modulate (amplify or attenuate) the signals of FSH and LH. This is one of the hottest areas of research in ovarian physiology today.

As an example, let us discuss further the story of the growth factor IGF-I in the ovary. IGF-I is emerging as one of the most important growth factors in the ovary. In humans, specific high-affinity IGF-I receptors have been identified on the granulosa cells of graafian follicles,[223] and quite high levels of IGF-I are found in the follicular fluid.[224] In tissue culture experiments, IGF-I receptors have been shown to be functionally coupled to both proliferation and cytodifferentiation. With respect to cytodifferentiation, physiologic levels of IGF-I are highly active in stimulating human granulosa estradiol production; in fact, IGF-I is as effective as or more effective than FSH or LH.[196] Significantly, IGF-I acts synergistically with both FSH and LH to increase and sustain maximal levels of E_2 synthesis by human granulosa cells.[196] This ability of IGF-I to stimulate $P450_{AROM}$ appears to be a characteristic of selected follicles.[196] Thus, the concept that IGF-I may play a role in selection in women is attractive.

In regard to this issue, a surprising finding is that the amount of FSH (3 to 5 mIU/ml) in the human dominant follicle (Table 17A-1) is ineffective by itself in stimulating $P450_{AROM}$ activity.[196] This suggests that the concentration of FSH in the microenvironment is too low to induce the extraordinarily high level of $P450_{AROM}$ expressed in human granulosa cells during selection. Importantly, IGF-I can render 3 to 5 mIU/ml FSH maximally effective in stimulating $P450_{AROM}$.[196] Thus, the IGF-I synergy with FSH may offer an explanation for the marked increases in estradiol synthesis by the dominant follicle in spite of relatively low levels of FSH in the microenvironment. It is noteworthy that a recent study in the rat demonstrated that only granulosa cells in healthy dominant follicles produce IGF-I.[210] Thus, all available data support the hypothesis that IGF-I plays a central role in the mechanism of follicle selection via an autocrine mechanism involving the granulosa cells.

There can be no doubt that growth factors have significant biological effects on human follicle cells in vitro. However, there are no data to indicate that growth factor actions actually occur in vivo. Certainly, until the in vitro results have been extrapolated to the in vivo situation, the novel idea that growth factors are key regulators of ovarian physiology must remain only a theory. Still, the data raise the intriguing possibility that growth factors, acting through autocrine/paracrine mechanisms, may be a fundamental part of ovarian physiology. If this theory is proved true, the clinical question must be raised, To what extent are disorders of ovarian function caused by alterations in ovarian growth factor production and/or mechanism of action?

CONCLUSION

Finally, it must be stressed that our current understanding of ovarian physiology leans heavily on research performed on rodent species. The methods and technology have been adopted by researchers working on the human ovary. The problem that is now evident is that although many physiologic, cellular, and molecular processes found in the rodent are also found in the human, many are not. A case in point is the expression of the estrogen receptor in developing follicles of the rat but not the primate. A difficulty in this situation is the tendency to generalize research findings to all animals. The conclusion is that it is dangerous to generalize from the laboratory animal to the human. Certainly much more needs to be learned before follicle growth and development can be understood. The more that is understood concerning this process in the human, the more likely we are to understand fertility and alleviate the afflictions of infertility.

REFERENCES

1. Reynolds SRM: The vasculature of the ovary and ovarian function. *Recent Prog Horm Res* 5:65, 1950.
2. Neilson D, Jones GS, Woodruff JD, Goldberg B: The innervation of the ovary. *Obstet Gynecol Surv* 25:84, 1970.
3. Owman CH, Rosengren E, Sjöberg N-O: Adrenergic innervation of human female reproductive organs: A histochemical and chemical investigation. *Obstet Gynecol* 30:763, 1967.
4. Walles B, Groschel-Stewart U, Owman CH, Sjöberg N-O, Unsicker K: Fluorescence histochemical demonstration of a relationship between adrenergic nerves and cells containing actin and myosin in the rat ovary with special reference to the follicle wall. *J Reprod Fertil* 52:175, 1978.
5. Condon WA, Black DL: Catecholamine-induced stimulation of progesterone by the bovine corpus luteum *in vitro*. *Biol Reprod* 15:593, 1976.
6. Veldhuis JD, Harrison TS, Hammond JM: β_2-Adrenergic stimulation of ornithine decarboxylase activity in porcine granulosa cells *in vitro*. *Biochem Biophys Res Commun* 627:123, 1980.
7. Bahr J, Kao L, Nalbandov AV: The role of catecholamines and nerves in ovulation. *Biol Reprod* 10:273, 1974.
8. Capps ML, Lawrence IE, Burden HW: Ultrastructure of the cells of the ovarian interstitial gland in hypophysectomized rats: The effects of stimulation of the ovarian plexus and of denervation. *Cell Tissue Res* 193:433, 1978.
9. Eshkol A, Lunenfeld B, Peters H: Ovarian development in infant mice: Dependence on gonadotropic hormones, in Butt WR, Crooke AC, Ryle M (eds): *Gonadotropins and Ovarian Development*. London, Livingstone, 1970, p 249.
10. Hisaw FL: Development of the graafian follicle and ovulation. *Physiol Rev* 27:95, 1947.
11. Ohno S, Klinger HP, Atkin NB: Human oogenesis. *Cytogenetics* 1:42, 1962.
12. Baker TG, Sum OW: Development of the ovary and oogenesis. *Clin Obstet Gynecol* 3:3, 1976.
13. Pyrse-Davis J, Dewhurst CJ: The development of the ovary and uterus in the foetus, newborn and infant: A morphological and enzyme histochemical study. *J Pathol* 103:5, 1971.
14. Mandl A, Zuckerman A: The relation of age to the number of oocytes. *J Endocrinol* 7:190, 1951.
15. Erickson GF, Magoffin D, Dyer CA, Hofeditz C: The ovarian androgen producing cells: A review of structure/function relationships. *Endocr Rev* 6:371, 1985.
16. Albertini DF, Anderson E: The appearance and structure of intercellular connections during the ontogeny of the rabbit ovarian follicle with particular reference to gap junctions. *J Cell Biol* 63:234, 1974.
17. Merk FB, Botticelli CR, Albright JT: An intercellular response to estrogen by granulosa cells in the rat ovary: An electron microscope study. *Endocrinology* 90:992, 1972.
18. Pitts JD, Finbow ME: The gap junction. *J Cell Sci [Suppl]* 4:239, 1986.
19. Burghardt RC, Anderson E: Hormonal modulation of gap junctions in rat ovarian follicles. *Cell Tissue Res* 214:181, 1981.
20. Burghardt RC, Anderson E: Hormonal modulation of ovarian interstitial cells with particular reference to gap junctions. *J Cell Biol* 81:104, 1979.
21. McNatty KP, Moore-Smith D, Osathanondh R, Ryan KJ: The human antral follicle: functional correlates of growth and atresia. *Ann Biol Anim Biochem Biophys* 19:1547, 1979.
22. Okamura H, Virutamacen P, Wright KH, Wallach EE: Ovarian smooth muscle in the human being, rabbit, and cat. *Am J Obstet Gynecol* 112:183, 1972.
23. Amsterdam A, Lindner HR, Groschel-Stewart U: Localization of actin and myosin in the rat oocyte and follicular wall by immunofluorescence. *Anat Rec* 187:311, 1977.
24. Ingram DL: Atresia, in Zuckerman S, Mandl AM, Eckstein P (eds): *The Ovary*. New York, Academic, 1962, vol 1, p 247.
25. Spanel-Borowski K: Morphological investigations on follicular atresia in canine ovaries. *Cell Tissue Res* 214:155, 1981.
26. Hay MF, Cran DG: Differential response of components of sheep follicles to atresia. *Ann Biol Anim Biochem Biophys* 18:453, 1978.
27. Byskov AG: Atresia, in Midgley AR, Sadler WA (eds): *Ovarian Follicular Development and Function*. New York, Raven, 1979, p 41.
28. Krafka J: Parthenogenic cleavage in the human ovary. *Anat Rec* 75:19, 1934.
29. Gondos B, Hobel CG: Interstitial cells in the human fetal ovary. *Endocrinology* 93:736, 1976.
30. Tsang BK, Moon YS, Simpson CW, Armstrong DT: Androgen biosynthesis in human ovarian follicles: Cellular source, gonadotropic control, and adenosine-3′,5′-monophosphate mediation. *J Clin Endocrinol Metab* 48:153, 1979.
31. Tsang BK, Armstrong DT, Witfield JF: Steroid biosynthesis by isolated human ovarian follicular cells *in vitro*. *J Clin Endocrinol Metab* 51:1407, 1980.
32. McNatty KP, Makris A, Osthanondh R, Ryan KJ: Effects of luteinizing hormone on steroidogenesis by thecal tissue from human ovarian follicles *in vitro*. *Steroids* 36:53, 1980.
33. Magoffin DA, Erickson GF: Primary culture of differentiating ovarian androgen-producing cells in defined medium. *J Biol Chem* 257:4507, 1982.
34. Mossman HW, Koering MJ, Ferry D Jr: Cyclic changes of interstitial gland tissue of the human ovary. *Am J Anat* 115:235, 1964.
35. Guraya SS: Function of the human ovary during pregnancy as revealed by histochemical, biochemical and electron microscope techniques. *Acta Endocrinol* 69:107, 1972.
36. Kawakami M, Kubo K, Yemura T, Nagase M, Hagashi R: Involvement of ovarian innervation in steroid secretion. *Endocrinology* 109:136, 1981.
37. Dyer CA, Erickson GF: Norepinephrine amplifies hCG-stimulated androgen biosynthesis by ovarian theca-interstitial cells. *Endocrinology* 116:1645, 1985.
38. Berger L: Sur l'existence de glandes sympathicotropes dans l'ovaire et le testicule humains: Leurs rapports avec la glande interstitielle du testicule. *C R Seances Acad Sci* 175:907, 1922.
39. Sternberg WH: The morphology, androgenic function, hyperplasia and tumors of the human ovarian hilus cells. *Am J Pathol* 25:493, 1949.
40. Merkow LP, Slifkin M, Acevedo HF, Greenberg WV: Ultrastructure of an interstitial (hilar) cell tumor of the ovary. *Obstet Gynecol* 37:845, 1971.
41. Schnoy N: Ultastructure of a virilizing ovarian Leydig cell tumor. *Virchows Arch [A]* 397:17, 1982.
42. Corral-Gallardo J, Acevedo HA, Salazr JLP, Loria M,

Goldzeiher JW: The polycystic ovary: VI. A hilus cell tumor of the ovary associated with PCO disease *in vivo* and *in vitro* studies. *Acta Endocrinol (Copenh)* 52:425, 1966.
43. Echt CR, Hadd HE: Androgen excretion patterns in a patient with a metastatic hilus cell tumor of the ovary. *Am J Obstet Gynecol* 100:1055, 1968.
44. Jeffcoate SL, Prunty FTG: Steroid synthesis *in vitro* by a hilar cell tumor. *Am J Obstet Gynecol* 101:684, 1968.
45. Jezova D, Vigas M: Testosterone response to exercise during blockade and stimulation to adrenergic receptors in man. *Horm Res* 15:141, 1981.
46. Corner GW Jr: The histological dating of the human corpus luteum of menstruation. *Am J Anat* 98:377, 1956.
47. Crisp TM, Dessouky DA, Denys FR: The fine structure of the human corpus luteum of early pregnancy and during the progestational phase of the menstrual cycle. *Am J Anat* 127:37, 1970.
48. Bramley TA, Ryan RJ: Interactions of gonadotropins with corpus luteum membranes: VII. Association of hCG-binding and adenylate cyclase activities with rabbit corpus luteum plasma-membranes. *Mol Cell Endocrinol* 12:319, 1978.
49. Gillim SW, Christensen AK, McLennan CE: Fine structure of the human menstrual corpus luteum at its stage of maximum secretory activity. *Am J Anat* 126:409, 1970.
50. Van Lennp EW, Madden LM: Electron microscopic observations on the involution of the human corpus luteum of menstruation. *Z Sellforsch* 66:365, 1965.
51. Miller WL: Molecular biology of steroid synthesis. *Endocr Rev* 9:245, 1988.
52. Strauss JF, Schuler LA, Rosenblum MF, Tanaka T: Cholesterol metabolism by ovarian tissue. *Adv Lipid Res* 18:99, 1981.
53. Gwynne JT, Strauss JF: The role of lipoproteins in steroidogenesis and cholesterol metabolism in steroidogenic glands. *Endocr Rev* 3:299, 1982.
54. Brown MS, Kovanen PT, Goldstein JL: Regulation of plasma cholesterol by lipoprotein receptors. *Science* 212:628, 1981.
55. Brown MS, Goldstein JL: Receptor-mediated endocytosis: Insights from lipoprotein receptor system. *Proc Natl Acad Sci USA* 76:3330, 1979.
56. Simpson ER: Cholesterol side-chain cleavage, cytochrome P-450, and the control of steroidogenesis. *Mol Cell Endocrinol* 13:213, 1979.
57. Bloom W, Fawcett DW: *A Textbook of Histology,* 10th ed. Philadelphia, Saunders, 1975.
58. The LV, Lachance YL, Labrie C: Full length cDNA structure and deduced amino acid sequence of human 3β-hydroxy-5-ene steroid dehydrogenase. *Mol Endocrinol* 3:1310, 1989.
59. Bara G, Anderson WA: Fine structural localization of 3β-hydroxysteroid dehydrogenase in rat corpus luteum. *Histochem J* 5:437, 1973.
60. Aono T, Kitamura U, Fukuda S, Matsumoto K: Localization of 4-ene-5α-reductase, 17β-ol-dehydrogenase and aromatase in immature rat ovary. *J Steroid Biochem* 14:1369, 1981.
61. Steinkamph MP, Mendelson CR, Simpson E: Regulation by follicle stimulating hormone of the synthesis of aromatase cytochrome P-450 in human granulosa cells. *Mol Endocrinol* 1:465, 1987.
62. Smith OW, Ofner P, Verra RL: In vitro conversion of testosterone-^{14}C to androgens of the 5α-androstene series by a normal human ovary. *Steroids* 24:311, 1974.
63. Hillier SG: Regulation of follicular oestrogen biosynthesis: A survey of current concepts. *J Endocrinol* 89:30, 1981.
64. Erickson GF: Primary cultures of ovarian cells in serum-free medium as models of hormone-dependent differentiation. *Mol Cell Endocrinol* 29:2, 1983.
65. Erickson GF, Hsueh AJW, Quigley ME, Reber RW, Yen SSC: Functional studies of aromatase activity in human granulosa cells from normal and polycystic ovaries. *J Clin Endocrinol Metab* 49:514, 1979.
66. Presl J, Pospisil J, Figarova V, Krabec Z: Stage dependent changes in binding of iodinated FSH during ovarian follicle maturation in rats. *Endocrinol Exp* 8:291, 1974.
67. Nimrod A, Erickson GF, Ryan KJ: A specific FSH receptor in rat granulosa cells: Properties of binding *in vitro. Endocrinology* 98:56, 1976.
68. Hild-Petito S, Stouffer RL, Brenner RM: Immunocytochemical localization of estradiol and progesterone receptors in the monkey ovary throughout the menstrual cycle. *Endocrinology* 123:2896, 1988.
69. McNatty KP, Smith DM, Ryan KJ: The human antral follicle: Functional correlates of growth and atresia. *Ann Biol Anim Biochem Biophys* 19:1547, 1979.
70. Gougeon A: Qualitative changes in medium and large antral follicles in the human ovary during the menstrual cycle. *Ann Biol Anim Biochem Biophys* 19:1461, 1979.
71. Gemzell C: Induction of ovulation with human gonadotropins. *Recent Prog Horm Res* 21:179, 1965.
72. Gospodarowicz D, Bialecki H: Fibroblast and epidermal growth factors are mitogenic agents for cultured granulosa cells of rodent, porcine, and human origin. *Endocrinology* 104:757, 1979.
73. Doody KJ, Lorence MC, Mason JI, Simpson ER: Expression of messenger ribonucleic acid species encoding steroidogenic enzymes in human follicles and corpora lutea throughout the menstrual cycle. *J Clin Endocrinol Metab* 70:1041, 1990.
74. Hillier SG, Harlow CR, Shaw HJ, Wickings EJ, Dixson AF, Hodges JK: Cellular aspects of preovulatory folliculogenesis in primate ovaries. *Hum Reprod* 3:507, 1988.
75. McFarland KC, Springel R, Phillips HS, Kohler M, Rosenblot N, Nikolics K, Segaloff DL, Seeburg PH: Lutropin-choriogonadotropin receptor: An unusual member of the G-protein-coupled receptor family. *Science* 145:494, 1989.
76. McNatty KP, Hunter WM, McNeilly AS, Sawers RS: Changes in the concentration of pituitary and steroid hormones in the follicular fluid of human graafian follicles throughout the menstrual cycle. *J Endocrinol* 64:55, 1975.
77. Oxberry BA, Greenwald GS: An autoradiographic study of the binding of ^{125}I-labeled FSH, LH, and prolactin to the hamster ovary throughout the estrous cycle. *Biol Reprod* 27:505, 1982.
78. Balboni GC, Vannelli GB, Barni T, Orlando C, Serio M: Transferrin and somatomedin C receptors in the human ovarian follicles. *Fertil Steril* 48:796, 1987.
79. Magoffin DA: Evidence that luteinizing hormone-stimulated differentiation of purified ovarian theca-interstitial cells is mediated by both type I and type II adenosine 3′-5′-monophosphate-dependent protein kinases. *Endocrinology* 125:1464, 1989.
80. Magoffin DA, Kurtz KM, Erickson GF: Insulin-like growth factor-1 selectively stimulates cholesterol side-chain cleavage expression in ovarian theca interstitial cells. *Mol Endocrinol* 4:489, 1990.
81. Farkash Y, Timberg R, Orly J: Preparation of antiserum to rat cytochrome P-450 cholesterol side chain cleavage and its use for ultrastructural localization of the immunoreactive enzyme by protein A-gold technique. *Endocrinology* 118:1353, 1986.
82. Mikhail G, Zander J, Allen WM: Steroids in human ovarian vein blood. *J Clin Endocrinol Metab* 23:1267, 1963.
83. Baird DT, Guevara A: Concentration of unconjugated estrone and estradiol in peripheral plasma in non-pregnant women throughout the menstrual cycle, castrate, and postmenopausal women and men. *J Clin Endocrinol* 29:149, 1969.
84. Abraham GE, Odell WD, Swerdloff RS, Hopper K: Simultaneous radioimmunoassay of plasma FSH, LH, progesterone, 17-hydroxyprogesterone and estradiol-17β during the menstrual cycle. *J Clin Endocrinol* 34:312, 1972.
85. Thorneycroft IH, Sribyatta B, Tom WK, Nakamura RM, Mishell DR: Measurement of serum LH, FSH, progesterone, 17α-hydroxyprogesterone and estradiol-17β level at 4-hour intervals during the periovulatory phase of the menstrual cycle. *J Clin Endocrinol Metab* 39:754, 1974.
86. Baird DT, Burger PE, Heavon-Jones GD, Scaramuzzi RJ:

The site of secretion of androstenedione in non-pregnant women. *J Endocrinol* 63:210, 1974.
87. Baird DT, Fraser IS: Blood production and ovarian secretion rates of estradiol-17β and estrone in women throughout the menstrual cycle. *J Clin Endocrinol Metab* 38:1009, 1974.
88. Huang WY, Pearlman WH: The corpus luteum and steroid hormone formation: II. Studies on the human corpus luteum *in vitro*. *J Biol Chem* 238:1308, 1963.
89. Hammerstein J, Rice RB, Savard K: Steroid hormone formation in the human ovary: I. Identification of steroids formed *in vitro* from acetate-1-^{14}C in the corpus luteum. *J Clin Endocrinol* 24:597, 1964.
90. Vande Wiele RI, Bogumil J, Dyrenfurth I, Ferin M, Jewelewicz R, Warren M, Rizkallah T, Mikhail G: Mechanisms regulating the menstrual cycle in women. *Recent Prog Horm Res* 26:63, 1970.
91. Lee CY, Coulam CB, Jiang NS, Ryan RJ: Receptors for luteinizing hormone in human corpora luteal tissue. *J Clin Endocrinol Metab* 36:148, 1973.
92. McNeilly AS, Kerin J, Swanston IA, Bramley TA, Baird DT: Changes in the binding of human chorionic gonadotropin/luteinizing hormone, follicle-stimulating hormone and prolactin to human corpora lutea during the menstrual cycle and pregnancy. *J Endocrinol* 87:315, 1980.
93. Rajaniemi HJ, Ronnberg L, Kauppila A, Ylostalo P, Jalkanen M, Saastamoinen J, Selander K, Paavo P, Vittko R: Luteinizing hormone receptors in human ovarian follicles and corpora lutea during menstrual cycle and pregnancy. *J Clin Endocrinol Metab* 108:307, 1981.
94. Dennefors BL, Hamberger L, Nilsson L: Influence of hCG in vivo on steroid formation and gonadotropin responsiveness of isolated preovulatory follicular cells. *Fertil Steril* 39:56, 1983.
95. Polan ML, Sen D, Tarlatzis B: Human chorionic gonadotropin stimulation of estradiol production and androgen antagonism of gonadotropin-stimulated responses in cultured human granulosa luteal cells. *J Clin Endocrinol Metab* 62:628, 1986.
96. Vega M, Devolo L, Navarro V, Castro O, Koheu P: In vitro net progesterone productions by human corpora lutea: Effects of human chorionic gonadotropin, dibutyryl adenosine 3′,5′-monophosphate, cholera toxin, and forskolin. *J Clin Endocrinol Metab* 65:747, 1987.
97. Rojas FJ, Moretti-Rojas IM, Balmaceda JP, Asch RH: Changes in adenyl cylase activity of the human and nonhuman corpus luteum during the menstrual cycle and pregnancy. *J Clin Endocrinol Metab* 68:379, 1989.
98. Polan ML, Lauter N, Dulgi AM, Tarlatzis BC, Hazeltine FP, Decherney AH, Behrman HR: Human chorionic gonadotropin and prolactin modulation of early function and luteinizing hormone receptor binding activity in cultured human granulosa luteal cells. *J Clin Endocrinol Metab* 59:773, 1984.
99. Jones GS: The luteal phase defect. *Fertil Steril* 27:351, 1976.
100. Wentz AC: Physiologic and clinical considerations in luteal phase defects. *Clin Obstet Gynecol* 22:169, 1979.
101. McNeely MJ, Soules MR: The diagnosis of luteal phase deficiency: A critical review. *Fertil Steril* 50:1, 1988.
102. Hunter MG, Baker TG: Effect of hCG, cAMP, and FSH on steroidogenesis by human corpora lutea in vitro. *J Reprod Fertil* 63:285, 1981.
103. Ohara A, Mori T, Taii S, Ban C, Narimoto K: Functional differentiation in steroidogenesis in two types of luteal cells isolated from mature human corpora lutea of the menstrual cycle. *J Clin Endocrinol Metab* 65:1192, 1987.
104. Ohara A, Taii S, Mori T: Stimulatory effects of purified human FSH on estradiol production in the human luteal phase. *J Clin Endocrinol Metab* 68:359, 1989.
105. Erickson GF, Garzo VG, Magoffin DA: Insulin-like growth factor I (IGF-1) regulates aromatase activity in human granulosa and granulosa luteal cells. *J Clin Endocrinol Metab* 69:716, 1989.
106. Fujita Y, Mori T, Suzuki A, Nihnobu K, Nishimura T: Functional and structural relationships in steroidogenesis *in vitro* by human corpora lutea during development and regression. *J Clin Endocrinol Metab* 53:744, 1981.
107. Hunter MG, Baker TG: Effect of hCG, cAMP and FSH on steroidogenesis by human corpora lutea *in vitro*. *J Reprod Fertil* 63:285, 1981.
108. Hoffman F: Unterschungen uber die hormonale Beeinflussung der Lebensdauer des corpus luteum in Zyklus der Frau. *Geburtshilfe Frauenheilkd* 20:1153, 1960.
109. Williams MT, Roght MS, Marsh JM, Lemaire WJ: Inhibition of human chorionic gonadotropin-induced progesterone synthesis by estradiol in human luteal cells. *J Clin Endocrinol Metab* 48:437, 1979.
110. Thibier M, El-Hassan N, Clark MR, Lemaire WJ, Marsh JM: Inhibition by estradiol of human chorionic gonadotropin-induced progesterone accumulation in isolated human luteal cells: Lack of mediation by prostaglandin F. *J Clin Endocrinol Metab* 50:590, 1980.
111. Depp R, Cox DW, Pion RJ, Conrad SH, Heinrichs WL: Inhibition of pregnenolone Δ^5-3β-hydroxysteroid dehydrogenase Δ^5-4-isomerase systems of human placenta and corpus luteum of pregnancy. *Gynecol Invest* 4:106, 1973.
112. Hagerman DD, Smith O, Day CF: Mechanism of the stimulatory effect of clomid on aromatization of steroids by human placenta *in vitro*. *Acta Endocrinol (Copenh)* 51:591, 1966.
113. McNatty KP, Sawers RS, McNeilly AS: A possible role for prolactin in control of steroid secretion by the human graafian follicle. *Nature* 250:5468, 1974.
114. Demura R, Ono M, Demura H, Shizume K, Oouchi H: Prolactin directly inhibits basal as well as gonadotropin-stimulated secretion of progesterone and 17β-estradiol in the human ovary. *J Clin Endocrinol Metab* 54:1246, 1982.
115. Clayton RN, Huhatniemi IT: Absence of gonadotropin-releasing hormone receptors in human gonadal tissue. *Nature* 299:56, 1982.
116. Casper RF, Erickson GF, Yen SSC: Studies on the effect of gonadotropin-releasing hormone and its agonist on human luteal steroidogenesis *in vitro*. *Fertil Steril* 42:39, 1984.
117. Tureck RW, Mastroianni L, Blasco L, Strauss JF: Inhibition of human granulosa cell progesterone secretion by gonadotropin-releasing hormone agonist. *J Clin Endocrinol Metab* 54:1078, 1982.
118. Casper RF, Erickson GF, Rebar RW, Yen SSC: The effect of luteinizing hormone-releasing factor and its agonist on cultured human granulosa cells. *Fertil Steril* 37:406, 1982.
119. Aten RF, Polan ML, Bayless R, Behrman HR: A GnRH-like protein in human ovaries: Similarity to the GnRH-like ovarian protein of the rat. *J Clin Endocrinol Metab* 64:1288, 1987.
120. Rao CV, Griffin LP, Carman FR: Prostaglandin $F_{2\alpha}$ binding sites in human corpora lutea. *J Clin Endocrinol Metab* 44:1032, 1977.
121. Challis JRG, Calder AA, Dilley S, Foster CS, Hillier K, Hunter DJS, Mackenzie IZ, Thorburn GD: Production of prostaglandin E and F2α by corpora lutea, corpora albicantes and stroma from the human ovary. *J Endocrinol* 68:401, 1975.
122. Swanston IA, McNatty KP, Baird DR: Concentration of prostaglandin $F_{2\alpha}$ and steroids in the human corpus luteum. *J Endocrinol* 73:115, 1977.
123. Richardson MC, Masson GM: Progesterone production by dispersed cells from human corpus luteum: Stimulation by gonadotropins and $PGF_{2\alpha}$: Lack of response to adrenaline and isoprenaline. *J Endocrinol* 87:247, 1980.
124. McKay DG, Hertig AT, Adams EC, Danziger SL: Histochemical observation on the germ cells of human embryos. *Anat Rec* 117:201, 1953.
125. Eddy EM, Clark JM, Gong D, Fenderson BA: Origin and migration of primordial germ cells in mammals. *Gamete Res* 4:333, 1981.
126. Wartenberg H: Development of the early human ovary and

the role of the mesonephros in the differentiation of the cortex. *Anat Embryol* 165:253, 1982.

127. Updahyay S, Luciani J, Zamboni L: The role of the mesonephros in the development of the indifferent gonads and ovaries of the mouse. *Ann Biol Anim Biochem Biophys* 19:1179, 1979.
128. Monk M, McLaren A: X-Chromosome activity in fetal germ cells of the mouse. *J Embryol Exp Morphol* 63:75, 1981.
129. Burgogne PS, Baker TG: Oocyte depletion in XO mice and their XX sibs from 12 to 200 days post partum. *J Reprod Fertil* 61:207, 1981.
130. Ruby JR, Dyer RF, Skalko RG: The occurrence of intercellular bridges during oogenesis. *J Morphol* 127:307, 1969.
131. Byskov AG: Regulation of meiosis in mammals. *Ann Biol Anim Biochem Biophys* 19:1251, 1979.
132. Bachvarova R: Gene expression during oogenesis and oocyte development in mammals, in Browder L (ed.): *Developmental Biology: A Comprehensive Synthesis,* vol I: *Oogenesis.* New York; Plenum, 1985, p 453.
133. Roller RJ, Kinloch RA, Hiraoka BY, Li SSC, Wassarman PM: Gene expression during mammalian oogenesis and early embryogenesis: Quantification of three messenger RNAs abundant in fully grown mouse oocytes. *Development* 106:251, 1989.
134. Bachvarova R, Baran MM, Tejblum A: Development of naked growing mouse oocytes *in vitro. J Exp Zool* 211:159, 1980.
135. Eppig JJ: A comparison between oocyte growth in coculture with granulosa cells and oocytes with granulosa cell-oocyte junctional contact maintained *in vitro. J Exp Zool* 209:345, 1979.
136. Gilula NB, Epstein ML, Beers WH: Cell-to-cell communication and ovulation. *J Cell Biol* 78:58, 1978.
137. Heller DT, Cahill DM, Schultz RM: Biochemical studies of mammalian oogenesis: Metabolic cooperativity between granulosa cells and growing mouse oocytes. *Dev Biol* 84:455, 1981.
138. Brower PT, Schultz RM: Intercellular communication between granulosa cells and mouse oocytes: Existence and possible nutritional role during oocyte growth. *Dev Biol* 90:144, 1982.
139. Wassarman PM: The biology and chemistry of fertilization. *Science* 235:553, 1987.
140. Wassarman PM: Fertilization in mammas. *Scientific American,* December 1988, p 78.
141. Nishimoto T, Mori T, Yamada I, Nishimura T: Autoantibodies to zona pellucida in infertile and aged women. *Fertil Steril* 34:552, 1980.
142. Sacco AG: Zona pellucida: Current status as a candidate antigen for contraceptive vaccine development. *Am J Reprod Immunol Microbiol* 15:122, 1987.
143. Millar SE, Chamow SM, Baur AW, Oliver C, Rubey F, Dean J: Vaccination with a zona pellucida peptide produces long term contraception in female mice. *Science* 246:935, 1989.
144. Tsuji K, Sowa M, Nakano R: Relationship between human oocyte maturation and different follicular sizes. *Biol Reprod* 32:413, 1985.
145. Eppig JJ, Downs SM: Chemical signals that regulate mammalian oocyte maturation. *Biol Reprod* 30:1, 1984.
146. Eppig JJ, Schroeder AC: Capacity of mouse oocytes from preantal follicle to undergo embryogenesis and development to live young after growth, maturation, and fertilization *in vitro. Biol Reprod* 41:268, 1989.
147. Testart J, Frydman R, Mouzon JD, Lassalle B, Belaisch JC: A study of factors affecting the success of human fertilization *in vitro:* I. Influence of ovarian stimulation upon the number and condition of oocytes collected. *Biol Reprod* 28:415, 1983.
148. Downs SM, Daniel SAJ, Eppig JJ: Induction of maturation of cumulus cell enclosed mouse oocytes by FSH and EGF: Evidence for a positive stimulus of somatic origin. *J Exp Zool* 245:86, 1987.
149. Banka C, Erickson GF: GnRH induces classical meiotic maturation in subpopulations of atretic preantral follicles. *Endocrinology* 177:1500, 1985.
150. Tsafriri A, Dekel N, Bar-Ami S: The role of OMI in follicular regulation of oocyte maturation. *J Reprod Fertil* 64:541, 1982.
151. Whittingham DG, Siracuse G: The involvement of calcium in the activation of mammalian oocytes. *Exp Cell Res* 113:311, 1978.
152. Takahashi M, Koide SS, Donahoe PK: Mullerian inhibiting substance as oocyte meiosis inhibitor. *Mol Cell Endocrinol* 47:225, 1986.
153. O W-S, Robertson DM, deKrester DM: Inhibin as an oocyte meiotic inhibitor. *Mol Cell Endocrinol* 62:307, 1987.
154. Moor RM: Role of steroids in the maturation of ovine oocytes. *Ann Biol Anim Biochem Biophys* 18:477, 1978.
155. Gougeon A, Chainy GBN: Morphometric studies of small follicles in ovaries of women at different ages. *J Reprod Fertil* 81:433, 1987.
156. Gougeon A: Dynamics of follicular growth in the human: A model from preliminary results. *Hum Reprod* 1:81, 1986.
157. Pedersen T: Follicular growth in the immature mouse ovary. *Acta Endocrinol (Copenh)* 62:117, 1969.
158. Krarup T, Pedersen T, Faber M: Regulation of oocyte growth in the mouse ovary. *Nature* 224:187, 1969.
159. Pedersen T, Peters H: Follicle growth and cell dynamics in the mouse ovary during pregnancy. *Fertil Steril* 22:42, 1971.
160. Peters H, Byskov AGS, Sorensen IN, Krarup T, Pedersen T, Faber M: The development of the mouse ovary after testosterone propionate injection on day 5, in Butt WR, Crooke AC, Ryle E (eds): *Gonadotropins and Ovarian Development.* London, Livingstone, 1970, p 351.
161. Lintern-Moore S: Effect of athymia on the initiation of follicular growth in the rat ovary. *Biol Reprod* 17:155, 1977.
162. Lintern-Moore S, Everitt AV: The effect of restricted food intake on size and composition of the ovarian follicle population in the Wistar rat. *Biol Reprod* 19:688, 1978.
163. Lintern-Moore S, Supasri Y, Parasuthpaisit K, Sobhon P: Acute and chronic morphine sulfate treatment alters ovarian development in prepubertal rats. *Biol Reprod* 21:379, 1979.
164. McFarland KC, Sprengel R, Phillips HS, Köhler M, Rosenblit N, Nikolics K, Segaloff DL, Seeburg PH: Lutropin-choriogonadotropin receptor: An unusual member of the G-protein-coupled receptor family. *Science* 245:494, 1989.
165. Shalgi R, Kraicer P, Rimon A, Pinto M, Soferman N: Proteins of human follicular fluid: The blood-follicle barrier. *Fertil Steril* 24:429, 1973.
166. Hillier SG, Van den Boogard AMJ, Reichert LE, Van Hall EV: Intraovarian sex steroid hormone interactions and the control of follicular maturation: Aromatization of androgens by human granulosa cells *in vitro. J Clin Endocrinol Metab* 50:640, 1980.
167. Erickson GF, Yen SSC: New data on follicle cells in polycystic ovaries: A proposed mechanism for the genesis of cystic follicles. *Semin Reprod Endocrinol* 2:231, 1984.
168. McNatty KP: Relationship between plasma prolactin and the endocrine microenvironment of the developing human antral follicle. *Fertil Steril* 32:433, 1979.
169. Hartman CG, Leathem JH: Oogenesis and ovulation, in: *Conference on Physiological Mechanisms Concerned with Conception.* New York, Pergamon, 1963, p 205.
170. Cajander S, Bjersing L: Fine structural demonstration of acid phosphatase in rabbit germinal epithelium prior to induced ovulation. *Cell Tissue Res* 164:279, 1975.
171. Takahashi M, Ford JJ, Yoshinaga K, Greep RO: Induction of ovulation in hypophysectomized rats by progesterone. *Endocrinology* 95:1322, 1974.
172. Marsh JM, Yang NST, Lemaire WJ: Prostaglandin synthesis in rabbit graafian follicles *in vitro:* Effect of luteinizing hormone and cyclic AMP. *Prostaglandins* 7:269, 1974.
173. Armstrong DT: Role of prostaglandins in follicular responses to luteinizing hormone. *Ann Biol Anim Biochem Biophys* 15:181, 1975.

174. Armstrong DT, Grinwich DL, Moon YS, Zamecnik J: Inhibition of ovulation in rabbits by intrafollicular injection of indomethacin and PGF antiserum. *Life Sci* 14:129, 1974.
175. Downs SM, Long FJ: An ultrastructural study of preovulatory development in mouse ovarian follicles: Effects of indomethacin. *Anat Rec* 205:159, 1983.
176. Beers WH, Strickland S, Reich E: Ovarian plasminogen activator: Relationship to ovulation and hormonal regulation. *Cell* 6:387, 1975.
177. Beers WH, Strickland S: A cell culture assay for follicle stimulating hormone. *J Biol Chem* 253:3877, 1978.
178. Beers WH: Follicular plasminogen and plasminogen activator and the effect of plasmin on ovarian follicle wall. *Cell* 6:379, 1975.
179. Erickson GF: An analysis of follicle development and ovum maturation. *Semin Reprod Endocrinol* 4:233, 1986.
180. Martin GG, Talbot P: The role of follicular smooth muscle cells in hamster ovulation. *J Exp Zool* 216:469, 1981.
181. Walles B, Falck B, Owman CH, Sjöberg N-O: Characterization of autonomic receptors in the smooth musculature of human graafian follicle. *Biol Reprod* 17:423, 1977.
182. Bronson RA, Bryant G, Balk MW, Emanuele N: Intrafollicular pressure within preovulatory follicles of the pig. *Fertil Steril* 31:205, 1979.
183. Jungman RA, Schweppe JS: Biosynthesis of sterols and steroids from acetate-^{14}C by human fetal ovaries. *J Clin Endocrinol Metab* 28:1599, 1968.
184. Bloch E: Metabolism of 4-^{14}C-progesterone by human fetal testis and ovaries. *Endocrinology* 74:833, 1964.
185. Taylor T, Coutts JRT, MacNaughton MC: Human foetal synthesis of testosterone from perfused progesterone. *J Endocrinol* 60:321, 1974.
186. Payne AH, Jaffe RB: Androgen formation from pregnenolone sulfate by the human fetal ovary. *J Clin Endocrinol Metab* 39:300, 1974.
187. Huhtaniemi I, Vinko R: Determination of unconjugated and sulfated neutral steroids in human fetal blood of early and midpregnancy. *Steroids* 16:197, 1970.
188. Wilson EA, Joe-Jowad M: The effect of trophic agents on fetal ovarian steroidogenesis in organ culture. *Fertil Steril* 32:73, 1979.
189. Pryse-Davies J, Dewhurst CJ: The development of the ovary and uterus in the foetus, newborn and infant: A morphological and enzyme histochemical study. *J Pathol* 103:5, 1971.
190. Valdes-Dapena MA: The normal ovary of childhood. *Ann NY Acad Sci* 142:597, 1967.
191. Peters H, Himelstein-Braw R, Faber M: The normal development of the ovary in childhood. *Acta Endocrinol (Copenh)* 82:617, 1976.
192. Himelstein-Braw R, Byskov AG, Peters H, Faber M: Follicular atresia in the infant human ovary. *J Reprod Fertil* 46:55, 1976.
193. Lintern-Moore S, Peters H, Moore GPM, Faber M: Follicular development in the infant human ovary. *J Reprod Fertil* 39:53, 1974.
194. Faiman C, Winter JSD: Gonadotropins and sex hormone pattern in puberty, in Grumbach MM, Grave GD, Mayer FE (eds): *The Control of the Onset of Puberty*. London, Wiley, 1974.
195. Bala RM, Lopatka J, Leung A, McCoy E, McArthur RG: Serum immunoreactive somatomedin levels in normal adults, pregnant women at term, children at various ages, and children with constitutionally delayed growth. *J Clin Endocrinol Metab* 52:508, 1981.
196. Erickson FG, Garzo VG, Magoffin DA: IGF-1 regulates aromatase activity in human granulosa and granulosa luteal cells. *J Clin Endocrinol Metab* 69:716, 1989.
197. Erickson GF, Magoffin DA, Jones KL: Theca function in polycystic ovaries of a patient with virilizing congenital adrenal hyperplasia. *Fertil Steril* 51:173, 1989.
198. Peters H: The development and maturation of the ovary. *Ann Biol Anim Biochem Biophys* 16:271, 1976.
199. Green SH, Zuckerman S: Quantitative aspects of the growth of the human ovum and follicle. *J Anat* 85:373, 1951.
200. Zeleznik AJ: Premature elevation of systemic estradiol reduces levels of FSH and lengthens the follicular phase of the menstrual cycle in rhesus monkeys. *Endocrinology* 109:352, 1981.
201. Dennefors BL, Hamberger L, Nilsson L: Influence of human chorionic gonadotropin in vivo on steroid formation and gonadotropin responsiveness of isolated preovulatory follicular cells. *Fertil Steril* 34:56, 1983.
202. Magoffin DA, Erickson GF: Mechanism by which 17β-estradiol inhibits ovarian androgen production in the rat. *Endocrinology* 108:962, 1982.
203. Magoffin DA, Erickson GF: Direct inhibitory effect of estrogen on LH-stimulated androgen synthesis by ovarian cells cultured in defined medium. *Mol Cell Endocrinol* 28:81, 1982.
204. Edwards RG: Studies on human conception. *Am J Obstet Gynecol* 117:587, 1973.
205. Carr BR, MacDonald PC, Simpson ER: The role of lipoproteins in the regulation of progesterone secretion by the human corpus luteum. *Fertil Steril* 38:303, 1982.
206. Mattingly RF, Huang W: Steroidogenesis of the menopausal and postmenopausal ovary. *Am J Obstet Gynecol* 103:679, 1969.
207. Asch RH, Greenblatt RB: Steroidogenesis in the postmenopausal ovary. *Clin Obstet Gynecol* 4:85, 1977.
208. Adashi EY, Resnick CE, D'Ercole AJ, Svoboda ME, Van Wyk JJ: Insulin like growth factors as intraovarian regulators of granulosa cell growth and function. *Endocr Rev* 6:400, 1985.
209. Gospodarowicz D, Ferrara N, Schweigerer L, Neufeld G: Structural characterization and biological functions of fibroblast growth factor. *Endocr Rev* 8:95, 1987.
210. Oliver AE, Aitman TJ, Powell JF, Wilson CA, Clayton RN: Insulin like growth factor-I gene expression in the rat ovary is confined to granulosa cells of developing follicles. *Endocrinology* 124:2671, 1989.
211. Voutilainer R, Miller W: Coordinate tropic regulation of mRNAs for insulin-like growth factor II and the cholesterol side chain cleavage enzyme $P450_{scc}$ in human steroidogenic tissue. *Proc Natl Acad Sci USA* 84:1590, 1987.
212. Ramasharma K, Li CH: Human pituitary and placental hormones control human insulin-like growth factor II secretion in human granulosa cells. *Proc Natl Acad Sci USA* 84:2643, 1987.
213. Suikkari A-M, Jalkanen J, Koistinen R, Bützow R, Ritvos O, Ranta T, Seppäla M: Human granulosa cells synthesize low molecular weight insulin-like growth factor binding protein. *Endocrinology* 124:1088, 1989.
214. Voutilainen R, Miller WL: Human Mullerian inhibitory factor mRNA is normally regulated in the fetal testes and adult granulosa cells. *J Mol Endocrinol* 1:604, 1987.
215. Ying S-Y: Inhibins, activins and follistatins: Gonadal proteins modulating the secretion of FSH. *Endocr Rev* 9:267, 1988.
216. Daughaday WH, Rotwein P: Insulin-like growth factors I and II: Peptide, messenger ribonucleic acid and gene structures, serum, and tissue concentrations. *Endocr Rev* 10:68, 1989.
217. Lobb DK, Kobrin MS, Kudlow JE, Dorrington JH: Transforming growth factor-alpha in adult bovine ovary: Identification in growing ovarian follicles. *Biol Reprod* 40:1087, 1989.
218. Downs SM, Daniel SAJ, Eppig JJ: Induction of maturation of cumulus cell enclosed mouse oocytes by FSH and epidermal growth factor: Evidence for a positive stimulus of somatic cell origin. *J Exp Zool* 245:86, 1988.
219. Kudlow JE, Korbin MS, Purchio AF, Twardzik DR, Hernandez ER, Asa SL, Adashi EY: Ovarian transforming growth factor α gene expression: Immunohistochemical localization to the theca interstitial cells. *Endocrinology* 121:1577, 1987.
220. Mondschein JS, Schomberg DW: Growth factors modulate

gonadotropin receptor induction in granulosa cell cultures. *Science* 211:1179, 1981.

221. Knecht N, Catt KJ: Modulation of cAMP-mediated differentiation in ovarian granulosa cells by EGF and PDGF. *J Biol Chem* 258:2789, 1983.

222. Magoffin DA, Gancedo B, Erickson GF: Transforming growth factor β promotes differentiation of ovarian theca interstitial cells but inhibits androgen production. *Endocrinology* 125: 1951, 1989.

223. Gates GS, Bayer S, Seibel M, Poretsky L, Flier JS, Moses AC: Characterization of insulin-like growth factor binding to human granulosa cells obtained during in vitro fertilization. *J Receptor Res* 7:885, 1987.

224. Eden JA, Jones J, Carter GD, Alagnband-Zadeh J: A comparison of follicular fluid levels of IGF-I in normal dominant and cohort follicles, polycystic and multicystic ovaries. *Clin Endocrinol (Oxf)* 29:327, 1988.

The Ovary: Basic Principles and Concepts

B. CLINICAL

Robert I. McLachlan
Neil McClure
David L. Healy
Henry G. Burger

In this section an approach to the management of the clinical disorders of ovarian function is outlined, based on the particular setting in which patients present to the clinician, i.e., in teenagers, young adults, and individuals of middle age.

OVARIAN DISORDERS IN TEENAGERS

Primary Amenorrhea

The time of menarche varies widely among racial groups and families but is normally thought to occur between 9 and 16 years of age. It is preceded by an acceleration of growth and some development of secondary sexual characteristics, normally by age 14. These changes reflect the rise in estrogen secretion from the pubertal ovary and the consequent increase in circulating somatomedin concentrations. In addition, the development of pubic hair, reflecting a rise in androgen production (adrenarche), precedes menarche by 1 to 3 years. Failure of menses to occur by age 16 years is termed *primary amenorrhea*. The clinical evaluation of a girl with primary amenorrhea commences with an assessment of her growth and development. The failure of normal growth and/or pubertal development (Fig. 17B-1) to occur by the age of 14, or of menses to occur by 16, should lead to investigation.

A wide variety of disorders of the hypothalamic-pituitary-ovarian axis can result in primary amenorrhea. It is more helpful to classify these conditions clinically according to the girl's stature and the degree, timing, and nature of pubertal change. The more common causes of primary amenorrhea are classified according to clinical presentation in Table 17B-1.

Short Stature and No Pubertal Development

Gonadal Dysgenesis

Turner's Syndrome Short stature, absence of a pubertal growth spurt, and absence of secondary sexual characteristics suggest the syndromes of gonadal dysgenesis which represent an important cause of primary amenorrhea. The most common is classic Turner's syndrome, a sporadic condition which affects approximately 1 in 3000 girls and results from a deficiency of one X chromosome, leading to a 45,XO karyotype. The müllerian duct derivatives and genitalia are female; however, the ovaries are represented by gonads devoid of primordial follicles. The characteristic phenotype includes short stature [>2.5 standard deviations (SD) below the mean for chronologic age, adult mean height <148 cm], infantile female genitalia, and absence of secondary sexual characteristics. Somatic abnormalities are usually but not invariably present and may include webbing of the neck, cubitus valgus, hypoplastic nails, a shieldlike chest with wide-spaced nipples, micrognathia, and external ear abnormalities. Investigation shows low estrogen secretion and elevated gonadotropin concentrations; a 45,XO karyotype is diagnostic. Cardiovascular assessment is indicated in view of a 10 to 20 percent incidence of coarctation of the aorta. Thyroid function should also be measured because of an increased incidence of autoimmune thyroid disease. Routine diagnostic imaging of the kidneys is performed in the initial evaluation because of the increased incidence of renal tract abnormalities, especially horseshoe kidney.

Lifelong estrogen replacement is essential in patients with Turner's syndrome. Significant acceleration of ulnar bone growth has been shown in short-

Breast Development

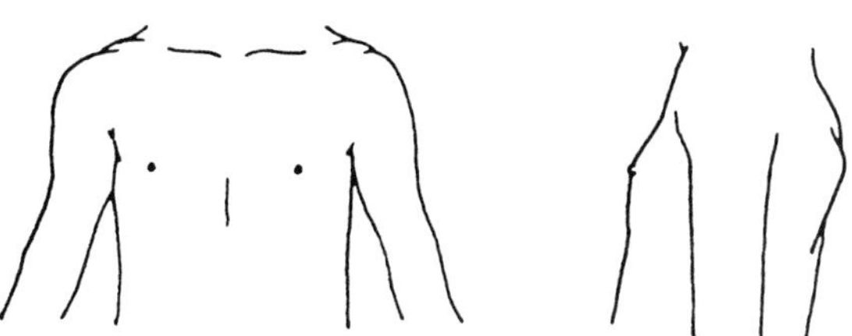

Stage 1 – prepubertal

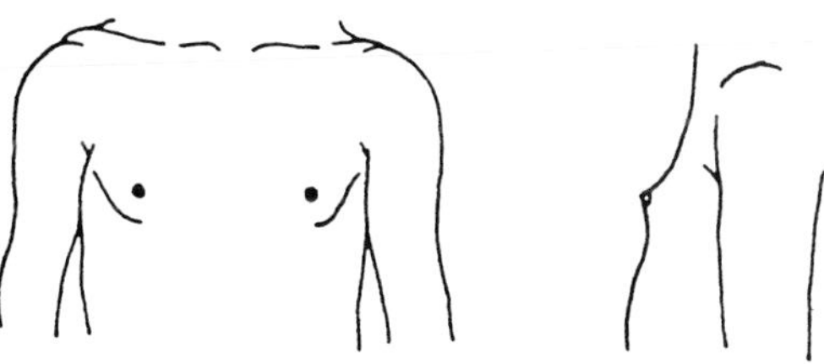

Stage 2 – elevation of breasts and papilla

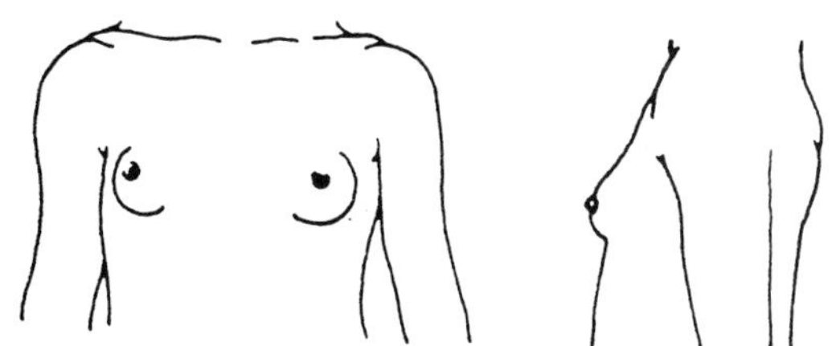

Stage 3 – further elevation and areola but no separation of contours

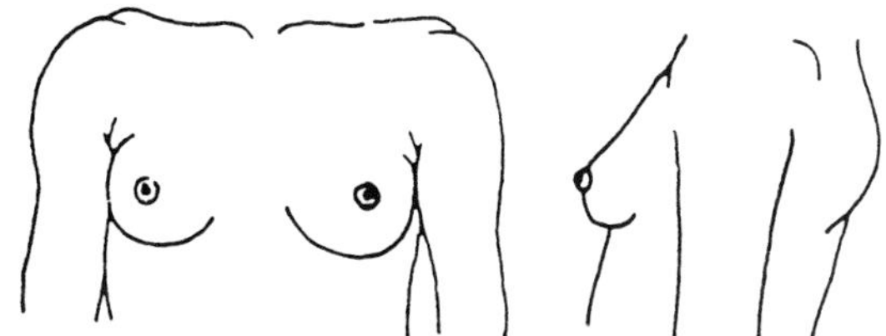

Stage 4 – areola and papilla form a secondary mound above level of the breast

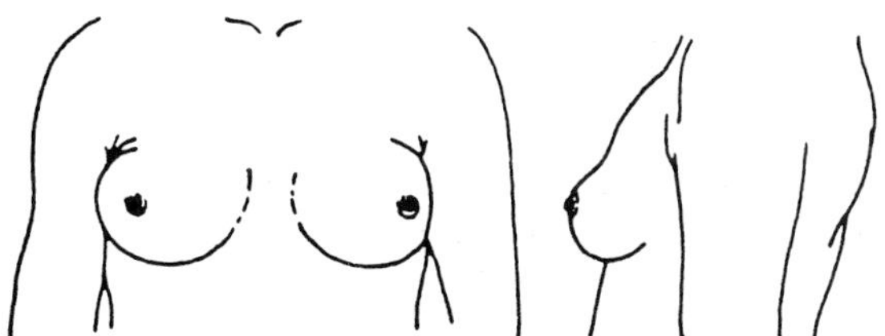

Stage 5 – areola recesses to the general contour of the breast

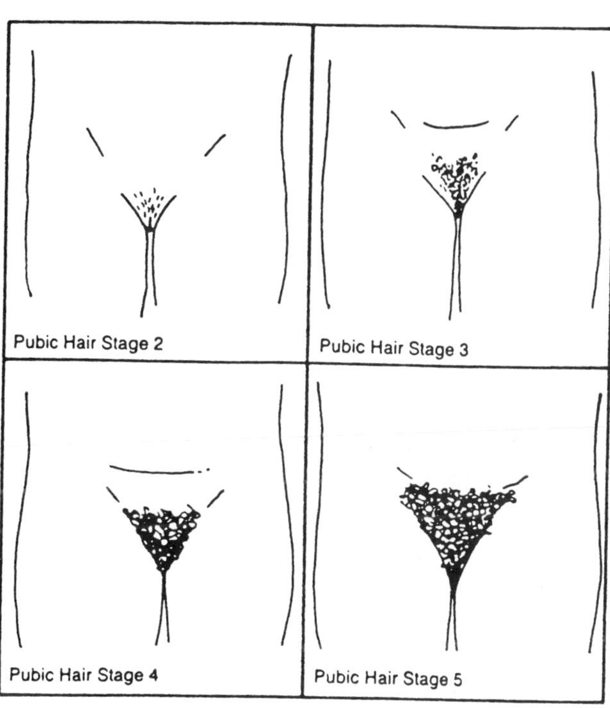

FIGURE 17B-1
STAGES OF PUBERTY
Pubertal staging is based on the degree of breast and pubic hair development. (Adapted from Tanner J, Davis PSW: *J Paediatrics* 107:317, 1985.)

Breast development: Stages 1–5 as shown.

Pubic hair

Stage 1. Preadolescent. The vellus over the pubes is not further developed than that over the abdominal wall, i.e., no pubic hair.

Stage 2. Sparse growth of long, slightly pigmented downy hair, straight or slightly curled, chiefly along labia.

Stage 3. Considerably darker, coarser, and more curled. The hair spreads sparsely over the junction of the pubes.

Stage 4. Hair now adult in type, but area covered is still considerably smaller than in the adult. No spread to the medial surface of thighs.

Stage 5. Adult in quantity and type with distribution of the horizontal (or classically "feminine") pattern. Spread to medial surface of thighs but not up linea alba or elsewhere above the base of the inverse triangle (spread up linea alba occurs late and is rated stage 6).

TABLE 17B-1 Clinical Classification of Primary Amenorrhea

Short stature, no pubertal development
Gonadal dysgenesis
Turner's syndrome (45,XO)*
Turner's mosaicism (e.g., 46,XX, 45,XO)
Abnormalities of X chromosome
Mosaicism 46,XX, 45,XO + Y variants
Pure gonadal dysgenesis
Hypopituitarism
Hypothalamopituitary dysfunction: idiopathic or associated with surgery, irradiation, trauma, tumor
Normal stature, no or minimal pubertal development
Hypogonadotropic hypogonadism (Kallmann's syndrome)
Idiopathic*
Organic lesions
Idiopathic delayed puberty*
Malnutrition, systemic disease, intensive exercise*
Normal stature and pubertal development
With adrenarche: müllerian (paramesonephric) duct-derivative abnormalities
Without adrenarche: testicular feminization
Virilization and/or anomalous genitalia
Miscellaneous rare disorders:
Partial testicular feminization
Inborn errors of testosterone biosynthesis or conversion to dihydrotestosterone
Untreated congenital adrenal hyperplasia

* Most common differential diagnoses.

term studies using low-dose estrogen replacement (5 μg ethinyl estradiol), while a dose of 10 μg ethinyl estradiol daily similarly accelerates bone growth but also induces breast budding.[1] Drug administration should be commenced at 10 to 12 years of age, and the dose should be gradually increased from 2.5 to 20 μg daily with cyclic progesterone (e.g., medroxyprogesterone acetate 10 mg daily for 10 to 12 days every month) when the ethinyl estradiol dose exceeds 10 μg daily. Whether this therapy augments eventual adult height is controversial, but it has the clinical advantage of inducing pubertal change, menses, and a pubertal growth spurt in line with that of the patient's peers. The maintenance of bone density and normal female lipid profiles (with a likely reduction in the risk of atherosclerotic vascular disease) are other important advantages of estrogen replacement.

Improvement in growth velocity and adult height are the major aims of treatment. Several studies have shown that recombinant human growth hormone (hGH) alone or in combination with androgens or estrogens can accelerate growth velocity and stimulate catch-up growth.[2–4] For example, hGH 1 IU/kg per week is commenced at 4 to 5 years and continued until completion of growth. If the initial response is poor and in patients presenting at 8 to 10 years of age, a low dose of an anabolic agent such as oxandrolone may be added. The anabolic agent is ceased when estrogen therapy is begun. Such treatment programs have substantially improved the probability of achieving a more normal adult height.

Although these subjects have no oocytes and have been regarded as sterile, with the advent of donor oocyte in vitro fertilization (IVF) programs, fertility is now possible. Thirty-five children or ongoing pregnancies have been achieved at Monash University, Australia, with a schedule of steroid replacement, oocyte donation, and embryo transfer in patients with no functioning ovaries.[5,6] Three of these patients have Turner's syndrome. Thus, a new optimism should permeate the paramedical and lay support groups for Turner's syndrome patients which are available in many centers for counseling of the patient, her parents, or her husband regarding the nature of this condition (see also Management of Premature Ovarian Failure, below).

Mosaicism Compared to the XO karyotype, the XO/XX karyotype is associated with taller stature, fewer somatic abnormalities, and occasionally menstruation and fertility. Pregnancies result in abortion 25 percent of the time and have 10 percent incidences of births with Down's and Turner's syndromes, dictating the need for counseling and amniocentesis. Rare variants of gonadal dysgenesis include abnormalities of the short or long arms of the X chromosome, resulting in a phenotypic spectrum of amenorrhea, short stature, and somatic abnormalities.

Disorders incorporating XO/XY mosaicism lead to a range of phenotypes from male to female. Predominantly female phenotypes usually present with amenorrhea and a degree of genital virilization. The 30 to 70 percent frequency of gonadal tumors, especially dysgerminoma, warrants prophylactic removal of these gonads in teenagers with proven gonadal dysgenesis (see Chap. 18).

Hypopituitarism

Conditions that diminish pituitary function are often associated with inadequate growth hormone and gonadotropin secretion, resulting in short stature and failure to enter puberty. Features of thyroid and adrenal deficiency may also be present. Often a history of head trauma, cranial tumor surgery, or irradiation is elicited, although the patient may present with primary amenorrhea reflecting an underlying and often idiopathic hypothalamopituitary disorder. Depressed levels of gonadotropins and other pituitary hormones, which may be unresponsive to their normal trophic stimuli, will be found. Computed tomography (CT) or magnetic resonance imaging (MRI) of the pituitary region is essential to exclude a neoplasm, especially a craniopharyngioma. Therapy involves treatment of the underlying cause and replacement of sex steroids and other deficient hormones.

Normal Stature and No or Minimal Pubertal Development

Hypogonadotropic Hypogonadism (Kallmann's Syndrome)

Delayed or absent pubertal change, particularly when associated with hyposmia or anosmia in a subject of normal height, suggests the possibility of idiopathic hypogonadotropic hypogonadism. This congenital, often familial condition results from an isolated deficiency of hypothalamic gonadotropin releasing hormone (GnRH) and therefore of gonadotropins (Fig. 17B-2). This deficiency appears to result from the failure of GnRH neurons to migrate from the olfactory placode into the hypothalamus. Associated somatic abnormalities include cleft lip and palate and congenital deafness. Deletion of the Xp 22.3 region of the X chromosome is associated with Kallmann's syndrome and occasionally with other congenital defects such as ichthyosis and chondromalacia punctata.[7] Laboratory features include low ovarian steroid production and low to low normal gonadotropin levels. The pituitary, chronically deprived of GnRH stimulation, generally responds poorly to acute GnRH infusion, although normal or exaggerated responses have been described. Basal and stimulated levels of other pituitary hormones are usually normal, although diminished prolactin secretion in response to thyrotropin releasing hormone (TRH) has been described in females. CT or MRI scanning of the hypothalamopituitary region is also indicated in view of the occasional occurrence of tumor, hamartoma, empty sella syndrome, and disorders of the rhinencephalon. Induction of pubertal changes and menses is achieved with exogenous estrogen and progesterone. Women with this syndrome are characteristically unresponsive to clomiphene. Fertility can be achieved with exogenous gonadotropin ovulation induction (see below) or with pulsatile GnRH infusion therapy. Pulsatile GnRH, either subcutaneous or intravenous, is preferable because of the low rate of multiple pregnancy.

FIGURE 17B-2 Clinical appearance of a 19-year-old female with hypogonadotropic hypogonadism. Note the normal height (152 cm) and absence of a female body habitus. There was no breast development in this patient.

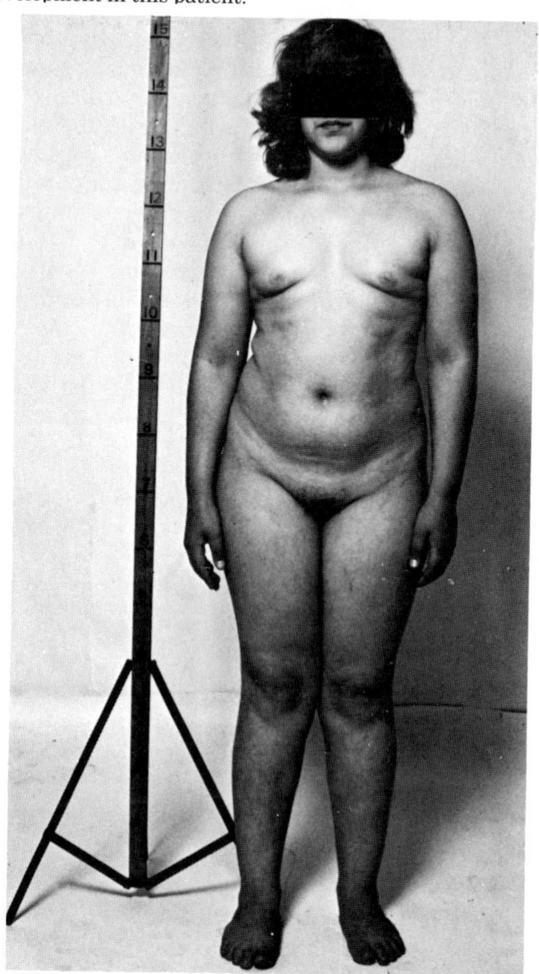

Idiopathic Delayed Puberty

A delay in menarche as a component of delayed puberty is a common cause of presentation with primary amenorrhea. Its differentiation from hypogonadotropic hypogonadism can be very difficult. Features supporting the diagnosis include a family history of delayed puberty, normal development in other respects, and usually some development and progression of pubertal changes by the time of consultation. These subjects are often short (3d to 10th percentile) with an appropriately delayed bone age. Serum gonadotropin and ovarian steroid secretion either is prepubertal or shows early pubertal changes corresponding to the degree of pubertal development. Neither GnRH infusion nor other tests, such as the prolactin response to TRH or metoclopramide, lead to confident diagnostic discrimination between delayed puberty and hypogonadotropic hypogonadism. Therefore, after other likely causes have been excluded, reassurance and review of these patients should be rewarded by spontaneous menses between ages 17 and 20 years. The pubertal growth spurt is also delayed, but adult height is usually normal. Pubertal development can be hastened, if desired by the patient, by estrogen replacement (as described above for Turner's syndrome) alone with intermittent withdrawal to observe the underlying state of the pituitary ovarian axis, at which time the possibility of hypogonadotropic hypogonadism can be readdressed.[8] It should be noted that hyperprolactinemia is an occasional cause of primary amenorrhea.

Malnutrition, Systemic Disease, or Intensive Exercise

Normal puberty can be interrupted by intercurrent problems such as the severe weight loss seen in starvation, anorexia nervosa, or severe systemic diseases. Intensive athletic training, particularly ballet and running, can be associated with decreased body weight, particularly fat content, along with menstrual disturbances including amenorrhea. Although more commonly a cause of secondary amenorrhea, such activities, when undertaken and maintained from early puberty, can produce primary amenorrhea. Restoration of good nutrition with weight gain or resolution of underlying illness should restore pubertal progression. In these settings serum gonadotropins show a prepubertal pattern of low levels [particularly of luteinizing hormone (LH)], lack of pulsatile secretion, and blunted response to GnRH.

Normal Stature with Normal Pubertal Development

Müllerian Duct–Derivative Abnormalities

Primary amenorrhea with normal growth and pubertal development to a stage where menses ought to be occurring suggests abnormalities of the müllerian duct–derived structures (uterine tubes, uterus, cervix, and upper vagina).[9] Ovarian function is normal, but menses do not occur because of an absence of normal endometrial tissue or the lack of a conduit for menstrual flow to the exterior. An imperforate vagina (often incorrectly diagnosed as an imperforate hymen) may lead to retention of menstrual fluid behind a membrane (hematocolpos) or cyclic abdominal pain from an accompanying hematosalpinx. The resultant mass may be sufficiently large to produce abdominal distension. Clinical examination, including examination under general anesthesia, will define these anatomic variations. Therapy will depend on the anatomy and may range from simple stellate incision of the vaginal membrane, drainage, and use of prophylactic antibiotics to laparotomy for excision of a noncommunicating uterine horn.

Testicular Feminization

A normal female phenotype, often with tall stature and breast development but absent or scanty pubic hair, suggests the possibility of testicular feminization. This is an X-linked dominant condition in which absent or defective cytosolic testosterone receptors result in androgen insensitivity in genetic males (46,XY). Analysis of the androgen receptor gene reveals a range of mutations (deletions, substitutions) which lead to androgen resistance.[10,11] Testes are present, but spermatogenesis does not occur and the testes lie in the inguinal canal or labia. This key examination feature underlines the importance of a thorough examination of the inguinal and labial region. External genitalia are female; however, the vagina is a short pouch and no müllerian duct derivatives are present. The absence of a uterus can be confirmed by vaginal and/or rectal examination and ultrasound. Diagnostic features include a serum testosterone level in the normal male range while serum LH concentration is raised, underlining the insensitivity of the pituitary gonadotrophs to testosterone feedback. Testicular estrogen production and conversion of testosterone to estradiol, in the absence of testosterone effects, lead to pubertal breast development (Fig. 17B-3). Cytosolic androgen receptors are absent or defective. Therapy includes reinforcement of the female gender identity and orchidectomy at any time in the presence of a gonadal hernia or otherwise after puberty in view of an increased incidence of testicular neoplasia. Lifelong estrogen replacement is then required, with or without added progestogens (see Hormonal Replacement Therapy under Postmenopausal Problems, below).

Virilization and/or Anomalous Genitalia

A range of rare disorders may present with amenorrhea and varying degrees of virilization and/or anomalous genitalia in a young girl. Partial testicular feminization occurs when the defect in the androgen receptor is incomplete. Some androgen effect therefore leads to labioscrotal fusion or clitoromegaly. Deficiency of the 5α-reductase enzyme is an autosomal recessive condition of genetic males in which there are normal testosterone levels but inadequate conversion to the more potent androgen dihydrotestosterone (DHT). Ambiguous genitalia (varying degrees of labioscrotal fusion) with a blind-ending vaginal pouch occur. Virilization occurs at puberty, while breast development fails. Finally, a range of inborn errors of the testosterone biosynthetic pathway are other rare causes of female or anomalous genitalia associated with amenorrhea in the genetic male. These conditions are outlined in

FIGURE 17B-3 Testicular feminization. Note the Tanner stage 5 breast development, resulting from testicular estrogen secretion, and the absence of axillary hair.

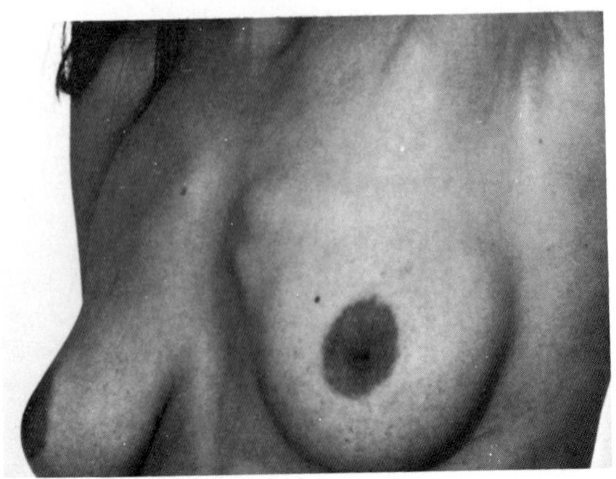

Chap. 16. They require extensive investigation of steroid metabolism and androgen receptor activity as well as anatomic delineation.

Menarcheal Menorrhagia

The mammalian uterus is a highly specialized fibromuscular and secretory organ in which the myometrium is elastic and contractile properties are responsive to a variety of hormonal regulators secreted both locally and distantly. In contrast, the inner lining of the uterus, the endometrium, is a distinctive tissue in both form and function. Throughout adult reproductive life in humans and other higher primates, the endometrium grows and is shed cyclically as a bloody discharge (i.e., the menstrual cycle) that typically recurs at about 28-day intervals. The temporal nature of this sequence (proliferation, differentiation, and sloughing of the endometrium) is the classic manifestation of an end organ response to the changing steroidal milieu imposed by the ovarian cycle. Until recently little attention was given to the endometrium as a source of hormone secretion. Accordingly, traditional emphasis on clinical disorders of the ovary can now usefully be widened to include endometrial secretion of hormones that may act both locally and distantly. Increasing evidence suggests that endometrial tissue may play a central role in the complement of endocrine signals governing female fertility.[12]

Cyclic ovarian function normally begins in adolescent girls soon after menarche. Before the attainment of gonadotropin secretory capabilities sufficient to support follicular maturation leading to ovulation, a limited degree of intermittent estrogen secretion results in endometrial proliferation and irregular vaginal bleeding; that is, variable degrees and intervals of hypoestrogenism are interspersed with transient elevations of blood estrogen levels. The initial ovulatory cycles in these young women are often characterized by abbreviated intermenstrual intervals and serum progesterone levels below those of the normal adult in the luteal phase. Clinically, these changes can be seen in a young teenager with heavy and irregular menses due to recurrent anovulation. In developed parts of the world menarche normally occurs between 11.5 and 15.5 years (mean 13.5 years, SD 1.0 year). Menstruation occurs regularly; cycles occur between 21 and 35 days apart (28.0 ± 3.5 days) and persist for 3 to 7 days. Studies by Baird and associates have proved that dysfunctional uterine bleeding in this age group is often associated with a defect in the positive feedback response to estradiol.[13]

Heavy menarcheal bleeding is not rare. If there is no possibility of pregnancy, the initial therapy should be medical, with progestogen treatment, such as 5 to 10 mg per day of norethindrone for 10 days (in the absence of cycles) or from day 5 to day 25 of the cycle, usually being effective since there has been sufficient estrogen secretion from the ovaries to induce progesterone receptors in the endometrium. If this has not occurred, it may be worth coadministering a conjugated estrogen preparation (e.g., Premarin) with a progestogen to induce this effect. In young teenagers curettage should be a last resort in attempting to control endometrial hemorrhage as well as in excluding rare diseases such as sarcoma botryoides. A hemorrhagic diathesis should always be excluded in a teenager who presents with catastrophic menarcheal bleeding. Fifty to 80 percent of patients with hemorrhagic diatheses have excessive menstrual blood loss.

OVARIAN DISORDERS IN YOUNG ADULTS

Secondary Amenorrhea

The cessation of menses for longer than 6 months in a patient who has previously menstruated is termed *secondary amenorrhea*. The most common cause is pregnancy, although a pregnancy beyond 12 weeks gestation should not be missed clinically by any doctor. Early pregnancy findings are minimal, and a pregnancy test therefore is essential in all patients with secondary amenorrhea. Serum gonadotropin assays in pregnancy may reveal a markedly elevated LH level, reflecting cross-reaction of hCG in most LH radioimmunoassays, while follicle stimulating hormone (FSH) concentration is low normal. Another important physiologic cause of amenorrhea is breast-feeding. This is associated with a period of ovarian inactivity, the duration of which depends on the frequency and duration of suckling. It is associated with elevated prolactin levels, failure of positive feedback of estradiol on LH and FSH secretion, and disturbances of pulsatile LH release. With decreased breast-feeding, ovarian function gradually returns, yielding periods of initially increased estradiol production without menses, menses without ovulation or with inadequate luteal function, and, finally, normal ovulatory cycles. Maternal undernutrition prolongs the period of lactational amenorrhea. Finally, the natural menopause generally occurs after age 40. The cessation of menses in the menopause can take the form of oligomenorrhea, menorrhagia, or abrupt cessation. Symptoms of estrogen deficiency (vaginal atrophy, hot flushes) are common, and gonadotropin levels are in the postmenopausal range. A family history in patients with early menopause is common. The most important clinical disorders, after the physiologic causes of secondary amenorrhea, are outlined in Table 17B-2.

Premature Ovarian Failure

Premature ovarian failure (POF) can be defined as the syndrome of amenorrhea, hypoestrogenism,

TABLE 17B-2 Clinical Classification of Secondary Amenorrhea

Physiologic
- Pregnancy
- Lactation
- Menopause

Premature ovarian failure
- Congenital
- Acquired
  - Autoimmune
  - Idiopathic
  - Chemotherapy, irradiation
  - Surgery, trauma
  - Infection

Hyperprolactinemia and/or galactorrhea
- Drug-associated
- Prolactinoma
  - Microadenoma
  - Macroadenoma
- Systemic illness (e.g., hypothyroidism)

Nutrition/exercise-associated
- Weight loss
  - Simple
  - Anorexia nervosa
  - Systemic illness
- Intensive exercise

Polycystic ovary syndrome

Rare conditions
- Uterine synechiae: postcurettage endometritis
- Pituitary deficiency
  - Tumors, especially after surgery or irradiation
  - Sheehan's syndrome
- Ovarian/adrenal neoplasia, empty sella syndrome

and elevated serum gonadotropin concentrations occurring before age 40 years. For practical purposes, 40 may reasonably be taken as the age after which cessation of menses is most likely to be due to spontaneous cessation of ovarian function. Cessation of ovarian function may occur in the teenage years as a rare cause of primary amenorrhea; most commonly it presents with secondary amenorrhea and accounts for about 5 percent of new cases.[14,15]

The clinical and hormonal features are similar to those of the normal menopause and commonly develop over a period of several years. Approximately half the subjects present with clinical features of hypoestrogenism (mainly vaginal dryness and hot flushes), while secondary sexual characteristics are usually normal. If the condition develops around the time of menarche, the secondary sexual characteristics may be underdeveloped. The combination of hot flushes and amenorrhea always warrants exclusion of POF. Serum gonadotropin concentrations are elevated and hyperresponsive to GnRH as after the normal menopause. As is also seen in the perimenopausal period, serum FSH levels may fluctuate in and out of the normal range and serum estradiol levels may rise to the midfollicular range. These fluctuations may be seen over a period of several years with a gradual trend toward established hypoestrogenic hypergonadotropic amenorrhea. The variable natural history of this transition was underlined by a study of 67 women suspected of having premature ovarian failure on the basis of an elevated FSH level.[16] Over one-quarter of these women resumed normal ovarian function in 1 to 5 years; six subjects conceived. Neither clinical features (e.g., age, mode of presentation) nor the degree of FSH concentration elevation predicted which subjects would resume ovarian function. Little is known about the natural history of POF, although spontaneous resumption of menses and fertility may occur in some women.

Etiologies of Premature Ovarian Failure

Genetic Chromosomal abnormalities, particularly variants of gonadal dysgenesis, may present with POF and secondary amenorrhea. The previous pattern of menses and physical findings may be normal and require that karyotyping be performed on nulliparous women under investigation for POF. Future management may be influenced by an abnormal karyotype, particularly one including a Y chromosome. The majority of subjects, however, have the normal 46,XX karyotype. A family history of POF is found in 10 percent of subjects. The pattern of inheritance is not clear, but reports of vertical transmission of the trait are consistent with autosomal dominant or sex-linked inheritance.[17]

Physical Agents Pelvic surgery and viral (especially mumps) oophoritis are rare causes of POF. Gonadal irradiation and/or chemotherapy (especially with cyclophosphamide or busulfan) for malignant conditions are also known to cause transient (especially with exposure before age 30) or permanent ovarian failure.[18] Finally, cigarette smoking, perhaps via an antiovarian action of polycyclic aromatic hydrocarbons, is associated with menopause 1 to 2 years earlier than in nonsmokers.

Autoimmune Premature Ovarian Failure Evidence for an autoimmune basis for some cases of POF is based on two observations. First, the association of POF with other autoimmune diseases, especially Hashimoto's thyroiditis and Addison's disease, has been reported. In a study of 33 women with POF, 39 percent had an associated autoimmune condition and 18 percent had a family history of such a condition.[19] Recently, another study of 24 patients demonstrated non-organ-specific autoantibodies (e.g., antinuclear) and various organ-specific autoantibodies (adrenal, gastric, pancreatic, ovarian) in 92 percent of subjects, although very few had associated disease states.[20] Second, the presence of antiovarian antibodies, including anti–zona pellucida antibodies, in the serum of some of these patients has been reported. The methodology for assessing the presence of antibodies is not universally accepted, and a direct pathogenic role for these antibodies has not been established. Overall, an autoimmune link with POF may be present in 20 to 50 percent of these patients. Consideration of possible autoimmune thyroid or adrenal disease should be given in initial assessment and intermittently during a review of patients with POF.

Occult Ovarian Failure

Occult ovarian failure is a term for a new syndrome of the clinical triad of infertility, regular menses, and hypergonadotropic hypogonadism.[21] Unlike POF, occult ovarian failure is not associated with impaired ovarian steroid synthesis. However, serum FSH and LH concentrations are elevated throughout the spontaneous menstrual cycle in these patients. In addition, autoantibodies to the ovary or the adrenal or thyroid glands are present in 50 percent of these individuals and antiovarian antibodies are detectable in 40 percent. In addition to ovarian estradiol and progesterone secretion equivalent to that seen in the spontaneous ovarian cycle, serum inhibin concentrations are also within the normal range in these patients. It is believed that occult ovarian failure represents a state of compensated granulosa cell failure where ovarian steroid and glycoprotein secretion is maintained by a compensatory increase in pituitary FSH secretion. Women with occult ovarian failure have an impaired response to ovarian hyperstimulation and may be at increased risk of developing polyglandular autoimmunity. A syndrome of "incipient ovarian failure" has also been described,[22] in which inhibin levels are below the normal range and FSH is more greatly elevated than in occult ovarian failure.

Management of Premature Ovarian Failure

The diagnosis of POF is confirmed by the finding of sustained gonadotropin elevation associated with depressed estrogen secretion. Weekly serum gonadotropin determinations and tests of urinary estrogen and progesterone excretion over a 6-week period will establish a true baseline estimate of any ovarian follicular activity. Karyotyping is performed in nulliparous patients.

Therapy for POF involves the replacement of cyclic estrogen and progesterone for the maintenance of normal secondary sex characteristics and libido and avoidance of the long-term sequelae of hypoestrogenism. Although achievement of fertility is unlikely, many spontaneous and therapy-associated pregnancies have been reported. Ovarian biopsy has been emphasized by some authors as necessary to differentiate oocyte depletion from the gonadotropin-resistant ovary syndrome, which allegedly is amenable to treatment. However, ovarian biopsy may not provide a representative tissue sample, and patients said to lack primordial follicles may subsequently ovulate. High-dose exogenous gonadotropin therapy has occasionally been associated with pregnancy, but the results of this expensive therapy have generally been disappointing.[14,15] The majority of POF subjects who subsequently conceive have been exposed to estrogen. In theory, estrogen may act to induce FSH receptors in the remaining follicles, prevent down regulation of ovarian gonadotropin receptors by suppressing circulating gonadotropin levels, or increase the biological activity of the gonadotropins.

None of these therapies for POF has been subjected to a proper prospective trial with due regard to the variable natural history of POF and the spontaneous pregnancy rate.[16,23,24] In view of these facts, POF patients requesting fertility are not routinely subjected to ovarian biopsy. Review of the underlying ovarian-pituitary axis during sex steroid replacement is undertaken every 3 to 6 months. The return of a normal serum FSH level may occur spontaneously even years after diagnosis, with the return of menses and fertility. Ovulation induction (see below) may be undertaken during the period of normal circulating FSH levels. Further studies of the natural history, autoimmunity, and ovarian histology of POF and prospective study of a range of therapies are needed to allow better categorization of POF and particularly to identify subgroups amenable to therapy.

At Monash University some patients with premature ovarian failure have been managed by applying IVF techniques and oocyte donation. Initially, such patients received a schedule of 6 weeks of steroid replacement[25] in an attempt to mimic the spontaneous ovarian cycle and create an artificial menstrual cycle. A replacement schedule of oral estradiol valerate up to 6 mg per day and up to 100 mg per day of vaginal progesterone suppositories was initially used to produce plasma levels of estradiol and progesterone within the normal range of the spontaneous ovulatory cycle. On day 21 of this replacement regimen, the endometrium from patients was consistent with the expected appearance according to the criteria of Noyes and associates.[26]

With the demonstration that steroid replacement schedules can be flexible in these subjects while still allowing development of a receptive endometrium, oral estradiol valerate is now administered at 2 mg/day in an unchanging schedule for up to 3 weeks before a donor oocyte becomes available for possible fertilization and then embryo transfer. After embryo transfer, more recent studies have shown that vaginal progesterone pessaries at 100 mg every 12 h produce serum progesterone concentrations closer to the median for the spontaneous ovarian cycle.

In these treatments, the oocyte donor has been either anonymous or known to the recipient. The general phenotypic characteristics of the recipient and donor have been matched in a fashion similar to the matching of phenotypic characteristics which occurs in programs of artificial insemination using donor semen. In some countries legislation has established registries of such oocyte donors so that the children born from these procedures may acquire nonidentifying information about the donors upon attaining adulthood.[6]

Hyperprolactinemia and Galactorrhea

Hyperprolactinemia is a common cause of female infertility, accounting for about 20 percent of cases, depending on the referral center. When sustained, hyperprolactinemia is usually associated with oligo- or amenorrhea and infertility. Impairment of reproductive capacity probably occurs at the hypothalamic level with disturbance of the dopaminergic control of pulsatile GnRH release. Defects in the positive feedback of sex steroids on the hypothalamus and a direct antiovarian action of prolactin have also been postulated. Galactorrhea is an important and frequent accompaniment of hyperprolactinemia. It is usually defined as any persistent milklike discharge from the nipple or overt lactation occurring in a nulliparous woman or a mother whose offspring has been weaned more than 6 months previously. It may be spontaneous or apparent only on manual expression. The majority of women with galactorrhea and secondary amenorrhea have hyperprolactinemia. Galactorrhea may, however, occur with normal prolactin concentrations and without menstrual disturbance. Such idiopathic galactorrhea was reported as the largest single category (32 percent) in 235 consecutive cases of galactorrhea.[27] The presence of galactorrhea always requires careful exclusion of the causes of hyperprolactinemia, as detailed below. Serial sampling is routinely performed at 20-min intervals for 2 h when a single elevated prolactin value is detected, as the prolactin may be elevated by the stress of venipuncture or a preceding breast examination.

Etiologies of Hyperprolactinemia

Drug-Related Phenothiazines and other psychotropic agents that act to antagonize hypothalamic dopaminergic pathways are associated with mild to moderate elevations of prolactin concentrations (up to four times normal).[28] Galactorrhea has been reported in one-quarter of female psychiatric patients on high doses of such medications. Amenorrhea in association is less common, occurring in 22 percent of patients with drug-induced galactorrhea. Many other medications are associated with hyperprolactinemia, including metoclopramide, H_2 histamine antagonists, calcium channel blockers, and α-methyldopa.[29] These symptoms generally resolve with the cessation of medication.

Estrogens stimulate prolactin synthesis and mitotic activity in pituitary lactotrophs. Estrogen therapy, particularly the oral contraceptives, may lead to a mild elevation (approximately a doubling) of serum prolactin concentration. Estrogen has been implicated in the development of prolactinoma in cases of postpill amenorrhea syndromes; however, most recent case-control studies have not supported this contention.[30]

Hypothalamic Disorders Pituitary prolactin secretion is under tonic inhibitory control by the hypothalamus via the postulated prolactin inhibitory factor(s) (PIF). Disruption of this system by a hypothalamic tumor, infiltrative disease (e.g., sarcoidosis), or surgical or traumatic stalk section can lead to a moderate elevation of prolactin concentration to four to six times normal. Galactorrhea and amenorrhea may result from the effect of elevated prolactin levels combined with interference with GnRH production in some cases.

Systemic Disease Primary hypothyroidism is associated with elevated hypothalamic TRH secretion, which enhances pituitary thyroid stimulating hormone (TSH) and prolactin secretion. It is therefore an uncommon but important cause of the amenorrheic galactorrhea syndrome and is easily excluded by clinical assessment and thyroid function tests. Renal failure and hepatic cirrhosis are additional causes of hyperprolactinemia that usually do not present a diagnostic problem.

Local Factors Repetitive nipple stimulation can be associated with hyperprolactinemia and galactorrhea; irritative chest wall diseases (thoracic scarring or herpes zoster) are rare causes.

Polycystic Ovary Syndrome Inappropriately enhanced estrogen feedback leading to increased pituitary lactotroph secretion probably explains the modest (up to fivefold) elevation of prolactin concentration commonly seen in polycystic ovary syndrome (PCOS). Disturbance in the normal dopaminergic control of GnRH release has also been described; this may further explain diminished PIF activity. Clinical features of hirsutism, obesity, and absence of galactorrhea assist in the differentiation from prolactinoma, although occasionally further biochemical and radiologic investigations are needed. The picture is somewhat confused by a purportedly increased risk of prolactinoma in PCOS.

Prolactinoma Pituitary prolactinoma accounts for approximately 50 percent of cases of hyperprolactinemia. Its diagnosis depends on the finding of the following:

1. Sustained hyperprolactinemia, often of marked degree.

2. Normal or suppressed serum gonadotropin levels and estrogen production, as are commonly seen in association with amenorrhea.
3. Radiologic abnormalities of the pituitary. High-resolution CT scanning[31] and MRI scanning (where available) are the essential examinations. The relative merit of the two scanning methods is unclear, but CT may be better at detecting small lesions within a normal or minimally enlarged gland. MRI is superior in visualizing structures adjacent to the pituitary, which is often the most significant issue.[32,33] Conventionally, tumors are classified as microadenomas (less than 1 cm in diameter) or macroadenomas. Macroadenomas are less common in women; these larger tumors may extend beyond the pituitary fossa superiorly (suprasellar), laterally (parasellar), or anteroinferiorly into the sphenoid sinus.

Clinically, oligo- or amenorrhea may develop in association with prolactinoma at any reproductive age. With the widespread use of oral contraceptives, the problem is frequently recognized when these agents are ceased. As was previously mentioned, an etiologic role for this estrogen therapy in the genesis of prolactinoma has been suggested but not proved. Galactorrhea occurs in approximately 50 percent of cases. Occasionally mild obesity and hirsutism are seen, again with the differential diagnostic problem of PCOS. Estrogen deficiency resulting in frictional dyspareunia and loss of libido may occur. All these symptoms generally resolve upon restoration of normal prolactin levels. Symptoms of tumor enlargement (headache, visual field defects) are uncommon in females but can occur with macroadenomas and are an especially important consideration during pregnancy (see below).

Idiopathic Hyperprolactinemia Idiopathic hyperprolactinemia is differentiated from prolactinoma by the failure to demonstrate a tumor on CT or MRI scanning. This distinction may be somewhat artificial in that the tumor may simply be too small to resolve even on the most sophisticated equipment. Therapeutically, the two conditions can be considered together. Various dynamic tests, such as the prolactin response to TRH or levodopa, have been suggested to differentiate tumorous from idiopathic hyperprolactinemia. None has been conclusively shown to be superior to the imaging techniques.

Management of Hyperprolactinemia

Therapeutic intervention may be indicated for the following reasons:

1. Tumor-related problems, particularly compressive features such as headache, visual field defects, and cranial nerve palsies.
2. Infertility.
3. Disabling galactorrhea.
4. Short-term symptoms and long-term side effects of chronic hypoestrogenemia, which may be avoided by restoration of normal menses and estrogen status. Bone density is reduced in chronic hyperprolactinemic amenorrhea and is improved by correction of hyperprolactinemia.[34,35]

Conservative therapy may be considered in selected cases.

Bromocriptine This dopamine agonist has been established as the drug of choice in the management of hyperprolactinemia, including in some patients with PCOS (see below). Control of hyperprolactinemia using bromocriptine is followed by restoration of ovulatory menses and fertility and abolition of galactorrhea in 78 to 85 percent of patients.[36] A dramatic reduction in tumor volume is seen in up to three-quarters of subjects with a demonstrable prolactinoma.[31] Bromocriptine therapy is initiated with 1.25 mg at night with food, and the dose is gradually increased over 2 weeks until control of symptoms and hyperprolactinemia is achieved, usually at 5.0 to 7.5 mg per day.[37] Side effects of nausea, vomiting, constipation, and postural hypotension are minimized with this gradual introduction. If side effects occur, a return to a lower dose will usually be tolerated, although a few patients are unable to tolerate any dosage. A long-acting injectable bromocriptine preparation has been reported which is both efficacious and well tolerated.[38] Other dopamine agonists (e.g., lisuride, pergolide) are also effective, but no advantage over bromocriptine has been shown. Recently a new long-acting dopamine agonist, CV205-502, has been reported to be effective in a once-daily dose and may be beneficial in patients who do not respond to bromocriptine.[39]

Bromocriptine can maintain control of hyperprolactinemia, often in low doses over long periods. The natural history of prolactinoma is poorly defined, but there is no evidence that long-term bromocriptine use adversely affects this. In a study of 15 subjects with micro- and macroadenomas, cessation of bromocriptine administration after 1.5 to 7 years of therapy was followed by a recurrence of symptoms and hyperprolactinemia, but tumor or gland size did not increase in 13, decreased in 1, and increased minimally in the other.[40]

When fertility is desired in hyperprolactinemic women, it can be achieved in 75 to 85 percent of patients using bromocriptine.[36] Therapy is ceased upon confirmation of pregnancy. Enlargement of a prolactinoma during pregnancy may occur; this probably relates to the trophic effect of high estrogen levels. A review of 16 studies indicated that tumor enlargement during pregnancy is uncommon in microadenomas or in a macroadenoma previously treated with x-ray or surgical therapy.[41] However, untreated macroadenoma is associated with an approximately 5 to 10 percent risk of tumor enlargement. The authors seek symptoms of enlargement and perform visual field estimations every 2 months during pregnancy in all patients with a macroadenoma. CT scanning and reinstitution of bromocriptine are performed if deteriorating vision occurs; control is usually achieved with bromocriptine. Adverse effects on the fetus have not been found when bromocriptine is ceased in the first few weeks of pregnancy or in more limited studies in which it was continued throughout pregnancy.[42]

There appears to be no adverse long-term effect of pregnancy or breast-feeding on the natural history of a prolactinoma. Serum prolactin concentration has been reported to fall by over 50 percent in one-third of patients 1 to 9 years post partum.[43]

Surgery Surgical management of prolactinoma has a limited role. Success of transsphenoidal surgery, as judged by short-term normalization of prolactin concentration and resolution of symptoms, has been claimed in 60 to 90 percent of microadenoma patients, while the cure rate is much lower with larger tumors. Recent studies have indicated a late relapse rate of up to 20 percent at 5 years in previously "cured" subjects.[44,45] In view of the efficacy of bromocriptine, the role of pituitary surgery is now seen as limited to subjects who are intolerant of or resistant to bromocriptine and those with tumors causing compressive symptoms, where bromocriptine has had an inadequate effect.

Nutritional Amenorrhea

Adequate nutrition is essential to the initiation and maintenance of reproductive capacity. Frisch and Revelle showed that the mean weight of normal girls at the time of menarche is 48 kg, independent of their age at sexual maturation.[46] Subsequently, it was postulated that a critical percentage of body weight (17 percent) must be present as fat for menarche to occur and that during puberty this percentage increases, stabilizing at approximately 28 percent in adulthood.[47] The maintenance of normal ovulatory cycles requires about 22 percent body weight as fat. In practical terms weight loss below 10 to 15 percent of ideal body weight is sufficient to interfere with reproductive capacity. Improved nutrition over the past century may therefore be related to the trend toward an earlier menarche. Undernutrition of any cause can be associated with diminished reproductive capacity, the severity of which is proportional to the degree of weight loss.

The mechanism by which body fat is related to reproductive state is obscure but probably is mediated through the hypothalamus and thus through pituitary gonadotropin release. There is a reversion toward a prepubertal pattern of diminished GnRH responsiveness and a decrease in levels of gonadotropins, particularly LH, which is proportional to the degree of fat loss (Fig. 17B-4).[48] Mediation of these effects by opiate peptide inhibition of GnRH secretion has been suggested; the opiate antagonist naloxone has been successful in restoring LH in weight loss–related amenorrhea.[49] Estrogen production by the ovary and from peripheral conversion of androgen in fat tissue is reduced to prepubertal levels in these women. Overall, these can be considered appropriate adaptive responses to starvation. Other hormonal changes have been described in anorexia nervosa, including diminished serum triiodothyronine (T_3) and prolactin concentrations and increased secretion of hydrocortisone and growth hormone.[50]

Etiologies of Nutritional Amenorrhea

The common etiologies of nutritional amenorrhea are summarized below. The endocrine changes outlined above are essentially common to all these etiologies.

Simple Weight Loss The most common presentation of secondary amenorrhea is that of a girl who complains of absence of menses without obvious cause, occurring either spontaneously or after discontinuation of the oral contraceptive pill. Careful questioning reveals a history of weight loss, often

FIGURE 17B-4 As the proportion of body fat decreases, a diminished gonadotropin responsiveness to GnRH occurs. *(Reproduced from Berg et al.,[48] with permission.)*

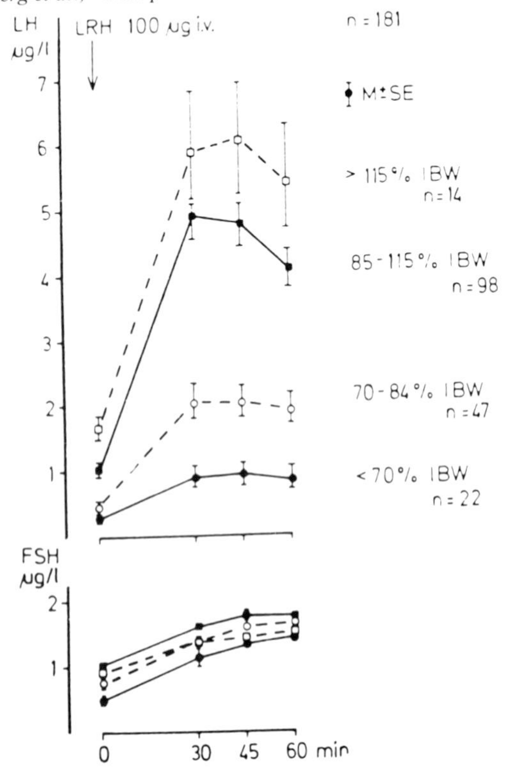

relatively rapid, of about 3 to 7 kg (7 to 15 lb), usually because of a conviction that she is somewhat overweight. There may be an accompanying history of fairly intensive exercise. Such weight loss may occur while the contraceptive pill is being taken, in which case the postpill amenorrhea may be falsely ascribed to an effect of the pill rather than the incidental weight loss. There are usually accompanying drops in the levels of LH and estradiol. Regain of weight commonly leads to restoration of the hormone levels to normal and reinitiation of cyclic menses.

Anorexia Nervosa This is a severe psychiatric condition featuring a distortion of body image and perceptions of feelings of hunger and satiety. Such patients are often adolescent girls with extremely manipulative personalities, making treatment difficult. Avoidance of carbohydrate-rich foods in particular is typical; binging and self-induced vomiting (bulimia) may occur. Amenorrhea occurs with reduction of body weight and fat; weight may be as low as 25 kg in severe cases. The causes of the psychological changes are unknown, but risk factors that have been suggested include a high-achieving personality, upper socioeconomic class, and careers requiring avoidance of obesity (e.g., dancing). The condition is more subtle in the early stages and should always be considered in underweight amenorrheic subjects. Treatment occasionally involves hospitalization for severe cachexia but primarily involves intensive psychotherapy. Rates of successful treatment vary but are improved by early diagnosis. Mortality rates of 0 to 19 percent have been reported.[51]

Exercise-Related Amenorrhea Intensive exercise programs require increased caloric intake for the maintenance of body weight. Weight loss, particularly a reduction in the percentage of body weight as fat, may occur if exercise programs are too severe and/or dietary intake is inadequate. In adolescent ballet dancers a delay in the age of menarche compared to normal students matched for career stress has been reported.[52] An increased incidence of secondary amenorrhea in athletes has also been reported.[53] Among 23 runners, the incidence of amenorrhea was highest in those who began running before age 30, those running more than 40 miles per week, and nulliparous compared with multiparous subjects.[54]

Management of Nutritional Amenorrhea

Resumption of menstruation and fertility usually accompanies the regain of weight. Improved nutritional status requires treatment of any underlying psychiatric problem and modification of inappropriate diets or exercise programs. Attempts at ovulation induction in the presence of severe weight loss are usually unsuccessful[55] and inadvisable with respect to maternal and fetal health. If weight gain is not practicable, consideration should be given to estrogen replacement therapy to avoid the long-term sequelae of hypoestrogenism, though such patients may be intolerant even of low-dose estrogen therapy. Exercise may not, as previously suspected, protect against the loss of bone density in amenorrheic runners.[56]

Polycystic Ovary Syndrome

The classic description of PCOS is of a syndrome that includes oligo- or amenorrhea, infertility, hirsutism, obesity, and enlarged polycystic ovaries. It is now recognized that PCOS is a heterogeneous group of disorders whose manifestations vary from the classic description to the isolated presence of one or more of the components. Assessment of its prevalence is difficult because of the lack of universally accepted diagnostic criteria. In the past, diagnosis was based on the typical clinical features associated with an elevated plasma LH/FSH ratio and elevated plasma androgen levels. Histologic confirmation of polycystic ovaries has not been widely available. With the advent of high-resolution ovarian ultrasound, ovarian anatomy can be assessed noninvasively; this tool promises to reorganize present classifications. Polycystic ovaries defined ultrasonically have been described in nonhirsute, regularly ovulating women.[57] There is a strong familial component to PCOS, with polycystic ovaries on ultrasound being common in asymptomatic first-degree relatives of patients presenting with PCOS.[58] Therefore, this common condition has heterogeneous clinical, anatomic, and biochemical features. Surprisingly little is known about the primary nature of the problem.

Clinical Features

A variety of clinical features are associated with PCOS (Table 17B-3). While patients may present with one or more features, additional ones are often apparent on assessment.[59]

Menstrual Disturbance

Menarche usually occurs normally in PCOS, but there is menstrual irregularity with oligo- or amenorrhea persisting into adulthood. PCOS is probably the most common cause of persistent menstrual disturbance. One study reported a 20 percent incidence of polycystic ovaries on ultrasound in a large group of unselected "normal" women.[60] Three-quarters of these PCOS women had a history of menstrual irregularity. Menstrual bleeding may be heavy and painful in view of the continuous unopposed estrogen effect (see below). Cycles are often anovulatory or associated with a deficient luteal phase. Patients may seek help for irregular cycles per se, dysfunctional uterine bleeding, or infertility. The prevalence of PCOS as a cause of infertility varies depending on

TABLE 17B-3 Clinical Features of 300 Women with Polycystic Ovary Syndrome Diagnosed by Ultrasound

	Presenting Features, %	Total, %*
Hirsutism	34	64
Acne	9	27
Obesity, BMI > 25 kg/m^2	10	35
Infertility	41	42
Amenorrhea	23	28
Oligomenorrhea/irregular cycle	38	52
Dysfunctional bleeding	6	14

* The total in the right-hand column refers to the total number of subjects who on history and/or examination were found to have the clinical abnormalities indicated. Ten women (3%) also had androgen-dependent alopecia, and two (1%) had acanthosis nigricans.

Source: Adapted from Franks.[59]

the referral center but has been reported in up to 50 percent of cases.[57]

Hirsutism

A degree of hirsutism varying from mild to severe (i.e., masculine pattern) is common in PCOS. It may be the primary reason for presentation or may have frustrated cosmetic attempts at management. Frequently acne is a troublesome accompaniment.

Obesity

Weight gain at the time of puberty causing mild to moderate obesity is common in PCOS, although many patients are of normal weight.

Pathophysiology

The complex question of the primary defect in PCOS remains unresolved, but the large body of knowledge available can be considered under the following headings. Figure 17B-5 depicts one schema for the pathogenesis of the PCOS, which may be outlined as follows:

1. Defects in ovarian function
   a. Folliculogenesis
   b. Sex steroid secretion
2. Defects in hypothalamic-pituitary function
3. Abnormal androgen metabolism

These defects exist concurrently and interact to produce a chronic anovulatory state with or without evidence of hyperandrogenemia. Whatever the primary defect, once these events are established, they are usually self-maintaining.

Defects in Ovarian Function

Folliculogenesis Polycystic ovaries contain numerous small cysts (usually 2 to 4 mm in diameter) and characteristically increased stromal tissue; the increased stromal tissue is primarily responsible for increased ovarian volume. Granulosa cells from these cysts have a normal appearance and respond to FSH stimulation in vitro.[61] However, there is a failure of one follicle to become dominant and to develop to a preovulatory state with suppression of other follicles. The nature of this defect in intraovarian regulation is unknown. Abnormal regulation of the steroidogenic enzyme cytochrome P450c17α within ovarian thecal cells may underlie their LH-induced hypersecretion of androgens.[62] Increased intraovarian androgen levels resulting from enhanced thecal cell secretion of androgen may impair FSH action and enhance follicular atresia.

Sex Steroid Secretion Estrogen secretion in the absence of a normal follicular development is acyclic with total estradiol levels in the early to midfollicular range. Increased ovarian and adrenal androgen secretion (see below) also bear directly on estrogen levels by acting as a substrate for extraovarian estrogen production (especially of estrone), primarily in fat tissue. Androgens also act to lower sex hormone–binding globulin (SHBG) levels, thereby increasing the free androgen and estrogen levels. Abnormal sex steroid profiles are therefore present to feed back on the hypothalamic-pituitary system.

Defects in Hypothalamic-Pituitary Function

Plasma LH levels are raised approximately two-fold, while plasma FSH levels are normal or depressed, leading to the characteristic though not invariable elevation in the LH/FSH ratio.[63] Chronic acyclic elevation of free estrogen levels in PCOS may explain this abnormal profile of gonadotropins. Unopposed estrogen feedback may enhance pituitary LH, but not FSH, release in response to GnRH exposure. Progesterone suppresses LH secretion, and its deficiency in anovulatory PCOS patients may also be important. Coordinated cyclic release of gonadotropins does not occur, and failure of normal folliculogenesis results. Higher LH levels are associated with higher androgen levels, a greater incidence of anovulation, and resistance to ovulation induction therapy. A primary hypothalamic problem independent of abnormal sex steroid feedback has been suggested by the finding of increased LH secretory pulse frequency in adolescent girls and adult PCOS subjects.[64,65] This may suggest alterations in hypothalamic GnRH pulsatility. However, other studies have shown normal LH pulse frequency in PCOS.[66]

Moderate elevation of serum prolactin concentration (one to five times normal) was apparent in 27 percent of 394 PCOS subjects in a review of several published series.[67] Increased LH sensitivity to dopamine inhibition in PCOS compared to the sensitivity in the early follicular phase in normal women

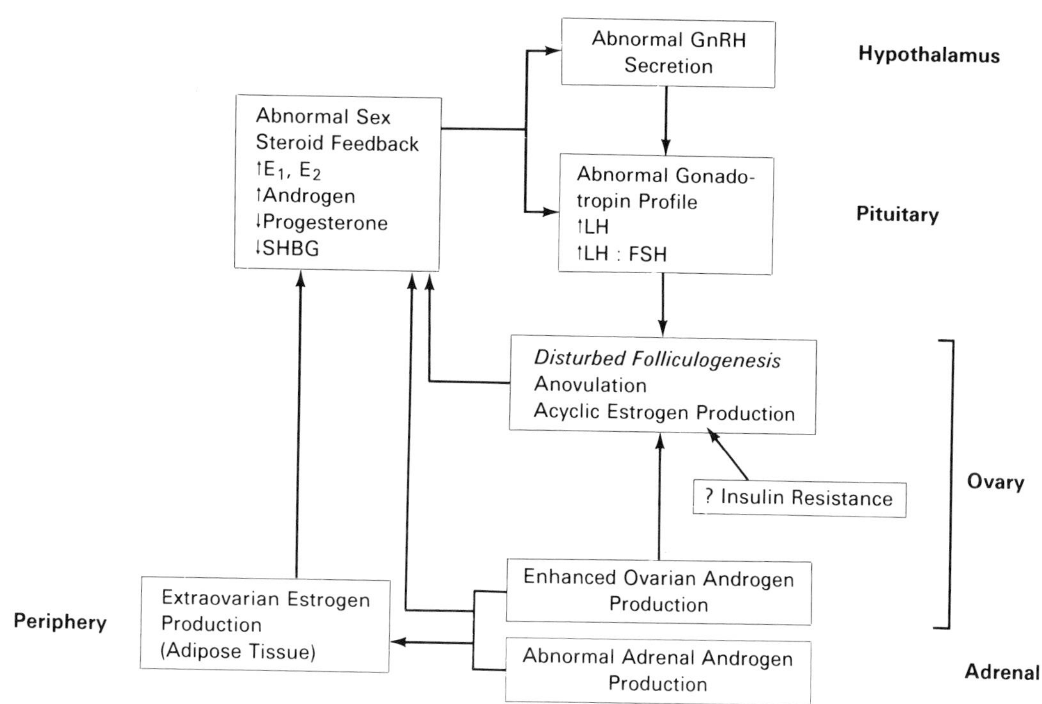

FIGURE 17B-5 Schema for the pathogenesis of the polycystic ovary syndrome.

has been reported,[68] but this has not been confirmed by others.[69] Whether unopposed estrogen action or abnormal hypothalamic dopamine metabolism is important in producing these elevations is unclear. It seems that most cases are due to a coexisting prolactinoma which occurs with increased frequency in PCOS, warranting careful exclusion of this tumor, particularly in patients with more marked elevations of prolactin concentration.[70]

Elevated serum levels of inhibin, a gonadal peptide which specifically acts to lower FSH secretion, do not appear important in the production of the abnormal gonadotropin profiles in PCOS. The level of inhibin immunoactivity in the serum of PCOS subjects was low, in the normal early follicular phase range.[71]

Abnormal Androgen Secretion

Controversy has existed in regard to whether the ovary or the adrenal is the principal source of hyperandrogenemia in PCOS. Approximately 50 percent of PCOS subjects have elevated levels of total testosterone (generally up to twice the normal level); with the suppression of SHBG seen in this condition, about 75 percent have elevated unbound levels.[72] The specific suppression of gonadotropins using GnRH analogues has been shown to suppress the elevated testosterone and androstenedione levels in PCOS, suggesting that the ovary is the primary source of these androgens. Dehydroepiandrosterone sulfate (DHEA-S) is predominantly an adrenal androgen, and its concentration is elevated in about 50 percent of PCOS subjects.[73]

It is apparent, therefore, that in most subjects both the adrenal and the ovary hypersecrete androgens, while in the remainder either or neither does so. The correlation is poor between total androgen levels and the severity of hirsutism, although free T levels and the 5α reduced urinary T metabolites tend to be higher in more hirsute subjects. It should be emphasized that hyperandrogenemia may be due to other causes, e.g., endocrine tumors or cryptic congenital adrenal hyperplasia, in which the elevation of the 17-hydroxyprogesterone level, especially after ACTH infusion, is characteristic. These diagnoses should therefore be considered.

The interaction of these components is shown in Fig. 17B-5. This self-perpetuating cycle of events can be followed, commencing at the pituitary. In response to elevated and acyclic estrogen exposure and possibly abnormal inhibin levels, pituitary LH release is enhanced, while the FSH/LH ratio is depressed and cyclic release of gonadotropins is abnormal. Orderly folliculogenesis fails to occur because of a relative lack of FSH and therefore of aromatase activity, and ovulation does not occur. Enhanced ovarian and/or adrenal androgen secretion provides the substrate for peripheral estrogen production, lowers the SHBG level, and produces hirsutism in some patients. It must be emphasized that not all components of this schema need always be present.

Insulin Resistance

Insulin resistance is common in PCOS[74] and has been attributed to defects in both receptor and postreceptor mechanisms. Obesity only partially explains the resistance. The severity of insulin resistance correlates with the degree of hyperandrogenemia.[74] Insulin sensitivity does not consistently improve with a reduction in androgen levels by ovariectomy[75] or GnRH agonist treatment, suggesting that it is one of the primary defects in PCOS. As insulin influences granulosa cell maturation, abnormal insulin action may be involved in the disturbance of folliculogenesis.

Management of Polycystic Ovary Syndrome

Indications for therapeutic intervention in PCOS can be summarized as follows:

Control of menstrual cyclicity and/or bleeding
Management of infertility
Management of hirsutism

Menstrual Cyclicity

The use of a combined oral contraceptive can control irregular cycles in PCOS. Heavy bleeding may occur in PCOS in view of the anovulatory state, with continuous unopposed estrogen exposure leading to thickening of the endometrial lining. A course of progestogen (norethindrone 5 to 10 mg daily for 10 days) will usually control this bleeding. A combined oral contraceptive or a regular cyclic progestogen alone can then be used to maintain menstrual control. Induction of regular menses is advisable in patients with anovulatory PCOS in view of the reported increased incidence of endometrial hyperplasia and neoplasia.[76,77]

Infertility

Clomiphene citrate has conventionally been used for the induction of ovulation. Its mechanism of action is presumed to occur by means of the temporary relief of estrogen feedback on gonadotropins, especially FSH. Follicular development is permitted, and the estrogen level increases to stimulate an LH surge. Ovulation can be induced in the majority (80 percent) of PCOS subjects, although the pregnancy rate is often reported as lower (39 percent).[78] In addition, there appears to be a high rate of spontaneous abortion in clomiphene-induced PCOS pregnancy: 40 percent compared with 25 percent in non-PCOS clomiphene-induced pregnancy. Nonetheless, clomiphene offers the most convenient form of ovulation induction for the majority of these subjects. Doses of 50 to 150 mg daily for 5 days commencing on day 5 of the cycle are suggested. The response is monitored by charting basal body temperature and with ovarian ultrasound and luteal-phase estimations of progesterone concentration.

For PCOS subjects who fail to ovulate with clomiphene, a range of therapies has been applied,[79] including the addition of hCG or glucocorticoids to clomiphene, although a clear benefit over clomiphene alone has not been shown. Bromocriptine has also been shown to induce ovulation in some PCOS women, especially when hyperprolactinemia is present.[80] Many of these patients require ovulation induction with gonadotropins, while they are generally resistant to therapy with pulsatile GnRH. Treatment using GnRH analogues to suppress endogenous gonadotropin secretion in combination with gonadotropin is a recent and increasingly common approach (see Ovulation Induction, below). Finally, electrocautery of the ovarian surface has recently been claimed to restore the ovulatory cycle and produce pregnancy rates similar to those with gonadotropin therapy.[81] The mechanism of action of electrocautery is obscure.

Virilization and Hirsutism

Clinical Assessment and Investigation

The number of advertisements offering the removal of superfluous hair suggests that hirsutism is a common disorder. It may be defined as the excessive growth of terminal hair in a male distribution, and it affects particularly the upper lip, chin, chest, sacral area, lower abdomen, and thighs. It is frequently perceived as being much more severe by the patient than by the doctor to whom she brings her complaint. In contrast, virilization is uncommon. It is manifested by male pattern baldness, clitoral hypertrophy, deepening of the voice, and increased muscularity in addition to hirsutism. The presence of virilization strongly suggests an underlying organic cause.

A variety of methods have been used to measure the degree of hirsutism and the rate of hair growth. From a practical viewpoint, the scoring system of Ferriman and Gallwey has achieved widespread popularity.[82] The degree of hair growth is graded on a scale of 0 to 4 on the upper lip, chin, chest, upper back, lower back, upper abdomen, lower abdomen, upper arm, and thigh, giving a maximal possible score of 36 with an upper limit of normal of 7. Forty percent of normal white women have a score of 0. More cumbersome objective methods of assessing the velocity of hair growth have been described.[83]

There is considerable variation among different ethnic groups in the amount of hair growth which is perceived as normal. In Australian immigrants, those coming from the Mediterranean area have much more body hair than do women of Anglo-Saxon origin or those coming from southeast Asian countries.

Hirsutism may be classified as increased hair growth occurring in otherwise apparently normal subjects, for example, at puberty or in the late teens or early twenties, during pregnancy, or at the time of menopause. It may also occur in response to the administration of certain drugs, including phenytoin, norgestrel, norethindrone, metronidazole, minoxidil, corticosteroids, anabolic steroids, androgens, and cyclosporin. Patients with hypothyroidism, acromegaly, and porphyria may develop increased hair growth, although the classic associations are with increased androgen production of either ovarian or adrenal origin. Ovarian causes include the polycystic ovary syndrome, hyperthecosis, and ovarian tumor; adrenal causes include tumors and congenital adrenal hyperplasia, particularly the late-onset adult type. Patients with Cushing's syndrome usually have some degree of hirsutism.

From a practical clinical viewpoint, by far the most common clinical varieties of hirsutism are the idiopathic form and PCOS. The terminology of the former is somewhat confused, as the majority of patients with idiopathic hirsutism actually have an increase at least in the androgen production rate, though the cause of this remains undefined. An alternative term for this disorder is *functional androgen excess*. The concentration of a peripheral metabolite of DHT, androstanediol glucuronide, has been reported to be markedly elevated in hirsute patients and correlates with the degree of hirsutism.[84]

Idiopathic hirsutism is often associated with a family history of excess hair growth in either male or female relatives and tends to come on in the late teens or early twenties. The hirsutism is usually mild to moderate in extent, and menstrual cycles usually remain regular and ovulatory. Nonetheless, many of these women probably have PCOS, as many have ultrasonographic evidence of ovarian enlargement. The PCOS classically has its onset just before or at the time of puberty and is associated with obesity, menstrual irregularity (either oligomenorrhea or amenorrhea, which may be primary or secondary), and infertility. Both idiopathic hirsutism and PCOS may be associated with acne and excessively oily skin. It has become increasingly recognized that a syndrome indistinguishable from PCOS may occur in previously normal women who gain excess weight, often associated with one or more pregnancies, and present in their late twenties or early thirties with obesity, hirsutism, and oligomenorrhea. In these patients, the obesity may be the primary disorder and restoration of menstrual periodicity and some decrease in hirsutism may accompany successful weight loss, though this is difficult to achieve. Other very rare associations of this disorder are insulin resistance and acanthosis nigricans (termed the HAIR-AN syndrome: *h*yper*a*ndrogenism, *i*nsulin *r*esistance, and *a*canthosis *n*igricans).[85]

Some authors report that between one-third and two-thirds of hirsute women have mild defects in adrenal steroidogenesis that are suggestive of late-onset congenital adrenal hyperplasia, based on measurements of basal and ACTH-stimulated levels of steroids in the androgen pathway.[86,87] The frequency with which this diagnosis is made probably varies with the ethnicity of the patients and the effort applied to studying their steroidogenesis.

The clinical assessment of patients presenting with hirsutism must include taking an appropriate history, including a family history, and paying particular attention to the rapidity of onset of the hirsutism: An abrupt onset suggests the possibility of organic lesions such as an adrenal or ovarian tumor. A careful menstrual history with attention to symptoms suggesting the presence of ovulation should be recorded. It is important to determine whether the patient is also complaining of infertility and whether she requires contraception. Physical examination should include an assessment of the severity of the hirsutism. Using the Ferriman and Gallwey hormonal score with a maximum score of 36, mild hirsutism may be regarded as a score of 8 to 12, moderate hirsutism as a score of 13 to 18, and severe hirsutism as a score of over 19.[88] Careful assessment should be made for evidence of accompanying virilization (e.g., clitoral hypertrophy) and for stigmata of rare causes of hirsutism such as Cushing's syndrome and hypothyroidism.

An area of significant concern and controversy is the question of what degree of investigation should be undertaken in patients presenting with apparently uncomplicated hirsutism. Although it is of theoretical interest to establish whether excessive androgen secretion is arising from the ovary or the adrenal, in practice this may not significantly affect the choice of management unless a specific adrenal lesion has been identified and suppressive therapy is contemplated.

Measurements which may be made include the plasma testosterone concentration, or, preferably, the free testosterone level, as total testosterone is occasionally normal despite significant hyperandrogenemia, in part as a result of lower SHBG levels. Salivary testosterone determination is an alternative approach to assessing the unbound steroid level. DHT, DHEA-S, and androstenedione concentrations may be measured, together with that of 17-hydroxyprogesterone. A marked elevation in plasma testosterone to around twice the upper limit of normal is compatible with the PCOS, but if testosterone is substantially above that level, the possibility of an ovarian tumor must be kept in mind and is best evaluated with pelvic examination and vaginal ultrasonography or CT scanning. A marked elevation in the DHEA-S concentration to more than twice the upper limit of normal suggests the possibility of an adrenal tumor, which should again be excluded by CT scanning. Androstenedione and DHEA-S together with testosterone levels are frequently moderately elevated in PCOS. An elevation in basal levels of 17-hydroxyprogesterone suggests late-onset congenital adrenal hyperplasia; in this disorder a stimulation test with ACTH may establish the diagnosis.[89] We have found late-onset congenital adrenal hyperplasia (CAH) to be most uncommon and screen for it only in severe or atypical cases or in patients with elevated basal levels of 17OH progesterone in additon to DHEA-S. As antiandrogen therapy is effective in most hirsute patients (see below), the cost-effectiveness of exhaustively investigating all subjects for more subtle abnormalities remains unproven, although this point is controversial.[90] Measurements of FSH, LH, and prolactin levels may also be diagnostically helpful, with an elevation of LH concentration and a high LH/FSH ratio being typical of PCOS. Prolactin-secreting pituitary adenomas may occasionally be associated with excess hair growth.

It is difficult to formulate satisfactory general rules for the degree of investigation which should be undertaken in an individual patient. As a general guide, in mild to moderate hirsutism with normal menses investigations are of extremely doubtful value. In mild to moderate hirsutism with menstrual irregularity, investigations may be directed toward establishing PCOS as the cause with measurements of FSH, LH, and total or, preferably, free testosterone levels. It is well recognized that the free testosterone fraction is much more frequently elevated in hirsutism than is total plasma testosterone, but this observation is of little practical value in terms of management.

In more severe hirsutism, levels of DHEA-S, testosterone, and 17-hydroxyprogesterone, with the latter's response to ACTH, should be assessed, and, where indicated, abdominal CT scanning or ultrasound should be undertaken to clarify the diagnosis.

When management with antiandrogens, particularly cyproterone acetate, is contemplated, it is also useful to measure baseline cholesterol and triglyceride levels, as cyproterone acetate may cause an increase in plasma lipid levels. In patients in whom spironolactone is to be used, basal renal function should be assessed.

Management

The overall approach to a hirsute patient should be one of empathy and understanding with emphasis on the fact that it is a lifelong disorder for which cosmetic approaches provide the cornerstone of management. The available measures include simple plucking, waxing, and shaving and the use of depilatory creams, all of which require long-term use. Permanent cure may be achieved with properly performed electrolysis, which is, however, tedious, uncomfortable, and expensive. In addition, in obese patients weight loss may have a favorable effect on hirsutism.

Medical measures include regimens of ovarian suppression (with a combination of estrogen and progestogen, e.g., the oral contraceptive) and adrenal suppression (with nocturnally administered corticosteroids such as prednisone 7.5 mg daily or dexamethasone 0.5 mg daily) if a defect in adrenal steroid synthesis has been shown. Results with such measures are slow to occur and often disappointing. More successful approaches have involved the use of antiandrogens, such as cyproterone acetate (given in reverse sequential fashion).

Cyproterone acetate has been extensively tried in Europe and Australia and has been found to be highly effective. It is administered in reverse sequential order with cyclic estrogen, e.g., cyproterone 50 to 100 mg daily on days 5 through 15 and ethinyl estradiol 30 to 50 μg daily on days 5 to 25 of each calendar month.[91] This treatment also provides effective contraception. A response is seen within 3 to 6 months. Both acne and hirsutism respond in about three-quarters of patients. The dose of cyproterone can often be gradually reduced to a maintenance dose of 2 mg daily. Spironolactone in a high dose (100 to 200 mg daily) is also useful but must be given with contraceptive cover and is probably less effective than cyproterone, although this has not been formally established.[92,93] Unfortunately, hirsutism almost always recurs when therapy is discontinued. It is mandatory that pregnancy be avoided during such therapy because of the risks of feminization of a male fetus.

Female Infertility: Diagnosis of Ovulatory Dysfunction

It has been estimated that 1 couple in 10 will experience difficulty with conception, with male and female factors being equally prevalent. Thus, it is important to see both partners together and to recognize that anxiety and depression are common in both. Eliciting these emotions is an integral part of the initial interview, and the physician must gain the patients' confidence before proceeding with any of the large number of investigations available, particularly in women with possible ovarian dysfunction. The number and outcome of previous pregnancies are also significant, as the prognosis for secondary infertility is better than that for primary infertility.

Previous medical treatments such as cytotoxic or psychopharmacologic agents or irradiation may have caused permanent or temporary damage to folliculogenesis. Surgery, including not only gynecologic procedures such as ovarian cystectomy and abdominal operations such as complicated appendectomy but also tissue handling at laparotomy, may cause adhesions to form in the pelvis and thus affect tubal function. Environmental and occupational factors, for example, frequent night shift work, may disturb ovarian function and also make intercourse in the fertile period less likely.

TABLE 17B-4 Ovulation-Inducing Agents

Category	Agents
Antiestrogens	Clomiphene
Dopamine agonists	Bromocriptine, CV 205-502
FSH, LH	hMG
Purified FSH	Metrodin
Surrogate LH	hCG
GnRH	
GnRH agonists	Buserelin, Nafarelin, Leuprolide, Goserelin

Abbreviations: hMG = human menopausal gonadotropin; hCG = human chorionic gonadotropin.

In a general physical examination use of a weight index such as the Garrow index (weight in kilograms divided by squared height in meters) is recommended. Hair distribution should be scored according to the definitions of Ferriman and Gallwey.[82] Excessive hair growth (bearing in mind the patient's ethnic background) may indicate excessive androgen secretion or action, and this may be associated with anovulation. Hypoestrogenism may be indicated by incomplete breast development and should be recorded by the appropriate Tanner stage.[94] Galactorrhea is detected by gentle sustained pressure on the areolae, but the secretion should not be brown or bloodstained, which would indicate organic breast disease, including malignancy. In ideal circumstances, galactorrhea should be confirmed by testing for lactose and by microscopic examination for fat globules.

There are a number of possible tests of ovulation: charting of mucous symptoms and/or basal body temperature, urinary LH monitoring, determination of luteal-phase plasma progesterone concentrations, ultrasonic ovarian follicle assessment, and luteal-phase endometrial biopsy. The emphasis placed on each of these tests will depend on the clinical facilities at hand. The authors use a plasma progesterone assay as a screening test of ovulation, drawing the blood sample on day 21 of an expected 28-day cycle or approximately 7 days before the next anticipated menses.

In patients in whom chronic anovulation appears to be the major cause of infertility, a large number of ovulation induction agents are now available for therapy (Table 17B-4 and Fig. 17B-6). Low plasma estradiol concentrations (< 100 p*M*) suggest that the response to antiestrogens, e.g., clomiphene citrate, will be inadequate. However, the progestogen withdrawal for estrogen priming of the endometrium does provide useful information, and withdrawal uterine bleeding should be assessed by giving 10 mg per day of a progestogen such as medroxyprogesterone acetate or 1.25 mg norethindrone orally for 5 days. If no vaginal bleeding occurs, the test is negative; any bleeding up to 1 week after the test is positive and suggests that there is sufficient circulating estrogen present for antiestrogen therapy to be beneficial.

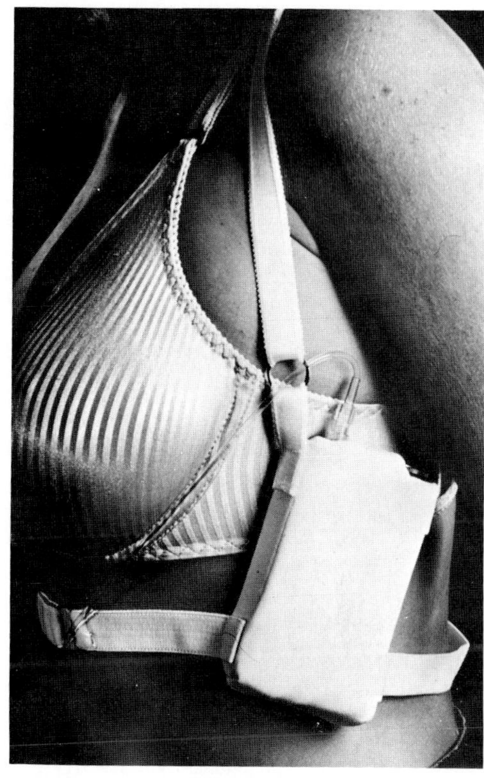

FIGURE 17B-6 Pulsatile GnRH infuser assembled to allow subcutaneous hormone administration in an ambulatory patient.

Antiestrogen Ovulation Induction

With the antiestrogen clomiphene citrate, treatment starts at 50 mg per day for 5 days and should be increased by 50-mg increments in each cycle, to a daily maximum of 250 mg or until ovulation occurs. Treatment is begun on day 1, 2, or 5 of the cycle, and ovulation is assessed by charting basal body temperature as well as measuring serum progesterone concentrations between days 21 and 24. Ovulation may occur anywhere from 5 to 10 days after the last clomiphene tablet. Theoretically, beginning therapy on days 1 or 2 leads to the recruitment of more follicles, while beginning on day 5 augments gonadotropin levels at the time of selection of the dominant follicle and enhances its particular development. The serum progesterone level should be above 25 n*M* per liter in the midluteal phase to support the occurrence of ovulation, but the date of the next menses is of obvious significance in ensuring that the progesterone estimate was made on the appropriate day.

Patients who fail to respond may benefit from the addition of continuous low-dose dexamethasone therapy (0.5 mg decreasing to 0.25 mg after 4 to 8 weeks) if androgen levels are elevated, or from an hCG bolus to induce ovulation where a leading follicle develops but fails to rupture.

Side effects from clomiphene citrate therapy are infrequent but include hot flushes, mood disturbance, bloating, breast tenderness, and very rarely visual disturbances. If eyesight is affected, therapy should cease immediately and not be repeated. Low multiple gestations are increased, and on higher doses ovarian enlargement may occur. Repeat cycles should be postponed until this has settled. Efforts are continuing to separate the two stereoisomers of clomiphene citrate for separate clinical use to optimize its efficacy.

Ovulation induction with clomiphene citrate in anovulatory women with no other additional cause for infertility should not usually continue beyond six (approximately a 60 percent prospect of pregnancy) to nine (75 percent prospect) ovulations without considering other options (see below).

Gonadotropic Ovulation Induction

Clinical use of human pituitary FSH resulting in pregnancy was first reported in 1958.[95] Human gonadotropins were initially prepared from cadaver pituitaries or derived from the urine of postmenopausal women. More recently, highly purified FSH/LH preparations from postmenopausal urine have been obtained. Pituitary gonadotropins have been withdrawn because of the reported transmission of Creutzfeldt-Jakob disease.[96]

Gonadotropins may be given in a fixed dosage regimen in which a predetermined dose of gonadotropin is administered in increasing concentrations in each cycle of treatment until a response occurs. Alternatively, the dose of gonadotropin may be tailored to the patient's response during treatment so that an effective dose is administered during each cycle. This has the advantage of yielding a smaller number of cycles per pregnancy, and in the authors' hands it has produced a pregnancy rate which is equivalent to the natural conception rate in the community, as assessed by life table analysis (Fig. 17B-7).[97]

We use a variable gonadotropin schedule, starting at 75 per day IU human menopausal gonadotropins. The dose increases every 7 days if there is no doubling of serum estradiol values. Monitoring is done by means of daily serum estradiol and ovarian vaginal ultrasonography.

With current human gonadotropin treatments, excessive stimulation of the ovaries is the major complication of therapy. This can be expressed either as the ovarian hyperstimulation syndrome (OHSS), which presents with a spectrum of clinical features varying from palpable ovarian cysts to its most severe form, which includes abdominal distension, nausea, hydrothorax, coagulopathy, and occasionally death, [98] or by multiple ovulation and multiple

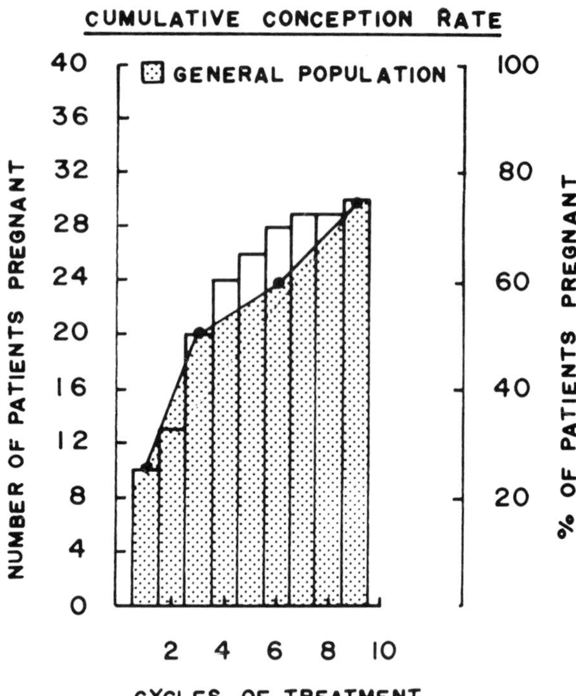

FIGURE 17B-7 Cumulative conception rate in a series of patients receiving human pituitary gonadotropin for ovulation induction. Stippled area shows the conception rate for the general population *(Reproduced from Healy et al.,[97] with permission.)*

pregnancy in up to 20 to 30 percent of patients. To decrease the incidence of these complications, cycles are monitored ultrasonically for follicular development and by serum estradiol levels. Multiple linear regression analysis has shown that the number of follicles greater than 10 mm in diameter at the time of the ovulatory hCG injection is predictive of both pregnancy and the number of fetuses but not of OHSS while the estradiol level at the same point is predictive for OHSS but not of pregnancy.[99]

Mean serum FSH and LH concentrations are markedly elevated during ovulation induction therapy with human gonadotropins.[100] Elevated FSH/LH ratios for more than 8 days provide unrelenting FSH exposure to the cohort of recruited follicles; this appears to be important in inducing the disordered multiple folliculogenesis in these patients. Two or more ovarian follicles develop in approximately 86 percent of gonadotropin-treated cycles, compared with only 23 percent of spontaneous cycles, and at least three follicles greater than 12 mm in diameter develop during 50 percent of gonadotropin-stimulated cycles (Table 17B-5).

Various permutations of human gonadotropin or GnRH therapy have been reported for the PCOS, where the treatment response is often unpredictable. Pulsatile administration of either human menopausal gonadotropin or FSH has been tried with or without GnRH agonist pituitary down regulation.[101] The re-

TABLE 17B-5 Results of Ovulation Induction by Gonadotropin Therapy*

	Percent with Follicles > 10 mm	
	2 Follicles	3 Follicles
Human gonadotropin-induced cycles (n = 28)	86	50
Spontaneous cycles (n = 13)	23	0

* Percent of cycles with two or three follicles developing to > 10 mm in diameter.

sults have varied between centers, but one of the larger trials has shown pulsatile FSH to produce a very low incidence of OHSS but also a disappointingly low pregnancy rate, while intramuscular pure FSH has a comparable pregnancy rate with human menopausal gonadotropin and an incidence of OHSS intermediate between the other two regimens.[102] GnRH agonist administration has been used in an attempt to induce pituitary down regulation and convert abnormal secretion of LH and FSH and aberrant LH/FSH ratios to more normal patterns (Fig. 17B-8) prior to gonadotropin therapy. Reports are variable, but the overall complication rate does seem decreased and the ovulation and pregnancy rates are similar to therapy without GnRH agonist suppression.[102] Larger groups of patients must be studied to be confident that these therapies offer a significant advantage over current methods of ovarian stimulation.

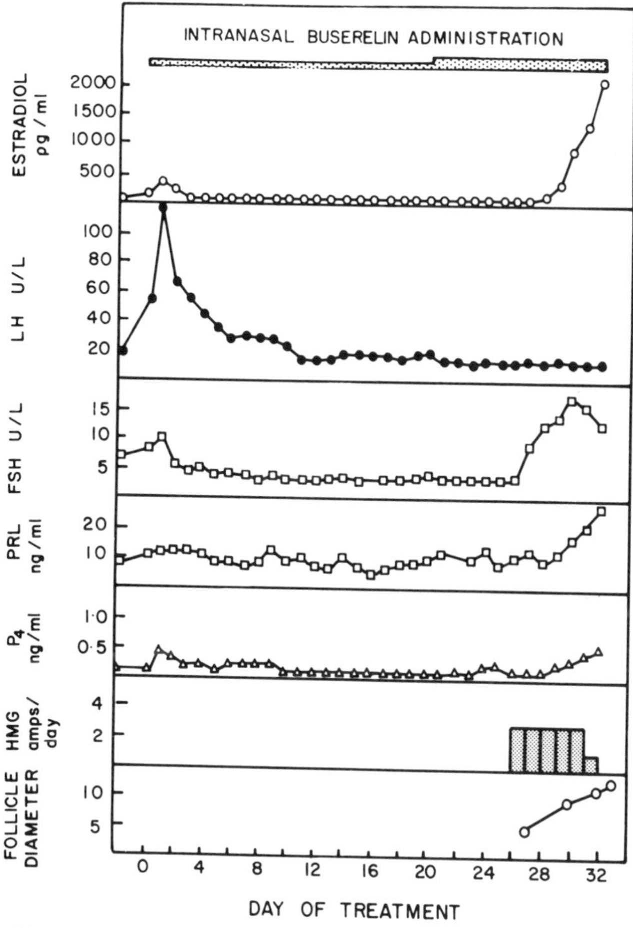

FIGURE 17B-8 Intranasal GnRH agonist (buserelin) administration to an anovulatory patient with polycystic ovary syndrome. Note the initial LH/FSH ratio, the suppression of plasma estradiol levels with buserelin therapy, the exponential increase in estradiol values when hMG treatment has begun, and the rapid increase in follicle growth.

Pulsatile GnRH Ovulation Induction

Leyendecker and colleagues were the first to report the pulsatile administration of GnRH in women with hypothalamic amenorrhea.[103] Since then it has been given by both the subcutaneous and intravenous routes (Fig. 17B-6). When endogenous gonadotropins are used, the normal pituitary-ovarian feedback mechanisms remain intact. Therefore, in comparison with gonadotropin therapy it requires less monitoring, both hormonal and ultrasonographic, and the incidences of multiple pregnancy and the ovarian hyperstimulation syndrome are reduced. Its disadvantages include the cost and inconvenience of the GnRH pump and delivery unit and, particularly with the intravenous route, the risk of local and systemic infection. In PCOS the therapy has been disappointing, though pretreatment with a GnRH agonist in a small series has improved the ovulation rates.[104]

The intravenous route provides a more physiologic profile than does the subcutaneous route and requires less drug. However, while ovulation is increased (90 percent vs. 75 percent), the conception rate per ovulatory cycle is the same (approximately 30 percent). As the subcutaneous route is more convenient and has a reduced risk of septicemia, it is arguable that the intravenous route should be reserved for patients who fail to respond to the subcutaneous therapy.

In the authors' clinic, we use 90-min subcutaneous pulses of GnRH, commencing at 5 μg per pulse and increasing by 5 μg every 7 to 14 days until a progressive rise in the urinary estrone glucuronide level is observed.[105] Twenty-three of the 30 ovulatory cycles with this therapy were induced with 10-μg pulses. There were 13 pregnancies in 14 subjects in our study.

The incidence of multiple pregnancy is lower with GnRH therapy compared with human gonadotropin treatment. In reported series, a multiple pregnancy rate of 8 percent occurred, although it is noteworthy that several cases of triplet pregnancies and one quadruplet pregnancy have been reported, as have other instances of ovarian hyperstimulation.

Menorrhagia and Dysmenorrhea

The clinical problems of menorrhagia and dysmenorrhea are among the most common which present to a gynecologist. To properly understand the basis of present clinical management of these disorders, a brief review of endometrial anatomy and physiology is necessary.

Endometrial Anatomy and Physiology

Normal endometrium consists of a simple columnar epithelium which contains estrogen-responsive and progesterone-dependent mucous glands on an underlying stroma. The endometrium is typically classified into a more superficial functional zone, which is supplied by coiled spiral arteries (Fig. 17B-9) and is shed at menstruation, and a deeper basal zone, which is supplied by straight arteries. This remains after menstruation and regenerates the endometrium. Moreover, the functional zone contains a superficial luminal zone (zone 1), an intermediate zone 2 where the glands are straight and widely separated by stroma, and a deeper layer, zone 3, where the glands are coiled and closely packed. These differences are clinically relevant, since the highest mitotic rates are observed in the upper third of human endometrium on days 8 to 10 of the cycle.

FIGURE 17B-9 Schematic representation of the interactions of the endometrium, pituitary, and ovaries during ovulatory menstrual cycles. *(Reproduced from Healy and Hodgen,[12] with permission.)*

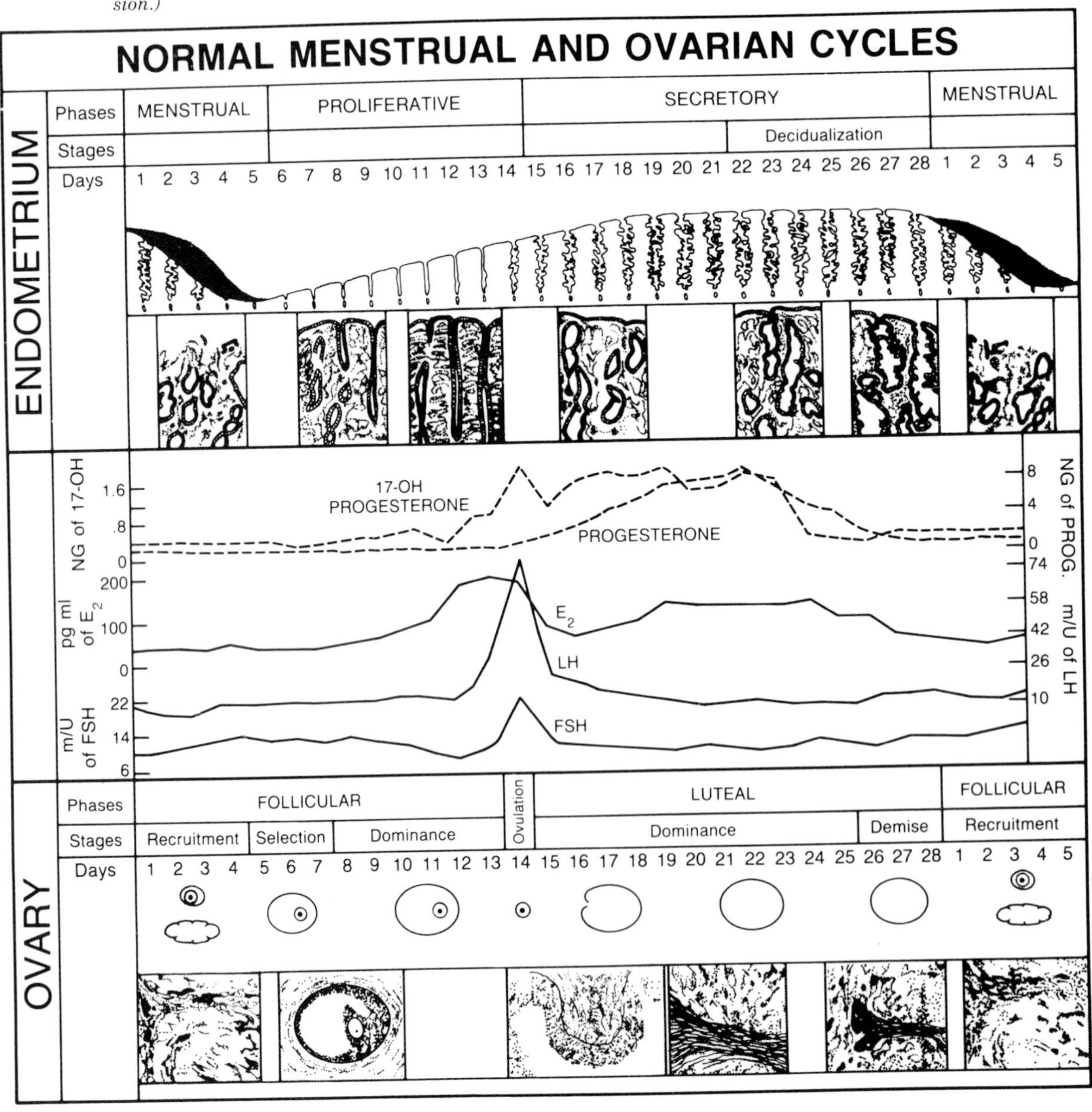

In 1950, Noyes, Hertig, and Rock established criteria for dating endometrial biopsies (Fig. 17B-10).[26] They found that the proliferative phase of the menstrual cycle was variable in length and the endometrial changes were too indistinct to permit day-to-day recognition or "dating" of the endometrium. They recognized early proliferative, midproliferative, and late proliferative endometrium (Fig. 17B-10). Through these phases, the endometrium thickens because of an increase in the number and size of the glands, which become tortuous. Glandular diameter and volume are directly related to plasma estradiol concentrations.

In contrast to the proliferative phase, Noyes and colleagues found that secretory-phase endometrium developed in such a characteristic rate and fashion after ovulation that daily changes were recognizable; the endometrium could therefore be dated. Basal or subnuclear vacuolation of the glandular epithelium was found 36 to 48 h after ovulation and was the first endometrial sign of luteinization. This change was prominent from days 16 to 19 of a typical menstrual cycle. From day 19, basal vacuoles disappeared as the glycogen-enriched secretion passed by the gland nuclei and into the lumen. The nuclei were thus seen at the base of the epithelial cells. From days 21 to 23 the spiral arterioles acquired a cuff of stromal cells with enlarged nuclei and cytoplasm. This constituted the earliest predecidual or pseudodecidual change. Predecidua extended to beneath the epithelium by day 25 and at day 27 appeared as solid sheets of decidua-like cells infiltrated by leukocytes. These predecidual cells underwent mitosis as well as hypertrophy. If conception occurs, further enlargement forms polygonal decidual cells in a highly vascular stroma. After implantation, the portion of the decidua between the placenta and myometrium is called the *decidua basalis*. The part covering the blastocyst is the *decidua capsularis*, which fuses with the part lining the remainder of the uterus, the *decidua parietalis*.

In a young adult, menstrual blood loss can be measured by collecting tampons and/or sanitary pads and extracting the iron or hemoglobin. Hallberg and associates found in 476 women that the volume of menstrual blood loss was not normally

FIGURE 17B-10 Morphologic changes in human endometrium during a normal menstrual cycle: (*A*) early proliferative; (*B*) midproliferative; (*C*) late proliferative. During the follicular phase, the endometrium thickens as a result of an increase in the number and size of the glands. Moderate tortuosity is seen as they become wider and longer. (*D*) Basal vacuolation of the gland epithelium is the earliest morphologic evidence of luteinization. Day 16 endometrium. (*E*) During the secretory stage, basal vacuoles disappear and nuclei are seen at the base of the epithelial cells. Note also stromal edema. Day 20 endometrium. (*F*) During the premenstrual stage, glands may present a pronounced sawtooth appearance. Day 25 endometrium (*G*) Stromal cells first show predecidual change around arterioles. Day 23 endometrium. (*H*) Just before menstruation, a compact layer of predecidual cells is formed. (*I*) During the menstrual phase, the endometrium typically crumbles away and is densely infiltrated with leukocytes.

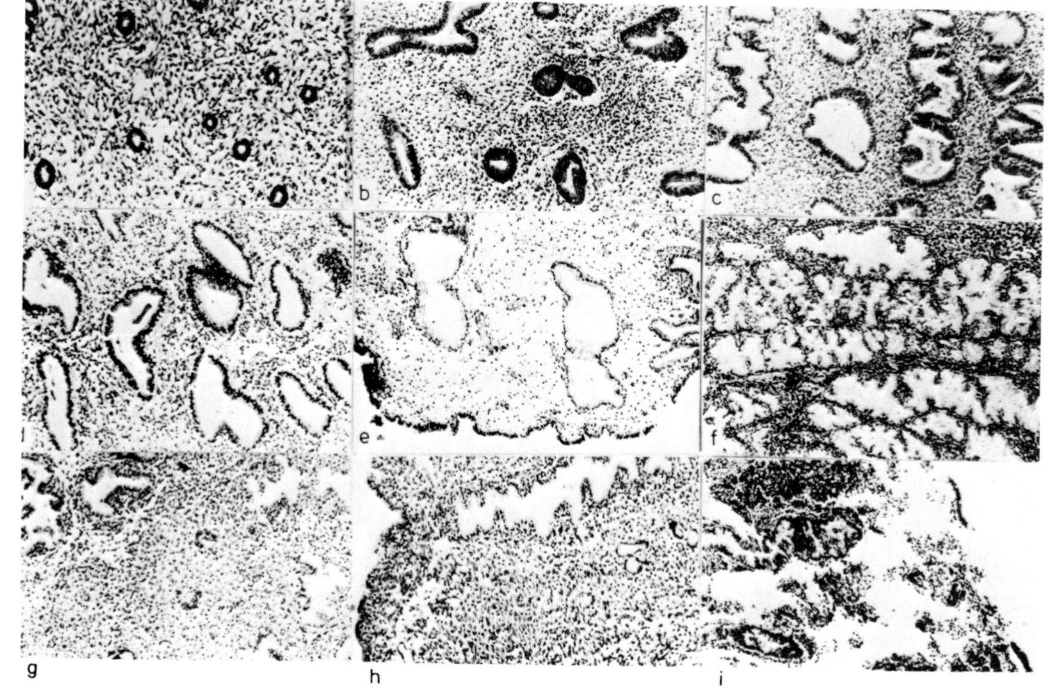

distributed but rather was skewed in distribution:[106] Median blood loss was 43 ml, and 90 percent of randomly selected women had menstrual blood losses less than 80 ml. Cole and colleagues examined 348 unselected women and confirmed a skewed distribution of menstrual blood loss.[107] In their study, median blood loss was 28 ml; in only 20 percent of these women was the difference in menstrual blood loss in consecutive periods greater than 20 ml. Menstrual blood loss increased with parity, perhaps because of an increased endometrial area or vascularity or both, but did not increase with age. Above 80 ml of menstrual blood loss, most women will probably develop iron-deficiency anemia.

Approximately 50 to 70 percent of the menstrual discharge is blood. The platelet count found in menstrual fluid is about 10 percent of that in blood. The remainder of the menses consists of fragments of endometrium and mucus. Normal menstrual blood does not readily clot. Although Buller reported that menstrual blood does not contain fibrin and that menstrual clots also contain no fibrin[108] and thus are not true clots, more recent studies by Bonnar and colleagues[109] found fibrin in 85 percent of normal menstrual clots and in 88 percent of patients with dysfunctional uterine bleeding. They found no fibrinogen in menstrual blood but did find large amounts of fibrin degradation products and suggested that thrombin and plasmin generation are central to menstrual hemostasis. This active fibrinolytic system seems to be confined to the endometrial glandular epithelium. Not surprisingly, therefore, antifibrinolytic drugs such as ϵ-aminocaproic acid and tranexamic acid, 1 g every 8 h for 3 days, have proved effective in decreasing menstrual blood loss.

Endometrial Prostaglandins

Since the discovery of an acidic lipid with oxytocic properties in menstrual fluid,[110] later shown to be $PGF_{2\alpha}$ and PGE_2, these substances have been implicated in normal and abnormal menstruation. Figure 17B-11 presents a scheme of the interrelations of the various prostaglandins (PGs) or prostanoids. Intrauterine PGs derive from arachidonic acid, originating predominantly from the essential fatty acid linoleic acid. Arachidonic acid is a polyunsaturated 20-carbon chain with four double bonds and no nitrogen and is liberated from cell membrane phospholipids by the enzyme phospholipase A_2 in response to many physical and hormonal stimuli. In the best-

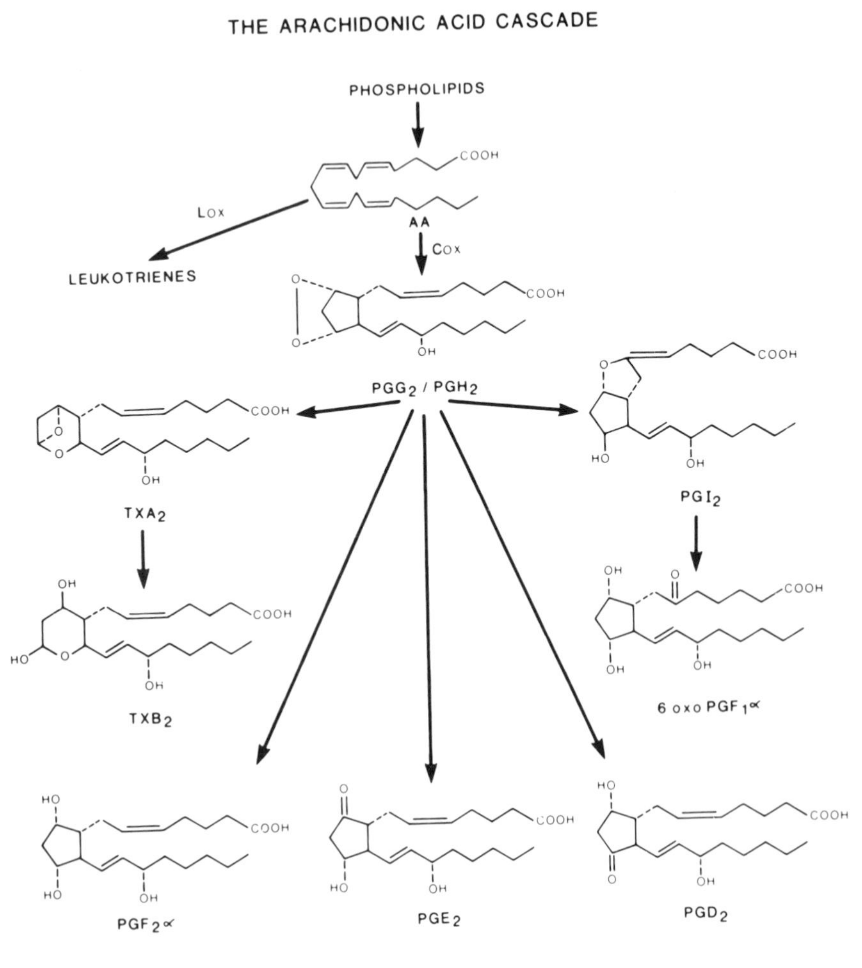

FIGURE 17B-11 The cyclooxygenase (COX) and lipoxygenase (LOX) cascade pathways of arachidonic acid (AA) metabolism. Note the pivotal position of the endoperoxide intermediates PGG_2 and PGH_2 in the production of the three classes of prostanoids, the thromboxanes (TXA_2 and TXB_2), prostacyclin (PGI_2), and the prostaglandins $PGF_{2\alpha}$, PGE_2, and PGD_2.

studied pathway, arachidonic acid is oxygenated rapidly by the enzyme PG synthetase or cyclooxygenase (COX) to form a family of prostaglandins; each contains only two double bonds. Later research discovered a second enzyme, lipoxygenase (LOX); its products, the *leukotrienes*, have a straight-chain conformation. *Eicosanoids* is the generic name for both COX and LOX products. In the COX path, the initial intermediates generated are two endoperoxides: PGG_2 and PGH_2. Both substances are pivotal in liberating at least three groups of prostanoids. $PGF_{2\alpha}$ and PGE_2 are among the most studied, in part because of their potency in the induction of myometrial contraction. $PGF_{2\alpha}$ and thromboxane A_2 (TXA_2) are potent vasoconstrictors; conversely, PGE_2 and especially prostacyclin (PGI_2) cause vasodilation. PGI_2 also dissociates platelets, while TXA_2 aggregates platelets. Both PGE_2 and TXA_2 are rapidly converted to more stable products, including 6-oxo-PGF_1 and TXB_2, respectively. Estrogen stimulates COX-mediated synthesis of endometrial $PGF_{2\alpha}$ and PGE_2 in women. In contrast, progesterone inhibits this production from proliferative and secretory-phase endometrium. The precise intracellular mechanisms controlling steroid induction of PG synthesis are unknown.

$PGF_{2\alpha}$ is quantitatively the major endometrial prostanoid liberated during the human menstrual cycle. As estrogen does stimulate COX activity, it is not surprising that prostaglandin production rates are high in the proliferative phase of the menstrual cycle. In early human pregnancy, decidua contains less $PGF_{2\alpha}$ than is found in secretory endometrium. This chronic suppression appears to be due to an inhibitor of COX which is identifiable in amniotic fluid and maternal serum. The origin and nature of this endogenous inhibitor of prostaglandin synthesis by amniochorion are unknown, though suppression by decidual prolactin or a metabolite is possible.[111]

Excessive menstrual blood loss may affect up to 20 percent of women. In the majority of individuals, no organic cause for this menorrhagia is found and the diagnosis of dysfunctional uterine bleeding is made. Clinically, it is important to realize that only approximately one-third of patients presenting with menorrhagia have excessive menstrual blood loss (> 80 ml).

It is now evident that excessive menstrual blood loss is associated with changes in PG production by the uterus. Endometrium from women with ovular dysfunctional uterine bleeding, which is common in young adults, synthesizes more PGE_2 than does endometrium from normal women, and the myometrial production of PGI_2 is markedly enhanced.[112] In women with anovular dysfunctional bleeding, excessive menstrual loss is associated with a relative deficiency of $PGF_{2\alpha}$ synthesis. There is, in fact, a direct relation between the $PGE_2/PGF_{2\alpha}$ ratio and the amount of blood loss; it may be, therefore, that menstrual loss is determined by the relative synthesis of PGs with mainly vasoconstrictive properties on the one hand ($PGF_{2\alpha}$) as opposed to those with vasodilatory properties (PGE_2 and PGI_2) on the other.

Conventional gynecologic management of menorrhagia in young adults in whom pregnancy is excluded consists of prescribing a progestogen in an attempt to induce a secretory and regressed endometrium. Drugs such as norethindrone 5 to 10 mg per day from days 5 to 25 of the cycle are suitable for this purpose. Note that the first menses on this treatment may still be heavy; the patient should be warned about this. For the majority of patients, this long administration of an androgenic progestogen will usually lead to endometrial atrophy sufficient to reduce the amount of menstrual bleeding. An alternative drug is medroxyprogesterone acetate 10 mg per day from days 5 to 25 of the cycle. Although it has been customary to state that oral progesterone is not clinically useful because of its erratic intestinal absorption, recent studies suggest that a dose of 300 mg of progesterone (in micronized form) per day, if absorbed satisfactorily, leads to normal progesterone concentrations and a normal secretory endometrium.[113] Because it does not have the powerful androgenic side effects of many synthetic progestogens, micronized progesterone is expected to have a major place in the management of menorrhagia in the near future.

COX inhibitors reduce menstrual blood loss as well as reducing the pain of primary dysmenorrhea by reducing the formation of $PGF_{2\alpha}$ and PGE_2. Drugs such as mefenamic acid should be prescribed in a relatively high dosage (1000 to 1500 mg per day) to prevent the generation of the prostaglandins that contribute to these two gynecologic disorders. The aim of treatment here is to prevent the synthesis of PGs; it is therefore important for the clinician to advise the patient to begin taking these tablets at the first sign of impending menstruation rather than to avoid taking medication until the pain becomes unbearable.

In an important double-blind, crossover clinical trial, Shan and colleagues demonstrated that the PG synthetase inhibitor ibuprofen, at 1200 mg per day beginning 3 days before the expected onset of menses through 3 days after the onset of menses, decreased by a factor of 3 to 4 both menstrual pain symptoms and $PGF_{2\alpha}$ concentrations measured in menstrual fluid.[114] In placebo cycles, there was a close correlation between the severity of menstrual pain as assessed daily by the patient and the level of $PGF_{2\alpha}$ released during the corresponding period.

Operative Hysteroscopy

Recent advances in hysteroscopic equipment have allowed new surgical treatments for menorrhagia and dysmenorrhea resistant to medical treatment while avoiding hysterectomy. These techniques aim to destroy not only the full thickness of the endometrium but also the adjoining 1 or 2 mm of myometrium to prevent endometrial regrowth and continuing menstrual ill health. The two operative methods are electrical hysteroscopy, using the resectoscope or "roller-ball" technique with a combination of cutting (100 W) and coagulation (50 W) current, and the use of laser energy to vaporize the endometrium. Although objective proof of decreased or absent menstrual blood loss after these procedures is often lacking, several series have reported 83 to 96 percent success of these operations for menorrhagia.[115]

It is of considerable interest that not only menorrhagia but also previously intractable dysmenorrhea may be effectively treated with operative hysteroscopy. Presumably, endometrial removal reduces the amount of PG production by the uterus, although this has not been proved.

Premenstrual Syndrome

There is no widely accepted definition of the common clinical entity of premenstrual syndrome (PMS), and the need exists for improved classification.[116] The incidence of PMS is not known, although 20 to 40 percent of menstruating women report some degree of recurrent mental or physical incapacitation prior to menses.[117] The range of symptoms commonly includes a disordered mood (irritability, depression), breast tenderness and abdominal bloating, headache, and altered appetite (especially carbohydrate craving) and libido. There have been many unsuccessful attempts to conclusively define clinical, menstrual, or hormonal parameters unique to PMS sufferers, including investigation of the sex steroid profile, the renin-angiotensin system, vitamin deficiency, glucose metabolism, and the opiate neuropeptides.[117,118] It has been suggested that ovulation occurs prematurely in PMS patients.[119] Although it may be a clinical disorder of the ovary, the PMS complex is still so imprecisely defined that other mechanisms are equally plausible. Social and psychological factors are important in the subjective assessment of PMS severity.[119,120] Not surprisingly, in view of the poorly defined pathophysiology, there are a large number of therapies available, commonly including relaxation therapy, pyridoxine hydrochloride, diuretics (including spironolactone), oral contraceptives, bromocriptine, and metronidazole, while "medical oophorectomy" using GnRH agonist therapy has been reported to be of benefit.[121] All may be of some benefit in selected cases. It has been suggested that a therapeutic trial be commenced using the most benign therapy, and if it is unsuccessful, other agents should be tried in line with the severity of symptoms and the patient's desire for intervention.

OVARIAN DISORDERS IN MIDDLE AGE

Endocrinology of the Menopause

The menopause is the permanent cessation of menstruation which results from loss of ovarian follicular activity. The term *perimenopause*, or *climacteric*, signifies the period of months when the endocrine, biological, and clinical features of declining ovarian function commence until the first year after menses have ceased (Fig. 17B-12). The postmenopause dates from the menopause but by convention cannot be determined until spontaneous amenorrhea has persisted for 12 months.[122] Uterine bleeding which recommences after 12 months of amenorrhea in a woman over age 40 years requires investigation to exclude endometrial cancer, although the most likely finding on endometrial sampling is an atrophic endometrium.

The median age at menopause is about 50 years for women of European origin in developed countries, but there is no generally agreed on range for this age, making the definition of premature menopause arbitrary. Cessation of ovarian function prior to age 40 years is regarded widely as consistent with the concept of a premature menopause (see Premature Ovarian Failure, above). Cigarette smoking is associated with a slightly reduced age at menopause.[123]

The most striking aspect of ovarian morphology as the menopause approaches is the accelerated loss of primordial follicles. While a gradual decline in follicular numbers is seen from the time of birth, the rate of decline increases markedly from about age 40. In an important study of Richardson et al.[124] the mean number of primordial follicles per ovary was 1392 ± 355 (SEM) in a group of women age 45 to 50 years who were still experiencing regular cycles. In a group that had entered a phase of cycle irregularity, the mean number fell to 142 ± 72, while in women who were postmenopausal, a single follicle was identified in one of four ovaries subjected to serial section. The overall decline in follicle numbers from both groups is illustrated in Fig. 17B-12.[124]

Endocrinologically, the major features of the loss of ovarian function are a marked fall (by 90 to 95 percent) in circulating estradiol level (from normal follicular-phase levels of 200 to 500 pM to 30 to 50 pM) and in inhibin, which becomes undetectable. There are marked elevations of FSH concentration (10- to 15-fold, from normal follicular-phase levels of 3 to 7 IU/L to 40 to 50 IU/L) and LH concentration (threefold, from 3 to 7 to 10 to 20 IU/L) (Fig. 17B-13). Progesterone secretion virtually ceases. The increase in gonadotropin levels results from loss of ovarian feedback both by estradiol and by inhibin. During the transition between normal menstrual cyclicity and the postmenopausal period, a variety of

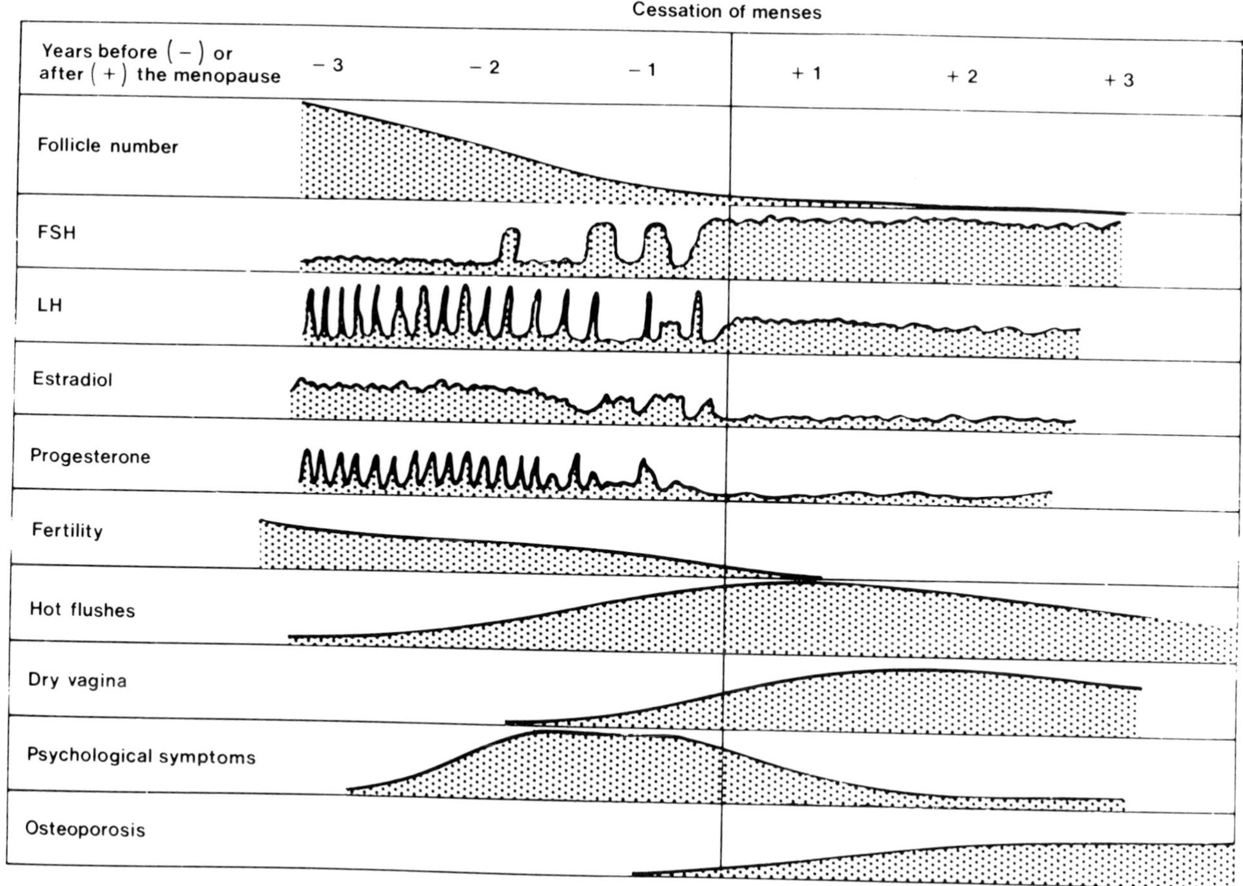

FIGURE 17B-12 Schematic representation of some clinical, biological, and endocrinologic features of the peri- and postmenopausal years.

hormonal patterns may be encountered. In women over age 45 who continue to have regular cycles, the follicular phase in particular may show moderate elevations in serum FSH levels and decreases in serum estradiol and particularly inhibin levels,[125] with LH and progesterone secretion remaining unchanged.[126] The menopausal transition is marked by considerable variability in menstrual cycle length; during this phase, apparently bizarre hormonal changes are found,[127] including elevation of levels of FSH or LH alone or FSH with LH and high or low levels of estrogens. In contrast to the decline in ovarian estrogen production, ovarian androgen production persists and there is little change in the circulating testosterone concentration after the menopause. This may be an important consideration when decisions are made regarding removal of the ovaries in peri- and postmenopausal women. Because of the variability in FSH and estradiol levels, the diagnosis of the menopausal state may not be made reliably by means of hormonal measurements alone, especially in women who have experienced lack of menses for only a few months. From a practical viewpoint, the possibility of fertility cannot be excluded until 1 year after the menopause; estimates of the annual risk of pregnancy are 10 to 20 percent for women age 40 to 44 and 2 to 3 percent for women age 45 to 49.[128] The finding of a clearly elevated serum FSH concentration and a serum estradiol level below 50 pM in a woman with 6 months or more of amenorrhea certainly makes the diagnosis of the postmenopausal state highly probable.

Climacteric Symptoms

Perimenopausal patients may seek medical advice regarding the desirability of hormone replacement therapy (HRT) when they are asymptomatic because of the widespread prominence given to such therapy in the media. Alternatively, vasomotor symptoms, psychological complaints, and/or loss of sexuality, often in the context of menstrual irregularity, are frequent reasons for presentation.

The most characteristic perimenopausal symptom is the hot flush (or flash), which was found in one study in 17 percent of women in the age range 42 to 62 years still experiencing regular cycles, 40 percent of those with irregular cycles, 65 percent of those in

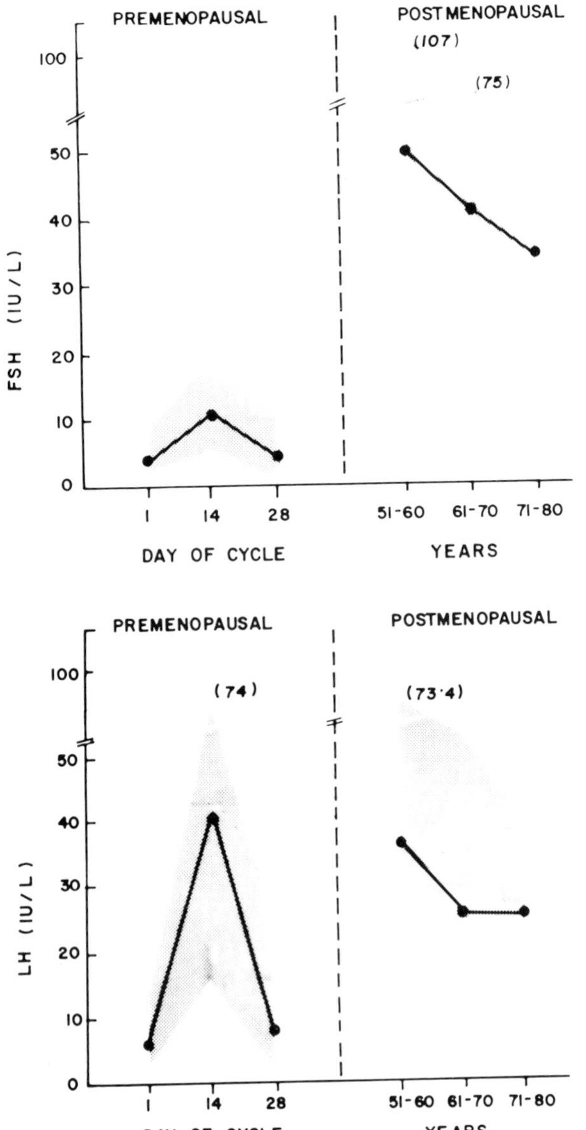

FIGURE 17B-13 Diagrammatic representation of serum FSH and LH concentrations during the follicular, periovulatory, and luteal phases of the normal menstrual cycle and during the postmenopausal period. Note that postmenopausal FSH levels greatly exceed those found during the menstrual cycle.

the 1 to 2 years after menopause, and 35 percent of those 5 to 10 years after menopause.[129] The symptom is described as a brief sensation of heat usually involving the face and upper trunk; it is accompanied by a rise in skin temperature (up to 4°C or more), peripheral vasodilation, transient increase in heart rate, and lowering of skin resistance.[130] There may be sweating, chills, nervousness, irritability, and headache. Flushes are thought to be due to a sympathetic discharge[131] and occur more or less simultaneously with pulses of LH secretion, though they are not a result of such pulses.[132] Thus, it is likely that a hypothalamic event in which there is a transient downward resetting of the central thermostat occurs at the same time as the episodic discharge of GnRH.

Flush frequency is variable; occurrence during the night leads to sleep disturbance. Estrogen therapy specifically relieves the symptom, providing strong evidence for the role of estrogen withdrawal in its occurrence. When specific transdermal estradiol replacement was used, a linear decline in flush frequency occurred as circulating estradiol levels increased.[133] Relief may also be afforded by the central alpha-adrenergic agonist drug clonidine and by progestogens such as medroxyprogesterone. Techniques such as continual recording of such symptoms now allow objective monitoring of flush frequency, permitting proper study of the efficacy of various treatment regimens.[134]

Controversy has surrounded the specificity of psychological symptoms in relation to the menopause; the degree to which symptoms such as fatigue, irritability, depression, and a general sense of feeling unwell are a reflection of "general lack of well-being" or of more specific psychological states such as depression is unclear, but there is substantial evidence that estrogen replacement will alleviate such symptoms, particularly in women who have no prior history of psychological disturbance.[135]

A decline in sexual interest of varying severity may occur after the menopause,[136] although the frequency of this problem has been questioned.[137] There may be associated vaginal dryness and dyspareunia, but correction of the dyspareunia with local or systemic estrogens often fails to restore sexual interest and enjoyment.

Urinary symptoms, such as frequency and urgency of micturition, may be experienced for the first time by peri- and postmenopausal women, but their association with estrogen deficiency has not been established clearly. In the absence of another underlying cause, a trial of vaginal or systemic estrogen therapy may be rewarding.

Alterations in appearance due to declining skin quality are common complaints in perimenopausal women, and the skin has been shown to contain estradiol receptors.[138] The postmenopausal state is associated with a decrease in skin collagen, which can be restored by HRT.[139]

The symptoms of flushes, psychological disturbances, and loss of sexuality are self-limited and respond satisfactorily to HRT. The presence of such symptoms constitutes a strong indication for at least short-term HRT for 6 to 12 months. During such a limited period the choice of estrogen is not a major issue, and oral therapy with a synthetic estrogen such as ethinyl estradiol (10 to 20 μg daily) or a natural estrogen [e.g., conjugated equine estrogens (Premarin) 0.625 to 1.25 mg daily or estradiol valerate 1 to 2 mg daily] is used conventionally. Although not mandatory with short-term therapy, it is prudent to add a cyclic progestogen (e.g., medroxyprogesterone 10 mg daily for 12 days per month) in order to avoid unexpected vaginal bleeding. Topical vaginal estrogen creams or tablets are valuable for the specific relief of vaginal dryness or dyspareunia. Conventional contraindications to estrogen therapy include a history of breast cancer or endometrial cancer, recent undiagnosed genital bleeding, liver disease, or a history of thromboembolism. There is, however, some controversy regarding the seriousness of these contraindications. For example, a patient who has no evidence of recurrence of breast cancer treated more than 5 years previously or who has had a stage 1 or 2 endometrial cancer treated can probably be given HRT without danger, especially if quality of life is taken into consideration. Relief of severe flushing or dyspareunia may be an overwhelming indication for HRT despite the theoretical concerns regarding reactivation of a treated malignancy. For patients with mild liver disease or a past history of thromboembolism, parenteral estrogen therapy (e.g., by transdermal patch) is almost certainly safe, as this route is not associated with significant effects on liver function, including levels of clotting factors.[133] For patients with loss of libido persisting despite adequate oral estrogen replacement, combined subcutaneous implants of estradiol (40 mg) and testosterone (50 mg) have proved efficacious.[140]

Postmenopausal Problems

Osteoporosis

Osteoporosis is defined as a reduction in the mass of bony tissue relative to the volume of anatomic bone. Conventionally, the reference value for normal bones is taken as that derived from a normal young (premenopausal) adult population; a significant reduction is to less than 2 SD below that mean. A variety of techniques are available for the measurement of bone mass, including CT and densitometry of the forearm, the os calcis, the spine, and the neck of the femur. There is a growing tendency to make such measurements in women in the peri- or postmenopausal period in order to identify those at increased risk for the later development of osteoporotic fractures, which especially affect the radius, spine, and femoral neck. Loss of cortical bone in particular predisposes women to radial and femoral fractures, while loss of trabecular bone leads to vertebral crush fractures. Assessment of bone density is the only reliable method for estimating the risk of fracture.[141]

The exact pathogenesis of postmenopausal osteoporosis is not understood; however, there is a clear association between cessation of ovarian function and loss of bone mass, and estradiol receptors have been identified in bone cells.[142] It is hypothesized that estrogens somehow have a protective effect on bone, opposing bony resorption induced by parathormone, vitamin D, or both. Controversy exists regarding the role of calcitonin; there is some evidence that its levels fall after menopause and are stimulated by estrogen. The mean daily calcium requirement to maintain calcium balance was shown to increase after the menopause from about 500 to about 1500 mg.[143] Despite this, rates of loss of bone after menopause appear to be independent of calcium uptake over a wide range of values.[144] There is a slight rise in serum calcium and phosphate levels after the menopause, as well as in urinary calcium and hydroxyproline levels.[145] Measurement of the fasting urinary calcium/creatinine ratio provides a useful index of the rate of loss of calcium in the urine.

The prevention of postmenopausal osteoporosis is a major reason to consider long-term HRT (further discussed below); three separate case-control studies have shown a risk ratio for fractures of about 2 to 3 in favor of estrogen therapy.[146–148] Ensuring an adequate calcium intake (about 1500 mg daily) and encouragement of physical exercise are useful general measures, although the role of calcium supplementation remains highly controversial.

The treatment of established osteoporosis remains an area of debate, but several approaches have shown promise. These include HRT,[149–151] cyclic disphosphonates,[152] and calcitonin.[153] The place of sodium fluoride therapy is uncertain, as some studies have failed to show any beneficial effect on fracture prevention despite an increase in radiologic bone density.[154] Supplementary vitamin D in physiologic replacement doses should be given to women whose diet is deficient or who have little exposure to sunlight.

Atherosclerotic Cardiovascular Disease

Because cardiovascular disease is a leading cause of death, its possible relation to cessation of ovarian function and its possible prevention by HRT assume great importance.[155] It has been shown that the menopause is associated with increases in levels of serum cholesterol and triglycerides, accepted risk factors for atherosclerotic vascular disease.[156–158] Two population studies have examined the relation between carefully defined cardiovascular disease and the menopause. In Goteborg, Sweden, systematic samples from birth cohorts of women were examined and classified on the basis of a past history of myocardial infarction, angina pectoris, and EKG evidence of ischemic heart disease.[158] The observed cases were compared to unaffected members of their cohort in three age groups, and those in all three affected groups were found to have undergone earlier menopause. In the Framingham Study, an increase in the incidence of coronary heart-disease and in the severity of the presenting syndrome was found to occur after menopause among the 2873 women who had been followed up for up to 24 years after initial assessment.[159] No premenopausal women developed myocardial infarction or died of coronary heart disease, whereas such events were commonly seen among postmenopausal women. Within each of the age groups 40 to 44, 45 to 49, and 50 to 54 years, coronary heart disease was more than twice as common in postmenopausal as in premenopausal women, whether the menopause was spontaneous or surgical. In a study of American nurses, those who had had bilateral oophorectomy before age 35 years had more than seven times the risk of having a nonfatal myocardial infarct compared with premenopausal women of the same age and with the same risk factors.[160] Although there are other data not supportive of these associations, it can reasonably be concluded that menopause is associated with an increase in the risks of morbidity and mortality from atherosclerotic cardiovascular disease.

Estrogen therapy alone given to postmenopausal women has beneficial effects on coronary risk factors, causing a fall in serum cholesterol and low-density lipoprotein levels and an increase in the concentration of high-density lipoprotein,[161,162] with variable effects on levels of plasma triglycerides. Synthetic progestogens tend to nullify these estrogen effects,[163] although their ability to do so varies with the dose and with the precise time during the treatment regimen at which lipid levels are measured. Although an initial report suggested that 17-acetoxyprogestogens are less potent in this regard than are 19-nor-progestogens, the doses of the latter used in that study were relatively much greater than those of medroxyprogesterone.[163] Whether progestogens in the lower doses currently recommended have long-term adverse effects on plasma lipids, in particular on morbidity or mortality from coronary artery disease, remains to be established (see below).[164] Effects of estrogen on blood coagulation factors are variable; dosage, route of administration, and the nature of the estrogen preparation are important. Thus, oral estrogens cause increases in levels of factors VII, IX, X, and X complex[165,166] and lower concentrations of anticoagulation factors such as antithrombin III. Percutaneously administered estradiol has no effect on antithrombin III.[167]

Whether estrogen therapy leads to an alteration in the actual occurrence of cardiovascular disease remains controversial.[168] At least one study of death from ischemic heart disease in a retirement community suggests a strong protective effect of oral estrogen (risk ratio with estrogen therapy 0.43).[169] A report from the Lipid Research Clinics Program follow-up study indicated a marked decrease in all-causes mortality in estrogen users compared with nonusers,[170] mainly as a result of reduced cardiovascular mortality.[171] Confirmatory reports have been published.[172] It is now clear that progestogen should be used routinely in patients who have intact uteri to protect against the risk of endometrial cancer arising from unopposed estrogen; however, no epidemiologic data are available which examine estrogen-progestogen combinations for their effect on heart disease. Studies in the cynomolgus monkey are reassuring in this regard, as the addition of progestogens failed to neutralize the beneficial effects of estrogens in protecting against the development of atherosclerotic lesions in animals that were fed a high-cholesterol diet.[173,174] This remains a major unanswered question in the overall assessment of risk/benefit ratios for HRT.

Long-Term Hormone Replacement Therapy

Modes of Administration

From a therapeutic viewpoint, estrogens are arbitrarily classified into those which occur in nature and those which are synthetic (Table 17B-6). Natural estrogens include estradiol and its esters, estrone sulfate (including its piperazine salt), estriol, and conjugated equine estrogens (Premarin, a mixture of estrone sulfate, equilin, and equilenin). The major synthetic estrogen is ethinyl estradiol; mestranol and diethylstilbestrol are additional examples. Estrogens may be given orally or parenterally; approximately equivalent doses of the commonly used preparations are listed in Table 17B-7. Although preparations differ in their relative potencies, depending on the assay end point, the doses listed are approximately equivalent in terms of FSH suppression.[175] The synthetic estrogens are relatively more potent than the natural estrogens in their hepatic effects.

The oral estrogens may be given cyclically (3 weeks on, 1 week off) in the belief that this will minimize the likelihood of development of endometrial hyperplasia, but there is no evidence that continuous oral administration results in a greater risk,[176] and some patients suffer recurrence of hot flushes during the week off therapy on the cyclic regimen.

Oral estrogen administration results in "first-pass" effects on the liver, with maximal opportunity

TABLE 17B-6 Types of Estrogen Available for Therapeutic Use

Natural
Estradiol
Estrone and estrone sulfate
Estriol
Conjugated (mixture of sodium estrone sulfate, sodium equilin sulfate, sodium equilenin sulfate, and sodium estradiol sulfate)
Synthetic
Ethinyl estradiol
Mestranol
Quinestrol
Diethylstilbestrol
Dienestrol

TABLE 17B-7 Oral Estrogen Preparations and Approximately Equivalent Doses

Preparation	Dose
Oral estrogens	
Conjugated equine estrogens	0.625–1.25 mg daily
Piperazine estrone sulfate	1.25–2.5 mg daily
Estradiol valerate	1–2 mg daily
Micronized estradiol	1–2 mg daily
Ethinyl estradiol	10–20 μg daily
Parenteral estrogens	
Transdermal estradiol	50 μg patch twice weekly
Percutaneous estradiol	3 mg daily
Subcutaneous estradiol implant	50 mg every 6 months

for effects on hepatic protein synthesis. Synthetic estrogens are particularly potent from this standpoint and produce significant increases in the synthesis of renin substrate, SHBG, corticosteroid-binding globulin, thyroxine-binding globulin, and lipoproteins.[177] This has led to the development of various parenteral estrogen preparations, e.g., subcutaneous estradiol implants, estradiol gels for application to the skin, estrogen-containing vaginal creams, and transdermal therapeutic systems.[178] These preparations have little if any effect on hepatic protein synthesis and may thus have at least theoretical advantages for long-term use. In addition, while all natural orally administered estrogens give rise to plasma levels of estrone markedly in excess of that of plasma estradiol, the parenteral preparations produce plasma levels of estradiol greater than those of estrone, mimicking the physiologic situation of the normal follicular phase of the menstrual cycle.[178–180]

In women with an intact uterus, cyclic administration of a progestogen for a minimum of 10 and preferably 12 to 13 days each month is mandatory in order to avoid the risk of estrogen-induced endometrial hyperplasia, which may progress to endometrial carcinoma.[181] Other possible beneficial effects of the added progestogen (e.g., possible reduction in the risk of occurrence of breast cancer, actual increase in bone mass) remain controversial, and the potential adverse effects (neutralization of the possible beneficial effects of estrogens) have not been well defined. The dose of progestogen required to protect against the development of endometrial hyperplasia and carcinoma varies with the type of progestogen.[182] Currently recommended regimens include the use of medroxyprogesterone acetate 5 to 10 mg daily or norethindrone 0.7 to 1.25 mg daily, most conveniently given on the first 12 calendar days of the month to facilitate patient compliance. A useful clinical indicator that the dose of progestogen is adequate is that induced menstrual bleeding occurs only after the 10th to 12th day of the month.[182] The occurrence of withdrawal bleeding as a result of cyclic progestogen administration is a major disincentive to some women in considering HRT. Several reports have provided early indications that an alternative therapeutic regimen that can lead to amenorrhea is the combined continuous administration of a standard dose of estrogen (either orally or parenterally) with a dose of progestogen lower than that required for cyclic therapy, e.g., medroxyprogesterone acetate 2.5 mg, norethindrone 0.35 to 0.7 mg, or norethisterone acetate 1 mg daily.[183] Although breakthrough bleeding in the first 3 to 4 months of such combined continuous therapy may occur in 40 to 50 percent of patients, amenorrhea is usually induced after 4 to 6 months. The long-term safety of this type of combined continuous therapy has not yet been established,[182] although the lack of adverse effects on cardiovascular risk factors and the beneficial effects on bone mineral density provide grounds for optimism. The use of progestogens in women who have had a hysterectomy is not regarded as necessary.[184] The development of "nonandrogenic" progestogens gives promise that HRT can be made even safer in the future.

Routine supervision of patients on long-term HRT should include blood pressure measurement, breast examination, and assessment of lipid levels, with endometrial sampling in any patient who develops unexpected uterine bleeding. Whether endometrial biopsy should be undertaken routinely before long-term HRT is instituted is controversial; in a patient previously untreated with estrogen, the procedure may be associated with significant discomfort, and if there is no history of abnormal uterine bleeding and a cyclic progestogen is used, endometrial biopsy is unlikely to yield clinically significant information. Especially in patients with a history of benign breast disease or a family history of breast cancer, routine mammography is desirable prior to initiating therapy and at intervals of 1 to 2 years thereafter.

Benefits and Risks

The major potential benefits of long-term HRT are the established benefit of its prevention of osteoporosis and hence of lowering the risk of osteoporosis-associated fracture, particularly of the femoral neck, and the theoretical benefit of the prevention of atherosclerotic cardiovascular disease. If the latter is established on the basis of further epidemiologic studies, it will be extremely important to consider using HRT more routinely in the community.

The major potential risks are of endometrial and breast cancer. Although it has been established that estrogen therapy without accompanying progestogen leads to a substantially increased risk of endometrial hyperplasia and carcinoma, this risk is abolished if regular cyclic progestogen is administered.[122,185] The question of whether HRT causes an increased risk of developing breast cancer is unresolved;[122,186] if a risk does exist, it is relatively small (risk ratio ≤ 2).[187] However, because breast cancer is an extremely frightening prospect for the individual patient, the risk must be taken into account in making a decision concerning long-term HRT. It has proved extremely difficult to arrive at an objective resolution of the benefit/risk ratio for HRT,[187] and the situation has become more complex because there are few epidemiologic data on the benefits (and risks) of long-term HRT using both estrogens and progestogens. Further, there are no comprehensive data on regimens of parenteral estrogen administration. The authors have adopted the approach of being ready to administer long-term HRT to any woman who seeks such therapy, provided that no contraindications are present and that she is willing to tolerate the inconvenience of monthly withdrawal bleeding. A regimen commonly used is oral estradiol valerate 1 to 2 mg or conjugated equine estrogen 0.625 to 1.25 mg daily continuously with medroxyprogesterone acetate 10 mg daily or norethindrone 1.25 mg daily for the first 12 calendar days each month. Patients are reviewed at 6- to 12-month intervals for assessment of blood pressure and breasts and for measurement of serum lipids. Endometrial biopsy is undertaken only when abnormal uterine bleeding is reported.

Parenteral estrogen administration has become increasingly popular in many parts of the world.

Postmenopausal Bleeding

Patients with or without HRT may develop bleeding more than 12 months after the cessation of their spontaneous menstrual cycles. Each patient with unanticipated postmenopausal bleeding must be thoroughly evaluated because of the increased incidence of endometrial adenocarcinoma, which in some series has reached 23 percent.[188]

Outpatient curettage using a Novak or Randall instrument or a suction device such as the Vabra aspirator has been reported to correlate with formal inpatient cervical dilatation and uterine curettage in approximately 90 percent of subjects.[189] Simpler sampling devices have been developed, such as the Pipelle cannula and Gynoscann,[190] and the use of endometrial sampling in women on HRT has been reviewed.[191] Where available, such outpatient procedures and office diagnostic hysteroscopy are now the diagnostic methods of choice for directed endometrial biopsy in patients with postmenopausal bleeding. In the 10 percent of outpatients in whom the endometrial cavity cannot be sounded or in whom repeated or persistent postmenopausal bleeding occurs, inpatient examination under anesthesia and curettage is mandatory. Gambrell and Greenblatt have emphasized the usefulness of progestogen and estrogen therapy to arrest heavy postmenopausal bleeding and the value of cyclic courses of progestogens to reverse hyperplasia of the endometrium.[192] Patients with any degree of endometrial hyperplasia must have repeat curettage after 3 months of progestogen treatment and hysterectomy if hyperplasia persists.

CHEMICAL CONTRACEPTION AND CONTRAGESTATION

Oral contraceptives are probably the most studied medicines in the history of therapeutics. Many international conferences, books, and reviews on chemical contraceptives can be found in the literature.[193,194] It is not the aim of this section to provide an exhaustive review of the last 30 years of oral contraceptives, which are now estimated to have been taken at some time by four out of every five western women in their midthirties. Rather, the aim is to briefly review the benefits and risks of oral contraceptives, describe recent advances in progestogen therapy, and review chemical contragestion by progesterone receptor antagonists such as Mifepristone.[195]

During the last three decades there have been major modifications to oral contraceptives. Initially, the amount of progestogen was markedly reduced by the introduction of norgestrel and subsequent isolation of its active isomer, levonorgestrel. This was also associated with a decrease of the estrogen component in 1973 to 30 μg of ethinylestradiol per day. In the 1980s, there were also attempts to further reduce the estrogen content of oral contraceptives with the introduction of the triphasic approach to oral contraception.

Studies over the past 30 years have shown a number of rare but serious adverse effects from chemical contraception, especially in the cardiovascular system. However, it is important to emphasize that current studies on cardiovascular effects, metabolic actions, and the incidence of various tumors tell us about only the previous generation of oral chemical contraceptives, not those in current use. As far as increased cardiovascular risk is concerned, this is mainly concentrated in women who are over 35 years old, smoke cigarettes, or have other risk factors such as obesity or diabetes. The most recent data indicate that healthy nonsmoking women age 35 to 45 years can continue to use oral contraceptives without an increased risk of cardiovascular disease.

A major benefit of the use of chemical contraception has been a clear reduction in the risk of various cancers. At least nine major studies indicate that oral contraceptives have a protective effect against endometrial cancer, the third most common cancer among women in the United States. This protective effect is greatest in women who have no children or only one child, and it is precisely these women who have the greatest risk of acquiring endometrial cancer. Ovarian cancer kills more women than all other genital malignancies combined. There are over 12 published reports indicating that the use of chemical contraception reduces the risk of ovarian cancer, in particular the most common types of epithelial ovarian cancer. As little as 6 months of oral contraceptive use provides protection, and this protective effect continues for at least 15 years after the use of chemical contraception stops (Table 17B-8).

Many studies have looked at the risk of breast cancer among users of chemical contraception. On balance, it is known that the rate of breast cancer is not increasing and that there does not appear to be an overall increase in the incidence of breast cancer in users of chemical contraception. Some studies have suggested that use of the contraceptive pill before age 25 years or before the first pregnancy does increase the risk of breast cancer in later life. However, other studies have not confirmed these suggested risks. In addition, there is evidence that breast-feeding for 1 year reduces the risk of breast cancer in later life by as much as one-third of the risk seen in women who have never lactated.

There have been reports that increased cervical intraepithelial neoplasia may be associated with chemical contraception. It is currently impossible to say whether this is a casual relation because of the confounding difficulties with other risk factors, such as the age of first intercourse, the number of sexual partners, and infection with papilloma or wart virus. There is a high correlation between oral contraceptive use and benign liver tumors. Such benign hepatocellular adenomas are rare in western countries, and although these tumors may become malignant, the rate of death from this disease has remained unchanged in the United States over the past 25 years, a period of time when millions of women have used chemical contraception. Furthermore, other tumors, including malignant melanoma and pituitary adenoma, are no more frequent among users of chemical contraception than among nonusers.

TABLE 17B-8 Benefits and Risks of Chemical Contraception

Benefits	Risks
Menstrual loss reduced	Hypertension
Iron deficiency anemia decreased	Arterial thromboembolism increased
Dysmenorrhea less	Venous thromboembolism increased
Benign ovarian cysts fewer	Gallbladder disease increased
Endometrial cancer decreased	
Ovarian cancer decreased	
Bone density increased	
Risk of ectopic pregnancy reduced	
Risk of endometriosis reduced	

New Progestogens

As part of a continuum in the development of chemical contraception, recent research has explored the potential usefulness of a new series of gonane progestogens related to levonorgestrel. The most studied of these newer derivatives are gestodene and desogestrel. Both molecules are derivatives of 19-norprogesterone and, like levonorgestrel, bind with higher affinity to the progesterone receptor than does the natural hormone. There was no affinity for the estrogen receptor and similar affinities with levonorgestrel to the androgen receptor. Gestodene and desogestrel bind three to five times more avidly to the aldosterone receptor than does levonorgestrel. Gestodene and desogestrel inhibit ovulation in doses of approximately 40 μg per day, which is similar to levonorgestrel and compares with an inhibitory action of progesterone at only 300 mg per day. Gestodene and desogestrel cause progestogenic transformation of endometrium at doses of only 2 mg per cycle compared with levonorgestrel (5 to 6 mg/cycle).[196]

The clinical interest in "third-generation" progestogens arises from data suggesting that the progesterone component of the combined oral contraceptive may contribute to the increased risk of stroke and ischemic heart disease in women taking these medicines. It has been suggested that the progestogen used in combined oral contraceptives modifies the estrogen effect on blood coagulation. It has been reported that these progestogens increase fibrinolytic activity and decrease platelet aggregation; this suggests that these new forms of chemical contraception will have fewer thrombogenic hazards than previous formulations did.

A second recent advance in chemical regulation of fertility has been the development of progesterone receptor antagonists such as Mifepristone (RU-486).[197] Progesterone receptor antagonists bind avidly to the progesterone receptor and glucocorticoid receptor and have essentially no binding to the mineralocorticoid, estrogen, or androgen receptors. Mifepristone also binds avidly to albumin, resulting in a half-life of approximately 24 h after oral administration.

Progesterone receptor antagonists can induce menstruation by a direct action on the endometrium.[198] This action is produced by the release of PGF_2 and PGE_2 and by a decrease in the metabolism of these eicosanoids.[199]

Baulieu has highlighted the use of progesterone

receptor antagonists as contragestives or antigestational agents.[197] Chemical contragestives regulate fertility by preventing or interrupting implantation and act regardless of whether fertilization has occurred. Ulmann[200] has reported that 600 mg of Mifepristone taken on day 27 of the cycle in women who had unprotected intercourse at midcycle resulted in menstruation within 72 h in all patients. However, of the 35 of 102 women who had conceived, 6 of these 35 pregnancies continued and required surgical termination. Further studies are required to establish whether progesterone receptor antagonists alone or in combination with other medicines will be clinically effective for occasional contragestion.

REFERENCES

1. Ross JL, Cassorla FG, Skerda NC, Valk IM, Loriaux DL, Cutler GB: A preliminary study of the effect of estrogen dose on growth in Turner's syndrome. *N Engl J Med* 309:1104, 1983.
2. Rosenfeld RG, Hintz RL, Johanson AJ, Sherman B, Brasel JA, Burstein S, Chernausek S, Compton P, et al: Three year results of a randomized prospective trial of methionyl human growth hormone and oxandrolone in Turner's syndrome. *J Pediatr* 113:393–400, 1988.
3. Takano K, Shizume K, Hibi I: Turner's syndrome: Treatment of 203 patients with recombinant human growth hormone for one year: A multicentre study. *Acta Endocrinology (Copenh)* 120:559–568, 1989.
4. Vanderschueren-Lodeweyckz M, Massa G, Maes M, Craen M, van Vliet G, Heinrichs C, Malvaux P: Growth-promoting effect of growth hormone and low dose ethinyl estradiol in girls with Turner's syndrome. *J Clin Endocrinol Metab* 70:122–126, 1990.
5. Lutjen P, Trounson AO, Leeton JF, Findlay JK, Wood EC, Renou P: The establishment and maintenance of pregnancy using in vitro fertilization and embryo donation in a patient with primary ovarian failure. *Nature* 307:174, 1984.
6. Cameron IT, Rogers PAW, Caro C, Harman J, Healy DL, Leeton JF: Oocyte donation: A review. *Br J Obstet Gynaecol* 96:893–899, 1989.
7. Ballabio A, Bardoni B, Carrozzo R, Andria G, Bick O, Campbell L, Hamel B, Ferguson-Smith MA, et al: Contiguous gene syndromes due to deletions in the distal short arm of the human X chromosome. *Proc Natl Acad Sci USA* 86:10001–10005, 1989.
8. Shalet SM: Treatment of constitutional delay in growth and puberty (CDGP). *Clin Endocrinol (Oxf)* 31:81–86, 1989.
9. Dewhurst CJ (ed): *Integrated Obstetrics and Gynaecology for Postgraduates*. London, Blackwell, 1981.
10. Brown TR, Lubahn DB, Wilson EM, Joseph DR, French FS, Migeon CJ: Deletion of the steroid-binding domain of the human androgen receptor gene in one family with complete androgen insensitivity syndrome: Evidence for further genetic heterogeneity in this syndrome. *Proc Natl Acad Sci USA* 85:8151–8155, 1988.
11. Marcelli M, Tilley WD, Wilson CV, Wilson JD, Griffin JE, McPhaul MJ: A single nucleotide substitution introduces a premature termination codon into the androgen receptor gene of a patient with receptor-negative androgen resistance. *J Clin Invest* 75:1522–1528, 1990.
12. Healy DL, Hodgen GD: The endocrinology of human endometrium. *Obstet Gynecol Surv* 38:509, 1983.
13. Fraser IS, Michie EA, Wide L, Baird DT: Pituitary gonadotropins and ovarian function in adolescent dysfunctional uterine bleeding. *J Clin Endocrinol Metab* 37:407, 1973.
14. Coulam CB: Premature ovarian failure. *Fertil Steril* 38:645, 1982.
15. Friedman CI, Barrows H, Kim MH: Hypergonadotropic hypogonadism. *Am J Obstet Gynecol* 145:360, 1983.
16. O'Herlihy C, Pepperell RJ, Evans JH: The significance of FSH elevation in young women with disorders of ovulation. *Br Med J* 281:1447, 1980.
17. Keelam CV, Stringfellow S, Frohoefnagel D: Evidence for a genetic factor in the etiology of premature ovarian failure. *Fertil Steril* 40:693, 1983.
18. Warne GL, Fairley KF, Hobbs JH, Martin FIR: Cyclophosphamide-induced ovarian failure. *N Engl J Med* 289:1159, 1973.
19. Alper MM, Garner PR: Premature ovarian failure: Its relationship to autoimmune disease. *Obstet Gynecol* 66:27, 1985.
20. Mignot MH, Shoemaker J, Kleingeld M, Ramanath Rao B, Drexhage HA: Premature ovarian failure: I. The association with autoimmunity. *Eur J Obstet Gynecol Reprod Biol* 30:59–66, 1989.
21. Cameron IT, O'Shea F, MacLachlan V, Healy DL: Occult ovarian failure: A clinical syndrome of regular menses, infertility and elevated FSH values shows an impaired response to superovulation. *J Clin Endocrinol Metab* 67:1190–1194, 1988.
22. Buckler HM, Evans CA, Mamtora H, Burger HG, Anderson DC: Gonadotropin, steroid, and inhibin levels in women with incipient ovarian failure during anovulatory and ovulatory rebound cycle. *J Clin Endocrinol Metab* 72:116–124, 1991.
23. Wright CSW, Jacobs HS: Spontaneous pregnancy in a patient with hypergonadotrophic ovarian failure. *Br J Obstet Gynaecol* 86:389, 1979.
24. Kreiner D, Droesch K, Navot D, Scott R, Rosenwaks Z: Spontaneous and pharmacologically induced remissions in patients with premature ovarian failure. *Obstet Gynecol* 72:926–928, 1988.
25. Lutjen PJ, Findlay JK, Trounson AO, Leeton JF, Chan CLK: Effects on plasma gonadotropins of cyclic steroid replacement prior to embryo transfer in women with premature ovarian failure. *J Clin Endocrinol Metab* 62:419, 1986.
26. Noyes RW, Hertig AT, Rock AJ: Dating the endometrial biopsy. *Fertil Steril* 1:3, 1950.
27. Kleinberg BL, Noel GL, Francz AG: Galactorrhea: A study of 235 cases, including 48 with pituitary tumours. *N Engl J Med* 296:589, 1977.
28. Hooper JH, Welch VC, Point P, Schackleford RT: Abnormal lactation associated with tranquilizing drug therapy. *JAMA* 178:506, 1961.
29. Katz E, Adashi EY: Hyperprolactinemic disorders. *Clin Obset Gynecol* 33:622–639, 1990.
30. Shearman RP (ed): *Clinical Reproductive Physiology*. Sydney, Blackwell, 1985.
31. Bonneville JF, Poulignot D, Cattin F, Couturier M, Mollet E, Dietmann JL: Computed tomographic demonstration of the effects of bromocriptine on pituitary microadenoma size. *Neuroradiology* 143:451, 1982.
32. Davis PC, Hoffman JC Jr, Spencer T, Tindall GT, Braun IF: MR imaging of pituitary adenoma: CT, clinical and surgical correlation. *AJNR* 148:797, 1987.
33. Stein AL, Levenick MN, Kletzky OA: Computed tomography versus magnetic resonance imaging for the evaluation of suspected pituitary adenomas. *Obstet Gynecol* 73:996, 1989.
34. Klibanski A, Neer RM, Beilins JZ, Ridgway EC, Zervas NT, McArthur JW: Decreased bone density in hyperprolactinemic women. *N Engl J Med* 303:1511, 1980.
35. Klibanski A, Greenspan SL: Increase in bone mass after treatment of hyperprolactinemic amenorrhea. *N Engl J Med* 315:542, 1986.
36. Pepperell RJ, Evans JH, Brown JB, Smith MA, Healy DL, Burger HG: Serum prolactin levels and the value of bromocriptine (CB154) in the treatment of anovulatory infertility. *Br J Obstet Gynaecol* 84:58, 1977.
37. Healy DL, Burger HG: Human prolactin. II. Recent advances in therapy. *Aust NZ J Obstet Gynaecol* 17:73, 1977.

38. Schettini G, Lombardi G, Merola B, Colao A, Miletto P, Caruso E, Lancranjan I: Rapid and long-lasting suppression of prolactin secretion and shrinkage of prolactinomas after injection of long-acting repeatable form of bromocriptine (Parlodel Lar). *Clin Endocrinol (Oxf)* 33:161–169, 1990.
39. Barnett PS, Dawson JM, Butler J, Coskeran PB, MacCabe JJ, McGregor AM: CV205-502, a new non-ergot dopamine agonist, reduces prolactinoma size in man. *Clin Endocrinol (Oxf)* 33:307–316, 1990.
40. Johnston BG, Hall K, Kendall-Taylor P, Patrick D, Watson M, Cook DV: The effect of dopamine agonist withdrawal after longterm therapy in prolactinomas. *Lancet* ii:187, 1984.
41. Molitch ME: Pregnancy and the hyperprolactinemic woman. *N Eng J Med* 312:1364, 1985.
42. Griffith RW, Turkal JI, Braun P: Pituitary tumours in pregnancy in mothers treated with bromocriptine. *Br J Clin Pharmacol* 7:393, 1979.
43. Rasmussen C, Berg HT, Nillius SJ, Wide L: The return of menstruation and normalization of prolactin in hyperprolactinemic women with bromocriptine-induced pregnancy. *Fertil Steril* 44:31, 1985.
44. Rodman EF, Molitch ME, Post KD, Boller BJ, Reichman S: Long-term followup of transsphenoidal selective adenomectomy for prolactinoma. *JAMA* 252:921, 1984.
45. Serri U, Rasio E, Beauregard H, Hardy J, Sommer AN: Recurrence of hyperprolactinemia after selective transphenoidal adenomectomy in women with prolactinoma. *N Engl J Med* 309:280, 1983.
46. Frisch RE, Revelle ER: Height and weight at menarche and a hypothesis of critical body weight and adolescent events. *Science* 169:397, 1970.
47. Van der Spuy ZM: Nutrition and reproduction. *Clin Obstet Gynecol* 12:579, 1985.
48. Berg HT, Nillius SJ, Wide L: Serum prolactin and gonadotrophin levels before and after luteinising hormone releasing hormone in the investigation of amenorrhoea. *Br J Obstet Gynaecol* 85:945, 1978.
49. McArthur JW, Bullen BA, Beitins IZ, Pagano M, Badger TM, Klibanski A: Hypothalamic amenorrhea in runners of normal body composition. *Endocr Res Commun* 7:13, 1980.
50. Herd HP, Palumbo PJ, Gharib H: Hypothalamic-endocrine dysfunction in anorexia nervosa. *Mayo Clin Proc* 51:711, 1977.
51. Hsu LKG: Outcome of anorexia nervosa. *Arch Gen Psychiatry* 37:1041, 1980.
52. Warren MP: The effects of exercise on pubertal progression and reproductive function in girls. *J Clin Endocrinol Metab* 51:1150, 1980.
53. Feicht CB, Johnston TS, Martin BJ, Sparkes KE, Wagner WW Jr: Secondary amenorrhoea in athletes. *Lancet* ii:1145, 1978.
54. Baker ER, Mathur RS, Kirk RS, Williamson HO: Female runners and secondary amenorrhea: Correlation with age, parity, mileage, and plasma hormonal and sex-hormone-binding globulin concentrations. *Fertil Steril* 36:183, 1981.
55. Marshall JC, Fraser TR: Amenorrhoea and anorexia nervosa: Assessment and treatment with clomiphene citrate. *Br Med J* 4:590, 1971.
56. Drinkwater BL, Nilson K, Chestnut CH, Bremner WJ, Shainholtz S, Southworth MB: Bone mineral content of amenorrheic and eumenorrheic athletes. *N Engl J Med* 311:277, 1984.
57. Franks S, Adams J, Mason H, Poulson D: Ovulatory disorders in women with polycystic ovary syndrome. *Clin Obstet Gynecol* 12:605, 1985.
58. Hague W, Adams J, Reeders S, Peto TEA, Jacobs HS: Familial polycystic ovaries: A genetic disease. *Clin Endocrinol (Oxf)* 29:593–606, 1988.
59. Franks S: Polycystic ovary syndrome: A changing perspective. *Clin Endocrinol (Oxf)* 31:87–120, 1989.
60. Polson DW, Adams J, Wadsworth J, Franks S: Polycystic ovaries—a common finding in normal women. *Lancet* 1:870–872, 1988.
61. Erickson GS, Hsueh AJW, Quigley ME, Rebar RW, Yen SSC: Functional studies of aromatase activity in human granulosa cells from normal and polycystic ovaries. *J Clin Endocrinol Metab* 49:514, 1979.
62. Rosenfield RL, Barnes RB, Cara JF, Lucky AW: Dysregulation of cytochrome P450c17α as the cause of polycystic ovarian syndrome. *Fertil Steril* 53:785–791, 1990.
63. Baird DT, Corker CS, Davidson DW, Hunter WN, Michie EA, Van Look PFA: Pituitary-ovarian relationships in polycystic ovary syndrome. *J Clin Endocrinol Metab* 45:798, 1977.
64. Zumoff B, Freeman R, Coupey S, Saenger P, Markowitz N, Krean J: A chronobiologic abnormality in luteinizing hormone secretion in teenage girls with the polycystic-ovary syndrome. *N Engl J Med* 309:1206, 1983.
65. Waldstreicher J, Santoro NF, Hall JE, Filicori M, Crowley WF Jr: Hyperfunction of the hypothalamo-pituitary axis in women with polycystic ovarian disease: Indirect evidence for partial gonadotroph desensitization. *J Clin Endocrinol Metab* 66:165–172, 1988.
66. Rebar J, Judd HL, Yen SSC: Characterization of the inappropriate gonadotropin secretion in polycystic ovary syndrome. *J Clin Invest* 57:1320, 1976.
67. Futterweit W: Pathologic anatomy of polycystic ovarian disease, in Futterweit W (ed): *Polycystic Ovarian Disease.* New York, Springer-Verlag, 1984, p 41.
68. Quigley ME, Rakoff JS, Yen SSC: Increased luteinizing hormone sensitivity to dopamine inhibition in polycystic ovary syndrome. *J Clin Endocrinol Metab* 52:231, 1981.
69. Barnes RB, Mileikowsky CN, Cha KY, Spencer CA, Lobo RA: Effects of dopamine and metoclopramide in polycystic ovary syndrome. *J Clin Endocrinol Metab* 65:506–509, 1986.
70. Futterweit W: Pituitary tumors and polycystic ovarian disease. *Obstet Gynecol* 62:74, 1983.
71. Buckler HM, McLachlan RI, MacLachlan VB, Healy DL, Burger HG: Serum inhibin levels in polycystic ovary syndrome: Basal levels and response to luteinizing hormone-releasing hormone agonist and exogenous gonadotrophin administration. *J Clin Endocrinol Metab* 55:798–803, 1988.
72. Lobo RA: Disturbances of androgen secretion and metabolism in polycystic ovary syndrome. *Clin Obstet Gynecol* 12:633, 1983.
73. Chang RJ, Loufer LR, Meldrum DR, De Fazio J, Lu JKH, Vale WW, Rivier JE, Hudd HL: Steroid suppression in polycystic ovarian disease after ovarian suppression by a long-acting gonadotropin-releasing hormone agonist. *J Clin Endocrinol Metab* 56:897, 1983.
74. Burghen GA, Givens JR, Kitabashi AE: Correlation of hyperandrogenism with hyperinsulinism in polycystic ovarian disease. *J Clin Endocrinol Metab* 50:113–116, 1980.
75. Givens JR, Kerber IJ, Wiser WL, Andersen RN, Coleman SA, Fish SA: Remission of acanthosis nigricans associated with polycystic ovarian disease and a stromal luteoma. *J Clin Endocrinol Metab* 38:347–355, 1974.
76. Chamlian DL, Taylor HB: Endometrial hyperplasia in young women. *Obstet Gynecol* 36:659, 1970.
77. Jackson RL, Docherty NB: The Stein-Leventhal syndrome: Analysis of 43 cases with special reference to association with endometrial carcinoma. *Am J Obstet Gynecol* 73:161, 1950.
78. Garcia JE, Jones GS, Wentz AC: The use of clomiphene citrate. *Fertil Steril* 28:707, 1977.
79. Kelly AC, Jewelewicz R: Alternate regimens for ovulation induction in polycystic ovarian disease. *Fertil Steril* 54:195–202, 1990.
80. Spruce BA, Kendall-Taylor P, Dunlop W, Anderson AJ, Watson MJ, Cook DB, Gray C: The effect of bromocriptine in the polycystic ovary syndrome. *Clin Endocrinol* 20:481, 1984.
81. Gadir AA, Mowafi RS, Alnaser HMI, Alrashid AH, Alonezi DM, Shaw RW: Ovarian electrocautery versus human meno-

pausal gonadotrophins and pure follicle stimulating hormone therapy in the treatment of patients with polycystic ovarian disease. *Clin Endocrinol (Oxf)* 33:585–592, 1990.
82. Ferriman D, Gallwey JD: The clinical assessment of body hair growth in women. *J Clin Endocrinol Metab* 21:1440, 1961.
83. Burgess CA, Edwards CRE: Hirsutography. *Br J Photography* 8:770, 1978.
84. Lobo RA, Groebelsmann U, Horton R: Evidence for the importance of peripheral tissue events in the development of hirsutism in polycystic ovary syndrome. *J Clin Endocrinol Metab* 57:393, 1983.
85. Barbieri MD, Ryan KJ: Hyperandrogenism, insulin resistance, and acanthosis nigricans syndrome: A common endocrinopathy with distinct pathophysiologic features. *Am J Obstet Gynecol* 147:90, 1983.
86. Siegel SF, Finegold DN, Lanes R, Lee PA: ACTH stimulation tests and plasma dehydroepiandrosterone sulfate levels in women with hirsutism. *N Engl J Med* 323:849–854, 1990.
87. Eldar-Geva T, Hurwitz A, Vecsei P, Pulti Z, Milwidsky A, Rusler A: Secondary biosynthetic defects in women with late-onset congenital adrenal hyperplasia. *N Engl J Med* 323:855–863, 1990.
88. Holdaway IM, Croxson MS, Frengley PA, Ibbertson HK, Sheehan A, Fraser A, Evans MC, Knox B, et al: Clinical and biochemical evaluation of patients with hirsutism. *Aust NZ J Obstet Gynaecol* 24:23, 1984.
89. Chetkowski RJ, DeFazio J, Shamonki I, Judd HL, Chang RJ: The incidence of late-onset congenital adrenal hyperplasia due to 21-hydroxylase deficiency among hirsute women. *J Clin Endocrinol Metab* 58:595, 1984.
90. Ehrmann DA, Rosenfield RL: Hirsutism—beyond the steroidogenic block. *N Engl J Med* 323:909–911, 1990.
91. Belisl S, Love EJ: Clinical efficacy and safety of cyproterone acetate in severe hirsutism: Results of a multicentered Canadian study. *Fertil Steril* 46:1015–1020, 1986.
92. Shapiro G, Evron S: A novel use of spironolactone: Treatment of hirsutism. *J Clin Endocrinol Metab* 51:429, 1980.
93. Barth JH, Cherry CA, Wojnarowski F, Dawber RP: Spironolactone is an effective and well tolerated systemic antiandrogen therapy for hirsute women. *J Clin Endocrinol Metab* 68:966–970, 1989.
94. Marshall WA, Tanner JM: Variations in pattern of pubertal changes in girls. *Arch Dis Child* 44:291, 1969.
95. Gemzell CA, Diczfalusy E, Tillinger KG: Clinical effect of human pituitary follicle stimulating hormone (FSH). *J Clin Endocrinol Metab* 18:1333, 1958.
96. Lazarus L: Suspension of the Australian human pituitary programme. *Med J Aust* 43:57–59, 1985.
97. Healy DL, Kovacs GT, Pepperell RJ, Burger HG: A normal cumulative conception rate with human pituitary gonadotropin. *Fertil Steril* 34:341, 1980.
98. Schenker JG, Polishuk WZ: Ovarian hyperstimulation syndrome. *Obstet Gynecol* 46:23, 1975.
99. Haning RV Jr, Boehalein LM, Carlson IH, Kuzma DL, Zweibel WJ: Diagnosis-specific serum 17β-estradiol upper limits for treatment with menotropins using a ^{125}I direct E_2 assay. *Fertil Steril* 42(6):882–889, 1984.
100. Healy DL, Burger HG: Serum follicle-stimulating hormone, luteinizing hormone and prolactin during the induction of ovulation with exogenous gonadotropin. *J Clin Endocrinol Metab* 56:474, 1983.
101. Fleming R, Haxton MJ, Hamilton MPR, McGune GS, Black WP, MacNaughton MC, Coutts JRT: Successful treatment of infertile women with oligomenorrhea using a combination of an LHRH agonist and exogenous gonadotrophins. *Br J Obstet Gynaecol* 92:369, 1985.
102. McFaul FB, Traub AI, Thompson W: Treatment of clomiphene citrate-resistant polycystic ovarian syndrome with pure follicle-stimulating hormone or human menopausal gonadotropin. *Fertil Steril* 53:792–797, 1990.
103. Leyendecker G, Struve T, Potz EJ: Induction of ovulation with chronic intermittent (pulsatile) administration of LHRH in women with hypothalamic and hyperprolactinaemic amenorrhea. *Arch Gynecol* 229:177, 1980.
104. Filicori M, Campaniello E, Michelacci L, Pareschi A, Ferrari P, Bolelli G, Flamigni C: Gonadotropin-releasing hormone (GnRH) analog suppression renders polycystic ovarian disease patients more susceptible to ovulation induction with pulsatile GnRH. *J Clin Endocrinol Metab* 66(2):327–333, 1988.
105. Hurley DM, Brian RJ, Burger HG: Ovulation induction with subcutaneous pulsatile gonadotropin-releasing hormone: Singleton pregnancies in patients with previous multiple pregnancies after gonadotropin therapy. *Fertil Steril* 40:575, 1983.
106. Hallberg L, Hogdahl IEM, Nilsson L, Rybog T: Menstrual blood loss—a population study. *Acta Obstet Gynecol Scand* 45:320, 1966.
107. Cole SK, Billewicz WZ, Thomson AM: Sources of variation in menstrual blood loss. *J Obstet Gynaecol Br Cwlth* 78:933, 1971.
108. Buller FJ: Observations on the clotting of menstrual blood and clot formation. *Am J Obstet Gynecol* 111:535, 1971.
109. Bonnar J, Shepherd VL, Dockerey CJ: The haemostatic system and dysfunctional uterine bleeding. *Res Clin Forum* 5:277, 1983.
110. Pickles VR, Hall WS, Best FA, Smith GN: Prostaglandins in endometrium and menstrual fluid from normal and dysmenorrhoeic subjects. *J Obstet Gynaecol Br Cwlth* 72:185, 1965.
111. Healy DL: The clinical significance of endometrial prolactin. *Aust NZ J Obstet Gynaecol* 24:111, 1984.
112. Smith SK, Abel MH, Kelly RW, Baird DT: A role for prostacyclin (PGI_2) in excessive menstrual bleeding. *Lancet* i:522, 1981.
113. Lane G, Sittle NC, Rider TA, Pryce-Davies J, Kine RJV, Whitehead MI: Dose-dependent effects of oral progesterone on the oestrogenised post-menopausal endometrium. *Br Med J* 287:1241, 1983.
114. Chan YW, Dawood MY, Fuchs F: Relief of dysmenorrhea with the prostaglandin synthetase inhibitor ibuprofen: The effect on prostaglandin levels in menstrual fluid. *Am J Obstet Gynecol* 135:102, 1979.
115. Garry R: Hysteroscopic alternatives to hysterectomy. *Br J Obstet Gynaecol* 97:199–207, 1990.
116. Freeman EW, Sondheimer S, Weinbaum PJ, Rickels K: Evaluating premenstrual symptoms in medical practice. *Obstet Gynecol* 65:500, 1985.
117. Reid RL, Yen SSC: Premenstrual syndrome. *Am J Obstet Gynecol* 139:85, 1981.
118. Bancroft J, Backstrom T: Premenstrual syndrome. *Clin Endocrinol (Oxf)* 22:247, 1985.
119. Wasp JSF, Butt WR, Edwards RL, Holder G: Hormonal studies in women with premenstrual tension. *Br J Obstet Gynaecol* 92:247, 1985.
120. Steege JF, Stout AL, Rupp SL: Relationships among premenstrual symptoms and menstrual cycle characteristics. *Obstet Gynecol* 65:398, 1985.
121. Muse KN, Cetel NS, Futterman LA, Yen SSC: The premenstrual syndrome: Effects of medical ovariectomy. *N Engl J Med* 311:1345, 1984.
122. Research on the menopause. Report of a WHO Scientific Group. World Health Organization technical report series 670, Geneva, 1981.
123. Kaufman DW, Slone D, Rosenberg L, Miettinen OS, Shapiro S: Cigarette smoking and age of natural menopause. *Am J Public Health* 70:420, 1980.
124. Richardson SJ, Senikas V, Nelson JF: Follicular depletion during the menopausal transition: Evidence for accelerated loss and ultimate exhaustion. *J Clin Endocrinol Metab* 65:1231–1237, 1987.
125. MacNaughton JA, Bangah M, McCloud PI, Hee J, Burger HG: Age related changes in follicle-stimulating hormone luteinising hormone, oestradiol and immunoreactive inhibin

in women of reproductive age. *Clin Endocrinol (Oxf)* 1992 (in press).
126. Sherman B, West JH, Korenman SG: The menopausal transition: Analysis of LH, FSH, estradiol, and progesterone concentrations during menstrual cycles of older women. *J Clin Endocrinol Metab* 42:629, 1976.
127. Metcalf MG, Donald RA, Livesey JH: Pituitary-ovarian function in normal women during the menopausal transition. *Clin Endocrinol (Oxf)* 14:245, 1981.
128. Gray RH: Biological and social interactions in the determination of late fertility. *J Biosoc Sci [Suppl]* 6:97, 1979.
129. Jaszmann L, van Lith ND, Zaat JCA: The perimenopausal symptoms. *Med Gynaecol Sociol* 4:268, 1969.
130. Tataryn IV, Lomax P, Bajorek JG, Chesarek W, Meldrum DR, Judd HL: Postmenopausal hot flushes: A disorder of thermoregulation. *Maturitas* 2:101, 1980.
131. Sturdee DW, Wilson KA, Pipili E, Crocker AD: Physiological aspects of menopausal hot flush. *Br Med J* 2:79, 1979.
132. Casper RF, Yen SSC, Wilkes MM: Menopausal flushes: A neuroendocrine link with pulsatile luteinizing hormone secretion. *Science* 205:823, 1979.
133. Chetkowski RJ, Meldrum DR, Steingold KA, Randle D, Lu JK, Eggena P, Hershman JM, Alkjaersig NK, et al: Biological effects of transdermal estradiol. *N Engl J Med* 314:1615, 1986.
134. Meldrum DR, Shamonki IM, Tataryn I, et al: Elevations in skin temperature of the finger as an objective index of postmenopausal hot flushes: Standardization of the technique. *Am J Obstet Gynecol* 135:713, 1979.
135. Dennerstein L, Burrows GD, Hyman GJ, Sharpe K: Hormone therapy and affect. *Maturitas* 1:247, 1979.
136. Hallstrom T: *Mental Disorder and Sexuality in the Climacteric.* Stockholm, Scandinavian University Books, Esselte Studium, 1973.
137. Youngs DD: Some misconceptions concerning the menopause. *Obstet Gynecol* 75:881–883, 1990.
138. Hasselquist MB, Goldberg N, Schroeter A, Spelsberg TC: Isolation and characterization of the estrogen receptors in human skin. *J Clin Endocrinol Metab* 50:76, 1980.
139. Brincat M, Wong Ten Yuen A, Studd JWW, Montgomery J, Magos AL, Savvas M: Response of skin thickness and metacarpal index to estradiol therapy in postmenopausal women. *Obstet Gynecol* 70:538, 1987.
140. Burger HG, Hailes J, Menelaus M, Nelson J, Hudson B, Balazs N: The management of persistent symptoms with oestradioltestosterone implants: Clinical, lipid and hormonal results. *Maturitas* 6:351, 1984.
141. Conference Report: Consensus Development Conference: Prophylaxis and treatment of osteoporosis. *Am J Med* 90:107–110, 1991.
142. Eriksen EF, Colvard DS, Berg NJ, Graham ML, Mann KG, Spelsberg TC, Riggs BL: Evidence of estrogen receptors in normal human osteoblast-like cells. *Science* 241:84, 1988.
143. Heaney RP et al: Calcium balance and calcium requirements in middle-aged women. *Am J Clin Nutr* 30:1603, 1977.
144. Stevenson JC, Whitehead MI, Padwick M, Endacott JA, Sutton C, Banks LM, Freemantle C, Spinks TJ, Hesp R: Dietary intake of calcium and postmenopausal bone loss. *Br Med J* 297:15–17, 1988.
145. Crilly RG, Francis RM, Nordin BEC: Steroid hormones, ageing and bone. *Clin Endocrinol Metab* 10:115, 1981.
146. Paganini-Hill A, Ross RK, Gerkins VR, Henderson BE, Arthur M, Mack TM: Menopausal estrogen therapy and hip fractures. *Ann Intern Med* 95:28, 1981.
147. Hutchinson TA, Polansky SM, Feinstein AR: Postmenopausal oestrogens protect against fractures of hip and distal radius. *Lancet* ii:705, 1979.
148. Weiss NS, Ure CL, Ballard JH, Williams AR, Daling JR: Decreased risk of fractures of the hip and lower forearm with postmenopausal use of estrogen. *N Engl J Med* 303:1195, 1980.
149. Lindsay R, Tohme JF: Estrogen treatment of patients with established postmenopausal osteoporosis. *Obstet Gynecol* 76:290–295, 1990.
150. Munk-Jensen N, Nielsen SP, Obel EB, Eriksen PB: Reversal of postmenopausal vertebral bone loss by oestrogen and progestogen: A double blind placebo controlled study. *Br Med J* 296:1150–1152, 1988.
151. Christiansen C, Riis BJ: 17β-Estradiol and continuous norethisterone: A unique treatment for established osteoporosis in elderly women. *J Clin Endocrinol Metab* 71:836–841, 1990.
152. Storm T, Thamsborg G, Steiniche T, Genant HK, Sorensen OH: Effect of intermittent cyclical etidronate therapy on bone mass and fracture rate in women with postmenopausal osteoporosis. *N Engl J Med* 322:1265–1271, 1990.
153. Civitelli R, Gonnelli S, Zacchei F, Bigazzi S, Vattimo A, Avioli LV, Gennari C: Bone turnover in postmenopausal osteoporosis: Effect of calcitonin treatment. *J Clin Invest* 82:1268–1274, 1988.
154. Riggs BL, Hodgson SF, O'Fallon WM, Chao EYS, Wahner HW, Muhs JM, Cedel SL, Melton LJ: Effect of fluoride treatment on the fracture rate in postmenopausal women with osteoporosis. *N Engl J Med* 322:802–809, 1990.
155. Bengtsson C, Lindquist O: Menopausal effects on risk factors for ischaemic heart disease. *Maturitas* 1:165, 1979.
156. Hjortland MC, McNamara PM, Kannel WB: Some atherogenic concomitants of menopause: The Framingham study. *Am J Epidemiol* 103:304, 1976.
157. Shibata H, Matsuzaki T, Hapana S: Relationship of relevant factors of atherosclerosis to menopause in Japanese women. *Am J Epidemiol* 109:420, 1979.
158. Bengtsson C: Ischemic heart disease in women. *Acta Med Scand [Suppl]* 549:75, 1973.
159. Gordon T, Kannell WB, Hjortland MC, McNamara PM: Menopause and coronary heart disease. The Framingham study. *Ann Intern Med* 89:157, 1978.
160. Rosenberg L, Hennekens CH, Rosner B, Belanger C, Rothman KJ, Speizer FE: Early menopause and the risk of myocardial infarction. *Am J Obstet Gynecol* 139:47, 1981.
161. Gustafson A, Svanborg A: Gonadal steroid effects on plasma lipoprotein and individual phospholipids. *J Clin Endocrinol Metab* 35:203, 1972.
162. Wallentin L, Larsson-Cohn V: Metabolic and hormonal effects of post-menopausal estrogen replacement: II. Plasma lipids. *Acta Endocrinol (Copenh)* 86:579, 1977.
163. Hirvonen E, Malkonen M, Manninen V: Effects of different progestogens on lipoproteins during postmenopausal replacement therapy. *N Engl J Med* 304:560, 1981.
164. Hunt K, Vessey M, McPherson K: Mortality in a cohort of long-term users of hormone replacement therapy: An updated analysis. *Br J Obstet Gynaecol* 97:1080–1086, 1990.
165. Von Kaulla E, Droegemuller W, Von Kaulla KN: Conjugated estrogens in hypercoagulability. *Am J Obstet Gynecol* 122:688, 1975.
166. Bonnar J, Haddon M, Hunter DH, Richards D, Thornton C: Coagulation system changes in postmenopausal women receiving oestrogen preparations. *Postgrad Med J* 52(Suppl 6):30, 1976.
167. Elkik F: Potency and hepato-cellular effects of oestrogens after oral, percutaneous, and subcutaneous administration, in van Keep PA, Utian WH, Vermeulen A (eds): *The Controversial Climacteric,* workshop 12. Lancaster, England, MTP, 1982.
168. Sitruk-Ware R, dePalacios I: Oestrogen replacement therapy and cardiovascular disease in post-menopausal women: A review. *Maturitas* 11:259–274, 1989.
169. Ross RK, Paganinni-Hill A, Mack TM, Arthur M, Henderson BE: Menopausal estrogen therapy and protection from ischaemic heart disease death. *Lancet* i:858, 1981.
170. Bush TL, Cowan LD, Barrett-Connor E, Criqui MH, Karon JM, Wallace RB, Al Tyroler H, Rifkind BM: Estrogen use and all-cause mortality. *JAMA* 249:903, 1983.
171. Bush TL, Barrett-Connor E, Cowan LD, Criqui MH, Wallace

RB, Suchindran CM, Tyroler HA, Rifkind BM: Cardiovascular mortality and noncontraceptive use of estrogen in women. *Circulation* 75:1102–1109, 1987.

172. Henderson BE, Paganini-Hill A, Ross RK: Decreased mortality in users of estrogen replacement therapy. *Arch Intern Med* 151:75–78, 1991.
173. Adams MR, Clarkson TB, Koritnik DR, Nash HA: Contraceptive steroids and coronary artery atherosclerosis in cynomolgus macaques. *Fertil Steril* 47:1010–1018, 1987.
174. Adams MR, Clarkson TB, Kaplan JR, Koritnik DR: Experimental evidence in monkeys for beneficial effects of estrogen on coronary artery atherosclerosis. *Transplant Proc* 21:3662–3664, 1989.
175. Mashchak CA, Lobo RA, Dozono-Takano R, Eggena P, Nakamura RM, Brenner PF, Mishell DR: Comparison of pharmacodynamic properties of various estrogen formulations. *Am J Obstet Gynecol* 144:511, 1982.
176. Schiff I, Seta HK, Cramer D, Tulchinsky D, Ryan KJ: Endometrial hyperplasia in women on cyclic or continuous estrogen regimen. *Fertil Steril* 37:79, 1982.
177. Mandel FP, Geola FL, Lu JKH, Eggena P, Sambhi MP, Hershman JM, Judd HL: Biological effects of various doses of ethinyl estradiol in postmenopausal women. *Obstet Gynecol* 59:673, 1982.
178. Steingold KA, Laufer L, Chetkowski RJ, de Fazio JD, Watt DW, Meldrum DR, Judd HL: Treatment of hot flushes with transdermal estradiol administration. *J Clin Endocrinol Metab* 61:627, 1985.
179. Yen SSC, Martin PL, Burnier AM, Czekala NM, Greaney Jr. MD, Callantine MR: Circulating estradiol, estrone and gonadotropin levels following the administration of orally active 17-beta-estradiol in postmenopausal women. *J Clin Endocrinol Metab* 40:518, 1975.
180. Englund DE, Johansson EDB: Pharmacokinetic and pharmacodynamic studies on estradiol valerianate administered orally to postmenopausal women. *Acta Obstet Gynecol Scand [Suppl]* 65:27, 1977.
181. Sturdee DW, Wade-Evans T, Paterson MEL, Thom M, Studd JWW: Relations between bleeding pattern, endometrial histology, and oestrogen treatment in menopausal women. *Br Med J* 1:575, 1978.
182. Whitehead MI, Hillard TC, Crook D: The role and use of progestogens. *Obstet Gynecol* 75:595, 1990.
183. Hovik P, Sundsbak HP, Gaasemyr M, Sandvik L: Comparison of continuous and sequential oestrogen-progestogen treatment in women with climacteric symptoms. *Maturitas* 11:75–82, 1989.
184. Editorial: Consensus statement on progestin use in postmenopausal women. *Maturitas* 11:175–177, 1988.
185. Gambrell RD Jr: The prevention of endometrial cancer in postmenopausal women with progestogens. *Maturitas* 1:107, 1978.
186. Hulka BS: When is the evidence for "no association" sufficient? *JAMA* 252:81, 1984.
187. Dupont WD, Page DL: Menopausal estrogen replacement therapy and breast cancer. *Arch Intern Med* 151:67–72, 1991.
188. Keirse MJNC: Aetiology of postmenopausal bleeding. *Postgrad Med J* 49:344, 1973.
189. Kahler VL, Creasy RK, Morris JA: Value of the endometrial biopsy. *Obstet Gynecol* 34:91, 1969.
190. Kovacs G, Burger HG, Hailes J, Medley G: A new method of endometrial sampling—the Gynoscann: A comparison with Vabra curettage. *Med J Aust* 148:498–503, 1988.
191. Kovacs GT, Burger HG: Endometrial sampling for women on perimenopausal hormone replacement therapy. *Maturitas* 10:259–262, 1988.
192. Gambrell RD, Greenblatt RV: Management of dysfunctional uterine bleeding with norgestrel-ethinyl estradiol. *Curr Med Dialogue* 42:80, 1975.
193. Shearman RP: Oral contraceptive agents. *Med J Aust* 144:180–192, 1986.
194. Mishell DR: Contraception. *New Engl J Med* 320:777–789, 1989.
195. Healy DL, Fraser HM: The antiprogesterones are coming: Menses induction, abortion, labour? *Br Med J* 290:580–581, 1985.
196. Elstein M (Ed.): A new specific progestogen for low dose oral contraception. New Jersey: Parthenon Publishing Group, 1989.
197. Baulieu EE, Segal S: The Antiprogestin-Steroid RU486 and Human Fertility Control. New York, Plenum, 1985.
198. Healy DL, Baulieu EE, Hodgen GD: Induction of menstruation by an antiprogesterone steroid (Mifepristone) in primates: site of action, dose response relationships and hormonal effects. *Fertil Steril* 40:253–260, 1983.
199. Kelly RW, Healy DL, Cameron IJ, Cameron IT, Baird DT: The stimulation of prostaglandin production by two antiprogesterone steroids in human endometrial cells. *J Clin Endocrinol Metab* 62:1116–1123, 1986.
200. Ulmann A: Use of RU486 for contragestion: An update. *Contraception* 36(suppl.): 27–31, 1987.

CHAPTER 18

Sexual Differentiation

Jeremy S. D. Winter
Robert M. Couch

Attempts to explain sexual dimorphism are as old as humankind itself, and countless theories have been promulgated to provide a rational basis for separate patterns of male and female development. Aristotle, with remarkable prescience, suggested that semen determines embryonic sex through its innate ability to impose maleness upon a process which otherwise tends to be female; the role of the female parent was seen to be essentially passive, providing the material and the environment for embryonic development. Two thousand years later light microscopy led to the description of spermatozoa, ova, and the events of fertilization. It was probably Mendel who first perceived that sex might be a genetic character, obeying the laws of inheritance, but, like many of his ideas, the notion remained buried until this century. In 1924 Painter provided direct evidence for the role of the male parent in human sex determination when he showed that human primary spermatocytes contain an unequal pair of chromosomes, termed X and Y, which segregate into different gametes during the first meiotic division,[1] a finding which has since been confirmed by modern techniques of chromosome analysis.

Sexual reproduction requires each parent to contribute equal (*haploid*) amounts of genetic material to the offspring, a mechanism which provides for rapid gene assortment, with an increased opportunity for favorable combinations of genes to develop and be selected in a changing environment. In higher organisms the parents are of different sexes, maintained separate and distinct by the actions of unpaired sex chromosomes which contain the genetic information for sex determination. One sex (in mammals XX, or female) is homogametic while the other (XY, or male) is heterogametic. The Y chromosome contains important male-determining factors that direct the embryo away from an otherwise predetermined course of female differentiation. Fisher has pointed out that it is not necessary for all male characters to be under the control of genes on the Y chromosome.[2] Rather, a single Y-linked gene need only cause male differentiation of the gonad; in turn, testicular hormones can activate or repress genes throughout the autosomal complement, a strategy which would allow any gene to become involved in producing sexual dimorphism.

The past quarter century has seen a flood of new information and new insights into both the initial genetic process of sex determination and the endocrine mechanisms which subsequently direct sexual differentiation; indeed, it is probable that no aspect of prenatal development is better understood. Vital clues about these events have been provided by patients with various anatomic abnormalities of sexual differentiation. It is therefore fitting that these insights have led to the development of rapid and exact techniques for diagnosis and specific forms of therapy which, if applied early and properly, can prevent much of the physical and psychological scarring which previously was the lot of these patients.

NORMAL SEX DETERMINATION AND SEXUAL DIFFERENTIATION

The appearance of a fertile adult with congruent secondary sexual characteristics and psychosexual orientation represents the denouement of a logical and ordered sequence which begins at conception with the establishment of *genetic sex*. In turn, the presence or absence of the male-determining portion of the Y chromosome defines *gonadal sex*, causing the indifferent embryonic gonad to become either a testis or an ovary. Subsequent differentiation of the internal genital ducts and the external genitalia follows a similar paradigm, in which indifferent common primordia show an innate tendency to feminize unless male patterns of development are imposed by secretions from the fetal testis. At birth the external genitalia provide the basis by which society assigns both gender role and legal sex. Later, during and after puberty, testicular or ovarian hormones induce secondary sexual characteristics which serve both to reinforce psychosexual identity and to signal adult reproductive capabilities. The six parameters of sexual dimorphism listed in Table 18-1 define the sum of what is meant by the terms *male* and *female*. In clinical situations of disordered sexual differentiation, the physician must be aware that complete diagnosis requires a definitive statement concerning each of these aspects of sexual development. In the absence of such information, the initiation of therapy, or even the assignment of sex of rearing, carries grave risk of a later psychosexual disaster.

Genetic Sex

In some fish and amphibians complete sex reversal can be caused by environmental influences such as hormones, but in mammals sex is solely and decisively determined by chromosomal mechanisms. All physicians are now familiar with the systematized array of metaphase chromosomes known as a *karyotype* (Fig. 18-1). The 22 pairs of autosomes and the unpaired (X and Y) sex chromosomes can each be characterized according to size, centromeric position, and a distinctive pattern of banding. Various techniques are used to demonstrate these bands, including fluorescent staining with quinacrine (Q banding) and several methods of Giemsa staining (G, C, or R banding). The chemical basis for specific bands is not entirely clear, but the bands appear to reflect not only variations in DNA base composition but also the nature and quantity of associated histone and nonhistone proteins. *An International System for Human Cytogenetic Nomenclature,* first developed in 1960 and revised at intervals, provides a standard method for the description of the regions and bands of both normal and structurally altered chromosomes.[3]

Chromosomal Errors

Chromosomal abnormalities include both deviations from the normal number (*aneuploidy*) and various structural changes in individual chromosomes.

Aneuploidy

During cell division a chromosome may be lost; this circumstance, known as *anaphase lag,* is more likely to occur if the chromosome is structurally abnormal. A more common mechanism for losing a chromosome (*monosomy*) or gaining extra chromosomes (*trisomy* or *polysomy*) is primary nondisjunction; in this case a pair of sister chromatids (during mitosis) or homologous chromosomes (during meiosis) fails to separate at metaphase, so that one daughter cell receives both members of the pair while the complementary cell receives none. If nondisjunction occurs during meiotic division, aneuploid gametes will ensue and the resulting embryo will contain a single aneuploid cell line. Nondisjunction occurring after fertilization during an early mitotic division will produce an individual with two or more cell lines. Such mosaicism, particularly for the sex chromosomes, is not uncommon and can be ruled out only by means of karyotype analysis of relatively large numbers of cells from a variety of tissues. *Mosaicism,* in which the different cell lines have the same genetic origin, must be differentiated from the much less common situation of *chimerism,* in which double fertilization of a binucleate ovum or fusion of two zygotes leads to a single embryo having two cell lines of different genetic origin (e.g., 46,XY/46,XX).

Structural Anomalies

Aberrations of chromosome structure arise through breakage, often followed by improper reunion of the fragments; these occurrences can lead to phenotypic abnormalities through a deficiency or duplication of genetic information or through a position effect. A simple *deletion* involves the loss of a portion of the short arm, designated *p* [e.g., 46,X,del(X)(p21), indicating deletion of the short arm of X distal to band Xp21], or of the long arm, designated *q*. *Ring chromosomes* occur after breaks in both the short and long arms, the ends of which then fuse, with loss of the acentric fragments [e.g., 46,X,r(X)]. *Duplications* may involve a portion of a single chromosome or *translocation,* in which genetic material is transferred from one chromosome to another. In translocation, although both chromosomes are structurally abnormal, the translocation may be balanced; however, an offspring receiving one of the translocation chromosomes without the other will be genetically unbalanced and presumably phenotypically abnor-

TABLE 18-1 Parameters of Sexual Dimorphism

	Determining factors		
	Female development	Male development	Identified by
Genetic sex	Homogametic (XX)	Heterogametic (XY)	Karyotype
Gonadal sex	Oocytes	Y-linked testis-determining factor (TDF)	Histology
Genital ducts	Innate tendency	Müllerian inhibiting substance; testosterone	Ultrasound
External genitalia	Innate tendency	Dihydrotestosterone	Examination
Gender role	Psychosocial factors	Psychosocial factors	Observation
Puberty	Estradiol	Testosterone	Hormone assay

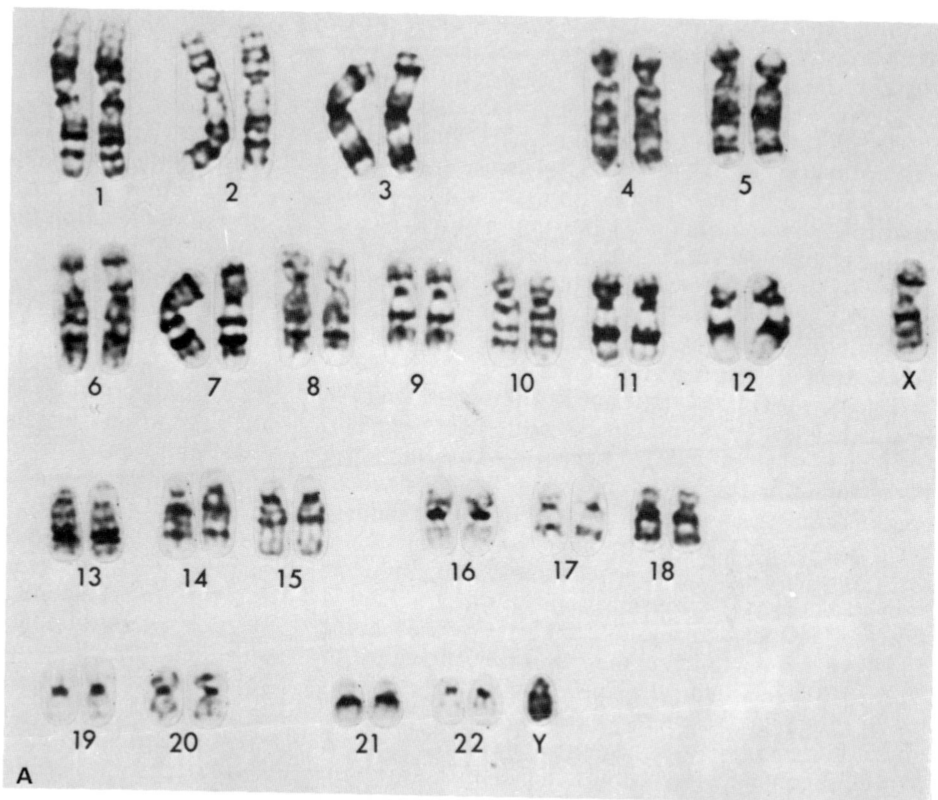

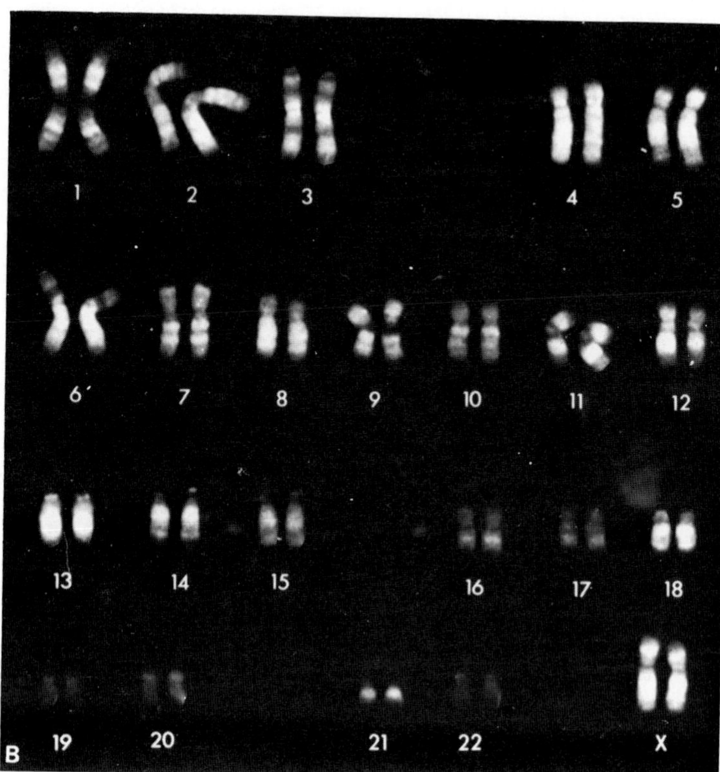

FIGURE 18-1 (*A*) Normal male karyotype (46,XY) pretreated with trypsin and Giemsa-stained to show characteristic banding patterns. (*B*) Normal female karyotype (46,XX) stained with quinacrine dihydrochloride to show fluorescent bands of differing intensity.

mal. *Isochromosomes* result from the loss of an entire arm with replication of the remaining one, so that the chromosome comes to have either two identical long arms [e.g., 46,X,iso(Xq)] or two short arms.

The frequency of chromosome abnormalities at conception has been estimated to be between 10 and 50 percent,[4] but most of these abnormalities terminate in early spontaneous abortion. Studies of human spermatozoa show abnormal chromosome complements in about 9 percent (range 0 to 28 percent in different donors), with aneuploidy and structural anomalies affecting every chromosome.[5] It is of interest that X-bearing sperm normally outnumber Y-bearing sperm by a ratio of 54:46, suggesting selective loss of the latter during gametogenesis. The incidence of significant abnormality involving the sex chromosomes is probably about 17 per 1000 conceptions;[6] most of these abnormalities, particularly those with a 45,X karyotype, lead to early abortion. Surveys of unselected liveborn infants indicate that sex chromosome abnormalities (mainly 47,XYY, 47,XXY, and 47,XXX) occur in 0.3 percent of males and 0.15 percent of females. The low incidence of 45,X newborns (about 0.01 percent) is in sharp contrast to the high frequency of this karyotype in spontaneous abortions.

The frequency of chromosome abnormalities in adult patients is naturally biased by preselection for reproductive disorders. For example, approximately 25 percent of young women with primary amenorrhea and 4 percent with secondary amenorrhea show an abnormal karyotype, usually 45,X or one of its variants.[7] About 10 percent of males with azoospermia show an abnormality. Similarly, one may expect to find a chromosomal abnormality such as reciprocal autosomal translocation or mosaicism for X chromosome aneuploidy in about 10 percent of couples with a history of recurrent abortion.[8]

The techniques of modern molecular biology, in particular the increasing availability of specific DNA probes for the sex chromosomes and for autosomal loci that regulate pituitary or gonadal hormone production, sex steroid action, and gametogenesis, have made possible the elucidation of point mutations and other minor genetic variants that may underlie reproductive dysfunction.

Properties and Functions of the Sex Chromosomes

It is probable that the X and Y chromosomes evolved from an ancestral pair of autosomes through translocation of sex-specific genes plus a mechanism to discourage crossing-over or gene exchange between the sex chromosomes during meiosis.

The Y Chromosome

The Y chromosome is the most specialized mammalian chromosome, being almost exclusively involved in the control of sex determination and fertility. By conventional cytogenetic methods, it contains a euchromatic portion that includes the entire short arm and the proximal long arm and a quinacrine-positive heterochromatic portion that includes the rest of the long arm and the centromeric region. In quinacrine-stained interphase cells this heterochromatic portion shows up as the fluorescent Y body, which usually is adjacent to the nuclear membrane (Fig. 18-2*A*) and which provides evidence of the number of Y chromosomes present. The occasional absence of the entire quinacrine-positive region in normal fertile males suggests that this region does not contain functional genes, being composed mainly of tandem DNA repeats.[9]

During male meiosis X/Y genetic exchange normally occurs only within the so-called pseudoautosomal region at the distal end of the short arm (Fig.

FIGURE 18-2 (*A*) A fluorescent Y chromatin mass (arrow) in an interphase nucleus, indicating the presence of the long arm of the Y chromosome. (*B*) An X chromatin mass in an interphase nucleus. In diploid lines the number of X chromatin bodies equals the number of X chromosomes minus one.

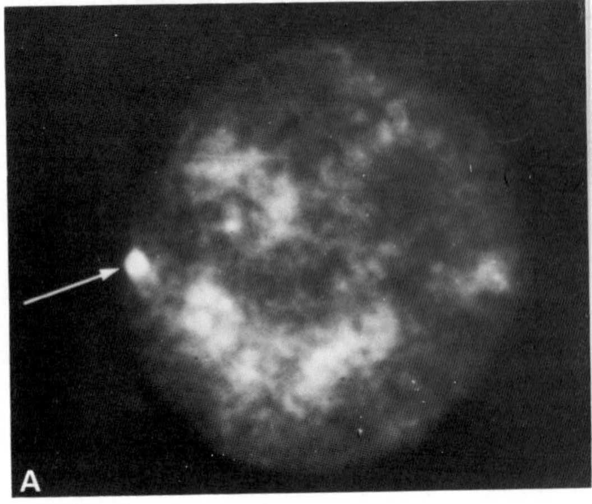

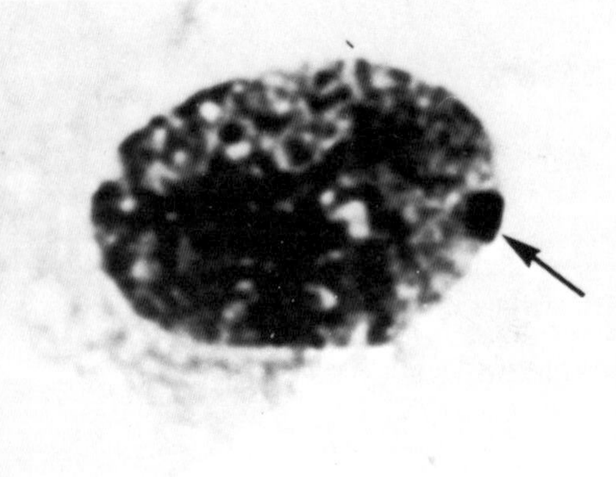

18-3); the only functional gene mapped to this region so far is MIC2, which encodes a cell-surface antigen of unknown function. The testis-determining gene, termed TDF in humans, is located on the distal short arm immediately adjacent to this pseudoautosomal region. A highly conserved gene has been identified here which is expressed only in the testis and encodes a protein with a potential DNA-binding domain.[10] Loss of this TDF gene causes XY gonadal dysgenesis, while its inappropriate exchange to the X chromosome during male meiosis results in an XX male.

There is considerable circumstantial evidence for the existence of other functional genes on the human Y chromosome. Some of these genes may be involved in the regulation of spermatogenesis and stature. Others appear to suppress the appearance of the somatic features of Turner's syndrome and to influence the predisposition to gonadoblastoma in the dysgenetic gonads of this disorder. H-Y antigen is a male-specific minor transplantation antigen found in all male tissues; there is evidence that its expression is controlled by a gene on the proximal long arm (Yq) of the Y chromosome.[11] A separate serologically detectable antigen, termed S_{xs} or H-Ys, which is expressed to a much greater extent in males, is probably encoded by a gene on chromosome 6. During the search for the testis-determining factor, Page et al.[12] identified a highly conserved gene termed ZFY on the short arm of the Y chromosome. Subsequently, it was established that this gene, which may encode a DNA-binding transcription factor, occurs also on the

FIGURE 18-3 Mapping of genes involved in sexual differentiation on the Y chromosome (*top*) and the X chromosome (*bottom*).

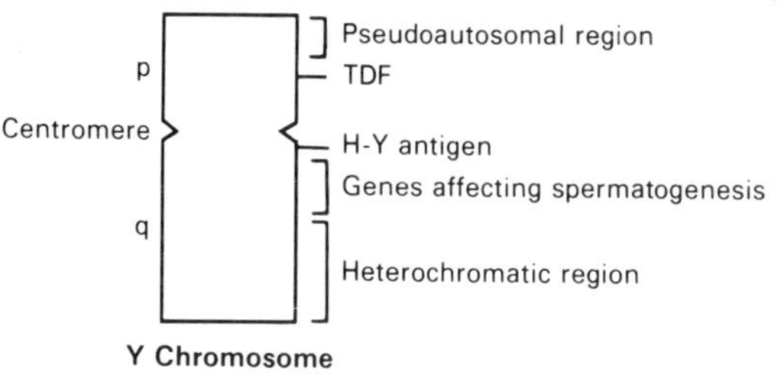

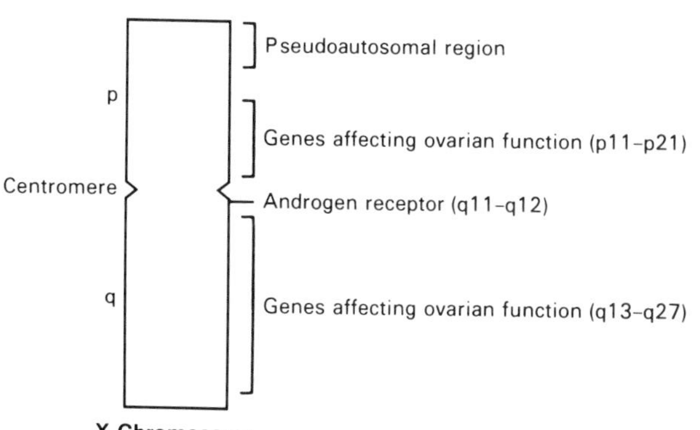

X chromosome and is autosomal in marsupials. Its true function is unclear, but it may be involved in germ cell differentiation.

Patients with structural abnormalities of the Y chromosome are usually normal but may show genital ambiguity or short stature. The abnormal Y chromosome is often lost through anaphase lag, in which case the patients demonstrate 45,X/46,XY mosaicism.

The X Chromosome

The X chromosome (Fig. 18-3) is a large metacentric chromosome which contains about 5 percent of the total DNA in a haploid set (22 autosomes plus the X). In sharp contrast to the Y chromosome, the X chromosome is involved in the function of every system in the body and contains at least 200 mapped genetic loci. These loci include genes that play important roles in the sexual differentiation of both males and females. The gene for the androgen receptor, which is essential in the male for both genital differentiation and secondary sexual characteristics, is located in band Xq11-12.[13] Male carriers of X-autosome translocations, regardless of the position of the break point on the X, usually are azoospermic or severely oligospermic, while ambiguous genitalia have been observed in males carrying a pericentric X inversion. Deletion mapping has shown that genes on the long arm of X (between bands Xq11 and Xq22) are involved in the expression of the stigmata of Klinefelter's syndrome. Such observations indicate the critical but still incompletely defined role that this chromosome plays in male reproductive function.[14]

There is a critical segment on the long arm of the X chromosome, lying between bands Xq13 and Xq27, which is essential for normal ovarian differentiation and function. Females with structural abnormalities or break points in this region present with premature follicular atresia leading to gonadal dysgenesis, primary or secondary amenorrhea, and infertility.[14] Although some deletions of the short arm (Xp) cause only short stature with normal sexual development, more severe abnormalities such as monosomy (45,X) or an isochromosome [46,X,iso(Xq)] give rise to the full Turner's syndrome, with gonadal dysgenesis, short stature, and somatic abnormalities.[15] It would appear, therefore, that determinants on both the short and long arms of the X chromosome are necessary for normal female growth and development.

The X chromosome also contains a large number of unpaired genes that are not present on the Y chromosome, defects of which cause disease in hemizygous males and females with monosomy X. Examples of these X-linked traits include color blindness, hemophilia A (factor VIII), hemophilia B (factor IX), and glucose-6-phosphate dehydrogenase deficiency, the loci for which are located on the long arm. The steroid sulfatase (STS) locus, which is involved in

X-linked ichthyosis and placental sulfatase deficiency, has been assigned to the distal part of the short arm.

Since normal 46,XX females obtain twice as many of these unpaired genes as do normal males, a dosage difference with effects similar to those of aneuploidy might be expected if there were not some mechanism for dosage compensation. This compensation is effected by inactivation of one X chromosome in the female early in development, so that the expressed dosage of X-linked genes is equivalent in males and females. This process is random but is fixed thereafter for each cell line; thus the female comes to be a mosaic of active paternal and maternal X chromosomes. Regardless of the number of X chromosomes present in a cell, all but one are inactivated. After inactivation, cell lines in which the active X is structurally abnormal may replicate less efficiently than do their normal counterparts, so that selection against this line may occur.

The inactive X chromosome can be identified during cell division in the presence of [^{3}H]thymidine by its asynchronous delayed pattern of DNA synthesis. In interphase cells this late-replicating X can be stained and visualized as an X chromatin, or Barr body, of about 1 μm diameter applied to the inner surface of the nuclear membrane (Fig. 18-2*B*). In smears of female buccal mucosa, X chromatin can be found in about 20 percent of cells. Sex chromatin also appears in the form of a drumstick-shaped accessory appendage on 1 to 15 percent of the nuclei of female polymorphonuclear leukocytes. The number of chromatin bodies in any diploid nucleus is one less than the total number of X chromosomes; thus the buccal smear of a 48,XXXY male will show two chromatin bodies, while that of a 45,X female will show none. Structural anomalies altering the size of the X chromosome may influence the size of the resulting mass of heterochromatin.

In recent years the concept of mammalian X inactivation and dosage compensation has been extended and modified to some degree.[16] In the embryo, even though X-linked genes become active in transcription as early as the two-cell stage, X inactivation does not occur until the early blastocyst stage. Thus very early female embryos show levels of X-linked enzyme activity twice as high as those of male embryos. The initiation of X inactivation seems to coincide with the beginning of cell differentiation and is seen first in the trophoderm, then in the primitive endoderm, and finally in the inner cell masses. Both somatic and germ cells appear to be derived from a common pool of X-inactivated cells. However, in females germ cells undergo genetic reactivation before entering meiosis so that both X chromosomes become active again in the primary oocytes of the fetal and postnatal ovary. This pattern is exactly the opposite of what occurs in the normal male during spermatogenesis, when the single active X chromosome undergoes apparent inactivation at the onset of meiosis.[17] These observations may underlie the accelerated oocyte degeneration seen in 45,X females and the azoospermia in 47,XXY males. In Turner's syndrome the lack of two active X chromosomes in the germ cell appears to accelerate follicular atresia; conversely, in Klinefelter's syndrome the extra, presumably active, X chromosome interferes with normal spermatogenesis.

In somatic cells and their descendants X inactivation affects all but a single X chromosome. It has therefore been difficult to explain the somatic abnormalities of 45,X and 47,XXY subjects. Indeed, in polysomy X the severity of the somatic anomalies correlates with the number of X chromosomes, a finding which suggests that dosage compensation as achieved by X inactivation is incomplete. Recent evidence has partially resolved this paradox by demonstrating that several loci, including those for the Xg^a red blood cell antigen and for microsomal STS, both of which are located at the distal end of the short arm, escape complete inactivation and are expressed by both X chromosomes. Therefore, X inactivation does not involve the entire chromosome and females normally express some gene loci in double dosage. Some inactivated genes may also be reactivated with aging.

The molecular basis of X chromosome inactivation is not entirely understood. Studies of X-autosome translocations have produced clear evidence that the process is initiated from an inactivation center on the X. Methylation of DNA cytosine residues plays a role since incorporation of 5-azacytidine to inhibit DNA methyltransferase can cause stable reactivation of loci on an inactive X chromosome. Some authors have suggested that similar processes of DNA methylation and demethylation are involved in all specialized tissue differentiation, but this has not been confirmed.[18]

Gonadal Sex

Although a person's genetic sex is determined at conception, for the first few weeks of fetal life the gonadal anlagen maintain a similar appearance in both sexes. This indifferent gonad forms at about 7 to 10 days in the mesenchyme at the ventral edge of the cranial medial part of the mesonephros and is invaded in turn by primordial germ cells and cells originating from the mesonephros and the coelomic epithelium. The large spherical germ cells probably arise in or close to the yolk sac endoderm; from there they migrate through the hindgut region and the dorsal mesentery to reach the gonadal ridge at around day 35 to 45, where they proliferate rapidly. The mesonephros itself contributes dense cell cords which in the male will form the rete testis and part of the epididymis and in the female will remain as the rete ovarii. It has been suggested that mesonephric cells within the gonad may give rise to Sertoli and granulosa cells, while Leydig cells, theca, and ovarian stroma arise from mesenchyme.[19] These findings emphasize that although the testis and ovary differentiate into dissimilar organs, they continue throughout life to show numerous homologies in their gametogenic and steroidogenic functions (Fig. 18-4).

Testicular Differentiation

The earliest sign of male differentiation is the appearance within the indifferent gonad of large numbers of Sertoli cells at about 6 to 7 weeks and the subsequent organization of seminiferous tubules containing Sertoli cells and primordial germ cells.[20] Selective destruction of germ cells before they reach the gonad confirms that these cells do not play a role in the initiation of testis differentiation. Rather, it appears that the TDF gene product acts autonomously to cause Sertoli cell differentiation and that all subsequent events reflect Sertoli cell activity.[21] Germ cells (gonocytes and spermatogonia) undergo mitotic division within the testicular cords as these structures grow in length, anastomose, and eventually become canalized. In contrast to the female, in the male meiosis does not occur before puberty.

At 8 weeks typical Leydig cells equipped with membrane receptors for human chorionic gonadotropin (hCG) and luteinizing hormone (LH) appear in the interstitium between the testicular cords; by 14 weeks they make up more than half the volume of the testis. These Leydig cells have the typical ultrastructural appearance of steroid-secreting cells and contain abundant amounts of steroidogenic enzymes. After the end of the fourth month the number of fetal Leydig cells decreases, and only a few are visible at term. The appearance and decline of fetal Leydig cells closely parallels the rise and fall of fetal serum hCG levels. Mean testis weight increases to about 850 mg at term and is greater than ovarian weight at every gestational age. The final stage of testis differentiation is descent through the inguinal canal to reach the scrotum at about 34 to 35 weeks gestation.

Ovarian Differentiation

In contrast to testicular development, which is independent of the presence of germ cells, differentiation of the ovary is largely defined in terms of germ cell maturation. At 7 to 9 weeks gestation clumps of oogonia undergoing mitotic division are scattered throughout the ovarian parenchyma. The first definitive sign of ovarian development is the onset of meiotic prophase in primary oocytes at around 10 to 11 weeks. The first meiotic division is arrested at the

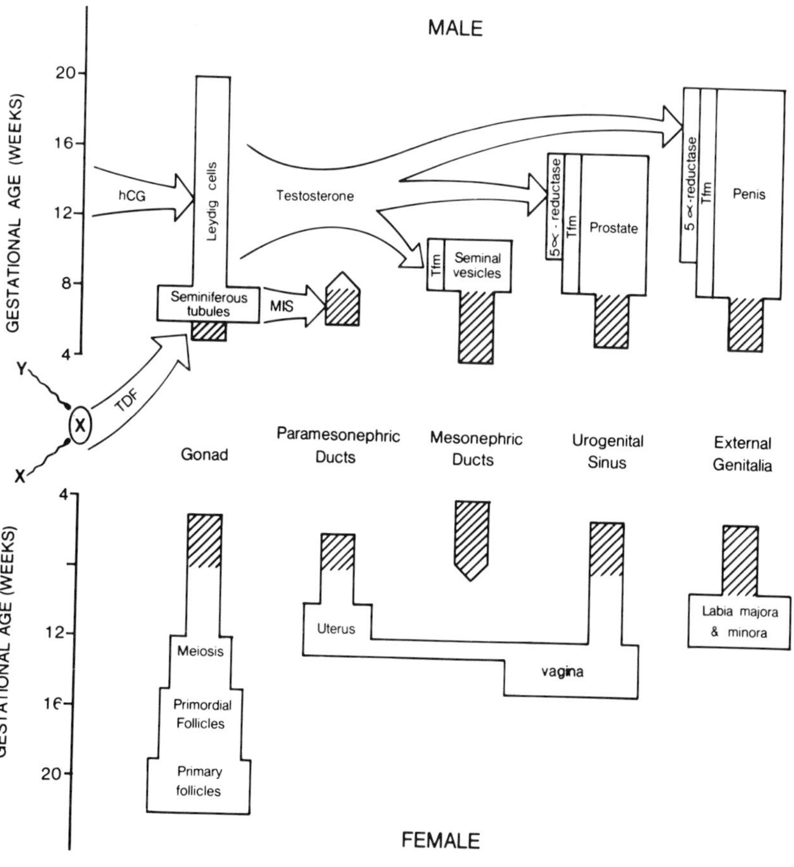

FIGURE 18-4 The major determinants of sexual differentiation, showing the cascade of genetic and endocrine effects and their timing in relation to fetal age in the male (*top*) and the female (*bottom*). The broad arrows show the sequential effects of the Y-linked testis-determining factor (TDF), human chorionic gonadotropin (hCG), müllerian inhibiting substance (MIS), and testosterone in directing male differentiation. Tfm indicates the target cell androgen receptor. The crosshatched segments refer to a sexually undifferentiated structure.

diplotene stage shortly before birth and is not completed until ovulation runs its course 12 to 40 years later. The peak number of germ cells is observed at midpregnancy, when the fetal ovary contains up to 7 million oogonia, oocytes, and degenerating cells. At about 13 weeks gestation oocytes become surrounded by follicular cells,[22] and by 17 weeks most oocytes are in primordial follicles. After 22 to 25 weeks multilayered and even a few antral follicles can be seen; the newborn ovary still contains mainly primary and primordial (single-layer) follicles, although small numbers of more mature and atretic forms occur. Although small amounts of steroid hormones can be produced by theca and interstitial cells, which are homologous with Leydig cells, their nature and local significance for oocyte maturation remain unclear.

The most remarkable phenomenon of ovarian development during the latter half of pregnancy and indeed during postnatal life is a decline in the total germ cell population as a result of atresia. By term the ovaries contain about 2 million germ cells, but only about 400 of these cells will survive to ovulate during a woman's reproductive life.

Preservation of a viable follicle requires an oocyte equipped with two active X chromosomes. Females with various chromosomal abnormalities show inadequate ovarian development and excessive loss of germ cells. Thus in 45,X Turner's syndrome, germ cells migrate to the gonad and undergo mitosis, but subsequently the rate of loss through degeneration is accelerated, leaving the neonate with only a few follicles. There is evidence that the genes necessary for normal follicular development are found on both the long and short arms of the X chromosome; the syndrome of autosomal recessive XX gonadal dysgenesis suggests that other genes are also involved.

Differentiation of the Genital Ducts

The mesonephric, or wolffian, ducts appear in the fetus at about 4 weeks gestation; they then grow caudally, become canalized, and open into the cloaca. The mesonophric nephrons, except for those contiguous with the rete system of the gonad, degenerate once the definitive kidney (metanephros) forms, but their ducts become incorporated into the genital system. The paramesonephric (müllerian) ducts originate at about 6 weeks gestation as solid cords of coelomic epithelial cells lateral to the mesonephric ducts which grow caudally and cross the epithelial cells ventrally to reach the urogenital sinus. These paired cords become canalized; caudally, where they meet in the midline, they fuse to form a single uterovaginal canal. Thus by 7 weeks gestation each fetus is equipped with the primordia of both male and female genital ducts (Fig. 18-5).

Female Internal Genital Development

In female fetuses the mesonephric ducts degenerate relatively early, leaving only remnants of tubules that can be identified later as the epoöphoron, paraoöphoron, and Gartner's duct. The partially fused paramesonephric ducts provide the paired fallopian tubes, the midline uterine primordium, and, in collaboration with tissue contributed by the urogenital sinus, the vaginal primordium. The development of these structures does not depend on hormonal or other influences from the ovary. However, it is contingent on the prior appearance of the mesonephric ducts; thus renal aplasia is commonly associated with agenesis of the fallopian tube, uterus, and vagina. Although the female internal genitalia differentiate morphologically somewhat later than do those of the male, there is evidence that they are functionally committed to become female by as early as 8 weeks gestation.

Male Internal Genital Development

The development of male internal genitalia involves two separate processes: regression of the paramesonephric ducts and stabilization of the mesonephric ducts. These processes are mediated by two secretions of the fetal testis: müllerian inhibiting substance (MIS), also called antimüllerian hormone, produced by the Sertoli cells and testosterone from the fetal Leydig cells (Fig. 18-4).

Müllerian Inhibiting Substance

Regression of the paramesonephric ducts begins at about 8 weeks gestation, initially adjacent to the caudal pole of the testis and then extending cranially and caudally. In the normal male only the cranial tip, which becomes the appendix testis, is spared. Close juxtaposition of the paramesonephric duct and the ipsilateral testis is necessary to initiate regression, but even large amounts of testosterone applied locally cannot duplicate the effect. Rather, paramesonephric regression is induced by the local paracrine action of MIS secreted by Sertoli cells of the ipsilateral testis.

MIS is a dimeric glycoprotein (molecular mass of 140,000 dalton) encoded by a gene in the short arm of chromosome 19.[23,24] It possesses interesting structural homologies with both transforming growth factor β (TGF-β) and the beta chain of inhibin and appears at around 7 weeks gestation, at the time of Sertoli cell differentiation. Secretion of MIS appears to be enhanced by cyclic AMP but is not regulated by known factors such as follicle stimulating hormone (FSH) or testosterone.[25,26] Regression of the paramesonephric ducts occurs in response to the paracrine effect of MIS from the ipsilateral testis. The mechanism of this action is not clear but may involve inhibition of phosphorylation of membrane protein.[27]

MIS is still detectable in males at birth and is secreted postnatally by juvenile and adult Sertoli cells, although levels are lower after the onset of puberty.[28] Circulating MIS is undetectable in females at birth, but some is secreted by postnatal ovarian granulosa cells. The functions of MIS in the

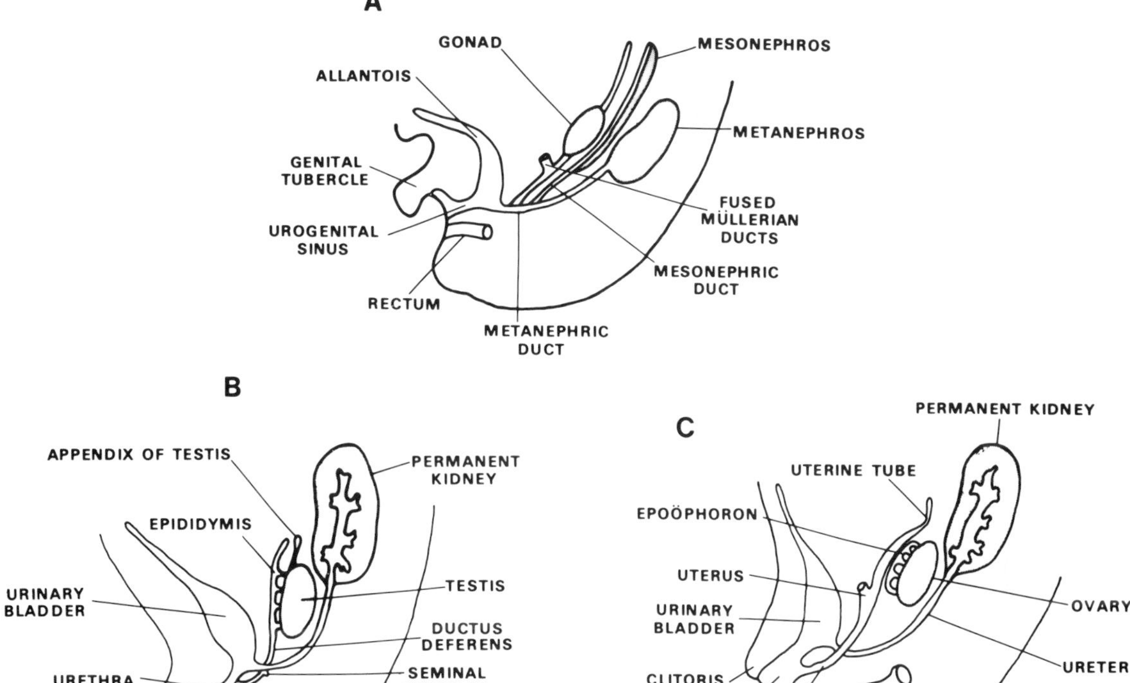

FIGURE 18-5 Diagrammatic sagittal sections of the internal genitalia of an 8-week fetus (*A*) and of male (*B*) and female (*C*) fetuses at 13 weeks gestation. [*From Smail P, Reyes FI, Winter JSD, Faiman C, in Kogan SJ, Hafez ESE (eds): Pediatric Andrology. The Hague, Martinus Nijhoff, 1981, p 11.*]

male after paramesonephric duct involution is not known; there is some evidence that in the female MIS may act as an inhibitor of oocyte meiosis.[29] Exposure of fetal ovaries to MIS causes inhibition of germ cell replication, suppression of aromatase activity, and the appearance of seminiferous tubulelike structures, suggesting that this factor may also play a role in normal testis development.[30–32] It is therefore possible to postulate a model of male development in which the TDF gene product triggers Sertoli cell differentiation and activates MIS gene expression. MIS could then act in an autocrine fashion to induce further differentiation of the Sertoli cell (which has MIS receptors) and thus could eventually influence Leydig cell differentiation, germ cell proliferation, seminiferous tubule formation, and even testicular descent.[33]

Testosterone

Stabilization and differentiation of the paired mesonephric ducts to form the vasa efferentia, epididymis, vasa deferentia, ejaculatory ducts, and seminal vesicles is dependent on local high concentrations of androgen from the ipsilateral testis. Androgen receptors in the ductal cells bind both testosterone and dihydrotestosterone; however, since only small amounts of the latter are synthesized by the testis and since the ductal cells themselves appear to lack 5α-reductase until after differentiation, it is generally assumed that testosterone is the active intracellular mediator that is primarily responsible.[34]

In patients with asymmetric gonadal differentiation, duct development on each side correlates closely with the degree of testicular development on the same side. Patients with enzymatic defects in testosterone biosynthesis or defective androgen receptors show rudimentary mesonephric duct structures, but in genetic 5α-reductase deficiency male genital ducts are normal. That this effect of testosterone is a local paracrine effect rather than a blood-borne endocrine effect is underscored by the failure of adrenal androgens to prevent normal regression of the mesonephric ducts in females with congenital adrenal hyperplasia.

Differentiation of the Urogenital Sinus and External Genitalia

For the first 2 months of prenatal development the external genitalia are identical in both sexes. They consist of a midline genital tubercle (*phallus*) and lateral labioscrotal swellings. Behind these structures lies the urogenital sinus, into which both the ureters and the internal genital ducts open.

Feminization of the External Genitalia

In females the phallus remains small and bends ventrally, the anogenital distance remains short, and the labioscrotal swellings and urethral groove do not fuse in the midline. The labioscrotal swellings become the labia majora, the separate genital folds become the labia minora, and the phallic part of the urogenital sinus becomes the vestibule (Fig. 18-6). The urogenital sinus is divided by downgrowth of a vaginal plate which approaches the perineum to provide separate urethral and uterovaginal access to the exterior. The contribution of paramesonephric duct tissue to the upper vagina is indicated by the abnormally shallow vagina of patients with complete testicular feminization, in whom the paramesonephric ducts regress. It appears that the development of female external genitalia is independent of ovarian influence, although prenatal exposure to diethylstilbestrol can cause persistence of müllerian-derived vaginal epithelium, with vaginal adenosis and a predisposition to malignant transformation.

Masculinization of the External Genitalia

During male differentiation the labioscrotal swellings and urethral folds fuse in the midline to form the scrotum and a penis enclosing the phallic urethra (Fig. 18-6). This process, which is imposed by testicular androgens, begins at 9 weeks and is complete by 14 weeks gestation. The urogenital sinus differentiates into the male urethra and the prostate. During the latter half of pregnancy the penis continues to enlarge, with a rate of growth three to four times that of the female clitoris.[35] During this same period the testes descend into the scrotum, a process that appears to be androgen-dependent, although other testicular factors may play a role.[33,36] In males with deficient testicular function the prostatic utricle, which is homologous to the female upper vagina, is commonly larger than normal.

Hormonal Sex: Differentiation of the Hypothalamic-Pituitary-Gonadal Axis

Gonadal Steroid Production

By the time Leydig cells can be recognized at 6 to 7 weeks fetal age the fetal testis contains the necessary enzymes for the synthesis of testosterone from various substrates, although the preferred substrate is probably circulating low-density lipoprotein cholesterol. Testicular concentrations of testosterone rise to a peak at 12 to 14 weeks gestation and then decline, a pattern which correlates closely with the growth and involution of fetal Leydig cells and with testicular mRNA levels for certain key steroidogenic

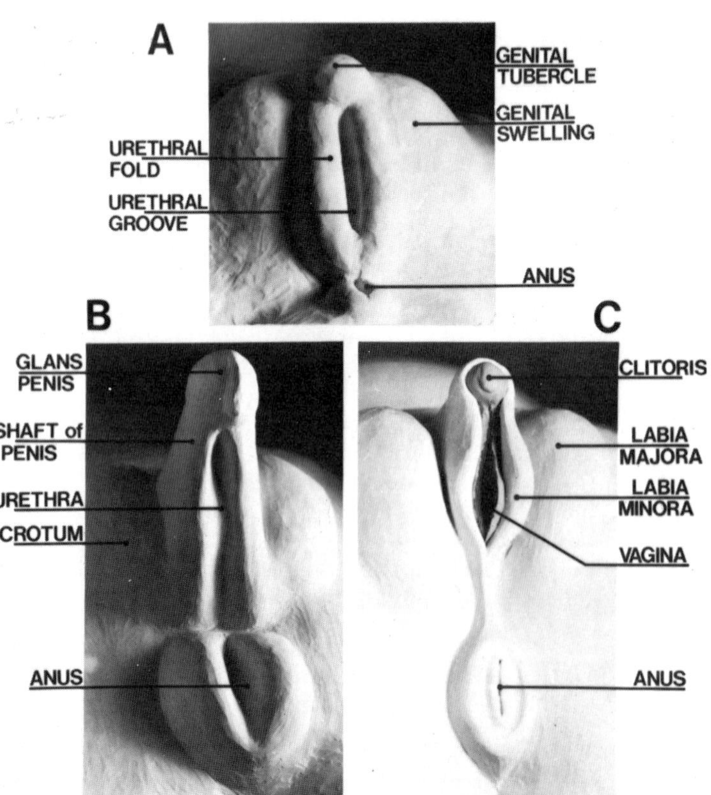

FIGURE 18-6 Models of the external genitalia in an 8-week undifferentiated fetus (*A*) and in male (*B*) and female (*C*) fetuses at 13 weeks gestation. [*From Smail P, Reyes FI, Winter JSD, Faiman C, in Kogan SJ, Hafez ESE (eds): Pediatric Andrology. The Hague, Martinus Nijhoff, 1981, p 12.*]

enzymes.[37,38] Although the fetal ovaries of some mammalian species contain enzymes for both the synthesis of androgens and their aromatization to estrogen, there is no evidence that the human fetal ovary secretes significant amounts of sex steroids, at least during the first half of pregnancy, when sexual differentiation is taking place.

Sex Steroids in the Fetal Circulation

The initial local or paracrine action of fetal testosterine is to stabilize development of the ipsilateral mesonephric duct and possibly to stimulate growth of the testis itself. Soon, however, male fetal serum testosterone concentrations begin to rise, reaching peak concentrations of 200 to 600 ng/dl (7 to 21 nmol/L) at 16 to 18 weeks gestation, values which are in the adult male range.[37] After midpregnancy, as Leydig cells involute male serum testosterone levels gradually decline, but they remain higher than female levels until term. At the same time the fetus is exposed to high concentrations of steroids from the placenta, notably estrogens and progesterone, and from the adrenal cortex, in particular dehydroepiandrosterone sulfate. There is no significant sex difference in serum concentrations of these steroids; presumably, therefore, they do not play a direct role in sexual differentiation, but they may influence the process through their effects on gonadal steroidogenesis, binding of steroids by serum proteins, and target cell receptor occupancy.

Serum levels of sex steroid–binding globulin (TeBG) are only about one-twentieth of those in maternal serum, and the human fetus does not appear to produce any other high-affinity androgen-binding protein. Although albumin serves as a low-affinity high-capacity carrier of many steroids, its concentration is also low in the fetal circulation. The effect of this low level of sex steroid binding is to increase the fraction of serum testosterone which is free and therefore presumably active.

Actions of Sex Steroids on the Genitalia

The changing patterns of testosterone concentrations in the fetal testis and circulation, in relation to the major events of male genital development, are summarized in Fig. 18-7. Testosterone appears first in high concentrations in the testis itself, where, by a local paracrine effect, it induces masculinization of the ipsilateral mesonephric duct. Subsequently, circulating testosterone levels become sufficiently high to initiate masculinization of the urogenital sinus and external genitalia.

In all these target cells specific high-affinity androgen receptors can be found prior to differentiation. Androgens bind to this nuclear receptor protein, and the steroid-receptor complex binds to specific chromatin acceptor sites to initiate transcription of new messenger RNA;[39] in turn, this RNA is processed and transported to cytoplasmic ribosomes, where it is translated for synthesis of andro-

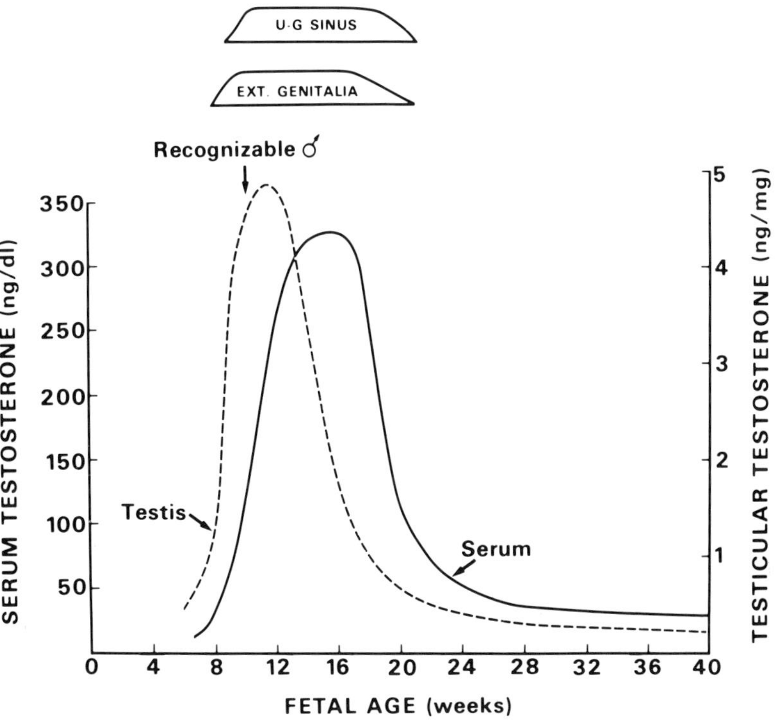

FIGURE 18-7 The relation of changes in mean testicular and serum testosterone concentrations to the time of development of the mesonephric ducts (W.D.) and virilization of the urogenital (U-G) sinus and external genitalia in male fetuses. (*From Winter et al.*[37])

gen-induced proteins. There is evidence that the actual target for these androgen effects is the mesenchyme of the genital anlagen, which in turn induces specific patterns of morphogenesis, cytodifferentiation, and functional activity in the overlying epithelium.[40]

The androgen receptor protein has a higher binding affinity and a slower rate of dissociation for dihydrotestosterone than for testosterone itself. The enzyme necessary for this intracellular conversion—5α-reductase—does not appear in the mesonephric ducts until development is already well advanced, but high local concentrations of testosterone are sufficient to accomplish masculinization. The urogenital sinus and external genitalia contain active 5α-reductase as soon as testosterone appears in the circulation; it therefore seems likely that masculinization of these structures is accomplished by lower concentrations of the more potent androgen dihydrotestosterone.

The androgen receptor (Tfm) gene has been cloned[41,42] and localized to band Xq11-12 of the X chromosome.[13] The 5α-reductase gene is autosomal. Thus, in normal circumstances both sexes can respond to circulating androgen; the direction of genital differentiation is determined solely by testicular testosterone production. Defects in testosterone synthesis, deficient 5α-reductase activity, and an ineffective androgen receptor will each prevent normal genital masculinization of the genetic male, although in 5α-reductase deficiency mesonephric duct development is normal. Conversely, exposure of a female fetus to high levels of circulating androgen does not induce mesonephric duct development but does inhibit separation of the vagina from the urogenital sinus and promotes labioscrotal fusion and clitoral hypertrophy.

Control of Fetal Gonadal Function

Chorionic Gonadotropin

There is considerable circumstantial evidence that testosterone synthesis by Leydig cells during the period of genital differentiation is dependent on hCG, although one cannot rule out the possibility that steroidogenesis in the very youngest testes may be initiated by other factors.[43] Thus hypopituitary males do not demonstrate genital ambiguity, although micropenis and cryptorchism are often observed. Chorionic gonadotropin appears in the maternal circulation immediately after implantation of the blastocyst; levels rise to a peak at about 10 weeks fetal age and then decline, although significant placental production continues until term. The pattern in the fetal circulation of both sexes is similar, but fetal hCG concentrations are only about one-thirtieth of those in the maternal compartment.[37]

Fetal Leydig cells, but not ovarian cells, have specific membrane receptors for LH and hCG; the number of these receptors increases to a maximum at 15 to 18 weeks gestation and then declines. Via a mechanism that appears to utilize cyclic AMP as the intracellular second messenger, hCG increases the number of low-density lipoprotein receptors, enhances de novo cholesterol synthesis, and stimulates mitochondrial cholesterol side-chain cleavage, all of which serve to increase the pool of available pregnenolone for androgen biosynthesis.[44]

Pituitary Gonadotropins

Although maternal pituitary gonadotropins do not cross the placental barrier, the fetal pituitary after about 9 weeks gestation produces significant amounts of FSH and LH. By 4 to 5 weeks fetal age the pituitary anlage has the ability to synthesize glycoprotein hormone α subunit, but gonadotropin releasing hormone (GnRH)–mediated hypothalamic stimulation is probably necessary for the synthesis of the hormone-specific β subunit and thus of intact FSH and LH.

Both gonadotropins appear in the fetal circulation at about 11 to 12 weeks and rise to peak concentrations at midpregnancy.[47] Serum FSH concentrations are much higher in female fetuses, in whom adult castrate values occur, than in male fetuses, in whom values are in the normal adult range. This sex difference demonstrates that a negative feedback mechanism mediated by testicular androgens is already operative by midgestation; in experimental animals, castration of the male fetus raises gonadotropin levels to the female range while castration of the female has no effect. After 28 weeks gestation serum gonadotropin levels decline in both sexes, a phenomenon that probably reflects maturation of placental estrogen–mediated feedback inhibitory mechanisms. The decline in Leydig cell testosterone production in the latter half of pregnancy would appear to result from the combined effects of a decline in circulating levels of hCG, FSH, and LH and direct inhibition of androgen biosynthesis by high levels of circulating placental estrogens.

The pattern of mean serum hCG and pituitary gonadotropin concentrations in the male fetus, in relation to changes in testicular morphology and function, is summarized in Fig. 18-8. While hCG is the major gonadotropin in the fetal circulation and clearly drives testosterone synthesis during genital differentiation, pituitary gonadotropins become relatively more significant in later gestation and influence such phenomena as phallic growth and testicular descent. The testes of anencephalic and hypogonadotropic fetuses show reduced numbers of Leydig cells. In addition, they may show reduced numbers of spermatogonia, suggesting that FSH- or possibly LH-mediated testosterone secretion plays a role in germ cell maturation.

The relationships between serum gonadotropins and ovarian development are summarized in Fig.

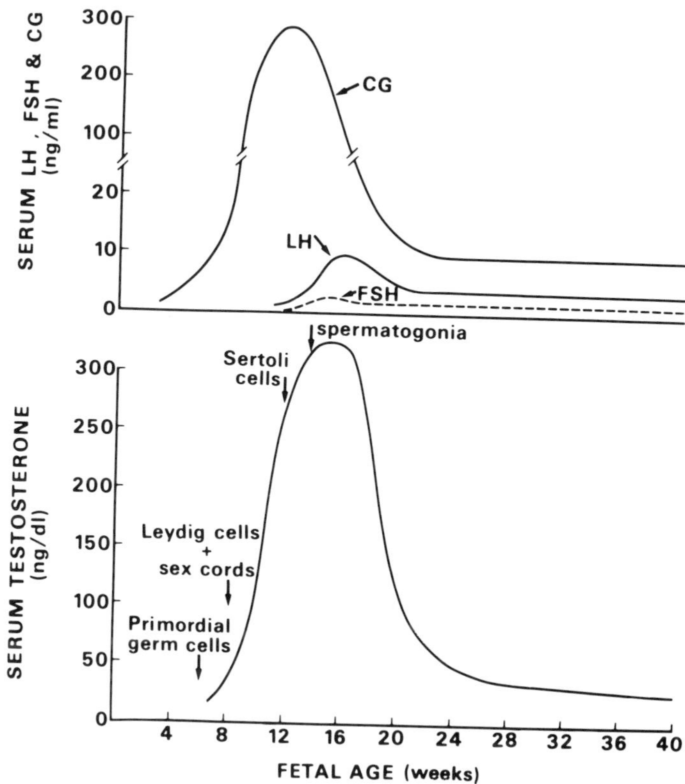

FIGURE 18-8 A schematic summary of the temporal relation between mean serum concentrations of hCG, LH, and FSH; mean serum testosterone concentrations; and morphologic development of the fetal testis. (*From Winter et al.*[37])

18-9. Ovarian development proceeds normally in anencephalic fetuses until about 32 weeks gestation; after this one observes reduced ovarian size and accelerated atresia with premature loss of germ cells and absence of antral follicles, suggesting inadequate granulosa cell proliferation and differentiation. This coincides with the timing of the appearance of FSH receptors in ovarian granulosa cells.

There is considerable evidence that fetal pituitary gonadotropin secretion is regulated by hypothalamic GnRH. Neurons expressing pro-GnRH mRNA appear in the nasal area of the brain by 5 weeks fetal age and migrate to the basal hypothalamus.[45] By 9 to 11 weeks GnRH-secreting neurons can be demonstrated which have their perikarya in the pericommissural, preoptic, lamina terminalis, and perimamillary regions; their axons end in the median eminence apposed to a capillary plexus which connects to the anterior pituitary, although a clearly defined hypothalamic-hypophyseal portal system develops later. Between 11 and 14 weeks gestation there is a 14-fold rise in hypothalamic GnRH content which parallels the increase in pituitary gonadotropin secretion.[46]

By midgestation the fetus demonstrates pulsatile GnRH release; both in vivo and in vitro fetal pituitary gonadotropin secretion is enhanced by GnRH administration[47] and blocked by specific GnRH antagonists.[48] The striking sex difference in circulating FSH and LH levels at midpregnancy suggests that testosterone in the male fetus suppresses gonadotropin release. Thus orchiectomy increases fetal FSH and LH levels, an effect that can be blocked by the administration of testosterone. As one would expect, fetal ovariectomy has no effect on gonadotropin levels. The subsequent decline in gonadotropin secretion in both sexes presumably reflects the appearance of specific estrogen receptors in the hypothalamus and pituitary and maturation of a feedback system mediated by placental estrogens.

Less is known about central nervous system (CNS) regulation of fetal hypothalamic GnRH release. Certainly by midgestation hypothalamic nuclei are developed and can produce significant amounts of potential regulators such as dopamine, norepinephrine, and serotonin. Observations that neurons in the arcuate-median eminence unit of the fetal hypothalamus contain β-endorphin and that fetal hypothalamic GnRH secretion in vitro is responsive to naloxone suggest the possibility that endogenous opiates exert a tonic inhibitory influence on GnRH release at this time.[49] In addition, material which immunologically resembles GnRH is produced by the placenta; its relevance for the regulation of fetal pituitary function is unclear, although it does appear to influence placental hCG synthesis.[50,51]

In addition to gonadotropins, other factors of placental or pituitary origin, such as growth hormone, may influence fetal gonadal growth and differentiation. The fetal testis shows significant expression of

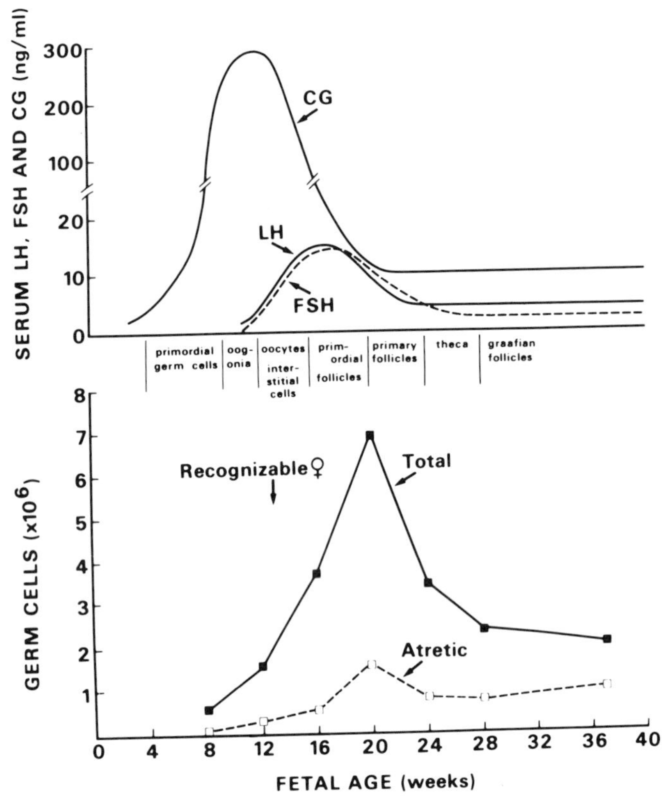

FIGURE 18-9 A schematic summary of the temporal relation between mean serum concentrations of hCG, LH, and FSH; morphologic development of the fetal ovary; and ovarian total content of germ cells. (*From Winter et al.*[37])

IGF-II.[52] Other local growth factors, including insulin-like growth factor I (IGF-I), fibroblast growth factor, epidermal growth factor, and (TGF-β), influence the development of other fetal systems and may well play a role in the developing gonad. Inhibin and activin are structurally related dimeric gonadal glycoproteins which may act to modulate both pituitary FSH secretion and various intragonadal processes. Inhibin levels are much higher in midtrimester fetal testes than in fetal ovaries,[53] and secretion of this glycoprotein appears to be stimulated by both FSH and hCG. The observation that inhibin/activin subunit synthesis begins later in the fetal ovary than in the testis may explain in part why FSH secretion declines earlier in male fetuses than it does in female fetuses.[54] Inhibin is also produced by the placenta, where it may be involved in the suppression of hCG secretion in late gestation.[55]

Perinatal Adaptations of the Reproductive Endocrine System

By term, the pituitary-gonadal axis of the human infant is structurally complete and capable of relatively mature function.[56] Circulating levels of placental sex steroids such as estrone (900 to 4000 ng/dl), estradiol (200 to 1600 ng/dl), estriol (1200 to 15,000 ng/dl), 17-hydroxyprogesterone (1000 to 7000 ng/dl), and progesterone (12,000 to 50,000 ng/dl) are extremely high. Surprisingly, the only visible effects of these hormones on the neonate are occasional breast enlargement and some degree of endometrial hyperplasia. However, the feedback effect of these steroids suppresses serum FSH and LH secretion in both sexes. At term, cord serum hCG levels range from 20 to 9000 mIU/ml (median 50 mIU/ml). The only hormonal sex difference is in serum testosterone, which is still slightly higher in males than in females. Parturition elicits a transient release of LH in the male, so that at birth circulating LH levels are higher than in the female.[57]

Immediately after birth, placental estrogens, progesterone, and 17-hydroxyprogesterone are cleared from the neonatal circulation. Concentrations of hCG fall more slowly, but by 4 days of age this gonadotropin is no longer detectable, while testosterone levels have become similar in both sexes. During the second week of life a remarkable phenomenon occurs in all normal infants, which can only be interpreted as an apparent onset of puberty. As the infant is released from the inhibitory influence of placental estrogens, there is brisk pulsatile secretion of pituitary gonadotropins, which is clearly driven by hypothalamic GnRH just as at adolescence.

In male infants serum gonadotropin levels rise until 1 month of age and then decline to prepubertal levels by 4 months. This rise is accompanied by a parallel rise in serum testosterone concentrations to a peak at 1 to 3 months of age (see Table 18-5). Although levels of sex hormone–binding globulin also increase, values of free testosterone are distinctly raised in normal male infants.[58] This neonatal activation of the pituitary-testicular axis may influence the timing and course of subsequent sexual development, since blockade with a GnRH agonist appears to cause a significant delay in the onset of puberty.[59]

In female or functionally hypogonadal infants, because of a relative lack of gonadal steroid feedback inhibition, serum FSH and LH levels continue to rise until 3 to 4 months of age and do not decline to their prepubertal nadir until age 3 to 4 years. The steroidogenic response of the infant ovary to this postnatal gonadotropin surge is neither so immediate nor so dramatic as that of the testis. There is usually an increase in the number of large antral follicles, which can be observed on pelvic ultrasonography, but only a variable, unsustained rise in serum estradiol levels. The major clinical correlate of these events is the common appearance of transient breast enlargement in girls 1 to 2 years of age, referred to as *benign premature thelarche*.

The most interesting aspect of these neonatal phenomena is the decline in pituitary gonadotropin secretion which occurs in both sexes, even in the absence of gonads. This clearly reflects maturation of a central mechanism for inhibition of pulsatile hypothalamic GnRH secretion. This prepubertal suppression of pituitary gonadotropin secretion is the penultimate stage in sexual differentiation—the final phase is puberty, with the appearance of sexually dimorphic secondary sex characteristics and eventual acquisition of full adult reproductive function.

Gender Role and Psychosexual Differentiation

Gender role encompasses a person's psychosexual self-identity, legal and social gender designation, external manifestations such as dress and social comportment, and erotic responsiveness to one sex or the other. For years a nature-versus-nurture controversy has raged regarding the potential significance of prenatal androgen exposure as an organizer of these postnatal phenomena. At one extreme is the concept that each infant is psychosexually neuter at birth and that gender identity is permanently imposed during the first few years of life by social and environmental influences. Numerous reports of persons raised in a sex discordant with their genetic or gonadal sex certainly testify to the importance of such influences, although it seems simplistic to assume that their effect is limited to infancy. More likely, gender role is continually reinforced through childhood and puberty by both external influences and awareness of one's genital and secondary sexual characteristics. The demonstration of spontaneous and successful gender role reversal in male pseudohermaphrodites after virilization at puberty[60] underscores the important influence of these sex hormone–mediated factors in later life.

The opposite viewpoint holds that postnatal behavior and intellectual function, to the extent that they are dimorphic, are programmed by sex steroids during a critical prenatal phase of neural differentiation. In its most extreme form this theory proposes that subtle deficiencies of androgen in genetic male fetuses can permit female organization of the brain and predispose to homosexuality.[61] Conversely, excess androgen in a genetic female might induce masculine postnatal behavior, homosexuality, and anovulatory infertility. It must be emphasized that this model invokes not just a direct and immediate activational effect of androgens, such as that upon energy expenditure and libido in adults, but also an organizational effect on neuronal growth and synaptogenesis which is permanent and is expressed for years after the actual hormone exposure. Such organizational effects can be readily demonstrated in female rodents, in which brief exposure to sex steroids at a critical time can permanently impose male-type acyclic gonadotropin secretion and copulatory behavior in later adult life. Gorski has described sexually dimorphic development of the preoptic area of rat brain which is dependent on the level of circulating androgens during brain differentiation,[62] but it is not clear to what extent these phenomena have a counterpart in human brain development.

The developing fetal brain expresses not only androgen receptor activity but also 5α-reductase and aromatase, suggesting that androgens can be transformed to products that could have greater or lesser biological activity.[63] Prenatal exposure of female primates to testosterone in amounts sufficient to masculinize the genitalia may induce increased postnatal aggressiveness and lead to aberrant adult sexual behavior but does not block normal ovulatory cycles. The human parallel of this situation might be congenital adrenal hyperplasia, but here any permanent organizational effect has been difficult to prove. Early reports of higher IQ scores in androgen-exposed females have not been confirmed. No studies of the behavior of children with such endocrine disorders have been able to correct adequately for postnatal variations in sex steroid levels or for the impact that awareness of the disease, its treatment, and its potential implications has on both self-image and parental perceptions of behavior. Prenatal exposure of females to the synthetic estrogen diethylstilbestrol may increase the likelihood of homosexuality,[64] but the observation that the great majority of such women are exclusively heterosexual suggests that other unidentified variables play a more important role in sexual orientation.

A reasonable viewpoint would suggest that prenatal androgen may play a role in the differentiation of human psychosexual behavior but is certainly not the decisive determinant. Successful differentiation of gender role appears to depend primarily on appropriate assignment of the sex of rearing plus continued unambiguous reinforcement by social interaction, concordant genital appearance, and appropriate secondary sexual characteristics. Even in adult life sex steroids continue to interact with psychological and sociocultural factors to maintain patterns of dimorphic behavior we identify as male and female. The implications of this concept for the management of children with disorders of sexual differentiation should be obvious.

ABNORMAL SEXUAL DIFFERENTIATION

Under normal circumstances genetic sex is defined at conception. Subsequently, unambiguous male or female differentiation is effected by the presence or absence of three key determinants: a testis-determining factor, müllerian inhibiting substance, and testosterone. The synthesis of each is regulated by specific genetic loci, and each requires specific receptor mechanisms which are normally present in the target cells of either sex. Disordered differentiation may occur at any stage in this process and result in inadequate masculinization of a genetic male or inappropriate virilization of a genetic female. Some relatively common situations which should alert the clinician to the possible presence of such a disorder are listed in Table 18-2. In these situations the diagnostic process is not merely an attempt to assign a label but rather a logical stepwise evaluation of the operation of each of the three key determinants until the clinician can define or rationally infer the status of each of the parameters of sexual dimorphism listed in Table 18-1.

TABLE 18-2 Clinical Features Suggestive of a Possible Disorder of Sexual Differentiation

In the neonate or infant
- Ambiguous external genitalia
- Cryptorchism and/or hypospadias
- Female with mass in the groin or labium majus pudendi
- Lymphedema or other stigmata of Turner's syndrome
- Family history of anomalous sexual development
- Maternal virilization or hormone ingestion

In the child or young adult
- Female with short stature or other stigmata of Turner's syndrome
- Female with sexual infantilism or precocious ovarian failure
- Male with small testes, gynecomastia, or other stigmata of Klinefelter's syndrome
- Unexplained virilization

Such an approach can also be applied to the classification of disorders of sexual differentiation, as summarized in Table 18-3.

Errors of Primary Sex Determination

Disorders of sex determination involve sex chromosome abnormalities and/or defective gonad formation. For completeness, the relatively common situations of trisomy X and XYY syndrome are included in this category, even though neither produces any consistent abnormality of gonadal structure or function.

Sex Chromosome Anomalies Associated with Functional Testes and Male Phenotype

Klinefelter's Syndrome

In 1942 Klinefelter and associates described in adult males a syndrome of seminiferous tubule dysgenesis characterized by small firm testes, azoospermia, eunuchoid body habitus, and gynecomastia.[65] Subsequent genetic studies disclosed that most of these patients had two X chromosomes; the term *Klinefelter's syndrome* is now usually restricted to persons with a 47,XXY karyotype, although variant forms with similar clinical features also occur.

The genetic abnormality arises from nondisjunction during the first or second meiotic division of gametogenesis. In 60 percent of cases the nondisjunctional error is maternal; therefore, the frequency of this disorder is maternal age–dependent. Testis formation, paramesonephric duct regression, and mesonephric duct development are normal and the external genitalia are male, although micropenis may occur. There does not appear to be any excess prenatal wastage of 47,XXY embryos; the frequency in unselected newborns is approximately 1 per 1000 males. As a group, 47,XXY infants have a tendency to lower birth weights and minor somatic anomalies such as clinodactyly, but a clinical diagnosis at this time is unusual. There is some evidence that cord serum testosterone concentrations may be lower than those of controls, but no data regarding the neonatal gonadotropin/testosterone surge are available.

During childhood many, but not all, patients with Klinefelter's syndrome show increased stature (above the 50th percentile), with relatively long legs, decreased head circumference, diminished verbal skills, emotional immaturity, and poor neuromuscular coordination. Penile length and testis volume are usually in the low-normal range. Before puberty the testes show reduced numbers of spermatogonia, but tubular hyalinization is not observed. Serum concentrations of FSH, LH, testosterone, and estradiol are in the normal prepubertal range, and responses to stimulation with GnRH and hCG are appropriate for age.[66]

TABLE 18-3 A Classification of Abnormal Sexual Development

I. Errors of primary sex determination
  A. Sex chromosome anomalies
    1. With testes and male phenotype
      a. Klinefelter's syndrome (47,XXY and variants)
      b. XYY syndrome
      c. XX males (X-Y interchange)
    2. With ovaries and female phenotype
      a. Trisomy X and variants
    3. With bisexual gonads
      a. True hermaphroditism (X-Y interchange)
      b. Chimeric (XX/XY) true hermaphroditism
      c. Mosaic (XX/XXY) true hermaphroditism
    4. With dysgenetic gonads
      a. Y chromosome anomalies (XYp−)
      b. Mixed gonadal dysgenesis (45,X/46,XY)
      c. Turner's syndrome (45,X and variants)
  B. Anomalies of gonadogenesis
    1. Defective ovary development
      a. XX gonadal dysgenesis
    2. Defective testis development
      a. XY gonadal dysgenesis
      b. Dysgenetic male pseudohermaphroditism
      c. Testicular regression syndromes (agonadism, rudimentary testis, anorchia)
II. Errors of sexual differentiation
  A. Inadequate masculinization of genetic male
    1. Defective paramesonephric duct regression
      a. Persistent paramesonephric ducts
    2. Defective genital virilization
      a. Leydig cell hypoplasia (LH/hCG receptor defect)
      b. Inborn errors of corticosteroid and testosterone synthesis
        (1) Cholesterol side-chain cleavage (20,22-desmolase) deficiency
        (2) 3β-Hydroxysteroid dehydrogenase deficiency
        (3) 17α-Hydroxylase deficiency
      c. Inborn errors of testosterone synthesis
        (1) 17,20-Desmolase deficiency
        (2) 17β-Hydroxysteroid dehydrogenase deficiency
      d. Inborn error of testosterone metabolism
        (1) 5α-Reductase deficiency
      e. Defective target cell response
        (1) Complete androgen insensitivity
        (2) Incomplete androgen insensitivity and variants
      f. Environmental feminization
        (1) Maternal ingestion of estrogen or progestin
      g. Multigenic/multifactorial
        (1) Isolated hypospadias and cryptorchism
        (2) Multiple congenital anomaly syndromes
  B. Virilization of genetic female
    1. Adrenal androgens (congenital adrenal hyperplasia
      a. 21-Hydroxylase deficiency
      b. 11β-Hydroxylase deficiency
      c. 3β-Hydroxysteroid dehydrogenase deficiency
    2. Environmental hormones
      a. Maternal virilizing disorders
      b. Iatrogenic virilization
    3. Teratologic malformation
      a. Abnormal development of vagina or uterus
      b. Multiple congenital anomaly syndromes

Secondary sex characteristics usually appear at the normal age. Testis size often increases initially, but growth usually ceases before midpuberty at an average volume of 3.5 ± 1.5 ml.[67] Coincident with the onset of puberty, serum gonadotropin values increase abruptly to abnormal levels (Fig. 18-10). Presumably this hypergonadotropic state reflects diminished testosterone production; in turn, it leads to progressive hyalinization and fibrosis of seminiferous tubules, clumping of Leydig cells, and enhanced testicular secretion of estrogen. Spermatogenesis is rarely present except in a few isolated tubules. Because of tubular shrinkage the Leydig cells appear hyperplastic, but in fact Leydig cell volume is not affected. Serum estradiol concentrations tend to be high-normal, while serum testosterone concentrations fail to rise above the low-normal adult range. In 50 to 75 percent of unselected patients, clinically apparent gynecomastia develops; in contrast to benign juvenile gynecomastia, this often persists into adult life.

Virtually all adult 47,XXY subjects are azoospermic; the occasional report of paternity may reflect hidden XY/XXY mosaicism or the appearance of a clone of XY spermatocytes through mitotic nondisjunction. Clinical problems possibly related to androgen deficiency include a eunuchoid body habitus, persistent gynecomastia, reduced lean body mass, decreased libido and seminal volume, and a lack of social drive and aggressiveness. It is not clear to what extent these physical and psychosexual handicaps can be prevented or ameliorated by supplementation with exogenous androgens from early puberty.

In addition to consistently elevated values of serum FSH and LH, adults with Klinefelter's syn-

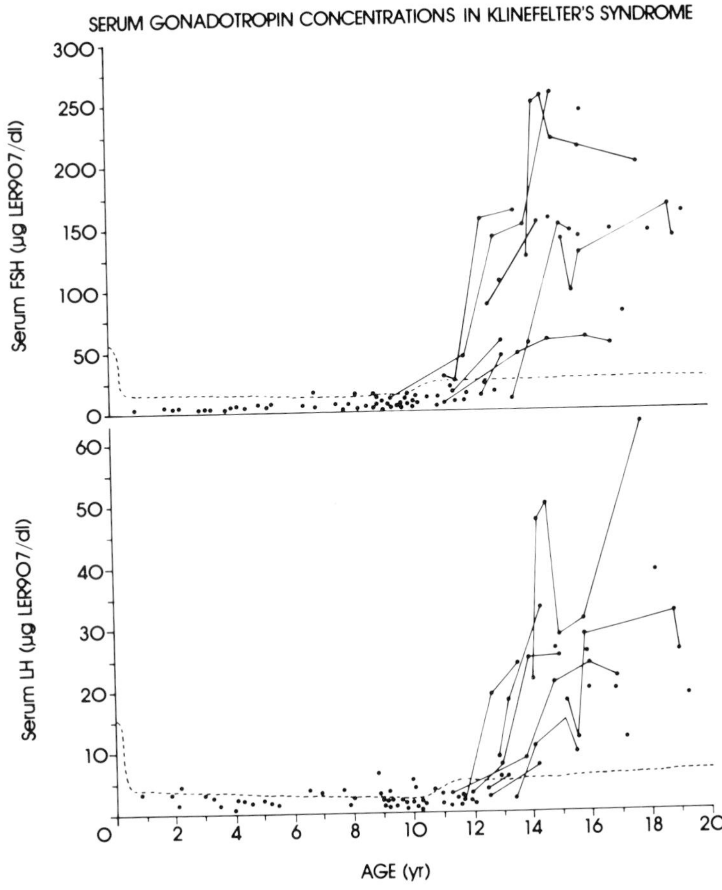

FIGURE 18-10 Basal serum FSH and LH concentrations in boys with Klinefelter's syndrome before and during puberty. The dotted lines show the upper limit of the normal male range. The gonadotropin values may be converted from micrograms of LER907 per deciliter to international units per liter by multiplying FSH by 0.5 and LH by 4.5. (*From Salbenblatt et al.*[66])

drome show reduced circulating levels of testosterone (276 ± 156 ng/dl) and dihydrotestosterone (28 ± 9.4 ng/dl) and increased levels of estradiol (2.8 ± 0.9 ng/dl); levels of adrenal androgens are not significantly different from normal. With advancing age, testicular function continues to decline, with a further decrease in serum testosterone levels and testosterone/estradiol ratios.

The prevalence of impaired glucose tolerance, chronic pulmonary disease, and varicose veins appears to be increased in adults with Klinefelter's syndrome. In addition, there is a predisposition to various neoplasms, including germ cell tumors, bronchogenic carcinoma, acute lymphocytic leukemia, and carcinoma of the breast. The frequency of breast cancer in Klinefelter's syndrome patients is about 20 times that in normal men.[68]

The diagnosis of Klinefelter's syndrome may be suspected on the basis of the traditional phenotype but should be considered in any male with hypergonadotropic hypogonadism. The diagnosis is supported by the finding of a chromatin-positive buccal smear but should always be confirmed by means of karyotype analysis.

The most common variant form of Klinefelter's syndrome is 46,XY/47,XXY mosaicism; these patients show lesser degrees of hypogonadism, may be fertile, and may not complain of androgen deficiency until the fourth or fifth decade of life. Patients with more severe sex chromosome anomalies such as 48,XXYY, 48,XXXY, 49,XXXYY, and 49,XXXXY have the typical features of Klinefelter's syndrome but also are mentally retarded and show a wide range of somatic anomalies, particularly radioulnar synostosis, epiphyseal dysplasia, and patent ductus arteriosus. The presence of testes in these syndromes of X polysomy demonstrates the power of the Y chromosome to direct male gonadal differentiation.

The treatment of Klinefelter's syndrome is amelioration of hypergonadotropic hypogonadism and the resulting poor self-image. Most patients benefit psychologically and socially from surgery to reduce gynecomastia and administration of full replacement doses of oral testosterone undecanoate or intramuscular testosterone esters, coupled with long-term counseling by an informed and sympathetic physician.

XYY Males

Strictly speaking, the 47,XYY karyotype, which occurs in about 1 in every 1000 males, does not produce a disorder of sexual differentiation, since testicular, internal genital, and external genital development is male. There are no consistent physical anomalies, but hypotonia, delayed speech, and poor neuromuscular coordination appear to be relatively common. Tall stature is often described but is not a consistent finding. Testicular size is usually normal, but up to 10 percent of these individuals may have small testes. Adolescent and adult testicular endocrine function is normal, with no evidence of hypergonadotropic hypogonadism. Although many XYY males are fertile and presumably have normal seminiferous epithelium, biopsy studies of institutionalized adult patients have described variable but often severe abnormalities of spermatogenesis. The XYY disorder initially gained notoriety when it was discovered that its incidence was increased in criminals with persistent violent or aggressive behavior. It is now generally recognized that various sex chromosome anomalies, including but not limited to XYY, may be associated with behavioral difficulties in children and adults, but the suggestion that criminality may be the inevitable result is both naive and simplistic.

XX Males

Although phenotypic males with a 46,XX karyotype occur only once in every 30,000 male infants, this situation provides a useful illustration of the central role played in male sexual differentiation by the testis-determining gene locus found on the Y chromosome. Even though these persons lack a Y chromosome, they have testes which resemble histologically those of XXY males. Recent studies have demonstrated that in XX males X-Y interchange has occurred during paternal gametogenesis, with the testis-determining segment and other DNA sequences normally located on the Y chromosome being translocated to the short arm of the X chromosome; in turn, the paternal X chromosome can be shown to have lost genetic material from its short arm.[69] Such X-Y translocation, which presumably occurs during the pairing of the pseudoautosomal regions in meiosis, does not always lead to the development of testes but may result in gonadal dysgenesis with a female phenotype if the testis-determining locus is not involved or is inoperative.[70]

Clinically, XX males resemble those with Klinefelter's syndrome, although they tend to be somewhat shorter (mean height 168 cm). Their internal and external genitalia are usually normal, but hypospadias, cryptorchism, or more severe genital ambiguity occurs in about 10 percent of cases. The testes are small and soft, with uneven hyalinization, peritubular fibrosis, and Leydig cell clumping after the onset of puberty. Spermatogonia are usually absent, possibly because of premature commitment of the XX germ cells to meiosis. It is of interest that while two functioning X chromosomes are essential to the survival of germ cells in the ovary, they are detrimental to survival in a testicular environment. One-third of these patients develop significant gynecomastia. The hormonal profile of adult XX males confirms their hypergonadotropic hypogonadism, with increased serum concentrations of FSH and LH and reduced levels of testosterone. Basal and GnRH-stimulated androgen levels may be normal during childhood, as in Klinefelter's syndrome.

Sex Chromosome Anomalies Associated with Ovaries and Female Phenotype

A 47,XXX karyotype occurs in about 1 per 1000 female infants, usually as a result of nondisjunction during maternal meiosis; thus, as in Klinefelter's syndrome, there is a maternal age effect. Sexual differentiation is female. No consistent pattern of somatic abnormalities is observed in this condition (*trisomy X*), but birth weight tends to be low and various minor anomalies have been reported.[71] Although one must be cautious regarding sampling bias due to investigation in institutions, triple-X females do seem to show a greater prevalence of mental retardation, cognitive dysfunction, and schizophreniform psychoses. There is a variable effect on oogenesis: about one-quarter of these patients experience some form of ovarian dysfunction, ranging from delayed menarche to premature ovarian failure, but fertility does occur. Naturally, the hormonal profile is dependent on the degree of ovarian dysfunction. Similar abnormalities, but usually associated with more severe somatic anomalies, have been described in association with 48,XXXX and 49,XXXXX karyotypes.

Sex Chromosome Anomalies Associated with Bisexual Gonadal Development

A person can be classified as a *true hermaphrodite* only if both testicular tissue with distinct tubules and ovarian tissue containing follicles or corpora albicantia are present. The more frequent finding of a dysgenetic gonad containing testicular elements plus fibrous stroma without follicles does not establish true hermaphroditism. About 30 percent of cases are classified as lateral, with a testis on one side and an ovary on the other; 50 percent have one ovotestis; and the rest have bilateral ovotestes containing distinct ovarian and testicular elements.[72]

Approximately two-thirds of true hermaphrodites show a 46,XX karyotype. In these individuals the most common genetic mechanism is X-Y interchange during paternal gametogenesis, as in the XX male. Thus interchange between the X and Y chromosomes may result in an XX male (with or without hypospadias), true hermaphroditism, or gonadal dysgenesis, depending presumably on the amount and efficacy of the translocated testis-determining DNA segment. Pedigrees containing both XX males and XX true hermaphrodites are thought to result from familial deletion of an X-linked locus or an autosomal recessive structural gene defect. The pathogenesis of the less common 46,XY form of true hermaphroditism is less clear but may involve undetected XX/XY chimerism. Such whole-body chimerism has been documented in several cases and presumably results from double fertilization (by an X and Y sperm) of a binucleate ovum or fusion of XX and XY zygotes. Finally, a few cases of XX/XXY mosaicism have been described as a result of the loss of a Y chromosome from a 47,XXY zygote at an early mitotic division. Thus, a variety of genetic mechanisms may be operative, but all have the same end result: variable expression of TDF within the developing gonad.

The clinical presentation of true hermaphroditism depends on the amount of functioning testicular tissue. In patients with a testis and an ovary, development of the mesonephric and paramesonephric ducts is consistent with the appearance of the ipsilateral gonad. With ovotestes, genital duct development is usually female. According to the level of circulating androgen, the external genitalia may appear female, may be ambiguous, or may be frankly masculine, although hypospadias and cryptorchism are common. Sometimes an inguinal hernia contains an ovotestis. At puberty virilization is variable. Breast development and menstruation are common, reflecting the low serum testosterone/estradiol ratio in most patients. If testicular function is minimal or if all testicular tissue has been removed, cyclical gonadotropin secretion, ovulation, and fertility may be observed. Spermatogenesis is rare, and male fertility has not been documented. Gonadal tumors, usually gonadoblastoma, dysgerminoma, or seminoma, occur in about 2 percent of true hermaphrodites.

The diagnosis of true hermaphroditism can be confirmed only by histologic examination of the gonads. In an infant the sex of rearing should be assigned according to the degree of virilization of the internal and external genitalia. Any discordant or dysgenetic gonadal tissue, together with inappropriate internal genital structures, should be removed, and plastic repair of the external genitalia should be undertaken. In children being raised as males it is probably wise to retain a testis only if it appears normal and is located in the scrotum, because of the risk of malignancy. Appropriate sex hormone replacement will usually be required at the age of puberty.

Sex Chromosome Anomalies Associated with Dysgenetic Gonads

Structural Anomalies of the Y Chromosome

Abnormalities of the Y chromosome may include ring formation, deletions, dicentrics, inversions, and isochromosomes. Patients with extensive deletions of the short arm of Y may present with gonadal dysgenesis, a female phenotype, and the somatic stigmata of Turner's syndrome. Conversely, if the short arm is intact, testes and male sexual differentiation may develop. However, the abnormal Y chromosome is frequently lost during an early mitotic division, producing a variable proportion of 45,X cells and some degree of gonadal dysgenesis. The clinical picture then becomes that of mixed gonadal dysgenesis.

Mixed Gonadal Dysgenesis

It is not uncommon for a Y chromosome, particularly one that is structurally abnormal, to be lost from a 46,XY zygote as a result of anaphase lag or mitotic nondisjunction. The karyotype will then show 45,X as well as 46,XY and/or 47,XYY cell lines in varying proportions, and the phenotype will depend on the amount of testicular tissue present. If no testicular development occurs, the clinical presentation will be that of a female with bilateral streak gonads, although short stature and the somatic anomalies of Turner's syndrome (see below) may be less obvious than in the pure 45,X patient.

The term *mixed gonadal dysgenesis* is applied to persons with 45,X/46,XY mosaicism in whom some prenatal virilization has occurred. These patients are TDF-positive and show either one dysgenetic testis (usually intraabdominal) and one streak gonad or bilateral testes, both usually dysgenetic to some degree. Internal genital differentiation depends on the functional integrity of the ipsilateral gonad, but usually one or both paramesonephric ducts fail to regress and a rudimentary uterus is present. Depending on the level of prenatal androgen secretion, the newborn patient may display isolated clitoral hypertrophy, ambiguous external genitalia, or even relatively normal male genitalia, with or without hypospadias.[73] Two-thirds of the reported patients have been raised as females.

The importance of identifying 45,X/46,XY mosaicism, regardless of the phenotype, lies in the potential for significant virilization at puberty and the propensity of the affected gonads to undergo malignant degeneration. In most cases there is fairly good correlation between the degree of genital masculinization and the secretion of testosterone at puberty; this can be assessed directly before puberty by observing the serum testosterone response to several days of hCG stimulation.

The risk of gonadal neoplasm, whether gonadoblastoma, dysgerminoma, or embryonal carcinoma, in patients with 45,X/46,XY mosaicism is approximately 20 percent overall and increases with age.[74] The risk of malignancy is probably highest in dysgenetic testes and lowest in streak gonads. The occurrence of spontaneous breast development nearly always signals the presence of an estrogen-secreting gonadoblastoma. Often a gonadal neoplasm can be detected with pelvic ultrasonography or computed tomography, but regardless of these findings or the clinical phenotype, it is a prudent policy to recommend prophylactic removal of streak gonads and undescended testes during the first decade in all children with 45,X/46,XY mosaicism. Occasionally in a phenotypic male, scrotal testes of normal consistency may be preserved under close and continuing observation.

Because of the continuum of genital differentiation seen in these patients, decisions regarding the sex of rearing should be based on the potential for normal genital function. In females, clitoroplasty and vaginoplasty should be undertaken in infancy. In males, all paramesonephric duct remnants should be removed, hypospadias repaired, and testicular prostheses placed in the scrotum. In either case, prophylactic gonadectomy is desirable, and appropriate sex steroid replacement will be needed at puberty.

Turner's Syndrome

Classic Turner's syndrome consists of bilateral gonadal dysgenesis with streak gonads, a female phenotype, and sexual infantilism plus short stature and a pattern of distinctive somatic stigmata (Fig. 18-11). The typical syndrome results from monosomy for the X chromosome (45,X), with or without mosaicism, but it may also be seen in patients with two sex chromosomes in which one (X or Y) is structurally defective, producing effective monosomy.

Comparison of the frequency of the 45,X karyotype in spontaneous abortions (approximately 1 in 15) and in live births (1 in 20,000) demonstrates that monosomy X is nearly always lethal in utero; surviving patients often show some degree of mosaicism, indicative of a postfertilization mitotic error. It is of interest that Turner's syndrome is more frequently associated with young maternal age.[75] In 80 percent of 45,X survivors the single X chromosome is of maternal origin, suggesting preferential loss of the paternal sex chromosome either before or after fertilization. Mosaic forms commonly result from postzygotic loss of a sex chromosome that is structurally abnormal. Monozygotic twinning appears to be more frequent in such mosaicism situations; the twins may be discordant for the Turner's syndrome phenotype because of heterogeneous distribution of the 45,X and other (usually XX, XY, or XXX) cell lines.

The indifferent gonad of the 45,X fetus forms normally and is seeded by germ cells which become incorporated into primordial follicles. However, the

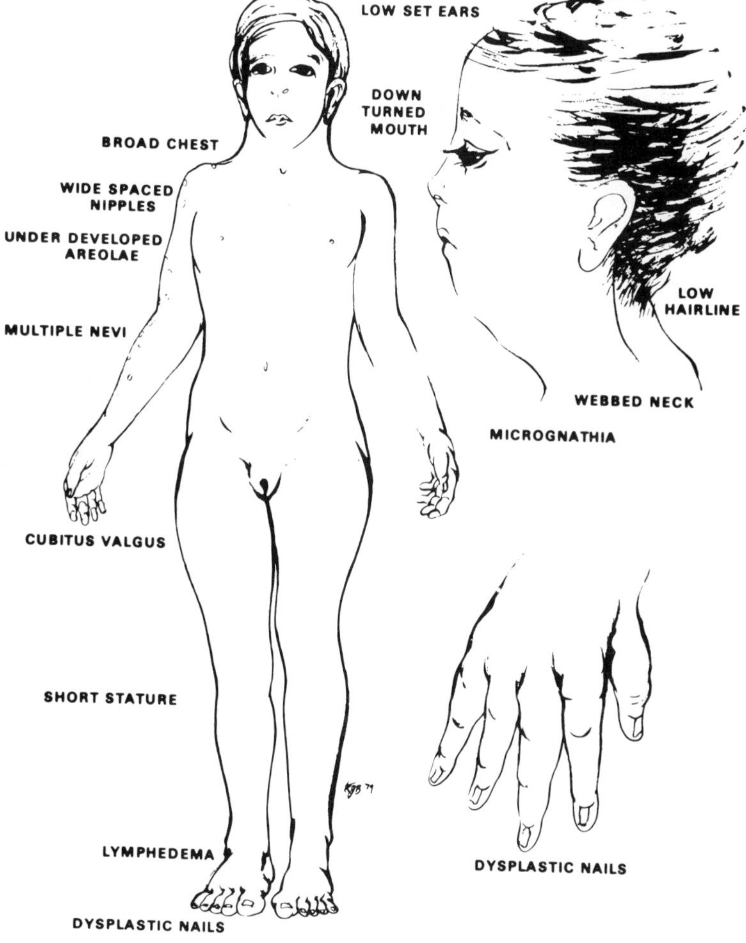

FIGURE 18-11 The major clinical features of a child with Turner's syndrome (45,X gonadal dysgenesis). [*From Dean HJ, Winter JSD, in Collu C, Ducharme JR, Guyda H (eds): Pediatric Endocrinology, 2d ed. New York, Raven, 1989, p 345.*]

rate of follicular atresia and degeneration is greatly increased, so that by birth only a few primary follicles remain. Almost always these, too, disappear before puberty, leaving fibrous streak gonads, the consequence of which is sexual infantilism and primary amenorrhea. As one would expect, the internal and external genitalia are female. Any sign of prenatal or postnatal virilization indicates the presence of a Y-bearing cell line and some testicular tissue (mixed gonadal dysgenesis).

Generalized lymphedema with hygromatous neck masses is characteristic of 45,X fetuses. In newborn infants this same lymphatic hypoplasia can produce the Bonnevie-Ullrich syndrome, with distal lymphedema, loose skin folds at the nape, ascites, and pleural effusion. Birth weight and length are usually low for gestational age.

During childhood the dominant clinical feature is short stature. Height is invariably below the third percentile for age, while growth velocity is less strikingly reduced (between the 10th and 25th percentiles). Because of the sexual infantilism, untreated patients show no pubertal growth spurt, and radiologic bone maturation becomes retarded after 11 years of age. The mean adult height is 143 cm, but height can range up to 155 cm, depending on parental stature.[76]

Accompanying this short stature is often a characteristic pattern of somatic abnormalities (Fig. 18-11). The skull is brachycephalic, and the facies are distinctive, with a triangular shape, a retruded mandible, epicanthal folds, ptosis, and a narrow high palate. The ears are low-set and often deformed. The nuchal hairline is low and the neck is short in most cases, but frank webbing of the neck (pterygium colli) occurs in only 40 percent. The chest is usually square or shield-shaped, the nipples are relatively wide spaced, and pectus excavatum may be present. There are commonly many pigmented nevi over the face, arms, and chest. Anomalies of the extremities include cubitus valgus (in about 50 percent), lymphedema or puffiness of the hands and feet, shortening of the fourth metacarpal, and hypoplastic nails. Kyphoscoliosis is not uncommon. Renal anomalies, including unilateral aplasia, horseshoe kidney, and ureteral duplication, are found in 60 percent of cases. Bicuspid aortic valve is the most common cardiovascular anomaly (34 to 50 percent), but coarctation of the aorta, ventricular septal defect, aortic stenosis, and aortic aneurysm also occur. Occasionally gastrointestinal bleeding may result from congenital intestinal telangiectasia. Strabismus is not uncommon, and there may be hearing loss due to a sensorineural deficit or recurrent otitis media. Although most 45,X patients have normal intelligence and the incidence of severe psychopathology is not increased, they frequently demonstrate social immaturity and specific perceptual disability in areas of directional sense and space-form recognition.[77]

Radiographic examination often discloses characteristic bony anomalies, including shortening of the fourth metacarpal, the "carpal sign," or a reduced angle in the proximal row of carpals,[78] basilar impression of the skull, hypoplasia of cervical vertebrae, and occasional areas of aseptic necrosis, particularly around the knee. In adults who have not received sex steroids, osteoporosis may become severe. Reactive enlargement of the pituitary fossa has also been described in adult patients with long-standing untreated hypergonadotropic hypogonadism. Excretory urography commonly discloses structural or positional abnormalities of the kidney, occasionally associated with significant ureteropelvic obstruction.

Several other disorders appear to be increased in patients with Turner's syndrome. Hypertension unrelated to aortic coarctation or renal disease occurs in about half of adult patients; although the initial rise in blood pressure occurs during the second decade, there does not seem to be an obvious relation to estrogen therapy. The risk of developing autoimmune endocrine disease, particularly of the thyroid, is considerably increased. Antithyroid antibodies indicative of chronic lymphocytic thyroiditis can be detected in about a third of these patients, and many of them in time develop goiter or become hypothyroid. Impaired carbohydrate tolerance can frequently be demonstrated, but frank diabetes mellitus is less common. Other autoimmune disorders, such as rheumatoid arthritis and inflammatory bowel disease, appear to be more frequent in Turner's syndrome. In addition to concern regarding possible gonadal neoplasms (see below), there is some evidence for an increased risk of developing nongonadal malignancy in these patients.

Phenotype-Karyotype Correlations The key genetic determinants which are absent in Turner's syndrome appear to be on the short arm of the X or Y chromosome, and the severity of the clinical presentation to some extent correlates with the amount of this loss. Patients with complete monosomy (45,X) or an isochromosome for the long arm [46,X,iso(Xq)] usually show the classic syndrome, with short stature, sexual infantilism, and multiple somatic stigmata. These patients are unlikely to show aortic coarctation or severe lymphedema but appear to be more at risk for developing autoimmune disorders such as Hashimoto's disease and diabetes mellitus. Patients with major deletions of the short arm [46,X(Xp−)] or a ring X chromosome [46,X,r(X)] tend to have fewer somatic stigmata, while those with deletions of the long arm [46,X(Xq−)] usually present with only sexual infantilism or primary amenorrhea, are of normal stature, and show none of the usual somatic stigmata. However, structurally abnormal sex chromosomes are frequently lost during an early mitotic division, leading to a variable proportion of 45,X cells, which will naturally confute phenotype-karyotype generalizations. For the same reason, the buccal smear may be chromatin-negative or chromatin-positive, depending on the relative proportion of 45,X and 46,XX cells in that tissue. Occasionally a clue to the presence of an isochromosome or major deletion may be provided by a sex chromatin body that is larger or smaller than normal.

There have been many reports of breast development, menses, and even fertility in patients with Turner's syndrome.[79] Most such patients show few physical stigmata and can be demonstrated to have 45,X/46,XX or 45,X/47,XXX mosaicism. If mosaicism cannot be detected in peripheral leukocytes, it may be impossible to determine whether this spontaneous ovarian function represents hidden mosaicism or the rare survival of a 45,X oocyte. To date most reported patients with 45,X/46,XX mosaicism with secondary amenorrhea have also had short stature, but it is not clear to what extent this represents sampling bias.

Several interesting patients have demonstrated either pericentric inversion or balanced X-X or X-autosome translocation; that is, breakage and structural rearrangement of segments of the X chromosome without any detectable loss of genetic material. These studies demonstrate that there is a critical segment on the long arm of X (between bands Xq13 and Xq27) which is essential for normal gonadal development.[80] Females with break points or rearrangements affecting this segment often suffer from primary or secondary amenorrhea; males with the same defect may show disturbed spermatogenesis.

As described previously, patients with 45,X/46,XY or 45,X/47,XYY mosaicism may show varying degrees of virilization, depending on the amount of functional testicular tissue. Not only may their genital development be female, ambiguous, or male, the degree of short stature and the frequency of somatic anomalies are also highly variable. At puberty they may be virilized because of Leydig cell activity, may remain sexually infantile because of gonadal dysgenesis, or may be feminized because of an estrogen-secreting gonadal neoplasm. Because of the propensity to develop gonadoblastoma or malignant germinoma, the risk of which approaches 20 percent in the second decade, the streak gonads or dysgenetic testes of any patient with 45,X/46,XY mosaicism should be removed. However, in classic Turner's syndrome patients with no apparent prenatal or pubertal virilization and no cytogenetic evidence of a Y-bearing cell line, prophylactic gonadectomy does not appear to be necessary.

Diagnosis and Treatment A definitive diagnosis of Turner's syndrome requires careful karyotype analysis, including banding and study of sufficient cells to confirm or exclude mosaicism. In equivocal situations, particularly when the presence of a Y-bearing or 45,X cell line is critical to patient management, consideration should be given to genetic analysis of additional tissues such as skin fibroblasts. Because of the relatively high proportion of patients with mosaicism, a buccal smear for sex chromatin is an inadequate diagnostic technique.

In the evaluation of females with short stature or late puberty, a clue to the presence of gonadal dysgenesis may be the finding of serum FSH concentrations which are above the age-specific normal range (Fig. 18-12). In contrast to the situation in Klinefelter's syndrome, children with gonadal dysgenesis will usually show high serum FSH levels[81] and exaggerated responses to stimulation with exogenous GnRH. Even though the absence of gonadal negative feedback leads to increased gonadotropin secretion, the pattern of serum gonadotropin values in agonadal children parallels that in normal girls, with higher values in infancy, a decline in midchildhood, and a rise to the postmenopausal range again at the normal time of puberty.

The short stature of patients with Turner's syndrome is due to a combination of intrauterine growth retardation, subnormal growth velocity during childhood, and lack of a pubertal growth spurt. Spontaneous and stimulated growth hormone levels are normal during childhood but may decline after age 9 years, presumably because of the absence of sex steroid. The current availability of biosynthetic growth hormone has led to numerous studies of its efficacy and safety.[82] Short-term results using doses higher than those used in growth hormone–deficient patients reveal an increase in growth rate. Combination therapy with growth hormone and low-dose oxandrolone results in an even greater increase in growth rate but may increase carbohydrate intolerance. Although both therapies are reported to increase predicted adult height, final data are awaited.

Patients with Turner's syndrome show normal serum levels of adrenal androgens and a normal adrenarchal rise in these values before the age of puberty; thereafter, because of deficient gonadal contribution, serum testosterone and androstenedione concentrations are slightly lower than in normal females.[83] Several studies have demonstrated improved growth velocity in patients treated with low doses of exogenous androgen (fluoxymesterone or oxandrolone, 0.1 to 0.3 mg/kg of body weight per day), but it has been difficult to ascertain whether such treatment has a significant effect on eventual adult size.[84] Low doses of ethinyl estradiol (100 ng/kg per day) can also increase short-term growth velocity,[85] but with longer periods of therapy skeletal maturation may be accelerated, with little effect on final height.[86] The addition of low-dose estrogen to growth hormone therapy in girls with Turner's syndrome does not appear to significantly increase growth velocity over that occurring with GH alone.[87,88] All patients with gonadal dysgenesis require sex steroid

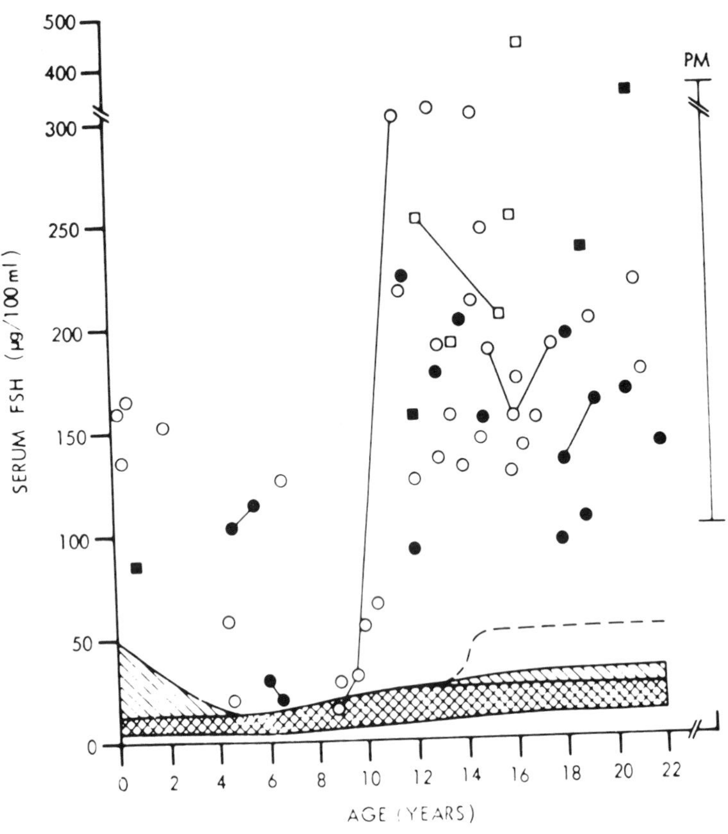

FIGURE 18-12 Serum FSH concentrations in agonadal subjects. The normal male and female ranges are shown by the hatched areas. The dotted line represents the adult female midcycle peak, and the bar (PM) represents the postmenopausal range. Patients with gonadal dysgenesis are shown by open circles. (*From Winter and Faiman.*[81])

therapy for normal secondary sex characteristics. Our approach has been to initiate estrogen replacement in low doses (ethinyl estradiol, 5 to 10 μg per day) at the age (usually 12 to 14 years) at which the patient's peers begin puberty. This will elicit gradual development of breasts and pubic hair and appears to induce at least a temporary acceleration of growth.[89] Because of the significant risk of developing endometrial hyperplasia and carcinoma in patients treated only with estrogen, it is essential that patients after 6 to 24 months be switched to a combination estrogen-progestin preparation administered in cyclic fashion. In our experience, satisfactory secondary sexual maturation and regular menses can be maintained in young adults with daily doses of ethinyl estradiol or mestranol of 50 μg or less in combination with a progestin; there is reason to believe that such a regimen does not carry an increased risk of abnormal endometrial histology or breast cancer.

Anomalies of Gonadogenesis without Chromosomal Abnormality

Defective Ovary Formation

Defective ovary formation is exemplified by *XX gonadal dysgenesis,* in which patients have bilateral streak gonads but normal stature, a 46,XX karyotype, and none of the somatic stigmata of Turner's syndrome. Their internal and external genitalia are normal female, and the diagnosis is not suspected until sexual infantilism and hypergonadotropic hypogonadism become apparent at the normal age of puberty. Familial aggregation is common, and siblings may show hypoplastic ovaries and precocious menopause, suggesting variable expression of the basic genetic disorder. In several families gonadal dysgenesis and sensorineural deafness were observed together, but it is not clear whether this represented varied expression of a single mutant gene or coincident occurrence of two genetic disorders. An occasional patient has shown signs of postpubertal virilization, which was thought to reflect hilus cell hyperplasia within the streak gonads in response to high circulating gonadotropin levels. Gonadal neoplasia does not seem to be a feature of XX gonadal dysgenesis.

The common finding of consanguinity in affected families points to the presence of a rare X-linked or autosomal recessive gene which must be present in double dose to prevent normal ovarian development. Genetic heterogeneity seems likely, since occasional patients have shown short stature or various neurologic deficits. The pathogenesis remains obscure, but presumably the mutant gene acts to impair oogonial maturation and follicle formation or to accelerate the rate of germ cell attrition, as in Turner's syndrome. Because of the genetic implications of this disorder, it is important to rule out 45,X/46,XX mosaicism with great care. Treatment of the hypergonadotropic hypogonadism is carried out with replacement estrogen and progestin, as in other forms of gonadal dysgenesis.

Defective Testis Formation

XY Gonadal Dysgenesis (Swyer Syndrome) If in spite of normal male genetic sex (46,XY) testes fail to develop, the phenotypic result will be XY gonadal dysgenesis with streak gonads, female internal and external genitalia, and sexual infantilism at the time of puberty. The short stature and somatic stigmata of Turner's syndrome are not features of this syndrome and, if present, probably indicate undetected 45,X/46,XY mosaicism. However, different pedigrees have been described in which XY gonadal dysgenesis was associated with other somatic anomalies, notably camptomelic dwarfism, interstitial nephritis or renal failure, and ectodermal and cardiac anomalies.[90]

This clinical variability underscores the genetic heterogeneity of this syndrome. Some cases are sporadic, while others appear to be due to a male-limited autosomal recessive defect. About 70 percent of reported cases appear to be X-linked recessive. Possible genetic defects include a deletion or point mutation in the Y-linked TDF locus and a defect in another chromosomal locus involved later in the cascade of male sexual development. This syndrome shows overlap with the clinical triad of XY dysgenetic pseudohermaphroditism, nephropathy, and Wilms' tumor.[91]

Regardless of the etiology, the usual clinical presentation is a phenotypic female with sexual infantilism and primary amenorrhea. Clitoromegaly can occur in untreated adults because of hyperstimulation of androgen-secreting hilus cells in the streak gonads. Spontaneous breast development does not occur unless an estrogen-secreting neoplasm appears.

As in other forms of defective testis development, there is a 20 to 30 percent risk of gonadal neoplasm, mainly gonadoblastoma or dysgerminoma. It is not clear whether the risk is higher in patients who are TDF-positive and therefore more likely to have foci of testicular tissue. Until this issue is clearer, it seems reasonable to suggest prophylactic gonadectomy for all patients with XY gonadal dysgenesis. Sex hormone replacement should be initiated in the same manner as in other forms of gonadal dysgenesis.

Dysgenetic Male Pseudohermaphroditism The term *dysgenetic male pseudohermaphroditism* does not define a distinct clinical entity but rather is a catch-all phrase to describe patients with a 46,XY karyotype who present with bilateral dysgenetic testes (usually intraabdominal), incomplete masculinization with ambiguous external genitalia, and variable persistence of paramesonephric duct structures. In most such patients the disorder is not familial. It seems likely that many of these patients have a subtle structural anomaly of the Y chromosome [e.g., 46,X(Yp−) or 46,X(Yp−)/46,XY mosaicism] or represent unrecognized cases of 45,X/46,XY mosaicism. The latter situation may prove impossible to detect if selective pressures mitigate against survival of the 45,X cell line in peripheral leukocytes or fibroblasts. Other patients may represent a less severe variant of XY gonadal dysgenesis with some testicular differentiation. A few pedigrees have been reported in which some members showed typical XY gonadal dysgenesis with bilateral streak gonads and a female phenotype, while others appeared to demonstrate an incomplete variant with one or two dysgenetic testes, ambiguous genitalia, and rudimentary paramesonephric duct derivatives. Most of these patients will show some virilization at puberty if their testes remain, and they are at high risk of developing a gonadoblastoma or germinoma. As in any intersex situation in which sterility is inevitable, sex of rearing should be assigned to provide the greatest opportunity for normal genital function. Because of the high risk of neoplasia, early prophylactic gonadectomy should be performed; appropriate sex steroid replacement will be necessary at the time of puberty.

A subset of patients with dysgenetic male pseudohermaphroditism appear to have a teratologic anomaly causing dysplasia of both the testes and the kidney.[92] In addition to ambiguous genitalia and persistent paramesonephric structures as a result of their dysgenetic testes, these infants have a constellation of renal abnormalities which may include hypertension, proteinuria and nephrotic syndrome, end-stage glomerulonephritis with renal failure, and Wilms' tumor. Several children have been described with bilateral aniridia (as well as cataracts or glaucoma), male pseudohermaphroditism (with hypospadias, cryptorchism, ambiguous genitalia, or gonadoblastoma), and early development of Wilms' tumor. Recent evidence[91] indicates that this syndrome is due to a defect in a gene on chromosome 11 (11p13) that is involved in mesenchymal-epithelial transition in the gonad and the genitourinary tract.

Testicular Regression Syndromes The general term *testicular regression syndrome* applies to a heterogeneous group of conditions in which, for largely undetermined reasons, there is a cessation of testicular function during fetal life. Obviously, the pathogenesis of these conditions is closely related to that of XY gonadal dysgenesis and dysgenetic male pseudohermaphroditism. As shown in Table 18-4, the clinical phenotype depends on the degree of testicular func-

TABLE 18-4 Clinical Features of Testicular Dysgenesis Syndromes

	XY gonadal dysgenesis	True agonadism	Rudimentary testes	Congenital anorchia
Genetic sex	46,XY	46,XY	46,XY	46,XY
Time of testis dysfunction (gestational)	Before 8 weeks	8–12 weeks	14–20 weeks	After 20 weeks
External genitalia	Female	Ambiguous	Micropenis	Male
Vagina	Complete	Blind pouch	Absent	Absent
Paramesonephric structures	Present	Rudimentary	Absent	Absent
Mesonephric structures	Absent	Absent	Present	Present
Gonads	Streak	Absent	Rudimentary testis	Absent

Source: Cleary, Caras, Rosenfield, and Young.[93]

tion and its duration during sexual differentiation. Any of these disorders may be familial; the occasional reports of coexistence of, for example, XY gonadal dysgenesis and congenital anorchia in the same family suggest that all these syndromes of testicular regression may represent variable expressions of a common genetic defect.

So-called true agonadism probably is a variant form of dysgenetic male pseudohermaphroditism in which there is some testicular function during early development, after which the testes disappear.[93] The external genitalia are ambiguous, with a phallus the size of an enlarged clitoris, partial labioscrotal fusion, and a persistent urogenital sinus; both paramesonephric and mesonephric ductal structures are absent. Stimulation testing with chorionic gonadotropin in later life may sometimes induce a slight rise in plasma testosterone, even though testes cannot be found. Associated craniofacial or vertebral anomalies have occasionally been observed, suggesting the action of a teratogen or an underlying connective tissue defect.

Bergada et al. have described a sibship in which the affected members were phenotypically male but had a micropenis and small testes (less than 1 cm in diameter) containing only a few tubules and occasional Leydig cells.[94] Suppression of paramesonephric structures was complete, suggesting that testicular function was relatively normal until around 14 weeks gestation.

Complete regression of the testes after 20 weeks gestation leads to congenital anorchia, in which male sexual differentiation is complete but testes are absent. This situation can be distinguished from cryptorchism by the finding of high levels of serum FSH[81] and a failure of serum testosterone to rise after stimulation with hCG.[95] The mechanism underlying this late regression of the testes is unknown but is thought to involve torsion or occlusion of the testicular vascular supply.

Errors of Sexual Differentiation

Once structurally normal gonads have been formed, it is still possible for sexual differentiation to be aberrant if the testes are unable to accomplish normal masculinization of a genetic male (male pseudohermaphroditism) or if an abnormal source of androgen induces inappropriate prenatal virilization of a genetic female (female pseudohermaphroditism).

Persistent Paramesonephric Ducts

A failure of paramesonephric (müllerian) duct regression, ranging from simple enlargement of the prostatic utricle to complete preservation of a uterus and tubes, is expected in disorders of testicular dysgenesis, in which case one also sees impaired testosterone-dependent differentiation.[96] However, more than 80 genetic males have been reported in whom normal male external genitalia were present but in whom at laparotomy or herniorrhaphy a cervix, a uterus, and fallopian tubes were found in addition to normal male mesonephric duct structures.[97] This situation, referred to as *persistent müllerian duct syndrome* or *hernia uteri inguinalis,* is commonly associated with cryptorchism. Developmental anomalies of the vasa deferentia, epididymis, or tunica albuginea have been reported. Testicular endocrine function appears to be normal at puberty, spermatogenesis occurs, and fertility appears to be possible. There may, however, be an increased propensity to neoplastic degeneration of the testis. The disorder is often familial, most likely sex-limited autosomal recessive. In one series of six patients, two were found to have normal MIS expression and activity while the others had detectable MIS mRNA but no detectable bioactive or immunoreactive MIS protein.[98] Therefore, in some cases the defect may be due to a defective MIS receptor while in others a deletion or mutation in the MIS gene is the likely cause. Therapy involves correction of undescended testes and hysterectomy, provided that the latter can be accomplished without damage to the vasa deferentia contained within the broad ligaments.

Defective Genital Virilization (Male Pseudohermaphroditism)

Leydig Cell Hypoplasia

Leydig cell agenesis or hypoplasia is thought to represent a genetic defect in the LH-hCG receptor, resulting in Leydig cell unresponsiveness to gonadotropic stimulation and inadequate testosterone production before and after birth. These are 46,XY patients with female external genitalia, absent paramesonephric duct structures, and small intraabdominal testes lacking any Leydig cells.[99] There is no serum testosterone response to exogenous hCG, and testicular membrane preparations show defective receptor binding of hCG. However, some Leydig cell function may occur in fetal life, since occasional patients show minimal posterior labial fusion and some development of mesonephric duct structures (epididymis and vas deferens).

Inborn Errors of Testosterone Biosynthesis

Of the five known inborn errors of testosterone synthesis, three also impair adrenal secretion of cortisol and therefore cause variant forms of congenital adrenal hyperplasia (Fig. 18-13). In all cases prenatal androgen deficiency in affected genetic males results in either a female external genetic phenotype or ambiguous genitalia; at puberty there is sexual infantilism in both males and females because of the inability to produce any sex steroids.

Cholesterol Side-Chain Cleavage (20,22-Desmolase) Deficiency Whether in the testis, ovary, or adrenal cortex, the initial and rate-limiting step in steroid hormone biosynthesis involves hydroxylation of cholesterol at the 20 and 22 positions followed by cleavage of the side chain at the C-20–C-22 bond to form pregnenolone. This step is catalyzed by a mitochondrial mixed-function oxidase, cytochrome $P450_{scc}$, which utilizes NADPH as an electron donor. The side-chain cleavage (SCC) complex is an electron transfer system composed of a flavoprotein (NADPH-adrenodoxin reductase), an iron sulfur protein (adrenodoxin), and a specific oxygenase (cytochrome $P450_{scc}$) which interacts with the substrate cholesterol. The role of trophic hormones such as LH/hCG and ACTH appears to be to enhance the availability and binding of free cholesterol to the $P450_{scc}$, which is the substrate-specific component of the complex.

Cytochrome $P450_{scc}$ is a large (molecular mass of 850,000 dalton) hemoprotein encoded by a single gene on chromosome 15; its transcription in gonads is regulated by gonadotropins acting via cyclic AMP. Although a clinical deficiency of SCC activity might result from abnormalities of adrenodoxin reductase or adrenodoxin or from abnormal binding of cholesterol to $P450_{scc}$, in at least one case the disorder was accompanied by a virtual absence of mitochondrial $P450_{scc}$ protein.[100] Patients with such a complete deficiency cannot synthesize any sex steroids, glucocorticoids, or mineralocorticoids; their adrenal glands are enlarged and laden with lipid, for which reason the disorder was formerly termed *congenital lipoid adrenal hyperplasia*. Without replacement therapy, most affected infants die of severe mineralocorticoid and glucocorticoid insufficiency, although survival has been reported in at least one untreated infant thought to have had a less severe variant.[101]

Affected males have either female or ambiguous external genitalia, hypoplastic mesonephric duct structures, and a blind vaginal pouch with no uterus or fallopian tubes. The testes appear normal and may be intraabdominal, inguinal, or in the labioscrotal area. Affected females have normal external and internal genitalia. Endocrine studies demonstrate low or negligible levels of glucocorticoids, mineralocorticoids, and sex steroids in the presence of high plasma levels of ACTH, renin activity, and gonadotropins. In genetic female infants it may be necessary to differentiate this condition from congenital adrenal hypoplasia by radiographic demonstration of hyperplastic adrenals. Therapy for SCC deficiency includes glucocorticoid and mineralocorticoid replacement and appropriate sex steroid replacement at puberty. To date, all affected genetic males have been assigned a female sex of rearing but have required prophylactic orchiectomy to obviate any possible virilism at puberty. In the future, with early neonatal diagnosis of this form of male pseudohermaphroditism, testosterone therapy in infancy to render the penis normal in size, followed by genital plastic surgery, may be a more appropriate course of action.

3β-Hydroxysteroid Dehydrogenase Deficiency All human biologically active steroid hormones, whether of adrenal or gonadal origin, have in common a Δ^4-3-keto configuration. The enzyme complex responsible for conversion of pregnenolone, 17-hydroxypregnenolone, and dehydroepiandrosterone to their respective Δ^4-3-keto forms (progesterone, 17-hydroxyprogesterone, and androstenedione) is 3β-hydroxysteroid dehydrogenase/isomerase, which utilizes NAD as a cofactor and is located in the smooth endoplasmic reticulum, with lesser amounts in mitochondria. A single gene encoding a protein with 3β-hydroxysteroid dehydrogenase (3β-HSD)/isomerase activities has recently been cloned and assigned to the short arm of chromosome 1.[102] One remarkable characteristic of this enzyme is its susceptibility to inhibition by micromolar concentrations of circulating or intraadrenal steroids. Changes in ambient steroid concentrations appear to account for shifts in adrenal 3β-HSD activity during development;[103] thus in fetal and adult life, 3β-HSD normally becomes a rate-limiting step in cortisol biosynthesis, and large amounts of dehydroepiandrosterone are secreted by the adrenal cortex.

Infants affected with autosomal recessive 3β-HSD deficiency typically present with ambiguous genitalia plus severe adrenal insufficiency. The genitalia of affected females may be normal or show mild clitoromegaly, presumably a result of peripheral

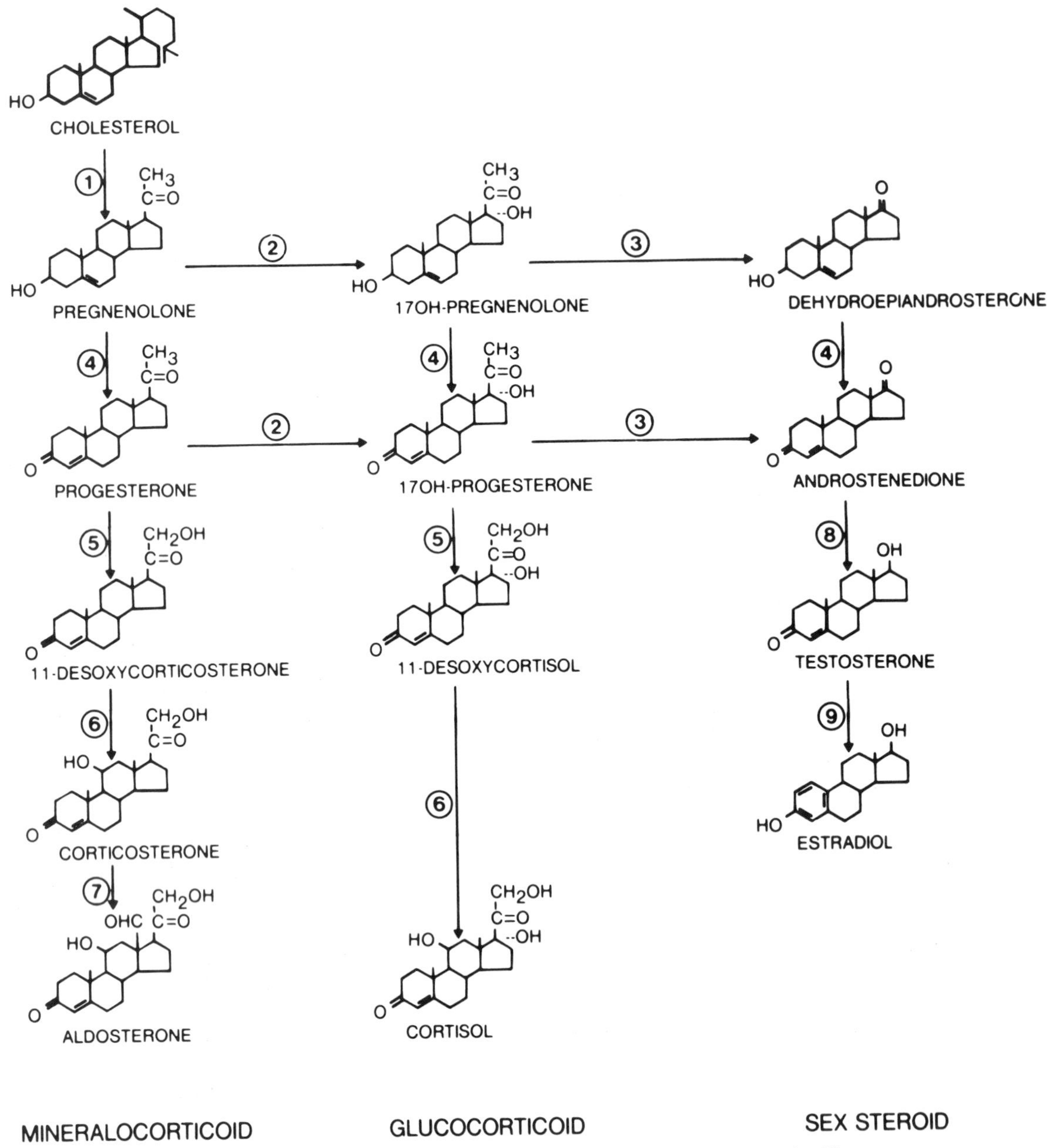

CHOLESTEROL
PREGNENOLONE
17OH-PREGNENOLONE
DEHYDROEPIANDROSTERONE
PROGESTERONE
17OH-PROGESTERONE
ANDROSTENEDIONE
11-DESOXYCORTICOSTERONE
11-DESOXYCORTISOL
TESTOSTERONE
ESTRADIOL
CORTICOSTERONE
ALDOSTERONE
CORTISOL

MINERALOCORTICOID GLUCOCORTICOID SEX STEROID

FIGURE 18-13 Pathways of steroidogenesis in the adrenal cortex and gonads. The enzymes involved include cytochrome $P450_{scc}$ (cholesterol side-chain cleavage) ①); cytochrome $P450_{C17}$ (responsible for both 17-hydroxylase ② and 17,20-desmolase ③); 3β-hydroxysteroid dehydrogenase/isomerase ④; cytochrome $P450_{C21}$ (21-hydroxylase ⑤); cytochrome $P450_{C11}$ (responsible for 11β-hydroxylase ⑥, 18-hydroxylase, and aldehyde synthetase ⑦); 17β-hydroxysteroid dehydrogenase ⑧; and cytochrome $P450_{arom}$ (aromatase ⑨).

transformation of adrenal dehydroepiandrosterone to testosterone. At puberty there is no spontaneous breast development. Affected males typically show a small hypospadic phallus, partially fused labioscrotal folds, and a urogenital sinus with a blind vaginal pouch. Paramesonephric duct structures are absent, but surprisingly, mesonephric duct structures are normal, indicating that the prenatal testis was capable of some androgen production. At the time of puberty males show hypergonadotropic hypogonadism, with gynecomastia, inadequate masculinization, and spermatogenic arrest.

The diagnosis of 3β-HSD deficiency requires demonstration of increased concentrations of Δ^5-3β-hydroxysteroids such as dehydroepiandrosterone, Δ^5-androstenediol, and 17-hydroxypregnenolone in serum or increased urinary excretion of their metabolites. During the neonatal period attention must be paid to the normally high excretion of Δ^5-3β-hydroxysteroids at this time. It is of interest that patients with 3β-HSD deficiency also characteristically show slightly increased serum levels of 17-hydroxyprogesterone and increased urinary pregnanetriol, presumably because of hepatic conversion of 17-hydroxypregnenolone. Therapy for this disorder requires glucocorticoid and mineralocorticoid replacement from birth and appropriate sex steroid replacement at puberty. Affected males should receive sufficient testosterone in infancy to correct the micropenis and permit satisfactory repair of hypospadias.

The clinical picture of severe adrenal insufficiency in a male pseudohermaphrodite represents the most severe form of 3β-HSD deficiency, but many patients with milder variants have been described. Some of this biochemical and clinical heterogeneity may reflect synthesis of a functional 3β-HSD enzyme which is unduly susceptible to the type of steroidal inhibition described above. Thus some patients show apparent preservation of aldosterone secretion,[104] since intraadrenal steroid concentrations are normally lowest in the zona glomerulosa. In addition, partial deficiencies of 3β-HSD have been documented in pubertal girls with clitoromegaly, hirsutism, and primary amenorrhea[105] and in males with hypospadias and pubertal gynecomastia.[106] Awareness of this genetic heterogeneity has not unreasonably led to the proposition that even more subtle defects which are apparent only after ACTH stimulation might cause postpubertal hirsutism or infertility resembling the polycystic ovary syndrome.[107]

No data are available to establish whether placental 3β-HSD activity is also deficient when the fetus is homozygous for severe deficiency. If the syncytiotrophoblast (also of fetal origin) is not affected, as one might assume from the fact that pregnancies with such fetuses proceed to term, this would imply that 3β-HSD deficiency does not represent a primary lack of enzyme protein (as in cholesterol SCC deficiency) but represents the synthesis of an enzyme which can be effective in the placental but not in the adrenal or gonadal intracellular milieu.

17α-Hydroxylase Deficiency Conversion of pregnenolone to 17-hydroxypregnenolone takes place in the adrenal cortex, testicular Leydig cells, and ovarian theca and granulosa cells. The enzyme complex, which is located in the smooth endoplasmic reticulum, is a typical mixed-function oxidase; NADPH is the preferred electron donor, and the electron transport system involves a flavoprotein which interacts directly with the terminal cytochrome P450. This cytochrome P450 (59,000 dalton) has been purified and shown to have not only 17α-hydroxylase but also 17,20-desmolase activity.[108] The gene for cytochrome $P450_{C17}$ has recently been assigned to chromosome 10 (10q24.3). In recent years several different molecular defects in the coding sequence of this gene have been described in patients with varying degrees of 17α-hydroxylase deficiency.[109–112]

In males, deficiency of 17α-hydroxylase results in variable genital ambiguity and mesonephric duct differentiation. The phenotype may vary from apparently female external genitalia with a blind vaginal pouch to a hypospadic male with micropenis (Fig. 18-14). The testes are normally formed and may be intraabdominal, inguinal, or in the labioscrotal folds. Affected females have normal internal and external development. Hypertension, with or without hypokalemic alkalosis, due to excessive adrenal secretion of mineralocorticoids such as deoxycorticosterone, becomes evident by 2 years of age.[113] In both sexes there is failure of sexual maturation at puberty, although untreated males usually develop gynecomastia.

The diagnosis of 17α-hydroxylase deficiency can be confirmed by demonstrating increased serum concentrations of pregnenolone, progesterone, corticosterone, and deoxycorticosterone, with increased urinary excretion of their metabolites. Plasma renin activity and serum aldosterone levels are usually suppressed,[114] but plasma ACTH is increased. Occa-

FIGURE 18-14 External genitalia of a male with 17-hydroxylase deficiency at 10 months of age. Testes were palpable in the labioscrotal folds. (*From Dean et al.*[113])

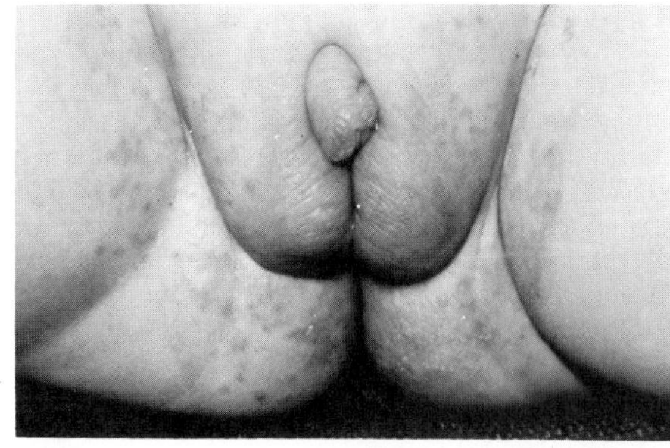

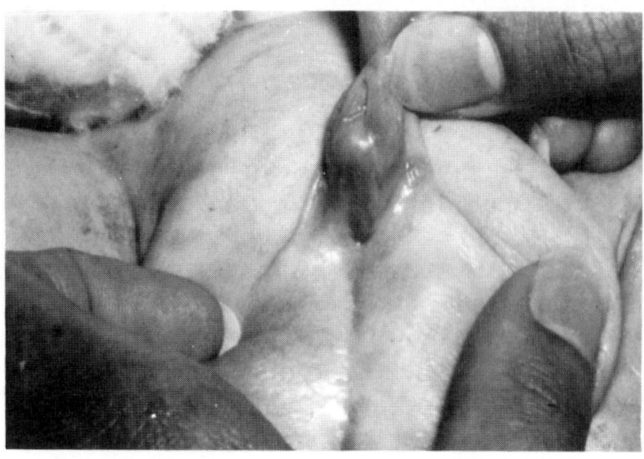

sionally circulating aldosterone levels are increased; such patients may appear to have primary hyperaldosteronism or dexamethasone-suppressible hyperaldosteronism. Affected males show low serum testosterone and cortisol values, with inadequate responses to hCG and ACTH. Serum FSH and LH levels are elevated into the age-specific agonadal range because of the lack of sex steroid–mediated feedback inhibition.

Replacement glucocorticoid therapy (cortisol, 10 to 20 mg/m^2 daily) suppresses corticosterone and deoxycorticosterone secretion and corrects the hypertension and hypokalemic alkalosis. Infant males should receive sufficient testosterone to produce a normal-sized penis, followed by surgical correction of the hypospadias.[113] In both sexes, appropriate sex steroid replacement is required at the time of puberty.

17,20-Desmolase Deficiency Synthesis of testosterone involves two enzymes—17,20-desmolase and 17β-HSD—which are not necessary for biosynthesis of cortisol or aldosterone (Fig. 18-13). Genetic deficiencies of these enzymes cause inadequate virilization of genetic males (male pseudohermaphroditism) without any associated adrenal insufficiency. They are autosomal recessive traits and should also present as sexual infantilism and primary amenorrhea in genetic females, since testosterone is a necessary precursor of estradiol biosynthesis. Few affected females have been described, presumably because of inadequate endocrine investigation of women presenting with hypergonadotropic hypogonadism.

If, as has been suggested, a single enzyme protein in both the gonad and the adrenal gland catalyzes both 17-hydroxylation and side-chain cleavage of pregnenolone and/or progesterone, it is difficult to understand isolated 17,20-desmolase deficiency. It seems likely that such patients have a mutant form of the gene for cytochrome $P450_{C17}$ in which 17-hydroxylation of C-21 steroids is maintained but subsequent cleavage to form C-19 steroids is impaired.[115] There are at least two genetic variants of this syndrome which differ in regard to the severity of the block in androgen biosynthesis.[116] Some affected genetic males present with female external genitalia and show little or no spontaneous pubertal development owing to an almost complete inability to secrete testosterone. Others present as undervirilized males with micropenis, perineal hypospadias, and a bifid scrotum; these patients may show some Leydig cell response to hCG and will virilize to some extent at puberty. The testes in either case appear histologically normal, although tubular atrophy and hyalinization have been described after puberty. In most patients mesonephric duct structures are present, but a uterus is uniformly absent. Very few 46,XX females with apparent 17,20-desmolase deficiency have been recognized.[117] They might be expected to present with sexual infantilism, amenorrhea, or possibly just infertility, depending on the capacity for ovarian estrogen production.

In vivo and in vitro studies confirm the inability of the gonad and adrenal cortex to convert pregnenolone or 17-hydroxypregnenolone to C-19 androgens, but secretion of cortisol and aldosterone is normal. Serum concentrations of testosterone, androstenedione, and dehydroepiandrosterone are subnormal, while levels of C-21 precursors such as pregnenolone, 17-hydroxypregnenolone, and 17-hydroxyprogesterone are inappropriately high; this discrepancy is accentuated on stimulation with hCG or ACTH. Patients with ambiguous genitalia excrete significant amounts of pregnanetriolone, a metabolite of 17-hydroxypregnenolone; conversely, patients with a female phenotype do not excrete pregnanetriolone, but some dehydroepiandrosterone is found in serum and urine.[115]

Patients who are identified at birth require plastic repair of the external genitalia and replacement therapy with testosterone. Those who have been raised as females and whose condition is not recognized until adolescence require castration and estrogen replacement therapy.

17β-Hydroxysteroid Dehydrogenase Deficiency The final step in the biosynthesis of testosterone is 17-keto reduction of androstenedione (Fig. 18-13). The enzyme which catalyzes this conversion, and also the conversion of estrone to estradiol, is 17β-HSD (also called *17-ketosteroid reductase*). The gene encoding this enzyme has recently been characterized and assigned to chromosome 17.[118]

Genetic males with 17β-HSD deficiency usually present with female external genitalia at birth (although a few show mild clitoromegaly or posterior labioscrotal fusion); thus the sex of rearing has almost always been female. The testes are usually inguinal or in the labioscrotal folds; in infancy such a condition may be misdiagnosed as testicular feminization. There is a blind vagina, and mesonephric duct structures are present.

The diagnosis is usually made at puberty, when, unless castration has already been performed, striking virilization occurs with marked enlargement of the phallus, hirsutism, acne, and deepening of the voice. Some breast enlargement may occur, but primary amenorrhea is constant. In some cases the degree of virilization has been such that successful transition to a male gender role has been possible.[119]

In vitro studies have confirmed reduced levels of 17β-HSD activity within the testis,[120] although there is some evidence that the activity in peripheral tissues is unimpaired, presumably owing to a different enzyme. The diagnostic hallmark of this disorder is a markedly elevated serum concentration of androstenedione after puberty or hCG stimulation, with low-normal levels of testosterone.[121] Serum estradiol values are normal, but estrone levels are increased. The reason for the discrepancy between the apparent lack of prenatal testosterone biosynthesis and the significant virilization which occurs at puberty is not clear. It may reflect postnatal peripheral conversion of androstenedione to testosterone, but in addition the abnormal testicular 17β-HSD may be affected by the high concentrations of placental steroids in the fetal circulation. There have been no studies of placental 17β-HSD activity in this syndrome, and it is not known to what extent placental estradiol synthesis is affected.

A deficiency of 17β-HSD should be considered in any male pseudohermaphrodite who has normal adrenal glucocorticoid and mineralocorticoid function and an absent uterus, particularly if virilization occurs at puberty. Since these patients have generally already been assigned a female gender, the appropriate therapy is usually castration followed by estrogen replacement at puberty. When a male gender role is assigned or feasible, the patient requires plastic repair of the external genitalia and supplementary testosterone therapy. Spermatogenesis would not be expected because of the lack of testicular testosterone.

Defects in Androgen Target Tissues

The bulk of testosterone in the circulation is bound to either sex hormone–binding globulin or albumin, although levels of both proteins are markedly reduced in the fetus at the time of sexual differentiation. Unbound testosterone enters target cells by passive diffusion and is then converted to the more potent androgen dihydrotestosterone through the action of the enzyme 5α-reductase. Both androgens bind to a specific high-affinity androgen receptor in the nucleus; the hormone-receptor complex binds to chromatin acceptor sites composed of DNA and nonhistone chromosomal protein. This interaction initiates transcription and processing of specific messenger RNAs which subsequently are translated to initiate ribosomal synthesis of new proteins. The androgen receptor is regulated by a gene on the X chromosome, while the gene for 5α-reductase is autosomal. Thus the cellular mechanisms for androgen action are present in target tissues of both sexes. There is evidence that dihydrotestosterone is the major androgen responsible for virilization of the external genitalia and the later appearance of male secondary sexual characteristics at puberty; testosterone itself appears to mediate differentiation of the mesonephric duct and possibly also spermatogenesis and feedback control of gonadotropin secretion in adult life. In some forms of male pseudohermaphroditism, testosterone synthesis and paramesonephric duct regression are normal, but prenatal masculinization of the external genitalia is inadequate because of target cell resistance to androgen. The molecular basis for such androgen resistance may include a defect in 5α-reductase, in the androgen receptor, or at one or more postreceptor loci.

Defective Androgen Metabolism: 5α-Reductase Deficiency Genetic males with a deficiency of 5α-reductase present with a clinical picture formerly termed *pseudovaginal perineoscrotal hypospadias.* Typical features at birth include a clitoris-sized phallus with a hooded prepuce, a ventral urethral groove, a variable chordee, and a urogenital sinus opening on the perineum.[122] Because paramesonephric duct regression is normal, there is a blind vaginal pouch opening into the urogenital sinus. The testes are normally formed and located in either the inguinal canal or the partially fused labioscrotal folds. Mesonephric duct structures (epididymis, vas deferens, seminal vesicle, and ejaculatory duct) are well differentiated and empty into the blind vagina. Most of these patients have been raised as females.

At puberty, if castration was not accomplished earlier, serum testosterone increases into the adult male range; variable virilization occurs, without gynecomastia. The phallus enlarges to as much as 8 cm in length, the testes enlarge and complete their descent, muscle mass increases, the voice deepens, and spermatogenesis may occur. However, prostatic enlargement, acne, growth of facial and body hair, and temporal hair recession, features which are dihydrotestosterone-dependent, do not occur. Many such patients spontaneously and successfully change to a male gender identity and role, in spite of unambiguous assignment of female gender throughout childhood.[123] Such occurrences demonstrate the powerful influence that self-perceptions of genital and secondary sexual development have on gender identity and cast serious doubts on the previous notion that core psychosexual identity is always permanently imprinted during a critical period in infancy and early childhood. Although most reported patients have chosen this postpubertal gender reassignment, some patients, particularly those with a relatively small phallus, have opted to retain their female psychosexual orientation.[124]

The absence of paramesonephric duct remnants differentiates 5α-reductase deficiency from disorders of gonadogenesis such as 45,X/46,XY mixed gonadal dysgenesis; however, detailed endocrine studies are necessary to rule out a disorder of testosterone biosynthesis or other forms of androgen resistance such as incomplete testicular feminization. Homozygous postpubertal males show normal or slightly increased levels of circulating FSH and LH. Serum testosterone concentrations are also normal or slightly elevated, but dihydrotestosterone concentrations remain relatively low; thus the testosterone/dihydrotestosterone ratio exceeds 35, in contrast to the normal adult male ratio of 8 to 16.[125] A similar pattern can be elicited in affected children after Leydig cell stimulation with hCG. Decreased conversion of ^{3}H-labeled testosterone to dihydrotestosterone has been confirmed in vivo. Study of urinary steroids shows diminished ratios of 5α-reduced to 5β-reduced C-19 and C-21 steroids (for example, a reduced androsterone/etiocholanolone ratio). Homozygous females show similar urinary steroid patterns but have no clinical manifestations; heterozygotes show intermediate 5α/5β steroid ratios. In vitro study of tissue slices or cultured genital skin fibroblasts may confirm the inability to convert [^{3}H]testosterone to 5α-reduced metabolites, but the wide variation observed in normal control preparations can make interpretation of the results problematic. The 5α-reductase activities of liver, nongenital skin, and genital skin may be due to separate enzymes;[126] the enzyme in nongenital skin appears to be induced by androgens, while that in genital tissues is independent of androgen exposure. It will be necessary to resolve these and other questions regarding the interpretation of in vitro 5α-reductase assays before issues such as genetic heterogeneity can be resolved.[127] In addition, it is necessary to differentiate primary genetic 5α-reductase deficiency from disorders, such as complete androgen insensitivity, porphyria, hypothyroidism, and Cushing's syndrome, in which secondary defects in hepatic or peripheral 5α-reductase activity may occur. Although plasma concentrations of 3α-androstenediol glucuronide appear to reflect 5α-reductase activity, they are reduced in both primary and secondary deficiencies of the enzyme.

If the diagnosis of 5α-reductase deficiency is suspected and confirmed during the neonatal period, the sex of rearing should be male. Androgen (testosterone or dihydrotestosterone) therapy can be used to enhance penile growth and facilitate surgical repair of the genitalia. In such patients virilization can be expected at puberty, and fertility is theoretically possible. Those who are diagnosed later and who have an unambiguous female gender identity should undergo orchiectomy and receive estrogen therapy at the time of puberty.

Androgen Insensitivity: Complete and Incomplete Testicular Feminization The clinical phenotype in genetic males with various forms of androgen insensitivity may range from female through genital ambiguity to male with hypospadias or infertility, presumably a reflection of the severity of the receptor or postreceptor defect. In all these disorders, regardless of phenotype, the affected males have a 46,XY karyotype and have testes capable of normal testosterone secretion.

The most common form of male pseudohermaphroditism is complete testicular feminization, an X-linked recessive disorder analogous to the Tfm mutation in the mouse.[128] Phenotypically, the hemizygous male presents with normal female external genitalia; a blind vaginal pouch with absent cervix, uterus, and tubes; and absent or vestigial mesonephric duct structures. The testes may be intraabdominal, inguinal, or labial.

During infancy and childhood, complete testicular feminization should be considered in any girl with an inguinal hernia, particularly if it contains a palpable gonad; 1 in 50 girls with a hernia has this disorder. The diagnosis is almost certain if the karyotype is 46,XY and ultrasonography fails to demonstrate a uterus but should be confirmed by in vitro study of androgen receptors. After puberty the presenting complaint is primary amenorrhea, which in up to 10 percent of cases may be due to testicular feminization. At puberty these patients acquire a normal female body habitus and well-developed breasts, but the clitoris remains small and pubic and axillary hair is absent or sparse.

The testes are characterized by small seminiferous tubules devoid of spermatogenic elements other than spermatogonia. After puberty varying degrees of Leydig cell hyperplasia, frequently in adenomatous clumps, can be observed. These patients are predisposed to develop germ cell tumors of the testis, of which seminoma is the most common malignant variety. The incidence of malignant degeneration ranges from 5 to 20 percent and is clearly related to the age of the patient. Clinically apparent neoplasm rarely occurs before the third decade, but studies of even prepubertal testes frequently show carcinoma in situ.[129]

The hypothalamus and pituitary of these patients are resistant to the feedback effects of androgen, although gonadotropin suppression by estrogens is normal.[130] After puberty serum LH concentrations are higher than in normal men, and as a result, levels of testosterone, dihydrotestosterone, and estradiol are also elevated. In spite of defective spermatogenesis, serum FSH concentrations are usually normal or only slightly increased.

Most patients with androgen insensitivity show markedly reduced androgen binding in cultured genital skin fibroblasts.[131] The genetic defects in such receptor-negative families may involve a deletion in the segment coding for the hormone-binding domain[132] or small deletions or point mutations that interfere with the expression of a functioning receptor protein.[133–135] Other, so-called receptor-positive patients in vitro show relatively normal levels of androgen binding,[136] but the receptor appears to be defective, forming a steroid-receptor complex which is thermolabile or readily dissociable.[137–139] These patients may have mutations of the androgen receptor gene in the DNA-binding domain or a defect in the genomic acceptor site.[140]

Therapy for androgen-insensitive patients requires positive reinforcement of the female gender identity, a process that will rarely be assisted by discussion of male chromosomes and gonads. The testes should probably be removed as soon as the diagnosis is made, particularly if herniorrhaphy is required. There seems to be little merit in retaining such testes in order to permit spontaneous puberty, since later prophylactic orchiectomy to prevent malignancy will be required as a second surgical procedure. Estrogen replacement therapy is required after castration to initiate and maintain secondary sex characters, but since no endometrium is present, there is no need to provide this in cyclic fashion. The blind vagina will usually permit normal sexual intercourse, but occasionally dilatation is required. In adult life the female gender identity remains firm, and marital and maternal attitudes are clearly feminine.

About 10 percent of patients with androgen insensitivity show some evidence of prenatal and adolescent virilization, and their condition is termed *incomplete testicular feminization*. Some of these patients show reduced levels of cytosol androgen binding, some have a defective androgen receptor, and some appear to have a postreceptor defect. In contrast to typical receptor-negative complete testicular feminization, there is considerable clinical heterogeneity even within the same pedigree. Furthermore, there is little if any correlation between the degree of virilization and the severity of the receptor abnormality demonstrable in vitro. In view of this clinical variability, there seems to be no reason to retain eponymic syndromes based on phenotype, such as those of Reifenstein, Rosewater, Gilbert-Dreyfus, and Lubs.[127]

All these patients are 46,XY, have testes, and lack paramesonephric duct structures. In some the genitalia are female, as in complete testicular feminization, but distinct mesonephric duct structures can be identified. More commonly the genitalia are ambiguous, with varying degrees of clitoromegaly and labioscrotal fusion and a short blind vagina (pseudovaginal perineoscrotal hypospadias). At puberty such patients show, in addition to gynecomastia and primary amenorrhea, significant virilization with clitoral enlargement, masculine body habitus, and growth of pubic and axillary hair. In most the gender identity is female, and therapy involves immediate orchiectomy, genital reconstruction as necessary, and estrogen replacement.

The term *Reifenstein syndrome* was formerly applied to less severe variants of X-linked partial androgen insensitivity in which affected individuals presented as phenotypic males with hypospadias, inadequate pubertal virilization, gynecomastia, and infertility.[141] Cryptorchism is common; the testes are small, with normal Leydig cells but arrested spermatogenesis. Some patients show defective mesonephric duct development, such as severe hypoplasia of the vas deferens. In one such pedigree, the only abnormality detected was a decreased concentration of the androgen receptor, but gene sequencing was not done.[142] More recently similar degrees of in vitro androgen sensitivity have been demonstrated in males presenting with only microphallus, simple penile hypospadias, or idiopathic infertility.[142]

It is obvious that with this wide spectrum of clinical phenotypes, the diagnosis of partial androgen insensitivity is problematic unless there is an obvious family history. Serum concentrations of FSH, LH, testosterone, and estradiol are normal or moderately elevated after puberty. The diagnosis may be suspected because of a poor clinical response to administered androgen but must be confirmed by in vitro study of androgen binding.

In patients with male sex of rearing, therapy is even more problematic in view of the limited response to testosterone. Any hypospadias or cryptorchism should be corrected surgically; mastectomy will often be required because of gynecomastia. There is no evidence that the risk of developing a gonadal neoplasm in this situation exceeds that in normal males with undescended testes.

Defective Virilization Due to Exogenous Sex Steroids

While normal exposure to placental estrogens and progesterone does not disturb fetal sexual differentiation, data derived from studies in experimental animals and some circumstantial epidemiologic evidence have raised the possibility that maternal ingestion of synthetic sex steroids may lead to hypospadias or more severe genital ambiguity.[143] Variable degrees of incomplete masculinization can be induced in rats and rabbits by prenatal exposure to high doses of progestational compounds such as the 19-nor- and 17α-ethinyl derivatives of testosterone. In addition, there has been an apparent increase in the incidence of hypospadias in industrialized countries during the past decade; this may relate to the use of such drugs for threatened abortion or as a pregnancy test or to inadvertent ingestion of contraceptive steroids during early pregnancy. Several retrospective studies of hypospadiac boys have demonstrated an increased rate of maternal sex steroid ingestion, with some correlation between the time of ingestion and the severity of the defect. However, prospective studies have failed to show an increased risk in the offspring of women exposed to synthetic progestogens in early pregnancy, perhaps because of the high incidence of spontaneous hypospadias.[144]

A case of male pseudohermaphroditism has been reported in which the mother received large doses of diethylstilbestrol during early pregnancy; in two surveys of boys similarly exposed, no increased incidence of hypospadias was found, although other genital anomalies, such as meatal stenosis, epididymal cyst, and testicular hypoplasia, were increased.[145] Estrogens are known to be potent inhibitors of the steroidogenic enzyme 3β-HSD, but there is no proof that exogenous estrogens, even in combination with the high levels produced by the placenta, could cause significant inhibition of fetal testosterone biosynthesis. Progesterone and the synthetic progestogen norethindrone have been shown to cause dose-dependent inhibition of 5α-reductase activity in genital skin fibroblasts,[146] but again, the concentrations required make it seem unlikely that this mechanism could explain any teratogenic effect. A direct relation between exogenous sex steroids and male pseudohermaphroditism cannot be said to have been confirmed, but the possibility remains that their influence may be significant in certain genetically predisposed persons.

Male Pseudohermaphroditism of Unknown Etiology

Multiple Malformation Syndromes The presence of ambiguous genitalia in a genetic male may alert the physician to the presence of associated somatic anomalies which require immediate therapy.[147] Such situations include the Smith-Lemli-Opitz syndrome, in which hypospadias is associated with mental retardation, short stature, and skeletal defects; the Najjar syndrome of ambiguous genitalia, cardiomyopathy, and mental retardation; and the genito-palato-cardiac (Gardner-Silengo-Wachtel) syndrome[148] of micrognathia, facial asymmetry, cleft palate, cardiac defects, and female external and internal genitalia. These situations probably represent defects in an autosomal gene involved in gonad development but are more readily ascertained in 46,XY individuals because of the discrepancy between genetic and genital sex.

Isolated Hypospadias Failure of fusion of the urethral folds is one of the most common congenital malformations, with an incidence of about 5 per 1000 live male births. In most cases there is no obvious underlying endocrine defect; indeed, nonendocrine factors are suggested by the frequent coexistence of associated genitourinary and other anomalies. In about one-quarter of cases another family member is affected. The overall risk factor for a subsequent male sibling has been estimated as 11 percent[149] but increases with more severe degrees of hypospadias, suggesting a multigenic form of inheritance. The concordance rate in identical twins is about 50 percent. Basal serum gonadotropin and testosterone concentrations are normal in unselected hypospadiac boys, but a slight diminution in mean testosterone levels has been reported in affected young adults.[150,151] More detailed testing even during childhood may reveal exaggerated FSH and LH responses to gonadotropin releasing hormone and reduced testosterone response to hCG stimulation, indicative of some degree of Leydig cell dysfunction.[152] Genital skin 5α-reductase activity appears to be normal in hypospadiac boys, but cytosol androgen receptor levels may be reduced.[153] These findings only underscore the heterogeneous nature of simple hypospadias and its multigenic-multifactorial etiology.

Cryptorchism The testes are frequently undescended in various forms of male pseudohermaphroditism and also in association with a number of multiple anomaly syndromes. In some of these latter situations, such as the Prader-Willi syndrome, the cryptorchism reflects hypogonadotropic hypogonadism. Because of the role of pituitary gonadotropins in the regulation of Leydig cell function during the latter half of pregnancy, the occurrence of microphallus and cryptorchism in an infant with otherwise normally formed genitalia should alert theclinician to a possible hypogonadotropic or hypopituitary condition. A high proportion of maldescended testes show abnormalities of germ cells, but it is not clear whether these abnormalities represent a cause or effect of the maldescent.[154]

Virilization of a Genetic Female (Female Pseudohermaphroditism)

Exposure of a female fetus to inappropriate levels of circulating androgen does not affect ovarian or uterine development but results in some virilization of the external genitalia, or so-called female pseudohermaphroditism. The degree of genital ambiguity present at birth, which may be graded according to the classification of Prader,[155] depends mainly on the timing of the androgen exposure. Late exposure, after 12 weeks gestation, causes only clitoral hypertrophy. However, exposure between 4 and 12 weeks gestation results in varying degrees of labioscrotal fusion; the urogenital sinus commonly opens on the perineum but occasionally may reach the tip of the phallus. The most common source of the offending androgens is the adrenal cortex because of an inborn error of cortisol biosynthesis, but occasionally a maternal source of androgen can be identified. In addition, several nonendocrine malformation syndromes affecting the female external genitalia may produce a similar clinical picture.

Congenital Adrenal Hyperplasia

The virilizing syndromes of congenital adrenal hyperplasia (CAH) have in common reduced adrenal capacity to secrete cortisol (and in some forms also aldosterone). This cortisol deficiency, which during fetal life is exacerbated by rapid placental clearance of cortisol, leads to compensatory hypersecretion of ACTH, adrenocortical hyperplasia, and excessive synthesis of steroids proximal to the enzymatic block (Fig. 18-3). These steroids, such as 17-hydroxyprogesterone, may be converted to testosterone and cause virilization. The impact after birth on salt and water handling depends on the specific enzymatic defect: thus in 11β-hydroxylase deficiency there is excessive secretion of steroids, such as 11-deoxycorticosterone, which have mineralocorticoid activity, but in 21-hydroxylase deficiency the predominant abnormal steroids, 17-hydroxyprogesterone and progesterone, have an antimineralocorticoid effect through their ability to compete for renal tubular aldosterone receptors.

These CAH syndromes are by far the most common cause of female pseudohermaphroditism and account for the majority of all neonates with ambiguous genitalia. Although it has been customary to consider each disorder, defined in vivo from its steroid secretion patterns, as a genetically distinct and homogeneous entity, recent evidence has demonstrated that there is remarkable phenotypic variation, which must reflect in part considerable genetic heterogeneity. It seems inevitable that future studies with cDNA probes will demonstrate many allelic variants at each steroidogenic gene locus, as has been shown for the globin genes.

It may be useful to examine the variables which interact to determine the age of onset and the severity of clinical abnormalities in any patient with CAH. These include both the factors which influence adrenal steroid secretion and those which regulate target cell responses. Obviously, the primary variable is the underlying genetic defect. This may be a major deletion which renders the gene incapable of transcription; such a defect has been suggested in at least one patient with cholesterol side-chain cleavage deficiency in whom there was complete absence of the mitochondrial cytochrome $P450_{scc}$.[100] However, in most cases it is likely that varying amounts of gene product are formed which are defective in terms of substrate or cofactor affinity, maximal activity per cell, or susceptibility to intracellular inhibitors. In addition, genetic defects may occur in mitochondrial or microsomal proteins which serve to orientate enzymatic complexes; such factors may regulate the relative activities of those enzyme proteins (such as 17-hydroxylase/17,20-desmolase or 11β-hydroxylase/18-hydroxylase) which appear to catalyze two steps in steroidogenesis. The activities of steroidogenic enzymes are also regulated by hormones such as ACTH and angiotensin, electrolytes such as potassium, and the modulating effects of ambient intracellular steroids.[103]

Since steroids show a significant gradient across the adrenal cortex and these intraadrenal concentrations change with age and adrenal growth,[156] they may influence the relative secretion of mineralocorticoid, glucocorticoid, and androgen in both normal and CAH patients at different stages of development. ACTH and various unidentified mitogenic peptides interact to regulate the total mass of adrenal steroidogenic tissue. The interaction of all these variables determines the daily secretion of cortisol, aldosterone, and various other steroids, some of which are metabolically active while others are available for peripheral conversion to active steroids. Finally, the biological effect of secreted cortisol or aldosterone may be altered by the presence of steroids which bind competitively to plasma proteins or target cell receptors. These variables are probably sufficient to explain phenotypic variation in CAH without the need to postulate multiple age-, zone-, and substrate-specific steroidogenic enzymes, each under separate genetic control.

Prenatal virilization of a genetic female can result from defects of adrenal 21-hydroxylase, 11β-hydroxylase, or 3β-HSD. The more proximal defects of cortisol biosynthesis, such as cholesterol side-chain cleavage and 17-hydroxylase, also impair androgen synthesis; thus virilization of the female is not a clinical feature. All these CAH variants demonstrate an autosomal recessive pattern of inheritance.

21-Hydroxylase Deficiency Over 90 percent of CAH patients have a deficiency of 21-hydroxylase. At least two clinical variants have been identified: the classic form, which causes prenatal and continuing postnatal virilization with varying degrees of apparent glucocorticoid and mineralocorticoid insufficiency, and a late-onset or attenuated form, which is expressed as hirsutism, virilism, or infertility during the second or third decade. The usual incidence of homozygous classic 21-hydroxylase deficiency detected by screening is 1 per 14,500 live births with a carrier frequency of 1 in 61; however, in one genetic isolate, the Yupik of Alaska, the incidence may reach 1 in 400 live births.[157]

The 21-hydroxylase complex, which is located in adrenal smooth endoplasmic reticulum, utilizes NADPH as cofactor, atmospheric oxygen, an intermediary flavoprotein, and a terminal substrate-specific cytochrome P450 of about 48,000 dalton. This single enzyme complex catalyzes 21-hydroxylation of both 17-hydroxyprogesterone and progesterone (Fig. 18-13), but the former is the preferred substrate. Extraadrenal 21-hydroxylation does not appear to involve the same enzyme and is not impaired in CAH.

Two 21-hydroxylase genes, termed $CYP_{21}A$ and $CYP_{21}B$, are located on the short arm of chromosome 6 between the loci for HLA-B and HLA-DR and adjacent to the two genes for the fourth component of complement (C_4A and C_4B). The two CYP_{21} genes are highly homologous, but only $CYP_{21}B$ encodes an active enzyme. The most common genetic defects in 21-hydroxylase deficiency include deletion of $CYP_{21}B$, gene conversion of $CYP_{21}B$ to a second $CYP_{21}A$ pseudogene, and various point mutations causing either defective transcription or abnormal mRNA splicing.[158]

Close linkage with histocompatibility and complement loci makes it possible to use extended HLA and complement haplotyping to trace the inheritance of a particular 21-hydroxylase gene (Fig. 18-

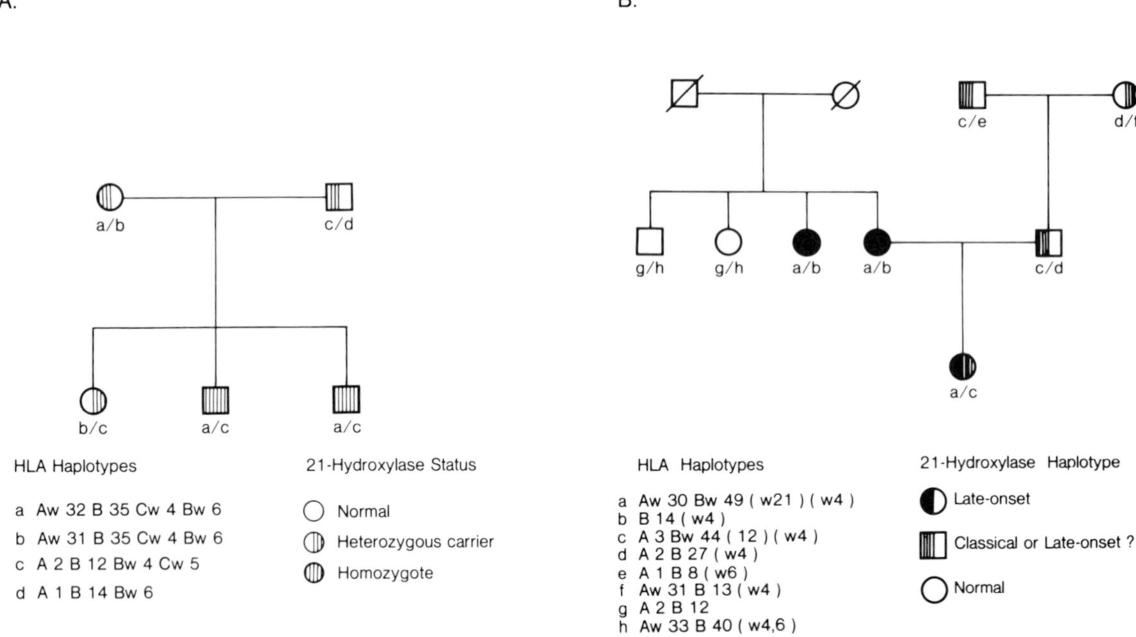

FIGURE 18-15 Application of HLA typing to the genotyping of 21-hydroxylase deficiency. (*A*) Classic 21-hydroxylase deficiency in a family with two affected sons and one heterozygous daughter. (*B*) Pedigree in which the mother is homozygous for late-onset 21-hydroxylase deficiency, the father is heterozygous for 21-hydroxylase deficiency, and the daughter appears to be a genetic compound, showing elevated serum 17-hydroxyprogesterone levels but no virilization.

15). HLA testing combined with careful analysis of basal and ACTH-stimulated 17-hydroxyprogesterone levels can define accurately subjects who are homozygous for classic or late-onset 21-hydroxylase deficiency, genetic compounds carrying both genes, or heterozygous carriers.[157]

This close linkage of 21-hydroxylase with the major histocompatibility locus should not be confused with the phenomenon of genetic linkage disequilibrium, in which the frequency of certain HLA haplotypes differs in affected subjects from that observed in normal persons in the same population. Thus among northern European groups the haplotype Bw47DR7 occurs with increased frequency in association with classic 21-hydroxylase deficiency, while the B8 haplotype frequency is reduced.[157] In the late-onset variant of 21-hydroxylase deficiency the frequency of the B14 haplotype appears to be increased.

The important clinical features of homozygous classic 21-hydroxylase deficiency are virilization and salt wasting. Their pathogenesis is summarized in Fig. 18-16. The primary impairment of cortisol synthesis causes increased pituitary secretion of ACTH, which in turn leads to excessive production of both 17-hydroxyprogesterone and progesterone. Side-chain cleavage of 17-hydroxyprogesterone produces androstenedione, which is then available for adrenal and peripheral conversion to the active androgen testosterone. In untreated patients plasma ACTH is moderately raised; levels of 17-hydroxyprogesterone, progesterone, androstenedione, testosterone, 21-deoxycortisol, and pregnenolone sulfate are markedly increased, with less striking increases in the levels of dehydroepiandrosterone and its sulfate conjugate. Even if basal serum cortisol levels are in the normal range, stress or ACTH testing may evoke

FIGURE 18-16 Pathogenesis of virilization and salt wasting in classic 21-hydroxylase deficiency, showing the close interrelation of these two aspects of the disease and the central importance of serum 17-hydroxyprogesterone (17OH-prog) and plasma renin activity for diagnosis and management. (*From Winter and Couch.*[159])

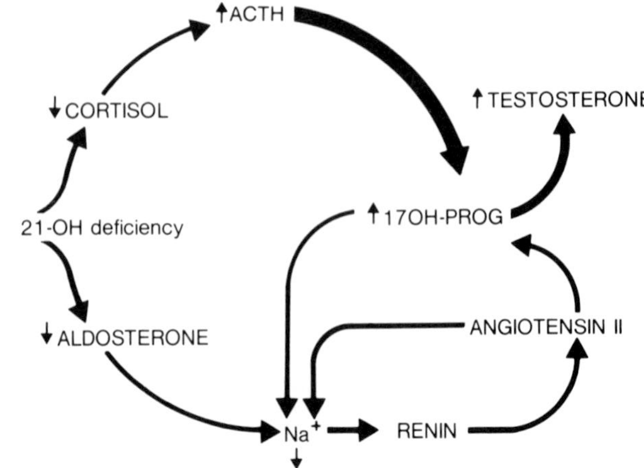

only a blunted rise in spite of a brisk increase in 17-hydroxyprogesterone. Metabolism of these abnormal steroids leads to increased urinary excretion of 17-ketosteroids and pregnanetriol.

Prenatal exposure to adrenal androgens has no effect on male sexual differentiation. The genitalia of affected males appear normal at birth, but continued androgen exposure becomes apparent by age 2 to 3 years, with rapid growth and skeletal maturation and precocious appearance of secondary sex characters in the absence of preceding testicular enlargement.

Genetic females who are homozygous for classic 21-hydroxylase deficiency have ambiguous external genitalia at birth (Fig. 18-17). Careful physical examination will demonstrate clitoromegaly, labioscrotal fusion without palpable testes, and a single urogenital sinus which opens usually on the perineum but occasionally on the phallus. By rectal examination one can usually palpate the cervix and thus confirm at once the presence of female paramesonephric structures. If appropriate therapy to suppress adrenal androgen production is not initiated, this virilism continues during childhood, causing further clitoromegaly, rapid growth, and the appearance of pubic hair, acne, and a masculine body habitus. Even though growth is accelerated, precocious epiphyseal fusion leads to an arrest of growth by about 10 years of age, with marked reduction of adult height. Continued androgen exposure after puberty causes anovular infertility and amenorrhea.

The late-onset or attenuated variant of 21-hydroxylase deficiency is characterized by low-level androgen exposure which does not produce clinically apparent disease until late childhood or adolescence. Affected males are rarely detected unless they present with premature adrenarche. Homozygous females have normal genitalia at birth; the disorder may be suspected in a child with premature adrenarche or a young woman with mild clitoromegaly, hirsutism, or anovular infertility.[160] These patients show moderately increased basal serum concentrations of 17-hydroxyprogesterone and testosterone, with an exaggerated response of 17-hydroxyprogesterone to ACTH stimulation.

FIGURE 18-17 External genitalia of a newborn female with classic 21-hydroxylase deficiency. No gonads were palpable, and the cervix was felt on rectal examination.

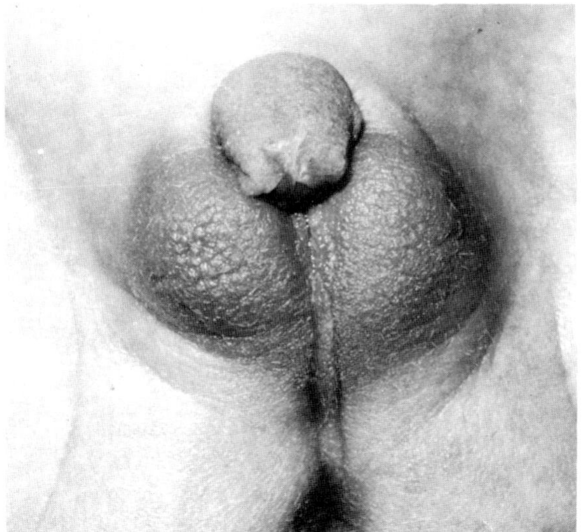

A few persons who represent genetic compounds for the classic and late-onset variants of 21-hydroxylase deficiency have been identified (Fig. 18-15). They have normal genitalia, and postnatal signs of androgen excess or even infertility do not usually occur, even though basal serum 17-hydroxyprogesterone levels are persistently increased. Heterozygous carriers for either variant are clinically normal and show normal basal serum concentrations of all adrenal steroids. Examination of basal and ACTH-stimulated 17-hydroxyprogesterone of 21-deoxycortisol values will usually permit appropriate categorization of individuals within an affected pedigree (Fig. 18-18).

Biochemical evidence of sodium depletion, as evidenced by increased levels of plasma renin activity or concentration, can be observed in virtually all untreated patients with homozygous classic 21-hydroxylase deficiency. However, clinically significant salt wasting develops in only about two-thirds of these patients,[161] usually during early infancy prior to diagnosis. In an affected neonate the first clues to an impending salt-losing crisis are hyperkalemia and rising levels of plasma renin activity, which are usually detectable by 1 week of age. If mineralocorticoid therapy is not initiated, progressive weight loss, vomiting, acidosis, hypoglycemia, and hyponatremic dehydration ensue, leading to peripheral vascular collapse by the third or fourth week. The clinical picture resembles that of hypertrophic pyloric stenosis except that in CAH, because of osmotic diuresis, urinary volume is often maintained in spite of obvious dehydration. The finding of hyponatremia and hyperkalemia in a dehydrated male (or virilized female) infant should lead immediately to investigation of adrenal function, including measurement of serum 17-hydroxyprogesterone levels. The differential diagnosis of a neonatal salt-losing crisis includes other forms of CAH, pyloric stenosis, congenital adrenal hypoplasia, and interstitial pyelonephritis.

Although 21-hydroxylase deficiency is certainly genetically heterogeneous, it is probably simplistic to assume that the presence or absence of a neonatal salt-losing crisis defines two genetically distinct disorders, a salt-losing variant and a simple virilizing variant. In later life most so-called salt losers show a persistent inability to tolerate sodium restriction, but some apparently gain the ability to conserve sodium relatively well.[162] Similarly, one may observe apparent discordance between HLA-identical sib-

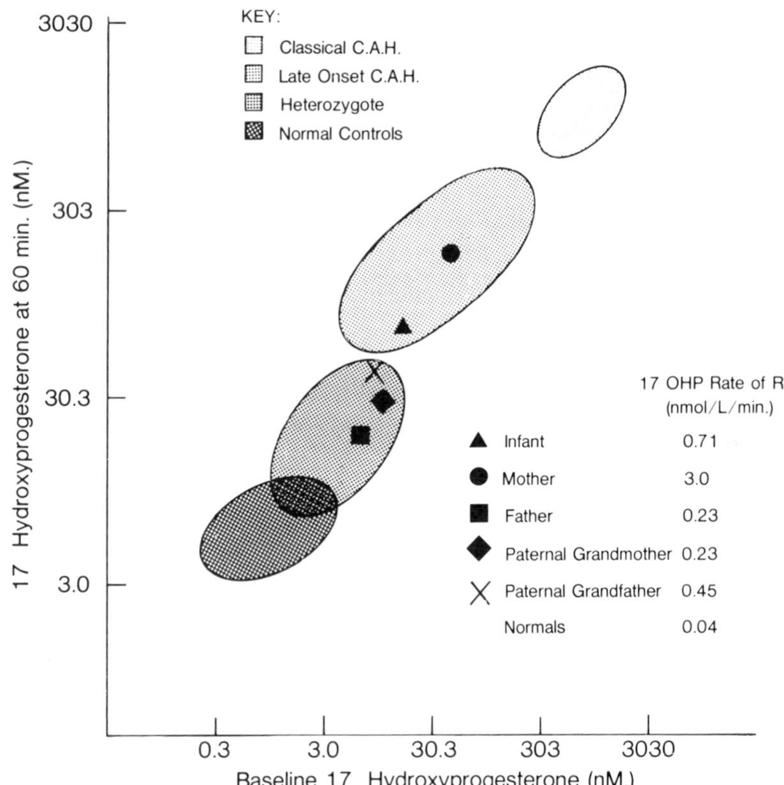

FIGURE 18-18 ACTH stimulation tests (Cortrosyn 0.2 mg/m^2 IV maximum 0.25 mg). The relation of baseline and 60-min ACTH-stimulated serum 17-hydroxyprogesterone concentrations in normal controls, heterozygous carriers, and patients with homozygous late-onset and homozygous classic forms of 21-hydroxylase deficiency. The application of the nomogram is illustrated, using data from individuals in pedigree B of Fig. 18-15. Data in nanomols per liter may be changed to nanograms per deciliter by multiplying by 33. (*Adapted from New et al.*[157])

lings as regards clinically significant salt wasting. It may be useful, therefore, to consider the variables which interact to determine whether and when a salt-losing crisis will occur.

One important determinant is the capacity to secrete aldosterone during sodium deprivation. Although all patients with 21-hydroxylase deficiency show evidence of an aldosterone biosynthetic defect and hypovolemia, those with clinically apparent salt wasting have reduced plasma aldosterone levels and aldosterone secretion rates relative to their plasma renin activities, with little response to sodium restriction; aldosterone levels in those who are not salt losers are typically above normal and may rise further with sodium restriction.[163] However, this distinction is not absolute, as clinical salt wasting has been reported in infants with high aldosterone levels. This variability in aldosterone secretory capacity appears to reflect the severity of the defect in 21-hydroxylation, since persistent salt losers show more striking prenatal virilization and a lower capacity to secrete cortisol and 11-deoxycorticosterone during ACTH stimulation. The observation that homozygous HLA Bw47 subjects are salt losers suggests that this haplotype is a marker for a more severe genetic defect, possibly a major deletion. The capacity to secrete aldosterone is also influenced by the total mass of the zona glomerulosa; although this aspect has not been carefully correlated with endocrine and genetic markers, it appears that salt-losing neonates show a deficient zona glomerulosa, while in older children with 21-hydroxylase deficiency this zone is usually hyperplastic.[164]

The second variable is the effect of high circulating levels of steroids such as 17-hydroxyprogesterone and progesterone, which bind to the renal tubular receptor for aldosterone and act as competitive inhibitors of mineralocorticoid action. This phenomenon greatly exacerbates salt wasting unless the patient can compensate with increased secretion of aldosterone. A salt-losing crisis tends to be self-accelerating (Fig. 18-16), since both ACTH and angiotensin levels rise, and both stimulate increased secretion of these antimineralocorticoid steroids.[165] Thus the glucocorticoid and mineralocorticoid abnormalities interact closely in this disorder: Suppression of ACTH with glucocorticoid therapy serves to ameliorate the salt wasting, while suppression of the renin-angiotensin system by salt, fluids, and mineralocorticoid is essential for normalization of 17-hydroxyprogesterone secretion.

The third variable includes various nonendocrine aspects of fluid and electrolyte balance, such as body fluid compartment size, renal function, dietary intake of salt and water, and intercurrent infection, which may predispose a young infant to a salt-losing crisis under circumstances which would be less threatening in later life. In summary, the burden of current evidence suggests that severe and persistent salt wasting may constitute evidence of a more profound genetic defect in 21-hydroxylation, but one cannot differentiate genotypes solely by whether a neonatal salt-losing crisis has been recognized. A distinction between salt losing and simple virilizing forms of homozygous classic 21-hydroxylase deficiency has little impact on therapy, since it is now customary to provide sufficient mineralocorticoid to all patients to ensure normalization of plasma renin activity.

The diagnosis of classic 21-hydroxylase deficiency should be considered in three clinical situations: (1) a newborn with ambiguous genitalia (including apparent males with bilateral cryptorchism and hypospadias), (2) a young infant with dehydration, hyponatremia, and hyperkalemia, and (3) a child with precocious virilization. Investigation begins with the immediate determination of serum 17-hydroxyprogesterone levels[166] at the same time that samples are being taken for karyotype analysis and assays of plasma renin activity. Umbilical-cord serum 17-hydroxyprogesterone values are high in normal infants (Table 18-5) but fall to below 200 ng/dl by 48 h (Fig. 18-19). Occasional values above 1000 ng/dl may be observed in sick or premature infants during the first week.[167] In classic 21-hydroxylase deficiency, serum 17-hydroxyprogesterone levels greatly exceed normal, ranging from 3000 to 100,000 ng/dl, and rise with age. Similar increases can be observed in levels of androstenedione, testosterone, progesterone, 21-deoxycortisol, and pregnenolone sulfate. Moderate increases in serum 17-hydroxyprogesterone are observed in 11β-hydroxylase deficiency, but in this disorder serum levels of 11-deoxycortisol are raised. Assays of urinary 17-ketosteroids and pregnanetriol were formerly used for the diagnosis of 21-hydroxylase deficiency, but the vagaries of neonatal steroid metabolism and urine collection can create serious errors of interpretation. Plasma renin activity is normal for the first few days of life, but by the fifth day all infants with classic 21-hydroxylase deficiency show elevated and rising values. There seems little merit in waiting to see if this signals a frank salt-losing crisis, and it is now customary to initiate mineralocorticoid therapy at this time.

Deficiency of 21-hydroxylase can be diagnosed prenatally after 14 weeks gestation through measurement of amniotic fluid concentrations of 17-hydroxyprogesterone[168–170] and confirmed by means of HLA typing or DNA analysis of amniocytes or chorionic villus tissue. Unfortunately, such a diagnosis does not permit antenatal treatment in time to prevent virilization of affected females. The fetal adrenal cortex can be effectively suppressed during the period of sexual differentiation through the administration of relatively large doses of dexamethasone (0.5 mg three times a day), provided that the therapy is begun by 4 to 5 weeks fetal age or as soon as pregnancy can be ascertained.[170] This treatment is then continued until the diagnosis of an affected 46,XX fetus can be determined by means of amniocentesis or chorionic villus biopsy; in such a circumstance, therapy is continued to term, but if the fetus is unaffected or male (seven of eight pregnancies), it is discontinued. At term, provided that dexamethasone therapy was started sufficiently early, the affected female will have normal genitalia and will not need corrective surgery. In circumstances where therapy was discontinued before midpregnancy, one does not observe significant pituitary-adrenal suppression in the neonate.

In many jurisdictions neonatal screening for 21-hydroxylase deficiency by means of radioimmunoassay (RIA) of 17-hydroxyprogesterone in blood spots is now routine since studies have demonstrated considerable unrecognized mortality, particularly in male probands with CAH[171]; the disorder has a relatively high incidence; and the screening test is rapid and inexpensive.[172] Neonatal screening demonstrates that many affected male infants show no clinical signs of salt wasting in spite of remarkable hyper-

TABLE 18-5 Normal Values of Hormones Commonly Used for the Diagnosis and Management of Congenital Adrenal Hyperplasia

	Serum					Plasma
	17-Hydroxyprogesterone, ng/dl	Androstenedione, ng/dl	Testosterone, ng/dl		Aldosterone, ng/dl	Renin activity, ng/ml per h
			Male	Female		
Cord	1100–6500	50–200	5–50	5–50	95 ± 10*	8 ± 2*
1-2 days	65–400	20–100	60–400	20–70	7–850	25 ± 8
3-6 days	60–250	10–100	15–25	10–25	35–210	12 ± 2
1-3 weeks	20–220	10–150	50–350	3–25	15–105	6 ± 2
1-12 months	5–150	5–50	5–350	3–20	5–95	6 ± 1
1-3 years	5–90	3–40	3–15	3–15	10–80	5 ± 2
3-6 years	5–90	3–40	3–15	3–15	10–70	3 ± 1
6-15 years	10–160	5–150	10–770	10–60	10–70	2 ± 0.3
Adult	10–285	50–200	260–1000	15–65	5–50	2 ± 0.4

* Mean ± standard error of mean.

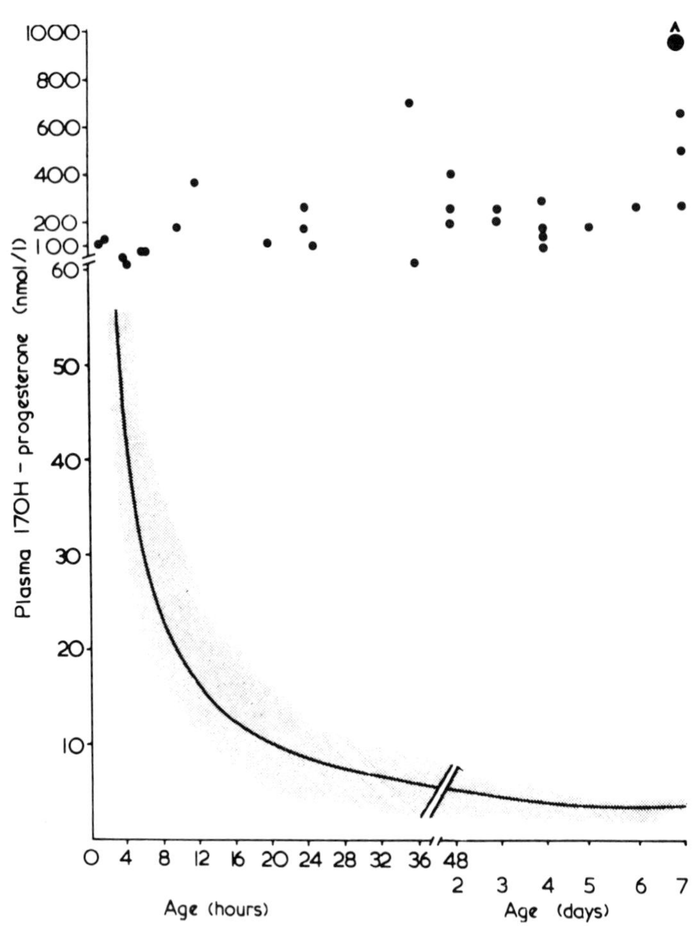

FIGURE 18-19 Plasma 17-hydroxyprogesterone concentrations in normal infants (shaded area indicates mean and range) and in untreated infants with classic 21-hydroxylase deficiency (individual dots) during the first 7 days of life. Values may be changed to nanograms per deciliter by multiplying by 33. (*From Hughes et al.*[167])

kalemia and thus may present as unexpected crib deaths. Unfortunately, because of the relative adrenocortical hyperplasia of normal neonates, even postmortem examination often fails to establish the correct diagnosis. Other benefits of neonatal screening, by comparison with the usual clinical screening,[173] include correct gender assignment in virilized girls and avoidance of significant morbidity resulting from delays in diagnosis.

The diagnosis of the late-onset or attenuated variant of 21-hydroxylase deficiency in patients with premature adrenarche, hirsutism, or infertility requires assessment of serum 17-hydroxyprogesterone concentrations before and after stimulation with ACTH.[157] In postmenarcheal females this test should be carried out in the early follicular phase to avoid ovarian midcycle and luteal secretion of 17-hydroxyprogesterone. Some investigators feel that the test is more discriminating if preceded by overnight adrenal suppression with dexamethasone.

Successful treatment of congenital adrenal hyperplasia depends on daily replacement of glucocorticoid and mineralocorticoid in the smallest doses sufficient to reduce pituitary ACTH secretion and the renin-angiotensin system to normal. If this is done correctly, an affected patient can achieve normal growth, healthy psychosexual adjustment, and normal adult reproductive function. Other cornerstones of modern therapy include education of the patient and family to ensure compliance and early perineal repair for affected females to provide normal genital appearance and function.

If the condition is diagnosed during a salt-losing crisis, treatment begins with intravenous fluids, initially with 5% glucose in saline (20 ml/kg of body weight in 1 h) to restore intravascular volume and then with a more gradual infusion of the same fluid or 3% saline to replace fluid and electrolyte losses. Hydrocortisone hemisuccinate (50 mg/m^2) is administered as an initial IV bolus, with a similar dose infused over the subsequent 24 h. If available, deoxycorticosterone acetate (1 to 3 mg IM every 12 h) or aldosterone (0.5 mg IV every 4 to 6 h) may be added, but mineralocorticoids tend to be relatively ineffective at first because of high levels of circulating 17-hydroxyprogesterone and other inhibitors. In small infants severe hyperkalemia may induce electrocardiographic changes and necessitate the use of rectal cation exchange resins.

Maintenance therapy seeks to provide sufficient glucocorticoid and mineralocorticoid to suppress adrenal 17-hydroxyprogesterone and androgen secretion without causing side effects such as growth failure and hypertension.[159] Irrespective of the presence or absence of a previous frank salt-losing crisis, sufficient mineralocorticoid to reduce plasma renin levels to the age-specific normal range should always be provided. In infancy 9α-fluorohydrocortisone (fludrocortisone) doses of 0.15 to 0.2 mg per day are frequently necessary, but in older children and adults the same effect can be achieved with 0.05 to 0.1 mg per day. To avoid hypertension, the dose of 9α-fluorohydrocortisone should always be reduced if the plasma renin activity falls below normal. With such a regimen there appears to be no need for salt supplementation, but patients should not be denied access to salt, particularly during hot weather. Older forms of mineralocorticoid replacement, such as IM injections and subcutaneous pellets of deoxycorticosterone, are ineffective, cumbersome, and potentially dangerous.

If plasma renin activity is normal, adrenal androgen secretion can be suppressed by the use of oral hydrocortisone (cortisol), 10 to 15 mg/m^2 daily in three divided doses. Cortisone acetate appears to be less effective, with reduced bioavailability; more potent glucocorticoids such as prednisone or dexamethasone are useful in adults but carry too great a risk of growth inhibition for use during childhood.

Therapy should be monitored by measurements of plasma renin activity and serum 17-hydroprogesterone and testosterone at least every 3 to 6 months. The goal should be to maintain serum 17-hydroxyprogesterone values below 200 ng/dl (6 nmol/L) and renin and testosterone values within the age- and sex-specific normal range (Table 18-5). The sensitivity of serum 17-hydroxyprogesterone to stress-induced fluctuations in ACTH release and its circadian rhythmicity demand careful attention to sampling details such as time of day, time since previous steroid administration, and successful initial venipuncture. Our approach for the past 15 years has been to measure plasma renin activity, serum 17-hydroxyprogesterone, and testosterone at 0900 h, just before the ingestion of medication, and the serum steroid levels again 3 h later. Assays of salivary 17-hydroxyprogesterone and testosterone show excellent correlation with serum levels and provide a noninvasive technique for serial home monitoring.[174] Serum 17-hydroxyprogesterone and testosterone concentrations closely parallel each other in prepubertal children and females (Fig. 18-20), but naturally they deviate in adolescent boys.[175] Serum androstenedione, 17-hydroxypregnenolone, or 21-deoxycortisol determinations also correlate with 17-hydroxyprogesterone and can be used for monitoring therapy; however, levels of dehydroepiandrosterone (and its sulfate conjugate) remain markedly reduced after long-term glucocorticoid therapy and therefore do not provide a sufficiently sensitive index of day-to-day ACTH suppression. Assays of urinary 17-ketosteroids and pregnanetriol were formerly used to monitor therapy in CAH; however, they provide no advantage and are considerably less sensitive and more cumbersome.

In addition, patients should be monitored carefully in regard to growth velocity and skeletal maturation, since there is no biochemical test for overtreatment. At all ages the smallest dose of cortisol which will normalize hormone levels should be used. During major infections the dose of cortisol should be doubled, and extra doses of oral or parenteral glucocorticoid should be provided before surgery requiring general anesthesia. It is our habit to instruct parents to repeat the previous medications any time the child vomits and to give IM cortisone acetate 25 to 100 mg if there is a second episode of vomiting; relatively large doses of cortisone acetate should be used, since this agent has been shown to have low bioavailability as a result of either poor absorption or incomplete conversion to cortisol.

Therapy for late-onset CAH requires only oral hydrocortisone in the same doses, without supplementary mineralocorticoid. Once growth is complete, satisfactory control and normal fertility can be achieved more easily with longer-acting agents such as dexamethasone.

Occasionally, if the diagnosis of classic CAH has been delayed or therapy has been inadequate, significant advance of both skeletal maturation and hypothalamic-pituitary maturation may occur, with physical signs and hormonal evidence of true precocious puberty. This complication may require adjunctive use of GnRH analogue therapy, as in other forms of true precocious puberty. From time to time other adjuncts, such as surgical or medical adrenalectomy (using aminoglutethimide), have been suggested to treat CAH. However, there is no evidence that such steps are necessary or even beneficial in patients who are compliant with standard glucocorticoid and mineralocorticoid replacement.

In all forms of female pseudohermaphroditism, including 21-hydroxylase deficiency, plastic repair of the external genitalia should be undertaken by 18 months of age so that the child is never aware of the deformity. The appropriate procedure includes vaginoplasty to provide labia majora and minora and separate urethral and vaginal communication to the perineum, plus clitoroplasty, in which the separated crura of the clitoris are placed under the symphysis pubis, leaving only the glans visible, with its vascular and nervous supply intact. Occasionally the connection between the upper vagina and the urogenital sinus is proximal to the external sphincter, so far from the perineum that it is necessary to delay creating the appropriate outlet to the perineum until after menarche. However, in all cases the external appearance of the genitalia should be made normal in infancy, with no further surgical interference during childhood. Vaginal dilatation may be necessary in

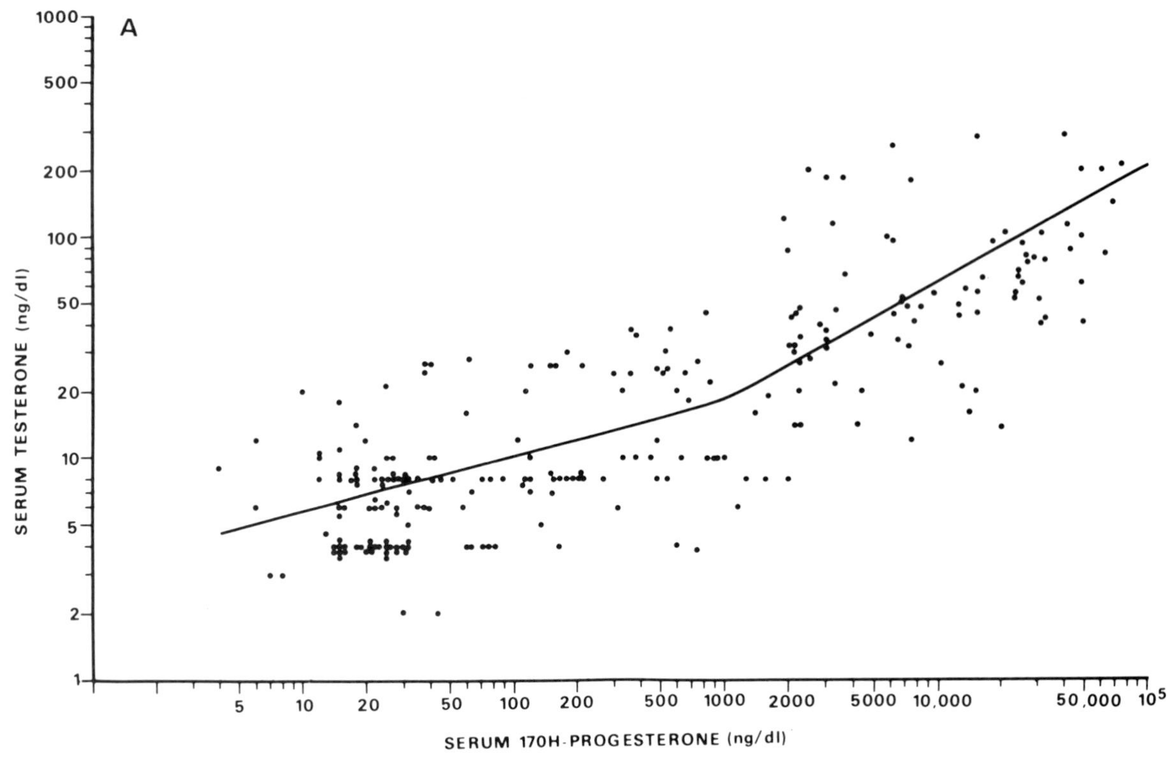

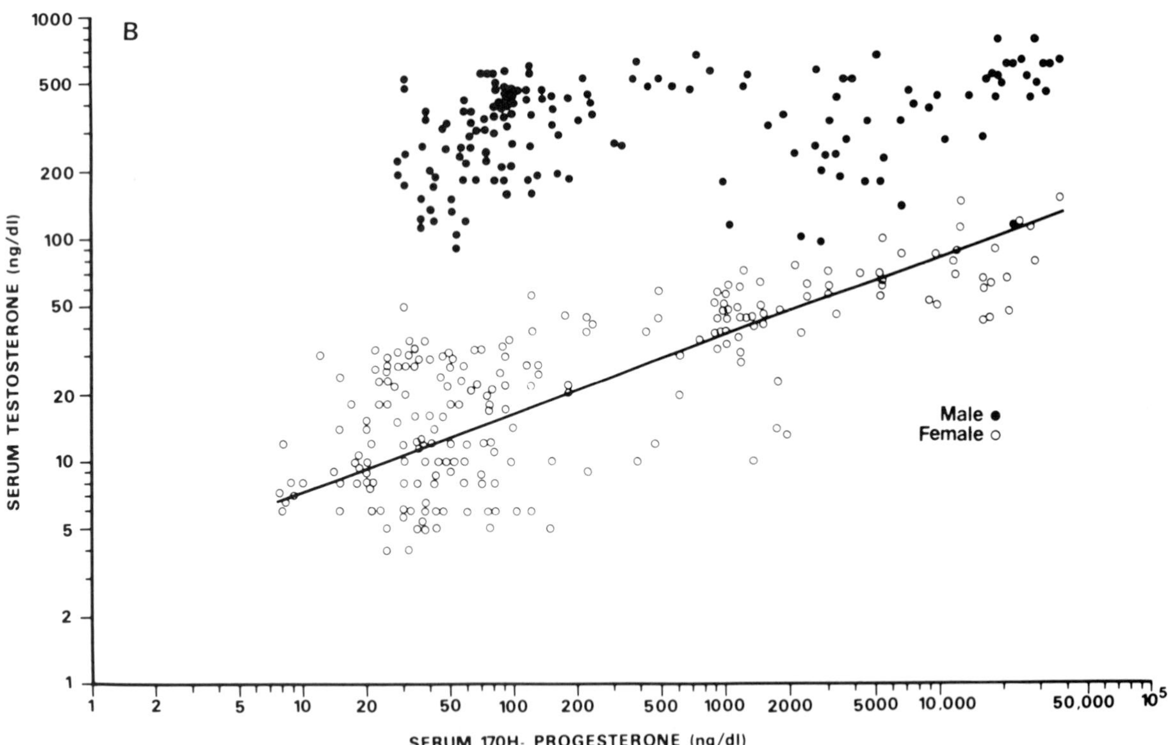

FIGURE 18-20 (*A*) Relation between log serum concentrations of 17-hydroxyprogesterone and testosterone in prepubertal patients with classic 21-hydroxylase deficiency. (*B*) Relation between log serum 17-hydroxyprogesterone and testosterone concentrations in adolescent male (closed circle) and female (open circle) patients with classic 21-hydroxylase deficiency. (*From Hughes and Winter.*[175])

young women who underwent vaginoplasty in infancy, but thereafter sexual function is completely normal. It is our custom to recommend cesarean section in women who have undergone this repair, as we have no information regarding the effects of vaginal delivery.

If the diagnosis of 21-hydroxylase deficiency is made soon after birth and appropriate medical care is maintained through childhood, one can expect normal growth, intellectual and psychosexual development, adolescence, and adult reproductive function. In young women regular ovulatory menstrual cycles do not occur unless serum testosterone and 17-hydroxyprogesterone levels are reduced to normal. Although apparent well-being and even normal spermatogenesis have been observed in occasional untreated adult males, it seems better to recommend lifelong therapy, since infertility due to suppression of gonadotropins is the more likely result of inadequate treatment.[176] Untreated adult males may also develop testicular tumors as a result of chronic ACTH stimulation of adrenal rest cells.

11β-Hydroxylase Deficiency The enzyme complex which catalyzes the conversion of 11-deoxycortisol to cortisol is a mitochondrial oxidase consisting of a flavoprotein, an adrenodoxin, and a substrate-specific cytochrome P450. Immunochemical studies indicate that this single cytochrome P450 catalyzes both 11β- and 18-hydroxylation.[177] The gene for 11β-hydroxylase is located on the long arm of chromosome 8.

Deficiency of 11β-hydroxylase is the second most common form of CAH; it accounts, however, for only 5 percent of all CAH cases, although it is relatively more common among Jews of north African origin. It is an autosomal recessive disorder in which the classic signs are virilization plus hypertension. Increased adrenal secretion of 11-deoxycorticosterone (DOC) and 11-deoxycortisol leads to ACTH-dependent hypertension of variable severity. Accumulation of steroids more proximal in the steroidogenic path (such as 17-hydroxyprogesterone) and their subsequent metabolism to androgens lead to prenatal masculinization of the external genitalia in genetic females, as in 21-hydroxylase deficiency.[178] Postnatally, untreated males and females show progressive virilization, with rapid skeletal maturation and eventual short stature. Prepubertal gynecomastia of uncertain pathogenesis has been reported in affected males. Severe virilization may occur without hypertension, but the reverse has not been observed. In addition to this classic form of 11β-hydroxylase deficiency, milder variants have been described, with onset of hirsutism, acne, amenorrhea, and variable hypertension in adolescence or even latter.[179] There is a separate defect in aldosterone synthesis, defined as 18-dehydrogenase or corticosterone methyl oxidase II deficiency, which presents at birth with hyponatremic dehydration and hyperkalemia; recent evidence shows that this is an allelic variant of 11β-hydroxylase deficiency due to mutation in the gene for $P450_{C11}$.[180]

In untreated patients with the classic disorder, hypervolemia suppresses plasma renin activity and aldosterone secretion. After glucocorticoid therapy and suppression of DOC production, plasma renin increases and there is a rise in aldosterone levels. However, the aldosterone response to sodium restriction is subnormal, and salt wasting may occur, particularly in infants, after the initiation of therapy.[181] In some cases the abnormal enzyme appears to be capable of 11β-hydroxylating 17-hydroxyprogesterone to form 21-deoxycortisol, the presence of which can mimic the hormonal pattern of 21-hydroxylase deficiency.[182]

The hallmark of 11β-hydroxylase deficiency is the presence of elevated serum concentrations of 11-deoxycortisol and DOC and their suppression by exogenous glucocorticoid. Urinary excretion of metabolites such as tetrahydro-11-deoxycortisol (THS) is usually increased but may be normal during early infancy. Prenatal diagnosis can be achieved by determining increased amniotic fluid concentrations of 11-deoxycortisol or increased maternal excretion of THS.[183] Therefore, prenatal therapy with dexamethasone should be feasible to prevent genital virilization in affected females. In obligate heterozygotes, however, basal and ACTH-stimulated 11-deoxysteroid levels cannot be distinguished from normal.[184]

Treatment of 11β-hydroxylase deficiency requires cortisol in doses similar to those used in other forms of CAH. With adequate treatment, virilization ceases and hypertension usually disappears; serum concentrations of DOC and 11-deoxycortisol fall to normal, while plasma renin activity rises to the normal range. Early vaginoplasty and clitoroplasty are required for prenatally virilized females.

3β-HSD Deficiency This disorder was discussed in detail earlier under Defective Genital Virilization (Male Pseudohermaphroditism), since it can cause genital ambiguity in both males and females. The originally described classic variant is an autosomal recessive disease which is not HLA-linked and which causes a major block in the biosynthesis of mineralocorticoid, glucocorticoid, androgens, and estrogens in both the adrenal cortex and the gonads (Fig. 18-13). Infant girls present with slight to moderate clitoral enlargement plus severe salt wasting; however, a few patients have been described who could maintain normal salt balance and apparently adequate aldosterone production by means of compensatory high renin-angiotensin stimulation. The virilization of affected females is presumably due to peripheral conversion of Δ^5-3β-hydroxysteroid precursors to androgen.

As in other forms of CAH, it is now recognized that 3β-HSD deficiency exists in several clinical variants, presumably reflecting underlying genetic heterogeneity. Genetic females with the milder late-onset variants have normal genitalia at birth and normal mineralocorticoid secretion; plasma renin activity may be normal or increased. They present during late childhood with premature adrenarche; during puberty with male-pattern hirsutism, acne, clitoromegaly, and primary amenorrhea; and in the older female with menstrual irregularity and infertility.[104] Obviously, this type of adrenal virilism can overlap with the presentation of polycystic ovary syndrome, particularly since adrenal androgens can produce the ovarian changes of polycystic ovary syndrome.

The diagnosis of 3β-HSD deficiency is indicated by the finding of high serum concentrations of dehydroepiandrosterone, pregnenolone, and 17-hydroxypregnenolone with their respective sulfate conjugates. Because of hepatic 3β-HSD activity, one may find increased serum levels of Δ^4-3-ketosteroids such as 17-hydroxyprogesterone and androstenedione, but these ketosteroids are never as markedly elevated as the Δ^5-3β-hydroxysteroids. There is a similar characteristic Δ^5/Δ^4 imbalance in the urinary excretion of Δ^5-pregnenetriol and pregnanetriol. In the classic variant, ACTH and hCG stimulation elicits little rise in circulating levels of cortisol and gonadal sex steroids. In the late-onset variants, basal hormone levels are frequently normal but a relative deficiency in 3β-HSD can be demonstrated by ACTH stimulation, which elicits a disproportionate increase in Δ^5-3β-hydroxysteroid levels.

Therapy for 3β-HSD deficiency requires replacement of cortisol, as in other forms of CAH, plus full mineralocorticoid replacement in any patient with elevated plasma renin activity or intolerance to sodium restriction. In addition, patients with the classic variant usually show defective pubertal development[185] and therefore require sex steroid (estrogen and progestin) replacement at the appropriate age. In the less severe variants, normal puberty and regular ovulatory menstrual cycles usually follow suppression of adrenal androgen secretion.

Prenatal Virilization by Environmental Hormones

Masculinization of the external genitalia of female infants can also occur if the mother ingests androgens or has a virilizing disorder such as an ovarian tumor (usually an arrhenoblastoma or hCG-dependent luteoma of pregnancy), adrenal neoplasm, or inadequately treated CAH. In addition, female pseudohermaphroditism of varying degrees has been observed in the offspring of women treated with synthetic progestins such as norethindrone, ethisterone, norethynodrel, and medroxyprogesterone.[186] Similar virilization may also occur after maternal ingestion of large doses of stilbestrol, perhaps because of inhibition of fetal adrenal 3β-HSD; such offspring would also be at risk for later development of adenocarcinoma of the cervix and vagina.

The only treatment necessary for this form of female pseudohermaphroditism is surgical repair of the external genitalia. There is no need for ongoing hormone replacement therapy, and subsequent physical and psychosexual development should be entirely normal.[187]

Teratologic Malformations of the External Genitalia

Genital abnormalities, occasionally presenting as female pseudohermaphroditism, are frequently observed in association with renal agenesis, imperforate anus, and other malformations of the urinary and intestinal tracts.[188] Usually the internal genitalia are absent or abnormal. Similar apparently nonendocrine masculinization of a female fetus has been observed in association with multiple malformation syndromes, including cryptophthalmos, middle and outer ear maldevelopment, meningoencephalocele, and cardiac malformations; there may be familial recurrence of these anomalies, most of which have been lethal. A familial association of vaginal agenesis, middle ear malformations, and renal hypoplasia has been described.[189] Apparent clitoral enlargement giving the appearance of female pseudohermaphroditism can also occur in neurofibromatosis.

CLINICAL APPROACH TO DISORDERS OF SEXUAL DIFFERENTIATION

The Newborn with Abnormal Genitalia

Genital ambiguity in a neonate presents a psychosocial crisis which demands rapid yet sophisticated investigation before therapy and sex assignment. Such infants should be transferred at once to a center capable of providing within days a definitive diagnosis in terms of genetic sex, gonadal and genital structure, and endocrine function. Although the resources and expertise of a team of physicians are required, a single person, usually the pediatric endocrinologist, should be responsible for communication with the parents in order to explain the problem and proposed investigations and to counsel them regarding the prognosis for health, psychosexual adjustment, and reproductive function. Naming of the child should be delayed until gender assignment is decided; under no circumstances should parents be encouraged to select purposely a sexually ambiguous name. When reassignment of the sex of rearing is necessary because of a previous incorrect diagnosis or ignorance of the principles that govern gender assignment, it becomes doubly important that the reasons for this decision be explained to the parents in simple terms by a physician who is familiar with their cultural, religious, and educational background.

An abnormality of sexual differentiation should be suspected not only in an infant with obviously ambiguous genitalia but also in apparent males with hypospadias, cryptorchism, or micropenis and in apparent females with partial labial fusion, clitoromegaly, or an inguinal mass. An abbreviated flowchart for the logical application of genetic and endocrine investigations in these circumstances is presented in Fig. 18-21. Only rarely will the genitalia be sufficiently distinctive to diagnose a particular disorder. Rather, examination of the external genitalia serves to document specific points, such as size of the phallus, location of the urethral meatus, number and location of ventral frenula on the phallus, degree of labioscrotal fusion, and presence or absence of palpable gonads. It is usually possible with careful rectal examination of the newborn to determine whether a cervix is present. Finally, a careful assessment should be made of any associated congenital malformations, dehydration, or hyperpigmentation. A careful review of both pregnancy history and family history is essential. Maternal virilization during pregnancy may suggest ovarian or adrenal disease with transplacental passage of maternal androgens. Parental consanguinity suggests the possible expression of an autosomal recessive disorder. A family history of genital ambiguity or infertility is often available when an X-linked condition presents.

Initial laboratory investigation in an infant without palpable gonads includes karyotype analysis (supplemented by sex chromatin if the karyotyping will be delayed) and assays of serum 17-hydroxyprogesterone levels. The infant's intake, weight, and serum electrolytes should be monitored daily to assess any salt wasting, but assays of plasma renin activity are best delayed until after 4 days of age. During this period ultrasonography should be performed to confirm the status of the paramesonephric duct structures. Genitography is occasionally necessary. The purpose of this approach is to identify the most common condition, 21-hydroxylase deficiency, before salt-losing complications appear. If, in a genetic female, the serum 17-hydroxyprogesterone concentrations are not significantly raised (over 3000 ng/dl) and rising by 5 days of age, one should consider other forms of female pseudohermaphroditism and assess serum levels of steroids such as 11-deoxycortisol, dehydroepiandrosterone, and 17-hydroxypregnenolone.

Any gonad felt in the labioscrotal or inguinal area almost certainly contains testicular tissue. If portions of it differ in consistency, one should consider a possible ovotestis or a gonad that has undergone neoplastic transformation. Absence of well-differen-

FIGURE 18-21 A simplified flowchart for the investigation and diagnosis of an infant with genital ambiguity.

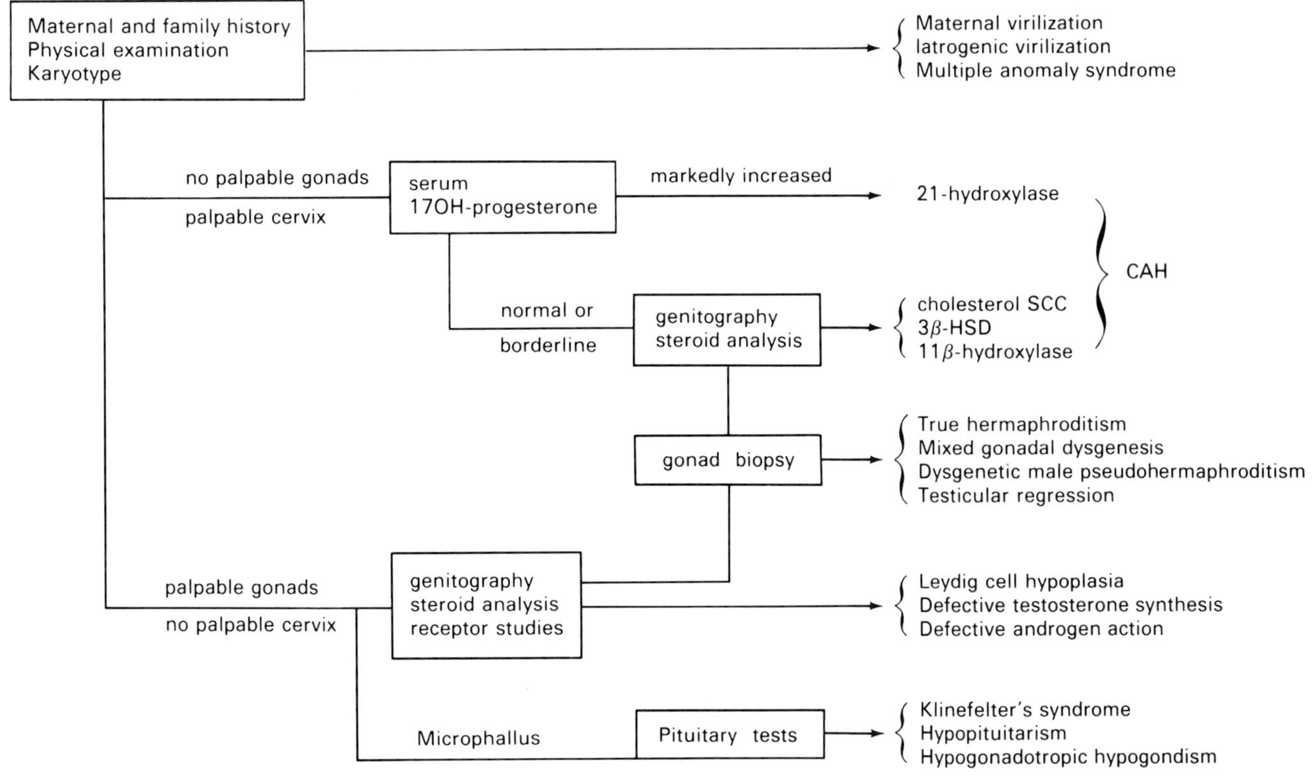

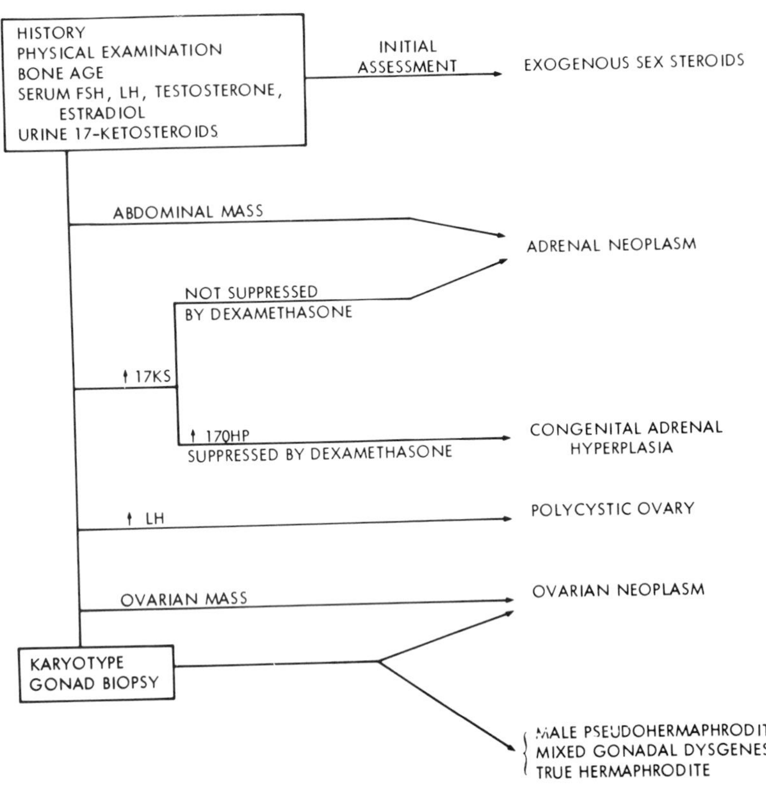

FIGURE 18-22 A flowchart illustrating a practical diagnostic approach to children with inappropriate virilization. [*From Dean HJ, Winter JSD, in Collu R, Ducharme JR, Guyda H (eds): Pediatric Endocrinology. New York, Raven, 1981, p 350.*]

tiated paramesonephric duct structures on one side provides further evidence that the ipsilateral gonad contains testicular tissue. Complete absence of these structures shown by genitography in a 46,XY infant with ambiguous genitalia suggests one of the several forms of male pseudohermaphroditism; further investigation requires detailed analysis of hCG-stimulated androgen biosynthesis and of target cell receptors and metabolism.

With increasing frequency, a family history of abnormal sexual differentiation raises the question of possible prenatal diagnosis during a subsequent pregnancy. Ultrasonography may permit visualization of the external genitalia after the fifth month of gestation, amniocentesis can often provide a biochemical diagnosis at 15 to 20 weeks, and chorionic villus biopsy offers an opportunity to assess genetic sex and HLA haplotype even earlier. These techniques have been used successfully to identify affected fetuses with 21-hydroxylase deficiency and permit prenatal treatment with dexamethasone given to the mother. Such an approach has resulted in the birth of affected females with normal or only minimally virilized genitalia.

In a female pseudohermaphrodite capable of normal fertility, it is obvious that the sex of rearing should be female. Similarly, in a male with 5α-reductase deficiency, the potential for dramatic virilization and adult male reproductive function requires that the infant be raised as male regardless of genital appearance. However, in most intersex disorders there is no chance for fertility, and the prime consideration for gender assignment should be the potential to achieve functional and cosmetically acceptable external genitalia with endocrine and surgical therapy. Genetic males with microphallus often benefit from a course of androgen therapy (testosterone cyclopentylpropionate 25 mg IM monthly for three doses) before any surgery. However, if a defect in androgen receptor activity has been demonstrated, such virilization is impossible and assignment of female gender is appropriate.

To ensure family acceptance and normal adjustment of the infant, reconstructive surgery to provide gender-compatible external genitalia should if possible be performed before 18 months of age. In females a type of vaginoplasty and clitoroplasty that preserves clitoral innervation and blood supply is most desirable. Thereafter, any further surgery should be delayed until late adolescence. In males the creation of a phallic urethra is more difficult and requires several procedures; if the testes are absent or have been removed, consideration should be given to the insertion of prostheses, usually during adolescence.

Where there is a significant risk of gonadal neoplasia, as in gonadal dysgenesis with a Y-bearing cell line, the gonads should be removed as early as is convenient. It has been customary in complete testicular feminization to leave the testes in place until after puberty, but when an infant is already under-

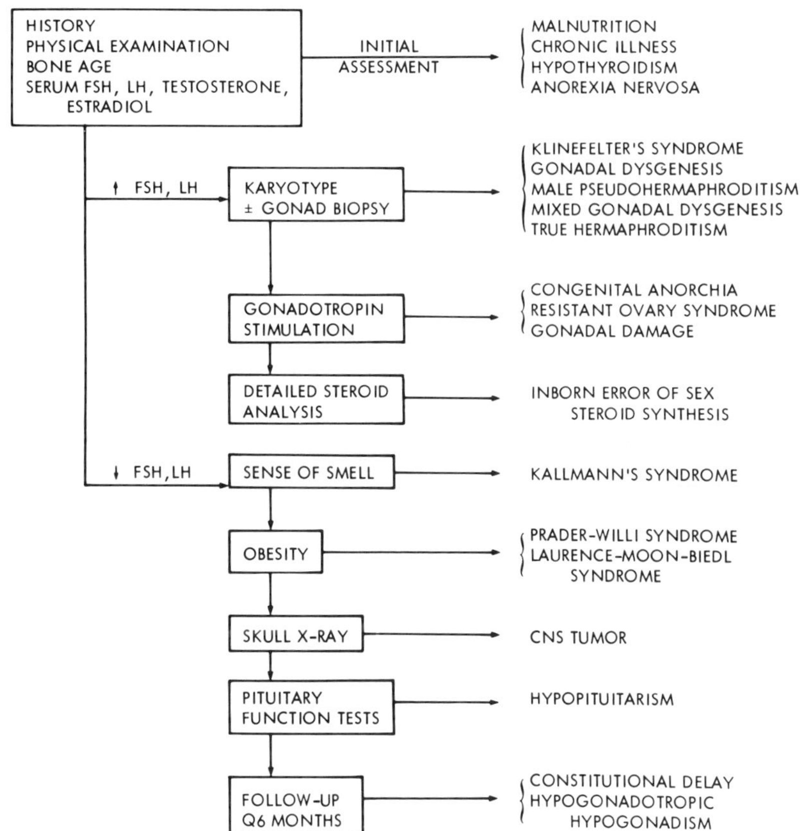

FIGURE 18-23 A flowchart illustrating a practical diagnostic approach to patients with delayed puberty. [*From Dean HJ, Winter JSD, in Collu R, Ducharme JR, Guyda H (eds): Pediatric Endocrinology. New York, Raven, 1981, p 333.*]

going repair of inguinal hernias, it is probably more reasonable to remove the testes and then to provide estrogen replacement at the time of puberty. If the sex of rearing is female and there is any risk of even partial virilization at puberty (as in incomplete testicular feminization), the gonads should be removed during childhood.

Virilization during Childhood or Adolescence

The precocious appearance of pubic hair and acne or inappropriate hirsutism, clitoral enlargement, or other sign of virilization deserves careful investigation, as outlined in Figure 18-22. A small but significant fraction of such patients will prove to have a late-onset variant of CAH (21-hydroxylase, 11β-hydroxylase, or 3β-HSD deficiency). Frequently ACTH stimulation and dexamethasone suppression testing are necessary to demonstrate the defect in steroidogenesis.

Delayed Puberty, Amenorrhea, and Infertility

The initial evaluation of a patient presenting with delayed or unsatisfactory pubertal development, primary or secondary amenorrhea, or unexplained infertility should include assessment of serum gonadotropin concentrations. Those with hypergonadotropic hypogonadism (Fig. 18-23) may turn out to have an unrecognized disorder of sexual differentiations. Females with gonadal dysgenesis may present early with pubertal failure or later with secondary amenorrhea and infertility. If an apparent female shows normal breast development, sparse sex hair, and primary amenorrhea, the likely diagnosis is testicular feminization.

REFERENCES

1. Painter TS: The sex chromosome of man. *Am Nat* 58:506, 1924.
2. Fisher RA: *The Genetical Theory of Natural Selection.* Oxford, Clarendon, 1930.
3. National Foundation for Birth Defects: *An International System for Human Cytogenic Nomenclature (1978). Birth Defects.* New York, 1978, vol 14, no 8; also *Cytogenet Cell Genet* 21:309, 1978.
4. Boué J, Boué A, Lazar P: Retrospective and prospective epidemiological studies of 1500 karyotyped spontaneous human abortions. *Teratology* 12:11, 1975.
5. Martin RH, Balkan W, Burns K, Rademaker AW, Lin CC, Rudd NL: The chromosome constitution of 1000 human spermatozoa. *Hum Genet* 63:305, 1983.
6. Jacobs PA: The incidence and etiology of sex chromosome abnormalities in man. New York, The National Foundation, 1979.

7. Opitz O, Zoll B, Hansmann I, Hinney B: Cytogenetic investigation of 103 patients with primary or secondary amenorrhea. *Hum Genet* 65:46, 1983.
8. Diedrich U, Hansmann I, Janke D, Opitz O, Probeck H-D: Chromosome abnormalities in 136 couples with a history of recurrent abortions. *Hum Genet* 65:48, 1983.
9. Muller U: Molecular biology of the human Y chromosome, in SS Wachtel (ed): *Evolutionary Mechanisms in Sex Determination.* Boca Raton, FL, CRC Press, 1989, pp 91–98.
10. Sinclair AH, Berta P, Palmer MS, Hawkins JR, Griffiths BL, Smith MJ, Foster JW, Frischauf AM, et al: A gene from the human sex-determining region encodes a protein with homology to a conserved DNA-binding motif. *Nature* 346:240, 1990.
11. Simpson E, Chandler P, Goulmy E, Disteche CM, Ferguson-Smith MA, Page DC: Separation of the genetic loci for H-Y antigen and for testis determination on human Y chromosome. *Nature* 326:876, 1987.
12. Page DC, Mosher RM, Simpson EM, Fisher EMC, Mardon G, Pollack J, McGillivray B, de la Chapelle A, Brown LG: The sex-determining region of the human Y chromosome encodes a finger protein. *Cell* 51:1091, 1987.
13. Brown CJ, Goss SJ, Lubahn DB, Joseph DR, Wilson EM, French FS, Willard HF: Androgen receptor locus on the human X-chromosomes: Localization to Xq11–12 and description of DNA polymorphism. *Am J Hum Genet* 44:264, 1989.
14. Wolf U: X-linked genes and gonadal differentiation. *Differentiation* 23 (suppl):S104, 1983.
15. Therman E, Denniston C, Sarro GE, Uber M: X chromosome constitution and the human female phenotype. *Hum Genet* 54:133, 1980.
16. Lyon MF: X-chromosome inactivation and the location and expression of X-linked genes. *Am J Hum Genet* 42:8, 1988.
17. Monesi V: Chromosome activities during meiosis and spermiogenesis. *J Reprod Fertil* 13:1, 1971.
18. Cooper DN: Eukaryotic DNA methylation. *Hum Genet* 64:315, 1983.
19. Byskov AG: Gonadal sex and germ cell differentiation, in Austin CR, Edwards RG (eds): *Mechanisms of Sex Differentiation in Animals and Man.* London, Academic, 1981, p 145.
20. Rabinovici J, Jaffe RB: Development and regulation of growth and differentiated function in human and subhuman primate fetal gonads. *Endocr Rev* 11:532, 1990.
21. Burgoyne PS: Role of mammalian Y chromosome in sex determination. *Philos Trans R Soc Lond [Biol]* 322:63, 1988.
22. Kurilo LF: Oogenesis in antenatal development in man. *Hum Genet* 57:86, 1981.
23. Cate RL, Mattalinao RJ, Hession C, Tizard R, Farber NM, Cheung A, Ninfa EG, Frey AZ, et al: Isolation of the bovine and human genes for Mullerian inhibiting substance and expression of the human genes in animal cells. *Cell* 45:685, 1986.
24. Cohen-Haguenauer O, Picard JY, Mattei MG, Serero S, Nguyen VC, deTand MF, Guerrier D, Hors-Cayla MC, et al: Mapping of the gene for antimullerian hormone to the short arm of human chromosome 19. *Cytogenet Cell Genet* 44:2, 1987.
25. Vigier B, Picard JY, Campargue J, Forest MG, Heyman Y, Josso N: Secretion of anti-Mullerian hormone by a competition-type radioimmunoassay: Lack of modulation by either FSH or testosterone. *Mol Cell Endocrinol* 43:141, 1985.
26. Voutilainen R, Miller WL: Human Mullerian inhibitory factor messenger ribonucleic acid is hormonally regulated in the fetal testis and in adult granulosa cells. *Mol Endocrinol* 1:604, 1987.
27. Donahoe PK, Cate RL, MacLaughlin DT, Epstein J, Fuller AF, Takahashi M, Coughlin JP, Ninfa EG, Taylor LA: Mullerian inhibiting substance: Gene structure and mechanism of action of a fetal regressor. *Recent Prog Horm Res* 43:431, 1987.
28. Baker ML, Metcalfe SA, Hutson JM: Serum levels of Mullerian inhibiting substance in boys from birth to 18 years, as determined by enzyme immunoassay. *J Clin Endocrinol Metab* 70:11, 1990.
29. Takahashi M, Koie SS, Donahoe PK: Mullerian inhibiting substance as oocyte meiosis inhibitor. *Mol Cell Endocrinol* 47:225, 1986.
30. Vigier B, Watrin F, Magre S, Tran D, Josso N: Purified bovine AMH induces a characteristic freemartin effect in fetal rat prospective ovaries exposed to it in vitro. *Development* 100:43, 1987.
31. Vigier B, Forest MG, Eychenne B, Bezard J, Garrigou O, Robel P, Josso N: Anti-Mullerian hormone produces sex reversal of fetal ovaries. *Proc Natl Acad Sci USA* 86:3684, 1989.
32. Behringer RR, Cate RL, Froelick GJ, Palmiter RD, Brinster RL: Abnormal sexual development in transgenic mice chronically expressing mullerian inhibiting substance. *Nature* 346:167, 1990.
33. Hutson JM, Donahoe PK: The hormonal control of testicular descent. *Endocr Rev* 7:270, 1986.
34. Siiteri PK, Wilson JD: Testosterone formation and metabolism during male sexual differentiation in the human embryo. *J Clin Endocrinol Metab* 38:113, 1974.
35. Feldman KW, Smith DW: Fetal phallic growth and penile standards for newborn male infants. *J Pediatr* 86:395, 1975.
36. Habenicht U-F, Newmann F: Hormonal regulation of testicular descent. *Adv Embryol Cell Biol* 81:1, 1983.
37. Winter JSD, Faiman C, Reyes FI: Sex steroid production by the human fetus: Its role in morphogenesis and control by gonadotropins, in Blandau RJ, Bergsma D (eds): *Morphogenesis and Malformation of the Genital System.* New York, Liss, 1977, pp 41–58.
38. Voutilainen R, Miller WL: Development expression of genes for the steroidogenic enzymes $P450_{scc}$(20,22-desmolase), $P450_{C17}$(17-alpha-hydroxylase/17,20-lyase) and $P450_{C21}$(21-hydroxylase) in the human fetus. *J Clin Endocrinol Metab* 63:1145, 1986.
39. Rundlett SE, Wu X-P, Miesfield RL: Functional characterizations of the androgen receptor confirm the molecular basis of androgen action is transcriptional regulation. *Mol Endocrinol* 4:708, 1990.
40. Cunha GR, Shannon JM, Neubauer BL, Sawyer LM, Fujii H, Taguchi O, Chung LWK: Mesenchymal-epithelial interactions in sex differentiation. *Hum Genet* 58:68, 1981.
41. Chang C, Kokontis J, Liao S: Molecular cloning of human and rat complementary DNA encoding androgen receptors. *Science* 240:324, 1988.
42. Lubahn DB, Joseph DR, Sullivan PM, Willard HF, French FS, Wilson EM: Cloning of human androgen receptor complementary DNA and localization to the X chromosome. *Science* 240:327, 1988.
43. Word RA, George FW, Wilson JD, Carr BR: Testosterone synthesis and adenylate cyclase activity in the early human fetal testis appear to be independent of human chorionic gonadotropin control. *J Clin Endocrinol Metab* 69:204, 1989.
44. Carr BR, Parker CR Jr, Ohashi M, MacDonald PC, Simpson ER: Regulation of human fetal testicular secretion of testosterone: Low density lipoprotein-cholesterol and cholesterol synthesized de novo as steroid precursor. *Am J Obstet Gynecol* 146:241, 1983.
45. Ronnekleiv OK, Resko JA: Ontogeny of gonadotropin-releasing hormone-containing neurons in early fetal development of rhesus macaques. *Endocrinology* 126:498, 1990.
46. Clements JA, Reyes FI, Winter JSD, Faiman C: Ontogenesis of gonadotropin-releasing hormone in the human fetal hypothalamus. *Proc Soc Exp Biol Med* 163:437, 1980.
47. Dumesic DA, Pohl H, Kamel F, Terasawa E: Increase in luteinizing hormone content occurs in cultured human fetal pituitary cells exposed to gonadotropin-releasing hormone. *J Clin Endocrinol Metab* 70:606, 1990.
48. Reyes FI, Winter JSD, Faiman C: Endocrinology of the fetal testis, in H. Burger and D. de Kretser (eds): *The Testis,* 2d ed. New York, Raven Press, 1989, pp 119–142.

49. Rasmussen DD, Liu JH, Wolf PL, Yen SSC: Endogenous opioid regulation of gonadotropin-releasing hormone release from the human fetal hypothalamus in vitro. *J Clin Endocrinol Metab* 57:881, 1983.
50. Kim SJ, Namkoong SE, Lee JW, Jung JK, Kang BC, Park JS: Response of human chorionic gonadotrophin to luteinizing hormone-releasing hormone stimulation in the culture media of normal human placenta, choriocarcinoma cell lines, and in the serum of patients with gestational trophoblastic disease. *Placenta* 8:257, 1987.
51. Iwashita M, Watanabe M, Adachi T, Ohira A, Shinozaki Y, Takeda Y, Sakamoto S: Effect of gonadal steroids on gonadotropin-releasing hormones stimulated human chorionic gonadotropin release by trophoblastic cells. *Placenta* 10:103, 1989.
52. Voutilainen R, Miller WL: Developmental and hormonal regulation of mRNAs for insulin-like growth factor II and steroidogenic enzymes in human fetal adrenals and gonads. *DNA* 7:9, 1989.
53. Sheth JJ, Sheth AR, Vin FK: Bioimmunoreactive inhibin-like substance in human fetal gonads. *Biol Res Pregnancy Perinatol* 4:110, 1983.
54. Albers N, Hart CS, Kaplan SL, Grumbach MM: Hormone ontogeny in the ovine fetus: XXIV. Porcine follicular fluid "inhibins" selectively suppress plasma follicle-stimulating hormone in the ovine fetus. *Endocrinology* 125:675, 1989.
55. Merson-Barg MS, Miller KF, Choi CM, Lee AC, Kim MH: Inhibin suppresses human chorionic gonadotropin secretion in term, but not first trimester, placenta. *J Clin Endocrinol Metab* 71:1294, 1990.
56. Winter JSD, Faiman C, Reyes FI: Sexual endocrinology of fetal and perinatal life, in Austin CR, Edwards RG (eds): *Mechanisms of Sex Differentiation in Animals and Man*. London, Academic, 1981, pp 205–253.
57. Corbier P, Dahennin L, Castanier M, Mebazaa A, Edwards DA, Roffi J: Sex differences in serum luteinizing hormone and testosterone in the human neonate during the first few hours after birth. *J Clin Endocrinol Metab* 7:1344, 1990.
58. Bolton NJ, Tapanainen J, Koivisto M, Vihko R: Circulating sex hormone-binding globulin and testosterone in newborns and infants. *Clin Endocrinol (Oxf)* 31:201, 1989.
59. Mann DR, Gould KG, Collins DC, Wallen K: Blockade of neonatal activation of the pituitary-testicular axis: Effect on peripubertal luteinizing hormone and testosterone secretion and on testicular development in male monkeys. *J Clin Endocrinol Metab* 68:600, 1988.
60. Imperato-McGinley J, Peterson RE, Gautier T, Sturla E: The impact of androgens on the evolution of male gender identity, in Kogan SJ, Hafez ESE (eds): *Pediatric Andrology*. The Hague, Martinus Nijhoff, 1981, pp 99–108.
61. Dorner G: Hormones, brain differentiation and the fundamental process of life. *J Steroid Biochem* 8:531, 1977.
62. Gorski RA: Sexual differentiation of the brain: Possible mechanisms and implications. *Can J Physiol Pharmacol* 63:577, 1985.
63. Sholl SA, Goy RW, Kim KL: 5α-Reductase, aromatase, and androgen receptor levels in the monkey brain during fetal development. *Endocrinology* 124:627, 1989.
64. Ehrhardt AA, Meyer-Bahlburg HFL, Rosen LR, Feldman JF, Veridiano NP, Zimmerman I, McEwen BS: Sexual orientation after prenatal exposure to exogenous estrogen. *Arch Sex Behav* 14:57, 1985.
65. Klinefelter HF Jr, Reifenstein EC Jr, Albright F: Syndrome characterized by gynecomastia, aspermatogenesis with a-leydigism, and increased excretion of follicle-stimulating hormone. *J Clin Endocrinol Metab* 2:615, 1942.
66. Salbenblatt JA, Bender BG, Puck MH, Robinson A, Faiman C, Winter JSD: Pituitary-gonadal function in Klinefelter syndrome before and during puberty. *Pediatr Res* 19:82, 1985.
67. Topper E, Dickerman Z, Prager-Lewin R, Kaufman H, Maimon Z, Laron Z: Puberty in 24 patients with Klinefelter syndrome. *Eur J Pediatr* 139:8, 1982.
68. Mies R, Fischer H, Pfeiff B, Winkelmann W, Wurz H: Klinefelter's syndrome and breast cancer. *Andrologia* 14: 317, 1982.
69. Page DC, Brown LG, de la Chapelle A: Exchange of terminal portions of X- and Y-chromosomal short arms in human XX males. *Nature* 328:437, 1987.
70. Page DC, Fisher EMC, McGillivray B, Brown L: Additional deletion in sex-determining region of human Y chromosome resolves paradox of X,t(Y;22) female. *Nature* 346:279, 1990.
71. Kohn G, Winter JSD, Mellman WJ: Trisomy X in three children. *J Pediatr* 72:248, 1968.
72. Van Kiekerk WA, Reitief AE: The gonads of human true hermaphrodites. *Hum Genet* 58:117, 1981.
73. Davidoff F, Federman DD: Mixed gonadal dysgenesis. *Pediatrics* 52:725, 1973.
74. Manuel M, Katayama KP, Jones HW Jr: The age of occurrence of gonadal tumors in intersex patients with a Y chromosome. *Am J Obstet Gynecol* 124:293, 1976.
75. Warburton D, Cline J, Stein Z, Susser M: Monosomy X: A chromosomal anomaly associated with young maternal age. *Lancet* i:167, 1980.
76. Lyon AJ, Preece MA, Grant DB: Growth curve for girls with Turner's syndrome. *Arch Dis Child* 60:932, 1985.
77. Bender B, Puck M, Salbenblatt J, Robinson A: Cognitive development of unselected girls with complete and partial X monosomy. *Pediatrics* 73:175, 1984.
78. Kosowicz J: The roentgen appearance of the hand and wrist in gonadal dysgenesis. *Am J Roentgenol Radium Ther Nucl Med* 93:354, 1965.
79. Reyes Fi, Koh KS, Faiman C: Fertility in women with gonadal dysgenesis. *Am J Obstet Gynecol* 126:668, 1976.
80. Krauss CM, Turksoy RN, Atkins L, McLaughlin C, Brown LG, Page DC: Familial premature ovarian failure due to an interstitial deletion of the long arm of the X-chromosome. *N Engl J Med* 317:125, 1987.
81. Winter JSD, Faiman C: Serum gonadotropin levels in agonadal children and adults. *J Clin Endocrinol Metab* 35:561, 1972.
82. Rosenfield RG: Update on growth hormone therapy for Turner's syndrome. *Acta Paediatr Scand [Suppl]* 356:103, 1989.
83. Apter D, Lenko HL, Perheentupa J, Soderholm A, Vihko R: Subnormal pubertal increases of serum androgens in Turner's syndrome. *Horm Res* 16:164, 1982.
84. Sybert VP: Adult height in Turner syndrome with and without androgen therapy. *J Pediatr* 104:365, 1984.
85. Ross JL, Cassorla FG, Skerda MC, Valk IM, Loriaux DL, Cutler GB Jr: A preliminary study of the effect of estrogen dose on growth in Turner's syndrome. *N Engl J Med* 309:1104, 1983.
86. Martinez A, Heinrich JJ, Domene H, Escobar ME, Jasper H, Moinuori, Bergada C: Growth in Turner's syndrome: Long term treatment with low dose ethinyl estradiol. *J Clin Endocrinol Metab* 65:253, 1987.
87. Ross JL, Cassorla F, Carpenter G, Long LM, Royster MS, Loriaux DL, Cutler GB: The effect of short term treatment with growth hormone and ethinyl estradiol on lower leg growth rate in girls with Turner's syndrome. *J Clin Endocrinol Metab* 67:515, 1988.
88. Vanderschueren-Lodeweyckx M, Massa G, Malraux P: Growth-promoting effect of growth hormone and low dose ethinyl estradiol in girls with Turner's syndrome. *J Clin Endocrinol Metab* 70:122, 1990.
89. Demetriou F, Emans SJ, Crigler JF Jr: Final height in estrogen-treated patients with Turner's syndrome. *Obstet Gynecol* 64:459, 1984.
90. Simpson JL: Genetic heterogeneity in XY sex reversal: Potential pitfalls in isolating the testis-determining factor (TDF), in Wachtel SS (ed): *Evolutionary Mechanisms in Sex Determination*. Boca Raton, FL, CRC Press, 1989, pp 265–277.
91. Pritchard-Jones K, Fleming S, Davidson D, Bickmore W,

Porteous D, Gosden C, Bard J, Buckler A, et al: The candidate Wilms' tumour gene is involved in genitourinary development. *Nature* 346:194, 1990.

92. Drash A, Sherman E, Hartmann WH, Blizzard RM: A syndrome of pseudohermaphroditism, Wilms' tumor, hypertension, and degenerative renal disease. *J Pediatr* 76:585, 1970.
93. Cleary RE, Caras J, Rosenfield RL, Young PCM: Endocrine and metabolic studies in a patient with male pseudohermaphroditism and true agonadism. *Am J Obstet Gynecol* 128:862, 1977.
94. Bergada C, Cleveland WW, Jones HW, Wilkins L: Variants of embryonic testicular dysgenesis: Bilateral anorchia and the syndrome of rudimentary testes. *Acta Endocrinol (Copenh)* 40:521, 1962.
95. Winter JSD, Taraska S, Faiman C: The hormonal response to hCG stimulation in male children and adolescents. *J Clin Endocrinol Metab* 34:348, 1972.
96. Josso N, Fekete C, Cachin O, Nezelogf C, Rappaport R: Persistence of mullerian ducts in male pseudohermaphroditism, and its relationship to cryptorchidism. *Clin Endocrinol (Oxf)* 19:247, 1983.
97. Brook CGD, Wagner H, Zachmann M, Prader A, Armendares S, Frank S, Aleman P, Najjar SS, et al: Familial occurrence of persistent mullerian structures in otherwise normal males. *Br Med J* 1:771, 1973.
98. Guerrier D, Tran D, Vanderwinden JM, Hideux S, Van Outryve L, Legeai L, Bouchard M, VanVliet G, et al: The persistent mullerian duct syndrome: A molecular approach. *J Clin Endocrinol Metab* 68:46, 1989.
99. Eil C, Austin RM, Sesterhenn I, Dunn JF, Cutler GB Jr, Johnsonbaugh RE: Leydig cell hypoplasia causing male pseudohermaphroditism: Diagnosis 13 years after prepubertal castration. *J Clin Endocrinol Metab* 58:441, 1984.
100. Koizumi S, Kyoya S, Mujawaki T, Kidani H, Funabashi T, Nakashima H, Naskamura Y, Ohta G, et al: Cholesterol side chain cleavage enzyme activity and cytochrome P450 content in adrenal mitochondria of a patient with congenital lipoid hyperplasia (Prader disease). *Clin Chim Acta* 77:301, 1977.
101. Camacho AM, Kowarski A: Congenital adrenal hyperplasia due to deficiency of one of the enzymes involved in biosynthesis of pregnenolone. *J Clin Endocrinol Metab* 28:153, 1968.
102. The VL, Lachance Y, Labrie C, Leblanc G, Thomas JL, Strickler RC, Labrie F: Full-length cDNA structure and predicted amino acid sequence of human placenta 3β-hydroxy-5-ene steroid dehydrogenase. *Mol Endocrinol* 3:1310, 1989.
103. Byrne GC, Perry YS, Winter JSD: Steroid inhibitory effects upon human adrenal 3β-hydroxysteroid dehydrogenase activity. *J Clin Endocrinol Metab* 62:413, 1986.
104. Pang S, Levine LS, Stoner E, Opitz JM, Pollack MS, Dupont B, New MI: Nonsalt-losing congenital adrenal hyperplasia due to 3β-hydroxysteroid dehydrogenase deficiency with normal glomerulosa function. *J Clin Endocrinol Metab* 56:808, 1983.
105. Rosenfield RL, Rich BH, Wolfsdorf JI, Cassorla F, Parks JS, Bongiovanni AM, Wu CH, Shackleton CHL: Pubertal presentation of congenital Δ^5-3β-hydroxysteroid dehydrogenase deficiency. *J Clin Endocrinol Metab* 51:345, 1980.
106. Martin F, Perheentupa J, Adlercreutz H: Plasma and urinary androgens and oestrogens in a pubertal boy with 3β-hydroxysteroid dehydrogenase deficiency. *J Steroid Biochem* 13:197, 1980.
107. Pang S, Lerner AJ, Stoner E, Levine LS, Oberfield SE, Engel I, New MI: Late-onset adrenal steroid 3β-hydroxysteroid dehydrogenase deficiency: A cause of hirsutism in pubertal and postpubertal women. *J Clin Endocrinol Metab* 60:428, 1985.
108. Kominami S, Shinzawa K, Takemori S: Purification and some properties of cytochrome P-450 specific for steroid 17α-hydroxylation and C17-C20 bond cleavage from guinea pig adrenal microsomes. *Biochem Biophys Res Commun* 109: 916, 1982.
109. Kagimoto M, Winter JSD, Kagimoto K, Simpson ER, Waterman MR: Structural characterization of normal and mutant human steroid 17α-hydroxylase genes: Molecular basis of one example of combined 17α-hydroxylase/17,20-lyase deficiency. *Mol Endocrinol* 2:564, 1988.
110. Yanase T, Kagimoto M, Matsui N, Simpson ER, Waterman MR: Combined 17α-hydroxylase/17,20-lyase deficiency due to a stop codon in the N-terminal region of 17α-hydroxylase cytochrome P450. *Mol Cell Endocrinol* 59:249, 1988.
111. Yanase T, Kagimoto M, Suzuki S, Hashiba K, Simpson ER, Waterman MR: Deletion of a phenylalanine in the N-terminal region of human cytochrome $P450_{17\alpha}$ results in partial combined 17α-hydroxylase/17,20-lyase deficiency. *J Biol Chem* 264:18076, 1989.
112. Yanase T, Sanders D, Shibata A, Matsui N, Simpson ER, Waterman MR: Combined 17α-hydroxylase/17,20-lyase deficiency due to a 7 base pair duplication in the N-terminal region of the cytochrome $P450_{17\alpha}$ (CYP17) gene. *J Clin Endocrinol Metab* 70:1325, 1990.
113. Dean HJ, Shackleton CHL, Winter JSD: Diagnosis and natural history of 17-hydroxylase deficiency in a newborn male. *J Clin Endocrinol Metab* 59:513, 1984.
114. Kater CE, Biglieri EG, Brust N, Chang B, Hirai J: The unique patterns of plasma aldosterone and 18-hydroxycorticosterone concentrations in the 17β-hydroxylase deficiency syndrome. *J Clin Endocrinol Metab* 55:295, 1982.
115. Zachmann M, Vollmin JA, Hamilton W, Prader A: Steroid 17,20-desmolase deficiency: A new cause of male pseudohermaphroditism. *Clin Endocrinol (Oxf)* 1:369, 1972.
116. Zachmann M, Werder EA, Prader A: Two types of male pseudohermaphroditism due to 17,20-desmolase deficiency. *Acta Endocrinol (Copenh)* 103:400, 1983.
117. Larrea F, Lisker R, Banuelos R, Bermudez JA, Herrara J, Rasilla VN, Perez-Palacios G: Hypergonadotrophic hypogonadism in an XX female subject due to 17,20-desmolase deficiency. *Acta Endocrinol (Copenh)* 103:400, 1983.
118. The VL, Labrie C, Zhao HF, Coriet J, Lachance Y, Simard J, Leblanc G, Cote J, et al: Characterization of cDNAs for human estradiol 17β-dehydrogenase and assignment of the gene to chromosome 17: Evidence of two mRNA species with distinct 5′-termini in human placenta. *Mol Endocrinol* 3:1301, 1989.
119. Imperato-McGinley J, Peterson RE, Stoller R, Goodwin WE: Male pseudohermaphroditism secondary to 17β-hydroxysteroid dehydrogenase deficiency: Gender role change with puberty. *J Clin Endocrinol Metab* 49:391, 1979.
120. Wilson SC, Oakey RE, Scott JS: Steroid metabolism in testes of patients with incomplete masculinization due to androgen insensitivity or 17β-hydroxysteroid dehydrogenase deficiency and normally differentiated males. *J Steroid Biochem* 29:649, 1988.
121. Wilson SC, Hodgins MB, Scott JS: Incomplete masculinization due to a deficiency of 17β-hydroxysteroid dehydrogenase: Comparison of prepubertal and peripubertal siblings. *Clin Endocrinol* 26:459, 1987.
122. Ivarsson SA, Nielsen MD, Lindberg T: Male pseudohermaphroditism due to 5α-reductase deficiency in a Swedish family. *Eur J Pediatr* 147:532, 1988.
123. Imperato-McGinley J, Peterson RE, Gautier T, Sturla E: Androgens and the evolution of male-gender identity among male pseudohermaphrodites with 5α-reductase deficiency. *N Engl J Med* 300:1233, 1979.
124. Cantu JM, Corona-Rivera E, Diaz M, Medina C, Esquinca E, Cortes-Gallegos V, Vaca G, Hernandez A: Post-pubertal female psychosexual orientation in incomplete male pseudohermaphroditism type 2 (5α-reductase deficiency). *Acta Endocrinol (Copenh)* 94:273, 1980.
125. Savage MO, Preece MA, Jeffcoate SL, Ransley PG, Rumsby G, Mansfield MD, Williams DI: Familial male pseudohermaphroditism due to deficiency of 5α-reductase. *Clin Endocrinol (Oxf)* 12:397, 1980.
126. Theintz GE, Steimer TJ, Sizonenko PC: Developmental pattern of 17β-hydroxysteroid dehydrogenase and 5α-reductase

activities in the foreskin of boys from birth to eight years of age. *Horm Res* 32:124, 1989.
127. Griffin JE, Wilson JD: The syndromes of androgen resistance. *N Engl J Med* 302:198, 1980.
128. Migeon BR, Brown TR, Axelman J, Migeon CJ: Studies of the locus for androgen receptor: Localization on the human X chromosome and evidence for homology with the Tfm locus in the mouse. *Proc Natl Acad Sci USA* 78:6339, 1981.
129. Müller J, Skakkebaek NE: Testicular carcinoma in situ testis in children with the androgen insensitivity (testicular feminization) syndrome. *Br Med J* 1:1419, 1984.
130. Faiman C, Winter JSD: The control of gonadotropin secretion in complete testicular feminization. *J Clin Endocrinol Metab* 39:631, 1974.
131. Keenan BS, Meyer WJ, Hadjian AJ, Jones HW, Migeon CJ: Syndrome of androgen insensitivity in man: Absence of 5α-dihydrotestosterone binding protein in skin fibroblasts. *J Clin Endocrinol Metab* 38:1143, 1974.
132. Brown TR, Lubahn DB, Wilson EM, Joseph DR, French FS, Migeon CJ: Deletion of the steroid-binding domain of the human androgen receptor gene in one family with complete androgen insensitivity syndrome: Evidence for further genetic heterogeneity in this syndrome. *Proc Natl Acad Sci USA* 85:8151, 1988.
133. Lubahn DB, Brown TR, Simental JA, Higgs HN, Migeon CJ, Wilson EM, French FS: Sequence of the intron/exon junctions of the coding region of the human androgen receptor and identification of a point of mutation in a family with complete androgen insensitivity. *Proc Natl Acad Sci USA* 86:9534, 1989.
134. Marcelli M, Tilley WD, Wilson CM, Wilson JD, Griffin JE, McPhaul MJ: A single nucleotide substitution introduces a premature termination codon into the androgen receptor gene of a patient with receptor-negative androgen resistance. *J Clin Invest* 85:1522, 1990.
135. Imperato-McGinley J, Ip NY, Gautier T, Neuweiler J, Gruenspan H, Liao S, Chang C, Balazs I: DNA linkage analysis and studies of the androgen receptor gene in a large kindred with complete androgen insensitivity. *Am J Med Genet* 36:104, 1990.
136. Amrhein JA, Meyer WJ III, Jones HW Jr, Migeon CJ: Androgen insensitivity in man: Evidence for genetic heterogeneity. *Proc Natl Acad Sci USA* 73:891, 1976.
137. Kaufman M, Pinsky L, Simard L, Wong SC: Defective activation of androgen-receptor complexes: A marker of androgen insensitivity. *Mol Cell Endocrinol* 25:151, 1982.
138. Griffin JE, Durrant JL: Qualitative receptor defects in families with androgen resistance: Failure of stabilization of the fibroblast cytosol androgen receptor. *J Clin Endocrinol Metab* 55:465, 1982.
139. Eil C: Familial incomplete male pseudohermaphroditism associated with impaired nuclear androgen retention. *J Clin Invest* 71:850, 1983.
140. Gyorki S, Warne GL, Khalid BAK, Funder JW: Defective nuclear accumulation of androgen receptors in disorders of sexual differentiation. *J Clin Invest* 72:819, 1983.
141. Amrhein JA, Klingensmith GJ, Walsh PC, McKusick VA, Migeon CJ: Partial androgen insensitivity: The Reifenstein syndrome revisited. *N Engl J Med* 297:350, 1977.
142. Aiman J, Griffin JE: The frequency of androgen receptor deficiency in infertile men. *J Clin Endocrinol Metab* 54:725, 1982.
143. Aarskog D: Maternal progestins as a possible cause of hypospadias. *N Engl J Med* 300:75, 1979.
144. Mau G: Progestins during pregnancy and hypospadias. *Teratology* 24:285, 1981.
145. Gill WB, Schumacher GFB, Bibbo M: Structural and functional abnormalities in sex organs of male offspring of mothers treated with diethylstilbestrol (DES). *J Reprod Med* 16:147, 1976.
146. Dean HJ, Winter JSD: The effect of five synthetic progestational compounds on 5α-reductase activity in genital skin fibroblast monolayers. *Steroids* 43:13, 1985.
147. Smith DW: *Recognizable Patterns of Human Malformation: Genetic, Embryologic and Clinical Aspects,* 3d ed. Philadelphia, Saunders, 1982.
148. Greenberg F, Gresik MW, Carpenter RT, Law SW, Hoffman LP, Ledbetter DH: The Gardner-Silengo-Wachtel or genito-palato-cardiac syndrome: Male pseudohermaphroditism with micrognathia, cleft palate and conotruncal cardiac defects. *Am J Med Genet* 26:59, 1987.
149. Bauer SB, Bull MJ, Retik AB: Hypospadias: A familial study. *J Urol* 121:474, 1979.
150. Svensson J, Eneroth P, Gustafsson J-A, Ritzen M, Stenberg A: Metabolism of androstenedione in skin and serum levels of gonadotrophins and androgens in prepubertal boys with hypospadias. *J Endocrinol* 76:399, 1978.
151. Raboch J, Pondelickova J, Starka L: Plasma testosterone values in hypospadias. *Andrologia* 8:255, 1976.
152. Nonomura K, Fujieda K, Sakakibara N, Terasawa K, Matsuno T, Matsuura N, Koyanagi T: Pituitary and gonadal function in prepubertal boys with hypospadias. *J Urol* 132:595, 1984.
153. Svensson J, Snochowski M: Androgen receptor levels in preputial skin from boys with hypospadias. *J Clin Endocrinol Metab* 49:340, 1979.
154. Müller J, Skakkebaek NE: Abnormal germ cells in maldescended testes: A study of cell density, nuclear size and deoxyribonucleic acid content in testicular biopsies from 50 boys. *J Urol* 131:730, 1984.
155. Prader A: Der Genitalbeffund beim Pseudohermaphroditismus feminus des Kongenitalen Adenogenitalen Syndroms. *Helv Paediatr Acta* 9:231, 1954.
156. Dickerman Z, Grant DR, Faiman C, Winter JSD: Intra-adrenal steroid concentrations in man: Zonal differences and developmental changes. *J Clin Endocrinol Metab* 59:1031, 1984.
157. New MI, White PC, Pang S, DuPont B, Speiser PW: The adrenal hyperplasias, in Scriver CR, Beudet AL, Sly WS, Valle D (eds): *The Metabolic Basis of Inherited Disease,* 6th ed. New York, McGraw-Hill, 1989, pp 1881–1917.
158. Owerbach D, Crawford YM, Dragnin MB: Direct analysis of CYP21B genes in 21-hydroxylase deficiency using polymerase chain reaction. *Mol Endocrinol* 4:125, 1990.
159. Winter JSD, Couch RM: Modern medical therapy of congenital adrenal hyperplasia: A decade of experience. *Ann NY Acad Sci* 458:165, 1985.
160. Blankstein J, Faiman C, Reyes FI, Schroeder M, Winter JSD: Adult-onset familial 21-hydroxylase deficiency. *Am J Med* 68:441, 1980.
161. Fife D, Rappaport EB: Prevalence of salt-losing among congenital adrenal hyperplasia patients. *Clin Endocrinol (Oxf)* 18:259, 1983.
162. Speiser PW, Agdere L, Ueshiba H, White PC, New MI: Aldosterone synthesis in salt-wasting congenital adrenal hyperplasia with complete absence of adrenal 21-hydroxylase. *N Engl J Med* 324:145, 1991.
163. Pham-Huu-Trung MT, Raux MC, Gourmelen M, Baron MC, Girard F: Plasma aldosterone concentrations related to 17α-hydroxyprogesterone in congenital adrenal hyperplasia. *Acta Endocrinol (Copenh)* 82:572, 1976.
164. Neville AM, O'Hare MJ: *The Human Adrenal Cortex.* Berlin, Springer-Verlag, 1982.
165. Schaison G, Couzinet B, Gourmelen M, Elkik F, Bougneres P: Angiotensin and adrenal steroidogenesis: Study of 21-hydroxylase-deficient congenital adrenal hyperplasia. *J Clin Endocrinol Metab* 51:1390, 1980.
166. Hughes IA, Winter JSD: The application of a serum 17OH-progesterone radioimmunoassay to the diagnosis and management of congenital adrenal hyperplasia. *J Pediatr* 88:766, 1976.
167. Hughes IA, Riad-Fahmy D, Griffiths K: Plasma 17OH-progesterone concentrations in newborn infants. *Arch Dis Child* 54:347, 1979.
168. Forest MG, Betuel H, Couillin P, Boue A, David M, Floret D,

Francois R, Guibaud P, et al: Prenatal diagnosis of congenital adrenal hyperplasia (CAH) due to 21-hydroxylase deficiency by steroid analysis in the amniotic fluid of mid-pregnancy: Comparison with HLA typing in 17 pregnancies at risk for CAH. *Prenat Diagn* 1:197, 1981.
169. Hughes IA, Laurence KM: Prenatal diagnosis of congenital adrenal hyperplasia due to 21-hydroxylase deficiency by amniotic fluid steroid analysis, *Prenat Diagn* 2:97, 1982.
170. Pang S, Pollack MS, Marshall RN, Immken L: Prenatal treatment of congenital adrenal hyperplasia due to 21-hydroxylase deficiency. *N Engl J Med* 322:111, 1990.
171. Thompson R, Seargeant L, Winter JSD: Screening for congenital adrenal hyperplasia: Distribution of 17α-hydroxyprogesterone concentrations in neonatal blood spot specimens. *J Pediatr* 114:400, 1989.
172. Pang S, Wallace MA, Hofman L, Thuline HC, Dorche C, Lyon ICT, Dobbins RH, Kling S, et al: Worldwide experience in newborn screening for classical congenital adrenal hyperplasia due to 21-hydroxylase deficiency. *Pediatrics* 81:866, 1988.
173. Thilen A, Larsson A: Congenital adrenal hyperplasia in Sweden 1969–1986. *Acta Paediatr Scand* 79:168, 1990.
174. Hughes IA, Read GF: Simultaneous plasma and saliva steroid measurements as an index of control in congenital adrenal hyperplasia: A longitudinal study. *Horm Res* 16:142, 1982.
175. Hughes IA, Winter JSD: The relationship between serum concentrations of 17OH-progesterone and other serum and urinary steroids in patients with congenital adrenal hyperplasia. *J Clin Endocrinol Metab* 46:98, 1978.
176. Wischusen J, Baker HWG, Hudson B: Reversible male infertility due to congenital adrenal hyperplasia. *Clin Endocrinol (Oxf)* 14:571, 1981.
177. Watanuki M, Tilley BE, Hall PF: Cytochrome P450 for 11β and 18-hydroxylase activities of bovine adrenocortical mitochondria: One enzyme or two? *Biochemistry* 17:127, 1978.
178. Rosler A, Leiberman E, Sack J, Landau H, Benderly A, Moses SW, Cohen T: Clinical variability of congenital adrenal hyperplasia due to 11β-hydroxylase deficiency. *Horm Res* 16:133, 1982.
179. Cathelineau G, Brerault J-L, Fiet J, Julien R, Dreux C, Canivet J: Adrenocortical 11β-hydroxylation defect in adult women with postmenarchial onset of symptoms. *J Clin Endocrinol Metab* 51:287, 1980.
180. Globerman H, Rosler A, Theodor R, New MI, White PC: An inherited defect in aldosterone biosynthesis caused by a mutation in or near the gene for steroid 11-hydroxylase. *N Engl J Med* 319:1193, 1988.
181. Zadik Z, Kahana L, Kaufman H, Benderli A, Hochberg Z: Salt loss in hypertensive form of congenital adrenal hyperplasia (11β-hydroxylase deficiency). *J Clin Endocrinol Metab* 58:384, 1984.
182. Finkelstein M, Litvin Y, Mizrachi Y, Neiman G, Rosler A: Apparent double defect in C11β and C21-steroid hydroxylation in congenital adrenal hyperplasia. *J Steroid Biochem* 19:675, 1983.
183. Rosler A, Weshler N, Leiberman E, Hochberg Z, Weidenfeld J, Sack J, Chemke J: 11β-hydroxylase deficiency congenital adrenal hyperplasia: Update of prenatal diagnosis. *J Clin Endocrinol Metab* 66:830, 1988.
184. Pang S, Levine LS, Lorenzen F, Chow D, Pollack M, Dupont B, Genel M, New MI: Hormonal studies in obligate heterozygotes and siblings of patients with 11β-hydroxylase deficiency congenital adrenal hyperplasia. *J Clin Endocrinol Metab* 50:586, 1980.
185. Zachman M, Forest MG, De Peretti E: 3β-Hydrosteroid dehydrogenase deficiency: Followup study in a girl with pubertal bone age. *Horm Res* 11:292, 1979.
186. Ishizuka N, Kawashima Y, Nakanishi T, Sugawa T, Nishikawa Y: Statistical observations on genital anomalies of newborns following the administration of progestin to their mothers. *Obstet Gynecol Surv* 19:496, 1964.
187. Lynch A, Mychalkiw W, Hutt SJ: Parental progesterone: I. Its effect on development and on intellectual and academic achievement. *Early Hum Dev* 2:305, 1978.
188. Franks RC, Northcutt R: Female pseudohermaphroditism and renal anomalies. *Am J Dis Child* 105:490, 1963.
189. Winter JSD, Kohn G, Mellman WJ, Wagner S: A familial syndrome of renal, genital, and middle ear anomalies. *J Pediatr* 72:88, 1968.

P A R T VI

Fuel Metabolism

C H A P T E R 19

The Endocrine Pancreas: Diabetes Mellitus*

Philip Felig

Michael Bergman

The histologic identification by Paul Langerhans in 1869 of the islet cells which constitute the endocrine portion of the pancreas preceded by 20 years the classic studies of Minkowski and Von Mering, which demonstrated that pancreatectomy results in diabetes. Fifty-two years later, the discovery of insulin as the internal secretion of the pancreas by Banting and Best heralded a new era in the treatment of diabetes. The significance of insulin secretion and action with respect to human disease is underscored by the ranking of diabetes mellitus as the third leading cause of death and the leading cause of blindness in the United States and its accentuation of the risk of coronary artery disease fourfold or more.[1] The role of diabetes in early mortality varies with the level of development in different parts of the world; in most countries it ranks between fourth and eighth as a cause of death.[2] Furthermore, the cost of medical care and disability associated with diabetes exceeds $40 billion per year in the United States.[3]

The islets of Langerhans consist of approximately 2 million clusters of pale-appearing cells dispersed among the pancreatic acinar (exocrine) cells. In the newborn, the islet cells constitute 20 percent of the volume of pancreatic tissue. With normal growth and development, the exocrine mass increases at a far greater rate than do the endocrine cells so that in adults the islets constitute only 1 to 2 percent of pancreatic mass. On the basis of histochemical, ultrastructural, and immunofluorescent techniques as well as the identification of their hormonal secretory products, the islet cells are recognized as consisting of four distinct cell types (Table 19-1): *alpha*, or A, cells, which produce glucagon; *beta*, or B, cells, which produce insulin; *delta*, or D, cells, which produce somatostatin; and PP cells, which produce pancreatic polypeptide. By light microscopy, beta cells can be identified by their positive staining with aldehyde fuchsin and lack of staining with silver nitrate. In contrast, alpha and delta cells are argyrophilic and do not stain with the aldehyde fuchsin. The various cells types also show specific ultrastructural characteristics with respect to their secretory granules (Fig. 19-1). In alpha cells, the granules have an electron-dense core and a paler periphery. Beta cells show crystalloid pleomorphic granules. In delta cells, less dense and uniform-appearing granules extend to the limiting membrane of the vesicle. The secretory granules of the PP cells are electron-dense and elongated.

The various islet cells show characteristics which have led to their being grouped, along with other secretory cells (e.g., thyroid C cells, adrenal medullary cells), in the family of cells designated the diffuse neuroendocrine system (DNES).[4] Initially these cell types were referred to the amine precursor uptake and decarboxylation (APUD) series. The APUD designation was also meant to convey a common ectodermal origin among the members of this series. However, allograft experiments have demonstrated that the pancreatic islet cells are of endodermal origin.

Of the various disease states associated with abnormalities of the endocrine pancreas, diabetes mellitus, a disorder characterized by an absolute or relative lack of insulin, is by far the most common; it forms the basis of this chapter. Abnormalities in the secretion of glucagon are frequently observed as a secondary phenomenon in diabetes and in very rare instances (e.g., the glucagonoma syndrome) may be the primary factor responsible for disturbances in metabolism. They too are discussed below. The consequences of excess somatostatin secretion are covered in Chap. 26. The clinical syndromes associated with insulin-producing beta cell tumors are discussed in Chap. 20.

* The authors acknowledge the contributions to this chapter by Eleazar Shafrir, which appeared in the second edition.

TABLE 19-1 Characteristics of Islet-Cell Types

Cell Type	Percentage of Total	Hormone	Secretory Granules
Alpha (α)	15	Glucagon	Dense core, pale periphery
Beta (β)	60	Insulin	Crystalloid, pleomorphic
Delta (δ)	10	Somatostatin	Low density, homogeneous, fill membrane
PP	15	Pancreatic polypeptide	Dense, elongated

PHYSIOLOGY OF FUEL METABOLISM

Diabetes mellitus is characterized by changes in the metabolism of each of the major body fuels (carbohydrate, fat, and protein) and is associated with primary or secondary disturbances in the secretion of and/or sensitivity to a variety of hormones [insulin, glucagon, catecholamines, growth hormone (GH), and cortisol]. The normal physiology of these substrates and hormones is therefore considered here.

Carbohydrate Metabolism

Carbohydrates are molecules of three or more carbon atoms combined with hydrogen and oxygen in a proportion of two hydrogen atoms per oxygen atom or

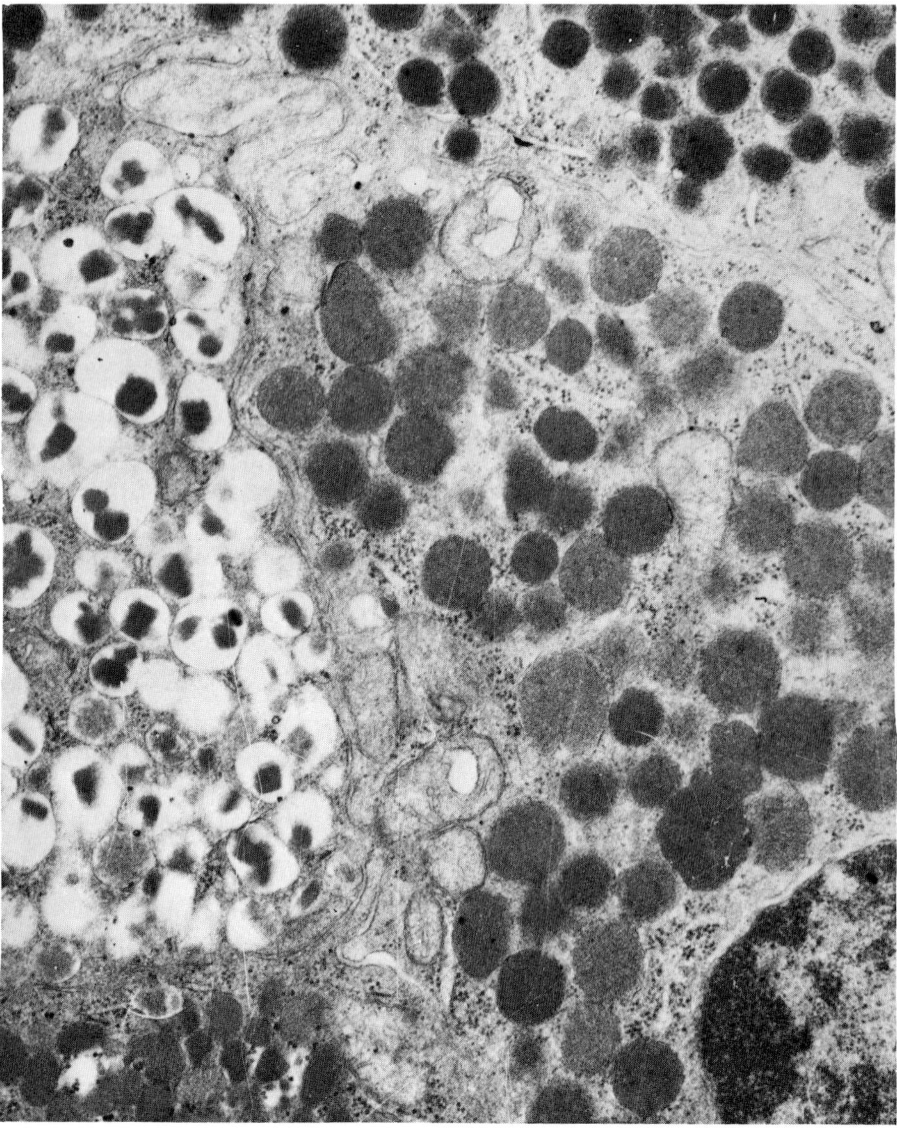

FIGURE 19-1 Electron micrograph of portion of normal human islet showing alpha, beta, and delta cells. In the alpha cell (upper right), the secretory granules show a dense core and a pale periphery. In the beta cells (left), there are pleomorphic granules with a crystalloid matrix. In the delta cell (center), the secretory granules are homogeneous and fill the vesicles.

simple derivatives of those basic molecules. Most Americans and Europeans obtain 40 to 45 percent of their dietary calories in the form of carbohydrate. Despite the diversity of forms and sources of dietary carbohydrate, the end products of digestion which are absorbed in the intestine are the hexoses glucose, fructose, and galactose. Of these simple sugars, glucose is by far the largest constituent.

Glucose Transport and Glucose Phosphorylation

The initial event in the cellular metabolism of glucose is its facilitative transport across the plasma membrane of cells. This step is catalyzed by a family of carrier proteins designated as glucose transporters.[5,5a] Using techniques of complementary DNA cloning, five structurally related glucose transporters (isoforms) have been identified which are encoded by specific genes, are expressed in specific tissues, and have distinct functional characteristics (Table 19-2). The transporter proteins consist of approximately 500 amino acids and show an amino acid identity of only 39 to 65 percent between isoforms within a species but up to 98 percent identity between human and rat for the same isoform. This interspecies conservation of isoform structure suggests the early appearance of tissue-specific transporter function in phylogenetic development. The numerical system used to identify each of the glucose transporter isoforms is based on the chronological order of identification of cDNA sequences.

The GLUT-1 and GLUT-3 isoforms are found primarily in erythrocytes and the brain. These low-K_m transporters facilitate glucose uptake and are essential for these tissues in the basal state. In contrast, the GLUT-2 transporter has a high K_m of approximately 15 to 20 m*M*. In the liver and kidney, this characteristic allows for the bidirectional transport of glucose in response to changes in the ambient glucose concentration. Thus, in circumstances of high glucose concentration (e.g., after food ingestion), glucose uptake by the liver is increased, while during periods of fasting, glucose is released by liver and, after prolonged starvation, by the kidney as well. In a beta cell, the high-K_m glucose transporter functions as an essential component of the glucose sensor that regulates insulin secretion. Underexpression of GLUT-2 in beta cells has been proposed as a component of diminished insulin secretion in insulin-dependent as well as non-insulin-dependent diabetes mellitus.[5a]

In the fat cells (adipocytes) as well as in muscle, the major glucose transporter is GLUT-4. This isoform has a K_m of 5, which is close to that of the normal plasma glucose concentration. Transport of glucose is rate-limiting for the metabolism of glucose in adipocytes and muscle. Insulin rapidly increases the uptake of glucose by these tissues by inducing the translocation of GLUT-4 transporters from intracellular storage sites to the plasma membrane. A reduction in GLUT-4 transporter function, particularly in adipocytes, has been implicated in the insulin resistance observed in non-insulin-dependent diabetes.[6]

Little if any free glucose is present as such inside cells, since glucose taken up by tissues undergoes rapid metabolic transformation (Fig. 19-2). The major fates of glucose after it enters the cells are (1) intermediate storage as glycogen, (2) anaerobic metabolism via the glycolytic pathway to pyruvate and lactate, (3) continued aerobic oxidation in the main energy-yielding pathway, the tricarboxylic acid (TCA, or Krebs) cycle, (4) conversion to fatty acids (*lipogenesis*) and storage as triglyceride, and (5) to a small extent, oxidation via the pentose pathway.

Regardless of its ultimate metabolic fate, the first intracellular reaction involving glucose is phosphorylation to glucose 6-phosphate (G6P) (Fig. 19-2). A family of hexose phosphorylating enzymes, the *hexokinases*, catalyze this process.[7] In mammals, four isoenzymes have been identified: hexokinase I, II, III, and IV. Hexokinase IV is also known as *glucokinase*. Glucokinase differs from the other isoenzymes by having a narrower range of hexose substrate specificity that is limited to glucose with a K_m of 5 m*M*, the physiologic glucose concentration, and a tissue distribution limited to liver and beta cells. In conjunction with GLUT-2 (Table 19-2), glucokinase thus serves as an integral part of the glucose sensor that regulates insulin secretion by beta cells. In the liver, glucokinase influences changes in intracellular glucose metabolism in response to the rise in blood glu-

TABLE 19-2 Facilitative Glucose Transporters

Glucose Transporter	Sites of Expression	K_m	Function
GLUT-1	Blood cells, brain	1–2	Basal uptake
GLUT-2	Liver	15–20	Bidirectional glucose flux
	Beta cell		Glucose sensor
	Kidney, gut		Glucose efflux
GLUT-3	Brain	1	Basal uptake
GLUT-4	Fat, muscle	5	Insulin-stimulated glucose uptake
GLUT-5	Jejunum	?	?

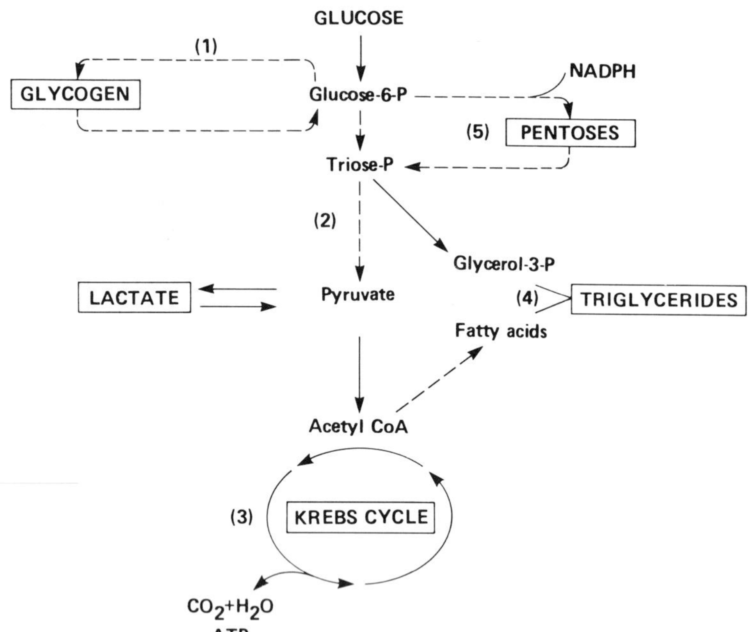

FIGURE 19-2 The major metabolic fates of glucose in humans. For delineation of the pathways, see the text.

cose after meal ingestion. Furthermore, glucokinase is an inducible enzyme that is under the control of insulin; its activity declines with fasting or in diabetes and rises on refeeding or insulin administration.

In contrast to glucokinase, the K_m of hexokinase I, II, and III is in the range of 0.1 to 0.0001 mM. In muscle and fat tissue, only the low-K_m hexokinases are expressed. In those tissues the rate-limiting step in glucose utilization is not phosphorylation but transport. This transport, as was noted above, is stimulated by insulin via the translocation of the GLUT-4 transporter to the cell membrane.

Glycogenesis and Glycogenolysis

Carbohydrate is stored inside cells in the form of *glycogen*, a branched, treelike, high-molecular-weight polysaccharide composed of glucose units linked in 1,4 bonds, with branch points of 1,6 glucosidic linkage (Fig. 19-3). The addition of glucosyl residues in 1,4 linkage constitutes the rate-limiting step in glycogen synthesis; it requires as a primer a polysaccharide chain of at least four glucose residues. This rate-limiting reaction depends on the activity of the enzyme *glycogen synthase*, which exists in two rapidly interconvertible forms: an active form (synthase I), and an inactive form (synthase D). Phosphorylation of glycogen synthase by a protein kinase inactivates the enzyme (forming synthase D), while dephosphorylation by a phosphatase activates the enzyme (forming synthase I). The interconversion of these two forms of glycogen synthase involves the net addition or removal of three phosphate groups.[8]

Hormonal inhibition of glycogen synthase is effected via stimulation of a cAMP-dependent protein kinase in the case of glucagon and a calcium-dependent kinase in the case of the catecholamines. These kinases phosphorylate the synthase. In circumstances of increased glucose availability (feeding), glycogen synthase activity is increased by mechanisms involving insulin as well as the direct substrate effects of glucose. In the liver, insulin is necessary for the maintenance of normal amounts of the glycogen synthase phosphatase enzyme while glucose has a direct effect in activating the phosphatase, increasing the availability of the active form of glycogen synthase. This direct effect of glucose in promoting glycogen storage in the liver is evident from studies in humans. Combined infusions of insulin and glucose resulting in hyperinsulinemia in the absence of hyperglycemia cause only a minimal net hepatic uptake of glucose. In contrast, increasing the rate of glucose infusion so as to induce hyperglycemia markedly augments net hepatic glucose uptake in the absence of a further elevation in plasma insulin.[9] Unlike the situation in the liver, in muscle tissue insulin rather than glucose is the major regulator of glycogen synthase activity. Polymorphism of the gene on chromosome 19 that regulates the expression of human glycogen synthase has recently been identified as a marker for a subgroup of patients with non-insulin-dependent (type II) diabetes[10] (see Etiology of Diabetes, below).

The initial step in the breakdown of glycogen involves the removal of glucose residues from the terminal 1,4 linkages by the action of *phosphorylase*, which splits off the glucose bond, inserting a phosphate at C-1 and releasing glucose 1-phosphate. Phosphorylase likewise exists in an inactive form which must be activated. However, in this case,

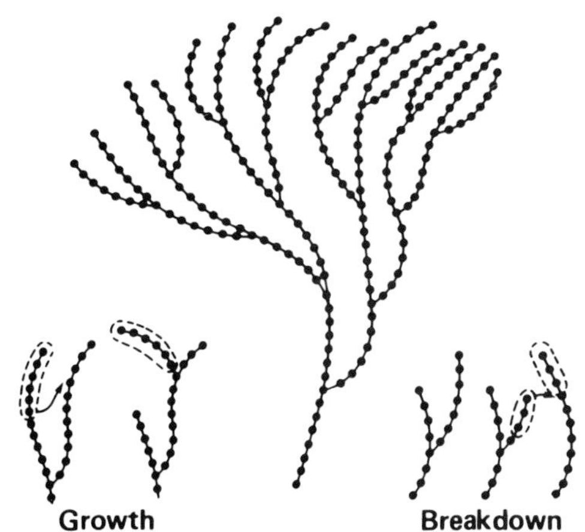

FIGURE 19-3 Part of an idealized glycogen particle represented as a continually branching tree without a main stem. Glucose residues (-●-) are linked in 1:4 glycoside bonds; branches are attached by 1:6 bonds. The ratio of 1:4 to 1:6 bonds varies from 12 to 18. *Growth*: *Glycogen synthase* successively transfers glucose residues from uridine diphosphate glucose (UDPG) to the outer branches of glycogen; a preexisting small glycogen particle is obligatory to prime the reaction. When the chain length reaches 10 to 12 residues, a group of 6 residues is transferred to a neighboring shorter chain to allow further elongation to take place. This is carried out by a "branching" enzyme, *amylo-1,4-→1,6-transglucosidase*, forming a 1:6 bond (*left*). Glycogen may attain a mass of 10^7 daltons in muscle and as much as 10^9 daltons in the liver. *Breakdown:* Phosphorylase degrades the 1:4 bonds on the outer branches of the glycogen particle, yielding glucose 1-phosphate, down to four glucose residues proximate to the 1:6 bonds. At this stage *α-1,4-α-1,4-glucan transferase* translocates the three-glucose segment to a neighboring chain, exposing the 1:6 bond to the "debranching" enzyme *amylo-1,6-glucosidase* (*right*). This is a specific hydrolytic cleavage yielding glucose, so that altogether up to 8 percent of the glycogen particle may be released as free glucose. The phosphorolysis of the branch may proceed after the removal of the 1:6 glucose stub.

phosphorylation of the enzyme by *phosphorylase kinase* (*ATP*) (Fig. 19-4) activates rather than inhibits the enzyme. The activation of phosphorylase involves a cascade of events activated by the binding of glycogenolytic hormones such as glucagon and epinephrine to cell surface receptors on the liver. After hormone binding, the membrane-associated enzyme *adenyl cyclase* catalyzes the formation of cyclic AMP. This process activates a cAMP-dependent protein kinase, *phosphorylase kinase*, which converts the inactive phosphorylase b to the active form, phosphorylase a. Stimulation of adenyl cyclase and protein kinase is a primary factor in expressing the effect of many hormones. In this instance, the classic phosphorylation cascade leading to the activation of phosphorylase is triggered by epinephrine or glucagon through β-adrenergic receptors. It should be noted, however, that epinephrine-mediated stimulation of glycogenolysis may also occur via α-adrenergic mechanisms, independent of changes in the concentration of cAMP. These α-adrenergic effects are mediated by increases in intracellular calcium concentration.[11] Muscle glycogenolysis induced by exercise is also mediated by a rise in intracellular calcium. In addition, the activities of phosphorylase and glycogen synthase can be influenced by alterations of the circulating glucose concentration independent of changes in the levels of hormones or cAMP.[8] Furthermore, in humans, so long as basal insulin concentrations are present, a rise in plasma glucose concentration of itself inhibits glycogenolysis, presumably via a decrease in the activity of phosphorylase.[12]

The glucose 1-phosphate released from glycogen is converted by the action of the freely reversible, bidirectional enzyme *phosphoglucomutase* to G6P, which may then enter the glycolytic pathway (see below) or be converted to free glucose. The latter reaction is catalyzed by the regulatory unidirectional enzyme G6Pase, which is present in liver but not in muscle. As a result, stimulation of glycogenolysis in muscle tissue results in the release of lactate and pyruvate as the end products of glycolysis, since the G6P formed in glycogenolysis cannot be converted to free glucose but instead enters the glycolytic pathway.

Glycolysis

The anaerobic catabolism of glucose to pyruvate and lactate is termed *glycolysis*. This catabolic pathway, with its enzymes and intermediate metabolites, was the first to be elucidated; it has been referred to as the *Embden-Meyerhof* pathway. By this pathway, the energy of glucose is made available for cellular processes in the form of high-energy phosphate bonds in ATP; the mechanism involves oxidation-reduction reactions which may occur in the absence of oxygen. Under such anaerobic circumstances the end product of glycolysis is lactate. In aerobic conditions pyruvate, after conversion to acetyl CoA, enters the TCA cycle and is oxidized to CO_2 (Fig. 19-5). The enzymes involved in glycolysis are located within the cytoplasm and are present in virtually all cells throughout the body. However, glycolysis is quantitatively a major route of glucose utilization in only specific cell types: (1) brain, which has limited access to substrates which do not cross the blood-brain barrier, (2) red blood cells, which lack the aerobic oxidative pathway, (3) skeletal muscle, particularly during vigorous exercise, and (4) heart muscle during circumstances of impaired perfusion (e.g., coronary artery disease). The overall glycolytic catabolism of glucose involves three simultaneously coordinated processes: (1) breakdown via a series of enzymatic steps of the 6-carbon skeleton of glucose, an aldehyde, to two molecules of a 3-carbon acid, pyruvic acid (or pyruvate), in equilibrium with lactic acid (or lactate), (2) transfer of energy by the net resynthesis of two molecules of ATP, and (3) transfer

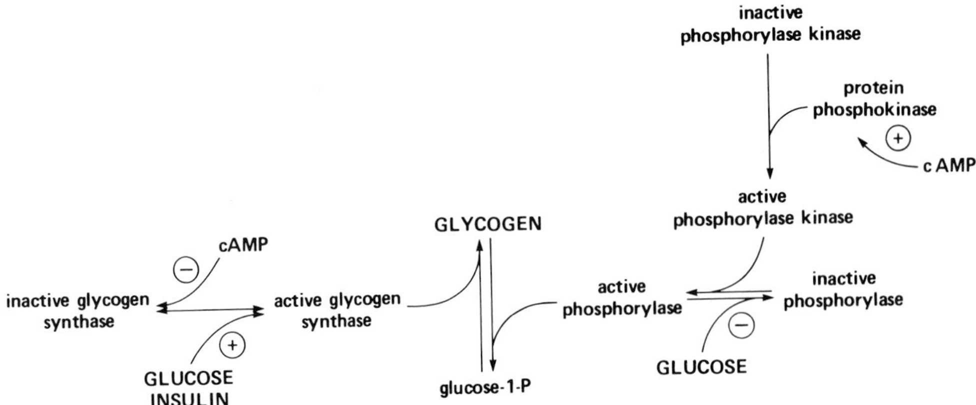

FIGURE 19-4 Regulation of glycogen synthesis and breakdown. Glycogen formation requires the activation of *glycogen synthase* and the inactivation of *glycogen phosphorylase*. These processes are stimulated by glucose and/or insulin. Glycogen breakdown requires activation of phosphorylase and inactivation of synthase. These processes are regulated in a reciprocal fashion by a fall in insulin concentration and by increased concentrations of glucagon and epinephrine which act via a cAMP-protein kinase mechanism.

of electrons via a sequence of oxidation-reduction reactions, resulting in a major ATP gain.

Of the 11 enzymatic steps involved in the conversion of glucose to lactate, only 3 are thermodynamically irreversible, nonequilibrium reactions and constitute regulatory points: the reactions catalyzed by (1) hexokinase or glucokinase, (2) phosphofructokinase, and (3) pyruvate kinase, which catalyzes the formation of pyruvate from phospho*enol*pyruvate (Fig. 19-5). The hexokinase/glucokinase reaction and its regulation were discussed above. A key position in glycolysis is the step at which 6-phosphofructo-1-kinase (PFK-1) catalyzes the conversion of fructose 6-phosphate (F6P) to fructose-1,6-bis(dihydrogen) phosphate (fructose-1,6-diphosphate, F1,6P_2).[13] The enzyme, 6-phosphofructo-2-kinase (PFK-2), tightly associated with this step, converts F6P to fructose-2,6-diphosphate (F2,6P_2), which is not a metabolic intermediate but a prominent intracellular regulator. F2,6P_2 acts as a potent allosteric effector of PFK-1 activity (Fig. 19-5).

The case of PFK-1 illustrates an important regulatory principle: A nonequilibrium, unidirectional reaction that is conditioned to magnify the flow of metabolites in one direction is coincidently reinforced by a reciprocal effect curtailing the flow in the opposite direction. This is accomplished by the same PFK-1 effector, F2,6P_2, which inhibits the activity of fructose 1,6-diphosphatase (FDPase-1) by allosterically raising its K_m for the substrate F1,6P_2. In this way, not only is efficient glycolysis secured, but the waste of ATP by cycling between F1,6P_2 and F6P is kept to a minimum. The potential for such "futile" cycling is not fortuitous; its existence provides a mechanism for rapidly switching, influenced by proximate cellular effectors, into a reverse direction whenever a physiologic need for glucose production arises.

FIGURE 19-5 Regulatory steps in glycolysis stressing the nonequilibrium sites of *glucokinase* + *hexokinase* (GK + HK), *6-phosphofructo-1-kinase* (PFK-1) and *fructose 1,6-diphosphatase* (FDPase-1), and *pyruvate kinase* (PK). For the mechanisms of inhibition and activation of *PFK-1* and *FDPase-1* by the regulatory activities of *PFK-2, FDPase-2*, and fructose 2,6-diphosphate (F-2,6-P_2), see the text.

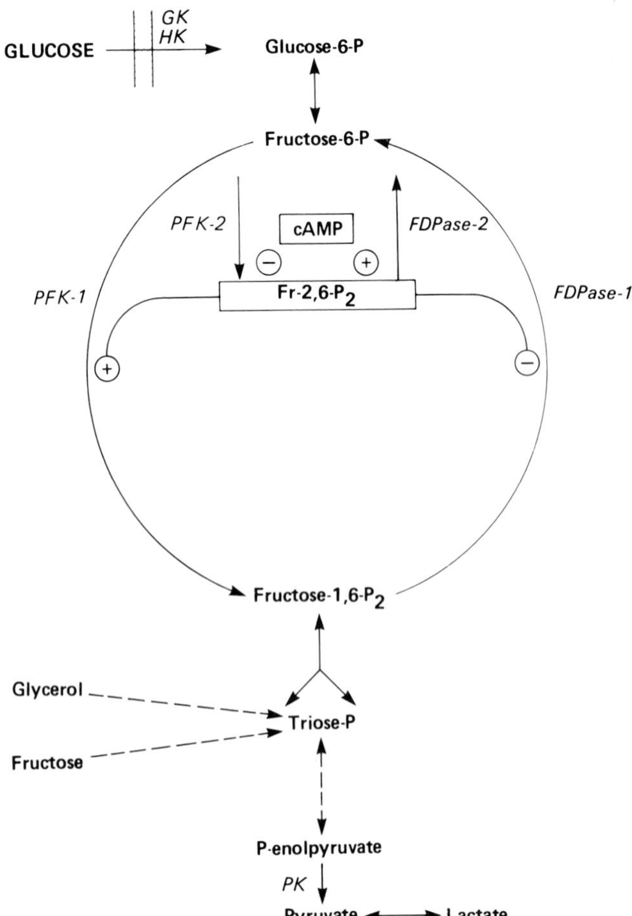

PFK-2 is a unique bifunctional enzyme acting also as FDPase-2 (fructose-2,6-bisphosphatase), which catalyzes the conversion of $F2,6P_2$ to F6P. Both activities are located on the same protein molecule, and their expression is regulated by cAMP-dependent protein phosphorylation (and modulated by F6P concentration). The phosphorylated enzyme performs as FDPase-2; the dephosphorylated enzyme performs as PFK-2. Thus, the expression and the direction of orientation of this regulatory enzyme are under control of hormones affecting the cellular cAMP content (insulin, epinephrine, and glucagon).

Pyruvate kinase is an enzyme with two mechanisms of regulatory adjustment. One form of control is rapid: alterations in activity are effected by protein phosphorylation/dephosphorylation or conformational changes[13]; the latter include both feed-forward activation by $F1,6P_2$, which accumulates during brisk glycolysis as a result of enhanced PFK-1 activity, and inhibition by alanine released from muscles on fasting. Glucagon and epinephrine inhibit pyruvate kinase via cAMP-dependent protein kinase–catalyzed phosphorylation of the enzyme.[13] The second aspect effects long-term regulation; it involves the acceleration of enzyme protein transcription. Insulin and diets rich in carbohydrate have distinct effects on this adaptive rise in enzyme level; in contrast, diabetes and starvation cause its decline. Pyruvate kinase is an enzyme with high activity, one of the highest among the 11 enzymes of glycolysis; it might thus appear to be unsuitable for the control of glycolytic flow. While its activation may be superfluous for the accommodation of the maximal rate of glycolysis dictated by glucokinase and PFK-1, it seems to be of value in the control of the glycolytic metabolism of other substrates, such as fructose, a hexose which enters the pathway below the PFK-1 step. The enzyme responsible for phosphorylation of fructose to fructose-1-phosphate, *fructokinase*, has a capacity several times higher than that of glucokinase and hexokinase combined.[14]

Control of pyruvate kinase is particularly important when a reversal of the metabolite flow toward glucose production is required (see Gluconeogenesis, below). To limit the wasteful breakdown of newly synthesized phospho*enol*pyruvate on its way to glucose, pyruvate kinase activity has to be severely restrained. cAMP-dependent phosphorylation, which is promoted by lack of insulin, and/or glucagon excess greatly reduces the enzyme's activity, as does allosteric inhibition by alanine and other amino acids when they become abundant during the need for gluconeogenesis.

The final step in glycolysis is the conversion of pyruvate to lactate by the enzyme *lactate dehydrogenase*. In this reductive reaction, NADH formed earlier in glycolysis (by the oxidation of glyceraldehyde 3-phosphate to 3-phosphoglycerate) is reconverted to NAD^+. The equilibrium of this reaction favors the formation of lactate, particularly in muscles and brain. The significance of this reaction is that it permits the continued breakdown of glucose by providing NAD^+ at this critical site, at the expense of lactate formation. The lactate formed in glycolysis diffuses freely from cells and enters the bloodstream, from which it is removed mainly by the liver.

Gluconeogenesis

Gluconeogenesis refers to the formation of glucose from noncarbohydrate sources. The principal precursor substrates from which glucose may be derived are pyruvate, lactate, glycerol, and amino acids. Most of the constituent amino acids in tissue proteins (except the "ketogenic" amino acids, leucine, isoleucine, and valine) can ultimately be converted to glucose. However, the pattern of amino acid uptake by the liver is such that alanine is the major gluconeogenic substrate released from peripheral protein reservoirs. Conversion of even-chain fatty acids (accounting for >95 percent of total fatty acid content) to glucose is not possible in the mammalian liver, because there is no mechanism for net glucose synthesis from their final 2-carbon oxidation product, acetyl CoA. A precursor for glucose must contain at least a 3-carbon chain. When odd-chain fatty acids are oxidized, the final product, propionyl CoA, may serve as a glucogenic substrate by conversion to methylmalonyl CoA and succinyl CoA. Recently, a metabolic pathway has been uncovered which can use another 3-carbon product of incomplete fatty acid oxidation, acetone, and convert it to lactate and glucose (see below).

With the exception of glycerol, each of the gluconeogenic precursors must be converted to pyruvate and/or oxaloacetate before the formation of glucose. The enzymatic steps involved in the formation of glucose from pyruvate differ from those involved in glycolysis, since they must bypass in the opposite direction the three irreversible steps of glycolysis outlined in Fig. 19-5. They involve (1) the synthesis of phospho*enol*pyruvate from pyruvate by the enzymes *pyruvate carboxylase* (PC) and *phospho-*enol*pyruvate carboxykinase* (PEPCK), (2) dephosphorylation of $F1,6P_2$ to F6P by FDPase-1, and (3) dephosphorylation of glucose 6-phosphate to glucose by *glucose 6-phosphatase* (G6Pase) (Fig. 19-6). These enzymes are unique to gluconeogenesis and are present in liver, kidney, and intestinal epithelium but not in muscle or heart. Quantitatively, the liver is the most important site of gluconeogenesis in physiologic circumstances such as fasting and exercise and in pathologic conditions such as diabetes. The kidney becomes an important gluconeogenic organ during prolonged starvation.[15]

The moment-to-moment regulation of gluconeogenesis depends on substrate availability, enzyme activity, and the hormonal milieu. In the postabsorptive state (e.g., overnight fast) and during short-term

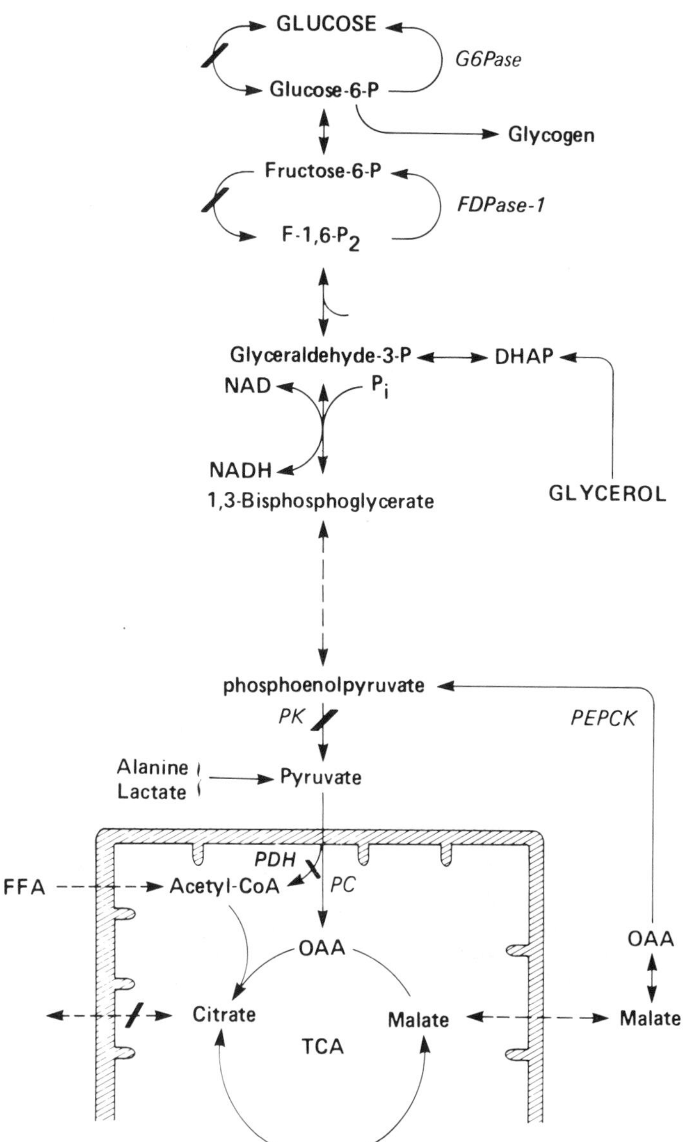

FIGURE 19-6 Regulatory steps in hepatic gluconeogenesis under the conditions of fasting and insulin deficiency. Pyruvate, mainly derived from extrahepatic lactate and alanine, enters the mitochondria to be carboxylated to oxaloacetate (OAA) by *pyruvate carboxylase* (PC) rather than converted to acetyl CoA by *pyruvate dehydrogenase* (PDH). The increased hepatic concentration of acetyl CoA, which arises from large FFA inflow, is instrumental in this change (see text). Citrate is formed from the OAA in the tricarboxylic acid cycle (TCA); however, its transport into the cytosol is reduced in this condition. By contrast, most of the OAA is exported, via malate, into the cytosol and converted to phospho*enol*pyruvate by *phospho*enol*pyruvate carboxykinase* (PEPCK) bypassing the *pyruvate kinase* (PK) reaction, which is strongly inhibited in this situation by alanine and cAMP-dependent protein phosphorylation. A further step on the route to glucose involves *phosphoglycerate kinase*. The direction of action of this enzyme is determined by the NADH/NAD$^+$ ratio, which in this situation favors glyceraldehyde 3-phosphate production because of an ample supply of NADH from increased fatty acid oxidation. Glycerol, derived from the enhanced lipolysis of adipose tissue triglycerides, joins the pathway of gluconeogenesis at this point, following phosphorylation by *glycerokinase* and oxidation to dihydroxyacetone phosphate (DHAP) by *glycerophosphate dehydrogenase*. The next regulatory points include the cleavage of F1,6P_2 by *FDPase-1* (see Fig. 19-5) and the final phosphorolysis of glucose 6-phosphate to free glucose by the microsomal *glucose 6-phosphatase* (G6Pase).

starvation, a reduction in serum insulin concentration enhances protein breakdown and amino acid mobilization, providing a supply of glucose precursors. However, as starvation continues for prolonged periods, the availability of precursor substrates becomes the rate-limiting process, as peripheral release of alanine is markedly reduced.[16]

Starvation, as well as diabetes, is characterized by massive mobilization of free fatty acids (FFA) from adipose tissue; FFA serve as a major oxidative substrate in the liver. As a consequence, the hepatic acetyl CoA concentration is markedly elevated while that of free coenzyme A is commensurately reduced. This change profoundly affects the activity of the two enzymes for which pyruvate is the substrate: *pyruvate dehydrogenase* (PDH) and PC. PDH is prevented from converting pyruvate to acetyl CoA by scarcity of CoA and is inhibited by acetyl CoA. PC is allosterically activated by acetyl CoA. Thus, pyruvate is preferentially channeled to oxaloacetate (Fig. 19-6).

These initial reactions related to gluconeogenesis occur in the mitochondria. The next step, entailing the combined decarboxylation and phosphorylation of oxaloacetate to phospho*enol*pyruvate, is carried out by PEPCK in the cytosol. Oxaloacetate does not readily cross the mitochondrial membrane; it is transported out via malate. Regulation of PEPCK activity is effected mainly by transcriptional changes in the synthesis of this enzyme, which has a rapid turnover rate.[17] Insulin deficiency in starvation or diabetes results in marked enzyme induction, whereas ingestion of a diet plentiful in carbohydrate or administration of insulin reduces the synthesis of

PEPCK. Insulin swiftly suppresses the synthesis of the enzyme protein, probably at the point of transcription initiation. The concentration of cAMP, which rises under glucagon stimulation or when glucose is in short supply, also has a strong promoting effect on PEPCK activity, not by protein kinase–mediated phosphorylation of the enzyme but by interfering with its synthesis at the mRNA level. PEPCK is also induced by glucocorticoid and thyroid hormones. These hormones also promote gluconeogenesis through their catabolic effects on tissue proteins, thus increasing the availability of gluconeogenic amino acid precursors.

Regulation of gluconeogenesis at the level of FDPase-1 is, as was noted above (see Glycolysis), influenced by the concentration of a key metabolic regulator: fructose-2,6-bisphosphate ($F2,6P_2$). In circumstances of insulin lack (starvation, diabetes) and/or glucagon or epinephrine excess, the level of $F2,6P_2$ is reduced by virtue of a phosphorylation reaction which activates FDPase-2. As a consequence of the decrease in $F2,6P_2$, the enzyme FDPase-1 is activated, facilitating the movement of carbon skeletons along the gluconeogenesis pathway toward glucose. The importance of FDPase-1 in the control of gluconeogenesis is underscored by the hypoglycemic effect of aicariboside, a potent inhibitor of FDPase-1.[18]

G6Pase controls the last step before glucose is released into the circulation. This enzyme is insoluble; it is linked to the endoplasmic reticulum. Its activity is determined by membrane translocation, giving it increased access to substrate within the cytosol, as well as by protein synthesis induction, abetted by insulin deficiency or glucocorticoid excess.

Integration of Glycolysis and Gluconeogenesis: The Lactate (CORI) and Alanine Cycles

While within a given tissue such as the liver the net movement of carbon atoms is in the direction of either glycolysis or gluconeogenesis, in the organism as a whole both glycolysis and gluconeogenesis generally proceed simultaneously, albeit in different tissues. Net glucogenic activity begins in the liver approximately 3 h after the ingestion of a carbohydrate-containing meal and continues as long as food is withheld. By contrast, lactate is continuously produced by the formed elements of the blood, resting muscle, and, to a much larger extent, exercising muscle. The combined activity of gluconeogenesis and glycolysis results in a cycling of carbon skeletons as glucose and lactate between liver and muscle known as the *Cori cycle* (Fig. 19-7). Glucose is released by the liver into the bloodstream and is taken up by muscle tissue. Within muscle the glucose undergoes glycolysis, and its carbon skeleton is released to the bloodstream as lactate and pyruvate.

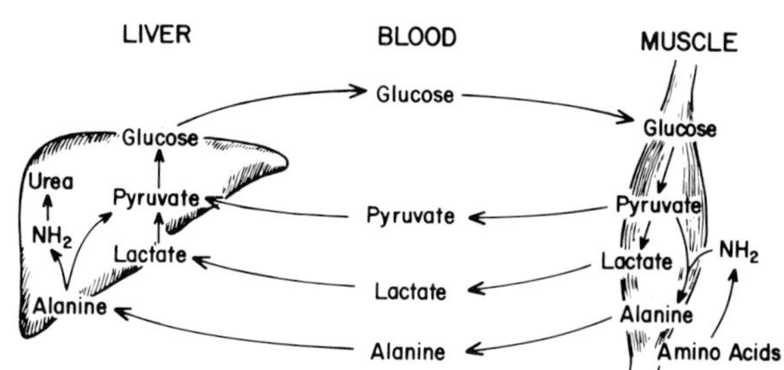

FIGURE 19-7 The lactate-glucose (Cori) and alanine-glucose cycles. In both cycles, glucose is taken up by muscle and converted to pyruvate and lactate. Some of the pyruvate undergoes transamination in muscle to form alanine. The glucose-derived lactate and alanine are released into the bloodstream and taken up by the liver, where they are reconverted to glucose.

Lactate is a means for the release of unused pyruvate, the endpoint of glycolysis, in tissues in which the oxidative capacity of the TCA cycle is lower than that of glycolysis. Alanine, which is produced by amination of pyruvate by *alanine aminotransferase*, is another end product of glycolysis released from muscles (the glucosine-alanine cycle[16] is further discussed under Amino Acid Metabolism, below). The liver extracts lactate, pyruvate, and alanine from the blood and, by the process of gluconeogenesis, reconverts those substrates to glucose and glycogen. The recycling of carbon skeletons between lactate and glucose has been estimated to account for 20 percent of the total turnover of each of these substrates.[16]

The Cori cycle does not appear to result in the net production of new glucose, although lactate may substantially contribute to hepatic glycogen repletion even in the early postprandial state, when glucose becomes available. It does, however, provide a means by which the end products of glycolysis may reenter the anabolic pathway rather than accumulate within the bloodstream or undergo further oxidation. Furthermore, the Cori cycle permits redistribution of glycogen stores from resting to exercised muscle in the recovery period after prolonged exercise.[19]

Despite the rapid turnover of glucose via the Cori and alanine cycles, the circulating levels of lactate are normally <1 m*M*. However, lactate accumulation occurs in circumstances of increased anaerobic glycolysis whether due to physiologic (e.g., exercise) or to pathologic stimuli (e.g., cardiovascular collapse due to hypovolemia, sepsis, or cardiogenic shock). Lactate also accumulates when the Cori cycle is interfered with by substances which suppress gluconeogenesis from pyruvate, such as ethanol. The antigluconeogenic effect of ethanol derives from a marked increase in the $NADH/NAD^+$ ratio incident to the metabolism of ethanol by the enzyme alcohol dehydrogenase. As a result of excessive accumulation of NADH, conversion of lactate to pyruvate is inhibited. Furthermore, the pyruvate formed from alanine is also rapidly sequestered as lactate and becomes unavailable for gluconeogenesis. In contrast, gluconeogenesis from glycerol or fructose, both of which enter the gluconeogenic pathway at the triose phosphate level (Fig. 19-4), is not inhibited by ethanol.

The Cori cycle may also be operative within the liver itself and may account for the *indirect synthesis* of glycogen from ingested glucose via gluconeogenic intermediates. A variety of studies have indicated that glycogen formation after glucose intake is not restricted to the direct pathway by which G6P is converted to G1P, which is then added to the glycogen skeleton (Fig. 19-3). As much as 30 to 50 percent of the glycogen formed after oral glucose intake may involve initial breakdown of the glucose via glycolysis to 3-carbon fragments (lactate, pyruvate) which are then reconverted to glucose via the gluconeogenic pathway.[20] Since neither peripheral (muscle) release nor intestinal release of lactate, pyruvate, and alanine is significantly increased by glucose ingestion, the liver itself may be the source of these gluconeogenic intermediates. Metabolic zonation may exist within the liver such that some of the ingested glucose is converted to lactate in the perivenous region and reconverted to glucose in periportal hepatocytes.[20,21]

Gluconeogenesis is not the sole metabolic fate of lactate released into the bloodstream. Within the liver and, to a much larger extent, the heart and kidneys, lactate undergoes oxidation to CO_2; it is also a good substrate for fatty acid synthesis in the liver.

Tricarboxylic Acid Cycle

The enzymatic process by which aerobic tissues utilize oxygen and produce CO_2 (i.e., undergo cellular respiration) is the TCA or Krebs cycle (Fig. 19-8). This sequence of metabolic conversions represents the final common pathway of aerobic oxidation and CO_2 formation for all substrates, carbohydrates, fatty acids, and amino acids. The enzymes catalyzing the TCA cycle are located within the mitochondria. Within those organelles they are in close association with the respiratory chain, a sequence of proteins which permits the energy liberated in the oxidation reactions of the TCA cycle products to be coupled with the formation of ATP, e.g., the process of oxidative phosphorylation. The TCA cycle thus is quantitatively the most important pathway for the generation of the energy inherent in various metabolic fuels.

The reaction linking the glycolytic pathway with the TCA cycle is the oxidative decarboxylation of pyruvate to acetate and the condensation of acetate with CoA to form acetyl CoA. This process is catalyzed by PDH. PDH is inhibited in the presence of high concentrations of ATP; in contrast, when the ATP level is reduced, the oxidation of pyruvate is accelerated. PDH activity is also regulated by phosphorylation/dephosphorylation of the enzyme protein, albeit not mediated by cAMP. Hormones affect this process, especially insulin; when insulin is abundant, the enzyme exists in a dephosphorylated, fully activated form.[22]

PDH activity is strongly influenced by the rate of FFA oxidation. Intramitochondrial elevation of acetyl CoA concentration deactivates the enzyme both by direct inhibition and by the trapping of free CoA necessary for enzyme function. In the liver this situation results in redirection of pyruvate flow back to glucose via PEPCK (Fig. 19-6), whereas in muscles it interferes with glucose oxidation (see The Glucose–Fatty Acid Cycle, below). An inhibitory effect of leucine (an amino acid catabolized to acetyl CoA) on glucose oxidation in muscle tissue has also been attributed to inhibition of PDH.

Acetyl CoA is the final carbon product of all metabolic fuels entering terminal oxidation in the TCA cycle. The cyclic nature of this pathway derives from the fact that the substrate combining with acetyl CoA in the first reaction of the cycle—oxaloacetate—is reconstituted in the final reaction. The product of this initial reaction is citrate, a tricarboxylic acid (hence the terms TCA and citric acid cycle).

The overall activity of the TCA cycle is determined by the availability of ATP and substrate, enzyme activities, and hormonal milieu. These controlling influences are largely interdependent. For example, when insulin levels are low and the gluconeogenic pathway is markedly activated, oxaloacetate may be increasingly siphoned to PEP so as to limit the activity of the TCA cycle.

The major determinant of TCA cycle enzyme activity is the relative concentrations of ATP, ADP, and AMP, which change according to general energy requirements and determine the respiratory chain activity; this in turn dictates the rate of TCA cycling. Fine regulation of the enzymes is dependent on relations among the intramitochondrial intermediates and various nucleotides. In circumstances of decreased ATP availability and increased levels of ADP, the activities of both *citrate synthase*, which catalyzes the condensation of acetyl CoA and oxaloacetate, and *isocitrate dehydrogenase* are increased. In contrast, these enzymes are inhibited when ATP levels are high and ADP levels are low. In this manner, the consumption of ATP by muscular contraction accelerates glucose oxidation, whereas in the resting state glucose oxidation by muscle is virtually nil.

Other Pathways of Glucose Metabolism

A number of alternative pathways of glucose metabolism exist; the activity of some is largely determined by the concentration of circulating glucose. These pathways include enzymes with a high K_m for glucose which are not insulin-dependent; their share

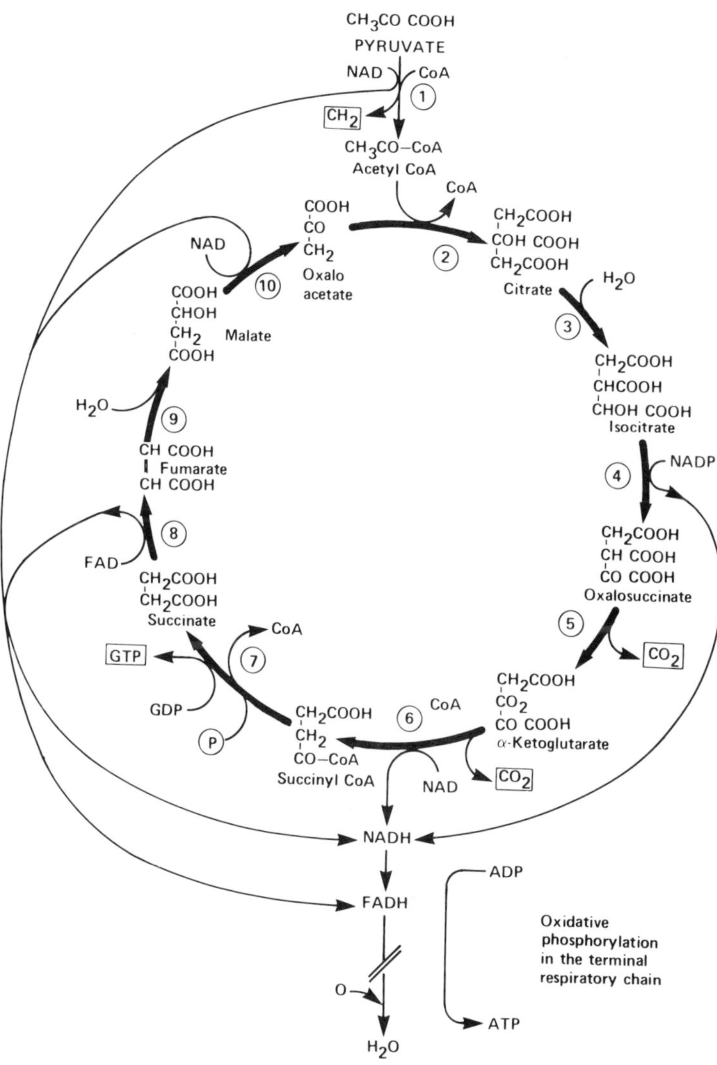

FIGURE 19-8 Enzymatic steps within the tricarboxylic acid cycle leading to the formation of NADH and FADH, which are oxidized along the tightly linked respiratory chain, coupled to phosphorylation of ADP. For each atom of oxygen consumed in oxidation of NADH, 3 mol of ATP is obtained. Oxidation of FADH results in 2 mol of ATP, since it starts at a second phosphorylation site. Overall, one turn of the cycle oxidizing a pyruvate molecule produces 15 high-energy phosphate bonds, whereas glycolysis to pyruvate results in net production of 2 mol ATP altogether.

$$CH_3COCOOH + \frac{1}{2}O_2 + 15P_i + 14ADP + GDP \rightarrow 3CO_2 + 2H_2O + 14ATP + GTP$$

Enzymes involved are (1) pyruvate dehydrogenase, (2) citrate synthase, (3) aconitase, (4,5) isocitrate dehydrogenase, (6) α-ketoglutarate dehydrogenase, (7) succinate thiokinase, (8) succinate dehydrogenase, (9) fumarase, (10) malate dehydrogenase.

in glucose metabolism may rise from <3 percent at normal glucose concentration to >15 percent in the presence of marked hyperglycemia and insulin deficiency (as occurs in uncontrolled diabetes).

Pentose Shunt

G6P, in addition to undergoing glycolysis and aerobic oxidation via the TCA cycle, may be metabolized via the *pentose shunt* pathway, in which it is oxidized by the $NADP^+$-dependent enzyme *glucose-6-phosphate dehydrogenase*, resulting in the formation of 6-phosphogluconate. The latter may then be converted via a sequence of intermediate reactions to the pentoses ribulose, ribose, and xylulose. The major purposes of this pathway are the formation of pentoses required for nucleic acid synthesis and the generation of reducing equivalents in the form of NADPH, which are necessary in the reductive synthesis of fatty acids and sterols. Consequently, the pentose pathway is of some importance in the metabolism of glucose both in liver, the major site of fatty acid biosynthesis in humans, especially in circumstances of glucose abundance when active lipogenesis proceeds, and adrenal tissue and testis (sites of sterol biosynthesis). In contrast, virtually no pentose pathway activity is demonstrable in muscle.

Polyol Pathway

Glucose may be converted to the polyhydroxy alcohol *sorbitol* by the enzyme *aldose reductase* (Fig. 19-9). Aldose reductase is present in most mammalian tissues, including some highly specialized ones that are prone to lesions in diabetes, such as nerves, lens, retina, and vascular endothelium.[23] Aldose reductase is relatively nonspecific, capable of converting several aldohexoses to their respective alcohols; this explains the general term *polyol pathway*. Sorbitol generally traverses cellular membranes poorly and tends to accumulate within the cells unless it is converted by *sorbitol dehydrogenase* to more readily passable fructose. The cellular retention of sorbitol is therefore dependent to a large extent on the relative

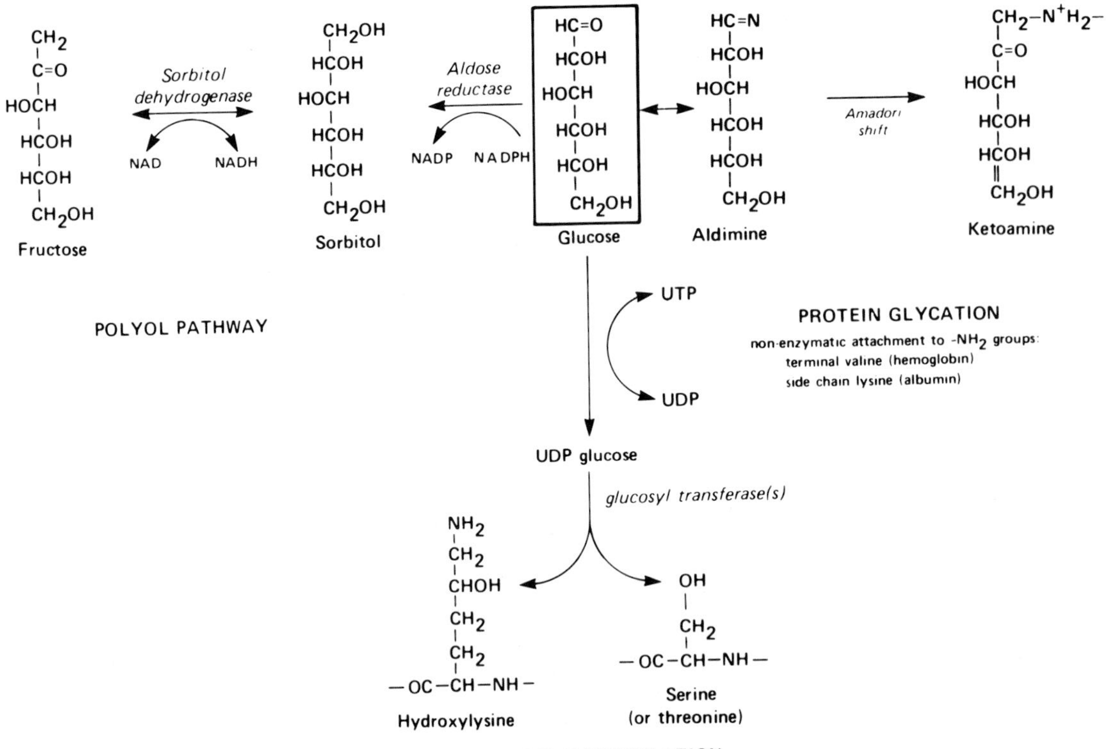

FIGURE 19-9 Glucose, especially at higher than normal concentrations, may enter several pathways apparently associated with deterioration of the function of the affected cell types or proteins.
Polyol pathway: NADP$^+$-dependent *aldose reductase* reduces aldohexoses to the corresponding polyhydroxy alcohols. The alcohols are trapped within the cells unless converted to freely diffusible fructose by a *polyol dehydrogenase*.
Protein glycation: In a two-stage mechanism, glucose reacts with exposed amino groups on proteins, resulting in conversion into ketohexoses, covalently attached for the life span of the protein molecule. This process occurs nonenzymatically.
Protein glycosylation: Glucose alone or together with other hexoses may be increasingly linked to the hydroxyl groups within a defined amino acid sequence on cellular proteins. The acceptor groups are mainly serine and threonine as well as 5-hydroxylysine, which is present mainly in collagen; the last arises as a result of posttranslational hydroxylation. Glycosylation involves prior formation of UDP-glucose from UTP and glucose 1-phosphate by a pyrophosphorylase reaction followed by the transfer of the glucose residue to the hydroxyl acceptor by a transferase.

activities of aldose reductase and sorbitol dehydrogenase. Increased accumulation of sorbitol is observed in Schwann cells and axons from diabetic patients and is accompanied by reduced levels of *myoinositol*.[23] The suggested mechanism of damage in cells accumulating sorbitol is inhibition of Na^+, K^+-ATPase activity probably linked to reduced uptake of *myoinositol*, a cyclic hexanol and precursor of phosphorylated cellular metabolism effectors and of membrane phospholipids, which are of importance in Schwann cells.[23] This suggestion led to attempts to prevent these complications, which are associated with protracted diabetic hyperglycemia, by the use of aldose reductase inhibitors[24,25] (see Diabetic Neuropathy, below).

Protein Glycation

The term *glycation* implies a nonenzymatic covalent bonding of glucose to the exposed amino groups in proteins, in distinction to *glycosylation*, which represents an enzymatic linkage of hexose molecules to hydroxyl groups on proteins; previously, the term *glycosylation* was widely and inaccurately used to describe nonenzymatic glucose bonding. At high concentrations, glucose forms first a reversible and unstable ketimine (Schiff base) in association with the amino group of terminal valine (in hemoglobin) or the ε-amino group of lysine (in albumin). The ketimine then undergoes a slow, spontaneous internal (Amadori) rearrangement, forming a stable covalent bond, involving a change from an aldo- to a ketohexose (Fig. 19-9).

The excessive glycation in the presence of hyperglycemia generally has a detrimental influence on the function of proteins as a result of both alterations in configuration and surface charge and susceptibility to degradation. Hemoglobin (Hb) was one of the first proteins reported to undergo glycation to glycohemoglobin (HbA_{Ic}).[26,27] Both the terminal valine on the beta chain and the intrapeptide lysines are glycated, but loss of the terminal amino group increases the electrophoretic and chromatographic mobility of Hb. The concentration of HbA_{Ic} is roughly proportional to blood glucose concentration and may be used as an indicator of therapeutic control of diabetic hyperglycemia[28,29] (see below). Albumin,[30] lipoproteins,[31,32] other plasma proteins, and cellular membranes including glomerular basement membrane proteins are also targets of glycation. Some of the covalent products of protein glycation undergo a series of chemical rearrangements involving cross-linking between or within proteins known as *advanced glycosylation end products* (AGEs).[33] Increased accumulation of AGEs has been seen in patients with diabetic nephropathy.[34]

Protein Glycosylation

Glycoproteins include a variety of proteins, including circulating plasma constituents (fibrinogen, immunoglobulins), hormones (gonadotropins), enzymes (ribonuclease B), mucous secretions, collagen, and basement membrane. The addition of hexoses or other carbohydrate components in covalent linkage with amino acids in the course of protein synthesis imparts a diversified structure and expands the capacity of the protein to perform specific functions. The attachment of various carbohydrate moieties to serine or threonine hydroxyl groups on the polypeptide chains involves initial reaction of the hexose with uridine triphosphate (UTP) to form the UDP derivative. Specific transferases then catalyze the transfer of carbohydrate to the polypeptide.

In the hyperglycemia of diabetes, excessive post-transcriptional glycosylation of proteins does occur, with presumed deleterious consequences for cell function; the glomerular basement membrane, collagen, and other cellular proteins are affected.[35,36]

The various pathways of glucose metabolism involving polyol formation, glycation, and glycosylation have been implicated in the microvascular complications—neuropathy, retinopathy, and nephropathy—which occur with long-standing diabetes[23,33,37,38] (see Pathogenesis of Diabetic Complications, below).

Fat Metabolism

Fatty acids are stored in adipose tissue and, to a lesser extent, in other cells as esters of the trihydroxy alcohol *glycerol*; hence the name triacylglycerols or, trivially, *triglycerides*. The triglycerides constitute the most important fuel depot in mammalian organisms, accounting for >80 percent of total energy stores.

Synthesis of Fatty Acids and Triglycerides

The precursor of fatty acids is acetyl CoA, which is derived mainly from glucose via pyruvate by the pyruvate dehydrogenase reaction (see above). Actually, the acetyl CoA formed by this reaction in the mitochondria is not directly available for fatty acid synthesis, which occurs in the cytosol; it has to be transferred out via citrate. Citrate is synthesized by condensation of acetyl CoA with oxaloacetate and transported into the cytosol, where it is cleaved to acetyl CoA by the enzyme *ATP-citrate lyase* (Fig. 19-10). Citrate, which becomes abundant in liver cells during the period of carbohydrate alimentation,

FIGURE 19-10 Hepatic fatty acid synthesis. The starting substrate for fatty acid synthesis is citrate, which is produced copiously in mitochondria from acetyl CoA and oxaloacetate whenever the rate of glycolysis after a carbohydrate-rich meal exceeds the energy requirements met by the TCA cycle. Citrate is actively transported out into the cytosol by a membrane transporter and cleaved by an insulin-induced enzyme, *ATP-citrate lyase* (CL). *Acetyl CoA carboxylase* (ACC) converts acetyl CoA to malonyl CoA by a rate-limiting process involving "fixation" of aqueous CO_2. The fatty acid chain is synthesized by a repetitive cyclic process catalyzed by several enzymes aggregated on an acyl-binding protein; it is termed *"fatty acid synthase"* (FAS). This "enzyme" is also insulin-dependent. Each cycle results in elongation by two carbon atoms. Reducing equivalents, particularly NADPH, are provided by the $NADP^+$-malate dehydrogenase and pentose shunt pathways. Fatty acid synthesis usually stops at 16 (14 to 18) carbon atoms; the fatty acyl CoA moieties are linked with glycerol 3-phosphate by an esterification system located on the endoplasmic reticulum, converted to triglycerides (or phospholipids), and transferred into the Golgi apparatus for secretion in plasma lipoproteins. Malonyl CoA exerts a feed-foward effect by preventing the entry of long-chain fatty acyl CoA into the mitochondria by inhibiting *carnitine acyltransferase* (CAT). Accumulation of long-chain fatty acyl CoA may have a feedback effect by inactivating ACC.

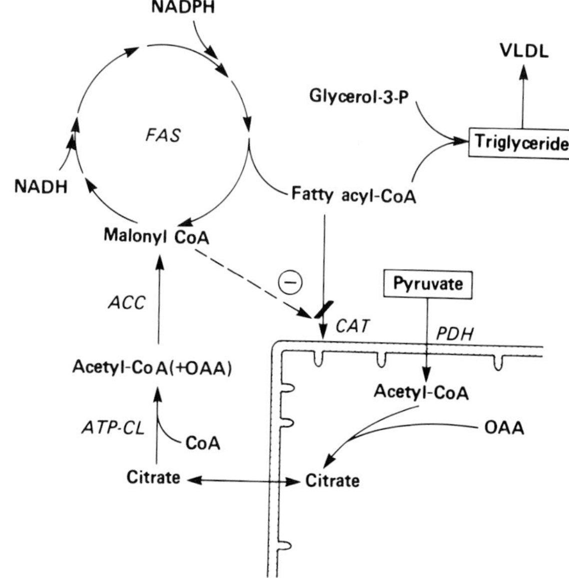

is not only the initial substrate but also an important effector of lipogenesis.

The first committed step in the pathway of fatty acid synthesis in the cytosol is the carboxylation of acetyl CoA to form *malonyl CoA*. The catalysis of this reaction, by *acetyl CoA carboxylase*, is the rate-limiting step in fat biosynthesis.[39] The enzyme requires biotin as a cofactor. The short-term regulation of its activity is effected by citrate (which promotes conversion of inactive monomers to the active tetrameric enzyme), by cAMP-dependent phosphorylation (which reduces activity), and by the end products of fatty acid synthesis, the long-chain fatty acyl derivatives (which may inactivate the enzyme). Long-term regulation of acetyl CoA carboxylase is dependent on insulin-modulated synthesis of the enzyme protein. Thus, the levels of the enzyme are decreased in starvation and diabetes and are increased during refeeding. Malonyl CoA, the product of acetyl CoA carboxylation, is in turn a potent inhibitor of fatty acid oxidation and ketogenesis.[40,41] By binding to regulatory sites, malonyl CoA is a potent inhibitor of carnitine palmitoyl transferase I (CPT-I), which is present on the outer membrane of mitochondria and facilitates the entry of long-chain fatty acyl CoA into the mitochondria.[42] In this manner a futile cycle, by which fatty acid synthesis and oxidation are simultaneously stimulated, is avoided.

For storage as fat droplets in cells and transport out of liver cells in lipoproteins, fatty acids must be esterified with *glycerol 3-phosphate* to form triglycerides. Glycerol 3-phosphate may be generated by the glycolytic breakdown of glucose to *dihydroxyacetone phosphate*, which can then undergo reduction in the presence of NADH. Alternatively, glycerol 3-phosphate may be formed from free glycerol (liberated in the breakdown of triglycerides) by the enzyme *glycerol kinase* (ATP). This enzyme is present in liver but is virtually absent in adipose tissue. Consequently, triglyceride formation and storage in adipose tissue require not only the availability of fatty acyl CoA esters (present in situ or derived from circulating lipoproteins) but also the uptake of glucose and its metabolism via the glycolytic pathway so as to generate glycerol 3-phosphate.

The enzymes required for fat synthesis are present in a variety of tissues, notably liver. In contrast to many other mammals, in humans adipose tissue exhibits low rates of glucose incorporation into fatty acids.[43] De novo lipogenesis in humans occurs largely in the liver, from which lipids are secreted as triglycerides in very low density lipoproteins (VLDL). VLDL transport triglycerides to adipose tissue; there, the insulin-dependent enzyme *lipoprotein lipase*, which is localized to the endothelium, catalyzes the hydrolysis of triglycerides to glycerol and FFA, which then enter the cell. The reesterification reaction within the adipose cells occurs between glucose-derived glycerol 3-phosphate and lipoprotein-derived fatty acids. The synthetic function of human adipose tissue is thus mainly confined to the formation of glycerol 3-phosphate (Fig. 19-11). Enzymes involved in fatty acid synthesis have been studied in fat cells. Fatty acyl CoA synthetase activity is reduced in the presence of noradrenaline, as is glycerol phosphate acyltransferase, which is responsible for catalyzing fatty acyl CoA conversion to phosphatidate. This is reversed in the presence of insulin.[44]

Mobilization of Fatty Acids

Although fat is transported for storage as VLDL-borne triglycerides, its uptake and combustion by tissues (heart, muscle, liver) require its release from depot stores as FFA, which are transported in the blood bound to plasma albumin (Fig. 19-11). The breakdown of triglycerides in adipose tissue is regulated by an intracellular tissue lipase which catalyzes the reaction

$$\text{Triglyceride} + 3H_2O \rightarrow 3\text{FFA} + \text{glycerol}$$

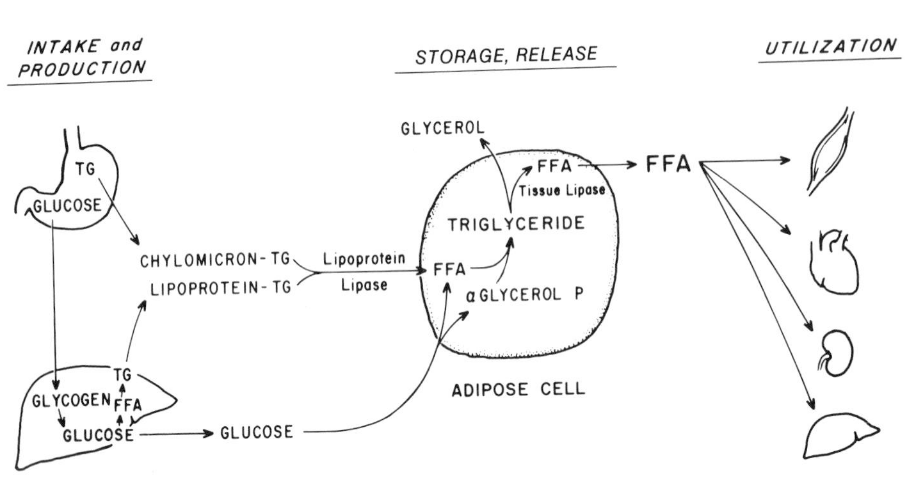

FIGURE 19-11 Fat homeostasis in humans. Fatty acids either enter the body as dietary triglyceride (TG) or are synthesized in the liver from glucose. Transport from the intestine and liver is in the form of chylomicrons and very low density lipoproteins, respectively. Uptake by the fat cell requires initially the action of endothelial lipoprotein lipase, which liberates free fatty acids (FFA). FFA enter the cell and are reesterified to triglycerides with endogenously elaborated glycerol 3-phosphate. Release from the fat cell is regulated by an intracellular hormone-sensitive tissue lipase. FFA may then be taken up by muscle, heart, kidney, liver, and other tissues.

This process, which is termed *lipolysis*, is under the regulation of a variety of hormones. The rate-limiting step is catalyzed by triacylglycerol lipase, which is regulated by insulin and other hormones potentially acting on a specific membrane carrier system.[45] Lipolysis is increased by epinephrine, glucagon, GH, adrenocorticotropic hormone (ACTH), or thyroid hormone and is reduced by insulin. Activation of triacylglycerol lipase by adrenaline, ACTH, and glucagon occurs through phosphorylation by cAMP-dependent protein kinase.[46] The relevant lipase is consequently often referred to as *hormone-sensitive lipase* (although other lipases are hormone-regulated too). In general, an increase in cAMP concentration accompanies the protein kinase–mediated activation of the lipase, while a decrease in cAMP concentration is associated with inactivation. From a physiologic viewpoint, epinephrine and, to a lesser extent, thyroid hormone are the most important activators of the hormone-sensitive lipase, while insulin is the most important inhibitor. Insulin reverses the increased phosphorylation of triacylglycerol lipase, resulting in a decreased lipolytic rate.[46,47] This corresponds to the decrease in cAMP-dependent protein kinase activity. It is unlikely that ACTH or glucagon contributes to the physiologic modulation of lipolysis; inordinately high concentrations of these hormones are required to increase lipase activity.

The net rate of FFA outflow is also influenced by glucose utilization in adipose tissue. As indicated in Fig. 19-11, triglycerides are retained by reesterification so long as an adequate supply of glycerol 3-phosphate is maintained. Since adipose tissue lacks glycerol kinase, the availability of glycerol 3-phosphate is determined by the rate of glycolysis. Consequently, in circumstances of increased glucose utilization, the outflow of FFA is reduced because of both increased substrate availability for esterification and a reduction in the activity of the hormone-sensitive lipase.

Oxidation of Fatty Acids

The process by which fatty acids are oxidized to provide high-energy phosphate in the form of ATP has been termed β *oxidation*, since it involves a series of consecutive oxidations of the β carbon to yield a β-ketoacid, which undergoes cleavage to produce acetyl CoA. In this process the fatty acid is shortened by two carbon atoms. The steps are repeated until the entire fatty acid has been oxidized to acetyl CoA, which enters the TCA cycle for oxidation to CO_2 (Fig. 19-12).

The initial step in the mitochondrial oxidation of fatty acids is their activation in the cytosol by the formation of the acyl CoA derivative. However, the long-chain fatty acyl CoA derivatives (12 or more carbons) cannot penetrate the mitochondrial membrane. Consequently, a carrier molecule, *carnitine* (γ-amino-β-hydroxybutyric acid trimethylbetaine), is required. The enzyme *carnitine palmitoyl transferase 1* (CPT-1) catalyzes the formation of the fatty acyl-carnitine derivative, which crosses the inner mitochondrial membrane. The fatty acyl group is transferred to intramitochondrial CoA by the action of the enzyme CPT-2. Free carnitine is regenerated and is thus available for the shuttling of additional fatty acyl residues into the mitochondria (Fig. 19-13). Data strongly indicate that CPT-1 is inhibited by malonyl CoA,[40,41] the first committed intermediate in the pathway of fatty acid biosynthesis (Fig. 19-10). Thus, mitochondrial β oxidation is controlled by three factors: (1) the rate of FFA supplied by fat-storing tissues (lipolysis), (2) the cytosolic concentration of malonyl CoA, and (3) the availability of carnitine. These factors are regulated in turn by insulin. An increase in insulin concentration prevents adipose tissue lipolysis, decreases carnitine availability, and promotes lipogenesis from glycolysis-derived acetyl CoA, thus increasing malonyl CoA levels and inhibiting CPT-1. Carnitine palmitoyl transferase may also be controlled by phosphorylation.[48] Furthermore, based on evidence from rat studies, it appears that CPT-1 is immunologically distinct from CPT-2 and that the activity of CPT-1 is dependent on its association with a membrane component.[49] Absence of insulin causes increased FFA mobilization, increased carnitine availability, and depression in lipogenesis, together with a decline in malonyl CoA concentration, effecting a rise in CPT-1 activity (Fig. 19-13). The latter two prerequisites for facilitation of mitochondrial entry of fatty acyl CoA are enhanced by the concomitant rise in glucagon concentration.[41] The regulatory relation between the intermediate of fatty acid biosynthesis (malonyl CoA) and fatty acid oxidation thus assures that in circumstances of anabolism (i.e., fat synthesis), there is a concomitant inhibition of catabolism (fat oxidation).

Ketogenesis and Ketone Utilization

When there is an unrestrained increase in FFA mobilization, the rate at which acetyl CoA is produced in the course of β oxidation may exceed the capacity of the TCA cycle. In such circumstances, the surplus of acetyl CoA is shifted into the production of acetoacetate, β-hydroxybutyrate, and acetone. A decline in malonyl CoA results in the increased synthesis of ketone bodies via β oxidation. Glucagon plays a pivotal role in the regulation of this pathway, among other ways by inhibiting acetyl CoA carboxylase, which catalyzes the formation of malonyl CoA. These substances are collectively termed *ketone bodies*. It should be emphasized that ketone bodies are products of incomplete fat oxidation. Only a fraction of the total ketone bodies can be used; excretion of the remainder constitutes a loss of energy. When produced in marked excess, as occurs in uncontrolled diabetes, acetoacetate and β-hydroxybutyrate cause metabolic acidosis (i.e., diabetic ketoacidosis, DKA).

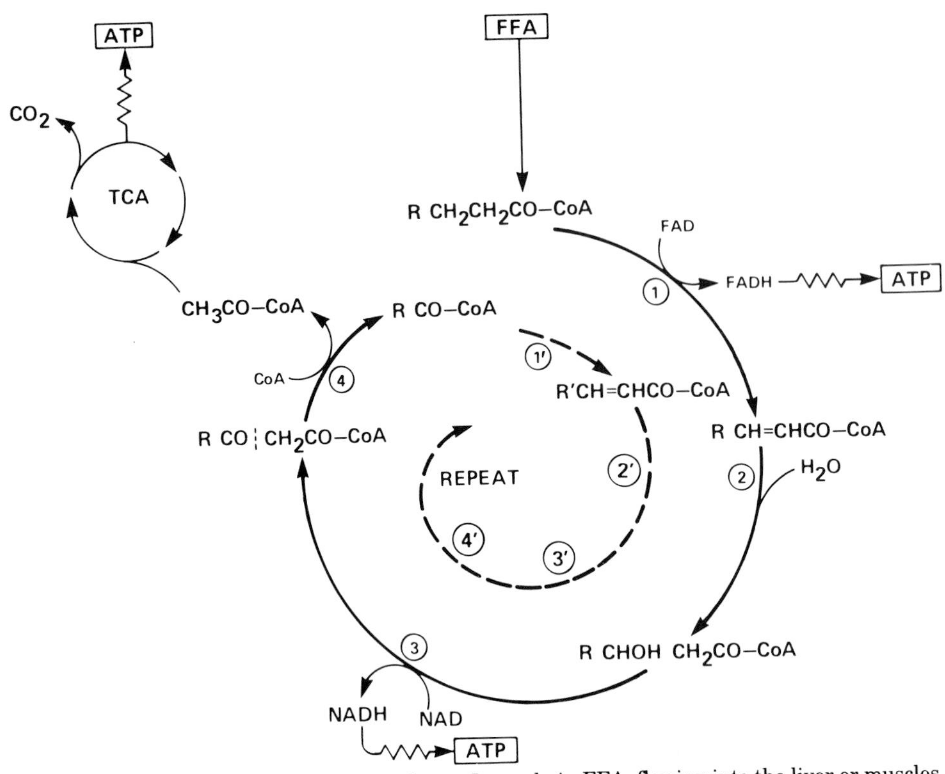

FIGURE 19-12 Fatty acid oxidation pathway. Long-chain FFA, flowing into the liver or muscles, are first acylated outside the mitochondria to form fatty acyl CoA esters by the enzyme *acyl CoA synthase* (thiokinase):

$$RCH_2CH_2COOH + ATP + CoA \rightarrow RCH_2CH_2COCoA + AMP + PP_i$$

Short-chain FFA (≤10 carbons) are acylated within the mitochondria. The fatty acid chain is rapidly shortened by two carbons in a four-step cycle by an enzyme complex collectively termed *"fatty acid oxidase"*: (1) desaturation by FAD^+-dependent acyl CoA dehydrogenase, (2) hydration by Δ^2-enoyl CoA hydratase, (3) dehydration by NADH-dependent β-hydroxyacyl CoA dehydrogenase, (4) cleavage by β-ketothiolase. The acetyl CoA produced is oxidized in the TCA cycle, whereas the shortened FFA goes through repeated deacylation cycles. Each turn of the cycle, tightly associated with the terminal respiratory chain, generates 5 ATP (2 from FADH and 3 from NADH); the oxidation of acetyl CoA in the TCA cycle yields 12 more ATP bonds.

The large quantities of acetone present in various forms of ketosis do not contribute to the metabolic acidosis but impart a characteristic fruity odor to the patient's breath.

The initial step in the formation of ketone bodies from acetyl CoA (Fig. 19-14) involves condensation of two molecules of acetyl CoA to form acetoacetyl CoA. The conversion of acetoacetyl CoA to acetoacetate requires conversion to β-hydroxy-β-methylglutaryl CoA, which is then cleaved to acetoacetate and acetyl CoA. Formation of β-hydroxybutyrate from acetoacetate involves a reversible oxidation-reduction employing NADH as the cofactor. Acetone is produced from acetoacetate by a nonenzymatic spontaneous decarboxylation.

Neither the esterification of FFA (for triglyceride formation) nor the rate of acetyl CoA oxidation via the TCA cycle is necessarily inhibited in a ketogenic liver. In fact, the hepatic triglyceride formation may be enhanced together with ketone production if FFA delivery is massive. As a consequence, a fatty, triglyceride-laden liver and an elevation of circulating VLDL concentrations are common findings in patients with poorly regulated diabetes. By contrast, synthesis of fatty acids from acetyl CoA is strongly inhibited in the ketogenic liver.

The acetoacetate and β-hydroxybutyrate produced in the liver enter the bloodstream and circulate in a ratio of approximately 1:3. The circulating ketones are oxidized by extrahepatic tissues and, in circumstances of prolonged starvation, are taken up and oxidized by the brain.[43] The first step in the pathway of ketone utilization involves oxidation of β-hydroxybutyrate to acetoacetate. Acetoacetyl CoA is then formed by a transferase-catalyzed reaction with succinyl CoA (Fig. 19-15). The enzymes re-

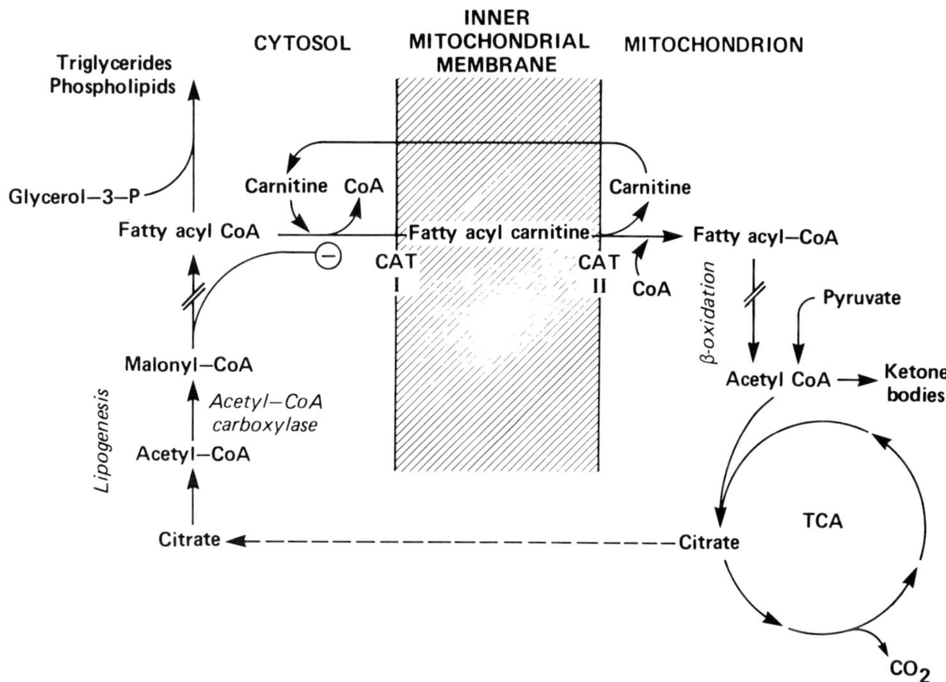

FIGURE 19-13 Fatty acid transport into mitochondria. The controlling step is the rate of transfer of fatty acyl CoA derivatives across the mitochondrial membrane, as determined by the activity of the transporter system composed of carnitine and carnitine palmitoyltransferases (CPT) 1 and 2. Carnitine, β-hydroxy-α-timethyl-ammonium butyrate, is synthesized in the liver but widely distributed among tissues, particularly muscles. Transfer of long-chain fatty acyl CoA is activated by an increased availability of free carnitine and a fall in the level of malonyl CoA, the latter reflecting reduced lipogenesis. CPT-1 on the outer side of the membrane, allows penetration by cleaving the CoA bond and forming an acylcarnitine complex. The activity of CPT-1 is thought to be modulated by competitive binding of fatty acyl CoA and malonyl CoA to the regulatory site of the enzyme. CPT-2, on the inner side, catalyzes the interaction of acylcarnitine with mitochondrial CoA. Fatty acyl CoA is re-formed, and the liberated free carnitine is transported in the opposite direction in synchrony with acylcarnitine. Activation of short-chain FFA (≤10 carbon atoms) occurs within the mitochondria independently of carnitine.

quired for these reactions are present in muscle, brain, and fetal liver but not in adult liver. In starvation, the utilization of ketone bodies by extrahepatic tissues appears to be proportional to the ketone body concentration in the blood; their utilization, in addition to glucose or FFA, contributes to fuel economy. Saturation occurs at ~70 mg/dl, at which level the ketones are mostly excreted in urine or exhaled.

Pathways for the metabolism of acetone have been outlined. Acetone may be converted to acetate and acetyl CoA[43a] and may also serve as a substrate for the synthesis of nonnegligible amounts of glucose in nondiabetic starving animals[50,51] or humans.[52] This pathway operates by conversion of acetone to pyruvaldehyde (methylglyoxal) in the liver or 1,2-propanediol in extrahepatic tissues (Fig. 19-15).

Interactions of Fat and Carbohydrate Medium

The convergence of pathways of fat and carbohydrate metabolism via a shared intermediate (acetyl CoA) and the effects of intermediates derived from one process on enzymatic reactions in other pathways result in a variety of regulatory relations between fat and carbohydrate metabolism. These relations are best illustrated by the effects of augmented carbohydrate utilization on fat metabolism and the effects of augmented fat utilization on carbohydrate metabolism. These interactions are summarized in Table 19-3.

When the supply of carbohydrate is increased (e.g., after a carbohydrate-containing meal) and glucose utilization is stimulated, changes are observed in fat metabolism with respect to lipolysis, ketogenesis, and lipogenesis. The increase in glucose uptake decreases FFA release from adipose tissue by enhancing the availability of glycerol 3-phosphate for FFA reesterification. In addition, the rise in circulating glucose concentration stimulates the secretion of insulin, which in turn suppresses the hormone-sensitive lipase in adipose tissue. Thus, the antilipolytic action of carbohydrate is both substrate- and hormone-mediated.

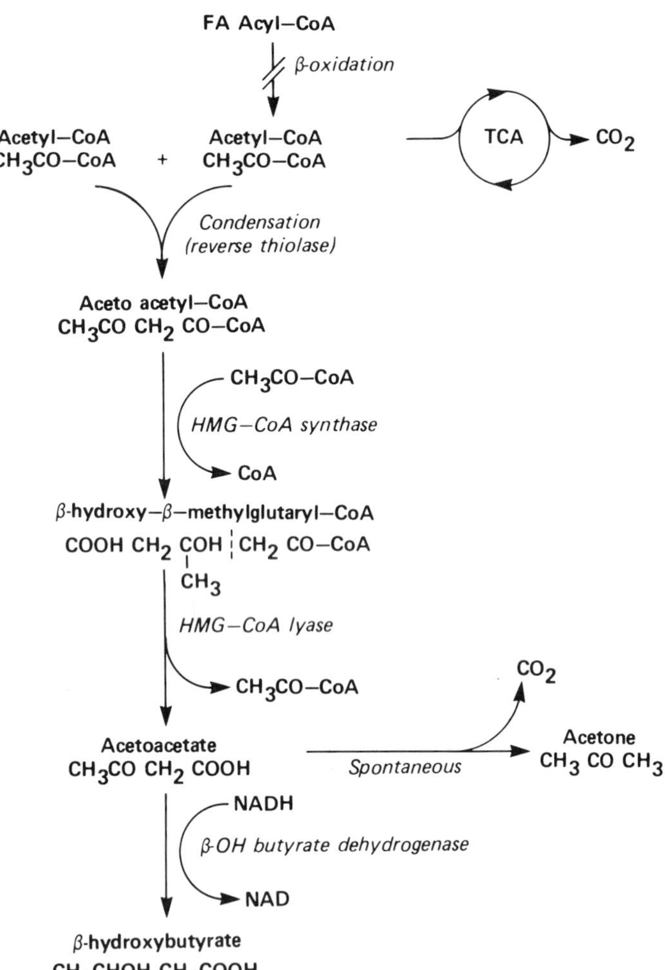

FIGURE 19-14 Ketogenesis pathway. In the presence of large amounts of acetyl CoA derived from excessive FFA oxidation, condensation into acetoacetyl CoA takes place in liver mitochondria. Earlier it was thought that during enhanced ketogenesis acetoacetate may be directly formed by deacylation of acetoacetyl CoA, an intermediate in the last stage of β oxidation. It is known today that the main pathway requires an additional condensation with acetyl CoA to form β-hydroxy-β-methylglutaryl CoA (HMG-CoA) catalyzed by *HMG-CoA synthase*. Acetoacetate is formed and released from the mitochondria after cleavage of HMG-CoA by *HMG-CoA lyase*, which also results in the recovery of acetyl CoA. Acetoacetate may be converted to β-hydroxybutyrate, which is quantitatively the predominant ketone body in the circulation, or decarboxylated to acetone. Neither of the above reactions is rate-limiting; FFA supply is the major determinant of ketogenesis.

The utilization of carbohydrate also promotes the net synthesis of long-chain fatty acids. The rate-limiting enzyme in fat biosynthesis, acetyl CoA carboxylase, is induced by carbohydrate feeding. This effect is mediated by hormonal changes (increased insulin concentration) as well as substrate-induced changes; the latter include augmented availability of citrate, which is an activator of the enzyme, and reduction in fatty acyl CoA esters, which inactivate the enzyme. The utilization of glucose along the pentose pathway also supplements the NADPH necessary for brisk fat biosynthesis.

Ketogenesis is also markedly inhibited by carbohydrate utilization. This effect is mediated via the inhibition of lipolysis, which decreases the supply of FFA for oxidation by the liver. As noted above, fatty acid oxidation is influenced not only by the rate of lipolysis but also by the activity of the enzyme CPT-1, which in turn is influenced by the availability of carnitine and malonyl CoA. Thus, augmented rates of ketogenesis in diabetes or starvation are a consequence of substrate delivery (lipolysis) as well as augmented intrahepatic fatty acid oxidation. The hormonal changes accompanying carbohydrate utilization (increased insulin and reduced glucagon concentrations) also reduce the availability of free carnitine necessary for the transport of fatty acid derivatives across the mitochondrial membrane.

When fat utilization is increased, as occurs with restriction of dietary carbohydrate intake, total starvation, and diabetes, changes in glucose production as well as utilization are observed. An increase in gluconeogenesis generally accompanies augmented fat utilization and ketogenesis. The mechanism by which fat oxidation stimulates gluconeogenesis is based in large measure on inverse modulation enzymes: activation of PC and inhibition of PDH. This causes the oxaloacetate to flow to phospho*enol*pyruvate (as the gluconeogenic intermediate) in the cytosol (Fig. 19-6). Thus, while fatty acids cannot generally provide carbon skeletons for glucose synthesis, their oxidation enhances gluconeogenesis through the regulation of enzyme activity.

Increases in fat oxidation are accompanied by inhibition of lipogenesis from acetyl CoA. Acetyl CoA carboxylase synthesis is reduced in the insulin-defi-

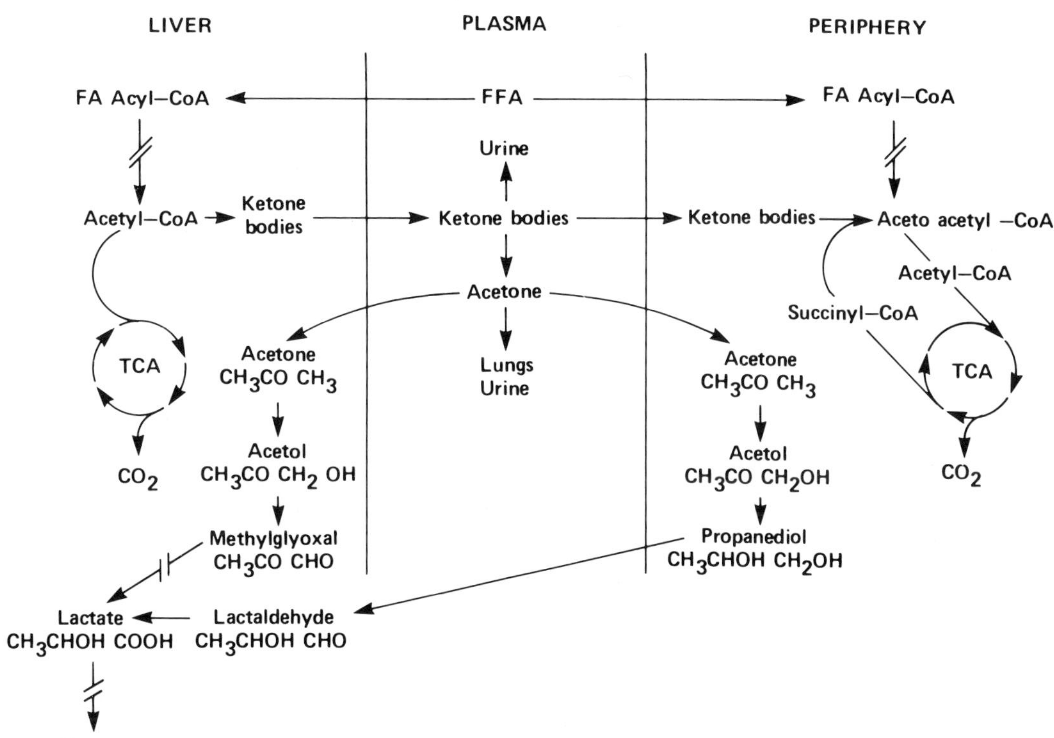

FIGURE 19-15 Distribution and utilization of ketone bodies. Ketone bodies are released from the liver into plasma. In uncontrolled diabetes large amounts may be excreted in urine. The volatile acetone may also be exhaled. In prolonged fasting, when ketone production is not excessive and glucose is scarce, there is an adaptation for ketone utilization in extrahepatic tissues. Acetoacetate is converted to acetoacetyl CoA in the mitochondria by a CoA transferase reaction using TCA cycle-derived succinyl CoA as a CoA donor. Direct acylation of acetoacetate by a thiokinase reaction is thought to be minimal. Acetoacetyl CoA is then cleaved into two acetyl CoA molecules by the action of *thiolase* and is catabolized in the TCA cycle. A fraction of acetone may be used for gluconeogenesis after conversion to 1-hydroxy-2-propanone (acetol) by the mitochondrial *NADPH-acetone monoxygenase*, an enzyme probably related to the respiratory chain. The activity of this enzyme was found to be elevated in fasting rats. Acetol is converted to pyruraldehyde (methylglyoxal) in the liver by NADPH-alcohol dehydrogenase and to lactate by a mechanism that is not well defined. In peripheral tissues 1-hydroxy-2-propanone is converted to 1,2-propanediol and then to lactaldehyde in the liver by NAD^+-aldehyde dehydrogenase.

cient hormonal milieu; this enzyme may be further inactivated by high intrahepatic levels of long-chain fatty acyl CoA.

In studies with muscles in vitro, an inhibitory effect of FFA on glucose utilization via glycolytic and aerobic pathways has been observed.[53,54] The points of inhibition of glucose utilization are the steps catalyzed by PFK and PDH. Citrate, a potential PFK inhibitor, accumulates in fat-utilizing heart muscle to levels which may affect the activity of PFK; the coincident increase in the acetyl CoA/free CoA ratio is detrimental to PDH activity. This relation has been termed by Randle and associates the *glucose–fatty acid cycle*[55]; they proposed that an elevation in circulating FFA interferes with glucose oxidation. Whether this relation applies to all muscles is unclear. For example, during exercise an *increase* in glucose utilization is observed together with a rise in FFA oxidation by the contracting muscles. Nevertheless, a reciprocal relation between fat and glucose oxidation serves to prevent superfluous glucose utilization in starvation or exercise, for the benefit of glucose-obligatory tissues (e.g., brain).

Amino Acid Metabolism

Maintenance of steady-state concentrations of circulating amino acids is dependent on the net balance between release from endogenous protein stores and utilization by various tissues. Since muscle accounts for >50 percent of the total body pool of free amino acids and the liver is the repository of the urea cycle enzymes necessary for nitrogen disposal, these two organs may be expected to play a major role in determining the circulating levels and turnover of amino acids.

TABLE 19-3 Interrelations between Fat and Carbohydrate Metabolism

Carbohydrate Utilization		Metabolic Effects and Changes in Enzyme Activity and Concentrations of Intermediates		Fat Utilization (Starvation, Diabetes)
↑		Glycolysis		↓
	↑	Phosphofructokinase-1	↓	
	↓	Fructose diphosphatase-1	↑	
	↑	$F2,6P_2$	↓	
	↑	Pyruvate kinase	↓	
	↑	Pyruvate dehydrogenase	↓	
↑		Lipogenesis and fat storage		↓
	↑	Acetyl CoA carboxylase	↓	
	↑	Hepatic citrate	↓	
	↑	VLDL production	↓	
	↑	TG esterification	↓	
	↑	Lipoprotein lipase	↓	
↓		Fat oxidation and ketogenesis		↑
	↓	Lipolysis and FFA release	↑	
	↓	Adipose tissue intracellular lipase	↑	
	↓	Carnitine acyltransferase	↑	
	↑	Malonyl CoA	↓	
	↑	Muscle glucose oxidation	↓	
↓		Gluconeogenesis		↑
	↓	Pyruvate carboxylase	↑	
	↓	Phospho*enol*pyruvate carboxykinase	↑	
	↓	Acetyl CoA and fatty acyl CoA	↑	
	↑	Free CoA	↓	

In the postabsorptive state (e.g., after a 12- to 14-h overnight fast), there is a net release of amino acids from muscle tissue (Fig. 19-16*A*). The pattern of this release is quite distinctive: The output of alanine and glutamine exceeds that of all other amino acids and accounts for >50 percent of total α-amino nitrogen release. Complementing the amino acid release from muscle tissue is the consistent uptake of amino acids across the splanchnic bed. As in the case of peripheral output, alanine and glutamine predominate in the uptake of amino acids by splanchnic tissues. In fact, there is a fairly close correspondence between the relative outputs of most amino acids from the periphery and their uptake by splanchnic tissues. Within the splanchnic bed, the liver is the site of uptake of alanine, while the large intestine is the site of utilization of glutamine. Most of the amino groups of the glutamine extracted by the large intestine are released as alanine or free ammonia. The major site of glutamine disposal is the kidney, where it provides nitrogen for ammoniagenesis.

The Glucose-Alanine Cycle

The primacy of alanine in the overall availability and uptake of amino acids by the liver and the rapidity with which the liver converts alanine to glucose indicate the importance of alanine as the key protein-derived glucose precursor. The predominance of alanine in the outflow of amino acids from muscle cannot be explained on the basis of its availability in constituent cellular proteins, since no more than 7 to 10 percent of the amino acid residues in muscle proteins is alanine. This discrepancy led to the recognition that alanine is synthesized de novo in muscle tissue by transamination of pyruvate and the formulation of the *glucose-alanine cycle.*[16,56,57] By this formulation alanine is synthesized in muscle by transamination of glucose-derived pyruvate and is transported to the liver, where its carbon skeleton is reconverted to glucose (Fig. 19-7). The branched-chain amino acids (valine, leucine, isoleucine) have been suggested as the origin of the amino groups for muscle alanine synthesis inasmuch as extrahepatic tissues, particularly muscle, have been demonstrated to be the sites of oxidation of these amino acids.

Studies using [^{14}C]glucose indicate that 60 percent of the carbon skeletons of alanine residues released by muscle are derived from endogenous glucose, while virtually none of the carbon skeletons are derived from the in situ catabolism of other amino acids.[57] Quantitatively, as end products of peripheral glucose utilization as well as precursors of hepatic glucose production, carbon skeletons are recycled

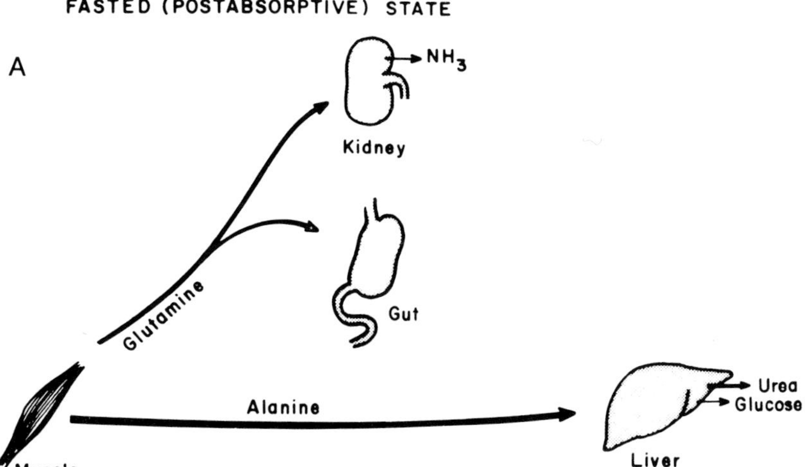

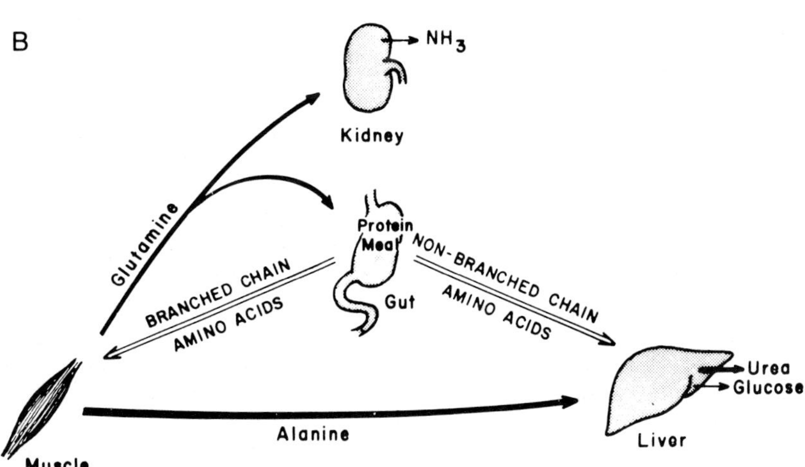

FIGURE 19-16 The effect of protein feeding on the exchange of amino acids between organs. In the fasted (postabsorptive) state there is net outflow of amino acids from muscle involving primarily alanine and glutamine (*A*). After a protein meal is eaten (*B*), the branched-chain amino acids (valine, leucine, and isoleucine) in the ingested protein are delivered to muscle tissue, where they are used for protein synthesis and as an oxidative fuel. In contrast, only a small proportion of all other amino acids are taken up by muscle; they are largely extracted by the liver, where they are converted to glucose, oxidized, or used for protein synthesis.

along the glucose-alanine cycle at a rate approximately 50 percent of that observed for the Cori (lactate) cycle.[16,57]

Although the glucose-alanine cycle does not yield new carbon skeletons for de novo glucose synthesis, it is of importance in glucose homeostasis as well as nitrogen and energy metabolism. A deficiency of alanine has been implicated in the accelerated starvation observed in pregnancy,[58] ketotic hypoglycemia of infancy,[59] and hypoglycemia of maple syrup urine disease.[60] Alanine also provides a nontoxic alternative to ammonia in the transfer of amino groups, derived from the catabolism of branched-chain amino acids in muscle, to the liver. Hyperalaninemia is observed in a variety of disorders of urea cycle enzymes, where it may moderate the hyperammonemia.[16]

The glucose-alanine cycle may also be useful with respect to ATP production. Conversion of glucose to alanine provides 8 mol of ATP compared with 2 mol provided by conversion to lactate. Furthermore, to the extent that alanine formation facilitates the oxidation of the branched-chain amino acids, an additional 30 to 40 mol ATP is generated per mol of amino acid oxidized.

Protein Repletion and Feeding

Since the nitrogen balance of muscle tissue in the fasting state is negative, repletion of muscle nitrogen depends on net uptake of amino acids in response to protein feeding. Ingestion of a protein meal (e.g., lean beef) is followed by a large output of amino acids, predominantly the branched-chain amino acids, from the splanchnic bed.[61] Valine, isoleucine, and leucine together account for 60 percent of the total of amino acids entering the systemic circulation, despite the fact that they contribute only 20 percent of the total amino acids in the protein meal. Simultaneous with the release of amino acids from the splanchnic bed, peripheral muscle exchange of most amino acids reverts from the net output observed in the basal state to net uptake. As in the case of splanchnic exchange, the uptake of amino acids across peripheral muscle tissue is most marked for the branched-chain amino acids.[61] Since the branched-chain amino acids constitute only 20 percent of the amino acid residues in muscle proteins, it is likely that these amino acids are not used solely for protein synthesis but are also metabolized within muscle.

These effects of protein feeding on interorgan amino acid exchange and the key role of the branched-chain amino acids are summarized in Fig. 19-16*B*. A nitrogen "shuttle" is observed in which branched-chain amino acids provide for nitrogen repletion in muscle tissue in the fed state. The nitrogen thus delivered is released as alanine and glutamine in the fed condition as well as the fasted condition. The elevation of circulating and intracellular levels of branched-chain amino acids induced by protein feeding may have importance beyond the delivery of nitrogen. The branched-chain amino acids, particularly leucine, may play a regulatory role in stimulating protein synthesis.[62] Furthermore, the overall uptake of branched-chain amino acids by muscle is regulated by insulin and is impaired in diabetic individuals.[61]

Insulin

History

Von Mering and Minkowski in 1889 showed that removal of the pancreas of dogs can cause serious disturbances of glucose metabolism, with elevation of the blood glucose concentration and the clinical picture of diabetes mellitus. The assumption that this effect is due to removal of a necessary hormone was confirmed in 1921, when Banting and Best prepared a pancreatic extract capable of lowering the blood glucose concentration. This substance, named *insulin*, was crystallized by Abel in 1926. Sanger determined the amino acid composition of insulin. However, synthesis of insulin was difficult because of an inability to direct its two component chains into proper alignment (Fig. 19-17). Nevertheless, in 1965 Katsoyannis succeeded in chemically synthesizing small amounts of insulin.

The three-dimensional structure of insulin was determined by x-ray diffraction techniques in 1969. *Proinsulin*, the larger biosynthetic precursor of insulin, was discovered by Steiner in 1967,[63] clearing the way for large-scale insulin production. In 1979, biosynthesis of insulin by bacteria was accomplished using the techniques of recombinant DNA.[64] This procedure is now employed in the commercial production of human insulin, which is increasingly used in clinical practice. Thus, insulin is the first protein hormone to be isolated, crystallized, sequenced, and synthesized; to have its precursor defined; and to be cloned.

Chemistry

The human insulin molecule consists of two polypeptide chains, designated *A* and *B*, connected by two disulfide bridges. There is in addition a disulfide bridge between the sixth and eleventh amino acid residues of the A chain (Fig. 19-17). The complete unit contains 51 amino acids and has a molecular weight of 5800 and an isoelectric pH of 5.35. By definition, 1 mg of the pure substance contains 24.0 international units (IU). The amino acid composition is constant among the various species except for residues number 4, 8, 9, and 10 of the A chain and residues 1, 2, 3, 27, 29, and 30 of the B chain. Porcine insulin differs from human insulin only in the presence of a terminal alanine rather than threonine in the B chain; there are two additional differences between bovine and human insulin, at positions 8 (alanine replaces threonine) and 10 (valine replaces isoleucine) (Fig. 19-17). According to x-ray crystallographic studies, the unit cell of crystalline porcine insulin consists of an insulin hexamer made up of thre dimers arranged around an axis on which lie two atoms of zinc; the zinc content of most crystalline preparations of insulin is 0.4 to 0.5 percent. In dilute

FIGURE 19-17 Amino acid sequence in human insulin. In porcine insulin alanine rather than threonine is the terminal amino acid in the B chain. Bovine insulin differs from human insulin in having an alanine at position 30 in the B chain, alanine (rather than a threonine) at position 8 in the A chain, and valine (rather than isoleucine) at position 10 in the A chain.

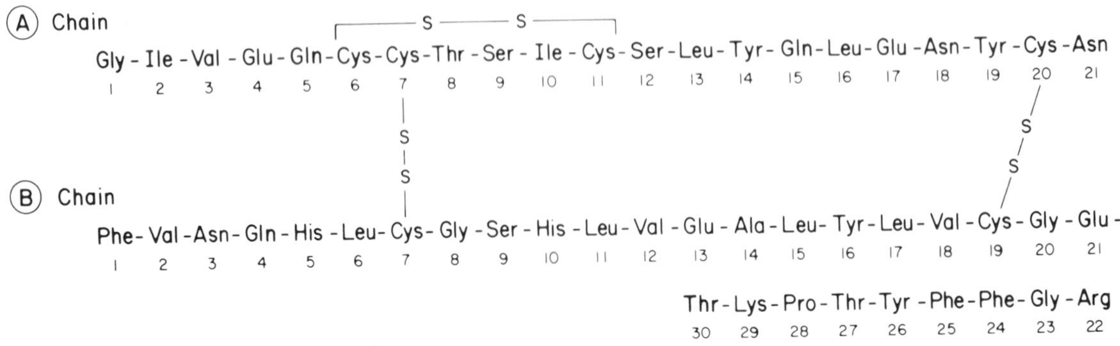

solution, insulin is adsorbed to glass or plastic [e.g., intravenous (IV) infusion sets]; adsorption can be minimized by the addition of albumin. Insulins derived from porcine and bovine pancreases were the most commonly used until biosynthetic human insulin became available.

Splitting of insulin into its constituent A and B chains by oxidation or reduction of the disulfide bridges results in complete loss of biological activity. In contrast, the activity of the insulin molecule is not appreciably affected by removal of the amide group from the asparagine on the carboxyl end of the A chain or removal of the carboxy-terminal alanine from the B chain. When the entire asparagine (or aspartate) residue is removed from the carboxyl terminal of the A chain and the alanine is removed from the analogous position on the B chain, ~95 percent of the activity is lost. Removal by trypsin digestion of eight amino acids (residues 23 through 30) from the carboxyl terminal of the B chain (deoctapeptide insulin) eliminates all detectable activity. The region between residues 22 and 26 of the B chain is considered of crucial importance in the binding of insulin to its receptor as well as in the overall action of insulin.[65]

Biosynthesis

Insulin is synthesized in the beta cells of the islets of Langerhans as a single-chain precursor, proinsulin, which has a molecular weight of ~9000.[63] Studies using cell-free systems indicate that the immediate translation product of proinsulin messenger RNA is a larger peptide of 11,500 daltons containing 23 additional amino acid residues at the amino terminal (Fig. 19-18). This precursor has been designated *preproinsulin*; it is converted to proinsulin by microsomal proteases within minutes of its synthesis. The peptide extension in preproinsulin is similar in size, partial amino acid composition, and amino-terminal location to the additional sequences found on the in vitro translation products of the mRNAs for a variety of hormones, such as proparathyroid hormone and GH, as well as nonhormonal proteins such as immunoglobulin light chains.[66]

The intracellular sites where preproinsulin is synthesized and rapidly cleaved to proinsulin are the polysomes of the rough endoplasmic reticulum (Fig. 19-18). Proinsulin is then transferred by an energy-dependent process to the Golgi apparatus. At the Golgi, packaging into smooth-surfaced microvesicles takes place so as to form storage or clathrin-coated secretory granules (Fig. 19-18). Beginning within the Golgi complex and continuing in the secretory granules, membrane-bound specific proteases cleave proinsulin into equimolar amounts of insulin and *C peptide*, the latter of which is composed of 26 to 31 amino acid residues, according to species. Cleavage involves two basic residues, and replacement of one of them with histidine results in incomplete conversion, leading to familial hyperproinsulinemia. The insulin, along with zinc, accumulates within the central core of the maturing secretory granule, which becomes progressively more electron-dense; the C peptide is localized in the peripheral clear space of the secretory granule.

In contrast to the minor differences in the amino acid sequences of A and B chains in various species, considerably greater variability is observed in the structure of the corresponding C peptides. Thus, human and porcine insulin differ by a single amino acid, whereas human C peptide, a 23-amino acid chain of 3021 daltons, differs from porcine C peptide by 10 residues and contains two fewer amino acids.[67,67a] This lack of interspecies homology is in keeping with the lack of a specific hormonal function of C peptide. Although proinsulin cross-reacts to a small degree with antibodies to insulin, it has only 3 to 7 percent of the biological effectiveness of native insulin. It is unsettled whether this small degree of biological activity is a genuine effect of proinsulin or a consequence of its conversion to insulin by target tissues. Compared with insulin, human proinsulin has been shown to have a relatively greater effect on hepatic than on peripheral glucose metabolism.

Release of the contents of the mature secretory granules involves progressive migration of the granules to the plasma membrane of the cell, followed by extrusion of insulin and C peptide. Within the cytosol of the beta cells, microtubules, 24-nm-diameter dimeric structures composed of 120,000-dalton subunits known as *tubulin*, act to guide granule movement to the plasma membrane. A series of microfilaments, 4- to 8-nm structures which are thought to be composed of the contractile protein *actin*, form a network near the plasma membrane and surround the secretory granules. The "final common path" of secretion is believed to involve the intracellular entry of calcium, resulting in contraction of the microfilaments.[68] As a result, the secretory granules are moved to the cell surface, where their membranes fuse with the plasma membrane and their contents are discharged into the extracellular space. This process of membrane fusion has been termed *emiocytosis*, a form of exocytosis.

The development of methods of chemical DNA synthesis, combined with recombinant DNA technology, has permitted the synthesis of human insulin by bacterial cells (*Escherichia coli*).[63,69] The synthetic plan involves either the reverse transcription of messenger RNA coding for proinsulin so as to obtain the complementary DNA (cDNA) for proinsulin or the chemical synthesis of smaller DNA fragments coding for the A and B chains of human insulin. The synthetic genes are then fused with a gene normally expressed in the *E. coli* host (e.g., the genes for penicillinase or β-galactosidase) so as to provide efficient transcription and translation to yield a stable precursor protein and (in the case of a periplasmic protein such as penicillinase) to facilitate transport outside the cell. The vectors used

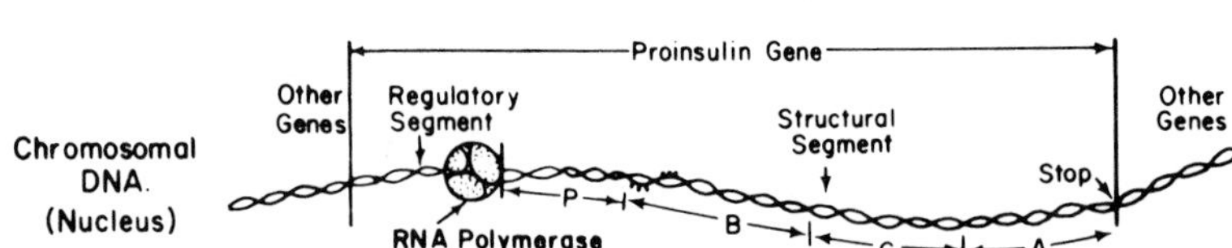

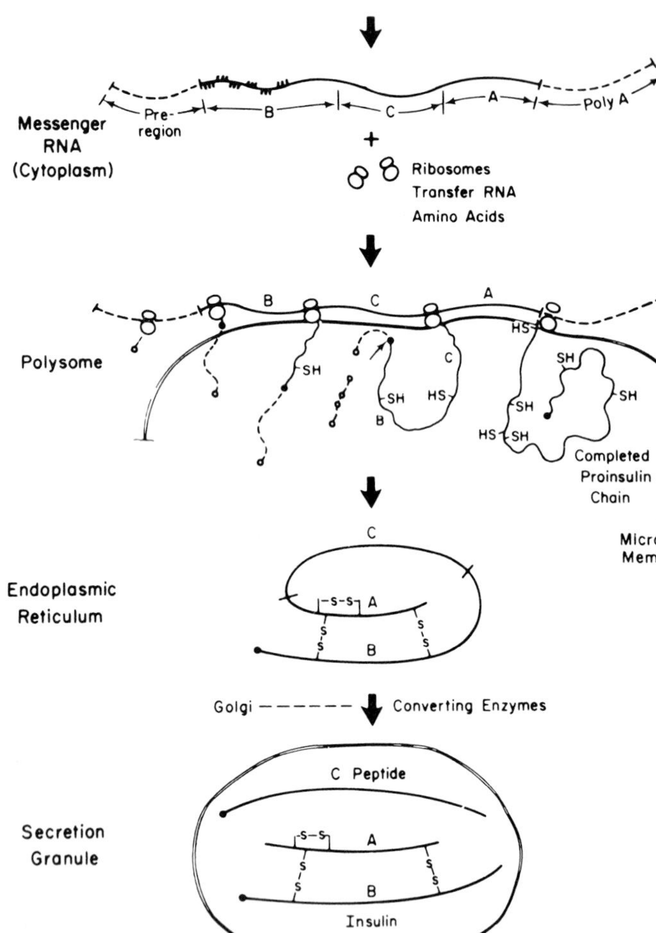

FIGURE 19-18 Schematic representation of the biosynthesis of proinsulin and its conversion to insulin and C peptide. The proinsulin gene is represented in the upper panel. These genes contain introns that are processed out in forming mature messenger RNA. The mRNA serves to guide the formation of preproinsulin chains on the polysomes. Preproinsulin, indicated as "completed proinsulin chain" on the right-hand side of the polysome band in the middle panel, is cleaved and folded into the proinsulin molecule. The single-chain proinsulin, kept in configuration with the aid of two disulfide bonds, is then transferred to the Golgi apparatus and inserted into secretory granules. During secretion, proinsulin is cleaved into two-chain, biologically active insulin by a protease specific to arginine and lysine bonds at positions 1 and 30 (Fig. 19-17). Together with insulin, there are equimolar amounts of a biologically inactive connecting peptide (C peptide) of 26 to 31 amino acids (lower panel). (*Adapted from Steiner.*[63])

for the transfer of the foreign and bacterial DNA into the bacterial cell are either bacteriophages or plasmids. The bacterium containing the plasmid transcribes its own gene as well as the inserted sequences, producing the desired polypeptide (Fig. 19-19). The fact that eukaryotic DNA sequences can be cloned and expressed in prokaryotic (bacterial) cells was successfully used in the production of human insulin, which may ultimately replace the current extraction procedures involving porcine or bovine pancreas (see below).

Insulin Secretion

Basal Concentrations

The concentration of insulin in peripheral venous or arterial plasma or serum in healthy subjects after an overnight fast is generally 10 to 20 μU/ml (0.4 to 0.8 ng/ml). As noted above, equimolar amounts of C peptide are released with insulin during the secretory process and are present in concentrations of 0.9 to 3.5 ng/ml in the fasting state. The relatively higher level of C peptide compared to insulin reflects the slower metabolic clearance of this substance.[67] Since the pancreatic islets drain into the portal vein and the liver removes 50 to 60 percent of the insulin presented to it, the portal/peripheral ratio of insulin in the basal state is 3:1. After bursts of secretion (e.g., in response to administration of glucose or amino acids), the portal/peripheral ratio of insulin may reach a value of 9:1. The higher concentration of insulin in the portal vein may in part account for the fact that small increments in insulin secretion alter hepatic glucose metabolism in the absence of changes in peripheral glucose utilization.[70]

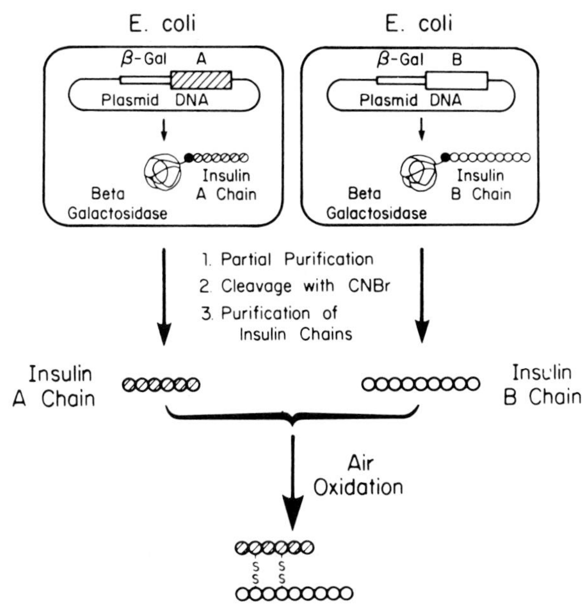

FIGURE 19-19 Schematic summary of the synthesis of the A and B chains of insulin by bacteria (*E. coli*) using recombinant DNA techniques. *(From Riggs A, Itakura K: Am J Hum Genet 31:531, 1979.)*

Although proinsulin may be found in peripheral plasma, it generally accounts for <15 percent of total circulating insulin immunoreactivity. The percentage of circulating proinsulin is decreased in the postprandial state compared to the fasting state. In *familial hyperproinsulinemia,* an asymptomatic genetic defect with autosomal dominant inheritance, 65 to 90 percent of total plasma insulin immunoreactivity is accounted for by proinsulin.[71] This defect probably represents an abnormality in an intermediate formed on cleavage of proinsulin. A mutation affecting the dibasic amino acids arginine and lysine, which link the C peptide to the A chain of insulin, impairs the conversion of proinsulin to insulin.[72] Patients with familial hyperproinsulinemia are euglycemic unless they are stressed, when they become hyperglycemic. The degree of manifest hyperinsulinemia is dependent on the cross-reactivity between the antiserum and proinsulin. Plasma levels of proinsulin are also relatively increased in patients with insulinoma (see Chap. 20), decompensated diabetes mellitus, and hypokalemia. Absolute increments in proinsulin are noted in obesity, pregnancy, growth hormone or glucocorticoid excess, and thyrotoxicosis. Elevations in proinsulin concentration in these conditions are generally proportional to those in insulin concentration.[73]

In insulin-treated diabetic patients the presence of antibodies precludes the measurement of circulating insulin concentration by conventional radioimmunoassay (RIA) techniques. In such circumstances the determination of C peptide provides a means of evaluating residual insulin secretory reserve as C peptide immunoassay does not cross-react with insulin antiserum;it does cross-react with proinsulin unless the latter has been removed previously.[67,67a] In patients with hypoglycemia and hyperinsulinemia, the measurement of C peptide concentration can indicate whether circulating insulin is of endogenous origin (high C peptide levels) or is due to surreptitious insulin administration (low C peptide levels). Plasma C peptide determinations may also be helpful in assessing the pancreatic insulin secretion capacity in young individuals suspected, on the basis of islet antibody findings, of developing type I diabetes (see below).

The insulin secretory rate necessary to maintain normal basal concentrations of insulin is in the range of 0.25 to 1.5 U/h. These basal rates of secretion are normally present in the intervals between meal ingestion; their significance is underscored by studies showing that programmed insulin infusion systems, which provide insulin in basal as well as premeal doses, are more effective in normalizing blood glucose concentrations in type I diabetes than are premeal insulin doses alone.[73]

Carbohydrate

Among the various factors capable of stimulating insulin secretion, glucose is physiologically the most important. This is reflected by the moment-to-moment fluctuations in plasma insulin concentration which accompany fluctuations in plasma glucose concentration (Fig. 19-20). The precise mechanism by which glucose acts on the beta cells to cause insulin release has not been entirely clarified. The preponderance of data indicates that glucose metabolism within the cell, rather than a signal from a membranal "glucose receptor," produces the stimulus for insulin release. Supporting this contention are the observations that (1) metabolizable sugars (hexoses or trioses) are more potent stimulators of insulin secretion than are nonmetabolizable carbohydrates (e.g., mannose), (2) glucose increases the concentration of glycolytic intermediates within islet cells, (3) compounds which inhibit glucose metabolism (mannoheptulose and 2-deoxyglucose) interfere with insulin secretion, and (4) the alpha anomer of glucose, a better substrate for glycolysis than the beta anomer, is more effective in stimulating insulin secretion. The stereospecificity resides at the level of the phosphoglucose isomerase or phosphoglucomutase reaction.[74] Glycolysis may promote insulin secretion via increases in cellular NADH and NADPH concentrations as well as H^+ concentration.[75]

In the context of a glucose metabolism initiation of insulin release, two aspects have been advocated: (1) glucokinase might function as the glucose sensor, being an enzyme that is rate-limiting for overall glycolysis at the point of entry, rate-potentiated by glucose concentration, insulin-inducible, and glucose-

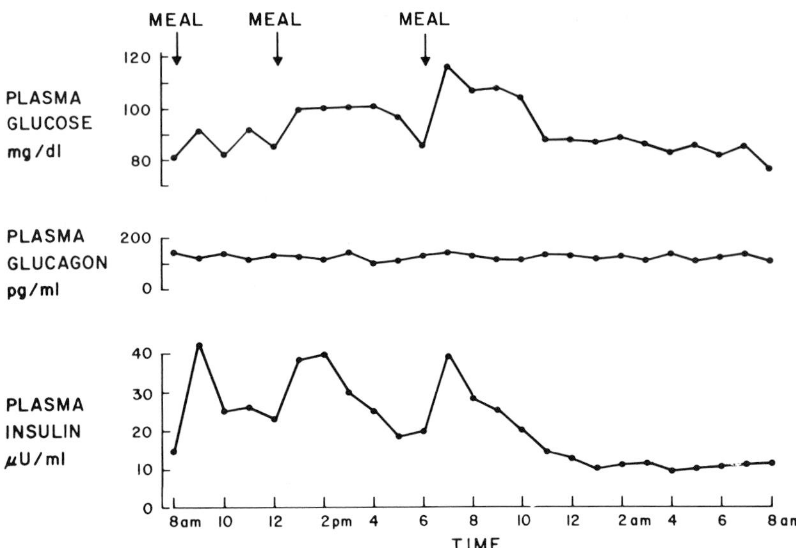

FIGURE 19-20 Fluctuations in plasma glucose, glucagon, and insulin concentrations over a 24-h period in normal healthy subjects ingesting mixed meals. The maximal excursion in plasma glucose concentration over 24 h is generally less than 30 mg/dl. The minimal degree of fluctuation of plasma glucose level is a consequence of the feedback relationship to insulin secretion and the enhancement of insulin secretion by gastrointestinal hormones in response to meal ingestion. In contrast to the changes in plasma insulin concentration, there is virtually no change in plasma glucagon level when mixed meals are fed. (*Modified from Tasaka et al: Horm Metab Res 7:205, 1975.*)

protected,[76,77] and (2) beta cell PFK-1 is highly activated by F2,6P_2 (see Fig. 19-5). A burst of the glycolytic cascade, in association with increased insulin outflow, occurs rapidly after the formation of F2,6P_2, subsequent to the extracellular availability of glucose.[78] Another hexose diphosphate, glucose, 1,6-diphosphate, formed by the action of phosphoglucomutase, also activates PFK-1 markedly, acting in concert with F2,6P_2.[78] These findings indicate that the activation of PFK-1 may represent another critical event in the regulation of the glycolytic rate in the beta cell which mediates the acceleration of insulin secretion.

As in the case of a large number of intracellular processes, cAMP participates in the insulin secretory process. cAMP is believed to act as a positive synergistic modulator of a glucose-sensitive secretory step. An increase in cAMP concentration is not of itself sufficient to stimulate insulin secretion, as indicated by the fact that theophylline (an inhibitor of phosphodiesterase) elevates cAMP concentration but has a weak stimulatory action on insulin secretion unless glucose is present.

As was noted above, an increase in intracellular calcium concentration is believed to be the final triggering mechanism by which glucose or other stimuli result in the release of insulin from beta cells. Glyceraldehyde, a weak stimulator of calcium release in vitro, was shown to increase free calcium concentrations in beta cells.[28] The increased calcium uptake appeared to be due to a decrease in potassium permeability, resulting in depolarization. These alterations in calcium concentration are a consequence of inhibition of calcium efflux by glucose and enhanced mobilization of stored intracellular calcium by cAMP. The importance of changes in intracellular calcium concentration is strongly supported by studies using ionophores, molecules that act as membrane carriers for ion transport. In the presence of A23187, a specific divalent cation ionophore which transports calcium across biological membranes, addition of calcium to beta cells results in a burst of insulin secretion in the absence of rises in glucose availability or intracellular cAMP concentration.[80]

It should also be noted that glucose, in addition to stimulating calcium entry, may under certain conditions lead to the intracellular sequestration and extrusion of calcium.[81] Therefore, high levels of glucose may paradoxically cause an inhibition of insulin release, which may be a factor in the low beta cell function noted in persons with poorly controlled type II diabetes. The role of calcium-independent mechanisms (e.g., GTP) of insulin secretion has also been investigated.[82]

The overall sequence of events leading to glucose-stimulated insulin secretion is summarized in Fig. 19-21. A characteristic kinetic feature of the insulin response to glucose is its biphasic nature (Fig. 19-22). An initial rapid secretory burst begins within 1 min of the presentation of a glycemic stimulus, reaches a peak within 2 min, and declines over the ensuing 3 to 5 min. A second phase, characterized by a more gradual increase in insulin levels, commences 5 to 10 min after the initiation of glucose infusion and continues over the next hour. In a perfused pancreas, puromycin, an inhibitor of protein synthesis, attenuates the second phase but has no effect on the early phase of insulin release. These observations have led to the concept that insulin exists within the beta cell in a two-pool system.[83] An immediately releasable pool consisting of preformed insulin is discharged rapidly during the early secretory phase. A continuing release pool that is composed of newly synthesized insulin and small amounts of proinsulin in addition to stored insulin is gradually discharged during the second phase. The

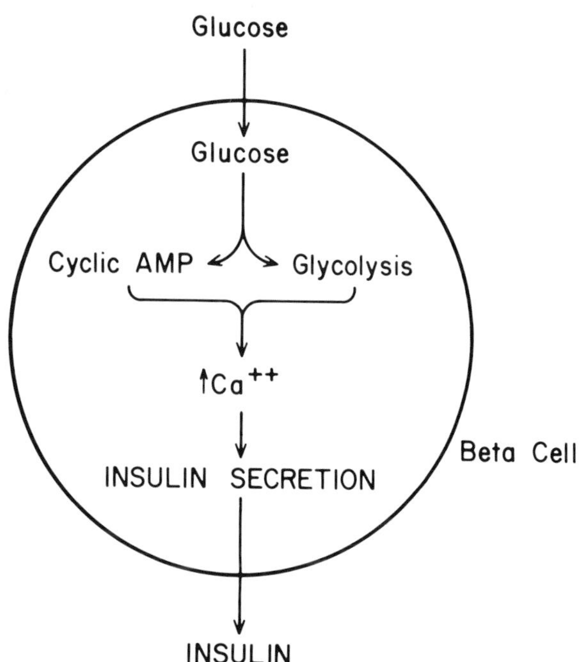

FIGURE 19-21 A simplified scheme of intracellular events underlying the stimulatory effect of glucose on insulin secretion by the beta cell. The entry of glucose into the beta cell is followed by an increase in glycolysis and a rise in cAMP concentration. These metabolic changes result in the accumulation of cytosolic calcium, rises in NADH and NADPH levels, and membrane depolarization, which are all involved in propelling the extrusion of insulin secretory granules.

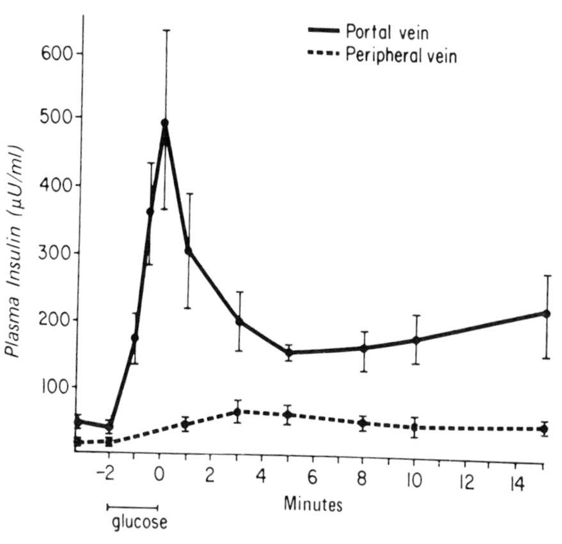

FIGURE 19-22 Plasma insulin concentrations in portal and peripheral venous blood before and after IV administration of glucose. The portal concentration of insulin is 3 times the peripheral level in the fasting state and may increase to 10 times the peripheral level immediately after glucose is infused. The changes in portal insulin concentration indicate the presence of a biphasic secretory response by the beta cell in which an acute rise in insulin release is followed by a slower, more sustained increment. *(From Blackard WG, Nelson NC: Diabetes 19:302, 1970.)*

mechanism by which glucose stimulates the synthesis of insulin is posttranscriptional; it is independent of new mRNA synthesis.[84]

Gastrointestinal Hormones

As early as 1906, Moore et al.[85] suggested that the duodenum provides "a chemical excitant for the internal secretion of the pancreas." Subsequently, La Barre demonstrated a hypoglycemic response to crude preparations of secretin and in 1926 postulated the existence of an "incretin," a factor produced by the gastrointestinal tract which stimulates the internal secretion of the pancreas. Interest in incretins was renewed with the demonstration that the plasma insulin response to an oral glucose load is two or more times greater than after an IV load despite lower or equal plasma glucose levels (Fig. 19-23).

The GI tract may influence insulin secretion via three mechanisms: (1) provision of high local nutrient concentrations upon absorption and entry into the systemic circulation, (2) release of GI hormones, and (3) emission of neurogenic signals induced by food ingestion (Fig. 19-24). The precise nature of the GI hormones which enhance glucose-stimulated insulin secretion has been the subject of extensive study.[86] To qualify as a physiologic regulator of insulin secretion, a polypeptide should meet two criteria: Its concentration must increase after nutrient ingestion, and it must stimulate glucose-mediated insulin release at physiologic concentrations (e.g., at plasma levels comparable to those observed after nutrient ingestion). Among the various gut hormones postulated to influence insulin secretion, only gastric inhibitory peptide (GIP) fulfills the necessary criteria. Neither secretin, cholecystokinin (CCK), nor vasoactive inhibitory polypeptide (VIP) shows an increment in plasma levels after oral glucose administration. CCK may, however, contribute to the incretin effect observed with oral glucose.

After an oral glucose load, serum levels of GIP increase before or simultaneously with the rise in serum insulin concentration.[87] IV infusion of purified GIP, in amounts resulting in plasma concentrations comparable to those observed after oral glucose administration (1 ng/ml), causes an enhancement of glucose-induced insulin secretion. Furthermore, an insulinotropic effect of endogenous GIP is suggested by the observation that ingestion of corn oil, a potent stimulus for GIP secretion, increases the insulin response to IV glucose. It is likely, however, that gut hormones other than GIP are insulinotropic. The augmented insulin response to oral glucose persists in patients after recovery from resection of the gastric antrum, duodenum, proximal jejunum, and head of the pancreas (Whipple's operation). Furthermore, injection of a potent GIP antiserum reduces but does

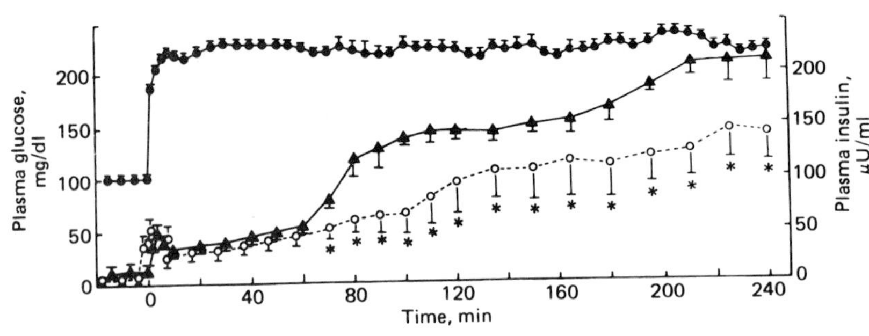

FIGURE 19-23 Enhancing effect of the oral route of glucose administration on the plasma insulin response to hyperglycemia. Hyperglycemia was induced and maintained constant (●) by a variable IV infusion of glucose. After 60 min, additional glucose was ingested by mouth while the plasma glucose level was maintained at the same hyperglycemic plateau. Despite the constancy of the plasma glucose level, there was a significantly greater rise in plasma insulin concentration after oral glucose (▲) than when hyperglycemia was maintained solely via the IV administration of glucose (○). (*From DeFronzo et al.*[9])

not abolish the exaggerated insulin response to intraduodenal glucose.[88] These findings suggest that several incretins may exist and may be produced in areas distal to the jejunum.

Amino Acids and Fat-Derived Substrates

Ingestion of protein or infusion of single or multiple amino acids stimulates insulin secretion. As in the case of glucose, stimulation of insulin secretion by orally ingested amino acids exceeds that of IV-administered amino acids, suggesting that enhancement of GI hormones takes place. Protein-stimulated secretion of GIP may mediate this effect.[89] Nonmetabolizable analogues of leucine and arginine have been shown to stimulate insulin secretion, suggesting that membrane recognition (receptor interaction) rather than intracellular metabolism may trigger insulin secretion in this case.[90]

"Redundant regulation" by fat-derived substances is an attractive concept. Accordingly, FFA or their oxidation products, the ketones, whose concentrations are initially elevated by insulin deficiency, subsequently sustain basal insulin secretion at low glucose concentration, to prevent unrestrained fat loss from adipose tissue. Evidence supporting this concept is available primarily from animal studies.[53,91] In obese human subjects, bolus injections of acetoacetate cause a small rise in plasma insulin concentration, but this is not observed in nonobese subjects.[92] A small increment in insulin levels has been observed in normal humans after ingestion of medium-chain triglycerides. However, more evidence is needed to establish the validity of an insulin-secretory role of ketones or FFA in humans.

Neural and Neurohumoral Regulation

The catecholamines epinephrine and norepinephrine inhibit glucose-stimulated insulin release via actions mediated by α-adrenergic receptors in the islet cells. That β-adrenergic receptors are present as well is indicated by the stimulatory effect of isoproterenol, which in turn is inhibited by the β-adrenergic blocking agent propranolol. Despite this dual receptor system in the beta cells, the

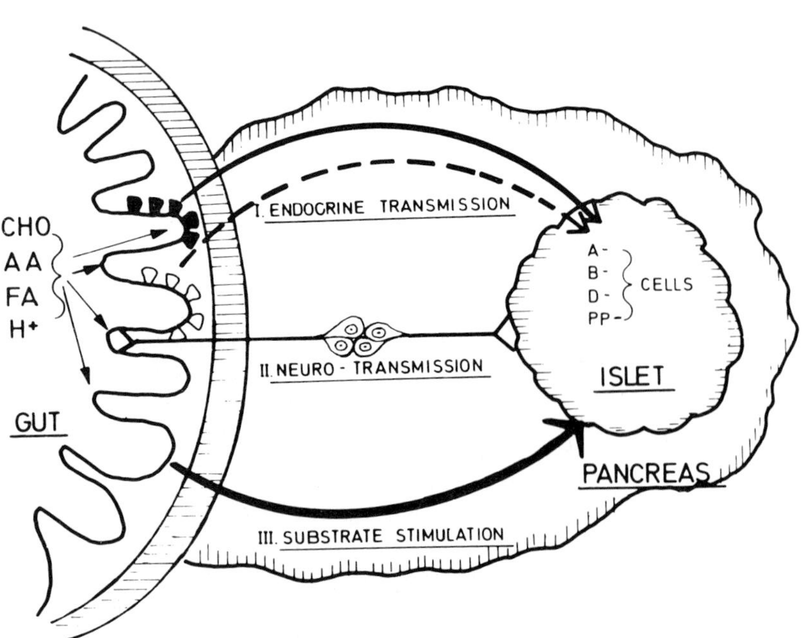

FIGURE 19-24 The enteroinsular axis. Entry of nutrients into the intestine influences the secretion of islet-cell hormones via three mechanisms: (1) endocrine transmission (e.g., release of gastric inhibitory polypeptide), (2) neurotransmission (e.g., vagal stimulation), and (3) substrate stimulation (e.g., glucose absorption resulting in hyperglycemia). CHO = carbohydrate; AA = amino acids; FA = fatty acids. (*From Creutzfeldt.*[86])

α-adrenergic action of epinephrine predominates; the net effect of epinephrine is therefore inhibition of glucose-stimulated insulin secretion, particularly the rapidly releasable pool. The adrenergic receptors in the islet cells appear to influence insulin secretion via alterations in intracellular cAMP concentration.[93]

The regulatory role of the autonomic nervous system and circulating catecholamines in the control of insulin secretion is manifested both in the physiologic hypoinsulinemia which accompanies exercise and in pathologic circumstances such as stress hyperglycemia. During moderate or severe exercise, plasma insulin levels decline in association with a rise in plasma catecholamine concentrations. In stress hyperglycemia (e.g., with severe body burns or compound fractures), the failure of basal insulin levels to rise in association with increases in blood glucose concentration is probably a consequence of catecholamine action. Catecholamines also contribute to the blunted insulin response observed in patients with pheochromocytoma. By contrast, very modest (two- to threefold) increments in plasma epinephrine concentration, as occur, e.g., with a mild viral illness, result in glucose intolerance by interfering with insulin action rather than by inhibiting secretion[94] (see below).

In contrast to the action of epinephrine, the result of stimulation of the parasympathetic nervous system (e.g., the vagus nerves) is increased insulin secretion. This effect of acetylcholine is glucose-dependent.[95] However, the effect of atropine administration on insulin secretion in humans is modest.

Participation of the central nervous system in the regulation of insulin secretion is indicated by the response to stimulation or destruction of hypothalamic nuclei. Stimulation of the ventromedial nuclei suppresses insulin release. This effect is reversed by adrenalectomy, suggesting that mediation occurs via adrenomedullary catecholamines. In contrast, destruction of the ventromedial nuclei leads to hyperinsulinism and hyperphagia.[96]

Other neurohumoral agents which have been identified within islet tissue and have also been shown to influence insulin secretion are serotonin and dopamine.[97] The response to serotonin is species-specific: serotonin stimulates or has no effect on insulin secretion in the dog and human; it inhibits insulin release in the golden hamster and rabbit. Dopamine has been shown to diminish insulin release in vitro.

An inhibitory effect of prostaglandin A on insulin secretion has been observed in dogs and humans. Diminished insulin secretion in type II diabetes may in part be mediated by prostaglandin synthesis.[98] The cyclooxygenase pathway has been found to exert an inhibitory effect on glucose-induced insulin secretion, whereas the lipooxygenase pathway stimulates insulin release.[99] Naturally occurring opioids (enkephalins, endorphins) may not in themselves stimulate insulin secretion but may potentiate the effect of glucose or glyceraldehyde.[100] This may occur by a mechanism involving an increase in cAMP level and calcium uptake. The endocrine pancreas appears to have several types of opioid peptide receptors.[100]

Somatostatin

Somatostatin is a tetradecapeptide originally isolated from the hypothalamus as a GH release inhibitory factor and subsequently identified by immunofluorescent techniques in pancreatic islet cells, stomach antrum, jejunal cells of the GI tract, and a variety of areas of the brain.[101] In addition to interfering with the release of GH, somatostatin is a potent inhibitor of both insulin and glucagon secretion. This effect of somatostatin on islet hormones represents a direct action which is demonstrable with in vitro techniques. Within the islets of Langerhans, somatostatin is localized to the delta cells located at the periphery of the islets. An increase in somatostatin-containing cells has been observed in rats rendered diabetic by streptozotocin and in some forms of genetic diabetes in experimental animals. High-affinity, specific somatostatin receptors have been characterized. Somatostatin analogues capable of displacing somatostatin from its binding sites are also capable of inhibiting insulin release[102]

In addition to altering islet-cell and GH secretion, somatostatin has been demonstrated to inhibit a variety of GI hormones, including gastrin, CCK, and secretin.[101] Diminished absorption of glucose and protein, decreased splanchnic blood flow,[103] and decreased gastrointestinal motility have also been noted. In addition, in patients with islet-cell tumors composed of somatostatin-containing cells (somatostatinomas), steatorrhea is a prominent symptom.[104]

A major unresolved question concerns the physiologic role of somatostatin in the regulation of insulin and glucagon secretion as well as nutrient absorption. A rise in somatostatin concentration has been reported after glucose or fat ingestion and has been proposed to be a modulator of nutrient absorption.[105] Somatostatin has also been proposed to regulate insulin and glucagon secretion by release into the interstitial environment of beta and alpha cells, a phenomenon which has been designated a paracrine effect. Undoubtedly, the myriad inhibitory effects of somatostatin on endocrine secretion and GI function (secretion, absorption, and motility) are at least in part pharmacologic in nature (Fig. 19-25).

Other Hormones

In GH-deficient dwarfs, diminutions in basal, glucose-stimulated, and arginine-induced insulin levels are observed. In contrast, hyperinsulinemia is a characteristic finding in acromegaly. A stimulatory action of glucagon on beta cell secretion has been

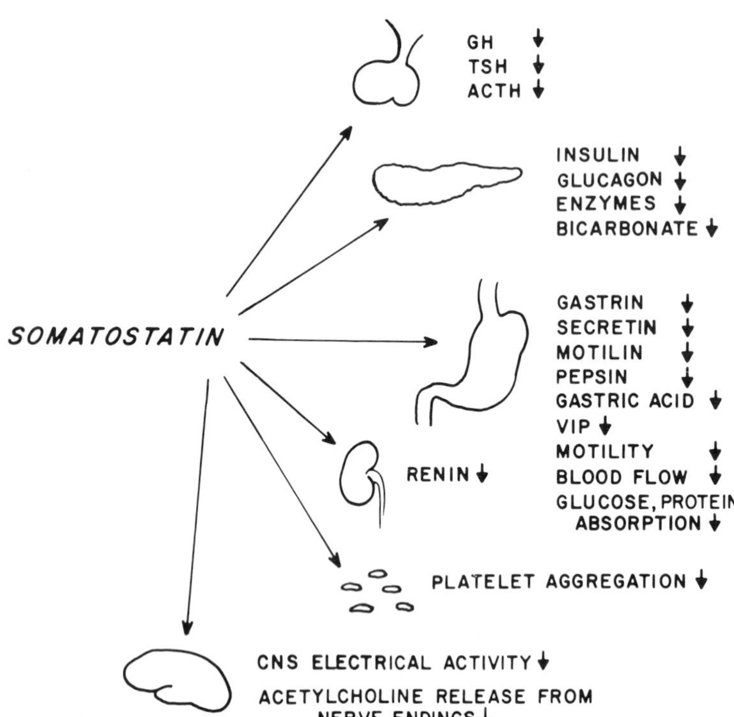

FIGURE 19-25 The multisystem inhibitory effects of somatostatin. In addition to inhibiting GH, insulin, and glucagon secretion, somatostatin has been shown to inhibit a variety of GI functions: Secretion of GI hormones and splanchnic blood flow are decreased, motility is inhibited, and absorption of glucose and amino acids is reduced.

demonstrated with the perfused pancreas. However, the small increments in plasma insulin concentration observed during in vivo infusions of glucagon in physiologic doses are probably a result of the accompanying rise in the plasma glucose concentration.

Hyperinsulinemia has been observed with exogenous administration or endogenous increments of adrenocorticosteroids, estrogens, progestins, and parathyroid hormone. Since glucose levels are not reduced and sometimes are even raised in these situations, it may be inferred that resistance to the effectiveness of insulin accompanies these hormonal changes. There is no convincing evidence that these hormones have a direct effect on insulin secretion. Alternatively, some feedback signal from the insulin-resistant tissues or hyperglycemia may provide the necessary insulinotropic stimulus to the beta cells.

Obesity

The most common hyperinsulinemic condition encountered in humans is obesity. High plasma insulin levels are observed in obese individuals in the basal state as well as after meal ingestion. That hyperinsulinemia is a consequence rather than a cause of obesity is indicated by the fact that loss of weight results in a fall in insulin level while gain in weight in previously lean individuals is followed by a rise in plasma insulin concentration. The various factors determining the magnitude of hyperinsulinemia in obesity include (1) the extent of adiposity, (2) the caloric and carbohydrate content of the meals ingested, and (3) the extent of physical activity. The correlation between plasma insulin levels and body weight is due to adiposity rather than augmented muscle mass (as in weight lifters). By contrast, a decrease in carbohydrate content of the diet or an overall reduction in caloric intake results in normalization of insulin levels well before ideal body weight has been attained. In addition, physical training may result in a fall in insulin level independent of weight loss.[106]

The precise signal responsible for basal and postmeal hyperinsulinemia in obese persons has not been established; hyperaminoacidemia has been suggested as a possible mechanism.[107] Inasmuch as obesity is not accompanied by hypoglycemia and in fact is associated with a tendency to develop type II diabetes (see below), the obese condition is clearly an insulin-resistant state.

Insulin Action

Insulin is the primary factor which controls the storage and metabolism of ingested metabolic fuels. After a meal, secretion of insulin facilitates the uptake, utilization, and storage of glucose, fat, and amino acids. Conversely, a reduction in the circulating insulin concentration leads to mobilization of endogenous fuels and reduced uptake of ingested nutrients. The action of insulin involves all three major metabolic fuels—carbohydrate, protein, and fat—and occurs in three principal tissues: liver, muscle, and adipose tisse. In each of these tissues there are anticatabolic as well as anabolic effects of insulin which act to reinforce each other (Table 19-4).

Carbohydrate Metabolism

The liver is a major site of insulin action in the disposal of an oral glucose load.[108–110] Since glucose is absorbed via the portal system, the extent to which an oral glucose load is available for uptake by peripheral tissues depends on its escape from the splanchnic bed. During the 3-h period following the ingestion of 100 g of glucose, 30 to 60 g is taken up by the liver and used for glycogen synthesis and triglyceride formation. Of the total ingested glucose, it appears that only ~10 percent is taken up on the first pass. Since the major portion of glucose in the portal vein is recirculating, the hepatic glucose uptake exceeds 50 percent of the total. In addition, ~15 percent of the hepatic glycogen is promptly synthesized from 3-carbon glucose precursors formed from peripheral and hepatic glucose degradation.[111]

The relative amount of glucose directly deposited as glycogen in the liver vs. the amount requiring resynthesis from the 3-carbon compounds can be inferred from randomization of labeled glucose carbons upon incorporation into glycogen. These estimates may vary with the species. The role of the liver as the primary site of glucose uptake was questioned when the proportion of directly vs. indirectly formed glycogen in fasting rats was found to be as low as ~1:2.[112] A similar proportion was obtained in another study in rats,[113] in which the ^{13}C-glucose labeling pattern was traced by NMR spectroscopy.

This randomization was assessed by trapping of carbons from UDP-glucose (the direct precursor of glycogen). Administration of diflunisal, a drug requiring hepatic glucuronidization for its excretion, and isolation of the UDP-glucose-derived glucuronide from the urine of humans receiving the labeled hexose permitted the estimate that 70 to 75 percent of hepatic glycogen is formed directly from glucose.[114]

In circumstances of mixed-meal intake, the blood glucose concentration in normal humans generally rises only by 30 to 40 mg/dl (1.7 to 3.4 m*M*) over 24 h (Fig. 19-20). This fine-tuning of blood glucose regulation is determined by the exquisite sensitivity of the liver to small changes in insulin secretion. When blood glucose concentration rises by only 10 to 15 mg/dl (0.6 to 0.8 m*M*), there is a 60 to 100 percent increase in peripheral insulin levels and virtually complete inhibition of hepatic glucose output (i.e., sparing of hepatic glycogen and cessation of gluconeogenesis) with no stimulation of peripheral glucose utilization.[70] Thus, compared with the liver, muscle and adipose tissues are less sensitive with respect to responses to small increases in the plasma insulin concentration. In fact, the plasma concentration of insulin necessary for half-maximal stimulation of peripheral glucose uptake is several times higher than that required for half-maximal inhibition of hepatic glucose output.[110] Nevertheless, with significant peripheral hyperinsulinemia, glucose uptake by fat and muscle tissues helps minimize the fluctuations in the systemic blood glucose level.

In view of the permeability of the hepatocyte to glucose, uptake of glucose by the liver is not rate-limiting. The first potential control point is initiation of glucose metabolism by phosphorylation to G6P. As was mentioned above, phosphorylation in the liver takes place under the influence of hexokinase and glucokinase. While hexokinase is saturated at physiologic glucose concentrations, glucokinase is only half saturated at the glucose concentration of 180 mg/dl (10 m*M*). Consequently, hepatic glucose uptake, by fully using glucokinase capacity, adjusts to the changing blood glucose concentration.

As was noted above (see Glycolysis), a second crucial step in the glycolytic pathway involves the phosphorylation of F6P by PFK-1 activated by F2,6P_2 (Fig. 19-5). When insulin is plentiful, this is efficiently accomplished and has significance not only with regard to stimulation of glycolysis but also with respect to inhibition of gluconeogenesis. In contrast, insulin deficiency results in reduced levels of F2,6P_2, decreased activity of PFK-1, and activation of FDPase. The net effect is a reversal of substrate flow from pyruvate (and alanine) to glucose, a catabolic process.

The glycogen content of the liver in patients with diabetic acidosis is significantly reduced but is

TABLE 19-4 Insulin Action on Liver, Adipose Tissue, and Muscle

	Liver	Adipose Tissue	Muscle
Anticatabolic effects	↓ Glycogenolysis	↓ Lipolysis	↓ Proteolysis
	↓ Gluconeogenesis		↓ Amino acid output
	↓ Ketogenesis		
Anabolic effects	↑ Glycogen synthesis ↑ Fatty acid synthesis	↑ Fatty acid uptake, synthesis, and esterification	↑ Amino acid uptake ↑ Protein synthesis ↑ Glycogen synthesis

promptly restored after insulin administration. This effect of insulin is due to its ability to activate glycogen synthase and reduce the activity of phosphorylase (Fig. 19-4) within a few minutes after it has been administered.

The salient effect of insulin on the output of glucose from the liver is not only promotion of glycogen synthesis but mainly inhibition of gluconeogenesis. The rate-limiting step in the gluconeogenic pathway lies between pyruvate and phospho*enol*pyruvate, which depends on the relative activities of PC and PEPCK on the one hand and pyruvate kinase on the other hand (Fig. 19-6). The activities of these enzymes are adjusted inversely either through rapid inhibition by specific metabolites or by slower, insulin-dependent induction/deinduction, as discussed above (see Fig. 19-6 and corresponding text).

In addition to influencing hepatic gluconeogenesis by altering FFA availability, it has been suggested that insulin diminishes gluconeogenesis by decreasing the supply of precursor amino acids. A number of studies, however, do not support this hypothesis. For example, exogenous insulin fails to inhibit the release of alanine, the key glucogenic amino acid, from peripheral muscle tissues. In like manner, plasma alanine levels show no consistent diminution after stimulation of endogenous insulin secretion. In contrast, glucose-stimulated insulin secretion results in a fall of hepatic alanine uptake despite unchanged arterial alanine levels. The bulk of the evidence thus indicates that insulin regulates gluconeogenesis primarily by altering intrahepatic processes rather than by influencing the rate of precursor supply.[108–110]

Inhibition of gluconeogenesis requires greater amounts of insulin than are necessary for inhibition of glycogenolysis. Thus, a 60 to 100 percent increase in plasma insulin concentration results in virtually complete inhibition of glycogenolysis, yet hepatic uptake and conversion of alanine, lactate, and pyruvate to glucose persist in the face of such minor increments of insulin concentration.[70,115] It should be noted that net liver glycogen storage has been suggested to occur in the face of active conversion of 3-carbon precursors to G6P.[112] Thus, gluconeogenesis need not always be accompanied by net output of glucose from the liver. Nonetheless, when the effect of basal insulin on gluconeogenesis is considered, insulin is found to inhibit this process considerably. The K_m for inhibition is below basal insulin levels so that small increases do not significantly affect the gluconeogenic rate, whereas decreases augment the rate considerably.[116]

A major question in the overall control of hepatic glucose metabolism concerns the relative importance of hyperinsulinemia and hyperglycemia as regulatory signals. Soskin and Levine in the 1940s proposed that blood glucose concentration is the primary stimulus that determines glucose uptake or glucose output by the liver. Support of this hypothesis derives from studies demonstrating that (1) glycogen synthase and phosphorylase are exquisitely sensitive to the ambient glucose concentration,[5] (2) hyperglycemia at constant insulin concentration inhibits hepatic glucose output from human[8] and rat liver,[117] and (3) in the absence of hyperglycemia, hyperinsulinemia fails to induce net uptake of glucose by the liver.[6] When the insulin concentration is raised between 400 to 600 μU/ml in euglycemic men, splanchnic uptake accounts for <8 percent of total glucose metabolism.[110] In contrast, other data emphasize the importance of insulin in regulating hepatic glucose output: (1) in insulin-deficient diabetic subjects, hyperglycemia induced by glucose infusion fails to inhibit hepatic glucose output,[118] (2) in perfused liver insulin activates glycogen synthase in the absence of added glucose,[118] and (3) much smaller increments in blood glucose concentration (10 to 15 mg/dl) effectively inhibit hepatic glucose output when accompanied by a rise in insulin concentration compared with the increments in arterial glucose concentration (60 mg/dl) required to inhibit hepatic glucose output when insulin concentrations are kept at basal levels. There is also evidence that even in the face of hyperglycemia and hyperinsulinemia, net uptake of glucose by the liver is relatively small (<15 percent of total glucose utilization) unless the glucose is administered orally[6] or via the portal vein.[119,120] It has been shown that net hepatic glucose uptake is enhanced with intraportal glucose delivery in the presence of basal or moderate elevations in glucose delivery.[121,122] It has also been suggested that in the postprandial phase dietary carbohydrate is converted into liver glycogen indirectly, mostly via lactate and alanine flowing in from the periphery. In this situation the G6P elaborated from pyruvate would be preferentially directed to glycogen rather than to glucose.[109]

The overall data thus indicate that hyperinsulinemia, hyperglycemia, and possibly signals from the GI tract, portal vein,[119,120] and glucogenic substrate flow contribute to the regulation of hepatic glucose balance. A rise in insulin concentration markedly increases the sensitivity of the liver to the inhibitory effects of glucose on hepatic glucose release. In like manner, a rise in glucose concentration facilitates and is probably essential for insulin-induced uptake of glucose by the liver. The net uptake of glucose by the liver is further stimulated when glucose is administered orally rather than IV.[9] A "portal factor" rather than a "gut factor" has been postulated to promote hepatic glucose uptake, since intraportal rather than peripheral delivery of glucose may cause greater hepatic uptake.[119,120,123]

Unlike the situation in a hepatocyte, the rate of entry of glucose into a muscle cell, at physiologic concentrations of plasma glucose, is the slowest (and therefore the rate-limiting) step. A major effect of insulin in this tissue is to control the transport of glucose across the cell membrane; the major end product of glucose uptake in nonexercising muscle is glycogen. The PFK system in muscle is also influenced by insulin via a mechanism similar to that in the liver, except that the reverse reaction, in the direction of glucose production, is of little significance in this tissue. It should be emphasized that glucose uptake by exercising muscle is not dependent on an increase in insulin secretion (see Exercise, below).

In the fat cell too, insulin acts primarily to stimulate the transport of glucose across the cell membrane. An effect is also observed on glycogen synthase and on PFK. The major end products of glucose metabolism in adipose cells are fatty acids and glycerol 3-phosphate. Glycerol 3-phosphate is important for fat storage because it provides the glycerol moiety necessary for triglyceride synthesis. As was noted above, most synthesis of carbohydrate-derived fatty acids in humans occurs in the liver rather than in adipose tissue (Fig. 19-11).

Amino Acid and Protein Metabolism

Insulin increases the transport of most amino acids into muscles, stimulates protein synthesis, and inhibits protein catabolism.[124] In intact humans, intrabrachial arterial infusion of insulin in physiologic amounts results in diminished output of amino acids from deep forearm tissues. This effect is particularly prominent with respect to the branched-chain amino acids leucine and isoleucine, as well as tyrosine and phenylalanine. The action of insulin on muscle amino acid exchange probably accounts for its ability to lower systemic amino acid levels. In the absence of adequate insulin, e.g., in a diabetic patient in ketoacidosis, elevations are observed in plasma levels of valine, leucine, and isoleucine. In addition, the uptake of these amino acids by muscle tissue after the ingestion of a protein meal is reduced in the absence of adequate amounts of insulin.[61,124] Thus, the stimulatory effect of ingested protein on insulin secretion (see above) serves to promote the uptake and anabolic utilization of the constituent amino acids. Insulin stimulates facilitated glucose uptake in muscle and adipose tissue via a carrier molecule. Muscle cells are less responsive to insulin upon attaining maximal glycogen stores (1 to 2 percent of its weight).[125]

In addition to its effect on protein synthesis, the overall anabolic action of insulin derives from its ability to inhibit protein catabolism. Insulin has been shown to inhibit the diabetes-induced rise in the activity of a protease bound to the myofibrils of skeletal muscle.[126,127] The oxidation of branched-chain amino acids by muscle tissue is also inhibited by insulin and is accelerated in the diabetic state. Insulin thus increases body protein stores via at least four mechanisms: (1) increased tissue uptake of amino acids, (2) increased protein synthesis, (3) decreased protein catabolism, and (4) decreased oxidation of amino acids. Insulin appears to have a greater inhibitory effect on proteolysis in liver than in muscle in vitro.

Fat Metabolism

In the liver, the synthesis of fatty acids is stimulated at a high insulin concentration. This effect reflects several actions: (1) The increased flow of substrate down the glycolytic pathway into the TCA cycle increases the availability of citrate, which stimulates the liposynthetic pathways, particularly the activity of acetyl CoA carboxylase (Fig. 19-10); (2) the reduction of FFA inflow removes the inhibitory influences which may be exerted on acetyl CoA carboxylase; (3) the availability of NADPH, which is a necessary hydrogen donor for the synthesis of fatty acids, is increased by insulin through the induction of pentose shunt and $NADP^+$-malate dehydrogenase enzymes; and (4) insulin directly stimulates acetyl CoA carboxylase both by promoting its synthesis and by preventing its phosphorylation. In the human, stimulation of hepatic lipogenesis is tantamount to stimulation of total body fat production, since the triglycerides are mostly liver-derived and VLDL-transported for deposition in adipose tissue; all these processes are insulin-dependent.

Insulin accelerates the removal of circulating triglycerides derived from exogenous or endogenous sources by inducing the synthesis of the adipose tissue "entry" enzyme, lipoprotein lipase (LPL). In addition, insulin is extremely effective in inhibiting the intracellular (hormone-sensitive) lipase which catalyzes the hydrolysis of stored triglycerides and the liberation of FFA. The antilipolytic effect occurs at concentrations of insulin below those needed to promote glucose transport; this is considered the most sensitive action of insulin. Furthermore, a large proportion of the glucose from insulin-promoted uptake in fat cells is used for the formation of glycerol 3-phosphate for FFA esterification. The net effect of these antilipolytic, glycerolgenic, lipogenic, and lipid-assimilating actions of insulin is to increase total fat.

Glucocorticoid and sex steroid hormones regulate adipose tissue metabolism as well. Intraabdominal fat accumulation may result from a high density of glucocorticoid receptors in this region, stimulating LPL activity. Progesterone and testosterone cause opposite effects.[128] Cushing's syndrome, menopause, polycystic ovary syndrome, aging in men, alcohol, and smoking are all associated with a hormonal imbalance resulting in a preponderance of abdominal fat distribution.[129]

In addition to affecting fatty acid metabolism, insulin has a profound suppressive effect on circulating blood ketone concentrations. The formation and accumulation of β-hydroxybutyrate and acetoacetate are consequences of three distinct metabolic events: (1) unrestrained mobilization of FFA from adipose tissue, (2) surplus of hepatic acetyl CoA due to excessive FFA oxidation; the acetyl CoA has to be converted to ketones because of TCA cycle saturation, and (3) a reduction in ketone utilization by peripheral tissues. As was already noted, insulin is a powerful antilipolytic hormone. In addition, insulin decreases the liver's capacity to oxidize fatty acids irrespective of substrate availability. This antiketogenic action of insulin is intimately related to both its regulation of hepatic carnitine levels and its stimulation of fatty acid synthesis, which increases malonyl CoA availability. These two factors are instrumental in rerouting fatty acyl CoA; they prevent it from entering the oxidative spiral in the mitochondria and redirect it into microsomal esterification to triglycerides (Figs. 19-10 and 19-13). The net result is a reduction in the ketogenic capacity of the liver. In addition, in the presence of insulin, the uptake and oxidation of ketone acids by muscle tissue are accelerated.[130]

The diverse effects of insulin on body fuel metabolism tend to reinforce each other (Table 19-4). Thus, the inhibition of gluconeogenesis spares amino acids for protein synthesis. Similarly, the inhibition of lipolysis decreases the availability of acetyl CoA needed for stimulation of gluconeogenic enzymes. Enhancement of fat synthesis increases the availability of malonyl CoA, an inhibitor of hepatic carnitine transferase, which antagonizes the oxidation of fatty acids; fatty acid concentration is also reduced by the antilipolytic effects of insulin.

Potassium and Sodium Metabolism

Insulin deficiency in diabetes is known to be associated with plasma cation losses due to increased use of cations for neutralizing organic acids, particularly ketoacids, thus enabling excretion of the acids. The drain affects particularly the total pools of body sodium and potassium (the latter is also released from tissues to meet the neutralization requirements). The administration of exogenous insulin or the stimulation of endogenous insulin secretion reverses the potassium outflow and results in a fall in the serum potassium concentration. This hypokalemic action of insulin is due to stimulation of potassium uptake by muscle and liver tissue, which may occur independently of changes in glucose metabolism. The regulatory role of insulin in potassium metabolism is underscored by the changes in serum potassium concentration which accompany a reduction in the basal insulin level. In association with a 50 percent decline in the fasting insulin level induced by somatostatin, the serum potassium concentration increases by 0.5 to 1.0 mEq/liter.[131] This hyperkalemic effect of modest insulinopenia is not due to altered renal handling of potassium. The sensitivity of body potassium homeostasis to minor changes in insulin secretion may in part explain the tendency of diabetic patients to develop hyperkalemia in the absence of uremia or acidosis.

Insulin has also been shown to influence sodium metabolism, although this action (in contrast to the effects on potassium) is a consequence of altered renal secretion of this cation.[132] After a physiologic increase in plasma insulin concentration, urinary sodium excretion falls in the absence of changes in the glomerular filtration rate (GFR) or aldosterone excretion. In contrast, inhibition of basal insulin secretion by somatostatin is accompanied by a 50 percent increase in urinary sodium excretion. The antinatriuretic effect of insulin may account for the edema which occasionally appears in hyperglycemic diabetic patients after blood glucose regulation by insulin treatment. Similarly, the refeeding edema observed after starved or malnourished subjects are refed and the diuresis which accompanies starvation may be mediated in part by altered secretion of insulin.

Insulin Receptors

Receptor Interaction and Structure

As in the case of other polypeptide hormones, insulin initially binds to a specific receptor on the plasma membrane of the cell. A model of the insulin receptor is depicted in Fig. 19-26. The receptor is a symmetric tetrameric protein composed of two α and two β subunits linked by disulfide bonds forming a $\beta\alpha\alpha\beta$ structure. The receptor is designed to carry out three functions:[133] (1) recognition of insulin by binding the hormone with high specificity, (2) transmission of a signal which results in activation of intracellular metabolic pathways, and (3) endocytosis of the complex leading to lysosomal proteolysis of insulin with recycling of the subunits to the membrane.

The α subunit (135,000 daltons) is the binding unit and exists in two isoforms (719 or 731 amino acids) derived from a common preproreceptor of 1370 or 1382 amino acids.[134]

The 95,000-dalton β subunit is the effector unit. It possesses an insulin-sensitive protein kinase activity, specifically phosphorylating tyrosine residues in proteins, and is responsible for signal transduction across the plasma membrane. Both subunits have been found to be glycoproteins, containing carbohydrate side chains which are involved in insulin binding.[135]

The physiologic essence of a hormone receptor is its specificity of binding and the close relation of this binding to the expression of hormone action. In studies involving over 40 insulin analogues, a direct relation has been demonstrated between the affinity of different insulins and insulin analogues for the receptor and the biological activity resulting from this interaction (Fig. 19-27).

The interaction between insulin and its receptor is not a simple, reversible bimolecular reaction with

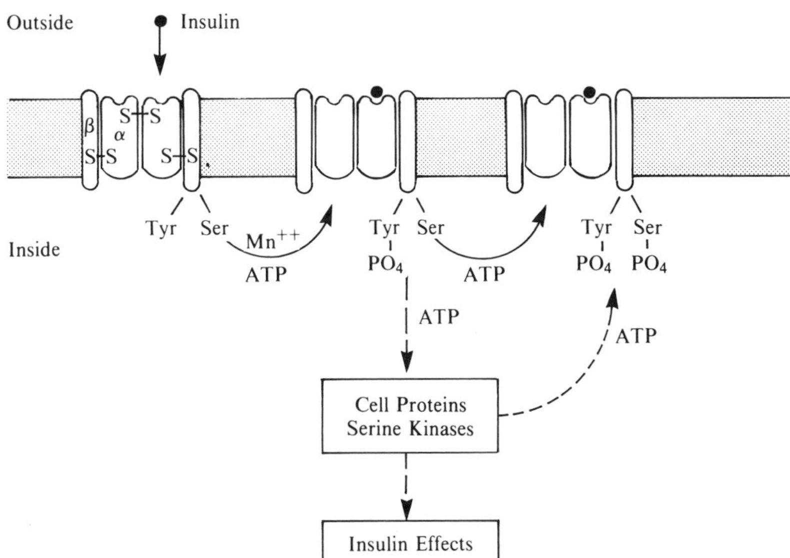

FIGURE 19-26 Model of the membranal insulin receptor and the intracellular transmission of the signal generated by insulin binding. Insulin binds to the external α subunit of the receptor. As a result, the tyrosine kinase activity on the internal segment of the β subunit becomes activated (left) and the insulin receptor undergoes autophosphorylation (middle). Three factors affect the activity of tyrosine kinase: (1) receptor-bound insulin, which increases V_{max}, (2) M_n^{2+}, which decreases the K_m toward ATP, and (3) the state of receptor phosphorylation, which sustains the activity after the removal of insulin. The activated receptor kinase is cytosol-oriented and most probably continues to phosphorylate other intracellular proteins and enzymes with regulatory function, thus propagating the insulin message. In addition, serine residues on the receptor are also phosphorylated (right) in the basal state; their phosphorylation increases in the course of signal transmission. (*From Kahn and Crettaz.*[133])

a single affinity or equilibrium constant; it is more complex, demonstrating heterogeneity of ligand affinity. This complexity is revealed by the curvilinear nature and upward concave shape of the plots obtained when insulin binding data are subjected to Scatchard analysis.[136] These findings have been interpreted as indicating the presence of "negative cooperativity," a phenomenon in which increasing occupancy of receptors results in decreased affinity for additional insulin molecules as a result of site-site-interactions.[137] Negative cooperativity can occur either by allosteric transformation of the second subunit after insulin has interacted with the first subunit or by alteration of receptor affinity resulting from the formation of receptor oligomers. The various steric forms of the receptor are postulated to be in equilibrium in the plasma membrane of the cell, changing with insulin concentration. Although strong evidence was submitted for the negative cooperativity model, other explanations for the Scatchard plot pattern exist. They are based on the presence of two distinct classes of receptors, one with high affinity and low capacity and the other with low affinity and high capacity.[138,139] The existence of different classes of binding sites is suggested by the evidence that there are high-molecular-weight oligomeric forms of the receptor,[140,141] which seem to involve complexes of α, β, or α and β subunits exhibiting decreased affinity for insulin. Formation of receptor oligomers could account for receptor aggregation, which may be important in modifying insulin action. Such a model of the insulin receptor has been compared to the association of adenyl cyclase with its receptor,[133] effecting the formation of cAMP from ATP. In both systems, linkage of the biologically active form of the receptor to an effector system results in increased molecular weight and decreased receptor affinity. Whereas in the insulin receptor the β (effector) subunit is linked to the α subunit by disulfide bridges, the G protein effector in the adenyl cyclase system is noncovalently bonded.[142]

FIGURE 19-27 The functional domains of the insulin receptor α subunit and β subunit. The functions of the different amino acid residues of the α subunit and β subunit are explained in the text. (*From Häring and Obermaier-Kursser.*[134])

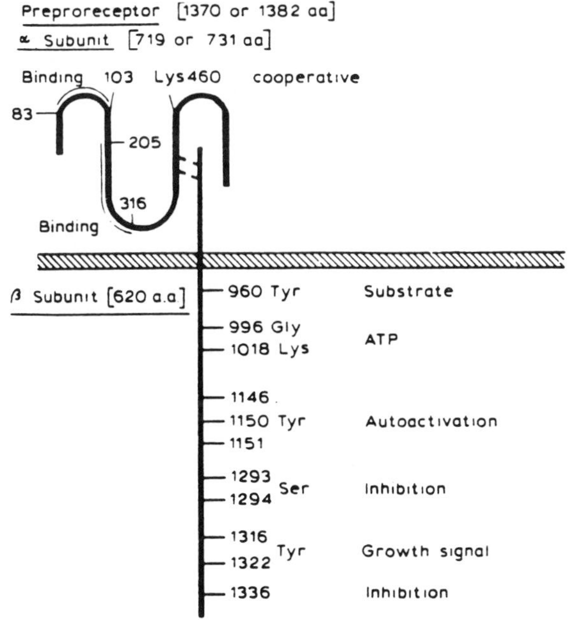

Functional domains of both α and β subunits have been described (Fig. 19-27). Amino acids 83 to 103 and enriched region (amino acids 205 to 316) are thought to be involved in binding.[143] Insulin receptor cooperativity is attributed to the lysine at amino acid

460,[144] while affinity and degradation are considered to be modulated by 12 amino acids residing at the C-terminal end.[145] Disulfide coupling of the α and β subunits is attributable to amino acid 435, 468, or 524.[146] Functional domains of the β subunit (containing 620 amino acids) consist of a 194-amino acid extracellular glycosylated domain,[147] a 23-amino acid transmembrane domain, a cytoplasmic tyrosine kinase domain, and a C-terminal tail, the function of which remains unclear. The ATP-binding region occurs about lysine 1018 and glycine 996.[148,149]

Insulin receptors have been found to be ubiquitous in mammals. They have been demonstrated in insulin-responsive tissues as well as in tissues and cells not directly responsive to insulin, such as the brain,[150] erythrocytes,[151] vascular endothelial cells,[152] gonadal cells,[153] and placenta.[154] Presence of receptors may signify a dependence on slow, long-term effects of insulin, e.g., growth. Insulin receptors may vary in structure, depending on the tissue in which they are found. Small differences have been found in molecular weight, nature of disulfide bonding of subunits, and state of receptor aggregation.

Insulin Receptor Turnover

Insulin receptors constantly turn over, as do other membrane proteins. The preproreceptor of 1370 or 1382 amino acids is converted into a partially glycosylated proreceptor of 190,000 daltons.[135] After further glycosylation and cleavage, the α and β subunits are inserted into the plasma membrane.[155] This takes 1.5 to 3h.

Electron microscopic studies have provided direct evidence that after the binding of insulin to its receptor, the hormone-receptor complex enters the cell by endocytosis, where the hormone and the subunits may be degraded in lysosomes[156] (Fig. 19-28). However, most of the internalized receptors are recycled back to the membrane.[157] Degradation is enhanced by exposure to insulin: the half-life of the receptor is 7 to 12 h, but this can be shortened to 2 to 3 h in the presence of insulin.[135] A single receptor makes several cycles before being degraded.[158] Studies have suggested that the hormone-receptor complex is concentrated in Golgi-enriched endosomes to a greater degree than in lysosomes.[159] The endosomes may function as a clearinghouse in which the hormone-receptor complex is dissociated; the hormone may then be directed to lysosomes and the receptor may be recycled back to the cell surface.[159] Alternatively, the receptor can be degraded by lysosomal proteolysis or remain sequestered. The proportion of receptors recycled, degraded, or sequestered determines the final receptor concentration and the amount found on the cell surface at any particular time, which varies with the type of tissue.[159,160]

A salient regulatory feature of the insulin receptor is its susceptibility to the ambient insulin concentration. In circumstances of hyperinsulinemia (e.g., obesity), the number of insulin receptors is reduced ("*down regulation*") while the reverse ("*up regulation*") occurs with hypoinsulinemia (e.g., starvation). These changes apply to the membrane concentration of the receptors, which are shifted to intracellular storage, sequestration, and/or degradation.[159,160] In addition, they may involve the formation or dissociation of oligomeric forms.

Insulin Receptor Phosphorylation

Phosphorylation, the process by which phosphate groups are transferred from high-energy donors

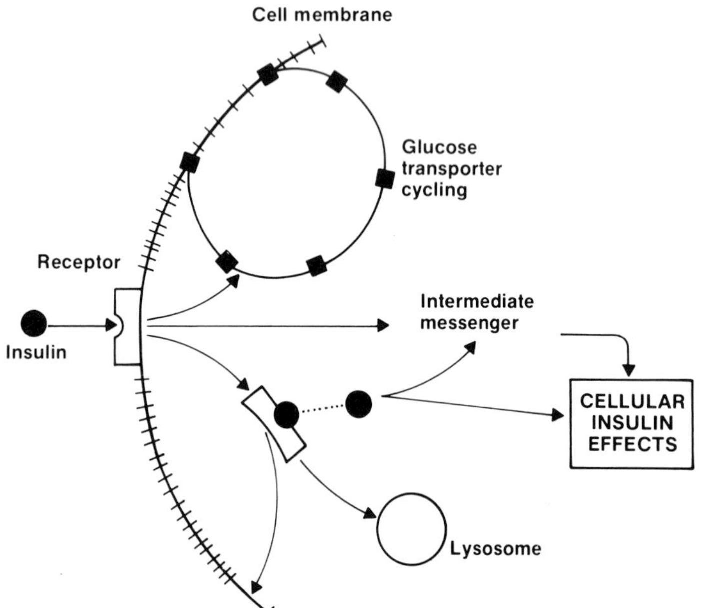

FIGURE 19-28 Events following the interaction of insulin with its receptor. Binding of insulin results are autophosphorylation and increased receptor kinase activity (as outlined in Fig. 19-26), which may transduce the insulin message by phosphorylating intracellular proteins. In addition, the generation of an intermediate "second messenger" was postulated to transmit the insulin signal to intracellular proteins regulating various metabolic and protein-synthetic pathways and to initiate nuclear synthetic events. After insulin binding there is increased internalization of the receptor translocating to the lysosomes and Golgi apparatus for degradation or recycling to the membrane. Intracellular actions of the activated receptor and of bound or dissociated insulin are possible. Furthermore, binding of insulin triggers a brisk movement of glucose transporters to the cell membrane, facilitating glucose entry into insulin-dependent cells.

(e.g., ATP) to hydroxyl acceptors on amino acid residues on proteins, is mediated by protein kinases. The binding of insulin to the receptor activates the tyrosine-specific protein kinase which effects receptor autophosphorylation.[161,162] It would appear that 6 of 13 tyrosine residues become phosphorylated, particularly residues 1146, 1150, and 1151, and this is related to kinase activity.[163,164] Phosphorylation of the latter three residues invokes a conformational change of the β subunit with subsequent influence on other substrates.[165,166] Although the precise physiologic role of the receptor tyrosine kinase activity is not fully established, it is likely that this activity is a transmembrane signal leading to the biological effects of insulin. The receptor kinase activity is probably reflected in continuing phosphorylation of intracellular proteins, some of them possibly with protein kinase activity. These kinases may in turn continue the phosphorylation cascade with resultant activity modulations of the phosphorylation-sensitive cellular metabolic systems.

The insulin receptor is also phosphorylated on serine residues[161,162] (Fig. 19-26) both in the basal state and in the course of insulin binding.

Serine phosphorylation is found largely in the basal state in intact cells. Tyrosine phosphorylation occurs within seconds after insulin stimulation, while serine phosphorylation follows within minutes. The latter serves to inhibit receptor kinase activity and perhaps to facilitate the insulin signal on other effector systems.[134] Several proteins have been demonstrated to be phosphorylated in intact cells, including a 46-kDa and 180-kDa protein in the plasma membrane, as well as a 185-kDa, 115-120-kDa, 60-kDa, and a 15-kDa protein in the cytosol.[167–169] Phorbol esters, which are known for their insulin-like action, have been recently found to promote the phosphorylation of serine residues on the receptor,[170,171] which probably extends to other proteins as well. Thus, one of the intracellular phosphorylation substrates of the receptor kinase could be protein kinase C, a Ca^{2+} and phospholipid-dependent serine-phosphorylating enzyme involved in the regulation of metabolic processes and cell growth and proliferation. The interaction of the tyrosine- and serine-specific kinases is not known; it has been suggested that they may mediate insulin action on metabolism and growth in dual or sequential modes.[162] It is pertinent that some receptors for insulin-like growth factors also undergo autophosphorylation upon the emergence of tyrosine kinase activity; they include epidermal growth factor,[172] platelet-derived growth factor,[173] and insulin-like growth factor-I (IGF-I, or somatomedin C)[174] (see below).

Insulin is known to stimulate the synthesis of certain phospholipids, especially diacylglycerol and 1,4,5-triphosphoinositol, as well as the activity of phospholipase C.[175] Insulin receptor itself has a phosphoinositol kinase activity.[176] These phospholipids are postulated to act as intracellular "second messengers" of insulin.[177,178] Diacylglycerol stimulates protein kinase C activity; diacylglycerol and insulin synergistically stimulate DNA synthesis and cell growth.[178] In addition, protein kinase C, in stimulating serine phosphorylation of the receptor (as it does elsewhere), may exert desensitizing feedback action, since excessive serine phosphorylation weakens the activity of tyrosine-phosphorylated receptors.[133]

Indirect evidence appears to also support the putative role of GTP binding in insulin signal transduction.[179]

Postreceptor Events

While the kinetic phenomena related to insulin-receptor interaction are reasonably characterized, the molecular mechanisms leading to the modification of cellular processes such as glucose transport, glycogen synthesis and breakdown, lipolysis proteolysis, enzyme transcription, and translation remain to be elucidated. Several studies[180–184] support the following concepts (Fig. 19-28):

1. The intracellular transport of glucose, early identified as a prominent effect of insulin, has now been shown to be carried out by membrane vesicles termed *glucose transporters*.[185,186] Within seconds of insulin binding to the receptor, translocation of the glucose transporters from an intracellular pool to the plasma membrane occurs, with acceleration of the cycling of transporters. These are probably the most immediate events in the receptor-mediated stimulation of glucose transport.

   Facilitative glucose transporters (energy-independent) are situated on virtually all cell surfaces. These are structurally related proteins which transport glucose down a concentration gradient and may play an etiologic role in diabetes mellitus.[187,188] Glucose transporters have been classified numerically according to their order of identification or concentration in various tissues (Table 19-2).[188–190] GLUT-1 transporter (erythrocyte) is ubiquitous and may provide for basal glucose requirements. GLUT-2 is the liver transporter but is also located in the kidneys, intestines, and beta cells of the pancreas. GLUT-4 is the principal transporter in insulin-sensitive tissues (muscle and fat). The roles of GLUT-3 and GLUT-5, which are present in brain and jejunum, respectively, have not been as clearly elucidated. Abnormalities in glucose transporters may be responsible for the defects observed in both insulin-dependent and non-insulin-dependent diabetes.[191–193]
2. Alterations in intracellular enzyme activities may be mediated by a cAMP-independent phosphorylation cascade subsequent to autophospho-

rylation at the membrane site by contact of receptor kinase with subcellular sites before or during internalization. It may be assumed that among the many affected proteins there are also certain protein phosphatases which become activated by phosphorylation. Thus, dephosphorylation, which is usually characteristic of the insulin-mediated switch from catabolic to anabolic processes (e.g., the inhibition of glycogen phosphorylase), would be actually accomplished by phosphorylation of regulatory proteins. Such effects would offset cAMP-dependent phosphorylations. Other cAMP-mitigating effects of insulin could be stimulation of phosphodiesterase[194] or direct inhibition of protein kinase activities.[195]

3. Generation of a family of cytoplasmic mediators of insulin action. These mediators could be low-molecular-weight peptides[181] or phospholipids.[182,196] They may interact with various enzyme systems directly[182] or may become phosphorylated independently of cAMP and/or carry out phosphorylations and dephosphorylations.[197,198]
4. The intracellular effects of insulin may be facilitated by internalization of the receptor-insulin complex. Contact with the microsomal and nuclear systems involved in protein synthesis could be made possible by dissociation of insulin from the internalized receptor. Which cellular actions (e.g., membrane function, enzyme dephosphorylation) are dependent on such internalization remains to be established.

The proposed mechanisms are not mutually exclusive. They could function in concert or amplify each other.

Insulin Resistance

Insulin resistance is generally recognized by diminished response to either endogenous insulin (e.g., hyperinsulinemia in association with normal or elevated blood glucose concentration) or exogenous insulin (e.g., diabetes requiring very large doses of insulin). Such resistance may be due to changes in insulin receptors, postreceptor events, or both. Although the number of insulin receptors per cell is estimated to vary between 50,000 (in adipocytes) and 250,000 (in hepatocytes), maximal biological effects depend on the occupation of a certain *number* of receptors, which may represent a small fraction (<10 percent) of those present. The functional correlate of the existence of "spare receptors" is that in circumstances of reduced numbers of receptors (e.g., obesity), if the insulin concentration is sufficiently elevated, the number of receptor-hormone complexes will ultimately reach the critical concentration necessary to trigger a biological event (i.e., the dose-response curve for insulin is shifted to the right). This type of receptor-mediated insulin resistance occurs without a change in the maximal response (i.e., maximal rates of glucose utilization do not change); it is termed decreased *insulin sensitivity*. In contrast, a decrease in the maximal tissue response (i.e., a reduction in the maximal rate of glucose utilization) may be observed when insulin resistance is due to a postreceptor defect. Such a downward shift in the insulin dose-response curve is termed decreased *insulin responsiveness* (Fig. 19-29). Whether the insulin dose-response curve shifts rightward or downward has thus been used to identify receptor-mediated or postreceptor-mediated mechanisms of insulin resistance; a mixed mechanism produces both rightward and downward shifts. In fact, in most cases of type II diabetes or obesity a mixed type of resistance is seen because of reduced insulin sensitivity and responsiveness.

Studies of insulin receptors in humans have been extensive.[199] Many of them assessed the binding of insulin to monocytes removed from the circulation, which were demonstrated to mirror insulin binding in target tissues of insulin action (liver, muscle, and fat tissue). How the conditions of tissue response vary with the availability of insulin in vivo is shown in Fig. 19-30.

Conditions characterized by altered sensitivity to insulin are outlined in Table 19-5. Some patients with lipoatrophic diabetes and patients with the syndrome of *acanthosis nigricans* exhibit extreme insulin resistance. In acanthosis nigricans, receptor function is decreased in some patients because of the presence of a circulating antireceptor antibody which interferes with insulin binding.[200] In other patients there is a genetically mediated decrease in receptor synthesis as well as an increase in receptor degradation.[201] The most common insulin-resistant

FIGURE 19-29 Types of resistance to insulin. Partial loss of high-affinity receptors or defective receptor function results in reduced binding due to decreased *sensitivity*. This is characterized by a shift of the dose-response curve to the right without a change in maximal response. In a postreceptor defect or in the absence of sufficient receptor-binding capacity, the maximal insulin effect is lower, causing decreased *responsiveness*. Often both receptor sensitivity and postreceptor responsiveness are reduced. (*From Kahn and Crettaz.*[133])

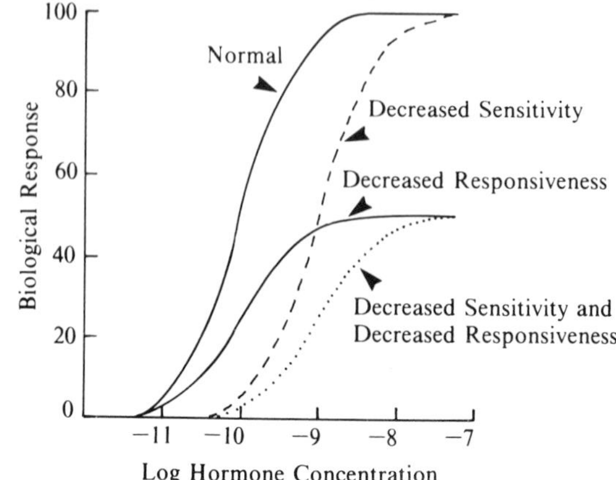

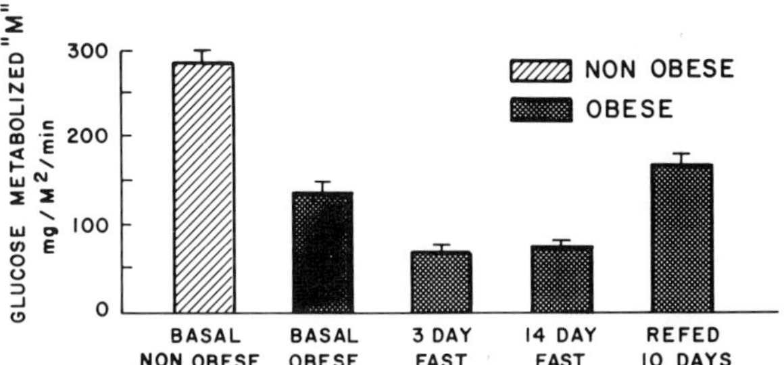

FIGURE 19-30 Insulin action in normal-weight and obese subjects in the basal (overnight-fasted) state and after 3- and 10-day fasts. Insulin action is indicated as the rate of glucose metabolized (M) during physiologic hyperinsulinemia achieved with the insulin clamp technique. In the basal state decreased insulin action in obesity is associated with a reduction in insulin binding, demonstrating that the receptor binding is a rate-limiting step in insulin action. In contrast, after fasting, insulin action is further reduced despite a rise in insulin binding, indicating that postreceptor events are rate-limiting. (*Based on data of DeFronzo R et al.*[211])

state is obesity, in which a decrease in insulin binding has been observed in monocytes, adipocytes, hepatocytes, and muscle cells. Altered receptor function has also been observed in hyperinsulinemic, nonobese type II diabetic patients. Receptor phosphorylation decreases concomitantly with the decrease in insulin binding, but several insulin-resistant individuals with virtually normal insulin binding but defective receptor kinase activity have also been identified.[202]

Insulin resistance thus may result from reduced insulin binding, reduced receptor kinase activity with normal binding, or a combination of defects. Defective receptor kinase activity has been demonstrated in skeletal muscle from patients with non-insulin-dependent diabetes mellitus.[203] The autoactivation cascade of insulin receptor kinase may be defective, thus resulting in reduced formation of triphosphorylated receptors.[204] At present it remains unclear whether the defect in kinase activity is a primary or secondary event caused by obesity and/or hyperinsulinemia.[205] Support for the latter comes from evidence for partial reversibility subsequent to weight loss.[206]

A decrease in insulin binding may not, however, be the sole or even major mechanism of insulin resistance for a given target cell. For example, in obesity, a defect in intracellular glucose oxidation is demonstrable at maximal concentrations of insulin and cannot be accounted for by a diminution in insulin binding.[206] A decrease in the number and/or function of glucose transporters (GLUT-4) may account for insulin resistance in a variety of insulin-resistant states (Fig. 19-31). A reduction in insulin-sensitive GLUT-4 transporters has been demonstrated in fat cells but not in muscle cells from patients with type II diabetes.[207] Postreceptor changes that mediate resistance to insulin may also involve tissue enzymes such as muscle glycogen synthase. This enzyme has been implicated in view of the evidence of a defect in insulin-mediated glycogen synthesis in muscle tissue in type II diabetes while muscle oxidative metabolism remains intact.[208] These findings indicate that insulin resistance may be a consequence of a variety of mechanisms at the receptor and/or postreceptor intracellular sites.

TABLE 19-5 Conditions Characterized by Altered Sensitivity to Insulin

Insulin resistance
Obesity
Type II diabetes
Severe insulin resistance and acanthosis nigricans
Growth hormone excess
Glucocorticoid excess
Lipoatrophic diabetes
Insulin hypersensitivity
Athletic training
Anorexia nervosa
Glucocorticoid deficiency

In contrast to obesity and type II diabetes, a number of conditions are characterized by increased sensitivity to insulin. Such increased sensitivity is observed in physically trained athletes, patients with anorexia nervosa, and patients with growth hormone or glucocorticoid deficiency. A postreceptor mechanism involving an increase in the number of GLUT-4 transporters has been demonstrated as the mechanism of enhanced insulin sensitivity after physical training.[209,210,211]

Insulin Degradation

The biological half-life of insulin is in the range of 6 to 10 min. The major site of insulin degradation is the liver, where 40 to 60 percent of the hormone is removed in a single passage. As noted above, insulin is internalized by liver cells after it binds to the receptor and is translocated to lysosomes, the intracellular site of a variety of degradative enzymes. At least two insulin-degrading enzymes have been identified. *Glutathione-insulin transhydrogenase* cleaves the disulfide bonds of insulin, releasing intact A and B chains. Proteases inactivate insulin by peptide bond cleavage.[212]

The kidney accounts for 15 to 20 percent of insulin degradation. The renal clearance of insulin is larger than the GFR, indicating that the hormone is removed from the blood by the tubules as well as by filtration. In patients with renal insufficiency, insulin uptake by the kidney may fall to ~9 percent.[213] This accounts in part for the diminished insulin requirements sometimes seen in patients with diabetic glomerulosclerosis. The kidney assumes increased importance in the degradation of exogenous insulin since subcutaneously injected insulin is absorbed via

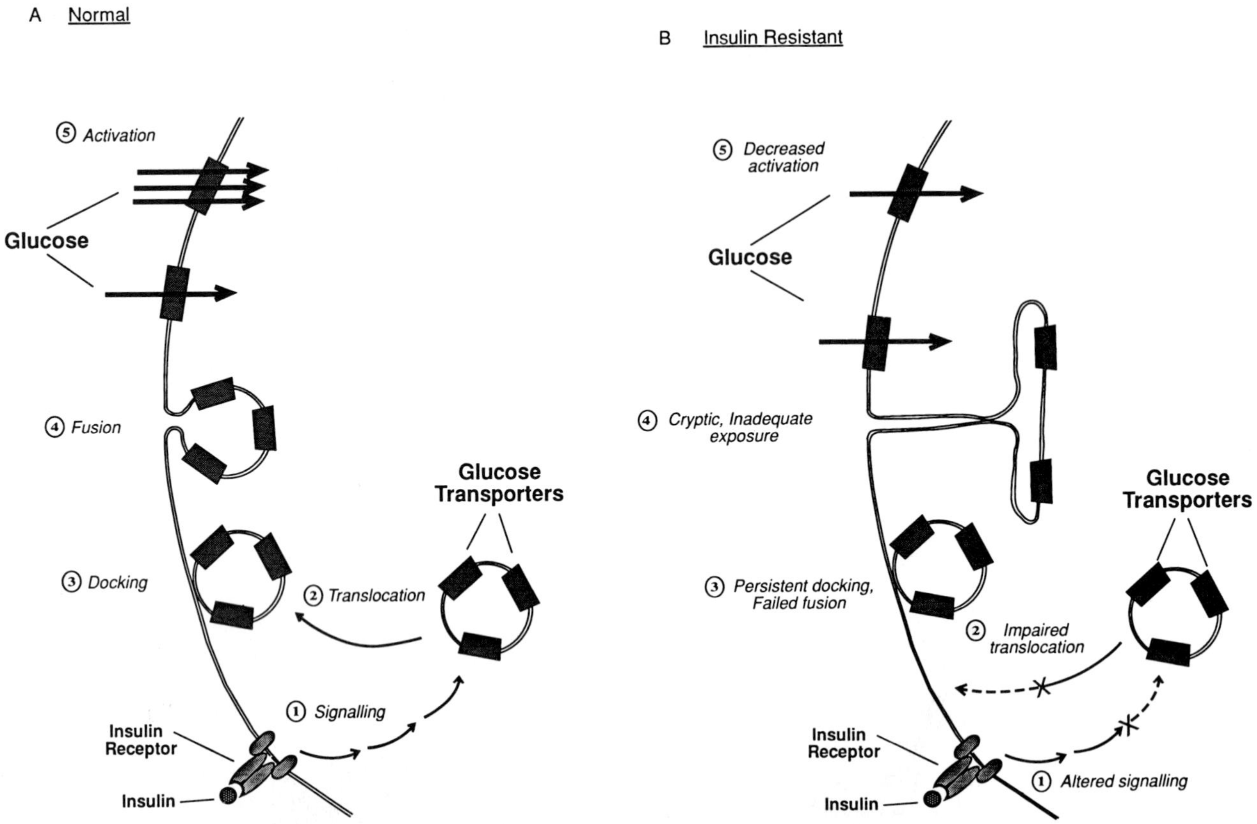

A Normal

B Insulin Resistant

⑤ Activation
Glucose
④ Fusion
Glucose Transporters
③ Docking
② Translocation
① Signalling
Insulin Receptor
Insulin

⑤ Decreased activation
Glucose
④ Cryptic, Inadequate exposure
Glucose Transporters
③ Persistent docking, Failed fusion
② Impaired translocation
Insulin Receptor
① Altered signalling
Insulin

FIGURE 19-31 (*A*) Sequence of events involved in insulin stimulation of glucose transport in muscle and adipose cells: (1) Insulin binding to its receptor in the plasma membrane initiates a cascade of signals resulting in (2) the translocation of glucose transporters from an intracellular pool associated with membrane vesicles to the plasma membrane, where they (3) dock, (4) fuse, and (5) are further activated. (*B*) Potential functional defects contributing to insulin-resistant glucose transport in muscle in diabetes, obesity, and other insulin-resistant states. Defects may involve (1) deficient signaling, (2) impaired translocation, (3) persistent "docking" without fusion, (4) partial fusion rendering transporters cryptic with inadequate exposure to the extracellular milieu, or (5) reduced activation of transporters. (*From Kahn.*[207])

the systemic circulation while endogenous insulin is released into the portal vein.

Glucagon

Chemistry and Biosynthesis

Glucagon is a polypeptide consisting of a single chain of 29 amino acids, with a molecular mass of 3485 daltons. Recent studies of structure-activity relations indicate that the terminal amino group is active in both binding and cellular action of the hormone. However, the terminal carboxyl group confers with high affinity of the hormone for its receptor, which permits hormone binding and action at physiologic concentrations. Unlike insulin, the amino acid sequence of glucagon is identical in all mammalian species examined.

The alpha cells of the islets of Langerhans are the site of glucagon biosynthesis. Immunofluorescent studies indicate that these cells are situated on the outer rim of the islets and constitute ~25 percent of the islet-cell population.[214] Within the islet cells, synthesis of glucagon involves the initial formation of a larger precursor: preproglucagon (a 180-amino acid protein), which is converted to proglucagon. Proglucagon is made up of 69 amino acid residues (9000 daltons) and is also referred to as *glicentin* or glucagon-like immunoreactivity (GLI)-1[215]; the secretory granules of alpha cells contain glucagon as the central core with glicentin in the outer band.[216] After cleavage of this molecule to glucagon, the contents of the secretory granules are discharged by the process of exocytosis (emiocytosis), which is analogous to that described for insulin.

GLI (enteroglucagon) resides in the carboxy-terminal section of glicentin. It has 10 to 20 percent of the potency of glucagon and binds to the glucagon receptor. GLI stimulates adenyl cyclase of the oxyntic mucosa of the stomach and inhibits gastric acid secretion.[217,218]

Circulating Glucagon

Advanced and specific immunoassay and gel filtration techniques have demonstrated that only 40 to 50 percent of human plasma glucagon represents biologically active hormone (i.e., of 3485 daltons). Most of the remaining glucagon immunoreactivity (of 160,000 daltons) elutes together with plasma proteins in the void volume. This fraction has been termed "*big plasma glucagon*" (BPG); it probably is devoid of biological activity. Two small additional fractions of ~9000 and ~2000 daltons have been identified in normal plasma. The biological significance of these fractions remains to be determined, although the 9000-dalton material is thought to represent proglucagon. The concentration of this fraction is increased in patients with chronic renal failure, presumably because of impaired renal removal.[219]

In pancreatectomized humans, glucagon has been reported to be absent from the circulation.[220] However, GLI polypeptides (of gut origin) may be capable of being converted to glucagon once they have entered the circulation.[221] This may account for the measurable glucagon levels after total pancreatectomy in humans. Extrapancreatic glucagon-containing cells may also be present in the digestive tract.[222,223] Although basal levels of immunoreactive glucagon (75 to 150 pg/ml) represent the biologically active and inactive components described above, alterations in circulating immunoreactivity in response to physiologic stimulation (e.g., by amino acids) or suppression (e.g., by glucose) generally reflect changes in the biologically active true pancreatic (3485-dalton) component of the immunoreactivity. Familial hyperglucagonemia is a rare asymptomatic autosomal dominant trait in which total plasma glucagon reactivity is increased 2 to 10 times, but 85 percent of this immunoreactivity consists of biologically inactive, high-molecular-weight components[224] (see below).

Secretion

Glucagon secretion does not markedly fluctuate throughout the day in normal subjects receiving mixed meals (Fig. 19-20). The relative constancy of glucagon concentration thus contrasts with the fluctuation of insulin concentration which accompanies mixed-meal ingestion or even minor changes (10 to 20 mg/dl) in blood glucose concentration (Fig. 19-20). The major physiologic stimuli of glucagon secretion in normal humans are protein ingestion, infusion of amino acids, and exercise, particularly if strenuous or prolonged.[225] β-Endorphins may also play a role in glucagon stimulation via the effects on adenylate cyclase activity.[226] Increases in glucagon secretion are also observed with acute hypoglycemia, after the infusion of large doses of epinephrine, and in association with hypercorticism.[225,227] Glucagon's dominant counterregulatory effect in hypoglycemia is confirmed by the inability of increased epinephrine secretion to compensate for its lack.[229] Impaired glucagon secretion has also been demonstrated in insulin-induced hypoglycemia in anorexia nervosa.[230] In type I diabetes, the stimulating effect of hypoglycemia on glucagon secretion is markedly reduced. Furthermore, significant improvement in glucose recovery subsequent to insulin-induced hypoglycemia was associated with improved glucagon secretion in type I diabetic recipients of pancreatic transplants.[231] Normalization of basal glucagon levels has also been demonstrated with renal subcapsular pancreatic islet-cell transplants in rats.[232] Prostaglandins may play a partial role in the impairment of both glucagon and epinephrine secretion in response to insulin-induced hypoglycemia.[233] The hyperglucagonemia observed with starvation is largely due to decreased catabolism rather than augmented secretion (see below). Hypoglycemia may provoke glucagon secretion by an α-adrenergic mechanism independent of insulin.[227]

Suppression of glucagon secretion occurs after the ingestion or infusion of glucose. The hypoglucagonemic effects of glucose may depend on insulin-mediated uptake of glucose by the alpha cells and/or the absence of marked hyperglycemia.[227] In diabetic patients glucose fails to inhibit glucagon secretion, but this effect is restored after insulin treatment.[228] As was noted above, somatostatin is a potent inhibitor of glucagon as well as insulin and GH secretion. In fact, the inhibitory action of somatostatin on alpha cell function has been the basis in part of its use as an adjunct in the management of insulin-dependent diabetes.[101]

Action

Although glucagon was discovered in the 1930s in crude insulin preparations as a "hyperglycemic-glycogenolytic factor," its physiologic role and mechanism of action have been elucidated only recently. Early studies were hampered by the inability to produce a pure glucagon-deficient state without concomitant insulin deficiency and the lack of data on circulating levels and secretory rates of glucagon.

It is now apparent that physiologic increments in glucagon concentration produce a rise in blood glucose concentration by stimulating hepatic glycogenolysis and gluconeogenesis (Fig. 19-32). In contrast, a fall in glucagon concentration to below basal level results in a decrease in hepatic glucose production.[234] However, when an increment in glucagon concentration is accompanied by a small (50 to 150 percent) rise in the circulating insulin concentration, hepatic glucose production remains unchanged. The latter phenomenon accounts for the importance of the bihormonal response (i.e., rise in glucagon concentration as well as insulin concentration) to the ingestion of a protein meal (Fig. 19-33). Glucagon has been shown to play a critical role in vivo in the

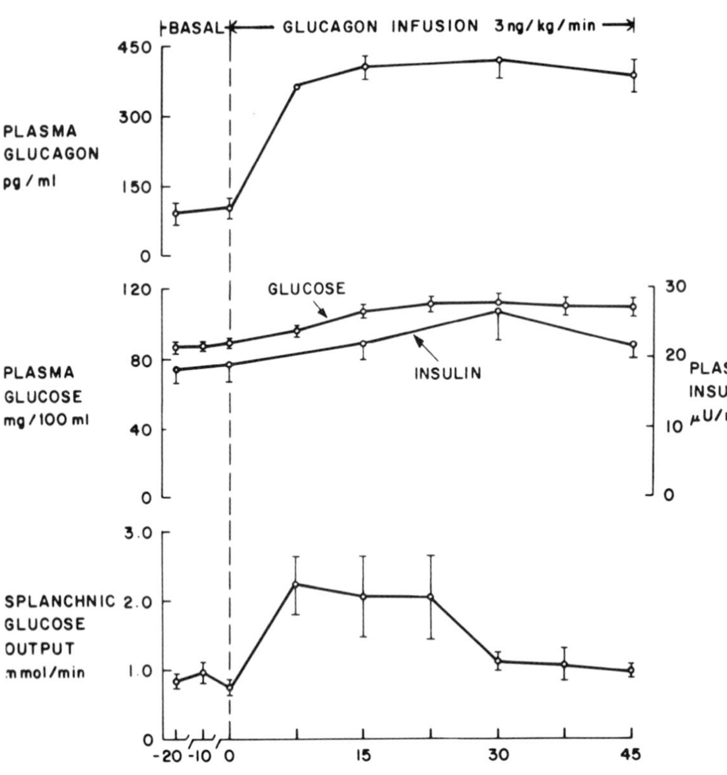

FIGURE 19-32 Stimulation by glucagon of hepatic (splanchnic) glucose production in normal humans. Physiologic hyperglucagonemia causes a prompt rise in hepatic glucose production. The effect is transient, however, lasting less than 45 min. The stimulatory action of glucagon on glucose production thus results from changes in concentrations of glucagon rather than absolute concentrations themselves. *(From Felig P et al.*[238]*)*

disposition of amino acids by increasing their inward transport, degradation, and conversion into glucose.[235] The insulin response engendered by the protein meal ensures the cellular uptake and utilization of amino acids contained in the meal. However, the rise in insulin concentration alone would inhibit hepatic glucose output, resulting in hypoglycemia. The simultaneous increase in glucagon concentration mitigates such an effect by ensuring that glucose production is maintained (Fig. 19-33). A speculation is that since mixed meals fail to alter glucagon levels (Fig. 19-20), glucagon's role in evolution may relate primarily to carnivorous populations that feed on infrequent but large protein meals.

In contrast to insulin, whose effects on various target tissues are ongoing so long as hypoglycemia does not occur, glucagon's stimulatory action on hepatic glucose production lasts only 30 to 60 min (Fig. 19-32).[225] However, once a given level of plasma glucagon concentration has been established, a further increase or decrease is followed, respectively, by a rise or fall in glucose production. Thus, hepatic glucose metabolism is influenced by *changes* in glucagon levels rather than by absolute glucagon concentration. The liver thus shows ongoing responsiveness to pulsatile alterations in circulating glucagon concentration, but the effect of any alteration is evanescent both in vivo[236] and in vitro.[237]

Because of the opposing actions of insulin and glucagon on the liver, and inasmuch as glucose sup-

FIGURE 19-33 Influence of protein feeding on plasma insulin and glucagon concentrations and on splanchnic (hepatic) glucose production in normal humans. The rise in glucagon concentration induced by protein feeding is necessary for the uptake and anabolic utilization of the amino acids contained in the protein meal. *(Based on the data of Wahren J, Felig P, Hagenfeldt, LJ: J Clin Invest 58:761, 1976.)*

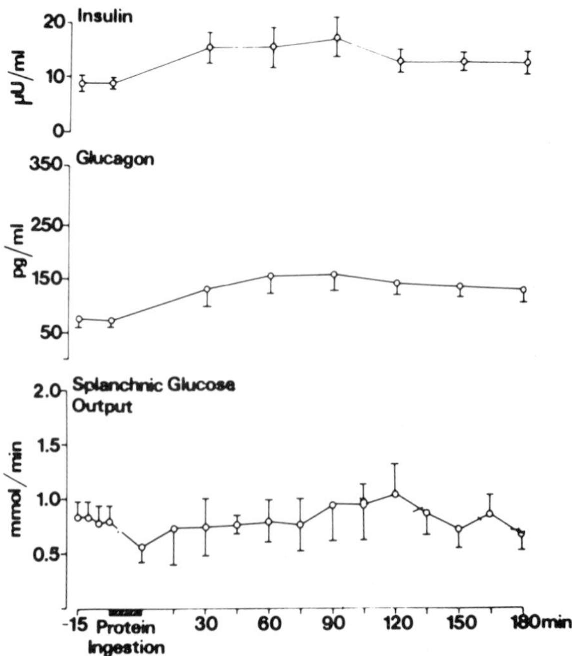

presses glucagon secretion while stimulating insulin secretion, Unger has suggested that the insulin/glucagon molar ratio (I/G) rather than the concentration of either hormone alone governs overall carbohydrate homeostasis.[227] The applicability of this bihormonal hypothesis to the intact organism has been seriously challenged in studies involving infusions of glucagon in physiologic doses.[238,239] Those studies demonstrated that high plasma glucagon levels of 300 to 400 pg/ml (comparable with those observed in a variety of hyperglucagonemic states) fail to alter glucose tolerance in normal subjects. This conclusion is supported by the finding that despite a marked fall in I/G (from 34:1 to 6:1) induced by glucagon infusion, no change in glucose tolerance occurs.[225] Glucagon-induced changes in glucose tolerance thus require an absolute deficiency of insulin, pharmacologic doses of glucagon, or in some circumstances the presence of a glucagon-producing tumor (see below). Furthermore, while glucose administration normally suppresses glucagon secretion, hypoglucagonemia is not necessary for normal glucose-disposal so long as insulin secretion is normal.[238,239]

Finally, recent in vitro data from human hepatocytes have shown that mobilization of glycogen stores is dependent on glucagon and is not due to a decline in glucose concentrations. Insulin was able to suppress both basal and glucagon-activated glycogenolysis.[240]

In addition to its action on carbohydrate metabolism, glucagon is involved in the regulation of ketogenesis. Livers obtained from rats given physiologic doses of glucagon display augmented ketone production from FFA.[40] In vivo, ketonemia may occur in the absence of glucagon, as in pancreatectomized patients.[220] However, in insulin-deficient diabetic patients, hyperglucagonemia increases the ketogenic capacity. It should be emphasized that glucagon's effects in raising blood glucose concentration and enhancing ketosis are entirely a consequence of its actions on the liver. Increases in FFA oxidation and ketogenesis result from glucagon's inhibitory effect on hepatic lipogenesis decreasing malonyl CoA availability rather than from stimulation of peripheral lipolysis.

The first step in the action of glucagon on the liver is interaction with a specific receptor on the cell membrane; this appears to be different from and somewhat simpler than signal transmission with insulin (Fig. 19-34). The structure of the glucagon receptor is not completely understood, although linkage to GTP-binding proteins and adenylate cyclase has been determined. It is not linked to tyrosine kinase as are the insulin and epidermal growth factor (EGF) receptors. If the glucagon receptor had multiple spanning regions similar to other GTP and cyclase-linked receptors, its mobility might be limited. Ligand receptor mobility is greater for insulin and EGF than for glucagon in the rat hepatocyte; this

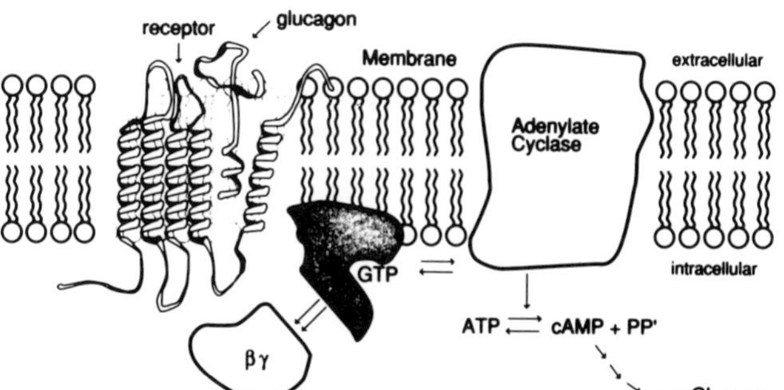

FIGURE 19-34 The glucagon-sensitive adenylate cyclase system. Glucagon interacts with its membrane-bound receptor protein in a specific topology such that the resulting complex induces the G_s protein to exchange GDP for GTP and promotes the dissociation of the α-GTP complex from the βγ subunits. Gα-GTP activates the catalytic subunit of adenylate cyclase, leading to cAMP and the cascade of events that subsequently produce a rise in blood glucose levels. (*From Unson et al.*[242])

may be due to the fact that the β subunits of the insulin and EGF receptor span the plasma membrane once and both undergo autophosphorylation.[241] It would appear that the substitution of aspartic acid in position 9 results in a reduction in transduction of the biological response which is uncoupled from binding. This may be due to interference of the electrostatic interaction involving the positively charged histidine and aspartic acid at position 9.[242] Binding to the receptor activates a coupled catalytic effector unit (E) containing the enzyme adenyl cyclase, which converts ATP to cAMP, the intracellular glucagon messenger. A GTP-dependent regulatory protein (G) mediates the cyclase activation.[243] Rodbell[244] suggested that the G protein may dissociate into smaller molecules upon the GTP and hormone activation; these molecules may serve as messengers of the hormone in addition to cAMP. At the same time the change in G protein may also transiently decrease the binding affinity of the receptor. The rise in cAMP concentration triggers several phosphorylation reactions, resulting in activation of glycogen phosphorylase and simultaneous inhibition of glycogen synthase (Fig. 19-4). Insulin antagonizes this action by reducing the activity of cAMP-dependent protein kinase[195,196] and/or augmenting the activity of phosphodiesterase responsible for cAMP degradation.[194] The glucagon-sensitive, cAMP-mediated steps in control of substrate flow toward gluconeogenesis are at the level of conversion of pyruvate to phospho*enol*pyruvate by induction of PEPCK synthesis and phosphorylation of pyruvate kinase as well as FDPase-2 (Figs. 19-5 and 19-6).

Administration of glucagon has been observed to lower serum potassium and calcium concentrations, decrease gastric acid and pancreatic enzyme secretion, raise serum GH secretion, and increase myocardial contractility. However, each of these effects requires pharmacologic doses of the hormone.

Degradation

In contrast to insulin, glucagon degradation is carried out primarily in the kidney rather than liver. As a result, plasma glucagon concentration is elevated in uremia despite the absence of hypersecretion.[225] Glucagon removal by the kidney normally exceeds the filtered load, suggesting that peritubular uptake contributes to renal clearance. A tubular catabolic mechanism has been suggested by data from isolated kidney experiments investigating ^{125}I-labeled human glucagon-like peptides 1 and 2.[245] A reduction in glucagon catabolism is also the major factor responsible for the hyperglucagonemia observed in short-term (3-day) starvation.[225] Although hyperglucagonemia is observed in cirrhosis patients, particularly when accompanied by portal hypertension, augmented secretion rather than diminished degradation is the major mechanism of the elevated plasma glucagon concentration in such patients.[246]

Catecholamines

Epinephrine and norepinephrine inhibit glucose-stimulated insulin secretion via an α-adrenergic effect. Studies in patients with cervical cord transections, however, indicate that increased rather than basal levels of plasma catecholamine concentrations and sympathetic nervous system activity are important in the regulation of basal or glucose-stimulated insulin secretion in the resting state.

Apart from altering insulin secretion, catecholamines raise the blood glucose concentration by at least five additional mechanisms: (1) activation of glycogenolysis, (2) stimulation of gluconeogenesis, (3) inhibition of insulin-mediated glucose uptake, (4) increased lipolysis, and (5) stimulation of glucagon secretion.

The glycogenolytic effect of epinephrine is considerably greater than that of norepinephrine and occurs in liver as well as muscle tissue. Since muscle lacks G6Pase, glycogen breakdown in muscle brings about a rise in blood glucose concentration via indirect mechanisms. Enhanced glycogenolysis in muscle is followed by an increase in glycolysis, resulting in the release of lactate. The lactate is transported to the liver, where it serves as a gluconeogenic substrate. The glycogenolytic effect of epinephrine in muscle tissue is mediated via β-adrenergic receptors and a rise in cAMP concentration (Fig. 19-4). However, in liver tissue glycogenolysis is not necessarily dependent on β-adrenergic receptors; it may be triggered by α-adrenergic receptors whose effects are mediated via a calcium-dependent protein kinase. In liver, epinephrine also interferes with glycogen synthesis.

In addition to stimulating glycogen breakdown, epinephrine interferes with insulin-mediated glucose uptake. A physiologic rise in plasma epinephrine concentration (500 pg/ml) results in a 60 to 90 percent fall in the rate of glucose disposal, induced by postprandial increments in plasma insulin concentration (100 μU/ml).[247] This effect is mediated via β-adrenergic receptors. The insulin-antagonistic action of epinephrine is also observed with minimal plasma elevations of epinephrine concentration (25 to 50 pg/ml), which are comparable to those accompanying a mild viral illness and are insufficient to interfere with insulin secretion.[94] The fall in glucose clearance (the rate of glucose uptake relative to the plasma glucose level) induced by epinephrine accounts for its having a substantially greater hyperglycemic effect than comparable doses of glucagon despite the fact that glucagon causes a greater rise in glucose production.[248]

Epinephrine is a potent lipolytic agent by virtue of its stimulation of cAMP-dependent lipase in adipose tissue. Decreased glucose uptake induced by epinephrine also limits the availability of glycerol 3-phosphate for reesterification.

In contrast to its inhibitory effects on insulin secretion, epinephrine stimulates the secretion of glucagon. The hyperglycemia after epinephrine administration thus represents a composite effect of two hormones; it is blunted when hyperglucagonemia is prevented by the concurrent administration of somatostatin. This effect of somatostatin persists when glucagon is given in replacement doses, suggesting that somatostatin may blunt the hepatic response to epinephrine independent of glucagon availability.[249]

The major stimuli of catecholamine secretion and augmented sympathoadrenal activity are exercise, trauma, fever, surgery, and hypoglycemia. The homeostatic responses to hypoglycemia are dependent on an intact sympathetic nervous system and are blunted in adrenalectomized patients.[250] In type I diabetes, glucagon secretion in response to hypoglycemia is attenuated. This leads to a greater dependence on catecholamines to counteract insulin-induced hypoglycemia.

Glucocorticoids

It has been recognized since the classic experiments of Long and Lukens and Houssay in the 1930s that the secretions of the adrenal cortex have a diabetogenic effect. Subsequent work has established that adrenal corticosteroids stimulate proteolysis while increasing gluconeogenesis and glycogen formation, hence the name *glucocorticoids*.

Glucocorticoids also raise blood glucose levels by decreasing the responsiveness of muscle and adipose tissue to insulin-stimulated glucose uptake. This effect of glucocorticoids is mediated at least in part by a decrease in the number of glucose transporters consequent to a reduction in transporter mRNA levels.[251] The insulin-antagonistic effect of cortisol is generally accompanied by hyperglycemia and a rise in serum insulin concentration. Thus, in Cushing's syndrome of spontaneous or iatrogenic origin, hyperinsulinemia and insulin resistance are characteristic findings. Whether such patients develop diabetes depends in part on the insulin-secretory capacity of their beta cells, which determines whether enough insulin can be released to withstand the long-lasting hyperglycemic stimulus and meet the demands of their insulin-resistant tissues.

In contrast to the insulin antagonism induced by epinephrine, which is demonstrable within minutes, the effects of glucocorticoids require hours to days to become fully manifest. This time course of action is due to selective modulations in the rates of synthesis of several enzymes and other proteins involved in the transport and metabolism of glucose.

Growth Hormone

GH decreases glucose utilization and storage while promoting the formation of tissue proteins and stimulating lipolysis. The antagonistic effects of GH on insulin-stimulated glucose uptake may be mediated by postreceptor events occurring largely in the liver.[252] In general, this action of GH results in a compensatory increase in insulin secretion so that glucose tolerance remains normal. However, if large enough increments in GH are observed either from the pituitary or by injection or if insulin secretion is impaired (e.g., a genetic tendency to diabetes), the blood glucose concentration may rise to abnormal levels or previously established diabetes may be aggravated.

During fasting, the blood glucose levels falls to strikingly lower concentrations in GH-deficient dwarfs than are observed in normal controls.[253] Growth hormone thus plays an important role in setting the basal blood glucose concentration ("glucostat" effect).

In contrast to the insulin-antagonizing effects of prolonged or repeated administration of GH, the early response to this hormone is characterized by a fall in blood glucose concentration and other insulin-like effects. This action of GH may derive from its induction of insulin-like growth factor-I.

Insulin-Like Growth Factors

Before the advent of RIA procedures, plasma insulin was bioassayed by measuring in vitro glucose uptake by rat epididymal adipose tissue or diaphragm. Subsequent determinations revealed that only ~10 percent of the total insulin-like activity measured by bioassay corresponds to true pancreatic insulin as determined by RIA. The remainder of the circulating insulin-like activity persists even after pancreatectomy or the precipitation of insulin by specific antibodies and was consequently termed nonsuppressible insulin-like activity (NSILA). NSILA has been shown to consist of two polypeptides which promote the growth of chick embryo fibroblasts (increase cell multiplication and DNA synthesis). These peptides have been termed insulin-like growth factors-I and -II (IGF-I and IGF-II) and are generically referred to as somatomedins.[254] An unexpected finding was the extensive homology between the primary structures of IGF-I and -II on the one hand and the A and B chains of insulin on the other.[255] Structural homology also exists with respect to tertiary structure, contributing to the cross-reactivity of IGFs with the insulin receptor.

In contrast to insulin, the C peptide region in circulating IGF-I and IGF-II is conserved and there is no resemblance in amino acid sequence in the C peptide region.[255]

The IGFs mimic many actions of insulin; insulin is more potent in producing metabolic effects, while the IGFs have greater growth-promoting effects (Table 19-6). IGF-II has greater insulin-like effects than does IGF-I. Two IGF plasma membrane receptors have been identified. The type I receptor has a structure homologous to the insulin receptor with α and β subunits, one responsible for hormone binding and the other undergoing tyrosine phosphorylation.[133] The type II receptor contains a single polypeptide chain and does not appear to have tyrosine kinase activity.[256] Insulin, IGF-I, and IGF-II have differing affinities for the three receptors. Insulin binds strongly to its own receptor, has a low affinity for the IGF-I receptor, and has virtually no affinity for the IGF-II receptor. The IGF-I receptor has considerably

TABLE 19-6 Properties of Insulin and Insulin-Like Growth Factors

	Source	No. Amino Acids	Mode of Secretion	Regulator(s)	Plasma Concentration, ng/ml	Plasma Carrier Protein	Half-Life	Physiologic Role
Insulin	Beta cells	51	Pulsatile	Glucose, amino acids	0.3–2.0	No	<10 min	Control of metabolism
IGF-I*	Liver	70	Constant	GH, nutrition	0.2	Yes	16 h	Skeletal and cartilage growth
IGF-II†	Diverse	67	Unknown	Unknown	0.6	Yes	Unknown	Unknown

* Also called somatomedin C.

† Also called multiplication-stimulating activity.

greater affinity for IGF-I than for IGF-II in most mammalian cells and the same affinity for both IGFs in chick cells. The IGF-II receptors preferably bind IGF-II, have a lower affinity for IGF-I, and do not bind insulin at all.

Another difference between IGFs and insulin is that IGFs are bound to specific proteins in the circulation whereas insulin is not. IGFs are bound to two proteins of ~50,000 and ~200,000 daltons; this binding provides a half-life of 4 h in the rat and 16 h in humans, in contrast to <10 min for insulin. Small amounts reach target organs in the dissociated form. Diurnal variations in IGF plasma concentrations have not been demonstrated.

In ordinary circumstances, IGF-I levels are regulated by GH. However, in disease states such as malnutrition, IGF-I deficiency occurs despite increased GH levels. Poorly regulated diabetes is also associated with relative or absolute IGF-I deficiency that is correctable with insulin therapy. Excess production of IGF-II has been implicated as the mechanism for extrapancreatic tumor hypoglycemia in some patients with mesenchymal tumors or hepatocellular carcinomas.[256]

Pancreatic Polypeptide

This 36-amino acid polypeptide originates in islet cells which are distinct from alpha, beta, and delta cells. Protein ingestion, fasting, exercise, and hyperglycemia raise the plasma levels of this polypeptide. Elevations have also been observed in diabetic patients and patients with a variety of pancreatic endocrine tumors.[257] The physiologic action of pancreatic polypeptide on nutrient metabolism has not been established.

Regulatory and Counterregulatory Hormones

The large number of hormones which influence body fuel metabolism may be categorized as favoring either the storage or the dissipation of energy. In this regard, insulin is unique because it favors the storage of each of the major body fuels (glucose, fat, and protein). In contrast, five hormones (epinephrine, glucagon, cortisol, GH, and thyroid hormone) promote the dissipation of body fat, glycogen, and/or protein. These hormones may also be classified with respect to the feedback effect of plasma glucose concentration on their secretion and in terms of their action on blood glucose concentration. Insulin is the only hormone whose secretion is influenced on a moment-to-moment basis by physiologic fluctuations in blood glucose concentration (Fig. 19-20) and which brings about a fall in the blood glucose concentration. In contrast, each of the energy-dissipating hormones (except for thyroid) causes a rise in the blood glucose concentration. Furthermore, an increase in their secretion requires either the development of frank hypoglycemia or the interposition of signals other than a change in blood glucose concentration (e.g., protein feeding, exercise, stress). Consequently, with respect to blood glucose control, insulin is generally considered the major regulatory hormone, while glucagon, catecholamines, cortisol, and GH are collectively referred to as *counterregulatory* hormones[258] (Table 19-7). The actions of the counterregulatory hormones in raising blood glucose concentration may result from coordinate effects on glycogen metabolism and/or gluconeogenesis or antagonism of insulin-mediated glucose uptake (Table 19-7).

Fuel-Hormone Interactions

The homeostasis of body fuels is dependent not only on the availability of enzymatically regulated pathways and a variety of hormonal signals but also on finely coordinated substrate-hormone interactions. These interactions are best understood by considering the changes which occur in conditions of fuel availability (the fed state), fuel need (starvation, exercise), or fuel imbalance ("stress" hyperglycemia). These perturbations, however, require an understanding of normal body composition (e.g., fuel stores) and the conditions which exist in the basal state.

Body Composition

The caloric composition of a typical American or western European diet consists of 40 to 45 percent carbohydrate, 40 percent fat, and 15 to 20 percent protein. The composition of the fuels stored in the human body is far different from that of fuels ingested in the diet (Table 19-8). Carbohydrate represents a calorically insignificant fuel store. The combined caloric value of liver glycogen (70 g), muscle glycogen (200 g), and circulating blood glucose (20 g) amounts to ~1200 kcal, well below the average caloric expenditure of a single day. Nevertheless, liver glycogen represents an important source of carbohydrate for the ongoing supply to the brain and the needs of muscle during exercise (see below). The teleologic basis of the limitation for storing carbohydrate derives not only from its low caloric density (4 kcal/g, compared with 9 kcal/g in fat) but also from the large amount of tissue water obligatory for the storage of glycogen (4 ml/g).

By far the largest reservoir of body fuel is fat, which is stored as triglyceride. In a nonobese subject, body fat amounts to ~20 percent of total body weight, representing 130,000 to 140,000 kcal and *accounting for 80 percent* of total body fuel depots. The compact nature of this large fuel depot is due to its caloric density and anhydrous nature. To store an equivalent amount of energy as carbohydrates would require more than eight times the weight of fat. The

TABLE 19-7 Regulatory and Counterregulatory Hormones in the Control of Blood Glucose Concentration

	Secretion Stimuli	Actions
Insulin	Moment-to-moment fluctuations in blood glucose concentration	↓ Blood glucose ↑ Glucose uptake ↑ Glycogen synthesis ↓ Glycogenolysis ↓ Gluconeogenesis
Counterregulatory hormones:	Frank hypoglycemia (blood glucose concentration <50 mg/dl), exercise, stress, protein feeding	↑ Blood glucose
Glucagon		↑ Glycogenolysis ↑ Gluconeogenesis
Catecholamines		↑ Glycogenolysis ↓ Glucose uptake
Cortisol		↑ Gluconeogenesis ↓ Glucose uptake
Growth hormone		↓ Glucose uptake

fat depot is sufficient to meet the caloric requirements for ~2 months. In obese subjects, fat tissue may provide for the storage of over 500,000 kcal. Regardless of the degree of adiposity, fat clearly represents the most expendable as well as the most plentiful fuel available to humans.

The major reservoir of body protein is in muscle tissue, amounting to 10 kg (exclusive of tissue water) or 40,000 kcal. Because of protein's indispensability in body structure, in muscle function, and as a catalytic agent (e.g., enzymes), loss of >50 percent of body protein is incompatible with survival despite residual mobilizable fat tissue. Death from starvation generally results not from hypoglycemia but from dissolution of protein stores: loss of respiratory muscle function leads to terminal pneumonia.

Of particular importance in considering the homeostatic response to the need for fuel is an understanding of the interchangeability of body fuels. Body protein (by virtue of its constituent amino acids other than leucine or valine) is readily converted to glucose (gluconeogenesis). Carbohydrate availabilty for glucose-dependent tissues (e.g., brain) thus does not cease with depletion of liver glycogen. In contrast, fatty acids cannot generally be converted to glucose, since mammalian tissue lacks the enzymatic capacity for net gluconeogenesis from substrates with less than three carbons, e.g., acetyl CoA. Thus, to the extent that glucose is terminally oxidized (by brain) and must be replenished by gluconeogenesis, there is an obligate dissolution of body protein stores in total starvation.

The Basal State

The basal or postabsorptive state, the condition which exists 6 to 12 h after food ingestion, represents the change from feeding to fasting. While this interval represents a nonsteady state, it is nevertheless a readily identifiable reference point with which various perturbations may be compared. In the postabsorptive condition, adipose tissue releases FFA to meet the fuel requirements of muscle and heart as well as parenchymal tissues (liver, kidney). The respiratory quotient of most muscles is close to 0.7, reflecting virtual dependence on fat oxidation. Carbohydrate utilization occurs primarily in the brain, which terminally oxidizes glucose at a rate of 50 to 100 g per day. Smaller amounts of glucose are uti-

TABLE 19-8 Body Composition and Fuel Reserves in a Normal 70-kg Human

Fuel	Tissue	Weight, kg	% Body Weight	Energy Value, kcal
Fat	Adipose tissue	11–17	15–25	100,000–150,000
Protein	Muscle (primarily)	8–12	12–17	32,000–48,000
Carbohydrate	Liver (glycogen)	0.070	<1	280
	Muscle (glycogen)	0.200	<1	800
	Blood (glucose)	0.020	<1	80

lized by resting muscle, by adipose tissue, and by obligate anaerobic tissues such as the formed elements of the blood and the renal medulla[259] (Fig. 19-35).

While several tissues contribute to glucose utilization, the production of glucose is virtually limited to the liver. Maintenance of euglycemia depends on the release of glucose from the liver at a rate equal to the combined utilization in brain and peripheral tissues (100 to 200 g per day, 2 to 2.5 mg/min per kilogram of body weight; ~75 percent of the glucose produced during an overnight fast is derived from glycogen, and the remainder is formed by gluconeogenesis from lactate, alanine, and, to a lesser extent, pyruvate and glycerol.[16] In the complete absence of hepatic glucose production, the blood glucose level would be halved in 40 to 60 min. The increased delivery of FFA to the liver results in the formation of ketone bodies. However, the rate of ketogenesis in the basal state is such that it maintains the concentration of circulating ketone acids at <0.5 m*M* only.

The hormonal signal which permits the initiation of glycogenolysis, gluconeogenesis, and ketogenesis in the basal state is the fall in plasma insulin concentration from the level observed in the fed state (30 to 100 μU/ml) to values of 10 to 200 μU/ml. Glucose utilization in the basal state is thus largely (~70 percent) non-insulin-dependent, occurring primarily in the brain. In contrast, the presence of basal insulin levels (and basal secretory rates of 0.25 to 1.5 U/h) ensures maximal efficiency in fuel economy by preventing excessive gluconeogenesis and unrestrained FFA mobilization and ketogenesis. There is an apparent "redundant regulation" of insulin secretion at low glucose levels, probably by FFA or the products of their oxidation. Thus, the rates of glucose and ketone production do not exceed the rates of glucose and ketone utilization, precluding the development of hyperglycemia and hyperketonemia. When there is no basal insulin secretion (as in type I diabetes) or if hormonal perturbations occur which interfere with basal insulin action (see Stress Hyperglycemia, below), the blood glucose and ketone concentrations rise.

Fuel Availability: The Fed State

The hormonal response to the fed state is determined in part by the nature of the ingested substrate (Table 19-9). If pure glucose is ingested, a multihormonal response ensues, involving a rise in insulin concentration and decreases in glucagon and GH concentrations. If pure protein is ingested, the multihormonal response consists of a rise in insulin as well as glucagon and GH concentrations. In contrast, when mixed meals are eaten (the usual dietary intake), only a rise in insulin level is observed. Regardless of the substrate ingested, the rise in insulin concentration is the key signal which shifts metabolism to the fed state by stimulating cellular uptake of glucose, amino acids, or both and inhibiting lipolysis. When the rise in insulin concentration is not accompanied by a rise in glucagon concentration (e.g., with

FIGURE 19-35 Glucose turnover in the postabsorptive and postprandial states. In the postabsorptive state (overnight fast, basal state), the liver is the sole site of the production of glucose by glycogenolysis (75 percent) and gluconeogenesis (25 percent). The brain is the major site of glucose utilization which is not insulin-dependent. Muscle provides gluconeogenic precursors in the form of lactate, alanine, and glutamine, while fat cells are a source of glycerol. In the postprandial state, glucose uptake is insulin-dependent and occurs in liver, muscle, and fat cells. Some of the glycogen stored in the liver is synthesized via the indirect (gluconeogenic) pathway. (*From Dineen et al.*[259])

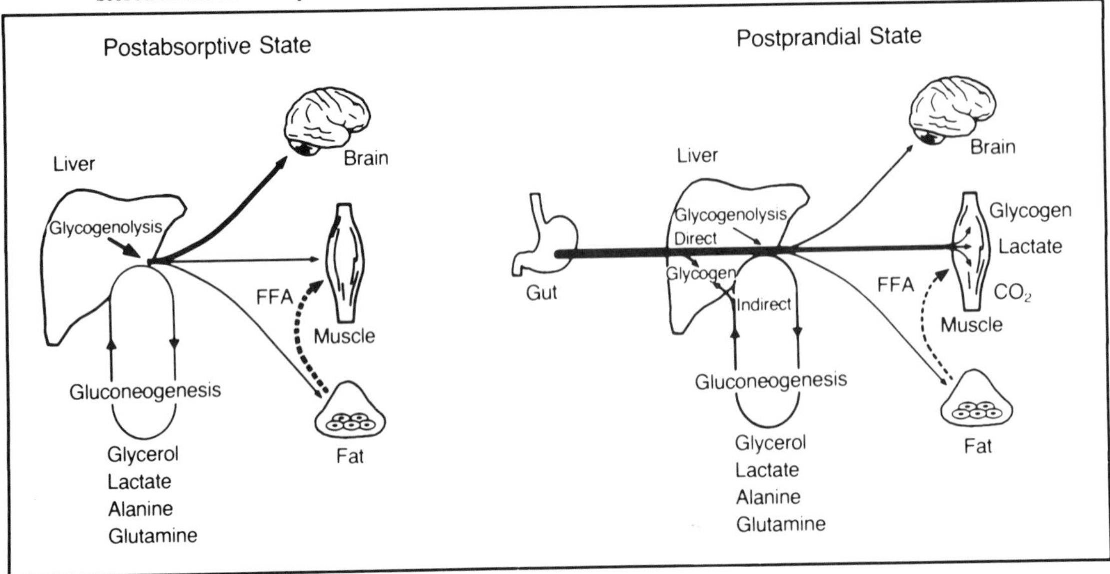

TABLE 19-9 Hormonal Response to Altered Fuel Availability or Need

Condition	Insulin	Glucagon	Growth Hormone	Epinephrine	Cortisol
Fuel availability					
Glucose ingestion	↑	↓	↓	±	±
Protein ingestion	↑	↑	↑	±	±
Mixed-meal ingestion	↑	±	±	±	±
Fuel need					
Starvation	↓	↑	↑ or ±	↑ or ±	↓
Acute hypoglycemia	↓	↑	↑	↑	↑
Exercise	↓	↑	↑	↑	↑

Abbreviations: ↑ = increased secretion; ↓ = decreased secretion; ± = unchanged.

glucose or mixed-meal ingestion), glucose output from the liver is inhibited and net hepatic uptake of glucose occurs. As was noted above (see Integration of Glycolysis and Gluconeogenesis), some hepatic gluconeogenesis may continue even during periods of net hepatic glucose storage by virtue of glycogen formation via the "indirect" (gluconeogenic) pathway[20] (Fig. 19-35). The fall in GH concentration, accompanying glucose ingestion may enhance insulin's antilipolytic effects.

When both insulin and glucagon levels rise (e.g., with protein feeding), glucose output from the liver is maintained at basal rates (Fig. 19-33). The importance of the latter derives from the fact that ingested protein cannot of itself provide for the fuel requirements of the brain. Note that feeding fails to alter abruptly the secretion of catecholamines or cortisol (Table 19-9).

Fuel Need

Starvation

If the basal state is not perturbed by the ingestion of food, the metabolic response progresses to one which characterizes starvation (starvation is considered in detail in Chap. 20). The major hormonal signals governing the fasting state are a fall in insulin concentration and, to a lesser extent, a rise in glucagon concentration. The progressive decline in insulin concentration is triggered by a small decline in blood glucose concentration but may be initiated by caloric lack per se. The hypoinsulinemia leads to an increase in lipolysis and hepatic fatty acid oxidation, resulting in a gradual increase in ketogenesis. The outflow of amino acids (particularly alanine) from muscle and the key rate-limiting enzymes involved in hepatic gluconeogenesis are stimulated. In this manner, hepatic glucose production is sustained despite the fact that liver glycogen stores are depleted within 24 h.

When starvation is prolonged for >3 weeks, the kidney, in addition to the liver, contributes to glucose production. Nevertheless, the total rate of gluconeogenesis as well as glucose utilization is markedly reduced. In this circumstance, ketones become an important substrate for the brain (replacing some glucose) and may provide the signal to muscle by which protein catabolism and alanine outflow are diminished.[260] Even some acetone may be converted to glucose, as was discussed earlier. Although growth hormone levels rise with starvation, the increment is transient and is not essential for the lipolytic or ketogenic response.

Exercise

A marked increase in fuel requirements occurs in either fed or fasted humans during muscular exercise. The major fuel consumed (carbohydrate or fat) depends on the duration as well as the intensity of the exercise performed[261] (Fig. 19-36). With very brief exercise (a run lasting only a few minutes), the major fuel consumed is muscle glycogen. With longer periods of exercise, extending to 1 to 2 h, blood-borne glucose accounts for ~40 percent of the increased fuel consumption, with the rest being provided by FFA. The rate of glucose uptake by muscle is stimulated up to 40 times the resting level, while total body glucose turnover may increase three- to fourfold. With very prolonged exercise, there is progressively less dependence on glucose and increased utilization of fat.

The stimulatory effect of exercise on glucose utilization occurs in the face of a declining insulin concentration. The multihormonal response to exercise (Table 19-9) is thus largely directed at providing a milieu which favors hepatic glycogenolysis and gluconeogenesis as well as lipolysis. The response to exercise is further discussed below (see Treatment of Diabetes).

Hypoglycemia

When the blood glucose level is suddenly lowered by the administration of insulin, there is an immediate need to restore circulating glucose levels so that brain function will not be irreversibly disturbed (see Chap. 20). The homeostatic response consists of a marked increase in the secretion of each of the counterregulatory hormones and inhibition of endogenous insulin secretion (Table 19-9). As a result,

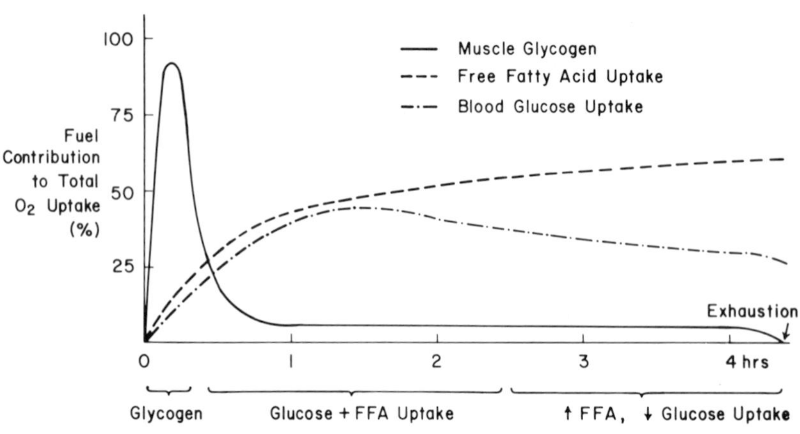

FIGURE 19-36 Pattern of fuel utilization by muscle during exercise of varying duration. During the initial few minutes of exercise, muscle glycogen is a major fuel for the production of ATP. Between 10 and 40 min of exercise, blood-borne glucose and FFA each account for 40 percent of total fuel oxidation. Thereafter (i.e., with very prolonged exercise), there is a progressive rise in the utilization of FFA and lessened uptake of blood glucose. Although muscle glycogen makes only a small contribution to fuel utilization in prolonged exercise, its total depletion is associated with the development of fatigue.

within 15 to 30 min of the bolus administration of insulin, a reversal of its inhibitory effects on hepatic glucose production is observed. The redundant nature of the counterregulatory hormone response to hypoglycemia is particularly important in diabetic patients. In such patients, the glucagon response to hypoglycemia may be blunted, increasing their dependency on catecholamines.[262] The lowered blood glucose level may of itself contribute to the reversal of insulin's action on the liver, independent of the rises in concentrations of counterregulatory hormones.[263]

Fuel-Hormone Imbalance

Stress Hyperglycemia

The hormonal response characteristic of acute fuel need (low insulin concentration and increased glucagon, catecholamine, cortisol, and GH concentrations) is occasionally observed in the absence of starvation, exercise, or hypoglycemia. In patients with various types of stress (extensive body burns, compound fractures, sepsis, etc.), high levels of counterregulatory hormones and a low plasma insulin concentration are often noted. In the absence of a stimulus for glucose utilization (e.g., exercise), such a hormonal pattern results in a rise in blood glucose concentration (*stress hyperglycemia*). This phenomenon involves overproduction as well as underutilization of glucose. It is due to synergistic interaction among the various counterregulatory hormones.[248,258] Thus, while glucagon, epinephrine, or cortisol causes only minor rises in the blood glucose concentration when elevated individually, the effect of a multihormonal response is far more than additive (Fig. 19-37). The synergism derives from the fact that while cortisol itself has little effect on glucose production, it converts the transient hepatic effect of glucagon or epinephrine to one of sustained glucose overproduction. In addition, epinephrine, by virtue of its suppressive effects on insulin secretion as well as its antagonism of insulin action, exaggerates the hyperglycemic response by decreasing glucose utilization. If insulin levels are already reduced, as in a diabetic patient, the effect of such a multihormonal response is to intensify the diabetic state.

DIABETES MELLITUS

History

The historical background of diabetes was reviewed by Mann.[264] The writings ascribed to the ancient Hindu Susruta (600 B.C.) contain what is probably the earliest recorded reference to diabetes mellitus: "When the doctor states that a man suffers from honey urine, he has declared him incurable." A more detailed clinical description, which included mention of the "melting down of the flesh into urine," excessive thirst, and increased urination, is provided in the works of Aretaeus of Cappadocia (A.D. 81–138).

With respect to the pathogenesis of diabetes, as early as 1682 Brunner noted that partial removal of a dog's pancreas made the animal drink and urinate copiously. A causal relation between human diabetes and lesions in the pancreas was suggested by Lancereaux in 1877 on the basis of studies in two patients. It remained, however, for Minkowski to demonstrate definitively in 1899 that pancreatic extirpation could produce diabetes. The histologic studies of Opie in 1901 suggested that the pancreatic lesion responsible for human diabetes is located in the islets of Langerhans. In 1920, Moses Barron hypothesized that the islets secrete a hormone which regulates carbohydrate metabolism. Finally, in December 1921, Banting and Best presented their findings that injection of an extract of pancreatic tissue obtained 6 to 8 weeks after ligation of the pancreatic duct resulted in reversal of the hyperglycemia and glucosuria of diabetic animals.

Definition and Classification

Diabetes mellitus is a chronic disorder of metabolism caused by an absolute or relative lack of insulin. It is

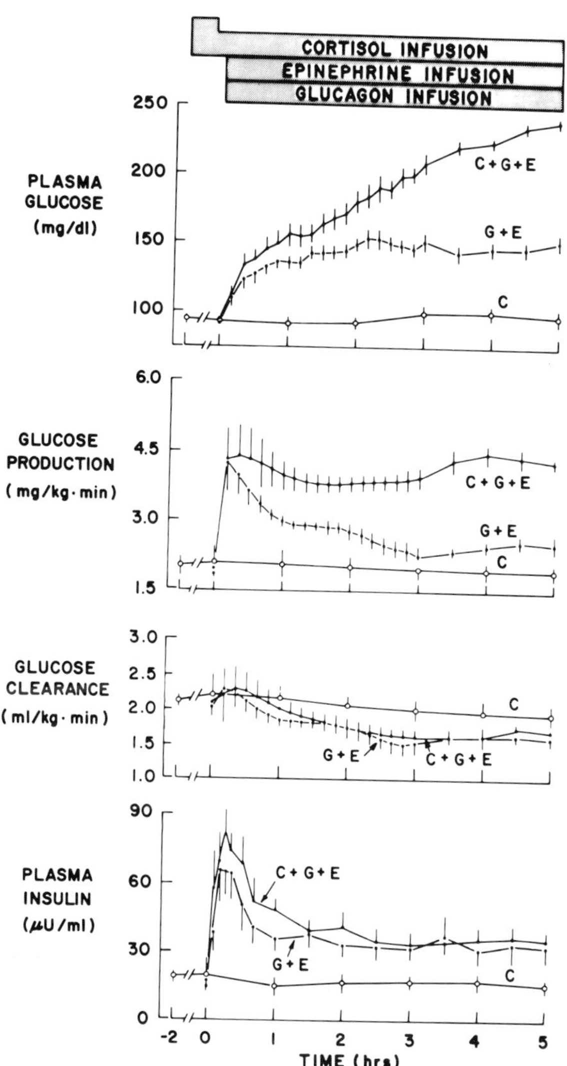

FIGURE 19-37 The synergistic effects of cortisol (C), glucagon (G), and epinephrine (E) in raising plasma glucose concentration, stimulating glucose production, and reducing glucose clearance. The hyperglycemic response to the triple hormone infusion (C + G + E) is far greater than the additive response to all three hormones given singly or the response to any combination of two hormones given together plus one hormone given singly. The development of "stress" hyperglycemia is a consequence of this hormonal synergism, which also includes GH. (*From Eigler et al.*[248])

characterized by hyperglycemia in the postprandial and/or fasting state, and in its most florid forms is accompanied by ketosis and protein wasting. When present for prolonged periods, the disease is complicated by the development of small-vessel disease (*microangiopathy*) involving particularly the retina and renal glomerulus, neuropathy, and accelerated atherosclerosis. Clinically, diabetes mellitus may vary from an asymptomatic disorder detected on the basis of an abnormal blood glucose level determined during a routine examination to a fulminant, potentially catastrophic condition in which there is shock and/or coma (e.g., DKA).

Diabetes had long been classified on the basis of specific clinical features (age of onset, insulin dependence) into two major types: juvenile-onset and maturity-onset diabetes. The large overlap of age of onset among insulin-dependent and non-insulin-dependent diabetic patients indicates that descriptive terms based solely on age of onset, though time-honored, are often inaccurate. Studies on the role of genetic and acquired factors in the etiology of diabetes indicate that primary diabetes is not a single disorder but a syndrome which is heterogeneous with respect to etiology as well as pathogenesis. These findings suggest that potential etiologic factors such as the presence of islet-cell antibodies and specific HLA (histocompatibility) haplotypes (see below) should be considered in the classification process. According to the classification recommended by the National Institutes of Health (NIH), five major diagnostic groups are recognized: spontaneous diabetes, either insulin-dependent or non-insulin-dependent; secondary diabetes; impaired glucose tolerance; and gestational diabetes (Table 19-10).

In over 90 percent of cases diabetes is a spontaneous disorder which cannot be ascribed to another, more primary disease process. Two major types of spontaneous diabetes are recognized: type I, or insulin-dependent, diabetes (formerly called juvenile-onset diabetes) and type II, or non-insulin-dependent,

TABLE 19-10 Classification of Diabetes Mellitus

Spontaneous diabetes mellitus
- Type I (insulin-dependent) diabetes (IDDM) (formerly called juvenile-onset diabetes)
- Type II (non-insulin-dependent) diabetes (NIDDM) (formerly called maturity-onset diabetes)

Secondary diabetes
- Pancreatic disease (pancreoprival diabetes, e.g., due to pancreatectomy, pancreatic insufficiency, hemochromatosis)
- Hormonal: excess secretion of counterregulatory hormones (e.g., acromegaly, Cushing's syndrome, pheochromocytoma)
- Drug-induced (e.g., potassium-losing diuretics, contrainsulin hormones, psychoactive agents, phenytoin)
- Associated with complex genetic syndromes (e.g., ataxia telangiectasia, Lawrence-Moon-Biedl syndrome, myotonic dystrophy, Friedreich's ataxia)

Impaired glucose tolerance (formerly called chemical diabetes, asymptomatic diabetes, latent diabetes, and subclinical diabetes): fasting plasma glucose concentration normal; 2-h value on glucose tolerance test >140 mg/dl but <200 mg/dl

Gestational diabetes: transient glucose intolerance which has its onset in pregnancy

Source: National Diabetes Data Group: *Diabetes* 28:1039, 1979.

diabetes (formerly called maturity-onset diabetes). The contrasting clinical, genetic, and immunologic characteristics of these two types of diabetes are summarized in Table 19-11. Insulin-dependent diabetes mellitus (IDDM) is characterized by an absolute requirement for insulin treatment, a marked tendency to ketosis, onset generally but not exclusively below age 40, absence in most patients of obesity and presence in 80 percent or more of patients of circulating islet-cell antibodies at the time of diagnosis. Non-insulin-dependent diabetes mellitus (NIDDM) generally appears after age 40, does not lead to ketosis, and often (but not always) does not require treatment with insulin; in 80 percent of cases the patients are obese and circulating islet-cell antibodies are not present. Even when insulin treatment is required in NIDDM, it is necessary not for the prevention of ketosis, as in IDDM, but for the management of hyperglycemia that is unresponsive to diet and oral hypoglycemic drugs. Fajans has called attention to a form of insulin-independent diabetes which he has designated maturity-onset diabetes of young people (MODY).[265] In this form of diabetes there is neither ketosis nor insulin dependence, but asymptomatic hyperglycemia is observed in children, adolescents, and young adults and is associated with autosomal dominant transmission. MODY-type diabetes is of particular interest with respect to its autosomal dominant mode of transmission. A gene responsible for MODY has been mapped to the long arm of chromosome 20 in a large American pedigree.[266] In addition, in a French pedigree, linkage has been observed between MODY and the locus on chromosome 7p that governs the expression of the enzyme glucokinase.[267] As noted above (see Glucose Transport and Glucose Phosphorylation), glucokinase, together with the GLUT-2 transporter, is believed to function as the glucose sensor that regulates insulin secretion by beta cells.

In clinical practice, occasional diabetic patients are observed who do not neatly fit into the type I or type II categories. For example, some patients may have experienced diabetic ketoacidosis yet are subsequently manageable with an oral hypoglycemic agent. Such cases are occasionally described as "type 1½ diabetes." Regardless of the type of spontaneous diabetes, there is a progressive increase in vascular and neuropathic complications as the disease continues.

Secondary diabetes (accounting for <5 percent of all cases) is that form of the disease which occurs in patients with primary pancreatic disease or hypersecretion of hormones antagonistic to insulin, after the administration of drugs which interfere with carbohydrate metabolism, or in association with complex genetic syndromes in whch hyperglycemia is a characteristic feature (Table 19-10). The clinical spectrum of these secondary forms of diabetes is quite variable, and an association with long-term complications may be more difficult to establish.

Those patients in whom an abnormality in carbohydrate homeostatis is demonstrable only on the basis of the findings on a glucose tolerance test (i.e., the fasting plasma glucose concentration is normal) and in whom the elevation in plasma glucose concentration at the 2-h point in the test is <200 but >140 mg/dl (<11.1 but >7.8 m*M*) are classified as having *impaired glucose tolerance* rather than overt diabetes. The basis for this separate classification (rather than inclusion in type II diabetes) is the observation that overt diabetes develops in such patients at a rate of only 1 to 5 percent per year and that such impairment in glucose tolerance in the absence of overt diabetes may not be associated with an increased risk of long-term microangiopathic and neuropathic complications. The criteria for the diagnosis of overt diabetes and impaired glucose tolerance are further discussed below (see Diagnosis). When im-

TABLE 19-11 Clinical, Genetic, and Immunologic Characteristics of Insulin-Dependent and Non-Insulin-Dependent Diabetes

	Insulin-Dependent Diabetes (Type I)*	Non-Insulin-Dependent Diabetes (Type II)†
Age of onset	Usually <30	Usually >40
Ketosis	Common	Rare
Body weight	Nonobese	Obese (80% of patients)
Prevalence	0.5%	4–5%
Genetics	HLA-associated; 25–35% concordance rate in twins	Non-HLA-associated; 95–100% concordance rate in twins
Circulating islet-cell antibodies	65–85%	<10%
Treatment with insulin	Necessary	Usually not required
Complications	Frequent	Frequent

* Formerly "juvenile-onset" diabetes.

† Formerly "maturity-onset" diabetes.

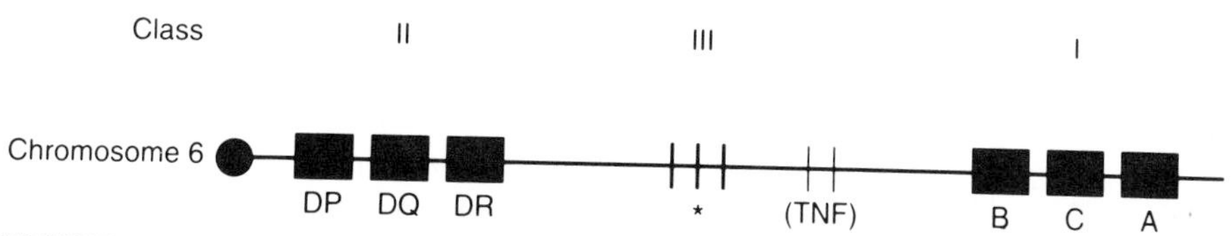

FIGURE 19-38 The human HLA complex gene regions on chromosome 6. The class I region contains genes for the HLA-A, HLA-B, and HLA-C antigens. The class II antigens include HLA-*DP*, *-DQ*, and *-DR* alleles. The class III region contains genes for the classic (C2, C4A, and C4B) and alternative (factor B) complement pathways, as indicated by the asterisk. Between the class III and the HLA-B regions are the genes for tumor necrosis factor (TNF). (*From Claman HN: JAMA 268:2790, 1992.*)

paired glucose tolerance or overt diabetes first appears in pregnancy, it is referred to as *gestational diabetes* (see Pregnancy and Diabetes, below).

Etiology

No single causative factor has been identified as the basis of the etiology of spontaneous diabetes. Increasing evidence has accumulated which indicates that diabetes is a heterogeneous group of disorders with varying etiologies. The major factors which have been identifed are inheritance, viral infections, autoimmunity, and nutrition.[268,269]

Genetics

A familial clustering of diabetes has long been recognized. In large population surveys, the prevalence of the disease among relatives of diabetic patients has been reported to be 4 to 10 times greater than in control subjects. In addition, diabetes may occur with unusually high frequency in certain ethnic groups (e.g., type II diabetes in the Pima group of Native Americans) or may occur infrequently in certain populations (e.g., type I diabetes is less common in the Japanese and in African blacks than it is in Europeans). Such aggregation may, however, reflect common environmental factors (e.g., diet) rather than inheritance. More compelling evidence for genetic transmission is provided by twin studies. Among monozygotic twins, the concordance rate for diabetes (whether type I or type II) is substantially greater than it is in dizygotic twins.[270] While inheritance is an important etiologic factor in both types of diabetes, the genetic basis of type I diabetes is clearly different from that of type II diabetes. When monozygotic twin pairs are segregated on the basis of age of onset of diabetes, a concordance rate of 92 percent is found among those in whom diabetes began at age 40 or more in the index twin, while the concordance rate is <50 percent when diabetes was diagnosed in the index twin before age 40.[271] The different concordance rate not only indicates a distinction between type I and type II diabetes with regard to genetic input but also suggests a relatively greater role for environmental (i.e., acquired) factors in the development of type I diabetes. That the two major types of diabetes have different genetic inputs is also indicated by the fact that the prevalence of type II diabetes in the ancestors of type I diabetic patients is no greater than it is in the families of nondiabetic individuals.

A second line of evidence indicating genetic differences between type I and type II diabetes patients derives from studies showing an association between specific HLA antigens and predisposition to type I diabetes but no association between HLA antigens and type II diabetes.[269,272] The HLA (human leukocyte antigen) system constitutes part of the major histocompatibility complex (MHC) located on the short arm of the sixth chromosome. The gene products of MHC include not only the HLA but also the C2 and C4 components of the complement system (also referred to as class III genes) and other proteins such as the adrenal enzyme 21-hydroxylase. The HLA region of the MHC is divided into loci designated as A, B, C, and D (Fig. 19-38). The alleles at the A, B, and C loci are described as class I genes and encode for single-chain glycoproteins expressed as surface antigens on all nucleated cells. The HLA-D region encodes for class II antigens [also referred to as Ia (immune-associated) or Ir (immune response) molecules], which are polymorphic dimers, each containing an A chain and a B chain. These antigens may be expressed on a variety of cells, particularly in response to various stimuli. Within the *D* region of the HLA complex, at least three loci (*DR, DP, DQ*) have been identified, at each of which several alleles have been identified. Among type I diabetic patients a significantly increased frequency of HLA antigens B8 and B15 was initially recognized. Subsequent studies demonstrated that the association with the B locus is secondary, the primary association being with the DR (D-related) locus, specifically the *DR3* and *DR4* alleles. The presence of one of the haplotypes increases the relative risk for type I diabetes five- to sixfold and 14-fold when both alleles (*DR3* and *DR4*) are present (Table 19-12). In fact, 90 percent or more of patients with newly detected type I diabetes carry either or both alleles.[272] Interestingly, the presence of the *DR2* or *DR7* allele appears to confer some protection against the development of type I diabetes. There is evidence that alleles at the

TABLE 19-12 Risk of Type I Diabetes for Various HLA Phenotypes Relative to the General Population

DR3	DR4	DR3 + DR4	DR2	DR7
5.0	6.8	14.3	0.1	0.1

Source: Wolf et al.: *Diabetologia* 24:224, 1983.

DQ locus may be even more tightly linked to susceptibility to type I diabetes than are those at the DR locus.[272] The absence or presence of an aspartate residue at the 57 position in the B chain of DQ antigens may be particularly important in determining increased susceptibility (asparate absent) or protection (aspartate present) with respect to the development of type I diabetes.

Concerning their role in the pathogenesis of diabetes, the various HLA alleles may not of themselves be responsible for the predisposition to diabetes; they appear to exist in linkage disequilibrium with other genes that are more directly related to diabetes susceptibility. The linkage of the HLA system to the specific immune response genes has raised the possibility that the diabetic genotype operates by permitting the interaction of a virus or other environmental insult (see below) with specific antigens on the beta cell membrane. It has also been postulated that viral infection or other environmental agents may trigger the expression of Type II HLA molecules (*DR* or *DQ* alleles) on endocrine epithelial cells, which may allow presentation of autoantigens to T cells, followed (in genetically predisposed individuals) by activation of autoreactive immunocytes.[269,272] (See Autoimmunity, below).

The discovery of the HLA population associations with type I diabetes has thus far failed to provide a clear-cut understanding regarding the mode of inheritance of this disorder. The relative rarity of type I diabetes in the siblings, parents, and offspring of affected patients (Table 19-13)[272] provides strong evidence against autosomal dominant transmission. Other modes of inheritance (e.g., autosomal recessive with two alleles, one normal and one diabetogenic) and more complex modes (e.g., two or more diabetogenic alleles in linkage disequilibrium with *DR3* and *DR4*, respectively, or multiple loci) have been suggested.[272] The preponderant evidence does not support simple autosomal inheritance via a single gene linked to HLA but favors two or more genes. First, the susceptibility to diabetes is substantially greater in *DR3DR4* heterozygotes than in *DR3DR3* and *DR4DR4* homozygotes or when either allele is present alone. Also, *DR3DR4* heterozygotes are twice as common in identical twin pairs concordant for type I diabetes as in identical twin pairs discordant for type I; in contrast, *DR3* or *DR4* homozygotes are not more common in concordant than in discordant pairs.

It has been postulated that a *DR3*-associated allele confers an autosomal recessive risk for type I diabetes while the *DR4* allele exists in linkage disequilibrium with a dominant disease form.[272] The synergism between these distinct genetic mechanisms results in the excessive risk observed in *DR3DR4* heterozygotes. An alternative proposal is that an additional non-HLA-linked gene or genes on loci other than the short arm of chromosome 6 influences susceptibility to type I diabetes. The far greater concordance rate for type I diabetes in identical twins (35 to 50 percent) compared with haploidentical nonidentical siblings underscores the importance of non-HLA-linked loci. Such a gene has not been identified in human IDDM, although recent interest has focused on genes on chromosome 11p near the insulin–IGF-II gene.[273] Regardless of the mode of inheritance, it is noteworthy that the risk of transmission of susceptibility to type I diabetes is far greater from an affected father (6 percent) than from an affected mother (1 percent) (Table 19-13).

In addition to genetic heterogeneity of type I diabetes as reflected by two or more susceptibility genes, phenotypic heterogeneity with respect to clinical, epidemiologic, and immunologic factors has also been suggested to exist. There is some evidence that type I diabetes in patients with the *DR4* haplotype may be clinically more severe at the time of onset and that *DR4* patients more often have a history of viral infection and are more apt to have raised antibody titers against Coxsackie B viruses. In contrast, *DR3* homozygotes are more likely to have associated autoimmune endocrinopathies (e.g., autoimmune thyroiditis, adrenal insufficiency). Determining HLA haplotype is not clinically useful in predicting susceptibility to the complications of diabetes.

The mode of inheritance in type II diabetes is also complex. Simple recessive inheritance is unlikely since only 30 to 50 percent of the offspring of two diabetic parents develop the disease. Incomplete penetrance cannot be invoked as the explanation of this phenomenon inasmuch as virtually 100 percent concordance rates are observed among homozygotic

TABLE 19-13 Familial Risk of Type I Diabetes Mellitus (IDDM)

Relation to Affected Patient	Risk for IDDM, %
Sibling	5–6
Identical twin	35–50
HLA identical	15
HLA haploidentical	5
HLA nonidentical	1
Parent	3
Offspring	
Affected father	6
Affected mother	1
General population	0.4–0.5

Source: Modified from Muir, Schatz, and Maclaren, 1992.[272]

twin pairs with type II diabetes (see above). Thus, it is likely that the transmission of type II diabetes is polygenic.

Attempts to identify specific genetic defects that cause type II diabetes have delineated specific mutations in only a small number of such patients.[274] Studies on the pathogenesis of type II diabetes indicating abnormalities in muscle glucose uptake, hepatic glucose production, and insulin secretion (see Pathogenesis, below) have focused on various candidate genes regulating these cellular functions. Mutant insulins and a variety of mutations in the insulin receptor have been identified in individual families with extreme hyperinsulinemia and severe insulin resistance, respectively. In contrast, in the vast majority of patients with type II diabetes, mutations have not been observed in the genes regulating the synthesis of the insulin molecule, the insulin receptor, the insulin-stimulated glucose transporter (GLUT-4) found in muscle cells, or the GLUT-2 transporter and glucokinase (which together function as the glucose sensor on beta cells). In contrast, polymorphism in the glycogen synthase gene has been observed in a Finnish population. A specific allele (*A2*) has been identified in 30 percent of type II patients compared with 8 percent of normal subjects.[275] Nevertheless, patients with the *A2* allele had normal amounts of glycogen synthase on muscle biopsy and accounted for a minority of the total population of type II patients. Thus, polymorphism of the gene for glycogen synthase may be important as a genetic marker for a subgroup of patients with type II diabetes than as a mechanism of insulin resistance.[275]

Studies examining the inheritance pattern of MODY[266] provide evidence for genetic transmission which differs from that observed in type I diabetes or the more typical adult-onset type II diabetes. In the families of MODY patients several features point to autosomal dominant inheritance: (1) There is vertical transmission of diabetes through three generations in almost half the families, (2) 85 percent of affected patients have an affected parent, and (3) one-half of the siblings are diabetic. As was noted above, a gene responsible for MODY has been mapped to the long arm of chromosome 20 in a large American pedigree.[266] In a French pedigree, linkage between MODY and the locus on chromosome 7p governing expression of the enzyme glucokinase has been reported.[267]

In summary, genetic factors contribute to the development of all clinical forms of spontaneous diabetes, but the mode of inheritance is distinct for each type. In MODY patients an autosomal dominant pattern involving mutations in glucokinase has been identified. In type I and type II patients complex patterns of inheritance have been determined, but it is clear that environmental factors are of great importance in type I diabetes. Furthermore, the inherited susceptibility for type I but not type II diabetes is linked to the HLA system; it is likely to involve at least two diabetogenic alleles and probably several loci, including one or more genes which are not HLA-linked.[269,272]

Environmental Factors in Type I Diabetes

The high frequency (50 to 65 percent) with which type I diabetes occurs in one member of a monozygotic twin pair but not in the other indicates a strong role for nongenetic, acquired factors in the etiology of type I diabetes. Among potential environmental causes, viral infections, toxins, and dietary constituents, particularly in early life, have been implicated.[276]

The histologic appearance of the islets in patients dying with type I diabetes is characterized by infiltration with mononuclear cells, particularly lymphocytes, and degeneration of islet cells (Fig. 19-39). The presence of this inflammatory response, termed *insulitis*, is compatible with a viral and/or autoimmune process. Further circumstantial evidence for a viral etiology is provided by the seasonal variation in the onset of type I diabetes; the peak incidence occurs in late summer or winter, and few cases appear in spring or early summer.

Mumps, rubella, Coxsackie B, and mengo- and encephalomyocarditis (EMC) virus have been implicated as possible etiologic agents. Diabetes has been observed in the congenital rubella syndrome with a frequency as high as 20 percent. However, it is noteworthy that in the decade after the institution of immunization against measles, mumps, rubella, and poliovirus, neither the incidence nor the age of onset of type I diabetes changed significantly in the United States. Coxsackievirus B4 was initially implicated on the basis of high titers of neutralizing antibodies in the sera of patients at the onset of diabetes. Subsequent studies demonstrated that mumps virus as well as Coxsackieviruses B3 and B4 were capable of replicating in human pancreatic beta cells maintained in cell culture. Furthermore, repeated passage of Coxsackievirus B4 in mouse beta cell cultures led to isolation of a diabetogenic strain which produced hyperglycemia when injected into intact mice. In contrast, case-control studies of antibodies to Coxsackievirus B antibodies have failed to show consistent evidence of an association with type I diabetes. The most convincing evidence for a viral etiology in some cases of type I diabetes is provided by reports of isolation of Coxsackievirus from islet tissue of infants or children with fatal diabetes; the virus isolated caused diabetes upon inoculation of mice.[277]

It is likely that overwhelming infection with a virus resulting in acute extensive beta cell destruction is only rarely the proximate cause of type I diabetes. In the vast majority of type I patients, beta cell destruction is initiated years before the clinical expression of the disease[268] (see Prediction and Preven-

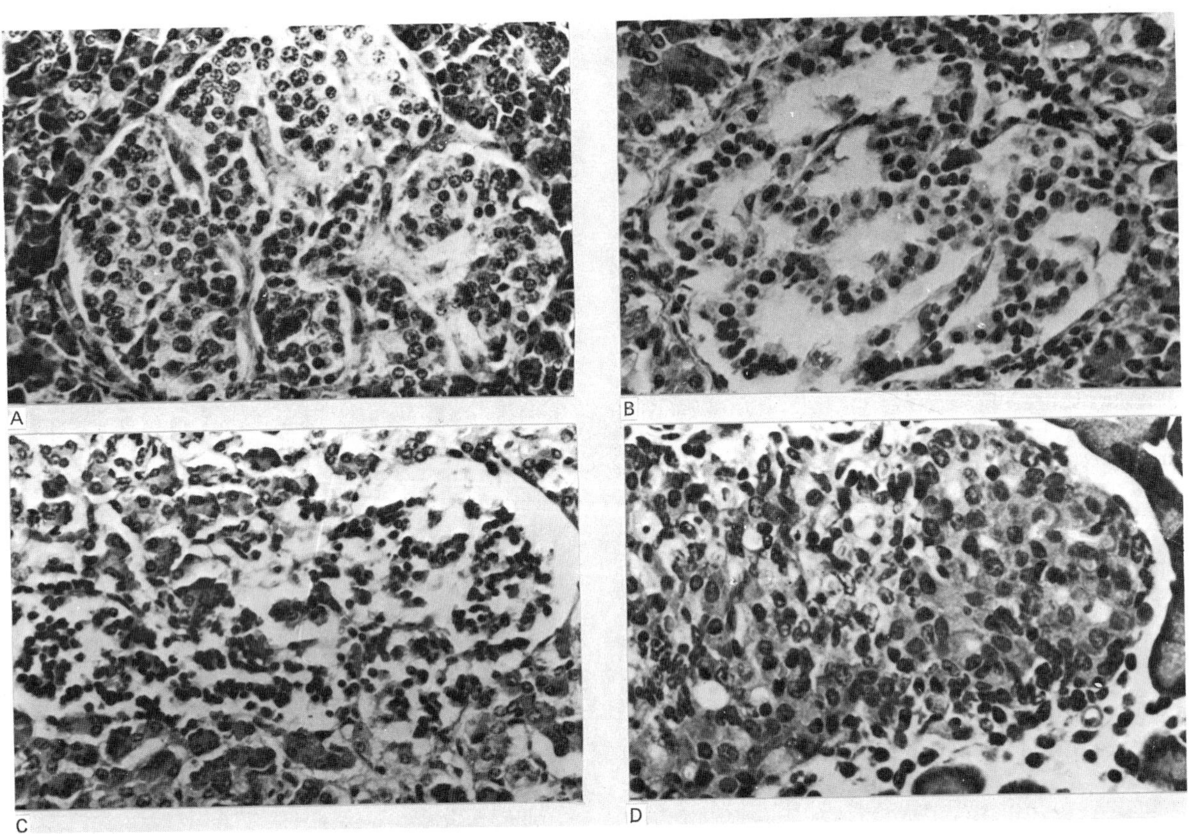

FIGURE 19-39 Insulitis in islet cells of a fatal case of virus-induced human diabetes. (*A*) Normal human pancreas with a single islet of Langerhans. Sections of pancreas from the patient (*B*) show moderate accumulation of inflammatory cells at the periphery of the islet and (*C*) an extensive inflammatory infiltrate with loss of normal islet architecture and islet-cell degeneration. (*D*) Section of pancreas from a mouse 7 days after infection with the human isolate, showing inflammatory cells and marked islet-cell degeneration. (*From Yoon et al.*[277])

tion, below). Thus, viral infections may play a role in the etiology of diabetes by triggering autoimmune-mediated destruction of beta cells in genetically predisposed individuals.[278] The mechanism of such viral triggering may involve the systemic release of various cytokines, including interferon-γ. The cytokines induce the expression of specific antigens (e.g., the 64-kDa antigen glutamic acid decarboxylase) on the surface of beta cells, thus exposing some of these cells to immune destruction. In addition, homology has been observed between amino acid sequences in the Coxsackievirus and glutamic acid decarboxylase (GAD) expressed in islet cells.[279] Antibodies induced by and directed at the Coxsackievirus may therefore induce islet-cell destruction via molecular mimickry.[279] Repeated, seemingly innocuous viral infections in a genetically predisposed host thus may result in sufficient immune-mediated beta cell destruction to result in clinically manifest type I diabetes.

Dietary constituents have also been implicated in the etiology of type I diabetes via direct toxic effects and/or via autoimmune mechanisms. In Iceland, ingestion of cured mutton containing *N*-nitroso compounds by mothers at the time of conception may play a role in the etiology of type I diabetes in their offspring. Ingestion in infancy of a more universally prevalent dietary constituent, *cow's milk*, has also been suggested as a possible triggering factor.[280] In genetically diabetes-prone rodents (BB rat), diabetes can be prevented by rearing offspring on a diet free of cow's milk. In humans, exclusive breast-feeding with delayed exposure to infant formula based on cow's milk reduced the risk of diabetes in Finnish children. The specific factor that has been incriminated in cow's milk is the whey protein bovine serum albumin (BSA), and an albumin peptide containing 17 amino acids (ABBOS) may be the reactive epitope. In newly discovered type I diabetes an elevation in anti-BSA antibodies has been observed, the bulk of which were specific for ABBOS.[280] Anti-ABBOS antibodies have also been shown to cross-react with a 69-kDa beta cell protein. It has been postulated that neonatal exposure to cow's milk in a genetically susceptible host establishes immune memory for ABBOS. Subsequent viral-induced expression of cross-reactive antigens on beta cells (e.g., 69-kDa antigen) may result in immune-mediated destruction of these cells by triggering anti-ABBOS antibody production. Thus, the cow's milk hypothesis allows for the interaction of genetic, viral, and early-life dietary factors in the etiology of type I diabetes. The data are not, however, sufficiently conclusive at this time to warrant recommending the elimination of cow's milk from the diets of infants considered to be at risk for type I diabetes.[276]

An additional environmental agent which has been implicated as a causative factor in the development of diabetes is the rodenticide pyriminil (Vacor), a nitrophenylurea derivative. Over 20 cases of insulin-dependent diabetes have been reported after the accidental ingestion of this poison. These observations are significant in that they raise the possibility that other chemicals in the environment may act as diabetogenic agents.

Autoimmunity in Type I Diabetes

The possibility that an autoimmune process is involved in the development of type I diabetes is indicated on the basis of several lines of evidence from human and animal studies:[268,269,272] (1) the presence of mononuclear cell infiltrates in the islets of newly discovered type I diabetes (insulitis), (2) the long-recognized clinical association of diabetes with autoimmune endocrinopathies (Addison's disease, Schmidt's syndrome, Graves' disease) and nonendocrine autoimmune disorders (myasthenia gravis, pernicious anemia), (3) the relation between diabetes and the HLA complex (see above), (4) the presence of circulating islet-cell antibodies (ICA) in newly discovered diabetic patients, and (5) the demonstration that intervention with cyclosporin A, a potent nonmyelotoxic immunosuppressant, may induce a remission in patients with newly discovered type I diabetes.[281,282]

Using immunofluorescent and/or complement-fixing techniques, ICA directed against cytoplasmic antigens have been detected in 60 to 98 percent of type I diabetic patients at the time of diagnosis; the percentage of patients with antibodies declines thereafter to only 20 percent after 3 years. By contrast, ICA were found in <10 percent of type II diabetic subjects and in only ~1 percent of the normal population. These antibodies are of the IgG class and are organ-specific, reacting with all types of islet cells. These antibodies are not directed at the islet hormones (insulin or glucagon) but at islet glycolipids and gangliosides. ICA directed at beta cell surface antigens [islet-cell surface antibodies (ICSA)] have also been observed in patients with newly detected type I diabetes. A cytotoxic effect on beta cells is generally demonstrable with ICSA but not with cytoplasmic ICA. Whereas the presence of these antibodies is usually a transient phenomenon closely related to the time of onset of diabetes, in patients with associated autoimmune polyendocrinopathy (Schmidt's syndrome), the antibody titer may remain persistently elevated.

More recently, an antibody directed at a 64-kDa islet-cell protein has been identified in new-onset type I diabetes and in healthy individuals years before the appearance of clinically overt type I diabetes.[268,269,272] The antigenic target of this antibody has been identified as GAD, the rate-limiting enzyme for the synthesis of the neurotransmitter γ-aminobutyric acid (GABA). Homology has been observed between the amino acid structure of GAD and the Coxsackie virus, which has been implicated in the pathogenesis of type I diabetes (see Environmental Factors, above). These findings raise the possibility that infection with Coxsackie virus in a susceptible host may trigger autoimmune destruction of islet cells by initiating the production of antibodies which, via molecular mimickry, react against islet GAD.[279]

In addition to islet-cell antibodies, insulin autoantibodies (IAA) are observed in 20 to 60 percent of type I patients at diagnosis and before the initiation of insulin treatment. IAA are often detectable before the appearance of overt diabetes and, together with ICA and anti-GAD antibody, may be useful in the prediction of type I diabetes among first-degree relatives of diabetic patients (see Prediction and Prevention of Diabetes, below).

Antipancreatic cell-mediated autoimmunity has also been described in type I diabetes on the basis of the leukocyte migration inhibition test. In 50 to 65 percent of patients, migration of leukocytes was inhibited when they were incubated with porcine or human pancreatic homogenates. Lymphocytes from diabetic patients have also been observed to lyse cultured human insulinoma cells. Alterations in the expression of adhesion molecules on monocytes have also been observed in new-onset diabetic patients.

The precise pathogenic role of ICA, anti-GAD antibodies, and cell-mediated immunity in the development of type I diabetes has not been established. Whether these autoimmune phenomena are primary events, secondary effects of beta cell damage due to another cause, or mediators of the histopathologic interactions between a genetically predisposed beta cell and some environmental agent (e.g., a virus) remains to be determined. Evidence for a pathogenic role in inducing diabetes derives from the observation that the appearance of anti-GAD antibodies and ICA precedes rather than follows the appearance of type I diabetes. A linear correlation between loss of beta cell function and elevated ICA titer was found.[283] However, first-degree relatives of individuals with type I diabetes may show transient increases in ICA titer and yet retain normal glucose tolerance. Furthermore, in the general population (as opposed to the relatives of diabetic patients), ICA have limited value in predicting diabetes.[284]

Perhaps the most compelling evidence for the autoimmune etiology of human type I diabetes derives from studies with cyclosporine Stiller et al.[281] and others[282] have shown that when initiated within a few weeks of the clinical onset of type I diabetes, treatment with cyclosporine induces a significantly higher rate of remission than treatment with placebo (18 to 24 percent vs. 0 to 10 percent after 12 months of cyclosporine administration).[282] These findings raise hopes for even greater success of immunosuppressive intervention during the "silent" prediabetic period, when the beta cell mass is not yet extensively destroyed (see Prediction and Prevention, below). The nephrotoxicity of long-term cyclosporine therapy precludes its use for the routine management of new-onset type I diabetes.

Obesity and Nutrition in Type II Diabetes

In contrast to viral and autoimmune agents implicated as potential etiologic factors in type I diabetes, obesity is the most important acquired factor that contributes to the development of the type II disorder. The prevalence of obesity among type II diabetic patients is >80 percent. Conversely, in the obese population the prevalence of diabetes is increased; diabetes in this group depends on the duration rather than the degree of obesity. Ingestion of carbohydrate has not been shown to increase the likelihood of diabetes except by virtue of contributing to excessive weight gain. The mechanism by which obesity predisposes to the development of diabetes is intimately related to the insulin resistance accompanying excessive weight gain (see below). Thus, in the genetically predisposed individual with a limited capacity for insulin secretion, the development of obesity engenders a demand for insulin that exceeds the beta cells' secretory capacity. The initial impairment of glucose tolerance may still be reversed by weight reduction. Gradually, fasting hyperglycemia and overt diabetes develop. These changes in insulin secretion and action in type II diabetes are discussed more fully below (see Pathogenesis). While obesity invariably precedes the development of diabetes, the possibility that the genetic input in type II diabetic patients includes a disordered mechanism of appetite regulation or energy expenditure has not been excluded. It has been suggested, for example, that the insulin resistance of type II diabetes may accelerate the development of obesity by interfering with the thermogenic response that normally accompanies overeating.

Summary of Etiologic Factors

Etiologically as well as clinically, diabetes is not a single disease entity. In type I diabetes a genetic predisposition linked to the HLA system (specifically the HLA *DR* and *DQ* alleles) is of importance but is not sufficient to bring about the disease. Acquired factors such as viral infection, early exposure to dietary constituents (e.g., cow's milk), and/or autoimmunity are of greater significance, since they are capable of causing diabetes in the genetically susceptible host only. Genetic predisposition involves a complex mode of inheritance mediated by several loci and alleles, at least two of which (linked to loci *DR3* and *DR4,* respectively) have a synergistic effect. A sequence of events which may be postulated is that in a genetically predisposed individual, repeated viral infections trigger an autoimmune process, leading to islet-cell damage (Fig. 19-40). In type II diabetes the mode of inheritance is also complex, but in contrast to type I diabetes, genetic predisposition rather than acquired beta cell injury is of the utmost importance. In this circumstance, most commonly, obesity leads to the clinical expression of insulin deficiency by augmenting insulin resistance, thus increasing the demand for insulin secretion from genetically impaired beta cells (Fig. 19-40).

Prediction and Prevention

The evidence of an autoimmune basis of type I diabetes and the efficacy of cyclosporine and azathioprine in inducing remissions in selected patients with new-onset type I diabetes raise the possibility that intervention before the clinical appearance of type I diabetes may prevent its clinical expression. As was noted above, a variety of autoantibodies (ICA, anti-GAD, and IAA) appear years before the development of overt IDDM. Furthermore, islet-cell function and mass are believed to decline progressively in the years before clinical diabetes is manifest (Fig. 19-41). Thus, the challenge is to identify individuals destined to develop type I diabetes and intervene with a safe and effective preventive therapy.

With respect to the prediction of diabetes, this is best achieved in first-degree relatives, particularly the siblings of known type I diabetic patients (Table 19-13). In nonaffected siblings, the presence of ICA and IAA (3 to 6 percent of siblings), a diminished first-phase insulin response to intravenous glucose, and a minimal increase in the fasting blood glucose concentration (>108 mg/dl) are predictive of overt type I diabetes mellitus within 1.5 years.[285] Current investigation is thus directed at determining whether immunotherapy will safely prevent the appearance of type I diabetes in such predisposed siblings.

For the general population, the presence of ICA does not provide the predictability observed among relatives of diabetic patients.[284] In addition, genetic markers associated with type I diabetes such as HLA-*DR3* and -*DR4* and the absence of aspartate at *DQB57* are observed in 20 to 50 percent of the general population, while the overall prevalence of type I diabetes is less than 0.5 percent. Thus, general population screening to identify candidates for interventional therapy to prevent type I diabetes is not

TYPE I DIABETES

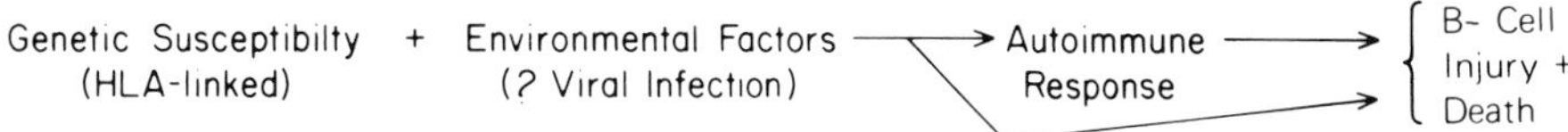

TYPE II DIABETES

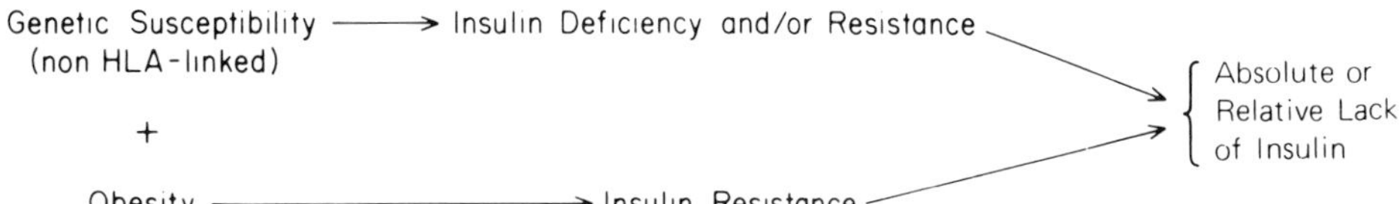

FIGURE 19-40 Etiologic factors in type I (insulin-dependent) and type II (non-insulin-dependent) diabetes. In type I diabetes genetic susceptibility (HLA-linked) plus acquired environmental factors are necessary. The latter may take the form of a viral infection which either directly or via an autoimmune response leads to beta cell defects. In type II diabetes genetic factors are of even greater importance than in type I diabetes. The genetic susceptibility entails a secretory disorder and/or resistance to insulin. Insulin resistance is intensified by obesity (present in 80 percent of cases), resulting in an absolute or relative deficiency of insulin.

yet feasible even on an investigational basis. The importance of finding techniques for the prediction of type I diabetes is underscored by the fact that 90 percent of new cases occur in individuals who do not have a close relative with the disease.[272,284]

Current guidelines indicate that immunosuppressive therapy with cyclosporine or other agents to induce a remission in new-onset type I diabetes or for the prevention of type I diabetes in high-risk subjects should be restricted to investigational use with informed consent.

Pathogenesis

The available data clearly indicate that failure of insulin secretion is the primary pathogenic factor in type I diabetes. Glucagon excess may exaggerate the effects of insulin lack in such patients. In type II diabetes changes in tissue sensitivity to insulin (i.e., insulin resistance) have been implicated. The pattern of insulin is heterogeneous; most commonly there is a relative deficiency in insulin secretion. However, resistance to insulin is often more prominent and apparent earlier than the low beta cell capacity.

FIGURE 19-41 Changes in beta cell mass in individuals with genetic susceptibility and progression to type I diabetes. The decline in beta cell mass follows the appearance of antibodies to a 64-KDa antigen present on beta cells (64KA), progresses with the appearance of insulin autoantibodies (IAA) and islet-cell antibodies (ICA), and precedes the earliest clinical manifestation of diabetes. *(Modified from Muir et al.[272])*

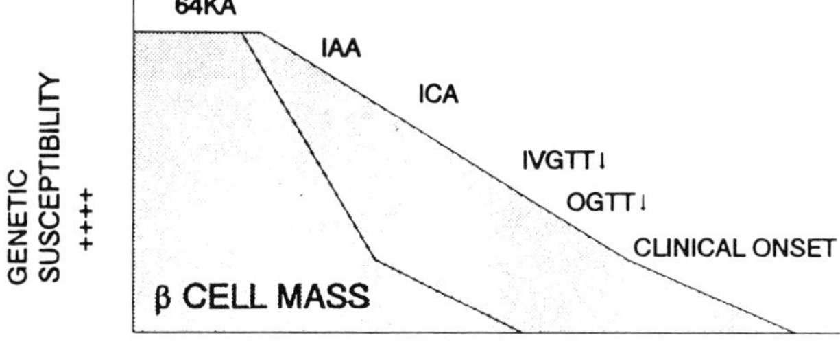

Insulin Secretion

The defect in insulin secretion in type I diabetes involves both the early and the late phases of insulin release; it rapidly progresses to nearly total secretory deficiency. As noted above, a specific loss of glucose-stimulated first-phase insulin secretion may antedate the clinical appearance of type I diabetes by more than a year.[268] In children with new-onset type I diabetes a transient remission often occurs, the so-called *honeymoon phase*, and is associated with a recovery of insulin secretory ability (Fig. 19-42). This transient recovery of beta cell function may be a consequence of the amelioration of hyperglycemia by exogenous insulin. Studies in experimental animals have suggested that chronic hyperglycemia may actually interfere with insulin secretion in the face of a diminished islet-cell mass, a phenomenon referred to as *glucose toxicity*.[286] Ultimately, an irreversible loss of insulin secretion occurs, and hyperglycemia returns. Nevertheless, the defect in insulin secretion in type I diabetic patients is generally not a complete failure of beta cell function. C peptide measurements have shown evidence of residual insulin secretion in some patients with long-standing insulin-treated diabetes. In fact, the persistence of endogenous insulin secretion may be a major determinant of the ease

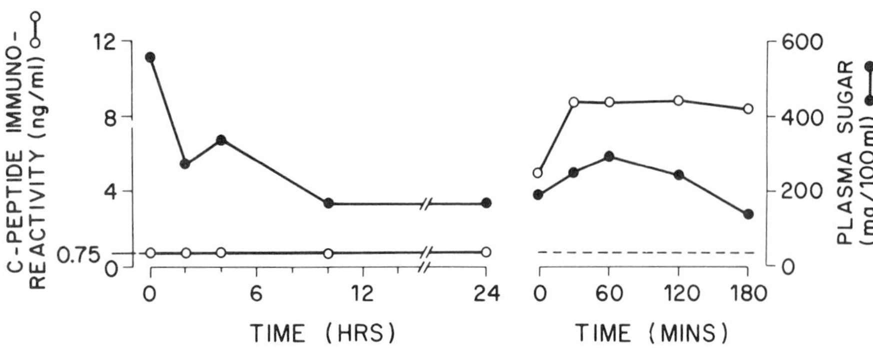

FIGURE 19-42 Changes in C peptide immunoreactivity during therapy for marked hyperglycemia in type I (insulin-dependent) diabetes (*left*) and in response to oral glucose and during a remission phase (*right*). The dotted line represents the lower limit of sensitivity of the C peptide assay. The data indicate the total absence of endogenous insulin secretion in patients with type I diabetes and moderate to severe hyperglycemia (*left*). A return of insulin secretion is seen in the transient remission phase (*right*). (*From Rubenstein AH et al: Arch Intern Med 137:625, 1977.*)

with which the blood glucose concentration can be regulated using exogenous insulin.

The absence of insulin secretion is evident with nonglucose stimuli as well. This lack of insulin responsiveness to all stimuli in type I diabetes represents a difference from type II diabetes, in which partial responsiveness to nonglucose stimuli is preserved.[287] With the onset of fasting hyperglycemia, the response to nonglucose stimuli deteriorates.

Insulin resistance also occurs to a certain extent in type I diabetes. Decreased disposal of glucose in the presence of normal and high insulin levels has been demonstrated in patients with poorly controlled type I diabetes.[288,289] The defect appears to be due to postreceptor unresponsiveness. It seems to be reversible upon insulin therapy, as suggested by experiments in dogs with alloxan-induced diabetes.[290,291] Hepatic glucose overproduction in type I diabetes is most probably due not to insulin resistance but to insulin deficiency abetted by glucagon excess.

In type II diabetes the situation with regard to insulin secretion is less clear-cut; it never involves the severe degree of hyposecretion observed in type I patients. Early reports that insulin concentrations in type II diabetic patients were increased or comparable to those in healthy individuals suggested that there is an impairment in insulin action rather than in secretion. Confounding the interpretation of fasting or postprandial insulin levels in type II diabetes are factors such as the frequent coexistence of obesity (>80 percent of patients), which of itself causes hyperinsulinemia, and the severity of diabetes as reflected by ambient blood glucose concentrations. The available data suggest that in the earliest stages of type II diabetes as reflected by a normal fasting blood glucose level (<120 mg/dl) and a 2-h postprandial glucose level in excess of 200 mg/dl, insulin secretion in the basal state and in response to glucose administration is often *increased* compared with secretion in weight-matched controls.[208,292] As diabetes progresses in severity and the fasting blood glucose level exceeds 120 to 140 mg/dl, insulin secretion progressively declines to values well below those observed in nondiabetic controls. The overall shape of the insulin secretory curve relative to fasting blood concentration in type II diabetes is thus an inverted U and is analogous to the Starling curve for cardiac contraction (Fig. 19-43). By contrast, in at least some patients with the earliest and mildest manifestations of type II diabetes (impaired glucose tolerance), a defect in the first phase of insulin secretion may account for the failure of suppression of hepatic glucose production which results in postprandial hyperglycemia.[293] The key implication of these observations is that while a defect in insulin secretion may or may not be the initiating event in the earliest stages of type II diabetes, it contributes importantly to the progressive development of fasting and postprandial hyperglycemia.

A failure of glucose recognition and/or metabolism despite the presence of an otherwise normal insulin-secretory process has been suggested to account for the hyposecretion of insulin in relation to ambient glucose concentration in most type II dia-

FIGURE 19-43 Relation between the insulin response during oral glucose tolerance testing (OGTT) and the fasting plasma glucose level in nonobese patients with impaired glucose tolerance and overt type II diabetes. As the fasting plasma glucose rises, there is an increase in the insulin response until the fasting plasma glucose level reaches levels of 120 to 140 mg/dl. With further increases in fasting hyperglycemia, the insulin response to ingested glucose declines. This inverted U-shaped curve is analogous to the Starling curve for cardiac contraction. (*From DeFronzo et al.*[208])

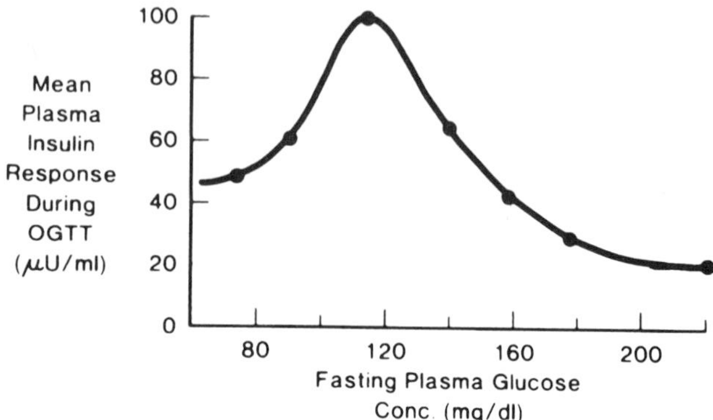

betic patients with fasting hyperglycemia. Evidence for such beta cell abnormality has come from studies demonstrating a loss of early (i.e., acute-phase) insulin secretion in response to glucose stimulation even though the secretory response to isoproterenol, secretin, and arginine remains normal.[287] That the decrease in glucose-stimulated insulin secretion may be mediated by the adrenergic nervous system is suggested by the improvement in secretion seen with α-adrenergic blockade and treatment with indomethacin, an inhibitor of prostaglandin synthesis.[98] Type II diabetic patients with severe fasting hyperglycemia (>250 mg/dl, or >14 m*M*) are generally severely insulinopenic and display abnormalities not only in fast-phase insulin release but in the second-phase response to glucose as well.[287] The hyperglycemia of type II diabetes may actually serve to enhance the insulin response to nonglucose stimuli, since reduction of plasma glucose concentration to normal levels results in a lowering of the acute-phase insulin response to a nonglucose stimulus.

The precise mechanism responsible for decreased insulin secretion in type II diabetes has not been defined. As noted above, in MODY-type diabetes, linkage has been observed with the gene governing the expression of glucokinase. This enzyme, together with the GLUT-2 transporter, has been implicated as a key component of the glucose sensor on the beta cell. In contrast, a genetic defect involving glucokinase, the GLUT-2 transporter, conversion of proinsulin to insulin, or the expression of the insulin molecule has not been detected in type II diabetes.[274] An alternative hypothesis involves the 37-amino acid peptide *amylin*, which was discovered in studies examining the accumulation of amyloid in pancreatic islet cells of type II diabetic patients. Amylin, which is structurally related to the calcitonin gene–related peptide, is packaged within beta cells and cosecreted with insulin. Increased pancreatic levels of amylin have been postulated to interfere with insulin secretion, while increased systemic levels of this peptide have been postulated to interfere with insulin action in type II diabetes.[294] However, studies evaluating the response to administered amylin or circulating amylin levels have failed to substantiate its role in altering insulin secretion or action in diabetes.[295]

The thesis has also been advanced that the defect in insulin secretion observed in type II diabetes is *secondary* to the hyperglycemia engendered by insulin resistance. This concept of *glucose toxicity* posits the inverted U-shaped or Starling curve of insulin secretion relative to glucose concentration that was noted above (Fig. 19-43). It derives support from observations in animals with experimental diabetes demonstrating that lowering of blood glucose levels by renal losses with the drug phloridzin improves insulin secretion. In addition, in human type II diabetes improved glycemic control, whether induced by diet, sulfonylureas, or exogenous insulin, is associated with improved endogenous insulin secretion.[296] Glucose toxicity thus may contribute to reduced insulin secretion in more advanced stages of type II diabetes. Nevertheless, a primary defect in insulin sensitivity in the absence of defective islet-cell function cannot of itself account for type II diabetes. This is clearly indicated by observations in obesity. Insulin resistance is uniformly observed in obesity, yet only a minority of obese individuals ultimately develop type II diabetes. The appearance of type II diabetes in obese subjects results from a failure of islet cells to keep pace with the increased demands for insulin secretion engendered by the obese state.

Insulin Resistance

The coexistence of hyperglycemia or normoglycemia with hyperinsulinemia suggests that insulin resistance is present. More direct evidence of insulin resistance is provided by demonstrating that the in vivo effectiveness of exogenous insulin in stimulating glucose uptake by various target tissues is reduced. On the basis of these criteria, obesity is clearly the most commonly encountered insulin-resistant state in humans. Its association with type II diabetes in >80 percent of cases underscores its importance in unmasking the metabolic consequences of a deficiency of beta cell function in such patients. However, even in the absence of obesity, insulin resistance is demonstrable in type II diabetes.

Insulin resistance includes a wide spectrum of reduced tissue sensitivity and/or reduced responsiveness to insulin. In its initial stages the enhanced insulin secretion may compensate for the reduced tissue sensitivity to insulin. Gradually, hyperglycemia may develop and prevail in the face of insufficient insulin secretion. Even in the absence of obesity, many type II diabetic patients are hyperinsulinemic in the face of hyperglycemia.[208] Further evidence of insulin resistance in such patients was provided by studies of Reaven et al.,[297] in which the response to exogenous insulin was measured. Endogenous insulin secretion was suppressed by a combined infusion of epinephrine and propranolol at a steady rate of insulin and glucose infusion. Since similar steady plasma insulin concentrations were achieved, the steady-state plasma glucose level (SSPG) could be taken as a measure of insulin resistance; the higher the SSPG, the greater the insulin resistance. In normal subjects these investigators found SSPGs of ~125 mg/dl compared with SSPG values of 200 to 350 mg/dl in patients with type II diabetes. An alternative approach, which avoids the infusion of epinephrine and propranolol (which may of themselves alter insulin sensitivity), is the "insulin clamp" technique. In this procedure, insulin is infused in physiologic doses and euglycemia is maintained by means of a variable glucose infusion. Since all the glucose infused must be metabolized, the rate of glucose infusion serves as an index of insulin-mediated glucose uptake. Using this procedure DeFronzo et al.[208,298] have shown a 30 to 40 percent decrease in insulin response in type II diabetes. Examination of the individual responses, however, indicates the heterogeneity of insulin resistance in this disorder. In about half the subjects tissue responsiveness to insulin is reduced, while in the remainder it is normal (Fig. 19-44). Of particular relevance to the pathogenesis of type II diabetes is the observation that decreased insulin action (as reflected by insulin clamp studies) was demonstrable in the offspring of two type II diabetic parents even before clinical diabetes was manifest.[299] These findings support a primary role for insulin resistance in the development of type II diabetes.

Tissue Sites of Insulin Resistance

The major sites of insulin action with respect to glucose metabolism are the liver and muscle tissue. In insulin-resistant states such as obesity and type II diabetes, both liver and muscle demonstrate a reduced sensitivity to insulin. With respect to liver, in nondiabetic obese subjects insulin-mediated suppression of hepatic glucose production is reduced. In type II diabetic patients, hepatic glucose uptake is diminished after oral glucose administration and contributes to postprandial hyperglycemia. Furthermore, basal hepatic glucose production is augmented in type II diabetic patients with fasting hyperglycemia >140 mg/dl in the face of normal or augmented plasma insulin levels.[300]

Resistance by muscle tissue to insulin action is also readily demonstrable in type II diabetes and obesity. As was noted above, using the euglycemic insulin clamp technique, decreased glucose turnover in response to insulin infusion is demonstrable in many patients with type II diabetes even in the absence of obesity. Under these conditions of the insulin clamp study, muscle tissue is the major site of glucose uptake. By combining arteriovenous catheterization with the insulin clamp, one can demonstrate a 40 to 50 percent decrease in muscle uptake of glucose.[208] Furthermore, studies involving indirect calorimetry, magnetic resonance imaging, and muscle biopsies have shown that the defect in muscle glucose utilization in lean and obese type II diabetic patients involves primarily nonoxidative rather than oxidative pathways of glucose utilization.[208,301] Specifically, incorporation of glucose into muscle glycogen is reduced in type II diabetes.

FIGURE 19-44 The heterogeneity of tissue sensitivity to insulin in insulin-independent (type II maturity-onset) diabetes (MOD). Insulin sensitivity is indicated as the rate of insulin-mediated glucose metabolism (*M*) during physiologic hyperinsulinemia induced by the insulin clamp technique. In the diabetic group, insulin sensitivity decreased in approximately half the subjects compared with healthy controls. (*From DeFronzo et al.*[298])

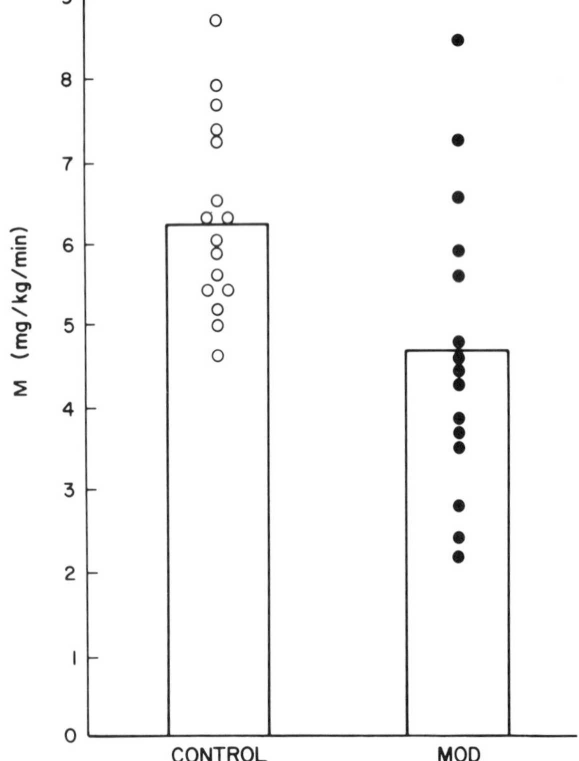

Insulin Receptors in Diabetes

In obesity, resistance to insulin is related to diminished insulin binding, as assessed by measurements on adipocytes as well as circulating monocytes.[206] In nonobese, hyperinsulinemic type II diabetic patients, a decrease in insulin binding has also been observed. This decrease is due to a fall in the number of insulin receptors per cell rather than a change in binding affinity. Interestingly, the decrease in insulin binding is observed only in hyperinsulinemic type II diabetes. As was noted previously, the ambient insulin concentration has been demonstrated to regulate the number of insulin receptors.[199] Thus, decreased insulin binding and the accompanying reduction in insulin response observed in type II diabetic patients may be a consequence of down regulation by the hyperinsulinemia rather than an initiating event. This concept received strong support as shown by the progressive decrease in both insulin sensitivity and responses in adipocytes cultured in the presence of insulin.

The more severe the postprandial hyperglycemia in type II diabetes, the greater the magnitude of insulin resistance.[302] In patients with mild fasting hyperglycemia (<115 mg/dl or 6.4 m*M*), a rightward shift in the glucose dose–insulin response curve has been demonstrated while the maximal response remains unaffected. This is consistent with a decrease in the number of high-affinity insulin receptors (i.e., lowered insulin sensitivity, Fig. 19-29). With more severe diabetes, both a greater rightward shift in the insulin response curve and a decrease in the maximal rate of glucose disposal (impaired sensitivity and responsiveness) are seen. These observations suggest the presence of a postreceptor defect in peripheral tissues in overt type II diabetes. In fact, other than in patients with very mild type II diabetes and patients with extreme insulin resistance and acanthosis nigricans (see below), decreased insulin binding to the receptor is not a major mechanism of insulin resistance in diabetes.

Postreceptor Defects

From a theoretical standpoint, resistance to insulin in the absence of a defect in insulin binding could be a consequence of a defect in intracellular signal transduction (insulin "second messenger"), in the number or action of glucose transporters, or in one or more key enzymes that regulate glucose metabolism. Although the precise identity of the insulin second messenger remains elusive, tyrosine kinase is believed to play a key role in the intracellular insulin signaling mechanism. A decrease in insulin receptor tyrosine kinase activity reversible with weight loss has been observed in obese type II diabetic patients.[206] A reduction in the insulin-sensitive GLUT-4 transporter has also been demonstrated in fat cells obtained from patients with type II diabetes. However, muscle tissue (the major site of insulin-mediated peripheral glucose disposal) shows normal levels of GLUT-4 mRNA and GLUT-4 protein in patients with type II diabetes. With respect to tissue enzymes, muscle glycogen synthase is a key candidate site for insulin resistance in view of the marked diminution in nonoxidative glucose metabolism (glycogen synthesis) observed in insulin-resistant muscle tissue. As was noted above, polymorphism for the gene regulating the expression of glycogen synthase may be a marker for a subgroup of patients with type II diabetes. However, a reduction in muscle glycogen synthase activity was not demonstrable in such patients.[275] Thus, the precise primary site of postreceptor insulin resistance in type II diabetes remains to be established.

Acanthosis Nigricans

Decreased insulin binding has also been shown to be of importance in some rare cases of extreme insulin resistance associated with acanthosis nigricans. This syndrome consists of skin lesions characterized by velvety hyperpigmentation in the back of the neck, axillae, and other intertriginous areas (under the breast, upper thighs). In patients with this disorder, insulin binding is reduced 50 to 100 percent. Analysis of clinical findings and receptor function permits the classification of these patients into two groups.[200,303] In type A, the patients are younger and glucose tolerance is only mildly impaired and frequently is accompanied by the polycystic ovary syndrome and virilization. In type B, the patients are older and manifest immunologic abnormalities, including a circulating antireceptor antibody which is responsible for the decrease in insulin binding. The hyperglycemia is more serve than that in type A patients but is not accompanied by ketosis. The decrease in receptor numbers observed in the type A syndrome was initially theorized to have been due to down regulation caused by the prevailing hyperinsulinemia. However, when type A patients fast, plasma insulin levels return to normal although insulin binding remains abnormal. In contrast, obese subjects who fast show an increase in insulin binding. More recent studies have shown a variety of mutations involving the insulin receptor gene in type A patients.[303] The skin changes in type A and type B patients may be a consequence of the very high circulating insulin levels interacting with the IGF-I receptor. From a clinical standpoint, most patients with acanthosis nigricans do not have extreme insulin resistance. Most commonly, the condition occurs in association with obesity, or it may signal the presence of an occult malignancy, such as a gastric carcinoma, particularly when the skin lesions first appear after age 50 to 55.

Syndrome X

In addition to obesity, type II diabetes is frequently associated with hypertension, hyperlipidemia (particularly hypertriglyceridemia), and coronary artery disease. Reaven[304] has termed the coexistence of these disorders "syndrome X." He and others have suggested that the presence of hyperinsulinemia and/or insulin resistance in each of these conditions may signify a common pathogenetic mechanism.[304,305] The presence of hyperinsulinemia has been recognized in hypertension even in the absence of obesity or diabetes.[306] Hyperinsulinemia may contribute to the development of hypertension by increasing renal sodium reabsorption, by augmenting catecholamine secretion, or through other, undetermined mechanisms. Hyperinsulinemia may play a role in hypertriglyceridemia by enhancing hepatic production of VLDL and may accelerate atherosclerosis by direct tropic effects on smooth muscle proliferation and/or plaque formation in the arterial wall. Regardless of the precise mechanisms involved, the central role of insulin resistance and/or hyperinsulinemia in each of these conditions underscores the importance of treatment modalities which enhance insulin sensitivity and lower plasma insulin levels. The syndrome X concept thus provides a rationale for the usefulness of weight reduction and/or exercise in the management of hypertension and hyperlipidemia and in the prevention of coronary artery disease, in addition to their established roles in the management of type II diabetes and obesity. Physical training has clearly been shown to reduce plasma insulin levels, enhance insulin sensitivity, prevent the development of type II diabetes, and reduce the risk of coronary artery disease.[307]

Glucagon Secretion

Unger[227] has suggested that the metabolic defects in diabetes are not due solely to insulin lack but that diabetes is a bihormonal disorder to which relative or absolute hyperglucagonemia is an essential contributor. Evidence that altered secretion of glucagon is important in the pathogenesis of diabetes is presented by a variety of observations. In diabetic patients, glucose fails to suppress glucagon secretion and the administration of protein or amino acids causes hypersecretion of glucagon[61] (Fig. 19-45). In contrast, the glucagon response to hypoglycemia is blunted in type I diabetic patients, suggesting a defect in a glucose receptor on the alpha cell.[308] In addition, in experimental animals, diabetes induced by pancreatectomy is accompanied by excessive extrapancreatic production of glucagon.[227] Furthermore, a reduction in plasma glucagon concentration induced by somatostatin results in amelioration of diabetic hyperglycemia.[101]

Despite the attractiveness of the bihormonal concept, other findings have cast serious doubt on the essentiality of glucagon or the presence of a primary defect in alpha cell function in spontaneous human diabetes.[238,239] So long as insulin is available, an elevation in plasma glucagon concentration (produced by infusion), which simulates the hyperglucagonemia of diabetes or other hyperglucagonemic states, fails to cause glucose intolerance in normal humans or to precipitate deterioration of glucose control in known diabetic patients.[239] In pancreatectomized humans, extrapancreatic glucagon is not produced, yet hyperglycemia and ketosis develop.[220] In like manner, prolonged suppression of glucagon and insulin secretion by somatostatin results in transient hypoglycemia that is followed by fasting hyperglycemia and glucose overproduction (i.e., a diabetic state) despite ongoing suppression of glucagon.[238] In insulin-dependent diabetic patients, in whom somatostatin substantially reduces postprandial hyperglycemia, the effect is largely a consequence of diminished carbohydrate and protein absorption rather than enhanced carbohydrate use.[103] Finally, treatment with insulin results in suppression of hyperglucagonemia in human diabetes and in the restoration of normal alpha cell function in experimentally induced animal diabetes.[228]

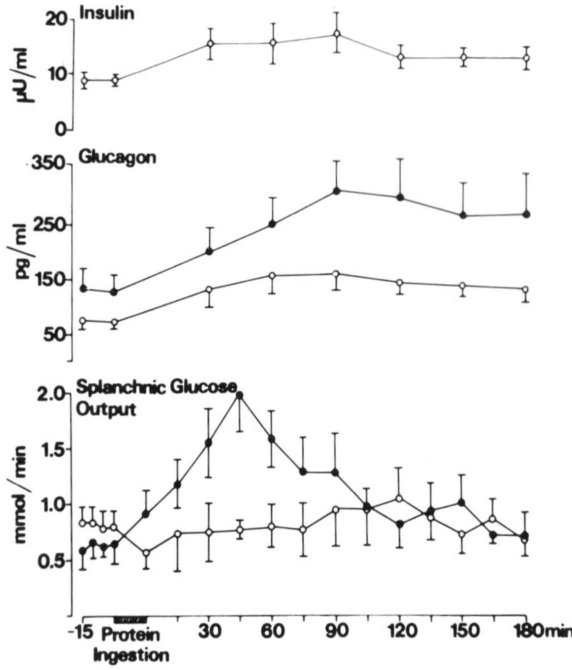

FIGURE 19-45 Effect of protein feeding on plasma glucagon concentration and splanchnic (hepatic) glucose production in normal subjects (○) and insulin-dependent (type I) diabetic patients (●). Plasma insulin concentration could not be measured in the diabetic patients because of prior treatment with insulin. The protein meal results in a marked increase in glucose production in the diabetic patients but not in normal individuals. This difference is due to the exaggerated rise in plasma glucagon level in a setting of absolute insulin deficiency. (*Based on the data of Wahren et al.*[61])

The major role of glucagon in diabetes is thus to intensify the consequences of insulin deficiency. Accordingly, meal-induced glucagon secretion in poorly controlled diabetes exaggerates the degree of postprandial hyperglycemia. In addition, the hyperglucagonemia enhances hepatic ketogenesis and gluconeogenesis.[41] A primary role for glucagon in the development of hyperglycemia has been observed in patients with the glucagonoma syndrome (see Endocrine-Associated Diabetes, below).

Other Hormones

Persistent hypersecretion of glucocorticoids (Cushing's syndrome) or GH (acromegaly) often results in secondary diabetes (see below). In both conditions hyperglycemia is a consequence of hormone-induced insulin resistance. In contrast, in primary spontaneous diabetes (either type I or type II), circulating levels of GH, cortisol, and catecholamines are usually normal. However, in DKA and in response to exercise in poorly controlled diabetes, marked increments of concentrations of each of the counterregulatory hormones are observed. The secondary nature of these abnormalities is suggested by the fact that normalization of plasma glucose concentration by insulin treatment restores normal testing and postexercise levels of the counterregulatory hormones.[309] Nevertheless, during surgery or other forms of stress, hypersecretion of counterregulatory hormones may cause a worsening of an already manifest diabetic state or the transient development of hyperglycemia in a previously normal patient (see Stress Hyperglycemia, above).

Pathophysiology

The metabolic alterations observed in diabetes primarily reflect the degree to which there is an abso-

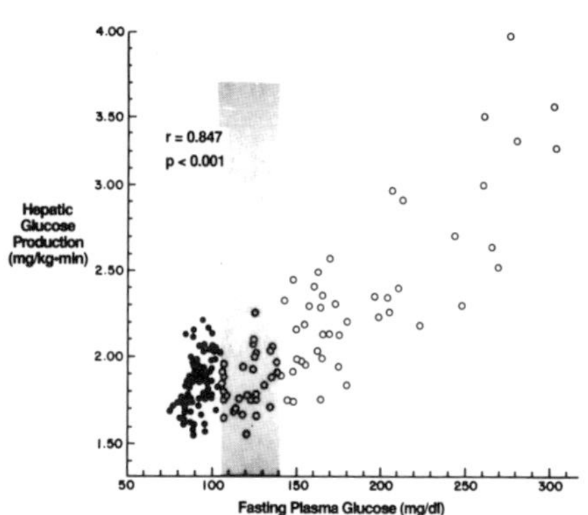

FIGURE 19-46 The relation between hepatic glucose production and fasting plasma glucose concentration in patients with type II diabetes (open circles) and healthy controls (closed circles). In the diabetic patients with fasting plasma glucose levels below 140 mg/dl (shaded area), hepatic glucose production was similar to that of controls. In the diabetic patients with fasting hyperglycemia in excess of 140 mg/dl there was a progressive rise in hepatic glucose production to values well above those seen in controls. (*From Defronzo et al.*[208,300])

lute or relative deficiency of insulin. Since insulin is the major storage hormone, minimal insulin deficiency results in diminished ability to increase the reservoir of body fuels because of inadequate disposal of ingested foodstuffs. With a major deficiency of insulin, not only is fuel accumulation hampered in the fed state, excessive mobilization of endogenous metabolic fuels (e.g., hyperglycemia, hyperaminoacidemia, and elevated FFA concentration) occurs in the fasting condition and even in the face of hyperphagia. In the most severe form of diabetes (DKA) there is overproduction of glucose and marked acceleration of catabolic processes (e.g., lipolysis, proteolysis).

Carbohydrate Metabolism

The mildest type of abnormality in carbohydrate metabolism related to diabetes is a decrease in glucose tolerance in association with a normal fasting blood glucose concentration. In this circumstance, ingested glucose fails to elicit an adequate insulin response (because of either a secretory defect or tissue resistance to insulin); glucose consequently escapes uptake by the liver and is more slowly metabolized by peripheral tissues.[310]

When absolute or relative insulin deficiency occurs in the basal state, an elevation in fasting blood glucose concentration ensues. In this situation, normal basal levels of insulin may be maintained, but only at the cost of developing fasting hyperglycemia. In patients with mild fasting hyperglycemia (140 to 180 mg/dl), glucose production (determined by either radioactive tracer techniques or splanchnic balance studies) is generally normal or only slightly increased,[300] while fractional glucose turnover (glucose utilization relative to plasma glucose concentration) is reduced (Fig. 19-46). In a normal individual even mild hyperglycemia is insufficient to inhibit hepatic glucose output (because of an accompanying rise in insulin concentration[64]); however, a diabetic patient with even mild fasting hyperglycemia is always in a state of relative or absolute glucose overproduction. As fasting plasma glucose levels rise to values of 200 mg/dl or above, an absolute increase in hepatic glucose production is observed (Fig. 19-46). Furthermore, the relative contribution of gluconeogenesis to total hepatic glucose output is increased twofold.[118] This enhancement of gluconeogenesis with a moderate deficiency of insulin is in keeping with the relatively greater amounts of insulin necessary to inhibit gluconeogenesis compared with glycogenolysis.[70,115] In addition, the failure of hepatic glucose uptake after feeding results in glycogen depletion.

With the progress to total beta cell failure, an ever-increasing fasting blood glucose level fails to elicit a beta cell secretory response. In the absence of the restraining influence exerted by insulin, glucose production by the liver increases to three or more times normal, largely as a consequence of accelerated gluconeogenesis. The clinical correlate of this sequence of events is severe hyperglycemia, as is observed in DKA or nonketotic hyperosmolar coma.

Although the kidney also possesses the enzymes necessary for gluconeogenesis, a significant addition of glucose to the bloodstream by the kidney has not been observed in compensated human diabetes[311]; renal production of glucose may, however, become substantial on prolonged fasting.[312] Renal gluconeogenesis plays an important physiologic role by regulating the ammonia ion supply in response to shifts in acid-base status. In the acidotic stage of diabetes, cations are extensively required in order to permit the excretion of ketoacids and other acids. The kidney responds by deaminating glutamine and glutamic acid, thus producing NH_4^+. This is achieved by direct activation of a phosphate-dependent glutaminase and adaptive induction of PEPCK. The enhanced gluconeogenesis actually serves as a removal pathway for carbon skeletons of glutamine. Thus, the renal mechanism for the alleviation of the acidemia involving oral and urinary cation loss in DKA carries the risk of aggravating the hyperglycemia.

Protein and Amino Acid Metabolism

Severe insulin deficiency is accompanied by negative nitrogen balance and marked protein wasting. In insulin-dependent diabetic patients, growth retardation is a frequent complication of poor diabetes control. Such changes are not surprising, since insulin, when present in normal amounts, stimulates protein synthesis and muscle amino acid uptake and inhibits protein catabolism and the output of amino acids from muscle. The changes in protein metabolism also involve gluconeogenesis, inasmuch as glucose overproduction in ketotic diabetic patients depends in part on augmented utilization of protein-derived precursors. The alterations in amino acid metabolism which characterize the diabetic state are, however, demonstrable even in the absence of severe insulin deficiency; they occur in the fasted (postabsorptive) state as well as the protein-fed state.

In an insulin-dependent diabetic patient with mild to moderate hyperglycemia, changes in circulating amino acid levels, hepatic amino acid uptake, and muscle output of amino acids are demonstrable. A reduction in the plasma concentration of alanine and elevations in branched-chain amino acid concentrations (valine, leucine, and isoleucine) have been repeatedly shown in spontaneous diabetes in humans[124] as well as in experimental diabetes in animals. Despite the reduction in plasma alanine concentration, uptake of glucogenic amino acids and other glucose precursors by the liver is increased twofold or more.[118] As a consequence of this increase in substrate uptake, gluconeogenesis can account for >30 percent of hepatic glucose production, compared with 15 to 20 percent in normal humans. Since circulating alanine levels are reduced in diabetic patients, augmented fractional alanine extraction by the liver is responsible for the increase in alanine uptake. In the absence of the normal restraining effect of insulin on gluconeogenesis, the liver acts as a sink, depleting arterial alanine.

In contrast to the decrease in circulating alanine level, elevations in plasma concentrations of branched-chain amino acids are demonstrable in the fasting state in diabetes. Studies in experimental animals indicate that oxidation of leucine, isoleucine, and valine, once they enter muscle tissue, is accelerated in the diabetic state.[313] Repletion of muscle nitrogen after protein feeding is also reduced in diabetic patients. In contrast to the large, persistent uptake of branched-chain amino acids by muscle tissue which follows the ingestion of a protein meal by normal subjects, in diabetic patients amino acid uptake is only transient. As a consequence, total amino acid uptake by muscle is decreased and the plasma levels of the branched-chain amino acids are abnormally elevated after protein feeding.[61,124] These observations are in keeping with the known stimulatory effect of insulin on muscle amino acid uptake, which is most marked for the branched-chain amino acids. The arterial accumulation and reduced uptake of amino acids after protein feeding indicate that diabetes is characterized by protein as well as glucose intolerance. The defect in protein metabolism in diabetic individuals is further accentuated by the fact that those amino acids which are taken up by muscle tissue are preferentially catabolized rather than incorporated into protein.

Protein-Carbohydrate Interactions

In addition to the abnormalities in amino acid metabolism, protein feeding exacerbates the changes in carbohydrate homeostasis characteristic of diabetes. In normal, healthy subjects after protein feeding, blood glucose levels and splanchnic glucose output remain unchanged despite an elevation in plasma insulin concentration (Figs. 19-33 and 19-45). This constancy of hepatic glucose production and blood glucose concentration is a consequence of protein-stimulated glucagon secretion which counteracts the effects of the concomitant rise in plasma insulin concentration. In marked contrast, in diabetic patients protein feeding results in a 150 percent increase in splanchnic glucose output (Fig. 19-45) as well as an exaggerated rise in plasma glucose concentration.[61] The stimulatory effect of protein feeding on hepatic glucose production is probably a consequence of the rise in plasma glucagon concentration; in diabetic patients the glucagon concentration increase is exaggerated and occurs in a setting of absolute insulin deficiency. However, despite ongoing hyperglucagonemia, the increase in hepatic glucose production in diabetic patients does not persist (Fig. 19-45). This transient hepatic response is in keeping with the only evanescent stimulatory effect of physiologic increments in glucagon concentration on hepatic glucose output.[236,238] Thus, the progressive increase in blood glucose concentration which accompanies a protein meal in insulin-deficient diabetic patients does not reflect ongoing glucagon-mediated stimulation of hepatic glucose production. Rather, the hyperglycemia reflects the persistent failure (engendered by insulin lack) to metabolize the increased amount of glucose which is delivered to the periphery as a consequence of a transient elevation in hepatic glucose output.

Fat Metabolism and Diabetic Hyperlipidemia

Elevation of plasma lipid concentration in diabetes is well documented. Mean levels of plasma triglycerides and cholesterol in individuals with various types of diabetes are higher than levels in nondiabetic subjects, reflecting an elevation in at least 50 percent of patients. However, the individual values vary widely depending on the severity of diabetes, its therapeutic control, and the composition of the diet.

In decompensated type I diabetic patients, the plasma FFA concentration is elevated as a result of increased FFA outflow from fat depots, where the balance of the FFA esterification–triglyceride lipolysis cycle is displaced in favor of lipolysis. The hepatic FFA inflow exceeds the energy requirement. One obvious outcome is increased ketone formation; the other entails reesterification of the FFA and reassembly of the triglycerides into VLDL, with return to the circulation.[314] Thus, the increased uptake of preformed FFA by the liver and their reexport as VLDL-borne triglycerides is one of the mechanisms leading to hyperlipidemia. This is not a strictly proportional relation; in severe insulin deficiency VLDL secretion may be retarded because of a disturbance in apolipoprotein synthesis, and the liver triglyceride content may increase considerably (diabetic "fatty liver").

Another mechanism leading to the retention in plasma of either VLDL elaborated in the liver or chylomicrons produced from exogenous fat in the small intestine is decreased uptake by peripheral tissues.[315] The low capacity for triglyceride storage can be attributed in large measure to the reduction in lipoprotein lipase, an enzyme specifically oriented to cleave VLDL- and chylomicron-borne triglycerides, located on the capillary endothelial walls. The low activity of this rapidly turning over enzyme in adipose tissue in experimental and human diabetes results from an absolute or relative insulin deficiency, since its synthesis is induced by insulin.[316] However, despite the importance of adipose tissue lipoprotein lipase in triglyceride removal, its overall contribution to diabetic hyperlipidemia must be viewed in the context that adipose tissue constitutes <15 to 25 percent of body weight and that substantial lipoprotein lipase activity resides in other tissues, notably heart and skeletal muscle. Generally, a reciprocal relation exists between adipose tissue and muscle lipoprotein lipase activity; the latter increases in conditions of insulin deficiency, exercise, and glucocorticoid-induced insulin antagonism.[317] Thus, even if the total body capacity to remove triglycerides is lowered somewhat, a redistribution in sites of triglyceride uptake occurs in diabetes, in keeping with the shift from triglyceride storage in adipose tissue to triglyceride utilization in muscles and other tissues.

Therefore, factors in addition to the suppression of adipose tissue lipoprotein lipase activity may be instrumental in eliciting the diabetic hyperlipidemia, e.g., alterations in apolipoprotein composition of VLDL and chylomicrons, notably a decrease in the apoprotein E component. This change is associated with delayed removal of these particles from the circulation, presumably as a result of an altered recognition pattern by tissue receptors.[318]

Plasma triglyceride (e.g., VLDL) concentration is elevated more frequently in diabetes than is the cholesterol level. When the total plasma cholesterol concentration is elevated, this often represents an increase in the VLDL cholesterol concentration. However, the presumption that the high-carbohydrate diet that has been advocated for the maintenance of diabetic patients may result in hypertriglyceridemia and deterioration of diabetes control has not been supported provided that total caloric intake is restricted.[319]

Hypertriglyceridemia is present in type II diabetes as well. However, in contrast to the increased FFA recirculation associated with insulinopenia, the hypertriglyceridemia in type II diabetes may be attributed to hyperinsulinemia (Fig. 19-47). This enhances de novo fatty acid and VLDL synthesis in the liver as well as transport and storage of triglycerides in the periphery. The combined impact of hyperglycemia and hyperinsulinemia promotes lipogenesis from carbohydrate, as insulin resistance at the hepatic level does not appear to affect the lipogenic pathway.[317] Thus, hypertriglyceridemia in most patients with type II diabetes is associated with increased adipose tissue mass leading to increased plasma FFA concentration[320]; the hepatic triglyceride synthesis is further aided by increased availability of performed FFA, which is characteristic of obesity. Studies of triglyceride turnover confirm the

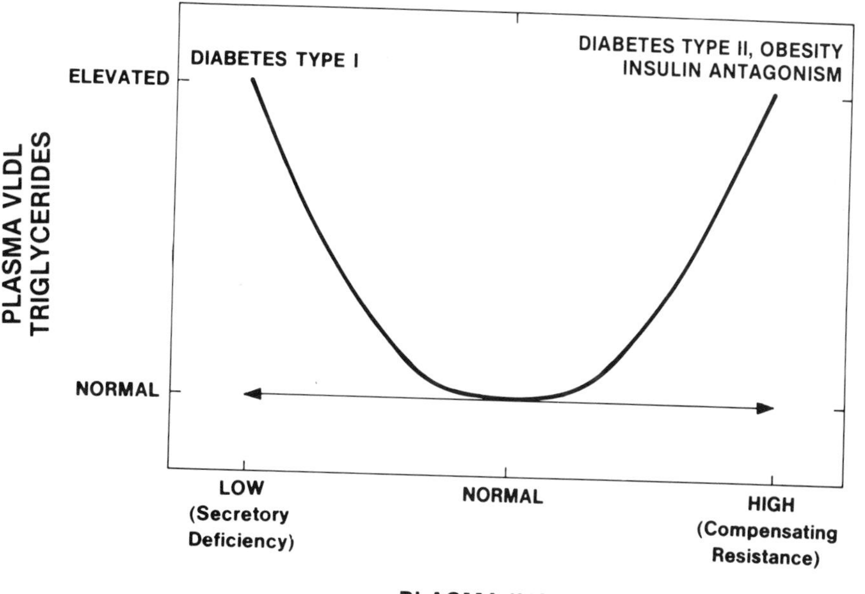

FIGURE 19-47 Summary representation showing that hypertriglyceridemia in diabetes may be elicited by both insulin deficiency and insulin excess. In type I diabetes low insulin availability causes an increased transfer of FFA from adipose tissue to the liver. The liver responds with esterification and return of a part of the preformed FFA surplus into the circulation as VLDL-borne triglycerides. In type II diabetes the liver responds to the elevated insulin and glucose concentrations in the circulation with stimulation of the lipogenic pathway, resulting in de novo lipogenesis, reduced FFA oxidation, and enhanced VLDL production.

existence of VLDL overproduction in type II diabetes. The defect in FFA turnover is potentially reversible with improved metabolic control.[321]

Both the frequency and the mechanism of plasma cholesterol concentration elevation in diabetes remain unsettled. A consistent relation between plasma glucose and serum cholesterol concentrations has not been observed. Furthermore, total sterol synthesis is not necessarily elevated in patients with poorly regulated diabetes. The complexity of cholesterol metabolism is illustrated by the stimulation of intestinal cholesterologenesis in diabetes,[322] while the hepatic cholesterol synthesis is uninfluenced or suppressed. Increased glycosylation of tissue collagen[323] and glycation of cholesterol-carrying low-density lipoproteins (LDL),[31] occurring under the conditions of hyperglycemia, lead to the retention of LDL cholesterol in the circulation because of delayed entry into the cells. In any event, hypercholesterolemia, together with hypertriglyceridemia, should be regarded as a factor contributing to accel erated atherosclerosis and the high incidence of coronary heart disease in the diabetic population. The enhanced atherosclerotic process may also be related to a decrease in plasma HDL and apoprotein A-I concentrations,[324–326] particularly in patients with suboptimal treatment and/or high VLDL levels.

Summary

Mild or moderate insulin lack is characterized by a failure to replete or augment body fuel stores in response to feeding (Fig. 19-48). Consequently, when a glucose-containing meal is eaten, failure of hepatic and muscle uptake of glucose results in hyperglycemia which is augmented by inadequate suppression of hepatic gluconeogenesis. When protein is ingested, insulin deficiency results in decreased amino acid uptake by muscle accompanied by hyperaminoacidemia. Hypersecretion of glucagon in response to the protein meal causes hyperglycemia. When a fat-containing meal is eaten, postprandial hypertriglyceridemia occurs because of inadequate removal of the circulating chylomicrons, mainly as a result of diminished activity of lipoprotein lipase. The hypertriglyceridemia is caused mainly by hepatic recirculation of the high levels of plasma FFA in the form of VLDL-borne triglycerides (in type I diabetes) or de novo lipogenesis in the liver (in type II diabetes).

With severe insulin lack, plasma elevations of concentrations of each of these fuels (glucose, amino acids, FFA) are observed in the fasted state as well as the fed state (Fig. 19-48). The increased levels of circulation substrates are due to accelerated breakdown of body fuel reserves through increased proteolysis and lipolysis as well as to overproduction of glucose and ketones from the respective precursors (amino acids and FFA).

Diagnosis

The diagnosis of diabetes rests on the demonstration of the presence of hyperglycemia. In a patient who is

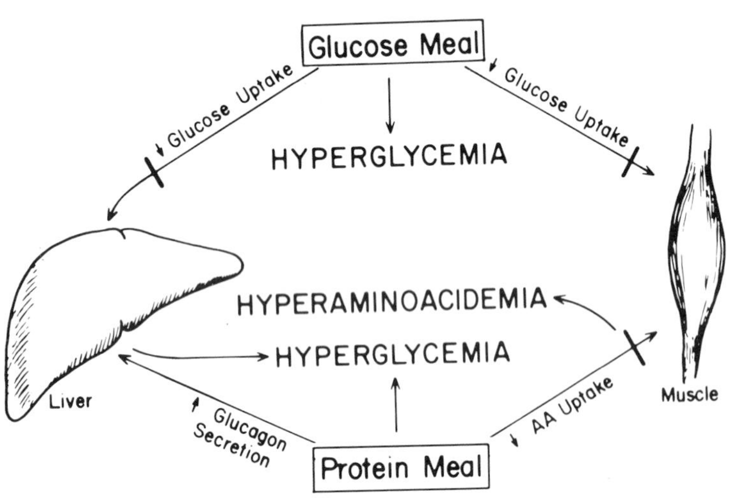

FIGURE 19-48 Pathophysiology of the metabolic abnormalities in insulin-deficient diabetic patients in the fed state. Failure of glucose uptake by liver and muscle results in hyperglycemia after a carbohydrate meal. After a protein meal hyperaminoacidemia occurs because of failure of amino acid (AA) uptake in muscle; hyperglycemia occurs because of the unopposed action of excessive increments in plasm glucagon concentration. After a fatty meal diminished activity of lipoprotein lipase results in decreased clearance of chylomicrons by adipose tissue, leading to hypertriglyceridemia. Increased production of triglycerides by the liver may also occur as a consequence of increased FFA delivery to the liver and recirculation of FFA in VLDL.

clearly symptomatic, with polydipsia, polyuria, polyphagia, and weight loss, hyperglycemia is likely to be present in the fasting state as well as the postprandial state. However, in an asymptomatic patient with a normal or nearly normal fasting plasma glucose level, the criteria for diagnosis and the indications for glucose tolerance testing have been the subject of debate.[327] Regardless of the criteria employed, a proper understanding of the technical and physiologic factors which influence the glucose concentration is necessary for the correct interpretation of laboratory data.

Since the introduction of automated laboratory methods, plasma or serum rather than whole blood has generally been employed for glucose measurement in the laboratory. In contrast, a drop of whole blood is employed when patients self-monitor blood glucose with reagent strips and a glucose meter. The lower glucose concentration within red cells compared with extracellular fluid accounts for the fact that glucose concentrations when measured in whole blood are ~85 percent of those observed in plasma.

Fasting Plasma Glucose Concentration

In normal subjects the fasting plasma glucose concentration generally is <110 mg/dl (<6 m*M*) after an overnight (10- to 14-h) fast. A fasting plasma glucose level of >140 mg/dl (>8 m*M*) is definitely abnormal; if documented on more than one occasion (to exclude the possibility that the patient has failed to recall having eaten breakfast or that an error has been made), such a plasma glucose level establishes the diagnosis of diabetes. Many of the factors discussed below which influence glucose tolerance (e.g., age, diet, activity) have little effect on the fasting plasma glucose level. By contrast, intercurrent disease, by virtue of its "stress" effects (see Stress Hyperglycemia, above), may cause fasting hyperglycemia which reverts to normal after resolution of the underlying disease process. Individuals with this type of hyperglycemia, however, may be prone to the subsequent development of permanent diabetes.

Oral Glucose Tolerance Testing

If the fasting plasma glucose concentration is not abnormally elevated (between 110 and 140 mg/dl or 6 to 8 m*M*), carbohydrate metabolism may nevertheless be abnormal as reflected by the plasma glucose response to an oral or IV glucose load. The procedure most commonly employed to evaluate carbohydrate metabolism is the oral glucose tolerance test. For proper interpretation of data, the testing conditions must be standardized. The test should be performed in the morning after an overnight, 10- to 14-h fast. The patient is seated or supine during the test and is not permitted to smoke. After a fasting blood sample is obtained, a glucose solution (generally a commercial cola-flavored preparation) is ingested over 5 min in a dose of 1.75 g glucose per kilogram of body weight up to a maximum dose of 100 g (the results do not differ if a maximum dose of 75 g is used). Thereafter, venous blood samples are obtained at 60, 90, and 120 min. In patients in whom the diagnosis of hypoglycemia is suspected, additional blood samples are obtained at 3, 4, and 5 h and at any time the patient notes the development of symptoms.

The ingestion of a diet rich in carbohydrate (300 g per day) for at least 3 days before glucose tolerance testing was recommended in the past as a necessary preparation to avoid the glucose intolerance associated with starvation-like conditions. However, a reduction in dietary carbohydrate intake to as little as 100 g per day fails to diminish glucose tolerance. Consequently, only if the patient has been following a severely restricted dietary regimen is any increase in carbohydrate intake necessary before testing.

Factors Affecting Glucose Tolerance

The ability to metabolize a glucose load is influenced by the patient's age, activity, and diet; drugs; and intercurrent disease (Table 19-14). Aging is recognized as one of the most important factors influencing performance on glucose tolerance tests.[328] Compared with younger individuals, a progressive rise in 1- and 2-h glucose concentration values is observed beyond age 50. A decrease in tissue sensitivity is the major factor responsible for the diminution in glucose tolerance.[328] Although physical inactivity and reduction in lean body mass may be contributory factors, the aging process per se contributes to the development of insulin resistance. In general, the 1- and 2-h values on the glucose tolerance test rise by 10 mg/dl for each decade beyond the fifth. Consequently, unless the diagnostic criteria (see below) are age-adjusted, as many as 70 percent of patients above age 70 will be labeled "diabetic."

TABLE 19-14 Factors Diminishing Performance in Glucose Tolerance Testing

- Age: blood glucose concentration increases 10 mg/dl per decade beyond the fifth decade
- Inactivity
- Diet (if <100 g carbohydrate per day)
- Drugs
  - Potassium-wasting diuretics
  - Phenytoin
  - Alcohol (large amounts)
  - Corticosteroids
  - Oral contraceptives
  - Psychoactive drugs
- Intercurrent disease
  - Endocrine abnormalities
  - Renal failure
  - Cirrhosis
  - Nonspecific severe stress
    - Myocardial infarction
    - Sepsis

Inactivity associated with prolonged bed rest (i.e., several weeks or more) also results in a rise in the postprandial plasma glucose level. As in the case of aging, the effect of inactivity is to diminish tissue response to insulin rather than insulin secretion. In contrast, a marked increase in physical activity (as in a trained athlete) enhances sensitivity to insulin. Very active individuals nevertheless show normal glucose concentration increments during glucose tolerance testing but only minimal elevations in plasma insulin concentration.[329] Circadian factors also influence carbohydrate metabolism; a mild decrease in glucose disposal is observed in the late afternoon and evening. As was noted above, severe restriction in dietary carbohydrate (<100 g per day) diminishes glucose tolerance.

A variety of drugs also may influence glucose tolerance. Consequently, where possible, their intake should be discontinued 3 days before testing. Large amounts of alcohol, thiazides, and other potassium-wasting diuretics (e.g., furosemide and chlorthalidone) and high doses of phenytoin (which interferes with insulin release) are associated with a lessening of glucose tolerance. The oral contraceptive agents (estrogen-progestins) cause a deterioration in glucose tolerance; this is due primarily to the estrogen component. Psychoactive agents such as phenothiazines and tricyclic antidepressants (amitriptyline, imipramine, nortriptyline) reduce glucose disposal. However, depression per se is associated with a fall in glucose tolerance, which is restored to normal with improvement in mood. A variety of endocrine disorders, such as acromegaly and spontaneous and iatrogenic Cushing's syndrome, as well as renal failure and hepatic cirrhosis are associated with an increased frequency of glucose intolerance. In renal failure, resistance to insulin, hyperglucagonemia, and augmented sensitivity to glucagon have been implicated as pathogenic factors.[225] In cirrhosis, portal-systemic shunting, resulting in failure of hepatic glucose uptake, resistance to insulin, decreased insulin secretion, and hyperglucagonemia, may be a contributory factor.[246] Glucose tolerance may also be diminished as a result of the nonspecific stress effects of any serious acute illness, e.g., myocardial infarction or sepsis (see Stress Hyperglycemia, above).

Diagnostic Criteria

The criteria for the diagnosis of diabetes on the basis of glucose tolerance testing varied widely in the past. However, over the past decade there has been increasing acceptance of the criteria proposed by the National Diabetes Data Group (NDDG). As shown in Table 19-15, in the absence of fasting hyperglycemia, overt diabetes is present if the 2-h glucose concentration is >200 mg/dl (11.1 m*M*) and one other value (at 30, 60, or 90 min) is also >200 mg/dl. Plasma glucose concentrations which are intermediate between normal and overt diabetes (2-h value 140 to 200 mg/dl plus one value at 30 to 90 min >200 mg/dl) are defined as *impaired glucose tolerance*. Such patients were previously described as having "chemical," "latent," or "subclinical" diabetes, terms which should be abandoned. In pregnancy substantially lower plasma glucose levels are employed for the diagnosis of gestational diabetes (see Pregnancy and Diabetes, below).

The observation that with less severe abnormalities in glucose metabolism (i.e., in individuals with impaired glucose tolerance), the microangiopathy (retinopathy or nephropathy) characteristic of overt diabetes is not observed supports the strict criteria of the NDDG for overt diabetes. Furthermore in highly diabetes-prone population groups such as the Pima, a bimodal distribution is observed on glucose testing: A 2-h value >200 mg/dl separates the diabetic group from the nondiabetic group and is predictive of a predisposition to the long-term complication of diabetes.[330] Nevertheless, compared with the general population, individuals in the intermediate category of impaired glucose tolerance are at increased risk for the development of overt diabetes (30 percent) as well as coronary artery disease.

TABLE 19-15 Criteria for the Diagnosis of Diabetes by Oral Glucose Tolerance Testing

		National Diabetes Data Group*
Time, min	Overt Diabetes	Impaired Glucose Tolerance
30		
60	1 value >200 (at 30, 60, or 90)	1 value >200 (at 30, 60, or 90)
90		
120	>200	>140† but <200

Note: All plasma glucose concentrations are given in mg/dl.

* National Diabetes Data Group: *Diabetes* 28:1039, 1979.

† In patients above age 50, add 10 mg/dl for each decade beyond the fifth.

The "Flat" Glucose Tolerance Curve

Frequently, patients are referred for consultation to the diabetologist for evaluation of a "flat" glucose tolerance curve, i.e., one in which a minimal elevation in blood glucose concentration is observed during the early part of the glucose tolerance test. Such patients occasionally are misdiagnosed as having hypoglycemia, "mild" diabetes, or malabsorption. It should be noted that after the administration of a 100-g glucose load, the 1-h glucose concentration value remains below 100 mg/dl (5.6 m*M*) in as many as 35 percent of normal subjects and does not exceed 90 mg/dl (5.0 m*M*) in 19 percent of cases.[331] In the absence of other corroborative evidence, such "flat" responses should not be interpreted as indicative of hypoglycemia, malabsorption, or glucose intolerance. A flat glucose curve may sometimes be indicative of a low renal threshold for glucose (normally at ~170 mg/dl, 9.4 m*M*); the presence of glucose in urine should then be examined during the test. Also, children and young persons exhibit high rates of tissue glucose uptake with rapid assimilation of the glucose load. Measurement of other parameters indicative of glucose absorption, such as plasma insulin and FFA concentration (a pronounced decrease at 1 to 2 h after glucose administration), may be helpful in the evaluation.

Indications for Glucose Tolerance Testing

In a patient with fasting hyperglycemia (>140 mg/dl), glucose tolerance testing is not necessary (or warranted) for the diagnosis of diabetes. In patients with normal fasting glucose levels, indiscriminate use of the test should also be avoided. While the glucose tolerance test in itself poses no direct risk to the patient, a variety of hazards of overdiagnosis of diabetes are now recognized. Overzealous diagnosis of diabetes may lead to employment discrimination, denial of insurance, mental anguish for the patient and family, and unnecessary treatment with antidiabetic drugs. The significance of these potential dangers is underscored by the observations that (1) a large proportion (up to 50 percent) of patients with impaired glucose tolerance on first testing revert to normal on subsequent testing and (2) intervention with sulfonylurea agents fails to lower the rate of progression to overt diabetes. Consequently, glucose tolerance testing should not be done as a mass or even individual screening procedure other than in pregnancy (see Pregnancy and Diabetes, below). In nonpregnant individuals it should be limited to situations in which some intervention is likely to be of benefit.

In obesity, the detection of glucose intolerance may provide a stimulus (to the patient as well as the physician) to implement a weight-reducing diet inasmuch as normalization of body weight generally results in improved metabolism of carbohydrates. In pregnancy (see below), proper management of gestational diabetes with diet and/or insulin leads to improved fetal mortality and morbidity. In patients with a strong genetic predisposition for diabetes (e.g., if both parents have overt diabetes), a normal glucose tolerance test may have prognostic value and relieve anxiety (<2 percent of patients with normal glucose tolerance develop frank diabetes over the ensuing 5 to 10 years). The glucose tolerance test may also be useful in evaluating patients with the nephrotic syndrome, peripheral neuropathy, or premature arteriosclerosis, since these syndromes may manifest themselves as complications of diabetes before the development of fasting hyperglycemia.

The Intravenous Glucose Tolerance Test

The IV glucose tolerance test is much less widely used than the oral procedure but is preferable in patients who develop nausea after an oral glucose load or who have GI disease with malabsorption. It has recently been used for the evaluation of residual beta cell function in persons suspected of developing type I diabetes. Glucose is administered IV as a 50% solution over 2 to 4 min in a standard 25-g dose or in a dose of 0.5 g per kilogram of ideal body weight. Blood samples are then obtained at 10-min intervals until 60 min.

Evaluation of the test is based on the assumption that the curve of glucose disappearance is logarithmic, as described by the equation

$$C_t = C_0 e^{-kt}$$

where C_0 = glucose concentration at time zero
C_t = glucose concentration at time t
k = rate constant or rate of fall of blood glucose concentration in percent/min

Calculation of k is simplified by determining $t_{1/2}$, or the time necessary for the glucose concentration to fall by one-half, using the formula

$$k = \frac{0.69}{t_{1/2}} \times 100$$

In normal subjects, $k > 1.2$. In instances of impaired glucose tolerance, $k < 1.0$.

Insulin Determination

Measurements of insulin concentration are frequently obtained during glucose tolerance tests as part of research studies concerned with insulin secretion and/or response. In clinical practice, insulin concentration provides little information to facilitate the diagnosis of diabetes or impaired glucose tolerance. This is particularly true because of the heterogeneity of insulin response in type II diabetes and the frequent coexistence in type II patients of obesity, which of itself raises insulin levels. Consequently, insulin determination should be restricted to research, to circumstances in which hypoglycemia due to an islet-cell tumor is suspected (see Chap. 20), or when flat glucose tolerance curves are encountered. Measurement of C peptide which reflects endogenous insulin secretion may also be helpful in patients whose clinical characteristics do not permit their precise categorization as type I or type II diabetic patients. A low C peptide level, particularly after provocative stimuli such as glucose or glucagon, points to type I diabetes as the correct diagnosis.

Urinary Glucose Determination

Clinical measurements of urinary glucose are made with paper strips impregnated with glucose-specific enzymes. The urinary glucose concentration does not, however, necessarily reflect the concentration of glucose in the plasma. The glucose in the glomerular filtrate is quantitatively reabsorbed until the maximum capacity of the tubules to remove glucose is exceeded. In normal humans this occurs at a concentration of 160 to 180 mg/dl, the renal threshold. This level varies from one person to another, however, and is also altered by changes in kidney function. In patients with a low renal threshold, glucose may appear in the urine even when the blood glucose concentration is within the normal range; in some patients with kidney disease even high blood glucose concentrations may not be associated with glucosuria. Moreover, the urine in the bladder at any given time reflects the blood concentration at the time the urine was excreted by the kidney, not at the time it is passed from the bladder. Therefore, when patients have not voided for several hours, the degree of glycosuria may bear little relation to the blood glucose concentration at the time of urination. The diagnosis of diabetes should never be established solely on the basis of a single or even multiple urine glucose determinations; diagnosis depends on measurement of plasma or blood glucose concentration. However, in a patient with known diabetes, the urinary glucose concentration provides an index for the assessment of blood glucose control. It is more useful when "second-voided" urine collected within 30 min of prior voiding is tested. Furthermore, urine glucose measurements are not nearly as useful as self-monitored blood glucose measurements in the assessment of control of diabetes.

Glycohemoglobin

The red cells of diabetic patients have an increased proportion of a component of hemoglobin which elutes on cation exchange chromatography or moves on electrophoresis before the main HbA peak; it is designated *glycohemoglobin* (HbA_{Ic}). This component is structurally identical to HbA except for the presence of hexose residues bound covalently to the terminal valine of the β chain and to the ε-amino lysine side chains. The formation of glycohemoglobin represents a posttranscriptional nonenzymatic modification of the hemoglobin protein (Fig. 19-9), which is dependent on the concentration of blood glucose. In poorly regulated diabetic patients HbA_{Ic} increases 12 to 15 percent of total Hb compared with 4 to 6 percent in normal subjects. Since the life span of the red cell is 15 weeks, glycated hemoglobin concentration provides a time-averaged index of the blood glucose level over a 5- to 10-week period rather than just at the time of blood sampling.[29] Consequently, measurements of glycohemoglobin provide a more reliable index of overall plasma glucose control than can be obtained from isolated blood glucose determinations.

Since plasma albumin likewise undergoes glycation during hyperglycemia[30] and since its half-life is markedly shorter than that of hemoglobin, measurement of the glycoalbumin level may provide a weekly integrative assessment of blood glucose control.[332] Whereas 1 week of intense insulin treatment of type 1 diabetes has been shown to reduce HbA_{Ic} by <10 percent of the original value, glycoalbumin has been found to fall by 18 percent at 1 week and by 40 percent after 17 days.[30]

HbA_{Ic} can be determined by affinity chromatography, ion-exchange chromatography, agarose gel electrophoresis, and high-performance liquid chromatography. Affinity chromatography is widely used; it is simple to apply using commercially available kits and has the advantage of being unaffected by associated hemoglobinopathies or the presence of the labile fraction of hemoglobin. Specimens may be stored up to 21 days at room temperature without affecting the HbA_{Ic} value.[333] More recently an immunoassay technique has become available which involves premixed reagents in a single-use cartridge. This technique permits office-based measurement of HbA_{Ic} within 9 min with precision and reliability comparable to those of affinity chromatography.[334]

The major usefulness of the measurement of glycohemoglobin is that it constitutes the most reliable means of assessing chronic blood glucose control over the prior 1 to 2 months from a single blood measurement. For detailed adjustment of insulin therapy, it does not take the place of self-monitored blood glucose levels. Rather, glycohemoglobin provides a means of verifying the reliability of self-monitored blood glucose levels. With respect to the initial diagnosis of diabetes, an abnormal elevation in glycohemoglobin has a specificity of >99 percent but a sensitivity of <50 percent.[28] Thus, a normal glycohemoglobin (particularly if it is just below the upper limits of normal) does not exclude the diagnosis of diabetes.

Summary of Diagnostic Criteria and Diagnostic Terms

The diagnosis of diabetes is dependent on the demonstration of fasting hyperglycemia (plasma glucose concentration >140 mg/dl or >7.8 m*M*) on more than one occasion or a 2-h plasma glucose level (plus one other value) >200 mg/dl (or >11.1 m*M*) during an oral glucose tolerance test. Two-hour values on the oral glucose tolerance test of 140 to 200 mg/dl indicate *impaired glucose tolerance*. Patients with this diagnosis develop overt diabetes at a rate of 1 to 5 percent per year and, in the absence of such progression, are not generally at risk of developing microangiopathy. The terms *chemical, latent,* and *asymptomatic* or *subclinical diabetes,* which previously were used to describe patients with impaired glucose tolerance, should be discarded. *Prediabetes* refers to entirely normal glucose tolerance in an individual who is predisposed to develop overt diabetes.

Because of the complexity and heterogeneity of the genetic and environmental factors diagnostically predictive for diabetes, the prediabetic state is usually hypothetical. Among first-degree relatives of type I diabetic patients a combination of immunologic markers (ICA, IAA, anti-GAD antibodies) and IV glucose responses is being used in research studies to identify prediabetes (see Prediction and Prevention, above). *Gestational diabetes* refers to generally transient diabetes or glucose intolerance which has its onset in pregnancy; this is discussed in detail below (see Pregnancy and Diabetes).

Prevalence

The prevalence of diabetes can only be estimated in view of the relatively arbitrary nature of the criteria employed for diagnosis. The overall prevalence of type II diabetes is estimated at 5 to 7 percent in the United States and Japan and 25 percent in Europe.[2] However, overt diabetes is present in only 2 to 3 percent of the population. The prevalence of insulin-dependent (type I) diabetes is approximately 0.5 percent.

The frequency with which diabetes is encountered is quite variable among different ethnic groups. Diabetes is virtually never seen in the Inuit (Eskimo). In contrast, the highest reported prevalence is among the Pima, where conventional interpretation of the oral glucose tolerance test results in a diagnosis of type II diabetes in 50 percent of the population. This is not a specifically Native American trait, because the Cocopah have a much lower incidence in spite of a roughly comparable level of obesity. As noted above, the Pima differ from other population groups by showing a bimodal distribution on glucose tolerance testing; the cutoff between nondiabetic individuals and diabetic patients ranges between 200 and 250 mg/dl (11.7 and 13.4 m*M*).[330] High prevalence rates of type II diabetes are also observed in Mexican-Americans, Asian Indians, and Polynesians. The risk factors identified in these population groups include obesity, particularly involving the upper body (as reflected by an elevated waist-to-hip ratio); physical inactivity; and increased dietary consumption of saturated fat.[335]

Pathology

Florid diabetes (with DKA) may exist in the absence of any pathognomonic lesions identifiable by histologic examination. This is particularly true in patients in whom diabetes has been present for a relatively brief period (a few months). However, in most patients dying with diabetes, histologic changes are observed in the islets of Langerhans; with long-standing diabetes pathognomonic lesions are observed in small blood vessels (microangiopathy) and peripheral nerves (neuropathy).

Islets of Langerhans

As discussed above (see Etiology), in patients who succumb to acute-onset type I diabetes a lymphocytic infiltration of the islets (insulitis) is frequently observed on autopsy, providing evidence for an autoimmune and/or viral etiology for type I diabetes (Fig. 19-40). In addition to the infiltrative changes, immunocytochemical studies reveal a reduction in the number of beta cells, while the numbers of alpha and delta cells remain unchanged.[336] By the time diabetes has been established for 5 years or more, the number of islets, the size of the islets, and the number of beta cells are reduced.

In patients with type II diabetes, hyaline degeneration of the islets, consisting of amorphous deposits with the staining characteristics of amyloid, is observed. The amyloid deposits in diabetic islets represent a concentrated and polymerized form of a 37-amino acid polypeptide known as *amylin* or islet amyloid–associated protein (IAAP).[294] This peptide, which has homology with the calcitonin gene–related peptides expressed in neural tissue, is synthesized by beta cells and cosecreted with insulin in response to glucose. Excess production of amylin has been implicated as the mechanism of amyloidogenesis in the islet cells of type II diabetic patients. A role for amylin overproduction in the pathogenesis of insulin resistance in type II diabetes has also been suggested but has not been established.[294,295]

Fibrosis occurs in about 25 percent of patients. It begins with thickening of the capsule and invasion of the islet with fibrous tissue; the fibrous tissue ultimately replaces the functioning cells completely. The process also extends outward from the islets so that the exocrine portion of the pancreas may also be extensively involved. Although hyalinization and fibrosis affect both the alpha and the beta cells, the beta cells are more heavily involved.

Glycogenosis of the islets occurs in a small percentage of patients. This appears as large vacuolated cells. These findings, formerly termed *hydropic degeneration*, are now unusual; they are generally a reflection of severe, persistent hyperglycemia.

In some patients with type II diabetes histologic examination of the islets reveals minimal or no changes. However, careful determination of islet volume reveals a decrease in the mass of islet cells in virtually all patients with diabetes.[336]

Blood Vessels

Arteriosclerosis occurs with a much greater frequency and at an earlier age in the diabetic population compared with the nondiabetic population.[1,2] However, in the case of coronary artery disease as well as large-vessel peripheral vascular disease (the two major areas resulting in clinical disease, myocardial infarction, and gangrene), the histologic appearance of the lesions (atheromatous plaque formation) is no different from that observed in the general population.

Diabetic patients are, however, also predisposed to microangiopathy. This term derives from the fact that the earliest lesions involve the capillaries and precapillary arterioles. The characteristic finding in early diabetic microangiopathy is a thickening of the capillary basement membrane (Fig. 19-49). On light microscopy this thickening is due to the accumulation of material which stains positively with periodic acid Schiff (PAS) reagent and is composed of glycoproteins. Basement membrane thickening may be observed in virtually all tissues (including skin and muscle) but is of particular importance when present in the renal glomerulus (diabetic nephropathy) and the retina (diabetic retinopathy). Contrary to initial reports, basement membrane thickening in muscle tissue is related to the duration of clinically overt diabetes; it is absent in unaffected monozygotic twins of individuals with known diabetes.[337]

The Kidney

In newly diagnosed type I diabetes, kidney size is increased (as determined by x-ray examination) and the volume of the glomerular tufts is increased on renal biopsy. A reduction to normal size is observed within a few months of the initiation of insulin treatment.

Thickening of the glomerular basement membrane and of basement membrane–like PAS-positive material in the mesangium (the interstitial tissue lying between gomerular capillaries) is demonstrable on electron microscopic examination of renal biopsy material obtained 2 years after the clinical onset of diabetes.[338] The thickening may progress so that the entire glomerulus is ultimately replaced by a sheet of amorphous material. Alternatively, it may coalesce into nodular masses, as first described by Kimmelstiel and Wilson, which are highly characteristic of diabetes mellitus. The Kimmelstiel-Wilson lesions consist of spherical hyaline masses within the glomerular tufts; they are acidophilic and PAS-positive (Fig. 19-50). Similar thickening, but of lesser degree, has been reported in rare instances before clinically detectable diabetes is present. This finding has been cited as providing evidence that the microvascular lesions are not caused by the carbohydrate defect, but the possibility cannot be excluded that such patients had mild fluctuations in glucose tolerance before the development of these lesions. Furthermore, as noted above, patients with overt diabetes show neither light microscopic nor electron microscopic evidence of basement membrane thickening until the metabolic abnormalities (e.g., hyperglycemia) have been present for at least 2 years.

FIGURE 19-49 Schematic representation of capillary basement membrane in the kidney glomerulus, skin, and muscle of normal individuals and diabetic patients. Thickening of the basement membrane is the earliest histologic evidence of diabetic microangiopathy. BM = basement membrane; END = endothelial cell; EP = epithelial cell; RBC = red blood cell. *(From Siperstein M: Adv Intern Med 18:325, 1972.)*

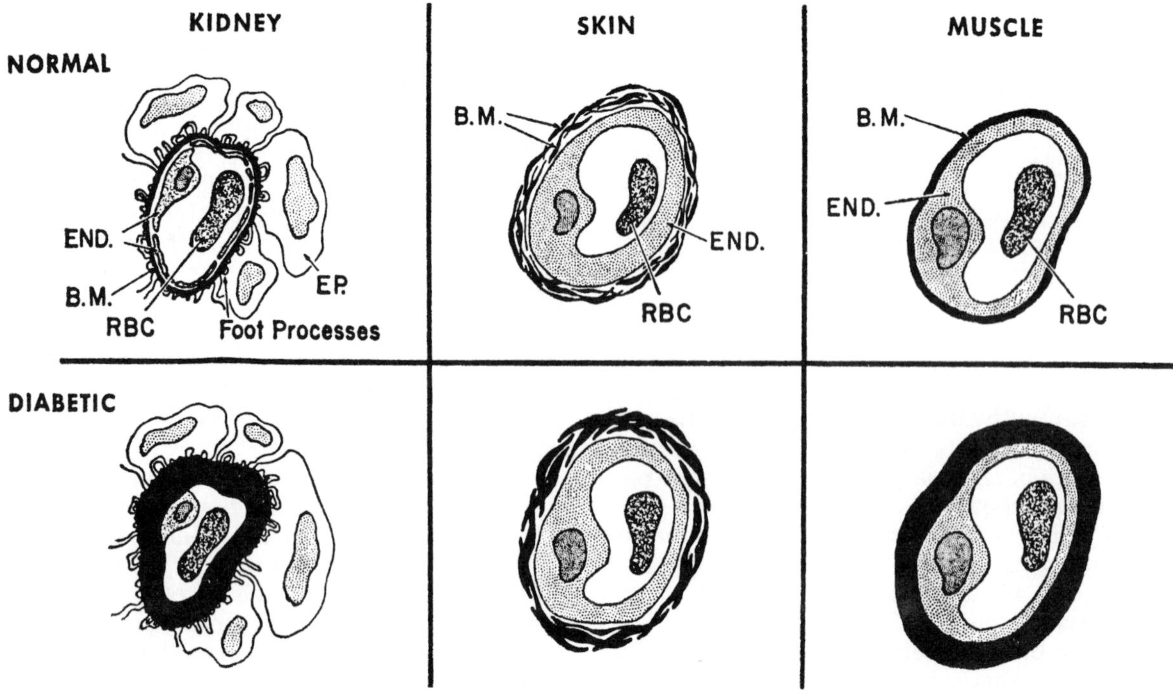

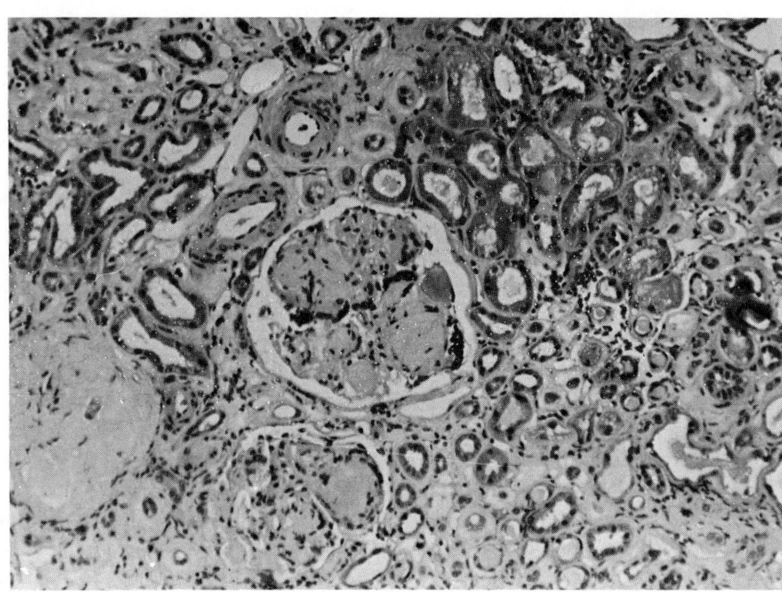

FIGURE 19-50 Section of kidney from a patient with type I (insulin-dependent) diabetes demonstrating the nodular intercapillary glomerulosclerosis (Kimmelstiel-Wilson lesions) characteristic of diabetic nephropathy. (*Courtesy of M Kashgarian.*)

The Eye

The earliest histologic changes in diabetic retinopathy are *microaneurysms*, globular or fusiform outpouchings of the capillary walls. These lesions are often associated with loss of pericytes (mural cells which normally surround the endothelial cells) and adjacent areas of occluded capillaries; whether the occlusions are a cause or a consequence of the microaneurysms has not been established. The *yellow exudates* observed on funduscopic examination consist of foci of extravasated lipid and protein in the deep layers of the retina. Hemorrhages are also observed in the deep layers (round) or superficial layers (flame-shaped) of the retina. *Proliferative retinopathy* is characterized by *neovascularization*, new vessel formation which undergoes repeated regression and scarring, resulting in a mass of fibrovascular tissue which forms adhesions with the vitreous body. Contraction of this scar tissue results in hemorrhage from these fragile vessels into the vitreous or detachment of the retina, the two major causes of blindness in diabetic retinopathy. Blindness may also occur when intraretinal hemorrhages destroy the macular region.

Nervous System

In patients with diabetic peripheral polyneuropathy there is segmental demyelination, proliferation of Schwann cells, and an increase in connective tissue elements, while the vasa nervorum remain patent and show no significant disease. In contrast, the pathologic basis of cranial nerve palsies and mononeuritis multiplex associated with diabetes consists of ischemic changes involving the nutrient vessels.

Other Tissues

Hepatomegaly due to marked fatty infiltration of the liver is often observed in poorly regulated diabetes. When accompanied by hypercholesterolemia and (in rare instances) evidence of portal hypertension, the term *Mauriac syndrome* has been applied.[339]

Osteopenia has been reported in diabetes.[340] However, the mechanism of the decrease in bone mass has not been established.

Clinical Manifestations

The symptoms and signs of diabetes can be divided into three groups: (1) those directly related to elevations in plasma glucose concentration (e.g., polydipsia and polyuria), (2) those arising from the specific long-term lesions of diabetes [e.g., microangiopathy (particularly in the eye and kidney) and neuropathy], and (3) those resulting from the acceleration of or increased predisposition to disease processes which occur in the general population (e.g., atherosclerosis and skin and urinary tract infections). In addition, the diabetic syndrome may be clinically silent; its recognition may result from the discovery of hyperglycemia or glucosuria in the course of a routine medical examination or during the evaluation of another disease process. Occasionally, the premature development of myocardial infarction or peripheral vascular disease calls attention to the presence of diabetes. In rare cases, retinopathy or nephropathy may constitute the first clinical manifestation of diabetes.

Symptoms of Hyperglycemia

When hyperglycemia is of sufficient magnitude to result in fairly consistent glucosuria (generally >180 mg/dl or 10.0 m*M* throughout the day and night), the "polys" characteristic of diabetes appear: polydipsia, polyuria, and polyphagia. Despite the increase in food intake, such patients lose weight because of the loss of glucose in the urine. In patients with a high renal threshold for glucose (as a consequence of reduced GFR caused by diabetic nephropathy or other forms of renal disease), hyperglycemia may be persistent and moderately severe yet fail to result in glucosuria. In such circumstances, poor control of diabetes cannot be invoked as the explanation for weight loss irrespective of the blood glucose level. The increase in hyperglycemia which occurs in the postprandial period accounts for the lethargy which individuals with poorly controlled diabetes often notice after meals.

The augmentation in gluconeogenesis which contributes to the development of fasting hyperglycemia results in protein wasting and increased urinary nitrogen loss. These changes in protein metabolism contribute to the growth failure observed in children with untreated or poorly regulated insulin-dependent diabetes. Protein wasting may also be responsible for muscle weakness and may contribute to poor wound healing.

Marked swings in blood glucose concentration may cause visual blurring. This is due to changes in the water content of the lens in response to alterations in plasma osmolarity. The visual symptoms may be particularly troublesome when insulin treatment is instituted. Consequently, the patient should be reassured that the visual disturbance is transient and is not due to retinopathy. In addition, refraction for the purpose of fitting corrective lenses should not be undertaken until the blood glucose level has been stabilized.

Persistent glucosuria in women is frequently accompanied by vulvovaginitis, which manifests itself as itching and a malodorous vaginal discharge. Recurrent or severe skin infections (furunculosis) and cellulitis may also call attention to the presence of hyperglycemia.

The clinical manifestations of DKA and nonketotic hyperosmolar coma are discussed below.

Diabetic Retinopathy

In addition to refractive errors associated with fluctuations in blood glucose concentration, visual impairment may occur in diabetes as a result of cataracts or glaucoma and most commonly as a consequence of retinal microangiopathy, generally referred to as diabetic retinopathy. The significance of diabetic retinopathy is underscored by the fact that diabetes is the leading cause of blindness in the United States. Among blind diabetic patients, 85 percent lose sight as a result of retinopathy.[341] Of those who are legally blind, diabetes is the reported etiology in ~8 percent. The absolute risk of retinopathy resulting in severe visual impairment is dependent on the age of onset as well as the duration of diabetes. If diabetes is diagnosed at age 20, the risk of blindness at age 40 is 23 times that of the nondiabetic population. If diagnosis is at age 40, by age 70 the risk of blindness is 15 times the risk for the general population. An estimated 40 percent of type I and 50 percent of type II patients ultimately may develop proliferative retinopathy. Overall, the rate of blindness among all diabetics is ~2 percent. The risk of severe visual impairment and blindness has, however, been substantially reduced since the advent of laser therapy.

Clinical evaluation of diabetic retinopathy is based on ophthalmoscopic examination of the fundus and, where indicated, slit lamp examination and fluorescein angiography of the retina. The retinal changes observed in diabetic patients are generally divided into *background* retinopathy and *proliferative* retinopathy.[342] This classification has prognostic as well as therapeutic implications. Background retinopathy represents the earliest ophthalmic manifestation of diabetes; it consists of microaneurysms, dot and blot hemorrhages, exudates, and retinal edema (Fig. 19-51). It is often not possible to be certain that small red dots observed on ophthalmoscopic examination in the posterior fundus represent microaneurysms rather than dot hemorrhages. The exudates present in diabetic patients may be the "hard" yellow type with discrete borders or the "fluffy" white "cotton wool" exudates, grayish white lesions with indistinct borders. The cotton wool exudates were previously thought to be a consequence of hypertension but are now recognized in normotensive diabetic patients. They correspond to areas of microinfarction of the superficial nerve fiber layer.

Background retinopathy generally fails to result in visual impairment unless retinal edema, a plaque of hard exudate, or an intraretinal hemorrhage occurs at the macula (maculopathy). Maculopathy may be more common in NIDDM patients than in the type I population. Background retinopathy is found with increasing frequency both as the patients become older and as the disease progresses. Thus, it occurs very rarely in patients whose diabetes was diagnosed before age 30 and who have had the disease <5 years. By contrast, the frequency approaches 50 percent in patients who have had diabetes 10 years or more, 65 percent in those with diabetes for 15 years, and over 80 percent in patients who have had diabetes >30 years, no matter how old they were at the time of diagnosis. The lesions of simple retinopathy are not fixed; when the patient is followed over the course of years, the lesions appear and disappear in an unpredictable fashion.

The more severe and dangerous form of retinal disease is proliferative retinopathy. This consists of neovascularization (see above) (Fig. 19-52). These vessels proliferate outside the retina (into the vitreous) and are prone to hemorrhage, particularly when present near the optic disk. This leads to the development of fibrous tissue extending into the vitreous. Vitreous hemorrhages may initially be small and

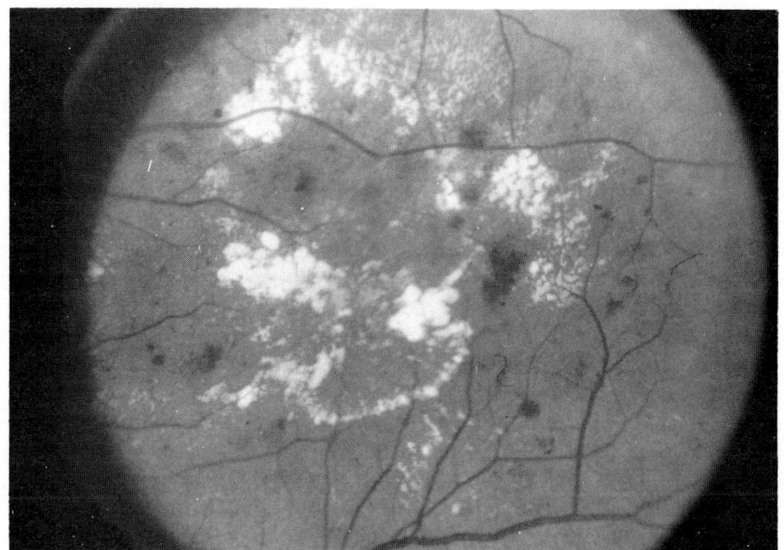

FIGURE 19-51 Fundus photograph demonstrating hemorrhages and exudates characteristic of background retinopathy in diabetes. The extensive degree of hemorrhages and exudates indicates a more severe form of background retinopathy designated as transitional retinopathy.

may be resorbed in days or weeks, causing only partial and temporary impairment of vision. However, severe visual loss occurs with massive hemorrhage or the contraction of fibrous bands leading to retinal detachment. This type of retinopathy occurs predominantly but not exclusively in insulin-dependent diabetes which begins in childhood. Thus, while only 15 percent of all diabetic patients are type I, ~50 percent of patients referred for the treatment of proliferative retinopathy developed diabetes before age 20 and only 15 percent developed it after age 50.

From the standpoint of clinical assessment and management, a major concern is the identification of patients who are at greatest risk of developing visual loss if left untreated.[342,342a] In some patients intraretinal hemorrhages occur in association with new vessel formation which is at the disk (NVD) or is severe in degree and located more than one disk diameter from the optic disk [new vessels elsewhere (NVE)]. A prospective study has revealed that in such patients the 2-year incidence of severe visual loss is increased from 3 to 4 percent to 25 to 35 percent.[342,343] These findings underscore the importance of fluorescein angiography in the evaluation of retinopathy, since this technique permits the identification of new vessels which often go undetected on ophthalmoscopic examination. In addition, a more advanced phase of background retinopathy termed *preproliferative retinopathy* can be identified by fluorescein angiography. Preproliferative retinopathy consists of large, extensive areas of capillary closure (usually associated with cotton wool exudates) or venous abnormalities in the form of dilated capillary shunt vessels. The presence of these findings sug-

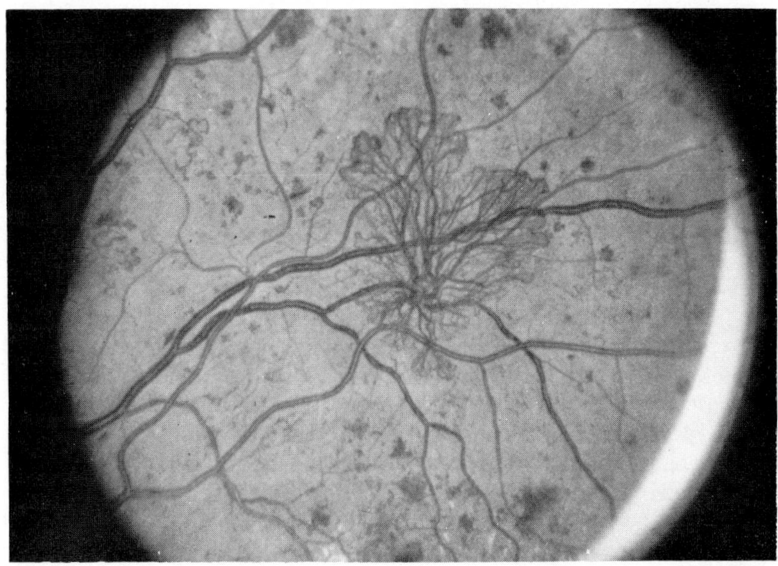

FIGURE 19-52 Fundus photograph demonstrating proliferative retinopathy as indicated by new vessel formation and scar tissue formation. (*Courtesy of J Puklin.*)

gests early progression to the proliferative state. A stage of retinopathy intermediate in severity between background and preproliferative retinopathy has been identified as *transitional retinopathy*. This category refers to the presence of significant blotch hemorrhages, soft exudates, or intraretinal microvascular abnormalities. In this categorization, background diabetic retinopathy is restricted to eyes with only microaneurysms or an occasional blotch hemorrhage or exudate. Patients may remain stable for years with transitional retinopathy, revert to background retinopathy with resorption of hemorrhages and resolution of exudates, or progress to preproliferative or proliferative retinopathy.

The most frequently employed method for the treatment of diabetic retinopathy is *photocoagulation*.[342,342b] The principle underlying this treatment is that absorption of light by pigmented retinal epithelium and its conversion to heat result in protein denaturation and a therapeutic burn (Fig. 19-53). After healing, points of vascular leakage are closed, areas of neovascularization may be obliterated, and further neovascularization is diminished, presumably by lessening the demand for oxygen in tissues where the vascular supply is compromised. The light source employed is either a xenon arc or an argon or krypton laser. The latter are two to three times more effective than the xenon arc in raising the temperature of retinal epithelium; they also permit greater safety in treating conditions in high-risk areas, such as neovascularization arising from the optic disk (NVD) and leaking microvascular abnormalities near the macula. A variety of studies have clearly documented the beneficial effects of panretinal photocoagulation in the treatment of proliferative diabetic retinopathy. In a large multicenter study in which patients with severe proliferative retinopathy received treatment in one eye only, the incidence of legal blindness over a 2-year follow-up was 16.3 percent in untreated eyes and 6.4 percent in treated eyes, a difference of 61 percent. On the basis of these results, photocoagulation is currently recommended in the following circumstances: (1) moderate or severe neovascularization extending from or close to the optic nerve, (2) mild neovascularization extending from the optic nerve with hemorrhage into the vitreous, (3) moderate peripheral neovascularization with a hemorrhage into the vitreous, (4) diabetic maculopathy, and (5) diabetic rubeosis of the iris (proliferation of vessels on the iris or in the angle). In the treatment of macular edema and rubeosis of the iris, focal rather than panretinal photocoagulation is employed. Because photocoagulation treatment is most effective when started early but is not without risk, a key issue is whether such treatment is beneficial in patients with mild to moderate background retinopathy. Data from the Early Treatment Diabetic Retinopathy Study indicate that the risks of photocoagulation outweigh the benefits in patients with mild to moderate background retinopathy.[342a,344] An effect of aspirin or other antiplatelet drugs (dipyridamole or ticlopidine) in preventing the progression of mild to moderate retinopathy to high-risk characteristics has not been consistently observed.[342a,345]

A second major advance in the treatment of diabetic retinopathy has been the development of vitrectomy.[342,342a] This procedure involves the surgical excision of the vitreous via an incision in the pars plana behind the lens. The development of tiny rotating cutting instruments which suck in vitreous, cut it off, and replace the lost volume with saline now permits the excision of the vitreous without the corneal and retinal complications which accompanied earlier techniques. Vitrectomy is indicated in patients who have sustained a massive vitreous hemor-

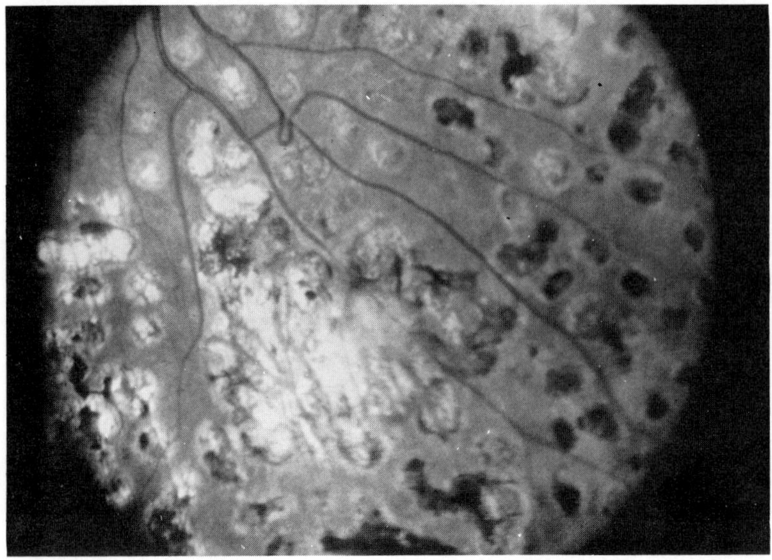

FIGURE 19-53 Fundus photograph demonstrating lesions produced by photocoagulation therapy for diabetic retinopathy. (*Courtesy of J Puklin.*)

rhage that fails to clear after several months. Before vitrectomy, ultrasonography and electroretinography are performed to ensure that the retina is attached and functioning well. The results to date indicate improvement of vision in 50 to 75 percent of cases. Vitrectomy is also frequently indicated for macular detachment since prolonged detachment may result in poor function even if the surgical outcome is good.[346]

The observation that a patient with severe retinopathy underwent remission after spontaneous infarction of the pituitary led to the hypothesis that ablation of the pituitary will bring about improvement or prevent progression of diabetic retinopathy. Hypophysectomy, either surgical or by some form of radiation (implantation of radioactive pellets or heavy-particle beam), and pituitary stalk section had their vogue in the 1960s. Both unoperated controls and patients with varying grades of hypophysectomy were studied. Microaneurysms, neovascularization, and hemorrhages were better controlled in some patients with maximal or severe pituitary destruction than in unoperated or mildly hypopituitary controls, but visual acuity was not significantly improved. Compared with photocoagulation, the hazards of hypophysectomy are far greater and the benefits are considerably less. Accordingly, hypophysectomy has been abandoned in the management of diabetic retinopathy.

The relation of control of blood glucose concentration to the progression of diabetic retinopathy is discussed below (see Pathogenesis of Complications). The recent findings of the Diabetes Control and Complications Trial clearly indicate a beneficial effect of near-normalization of blood glucose control in reducing the risk of development of retinopathy (see below, Treatment of Diabetes). Treatment of coexisting hypertension is particularly important in modifying the development of retinopathy. In patients at high risk for the development of vitreous hemorrhage, aspirin and nonsteroidal anti-inflammatory drugs (NSAID) should generally be avoided.

Diabetic patients are prone to the development of glaucoma. This may take the form of narrow-angle glaucoma due to neovascularization of the iris (rubeosis of the iris). In addition, primary open-angle glaucoma is more prevalent in diabetic patients, particulary patients who are free of proliferative retinopathy.

Senile cataracts observed in diabetic patients are indistinguishable from those occurring in the general population, but they occur at an earlier age and progress more rapidly. One particular type of cataract, the "snowflake," or metabolic, cataract, is characteristic of diabetes and is most commonly observed in children or adolescents with "brittle" diabetes. Similar "sugar" cataracts develop in rats with experimentally induced hyperglycemia and can be produced in vitro when rabbit lenses are maintained in organ culture with high concentrations of glucose. These cataracts are believed to be associated with sorbitol accumulation within the lens.

Current guidelines indicate that diabetic patients should have an ophthalmologic examination (by an ophthalmologist through a dilated pupil) within 5 years of the onset of type I diabetes beginning in childhood or in the teen years and at the time of onset in older patients with either type I or type II diabetes. Follow-up examinations should be obtained at yearly intervals in patients without significant retinopathy and at intervals of 4 to 6 months in patients with significant retinopathy.

Diabetic Nephropathy

Microangiopathy involving the kidney (diabetic nephropathy) is a major cause of morbidity and mortality in the diabetic population. Among type I diabetic patients, clinically detectable proteinuria develops in 30 to 40 percent of cases after 20 years and renal failure is responsible for 40 to 50 percent of deaths. In most patients with type II diabetes, proteinuria is seen within 10 years of clinical diagnosis; in type I, by contrast, it generally occurs after ~15 years of disease. Approximately 10 percent of type II patients develop clinically overt diabetic nephropathy. A family history of hypertension, prior hypertension in the patient, poor glycemia control, and cigarette smoking are associated with a higher prevalence of nephropathy.[347] Unlike retinopathy, the risk of which increases with the duration of diabetes, the risk of nephropathy increases until a duration of 20 years and then declines. Diabetes accounts for ~25 percent of new cases of end-stage renal disease in the United States. As noted above, the histologic lesions specific to diabetic renal disease consist of thickening and accumulation of basement membrane material and mesangium, which may form nodular deposits described as Kimmelstiel-Wilson lesions (Fig. 19-50). The functional correlates of these morphologic changes are increased glomerular permeability resulting in proteinuria, followed by a progressive reduction in GFR and overall renal function.

In the earliest stages of type I diabetes, both renal size (as assessed by radiographic or ultrasound studies) and GFR are increased.[348,349] The increase in GFR is a consequence of an elevation in renal plasma flow and in the glomerular transcapillary hydraulic pressure difference.[350,351] These changes in intrarenal hemodynamics can be reversed by restoration of normal or nearly normal blood glucose concentrations.[352] The increases in glomerular pressure and flow have been proposed to be the basis for the increased glomerular passage of protein, leading to proteinuria (*hyperfiltration hypothesis*). Mesangial protein accumulation occurs as well; this is a postulated forerunner of glomerular sclerosis. Independent of increased perfusion, the increase in renal size and/or changes in the chemical structure of the basement membrane may also be of importance in the pathogenesis of diabetic nephropathy.[353] An increase in hydroxylysine and hydroxyproline content, greater amounts of glucose and galactose, a decrease in the number of sialic acid residues, and reduced sulfation of glycosaminoglycans have been observed in diabetic glomerular basement membrane compared with control material from nondiabetic persons.[354–356] The reduction in negatively charged sialic acid and sulfate residues may impede the normal charge-dependent barrier to filtration of negatively charged macromolecules (e.g., albumin), thus leading to proteinuria. The increased hexose content of the basement membrane proteins may alter the tridimensional shape and packaging and affect membrane permeability. The possibility also exists that nephromegaly, excessive perfusion, and alterations in the chemical structure of basement membrane act in concert to produce diabetic nephropathy.

The earliest clinical manifestation of renal disease is the development of proteinuria. Interestingly, histologic evidence of diabetic nephropathy may be present for years before the appearance of proteinuria.[357] Although gross proteinuria (>300 to 500 mg/24 h) has long been recognized as a hallmark of diabetic nephropathy, recent studies have focused on the presence of *microalbuminuria* which appears earlier in the development of renal disease. Microalbuminuria is defined as an increase in urinary albumin measurable by RIA (20 to 450 mg/24 h or 15 to 300 μg/min) but undetectable by conventional dipstick assay (<500 mg/24 h or 300 μg/min). Microalbuminuria (particularly when accompanied by markedly increased perfusion) has predictive significance for clinically overt nephropathy (gross proteinuria) and its possible reversal by the restoration of normal or nearly normal blood glucose concentration.[358] Consequently, the presence of microalbuminuria has been suggested as identifying a stage of diabetic renal disease designated as *incipient diabetic nephropathy*. Further progression from incipient to clinically overt diabetic nephropathy can be prevented or slowed by strict maintenance of euglycemia, as recently reported in the Diabetes Control and Complications Trial (see below, Treatment of Diabetes).

In 20 to 40 percent of type I diabetic patients progression to gross proteinuria occurs. In such patients there is an inexorable deterioration culminating in renal failure within 5 to 7 years. The institution of intensive insulin therapy and the restoration of euglycemia generally fail to alter progression at this stage.[359] Proteinuria in excess of 500 mg/24 h may, however, persist for years in type II diabetic patients without progressing to renal failure. The proteinuria may reach massive proportions, resulting in the nephrotic syndrome, characterized by hypoalbuminemia and edema. Classically, a diabetic patient with the nephrotic syndrome also shows hypertension and hyperlipidemia. Patients in whom the level of serum creatinine has reached 8 mg/dl survive (in the absence of treatment with hemodialysis or transplantation) for an average of 7 months. In type I patients who develop renal failure, the interval from the diagnosis of diabetes to the appearance of an elevation in blood urea nitrogen (BUN) concentration is 12 to 15 years; this interval varies from 8 to 21 years among insulin-dependent diabetic patients and from 2 to 35 years among non-insulin-dependent diabetic patients.[360] Once azotemia is present, progression to frank uremia generally occurs in 3 to 4 years, but in some patients dialysis may not be required for 6 years or more.

The course of diabetic nephropathy is complicated by the presence of hypertension in over 70 percent of patients. In the large majority of cases the hypertension follows rather than precedes the development of renal insufficiency. Low plasma renin concentration is often observed in diabetic patients, suggesting that the hypertension is not due to increased activity of the renin-angiotensin system but may be due to increased fluid volume. In addition to hypertension and the nephrotic syndrome, fluid overload is also frequently manifested as recurrent pulmonary edema. Diabetic retinopathy is almost invariably present; it often deteriorates rapidly, perhaps as a consequence of accompanying hypertension and possibly as a result of the use of heparin during hemodialysis treatment. However, patients occasionally display only mild background retinopathy. Severe neuropathy is also frequently present in patients with renal failure. Differentiation of uremic from diabetic neuropathy in such patients is often not possible. *Hyperkalemia* is not uncommonly observed in diabetic patients in the presence of only moderate azotemia (BUN < 60 mg/dl) and in the absence of acidosis. Several mechanisms have been advanced to account for this syndrome of nonacidotic, nonuremic hyperkalemia of diabetes.[132] Hyporeninemic hypoaldosteronism, presumably due to interstitial nephritis, is demonstrable in some patients. Alternatively, in view of the importance of basal insulin levels for maintaining potassium homeostasis, hypoinsulinemia per se may predispose to the accumulation of serum potassum in circumstances of compromised renal function. Diabetic patients with renal disease are at particular risk of developing *drug-induced hyperkalemia*. Increases in serum potassium may be observed in such patients in association with the administration of angiotensin-converting enzyme (ACE) inhibitors (e.g., captopril), beta-adrenergic blockers, NSAIDs (which may also intensify azotemia), and potassium-sparing diuretics (e.g., spironolactone, triamterene, amiloride).

Since diabetic patients are susceptible to all the other diseases of the kidney which may afflict nondiabetic individuals, many diabetic patients have glomerular nephritis, chronic pyelonephritis, and other kidney diseases which may lead to the nephrotic syndrome. Asymptomatic bacteruria is particularly common in diabetic patients. Renal papillary necrosis, a lesion which is almost never observed in the nondiabetic population, is also only rarely diagnosed among patients with diabetes (in only 1 percent of diabetic patients with end-stage renal failure). However, it is likely that many cases of papillary necrosis go unrecognized during life, since as many as 10 percent of diabetic patients show such lesions at autopsy.

Although renal biopsy is the only definitive means of being certain of the presence of diabetic nephropathy, the procedure is rarely necessary in a diabetic patient with severe or end-stage renal disease. Diagnostic procedures should be directed at the detection of reversible lesions, such as bacterial infection or obstructive uropathy, which frequently complicate diabetic nephropathy. Caution should be applied in the use of the IV pyelogram. In diabetic patients with a serum creatinine concentration in excess of 4 to 6 mg/dl, irreversible deterioration of renal function and oliguria may follow IV pyelography or angiography.

A common observation in patients with advanced diabetic nephropathy and uremia is their tendency to require less insulin than they did before the onset of renal failure. Careful examination of large numbers of patients with this complication, however, shows that as many patients have an increased insulin requirement as have a decreased one; it is therefore impossible to justify a blanket statement that advanced renal disease reduces the insulin requirement. It is quite likely that when the reduced insulin requirement occurs, it is a result of anorexia and decreased caloric intake as well as loss of the insulin-degradative function of the kidneys.[213]

Before the development of frank uremia, the management of diabetic renal disease is directed at control of blood pressure with antihypertensive agents, use of diuretics for the management of edema, and restriction of dietary salt and, where appropriate, protein. Dietary protein restriction may slow the progression of azotemia in patients with manifest renal insufficiency. A reduction in dietary protein has also been suggested for patients with incipient nephropathy (microalbuminuria) as a means of preventing progression to gross proteinuria and azotemia. The rationale for these dietary changes is based largely on data in experimental animals with a reduced renal mass indicating that a restriction in dietary protein intake may prevent hyperfiltration and progressive renal deterioration. Whether dietary protein restriction has such protective effects in human diabetes has not been established. Furthermore, as dietary protein is reduced, carbohydrate content is increased and control of blood glucose may become more difficult.

Although improved metabolic control delays the onset of nephropathy or may reverse microalbuminuria in some patients (see Pathogenesis of Complications, above), once gross proteinuria has developed, the clinical course is unlikely to be altered significantly by improved blood glucose control. In marked contrast, control of hypertension is of crucial importance in slowing the progression of renal disease in patients with manifest nephropathy.[361] Antihypertensive therapy is effective in retarding the decline in GFR, reducing proteinuria, and delaying the requirement for renal replacement therapy (Fig. 19-54). The efficacy of antihypertensive therapy in preventing the progression of diabetic nephropathy has been demonstrated with a variety of drugs. A special role for ACE inhibitors has been proposed on the basis of their ability to lower intraglomerular pressure and preserve renal function in diabetic rats.[351,362] A recent multicenter trial has, in fact, shown that treatment with an ACE inhibitor (Captopril) in insulin-dependent diabetic patients with gross proteinuria ($>$ 500 mg per day) and serum cre-

FIGURE 19-54 Effect of antihypertensive therapy in slowing the rate of decline in glomerular filtration rate (GFR) and reducing albuminuria in patients with overt diabetic nephropathy. (*From Parving et al.*[361])

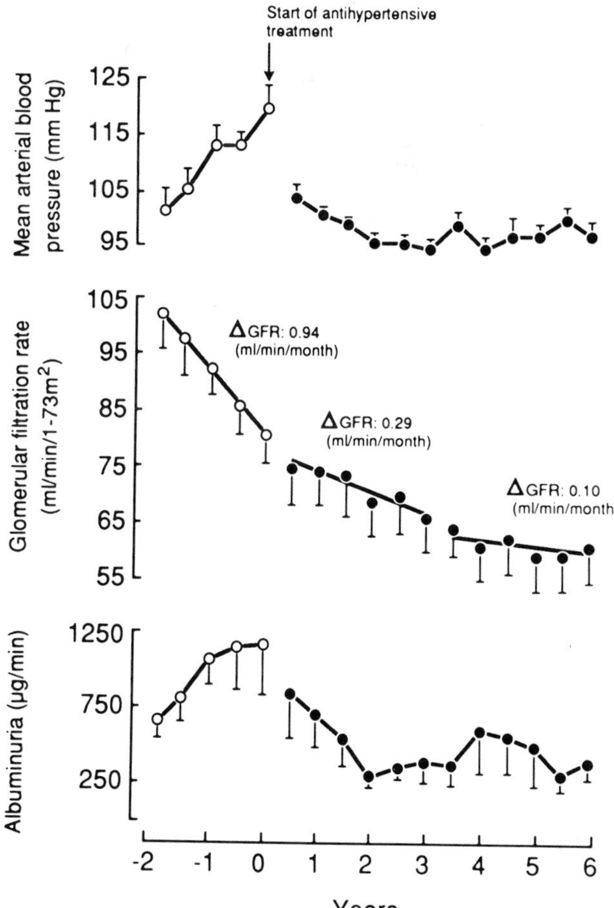

atinine < 2.5 mg/dl slows the progression of diabetic nephropathy. This effect was independent of control of blood pressure.[362a] These findings indicate that an ACE inhibitor should be administered to diabetic patients with gross proteinuria even in the absence of hypertension. In limited human studies, treatment of *normotensive* diabetic patients with microalbuminuria with an ACE inhibitor or calcium channel blocker resulted in stabilization of microalbuminuria and lowered the rate of progression to gross proteinuria.[363,364] Whether such treatment of normotensive diabetic patients prevents or delays renal structural damage and a decline in GFR remains to be established. Thus, the use of ACE inhibitors or calcium channel blockers in normotensive diabetic patients with microalbuminuria remains investigational at this time. In contrast, as noted above, ACE inhibitors have been established as having a special protective role in diabetic patients with gross proteinuria.

Ultimately, consideration must be given to dialysis or transplantation. The 3-year survival rate for patients receiving hemodialysis or transplantation is now reported to exceed 50 percent. Which of the two modalities is the preferred method of treatment and the precise degree of renal impairment (adjudged by serum creatinine concentration or creatinine clearance) at which hemodialysis should be instituted have not been established. Continuous ambulatory peritoneal dialysis has also been shown to be an effective alternative to hemodialysis.[365] It should be noted that histologic changes compatible with diabetic vascular disease have been observed in normal kidneys 2 to 4 years after transplantation into patients with diabetes.[366] However, a functional renal transplant offers improved quality of life compared with dialysis. As many as 88 percent of renal transplant patients and 82 percent of grafts survive for 2 years, regardless of donor source; of those receiving transplants for HLA-identical siblings, 100 percent survive for 2 years.[367,368]

The relation of control of hyperglycemia in diabetes to diabetic nephropathy is discussed below (see Pathogenesis of Complications).

Diabetic Neuropathy

Involvement of the nervous system in diabetes may take the form of clinical syndromes due to lesions specific for diabetes (e.g., symmetric distal polyneuropathy) or may be a consequence of accelerated atherosclerosis leading to infarction of a spinal or cerebral artery and the resultant focal neurologic deficit (e.g., paraplegia). Those syndromes resulting from disordered function of somatic or autonomic nerves are collectively referred to as *diabetic neuropathy*. The true prevalence of neuropathy in the diabetic population is not known; it depends in part on the criteria employed for diagnosis. For example, on the basis of laboratory examination of nerve conduction velocity, 71 percent of a group of unselected diabetic patients showed impaired function.[369] The prevalence of clinically overt neuropathy is substantially lower and does not constitute the potentially life-threatening situation observed with diabetic renal disease. Nevertheless, neuropathy may cause severe disability in the form of pain, motor weakness, or abnormal bowel and bladder function. In addition, it may result in repeated trauma to the legs and feet (because of sensory loss), resulting in nonhealing ulcers that ultimately necessitate amputation.

The various forms of neuropathy may be divided into three major categories, depending on whether there is involvement of multiple peripheral nerves in symmetric fashion (symmetric peripheral polyneuropathy), one or several specific nerve trunks (mononeuropathy, mononeuritis multiplex), or the autonomic nervous system (autonomic neuropathy). These syndromes differ with regard to clinical manifestations, histologic findings, and prognosis. A finding common to all forms of diabetic neuropathy is an elevation in the protein content of cerebrospinal fluid, which may precede the clinically overt neuropathy in diabetic patients.

Symmetric Peripheral Polyneuropathy

Symmetric peripheral polyneuropathy is the most common form of diabetic neuropathy. It is characterized by the development of symmetric sensory loss which is most marked in the distal portions of the lower extremities; motor loss and involvement of the upper extremities are less frequently observed. The symptoms, which often begin insidiously, consist of numbness, tingling, and, later, paresthesias, burning, and sharp, shooting pains; the pain is particularly severe at night. In spite of numbness, hyperesthesia is also often present. Consequently, even the light touch of bedclothes rubbing against the skin may evoke a severe burning sensation. Ambulation may result in clinical improvement; this can be helpful in differentiating neuropathy from vascular insufficiency (claudication). On physical examination, the earliest findings are loss of vibratory sensation and absence of the ankle jerk reflex. Ultimately, there may be loss of all sensory modalities (light touch, pain, position) in a stocking type of distribution.

When sensory loss due to polyneuropathy is severe, secondary changes may develop as a result of repeated unrecognized trauma to the feet. *Neuropathic ulcers* may appear in the area of callus formation; they are often deep and penetrating. *Charcot's joints* (neuropathic arthropathy) occur at the ankle or in the foot at the tarsometatarsal or metatarsophalangeal joints. Unilateral painless swelling and erythema of the ankle and/or foot in association with joint instability and radiographic evidence of disruption of articular surfaces and bone demineralization are the characteristic findings. Neuropathy also contributes to the disability associated with peripheral vascular disease (see below) because of the greater likelihood of repeated foot trauma in a patient who has lost sensation (e.g., skin burns resulting from the use of excessively hot water for bathing or penetrating infection after stepping on a tack).

The pathogenesis of neuropathy (as well as other diabetic complications), particularly with respect to the polyol pathway and low cellular inositol content is discussed in detail below.[22] Metabolic changes observed in diabetic nerves include an increase in sorbitol, a decrease in myoinositol, and a reduction in Na^+,K^+-ATPase. The latter may in turn be a consequence of the reduction in myoinositol.[23] Autoimmune factors have also been implicated. Autoantibodies to GAD, a key enzyme in the synthesis of the neurotransmitter GABA, have been observed before and at the onset of type I diabetes. The persistence of anti-GAD antibodies has been associated with the presence of neuropathy.[279] Finally, vascular factors also may play a role, as reflected by closure of the vasa nervorum. Such closure is of particular importance in mononeuropathy (see below). As previously noted, the histologic changes in peripheral polyneuropathy generally consist of segmented demyelination despite intact vasa nervorum. The factors contributing to the pathogenesis of diabetic neuropathy are summarized in Fig. 19-55.

With respect to the treatment of diabetic neuropathy, subclinical polyneuropathy in the form of decreased nerve conduction velocity, which may be present in type I diabetic patients at the time of initial diagnosis, reverts to normal with the institution of insulin treatment.[370] An effect of insulin treatment on preventing clinically overt neuropathy has been observed in the Diabetes Control and Complications Trial (see below, Treatment of Diabetes). Treatment of polyneuropathy is symptomatic and is directed at pain relief.[371] Initially, treatment should be attempted with simple analgesics such as aspirin, acetaminophen, and NSAIDs. The possible adverse effect of NSAIDs on coexistent diabetic nephropathy (see above) may, however, limit their usefulness. In patients with burning dysesthesias, topical treatment with capsaicin (Zostrix) may be helpful. If topical measures or simple analgesics are ineffective, tricyclic antidepressants such as amitriptyline (in a starting dose of 25 to 50 mg hs) and nortriptyline (starting at 10 to 24 mg hs) may be given alone or in combination with a phenothiazine (e.g., fluphenazine 1 to 2 mg hs). Side effects which may limit the usefulness of such measures include dry mouth and drowsiness. Alternatively, a trial of carbamazepine (Tegretol), clonodine (Catapres), clonazepam (Clonopin), or mexiletine (Mexitil) may be attempted.[371] Clinical studies with various aldose reductase inhibitors have failed to show enough efficacy or safety to warrant their approval.[23,371] Unfortunately, neuropathic pain may be resistant to each of these measures, necessitating treatment with opioid analgesics. Nevertheless, in the vast ma-

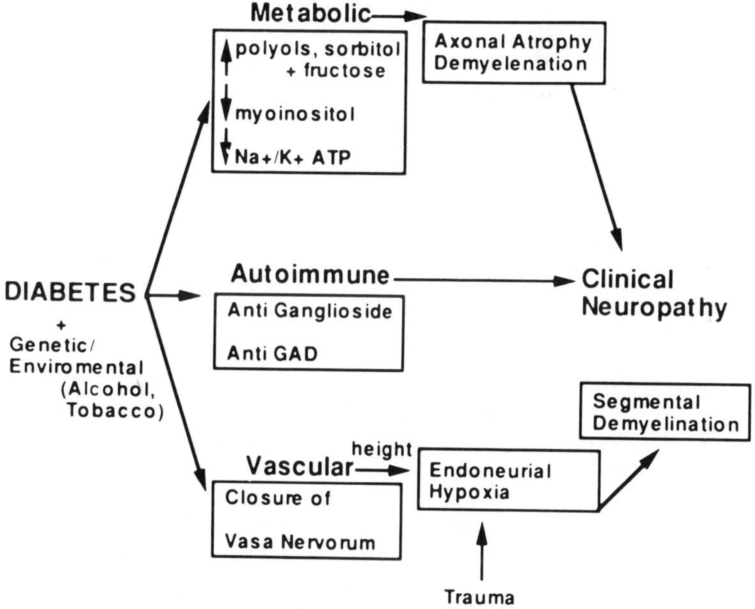

FIGURE 19-55 Pathogenetic factors (metabolic, autoimmune, and vascular) in the development of diabetic neuropathy. (*From Vinik et al.*[371])

jority of patients, the pain and dysesthesias spontaneously subside after 6 to 18 months, probably reflecting progressive denervation. The importance of diabetic foot care in minimizing the morbidity from peripheral neuropathy and/or vascular disease is discussed below (see Peripheral Vascular Disease: The Diabetic Foot).

Mononeuropathy

Disease of the nervous system may involve a single, clinically identifiable nerve trunk or several specific nerve trunks. In the latter circumstance, the term *mononeuritis multiplex* is applied. The peripheral nerves most commonly affected are the femoral, obturator, and sciatic nerves in the lower extremity and the median and ulnar nerves in the upper extremity. The external pressure points are the sites involved, or an entrapment type of syndrome (e.g., the median nerve in the carpal tunnel) may arise. Onset is abrupt, consisting of weakness, pain, and muscle atrophy. The distribution of weakness reflects the nerve trunk involvement (e.g., wrist drop with ulnar nerve involvement). Entrapment syndromes frequently can be remedied only by surgical decompression. *Diabetic amyotrophy* is a syndrome affecting the pelvic girdle or, less commonly, the shoulder muscles. In it there is severe weakness, atrophy, fasciculations, and pain, but no clinically overt sensory loss.

Mononeuropathy may also take the form of isolated or multiple cranial nerve palsies. The third, sixth, and fourth nerves (in descending order of frequency) are the most commonly affected.

In contrast to the demyelinative changes observed with symmetric peripheral polyneuropathy, the mononeuropathies are felt to be vascular in origin.[371] Attempts to "improve" blood glucose control have had no influence on the course of the disorder. The prognosis is nevertheless generally good, with recovery of function and resolution of pain over 6 to 18 months. Symptomatic measures, as discussed in the section on peripheral polyneuropathy, may be tried for pain relief.

Autonomic Neuropathy

Abnormalities of the autonomic nervous system commonly occur in long-standing diabetes, particularly in patients with peripheral polyneuropathy. Impairment in the regulation of heart rate and blood pressure and in genitourinary and gastrointestinal function are the consequences of such involvement. A resting tachycardia of >100 beats/min may reflect autonomic dysfunction. A simple bedside test of parasympathetic function involves measuring the heart rate response to deep breathing by comparing the longest RR interval in expiration with the shortest during inspiration. With the patient breathing at 6 breaths/min, a difference in heart rate (maximal vs. minimal) of >15 beats/min is considered normal while a difference of <10 beats/min is considered abnormal.[371] Computerized ECG techniques for assessing RR variability relative to respiration are now available. Heart rate can also be determined while performing the Valsalva maneuver or on standing up. Papillary light reflex may also be defective in the presence of autonomic neuropathy.[372] *Orthostatic hypotension* reflects the loss of normal vasomotor tone on assuming the upright posture as well as failure of stimulation of plasma renin release. Decreased sweating in the lower extremities accompanied by excessive sweating in the upper half of the body is another frequent finding. Some patients experience increased sweating with food ingestion (gustatory sweating).

Urogenital dysfunction takes the form of impotence (present in as many as 40 to 50 percent of diabetic patients), retrograde ejaculation (reflecting incompetence of the internal vesicle sphincter), urinary incontinence, and failure to empty the bladder fully. The resulting dilated, flaccid bladder may be a contributory factor in the development of chronic urinary tract infections. Treatment includes the use of parasympathomimetics (e.g., bethanechol) and, if necessary, repeated self-catheterization.

GI involvement is manifested as either subclinical or clinical disturbances of motility. Esophageal motility is frequently abnormal; emptying time is delayed, and primary esophageal contractions are poor or absent. Retention of gastric contents is also quite common; at times, this complication may cause retention of large volumes of fluid in the dilated stomach (*gastroparesis diabeticorum*). Comparable distention of the gallbladder also occurs quite commonly. These abnormalities of motility are usually asymptomatic but may be responsible for nausea, vomiting, or dysphagia. Frequent small feedings and the use of the motility-increasing agents metoclopramide or cisapride may provide symptomatic relief. The small intestine and colon also suffer from abnormalities of motility, but in these organs increased activity associated with diarrhea is the common pattern. Characteristically, the diarrhea is worse at night and may be associated with fecal incontinence. Intestinal stasis permits the development of abnormal bacterial flora in the upper jejunum in some patients, and a pattern reminiscent of the "blind loop" syndrome may occur. Steatorrhea is a common problem in association with diabetic diarrhea, but in most cases pancreatic exocrine function is unimpaired, and the histologic appearance of the mucosa and muscular and vascular apparatus is normal. Since diabetic diarrhea is usually associated with malabsorption, vitamin supplementation may be helpful. The use of pancreatic enzymes is not usually helpful. In some patients, the administration of a broad-spectrum antibiotic (tetracycline, metronidazole) may cause improvement in the diarrhea and the malabsorption. Celiac disease is also more common in the diabetic population, resulting from a shared predisposing HLA haplotype.

In occasional patients with combined peripheral and autonomic neuropathy, marked weight loss may be observed. This syndrome, which has been described as *diabetic neuropathic cachexia*, generally is self-limited and may suggest the presence of a malignant tumor. There is usually spontaneous improvement in symptoms and gain in weight after 6 to 18 months.[373]

Coronary Artery Disease

Atheromatous disease involving the coronary arteries occurs more frequently and at an earlier stage in diabetic patients compared with the general population; studies have shown an excess mortality rate from "sudden death" and myocardial infarction. The risk of a fatal myocardial infarction is also greater in diabetic patients than in nondiabetic individuals. The greater risk of experiencing a myocardial infarction holds particularly for diabetic women before age 40, contrary to the "protection" against coronary disease characteristic of the female gender. It has been suggested that chest pain is less frequent and less intense in diabetic patients than in nondiabetic individuals at the time of infarction. However, objective evidence documenting a greater prevalence of "silent" myocardial infarction among diabetic patients has not been reported.

The factors responsible for the accelerated atherosclerosis in the diabetic population have not been entirely identified. As was discussed earlier (see Pathophysiology), hypercholesterolemia and hypertriglyceridemia are more common in diabetics, and are associated with increased concentrations of VLDL and LDL and reduced concentrations of HDL. Current theories of the pathogenesis of atherosclerosis ascribe an important role to platelet adherence and aggregation at the site of endothelial damage.[374] Abnormalities in platelet function (increased adhesiveness and sensitivity to aggregating agents) have been observed in diabetic patients and may contribute to accelerated atherogenesis. Glycation of VLDL, LDL, and HDL apolipoproteins[31,32] and other compositional changes in lipoproteins[318,375] may result in defective clearance and metabolism of these particles; this would establish a favorable milieu for atherogenesis. As noted previously,[323] glycation can also alter the properties of collagen, thus contributing to vascular abnormalities by binding LDL and VLDL remnants. In patients with type II diabetes, hyperinsulinemia has been implicated as a risk factor for atherosclerosis, perhaps by stimulating vascular smooth muscle proliferation.[305] Regardless of the precise mechanism, in view of the markedly increased risk for coronary disease, prudence dictates that diabetic patients restrict the cholesterol and saturated fat content of their diets (see Diet, below).

An increased predilection for heart disease in diabetes may also take the form of *diabetic cardiomyopathy*. In such patients, decreased myocardial function is observed in the absence of significant coronary artery disease or other etiologic factors, such as hypertension, valvular disease, and alcoholism.[376] A variety of histologic changes, including capillary basement membrane thickening typical of diabetic microangiopathy in other organs, arteriolar thickening, and interstitial fibrosis, have been observed. Decreased formation of myocardial fibrillar protein secondary to the altered metabolic milieu characteristic of diabetes also may be a contributory factor. Clinically, diabetic cardiomyopathy may manifest as congestive heart failure or, in less severe cases, a decrease in the exercise-induced ventricular ejection fraction on radionuclide ventriculography.[376]

Peripheral Vascular Disease: The Diabetic Foot

Besides coronary artery disease, the second major site of clinically overt arteriosclerosis in diabetic patients is in the vasculature of the lower extremity. The major syndromes resulting from vascular impairment in the leg and/or foot are intermittent claudication, foot ulcer, and gangrene; the last is >50 times more frequent in diabetic patients than in nondiabetic individuals. Peripheral vessel disease may lead to intermittent claudication and, in more severe cases, pain at rest and necrosis. The sites of occlusion in diabetic patients are often smaller (tibial and popliteal arteries) than in nondiabetic individuals (in whom iliac and femoral arteries are involved), and the affected segments are often longer, making reconstructive surgery more difficult.

Foot ulcers develop as a consequence of ischemia, peripheral polyneuropathy, or, more commonly, a combination of the two. Ulceration may be followed by the development of gangrene and/or infection. Infected necrotic lesions may show evidence of gas on x-ray examination. Gas does not necessarily signify the presence of clostridia; it may be a result of *Escherichia coli*, anaerobic streptococci, or *Bacteroides* sp. infection. Treatment of the diabetic foot ulcer depends on an initial assessment of whether the ulcer is superficial or deep. If the ulcer is superficial and is not accompanied by significant cellulitis, hospitalization is not required and management consists of an oral broad-spectrum antibiotic, avoidance of weight bearing, debridement, and local dressings. If the ulcer is deep and/or is accompanied by evidence of cellulitis, hospitalization is necessary for the administration of intravenous antibiotics (e.g., Unasyn [ampicillin/sulbactam]), radiolabled white cell studies to search for osteomyelitis, bed rest, and surgical debridement. Since failure to respond may lead to generalized septicemia and death, it necessitates amputation. The general principle applied in amputation is preservation of as much limb as feasible while ensuring healing of the stump.

In most instances gangrenous lesions and/or ulcers develop as a result of avoidable, seemingly trivial, and (because of accompanying neuropathy) unrecognized episodes of trauma. Vigorous care and protection of the feet thus constitute an extremely important aspect of the day-to-day management of the diabetic patient. The principles of diabetic foot care to be followed by the patient are (1) inspect the foot daily for ulceration, discoloration, or cracking of callus; (2) avoid poorly fitting shoes which cause pressure sores; (3) never walk barefoot; (4) apply skin lubricant daily to prevent or reduce callus formation; (5) cut toenails straight across (to avoid ingrown toenails) and, where necessary (e.g., when vision is impaired), have it done by a podiatrist. Patients should be advised to refrain from smoking since this may aggravate the existing vascular disease. The most important principle to be followed by the physician is to be certain to examine the patient's feet at regular intervals.

The Skin

Skin changes may be observed in diabetes as a consequence of large- or small-vessel disease, as a direct result of metabolic abnormalities (e.g., hypertriglyceridemia), and as a result of infection.[377]

Necrobiosis lipoidica diabeticorum is an uncommon but highly characteristic lesion consisting of a sharply demarcated plaque with an erythematous border and a red-brown, shiny center that becomes yellow as lipids (including carotene) are deposited (Fig. 19-56). Ulcerations with crusts and dilated blood vessels frequently occur in the central portions of the lesions. The plaques vary in size from 0.5 to 15 cm and often begin as flat erythematous areas which slowly expand. In >90 percent of cases the lesions are located in the shin (pretibial) area. They occur three times more often in women than in men. The histopathologic changes accompanying necrobiosis lipoidica diabeticorum are characteristic of the microangiopathy observed in other tissues. There is an accompanying secondary necrosis of collagen. In occasional patients the skin lesions antedate the appearance of clinical diabetes, and in rare instances no abnormalities of glucose tolerance are observed.

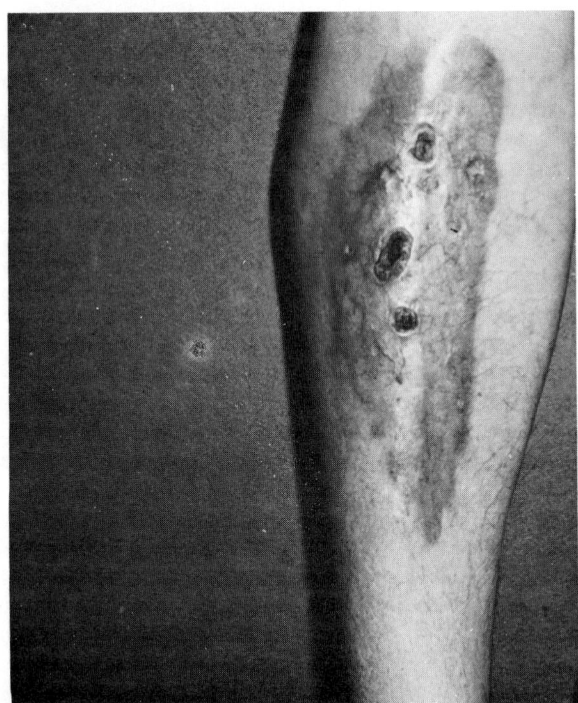

FIGURE 19-56 Necrobiosis lipoidica diabeticorum. The lesions consist of plaquelike areas in the pretibial region with a shiny atrophic surface, a red brown center that becomes yellow, telangiectatic vessels, and areas of ulceration with crusts. (*Courtesy of I. Braverman.*)

Diabetic dermopathy, or shin spots, are circumscribed, atrophic, hyperpigmented, scaly patches which begin as red-brown papules. The lesions are almost always located in the pretibial area. Whether these skin findings are a consequence of microangiopathy has not been established. *Diabetic bullae* are blisters which may appear in the absence of trauma, particularly on the feet.

Eruptive xanthomas may develop in diabetic patients with marked hypertriglyceridemia. The lesions are no different from those observed in familial or primary hypertriglyceridemic states without diabetes; they consist of red-yellow papules with an erythematous base, located primarily in the elbow, buttocks, and posterior thigh areas. Diabetic patients with these lesions usually have very poor metabolic control (marked hyperglycemia and weight loss) and may display *lipemia retinalis* as a further manifestation of their hypertriglyceridemia. Generally, elevation in plasma cholesterol concentration with normal triglyceride concentrations (e.g., an increase in LDL concentration only) does not give rise to eruptive xanthomas.

Infectious Complications

Infections of various types come to clinical attention more often in diabetic patients not because invasion by bacteria is more common among these patients, but because they handle the invaders less well than do nondiabetic individuals. For example, sporadic furuncles occur in most normal individuals but do not usually progress to carbuncles or disseminated furunculosis, whereas in diabetic patients this course is common. The incidence of asymptomatic bacteriuria is no greater in diabetic patients than in control groups whether the study is conducted in hospital populations or in otherwise healthy ambulatory subjects, but the most rapidly advancing phase of pyelonephritis, *necrotizing papillitis*, is almost unknown except in diabetic patients and patients with urinary tract obstruction. Bacteremia is more common as a complication of urinary tract infections in diabetic patients than in nondiabetic individuals.

Infections with relatively benign organisms may assume progressive and threatening forms in diabetic patients. For example, *E. coli* may present the picture of gas gangrene. Tuberculosis progresses more rapidly in diabetic than in nondiabetic patients, and the course of the tuberculous infection is not greatly altered by the treatment of diabetes as long as ketoacidosis is prevented. In spite of the improved control provided by antituberculous treatment, the prognosis for the diabetic patient is worse than that for the nondiabetic patient. Malignant otitis externa caused by *Pseudomonas aeruginosa* may be seen in elderly diabetic patients. This can result in osteomyelitis of the base of the skull, cranial nerve paralysis, brain abscess, and meningitis. Cellulitis may be caused by mixed pathogens, including *Staphylococcus aureus*, streptococci, and *Proteus* and *Pseudomonas* spp. Gas-forming anaerobes may be involved as well.

Saprophytic fungi of the order Mucorales, which rarely cause disease in normal subjects, may produce a progressive and usually fatal mucormycosis infection in diabetic patients. The process usually begins in the nasal sinuses and invades the orbit and cranial cavity, causing neurologic disorders and ultimately death. It is associated initially with purulent nasal discharge and gangrene of the nasal mucous membrane; later, unilateral ophthalmoplegia and exophthalmos herald involvement of the orbit. In about one-third of these patients late blood-borne involvement of the heart, kidneys, and other organs occurs. The fungus may also infect the lungs (where it is usually an airborne infection) or the skin. The infection can sometimes be controlled by treatment with amphotericin B and careful control of the diabetes.

With respect to the mechanisms by which infectious processes may be more severe in diabetes, there is no evidence of defective antibody formation, but mobilization of inflammatory cells is defective, and phagocytosis is clearly impaired in the white cells of diabetic patients with ketoacidosis.[378] Even in the absence of ketosis, there is defective phagocytosis and killing by polymorphonuclear leukocytes in diabetic patients. Such cells also show decreased production of prostaglandins, thromboxanes, and leukotrienes. As to the mechanism of decreased leukocyte function, hyperosmolar solutions interfere in vitro with phagocytosis, but the degree of hyperosmolarity required is so large (~400 mOsm or 700 mg/dl of glucose) that this factor has usually been discounted. Undoubtedly, acidosis and dehydration, when present, also play a part. These observations justify the conclusion that the progression of infection can probably be reduced by careful control of the blood glucose concentration.

Joint Disease

In addition to neuropathic arthropathy (Charcot's joints), diabetic patients show an increased predilection for osteoarthritis, Dupuytren's contracture (thickening of the subcutaneous tissue in the palms), carpal tunnel syndrome, flexor tenosynovitis of the hand ("trigger finger"), and adhesive capsulitis of the shoulder. As opposed to the marked male predominance observed when Dupuytren's contracture occurs in the general population, women with diabetes are affected as frequently as are male diabetic patients.

Limited joint mobility (LJM) is a form of arthropathy that is believed to occur exclusively in diabetes.[379] It is characterized by painless, noninflammatory limitation of the hand and wrist joints, particularly the metacarpal-phalangeal (MP) and interphalangeal (IP) joints of the fifth finger. LJM may be clinically detected by the inability of the patient to approximate the palmar surfaces of the MP and IP joints with the fingers fanned ("prayer position").

Although LJM does not cause clinically significant disability, its appearance in children with type I diabetes may be predictive of increased risk for the subsequent development of diabetic retinopathy or nephropathy.[379]

Pathogenesis of Diabetic Complications

One of the most important unresolved questions in diabetes mellitus concerns the pathogenesis of the long-term microvascular and neuropathic complications. In general, two schools of thought regarding pathogenesis have emerged. One school holds that microangiopathy and neuropathy are a consequence of hyperglycemia and/or other metabolic abnormalities resulting from insulin lack ("metabolic" hypothesis). The second school holds that these lesions are genetically determined abnormalities that occur independently of elevations in blood glucose concentration and/or insulin deficiency and may in fact precede any of the metabolic changes ("genetic" hypothesis).[380] This controversy is of more than academic significance because it is intimately related to concepts of the management of diabetes. Proponents of the metabolic theory generally believe that control of hyperglycemia prevents or minimizes diabetic complications; they consequently favor tight control of insulin-dependent diabetes. In contrast, advocates of the genetic theory favor "loose" control, since by their formulation the magnitude of hyperglycemia does not influence the development of complications. A host of data have been accumulated in recent years on both sides of the argument, based on the investigation of tissue biopsies, metabolic studies in target tissues, and evaluation of the effect of treatment on the development of complications. On balance, the data currently favor strongly the conclusion that metabolic factors are primarily responsible for the initiation and development of complications in most diabetic patients. A role for a genetic predisposition to certain complications is also suggested but remains to be firmly established.

Biopsy Studies

As was noted previously, basement membrane thickening is present in diabetes in skin and muscle tissue as well as in the target sites of diabetic complications such as the renal glomerulus and retina (Fig. 19-50). The accessibility of muscle tissue for needle biopsy has permitted studies of capillary basement membrane in normal subjects, in patients who are predisposed to the development of diabetes but have normal glucose tolerance, and in diabetic patients after varying durations of overt hyperglycemia. With this approach, Siperstein et al.[381] reported electron micrographic evidence of thickened basement membranes in the offspring of two diabetic parents ("prediabetics") despite normal glucose tolerance in the biopsied subjects. In contrast, Kilo et al. have shown that muscle capillary basement membrane thickening in patients with overt diabetes depends on the duration of hyperglycemia.[382] Furthermore, in monozygotic twin pairs discordant for diabetes, the basement membrane was thickened in the diabetic twin and normal-sized in the nondiabetic twin in most pairs.[383] Studies in the Pima also favor the conclusion that muscle capillary basement membrane thickening follows rather than precedes the development of overt diabetes.[384] This view is further supported by observations in individuals who have ingested pyriminil (Vacor).[385] These hyperglycemic patients exhibited a thickening of muscle capillary basement membrane, to an extent comparable with that of a group of type I diabetic patients, in frequent association with retinopathy and proteinuria. Thus, hyperglycemia of nongenetic origin can cause microvascular abnormalities.

Regardless of the state of basement membrane in muscle capillaries, it is well recognized that clinical evidence of retinal and glomerular capillary involvement is related to the duration of diabetes. Biopsy studies also show that histologic changes in the kidney are absent for at least the first 2 years after the onset of insulin-dependent diabetes.[338,357] Important evidence in favor of the metabolic theory is also derived from studies in patients with secondary diabetes (chronic pancreatitis) and patients with primary diabetes who have received a kidney transplant from a nondiabetic donor. In patients with chronic pancreatitis and secondary diabetes, nodular and diffuse glomerulosclerosis has been observed[386]; in normal kidneys transplanted in diabetic patients, hyalinosis of arterioles is more common than it is in nondiabetic transplant recipients.[366] Of particular interest are histologic studies of the transplanted kidney in diabetic patients undergoing successful combined pancreatic and kidney transplantation. In such patients, such restoration of normal glucose metabolism was associated with preservation of normal glomerular basement membrane structure in the donor kidney on biopsy 2 to 3 years after transplantation.[387] Thus, the histologic response of a kidney transplanted from a nondiabetic individual to a diabetic patient favors the concept that diabetic glomerulopathy is a consequence of the abnormal metabolic milieu characteristic of the diabetic state.

Metabolic Studies

A second approach to determining the pathogenesis of complications in diabetes involves metabolic studies of target tissues (e.g., basement membrane, peripheral nerve). Such investigations are directed at providing the metabolic link between insulin deficiency and/or hyperglycemia and diabetic complications. As discussed above (see Diabetic Nephropathy), fine polar and configurational changes in the diabetic glomerular basement membrane appear to alter its filtration characteristics, shape, and packing. Furthermore, since the entry of glucose into the kidney cells is not insulin-dependent, these changes, which are related at least in part to excessive glycosylation, would be expected to depend on substrate concentration and to increase with cellular hyperglycemia. It is pertinent that no complications are seen in tissues with insulin-obligated glucose transport. Two general concepts of metabolic abnormality in the pathogenesis of diabetic complications have been the focus of particular attention: (1) the polyol pathway and (2) protein glycation.

With respect to the polyol pathway, initial studies demonstrated an increase in the sorbitol content in nerve tissue from diabetic animals. Excess sorbitol formed from glucose by the enzyme aldose reductase was postulated to interfere with nerve function via an osmotic effect that causes nerve swelling. While such an osmotic effect of sorbitol can account for metabolic cataracts in diabetic patients, the postulated changes in nerve tissue water content have not been substantiated.[23,37]

The role of the polyol pathway in diabetic complications may, however, be mediated by the decreases in myoinositol which accompany the accumulation of sorbitol.

As shown first in the nerve[388,389] but also in the glomerulus and retina, the accumulation of sorbitol is associated with a secondary decrease in the cellular myoinositol content, whereas plasma myoinositol concentration is not appreciably affected. The increased operation of the polyol pathway is causally related to the depletion of a small but specific pool of myoinositol within the cell, which is important for the regulation of Na^+,K^+-ATPase activity.[23] Na^+,K^+-ATPase is a membrane transport enzyme, the energy of hydrolysis of an ATP molecule being used to translocate 3 Na^+ ions from and 2 K^+ ions into the cytosol. The activity of Na^+,K^+-ATPase is thus electrogenic and, importantly, contributes to the maintenance of a proper membrane potential. A decrease in ATPase activity was found in the three complication-susceptible tissues, in association with the decline in myoinositol content and the increased flow through the polyol pathway.

In the nerve, the maintenance of an axoplasmic transmembrane ion gradient is essential for the generation of the normal action potential. Decreased ATPase activity, failing to extrude the axoplasmic Na^+, is thus involved in the causation of the reduced nerve conduction velocity in diabetes.

In the kidney, the early hemodynamic defect in the afferent/efferent arterioles and the mesangium, rather than metabolic abnormalities, has been proposed as the critical determinant of the initiation of hyperfiltration and its progress to nephropathy (see above). However, the hemodynamic effect which stems from hyperglycemia appears to be initially associated with elevated intracellular Na^+ concentration, reduced Na^+,K^+-ATPase activity, and low myoinositol content. In experimental animals with diabetes, treatment with aldose reductace inhibitors, a myoinositol-rich diet, or vigorous control of hyperglycemia prevents the increase in GFR, glomerular hypertension, and mesangial permeability, similar to the prevention of the decrease in conduction velocity in the peripheral nerve.[390,391]

In the retina an early functional derangement is likewise demonstrable in human and animal type I diabetes, manifested by vitreous fluorescein retention on IV injection. It is due to the increase in permeability of the pigmented epithelium, a component in the blood-retina barrier regulating the composition of the retinal fluid. This abnormality results from delayed outward transport of the ions and metabolites which appear to be responsible for the elevated Na^+ content as a result of the decreased activity of Na^+,K^+-ATPase, retinal edema, and consequent vascular disease. It is likewise preventable by control of hyperglycemia, inhibition of aldose reductase, or dietary myoinositol supplementation.

A novel regulatory system appears to be involved in the modulation of the electrogenic Na^+,K^+-ATPase activity as well as of other cellular processes. The effector arm is phosphatidylinositol (PI) derived from myoinositol and a specific diglyceride by the action of CDP diacylglyceride phosphotransferase. The system also includes products of PI phosphorylation, i.e., phosphatidylinositol phosphate and diphosphate, and of PI hydrolysis, i.e., diacylglycerol (DAG) and inositol 1,4,5-triphosphate. These compounds affect cellular Ca^{2+} concentrations and protein kinase C–catalyzed (cAMP-independent) phosphorylation, the latter of which may be instrumental in maintaining ATPase activity. The relation between the polyol pathway and the activity of protein kinase C (PKC) is, however, complex and tissue-specific. In nerve tissue, a decrease in myoinsitol is accompanied by the predicted decrease in the content of DAG and the activity of PKC.[23,37] In contrast, in retinal and renal tissue, increased accumulation of DAG and increased activity of PKC can be induced by hyperglycemia.[37] Regardless of the precise mechanisms involved, diabetes is associated with activation of the polyol pathway in nerve, retinal, and renal tissue. This activation involves an increase in sorbitol content, a decrease in myoinositol (in specific subcellular pools), decreased activity of Na^+,K^+-ATPase, and tissue-specific alterations in PKC activity.

The second general biochemical mechanism proposed as a link between hyperglycemia and the complications of diabetes involves protein glycation. As discussed above (see Protein Glycation), the term *glycation* refers to the nonenzymatic covalent bonding of glucose to the exposed amino groups in proteins (Fig. 19-9). In a variety of proteins, glycation has been observed to alter function as well as structure. The most extensively studied glycated protein is glycohemoglobin, which provides a useful clinical index of glycemic control. In addition, glycation of hemoglobin results in enhanced oxygen binding, as is evident from the rightward shift in the O_2 dissocation curve. The decreased release of oxygen to the peripheral tissues may not be sufficient to cause local ischemia in normal situations but may become critical when the oxygen demand is increased in infected, hyperemic, or injuried body regions. It may be of importance in slow wound healing in diabetic patients.

Glycation of the lysine residues in proteins may interfere with the recognition of glycoproteins by hepatic cells,[392] enhance albumin's passage through the endothelial membranes, and reduce its affinity for small molecules. Glycation of clotting factor VIII has been shown to be related to the increased tendency toward platelet aggregation in diabetes.[393] Glycation of immunoglobulins may impair their antibody functions.[394] Glycation of lipoproteins alters their biological behavior, decreasing (LDL)[30] or increasing (HDL) their catabolism. Further evidence that protein turnover is altered by glycation is provided by the finding that glycated fibrinogen produces clots that are more resistant to fibrinolysis by the enzyme plasmin.[395] This may be instrumental in producing tissue fibrin deposits in diabetes.

Glycation with or without glycosylation of serine and threonine residues of structural tissue proteins has also been reported to result in untoward functional alterations. The glycated crystalline proteins of the lens[396] seem liable to form cross-linking disulfide bridges. This increases their particle size and renders their structure more compact and less transparent, leading to cataract formation.[27] Glycosylation of tissue collagen, apart from causing basement membrane thickening in kidney glomeruli, may have deleterious effects in other tissues as well.

These effects include trapping of lipoproteins in vascular walls and reduction of skin collagen solubility and digestibility by collagenase,[397] thus prolonging its biological turnover time. In contrast, glycosylation and/or glycation of the cell membrane appears to reduce the life span of red cells. This membrane modification also decreases red cell capability for shape adaptation, resulting in tendency to sludge in capillaries, which is probably connected to diabetic peripheral ischemia.[398]

The typical functions of leukocytes, such as chemotaxis, phagocytosis, and bactericidal potency,[399] are adversely affected by membrane rigidity resulting from excessive glycosylation and/or glycation. Finally, glycosylated tissue proteins may present a new, "foreign" epitope to the immunoprotective systems of the body and stimulate the formation of autoantibodies, as demonstrated in the case of glycosylated collagen.[400] This finding is of potential importance. If expanded, it could represent a link between hyperglycemia and the immune complications in diabetes; such complications are evident from the deposition of antibody complexes in diabetic tissues, particularly in the kidney.

The covalent products of protein glycation which are formed relatively quickly are known to undergo degradation into various highly reactive compounds which react again with free amino groups on protein, resulting in the more gradual appearance of cross-linked proteins known as advanced glycosylation end products (AGEs).[33] While the precise chemical structure of only some AGEs has been elucidated, they may be responsible for qualitative and quantitative changes in intracellular matrix proteins such as type IV collagen and laminin. They also may impair endothelial cell and macrophage function by interacting with specific receptors, resulting in matrix overaccumulation, cellular proliferation, and focal thrombosis. The ability of aminoguanidine, an inhibitor of AGE formation, to prevent retinal, renal, and nerve changes in experimental diabetes provides support for a pathogenetic role of AGE formation in the complications of diabetes.[33]

Effect of Treatment

A major corollary of the metabolic hypothesis is that treatment of diabetes resulting in normalization of blood glucose concentration prevents the vascular and neurologic complications. Retrospective studies have been published suggesting that by comparison with long-term insulin therapy, multiple short-acting insulin injections and better control of hyperglycemia are associated with a lower incidence of some complications.[401,402] With respect to prospective studies, data demonstrating the beneficial effects of insulin treatment on complications in experimentally diabetic animals have been more consistent than data from humans. In dogs with alloxan-induced diabetes, insulin therapy has been shown to reduce the incidence of retinopathy.[403] In rats with streptozotocin-induced diabetes, renal glomerular lesions regress after islet-cell transplants.[404] In genetically diabetic *dbdb* mice, metabolic control by several pharmacologic and dietary means results in improvement of glomerular abnormalities. Nerve conduction is also ameliorated in diabetic animals after insulin treatment.

Of particular interest is the observation in dogs with alloxan-induced diabetes in which intervention with strict diabetic control was initiated after an initial 2½-year period of poor diabetic control.[405] Although retinopathy was not yet present in the dogs at the time when strict control was initiated, over the ensuing 2½-year period of nearly normal glucose homeostasis, diabetic retinopathy developed which was comparable to that observed in diabetic dogs maintained on poor glycemic control for the entire 5-year period. In contrast, retinopathy was prevented in dogs in which strict control was initiated at the outset of diabetes and was continued for the entire 5-year period. These observations suggest that failure to institute nearly normal glucose homeostasis during a critical interval in the earliest stages of diabetes may ultimately result in the development of diabetic complications despite the institution of strict control before the clinical appearance of such complications.

With respect to prospective human interventional trials, a number of studies involving observations of limited numbers of patients (40 to 100) for periods of 8 months to 5 years have shown an initial worsening of diabetic retinopathy compared with controls during the first year of nearly normal glycemia induced by insulin pump therapy or multiple daily injections.[342,406–408] By 3 years of observation, the control groups and intensively treated groups were comparable. The data available at 5 years showed a trend toward less retinopathy.[408]

Of particular importance are the data which have emerged from the Diabetes Control and Complications Trial (DCCT). This prospective randomized trial involved over 1400 patients assigned either to conventional or to intensive control.[409] Patients were followed for an average of 7 years and achieved A_{Ic} hemoglobin levels of 7.2 percent with a mean blood glucose of 155 mg/dl in the intensively treated group and respective values of 8.9 percent and 231 mg/dl in the conventionally treated group. By 3 years of observation, a beneficial effect of intensive control was not demonstrable. However, after 5 to 7 years of treatment, the intensively managed group demonstrated a 50 to 70 percent reduction in the risk of progression to clinically significant retinopathy, a 45 percent decrease in the requirement for laser therapy, and comparable reductions of 50 to 60 percent in the rate of development of nephropathy (proteinuria) and neuropathy.[409a] These data thus provide clear-cut evidence that treatment directed at achieving normal or nearly normal blood glucose levels has long-term beneficial effects in preventing the complications of diabetes. Of note, however, is the equally strong evidence that these benefits are not achieved without the risk of severe hypoglycemia. The frequency of severe hypoglycemia (e.g., loss of consciousness) in the intensively treated patients was threefold greater than in conventionally treated patients.[409a,410] Thus, the beneficial effects of intensive diabetic control in preventing diabetic retinopathy, nephropathy, and neuropathy which are manifest after 5 to 7 years of therapy must be weighed against the risk of an increased frequency of severe hypoglycemia throughout the treatment period.

With regard to nephropathy, continuous subcutaneous insulin infusion (CSII) treatment evoked significant improvement in patients with microalbuminuria of <500 mg/24 h but failed to produce improvement in renal function in patients with gross proteinuria.[411] As noted above, in the DCCT study, intensive treatment significantly reduced progression from microalbuminuria to gross proteinuria.[409a] Furthermore, beneficial effects of intensified treatment on neuropathy[412] and capillary basement membrane thickening,[413] as well as growth abnormalities in juvenile diabetic patients, have been reported for CSII treatment.

Summary

A wealth of data indicates that microvascular lesions in the retina and kidney follow (by 3 to 5 years) rather than precede the development of overt diabetes mellitus. Similar lesions occur in secondary diabetes and in normal kidneys transplanted into diabetic patients.[414] Conversely, normal donor kidneys are protected from diabetic complications by simultaneous pancreatic transplantation.[387] A variety of biochemical abnormalities, including nonenzymatic and enzymatic incorporation of glucose into soluble and structural proteins as well as changes in polyol and myoinositol metabolism, may constitute the metabolic link between hyperglycemia with or without insulin deficiency and the development of diabetic complications. The results of a prospective trial evaluating the effect of restoration of nearly normal glucose metabolism on the development of complications (DCCT study) are emerging which provide strong evidence for a role of intensive treatment in preventing diabetic complications.[409a] Such treatment does, however, confer an increased risk of severe hypoglycemia.[410] It should also be noted that the metabolic and genetic hypotheses may not be mutually exclusive. In diabetic patients followed for 25 to 30 years, microangiopathy progressively increases, reaching a peak prevalence of 80 percent.[415] The 20 percent of patients who escape these complications are no different with respect to clinical control of their diabetes but may differ from other diabetic patients with respect to genetic predisposition to complictions. Possibly, a genetic component necessary for the development of complications may be lacking or a genetic factor conferring protection may be present in these patients. In contrast, in the remaining 80 percent of patients, metabolic changes such as the presence of hyperglycemia and/or other consequences of insulin deficiency may be necessary initial steps for the clinical expression of their genetic predisposition to the development of microangiopathy and neuropathy. Unfortunately, patients who are protected from the development of complications cannot be identified in advance at the present time. Consequently, in the light of current knowledge, the implication with regard to therapy is to recommend the restoration of as normal a metabolic milieu as possible while minimizing the risk of hypoglycemia or impairing psychosocial adaptation.

Mortality

Over the past 50 to 60 years there has been a striking change in the life expectancy as well as causes of death among diabetic patients. In the preinsulin era, the survival of insulin-dependent diabetic patients was measured in months after diagnosis, and death in >40 percent of cases was due to DKA. At present, ketoacidosis and hyperosmolar coma account for <1 percent of deaths among diabetic patients; the major causes of death are renal failure in type I diabetic patients and coronary artery disease in type II diabetic patients. Ischemic heart disease is involved in ~25 percent. Of deaths related to diabetes, ~75 percent occur at 65 or older and ~46 percent occur after the age of 75. The 20-year survival rate after the diagnosis of diabetes is 50 to 80 percent of the expected survival rate in the general population; ~12 percent of individuals with type I diabetes die within 20 years after the onset of the disease.[416]

Treatment

Management of diabetic patients has as its optimal goals (1) normalization of carbohydrate, fat, and protein metabolism, (2) prevention of long-term systemic complications, (3) normal psychosocial adaptation, and (4) avoidance of hypoglycemia or other complications of treatment. The application of intensive programs of insulin therapy involving self-monitoring of blood glucose concentration (see below) has increased the success rate with which normal or nearly normal blood glucose concentrations can be achieved.[417–419]

The principle underlying all forms of treatment of diabetes is the recognition that an imbalance exists between the availability of insulin from endogenous sources (i.e., beta cell secretion) and the amount of insulin required by target tissues to maintain normal disposal and mobilization of glucose, fat, and protein. Normalization of these metabolic processes requires equalization of the supply of and demand for insulin. In type II diabetic patients, among whom >80 percent are obese and insulin-resistant, the demand for insulin is increased in the face of a diminished (but not exhausted) beta cell capacity for insulin secretion. Treatment is thus directed at reducing the demand for insulin by dietary management involving a low intake of calories aimed at reducing body weight. If dietary measures fail or are insufficient, stimulation of endogenous insulin secretion by sulfonylurea agents may be helpful. In contrast, the insulin-dependent, ketosis-prone, nonobese type I diabetic patient is characterized by virtually absolute secretory deficiency of insulin which is not improved by sulfonylurea administration or sufficiently mitigated by dietary management. In such patients treatment with insulin is the mainstay of management.

The therapy for the various complications of diabetes (e.g., photocoagulation for retinopathy, hemodialysis for renal failure) has been covered above.

Insulin Therapy

Among the total population of diabetic patients, only a minority (15 to 25 percent) require insulin treatment. This category includes (1) insulin-dependent, ketosis-prone (type I) diabetic patients, regardless of age of onset, (2) maturity-onset NIDDM (type II) patients not responsive to dietary measures and/or sulfonylurea agents, (3) type II diabetic patients during periods of intercurrent stress (surgery, acute inflammation, etc.) in which a transient deterioration in metabolic homeostasis is observed, and (4) gestational diabetic patients in whom postprandial or fasting hyperglycemia is present during pregnancy (see Pregnancy and Diabetes, below). Proper management of such patients requires familiarity with the types of insulin preparations available, knowledge of the techniques of intensive management programs, and recognition of the need for individualization of treatment so as to meet the metabolic, psychological, and social needs of the patient.

Insulin Preparations

The most widely used preparations are intermediate-acting isophane insulin suspension (NPH) and insulin zinc suspension (lente insulin) and the rapid-acting regular insulin and (semilente) insulin zinc suspension (Table 19-16). In addition, long-acting (ultralente) insulin zinc suspension is occasionally used to prolong the action of lente insulin. These insulins, used singly or in combination, can generally provide for the needs of virtually all insulin-dependent diabetic patients. Protamine zinc suspension and globin insulin have little application in current clinical practice. Animal insulin preparations currently available are derived from porcine or bovine sources and are highly purified. Human insulin, manufactured either by recombinant DNA technology or semisynthetically (removal of alanine from porcine insulin), is also available for clinical use. The desired advantage of using human insulin—avoiding immunogenicity (i.e., elicitation of insulin antibodies)—has not been borne out.[420] Nevertheless, such preparations guarantee an ongoing supply of insulin irrespective of the availability of animal pancreases.

The approximate time course of activity of the various insulin preparations currently used is shown in Table 19-16. While the values shown apply to most patients, it is not uncommon for some diabetic patients to experience a slower onset and longer duration of action than expected. This effect is at least in part a consequence of the development of insulin antibodies. Thus, the pharmacokinetics of a particular preparation should be evaluated on an individual basis. Furthermore, the duration of action of insulin varies according to the insulin dose employed. The larger the quantity of insulin administered, the longer are critical levels of insulin present at receptor sites.

Human insulin activity may have a somewhat altered time course. NPH human insulin may be slightly shorter-acting than its animal-derived counterpart, and the regular form of human insulin may be more rapid-acting than bovine or porcine regular insulin. This may require a modification of existing insulin regimens when patients are switched to human insulin from bovine or porcine insulins. The differences in the absorption pattern between porcine and human insulins subsequent to subcutaneous injection are due to disparities in the dissociation of their respective hexamers. Monomeric or dimeric insulin analogues with a reduced tendency to self-

TABLE 19-16 Insulin Preparations

Insulin Preparation	Action	Peak Activity, h	Duration, h	Buffer	Protein
Regular (neutral)	Rapid	1–3	5–7	None	
Semilente	Rapid	3–4	10–16	Acetate	
NPH	Intermediate	6–14	18–28	Phosphate	Protamine
Lente	Intermediate	6–14	18–28	Acetate	
Ultralente	Prolonged	18–24	30–40	Acetate	

associate are more rapidly absorbed, which may minimize postprandial hyperglycemia and hypoglycemia in the postabsorptive state.[421]

Whereas the intermediate-acting insulins are generally capable of preventing marked hyperglycemia through much of the day, their peak action does not coincide with the increases in blood glucose concentration occurring with each meal; they therefore preclude (in most patients) complete elimination of postprandial hyperglycemia. Glucoregulation can be improved by the use of insulin mixtures (rapid- plus intermediate-acting insulin), split doses (a morning dose and an evening dose of insulin), or combined split doses (morning and evening doses, each consisting of mixtures of intermediate- and rapid-acting insulin).

Although not available commercially, proinsulin was initially thought to be potentially advantageous in the treatment of diabetes because of its unique biological properties. Synthetic human proinsulin, despite its low activity, has a more prolonged hypoglycemic effect than does regular insulin. Furthermore, it suppresses hepatic glucose output to a relatively greater extent than it stimulates peripheral glucose disposal. This is important for suppression of hepatic glucose output in patients with fasting hyperglycemia.[422] However, the relative hepatospecificity of human proinsulin failed to evoke clinical efficacy in multicenter trials. Furthermore, concern about potential atherogenicity and an increased incidence of myocardial infarction in one study led to the discontinuation of additional studies with proinsulin.[423] Recent studies have raised the possibility that C peptide may have unique properties in reversing the glomerular hyperfiltration observed early in the course of type I diabetes.[423a]

Types of Diabetes Control

Treatment of patients with insulin-dependent diabetes can now be defined on the basis of the techniques used to monitor, control, and adjust the dose of insulin rather than on the basis of therapeutic goals (e.g., tight vs. loose control). Management of an ambulatory patient with diabetes may be characterized as either conventional or intensive. Conventional treatment involves one or two injections of insulin per day. Blood glucose levels are monitored by the patient once or twice daily, and blood glucose and/or glycohemoglobin determinations are made by the physician at various intervals during office visits. Intensive management consists of self-monitoring of blood glucose levels by the patient generally four or more times per day and adjustment of insulin doses on the basis of the determinations. The insulin is injected manually twice or more per day or administered by CSII with a portable pump.

Initiating Insulin Treatment Insulin therapy may be initiated either in the hospital or in an outpatient setting, depending on the severity of the metabolic disorder, the prior medical condition of the patient, and the availability of instructional personnel. In the absence of severe metabolic decompensation (e.g., diabetic ketoacidosis), hospitalization is generally not necessary for the initiation of insulin treatment. There is no way of knowing in advance the necessary dose or doses of insulin; the treatment programs thus must be worked out empirically. Care should be taken to rule out factors which may precipitate diabetes, the correction of which might obviate the need for insulin, e.g., Cushing's disease, pheochromocytoma, acromegaly, and hypokalemia. With the advent of capillary blood glucose monitoring (see below), the use of urine testing for determining control of diabetes is much less widely employed. Patients with stable hyperglycemia (without acidosis) may be started on a single dose of 15 to 20 U of intermediate-acting insulin (NPH or lente) administered 30 min before breakfast. In patients with severe hyperglycemia or ketosis, supplementary short-acting insulin should be given in the morning and evening until adequate doses of intermediate-acting insulin are reached.

Blood glucose monitoring should be performed before meals and at bedtime (before snack). Measurements must be taken with sufficient frequency during the course of a given week to allow adequate assessment and adjustment in the insulin dosage (see Intensive Insulin Treatment: Self-Monitoring of Blood Glucose Concentration, below). At a minimum, plasma glucose concentration is measured before breakfast and before the evening meal. The dose of intermediate-acting insulin is increased 2 to 4 U every other day until the blood glucose values remain consistently in the range of 150 mg/dl or below. Optimal doses of intermediate-acting insulin are eventually achieved by gradual dosage adjustment at a time when the patient has resumed his or her daily activities (outside the hospital).

When the maximal glucoregulatory effect is achieved during the daytime, it is important to determine whether a single dose of intermediate-acting insulin is capable of sustaining the effect throughout the night. In many patients, nocturnal and early-morning hyperglycemia cannot be controlled by a single dose of intermediate-acting (NPH) or lente insulin without causing afternoon or early evening hypoglycemic reactions. Such patients should receive a second dose of intermediate-acting insulin at 5 to 6 P.M. or before bedtime. NPH or lente insulin is given before breakfast (65 to 90 percent of the total dose), and the remainder of the dose (10 to 35 percent) is given as a second dose before the evening meal. The need for rapid-acting insulin is based on blood glucose concentrations in the late morning and at bedtime. Generally, patients without significant residual insulin secretion require a twice-daily schedule of combined rapid- and intermediate-acting insulin. Often the dose of intermediate-acting insulin must be given at bedtime (with a snack) while the short-acting insulin is administered before the evening meal. This is desirable to avert early-morning hyperglycemia, probably caused by the dawn phenomenon (see below); during this time excessive secretion of counterregulatory hormones occurs, involving GH in particular.[424,425]

Initiation of insulin therapy is not complete without an effort toward patient education. Instruction in the technical and medical aspects of diabetes and in dietary principles and practice is particularly useful at this time. Insulin treatment will not be successful if dietary intake is haphazard or if faulty injection techniques are employed. Periodic instruction is strongly advisable, even in patients who are seemingly knowledgeable.

Once the dose of insulin has been established, it is important that the patient continue blood glucose monitoring (the frequency of testing will depend on the severity of the diabetes and the insulin preparations used) and that glycohemoglobin levels be checked every 2 to 3 months. Generally, the patient's insulin needs are not fixed, so that periodic reevaluation is essential. A variety of factors may induce changes in the patient's insulin requirements over time. The development of anti-insulin antibodies may prolong the duration of action from that observed at the initiation of treatment. A marked increase in physical activity may necessitate a reduction in insulin dosage or an increase in snacks to prevent hypoglycemia (see Exercise, below). Normal adolesence is frequently accompanied by a marked increase in insulin requirements. Finally, progressive deterioration in renal function, reducing insulin degradation, may lead to lowering of the insulin dose.[213] Unfortunately, the clinician's ability to assess the adequacy of diabetes control with random urinary and blood glucose concentration measurements can only give small glimpses of the actual metabolic status of the patient. Assays of glycohemoglobin (see above) permit a more complete assessment of glucoregulation and are particularly helpful in a patient with wide fluctuations from day to day (or within a given day) in blood and/or urinary glucose concentration.

Some patients have erratic, unpredictable, and unexplained swings of blood glucose concentration, varying from severe hyperglycemia to normal or even hypoglycemic levels, regardless of the insulin regimen employed. It is not clear why this pattern of "brittle" diabetes occurs. In some cases, erratic eating habits may produce an unpredictable variation between the amount of insulin available and the amount of carbohydrate entering the blood. In these cases, careful control of the pattern of eating may help. For example, the addition of a between-meals snack may eliminate hypoglycemia and subsequent reactive hyperglycemia (see Somogyi Phenomenon, below). Sometimes the lability can be explained by emotional problems which incite excessive secretion of catecholamines. In this situation the use of beta-adrenergic blocking agents has been recommended; however, the overall experience with these drugs has been disappointing. One explanation for the "brittle" state derives from the observation that many insulin-dependent diabetic patients continue to secrete some endogenous insulin, as reflected by plasma levels of C peptide. The lack of or variation in this residual endogenous insulin may contribute to a more brittle state. In some type I diabetic patients, frequent, severe episodes of hypoglycemia may be a consequence of the loss of normal sympathoadrenal mechanisms for counterregulating insulin-induced hypoglycemia.[424] This may manifest as a loss of the typical warning signs of hypoglycemia, such as sweating and palpitations (*hypoglycemia unawareness*), with sudden obtundation. This appears to be unrelated to the species of insulin (human or porcine) administered.[426,427] This predisposition to hypoglycemia may occur in the absence of other evidence of autonomic dysfunction. For whatever reason, some diabetic patients appear never to reach a stable state; they present very difficult problems in designing proper control regimens. In these patients it may be necessary to accept less rigid control standards than might otherwise be preferred in order to prevent severe hypoglycemic reactions.

Intensive Insulin Treatment: Self-Monitoring of Blood Glucose Concentration A major limitation in the use of urine glucose measurements in the management of diabetic patients is the poor correlation between blood and urinary glucose concentration values. This discrepancy is a consequence of the variability of the renal threshold for glucose, the variation in interval over which the urine sample may have accumulated before being voided, and the semiquantitative nature of the urinary glucose determination. Furthermore, at blood glucose concentrations below the renal threshold (~160 mg/dl, 8.9 m*M*), a zero urinary value cannot distinguish between a normal blood glucose concentration, moderate hyperglycemia, and hypoglycemia. To overcome these deficiencies, the procedure of self-monitoring of blood glucose levels was introduced in the late 1970s.

To monitor the blood glucose level, the patient measures the concentration in a capillary blood sample obtained by pricking the finger or earlobe. A drop of capillary blood is placed on a reagent-treated test strip which is read on a reflectance meter or by visual comparison with a color chart. There is no consensus on the frequency of capillary blood testing needed to optimize diabetic regulation. Some investigators favor obtaining one fasting sample and one other value on 6 days of the week, with a complete profile (fasting, pre-, and postprandial determinations, and one at night) determined on the seventh day. Others have suggested six daily measurements. A favored approach consists of four determinations daily (before the main meals and at bedtime) plus occasionally sampling during the night (at about 3 A.M.) to diagnose nocturnal hypoglycemia.[425,428,429] In some patients, monitoring is required only twice daily to achieve excellent blood glucose control. The practitioner should be aware that patients do not always reliably report results of blood glucose level monitoring.[419] Recommended target fasting and preprandial blood glucose concentration values are between 80 and 125 mg/dl (4.4 and 7.0 m*M*); target 2-h postprandial level is <180 mg/dl (8.5 m*M*). Target values such as these or similar ranges are appropriate for healthy individuals but are not advisable for patients with hypoglycemia unawareness, angina pectoris, cerebrovascular disease, or the presence of other complications.[430] Performance of self-monitoring should occasionally be compared with simultaneously obtained laboratory determinations to ensure accuracy in the performance and interpretation of patient-determined values.

It is essential that patients be properly instructed in all facets of this methodology, including basic techniques in resolving technical problems. The precision of devices for monitoring is dependent on user variability, hematocrit (e.g., anemia or polycythemia may affect their reliability), the presence of hypoglycemia or severe hyperglycemia, and defects in the instrument and/or reagent strips.[431]

Central to all programs of self-monitoring of the blood glucose level is the administration of at least two doses of insulin per day and modification of the insulin dose on the basis of the blood glucose determinations. The use of a pen-injecting device may be particularly helpful to patients requiring premeal insulin injections when not at home (e.g., when at work or at a restaurant). The dose adjustments are carried out through frequent contact with the physician and by providing the patient with instructions or rules to be followed when the blood glucose level falls outside the desired range; for example, if the fasting blood glucose level exceeds 150 mg/dl, the evening doses of NPH or lente insulin should be increased by 2 U (Table 19-17). The types of rules used have ranged from relatively simple instructions to complex algorithms. The involvement of the patient in the management of his or her disease is consequently crucial to the success of the regimen. In particular, patients should be aware of the relation between blood glucose levels at particular times of the day and specific insulin doses (e.g., the fasting glucose level is controlled by evening dose of NPH) (Table 19-16).

The effectiveness of such treatment regimens in lowering the blood glucose level to nearly normal concentration and in restoring a nearly normal concentration of glycohemoglobin has been documented in many but not all patients. The recent findings from the DCCT study indicate that restoration of near-normal blood glucose levels (glycohemoglobin on average of 7.2) prevents or retards the complications of diabetes.[409a] If such glycohemoglobin levels can be achieved with one or two injections of insulin per day and with no more than twice daily blood monitoring, the use of a more intensive regimen is not warranted.

Intensive management of type I diabetes is not without risk. The hazards include the precipitation of hypoglycemia, adverse psychological effects due to preoccupation with the care of diabetes, and increased costs. The multicenter DCCT has reported a 3.1-fold increased risk of severe hypoglycemia in intensively treated patients in contrast to conventional therapy.[410] Nocturnal hypoglycemia, which

TABLE 19-17 Intensive Insulin Treatment: Protocol and Rules for Adjustments

Goal: Fasting, preprandial, and bedtime blood glucose concentration 80 to 125 mg/dl
Protocol: NPH or lente plus regular insulin in the morning (7 to 8 A.M.) and evening (5:30 to 6:30 P.M.)

Adjustments

1. If blood glucose concentration is too high (>150 mg/dl) on two consecutive days,	
Before breakfast:	Increase evening dose of NPH or lente*
Before lunch:	Increase morning dose of regular insulin
Before dinner:	Increase morning dose of NPH or lente
Before bed:	Increase evening dose of regular insulin
2. If blood glucose concentration is too low (<60 mg/dl),	
Between breakfast and lunch:	Decrease morning dose of regular insulin†
Between lunch and dinner:	Decrease morning dose of NPH or lente
Between dinner and bedtime:	Decrease evening dose of regular insulin
During the night or early morning:	Decrease evening dose of NPH or lente

* Insulin dose should be increased by 2U; adjust only one insulin type at a time.

† Reduce dose by 2 U, depending on severity of reaction.

Source: Felig and Bergman,[432] as modified from Judd S, Sonksen PH: *Diabetes Care* 3:134, 1980.

may occur in 30 percent of patients, may pose the greatest risk because of the patient's unawareness. Intensive diabetes control per se may also contribute to the susceptibility to hypoglycemia by reducing the threshold for the release of counterregulatory hormones.[431a] Transient worsening of diabetic retinopathy has been reported which is obviated with extended improved control.[407,408] Consequently, intensive diabetic control is not indicated for all insulin-treated diabetic patients. It should be strongly encouraged in the management of diabetes occurring during pregnancy; for growing, adolescent diabetic patients; for those with brittle diabetes; for young diabetic patients who are free of complications; and for most diabetic patients who do not have a history of severe hypoglycemia. It should always be employed in patients treated with a portable insulin infusion pump. It is unwarranted in patients who already have severe nephropathy and are not undergoing a renal transplant and patients who are free of microvascular disease but have a limited life expectancy (e.g., those of advanced age or with severe coronary artery disease). Intensive therapy may be ill advised as well for individuals who are technically unable to learn or apply the necessary measures resulting in optimal control (e.g., psychological instability, unreliability, noncompliance). For the remainder of the type I diabetic population, self-monitoring of blood glucose concentration together with an intensive program of insulin administration should be offered as a therapeutic option. Finally, it should be emphasized that the goal of treatment should not be the achievement of the most intensive and complicated treatment protocol feasible but the normalization of the metabolic milieu in the manner that is least hazardous and intrusive for the patient. Thus, patients who are able to achieve A_{Ic} hemoglobin levels in the range of 7.2 to 7.5 percent and/or mean blood glucose levels of 150 to 160 mg/dl with regimens involving one or two insulin injections a day and blood testing only once or twice daily need not employ a more intensive regimen of more frequent injections or blood testing. The data from the DCCT study[409a] clearly show that such patients, by virtue of the status of their metabolic control, are at reduced risk for diabetes complications.

Devices for Insulin Delivery

The development of insulin delivery devices for the normalization of blood glucose concentration has involved two types of systems, designated *closed-loop* and *open-loop* devices.[432] The closed-loop types consist of a feedback circuit in which the insulin delivery rate is variable and is automatically dictated by continuous monitoring of the blood glucose concentration. Such systems, however, require the continuous withdrawal of small amounts of blood for glucose determination and are bulky; they are thus limited to inpatient use for 24- to 48-h periods. More practical use of closed-loop systems must await the development of an implantable long-lasting glucose sensor, which remains an elusive goal.

The open-loop systems involve the use of a preprogrammed portable infusion pump which delivers insulin at basal, between-meals rates and which, upon activation by the patient, increases the insulin delivery rate before meals (CSII). This permits greater flexibility, as the premeal boluses can be modified according to the timing and size of meals. In addition to eliminating the need for a glucose sensor, they employ a subcutaneous rather than IV access route, thus reducing the possibility of problems with infection and thrombosis. Pickup and colleagues in Great Britain[433] and Tamborlane et al. at Yale[73,434,435] first demonstrated the efficacy of such systems when continuously employed for periods of 2 weeks to several months. Virtually complete normalization of concentrations of plasma glucose, lipids, and branched-chain amino acids have been observed. Furthermore, the exaggerated rise in concentrations of counterregulatory hormones induced by exercise in conventionally treated patients is returned to normal after 1 to 2 weeks of pump treatment.

The diurnal profiles of glycemic control during long-term use of CSII have been shown to approximate closely the upper limits of glucose fluctuation found in normal individuals.[436] Insulin pumps capable of providing variable basal rates of infusion may facilitate control during the overnight period, when insulin requirements are increased as a result of the dawn phenomenon.[437,438] Delivery of insulin at a basal rate has also been successfully applied in the management of diabetes during hyperalimentation.[437] Although CSII provides insulin levels that are significantly higher than those found in individuals without diabetes, the concentrations are similar compared with a conventionally treated diabetic population.[436,439]

As in the case of intensive regimens of insulin therapy involving multiple manual injections, the key to successful treatment with an insulin pump is proper use of self-monitoring of the blood glucose concentration (see above). The indications and contraindications for insulin pump therapy are similar to those discussed above for self-monitoring of blood glucose concentration.

CSII therapy may result in a number of complications.[439a,439b] The rate of occurrence of DKA may be higher than during conventional insulin therapy and appears to be independent of simple instrument failure; it may be a consequence of needle dislodgement. Other causes, such as minor stress or emotional upset, may be responsible.[440] The frequency of localized infections at infusion sites is greater with CSII than with depot injections. The rate of localized infection is influenced by factors such as hygiene, antiseptic precautions, and the frequency with which infusion sites are changed. Another consideration is the insulin preparation used for CSII. Buffered purified porcine insulin has been shown to cause less infusion-site inflammation and obstruction of the catheter and/or needle than unbuffered bovine-porcine insulin mixture. Chemical changes in the insulin solution may occur as a result of prolonged exposure before the infusion.[441–443] However, there is no evidence of excess mortality with CSII compared with conventional therapy.

Although the precise place for CSII has yet to be defined, the critical role of blood glucose monitoring remains fundamental for all systems of intensified therapy.[445] Studies on the impact of CSII on the complications of diabetes compared with conventional treatment suggest that microalbuminuria, a predictor of clinical nephropathy, may decline.[446] By contrast, gross proteinuria is unaffected by CSII.[359] Furthermore, retinopathy has been found in some studies to deteriorate, although the worsening is transient and occurs in patients presenting with more severe retinal disease at the start of insulin pump therapy.[446,447] The results of the recently completed NIH multicenter diabetes control and complications trials have clearly shown that long-term intensive control results in less microvascular disease than is found in conventionally treated patients.[409,409a]

Implantable pumps for the IV or intraperitoneal administration of insulin have been employed in limited numbers of patients.[447] The use of such devices is limited at present for investigational purposes, due to the lack of an implantable glucose sensor (see Future Treatment, Implantable Insulin Pumps, below). Intraperitoneal insulin infusion is utilized in patients undergoing chronic ambulatory peritoneal dialysis. The peritoneum allows insulin direct access to the portal circulation. Pen or jet injectors have also been introduced into therapy. The pen injector simplifies insulin administration when patients require premeal insulin injections when at work or in a restaurant.A potiential application of jet injectors resides in adult patients with phobia of insulin injections.[448] Their efficacy with regard to blood glucose control in contrast to CSII and multiple injections appears to be comparable in the elderly as well.[449,450] An improvement in quality of life in pen users has been reported. [451]

Complications of Insulin Treatment

Hypoglycemia The most common and potentially most serious complication of insulin treatment is hypoglycemia. Hypoglycemia may be produced with any dose or preparation of insulin if the amount of insulin administered is excessive relative to the availability of glucose from endogenous and exogenous (e.g., dietary) sources. The time at which hypoglycemia occurs depends on the circumstances precipitating the attack. Overdoses of intermediate-acting insulin usually produce hypoglycema in the late afternoon or evening; rapid-acting insulin causes this complication about 3 h after administration, and with long-acting insulin it is a hazard during the early hours of the morning. Exercise may produce its effect within an hour, although delayed postexercise hypoglycemia may be more common than was originally realized. Insulin-induced hypoglycemia is experienced at some time by virtually all type I diabetic patients. In some series, severe hypoglycemia (necessitating hospitalization or assistance from another person) has been observed in 25 percent of patients over a 1-year period.[452] In addition, hypoglycemia accounts for 3 to 7 percent of deaths in patients with type I diabetes.[453]

The symptoms of hypoglycemia may be divided into two categories: the effect of low blood glucose concentration itself, which results mainly in symptoms in the central nervous system (confusion, bizarre behavior, depression, neurologic manifestations, convulsions, and coma), and the effects of the response of the body to hypoglycemia, which include secretion of epinephrine with resulting vasoconstriction, tachycardia, piloerection, perspiration, and subjective tension or a feeling of impending disaster. A rapid fall of blood glucose concentration is more likely to call forth the typical sympathetic discharge. When hypoglycemia occurs during sleep, the only symptoms may be nightmares, sweating, and a headache on awakening in the morning. Symptomatic nocturnal hypoglycemia (plasma glucose concentration <36 mg/dl or <2.0 m*M*) may occur in as many as 30 to 40 percent of insulin-treated diabetic patients.[454]

Patients with specific areas of reduced cerebral blood flow (a common problem since diabetic patients often have atherosclerosis) may experience localized neurologic defects during hypoglycemia, such as hemiplegias, visual disturbances, and temporal or frontal lobe syndromes. These aberrations usually are transient but may persist if the blood glucose concentration remains depressed long enough to cause irreversible damage to certain brain cells. Hypothermia is common during hypoglycemia and may be helpful as a diagnostic sign in a comatose patient. In view of the ability of the heart to subsist on substrates other than glucose, it is not surprising that hypoglycemia may be well tolerated in patients with arteriosclerotic heart disease, although the reactive secretion of epinephrine may precipate arrhythmias, pulmonary edema, angina, or myocardial infarction.

Symptoms subjectively indistinguishable from those caused by absolute hypoglycemia may sometimes occur when the plasma glucose level is not markedly below the normal range (e.g., 60 to 120 mg/dl or 3.3 to 6.7 m*M*). Presumably, these symptoms result from a rapid rate of fall of blood glucose concentration from high levels. Whereas normal subjects must become frankly hypoglycemic (<50 mg/dl or <2.7 m*M*) to elicit an adrenergic discharge, in chronically hyperglycemic diabetic patients plasma catecholamine concentrations rise when plasma glucose concentration rapidly declines to values of 100 mg/dl.[455] It is important to document a fall in plasma glucose concentration if the symptoms are equivocal, since an inappropriate reduction in insulin dose or an increase in dietary carbohydrate may make overall control more difficult.

Although a single attack of hypoglycemia is uncomfortable or even hazardous, the major risk is from repeated attacks, which can cause serious, though subtle, cerebral deterioration with reduction of intelligence and a tendency to cerebral dysrhythmias. Unfortunately, data are not available regarding the prevalence of brain damage due to hypoglycemia in insulin-treated diabetic patients. In animals, hypoglycemia results in brain damage only when it is of sufficient severity to cause an arrest of brain wave activity.

The occurrence of hypoglycemia in insulin-treated diabetic patients depends in part on the adequacy of counterregulatory hormone secretion and the intensity of the treatment program. A deficiency of glucagon secretion in response to hypoglycemia is frequently observed in type I diabetes but does not of itself increase vulnerability to insulin-induced hypoglycemia.[432] However, diabetic patients in whom epinephrine deficiency is combined with glucagon deficiency are severely predisposed to insulin-induced hypoglycemia.[432] Such combined deficiencies are often, but not always, accompanied by clinical evidence of autonomic neuropathy. Other factors which predispose to the development of insulin-induced hypoglycemia include a marked increase in physical activity (i.e., exercise), faulty injection technique, a decrease in food intake (skipped meals, low-calorie diet, or fasting), and a decrease in insulin turnover (e.g., renal failure). A questionnaire survey indicated that exercise was the most common daytime cause of hypoglycemia in children.[456]

Patients who are prone to exercise-induced hypoglycemia may be instructed to consume extra carbohydrate before exercise, to use a nonexercised injection site such as the abdomen (see Exercise, below), or to reduce the insulin dose before exercise. Faulty injection technique (e.g., failure to agitate the insulin vial properly before use), errors in the preparation of insulin mixtures, accidental injection into muscle, or injection into sites where insulin absorption is irregular (e.g., lipodystrophy) may be uncovered when the history is taken and can be eliminated by instruction by a trained nurse. Insulin infusion techniques for evaluating the adequacy of sympathoadrenal counterregulatory mechanisms have been described,[457] but their practical usefulness has not been established. The sudden onset of frequent hypoglycemic episodes may also result from (1) failure to reduce insulin dosage after resolution of stress or illness, (2) onset of diseases associated with increased insulin sensitivity (e.g., adrenal or pituitary insufficiency), and (3) onset of pregnancy.

The immediate treatment of hypoglycemia consists of the administration of carbohydrate, preferably as a sweetened drink or food or commercially prepared, premeasured glucose tablets; in an emergency, IV injection of 50 ml or more of a 50% glucose solution can be used. For occasions when glucose is unavailable or IV injection (e.g., by the patient's spouse) is not feasible, 1 mg of glucagon injected intramuscularly is effective; the small volume in which it is dissolved makes it convenient for inclusion in a physician's bag. If a single dose of glucagon is not effective within 15 min, it is unlikely that a second dose will help. Therefore, if glucagon fails, treatment with IV glucose is mandatory. Patients may experience nausea, vomiting, a transient increase in blood pressure, and rebound hyperglycemia in response to glucagon administration. Once the patient is aroused, food should be taken to avoid potential waning of glucagon's effect, given its short half-life.

Insulin-treated diabetic patients should be instructed to have at all times immediate access to (or carry) a source of carbohydrate (e.g., glucose tablets, hard candies) and to carry identification noting their diabetic status. They should become familiar with symptoms resulting from the gradual onset of hypoglycemia (loss of ability to concentrate, aberrant behavior, or other mental dysfunction) and the signs of hypoglycemia while asleep (nightmares, morning headache, or bedsheets drenched with sweat), in addition to the more commonly appreciated autonomic symptoms resulting from acute hypoglycemia (sweating, shakiness, and palpitations). The patient's spouse or parent should also be instructed about the symptoms of hypoglycemia and the use of glucagon in the event of hypoglycemic coma.

Somogyi Phenomenon Hyperglycemia and ketonuria may paradoxically occur after excessive insulin administration. Rebound or reactive hyperglycemia, otherwise known as the *Somogyi phenomenon*, results from the release of catecholamines, cortisol, and GH in response to acute hypoglycemia; this phenomenon may be responsible for worsening of diabetes. Of the various counterregulatory hormones contributing to reactive hyperglycemia, epinephrine appears to be the most important.[458–460] The rebound hyperglycemia may be further aggravated by excessive food intake in response to the symptoms of hypoglycemia. Patients exhibiting the Somogyi phenomenon are usually type I diabetic patients whose diabetes is difficult to control with single doses of insulin. If the Somogyi phenomenon is suspected, the patient's insulin dose should be reduced under careful supervision and/or additional carbohydrate should be added in the form of a late-evening snack.

Improvement in control despite a reduction in insulin dose provides strong presumptive evidence of the Somogyi phenomenon. In general, fasting hyperglycemia is likely to be a consequence of dissipation of insulin action (reflecting a need for a larger evening dose of intermediate-acting insulin) rather than a result of reactive hyperglycemia (reflecting a need for less evening insulin).

Dawn Phenomenon An early-morning increase in blood glucose concentration may, of course, be observed in insulin-treated type I diabetic patients in the absence of antecedent hypoglycemia. Dissipation of the action of previously injected insulin is by far the most common cause of such early-morning hyperglycemia.[461] By contrast, in occasional patients there is an early-morning rise in blood glucose concentration despite ongoing CSII; this occurrence has been termed the *dawn phenomenon*. In this circumstance the waning of previously injected insulin cannot be invoked as an explanation.[462] A nocturnal increase in GH secretion appears to be the mechanism responsible for the dawn phenomenon,[463] raising the possibility that late-evening administration of a long-acting somatostatin analogue, octreotide, which prevents nocturnal increases in GH secretion may improve blood glucose regulation in some diabetic patients. The importance of the dawn phenomenon in children and adolescents has been questioned, however.[464] A clinical role for octreotide in diabetes management has not been established.

Insulin Lipodystrophy Insulin lipodystrophy is a distressing, although benign, complication of insulin treatment which may take the form of hypertrophy or atrophy of subcutaneous tissues. The fibrous masses that develop are hypoesthetic; the problem is therefore often perpetuated (particularly in young diabetic patients), since these sites are favored for injection. Unfortunately, the absorption of insulin from these sites is often erratic and incomplete, thus leading to a deterioration in the control of diabetes. The development of insulin preparations which are >98 percent pure has markedly reduced the incidence of this complication. The use of human insulin may also be advantageous in this circumstance. Lipoatrophic areas should be injected gradually from the periphery toward the center of the "crater" until they are completely filled in.

Insulin Allergy Insulin allergy has been less of a problem since purified animal and human insulins have been introduced. It is thought that intermittent administration of insulin, particularly with bovine-porcine or bovine insulins, might serve as a potent immunogenic stimulus if the same insulin were administered again at a later time. Although human insulin of recombinant DNA origin is somewhat less immunogenic than porcine or bovine insulin, low-titer antibody formation may still occur, resulting in insulin allergy in rare patients.

Allergic reactions to insulin may be localized or systemic. Localized allergic reactions are manifested as induration, pruritus, erythema, or pain at the injection site. The symptoms appear 30 min to 4 h or more after the injection. The usual onset is within the first week or month of the initiation of insulin treatment. The immediate type of local allergy (within 30 to 120 min) is IgG-mediated. In most patients the reactions disappear spontaneously after several weeks. Improvement may occur by switching to monospecies insulin (e.g., pure porcine), to human insulin, or to the local use of small doses of glucocorticoids.

Systemic allergy may be manifested as generalized pruritus and urticaria, angioedema, or acute anaphylaxis; such anaphylaxis, fortunately, is extremely rare. Sixty percent of patients with systemic allergy have a history of discontinuation of treatment with insulin and recent reinstitution of insulin therapy. The systemic allergic reaction is thought to be mediated by IgE antibody. Treatment consists of desensitization with human or porcine insulin at an initial dose of 0.001 U.

The clinical advantages of human insulin compared to purified porcine insulin remain uncertain, particularly with regard to circulating levels of insulin antibodies. Alterations in the T lymphocyte subsets independent of changes in antibody levels may proffer an advantage.[465] Furthermore, transferring patients allergic to pork or bovine insulin to human insulin may be beneficial.[466]

Insulin Resistance The normal 24-h insulin output from the islets of Langerhans has been estimated at 20 to 40 U per day. Consequently, patients requiring a greater amount of insulin have some degree of insensitivity to insulin. The most common cause of resistance to insulin is obesity; intercurrent stress and illness may also increase insulin requirements through a variety of mechanisms. From a practical standpoint, clinical insulin resistance has been defined as the requirement for 200 U or more of insulin per day for several days in the absence of ketoacidosis, intercurrent infection, or associated endocrine disease (acromegaly, Cushing's syndrome). In a nonobese patient, various mechanisms may be reponsible for clinical insulin resistance: circulating antibodies to insulin, abnormalities of insulin receptors, increased local destruction of insulin, or secretion of abnormal insulin.

Immunogenic insulin insensitivity results from a higher titer of circulating IgG antibodies directed at bovine insulin and, to a lesser extent, porcine or human insulin. While all patients develop antibodies to insulin, in only a small proportion of patients is the titer sufficiently high to necessitate daily doses of >200 U of insulin. Most of these patients are adults who have been treated with insulin for long periods (>15 years); however, insensitivity may sometimes arise after several weeks. Insulin allergy usually does not accompany insulin insensitivity. Treatment consists initially of switching to pure porcine insulin or, preferably, human insulin. If human insulin fails, systemic steroids (60 to 80 mg of prednisone per day for 10 days) generally result in a marked reduction in insulin requirements.

A rare form of insulin resistance in which titers of circulating insulin antibodies are not increased is that encountered in young women who also have acanthosis nigricans. As was discussed earlier (see Acanthosis Nigricans, above), this syndrome has been subdivided into two types, in both of which there appear to be abnormalities in insulin receptors. In type A, there is a decrease in the number of insulin receptors and the patients show virilization and accelerated growth. In type B, circulating antibodies to the insulin receptor are demonstrable and evidence of an autoimmune disorder is present.

A limited number of patients have been observed who respond poorly to subcutaneous insulin but are quite sensitive to IV insulin.[463] Localized destruction of insulin has been postulated to account for this unusual disturbance. The use of aprotinin, a nonspecific protease inhibitor, or lidocaine has not been uniformly successful in the treatment of this syndrome. Furthermore, when studied carefully, so-called peripheral insulin resistance has been found in the majority of patients with this syndrome to be of factitious origin (e.g., failure to administer insulin). Close attention should be given to this possibility. However, since true resistance to peripherally but not intravenously administered insulin has been documented, either IV or intraperitoneal insulin administration can be attempted.[467]

Insulin resistance is also encountered in a rare form of diabetes, lipoatrophic diabetes (see below).

Insulin-Induced Edema Edema is a rare complication observed in patients with poorly regulated diabetes in whom glycemic control is restored by insulin. While sodium and fluid retention may in part be related to correction of volume reduction induced by glucosuria, insulin may have a direct effect in reducing urinary sodium excretion. Infusions of insulin in the upper physiologic range (without changes in blood glucose concentration) markedly reduce urinary sodium excretion in the absence of changes in the filtered load of glucose, GFR, renal blood flow, or aldosterone concentration.[131] Insulin-induced edema thus may be analogous to the refeeding edema observed in concentration camp survivors after they were placed on a normal caloric intake.

Goals of Insulin Treatment

In the past there was controversy between proponents of tight and loose control in the management of type I diabetes, which in part lies in differences of opinion about the pathogenesis of the *onset* of diabetic complications. As was discussed above, although neither the metabolic nor the genetic hypothesis can be proved at present, the preponderance of evidence clearly favors a metabolic pathogenesis. Evidence that restoration of a normal or nearly normal blood glucose concentration prevents or retards the development of diabetic complications, as shown in the DCCT trial,[409,409a] provides a scientific rationale for attempting to achieve nearly normal blood glucose levels. The overall philosophy to which virtually all diabetologists subscribe is that insulin treatment should be directed at restoring the plasma glucose concentration to as close to normal as possible (i.e., glycohemoglobin of 7 to 8, average blood glucose of ~150 mg/dl) without causing hypoglycemia or impairing the patient's psychosocial adaptation. The real issue is thus not the goal of treatment but the manner of implementation, i.e., whether to employ an intensive program of insulin administration. The indications and contraindications for such programs have already been discussed (see Intensive Insulin Treatment: Self-Monitoring of Blood Glucose Concentration, above). It should, however, be recognized that acceptance by the patient of an intensive regimen is likely to be influenced by the enthusiasm and zeal demonstrated by the physician, which in turns derives from the extent to which the metabolic hypothesis is embraced. Furthermore, an appreciation of the psychodynamic features underlying various behavior patterns encountered in the clinical setting may result in the achievement of far-ranging goals.[467a]

Diet Therapy

Dietary management forms the cornerstone of the treatment of all diabetic patients. This is true in circumstances in which insulin or oral hypoglycemic agents are used as well as in patients in whom dietary measures are the sole form of therapy. Despite its paramount importance, successful implementation of dietary management is achieved in only occasional patients.[468] The reasons for this frequent failure largely relate to a failure on the part of the physician and the patient to understand the goals, principles, and specific strategies of treatment. Whereas the purpose of insulin and oral agent treatment involves primarily the normalization of blood glucose concentration, the goals of diet therapy are two: normoglycemia and ideal body weight. These aims are achieved on the basis of three principles: (1) regulation of caloric intake, (2) selection of carbohydrate foods less likely to cause marked increases in blood glucose concentration without reducing total carbohydrate content, and (3) maintenance of frequent food intake in small portions.

Regulation of total caloric intake is directed at the achievement of ideal body weight. For type II diabetic patients (among whom, as already noted, the frequency of obesity is >80 percent), this generally entails a reduction in caloric intake. The importance of weight reduction in these patients is based on the fact that obesity results in resistance to endogenous insulin, which is reversed by a return to ideal weight[469]; with restoration to normal weight, the demand for endogenous insulin is reduced and improvement in glucose tolerance ensues. In contrast to the obese type II diabetic patient, a high caloric intake is indicated in the wasted type I diabetic patient, particularly in childhood. Such patients require an increase in calories to restore body fat and protein and permit normal growth.

The total carbohydrate content of the diet should not be disproportionately restricted. There is no compelling evidence that reduction in the carbohydrate content to 30 percent without reducing total caloric intake results in improvement of the diabetic state. Such an approach may in the long run be deleterious, since the calories not taken in as carbohydrate are generally made up in the form of fat; a high fat intake may have an adverse effect by accelerating atherosclerosis. Furthermore, an increase in the proportion of carbohydrate in the diet may improve glucose tolerance.

Once the appropriate caloric intake has been determined, 45 to 55 percent of the calories should be provided in the form of carbohydrate. An exception is the diabetic patient with a carbohydrate-inducible (type 4 or 5) form of hyperlipidemia characterized by hypertriglyceridemia, in whom a low-carbohydrate, low calorie intake may be indicated. The classic dietary recommendations for choice of carbohydrate-containing foods have called for avoidance by diabetic patients of concentrated sweets (e.g., table sugar, candies, pastries). The basis for this recommendation is the notion that foods containing preformed mono- or disaccharides are more likely to cause a marked rise in blood glucose concentration than are equivalent amounts of carbohydrate present as a starch (e.g., potato). Studies indicate, however, that such simple rules may not adequately predict the "glycemic index" of foods.[470] For example, the glycemic index of mashed potatoes is substantially greater than that of ice cream, sucrose, or fructose.[470] Sucrose (or fructose)-rich diets are not recommended in general, even if the postprandial glucose and insulin elevations they elict may be lower in comparison with other carbohydrates.[471,472] There is a metabolic tendency of fructose to be preferentially converted to lipids, mainly as a result of obligatory hepatic fructose metabolism with consequent hyperlipogenesis.[14] Excessive fructose consumption (as in diets rich in fruit content) should in fact be considered as an accessory risk factor in diabetes. The emerging data on blood glucose concentration responses to specific foods should thus permit a dietary selection process which contributes substantially to improving the overall control of the blood glucose level.

Day-to-day regularity of food intake with respect to total consumption of calories and carbohydrates and with regard to the timing of meals and snacks is of importance in insulin-treated diabetic patients to prevent insulin-induced hypoglycemia. The regularity and frequency of feedings are predicted on the fact that in contrast to the normal subject, in whom insulin secretion is dictated by food ingestion, the insulin-dependent diabetic patient must match food intake to the continuing action of injected insulin. Since insulin is being released continuously from injection sites, ideally the patient should eat sparingly but frequently rather than allow long intervals between large meals. Consistency in the pattern of food ingestion does not apply on days in which there is a marked increase in caloric expenditure as a consequence of moderate to intense exercise. In normal subjects, exercise causes a fall in endogenous insulin level which permits an increase in hepatic glucose output. In the diabetic subject receiving insulin injections, such homeostatic changes in circulating insulin levels do not happen; in fact, rapid insulin mobilization from the injection site may occur in response to exercise (see below). In such circumstances, extra food should be taken to meet the needs of contracting muscles and prevent hypoglycemia.

The recommended dietary allowance for protein is 0.8 g/kg body weight, which may need to be reduced further in the presence of renal disease. As was discussed above (see Diabetic Nephropathy), a role for protein-restricted diets in *preventing* diabetic nephropathy has not been established. Total fat should be restricted to <30 percent of total calories, including <300 mg per day of cholesterol. Saturated fats should be replaced by unsaturated fats, particularly monosaturated fats. Sodium intake not to exceed 3000 mg/day is also suggested in nonhypertensive patients.

Despite the simplicity of many of these principles, <50 percent of the diabetic population adheres to the recommended dietary regimen. Poor understanding on the part of the patient as well as the physician with respect to dietary goals and tactics is frequently responsible for failures. Often, the basic prescription is clearly in error and unsuitable for the specific patient. For example, to many physicians a "diabetic diet" almost by definition means an 1800-calorie intake. Such a diet in a vigorous, nonobese 160-lb (73-kg) type I diabetic patient is obviously too restricted and is likely to have one of two adverse consequences. Either the patient does not follow the diet and supplements his or her intake, generally with concentrated sweets, resulting in marked swings in the blood glucose concentration, or the patient sticks to the diet but develops hypoglycemic episodes and/or loses weight. An 1800-calorie diet is equally inappropriate in a 180-lb (82-kg), 5-ft 2-in

(158-cm), 50-year-old sedentary II diabetic woman; in such a patient the major objective should be weight reduction by means of a more limited caloric intake.

Dietary management thus must begin with a precise diet prescription which is meaningful to the dietician as well as the patient. This necessarily involves tailoring the diet to the individual patient. For example, in type II diabetic patients the most important consideration is caloric restriction. This should be emphasized to the patient and communicated to the dietitian in terms of total caloric content. In contrast, in the nonobese type I diabetic patient, regularity of food intake, use of between-meals snacks, and selectivity concerning the types of carbohydrate-containing foods are of higher priority than total caloric intake.

In all forms of diabetes the importance of patient education in the implementation of dietary management cannot be overstated. Of great importance is making certain that the patient understands the goals and strategies of the diet and that the dietary prescription takes into account the habits, behavior, and specific requirements of the individual patient. Initial referral and frequent follow-up by a competent dietitian or detailed discussion with the physician is essential to reinforce the importance of dietary complicance.

The combination of a very low calorie diet for 8 weeks in conjunction with behavior modification has been shown to have a salutary effect in very obese type II diabetic patients on glycemic control through 1-year follow up. Despite an initial weight loss achieved by week 20, overall weight loss from pretreatment to 1 year did not differ from the control group. Nonetheless, HbA_1 levels showed a greater improvement in the very low calorie diet group. The benefit was possibly attributable to increased endogenous insulin secretion.[473]

Many studies have been performed showing that addition to the diet of fiber (nonabsorbable carbohydrate) decreases postprandial hyperglycemia[470,474] and lowers lipid levels.[475] The ingestion of guar gum (a storage polysaccharide obtained from the cluster bean) or pectin (a structural polysaccharide obtained from apples and citrus fruits), together with meals containing absorbable carbohydrates, slows or reduces carbohydrate absorption as well as plasma insulin response[476] in normal and diabetic subjects. Studies of peripheral insulin sensitivity have shown no increase after fiber ingestion, suggesting that its major effect in reducing postprandial hyperglycemia is via effects on the GI handling of carbohydrate-containing foods.[477] Since relatively large amounts of fiber (40 g of fiber per day vs. 25 g/1000 kcal of food intake)[478] are required to achieve an effect, and inasmuch as the palatability of such diets is poor, the overall practicability and long-term efficacy of high-fiber diets in the routine management of diabetes remain to be established. Nevertheless, fiber supplementation appears to be efficacious if 50 percent of the diet contains carbohydrates. Sources of palatable fiber include fruits, legumes, lentils, green leafy vegetables, and whole grain cereals. Fiber-containing foods should be consumed raw and not purèed. The long-term safety of fiber is not known, and therefore individuals at risk for deficiencies (e.g., the elderly, growing children) may benefit from vitamin and mineral supplementation.

Oral Hypoglycemic Agents

Since the introduction of the sulfonylureas in the 1950s, the management of many patients with type II diabetes has included the use of oral hypoglycemic agents. The two classes of hypoglycemic drugs which have been employed are the sulfonylurea and biguanide compounds. These compounds differ with regard to structure, action, and clinical usefulness.

The Sulfonylureas

The sulfonylurea drugs share a basic molecular structure but differ in substituents on the benzene and urea groups.[479] These substitutions account for differences in the potency, metabolism, and duration of action of the sulfonylureas (Table 19-18). Sulfonylureas reduce blood glucose concentration mainly by augmenting the amount of endogenous insulin released by directly affecting the pancreatic islets. It has been hypothesized that by binding to the plasma membrane, ATP-sensitive K^+ channels are closed, leading to depolarization, facilitating Ca^{2+} entry, which results in stimulation of insulin release.[480] IV administration of sulfonylureas produces abrupt release of insulin, and the insulin response to feeding is increased after short-term sulfonylurea therapy. This concept is further supported by evidence that these drugs fail to reduce blood glucose concentration in pancreatectomized animals or in type I diabetic patients without residual endogenous insulin and produce rapid release of insulin from isolated islet-cell systems. The second-generation oral agents glipizide and glyburide are substantially more potent than the first-generation sulfonylureas in facilitating insulin release.[481,482] While these data convincingly demonstrate that sulfonylureas are effective insulin secretagogues, the persistent hypoglycemic action of these drugs may not be mediated solely via changes in insulin secretion. In fact, insulin secretion is actually reduced after several months of treatment despite improvement in glucose tolerance. The reduction in insulin secretion may, however, be more apparent than real; it may reflect the lower ambient blood glucose levels and improved metabolic control achieved with the sulfonylurea agents. Thus, if the plasma glucose level is raised to the pretreatment value, the insulin secretory response is greater than it was before treatment.[482] Additional evidence supporting an extrapancreatic

TABLE 19-18 Properties of Sulfonylurea Agents

Characteristic	Tolbutamide	Tolazamide	Chlorpropamide	Glipizide	Glyburide
Relative potency	1	5	6	100	150
Duration of action (h)	6–10	16–24	24–72	16–24	18–24
Protein binding					
Type	Ionic/nonionic	Ionic/nonionic	Ionic/nonionic	Nonionic	Nonionic
Extent (%)	98	98	95	98	98
Activity of hepatic metabolites	Weak	One active, others nonactive	Weak	Weak	One active, others nonactive
Dose (mg)					
Range	500–3000	100–1000	100–500	2.5–40	1.25–20
Average	1500	250	250	10	7.5
Doses per day (no.)	2–3	1–2	1	1–2	1–2
Usual initial daily dose (mg)	500	100	100	5	2.5
Dosage forms available (mg)	250, 500	100, 250, 500	100, 250	5, 10	1.25, 2.5, 5
Diuretic	Yes	Yes	No	No	Yes
Antidiuretic	Yes	No	Yes	No	No
"Disulfiram effect"	No	No	Yes	No	No
Frequency of severe hypoglycemia (%)	1	1	4–6	2–4	4–6
Overall frequency of side effects (%)	3	4	9	6	7

Modified from Gerich.[479]

effect of sulfonylureas is provided by studies demonstrating an increase in peripheral sensitivity to insulin.[483] However, those effects may also be secondary to enhanced insulin secretion and improved control of blood glucose concentration, inasmuch as intensive treatment of type II diabetic patients with sulfonylureas[484] or exogenous insulin[485] reduces insulin resistance, increases basal insulin levels, and causes a drop in fasting plasma glucose levels, most probably by restraining hepatic glucose production. In a comparison of treatments with exogenous insulin and tolazamide,[486] similar lowering of glycohemoglobin levels and glucose production was obtained. Since no change in insulin binding was seen, these improvements were achieved by increasing the maximal insulin response. All curves were shifted, however, to the right of normal, indicating a residual, postbinding defect in insulin action, which could not be reversed either by tolazamide or by insulin.

Sulfonylurea Preparations The various sulfonylurea agents differ primarily with respect to duration of action and potency (Table 19-18). The differences in duration of action reflect differences in drug metabolism.[479,487,488] Tolbutamide, the shortest-acting drug and the least potent, is metabolized by the liver to metabolically inert products (hydroxytolbutamide, carboxytolbutamide). Acetohexamide and tolazamide are also metabolized by the liver, but their metabolic products retain hypoglycemic activity; this may account for the more prolonged action of these drugs. The principal metabolic product of acetohexamide metabolism, hydroxyhexamide, is a particularly potent hypoglycemic agent; like other active metabolites, it is removed by the kidney. Unlike other sulfonylureas, the metabolite is more active than the parent compound. Hydroxyhexamide may accumulate and result in hypoglycemia in the presence of renal failure. Chlorpropamide is bound to plasma proteins (a property which probably accounts for its long duration of action) and is excreted either unchanged via the kidney or after hepatic metabolism. Metabolites of chlorpropamide retain some hypoglycemic activity. Steady-state levels are not attained for 7 to 10 days. Hence, dose alterations must be performed only once a week.

The second-generation sulfonylureas glipizide and glyburide differ from the first-generation ones in their structure and potency. Glipizide has the most rapid and short-acting effect because of its rapid absorption, distribution, and elimination.[489,490] In these agents the aliphatic side chains of tolbutamide and chlorpropamide have been replaced by a cyclohexyl group, with another ring structure added to the opposite side. Glipizide and glyburide are 50 to 100 times more potent than chlorpropamide and are effective at nanomolar rather than micromolar blood levels. Glipizide is usually administered in divided doses if more than 15 mg is required; the glyburide dose is split if more than 10 mg daily is indicated. Hepatic metabolites of glipizide are inactive, whereas the 4-hydroxyglyburide metabolite of glyburide retains moderate activity.

Clinical Effects The clinical usefulness of the sulfonylureas is limited by the requirement for beta cell reserve to ensure endogenous production of insulin in substantial amounts. This is true whether the agents act solely by enhancing insulin secretion or via an action on insulin sensitivity as well. The drugs are consequently ineffective in type I diabetic patients. Their chief value is in patients with type II diabetes who have little tendency to develop ketoacidosis. Even in this group, 15 to 40 percent do not respond. Moreover, of those whose diabetes is reasonably well controlled for a month or more, 25 to 40 percent ultimately escape from control (secondary failure), presumably because of progression of beta cell secretory failure. The tendency to develop secondary failure is greater in women than in men and in patients with diabetes for >1 year before treatment was started compared with those given treatment within the first year after recognition of the disease. Thus, continuous satisfactory control is exercised in no more than 30 percent.[487,488] Despite the increased potency of the second-generation agents, their efficacy is no greater than that of the first-generation compounds.[481]

Favorable responses to sulfonylureas have been attributed to the following factors: (1) age of onset >40 years, (2) duration of diabetes <5 years, (3) normal or excessive weight, and (4) lack of previous treatment with insulin or insulin requirement <40 U per day. While exhaustion of islet-cell function cannot be attributed to sulfonylurea agents, there is also no compelling evidence that prophylactic treatment of asymptomatic glucose intolerance with oral hypoglycemic agents either restores carbohydrate tolerance to normal or prevents its deterioration to overt diabetes.

With tolbutamide, it is preferable to give the drug in divided doses because of the short period of effectiveness. If chlorpropamide is used, a single dose once a day is adequate. There is no advantage in exceeding the maximum dosage recommended (Table 19-18), since no increase of effect is to be expected from doses larger than the maximum indicated.

Toxicity Sulfonylureas may on occasion induce profound and sustained hypoglycemia. These hypoglycemic episodes are generally associated with a condition which delays the metabolism or excretion of the sulfonylureas. Thus, they must be used with caution in the presence of liver and/or renal dysfunction, with renal dysfunction being particularly common in elderly diabetic patients. Because of their long duration of action, chlorpropamide and glyburide may be especially prone to cause hypoglycemia. Glyburide may be more likely to provoke long-lasting hypoglycemia than glipizide, perhaps because of its greater propensity to suppress hepatic glucose production.[491,492] In addition, certain drugs have been shown to potentiate the effects of sulfonylureas by (1) interfering with hepatic metabolism, e.g., sulfisoxazole and dicumarol, (2) reducing urinary excretion, e.g., phenylbutazone and acetohexamide, or (3) possessing an additive hypoglycemic action, e.g., salicylates. In contrast to the first-generation sulfonylureas, the second-generation sulfonylureas are nonionically bound to plasma proteins. Consequently, less variation in their bioavailability because of displacement from plasma proteins by other charged drugs may be expected.[487,488]

Another complication of sulfonylurea treatment is the development of hyponatremia.[493,494] While other sulfonylureas are potentially capable of impairing water excretion, clinically this syndrome is almost exclusively observed with chlorpropamide treatment. This is probably a consequence of chlorpropamide's long half-life and the resultant inability to escape from its effects. The hyponatremia is believed to result from chlorpropamide's ability to enhance the action of antidiuretic hormone (ADH). An additional factor may be the failure of ADH secretion to be completely suppressed in the face of a decline in serum osmolarity.[493] In one study, the prevalence of hyponatremia [serum $(Na^+) < 129$ mEq/liter] was 6.3 percent in chlorpropamide-treated patients during a mean follow-up period of 7.4 years; in contrast, only 0.6 percent of patients treated with either tolbutamide or glyburide developed this complication. Risk factors for the development of hyponatremia in patients treated with chlorpropamide include older age and coadministration of thiazide diuretics.[494]

In rare instances, patients may develop skin rashes, leukopenia, anemia, thrombocytopenia, jaundice due to allergic hepatitis, or the nephrotic syndrome.[495] Gastrointestinal complaints including nausea, vomiting, dyspepsia, abnormal liver function tests, and cholestosis can be seen in 1 to 3 percent of patients.[496] In some patients chlorpropamide administration is associated with the development of an intensive flush after the consumption of alcohol [chlorpropamide-alcohol flush (CPAF)] which is reminiscent of that observed with disulfiram (Antabuse). Although it has been hypothesized that CPAF may represent a genetic marker for a subtype of type II diabetes,[497] this has been refuted by evidence demonstrating that CPAF may be present in both type I diabetic patients and nondiabetic individuals with the same frequency as it occurs in type II diabetic patients.[498] The suggestion that CPAF patients may be protected against developing microvascular complications of diabetes has not been uniformly substantiated. This may be due to the lack of clarity in defining CPAF, since it is affected by a number of variables, including plasma chlorpropamide levels, ethanol, dose ambient temperature, basal facial skin temperature, response to ethanol alone, and activity of acetaldehyde dehydrogenase. The combined prevalence of all these complications of sulfonylurea treatment is <5 percent.

The most important question regarding the toxicity of the sulfonylurea drugs relates to the findings of the UGPD study.[499] The UGDP study, which was originally conceived to evaluate the relative effectiveness of tolbutamide, phenformin, and insulin in reducing vascular complications in type II diabetes, led to the unexpected observation that cardiovascular mortality was actually increased in subjects receiving tolbutamide and phenformin compared with placebo- and insulin-treated groups. These results incited an extensive debate among diabetologists and statisticans who maintained that (1) the mortality was concentrated in only a few of the treatment centers, (2) cardiovascular risk factors were not adequately evaluated (smoking and drug histories were not adequately obtained), (3) the treatment schedule for oral agents was fixed, and therefore no attempt was made to adjust the dose of the drug to the prevailing hyperglycemia (as is done in practice), and (4) the standards used to diagnose diabetes were inadequate, including subjects with age-related glucose intolerance. Arguments have also been made suggesting that the increased incidence of cardiovascular events in the tolbutamide-treated group was related to lowering of plasma HDL levels. Serious questions regarding the validity of the study thus continue to be raised. Other studies did not support the UGDP findings. In one trial, tolbutamide was found to improve survival among patients experiencing a myocardial infarction.[500] A retrospective analysis of over 2000 patients found no difference in cardiovascular survival among those treated with diet, insulin, and sulfonylurea, with overall survival greatest in the sulfonylurea group.[501]

Indications for Use Given the uncertainty regarding the UGDP findings, the sulfonylurea drugs are widely used in type II diabetics. Nevertheless, certain considerations hold:

1. The treatment of choice, whether an oral agent or exogenous insulin, should not be based on amelioration of insulin resistance but on the capacity to lower adequately the blood glucose levels, in view of the general noxious effects of hyperglycemia.
2. Sulfonylureas are adjuncts to the dietary management of type II diabetes, not a replacement for dietary therapy.
3. The addition of sulfonylurea to insulin therapy may reduce hyperglycemia, the insulin dose, or both although long-term benefits from this combination are uncertain.[502] Patients apt to benefit from combination therapy are slightly obese, have a short duration of NIDDM, and have preserved beta-cell function. This may result in more effective suppression of hepatic glucose production. The most notable side effect is an increased frequency of mild hypoglycemia.[503]
4. The continuous satisfactory control rate with these agents is ~30 percent.
5. Many patients receiving sulfonylureas for prolonged periods have no improvement in blood glucose concentration; consequently, it is recommended that sulfonylurea agents be administered to type II diabetic patients only when vigorous attempts to achieve glucose control with dietary measures alone have failed.
6. Sulfonylureas should be given cautiously and in reduced doses in patients with liver disease or renal disease.
7. Since only small amounts of tolbutamide and glipizide are excreted in the urine and their metabolites retain little activity, these are preferable for use in moderate-to-severe renal insufficiency.

The Biguanides

The mechanism of action of the biguanides (phenformin and metformin) is not established but it is clearly independent of altered insulin secretion. Improvement in blood glucose control may occur independently of effects on insulin binding or internalization.[504] An increase in insulin sensitivity has been postulated for metformin as a result of actions at the postreceptor level. It has been suggested that phenformin acts via stimulation of anaerobic glycolysis and inhibition of gluconeogenesis. However, the doses required to produce these effects in vitro generally exceed those used in clinical practice. More recently, it has been demonstrated that phenformin inhibits gastrointestinal absorption of glucose.[505] This effect, coupled with its anorexigenic properties, may largely account for the drug's weak hypoglycemic action.

Phenformin is capable of inducing lactic acidosis in a diabetic patient.[506] This rare but frequently fatal complication of phenformin treatment may derive from the drug's stimulatory effect on anaerobic glycolysis (augmenting the production of lactate) as well as its inhibition of gluconeogenesis (reducing lactate utilization). Lactic acidosis is particularly likely to occur in circumstances leading to reduced drug metabolism. The presence of renal and/or hepatic disease (phenformin is both excreted unchanged in the urine and metabolized by the liver) markedly increases the risk of lactic acidosis. Patients receiving phenformin are also particularly susceptible to lactacidemia in the presence of conditions known to augment lactic acid production (hypoxia) or reduce lactate utilization (alcohol use). Because of the substantial incidence of lactic acidosis, the U.S. Food and Drug Administration has withdrawn phenformin from the market in the United States. Metformin, however, has rarely resulted in lactic acidosis and is available for use in Europe and Canada; it is currently under clinical investigation in the United States. A problem associated with the use of metformin is the occurrence of severe diarrhea with incontinence.[507]

Biguanides (metformin) and sulfonylureas have

been used in combination, taking advantage of their different modes of action. Satisfactory diabetes control may be achieved with subsequent postponement or avoidance of insulin therapy. Combined use does not increase the incidence of side effects beyond those seen with monotherapy. However, additional data are needed before it will be possible to define more clearly their role in the treatment of NIDDM.[508] Metformin therapy has also been demonstrated to decrease triglycride levels and increase concentrations of HDL cholesterol.[504]

Investigational Drugs

A number of orally active compounds are currently under investigation for the management of diabetes. These agents include several classes of drugs.

Intestinal α-Glycosidase Inhibitors Starch, a polysaccharide, undergoes hydrolysis to monosaccharides at the (1-4) linkages by α-amylase of pancreatic and salivary origins as well as at the (1-6) linkages by α-glycosidase in the small intestine. Inhibition of these enzymes prevents hydrolysis and therefore attenuates postprandial hyperglycemia. Acarbose and miglitol, compounds that inhibit α-glycosidase, reduce postprandial hyperglycemia in patients with IDDM and NIDDM.[509,510] When administered with insulin, miglitol was more effective than insulin alone in controlling postprandial hyperglycemia in patients with type I diabetes. Furthermore, insulin could be given immediately before meals in conjunction with miglitol. This may be of practical importance given the usual necessity of delaying food intake after subcutaneous injection to avoid hypoglycemia resulting from differences in timing between peak food and insulin absorption.[511,512] After 8 weeks of treatment with miglitol in patients with type II diabetes, in addition to a reduction in postprandial hyperglycemia, a decrease in postprandial C peptide and an improvement in triglyceride levels were observed. Basal hepatic glucose output was not affected, consistent with the lack of notable changes in fasting blood glucose levels.[513] Side effects of α-glycosidase inhibitors include abdominal pain, borborygmus, flatulence, and diarrhea.[514]

Inhibitors of Lipolysis, Fatty Acid Oxidation, and Gluconeogenesis Elevations in circulating fatty acid levels and in lipid oxidation may be of pathogenetic significance in the insulin resistance and increased gluconeogenesis which characterize type II diabetic patients with fasting hyperglycemia. Consequently, drug discovery efforts have been directed at developing safe and effective inhibitors of lipolysis and/or fatty acid oxidation.[515] Drugs which decrease the release of fatty acids from adipocytes include nicotinic acid and its long-acting analogue acipimox. The usefulness of nicotinic acid is limited by a variety of side effects, including flushing, adverse effects on liver function, and, in some patients, exacerbation of hyperglycemia. Acipimox has been shown to be better tolerated and to have hypoglycemic effects in type II diabetic patients.[516]

Drugs which interfere with fatty acid oxidation may lower blood glucose by inhibiting hepatic gluconeogenesis via a decrease in the availability of acetyl CoA required for the activation of the key gluconeogenic enzyme pyruvate carboxylase. Augmented glucose utilization by muscle may also contribute to the hypoglycemic effects of such agents. A number of drugs are in development which interfere with fatty acid oxidation by inhibiting CPT, a rate-limiting step in long-chain fatty acid oxidation. The first drug in the class to be evaluated, methyl 2-tetradecylglycidate, had to be abandoned because of cardiac hypertrophy observed in animal toxicology studies. Clomoxir (POCA) and etomoxir are oxirane carboxylates which inhibit CPT-1. These agents suppress ketogenesis as well as gluconeogenesis and have had hypoglycemic effects in preliminary studies in type II diabetic patients.[515] The safety of these agents, particularly with respect to cardiac hypertrophy, remains to be established. SDZ 51-641 is an agent in early development which specifically inhibits fatty acid oxidation in the liver without affecting fat metabolism in muscle tissue. The specificity of this agent with respect to liver tissue may confer safety advantages compared with the oxirane carboxylates clomoxir and etomoxir.[515]

Interference with gluconeogenesis is also induced by inhibition of FDPase-1, an enzyme necessary for the movement of carbon skeletons along the gluconeogenic pathway. Aicariboside, a potent inhibitor of FDPase-1, has a hypoglycemic effect in rodents[18] and may be useful in diabetes.

Insulin Secretagogues Nonsulfonylurea insulin secretagogues include the pyridine compounds linogliride, pirogliride, and midaglizole. Linogliride and pirogliride potentiate glucose-stimulated insulin release. However, their primary site of action may be peripheral in stimulating oxidative glucose metabolism. Clinical studies were suspended because of seizure activity in dogs treated with linogliride.[516] Midaglizole appears to inhibit glucagon secretion and stimulate insulin secretion by blocking α_2-adrenoreceptor inhibition of insulin secretion. It is comparable to the sulfonylureas but most effective in patients with modest fasting hyperglycemia. Side effects include diarrhea and soft stools.[517]

β_3-Adrenoreceptor Agonists β_3-adrenoreceptor agonists may provide a link between increased glucose uptake and thermogenesis. By stimulating thermogenesis, they may have therapeutic potential for obesity as well as diabetes. Glucose tolerance in experimental animals has been demonstrated to improve with chronic administration of such agents and is linked to their thermogenic effects.[518,519] An increase in glucose transporter number has also been observed in brown adipose tissue of mice as a consequence of treatment with a thermogenic agent.[520] The key problem with such agents is dissociating their effects on adipose tissue from their cardiac effects (e.g., tachycardia).

Potentiators of Insulin Action Since insulin resistance is of major importance in the pathogenesis of type II diabetes, drugs which enhance tissue sensitivity to insulin are potentially useful as hypoglycemic agents. The thiazolidinediones are a new class of orally active agents which potentiate the action of insulin by enhancing peripheral glucose uptake.[521] The first of these agents to be identified, ciglitazone, has been abandoned because of toxicity in humans. However, the development of other drugs in this class, including pioglitazone, englitazone, and CS045 is being pursued. These agents are of particular interest in view of the evidence that the reduced number of GLUT-4 transporters observed in adipocytes of insulin-resistant mice is restored to normal by pioglitazone.[521] Despite the attractiveness of the mechanism of action of the thiazolidinediones, their safety and efficacy in human diabetes have not been established.

Exercise

Exercise has long been recommended as part of the overall management of diabetic patients. In the preinsulin era Allen observed that exercise has a blood glucose concentration-lowering effect. In fact, in type I diabetic patients exercise may provoke hypoglycemia in some circumstances or intensify hyperglycemia, depending in part on the nature of the patient's blood glucose concentration control in the resting state, dietary intake, and the timing of the exercise relative to insulin administration and food intake. In addition, repeated exercise (i.e., physical training) may alter tissue sensitivity to insulin. The overall interaction between exercise and diabetes is understood best in the context of the normal response of body fuel metabolism to exercise.[522,523]

Carbohydrate Metabolism during Exercise in Normal Humans

Glucose Utilization In the resting state, muscle satisfies most of its fuel requirements by oxidizing fatty acids; glucose accounts for <10 percent of total oxygen consumption. In contrast, during exercise, muscle glycogen and blood-borne glucose are major fuels for contracting muscle. During the earliest phase of exercise, muscle glycogen constitutes the major fuel consumed. The rate of glycogenolysis in muscle is most rapid in the first 5 to 10 min of exercise. As exercise continues and blood flow to muscle increases, blood-borne substrates become increasingly important sources of energy. During exercise lasting 10 to 40 min, glucose uptake by muscle rises 7- to 40-fold, increasing in proportion to the intensity of the work performed. The rise in glucose utilization is sufficient to account for 30 to 40 percent of the total oxygen consumption by muscle. The dependence of muscle on blood glucose concentration is thus comparable to the dependence on FFA, which provide an additional 40 percent of the oxidizable fuels.

As exercise is continued beyond 40 min, the rate of glucose utilization progressively increases, reaching a peak at 90 to 180 min and then declining slightly. In contrast to this late decline in glucose consumption, FFA utilization progressively increases in prolonged exercise. As a consequence, after 4 h of continuous exercise, the relative contribution of FFA to total oxygen utilization is twice that of carbohydrate. This increase in the uptake of FFA is in direct proportion to the delivery of FFA, as determined by the product of arterial concentration and plasma flow. Amino acid catabolism also occurs in exercise, but its overall contribution accounts for <5 percent of the total energy used.[524]

The overall pattern of fuel use during mild to moderate exercise extending for prolonged periods may thus be characterized as a triphasic sequence in which muscle glycogen, blood glucose, and FFA successively predominate as the major energy-yielding substrate. With exercise at heavy workloads, there is a more persistent dependence on muscle glycogen. This is suggested by the observation that exhaustion coincides with depletion of muscle glycogen but is not accompanied by significant changes in other physiologic parameters, such as heart rate, blood pressure, blood level of glucose, and concentrations of lactate or muscle electrolytes. It is unclear, however, why glycogen depletion should coincide with fatigue when large amounts of circulating substrate in the form of FFA are still available. It may be added that as a result of long-range homeostatic adjustment to physical training in type II diabetic patients, there is a decrease in concentrations of circulating lipids along with the improvement in glucose tolerance.[525]

Blood Glucose Concentration During the marked increase in glucose uptake by muscle, there is little change in blood glucose concentration during exercise of brief duration. With strenuous exercise an increment in blood glucose concentration of 20 to 30 mg/dl may be observed. When exercise is continued for 90 min or more, a decline in blood glucose concentration by 20 to 40 mg/dl is observed. Frank hypoglycemia (<50 mg/dl) is observed occasionally with very prolonged exercise in normal subjects. However, exercise performance may remain unimpaired in the face of hypoglycemia, nor is it necessarily improved by glucose administration.[522] The asymptomatic hypoglycemia of prolonged exercise in normal subjects contrasts markedly with the severe symptomatic hypoglycemia which may be precipitated by exercise in insulin-treated diabetic patients (see below).

Glucose Production In view of the stimulation of glucose utilization which characterizes exercise, ongoing repletion of the blood glucose pool can be achieved only by an exercise in glucose production. During short-term exercise, hepatic glucose output increases two- to fivefold, depending on the intensity of the work performed, and keeps pace with the increment in glucose utilization by muscle tissue. This increase in glucose production is almost entirely a consequence of augmented glycogenolysis, inasmuch as uptake of gluconeogenic precursors remains unchanged from the resting state, save for a transient rise in lactate consumption. The total amount of glucose released from the liver during 40 min of heavy work is estimated to be 18 g, representing 20 to 25 percent of the total hepatic glycogen stores in the postabsorptive state.

As exercise extends beyond 40 min, a slight imbalance between hepatic production and peripheral utilization of glucose and an increasing reliance on hepatic gluconeogenesis are observed. During prolonged mild exercise, glucose output doubles in the first 40 min and thereafter remains constant for the ensuing 3 to 4 h. Since glucose utilization continues to rise for 90 min or more, glucose production fails to keep pace with utilization, and a modest decline in blood glucose concentration is observed. The relative contribution from gluconeogenesis to overall hepatic glucose output (as inferred from substrate balances across the splanchnic bed) increases from 25 percent in the basal state to 45 percent during prolonged exercise, representing a threefold rise in the absolute rate of gluconeogenesis. These increments in the hepatic uptake of glucose precursors are largely a result of augmented fractional extraction. In the case of alanine, the major gluconeogenic precursor, fractional extraction by the splanchnic bed increases from resting levels of 35 to 50 percent to almost 90 percent in prolonged exercise, a rate well in excess of the 50 to 70 percent extraction rates observed in other circumstances of increased gluconeogenesis, such as diabetes, obesity, and starvation. The overall importance of gluconeogenesis in prolonged exercise is underscored by the estimation that 50 to 60 g of liver glycogen is mobilized in 4 h of exercise, representing a depletion of 75 percent of total liver glycogen stores.

Glucoregulatory Hormones The hormonal response to exercise is characterized by a fall in plasma insulin concentration and an increase in plasma glucagon concentration. These findings are especially pronounced in prolonged or severe exercise. The decrease in insulin concentration is particularly noteworthy in intensive exercise, in which circumstance hypoinsulinemia occurs despite a modest rise in blood glucose concentration. These findings suggest an inhibition of insulin secretion, probably mediated by the adrenergic nervous system and/or circulating catecholamines. Other hormonal changes occurring in exercise include elevations in plasma GH, cortisol, epinephrine, and norepinephrine levels.

The stimulatory effect of exercise on glucose uptake in the face of hypoinsulinemia indicates that such enhancement of glucose consumption is not dependent on an increase in insulin secretion. In fact, the presence of even minimal concentrations of insulin may not be necessary for the exercise-induced increases in glucose utilization.[526] Experiments with isolated muscles have established that the work-induced increment in glucose uptake is non-insulin-dependent. The physiologic significance of the altered hormonal milieu in exercise relates more to the stimulation of hepatic glucose production than to glucose utilization. The exquisite sensitivity of human hepatic glycogenolysis to the inhibitory action of small increments in insulin concentration has been demonstrated.[261] The importance of the hypoinsulinemia of exercise is thus manifested by its effect on hepatic glycogenolysis. In prolonged or severe exercise, the rises in glucagon, GH, and catecholamine concentrations also contribute to the glycogenolytic and gluconeogenic response. The overall substrate and hormone response to exercise is summarized in Fig. 19-57.

Exercise-Induced Hypoglycemia

For the type I diabetic patient exercise-induced hypoglycemia is a well-recognized complication of treatment with insulin. The tendency of these patients to develop hypoglycemia derives from the failure of their plasma insulin levels to decrease during exercise. In addition, some patients are deficient in catecholamine as well as in the glucagon secretion that is necessary for protection against hypoglycemia.[526] Thus, if exercise occurs at a time when insulin is being released from injection sites in amounts that exceed normal basal plasma levels, hypoglycemia is likely to occur. The presence of insulin levels higher than basal leads to excessive glucose utilization coupled with decreased glucose production. In the presence of deficient catecholamine and glucagon response as well, the patient is unable to overcome the effects of an insulin level that is inappropriately high for brief exercise.

The factors influencing the occurrence of exercise-induced hypoglycemia include (1) the timing of exercise in relation to the peak action of insulin, (2) the intensity of the exercise, (3) the training status of the patient (see below), (4) the timing and magnitude of meal and/or snack ingestion, (5) the use of pump vs. manual injection of insulin, and (6) the site of

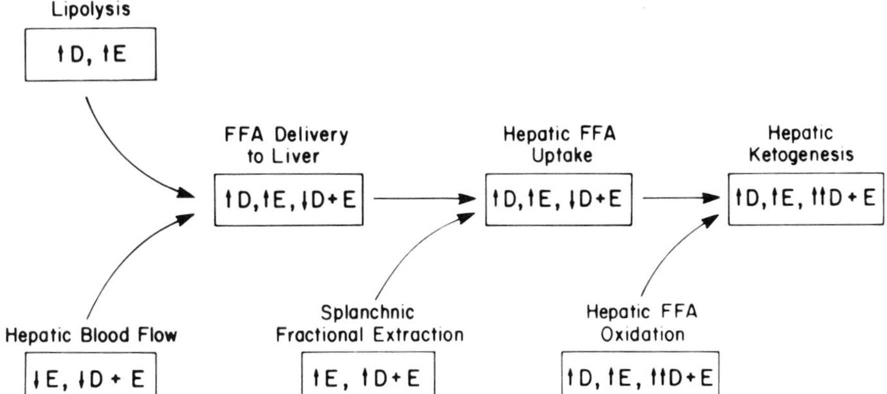

FIGURE 19-57 Regulatory sites in the control of ketogenesis in diabetes (D), with exercise (E), and during exercise in diabetic patients (D + E). ↑ = Increase; ↑↑ = marked increase; ↓ = decrease. (*From Wahren et al.*[530])

insulin injection. Clearly, exercise should be undertaken at times which do not coincide with the peak effect of previously injected rapid- or intermediate-acting insulin. Exercising after prolonged intervals without food ingestion (e.g., 3 to 4 h or more after lunch) may also increase the risk of hypoglycemia. If hypoglycemia is not prevented by appropriately timing the activity, a snack before or during the exercise should be tried. Avoidance of the use of exercised areas as an injection site (e.g., the abdominal wall or legs) helps prevent the accelerated insulin absorption which may occur from these areas.[522] The use of a portable pump has also been shown to lessen somewhat the tendency to develop exercise-induced hypoglycemia. If other approaches fail, the insulin dose should be reduced. Unfortunately, neither the amount of extra dietary carbohydrate nor the amount of insulin to be reduced can be predicted in advance; both must be determined by trial and error.

Exercise-induced hypoglycemia may also occur hours after the completion of the exercise. This phenomenon reflects the increase in insulin sensitivity observed in the postexercise recovery period, presumably as a result of the depletion of muscle glycogen.

Despite the potential danger of hypoglycemia, insulin treatment is by no means incompatible with a vigorous life in which exercise is a frequent pasttime. In fact, there are a number of professional athletes for whom the treatment of type I diabetes and the associated risk of exercise-induced hypoglycemia have not interfered with vigorous daily routines and the attainment of superstar status.

Exercise-Induced Hyperglycemia and Hyperketonemia

In some circumstances, exercise may actually worsen hyperglycemia and increase ketogenesis in diabetic patients.[528–530] This is true in patients with poorly regulated diabetes. When moderate to severe hyperglycemia (>300 mg/dl or >17 m*M*) and hyperketonemia (>2 m*M*) are present in the resting state, acute exercise causes a further rise rather than a fall in blood glucose concentration. Contributing to the rise in blood glucose concentration are inappropriate increments in levels of counterregulatory hormones (GH, epinephrine, and norepinephrine).[309]

An exaggerated ketogenic response to exercise is observed in diabetic patients, particularly if there is poor diabetic control before exercise. This ketogenesis is a result of increased fractional extraction of FFA by the liver as well as a marked increase in intrahepatic conversion of FFA to ketones[529] (Fig. 19-57). Despite the increase in ketogenesis which occurs during exercise, the hyperketonemic effect of exercise is not apparent until the postexercise recovery period. This is the case because the augmented ketogenesis of the diabetic patient is accompanied by increased muscle utilization of ketones. However, immediately after exercise, ketone utilization falls abruptly while ketone overproduction is sustained into the recovery period in poorly regulated diabetes.[529,530] The largest increment in concentrations of circulating ketones observed in poorly regulated diabetes occurs during recovery.[529,530] The important clinical implication of these observations is that exercise cannot be viewed as an alternative but should instead be viewed as an adjunct to proper control of blood glucose concentration with insulin.

Exercise-Induced Alterations in Insulin Action

In well-trained athletes (e.g., long-distance runners), the plasma insulin response to an IV glucose load is diminished in the face of normal glucose tolerance, suggesting enhanced tissue response to insulin. More direct evidence of increased insulin response is derived from studies involving the insulin clamp procedure. With this technique, insulin-mediated glucose uptake has been shown to increase in previously untrained healthy subjects after a 6-week training program. This increment in insulin sensitivity occurs in the absence of changes in body weight.[526] Recent studies indicate that this effect of physical training is accompanied by an increase in GLUT-4 transporters.[209]

Despite these findings in normal subjects, in the diabetic population a clinically useful effect of physical training in improving blood glucose concentration control has not been as readily demonstrable. Exercise in conjunction with increased self-monitoring of blood glucose and insulin adjustment may significantly improve overall metabolic control in type I diabetes.[531] Regular exercise in type II diabetic patients lowers the plasma insulin level and enhances insulin sensitivity. However, a consistent improvement in blood glucose concentration regulation has not been demonstrated.[532] The failure to observe an enhancement of blood glucose level control in type II diabetes may reflect the fact that while muscle response to insulin is increasing, insulin secretion falls and hepatic sensitivity to insulin fails to increase after physical training.[533] Thus, the net effect is often a reduction in hyperinsulinemia without an accompanying improvement in the control of blood glucose concentration. Similarly, in type I diabetic patients physical training results in an increase in sensitivity to insulin without an overall improvement in glucoregulation.[533] Nevertheless, to the extent that hyperinsulinemia may of itself be a risk factor for atherosclerosis, physical training may be useful in improving longevity. Physical activity has also been demonstrated to reduce the occurrence of NIDDM, particularly in individuals at highest risk for its development (e.g., high body mass index, family history). Vigorous activity such as swimming, tennis, and running may be more beneficial than milder forms of exercise.[307]

Summary: Risks and Benefits of Exercise in Diabetes

Exercise produces complex metabolic effects, in part immediately manifested in blood glucose concentration and in part more sustained on tissue response to insulin. The benefits of exercise may be summarized as follows:

1. Decrease in cardiovascular risk factors. Exercise decreases plasma insulin concentration in type II diabetes and the need for exogenous insulin in type I diabetes, increases plasma HDL concentration and lowers LDL levels, increases myocardial vascularity and work efficiency, increases pulmonary function, and decreases both systolic and diastolic blood pressure. These benefits, however, do not persist when training is discontinued.
2. Achievement of weight loss as an adjunct to diet in type II diabetes. Exercise results in increased energy expenditure but does not by itself usually lead to significant weight loss. Exercise alters body composition by increasing muscle mass and decreasing body fat content. Therefore, by improving self-image, this may provide motivation for increasing dietary compliance.
3. Potential improvement in glucose tolerance in some patients as a result of increased glucose utilization and an increased response to insulin. This may result in a reduction in insulin or oral hypoglycemic agent dosage.
4. Increased work capacity.
5. Increased sense of well-being and enrichment of quality of life.
6. Preventive effect, particularly in individuals at increased risk for type II diabetes.

The following risks have been found to be associated with exercise and diabetes:

1. Potentiation of the hypoglycemic effect of insulin or oral hypoglycemic agents in prolonged and/or vigorous exercise
2. Deterioration of metabolic control in poorly controlled diabetes (blood glucose concentration <300 mg/dl)
3. Worsening of musculoskeletal complications associated with neuropathy, retinopathy (e.g., vitreous hemorrhage), and nephropathy (e.g., increased proteinuria with exercise)

These observations indicate that exercise is a useful adjunct but not a substitute for proper glucoregulation with insulin and/or diet. Exercise should be encouraged as a means of decreasing risk factors for cardiovascular disease and possibly improving glucose homeostasis provided that no contraindications exist. The current state of knowledge, however, does not permit the formulation of a precise exercise prescription as part of the management of a diabetic patient. It is critical that diabetic patients who want to participate in an exercise program undergo a rigorous evaluation to determine the presence of undiagnosed retinopathy, neuropathy, nephropathy, hypertension, or cardiac disease. An exercise-stress test is recommended for patients >40 years old. Self-monitoring of glucose levels during exercise is suggested.

Future Treatment

As was noted above, even under optimal conditions complete normalization of blood glucose concentration is difficult to achieve with conventional or intensive therapy. Recognition of the inadequacy or difficulty of implementation of current treatment regimens and, more important, their unproven ability to prevent vascular and neurologic complications of diabetes have led to a search for newer approaches to treatment. Current investigative efforts are directed at three possible modalities: (1) immunosuppression as a means of inducing remission or preventing the appearance of type I diabetes, (2) transplantation of whole pancreas or islet cells, and (3) implantable insulin pumps.

Immunosuppression

As discussed above, a variety of findings provide compelling evidence that humoral and cell-mediated autoimmune processes are central to the etiology and pathogenesis of type I diabetes. Such observations make it probable that intervention with immunosuppressive agents may prevent, attenuate, or retard the onset of type I diabetes or induce a remission in patients in whom the disease is already manifest. Since it is possible only with specialized techniques to identify with near certainty first-degree relatives of type I diabetic patients who are likely to develop diabetes, immune intervention before the onset of symptoms should be considered only in the context of defined research studies. Standardized methods determined to be useful include oral and intravenous tolerance tests for assessing first-phase insulin response, islet-cell antibodies, and insulin autoantibodies. Their measurements should also be conducted within established research programs.[534] With advances in the identification and characterization of the specific antigenic factor(s) leading to islet-cell destruction, preventive immunosuppressive regimens are currently under investigation[268,269,282] (see Prediction and Prevention, above). In patients with long-standing disease, beta cell destruction is of such an advanced degree that recovery of function and an accompanying clinical remission cannot be expected. In contrast, newly discovered type I diabetes often enters a clinical remission or "honeymoon" phase in which insulin requirements decline and there is a partial, although transient, recovery of endogenous insulin secretion. Based on these findings and the observation that cyclosporine, a nonmyelotoxic immunosuppressive agent, is capable of preventing diabetes in the BB rat and the NOD mouse[535,536] (models of immunogenic type I diabetes), the effects of cyclosporine on human type I diabetes have been investigated. In two independent studies, cyclosporine was demonstrated to induce complete remissions (defined as normal glycohemoglobin levels in the absence of insulin therapy) in 24 to 37 percent of patients in whom treatment was initiated within a few weeks of clinical recognition of type I diabetes.[281,282] These remissions were accompanied by recovery of endogenous insulin secretory rates which were within the normal range and suppression of anti–beta cell autoimmunity. Since the frequency of spontaneous complete remission in type I diabetes is reported to be <6 percent, these findings suggest that the immunosuppressive treatment was in fact responsible for the recovery of beta cell function in the treated patients.

A number of important issues regarding the role of immunosuppression in type I diabetes remain to be clarified. First, remissions have been maintained for periods of 1 year while immunosuppression is continued, but cessation of cyclosporine therapy is associated with recurrence of insulin dependence. The observation that autoimmune destruction of beta cells may be retriggered as long as 20 years after the initial manifestation of diabetes[537] suggests that lifelong immunosuppression may be required to protect the beta cells, rather than a 1- to 2-year course of therapy. Also, the risk/benefit ratio of long-term cyclosporine therapy in type I diabetes remains to be established. Although the incidence of tumors in patients receiving cyclosporine for transplant or other autoimmune indications is extremely low,[538,539] the danger of nephropathy cannot be discounted. Consequently, the use of cyclosporine in type I diabetes is now limited to investigational trials in new-onset diabetic patients or patients with strong evidence for predicting the iminent onset of type I diabetes.[285,540]

Pancreatic and Islet-Cell Transplants

Whole-pancreas transplants have generally been undertaken in type I diabetes in conjunction with renal transplants which would otherwise necessitate the use of immunosuppressive agents. The procedures used in pancreas transplantation involve grafting of the whole pancreas together with the duodenum, the whole pancreas alone, or only a segment of the pancreas; the last is the procedure generally used at present. Cadaver grafts and segmental grafts from living related donors have been employed. A number of approaches also have been used to deal with the exocrine secretions of the pancreas, including cutaneous, ureteral, intraperitoneal, and enteral drainage. The most physiologic approach involving enteric drainage increases the incidence of sepsis and also obviates the ability to monitor exocrine secretions. Bladder drainage is less complicated and permits direct measurement of pancreatic exocrine function. Pancreatic biopsy can be performed via a transcystoscopic approach.[541–543] The most popular approach involves exocrine suppression by injecting the duct with synthetic polymers.[544] This procedures results in duct occlusion and atrophy of exocrine tissue in the transplant with progressive fibrosis.

The current 1-year actuarial patient survival rate is 88 percent, and the functional graft survival rate is 55 percent for all centers reporting to the international Pancreas Transplant Registry.[545] Individual centers have achieved patient survival rates of >90 percent and graft survival rates >80 percent at 1 year. To date, over 2000 transplants have been performed worldwide. In addition to elimination of exogenous insulin, evidence of pancreatic islet function in these patients has included the restoration of normal insulin secretory responses to meal ingestion, normal suppressibility of glucagon secretion by glucose ingestion, and normal glycohemoglobin levels.[432] Persistent metabolic abnormalities (response to glucose tolerance tests) may be due to steroids and cyclosporine immunosuppression.[546] The causes of failure in 165 transplants with >1 year of function included rejection and technical problems such as thrombosis (vascular complications), ascites, infection, abscess, hemorrhage, leakage, and pancreaticocutaneous fistules. Refined surgical techniques, including alignment of venous anastomoses, improved organ preservation, and modest anticoagulation with antiplatelet agents and low-dose heparin, have decreased the incidence of graft thrombosis.[543]

Pancreas transplantation requires, of course, the ongoing use of immunosuppressive agents and their attendant risks. Consequently, pancreatic transplantation has generally been restricted to patients requiring immunosuppression for concurrent renal transplantation. However, the available evidence suggests that when pancreas transplantation is performed before the onset of irreversible pathologic changes, complications may be prevented.[543]

Islet transplantation has been studied extensively in animals but thus far has been of quite limited application in humans. Islet grafts have the potential advantage of greater safety: they avoid many of the technical complications associated with the more extensive surgery and need for drainage of exocrine secretions which are associated with pancreas grafts. In addition, islets have the potential for manipulation (e.g., in tissue culture), which may reduce antigenicity. The donor islets are prepared by dispersion of adult cadaveric pancreas tissue. The transplant method most widely used is intraportal injection. The experience to date clearly indicates that islet transplantation is a safe procedure; no deaths have been attributed to the procedure. However, except in rare instances, it has been ineffective in restoring insulin secretion. The problems encountered have included low yield of islets from donor pancreas, lack of viability of the isolated islets, and rejection. Studies with islet transplants in experimental animals have provided possible approaches to preventing the rejection process. Immunoalteration permits the in vitro elimination of donor immune cells, whereas *immunoisolation* protects islets by various membranes at the time of transplantation.[543,547] Successful transplantation of islet allografts and even xenografts in nonimmunosuppressed rodent recipients has been achieved when the donor islets were cultured at 24°C or in 95% O_2 before transplantation and treatment with antibodies was directed against the antigen-presenting immune cells and ultraviolet light. The effectiveness of organ culture in prolonging graft survival is attributed to a loss of stimulator cells or passenger lymphocytes before transplantation. By contrast, studies in nonimmunosuppressed patients receiving live donor segmental pancreatic isografts (i.e., between identical twins) have shown recrudescence of diabetes after transient amelioration. The reappearance of diabetes in the recipients is due to reactivation of an autoimmune process consequent to the presentation of islet cells and their associated antigens.[537] Thus, immunosuppression may be necessary in transplant recipients not only to prevent rejection but to prevent recurrence of the autoimmune process initially responsible for beta cell destruction and type I diabetes.

Immunoisolation involves the encapsulation of islet cells in hollow fiber chambers which permit ongoing functioning of the donor islets without the need for immunosuppression. The chambers are designed to permit the inward diffusion of glucose and the outward diffusion of insulin yet protect against immune rejection of the encapsulated islets. In preliminary studies, a diffusion-based hybrid pancreas involving dog islet allografts encapsulated in acrylic membranes was shown to result in blood glucose control without a requirement for exogenous insulin in three of six pancreatectomized dogs.[548]

In summary, transplantations of whole pancreas and of isolated islets have been performed in a limited number of diabetic patients. The need for immunosuppression and its attendant risks have generally resulted in restricting transplantation to patients requiring immunosuppression on other grounds (e.g., patients requiring kidney transplants). Potential benefit regarding the development of recurrent diabetic nephropathy in previously or simultaneously transplanted kidneys and less definitive results concerning retinopathy and neuropathy suggest that earlier transplantation be given future consideration. Safer and more effective immunosuppression or immunoisolation also needs to be developed before early transplantation is contemplated.[549,550]

Implantable Insulin Pumps

The use of external pumps for CSII is now an established form of management for type I diabetes.[439a] Implantable insulin pumps which duplicate the insulin delivery and glucose-sensing capabilities of normal islet cells (a true artificial pancreas) remain an elusive goal. As of 1989, a total of 280 insulin pumps were implanted in diabetic patients. Few of these pumps have been programmable; thus, they do not permit the multiple rates of insulin delivery necessary for the normalization of blood glucose control. Furthermore, none of the devices currently under investigation in diabetic patients have a glucose sensor. Thus, self-monitoring of blood glucose remains necessary in the recipients of such implanted devices. Progress has been reported in the use of a variable-rate implanted insulin pump with catheters placed in the peritoneum or inferior vena cava and operated via a hand-held programmer. This device was demonstrated to provide excellent blood glucose control with a reduced risk of severe hypoglycemia compared with CSII involving an external pump.[551] Nevertheless, extensive application of implanted insulin pumps in the management of type I diabetes must await the development of an implantable glucose sensor.

Hyperglycemic-Ketoacidotic Emergencies

Although diabetes mellitus is generally manifested as a chronic disorder, in certain circumstances large increases in concentrations of plasma glucose and/or ketoacids may pose a life-threatening emergency. In clinical practice a spectrum of disorders is observed in which either glucose or ketones or both accumulate, either alone or in combination with lactic acid. Consequently, the major syndromes encountered are DKA (glucose plus ketone accumulation), alcoholic ketoacidosis (ketone accumulation with hyperglycemia), hyperosmolar nonketotic coma (glucose accumulation without ketonemia), and finally, any of these disorders plus lactic acidosis. These disorders require special attention because of the need for prompt, accurate diagnosis and treatment so that the condition does not rapidly progress to death.

Diabetic Ketoacidosis

The most severe clinical manifestation of insulin lack is the development of DKA. Since the advent of insulin therapy <60 years ago, the importance of DKA as a cause of death in the diabetic population has progressively declined. Nevertheless, this condition is encountered frequently. It may be a recurrent disorder, particularly in patients of limited educational background and lower socioeconomic class who are followed in hospital clinics rather than by a personal physician.[552] Furthermore, it is a potentially lethal disorder, particularly in elderly patients; the mortality rate remains at ~5 percent.[553,554]

In most circumstances death is due not to DKA per se but to some intercurrent catastrophic event (e.g., sepsis, myocardial infarction, pancreatitis) which may have precipitated or complicated the course of DKA.

Pathogenesis

From a metabolic standpoint, the major findings in DKA are the accumulation of the organic acids acetoacetate and β-hydroxybutyrate, elevation in serum acetone concentration, a marked increase in blood glucose concentration, and a serious cation loss in urine. Clinically, the major life-threatening abnormalities are metabolic acidosis (due to the hyperketonemia), hyperosmolarity (due to hyperglycemia and water loss), and dehydration (due to the osmotic diuresis accompanying hyperglycemia and the vomiting which generally accompanies severe metabolic acidosis). The hyperosmolarity is in fact more important than acidosis in causing obtundation and coma.[555] All these abnormalities may be traced directly to an absolute or relative lack of insulin which may develop over a period of several hours or days. A deficiency of insulin may result from failure of endogenous insulin secretion (as in an individual with newly discovered diabetes), inadequate administration of exogenous insulin (in a patient with known insulin dependent diabetes), or increased requirements for insulin engendered by the stress associated with an intercurrent infectious, inflammatory, traumatic, or endocrinologic disorder. The increased insulin requirements in such disorders may be attributed to the augmented secretion of hormones with an action antagonistic to insulin (e.g., epinephrine, cortisol, glucagon, and GH).

Severely decreased tissue utilization of glucose and glucose overproduction by the liver (and kidney in this condition) characterize the insulin-deficient state. Whereas glucose is released by the liver at a rate of 150 to 200 mg/min (2 to 3 mg per kilogram of body weight per min) in normal postabsorptive subjects, in DKA the rate of glucose production may rise to 600 mg/min. The kidney contributes to the hyperglycemia by acidosis-stimulated gluconeogenesis, as was discussed earlier. Hyperglycemia thus does not depend on failure to metabolize ingested carbohydrate but results from excessive production of glucose from endogenous precursors. Consequently, a diabetic patient may have had no intake of carbohydrate or other food for 12 to 24 h yet manifest hyperglycemia of 500 mg/dl (28 m*M*). Since protein-derived amino acids are the major precursors for de novo glucose synthesis, implicit in this increase in gluconeogenesis are dissolution of body protein stores and the development of negative nitrogen balance. Massive mobilization of fat from adipose tissue in the form of FFA (ketone precursors) and glycerol (a glucogenic substrate) causes an additional loss of body weight. In a juvenile insulin-dependent diabetic patient, repeated episodes of DKA may thus interfere with normal growth. A more immediate threat to the patient, however, is the osmotic diuresis which accompanies severe hyperglycemia. This leads to dehydration as a result of urinary losses of water and sodium and to the development of hyperosmolarity.

Coincident with the increase in blood glucose concentration, acetoacetate, β-hydroxybutyrate, and acetone progressively accumulate in blood, reaching levels of 8 to 15 m*M*. Insulin deficiency is responsible for the unrestrained FFA outflow from adipose tissue, as was discussed earlier. The increased hepatic ketogenesis not only is the outcome of the sheer mass of FFA but is also due to the regulatory adjustments within the liver. As illustrated in Fig. 19-13, the entry of fatty acyl CoA into the mitochondria, with the consequent β oxidation, is preferred over esterification of fatty acyl CoA with glycerol 3-phosphate because of the decrease in malonyl CoA concentration upon the cessation of de novo lipogenesis. The reduction in malonyl CoA concentration removes the inhibition of CAT 1, the enzyme responsible for intramitochondrial transfer of long-chain fatty acyl CoA,[40] resulting in excessive acetyl CoA production. The superfluity in acetyl CoA exceeds the capacity for its oxidation to CO_2 via the Krebs cycle, resulting in condensation of acetyl CoA to ketone acids (Fig. 19-14). An ancillary elevation in glucagon concentration potentiates the hepatic ketogenesis. Hyperglucagonemia increases the level of carnitine, decreases the concentration of malonyl CoA, and increases the activity of CAT in excess of that attributable to insulin deficiency alone. As a consequence, in pancreatectomized patients in whom glucagon as well as insulin is lacking, the magnitude of hyperketonemia is less than that observed in those with spontaneous diabetes.[220] Furthermore, in type I diabetic patients who have been taken off insulin therapy and rendered hypoglucagonemic by the administration of somatostatin, hyperketonemia is diminished although not entirely prevented.[101]

In addition to increased ketone production, hyperketonemia in diabetes is a consequence of decreased utilization of the ketoacids by muscle tissue. Even in patients with mild insulin lack, a diminution in the ability to dispose of ketones is demonstrable; this diminished disposal becomes increasingly important as serum ketone levels reach 10 m*M*.[556]

The ketone acids are generally present in plasma in a ratio of 3:1, favoring β-hydroxybutyrate. Acetone is also formed (by the spontaneous decarboxylation of acetoacetate) and circulates in a concentration which may reach 10 to 15 m*M*. Because of its low vapor pressure, excretion by the lungs, and characteristic fruity odor, the presence of acetone may be detected on the patient's breath and may serve as a useful diagnostic clue.

In addition to changes in glucose and fat metabolism, DKA is characterized by fluid and electrolyte losses. The severe hyperglycemia causes osmotic diuresis, resulting in large urinary losses of water and electrolytes. (Compared with plasma, the urine in osmotic diuresis is always hypotonic with respect to sodium concentration.) Cation losses are aggravated by the need to neutralize the organic acids before excreting them in urine. Insulin deficiency may of itself (independent of the osmotic diuresis) also contribute to renal sodium losses. Insulin administration has been shown to have an antinatriuretic effect, whereas an acute reduction in insulin concentration results in natriuresis.[131] If fluid intake is reduced, often because of nausea and vomiting, which are early harbingers of DKA, dehydration proceeds rapidly; blood volume drops, peripheral resistance is reduced, blood pressure falls, and renal function is impaired. Loss of water into vomitus and urine dehydrates the intracellular space. In fully developed DKA, therefore, all body compartments are dehydrated, and there are absolute deficiencies of water, sodium, potassium, magnesium, chloride, and bicarbonate. The hypovolemia may in turn aggravate the ketosis, perhaps by acting as a stimulus for the secretion of epinephrine. Contrariwise, if fluids and electrolytes are given to diabetic patients from whom insulin treatment has been withdrawn, hyperketonemia is delayed or reduced even in the absence of insulin administration.

The presence of large amounts of ketone bodies, which are moderately strong acids, causes an increase in the hydrogen ion concentration of the body fluids. As a result, there is a fall in the concentration of serum bicarbonate and an increase in the anion gap (i.e., the difference between the serum sodium concentration and the sum of chloride plus bicarbonate exceeds the normal range of 10 to 12 mEq/liter).

Clinical Manifestations

The major symptoms of DKA are nausea, vomiting, labored breathing, and depressed mental function which may vary from mild drowsiness to severe coma. On physical examination the patient appears dehydrated, as reflected by dry mucous membranes and decreased skin turgor. There is a characteristic fruity odor on the breath, and air hunger (Kussmaul's breathing, or rapid deep respiration) is observed. Blood pressure is often reduced, and there is an accompanying tachycardia. In some patients the GI symptoms are quite severe and include abdominal pain which may simulate an acute surgical abdomen (e.g., appendicitis).

The characteristic laboratory findings in DKA are an elevation in plasma glucose concentration, reductions in serum bicarbonate concentration and arterial pH, increase in anion gap, and large amounts of ketones in undiluted plasma. Because specific enzymatic techniques are cumbersome, reliance is placed on the semiquantitative reagent strip or tablet (nitroprusside) test for urinary ketone determinations. Unfortunately, the test measures only acetoacetate and acetone but not β-hydroxybutyrate concentration. Consequently, when acetoacetate accounts for <25 percent of the total ketone acids (as in combined DKA and lactic acidosis or in alcoholic ketoacidosis), the test may give a spuriously low value. Conversely, a spuriously high value is obtained after insulin treatment has been instituted because the β-hydroxybutyrate component falls before any change is observed in acetoacetate concentration.

Elevations in serum amylase concentration and in the amylase/creatinine clearance ratio are not uncommon in DKA. Although in some patients hyperamylasemia may signify accompanying pancreatitis, in most circumstances there is no clinical evidence of pancreatitis. The data suggest that the elevated amylase concentrations in DKA are of salivary rather than pancreatic origin.[557] The mechanism of this change in the release and renal clearance of amylase remains to be established.

In dehydration, in addition to the increased hematocrit, the hemogram usually shows leukocytosis, frequently with increased numbers of young polymorphonuclear leukocytes. Sometimes this finding reflects the precipitating cause of acidosis, such as infection, but even in the absence of such a complication, leukocytosis may be present, probably as a reflection of the severe hypertonicity of the plasma.

Diagnosis

Prompt diagnosis of DKA requires a high index of suspicion in patients with obfuscation, dehydration, hyperpnea, vomiting, and abdominal pain or with an acetone odor on the breath. The diagnosis can be rapidly established even before the serum bicarbonate concentration is reported by examining four parameters: (1) blood and/or urinary glucose concentration, (2) urinary ketone concentrations, (3) arterial blood pH and blood gases, and (4) serum ketone concentration. The diagnosis of DKA is established if all the following findings are present: (1) blood glucose concentration >200 mg/dl and/or 4+ glucosuria, (2) strong reaction for ketones in urine, (3) arterial pH below 7.3 with a P_{CO_2} of 40 mmHg or less, and (4) a strongly positive ketone reaction in serum.

The differential diagnosis includes all types of metabolic acidosis and coma. An accumulation of ketone acids sufficient to cause metabolic acidosis may be seen in the absence of diabetes in poorly nourished alcoholic patients with repeated bouts of vomiting.[558] In such cases of *alcoholic ketoacidosis*, treatment consists of glucose infusion (insulin is not required); blood glucose levels are <200 mg/dl (in 30 percent of cases frank hypoglycemia is present), and urine tests do not show a 4+ reaction for glucose. In addition, the plasma ketone reaction is generally only mildly or moderately positive since the ratio of β-hydroxybutyrate to acetoacetate is increased. The change in this ratio reflects the ability of alcohol to increase cellular levels of NADH. Often, it is not possible to separate the effects of ingested alcohol from those of diabetes, and patients may have combined diabetic and alcoholic ketoacidoses.

Acidosis of uremia or of various types of poisoning may present problems, especially since patients with diabetic acidosis may also have impaired renal function due to diabetic nephropathy as well as prerenal azotemia as a consequence of dehydration. Ketosis, however, is not present in uncomplicated uremic acidosis or methanol toxicity.

Hypoglycemia may also cause coma, but differentiation from DKA with coma is usually not difficult. In DKA, the onset is gradual and signs of acidosis are present, including hyperventilation, dehydration, hypotension, and tachycardia. In contrast, hypoglycemia occurs relatively rapidly and the patient is not dehydrated or hyperventilating. In spite of these differences, if there is uncertainty, the physician should draw a blood sample for determination of glucose and electrolyte concentrations and administer IV glucose (25 g) while awaiting the laboratory report. Coma may also occur with severe hyperglycemia without ketoacidosis; this syndrome—*nonketotic hyperosmolar coma*—is discussed below. Severe metabolic acidosis and coma may be present in the absence of ketosis in patients with lactic acidosis. The latter condition (also discussed below) is characterized by a reduction in arterial pH and serum bicarbonate concentration in the absence of a positive plasma ketone determination. However, a mildly positive reaction for ketones in a hyperglycemic patient with anion gap acidosis may signify the coexistence of DKA and lactic acidosis or combined alcoholic and diabetic acidoses.

Treatment

The immediate and long-term therapeutic goals are provision of adequate insulin to normalize intermediary metabolism, restoration of water and electrolyte losses, and identification (when possible) of precipitating factors (infection, medication errors, psychosocial stresses, etc.) to prevent the recurrence of DKA and facilitate the response to management. Coincident with the initiation of treatment, a diabetes flow sheet is constructed on which vital signs, laboratory data (blood glucose, ketone, and electrolyte concentrations, pH, urine volume, and content of glucose and ketones), and treatment (insulin, fluids, and electrolytes) are sequentially recorded.

Catheterization of the bladder should not be routinely performed but should be reserved for patients who fail to produce a urine sample after 3 to 4 h of treatment. Similarly, gastric lavage and aspiration should be undertaken only in mentally obtunded patients who repeatedly vomit or have evidence of gastric dilatation.

Insulin All patients with DKA have an immediate need for insulin. Accordingly, only rapid-acting insulin should be employed. The time-honored approach has involved intermittent administration of 50 to 100 U of insulin at 2- to 4-h intervals (high-dose insulin). Over the past 15 years studies have shown that the administration of 6 to 10 U of insulin per hour by continuous IV infusion or by intermittent intramuscular or subcutaneous injection (low-dose insulin) is equally effective.[559,560] It is clear that both techniques are successful provided that clinical and laboratory parameters are carefully monitored and treatment is individualized in accordance with the data obtained in monitoring the patient. The low-dose regimens may be more advantageous in that they lead to a lower incidence of hypoglycemia and hypokalemia.[559,560]

Regardless of the insulin dose, it is advantageous to give all insulin IV in the initial phases of treatment, since impaired circulation may prevent the absorption of subcutaneously or intramuscularly administered hormone. An initial loading dose of 6 to 10 U by bolus administration, followed by a continuous infusion of 6 U/h until the plasma glucose concentration falls to 250 mg/dl, is recommended. In children a dose of 0.1 U per kilogram of body weight per hour may be used. The low-dose continuous insulin infusion procedure as initially introduced involved the use of an infusion pump (to ensure delivery rates) and the use of serum albumin (to prevent adsorption of insulin to tubing or glassware). Subsequent experience has indicated that simpler procedures in which neither the pump nor albumin is employed are equally successful.

The response to treatment is assessed by monitoring the plasma glucose and serum electrolyte concentrations, arterial pH, and urinary glucose and ketone levels at 2- to 4-h intervals. Frequent arterial blood gas determinations may not be warranted if CO_2 levels are adequately followed. Following both parameters is usually redundant in determining the clinical strategy. If the plasma glucose level does not decline by 30 percent in the first 2 to 4 h or by 50 percent in 6 to 8 h, the insulin dose should be doubled. If hyperglycemia persists, the rate should be doubled at 2-h intervals. Once the plasma glucose level falls to 250 mg/dl (14 m*M*), the insulin infusion is discontinued and infusion of a 5% glucose solution is started. Intermittent small doses (10 U) of rapid-acting insulin are administered subcutaneously thereafter as necessary to control glucosuria. The arterial pH and serum bicarbonate level and the plasma glucose concentration should be used as indexes to determine when to stop the insulin infusion. If the plasma glucose level has fallen below 250 mg/dl but the arterial pH remains below 7.3, the serum (or plasma) ketone determination should be repeated. If large or moderate amounts of ketones are present (in undiluted serum), insulin (6 U/h) together with glucose (200 ml/h of 5% glucose) should be administered. This lag in the clearance of ketones may reflect a slower turnover compared with glucose. A common temptation involves the premature disruption of adequate insulin administration during the resolution of ketoacidosis owing to fear of inducing hypoglycemia or anticipation of continued rapid clearance of ketones. This often results in delaying complete reversion to metabolic stability or an inadvertent iatrogenically precipitated recurrence of ketoacidosis. Hence, the need for adequate insulin therapy on an ongoing basis (with or without concomitant administration of glucose) cannot be emphasized too strongly. If the ketone reaction is negative or only faintly positive, the findings (euglycemic, nonketotic metabolic acidosis) suggest the development of an accompanying lactic acidosis requiring treatment with sodium bicarbonate.

Intermediate-acting insulin should not be given until the clinical situation has stabilized and the patient is taking food and/or fluids by mouth. However, in patients whose clinical pattern is known to consist of brief episodes of DKA which respond rapidly to small amounts of extra insulin, there may be an advantage in giving intermediate-acting insulin early in the course of treatment.

Fluids In most patients the total fluid deficit is ~6 and rarely >10 liters. Since dehydration is a consequence of osmotic diuresis, the loss of water is relatively greater than that of salt. Fluid replacement (in the absence of hypotension) should thus be in the form of hypotonic saline administered IV as 0.45% sodium chloride (half-isotonic), or, alternatively (to avoid the unlikely possibility of hemolysis from infusion of dilute solutions), sodium-free water may be infused in the form of 2.5% fructose in 0.45% saline. In the first hour of treatment, 1 liter of fluid should be infused; thereafter, fluids should be administered at the rate of 300 to 500 ml/h. In patients in shock, the most important goal is expansion of intravascular fluid. Consequently, isotonic saline should be used.

After 4 to 6 h of treatment, or sooner if the blood glucose concentration falls below 250 mg/dl, the IV infusion should be changed from saline to 5% glucose. The purpose of administering glucose is not only to prevent hypoglycemia but also to reduce the likelihood of the development of cerebral edema. Cerebral edema is a complication (see below) which may accompany rapid insulin-induced reductions in plasma glucose concentration to levels below 250 mg/dl.[561] In patients with severe fluid depletion or persistent vomiting, 5% glucose in 0.45% saline should be administered. The overall rate of administration and the choice of IV fluids are facilitated by placement of a central venous catheter, particularly in elderly persons and patients with cardiac or renal impairment. Total fluid replacement in the first 12 h generally approximates 5 liters.

Bicarbonate Since acetoacetate and β-hydroxybutyrate are metabolizable anions, their oxidation (in a setting in which further production has been inhibited by insulin administration) results in the production of bicarbonate, resulting in a rise in serum bicarbonate concentration toward normal even in the absence of treatment with alkali-containing solutions. Consequently, infusion of bicarbonate in amounts sufficient to restore as little as 50 percent of the calculated base deficit (estimated on the basis of the reduction in serum bicarbonate concentration and 50 percent of body weight) often results in mild metabolic alkalosis. Theoretical objections to the routine use of bicarbonate may also be raised on the grounds that a rapid elevation in arterial pH may be accompanied by an exaggerated fall in cerebrospinal fluid pH and attendant worsening of CNS function. In addition, the shift to the left in the oxygen dissociation curve brought by alkalinization may limit tissue oxygen delivery, since red cell 2,3-diphosphogylcerate concentration is reduced in DKA and is not immediately restored by insulin treatment. Furthermore, retrospective analysis has not shown an improved outcome in patients receiving bicarbonate.[562] By contrast, severe reductions in arterial pH may impair myocardial contractility and may directly contribute to CNS depression. Accordingly, treatment with bicarbonate should be restricted to patients with severe metabolic acidosis as indicated by an arterial pH of 7.1 or less or a bicarbonate level of <5 mEq/liter. In such circumstances 88 to 100 mEq of sodium bicarbonate (132 mEq if pH < 7.0) should be added to the initial liter of hypotonic saline. Additional bicarbonate is given only so long as blood pH (measured 2 h after the institution of treatment) remains <7.25. To avoid the possibility of aggravating cellular dehydration by the infusion of a hypertonic solution, it is important to add the bicarbonate to a hypotonic 0.45% solution of sodium chloride rather than infuse it with isotonic (0.9%) saline. Since blood lactate levels tend to be slightly elevated in ketoacidotic patients, there is no justification for infusion of sodium lactate in preference to bicarbonate.

Potassium As a consequence of the ketonuria, diuresis, and frequent vomiting, body potassium stores are depleted by 5 to 10 mEq per kilogram of body weight. Nevertheless, the serum potassium concentration is generally normal or even elevated in DKA because of the shift in potassium from intracellular to extracellular fluid which accompanies an increase in hydrogen ion concentration. With correction of the acidosis and stimulation of cellular uptake of glucose, serum potassium levels decline. Accordingly, potassium chloride should be administered 3 h after the initiation of therapy (provided that the patient is not anuric) in a dose of 40 mEq/liter of IV fluid. A total of 120 to 160 mEq is generally infused in the first 12 to 18 h. In rare patients (<5 percent of cases) in whom hypokalemia is present at the outset, potassium supplements (40 to 60 mEq of KCl per liter) are added to the initial IV infusion. Monitoring of the electrocardiogram may be useful in detecting hypokalemia or hyperkalemia but should not replace frequent measurement of serum potassium concentration (at intervals of 2 to 4 h) in determining the need for, and the rate of, administration of potassium supplements.

Since body phosphate stores are reduced in DKA, there may be some theoretical advantage in administering potassium as the phosphate rather than the chloride salt. However, the administration of phosphate fails to accelerate improvement in clinical or biochemical parameters and may precipitate hypocalcemia.[563] Phosphate administration in the presence of decreased renal function may also culminate in hyperphosphatemia. It is therefore preferable to measure phosphate levels before its administration. Acute normalization of serum phosphate is generally unnecessary, as this comes about naturally with appropriate therapy and the resumption of feeding. In view of the long experience with potassium chloride, this remains the choice for potassium repletion.

Complications

In most cases a fatal outcome in DKA is attributable to a severe underlying illness such as myocardial infarction, overwhelming sepsis, or acute pancreatitis rather than DKA per se. Three complicating and potentially fatal situations that may occur in the absence of intercurrent illness are *shock, cerebral edema*, and *adult respiratory distress syndrome* (RDS).

Shock may develop as a consequence of severe hypovolemia, reduced myocardial contractility secondary to acidosis, and, possibly, decreased peripheral resistance. In hypotensive patients a central venous catheter should be placed, followed by rapid infusion of large volumes of isotonic (rather than hypotonic) saline. Failure to respond to saline may necessitate treatment with blood or plasma volume expanders. The efficacy of vasoconstrictor drugs (metaraminol and norepinephrine) or dopamine in such patients has not been established.

Attention has been called to the problem of irreversible fatal cerebral edema complicating DKA. The clinical picture is generally one of an adolescent diabetic patient with no underlying illness in whom progressive deterioration in consciousness develops after an initial period (3 to 10 h) of treatment characterized by improving laboratory test results. Papilledema, elevated cerebrospinal fluid pressure, dilated pupils of unequal size, hyperpyrexia, and occasionally diabetes insipidus may be observed in such cases.

Studies in hyperglycemic dogs and rabbits have shown that a sharp drop in blood glucose concentration to <250 mg/dl by rapid infusion of saline or administration of insulin results in gross brain edema.[561] The imbibition of water by the brain is due to a disequilibrium between brain and plasma osmolarity. The possibility that glucose-induced injury to brain capillaries may contribute to brain swelling has been suggested.[564] Cerebral edema is not observed in hyperglycemic experimental animals until the blood glucose concentration falls to <250 mg/dl. Similarly, in the clinical setting cerebral edema generally has not been shown to occur until the plasma glucose concentration has reached normal or nearly normal levels. Accordingly, when one is treating DKA or hyperosmolar coma, insulin treatment should be reduced or discontinued and glucose-containing fluids should be administered when the plasma glucose concentration has fallen to 250 mg/dl.

Survival in patients developing cerebral edema is dependent on early recognition and suspicion of impending events. Early premonitory features of neurologic deterioration observed in ~50 percent of patients, include severe headache, incontinence, alteration in arousal or behavior, pupillary and blood pressure changes, seizure, bradycardia, and disturbed temperature regulation. Patients need to be followed carefully in a closely monitored environment.[565]

Although successful treatment of cerebral edema has been infrequently recorded (spontaneous reversal has been noted), the use of mannitol or large doses of corticosteroids may be of some value in reducing cerebral swelling. It has been recommended that mannitol be placed at the bedside for the initial 24-h treatment period.[566] However, mannitol may aggravate hypertonicity and precipitate kidney damage and cause a rebound increase in intracranial pressure, and intubation and hyperventilation have been recommended as initial measures before infusing mannitol.[565,567] The most effective treatment of this crisis consists of the prevention of DKA.[565] Fortunately, the overall incidence of clinically overt cerebral edema is quite low; not a single case was recognized in one series of 257 patients.[568] However, subclinical brain swelling detectable by cranial CT scan is commonly observed during the course of treatment of DKA.[569]

In one report, *adult RDS* was observed in patients with DKA as well as hyperosmolar nonketotic coma.[570] The findings are those of dyspnea, hypothermia, chest x-ray findings suggestive of pulmonary edema, and normal capillary wedge pressure. Mortality is high in such patients.

Hyperosmolar Nonketotic Coma

Impaired consciousness may occur in a diabetic patient as a consequence of severe hyperglycemia, hyperosmolarity, and dehydration in the absence of keotacidosis. In hyperosmolar nonketotic coma, by definition, blood ketone acid concentrations are normal or only mildly elevated. Typically, this syndrome develops in middle-aged or elderly patients as either the first manifestation of diabetes or in a setting of previously mild type II diabetes. Symptoms of polydipsia and polyuria generally develop over a period of several (usually 7 to 10) days, culminating in disturbances of consciousness which often cause the patient to come to medical attention. As in DKA, mental obtundation varying from lethargy to coma occurs. However, in contrast to DKA, patients with hyperosmolar coma often have focal or generalized seizures.[571] In many instances the syndrome is temporally (and perhaps causally) related to the prior administration of drugs such as diuretics, glucocorticoids, immunosuppressive agents, and phenytoin. In as many as 25 percent of patients there is clinical and/or autopsy evidence of acute pancreatitis.

The laboratory findings consist of marked hyperglycemia (>600 mg/dl or 33 m*M*), hyperosmolarity (generally >310 mOsm), azotemia, and, by definition, the absence of hyperketonemia. The degree of azotemia is on average greater than that observed in DKA (BUN 70 to 90 mg/dl, compared with 40 mg/dl in DKA).[572] The serum sodium concentration may be normal, elevated, or even reduced. The failure to observe a consistent elevation of serum sodium concentration in the face of marked dehydration is a consequence of the redistribution of body fluids from the intracellular to the extracellular compartment engendered by hyperglycemia. The expected reduction in serum sodium concentration brought about by hyperglycemia may be calculated as 1.6 mEq/liter for each 100-mg/dl increment in serum glucose concentration above normal.[573] Thus, in a patient with a markedly elevated blood glucose level and a normal or elevated serum sodium concentration, a severe state of dehydration is likely to be present.

The pathogenesis of the syndrome of nonketotic hyperosmolar coma remains somewhat unclear. Two factors require explanation: the presence of hyperglycemia which exceeds that generally observed in DKA and the absence of ketoacidosis. With respect to the former, the diminution in renal function may limit the extent to which glucose can be excreted in the urine, thus resulting in the progressive accumulation of glucose in the blood. Supporting this possibility is the observation that alloxan-treated animals develop nonketotic hyperosmolar coma if the ureters are tied and glucocorticoids are administered.[574] The presence of small amounts of insulin sufficient to inhibit lipolysis (but not hyperglycemia) has been postulated to account for the failure to develop ketoacidosis. C peptide levels tend to be higher in hyperosmolar nonketotic coma than in DKA.[575] Hyperosmolarity per se has been shown to interfere with lipolysis and thus may play a role in preventing ketogenesis.[576] Plasma FFA levels tend to stay low in patients with hyperosmolar nonketotic coma.[575] Animal studies have shown that an increase in liver glycogen diminishes ketogenic capacity. The provocative effect of glucocorticoids in the pathogenesis of experimental or spontaneous hyperosmolar coma and the contributory role of excess carbohydrate intake in the experimental syndrome[577] support a role for increased liver glycogen content in the inhibition of ketogenesis.

Treatment consists of continuous IV infusion of insulin in low doses (6 to 10 U/h), together with large amounts of fluids as hypotonic saline (unless the patient is in shock, in which case isotonic saline is infused) and repletion of body potassium.[560]

The mortality rate has been reported to vary from 5 to 40 percent. Many of the fetal cases have accompanying lactic acidosis (see below), as reflected by reduced arterial pH and a large anion gap. In many instances death is due to a underlying disease process such as pancreatitis or sepsis.

Lactic Acidosis

Severe metabolic acidosis due to the accumulation of lactate (and to a much smaller extent pyruvate) may be observed in the diabetic as well as the nondiabetic population.[578] Among diabetic patients, lactic acidosis may develop in a variety of circumstances: (1) in association with DKA (~10 percent of patients with DKA have an accompanying lactic acidosis), (2) in association with hyperosmolar nonketotic coma (as many as 40 to 60 percent of such patients also have lactic acidosis), (3) as a complication of phenformin therapy, (4) in association with inadequate tissue perfusion due to cardiogenic, septic, or hypovolemic shock, and (5) as a spontaneous disorder.

The clinical manifestations are deep labored breathing, dehydration, abdominal pain, and depression of the sensorium ranging from lethargy to coma. The laboratory diagnosis is based on the presence of an arterial pH < 7.3 in the face of normal or reduced P_{CO_2}, reduction in serum bicarbonate concentration with an increased anion gap not attributable to ketonemia (as reflected by no more than trace amounts of serum ketones), and the absence of uremia or a history of the ingestion of salicylates or methanol. The definitive diagnosis rests on the demonstration of an increase in the plasma lactate concentration, generally to >5 m*M*.

The pathogenesis of lactic acidosis in patients with DKA, hyperosmolar coma, or various types of shock probably relates to disturbances in tissue perfusion, resulting in failure of hepatic uptake and metabolism of lactate and, possibly, increased production of lactate in muscle.[578] The basis for the increased tendency to develop spontaneous lactic acidosis among diabetic patients remains unexplained, however. The association with diabetes is particularly surprising, since hepatic uptake and utilization of lactate for gluconeogenesis are increased in diabetic patients.[118]

As in all forms of lactic acidosis, treatment consists of the administration of large volumes of saline and bicarbonate. In patients with plasma glucose concentration >250 mg/dl, administration of small doses of insulin may be helpful even in the absence of ketoacidosis or severe hyperosmolarity.[579]

Pregnancy and Diabetes

The interaction of pregnancy and diabetes requires special consideration because of the increased risks to the well-being of the fetus when the mother is diabetic and because the presence of the conceptus (fetus and placenta) alters substrate and hormone metabolism in the mother. The net result is that various aspects of the diagnosis and management of diabetes are altered or require emphasis when one is dealing with a pregnant diabetic patient.[580] Furthermore, it is now recognized that normalization of maternal fuel metabolism, which previously had been emphasized in late pregnancy to prevent perinatal mortality and morbidity, must be attempted at conception and during early pregnancy (i.e., during the earliest stages of embryogenesis) in order to lower rates of congenital malformation.

Maternal and Fetal Fuel Metabolism

The overall metabolic influence of pregnancy in normal subjects is the sum of two seemingly opposite phenomena: (1) the presence of "accelerated starvation," resulting in a tendency to develop fasting hypoglycemia and hyperketonemia,[581] and (2) the presence of insulin resistance, resulting in a tendency toward postprandial hyperglycemia. Which of these influences predominates depends on the stage of pregnancy (first or second half) and nutritional condition (fasted or fed).

Accelerated Starvation

The impact of pregnancy on metabolism in the postabsorptive or fasted condition is to lower plasma glucose and insulin levels while causing increased concentrations of ketones and FFA. The hormonal and substrate milieu after an overnight, 12- to 14-h fast in pregnancy is thus comparable to that observed after a 24- to 36-h fast in the nongravid state, hence the term "accelerated starvation."[581] This exaggerated response to fasting occurs in a setting of continuous siphoning of glucose and amino acids from the maternal to the fetal circulation (Fig. 19-58).

The conceptus is an obligate glucose-consuming organism whose utilization of glucose is not dependent on the availability of maternal insulin. In fact, maternal insulin and glucagon fail to cross the placenta, while glucose is readily transferred by a process of facilitated diffusion (Fig. 19-58). The rate of glucose utilization by the fetus at term is estimated at 6 mg per kilogram of body weight per minute, which is two to three times greater than in normal adult subjects. While maternal insulin does not reach the fetus, the fetal islets produce insulin by 12

FIGURE 19-58 Maternal-fetal fuel and hormone exchange in normal pregnancy. Glucose readily traverses the placenta and is continuously siphoned by the fetus from the mother. Active transport of amino acids and transfer of ketones to the fetus also occur. Free fatty acids (FFA) and triglycerides (TG) do not cross directly but are retained by the placenta and slowly released on the fetal side. In contrast, maternal insulin and glucagon do not reach the fetal circulation. Excessive fetal levels of glucose and amino acids elicit local hyperinsulinemia in the fetus.

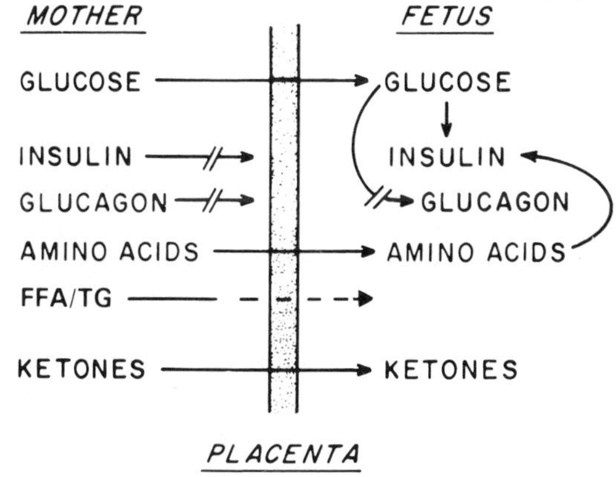

weeks of gestation; this hormone is a key growth factor in intrauterine life.

In addition to glucose, amino acids are transferred to the fetus by a process of active transport. Besides their utilization for protein synthesis, amino acids may also be catabolized and serve as an energy-yielding fuel. Regardless of their ultimate metabolic fate, the transfer of amino acids to the fetus results in maternal hypoaminoacidemia and therefore decreased availability of amino acids (particularly alanine) for maternal gluconeogenesis.

The sequence of events resulting in accelerated starvation is thus initiated by fetal glucose utilization. An increase in the maternal glucose dilution space may also contribute to the reduction in maternal plasma glucose concentration.[580] As a consequence, plasma insulin levels fall, resulting in augmented lipolysis and hyperketonemia. Simultaneously, the reduced availability of amino acids in the maternal circulation perpetuates and exaggerates the hypoglycemic state by limiting maternal gluconeogenesis.

FFA and triglycerides cross the placenta indirectly to a limited extent.[582] The transfer is increased in diabetes[583] as a result of maternal hyperlipidemia, producing a steep maternal-fetal triglyceride and FFA gradient. Even in gestational diabetes or in a controlled diabetic pregnancy, increased transfer to the fetus is evident from a rise in the placental lipid content.[584] However, from a clinical standpoint the important immediate consideration in fasting or diabetes is the elevation in blood ketone concentrations since the ketones cross the placenta freely. On the fetal side they are available for oxidation even by the fetal liver and brain.[585] Ketone utilization may, however, have an adverse effect on psychoneurologic development. Maternal ketonemia, whether due to starvation or to diabetes, has been shown in some studies to be associated with a significant reduction in IQ in offspring studied at ages 3 to 5.[586–588] Consequently, strict attention to management is required during pregnancy to avoid starvation ketosis (by frequent feeding and the maintenance of an adequate caloric and total carbohydrate intake) and prevent diabetic hyperketonemia due to inadequate insulinization.

Postprandial Hyperglycemia

In contrast to the tendency of *fasting* plasma glucose levels to be lower, in the *postprandial* condition plasma glucose concentration tends to be higher in pregnant compared with nonpregnant subjects. Large population studies have shown that unless the criteria for glucose tolerance are adjusted upward (by 25 mg/dl, or 1.4 m*M*, for the 2-h plasma glucose concentration), an inordinate number of women are diagnosed as having glucose intolerance in pregnancy.[589] Furthermore, even with such an adjustment in criteria, a substantial number of pregnant women are observed to have glucose intolerance which reverts to normal after delivery ("gestational diabetes"). The basis for these postprandial elevations in plasma glucose concentration is not a lack of insulin in normal pregnancy but the physiologic development of insulin resistance.

The plasma insulin response to glucose or protein ingestion is exaggerated in pregnancy, particularly in the second and third trimesters. The coexistence of hyperinsulinemia and normal or high glucose levels suggests tissue resistance to insulin. Studies of plasma insulin response to hyperglycemia maintained at a fixed level (glucose clamp technique) have indicated that tissue response to insulin is reduced in normal pregnancy by as much as 80 percent.[590] The basis of this insulin resistance is not entirely established; it may be related to the influence of placental hormones (lactogen, estrogen, progesterone, and prolactin), which antagonize the action of insulin and may have stimulatory effects on insulin secretion as well.

Human placental lactogen [HPL, also referred to as chorionic somatomammotropin (hCS)] is a polypeptide hormone produced by the syncytiotrophoblast. Chemically and immunologically it is similar to GH. However, HPL circulates at term in a concentration 1000 times that of GH. In addition to having an anabolic effect on protein metabolism and a lipolytic action, it is both mammotropic and luteotropic. A mild but definite impairment in glucose tolerance has been observed after a single infusion of HPL in nonpregnant subjects over periods of 5 to 12 h.[591] This is manifested as a small decrease in the rate of glucose utilization despite an increase in the circulating insulin level. Despite the known anti-insulin effects of this hormone, it is noteworthy that a consistent relation has not been observed between maternal HPL levels and insulin requirements during diabetic pregnancy.[592] Furthermore, maternal HPL levels are not altered by physiologic fluctuations in blood glucose concentration.

Pregnancy is characterized, in addition to increasing levels of HPL, by increasing placental secretion of estrogen and progesterone; these hormones readily enter the maternal circulation. Consensus regarding the effects of estrogen on carbohydrate metabolism is lacking. Synthetic estrogens may well produce greater anti-insulin effects than do natural estrogens. Thus, while estradiol administration results in hyperinsulinemia, it is accompanied by improvement rather than deterioration in glucose tolerance. These findings are in agreement with the ameliorative effect of natural estrogen on diabetes in partially pancreatectomized animals. Thus, it is clear that estrogen may contribute to hyperinsulinemia but probably is not a major factor in the insulin resistance of pregnancy. Progesterone may be a more important contributor to tissue insensitivity to insulin.

Pituitary prolactin concentration also increases markedly during pregnancy. Studies on women with prolactin-producing pituitary adenomas have revealed fasting and glucose-induced hyperinsulinemia, elevation in the glucose tolerance test curve, and augmented suppression of glucagon in response to hyperglycemia, similar to the responses observed in human pregnancy.[593,594]

Pregnancy is regarded as a diabetogenic condition on several grounds. For one thing, the tissue response to insulin is diminished in the fed state in normal pregnant subjects (as reflected by postprandial hyperinsulinemia). Also, pregnancy (particularly in the second and third trimesters) produces a transient gestational diabetes in some previously healthy women or a transient increase in insulin requirements in women with already manifest diabetes (see below). However, the presence of increasing insulin resistance in pregnancy cannot be equated with increased brittleness of the diabetic state. Brittleness of diabetes refers to variability and unpredictability of, and hence wide swings in, circulating glucose levels, which render clinical control of glycemia very difficult. In pregnant diabetic individuals brittleness may decline compared to the nonpregnant state despite the increase in insulin resistance.[595]

Diagnosis

The diagnosis of diabetes requires special emphasis in dealing with pregnancy, because the fetal mortality rate may be increased by glucose intolerance in the absence of overt diabetes and may be improved in such patients by insulin treatment.[596] Thus, there are more indications for performing a glucose tolerance test in the pregnant state compared with the nonpregnant state. Diagnosis is also especially important in pregnant women because, as was discussed above, the criteria for the diagnosis of glucose tolerance require adjustment in pregnancy. In addition, the normal tendency to renal glucosuria in pregnancy may lead to overdiagnosis of diabetes.

Because gestational diabetes may be present in the absence of known risk factors, it is recommended to perform a 1-h screening test with a 50-g glucose load at 26 to 28 weeks of gestation *in all pregnant women*. If the serum or plasma glucose level is ⩾140 mg/dl (7.8 m*M*), a full 100-g, 3-h oral glucose tolerance test should be done. The criteria for the diagnosis of diabetes in pregnancy by glucose tolerance testing as recommended by the NDDG are shown in Table 19-19. These differ somewhat from those employed in diagnosing impaired glucose tolerance in the nonpregnant state (Table 19-15) in that the upper limit of normal for the fasting plasma glucose is lower than is acceptable in the nongravid state (105 vs. 125 mg/dl) and the 1-h value is higher than that in the nongravid state (165 vs. 140 mg/dl). Carpenter and Coustan have proposed modified criteria which lower the acceptable limits of normal in pregnancy by 5 to 10 mg/dl at each time point compared to the NDDG criteria[597] (Table 19-19). Using the modified criteria, 50 percent more cases of gestational diabetes are diagnosed (5.0 percent vs. 3.2 percent of pregnancies), and nearly as much of an increase in perinatal morbidity (e.g., macrosomia, resuscitation at delivery) is observed compared with diagnosis by the NDDG criteria.[598] Thus, the Carpenter and Coustan criteria are probably more suitable than the NDDG criteria for identifying patients with gestational diabetes.

TABLE 19-19 Criteria for the Diagnosis of Gestational Diabetes by Oral Glucose Tolerance Test*

Hour	NDDG†, mg/dl	Modified‡, mg/dl
0	105	95
1	190	180
2	165	155
3	145	140

* Any two values equal to or greater than the values shown constitute a positive diagnosis.

† National Diabetes Data Group criteria (*Diabetes* 28:1039, 1979).

‡ Modified criteria proposed by Carpenter and Coustan (*Am J Obstet Gynecol* 144:768, 1982).

Classification

Gestational Diabetes

Gestational diabetes refers to overt diabetes or abnormal glucose tolerance which first appears or is diagnosed during pregnancy. Identification of gestational diabetes is important because the risks of congenital malformations, perinatal death,[596] fetal macrosomia, and neonatal hypoglycemia are higher in these women than in the general population. Furthermore, the diagnosis of gestational diabetes has important prognostic implications for the mother. Although most women with gestational diabetes revert to normal after delivery, permanent diabetes develops in ~35 percent within 16 years.[599] The presence of islet-cell antibodies in the plasma of gestational diabetic patients may predict those cases in which permanent diabetes will later develop or persist after delivery[600] and may predict that women with antepartum fasting plasma glucose concentrations >130 mg/dl are extremely likely to have permanent diabetes. Obesity confers a further substantial risk for the development of NIDDM, although many women of ideal weight demonstrate abnormal responses to a glucose challenge.[601]

In 1948, Priscilla White introduced a classification system specifically designed for pregnant diabetic patients. The various classes take into account the duration as well as the severity of diabetes, as indicated by the presence of microangiopathic complications in the form of retinopathy or nephropathy. Class A diabetic patients, as proposed by White, are the patients with "chemical diabetes only, with abnormal blood glucose levels when tested by a glucose load, but fasting values normal or near normal."[291] A more precise definition, which is preferable, is to classify patients as having gestational or pregestational diabetes. Among pregestational diabetic patients, class B individuals are patients with overt diabetes with onset after age 20 and duration >10 years. In class C, overt diabetes has been present for >10 years with onset before age 20. In classes D, F, and R, there is evidence of, respectively, benign retinopathy, nephropathy, or proliferative retinopathy. In general, the incidence of fetal wastage (stillbirths and neonatal deaths) increases in proportion to the severity of diabetes, as indicated by White's classification. In contrast, excessive birth weight (fetal macrosomia) is more common in classes A through C than in classes D through R.

Effect of Pregnancy on the Course of Diabetes

The effect of gestation on the clinical course of diabetes is quite variable, depending primarily on whether pregnancy is in an early or a late state. It is useful to divide pregnancy into first and second halves rather than trimesters in assessing its influence on diabetes.

During the early stages of pregnancy the dominant factor contributing to altered carbohydrate homeostasis is the transfer of maternal glucose to the fetus. This siphoning of glucose by the fetus results in a tendency toward maternal hypoglycemia; the hypoglycemia may be symptomatic and frequently necessitates a reduction in insulin dosage if the diabetes has previously been well controlled. A diminution in food intake as a consequence of the nausea and vomiting of early pregnancy may also contribute to a decrease in insulin requirements. The decreased need for insulin thus does not reflect a change in tissue sensitivity; rather, it is a consequence of lessened availability of circulating carbohydrate.

In the second half of pregnancy, the diabetogenic actions of placental hormones and prolactin outweigh the effects of continuous siphoning of glucose by the fetus. As a consequence, the demand for insulin is increased, necessitating an increase in insulin dosage. Quantitative assessment of the progressive rise in insulin requirement has been particularly feasible with the advent of portable pumps that permit the continuous subcutaneous delivery of insulin and produce normal or nearly normal glucose concentrations[602,603] (Fig. 19-59). Coincident with diminished effectiveness of insulin, the tendency to ketoacidosis is increased. The recognition of DKA in pregnancy is often more difficult because plasma glucose levels are generally not markedly elevated. In addition, ketonuria may reflect starvation ketosis rather than DKA, indicating that glucose rather than insulin is needed. The absence of hyperglycemia suggests the presence of starvation rather than diabetic ketosis.

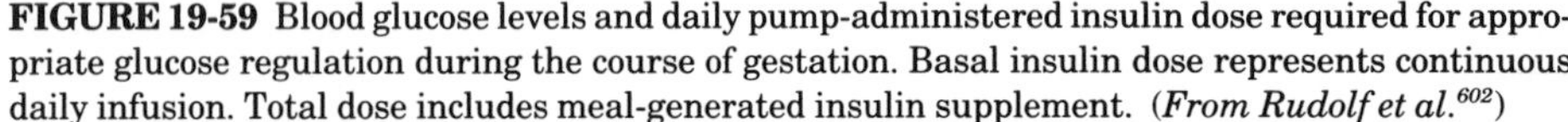

FIGURE 19-59 Blood glucose levels and daily pump-administered insulin dose required for appropriate glucose regulation during the course of gestation. Basal insulin dose represents continuous daily infusion. Total dose includes meal-generated insulin supplement. *(From Rudolf et al.*[602]*)*

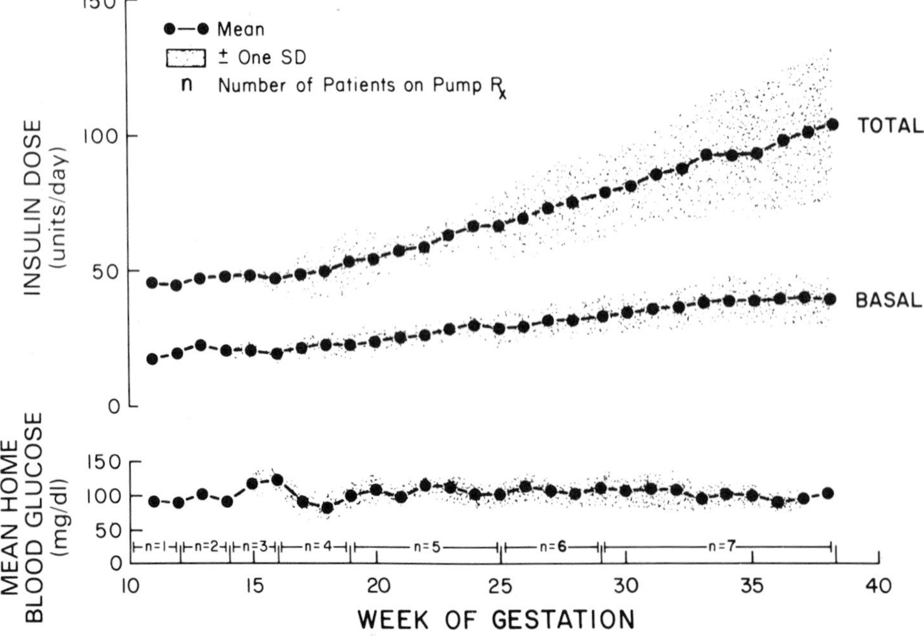

After delivery, the rapid fall in the concentrations of HPL, prolactin, estrogen, and progesterone, plus the continued suppression of GH secretion, which persists for 1 to 2 days after delivery, results in a reduction in maternal insulin requirement, frequently to levels below the prepregnant dose. Some patients experience a remarkable postpartum remission and gradually return to the prepregnancy course over the ensuing 3 to 6 weeks.

Effect of Diabetes on the Outcome of Pregnancy

The presence of diabetes in the mother continues to impose an increased risk for the developing fetus (Table 19-20). Perinatal mortality in diabetic pregnancy has progressively declined from rates of ⩾30 percent 20 to 30 years ago to current rates of 5 to 10 percent. Even with ideal management, fetal and neonatal death rates are at least twice those reported in pregnancies uncomplicated by diabetes. The major causes of fetal and neonatal wastage at present fall into three categories: congenital malformation, RDS, and intrauterine stillbirths.

Congenital Anomalies

The single largest perinatal problem in the 1980s was the two- to threefold increase in the incidence of congenital anomalies in infants of diabetic mothers. Birth defects are currently the major cause of perinatal mortality in diabetic pregnancy, accounting for 20,[604,605] 33,[606] or 50 percent[607,608] or more of all perinatal losses. Birth defects that occur with increased frequency in the offspring of diabetic mothers most commonly involve the heart and the nervous and skeletal systems. The caudal regression syndrome, which includes partial or complete agenesis of sacral vertebrae, is particularly common.

Studies in experimental animals as well as humans suggest that these abnormalities are a consequence of poor metabolic control during the period of organogenesis in early gestation. High levels of glucose in embryo culture medium have been associated with neural tube malformation,[609] as well as other anomalies.[609–611] Lumbosacral defects occurred in 17 percent of rat fetuses whose streptozotocin-diabetic mothers were not treated but in only 5 percent of those whose mothers were treated with insulin during the period of organogenesis.[612] When insulin-treated streptozotocin-induced diabetic pregnant rats underwent 2 days of insulin withdrawal during the first 7 days of gestation, increased skeletal malformations resulted in their embryos; however, if insulin was withdrawn for a 2-day period at 8 or more days of gestation, no such anomalies occurred.[613] Human studies also point out the causal role of inadequate metabolic control in teratogenesis. The demonstration that anomalies must have occurred before the seventh week of gestation, given the known times during gestation at which organ development occurs,[614] led to a focusing of investigation on the periconceptual period. Elevation in maternal glycohemoglobin at the end of the first trimester has been correlated with an increased incidence of major congenital malformations.[615–617] These observations suggest that any further reduction in perinatal mortality may require the restoration of a normal metabolic milieu in the diabetic mother from the time of conception.

Recent research has also focused on the role of hypoglycemia as a risk factor in fetal development, as stringent control of diabetes during pregnancy may result in frequent exposure to hypoglycemia.[618] Abnormal neural development in mouse embryos was demonstrated when the embryos were exposed to low glucose levels in culture.[619] Using an in vitro avian limb bud tissue culture system, proteoglycan core protein expression and reduced accumulation of proteoglycans during chondrogenesis were demonstrated with both high and low glucose levels, suggesting that both hyper- and hypoglycemia may be deleterious to skeletal development.[620] Nonetheless, until additional clinical studies confirm these findings, optimized control of diabetes during pregnancy is warranted. Excess malformation was not found despite the occurrence of hypoglycemia in 60 percent of women during embryogenesis.[621] Another study of the effect of intensified prepregnancy care resulting in a lower hemoglobin A_{Ic} concentration in the first trimester culminated in fewer congenital abnormalities despite more frequent hypoglycemic episodes.[622]

TABLE 19-20 Fetal Mortality and Morbidity in Diabetic Pregnancy

Perinatal mortality
Congenital anomalies
Respiratory distress syndrome
Stillbirths
Fetal morbidity
Congenital anomalies
Respiratory distress syndrome
Macrosomia
Hypoglycemia
Hyperbilirubinemia
Hypocalcemia

Respiratory Distress Syndrome

Although RDS was previously the major cause of neonatal death, its incidence has been reduced from ~30 percent to current rates of >10 percent of births, mainly because of the use of sophisticated methods of measuring fetal pulmonary maturity. In one series, RDS complicated 6 percent of births at 36.5 to 38.5 weeks of gestation in healthy pregnancies but affected 19 percent of infants born to diabetic mothers.[623] Neonatal death from RDS has become increasingly rare among infants of diabetic mothers because of the diminished incidence of RDS and improvements in the management of this clinical entity.

The pathophysiologic relation between maternal diabetes and RDS has not been fully elucidated. Pulmonary maturation in the fetus is largely dependent on the ability of the fetal lung to synthesize surfactant, a surface-active material which lines the alveoli and lowers surface tension, preventing alveolar collapse (atelectasis). Lecithin is the major surface-active material; in RDS, lecithin is deficient. The lecithin/sphingomyelin ratio may, however, be unreliable in determining pulmonary maturation in diabetic pregnancies.[624] Ammiotic determinations of phosphatidylcholine or phosphatidylglycerol are potentially better predictors of fetal lung maturation.[625] The synthesis of lecithin is dependent in part on an elevation in fetal glucocorticoid secretion late in gestation. In diabetic pregnancy, particularly in class A to C diabetic patients, pulmonary maturation is delayed.[626] Interestingly, insulin has been shown to be an antagonist of cortisol-induced synthesis of lecithin by fetal lung cells.[627] Thus, as in the case of fetal macrosomia (see below), maternal hyperglycemia leading to fetal hyperinsulinism may provide the explanation for the higher incidence of RDS in infants of diabetic mothers. Higher maternal levels of glycosylated hemoglobin were associated with the development of RDS.[628] Such an association thus provides an impetus for minimizing maternal hyperglycemia during pregnancy and for accurately assessing pulmonary maturation when the timing of delivery is gauged (see below).

Intrauterine Fetal Death

A remarkable reduction in the proportion of stillbirths among pregnant diabetic patients has occurred in recent years. From 1958 through 1969, in New York State exclusive of New York City, 12.3 percent of pregnancies in diabetic patients ended with intrauterine fetal death.[629] Large series from tertiary medical centers indicate stillbirth rates ranging from 0 to 4 percent.[630–632] The reasons for this dramatic decline in fetal mortality have not been proved, primarily because the causes of sudden intrauterine fetal death in diabetic pregnancy are poorly understood. Some deaths are due to poorly controlled diabetes with ketoacidosis,[633] and it is probable that intensive metabolic control has contributed greatly to the improvement in outcome. Indeed, it was demonstrated that fetal hyperglycemia and hyperinsulinemia may be associated with hypoxia, lactic acidosis, and fetal death.[634] Similarly, when hypertonic glucose solutions are administered to pregnant diabetic women in preparation for delivery, fetal acidosis may result.[635,636] In addition, placental insufficiency in a diabetic mother with vasculopathy may now be detected with the modern perinatal armamentarium of ultrasound and antepartum monitoring, leading to timely delivery before intrauterine death can occur.

Neonatal Morbidity

In addition to congenital anomalies and RDS, the major factors responsible for neonatal morbidity (Table 19-20) are fetal macrosomia, hypoglycemia, hypocalcemia, and hyperbilirubinemia. Fetal macrosomia refers to excessive fetal size for gestational age; it is much more common in class A to C diabetic patients than in class D through R diabetic patients. The increase in body weight is not due to edema; it is a consequence of increased deposition of fat and glycogen as well as visceromegaly. Pedersen in the 1930s was the first to ascribe these findings to maternal hyperglycemia leading to fetal hyperinsulinism and its resultant stimulation of fetal anabolism. Subsequent measurements of fetal insulin levels have substantiated this theory.[637] However, macrosomia is due not solely to the growth-promoting effect of fetal hyperinsulinemia but also to the plethora of glucose, fatty acids, and amino acids in the circulation of diabetic mothers mobilized in excess and reaching the fetus in overabundant amounts.

Neonatal hypoglycemia also stems from persisting fetal hyperinsulinemia, after the glucose source has been cut off at birth. It occurs in as many as 30 to 60 percent of infants of diabetic mothers. Suppression of fetal glucagon secretion during the course of a diabetic pregnancy has also been suggested as a contributory factor.[638] In addition to hypoglycemia, hypocalcemia also occurs fairly frequently and may be a consequence of suppression of fetal parathyroid secretion. Polycythemia resulting from minor degrees of hypoxia and increased blood viscosity may result in thrombosis of placental or fetal blood vessels.[639]

Diabetes has an impact on the mother. Diabetic pregnancies are associated with an increased risk of polyhydramnios and hypertensive disorders, including preeclampsia, edema, and pyelonephritis.[580] There is some evidence that preeclampsia is particularly increased in diabetic women with poor metabolic control.[640]

Postnatal Effects

Evidence from experimental animal studies suggests that uncontrolled maternal diabetes may have a protracted modifying effect on the pancreatic function of the offspring.[641] The impact of impaired glucose tolerance during intrauterine life is expressed as retarded growth and glucose intolerance in stressful conditions in adult life. Gestational diabetes is seen in females of the second generation; thus, the defect may be carried over to further generations. Long-term effects of gestational diabetes mellitus in the offspring of Pima Indian mothers include a higher frequency of poor glucose tolerance.[642] A slight increase in the incidence of IDDM in the children of diabetic mothers after 25 years was also demonstrated.[643] Furthermore, growth delay as defined by crown-rump length in the first trimester was predictive of worsened psychomotor outcome by age 4.[644] These findings lend emphasis to the importance of early and dedicated management of glucose intolerance in pregnancy.

Treatment

The principles of management in pregnant diabetic patients include (1) frequent evaluation of the patient, (2) close liaison between obstetrician and internist and, at the time of delivery, the pediatrician, and (3) most important, emphasis on intensive metabolic control, which optimally should be initiated before conception. The primary medical concern is adequate control of diabetes to minimize the incidence of fetal mortality and morbidity. The major obstetric decision concerns timing the delivery to avoid the risk of intrauterine death while delivering an infant with sufficient pulmonary maturity who will not succumb to RDS.

Insulin Pregnancy constitutes a major indication for intensive management of diabetes with self-monitoring of blood glucose concentration and either multiple manual injections of insulin or the use of an insulin infusion pump[602,645] (see Intensive Insulin Therapy, above). Such a treatment program should be instituted before conception in women who are contemplating pregnancy. As was indicated above, fetal anomalies are the single most important problem facing diabetic women undergoing pregnancy. It is most likely that poor metabolic control during organogenesis is in some way responsible for these anomalies. A program of intensive preconceptional metabolic control in diabetic women was shown to reduce the birth defect rate to 1.1 percent as opposed to 6.6 percent among diabetic women presenting for their care after the ninth week of gestation.[646] In keeping with those observations, the incidence of fetal anomalies is higher among diabetic pregnancies in which glycohemoglobin is elevated during the first trimester.

CSII has recently become popular for the management of diabetes in pregnancy. However, use of the pump requires a highly motivated individual. In a randomized trial of insulin pump vs. intensive conventional insulin therapy in pregnant diabetic women, there was no distinct advantage of either method.[645]

Although there is little evidence that insulin-induced maternal hypoglycemia has a detrimental effect on the fetus, this possibility has often been cited as a reason to avoid meticulous attempts to achieve euglycemia in pregnant diabetic patients. The impact of hypoglycemia on the development of congenital malformations was alluded to earlier. The Collaborative Perinatal Project demonstrated no adverse effect of maternal insulin reaction on subsequent mental and motor function tests of the offspring of diabetic mothers up to age 4 years.[647]

In the case of the gestational diabetic patient, management may take the form of strict dietary control or the administration of small amounts (15 to 20 U per day) of intermediate- and rapid-acting insulin. A gestational diabetic patient should do self-monitoring of blood glucose at least four times daily. If the fasting plasma glucose concentration exceeds 100 mg/dl or if any of the postprandial values exceeds 120 mg/dl or both, insulin therapy should be begun (or the previously instituted prophylactic dose should be increased). Gestational diabetic women whose circulating glucose concentrations remain below the above thresholds may be managed by diet alone. In pregestational diabetic patients, blood glucose control should be optimized to remain below values of 100 mg/dl in the fasting state and 120 mg/dl after meals. These criteria are ideal and require liberalization in women experiencing repeated hypoglycemia. The highly purified animal species or human insulin preparations are preferable in gestational diabetic patients, since they are less immunogenic.

Diet Dietary management of normal pregnancy for many years involved emphasis on curtailment of weight gain, generally to no more than 18 to 20 lb (8 to 9 kg). However, studies have shown that an average gain of 27.5 lb (12.5 kg) during the course of pregnancy is associated with the lowest overall incidence of preeclampsia, prematurity, and prenatal mortality. The Committee on Maternal Nutrition of the National Research Council recommends a slightly lower average weight gain of 24 lb (11 kg) and strongly condemns severe caloric restriction or weight reduction programs during normal pregnancy. The importance of avoiding calorie restriction is apparent from the data presented above regarding the acceleration of starvation ketosis in pregnancy and the adverse effects of ketones on fetal development.[648]

In the insulin-dependent pregnant diabetic patient the principles applying to the nongravid diabetic patient and those applying to normal pregnancy must be harmonized. This is achieved by recognizing that a weight gain of 24 lb is a physiologic component and a desirable goal of pregnancy in the diabetic patient as well as the nondiabetic subject; reduction in body weight to the ideal norm or limitation of weight gain to 20 lb (9 kg) should not be pursued during pregnancy. Accordingly, the recommended diet contains 30 to 35 kcal per kilogram of actual body weight. Of the total number of kilocalories, 45 percent, equivalent to a minimum of 200 g, is provided in the form of carbohydrate. The daily protein intake is generally 2 g per kilogram of body weight (100 to 200 g total); the remainder of the calories are provided as fat (45 to 60 g total). In patients with marked renal glucosuria, an additional 50 g or more of carbohydrate may have to be provided to make up for urinary losses. As in the nongravid diabetic patient, regularity and spacing of food intake are essential when insulin is administered. An evening snack is recommended to avoid morning ketosis in the presence of accelerated starvation. Adequate fiber, calcium, and vitamin intake should be ensured, including folate and iron supplements. When hyperemesis gravidarum occurs, early hospitalization with intravenous fluid administration is critical to prevent dehydration, malnutrition, and unstable metabolic control.

Although some clinics have found oral hypoglycemic agents useful in pregnancy, patients not responding to dietary control should be treated with insulin. The administration of sex steroids (estrogen and progesterone) has been recommended by some researchers but has not been generally adopted inasmuch as the evidence of a gestational hormonal deficiency in diabetes has not been convincing.

Delivery

Classically, the major dilemma in the time of delivery has been the avoidance of an intrauterine stillbirth, the likelihood of which is increased by delaying delivery too long, while minimizing the risks of RDS (the likelihood of which is increased by delivery before the development of pulmonary maturity). With current medical and obstetrical practice the risk of stillbirth is quite low. The advent of biochemical assays of amniotic fluid for fetal lung maturity has added another dimension to the ability to individualize the timing of delivery in these pregnancies. As previously indicated, the presence of a mature L/S (lecithin/sphingomyelin ratio) or, better yet, adequate phosphatidylglycerol concentration assures the obstetrician that RDS is unlikely to develop if the baby is delivered. Furthermore, with intensive management of diabetes, the likelihood of intrauterine death or deterioration of fetal status necessitating early delivery is unusual. Consequently, if the patient's diabetes is in good control, no obstetric or medical complications are present, and fetoplacental function testing indicates good fetal health, amniocentesis should be performed for pulmonary maturity at 38 weeks or beyond, depending on the state of the cervix.

It is uncertain whether premature labor occurs more frequently in diabetic pregnancies, although 5 percent are complicated by its occurrence.[649,650] The use of tocolytic agents (i.e., ritodrine, terbutaline) may result in deterioration of diabetes control or may unmask the presence of gestational diabetes.[650] Intravenous magnesium sulfate may be preferable as it does not affect glucose control. Potential complications of magnesium sulfate tocolysis include pulmonary edema, lethargy, muscle weakness, chest pain, and body warmth. Overdosage can result in respiratory difficulties, and levels need to be measured carefully, particularly in the presence of impaired renal function.

The route of delivery should be vaginal unless obstetrical indications for cesarean section are present. Management of diabetes on the day of delivery depends on the prior state of metabolic control as well as whether labor is to be induced, the patient is in spontaneous labor, or cesarean section is to be performed.[589] If labor is to be induced, insulin may be withheld on the morning of induction and a slow infusion of IV glucose may be administered. Rapid-acting insulin is infused only if the blood glucose concentration (monitored every 1 to 2 h) is 120 mg/dl. If the patient is in spontaneous labor, a similar approach of constant glucose infusion plus insulin (as necessary) is employed. If an elective cesarean section is to be performed, it should be done at breakfast time. Food is withheld on the morning of surgery, and (if the diabetes is well controlled) no insulin is given. IV saline is infused until after delivery.

Effect of Pregnancy on Complications of Diabetes

Severe worsening of retinopathy may occur during pregnancy in women with previous advanced background or untreated proliferative retinopathy. Deterioration of retinal status does not generally occur if prior retinopathy has been stabilized by prior laser therapy. Retinopathy has also been reported to progress with rapid improvement of blood glucose control, perhaps related to retinal hypoperfusion.[651] Hence, prepartum counseling and evaluation of pregestational diabetic patients should include a detailed retinal evaluation by a qualified specialist. Furthermore, glycosylated hemoglobin levels and, to a lesser extent, diastolic blood pressure are also related to the progression of retinopathy, although pregnancy per se appears to be the primary independent risk factor. Patients with hypertension and proliferative retinopathy should therefore be examined more frequently.[651]

Deterioration of renal function during gestation is unusual, although proteinuria may increase twofold to fourfold by the third trimester, followed by a postpartum decline. A decrease in GFR may also occur in some women. The presence of nephropathy is associated with a higher incidence of preeclampsia, premature delivery, and neonatal morbidity, particularly in the presence of hypertension.[651]

Lipoatrophic Diabetes

Lipoatrophic diabetes is a rare syndrome characterized by partial or complete absence of body fat, insulin-resistant diabetes, hypermetabolism in association with normal thyroid function, and hepatomegaly which often progresses to cirrhosis. The syndrome may be present at birth, in which circumstance the absence of fat tissue predates the development of diabetes by 10 to 12 years. Congenital occurrence includes the Dunnigan syndrome, which is rare and dominantly inherited, and the Seip-Berardinelli syndrome, which is more frequent and is of autosomal recessive inheritance. The congenital variant accounts for ~60 percent of cases of lipoatrophic diabetes. Associated conditions include intracerebral disorders and abnormalities involving the heart, kidneys, and ovaries. Mental retardation and psychiatric disturbance are also seen with the congenital variant. Acanthosis nigricans and cirrhosis are usually milder than in the acquired form. Alternatively, in the acquired form (Lawrence syndrome), the diabetes may appear first, the lipoatrophy not becoming manifest until late childhood or adult life, often following an acute viral illness. Associated findings are muscle hypertrophy (which may be more apparent than real, because of the lack of adipose tissue), accelerated growth, acanthosis nigricans, acromegaloid features with thick curly hair, hyperhidrosis, and clitoromegaly. This syndrome occurs twice as frequently in females as in males. Death is generally due to liver failure, although patients with retinopathy and nephropathy have occasionally been observed. Cirrhosis can progress to portal hypertension with splenomegaly; splenomegaly may, however, occur in the absence of cirrhosis.

The etiology of this syndrome remains unexplained. The presence of lipid-mobilizing factor isolated from the urine and abnormalities in pituitary releasing factor have been suggested but remain unproved. An increase in the basal metabolic rate, particularly after meals, has been described in lipoatrophic diabetes, although the exact mechanism is not known; thyroid hormone levels are normal. This condition is also characterized by very high basal insulin levels in the postabsorptive state but normal increases in insulin concentration after various beta cell stimuli, with a normal proinsulin/insulin ratio. The pathogenesis of insulin resistance is heterogeneous; it may involve both receptor and postreceptor abnormalities. Insulin receptor studies have shown decreased, normal, or increased binding.[651a] Increased insulin clearance has been proposed as a prereceptor defect.[652] Glucagon levels in lipoatrophic patients have been reported to be either normal or elevated. Gonadotropin levels are normal, although polycystic ovaries have been described in some cases of congenital lipoatrophic diabetes. Adrenal function is also reported to be normal. Acromegaloid features are present in some patients, but GH concentrations vary.

Radiographic studies show loss of subcutaneous fat and fat surrounding internal organs. Osteosclerosis of long bones appears commonly in this syndrome; it may be related to the replacement of hematopoietic marrow by fat. Marrow fat in turn may be transformed into osteogenic cells. Cardiomegaly may occur as a result of increased cardiac output resulting from the chronic hypermetabolic state.

The clinical distinction between lipoatrophic diabetes and poorly regulated insulin-dependent diabetes with wasting is generally not difficult. Differentiation is based on the lack of ketosis, the requirement for enormous doses of insulin, and the presence of hypermetabolism as well as the associated findings enumerated above. Treatment with U-500 insulin may be worth considering.

Partial lipoatrophy, although rare, is more common than is generalized lipoatrophy. Females are primarily involved, and rarely does it evolve into the generalized form. Loss of body fat tends to occur above the waist, but adiposity is normal below it. Partial lipoatrophy may be a variant of the generalized type, with accompanying glucose intolerance, insulin resistance, and hypermetabolism. This condition is associated with an increased incidence of brain tumors and membranoproliferative glomerulonephritis.

Secondary Diabetes

Diabetes may develop as a consequence of destructive lesions or surgical removal of the pancreas (pancreoprival diabetes); it also may result from hypersecretion of hormones which have actions antagonistic to insulin or which interfere with insulin secretion (endocrine-associated diabetes). Glucose intolerance is also observed fairly frequently in some nonendocrine disorders (uremia, cirrhosis).

In each of these conditions the possibility that a genetic predisposition to spontaneous diabetes is also playing a role (for example, in increasing the likelihood that a given amount of pancreatic destruction or counterregulatory hormone secretion will result in hyperglycemia) cannot be excluded.

Pancreoprival Diabetes

The surgical removal of more than two-thirds of the pancreas or pancreatic destruction resulting from chronic relapsing pancreatitis results in the development of diabetes. Clinically, such patients differ from those with spontaneous insulin-dependent diabetes by their greater tendency to develop insulin-induced hypoglycemia, lessened tendency to have ketosis, and requirement (in most instances) of no more than 20 to 40 U of insulin per day.[220] These characteristics may be related to the lack of glucagon secretion, which contrasts with the hyperglucagonemia observed in spontaneous diabetes. These patients are of interest from a theoretical standpoint because they demonstrate that (1) glucagon is not essential for the development of diabetes but, when present, accentuates the effects of insulin lack and (2) microangiopathy may occur in the absence of a genetic predisposition to diabetes, thus supporting the metabolic theory with regard to the pathogenesis of diabetic complications.[386]

Hemochromatosis is so often associated with diabetes that it is sometimes called "bronze diabetes." In one series of 115 patients, 72 had clinical diabetes and 14 others had abnormal results of glucose tolerance tests.[653] All 86 had an exaggerated insulin response like that seen in cirrhosis of the liver, which may be one of the causes of the diabetes in this disease. In addition, a family history of diabetes was present in 25 percent of those with diabetes and hemochromatosis. The usual complications of diabetes were quite common in this group of patients. It appears, therefore, that the diabetes of hemochromatosis can be explained as a combination of the effects of inheritance, cirrhosis, and, perhaps, the noxious effects of iron deposits in the pancreas. In this group of patients, 40 percent of the diabetic patients had some improvement of the carbohydrate abnormality after repeated phlebotomy had depleted the iron stores.[653]

Endocrine-Associated Diabetes

Sustained hypersecretion of hormones which have actions antagonistic to insulin (e.g., GH, glucocorticoids, epinephrine) or which interfere with insulin secretion (e.g., epinephrine, norepinephrine) is often associated with glucose intolerance of varying degrees of severity. Features common to virtually all forms of such endocrine-associated diabetes are reversibility of the hyperglycemia with cure of the underlying endocrine disorder and absence (in most patients) of ketosis. The latter characteristic probably reflects the ongoing availability of endogenous insulin.

Acromegaly

Growth hormone elevations seen in diabetes should not be confused with acromegaly. GH interferes with insulin-mediated glucose uptake while stimulating lipolysis. In most acromegalic patients hyperinsulinemia is present in the basal state and in response to meal ingestion. Diabetes generally occurs several years after the initial manifestation of acromegaly. Growth hormone levels tend to be higher in patients with abnormal carbohydrate tolerance.[654] The hyperinsulinemia may be sufficient to compensate for the insulin resistance so that carbohydrate metabolism remains intact. The prevalence of glucose intolerance in acromegaly is as high as 60 percent. Overt diabetes and impaired glucose tolerance (IGT) may occur with similar frequency. However, fasting hyperglycemia is observed in only 15 to 30 percent of the patients, and less than 10 percent require insulin therapy. The defect in insulin sensitivity in such patients may be mediated by a reduction in the binding of insulin to its receptor.[200]

Cushing's Syndrome

The administration of glucocorticoids in pharmacologic doses results in the development of hyperinsulinemia and insulin resistance in as short a period as 3 days.[655] With more sustained periods of hyperadrenalism, glucose intolerance generally appears. Fasting hyperglycemia is encountered in only 20 to 25 percent of patients with Cushing's syndrome; ketosis is unusual. In addition to stimulating gluconeogenesis, the increase in glucocorticoid concentrations interferes with insulin-mediated glucose uptake. The gluconeogenic action of glucocorticoids may be influenced by concomitant hyperglucagonemia.[656]

Pheochromocytoma

Excessive secretion of catecholamines may interfere with insulin secretion and/or action. The prevalence of IGT may reach 75 percent in patients with pheochromocytoma.[657] In tumors producing primarily norepinephrine, inhibition of insulin secretion is the major factor resulting in glucose intolerance. By contrast, hypersecretion of epinephrine results in interference with insulin-mediated glucose uptake as well as hypoinsulinemia.[247,248] Glucose load tests tend to show a diabetic pattern with a sudden drop in plasma glucose concentration at 60 to 90 min, probably as a result of the hyperglycemia-induced breakthrough in insulin secretion, after the initial blockade.[658] The degree of fasting hyperglycemia is usually mild in patients with pheochromocytoma. Abnormal carbohydrate metabolism may persist in some cases for weeks to months after tumor resection because of ongoing resistance to insulin.

Glucagonoma

Glucagon-secreting tumors of the alpha cells of the islets of Langerhans are rare tumors associated with glucose intolerance or fasting hyperglycemia, weight loss, diarrhea, an erythematous bullous skin eruption (necrolytic migratory erythema) frequently involving the trunk and perineum, angular stomatitis, glossitis, anemia, and hypokalemia.[659] Plasma glucagon levels generally are as high as 1000 to 2000 pg/ml, compared with values of 75 to 100 pg/ml in normal subjects and only moderate elevations (150 to 200 pg/ml) in patients with spontaneous diabetes. The increment in immunoreactive plasma glucagon concentration has been shown to be heterogeneous, consisting of four components: BPG, of ~150,000 daltons; "large plasma glucagon," of ~9000 daltons, which corresponds to proglucagon; pancreatic glucagon (~3500 daltons); and "small glucagon" (~2000 daltons). Studies using agents known to stimulate and suppress glucagon secretion have shown parallel changes in the levels of the three components other than BPG, which tends to remain constant.[660] Hyperglucagonemia has been observed in clinically unaffected family members of a patient with an alpha cell tumor.[224] However, the elevation in circulating glucagon immunoreactivity in family members was due not to pancreatic glucagon but to the larger molecular species, such as proglucagon and BPG.

Plasma insulin concentrations are generally elevated, accounting for the mildness of diabetes and the absence of ketosis despite the severe degree of hyperglucagonemia. The tumors may produce a variety of islet-cell hormones (e.g., insulin, somatostatin, pancreatic polypeptide) in addition to glucagon. Furthermore, the glucagonoma syndrome has appeared in patients with a prior history of clinically manifest insulinoma.[661]

Marked reductions in plasma amino acid concentrations are observed in glucagonoma patients. The hypoaminoacidemia is due to the hyperglucagonemia per se as well as to the weight loss, diarrhea, and protein loss from the skin lesions. Restoration of normal circulating amino acid levels by IV administration of amino acids has been accompanied by complete clearing of the skin rash.[662] In contrast to insulinomas, alpha cell tumors are often large enough to be detected by diagnostic imaging (i.e., CT scans) by the time they are suspected clinically.[663] Thromboembolic disease is frequently a cause of death. Treatment includes surgical resection and, in metastatic disease, administration of streptozotocin. A remarkable improvement in skin lesions has been observed after the administration of zinc or somatostatin[664] and Sandostatin (octreotide), the long-acting somatostatin analogue.[665]

Multiple Endocrine Deficiency

In some patients diabetes may coexist with adrenal failure and/or hypothyroidism. The simultaneous presence of more than one hormone deficiency state (unrelated to pituitary failure) is referred to as *Schmidt's syndrome,* or multiple endocrine deficiency (see Chap. 28). Such patients are characterized by the presence of circulating antibodies to islet cells as well as high titers of thyroid and adrenal antibodies. The diabetes is generally insulin-dependent. Diabetes may antedate or follow the other endocrine deficiencies. It is more commonly observed in women than in men. In contrast to most patients with insulin-dependent diabetes, in whom islet-cell antibodies disappear within months to a year after the onset of the diabetes, in patients with multiple endocrine deficiency titers of ICA may remain persistently elevated. Clinically, such patients are often difficult to manage because their lack of endogenous adrenal function predisposes them to severe insulin hypoglycemia even in the face of replacement doses of glucocorticoids.

Glucose Intolerance in Nonendocrine Disease

The pathogenesis of stress hyperglycemia in association with acute illness such as sepsis, myocardial infarction, and the postoperative state has been discussed above. In such circumstances tests of glucose tolerance (if indicated) should not be performed until the patient has recovered for several weeks to months after the acute event. In contrast, in certain disease states chronic abnormalities of glucose tolerance are frequently observed even in the absence of acute deterioration in the underlying primary disease process. In *uremia,* postprandial hyperglycemia and mild fasting hyperglycemia occur in a setting of hyperinsulinemia and hyperglucagonemia. Resistance to insulin, and hypersensitivity to glucagon are the major pathogenic factors responsible for hyperglycemia.[666] In addition, it is possible that a low-molecular-weight peptide unique to uremia induces insulin resistance by a protein synthesis–dependent mechanism.[667]

In *cirrhosis,* particularly when accompanied by portal hypertension, glucose intolerance is a frequent occurrence. Hyperinsulinemia and hyperglucagonemia have been noted. Decreased hepatic responsiveness to glucagon in cirrhosis suggests that insulin resistance may be the more important pathogenic factor in the derangement in carbohydrate metabolism.[246] The insulin resistance in human cirrhosis may be due to combined receptor and postreceptor defects.[668]

REFERENCES

1. Harris M, Entmacher PS: Mortality from diabetes, in *Diabetes in America,* NIH Publication 85-468. Washington, D.C., U.S. Government Printing Office, 1985.
2. WHO Study Group: *Diabetes Mellitus.* World Health Organization technical report series 727, Geneva, 1985.
3. Bransome E, Jr: Improving the financing of diabetes care in the 1990's. *Diabetes Care* 15(Suppl 1):66, 1992.
4. Pearse AGE: Neuroendocrine systems dispersed: APUD, in Adelman G (ed): *Encyclopedia of Neuroscience,* vol 2. Boston, Birkhauser, 1987, p 777.
5. Deuaskar SU, Mueckler MM: The mammalian glucose transporters. *Pediatr Res* 31:1, 1992.

5a. Kahn BB: Facilitative glucose transporters: Regulatory mechanisms and dysregulation in diabetes. *J Clin Invest* 83:1367, 1992.

6. Bell GI: Molecular defects in diabetes mellitus. *Diabetes* 40:413, 1991.
7. Middleton RJ: Hexokinases and glucokinases. *Biochem Soc Trans* 18:180, 1990.
8. Nuttal FQ, Gilboe DP, Gannon MC, et al: Regulation of glycogen synthesis in the liver. *Am J Med* 85:77, 1988.
9. DeFronzo R, Ferrannini E, Hendler R, et al: Influence of hyperinsulinemia, hyperglycemia and the route of glucose administration on splanchnic glucose exchange. *Proc Natl Acad Sci USA* 75:5173, 1978.
10. Groop LC, Kankuri RT, Sehalin-Jantti C, et al: Association between polymorphism of the glycogen synthase geno and non-insulin dependent diabetes mellitus. *N Engl J Med* 328:10, 1993.
11. Exton JH: Mechanisms involved in alpha adrenergic phenomena: Role of calcium ions in action of catecholamines in liver and other tissues. *Am J Physiol* 238:E3, 1980.
12. Sacca L, Hendler R, Sherwin RS, et al: Hyperglycemia inhibits glucose production in man independent of changes in

glucoregulatory hormones. *J Clin Endocrinol Metab* 47: 1160, 1978.
13. Pilkis SJ, Claus TH: Hepatic gluconeogenesis/glycolysis: Regulation and structure/function relationships of substrate cycle enzymes. *Annu Rev Nutr* 11:465, 1991.
14. Shafrir E; Effect of sucrose and fructose on carbohydrate and lipid metabolism and the resulting consequences, in Beitner R (ed): *Regulation of Carbohydrate Metabolism.* Boca Raton, CRC, 985, vol 2, p 96.
15. Owen OE, Felig P, Morgan AP, et al: Liver and kidney metabolism during prolonged starvation. *J Clin Invest* 48:574, 1969.
16. Felig P: The glucose-alanine cycle. *Metabolism* 22:179, 1973.
17. Granner DK, Andreone TL: Insulin modulation of gene expression, in DeFronzo RA (ed): *Diabetes/Metabolism Reviews.* New York, Wiley, 1985, vol 1, p 139.
18. Vincent MF, Gruber HE, Van Den Berghe G: Hypoglycemic effect of aicariboside in mice. *Diabetes* 40:1259, 1991.
19. Ahlborg G, Wahren J, Felig P, et al: Splanchnic and peripheral glucose and lactate metabolism during and after prolonged arm exercise. *J Clin Invest* 77:690, 1986.
20. Magnusson I, Shulman GI: Pathways of hepatic glycogen synthesis in humans. *Med Sci Sports Exerc* 23:939, 1991.
21. Cline G, Shulman GI: Quantitative analysis of pathways in glycogen repletion in periportal and perivenous hepatocytes *in vivo. J. Biol Chem* 266:4094, 1991.
22. Laker ME, Mayes PA: Investigations into the direct effects of insulin on hepatic ketogenesis, lipoprotein secretion and pyruvate dehydrogenase activity. *Biochim Biophys Acta* 795:4, 1984.
23. Greene DA, Sima AAF, Stevens MJ, et al: Complications: Neuropathy, pathogenetic considerations. *Diabetes Care* 15:1902, 1992.
24. Greene DA, Lattimer SA: Action of Sorbinil in diabetic peripheral nerve: Relation of polyol (sorbitol) pathway to a myoinositol mediated defect in sodium-potassium ATPase activity. *Diabetes* 33:712, 1984.
25. Sima AAF, Prashar A, Zhang W-X, et al: Preventive effect of long term aldose reductase inhibition (Ponalrestat) on nerve conduction and sural nerve structure in the spontaneously diabetic BB rat. *J Clin Invest* 85:1410, 1990.
26. Fluckiger R, Winterhalter KH: Glycosylated hemoglobins, in Caughey WS (ed): *Biochemical and Clinical Aspects of Hemoglobin Abnormalities.* New York, Academic Press, 1978, p 205.
27. Cerami A, Stevens VJ, Monnier VM: Role of nonenzymatic glycosylation in the development of the sequelae of diabetes mellitus. *Metabolism* 28(Suppl 1):431, 1979.
28. Singer DE, Coley CM, Samet JH, et al: Tests of glycemia in diabetes mellitus: Their use in establishing a diagnosis and in treatment. *Ann Intern Med* 110:125, 1989.
29. Larsen ML, Horder M, Mogensen EF: Effect of long-term monitoring of glycosylated hemoglobin levels in insulin-dependent diabetes mellitus. *N Engl J Med* 323:1021, 1990.
30. Dolhofer R, Brenner R, Wieland OH: Different behavior of hemoglobin A_{1c} and glycosyl-albumin levels during recovery from diabetic ketoacidosis and nonacidotic coma. *Diabetologia* 21:211, 1981.
31. Witzum JL, Mahoney EM, Branks MS, et al: Nonenzymatic glucosylation of low-density lipoprotein alters its biological activity. *Diabetes* 31:283, 1982.
32. Witzum JL, Fisher M, Pietro T, et al: Nonenzymatic glucosylation of high-density lipoprotein accelerates its metabolism in guinea pigs. *Diabetes* 31:1029, 1982.
33. Brownlee M: Glycation products and the pathogenesis of diabetic complications. *Diabetes Care* 15:1835, 1992.
34. Makita Z, Radoff S, Rayfield EJ, et al: Advanced glycosylation end products in patients with diabetic nephropathy. *N Engl J Med* 325:836, 1991.
35. Kohn RR, Schnider SL: Glucosylation of human collagen. *Diabetes* 31(Suppl 3):47, 1982.
36. Rahbrach DH, Hassell JR, Kleinman HK, et al: Alterations in the basement membrane (heparan sulfate) proteoglycan in diabetic mice. *Diabetes* 31:185, 1982.
37. Mandarino LJ: Current hypotheses for the biochemical basis of diabetic retinopathy. *Diabetes Care* 15:1892, 1992.
38. Ruderman NB, Williamson JR, Brownlee M: Glucose and diabetic vascular disease. *FASEB J* 6:2905, 1992.
39. Wakil SJ, Stoops JK, Joshi VC: Fatty acid synthesis and its regulation. *Annu Rev Biochem* 52:537, 1983.
40. McGarry JD, Foster DW: Regulation of hepatic fatty acid oxidation and ketone body production. *Annu Rev Biochem* 49:395, 1980.
41. Foster DW: From glycogen to ketones and back. *Diabetes* 33:1188, 1984.
42. Murthy MSR, Pande SV: Malonyl-CoA binding sites and the overt carnitine palmitoyl transferase activity reside on the opposite sides of the outer mitochondrial membrane. *Proc Natl Acad Sci USA* 84:378, 1987.
43. Owen OE, Reichard GA Jr; Fuels consumed by man: The interplay between carbohydrates and fatty acids. *Prog Biochem Pharmacol* 6:177, 1971.
43a. Kosugi K, Scofield RF, Chandramouli V, et al: Pathways of acetone's metabolism in the rat. *J Biol Chem* 261:3952, 1986.
44. Saggerson ED, Carpenter CA: Effects of streptozotocin-diabetes and insulin administration *in vivo* or *in vitro* on the activities of five enzymes in the adipose tissue triacylglycerol synthesis pathway. *Biochem J* 243:289, 1987.
45. Abumurad NA, Perry RR, Whitesell RR: Stimultion by epinephrine of the membrane transport of long chain fatty acids in the adipocyte. *J Biol Chem* 260:9969, 1985.
46. Stralfors P, Bjorgell P, Belfrage P: Hormonal regulation of hormone-sensitive lipase in intact adipocytes: Identification of phosphorylated sites and effects on the phosphorylation by lipolytic hormones and insulin. *Proc Natl Acad Sci USA* 81:3317, 1984.
47. Londos C, Honner RC, Dhillon GS: cAMP-dependent protein kinase and lipolysis in rat adipocytes: III. Multiple modes of insulin regulation of lipolysis and regulation of insulin responses by adenylate cyclase regulators. *J Biol Chem* 261:15139, 1985.
48. Harano Y, Kashigawa A, Kojima H, et al: Phosphorylation of carnitine palmitoyl transferase and activation by glucagon in isolated rat hepatocytes. *FEBS Lett* 188:267, 1985.
49. Woeltje DF, Kowajima M, Foster DW, McGarry JD: Characterization of the mitochondrial carnitine palmitoyltransferase enzyme system. II. Use of detergents and antibodies. *J Biol Chem* 262:9822, 1987.
50. Casazza JP, Felver ME, Veech RL: The metabolism of acetone in rats. *J Biol Chem* 259:231, 1984.
51. Hetenyi G Jr, Ferrarotto C: Gluconeogenesis from acetone in starved rats. *Biochem J* 231:151, 1985.
52. Reichard GA Jr, Hoff AC, Skutches CL et al: Plasma acetone metabolism in the fasting human. *J Clin Invest* 63:619, 1979.
53. Ruderman NB, Toews CJ, Shafrir E: The role of free fatty acids in glucose homeostasis. *Arch Intern Med* 123:299, 1968.
54. Rennie MJ, Holoszy JD: Inhibition of glucose uptake and glycogenolysis by availability of oleate in well-oxygenated perfused skeletal muscle. *Biochem J* 168:161, 1977.
55. Randle PT, Garland PB, Hales CN, et al: Glucose fatty acid cycle. *Lancet* 1:785, 1963.
56. Felig P, Pozefsky T, Marliss E, Cahill GF Jr: Alanine: Key role in gluconeogenesis. *Science* 167:1003, 1970.
57. Felig P: Amino acid metabolism in man. *Annu Rev Biochem* 44:933, 1975.
58. Felig P, Kim YJ, Lynch V, Hendler R: Amino acid metabolism during starvation in human pregnancy. *J Clin Invest* 51:195, 1972.
59. Haymond MW, Karl IE, Pagliara AS: Ketotic hypoglycemia: An amino acid substrate-limited disorder. *J Clin Endocrinol Metab* 38:521, 1974.

60. Haymond MW, Ben-Galim E, Strobel KE: Glucose and alanine metabolism in children with maple syrup urine disease. *J Clin Invest* 62:398, 1978.
61. Wahren J, Felig P, Hagenfeldt L: Effect of protein ingestion on splanchnic and leg metabolism in normal man and in diabetes mellitus. *J Clin Invest* 57:987, 1976.
62. Buse MG, Reid SS: Leucine. A possible regulator of protein turnover in muscle. *J Clin Invest* 56:1250, 1975.
63. Steiner D: Insulin today. *Diabetes* 26:322, 1977.
64. Goeddel DV, Kleid DG, Bolivar F, et al: Expression in *Escherichia coli* of chemically synthesized genes for human insulin. *Proc Natl Acad Sci USA* 76:106, 1979.
65. Weitzer G, Eisele K, Schulz V, Stock W: Structure and activity of insulin: XII. Further studies on biologically active synthetic fragments of B-chain. *Hoppe Seylers Z Physiol Chem* 354:321, 1973.
66. Chan SJ, Keim P, Steiner DF: Cell-free synthesis of rat preproinsulins: Characterization and partial amino acid sequence determination. *Proc Natl Acad Sci USA* 73:1964, 1976.
67. Bonser AM, Garcia-Webb P: C-peptide measurement: Methods and clinical utility. *CRC Crit Rev Clin Lab Sci* 19:297, 1984.
67a. Polonsky K, Frank B, Pugh W, et al: The limitations to and valid use of C-peptide as a marker of the secretion of insulin. *Diabetes* 35:379, 1986.
68. Gerich JE, Charles MA, Grodsky GM: Regulation of pancreatic insulin and glucagon secretion. *Annu Rev Physiol* 38:353, 1976.
69. Villa-Komaroff L, Efstratiadis A, Broome S, et al: A bacterial clone synthesizing proinsulin. *Proc Natl Acad Sci USA* 75:3727, 1978.
70. Felig P, Wahren J: Influence of endogenous insulin secretion on splanchnic glucose and amino acid metabolism. *J Clin Invest* 50:1702, 1971.
71. Gabbay KH, DeLuca K, Fisher JN Jr, et al: Familial hyperproinsulinemia: An autosomal dominant defect. *N Engl J Med* 294:911, 1976.
72. Robbins DC, Shoelson SE, Rubenstein AH, Tager HS: Familial hyperproinsulinemia: Two families secreting indistinguishable type II intermediates of proinsulin conversion. *J Clin Invest* 73:714, 1984.
73. Tamborlane WV, Sherwin RS, Genel M, Felig P: Reduction to normal of plasma glucose in juvenile diabetes by subcutaneous administration of insulin with a portable infusion pump. *N Engl J Med* 300:573, 1979.
74. Malaisse-Lagae F, Sener A, Malaisse WJ: Phosphoglucomutase: Its role in the response of pancreatic islets to glucose epimers and anomers. *Biochimie* 64:1059, 1982.
75. Malaisse WJ, Hutton JC, Kawazu S, et al: The stimulus-secretion coupling of glucose-induced release: XXXV. The links between metabolic and cationic events. *Diabetologia* 16:331, 1979.
76. Meglasson MD, Matschinsky FM: Pancreatic glucose metabolism and regulation of insulin secretion, in DeFronzo RA (ed): *Diabetes/Metabolism Reviews*. New York, Wiley, 1986, vol 2, p 163.
77. Meglasson MD, Burch PT, Benner DK, et al: Identification of glucokinase as an alloxan-sensitive glucose sensor of the pancreatic beta-cell. *Diabetes* 35:1163, 1986.
78. Malaisse WJ, Malaisse-Lagae F, Sener A: The glycolytic cascade in pancreatic cells. *Diabetologia* 23:1, 1982.
79. Hellman B: B-cell cytoplasmic Ca^{2+} balance as a determinant for glucose-stimulated insulin-release. *Diabetologia* 28:494, 1985.
80. Charles MA, Laweck J, Pictet R, Grodsky GM: Insulin secretion: Interrelationships of glucose, cyclic adenosine 3′5′-monophosphate and calcium. *J Biol Chem* 250:6134, 1976.
81. Wollheim CB, Pozzan T: Correlation between cytosolic free Ca^{2+} and insulin release in an insulin-secreting cell line. *J Biol Chem* 259:2262, 1984.
82. Wollheim CB, Ullrich S, Meda P, Vallar L: Regulation of exocytosis in electronically permeabilized insulin-secreting cells: Evidence for Ca^{++} dependent secretion. *Biosci Rep* 7:443, 1987.
83. Porte D Jr, Pupo AA: Insulin responses to glucose: Evidence for a two-pool system in man. *J Clin Invest* 48:2309, 1969.
84. Permutt MA: Effect of glucose on initiation and elongation rates in isolated rat pancreatic islets. *J Biol Chem* 248:2738, 1974.
85. Moore B, Edie ES, Abram JH: On the treatment of diabetes mellitus by acid extract of duodenal mucous membrane. *Biochem J* 1:28, 1906.
86. Creutzfeldt W: The incretin concept today. *Diabetologia* 16:75, 1979.
87. Ebert R, Creutzfeldt W: Influence of gastric inhibitory polypeptide antiserum on glucose-induced insulin secretion in rats. *Endocrinology* 111:1601, 1982.
88. Anderson DK: Physiological effects of GIP in man, in Bloom SR, Polak JM (eds): *Gut Hormones*. Edinburgh, New York, Churchill Livingstone, 1981, p 256.
89. Mazzaferri EL, Ciofalo L, Waters LA, et al: Effects of gastric inhibitory polypeptide on leucine and arginine-stimulated insulin release. *Am J Physiol* 245:E114, 1983.
90. Sener A, Malaisse-Lagae F, Malaisse WJ: Stimulation of pancreatic islet metabolism and insulin release by a nonmetabolizable amino acid. *Proc Natl Acad Sci USA* 78:5460, 1981.
91. Crespin SR, Greenough WB III, Steinberg D: Stimulation of insulin secretion by long-chain free fatty acids: A direct pancreatic effect. *J Clin Invest* 52:1979, 1973.
92. Owen OE, Reichard GA Jr, Markus H, et al: Rapid intravenous sodium acetate infusion in man: Metabolic and kinetic responses. *J Clin Invest* 52:2606, 1973.
93. Porte D Jr, Smith PH, Ensinck JW: Neurohumoral regulation of the pancreatic islet A and B cells. *Metabolism* 25(Suppl 1):1453, 1976.
94. Hamburg S, Hendler R, Sherwin RS: Epinephrine: Exquisite sensitivity to its diabetogenic effects in normal man. *Clin Res* 27:252A, 1979.
95. Bergman RN, Miller RE: Direct enhancement of insulin secretion of vagal stimulation of the isolated pancreas. *Am J Physiol* 225:481, 1973.
96. Martin JM, Konijnendijk W, Bouman PR: Insulin and growth hormone secretion in rats with ventromedial hypothalamic lesions maintained on restricted food intake. *Diabetes* 23:203, 1974.
97. Lebovitz HE, Feldman JM: Pancreatic biogenic amines and insulin secretion in health and disease. *Fed Proc* 32:1797, 1973.
98. Robertson RP, Chem M: A role for prostaglandin E in defective insulin secretion and carbohydrate intolerance in diabetes mellitus. *J Clin Invest* 60:747, 1977.
99. Metz SA, Murphy RC, Fujimoto W: Effects of glucose-induced insulin secretion of lipoxygenase-derived metabolites of arachidonic acid. *Diabetes* 33:119, 1984.
100. Green IC, Perrin D, Penman E, et al: Effect of dynorphin on insulin and somatostatin secretion: Calcium uptake and cAMP levels in isolated rat islets of Langerhans. *Diabetes* 32:685, 1983.
101. Gerich JE, Raptis S, Rosenthal J: Somatostatin symposium. *Metabolism* 27(Suppl 1):1, 1978.
102. Sullivan SJ, Schonbrunn A: Characterization of somatostatin receptors which mediate inhibition of insulin secretion in RINm5F cells. *Endocrinology* 121:544, 1987.
103. Wahren J, Felig P: Influence of somatostatin on carbohydrate disposal and absorption in diabetes mellitus. *Lancet* 2:1213, 1976.
104. Krejs GJ, Orci L, Conlon JM, et al: Somatostatinoma syndrome: Biochemical, morphologic and clinical features. *N Engl J Med* 301:285, 1979.
105. Ipp E, Dobbs E, Arimura A, Unger RH: Release of immunoreactive somatostatin from the pancreas in response to glu-

cose, amino acids, pancreozymin-cholecystokinin and tolbutamide. *J Clin Invest* 60:760, 1977.

106. Bjorntorp P, de Jounge C, Sjostrom L: The effect of physical training on insulin production in obesity. *Metabolism* 19:631, 1970.
107. Felig P, Marliss E, Cahill GF Jr: Plasma amino acid levels and insulin secretion in obesity. *N Engl J Med* 281:811, 1969.
108. Felig P, Wahren J, Hendler R: Influence of oral glucose ingestion on splanchnic glucose and amino acid metabolism. *Diabetes* 24:468, 1975.
109. Katz J, McGarry JD: The glucose paradox. Is glucose a substrate for liver metabolism? *J Clin Invest* 74:1901, 1981.
110. DeFronzo RA, Ferrannini E, Hendler R, et al: Regulation of splanchnic and peripheral glucose uptake by insulin and hyperglycemia in man. *Diabetes* 32:35, 1983.
111. Radziuk J: Glucose and glycogen metabolism following glucose ingestion in man: A turnover method, in Cobelli C, Bergman RN (eds): *Carbohydrate Metabolism.* New York, Wiley, 1981, p. 239.
112. Newgard CB, Moore SV, Foster DW, McGarry JD: Efficient hepatic glycogen synthesis in refeeding rats requires continued carbon flow through the gluconeogenic pathway. *J Biol Chem* 259:6958, 1984.
113. Shulman GI, Rothman DL, Smith D, et al: Mechanism of liver glycogen repletion in vivo by nuclear resonance spectroscopy. *J Clin Invest* 76:1229, 1985.
114. Magnusson I, Chandramouli V, Schumann WC, et al: Direct versus indirect pathways of glucose conversion to glycogen in humans. *Clin Res* 34:726A, 1986.
115. Chiasson JL, Liljenquist JE, Finger FE, Lacy WW: Differential sensitivity of glycogenolysis and gluconeogenesis to insulin infusions in dogs. *Diabetes* 25:283, 1976.
116. Davis SN, McGuinness OP, Cherrington AD: Insulin action in vivo, in Alberti KGMM, Krale LP (eds): *The Diabetes Annual/5.* New York, Elsevier, 1990, pp 585–614.
117. Bergman RN: Integrated control of hepatic glucose metabolism. *Fed Proc* 36:256, 1977.
118. Wahren J, Felig P, Cerasi E, Luft R: Splanchnic and peripheral glucose and amino acid metabolism in diabetes mellitus. *J Clin Invest* 51:1870, 1972.
119. Bergman RN, Beir JR, Hourigan PM: Intraportal glucose infusion matched to oral glucose absorption: Lack of evidence for "gut factor" involvement in hepatic glucose storage. *Diabetes* 31:27, 1982.
120. Ishida T, Chap Z, Chou J, et al: Differential effects of oral peripheral intravenous and intraportal glucose on hepatic glucose uptake and insulin and glucagon extraction in conscious dogs. *J Clin Invest* 72:590, 1983.
121. Adkins BA, Myers SR, Hendrick GK, Stevenson RW, Williams PE, Cherrington AD: Importance of the route of intravenous glucose delivery to hepatic glucose balance in the conscious dog. *J Clin Invest* 79:557, 1987.
122. Adkins-Marshall BA, Myers SR, Hendrick CK, Williams PE, Triebwasser K, Floyd B, Cherrington AD: Interaction between insulin and glucose delivery route in the regulation of net hepatic glucose uptake in conscious dogs. *Diabetes* 39:87, 1990.
123. Myers SR, Biggers DW, Neal DW, Cherrington AD: Intraportal glucose delivery enhances the effects of hepatic glucose load on net hepatic glucose uptake *in vivo. J Clin Invest* 88:158, 1991.
124. Felig P, Wahren J, Sherwin RS, Palaiologos G: Protein and amino acid metabolism in diabetes mellitus. *Arch Intern Med* 137:507, 1977.
125. Domalik LJ, Feldman JM: Carbohydrate metabolism and surgery, in Bergman M, Sicard GA (eds): *Surgical Management of the Diabetic Patient.* New York, Raven Press, 1991, pp 3–16.
126. Mayer M, Shafrir E: Glucocorticoid- and insulin-mediated reguation of skeletal muscle protein catabolism, in Shafrir E, Renold AE (eds): *Lessons from Animal Diabetes.* London, Libbey, 1984, p 235.
127. Dahlman B, Schroeter C, Herbertz L, Reinauer H: Myofibrillar protein degradation and muscle proteinase in normal and diabetic rats. *Biochem Med* 21:33, 1979.
128. Björntorp P, Ottosson M, Rebuffé-Scrive M, Xu X: Regional obesity and steroid hormonal interactions in human adipose tissues, in Bray G, Ricquier D, Spiegelmanon B (eds): *Obesity: Towards a Molecular Approach.* UCLA symposia. New York, Liss, 1990, p 147.
129. Björntorp P: Obesity and diabetes, in Alberti KGMM, Krall LP (eds): *The Diabetes Annual/5.* Amsterdam, Elsevier, 1990, pp 373–395.
130. Sherwin RS, Hendler RG, Felig P: Effect of diabetes mellitus and insulin on the turnover and metabolic response to ketones in man. *Diabetes* 25:776, 1976.
131. DeFronzo RA, Sherwin RS, Dillingham M et al: Influence of basal insulin and glucagon secretion on potassium and sodium metabolism: Studies with somatostatin in normal dogs and in normal and diabetic human beings. *J Clin Invest* 61:426, 1978.
132. DeFronzo RA: The effect of insulin on renal sodium metabolism: A review with clinical implications. *Diabetologia* 21:165, 1981.
133. Kahn CR, Crettaz M: Insulin receptors and the molecular mechanism of insulin action, in DeFronzo RA (ed): *Diabetes/Metabolism Reviews.* New York, Wiley, 1985, vol 1, p 5.
134. Häring H, Obermaier-Kusser B: The insulin receptor: Its role in insulin action and in the pathogenesis of insulin resistance, in Alberti KGMM, Krall LP (eds): *The Diabetes Annual/5*, Amsterdam, Elsevier, 1990, pp 537–567.
135. Hedo JA, Kasuga M, Van Obberghen E, et al: Direct demonstration of glycosylation of insulin receptor subunits by biosynthetic and external labeling: Evidence of heterogeneity. *Proc Natl Acad Sci USA* 78:4791, 1981.
136. Kahn CR, Freychet P, Neville DM Jr, Roth J: Quantitative aspects of the insulin-receptor interactions in liver plasma membranes. *J Biol Chem* 249:2249, 1984.
137. DeMeyts P, Bianco AR, Roth J: Site-site interactions among insulin receptors. Characterization of the negative cooperativity. *J Biol Chem* 251:1187, 1976.
138. Olefsky JM, Chang H: Insulin binding to adipocytes: Evidence for functionally distinct receptors. *Diabetes* 27:946, 1978.
139. Pollet RJ, Kampner ES, Standaert ML, Haase BA: Structure of the insulin receptor of cultured human lymphoblastoid cells IM-9: Evidence suggesting that two subunits are required for insulin binding. *J Biol Chem* 257:894 1982.
140. Massague J, Pilch PF, Czech MP: Electrophoretic resolution of three major insulin receptor structures with unique subunit stoichiometries. *Proc Natl Acad Sci USA* 77:7137, 1980.
141. Crettaz M, Jialal I, Kasuga M, Kahn CR: Insulin receptor regulation and desensitization in rat hepatoma cells: The loss of the oligomeric forms of the receptor correlates with the change in receptor affinity. *J Biol Chem* 259:11542, 1984.
142. Spiegel AM, Grerschik P, Levine MA, Downs AW Jr: Clinical implication of guanine nucleotide-binding proteins as receptor-effector couplers. *N Engl J Med* 312:26, 1985.
143. Yip CC, Hsu H, Hawley DM, Maddox BA, Goldfine ID: Localization of the insulin-binding site to the cysteine-rich region of the insulin-receptor α-subunit. *Biochem Biophys Res Comun* 157:321, 1988.
144. Kadowaki H, Kadowaki T, Marcus-Samuels B, Cama A, Rovina A, Taylor SI: Site-directed mutagenesis of position 460 in the α-subunit of the insulin receptor alters cooperative site-site interactions in insulin binding. *Diabetes* 38:A8, 1988.
145. McClair D, Mosthaf U, Ullrich A: Properties of the two naturally occurring alternative forms of the insulin receptor. *Diabetes* 38:A1, 1989.
146. Frias I, Waugh SM: Probing the α-α subunit interface re-

gion in the insulin receptor, location of interhalf disulfide(s). *Diabetes* 38:A238, 1989.

147. Hedo AJ, Kasuga M, Van Oberghen E, Roth J, Kahn CR: Direct demonstration of glycosylation of insulin receptor subunits by biosynthesis and external labelling: Evidence for heterogeneity. *Proc Natl Acad Sci USA* 78:4791, 1981.
148. Ebina Y, Araki E, Taira M, Shimada F, Craik CS, Siddle K, Pierce SB, Roth RA, Rutter WJ: Replacement of lysine residue 1030 in putative ATP-binding region of the insulin receptor abolishes insulin and antibody-stimulated glucose uptake and receptor kinase activity. *Proc Natl Acad Sci USA* 84:704, 1987.
149. Odawara M, Yamamoto R, Kadowaki T, Shiba P, Shibaski Y, Mikami Y, Metsuura N, Tabakaku F, et al: Mutation in ATP-binding site of insulin receptor in an insulin resistant patient. *Diabetes* 38:A66, 1989.
150. Hiedenreich KA, Zahniser NR, Berhanu P, et al: Structural differences between insulin receptors in the brain and peripheral target tissues. *J Biol Chem* 258:8527, 1983.
151. Jeong-Hyok I, Meezan E, et al: Isolation and characterization of human erythrocyte insulin receptors. *J Biol Chem* 258:5021, 1983.
152. King GL, Buzney SM, Kahn CR, et al: Differential responsiveness to insulin of endothelial and support cells from micro- and macrovessels. *J Clin Invest* 71:974, 1983.
153. Saucier J, Dube JY, Tremblay RR: Specific insulin binding sites in rat testis: Characterization and variations. *Endocrinology* 190:2220, 1981.
154. Posner BI: Insulin receptors in human and animal placental tissue. *Diabetes* 23:209, 1974.
155. Hedo JA, Kahn CR, Hayashi M, et al: Biosynthesis and glycosylation of the insulin receptors: Evidence for a single polypeptide precursor of the two major subunits. *J Biol Chem* 258:10020, 1983.
156. Carpentier J-L, Gorden P, Freychet P, et al: Lysosomal association of internalized ^{125}I-insulin in isolated hepatocytes: Direct demonstration by quantitative electron microscopic autoradiography. *J Clin Invest* 63:1249, 1979.
157. Marshall S: Kinetics of insulin receptor biosynthesis and membrane insertion: Relationship to cellular function. *Diabetes* 32:319, 1983.
158. Marshall S, Olefsky JM: Separate intracellular pathways for insulin receptor recycling and insulin degradation in isolated rat adipocytes. *Cell Physiol* 117:195, 1983.
159. Posner BI, Kahn MN, Bergeron JJM: Internalization of insulin: Structures involved and significance, in Vranic M, Hollenberg CH, Steiner G (eds): *Comparison of Type I and Type II Diabetes*. New York, Plenum, 1985, p. 159.
160. Kalant N, Osaki H, Mackubo B, et al: Downregulation of insulin binding by human and rat hepatocytes in primary cultures: The possible role of insulin internalization and degradation. *Endocrinology* 114:37, 1984.
161. Kasuga M, Zick Y, Blithe OL, et al: Insulin stimulation of phosphorylation of the β-subunit of the insulin receptor: Formation of both phosphoserine and phosphotyrosine. *J Biol Chem* 257:9891, 1982.
162. Gammeltoft S, Van Obberghen E: Protein kinase activity of the insulin receptor. *Biochem J* 235:1, 1986.
163. Tornquist HE, Pierce MW, Frackelton AR: Identification of insulin receptor tyrosine kinase residues autophosphorylated in vitro. *J Biol Chem* 262:10212, 1987.
164. Tornquist HE, Avruch J: Relationship of site-specific β subunit tyrosine autophosphorylation to insulin activation of the insulin receptor (tyrosine) protein kinase activity. *J Biol Chem* 263:4593, 1988.
165. Schenker E, Kohanski RA: Conformational states of the insulin receptor. *Biochem Biophys Res Commun* 157:140, 1988.
166. Rosen OM: After insulin binds. *Science* 237:1452, 1987.
167. White M, Tayakama Y, Kahn CR: Differences in the sites of phosphorylation of the insulin receptor in vivo and in vitro. *J Biol Chem* 260:9470, 1985.
168. Häring HU, White MF, Machicao F, Ermel B, Schleicher B, Obermaier B: Insulin rapidly stimulates phosphorylation of a 46 KDa membrane protein on tyrosine residues as well as phosphorylation of several soluble proteins in intact fat cells. *Proc Natl Acad Sci USA* 84:113, 1987.
169. Machicao F, Häring HU, White MF, Carrascosa JM, Obermair B, Wieland OH: A 180,000 molecular weight protein is an endogenous subrate for the insulin receptor associated tyrosine kinase in human placenta. *Biochem J* 243:787, 1987.
170. Jacobs S, Sahyoun NE, Saltiel AR, Cuatrecasas P: Phorbol esters stimulate the phosphorylation of receptors for insulin and somatomedin C. *Proc Natl Acad Sci USA* 80:6211, 1983.
171. Takayama S, White MF, Lauris V, Kahn CR: Phorbol esters modulate insulin receptor phosphorylation and insulin action in cultured hepatoma cells. *Proc Natl Acad Sci USA* 81:7797, 1984.
172. Cohen S, Ushiro H, Stoscheck C, Chinkers M: A native 170,000 epidermal growth factor receptor-kinase complex from shed plasma membrane vesicles. *J Biol Chem* 257: 1523, 1982.
173. Ek B, Heldin CH: Characterization of a tyrosine-specific kinase activity in human fibroblast membranes stimulated by platelet-derived growth factor. *J Biol Chem* 257:10486, 1982.
174. Jacobs S, Kull FC Jr, Earp HS, et al: Somatomedin-C stimulates the phosphorylation of the subunit of its own receptor. *J Biol Chem* 258:9581, 1983.
175. Koepfer-Hobelsberger B, Wieland OH: Insulin activates phospholipase C in fat cells: Similarity with the activation of pyruvate dehydrogenase. *Mol Cell Endocrinol* 36:1123, 1984.
176. Sale G, Fujita-Yamaguchi Y, Kahn CR: Evidence that the insulin receptor is associated with phosphatidylinositol kinase activity. *Eur J Biochem* 155:345, 1986.
177. Berridge MJ: Inositol triphosphate and diacylglycerol as second messengers. *Biochemistry* 220:345, 1984.
178. Rozengurt E, Rodriguez-Pena A, Coombs M, Sinnett-Smith J: Diacylglycerol stimulates DNA synthesis and cell division in mouse 3T3 cells: Role of Ca^{2+}-sensitive phospholipid-dependent protein kinase. *Proc Natl Acad Sci USA* 81:5748, 1984.
179. Obermaier-Kusser B, Häring HU, Muhlbacher CH: Insulin increases the binding of λS-GTP to isolated plasma membrane in rat skeletal muscle and rat fat cells. *Diabetes* 38:172, 1989.
180. Levine R: Insulin: The effects and mode of action of the hormone. *Vitam Horm* 39:145, 1982.
181. Larner J: Mediators of postreceptor insulin action. *Am J Med* 74:38, 1983.
182. Gottschalk WK, Jarett L: Intracellular mediators of insulin action, in DeFronzo RA (ed): *Diabetes/Metabolism Reviews*. New York, Wiley, 1985, p 229.
183. Czech MP, Kim-Tak Y, Lewis RF, et al: Insulin receptor kinase and its mode of signaling membrane components, in DeFronzo RA (ed): *Diabetes/Metabolism Reviews*. New York, Wiley, 1985, p 59.
184. Horuk R, Olefsky JM: Postbinding effects of insulin action, in DeFronzo RA (ed): *Diabetes/Metabolism Reviews*. New York, Wiley, 1985, p 33.
185. Susuki K, Kono T: Evidence that insulin causes translocation of glucose transport activity to the plasma membrane from an intracellular storage site. *Proc Natl Acad Sci USA* 77:2542, 1980.
186. Cushman SW, Wardzala LJ: Potential mechanisms of insulin action on glucose transport in the isolated rat adipose cell: Apparent translocation of intracellular transport systems to the plasma membrane. *J Biol Chem* 255:4758, 1980.
187. Unger RH: Diabetic hyperglycemia: Link to impaired glucose transport in pancreatic β cells. *Science* 251:1200, 1991.

188. Gluts and diabetes (editorial). *Lancet* 337:1517, 1991.
189. Bell GI, Kayamo T, Buse JB, et al: Molecular biology of mammalian glucose transporters. *Diabetes Care* 13:198, 1990.
190. Pilch PF: Glucose transporters: What's in a name? *Endocrinology* 126:3, 1990.
191. Bourey RE, Koranyi L, James DE, Mueckler M, Permutt MA: Effects of altered glucose homeostasis on glucose transporters expression in skeletal muscle in the rat. *J Clin Invest* 86:542, 1990.
192. Orci L, Ravazzola M, Baetens D, et al: Evidence that down regulation of β cell glucose transporters in non-insulin dependent diabetes may be the cause of diabetic hyperglycemia. *Proc Natl Acad Sci USA* 87:9953, 1990.
193. Johnson JH, Crider BP, McCorkle K, Alford M, Unger GH: Inhibition of glucose transport into rat islet cells by immunoglobulins from patients with new-onset insulin-dependent diabetes mellitus. *N Engl J Med* 322:653, 1990.
193a. Cushman SW, Wardzala LJ, Simpson IA, et al.: Insulin-induced translocation of intracellular glucose transporters of the isolated rat adipose cell. *Fed Proc* 43:2251, 1984.
194. Denton RM, Brownsey RW, Belsham GJ, et al: A partial view of the mechanism of insulin action. *Diabetologia* 21:347, 1981.
195. Gabbay RA, Lardy HA: Site of insulin inhibition of cAMP-stimulated glycogenolysis: cAMP-dependent protein kinase is affected independent of cAMP changes. *J Biol Chem* 259:6052, 1984.
196. Mato JM, Kelly KL, Abler A, Jarett L: Identification of a novel insulin-sensitive glycophospholipid from H35 hepatoma cells. *J Biol Chem* 262, 1987.
197. Alexander MC, Kowaloff EM, Witters LA, et al: Purification of a 123,000 dalton hormone-stimulated ^{32}P-peptide and its identification as ATP-citrate lyase. *J Biol Chem* 254:8052, 1979.
198. Seals JR, Czech MP: Characterization of a pyruvate dehydrogenase activator released by adipocyte plasma membranes in response to insulin. *J Biol Chem* 256:6529, 1981.
199. Roth J, et al: Receptors for insulin, NSILA-S and growth hormone: Applications to disease states in man. *Recent Prog Horm Res* 31:95, 1975.
200. Flier JS, Kahn CR, Roth J: Receptors, antireceptor antibodies and mechanisms of insulin resistance. *N Engl J Med* 300:413, 1979.
201. Hedo JA, McElduff A, Taylor SI: Defects in receptor biosynthesis in patients with genetic forms of extreme insulin resistance. *Trans Assoc Am Physicians* 97:151, 1984.
202. Greenberger G, Zick Y, Gorden P: Defect in phosphorylation of insulin receptors in cells from an insulin resistant patient with insulin binding. *Science* 223:932, 1984.
203. Arner P, Pollare T, Lithell H, Livingston JN: Defective insulin receptor tyrosine kinase in human skeletal muscle in obesity and type 2 (non-insulin dependent) diabetes mellitus. *Diabetologia* 30:437, 1987.
204. Brillon DJ, Freidenberg GR, Henry RR, Olefsky JM: Mechanism of defective insulin-receptor kinase activity in NIDDM: Evidence for two receptor populations. *Diabetes* 38:397, 1989.
205. Obermaier-Kusser B, White MF, Pongratz D, Su Z, Ermel B, Mühlbacher CM, Häring HU: A defective intramolecular autoactivation cascade may cause the reduced kinase activity in the skeletal muscle insulin receptor from patients with non-insulin dependent diabetes mellitus. *J Biol Chem* 264:9497, 1989.
206. Freidenberg DR, Reichart D, Olefsky JM, Henry RR: Reversibility of defective adipocyte insulin receptor kinase activity in non-insulin dependent diabetes mellitus. *J Clin Invest* 82:1398, 1988.
206a. Olefsky JM: The insulin receptor: Its role in the insulin resistance of obesity and diabetes. *Diabetes* 25:1154, 1976.
207. Kahn BB: Facilitative glucose transporters: Regulatory mechanisms and dysregulation in diabetes. *J Clin Invest* 89:1367, 1992.
208. DeFronzo RA, Bonadonna RC, Ferrannini E: Pathogenesis of NIDDM: A balanced overview. *Diabetes Care* 15:318, 1992.
209. Houmard JA, Egan PC, Neufer PD, et al: Elevated skeletal muscle glucose transporter levels in exercise trained middle-aged men. *Am J Physiol* 261:E437, 1991.
210. Douen AG, Ramlal T, Rastagi S, et al: Exercise induces recruitment of the "insulin-responsive glucose transporter." *J Biol Chem* 265:13427, 1990.
211. DeFronzo RA, Soman V, Sherwin RS, et al: Insulin binding to monocytes and insulin action in human obesity, starvation and refeeding. *J Clin Invest* 62:204, 1978.
212. Duckworth WC, Stentz FB, Heinemann M, Kitabchi AE: Initial site of insulin cleavage by insulin protease. *Proc Natl Acad Sci USA* 76:635, 1979.
213. Rabkin R, Simon N, Steiner S, Colwell JA: Effect of renal disease on renal uptake and excretion of insulin in man. *N Engl J Med* 282:182, 1970.
214. Orci L: The microanatomy of the islets of Langerhans. *Metabolism* 25:1303, 1976.
215. Moody AJ, Frandsen EK, Jacobson H, et al: The structural and immunologic relationship between gut GLI and glucagon. *Metabolism* 25(Suppl 1):1336, 1976.
216. Ravazzola M, Orci L: Glucagon and glicentin immunoreactivity are topographically segregated in the A granule of the human pancreatic cell. *Nature* 284:66, 1980.
217. Unger RH: Glucagon in diabetes, in Alberti KGMM, Krall LP (eds): *The Diabetes Annual*. New York, Elsevier, 1985, p 480.
218. Moody AJ, Thim L: Glucagon, glicentin and related peptides, in Lefebvre PJ (ed): *Glucagon*. Berlin, Springer-Verlag, 1983, p 139.
219. Kuku SF, Jaspan JB, Emmanouel DS, et al: Heterogeneity of plasma glucagon. *J Clin Invest* 58:742, 1976.
220. Barnes AJ, Bloom SR, Alberti KGMM, et al: Ketoacidosis in pancreatectomized man. *N Engl J Med* 296:1250, 1977.
221. Koranyi F, Peterfy F, Szabo J, et al: Evidence for transformation of glucagon-like immunoreactivity of gut into pancreatic glucagon *in vivo*. *Diabetes* 30:792, 1981.
222. Holst JJ, Holst-Pedersen J, Baldissera F, Stadil F: Circulating glucagon after total pancreatectomy in man. *Diabetologia* 25:396, 1983.
223. Geraud JC, Elroy R, Moody AJ, et al: Glucagon-glicentin immunoreactive cells in the lumen of the digestive tract. *Cell Tissue Res* 213:121, 1980.
224. Boden G, Owen OE: Familial hyperglucagonemia—an autosomal dominant trait. *N Engl J Med* 296:534, 1977.
225. Sherwin RS, Felig P: Glucagon physiology in health and disease, in McCann SM (ed): *International Review of Physiology*, vol. 16: *Endocrine Physiology*. Baltimore, University Park, 1977, p 151.
226. Giugliano D, Cozzolino D, Ceriello A, Salvatore T, Paolisso G, Torella R: Beta endorphin and islet hormone release in humans: Evidence for interference with cAMP. *Am J Physiol* 256:E361, 1989.
227. Unger RH: Glucagon physiology and pathophysiology in the light of new advances. *Diabetologia* 28:574, 1985.
228. Raskin P, Pietri A, Unger RH: Changes in glucagon levels after four to five weeks of glucoregulation by portable insulin infusion pumps. *Diabetes* 28:1033, 1979.
229. DeFeo P, Perriello G, Torlone E, Fanelli C, Ventura MM, Santeusanio F, Brunetti P, Gerich JS, Boll GB: Evidence against important catecholamine compensation for absent glucagon counterregulation. *Am J Physiol* 260:E203, 1991.
230. Fujii S, Tamai H, Kumia M, Takaichi Y, Nakasawa T, Aoki TT: Impaired glucagon secretion to insulin-induced hypoglycemia in anorexia nervosa. *Acta Endocrinol (Copenh)* 120:610, 1989.
231. Diem P, Redman JB, Abid M, Moran A, Sutherland DB, Halter JB, Robertson RP: Glucagon, catecholamine and pancreatic polypeptide secretion in Type I diabetic recipients of pancreas allografts. *J Clin Invest* 86:2008, 1990.

232. Ar'Rajab, Ahren B, Alumets J, Bengmonk S: Islet transplantation to the renal subcapsular space in streptozotocin diabetes in rats: Long-term effects on insulin and glucagon secretion. *Acta Chir Scand* 155:503, 1989.
233. Patel DG, Skau KA: Effects of chronic sodium salicylate feedings on the impaired glucagon and epinephrine responses to insulin-induced hypolgycemia in streptozotocin-diabetic rats. *Diabetologia* 32:61, 1989.
234. Cherrington AD, Chiasson JL, Liljenquist JE, et al: The role of insulin and glucagon in the regulation of basal glucose production in the postabsorptive dog. *J Clin Invest* 58:1407, 1976.
235. Boden G, Tappy L, Jadali F, Hoeldtke RD, Rezvani I, Owen OS: Role of glucagon in disposal of an amino acid load. *Am J Physiol* 259:E225, 1990.
236. Fradkin J, Shamoon H, Felig P, Sherwin RS: Evidence for an important role of changes in rather than absolute concentrations of glucagon in the regulation of glucose production in man. *J Clin Endocrinol Metab* 50:698, 1980.
237. Komjati M, Bratusch-Marrain P, Waldhausl W: Superior efficacy of pulsatile versus continuous hormone exposure on hepatic glucose production in vitro. *Endocrinology* 118:312, 1986.
238. Felig P, Wahren J, Sherwin RS, Hendler R: Insulin, glucagon and somatostatin in normal physiology and diabetes mellitus. *Diabetes* 25:1091, 1976.
239. Sherwin RS, Fisher M, Hendler R, Felig P: Hyperglucagonemia and blood glucose regulation in normal, obese and diabetic subjects. *N Engl J Med* 294:455, 1976.
240. Lopez MP, Gomez-Lechon MJ, Castell JV: Role of glucose, insulin and glucagon in glycogen mobilization in human hepatocytes. *Diabetes* 40:263, 1991.
241. DeDiego JG, Gorden P, Carpentier J-L: The relationship of ligand receptor mobility to internalization of polypeptide hormones and growth factors. *Endocrinology* 128:2136, 1991.
242. Unson CG, MacDonald D, Ray K, Durrah TL, Merrifield RB: Position G replacement analogs of glucagon uncouple biological activity and receptor binding. *J Biol Chem* 266:2763, 1991.
243. Rodbell M: The actions of glucagon at its receptor: Regulation of adenylate cyclase, in Lefebvre P (ed): *Glucagon.* Berlin, Springer-Verlag, 1983, p. 263.
244. Rodbell M: Programmable messengers: A new theory of hormone action. *Trends Biochem Sci* 10:461, 1985.
245. Ruiz-Grande C, Pintado J, Alarcon C, Castilla C, Valverde I, Lopez-Novoa JM: Renal catabolism of human glucagon-like peptides 1 and 2. *Can J Physiol Pharmacol* 68:1568, 1990.
246. Sherwin RS, Fisher M, Bessoff J, et al: Hyperglucagonemia in cirrhosis: Altered secretion and sensitivity to glucagon. *Gastroenterology* 74:1224, 1978.
247. Deibert DC, DeFronzo RA: Epinephrine-induced insulin resistance in man. *J Clin Invest* 65:717, 1980.
248. Eigler N, Sacca L, Sherwin RS: Synergistic interactions of physiologic increments of glucagon, epinephrine, and cortisol in the dog: A model for stress-induced hyperglycemia. *J Clin Invest* 63:114, 1979.
249. Sacca L, Sherwin R, Felig P: Influence of somatostatin on glucagon- and epinephrine-stimulated hepatic glucose output in the dog. *Am J Physiol* 236:E113, 1979.
250. Gerich J, Davis J, Lorenzi M, et al: Hormonal mechanisms of recovery from insulin-induced hypoglycemia in man. *Am J Physiol* 236:E380, 1979.
251. Garvey WT, Huecksteadt TB, Lima FE, et al: Expression of a glucose transporter gene cloned from cellular models of insulin resistance: Dexamethasone decreases transporter mRNA in primary cultured adipocytes. *Mol Endocrinol* 3:1132, 1989.
252. Orskov L, Schmitz O, Jorgensen JO, et al: Influence of growth hormone on glucose-induced glucose uptake in normal men as assessed by the hyperglycemic clamp technique. *J Clin Endocrinol Metab* 68:276, 1989.
253. Merimee TJ, Felig P, Marliss E, et al: Glucose and lipid homeostasis in the absence of human growth hormone. *J Clin Invest* 50:574, 1971.
254. Daughaday WH, Hall K. Salvion WD Jr, et al: On the nomenclature of the somatomedins and insulin-like growth factors. *J Clin Endocrinol Metab* 65:1075, 1987.
255. Froesch ER, Zapf J: Insulin-like growth factors and insulin: Comparative aspects. *Diabetologia* 28:485, 1985.
256. Daughaday WH, Emanuell UA, Brooks MH, et al: Synthesis and secretion of insulin-like growth factor II by a leiomyosarcoma with associated hypoglycemia. *N Engl J Med* 319:1434, 1988.
257. Adrian TE, Uttenthal LO, Williams SJ, et al: Secretion of pancreatic polypeptide in patients with pancreatic endocrine tumors. *N Engl J Med* 315:287, 1986.
258. Felig P, Sherwin RS, et al: Hormonal interactions in the regulation of blood glucose. *Recent Prog Horm Res* 35:501, 1979.
259. Dineen S, Gerich J, Rizza R: Carbohydrate metabolism in non-insulin dependent diabetes mellitus. *N Engl J Med* 327:707, 1992.
260. Felig P: The metabolic events of starvation. *Am J Med* 60:117, 1976.
261. Felig P, Wahren J: Fuel homeostasis in exercise. *N Engl J Med* 293:1078, 1975.
262. Cryer PE, Gerich JE: Glucose counterregulation, hypoglycemia and intensive insulin therapy of diabetes mellitus. *N Engl J Med* 313:232, 1985.
263. Sacca L, Sherwin R, Hendler R, Felig P: Influence of continuous physiologic hyperinsulinemia on glucose kinetics and counterregulatory hormones in normal and diabetic humans. *J Clin Invest* 63:849, 1979.
264. Mann RJ: Historical vignette: "Honey urine" to pancreatic diabetes: 600 B.C.–1922. *Mayo Clin Proc* 46:56, 1971.
265. Fajans SS: Scope and heterogenous nature of MODY. *Diabetes Care* 13:49, 1990.
266. Cox NJ, Xiang K-S, Fajans SS, Bell GI: Mapping diabetes susceptibility genes: Lessons learned from research for a DNA marker for maturity onset diabetes of the young. *Diabetes* 41:401, 1992.
267. Froguel P, Vaxillaire M, Sun F, et al: Close linkage of glucokinase locus on chromosome 7p to early onset non-insulin dependent diabetes mellitus. *Nature* 256:162, 1992.
268. Thai A-C, Eisenbarth GS: Natural history of IDDM. *Diabetes Rev* 1:1, 1993.
269. Rossini AA, Greiner DL, Freidman HP, et al: Immunopathogenesis of diabetes mellitus. *Diabetes Rev* 1:43, 1993.
270. Zonana J, Rimoin DL: Current concepts in genetics: Inheritance of diabetes mellitus. *N Engl J Med* 295:603, 1976.
271. Olmos R, A'Hern R, Heaton DA, et al: The significance of the concordance rate for Type I (insulin dependent) diabetes in identical twins. *Diabetologia* 31:747, 1989.
272. Muir A, Schatz DA, Maclaren NK: The pathogenesis, prediction and prevention of insulin-dependent diabetes mellitus. *Endocrinol Metab Clin North Am* 21:199, 1992.
273. Julier C, Hyer RN, Davies J, et al: Insulin-IGF 2 region on chromosome 11p encodes a gene implicated in HLA-DR4 dependent diabetes susceptibility. *Nature* 354:155, 1991.
274. Leahy JL, Boyd AE: Diabetes genes in non-insulin dependent diabetes mellitus. *N Engl J Med* 328:56, 1993.
275. Groop LC, Kankuri M, Schalin-Jantti, et al: Association between polymorphism of the glycogen synthase gene and non-insulin dependent diabetes mellitus. *N Engl J Med* 328:10, 1993.
276. Maclaren N, Atkinson M: Is insulin-dependent diabetes mellitus environmentally induced? *N Engl J Med* 327:348, 1992.
277. Yoon JW, Austin M, Onodera T, Notkins AL: Virus-induced diabetes mellitus: Isolation of a virus from the pancreas of a child with diabetic ketoacidosis. *N Engl J Med* 300:1173, 1979.
278. Schattner A, Rager-Zisman B: Virus-induced autoimmunity. *Rev Infect Dis* 12:204, 1990.

279. Kaufman DL, Erlander MG, Clare-Salzer M, et al: Autoimmunity to two forms of glutamate decarboxylase in insulin-dependent diabetes mellitus. *J Clin Invest* 89:283, 1992.
280. Karjalainen J, Martin J, Knip M, et al: A bovine albumin peptide as a possible trigger of insulin-dependent diabetes mellitus. *N Engl J Med* 327:302, 1992.
281. Stiller CR, Dupre J, Gent M, et al: Effects of cyclosporine immunosuppression in insulin-dependent diabetes of recent onset. *Science* 223:1362, 1985.
282. Skyler JS, Marks JB: Immune intervention in type I diabetes mellitus. *Diabetes Rev* 1:15, 1993.
283. Srikanta S, Ganda OP, Gleason RE, et al: Pre-type I diabetes: Linear loss of beta cell response to intravenous glucose. *Diabetes* 33:717, 1984.
284. Bingley PJ, Bonifacio E, Shattock M, et al: Can islet cell antibodies predict IDDM in the general population? *Diabetes Care* 16:45, 1993.
285. Bleich D, Jackson RA, Soeldner JS, et al: Analysis of metabolic progression to Type I diabetes in ICA + relatives of patients with Type I diabetes. *Diabetes Spect* 4:204, 1991.
286. Rossetti L, Giaccari A, DeFronzo RA: Glucose toxicity. *Diabetes Care* 13:610, 1990.
287. Pfeifer MA, Halter JB, Porte D Jr: Insulin secretion in diabetes mellitus. *Am J Med* 70:579, 1981.
288. DeFronzo RA, Hendler R, Simonson D: Insulin resistance is a prominent feature of type 1 (juvenile-onset) diabetes mellitus. *Diabetes* 31:795, 1982.
289. Proietto J, Nankervis A, Aitken P, et al: Glucose utilization in type 1 (insulin-dependent) diabetes: Evidence for a defect not reversible with acute duration in insulin. *Diabetologia* 25:331, 1983.
290. Pedersen O, Hjolland E: Insulin receptor binding to fat and blood cells and insulin action in fat cells from insulin dependent diabetes. *Diabetes* 31:706, 1982.
291. Caruso G, Proietto J, Calenti A, Alford F: Insulin resistance in alloxan-diabetic dogs: Evidence for reversal following insulin therapy. *Diabetologia* 25:273, 1983.
292. Warram JH, Martin BC, Krolewski AS, et al: Slow glucose removal rate and hyperinsulinemia precede the development of type II diabetes in the offspring of diabetic parents. *Ann Intern Med* 113:909, 1990.
293. Mitrakou A, Kelley D, Mokan M, et al: Role of reduced suppression of glucose production and diminished early insulin release in impaired glucose tolerance. *N Engl J Med* 326:22, 1992.
294. Johnson KH, O'Brien T, Betsholtz C, Westermark P: Islet amyloid polypeptide: Mechanisms of amyloidogenesis in the pancreatic islets and potential roles in diabetes mellitus. *Lab Invest* 66:522, 1990.
295. Steiner DF, Ohagi S, Nagamatsu S, et al: Is islet amyloid polypeptide a significant factor in pathogenesis or pathophysiology of diabetes? *Diabetes* 40:305, 1991.
296. Kosaka K, Kuzuya T, Akanuma Y, et al: Increase in insulin response after treatment of overt maturity onset diabetes mellitus is independent of the mode of treatment. *Diabetologia* 18:23, 1980.
297. Reaven GM, Bernstein R, Davis B, Olefsky JM: Nonketotic diabetes mellitus: Insulin deficiency or insulin resistance. *Am J Med* 60:80, 1976.
298. DeFronzo RA, Deibert D, Felig P, Soman V: Insulin sensitivity and insulin binding to monocytes in maturity onset diabetes. *J Clin Invest* 63:939, 1979.
299. Gulli G, Ferrannini E, Stern M, et al: The metabolic profile of NIDDM is fully established in glucose tolerant offspring of two Mexican-American NIDDM parents. *Diabetes* 41: 1575, 1992.
300. DeFronzo RA, Ferrannini E, Simonson DC: Fasting hyperglycemia in non-insulin dependent diabetes mellitus: Contributions of excessive hepatic glucose production and impaired glucose uptake. *Metabolism* 38:387, 1989.
301. Shulman GI, Rothman DL, Jue T, et al: Quantitation of muscle glycogen synthesis in normal subjects and subjects with non-insulin dependent diabetes by 13 C nuclear magnetic resonance spectroscopy. *N Engl J Med* 322:223, 1990.
302. Kolterman OG, Gray RS, Griffin J, et al: Receptor and postreceptor defects contribute to the insulin resistance in noninsulin-dependent diabetes mellitus. *J Clin Invest* 68:957, 1981.
303. Taylor SI, Cama A, Accili D, et al: Genetic basis of endocrine disease: I. Molecular genetics of insulin resistant diabetes mellitus. *J Clin Endocrinol Metab* 73:1158, 1991.
304. Reaven GM: Role of insulin resistance in human disease. *Diabetes* 37:1595, 1988.
305. DeFronzo RA, Ferrannini E: Insulin resistance: A multifaceted syndrome responsible for NIDDM, obesity, hypertension, dyslipidemia and atherosclerotic cardiovascular disease. *Diabetes Care* 14:173, 1991.
306. Ferrannini E, Buzzigoli G, Bonadonna R, et al: Insulin resistance in essential hypertension. *N Engl J Med* 317:350, 1987.
307. Helmrich SP, Ragland DR, Leung RW, et al: Physical activity and reduced occurrence of non-insulin dependent diabetes mellitus. *N Engl J Med* 325:147, 1991.
308. Gerich JE, Langlois M, Noacco C, et al: Lack of glucagon responses to hypoglycemia in diabetes: Evidence for an intrinsic alpha cell defect. *Science* 182:171, 1973.
309. Tamborlane WV, Sherwin RS, Koivisto V, et al: Normalization of the growth hormone and catecholamine response to exercise in juvenile onset diabetics treated with a portable insulin infusion pump. *Diabetes* 28:785, 1979.
310. Felig P, Wahren J, Hendler R: Influence of maturity onset diabetes on splanchnic glucose balance after oral glucose ingestion. *Diabetes* 27:121, 1978.
311. Felig P, Wahren J: Renal substrate exchange in human diabetes. *Diabetes* 24:730, 1975.
312. Owen OE, Felig P, Morgan AP, Wahren J, Cahill GF Jr: Liver and kidney metabolism during prolonged starvation. *J Clin Invest* 48:574, 1969.
313. Buse MG, Hertong HF, Wiegand DA: The effect of diabetes, insulin and the redox potential on leucine metabolism by isolated rat hemidiaphragm. *Endocrinology* 98:1166, 1976.
314. Murthy VK, Shipp JC: Regulation of hepatic triglyceride synthesis in diabetic rats. *J Clin Invest* 67:923, 1981.
315. Brunzell JD, Chait A, Bierman EL: Plasma lipoproteins in human diabetes mellitus, in Alberti KGMM, Krall LP (eds): *Diabetes Annual*. New York, Elsevier, 1985, p 463.
316. Garfinkel AS, Nilsson-Ehle P, Schotz MC: Regulation of lipoprotein lipase induction by insulin. *Biochim Biophys Acta* 424:265, 1976.
317. Krausz Y, Bar-On H, Shafrir E: Origin and pattern of glucocorticoid-induced hyperlipidemia in rats: Dose-dependent bimodal changes in serum lipids and lipoproteins in relation to hepatic lipogenesis and tissue lipoprotein lipase activity. *Biochim Biophys Acta* 663:69, 1981.
318. Levy E, Shafrir E, Ziv E, Bar-On H: Composition, removal and metabolic fate of chylomicrons derived from diabetic rats. *Biochim Biophys Acta* 834:376, 1985.
319. Hollenbeck CB, Connor WE, Riddle MC, et al: The effects of a high-carbohydrate, low-fat cholesterol-restricted diet on plasma lipid, lipoproteins, and apoprotein concentrations in insulin-dependent (type I) diabetes mellitus. *Metabolism* 34:559, 1985.
320. Fraze E, Donner CC, Swislock A, et al: Ambient plasma free fatty acid concentrations in noninsulin dependent diabetes mellitus: Evidence for insulin resistance. *J Clin Endocrinol Metab* 61:807, 1985.
321. Taskinen MR, Bogardus C, Kennedy A, Howard BV, Multiple disturbances of free fatty acid metabolism in noninsulin-dependent diabetes. *J Clin Invest* 76:637, 1985.
322. Feingold KR, Lear SR, Moser AH: De novo cholesterol synthesis in three different animal models of diabetes. *Diabetologia* 26:234, 1984.
323. Brownlee M, Vlassara H, Cerami A: Nonenzymatic glycosylation products of collagen covalently trap low-density lipoprotein. *Diabetes* 34:938, 1985.

324. Bergman M, Gidez LI, Eder HA: High density lipoprotein subclasses in diabetes. *Am J Med* 81:488, 1986.
325. Bergman M, Gidez LI, Eder HA: The effect of glipizide on HDL and HDL subclasses. *Diabetes Res* 3:245, 1986.
326. Laakso M, Voutilainen E, Pyörälä K, Sarlund H: Association of low HDL and HDL_2 cholesterol with coronary heart disease in noninsulin-dependent diabetics. *Arteriosclerosis* 5:653, 1985.
327. Sherwin RS: Limitations of the oral glucose tolerance test in the diagnosis of early diabetes. *Primary Care* 44:255, 1977.
328. Davidson MB: The effect of aging carbohydrate metabolism: A review of the English literature and a practical approach to the diagnosis of diabetes mellitus in the elderly. *Metabolism* 28:688, 1979.
329. Lohmann D, Liebold F, Heilmann W: Diminished insulin response in highly trained athletes. *Metabolism* 27:521, 1978.
330. Bennett PH: Epidemiologic studies of diabetes in the Pima Indians. *Recent Prog Horm Res* 31:333, 1976.
331. Sisk CW, Burnham CE, Stewart J, McDonald GW: Comparison of the 50 and 100 gram oral glucose tolerance test. *Diabetes* 19:852, 1970.
332. Schleicher ED, Gerbitz KD, Dolhofer R, et al: Clinical utility of nonenzymatically glycosylated blood proteins as an index of glucose control. *Diabetes Care* 7:548, 1984.
333. Little RR, England JD, Wiedmeyer HM, Goldstein DE: Glycosylated hemoglobin measured by affinity chromatography: Microsample collection and room temperature storage. *Clin Chem* 29:1080, 1983.
334. Marrero DG, Vandagriff JL, Gibson R, et al: Immediate HbA_{1c} results: Performance of new HbA_{1c} system in pediatric outpatient population. *Diabetes Care* 15:1045, 1992.
335. Zimmet P: Kelly West lecture 1991: Challenges in diabetes epidemiology—from West to the rest. *Diabetes Care* 15:232, 1992.
336. Gepts W: Sequential changes in the cytological composition of the pancreatic islets in juvenile diabetes, in Bajaj JS (ed): *Diabetes,* International Congress Series. Amsterdam, Excerpta Medica, 1977, p 299.
337. Karam JH, Rosenthal M, O'Donnell JL, et al: Discordance of diabetic microangiopathy in identical twins. *Diabetes* 25:24, 1976.
338. Kalant N: Diabetic glomerulosclerosis: Current status. *Can Med Assoc J* 119:146, 1978.
339. Bronstein HD, Kantrowtiz P, Schaffner R: Marked enlargement of the liver and transient ascites associated with the treatment of diabetic acidosis. *N Engl J Med* 261:1314, 1959.
340. Levin ME, Boisseau AV, Avioli LV: Effects of diabetes mellitus on bone mass in juvenile and adult onset diabetes. *N Engl J Med* 294:241, 1976.
341. L'Esperance F: Diabetic retinopathy. *Med Clin North Am* 62:767, 1978.
342. Davis MD: Diabetic retinopathy: A clinical overview. *Diabetes Care* 15:1844, 1992.
342a. Raskin P, Arauz-Pacheco C: The treatment of diabetic retinopathy. A view for the internist. *Ann Intern Med* 117:226, 1992.
342b. Ferris FL: How effective are treatments for diabetic retinopathy. *JAMA* 269:1290, 1993.
343. The Diabetic Retinopathy Study Group: Four risk factors for severe visual loss in diabetic retinopathy. *Arch Ophthalmol* 97:654, 1979.
344. Early Treatment Diabetic Retinopathy Study Research Group: Early photocoagulation for diabetic retinopathy: Early Treatment Diabetic Retinopathy Study Report Number 9. *Ophthalmology* 98(suppl):766, 1991.
345. Early Treatment Diabetic Retinopathy Study Research Group: Effects of aspirin treatment on diabetic retinopathy: Early Treatment Diabetic Retinopathy Study Report Number 8. *Ophthalmology* 98(suppl):757, 1991.
346. Charles S: Pars plana vitrectomy for traction retinal detachment, in Little HL et al (eds): *Diabetic Retinopathy.* New York, Thieme-Stratton, 1984, p 305.
347. Krolewski AS, Caness M, Warram J, et al: Predisposition to hypertension and susceptibility to renal disease in insulin dependent diabetes mellitus. *N Engl J Med* 318:140, 1988.
348. Christiansen JS, Gammelguard J, Troneir B, et al: Kidney function and size in diabetes before and during insulin treatment. *Kidney Int* 21:683, 1982.
349. Hostetter TH, Troy JL, Brenner BM: Glomerular hemodynamics in experimental diabetes mellitus. *Kidney Int* 19:410, 1981.
350. Hostetter TH, Rennke HG, Brenner BM: The case for intrarenal hypertension in the initiation and progression of diabetic and other glomerulopathies. *Am J Med* 72:375, 1982.
351. Zatz R, Meyer TW, Rennke HG, Brenner BM: Predominance of hemodynamic rather than metabolic factors in the pathogenesis of diabetic glomerulopathy. *Proc Natl Acad Sci USA* 82:5967, 1985.
352. Wiseman MJ, Saunders AJ, Keen H, Viberti GC: Effect of blood glucose control on increased glomerular filtration rate and kidney size in insulin-dependent diabetes. *N Engl J Med* 312:617, 1985.
353. Mauer SM, Steffes MW, Ellis EN, et al: Structural-functional relationship in diabetic nephropathy. *J Clin Invest* 74:1143, 1984.
354. Beisswenger PJ, Spiro RG: Studies on the human glomerular basement membrane: Composition, nature of the carbohydrate units and chemical changes in diabetes mellitus. *Diabetes* 22:180, 1973.
355. Schober E, Pollak A, Coradello H, Lubec G: Glycosylation of glomerular basement membrane in type I (insulin-dependent) diabetic children. *Diabetologia* 23:485, 1982.
356. Cohen MP, Surma ML: [^{35}S]Sulfate incorporation into glomerular basement membrane glycosaminoglycans is decreased in experimental diabetes. *J Lab Clin Med* 98:715, 1981.
357. Osterby R: Early phases in the development of diabetic glomerulopathy. A quantitative electron microscopic study. *Acta Med Scand* [Suppl.] 574:3, 1974.
358. Mogensen CE, Christensen CK: Predicting diabetic nephropathy in insulin-dependent patients. *N Engl J Med* 311:89, 1984.
359. Viberti GC, Bilous RW, Mackintosh D: Long term correction of hyperglycemia and progression of renal failure in insulin dependent diabetes. *Br Med J* 286:598, 1983.
360. Goldstein DA, Massry SG: Diabetic nephropathy: Clinical course and effect of hemodialysis. *Nephron* 20:286, 1978.
361. Parving H-H, Andersen AR, Smidt UM, et al: Effect of antihypertensive treatment on kidney function in diabetic nephropathy. *Br Med J* 294:1443, 1987.
362. Zatz R, Dunn BR, Meyer TW, Brenner B: Prevention of diabetic glomerulopathy by pharmacological amelioration of glomerular capillary hypertension. *J Clin Invest* 77:1925, 1986.
362a. Lewis EJ, Hunsicker LG, Bain RP, Rohde RD, et al.: The effect of angiotensin-converting-enzyme inhibition on diabetic nephropathy. *N Engl J Med* 329:1456; 1993.
363. Mathiesen ER, Hommel E, Giese J, Parving HH: Efficacy of captopril in postponing nephropathy in normotensive insulin-dependent diabetic patients with microalbuminuria. *Br Med J* 303:81, 1991.
364. Jerums G, Allen TJ, Tsalamandris C, et al: Angiotensin converting enzyme inhibition and calcium channel blockade in incipient diabetic nephropathy. *Kidney Int* 41:904, 1992.
365. Amair P, Khanna R, Leibel B, et al: Continuous ambulatory peritoneal dialysis in diabetics with end-stage disease. *N Engl J Med* 306:625, 1982.
366. Mauer MS, Barbosa J, Vernier RL, et al: Development of diabetic vascular lesions in normal kidneys transplanted into patients with diabetes mellitus. *N Engl J Med* 295:916, 1976.

367. Sutherland DER, Morrow CE, et al: Improved patient and primary renal allograft survival in uremic diabetic recipients. *Transplantation* 34:319, 1982.
368. Khauli RB, Norick AC, Brawn WE, et al: Improved results of cadaver renal transplantation in the diabetic patient. *J Urol* 130:867, 1983.
369. Braddom RL, Hollis JB, Castell DO: Diabetic peripheral neuropathy: A correlation of nerve conduction studies and clinical findings. *Arch Phys Med Rehabil* 58:308, 1977.
370. Ward JD, Fisher DJ, Barnes CG, et al: Improvements in nerve conduction following treatment in newly diagnosed diabetics. *Lancet* 1:428, 1971.
371. Vinik AI, Holland MT, LeBeau JM, et al: Diabetic neuropathies. *Diabetes Care* 15:1926, 1992.
372. Smith SA, Smith SE: Reduced papillary light reflexes in diabetic autoimmune neuropathy. *Diabetologia* 24:330, 1983.
373. Ellenberg M: Diabetic neuropathic cachexia. *Diabetes* 23: 418, 1974.
374. Saunders RN: Platelets and atherosclerosis. *Prog Drug Res* 24:49, 1985.
375. Curtiss LK, Witztum JL: Plasma apolipoproteins AI, AII, B, C, and E are glucosylated in hyperglycemic diabetes subjects. *Diabetes* 34:452, 1985.
376. Fein FS, Sonnenblick EH: Diabetic cardiomyopathy. *Prog Cardiovasc Dis* 27:255, 1987.
377. Braverman IM: Cutaneous manifestations of diabetes mellitus. *Med Clin North Am* 55:1019, 1971.
378. Bagdade JD, Nielson K, Root R, Bulger R: Host defense in diabetes mellitus: The feckless phagocyte during poor control and ketoacidosis. *Diabetes* 19:364, 1970.
379. Rosenbloom AL, Silverstein JH, Lezotte DC, et al: Limited joint mobility in childhood diabetes indicates increased risk for microvascular disease. *N Engl J Med* 305:191, 1981.
380. Siperstein MD, Foster DW, Knowles HC, et al: Control of blood glucose and diabetic vascular disease. *N Engl J Med* 296:1060, 1977.
381. Siperstein MD, Unger RH, Madison LL: Studies of muscle capillary basement membranes in normal subjects, diabetic and prediabetic patients. *J Clin Invest* 47:1973, 1968.
382. Kilo C, Vogler N, Williamson JR: Muscle capillary basement membrane changes related to aging and to diabetes mellitus. *Diabetes* 21:881, 1972.
383. Steffes MW, Sutherland DER, Goetz FC: Studies of kidney and muscle biopsy specimens from identical twins discordant for type I diabetes mellitus. *N Engl J Med* 312:1282, 1985.
384. Bennett PH: The basement membrane controversy. *Diabetologia* 16:280, 1979.
385. Feingold KR, Lee TH, Chung MY, Siperstein MD: Muscle capillary membrane width in patients with Vacor-induced diabetes mellitus. *J Clin Invest* 78:102, 1986.
386. Ireland JT, Patnaik BK, Duncan LJP: Glomerular ultrastructure in secondary diabetes and normal subjects. *Diabetes* 16:628, 1967.
387. Bonman SO, Tyden G, Wilcek H, et al: Prevention of kidney graft diabetic nephropathy by pancreas transplantation in man. *Diabetes* 34:306, 1985.
388. Simmonds DA, Winegrad AI, Martin DB: Significance of tissue myoinositol concentrations in metabolic regulation in nerve. *Science* 217:848, 1982.
389. Finegold D, Lattimer SA, Nolle S, et al: Polyol pathway activity and myo-inositol metabolism: A suggested relationship in the pathogenesis of diabetic neuropathy. *Diabetes* 32:988, 1983.
390. Gillon RKW, Hawthorne JN, Tomlinson DR: Myo-inositol and sorbitol metabolism in relation to peripheral nerve function in experimental diabetes in the rat: The effect of aldose reductase inhibition. *Diabetologia* 25:365, 1983.
391. Green DA, Lattimer SA: Impaired rat sciatic nerve sodium-potassium adenosine triphosphatase in acute streptozotocin diabetes and its correction by dietary myo-inositol supplementation. *J Clin Invest* 72:1058, 1983.
392. Summerfield JA, Vergalla J, Jones EA: Modulation of a glycoprotein recognition system on rat hepatic endothelial cells by glucose and diabetes mellitus. *J Clin Invest* 69:1337, 1982.
393. Jones RL, Peterson CM: Hematologic alterations in diabetes mellitus. *Am J Med* 70:339, 1981.
394. Dolhofer R, Siess EA, Wieland OH: Nonenzymatic glycation of immunoglobulins leads to an impairment of immunoreactivity. *Biol Chem Hope Seylers* 366:361, 1985.
395. Brownlee M, Vlassara H, Cerami A: Nonenzymatic glycosylation reduces the susceptibility of fibrin to degradation by plasma. *Diabetes* 32:680, 1983.
396. Liang JN, Hershorin LL, Chylack LT Jr: Non-enzymatic glycosylation in human diabetic lens crystellins. *Diabetologia* 29:225, 1986.
397. Schnider SL, Kohn RR: Effects of age and diabetes mellitus on the solubility and nonenzymatic glucosylation of human skin collagen. *J Clin Invest* 67:1630, 1981.
398. McMillan DE, Utterback NG, La Puma J: Reduced erythrocyte deformability in diabetes. *Diabetes* 27:895, 1978.
399. Tan JS, Anderson JL, Watanakunakorn C, et al: Neutrophil dysfunction in diabetes mellitus. *J Lab Clin Med* 85:26, 1975.
400. Bassiouny AR, Rosenberg H, McDonald TL: Glucosylated collagen is antigenic. *Diabetes* 32:1182, 1983.
401. Pirart J: Diabetes mellitus and its degenerative complications: A prospective study of 4400 patients observed between 1947 and 1973. *Diabetes Care* 1:168, 1:252, 1978.
402. Eschwege E, Job D, Guyot-Argenton C, et al: Delayed progression of diabetic retinopathy by divided insulin administration: A further followup. *Diabetologia* 16:131, 1979.
403. Engerman R, Bloodworth JMB Jr, Nelson S: Relationship of microvascular disease in diabetes to metabolic control. *Diabetes* 26:760, 1977.
404. Bretzel RG, Brocks DG, Federlin KF; Reversal and prevention of nephropathy by islet transplantation in diabetic rats, in Shafrir E, Renold AE (eds): *Lessons from Animal Diabetes*. London, Libbey, 1984, p 425.
405. Engerman R, Kern T: Progression of incipient diabetic retinopathy during good glycerine control. *Diabetes* 36:808, 1987.
406. Lauritzen T, Frost-Larsen K, Larsen HW, Deckert T: Two year experience with continuous subcutaneous insulin infusion in relation to retinopathy and neuropathy. *Diabetes* 34:74, 1985.
407. Brinchman-Hansen D, Dahl-Jorgensen K, Hannsen KF, Sandvik L, et al: The response of diabetic retinopathy to 41 months of multiple insulin injections, insulin pumps and conventional insulin therapy. *Arch Ophthalmol* 106:1242, 1988.
408. Reichard P, Nilsson BY, Rosenquist U: The effect of long term intensified insulin treatment on the development of microvascular complications of diabetes mellitus. *N Engl J Med* 329:304, 1993.
409. Protocol for the clinical trial to assess the relationship between metabolic control and early vascular complications of insulin-dependent diabetics. *Diabetes* 31:1132, 1982.
409a. DCCT Research Group: The effect of intensive treatment of diabetes on the development and progression of long-term complications in insulin-dependent diabetes mellitus. *N Engl J Med* 329:977, 1993.
410. DCCT Research Group: Epidemiology of severe hypoglycemia in the Diabetes Control and Complications Trial. *Am J Med* 90:450, 1991.
411. Tamborlane WV, Puklin J, Bergman M, et al: Long-term improvement of metabolic control with the insulin pump does not reverse diabetic microangiopathy. *Diabetes Care* 5(suppl 1):58, 1982.
412. Holman RR, Dornan TL, Mayor-White V, et al: Prevention of deterioration of renal and sensory nerve function by more intensive management of insulin-dependent diabetic patients: A two-year randomized prospective study. *Lancet* 1:204, 1983.

413. Raskin P, Pietri AO, Unger R, et al: The effect of diabetic control on the width of skeletal-muscle capillary basement membrane in patients with type I diabetes mellitus. *N Engl J Med* 309:1546, 1983.
414. Mauer SM, Miller K, Goetz FC, et al: Immunopathology of renal extracellular membranes in kidneys transplanted into patients with diabetes mellitus. *Diabetes* 25:709, 1976.
415. Knowles H: Long-term juvenile diabetes treated with unmeasured diet. *Trans Assoc Am Physicians* 85:95, 1971.
416. Dorman JS, LaPorte RE: Mortality in insulin-dependent diabetes, in *Diabetes in America,* NIH publication 85-1468. Washington, D.C., U.S. Government Printing Office, 1985.
417. Felig P, Bergman M: Insulin pump treatment of diabetes. *JAMA* 250:1045, 1983.
418. Tattersall RB: Self-monitoring of blood glucose 1978–1984, in Alberti KGMM, Krall LP (eds): *Diabetes Annual.* New York, Elsevier, 1985, vol. 1.
419. Mazze RS, Shammoon H, Pasmantier R, et al.: Reliability of blood glucose monitoring by patients with diabetes mellitus. *Am J Med* 77:211, 1984.
420. Fineberg SE, Galloway JA, Fineberg NS, et al: Immunogenicity of recombinant DNA human insulin. *Diabetologia* 25:465, 1983.
421. Kang S, Creagh FM, Peters JR, et al: Comparison of subcutaneous soluble human insulin and insulin analogues (Asp^{B9} Glu^{B27} Asp^{B10} Asp^{B28}) on meal-related plasma glucose excursions in type 1 diabetic subjects. *Diabetes Care* 14: 571, 1991.
422. Revers RR, Henry R, Schmeiser L, et al: The effects of biosynthetic human proinsulin on carbohydrate metabolism. *Diabetes* 33:762, 1984.
423. Galloway JA: Treatment of NIDDM with insulin agonists or substitutes. *Diabetes Care* 13:1209, 1990.
423a. Johannsson B-L, Linde B, Wahren J: Effects of C-peptide on blood-flow and capillary diffusion capacity in exercising forearm in young IDDM patients. *Diabetes* 41(Suppl 1):195A, 1992.
424. Cryer PE, Gerich JE: Glucose counterregulation, hypoglycemia, and intensive insulin therapy in diabetes mellitus. *N Engl J Med* 25:232, 1985.
425. Campbell PJ, Bolli GB, Cryer PE, Gerich JE: Pathogenesis of the dawn phenomenon in patients with insulin-dependent diabetes mellitus. *N Engl J Med* 312:1473, 1985.
426. Jones TW, Caprio S, Diamond MP, Hallarman L, Boulware SD, Sherwin AS, Tamborlane WV: Does insulin species modify counterregulatory hormone response to hypoglycemia? *Diabetes Care* 14:728, 1991.
427. Patrick AW, Bodmer CW, Tieszen KI, et al: Human insulin and awareness of acute hypoglycemic symptoms in insulin-dependent diabetes. *Lancet* 338:528, 1991.
428. Bergman M, Felig P: Self-monitoring of blood glucose levels in diabetes: Principles and practice. *Arch Intern Med* 144: 2029, 1984.
429. Felig P, Bergman M: Intensive ambulatory treatment of insulin-dependent diabetes. *Ann Intern Med* 97:225, 1982.
430. Hirsch IB, Farkas-Hirsch R, Skyler JS: Intensive insulin therapy for treatment of type 1 diabetes. *Diabetes Care* 13:1265, 1990.
431. Self-monitoring of blood glucose: Clinical practice recommendations: American Diabetes Association, 1990–1991. *Diabetes Care* 14(Suppl 2):57, 1991.
431a. Amiel SA, Sherwin RC, Simonson DC, Tamborlane WV: Effect of intensive insulin therapy on glycemia thresholds for counterregulatory hormone release. *Diabetes* 37:901, 1988.
432. Felig P, Bergman M: Newer approaches to the control of the insulin-dependent diabetic patient. *Dis Mon* 29:, No. 7, 1983.
433. Pickup JC, White MC, Keen H, et al: Long-term continuous subcutaneous insulin infusions in diabetics at home. *Lancet* 2:870, 1979.
434. Tamborlane WV, Sherwin RS, Genel H, Felig P: Restoration of normal lipid and amino acid metabolism in diabetic patients treated with a portable insulin infusion pump. *Lancet* 1:1258, 1979.
435. Tamborlane WV, Sherwin RS, Genel M, Felig P: Outpatient treatment of juvenile-onset diabetes with a preprogrammed portable subcutaneous insulin infusion system. *Am J Med* 68:190, 1980.
436. Conference on Insulin Pump Therapy in Diabetes: Multicenter Study of Effect on Microvascular Disease. Wilson RN (ed): *Diabetes* 35(Suppl 3), 1985.
437. Clarke W, Haymond M, Santiago J: Overnight basal insulin requirements in fasting insulin-dependent diabetes. *Diabetes* 29:78, 1980.
438. Service F, Rizza R, Westand R, et al: Considerations for the programming of an open-loop insulin infusion device from the biostator glucose controller. *Diabetes Care* 3:278, 1980.
439. Buysschaert M, Marchand E, Ketelslagers JM, Lambert AE: Comparison of plasma glucose and plasma free insulin during CSII and intensified conventional insulin therapy. *Diabetes Care* 6:1, 1983.
439a. Continuous subcutaneous insulin infusion: Clinical practice recommendations: American Diabetes Association 1992–1993. *Diabetes Care* 16(Suppl 2):35, 1993.
439b. Home PD, Alberti KGMM: Insulin Therapy, in Alberti KGMM, DeFronzo R, Keen H, Zimmet P (eds): *International Textbook of Diabetes Mellitus.* Chichester, Wiley 1992, pp 831–863.
440. Peden NR, Braaten JT, McKendry JBR: Diabetic ketoacidosis during long-term treatment with continuous subcutaneous insulin infusion. *Diabetes Care* 7:1, 1984.
441. Lougheed WD, Woulfe-Flanagan H, Clement JR, Albisser AM: Insulin aggregation in artificial delivery systems. *Diabetologia* 19:1, 1980.
442. Freedman DJ, Wolfe BM, Mascarennas M: Ketoacidosis resulting from precipitation of insulin in syringe used for delivery of constant subcutaneous insulin infusion. *Lancet* 1:828, 1983.
443. Mecklenburg RS, Guinn TS: Complications of insulin pump therapy: The effect of insulin preparation. *Diabetes Care* 8:367, 1985.
444. Teutsch SM, Herman WH, Dweyer DM, Lane JM: Mortality among diabetic patients using continuous subcutaneous insulin infusion. *N Engl J Med* 310:361, 1984.
445. Zinman B: The physiological replacement of insulin: An elusive goal. *N Engl J Med* 321:363, 1989.
446. Beck-Neilsen H, Richelson B, Mogensen CE, et al: Effect of insulin pump treatment for one year on renal function and retinal morphology in patients with IDDM. *Diabetes Care* 8:585, 1985.
447. Lauritzen T, Frost-Larsen K, Larsen HW, Deckut T, the Steno Study Group: Continuous subcutaneous insulin. *Lancet* 1:1445, 1983.
447a. Saudek CD, Duckworth WC, Veterans Affairs Study Group: The Department of Veterans Affairs Implanted Insulin Pump Study. *Diabetes Care* 15:567, 1992.
448. Jet injectors: Clinical practice recommendations: American Diabetes Association, 1990–1991. *Diabetes Care* 14(Suppl 2):50, 1991.
449. Reinaver K-M, Jokoch G, Renn W, et al: Insulin pens in elderly patients (letter). *Diabetes Care* 13:1136, 1990.
450. Murray DP, Keenan P, Gayer E, et al: A randomized trial of the efficacy and acceptability of a pen injector. *Diabetic Med* 5:750, 1988.
451. Tallroth G, Karlson B, Nilsson A, et al: The influence of different insulin regimens on quality of life and metabolic control in insulin dependent diabetes. *Diabetes Res Clin Pract* 6:37, 1989.
452. Goldgewicht C, Slama G, Papoz L, Tchobroutsky G: Hypolgycaemic reactions in 172 type I (insulin-dependent) diabetic patients. *Diabetologia* 24:95, 1983.
453. Turnbridge WMG: Factors contributing to deaths of diabetics under fifty years of age. *Lancet* 2:569, 1981.

454. Gale EAM, Tattersall RB: Unrecognized nocturnal hypoglycemia in insulin-treated diabetics. *Lancet* 1:1049, 1979.
455. DeFronzo R, Hendler R, Christensen N: Stimulation of counterregulatory hormonal responses in diabetic man by a fall in glucose concentration. *Diabetes* 29:125, 1980.
456. MacFarlane PI, Smith S: Perceptions of hypoglycemia in childhood diabetes mellitus: A questionnaire study. *Prac Diabetes* 5:56, 1988.
457. Bolli GB, De Feo P, De Cosmo S, et al: A reliable and reproducible test for adequate glucose counterregulation in type I diabetes mellitus. *Diabetes* 33:732, 1984.
458. Bolli GB, Gottesman IS, Campbell PI, et al: Glucose counterregulation and waning of insulin in the Somogyi phenomenon (posthypoglycemic hyperglycemia). *N Engl J Med* 311:1214, 1984.
459. Cherrington AD, Fuchs H, Stevenson RW, et al: Effect of epinephrine on glycogenolysis and gluconeogenesis in conscious overnight-fasted dogs. *Am J Physiol* 247:E362, 1984.
460. Gale EAM, Kurtz AB, Tattersall RB: In search of the Somogyi effect. *Lancet* 2:279, 1980.
461. Porte D Jr: Sympathetic regulation of insulin secretion: Its relations to diabetes mellitus. *Arch Intern Med* 123:252, 1969.
462. Campbell PJ, Gerich JE: Occurrence of dawn phenomenon without change in insulin clearance in patients with insulin-dependent diabetes mellitus. *Diabetes* 35:749, 1986.
463. Dandona P, Foster M, Healey F, et al: Low dose insulin infusions in diabetic patients with high insulin requirements. *Lancet* 2:283, 1978.
464. Marin G, Rose SR, Kibarian M, et al: Absence of dawn phenomenon in normal children and adolescents. *Diabetes Care* 11:393, 1988.
465. Eichner HL, Lajritano AA, Woertz LL, Selam J-L, Gupta S, Charles MA: Cellular immune alterations with human insulin therapy. *Diabetes Res* 8:111, 1988.
466. Bruni B, Barolo P, Blatto A, Carlins M, Ansaldi SG, Grassi G: Treatment of allergy to heterologous monocomponent insulin with human semisynthetic insulin: Long-term study. *Diabetes Care* 11:59, 1988.
467. Schade DA, Drumm DA, Eaton RP, Sterling WA: Factitious brittle diabetes mellitus. *Am J Med* 78:777, 1985.
467a. Bergman M, Akin SB, Felig P: Understanding the diabetic patient from a psychological dimension: Implications for the patient and provider. *Am J Psychoanal* 50:25, 1990.
468. West KM: Diet therapy of diabetes: An analysis of failure. *Ann Intern Med* 79:425, 1973.
469. Archer JA, Gorden P, Roth J: Defect in insulin binding to receptors in obese man: Amelioration with caloric restriction. *J Clin Invest* 55:166, 1976.
470. Jenkins DJA: Lente carbohydrate: A new approach to the dietary management of diabetes. *Diabetes Care* 5:634, 1982.
471. Crapo PA, Scarlett JA, Kolterman OG: Comparison of the metabolic responses to fructose and sucrose sweetened foods. *Am J Clin Nutr* 36:256, 1982.
472. Bantle JP, Laine DC, Castle GW, et al: Postprandial glucose and insulin responses to meals containing different carbohydrates in normal and diabetic subjects. *N Engl J Med* 309:7, 1983.
473. Wing RR, Marcus MD, Salata R, et al: Effects of a very low-calorie diet on long-term glycemic control in obese type 2 diabetic subjects. *Arch Intern Med* 151:1334, 1991.
474. Anderson JW, Ward K: High carbohydrate, high fiber diets for insulin-treated men with diabetes mellitus. *Am J Clin Nutr* 32:2312, 1979.
475. Anderson JW, Chen WL: Plant fiber carbohydrate and lipid metabolism. *Am J Clin Nutr* 32:346, 1979.
476. Crapo PA, Reaven G, Olefsky J: Post-prandial plasma-glucose and insulin responses to different complex carbohydrates. *Diabetes* 26:1178, 1977.
477. Wahren J, Juhlin-Dannfelt A, Bjorkman O, et al: Influence of fibre ingestion on carbohydrate utilization and absorption. *Clin Physiol* 2:315, 1982.
478. Nutritional recommendations and principles for individuals with diabetes mellitus. *Diabetes Care* 14(Suppl 2):20, 1991.
479. Gerich JE: Oral hypoglycemic agents. *N Engl J Med* 321:1231, 1989.
480. Malaisse WJ, LeBrun P: Mechanisms of sulfonyluria-induced insulin release. *Diabetes Care* 13(Suppl 3):9, 1990.
481. Kreisberg RA: The second-generation sulfonylureas: Change or progress? *Ann Intern Med* 102:125, 1985.
482. Pfeifer MA, Halter JB, Judzewitsch RG, et al: Acute and chronic effect of sulfonylurea drugs on pancreatic islet function in man. *Diabetes Care* 7(Suppl 1):25, 1984.
483. Olefsky JM, Reaven GM: Effects of sulfonylurea therapy on insulin binding to mononuclear leukocytes of diabetic patients. *Am J Med* 60:89, 1976.
484. Judzewitsch RG, Pfeifer MA, Best JD, et al: Chronic chlorpropamide therapy of noninsulin-dependent diabetes augments basal and stimulated insulin secretion by increasing islet sensitivity to glucose. *J Clin Endocrinol Metab* 55:321, 1982.
485. Scarlett JA, Gray RS, Griffin J, et al: Insulin treatment reverses the insulin resistance of type II diabetes mellitus. *Diabetes Care* 5:353, 1982.
486. Firth RG, Bell PM, Rizza RA: Effects of tolazamide and exogenous insulin on insulin action in patients with non-insulin-dependent diabetes mellitus. *N Engl J Med* 314: 1280, 1986.
487. Jackson JE, Bressler R: Clinical pharmacology of sulfonylurea hypoglycemic agents. *Drugs* 22:211, 22:295, 1981.
488. Skillman TG, Feldman JM: The pharmacology of sulfonylureas. *Am J Med* 70:361, 1981.
489. Groop L, Luzl L, Melander A, Groop P-H, Rafhesser K, Simonson DC, DeFronzo RA: Different effects of glyburide and glipizide on insulin secretion in normal and NIDDM subjects. *Diabetes* 36:1320, 1987.
490. Melander A, Bitzen P-O, Faber O, Groop L: Sulphonylurea antidiabetic drugs: An update of their clinical pharmacology and rational therapeutic use. *Drugs* 37:58, 1989.
491. Groop L, Groop P-H, Stenman S, Saloranta C, Tötterman K-J, Fyrquist F, Melander A: Comparison of pharmacokinetics, metabolic effects and mechanism of action of glyburide and glipizide during long-term treatments. *Diabetes Care* 10:671, 1987.
492. Seltzer HS: Drug-induced hypoglycemia: A review of 1418 cases. *Endocrinol Metab Clin North Am* 18:163, 1989.
493. Moses AM, Numann P, Miller M: Mechanisms of chlorpropamide-induced antidiuresis in man: Evidence for release of ADH and enhancement of peripheral action. *Metabolism* 22:59, 1973.
494. Kadowaki T, Hagura R, Kajin H, et al: Chlorpropamide-induced hyponatremia: Incidence and risk factors. *Diabetes Care* 6:468, 1983.
495. Appel GB, D'Agati V, Bergman M, Pirani CL: Nephrotic syndrome and immune complex glomerulonephritis associated with chlorpropamide therapy. *Am J Med* 74:377, 1983.
496. Jackson JE, Bressler R: Clinical pharmacology of sulfonylurea hypoglycaemic agents. *Drugs* 22:211, 1981.
497. Johnston C, Wiles PG, Pyke DA: Chlorpropamide-alcohol flush: The case in favour. *Diabetologia* 26:1, 1981.
498. Hillson RM, Hockaday TNR: Chlorpropamide-alcohol flush: A critical reappraisal. *Diabetologia* 26:6, 1984.
499. The University Group Diabetes Program: A study of the effects of hypoglycemic agents on vascular complications in patients with maturity-onset diabetes. *Diabetes* 19(Suppl 2):747, 1970.
500. Paasikivi J, Wahlberg F: Preventive tolbutamide treatment and arterial disease in mild hyperglycemia. *Diabetologia* 7:323, 1971.
501. Ohneda A, Maruhama Y, Itabashi H, et al: Vascular complications and long-term administration of oral hypoglycemic agents in patients with diabetes mellitus. *Tokoku J Exp Med* 124:205, 1978.

502. Genuth S: Insulin use in NIDDM. *Diabetes Care* 13:1240, 1990.
503. Groop LC, Groop P-H, Stenman S: Combined insulin-sulfonylurea therapy in treatment of NIDDM. *Diabetes Care* 13(Suppl 3):47, 1990.
504. Wu M-S, Johnston P, Sheu W-H-H, et al: Effect of metformin on carbohydrate and lipoprotein metabolism in NIDDM patients. *Diabetes Care* 13:1, 1990.
505. Natrass M, Todd PG, Hinks L: Comparative effects of phenformin, metformin, and glibenclamide on metabolic rhythms in maturity-onset diabetics. *Diabetologia* 13:145, 1977.
506. Conlay LA, Karam JH, Matin SB, Lowenstein JE: Serum phenformin-associated lactic acidosis. *Diabetes* 26:628, 1977.
507. Dandona P, Fonseca V, Mier A, Beckett AG: Diarrhea and metformin in a diabetic clinic. *Diabetes Care* 6:472, 1983.
508. Hermann LS: Biguanides and sultomylineas as combination therapy in NIDDM. *Diabetes Care* 13(Suppl 3):37, 1990.
509. Dimitriadis G, Karaiskos C, Raptis S: Effects of prolonged (6 months) α-glycosidase inhibition on blood glucose control and insulin requirements in patients with insulin-dependent diabetes mellitus. *Horm Metab Res* 18:253, 1986.
510. Johansen K: Acarbose treatment of sulfonylurea-treated non-insulin dependent diabetes: A double-blind, cross-over comparison of an α-glycosidase inhibitor with metformin. *Diabetes Metab* 10:219, 1989.
511. Dimitriadis G, Hatziagellaki E, Alexopoulos E, et al: Effects of α-glucosidase tolerance and timing of insulin administration in patients with type 1 diabetes mellitus. *Diabetes Care* 14:393, 1991.
512. Dimitriadis G, Gerich E: Importance of timing of preprandial subcutaneous insulin administration in the management of diabetes mellitus. *Diabetes Care* 6:374, 1983.
513. Schnack C, Prager RJF, Winkler J, et al: Effects of 8-week α-glucosidase inhibition on metabolic control, C peptide secretion, hepatic glucose output, and peripheral insulin sensitivity in poorly controlled type II diabetic patients. *Diabetes Care* 12:537, 1989.
514. Clissold SP, Edwards G: Acarbose: A preliminary review of its pharmacodynamic and pharmacokinetic properties and therapeutic potential. *Drugs* 35:214, 1988.
515. Foley JE: Rationale and application of fatty acid oxidation inhibitors in treatment of diabetes melliltus. *Diabetes Care* 15:773, 1992.
516. Sherratt HSA, Alberti KGMM: New oral hypoglycaemic drugs, in Alberti KGMM, Krall LP (eds): *The Diabetes Annual/5* Amsterdam, Elsevier, 1990, pp 125–151.
517. Kawazu S, Suzuki M, Negishi K, et al: Initial phase II clinical studies of midaglizole (DG-5128). *Diabetes* 36:221, 1987.
518. Sennitt MV, Arch JRS, Levey AL, et al: Antihyperglycaemic action of BRL 26830, a novel β-adrenoreceptor agonist. *Biochem Pharmacol* 34:1279, 1985.
519. Carrol MJ, Lister CA, Sennitt MV, et al: Improved glycemic control in c57/B1 KsJ (db/db) mice after treatment with the thermogenic β adrenoreceptor agonist BRL 26830. *Diabetes* 34:1198, 1985.
520. Le Marchand-Brustel Y, Olichon-Berltre C, Grémbaux T, et al: Glucose transporter in insulin sensitive tissues of lean and obese mice: Effect of the thermogenic agent BRL 26830A. *Endocrinology* 127:2687, 1990.
521. Hoffman CA, Colca JR: New oral thiazolidinedione antidiabetic agents act as insulin sensitizers. *Diabetes Care* 15:1075, 1992.
522. Calles-Escandon J, Felig P: Symposium on exercise: Physiology and clinical applications: Fuel-hormone metabolism during exercise and after physical training. *Clin Chest Med* 5, 1984.
523. Bergman M, Felig P: Exercise, in DeGroot L, Cahill GF Jr, et al (eds): *Endocrinology*, 2d ed. New York, Grune & Stratton, 1987.
524. Calles-Escandon J, Cunningham JJ, Snyder P, et al: Influence of exercise on urea, creatinine, and 3-methylhistidine excretion in normal human subjects. *Am J Physiol* 246:E334, 1984.
525. Ruderman NB, Ganda OP, Johansen K: The effect of physical training on glucose tolerance and plasma lipids in maturity onset diabetes. *Diabetes* 28(Suppl 1):89, 1979.
526. Richter EA, Ploug-Gulbo H: Increased muscle glucose uptake after exercise: No need for insulin during exercise. *Diabetes* 34:1071, 1985.
527. Koivisto V, Felig P: Effects of acute exercise on insulin absorption in diabetic patients. *N Engl J Med* 298:79, 1978.
528. Felig P, Ali-Cherif MS, Minagawa A, et al: Hypoglycemia during prolonged exercise in normal man. *N Engl J Med* 306:895, 1982.
529. Wahren J, Sato Y, Ostman J, et al: Turnover and splanchnic metabolism of free fatty acids and ketones in insulin-dependent diabetics at rest and in response to exercise. *J Clin Invest* 73:1367, 1984.
530. Wahren J, Felig P, Hagenfeldt L: Physical exercise and fuel homeostasis in diabetes. *Diabetologia* 14:213, 1978.
531. Stratton R, Wilson DP, Enders RK, Goldstein DE: Improved glycemic control after supervised 8-week exercise program in insulin-dependent diabetic adolescents. *Diabetes Care* 10:589, 1987.
532. Wallberg-Henriksson W, Gunnarsson R, Henriksson J, et al: Increased peripheral insulin sensitivity and muscle mitochondrial enzymes but unchanged blood glucose control in type I diabetics after physical training. *Diabetes* 31:1044, 1982.
533. Zawalich W, Maturo S, Felig P: Influence of physical training on insulin release and glucose utilization by islet cells and liver glucokinase activity in the rat. *Am J Physiol* 243:E464, 1982.
534. Prevention of type 1 diabetes mellitus: Clinical practice recommendations: American Diabetes Association 1990–1991. *Diabetes Care* 14(Suppl 2):14, 1991.
535. Laupacis A, Stiller CR, Gardell C, et al: Cyclosporin prevents diabetes in BB Wistar rats. *Lancet* 1:10, 1983.
536. Mori Y, Suko M, Okudaiva H, et al: Preventive effects of cyclosporin on diabetes in NOD mice. *Diabetologia* 29:244, 1986.
537. Sutherland DER, Sibley R, Xu X-Z, et al: Twin-to-twin pancreas transportation: Reversal and reenactment of the pathogenesis of type 1 diabetes. *Trans Assoc Am Physicians* 97:80, 1984.
538. Dhein B, Bartell L, Ferguson RM: Infectious complications and lymphomas in cyclosporine patients. *Transplant Proc* 15(Suppl 1/2):3162, 1983.
539. Rosenthal JT, Iwatsuki S, Starzl TE, et al: Histiocytic lymphoma in renal transplant patients receiving cyclosporine. *Transplant Proc* 15(Suppl 1/2):2805, 1983.
540. Ziegler AG, Herskowitz RD, Jackson RA, et al: Predicting type I diabetes. *Diabetes Care* 13:762, 1990.
541. Sullinger HW, Stratta RJ, D'Alessandro AM, Kalayoglu M, Pirsch JD, Belzer FO: Experience with simultaneous pancreas and kidney transplantation. *Ann Surg* 208:475, 1988.
542. Perkins JD, Engers DE, Munn SR, Barr D, Marsh CL, Carpenter HA: The value of cystoscopically-directed biopsy in human pancreatic duodenal transplantation. *Clin Transplant* 3:306, 1989.
543. McCullough CS, Scharp DW: Pancreas and islet transplantation for the treatment of type 1 diabetes mellitus, in Bergman M, Sicard GA (eds): *Surgical Management of the Diabetic Patient,* New York, Raven Press, 1991, pp 349–361.
544. Sutherland DER: Pancreas and islet transplantation: I. Experimental studies. *Diabetologia* 20:161; II. Clinical trials. *Diabetologia* 20:435, 1981.
545. Sutherland DER, Mondry-Munns KC: International Pancreas Transplant Registry Report, in Terasakai PI (ed): *Clinical Transplants 1988,* Los Angeles, UCLA Tissue Typing Laboratory, 1988, pp 53–64.

546. Katz H, Homan M, Velosa J, et al: Effects of pancreas transplantation on postprandial glucose metabolism. *N Engl J Med* 325:1278, 1991.
547. Fan MY, Lum ZP, Fu XW, Levesque L, Tai IT, Sun AM: Reversal of diabetes in BB rats by transplantation of encapsulated pancreatic islets. *Diabetes* 39:519, 1990.
548. Lanza RP, Borland KM, Lodge P, et al: Treatment of severely diabetic pancreatectomized dogs using a diffusion based hybrid pancreas. *Diabetes* 41:886, 1992.
549. Bilous RW, Mauer SM, Sutherland DER, Najarian JS, Goetz FC, Steffes MW: The effects of pancreas transplantation on glomerular structure of renal allografts: Patients with insulin-dependent diabetes. *N Engl J Med* 321:80, 1989.
550. Kennedy WR, Navarro X, Goetz FC, Sutherland DER, Najarian JS: Effects of pancreatic transplantation on diabetic neuropathy. *N Engl J Med* 322:978, 1990.
551. Selam J-L, Micossi P, Dunn FL, et al: Clinical trial of programmable implantable insulin pump for type I diabetes. *Diabetes Care* 15:877, 1992.
552. Flexner CW, Weiner JP, Saudek CD, Dans PE: Repeated hospitalization for diabetic ketoacidosis: The game of "Sartoris." *Am J Med* 76:691, 1984.
553. Faich GA, Fishbein HA, Ellis SE: The epidemiology of diabetic acidosis: A population-based study. *Am J Epidemiol* 117:551, 1983.
554. Ellemann K, Soerensen JN, Pedersen L, et al: Epidemiology and treatment of diabetic ketoacidosis in a community population. *Diabetes Care* 7:528, 1984.
555. Siperstein MD: Diabetic ketoacidosis and hyperosmolar coma. *Endocrinol Metab Clin North Am* 21:415, 1992.
556. Fery F, Balasse EO: Ketone body production and disposal in diabetic ketosis: A comparison with fasting ketosis. *Diabetes* 34:326, 1985.
557. Vinicor F, Lehrner LM, Karn RG, Merritt AD: Hyperamylasemia in diabetic ketoacidosis: Sources and significance. *Ann Intern Med* 91:200, 1979.
558. Levy LJ, Duga J, Girgis M, Gordon EE: Ketoacidosis associated with alcoholism in nondiabetic subjects. *Ann Intern Med* 78:213, 1978.
559. Fisher JN, Shahshahani MN, Kitabchi AE: Diabetic ketoacidosis: Low dose insulin therapy by various routes. *N Engl J Med* 297:238, 1977.
560. Carol P, Matz R: Uncontrolled diabetes mellitus in adults: Experience in treating diabetic ketoacidosis and hyperosmolar nonketotic coma with low-dose insulin and a uniform treatment regimen. *Diabetes Care* 6:579, 1983.
561. Arieff AL, Kleeman CR: Cerebral edema in diabetic comas: II. Effects of hyperosmolarity, hyperglycemia and insulin in diabetic rabbits. *J Clin Endocrinol Metab* 38:1057, 1974.
562. Lever E, Jaspan JB: Sodium bicarbonate therapy in severe diabetic ketoacidosis. *Am J Med* 75:263, 1983.
563. Fisher JN, Kitabchi AE: A randomized study of phosphate therapy in the treatment of diabetic ketoacidosis. *J Clin Endocrinol Metab* 57:177, 1983.
564. Winegrad AL, Kern EFO, Simmons DA: Cerebral edema in diabetic ketoacidosis. *N Engl J Med* 312:1184, 1985.
565. Rosenbloom AL: Intracerebral crises during treatment of diabetic ketoacidosis. *Diabetes Care* 13:22, 1990.
566. Duck SC, Wyatt DT: Factors associated with brain herniation in the treatment of diabetic ketoacidosis. *J Pediatr* 113:10, 1988.
567. Krane EJ: Diabetic ketoacidosis. *Pediatr Clin North Am* 34:935, 1987.
568. Beigelman PM: Severe diabetic ketoacidosis (diabetic "coma"), 482 episodes in 257 patients: Experience of three years. *Diabetes* 20:490, 1971.
569. Krane EJ, Rockoff MA, Wallman JK, Wolfsdorf JI: Subclinical brain swelling in children during treatment of diabetic ketoacidosis. *N Engl J Med* 312:1147, 1985.
570. Carroll P, Matz R: Adult respiratory distress syndrome complicating severely uncontrolled diabetes mellitus. *Diabetes Care* 5:574, 1982.
571. Guisado R, Arieff AL: Neurologic manifestations of diabetic comas: Correlation with biochemical alterations in the brain. *Metabolism* 24:665, 1975.
572. Arieff AL, Carrol JH: Non-ketotic hyperosmolar coma with hyperglycemia: Clinical features, pathophysiology, renal function, acid-base balance, plasma-cerebrospinal fluid equilibria and the effects of therapy. *Medicine (Baltimore)* 51:73, 1972.
573. Katz JA: Hyperglycemia-induced hyponatremia: Calculation of expected serum sodium depression. *N Engl J Med* 289:843, 1973.
574. Bavli S, Gordon EE: Experimental diabetic hyperosmolar coma in rats. *Diabetes* 20:92, 1971.
575. Malchoff CD, Pohl SL, Kaiser DL, Carey RM: Determinants of glucose and ketoacid concentrations in acutely hyperglycemic diabetic patients. *Am J Med* 77:275, 1984.
576. Turpin P, Duckworth WC, Solomon SS: Simulated hyperglycemic hyperosmolar syndrome: Impaired insulin and epinephrine effects upon lipolysis in the isolated rat fat cell. *J Clin Invest* 63:403, 1979.
577. Joffe BI, Seftel HC, Goldberg R, et al: Factors in the pathogenesis of experimental nonketotic and ketoacidotic diabetic stupor. *Diabetes* 22:653, 1973.
578. Cohen RD: Disorders of lactic acid metabolism. *Clin Endocrinol Metab* 5:613, 1976.
579. Dembo A, Marliss EB, Halperin ML: Insulin therapy in phenformin-associated lactic acidosis: A case report, biochemical considerations and review of the literature. *Diabetes* 24:28, 1975.
580. Coustan DR, Felig P: Diabetes mellitus, in Burrow GN, Ferris TF (eds): *Medical Complications During Pregnancy,* 3d ed. Philadelphia, Saunders, 1986.
581. Freinkel N: Of pregnancy and progeny. *Diabetes* 29:1023, 1980.
582. Hull D, Elphick MC: Evidence for fatty acid transfer across the human placenta, in Beard RW, Hoet JJ (eds): *Pregnancy Metabolism, Diabetes and the Fetus*, Ciba Foundation Symposium no. 63. New York, Excerpta Medica, 1979, p.71.
583. Shafrir E, Khassis S: Maternal-fetal rat transport versus new fat synthesis in the pregnant diabetic rat. *Diabetologia* 22:111, 1982.
584. Diamant YZ, Metzger GE, Freinkel N, Shafrir E: Placental lipid and glycogen content in human and experimental diabetes mellitus. *Am J Obstet Gynecol* 144:5, 1982.
585. Shambaugh GE III: Ketone body metabolism in development, in Meisami E, Tamiras PS (eds): *CRC Handbook of Human Growth and Development Biology,* vol 2. Boca Raton, CRC, 1987.
586. Churchill JA, Berendes HW, Nemore J: Neuropsychological deficits in children of diabetic mothers. *Am J Obstet Gynecol* 105:257, 1969.
587. Naeye RL, Chez RA: Effects of maternal acetonuria and low pregnancy weight gain on children's psychomotor development. *Am J Obstet Gynecol* 139:189, 1981.
588. Stehbens JA, Baker GL, Kitchell M: Outcome at age 1, 3 and 5 years of children born to diabetic women. *Am J Obstet Gynecol* 127:408, 1977.
589. O'Sullivan JB, Mahan CM: Criteria for the oral glucose tolerance test in pregnancy. *Diabetes* 13:278, 1964.
590. Fisher PM, Sutherland HW, Bewsher PD: Insulin response to glucose infusion in normal human pregnancy. *Diabetologia* 19:15, 1980.
591. Kalkhoff RK, Richardson BL, Beck P: Relative effects of pregnancy, human placental lactogen and prednisone on carbohydrate tolerance in normal and subclinical diabetic subjects. *Diabetes* 18:153, 1969.
592. Spellacy WN, Cohen JE: Human placental lactogen levels and insulin requirement in patients with diabetes mellitus complicating pregnancy. *Obstet Gynecol* 42:330, 1973.
593. Gustafson AB, Banasiak ME, Kalkhoff RK, et al: Correlation of hyperprolactinemia with altered plasma insulin and

glucagon: Similarity to effects of late human pregnancy. *J Clin Endocrinol Metab* 51:242, 1980.

594. Landgraf R, Landgraf-Leurs MMC, Weissman A, et al: Prolactin: A diabetogenic hormone. *Diabetologia* 13:99, 1977.
595. Lev-Ran A, Goldman JA: Brittle diabetes in pregnancy. *Diabetes* 26:926, 1977.
596. O'Sullivan JB, Charles D, Mahan CM, Dandrow RV: Gestational diabetes and perinatal mortality rate. *Am J Obstet Gynecol* 116:901, 1973.
597. Carpenter MW, Coustan DR: Criteria for screening tests for gestational diabetes. *Am J Obstet Gynecol* 144:765, 1982.
598. Magee MS, Walden CE, Benedetti TJ, et al: Influence of diagnostic criteria on the incidence of gestational diabetes and perinatal morbidity. *JAMA* 269:609, 1993.
599. O'Sullivan JB, Mahan CM: Insulin treatment and high risk groups. *Diabetes Care* 3:482, 1980.
600. Metzger BE, Bybee DE, Freinkel N, et al: Gestational diabetes mellitus: Correlations between the phenotypic and genotypic characteristics of the mother and abnormal glucose tolerance during the first year postpartum. *Diabetes* 34(Suppl 2):111, 1985.
601. Efendic J, Hanson V, Persson B, et al: Glucose tolerance, insulin release, and insulin sensitivity in normal-weight women with previous gestational diabetes mellitus. *Diabetes* 36:413, 1987.
602. Rudolf MCJ, Coustan DR, Sherwin RS, et al: Efficacy of the insulin pump in the home treatment of pregnant diabetics. *Diabetes* 30:891, 1981.
603. Coustan DR, Reece EA, Sherwin RS, et al: A randomized trial of the insulin pump and intensive conventional therapy in diabetic pregnancies. *JAMA* 255:631, 1986.
604. Drury MI, Greene AT, Stronge JM: Pregnancy complicated by clinical diabetes mellitus. *Obstet Gynecol* 49:519, 1977.
605. Kitzmiller JL, Cloherty JP, Younger MD, et al: Diabetic pregnancy and perinatal morbidity. *Am J Obstet Gynecol* 131:560, 1978.
606. Dooley SL, Depp R, Socol ML, et al: Urinary estriols in diabetic pregnancy: A reappraisal. *Obstet Gynecol* 64:469, 1984.
607. Coustan DR: Recent advances in the management of diabetic pregnant women. *Clin Perinatol* 7:299, 1980.
608. Soler NG, Soler SM, Malins JM: Neonatal morbidity among infants of diabetic mothers. *Diabetes Care* 1:340, 1978.
609. Ultrastructural analysis of malformations of the embryonic neural axis induced by *in vitro* hyperglycemic conditions. *Teratology* 32:363, 1985.
610. Eriksson UJ: Congenital malformations in diabetic animal models—a review. *Diabetes Res* 1:57, 1984.
611. Ornoy A, Zusman I, Cohen AM, Shafrir E: Effects of sera from Cohen, genetically determined diabetic rats, streptozotocin diabetic rats and sucrose fed rats on *in vitro* development of early somite rat embryos. *Diabetes Res* 3:43, 1986.
612. Baker L, Egler JM, Klein SH, Goldman AS: Meticulous control of diabetes during organogenesis prevents congenital lumbosacral defects in rats. *Diabetes* 305:955, 1981.
613. Eriksson UJ, Dahlstrom E, Hellerstrom C: Diabetes in pregnancy: Skeletal malformations in the offspring of diabetic rats after intermittent withdrawal of insulin in early gestation. *Diabetes* 32:1141, 1983.
614. Mills JL, Baker L, Goldman AS: Malformations in infants of diabetic mothers occur before the seventh gestational week. *Diabetes* 28:292, 1979.
615. Leslie RDG, John PN, Pyke SA, White JM: Haemoglobin A_1 in diabetic pregnancy. *Lancet* 2:958, 1978.
616. Miller E, Hare JW, Cloherty JP, et al: Elevated maternal hemoglobin A_{1c} in early pregnancy and major congenital anomalies in infants of diabetic mothers. *N Engl J Med* 304:1131, 1981.
617. Ylinen K, Aula P, Stenman UH, et al: Risk of minor and major fetal malformations in diabetics with high haemoglobin A1C values in early pregnancy. *Br Med J* 289:345, 1984.
618. Bergman M, Seaton TB, Auerhahn CC, Aaron-Young C, Glasser M, Shapiro LC: The incidence of gestational hypoglycemia in insulin-dependent (type 1) and noninsulin dependent (type 2) diabetic women. *NY State J Med* 86:174, 1986.
619. Sadler TW, Hunter ES: Hypoglycemia: How little is too much for the embryo. *Am J Obstet Gynecol* 157:190, 1987.
620. Leonard CM, Bergman M, Franz DA, MacCreery LA, Newman SA: Abnormal ambient glucose levels inhibit core protein gene expression and reduced proteoglycan during chondrogenesis: Possible mechanism for teratogenic effects of maternal diabetes. *Proc Natl Acad Sci USA* 86:10113, 1989.
621. Kitzmiller JL, Gavin LA, Gin GD, Jovanovich-Pederson L, Main EK, Zigrang WD: Preconception care of diabetes: Glycemic control prevents congenital anomalies. *JAMA* 265:731, 1991.
622. Steel JM, Johnstone FD, Hepburn DA, et al: Can prepregnancy care of diabetic women reduce the risk of abnormal babies? *Br Med J* 301:1070, 1990.
623. Minouni F, Miodovnik M, Whitesett SA, Horodye JC, Siddiqi T, Tsang R: Respiratory distress syndrome in infants of diabetic mothers in the 1980s: No direct adverse effect of maternal diabetes with modern management. *Obstet Gynecol* 69:191, 1987.
624. James DK, Chiswick ML, Harkes A, Williams M, Tindall VR: Maternal diabetes and neonatal respiratory distress: I Maturation of fetal surfactant. *Br J Obstet Gynecol* 91:316, 1989.
625. James DK, Chiswick ML, Harkes A, Williams M, Tindall VR: Maternal diabetes and neonatal respiratory distress: II. Prediction of fetal lung maturity. *Br J Obstet Gynecol* 91:325, 1989.
626. Gluck L, Kulovich MV: Lecithin/sphingomyelin ratios in amniotic fluid in normal and abnormal pregnancy. *Am J Obstet Gynecol* 115:539, 1973.
627. Smith BT, Giroud CJP, Robert M, Avery ME: Insulin antagonism of cortisol action on lecithin synthesis by cultured fetal lung cells. *J Pediatr* 87:953, 1975.
628. Ylinen K: Higher maternal levels of haemoglobin A_1C associated with delayed lung maturation in insulin dependent diabetic pregnancies. *Acta Obstet Gynecol Scand* 66:263, 1987.
629. North AF, Mazumdar S, Logrillo VM: Birth weight, gestational age, and perinatal deaths in 5471 infants of diabetic mothers. *Pediatrics* 90:444, 1977.
630. Jovanovic L, Druzin M, Peterson CM: Effect of euglycemia on the outcome of pregnancy in insulin-dependent diabetic women as compared with normal control subjects. *Am J Med* 71:921, 1981.
631. Olofsson P, Sjoberg NO, Solum T, Svenningsen NW: Changing panorama of perinatal and infant mortality in diabetic pregnancy. *Acta Obstet Gynecol Scand* 63:467, 1984.
632. Tevaarwerk GJM, Harding PGR, Miline KJ, et al: Pregnancy in diabetic women: Outcome with a program aimed at normoglycemia before meals. *Can Med Assoc J* 125:435, 1981.
633. Delaney JJ, Ptacek J: Three decades of experience with diabetic pregnancies. *Am J Obstet Gynecol* 106:550, 1970.
634. Widness JA, Susa JB, Garcia JF, et al: Increased erythropoiesis and elevated erythropoietin in infants born to diabetic mothers and in hyperinsulinemic rhesus fetuses. *J Clin Invest* 67:637, 1981.
635. Kenepp NB, Kumar S, Shelley WC, et al: Fetal and neonatal hazards of maternal hydration with 5% dextrose before cesarean section. *Lancet* 1:1150, 1982.
636. Lawrence GF, Brown VA, Parsons RJ, Cooke ID: Fetomaternal consequences of high-dose glucose infusion during labour. *Br J Obstet Gynaecol* 89:27, 1982.

637. Sosenko IR, Kitzmiller JL, Loo SW, et al: The infant of the diabetic mother: Correlation of increased cord C-peptide levels with macrosomia and hypoglycemia. *N Engl J Med* 301:859, 1979.
638. Bloom SR, Johnston DI: Failure of glucagon release in infants of diabetic mothers. *Br Med J* 4:453, 1972.
639. Lowey C: Pregnancy and diabetes mellitus, in Pickup J, Williams G (eds): *Textbook of Diabetes*. Oxford, Blackwell 1991, pp 835–850.
640. Bromham DR: The increased risk of pre-eclampsia in pregnant diabetics. *J Obstet Gynaecol* 3:212, 1983.
641. Aerts L, Van Assche FA: Transmission of experimentally induced diabetes in pregnant rats to their offspring in subsequent generations. A morphometric study of maternal and fetal endocrine pancreases at histological and ultrastructural level, in Shafrir E, Renold AE (eds): *Lessons from Animal Diabetes*. London, Libbey, 1984, p 705.
642. Pettit DJ, Bennett PH, Knowler WC, Baird HR, Alick KA: Gestational diabetes mellitus and impaired glucose tolerance during pregnancy: Long-term effects on obesity and glucose tolerance in the offspring. *Diabetes* 34(Suppl 2):119, 1985.
643. Persson B: Long-term morbidity in infants of diabetic mothers. *Acta Endocrinol (Copenh)* 277:156, 1986.
644. Bloch-Petersen M, Pederson SA, Greisen G, Fog-Pedersen J, Molsted-Pedersen L: Early growth delay in diabetic pregnancy: Relation to psychomotor development at age 4. *Br Med J* 296:598, 1988.
645. Cohen AW, Liston RM, Mennuti MT, Gabbe SG: Glycemic control in pregnant diabetic women using a continuous subcutaneous insulin infusion pump. *J Reprod Med* 10:651, 1982.
646. Fuhrmann K, Reiher H, Semmler K, Glockner E: The effect of intensified conventional insulin therapy before and during pregnancy on the malformation rate in offspring of diabetic mothers. *J Exp Clin Endocrinol* 83:173, 1984.
647. Churchill JA, Berendes HW: Intelligence of children whose mothers had acetonuria during pregnancy, in *Perinatal Factors Affecting Human Development,* scientific publication no. 185. Washington, D.C., Pan American Health Organization, 1969.
648. Felig P: Maternal and fetal fuel homeostasis in pregnancy. *Am J Clin Nutr* 26:998, 1973.
649. Mimouni F, Miodovnik M, Siddiqi TA, Berk MA, Wittekind C, Tsang R: High spontaneous premature labor rate in insulin dependent diabetic pregnant women: An association with poor glycemic control and urogenital infection. *Obstet Gynecol* 72:175, 1988.
650. Coustan DR: Diabetes and pregnancy, in Bergman M, Sicard GA (eds): *Surgical Management of the Diabetic Patient.* New York, Raven Press, 1991, Vol 11, p 363.
651. Persson B, Hanson U, Lunell N-U: Diabetes mellitus and pregnancy, in Alberti KGMM, DeFronzo RA, Keen H, Zimmet P (eds): *International Textbook of Diabetes Mellitus.* Chichester, Wiley, 1992, pp 1085–1101.
651a. Magré J, Reynet C, Capeau J, et al: In vitro studies of insulin resistance in patients with lipoatrophic diabetes: Evidence for heterogeneous postbinding detects. *Diabetes* 37:421, 1988.
652. Golden MP, Charles MA, Arquilla ER, et al: Insulin resistance in total lipodystrophy: Evidence for a prereceptor defect in insulin action. *Metabolism* 34:330, 1985.
653. Dymock IW, Cassar J, Pyke DA, Oakley WG, Williams R: Observations on the pathogenesis, complications and treatment of diabetes in 115 cases of hemochromatosis. *Am J Med* 52:203, 1972.
654. Jadresic A, Banks LM, Child DF, Diamant L, Doyle FM, Fraser TR, Joppla GF: The acromegaly syndrome: Relation between clinical features, growth hormone values and radiological characteristics of the pituitary tumors. *Q J Med* 202:189, 1982.
655. Perley M, Kipnis DM: Effect of glucocorticoids on plasma insulin. *N Engl J Med* 274:1237, 1986.
656. Wise JK, Hendler R, Felig P: Influence of glucocorticoids on glucagon secretion and amino acid concentrations in man. *J Clin Invest* 52:2774, 1973.
657. MacFarlane IA: Diabetes mellitus and endocrine disease, in Pickup J, Williams G (eds): *Textbook of Diabetes*. Oxford, Blackwell, 1991, pp 263–275.
658. Chowers I, Shapiro M, Pfau A, Shafrir E: Serum glucose and free fatty acid responses in pheochromocytoma. *Isr J Med Sci* 2:697, 1966.
659. Leichter SB: Chemical and metabolic aspects of glucagonoma. *Medicine (Baltimore)* 59:100, 1980.
660. Tanaka K, Watabe T, Shimizu N, et al: Immunologic characterization of plasma glucagon components in a patient with malignant glucagonoma. *Metabolism* 33:8, 1984.
661. D'Arcangues CM, Awoke S, Lawrence GD: Metastatic insulinoma with long survival and glucagonoma syndrome. *Ann Intern Med* 100:233, 1984.
662. Norton JA, Kahn CR, Schiebinger R, et al: Amino acid deficiency and the skin rash associated with glucagonoma. *Ann Intern Med* 91:213, 1979.
663. Breatnach ES, Han SY, Rahatzad MT, Stanley RJ: CT evaluation of glucagonomas. *J Comput Assist Tomogr* 9:25, 1985.
664. Elsbor L, Glenth A: Effect of somatostatin in necrolytic migratory erythema and glucagonoma. *Acta Med Scand* 218:245, 1985.
665. Ch'ng JLC, Anderson JV, Williams SI, et al: Remission of symptoms during chronic treatment of metastatic endocrine tumours with a long acting somatostatin analogue. *Br Med J* 292:981, 1986.
666. Sherwin RS, Bastl C, Finkelstein FO, et al: Influence of uremia and hemodialysis on the turnover and metabolic effects of glucagon. *J Clin Invest* 57:722, 1976.
667. McCaleb ML, Izzo MS, Lockwood DH: Characterization and partial purification of a factor from uremic human serum that induces insulin resistance. *J Clin Invest* 75:391, 1985.
668. Cavallo-Perin P, Cassader M, Bozzo C, et al: Mechanism of insulin resistance in human liver cirrhosis. *J Clin Invest* 75:1659, 1985.-

CHAPTER 20

Hypoglycemia

Harry Shamoon

Blood glucose concentration normally is regulated within exceedingly narrow limits, reflecting the virtually complete dependence of the brain on glucose for energy metabolism. In healthy individuals the plasma glucose concentration remains between 60 and 90 mg/dl (3.3 and 5.0 mmol/L) after overnight fasting and only transiently increases to 120 to 130 mg/dl (6.7 to 7.2 mmol/L) after a mixed meal. Since the total amount of intracellular (free) glucose in humans is relatively small and the largest pool is confined to the extracellular space, overlapping mechanisms exist to ensure precise homeostasis. Disruption of this system may lead to hypoglycemia severe enough to be catastrophic or mild enough to escape clinical attention. This wide range of nonspecific manifestations leads to difficulties in diagnosis. Nevertheless, recent advances in the understanding of glucose regulation at a physiologic and molecular level has provided powerful tools that enable the clinician to arrive at the underlying causes of hypoglycemic states.

DEFINITION

Much of the difficulty in the diagnosis of hypoglycemia stems from the confusion of biochemical abnormalities and clinical symptoms. Both factors must be taken into consideration since the apparent severity of symptoms and their episodic nature do not always correlate with plasma glucose values. Although the symptoms of hypoglycemia are usually relieved by ingestion of carbohydrate, the diagnosis should never be made on the basis of this observation alone. Although it is generally agreed that a plasma glucose concentration below 50 mg/dl (2.8 mmol/L) in adults is significant, no absolute level can be reliably established because women who are otherwise healthy may have a plasma glucose nadir as low as 25 to 30 mg/dl (1.4 to 1.7 mmol/L) after a 72-h fast.[1,2] In children, the diagnosis is complicated by difficulty in appreciating hypoglycemic symptoms, and plasma glucose levels as low as 30 mg/dl (1.7 mmol/L) in newborns once were considered normal.[3] Most authorities, however, agree that a child or infant who has a plasma glucose level below 50 mg/dl (2.8 mmol/L) should be observed carefully and that diagnostic evaluation and therapeutic intervention should begin at concentrations below 40 mg/dl (2.24 mmol/L).[4]

Whether the symptoms result from a given reduction in the plasma glucose concentration and the severity of those symptoms depend on other factors, including (1) the age of the patient, (2) the glucose threshold at which counterregulatory responses are triggered, (3) prior glucose concentrations in the individual, and (4) the availability of ketones for brain metabolism. Older persons and those with underlying central nervous system (CNS) disorders may exhibit focal neurologic deficits, an altered mental state, or seizures at plasma glucose concentrations seemingly well tolerated by others.[5] The plasma glucose threshold for release of counterregulatory hormones in healthy persons ranges between 50 and 70 mg/dl (2.8–3.9 mmol/L), although in some patients with diabetes or a chronic hypoglycemic state (e.g., insulinoma) these thresholds may be reduced.[6–8] The perception of hypoglycemia and counterregulatory hormone responses appear to occur at plasma glucose levels below 50 mg/dl (2.8 mmol/L) in intensively treated patients with type I diabetes.[7] Conversely, poorly controlled subjects with type I diabetes appear to exhibit both symptoms and counterregulatory hormone release at higher than normal thresholds,[9] suggesting that antecedent elevations in the plasma glucose concentration may influence subsequent reduction of the plasma glucose level. It has also been observed that persons who have fasted for several weeks are better able to tolerate the effects of hypoglycemia. This has been attributed to the increased circulating concentrations of ketones, and perhaps to augmented brain capacity to utilize ketones.[10]

SIGNS AND SYMPTOMS

The extensive symptomatology of hypoglycemia was not fully appreciated until the advent of insulin treatment for patients with diabetes. Although insulin-induced hypoglycemia is the only experimental model which can be studied in humans, it remains uncertain whether patients with hypoglycemia not due to hyperinsulinemia suffer from the same clinical symptoms and signs. Thus, it is apparent that the CNS and the sympathetic nervous system give rise to most of the symptoms and signs of hypoglycemia. Since many of these manifestations are nonspecific, confusion with various functional complaints may lead to overdiagnosis of hypoglycemia.

Neuroglycopenia

Changes in cerebral function probably accompany all levels of hypoglycemia, though subtle degrees of dysfunction may not be apparent at plasma glucose concentrations above 50 mg/dl. Experiments using sensory evoked potentials have indicated that some neurologic parameters, such as reaction time and cognitive function, may be slowed in healthy subjects at arterial plasma glucose levels of 60 mg/dl (3.3 mmol/L) and that recovery of function may lag 30 to 60 min after the restoration of euglycemia.[11,12] Overall brain energy metabolism and glucose utilization appear to be normal at this level of hypoglycemia, in keeping with the known kinetic characteristics of the glucose transport system.[13,14] A critical level of plasma glucose for the development of overt neurologic signs in most mammalian species appears to be ~2 mmol/L (~36 mg/dl).[13] This is also the threshold at which changes in behavior and slowing of alpha waves and increased delta waves in the electroencephalogram (EEG) can be discerned in humans.[15,16] Finally, this glucose concentration is also approximately that at which brain glucose transport becomes limiting; intracellular glucose concentrations approach zero when arterial plasma glucose falls below 2 mmol/L.[15]

The mechanisms underlying neural dysfunction and the possibility that regional brain metabolism may make certain areas of the brain more vulnerable have not been clarified. However, most of the neurologic signs and symptoms that accompany severe hypoglycemia can be reversed within a few minutes after restoration of euglycemia. Thus, the term *neuroglycopenia* has been used to denote manifestations of cellular glucose deficiency, including inability to concentrate, fatigue, headache, irrational behavior, amnesia, and confusion. In infants and children, irritability, feeding difficulties, lethargy, cyanosis, and tachypnea may be the only findings. At the most severe extreme, grand mal or focal seizures, hemiparesis (in older adults), and coma may occur.

It should be emphasized that the behavioral and cognitive dysfunction may be extremely subtle, particularly in patients with hypoglycemia unawareness. Such patients may exhibit no obvious sign of hypoglycemia except negativism, which may lead to the denial of the symptoms or to the refusal of assistance from others. Since these patients may be combative or abusive or display inappropriate responses, hypoglycemia may be mistaken for drug or ethanol intoxication, on occasion with devastating medical or legal consequences as a result of a delay in diagnosis.

A catastrophic result of severe and/or prolonged hypoglycemia is the development of irreversible coma. Experiments in nonhuman primates indicate that the plasma glucose concentration must fall to 1.1 mmol/L (20 mg/dl) for hypoglycemia to produce brain damage.[17] However, coexisting hypotension or hypoxemia can provoke the same changes at higher plasma glucose levels. Since most of the neuropathologic changes associated with severe hypoglycemia resemble those induced by cellular ischemia, differentiation from other causes may be difficult. Cerebral edema may also play a role in the development of irreversible coma. In patients who have survived for more than a few months, cortical atrophy and enlargement of the ventricular system may be seen. In some patients with repeated hypoglycemic episodes, a distal, symmetric peripheral neuropathy may develop.[18] This entity is most often reported in patients with islet-cell tumors who have experienced prolonged periods of hypoglycemia.[19] Motor neuron involvement is somewhat more common than sensory findings.

Sympathoadrenal Symptoms

The symptoms resulting from stimulation of the sympathoadrenal system consist of anxiety, tremulousness, perspiration, palpitations, and hunger. These symptoms often constitute the warning signs of hypoglycemia since they are likely to precede overt impairment of cortical function. The patient can therefore usually prevent a further deepening of hypoglycemia by ingesting carbohydrate. However, this should not be assumed to be an automatic response and must be taught to patients who are at the highest risk of suffering hypoglycemia.

Other Symptoms and Signs

Apart from its effects on the CNS and on the secretion of counterregulatory hormones, acute hypoglycemia has a number of other physiologic sequelae. Hemodynamic changes include tachycardia, a widened pulse pressure, and a dramatic increase in cardiac output. Changes in the electrocardiogram are common and include ST segment depression, T wave flattening, and prolongation of the Q-T interval.[20] Dysrythmias are also common, especially ectopic atrial or ventricular beats. These hemodynamic changes are responsible for the occurrence of angina or myocardial infarction in susceptible persons.[21]

Thermogenesis is increased during hypoglycemia[22] but is not usually accompanied by a rise in body temperature. In fact, comatose or severely obtunded patients with hypoglycemia may present with hypothermia. This is especially true in patients with alcohol-induced hypoglycemia. As with many of the signs of this entity, hypothermia is not specific for hypoglycemia since it can be encountered in all forms of shock, in sepsis, after cold exposure, and in severe myxedema.

Biochemical changes during hypoglycemia are multitudinous but depend somewhat on the inciting cause. These changes include decreases in plasma potassium, inorganic phosphate, free fatty acids (FFA), and ketones. All these changes are due to the prevailing hyperinsulinemia rather than to hypoglycemia per se; within 60 to 90 min of acute hypoglycemia, plasma FFA and blood ketone concentrations increase severalfold. Abnormalities of platelet function have been noted during insulin-induced and spontaneous hypoglycemia.[23] Plasma cAMP levels and urinary cAMP excretion also rise during acute hypoglycemia.[24] Lymphocytosis followed by neutrophilia has also been reported.[25]

Two features of hypoglycemia may complicate the diagnosis. The first is the episodic nature of hypoglycemic symptoms. Although these symptoms may recur, they usually last for periods of minutes to hours. The reason for this relatively brief duration is that endogenous glucose counterregulatory mechanisms or the ingestion of carbohydrate will restore the plasma glucose concentration to normal. Without these occurrences, the plasma glucose concentration will continue to decline to levels resulting in loss of consciousness, seizures, or coma. Thus, when patients complain of prolonged fatigue, lassitude, or inability to concentrate lasting for several hours or days, hypoglycemia is not likely to be the cause of these symptoms.

The second feature of hypoglycemia which may lead to an incorrect diagnosis is the misconception that reversal of symptoms after the ingestion of carbohydrate denotes underlying hypoglycemia. *Symptomatic relief associated with glucose ingestion as such does not constitute a specific sign of hypoglycemia.* A variety of symptoms associated with anxiety states may be relieved by eating. Thus, a low plasma glucose concentration must be documented before the administration of glucose to establish the presence of hypoglycemia. When such documentation is not available and the patient is suffering from neuroglycopenia, however, prompt reversal of the symptoms with glucose or glucagon is advisable.

TESTS FOR EVALUATION OF HYPOGLYCEMIA

Plasma Insulin

Accurate determination of plasma insulin by means of radioimmunoassay (RIA) is easily obtainable and should be included in the initial evaluation of all patients with fasting hypoglycemia. After an overnight fast plasma insulin concentrations are generally below 20 μU/ml, but higher values may be seen in simple obesity or after glucose infusion. In certain RIAs unheparinized serum should be employed since the heparin anticoagulant may affect the test adversely. Insulin antibodies can variably interfere with the RIA, spuriously raising or lowering the measured insulin value. In assays which employ charcoal or other substances to separate the free fraction, antibodies tend to raise the value falsely; in assays which employ a second ("double") antibody or polyethylene glycol to separate the bound fraction, insulin values are falsely low. Most commercially available RIAs are of the double-antibody type. Maneuvers to detect insulin antibodies in the patient's plasma include measurement of precipitable insulin tracer in a tube to which no antibody is added, the pretreatment of plasma with polyethylene glycol to precipitate insulin antibody before the RIA, and the use of high-performance liquid chromatography (HPLC) to resolve insulin-antibody complexes from free insulin. An important clue to the presence of interfering antibodies is the apparent monotony of plasma insulin values when determined over time in the subject.

Of greater importance than the isolated plasma insulin concentration is the relation between plasma insulin and plasma glucose determined simultaneously, preferably in the same sample of blood. Since the plasma glucose concentration normally exerts the major negative feedback on insulin secretion, low plasma glucose should be associated with a relatively suppressed plasma insulin concentration. This can be expressed as a fasting insulin (μU/ml): glucose (mg/dl) ratio (I/G ratio). An I/G ratio above 0.3 is highly suggestive of hyperinsulinism.[26] When both plasma insulin and glucose are determined repetitively during supervised fasting (see below), the likelihood of documenting inappropriate hyperinsulinemia is considerably enhanced.

In addition to the concentration of insulin in plasma, it may be useful to determine the species of insulin in order to distinguish endogenous insulin from surreptitious (animal species) insulin administration. Bovine or porcine insulin can be distinguished from human insulin by means of HPLC[27] or species-specific insulin antisera.[28]

C Peptide

C peptide determinations are readily available by means of RIA and are essential in differentiating endogenous from exogenous hyperinsulinism. Since (1) insulin and the C peptide fragment are secreted in equimolar amounts from the beta cell, (2) the peptides are immunologically distinct, and (3) the metabolic clearance rate of C peptide is slower than that of insulin, elevated C peptide values in the fasting state almost always indicate increased beta cell activity.[28,29] When combined with exogenous insulin infusion to induce hypoglycemia (C peptide suppression test), the presence of C peptide concentrations above 0.5 ng/ml suggests the presence of an unregulated islet-cell tumor. This test is best reserved for difficult diagnostic problems and should not precede the use of fasting plasma insulin and glucose measurements.

Proinsulin

Normally, proinsulin represents less than 20 percent of total insulin immunoreactivity in plasma.[28,29] In certain conditions, including islet-cell tumors, proinsulin makes up as much as 70 percent of the circulating insulin.[29] This measurement cannot be relied on as the sole means of distinguishing these patients. Proinsulin levels are significantly elevated in patients with renal failure and in members of families with benign hyperproinsulinemia.[30] It should be noted that proinsulin cross-reacts with C peptide in most RIAs for the C peptide and that proinsulin determination with HPLC is more specific.

Supervised Prolonged Fasting

The most reliable test for a diagnostic evaluation of fasting hypoglycemia is a prolonged fast (up to 72 h) in the supervised, controlled setting of a hospital. The onset of the fast and the sampling intervals should be timed carefully to coincide with the most likely time of occurrence of hypoglycemia. For example, in a patient with spontaneous episodes occurring after fasting for more than 8 h, the fast should be initiated in the early morning and samples should be obtained every 2 h. As noted below, rarely will patients require a full 72 h of fasting to provoke hypoglycemia. A practical sampling interval in the first 24 to 48 h may be every 4 h and whenever symptoms appear. The patient should be permitted to drink water, and sampling from an indwelling catheter is convenient and provides ready intravenous access for glucose infusion, if necessary. Blood should be drawn for glucose, insulin, and C peptide determinations, but only plasma glucose should be determined immediately. Urinary ketones, if present, are helpful in documenting that the patient is fasting and will be suppressed in the face of persistent insulin secretion. The blood samples should be carefully labeled with the time and day to allow subsequent assays in the proper sequence. This is especially important when frank symptomatic hypoglycemia does not develop during the fast; under these circumstances, a pattern of unchanging (or rising) plasma insulin concentrations in the face of declining plasma glucose levels may be diagnostic. Generally, however, the fast should be considered diagnostic when symptoms occur simultaneously with low plasma glucose (see below). An additional sample should be drawn at that moment for determinations of cortisol and growth hormone, and the patient should then be fed. Repeated plasma glucose values below 45 to 50 mg/dl (2.5–2.8 mmol/L) with strongly suggestive symptoms of hypoglycemia will increase the diagnostic yield. However, if neuroglycopenic symptoms develop, blood sampling at that time should be followed immediately by intravenous glucose infusion and feeding.

A common occurrence in the hospital setting is for a patient suspected of having a hypoglycemic disorder to receive parenteral glucose infusion. One can obtain semiquantitative information from the effect of this glucose infusion and the prevailing plasma glucose values. Thus, in an adult in whom euglycemia is maintained only at the expense of glucose infusion rates exceeding 2 mg/kg per minute, one can infer that there may be abnormal glucose homeostasis (i.e., an increase in glucose consumption, an impairment in glucose production, or both). However, in the face of unmonitored glucose administration in a hospital setting, an elevated plasma insulin concentration may not reflect abnormal insulin secretion. Only after several hours' withdrawal from parenteral glucose should the diagnostic fast be initiated.

Oral Glucose Tolerance Test

Unfortunately, this is probably the most overused test in the diagnostic evaluation of hypoglycemia and the one with the lowest degree of specificity. The oral glucose tolerance test (OGTT) is rarely helpful in the diagnosis of fasting hypoglycemia, yet it is likely to have been performed at an early stage of the patient's evaluation. In the diagnosis of reactive hypoglycemia, a 5- to 6-h test is advised. The patient should be fasted overnight and should refrain from ethanol, smoking, and severe exertion before the test. The test should not be performed if the patient is ill (even with a mild upper respiratory infection), but prior preparation with adequate carbohydrate intake as necessary for the diagnosis of diabetes is not required. An indwelling catheter for blood sampling will markedly reduce the likelihood of artifactual symptoms. After a sample for glucose and inulin determinations has been obtained, an oral load of 75 g glucose is administered. Blood samples should be withdrawn at 30-min intervals during the entire test, and a competent observer should be present to record the patient's reported symptoms and perform a repeat determination when severe symptoms occur. Frequently, the "symptoms" reported will be due to nausea after the ingestion of glucose or vasovagal complaints associated with frequent venipuncture.

Other Tests

Provocative tests involving the administration of oral arginine or leucine[31,32] or IV tolbutamide,[31,32] glucagon,[33] or calcium[34] generally have limited utility in the usual differential diagnosis. In the case of islet-cell tumors, false-negative tests occur in 25 percent or more of cases. Intravenous tolbutamide appears to yield the greatest sensitivity, but the risk of hypoglycemia as a result of the persistent hyperinsulinemia induced by this agent has rendered the test obsolete. Oral leucine (150 mg/kg) in patients with insulin-producing tumors increases insulin secretion and produces hypoglycemia which is generally milder than that induced by tolbutamide. In the rare leucine-sensitive child, ingestion of leucine also provokes hyperinsulinemia and severe hypoglycemia, but the amino acid produces small changes in plasma insulin concentrations (5 to 10 μU/ml) and plasma glucose (5 to 10 mg/dl) in normal subjects.[32]

Glucagon is a direct insulin secretagogue only in high concentrations (as a paracrine factor); physiologic concentrations induce insulin secretion secondary to hyperglycemia. Islet-cell tumors are especially responsive to glucagon (in contrast to glucose) in vitro, and some workers have exploited this aberrant response to design a rapid outpatient test.[31,33] Patients with an insulinoma may display an exaggerated plasma insulin response (with or without subsequent hypoglycemia) after IV injection of 1 mg glucagon. The maximal plasma insulin concentration 5 min after injection is normally below 150 μU/ml and may be severalfold greater in some patients with islet-cell tumors. Similarly, calcium infusion (5 mg/kg per hour infused over 2 h) induces hyperinsulinemia in such patients.[31,34] Neither test, however, has the required sensitivity or reproducibility to be recommended for inclusion in the routine diagnostic battery.

CLASSIFICATION

Hypoglycemia is not a diagnosis per se; rather, it is a marker for an underlying disorder of glucose homeostasis. Once it has been established as the cause of a patient's symptoms, the etiology of hypoglycemia should be established. The most useful diagnostic classification is one which divides hypoglycemia into the three major categories in which this disease presents: fasting hypoglycemia, reactive hypoglycemia, and induced hypoglycemia (Table 20-1).

While patients with fasting hypoglycemia may also have postprandial symptoms, individuals with reactive hypoglycemia should *never* have symptoms in the fasting state. Another useful clinical distinction is the fact that fasting hypoglycemic episodes almost never reverse without intervention whereas individuals with reactive symptoms always recover spontaneously without further food ingestion.

TABLE 20-1 Classification of Hypoglycemias

I. Fasting hypoglycemia
  A. Endocrine
    1. Excess insulin or insulin-like factors
      a. Insulin-producing islet-cell tumors
      b. Islet hyperplasia (adenomatosis, nesidioblastosis, etc.)
      c. Extrapancreatic tumors
    2. Deficiency of anti-insulin hormones
      a. Hypopituitarism
      b. Isolated ACTH or growth hormone deficiency
      c. Addison's disease
  B. Hepatic
    a. Glycogen storage diseases
    b. Congenital deficiencies of gluconeogenic enzymes
    c. Acute hepatic necrosis
      (1) Toxins
      (2) Viral hepatitis
      (3) Reye's syndrome
    d. Congestive heart failure
  C. Gluconeogenic substrate defects
    a. Pregnancy and lactation
    b. Ketotic hypoglycemia of infancy
    c. Chronic renal failure
    d. Severe malnutrition
    e. Maple syrup urine disease
  D. Miscellaneous
    a. Insulin autoimmune syndromes
    b. Systemic carnitine deficiency
II. Reactive hypoglycemia
  A. Reactive "functional"
  B. Alimentary
III. Induced hypoglycemia
  A. Insulin and sulfonylureas
    a. Diabetes mellitus
    b. Factitious
  B. Alcohol-induced
  C. Drug-induced

Fasting Hypoglycemia

These entities are characterized by unbalanced glucose homeostasis resulting in hypoglycemia when food is withheld. Although some reactive and induced hypoglycemias may present with hypoglycemia in the fasting state, the following disorders have in common the absence of factors inciting hypoglycemia such as food, drugs, and toxins. *Fasting hypoglycemia is always pathologic.* The response to prolonged fasting in normal humans can provide a framework for understanding the pathophysiology of these diseases.

Glucose Homeostasis during Fasting and Exercise

The remarkable degree of glucose control in humans occurs despite glucose input and outflow from a relatively small glucose pool of ~15 to 20 g (80 to 110 mmol), a fasting glucose turnover rate in adults of ~150 mg/min, and the addition of a glucose load up to 10 times larger than this pool during a meal. Humans, like most large mammals, feed intermittently. Between meals, a constant supply of glucose is maintained by hepatic production of glucose via combined glycogenolysis and gluconeogenesis. The more prolonged the period of fasting, the more dramatic the adaptive changes required and the greater the stress on the organism. Thus, brief periods of fasting which occur routinely (e.g., during sleep) are not accompanied by a detectable fall in plasma glucose in healthy humans. Longer-term fasting (12 to 72 h), by contrast, does produce a gradual decline in circulating glucose and tissue adaptation to the utilization of alternative fuels.

The dynamics of glucose metabolism after overnight fasting are well documented. In healthy subjects, glucose production is almost entirely derived from hepatic glycogenolysis (~75 percent) and gluconeogenesis (~25 percent). Of the total glucose flux averaging 2 mg/kg of body weight per minute, 70 to 80 percent is taken up by non-insulin-requiring uptake processes, predominantly in the brain. Other insulin-requiring tissues, such as resting muscle and adipose tissue, mainly consume FFA as an energy source. The major substrates for gluconeogenesis by the liver include lactate, pyruvate, amino acids (mainly alanine), and glycerol. The balanced rates of glucose production and uptake under normal conditions result in no net change in the plasma glucose concentration (Fig. 20-1).

The major hormonal signals which regulate these processes are insulin (acting on hepatic and extrahepatic tissues) and glucagon (acting on the liver). The decline in peripheral circulating insulin concentrations from peak values (50 to 100 μU/ml) 1 to 3 h after meal ingestion to basal values of 10 to 20 μU/ml removes the restraint on hepatic glucose production, which is supported primarily by glucagon. The decline in peripheral plasma insulin serves to limit glucose uptake in extrahepatic insulin-sensitive tissues and promotes the flux of gluconeogenic substrates such as lactate, amino acids, and glycerol from these sites.

FIGURE 20-1 The hormonal and substrate changes by which euglycemia is maintained (and hypoglycemia is prevented) in normal subjects during a fast. The fall in plasma insulin concentration is the key hormonal change resulting in increased glucose production and decreased glucose utilization. The decline in plasma insulin level is in turn a result of a small decrease in plasma glucose concentration (5 to 10 mg/dl) and/or a decrease in caloric intake per se.

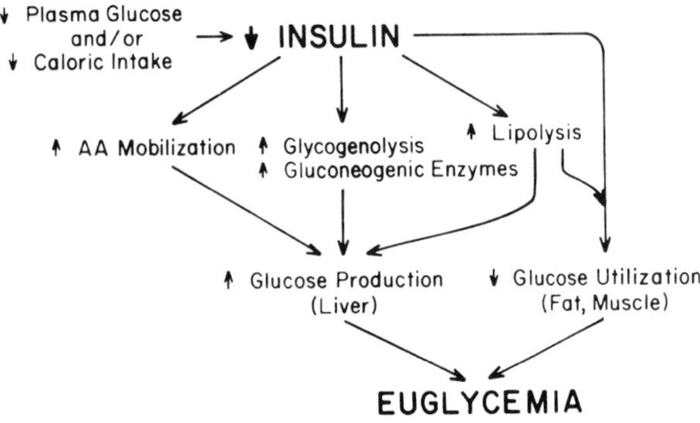

More prolonged fasting begins to deplete hepatic glycogen stores (within 24 h), and glucose production shifts progressively to gluconeogensis. A gradual decline in plasma glucose concentration (by ~25 percent after 3 days) invariably accompanies a 72-h fast under controlled conditions. Peripherally derived substrate availability becomes more critical and is enhanced by a further decline in plasma insulin concentrations from basal values to levels below 5 to 10 μU/ml. This relative hypoinsulinemia leads to increased mobilization of alanine from muscle and FFA from adipose tissue as lipolysis is stimulated. This process allows for sparing of glucose for the brain as increased fatty acid uptake provides a greater proportion of energy for muscle. The liver is another important site for fatty acid metabolism since conversion to glucose in the liver occurs pari passu with enhanced β oxidation of fatty acids to ketone bodies.

Plasma glucagon levels also begin to increase as fasting is extended, in part because of the small decline in plasma glucose concentration and perhaps as a result of direct neural sympathetic stimulation and/or the effect of decreased insulin secretion. Hyperglucagonemia further enhances the gluconeogenic and ketogenic effects of hypoinsulinemia. Other counterregulatory factors appear to be increased during prolonged fasting, including growth hormone, cortisol, and sympathoadrenal hormones. It is unlikely that all these effects are mediated by the small decrease in plasma glucose, but experimental and clinical data suggest that these hormonal and metabolic changes prevent the development of severe hypoglycemia. For example, the persistence of basal insulin infusion in fasting insulin-dependent diabetics will eventually produce hypoglycemia.

Exercise has been used as another modality for inducing hypoglycemia during evaluation for islet-cell tumors. In 72-h fasted subjects who have not developed clear-cut hypoglycemia, a 30-min bout of exercise frequently produces a further, and diagnostic, decline in plasma glucose concentrations. Glucose homeostasis during even brief exercise bears some resemblance to that in the fasting state; both a decline in portal venous insulin levels and an increase in glucagon secretion seem to be necessary signals for hepatic glucose output to increase sufficiently to match the augmented demands of exercising muscle. Exercise in the face of fixed basal insulin concentrations will result in hypoglycemia.

Glucose Counterregulation

Experimental data in animals and humans suggest that glucose counterregulatory hormone secretion is triggered at plasma glucose concentrations higher than the level which produces symptoms of hypoglycemia. This observation highlights the clinical concern that symptoms of "hypoglycemia" may not be accompanied by the presence of a low plasma glucose level and establishes the relative importance of glucose counterregulatory mechanisms in *preventing* a dangerous decline in blood glucose to levels which threaten the brain. Impaired glucose counterregulation may be defined as the failure to restore plasma glucose concentrations to normal or to prevent further decline.[35]

Counterregulatory hormone secretion during hypoglycemia has been studied extensively in humans during experimental insulin-induced reduction of the plasma glucose concentration.[35,36] It should be emphasized that dissipation of insulin action is an essential component of the recovery of plasma glucose. The suppression of hepatic glucose release and the increased peripheral utilization of glucose induced by insulin—the inciting factors leading to hypoglycemia—are reversed in part by declining plasma insulin concentrations. This mechanism is critical to the restoration of the plasma glucose concentration after hypoglycemia in patients with insulin-treated diabetes.[36,37] Counterregulatory hormones can overcome the effects of insulin even under conditions in which the plasma insulin concentration does not decrease.[38] Among the counterregulatory hormones, epinephrine (released from the adrenal medullae) and glucagon (secreted by the alpha cells of the islets of Langerhans) appear to be the most potent insulin antagonists. These hormones are secreted promptly after plasma glucose levels fall, and both induce a rapid increase in hepatic glucose production.[39] The independent contribution of each of these hormones to hepatic glucose production appears to be similar; hence, a deficient response of either hormone alone does not impair glucose counterregulation. This is best demonstrated in patients with type I diabetes, most of whom have a marked reduction in glucagon secretion during hypoglycemia[37] but counterregulate appropriately if epinephrine is not deficient. Conversely, glucose counterregulation appears to be normal in patients after adrenalectomy who are given adequate glucocorticoid replacement and in subjects receiving combined alpha- and beta-adrenergic blockade.[35,40] Finally, in many patients with insulin-dependent diabetes of greater than a few years' duration, failure of epinephrine secretion in response to hypoglycemia develops; the combined deficiencies of glucagon and epinephrine are most likely responsible for the greater propensity to severe and/or prolonged hypoglycemia in such patients[35–38,41] (Fig. 20-2).

The contributions of the other major counterregulatory hormones seem to be less critical in the initial glycemic recovery (<30 to 60 min) but are nonetheless important in the latter stage of glucose

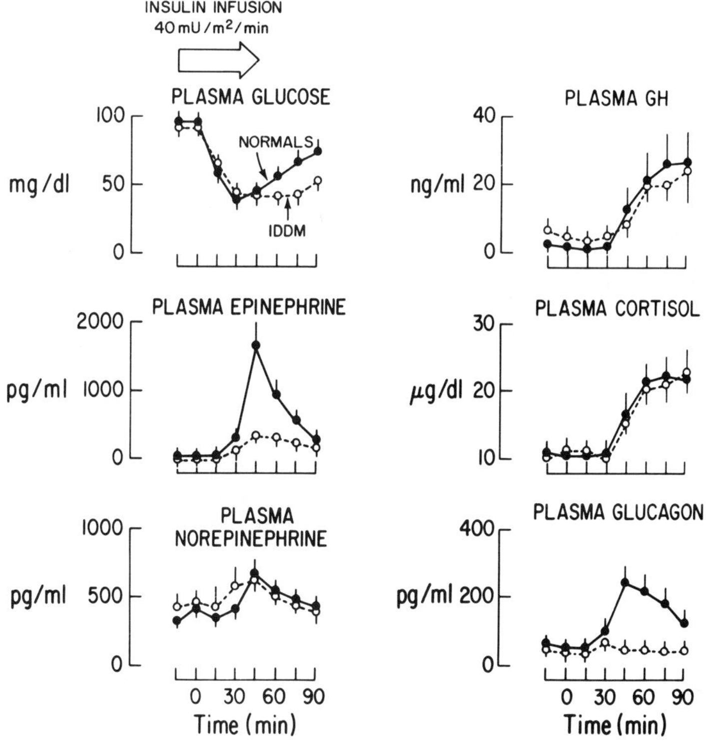

FIGURE 20-2 Hormonal responses to insulin-induced hypoglycemia in normal subjects (solid circles) compared with patients with insulin-dependent diabetes mellitus (IDDM) (open circles). The subjects received a 40 mU/m^2 per minute insulin infusion to induce equivalent hypoglycemia, yet the recovery of plasma glucose was significantly retarded in the patients with IDDM. With a mean duration of 10 years of diabetes, the IDDM patients displayed blunted secretion of epinephrine as well as glucagon. (*From Hirsch BR, Shamoon H, Diabetes 36:20, 1987, by permission of American Diabetes Association, Inc.*)

stabilization. Cortisol and growth hormone both have significant late effects on the ability of the liver to sustain glucose output in the face of hyperinsulinemia.[42,43] In addition, these hormones reduce peripheral glucose utilization during recovery from hypoglycemia, an action shared by epinephrine.[44] These effects are both direct and indirect (e.g., by stimulation of FFA release). In patients with insulin-dependent diabetes and impaired hepatic glucose release, the reduction in peripheral glucose uptake is vital in glycemic recovery from hypoglycemia.[41] Finally, chronic glucocorticoid and growth hormone deficiency can cause severe hypoglycemia. In particular, patients with hypopituitarism who suffer from these combined hormonal deficiencies may present with profound hypoglycemia despite the absence of hyperinsulinemia or known abnormalities in glucagon or epinephrine secretion.[45,46]

Other counterregulatory factors are known to exist, but their contribution is of uncertain importance. For example, it is likely that glucose per se exerts feedback control on its own production by the liver either directly (so-called autoregulation) or via neural pathways originating in the CNS.[47] Also, norepinephrine is known to activate glucose production and impair glucose utilization, but its concentrations in plasma during hypoglycemia do not achieve the levels required to affect glucose metabolism.[48] The secretion of a variety of other hormones and neurotransmitters is induced by hypoglycemia (e.g., vasopressin, angiotensin, prolactin, and pancreatic polypeptide), but none of these substances seem to possess major glucoregulatory actions.

Impaired glucose counterregulation has emerged as a clinical syndrome of considerable importance in patients who are the most likely to suffer hypoglycemia: those with insulin-dependent diabetes. As noted above, combined defects in the secretion of glucagon and epinephrine lead to inadequate hepatic glucose production during recovery from insulin-induced hypoglycemia. The etiology of these hormonal defects is uncertain. Although some affected patients clearly suffer from autonomic neuropathy (which has been implicated in defective adrenergic responses to hypoglycemia), most patients with impaired glucose counterregulation do not exhibit other clinical symptoms of autonomic neuropathy.[41,49,50] There is evidence that the defect in both glucagon and epinephrine release in diabetics may be specific to the hypoglycemic stimulus per se and that these hormones can be secreted in response to other stimuli.[50,51] The observation that intensive insulin therapy in diabetic patients further impairs epinephrine secretion (as well as the secretory responses of cortisol and growth hormone) suggests that "functional" defects in hormonal responses to hypoglycemia may be common.[7,52] Indeed, other syndromes of hypoglycemia may share such defects in glucose counterregulation. Some patients with islet-cell tumors have been shown to have reduced secretion of the major counterregulatory hormones,[6,8,53] and in one such patient reversal of this phenomenon occurred after surgical cure.[8] A clinical hallmark of impaired glucose counterregulation is "hypoglycemic unawareness."[36,37] As a result of the deficient epinephrine response in such patients, lack of adrenergic warning symptoms and impaired glucose production exacerbate the risk of developing prolonged and/or more severe hypoglycemia. It is of interest that not all the adrenergic symptoms of hypoglycemia can be attributed to epinephrine secretion,[54,55] suggesting that there may be defects other than reduced adrenomedullary epinephrine secretion.

From this discussion it is apparent that the maintenance of euglycemia in the fasting state is dependent on three factors: (1) a hormonal milieu characterized by basal or reduced insulin secretion and increased secretion of glucagon, growth hormone, and cortisol; (2) intact glycogenolytic and gluconeogenic processes in the liver; and (3) substrate availability for hepatic gluconeogenesis as well as sparing of glucose utilization in the periphery. Severe impairment of any of these defenses (or, usually, generalized partial defects in more than one) will result in fasting hypoglycemias (Table 20-1). In addition, impairment of glucose counterregulatory mechanisms may exacerbate and prolong hypoglycemia.

Insulin-Producing Islet-Cell Tumors

Clinical Characteristics

Insulin-producing tumors of the islet are rare, with an estimated annual incidence of 1 to 2 per million persons.[36,56] While the majority of these tumors are benign, 10 to 15 percent are malignant as defined by the presence of metastases. Malignant insulinomas may secrete human chorionic gonadotropin (hCG), a sensitive test for which is measurement of the α subunit of hCG.[57] Multiple benign tumors occur in about 10 percent of cases, usually in association with type 1 multiple endocrine neoplasia (MEN 1).[58] In such families the incidence of multiple adenomas may be as high as 50 percent. The average age at diagnosis of an insulinoma is 42 years, though patients have been reported from birth to the ninth decade. In prepubertal children with this diagnosis, a careful search for endocrine neoplasia in the patient and family members is necessary to uncover MEN 1. Malignant insulinoma has been reported in a 9-year-old child.[59]

Most insulinomas are small (<2 cm) and evenly distributed throughout the pancreas. They are usually, but not invariably, vascular and palpable at the time of surgery. The histologic appearance is usually that of clusters of normal β-cells, though secretory granules may not be demonstrable with traditional staining methods. Immunohistochemical stains or electron microscopy generally reveals insulin-containing granules, though some tumors are associated with other secretory products, such as adrenocorticotropic hormone (ACTH) and calcitonin. Coexisting islet-cell adenomatosis has been reported,[26,59,60] and normal islet tissue is usually not atrophic. Differentiation between benign and malignant tumors cannot be made on the basis of histologic criteria but rather on the finding of regional lymph node or hepatic metastases. Ectopic insulin-secreting tumors are extremely rare but can occur at sites in which pancreatic rests occur, including the wall of the duodenum, the porta hepatis, and the pancreatic bed.

The clinical presentation of patients with insulinomas includes psychiatric symptomatology, organic brain syndrome, suspected brain tumor, epilepsy, and intoxication. The duration of symptoms may be as short as a few weeks to as long as 30 years, though in some series most patients had symptoms of less than 12 months' duration.[26,59] The history suggests episodes of neuroglycopenia of increasing frequency provoked by abstinence from food, therapeutic dieting, or exercise. In rare cases, preexisting diabetes mellitus may gradually "improve" and insulin requirement may disappear. Between episodes, patients are likely to feel well; only about 30 percent of these patients develop obesity. Many patients are not aware of the connection between their symptoms and fasting or of the relief experienced after eating.

The mechanism underlying hypoglycemia in such patients is absolute or relative hyperinsulinemia. The normal suppression of insulin secretion as plasma glucose levels decline ensures that hepatic glucose production will increase as hypoglycemia develops. β-Cell tumors lack this negative feedback control on insulin secretion. Thus, earlier in the course of the disease glucose homeostatic mechanisms which tend to fail depend on a decrease in fasting plasma insulin (e.g., during exercise or after prolonged fasting), whereas absolute hyperinsulinemia tends to characterize long-standing disease.

Increased glucose utilization in insulin-sensitive tissues has not been a prominent feature in carefully studied patients. Indeed, patients with insulinoma may be insulin-resistant, presumably as a result of the down regulation of insulin action mediated by peripheral hyperinsulinemia. Insulin resistance, especially when combined with the reduced responsiveness of insulinoma tissue to glucose, may result in carbohydrate intolerance in some patients.

Diagnosis

A history suggestive of the recent onset of episodic confusion, bizarre behavior, or neurologic symptoms relieved by eating should prompt evaluation with fasting plasma glucose and insulin measurements. If hypoglycemia is present in the face of unequivocal hyperinsulinemia in an adult, the diagnosis of islet-cell tumor is almost certain. A repeat evaluation, however, may be necessary to confirm the biochemical diagnosis before one proceeds to localizing procedures. Since insulinomas may secrete insulin only intermittently, patients with suspicious symptoms may also require periodic reevaluation.

Various series have reported on the duration of the supervised fast required to detect the presence of hypoglycemia. Almost half of all patients with islet-cell tumors have a fasting plasma glucose concentration below 60 mg/dl (3.4 mmol/L) and a plasma insulin level above 20 μU/ml after overnight fasting.[61] The simple maneuver of prolonging the fast to a total period of 14 to 18 h will result in the development of diagnostic hypoglycemia in over 90 percent of patients.[61] Only a minority of patients will need to undergo the full 72-h fast, and an even smaller number will require the addition of exercise after the 3-day fast to provoke hypoglycemia. Under these extreme conditions, less than 2 percent of reported patients fail to exhibit hypoglycemia or neuroglycopenia.[62]

It is important to note the pattern of plasma insulin concentrations and the concomitant plasma glucose values obtained during fasting, particularly in patients who do not exhibit absolute hyperinsulinemia or clear-cut evidence of neuroglycopenia (Fig. 20-3). The lack of a decline in plasma insulin concentrations over time, if associated with decreasing plasma glucose levels, may be diagnostic. Supporting evidence for the presence of unrestrained β-cell secretion is provided by C peptide measurements. In a few patients the diagnosis of abnormal insulin secretion has required additional tests (see above). While data on the specificity of such ancillary tests is not available, the C peptide suppression test may be the most likely to yield unequivocal results.

Establishing the biochemical diagnosis is important in view of the current limitations of localizing procedures. Imaging studies should not be performed in lieu of diagnostic tests but should be reserved for the management stage of the work-up. Because of the unavoidability of false-negative findings with many of the procedures noted below, these tests should generally be undertaken after a decision to operate has been made (or when evidence of malignant metastases is sought).

Computerized tomography (CT) and ultrasound are generally safe but, because of the small size of tumors, yield localizing information in less than half the cases. Magnetic resonance imaging (MRI) has not altered this yield dramatically, though the technique is relatively new.[63] In the hands of a skilled radiologist, selective arteriography is often helpful. Most tumors located with this technique have been vascular, yet many avascular lesions have been reported using other localizing methods. Nonselective celiac angiography is less sensitive and probably no better than CT.[64] Intraoperative sonography has yielded helpful localizing information (see below).

Selective percutaneous transhepatic venous sampling combined with plasma insulin determinations

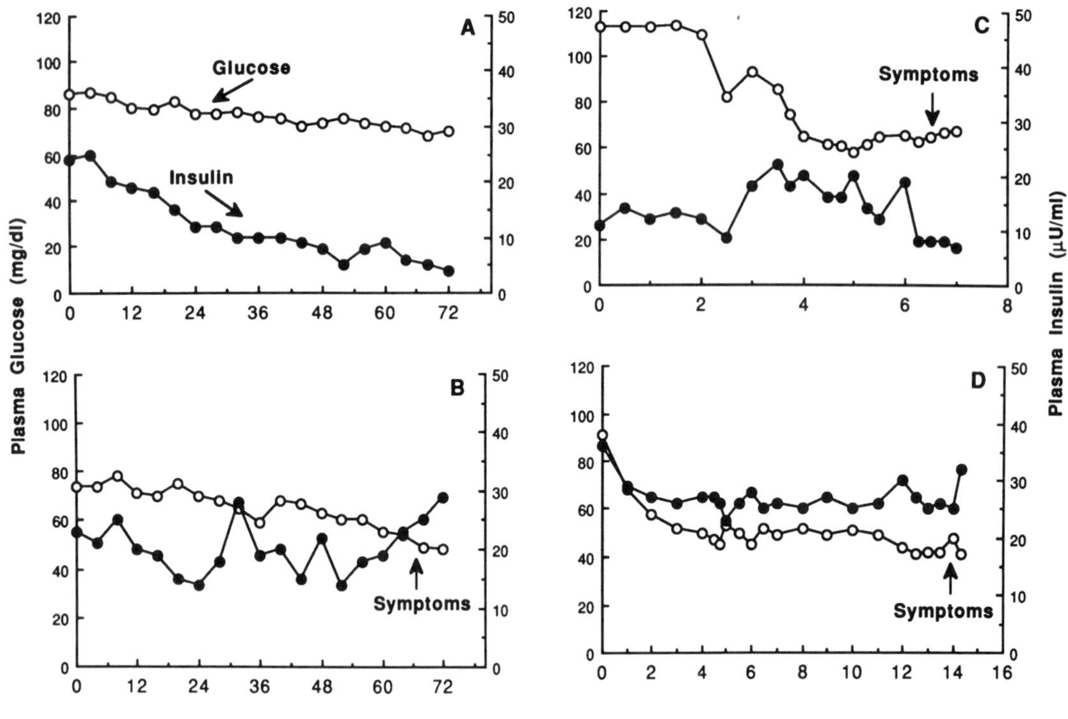

FIGURE 20-3 Examples of the response of plasma glucose and insulin to fasting in a normal atient and in three patients with islet-cell tumors and mild hyperinsulinemia. (*A*) A 72-h fast in a normal man results in a progressive decline in plasma insulin to the limits of detection together with a roughly parallel decrease in plasma glucose without symptoms of neuroglycopenia. (*B*) In a patient found to have a benign insulinoma and mild hyperinsulinemia, symptoms did not appear until late in the 3-day fast. (*C*) A patient with a malignant islet-cell tumor requiring intravenous glucose infusion to maintain plasma glucose levels. Only after a lag of several hours after discontinuation of the glucose infusion did plasma glucose fall to symptomatic levels. Sequential insulin values taken during hours 2 to 4 of the fast suggested unregulated insulin secretion. (*D*) Despite the initial decline in plasma glucose, this patient experienced symptoms coinciding with rising plasma insulin and falling glucose after 15 h of fasting. A benign islet-cell tumor was resected. Note the shorter time frames in (*C*) and (*D*) compared with (*A*) and (*B*).

to detect a gradient in insulin levels has been employed to definitively localize hyperinsulinism to the head, body, or tail of the pancreas.[65] However, four factors make this test problematic. First, considerable experience in selective venous catheterization is required on the part of the radiologist. Second, morbidity from the procedure includes intraperitoneal hemorrhage, infection, and bile leakage. Third, it is probable that adequate surgical exploration will suffice in the majority of first operations, and it is uncertain whether unusual cases (e.g., multiple adenomas and concomitant hyperplasia) are readily localizable with this technique. Since sampling takes place along the splenic and portal venous systems, where blood flow rates are relatively high, dilution of samples may yield falsely low plasma insulin values. Fourth, agents which inhibit insulin secretion generally must be discontinued for at least 24 h before sampling and can expose the patient to recurrent hypoglycemia. Consequently, this procedure should probably be reserved as a test to reevaluate patients in whom initial surgery was unsuccessful.

Intraoperative ultrasound may add a significant benefit during surgical exploration. This approach involves the application of an ultrasound probe directly to the pancreas during laparotomy to differentiate tumors from normal tissue.[66] Since surgery is the treatment of choice for most patients, the utility of this technique should be determined in the near future.

Treatment

Initial medical management with dietary measures may be entirely effective in alleviating symptoms in some patients; certainly, all patients should be instructed to increase the frequency of feedings, particularly at night. Carbohydrates should not be restricted, and more slowly absorbed complex forms (e.g., bread, potatoes, rice) are preferable. During hypoglycemic episodes, more rapidly absorbed carbohydrates (e.g., fruit juices and sucrose) should be used.

In patients with severe, refractory hypoglycemia, a continuous IV glucose infusion may be required to supplement oral feeding. At glucose infusion rates above 10 g/h (which would roughly approximate hepatic glucose delivery rates in a resting normal-weight adult), concentrations of 10% or higher of dextrose infusate will be needed, preferably delivered via a large-caliber vein.

In the hands of an experienced surgeon, cure of insulinomas is likely in the majority of benign cases. In the Mayo Clinic series, 154 patients underwent surgery, with 5.4 percent mortality.[67] Surgery was successful in removing a tumor in 85 percent of all patients and in 93 percent of patients with adenomas, though in some patients in whom no definite tumor was found a blind resection of the body and tail of the pancreas was performed. The success rate in patients with carcinomas was much lower, with only 50 percent found at surgery. The remainder manifested as metastases from a primary tumor which was too small to be identified at the time of the original surgery. It is often possible to detect an abrupt, intraoperative rise in plasma glucose after successful surgery. Although the response to surgical resection may vary and other factors can alter blood glucose levels in this setting, determinations of plasma glucose after presumed surgical resection can provide reassurance with relatively little risk.

Nonsurgical treatment of insulinomas plays a limited but important role. The oral drug with the greatest clinical utility—diazoxide—is a potent inhibitor of insulin secretion and can thus ameliorate the symptoms of hyperinsulinism. The dose needed ranges from 100 to 200 mg two to three times per day (12 mg/kg of body weight in children), with maintenance doses generally being lower than initial requirements. Diazoxide frequently causes sodium and water retention, resulting in edema, and so the drug should be used cautiously in persons with impaired cardiovascular function or should be combined with diuretic treatment. Occasional side effects include anorexia, tachycardia, and hirsutism (after prolonged use). In general, however, this agent is safe enough to be considered in the interim management of patients awaiting localizing tests or surgery and patients who are not candidates for surgery or have functional malignant metastases. Other drugs which may provide adjunctive treatment of hyperinsulinism include phenytoin (diphenylhydantoin), adrenocorticosteroids, and calcium-channel antagonists, including verapamil and diltiazem.[61]

Somatostatin is a potent inhibitor of insulin secretion, but its short half-life has made it impractical as a clinically useful agent. The recent approval for use of the long-acting somatostatin analogue octreotide in certain hormone-producing tumors has provided a potential alternative in the medical management of insulinomas. Since this octapeptide has a half-life of 90 to 120 min, subcutaneous injections given several times daily have sustained effects on the secretion of some hormones. Unfortunately, most patients do not appear to experience adequate or long-term suppression of insulin secretion that would justify the use of this agent alone.[68] There have been reports of successful use of this agent administered by continuous subcutaneous infusion.[69] It may also act synergistically with diazoxide treatment or be employed as a second agent in patients with unremitting side effects of higher doses of diazoxide. A recent application of octreotide is the use of a [125]-Tyr^3-labeled compound as a scanning agent to localize islet-cell tumors and their metastases which possess specific somatostatin receptors. Whether such procedures will become helpful in preoperative tumor localization (particularly of insulinomas which respond clinically to octreotide) remains to be elucidated.

In patients with inoperable or malignant insulinoma, streptozocin (streptozotocin; STZ) has been employed because of its relative affinity for neuroendocrine cells and its β-cytolytic properties in animals. This drug, however, has significant toxicity when given systemically, including transient nausea and vomiting, renal tubular damage, and hepatotoxicity. Although it has been reported to have some benefit in metastatic islet-cell carcinomas in general, STZ has relatively disappointing potency in the treatment of insulin-producing tumors. This is true both for reduction of the frequency of hypoglycemia and for tumor size and the survival of patients. Regimens for the palliative treatment of malignant insulinomas include combined STZ and 5-fluorouracil, mithramycin, doxorubicin, and interferon-α, all of which have been used with dismal results.[70]

Non-Islet-Cell Tumor Hypoglycemia

The relative frequency of non-islet-cell tumors that cause hypoglycemia is difficult to ascertain since nutritional hypoglycemia may accompany the late stages of malignancy and because such patients may not be referred for evaluation unless their hypoglycemia is severe and unremitting. However, it has become increasingly clear that a variety of nonpancreatic tumors are associated with hypoglycemia and suppressed plasma insulin concentrations. These tumors include retroperitoneal fibrosarcomas, hepatomas, gastrointestinal tumors, mesotheliomas, adrenal cortical carcinomas, and hypernephromas. Since many of these tumors are large (some mesenchymal tumors weighing several kilograms have been reported), the clinical presentation is usually obvious with tumor in the abdominal or thoracic areas. However, some common malignancies have rarely been associated with hypoglycemia (e.g., breast carcinoma, prostate carcinoma, and lymphoma).

Based on occasional reports of substantial glucose uptake as measured across the tumor bed, excess tumor consumption of glucose has been one postulated mechanism for the hypoglycemia of extrapancreatic tumors.[71] The increased uptake of glucose by the tumor may be mediated by activated oncogenes which enhance the activity of the glucose transporter system within the tumor mass.[72] Other studies have suggested that in over 50 percent of such patients there are elevated plasma concentrations of an insulin-like peptide.[73] Classical RIAs for insulin-like growth factor I (IGF-I) or IGF-II have been less helpful than radioreceptor assays in establishing the presence of these peptides. A number of technical considerations cloud the interpretation of the conflicting data.[73,74] Results from two independent laboratories, however, have shown the presence of IGF-II mRNA in tumors associated with clinical hypoglycemia.[75,76] These observations cannot be considered conclusive since the relatively modest IGF-II elevations in the plasma of most reported patients cannot account for the hypoglycemia. It is unclear whether IGF-I- or IGF-II-mediated tumor hypoglycemia results from the activation of the insulin receptor by the peptide, whether the IGF receptor mediates these hypoglycemic effects, or whether high local concentrations of the IGF in the tumor itself may be responsible for the increased rates of glucose removal. An interesting associated finding in some patients is the concomitant absence of a growth hormone (GH) response to hypoglycemia.[76] The return of the GH response after successful tumor resection is taken to indicate that the tumor caused IGF-II-mediated feedback inhibition of pituitary GH secretion. Thus, some impairment in glucose counterregulatory hormones may also play a role in the pathogenesis of hypoglycemia. Finally, it should be pointed out that other cytokines released by tumors or macrophages activated by tumors can affect glucose metabolism, including interleukin-1, interferon-α, and tumor necrosis factor, though the role of such factors in hypoglycemia is far from settled.[73]

Diagnostic evaluation in such patients is limited by the lack of understanding of the cause of hypoglycemia and the absence of clinically available assays for the putative hormonal mediators of hypoglycemia. Certainly, hypoglycemia associated with low plasma insulin levels in a patient with a mesenchymal tumor is highly suggestive of the diagnosis. Treatment of hypoglycemia associated with non-islet-cell tumors is directed at the tumor itself, e.g., surgery or chemotherapy. Since hypoglycemia in such patients is accompanied by hypoinsulinemia, therapy directed at reducing insulin secretion (e.g., diazoxide) is not indicated. Anecdotal reports also fail to suggest a prominent role for octreotide in such patients.

Hypoglycemia in Endocrine Deficiency States

As was discussed above, the prevention and reversal of hypoglycemia involve both attenuation of insulin secretion and secretion of cortisol, GH, glucagon, and catecholamines. Hypoglycemia may be the presenting symptom in patients with hypopituitarism with multiple deficiencies (e.g., in Sheehan's syndrome with combined ACTH and GH deficiency) or isolated deficiencies (e.g., in isolated GH deficiency). Hypoglycemia may also occur in Addison's disease. The occurrence of hypoglycemia may be more common in children, perhaps because the relatively greater rate of glucose turnover places a greater demand on the liver for glucose production.[77] In all these clinical conditions hypoglycemia is accompanied by an appropriate reduction in plasma insulin concentration and an increase in urinary ketones. The diagnostic evaluation depends on tests of pituitary and/or adrenal function (discussed in Chapters 8 and 12). Although glucagon is clearly important in the maintenance of glucose production and its absence contributes to insulin-induced hypoglycemia in patients with diabetes, a clinical syndrome of hypoglycemia due to glucagon deficiency per se in nondiabetic individuals has not been convincingly documented.

Hepatic Disease

Fasting hypoglycemia occurs only when there is widespread damage to hepatic parenchyma, but the level of the fasting plasma glucose does not correlate with the degree of liver dysfunction reflected in standard laboratory tests.[78] Patients with cirrhosis, hepatitis, or metastatic liver disease rarely display hypoglycemia (though portacaval shunting may increase the likelihood of developing hypoglycemia). Fulminant hepatitis due to infectious or toxic agents, however, may be associated with severe hypoglycemia. In infectious hepatitis, about 10 percent of individuals progress to a stage of fulminant hepatic failure and account for most of the hypoglycemia observed in these disorders. A variety of drugs causing hepatic failure [acetaminophen, isoniazid, valproic acid (sodium valproate), methyldopa, tetracycline, halothane] as well as chemical toxins (carbon tetrachloride, phosphorus, urethan) may be associated with hypoglycemia. Parenteral glucose infusions must be used in the acute stages of such disorders, and if the clinical condition improves, a gradual transition to frequent oral feedings is indicated. Intravenous glucagon is usually not useful in counteracting acute hypoglycemia in such cases.

Severe right-sided congestive heart failure with hepatomegaly in both children and adults can be associated with hypoglycemia. Since most of these patients exhibit signs of cardiac cachexia and since there is little evidence of hepatic parenchymal necrosis, the mechanism underlying hypoglycemia may be nutritional.[79] Once heart failure has been treated, however, hypoglycemia usually remits.

Infiltrative diseases such as amyloidosis, sarcoidosis, and hemochromatosis rarely produce sufficient parenchymal loss to cause hypoglycemia. However, hypoglycemia is a frequent concomitant of the rare acute fatty liver that occurs in late pregnancy.[80] A brief illness characterized by nausea, vomiting, epigastric pain, and jaundice precedes the development of hypoglycemia. Hemolysis, thrombocytopenia, and renal failure may ensue as terminal events. Appropriate treatment of hypoglycemia may reduce the incidence of encephalopathy and permit continued supportive management.

Hypoglycemia due to Substrate Deficiency

A diverse group of clinical entities is characterized by deficiency in gluconeogenic precursors with consequent hypoglycemia upon prolonged fasting. In childhood, the demands on glucose production by the liver may be outstripped because of the relatively larger brain weight (glucose uptake) and smaller muscle mass (source for gluconeogenic precursors). Glucose-6-phosphatase deficiency [glycogen storage disease (GSD), type 1] is due to a defect in the final common pathway for hepatic glucose release resulting from both glycogenolysis and gluconeogenesis. As such, it is one of the forms of GSD associated with hypoglycemia. As in the fructose-1,6-diphosphatase deficiency syndrome, plasma insulin concentrations are low and the child consequently presents with ketosis. Other, even rarer inborn errors resulting in hypoglycemia may present with a similar picture.[77] In children with defective gluconeogenesis, continuous nocturnal gastric infusions of glucose supplementing frequent feeding during the waking hours have been employed successfully.

Defects in gluconeogenic amino acid metabolism also cause hypoglycemia, as one would predict. In patients with maple syrup urine disease, an enzymatic defect in the decarboxylation of the α-ketoacids of leucine, isoleucine, and valine associated with profound hypoglycemia is due to decreased alanine production by muscle. In ketotic hypoglycemia of infancy and childhood, alanine deficiency has also been implicated in the pathogenesis of hypoglycemia.[81,82] Although these children are frequently small for age, the mechanism of the hypoalaninemia is unknown. Clinical hypoglycemia tends to become exaggerated during periods of stress or caloric deprivation and responds to feeding. The disorder remits by 8 to 9 years of age and has become increasingly uncommon.[81]

In adults, alanine deficiency has been the postulated mechanism to explain spontaneous hypoglycemia associated with renal failure. As in other patients with defective gluconeogenesis, these patients are generally calorie-deprived, but the precise pathogenesis of the disorder remains uncertain.

Finally, systemic carnitine deficiency is associated with hypoglycemia. As a result of the generalized carnitine-dependent defect in the transport of long-chain fatty acid into mitochondria, this disorder results in skeletal muscle weakness, hepatic dysfunction, and cardiomyopathy as well. Hypoglycemia is due to decreased hepatic synthesis coupled with greater muscle dependence on glucose for oxidative energy. Since ketogenesis is also impaired in these patients, this syndrome presents with hypoinsulinemic hypoglycemia without ketosis.[83] Treatment consists of frequent high-carbohydrate feeding and dietary administration of medium-chain triglycerides which do not depend on carnitine for oxidation.

Insulin Autoimmune Hypoglycemia

Several rare syndromes in which autoimmunity is associated with fasting hypoglycemia have been identified. These syndromes are caused by the presence of autoantibodies to the insulin receptor or to insulin itself.

Antibodies to the insulin receptor were first discovered in patients with extreme insulin resistance and hyperglycemia.[84] However, fasting hypoglycemia developed in some patients whose diabetes resolved. In addition, several patients with anti-insulin receptor antibodies have been reported in whom severe fasting hypoglycemia was not preceded by a history of diabetes.[85] Potential mechanisms include the insulinomimetic effect of the antibody and reduced insulin clearance from plasma. The latter explanation is consistent with the fact that the major mechanism for the removal of insulin from plasma is receptor-mediated endocytosis, which is reduced in patients with antireceptor antibodies. Diagnosis in these patients is a challenge because plasma insulin concentrations are usually elevated disproportionately to plasma C peptide levels[85] and because determinations of antireceptor antibody are not reliable unless performed in a research laboratory. Treatment of these patients has involved the use of corticosteroids, immunosuppressive drugs, and plasmapheresis while the disease is active; in most reported patients, antireceptor antibody titers declined over time.

Another form of autoimmune hypoglycemia is that associated with insulin autoantibodies. This syndrome must be distinguished from the more commonly occurring surreptitious use of exogenous insulin by the patient. The majority of cases of the so-called autoimmune insulin syndrome have been reported from Japan, and most of these patients have had associated autoimmune diseases [e.g., Graves' disease, systemic lupus erythematosus (SLE), or rheumatoid arthritis]. Both fasting and reactive patterns of hypoglycemia have been reported.[86] The presence of insulin autoantibodies will interfere with insulin RIAs (see above), although the "total" insulin concentration in the plasma in such patients is clearly elevated. The hypoglycemia in most of these patients has been mild and self-limited, with symptoms resolving within a year. Supportive therapy with frequent small feedings usually suffices; a few patients have required glucocorticoids.

The pathophysiology of hypoglycemia in these patients is obscure. Because of the large pool of antibody-bound insulin (which is in equilibrium with free insulin in plasma), inappropriate hyperinsulinism may occur at unpredictable times of the day. It is also hypothesized that insulin antibodies per se mimic insulin at the receptor (anti-idiotypic antibody) or that the antibodies may potentiate insulin action.

Reactive Hypoglycemias

A great deal of controversy surrounds the subject of reactive or "functional" hypoglycemia. The debate centers not on whether reactive symptoms associated with low blood glucose can be produced under the appropriate conditions but on whether spontaneous reactive hypoglycemia represents a common clinical entity. The recognition that fasting hypoglycemia, as discussed above, may be associated with disastrous sequelae has unfortunately resulted in more attention being paid to its poor cousins, the reactive hypoglycemias. Indeed, it is not uncommon to find that an evaluation for the symptoms of fasting hypoglycemia was initiated incorrectly with an OGTT.

Definition

It is well known that the ingestion of large amounts of glucose is often followed by a transient decline in plasma glucose below the fasting concentration.[87] The decline in plasma glucose during the later (3 to 5 h) stage of a 75-g OGTT is also associated with a small but detectable increase in the secretion of counterregulatory hormones.[87] Thus, reactive hypoglycemia has probably been overdiagnosed as a result of indiscriminate use of the OGTT. In fact, an international group has defined reactive hypoglycemia as a clinical disorder in which the patient has postprandial symptoms which are accompanied by a plasma or serum glucose below 45 to 50 mg/dl (2.5–2.8 mmol/L) in an arterialized specimen.[88] This definition requiring that symptoms be associated with documented chemical evidence of hypoglycemia under normal feeding conditions has rarely been met in various series reporting reactive hypoglycemia; thus, many patients with hypoglycemic-type symptoms in fact have "nonhypoglycemia."[89] Indeed, in a recent study of 28 patients with suspected postprandial hypoglycemia in whom capillary blood was collected at the time of symptoms, it was found that almost 50 percent of patients experienced symptoms at glucose levels higher than 3.3 mmol/L (~60 mg/dl). There was no correlation found between the plasma glucose values during oral glucose administration and the levels measured during symptoms.[90]

FIGURE 20-4 Flow sheet for the evaluation of a patient with suspected reactive (postprandial) hypoglycemia. "Mixed meal test" refers to the determination of the response of the plasma glucose concentration to mixed meals.

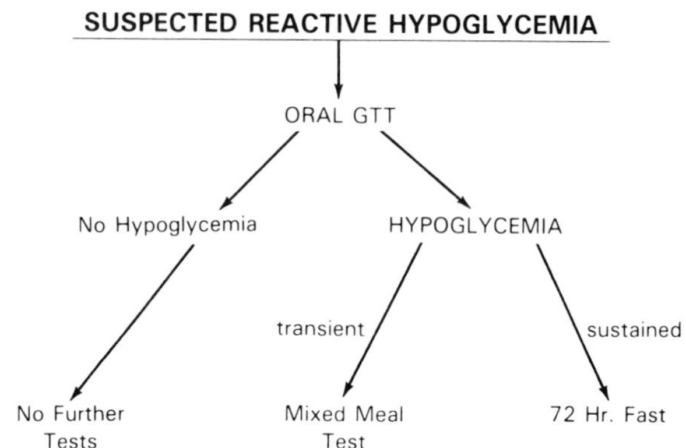

Symptoms

In contrast to fasting hypoglycemia, neuroglycopenia is rarely observed in patients who experience only postprandial symptoms. Glucose concentrations generally do not decline below 40 mg/dl (2.2 mmol/L), and the hypoglycemic period is also usually brief. Adrenergic symptoms accompany the transient decrease in blood glucose in the late stage of the OGTT, though a wide array of nonspecific symptomatology may be reported in patients allegedly suffering from this syndrome (Fig. 20-4).

Alimentary Hypoglycemia

Alimentary hypoglycemia represents one of the diverse pathologic causes of reactive hypoglycemia. Some patients who have undergone gastric surgery display an exaggerated early increase in both plasma glucose and insulin after oral glucose administration, followed by a rapid decline to hypoglycemic levels by 3 h. The symptoms accompanying this hypoglycemia tend to be predominantly of the adrenergic type, though loss of consciousness and seizures have been reported. These reactive symptoms can usually be distinguished from those due to the "dumping" syndrome since those symptoms tend to occur within 1 h of feeding and are generally associated with nausea and epigastric fullness induced by the rapid transit of a large osmotic and fluid load.

The mechanism underlying alimentary hypoglycemia has not been established with certainty. Rapid gastric emptying resulting from a reduced gastric pouch size (e.g., partial gastrectomy) or caused by vagal interruption has been postulated to result in rapid, early glucose absorption which in turn leads to excessive hyperglycemia and hyperinsulinemia. Augmentation of insulin secretion as a result of increased gastric inhibitory peptide (GIP) and other gut hormones may also play a role.

Reactive Hypoglycemia in Diabetes

A reactive pattern of hypoglycemia has long been noted in patients who have subsequently developed diabetes.[91] It is unclear whether this is a true association or simply a coincidence in which a common disease (diabetes) is combined with the overdiagnosed "idiopathic" hypoglycemia. Postprandial hypoglycemia has also been reported in patients with obesity, renal glycosuria, hypothyroidism, and congenital adrenal hyperplasia.

Treatment

Carbohydrate restriction, especially limitation of simple sugars in the diet, has been the empirical approach to the treatment of most of these patients. Although controlled studies of such dietary changes are not available, most patients experience relief and only rare patients require other modalities (e.g., drugs, reoperation on the gastric stoma). Patients with milder symptoms may need only minimal dietary interventions (such as the avoidance of simple sugars), whereas certain patients will require a carefully designed diet containing only 120 to 150 g per day of total carbohydrate and supervised by a qualified nutritionist. Meal size should be reduced, and the frequency of feedings should be increased as needed.

In patients who fail to respond to dietary manipulations, the physician should be concerned about the possibility of the patient having fasting hypoglycemia or make sure that hypoglycemia is not responsible for the symptoms. Pharmacologic interventions which may be attempted include anticholinergics, especially in patients with alimentary hypoglycemia.[92] Long-acting somatostatin analogues have been successful in a few patients.

Induced Hypoglycemias

Drug-induced hypoglycemias (Table 20-2) are the most common because of the complications associated with insulin and sulfonylurea use in patients with diabetes. However, a wide variety of other drugs have been reported to cause severe hypoglycemia, and over 50 individual agents have been implicated in published reports.[93] Treatment must include discontinuation of the agent when possible and supportive therapy for the hypoglycemia. The counterregulatory responses triggered by insulin-induced hypoglycemia and the syndrome of hypoglycemia unawareness are discussed in Glucose Counterregulation.

Sulfonylureas

These drugs account for a substantial proportion of drug-induced hypoglycemia. Because of their widespread clinical use, it is difficult to assess the true incidence of sulfonylurea hypoglycemia in patients with diabetes. The majority of reported cases of severe hypoglycemia have occurred in patients given chlorpropamide or glyburide. However, severe episodes characterized by coma have been reported with all the agents in common use (Table 20-2). In part, the hypoglycemic potential of an agent is related to its potency, its plasma and biological half-lives, and the use of concomitant substances. For example, liver disease prolongs the hypoglycemic actions of tolbutamide, acetohexamide, glyuburide, and glipizide, since these drugs are normally metabolized in the liver. The effects of chlorpropamide and acetohexamide are accentuated in patients with renal insuffiency, though even older patients without overt renal disease may suffer severe and prolonged hypoglycemia. Chlorpropamide may also cause hypoglycemia in patients treated for diabetes insipidus or when it has been mistakenly prescribed or dispensed.

In addition to the inherent potential of these drugs to lower plasma glucose, they may interact with other agents to produce severe hypoglycemia. The additive (or possibly synergistic) effects during combined insulin and sulfonylurea therapy account for an increasing number of such episodes. Drugs which interfere with sulfonylurea metabolism or compete for circulating plasma protein binding with sulfonylureas can also potentiate these effects (Table 20-2). Important among these agents is coumarin (heparin, warfarin, and phenindione do not possess these effects).

TABLE 20-2 Causes of Induced Hypoglycemia

1. Hypoglycemic drugs
   a. Insulin
   b. Sulfonylureas
   c. Biguanides
2. Nonhypoglycemic therapeutic agents
   a. Salicylates
   b. Propranolol
   c. Phenylbutazone
   d. Sulfonamides
   e. Dicumarol (bishydroxycoumarin)
   f. Quinine
   g. Pentamidine isethionate
   h. Ritodrine and β_2 agonists
   i. Disopyramide
3. Ethanol
4. Toxins
   a. Hypoglycine A (akee fruit)
   b. Pyriminil (Vacor)

Pentamidine Isethionate

The earliest report of hypoglycemia associated with the use of this drug appeared in 1977.[94] Since then, the widespread use of this agent in the treatment of *Pneumocystis carinii* infection in immunocompromised hosts has resulted in over 30 reported cases of severe hypoglycemia in patients with the acquired immunodeficiency syndrome (AIDS).[93] Although pentamidine is a biguanide derivative, the mechanism of the hypoglycemia is not clear. It is most likely that this agent causes beta cell injury with leakage of insulin, since plasma insulin concentrations during hypoglycemia may be increased and since diabetes has ultimately developed in a few patients.

Ethanol

Ethanol ingestion is a recognized cause of hypoglycemia among all age groups. Most of these patients have a history of chronic alcoholism and/or poor nutrition, but accidental ingestion in healthy children and binge drinking among adults also have been reported in association with hypoglycemia. The diagnosis may be obscured by the absence of signs of acute inebriation, although blood alcohol levels are usually detectable. Ketonuria is often present, in keeping with the reduction in insulin secretion; liver function tests and amylase and phosphate levels are usually normal. While plasma glucagon concentrations are appropriately increased, a hallmark of the disease is that exogenous glucagon administration has little effect on blood glucose.

The mechanism underlying this disorder most likely involves disruption of gluconeogenesis at the liver. This is suggested by the observation that hypoglycemia occurs when healthy volunteers are given ethanol after fasting for 36 to 72 h (at which time liver glycogen is depleted) but not after overnight fasting. During the hepatic oxidation of ethanol to acetaldehyde and acetate, nicotinamide-adenine dinucleotide (NAD) is reduced to NADH. The increased NADH/NAD ratio results in a redox state which does not promote the oxidation of substrates for gluconeogenesis such as lactate.[95] The levels of pyruvate fall, oxaloacetate and phosphoenolpyruvate are not formed, and gluconeogenesis is hampered. Hypoglycemia results when hepatic glycogen stores are also depleted, hence the relation to the nutritional state of the patient. Alcohol consequently also potentiates the hypoglycemic actions of insulin and sulfonylurea agents. It is particularly important to emphasize this risk for insulin-dependent diabetes patients since death and irreversible brain damage have been attributed to hypoglycemia induced by the combination.[96]

Diagnostic and Therapeutic Approach to Fasting Hypoglycemia

In the majority of patients historical clues (symptoms arising from neuroglycopenia) will point to the presence of fasting hypoglycemia. In some circumstances a diagnostic evaluation will be required not because of the patient's symptoms but by reason of laboratory (e.g., plasma glucose) or radiologic tests performed for other reasons (e.g., abdominal CT). Thus, in this latter instance, establishing the *presence* of fasting hypoglycemia is critical.

If postprandial hypoglycemia is considered on clinical grounds, only a 5-h OGTT is required (Fig. 20-4). The reactive hypoglycemias may be excluded if hypoglycemia fails to develop or if symptoms do not occur despite a fall in plasma glucose concentrations to a level below 50 mg/dl (2.8 mmol/L). If biochemical hypoglycemia or symptomatic hypoglycemia is observed, it is usually not necessary to test for fasting hypoglycemia unless the hypoglycemia is sustained. It is important, however, to determine whether the hypoglycemia is also provoked by the usual mixed meal before embarking on a therapeutic regimen.

In patients suspected of having fasting hypoglycemia, a supervised fast is mandatory (Fig. 20-5). Of course, patients with hypoglycemia after brief periods of fasting (12 to 18 h) should not be subjected to a full 72-h fast. Conversely, it may be sufficient for the patient to undergo an 18-h fast as an outpatient by merely skipping breakfast and giving a blood sample for plasma glucose and insulin before lunch. If plasma glucose remains above 70 mg/dl (3.9 mmol/L), further studies may not be warranted. If plasma glucose falls below 50 to 60 mg/dl (2.8–3.4 mmol/L), insulin levels should be obtained.

The development of hypoglycemia during a brief or prolonged fast is the sine qua non of diagnosis (Fig. 20-5). In contrast, hyperinsulinemia without concomitant hypoglycemia indicates neither the presence of an islet-cell tumor nor that of another hypoglycemic disorder. The most common form of nonhypoglycemic hyperinsulinemia is obesity. The concurrence of symptomatic hypoglycemia with relative or absolute hyperinsulinemia provides the highest degree of confidence in the clinical diagnosis of islet-cell pathology. No further tests are warranted in a patient who does not develop hypoglycemia after a prolonged fast. Long-term observation may, however, be necessary to reevaluate a patient with suspicious symptoms. A repeated fast with the addition of a bout of exercise in the last hour may be helpful in eliciting symptomatic hypoglycemia.

In a patient with both hypoglycemia and hyperinsulinemia, plasma C peptide determinations should help distinguish factitious or iatrogenic hypoglycemia caused by exogenous insulin. However, hypoglycemia due to sulfonylurea drugs cannot be excluded by the C peptide assay; detection of these agents in urine may be necessary.

When hypoglycemia is found in the presence of *low* plasma insulin concentrations, underlying hepatic or renal dysfunction is the most probable cause. However, these conditions are not likely to escape detection in a routine clinical evaluation. In other cases a careful search for an undetected endocrine

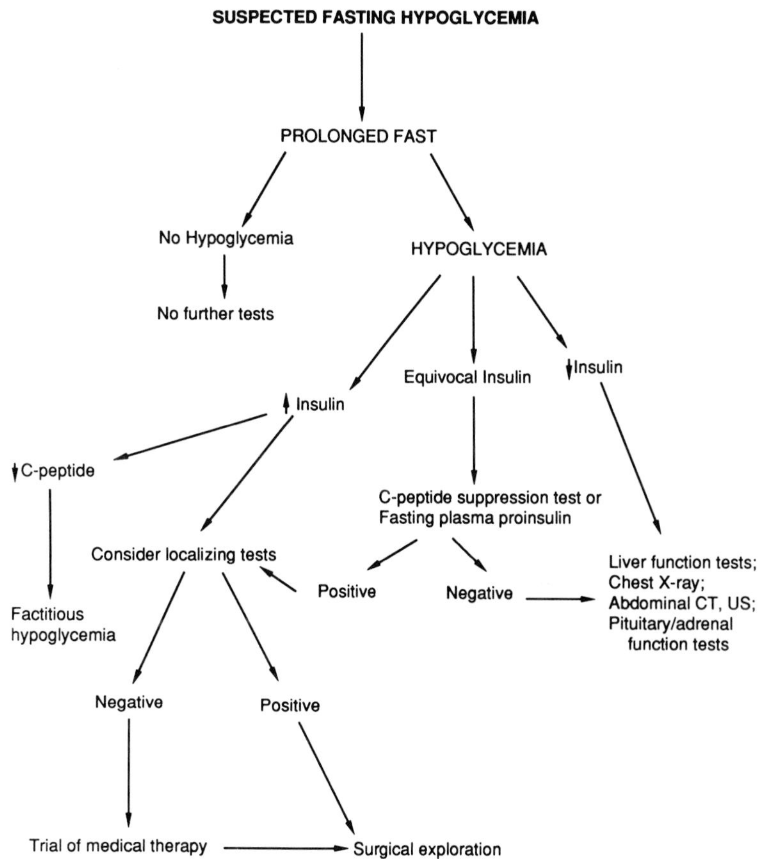

FIGURE 20-5 Approach to the diagnosis of fasting hypoglycemia (see text for details).

deficiency or occult extrapancreatic malignancy is warranted.

If the plasma insulin concentration is equivocal, additional examinations such as a C peptide suppression test or proinsulin determinations should be considered. If these examinations are abnormal, the diagnosis of an islet-cell lesion should be pursued (Fig. 20-5).

Only after unequivocal demonstration of fasting hypoglycemia and relative or absolute hyperinsulinemia should one consider tests to localize an islet-cell tumor. Since the frequency of false-negative imaging studies is substantial and reliance on the operative findings will be critical, a surgical consultation should be obtained. A trial of medical therapy with dietary and pharmacologic intervention (diazoxide and/or octreotide) should be considered at this stage. This is especially important if a tumor cannot be found at the time of laparotomy (estimated to occur in 10 percent of patients with biochemical evidence of autonomous insulin secretion). Before subjecting the patient to the risk of a partial or subtotal blind resection of the distal pancreas, one can let the preoperative response to medical therapy direct the appropriate course of action. In addition, one may choose to defer definitive surgery until more invasive tests (i.e., pancreatic venous sampling) allow better localization of pancreatic pathology.

REFERENCES

1. Merimee TJ, Tyson JE: Stabilization of plasma glucose during fasting. Normal variations in two separate studies. *N Engl J Med* 291:1275, 1979.
2. Field JB: Hypoglycemia, definition, clinical presentations, classification, and laboratory tests. *Endocrinol Clin North Am* 18:27, 1989.
3. Cornblath M, Schwartz R: *Disorders of Carbohydrate Metabolism in Infancy,* 2d ed. Philadelphia, Saunders, 1976.
4. Haymond MW, Karl E, Clark WL, Pagliara AS, Santiago JV: Differences in circulating gluconeogenic substrates during short-term fasting in men, women, and children. *Metabolism* 31:34, 1982.
5. Marks V, Rose FC: *Hypoglycaemia,* 2d ed. Oxford, Blackwell, 1981.
6. Marks V, Greenwood FC, Howorth PJN, Samols E: Plasma growth hormone levels in spontaneous hypoglycemia. *J Clin Endocrinol Metab* 27:523, 1967.
7. Amiel SA, Sherwin RS, Simonson DC, Tamborlane WV: Effect of intensive insulin therapy on glycemic thresholds for counterregulatory hormone release. *Diabetes* 37:901, 1988.
8. Davis MR, Shamoon H: Deficient counterregulatory hormone responses during hypoglycemia in a patient with insulinoma. *J Clin Endocrinol Metab* 72:788,1991.
9. Boyle P, Schwartz NS, Shah, Clutter WE, Cryer PE: Plasma glucose concentrations at the onset of hypoglycemic symp-

toms in patients with poorly controlled diabetes and in nondiabetics. *N Engl J Med* 318:1487, 1988.
10. Owen OE, Morgan AO, Kemp HG, Sullivan JM, Herrera MG, Cahill GF Jr: Brain metabolism during fasting. *J Clin Invest* 46:1589, 1967.
11. Holmes CS, Hayford JT, Gonzalez JL, Weydert JA: A survey of cognitive functioning at different glucose levels in diabetic persons. *Diabetes Care* 6:180, 1983.
12. Herold KC, Polonsky KS, Cohen RM, Levy J, Douglas F: Variable deterioration in cortical function during insulin-induced hypoglycemia. *Diabetes* 34:677, 1985.
13. Siejo BK: Hypoglycemia, brain metabolism, and brain damage. *Diabetes Metab Rev* 4:113, 1988.
14. Bryan RM Jr, Keefer KA, MacNeill C: Regional cerebral glucose utilization during insulin-induced hypoglycemia in unanesthetized rats. *J Neurochem* 46:1904, 1986.
15. Ferrendelli JA: Hypoglycemia and the CNS, in Ingrar DH, Lassen NA (eds): *Brain Work: The Coupling of Function, Metabolism and Blood Flow in the Brain.* Copenhagen, Munksgaard, 1975, p 298.
16. Horton RW, Meldrum BS, Bachelard HS: Enzymic and cerebral metabolic effects of 2-deory-D-glucose. *J Neurochem* 21:507, 1973.
17. Myers RE, Kahn KJ: Insulin-induced hypoglycemia in the nonhuman primate: II. Long-term neuropathological consequences, in Brierley JB, Meldrum BS (eds): *Brain Hypoxia.* Clinics in Developmental Medicine 39/40. London, Heinemann, 1971, p 195.
18. Danta G: Hypoglycemic peripheral neuropathy. *Arch Neurol* 21:121, 1969.
19. Bertoye A, Bourrat C, Bolot JF, Robert D: Neuropathie amyotrophique quadridistale par hyperinsulinisme. *Rev Neurol (Paris)* 126:220, 1972.
20. Lloyd-Mostyn RH, Oram S: Modification by propranolol of cardiovascular effects of induced hypoglycemia. *Lancet* i:1213, 1975.
21. Pladziewicz DS, Nesto RW: Hypoglycemia-induced silent myocardial ischemia. *Am J Cardiol* 63:1531, 1989.
22. Bennett T, Gale EAM, Green JH, MacDonald IA, Walford S: The influence of beta-adrenoceptor antagonists on thermoregulation during insulin induced hypoglycemia. *J Physiol* 308: 26, 1980.
23. Hutton RA, Mikhailidis D, Dormandy KM, Ginsburg J: Platelet aggregation studies during transient hypoglycemia. *J Clin Pathol* 32:434, 1979.
24. Brodows RG, Ensinck JW, Campbell RG: Mechanism of plasma cyclic AMP response to hypoglycemia in man. *Metabolism* 6:659, 1976.
25. Frier BM, Corrall RJM, Davidson NM, Webber RG, Dewar A, French EB: Peripheral blood cell changes in response to acute hypoglycemia in man. *J Clin Invest* 13:33, 1983.
26. Fajans S, Floyd JC: Fasting hypoglycemia in adults. *N Engl J Med* 294:766, 1976.
27. Shoelson SE, Polonsky KS, Zeidler A, Rubenstein AH, Tager HS: Human insulin B24(PHE—SER): Secretion and metabolic clearance of the abnormal insulin in man and in a dog model. *J Clin Invest* 73:1351, 1984.
28. Rubenstein AH, Steiner DF, Horwitz DL, Mako ME, Block MB, Starr JI, Kuzaya H, Melani F: Clinical significance of circulating proinsulin and C-peptide. *Recent Prog Horm Res* 33:435, 1977.
29. Gorden P, Sherman B, Roth J: Proinsulin-like component of circulating insulin in the basal state and in patients and hamsters with islet cell tumors. *J Clin Invest* 50:2113, 1971.
30. Gabbay KH, De Luca K, Fisher JN Jr, Mako ME, Rubenstein AH: Familial hyperproinsulinemia: An autosomal dominant defect. *N Engl J Med* 294:911, 1976.
31. Johansen K: Insulinoma: Clinical manifestation, diagnosis and treatment. *J Endocrinol Invest* 2:285, 1979.
32. Floyd JC, Fajans SS, Knopf RF, Conn JW: Plasma insulin in organic hyperinsulinism: Comparative effects of tolbutamide, leucine and glucose. *J Clin Endocrinol Metab* 24:747, 1964.
33. Marks V, Samols E: Glucagon test for insulinoma: A chemical study in 25 cases. *J Clin Pathol* 21:346, 1968.
34. Roy BK, Abuid J, Wendorff H, Nitiyanant W: Insulin release in response to calcium in the diagnosis of insulinoma. *Metabolism* 28:1029, 1975.
35. Cryer PE: Glucose counterregulation in man. *Diabetes* 30:261, 1981.
36. Gerich JE, Campbell PJ: Overview of counterregulation and its abnormalities in diabetes mellitus and other conditions. *Diabetes Metab Rev* 4:93, 1988.
37. Cryer PE, Gerich JE: Glucose counterregulation, hypoglycemia and intensive insulin therapy in diabetes mellitus. *N Engl J Med* 313:232, 1985.
38. Bolli G, De Feo P, Compagnucci P, Cartechini MG, Angeletti G, Santeusanio F, Brunetti P, Gerich JE: Abnormal glucose counterregulation in insulin-dependent diabetes mellitus: Interaction of anti-insulin antibodies and impaired glucagon and epinephrine secretion. *Diabetes* 32:134, 1983.
39. Shamoon H, Hendler R, Sherwin R: Synergistic interactions among anti-insulin hormones in the pathogenesis of stress hyperglycemia in hormones. *J Clin Endocrinol Metab* 52: 1235, 1981.
40. Gerich JE, Rizza R, Haymond M, Cryer PE: Hormone mechanisms in acute glucose counterregulation: The relative roles of glucagon, epinephrine, nonepinephrine growth hormones and cortisol. *Metabolism* 29(Suppl 1):1164, 1980.
41. Kleinbaum J, Shamoon H: Impaired counterregulation of hypoglycemia in insulin-dependent diabetes mellitus. *Diabetes* 32:493, 1983.
42. De Feo P, Perriello G, Torlone E, Ventura MM, Fanelli C, Santeusanio F, Burnetti P, Gerich JE, Bolli GB: Contribution of cortisol to glucose counterregulation in humans. *Am J Physiol* 20:E35, 1989.
43. De Feo P, Perriello G, Torlone E, Ventura MM, Santeusanio F, Brunetti P, Gerich JE, Bolli GB: Demonstration of a role for growth hormone in glucose counterregulation. *Am J Physiol* 19:E835, 1989.
44. Rizza R, Cryer P, Haymond M, Gerich JE: Adrenergic mechanisms for the effects of epinephrine on glucose production and clearance in man. *J Clin Invest* 65:682, 1980.
45. Hopwood NJ, Forsham PJ, Kenny FM, Drash AL: Hypolycemia in hypopituitary children. *Am J Dis Child* 129:918, 1975.
46. Smallright RC, Corrigan DF, Thomason AM, Blue PW: Hypoglycemia in pregnancy: Occurrence due to adrenocorticotropic hormone and growth hormone deficiency. *Arch Intern Med* 140:564, 1980.
47. Sacca L, Sherwin RS, Hendler R, Felig P: Influence of continuous physiologic hyperinsulinemia on glucose kinetics and counterregulatory hormones in normal and diabetic humans. *J Clin Invest* 63:849, 1979.
48. Silverberg AB, Shah SD, Haymond MW, Cryer PE: Norepinephrine: Hormone and neurotransmitter. *Am J Physiol* 234:E252, 1978.
49. Polonsky K, Bergenstal R, Pons G, Schneider M, Jaspan J, Rubenstein AH: Relation of counterregulatory response to hypoglycemia in type I diabetics. *N Eng J Med* 307:1106, 1982.
50. Hirsch BR, Shamoon H: Defective epinephrine and growth hormone responses in IDDM are stimulus-specific. *Diabetes* 36:20, 1987.
51. Gerich JE, Langlois M, Noacco C, Karam JH, Forsham PH: Lack of glucagon response to hypoglycemia in diabetes: Evidence for an intrinsic pancreatic alpha-cell defect. *Science* 182:171, 1973.
52. Simonson DC, Tamborlane WV, DeFronzo RA, Sherwin RS: Intensive insulin therapy reduces counterregulatory hormone responses to hypoglycemia in patients with type I diabetes. *Ann Intern Med* 103:184, 1985.
53. Cloutier MG, Pek S, Crowther RL, Floyd JC Jr, Fajans SS: Glucagon-insulin interactions in patients with insulin producing pancreatic islet lesions. *J Clin Endocrinol Metab* 48:201, 1979.

54. French EB, Kilpatric R: Role of adrenaline in hypoglycaemic reactions in man. *Clin Sci* 14:639, 1955.
55. Ginsburg J, Paton A: Effects of insulin after adrenalectomy. *Lancet* ii:491, 1965.
56. Marks V, Samols E: Insulinoma: Natural history and diagnosis. *Clin Gastroenterol* 3:559, 1974.
57. Kahn CR, Rosen SW, Weintraub BD, Fajans SS, Gorden P: Ectopic production of chorionic gonadotrophin and its subunits by islet-cell tumors. *N Engl J Med* 297:565, 1977.
58. Anderson A, Bergdahl L: Insulinomas and multiple endocrine neoplasia. *Acta Chir Scand* 142:297, 1976.
59. Stefanini P, Carboni M, Patrassi N, Basoli A: Beta-islet cell tumors of the pancreas: Results of a study on 1,067 cases. *Surgery* 75:597, 1974.
60. Tibaldi JM, Lorber D, Shamoon H, Lomasky S, Steinberg JJ, Reisman R: Postprandial hypoglycemia in islet beta cell hyperplasia with adenomatosis of the pancreas. *J Surg Onc*.
61. Fajans SS: Insulin-producing islet cell tumors. *Endocrinol Metab Clin North Am* 18:45, 1989.
62. Merimee TJ, Tyson JE: Hypoglycemia in man: Pathologic and physiologic variants. *Diabetes* 24:161, 1977.
63. Stark D, Moss AA, Goldberg HI, Deveney CW, Way L: Computed tomography and nuclear magnetic resonance imaging of pancreatic islet cell tumors. *Surgery* 94:1024, 1983.
64. Fulton RE, Sheedy PF, McIlrath DC, Ferris DO: Preoperative angiographic localization of insulin-producing tumors of the pancreas. *AJR* 123:367, 1975.
65. Roche A, Raissonnier A, Gillon-Savouret M-C: Pancreatic venous sampling and arteriography in localizing insulinomas and gastrinomas: Procedure and results in 55 cases. *Radiology* 145:621, 1982.
66. Grant CS, Van Heerden J, Charboneau JW, James EM, Reading CC: Insulinoma: The value of intraoperative ultrasonography. *Arch Surg* 123:843, 1988.
67. Laroche GP, Ferris DO, Priestly JT, Scholz DA, Dockerty MB: Hyperinsulinism: Surgical results and management of occult functioning islet cell tumors: Review of 154 cases. *Arch Surg* 96:763, 1968.
68. Laron Z: Somatostatin analogues in the management of benign insulinomas. *Isr J Med Sci* 26:1, 1990.
69. Glaser B, Rosler A, Halperin Y: Chronic treatment of a benign insulinoma using the long-acting somatostatin analogue SMS 201-995. *Isr J Med Sci* 26:16, 1990.
70. Comi RJ, Gorden P, Doppman J, Norton J: Insulinoma, in Go VLW (ed): *The Exocrine Pancreas: Biology, Pathobiology and Diseases*. New York, Raven Press, 1986, p 745.
71. Chowdhury F, Bleicha JJ: Studies of tumor hypoglycemia. *Metabolism* 22:663, 1973.
72. Flier JS, Mueckler MM, Usher P, Lodish HF: Elevated levels of glucose transport and transporter messenger RNA are induced by ras or src oncogenes. *Science* 235:1492, 1987.
73. Daughaday WH: Hypoglycemia in patients with non-islet cell tumors. *Endocrinol Metab Clin North Am* 18:91, 1989.
74. Merimee TJ: Insulin-like growth factors in patients with non-islet cell tumors and hypoglycemia. *Metabolism* 35:360, 1986.
75. Daughaday WH, Emanuele MA, Brooks MH, Barbato AL, Kapadia M, Rotwein P: Synthesis and secretion of insulin-like growth factor II by a leiomyosarcoma with associated hypoglycemia. *N Engl J Med* 319:1434, 1988.
76. Axelrod L, Ron D: Insulin-like growth factor II and the riddle of tumor-induced hypoglycemia. *N Engl J Med* 319:1477, 1988.
77. Bier D, Rosemary DL, Haymond MW, Arnold KJ, Gruenke LD, Sperling MA, Kipnis DM: Measurement of "true" glucose production rates in infancy and childhood with 6,6-dideuteroglucose. *Diabetes* 26:1016, 1977.
78. Comi RJ, Gorden P: Approach to hypoglycemia in adults. *Compr Ther* 13:38, 1987.
79. Block MB, Gambetta M, Resnekov L, Rubenstein AH: Spontaneous hypoglycemia and congestive heart-failure. *Lancet* ii:736, 1972.
80. Breen KJ, Penkins KW, Mistilis SP, Shearman R: Idiopathic acute fatty liver of pregnancy. *Gut* 11:82, 1970.
81. Haymond MW: Hypoglycemia in infants and children. *Endocrinol Metab Clin* 18:211, 1989.
82. Haymond MW, Pagliara AS: Ketotic hypoglycemia. *Clin Endocrinol Metab* 12:447, 1983.
83. Rebouche CJ, Engel AG: Carnitine metabolism and deficiency. *Mayo Clin Proc* 58:533, 1983.
84. Kahn CR, Flier JS, Bar RS, Archer JA, Gorden P, Martin MM, Roth J: The syndromes of insulin resistance and acanthosis nigricans: Insulin-receptor disorders in man. *N Engl J Med* 294:739, 1976.
85. Taylor SI, Grunberger G, Marcus-Samuel B, Underhill LH, Dons RF, Ryan J, Roddam RF, Rupe CE, Gorden P: Hypoglycemia associated with antibodies to the insulin receptor. *N Engl J Med* 307:1422, 1982.
86. Hirata Y: Autoimmune insulin syndrome, in Andreani D, Marks V, Lefebvre PJ (eds): *Hypoglycemia*. New York, Raven Press, 1987, p 105.
87. Kleinbaum J, Shamoon H: Selective counterregulatory hormone responses after oral glucose in man. *J Clin Endocrinol Metab* 55:787, 1982.
88. Lefebvre PJ, Andreani D, Marks V: Statement on "postprandial" or reactive hypoglycemia, in Andreani D, Marks V, Lefebvre PJ (eds): *Hypoglycemia*. New York, Raven Press, 1987, p 79.
89. Cahill GF, Soeldner JS: A non-editorial on non-hypoglycemia. *N Engl J Med* 291:905, 1974.
90. Palardy J, Havrankova J, Lepage R, Matte R, Bélanger R, D 'Amour P, Ste Marie LG: Blood glucose measurements during symptomatic episodes in patients with suspected postprandial hypoglycemia. *N Engl J Med* 321:1421, 1989.
91. Seltzer HS, Fajans SS, Conn JW: Spontaneous hypoglycemia as an early manifestation of diabetes mellitus. *Diabetes* 5:437, 1956.
92. Permutt MA: Postprandial hypoglycemia. *Diabetes* 25:719, 1976.
93. Seltzer HS: Drug-induced hypoglycemia: A review of 1418 cases. *Endocrinol Metab Clin* 18:163, 1989.
94. Grant AM, Sandler RM, Carrell RW: Hypoglycaemic effect of pentamidine detected by glucose screen. *Lancet* ii:510, 1977.
95. Krebs HA, Freedland RA, Hems R, Stubbs M: Inhibition of hepatic gluconeogenesis by ethanol. *Biochem J* 112:117, 1969.
96. Arky R, Veverbrants E, Abramson EA: Irreversible hypoglycemia: A complication of alcohol and insulin. *JAMA* 206:575, 1968.

CHAPTER 21

Obesity

John M. Amatruda

Stephen Welle

DEFINITION AND DIAGNOSIS OF OBESITY

Obesity is a chronic metabolic disorder characterized by an excess of body fat. This distinguishes obesity from *overweight*, which is defined as excess weight in reference to an arbitrary standard, usually a "desirable weight" from height-weight tables. A body builder will probably be overweight for his or her height but will be very lean and therefore not obese. Generally, normal females have 18 to 30 percent body fat and normal males have less than 25 percent body fat.

There are currently several methods of assessing fatness, all of which have certain advantages and disadvantages (Table 21-1). These techniques were extensively reviewed by Forbes.[1]

Underwater weighing to determine body density is considered the gold standard and requires few assumptions. This method, however, requires a specialized tank and the ability to measure residual lung volumes accurately. Furthermore, it requires substantial cooperation since in most cases the patient must be completely submerged. For these reasons, it is largely a research tool. Total body water and other ion dilution measurements require the administration of radioactive or stable isotopes of hydrogen, oxygen, or other elements and assume that a constant percentage of lean body mass is composed of water. This percentage can vary, potentially introducing error. This method is also expensive and is currently used primarily as a research tool. A third method is potassium 40 (^{40}K) measurement. Since potassium is distributed in fat-free mass, measuring total body potassium allows one to estimate lean body mass. This is another research tool requiring expensive and not widely available equipment, and it depends on assumptions about the potassium content of lean tissue. A simpler and far less expensive method of estimating lean body mass (and, by subtraction, fat) is to measure the 24-h excretion of creatinine (Cr). Forbes and Bruining[2] found that on an ad lib diet, lean body mass in kilograms = 0.0291 Cr (mg/day) + 7.38, with an r value of 0.97. This technique gives different results depending on the amount of meat in the diet and varies with day-to-day variation in creatinine excretion. Recently, electrical impedance has shown promise in measuring lean body mass, with correlation coefficients from 0.9 to 0.97 between fat-free mass by densitometry and by impedance.[3] This technique is easy to perform and relatively inexpensive, although one must be cautious if weight is changing[4,5] since changes in bioelectrical impedance may reflect changes in total body water rather than lean body mass.

Another measure of fatness is skin fold measurements, or anthropometry.[1] Skin fold measurements measure mostly subcutaneous fat and are usually made over the triceps at the tip of the scapula. Because the thickness of fat varies in different depots and because subcutaneous fat may not reflect total body fat, these measurements are not accurate.

Although it is not a true measure of fatness, the most commonly used indirect measure of obesity is body mass index [BMI = weight (kg)/height^2(m)]. While normal ranges for this index from Metropolitan Life Insurance Tables correlate with percentile values from height-weight tables from the National Health and Nutrition Survey in 1982 and body fat in some studies, they do not necessarily reflect body fat. BMIs for the midpoint of medium-frame men of all heights from the Metropolitan Life Insurance Tables, after adjusting for shoes and clothes, are 22 kg/m^2, which equals a Metropolitan relative weight of 100. The range of the midpoint for all heights and frames is 19.8 to 25.7 kg/m^2. The midpoint for medium-frame females of all heights is 21.5 kg/m^2, and the range of midpoint values for females of all heights and frames is 19 to 26 kg/m^2.[6]

Height-weight tables are based on the levels of overweight associated with excess mortality.[7] The most commonly used tables are the Metropolitan Life Insurance Tables (Table 21-2), which are based on the 1979 Build Study published by the Society of Actuaries and the Association of Life Insurance Medical Directors. These tables give relative body

TABLE 21-1 Body Composition Measurement Techniques: Advantages and Disadvantages

	Advantages	Disadvantages
Density	Apparatus inexpensive	Subject cooperation necessary for underwater weighing
	Estimates Lean Body Mass and fat simultaneously	Unsuitable for young children and the elderly
	Nonhazardous	Error from intestinal gas
	Can be repeated frequently	
Total body water and ion dilution	Estimate body fluid volumes Inexpensive Great variety: Na, K, Cl(Br), H_2O	Radiation exposure (some materials) Blood samples needed for some materials (some require several samples) Incomplete equilibration Na, K; overestimation by D_2O, 3 H_2O; value for extracellular fluid depends on method used; ^{18}O assay requires elaborate equipment
^{40}K counting	No hazard Minimal subject cooperation Can be repeated frequently	Instrument expensive Proper calibration necessary Problem in interpretation in subjects with K deficiency
Creatinine excretion	No hazard Estimate of muscle mass	Meticulous subject cooperation Influenced by diet; collection time critical Day-to-day variation (5 to 10%)
Electrical impedance	Noninvasive Easy to perform Minimal patient cooperation Quick	Inaccurate when weight or body H_2O is changing
Anthropometry (skin fold)	Cheap Direct estimate of body fat and muscle mass	Poor precision in obese subjects and those with firm subcutaneous tissue Regional variation in subcutaneous fat layer; uncertainty about the ratio of subcutaneous fat to total fat
Metabolic balance	No hazard Suitable for many elements Can detect small changes in body content (<1%) Many laboratory analyses needed	Measures only the change in body composition Meticulous subject cooperation Metabolic ward expensive Error from unmeasured skin losses
Neutron activation	Minimal subject cooperation Body content Ca, P, N, Na, Cl	Apparatus very expensive Calibration very difficult Radiation exposure
Fat-soluble gases	Direct estimate of body fat	Cyclopropane, xenon, ^{85}Kr Apparatus expensive Long equilibration time
Ultrasound	Organ size No hazard	Poor definition of subcutaneous fat layer
3-Methylhistidine excretion	Estimate of muscle mass	Meat-free diet 2 days before collection Subject cooperation Variable contribution from gastrointestinal tissue (?) Magnitude of day-to-day variations (?)
Functions of height and weight (BMI)	Easy Quick Cheap	Not an accurate measure of body composition

Source: Modified from Forbes,[1] with permission.

weights which do not necessarily reflect adiposity. The Build Study was flawed in many ways in its attempt to relate relative weight to mortality. It disproportionately included men, whites, people under 60 years old, and the middle and upper classes. Furthermore, the unit of analysis was the insurance policy, not the person. Thus, a person who had more than one policy was included more than once. A per-

TABLE 21-2 Life Insurance Table of Desirable Body Weights

Men					Women				
Height		Small	Medium	Large	Height		Small	Medium	Large
Ft	In	Frame	Frame	Frame	Ft	In	Frame	Frame	Frame
5	2	128–134	131–141	138–150	4	10	102–111	109–121	118–131
5	3	130–136	133–143	140–153	4	11	103–113	111–123	120–134
5	4	132–138	135–145	142–156	5	0	104–115	113–126	122–137
5	5	134–140	137–148	144–160	5	1	106–118	115–129	125–140
5	6	136–142	139–151	146–164	5	2	108–121	118–132	128–143
5	7	138–145	142–154	149–168	5	3	111–124	121–135	131–147
5	8	140–148	145–157	152–172	5	4	114–127	124–138	134–151
5	9	142–151	148–160	155–176	5	5	117–130	127–141	137–155
5	10	144–154	151–163	158–180	5	6	120–133	130–144	140–159
5	11	146–157	154–166	161–184	5	7	123–136	133–147	143–163
6	0	149–160	157–170	164–188	5	8	126–139	136–150	146–167
6	1	152–164	160–174	168–192	5	9	129–142	139–153	149–170
6	2	155–168	164–178	172–197	5	10	132–145	142–156	152–173
6	3	158–172	167–182	176–202	5	11	135–148	145–159	155–176
6	4	162–176	171–187	181–207	6	0	138–151	148–162	158–179

Weights at ages 25 to 59 based on lowest mortality, weight in pounds according to frame (in indoor clothing weighing 3 lb, shoes with 1-in. heels).

Source: 1979 Build Study, Society of Actuaries and Association of Life Insurance Medical Directors of America, 1980.

son with more than one policy would obviously disproportionately affect the mortality data whether that person lived or died. The length of time a person was followed depended on how long that person was insured. The average length of follow-up was only 6.6 years, which minimizes the ability to see the effect of weight on mortality. Smoking and other variables were not considered. Also, frame size was not actually measured, and patients were weighed with their shoes and clothes. Among approximately 4.2 million subjects, only 100,000 (2.5 percent) died during the course of the study. Finally, 10 percent of the heights and weights were self-reported. Other studies relating mortality to weight, including the Framingham, American Cancer Society, and National Health and Nutrition Examination Survey (NHANES) studies, all suffer from one or more of these problems, limiting the usefulness of height-weight tables. Of great importance is the fact that none of these studies considered the distribution of the body fat by measuring the waist/hip ratio, which has recently been shown to be predictive of multiple complications of obesity.

In summary, the usual method to assess the fatness of patients—height-weight tables—does not measure fatness, and the data bases on which risk is assessed are either inadequate or flawed. Nevertheless, these measurements are easy to acquire, and most evidence indicates that assigning a patient as obese on the basis of these data, while not quantitatively accurate, is usually qualitatively correct. Furthermore, there are ample data relating obesity based on height-weight tables to morbidity and mortality and demonstrating that weight loss lessens risk by reducing concomitant risk factors such as hypertension. Furthermore, supplementing height and weight measurements with waist/hip ratios may be extremely useful. Until inexpensive, easy to use, precise, and accurate methods for measuring adiposity become available, the current height-weight measurements, supplemented with waist and hip measurements, are useful if not ideal.

MEDICAL COMPLICATIONS OF OBESITY (Table 21-3)

The relation between body weight and mortality has been reviewed.[8] Data from the Framingham study[9] evaluated mortality in men followed for 30 years from the date of entry. These data and those from the 1979 Build Study[6,10] indicate that the effects of obesity on mortality are delayed by approximately 10 years (Fig. 21-1). Framingham data (Fig. 21-1) also indicate that in both nonsmokers and smokers the effects of obesity on mortality are demonstrable in each age decade, with the lowest mortality in men who are 100 to 109 percent of ideal body weight (IBW). In smokers, mortality curves are J-shaped, with those below IBW having a higher mortality than do those at IBW. In nonsmokers the mortality curves are also J-shaped, but there are an inadequate number of men who are underweight to evalute mortality risk in this group. Overweight nonsmoking men age 30 to 39 at entry have mortality rates before age 70 which are 3.9 times those of nonsmoking men who are 100 to 109 percent of IBW. The relative risk is 8.8 for smoking men and 9.8 for overweight smoking men, indicating that the risk of

TABLE 21-3 Medical Complications of Obesity

Cardiovascular
- Coronary artery disease
- Myocardial infarction
- Congestive heart failure
- Sudden death
- Cerebrovascular accidents
- Hypertension
- Left ventricular hypertrophy

Metabolic
- Hyperlipidemia
- Insulin resistance
- Non-insulin-dependent diabetes mellitus
- Cholesterol gallstones

Cancer
- Males: colon, rectum, prostate
- Females: breast, ovary, endometrium, cervix, gallbladder, bile ducts

Hormonal
- Menstrual abnormalities
- Hyperandrogenism
- Hirsutism
- Acanthosis nigricans
- Polycystic ovaries
- Decreased sex hormone-binding globulin
- Increased estrogens
- Decreased testosterone in males
- Decreased growth hormone
- Decreased prolactin responsiveness
- Enhanced cortisol production

Rheumatic
- Osteoarthritis

Pulmonary
- Decreased functional residual capacity, expiratory reserve volume, total lung capacity
- Increased residual volume and diffusing capacity
- Decreased maximum expiratory flow rate in males
- Sleep apnea and obesity hypoventilation syndrome

smoking far exceeds that of obesity.[11] The 1979 Build Study[6,10] was conducted from 1950 to 1972 and included approximately 4 million people. The lowest mortality in men, adjusted for length of follow-up, was at 25 percent below to 5 percent above average weight, and in females it was from 15 percent below to 5 percent above average weight. Similar data were obtained in the American Cancer Society study,[6,12] with the lowest mortality occurring in nonsmoking persons 80 to 89 percent of average weight adjusted for height. When cigarette smoking and duration of obesity are taken into consideration, obesity is clearly a risk factor for early death. Studies of insured persons show that underweight people have a high initial mortality which decreases with time, while obese individuals have a low initial mortality which increases with time. Thus, epidemiologic studies consistently show that the lowest mortality occurs at slightly below average weight for both sexes and that mortality increases both above and below the "optimal" weight.

Cardiovascular Disease

There has been substantial controversy about the relation between obesity and coronary artery disease.[13] Autopsy studies in general do not show an association between coronary artery disease and obesity, whereas epidemiologic studies do. Most notable is the Framingham Study,[14] which showed a positive relation between obesity as an independent risk factor for the 26-year incidence of cardiovascular disease, particularly among women (Fig. 21-2). The percentage of desirable weight on initial examination predicted the 26-year incidence of coronary disease, coronary death, and congestive heart failure in men independent of other risk factors. In women, relative weight was positively and independently associated with coronary disease, stroke, congestive failure, and death from coronary and cardiovascular disease. For example, in men below 50, the 26-year incidence of coronary heart disease per 1000 subjects was 177 for a Metropolitan relative weight less than 110 percent and 350 for a Metropolitan relative weight greater than 130 percent. In women below 50 years old, the 26-year incidence was 76 per 1000 for women less than 110 percent and 179 per 1000 for women greater than 130 percent. For myocardial infarction in men below 50, the 26-year incidence was 110 per 1000 for men less than 110 percent of Metropolitan relative weight and 187 per 1000 for men greater than 130 percent of Metropolitan relative weight. In women who were below 50 years old upon entering the study, the 26-year incidence was 24 per 1000 if less than 110 percent of IBW and 59 per 1000 if greater than 130 percent of IBW. Similar differences were observed for sudden death, congestive heart failure, and cerebrovascular accidents. Perhaps of greatest interest is the fact that the relative odds of developing cardiovascular disease were related to the degree of change of Metropolitan relative weight before age 25 years and entry into the Framingham Study. The men and women who lost weight decreased their relative odds, while those who gained weight increased their relative odds (Fig. 21-3).[14] Similarly, the American Cancer Society[12] and Manitoba studies[15] showed positive relations between the percent overweight or BMI and mortality from or incidence of coronary heart disease. Several other studies, however, have shown no such relation.[13] These studies are all subject to significant problems such as failure to consider smoking, to exclude people with health problems at entry, and to consider cultural and socioeconomic variability.

In a review of 25 major prospective studies evaluating the association of body weight and longevity, Manson et al. noted that all the studies suffer from at least one of three major biases: failure to consider cigarette smoking, inappropriate control of complications of obesity such as hypertension and diabetes, and failure to control for weight loss and subclinical

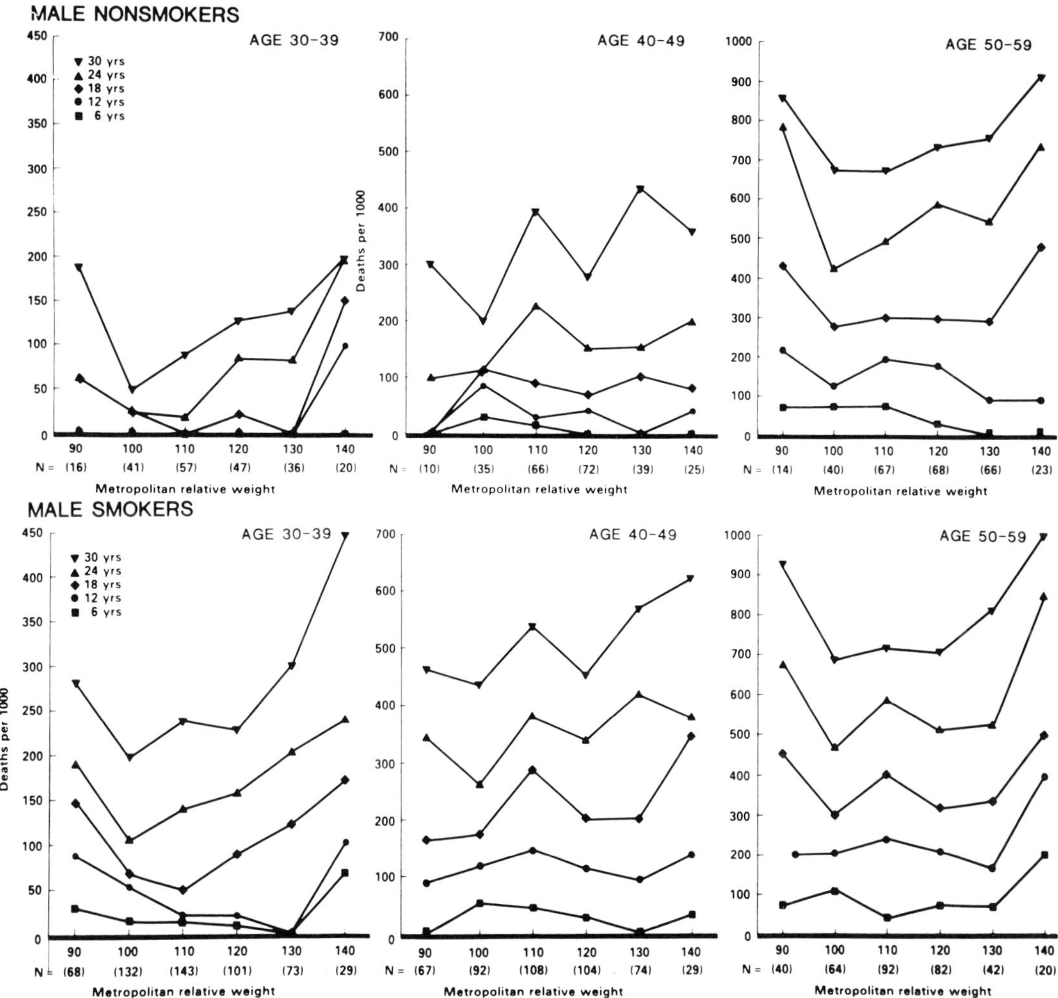

FIGURE 21-1 Cumulative death rates per 1000 male nonsmokers (top graphs) and smokers (bottom graphs) according to age group and duration of follow-up in 6-year intervals (6, 12, 18, 24, and 30 years). *(From Feinleib,[9] with permission.)*

disease.[8] Separating obesity from other risk factors such as cholesterol, systolic blood pressure, left ventricular hypertrophy, and glucose intolerance can be difficult. In the Framingham Study, only 8 percent of males and 18 percent of females in the highest weight class were free of risk factors. These conditions are effects of obesity with complex interrelationships, not confounding variables.[8,16] If obesity is directly causal for these factors, then obesity may exert its influence on longevity through them, and controlling for them will produce an independent but not a true effect of obesity on longevity. Manson et al. also pointed out that of the 25 studies reviewed, only 4 had enough deaths to have 90 percent statistical power to detect a 20 percent or greater difference in mortality between quintiles of weight groups.[8]

Of great importance and of considerable recent interest and attention has been the issue of body fat distribution and the metabolic complications of obesity. Jean Vague drew attention to "android" (waist-predominant) and "gynoid" (hip-predominant) obesity and the association of android obesity with diabetes and atherosclerosis.[17] The relation between the metabolic complications of obesity and the distribution of body fat was greater than the relation with weight alone.

Subsequent studies have confirmed and extended these observations. Hartz et al. evaluated data on 2,165 women 40 to 59 years of age and 11,791 women 20 to 39 years of age who were enrolled in a weight-reduction program.[18] They found that the ratio of waist girth to hip girth was significantly associated with diabetes (Fig. 21-4), hypertension (Fig. 21-5), and gallbladder disease in women age 40 to 59 and with menstrual abnormalities in women age 20 to 39. The distribution of fat was associated with a higher disease prevalence even among women with comparable total body fat. In the study of Kissebah et al., plasma glucose and insulin levels during oral glucose loading as well as fasting plasma triglycer-

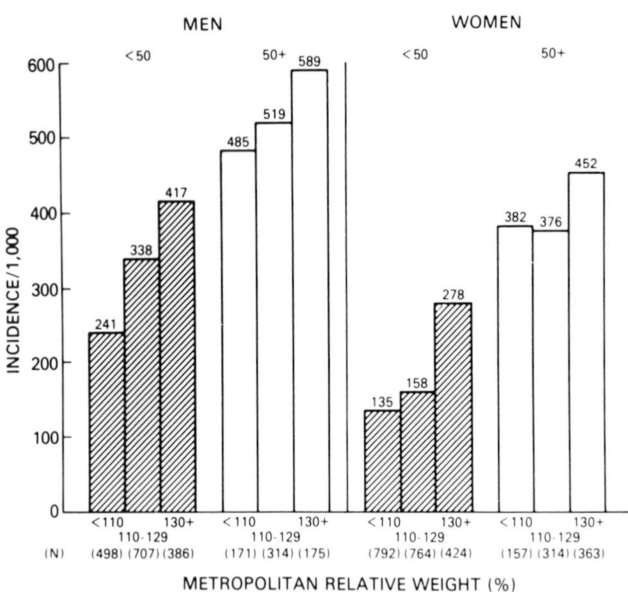

FIGURE 21-2 Twenty-six-year incidence of coronary heart disease from the Framingham Heart Study by Metropolitan Relative Weight at entry among men and women less than or more than 50 years old. N = number at risk. The numbers over the bars indicate incidence rate per 1000. (*From Hubert et al.,*[14] *with permission.*)

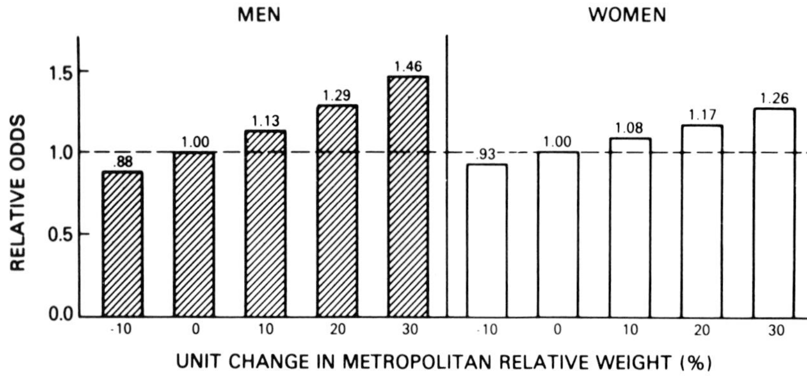

FIGURE 21-3 The relative odds of developing cardiovascular disease corresponding to the percent change in Metropolitan Relative Weight between age 25 and entry into the Framingham Heart Study. (*From Hubert et al.,*[14] *with permission.*)

ides were significantly higher in women with predominately upper body obesity.[19] Krotkiewski et al. studied 930 obese men and women and found similar relations.[20] Peiris et al. demonstrated in a group of 33 healthy but modestly obese women that visceral fat distribution assessed by computed tomography accounts for a greater degree of variance than does total body fat mass in regard to cumulative insulin levels during a glucose tolerance test, triglyceride levels, and systolic and diastolic blood pressure.[21] Evans et al. demonstrated that an increase in the percentage of free testosterone in women was associated with an increasing waist/hip ratio, increased plasma glucose and insulin levels, and diminished insulin sensitivity.[22] This group also showed insulin resistance in muscle in subjects with higher waist/hip ratios as well as a decreased hepatic extraction of insulin.[23,24] Others[25,26] have shown similar relations between abdominal obesity and insulin, triglycerides, hypertension, and low-density lipoprotein (LDL) and high-density lipoprotein (HDL) cholesterol levels. Among epidemiologic studies, the Goth-

FIGURE 21-4 The prevalence of diabetes according to relative weight and body fat distribution in 20,325 women. (*From Hartz et al.,*[18] *with permission.*)

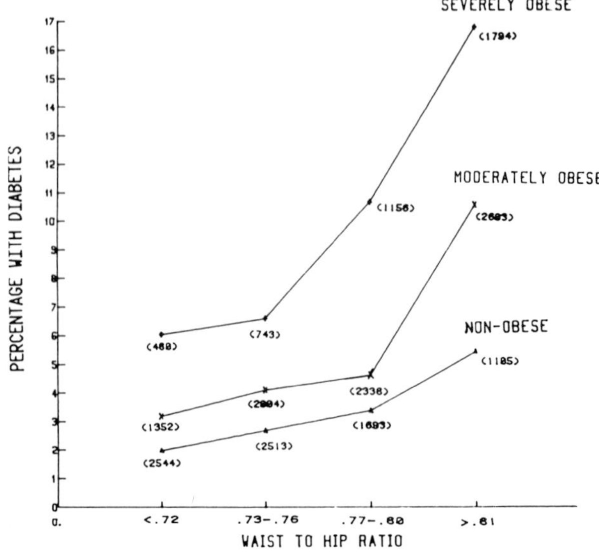

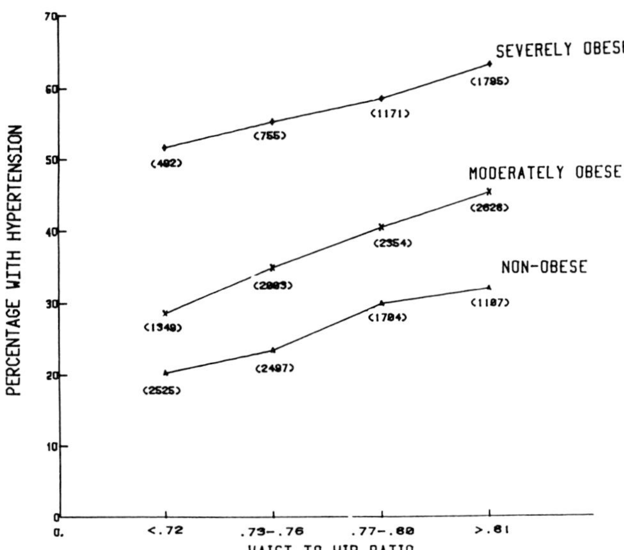

FIGURE 21-5 The prevalence of hypertension according to relative weight and body fat distribution in 20,380 women from 40 to 59 years old. (*From Hartz et al.,*[18] *with permission.*)

enberg study[27] followed 792 men born in 1913 for 13 years and found statistically significant associations between the ratio of waist to hip circumference and the occurrence of stroke and ischemic heart disease. Among 1452 women in Gothenberg followed for 12 years,[28] there was a significant positive association between the ratio of waist to hip circumference and the 12-year incidence of myocardial infarction, angina, stroke, and death. In a multivariate analysis, the association of the waist/hip ratio with myocardial infarction remained.

The mechanism of the relation between the waist/hip ratio and the metabolic complications of obesity is unknown. Obese individuals with high waist/hip ratios have decreased hepatic extraction of insulin, higher posthepatic insulin levels, and more insulin resistance.[23] This has led to the suggestion that enhanced free fatty acid delivery to the liver from intraabdominal stores may decrease insulin uptake by the liver and lead to peripheral hyperinsulinemia. This might explain the association of increased intraabdominal fat with conditions associated with hyperinsulinemia, such as non-insulin-dependent diabetes (NIDDM), hypertension, hyperlipidemia, and atherosclerosis. The combination of obesity, hyperinsulinemia, insulin resistance, hypertension, and a predisposition to NIDDM has been postulated to be part of a common metabolic abnormality caused by a combination of hyperinsulinemia and insulin resistance.[29] Finally, cigarette smoking, an important risk factor for cardiovascular disease, is associated with an increased waist/hip ratio in a dose-dependent manner.[30] This is independent of BMI, and while it was seen in both sexes, the association was stronger in women. This stronger association has been postulated to be due to the enhanced adrenal androgen levels associated with cigarette smoking.

Metabolic Disorders

The well-established association between obesity and NIDDM is discussed in Chap. 19. Insulin resistance and hyperinsulinemia are characteristic features of human obesity.[31–39] This resistance is especially pronounced at physiologic concentrations of insulin in patients with normal glucose tolerance,[35] is closely related to plasma insulin levels,[40] and involves glucose storage and oxidation.[33,41] Both glucose storage and glucose oxidation are directly related to glucose uptake during euglycemic hyperinsulinemia, but glucose storage makes a progressively greater contribution to glucose uptake from the most to the least insulin-resistant subjects with normal glucose tolerance. The degree of insulin resistance associated with obesity and whether resistance occurs at both maximal and submaximal insulin concentrations vary from study to study.[32,34,35,37,39] The reasons for such variability could include the use of height-weight tables or BMI[32–35,38,42] rather than true measures of the percentage of fat,[36,37,40,41] the lumping together of upper and lower body obese patients,[31–37,39–42] and the inclusion of obese patients with impaired glucose tolerance.[32,34,39,42,43] Peiris et al. performed multiple-dose euglycemic clamp studies on 10 females with lower and upper body obesity and found significant reductions in glucose utilization with the 300 $mU/m^2/min$ clamp only in the group with upper body obesity (waist/hip ratio > 0.85).[38] These authors did not measure the percentage of body fat directly, and their obese subjects did not have glucose tolerance tests. Some studies have included only patients with normal glucose tolerance,[33,35–37,41] and some have included patients with impaired glucose tolerance.[32,34,39,42,43] Only a few have studied patients with both normal glucose tolerance and measured the percentage of fat,[36,37,41] and several have done neither.[23,32,34,42] In the Pima Indian population, the degree of obesity does not account for the distribution of insulin action, which is a mixture of three normal distributions. However, a greater proportion of the more obese Pimas are in the more insulin-resistant groups.[40] Pima Indians who carry the gene for insulin resistance are more likely to become obese. This is consistent with the strong association between obesity and NIDDM and the paucity of studies of obese subjects with normal glucose tolerance. To our knowledge, a study of obese Caucasians prior to weight gain or after weight loss to IBW to evaluate the hypothesis that insulin resistance predisposes individuals to obesity has never been conducted. One could postulate that a defect in glucose storage in muscle would lead to hyperinsulinemia, which could lead to increased storage of calories as fat or lean body mass as a result of normal or enhanced insulin action in areas such as lipoprotein lipase or protein synthesis and insulin resistance in other areas, i.e., glucose oxidation and storage and apolipoprotein B secretion.[44] Indeed, there are many examples of differential insulin resistance in the same and different tissues.[44–47] Insulin resistance has been implicated in the etiology of NIDDM, hypertension, and hypertriglyceridemia.[29,44,48–52] It is possible that insulin resistance is also etiologic in the development of obesity. In recent studies of Pima Indians, however, most insulin resistance was associated with lower rates of weight gain.[53]

The primary mechanism of insulin resistance in human obesity is unknown, although several cellular abnormalities have been identified.[47,54,55] Some authors have postulated that since insulin action is closely correlated with glycogen storage[33] and glycogen synthase activity, a genetic defect in the step between the insulin receptor and glycogen synthase may be responsible for insulin resistance.[40,52] It is not clear whether the decrease in glycogen synthase or phosphatase activity is a primary genetic event or secondary to insulin resistance. Increased free fatty acids could also induce insulin resistance.[56,57] In subjects with impaired glucose tolerance, lowering free fatty acid levels with a nicotinic acid derivative improved glucose tolerance.[57] However, other investigators found that intralipid and heparin infusions in obese subjects with normal glucose tolerance did not inhibit insulin-mediated glucose disposal but did induce hepatic insulin resistance.[58] These authors postulated that since obesity is already an insulin-resistant state with high circulating free fatty acid levels and increased rates of whole body lipid oxidation, a further increase in free fatty acid levels will not cause a further impairment in glucose oxidation. In Pima Indians, however, there is no correlation between basal free fatty acid concentration or turnover, basal lipid oxidation or lipid oxidation during euglycemic hyperinsulinemia, and body fat.[36] Other proposed mechanisms of insulin resistance are decreased capillary density,[52] a decreased ability of insulin to increase blood flow,[59] and decreased physical fitness as reflected in a decreased $V_{O_{2max}}$.[39,60] High-fat diets may also contribute.

Obesity is frequently associated with hypertriglyceridemia, and plasma triglyceride levels and the very low density lipoprotein (VLDL) production rate are related to insulin levels[61–64] and the percentage of body weight that is fat.[65] It has been postulated that this hypertriglyceridemia is due to hyperinsulinemia.[29,66] However, in studies in humans[67,68] and in human[69] and rat hepatocytes,[70,71] insulin acutely inhibited both apolipoprotein B and VLDL triglyceride secretion from the liver. This is due to both direct mechanisms at the level of the liver cell and the ability of insulin to decrease free fatty acids released from adipose tissue, which decreases the substrate supply for VLDL triglyceride synthesis.[44,65] It is possible that an inability of insulin to elicit these effects—i.e., insulin resistance—causes the hypertriglyceridemia of obesity.[44,72,73] Alternatively, the acute and chronic effects of insulin might be different. That is, the acute effects lead to enhanced intracellular degradation of apolipoprotein B and decreased secretion,[71] while the chronic effects lead to enhanced synthesis of apolipoprotein B. There is also substantial variability in lipoprotein lipase levels in obese subjects, and it is likely that the balance between VLDL triglyceride production and triglyceride clearance determines whether an obese subject will have hypertriglyceridemia.[65] In fact, patients with hypertriglyceridemia have been shown to be insulin-resistant,[29,72–74] and subjects with high insulin levels have higher blood pressure and serum triglycerides. HDL cholesterol levels are also lower in obese individuals,[64,75] consistent with their hypertriglyceridemia.[64] Weight loss generally leads to favorable changes in plasma lipids and lipoproteins.[76,77]

Changes in insulin secretion and/or action have also been implicated in the pathogenesis of hypertension, another common complication of obesity.[73,74,78–80] Hypertension has been shown to be related to insulin resistance.[48,73,74,80,81] In young, healthy, nonobese, nondiabetic hypertensive subjects, stimulation of nonoxidative glucose disposal is impaired, and the severity of insulin resistance is closely related to the increase in blood pressure.[48] There are several possible mechanisms by which insulin might produce hypertension.[73] Insulin increases sodium reabsorption in both the proximal and distal tubules.[82–85] Indeed, obese individuals have normal responsiveness to the sodium-retaining effects of insulin.[86] Obese patients have increased total body sodium,[87–89] and weight loss leads to a natriuresis and dramatic decreases in blood pressure and insulin levels.[90–92] A second postulated mechanism of hypertension in obesity involves activation of the sympathetic nervous system.[64,73,93] In this regard, hyperinsulinemia increases the activity of the sympathetic nervous system.[94,95] As expected, weight reduction leads to sodium losses and decreases in sympathetic nervous system activity.[86,91,96–98] Rocchini et al. studied 60 obese adolescents and found an increased sensitivity of blood pressure to sodium restriction compared with nonobese adolescents.[99] This sensitivity to sodium disappeared with weight reduction and was not closely associated with decreases in insulin, norepinephrine, and aldosterone levels. These authors postulated that the sodium sensitivity of hypertensive obese individuals may be due to a combination of hyperinsulinemia, hyperaldosteronism, and increased activity of the sympathetic nervous system. Obese individuals also have increased plasma volume[73,86,87] and increased thickness of the left ventricular wall.[100] Weight loss leads to reduction in both parameters. Visceral obesity, which is associated with hyperinsulinemia and insulin resistance, is also associated with a higher incidence of hypertension,[18,27,101,102] increasing the association between hyperinsulinemia, activation of the sympathetic nervous system, obesity, and hypertension. It is not known, however, what effect, if any, obesity has on the ability of insulin to activate the sympathetic nervous system.

The sodium-hydrogen exchanger, which is equivalent to the sodium-lithium cotransport system, has been implicated in the pathogenesis of essential hypertension. While it has been postulated that this exchanger is also implicated in the hypertension of hyperinsulinemic states such as obesity, this postulate is unproven.[73]

Thus, obesity is associated with an expanded plasma volume, hyperinsulinemia which increases sodium resorption by the kidney and activates the sympathetic nervous system, and increased sensitivity of blood pressure to changes in body sodium. Variable sensitivities to any of these factors could explain why some obese subjects are hypertensive and others are normotensive. Additionally, it should be kept in mind that not all obese subjects become normotensive with weight reduction and that not all hyperlipidemic obese subjects become normolipidemic with weight loss. Thus, some obese subjects have underlying essential hypertension.

There is a strong association between obesity and cholesterol gallstones. In a recent study the risk was linearly related to weight and increased with age. A person approximately 50 percent above IBW has an approximately sixfold increase in the incidence of symptomatic gallstones.[103,104] Obesity and overnutrition both increase biliary secretion of cholesterol.[105,106] Total body cholesterol synthesis is increased in obesity,[107–109] and hepatic cholesterol synthesis is increased in patients with gallstones[110] and is enhanced by insulin.[111] The Pima Indians have an extremely high incidence of cholesterol gallstones, affecting approximately 80 percent of Pima women.[112] In addition to enhanced cholesterol secretion in bile as a result of obesity, Pima Indians also have decreased bile acid pool sizes.[113] Together, these factors lead to supersaturation of bile. Such a defect has not been demonstrated in Caucasians. Thus, obesity is associated with increased hepatic cholesterol synthesis, increased biliary cholesterol secretion, and gallbladder bile supersaturation with cholesterol.

Cancer

Obesity is also associated with a higher incidence of cancer. Obese males have higher mortality from cancer of the colon, rectum, and prostate, and obese females have higher mortality from cancer of the gallbladder, bile ducts, breast, endometrium, cervix, and ovaries.[64,114–118] The mechanism of the enhanced risk of cancer in obese patients is unknown. Recent studies have cast doubt on the relation between dietary fat and breast and colon cancer.[119,120] As recently reviewed by Grundy, however, the role of diet has not been excluded.[64] Since androgens are converted to estrogens in adipose tissue, a role for increased estrogen levels in the development of breast and uterine cancer is a possibility.[121] It is well known that adipose tissue aromatizes androgens to estrogens.[122–126] Furthermore, body weight and the percentage of conversion of androstenedione to estrone are highly correlated in women.[127] In obese postmenopausal women, estrogen levels are also increased.[128]

Endocrine Disorders

Obesity,[129] especially abdominal obesity,[18] is associated with menstrual abnormalities. Rogers and Mitchell reported that among 100 patients with menstrual disorders, 43 were 20 percent or more above IBW.[130] In the control group of women of similar age with normal menstrual periods, the overall incidence of obesity was 13 percent. In a subsequent study these authors reported that 13 of 15 patients who lost weight had a return of menstrual function.[131] Hartz et al. also reported a higher incidence of menstrual abnormalities as well as hirsutism in obese women.[132] Hyperandrogenism is also associated with menstrual abnormalities in obese women and frequently with acanthosis nigricans.[133,134] Flier et al. reported that acanthosis nigricans occurred in 5 percent of patients being evaluated for hyperandrogenism and that all these patients were obese and insulin-resistant.[135] Compared with hyperandrogenized women of similar body weight, patients with acanthosis nigricans were more hyperinsulinemic and insulin-resistant. With weight loss, acanthosis nigricans remitted as insulin resistance improved.

The polycystic ovary syndrome consists of anovulation, hyperandrogenemia, and obesity. Obesity is present in 40 percent of patients with polycystic ovaries.[136] As reviewed by Barnes and Rosenfield, obesity may contribute to the insulin resistance in the polycystic ovary syndrome; however, nonobese women with polycystic ovaries are also insulin-resistant.[136] The insulin resistance in the polycystic ovary syndrome correlates with the degree of hyperandrogenemia and in some but not all studies decreases with a reduction of androgen levels. It is likely that the hyperinsulinemia associated with insulin resistance is the cause of polycystic ovarian syndrome rather than the result of it. In obese women with this syndrome, weight loss reduces estrone levels and returns gonadotropin secretion to normal with resumption of regular menstrual cycles.[137,138] Also, since there is no improvement in insulin resistance with ovariectomy[139] or medical reduction of androgens,[140] it is possible that hyperinsulinemia is at least in part causal for hyperandrogenism. Evidence for this includes the fact that there are insulin and IGF-I receptors on granulosa cells and other cells in the ovary; the fact that insulin and IGF-I stimulate steroidogenesis in granulosa, thecal, and stromal cells; the fact that insulin and IGF-I act synergistically with luteinizing hormone (LH) or follicle stimulating hormone (FSH) to increase steroidogenesis in vitro; and the fact that insulin increases LH receptors and IGF-I enhances FSH induction of LH receptors in granulosa cells.[141] Further supporting a role for insulin in the hyperandrogenism of obese women with polycystic ovaries, Nestler et al. reduced serum insulin levels with diazoxide for 10 days and observed significant reductions in serum total testosterone and unbound testosterone.[142] McKenna has proposed that the development of the polycystic ovary syndrome in obese patients may be caused by abnormal gonadotropin secretion induced by increased levels of estrone and by amplification of the action of LH on the ovary in the presence of insulin.[138]

Hirsute women with the polycystic ovary syndrome have higher insulin levels than do women with this syndrome alone, and there is a significant correlation between plasma insulin and plasma testosterone or androstenedione. The hyperandrogenism can be due to the effects of insulin on granulosa cells or possibly to the effect of insulin to increase gonadotropin secretion.[143,144] Adipose tissue can also convert preandrogens to testosterone, and obesity is associated with the reduced sex hormone–binding globulin concentrations characteristic of hyperandrogen states.[143] Finally, it has been proposed that hyperandrogenemia may be responsible for the upper body fat localization in women with high waist/hip ratios (android obesity)[22] and decreased hepatic extraction of insulin.[145]

In obese (more than 160 percent of IBW) men, decreased plasma testosterone and decreased sex hormone–binding globulin levels have been reported.[146,147] Free testosterone levels are decreased in only some morbidly obese men who are more than 200 percent of IBW. The normal free testosterone level in most obese males is reflected in their normal masculinization, libido, potency, and spermatogenesis.[146,147] In morbidly obese men, the hypothalamic-hypophyseal-gonadal axis is normal as determined by the testicular response to human chorionic gonadotropin (hCG), the pituitary response to gonadotropin releasing hormone (GnRH), and the hypothalamic pituitary testicular response to clomiphene.[147,148] As in women, estrogen levels rise with increasing obesity in men and decrease after weight reduction.[147]

Despite enhanced growth, growth hormone levels are reduced in obesity; and growth hormone responses to GnRH, sleep, exercise, fasting, protein, and pharmacologic stimuli such as L-dopa, L-dopa plus propranolol, glucagon plus propranolol, insulin, arginine, and other drugs are blunted.[147] Weight loss improves the growth hormone response. Despite decreased growth hormone levels, somatomedin levels are normal to increased. It has been proposed that hyperinsulinemia or increased nutrition may enhance somatomedin production, which might have a negative feedback effect on growth hormone secretion. Prolactin levels are normal in obesity, but the response to pharmacologic stimuli such as thyrotropin releasing hormone (TRH) and chlorpromazine is blunted.[147,148] The significance of this is currently unknown.

Other endocrine abnormalities in obesity include enhanced cortisol production and clearance rates with normal cortisol levels, a normal pituitary response to corticotropin releasing factor (CRF), and a normal adrenal responsiveness to ACTH.[147,149] The overnight 1-mg dexamethasone suppression is usually normal in obese subjects, although 13 percent of obese control subjects have false-positive tests.[149] While urinary 17-hydroxycorticosteroids are increased in 27 percent of obese subjects, urinary free cortisol levels are normal.[147,149]

Skeletal Disorders

Osteoarthritis has been associated with obesity in several cross-sectional studies. Recently, Felson et al., in reviewing Framingham data, found a strong association between being obese in 1948–1952 and having either symptomatic or asymptomatic knee osteoarthritis approximately 36 years later.[150] The association was stronger for women and persisted after controlling for other risk factors. The cause in obese subjects may be related to the increased force on cartilage, increased subchondral bony stiffness, and obesity-related metabolic abnormalities.

Obesity is protective for osteoporosis.[151–153] In a recent study, weight was positively correlated with midshaft radius, lumbar spine, and femoral neck bone densities, yet risk factors alone were poor predictors of bone mass.[153] Other studies have shown normal[154] and increased[155] bone mass in obese individuals. Both increased estrogens and increased weight bearing in obese women have been postulated as etiologic in protecting against osteoporosis.[64,154]

In addition, and similar to black individuals, obese subjects have elevated PTH, 1,25-dihydroxyvitamin D, osteocalcin, and urinary cyclic AMP with lower 25-hydroxyvitamin D and urinary calcium, consistent with secondary hyperparathyroidism.[156] Parathyroid hormone levels fall with weight loss.[157] This is consistent with the postulate that increased bone mass results because increased muscle mass diminishes the skeletal response to PTH.[156,158]

Pulmonary Disorders

Obesity is also associated with abnormalities in pulmonary function. These abnormalities were recently studied by Rubenstein et al. in 103 obese nonsmokers without cardiopulmonary disease compared with 190 healthy, nonobese nonsmokers.[159] These authors found that obese patients had lower functional residual capacity, expiratory reserve volume, and total lung capacity than did nonobese controls. In addition, residual volume and diffusing capacity were higher in obese patients. Obese men, but not women, had a reduced maximum expiratory flow rate at 15 to 75 percent of exhaled vital capacity. As reviewed by Rubenstein et al., obesity adversely affects chest wall mechanics and causes a decrease in total respiratory compliance, perhaps as a result of deposition of subcutaneous adipose tissue.[159] In addition, respiratory muscle function may also be impaired as a result of the mechanical disadvantage of the chest wall configuration, fat deposition, and the increased energy expenditure needed to expand the lungs. Decreased peripheral airway size may be due to increased pulmonary blood volume, congestion of bronchial vessels in the submucosa, and narrowing of the airway wall.[159] The decrease in peripheral airway dimensions in morbidly obese men can predispose them to chronic airflow limitation or to rapid deterioration in airway function if they are exposed to cigarette smoke or respiratory infections which could contribute to airway narrowing.

Severe obesity is associated with obstructive sleep apnea and the obesity hypoventilation syndrome. Sleep apnea syndrome[160,161] is associated with loud snoring, frequent nocturnal awakening, daytime somnolence, and nocturnal oxyhemoglobin desaturation. Sleep apnea can be obstructive, central, or mixed. The obstructive type is the most common. Frequently, patients fall asleep during the day, as in the Pickwickian syndrome. Other associated problems include morning headaches, loss of libido, intellectual deterioration, systemic and pulmonary hypertension, congestive heart failure, and cardiac arrhythmias.[160,161] Patients with severe sleep apnea have a higher rate of automobile accidents.[162] The etiology of obstruction of the upper airway during sleep in obese patients is not completely understood,[160,161] but this condition probably is not due to excessive fat deposition.[163] The arrhythmias associated with sleep apnea may be related to increased plasma catecholamines, which are directly related to oxygen saturation.[164] Sleep apnea may also be an independent risk factor for myocardial infarction.[165]

In obese subjects with obstructive sleep apnea syndrome, weight loss is the treatment of choice. Relatively small amounts of weight loss can lead to significant improvement,[163] and the relation between apneic episodes per hour and body weight was shown to be a logarithmic function in one study.[166] Thus, relatively small changes in weight, such as 10 to 20 kg, can lead to marked changes in sleep apnea.[163,166] Other treatments for sleep apnea include sleeping in a lateral position and avoiding sedatives and alcohol. Various pharmacologic approaches have been tried with mixed results,[160,161] including protriptyline, progesterone, and acetazolamide. Continuous positive airway pressure is frequently effective but often is not well tolerated. Surgical procedures include tracheostomy, removal of a discrete obstruction, uvulopalatopharyngoplasty, and sectioning of the hyoid.[160,161] In morbidly obese patients, gastric bypass should be considered.[167] In one study comparing conservative treatment—weight loss—to tracheostomy, the conservatively treated group had more extreme daytime somnolence and greater vascular morbidity after 7 years of follow-up.[168]

Miscellaneous Disorders

Obesity is also associated with an increased history of pregnancy-associated hypertension and a previous stillborn infant as well as increased frequencies during current pregnancies of hypertension, gestational diabetes, multiple gestation, inadequate weight gain, and anemia.[169] In addition, morbid obesity can be associated with the nephrotic syndrome.[170] Anecdotally, morbid obesity has been associated with esophageal reflux, but this is difficult to document experimentally.[171]

ETIOLOGY OF OBESITY

Obesity results from positive energy balance, i.e., energy intake exceeding energy expenditure. All people are in a state of positive energy balance as growing children. As adults, lean individuals maintain energy balance close to zero over the long run, but even lean adults often go through periods of positive or negative energy balance. Obese adults also maintain their energy balance close to zero for prolonged periods, although at a higher level of energy stores. Because obesity may develop over many years, only small differences in energy intake and expenditure are required, and these differences may be impossible to detect with current methods. The cause of the excessive positive energy balance in obesity has not been clearly defined. It is likely that there are numerous causes of obesity, including metabolic, psychological, hormonal, and socioeconomic factors. It may never be possible to point to a single factor as being the predominant cause of obesity. Thus, the following discussion covers a variety of potential influences on the development of obesity, any of which may have a role in a particular obese patient.

Genetic Factors

There is no question that obesity tends to run in families. However, this observation does not indicate whether this familial clustering is genetic or is related to the similarity of environmental influences on members of the same family. The strongest evidence for a significant genetic influence comes from studies of adoptees in Denmark[172] and twins who were reared in separate families in Sweden.[173] The BMI of adoptees was closely related to that of their biological parents but not that of their adoptive parents (Fig. 21-6). An overweight adoptee was more than twice as likely to have an overweight biological mother than was a thin adoptee and 40 percent more likely to have an overweight biological father. In 93 pairs of identical twins who were reared apart, the intrapair correlation coefficient for BMI was 0.70 for men and 0.66 for women. Identical twins reared together had very similar intrapair correlations for BMI (0.74 in men and 0.66 in women). Dizygotic twins reared apart or together had intrapair correlations that were less than half the values observed in monozygotic twins. There was no evidence that sharing the same childhood environment contributed to the similarity in BMI later in life.

Most studies of the genetic transmission of obesity have used indirect indexes of obesity, such as BMI or percentage of IBW. However, in one study of Canadian subjects, fat mass and percentage of body fat were measured directly using the underwater weighing method.[174] Based on consideration of nine different types of family relationships in these subjects, it was concluded that about half the variance in fatness was transmissible, with 25 percent being genetic transmission and 30 percent being cultural transmission.

First-degree relatives of obese patients whose obesity first became evident in childhood are more likely to be obese than are relatives of obese patients whose obesity began later in life.[175] After controlling for gender, degree of obesity, and family size, the relatives of those with childhood-onset obesity are about twice as likely to be obese as are relatives of those with adult-onset obesity.

The predisposition to obesity could result from inheritance of a high metabolic efficiency or of a tendency to eat more food than lean individuals eat. The resting metabolic rate, which accounts for more than half of total energy expenditure, appears to have a significant genetic component (Fig. 21-7).[176,177] For example, it has been estimated that after the resting metabolic rate is adjusted for fat-free mass, age, and gender, 40 percent of the remaining variance is explained by genetic factors. Similar heritability estimates were made for the increase in energy expenditure associated with meals and low-intensity exercise.[177] A low resting metabolic rate and a low 24-h energy expenditure in a respiration chamber were associated with an increased risk of gaining a significant amount of weight in a prospective study of a group of southwestern American Indians.[178] However, it seems unlikely that inheritance of a low energy expenditure explains most cases of obesity, because obese individuals usually do not have a low metabolic rate. This issue will be discussed below.

Although there is familial resemblance in food intake, it is controversial whether this is entirely environmental or whether genetic influences play a role.[179,180] If the children of obese parents inherit a gene (or set of genes) that causes them to consume too much food, the nature of this genetic factor is unknown. As will be discussed later, the regulation

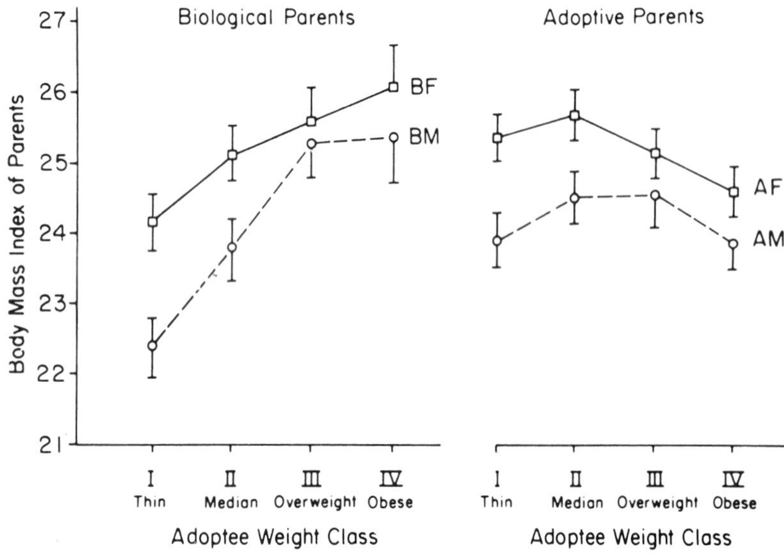

FIGURE 21-6 Mean body mass index (BMI) (±SEM) of biological fathers (BF), biological mothers (BM), adoptive fathers (AF), and adoptive mothers (AM) as a function of the weight class of adoptees (class I = thin with BMI in lowest 25 percent; class II = medium with BMI in the 26th through 91st percentile; class III = overweight with BMI in the 92d to 96th percentile; class IV = obese with BMI above the 96th percentile). (*From Stunkard et al.,*[173] *with permission.*)

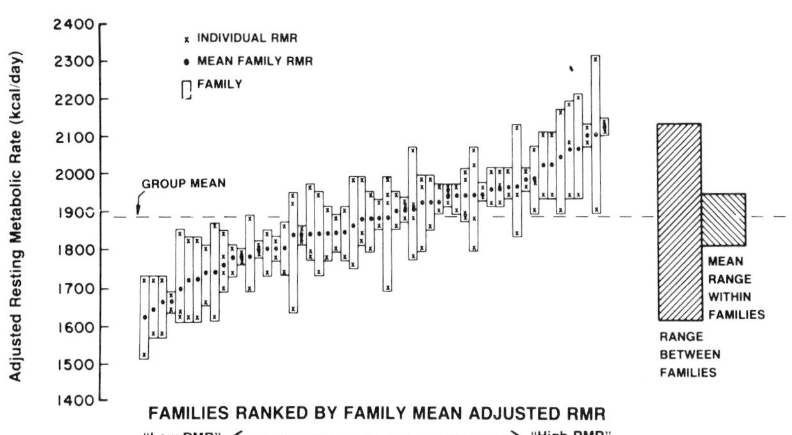

FIGURE 21-7 Mean family and individual resting metabolic rates in Pima Indians adjusted for the covariances of fat-free mass, age, and sex. *(From Bogardus et al.,[176] with permission.)*

of energy intake is extremely complex, and numerous metabolic and/or psychological factors may be involved.

In considering the genetics of obesity, it should be noted that throughout most of human evolution famine was very common. Those who were able to store energy efficiently as body fat when food was available would have been more likely to survive periods of famine and pass along their genes to offspring. Thus, obesity should not necessarily be viewed as a genetic abnormality but a predictable consequence of natural selection. Only when the obese genotype is placed in a situation of a constant supply of food which does not require much physical effort to obtain is the obese phenotype expressed.

Environmental Factors

Genetic makeup only determines the tendency to become obese. The interactions between genes and the environment determine whether obesity actually develops. For example, if food is scarce because of poverty or regional famine, even those who are highly predisposed toward obesity will not become obese.

Cultural factors may play a significant role in determining the prevalence of obesity. In developed societies there is an inverse relation between socioeconomic status and obesity in women; i.e., women with a low socioeconomic status are much more likely to be obese.[181] However, in underdeveloped countries women with a high socioeconomic status are more likely to be obese.[181] The most likely explanation for this discrepancy is that obesity signifies the desirable traits of wealth and sexual attractiveness in poorer societies with limited access to food. In contrast, obesity often is looked upon as a sign of low intelligence or lack of self-control in wealthy nations.

Among children, the prevalence of obesity is related to the amount of time spent watching television.[182] This relation may be explained by a lower rate of energy expenditure during television viewing than during alternative activities or by snacking during television viewing. Moreover, the large amount of food advertising may lead children to eat more even when not watching television.

Among children there are regional and seasonal influences on the prevalence of obesity. In the United States (data from 1963 to 1965), obesity was much more common in the northeast than in the western part of the country and was more prevalent in the winter than in the summer in all regions.[183]

Exposure to a high-fat diet may increase one's probability of becoming obese. A high percentage of fat in the diet is associated with adiposity, probably because a high-fat diet is associated with an increase in energy intake (Table 21-4).[184] Thus, a person who would not become obese on a high-carbohydrate diet, as is consumed by most of the world's population, may become obese when exposed to the typical high-fat western diet.

Energy Expenditure

One popular theory[185] of obesity is that preobese individuals have a low rate of energy expenditure. According to this theory, preobese persons with low energy expenditure eat the same amount of food as do individuals with normal energy expenditure. Total energy expenditure then increases as weight is

TABLE 21-4 Effect of a High- or Low-Fat Diet on Spontaneous Food Intake of Normal-Weight Young Men

	Low-Fat Diet	High-Fat Diet
Energy intake (kcal/day)	2987 ± 421	4135 ± 484*
Protein (g)	111 ± 13	122 ± 14
Fat (g)	73 ± 8	245 ± 28*
Carbohydrate (g)	488 ± 86	358 ± 59*

* $p < 0.01$. Values are mean ± SD of measured intake over 2 days.

Source: From Tremblay et al.[184]

gained because of the increased energy cost of maintaining and moving a larger body. Eventually energy expenditure matches energy intake, and body weight stabilizes at an obese level, with both energy intake and energy expenditure being "normal." This theory is attractive because many studies have indicated that obese subjects do not consume more energy than lean subjects consume.[186–189]

The major problem with this theory is that numerous studies have demonstrated that the average total energy expenditure is higher in obese subjects than in lean subjects (Fig. 21-8). Increased energy expenditure in obesity has been demonstrated using precise calorimetry chambers,[190–195] has been inferred from the increased weight-maintenance energy requirements of obese patients living in metabolic wards[196,197] and from measurements of the energy costs of various activities in lean and obese subjects,[198] and has been demonstrated under free-living conditions using the doubly labeled water method.[199–201] These studies indicate that the normal or low self-reported intake of groups of obese subjects results from underreporting of food intake. Nevertheless, there were a few obese individuals in these studies whose energy expenditure was in the range of values observed in lean subjects. Such individuals probably had a subnormal energy expenditure before they became obese, since energy expenditure increases as weight is gained. Of course, the finding that energy expenditure generally is increased in obesity only demonstrates that increased energy intake is usually needed to maintain the obese state. It does not prove that energy expenditure was not subnormal before obesity developed.

FIGURE 21-8 Total (top) and basal (bottom) energy expenditure in obese and lean subjects as a function of body weight. Total energy expenditure was measured by the doubly labeled water method. *(From Welle et al.,[199] with permission.)*

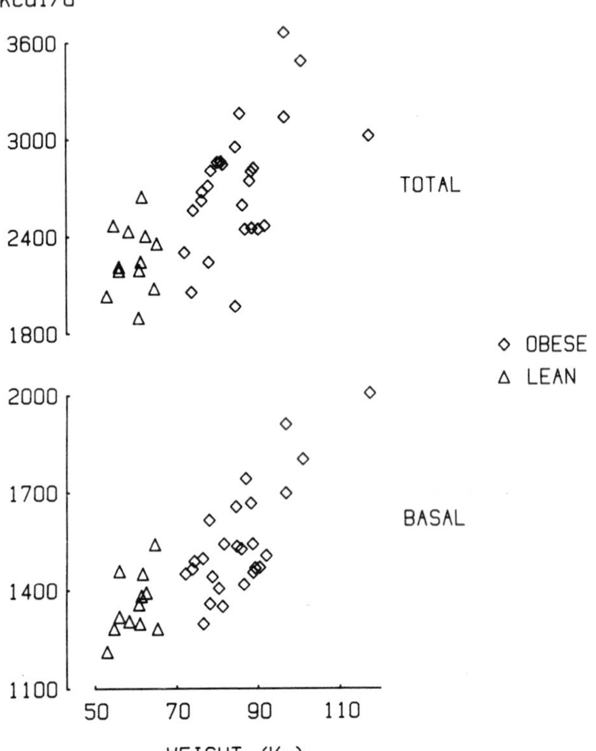

The doubly labeled water method has been used to study the free-living energy expenditure of infants born to lean and obese mothers.[202] Among six infants of lean mothers, none became obese in the first year of life, whereas six of 12 infants of overweight mothers became obese within the first year. The energy expenditure of the infants was measured when they were 3 months old, a time when the mean body weights and energy intakes of the different groups were similar. The mean total energy expenditure of the six infants who later became obese was 20 percent lower than that of the other groups. However, their mean resting metabolic rate was not low, indicating that their low energy expenditure was related to reduced physical activity. Only three of these six infants were considered to be obese when the follow-up period ended at 1 year, and so the question remains whether infants with a low energy expenditure will be plagued with obesity throughout life. Among normal-weight children 4 to 5 years old it was found that the averge resting metabolic rate of those with an obese parent was 16 percent lower than that of children whose parents had always been of normal weight.[203] The total daily energy expenditure of the group with obese parents was 22 percent lower than the energy expenditure in the group with lean parents. Although total expenditure was estimated with the imprecise heart rate method, these data suggest that those predisposed to obesity may have a reduced energy expenditure early in life. Unfortunately, no long-term follow-up was done to determine whether these children had an increased incidence of obesity later in life.

One approach to defining the energy expenditure of preobese people is to study reduced-obese subjects, assuming that their metabolic state reverts to its preobese condition when weight is normalized (although this assumption could be incorrect). Numerous studies have documented the fact that energy expenditure declines during weight loss in obese patients.[204–206] However, these subjects have an elevated metabolic rate before weight loss, and so a reduction in energy expenditure does not demonstrate that reduced-obese subjects are hypometabolic relative to normal-weight subjects. There is extremely little information regarding the energy expenditure of obese subjects who were reduced and stabilized at a normal body weight. The most convincing evidence for reduced energy expenditure in reduced-obese subjects comes from a study of 16 reduced-obese women and 16 normal-weight controls whose 24-h energy expenditure was measured in a respiration chamber at three different levels of activity.[207] At all activity levels, the reduced-obese women had metabolic rates about 15 percent lower than those of the normal-weight women. A similar study with fewer subjects did not confirm this finding, although total energy expenditure did tend to be lower (mean 6.5 percent) in reduced-obese subjects.[208]

Other investigations of the energy expenditure of reduced-obese subjects have involved subjects who were still overweight after their weight loss. Twenty-nine women who had lost some weight but who claimed that they could not lose any more on a low-energy diet (1000 to 1500 kcal/day) were isolated in a country house and fed 1500 kcal/day for 3 weeks.[209] One of them gained more than 1 kg, and nine maintained their weight within 1 kg. Their expected weight-maintenance requirement would be in excess of 2000 kcal/day, suggesting that a low metabolic rate contributed to their obesity. Unfortunately, body composition was determined by the imprecise skin fold thickness method, and so changes in energy stores during the study could not be calculated accurately. A change in body weight of 1 kg over 3 weeks could represent a change in energy stores of several hundred kilocalories per day. In another study the weight-maintenance energy intake of 26 reduced-obese patients who were given a liquid formula diet in a metabolic ward was compared with that of age- and sex-matched controls who had never been obese.[196] The reduced-obese subjects had a mean energy requirement that was slightly less than that of the normal-weight subjects, even though they were still 60 percent heavier. When energy requirements were expressed per square meter of surface area, the reduced-obese subjects had an energy requirement that was 25 percent below normal. Because the lean body mass was not determined, it is impossible to know if the difference could be explained by a lower active cell mass in the reduced-obese subjects. Body cell mass is the primary determinant of the resting metabolic rate, which is the primary determinant of total energy expenditure under sedentary conditions. In a similar experiment, the energy requirements of 10 reduced-obese patients were 18 percent below those of weight-matched subjects who had never dieted.[210] Both the reduced-obese and the control subjects were obese, suggesting that the weight loss itself rather than the predisposition to obesity was the main factor associated with reduced expenditure. The resting metabolic rate was normal when adjusted for lean body mass, suggesting that reduced physical activity could explain the lower energy requirement of the reduced-obese subjects. In contrast to these studies, other investigators have failed to find subnormal resting metabolic rates or total energy expenditure in obese subjects who had lost a substantial amount of weight.[204,211,212]

The *thermic effect* of food is the increase in metabolic rate that follows meals. The increase persists for several hours, and in an average person the thermic effect of food accounts for about 8 percent of total energy expenditure. Several studies have indicated that the thermic effect of food is reduced in obese subjects.[213–218] However, others have failed to find a reduced thermic effect in obesity.[219–221] A reduction in the thermic effect of food (or at least carbohydrate) may be related more to impaired glucose tolerance than to obesity per se.[222,223] This suggests that a reduced thermic response may be a result rather than a cause of obesity, but it has been reported that the thermic response to a glucose meal or a mixed meal remains low after weight loss.[211,224] The argument is often put forth that even though the decrease in the thermic effect of food amounts to only a few percent of total energy requirements, it can lead to obesity because even a positive energy balance of only 50 kcal/day will cause a weight gain of 5 pounds in a year. This argument is flawed because the basal metabolic rate and the energy cost of activity increase as weight is gained, so that the initial weight gain associated with a reduced thermic effect of food would quickly be offset by the increase in total energy expenditure. Hence, it is unlikely that a low thermic effect of food has more than a minor role in the development of obesity.

Inactivity has been described in obese children and adults.[225–229] However, the energy required to perform all types of activities is elevated in obese subjects, so that the actual amount of energy used for physical activity is slightly higher in obese than in lean individuals.[199–201] It is likely that the increased effort needed to perform activities causes obese people to limit their activity, and this could help perpetuate obesity. Reduced physical activity in preobese or reduced-obese subjects could contribute to a lower total energy expenditure. This decrease would eventually be offset by an increase in the basal metabolic rate and an increase in the energy cost of activity as weight is gained, but only after the subjects had become overweight. The extent of inactivity in preobese or reduced-obese individuals is not clear. A study of total energy expenditure of preobese infants[202] which was discussed earlier indicated that their lower energy expenditure was related to inactivity. In obese adults who had lost an average 21.5 percent of their body weight, the nonresting energy expenditure (estimated as the difference between weight-maintenance intake and resting metabolic rate) was several hundred kilocalories per day below the level observed in moderately obese patients who had not lost weight.[210] These results suggest that inactivity may contribute to the rebound in body weight usually seen after weight loss in obese patients.

Patients with the Prader-Willi syndrome usually are obese. It has been reported that such patients have a total energy expenditure, estimated with the doubly labeled water method, 47 percent lower than that of weight-matched controls.[230] When the data are normalized for their lower lean body mass, the difference is only 14 percent and the basal metabolic rate is normal.

Some obese patients claim that they cannot lose weight in spite of consuming only a very low energy diet, often less than 1000 kcal/day. We have measured the basal metabolic rates of many such patients and have not found one with an abnormally low basal metabolism. Usually the basal metabolic rate is higher than the self-reported total energy intake. Hence, the accuracy of self-reported very low energy requirements in obese patients should be viewed with suspicion. Treatment based on the assumption of hypometabolism should be undertaken with caution in the absence of direct evidence of low energy expenditure.

Regardless of whether energy expenditure is below normal in preobese individuals, it is clear that energy intake must exceed energy expenditure for obesity to develop. It has been pointed out that when subjects voluntarily overeat, there is considerable variability in the ease with which weight is gained.[231,232] The variability in weight gained observed in the famous Vermont overfeeding study[231] resurrected the notion of "luxuskonsumption," or the wastage of excess energy as heat during periods of overeating. If some subjects increase their thermogenesis more than others do when they overeat, they should be less susceptible to becoming obese. Unfortunately, this hypothesis was not tested by direct measurements of energy expenditure in the Vermont study. More recently, a correlation was found within twin pairs for weight gain during prolonged experimental overfeeding, suggesting a genetic component to the susceptibility to weight gain.[232] Although increased metabolic rates have been documented in overfeeding studies,[233–235] they are never great enough to prevent weight gain completely during periods of overeating. Thus individual differences in overfeeding-induced thermogenesis can explain only differences in the degree of obesity and are not sufficient to explain why some individuals become obese and others remain lean.

Food Intake

Because energy expenditure tends to be higher in weight-stable obese subjects, obese subjects generally must eat more food to maintain the obese state. In most cases it is likely that this increased food intake is the primary cause of obesity. Body weight then stabilizes at a high level of food intake because energy expenditure increases as weight is gained. These statements contradict the many studies indicating that the self-reported food intake of obese subjects is not increased.[186–189] However, the consistency with which increased energy expenditure is observed in obese patients necessitates acceptance of the fact that many obese patients underreport their intake. This fact, along with the poor accuracy of self-reported intake even in normal-weight subjects, makes studies of food intake under free-living conditions extremely difficult. Many investigations have been done of food intake in the laboratory or in metabolic wards, but the extent to which these studies reflect the regulation of food intake under actual living conditions is uncertain. Thus, it is very difficult to compare the regulation of food intake in lean and obese subjects.

It is often stated that obese individuals have a higher "set point" for body weight than do lean individuals. This concept suggests that some comparator exists in the central nervous system (CNS) that causes a person to eat more when weight is below the set point and eat less when weight is above the set point. The comparator presumably senses either body weight or body fat (the lipostatic theory). At this point, the nature of the presumed signal has not been elucidated. If there is a set point comparator, it appears to be located in the hypothalamus, according to studies done in rats and other animals. When lesions are made in the lateral hypothalamus (LH), a rat will become hypophagic but will usually survive (if postoperative care is intense enough) and maintain its weight at a subnormal level. However, if the rat is reduced to a weight below this reduced set point level before the LH lesion is made, it will actually become hyperphagic and gain weight after the lesion to reach the new set point.[236] In contrast, rats with lesions of the ventromedial hypothalamus (VMH) become obese and appear to defend an elevated body weight.[237] Obesity caused by hypothalamic damage is very rare in humans, and there is no evidence for any subtle anatomic or neurochemical abnormality in the hypothalamus of obese patients. It should be noted that neither normal nor VMH-lesioned rats defend their body weight very avidly. If normal animals are given a highly palatable diet, they become hyperphagic and obese,[238] and if VMH-lesioned rats are given an unpalatable diet, they lose weight.[239] Likewise, obese humans do not maintain their body weight when placed on a monotonous liquid diet even though they are allowed to eat ad libitum.[240] Obese subjects also fail to maintain a constant food intake when the energy density of the diet is covertly reduced with sugar or fat substitutes[241,242] and fail to increase energy intake when expenditure is increased by additional exercise.[243] These studies suggest that if a hypothalamic set point for weight or fat does exist, obese patients generally are above this set point and will go into negative energy balance under a variety of conditions.

Since the early work on LH and VMH lesions, a vast amount of research has been done to elucidate the finer details of the anatomic and neurochemical regulation of feeding in the CNS of animals, mostly rodents. Not only the hypothalamus but many nuclei in the hindbrain and forebrain are involved in regulating food intake, as are ascending and descending pathways that traverse the hypothalamus. Since no anatomic or biochemical CNS lesion is apparent in human obesity, such research has not succeeded in elucidating the specific etiology of obesity in humans. However, in the future the use of positron emission tomography (PET) scans may uncover changes in human obesity in areas of the brain that regulate food intake. It is worth noting that animal studies have demonstrated a key role for monoaminergic neurons (containing norepinephrine, dopamine, or serotonin) in regulating food intake. This may explain the fact that the available appetite suppressants used to treat obesity are sympathomimetics that cause the release of or inhibit the deactivation of catecholamines and serotonin (e.g., amphetamines, phenteremine, mazindol, fenfluramine, phendimetrazine, diethylpropion, and phenylpropanolamine hydrochloride).

Whether there is a set point comparator that is altered in human obesity and whether there is a signal emanating from adipose tissue that influences food intake are questions that will continue to be explored. The fact that obese patients almost always regain weight after losing weight and that lean subjects who are experimentally overfed return to their original weight by reducing food intake[244] makes the set point concept attractive. However, explanations other than a set point can account for these observations. Lean subjects who are overfed may consciously reduce their intake to lose weight. If reduced-obese subjects return to their former eating habits they also will return to their former weight simply because a certain level of food intake will support a certain amount of body weight.

If there is no physiologic set point that is avidly defended, it follows that short-term hunger and satiety cues are the primary determinants of food intake. There does not appear to be a single overriding signal that determines meal onset or termination. Thus, the probability of starting or ending a meal can be influenced by numerous neural, hormonal, metabolic, psychological, and environmental factors.

Because glucose ordinarily provides all the brain's energy, the role of glucose in the regulation of feeding has been an important area of investigation. The glucostatic theory holds that hunger is related to the circulating glucose concentration, or the rate of glucose metabolism in some critical area of the CNS.[245] Glucoreceptors also exist in the liver, which may relay information regarding hepatic glucose metabolism to the brain through vagal afferents.[246] Hypoglycemia induced by insulin or the inhibition of glucose metabolism with 2-deoxy-D-glucose can induce an intense craving for food. However, the degree of glucoprivation with these stimuli is much greater than that which ordinarily occurs between meals. Obese subjects tend to have higher rather than lower glucose levels, and this, according to the glucostatic theory, would tend to suppress food intake rather than stimulate it. Even though obese subjects tend to have glucose intolerance as a result of insulin resistance, the brain does not require insulin for glucose uptake and metabolism. Thus, it is unlikely that the hyperphagia of obesity is related to altered CNS glucose metabolism.

It has been proposed that the rate of tryptophan or tyrosine uptake into the brain is a determinant of appetite. These amino acids are precursors of dopamine and norepinephrine (tyrosine) and serotonin (tryptophan). The large neutral amino acids (LNAAs) compete with one another for uptake into the brain via a competitive transport system. Hence, the ratio of a particular LNAA to the others, not their absolute concentrations, can determine the availability of the precursors for monoanime synthesis, which apparently can influence concentrations of these neurotransmitters in the brain.[247,248] The ratio of tryptophan to total LNAA concentrations was reported to be lower than normal in obese subjects after a carbohydrate meal.[249] The obese subjects were classified as carbohydrate cravers, and it was suggested that the reduced Trp/LNAA ratio caused reduced appetite suppression because of reduced CNS serotonin synthesis. The reduced Trp/LNAA ratio probably resulted from the insulin resistance of obesity, which led to hyperinsulinemia and subsequently to an altered amino acid pattern. Thus, the proposed mechanism may explain why obese carbohydrate cravers have an increased food intake after they become hyperinsulinemic, but there is no evidence that preobese individuals have abnormal patterns of LNAAs that can explain the hyperphagia that eventually causes obesity. Nevertheless, the idea that a subgroup of obese subjects may overeat carbohydrates because of a need to increase serotonergic transmission in the CNS deserves further study.[250]

The fact that a high-fat diet tends to promote obesity raises the question of whether fat is less satiating than are other macronutrients. Fat has been reported to be as effective in reducing subsequent food intake and hunger ratings as other nutrients in single-meal studies.[251,252] When subjects were allowed to eat ad lib for 2 days in a laboratory setting, their energy intake was 38 percent greater with a high-fat diet (54 percent of energy as fat) than with a low-fat diet (22 percent of energy as fat) (Table 21-4).[184] Moreover, self-reported energy intake was greater in men with high-fat diets (45 ± 4 percent of energy) than in men with low-fat diets (30 ± 5 percent of energy), and the body fat content of the men on high-fat diets was 5 kg greater.[184] Obese subjects consume a greater percentage of their calories from fat, according to self-reports, but in these same studies there was no relation between obesity and self-reported energy intake.[253,254] Because a high-fat diet can promote obesity only by increasing energy intake or reducing energy expenditure, these studies are difficult to interpret. There is no good evidence that a high-fat diet increases energy efficiency in humans[255] apart from the slightly lower thermic effect of fat than of carbohydrate or protein.[256] Moreover, as was discussed earlier, there is ample evidence that obese subjects expend more energy than lean subjects do. Thus, if obese subjects underreport their energy intake, the accuracy of their self-reported diet composition must be questioned. The available evidence suggests that the high-fat diet consumed in western societies increases the prevalence of obesity, but there are many individuals who remain lean in spite of a high-fat diet and many who become obese with a dietary fat composition similar to that of lean individuals.

Adipose tissue lipoprotein lipase (LPL) activity is greater in obese subjects than in lean subjects.[257–261] This enzyme is responsible for hydrolyzing triglycerides in chylomicrons and circulating VLDLs to free fatty acids for uptake into adipocytes. The finding of higher activity of an enzyme that promotes the filling of adipocytes with fat is of obvious interest. However, as has been emphasized throughout this discussion, obesity can be understood only in terms of factors that increase energy intake or reduce energy expenditure. Since there is no reason to suspect that increased LPL activity reduces energy expenditure, this increased activity must increase energy intake to cause obesity. Because increased LPL activity enhances the storage of fat in adipocytes, less fat may be available to "feed" other tissues and increased food intake could result. The most attractive aspect of the theory that increased LPL activity is involved in the etiology of obesity is that adipose tissue LPL activity is unchanged or even increased after weight loss,[257–259,262,263] although a few studies have shown a decrease after weight loss.[260,264,265] Thus, increased adipose tissue LPL activity may be an inherent characteristic of obese subjects rather than a secondary consequence of obesity.

The role of insulin in regulating food intake is of obvious interest, given the hyperinsulinemia of obesity. It is known that insulin levels in the CSF are proportional to peripheral circulating insulin levels and that there are insulin receptors in certain areas of the brain.[266,267] In baboons, intracerebroventricular infusion of insulin suppresses food intake and body weight, suggesting that insulin is a satiety hormone.[266] However, it is well known that animals become hyperphagic if they receive sufficiently large doses of insulin peripherally. This effect often is assumed to be caused by the hypoglycemia induced by insulin. However, human subjects report increased hunger and increased palatability of sweet solutions and consume more of a liquid meal during peripheral hyperinsulinemia even when euglycemia is maintained by means of intravenous glucose infusion.[268] This finding suggests that hyperinsulinemia can contribute to hyperphagia. If this is true, the hyperinsulinemia of obesity could contribute to the maintenance of the obese state. However, there is no evidence that hyperinsulinemia precedes obesity, and it is therefore unknown whether it is a primary cause of the overeating that initially leads to obesity.

Endogenous opioids have been implicated in the control of food intake. It has long been known that opiate agonists stimulate hunger, and more recently it has been shown that opioid antagonists can inhibit food intake in certain situations.[269–271] Concentrations of the endogenous opioid agonist β-endorphin have been reported to be increased in the blood and CSF of obese humans.[270] However, it was reported that elevated plasma β-endorphin levels occur in obese women but not in obese men.[272] Several trials of the effects of opioid antagonists on the food intake and body weight of obese subjects have been published.[269,270] Although some inhibitory effects of naloxone on food intake have been observed in short-term studies, long-term controlled studies of naltrexone have demonstrated little or no inhibitory effects on food intake or body weight. (Naloxone must be given intravenously and therefore is not useful for long-term studies in humans.) Hence, it appears that even if opioids are involved in regulating short-term food intake, over longer periods other factors predominate in determining body weight in obese humans. However, this area of research must be reevaluated periodically as newer antagonists that act on specific opiate receptor subtypes are developed.

Satiety is mediated by numerous factors, including gastric distension, gut peptides (cholecystokinin, bombesin), and receptors that relay information from the large intestine and liver to the brain through the vagus nerve. These factors are important in terminating meals but probably are not very important in regulating food intake over long periods. It is not known whether obese humans respond differently to these signals than lean subjects do. These short-term satiety cues could be involved in the etiology of obesity only if long-term food intake or body weight itself were poorly regulated.

Sensory, cognitive, and psychological factors may override the physiologic regulation of food intake and contribute to obesity in some individuals. Although both lean and obese people tend to eat more food when it is very palatable, this effect appears to be exaggerated among obese subjects.[273] Obese people also may be more likely to prefer food with a higher fat content,[274] which tends to cause increased food intake. Obese subjects have been shown to be unusually responsive to nonphysiologic stimuli, such as time of day and level of anxiety, and less responsive to internal physiologic cues in determining their food intake.[273,275,276] However, many studies of the nonphysiologic factors that influence food intake in lean and obese subjects must be interpreted cautiously because they used contrived laboratory settings, did not carefully define obesity, and studied intake at only a single meal.[276]

Although many obese individuals suffer from psychologic problems, it is difficult to evaluate the extent to which such problems are the result rather than the cause of obesity. At this point there is no evidence for a common underlying psychological disturbance or personality trait that is typical of obese individuals.[273] However, it is possible that a significant proportion (30 percent) of obese subjects engage in binge eating, a form of compulsive behavior.[277]

Endocrine Systems and the Autonomic Nervous System

The thyroid hormones are the most important regulators of energy expenditure. Untreated hypothyroid individuals may have basal metabolic rates that are only 50 percent of normal, yet weight gain is not always present with this condition and obesity very rarely is caused by hypothyroidism.[278] Thyroid hormone levels are almost always within normal ranges in obese subjects, although it has been reported that the nuclear binding capacity for T_4 and T_3 is reduced in the monocytes of obese subjects.[279] As was discussed earlier, there is no strong evidence that low energy expenditure is a common cause of obesity, and so it is unlikely that obese subjects have a generalized thyroid hormone receptor defect that leads to low energy expenditure in spite of normal thyroid hormone levels.

Over the years there has been interest in the possible role of adrenal steroids in the etiology of obesity. Experimental obesity in animals is reversed or attenuated by adrenalectomy, an effect that appears to be mediated by the removal of the adrenal cortex.[280] Adrenalectomy normalizes body weight in obese animals by both reducing food intake and increasing energy expenditure.[280] However, the relevance of these animal models to human obesity is tenuous. Although the cortisol excess seen in Cushing's syndrome leads to a characteristic deposition of excess fat in the face, interscapular area, and mesenteric bed, there is no good evidence that the excess body fat in primary obesity is caused by high cortisol levels. Some early studies suggested that obese subjects hypersecrete cortisol, but later studies have not supported these results.[281] Even if some obese patients have slightly elevated cortisol production, this does not prove that high cortisol levels are the cause rather than the result of obesity. Dehydroepiandrosterone (DHEA) is an adrenal steroid that in high doses has an antiobesity effect in animals.[282,283] A negative correlation between the percentage of excess body weight and DHEA excretion has been observed.[284] However, circulating levels of DHEA and DHEA sulfate are normal in obese subjects in spite of increased DHEA production.[285,286] Large doses of DHEA given to obese men for 28 days had no effect on body weight.[287]

Insulin and β-endorphin were discussed earlier in this chapter in the context of the regulation of food intake. It also is possible that these hormones influence energy balance through effects on energy expenditure. Although insulin appears to have no thermogenic effect per se, it indirectly increases energy expenditure through its stimulatory effect on glycogen synthesis and lipogenesis. Opiates may increase energy expenditure.[270] However, it should be noted that the high levels of insulin and β-endorphin in obese subjects would tend to increase rather than reduce energy expenditure and therefore would tend to attenuate rather than promote weight gain. Thus, these hormones could contribute to obesity only through their effects, if any, on food intake.

As discussed earlier in this chapter, obesity is associated with a number of changes in endocrine systems. From the standpoint of the etiology of obesity, only changes that are present before the onset of obesity (which may be reflected by their persistence after weight loss) can be causative. Endocrine abnormalities that disappear when weight is normalized are unlikely to be involved in the development of obesity. In the vast majority of cases there is no evidence for any endocrine abnormality that is the cause of obesity.

Catecholamines (epinephrine and norepinephrine) are thermogenic hormones, and reduced sympathetic nervous system activity therefore could lead to reduced energy expenditure. Epinephrine and norepinephrine are secreted from the adrenal medulla, and norepinephrine is released from sympathetic nerves. (Most of the circulating norepinephrine comes from sympathetic nerves and reflects spillover from the synapses; thus, norepinephrine should be regarded more as a neurotransmitter than as a hormone.) Genetic obesity in *ob/ob* mice has been related to reduced sympathetic nervous system activity, especially in the nerves innervating brown adipose tissue,[288,289] but the relevance of this animal model to human obesity is questionable.

It has been reported that plasma norepinephrine and epinephrine levels were inversely related to body fat in a select group of healthy men with body fat ranging from 5 to 50 percent.[290] Other measures of sympathetic and parasympathetic activity also were inversely related to the percentage of body fat.[290] However, other data do not support the concept that obese or postobese subjects have impaired autonomic activity.[291] Our own data[292] and several other reports in the literature show a tendency for higher rather than lower norepinephrine levels in obese subjects. In view of the lack of data supporting the notion that impaired thermogenesis is an important causal factor in obesity (as discussed above), it seems unlikely that abnormal sympathetic nervous system activity plays a significant role in the pathogenesis of this condition.

Summary

The predisposition to become obese is inherited, but genetic factors apparently interact with environmental influences in complex ways to determine the body weight phenotype. Most obese subjects consume more energy than lean subjects do to maintain their obese condition, and it seems likely that this hyperphagia also is the primary cause of obesity. Although some obese individuals do not consume more energy than does the average lean person, they are hyperphagic in the sense that they consume more energy than they require to maintain a healthy body weight. Numerous factors that can influence food intake have been identified, but there is no evidence that an abnormality in any of these factors is a common cause of obesity. The mechanism by which energy intake is linked to either energy expenditure or body energy stores has not been elucidated. Thus, while it can be said that obesity definitely results from positive energy balance, it is not understood why some individuals are much more likely than others to go through periods of positive energy balance. Obesity is probably a multifactorial process with complex interactions among genetic, metabolic, hormonal, and psychological factors. It may be unrealistic to think that a single overriding cause will ever be identified.

Other Causes of Obesity

In the evaluation of an obese patient, secondary causes such as hypothyroidism, glucocorticoid excess, hypopituitarism, hypogonadism, and insulinoma should be considered. The signs and symptoms as well as the evaluation of these conditions are discussed in other chapters. Drugs such as phenothiazines and tricyclic antidepressants should also be considered.

Hypothalamic obesity can be caused by trauma, granulomatous disease, tumors, aneurysms, acute leukemia, and pseudotumor cerebri. This type of obesity is usually mild (5 to 15 kg overweight), although more severe obesity can occur with a sudden onset and can be associated with other symptoms of a space-occupying lesion, such as headache, impaired vision, hypogonadism, diabetes insipidus, impaired growth, seizures, and behavioral changes.[293,294]

Genetic syndromes associated with obesity include Prader-Willi syndrome, the Laurence-Moon-Biedl and Bardet-Biedl syndromes,[295] Cohen syndrome,[296] and Blount disease.[297] Prader-Willi syndrome is characterized by infantile hypotonia, mental deficiency, obesity, hypogonadism, behavioral abnormalities, and dysmorphic features.[298,299] Approximately 60 percent of these patients have a partial deletion of chromosome 15, 37 percent have normal chromosomes, and 3.6 percent have other abnormalities of chromosome 15.[300] Inheritance of both chromosome 15s from the mother may be causal in patients with normal chromosomes.[301] Treatment with both fluoxetine[302] and fenfluramine[303] has been reported.

TREATMENT OF OBESITY

Despite the numerous health and social problems associated with obesity as well as the physical limitations it imposes, the treatment of obesity is frustrating and usually unsuccessful. In a classic study, Stunkard and McLaren-Hume reviewed the literature on the treatment of obesity in 1959[304] and reported that less than 5 percent of patients were successful in losing 18 kg or more. The results of this study, as well as the experience of physicians in treating obese patients, have led to numerous strategies to treat obesity, including hypocaloric-balanced diets, "fad" diets, drugs, surgery, total starvation, jaw wiring, behavioral modification, exercise programs, very low calorie diets, and combinations of these treatments. Most of these treatments used alone are ineffective, and some are associated with significant side effects, are only transiently effective, or are dangerous.

Because of the frustrating nature of the treatment of obesity and the lack of a simple cure, misinformation and misinterpretation of information are rampant. Also, in a quest for a "cure," patients are susceptible to gimmicks and fad diets. The medically acceptable treatments for obesity are prevention, some diets, exercise, behavioral modification, surgery, and some drugs. The AMA Council on Scientific Affairs has recently reviewed the treatment of obesity in adults.[305]

Prevention

Prevention of obesity is obviously the best treatment. Unfortunately, the prevalence of obesity in children, adolescents, and adults in the United States is increasing.[306] Depending on the criteria used, from 23 to 25 percent of the American population either exceeds ideal body weight or is more than 20 percent above ideal body weight, and from 30 to 35 percent of women meet these criteria.[307–309] By comparing NHANES statistics of the 1963–1970 and 1976–1980 periods, Gortmaker et al. found a 39 to 54 percent increase in obesity in children age 12 to 17 and 6 to 11, respectively.[308] Williamson et al. estimated the 10-year incidence of weight gain, defined as an increase in BMI of ≥ 5 kg/m^2, and overweight, defined by a BMI of ≥ 27.8 for men and 27.3 for women, in U.S. adults using the 1971–1975

NHANES.[310] Follow-up included all adults whose age at baseline was 25 to 74 years in 1981 and 1984. Almost 10,000 people were restudied. The incidence of major weight gain was highest in persons age 25 to 34 years at 3.9 percent for men and 8.4 percent for women. Overweight women age 25 to 44 had the highest incidence of major weight gain at 14.2 percent. Among the approximately 7000 persons who were not overweight at baseline, the incidence of becoming overweight was highest in those age 35 to 44 years at 16.3 percent for men and 13.5 percent for women. These authors concluded that obesity prevention should begin among adults in their early twenties, with special emphasis on young women who are already overweight.

While the 1988 Surgeon General's Report on Nutrition and Health and the NIH Consensus Conference on the Health Implications of Obesity[311] both recommend that obesity be treated because of increased morbidity and mortality, it is important that health professionals not promote an excessive preoccupation with weight and dieting which might provoke eating disorders in susceptible individuals.[312] Some longitudinal studies have shown that obese babies do not necessarily become obese children.[313] This is in contrast to the generally accepted concept that fat children grow into fat adults.[314,315] The most important risk factor for obesity in children is parental obesity,[316] with both genetic[172,173,176,232,317] and environmental[318,319] factors. Because of the importance of parental modeling and supportive behaviors, Epstein and Cluss evaluated a program incorporating behavioral change reinforced by child and parent groups for the treatment of childhood obesity.[319] The 10-year follow-up of this program indicated that the techniques used were effective in achieving and maintaining long-term weight loss over a 10-year period.[320,321] This program involved several behavioral procedures, including contracting, self-monitoring, social reinforcement and modeling, and contingency management. If confirmed in other studies, this approach may be extremely useful in limiting obesity in adulthood. It should be mentioned that this treatment limited but did not prevent obesity. Patients in the child and parent treatment group were still approximately 35 percent overweight 10 years after intervention. This is in contrast to the nonspecific group, which was heavier 10 years later and was approximately 60 percent overweight.[321] In children, it is important that intervention not interfere with normal growth or promote the development of eating disorders.[306] It is recommended by the American Dietetic Association that intervention programs (1) be adaptable to individual needs, (2) include nutritionally sound and sensible eating patterns, (3) use psychologically sound family-oriented approaches and bring about positive behavioral modification, (4) be supportive of social needs, (5) include physical activity components, (6) be coordinated with medical care, (7) continue long enough to establish attitudinal and behavioral changes, (8) promote a positive attitude toward life and self, and (9) recognize that there is a wide range of acceptable body sizes and shapes.

Work site programs are often the most effective community approaches to weight control. As reviewed by Stunkard, weight-loss competitions are often extremely effective and attractive to groups that often ignore health promotion programs, such as men and blue-collar workers.[322] The effective elements of weight-loss competitions appear to be a combination of competition and cooperation since neither cooperation nor individual competition alone is effective. The advantage of such cooperative competition against natural competitors such as business rivals is its very low cost. As outlined by Stunkard, the cost of work site competition is less than a dollar per 1 percent reduction in percentage overweight as opposed to $6.30 for commercial programs and $89.20 for a university clinic.[322]

A primary objective for health care professionals should be the prevention of obesity in children and adults through nutrition and health education. Optimal weight should be determined by considering health risks, heredity, age, sex, percentage of body fat, and realistic goal setting. Children should not be placed on restricted-calorie diets but should be encouraged to be physically active and eat a well-balanced diet. Parents should be included in programs for children. Finally, weight-control programs should include behavioral management techniques for food intake, exercise, stress, and improved self-esteem. These programs should focus on the avoidance of repeated diet failures.[306] For adults, the inclusion of partners in weight-loss programs may facilitate weight loss and improve long-term maintenance of weight reduction for the patient while also promoting weight loss in the partner. Patients with normal-weight partners tend to lose more weight than do those with overweight partners; however, the body weight of overweight partners significantly decreases over time.[323,324] Commercial groups such as Weight Watchers and Tops can be extremely effective, but the attrition rates in these programs are very high.[325] Community programs for weight reduction have generally been ineffective.[326]

Exercise

Based on epidemiologic evidence and randomized trials supporting the association between exercise and weight control,[327] the report for the US Preventive Services Task Force[328] has stated that the efficacy of exercising in the prevention of obesity warrants a category A recommendation; i.e., there is good evidence to support the recommendation that the conditions be specifically considered in a periodic health examination. Based on a careful review of the literature, this report recommends the guidelines for physician action counseling outlined in Table 21-5.

Even small amounts of exercise may be beneficial, including weight training.[328] As reviewed by Wanger and Bell,[329] improvement in cardiovascular fitness can be achieved at relatively low levels of exercise intensity and is graded from intensities of 50 to 100 percent V_{O_2max}, frequencies of two to four times per week, and a duration of 15 to 45 min. Low-intensity exercise can be especially efficacious in the elderly and in persons with poor baseline fitness.[328] Also, low-intensity exercise (50 to 70 percent V_{O_2max}) over a longer period (35 to 45 min) can have an effect equal to or greater than that of higher-intensity (90 to 100 percent V_{O_2max}) exercise over a shorter period (25 to 35 min).[329]

An exercise prescription should take into account the patient's cardiopulmonary status, illnesses, exercise tolerance, and current lifestyle. As with most lifestyle changes, including diet, the smaller the increment in the change and the less radical the change, the more likely it is to be accepted by the patient. Intervention should be achieved in small increments. While the initial motivation for exercise is health-related, the motivation for continuing includes enjoyment, convenience, cost, and social support of the exercise. Low-intensity exercise has a greater compliance rate.[330] Few people over age 35 who are not currently exercising are likely to take on a program of vigorous exercise.[330] Physicians can have a significant impact on whether a patient exercises[328] and should focus on the reasons for recommending exercise and encouraging social support. Brisk walking is an excellent additional recommendation since it is weight-bearing; improves cardiovascular fitness; is convenient; has little perceived discomfort; can be done at flexible times and locations; has the potential for social interactions; can be

TABLE 21-5 Guidelines for Physical Activity Counseling

1. Incorporate questions regarding the physical activity level of patients into history taking during routine health care visits.
2. Identify inactive patients who do not appear to meet the minimal level of physical activity associated with gains in cardiorespiratory fitness: intensity of 50 to 100% V_{O_2max},* duration of 15 to 45 min, and frequency of 2 to 4 times per week.
3. Attempt to interest patients in adopting a program of regular physical activity by discussing the role of physical activity in disease prevention and addressing each patient's individual risk of conditions associated with inactivity and perceived health status.
4. Guide patients in choosing an appropriate type of physical activity that will be efficacious for health—such as an activity that is predominantly weight-bearing, results in energy expenditure, contributes to cardiorespiratory fitness, and has a low potential for adverse effects—and effective for adherence—such as an activity with moderate intensity; low perceived exertion; low cost; convenience; proximity to home; flexible time and location; lack of need for specialized facilities, equipment, skills, or formal programs; opportunity for simultaneous social interaction; and the potential to be incorporated into the patient's usual daily activities. Walking is the optimal activity in most cases.
5. Guide the patient to choose an appropriate level of participation in terms of intensity, duration, and frequency. The initial level should be only a small increment above baseline status. Gradual progression should be made over a period of several months, with a goal of reaching the minimum level outlined above. Familiarize the patient with measuring the pulse rate during exercise and set appropriate goals for intensity based on estimating the V_{O_2max} on the basis of the heart rate. (An intensity of 50 to 85% of the V_{O_2max} corresponds to 65 to 90% of the maximal heart rate. The maximal heart rate can be crudely estimated by subtracting one's age in years from 220.) Encourage patients at each visit to set at least one specific goal in terms of intensity, duration, and frequency that can be built on in the future. An exercise diary may be useful for this purpose.
6. Monitor compliance with physical activity and provide positive reinforcement during future health care visits.
7. Large increments in the physical activity level should be discouraged because of increased risk of injury and adverse effects as well as increased noncompliance. Patients should be told to consult a physician if they encounter persistent injury or adverse effects.
8. Encourage the social support of significant others.
9. Identify barriers that arise to optimal adherence and discuss strategies for overcoming them.
10. Encourage adherence to activity, particularly after major lifestyle transitions such as graduation from high school or college, marriage, job change, residence change, and recovery from illness or injury.
11. An exercise ECG is not necessary for asymptomatic, generally healthy persons planning to increase their level of physical activity. Patients needing specific medical attention and those in whom exercise is contraindicated should be identified.

*V_{O_2max} indicates maximal uptake.

Source: Modified from Harris et al.,[328] with permission.

incorporated into usual daily activities, making it less disruptive; and requires no special facilities, equipment, or skills.

Exercise could theoretically improve weight loss and help maintain a reduced weight by increasing caloric expenditure, decreasing energy intake, or making changes in lifestyle that promote better adherence to a diet. Exercise alone has led to little or no change in weight in most studies, although in one study exercise led to significant decreases in weight and body fat.[331–333] Woo et al. have presented evidence that obese individuals do not increase intake to compensate for increased energy expenditure, while lean individuals do.[334,335] The obese individuals did not, however, lose a significant amount of weight.[334] Exercise plus a weight-reducing diet leads to no or small, i.e., 2 to 2.5 kg, increases in weight loss over 4 to 12 weeks[331] compared with diet alone.[336–338] Increments in fat loss were not different compared with diet alone[337,338] in some studies but were greater in others,[332,339] with greater increases in $V_{O_{2max}}$.[332,337,338] Obviously, the effects of exercise on weight loss and body composition depend on the intensity, duration, and type of exercise. The greater the intensity and duration, the more calories are used, and the more resistance training is done, the more lean body mass (LBM) is preserved.[340] The greatest effect of exercise, however, is on the ability to maintain weight loss.[341] The more lean body mass can be preserved, the less the decrease is in resting energy expenditure, and the more total energy that is expended in exercise, the greater the weight loss will be. It is likely, however, that an exercise program in most middle-aged obese individuals represents a substantial lifestyle change.

As mentioned earlier, the major effect of exercise is in the maintenance of weight reduction. In one study subjects who exercised during weight reduction and continued to exercise afterward maintained their weight loss over an 18-month follow-up, whereas those who never exercised or stopped exercising regained most or all of their weight.[341] As shown in Fig. 21-9, among 52 subjects who lost an average of approximately 10 kg without exercise and were followed for 18 months after the diet, 47 who continued to abstain from exercise regained all their weight, while 5 subjects who began exercising after weight gain lost weight to approximately their original weight loss. Among the subjects who exercised during weight loss, all 36 who continued to exercise maintained their weight loss for 18 months. Those who stopped exercising regained most or all of their weight loss (Fig. 21-9). The authors concluded that treatment programs must be multidisciplinary and include a supervised exercise component, that exercise instruction alone is insufficient, that maintenance of weight loss requires a continuation of exercise at a level of at least three times weekly for a total of approximately 1500 calories per week, and that maintenance exercise need not be supervised if the treatment phase is conducted properly.

It can be concluded that exercise is a critical component of any weight-loss program and that emphasis should be placed on lifestyle changes that will lead to continued exercise after weight has been lost. Patients should exercise three to four times per week at activities they enjoy in order to avoid burnout. They should plan ahead and develop realistic exercise patterns that can be sustained in the future. The physician should provide reinforcement and encouragement and emphasize lifestyle changes. Exercise focuses patients on leading a healthy lifestyle, which includes attention to diet and body image. This may be more important in sustaining weight loss than is the increase in caloric expenditure induced by exercise. Other potential actions of exercise, such as effects on resting energy expenditure, modifying the thermic effect of food, and sustaining increased en-

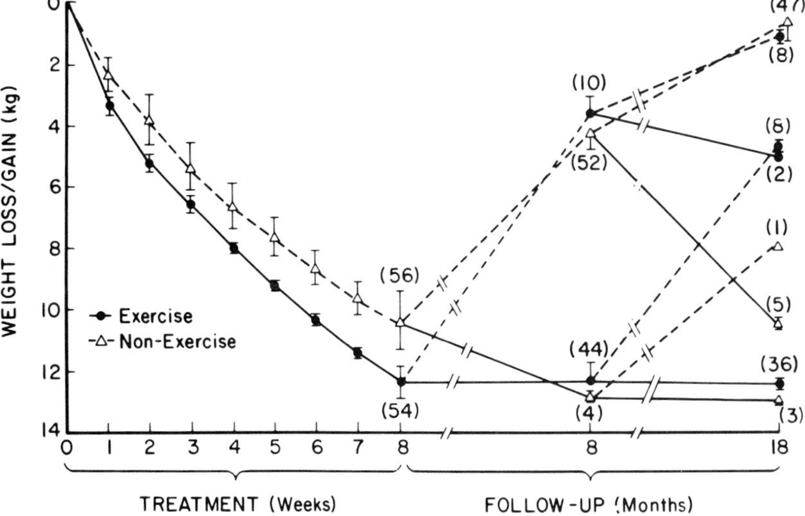

FIGURE 21-9 Weight loss or gain in exercise and nonexercise groups during an 8-week diet period and 18 months of follow-up. There was a small increase in weight loss in the exercise group during the first 8 weeks; however, the main difference was in weight maintenance. Subjects who continued to exercise (solid lines) maintained weight loss; those who discontinued exercise (dashed lines) gained weight. Subjects who never exercised regained their weight, whereas the poststudy introduction of exercise had a positive effect. (*From Pavlou et al.,*[341] *with permission.*)

ergy expenditure, along with the possible benefits of exercise before or after a meal, are of minor significance.[215,217,342–349]

Behavioral Modification

An organized behavioral modification program is critical to successful weight reduction and maintenance.[350] Without significant changes in lifestyle and eating habits, along with group support, a weight-reduction program is likely to fail. A successful behavioral modification program will describe the behavior to be changed, set goals for behavioral change and outcomes, modify the stimuli that precede eating, and modify the consequences of eating inappropriate foods. Such a program involves (1) setting goals for caloric intake, weight loss, and exercise and (2) keeping a diary to help recognize the cues that trigger eating behavior and develop appropriate responses to these cues. Patients should record the feelings that lead to eating behavior and list alternative behaviors related to what they are feeling at the time. Eventually, eating responses will be replaced by more productive behavior. This process of deconditioning old behavior and reconditioning new behavior does not occur rapidly and requires patience and repeated reinforcement. It is important to help patients realize that eating is often not done out of physical need. One should emphasize the importance of eating only three meals per day, since snacking behavior can lead to large increases in caloric intake, and to be aware of the potential caloric intake from beverages. Patients are instructed in how to slow down eating to prolong a meal and how to have only one place in the house where they eat to avoid eating while engaging in activities such as watching television and driving.

Diet

Any treatment for obesity will require a diet. As was mentioned above, exercise alone is usually not effective unless it involves extreme exertion, which is unlikely for the vast majority of obese patients. The standard or conventional hypocaloric diets (1000 to 1500 cal/day) when used alone are usually ineffective primarily because patients are hungry and their weight loss is slow. For example, a 5 foot, 2 inch woman who does not exercise would be expected to utilize a minimum of 1500 to 1700 kcal/day. On a 1000-calorie diet she would lose approximately 1 to 1.3 lb/week. If she weighed 180 lb and wanted to achieve an IBW of 110 lb, this would require from 54 to 70 weeks of dieting without ever exceeding 1000 cal/day, a nearly impossible task. For modest weight reduction, such an approach through an inexpensive, organized, reputable program such as Weight Watchers, Diet Workshop, or TOPS is reasonable. These programs all have organized behavioral modification programs and long-term follow-up. To be successful, however, patients must stay in the program, and this is often not the case. Volkmar et al. found that 50 percent of the members of commercial weight-reduction programs dropped out in 6 weeks and 70 percent in 12 weeks.[325] For patients with large amounts of weight to lose (more than 30 percent above IBW) a low-energy diet (<800 to 1000 cal/day) should be considered, but only after failure of the methods listed above. Patients should be given a chance with a commercial diet program first, with encouragement and a scientific explanation of expected weight loss on such a diet. Patients should also be instructed in the importance of weighing and measuring food. Most patients underestimate their caloric consumption by an average of 23 percent.[188]

Very low energy diets (400 to 600 cal/day) have recently been reviewed.[351] The liquid protein diets popularized in the 1970s proved to be unsafe. Based on research observations that 55 g of protein per day is accompanied by minimal negative nitrogen balance during the first week of a fast with subsequent return to equilibrium,[352] numerous investigators added protein to a total fast to reduce the protein loss associated with total fasting. While these research diets contained high-quality protein with some mineral and vitamin supplementation,[351,353] many commercial very low calorie or liquid protein diets consisted of collagen hydrolysates and lacked necessary minerals and micronutrients. In 1977, based on the book *The Last Chance Diet*,[354] it was estimated that over 100,000 people used this 300-cal hydrolyzed collagen diet exclusively for at least 1 month. In the same year at least 60 deaths were reported among persons who used these formulations. Among the 60 deaths between July 1977 and January 1978, Isner and colleagues[355] reported on 17 patients who were healthy prior to initiation of the diet and had detailed clinical information, autopsy data, or both at the time of death. All 17 patients had serious cardiac arrhythmias prior to death, including ventricular tachycardia, and autopsy findings showed significant cardiac muscle wasting compatible with cachexia.

In 1980 we published a detailed study of six patients ingesting a very low energy diet, similar to those which were commercially available, for 6 weeks in a controlled clinical research center setting.[356] This study demonstrated potentially life-threatening arrhythmias in three of six patients who were observed as early as 10 days after the start of the diet and increased in frequency and complexity as the diet continued. These arrhythmias were not seen on routine electrocardiograms but were detectable only by 24-h ambulatory ECG monitoring. Despite numerous balance studies, we could not find an association between the cardiac arrhythmias and imbalances of nitrogen or minerals. In 1983 we published a follow-up report in which obese subjects were given a highly supplemented 420-kcal diet under the same controlled conditions.[357] With this highly supplemented diet, no cardiac arrhythmias or significant mineral depletions were detected. We concluded that a vigorously supplemented, very low energy diet under proper medical supervision can be used safely. In a subsequent study we evaluated patients with obesity and NIDDM, again using a highly supplemented very low energy diet.[91] This study demonstrated that in a controlled clinical research center environment such a diet is both safe and efficacious in patients with complicated obesity and is highly effective in reducing blood glucose, cholesterol, triglycerides, and blood pressure in patients with type II diabetes. Cholesterol declined from a mean of 6.38 ± 0.51 mmol/L (247 ± 55 mg/dl) to 4.49 ± 0.32 mmol/L (174 ± 12.5 mg/dl), triglycerides declined from 3.01 ± 0.62 mmol/L (267 ± 55 mg/dl) to 1.58 ± 0.16 mmol/L (150 ± 15 mg/dl), and blood pressure declined from a mean of 136 ± 9/81 ± 2 to 116 ± 8/71 ± 2. We concluded that such diets under proper medical supervision are the initial treatment of choice for patients with type II diabetes who are 30 percent or more above IBW.

Very low energy diets, as they are used today, provide 420 to 600 kcal/day in the form of dietary protein alone or in combination with carbohydrate and fat. They contain 45 to 70 g of protein, 30 to 50 g of carbohydrate, and approximately 2 g of fat per day. Most diets use a milk- or egg-based protein formula served as a liquid diet. These diets contain the minimum daily requirements of vitamins, minerals, and trace elements. For some trace elements minimum daily requirements have not been established, and in such cases supplements are usually based on average daily intake. Because of the significant potassium losses that can occur, potassium supplements are frequently necessary, especially if patients are losing weight very rapidly, were on diuretics before starting the diet, or have low or low normal serum potassium. Some diets use animal protein in food form, i.e., meat, fish, or fowl. Proponents of these diets argue that patients learn to successfully handle conventional foods and can make the transition from a very low energy diet to a weight-maintenance diet more easily. Those who favor liquid formula diets argue that they promote better dietary adherence by simplifying the diet and removing food choices. Both diets produce similar weight loss, but there have been no controlled studies comparing the merits of the two diets for long-term maintenance.

Since the advent of commercially available very low energy diets which contain high-quality protein; daily minimum requirements of vitamins, minerals, and trace elements; and 45 to 70 g of protein per day, there have been no reports of sudden death attributable to these diets when used under medical supervision. Based on this information and studies in the literature directly demonstrating safety,[91,357] it is reasonable to conclude that these diets are safe when medically supervised and used for a short period in a properly selected group of patients.

The major advantages of very low energy diets compared with standard hypocaloric diets (over 800 to 1000 cal/day) are the more rapid rate of weight loss and the suppression of hunger. As noted above, a 5 ft, 2 in. woman on a 1200-cal diet would be expected to lose approximately 1 lb per week assuming that she weighed and measured all food accurately, exercised as she lost weight, and never exceeded 1200 cal each day. For such a woman to lose from a weight of 180 to 120 lb would take approximately 60 weeks of faithful dieting. In most people this is unrealistic, especially since people on such diets are always hungry. With a very low energy diet such a person would lose approximately 40 pounds within 12 weeks and, assuming compliance, would not be hungry.

Weight loss on a very low energy diet varies substantially depending primarily on the initial weight of the patient, complicating medical illnesses and medications, and the sex of the patient. During the first week of a very low energy diet the majority of the weight loss is related to fluid loss. Thus, a patient who is fluid-depleted as a result of diuretic use or hyperglycemia secondary to poorly regulated diabetes mellitus may lose less weight in the first 1 or 2 weeks. For example, the correlation coefficient between the percentage weight loss over 6 weeks and initial fasting plasma glucose level was $r = -0.98$.[91] The initial fluid loss is related to decreasing insulin levels that lead to decreased sodium resorption by the kidney, increased ketone body production resulting in sodium and water loss, and the utilization of carbohydrate stores, which, unlike lipid, must be stored in hydrated form. Obese patients without diabetes lose approximately 13 percent of their initial weight in the first 6 weeks of a very low energy diet,[357,358] while patients with hyperglycemia and type II diabetes lose approximately 10 percent of their initial body weight in the first 6 weeks.[91]

Obese women expend an average of approximately 32 calories per kilogram of total body weight.[199] Thus, the expected weight loss in subsequent weeks can be easily calculated, taking into account the fact that the metabolic rate falls approximately 15 percent on restrictive diets. A 5 foot, 2 inch, 180 lb woman would be expected to lose approximately 38 lb in 12 weeks: 13 percent in the first 6 weeks and 2 to 3 lb/week thereafter depending on her exercise level. Because of increased lean body mass in males, the metabolic rate is higher than it is in females of comparable height. Thus, males on average will lose more weight than females. Finally, obese individuals have more lean body mass than do normal individuals of comparable height, and consequently, the resting metabolic rate in obese individuals is increased since the resting metabolic rate is closely related to lean body mass.[199] Since total energy expenditure is best correlated with body weight, obese individuals have greater total energy expenditure than do lean individuals. Thus, the more a patient weighs, the greater that patient's resting and total energy expenditure and the faster that patient would be expected to lose weight.

The metabolic changes which occur with very low energy diets include decreases in blood pressure, plasma glucose, cholesterol, triglycerides, and edema and dramatic improvements in pulmonary function.[91,356–359] Sleep apnea syndrome frequently resolves within a few weeks.[163] In most patients plasma glucose declines very rapidly in the first week and subsequently declines more slowly.[91] Cardiac performance and exercise tolerance also improve.[91] Other benefits of weight reduction frequently include changes in body image and sense of well-being as well as improvements in joint and low back pain and frequently regulation of menses and enhanced fertility.

Unfortunately, there have been no long-term follow-up studies of these metabolic and clinical parameters in patients who have been treated with very low energy diets for the standard period of 12 weeks or longer. Studies evaluating long-term follow-up of glucose, blood pressure, pulmonary function, lipids, and other parameters are necessary to evaluate the long-term benefit of very low energy diets in complicated obesity. The paucity of long-term studies evaluating success at maintaining a reduced weight is also remarkable. However, several published reports have demonstrated the importance of behavioral modification in long-term success[360] as well as the importance of exercise.[341] It is likely that future studies will establish that the patients who are successful will be those who take the behavioral modification seriously, attend the behavioral modification classes, remain in long-term maintenance groups, and exercise. These measures help patients focus on a healthy lifestyle and long-term behavioral changes. As with weight loss on conventional diets, the people with diabetes who remain euglycemic will probably be those with diabetes of shorter duration, i.e., less than 5 to 10 years.[359,361] Those who are hypertensive secondary to obesity will have permanent resolution of blood pressure with persistent weight reduction. Those whose hypertension is only exacerbated by obesity will not have normalization of blood pressure. Similarly, secondary hyperlipidemias due to diet and obesity are corrected, whereas patients with primary hyperlipidemia will still have lipid abnormalities after weight reduction.

The complications of very low energy diets are generally minor and include fatigue, orthostatic dizziness, inability to concentrate, feelings of euphoria, constipation or diarrhea, dry skin, hair loss and cold intolerance, menstrual irregularities, and rarely muscle cramps. Rarely, patients complain of loss of libido, and a few patients have complained of worsening of migraine or the appearance of ocular migraine.[362] On carefully controlled refeeding, cholelithiasis and pancreatitis are rare. However, they can be a complication of binge eating on a very low energy diet. Hyperuricemia is common, but gout is rare. Some patients also experience problems with self-identity and body image, but serious psychiatric problems are rarely encountered. The two most frequent problems—constipation and orthostatic hypotension—are usually easily treated with fiber and bouillon, respectively.

Of recent interest and some concern has been the appearance of gallstones while patients are ingesting a very low energy diet.[363,364] It has been known for some time that weight-reducing diets are associated with decreased bile acid output, decreased cholesterol saturation of bile, decreased contraction of the gallbladder, increased biliary glycoproteins, and increased bile prostaglandin E_2 concentrations. In the study of Mok et al., bile acid pools in obese subjects decreased on caloric restriction to 1000 kcal/day.[365] In patients on a 520-cal/day diet,[364] bile saturation increased after 4 weeks, and this was associated with an increase in percent cholesterol, a decrease in percent bile acids, and a decrease in percent phospholipids. In addition, prostaglandin E_2 increased significantly. Total parenteral nutrition and gastric and ileal bypass surgery are also associated with an increased incidence of gallstones.[366–368] It has been proposed that decreased bile acid flow and gallbladder stasis may be important etiologic events. On very low energy diets, 5 of 19 patients developed gallstones in one study[364] and 13 of 51 subjects did so in another study.[363] In patients with gallstones who do not require surgery, 33 to 40 percent still have gallstones 6 to 36 months after completion of the diet. In one study, ursodeoxycholic acid was used to prevent the supersaturation of bile during weight reduction and aspirin was used to decrease prostaglandin-dependent glycoprotein formation.[364,369–372] Two of 21 subjects on aspirin developed gallstones; however, both patients had low salicylate levels. In the ursodeoxycholate-treated groups[364] only one patient developed cholesterol crystals.

The safety and efficacy of very low energy diets depend on proper patient selection, careful medical supervision, and the availability of an organized program which includes the participation of physicians, behaviorists, and nutritionists. It is mandatory to include an organized long-term maintenance program. Since exercise tolerance and exercise preferences vary substantially among individuals, it is difficult to include an exercise program as part of a weight-loss program. Nevertheless, to facilitate maintenance of weight loss, all patients should be required to enter into an exercise program of their choosing. The exercise should be something they enjoy and something that can be sustained for long periods. Patients should be encouraged to exercise 3 to 4 days per week and should be discouraged from developing unrealistic expectations about exercise. They should not plan on exercising vigorously only while losing weight and should expect to continue exercising after weight loss has been achieved.

Proper patient selection is critical. Patients must be at least 30 percent above IBW and should be less than 60 years old. As patients approach IBW, the proportion of weight loss which is lean body mass increases.[373] This is accelerated even more by a very low energy diet. It is therefore critical that patients who are below 120 percent of IBW not be maintained on a very low energy diet. Normal body composition can be achieved at IBW if caloric intake is increased to 800 calories when body weight has fallen to 120 percent above and gradually increased to maintenance calories when IBW has been achieved.

Generally, while most programs do not accept patients with serious underlying illnesses, the patients who have the most serious complications of obesity are the ones most likely to benefit from weight reduction. It is critical, however, that if such patients are accepted, they be monitored by a physician who is skilled in caring for patients on very low energy diets. Definite contraindications include cancer, cerebrovascular disease, a recent myocardial infarction, hepatic disease, a serious untreated psychiatric disease, and pregnancy. Any patient with psychiatric disease who is accepted into a program should have clearance from the psychiatrist or psychologist who is treating the illness. Patients who are over 50 years old or who have obesity complicated by cardiac disease, diabetes, pulmonary disease, or another significant illness should have a 24-h avionics which should demonstrate the absence of such problems as bigeminy, trigeminy, ventricular tachycardia, second- or third-degree heart block, ischemia, and a prolonged O-T interval. Patients over 60, less than 30 percent above IBW, with abnormal avionics, or with significant cardiopulmonary disease should be treated with a minimum of 800 cal/day. Patients with type I diabetes can be treated with very low energy diets if great care is given to the decreased insulin requirements. It should be required that all patients with insulin-treated diabetes use home glucose monitoring. Obese patients with renal failure can be treated, but it must be recognized that these patients usually have other serious medical problems and should not generally be treated with less than an 800-cal formula diet or a 1000-cal food diet.

During the initial evaluation for treatment with very low energy diets an ECG is usually obtained, although an ECG may not be reliable in picking up abnormal rhythms.[356,358] We therefore recommend a 24-h avionics in the situations outlined above. The physician should explain to the patient the physiologic basis for recommending the diet program and emphasize possible side effects and the importance of behavioral modification, exercise, and a long-term maintenance group in sustaining the reduced weight. These points should be reinforced by a lecture or tape dealing with the history and theory of low-energy diets as well as the issues mentioned above. Weekly visits include a physician visit and a behavioral modification class. For patients in whom exercise may constitute a risk, referral to a cardiac rehabilitation program may be indicated.

During the first visit prior to starting a very low energy diet, the physician and patient set a weight goal which is achievable and realistic for the time the patient is to be in the program. Long-term weight goals can also be established. Patients should sign a contract which includes the goal weight and very specific program rules. The criteria for expulsion from the program are specified, as is the warning system for expulsion. It is important that patients abide by these rules both to ensure the safety of the program and to maximize the chances of long-term success. The points to be emphasized include (1) eating the diet and supplement as three meals per day to extinguish snacking behavior and (2) the importance of the avoidance of eating food.[351] Most patients who eat food while on a very low energy diet are not successful in achieving their weight-loss goal. Patients are encouraged to keep a diary and take the behavioral modification seriously.

Patients with potassium below 4 mEq/dl and those who have been taking diuretics are started on a potassium supplement. For patients with type II diabetes, oral antidiabetic agents are discontinued. If a patient with type II diabetes is on less than 40 U/day of insulin, it is discontinued. If the patient is on more than 40 U/day of insulin, the insulin is decreased by 50 percent, blood sugars are followed by home glucose monitoring, and insulin is decreased appropriately. In most patients with type II diabetes insulin can be discontinued at the onset of the program. Antihypertensives are usually either discontinued or tapered at the first visit, depending on the level of hypertension and the number of antihypertensive agents. With rare exceptions, diuretics are discontinued. Since the vast majority of the weight loss in the first 1 to 2 weeks of a very low energy diet is fluid loss, except in unusual cases, diuretics are unnecessary and will exacerbate potassium wasting and lead to postural hypotension. Patients are informed that the weight loss during the first 1 to 2 weeks will be substantially greater than the subsequent weight loss.

In some programs patients are given a 1200-kcal balanced food diet for the initial week to 2 weeks. This introductory phase is optional. Most programs involve three phases. Phase I is the reduced-energy diet phase using the formula diet of 420 to 800 cal.

This phase usually lasts up to 12 weeks. Phase II is a refeeding phase, and phase III is a maintenance phase.

Once the diet is begun, the physician sees the patient each week and reviews the patient's weight loss, compliance, blood pressure, blood sugars if appropriate, medication lists, and any problems or complications the patient is having. Adjustments are made as necessary. Electrolytes, glucose, and blood urea nitrogen (BUN) are obtained on weeks 2 and 4 and every 4 weeks thereafter in phase I. The use of excessive laboratory testing is discouraged. For example, cholesterol and triglyceride levels will fall on a very low energy diet. There is generally no need to repeat cholesterol and triglyceride levels until after the patient is on a maintenance diet. At that time, if additional intervention other than weight loss is indicated (e.g., hypolipidemia drugs), appropriate measures can be taken. Similarly, there is no known indication for doing repetitive urinalyses. We have not detected significant changes in liver function studies or other routine tests,[91,357,358] and repetitive routine screening panels are also discouraged. Uric acid levels may rise on a very low energy diet because of the competition between ketones and uric acid for renal excretory mechanisms. In patients who do not have elevated uric acid before entering the program or a history of gout, complications related to the increase in uric acid observed during the program are extremely rare. It is important, however, to obtain electrolytes and a BUN, with special attention paid to serum potassium since patients may become potassium-depleted. Routine ECGs are also recommended in many programs. In our studies evaluating the cardiac effects of incomplete, unsupplemented very low energy diets, we detected arrhythmias only on 24-h avionics. Even in patients with abnormal 24-h avionics, the routine ECG was always within normal limits. While many programs require routine ECGs, in noncomplicated obesity repeated routine ECGs should be considered optional.

Most programs continue a 420-calorie supplement until the 12-week very low energy portion of the diet is complete. We recommend placing patients on either an 800-calorie formulation or the 420-calorie formulation plus 1 pint of 2% milk every sixth week. This is done because carefully controlled inpatient studies on safety have not been conducted beyond 6 weeks and outpatient studies on safety are unreliable because of the potential for noncompliance. The extra calories and fat provided by the milk supplement may also aid in gallbladder contraction. On weeks 8 and 12 electrolytes, BUN, and glucose are again obtained. Patients can stay on very low energy diets, cycling between the 420- and 800-cal formulations, for a maximum of 24 weeks or until they are 9 to 15 lb above the goal weight or 20 percent above IBW, at which time they are automatically placed in the refeeding phase. As was stated above, this is done because muscle catabolism accelerates in patients on very low energy diets as they approach IBW. Also, during the refeeding phase patients are expected to continue to lose weight. For individuals who consistently lose more than 5 lb/week, an 800-cal formulation should be used.

During the second phase the supplement is gradually decreased as food is increased. Patients continue in the weekly behavioral modification classes during this period and meet regularly with the dietitian on an individual basis and less frequently with the physician. Food is introduced slowly to prevent the complications of rapid refeeding, allow for continued weight reduction, and give patients time to apply behavioral modification techniques to their eating. The reintroduction of food usually makes patients apprehensive, and considerable encouragement is needed during this phase. It is again reemphasized that patients should continue the exercise program.

The maintenance phase consists of group support sessions. The group sessions are led by the behaviorist and a dietitian. After 3 months blood studies, including a lipid profile, are repeated.

Patients who still have substantial weight to lose after successful completion of 3 months of maintenance may reenter phase I. Despite patients' firm conviction that they can do this, however, it is very difficult for patients to go back on a very low energy diet, and a longer period of weight maintenance may be indicated. Long-term maintenance is encouraged, and it often takes several years before patients feel comfortable and in control of their eating. If patients regain weight, they can be allowed to reenter phase I only if they have regained less than 50 lb and are 30 percent above IBW.

In patients who have known gallstones or have symptoms of gallstones, ultrasonography is performed before the diet is started. If gallstones are confirmed, patients should not be enrolled in the program or should take ursodeoxycholic acid (8 to 10 mg/kg per day) during the weight-loss phase. Note that ursodeoxycholate is very expensive. Follow-up ultrasonography should be performed on the eighth week of the low-energy diet or any time the patient develops symptoms. Routine ultrasonography or treatment with ursodeoxycholate acid is not recommended at this time for patients who have neither symptoms nor a history of gallbladder disease. Aspirin use is still considered experimental, although it appears to be very promising (see above).

Weight-reduction programs and behavioral modification classes are not intended to be psychotherapy sessions and cannot address an individual's specific problems. When a patient shows signs of psychological difficulty, the issue should be addressed immediately. This usually involves referral for proper help.

A continuing problem in very low energy diet programs is the long-term success of patients, which unfortunately is quite low. Published studies have found that exercise and behavioral modification are critical to weight maintenance.[341,360] There have been no published studies, however, looking at weight maintenance several years later. It is critical that new methods be developed to help patients maintain weight loss. Additional long-term studies of different interventions such as drug treatment after weight loss, the intermittent use of very low energy diets, and the use of a combination of supplements and food will be important areas for future research.

Four issues frequently arise with regard to weight loss: caloric utilization, plateaus in weight loss, whether the decrease in energy expenditure with dieting hinders weight loss, and the possible danger of repeated weight fluctuations or "yo-yo" dieting. The first issue relates to patients who state that they eat very little food and yet either gain weight or cannot lose weight. Studies using metabolic chambers and studies measuring the ambulatory metabolic rate in adolescents and in women with postpartum obesity, as well as our own studies,[199] indicate that obesity is generally associated with increased caloric utilization. While there is some overlap between obese and lean individuals in ambulatory metabolic rate, there are no obese individuals who utilize fewer calories than lean individuals do. Reports by obese individuals that they gain or maintain weight on a reduced caloric intake must be considered suspect. We have noted that in a clinical research center setting, when obese patients are fed three meals a day at isocaloric levels, they routinely claim that they are getting too much food to eat. We believe that this is related to their usual eating habits, which include frequent snacking which never gives them the sense of fullness that comes with eating three meals a day. For this reason, modifying behavior to eat only three meals a day is important.

The second issue concerns the commonly held belief that plateaus in weight loss are due to a decreased metabolic rate secondary to the diet. It is true that patients lose substantially more weight during the first week or two of any diet as a result of fluid loss. Thereafter, weight loss continues at a predictable level, with some variations from week to week that are primarily dependent on the patient's fluid status. It is possible that premenstrually a patient could retain enough fluid to offset a week's weight loss, but if energy expenditure and energy intake remain constant, the body is using fat stores for energy and the patient will be losing fat and lean tissue at a predictable rate. Problems arise when patients weigh themselves too often since the weight loss from day to day may not be apparent on home scales or may be obliterated by fluid shifts. We encourage patients to weigh themselves only once a week.

The third question which frequently arises is whether the decrease in energy expenditure associated with very low energy dieting significantly hinders weight loss. The resting metabolic rate does decrease with severe caloric restriction and also decreases with weight loss as a result of decreases in lean body mass.[204,374] Upon refeeding, the resting metabolic rate rises, as one would expect, based on body composition and is not altered in a pathologic way.

Finally, repeated cycles of weight loss and regain have been reported to lead to more rapid weight gain and a lower metabolic rate.[375] Unfortunately, most of these studies in animals and people have failed to measure body composition adequately. In studies of people[376] and animals,[377] when body composition is carefully measured, repeated weight loss and regain do not lead to excessive fatness, a decreased rate of weight loss, an increased rate of weight gain, or a decrease in the metabolic rate.[378] Fluctuations in body weight may, however, increase the risk for coronary heart disease and death comparable to the risk of being obese.[379] Additional studies will be necessary to confirm this observation, especially in the absence of a clear hypothesis as to why this should be true.

Fad Diets

Fad diets, such as the grapefruit diet, should be discouraged since they frequently do not provide adequate nutrition, have severe side effects, and are not based on sound scientific principles.[380] Patients with a disease understandably are looking for a cure, and most of these subjects, frustrated with numerous past attempts, are vulnerable to so-called experts who promote fad diets that are "nutritional nonsense."[380] A good example of promoting a diet by inappropriately quoting the literature is the book *The Last Chance Diet*,[354] which promoted a collagen hydrolysate diet on the basis of research done with other sources of nutrients. The result was sudden death in over 60 people.[356] It is important to warn patients about fad diets and provide counseling about safe alternatives. Without safe alternatives, patients may seek unproven and unsafe diets.

Drugs

Drugs to treat obesity have had a history of failure, weight regain, drug abuse, adverse side effects, and inappropriate use. Nevertheless, several agents have limited or no potential for abuse and have been shown to be effective in enhancing weight reduction over short periods. In over 200 studies using amphetamine-like drugs which included almost 10,000 patients, active drugs produced more weight loss than did placebo in over 90 percent of the studies.[381] However, in 160 trials comparing placebo and active drugs, patients receiving active drug lost significantly more weight than patients receiving placebo in only 40 percent of the studies. The dropout rate at the end of the studies was 49 percent for placebo-treated patients and 47.9 percent for patients receiving active drug. Anorexic drugs enhanced weight loss by an average of 0.56 lb per week more than placebo. On the basis of these data, the FDA has approved several amphetamine-like drugs for marketing on the basis of their short-term efficacy. Amphetamine-like drugs led to a weight loss of at least 1 lb/week in 44 percent of subjects taking active drugs, compared with 26 percent of subjects taking placebo.[381] There was no significant difference between any of the active drugs. As reviewed by Weintraub and Bray,[382] weight loss occurs at a decelerating rate, stabilizing while patients are on active drug and increasing with discontinuation of drug.

Phentermine, an amphetamine-like drug with low addictive potential, is effective in inducing weight loss.[383] With dropouts included, average weight loss over 24 weeks (16 weeks of drugs) was 10.0 kg in the phentermine group and 4.4 kg in the placebo group. The group treated with fenfluramine, which stimulates serotonin release from nerve endings, lost 7.5 kg over 24 weeks. Combining the drugs to take advantage of the stimulatory effects of phentermine by giving one-half the usual dose in the morning and the sedative effects of fenfluramine by giving one-half the usual dose before supper led to a weight loss of 8.4 kg. All active treatment groups lost significantly more weight than the placebo group did. Adverse effects were less common with the combination group than with either phentermine or fenfluramine alone. Again, however, the difference in weight loss between placebo and active drug was small: 3.1 vs. 5.6 kg over the course of the study with a plateau in weight loss.

Since the *d* isomer of fenfluramine is the active isomer, recent studies have evaluated the effects of dexfenfluramine in obese subjects. A recent European cooperative study[384] of 822 obese patients evaluated dexfenfluramine in a placebo-controlled, double-blind fashion for 1 year. At 12 months, mean weight loss was 9.82 kg in the dexfenfluramine group and 7.15 kg in the placebo group. This represented 10.26 percent and 7.18 percent of initial weight, respectively. Again, 1 year of medication for a 2.7-kg differential in weight loss does not appear to be a cost-effective option. It is of interest that weight loss in the placebo and drug-treatment groups plateaued between the fourth and sixth months and increased slightly thereafter. An over-the-counter drug, phenylpropanolamine hydrochloride, leads to a weight loss of approximately 0.25 kg/week more than with placebo in short-term studies, not different from prescription appetite suppressants.[383]

Recently, a new class of atypical β-adrenergic receptor agonist (β_3 agonist) which stimulates thermogenesis in brown adipose tissue and muscle[385,386] has been described. One of these drugs, BRL 26830A, has been studied in obese humans for 18 weeks.[387] Mean weight loss was 15.4 kg in obese subjects and 10.0 kg in subjects who were given placebo. This was significant at week 18 only and represents a difference of 0.3 kg/week, not unlike all the other drugs tested. No adverse effects were detected on blood pressure, lipids, glucose, or other parameters. The only side effect regularly observed was tremulousness. Tremors should be less common with the newer β_3 agonists which are currently being tested and are reported to be more specific. Of interest is that BRL 26830A did increase energy expenditure 2 h after an oral dose but did not affect the resting metabolic rate. The effect on 24-h energy expenditure is not known.

Other drugs used to treat obesity, such as hCG,[388] opioid antagonists, and phenytoin, are ineffective and have no place in current therapy.[382] Thyroid hormone has been used, but it enhances the loss of lean body mass and its use is subject to all the complications associated with hyperthyroidism. It also has no place in the treatment of obesity. Bile acid resins are ineffective. α-Amylase inhibitors[389] have been shown to lower postprandial glucose levels, but long-term studies on weight loss have not been performed, and at doses which might be effective it is likely that the gastrointestinal (GI) side effects would be excessive. The data on sucrose polyester (Olestra) indicate that it reduces serum cholesterol but has minimal or no effects on body weight beyond that caused by diet alone.[390,391] Fiber added to a weight-reducing diet has been shown to lead to small increases in weight loss (mean = 1.8 kg over 12 weeks).[392]

Growth hormone has been used in conjunction with diets of 24 cal/kg[393] and 18 cal/kg.[394] These studies have demonstrated that short-term growth hormone administration is effective in decreasing loss of LBM. However, loss of LBM is a normal accompaniment of weight reduction since lean individuals have less LBM than do obese individuals. Body composition at reduced weight is normal in subjects treated with low-energy diets. Thus, growth hormone would be an expensive method to alter body composition, a situation which will probably change when growth hormone is discontinued. The more cost-effective and physiologic approach would be exercise with a resistance component. An inhibitor of pancreatic lipase, tetrahydrolipstatin, is derived from lipstatin, a lipid produced by *Streptomyces toxytricini*, and inhibits other lipases as well.[395] Tetrahydrolipstatin decreases triglyceride absorption but not free fatty acid absorption in animals in a dose-dependent manner. In animals with diet-induced obesity, tetrahydrolipstatin induces weight loss. Food intake is actually increased in treated animals, while fat absorption is decreased by 76 percent. Studies in people will be necessary to detemine if the symptoms of fat malabsorption limit the usefulness of this approach.

Endogenous cholecystokinin has been postulated to be a mediator of postprandial satiety. Recent studies in animals using antagonists to brain-type and peripheral-type cholecystokinin demonstrated that a brain-type cholecystokinin antagonist was 100 times more potent than a peripheral-type antagonist in increasing food intake in partially satiated animals and in postponing the onset of satiety.[396] These studies support the role of endogenous cholecystokinin in mediating satiety through central mechanisms. The usefulness of cholecystokinin or potential cholecystokinin agonists in the treatment of human obesity is unknown.

In patients with obesity and type II diabetes, the biguanide metformin decreases blood glucose and body weight, probably by inhibiting glucose absorption from the GI tract. Fluoxetine is a widely used antidepressant which is an inhibitor of serotonin reuptake in the CNS. Obese patients given fluoxetine at doses of 60 to 65 mg/day lose a mean of approximately 4 kg over 8 weeks.[397,398] In neither study were patients prescribed a diet. Furthermore, the doses given are approximately three times those used for depression. A 52-week study found that patients given fluoxetine 60 mg/day plus behavioral modification and diet individualized to produce a weight loss of approximately 1 lb/week lost a mean of 13.9 kg, while placebo-treated patients at 52 weeks gained 0.6 kg.[399] Most of the weight loss in the fluoxetine-treated group occurred by week 20, 11.2 kg vs. 2.1 kg in the placebo-treated group. Because fluoxetine may be useful in treating bulimia nervosa, because many obese patients are binge eaters, and because these patients do poorly in weight-loss programs, a group of obese binge eaters was included in the study. There was no difference in weight loss between binge eaters and nonbinge eaters treated with fluoxetine. Only approximately 50 percent of the subjects completed the study. Thus, fluoxetine shows promise as a useful adjunct in the management of obesity.

Surgery for Morbid Obesity

Morbid obesity is defined as either 100 lb or 100 percent above IBW. The excess mortality associated with morbid obesity comes largely from extrapolated data.[400] However, Drenick et al. compared a group of 200 morbidly obese men followed for a mean of 7.5 years with mortality statistics for men in the general population.[401] Complete follow-up data were available on 185 men. Fifty of the 200 morbidly obese men died during the course of the study, which was a 12-fold excess in the age group from 25 to 34 years of age and a sixfold excess in the age group from 35 to 45 years of age. Excess frequencies of cardiovascular disease, diabetes, and accidents as the cause of death were found in the morbidly obese men. It is of interest that the excess mortality of morbidly obese men over 65 years old diminished to approximately twofold.

Because of the marked excess mortality associated with morbid obesity as well as the other conditions associated with obesity and because of the failure of morbidly obese patients to respond to conventional modalities for the treatment of obesity,[400] various surgical techniques to induce weight reduction have been developed. In 1985 a task force of the American Society of Clinical Nutrition[402] developed guidelines for selection of patients for the surgical treatment of obesity. These criteria are listed in Table 21-6. The surgeon should be knowledgeable in the fields of obesity surgery, gastroenterology, and nutrition and should regularly perform such operations with a commitment to postoperative care and long-term follow-up. The governing body of the medical staff should review and update standards relating to obesity surgery and assure that the standards are maintained, audit the records, ensure the adequacy and accuracy of data collection, recommend changes when appropriate, and monitor postoperative care. Finally, the surgeon should ensure that the patient receives an adequate explanation of the oper-

TABLE 21-6 Guidelines for Selection of Patients for the Surgical Treatment of Obesity

The patient should
1. Be 100 lb or 100% above IBW or have one or more serious medical conditions related to severe refractory obesity
2. Have a history of repeated failures to lose weight by acceptable nonsurgical methods
3. Have been in the eligible weight range for 3 to 5 years
4. Be able to tolerate the surgical procedure
5. Have no alcoholism, drug addiction, or other psychopathology that would compromise cooperation
6. Sign an informed consent after an adequate explanation of the operation, its risk and benefits, and the long-term results and complications based on the experience of the surgeon
7. See a psychiatrist prior to surgery.

The program should have
1. Guaranteed standards of preoperative, operative, and postoperative care
2. A nutritional support program
3. An experienced surgeon with proper resources and commitment
4. A governing body in the hospital with a commitment to adopt standards for patient evaluation, treatment, and long-term follow-up and audit records to ensure compliance.

Source: Adopted from The Task Force of the American Society for Clinical Nutrition.[402]

ation and its risks and benefits as well as the effects on everyday life. Patients should be encouraged to talk to other patients and should sign a consent form which describes the procedure and its risks and long-term complications, the importance of postoperative follow-up, and the benefits to be expected based on the experience of the surgeon. It is also recommended that patients should be evaluated by a psychiatrist prior to surgery to assess motivation and the possibility of unrealistic expectations, to evaluate psychopathology and the extent to which it may interfere with cooperation, and to educate these patients.

With this in mind, several operations have been used to treat morbid obesity.[403,404] In reviewing the literature, one must keep in mind the way in which the data are reported and the way in which patients who are lost to follow-up are included in the data.[405] Zollinger et al. reported an analysis of 93 patients who had jejunoileal bypass surgery.[406] Thirty-six patients were not included in the data analysis because 26 patients were lost to follow-up and 10 had the procedure within 8 months of the writing of the manuscript. The average follow-up was 31 months, but there was no breakdown of patients by duration of follow-up. The average excess weight loss was between 61 and 75 percent depending on the procedure used. Complications included nephrolithiasis (8 percent), herniorrhaphy (7 percent), hemorrhoidectomy (7 percent), electrolyte imbalances (6 percent), wound abscesses (4 percent), intussusception (2 percent), and gallstones (3 percent). Six percent required reversal of the procedure. Hocking et al. reported "late" follow-up of 100 patients with jejunoileal bypass surgery.[407] Actually, 201 patients had been operated on 5 or more years earlier, but the data on 101 patients were not included because 22 patients required reversal, 12 patients died, and 67 patients had inadequate follow-up. For the 100 patients who were reported on, the mean weight loss was 33 percent and the complications included diarrhea in 58 percent, hypokalemia in 39 percent, hypomagnesemia in 33 percent, decreased vitamin B_{12} or folate in 88 percent, nephrolithiasis in 21 percent, cholecystectomy in 20 percent, hepatic changes on biopsy in 29 percent, and cirrhosis in 7 percent. Other complications included intussusception, gastric ulcers, and arthritis. The mechanisms involved in causing these complications have been studied extensively.[407–409] Patients did have improvement in hypertension, glucose tolerance, sleep apnea, congestive heart failure, angina, lipid levels, and venous disease. Owing to the multiple problems, however, jejunoileal bypass surgery has generally fallen out of favor.

With the decrease in interest in jejunoileal bypass surgery, various operations to restrict the size of the stomach came into favor. The first such operation was a horizontal gastroplasty. Thousands of these operations were performed before it was realized that the procedure failed to produce significant long-term weight reduction.[405] Because of this high failure rate, the vertical banded gastroplastic procedure was developed by Fabito, Eckhout, and Laws in 1979.[404] Initial reports of this procedure were also very favorable, with mean weight losses of approximately 36 percent in 2 years and minimal complications.[410] Eckhout et al. reported that "weight loss two years postoperatively was 25.5% for the chronic ring vertical gastroplasty, 29.9% for the covered silastic ring vertical gastroplasty group, and 36.7% for the uncovered silastic ring."[411] Unfortunately, there were no actual data reported for the 1,463 patients who were operated on. Makarewicz et al. followed 11 patients through 30 months of follow-up.[412] Six of the 11 patients started to gain weight, and in 2 of them weight loss was under 30 percent. Only three patients were doing well with regard to weight loss. These authors concluded that the data on the vertical banded gastroplasty approached the data on the horizontal banded gastroplasty, but the onset of failures was delayed.

Makarewicz et al. also noted that thousands of vertical banded gastroplasties were performed before it became evident that the long-term results were unsatisfactory and that there were more articles on "new" vertical banded gastroplasty techniques than weight loss data on the techniques originally described.[412] Makarewicz et al. pointed out that there were no long-term follow-up data and that patients lost to follow-up were not included. These authors stated that bariatric surgeons should do follow-up studies or cease performing the operation and have an obligation to publish their long-term follow-up data. Of interest also is the lack of animal data on these operations. Ravitch, in the presidential address of the American Surgical Association in 1984, reported, "We are now still in the era of various types of gastric bypasses and compartmentation procedures. What has chiefly distinguished these is what one might call the 'operation of the year.' This is the phenomenon of a large and carefully studied series of patients operated upon by a given technique, reported in a paper at the end of which the author states, 'because of some concern over these factors (risks, complications, unpredictable weight loss, gradual return of the weight that has been lost . . .), we have begun employing a new modification which consists of the following. . . . The early results are extremely promising.' The following year an entirely similar paper is written about the new procedure. The complications and the dissatisfaction with it are perhaps different, and still another procedure is proposed."[413]

The most commonly used gastric bypass procedure is the Roux-en-Y gastric bypass with stomach stapling. Thompson et al. reported on 13 studies, including their own, with patient numbers ranging from 17 to 700 and duration of follow-up ranging from 12 months to 60 months.[414] Among almost 3000 patients reported to have gastric bypass surgery before the date of publication, only 71 patients had been followed for 48 months and 44 patients had been followed for 60 months. Flickenger et al. reported on 397 patients followed for as long as 6 years.[415] There was a clear trend toward regaining weight after 2 years. Of the 397 patients studied, the mortality rate was 0.8 percent, with 16 percent of patients having nausea and vomiting and 71 percent dumping. Iron, B_{12}, or folate deficiencies were present in 15 percent, 27 percent, and 9 percent, respectively. Gastritis was present in 9 percent in the proximal pouch and in 97 percent in the distal pouch. Peptic ulcers occurred in less than 2 percent.

Benotti et al. reported results on gastric bypass and vertical banded gastroplasty, again showing a trend toward weight gain after the third year.[416] Sugerman et al. compared the Roux-en-Y gastric bypass with the vertical banded gastroplasty and demonstrated that after 3 years of follow-up the gastric bypass led to significantly greater weight loss.[417] These authors also showed that vertical banded gastroplasty patients who were "sweet eaters" tended to lose less weight than did those who were not, whereas there was no difference in patients who had the gastric bypass procedure.[418] In a comparison of gastroplasty vs. gastric bypass, the failure rate for gastroplasty patients at 2 years of follow-up was approximately 45 percent, whereas for gastric bypass patients it was only approximately 10 percent.[419] Fobi et al. discussed the early and late complications of the two procedures, with stomal obstruction being more common earlier in the vertical banded gastroplastic group and vitamin B_{12} deficiency, dumping syndrome, and transient neuropathy being more common as late complications in the gastric bypass group.[420] The neurologic syndromes following gastric surgery for morbid obesity include polyneuropathy.[421,422] Other operations, such as the biliopancreatic bypass and the duodenoileal bypass/biliointestinal bypass,[404] have not been adequately studied.

In 1987 a group of experts was asked if vertical banded gastroplasty constitutes safe and effective adjunctive therapy for the treatment of resistant cases of morbid obesity.[423] Fifty-one percent of those responding stated that safety was established, 38 percent felt that the procedure was investigational from a safety standpoint, 5 percent felt it was unacceptable, and 3 percent felt it was indeterminant. With regard to effectiveness, 46 percent felt it was established, 41 percent felt it was investigational, and 13 percent felt it was unacceptable or indeterminant. The same experts were asked if a Roux-en-Y gastrojejunostomy was safe and effective. With regard to safety, 42 percent felt it was established, 40 percent felt it was investigational, and 18 percent felt it was unacceptable or indeterminant. For effectiveness, 45 percent felt it was established, 42 percent felt it was investigational, and 13 percent felt it was unacceptable or indeterminant. Despite the limitations of both procedures, most patients feel better both physically and psychologically[424–427] after the surgical treatment of morbid obesity. Unfortunately, long-term follow-up studies have not been performed.

In summary, the surgical procedure of choice is the Roux-en-Y gastric bypass procedure. This procedure should not be performed without enforcement of the guidelines outlined by the task force of the American Society of Clinical Nutrition in 1985 (Table 21-6). If patients are refractory to all other forms of treatment, if the patient's health demands a radical treatment of obesity, and if an established program which meets these guidelines is operative, one should consider this procedure.

Summary

The treatment of obesity begins with prevention and good diet and exercise habits. A well-balanced hypocaloric diet should be combined with an established behavioral modification program and long-term maintenance. In more refractory cases and especially in patients with complications of obesity, very low energy diets should be considered, but only in conjunction with an established program, behavioral modification, and a long-term maintenance group. To ensure safety and maximize long-term success, the program should conform to the standards discussed above. There is no cost-effective pharmacologic approach to obesity at the present time, although many drugs can enhance weight loss a small amount and, if continued, help sustain the loss. Surgery is recommended only for morbid obesity, and the program should conform to the guidelines of the task force of the American Society of Clinical Nutrition (Table 21-6).[402]

Acknowledgments We wish to acknowledge the secretarial assistance of Ms. Sandy Webster and Ms. Liz Skeleton. This work was supported by NIH grants DK20948, DK40816, RR00044, and DK39063.

REFERENCES

1. Forbes GB: Techniques for estimating body composition, in *Human Body Composition.* New York, Springer-Verlag, 1987, pp 5–100.
2. Forbes GB, Bruining GJ: Urinary creatinine excretion and lean body mass. *Am J Clin Nutr* 29:1359, 1976.
3. Gray DS, Bray GA, Gemayel N, Kaplan K: Effect of obesity on bioelectrical impedance. *Am J Clin Nutr* 50:255, 1989.
4. Gray DS: Changes in bioelectrical impedance during fasting. *Am J Clin Nutr* 48:1184, 1988.
5. Kushner RF, Kunigk A, Alspaugh M, Andronis PT, Leitch CA, Schoeller DA: Validation of bioelectrical-impedance

analysis as a measurement of change in body composition in obesity. *Am J Clin Nutr* 52:219, 1990.
6. Simopoulos AP, VanItallie TB: Body weight, health, and longevity. *Ann Intern Med* 100:285, 1984.
7. Harrison GG: Height-weight tables. *Ann Intern Med* 103: 989, 1985.
8. Manson JE, Stampfer MJ, Hennekens CH, Wilett WC: Body weight and longevity: A reassessment. *JAMA* 257:353, 1987.
9. Feinleib M: Epidemiology of obesity in relation to health hazards. *Ann Intern Med* 103:1019, 1985.
10. Build study, 1979. Chicago, Society of Actuaries and Association of Life Insurance Medical Directors, 1980.
11. Garrison RJ, Castelli WP: Weight and thirty-year mortality of men in the Framingham Study. *Ann Intern Med* 103:1006, 1985.
12. Lew EA: Mortality and weight: Insured lives and the American Cancer Society Studies. *Ann Intern Med* 103:1024, 1985.
13. Barrett-Conner EL: Obesity, atherosclerosis, and coronary artery disease. *Ann Intern Med* 103:1010, 1985.
14. Hubert HB, Feinleib M, McNamara PM, Castelli WP: Obesity as an independent risk factor for cardiovascular disease: A 26-year follow-up of participants in the Framingham Heart Study. *Circulation* 67:968, 1983.
15. Rabkin SW, Mathewson FAL, Hsu PH: Relation of body weight to development of ischemic heart disease in a cohort of young North American men after a 26 year observation: The Manitoba Study. *Am J Cardiol* 39:452, 1977.
16. Stallones RA: Epidemiologic studies of obesity. *Ann Intern Med* 103:1003, 1985.
17. Vague J: The degree of masculine differentiation of obesities: A factor determining predisposition to diabetes, atherosclerosis, gout and uric calculous disease. *Am J Clin Nutr* 4:20, 1956.
18. Hartz AJ, Rupley DC, Rimm AA: The association of girth measurements with disease in 32,856 women. *Am J Epidemiol* 119:71, 1984.
19. Kissebah AH, Vydelingum N, Murray R, Evans DJ, Hartz AJ, Kalkhoff RK, Adams PW: Relation of body fat distribution to metabolic complications of obesity. *J Clin Endocrinol Metab* 54:254, 1982.
20. Krotkiewski M, Björntorp P, Sjöström L, Smith U: Impact of obesity on metabolism in men and women: Importance of regional adipose tissue distribution. *J Clin Invest* 72:1150, 1983.
21. Peiris AN, Sothmann MS, Hoffmann RG, Hennes MI, Wilson CR, Gustafson AB, Kissebah AH: Adiposity, fat distribution, and cardiovascular risk. *Ann Intern Med* 110:867, 1989.
22. Evans DJ, Hoffman RG, Kalkhoff RK, Kissebah AH: Relationship of androgenic activity to body fat topography, fat cell morphology, and metabolic aberrations in premenopausal women. *J Clin Endocrinol Metab* 57:304, 1983.
23. Evans DJ, Murray R, Kissebah AH: Relationship between skeletal muscle insulin resistance, insulin-mediated glucose disposal, and insulin binding: Effects of obesity and body fat topography. *J Clin Invest* 74:1515, 1984.
24. Peiris AN, Mueller RA, Smith GA, Struve MF, Kissebah AH: Splanchnic insulin metabolism in obesity. *J Clin Invest* 78:1648, 1986.
25. Haffner SN, Fong D, Hazuda HP, Pugh JA, Patterson JK: Hyperinsulinemia, upper body adiposity, and cardiovascular risk factors in non-diabetics. *Metabolism* 37:338, 1988.
26. Anderson AJ, Sobocinski KA, Freedman DS, Barboriak JJ, Rimm AA, Gruchow HW: Body fat distribution, plasma lipids, and lipoproteins. *Arteriosclerosis* 8:88, 1988.
27. Larsson B, Svardsudd K, Welin L, Wilhelmsen L, Björntorp P, Tibblin G: Abdominal adipose tissue distribution, obesity, and risk of cardiovascular disease and death: 13 year follow-up of participants in the study of men born in 1913. *Br Med J* 288:1401, 1984.
28. Lapidus L, Bengtsson C, Larsson B, Pennert K, Rybo E, Sjöström L: Distribution of adipose tissue and risk of cardiovascular disease and death: A 12 year follow-up of participants in the population study of women in Gothenburg, Sweden. *Br Med J* 289:1257, 1984.
29. Reaven GM: Role of insulin resistance in human disease. *Diabetes* 37:1595, 1988.
30. Barrett-Connor E, Khaw K-T. Cigarette smoking and increased central adiposity. *Ann Intern Med* 111:783, 1989.
31. Rabinowitz D, Zierler KL: Forearm metabolism in obesity and its response to intraarterial insulin: Characterization of insulin resistance and evidence for adaptive hyperinsulinism. *J Clin Invest* 41:2173, 1962.
32. Kolterman OG, Insel J, Saekow M, Olefsky JM: Mechanisms of insulin resistance in human obesity: Evidence for receptor and postreceptor defects. *J Clin Invest* 65:1272, 1980.
33. Felber J-P, Ferrannini E, Golay A, Meyer HU, Theibaud D, Curchod B, Maeder E, Jequier E, et al: Role of lipid oxidation in pathogenesis of insulin resistance of obesity and Type II diabetes. *Diabetes* 36:1341, 1987.
34. Prager R, Wallace P, Olefsky JM: Hyperinsulinemia does not compensate for peripheral insulin resistance in obesity. *Diabetes* 36:327, 1987.
35. Bonadonna RC, Groop L, Kraemer N, Ferrannini E, Del-Prato S, DeFronzo RA: Obesity and insulin resistance in humans: A dose-response study. *Metabolism* 39:452, 1990.
36. Lillioja S, Bogardus C, Mott DM, Kennedy AL, Knowler WC, Howard BV: Relationship between insulin-mediated glucose disposal and lipid metabolism in man. *J Clin Invest* 75:106, 1985.
37. Bogardus C, Lillioja S, Mott D, Reaven GM, Kashiwagi A, Foley JE: Relationship between obesity and maximal insulin-stimulated glucose uptake in vivo and in vitro in Pima Indians. *J Clin Invest* 73:800, 1984.
38. Peiris A, Struve MF, Mueller RA, Lee MB, Kissebah AH: Glucose metabolism in obesity: Influence of body fat distribution. *J Clin Endocrinol Metab* 67:760, 1988.
39. Devlin JT, Horton ES: Effects of prior high-intensity exercise on glucose metabolism in normal and insulin-resistant men. *Diabetes* 34:973, 1985.
40. Bogardus C, Lillioja S, Nyomba BL, Zurlo F, Swinburn B, Esposito-Del Puente A, Knowler WC, Ravussin E, et al: Distribution of in vivo insulin action in Pima Indians as mixture of three normal distributions. *Diabetes* 38:1423, 1989.
41. Lillioja S, Mott DM, Zawadzki JK, Young AA, Abbott WG, Bogardus C: Glucose storage is a major determinant of in vivo "insulin resistance" in subjects with normal glucose tolerance. *J Clin Endocrinol Metab* 62:922, 1986.
42. Laasko M, Edelman SV, Brechtel G, Baron AD: Decreased effect of insulin to stimulate skeletal muscle blood flow in obese man. *J Clin Invest* 85:1844, 1990.
43. Kida Y, Esposito-Del Puente A, Bogardus C, Mott DM: Insulin resistance is associated with reduced fasting and insulin-stimulated glycogen synthase phosphatase activity in human skeletal muscle. *J Clin Invest* 85:476, 1990.
44. Amatruda JM, Salhanick AI: Insulin and steatonecrosis: Are they related? *Hepatology* 10:1024, 1989.
45. Cech JM, Freeman RB, Caro JF, Amatruda JM: Insulin action and binding in isolated hepatocytes from fasted, streptozotocin-diabetic, and older, spontaneously obese rats. *Biochem J* 188:839, 1980.
46. Amatruda JM, Salhanick AI, Chang CL: Hepatic insulin resistance in non-insulin-dependent diabetes mellitus and the effects of a sulfonylurea in potentiating insulin action. *Diabetes Care* 7(suppl 1):47, 1984.
47. Amatruda JM, Livingston JN, Lockwood DH: Cellular mechanisms in selected states of insulin resistance: Human obesity, glucocorticoid excess, and chronic fetal failure. *Diabetes Metab Rev* 1:293, 1985.
48. Ferrannini E, Buzzigoli G, Bonadonna R, Giorico MA, Oleggini M, Graziadei L, Pedrinelli R, Brandi L, et al: Insulin resistance in essential hypertension. *N Engl J Med* 317:350, 1987.
49. Zavaroni I, Bonora E, Pagliara M, Dall'Aglio E, Luchetti L,

Buonanno G, Bonati PA, Bergonzani M, et al: Risk factors for coronary artery disease in healthy persons with hyperinsulinemia and normal glucose tolerance. *N Engl J Med* 320:702, 1989.
50. Haffner SM, Stern MP, Hazuda HP, Mitchell BD, Patterson JK: Increased insulin concentrations in nondiabetic offspring of diabetic parents. *N Engl J Med* 319:1297, 1988.
51. Laakso M, Sarlund H, Mykkänen L: Insulin resistance is associated with lipid and degrees of glucose tolerance. *Arteriosclerosis* 10:223, 1990.
52. Lillioja S, Bogardus C: Insulin resistance in Pima Indians. *Acta Med Scand (suppl)*723:103, 1990.
53. Swinburn BA, Nyomba BL, Saad MF, Zurlo F, Raz I, Knowlder WC, Lillioja S, Bogardus C, et al: Insulin resistance associated with lower rates of weight gain in Pima Indians. *J Clin Invest* 88:168, 1991.
54. Garvey WT, Maianu L, Huecksteadt TP, Birnbaum MJ, Molina JM, Ciaraldi TP: Pretranslational suppression of a glucose transporter protein causes insulin resistance in adipocytes from patients with non-insulin-dependent diabetes mellitus and obesity. *J Clin Invest* 87:1072, 1991.
55. Freidenberg GR, Reichart D, Olefsky JM, Henry RR: Reversibility of defective adipocyte insulin receptor kinase activity in non-insulin-dependent diabetes mellitus: Effect of weight loss. *J Clin Invest* 82:1398, 1988.
56. Ferrannini E, Barrett EJ, Bevilacqua S, DeFronzo RA: Effect of fatty acids on glucose production and utilization in man. *J Clin Invest* 72:1737, 1983.
57. Meylan M, Henny C, Temier E, Jequier E, Felber JP: Metabolic factors in the insulin resistance in human obesity. *Metabolism* 36:256, 1987.
58. Bevilacqua S, Bonadonna R, Buzzigoli G, Boni C, Ciociaro D, Maccari F, Giorico MA, Ferrannini E: Acute elevation of free fatty acid levels leads to hepatic insulin resistance in obese subjects. *Metabolism* 36:502, 1987.
59. Laasko M, Edelman SV, Brechtel G, Baron AD: Decreased effect of insulin to stimulate skeletal muscle blood flow in obese man. *J Clin Invest* 85:1844, 1990.
60. Rosenthal M, Haskell WL, Solomon R, Widstromo A, Reaven GM: Demonstration of a relationship between level of physical training and insulin-stimulated glucose utilization in normal humans. *Diabetes* 32:408, 1983.
61. Olefsky JM, Farquhar JW, Reaven GM: Reappraisal of the role of insulin in hypertriglyceridemia. *Am J Med* 57:551, 1974.
62. Grundy SM, Mok HYI, Zech L, Steinberg D, Berman M: Transport of very low density lipoprotein triglycerides in varying degrees of obesity and hypertriglyceridemia. *J Clin Invest* 63:1274, 1979.
63. Olefsky J, Reaven GM, Farquhar JM: Effects of weight reduction and obesity on lipid and carbohydrate metabolism in normal and hyperlipoproteinemic subjects. *J Clin Invest* 53:64, 1974.
64. Grundy SM, Barnett JP: Metabolic and health complications of obesity. *Dis Mon* 36:645, 1990.
65. Equsa G, Beltz WF, Grundy SM, Howard BV: Influence of obesity on metabolism of apolipoprotein B in humans. *J Clin Invest* 76:596, 1985.
66. Kazumi T, Vranic M, Steiner G: Changes in very low density lipoprotein particle size and production in response to sucrose feeding and hyperinsulinemia. *Endocrinology* 117: 1145, 1985.
67. Dunn FL, Carroll PB, Beltz WF: Treatment with artificial β-cell decreases very-low-density lipoprotein triglyceride synthesis in Type I diabetes. *Diabetes* 36:661, 1987.
68. Rosenstock J, Vega GL, Raskin P: Effect of intensive diabetes treatment on low-density lipoprotein apolipoprotein B kinetics in Type I diabetes. *Diabetes* 37:393, 1988.
69. Salhanick AI, Schwartz SI, Amatruda JM: Insulin inhibits apolipoprotein B secretion in isolated human hepatocytes. *Metabolism* 40:275, 1991.
70. Sparks CE, Sparks JD, Bolognino M, Salhanick AI, Strumph PS, Amatruda JM: Insulin effects on apolipoprotein B lipoprotein synthesis and secretion by primary cultures of rat hepatocytes. *Metabolism* 35:1128, 1986.
71. Jackson TK, Salhanick AI, Elovson J, Deichman ML, Amatruda JM: Insulin regulates apolipoprotein B turnover and phosphorylation in rat hepatocytes. *J Clin Invest* 86:1746, 1990.
72. Yki-Järvinen H, Taskinen M-R: Interrelationships among insulin's antilipolytic and glucoregulatory effects and plasma triglycerides in nondiabetic and diabetic patients with endogeneous hypertriglyceridemia. *Diabetes* 37:1271, 1988.
73. DeFronzo RA, Ferrannini E: Insulin resistance: A multifaceted syndrome responsible for NIDDM, obesity, hypertension, dyslipidemia, and atherosclerotic cardiovascular disease. *Diabetes Care* 14:173, 1991.
74. Reaven GM: Insulin resistance, hyperinsulinemia, hypertriglyceridemia and hypertension: Parallels between human disease and rodent models. *Diabetes Care* 14:195, 1991.
75. Garrison RJ, Wilson PW, Castelli WP, Feinleib M, Kannel WB, McNamara PM: Obesity and lipoprotein cholesterol in the Framingham offspring study. *Metabolism* 29:1053, 1980.
76. Follick MJ, Abrams DB, Smith TW, Henderson LO, Herbert PN: Contrasting short- and long-term effects of weight loss on lipoprotein levels. *Arch Intern Med* 144:1571, 1984.
77. Wood PD, Stefanick ML, Dreon DM, Frey-Hewitt B, Garay SC, Williams PT, Superko HR, Fortmann SP, et al: Changes in plasma lipids and lipoproteins in overweight men during weight loss through dieting as compared with exercise. *N Engl J Med* 319:1173, 1988.
78. Dustan HP: Obesity and hypertension. *Ann Intern Med* 103:1047, 1985.
79. Stamler R, Stamler J, Riedlinger W, Algera G, Roberts RH: Weight and blood pressure findings in hypertension screening of 1 million Americans. *JAMA* 240:1607, 1978.
80. Modan M, Halkin H, Almog S, Lusky A, Eskol A, Shefi M, Shitrit A, Fuchs Z: Hyperinsulinemia: A link between hypertension, obesity and glucose intolerance. *J Clin Invest* 75:809, 1985.
81. Pollare T, Lithell H, Berne C: Insulin resistance is a characteristic feature of primary hypertension independent of obesity. *Metabolism* 39:167, 1990.
82. DeFronzo RA, Cooke CR, Andres R, Faloona GR, Davis PJ: The effect of insulin on renal handling of sodium, potassium, calcium and phosphate in man. *J Clin Invest* 55:845, 1975.
83. DeFronzo RA, Goldberg M, Agus ZS: The effects of glucose and insulin on renal electrolyte transport. *J Clin Invest* 58:83, 1976.
84. Skott P, Hother-Nielsen O, Bruun NE, Giese J, Nielsen MD, Beck-Nielsen H, Parving HH: Effects of insulin on kidney function and sodium excretion in healthy subjects. *Diabetologia* 32:694, 1989.
85. Baum M: Insulin stimulates volume absorption in the rabbit proximal convoluted tubule. *J Clin Invest* 79:1104, 1987.
86. Rocchini AP, Katch V, Kveselis D, Moorehead C, Martin MN, Lampman R, Gregory M: Insulin and renal sodium retention in obese adolescents. *Hypertension* 14:367, 1989.
87. Dustan HP: Mechanisms of hypertension associated with obesity. *Ann Intern Med* 98:860, 1983.
88. Mujais SK, Tarazi RC, Dustan HP, Fouad FM, Bravo EL: Hypertension in obese patients: Hemodynamic and volume studies. *Hypertension* 4:84, 1982.
89. Frohlich ED: Mechanisms contributing to high blood pressure. *Ann Intern Med* 98:709, 1983.
90. Singler MH: The mechanism of natriuresis of fasting. *J Clin Invest* 55:377, 1975.
91. Amatruda JM, Richeson JF, Welle SL, Brodows RG, Lockwood DH: The safety and efficacy of a controlled low-energy ('very-low-calorie') diet in the treatment of non-insulin-dependent diabetes and obesity. *Arch Intern Med* 148:873, 1988.
92. Tuck ML, Sowers J, Dornfeld L, Kledzik G, Maxwell M: The

effect of weight reduction on blood pressure, plasma renin activity and plasma aldosterone levels in obese patients. *N Engl J Med* 304:930, 1981.
93. Landsberg L, Krieger DR: Obesity, metabolism, and the sympathetic nervous system. *Am J Hypertens* 2:1255, 1989.
94. Rowe JW, Young JB, Minaker KL, Stevens AL, Pallotta J, Landsberg L: Effect of insulin and glucose infusions on sympathetic nervous system activity in normal man. *Diabetes* 30:219, 1981.
95. Liang C-S, Doherty JU, Faillace R, Maekawa K, Arnold S, Gavras H, Hood WB Jr: Insulin infusion in conscious dogs: Effects on systemic and coronary hemodynamics, regional blood flows, and plasma catecholamines. *J Clin Invest* 69:1321, 1982.
96. DeHaven J, Sherwin R, Hendler R, Felig P: Nitrogen and sodium balance and sympathetic-nervous-system activity in obese subjects treated with a low-calorie protein or mixed diet. *N Engl J Med* 302:477, 1980.
97. Jung RT, Shetty PS, Barrand M, Callingham BA, James WPT: Role of catecholamines in hypotensive response to dieting. *Br Med J* 1:12, 1979.
98. Sowers JR, Whitfield LA, Catania RA, Stern N, Tuck ML, Dornfeld L, Maxwell M: Role of sympathetic nervous system in blood pressure maintenance in obesity. *J Clin Endocrinol Metab* 54:1181, 1982.
99. Rocchini AP, Key J, Bondie D, Chico R, Moorehead C, Katch V, Martin M: The effect of weight loss on the sensitivity of blood pressure to sodium in obese adolescents. *N Engl J Med* 321:580, 1989.
100. MacMahon SW, Wilcken DEL, MacDonald GH: The effect of weight reduction on left ventricular mass. *N Engl J Med* 314:334, 1986.
101. Krotkiewski M, Björntorp P, Sjöström L, Smith U: Impact of obesity on metabolism in men and women: Importance of regional adipose tissue distribution. *J Clin Invest* 72:1150, 1983.
102. Blair D, Habicht J-P, Sims EAH, Sylwester D, Abraham S: Evidence for an increased risk for hypertension with centrally located body fat and the effect of race and sex on the risk. *Am J Epidemiol* 119:526, 1984.
103. Maclure KM, Hayes KC, Colditz GA, Stampfer M, Speizer FE, Willett WC: Weight, diet, and the risk of symptomatic gallstones in middle-aged women. *N Engl J Med* 321:563, 1989.
104. Bennion LJ, Grundy SM: Risk factors in the development of cholelithiasis in man. *N Engl J Med* 299:1161, 1221, 1978.
105. Bennion LJ, Grundy SM: Effects of obesity and caloric intake on biliary lipid metabolism in man. *J Clin Invest* 56:996, 1975.
106. Mabee TM, Meyer P, DenBesten L, Mason EE: The mechanism of increased gallstone formation in obese human subjects. *Surgery* 79:460, 1976.
107. Shaffer EA, Small DM: Biliary lipid secretion in cholesterol gallstone disease: The effect of cholecystectomy and obesity. *J Clin Invest* 59:828, 1977.
108. Miettinen TA: Cholesterol production in obesity. *Circulation* 44:842, 1971.
109. Nestel PJ, Schreibman PH, Ahrens EH Jr: Cholesterol metabolism in human obesity. *J Clin Invest* 52:2389, 1973.
110. Salen G, Nicholan G, Shefer S, Mosbach EH: Hepatic cholesterol metabolism in patients with gallstones. *Gastroenterology* 69:676, 1975.
111. Nepokroeff CM, Lakshmanan MR, Ness GC, Dugan RE, Porter JW: Regulation of diurnal rhythm of rat liver β-hydroxy-β-methylglutaryl coenzyme A reductase activity by insulin, glucagon, cyclic AMP and hydrocortisone. *Arch Biochem Biophys* 160:387, 1974.
112. Sampliner RE, Bennett PH, Comess LJ, Rose FA, Burch TA: Gallbladder disease in Pima Indians: Demonstration of high prevalence and early onset by cholecystography. *N Engl J Med* 283:1358, 1970.
113. Grundy SM, Metzger AL, Alder RD: Mechanisms of lithogenic bile formation in American Indian women with cholesterol gallstones. *J Clin Invest* 51:3026, 1972.
114. Willett WC, Browne ML, Bain C, Lipnick RJ, Stampfer MJ, Rosner B, Colditz GA, Hennekens CH, et al: Relative weight and risk of breast cancer among premenopausal women. *Am J Epidemiol* 122:731, 1985.
115. London SJ, Colditz GA, Stampfer MJ, Willett WC, Rosner B, Speizer FE: Prospective study of relative weight, height, and risk of breast cancer. *JAMA* 262:2853, 1989.
116. Wolff GL: Body weight and cancer. *Am J Clin Nutr* 45:168, 1987.
117. Snowdon DA, Phillips RL, Choi W: Diet, obesity, and risk of fatal prostate cancer. *Am J Epidemiol* 120:244, 1984.
118. Willett WC: Implications of total energy intake for epidemiological studies of breast and large-bowel cancer. *Am J Clin Nutr* 45:354, 1987.
119. Willett WC, Stampfer MJ, Colditz GA, Rosner BA, Hennekens CH, Speizer FE: Dietary fat and the risk of breast cancer. *N Engl J Med* 316:22, 1987.
120. Kolonel LN: Fat and colon cancer: How firm is the epidemiologic evidence? *Am J Clin Nutr* 45:336, 1987.
121. Simopoulos AP: Obesity and carcinogenesis: Historical perspective. *Am J Clin Nutr* 45:271, 1987.
122. Nimrod A, Ryan KJ: Aromatization of androgens by human abdominal and breast fat tissue. *J Clin Endocrinol Metab* 40:367, 1975.
123. Edman CD, MacDonald PC: Effect of obesity on conversion of plasma androstenedione to estrone in ovulatory and anovulatory young women. *Am J Obstet Gynecol* 130:456, 1978.
124. Loncope C, Pratt JH, Schneider SH, Fineberg SE: Aromatization of androgens by muscle and adipose tissue in vivo. *J Clin Endocrinol Metab* 46:146, 1978.
125. Cleland WH, Mendelson CR, Simpson ER: Aromatase activity of membrane fractions of human adipose tissue stromal cells and adipocytes. *Endocrinology* 113:2155, 1983.
126. Schindler AE, Ebert A, Friedrich E: Conversion of androstenedione to estrone by human tissue. *J Clin Endocrinol Metab* 35:627, 1972.
127. Sitteri PK, MacDonald PC: Role of extraglandular estrogen in human endocrinology, in Greep RO (ed): *Handbook of Physiology*. Washington, D.C., American Physiological Society, 1973, p 615.
128. Klinga K, VonHolst T, Runnebaum B: Influence of severe obesity on peripheral hormone concentrations in pre-menopausal and postmenopausal women. *Eur J Obstet Gynecol Reprod Biol* 15:103, 1983.
129. Bray G: Complications of obesity. *Ann Intern Med* 103:1052, 1985.
130. Rogers J, Mitchell GW: The relation of obesity to menstrual disturbances. *N Engl J Med* 247:53, 1952.
131. Mitchell GW, Rogers J: The influence of weight reduction on amenorrhea in obese women. *N Engl J Med* 249:835, 1953.
132. Hartz AJ, Barboriak PN, Wong A, Katayama KP, Rimm AA: The association of obesity with infertility and related menstrual abnormalities in women. *Int J Obes* 3:57, 1979.
133. Glass AR, Dahms WT, Abraham G, Atkinson RL, Bray GA, Swerdloff RS: Secondary amenorrhea in obesity: Etiologic role of weight-related androgen excess. *Fertil Steril* 30:243, 1978.
134. Barbieri RL, Ryan KJ: Hyperandrogenism, insulin resistance, and acanthosis nigricans syndrome: A common endocrinopathy with distinct pathophysiologic features. *Am J Obstet Gynecol* 147:90, 1983.
135. Flier JS, Eastman RC, Minaker KL, Matteson D, Rowe JW: Acanthosis nigricans in obese women with hyperandrogenism: Characterization of an insulin-resistant state distinct from the Type A and B syndromes. *Diabetes* 34:101, 1985.
136. Barnes R, Rosenfield RL: The polycystic ovary syndrome: Pathogenesis and treatment. *Ann Intern Med* 110:386, 1989.
137. Harlass FE, Plymate SR, Fariss BL, Belts RP: Weight loss is associated with correction of gonadotropin and sex steroid

abnormalities in the obese anovulatory female. *Fertil Steril* 42:649, 1984.
138. McKenna TJ: Pathogenesis and treatment of polycystic ovary syndrome. *N Engl J Med* 318:558, 1988.
139. Annos T, Taymor ML: Ovarian pathology associated with insulin resistance and acanthosis nigricans. *Obstet Gynecol* 58:662, 1981.
140. Geffner ME, Kaplan SA, Bersch N, Golden DW, Landaw EM, Chang R: Persistance of insulin resistance in polycystic ovarian disease after inhibition of ovarian steroid secretion. *Fertil Steril* 45:327, 1986.
141. Poretsky L, Kalin MF: The gonadotropic function of insulin. *Endocr Rev* 8:132, 1987.
142. Nestler JE, Barlascini CO, Matt DW, Steingold KA, Plymate SR, Clore JM, Blackard WG: Suppression of serum insulin by diazoxide reduces serum testosterone levels in obese women with polycystic ovary syndrome. *J Clin Endocrinol Metab* 68:1027, 1989.
143. Rittmaster RS, Loriaux DL: Hirsuitism. *Ann Intern Med* 106:95, 1987.
144. Adashi EY, Hsueh HW, Yen SSC: Insulin enhancement of luteinizing hormone and follicle stimulating hormone release by cultured pituitary cells. *Endocrinology* 108:1441, 1981.
145. Peiris AN, Mueller RA, Struve MF, Smith GA, Kissebah AH: Relationship of androgenic activity to splanchnic insulin metabolism and peripheral glucose utilization in premenopausal women. *J Clin Endocrinol Metab* 64:162, 1987.
146. Amatruda JM, Harman SM, Pourmotabbed G, Lockwood DH: Depressed plasma testosterone and fractional binding of testosterone in obese males. *J Clin Endocrinol Metab* 47:268, 1978.
147. Glass AR: Endocrine aspects of obesity. *Med Clin North Am* 73:139, 1989.
148. Amatruda JM, Hochstein M, Hsu T-H, Lockwood DH: Hypothalamic and pituitary dysfunction in obese males. *Int J Obes* 6:183, 1981.
149. Crapo L: Cushing's syndrome: A review of diagnostic tests. *Metabolism* 28:955, 1979.
150. Felson DT, Anderson JJ, Naimark A, Walker AM, Meenan RF: Obesity and knee osteoarthritis: The Farmington Study. *Ann Intern Med* 109:18, 1988.
151. Kreiger N, Kelsey JL, Holford TR, O'Connor T: An epidemiologic study of hip fracture in postmenopausal women. *Am J Epidemiol* 116:141, 1982.
152. Kelsey JL, Hoffman S: Risk factors for hip fracture. *N Engl J Med* 316:404, 1987.
153. Slemenda CW, Hui SL, Longcope C, Wellman H, Johnston CC: Predictors of bone mass in premenopausal women: A prospective study of clinical data using photo absorptiometry. *Ann Intern Med* 112:96, 1990.
154. Teitelbaum SL, Halverson JD, Bates M, Wise L, Haddad WG: Abnormalities of circulating 25-OH vitamin D after jejunal bypass for obesity: Evidence of an adaptive response. *Ann Intern Med* 86:289, 1977.
155. Dalen N, Hallberd D, Lamke B: Bone mass in obese subjects. *Acta Med Scand* 197:353, 1975.
156. Bell NH, Epstein S, Greene A, Shary J, Oexmann MH, Shaw S: Evidence for alteration of the vitamin D-endocrine system in obese subjects. *J Clin Invest* 76:370, 1985.
157. Atkinson RL, Dahms WT, Bray GA, Schwartz AA: Parathyroid hormone levels in obesity: Effects of intestinal bypass surgery. *Miner Electrolyte Metab* 1:315, 1978.
158. Cohen SH, Abesamis C, Yasamura S, Aloia JF, Zanzi I, Ellis KJ: Comparative skeletal mass and radial bone mineral content in black and white women. *Metab Clin Exp* 26:171, 1977.
159. Rubinstein I, Zamel N, DuBarry L, Hoffstein V: Airflow limitation in morbidly obese, nonsmoking men. *Ann Intern Med* 112:828, 1990.
160. Kaplan J, Staats BA: Obstructive sleep apnea syndrome. *Mayo Clin Proc* 65:1087, 1990.
161. Prowse K, Allen MB: Sleep apnoea. *Br J Dis Chest* 82:329, 1989.
162. Findley LJ, Fabrizio M, Thommi M, Suratt PM: Severity of sleep apnea and automobile crashes. *N Engl J Med* 320:868, 1989.
163. Smith PL, Gold AR, Meyers DA, Haponik EF, Bleecker ER: Weight loss in mildly to moderately obese patients with obstructive sleep apnea. *Ann Intern Med* 103:850, 1985.
164. Eisenberg E, Zimlichman R, Lavie P: Plasma norepinephrine levels in patients with sleep apnea syndrome. *N Engl J Med* 322:932, 1990.
165. Hung J, Whitford EG, Parsons RW, Hillman DR: Association of sleep apnoea with myocardial infarction in men. *Lancet* 336:261, 1990.
166. Browman CP, Sampson MG, Yolles SF, Gujavarty KS, Weiler SJ, Walsleben JA, Hahn PM, Mitler MM: Obstructive sleep apnea and body weight. *Chest* 85:434, 1984.
167. Charuzi I, Ovnat A, Peiser J, Saltz H, Weitzman S, Lavie P: The effect of surgical weight reduction on sleep quality in obesity-related sleep apnea syndrome. *Surgery* 97:535, 1985.
168. Partinen M, Guilleminault G: Daytime sleepiness and vascular morbidity at seven-year follow-up in obstructive sleep apnea patients. *Chest* 97:27, 1990.
169. Gross T, Sokol RJ, King KC: Obesity in pregnancy: Risks and outcome. *Obstet Gynecol* 56:446, 1980.
170. Weisinger JR, Kempson RL, Eldridge FL, Swenson RS: The nephrotic syndrome: A complication of massive obesity. *Ann Intern Med* 81:440, 1974.
171. O'Brien TF, Stroop EM: Lower esophageal sphincter pressure (LESP) and esophageal function in obese humans. *J Clin Gastroenterol* 2:145, 1980.
172. Stunkard AJ, Sorensen TIA, Hanis C, Teasdale TW, Chakraborty R, Schull WJ, Schulsinger F: An adoption study of human obesity. *N Engl J Med* 314:193, 1986.
173. Stunkard AJ, Harris JR, Pedersen NL, McClearn GE: The body-mass index of twins who have been reared apart. *N Engl J Med* 322:1483, 1990.
174. Bouchard C: Current understanding of the etiology of obesity: Genetic and nongenetic factors. *Am J Clin Nutr* 53:1561S, 1991.
175. Price RA, Stunkard AJ, Ness R, Wadden TH, Heshka S, Kanders B, Cormillot A: Childhood onset (age <10) obesity has high familial risk. *Int J Obes* 14:185, 1989.
176. Bogardus C, Lillioja S, Ravussin E, Abbott W, Zawadzki JK, Young A, Knowler WC, Jacobowitz R, et al: Familial dependence of the resting metabolic rate. *N Engl J Med* 315:96, 1986.
177. Bouchard C, Tremblay A, Nadeau A, Despres JP, Theriault G, Boulay MR, Lortie G, Leblanc C, Fournier G: Genetic effect in resting and exercise metabolic rates. *Metabolism* 38:364, 1989.
178. Ravussin E, Lillioja S, Knowler WC, Christin L, Freymond D, Abbott WGH, Boyce V, Howard BV, et al: Reduced rate of energy expenditure as a risk factor for body-weight gain. *N Engl J Med* 318:467, 1988.
179. Wade J, Milner J, Krondl M: Evidence for a physiological regulation of food selection and nutrient intake in twins. *Am J Clin Nutr* 34:143, 1981.
180. Perusse L, Tremblay A, Leblanc C, Cloninger CR, Reich T, Rice J, Bouchard C: Familial resemblance in energy intake: Contribution of genetic and environmental factors. *Am J Clin Nutr* 47:629, 1988.
181. Sobal J, Stunkard AJ: Socioeconomic status and obesity: A review of the literature. *Psychol Bull* 105:260, 1989.
182. Dietz WH, Gortmaker SL: Do we fatten our children at the television set? Obesity and television viewing in children and adolescents. *Pediatrics* 75:807, 1985.
183. Dietz WH, Gortmaker SL: Factors within the physical environment associated with childhood obesity. *Am J Clin Nutr* 39:619, 1984.
184. Tremblay A, Plourde G, Despres J-P, Bouchard C: Impact of dietary fat content and fat oxidation on energy intake in humans. *Am J Clin Nutr* 49:799, 1989.

185. James WPT, Trayhurn P: An integrated view of the metabolic and genetic basis for obesity. *Lancet* 2:770, 1976.
186. McCarron DA, Morris CD, Henry HJ, Stanton JL: Blood pressure and nutrient in the United States. *Science* 224:1391, 1984.
187. Myers RG, Klesges RC, Eck LH, Hanson CL, Klem ML: Accuracy of self-reports of food intake in obese and normal-weight individuals: Effects of obesity on self-reports of dietary intake in adult females. *Am J Clin Nutr* 48:1248, 1988.
188. Romieu I, Willett WC, Stampfer MJ, Colditz GA, Sampson L, Rosner B, Hennekens CH, Speizer FE: Energy intake and other determinants of relative weight. *Am J Clin Nutr* 47:406, 1988.
189. Lissner L, Habicht J-P, Strupp BJ, Levitsky DA, Haas JD, Roe DA: Body composition and energy intake: Do overweight women overeat and underreport? *Am J Clin Nutr* 49:320, 1989.
190. Irsigler K, Veitl V, Sigmund A, Tschegg E, Kunz K: Calorimetric results in man: Energy output in normal and overweight subjects. *Metabolism* 28:1127, 1979.
191. Ravussin E, Burnard B, Schutz Y, Jequier E: Twenty-four-hour energy expenditure and resting metabolic rate in obese, moderately obese, and control subjects. *Am J Clin Nutr* 35:566, 1982.
192. Bessard T, Schutz Y, Jequier E: Energy expenditure and postprandial thermogenesis in obese women before and after weight loss. *Am J Clin Nutr* 38:680, 1983.
193. Ravussin E, Lillioja S, Anderson TE, Christin L, Bogardus C: Determinants of 24-hour energy expenditure in man. *J Clin Invest* 78:1568, 1986.
194. DeBoer JO, VanEs AJH, VanRaaij JMA, Hautvast JGAJ: Energy requirements and energy expenditure of lean and overweight women, measured by indirect calorimetry. *Am J Clin Nutr* 46:13, 1987.
195. Lean MEJ, James WPT: Metabolic effects of isoenergetic nutrient exchange over 24 hours in relation to obesity in women. *Int J Obes* 12:15, 1988.
196. Leibel RL, Hirsch J: Diminished energy requirements in reduced-obese patients. *Metabolism* 33:164, 1984.
197. Forbes GB, Brown MR: Energy need for weight maintenance in human beings: Effects of body size and composition. *J Am Diet Assoc* 89:499, 1989.
198. Blair D, Burkirk ER: Habitual daily energy expenditure and activity levels of lean and adult-onset and child-onset obese women. *Am J Clin Nutr* 45:540, 1987.
199. Welle S, Forbes GB, Statt M, Barnard RR, Amatruda JM: Energy expenditure under free-living conditions in normal-weight and overweight women. *Am J Clin Nutr* 55:14, 1992.
200. Prentice AM, Black AE, Coward WA, Davies HL, Goldberg GR, Murgatroyd PR, Ashford J, Sawyer M, Whitehead RG: High levels of energy expenditure in obese women. *Br Med J* 292:983, 1986.
201. Bandini LG, Schoeller DA, Dietz WH: Energy expenditure in obese and nonobese adolescents. *Pediatr Res* 27:198, 1990.
202. Roberts SV, Savage J, Coward WA, Chew B, Lucas A: Energy expenditure and intake in infants born to lean and overweight mothers. *N Engl J Med* 318:461, 1988.
203. Griffiths M, Payne PR: Energy expenditure in small children of obese and non-obese parents. *Nature* 260:698, 1976.
204. Welle SL, Amatruda JM, Forbes GB, Lockwood DH: Resting metabolic rates of obese women after rapid weight loss. *J Clin Endocrinol Metab* 59:41, 1984.
205. Weigle DA: Contribution of decreased body mass to diminished thermic effect of exercise in reduced-obese men. *Int J Obes* 12:567, 1988.
206. Elliot DL, Goldberg L, Kuehl KS, Bennett WM: Sustained depression of the resting metabolic rate after massive weight loss. *Am J Clin Nutr* 49:93, 1989.
207. Geissler CA, Miller DS, Shah M: The daily metabolic rate of the post-obese and the lean. *Am J Clin Nutr* 45:914, 1987.
208. McNeill G, Bukkens SGF, Morrison DC, Smith JS: Energy intake and energy expenditure in post-obese women and weight-matched controls. *Proc Nutr Soc* 49:1190, 1990.
209. Miller DS, Parsonage S: Resistance to slimming adaptation or illusion? Lancet 1:773, 1975.
210. Weigle DA, Sande KJ, Iverius P-H, Monsen ER, Brunzell JD: Weight loss leads to a marked decrease in nonresting energy expenditure in ambulatory human subjects. *Metabolism* 37:930, 1988.
211. Bessard T, Schutz Y, Jequier E: Energy expenditure and postprandial thermogenesis in obese women before and after weight loss. *Am J Clin Nutr* 38:680, 1983.
212. Dore C, Hesp R, Wilkins D, Garrow JS: Prediction of energy requirements of obese patients after massive weight loss. *Hum Nutr Clin Nutr* 36C:41, 1982.
213. Kaplan ML, Leveille GA: Calorigenic response in obese and nonobese women. *Am J Clin Nutr* 29:1108, 1976.
214. Shetty PS, Jung RT, James WPT, Barrand MA, Callingham BA: Postprandial thermogenesis in obesity. *Clin Sci* 60:519, 1981.
215. Segal KR, Gutin B: Thermic effects of food and exercise in lean and obese women. *Metabolism* 32:581, 1983.
216. Schutz Y, Bessard T, Jequier E: Diet-induced thermogenesis measured over a whole day in obese and nonobese women. *Am J Clin Nutr* 40:542, 1984.
217. Segal KR, Gutin B, Nyman AM, Pi-Sunyer X: Thermic effect of food at rest, during exercise, and after exercise in lean and obese men of similar body weight. *J Clin Invest* 76:1107, 1985.
218. Segal KR, Gutin B, Albu J, Pi-Sunyer X: Thermic effects of food and exercise in lean and obese men of similar lean body mass. *Am J Physiol* 252:E110, 1987.
219. Nair KS, Halliday D, Garrow JS: Thermic response to isoenergetic protein, carbohydrate or fat meals in lean and obese subjects. *Clin Sci* 65:307, 1983.
220. Felig P, Cunningham J, Levitt M, Hendler R, Nadel E: Energy expenditure in obesity in fasting and postprandial state. *Am J Physiol* 244:E45, 1983.
221. D'Alessio DA, Kavle EC, Mozzoli MA, Smalley KJ, Polansky M, Kendrick ZV, Owen LR, Bushman MC, et al: Thermic effect of food in lean and obese men. *J Clin Invest* 81:1781, 1988.
222. Ravussin E, Acheson KJ, Vernet O, Danforth E, Jequier E: Evidence that insulin resistance is responsible for the decreased thermic effect of glucose in human obesity. *J Clin Invest* 76:1268, 1985.
223. Nair KS, Webster J, Garrow JS: Effect of impaired glucose tolerance and type II diabetes on resting metabolic rate and thermic response to glucose meal in obese women. *Metabolism* 35:640, 1986.
224. Schutz Y, Golay A, Felber J-P, Jequier E: Decreased glucose-induced thermogenesis after weight loss in obese subjects: A predisposing factor for relapse of obesity? *Am J Clin Nutr* 39:380, 1984.
225. Chirico A-M, Stunkard AJ: Physical activity and human obesity. *N Engl J Med* 263:935, 1960.
226. Hutson EM, Cohen NL, Kunkel ND, Steinkamp RC, Rourke MH, Walsh HE: Measuresof body fat and related factors in normal adults. *J Am Diet Assoc* 47:179, 1965.
227. Bloom WL, Eidex MF: Inactivity as a major factor in adult obesity. *Metabolism* 16:679, 1967.
228. Stefanik PA, Heald FP, Mayer J: Caloric intake in relation to energy output of obese and non-obese adolescent boys. *Am J Clin Nutr* 7:55, 1959.
229. Bullen BA, Reed RB, Mayer J: Physical activity of obese and nonobese adolescent girls appraised by motion picture sampling. *Am J Clin Nutr* 14:211, 1964.
230. Schoeller DA, Levitsky LL, Bandini LG, Dietz WW, Walczak A: Energy expenditure and body composition in Prader-Willi syndrome. *Metabolism* 37:115, 1988.
231. Sims EAH: Experimental obesity, dietary-induced thermogenesis, and their clinical implications. *Clin Endocr Metab* 5:377, 1976.
232. Bouchard C, Tremblay A, Despres J-P, Nadeau A, Lupien PS, Theriault G, Dussault J, Moorjan S, et al: The response

to long-term overfeeding in identical twins. *N Engl J Med* 322:1477, 1990.
233. Welle S, Campbell RG: Stimulation of thermogenesis by carbohydrate overfeeding. *J Clin Invest* 71:916, 1983.
234. Norgan NG, Durnin VGA: The effect of 6 weeks of overfeeding on the body weight, body composition, and energy metabolism of young men. *Am J Clin Nutr* 33:978, 1980.
235. Ravussin E, Schutz Y, Acheson KJ, Dusmt M, Bourquin L, Jequier E: Short-term, mixed-diet overfeeding in man: No evidence for "luxuskonsumption." *Am J Physiol* 249:E470, 1985.
236. Powley RL, Keesey RE: Relationship of body weight to the lateral hypothalamic feeding syndrome. *J Comp Physiol Psychol* 70:25, 1970.
237. Hoebel BG, Teitelbaum P: Weight regulation in normal and hypothalamic hyperphagic rats. *J Comp Physiol Psychol* 61:189, 1966.
238. Sclafani A, Springer D: Dietary obesity in adult rats: Similarities to hypothalamic and human obesity syndromes. *Physiol Behav* 17:461, 1976.
239. Sclafani A, Springer D, Kluge V: Effects of quinine adulterated diets on the food intake and body weight of obese and non-obese hypothalamic hyperphagic rats. *Physiol Behav* 16:631, 1976.
240. Campbell RG, Hashim SA, VanItallie TB: Studies of food-intake regulation in man. *N Engl J Med* 285:1402, 1971.
241. Porikos KP, Booth G, VanItallie TB: Effect of covert nutritive dilution on the spontaneous food intake of obese individuals: A pilot study. *Am J Clin Nutr* 30:1638, 1977.
242. Glueck CJ, Hastings MM, Allen C, Hogg E, Baehler L, Gartside PS, Phillips D, Jones M, et al: Sucrose polyester and covert caloric dilution. *Am J Clin Nutr* 35:1352, 1982.
243. Pi-Sunyer FX: Exercise effects on calorie intake. *Ann NY Acad Sci* 499:94, 1987.
244. Roberts SB, Young VR, Fuss P, Fiatarone MA, Richard B, Rasmussen H, Wagner D, Joseph L: Energy expenditure and subsequent nutrient intakes in overfed young men. *Am J Physiol* 259:R461, 1990.
245. Mayer J: Regulation of energy intake and body weight: The glucostatic theory and the lipostatic hypothesis. *Ann NY Acad Sci* 63:15, 1955.
246. Novin D, VanderWeele DA: Visceral involvement in feeding: There is more to regulation than the hypothalamus, in Sprague JM, Epstein AN (eds): *Progress in Psychobiology and Physiological Psychology*. New York, Academic, 1977, p 193.
247. Fernstrom JD: Effects of tryptophan and the diet on brain serotonin formation and brain function, in Beers RF, Bassett EG (eds): *Nutritional Factors: Modulating Effects on Metabolic Processes*. New York, Raven, 1981, p 217.
248. Gibson CJ: Nutritional control of catecholamine synthesis, in Beers RF, Bassett EG (eds): *Nutritional Factors: Modulating Effects on Metabolic Processes*. New York, Raven, 1981, p. 217.
249. Caballero B, Finer N, Wurtman RJ: Plasma amino acids and insulin levels in obesity: Response to carbohydrate intake and tryptophan supplements. *Metabolism* 37:672, 1988.
250. Wurtman JJ: The involvement of brain serotonin in excessive carbohydrate snacking by obese carbohydrate cravers. *J Am Diet Assoc* 84:1004, 1984.
251. Geliebter AA: Effects of equicaloric loads of protein, fat, and carbohydrate on food intake in the rat and man. *Physiol Behav* 22:267, 1979.
252. Rolls BJ, Kim S, McNelis AL, Fischman MW, Foltin RW, Moran TH: Time course of effects of preloads high in fat or carbohydrate on food intake and hunger ratings in humans. *Am J Physiol* 260:R756, 1991.
253. Miller WC, Lindeman AK, Wallace J, Niederpruem M: Diet composition, energy intake, and exercise in relation to body fat in men and women. *Am J Clin Nutr* 52:426, 1990.
254. Dreon DM, Frey-Hewitt B, Ellsworth N, Williams PT, Terry RB, Wood PD: Dietary fat: Carbohydrate ratio and obesity in middle-aged men. *Am J Clin Nutr* 47:995, 1988.
255. Hill JO, Peters JC, Reed GW, Schlundt DG, Sharp T, Greene HL: Nutrient balance in humans: Effects of diet composition. *Am J Clin Nutr* 54:10, 1991.
256. Schwartz RS, Ravussin E, Massari M, O'Connell M, Robbins DC: The thermic effect of carbohydrate versus fat feeding in man. *Metabolism* 34:285, 1985.
257. Smolin LA, Grosvenor MB, Handelsman DJ, Brasel JA: Diet composition and lipoprotein lipase (EC 3.1.1.34) activity in human obesity. *Br J Nutr* 58:13, 1987.
258. Schwartz RS, Brunzell JD: Increased adipose-tissue lipoprotein-lipase activity in moderately obese men after weight reduction. *Lancet* 1:1230, 1978.
259. Schwartz RS, Brunzell JD: Increse of adipose tissue lipoprotein lipase activity with weight loss. *J Clin Invest* 67:1425, 1981.
260. Reitman JS, Kosmakos FC, Howard BV, Taskinen M-R, Kuusi T, Nikkila EA: Characterization of lipase activities in obese Pima Indians. *J Clin Invest* 70:791, 1982.
261. Ong JM, Kern PA: Effect of feeding and obesity on lipoprotein lipase activity, immunoreactive protein, and messenger RNA levels in human adipose tissue. *J Clin Invest* 84:305, 1989.
262. Eckel RH, Yost TJ: Weight reduction increases adipose tissue lipoprotein lipase responsiveness in obese women. *J Clin Invest* 80:992, 1987.
263. Kern PA, Ong JM, Saffari B, Carty J: The effects of weight loss on the activity and expression of adipose tissue lipoprotein lipase in very obese humans. *N Engl J Med* 322:1053, 1990.
264. Taskinen M-R, Nikkila EA: Basal and postprandial lipoprotein lipase activity in adipose tissue during caloric restriction and refeeding. *Metabolism* 36:625, 1987.
265. Rebuffe-Scrive M, Basdevant A, Guy-Grand B: Nutritional induction of adipose tissue lipoprotein lipase in obese subjects. *Am J Clin Nutr* 37:974, 1983.
266. Woods SC, Lotter EC, McKay LD, Porte D Jr: Chronic intracerebroventricular infusion of insulin reduces food intake and body weight of baboons. *Nature* 282:503, 1979.
267. Ciaraldi T, Robbins R, Leidy JW, Thamm P, Berhanu P: Insulin receptors on cultured hypothalamic cells: Functional and structural differences from receptors on peripheral target cells. *Endocrinology* 116:2179, 1985.
268. Rodin J, Wack J, Ferrannini E, DeFronzo RA: Effect of insulin and glucose on feeding behavior. *Metabolism* 34:826, 1985.
269. Alger SA, Schwalberg MD, Bigaouette JM, Michalek AV, Howard LJ: Effect of a tricyclic antidepressant and opiate antagonist on binge-eating behavior in normoweight bulimic and obese, binge-eating subjects. *Am J Clin Nutr* 53:865, 1991.
270. Atkinson RL: Opioid regulation of food intake and body weight in humans. *Fed Proc* 46:178, 1987.
271. Fantino M, Hosotte J, Apfelbaum M: An opioid antagonist, naltrexone, reduces preference for sucrose in humans. *Am J Physiol* 251:R91, 1986.
272. Ritter MM, Sönnichsen AC, Mohrle W, Richter WO, Schwandt P: β-endorphin plasma levels and their dependence on gender during an enteral glucose load in lean subjects as well as in obese patients before and after weight reduction. *Int J Obes* 15:421, 1991.
273. Rodin J, Schank D, Striegel-Moore R: Psychological features of obesity. *Med Clin North Am* 73:47, 1989.
274. Drewnowiski A, Brunzell JD, Sande K, Iverisu PH, Greenwood MRC: Sweet tooth reconsidered: Taste responsiveness in human obesity. *Physiol Behav* 35:617, 1985.
275. Schachter S: Obesity and eating. *Science* 161:751, 1968.
276. Leon GR, Roth L: Obesity: Psychological causes, correlations, and speculations. *Psychol Bull* 84:117, 1977.
277. Loro A, Orleans C: Binge eating in obesity: Preliminary findings and guidelines for behavioral analysis and treatment. *Addict Behav* 6:155, 1981.
278. Werner SC: Hypothyroidism: Introduction, in Werner SC,

Ingbar SH (eds): *The Thyroid,* 3d ed. New York, Harper & Row, 1971, p 715.

279. Burman KD, Latham KR, Djuh Y-Y, Smallridge RC, Tseng Y-CL, Lukes YG, Maunder R, Wartofsky L: Solubilized nuclear thyroid hormone receptors in circulating human mononuclear cells. *J Clin Endocrinol Metab* 51:106, 1980.
280. Bray GA: Obesity—a disease of nutrient or energy balance? *Nutr Rev* 45:33, 1987.
281. Rivera MP, Svec F: Is cortisol involved in upper-body obesity? *Med Hypotheses* 30:95, 1989.
282. Clearly MP: Antiobesity effect of dehydroepiandrosterone in the Zucker rat, in Lardy H, Stratman F (eds): *Hormones, Thermogenesis, and Obesity.* New York, Elsevier, 1989, p 365.
283. MacEwen EG, Kurzman ID, Haffa ALM: Antiobesity and hypocholesterolemic activity of dehydroepiandrosterone (DHEA) in the dog, in Lardy H, Stratman F (eds): *Hormones, Thermogenesis, and Obesity.* New York, Elsevier, 1989, p 399.
284. Lopez-S A, Krehl WA: A possible interrelation between glucose-6-phosphate dehydrogenase and dehydroepiandrosterone in obesity. *Lancet* 2:485, 1967.
285. Barrett-Connor E, Khaw K-T, Yen SSC: A prospective study of dehydroepiandrosterone sulfate, mortality, and cardiovascular disease. *N Engl J Med* 315:1519, 1986.
286. Kurtz BR, Givens JR, Komindr S, Stevens MD, Karas JG, Bittle JB, Judge D, Kitabchi AE: Maintenance of normal circulating levels of Δ^4-androstenedione and dehydroepiandrosterone in simple obesity despite increased metabolic clearance rates: Evidence for a servo-control mechanism. *J Clin Endocrinol Metab* 64:1261, 1987.
287. Usiskin KS, Butterworth S, Clore JN, Arad Y, Ginsberg HN, Blackard WG, Nestler JE: Lack of effect of dehydroepiandrosterone in obese men. *Int J Obes* 14:457, 1990.
288. Knehans AW, Romsos DE: Reduced norepinephrine turnover in brown adipose tissue of ob/ob mice. *Am J Physiol* 242:E253, 1982.
289. Young JB, Landsberg L: Diminished sympathetic nervous system activity in genetically obese (ob/ob) mouse. *Am J Physiol* 245:E148, 1983.
290. Peterson HR, Rothschild M, Weinberg CR, Fell RD, McLeish KR, Pfeifer MA: Body fat and the activity of the autonomic nervous system. *N Engl J Med* 318:1077, 1988.
291. Jung RT, Shetty PS, James WPT, Barrand MA, Callingham BA: Plasma catecholamines and autonomic responsiveness in obesity. *Int J Obes* 6:131, 1982.
292. Welle SL, Campbell RG: Normal thermic effect of glucose in obese women. *Am J Clin Nutr* 37:87, 1983.
293. Bray GA, Gallagher TF Jr: Manifestations of hypothalamic obesity in man: A comprehensive investigation of eight patients and a review of the literature. *Medicine (Baltimore)* 54:301, 1975.
294. Bray GA: Syndromes of hypothalamic obesity in man. *Pediatr Ann* 13:525, 1984.
295. Green JS, Parfrey PS, Harnett JD, Farid NR, Cramer BC, Johnson G, Heath O, McManamon PJ, et al: The cardinal manifestations of Bardet-Biedl syndrome, a form of Laurence-Moon-Biedl syndrome. *N Engl J Med* 321:1002, 1989.
296. Goecke T, Majewski F, Kauther KD, Sterzel U: Mental retardation, hypotonia, obesity, ocular, facial, dental, and limb abnormalities (Cohen Syndrome). *Eur J Pediatr* 138:338, 1982.
297. Dietz WH, Gross WL, Kirkpatrick JA: Blount disease (tibia vara): Another skeletal disorder associated with childhood obesity. *J Pediatr* 101:735, 1982.
298. Cassidy SB, Ledbetter DH: Prader-Willi Syndrome. *Neurol Clin* 7:37, 1989.
299. Aughton DJ, Cassidy SB: Physical features of Prader-Willi syndrome in neonates. *Am J Dis Child* 144:1251, 1990.
300. Ledbetter DH, Greenberg F, Holm VA, Cassidy SB: Conference report: Second annual Prader-Willi syndrome scientific conference. *Am J Med Genet* 28:779, 1987.
301. Nicholls RD, Knoll JHM, Butler MG, Karam S, Lalande M: Genetic imprinting suggested by maternal heterodisomy in non-deletion Prader-Willi syndrome. *Nature* 342:281, 1989.
302. Dech B, Budow L: The use of fluoxetine in an adolescent with Prader-Willi syndrome. *J Am Acad Child Adolesc Psychiatry* 30:298, 1991.
303. Selikowitz M, Sunman J, Pendergast A, Wright S: Fenfluramine in Prader-Willi syndrome: A double blind, placebo controlled trial. *Arch Dis Child* 65:112, 1990.
304. Stunkard A, McLaren-Hume H: The results of treatment for obesity: A review of the literature and report of a series. *Arch Intern Med* 103:79, 1959.
305. AMA Council on Scientific Affairs; Treatment of obesity in adults. *Conn Med* 53:21, 1989.
306. Position of the American Dietetic Association: Optimal weight as a health promotion strategy: ADA Reports. *J Am Diet Assoc* 89:1814, 1989.
307. *Obese and Overweight Adults in the United States.* DHHS Publication 83-1680 (Vital and Health Statistics: Series II, 230). Washington D.C.: U.S. Government Printing Office, 1983.
308. Gortmaker SL, Dietz WH, Sobol AM, Wehler CA: Increasing pediatric obesity in the United States. *Am J Dis Child* 141:535, 1987.
309. Simopoulos AP: Obesity and body weight standards. *Annu Rev Public Health* 7:481, 1986.
310. Williamson DF, Kahn HS, Remington PL, Anda RF: The 10-year incidence of overweight and major weight gain in U.S. adults. *Arch Intern Med* 150:665, 1990.
311. National Institutes of Health Consensus Development Conference Statement: Health implications of obesity. *Ann Intern Med* 103:1073, 1985.
312. Health and Public Policy Committee, American College of Physicians: Eating disorders: Anorexia nervosa and bulimia. *Ann Intern Med* 105:790, 1986.
313. Shapiro LR, Crawford PB, Clark MJ, Pearson DL, Raz J, Huenemann RL: Obesity prognosis: A longitudinal study of children from the age of 6 months to 9 years. *Am J Public Health* 74:968, 1984.
314. Sorensen TIA, Sonne-Holm S: Risk in childhood of development of severe adult obesity: Retrospective population-based care-cohort study. *Am J Epidemiol* 127:104, 1988.
315. Stark O, Atkins E, Wolff OH, Douglas JWB: Longitudinal study of obesity in the National Survey of Health and Development. *Br Med J* 283:13, 1981.
316. Garn SM, Clark DC: Trends in fatness and the origins of obesity. *Pediatrics* 57:433, 1976.
317. Stunkard AJ, Foch TT, Hrubel Z: A twin study of human obesity. *JAMA* 256:51, 1986.
318. Epstein LH, Wing RR: Behavioral treatment of childhood obesity. *Psychol Bull* 101:331, 1987.
319. Epstein LH, Cluss PA: Behavioral genetics of childhood obesity. *Behav Ther* 17:324, 1986.
320. Epstein LH, Valoski A, Wing RR, McCurley J: Ten-year follow-up of behavioral, family-based treatment for obese children. *JAMA* 264:2519, 1990.
321. Stunkard AJ, Berkowitz RI: Treatment of obesity in children. *JAMA* 264:2550, 1990.
322. Stunkard AJ: Some perspectives on human obesity: Treatment. *Bull NY Acad Med* 64:924, 1988.
323. Black DR, Threfall WE: Partner weight status and subject weight loss: Implications for cost-effective programs and public health. *Addict Behav* 14:279, 1989.
324. Brownell KD, Stunkard AJ: Couples training pharmacotherapy and behavior in the treatment of obesity. *Arch Gen Psychiatry* 38:1224, 1981.
325. Volkmar FR, Stunkard AJ, Woolston J, Bailey RA: High attrition rates in commercial weight reduction programs. *Arch Intern Med* 141:426, 1981.
326. Brownell KD: Public health approaches to obesity and its management. *Annu Rev Public Health* 7:521, 1986.
327. Epstein LH, Wing RR: Aerobic exercise and weight. *Addict Behav* 5:371, 1980.

328. Harris SS, Caspersen CJ, DeFriese GH, Estes FH: Physical activity counseling for healthy adults as a primary preventive intervention in the clinical setting: Report for the US Preventive Services Task Force. *JAMA* 262:2094, 1989.
329. Wanger HA, Bell GJ: The interactions of intensity, frequency and duration of exercise training in altering cardiovascular fitness. *Sports Med* 3:346, 1986.
330. Sallis JF, Haskell WL, Fortmann SP, Vraiult KM, Taylor CB, Solomon DS: Predictors of adaption and maintenance of physical activity in a community sample. *Prev Med* 15:331, 1986.
331. Krotkiewski M, Mandroukas K, Sjöström L, Sullivan L, Wetterqvist H, Björntorp P: Effects of long-term physical training on body fat, metabolism, and blood pressure in obesity. *Metabolism* 28:650, 1979.
332. Hagan RD, Upton SJ, Wong L, Whittam J: The effects of aerobic conditioning and/or caloric restriction in overweight men and women. *Med Sci Sports Exerc* 18:87, 1986.
333. Leon AS, Conrad J, Hunninghake DB, Serfass R: Effects of a vigorous walking program on body composition, and carbohydrate and lipid metabolism of obese young men. *Am J Clin Nutr* 32:1776, 1979.
334. Woo R, Garrow JS, Pi-Sunyer FX: Effect of exercise on spontaneous calorie intake in obesity. *Am J Clin Nutr* 36:470, 1982.
335. Woo R, Pi-Sunyer FX: Effect of increased physical activity on voluntary intake in lean women. *Metabolism* 34:836, 1985.
336. Phinney SF, LaGrange BM, O'Connell M, Danforth E: Effects of aerobic exercise on energy expenditure and nitrogen balance during very low calorie dieting. *Metabolism* 37:758, 1988.
337. VanDale D, Saris WHM, Schoffelen PFM, TenHoor F: Does exercise give an additional effect in weight reduction regimens? *Int J Obes* 11:367, 1987.
338. Lennon D, Nagle F, Stratman F, Shrago E, Dennis S: Diet and exercise training effects on resting metabolic rate. *Int J Obes* 9:39, 1985.
339. Pavlou KN, Whatley JE, Jannace PW, DiBartolomeo JJ, Burrows BA, Duthie EAM, Lerman RH: Physical activity as a supplement to a weight-loss dietary regimen. *Am J Clin Nutr* 49:1110, 1989.
340. Ballor DL, Katch VL, Becque MD, Marks CR: Resistance weight training during caloric restriction enhances lean body weight maintenance. *Am J Clin Nutr* 47:19, 1988.
341. Pavlou KN, Krey S, Steffee WP: Exercise as an adjunct to weight loss and maintenance in moderately obese subjects. *Am J Clin Nutr* 49:1115, 1989.
342. Henson LC, Poole DC, Donahoe CP, Heber D: Effects of exercise training on resting energy expenditure during caloric restriction. *Am J Clin Nutr* 46:893, 1987.
343. Freedman-Akabas S, Colt E, Kissileff HR, Pi-Sunyer FX: Lack of sustained increase in VO_2 following exercise in fit and unfit subjects. *Am J Clin Nutr* 41:545, 1985.
344. Bielinski R, Schutz Y, Jequier E: Energy metabolism during the postexercise recovery in man. *Am J Clin Nutr* 42:69, 1985.
345. Segal KR, Presta E, Gutin B: Thermic effect of food during graded exercise in normal weight and obese men. *Am J Clin Nutr* 40:995, 1984.
346. Dallosso HM, James WPT: Whole-body calorimetry studies in adult men. *Br J Nutr* 52:65, 1984.
347. Brehm BA, Gutlin B: Recovery energy expenditure for steady state exercise in runners and nonexercisers. *Med Sci Sports Exerc* 18:205, 1986.
348. Segal KR, Pi-Sunyer FX: Exercise and obesity. *Med Clin North Am* 73:217, 1989.
349. Welle S: Metabolic responses to a meal during rest and low-intensity exercise. *Am J Clin Nutr* 40:990, 1984.
350. Brownell KD, Kramer FM: Behavioral management of obesity. *Med Clin North Am* 73:185, 1989.
351. Amatruda JM: Very low energy diets for the treatment of simple and complicated obesity. *Endocrinologist* 1:171, 1991.
352. Apfelbaum M: The effects of very restrictive high protein diets. *Clin Endocr Metab* 5:417, 1976.
353. Bistrian BR, Blackburn GL, Flatt JP, Sizer J, Scrimshaw NS, Sherman M: Nitrogen metabolism and insulin requirements in obese diabetic adults on a protein-sparing modified fast. *Diabetes* 25:494, 1976.
354. Linn R, Stuart SL: *The Last Chance Diet*. Secaucus, NJ, Lyle Stuart, 1976.
355. Isner JM, Sours HH, Paris AL, Ferraus VJ: Sudden unexpected death in avid dieters using the liquid-protein-modified-fast diet: Observations in 17 patients and the role of the prolonged QT interval. *Circulation* 60:1401, 1979.
356. Lantigua RA, Amatruda JM, Biddle TL, Forbes GB, Lockwood DH: Cardiac arrhythmias associated with a liquid protein diet for the treatment of obesity. *N Engl J Med* 303:735, 1980.
357. Amatruda JM, Biddle TL, Patton ML, Lockwood DH: Vigorous supplementation of a hypocaloric diet prevents cardiac arrhythmias and mineral depletion. *Am J Med* 74:1016, 1983.
358. Amatruda JM, Brodows RG, Lockwood DH: Very low calorie diets: Efficacy, cardiac arrhythmias, nitrogen sparing mineral depletion, and hormone and substrate levels. *J Obes Weight Regul* 3:3, 1984.
359. Henry RR, Schaeffer L, Olefsky JM: Glycemic effects of intensive caloric restriction and isocaloric feeding in noninsulin-dependent diabetes mellitus. *J Clin Endocrinol Metab* 61:917, 1985.
360. Wadden TA, Stunkard AJ: Controlled trial of very low calorie diet, behavioral therapy, and their combination in the treatment of obesity. *J Consult Clin Psychol* 54:482, 1986.
361. Nagulesparan M, Savage PJ, Bennion LJ, Unger RH, Bennett PH: Diminished effect of caloric restriction on control of hyperglycemia with increasing known duration of type II diabetes mellitus. *J Clin Endocrinol Metab* 53:560, 1981.
362. Lockwood DH, Amatruda JM: Very low calorie diets in the management of obesity. *Annu Rev Med* 35:373, 1984.
363. Liddle RA, Goldstein RB, Saxton J: Gallstone formation during weight-reduction dieting. *Arch Intern Med* 149:1750, 1989.
364. Broomfield PH, Chopra R, Sheinbaum RC, Bonorris GG, Silverman A, Schoenfield LJ, Marks JW: Effects of ursodeoxycholic acid and aspirin on the formation of lithogenic bile and gallstones during loss of weight. *N Engl J Med* 319:1567, 1988.
365. Mok HY, Von Bergmann K, Crouse JR, Grundy SM: Biliary lipid metabolism in obesity: Effects of bile acid feeding before and during weight reduction. *Gastroenterology* 76:556, 1978.
366. Roslyn JJ, Pitt HA, Mann LL, Ament ME, DenBesten L: Gallbladder disease in patients on long term parenteral nutrition. *Gastroenterology* 84:148, 1983.
367. Wattchow DA, Hall JC, Whiting MJ, Bradley B, Iannos J, Watts JM: Prevalence and treatment of gallstones after gastric bypass surgery for morbid obesity. *Br Med J* 286:763, 1983.
368. Hocking MP, Duerson MC, O'Leary P, Woodward ER: Jejunoileal bypass for morbid obesity: Late follow-up in 100 cases. *N Engl J Med* 308:995, 1983.
369. Carey MC, Cahalane J: Whither biliary sludge? *Gastroenterology* 95:508, 1988.
370. Gallinger S, Tayler RD, Harvey PR, Petrunka CN, Strasberg SM: Effect of mucous glycoprotein on nucleation time of human bile. *Gastroenterology* 89:648, 1985.
371. Lee SP, LaMont JT, Carey MC: Role of gall bladder mucus hypersecretion in the evolution of cholesterol gallstones: Studies in the prairie dog. *J Clin Invest* 67:1712, 1981.
372. Lee SP, Carey MC, LaMont JT: Aspirin prevention of cholesterol gallstone formation in prairie dogs. *Science* 211:1429, 1981.
373. Forbes GB: Lean body mass-body fat interrelationships in humans. *Nutr Rev* 45:225, 1987.
374. Wadden TA, Foster GD, Leitzia KA, Mullen JL: Long-term

effects of dieting on resting metabolic rate in obese outpatients. *JAMA* 264:707, 1990.
375. Steen SN, Oppliger RA, Brownell KD: Metabolic effects of repeated weight loss and regain in adolescent wrestlers. *JAMA* 260:47, 1988.
376. vanDale D, Saris WHM: Repetitive weight loss and weight regain: Effects on weight reduction, resting metabolic rate, and lipolytic activity before and after exercise and/or diet treatment. *Am J Clin Nutr* 49:409, 1989.
377. Gray DS, Fisler JS, Bray GA: Effects of repeated weight loss and regain on body composition in obese rats. *Am J Clin Nutr* 47:393, 1988.
378. Bouchard C: Is weight fluctuation a risk factor? *N Engl J Med* 324:1887, 1991.
379. Lissner L, Odell PM, D'Agostino RB, Stokes J, Kreger BE, Belanger A, Brownell KD: Variability of body weight and health outcomes in the Framingham population. *N Engl J Med* 324:1839, 1991.
380. Mirkin GB, Shore RN: The Beverly Hills diet. *JAMA* 246:2235, 1981.
381. Scoville BA: Review of amphetamine-like drugs by the Food and Drug Administration: Clinical data and value judgments, in Bray GA (ed): *Obesity in Perspective*. DHEW (NIH) 75-708. Bethesda, MD, National Institutes of Health, 1975, p 441.
382. Weintraub M, Bray GA: Drug treatment of obesity. *Med Clin North Am* 73:237, 1989.
383. Weintraub M, Hasday JD, Mushlin AI, Lockwood DH: A double-blind clinical trial in weight control: Use of fenfluramine and phentermine alone and in combination. *Arch Intern Med* 144:1143, 1984.
384. Guy-grand B, Apfelbaum M, Crepaldi G, Gries A, Lefebvre P, Turner P: International trial of long-term dexfenfluramine in obesity. *Lancet* 2:1142, 1989.
385. Thurlby PL, Ellis RDM: Differences between the effects of noradrenaline and the β-adrenoceptor agonist BRL 28410 in brown adipose tissue and hind limb of the anaesthetized rat. *Can J Physiol Pharmacol* 64:1111, 1986.
386. Cunningham S, Leslie P, Hopwood D, Illingworth P, Jung RT, Nicholls DG, Peden N, Rafael J, et al: The characterization and energetic potential of brown adipose tissue in man. *Clin Sci* 69:343, 1985.
387. Connacher AA, Jung RT, Mitchell PEG: Weight loss in obese subjects on a restricted diet given BRL 26830A, a new atypical β adrenoceptor agonist. *Br Med J* 296:1217, 1988.
388. Greenway FL, Bray GA: Human chorionic gonadotropin (HCG) in the treatment of obesity. *West J Med* 127:461, 1977.
389. Samad AHB, Willing TST, Alberti KGMM, Taylor R: Effects of BAYm 1099, new α-glucosidse inhibitor, on acute metabolic responses and metabolic control in NIDDM over 1 mo. *Diabetes Care* 11:337, 1988.
390. Glueck CJ, Jandacek R, Hogg E, Allen C, Baehler L, Tewksbury M: Sucrose polyester: Substitution for dietary fats in hypocaloric diets in the treatment of familial hypercholesterolemia. *Am J Clin Nutr* 37:347, 1983.
391. Mellies MJ, Vitale C, Jandacek RJ, Lamkin GE, Clueck CJ: The substitution of sucrose polyester for dietary fat in obese, hypercholesterolemic outpatients. *Am J Clin Nutr* 41:1, 1985.
392. Solum TT, Ryttig KR, Solum E, Larsen S: The influence of a high-fibre diet on body weight, serum lipids and blood pressure in slightly overweight persons. *Int J Obes* 11(Suppl 1):67, 1987.
393. Clemmons DR, Snyder DK, Williams R, Underwood LE: Growth hormone administration conserves lean body mass during dietary restriction in obese subjects. *J Clin Endocrinol Metab* 64:878, 1987.
394. Snyder DK, Clemmons DR, Underwood LE: Treatment of obese, diet-restricted subjects with growth hormone for 11 weeks: Effects on anabolism, lipolysis, and body composition. *J Clin Endocrinol Metab* 67:54, 1988.
395. Hogan S, Fleury A, Hadvary P, Lengsfeld H, Meier MK, Triscari J, Sullivan AC: Studies on the antiobesity activity of tetrahydrolipstatin, a potent and selective inhibitor of pancreatic lipase. *Int J Obes* 11(Suppl 3):35, 1987.
396. Dourish CT, Rycroft W, Iversen SD: Postponement of satiety by blockade of brain cholecystokinin (CCK-B) receptors. *Science* 245:1509, 1989.
397. Ferguson JM, Feighner JP: Fluoxetine-induced weight loss in overweight non-depressed humans. *Int J Obes* 11(Suppl 3):163, 1987.
398. Levine LR, Enas GG, Thompson WL, Byyny RL, Dauer AD, Kirby RW, Kreindler TG, Levy B, et al: Use of fluoxetine, a selective serotonin-uptake inhibitor, in the treatment of obesity: A dose-response study. *Int J Obes* 13:635, 1989.
399. Marcus MD, Wing RR, Ewing L, Kern E, McDermott M, Gooding W: A double-blind, placebo-controlled trial of fluoxetine plus behavior modification in the treatment of obese binge-eaters and non-binge-eaters. *Am J Psychiatry* 147: 876, 1990.
400. VanItallie TB: "Morbid" obesity: A hazardous disorder that resists conservative treatment. *Am J Clin Nutr* 33:358, 1980.
401. Drenick EJ, Gurunanjappa SB, Seltzer F, Johnson GA: Excessive mortality and causes of death in morbidly obese men. *JAMA* 243:443, 1980.
402. VanItallie TB, Bray GA, Connor WE, Faloon WW, Kral JG, Mason EE, Stunkard AJ: Guidelines for surgery for morbid obesity. *Am J Clin Nutr* 42:904, 1985.
403. Kral JG: Malabsorptive procedures in surgical treatment of morbid obesity. *Gastroenterol Clin North Am* 16:293, 1987.
404. Linner JH: Overview of surgical techniques for the treatment of morbid obesity. *Gastroenterol Clin North Am* 16:253, 1987.
405. Brolin RE: Results of obesity surgery. *Gastroenterol Clin North Am* 16:317, 1987.
406. Zollinger RW, Coccia MR, Zollinger RW II: Critical analysis of jejunoileal bypass. *Am J Surg* 146:626, 1983.
407. Hocking MP, Duerson MC, O'Leary JP, Woodward ER: Jejunoileal bypass for morbid obesity. *N Engl J Med* 308:995, 1983.
408. Parfitt AM, Chir B, Miller MJ, Frame B, Villaneuva AR, Rao DS, Oliver I, Thomson DL: Metabolic bone disease after intestinal bypass for treatment of obesity. *Ann Intern Med* 89:193, 1978.
409. Chadwick VS, Modha K, Dowling RH: Mechanism for hyperoxaluria in patients with ileal dysfunction. *N Engl J Med* 289:172, 1973.
410. Willbanks OL: Long-term results of silicone elastomer ring vertical gastroplasty for the treatment of morbid obesity. *Surgery* 101:606, 1986.
411. Eckhout GV, Willbanks OL, Moore JT: Vertical ring gastroplasty for morbid obesity. Five year experience with 1,463 patients. *Am J Surg* 152:713, 1986.
412. Makarewicz PA, Freeman JB, Burchett H, Brazeau P: Vertical banded gastroplasty: Assessment of efficacy. *Surgery* 98:700, 1985.
413. Ravich M: Presidential address, American Surgical Association. *Ann Surg* 200:231, 1984.
414. Thompson WR, Amaral JF, Caldwell MD, Martin HF, Randall HT: Complications and weight loss in 150 consecutive gastric exclusion patients. *Am J Surg* 146:602, 1983.
415. Flickinger EG, Sinar DR, Swanson M: Gastric bypass. *Gastroenterol Clin North Am* 16:283, 1987.
416. Benotti PN, Hollingshead J, Mascioli EA, Bothe A Jr, Bistrian BR, Blackburn FL: Gastric restrictive operations for morbid obesity. *Am J Surg* 157:150, 1989.
417. Sugerman JH, Starkey JV, Birkenhauer R: A randomized prospective trial of gastric bypass versus vertical banded gastroplasty for morbid obesity and their effects on sweets versus non-sweets eaters. *Ann Surg* 205:613, 1987.
418. Sugerman HJ, Londrey GL, Kellum JM, Wolf L, Liszka T, Engle KM, Birkenhauer R, Starkey JV: Weight loss with

vertical banded gastroplasty and roux-Y gastric bypass for morbid obesity with selective versus random assignment. *Am J Surg* 157:93, 1989.

419. Linner JH: Treatment of morbid obesity. *Arch Surg* 117: 697, 1982.
420. Fobi MAL, Fleming AW: Vertical banded gastroplasty vs gastric bypass in the treatment of obesity. *J Natl Med Assoc* 78:1091, 1986.
421. Pasulka PS, Bistrian BR, Benotti PN, Blackburn GL: The risks of surgery in obese patients. *Ann Intern Med* 104:540, 1986.
422. Abarbanel JM, Berginer VM, Osimani A, Solomon H, Charuzi I: Neurologic complications after gastric restriction surgery for morbid obesity. *Neurology* 37:196, 1987.
423. Batson E: Diagnostic and therapeutic technology assessment (DATTA). *JAMA* 261:1491, 1989.
424. Saltzstein EC, Gutmann MC: Gastric bypass for morbid obesity. *Arch Surg* 115:21, 1980.
425. Stunkard AJ, Stinnett JL, Smoller JW: Psychological and social aspects of the surgical treatment of obesity. *Am J Psychiatry* 143:417, 1986.
426. Solow C, Silberfarb PM, Swift K: Psychosocial effects of intestinal bypass surgery for severe obesity. *N Engl J Med* 290:300, 1974.
427. Halmi KA, Stunkard AJ, Mason EE: Emotional responses to weight reduction by three methods: gastric bypass, jejunoileal bypass, diet. *Am J Clin Nutr* 33:446, 1980.

C H A P T E R 22

Disorders of Lipid Metabolism*

D. Roger Illingworth

P. Barton Duell

William E. Connor

Hyperlipidemia warrants special concern and interest because it is found with exceptional frequency in the American population. Ten percent of children and at least 25 percent of adults in the United States, Canada, and western Europe have lipid values that put them at increased risk of developing premature cardiovascular disease. Although most affected individuals have hyperlipidemia secondary to dietary factors or other metabolic disorders, some have genetic causes of hyperlipidemia. These are estimated to be among the most common hereditary disorders seen in adult medical practice. Thus, asymptomatic hyperlipidemia may be detected both in so-called healthy people and in patients seeking medical attention for a variety of other problems. Hyperlipidemia is especially noted today because plasma cholesterol and triglyceride concentrations are so frequently determined in the course of routine chemical screening.

Hyperlipidemia involves an elevation of plasma lipid levels, cholesterol, and triglyceride, singly or in combination. Because these lipids are transported in the plasma as components of lipoprotein molecules, hyperlipidemia implies an associated lipoprotein abnormality as well.

There are four important clinical reasons for concern about the correct diagnosis and treatment of hyperlipidemia. The first reason is the strong causative relation between hyperlipidemia and atherosclerotic vascular disease: coronary heart disease, stroke, visceral atherosclerosis, and peripheral vascular disease. The second is the direct correlation of hyperlipidemia with the occurrence in the skin and tendons of xanthomas, which should be regarded as external manifestations of lipid deposits in tissues that are analogous to similar deposits occurring internally in the arteries. Xanthomas present cosmetic problems and because of their unique characteristics may be of value in the differential diagnosis of the exact type of hyperlipidemia. Both atherosclerosis and xanthomas will be the subject of more extensive discussion in subsequent sections of this chapter.

The third reason relates to the diagnosis of obscure abdominal distress and even acute abdominal pain. In some patients, the episode of abdominal pain may progress to acute pancreatitis. Many hyperlipidemic patients with abdominal pain on the basis of a lipemic state have even been surgically explored for the presence of an acute abdomen. Thus, hyperlipidemia should be considered as a possible cause of both acute pancreatitis and obscure abdominal pain.

The fourth reason for clinical concern is that the occurrence of hyperlipidemia may point to another disease to which the hyperlipidemia is secondary. In many cases the primary condition may be obvious, but in others the hyperlipidemia may alert one to the possibility of hypothyroidism, for example.

THE PLASMA LIPOPROTEINS

The plasma of all vertebrates, including human beings, contains lipids which are transported as soluble complexes called *lipoproteins*. Individually such lipids have very limited solubility in aqueous environments, whereas as lipoprotein complexes they are readily held in solution. It is the lipid moieties with hydrated densities of 0.8 to 0.9 g/ml which give lipoproteins a unique density range that is lighter than that of the other plasma proteins. Notable landmarks in the separation of lipoproteins have been the development of ultracentrifugal flotation by Gofman and coworkers[1] and the development of electrophoretic separation techniques by Lees and Hatch.[2]

* This work was supported by Public Health Service Research Grant HL28399, National Heart, Lung and Blood Institute, by the General Clinical Research Centers Program (RR334) of the Division of Research, Resources, National Institutes of Health, and by the Clinical Nutrition Research Unit (P30 DK 40566).

Lipoprotein Classification

The separation of different lipoproteins has been achieved by means of two principal techniques—electrophoresis and ultracentrifugation in salt solutions—and their classification is most commonly expressed in operational terms. On the basis of ultracentrifugal separation of plasma, four lipoprotein classes are recognized: chylomicrons, very low density lipoproteins (VLDL), low-density lipoproteins (LDL), and high-density lipoproteins (HDL). The relation between this ultracentrifugal classification and the size and electrophoretic mobility of lipoproteins is shown in Fig. 22-1. Further refinements in these density classes have been made and are a topic of considerable current interest. Low-density lipoproteins may be separated into two or more fractions: LDL_1 [also commonly referred to as intermediate-density lipoprotein, IDL; density (*d*) 1.006 to 1.019] and LDL_2 (*d* 1.019 to 1.063). High-density lipoproteins may be similarly divided into HDL_2 (*d* 1.063 to 1.125) and HDL_3 (*d* 1.125 to 1.21). A fifth lipoprotein, lipoprotein (a), is present in plasma and has a hydrated density between 1.06 and 1.08 g/ml.[3] Lp(a) is usually a minor constituent of lipoproteins isolated by ultracentrifugation. Lp(a) consists of an LDL particle to which an additional protein termed apo (a) is covalently bound.[3]

In addition to this operational classification, Alaupovic has proposed a concept of lipoprotein families, each of which is distinguished by its apoprotein moiety.[4] These moieties are designated alphabetically as apo-A, apo-B, apo-C, apo-D, and apo-E. The apo-A family in turn contains three separate apoproteins designated A-I, A-II, and A-IV, and the C family also has three: C-I, C-II, and C-III. The distribution of these apoproteins within the four operational density classes is shown in Table 22-1. It is evident that when lipoproteins are classified according to their density, each class represents a polydisperse system of particles which differ in size, hydrated density, and constituent apoproteins. In contrast, the lipoprotein family classification[5,6] defines five families, each of which consists of a polydisperse system of lipid-apoprotein associations characterized by the presence of a single distinct apoprotein or its constituent polypeptides. We shall rely on the operational definition in this review.

FIGURE 22-1 Diagrammatic representation of the major classes and properties of human lipoproteins separated by electrophoresis and ultracentrifugation.

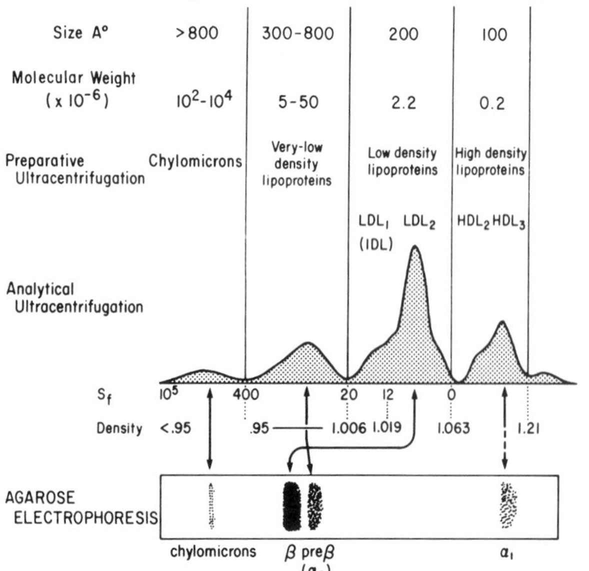

Lipoprotein Composition

Chylomicrons

Chylomicrons are the largest of the lipoprotein particles whose primary role in the transport of exogenously derived fat from the intestine is well defined. Their size varies from 800 to 10,000 Å, with larger particles being produced under conditions of high dietary fat intake. The larger particles contain relatively more triglycerides and less polar phospholipids and free cholesterol than do their smaller counterparts. Typical values for the composition of plasma chylomicrons are shown in Table 22-2. After a lipid-rich meal, the fatty acid composition of chylomicron triglycerides generally resembles that of consumed dietary fat, although with lower fat intakes the proportions of linoleic acid, which is derived from biliary lecithin, are higher. The large size and high triglyceride content of chylomicrons are responsible for the lactescent appearance of plasma with a high content of these particles. When present, a chylomicron layer will float to the surface of plasma stored overnight at 4°C. Despite their low content of protein, the A, B, and C apoproteins all appear to be integral components of chylomicrons. Human chylomicrons contain a unique form of apoprotein B (B-48) which is synthesized in the intestinal mucosal cells. Recent studies have demonstrated that B-48 represents a unique intestine-derived form of apoprotein B which consists of the amino-terminal 2,152 amino acids of the normal hepatic apo-B-100, which is 4,536 amino acids in length.[7,8] Apo-B-48 is produced from the apo-B-100 gene by a novel mechanism involving the editing of message RNA in the intestine which results in insertion of a stop codon (UAA) in place of the normal CAA, with a resultant termination of protein synthesis at amino acid number 2,152. Why the intestinal mucosal cells have evolved to synthesize this unique form of apoprotein B is not clear; possibilities include a more rapid adaptation to increase fat intake with a greater and more rapid synthetic capacity than would be observed for a longer protein (B-100) or the possibility that apo-B-48 containing chylomicrons can accommodate more apo-E

TABLE 22-1 Apoprotein Content of Human Plasma Lipoproteins

Chylomicrons	VLDL	LDL	Lp(a)	HDL
Major apoproteins				
Apo-B-48	Apo-B-100	Apo-B-100	Apo-B-100	Apo-A-I
Apo-C-I	Apo-C-I		Apo(a)	Apo-A-II
Apo-C-II	Apo-C-II			
Apo-C-III	Apo-C-III			
Apo-E	Apo-E			
Minor apoproteins				
Apo-A-I	Apo-D			Apo-C-I
Apo-A-II				Apo-C-II
Apo-A-IV				Apo-C-III
Apo-D				Apo-D
				Apo-E

Note: Apoproteins A-I, A-II, and A-IV each constitute 5 to 10 percent of the apoproteins in lymph chylomicrons but are minor components of the chylomicron particles present in plasma.

molecules per particle than can apo-B-100 containing lipoproteins, which in turn may enhance their subsequent uptake by the liver. Because of apoprotein transfer reactions, the C-apoprotein content of chylomicrons isolated from plasma is higher than that of similar particles isolated from thoracic duct lymph. The reverse situation is true for apoproteins A-I, A-II, and A-IV, whose concentrations are higher in chylomicron particles isolated from lymph compared with their plasma counterparts. As will be discussed later, such a transfer is physiologically important in the activation of lipoprotein lipase and the subsequent hydrolysis of chylomicron triglycerides.

Very Low Density Lipoproteins

Very low density lipoproteins, which are the major transport vehicle for endogenous triglycerides in plasma, are smaller than chylomicrons and constitute a heterogeneous series of particles ranging in diameter from 300 to 800 Å. Typical values for VLDL composition are shown in Tables 22-1 and 22-2. The size of VLDL particles is sufficient to scatter transmitted light and gives plasma containing these particles a turbid appearance. However, in contrast to lipemia due to chylomicrons, the turbidity due to VLDL does not separate after storage of plasma for 12 to 18 h at 4°C. Various methods have been used to show that the size heterogeneity of VLDL particles is paralleled by variations in both their lipid composition and their protein composition. Larger particles contain relatively more of the nonpolar triglycerides and less phospholipid and cholesterol than do their smaller counterparts. Thus, as a VLDL particle gets smaller, its relative content of both free and esterified cholesterol is increased. The proportion of apo-C present is also directly related to the size and triglyceride content of the VLDL particle, whereas the apo-B content shows an inverse relation with these parameters. VLDL particles contain the higher-molecular-weight form of apoprotein B termed *B-100,* which is the same apoprotein B present in LDL but is different from the B-48 protein present in chylomicrons.[8]

TABLE 22-2 Composition of Human Plasma Lipoproteins

	Chylomicrons	VLDL	LDL	HDL
Protein	2	8	21	50
Phospholipid	7	19	22	23
Cholesterol-free	2	7	8	4
Cholesterol ester	5	13	37	18
Triglyceride	84	51	11	4
Nonesterified fatty acid		2	1	1

Note: Values are expressed as percent total dry weight of the lipoprotein.

Low-Density Lipoproteins

Low-density lipoproteins (β-lipoproteins) are the major carrier of cholesterol, cholesteryl ester, and phospholipid in human plasma. A typical LDL molecule has a molecular weight of 2.2×10^6 and is composed of 20 to 25 percent protein and 75 to 80 percent lipid (Tables 22-1 and 22-2). A single molecule of apo-B-100 constitutes more than 95 percent of the protein content of LDL, with trace quantities of A, C, and E apoproteins also being present. Lower-density fractions of LDL do, however, contain higher proportions of apo-E and C, but apo-B-100 still contributes more than 90 percent of the total protein.

High-Density Lipoproteins

High-density lipoproteins (α-lipoproteins) are the heaviest (*d* 1.063 to 1.21) and smallest (diameter 90 to 120 Å) of the human lipoproteins and contain about equal proportions of lipid and protein (Table 22-2). Apo-A-I (55 percent) and apo-A-II (30 percent) constitute the major apoproteins in HDL, with smaller quantities of apo-C, apo-D, and apo-E also being present. The lipoproteins isolated in the HDL density range have frequently been further separated into HDL_2 (d 1.063 to 1.125) and HDL_3 (d 1.125 to 1.21). The latter are smaller and contain relatively more apo-A-I and apo-A-II and less apo-C and apo-E. Although the significance of HDL_2 and HDL_3 in physiologic terms remains unclear, the concentration of HDL_2 is some three times higher in premenopausal women than in men. Perturbations in HDL levels caused by factors such as increased exercise also seem to specifically increase the concentrations of HDL_2 in plasma. Based on the apoprotein content, HDL may also be separated into particles containing only apo A-I (Lp:A-I) or both apo A-I and A-II (Lp: A-I/A-II). It has been hypothesized that Lp:A-I and Lp:A-I/A-II particles are functionally distinct.

Lipoprotein (a)

Lipoprotein (a) is an LDL-like particle which contains cholesterol, phospholipid, triglycerides, and apo-B-100, which is linked via a single disulfide bond to a second large protein termed apolipoprotein (a) [apo (a)].[9] Lp(a) can be isolated by ultracentrifugation between the density of 1.06 and 1.08 g/ml, but unlike HDL, Lp(a) is precipitated by heparin manganese, and in this respect it resembles LDL. The structure of apo (a) is very similar to that of plasminogen and contains a number of pretzellike structures which have been termed "kringles." Considerable variability exists in the number of kringle IV repeats present in Lp(a) particles isolated from the plasma of different patients, and this variability is one of the factors responsible for the differences in molecular weight and plasma concentrations of Lp(a) observed in the plasma of different subjects. The size of apo (a) ranges between 450,000 and 750,000 daltons, and the relation between molecular mass and plasma concentrations is an inverse one, with the highest plasma concentrations being observed in patients with the lowest-molecular-weight forms of apo (a).[10] Increased plasma concentrations of Lp(a) greater than 20 to 30 mg/dl are associated with an increased risk of atherosclerosis, but the precise physiologic function of Lp(a) remains unknown.[11]

Abnormal Lipoproteins

Certain pathologic conditions may be associated with the presence of abnormal lipoprotein particles in plasma. This is most commonly seen in patients with cholestasis in which an abnormal cholesterol-rich lipoprotein termed lipoprotein X (LPX) is present in plasma.[12] Lipoprotein X appears as bilamellar discoidal structures measuring 40 to 60 nm in diameter and 10 nm in thickness when studied under electron microscopy. Lipoprotein X contains phospholipid and free cholesterol in a 1:1 molar ratio and albumin and apoproteins C-I, C-II, and C-III as the protein moieties. The cholesteryl ester content is low. The lecithin contained in LPX contains fatty acid moieties of similar composition to those of biliary lecithin, and this lipoprotein is believed to contain phospholipid and cholesterol which are transported into plasma when their normal route of excretion in bile is impaired. Similar lipoprotein particles also occur in the plasma of patients with lecithin cholesterol acyltransferase deficiency.[13]

The Apoproteins

Structure

The apoprotein moieties of plasma lipoproteins have in common the requirement that they bind and transport lipid in the bloodstream. During the past decade, major advances have occurred which have delineated the synthesis, structure, and function of these unique proteins. Eleven apoproteins—A-I, A-II, A-IV, B-48, B-100, C-I, C-II, C-III, D, E, and apo (a)—have been sequenced, and the genes responsible for their synthesis have been mapped in the human genome.[14,15] With the exception of apo (a), these apoproteins have one common structural feature: a domain containing an amphipathic helix.[16] The amino acid sequences of these regions of the protein are such that hydrophobic amino acids are arranged on one side of the helix and hydrophilic polar amino acids form the other side. The hydrophobic face of the helix is thought to interact with the acyl chains of phospholipids, whereas the hydrophilic region faces the polar region of phospholipid head groups. With the exception of apo-B-48, apo-B-100, and apo (a), all of the apoproteins appear to be capable of dissociating from one lipoprotein particle and moving to another. This movement of apoproteins between lipoproteins not only serves to enhance metabolic processing of given lipoprotein particles but it also prolongs the residence time of the apoproteins in plasma.

Studies of the biosynthesis of several apoproteins have indicated that the apoproteins are initially synthesized as preapolipoproteins or preproapolipoproteins, with pre and pro segments of the apolipoprotein being cleaved posttranslationally within the cell or after secretion of the proapolipoprotein into plasma.[17,18] The gene locations of the major apoproteins have been delineated; examples include apo-B on chromosome 2; apo (a) on chromosome 6; apo-A-I, A-IV, and C-III on chromosome 11; and apo-C-II, apo-E, and the LDL receptor gene on chromosome 19.[15] Application of the techniques of modern molecular biology to plasma apolipoproteins has resulted in the identification of regulatory and structural mutations in the genes for these apoproteins, several of which appear to predispose individuals to dyslipoproteinemias and the premature development of atherosclerosis. Different allelic forms of apoprotein E resulting from amino acid substitutions in the receptor-binding region of this apoprotein have been described and underlie susceptibility to type III hyperlipoproteinemia. Mutations in apo-B have been identified which result in hypercholesterolemia, in the case of familial defective apo-B-100, or hypocholesterolemia in the case of mutations resulting in truncated forms of apo-B.[8,14,15] A variety of apolipoprotein A-I isoproteins resulting from amino acid substitutions have also been described, and it is likely that many more variations will be identified in the future. In addition to alterations in apoprotein composition caused by amino acid substitutions resulting from structural gene mutations, differences in the sialic acid content of apoproteins also contribute to the apparent variations detected on isoelectric focusing. For example, three forms of apoprotein C-III can be resolved by means of isoelectric focusing; apoprotein C-III_0 contains no sialic acid, apoprotein C-III_1 has 1 mol of sialic acid per mole of protein, and apoprotein C-III_2 has 2 mol.[19] Various dietary and hormonal manipulations have been shown to alter the degree of sialation of apo-C-III.[20]

The major sites of biosynthesis of apolipoproteins are the liver and the intestinal mucosal cells; both organs appear to contribute to the plasma pool of apoproteins of the A and C families as well as apoprotein E.[21] Current data[8] indicate that the biosynthesis of human apoprotein B-48 occurs exclusively in the intestine, whereas apoprotein B-100 appears to be almost exclusively of hepatic origin. The biosynthesis of apoprotein E occurs in many nonhepatic tissues,[22] including muscle and macrophages; muscle tissue also appears capable of synthesizing apolipoprotein A-I.[21]

Function

In addition to their structural role in maintaining lipoprotein stability, several apolipoproteins are known to play distinct roles in the intravascular metabolism and cellular uptake of lipoproteins (Table 22-3). Apolipoprotein C-II serves as a cofactor for lipoprotein lipase, the enzyme which hydrolyzes the triglycerides in plasma chylomicrons and VLDL,[23] and a deficiency of apo-C-II is associated with severe hypertriglyceridemia.[24] The infusion of normal plasma or isolated apo-C-II fractions dramatically reduces the hypertriglyceridemia seen in patients with apo-C-II deficiency.[24,25] Apolipoprotein A-I, the major apoprotein in HDL, is a cofactor for lecithin cholesterol acyltransferase (LCAT), a plasma enzyme that catalyzes the conversion of cholesterol and phosphatidylcholine to cholesteryl esters and lysophosphatidylcholine.[14,26] Apo-C-I may also serve as an activator of LCAT. Apoproteins A-I, A-II, and A-IV are ligands for the candidate HDL receptor protein.

Distinct roles for apoprotein E and apoprotein B-100 in the cellular uptake of lipoprotein particles have been well established. The uptake of chylomicron and VLDL remnant particles is dependent on a specific hepatic receptor which has been termed the LDL receptor–related protein (LRP), which recognizes the apoprotein E moieties contained in these lipoprotein particles, and facilitates their uptake from plasma.[27,28] A single amino acid substitution between residues 140 and 160 of the 299-amino acid sequence of apoprotein E can profoundly affect receptor binding, and a substitution of cysteine for arginine at residue 158 is primarily responsible for the decreased receptor binding of apoprotein E-2 which is believed to underlie the clinical development of type III hyperlipoproteinemia.[29] The synthesis of apoprotein B-48 within intestinal mucosal cells and of apoprotein B-100 within the liver appears to be necessary for the normal formation of chylomicron and VLDL-LDL particles, respectively.[8] Although the hepatic uptake of chylomicron remnants does not require the interaction of apo-B-48 with hepatic receptors, the removal of LDL particles from plasma is facilitated by binding domains present in the C-terminal portion of apo-B-100 which are recognized by specific high-affinity LDL receptors.[8] Monoclonal antibodies directed against epitopes on apo-B-100 located between amino acids 2,980 and 3,780 completely block the specific binding of LDL parti-

TABLE 22-3 Metabolic Functions of Plasma Apoproteins

Apoprotein	Molecular Weight	Metabolic Role
A-I	28,000	Activates LCAT, ligand for putative HDL receptor
A-II	17,500	Activated hepatic lipase; may inhibit LCAT
A-IV	46,000	Unknown; has been tentatively linked to satiety in rats
B-48	210,000	Transport of lipids from the gut as chylomicrons
B-100	350,000	Transport of lipids from the liver as VLDL and LDL; recognized by cellular LDL receptors
C-I	7,000	Activates LCAT
C-II	9,000	Activates lipoprotein lipase
C-III	9,000	May inhibit activation of lipoprotein lipase by apo-C-II
D	22,000	May be involved in lipid transfer between lipoproteins
E	34,000	Recognized by hepatic apo-E receptors and cellular LDL receptors; recognition facilitates hepatic uptake of chylomicron and VLDL remnants
Transfer proteins	Variable	Facilitate the transfer of triglycerides, phospholipids, and cholesteryl esters between lipoproteins

cles to the LDL receptor and indicate that this region of apoprotein B contains the receptor-binding domain. These studies are also consistent with the observation that patients with familial defective apo-B-100, in which the amino acid glutamine is substituted for the normal arginine at position 3,500, exhibit increased plasma concentrations of LDL particles that bind poorly to the LDL-receptor.[8] Chemical modification of LDL with agents that block the charge on lysine or arginine residues inhibits the recognition of LDL by specific high-affinity LDL receptors and blocks this receptor-mediated pathway of cellular LDL uptake without having an apparent effect on receptor-independent pathways.[30]

Lipoprotein Structure

When viewed under the electron microscope, all normal mature lipoproteins appear as spherical particles without any discernible subunit structure.[26] The nonpolar triglycerides and cholesteryl esters are found in the central core of the lipoprotein particle, and the more polar phospholipids and free cholesterol are found at the surface. The apoproteins are also thought to be primarily located in an alpha-helical arrangement at the surface, although apolar regions of the protein chain may extend into the milieu of the lipid core. This lipid core model is consistent with the greater exchange of phospholipids and free cholesterol compared with the exchange of triglyceride and cholesteryl esters between lipoproteins.[26] A diagrammatic representation of the structure of LDL is shown in Fig. 22-2.[31]

FIGURE 22-2 Schematic structure of low-density lipoprotein indicating the location of apoprotein B-100. The locations of two sites where thrombin cleaves apoprotein B (residues 1297 and 3249) are indicated. The locations of the sixteen *N*-linked carbohydrates (CHO ○), cysteine residues (●), and disulfide bridges (=) are also shown. The five hypothetical domains of apo-B are indicated by roman numerals and separated by dashed lines. *(Reproduced from Yang et al.[31] with permission.)*

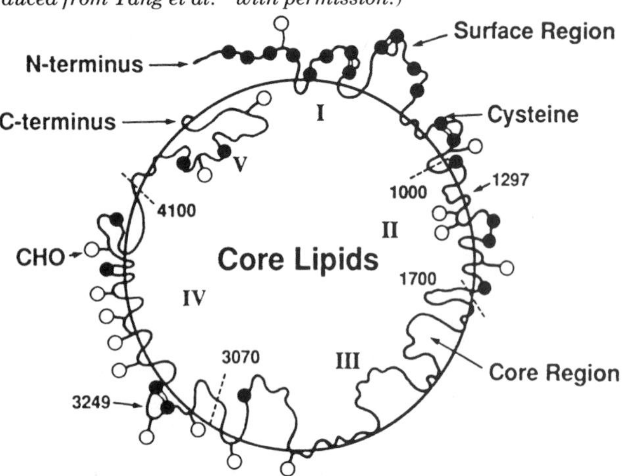

SYNTHESIS AND CATABOLISM OF LIPIDS AND LIPOPROTEINS

Lipids

Cholesterol

In the schemata for the cholesterol balance of the body (Table 22-4), cholesterol is synthesized from acetate by the liver and intestinal mucosa and released into the plasma in lipoproteins. Cholesterol biosynthesis is regulated in the liver by the enzyme 3-hydroxy-3-methylglutaryl coenzyme A reductase (HMG CoA reductase). This enzyme catalyzes the production of mevalonic acid, which is converted to cholesterol. Cholesterol absorbed from the diet also enters the body pool of cholesterol and thus provides a second major source of cholesterol which circulates in the plasma. Only about 40 percent of dietary cholesterol is absorbed by the intestine. While all cells in the body have the capacity to synthesize cholesterol, in most cells the locally synthesized cholesterol is utilized for membrane formation within the cell and does not contribute en masse to the plasma cholesterol concentration.

A variety of circumstances favor cholesterol biosynthesis, including excessive calories in the diet, saturated fat in the diet, and perhaps the total fat content of the diet. Cholesterol synthesis is depressed with hypocaloric and starvation diets. As will be indicated in the section on Pharmaceutical Agents, some of the lipid-lowering drugs act by altering cholesterol biosynthesis, although in general earlier agents such as triparanol, which inhibited a late stage in cholesterol biosynthesis, were too toxic for therapeutic use.

Cholesterol synthesis may also be inhibited by the presence of cholesterol in the liver cells; this is known as *feedback inhibition.* Likewise, the presence of bile acids through feedback inhibition tends

TABLE 22-4 The Cholesterol Balance of the Body

	Milligrams per day
Input	
From synthesis	500–1000
Absorbed from the diet	0–400
	500–1400
Output	
Excretion in the bile (cholesterol and bile acids) and subsequently in the feces	400–1300
Skin excretion	80–100
Synthesis of steroid hormones	Variable
Losses during pregnancy and lactation	Variable
Storage in the tissues	Variable
	500–1400

to inhibit the synthesis of additional bile acids from cholesterol. In humans, however, the inhibition of cholesterol biosynthesis is insufficient to prevent a rise in plasma cholesterol concentrations when a large quantity of cholesterol is present in the diet.

Besides the efflux of cholesterol from the plasma as carried by LDL to supply cholesterol for membranes in growing cells, cholesterol from the plasma may be utilized for the synthesis of the steroid hormones and bile acids.

The primary route of excretion of cholesterol from the body begins in the liver, where cholesterol and bile acids synthesized from cholesterol are secreted in the bile. Thus, the chief pathway of excretion of cholesterol from the body ultimately occurs via the feces, where this steroid nucleus appears either as cholesterol or as its bacterially altered products coprosterol (coprostanol) and coprostanone and as bile acids. The bile acids in the stool represent the small fraction excreted in the bile and not absorbed by the enterohepatic circulation. The usual output of cholesterol from the body is approximately 600 to 1000 mg per day. About 60 percent of the output is as cholesterol (or coprostanol), and the other 40 percent is as the secondary bile acids.

Cholesteryl ester is the predominant circulating form of cholesterol, with some 70 to 80 percent of the total plasma cholesterol being esterified through the action of the LCAT enzyme, as will be discussed subsequently. The predominant cholesteryl ester is cholesteryl linoleate, followed by cholesteryl oleate, cholesteryl palmitate, and cholesteryl stearate. Some arachidonic acid is also transported as a cholesteryl ester. The cholesterol of the bodily tissues is largely in the free form, except for the storage of cholesteryl ester in the adrenal glands and other steroid-synthesizing endocrine glands, where it becomes readily available for the synthesis of steroid hormones under conditions of rapid need. Some cholesteryl ester is also present in the liver, but in general normal tissues contain only free cholesterol, which is present primarily in cell membranes; of course, cholesteryl ester predominates in atheroma and xanthoma. Finally, it must be appreciated that cholesterol is unique in that once it is present in the body, it remains until it is excreted. The steroid nucleus cannot be broken down by the tissues, unlike lipids such as triglyceride.

Triglyceride

Like cholesterol, the triglyceride of the plasma lipoproteins is synthesized either by the intestinal tract (from absorbed fatty acids) or by the liver from both acetate and fatty acids and enters the plasma in the form of one of the four major lipoprotein classes: chylomicrons, VLDL, LDL, and HDL. Plasma triglyceride constitutes a readily available source of energy for the body, again through the action of lipoprotein lipase at the cellular level. The free fatty acid produced from the hydrolysis of triglyceride is then taken up by the cells of the body either for storage, as in adipose tissue, or for oxidation by muscle cells. Thus, hypertriglyceridemia can result from oversynthesis, impaired catabolism, or a combination of both circumstances. Caloric excess and adiposity apparently favor both increased synthesis of triglycerides in liver and gut and impaired removal by the peripheral tissue.

Phospholipids

The plasma phospholipids are derived almost entirely from synthesis in the liver and intestinal mucosa but can be synthesized by most body tissues. Dietary phospholipids are not absorbed as such and undergo hydrolysis by phospholipases in the intestinal juices with formation of both lysophosphatides and the basic constituent phosphorus-containing amine, 2 mol of fatty acids, and glycerol. Phospholipids are catabolized as components of their respective lipoproteins and also readily exchange between lipoproteins and cell membranes. Catabolism of individual phospholipids may proceed to their basic constituents or may undergo deacylation-reacylation reactions during which the fatty acid composition is altered. Lysolecithin may be formed by tissue phospholipases or may be formed in plasma by LCAT, and this somewhat toxic molecule is rapidly metabolized.

Enzymes and Transfer Proteins Active in Lipoprotein Metabolism

Three enzymes—lipoprotein lipase (LPL), hepatic lipase (HL), and LCAT—the activities of which can all be measured in plasma, are of physiologic importance in lipoprotein metabolism. In addition, a specific transfer protein, cholesteryl ester transfer protein (CETP), facilitates the interchange of cholesteryl esters between HDL and triglyceride-rich lipoproteins.

Lecithin Cholesterol Acyltransferase

The enzyme LCAT catalyzes the transfer of fatty acid from the 2 position of phosphatidylcholine to cholesterol with the formation of cholesteryl ester and lysophosphatidyl choline[32,33] (Fig. 22-3). Current evidence suggests that this enzyme is responsible for the formation of most of the esterified cholesterol present in plasma, although lesser amounts of cholesteryl ester also enter plasma as native constituents of VLDL and probably as chylomicrons. Phosphatidylcholine and free cholesterol present on HDL are the preferred substrate for LCAT, for which apo-A-I, the major apoprotein of HDL, and apo-C-I act as specific activators. The enzyme itself is secreted by the liver and is present in plasma, lymph, and cerebrospinal fluid. LCAT shows fatty acid specificity, which results in the preferential formation of cho-

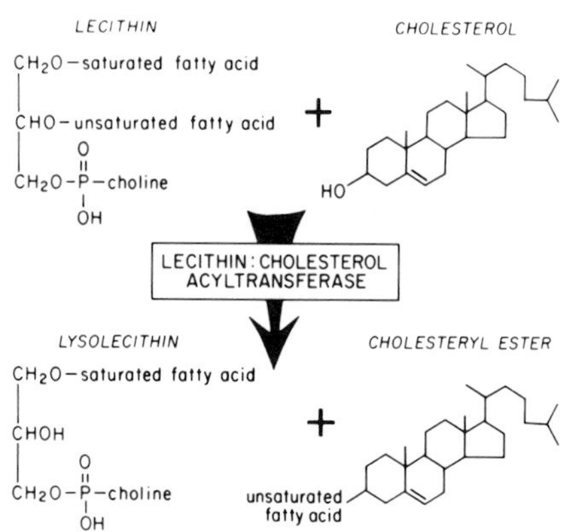

FIGURE 22-3 Lipid reactants in the plasma lecithin cholesterol acyltransferase reaction. (*Reproduced from Glomset et al.*[32] *with permission.*)

lesteryl linoleate. The absence of LCAT has been described in a rare disease which will be discussed later.

Lipoprotein Lipase

Lipoprotein lipase is an important enzyme which is present in a number of tissues, including muscle, adipose tissue, lung, brain, and breast tissue.[34] This enzyme is present primarily on endothelial cells in tissue capillary beds, where it is bound to heparan-sulfate proteoglycans present as components of the glycocalyx on the plasma membrane. The enzyme is present in very low concentrations in plasma but may be released by the injection of heparin. Physiologically, LPL acts in capillary beds to hydrolyze triglycerides present in chylomicrons and VLDL particles, with subsequent liberation of free fatty acids and monoglycerides. Apoprotein C-II functions as a specific activator for LPL, and defects in the synthesis or activity of either LPL or apo-C-II result in impaired triglyceride catabolism and severe hypertriglyceridemia. Classically, the deficiency of LPL is present in patients with familial type I hyperlipidemia. The activity of LPL in adipose tissue is increased in response to insulin and is reduced by fasting.[34] The activity of LPL increases in breast tissue during lactation, and this enzyme facilitates the provision of free fatty acids to this tissue. Lipoprotein lipase deficiency has been associated with a reduced content of essential fatty acids in breast milk.[35]

Hepatic Lipase

Hepatic lipase is a distinct lipolytic enzyme which is synthesized in hepatocytes and is also released into plasma by the intravenous injection of heparin.[36] Hepatic lipase does not require an apoprotein activator and appears to function in the hydrolysis of triglycerides present on VLDL and VLDL remnant particles, enhancing their conversion to LDL. Deficiency of HL has been associated with the accumulation of small triglyceride-rich VLDL particles in plasma as well as an increase in the concentration of HDL_2.[37] Kinetic studies of VLDL metabolism in a patient with hepatic lipase deficiency have indicated that the deficiency results in impaired conversion of small VLDL particles into LDL but that the initial delipidation of VLDL is normal.[38] These studies indicate that LPL and HL play complementary roles in the intravascular catabolism of triglyceride-rich lipoproteins.

Cholesteryl Ester Transfer Protein

Cholesteryl ester transfer protein mediates the transfer of cholesteryl esters from HDL particles to VLDL, with a reciprocal transfer of triglycerides from VLDL to HDL.[39] Deficiency of CETP has been associated with marked increases in the plasma concentrations of HDL cholesterol, and this deficiency supports the view that CETP is important in the normal physiology of lipid transport.[40] CETP activity has been shown to be increased in hypertriglyceridemia and in patients with diabetes or hypothyroidism but is decreased in response to alcohol consumption.[39] Whether reductions in CETP activity, which may lead to increases in HDL cholesterol, should be viewed as beneficial is unclear.

Lipoprotein Metabolism

Chylomicrons

Chylomicrons are synthesized by the small intestine, principally the jejunum, in response to the absorption of dietary fat. After a fat-rich meal, lipids are hydrolyzed in the intestinal lumen; the digestive products are then absorbed and utilized in the synthesis of triglycerides, cholesteryl esters, and phospholipids within the mucosal cell. Synthesis of apoproteins A-I, A-II, A-IV, and B-48 and possibly some C and E apoproteins occurs concurrently, and the resultant chylomicron particle is subsequently released from the mucosal cell into the lacteals, from where it progresses to enter the systemic circulation via the thoracic duct. Fatty acids with a chain length less than 12 carbon atoms are transported in the portal blood.

Upon entry into the systemic circulation, chylomicrons are metabolized rapidly with a half-life of 5 to 15 min. Transfer of apo-A-I and A-II to HDL and reciprocal transfers of C and E apoproteins from HDL serve to enhance the hydrolysis of chylomicron triglycerides by LPL and provide a source of chylomicron surface components which act as a precursor of nascent HDL particles. Hydrolysis of chylomicron triglycerides by this enzyme occurs at the endothelial cell surface and results in chylomicron remnants that are relatively enriched in cholesterol. These particles are taken up by the liver via a specific apo-E receptor, probably LRP,[27] but this uptake may also involve the apo-B or LDL receptor. As was previously discussed, apo-E is the apoprotein responsible for receptor-mediated clearance of chylomicron (and VLDL) remnants by the liver. Such uptake results in an increased hepatic cholesterol content and is associated with a decrease in de novo cholesterol synthesis.

Very Low Density Lipoproteins

The liver is the major site of synthesis of VLDL, with a minor contribution being derived from the intestine. Transport of endogenous triglyceride from the liver to peripheral tissues is probably the principal function of VLDL, but it also serves as the major precursor of LDL (Fig. 22-4). Many factors, including the basal diet; time of day; levels of insulin, glucagon, and epinephrine in plasma; and degree of adiposity, appear to modulate the rate of secretion of hepatic VLDL. Apo-B-100 appears to be essential for VLDL synthesis. Like chylomicrons, newly secreted VLDL rapidly acquire some C and possibly E apoproteins from HDL in plasma; this gain in apo-C-II in turn increases their susceptibility to hydrolysis by LPL. Clearance of VLDL is slower than that of chylomicrons, and their half-life in plasma is 6 to 12 h. Hydrolysis of VLDL triglycerides and phospholipids by LPL and HL results in a progressively smaller particle with lower S_f but with a constant content of apoprotein B-100. The content of C and E apoproteins in VLDL, however, decreases as the particle is metabolized and these proteins are transferred back to HDL. The catabolism of VLDL remnant particles by the liver is facilitated by their binding to high-affinity LDL receptors as well as possibly to the LDL receptor–related protein[27,28]; this process is abnormal in patients with apo-E variants (e.g., E-2) that have reduced receptor binding. HDL functions as a reservoir for the C apoproteins, and such transfer reactions between VLDL and HDL serve an economic role and prolong the half-life of the C apoproteins in plasma. In normolipidemic humans, virtually all the B apoprotein that enters plasma as a constituent of VLDL is preserved as the particle is metabolized to intermediate-density lipoproteins (IDL) and eventually to LDL. In contrast, in patients with severe hypertriglyceridemia, most of the VLDL particles are removed before conversion to LDL, and LDL concentrations are low. In addition to apo-B, a considerable proportion of the phospholipid, free cholesterol, and some of the cholesteryl esters of the plasma VLDL are retained during metabolism of VLDL to LDL. This precursor-product relation between VLDL and LDL may be seen clinically in patients with type IV hyperlipidemia who are treated with either diet or drugs. In such cases, initial falls in VLDL are not uncommonly accompanied by reciprocal rises in LDL.

Low-Density Lipoproteins

In humans, most of the LDL in plasma are derived from the intravascular catabolism of VLDL; LDL may therefore be regarded as the end product of VLDL metabolism (Fig. 22-4). Catabolism of LDL occurs in both peripheral cells and the liver (the liver is the major site of removal) and is facilitated by both receptor-mediated and non-receptor-mediated pathways.[41,42] The turnover of LDL is considerably slower than that of VLDL; the half-life in normal humans is from 3 to 4 days and is prolonged in patients with familial hypercholesterolemia. Based largely on the elegant studies of Goldstein and Brown, a variety of cells have been shown to contain specific receptors for LDL.[41,42] The uptake of LDL by cells results in suppression of endogenous cholesterol biosynthesis, an enhanced rate of intracellular cholesterol esterification, and a reduction in the number of high-affinity LDL receptors expressed on the cell surface (Fig. 22-5). Functional high-affinity LDL receptors are absent from the cells of most patients with homozygous familial hypercholesterolemia. Although the liver is quantitatively the most important organ for the removal of LDL from plasma, the *relative* rate of uptake is greatest in certain endocrine tissues (e.g., adrenal cortex and corpus luteum of the ovary) which have a high capacity for the synthesis of ste-

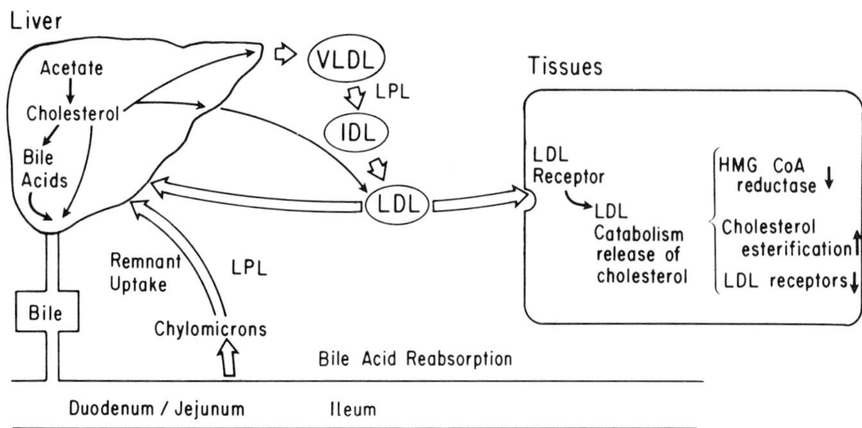

FIGURE 22-4 Metabolism and transport of lipoproteins in humans and the cellular changes that result from receptor-mediated uptake of low-density lipoproteins.

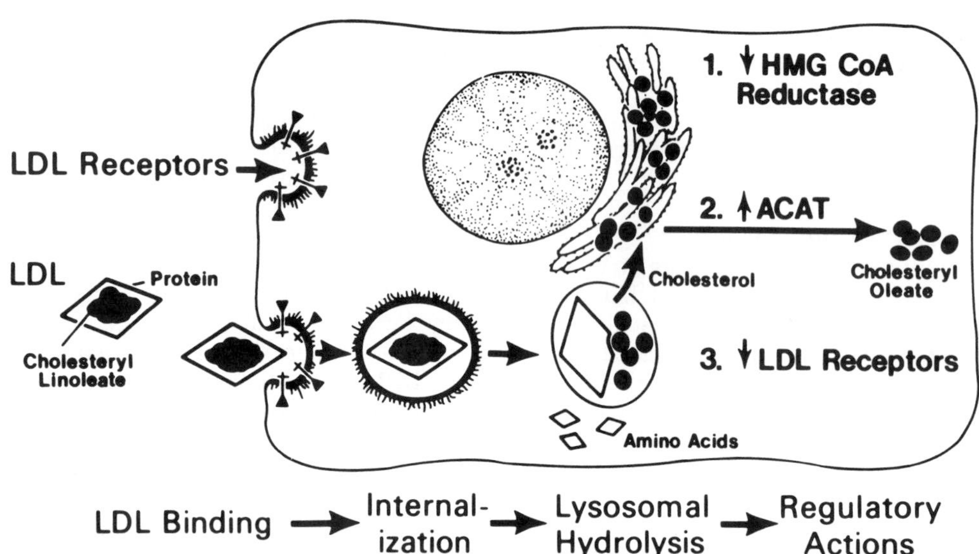

FIGURE 22-5 Sequential steps in the pathway of LDL metabolism in cultured human fibroblasts. The central role of the LDL receptor in controlling the binding, uptake, lysosomal hydrolysis, and regulation of cholesterol synthesis and cholesteryl ester formation is illustrated. (*Reproduced from Goldstein and Brown*[103] *with permission.*)

roid hormones for which cholesterol contained in LDL serves as an important precursor.[43,44] Clinical and epidemiologic studies have shown a strong positive relation between elevated levels of LDL cholesterol and an increased risk of cardiovascular morbidity and mortality.

High-Density Lipoproteins

The synthesis and secretion of HDL from the liver are well documented.[45] In addition, some HDL particles are also derived from the surface components of chylomicrons and VLDL particles during lipolysis (Fig. 22-6). This dual etiology for HDL explains the inverse correlation between plasma triglycerides and HDL as well as the known presence of HDL in patients with abetalipoproteinemia (who do not form chylomicrons and VLDL). Newly secreted

FIGURE 22-6 Diagrammatic representation of the origin and intravascular metabolism of high-density lipoproteins.

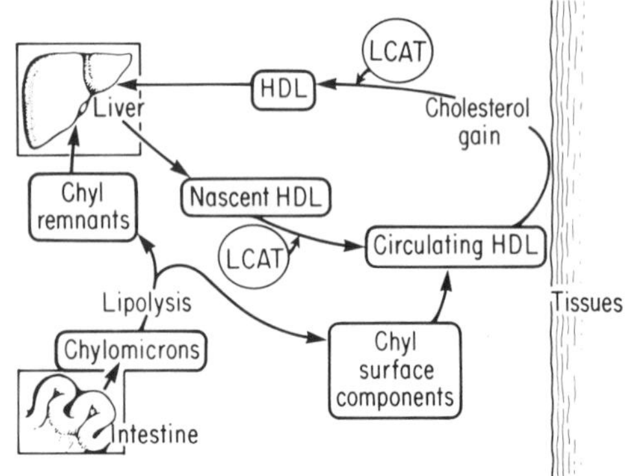

HDL appears as flat, disk-shaped structures containing predominantly protein, phospholipid, and free cholesterol. When exposed to the action of LCAT, these particles are converted to spherical particles that are enriched in cholesteryl esters. Indeed, the formation of cholesteryl esters in plasma catalyzed by LCAT appears to be an important function of HDL. HDL also provides a reservoir for C apoproteins which transfer to chylomicrons and VLDL during alimentary lipemia and subsequently move back to HDL with clearance of the larger fat-rich particles from plasma. The half-life of HDL, as assessed by that of apo-A-I and A-II, is from 4 to 6 days and is influenced by both diet and drugs. Thus, diets high in carbohydrate which raise VLDL cause a lowering of HDL and an enhanced HDL turnover. Similarly, nicotinic acid, which depresses VLDL synthesis, raises HDL levels and prolongs the half-life. Both effects on HDL metabolism probably are a consequence of changes in both the synthesis of VLDL and the catabolic rate of HDL[46] and support the general view that VLDL and HDL levels change reciprocally. On the basis of animal experiments, it has been concluded that the major sites of HDL catabolism are the liver and kidney, although evidence to support this view in humans is not available. Glomset and Norum[13] have proposed that an additional major function of HDL is to transport cholesterol from peripheral tissues back to the liver.[13] Thus, high levels of HDL may enhance removal of cholesterol from tissues, including the arterial wall, and protect against the development of atherosclerosis. Several factors have been shown to increase the concentrations of HDL in plasma,[47,48] and fluctuations in total

HDL concentrations are usually due to alterations in the levels in the higher HDL_2 subfraction. Variations in the concentration of HDL_2 also show the strongest inverse correlation with cardiovascular risk; thus, increased concentrations of HDL_2 are viewed as protective, whereas low concentrations may be detrimental.[49] Factors which have been shown to increase the concentrations of HDL include moderate ethanol consumption,[48] sustained regular exercise, correction of hypertriglyceridemia, and certain drugs, including phenobarbital, phenytoin, clofibrate, estrogens, nicotinic acid, and gemfibrozil.[47,49,50] Decreases in the plasma concentrations of HDL may be seen in association with weight gain, cigarette smoking, hypertriglyceridemia, and the use of probucol.

Free Fatty Acids

Free fatty acids (FFA) constitute the fifth class of lipoproteins. They consist of long-chain fatty acids bound to albumin, occupying up to two high affinity binding sites on the albumin molecule; if FFA levels are elevated, additional lower affinity binding sites are then occupied. FFA constitute a major metabolic fuel of the body. They are derived in part from lipolysis of triglycerides stored in the adipose tissue cell. The tissue lipase in these cells is under neuroendocrine control and operates through the adenyl cyclase system. A second origin of FFA is through the hydrolysis of plasma triglyceride present in chylomicrons and VLDL through the action of LPL.

FFA have a very short half-life of 4 to 8 min and are readily taken up from plasma by the muscle cells of the body. A second pathway for their catabolism is uptake by the liver and resynthesis into triglyceride, which then may be transported from the liver in VLDL, or oxidation to acetyl CoA. Physiologically, FFA levels may rise and fall in the blood with great rapidity in order to meet the body's needs for this form of energy. Levels tend to be low after the absorption of carbohydrate associated with increased insulin secretion but rise postprandially as blood glucose falls. In the fasting state, levels of 400 to 600 μEq/L are common; with a prolonged fast of 24 to 72 h, the levels of FFA may range from 1000 to 1500 μEq/L. Glucagon, epinephrine, growth hormone, and adrenocorticotropic hormone (ACTH) may also increase FFA levels. The major physiologic regulators of the plasma FFA are insulin and epinephrine.

The chief fatty acids of the plasma FFA fraction are oleic, palmitic, linoleic, and stearic acids, which reflect in most instances the composition of the adipose tissue triglyceride. Three of these four fatty acids (oleic, palmitic, and stearic acids) may be synthesized by the body from acetate. Linoleic acid is unique in being an essential fatty acid which cannot be synthesized in humans but is necessary for the body's growth and for membrane formation. The syndrome of essential fatty acid deficiency results when linoleic acid accounts for less than 1 percent of the total calories in the diet, as occurs after prolonged total parenteral nutrition. Linoleic acid is of special importance as the precursor substance for arachidonic acid, which in turn has multitudinous functions, of which a most important one is as a precursor for prostaglandin formation. Linolenic (18:3) and other omega-3 fatty acids are also components of adipose tissue and the plasma FFA. Deficiency states of omega-3 fatty acids occur with fat-free diets. Linolenic acid is the substrate for the synthesis of eicosapentaenoic acid and docosahexaenoic acid of this series, which are important in membrane formation, especially for the brain and retina, and in eicosanoid metabolism.

Atherogenicity of Individual Lipoprotein Particles

The lipoprotein particles in human plasma all contain cholesterol, but the extent to which elevated levels of each of these particles may contribute to the development of atherosclerosis differs widely (Table 22-5). Increased plasma concentrations of LDL, Lp(a), and cholesterol-rich remnant particles, the latter of which accumulate in the plasma of patients with type III hyperlipidemia, are all highly athero-

TABLE 22-5 Relative Atherogenicity of Individual Lipoprotein Particles

Lipoprotein	Atherogenicity	Typical Associated Dyslipoproteinemia
Chylomicrons (lipoprotein lipase deficiency)	0	Type I
VLDL	+	Type IV (familial hypertriglyceridemia)
Chylomicron and VLDL remnants	+++	Type III (dysbetalipoproteinemia)
LDL	++++	Type II (familial hypercholesterolemia)
Lp(a)	++++	Various
HDL	Negatively correlated with atherosclerosis	Familial hyperalphalipoproteinemia

genic,[8,9,11,29] whereas increased levels of HDL cholesterol appear to afford protection from atherosclerosis.[49]

Plasma concentrations of the major LDL apoprotein (apoprotein B) may provide a better prediction of the risk of coronary artery disease than does measurement of LDL cholesterol.[51] Similarly, plasma concentrations of the major HDL apoproteins (A-I and A-II) may be better discriminators for cardiovascular risk associated with low concentrations of HDL particles than are measurements of HDL cholesterol.[51,52] Hyperchylomicronemia as an isolated entity (e.g., that seen in patients with LPL deficiency) does not appear to be associated with an increased risk of atherosclerosis,[53] but concurrent or isolated elevations of VLDL do appear to be moderately atherogenic, as do lipoprotein particles produced from the intravascular hydrolysis of triglycerides from VLDL and chylomicrons.[54]

Modifications in lipoproteins, particularly oxidation of LDL, markedly enhance the uptake of these lipoproteins by macrophages when studied under in vitro conditions[55–57] and lead to foam cell development. It is believed that oxidation of LDL particles occurs in atherosclerotic plaques, but local oxidation of LDL may occur under conditions of endothelial cell injury and potentially under other circumstances in which plasma concentrations of natural antioxidants are reduced. The potential role of modified lipoproteins in the pathogenesis of atherosclerosis in humans is currently a subject of intense research, as is the potential role of antioxidants in the prevention of atherosclerosis.

TABLE 22-6 Classification of Hyperlipidemias Based on Lipoprotein Concentrations

Type	Lipoprotein Abnormality	Lipid Profiles	Typical Values, mg/dl
I	Chylomicrons markedly ↑, VLDL and LDL both normal or low	Chol ↑ Tg ↑↑	320 4000
IIa	LDL ↑, VLDL normal	Chol ↑ Tg N	370 90
IIb	LDL ↑, VLDL ↑	Chol ↑ Tg ↑	350 400
III	Abnormal cholesterol-enriched VLDL remnants (IDL) present in excess	Chol ↑ Tg ↑	500 700
IV	VLDL ↑, LDL normal	Chol N Tg ↑	220 400
V	Chylomicrons markedly ↑, VLDL ↑, LDL normal or low	Chol ↑ Tg ↑↑	700 5000

Source: Based on Fredrickson, Levy, and Lees[58] and the WHO committee.[59]

THE HYPERLIPIDEMIAS

Classification of Hyperlipidemias

Classification of hyperlipidemias on the basis of plasma lipoprotein patterns, as originally proposed by Fredrickson, Levy, and Lees[58] and modified by the WHO,[59] is the most widely used system of nomenclature. As shown in Table 22-6, the six types are classified with respect to increased levels of chylomicrons, VLDL, IDL, and LDL. Although this classification provides a simple way in which to categorize increases in the concentrations of given lipoproteins, it does not provide any information about the etiology of the abnormality. Thus, a given phenotype may occur as a primary genetic disorder or may be secondary to a variety of associated conditions. Similarly, this classification system does not consider variations in HDL concentrations as an independent variable. Despite these limitations, the Fredrickson classification provides a useful basis for describing most hyperlipoproteinemias.

Determination of the plasma concentrations of cholesterol and triglycerides, with a concurrent determination of the concentrations of HDL cholesterol, remains the basic lipid profile necessary for the diagnosis of most hyperlipidemias. Despite the fact that a number of dyslipidemias are now characterized on the basis of apoprotein abnormalities, apoprotein measurements are not in routine clinical use and are available only in specialized centers with a major interest in lipoprotein disorders. To avoid the postprandial increase in plasma triglycerides, it is advisable to request that patients fast for 12 to 15 h before venipuncture. In contrast, plasma cholesterol concentrations are minimally affected by eating, and nonfasting blood samples are adequate for the determination of total plasma cholesterol concentrations. The importance of determining plasma lipid and lipoprotein concentrations under steady-state conditions cannot be overemphasized; concentrations of cholesterol and triglyceride both decrease during periods of weight loss and commonly fall for 2 to 3 months after a myocardial infarction.

Hyperlipidemia can be divided into four basic patterns (Fig. 22-7) based on the initial determination of total plasma (or serum), cholesterol, and triglyceride concentrations: (1) hypercholesterolemia with normal concentrations of triglycerides (type IIa phenotype), (2) combined elevation of cholesterol and triglyceride in which the plasma triglyceride concentrations are one to three times higher than the cholesterol concentration (phenotypes IIb and III), (3) a primary elevation of triglycerides in which cholesterol concentrations are normal or only slightly increased (type IV phenotype), and (4) moderately to markedly elevated levels of cholesterol (>300 mg/dl) with a simultaneous marked increase in plasma tri-

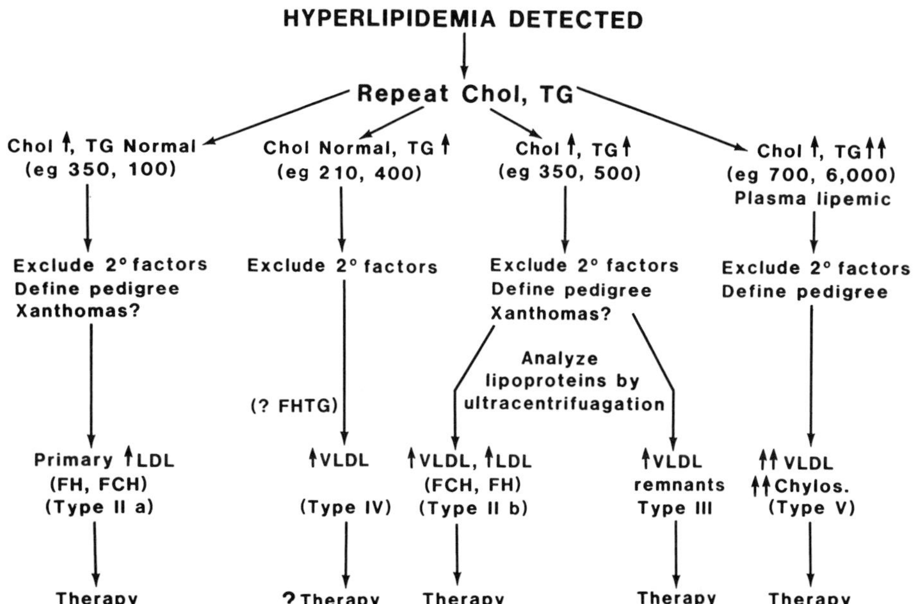

FIGURE 22-7 Algorithm for the progressive characterization and delineation of hyperlipidemia after its initial detection.

glycerides (>1000 mg/dl), in which the plasma appears lipemic (type I and type V phenotypes). In adult patients, such severe hypertriglyceridemia is invariably associated with increased plasma concentrations of both chylomicrons and VLDL particles. A fifth category of patients with dyslipidemia, who would not be identified on the basis of measurements of cholesterol and triglycerides alone, are patients with very low concentrations of HDL cholesterol who may also be at increased risk for developing coronary artery disease.[60] Disorders associated with variations in the plasma concentrations of HDL will be discussed later in this chapter.

Criteria for the Diagnosis of Hyperlipoproteinemia

In assessing the concentrations of lipids and lipoproteins in a given patient, it is important to consider the age of the patient and be familiar with the average concentrations of lipids and lipoproteins for that age and sex, in addition to the cutpoints recommended by expert panels for potential therapeutic intervention (Table 22-7).[61] Criteria for the diagnosis of hypercholesterolemia, with a particular emphasis on increased concentrations of LDL cholesterol, have been established, but these cutpoints are somewhat arbitrary and take into account the curvilinear relation between increased plasma concentrations of total and LDL cholesterol and the risk of coronary artery disease, which increases substantially when plasma cholesterol concentrations exceed 240 mg/dl or when LDL cholesterol concentrations exceed 160 mg/dl. The relation between serum cholesterol concentrations and the 6-year risk of coronary artery disease in 362,000 men studied in the MRFIT Study is illustrated in Fig. 22-8.[62]

The Consensus Conference on Lowering Blood Cholesterol to Prevent Heart Disease recommended that dietary modifications and potential drug therapy should be considered in adult patients in whom plasma concentrations of total cholesterol exceed the 90th percentile.[63] In this report, moderate hypercholesterolemia was defined as plasma cholesterol concentrations between the 75th and 90th percentiles. More recently, several expert panels in the United States,[64] Europe,[65] the United Kingdom,[66] and Canada[67] have defined more specific cutpoints for the diagnosis of hypercholesterolemia in adults and have made recommendations concerning concentrations of LDL cholesterol above which diet and drug therapy should be considered. The expert panels have concluded that desirable levels of total cholesterol for adults in western societies are under 200 mg/dl, and for most patients in this category further characterization of lipoproteins is not generally advocated. With the caveat that these recommendations will fail to detect patients with atypically low concentrations of HDL cholesterol in whom total cholesterol concentrations remain below 200 mg/dl, the latter value is an appropriate goal of therapy for patients who do not have evidence of coronary or peripheral vascular disease and who do not have a family history of premature atherosclerosis.

The Expert Panel of the National Cholesterol Education Program recommended determination of total cholesterol concentrations in serum or plasma for all adult patients in the United States.[64] Further decisions are based on the initial total plasma cholesterol concentrations and take into account the

TABLE 22-7 Average Values for Lipids and Lipoproteins in American Men and Women*

Age, years	Total Plasma Cholesterol	LDL Cholesterol	HDL Cholesterol	Total Plasma Triglyceride
		Men		
20–24	162 (212)†	103 (147)	45 (63)	89 (165)
25–29	179 (234)	117 (165)	45 (63)	104 (204)
30–34	193 (258)	126 (185)	46 (63)	122 (253)
35–39	201 (267)	133 (189)	43 (62)	141 (316)
40–44	205 (260)	136 (186)	44 (67)	152 (318)
45–49	213 (275)	144 (202)	45 (64)	143 (279)
50–54	213 (274)	142 (197)	44 (63)	154 (313)
		Women		
20–24	162	98	52	68
25–29	174 (22)	106 (151)	56 (81)	71 (128)
30–34	174 (220)	109 (148)	55 (75)	74 (138)
35–39	186 (251)	119 (173)	56 (82)	89 (174)
40–44	196 (253)	125 (174)	57 (87)	92 (179)
45–49	205 (167)	130 (188)	58 (86)	105 (192)
50–54	222 (292)	145 (214)	60 (89)	112 (214)
55–59	231 (296)	150 (212)	60 (86)	132 (280)

* Data obtained from 11 communities across the United States.[61]

† Values given in milligrams per deciliter are means and 95th percentiles (in parentheses) for white men and women.

presence or absence of atherosclerosis and other cardiovascular risk factors in determining the recommendations for specific therapy. Measurement of lipoprotein concentrations (LDL and HDL cholesterol) were advocated in patients with known cardiovascular disease or in those with two or more established cardiovascular risk factors in whom total cholesterol levels ranged between 200 and 239 mg/dl and were recommended in all patients in whom initial concentrations of total cholesterol exceeded 240 mg/dl. The NCEP Panel considered desirable concentrations of LDL cholesterol to be <130 mg/dl, borderline elevations to be between 130 and 159 mg/dl, and high-risk concentrations of LDL cholesterol to be greater than 160 mg/dl.[64] Some authorities have recommended an additional classification of "severe hypercholesterolemia" to identify patients in need of the most aggressive intervention.[68] This is illustrated in Table 22-8. The second revision of the NCEP Guidelines was published in 1994.[64]

The NCEP Expert Panel has provided a guideline for the concentrations of total and LDL cholesterol above which diet and drug therapy are recommended (Table 22-9). These recommendations should be considered as guidelines, and in specific patients a more or less aggressive approach may be justified depending on the age, the family history, and the potential benefit to be derived from diet and drug therapy. A particularly aggressive approach is indicated in patients with known coronary atherosclerosis in whom concentrations of LDL cholesterol less than 100 mg/dl may be necessary if no further progression of atherosclerosis and, potentially, some regression are to occur.[69,70]

Despite a broad consensus on the criteria for the diagnosis and potential treatment of hypercholesterolemia, the significance and treatment of isolated

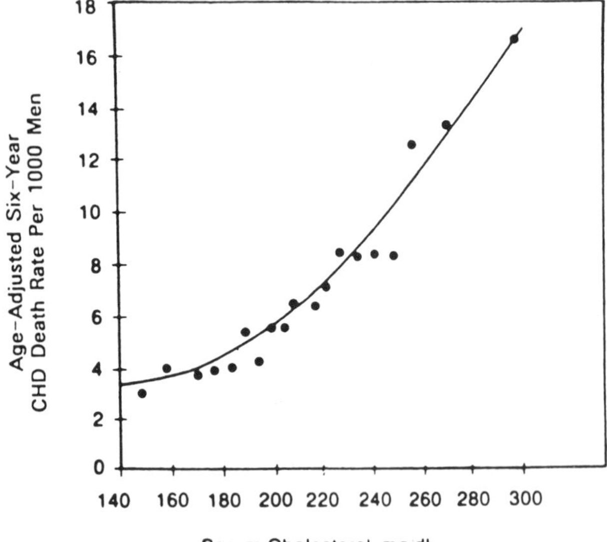

FIGURE 22-8 Relation between serum cholesterol concentrations and death from coronary artery disease in 361,662 men age 35 to 57 during an average follow-up of 6 years in MRFIT screens. Each point represents a medium value for 5 percent of the population. *(From Ref. 62.)*

TABLE 22-8 Classification of Plasma Total and LDL Cholesterol

	Total Cholesterol, mg/dl	LDL Cholesterol, mg/dl	Relative CHD Risk
Desirable serum cholesterol	<200	<130	<1.0
Borderline-high serum cholesterol	200–239	130–159	1.0–2.0
High serum cholesterol	>240	>160	
Moderate hypercholesterolemia	240–289	160–209	2.0–4.0
Severe hypercholesterolemia	>290	>210	>4.0

LDL = low density lipoprotein; CHD = coronary heart disease.

Source: Adapted from Grundy.[68]

hypertriglyceridemia remains controversial.[71,72] Two consensus conferences on hypertriglyceridemia[73,74] have concluded that borderline hypertriglyceridemia occurs in patients with plasma triglyceride concentrations between 250 and 500 mg/dl and that distinct (overt) hypertriglyceridemia occurs in patients in whom triglyceride concentrations exceed 500 mg/dl. Severe hypertriglyceridemia can be considered to be present when plasma triglyceride concentrations exceed 1000 mg/dl. A significant relation has been observed between hypertriglyceridemia and increased risk for coronary artery disease in some, but not all, studies in which multivariate statistical analysis have been performed and in which concentrations of total and LDL cholesterol have been controlled. However, in studies that have also controlled for HDL cholesterol concentrations, this association has often disappeared, particularly in studies involving men. In contrast, studies in women and in patients with diabetes have demonstrated significant positive univariate relations between plasma triglyceride concentrations and the risk for premature development of atherosclerosis.[75] Treatment guidelines for the institution of diet and drug therapy in patients with hypertriglyceridemia have not been precisely formulated, but in the opinion of the authors, dietary therapy is appropriate for patients with triglyceride concentrations which exceed 250 to 300 mg/dl and drug therapy should be considered in patients without cardiovascular disease or diabetes in whom the levels of triglycerides exceed 800 to 1000 mg/dl, with a goal of therapy being to reduce the increased risk of hepatic steatosis and, potentially, pancreatitis. Drug therapy may also be appropriate in individual patients with more modest degrees of hypertriglyceridemia in the setting of familial combined hyperlipidemia or in patients with known cardiovascular disease who concurrently have low levels of HDL cholesterol. An aggressive approach to the treatment of hypertriglyceridemia in patients with diabetes also appears to be justified, although clinical trials to document benefit from such therapy have not been conducted.

The recent report of the expert panel on blood cholesterol levels in children and adolescents has defined concentrations of total and LDL cholesterol which should be considered as acceptable, borderline, and high.[76] Acceptable concentrations of total and LDL cholesterol were defined as less than 170 and 110 mg/dl, respectively, and borderline elevations were considered to be present when the total cholesterol ranged between 170 and 199 mg/dl, with LDL values between 110 and 129 mg/dl, whereas hypercholesterolemia was considered to be present in children whose total plasma cholesterol concentrations exceeded 200 mg/dl and in whom LDL exceeded 130 mg/dl. The panel did not establish guidelines for the diagnosis of hypertriglyceridemia. The pediatric panel recommended that dietary therapy be the mainstay of treatment in children but that drug therapy be considered in children age 10 years or older in whom, after adequate trials of dietary

TABLE 22-9 Treatment Decisions Based on LDL Cholesterol

	Initiation Level, mg/dl	Minimal Goal, mg/dl
Dietary treatment		
Without CHD and <2 other risk factors	>160	<160
Without CHD but with >2 other risk factors	>130	<130
With CHD	>100	<100
Drug therapy		
Without CHD and <2 other risk factors after diet	>190	<160
Without CHD but with ≥2 other risk factors after diet	>160	<130
With CHD after diet	>130	<100

Source: Adapted from The Second Report of the National Cholesterol Education Program Expert Panel on Detection, Evaluation, and Treatment of High Blood Cholesterol in Adults.[64]

therapy, LDL cholesterol concentrations remained greater than 190 mg/dl in children with fewer than two cardiovascular risk factors or greater than 160 mg/dl in those with a strongly positive family history of coronary artery disease or two or more risk factors. In the opinion of the authors, these guidelines for drug therapy are too aggressive and, if widely instituted, would lead to the excessive use of hypolipidemic drugs in this population. We believe that additional factors, including the sex of the child (treat boys more aggressively than girls) and plasma concentrations of Lp(a), should be taken into consideration before the institution of drug therapy in children whose LDL cholesterol concentrations remain less than 220 to 250 mg/dl on dietary therapy.

In addition to criteria for the diagnosis of hyperlipidemia in children and adults, the NCEP panel and the recent Consensus Conference on Hypertriglyceridemia have both recommended that concentrations of HDL cholesterol below 35 mg/dl should be considered abnormally low. Hygienic measures are the cornerstone of therapy for patients with low concentrations of HDL cholesterol which frequently coexists with hypertriglyceridemia. Current data do not support the use of drugs aimed solely at increasing plasma concentrations of HDL cholesterol in the absence of concurrent elevated levels of LDL cholesterol or, in selected patients, hypertriglyceridemia.

Secondary Hyperlipidemias

Dietary

The majority of hyperlipidemias in western societies are secondary to other conditions. Among the secondary hyperlipidemias (Table 22-10), the most common cause is dietary. Dietary hypercholesterolemia affects an appreciable proportion of the American population and begins early in life, as witness the much higher plasma cholesterol concentrations in American children compared with children in other cultures. American children have a mean plasma cholesterol level of 168 mg/dl, compared with the Mexican Tarahumara Indian children, who consume a low-fat diet and have cholesterol levels of 118 mg/dl.[77] Tarahumara adults have values that are only a little higher than the levels in children (136 mg/dl). In contrast, among Americans, there is a much greater rise with age—a mean value of about 250 mg/dl among adults (Fig. 22-9) which continues to at least age 55 to 60 years.[78] This rise of plasma cholesterol with age is believed to be caused by a functional impairment of the LDL receptor.[79] As a group, American children and adults have much higher levels of blood cholesterol than are observed in many nonwestern societies. A major cause of this difference is the increased amount of fat, cholesterol, and excess calories in the American diet. This relation in adults is illustrated in Fig. 22-10.[61,64]

The factors that contribute to dietary hyperlipidemia include the intake of total fat, saturated fat, dietary cholesterol, and excessive calories. Among these dietary factors, the intake of total fat and saturated fat appears to exert the greatest influence on the serum cholesterol level. Dietary cholesterol is the next most important factor, particularly when the total intake is less than 300 to 400 mg per day, as shown in Fig. 22-25. Excessive caloric intake is typically manifested as obesity. Dietary deficiency of fiber is a minor contributor to hyperlipidemia. These factors are discussed further in the section on the dietary treatment of hyperlipidemia.

TABLE 22-10 Primary versus Secondary Hyperlipidemia

Primary: Genetic
Secondary
Diet; excessive saturated fat, cholesterol, or calories
Diabetes mellitus
Alcohol
Drug-induced: corticosteroids, estrogens, thiazides, beta blockers, 13-*cis*-retinoic acid (isotretinoin, Accutane)
Hypothyroidism
Nephrotic syndrome
Chronic renal failure
Biliary obstruction; primary biliary cirrhosis
Cushing's syndrome
Acromegaly
Dysglobulinemia; multiple myeloma
Autoimmune disease
Glycogen storage disease
Acute intermittent porphyria
Anorexia nervosa
Hepatoma

Diabetes

The next most common cause of secondary hyperlipidemia is diabetes mellitus. The hyperlipidemia associated with diabetes appears to be due in part to insulin deficiency (relative or absolute) and/or insulin resistance. Consequently, individuals with impaired glucose tolerance who have hyperinsulinemia without significant hyperglycemia may exhibit a pattern of hyperlipidemia that is typical for diabetic patients.

Patients with diabetes mellitus have a two- to sixfold increase in the risk of developing atherosclerosis. Part of this risk is attributable to the associated hyperlipidemia, but other risk factors are also contributory. Thus, diabetic patients deserve careful monitoring and treatment of other risk factors for atherosclerosis, including hypertension, smoking, obesity, and dietary excesses of saturated fat, cholesterol, and calories. The risk of atherosclerosis is severely accelerated in patients with proteinuria and possibly in those with microalbuminuria. The risk of atherosclerosis in women with diabetes appears to be nearly identical to the risk in diabetic men despite

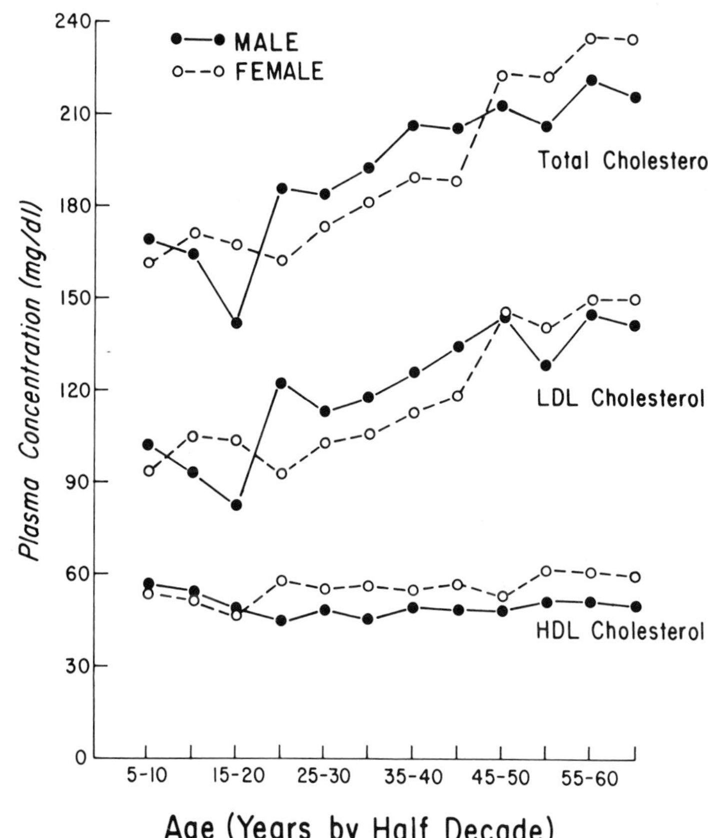

FIGURE 22-9 Age-related changes in the plasma concentrations of total, high-density, and low-density lipoprotein cholesterol in men and women age 6 to 65 years. Data derived from lipid analyses on 619 subjects residing in Portland, Oregon. (*Reproduced from Connor et al.*[78] *with permission.*)

FIGURE 22-10 Estimated effect of conversion to a phase I diet. Curve A represents the typical distribution of cholesterol levels among middle-aged (40 to 44 years) American men.[61] Curve B represents the hypothetical effects of conversion of all individuals from a typical American diet (about 37% fat, 400 mg cholesterol) to a phase I American Heart Association diet (<30% fat, <300 mg cholesterol).[64] For women in the same age group, curves A and B are shifted to the left by about 10 mg/dl.

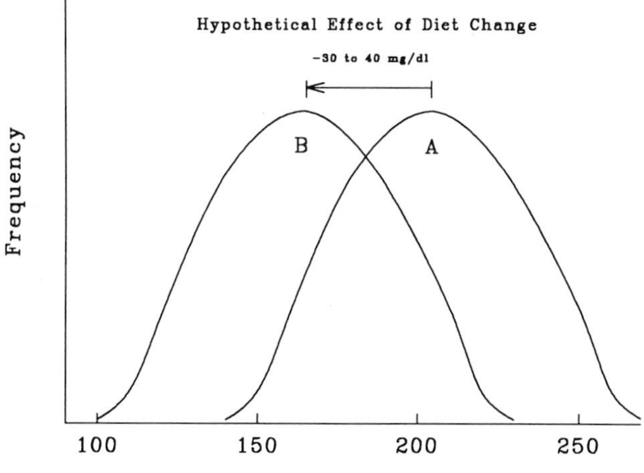

the relative resistance to atherosclerosis that is observed in nondiabetic women.

Because the abnormalities in lipid metabolism in diabetes include both qualitative (i.e., functional) and quantitative (e.g., hypertriglyceridemia) changes, the term *dyslipidemia* is often applied to this syndrome. The severity of dyslipidemia in diabetic patients is influenced by the type of diabetes, [non-insulin-dependent (NIDDM) or insulin-dependent diabetes mellitus (IDDM)], the severity of hyperglycemia, the degree of insulin deficiency, and the underlying genetic predisposition to hyperlipidemia.

Diabetic patients with dyslipidemia may be divided into the following groups:

IDDM with Ketoacidosis

Diabetic ketoacidosis (DKA) is associated with an overproduction of VLDL and impaired clearance of VLDL and chylomicrons from plasma. In some patients, this may lead to a type IV or V pattern of hyperlipidemia.

The overproduction of triglyceride and VLDL is primarily the result of an increased flux of FFA from insulin-deficient adipocytes to the liver. The extremely high circulating levels of FFA (800 to 1600 mEq/L) are derived from lipolysis of adipose tissue triglyceride and correlate directly with the blood glucose levels. When glucose cannot enter the cells because of absolute or relative insulin deficiency, the endocrine and biochemical effects are those of starvation. Triglyceride in adipose tissue cells undergoes lipolysis, and plasma FFA levels increase greatly to provide this alternative source of energy for the working cells of the body. FFA elevations may also promote vascular damage and platelet aggregation, although the clinical significance of this tendency to thrombosis has not been elucidated.

The decrease in the clearance of VLDL and chylomicrons in DKA occurs because the activity of the enzyme LPL, which is responsible for the clearance of triglyceride from VLDL and chylomicrons, is diminished in insulin-deficient states. When DKA occurs in a patient with baseline hypertriglyceridemia greater than 400 to 500 mg/dl (4.52 to 5.65 mmol/L), the triglyceride level may increase to over 5000 to 10,000 mg/dl (56.5 to 112.9 mmol/L) and lead to pancreatitis.

Correction of the ketoacidotic state by administering insulin will promptly ameliorate the hyperlipidemia. Since DKA is a temporary state, it does not present a long-term management problem.

Poorly Controlled Diabetes

Poorly controlled IDDM or NIDDM is an insulin-deficient state that can be associated with persistent combined hyperlipidemia that is similar to the type observed in DKA. The predominant lipoprotein abnormality is hypertriglyceridemia, which reflects the increased levels in plasma of VLDL and VLDL remnants. The reason for the hyperlipidemia relates both to insulin deficiency at the cellular level, with impaired LPL action and reduced clearance of VLDL triglyceride, and to increased production of triglyceride, the latter propagated both by elevated concentrations of FFA and by excessive caloric intake. Increased synthesis of cholesterol and its accumulation in LDL also occurs in such patients.[80] The qualitative abnormalities in these patients, particularly those with NIDDM, may include the presence of small dense VLDL, increased IDL (including remnants of VLDL and chylomicrons), small dense LDL (with or without an increase in the level of LDL cholesterol), decreased levels of HDL_2, and possibly increased levels of Lp(a). Each of these abnormalities is atherogenic.

Well-Controlled Diabetes

Patients with well-controlled IDDM tend to be normolipidemic or may have slightly increased levels of HDL cholesterol. In contrast, patients with well-controlled NIDDM tend to have persistent qualitative lipoprotein abnormalities, although the hyperlipidemia is improved compared with the uncontrolled diabetic state. The activity of LPL tends to be normal and the production of VLDL is only mildly elevated, but the stigmata of diabetes-associated dyslipidemia may be present. These abnormalities may include the presence of small dense VLDL, increased IDL, small dense LDL, and decreased HDL_2.

Several other abnormalities in lipoprotein metabolism may be present. Nonenzymatic glycation of apoproteins in LDL and HDL occurs in the hyperglycemic state[81] and may be associated with potentially atherogenic functional abnormalities in these lipoproteins.[82,83] The results of other preliminary studies have suggested that the diabetic state may also be associated with the following conditions: abnormalities in CETP activity and reverse cholesterol transport, a possibly increased tendency for oxidative modification of LDL, increased trapping of LDL in the subendothelial space, and enhanced accumulation of cholesteryl ester from LDL by macrophages in the artery wall. Further studies must be done to confirm the validity and significance of these observations.

Diet-Induced Hyperlipidemia

The typical diet of high fat, high saturated fat, high cholesterol, and relatively low carbohydrate still in use in some diabetic patients may result in hypercholesterolemia. While there has been some moderation of this dietary approach, there still is a tendency to shun carbohydrate in the diet and to prefer a diet high in animal fat. This may lead to increased LDL production and levels. The underlying etiology of the profound atherosclerotic complications of diabetes is thus not appropriately recognized.

Coexisting Genetic Hyperlipidemia

A further cause of hyperlipidemia in diabetic patients is the coexistence with diabetes of primary genetic hyperlipidemias, the most common of which are familial hypertriglyceridemia and familial combined hyperlipidemia. Thus, the abnormalities which may be found in diabetic patients with dyslipidemia are diverse and include both qualitative and quantitative abnormalities. Increases in chylomicrons, VLDL, remnants and IDL, small dense LDL, Lp(a), and FFA may occur, and HDL levels are frequently decreased. The characteristics of dyslipidemia in diabetes are influenced by the type of diabetes, the severity of insulin deficiency and hyperglycemia, and underlying genetic and environmental factors. Diabetic patients with a coexisting genetic cause of hyperlipidemia usually have the most severe hyperlipidemia.

Hypothyroidism

Apart from diabetes, hypothyroidism constitutes the most frequently seen endocrine disorder associated with secondary hyperlipidemia. The results of several studies, including a review of patients in the Lipid Disorders Clinic at the Oregon Health Sciences

University, have suggested that 2 to 4 percent of patients with hyperlipidemia have hypothyroidism.[84,85] The majority of these patients were not identified as clinically hypothyroid, despite thyroid stimulating hormone (TSH) levels over 20 μU/ml.

Any of the lipoprotein phenotypes may occur in hypothyroidism, but elevations of plasma cholesterol in the range of 250 to 600 mg/dl (6.5 to 15.5 mmol/L) with or without associated triglyceride elevation occur most commonly, i.e., a IIa or IIb pattern. Types IV, III, and V occur with decreasing frequency. The degree of hyperlipidemia shows a positive correlation with the severity of hypothyroidism. If hypothyroidism occurs concurrently with familial hyperlipidemia, the plasma lipid elevations are more extreme. Indeed, young patients with the heterozygous form of familial hypercholesterolemia and hypothyroidism may present with lipid values and xanthomas resembling those seen in homozygous familial hypercholesterolemia.[86]

The mechanisms responsible for the hyperlipidemia of hypothyroidism include reduced high-affinity receptor-mediated catabolism of LDL,[87] lower biliary excretion of cholesterol and bile acids, and decreased LPL activity. These factors more than counteract a concomitant decrease in cholesterol biosynthesis.

The dramatic lipid-lowering response which accompanies thyroid hormone replacement is particularly gratifying. Plasma cholesterol values as high as 350 mg/dl (9.05 mmol/L) frequently return to normal within 4 to 6 weeks of full-replacement doses of thyroxine and begin to decline within days of the initiation of therapy. It is the authors' practice and recommendation to screen most hyperlipidemic patients for hypothyroidism in order not to overlook this rewarding but easily missed diagnosis.

Renal Disease

Hyperlipidemia is common in renal disease and may be manifested by a variety of lipid and lipoprotein abnormalities.[88] Three categories of hyperlipidemic renal patients may be observed: uremic patients undergoing dialysis; renal-transplant patients receiving immunosuppressive therapy with corticosteroids, azathioprine, and/or cyclosporine; and nephrotic patients.

The characteristic abnormality in patients undergoing dialysis is hypertriglyceridemia with an increase in VLDL resulting in a type IV pattern. These patients have reduced clearance of triglyceride from the plasma, presumably because LPL activity is reduced. Transplant patients most frequently have an elevation of LDL cholesterol with a type IIa pattern but commonly also show elevated levels of VLDL cholesterol and triglycerides with a type IV or IIb phenotype. Rarely, patients with type V hyperlipidemia have been observed after transplantation. While no mechanism for transplant hyperlipidemia has been described, it presumably is related to increased appetite, weight gain, and the use of corticosteroids. Cyclosporine is an additional cause of increased levels of LDL and total cholesterol.

Patients with the nephrotic syndrome frequently have a mixed form of hyperlipidemia with elevation of both plasma cholesterol and triglyceride levels (type IIb is the most common). The hyperlipidemia is roughly related to the severity of hypoalbuminemia associated with this syndrome. Remission of the nephrotic state invariably brings about correction of the hyperlipidemia.

The numbers of patients with renal hyperlipidemia have dramatically increased in the last few decades, with the development of dialysis and transplantation programs resulting in prolonged survival of patients with end-stage kidney disease. The major cause of death in these patients is atherosclerotic coronary heart disease. Carotid and aortoileofemoral atherosclerosis is also common and emphasizes the fact that therapeutic attention to the hyperlipidemic state is of great importance. The authors' experience indicates that the same principles of dietary management should be applied to patients with hyperlipidemia secondary to renal disease, especially among those with renal transplants. Hyperlipidemic transplantation patients should be offered the maximum in dietary treatment. In those in whom satisfactory control of hyperlipidemia has not been achieved, the use of lipid-lowering drugs is appropriate. The HMG CoA reductase inhibitors[89] or niacin may be efficacious in these patients.

An additional potential contributor to accelerated atherosclerosis in patients with renal failure may be the atherogenic particle lipoprotein (a) [Lp(a)]. The plasma level of Lp(a) is significantly elevated by unknown mechanisms in uremic patients. Levels of Lp(a) greater than from 20 to 30 mg/dl are associated with an increased risk of stroke, myocardial infarction, and peripheral vascular disease. Niacin appears to be the only medication that may reduce the level of Lp(a), but the benefits of a reduced level of Lp(a) remain unproven.

Bile Duct Obstruction, Alpha$_1$ Antitrypsin Deficiency

Hyperlipidemia invariably occurs when the flow of bile is impeded. This secondary hyperlipidemia is commonly seen in biliary cirrhosis and biliary atresia, with plasma cholesterol values over 1500 mg/dl not being unusual. Planar xanthomas frequently occur as a result of the severe hyperlipidemia. Less strikingly, a similar hyperlipidemia is also seen in biliary obstruction arising from other causes, such as obstruction of the common bile duct by a stone or tumor. This secondary hyperlipidemia typically remits as hepatocellular function becomes progressively impaired as a result of a diminished capacity for hepatic synthesis of lipoproteins. Hyperlipidemia has also occurred in a child with severe liver disease present at birth associated with $alpha_1$ antitrypsin deficiency.[90] Lipoprotein X was present, but the bilirubin was only midly elevated. Thus, liver disease per se in the absence of biliary obstruction may be a rare cause of the same lipoprotein abnormality seen with biliary obstruction.

The lipoprotein abnormality associated with biliary obstruction is a characteristic one that is termed *lipoprotein X*. This lipoprotein has beta-electrophoretic mobility but has an unusual lipid composition consisting of predominantly free cholesterol with greatly reduced cholesteryl esters. Although it is not routinely determined, plasma phospholipid is also greatly increased, whereas plasma triglyceride is only moderately elevated. Lipoprotein X can be characterized by immunologic techniques and is often diagnostic of biliary obstruction, but it may also be associated with rare forms of LCAT deficiency.

The etiology of this hyperlipidemia is related to impaired excretion of bile acids (and probably cholesterol) into bile. The level of serum bile acids becomes elevated, and the conversion of cholesterol to bile acids in the liver is decreased. The activity of the enzyme LCAT is also reduced and probably contributes to the reduced level of cholesteryl ester in plasma. Abnormal HDL particles which appear as disks instead of spheres under electron microscopy are present; the changed shape is believed to be due to the reduced content of cholesteryl ester. Cholestyramine may be used to control the itching these patients invariably have and may also reduce plasma lipid levels, but therapy is aimed primarily at correcting the underlying hepatic disease of biliary obstruction. Plasmapheresis may be useful to remove cholesterol in patients with xanthomatous neuropathy.

Alcohol

A common cause of hypertriglyceridemia in western societies is excessive alcohol intake.[88] Considerable variation exists in the plasma lipid response of a given individual to alcohol, as is discussed later, and only about 10 percent of patients who habitually abuse alcohol develop hyperlipidemia, usually with a type IV phenotype. Combined elevations of cholesterol and triglycerides (type IIb) also occur, as do cases with more severe hypertriglyceridemia and a type V phenotype. The latter pattern is most apt to occur in chronic alcohol abusers during periods of high fat intake and may lead to pancreatitis. Alternatively, patients with baseline plasma triglyceride levels of 600 to 1000 mg/dl (6.8 to 11.2 mmol/L) may develop severe chylomicronemia (type V) and pancreatitis after a brief period of high-volume alcohol consumption.

The mechanisms of alcohol-induced hyperlipidemia are complex and are related in part to the high caloric content. When alcohol is taken with food, the magnitude and duration of alimentary lipemia are increased; this increase appears to be due to an enhanced secretion of VLDL which occurs concomitantly with postprandial hyperchylomicronemia and results in a prolonged clearance of both particles. In the fasting state, alcohol also enhances hepatic synthesis and secretion of VLDL and is the main factor responsible for the development of the type IV phenotype. This occurs because the increased levels of nicotinamide adenine dinucleotide (NADH) which are produced during the metabolism of ethanol by alochol dehydrogenase inhibit oxidation of FFA and result in an enhanced synthesis of triglycerides and VLDL. Alcohol may also promote the induction of hepatic microsomal enzymes with a separate stimulatory effect on lipoprotein synthesis.

Drug-Induced Hyperlipoproteinemia

A number of drugs and hormones have been reported to have an adverse effect on plasma lipoprotein concentrations in humans (Table 22-11). In the case of glucocorticoids,[91,92] estrogen,[93] and 13-*cis*-retinoic acid (isotretinoin, Accutane),[98,99] the primary effect appears to be stimulation of VLDL production and an increase in the concentrations of triglyceride-rich lipoproteins. In patients with underlying familial hypertriglyceridemia, familial combined hyperlipidemia, or diabetes-associated hypertriglyceridemia, the use of these agents may result in a profound elevation in the concentration of serum triglyceride. In some patients, the triglyceride level may increase from a baseline of 600 to 800 mg/dl (6.8 to 9.0 mmol/L) to over 5000 mg/dl (56.5 mmol/L), resulting in clinical symptoms of abdominal pain, pancreatitis, and the development of eruptive xanthomas. The thiazide diuretics have also been reported

TABLE 22-11 The Influence of Drugs on Plasma Lipids and Lipoproteins

	Lipid/Lipoprotein				
Drug	Total Chol	TG	LDL Chol	HDL Chol	Reference
Corticosteroids	↑	↑↑	±↑	±↑	91,92
Estrogens	↑	↑	↓	↑	93
Progestins	±↑	±↑	±↑	↓	94
Androgens	↓	—	±↑	↓	95
Beta blockers (without ISI)	↑	↑	±↑	↓	96,97
Thiazide diuretics	↑	↑	±↑	↓	96,97
Vitamin A derivatives	±↑	↑↑	↓	↓	98,99
Cimetidine	±↑	↑	↓	↓	100
Cyclosporin	↑	—	↑	—	101
Phenytoin	↑	—	—	↑	102
Barbiturates		—	—	↑	102

TG = triglycerides; chol = cholesterol; ISI = intrinsic sympathomimetic activity.

to increase the concentrations of cholesterol and triglyceride, an effect that is attributable to increased concentrations of VLDL and LDL particles in plasma.[96,97] Beta-blocking agents such as propranolol may also cause plasma triglyceride concentrations to increase and may concurrently reduce HDL cholesterol levels.[96,97] Beta-blocking agents with intrinsic sympathomimetic activity (e.g., pindolol and labetalol) do not cause hyperlipidemia. Therapy with thiazide diuretics and beta blockers should be avoided in patients with known hyperlipidemia if other avenues of therapy are available.

HYPERCHOLESTEROLEMIA

Elevated levels of plasma cholesterol in the setting of normal triglyceride concentrations are usually attributable to an increased number of LDL particles in plasma. Less commonly, hypercholesterolemia reflects cholestasis in which an abnormal lipoprotein (LPX) accumulates or is seen in the occasional patient with an atypically high level of HDL cholesterol; in this case, no treatment is indicated (see Familial Hyperalphalipoproteinemia under Disorders of High-Density Lipoproteins). The causes of hypercholesterolemia may be divided into primary (genetic) etiologies, secondary causes, and a combination of the two. Evaluation of a patient with hypercholesterolemia should therefore include satisfactory exclusion of secondary factors and a detailed family history. The potential value of identifying asymptomatic children and young adults with primary hypercholesterolemia cannot be overemphasized if preventive therapeutic measures to minimize the future development of atherosclerosis are to be successful. Increased concentrations of LDL cholesterol with normal triglycerides can be seen in patients with familial hypercholesterolemia, familial combined hyperlipidemia, familial defective apolipoprotein B-100, and so-called polygenic hypercholesterolemia. Polygenic hypercholesterolemia is a poorly characterized disorder of unknown etiology in which affected adults display moderate hypercholesterolemia (220 to 280 mg/dl) without evidence of tendon xanthomas. Whether it is a distinct disorder has not been established.

Familial Hypercholesterolemia

Definition

This condition (synonyms: familial xanthomatous hypercholesterolemia, type IIa and IIb hyperlipoproteinemia, hyperbetalipoproteinemia) is characterized by increased LDL, or β-lipoproteins, which are the chief carriers of cholesterol and cholesteryl ester in the plasma. Consequently, the plasma cholesterol concentration is always moderately to profoundly elevated, with plasma triglyceride levels usually normal or low (type IIa) but at times elevated (type IIb). The cause of the hypercholesterolemia is related to a deficiency of LDL receptor function in the cells of the body, with the result that there is impairment of LDL removal from the plasma. Of all the hyperlipidemias, familial hypercholesterolemia especially is characterized clinically by premature atherosclerosis and coronary heart disease as well as by the occurrence of tuberous and tendon xanthomas.[103]

Clinical Characteristics

The heterozygous form of familial hypercholesterolemia represents one of the most common genetic causes of moderate to severe hypercholesterolemia in North America.[103] The disorder may be found at any age in either sex and may be diagnosed in the homozygous state during intrauterine life.[104] The chief clinical manifestations of this disease are the occurrence of xanthomatous deposits in the skin and tendons and greatly accelerated rates of atherosclerosis. The homozygous form of familial hypercholesterolemia is usually detected in childhood; affected patients have planar, tuberous, and tendon xanthomas during the first 5 years of life and in some cases may even be born with these skin manifestations. Plasma cholesterol concentrations in these patients are generally in excess of 600 to 700 mg/dl. Because of their inherently lower levels of total (240 to 450 mg/dl) and LDL cholesterol (160 to 400 mg/dl), children and young adults with heterozygous familial hypercholesterolemia frequently have no physical abnormalities.[105] Small planar xanthomas (slightly raised yellow lesions) may occasionally be seen in the digital webs or behind the knees. Recurrent episodes of Achilles tendonitis, usually exercise-related, occur in 50 to 75 percent of heterozygotes and frequently have their onset in the patient's late teens or early twenties.[106] These episodes are a reflection of the insidious deposition of LDL cholesterol in the tendons of patients with familial hypercholesterolemia and often precede clinical evidence of thickening or xanthomatous deposits in the Achilles tendons. These nodular lipid-rich lesions have a mild inflammatory tissue reaction and an associated collagen accumulation. Tendon xanthomas, which are the hallmark of familial hypercholesterolemia, become more prominent as the patient gets older, and their development is often accelerated by local trauma. In the experience of the authors, tendon xanthomas are also more prominent in patients with heterozygous familial hypercholesterolemia who concurrently have increased plasma concentrations of Lp(a). In adult patients with heterozygous familial hypercholesterolemia who are over age 30 to 35, tendon xanthomas are usually detectable by means of clinical examination. Tendon xanthomas characteristically involve the extensor tendons of the hands

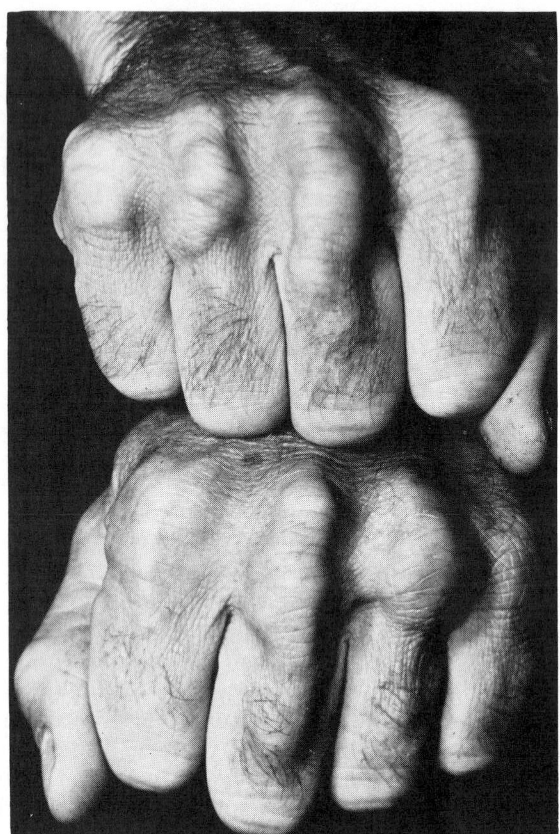

FIGURE 22-11 Tendon xanthomas in a patient with heterozygous familial hypercholesterolemia.

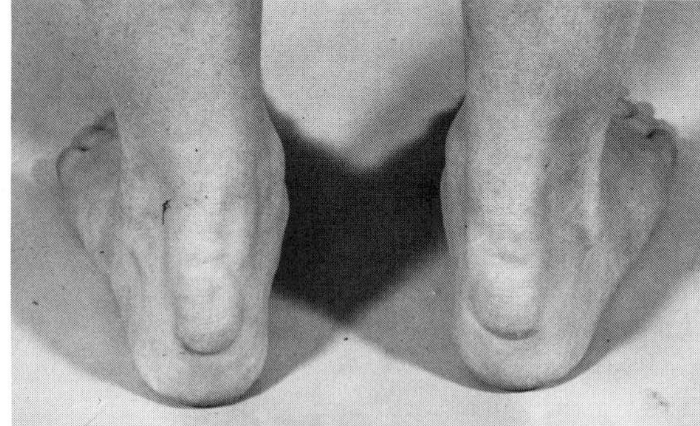

FIGURE 22-13 Xanthomas of the Achilles tendons in a patient with heterozygous familial hypercholesterolemia.

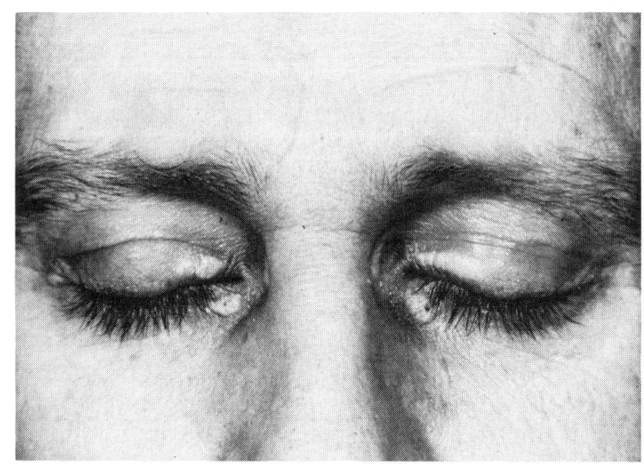

FIGURE 22-14 Xanthelasma in a patient with heterozygous familial hypercholesterolemia.

(Figs. 22-11 and 22-12), the olecranon tendon, the patellar tendon, and the Achilles tendon (Fig. 22-13). An increased thickening and nodularity of the Achilles tendon is often noted on palpation. Xanthelasmas (Fig. 22-14) are present in less than 20 percent of older patients[107] but are not specific for familial hypercholesterolemia, occurring frequently in patients with normal lipid values.[105] The presence of a corneal arcus (Fig. 22-15) in patients under age 35 years constitutes another external hallmark of familial hypercholesterolemia[105] but is surprisingly absent in some patients with severe hypercholesterolemia. In many patients, however, a long latent period with

FIGURE 22-12 The appearance of tendon xanthomas before surgical removal in a patient with heterozygous familial hypercholesterolemia.

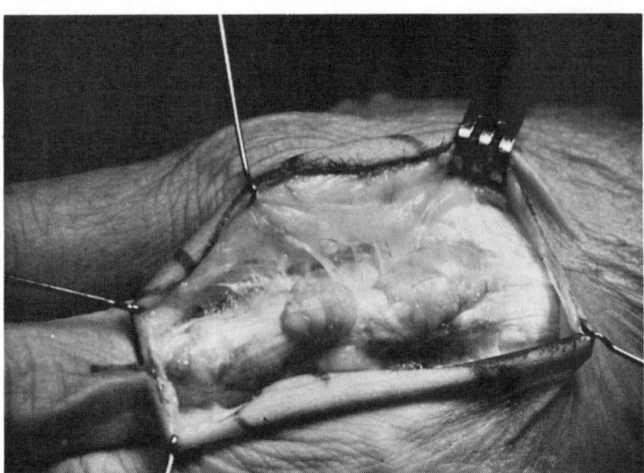

FIGURE 22-15 Corneal arcus in a young woman with heterozygous familial hypercholesterolemia.

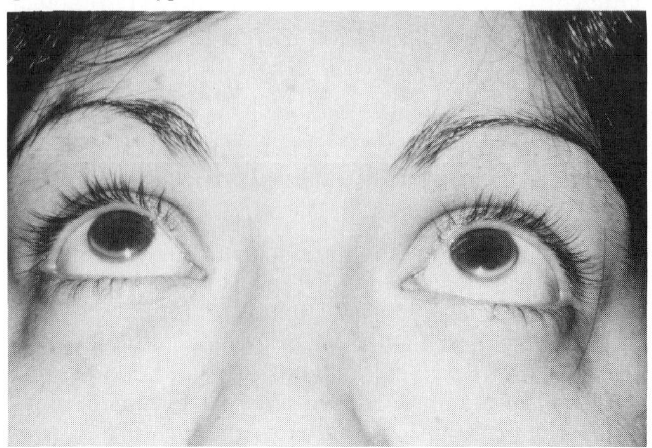

only hypercholesterolemia precedes the clinical manifestations of cholesterol accumulation in the tendons, skin, and arterial walls. Lipid accumulation in these tissues, however, tends to proceed in parallel, and manifestations of cardiovascular disease are more likely to be present in patients with prominent tendon xanthomas than in patients in whom such lesions are less conspicuous.[108]

The high incidence of premature coronary artery disease in patients with familial hypercholesterolemia has been well documented.[105,108–112] Homozygotes are the most severely affected individuals and develop symptoms of coronary atherosclerosis by 10 to 15 years of age.[103] Myocardial infarction has been reported at 1½ and 3 years of age.[113,114] In addition to precocious coronary artery disease, patients with homozygous familial hypercholesterolemia are also predisposed to both valvular and supravalvular aortic stenosis[115,116] and to atherosclerosis of the carotid and femoral arteries. Premature coronary artery disease is also characteristic of patients with heterozygous familial hypercholesterolemia; it is influenced by the magnitude of hypercholesterolemia, family history, and other cardiovascular risk factors and is also higher in patients who concurrently have increased plasma concentrations of Lp(a).[117,118] Unlike the situation in homozygotes, among whom vascular complications appear to be similar in men and women, the predilection for atherosclerosis is greater in men. The average age of onset for symptomatic coronary artery disease is 40 to 45 years in men and 50 to 60 years in women with heterozygous familial hypercholesterolemia (Table 22-12). Angiographic studies have also disclosed a higher than expected incidence of proximal lesions of the coronary arteries, including left main coronary artery disease, in patients with familial hypercholesterolemia.[119,120]

Diagnostic Laboratory Features

It must be stressed that many individuals with hypercholesterolemia resulting from elevated plasma levels of LDL will not have a distinctly definable genetic disorder and will have hypercholesterolemia on the basis of dietary or other secondary factors. These patients in general have plasma cholesterol concentrations which are lower than those of the genetically affected individuals, although severe hypercholesterolemia may be seen in association with both hypothyroidism and renal disease. Patients with familial hypercholesterolemia in the heterozygous form usually present with elevated levels of total and LDL cholesterol and normal levels of plasma triglycerides. Concentrations of HDL cholesterol are infrequently reduced by 5 to 10 mg/dl in heterozygotes and are even lower in homozygotes.[121] Plasma cholesterol levels in heterozygous patients generally range from 280 to 550 mg/dl in adults, and in homozygous patients they generally exceed 600 mg/dl during childhood. These increases correlate with increased concentrations of LDL cholesterol. Although not associated with other metabolic disorders, the concurrent presence of familial hypercholesterolemia with obesity, diabetes, or renal disease often results in increased triglyceride levels and the expression of a type IIb phenotype. Similarly, the coexistence of heterozygous familial hypercholesterolemia and another primary disorder of lipid metabolism (e.g., familial combined hyperlipidemia),[122] type III hyperlipoproteinemia,[123] or a secondary disorder such as hypothyroidism or the nephrotic syndrome may lead to more profound elevations of total cholesterol (often exceeding 500 to 600 mg/dl) than are usually seen in patients with heterozygous familial hypercholesterolemia alone.

TABLE 22-12 Coronary Artery Disease in Familial Hypercholesterolemia

	Mean Age for Onset of Coronary Artery Disease	Chance of Myocardial Infarction Before		
		Age 30, %	Age 50, %	Age 60, %
Men	40	5	50	85
Women	55	<1	15	50

Source: Data from Refs. 105, 108–112.

Pathophysiology

Major insights into the biochemical basis of familial hypercholesterolemia have been provided by the elegant studies of Goldstein and Brown. These investigators have proceeded from the initial demonstration of specific membrane receptors for LDL on normal cultured fibroblasts and their absence in cells cultured from patients with homozygous familial hypercholesterolemia to delineation of the molecular heterogeneity of the cellular abnormalities in familial hypercholesterolemia[124] and, most recently, delineation of the precise gene defects in cells from different patients with homozygous familial hypercholesterolemia.[125] The structure and functional domains of the human LDL-receptor are illustrated in Fig. 22-16. Specific mutations which have been identified in the LDL-receptor gene and result in impaired LDL-receptor function with a concurrent clinical phenotype of familial hypercholesterolemia are illustrated in Fig. 22-17. As previously discussed, specific high-affinity LDL receptors appear to be present on virtually all cells, including hepatocytes and mononuclear leukocytes. From the pathophysiologic point of view, the inability of cells in the body to incorporate LDL via the specific receptor pathway has a number of consequences, including an elevation in the concentration of LDL in plasma and an inappropriately higher rate of cellular cholesterol biosynthesis and LDL production from the liver. Pa-

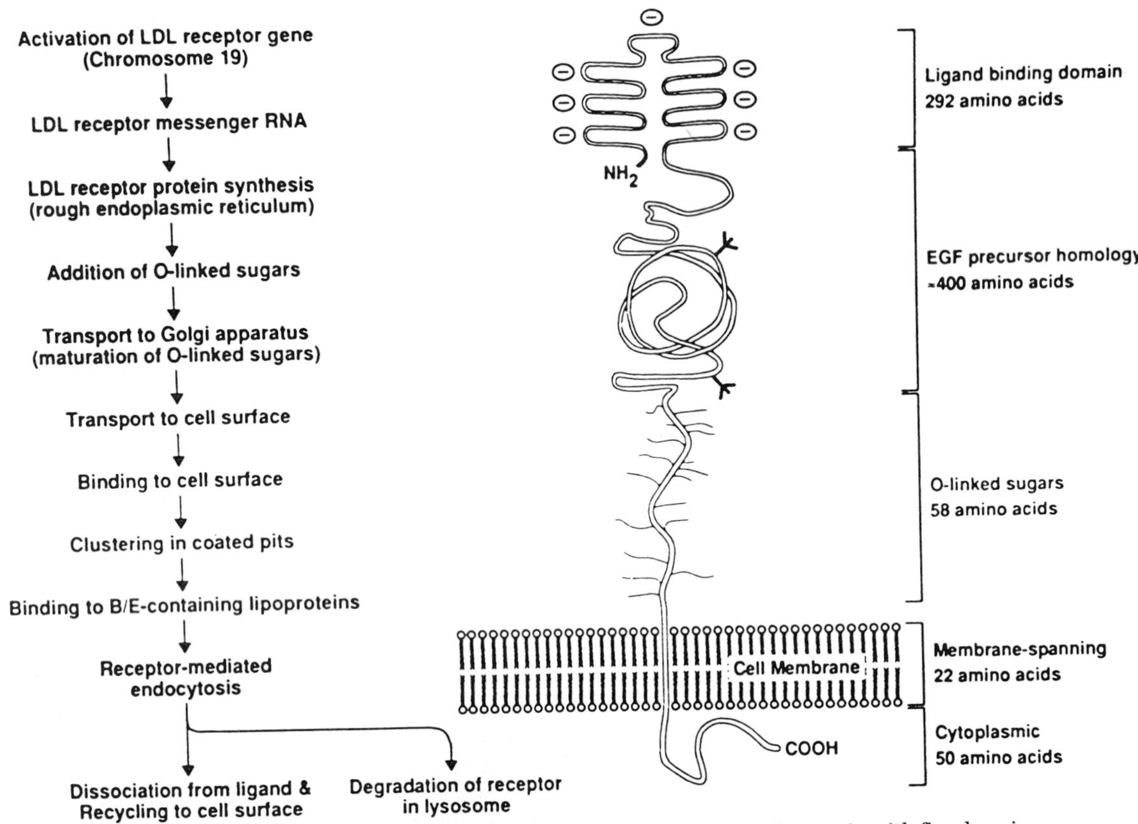

FIGURE 22-16 Structure of the mature human LDL receptor, a single protein with five domains. The pathway of synthesis, intracellular transport, and degradation of the LDL receptor is shown on the left, and the five different domains of the LDL receptor structure are shown on the right. *(Reproduced from Grundy and Vega[418] with permission.)*

tients with familial hypercholesterolemia show a decrease in the fractional rate of catabolism of LDL which is most marked in the homozygous state.[126] The biosynthesis of LDL, however, is normal or only modestly increased in heterozygotes but is two to three times greater than normal in homozygous patients.[126] Although genetic defects which reduce the number or functional capacity of LDL receptors explain the marked hypercholesterolemia in patients with familial hypercholesterolemia, the high rate of atherosclerosis which occurs in these patients clearly indicates that other non-receptor-mediated pathways must exist in which LDL cholesterol can be incorporated into cells. Such non-receptor-mediated pathways may be more important for the entry of LDL into certain cells (including macrophages)[127] and may contribute to the deposition of lipid in the arterial wall.

Genetics

Familial hypercholesterolemia is transmitted by an autosomal dominant mode of inheritance. Because this disorder is seldom lethal in the heterozygous form until after or during the childbearing period, the passage of the disorder from one generation to the next readily explains the large pedigrees of the disorder which have been described. The homozygous form may be diagnosed in utero by tissue culture studies of the LDL receptor in cells derived from the amniotic fluid[104] as well as in children or adults by means of skin biopsies with subsequent studies of the LDL-receptor mechanism in cultured skin fibroblasts or in patients in whom the precise gene defect is known by amplification of DNA obtained from white blood cells by the polymerase chain reaction and subsequent hybridization studies.[125] However, in most patients, this technique is not necessary; the diagnosis can be made on the basis of clinical and usual laboratory features. Only in the homozygote is such precise characterization desirable from the point of view of the demonstration of deficient LDL receptors.

To facilitate the detection of couples at risk for having a child with homozygous familial hypercholesterolemia, it is advisable to check lipid values in the spouses or future spouses of all young patients with known familial hypercholesterolemia. The incidence of heterozygous familial hypercholesterolemia is about 1 in 500 in Europe and North America but appears to be higher in certain population groups, most notably in the Afrikaans (Dutch) population of South Africa,[128] in Quebec, and in Lebanon.[129]

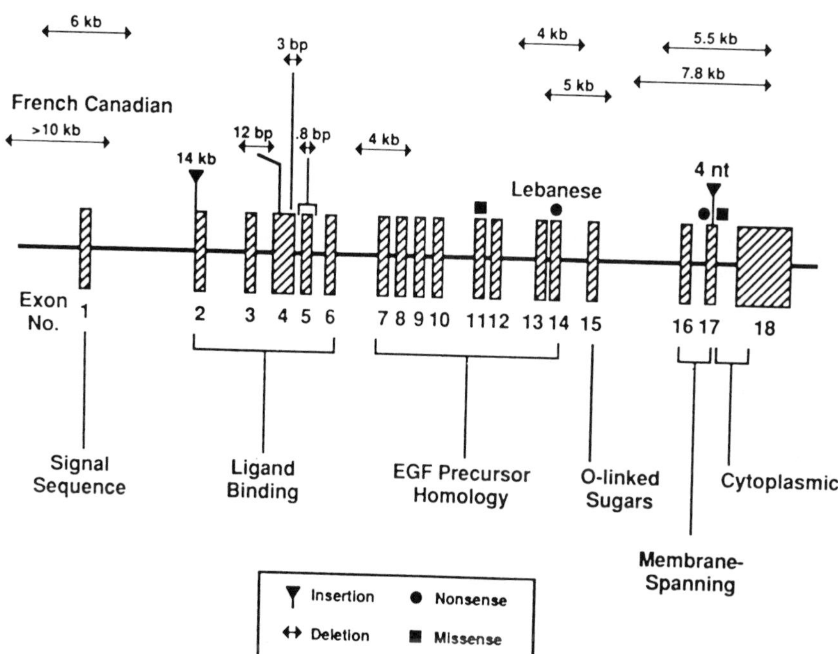

FIGURE 22-17 Location of mutations in the LDL receptor gene which cause familial hypercholesterolemia. Exons are represented by hatched boxes, and introns by lines between boxes. The sites of 16 mutations are indicated, and the key for the symbols is given in the box. (*Reproduced from Russell et al.[419] with permission.*)

Treatment

The increased predilection for premature coronary artery disease which occurs in patients with both heterozygous and homozygous familial hypercholesterolemia justifies the use of intensive treatment regimens to lower plasma LDL cholesterol concentrations with a view to preventing the premature development of atherosclerosis. Treatment in all patients should initially consist of the low-cholesterol, low-fat diet described in Dietary Treatment of Hyperlipidemia. In patients in whom plasma concentrations of total cholesterol are greater than 250 to 300 mg/dl, the response to dietary treatment may be most gratifying. However, in the vast majority of adult patients with heterozygous familial hypercholesterolemia, drug therapy in addition to intensive dietary treatment is almost always necessary. In the opinion of the authors, the goal of such therapy is to reduce the concentrations of LDL cholesterol to less than 130 to 160 mg/dl in adult patients with heterozygous familial hypercholesterolemia who do not have evidence of coronary artery disease and to less than 100 mg/dl in patients with evidence of atherosclerosis.

The development of specific competitive inhibitors of the rate-limiting enzyme in cholesterol biosynthesis, HMG CoA reductase, has provided an important and effective new avenue of therapy for adult patients with heterozygous familial hypercholesterolemia. At the present time, three of these drugs—lovastatin, simvastatin, and pravastatin—have been approved in North America, and one or more of these drugs is available in other countries throughout the world. As a class, the HMG CoA reductase inhibitors are the most effective agents available for the treatment of patients with elevated levels of LDL cholesterol. In patients with heterozygous familial hypercholesterolemia, lovastatin has been shown to reduce concentrations of LDL cholesterol by 17 to 40 percent at doses of 10 to 80 mg per day.[130,131] At the maximum dose of 40 mg per day, simvastatin has been shown to reduce LDL cholesterol concentrations by 37 to 44 percent,[132,133] whereas the same dose of pravastatin resulted in a mean decrease of 28 percent in the concentrations of LDL cholesterol in 40 patients with heterozygous familial hypercholesterolemia.[134] Considerable individual variability exists, however, in the magnitude of the LDL reduction attained in individual patients treated with HMG CoA reductase inhibitors.[130,132] To address the question "How effective is lovastatin as monotherapy in the treatment of adult patients with heterozygous familial hypercholesterolemia?" the efficacy of this drug at doses of 40 and 80 mg per day has been evaluated in patients attending our Lipid Disorders Clinic. In 69 men, mean concentrations of LDL cholesterol decreased from 301 mg/dl to 212 mg/dl during treatment, with 40 mg per day of lovastatin. However, the concentrations of LDL cholesterol remained above 200 mg/dl in 50.7 percent of the patients and fell to less than 160 mg/dl in only 11.6 percent and to less than 130 mg/dl in only 4.3 percent. Similar data from 83 women treated with the same dose of lovastatin indicated that mean concentrations of LDL cholesterol decreased from 294 mg/dl on diet to 196 mg/dl on lovastatin; 41 percent of the female patients had LDL concentrations exceeding 200 mg/dl, while the LDL values fell to under

160 mg/dl in 19.3 percent of the patients and to under 130 mg/dl in 7.2 percent. Similar analyses in patients treated with 80 mg per day of lovastatin indicated that as a group, female patients with heterozygous familial hypercholesterolemia responded better than their male counterparts but that in both groups of patients more than one-third maintained LDL cholesterol concentrations above 250 mg/dl during treatment with the maximum approved dose of lovastatin. These results indicate that single-drug therapy with maximal doses of lovastatin fails to achieve optimal control of hypercholesterolemia in the majority of adult patients with heterozygous familial hypercholesterolemia. However, these are the most effective agents available for the treatment of this disorder and, in the opinion of the authors, are an appropriate first-choice therapy to use in adult patients with heterozygous familial hypercholesterolemia; however, they should not be used in women who plan to have children in the near future or during pregnancy and lactation. The use of this class of drugs in pediatric patients with heterozygous familial hypercholesterolemia is investigational, and the drugs cannot be recommended for general use in the pediatric age group.

The bile acid–binding resins cholestyramine and colestipol are also drugs of first choice for the treatment of patients with heterozygous familial hypercholesterolemia. Notable exceptions include patients with a concurrent elevation in plasma triglyceride levels and patients with a history of severe constipation. Cholestyramine and colestipol are not absorbed and, in the opinion of the authors, are the drugs of first choice (if drug therapy is warranted) for pediatric patients with heterozygous familial hypercholesterolemia; such therapy should not be begun before 5 to 6 years of age and is most appropriate for patients with LDL concentrations exceeding 220 mg/dl on maximum dietary therapy. The dose response curves for both cholestyramine and colestipol are nonlinear, but in compliant patients these drugs reduce concentrations of LDL cholesterol by 23 to 36 percent when given at doses of 16 and 24 g per day in the case of cholestyramine or 20 to 30 g per day in the case of colestipol. An analysis of the hypolipidemic effect of colestipol as monotherapy (mean dose 21 g per day) in 38 patients with heterozygous familial hypercholesterolemia treated in our Lipid Disorders Clinic indicated that mean concentrations of LDL were reduced by 30 percent but that LDL concentrations remained greater than 190 mg/dl in 25 of the 38 patients and decreased to less than 160 mg/dl in only 3. These results indicate that in adult patients with heterozygous familial hypercholesterolemia, single-drug therapy with a bile acid sequestrant fails to achieve optimal concentrations of LDL cholesterol in the vast majority of cases.

Nicotinic acid (niacin) at doses of 3 to 6 g per day, taken in divided doses, is also an effective drug for adult patients with heterozygous familial hypercholesterolemia and is most appropriate to use as monotherapy in patients with concurrent hypertriglyceridemia. In the opinion of the authors, nicotinic acid should not be used in pediatric patients with heterozygous familial hypercholesterolemia. When used as monotherapy, nicotonic acid in doses of 3 to 8 g per day results in 15 to 40 percent decreases in the plasma concentrations of LDL cholesterol, with a modest increase in HDL concentrations. In 12 adult patients with heterozygous familial hypercholesterolemia treated in our Lipid Disorders Clinic who received a mean dose of 4.5 g per day (range: 3 to 6 g per day), concentrations of LDL cholesterol decreased from 318 mg/dl to 220 mg/dl (−30.8 percent), but in the group as a whole, they remained above 190 mg/dl in 9 of the 12 patients and decreased to under 160 mg/dl in only 1.[132]

Probucol is a modestly effective drug in the treatment of adult patients with heterozygous familial hypercholesterolemia and, at the recommended dose of 500 mg bid, reduces LDL cholesterol concentrations by 8 to 15 percent.[135] Individual patient response to probucol is, however, quite variable, and the use of this drug appears to be more effective in patients with homozygous familial hypercholesterolemia than it is in heterozygotes.[136] Despite a modest ability to lower LDL concentrations, however, probucol has been shown to cause regression of tendon xanthomas in patients with both homozygous and heterozygous familial hypercholesterolemia.[137]

Gemfibrozil and clofibrate have been shown to reduce concentrations of LDL cholesterol by less than 10 percent in patients with heterozygous familial hypercholesterolemia and cannot be recommended for general use in this disorder. Newer fibrate drugs, including fenofibrate, bezafibrate, and ciprofibrate, are, however, more effective, and with these three drugs, decreases in LDL cholesterol concentrations ranging from 18 to 30 percent have been observed.[132]

The effectiveness of a number of combined drug regimens which take advantage of the different mechanisms of action of the most effective LDL-lowering drugs have been evaluated in a number of clinical trials in adult patients with heterozygous familial hypercholesterolemia. The majority of these studies have utilized combinations which include one of the bile acid sequestrants (which act to increase sterol excretion) in combination with drugs that act to reduce the synthesis of VLDL and/or LDL (e.g., nicotinic acid) or agents which inhibit hepatic cholesterol biosynthesis (e.g., lovastatin, simvastatin, and pravastatin). Referral to a lipid specialist is appropriate for the optimal management of patients with severe heterozygous familial hypercholesterolemia in whom combination drug therapy is required. The efficacy of the combined drug regimens in the treatment of adult patients with heterozygous familial hypercholesterolemia is summarized in Table 22-13.

A number of surgical techniques have been used to treat patients with both heterozygous and homozygous familial hypercholesterolemia, but none can be generally recommended. In patients with heterozygous familial hypercholesterolemia, distal ileal bypass surgery, with surgical resection of the distal 200 cm of the ileum, has been reported to reduce concentrations of LDL cholesterol by 30 to 40 percent,[145] but this operation is ineffective in patients with homozygous familial hypercholesterolemia.[146] Distal ileal bypass surgery may be an appropriate treatment option for selected patients with heterozygous familial hypercholesterolemia who are intolerant to bile acid sequestrant therapy and in whom additional drug therapy with lovastatin may lead to overall reductions in LDL cholesterol greater than 50 percent.[147] Recent data have indicated that ileal bypass surgery leads to a reduction in cardiovascular morbidity and mortality,[148] but the individual hypolipidemic response to this surgical procedure is variable, and in the opinion of the authors, it cannot be generally recommended. LDL-apheresis may be appropriate for selected patients with severe heterozygous familial hypercholesterolemia in whom optimal drug therapy fails to reduce LDL cholesterol concentrations to less than 160 mg/dl.[149]

Intensive therapeutic intervention is necessary to reduce the severely elevated plasma concentrations of total and LDL cholesterol in patients with homozygous familial hypercholesterolemia. However, these patients, particularly those who are true homozygotes with no functional LDL receptors, respond poorly to single-drug therapy or combination drug therapy and invariably require other adjunctive measures to optimally reduce their LDL cholesterol concentrations. At the present time, LDL-apheresis is the treatment of choice for patients with homozygous familial hypercholesterolemia, and this techiques affords an opportunity to reduce plasma concentrations of LDL cholesterol by 80 to 90 percent in the immediate postapheresis period, with average reductions of 50 to 60 percent between treatments when the procedure is performed at weekly intervals.[149] The rate of increase in the plasma concentrations of LDL cholesterol can be reduced by concurrent therapy with lipid-lowering drugs, particularly HMG CoA reductase inhibitors or nicotinic acid.[150,151] Treatment of patients with homozygous familial hypercholesterolemia by plasmapheresis has been shown to favorably affect the natural history of the premature coronary artery disease which occurs in these patients.[152] Liver transplantation has been the most effective of the surgical procedures used in the treatment of homozygous familial hypercholesterolemia but is associated with all the complications of long-term immunosuppressive therapy. Liver transplantation, however, offers the advantage of providing functional LDL receptors in the transplanted liver; this procedure reduced concentrations of LDL cholesterol by 81 and 83 percent, respectively, in two children with homozygous familial hypercholesterolemia.[153,154] The National Institutes of Health recently approved gene replacement therapy for the treatment of homozygous familial hypercholesterolemia, and this technique may afford the potential to provide functional LDL receptors to the liver without the complications associated with liver transplantation.

TABLE 22-13 Efficacy of Combined Drug Regimens in Heterozygous Familial Hypercholesterolemia

Drug Combination	% Decrease in LDL Cholesterol	No. Patients Studied	References
Cholestyramine + NA	−48	6	Packard et al., 1980[138]
Colestipol + NA	−47	11	Illingworth et al., 1981[139]
Colestipol + lovastatin	−54	10	Illingworth, 1984[140]
Cholestyramine + simvastatin	−54	13	Lintott et al., 1989[141]
Cholestyramine + pravastatin	−45	30	Hoogerbrugge et al., 1990[142]
Cholestyramine + bezafibrate	−31	18	Curtis et al., 1988[143]
Lovastatin + NA	−49	8	Illingworth and Bacon, 1989[132]
Lovastatin + Colestipol + NA	−67	21	Malloy et al., 1987[144]

NA = Nicotinic acid (niacin)

Familial Defective Apolipoprotein B-100

Definition

Familial defective apolipoprotein B-100 (FDB) is an autosomal dominant disorder in which substitution of the amino acid glutamine for arginine at residue 3,500 in apoprotein B-100 results in LDL particles which have defective binding to the LDL receptor. This results in hypercholesterolemia; all patients identified to date have been heterozygous for FDB, and their plasma contains both normal and defective binding LDL particles. The diagnosis of FDB is based on an analysis of DNA and the demonstration of the G to A substitution at nucleotide 10,699 by polymerase chain reaction techniques.

Clinical Characteristics

Initial studies in which FDB was identified in patients with moderate hypercholesterolemia suggested that this disorder is not associated with any ocular, cutaneous, or tendon manifestations of hypercholesterolemia.[155] However, more recent studies in which patients with hypercholesterolemia attending specialty lipid clinics have been screened for FDB have indicated that the clinical phenotype mirrors that seen in patients with heterozygous familial hypercholesterolemia and that patients with FDB may have a premature corneal arcus and frequently have tendon xanthomas.[155–157] The development of tendon xanthomas in patients with FDB appears to increase with increasing age and may be higher in patients with more severe degrees of hypercholesterolemia. Figure 22-18 illustrates the frequency of tendon xanthomas in male and female patients with FDB identified in the Lipid Disorders Clinic at Oregon Health Sciences University when stratified according to the age of individual patients and plasma concentrations of LDL cholesterol obtained on diet only. Deposition of LDL-derived cholesterol in the tendons of patients with FDB also appears to be paralleled by an increased risk of coronary and, potentially, carotid artery disease. The incidence of coronary atherosclerosis is clearly increased and, on the basis of data from patients identified in Oregon and Europe, parallels that seen in patients with heterozygous familial hypercholesterolemia.[156–158]

Genetics

FDB is inherited as an autosomal dominant trait which shows complete penetration in children and young adults. The gene frequency of FDB varies among different populations but has an estimated frequency of 1 in 700 in the United Kingdom, Germany, and North America.[156,157,159] FDB was present in 3 percent of patients with a clinical phenotype consistent with heterozygous familial hypercholesterolemia attending a lipid clinic in Munich, Germany, and represents 8 percent of this patient population attending our Lipid Disorders Clinic in Portland, Oregon.[156,158]

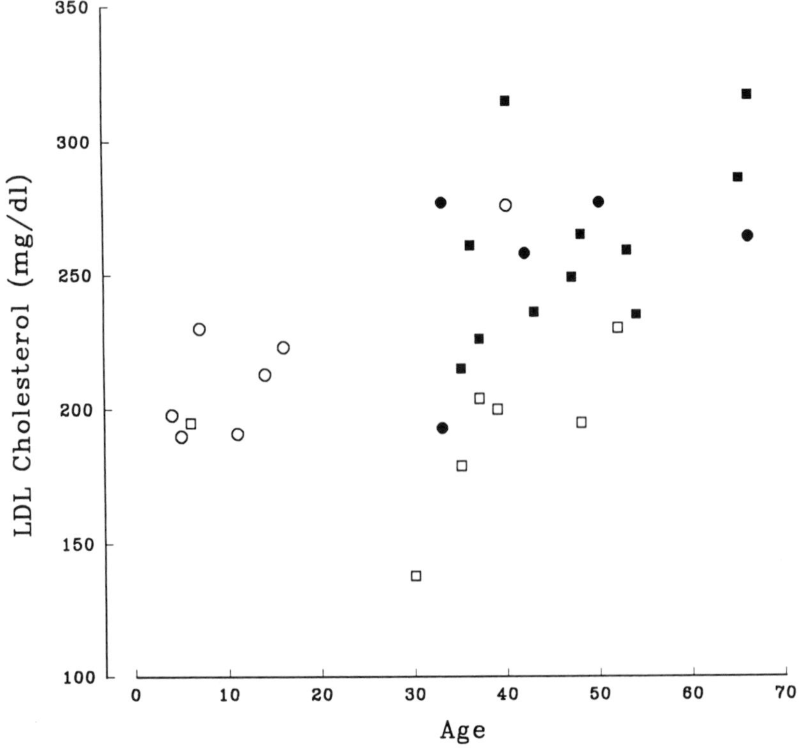

FIGURE 22-18 Plasma LDL concentrations in patients with familial defective apolipoprotein B-100 plotted as a function of age. The data are from patients identified to have this disorder attending the Lipid Disorders Clinic at Oregon Health Sciences University. Note that with increasing age, the number of patients who have tendon xanthomas increases. ○, Male, no xanthoma; □, female, no xanthoma; ●, male, with xanthoma; ■, female, with xanthoma.

Diagnostic Laboratory Features

The diagnosis of FDB is based on demonstration of the G → A mutation at nucleotide 10,699 in the apolipoprotein B gene by means of amplification of genomic DNA and subsequent hybridization with allele-specific oligonucleotide probes.[156,160] The presence of defective binding LDL particles isolated from the plasma of patients with FDB can also be demonstrated by competitive binding studies with ^{125}I-labeled LDL and cultured human fibroblasts, but the latter technique is more labor-intensive and less specific. It is likely that other amino acid substitutions in the apolipoprotein B molecule exist, and the latter technique would serve to identify these before precise delineation of the molecular defect in the apo-B gene. To date, all patients with FDB have been heterozygous for this disorder, and their plasma contains both defective binding and normal LDL particles in a ratio of approximately 7:3.[159] Despite a similar genetic etiology for hypercholesterolemia, the magnitude of LDL elevation observed in patients with FDB is quite variable (Fig. 22-18), although in the majority of patients, LDL cholesterol concentrations exceed 190 mg/dl. Plasma triglyceride concentrations are generally normal, and in contrast to the situation in patients with heterozygous familial hypercholesterolemia, in whom concentrations of HDL cholesterol are reduced, HDL cholesterol concentrations appear to be normal in patients with FDB.[156,159]

Pathophysiology

The initial identification of a patient with defective binding of LDL was made during kinetic studies of homologous and autologous LDL metabolism in patients with primary hypercholesterolemia in which it was observed that the fractional catabolic rate of ^{125}I LDL isolated from one patient was impaired irrespective of whether the LDL was injected into the patient himself or into another patient with primary hypercholesterolemia. Subsequent studies have indicated that LDL particles isolated from the plasma of patients with FDB exhibit extremely poor binding to the LDL receptor on cultured human fibroblasts.[161] Thus, the hypercholesterolemia in patients with FDB results from an impairment in high-affinity receptor-mediated catabolism of the abnormal LDL particles present in the plasma of these patients. Predictably, patients with FDB show abnormalities only in the concentrations of LDL and do not have hypertriglyceridemia or accumulate increased plasma concentrations of remnant lipoproteins. On theoretical grounds, we predict that the magnitude of hypercholesterolemia in patients with FDB will be exacerbated by factors known to increase the production of VLDL apoprotein B and that double heterozygotes for FDB and heterozygous familial hypercholesterolemia will exhibit more severe hypercholesterolemia and be more refractory to hypolipidemic therapy.

Treatment

The goals of therapy in patients with FDB are to reduce the plasma concentrations of LDL cholesterol and, in patients with concurrent increased levels of Lp(a), to reduce the plasma concentrations of this lipoprotein as well. Data on the response to specific dietary interventions in patients with FDB are unavailable, but it may be predicted that factors which would either decrease hepatic VLDL and LDL synthesis or enhance LDL receptor expression would promote reductions in the synthesis of LDL particles in the plasma of these patients and concurrently enhance the catabolism of the normal LDL particles. Although an initial report[162] in two patients with FDB suggested that they were hyporesponders to simvastatin, studies in a larger number of patients[158] have indicated that the overall response to lovastatin in patients with FDB is similar to that seen in patients with other primary causes of hypercholesterolemia, but the individual magnitude of LDL reduction is heterogeneous. Surprisingly, patients with FDB appear to be as responsive to treatment with bile acid sequestrants as are patients with heterozygous familial hypercholesterolemia[163] (and unpublished observations). The ability of these drugs to reduce LDL concentrations in patients with FDB seems unlikely to be due to an enhanced metabolism of LDL particles in the plasma of these patients but may reflect an increase in hepatic catabolism of VLDL remnants, thereby reducing the ultimate production of LDL particles with defective binding present in the plasma of FDB patients. Recent studies have demonstrated a 24 percent decrease in LDL cholesterol concentrations in patients with FDB treated with 3 g per day of niacin compared with a mean reduction of 14 percent in patients with heterozygous familial hypercholesterolemia treated with the same dose.[164] These results suggest that nicotinic acid may be a particularly effective drug in the treatment of patients with FDB.

Combined Hypercholesterolemia and Hypertriglyceridemia

Combined elevations of cholesterol and triglyceride can be due to the presence of an increased number of VLDL and LDL particles of normal composition (type IIb phenotype) or may reflect the presence of abnormal chylomicron and VLDL remnant particles that are typical of dysbetalipoproteinemia (type III hyperlipoproteinemia). It is in this group of patients with total plasma cholesterol values ranging between 280 and 700 mg/dl and concurrent triglyceride values ranging between 300 and 1500 mg/dl that more detailed studies should always be undertaken to precisely define the lipoprotein phenotype. Differentiation between patients with increased concentrations of VLDL and LDL (type IIb phenotype) and patients with type III hyperlipoproteinemia requires ultracentrifugal separation of VLDL in order to document the abnormal cholesterol-rich particles which are present in the plasma of patients with type III hyperlipoproteinemia. The detection of beta-VLDL by agarose gel electrophoresis and the identification of the abnormal apoprotein E-2/E-2 phenotype can help confirm the diagnosis of type III hypolipoproteinemia.

Increased concentrations of LDL in the presence of concurrent hypertriglyceridemia (phenotypic type IIb) may be secondary to other disorders (Table 22-10) or may be attributable to familial hypercholesterolemia, familial combined hyperlipidemia, or other genotypically less well defined causes. The elevated levels of VLDL present in the plasma of these patients are commonly accompanied by reduced levels of HDL cholesterol.[121] In many patients with phenotypic type IIb hyperlipidemia, the presence of a primary genetic disorder may be exacerbated by concurrent secondary disorders such as non-insulin-dependent diabetes mellitus, obesity, excessive alcohol intake, and medications. Thus, attainment of ideal weight, restricted use of alcohol, and control of other causes of secondary hyperlipidemia should be strongly encouraged in these patients. Because weight gain can cause a marked exacerbation of hypertriglyceridemia, patients should be cautioned to strive for modest levels of maintainable weight loss. More extreme weight loss is frequently associated with subsequent weight gain, potentially leading to chylomicronemia and pancreatitis.

The presence of tendon xanthomas and/or primary hypercholesterolemia in children within a given family indicates an underlying genotypic diagnosis of familial hypercholesterolemia, whereas in a family with multiple different phenotypes and an autosomal dominant pattern of inheritance, the genotypic diagnosis is most likely to be familial combined hyperlipidemia. The risk of premature cardiovascular disease is increased in patients with these hereditary disorders (type IIa or IIb phenotype).

Familial Combined Hyperlipidemia

Definition

Familial combined hyperlipidemia is an autosomal dominant inherited disorder in which affected family members may display different phenotypic forms of hyperlipidemia. The disorder appears to be due to an inherent overproduction of apoprotein B and the apoprotein B–containing lipoproteins, VLDL and LDL, by the liver. This defect may result in the expression of increased levels of LDL cholesterol (type IIa phenotype), combined elevations of VLDL and LDL cholesterol (type IIb phenotype), or singular elevation in the concentration of VLDL (type IV phenotype).

Clinical Characteristics

There are no typical physical findings associated with the underlying presence of familial combined hyperlipidemia. Tendon xanthomas are usually but not invariably absent in patients with this disorder, and the absence of tendon xanthomas in patients with primary hypercholesterolemia serves as a useful distinction between this disorder and familial hypercholesterolemia, although it must be emphasized that not all patients with familial hypercholesterolemia have tendon xanthomas. Severe hypertriglyceridemia with the development of eruptive xanthomas may occur in patients with familial combined hyperlipidemia who concurrently develop diabetes or other secondary disorders, whereas patients who are homozygous for apoprotein E-2 may present clinically with tuberous xanthomas and a type III phenotype. In patients with familial combined hyperlipidemia who have elevated levels of only LDL cholesterol, the total plasma cholesterol concentration usually ranges from 250 to 350 mg/dl (6.47 to 9.05 mmol/L), with LDL cholesterol ranging from 180 to 300 mg/dl (4.65 to 7.76 mmol/L).

Because familial combined hyperlipidemia shows incomplete penetration in children and young adults, lipid values in affected patients often do not increase substantially until the third or fourth decade of life. This, together with the lower absolute lipid values usually seen in familial combined hyperlipidemias compared with familial hypercholesterolemia, may explain the lower incidence of premature coronary artery disease in patients with familial combined hyperlipidemia. The typical age of onset for symptomatic coronary artery disease in men with familial combined hyperlipidemia is approximately 50; it occurs 10 to 15 years later in women patients.[166]

Genetics

Familial combined hyperlipidemia is a heterogeneous disorder that is inherited as an autosomal dominant trait with incomplete penetration in children and young adults. It is a common genetic disease, with an estimated frequency of 1 or 2 in 200 in North America. Because no specific marker for familial combined hyperlipidemia exists, it is likely that many patients with moderate inherited hypercholesterolemia who do not have tendon xanthomas have familial combined hyperlipidemia. Heterozygous deficiency of LPL may constitute one subtype of this disorder.[167] In another recent study, familial combined hyperlipidemia was linked to the apoprotein A-I-C-III-A-IV gene cluster on chromosome 11q23-q24 in 16 unrelated probands of nothern European origin.[168] Further studies are required to better delineate the genetic determinants of this heterogeneous disorder.

Diagnostic Laboratory Features

Patients with familial combined hyperlipidemia may present with primary hypercholesterolemia, primary hypertriglyceridemia, or combined elevations of cholesterol and triglyceride. Because the expression of this disorder appears to be exacerbated by factors such as weight gain and increasing age, the diagnosis of familial combined hyperlipidemia rests on a demonstration of multiple different lipoprotein phenotypes in different family members with an autosomal dominant pattern of inheritance. The detection of an elevated level of apoprotein B is consistent with this disorder but is not diagnostic. Some patients with familial combined hyperlipidemia appear to have proportionally higher levels of LDL apoprotein B than would be expected from their LDL cholesterol concentrations.[169] Studies by Sniderman and colleagues[170] suggest that these patients with high levels of apoprotein B also have an increased incidence of premature cardiovascular disease even when the LDL cholesterol level is not elevated.

Pathophysiology

Lack of a specific marker for familial combined hyperlipidemia has hindered investigations of the biochemical causes of this disorder(s). Kinetic studies in which radioiodinated lipoproteins have been injected into patients with familial combined hyperlipidemia have shown an inherently high production rate of apoprotein B, VLDL, and LDL in these patients. In contrast to the low fractional catabolic rate of LDL seen in patients with familial hypercholesterolemia, the rate of catabolism of LDL is normal in patients with familial combined hyperlipidemia, and the expression of LDL receptors in cells from these patients is also normal.[171] By current diagnostic criteria, familial combined hyperlipidemia undoubtedly represents a heterogeneous group of disorders in which the hepatic production of apoprotein B-100 is increased. Further insights into the causes of this defect should be rapidly forthcoming now that the gene for apoprotein B has been cloned.[172,173]

Treatment

The primary goal of therapy for patients with familial combined hyperlipidemia is to reduce the levels of LDL cholesterol and apoprotein B in plasma. Because hepatic production of VLDL and LDL may be increased by secondary factors such as obesity, type II diabetes, and excessive alcohol intake, correction of secondary predisposing factors should be attempted in all patients with this disorder. Knowledge about the pathophysiology of familial combined hyperlipidemia suggests that lipid-lowering agents which primarily inhibit the synthesis of apoprotein B, VLDL, and LDL may be the most effective therapy in patients with this disorder. Based on these criteria, nicotinic acid is the drug of choice for patients with familial combined hyperlipidemia. The bile acid–binding resins cholestyramine and colestipol are second-choice agents but can be useful in combination with niacin or HMG CoA reductase inhibitors. The use of bile acid–binding resins as single-drug therapy can exacerbate preexisting hypertriglyceridemia and should be avoided.[174] Gemfibrozil and probucol are third-choice drugs that are variably effective in this disorder. The results of a recent angiographic study of men with presumed familial combined hyperlipidemia showed that net regression of established coronary artery disease could be detected after 2½ years of aggressive treatment [LDL cholesterol reduced to less than 100 mg/dl (2.59 mmol/L)] with diet and colestipol combined with niacin or lovastatin.[69]

Primary Type III Hyperlipoproteinemia

Definition

Type III hyperlipoproteinemia, also referred to as broad-beta disease, floating beta disease, and dysbetalipoproteinemia, is a rare disorder characterized by the presence in plasma of abnormal VLDL remnants and intermediate-density lipoprotein (*d* 1.006 to 1.019) particles with an abnormally high ratio of cholesterol to triglyceride and beta mobility on electrophoresis. Patients with this disorder are usually homozygous for the abnormal apoprotein E-2. Plasma lipid values vary widely but generally reveal cholesterol levels in the range of 300 to 600 mg/dl with triglyceride levels of 400 to 800 mg/dl.

Clinically, patients with type III hyperlipidemia commonly have palmar and tuberous xanthomas and display an increased incidence of both coronary and peripheral vascular disease.

Clinical Characteristics

The initial recognition of type III hyperlipidemia was as "xanthoma tuberosum" by Goffman and colleagues[175] over 40 years ago. Although the physical findings in patients with type III vary widely, certain features are strongly suggestive of this diagnosis.[176] The most characteristic and common[177] xanthomas seen in type III, termed xanthoma striatum palmare or palmar xanthomas, are present on the hands. These lesions, which may be the only skin manifestation of the disorder, vary from a yellow-orange discoloration of the palmar creases of both hands to more advanced lesions with planar elevation of the skin and eventually, in the most severe form, to raised tuberous xanthomas on the palms and fingers (Fig. 22-19). Palmar xanthomas occur in less than 50 percent of patients with this disorder but are considered diagnostic of type III hyperlipidemia when present.

Tuberoeruptive xanthomas (Fig. 22-20), which consist of raised erythematous nodular lesions 0.5 cm or greater in diameter which commonly coalesce into

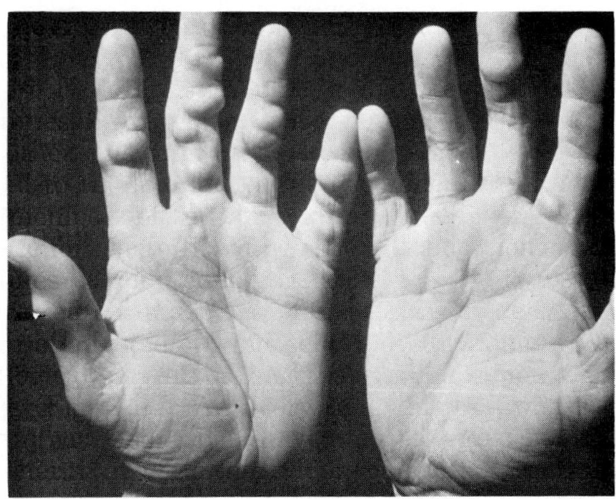

FIGURE 22-19 Tuberous palmar xanthomas in a patient with type III hyperlipoproteinemia.

larger lesions, are also typical of type III. They have a tendency to occur in areas of pressure, most notably the extensor surface of the elbows and knees and on the buttocks. Tuberous xanthomas were present in 51 percent of the patients studied by Morganroth and associates,[177] whereas in other series their incidence has varied from 35 to 100 percent. Xanthelasmas and corneal arcus are uncommon, but tendon xanthomas are present in about 10 percent of patients with type III. Patients with type III have an increased incidence of premature coronary and peripheral vascular disease, both of which have been present in 20 to 40 percent of the patients studied in most reports.[178] The likelihood of both complications is higher in patients who present with advanced tuberous xanthomas than in those with less severe skin lesions.

FIGURE 22-20 Tuberoeruptive xanthomas on the buttocks of a patient with type III hyperlipoproteinemia. The lesions regressed with hypolipidemic therapy.

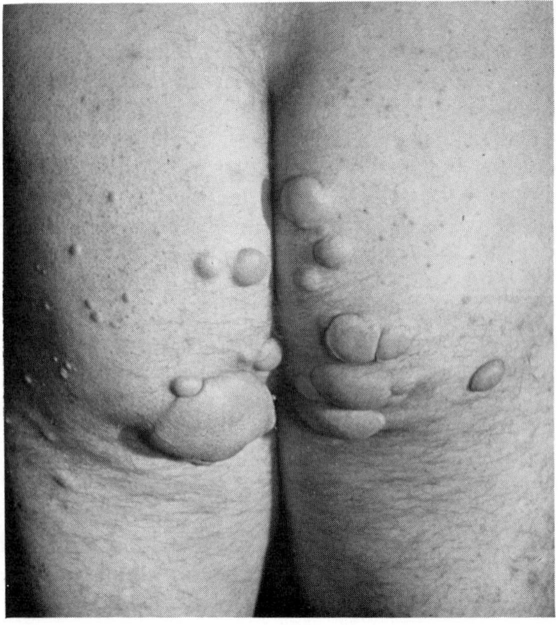

To date, fewer than 10 cases of phenotypic type III have been described in patients under 20 years of age, and these have frequently been associated with coexisting hypothyroidism. Phenotypic expression of the type III disorder in older patients is also commonly associated with obesity, hypothyroidism, diabetes mellitus, or a coexistent separate familial hyperlipidemia. By far the most common of these factors is obesity, which is present in up to 75 percent of cases. Thorough screening of the family members of a patient with type III hyperlipidemia should be a mandatory part of the evaluation. Because the pattern of inheritance is autosomal recessive, other family members may be normolipidemic or may show indications of other primary disorders of lipid metabolism. Phenotypic expression of the type III disorder is more common in men than in women.

Delineation of the autosomal recessive pattern of inheritance of type III hyperlipoproteinemia has been clarified by the recognition that apoprotein E exists in three common allelic forms—apoproteins E-2, E-3, and E-4—and that the vast majority of patients with this disorder are homozygous for apoprotein E-2.[179] The different allelic forms of apoprotein E can be identified by isoelectric focusing or can be confirmed by analysis of DNA samples obtained from peripheral white blood cells. The frequency of homozygosity for apoprotein E-2 has been estimated at 1 percent of the population,[178] whereas heterozygosity occurs in approximately 15 percent of the population. As discussed below, however, only about 1 percent of patients who are homozygous for apoprotein E-2 actually develop hyperlipidemia. Thus, the prevalence of the type III phenotype has been estimated at 1 or 2 in 10,000. The majority of patients who are homozygous for the apoprotein E-2 phenotype are actually mildly hypolipidemic, but all these individuals show an abnormal ratio of VLDL cholesterol to triglyceride and the accumulation of abnormal beta-VLDL in plasma. Type III hyperlipidemia ensues only when a second disorder associated with overproduction of VLDL (e.g., hypothyroidism, menopause, diabetes, familial combined hyperlipidemia) is present. Rare forms of type III hyperlipidemia may be inherited in an autosomal dominant mode.

Diagnostic Laboratory Features

Lipid values in patients with the type III phenotype vary widely but frequently show cholesterol levels in the range of 300 to 600 mg/dl with triglycerides of 400 to 800 mg/dl. These parameters alone, however, are not diagnostic, since similar values may occur in patients with type IIb hyperlipidemia. Determination of the ratio of VLDL cholesterol to the total plasma triglyceride concentration is the most readily available method for the diagnosis of type III hyperlipoproteinemia.[180] A ratio greater than 0.30 is regarded as diagnostic, whereas values of 0.25 to 0.30 should be considered suggestive. This method is reliable at triglyceride values of 150 to 1000 mg/dl, above which spuriously low ratios may be obtained because of the contribution of chylomicrons to the calculated ratio. An older and less optimal criterion for the diagnosis of type III is based on the demonstration of a beta-migrating band on agarose gel electrophoresis of isolated VLDL. The presence of such a slow-moving band in VLDL is, however, not specific and may be seen in patients with the type IV phenotype.

Although still available primarily in research laboratories, separation of the apoprotein E isoproteins by isoelectric focusing is a reliable method for the diagnosis of most patients with type III hyperlipoproteinemia.[178,179] These studies have disclosed that the vast majority of patients with type III hyperlipoproteinemia are homozygotes for apoprotein E-2 and lack apoproteins E-3 and E-4. This disorder may also occur in patients with a complete deficiency of apoprotein E[181] and is likely to be found in patients with aberrant hepatic receptors for apoprotein E[182] and patients with other amino acid substitutions in the apoprotein E receptor-binding domain which do not affect the isoelectric point of the variant. The analysis of the apoprotein E gene in DNA isolated from 10 ml of EDTA-anticoagulated blood can be accomplished using the polymerase chain reaction and specific probes. This sophisticated method of analysis is available at only a limited number of research laboratories.

Pathophysiology

Type III hyperlipoproteinemia is an inherited disorder in which the phenotypic expression requires the presence of secondary factors such as obesity, hypothyroidism, and concomitant familial hyperlipidemia. Studies of the binding of apoprotein E–containing lipoproteins to receptors of various cells have shown that apoprotein E-2 has a markedly reduced binding affinity to the B,E (LDL) receptor and the hepatic apoprotein E receptor. The normal interaction of apoprotein E with its receptor depends on the presence of specific lysine and arginine residues situated between amino acids 140 and 160 in the apoprotein E molecule. This decrease in the binding affinity of apoprotein E-2 is commonly due to a substitution of cysteine for the positively charged amino acid arginine at residue 158 in the apoprotein E molecule. The difference in isoelectric point between apoproteins E-3 and E-4 reflects a substitution of cysteine for arginine at residue 112; however, this does not affect receptor binding, and the affinity of apoproteins E-3 and E-4 for the receptor is similar. In patients with type III hyperlipoproteinemia who are homozygous for apoprotein E-2, the reduced binding affinity of chylomicron and VLDL remnant particles to the hepatic apoprotein E receptor results in delayed clearance of these particles from plasma. This leads to the accumulation in plasma of remnant lipoproteins (e.g., beta-VLDL) which are relatively enriched in cholesterol (they are triglyceride-depleted). Such remnant lipoproteins accumulate in the plasma of all patients who are homozygous for apoprotein E-2, but the development of hyperlipidemia requires the concurrent presence of a second disorder leading to overproduction of VLDL (Fig. 22-21). Subjects who are homozygous for apoprotein E-2 but do not overproduce VLDL have beta-VLDL particles detectable in plasma and tend to have low levels of total and LDL cholesterol. This is presumably attributable to the impaired conversion of VLDL to LDL and to possible increases in the rate of catabolism of LDL.[179,182] The concurrent presence of an enhanced rate of production of VLDL, as seen in patients with familial combined hyperlipidemia or in obesity, leads to accentuation of the accumulation of beta-VLDL remnant particles and the development of clinical type III hyperlipoproteinemia. The accelerated atherosclerosis which develops in patients with type III hyperlipoproteinemia is believed to be due to the uptake of cholesterol-rich beta-VLDL particles by macrophages and possibly by smooth muscle cells in the arterial wall.

Treatment

Patients with type III hyperlipidemia respond very well to therapy. As will be discussed later, we favor a unified approach to dietary treatment of hyperlipidemias and encourage a low-fat (20 percent), 100-mg-cholesterol diet together with caloric restriction to achieve ideal body weight. As with all forms of hyperlipidemia, elimination of secondary causes is mandatory. Thus, appropriate studies to evaluate the percentage of ideal body weight and exclude hypothyroidism, excessive alcohol consumption, diabetes mellitus, and a concomitant second familial hyperlipidemia should be undertaken in all patients. Reduction of caloric intake to achieve ideal body weight in obese patients is extremely beneficial and by itself was successful in achieving normal lipid values in 25 of 29 patients treated by Morganroth and associates.[177] In the absence of a contraindica-

FIGURE 22-21 Diagrammatic representation of the factors contributing to clinical expression of type III hyperlipoproteinemia.

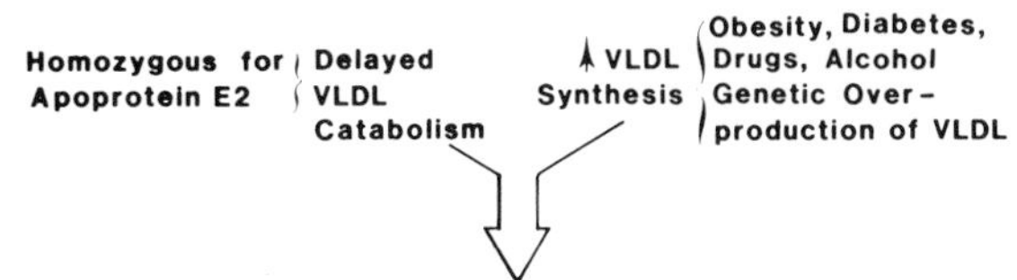

tion such as breast cancer, estrogen replacement therapy should be given to women who are post-menopausal or are otherwise estrogen-deficient.

In patients whose response to diet is less than adequate, drug therapy is usually highly effective. Despite reservations about the use of clofibrate as therapy for other disorders of lipid metabolism, this drug is extremely effective in patients with type III hyperlipoproteinemia, for which it is the drug of choice. Therapy with 1 g twice daily usually results in rapid decreases in the concentrations of cholesterol and triglyceride (Fig. 22-22), and in some cases patients can be maintained on lower doses (e.g., 500 mg twice daily) with equal efficacy. Nicotinic acid 3 to 6 g per day, gemfibrozil 600 mg twice daily, and lovastatin 20 to 40 mg twice daily are also effective. Refractory patients, particularly those in whom the expression of type III hyperlipoproteinemia occurs as a consequence of underlying familial combined hyperlipidemia, may be treated with a combination of clofibrate and nicotinic acid. Patients receiving this combination should be monitored closely because of the increased risk of hepatic dysfunction. Women patients who are unable to take any of these medications may also respond to treatment with ethinyl estradiol (1 μg per kilogram per day).[183] Although this paradoxic effect of estrogen may in part explain the higher prevalence of type III hyperlipoproteinemia in men, such therapy is not generally advocated and probably should be reserved for selected women patients in whom dietary treatment alone is unsuccessful and who are unable to take clofibrate or nicotinic acid. The bile acid–binding resins and probucol are contraindicated in patients with type III hyperlipidemia. The use of bile acid–binding resins will exacerbate this disorder, as will distal ileal bypass surgery.

FIGURE 22-22 The effects of an isocaloric < 300 mg cholesterol diet plus clofibrate (2 g per day) on the plasma cholesterol, triglyceride, and peak reactive hyperemic blood flow (RHBF) in six patients with type III hyperlipoproteinemia. (*Adapted from Zelis et al.*[184])

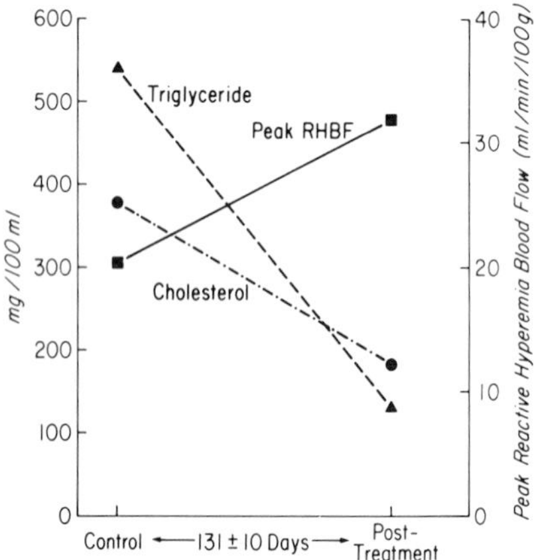

Response to diet and drug therapy is usually dramatic, and, as occurred with the patient shown in Figs. 22-19 and 22-20, regression of xanthomas frequently occurs in less than 1 year. Marked improvement in the symptoms of angina pectoris and intermittent claudication have also been noted and suggest that regression of xanthomas may be paralleled by similar changes in lesions of the arterial wall. Objective evidence of such changes was obtained by Zelis and associates[184] (Fig. 22-22), who noted a 55 percent improvement in maximal blood flow in patients with type III treated with diet plus clofibrate. The excellent therapeutic response found in patients with type III hyperlipidemia justifies an aggressive approach to both the diagnosis and the treatment of this interesting disorder.

Hepatic Lipase Deficiency

Combined hyperlipidemia with elevated plasma concentrations of cholesterol (260 to 1500 mg/dl) and triglyceride (395 to 8200 mg/dl) has been ascribed to a deficiency of hepatic lipase in two Canadian patients.[185] Clinically, the index patient had palmar and tuberoeruptive xanthomas and was noted to have a corneal arcus at age 38. Lipoprotein studies demonstrated the accumulation of small VLDL particles with beta mobility, but no abnormality in apoprotein E could be demonstrated. After intravenous injection of heparin, concentrations of HL in plasma were less than 5 percent of normal whereas LPL activity was not reduced. The ratio of VLDL cholesterol to total plasma cholesterol (which is generally greater than 0.3 in patients with type III hyperlipoproteinemia) ranged between 0.16 and 0.22 in patients with HL deficiency, whereas analysis of the composition of LDL disclosed a characteristic enrichment of these particles with triglyceride (28 percent of LDL by weight; normal, 6 percent). Dietary restriction of calories, total fat, and cholesterol was effective in reducing plasma lipid values in this disorder, but clofibrate appeared to be ineffective.

Hypertriglyceridemia

Hyperchylomicronemia: Types I and V Hyperlipoproteinemia, Familial Apoprotein C-II Deficiency

Definition

An abnormal accumulation of chylomicrons in plasma is characteristic of both type I and type V hyperlipidemia and justifies discussing them together. In type I hyperlipidemia, chylomicronemia is detectable in plasma obtained after an overnight (12 to 16 h) fast, and levels of VLDL are normal; in the type V phenotype, chylomicronemia is accompanied by a concomitant increase in concentrations of VLDL. Both phenotypes may occur as primary familial disorders or secondary to a variety of associated conditions. The biochemical defect in type I is due to a functional deficiency or absence of the enzyme LPL; in type V, impaired clearance of chylomicrons has not been correlated with lipolytic activity, and the nature of the deficit or deficits is not known. In familial apoprotein C-II deficiency, the clearances of both chylomicrons and VLDL are impaired since C-II is a cofactor for LPL activation. The clinical aspects of this rare apoprotein disorder are identical to those of type I hyperlipidemia due to LPL deficiency.[186]

Clinical Features

Both the type I and type V phenotypes may occur as primary familial disorders or may be secondary to a number of associated underlying conditions (Table 22-10). In children the disorder is most likely to be familial, whereas in adults secondary causes constitute the most common etiology. In many cases, however, secondary factors are the provoking stimulus which exacerbates the expression of an underlying familial hyperlipidemia and brings it to clinical attention. The clinical features of both type I and type V are similar and are attributable to the presence of hyperchylomicronemia.[186–189] The age of presentation, however, is different, and in most cases type I is detected in childhood. In a review of 32 cases, Fredrickson and Levy noted that the diagnosis was made before age 10 in 22 patients and prior to age 1 in 7.[187] In contrast, patients with type V usually, although not invariably,[190] are detected after age 20 and generally do not have severe hyperchylomicronemia in childhood.

Abdominal pain is the most frequent symptom which brings the patient to medical attention. The pain may be mild to severe and may mimic an "acute abdomen." The pain may be generalized or localized to the upper abdomen and frequently radiates to the back. Associated tenderness of the liver or spleen is common and is accompanied by hepatomegaly, splenomegaly, or both in over 50 percent of cases. The abdominal pain may proceed to acute pancreatitis. In the series of 32 patients with type I reported by Fredrickson and Levy, 24 reported abdominal pains and 12 had episodes of pancreatitis, with the latter being responsible for four fatalities.[187] Similarly, in reports of patients with type V hyperlipidemia, abdominal pain has been noted in up to 70 percent, with pancreatitis seen in 50 percent.[191,192] Because chylomicrons may interfere with the chemical determination of amylase and result in falsely low readings, such assays should be performed on diluted or chylomicron-free plasma, or alternatively, the serum lipase level or the amylase creatinine clearance ratios should be determined on urine samples.[193] Values over 0.04 are suggestive of pancreatitis. The mechanism by which hyperchylomicronemia produces abdominal pain and pancreatitis remains an enigma. Stretching of the hepatic and splenic capsule secondary to enlargement of these organs from the infiltration of fat seems a likely cause of the pain and tenderness of these organs, especially the liver. It has been postulated that the chylomicronemic state leads to occlusion of the microvasculature of the pancreas; with the resultant ischemia and necrosis, pancreatic enzymes are released locally to induce pancreatitis.

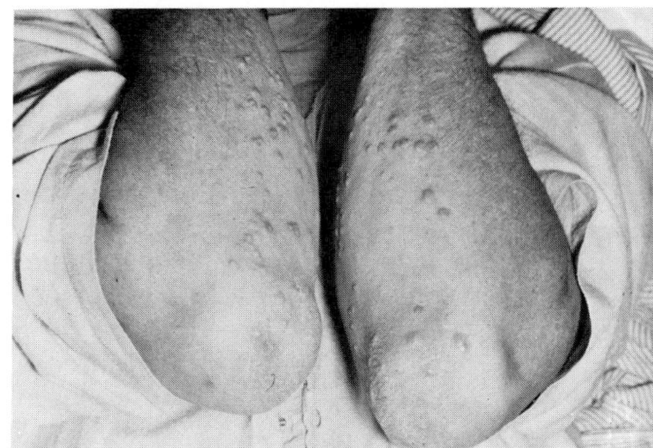

FIGURE 22-23 Eruptive xanthomas on the arms of a patient with severe hypertriglyceridemia and phenotypic type V hyperlipoproteinemia.

Two physical findings—lipemia retinalis and eruptive xanthomas—are diagnostic of severe hyperchylomicronemia. Eruptive xanthomas appear as 1- to 5-mm yellow papules on an erythematous base. The lesions are nonpruritic and characteristically appear on the trunk and the extensor surfaces of the arms, buttocks, and thighs (Figs. 22-23 and 22-24) over a period of several weeks. Their presence implies severe hyperchylomicronemia (triglycerides usually greater than 4000 mg/dl). After therapeutic reduction of the hyperchylomicronemia, eruptive xanthomas gradually disappear over a 4- to 12-week period. In lipemia retinalis, the other hallmark of hyperchylomicronemia, the retinal arteries and veins have a salmon-pink color on funduscopic examination. This also disappears with treatment.

FIGURE 22-24 Eruptive xanthomas on the buttocks of a patient with severe hypertriglyceridemia and phenotypic type V hyperlipoproteinemia.

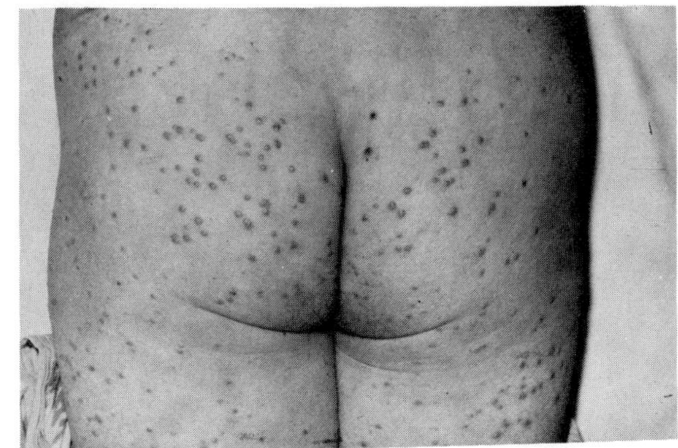

The type I phenotype is rarely associated with hyperglycemia or abnormal glucose tolerance, and affected patients are usually of normal body weight. In contrast, patients with the type V phenotype have a high incidence of hyperglycemia with hyperinsulinism and are frequently above ideal body weight. Although the relation between these abnormalities is complex, a positive correlation has been documented between the degree of hypertriglyceridemia and both body weight and hyperglycemia.[191] Type I hyperlipidemia does not appear to be associated with an increased incidence of atherosclerotic vascular disease.[186,187,189]

In patients with type V hyperlipidemia, by contrast, there is a high incidence of atherosclerotic disorders, including coronary, cerebral, and peripheral atherosclerosis (Table 22-14). A comparison of the incidence of atherosclerotic disorders in type V patients and in patients with familial hypercholesterolemia (type IIa) reveals a remarkable similarity. The numbers of type V and type IIa patients were 83 men and women in both groups, age- and sex-matched from our lipid clinic patients. Forty-three percent of the type V patients seen in our lipid clinic had clinical atherosclerotic disease, compared with 44.6 percent in patients with type IIa hyperlipidemia. As will be stressed subsequently, type V patients have particularly low LDL concentrations as well as low HDL. The predominant lipoproteins are chylomicrons, VLDL, and the remnant particles, which are particularly atherogenic. This is in contrast to the predominant lipoprotein LDL in the type IIa patients.

Genetics

Familial lipoprotein lipase deficiency (type I hyperlipoproteinemia) is inherited as an autosomal recessive trait. Obligate heterozygotes may have combined hyperlipidemia but have reduced levels of adipose tissue lipoprotein lipase.[25,167,194] Many different molecular defects result in a deficiency of lipoprotein lipase. The identification of the lipoprotein lipase gene has offered the possibility of determining the different mutations of this condition.[195]

TABLE 22-14 Incidence of Atherosclerosis in Patients with Type V Hyperlipidemia and in Familial Hypercholesterolemia (Type IIa) (percent of the total number)

	Type V (n = 83)*	Type IIa (n = 83)*
Coronary heart disease	32.5	38.6
Peripheral atherosclerosis	15.7	18.2
Cerebral vascular disease	7.2	6.8
Any atherosclerotic disease	43.4	44.6

* There were 44 men and 39 women in both groupings

The genetics of type V hyperlipoproteinemias are not well characterized, in part because of the heterogenous etiologies of these disorders. Family members of an index patient with phenotypic type V hyperlipoproteinemia show a high incidence of both the type IV and type V phenotypes, the frequencies of which both increase with age. In the largest study to date,[191] the distribution of lipoprotein phenotypes in 181 first-degree relatives from 32 patients with familial type V revealed 57 percent to be normal, 11 percent with type II phenotype, 15 percent with type IV, and 16 percent with type V. Fallat and Glueck noted an even higher incidence of type IV and type V phenotypes in first-degree relatives and concluded that the inheritance was consistent with an autosomal dominant mode of transmission.[192] These studies are consistent with the view that patients with the type V phenotype represent a heterogeneous population in which most appear to have familial hypertriglyceridemia or familial combined hyperlipidemia as the underlying genetic disorder.[189] Familial apoprotein C-II deficiency is inherited as an autosomal recessive trait.[24,186]

Diagnostic Laboratory Features

The determinations of cholesterol and triglyceride in plasma obtained after a 12- to 14-h fast, together with the visual inspection of a plasma sample that has been allowed to stand for 12 to 18 h at 4°C for the presence of chylomicronemia, will permit diagnosis of the type I or type V phenotype in most cases. In type I hyperlipidemia, increases in triglyceride are paralleled by a much smaller rise in cholesterol such that the triglyceride/cholesterol ratio is usually greater than 10:1 (e.g., triglyceride 4200 mg/dl, cholesterol 320 mg/dl). Upon refrigeration, the chylomicron layer is seen to overlay a clear subnatant which does not contain increased concentrations of VLDL. The levels of both LDL and HDL in type I hyperlipidemia are low, typically averaging 50 percent of normal. Lipid values in the type V phenotype reflect the combined increase in both VLDL and chylomicrons; the triglyceride/cholesterol ratio is therefore lower than in type I and usually ranges from 5:1 to 8:1 (e.g., triglyceride 4800 mg/dl, cholesterol 730 mg/dl). Concentrations of LDL and HDL in type V are 50 percent or more lower than normal and reflect the impaired catabolism of both VLDL and chylomicrons to smaller particles in this disorder. As previously discussed, hyperglycemia frequently coexists in patients with the type V phenotype but does not occur at increased frequency in patients with the type I disorder. Documentation of very low or absent levels of lipoprotein lipase mass and/or activity either in adipose tissue or in plasma after the intravenous injection of heparin remains the sine qua non for the diagnosis of type I hyperlipidemia. In contrast, the activity of both HL and LPL is usually normal in patients with type V hyperlipidemia.

Pathophysiology

The biochemical defect in type I hyperlipidemia involves an abnormality in the synthesis, storage, or, less likely, release of lipoprotein lipase. Abnormalities in chylomicrons obtained from patients with type I have not been demonstrated, and such particles are metabolized at a normal rate when infused into control subjects or used as a substrate for LPL in vitro. The profound impairment in chylomicron metabolism which occurs in patients with type I clearly illustrates the key role of LPL in normal chylomicron metabolism. It is also not clear why only chylomicrons accumulate in patients with type I, when in fact both chylomicrons and VLDL are thought to require LPL for hydrolysis of their triglycerides. The etiologic factors responsible for the development of phenotypic type V hyperlipidemia remain poorly understood. Most patients have an underlying hereditary disorder associated with enhanced VLDL production (familial hypertriglyceridemia or familial combined hyperlipidemia) plus a secondary factor which concurrently stimulates triglyceride synthesis (e.g., diabetes or estrogen therapy).[189] The activities of both LPL and HL are normal in most patients with type V[196] and do not explain the impaired triglyceride clearance found in this disorder. Enhanced production of VLDL has been demonstrated in some patients with type V and may, in the presence of a high fat intake, lead to overload of the normal lipolytic pathway, with resultant elevation of both VLDL and chylomicrons. Impaired chylomicron and VLDL catabolism occurs concomitantly and is responsible for the low levels of LDL and HDL which typically occur. A deficiency of apo-C-II, the apoprotein activator of lipoprotein lipase, has been reported in several families, with one family member being originally diagnosed as type V.[24,37]

Treatment

In both the type I and the type V phenotypes, elimination of secondary factors is important if a readily treatable etiology is not to be overlooked (Tables 22-10 and 22-11). Lipid values in first-degree relatives should also be determined and are valuable both for verification of a familial pattern and to detect other hyperlipidemic family members. Therapy for both type I and type V hyperlipidemia is primarily aimed at reduction or elimination of hyperchylomicronemia so that episodes of abdominal pain and pancreatitis can be prevented. Correction of hyperchylomicronemia is accomplished by means of a reduction in dietary fat and total calories, as described in Dietary Treatment. Alcohol is contraindicated. Fish oils and fatty fish may be useful in the type V disorder and possibly also in type I, as will be amplified later. Hypolipidemic drugs have no place in therapy for type I. In the authors' experience, gemfibrozil (Lopid) is especially helpful in patients with type V hyperlipidemia.[197] Niacin is of some value; other drugs have not been useful. Infusions of normal plasma containing apoprotein C-II will temporarily correct the defect in familial apoprotein C-II deficiency.[24,37] This may be helpful during episodes of acute pancreatitis.

The response to the appropriate treatment in type V patients is dramatic. Triglyceride values of 4000 to 8000 mg/dl may decrease to 300 to 400 mg/dl within 2 weeks with a 10 percent fat diet, weight loss, and gemfibrozil. Frequently, type V patients develop a lipoprotein pattern characteristic of type IV patients. Unfortunately, relapse is common as the patients regain weight and consume a high-fat diet again.

Hypertriglyceridemia in Pregnancy

As is well known, there are pronounced increases in plasma triglyceride and cholesterol concentrations during pregnancy, presumably because of the hormonal effects along with weight gain.[198] The hyperlipidemia reaches a peak during the third trimester of pregnancy. In some women who have prepregnant hypertriglyceridemia, the pregnant state may bring on severe hypertriglyceridemia with the occurrence of the chylomicronemia syndrome. There is both increased production of triglyceride and VLDL and decreased removal because of lower LPL activity. Acute pancreatitis may develop as a most severe complication in hypertriglyceridemic pregnant women.

There are two aspects to the management of this condition. The very low fat diet can be employed; dietary fat is restricted to less than 10 percent of total calories. If this first step is not successful, omega-3 fatty acids in a dose of 10 to 15 g per day can be utilized. Such administration decreases the synthesis of triglyceride in the liver and also promotes clearance. This has been successfully employed in one pregnant woman to avoid acute pancreatitis (Farquhar J, personal communication). The second method of management utilized in a recent clinical report is the hospitalization of the patient and the provision of intravenous glucose feeding.[199] Calories can be administered via this modality without stimulating triglyceride synthesis, whereas carbohydrate taken orally may in some instances further aggravate the problem.[200] Successful conclusion of the pregnancy resulted with this treatment.[199] Also, the relative reduction of caloric intake will reduce triglyceride synthesis.

Type IV Hyperlipoproteinemia

Definition

Type IV hyperlipidemia, also called hyperprebetalipoproteinemia, is characterized by an increased concentration of VLDL in plasma without the concomitant presence of chylomicrons or increased levels of LDL. The disorder may be secondary to a number of associated conditions or may result from primary familial disorders, most notably familial hypertriglyceridemia and familial combined hyperlipidemia. Lipid values obtained after a 12- to 14-h fast characteristically reveal elevated triglyceride levels greater than 140 mg/dl, usually above 200 mg/dl and under 1000 mg/dl, without chylomicronemia. Cholesterol levels are average or only mildly elevated. HDL is usually decreased.

Clinical Characteristics

The clinical presentation of type IV hyperlipidemia varies markedly. The disorder may be primary or, more commonly, secondary.[201] Most patients are asymptomatic, and the abnormality is frequently detected on a routine multichannel chemistry screen. Xanthomas are seldom seen. Xanthelasmas are likewise uncommon; their presence in patients with increased triglycerides is more suggestive of the type IIb phenotype. Vascular disease, particularly coronary heart disease, is a frequent complication in patients over age 45 with type IV hyperlipidemia, particularly those with genotypic familial combined hyperlipidemia. Peripheral vascular disease is less common. The importance of type IV hyperlipidemia as a risk factor in coronary heart disease was illustrated in a study of 500 survivors of myocardial infarction,[202] among whom this phenotype was present in 15 percent. Secondary causes should be sought in all patients who present with a type IV phenotype. Obesity, chronic renal failure or nephrotic syndrome, diabetes mellitus, and hypothyroidism together with excessive consumption of alcohol are the most commonly associated conditions. It must be stressed that the vast majority of patients with type IV are overweight. Only in families with endogenous familial hypertriglyceridemia or familial combined hyperlipidemia is obesity not common. Included in this group are children and slender individuals with type IV. A variety of medications, most notably estrogen-containing oral contraceptives, β-adrenergic blocking agents, and thiazide diuretics, have also been implicated.

Genetics

In addition to secondary causes, the type IV phenotype may occur in patients with endogenous familial hypertriglyceridemia and in familial combined hyperlipidemia. The distinction between the two is dependent on the lipid values in first-degree family members. In the former, the proband comes from a family in which all affected relatives have isolated hypertriglyceridemia with increased levels of VLDL. In familial combined hyperlipidemia, the affected relatives are heterogeneous and may have isolated hypercholesterolemia (IIa), hypertriglyceridemia (IV or V), or both (IIb).[166] Both disorders appear to be inherited as an autosomal dominant trait which frequently shows penetrance only after the first two decades of life.

Diagnostic Laboratory Features

The hallmark of type IV hyperlipidemia is an elevation of endogenously synthesized VLDL. The criteria for the diagnosis of this disorder are not absolute and are influenced by the race, age, sex, and diet of the patient and by the reliability of the available lipid determinations. For North American adults over age 45, the combination of a plasma cholesterol level lower than 240 mg/dl with a triglyceride level higher than 200 mg/dl without chylomicrons present may be considered diagnostic. Visualization of turbid plasma without chylomicrons together with an increased triglyceride level and a slightly elevated cholesterol level is all that is required in the diagnosis of type IV (see Laboratory Tests). Frequently, HDL will be low; this is probably partly responsible for the vascular disease in these patients. Associated laboratory abnormalities commonly seen in patients with type IV include hyperuricemia, hyperglycemia, and an abnormal glucose tolerance test.

Pathophysiology

The accumulation of endogenously synthesized VLDL may result from enhanced synthesis of this lipoprotein with overload of the normal removal mechanism or, alternatively, from impaired removal in the presence of normal rates of synthesis. In some cases, both mechanisms may be operative together. The secondary forms of hypertriglyceridemia, particularly those associated with obesity and hyperinsulinism, excessive alcohol intake, and the use of oral contraceptives, are associated with enhanced synthesis of VLDL; this seems to be the primary factor responsible for the type IV phenotype. In contrast, both increased synthesis and decreased catabolism may occur in obese patients and in poorly controlled insulin-dependent diabetics. The primary mechanism underlying VLDL accumulation in the familial hypertriglyceridemias has not been clearly established but may involve increased synthesis of VLDL. Enhanced hepatic VLDL and triglyceride synthesis, possibly mediated by an increased responsiveness to insulin, has been proposed to explain the lipid abnormalities in patients with endogenous familial hypertriglyceridemia.[203]

Treatment

Because of the common association of the type IV phenotype with obesity, adult-onset diabetes mellitus, and excessive alcohol intake, correction of secondary predisposing factors should be attempted in all patients. Thus, the attainment of ideal weight and restricted use of alcohol should be strongly encouraged; caloric restriction is essential if the patient is overweight. Estrogens, unless prescribed for a compelling medical reason, should be withdrawn or changed to a transdermal preparation in patients with type IV. As discussed elsewhere, we favor a single dietary approach to the treatment of hyperlipidemias and recommend a low-cholesterol (100-mg) diet in which the fat content is reduced to 20 percent of total calories, with an emphasis on restriction of saturated fat.

Drug therapy for type IV should be reserved for patients in whom an adequate trial of dietary therapy (6 to 8 months) and correction of secondary factors have failed to reduce the elevated VLDL levels. Drug therapy should be regarded as an adjunct to, rather than a substitute for, dietary therapy. Gemfibrozil 600 mg twice daily is the most widely accepted and most tolerated drug for therapy for type IV (see Pharmaceutical Agents). Gemfibrozil is successful in reducing triglyceride and VLDL levels in most patients. In some cases, however, decreases in VLDL are not paralleled by reductions in total cholesterol, which may actually increase.[174] This paradox is attributable to enhanced conversion of VLDL to LDL and to mild increases in HDL and may on occasion convert a type IV phenotype to a mild type IIa pattern. Strict control of dietary cholesterol and saturated fat will frequently correct the increase in LDL cholesterol, but if this does not occur, serious thought should be given to the discontinuation of gemfibrozil or the addition of a second drug effective in type IIa. Nicotinic acid is probably more effective than gemfibrozil in reducing VLDL triglyceride and apoprotein B levels and rarely produces a paradoxic increase in LDL. As discussed in Pharmaceutical Agents, side effects are much more common with this medication and result in much poorer patient compliance. Bile acid sequestrants (cholestyramine and colestipol), HMG CoA reductase inhibitors (e.g., lovastatin), and probucol (Lorelco) have no place in the treatment of type IV hyperlipidemia.

DISORDERS OF HIGH-DENSITY LIPOPROTEINS

A number of epidemiologic studies conducted over the last three decades have established a strong inverse relation between the concentrations of HDL cholesterol in plasma and the incidence of coronary heart disease observed in western populations.[204–206] Although these studies support the view that HDL may facilitate the transport of cholesterol from peripheral tissues back to the liver, the precise role of HDL in the pathogenesis of the atherosclerotic process has not been clarified. Thus, it is not clear whether high levels of HDL are themselves protective or whether they are simply a marker for other, more fundamental differences in lipoprotein metabolism (for example, more efficient lipolysis and hepatic uptake of triglyceride-rich lipoproteins) which occur in patients with high levels of HDL cholesterol. Concentrations of HDL cholesterol are low (25 to 30 mg/dl) in some societies habituated to a very low fat, low-cholesterol diet in which the incidence of coronary heart disease is also very low.[78] Notably, concentrations of LDL are also low in these populations, suggesting that the inverse correlations noted between low concentrations of HDL cholesterol and high rates of coronary heart disease in western societies may require the concurrent presence of a permissive level of LDL cholesterol (e.g., >120 mg/dl) which is not normally present in more "primitive" societies.

Despite strong epidemiologic associations between low levels of HDL cholesterol and an increased incidence of coronary heart disease, it is not clear whether therapeutic measures to increase HDL cholesterol levels in individuals in whom these are low are of therapeutic benefit.[74] The use of pharmaceutical agents or alcohol which are intended *solely* to increase HDL cholesterol levels cannot therefore be recommended. In contrast, the use of other measures (e.g., diet, weight loss, increase in exercise, and cessation of cigarette smoking) which may raise HDL cholesterol levels as a secondary phenomenon should be encouraged.

Reduced levels of HDL cholesterol may occur in association with several secondary factors (Table 22-15), including hypertriglyceridemia, obesity, cigarette smoking, and physical inactivity, and are 10 mg/dl lower in men than in premenopausal women.[61] The plasma levels of HDL cholesterol are identical in prepubertal boys and girls, but the levels decrease during puberty in boys,[207] and remain depressed throughout life. This effect is mediated by testosterone. Reductions in plasma concentrations of HDL cholesterol may also be seen in patients receiving probucol[208] and during the administration of anabolic steroids.

A number of secondary factors have been shown to increase concentrations of HDL cholesterol in human plasma (Table 22-15). These include exercise,

TABLE 22-15 Secondary Factors That Influence HDL Cholesterol Concentrations

Decrease	Increase
Hypertriglyceridemia	Exercise
Obesity	Ethanol consumption
Cigarette smoking	Weight loss
Androgens	Cessation of cigarette smoking
Puberty in boys	Estrogens
NIDDM (type II diabetes mellitus)	Lipid-lowering drugs
Physical inactivity	Niacin (most potent)
Probucol	Fibric acid derivatives
Low-fat diet	HMG CoA reductase inhibitors
	Bile acid–binding resins
	Phenytoin
	Barbiturates
	High-fat diet

moderate consumption of alcohol, cessation of cigarette smoking, and correction of hypertriglyceridemia. Several medications, including estrogens, phenytoin, and barbiturates, are also known to increase plasma concentrations of HDL cholesterol. The consumption of a high-fat diet is associated with an increase in the HDL cholesterol level, but any potential benefit from the increased HDL is overshadowed by a disproportionate increase in the level of LDL cholesterol.

A number of familial syndromes in which HDL cholesterol levels are reduced below the 10th percentile in the absence of severe hypertriglyceridemia have been described. These disorders include familial apo-A-I and -C-III deficiency,[209–211] familial apo-A-I, C-III, A-IV deficiency,[209,212] Tangier disease,[213,214] HDL deficiency with planar xanthomas,[215,216] LCAT deficiency,[217,218] fish eye disease,[219,220] apo-A-I variants (Milano, Glessen, Marburg, Munster 1-3),[221–224] familial hypoalphalipoproteinemia,[225,226] and some individuals with familial hypertriglyceridemia.[166] In addition to these disorders of HDL deficiency, increased plasma concentrations of HDL cholesterol and a low risk of atherosclerosis have been described in familial hyperalphalipoproteinemia.[227] In the following section, the salient features of these disorders will be briefly reviewed. Distinguishing clinical and biochemical features of the familial HDL deficiency disorders are outlined in Table 22-16.

Familial Apolipoprotein A-I and C-III Deficiency

Three patients from two separate kindreds have been described with a marked reduction in the concentrations of HDL cholesterol (1 to 6 mg/dl) and a virtual absence of apoproteins A-I and C-III from plasma.[209,210] Corneal opacification was noted in all three patients, and prominent planar xanthomas were present on the trunk, neck, and eyelids of the two sisters from the second family. Coronary atherosclerosis was present in one patient by age 40 and was present in the other two by their late twenties. Reduced concentrations of HDL cholesterol (25 to 35 mg/dl) were found in obligate heterozygotes from both kindreds, but of 17 heterozygotes in one kindred, none developed premature coronary artery disease before age 40 and only 2 did so before age 60. Thus, the heterozygous form of this disorder does not appear to be associated with a marked increase in premature coronary artery disease. The defect in this disease appears to be an inability to synthesize apoproteins A-I and C-III because of a DNA insertion in the coding region of the apo-A-I gene.[211] Although it is of unproven efficacy in this rare disorder, it would seem prudent to attempt to reduce the LDL cholesterol concentrations with a view to reversing the tendency for accelerated atherosclerosis and possibly causing regression of the cutaneous xanthomas.

TABLE 22-16 Clinical and Biochemical Findings in Familial HDL Deficiency Disorders

	Familial Apo-A-I, C-III Deficiency	Familial Apo-A-I, C-III, A-IV Deficiency	Tangier Disease	HDL Deficiency with Planar Xanthomas	Apo-A-I Variants (e.g., Milano)	LCAT Deficiency	Fish Eye Disease	Familial Alphalipo-proteinemia
Corneal opacities	+	+	+	+	—	+++	+++	—
Planar xanthomas	+	—	—	+	—	—	—	—
Abnormal tonsils	—	—	+	—	—	—	—	—
Neuropathy	—	—	+	—	—	—	—	—
Hepatosplenomegaly	—	—	+	+	—	—	—	—
Premature CAD	+++	+++	+	++	—	—	—	+++
Plasma cholesterol (mg/dl)								
Total	138	111	65	260	182	170–500	207	165
LDL	120	106	42	134	137	225	199	115
HDL	6	1	2	3	18	5–15	7	26
Plasma triglycerides (mg/dl)	62	62	200	290	188	105–1800	424	113
Apo-A-I	ND	ND	1.3	2	74	51	38	65

CAD = coronary artery disease; ND not detectable.

For premature CAD, +++ indicates onset before age 40, ++ before age 50, and + before age 60. Patients with apo-A-I Milano and familial hypoalphalipoproteinemia are heterozygous, whereas for the other disorders, the description refers to homozygotes.

Source: Modified from Schaefer[228] and Breslow.[230]

Familial Apo-A-I, C-III, A-IV Deficiency

This rare disorder was first described in 1982 in a 45-year-old woman who had mild corneal opacifications, severe coronary artery disease, normal tonsils, and no xanthomas.[209,212] The level of LDL cholesterol was normal, but the levels of VLDL cholesterol and apoprotein C-II were reduced and the HDL cholesterol concentration was severely diminished. Apolipoproteins A-I and C-III were undetectable, and the apoprotein A-II level was decreased 90 percent. The activity and mass of the LCAT enzyme were 40 percent of normal. Seventeen heterozygotes were identified in the kindred and had levels of HDL cholesterol and apoproteins A-I, C-III, and A-IV that were 50 percent of normal. The frequency of coronary artery disease was increased among the heterozygotes. The molecular defect in this disorder may be due to a major deletion in the apoprotein A-I, C-III, A-IV gene complex.

HDL Deficiency with Planar Xanthomas

This disorder of unknown etiology[215,216] has been described in one Swedish woman who presented with an HDL cholesterol of 3 mg/dl and extensive cutaneous planar xanthomas. The patient developed coronary artery disease in her late forties, and apoprotein analyses disclosed a marked decrease in the concentrations of apo-A-I, with concentrations of apo-C-III that were slightly above normal. Corneal opacification was also observed, but the patient's tonsils were normal. The molecular defect responsible for this disorder has not been determined.

Lecithin Cholesterol Acyltransferase Deficiency

This disorder is discussed in further detail in Other Lipoprotein Disorders.

Fish Eye Disease

Severe corneal opacification and low concentrations of HDL cholesterol (7 mg/dl) have been reported in two Swedish kindreds, and this abnormality has been termed *fish eye disease* because of the ocular findings.[219,220] Despite modest elevations in the concentrations of LDL cholesterol and modest hypertriglyceridemia, the reported patients did not develop coronary artery disease before the sixth decade of life. Concentrations of apo-A-I and A-II were reduced in the homozygous patients, and concentrations of HDL cholesterol were approximately 50 percent of normal in heterozygotes. The metabolic defect in this disorder has not been determined, but it appears to be related to a selective deficiency in α-LCAT-mediated esterification of cholesterol in HDL.[217]

Familial Apo-A-I Variants

Eleven distinct structural variants of the apoprotein A-I molecule have been identified, primarily by isoelectric focusing. Each of these variants is associated with a point mutation in the apoprotein A-I gene, resulting in a single amino acid substitution. Apoprotein A-I Milano was initially reported in an Italian man who had low levels of HDL cholesterol (11 mg/dl) with no clinical evidence of coronary artery disease. The low concentrations of HDL cholesterol were due to heterozygosity for a substitution of cysteine for arginine at residue 173 in apo-A-I; this resulted in an enhanced rate of catabolism of these lipoprotein particles from plasma.[221,229] Corneal opacification, xanthomas, and hepatosplenomegaly were not reported in this patient, and there was no family history of premature coronary artery disease. The other variants include apoproteins Gleesen, Marburg, and Munster 1-3.[222–224] All of these were identified as heterozygous defects. None of these apoprotein A-I variants have been associated with coronary artery disease or other clinical abnormalities despite the exceptionally low levels of HDL cholesterol.

Familial Hypoalphalipoproteinemia

Familial hypoalphalipoproteinemia is a relatively common autosomal dominant inherited trait which is associated with concentrations of HDL cholesterol below the 10th percentile (less than 30 mg/dl in men; less than 35 mg/dl in women) and an accelerated rate of premature coronary artery disease.[225,226] There are no specific clinical findings, and corneal opacities are not characteristic of this disorder. Recent studies suggest that familial hypoalphalipoproteinemia may have a gene frequency as common as 1 in 400 in the United States. Although the cause of this disorder is not known, patients with familial hypoalphalipoproteinemia appear to have a 15-fold increase in the frequency of a restriction enzyme polymorphism after DNA digestion with the restriction enzyme PstI.[230] Familial hypoalphalipoproteinemia has also been associated with an increased incidence of stroke in children.[231] Therapy for patients with familial hypoalphalipoproteinemia should aim to minimize other potential risk factors for cardiovascular disease and maintain the level of LDL cholesterol below 100 mg/dl. Whether pharmaceutical measures which raise HDL cholesterol levels have any benefit in this disorder is not known, but therapy with nicotinic acid would be an attractive strategy to reduce LDL and increase HDL cholesterol levels.

Tangier Disease

Definition

Tangier disease is a rare disorder characterized by severe deficiency of normal HDL in plasma and the accumulation of cholesteryl esters in many tissues throughout the body, including the characteristic deposition in the tonsils. The disorder takes its name from Tangier Island, Virginia, where the first cases were reported. To date, fewer than 50 cases have been reported in North America, Japan, Europe, and Australia.[213,214]

Clinical Features

Suspicion of Tangier disease is most commonly aroused by the unique appearance of the tonsils. Oral pharyngeal examination reveals large lobulated tonsils which have a distinctive orange or yellow color that is attributable to deposits of cholesteryl esters within the tissue. Deposition of this lipid in other tissues frequently results in splenomegaly (80 percent), hepatomegaly (30 percent), and lymphadenopathy (20 percent) and may provoke suspicion of a malignancy. Cholesteryl esters are also deposited in the rectal mucosa, which shows 1- to 2-mm orange and brown spots on proctosigmoidoscopic examination. Rectal biopsy reveals foamy cholesteryl ester–laden histiocytes in the mucosa and submucosa. Corneal infiltration is usually detectable by means of slit-lamp examination in patients over age 40 years but does not impair vision. A variety of neurologic symptoms occur in patients with Tangier disease, and these symptoms may constitute the initial reason for seeking medical attention. Symptoms include weakness, paresthesias, diplopia, and increased sweating. Objectively, reduced muscle strength with wasting, decreased tendon reflexes, ocular palsies, and selective loss of pain and temperature sensation have been described. Electromyography (EMG) reveals signs of denervation in affected muscles, but nerve conduction is normal. No episodes of premature coronary artery disease or cerebral vascular disease have been noted in homozygous or heterozygous patients with Tangier disease before age 40. However, among eight homozygotes over age 40, five had evidence of coronary artery disease or cerebral vascular disease,[232] whereas the other three are alive and well in their fifth and sixth decades. Thus, although patients homozygous for Tangier disease may be at increased risk for the premature development of atherosclerosis, this risk is clearly lower than it is in several other disorders which are associated with a similar marked deficiency of HDL but in which LDL cholesterol concentrations are generally higher.

Genetics

Full expression of Tangier disease occurs in patients homozygous for this disorder and is consistent with an autosomal dominant mode of transmission.[213,214] Heterozygous patients frequently have reduced levels of HDL cholesterol (25 to 30 mg/dl) and reduced concentrations of apoprotein A-I but do not have any of the tonsillar or neuropathic findings noted in the homozygous form and remain asymptomatic. Because of their reduced concentration of HDL cholesterol, heterozygous patients may be at increased risk for the premature development of coronary artery disease.[233]

Diagnostic Laboratory Features

The plasma lipid profile of patients who are homozygous for Tangier disease is characterized by a low concentration of cholesterol (60 to 100 mg/dl) with moderately increased triglyceride levels (100 to 300 mg/dl). Lipoprotein fractionation discloses a marked reduction in the concentration of HDL cholesterol (1 to 3 mg/dl). Plasma concentrations of apoprotein A-I and A-II are reduced to 1 percent and 9 percent of normal, respectively, and concentrations of other major apoproteins are 50 to 80 percent of normal. Patients who are heterozygous for Tangier disease have plasma concentrations of HDL cholesterol, apo-A-I, and apo-A-II that are approximately 50 percent of normal. The laboratory findings taken in conjunction with the usual clinical picture permit a definitive diagnosis of Tangier disease to be made in virtually all cases.

Pathophysiology

The biochemical defects underlying the lipoprotein abnormalities and presumed secondary storage of cholesteryl esters in Tangier disease have not been fully elucidated. Studies utilizing apoprotein A-I isolated from the plasma of patients with Tangier disease have demonstrated an increased content of proapo-A-I,[234] which has a reduced affinity to associate with HDL particles.[233] The amino acid composition of apo-A-I Tangier may also differ slightly from that of normal apoprotein A-I.[235] Kinetic studies have indicated an enhanced fractional catabolic rate for proapoprotein A-I in patients with Tangier disease, but the activity of the converting enzyme responsible for the formation of apo-A-I from proapo-A-I is normal. Thus, despite considerable progress and the application of the newer tools of molecular biology, the precise defects responsible for the apparent hypercatabolism of apoprotein A-I in this disorder remain unknown. The increased catabolism of apoprotein A-I is, however, presumably responsible for the uptake of cholesteryl ester–rich chylomicron remnants by macrophages of the reticuloendothelial system, which results in the selective storage of this lipid in these tissues from homozygous patients with Tangier disease.

Treatment

There is no treatment for Tangier disease. Dietary restriction of fat in order to minimize the formation of chylomicron remnants has been advocated by some authors; although of unproven benefit, such a regimen would seem prudent until further evidence becomes available.

Familial Hyperalphalipoproteinemia

Familial hyperalphalipoproteinemia is characterized by distinct elevations in the concentrations of HDL cholesterol in association with normal levels of LDL and VLDL cholesterol and normal plasma triglyceride concentrations.[227] When adjusted for age and sex, total cholesterol concentrations are mildly elevated and typically lie in the range of 230 to 280 mg/dl. The condition is of interest largely because it is the only known hyperlipidemia which actually appears to be beneficial to the patient. As with familial hypobetalipoproteinemia, patients with this disorder have a low incidence of cardiovascular disease and show increased longevity. Familial hyperalphalipoproteinemia should be suspected when the HDL cholesterol level is in excess of 70 mg/dl in male patients and in excess of 85 to 90 mg/dl in female patients in whom secondary causes of HDL elevation have been excluded. Genetic studies by Glueck and associates have indicated that familial hyperalphalipoproteinemia is inherited as an autosomal dominant trait with full penetrance in neonates and children.[236] The incidence of this condition in the general population is not known but is probably greater than 1 in 3000. The condition is benign, and no treatment is indicated. Marked familial hyperalphalipoproteinemia (HDL cholesterol over 150 mg/dl) has been identified in Japanese patients with cholesteryl ester transfer protein deficiency.[237,238]

OTHER LIPOPROTEIN DISORDERS

Abetalipoproteinemia

Definition

The term *abetalipoproteinemia* refers to a group of disorders characterized by a complete absence of apoprotein B-100, the protein essential for the formation of LDL and VLDL, from plasma.[239] To date, three distinct genetic conditions have been described in which there is a complete absence of VLDL and LDL from plasma. In classic abetalipoproteinemia and homozygous hypobetalipoproteinemia there is a concurrent absence of apoprotein B-48–containing chylomicron particles from plasma, whereas in normotriglyceridemic abetalipoproteinemia the intestinal production of apoprotein B-48–containing chylomicron particles is normal and hepatic production of apoprotein B-100 in VLDL and LDL is impaired.[240,241] Patients with these disorders have profound hypocholesterolemia (20 to 40 mg/dl), which in classic abetalipoproteinemia and homozygous hypobetalipoproteinemia is accompanied by marked hypotriglyceridemia (5 to 10 mg/dl).

Clinical Characteristics

Patients with phenotypic abetalipoproteinemia due to the classic form of this disorder or to homozygous hypobetalipoproteinemia show similar clinical features. Such patients manifest steatorrhea from birth which is attributable to the block in mucosal formation of chylomicron particles, with a resulting impairment of fat absorption. There is concomitantly an impairment of the absorption of the fat-soluble vitamins (A, D, E, and K) and of essential fatty acids and cholesterol. Biopsies of intestinal mucosal cells show intense engorgement of fat within the enterocytes. Because of the malabsorption of fat-soluble vitamins, patients with abetalipoproteinemia may manifest vitamin A and vitamin K deficiency at a young age[242] and clearly develop profound vitamin E deficiency.[243,244] This results from two factors. First, absorption of vitamin E is impaired, as is absorption of all other fat-soluble vitamins, because of the blockade of chylomicron formation. Second, plasma transport of vitamin E is greatly disturbed because the chief transport form—LDL—is not present at all. Thus, vitamin E deficiency in humans may be most clearly seen in patients with abetalipoproteinemia.

Steatorrhea and, in patients who remain undiagnosed, a general failure to thrive may be the only manifestations of the disease for the first 5 to 7 years of life. Subsequent to this, in untreated patients there is progressive development of neurologic and retinal dysfunction, which if unrecognized ultimately will prove profoundly disabling. Initially, deep tendon reflexes disappear and there is mild impairment of sensation. Signs of abnormal cerebellar, posterior column, and peripheral nerve function together with muscle weakness progress if the disease is not recognized, and in untreated patients severe ataxia is present by the second decade of life. Retinal dysfunction is manifested by the insidious development of retinitis pigmentosa with loss of night vision and progressive visual impairment. Although some of the visual loss may reflect vitamin A deficiency, treatment with vitamin A alone does not halt further progression of disease, suggesting that vitamin E deficiency may be the primary insult responsible for these retinal abnormalities.

The abnormal lipoprotein environment also affects the erythrocytes, and the peripheral smear reveals large numbers of acanthocytes, which form because of the abnormal cholesterol and phospholipid composition of the erythrocyte membranes. These patients do not, however, generally develop anemia as a result of the abnormal red cell membranes.

Because of the important role of LDL in delivering cholesterol to steroid hormone–producing tissues, the question of whether corticosteroid or progesterone production may be impaired in abetalipoproteinemia has been addressed. Studies of the adrenal response to prolonged ACTH infusion have documented a modest impairment in corticosteroid production which is probably not of clinical significance.[245,246] Reduced progesterone levels were reported in one patient with homozygous hypobetalipoproteinemia[247] who was followed through pregnancy. Although pregnancy proceeded normally in this patient without the need for exogenous progesterone, such a supplement may be necessary in other patients.

Recognition of the key role of vitamin E deficiency in the pathogenesis of the neurologic abnormalities in abetalipoproteinemia has radically changed the prognosis for patients with this disorder. Current data strongly suggest that with appropriate therapy, the disabling neurologic and visual deterioration can be totally prevented.[248–250]

Reported findings in normotriglyceridemic abetalipoproteinemia have included hypocholesterolemia (25 mg/dl) with plasma triglyceride concentrations of 25 to 35 mg/dl, a lack of significant steatorrhea, and the presence of acanthocytes on peripheral blood smears.[240,241] In one patient[240] neurologic symptoms of ataxia were present at 8 years of age, suggesting that even in the presence of normal chylomicron formation, and therefore normal absorption of vitamin E, transport of this vitamin in plasma and its subsequent delivery to tissues are severely compromised when apoprotein B-100–containing lipoproteins are absent.

Genetics

The inherited pattern of phenotypic abetalipoproteinemia takes two forms. The most common disorder (classic abetalipoproteinemia) is inherited as an autosomal recessive trait for which affected patients are homozygotes. Obligate heterozygous parents have normal concentrations of plasma lipids and lipoproteins, and the carrier state cannot be identified. In the second form, phenotypic abetalipoproteinemia represents the homozygous form of hypobetalipoproteinemia, which is inherited as an autosomal dominant trait. Fewer than 10 cases of homozygous hypobetalipoproteinemia have been reported, and obligate heterozygotes show LDL cholesterol concentrations ranging from 15 to 40 mg/dl.[251] Normotriglyceridemic abetalipoproteinemia appears to be inherited as an autosomal recessive trait, and obligate heterozygous parents have normal plasma lipid values.[241]

Laboratory Findings

Patients with phenotypic abetalipoproteinemia show extremely low levels of plasma cholesterol (20 to 30 mg/dl), and their levels of triglycerides are generally lower than 10 mg/dl. Lipoprotein fractionation studies disclose a total absence of chylomicrons, VLDL, and LDL, and plasma concentrations of HDL are reduced approximately 50 percent. A fatty meal does not result in the appearance of chylomicrons in the blood or elevation of the plasma triglyceride concentrations. In untreated patients, plasma concentrations of carotene and vitamin A are very low whereas vitamin E levels are usually undetectable. Because of vitamin K deficiency, the vitamin K–dependent coagulation factors may be reduced, resulting in a prolonged prothrombin time; hemorrhagic bleeding has been the initial presentation in several cases.[242] The synthesis of vitamin D in the skin appears to be adequate to compensate for the presumed decrease in the absorption of vitamin D, and rickets is not described as a complication of abetalipoproteinemia. The content of linoleic acid and linolenic acid as well as the long-chain polyunsaturated fatty acids derived from these two essential fatty acids is reduced in the plasma lipids of patients with abetalipoproteinemia, and this reduction is also reflected in reduced levels in adipose tissue, erythrocytes, and breast milk.[252] Mild elevations in alkaline phosphatase, lactic acid dehydrogenase (LDH), and serum glutamic oxaloacetic transaminase (SGOT) have been observed in some patients and are presumed to reflect hepatic steatosis.

Pathophysiology

Considerable progress in elucidating the biochemical defects responsible for abetalipoproteinemia have occurred since the cloning and characterization of apoprotein B. Studies in patients with classic abetalipoproteinemia have failed to detect any abnormalities in the apo-B gene,[253] and in two patients, concentrations of mRNA in liver biopsies were increased fivefold to sixfold, suggesting that apo-B-100 is inducible and that the defect in this disorder does not involve a transcriptional abnormality. Immunofluorescence for apoprotein B-100–like material has also been detected in liver biopsies, suggesting that in these particular patients, the disorder resulted from a posttranslational defect in the assembly or secretion of apoprotein B–containing lipoprotein from hepatocytes. It seems likely that multiple molecular defects result in the clinical phenotype in abetalipoproteinemia. In contrast to abetalipoproteinemia, studies in patients with hypobetalipoproteinemia have indicated that this disorder results from a series of mutations in the apo-B gene which result in premature termination of apo-B synthesis and lead to the synthesis of truncated species of apoprotein B which are unable to associate adequately with lipids and are rapidly catabolized.[239,254,255] In a series of elegant experiments, Hardman and associates demonstrated that the molecular defect in normotriglyceridemic abetalipoproteinemia results from the synthesis of a truncated form of apo-B-100 (B-50), which is secreted into plasma as a VLDL-like particle but is rapidly catabolized without any subsequent production of LDL particles.[256] Current data[248–250] strongly support the view that the acquired neurologic and retinal degeneration which occurs in untreated patients with abetalipoproteinemia represents a manifestation of vitamin E deficiency. A current hypothesis suggests that the formation of peroxides in the face of low levels of vitamin E may create damage to certain tissues (the retina and the posterior columns of the spinal cord) which are rich in long-chain polyunsaturated fatty acids. Symptoms of deficiency of essential fatty acids have not been reported in patients with abetalipoproteinemia despite profound fat malabsorption and low concentrations of linoleic acid in plasma and adipose tissues.

Treatment

Steatorrhea in patients with phenotypic abetalipoproteinemia can be readily controlled with a very low fat diet (5 to 10 percent of total calories as fat). The degree of fat restriction necessary to prevent steatorrhea is greater in infants and children than in adults, in whom a diet with 15 to 20 percent of calories derived from fat is usually well tolerated. Deficiencies of fat-soluble vitamins can be completely corrected by the administration of water-soluble forms of vitamin A (Aquasol A) 10,000 to 25,000 U daily and vitamin K (Synkayvite) 5 mg weekly. Plasma levels of vitamin E can never be restored to normal, but high-dose vitamin E therapy has been shown to result in normal tissue concentrations of vitamin E in both adults and children[257,258] and clinical improvement and lack of further deterioration in newly diagnosed patients. We recommend that vitamin E be administered at 200 mg per kilogram of body weight per day in single or divided doses.[244] Treatment of patients with normotriglyceridemic abetalipoproteinemia is aimed at providing adequate intake of the fat-soluble vitamins, particularly vitamin E, but the ability of these patients to form chylomicrons allows the use of lower doses (400 U per day). The use of medium-chain triglycerides should be regarded as contraindicated in all patients with abetalipoproteinemia.[259] In the face of defective hepatic triglyceride secretion, medium-chain triglycerides may result in the accumulation of two-carbon fragments in the liver and may lead to the development of cirrhosis.

Hypobetalipoproteinemia

Reduced plasma concentrations of LDL cholesterol in the absence of hypertriglyceridemia (less than 40 mg/dl) can be seen in association with hyperthyroidism, malabsorption, and resection of the ileum and can also be seen in patients with autoantibodies directed against apoprotein B.[260] Low plasma concentrations of LDL may also occur in patients with heterozygous familial hypobetalipoproteinemia, which represents a heterozygenous group of disorders characterized by the synthesis of abnormal truncated forms of apoprotein B, which undergo rapid catabolism in plasma.[239,254,255] These disorders are inherited as autosomal dominant traits and show full phenotypic expression in childhood.[261,262] Heterozygous familial hypobetalipoproteinemia has an estimated gene frequency of 1 in 1000 to 1 in 2000,[263] and because of the low risk of coronary heart disease, it is associated with an overall increase in longevity.[264] Patients with heterozygous familial hypobetalipoproteinemia usually have no clinical abnormalities but occasionally may develop neuromuscular symptoms suggestive of vitamin E deficiency; in these cases, supplemental treatment with vitamin E is advisable. Additional supplementation with vitamin A and vitamin K should be dictated based on serum concentrations of vitamin A and the prothrombin time. In a family where two patients with heterozygous hypobetalipoproteinemia are to marry, the risk of having a child homozygous for this disorder will be one of four, and such a child will have the clinical features of abetalipoproteinemia.

Chylomicron Retention Disease

Several patients have been reported in whom fat malabsorption and lipid storage in enterocytes appear to be due to an inability to synthesize or secrete chylomicrons in response to oral intake of fat.[239] These patients have all presented with severe diarrhea in childhood and have concurrently had low levels of total and LDL cholesterol but a total absence of chylomicrons and lack of a rise in plasma triglycerides after an oral fat challenge. Apoprotein B was detectable immunologically in the enterocytes obtained from patients with chylomicron retention disease, suggesting that the disorder is due to an undefined abnormality in the formation or secretion of chylomicrons. Chylomicron retention disease appears to be inherited as an autosomal recessive trait. Absorption of other fat-soluble vitamins is impaired, and these patients should concurrently receive supplemental vitamin E and, potentially, vitamins A and K. In addition to fat-soluble vitamin supplementation, treatment is directed at maintaining adequate caloric intake in the setting of a low-fat diet to prevent steatorrea.

Familial Lecithin Cholesterol Acyltransferse Deficiency

Absence of the enzyme LCAT is a rare disorder characterized by moderately increased total cholesterol and triglyceride levels with markedly reduced levels of cholesteryl ester and lysolecithin and an increased level of free cholesterol in plasma. Clinically, these patients have corneal opacities and normochromic anemia and develop progressive renal insufficiency.[33]

Clinical Features

Corneal opacities develop in early childhood and consist of numerous gray dots in the corneal stroma, especially in the periphery, resembling an arcus senilis. They are the most consistent and sometimes the only abnormal physical findings in patients with LCAT deficiency. The disorder is associated with premature atherosclerosis and progressive renal dysfunction, both of which are commonly present in the third and fourth decades.[33]

Genetics

Familial LCAT deficiency appears to be an autosomal recessive disorder, the clinical expression of which occurs only in homozygotes. Obligate heterozygotes typically have normal levels of both plasma LCAT and esterified cholesterol and do not develop corneal opacities. However, in one kindred the heterozygotes had low levels of plasma LCAT activity, HDL cholesteryl ester, and apoprotein A-I and higher levels of triglyceride and apoprotein B, but without a detectable increased risk of developing atherosclerosis.[265]

Diagnostic Laboratory Features

The plasma lipid profile in patients with LCAT deficiency is variable but generally reveals total cholesterol of 250 to 400 mg/dl and triglycerides of 250 to 800 mg/dl. Chromatographic separation of plasma lipids reveals 85 to 90 percent of the cholesterol to be in the free form, with only 10 to 15 percent esterified. Various lipoprotein abnormalities can be demonstrated; paper electrophoresis reveals a prominent beta band with faint or absent prebeta and alpha bands, whereas ultracentrifugal separation shows reduced HDL levels. Documentation of the absence of LCAT remains the key to diagnosis. Some other disorders, notably obstructive jaundice, primary biliary cirrhosis, and $alpha_1$ antitrypsin deficiency, may be associated with marked elevations in free cholesterol and the presence of an abnormal low-density lipoprotein, termed LPX, similar to that seen in LCAT deficiency. Such conditions, however, are usually evident clinically and are not associated with a total deficiency of LCAT. Laboratory findings in patients with LCAT deficiency frequently include a normochromic anemia with hemoglobin concentrations of 10 g/dl and target cells visible on peripheral smear. Proteinuria of 1 to 2 g/24 h is also commonly seen and increases as renal function deteriorates. Bone marrow aspiration has revealed foam cells which stain as sea-blue histiocytes on Giemsa stain.

Pathophysiology

The primary defect in this disease is a failure in the hepatic synthesis or secretion of the enzyme LCAT. This in turn leads to above-normal concentrations of free cholesterol and phosphatidylcholine in plasma and is manifested by a variety of abnormal lipoproteins. Although the precise pathophysiologic mechanisms by which these lipids affect blood vessels and the renal glomerulus and are responsible for the pathologic features of LCAT deficiency are not known, these may be mediated by an enhanced transfer of free cholesterol from plasma lipoproteins to cell plasma membranes or, alternatively, by a reduction in the normal egress of this lipid from the cells to the plasma.

Treatment

At present, there is no specific therapy for patients with LCAT deficiency. Restriction of fat and cholesterol has been advocated and seems efficacious in lowering both cholesterol and triglyceride levels. Progressive renal disease has been managed with hemodialysis and transplantation, but both maneuvers must be regarded as palliative rather than curative.

STEROL STORAGE DISEASES

Atherosclerosis

The common atherosclerotic lesions of the coronary arteries, the extracranial arteries of the head, and the distal aorta and arteries of the lower extremities represent fundamentally a biochemical storage disease with a tremendous accumulation of cholesterol, particularly cholesteryl ester.[266] This great storage of sterol initially occurs intracellularly but later occurs mainly extracellularly. There is associated proliferation of smooth muscle cells and macrophages which become foam cells as a result of the storage of cholesteryl ester. A second biochemical event is the synthesis of collagen, which occurs as a reaction to the presence of cholesterol in the arterial intima. Thrombosis and platelet aggregation are important late events that occur after the endothelial surface of the growing atheromatous plaque has been disrupted.

This storage of cholesteryl ester and free cholesterol in the intima of the arteries has its counterpart in only a few other conditions. A similar storage occurs in xanthomatous lesions, whose chemistry will be discussed later in this chapter. An accumulation of free cholesterol clearly occurs in cholesterol gallstones, with the cholesterol content being 60 to 80 percent by weight. Large quantities of cholesteryl ester under physiologic circumstances are stored in the steroid-secreting endocrine glands as precursors for hormonal synthesis. Cholesteryl ester, of course, circulates physiologically in the blood as a vital constituent of lipoproteins. In only the latter two circumstances is the presence of cholesteryl ester other than pathologic.

The majority of the cholesterol in atherosclerotic plaques originates from the circulating plasma. While the arterial wall has a small capacity to synthesize cholesterol, its synthetic rate is insufficient to account for the tremendous mass of cholesterol present. Cholesterol enters the arterial wall as a part of the LDL molecule or other atherogenic lipoproteins. The mechanisms by which LDL induces cholesterol uptake in macrophages leading to foam cell formation remain unclear. Native LDL cannot stimulate foam cell formation in vitro, but LDL modified by malondialdehyde, acetylation, or oxidation, is avidly taken up by macrophages. Thus, it is hypothesized that LDL must be modified first possibly by oxidation in the artery wall to "activate" its atherogenic potential. There is mounting evidence to support this feasible hypothesis.

With hypercholesterolemia and concomitant increases in LDL cholesterol, the arterial wall picks up the modified LDL molecule and its cholesterol load at an accelerated rate which is greater than the amount of cholesterol which is exchanged back into the plasma and picked up by the HDL molecule for transport to the liver. Thus, the physiologic disposal system for excess cholesterol in any tissue, but particularly in the arterial intima, becomes overloaded when the plasma LDL cholesterol concentration is high.

This concept of cholesterol transport and storage in the artery has been greatly clarified by tissue-culture experiments in which a variety of cells from animals and humans have been incubated with both LDL and HDL. When modified LDL is in high concentration, there is a tremendous uptake of cholesterol, particularly cholesteryl ester. The resultant mass accumulation within the cell may be reversed by incubation of the cells in a medium containing HDL.

After the uptake of LDL and modified LDL by cultured cells, there is intracellular digestion of the LDL molecule, and its load of cholesterol, especially cholesteryl ester, is left within the cell in a storage form which the cell is unable to excrete as long as the medium contains a high content of LDL (Fig. 22-5). Some internal rearrangement with further esterification of free cholesterol taken up by the cell may also be occurring.[41] Note that the cholesterol molecule cannot be broken down by the cells of the arterial intima; hence, storage and excretion are the only possible metabolic pathways. It has been suggested that there is a relative enzymatic deficiency of cholesteryl ester hydrolase in the arterial wall which would tend to promote the accumulation of cholesteryl ester which has come into the wall carrried by LDL. This cellular uptake of cholesteryl ester from the medium may be considered as a model system for the uptake of cholesterol and cholesteryl ester by the arterial wall in atherosclerosis and by the skin and tendons in xanthomatosis. Thus, the lifetime accumulation of cholesterol in countless numbers of smooth muscle cells and macrophages and in the extracellular milieu brings about the atherosclerotic process.

The pathogenicity of other lipoproteins for the development of atherosclerosis varies greatly (see Table 22-5). Epidemiologically, many studies reveal an association between VLDL and triglyceride levels and the development of coronary heart disease, especially in older women.[267] Clinically, premature coronary heart disease has been observed in families with type IV hyperlipidemia. The VLDL molecule, unlike HDL, can be picked up by tissue-culture cells and does contain apoprotein B. Furthermore, it carries a considerable amount of cholesterol, albeit less than does LDL. Thus, a moderate view would acknowledge that VLDL in excess may be associated with an increased risk for developing coronary heart disease in some patients. IDL, which is found in type III hyperlipoproteinemia, has an undisputed relation with both atherosclerosis and xanthomatosis. Both coronary heart disease and peripheral atherosclerosis occur at an accelerated rate with IDL elevation.

Chylomicrons would appear to have a minimum of atherogenicity because of the large size of the particle. Atherosclerosis is reportedly rare in type I hyperlipoproteinemia with an absence or deficiency of lipoprotein lipase. However, there is considerable evidence that the chylomicron remnant, which is produced during the action of the tissue enzyme lipoprotein lipase on chylomicron triglycerides, is very atherogenic. The chylomicron remnant is less rich in triglyceride and richer in cholesterol and cholesteryl ester than is the original chylomicron. In type V hyperlipidemia, with poor clearing of chylomicrons, a great accumulation of remnants and VLDL, and low HDL, atherosclerosis and coronary heart disease certainly do occur. The remnant of chylomicron metabolism may be analogous to the remnant—IDL—from VLDL metabolism.

However, HDL has a negative relation to atherosclerosis.[268] The data from all sources place HDL as having a protective role against the development of atherosclerosis. This applies particularly to American women before menopause, who have an attack rate for coronary heart disease much lower than that for similarly aged men and in whom HDL levels are 10 to 15 mg/dl higher. As has already been stressed,[47] the current thinking about HDL in this connection is that HDL may be a transport mechanism to carry cholesterol from the tissues back to the liver. Animals, for example, that have high HDL levels are relatively resistant to atherosclerosis, e.g., the rat and the dog. In tissue-culture systems, HDL does not induce the deposition of cholesteryl ester. Instead, its presence in the medium seems to prevent this occurrence and actually produce regression of cholesteryl esters in cells previously incubated in LDL. Both autopsy and, more recently, coronary angiographic evidence afford further confirmation of these concepts about the atherogenicity of various lipoproteins and plasma lipids.

Xanthomas

In this discussion of the various types of hyperlipidemia, considerable emphasis has been placed on xanthomas as one of the chief and cardinal clinical manifestations. In this section, emphasis will be placed on their collective characteristics, particularly as representing another disorder of lipid storage. Tendon and tuberous xanthomas represent sterol (ester) storage,[266] but in eruptive xanthomas of the skin, triglyceride (from chylomicrons) is the chief constituent.

Ordinarily xanthomas represent a clinical manifestation of severe hyperlipidemia. The more severe the hyperlipidemia, the earlier in life the xanthomas appear. This concept is expressed most fully in the homozygote of familial hypercholesterolemia when the xanthomas appear in the first decade of life or at birth.

While the appearance of xanthomas is usually related to the duration and level of hypercholesterolemia, important exceptions occur. These include several other sterol storage diseases: cerebrotendinous xanthomatosis (the CTX syndrome) and "sitosterolemia and xanthomatosis." The presence of other sterols in the blood and in the tissues, cholestanol (CTX syndrome) and the plant sterols (sitosterolemia and xanthomatosis), potentiates greatly the development of xanthomas, particularly tendon xanthomas, as will be discussed subsequently.

Xanthomas may be regarded as the outward manifestation of sterol and lipid storage, analogous to the internal sterol storage occurring in developing atherosclerotic lesions or in other tissues; xanthomas have been found in the lung and the soft tissues of the buttocks.[269] These two manifestations generally can be correlated, and when xanthomas are present, suspicion of underlying latent atherosclerosis must always be entertained. Xanthomas may also provide a clue to the diagnosis of a particular hyperlipidemia. Eruptive xanthomas indicate the presence of type I or type V hyperlipidemia with chylomicronemia. Tuberous xanthomas may indicate type II familial hypercholesterolemia or type III. Tendon xanthomas are also found in these two conditions. Xanthelasmas have no absolute predilection for a given form of hyperlipidemia, although they are most commonly seen in association with hypercholesterolemia and patients homozygous for apoprotein E-2 without hyperlipidemia. The fact that many patients with severe familial hypercholesterolemia may not have xanthelasmas at all is also puzzling. The appearance of corneal arcus, another lipid storage entity, is certainly not predictable on the basis of hyperlipidemia: It may or may not be present. However, when it is found early in life without there having been injury to the eye, the presence of a profound corneal arcus is highly suggestive of severe hypercholesterolemia.

As is the case with early atherosclerotic plaques, xanthomas are composed principally of foam cells laden with cholesteryl esters, a mild inflammatory reaction with the presence of Touton giant cells, and some increased collagen. Cholesteryl ester is the chemical constituent most characteristically increased.[266,270] It is presumed that LDL [or Lp(a) or IDL] is taken up by the cells of the tendons and skin, much in the same way that these lipoproteins are taken up from the plasma into the atherosclerotic plaque.

It is worth emphasizing the potential reversibility of all xanthomas in response to decreases in plasma lipid concentrations because xanthoma cholesterol exchanges with plasma cholesterol.[270] Reversibility has occurred most dramatically with regard to the eruptive xanthomas of types I and V hyperlipidemia. These lesions may disappear completely in a month. Xanthelasmas and tuberous xanthomas have been observed to disappear over a period of 1 to 2 years with pronounced plasma lipid lowering. Tendon xanthomas are slower to regress, and significant changes take 2 or more years of effective therapy to become evident.

The surgical removal of xanthomatous lesions, usually for cosmetic reasons, is almost invariably succeeded by their recurrence unless attention is paid to concomitant lowering of plasma lipids. This has occurred especially in regard to xanthelasmas but also for surgically removed tendon and tuberous xanthomas.

Acid Cholesteryl Ester Hydrolase Deficiency

Two other sterol storage diseases—Wolman disease and cholesteryl ester storage disease—in which cholesteryl esters and triglycerides accumulate in lysosomes have been described[271] and appear to be allelic. In both inherited disorders, the biochemical defect involves the deficiency of a lysosomal esterase which at optimal acidic pH is capable of the hydrolysis of both cholesteryl esters and triglycerides. Etiologically, both diseases appear to be similar to other lysosomal storage diseases associated with catabolic enzyme deficiencies, such as the sphingolipidoses and gangliosidoses.

Wolman Disease

Wolman disease is usually detected within the first few weeks of life. Symptoms include vomiting, abdominal distension, steatorrhea, and a general failure to thrive.[271] Examination reveals hepatosplenomegaly with normal tonsils. Calcification of the adrenal glands is usually apparent on x-ray, and the plasma lipids are normal or low. Bone marrow aspiration reveals foam cells laden with cholesteryl esters and triglycerides; at autopsy, increased concentrations of these lipids are found throughout the body, most notably in the liver, spleen, and lymph nodes. A definitive diagnosis is based on the clinical picture together with a demonstrable absence of acid cholesteryl esterase in cultured fibroblasts or peripheral leukocytes. Studies of the known cases suggest that the disorder is inherited as an autosomal recessive trait; obligate heterozygotes may have reduced acid esterase activity but are clinically normal. Treatment is supportive, and the disease is fatal within the first year of life.

Cholesteryl Ester Storage Disease

Clinically less severe than Wolman disease, cholesteryl ester storage disease is usually but not invariably detected in childhood.[271] Affected infants are usually asymptomatic, and the only consistent finding on physical examination has been hepatomegaly, which may be associated with splenomegaly in older subjects. Adrenal calcification is unusual in children but may occur in older subjects. Portal hypertension and esophageal varices have been reported secondary to hepatic fibrosis and cirrhosis in some of the reported cases. Plasma lipid values have shown moderate hypercholesterolemia (250 to 400 mg/dl) with increased levels of VLDL and LDL and low levels of HDL. Xanthomas have not been reported, but there is autopsy evidence for premature atherosclerosis in two subjects.

The diagnosis of this autosomal recessive disorder is based on clinical findings together with enzyme studies similar to those in Wolman disease, which reveal a virtual absence of lysosomal cholesteryl esterase. In addition to dietary restriction of fat and cholesterol, recent studies have suggested that treatment of patients with cholesteryl ester hydrolase deficiency with lovastatin or simvastatin reduces plasma concentrations of total and LDL cholesterol and also leads to a diminution in liver size[272,273]; the latter observation suggests that this treatment reduces the storage of cholesteryl esters within the liver. Favorable effects were not, however, observed in response to lovastatin treatment in three patients with cholesteryl ester hydrolase deficiency evaluated at the NIH.[274] Use of lovastatin or simvastatin in patients with cholesteryl ester hydrolase deficiency must be regarded as investigational, and long-term follow-up of the patients currently being treated will be necessary to objectively assess whether such therapy is beneficial.

Lp(a) Hyperlipidemia

Increased plasma concentrations of Lp(a) have been associated with an increased risk of premature atherosclerosis in western societies.[9,11] The plasma concentrations of Lp(a) do not show a normal distribution, and the majority of the population exhibits Lp(a) concentrations between 5 and 20 mg/dl. Although the definition is arbitrary, plasma concentrations of Lp(a) which exceed 30 mg/dl should be considered abnormally high. As previously discussed in the section on familial hypercholesterolemia, the incidence of coronary artery disease in patients with that disorder appears to be higher in individuals who concurrently have increased plasma concentrations of Lp(a).[117,118] Tendon xanthomas may be particularly prominent in patients with heterozygous familial hypercholesterolemia who concurrently have high plasma concentrations of Lp(a).

Data on proof of benefit from reducing plasma concentrations of Lp(a) in individuals in whom the levels are increased are incomplete, but in view of the evidence linking high plasma concentrations of Lp(a) with an increased risk of atherosclerosis and, potentially, thrombosis, strategies to reduce elevated plasma concentrations of this lipoprotein seem to be appropriate in selected patients. Plasma concentrations of Lp(a) do not appear to change appreciably in response to different dietary perturbations[275]; treatment with a number of lipid-lowering drugs, including bile acid sequestrants,[276] fibrates,[174] and lovastatin or simvastatin,[277,278] also fails to alter concentrations of Lp(a). In contrast, treatment with nicotinic acid has been shown to reduce plasma Lp(a) concentrations.[279] Estrogen replacement therapy in postmenopausal women has also been shown to reduce plasma concentrations of Lp(a).[280]

FAMILIAL DISEASES WITH STORAGE OF STEROLS OTHER THAN CHOLESTEROL

This section describes two lipid storage diseases characterized by the accumulation of unusual sterols in the blood and tissue. In cerebrotendinous xanthomatosis (CTX syndrome), cholestanol (dihydrocholesterol) accumulates in the blood and tissues. The second disease, sitosterolemia and xanthomatosis, involves the accumulation of plant sterols, particularly sitosterol, in the blood and tissues, notably in the tendons. Xanthomas can occur in the absence of hypercholesterolemia in both disorders.[281,282] In both, premature coronary heart disease also occurs.

Cerebrotendinous Xanthomatosis

Cerebrotendinous xanthomatosis is a rare familial disease characterized by xanthomas of the tendons, lungs, and brain in spite of normal or low plasma cholesterol levels.[281,282] The other clinical manifestations include cataracts, subnormal intelligence, progressive cerebellar ataxia, dementia, and spinal cord paresis. Cholestanol accumulates in the white matter of the cerebrum and cerebellum and in xanthomas. The plasma cholestanol concentration is increased. The disease appears to be inherited according to an autosomal recessive mode; the basic inheritable defect is due to a lack of the hepatic enzyme 26-hydroxylase.

Clinical Manifestations

The onset of CTX is insidious and unpredictable. Dementia has been observed at age 10 years, cataracts by age 15, tendon xanthomas at age 15, and ataxia by age 18 years.

The course may be divided into several time phases. The initial stage usually begins in childhood, when borderline intelligence, mental retardation, mental deterioration, or even dementia may be found. This is not invariable, however, and in some patients mentation has been found to be normal even in the third and fourth decades of life.

During adolescence and young adulthood, spasticity and at times ataxia develop and become progressively more severe. Juvenile cataracts and tendon xanthomas are frequently observed in this second stage of disease and are usually well developed by young adulthood. The Achilles tendon is the most common site of xanthoma formation, but xanthomas also may occur in the triceps, the tibial tuberosities, and the extensor tendons of the fingers. These lesions are similar in appearance to those seen in familial hypercholesterolemia. Tuberous xanthomas and xanthelasmas (palpebral xanthomas) may also be present.

In the third stage of CTX, enlargement of xanthomas and neurologic deterioration with spasticity, ataxia, difficulties of speech, tremors, and atrophy of the distal musculature become prominent. There may be bilateral Babinski signs and loss of pain and vibratory sensation. The disease follows a deteriorating course characterized by cerebellar ataxia, systemic spinal cord involvement, and finally a phase of pseudobulbar paresis leading to death. Four of the ten deaths reported so far, however, resulted from acute myocardial infarction. In the others, death presumably resulted from neurologic dysfunction. Death has usually occurred between the fourth and sixth decades.

Laboratory and Pathologic Findings

In most patients, the plasma cholesterol and triglyceride levels have been within the normal range, i.e., 117 to 220 mg/dl. The plasma cholestanol (5α-cholestan-3β-ol) is elevated (i.e., to 4 mg/dl vs. a normal level of less than 0.6 mg/dl). Cholestanol is a saturated sterol which differs from cholesterol by the absence of the 5,6 double bond. Cholestanol is normally present in small amounts in tissues and plasma and occurs in both the free and the ester forms.

Cholestanol is normally excreted in trace amounts in the bile, but in the CTX syndrome its excretion is greatly increased (4 to 11 percent of total sterols). Abnormalities of the secretion of bile acid occur concomitantly and reveal decreased concentrations of chenodeoxycholic acid with an increase in cholic acid, to about 80 percent of the total bile acids. Allocholic acid, which is formed from cholestanol, is also increased and represents the other bile acid abnormality.

In the CTX syndrome, large quantities of cholestanol are found in the tissues throughout the body. This phenomenon is particularly manifest in the nervous system, where cholestanol may constitute up to 25 percent of the total sterols. Although in the tendon xanthomas cholestanol may constitute up to 11 percent of the total sterols, cholesterol is still the predominant steroid present. Considerable amounts of cholestanol may be found in any tissue examined, including that of the skin, lung, liver, spleen, adipose tissue, and muscle. Large ectopic xanthomas that are particularly rich in cholestanol may be found internally, particularly in the lung and brain.

Pathophysiology

The origin of the great increase of tissue cholestanol hypothetically includes increased local synthesis, influx from the blood after synthesis elsewhere, absorption from the diet, or a block in catabolism or excretion from the tissues. The underlying biochemical defect in the CTX syndrome is a lack of the liver enzyme 26-hydroxylase, which is necessary for the normal synthesis of bile acids, especially chenodeoxycholic acid.[282,283] In this disorder, as already indicated, there is decreased synthesis of chenodeoxycholic acid. Thus, many intermediate metabolites that occur in bile acid synthesis are excreted in the bile, the feces, and the urine. At least part of the excess cholestanol in CTX patients may be formed from these accumulated intermediates in bile acid synthesis. There is also increased synthesis of both cholestanol and cholesterol.

Treatment

Since cholestanol is present in certain foods of animal origin, mainly eggs and dairy products, reduction in or elimination of their consumption in a very low cholesterol diet has led to a lowering of plasma cholestanol levels. The logical drug treatment has been chenodeoxycholic acid administered orally. This treatment has increased the bile acid pool and produced normal concentrations of chenodeoxycholic acid in bile. The abnormally present bile acid precursors disappear from bile, and levels of cholestanol in the plasma are reduced. Whether this treatment will ultimately change the course of this progressively deteriorating disorder is not yet certain, but the prospect is certainly exciting.[284]

Sitosterolemia and Xanthomatosis

This rare familial disease was initially described in two sisters[285] and has now been verified in a number of other patients.[282] It is characterized by the accumulation of plant sterols, particularly sitosterol, in the blood and tissues. The prominent clinical manifestations of the disease reported to date are xanthomas of tendons and skin, which appear in childhood despite normal or only slightly elevated plasma cholesterol concentrations.

The metabolic defects that cause the disease are twofold: greatly increased intestinal absorption of all dietary sterols, including sitosterol and other plant sterols which are normally absorbed only in minute amounts, and impaired excretion of sitosterol from the body. The exact nature of these metabolic defects is not known. The disease appears to be inherited as an autosomal recessive trait.

Clinical Features

In the patients in the initial report, xanthomas were first noted in childhood in the extensor tendons of both hands; over the years, they subsequently developed in the patellar, plantar, and Achilles tendons. The plant sterols—sitosterol, campesterol, and stigmasterol—are present in high concentrations in the blood and tissues. Cholestanol levels are also increased.

As might be expected from the extensive tendon xanthomas found in this disease, severe atherosclerosis also occurs at an early age. Indeed, the severity of the atherosclerotic disease mirrors that found in familial hypercholesterolemia. Altogether, three males have died of coronary atherosclerosis at ages 13, 18, and 42 years and one female has died at age 39.[282] Three living patients have sustained myocardial infarction; one had coronary bypass surgery, and two other patients had severe coronary atherosclerosis demonstrated by angiography. The postmortem examination of the 18-year-old male, who died suddenly of acute myocardial infarction, revealed diffuse and extensive coronary atherosclerosis in the proximal left main and proximal right coronary arteries as well as in the right and left anterior descending and circumflex arteries.[286] The thoracic and abdominal aorta and illiac vessels also had severe atherosclerosis.

Since most of these patients have average plasma cholesterol levels for western populations, the cause of the severe atherosclerosis cannot be just cholesterol carried in the LDL molecule. The presence of the plant sterols in the lipoproteins somehow increases the propensity to foam cell formation both in the tendons as xanthoma and in the medium- and large-size arteries as atherosclerosis. Biochemical examination of the tendon xanthomas has revealed a higher cholesterol/plant sterol ratio than is found in the blood. A uterine artery removed at the time of elective surgery in one of the sitosterolemic patients revealed the presence of plant sterols as well as cholesterol in the arterial wall.[287] Sitosterolemia should be considered in the differential diagnosis of any patient with myocardial infarction before age 40.

Although the red cell membranes contain the characteristic plant sterols of sitosterolemia, anemia has not been a problem in the majority of these patients. However, in four patients hemolysis and chronic hemolytic anemia have been described, along with hypersplenism and platelet abnormalities.[282] These findings of an autoimmune state may be accompanied by arthritis and a positive ANA test. It may well be that sitosterolemia does not represent a single gene defect and may express itself in several clinical entities, one of which leads to hemolytic anemia.

Chemistry, Absorption, and Metabolism of Plant Sterols in Humans

The three plant sterols—sitosterol, campesterol, and stigmasterol—are usually found only in the lipids of plants and thus are particularly plentiful in vegetable oils, nuts, and fat-rich vegetables and fruits. In chemical structure, the three plant sterols resemble cholesterol except for minor differences in their side chains.

Plant sterols are habitually consumed by human beings in the usual diet. A typical American diet may contain up to 250 mg of these sterols per day, of which sitosterol makes up to 75 percent of the total, with lesser proportions of campesterol and stigmasterol.

Intestinal absorption of plant sterols in humans is normally less than 5 percent of the amount in the diet and is responsible for their low plasma concentration (0.3 to 1.73 mg/dl). However, during infancy, considerable amounts of sitosterol can be found in the blood (up to 9 mg/dl) and also in the aortas of infants fed vegetable oil–rich formulas. Twenty percent of the absorbed dietary sitosterol is converted to bile acids, and the remainder is excreted in the bile as free sterol.

Laboratory Abnormalities

High concentrations of sitosterol and the other two plant sterols in the plasma are the chief characteristic of sitosterolemia and xanthomatosis. Sitosterol predominates in concentrations ranging between 12 and 27 mg/dl. The campesterol concentration is 6 to 10 mg/dl, while less than 1 mg/dl of stigmasterol is present. About 60 percent of the plasma sitosterol and campesterol is esterified. The plasma plant sterols are distributed between the low-density (about 70 percent of the total) and high-density lipoproteins. The very low density lipoproteins carry only trace amounts. Hypercholesterolemia is a variable feature that is most prominent in children with sitosterolemia who are also consuming and hyperabsorbing a high-cholesterol diet. Cholestanol may also be increased.

Erythrocytes also contain unesterified plant sterols. The ratio of cholesterol to sitosterol in these cells is similar to that in the plasma and suggests that free exchange of both sterols occurs.

Considerable accumulation of plant sterols, mainly unesterified sitosterol, occurs in the tendon xanthomas. However, despite the high content of plant sterols, cholesterol is still the predominant sterol, constituting 73 to 88 percent of the total. Histologically, these xanthomatous lesions are indistinguishable from the tendon xanthomas found in hyperlipoproteinemia and CTX.

The subcutaneous adipose tissue and the skin of patients also have been found to contain plant sterols. Other tissues of the body also probably contain them in abnormal amounts.

Pathophysiology

The principal metabolic defect in sitosterolemia and xanthomatosis appears to be the greatly increased intestinal absorption of dietary sitosterol and other sterols including cholesterol, but the exact mechanism is not known. One hypothesis is that the esterification of plant sterols is abnormally enhanced and that this in turn promotes absorption. The biliary excretion of sitosterol as neutral sterol or as bile acid is critically limited, resulting in slow turnover of sitosterol.

The accumulation of sitosterol and the other two plant sterols in smaller amounts in the tendons implies that the plant sterols probably produce the major manifestations of the disease and initiate xanthoma formation. Analogous to the situation in CTX, it is noteworthy that despite high concentrations of sitosterol in the xanthomas, the increase in the xanthoma cholesterol is quantitatively more important. It has been hypothesized that the incorporation of the plant sterols into the plasma lipoproteins affects the stability of the lipoprotein complexes, favoring deposition of sterols generally into the tissues.

In this context, a role of plant sterols in the development of atherosclerotic vascular disease should also be considered. Plant sterols favor deposition of cholesterol in the arterial wall and lead to premature atherosclerotic lesions. The development of overt coronary disease in patients with sitosterolemia and xanthomatosis provides evidence in support of this view.

Diagnosis

Sitosterolemia and xanthomatosis should be considered in every patient who has developed xanthomas in childhood and does not have either familial hypercholesterolemia or the CTX syndrome. The diagnosis of this disease can be established by analyzing the sterols of the plasma by means of gas-liquid chromatography. The variable hypercholesterolemia which some of these patients manifest is noteworthy. There should be a high index of suspicion that sitosterolemia may be the underlying diagnosis in any young person with xanthomas whose cholesterol level is normal or elevated to the range of 300 to 500 mg/dl. Some of these hypercholesterolemic sitosterolemia patients have been termed pseudohomozygotes of familial hypercholesterolemia because their parents were completely normal. Restudied with plasma sterols determined, they were found to have sitosterolemia.[282]

Treatment

The logical treatment for this sterol storage disease is a diet low in or devoid of plant sterols, since the excessive plant sterols in the body originate from the diet. The results of such treatment in two patients revealed a 29 percent decrease in the level of plasma sitosterol. Presumably the great stores of plant sterols in the tissues are in equilibration with the plant sterols of plasma, and prolonged dietary treatment is required to reduce the plasma sitosterol level to normal.

The guiding principles in the formulation of a diet with a low content of plant sterol are to (1) eliminate all sources of vegetable fats such as vegetable oil, shortenings, and margarines, (2) eliminate all plant foods with a high fat content such as nuts, seeds, chocolate, olives, and avocado, and (3) use only refined cereal products which have the germ (rich in fat and plant sterols) removed. In general, foods which have a high content of vegetable fat will also have a high content of plant sterols. The detailed composition of such a diet has been published elsewhere.[281] The diet should be low in cholesterol and shellfish sterols, since all sterols are hyperabsorbed.

Theoretically, drugs that may interfere with the intestinal absorption of plant sterols may prevent the expression of sitosterolemia and xanthomatosis. No such drug trial has been conducted. However, two drugs have been found to be useful in greatly reducing the plasma levels of all sterols, including the plant sterols as well as cholestanol and cholesterol. These agents are the bile acid–binding resins such as cholestyramine and the HMG CoA reductase inhibitors of cholesterol biosynthesis. These include lovastatin, which has an effective sterol-lowering action in some patients with sitosterolemia.

DIETARY TREATMENT OF HYPERLIPIDEMIA

The cornerstone in the treatment of hyperlipidemia is dietary alteration. This is true regardless of the degree to which primary genetic abnormalities are partly or completely responsible for the development of the hyperlipidemia. Dietary factors in the American population inevitably exacerbate any genetic abnormality when this is largely responsible for the hyperlipidemic state. Dietary treatment will almost always result in some improvement of the condition. Therapy has been simplified by the concept that a single basic diet may be used initially in the treatment of all forms of hyperlipidemia.[288] This single diet is low in cholesterol and low in total and saturated fat; it is high in complex carbohydrate. It is of low caloric density and provides only enough calories to achieve and maintain ideal body weight.

The aim of the dietary treatment of hyperlipidemia is straightforward: the achievement of "normal" plasma cholesterol and triglyceride concentrations. Dietary treatment should be initiated when the plasma cholesterol concentration is above 200 mg/dl in older adults and 180 mg/dl in young adults and children; the upper limit for plasma triglyceride concentration is 140 mg/dl.

The recommended dietary treatment is appropriate and safe for both adults and children. Such treatment must clearly answer all the nutritional needs of the body and at the same time have beneficial effects on the elevated plasma lipid and lipoprotein concentrations. These criteria have been satisfied both theoretically and practically.[288]

The Effects of Specific Nutrients on the Plasma Lipids and Lipoproteins

Historically and to the present time, a vast amount of evidence in both humans and animals has pointed to certain dietary factors which have hyperlipidemic effects (Table 22-17). Some have a hypolipidemic action. Many other factors have no or minimal effects. These nutritional factors will be discussed briefly to provide a theoretical and practical basis for dietary prescription in the treatment of hyperlipidemia. It must also be appreciated that certain dietary factors can affect thrombosis, an event which adds greatly to the organ ischemia produced by atherosclerotic blockage of blood flow.

TABLE 22-17 Dietary Effects on Plasma Lipids and Lipoproteins in Humans

Hyperlipidemic dietary factors
1. Dietary cholesterol
2. Saturated fat
3. *Trans* fatty acids
4. Total fat
5. Total calories with adiposity
6. Alcohol (in some individuals)

Hypolipidemic dietary factors
7. Polyunsaturated fat: omega-6-rich vegetable oils[a] and omega-3-rich fish and fish oils
8. Monounsaturated fat*
9. Soluble fibers (pectin, guar gum)
10. Carbohydrate as starches replacing fat
11. Possibly vegetable protein or other substances from vegetables

Dietary factors with no discrete long-term effects
12. Protein generally
13. Vitamins and minerals
14. Lecithin

* Very high amounts of polyunsaturated or monounsaturated vegetable fat, while resulting in a hypocholesterolemic effect overall, would produce postprandial hypertriglyceridemia and increased remnant formation.

Cholesterol

Cholesterol in the diet has important effects on lipid metabolism.[289] Cholesterol-rich diets have regularly caused hypercholesterolemia, atherosclerosis, and even at times myocardial infarction in a large number of species of experimental animals, including primates.[290,291] Dietary cholesterol enters the body by way of the chylomicron pathway and is removed from the plasma by the liver as a component of chylomicron remnants. Only about 40 percent of ingested cholesterol is absorbed; the remaining 60 percent passes out in the stool. Dietary cholesterol is thus added to the cholesterol synthesized by the body, since feedback inhibition of cholesterol biosynthesis in the body only partially occurs in humans, even when a large amount of dietary cholesterol is ingested.[292] Because the ring structure of the sterol nucleus cannot be broken down by the tissues of the body, as occurs with fat, protein, and carbohydrate, cholesterol must be either excreted or stored. Thus, it is easy to see how the body or a particular tissue (i.e., a coronary artery) can become overloaded with cholesterol if there are limitations in cholesterol excretion from the body. Cholesterol is excreted in the bile and ultimately in the stool, either as cholesterol or as bile acids, synthesized in the liver from cholesterol. Both pathways of excretion are limited, and furthermore, much of what is excreted in the bile is returned to the body by the very efficient enterohepatic reabsorption.

Dietary cholesterol does not directly enter into the formation of the very low density lipoproteins and low-density lipoproteins synthesized in the liver because it is removed by the liver as a component of the chylomicron remnants. It can, however, profoundly affect the catabolism of LDL as mediated through the LDL receptor. Because dietary cholesterol ultimately contributes to the total amount of hepatic cell cholesterol, it can affect the biosynthesis of both cholesterol and LDL receptors in the liver. In particular, an increase in hepatic cell cholesterol will decrease the synthesis of mRNA for the LDL receptor, which decreases the number of LDL receptors and subsequently, as in other conditions that decrease LDL receptors, will cause an *increase* in the plasma level of LDL cholesterol.[293–296] Conversely, a drastic decrease in dietary cholesterol will increase the number of LDL receptors in the liver, enhance LDL removal, and hence lower plasma LDL levels. The effects of dietary cholesterol follow.

1. Increased chylomicrons and remnants
2. Increased hepatic cell cholesterol, which has the following consequences:
   a. Decreased cholesterol biosynthesis

b. Partial compensation in excretion of biliary cholesterol and bile acids to lessen hepatic cholesterol
c. Decreased synthesis of LDL receptors
d. Increased plasma LDL
3. Increased plasma LDL and deposition of cholesterol into the arterial wall

Over the past 30 years, 26 separate metabolic experiments involving 196 human subjects have demonstrated that dietary cholesterol exerts decisive effects on plasma cholesterol and LDL levels.[297–299] However, as was pointed out years ago, the doubling or tripling of the amount of dietary cholesterol will not necessarily increase the plasma levels if the initial amount of dietary cholesterol is already substantial (e.g., an increase in intake from 475 mg per day to 950 mg per day).[298] This phenomenon is restudied from time to time and mistakenly interpreted as showing that dietary cholesterol has no effect on the plasma levels, as will be explained later. For those who wish to explore the subject more fully, the results of various cholesterol feeding studies have been reviewed.[300]

The effects on the plasma cholesterol levels as the amount of dietary cholesterol is gradually increased are depicted in Fig. 22-25. These data are supported by both animal and human experiments. With a baseline cholesterol-free diet, the amount of dietary cholesterol necessary to produce an increase in the plasma cholesterol concentration is referred to as the *threshold amount.* Then, as the amount of dietary cholesterol is increased, the plasma cholesterol increases until the second important point on this curve—the *ceiling amount*—is reached. Further increases in dietary cholesterol do not lead to higher levels of plasma cholesterol even though phenomenally high amounts may be ingested. Each animal or human being probably has its own distinctive threshold and ceiling amounts. Generally speaking, however, and again based on the experimental literature, we suggest that an average threshold amount for human beings is 100 mg per day; an average ceiling amount of dietary cholesterol is in the neighborhood of 300 to 400 mg per day. Further experiments are necessary to provide more precise information about the ceiling. Thus, a baseline dietary cholesterol intake of 500 mg per day from two eggs would already exceed the ceiling for most individuals. The addition of two more egg yolks, for a total dietary cholesterol intake of 1000 mg per day, would not then further increase the plasma cholesterol concentration. Yet beginning with a baseline very low cholesterol diet under 100 mg per day and adding the equivalent of two egg yolks, or 500 mg, to this baseline amount would produce a striking increase in plasma cholesterol concentrations, perhaps, as shown in many experiments, by up to 60 mg/dl.

FIGURE 22-25 The effects of gradually increasing amounts of dietary cholesterol on the plasma cholesterol levels of human subjects whose background diet is very low in cholesterol content. (See text for a discussion of threshold and ceiling concepts.)

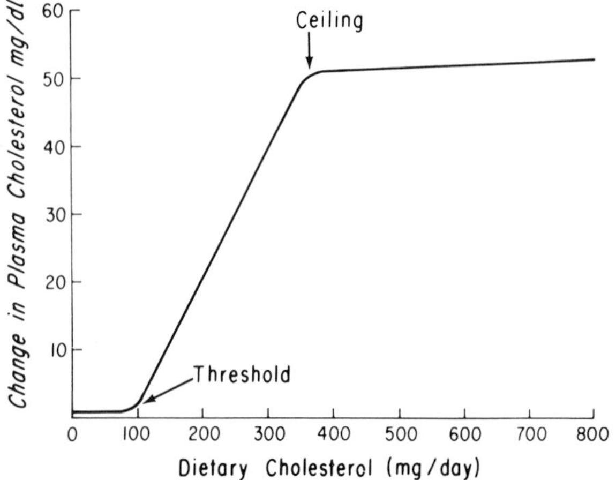

Dietary surveys indicate that the average American intake of dietary cholesterol is about 400 mg per day for women and 500 mg per day for men.[301] Decreasing these amounts of dietary cholesterol to 100 mg per day, as would take place in the therapeutic and preventive diets, would then have a profound effect on plasma cholesterol concentrations, because, as shown in Fig. 22-25, operationally one would be on the descending limb of the curve.

Dietary Fat, Amount and Saturation, Kinds of Polyunsaturation

The amount and kind of fat in the diet have a well-documented effect on plasma lipid concentrations. The *total* amount of dietary fat is important because the formation of chylomicrons in the intestinal mucosa and their subsequent circulation in the blood are directly proportional to the amount of fat that has been consumed in the diet. A fatty meal will result in the production of large numbers of chylomicrons and will impart the characteristic lactescent appearance to postprandial plasma that is observed some 3 to 5 h after meal consumption. A typical American diet containing 110 g of fat will produce 110 g of chylomicron triglyceride per day. *Remnant* production from chylomicrons is proportional to the number of chylomicrons synthesized. Chylomicron remnants resulting from the action of lipoprotein lipase are cholesterol-rich and are atherogenic particles.[54]

Postprandial lipemia is, of course, intense after the usual American diet and may be present for many hours before being cleared. Not only is this lipemia (the composite of chylomicrons and remnants) suspected to be atherogenic, it may also promote thrombosis. Postprandial lipemia is lessened by physical activity and by a diet low in fat and/or containing omega-3 fatty acids from fish. It is worse and very prolonged in patients with fasting hypertriglyceridemia whose clearance mechanisms are already impaired.

Different types of fat have different effects on plasma lipids and lipoproteins. Fats may be divided into three major classes identified by saturation and unsaturation characteristics. Long-chain saturated fatty acids have no double bonds, are not essential nutrients, and may be readily synthesized in the body from acetate. Dietary saturated fatty acids typically have a profound hypercholesterolemic effect, increase the concentrations of LDL, and are thrombogenic. All animal fats are highly saturated (30 percent or more of the fat is saturated) and contains little polyunsaturated fatty acid. The molecular basis for the effects of dietary saturated fat on the plasma cholesterol level is now well understood. It rests on the influence of saturated fat on the LDL receptor activity of liver cells as described by Brown and Goldstein.[293] Dietary saturated fat suppresses mRNA synthesis for the LDL receptor, which decreases hepatic LDL receptor activity, decreases the removal of LDL from the blood, and thus increases the concentration of LDL cholesterol in the blood.[294–296] Cholesterol in this diet augments the effect of saturated fat by further suppressing hepatic LDL receptor activity and raising the plasma LDL cholesterol level. Conversely, a decrease in dietary cholesterol and saturated fat increases the LDL receptor activity of the liver cells, enhances the hepatic pickup of LDL cholesterol, and lowers the concentration of LDL cholesterol in the blood.[294] Some saturated fats, such as coconut oil, increase the synthesis of cholesterol and LDL in the liver. Metabolic studies suggest that one can expect an average plasma cholesterol decrease of 20 percent by maximally decreasing dietary cholesterol and saturated fat.

Besides natural sources of saturated fats, the hydrogenation of liquid vegetable oils can saturate the unsaturated fatty acids. Soft margarines and shortenings are lightly hydrogenated. The softer a margarine is at room temperature, the less hydrogenated it is. Peanut butter is so lightly hydrogenated that its fatty acid composition is little affected. Large quantities of highly hydrogenated fat should be avoided to keep the total saturated fat low. The daily use of small quantities of soft margarines is acceptable in the context of a low-fat diet. Monounsaturated *trans* fatty acids, isomers of the *cis* oleic acid, are important byproducts of this process. *Trans* fatty acids are oxidized for energy, as are other fatty acids. In a recent study in which large amounts of *trans* fatty acids were consumed, the plasma LDL cholesterol level was significantly elevated.[302] However, the presence of small amounts of *trans* fatty acids in lightly hydrogenated margarines (those in which a liquid vegetable oil is listed as the first ingredient) does not appear to constitute a problem in the diet for the treatment of hyperlipidemia.

Attention has been called to the fact that some saturated fats do not seem to cause hypercholesterolemia. Medium-chain triglycerides (C8 and C10 saturated fatty acids) are water-soluble and are handled metabolically more like carbohydrate than like fat. They are transported to the liver in portal vein blood rather than as chylomicrons. These fatty acids do not elevate the plasma cholesterol concentration.

Stearic acid, an 18-carbon saturated fatty acid, also has a limited effect on the plasma cholesterol concentration. Excessive stearic acid from the diet is converted into oleic acid, a monounsaturated fatty acid, by a desaturase enzyme. Feeding animals large quantities of stearic acid does not result in the deposition of stearic acid in the adipose tissue, as would occur with mono- and polyunsaturated fat feeding. This is due to the action of the desaturase enzyme. The practical importance of these observations about stearic acid is limited because stearic acid is present in foods that also contain appreciable amounts of other fatty acids that cause hypercholesterolemia. Palmitic acid is the most common saturated fat found in our food supply. It has 16 carbons and is intensely hypercholesterolemic. Myristic acid and lauric acid, with 14 and 12 carbons, respectively, also are intensely hypercholesterolemic. It is these fatty acids present in "saturated" dietary fats that cause their untoward effects. Amounts of stearic acid in the American diet are not great compared with amounts of palmitic acid.

The second class of dietary fats consists of the characteristic monounsaturated fatty acids that are present in all animal and vegetable fats. For practical purposes, oleic acid, which has one double bond at the omega-9 position, is the only significant dietary monounsaturated fatty acid. In general, the effects of dietary monounsaturated fatty acids on the plasma lipids are neutral, neither raising nor lowering their concentrations. They are, however, cholesterol-lowering compared to saturated fat. Reports that Mediterranean basin populations that consume olive oil in large quantities have fewer heart attacks than do people in the United States have led to further investigations of the antiatherogenic properties of the monounsaturates. Studies have shown that large amounts of monounsaturated fat, like polyunsaturated oils, lower plasma total and LDL cholesterol levels compared with saturated fat.[303] Furthermore, unlike polyunsaturated oils, monounsaturated fat did not lower the plasma HDL cholesterol level.

There are several additional points to be made in regard to these recent studies:

1. The "Mediterranean diet" is also rich in fish, beans, fruits, and vegetables and is *low* in both saturated fat and cholesterol. These could be the decisive factors that influence the lessened incidence of coronary disease and lower plasma cholesterol levels.

2. Olive oil is low in saturated fatty acids, which raise plasma cholesterol levels; this is why recent metabolic experiments have shown some cholesterol lowering as a result of large amounts of monounsaturated fat in the diet.
3. Large amounts of any kind of fat should be avoided to lower the risk of other diseases, such as colon or breast cancer and obesity. In addition, all fats, after absorption as chylomicrons, are acted on by LPL to form remnant particles that circulate in the blood. These are atherogenic.

Based on these considerations, it is prudent to include monounsaturated fat as part of a general lower-fat eating style but not to consider them as particularly antiatherogenic or hypolipidemic.

The third class of fatty acids—the polyunsaturated fatty acids—are vital constituents of cellular membranes and serve as prostaglandin precursors. Because they cannot be synthesized by the body and can be obtained only from the diet, they are "essential" fatty acids.[304] The two classes of essential fatty acids are the omega-6 and omega-3 fatty acids (Fig. 22-26). The most common examples of omega-6 fatty acids are arachidonic acid, 20 carbons in length with four double bonds, and its dietary precursor, linoleic acid. Linoleic acid is converted to arachidonic acid in the liver. Since the basic structure of omega-6 fatty acids cannot be synthesized by the body, 2 to 3 percent of the total energy in the diet must consist of linoleic acid to meet the metabolic requirements for the omega-6 structure.

Omega-3 fatty acids differ in the position of the first double bond. Counting from the methyl end of the molecule, this double bond is at the third rather than the sixth carbon. Omega-3 fatty acids are also "essential." They constitute important membrane components of the brain, retina, and sperm.[304,305] Omega-6 and omega-3 fatty acids are not interconvertible. The dietary sources of omega-6 fatty acids are plant foods, some but not all vegetable oils, and leafy vegetables. Fish and shellfish are especially rich in omega-6 fatty acids. Linolenic acid, C18:3, is obtained from vegetable products. Eicosapentaenoic acid (EPA), C20:5, and docosahexaenoic acid (DHA), C22:6, are derived from fish, shellfish, and phytoplankton. They are highly concentrated in fish oils. Like omega-6 fatty acids, omega-3 fatty acids are viewed as essential nutrients, and a safe intake would be 0.4 to 0.6 percent of total calories. Once either the omega-3 or omega-6 structure comes into the body as the 18-carbon linoleic or linolenic acid, the body can synthesize the longer-chain and more highly polyunsaturated omega-6 or omega-3 fatty acids (20 and 22 carbons, respectively).

EPA and DHA are present in the diet in two forms: as triglyceride in the adipose tissue of fish, usually present between muscle fibers, and as membrane phospholipids of the muscle of fish. These highly polyunsaturated fatty acids occupy the middle position of the glycerol skeleton for both triglycerides and phospholipids. In either of these dietary forms, EPA and DHA are efficiently absorbed from the intestinal tract. After absorption, EPA and DHA readily associate with membranes and are found in all four lipid classes: triglycerides, FFA, cholesteryl esters, and phospholipids. Ultimately, they are stored in the adipose tissue, and in experimental animals they even reach the brain and the retina.

Polyunsaturated fatty acids in large amounts, either the omega-6 or omega-3 structure, reduce plasma total and LDL cholesterol concentrations in normal and hypercholesterolemic individuals.[306,307] The situation is somewhat different in hypertriglyceridemic individuals or in those with combined hyperlipidemia. Only the omega-3 fatty acids from fish and fish oil have a decided hypotriglyceridemic effect. VLDL in particular is decreased by the omega-3 fatty acids[308] (Fig. 22-27). Isotopic studies have shown that the hypotriglyceridemic effect of omega-3 fatty acids occurs as a result of the depression of triglyceride and VLDL synthesis in the liver and

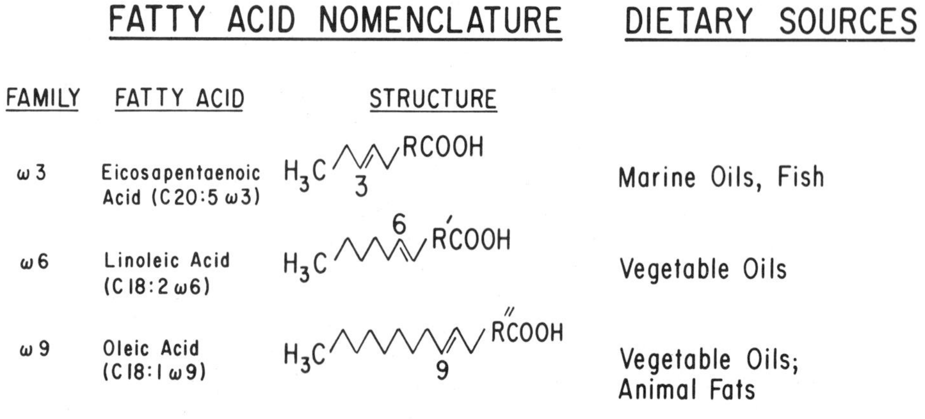

FATTY ACID NOMENCLATURE			DIETARY SOURCES
FAMILY	FATTY ACID	STRUCTURE	
ω3	Eicosapentaenoic Acid (C20:5 ω3)	H_3C (3) RCOOH	Marine Oils, Fish
ω6	Linoleic Acid (C18:2 ω6)	H_3C (6) RCOOH	Vegetable Oils
ω9	Oleic Acid (C18:1 ω9)	H_3C (9) RCOOH	Vegetable Oils; Animal Fats

FIGURE 22-26 The structure and sources of dietary fatty acids. Fatty acids can be organized into families according to the position of the first double bond from the terminal methyl group. The omega-3 fatty acids all have three carbons between the methyl end and the first double bond. Fatty acids in this family include eicosapentaenoic acid (C20:5), linolenic acid (C18:3), and docosahexaenoic acid (C22:6). Linoleic acid (C18:2) and arachidonic acid (C20:4) are the most important omega-6 fatty acids, while oleic acid (C18:1) is the most common fatty acid in the omega-9 family.

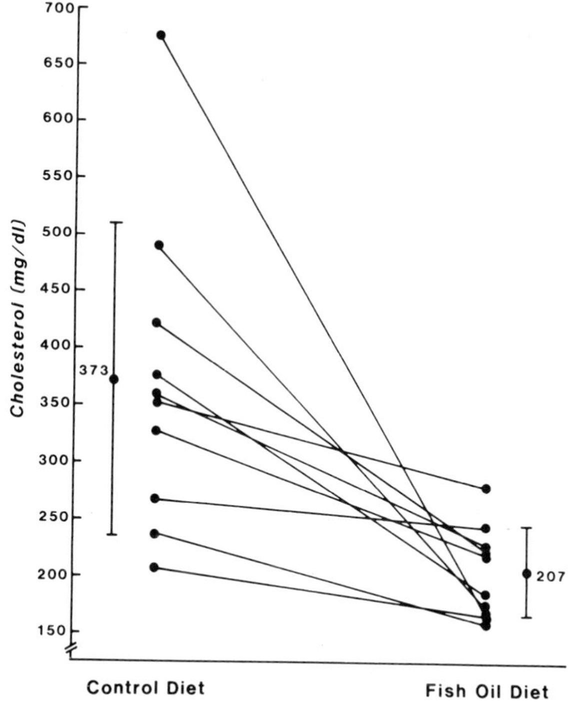

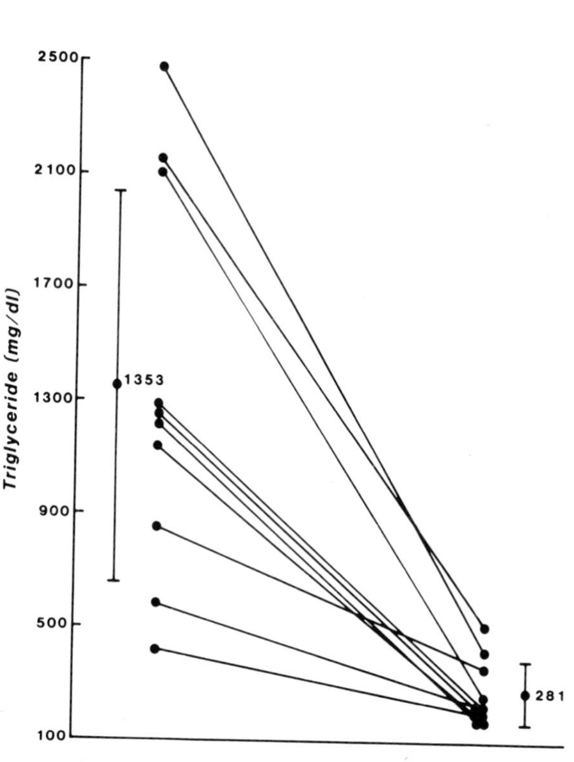

from the accelerated catabolism of VLDL from the plasma. In some patients with type IV hypertriglyceridemia and in some patients with combined hyperlipidemia, there have been reports of an increase in LDL as the plasma triglycerides fall. This also occurs when gemfibrozil is given to these patients. In severely hypertriglyceridemic type V patients, however, large doses of fish oil (10 to 15 g/day) produce a dramatic clearing of chylomicronemia and lower both triglyceride and cholesterol concentrations. Fish oil also seems to promote the clearing of chylomicrons after the administration of a fatty meal. This would be of particular benefit in type V patients in whom there is great difficulty in clearing chylomicrons. Most experiments have not shown plasma triglyceride lowering from the omega-6 vegetable oils.

It is not known exactly how the intake of dietary omega-3 fatty acids should be altered to achieve the optimum effect. One study from The Netherlands indicated that men who included fish in their diet twice a week had fewer deaths from heart disease. A similar protective effect from eating fish was demonstrated in Japan. In a prospective trial in Wales, the prescription of two fish meals per week led to a reduction in both total mortality and the number of coronary events.[309] Even very low fat seafood contains an appreciable amount of omega-3 fatty acids, up to 40 or more percent of total fatty acids. Eating a total of 12 oz of a variety of fish and shellfish each week would provide 3 to 5 g of omega-3 fatty acids as well as protein, vitamins, and minerals. The fish can be fresh, frozen, or canned without affecting the quantity of omega-3 fatty acids. The beneficial effects from following this dietary advice are especially evident if the fish replaces meat in the diet, meat being a major source of saturated fat. Also to be considered are the antithrombotic actions of fish oil, which seem to be mediated through the inhibition of the thromboxane A_2 in platelets,[305] and the enhanced clearance of chylomicrons.[310,311] Other effects of fish oil include inhibition of platelet-derived growth factor, alteration of leukocyte function, reduction of blood viscosity, increased fibrinolysis, and the inhibition of intimal hyperplasia in vein grafts used for arterial bypass. Thus, fish oils not only influence plasma lipids and lipoproteins, they also affect the thrombotic process.

FIGURE 22-27 The hypocholesterolemic and hypotriglyceridemic effects of fish oils rich in omega-3 fatty acids in patients with phenotypic type V hyperlipoproteinemia. Changes in the plasma concentrations of total cholesterol, $\Delta = -166$ mg/dl, $p < 0.01$ (*A*) and triglyceride, $\Delta = -1072$ mg/dl, $p < 0.001$ (*B*) from 10 patients fed a fish oil–supplemented diet containing 20 to 30 g of omega-3 fatty acids. (*Reproduced from Phillipson et al.*[308] *with permission.*)

Calories and Obesity

Excessive caloric intake from any source (fat, carbohydrate, protein, or alcohol) promotes hyperlipidemia (especially hypertriglyceridemia) in some individuals. Plasma triglyceride levels rise, and levels of high-density lipoprotein fall. The immediate metabolic consequence of excessive calories is an increased substrate for triglyceride synthesis in the liver, with subsequent elevated plasma VLDL triglyceride.[312] Furthermore, overproduction of VLDL triglyceride combined with reduced clearance of VLDL triglyceride from the blood may be responsible in part for the hypertriglyceridemia of obesity. The enlarged adipose tissue cells, because of their lessened sensitivity to the circulating insulin that stimulates lipoprotein lipase, the "clearing factor" enzyme, may have a reduced capacity to remove circulating triglyceride from the plasma.

In hypertriglyceridemic overweight patients, there is usually an associated hypercholesterolemia, partly because of the increased intake of dietary cholesterol and saturated fat that occurs in the obese but also because the VLDL that carries the increased triglyceride content transports cholesterol as well. The lower HDL concentrations apparently reflect the shunting of HDL apoproteins into the VLDL molecule. Moderate reduction of caloric intake in hypertriglyceridemic overweight patients and the subsequent loss of adiposity invariably lead to lower plasma triglyceride levels, often to a normal range. Plasma cholesterol levels concomitantly fall; HDL levels reciprocally rise.[312,313]

While caloric control is the most important consideration for these hypertriglyceridemic patients, the source of the calories in weight-loss diets is of some importance in the establishment of patterns of food consumption that will be useful when a more ideal weight has been achieved. Many patients have combined hyperlipidemia (i.e., type IIb), and whatever hypercholesterolemia remains after both body weight and plasma triglyceride stabilize at lower levels will require attention in regard to the reduction of dietary cholesterol and saturated fat. Furthermore, the pattern of food intake should then be such that future weight gain will be avoided. The low-fat, high-complex-carbohydrate diet concept can be useful for both the period of weight reduction and the subsequent period of stabilization of body weight.

When excessive dietary cholesterol and fat are combined with excessive calories, a particularly potent hyperlipidemic effect occurs. Such a "holiday" diet occurs in the United States between Thanksgiving and New Year's day. The effects of such dietary excesses were studied in the Tarahumara Indians of Mexico, a people habitually accustomed to a very low fat diet.[314] After a suitable baseline period in which they consumed their typical diet, Tarahumara Indians were given a diet high in cholesterol, fat, and calories. Within 2 weeks, their plasma lipids had increased tremendously: total cholesterol 31 percent, LDL 39 percent, HDL 31 percent, and a plasma triglyceride 18 percent. Body weight gain averaged 7 to 8 lb for each individual. The composite effect of these potent dietary hyperlipidemic factors (fat, cholesterol, calories) was greater than that of any one of them alone.

Carbohydrate

If the total fat content of a hypolipidemic diet is reduced from the current American fat intake of 40 percent of total calories to only 20 percent and if the protein in the diet is kept constant, the difference in caloric intake between a high-fat diet and a low-fat diet must be made up by increasing the carbohydrate content of the diet. Epidemiologic evidence buttresses this basic concept, since populations ingesting a high-carbohydrate diet from complex carbohydrates have low plasma cholesterol levels and a low incidence of coronary disease. Are there harmful effects from a high-carbohydrate diet? It was demonstrated more than 25 years ago that a sudden increase in the amount of dietary carbohydrate in Americans accustomed to a high-fat diet can dramatically increase the plasma triglyceride concentration. After many weeks of the new diet, however, adaptation occurs and the hypertriglyceridemia subsides. If the dietary carbohydrate is gradually increased as fat is reduced, hypertriglyceridemia does not occur. Thus, high dietary carbohydrate need not be regarded as a problem but rather as a caloric replacement for the saturated fat removed from the diet. For example, we recently increased the dietary carbohydrate intake gradually from 45 percent kcal to 65 percent kcal over a 28-day period in eight mildly hypertriglyceridemic subjects. There was a significant fall in the mean plasma cholesterol level, from 232 to 198 mg/dl. The mean plasma triglyceride level remained constant, at 213 to 230 mg/dl.[315]

In the low-fat, high-carbohydrate diet described earlier, the majority of the carbohydrate is in the form of cereals and legumes, not in the form of sucrose or other simple sugars. Americans commonly consume about 20 percent of their total calories, half of their carbohydrate intake, as sucrose or other simple sugars. In the dietary changes being suggested, simple sugars fall to about 10 percent of the total. Sucrose, in large quantities, is hypertriglyceridemic. The primary point is that all simple sugars, including sucrose, are potent promoters of obesity; they are extremely low in bulk and have a high caloric density. Thus, in substituting carbohydrate for fat, a hypolipidemic effect can be expected only to the extent that total caloric intake is not increased and simple sugars are restricted.

Fiber, Saponins, and Antioxidants

Dietary fiber is a broad and nondescript term that includes several carbohydrates thought to be indigestible by the human gut. These include cellulose, hemicellulose, lignin, pectin, and beta glucans. Dietary fiber is found only in plants and is commonly present in unprocessed cereals, legumes, vegetables, and fruits. In ruminant animals, dietary fiber is completely digested by the microbial flora of the rumen; in these animals, fiber provides a major source of energy. In humans, however, dietary fiber contributes little to the caloric content of the diet but promotes satiety through its bulk. The bulk also greatly affects colonic function. A high-fiber diet produces larger stools and a more rapid intestinal transit, factors that may prevent certain diseases of the colon (i.e., diverticulitis, colon cancer).

Interest in the hypolipidemic effects of fiber dates back at least 30 years. Fiber added to semisynthetic diets fed to rats usually has a plasma cholesterol–lowering effect. Feeding fiber, predominantly in an insoluble form such as wheat bran, does not have a hypocholesterolemic effect in humans. Soluble fiber may be different. Large amounts of soluble fiber (17 g/2000 kcal), such as that contained in oat bran or beans, produced a 20 percent reduction of the plasma total and LDL cholesterol levels.[316] These decreases were, at least in part, a result of concurrent weight loss. Rich sources of soluble fiber include fruits, oats and some other cereals, legumes, and vegetables. One way in which soluble fiber acts to lower cholesterol is by binding bile acids in the gut and preventing their reabsorption. This is the same mechanism used by bile acid–binding resins such as cholestyramine. Soluble fibers also may reduce cholesterol absorption.

A high-fiber diet is certainly an integral part of the dietary concept for the treatment of hyperlipidemia. The consumption of more foods from vegetable sources will automatically mean a higher consumption of both total and soluble fiber. Such foods are bulky and have a lower caloric density, which is helpful for overweight patients. A feeling of satiety occurs from the consumption of high-fiber foods that also are low in calories. If oat bran is consumed in place of bacon and eggs for breakfast, this high-fiber food will also have a beneficial effect indirectly, since it has replaced foods high in cholesterol and saturated fat. Finally, plant foods rich in fiber also may contain other hypocholesterolemic substances. One of these substances is a group of compounds called saponins, which in monkeys have a hypocholesterolemic action.[317] Saponins bind cholesterol in the gut lumen and prevent its absorption.

Other dietary factors contained in fruits, vegetables, grains, and beans which may be important in the prevention of the atherogenic process are the antioxidants. The antioxidants may block the oxidation of LDL, which is believed to be central to the atherosclerotic process.[318,319] The antioxidant factors in plant foods include beta carotene, ascorbic acid (vitamin C), and alpha tocopherol (vitamin E). There is little evidence that consuming these vitamins in the form of vitamin supplements has an antiatherogenic effect. The important point is that when dietary fat is reduced, the consumption of fruits, vegetables, and beans is enhanced, which will increase the intake of the desirable antioxidants in a more natural and physiologic fashion.

Alcohol

In the past few years, there has been confusion about the relation between alcohol consumption and factors related to coronary heart disease. Alcohol consumption correlates well with higher values of HDL in the blood and reduced mortality from coronary heart disease.[320–323] Since HDL plays a role in "reverse" cholesterol transport, this finding has encouraged some researchers to conclude that drinking ethanol is "good for the heart." The findings related to alcohol, HDL, and coronary disease, however, are too scanty, contradictory, and complex to lead to any definite conclusions. From a clinical point of view, the typical patient attending a lipid clinic who is overweight and consumes two or more drinks a day could have a problem directly related to alcohol consumption. Usually such patients are hypertriglyceridemic and have low HDL concentrations.[324] A key aspect of the treatment for hypertriglyceridemia is to reduce alcohol consumption or even stop it completely, since alcohol increases hypertriglyceridemia. Alcohol also has a high caloric content of 140 kcal per drink. Two to three drinks a day can contribute 300 to 400 kcal to an already hypercaloric state, stimulating further the synthesis of triglyceride and VLDL by the liver. We therefore generally suggest that alcohol consumption in hyperlipidemic patients be restricted to no more than two to four drinks per week in order to avoid adverse effects on the plasma lipids and lipoproteins. However, if this amount of alcohol produces hyperlipidemia, the use of alcohol should be completely discontinued. The use of alcohol is clearly precluded in type I and type V patients who have had pancreatitis. If liver disease and hyperlipidemia occur together, alcohol should not be used in any circumstances. The use of alcohol as a means of elevating HDL concentrations is not to be recommended. Evidence that benefit would result is flimsy, and the diseases and social calamities that can result from excessive alcohol consumption are problems that are just as serious as hyperlipidemia.

Protein

Dietary protein has been studied extensively for possible effects on plasma lipid concentrations. These studies have utilized both single protein sources and mixtures of different proteins with range of protein intake from 25 to 150 g per day. No changes in the plasma cholesterol and triglyceride concentrations have resulted from these different amounts of protein, provided that at least the minimum amounts of essential amino acids were ingested. It has been suggested on the basis of animal studies that animal protein (such as casein from milk) is hypercholesterolemic and that vegetable protein (such as soybean protein) has a hypocholesterolemic effect. Well-designed experiments in humans to test the differential effects of casein and soy protein have not been conclusive. However, the rabbit experiments are not completely translatable to humans. Many human studies used formula diets with casein as the sole protein source. Since these diets were also free of cholesterol, plasma lipid levels fell greatly; this suggests that casein is probably not hypercholesterolemic. While the single-diet concept makes extensive use of proteins from vegetable sources, it does contain casein and is not a vegetarian diet. Thus, the inclusion of more protein from vegetable sources may confer some benefit to hyperlipidemic patients.

Lecithin

This phospholipid derived from soybeans is commonly sold in health food stores and is widely publicized as a popular remedy for hypercholesterolemia. Aside from its high content of linoleic acid, the consumption of lecithin is irrational, since this lipid is not absorbed as such from the digestive tract but is hydrolyzed into its constituent fatty acids, glycerol and choline. A higher content of linoleic acid in the diet can therefore be obtained much more inexpensively from a liquid polyunsaturated vegetable oil. There are no practical or theoretical reasons for the discrete use of lecithin, but no harm occurs.

Minerals and Vitamins

Assuming that the minimum daily requirements for minerals and vitamins have been met in the diet, there is no information to indicate that additional vitamins and minerals will have any effect on the plasma lipid concentrations. Recent information suggests that the antioxidant vitamins such as betacarotene, vitamin E, and vitamin C may be antiatherogenic.[319] The consumption of fruits, vegetables, grains, and beans would enhance the consumption of all vitamins and minerals. There is little evidence that adding vitamins as supplements to the low-fat, high-complex-carbohydrate diet would have an additional benefit. Excessive amounts of vitamin D cause hypercalcemia and hence would promote atherogenesis. The one exception is niacin (vitamin B_3), which, when given as a drug in a dose 50 times its requirement as a vitamin, does have a hypolipidemic effect. In this instance, niacin is used as a pharmaceutical preparation, not as a nutrient.

Coffee and Tea

Because of the enjoyment people derive from drinking coffee, there is great interest in the conflicting reports on the relation between coffee and coronary heart disease. Most of the reports are contradictory. One study from Europe does make some sense in that boiled coffee, in which most of the ingredients that might have an effect on health are extracted, is positively associated with the incidence of coronary heart disease.[325] The methods of coffee preparation in the United States are generally different (instant coffee, percolated coffee, filtered coffee). In a recent U.S. study, only the consumption of 720 ml of filtered caffeinated coffee raised the plasma cholesterol slightly (both LDL and HDL alike), in contrast to no effect from the same amount of decaffeinated coffee.[326] A theoretical reason why larger quantities of coffee may be harmful relates to the caffeine content. Caffeine stimulates the release of epinephrine, which increases FFA concentrations. The production of VLDL and triglyceride would be expected to increase as a consequence. No one has defined precisely what an excessive intake of coffee is. When patients ask, we generally suggest no more than four cups per day. Tea, by contrast, has not been associated with heart disease. In fact, tea drinkers, if anything, seem to have less coronary heart disease. Whether a patient chooses to drink decaffeinated or regular coffee or tea is a matter of personal choice.

Implementation of the Single-Diet Concept for the Treatment of Hyperlipidemia

Instead of multiple diets, each for a different form of hyperlipidemia, we favor a "single-diet" concept for the treatment of hyperlipidemia. The chemical formulation of the single diet, low in total and saturated fat and cholesterol and high in complex carbohydrates and fiber, is presented in terms of major components, as follows. Of course, the ultimate and optimal objectives in terms of a diet to produce maximal plasma lipid lowering will be achieved in a series of phases which have been fully described in detail, with appropriate menu planning and recipes, in recent publications.[327–329]

Dietary cholesterol is reduced from the usual American intake of 500 mg per day to 100 mg per day. This change will lower LDL cholesterol, which is elevated in types IIa and IIb hyperlipidemia, and also both VLDL and intermediate-density lipoproteins in types IV and III hyperlipidemias, respectively (Table 22-18). In many patients with "diet-induced" IIa or IIb hypercholesterolemia, a reduction of dietary cholesterol to 100 mg per day will lower the plasma lipids to "normal" values (plasma cholesterol level below 220 mg/dl). Frequently, hyperlipidemic patients are also overweight. For overweight patients, the same diet at a hypocaloric level should be prescribed initially until the patient attains optimum weight. At that time,

TABLE 22-18 Dietary Factors in the Causation and Correction of Lipoprotein Abnormalities

Lipoprotein Abnormality	Cause	Dietary Factor Increasing Lipoprotein Synthesis	Dietary Correction
Increased Chylomicrons (types I and V)	Impaired removal	Fat, except for omega-3 fatty acids from fish	Reduction of dietary fat to 5–10% of total calories*
Increased VLDL (types IV and IIb) and IDL (type III)	Impaired removal (obesity) and/or increased synthesis	Excessive calories from any source Dietary cholesterol and saturated fat	A hypocaloric 20% fat diet to induce loss of excess adiposity; reduction of dietary cholesterol and saturated fat
Increased LDL (types IIa and IIb)	Increased synthesis and impaired removal	Dietary cholesterol, saturated fat, and total fat	Reduction of dietary cholesterol to 100 mg, saturated fat to 5% of total calories, and total fat to 20%
Decreased HDL	Utilization of HDL apoproteins in triglyceride-carrying lipoproteins in types I, V, IV, IIb, and III hyperlipidemias	Excessive calories with adiposity	Correction of obesity as noted above

* All overweight hyperlipidemic patients should have the appropriate dietary factor modified as above and should be provided with a hypocaloric diet to help in the attainment of normal body weight. For an insulin-dependent diabetic, appropriate use of insulin may also aid in the correction of the hyperlipidemia. The omega-3 fatty acids from fish may help reduce plasma VLDL and triglyceride levels.

the low-fat, high-complex-carbohydrate diet at a eucaloric level is prescribed.

In patients with genetically determined severe hypercholesterolemia, normal plasma cholesterol levels cannot be achieved by means of diet alone; combined diet plus drug therapy is needed. Restrictions on dietary cholesterol and saturated fat are nevertheless critically important in severe type IIa patients.

Dietary fat content is lowered to 20 percent of total calories compared with the usual American fat intake of 40 percent of total calories. Most of this decrease is in saturated fat, which is reduced to no more than 5 percent of total calories. This change in total fat content and composition has a beneficial effect in all forms of hyperlipidemia for reasons already discussed but especially in type II and types I and V hyperlipidemia (Table 22-18). In the latter two cases, when dietary fat is reduced to a minimum, the chylomicrons present in the blood gradually clear and the plasma triglycerides fall. Plasma cholesterol levels also decline, and HDL and LDL, both very low, rise. This "minimum" of dietary fat varies from patient to patient with hyperchylomicronemia; the exact level necessary for chylomicron clearance can be ascertained only by means of a trial of several diets with a fat content varying from 5 to 20 percent.[330]

In some patients with extreme chylomicronemia who are in danger of acute pancreatitis, a 1 percent fat or fat-free formula diet (protein, glucose, minerals, and vitamins) can be employed to promote maximal chylomicron lowering. Another simple but effective approach is the use of fruit juices for a few days of initial therapy. In both cases, triglyceride levels fall rapidly (Fig. 22-28).

While the basic problem in types I and V hyperlipidemia is not an excess of dietary cholesterol and while the suggested diets need not restrict cholesterol per se, they are lower in cholesterol content because most foods that contain cholesterol are also high in fat. However, shellfish, which are relatively high in cholesterol content, are low in fat content and in saturated fat. Consequently, shellfish and fish can be freely used by patients with types I and V hyperlipidemia.

Omega-3 fatty acids derived from fish may be added to the low-fat diet in order to achieve a specific hypolipidemic effect over and above what can be obtained from the dietary measures suggested in the single-diet concept. The omega-3 fatty acids from fatty fish, or even fish oil used experimentally, will have a pronounced plasma triglyceride (VLDL)–lowering action in hypertriglyceridemic patients with an exaggerated synthesis of VLDL. The result of giving omega-3 fatty acids to type V patients is illustrated in Fig. 22-27.[308] Polyunsaturated vegetable oil, as is well known, raises triglyceride levels in type V patients, and its use is therefore contraindicated. Fatty fish such as salmon, mackarel, and sardines may be particularly effective. Fish oil in doses of 15 g per day or more may also be used in type V patients.

Saturated fat in the diet is reduced greatly to maximize the lowering of LDL in types IIa and IIb. The polyunsaturated fat content remains little

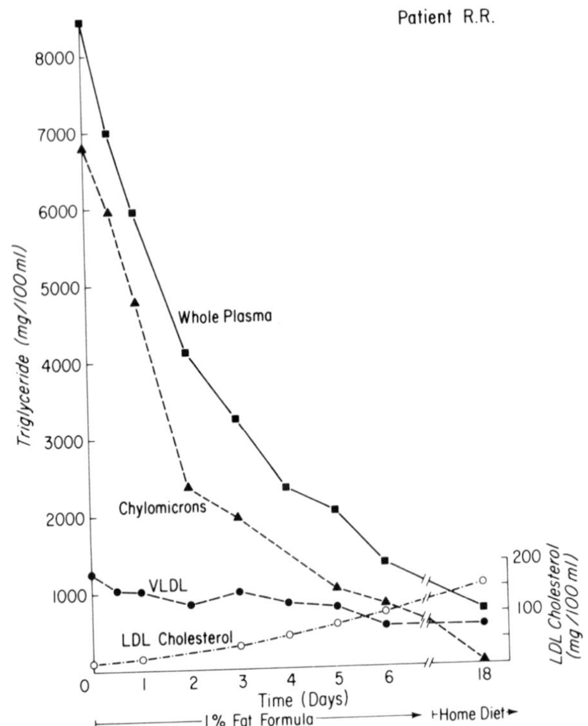

FIGURE 22-28 Reduction in chylomicronemia by means of a 1 percent fat formula diet plus insulin replacement in a patient with adult-onset diabetes mellitus and phenotypic type V hyperlipoproteinemia. Note that the fall in chylomicron and VLDL levels is associated with a reciprocal rise in LDL cholesterol. Concentrations of HDL cholesterol also rose (not shown).

changed from the usual American intake of 6 to 8 percent of total calories. Most of the reduction of the total fat from 40 percent of total calories to 20 percent is accomplished by cutting down on foods which are rich in saturated fatty acids.

Of particular importance is the decrease in the HDL cholesterol level that occurs with a low-fat, low-cholesterol diet. Populations that eat low-fat diets have been observed to have low HDL cholesterol levels.[331,332] Since these populations have low LDL cholesterol levels and little coronary heart disease, the low HDL cholesterol level is not a risk factor. The physiologic response to a low-fat diet is a 10 to 20 percent decrease in the HDL cholesterol level.[330] Since LDL cholesterol is lowered even more, the LDL to HDL ratio is little changed or even improved. Also, a lower HDL cholesterol level resulting from a low-fat, high-complex-carbohydrate diet is different from a genetically low HDL cholesterol level in that the coronary risk is not enhanced.[333]

The Cholesterol–Saturated Fat Index of Foods

The major plasma cholesterol–elevating effects of a given food reside in its content of cholesterol and saturated fat. To understand the contribution of these two factors in a single food item and to compare one food with another, we have computed a cholesterol–saturated fat index (CSI) for selected foods.[334,335] The formula for the CSI is CSI = $(1.01 \times \text{g saturated fat}) + (0.05 \times \text{mg cholesterol})$, where the amounts of saturated fat and cholesterol in a given amount of a food item are entered into this equation. The higher the CSI of a food, the greater the hypercholesterolemic and atherogenic effect. This index is a representation of how much a given food will decrease the activity of the LDL receptor and hence raise the level of LDL cholesterol in plasma.

In this context, it is particularly instructive to compare the CSI of fish with that of moderately fatty beef. An 85-g portion of cooked fish contains 51 mg of cholesterol and 0.14 g of saturated fat. This contrasts to 80 mg of cholesterol and 11.3 g of saturated fat in 30 percent fat beef. The CSI for 85 g (3 oz) of fish is 3; that of 85 g of beef is 15. The caloric value of these two portions also differs greatly (71 for fish and 323 for beef). The CSI of cooked chicken and turkey (without the skin) is also lower than that of beef and other red meats. The total fat content is considerably lower. The saturated fat in an 85-g serving is 1.6 g, and the cholesterol is 71 mg. The CSI of poultry is 5. Table 22-19 lists the CSI for various foods. Shellfish have a low CSI because their saturated fat content is extremely low despite the fact that their cholesterol content is 2.5 to 3 times higher than that of fish, poultry, or red meat. Shellfish have a CSI of 3. This means that when one is considering both cholesterol and saturated fat, shellfish, like poultry, is a better choice than even the leanest red meats. Salmon also has a low CSI and is preferred to meat. The CSI of 1000 foods, as well as information about selection for categories of foods and over 300 recipes with low CSIs, can be found in *The New American Diet System*.[329]

The *protein* intake is kept at an amount similar to what Americans commonly eat: about 15 percent of total calories. The decrease in fat content is thus offset by a reciprocal increase in dietary *carbohydrate,* ultimately to 65 percent of total calories. This is provided primarily in terms of complex carbohydrate ordinarily associated with protein. Other constituents of the diet are not reduced or are enhanced in terms of nutritional adequacy.

Caloric control is vitally important in overweight patients for decreasing the VLDL of types IIb and IV and the IDL of type III hyperlipidemia and in improving the chylomicron clearance in type V hyperlipidemia (Table 22-18). These overweight patients have elevated plasma triglyceride levels, often with concomitant adult-onset diabetes. Such hyperlipidemias are particularly sensitive to the state of caloric balance. Dietary factors operate indirectly but crucially in supplying the substrate for triglyceride synthesis. Type III hyperlipidemia is rare, and be-

TABLE 22-19 The Cholesterol–Saturated Fat Index (CSI) and Kilocalorie Content of Selected Foods

	CSI*	Calorie, kcal*
Fish, poultry, red meat [3oz (85 g) cooked]		
Shellfish (oysters, scallops, clams)	3	100
Whitefish (snapper, perch, sole, cod, halibut, etc.)	3	100
Salmon	5	168
Shellfish (shrimp, crab, lobster)	5	85
Poultry, no skin	5	154
Beef, pork and lamb		
10 percent fat (ground sirloin, flank steak)	7	170
15 percent fat (ground extra lean, round steak, pork chop)	9	215
25 percent fat (ground lean, rump roasts)	12	278
30 percent fat (typical ground beef, ground lamb, steaks, ribs, lamb chops, pork sausage, roasts)	15	323
Cheese [1 oz (28g)]		
Low-fat ricotta, tofu (bean curd), Dorman's Light†, Alpine Lace Free N Lean, Kraft Free Singles	<1	53
Imitation mozzarella†, Hickory Farms Lyte†, Heart Beat Sharp Cheddar†	1	74
Lite-line, part-skim ricotta, Reduced Calories Laughing Cow, lite part-skim mozzarella, Mini Chol (Swedish low fat)†	2	62
Lite n'Lively, Olympia's Low Fat, Green River Part-Skim, Kraft Light Naturals, Light cream cheese, Heidi Ann Low Fat Ched-Style, Lappi, String, part-skim mozzarella	4	73
Cheese spreads (jars), Neufchatel (lower-fat cream cheese), Velveeta, Brie, Swiss, gruyere	6	93
Cheddar, roquefort, jack, American, cream cheese, havarti, feta	8	111
Eggs		
Whites (two)	0	32
Egg substitute (equivalent to two eggs)	0	98
Whole (two)	25	158
Fats (1/4 cup or 4 tablespoons)		
Peanut butter	6	380
Mayonnaise, fat free, cholesterol free	trace	48
Mayonnaise, Light	3	200
Mayonnaise, regular	8	404
Most vegetable oils	7	491
Olive oil	8	486
Soft vegetable margarines	8	405
Soft shortenings	13	464
Bacon grease	20	464
Butter	36	432
Coconut oil, palm oil	37	491
Frozen desserts (1 cup)		
Fruit ices, sorbets	0	255
Nonfat frozen yogurt	trace	224
Sherbet or frozen yogurt (low-fat)	3	249
Ice milk	4	224
Ice cream, 10% fat	15	329
Rich ice cream, 12% fat	19	480
Specialty ice cream, 18% fat	30	580
Milk products (1 cup)		
Skim milk or powdered nonfat	1	85
1% milk, buttermilk	2	100
2% milk	4	122
Whole milk (3.5% fat)	7	149
Cottage cheese, low-fat (2%)	4	204
Cottage cheese, regular	8	222
Liquid nondairy creamers: soybean oil	4	326
Liquid nondairy creamers: coconut oil	23	326
Sour cream	36	468
Imitation sour cream (IMO)	40	480

* Averages.

† Cheeses made with skim milk and vegetable oils.

cause its dietary treatment is similar to that for type IV, it will not be referred to specifically in the subsequent comments other than to emphasize the extreme importance of weight control.

Reduction of excess body weight is the most important measure for the correction of type IV hyperlipidemia. We stress gradual rather than sudden weight loss so that the weight-loss diet will be balanced in nutrients and will not have untoward effects. For overweight patients, the caloric content of the diet can be reduced to one-third or two-fifths of the patient's caloric requirements. We then expect a gentle weight loss of about 2 lb per week.

The plasma triglyceride and cholesterol response to caloric restriction and weight loss is prompt and dramatic. Within 1 to 2 weeks, the plasma triglyceride and cholesterol levels decrease, and they remain lower as long as weight loss continues. With the achievement of normal weight, the plasma triglyceride level usually is in the normal range. Glucose intolerance and the associated diabetic state may also disappear with the hypertriglyceridemia.

The special case of overweight type IIb patients warrants further comment. After the excessive plasma triglyceride levels are corrected by means of weight loss, such patients will be left with some hypercholesterolemia carried by LDL. Particular attention will have to be directed toward the restriction of dietary cholesterol and fat when the eucaloric diet to maintain weight is initiated.

It should be noted that in some hypertriglyceridemic patients, caloric control and a reduction in serum triglycerides will not be achieved unless dietary carbohydrate is restricted. This reduction in dietary carbohydrate should be accompanied by a decrease in dietary fat.

A Phased Approach to the Dietary Treatment of Hyperlipidemia

A realistic view is that even highly motivated patients have difficulty making abrupt changes in their dietary habits. It may take many months and even years to change patterns of food consumption. Therefore, the changes recommended from the current American diet of most hyperlipidemic patients should be approached in a gradual manner, with each of three phases introducing more changes toward the eating pattern ultimately required for maximal therapy.

The goal of phase I is to modify the customary consumption of foods very high in cholesterol and saturated fat (Table 22-20). This can be accomplished by deleting egg yolk, butterfat, lard, and organ meats from the diet and by using substitute products when possible: soft margarine for butter, vegetable oils and shortening for lard, skim milk for whole milk, and egg whites for whole eggs.

In phase II, a reduction in meat consumption is the goal, with a gradual transition from the presumed American ideal of up to a pound of meat a day to no more than 6 to 8 oz per day (Table 22-20). Meat can no longer be the center of the meal, particularly for two or three meals a day. Some ideas for lunch with and without sandwiches have been detailed in sample menus and recipes.[327–329] In addition, in phase II we propose the use of less fat and cheese.

Substitute recipes have been developed to replace recipes which are centered on meat or high-fat dairy products (cream cheese, butter, sour cream, cheese) as the principal ingredients. Since these foods are to be eaten in smaller amounts or even omitted (butterfat), the patient needs to find recipes which use larger amounts of grains, legumes, vegetables, and fruits. Examples of such recipes are included in Refs. 327 through 329.

In phase III, the maximal diet for the treatment of hyperlipidemia is attained (Table 22-20). The cholesterol content of the diet is reduced to 100 mg per day, and saturated fat is lowered to 5 to 6 percent of total calories. Since cholesterol is contained only in foods of animal origin, these changes mean that meat consumption in particular must be further reduced. Meat, fish, and poultry should be used as "condiments" rather than "aliments." With this philosophy, the meat dish will no longer occupy the center of the table. Instead, meat in smaller quantities will spice up dishes based on vegetables, rice, cereal, and legumes, much as Asian, Indian, and Mediterranean cookery has been doing for eons. The total of meat and poultry should average 3 to 4 oz per day, but the use of poultry should be stressed because of its lower content of saturated fat. The use of fish is also preferred. Note the low CSI of fish in Table 22-19, shared also by shellfish, as alluded to subsequently. Because of a low CSI, up to 6 oz of fish can

TABLE 22-20 Summary of the Suggested Dietary Changes in the Different Phases of the Diet

Phase I
- Avoid foods very high in cholesterol and saturated fat
  - Delete egg yolk, butterfat, lard, and organ meats
- Substitute soft margarine for butter, vegetable oils and shortening for lard, skim milk for whole milk, egg whites for whole eggs

Phase II
- Gradually use less meat and more fish, chicken, and turkey
  - No more than 6–8 oz a day
  - Use less fat and cheese
  - Acquire new recipes

Phase III
- Eat mainly cereals, legumes, fruits, and vegetables
  - Use meat as a condiment
  - Use low-cholesterol cheeses
- Save these foods for use only on special occasions: extra meats, regular cheese, chocolate, candy, and coconut

be used in place of meat during phase III of the diet. All fish contain omega-3 fatty acids.

Shellfish are divided into two groups: high-cholesterol shellfish (shrimp, crab, and lobster) and low-cholesterol shellfish (oysters, clams, and scallops). Both groups contain omega-3 fatty acids and have a low fat content. Because of these differences, high-cholesterol shellfish are more restricted in the daily diet than are low-cholesterol shellfish, i.e., 3 oz vs. 6 oz per day. The low-cholesterol shellfish contain other sterols (e.g., brassicasterol) that are more analogous to plant sterols. These are poorly absorbed by humans.

The use of special low-cholesterol cheeses is an important component of phase III (Table 22-19). The sample menus in Refs. 327 through 329 give some idea about the eating pattern in phase III.

A new eating habit questionnaire, the Diet Habit Survey, can be used to classify the diet into the typical U.S. diet and into phases I, II, and III of the low-fat, high-complex-carbohydrate diet.[336] The Diet Habit Survey is related to plasma cholesterol change, measures eating habits directly, reflects nutrient composition indirectly, is quick to administer, and is inexpensive to analyze. Thus, it is useful as a research questionnaire and helpful in the dietary management of patients with hyperlipidemia and coronary heart disease.

The Chemical Composition of the Low-Fat, High-Complex-Carbohydrate Diet

The American diet contains approximately 500 mg of cholesterol per day. This is decreased in phase I to 300 mg, in phase II to 200 mg, and in phase III to 100 mg. The fat content decreases from 40 percent of calories in the American diet to 30 percent in phase I, 25 percent in phase II, and 20 percent in phase III, with special consideration given to the decrease in saturated fat. To provide sufficient calories to meet body needs, the carbohydrate content should be increased as the fat content is decreased, with emphasis on the use of the fiber-containing complex carbohydrates contained in whole grains, cereal products, and legumes. The carbohydrate content increases from 45 percent of the calories in the American diet to 55 percent in phase I, 60 percent in phase II, and 65 percent in phase III. The bulk or fiber in the diet is enhanced considerably, a feature which induces satiety sooner per unit of calories and helps promote weight loss. The dietary fiber content increases from 18 to 45 g per day.

Predicted Plasma Cholesterol Lowering from the Three Phases of the Low-Fat, High-Complex-Carbohydrate Diet

As has been emphasized, both dietary cholesterol and saturated fat elevate plasma cholesterol levels, whereas monounsaturated and polyunsaturated fats have a mild depressing effect. In stepwise fashion, the cholesterol and saturated fat of each phase of the diet are successively reduced, with phase III providing for the lowest intakes. According to calculations derived from Hegsted and coworkers,[337] phase III of the diet would provide for maximal plasma cholesterol lowering, an estimated average change of 20 percent. Phase II would produce a lowering of 14 percent; and phase I, 7 percent. These plasma cholesterol changes for all phases offer the possibility of improved plasma lipids, depending on the amount of dietary modifications, with phase III as the ultimate goal.

The Use of the Low-Fat, High-Complex-Carbohydrate Diet in Diabetic Patients, Pregnant Patients, Children, and Hypertensive Patients

The approach to diabetic patients who are also hyperlipidemic involves the same dietary considerations for the treatment of the hyperlipidemia. Phase III of the diet has been used successfully in both juvenile-onset and maturity-onset diabetic patients, insulin-dependent and non-insulin-dependent. Clearly involved in this treatment is the appropriate control of carbohydrate as well as lipid metabolism by means of adequate amounts of insulin and weight reduction when the patient is overweight. The great propensity of diabetic patients to atherosclerotic vascular disease makes control of their hyperlipidemia of particular importance. The principles we have outlined can be utilized fully with benefit to the patient.

Pregnancy constitutes a particularly difficult situation, because in most pregnant women there will be a 40 to 50 percent increase in plasma lipids and lipoproteins (chiefly LDL) in physiologic circumstances. A hyperlipidemic patient who becomes pregnant should continue on the same diet recommended previously for the treatment of her hyperlipidemia, supplemented by vitamins and minerals as is usual in pregnancy. In patients with familial hypercholesterolemia, the phase III diet is utilized as before, with some increase in calories to permit the desired weight gain. In type I or V hypertriglyceridemic pregnant patients, there is apt to be a profound augmentation of the usual hyperchylomicronemia, and strict adherence to the 5 to 10 percent fat diet is often necessary to avoid pancreatitis.

The single-diet concept for the treatment of hyperlipidemic children can be applied as for adults, with the exception that a child up to 4 years of age is allowed less cholesterol than an older child. Above age 4 years, no more than 3 oz of meat per day is the goal. Egg yolk, organ meat, and butterfat are eliminated from the diet, even for infants. Dietary iron is supplemented from fortified cereals. Human breast milk or whole cow's milk is recommended before weaning or until the infant eats enough table food to provide adequate calories for growth. This is usually from 1 to 2 years. From that time on, the child should drink skim milk.

For the rare infant with type I hyperlipidemia, the fat content of the usual human breast or cow's milk is much too high. A basic skim milk formula will have to be used to avoid the abdominal pain and episodes of pancreatitis to which these patients are so prone. The main objective of such therapy is the provision of sufficient amounts of essential fatty acids, which can be prescribed separately as canola or soybean oil, to yield at least 2 to 4 percent of the total calories. Such oils will provide both omega-6 and omega-3 fatty acids. In this way much of the fat intake will be from linoleic and linolenic acids, and very little other fat will be taken in. Success in several infants with the type I disorder has been achieved using this dietary approach, resulting in the abolition of episodes of abdominal pain.

Special attention must be given to hypertensive, hyperlipidemic patients for several reasons. First, coronary heart disease and atherosclerotic brain disease are common causes of death in hypertensive patients. Second, some diuretic agents (thiazides) and β-adrenergic blocking agents are hyperlipidemic in themselves so that the usual hypertensive patient will have an increase in plasma lipids from the use of these agents alone. Thus, hypertensive individuals who are given thiazides or β-adrenergic blocking agents should have additional dietary therapy in the form of the single-diet approach. Furthermore, the genetic syndrome of both hypertension and hypertriglyceridemia requires simultaneous treatment of both conditions. Finally, a salt-restriction program can readily be incorporated to provide for the additional treatment of the essential hypertension as this is desired by the physician. The correction of obesity and lessening of alcohol intake may also have blood-pressure-lowering effects. To combine the dietary treatment of hypertension and that of hyperlipidemia in a single diet, a stepwise reduction in salt use is also advocated and incorporated into the different phases.[328]

Interrelations Between Dietary and Pharmaceutical Therapy of Hyperlipidemic States

Although dietary therapy remains the cornerstone in the treatment of hyperlipidemia, many patients require pharmaceutical treatment to attain the therapeutic objectives. In this connection, some patients may believe that once they are started on drug therapy, they no longer need to pay as much attention to their diet. Nothing could be farther from the truth. The two modes of therapy are not mutually exclusive but are complementary. Maximum dietary treatment may lower plasma LDL and total cholesterol as much as 15 to 20 percent. This will continue to be the case when pharmaceutical treatment is added.

The complementary nature of diet and drugs is easily noted during the holiday period from Thanksgiving to New Year's day, when weight gain and additional intake of cholesterol and saturated fat from holiday foods occur. When patients were given a diet high in cholesterol and saturated fat while still maintaining the usual dose of lovastatin, the plasma cholesterol level increased from 246 to 289 mg/dl, a 17.5 percent increase. LDL cholesterol increased 20 percent. When it is considered that dietary cholesterol and saturated fat decrease LDL receptor activity[294] and that lovastatin increases LDL receptor activity,[293] it becomes apparent that a diet high in cholesterol and saturated fat may nullify some of the beneficial effects of lovastatin.

Similar responses may occur in patients with type IV or type V hyperlipidemia. Weight gain and a high-fat diet or an increase in carbohydrate intake can nullify the effects of gemfibrozil in maintaining lower plasma triglyceride concentrations. When a patient whose lipid values have previously been under good control with diet and medication has a deterioration in lipid values, it is reasonable to question whether the previous dietary lifestyle changes have been disregarded. In diabetic hypertriglyceridemic patients, the dietary deviations will upset glycemic control as well. When this matter is explained to the patient, he or she is then able to return to the previous excellent dietary lifestyle, with a concomitant decrease in the plasma triglyceride levels and, if the patient is diabetic, better glucose control.

PHARMACEUTICAL AGENTS FOR THE TREATMENT OF HYPERLIPOPROTEINEMIA

The rationale for the treatment of hyperlipoproteinemia is based on the premise that a successful reduction in lipid levels will lead to slowing of the rate of progression of atherosclerosis or, potentially, a reversal of this process with a subsequent reduction in cardiovascular morbidity and mortality. A substantial body of evidence now supports the view that reductions in the plasma concentrations of LDL cholesterol and, possibly, concurrent decreases in Lp(a) and increases in HDL cholesterol are associated with a reduction in coronary morbidity and mortality in middle-aged men studied in prospective primary prevention trials.[338,339] An increased frequency of regression and less progression of coronary artery disease[69,70,340,341] is observed in patients with established coronary disease treated with lipid-lowering drugs. Treatment of patients with severe hypertriglyceridemia is aimed at the prevention of medical complications (abdominal pain and pancreatitis) resulting from severe hyperchylomicronemia and concurrently at a reduction of the long-term risks of atherosclerosis. Because hyperlipoproteinemia is a lifelong disorder, the decision to begin drug therapy should be made only after satisfactory exclusion of secondary factors and after an adequate trial of diet has failed to achieve satisfactory lipid levels. It must be emphasized that once drugs are used to treat hyperlipoproteinemia, dietary therapy should be stressed again at the same time. The response to therapy generally will be maximized when this twofold approach is employed. A limited number of drugs are available, and their clinical indications will be reviewed in this section. Several reviews have been published recently.[342,343]

Bile Acid Sequestrants

Two products are currently available: cholestyramine (Questran) and colestipol (Colestid). Both are high-molecular-weight polymers to which anionic bile acids are ionically bound in exchange for chloride ions. These bile acid–binding resins are not absorbed, and their activities are based entirely on sequestration of bile acids in the intestinal lumen. The bile acid–resin complex is excreted in the stools.

Mechanism of Action

The primary action of both cholestyramine and colestipol is to bind bile acids in the intestinal lumen. This in turn results in an interruption of the enterohepatic circulation of bile acids and a markedly increased excretion of these steroids in the feces. The size of the bile acid pool is decreased, and this reduction stimulates increased hepatic synthesis of bile acids from cholesterol. Depletion of the hepatic pool of cholesterol results in two compensatory changes: an increase in cholesterol biosynthesis and an increase in the number of specific high-affinity receptors for LDL on the hepatocyte membrane.[344,345] The increased number of hepatic LDL receptors stimulates the rate of LDL catabolism from plasma and thus lowers the concentration of this lipoprotein. The selective stimulation of hepatic LDL receptors explains why concentrations of LDL are selectively reduced during therapy with a bile acid sequestrant. Bile acid sequestrants are ineffective in patients with homozygous familial hypercholesterolemia who lack the ability to make more high-affinity LDL receptors. The increase in hepatic cholesterol biosynthesis which occurs during therapy with a bile acid sequestrant may be paralleled by an increase in hepatic VLDL production and often results in a slight increase in plasma concentrations of triglyceride and VLDL.

Side Effects

The most common side effects of cholestyramine and colestipol consist of changes in bowel function, including constipation, bloating, epigastric fullness, nausea, and flatulence. Constipation, which is the most frequent side effect, may be relieved with stool softeners, but the gritty nature of these medications may exacerbate hemorrhoids. Patients frequently complain that these medications are bulky, and some find the sandy or gritty texture unpleasant. Rare side effects have included intestinal obstruction and the development of hyperchloremic acidosis. Decreased absorption of fat-soluble vitamins and folic acid may occur with prolonged high doses of both medications, and oral supplementation with these vitamins may be advisable in children. Because of their avidity for anionic molecules, cholestyramine and colestipol may interfere with the absorption of other drugs, and it is advisable to take other medications 1 h before or 4 h after taking the resin. Such effects have been reported with digoxin, thyroxine, warfarin, pravastatin, and thiazides and may occur with any anionic drug. Biochemical side effects include a modest increase in plasma triglyceride concentrations in many patients; mild increases in alkaline phosphatase and transaminases have also been reported.

Indications and Dosage

Cholestyramine is available in 9-g packets (Questran), which contain 4 g of cholestyramine and 5 g of orange flavoring, and in cans that contain 378 g. A second preparation of this drug (Questran Lite) contains the same 4 g of cholestyramine but 1 g of orange flavoring, which is sweetened with Nutrasweet. This preparation is available in 5-g packets and 210-g cans. Colestipol is available in 5-g packets and 500-g bottles; this formulation contains no additives. The cholesterol-lowering effects of 4 g of cholestyramine appear to be equivalent to those obtained with 5 g of colestipol. Both medications must be mixed with water or juice and are taken in two (or occasionally three) divided doses with or just after meals. The total daily dose of cholestyramine is 8 to 24 g a day, and the daily dose of colestipol is 10 to 30 g; however, the benefits of increasing the dose above 16 g of cholestyramine or 20 g of colestipol per day must be balanced against the high incidence of gastrointestinal side effects and poorer patient compliance at these higher doses.

As was discussed in Hypercholesterolemia, bile acid sequestrants are among the drugs of choice for patients with primary elevations in the concentrations of LDL cholesterol who do not have concurrent hypertriglyceridemia. These agents have no place in the treatment of other hyperlipidemias and may in fact aggravate the hypertriglyceridemia seen in patients with type III hyperlipoproteinemia and patients with chylomicronemia. The response to therapy in patients with primary hypercholesterolemia is variable, but 15 to 25 percent reductions in concentrations of LDL cholesterol may be achieved with 16 g a day of cholestyramine or 20 g of colestipol.[132] The addition of nicotinic acid to this regimen may result in further decrements of 20 to 25 percent, and this combination remains one of the most effective for patients with severe type IIa hypercholesterolemia (Table 22-13). This is illustrated in Fig. 22-29. Combined drug therapy with a bile acid sequestrant and probucol[346] or gemfibrozil is sometimes effective in patients who are unable to take nicotinic acid. Combined drug therapy with an inhibitor of HMG CoA reductase plus a bile acid sequestrant is the most consistently effective regimen available, resulting in a greater than 50 percent reduction in the concentrations of LDL cholesterol in patients with familial hypercholesterolemia (Table 22-13).

Cholestyramine was the drug used in the Lipid Research Clinic's Primary Prevention Trial.[338] The results from this large clinical trial have established the long-term safety and efficacy of bile acid sequestrants and have provided conclusive proof that reduction of LDL cholesterol reduces morbidity and mortality from cardiovascular disease. Because they are not absorbed, bile acid sequestrants are the only drugs safe for use in the treatment of children with heterozygous familial hypercholesterolemia; if clinically indicated, these drugs can also be used for the treatment of patients with severe type II hypercholesterolemia during pregnancy.

Nicotinic Acid

The hypolipidemic action of nicotinic acid, or niacin, has been recognized for 30 years[347] and appears to be unrelated to its action as a coenzyme in intermediary metabolism. It is well absorbed from the gastrointestinal tract and is excreted in the urine.

FIGURE 22-29 The effects of sequential therapy with diet, colestipol, and colestipol plus nicotinic acid on the plasma concentrations of cholesterol and triglycerides in 13 patients with heterozygous familial hypercholesterolemia. (*Redrawn from Illingworth et al.*[139])

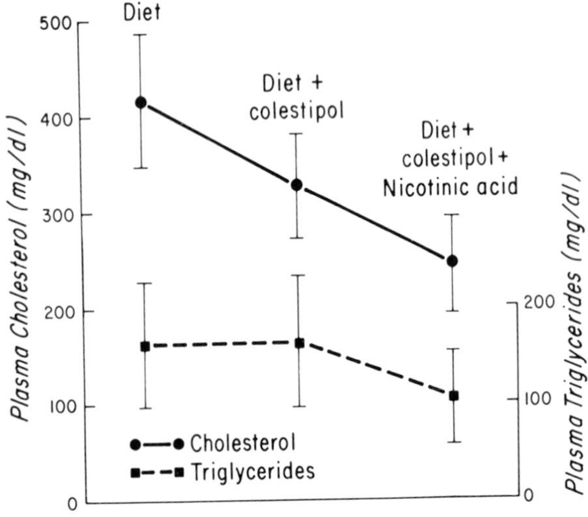

Mechanism of Action

The precise mechanism of action of nicotinic acid at the cellular level that is responsible for reducing plasma concentrations of VLDL and LDL is not known. Considerable evidence, however, points to an effect in reducing the hepatic synthesis of VLDL,[348] which in turn leads to a reduction in LDL synthesis. Factors responsible for the decreased hepatic production of VLDL include inhibition of lipolysis with a concomitant decrease in FFA levels in plasma, decreased hepatic esterification of triglycerides, and possible effects on the hepatic production of apoprotein B.

Side Effects

The main side effects of nicotinic acid involve the skin and gastrointestinal tract. Cutaneous flushing occurs 15 min to 2 h after a patient takes the medication, but the duration and magnitude usually diminish with prolonged therapy and can be minimized by starting at a low dose and always taking the medication after the ingestion of food. The flushing appears to be mediated by prostaglandins and can be reduced by means of the concurrent administration of 150 to 325 mg of aspirin.[349] Nausea, abdominal discomfort, and diarrhea constitute the most common gastrointestinal side effects, and the drug is contraindicated in patients with active liver disease, peptic ulcer disease, or hyperuricemia. Less common side effects include itching, development of rash, hyperpigmentation of the skin with development of acanthosis nigricans, and blurred vision due to macular edema; blurred vision is not common but will necessitate the discontinuation of therapy. Other side effects have included activation of peptic ulcer disease and exacerbation of both hyperuricemia and diabetes. Laboratory disturbances noted in patients on nicotinic acid are more common with higher doses (>3 g per day) and include increases in alkaline phosphatase and transaminases and elevation of uric acid and glucose. The incidence of elevated transaminases and alkaline phosphatase is higher in patients receiving time-release formulations of niacin,[350] and patients should be advised not to change from regular to sustained-release formulations of this drug because of the increased risk of hepatotoxicity at the same daily dose.[351] Liver function tests and uric acid should be monitored during the initiation of nicotinic acid and should be checked periodically once an appropriate dosage regimen has been established.

Indications and Dosage

Nicotinic acid is available in tablets containing 100, 250, or 500 mg and in time-release preparations containing 125, 250, or 500 mg. The authors do not recommend the time-release forms of nicotinic acid, which increase the risk of abnormal liver function. Niacinamide, which is widely available in health food stores, has no effect on lipid or lipoprotein concentrations. Therapy with nicotinic acid is best initiated with a low-dose regimen (e.g., 100 to 250 mg once to three times daily with or just after meals), with the dose then being gradually increased at 7- to 14-day intervals to a total dose of 3 g per day. Lipid values as well as tests of liver function, blood glucose, and uric acid should be assessed at this point; if a satisfactory reduction in plasma lipids has not been achieved, the dose should be increased a further 1.5 g per day. Periodic increases in the dose up to a maximum of 7.5 to 8 g per day may be administered, but the increased hypolipidemic effect of such higher doses must be balanced against the higher incidence of side effects noted at doses above 4.5 g per day. Nicotinic acid is useful in the treatment of all hyperlipoproteinemias except those due to familial LPL deficiency. The drug is used chiefly in the treatment of primary hypercholesterolemia; when used by itself, it results in 15 to 30 percent decreases in concentrations of LDL cholesterol with a concurrent 10 to 20 percent rise in HDL levels.[132] In addition to reducing LDL concentrations, nicotinic acid at a dose of 4 g per day has been reported to reduce Lp(a) concentrations by 30 percent.[279] Forty to eighty percent reductions in the concentrations of plasma triglycerides may be obtained with nicotinic acid, and this drug is effective in reducing both VLDL and LDL levels in patients with phenotypic type IIb hyperlipidemia. Nicotinic acid is a second-choice drug for patients with type III hyperlipoproteinemia (clofibrate is the drug of choice) and is a good second-choice drug for patients with severe hypertriglyceridemia (type V phenotype), in whom gemfibrozil is currently the drug of choice. As was discussed previously, combined treatment with nicotinic acid and a bile acid sequestrant is an effective therapy for patients with severe hypercholesterolemia and LDL concentrations greater than 300 mg/dl. Although combination therapy with nicotinic acid and an HMG CoA reductase inhibitor (e.g., lovastatin) may also be an effective regimen, the use of these two drugs together cannot be generally recommended because of an increased risk of myopathy.[352]

HMG CoA Reductase Inhibitors

The recent development of specific competitive inhibitors of HMG CoA reductase, the rate-limiting enzyme in cholesterol biosynthesis, has provided an important therapeutic approach to the treatment of hypercholesterolemia and combined hyperlipidemia.[342] Lovastatin, the first agent in this class to become available, was approved for prescription use in the United States in 1987, and two other agents in this class, simvastatin and pravastatin, have recently become available. Other drugs in this class (e.g., Fluvastatin and Dalvastatin) remain in clinical trials.

Mechanism of Action

The structure of the currently available and some of the investigational HMG CoA reductase inhibitors is shown in Fig. 22-30. Lovastatin is made by a soil fungus (*Aspergillus terrius*), and simvastatin is a methylated derivative of this drug. Pravastatin is produced by microbial transformation of mevastatin. Lovastatin and simvastatin are administered as prodrugs (lactones), and conversion to the open acid occurs after gastrointestinal absorption; in contrast, pravastatin is administered orally as the open acid formulation. Studies in animals and in tissue culture on the relative rates of uptake of these drugs by the liver and by peripheral tissues are contradictory,[353–355] and further work is needed to assess whether the greater hydrophilicity of pravastatin compared with simvastatin and lovastatin results in lower rates of uptake of this drug in peripheral tissues. At the present time, any clinical advantage of pravastatin resulting from potential "tissue selectivity" activity remains to be demonstrated.[356] At clinically effective doses, all these drugs are primarily taken up by the liver and exert their hypolipidemic effects by inhibiting hepatic HMG CoA reductase. Lovastatin and simvastatin reduce the 24-h rates of excretion of mevalonic acid (the product of HMG CoA reductase) by 30 to 40 percent at doses of 40 mg per day in patients with heterozygous familial hypercholesterolemia.[357,358] Reduced formation of mevalonic acid leads to a corresponding decrease in hepatic cholesterol biosynthesis and a reduction in the cellular pool of cholesterol. This leads to a compensatory increase in the number of high-affinity LDL receptors expressed on the cell surface, and this in turn stimulates an increase in receptor-mediated catabolism of VLDL remnant particles and LDL.[342] Hepatic synthesis of VLDL and LDL may be concurrently reduced in response to drug therapy with HMG CoA reductase inhibitors.[359]

Side Effects

HMG CoA reductase inhibitors have been well tolerated, and side effects in both short-term and more extended (up to 9 years) use have been fairly uncommon.[360–362] The reported side effects include changes in bowel function, headache, nausea, fatigue, insomnia, and skin rashes. Less common but more severe side effects include myopathy and hepatitis, with elevated liver enzymes. The development of myopathy does not appear to be due to an unusual susceptibility to the inhibition of mevalonic acid production by lovastatin,[363] and the etiologic factors responsible for this remain to be better defined. Fortunately, myopathy is uncommon in patients treated with lovastatin, simvastatin, or pravastatin as monotherapy and appears to be dose-dependent. The incidence of myopathy is, however, increased in patients treated with lovastatin who are also receiving cyclosporin, nicotinic acid, gemfibrozil, or erythromycin.[352] Until proved otherwise, these drug interac-

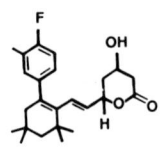

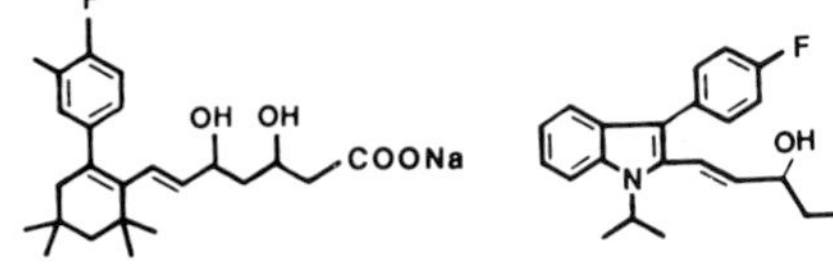

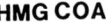

FIGURE 22-30 Structure of HMG CoA and the HMG CoA reductase inhibitors that are available for prescription use or are currently in clinical trials.

tions should be regarded as a class effect, not specifically limited to lovastatin. HMG CoA reductase inhibitors should be used very cautiously in combination with these other drugs; combined therapy with gemfibrozil or niacin cannot be recommended.[364] HMG CoA reductase inhibitors do not exert any adverse effects on steroid hormone biosynthesis.[365] Biochemical tests to monitor the safety of these drugs should be assessed at 6- to 8-week intervals for the first 9 or 12 months of therapy, and at 3- to 6-month intervals thereafter. These should include assessment of liver and muscle function in addition to an assessment of efficacy. Although initial studies in dogs indicated that HMG CoA reductase inhibitors occasionally cause cataracts when administered at doses 30 to 60 times the maximal human dose, subsequent studies in patients treated with these drugs for periods of 3 to 9 years have failed to document any increased frequency of lenticular opacities; the FDA does not currently require slit-lamp examinations during the treatment of patients with this class of drugs. Lovastatin, simvastatin, and their metabolites are excreted primarily in bile, and toxic levels can easily be reached if these drugs are given to patients with cholestasis or other disorders in which hepatic excretion and metabolism are significantly compromised. Renal excretion and hepatic metabolism appear to be important mechanisms for the elimination of pravastatin.[366]

Indications and Dosage

Lovastatin is available in 10-, 20-, and 40-mg tablets, whereas simvastatin and pravastatin are available in 5-, 10-, 20-, and 40-mg tablets. The hypocholesterolemic effects of lovastatin in doses of 10 to 80 mg per day and those of pravastatin and simvastatin at doses of 10 to 40 mg per day have been extensively investigated, and all three drugs have been found to be effective in patients with heterozygous familial hypercholesterolemia, familial combined hyperlipidemia, and moderate primary hypercholesterolemia.[130,360,367] The dose-response relations between changes in LDL cholesterol concentrations and the daily dose of lovastatin, pravastatin, and simvastatin in patients with heterozygous familial hypercholesterolemia, studied in separate clinical trials, are presented in Table 22-21. Based on these studies in different patients, it appears that on a milligram for milligram basis, lovastatin and pravastatin are of equal efficacy, whereas simvastatin is twice as potent. Single-drug therapy with lovastatin, simvastatin, and pravastatin has been associated with a 10 to

TABLE 22-21 Comparative Hypolipidemic Effects of HMG CoA Reductase Inhibitors in Patients with Heterozygous FH

Daily Dose, mg	Percent decrease in LDL cholesterol				
	Lovastatin		Simvastatin		Pravastatin
	a	b	c	d	e
10	20 (13)	17 (20)	28 (8)	ND	ND
20	28 (13)	25 (20)	30 (4)	38 (10)	21 (40)
40	35 (13)	31 (20)	37 (7)	44 (10)	28 (40)
80	38 (13)	40 (20)	—	—	—

LDL = low density lipoprotein; ND = not determined; FH = familial hypercholesterolemia.

Drugs given twice daily; a = Illingworth and Sexton[130]; b = Havel et al.[131]; c = Mol et al.[133]; d = Illingworth and Bacon[132]; e = Wiklund et al.[134]

30 percent dose-dependent decrease in plasma triglycerides and an overall tendency for HDL cholesterol to increase by 2 to 15 percent.[130,342]

In the opinion of the authors, HMG CoA reductase inhibitors are among the drugs of first choice for the treatment of adult patients with primary hypercholesterolemia and are also effective in the treatment of patients with combined hyperlipidemia and type III hyperlipidemia. They may also be useful in selected patients with secondary causes of hyperlipidemia, including the nephrotic syndrome, and in some patients with diabetes, particularly those who do not have marked hypertriglyceridemia. The usual starting dose of lovastatin is 20 mg once daily in the evening, but at doses above this level, the drug is more effective in a twice-daily regimen. In contrast, simvastatin and pravastatin are equally effective given as single doses in the evening; it is usually recommended that simvastatin be taken with dinner, whereas pravastatin is taken at bedtime. In humans, cholesterol biosynthesis increases at night, and this may explain the greater efficacy of HMG CoA reductase inhibitors when given as a single dose in the evening, compared with the same dose given in the morning.[368,369] HMG CoA reductase inhibitors do not influence plasma concentrations of Lp(a)[277,278] and should not be used for the treatment of severe hypertriglyceridemia.[370]

The hypocholesterolemic effects of HMG CoA reductase inhibitors can be enhanced by using these drugs in combination with bile acid sequestrants, and low doses of both drugs may be a particularly efficacious and cost-effective means of treating moderately severe hypercholesterolemia[371] (Fig. 22-31). As illustrated in Table 22-13, the combination of lovastatin, colestipol, and nicotinic acid has been shown to reduce LDL concentrations by 60 to 70 percent in patients with heterozygous familial hypercholesterolemia. Certain drug combinations cannot be recommended because of a lack of efficacy or the potential

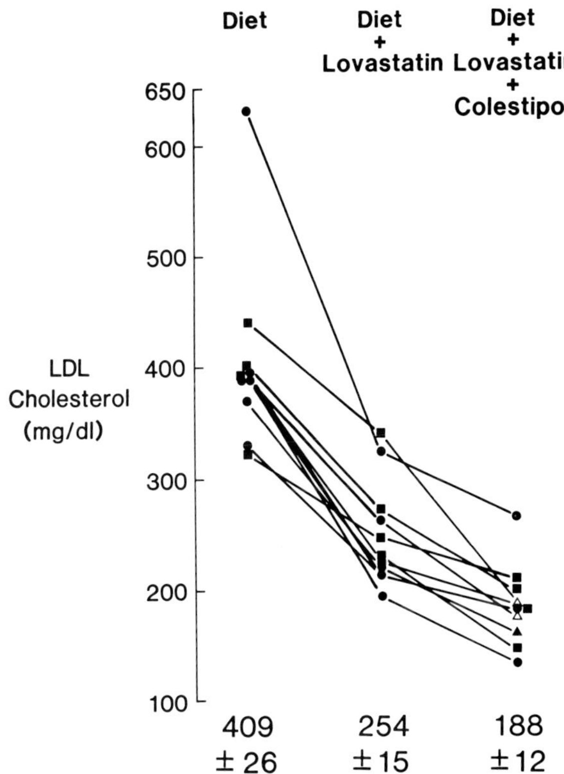

FIGURE 22-31 Changes in concentrations of low-density lipoprotein cholesterol in 10 patients with heterozygous familial hypercholesterolemia during sequential therapy with diet, lovastatin (80 mg per day), and lovastatin plus colestipol (15 to 20 g per day). (*Reproduced from Illingworth[140] with permission.*)

for increased toxicity. These include therapy with an HMG CoA reductase inhibitor and probucol[372] or gemfibrozil.[373] Although the latter combination may have potential therapeutic appeal in patients with combined hyperlipidemia, it does not exert a significant further LDL-lowering effect compared with lovastatin alone in patients with heterozygous familial hypercholesterolemia and is associated with an increased risk of myopathy.[364,373]

Probucol

Probucol (Lorelco) is a second-line drug for the treatment of primary hypercholesterolemia. Less than 10 percent of probucol is absorbed in the intestinal tract, and the hydrophobic nature of this drug contributes to its prolonged storage in adipose tissue. When used as a single agent, probucol has been shown to reduce plasma LDL cholesterol concentrations 8 to 15 percent and concurrently to lower HDL levels up to 25 percent.[135]

Mechanism of Action

The mechanism by which probucol influences plasma lipoprotein levels has not been completely defined.[135] The drug has been shown to increase the fractional rate of clearance of LDL[374] and to increase biliary secretion of cholesterol. The increased removal of LDL may be due to an increase in nonreceptor-mediated pathways, and this would explain the modest efficacy of probucol in patients with homozygous familial hypercholesterolemia who lack LDL receptors. The decrease in HDL levels seen with probucol is due to a decrease in apoprotein A-I synthesis, a decrease in lipoprotein lipase, and an increase in cholesterol ester transfer protein activity.[375,376]

Side Effects

Probucol is well tolerated and appears to have minimal side effects; in order of decreasing frequency, these include diarrhea (10 percent of patients), flatulence, abdominal pain, and nausea and vomiting.[135] Less common side effects have included hyperhidrosis, fetid sweat, and angioneurotic edema. With the possible exception of mild eosinophilia, no consistent biochemical abnormalities have been reported. Probucol causes prolongation of the QT interval, and although no arrhythmias have been attributed to its use in humans, the drug should probably be regarded as contraindicated in patients with electrocardiographic (ECG) findings suggestive of ventricular irritability.[135] Probucol is stored in adipose tissue, and blood levels fall slowly after therapy is discontinued. For this reason, the drug should not be given to women who plan to have children in the near future or to children.

Indications and Dosage

Probucol is available in 500-mg tablets. The recommended dose is 500 mg twice daily with the morning and evening meals. Probucol should be regarded as a second-line drug for the treatment of primary hypercholesterolemia, and 8 to 15 percent reductions in plasma concentrations of LDL can be expected. The drug concurrently lowers HDL levels up to 25 percent and may adversely affect the ratio of LDL to HDL. Probucol has been shown to cause regression of tendon xanthomas in patients with familial hypercholesterolemia[137] and may exert other potentially beneficial effects on lipoproteins, including inhibition of LDL oxidation[56] and an increase in reverse cholesterol transfer.[376] Probucol has not been used in any primary or secondary prevention trials published to date, and it is unclear whether the antioxidant effects of this drug may contribute to a reduction in atherosclerosis in humans. Probucol has no role in the treatment of hypertriglyceridemia.

Clofibrate

Clofibrate (Atromid-S) is the ethyl ester of *p*-chlorophenoxyisobutyrate and is well absorbed from the gastrointestinal tract. In plasma, the ester bond is hydrolyzed and the free acid is transported bound to albumin. The plasma half-life is 12 to 15 h. The drug is excreted in the urine, and its clearance is decreased in patients with chronic renal failure.

Mechanism of Action

The mechanism of action of clofibrate at the molecular level is not known. The most important effect, however, is to increase the rate of metabolism of triglyceride-rich lipoproteins as a result of increases in the activity of lipoprotein lipase.[174] Small and variable reductions in the synthesis and/or secretion of hepatic VLDL into plasma may also occur; these may be mediated by a number of mechanisms, including decreases in the hepatic synthesis of cholesterol and fatty acids and enhanced biliary excretion of cholesterol.

Side Effects

Clofibrate is generally well tolerated and has a low incidence of side effects. Nausea, abdominal discomfort, and in men decreased libido and breast tenderness are the most commonly reported. Less common side effects include dry skin, alopecia, and the development of a myositis-like syndrome with muscle tenderness and increased creatine phosphokinase (CPK).[174] The latter syndrome is more likely to occur in patients with hypoalbuminemia or impaired renal function. Rarely, ventricular arrhythmias and a lupuslike syndrome have been associated with clofibrate therapy. Biochemical abnormalities have included a decrease in alkaline phosphatase and transient increases in transaminases. Two long-term clinical trials, The Coronary Drug Research Project[377] and the WHO Primary Prevention Trial,[378] have provided data concerning the long-term safety and efficacy of clofibrate. In both studies there was an increased incidence of gallstones, whereas in the WHO study clofibrate-treated patients had a higher noncardiac mortality rate than did control subjects. This was mainly attributable to an increased incidence of malignant neoplasms and complications resulting from cholecystectomy. The increased incidence of noncardiac deaths did not persist after discontinuation of clofibrate therapy.[379,380] The increased incidence of noncardiac deaths in the WHO trial has led to a marked reduction in the use of clofibrate in the treatment of hyperlipidemia. Drug interactions may occur with clofibrate and other albumin-bound drugs, most notably warfarin (Coumadin).

Indications and Dosage

Clofibrate is available in 500-mg capsules; the usual dose is 1 g twice daily. Clofibrate is one of the drugs of choice for patients with type III hyperlipoproteinemia and should be regarded as a second-choice drug for patients with severe hypertriglyceridemia (type V phenotype) who are unable to take gemfibrozil or nicotinic acid. In patients with type III hyperlipoproteinemia, clofibrate therapy frequently reduces cholesterol and triglyceride concentrations 50 to 80 percent and leads to the regression of xanthomas. When given to patients with primary hypertriglyceridemia, clofibrate lowers VLDL cholesterol and plasma triglyceride concentrations up to 50 percent but frequently results in increased concentrations of LDL cholesterol. The drug is generally ineffective in patients with primary hypercholesterolemia and has no role in the treatment of disorders associated with increased plasma concentrations of LDL cholesterol. The drug is contraindicated in patients with chronic renal disease or the nephrotic syndrome; use in this population frequently results in the development of muscle tenderness and a myositis-like syndrome.

Gemfibrozil

Gemfibrozil (Lopid) is a fibric acid derivative that is structurally related to clofibrate. The drug is well absorbed from the intestinal tract and is transported, in part, bound to albumin. Although gemfibrozil undergoes enterohepatic circulation, the primary route of excretion is in urine.[174]

Mechanism of Action

The hypotriglyceridemic effect of gemfibrozil results primarily from a reduction in VLDL triglyceride and, to a lesser extent, apoprotein B synthesis with a concurrent increase in the rate of removal of triglyceride-rich lipoproteins from plasma.[174] The latter effect is believed to result from an increased activity of lipoprotein lipase, but the ability of gemfibrozil to inhibit VLDL triglyceride production appears to be much greater than that seen with clofibrate. Although gemfibrozil has also been shown to reduce the rate of synthesis of LDL apoprotein B,[381] this may simply be a reflection of a reduced rate of synthesis of VLDL, the precursor for LDL, in plasma.

Side Effects

Gemfibrozil is well tolerated in most patients; the most frequent side effects are changes in bowel function, abdominal pain, diarrhea, and occasionally nausea. These effects occur in 3 to 5 percent of patients and may necessitate the discontinuation of gemfibrozil. Less common side effects include muscle tenderness and skin rash. Biochemical changes are uncommon; they include eosinophilia, decreases in the plasma concentration of alkaline phosphatase, and occasionally rises in transaminases. Like clofibrate, gemfibrozil potentiates the effects of oral anticoagulants and may increase biliary lithogenicity, with a predicted long-term increase in the incidence of gallstones.

Indications and Dosage

Gemfibrozil is available in 600-mg tablets; the usual dose is 600 mg twice daily. Gemfibrozil has been shown to reduce the incidence of coronary artery disease in middle-aged men with primary hyperlipidemia,[339] and in this study, the greatest benefit was noted in patients with combined hyperlipidemia. In these patients, gemfibrozil reduced concentrations of total cholesterol and triglycerides as well as the level of LDL cholesterol and resulted in an increase in the levels of HDL cholesterol.[339] Debate continues on which factor was most influential in reducing coronary artery disease in this study, although it is noteworthy that the beneficial effects of gemfibrozil were limited to patients without coronary artery disease at the outset and that no benefit was observed in patients with preexistent coronary artery disease. Gemfibrozil is the drug of choice for patients with severe hypertriglyceridemia (type V phenotype) and in the authors' experience is superior to clofibrate in treating this disorder. Reductions of 75 to 90 percent in plasma concentrations of triglycerides may be seen in patients with severe hypertriglyceridemia; in this population, the drug may be effective in reducing the risk of pancreatitis and, on a long-term basis, the risk of atherosclerosis. Gemfibrozil should be regarded as a potential first-choice drug for patients with type III hyperlipoproteinemia, but it is inconsistently effective in patients with primary hypercholesterolemia and elevated concentrations of LDL cholesterol.[174] In the latter group of patients, particularly those unable to take nicotinic acid, combined drug therapy with gemfibrozil and a bile acid sequestrant is often quite effective. In the authors' experience, 25 to 45 percent reductions in concentrations of LDL cholesterol can be achieved in some patients on this regimen, whereas in other patients no additional LDL-lowering effect is seen with the addition of gemfibrozil. Concentrations of HDL cholesterol increase 10 to 20 percent during therapy with gemfibrozil, and even greater increases may be seen in patients with severe hypertriglyceridemia. As was discussed previously, combination drug therapy with gemfibrozil and HMG CoA reductase inhibitors may be associated with an increased risk of myopathy and cannot be recommended.

Miscellaneous Agents

A number of other drugs may be of value in specific situations, but these agents are not recommended for general use and will be discussed only briefly.

Neomycin

The nonabsorbable aminoglycoside antibiotic neomycin, at a dose of 1 g twice daily, has been shown to reduce LDL cholesterol concentrations by 10 to 15 percent in patients with primary hypercholesterolemia.[382] Neomycin appears to reduce the absorption of cholesterol from the small intestine and increases fecal excretion of neutral steroids. This enhanced sterol loss is presumed to increase the expression of high-affinity LDL receptors on hepatocyte membranes, which in turn stimulates an increased rate of LDL catabolism. Side effects, including diarrhea and abdominal cramps, limit the usefulness of neomycin, and the drug has the potential for ototoxicity and nephrotoxicity. Although combination drug therapy with neomycin and nicotinic acid has been shown to reduce LDL cholesterol concentrations by 45 percent in patients with primary hypercholesterolemia,[383] better drug combinations are available; in the opinion of the authors, the use of neomycin cannot be generally recommended.

Dextrothyroxine

Dextrothyroxine, the optical isomer of L-thyroxine, has been shown to reduce plasma concentrations of LDL cholesterol by 10 to 15 percent, but it does so at the expense of making the patient modestly hyperthyroid.[384] Use of dextrothyroxine in the Coronary Drug Project was associated with an increased incidence of cardiac arrhythmias, and the drug should be regarded as contraindicated in patients with known or potential coronary artery disease. In the opinion of the authors, dextrothyroxine has no role as a hypolipidemic drug in the 1990s.

Anabolic Steroids

The anabolic steroid oxandrolone 7.5 mg per day has been shown to reduce VLDL and chylomicron levels and to increase postheparin lipolytic activity.[385] Oxandrolone concurrently reduces the concentrations of HDL cholesterol. The drug may be potentially useful in certain male patients with severe hypertriglyceridemia who have not responded to conventional therapy.

Progestational Agents

The use of norethindrone acetate (Norlutate) 5 mg per day has been shown to reduce triglyceride levels in women patients with severe hypertriglyceridemia and the type V phenotype.[386] The drug appears to increase postheparin lipolytic activity and results in an enhanced clearance of triglyceride-rich lipoproteins from plasma. Norethindrone acetate may be useful in women patients with severe hypertriglyceridemia who fail to respond to other therapeutic regimens.

Estrogens

Concentrations of LDL cholesterol are known to increase in women after menopause; the magnitude of this increase is greatest in women with preexistent hypercholesterolemia (e.g., heterozygous familial hypercholesterolemia). Estrogen deficiency has also been associated with the phenotypic expression of type III hyperlipidemia in women homozygous for apoprotein E-2. In both of these situations, estrogen therapy significantly reduces the magnitude of hyperlipidemia and may minimize the need for concurrent hypolipidemic drug therapy. Although estrogens increase concentrations of HDL cholesterol, they also stimulate VLDL synthesis and may lead to severe hypertriglyceridemia in patients with preexisting hypertriglyceridemia. In the authors' experience, the use of transdermal preparations of estradiol minimizes the tendency to exacerbate hypertriglyceridemia and can be effective in women in whom hormone replacement therapy is advocated for other reasons (e.g., prevention of osteoporosis). Estrogens have no role as lipid-modifying agents in men, and in the Coronary Drug Project, the use of both 2.5-mg and 5-mg doses of Premarin in men was associated with an increased incidence of morbid cardiovascular events which led to premature termination of this part of the study.[387]

Future Advances

Fibric Acid Derivatives

Two fibric acid derivatives—clofibrate and gemfibrozil—have been approved for clinical use in the United States, and several other derivatives are currently undergoing clinical trials or have been approved for general use in Europe. These drugs, which include bezafibrate, fenofibrate, and ciprofibrate, are considerably more effective than either clofibrate or gemfibrozil in reducing LDL concentrations in patients with primary hypercholesterolemia.[174] Fenofibrate and ciprofibrate seem to be the most effective, and both have been shown to reduce levels of LDL cholesterol 20 to 25 percent in patients with heterozygous familial hypercholesterolemia (Table 22-22). The hypocholesterolemic effects of these drugs appear to be mediated by an enhanced rate of receptor-mediated clearance of LDL from plasma.[174]

Nicotinic Acid Derivatives

Several derivatives of nicotinic acid have been developed in an attempt to maintain the lipid-modifying effects of nicotinic acid with a concurrent reduction in the side effect profile, particularly cutaneous flushing. Several esters of nicotinic acid, including xanthinol nicotinate and niceritrol, have been evaluated, and both preparations show a hypolipidemic profile similar to that of the parent compound, but with fewer side effects.[394] Etofibrate is an interesting derivative of nicotinic acid in which the nicotinic acid moiety is esterified to clofibrate. Etofibrate has been shown to reduce plasma triglyceride and cholesterol concentrations in patients with hypercholesterolemia and enhance catabolism of LDL via the LDL-receptor pathway.[395] Perhaps the most interesting of the nicotinic acid derivatives is acipi-

TABLE 22-22 Comparative Efficacy of Fibric Acid Derivatives in Decreasing LDL Cholesterol Concentrations in Patients with Heterozygous Familial Hypercholesterolemia

Drug	Dose, g/day	Initial LDL Cholesterol, mg/dl	No. Patients Studied	% Decrease in LDL Cholesterol	References
Clofibrate	2.0	286	10	4.6	Levy et al., 1972[388]
Gemfibrozil	1.2	309	9	9.6	Meinertz, 1987[389]
Bezafibrate	0.6	313	12	28.0	Eisenberg et al., 1987[390]
Bezafibrate	0.6	262	18	18.3	Curtis et al., 1988[143]
Ciprofibrate	0.1	293	10	24.0	Illingworth et al., 1982[391]
Ciprofibrate	0.1	336	20	19.5	Rouffy et al., 1985[392]
Ciprofibrate	0.2	336	20	27.0	Rouffy et al., 1985[392]
Fenofibrate	0.3	309	9	24.0	Weisweiler et al., 1984[393]
Fenofibrate	0.3	309	21	25.0	Rouffy et al., 1985[392]
Fenofibrate	0.4	309	21	31.0	Rouffy et al., 1985[392]

mox, which at a dose of 250 mg three times daily has been shown to reduce LDL cholesterol concentrations by 11 percent, with a concurrent 20 percent increase in concentrations of HDL cholesterol.[396] In contrast to nicotinic acid, which exacerbates hyperglycemia, acipimox exerts a hypoglycemic effect, making this agent potentially useful for the treatment of lipid disorders in diabetics.

Agents which Reduce Cholesterol Biosynthesis

The clinical utility of drugs which inhibit HMG CoA reductase inhibitors as hypocholesterolemic agents has been well demonstrated, and three drugs in this class—lovastatin, simvastatin, and pravastatin—have been approved by regulatory authorities in different countries. These three drugs are effective in doses ranging from 5 to 80 mg per day, and preliminary information indicates that at least two of the newer agents in this class, Fluvastatin and Dalvastatin, are likely to have a similar potency. In contrast, a new synthetic inhibitor of HMG CoA reductase, BAY w 6228, has been shown to be 110 times more potent that lovastatin in in vitro assays and is likely to have clinical applicability with doses of 50 to 300 μg per day.[397] However, despite this increased potency, it seems unlikely that the magnitude of hypolipidemic effects observed with different HMG CoA reductase inhibitors will differ, and the newer agents seem unlikely to afford any additional benefit over the available drugs whose safety profile has been well characterized.

The clinical efficacy of the HMG CoA reductase inhibitors indicates that inhibition of other enzymes in the cholesterol biosynthetic pathway may have clinical utility in the treatment of hypercholesterolemia. Inhibition of late steps in sterol biosynthesis has resulted in the accumulation of lipid-soluble precursors in tissues and has been associated with the development of cataracts and icthyosis. Inhibition of squalene synthase is a particularly attractive therapeutic target, since this enzyme represents the first committed step in cholesterol biosynthesis, and the substrate for this enzyme—farnesyl pyrophosphate—can be metabolized to other water-soluble products which would not be expected to accumulate and lead to toxicity. Three structurally related fungal metabolites which are potent inhibitors of squalene synthase have been identified, and the structure of these compounds resembles that of presqualene pyrophosphate. The compounds identified have been named either "Zaragozic Acids"[398] or "Squalestatin"[399]; despite these different names, the structures of these products are similar, and they are effective in inhibiting squalene synthase in nanomolar concentrations. These agents represent an important new class of fungal metabolites which inhibit cholesterol biosynthesis and have potential as clinically effective hypocholesterolemic agents in humans.

Inhibitors of Acyl Coenzyme A Cholesterol Acyltransferase

The enzyme acyl coenzyme A cholesterol acyltransferase (ACAT) catalyzes the esterification of cholesterol and is present in intestinal mucosal cells, liver, and monocytes and macrophages. A number of inhibitors of this enzyme have been synthesized,[400] and these agents exert hypocholesterolemic effects in cholesterol-fed animals. Their potential as hypolipidemic agents in humans is based on their ability to reduce cholesterol esterification in the small intestine, reducing cholesterol absorption, and potentially to influence cholesterol esterification in the liver, with a concurrent reduction in VLDL production. At the present time, ACAT inhibitors remain investigational and do not appear to be effective as hypocholesterolemic agents in humans.[401] The potential adverse effects of ACAT inhibitors, including impairment of cholesterol esterification in steroid hormone–producing tissues, remain to be better defined; in the opinion of the authors, the therapeutic potential of ACAT inhibitors is limited.

THE SURGICAL TREATMENT OF HYPERLIPOPROTEINEMIA

A variety of surgical procedures have been performed on patients with familial hypercholesterolemia in an attempt to reduce plasma concentrations of total and LDL cholesterol. The distal ileal bypass operation is the most widely used surgical procedure for the treatment of severe hypercholesterolemia but is less effective than combined drug therapy in lowering LDL cholesterol concentrations; thus, this surgical procedure cannot be generally recommended. The operation bypasses 200 cm of the distal ileum, leaving a blind loop, and in experienced hands has an operative mortality rate under 1 percent. This surgical procedure interrupts the normal enterohepatic circulation of bile acids; the mechanism of action is similar to that of the bile acid–binding resins discussed earlier. In patients with heterozygous familial hypercholesterolemia, reductions of 30 to 40 percent in concentrations of LDL cholesterol can be attained.[145] In a 10-year follow up of 27 patients treated with this operation, only 2 patients achieved normal lipid values, indicating that even in patients who undergo distal ileal bypass surgery, other medical measures are necessary to achieve optimal lipid values.[402] Lovastatin appears to be particularly well suited for this purpose.[147] Complications of distal ileal bypass surgery include diarrhea, bowel obstruction, vitamin B_{12} deficiency, and an increased risk of hyperoxaluria and oxalate kidney stones. Patients frequently need to take bile acid sequestrants to control diarrhea, which is caused by increased fecal excretion of unbound bile acids, and require lifelong injections of vitamin B_{12}. Because of unknown effects on growth and development, distal ileal bypass surgery should not be considered for children. The operation has no role in other forms of hyperlipoproteinemia, nor is it effective in patients with homozygous familial hypercholesterolemia.

Portacaval shunt surgery has also been performed in patients with heterozygous familial hypercholesterolemia,[403] but in these patients the operation must be regarded as an investigational procedure and cannot be recommended.

Surgical Procedures in Homozygous Familial Hypercholesterolemia

A variety of surgical procedures have been performed in patients with homozygous familial hypercholesterolemia in an attempt to reduce their markedly elevated LDL cholesterol concentrations. Distal ileal bypass surgery and total biliary diversion do not work in these patients because of compensatory increases in cholesterol biosynthesis which nullify the increased excretion of bile acid.[146] Portacaval shunt surgery has been shown to be effective in some patients,[404] but the 25 to 40 percent decrease in LDL cholesterol concentrations achieved after this procedure still leaves these patients markedly hypercholesterolemic. Liver transplantation has been successful in two patients.[153,154] By providing a liver which is able to express high-affinity LDL receptors, this operation is physiologically the most attractive. At the present time, however, all surgical procedures employed in patients with homozygous familial hypercholesterolemia must be regarded as experimental.

Treatment of Special Patient Populations

The criteria for the diagnosis of hyperlipoproteinemia in both adults and children were discussed earlier in this chapter. Although clinical trials of hypolipidemic drugs have demonstrated a decreased incidence of cardiovascular events in middle-aged men with primary hypercholesterolemia, they lacked sufficient power to demonstrate a reduction in total mortality. For this reason, controversy continues to surround the use of lipid-lowering drugs in certain populations, particularly, the elderly, women, and children.[380] Treatment of these special patient populations is discussed below.

Hyperlipidemia in Women

The primary and secondary intervention trials of diet or drug treatment of hyperlipidemia have focused on middle-aged men, and proof of benefit from treatment of hyperlipidemia in women therefore has not been clearly documented. With the exception of patients with major genetic lipid disorders such as familial hypercholesterolemia, men typically develop coronary artery disease in their fifties and sixties, whereas women are more often affected in their late sixties and seventies, when they are postmenopausal.[405] In women who do not receive estrogen replacement therapy, the postmenopausal period is associated with a decrease in LDL-receptor activity and a rise in the plasma concentrations of LDL cholesterol.[406] Although some investigators have questioned whether high concentrations of LDL cholesterol represent risk factors in women,[407] data from the Honolulu Heart Study and several other epidemiologic studies have indicated that women have the same risk factors for coronary artery disease that men have, including elevated plasma concentrations of total and LDL cholesterol, reduced concentrations of HDL cholesterol, and hypertriglyceridemia.[408,409] Despite the fact that women develop coronary artery disease at a later age than do men, the absolute number of men and women who die from coronary heart disease (CHD) is quite similar, and CHD represents the number one cause of death among American women.[408] Data from a number of epidemiologic studies support the view that women can benefit from cholesterol management guidelines such as those recommended by the National Cholesterol Education Program.[410] Indeed, aggressive lipid lowering with combination drug treatment in patients with heterozygous familial hypercholesterolemia was associated with greater degrees of angiographic regression in women than was observed in men[340] and supports the view that in selected high-risk patients drug therapy does retard the progression of atherosclerosis and that these effects may be more readily attainable in women than in men.

The decision to use lipid-lowering drugs aimed at the primary prevention of coronary artery disease in women must take into account a number of factors, of which a family history of atherosclerosis and the presence of other risk factors [e.g., low concentrations of HDL, increased levels of Lp(a), concurrent presence of diabetes] are the most important. With the exception of women with heterozygous familial hypercholesterolemia, it may be reasonable to postpone drug therapy until the postreproductive years or even until the menopause if LDL concentrations do not exceed 210 to 220 mg/dl on dietary therapy. Even in women with heterozygous familial hypercholesterolemia who have LDL cholesterol values below 220 mg/dl, there is little urgency to commence drug therapy during adolescence or in the early twenties, and in women who plan to have children, the use of systemically acting drugs should be avoided. Aggressive measures to reduce concentrations of atherogenic lipoproteins are indicated in women who have developed premature coronary artery disease, in whom the goal of therapy should be to reduce LDL concentrations to under 100 mg/dl.

Hyperlipidemia in Older Patients

Coronary artery disease remains the leading cause of mortality in men and women over age 65; the prevalence of hypercholesterolemia and coronary artery disease is also highest in this age group.[411] In the Honolulu Heart Program, the incidence of coronary artery disease was twofold higher in subjects age 65 to 75 years old whose total cholesterol concentrations exceeded 240 mg/dl compared with participants whose values were under 190 mg/dl.[412] Despite a lack of controlled trials of lipid-lowering interventions in this population, hypolipidemic drugs are widely prescribed for both men and women over age 60.[413] A prospective 7-year trial, the Cholesterol Reduction in Senior People (CRISP) trial of diet and drug treatment, has been proposed by the NIH to examine this important question, but results are not expected to be available until the end of the century.

We do not believe older patients without evidence of coronary or peripheral vascular disease who are in relatively good health should be excluded from testing and possible therapy for hyperlipidemia. If moderate dietary changes fail to produce the desired goals of LDL reduction, the risk of drug therapy must be weighed carefully against the expected benefits. In the opinion of the authors, drug therapy should be reserved for patients in whom the potential benefit can reasonably be expected to outweigh the potential side effects and increased medical costs.[411] In our Lipid Disorders Clinic, we rely heavily on family history and the personal wishes of the patient in deciding which patients should be treated with lipid-lowering medications. The NCEP guidelines provide a broad framework for cutpoints above which medications could be considered after satisfactory exclusion of potentially exacerbating secondary factors. Side effects associated with bile acid sequestrant therapy and nicotinic acid may be more commonly observed in older patients, and for this reason, the HMG CoA reductase inhibitors are preferred as the initial therapeutic agents. In many older patients, 10 or 20 mg per day of lovastatin will achieve the desired result. It has been the policy of the authors not to discontinue hypolipidemic drug therapy in patients with genetic lipid disorders on the basis of increasing age unless another life-limiting illness is diagnosed. For older patients who have evidence of coronary or peripheral vascular disease and who concurrently have hypercholesterolemia, benefits from hypolipidemic drug therapy can be seen in as little as 2 years, and an aggressive approach toward treating these patients seems justified, particularly if it can be accomplished without adversely affecting the quality of life.[70]

Hyperlipidemia in Children

Criteria for the diagnosis of hypercholesterolemia in children have been formulated by the Pediatric Expert Panel of the National Cholesterol Education Program,[76] and there is uniform agreement that once the secondary causes of hyperlipidemia have been excluded, dietary therapy is the cornerstone of treatment in this patient population. As discussed previously, we believe that the guidelines advocated by the pediatric panel are too aggressive in terms of the cutpoints for drug therapy in children with heterozygous familial hypercholesterolemia and, as with women, recommend individual therapy with particular emphasis being given to a family history of premature coronary artery disease in deciding which children should be treated with lipid-lowering medications in addition to diet. At the present time, only the bile acid sequestrants (cholestyramine and colestipol) can be recommended, based on their proven efficacy and safety.[414] Depending on the age of the child and the magnitude of hypercholesterolemia, one or two (rarely, up to four) packets or scoops of a bile acid sequestrant may be used. Supplements of folic acid and fat-soluble vitamins are advisable in children who are maintained on long-term therapy with these drugs. Insufficient data are available concerning the efficacy and long-term safety of HMG CoA reductase inhibitors or fibrates to recommend their use in children with heterozygous familial hypercholesterolemia; the use of any systemically acting drugs in this population should be considered investigational at the present time. Referral to a center specializing in lipid disorders is recommended for pediatric patients in whom drug therapy is being considered and is mandatory for the effective management of the rare child with homozygous familial hypercholesterolemia.

LABORATORY TESTS IN THE DIAGNOSIS OF HYPERLIPIDEMIAS

The accurate determination of cholesterol, triglyceride, lipoproteins, and in selected patients apoproteins remains the cornerstone for the diagnosis of hyperlipidemia. In this section, we shall briefly discuss factors which can interfere with determinations as well as the indications and methods available for lipoprotein quantification. Mention will also be made of provocative tests which may aid in the diagnosis of hyperlipidemias. Detailed reviews have been published.[415,416]

Collection and Handling of the Sample

Lipid and lipoprotein determinations may be performed on serum or plasma, but plasma is preferable, since it allows for more rapid cooling and separation of plasma and red cells. Ethylenediaminetetraacetic acid (edetic acid, EDTA) is the preferred anticoagulant. Lipid values in plasma are about 3 percent lower than in similar samples of serum obtained simultaneously from the same subject. Because of increases in the plasma volume which occur when subjects change from a standing to a recumbent posture, lipid values may be 5 to 10 percent lower when taken from patients in a supine position. Much smaller changes occur with sitting, and this is the position we recommend for venipuncture. Fluid shifts may also occur with prolonged venous occlusion and may result in erroneously increased lipid values.

Separation of red cells should occur promptly; in the interim, the sample should be stored at 4°C. For determinations of total cholesterol and triglyceride, plasma samples can be frozen or stored at 4°C for up to 1 week. When lipoproteins are to be separated, the plasma should not be frozen and the samples should be handled promptly. The addition of SH inhibitors to such samples is advisable to minimize the lipid changes which may occur before lipoprotein separation. Plasma triglyceride concentrations increase postprandially, and for this reason accurate determinations of triglyceride require the patient to have fasted 12 to 16 h before venipuncture. In contrast, cholesterol levels are minimally affected by eating, and casual blood samples are quite satisfactory if only cholesterol is to be determined.

Lipid Determinations

Multichannel automated systems constitute the most commonly available methods for cholesterol and triglyceride determination by either enzymatic or colorimetric methods. Extraction of the samples with isopropanol before colorimetric assay of cholesterol is more tedious; this was the method used by the Lipid Research Clinics. The measurement of the cholesterol level in capillary blood samples obtained from a finger prick has become popular because of convenience and ease of use for screening programs. However, the results of these tests can be highly variable and misleading (we have seen measurement errors as large as 80 mg/dl in individual patients). Thus, this convenient method cannot be used to reliably classify patients with hypercholesterolemia.

Lipoprotein Separations

Indications

Determination of plasma concentrations of LDL cholesterol and HDL cholesterol provides more detailed information about cardiovascular risk in patients with normal concentrations of plasma triglycerides (less than 200 mg/dl) and plasma cholesterol values in excess of 220 to 240 mg/dl. Determination of LDL and HDL concentrations is also appropriate in patients with premature cardiovascular disease (before age 50) and in any patient with xanthomas of the skin suggestive of a possible underlying lipid abnormality. In patients with elevated levels of both cholesterol and triglyceride in whom the distinction between phenotypic type IIb and type III hyperlipoproteinemia cannot be made, ultracentrifugal flotation of VLDL with determination of the ratio of VLDL cholesterol to total triglycerides is the method of choice. This will indicate that an abnormal cholesterol-rich VLDL particle is present in the plasma of patients with type III hyperlipoproteinemia. This method is more specific and is preferable to the electrophoretic demonstration of a beta-migrating band, which has also been considered diagnostic of type III hyperlipidemia. The diagnosis of type III hyperlipidemia can be confirmed by apoprotein E phenotyping by isoelectric focusing or apoprotein E gene analysis.

Demonstration of chylomicronemia does not generally require lipoprotein separations and can be visually documented by means of inspection of plasma which has been stored for 12 to 18 h at 4°C or has been centrifuged for 20 min at 3000 g in a refrigerated centrifuge. When the triglyceride level is about 1000 mg/dl (11.3 mmol/L), the plasma has an appearance resembling skim milk. Chylomicrons are invariably present when the triglyceride level is greater than or equal to 1000 mg/dl (11.3 mmol/L) and cause turbidity as a result of efficient light scattering. A creamy appearance of the plasma is indicative of severe chylomicronemia with triglyceride levels over 2000 to 4000 mg/dl (22.6 to 45.2 mmol/L) and a high risk of pancreatitis.

It is the authors' belief that current indications for electrophoresis of whole plasma are minimal and that the usefulness of this procedure is small. With the growing awareness of apoprotein abnormalities as causal factors in the pathogenesis of dyslipoproteinemias, it is likely that apoprotein determinations will become more readily available outside academic institutions in the coming years. At the present time, however, reliable commercial assays for apoproteins are not generally available and patients with suspected dyslipoproteinemias due to apoprotein abnormalities should be referred to medical centers with a specialized interest in lipid disorders where these assays are routinely performed.

Available Methods

Three methods are available for lipoprotein separation: electrophoresis, ultracentrifugation, and precipitation. Electrophoresis is usually carried out on paper, cellulose acetate, or agarose, but the method is imprecise and not easily quantitated in terms of the lipid content of a given lipoprotein. Ultracentrifugal separation of plasma is the most precise method but is time-consuming and requires an ultracentrifuge. Detailed information on the methods used for isolation of VLDL, LDL, and HDL have been published[416] and are beyond the scope of this chapter. Precipitation methods which rely on the interaction between lower-density lipoproteins (VLDL and LDL), sulfated polysaccharides, and divalent cations have gained in acceptance and are widely used. For example, the supernatant obtained after precipitation of VLDL and LDL by heparin-manganese contains only HDL and may be used for determination of the cholesterol content of the lipoprotein. Two additions to this method have been used to provide extra data. In the first, VLDL is removed by ultracentrifugation from the *d* 1.006 subnatant containing LDL and HDL. Determination of the lipid content of whole plasma, the heparin-manganese supernatant from whole plasma (HDL), and the VLDL and LDL plus HDL fractions from ultracentrifugation allows for quantification of VLDL, LDL, and HDL. A second, simpler method which does not require an ultracentrifuge has been widely used and gives indirect values for VLDL and LDL and direct values for HDL. This procedure relies on the assumption that the total plasma triglycerides divided by 5 approximates the value for VLDL cholesterol. Lipid values for whole plasma and for the heparin-manganese supernatant (HDL) are determined, and concentrations are calculated as follows:

$$\text{HDL cholesterol} = \text{cholesterol in heparin-manganese supernatant} \quad (22\text{-}1)$$

$$\text{VLDL cholesterol} = \text{total plasma triglyceride} \div 5 \quad (22\text{-}2)$$

$$\text{LDL cholesterol} = \text{total plasma cholesterol} - (\text{HDL cholesterol} + \text{VLDL cholesterol}) \quad (22\text{-}3)$$

In many patients this method yields reliable results that are comparable to the values obtained with the ultracentrifugation procedure. However, this method is not reliable at triglyceride concentrations greater than 400 mg/dl or in the presence of either chylomicrons or the IDL seen in type III.

Additional Laboratory Tests

A number of additional laboratory tests may aid in the precise characterization of patients with rare disorders of lipoprotein metabolism. Specific assays for Lp(a), LCAT, lipoprotein lipase, and hepatic lipase are available in many research laboratories but are not generally available, and it is probably preferable to send samples to centers where these assays are performed regularly. Reliable commercial assays for apoproteins are not widely available, and accurate diagnosis of the major HDL deficiency disorders and apoprotein C-II deficiency or confirmation of apoprotein E-2 homozygosity in a patient with suspected type III hyperlipoproteinemia depends on the availability of assays in medical centers which specialize in lipoprotein metabolism. The precise diagnosis of homozygous familial hypercholesterolemia has historically required the determination of high-affinity LDL receptor activity on cultured fibroblasts, which can be obtained by means of amniocentesis in the case of prenatal diagnosis[417] or skin biopsy in a suspected case.[103,153] Determination of the number of high-affinity LDL receptors requires culture of the fibroblasts and subsequent measurement of the binding, internalization, and degradation of radiolabeled low-density lipoprotein. Consultation with a medical center or research laboratory that routinely performs this assay should be obtained before obtaining the fibroblast sample so that the cells will remain viable and the assay will be run with appropriate controls.

With the advent of modern molecular genetic analytic techniques, including the polymerase chain reaction for amplification of DNA, restriction fragment length polymorphism analysis, and the cloning and sequencing of numerous normal and defective genes, many lipoprotein disorders can be definitively identified by means of DNA analysis. The amount of DNA present in the buffy coat of 10 ml of EDTA-anticoagulated blood is usually sufficient to permit this type of analysis.

REFERENCES

1. Goffman JW, Lindgren FT, Elliot M: Ultracentrifugal studies of lipoproteins of human plasma. *J Biol Chem* 179:973, 1949.
2. Lees RS, Hatch FT: Sharper separation of lipoprotein species by paper electrophoresis in albumin containing buffer. *J Lab Clin Med* 61:418, 1963.
3. Utermann G: The mysteries of lipoprotein (a). *Science* 246:904, 1989.
4. Alaupovic P: Apoproteins and lipoproteins. *Atherosclerosis* 13:141, 1971.
5. McConathy WJ, Koren K, Wieland H, Campos EM, Lee DN, Kloer HU, Alaupovic P: Evaluation of immunoaffinity chromatography for isolated human lipoproteins containing apoprotein B. *J Chromatogr* 342:47, 1985.
6. Agnani G, Bard JM, Candelier L, DeLatere PS, Fruchart JC, Clavey V: Interaction of LpB, LpB:E, LpB:CIII and LpB:C-III:E lipoproteins with the low density lipoprotein receptor of HeLa cells. *Arteriosclerosis Thromb* 11:1021, 1991.
7. Powell LM, Wallace SC, Pease RJ, Edwards YH, Knott TJ, Scott J: A novel form of tissues specific RNA processing produces apolipoprotein B-48 in intestine. *Cell* 50:831, 1987.
8. Young SG: Recent progress in understanding apolipoprotein B. *Circulation* 82:1574, 1990.
9. Rader DJ, Brewer HB, Jr.: Lipoprotein (a): Clinical approach to a unique atherogenic lipoprotein. *JAMA* 267:1109, 1992.
10. Scott J: Thrombogenesis linked to atherogenesis at last? *Nature* 341:22, 1989.
11. Scanu AM, Lawn RM, Berg K: Lipoprotein (a) and atherosclerosis. *Ann Intern Med* 115:209, 1991.
12. Sabesin SM: Cholestatic lipoproteins: Their pathogenesis and significance. *Gastroenterology* 83:704, 1982.
13. Glomset JA, Norum KR: The metabolic role of lecithin cholesterol acyltransferase: Perspective from pathology. *Adv Lipid Res* 11:1, 1973.
14. Schonfeld G: The genetic dyslipoproteinemias: Nosology Update 1990. *Atherosclerosis* 81:81, 1990.
15. Breslow JL: Lipoprotein transport gene abnormalities underlying coronary heart disease susceptibility. *Ann Rev Med* 42:357, 1991.
16. Segrest JP: A molecular theory of lipid protein interactions in the plasma lipoproteins. *FEBS Lett* 38:247, 1974.
17. Gordon JL, Bisgaier CL, Sims HF, Sachdev OP, Glickman RM, Strauss AW: Biosynthesis of human preapolipoprotein AIV. *J Biol Chem* 259:468, 1984.
18. Blaufuss MC, Gordon JL, Schonfeld G, Strauss AW, Alpers DH: Biosynthesis of apolipoprotein CIII in rat liver and small intestinal mucosa. *J Biol Chem* 259:2452, 1984.
19. Vaith P, Hassman G, Uhlenbreck G: Characterization of the oligosaccharide side chain of apolipoprotein CIII from human plasma very low density lipoproteins. *Biochim Biophys Acta* 541:234, 1978.
20. Patsch W, Schonfeld G: Degree of sialation of apo CIII is altered by diet. *Diabetes* 30:530, 1981.
21. Zannis VI, Cladaras C, Zanni EE: Apolipoprotein and lipoprotein synthesis and modifications. *Curr Opinion Lipidol* 2:149, 1991.
22. Basu SK, Goldstein JL, Brown MS: Independent pathways for secretion of cholesterol and apolipoprotein E by macrophages. *Science* 219:871, 1983.
23. Jackson RL, Pattus F, deHaas G: Mechanism of action of milk lipoprotein lipase at substrate interphases: Effects of apolipoproteins. *Biochemistry* 19:373, 1980.
24. Breckenridge WC, Little JA, Steiner G, Chow A, Poast M: Hypertriglyceridemia associated with a deficiency of apolipoprotein CII. *N Engl J Med* 298:1265, 1978.
25. Miller NE, Rao SN, Alaupovic P, Nobel N, Slack J, Brunzell JD, Lewis B: Familial apolipoprotein CII deficiency: Plasma lipoproteins and apolipoproteins in heterozygous and homozygous subjects and the effects of plasma infusion. *Eur J Clin Invest* 11:69, 1981.
26. Havel RH, Kane JP: Lipoprotein and lipid metabolism disorders, in Scriver CR, Beaudet AL, Sly WS, Valle D (eds): *The Metabolic Basis of Inherited Disease,* 6th ed. New York, McGraw-Hill, 1989, p 1129.
27. Brown MS, Herz J, Kowal RC, Goldstein JL: The LDL receptor related protein (LRP): Double agent or decoy: *Curr Opinion Lipidol* 2:65, 1991.
28. Mahley RW, Hussain MM: Chylomicron and chylomicron remnant catabolism. *Curr Opinion Lipidol* 2:170, 1991.
29. Mahley RW, Rao SC Jr: Type III hyperlipoproteinemia (dysbetalipoproteinemia): The role of apolipoprotein E in normal and abnormal lipoprotein metabolism, in Scriver CR, Beaudet AL, Sly WS, Valle D (eds): *The Metabolic Basis of Inherited Disease,* 6th ed. New York, McGraw-Hill, 1989, p 1195.
30. Mahley RW, Innerarity TL, Pitis RE, Weisgraber KH, Brown HJ, Gross E: Inhibition of lipoprotein binding to cell surface receptors of fibroblasts following selective modification of arginyl residues in arginine rich and B apoproteins. *J Biol Chem* 252:7279, 1977.
31. Yang CY, Gu CW, Weng SA, Kim TW, Chen SH, Pownall HJ, Sharp PM, Liu SW, et al: Structure of apolipoprotein B-100 of human low density lipoproteins. *Arteriosclerosis* 9:96, 1989.
32. Glomset JA, Norum KR, Gjone E: Familial lecithin cholesterol acyl transferase deficiency, in Stanbury JB, Wyngaarden JB, Fredrickson DS, Goldstein JL, Brown MS (eds): *The Metabolic Basis of Inherited Disease,* 5th ed. New York, McGraw-Hill, 1983, p 643.
33. Norom KR, Gjone E, Glomset JA: Familial lecithin cholesterol acyl transferase deficiency including fish eye disease, in Scriver CR, Beaudet AL, Sly WS, Valle D (eds): *The Metabolic Basis of Inherited Disease,* 6th ed. New York, McGraw-Hill, 1989, p 1181.
34. Eckel RH: Lipoprotein lipase: A multifunctional enzyme relevant to common metabolic diseases. *N Engl J Med* 320:1060, 1989.
35. Steiner G, Myher JJ, Kuksis A: Milk and plasma composition in a lactating patient with Type I hyperlipoproteinemia. *Am J Clin Nutr* 41:121, 1985.
36. Olivecrona T, Bengtsson-Olivecrona G: Lipoprotein lipase and hepatic lipase. *Curr Opinion Lipidol* 1:222, 1990.
37. Breckenridge WC, Little JA, Alaupovic P, Wang CS, Kuksis A, Lundgren A, Gardiner G: Lipoprotein abnormalities associated with a familial deficiency of hepatic lipase. *Atherosclerosis* 45:161, 1982.
38. Demant T, Carlson LA, Holmquist L, Karpe F, Nilsson-Ehel P, Packard CJ, Shepherd J: Lipoprotein metabolism in hepatic lipase deficiency: Studies on the turnover of apolipoprotein B and on the effect of hepatic lipase on high density lipoprotein. *J Lipid Res* 29:1603, 1988.
39. Cholesterol ester transfer protein (editorial). *Lancet* 338:666, 1991.
40. Inazu A, Brown ML, Hesler CB, Agellon LB, Koizumi J, Takata K, Maruhama Y, Mabuchi H, Tall AR: Increased high density lipoprotein levels caused by a common cholesterol ester transfer protein gene mutation. *N Engl J Med* 323:1234, 1990.
41. Goldstein JL, Brown MS: Low density lipoprotein pathway and its relationship to atherosclerosis. *Annu Rev Biochem* 46:897, 1977.
42. Goldstein JL, Brown MS: The LDL receptor defect in familial hypercholesterolemia: Implications for pathogenesis and therapy. *Med Clin North Am* 66:355, 1982.
43. Carr BR, Simpson ER: Lipoprotein utilization and choles-

terol synthesis by the human fetal adrenal gland. *Endocr Rev* 2:306, 1991.
44. Gwynne JJ, Strauss JF III: The role of lipoproteins in steroidogenesis and cholesterol metabolism in steroidogenic glands. *Endocr Rev* 3:299, 1982.
45. Eisenberg S: High density lipoprotein metabolism. *J Lipid Res* 25:1017, 1984.
46. Brinton EA, Eisenberg S, Breslow JL: A low-fat diet decreases HDL cholesterol levels by decreasing HDL apolipoprotein transport rates. *J Clin Invest* 85:144, 1990.
47. Krauss RM: Regulation of high density lipoprotein levels. *Med Clin North Am* 66:403, 1982.
48. Williams PJ, Krauss RM, Wood PD, Albers JJ, Dreon D, Ellswort N: Association of diet and alcohol intake with high density lipoprotein subclasses. *Metabolism* 35:524, 1985.
49. Gordon DJ, Rifkind BM: High density lipoprotein: The clinical implications of recent studies. *N Engl J Med* 321:1311, 1989.
50. Henkin Y, Como JA, Oberman A: Secondary dyslipidemia: Inadvertent effects of drugs in clinical practice. *JAMA* 267:961, 1992.
51. Reinhart RA, Gani K, Arndt MR, Broste SK: Apolipoproteins AI and B as predictors of angiographically defined coronary artery disease. *Arch Intern Med* 150:1629, 1990.
52. Avogaro P, Pittle BG, Cazzolato G: Are apolipoproteins better discriminators than lipids for atherosclerosis? *Lancet* 1:901, 1979.
53. Santamarina-Fojo S, Brewer HB Jr.: The familial hyperchylomicronemia syndrome: New insights into underlying genetic defects. *JAMA* 265:904, 1991.
54. Zilversmit DB: Atherosclerosis: A postprandial phenomenon. *Circulation* 60:473, 1979.
55. Fredrickson DS, Goldstein JL, Brown MS: The familial hypercholesterolemias, in Stanbury JD, Wyngarden JB, Fredrickson DS (eds): *The Metabolic Basis of Inherited Disease,* 3d ed. New York, McGraw-Hill, 1978, p 604.
56. Steinberg D, Parthasarathy S, Carew TE, Khoo JC, Witztum JL: Beyond cholesterol: Modifications of low density lipoprotein that increase its atherogenicity. *N Engl J Med* 320:915, 1989.
57. Leake DS: Effects of mildly oxidized low density lipoprotein on endothelial cell function. *Curr Opinion Lipidol* 2:301, 1991.
58. Fredrickson DS, Levy RI, Lees RS: Fat transport in lipoproteins: An integrated approach to mechanisms and disorders. *N Engl J Med* 276:32, 1967.
59. Beaumont JL, Carlson LA, Cooper GR, Fejfar Z, Fredrickson DS, Strasser T: Classification of hyperlipidemias and hyperlipoproteinemias. *Bull WHO* 43:891, 1970.
60. Miller M, Mead LA, Kwiterovich PO, Pierson TA: Dyslipidemias with desirable plasma total cholesterol levels and angiographically demonstrated coronary artery disease. *Am J Cardiol* 64:1, 1990.
61. Lipid Research Program: *The Lipid Research Clinics Population Studies Data Book.* Bethesda, Md., NIH Publication No. 80:1527, vol 1, 1980.
62. Multiple Risk Factor Intervention Trial Research Group: Multiple risk factor intervention trial: Risk factor changes and mortality results. *JAMA* 248:1465, 1982.
63. Consensus Conference: Lowering blood cholesterol to prevent heart disease. *JAMA* 253:2080, 1985.
64. National Cholesterol Education Program. Second report of the expert panel on detection, evaluation and treatment of high blood cholesterol in adults. *Circulation* 89:1329, 1994.
65. European Atherosclerosis Society. Prevention of coronary heart disease, scientific background and new clinical guidelines. *Nutr Metab Cardiovasc Dis* 2:113, 1992.
66. Betteridge DJ, Dodson PM, Durrington PN. Management of hyperlipidemia. Guidelines of the British Hyperlipidemia Association. *Postgrad Med J* 69:359, 1993.
67. Basinki A, Frank JW, Naylor CC, Rachlas MM: Detection and management of asymptomatic hypercholesterolemia: A policy document by the Toronto Working Group on Cholesterol Policy. Toronto, Ontario Ministry of Health, 1989.
68. Grundy SM: Multifactorial etiology of hypercholesterolemia: Implications for prevention of coronary heart disease. *Arteriosclerosis Throm* 11:1619, 1991.
69. Brown G, Albers JJ, Fisher LD, Schaefer SM, Lin JT, Kaplan C, Zhao XQ, Bisson BD, et al: Regression of coronary artery disease as a result of intensive lipid-lowering therapy in men with high levels of apolipoprotein B. *N Engl J Med* 323:1289, 1990.
70. Cashin-Hemphill L, Mack WJ, Pagoda JM, SanMarco ME, Azen SP, Blankenhorn DH: Beneficial effects of colestipol niacin on coronary atherosclerosis: A four-year follow-up. *JAMA* 264:3013, 1990.
71. Grundy SM, Vega GL: Two different views of the relationship of hypertriglyceridemia to coronary artery disease: Implications for treatment. *Arch Intern Med* 152:28, 1992.
72. Hulley SB, Avins AL: Asymptomatic hypertriglyceridemia: Insufficient evidence to treat. *Br Med J* 304:395, 1992.
73. National Institutes of Health Consensus Conference: Treatment of hypertriglyceridemia. *JAMA* 251:1196, 1984.
74. National Institutes of Health Consensus Conference: Triglycerides, high density lipoprotein and coronary artery disease *JAMA* 269:505, 1993.
75. Austin MA: Plasma triglyceride and coronary heart disease. *Arteriosclerosis Throm* 11:2, 1991.
76. The Expert Panel: Report of the Expert Panel on blood cholesterol levels in children and adolescents. *Pediatrics* 89(Suppl 2):525, 1992.
77. Connor SL, Connor WE, Sexton G, Calvin L, Bacon S: The effects of age, body weight and family relationships on plasma lipoproteins and lipids in men, women and children of randomly selected families. *Circulation* 65:1290, 1982.
78. Connor WE, Cerquiera MT, Connor RW, Wallace RB, Malinow MR, Casdorph HR: The plasma lipids, lipoproteins and diet of the Tarahumara Indians of Mexico. *Am J Clin Nutr* 31:1131, 1978.
79. Grundy SM, Vega GL, Bilheimer DW: Kinetic mechanism determining variability in low density lipoprotein levels and rise with age. *Arteriosclerosis* 5:623, 1985.
80. Brunzell JB, Chait A: Lipoprotein pathophysiology and treatment, in Rifkin H, Porte D, Jr (eds): *Diabetes Mellitus: Theory and Practice,* 4th ed. New York, Elsevier, 1990, pp 756–767.
81. Curtiss LK, Witztum JL: Plasma apolipoproteins AI, AII, B, CI and E are glucosylated in hyperglycemic diabetic subjects. *Diabetes* 34:452, 1985.
82. Duell PB, Oram JF, Bierman EL: Nonenzymatic glycosylation of HDL resulting in inhibition of high-affinity binding to cultured human fibroblasts. *Diabetes* 39:1257, 1990.
83. Duell PB, Oram JF, Bierman EL: Nonenzymatic glycosylation of HDL and impaired HDL-receptor-mediated cholesterol efflux. *Diabetes* 40:377, 1991.
84. Glueck C, Lang J, Tracy T, Spers J: High prevalence of hypothyroidism in patients with hyperlipoproteinemia. *Clin Chim Acta* 201:113, 1991.
85. Ball MJ, Griffiths D, Thorogood M: Asymptomatic hypothyroidism in hypercholesterolemic patients. *J R Soc Med* 84:527, 1991.
86. Illingworth DR, McClung MR, Connor WE, Alaupovic P: Familial hypercholesterolemia and primary hypothyroidism: Coexistence of both disorders in a young woman with severe hypercholesterolemia. *Clin Endocrinol (Oxf)* 14:145, 1981.
87. Chait A, Bierman EL, Albers JJ: Regulatory role of triiodothyronine in the degradation of low density lipoprotein by cultured human skin fibroblasts. *J Clin Endocrinol Metab* 48:887, 1979.
88. Lewis B: *The Hyperlipidemias: Clinical and Laboratory Practise.* Oxford, Blackwell, 1976, p 292.
89. Golper TA, Illingworth DR, Morris CD, Bennett WM: Lova-

statin in the treatment of multifactorial hyperlipidemia associated with proteinuria. *Am J Kidney Dis* 13:312, 1989.

90. DeLiberti JH, McMurry MP, Connor WE, Alaupovic P: Hypercholesterolemia associated with alpha-I antitrypsin deficiency and hepatitis: Lipoprotein and apoprotein determinations, sterol balance and treatment. *Am J Med Sci* 288:81, 1984.
91. Ettinger WH, Hazzard WR: Prednisone increases very low density lipoprotein and high density lipoprotein in healthy men. *Metabolism* 36:1055, 1988.
92. Shaboury AM, Hayes TM: Hyperlipidemia in asthmatic patients receiving long term steroid therapy. *Br Med J* 1:85, 1973.
93. Molitch ME, Oill P, Odell WD: Massive hyperlipidemia during estrogen therapy. *JAMA* 227:522, 1974.
94. Crook D, Godsland I, Winn V: Oral contraceptives and coronary heart disease: Modulation of glucose tolerance and plasma lipids by progestins. *Am J Obstet Gynecol* 158:1612, 1988.
95. Burry KA, Patton PE, Illingworth DR: Metabolic changes during medical treatment of endometriosis: Nafarelin acetate *vs.* Danazol. *Am J Obstet Gynecol* 160:1454, 1989.
96. Lardinois CK, Newman SL: The effects of antihypertensive agents on serum lipids and lipoproteins. *Arch Intern Med* 148:1280, 1988.
97. Krone W, Nagele H: Effects of antihypertensives on plasma lipids and lipoprotein metabolism. *Am Heart J* 116:1729, 1988.
98. Bershad S, Rubenstein A, Paterniti JR Jr, et al: Changes in plasma lipids and lipoproteins during isotretinoin therapy for acne. *N Engl J Med* 313:981, 1985.
99. Katz RA, Jorgensen H, Nigra TP: Elevation of serum triglyceride levels from oral isotretinoin in disorders of keratinization. *Arch Dermatol* 116:1369, 1980.
100. Iverius PH, Brunzell JD: Chylomicronemia induced by cimetidine. *Gastroenterology* 89:664, 1985.
101. Ballantyne CM, Podet EJ, Patsch WP, et al: Effects of cyclosporine therapy on plasma lipoprotein levels. *JAMA* 262:53, 1989.
102. Wallace RB, Hunninghake DB, Reiland S, et al: Alterations of plasma high density lipoprotein cholesterol levels associated with consumption of selected medications. *Circulation* 62(Suppl 4):77, 1980.
103. Goldstein JL, Brown MS: Familial hypercholesterolemia, in Scriber CR, Beaudet AL, Sly WS, Valle D (eds): *The Metabolic Basis of Inherited Disease,* 6th ed. New York, McGraw-Hill, 1989, p 1215.
104. Brown MS, Kovanen PT, Goldstein JL, Eeckles R, Vandenberg K, Vandenberg H, Fryns JP, Cassiman JJ: Prenatal diagnosis of homozygous familial hypercholesterolemia. *Lancet* 1:526, 1978.
105. Gagne C, Moorjani S, Grun D, Doussaint M, Lupen PJ: Heterozygous familial hypercholesterolemia: The relationship between plasma lipids, lipoproteins, clinical manifestations, and ischemic heart disease in men and women. *Atherosclerosis* 34:13, 1979.
106. Shapiro JR, Fallet RW, Tsang RC, Glueck CJ: Achilles tendonitis and tenosinovitis: A diagnostic manifestation of familial Type II hyperlipoproteinemia in children. *Am J Dis Child* 128:486, 1974.
107. Watanabe A, Yoshimura A, Wacasugi T, Tatami R, Takada R: Serum lipids, lipoproteins and coronary heart disease in patients with xanthelasma palpebrarum. *Atherosclerosis* 38:283, 1981.
108. Mabuchi M, Ito S, Haba T: Achilles tendon thickness and ischemic heart disease in familial hypercholesterolemia. *Metabolism* 27:1672, 1978.
109. Jensen D, Blankenhorn DH, Kornerup V: Coronary disease in familial hypercholesterolemia. *Circulation* 36:77, 1967.
110. Stone NY, Levy RI, Fredrickson DS, Vetter J: Coronary artery disease in 116 kindred with familial Type II hypercholesterolemia. *Circulation* 49:476, 1974.
111. Slack J: Risks of ischemic heart disease in familial hypercholesterolemia. *Lancet* 2:1380, 1969.
112. Hale JS, Hayden NR, Frohlich J, Pritchard PH: Genetic and environmental factors affecting the incidence of coronary artery disease in heterozygous familial hypercholesterolemia. *Arteriosclerosis Thromb* 11:290, 1991.
113. Coetze GA, VanderWesthuyzen DR, Berger JMB, Henderson HE, Gevers W: Low density lipoprotein metabolism in cultured fibroblasts from a new group of patients presenting clinically with homozygous familial hypercholesterolemia. *Arteriosclerosis* 2:303, 1982.
114. Rose V, Wilson G, Steiner G: Familial hypercholesterolemia: Report of coronary death at age 3 in a homozygous child and prenatal diagnosis in a heterozygous sibling. *J Pediatr* 100:757, 1982.
115. Allen JM, Thompson GR, Myant MB, Steiner R, Oakley MC: Cardiovascular complications of homozygous familial hypercholesterolemia. *Br Heart J* 44:361, 1980.
116. Forman MB, Kinsley RH, Duplessis JP, Danskey R, Milner S, Levine SE: Surgical correction of combined supravalvular and valvular aortic stenosis in homozygous familial hypercholesterolemia. *S Afr Med J* 61:579, 1982.
117. Seed M, Hoppichler F, Reaveley D, Thompson GR: Relation of serum lipoprotein (a) concentration and apolipoprotein (a) phenotype to coronary heart disease in patients with familial hypercholesterolemia. *N Engl J Med* 322:1494, 1990.
118. Wiklund O, Angelian B, Olofsson SO, Eriksson M, Fajer G, Berglund L, Bondjers G: Apolipoprotein (a) and ischemic heart disease in familial hypercholesterolemia. *Lancet* 335:1360, 1990.
119. Bloch A, Dinsmore RE, Lees RS: Coronary angiographic findings in Type II and Type IV hyperlipoproteinemia. *Lancet* 1:928, 1976.
120. Sugrue DD, Thompson GR, Oakley CM, Trainer IM, Steiner RE: Contrasting patterns of coronary atherosclerosis in normocholesterolemic smokers and patients with familial hypercholesterolemia. *Br Med J* 283:1358, 1981.
121. Streja D, Steiner G, Kwiterovich PO: Plasma high density lipoproteins in ischemic heart disease: Studies in a large kindred with familial hypercholesterolemia. *Ann Intern Med* 89:871, 1978.
122. Ginsberg H, Davidson N, Le NA, Gibson J, Ahrens EH, Brown WV: Marked overproduction of low density lipoprotein apoprotein B in a subject with heterozygous familial hypercholesterolemia. *Biochim Biophys Acta* 712:250, 1982.
123. Hazzard WR, Albers JJ, Caron P, Lewis B: Association of isoapolipoprotein EIII deficiency with heterozygous familial hypercholesterolemia: Implications for lipoprotein physiology. *Lancet* 1:298, 1981.
124. Tolleshaug H, Hopgood KK, Brown MS, Goldstein JL: The LDL receptor locus in familial hypercholesterolemia: Multiple mutations disrupt transport and processing of a membrane receptor. *Cell* 32:941, 1983.
125. Hobbs HH, Russell DW, Brown MS, Goldstein JL: The LDL receptor locus in familial hypercholesterolemia: Mutational analysis of a membrane protein. *Annu Rev Genet* 24:133, 1990.
126. Bilheimer DW, Stone NJ, Grundy SM: Metabolic studies in familial hypercholesterolemia: Evidence for a gene dosage effect *in vivo*. *J Clin Invest* 64:524, 1979.
127. Fogelman AM, Hokam MM, Haberland ME, Tanaka RD, Edwards PA: Lipoprotein regulation of cholesterol metabolism in macrophages derived from human monocytes. *J Biol Chem* 258:14081, 1982.
128. Seftel HC, Baker CG, Sundler MP: A host of hypercholesterolemic homozygotes in South Africa. *Br Med J* 281:633, 1980.
129. Khachadurian AK, Uthman SM: Experiences with homozygous cases of hypercholesterolemia: A report of 52 patients. *Nutr Metab* 15:132, 1973.
130. Illingworth DR, Sexton GJ: Hypocholesterolemic effects of mevinolin in patients with heterozygous familial hypercholesterolemia. *J Clin Invest* 74:1972, 1984.

131. Havel RG, Hunninghake DB, Illingworth DR, Stein EA: Lovastatin (mevinolin) in the treatment of heterozygous familial hypercholesterolemia: A multicenter study. *Ann Intern Med* 107:609, 1987.
132. Illingworth DR, Bacon S: Treatment of heterozygous familial hypercholesterolemia with lipid-lowering drugs. *Arteriosclerosis* 9(Suppl 1):1–121, 1989.
133. Mol MJTM, Erkelens DW, Gevers-Leuven JA: Effects of synvinolin (MK 733) on plasma lipids in familial hypercholesterolemia. *Lancet* 2:936, 1986.
134. Wiklund O, Angelin B, Fager G: Treatment of familial hypercholesterolemia: A controlled trial of the effects of pravastatin or Cholestyramine therapy on lipoprotein and apoprotein levels. *J Intern Med* 228:241, 1990.
135. Buckley MMT, Goa KL, Price AH, Brogden RN: Probucol: A reappraisal of its pharmacological properties and therapeutic use in hypercholesterolemia. *Drugs* 37:761, 1989.
136. Baker SG, Joffe BI, Mendelsohn D, Seftel HC: Treatment of homozygous familial hypercholesterolemia with Probucol. *S Afr Med J* 62:7, 1982.
137. Yamamota A, Matsuzawa Y, Yokoyama S: Effects of Probucol on xanthoma regression in familial hypercholesterolemia. *Am J Cardiol* 57:29H, 1986.
138. Packard CJ, Stewart JM, Morgan HG, Shepherd J: Combined drug therapy for familial hypercholesterolemia. *Artery* 7:281, 1980.
139. Illingworth DR, Phillipson BE, Rapp JH, Connor WE: Colestipol plus nicotinic acid in treatment of heterozygous familial hypercholesterolemia. *Lancet* 1:296, 1981.
140. Illingworth DR: Mevinolin plus Colestipol in therapy for severe heterozygous familial hypercholesterolemia. *Ann Intern Med* 101:598, 1984.
141. Lintott CJ, Scott RS, Nye ER, Sutherland EW: Simvastatin (MK 733): An effective treatment for hypercholesterolemia. *Aust N Z J Med* 19:317, 1989.
142. Hoogerbrugge N, Mol NJTM, van Dormaal JJ: The efficacy and safety of pravastatin compared to and in combination with bile acid-binding resins in familial hypercholesterolemia. *J Intern Med* 228:261, 1990.
143. Curtis LD, Dixon AC, Ling KLE, Betteridge J: Combination treatment with Cholestyramine and Bezafibrate for heterozygous familial hypercholesterolemia. *Br Med J* 297:173, 1988.
144. Malloy MJ, Kane JP, Kunitake ST, Havel RJ: Complimentarity of Colestipol, niacin and lovastatin in treatment of severe familial hypercholesterolemia. *Ann Intern Med* 107:616, 1987.
145. Spengel FA, Jadhav A, Duffield RGM, Wood CB, Thompson GR: Superiority of partial illeal bypass over Cholestyramine in reducing cholesterol in familial hypercholesterolemia. *Lancet* 2:768, 1981.
146. Buchwald H, Moore RB, Varco RL: Surgical treatment of hyperlipidemia. *Circulation* 49(Suppl 1):1, 1974.
147. Illingworth DR, Connor WE: Hypercholesterolemia persisting after distal ileal bypass: Response to mevinolin. *Ann Intern Med* 100:850, 1984.
148. Buchwald H, Varco RL, Matts JP, et al: Effect of partial ileal bypass surgery on mortality and morbidity from coronary heart disease in patients with hypercholesterolemia: Report of the Program on the Surgical Control of the Hyperlipidemias. *N Engl J Med* 323:946, 1990.
149. Keller C: LDL apheresis: Results of long-term treatment and vascular outcome. *Atherosclerosis* 86:1, 1991.
150. Thompson GR, Barbir M, Okabayashi K: Plasmapheresis in familial hypercholesterolemia. *Arteriosclerosis* 9(Suppl 1): 152, 1989.
151. Eisenhauer T, Armstrong VW, Wieland H, Fuchs C, Scheler F, Seidel D: Selective removal of low density lipoprotein by precipitation at low pH: First clinical application of the HELP System. *Klin Wochenschr* 65:1, 1987.
152. Thompson GR, Miller JP, Breslow JL: Improved survival of patients with homozygous familial hypercholesterolemia treated by plasma exchange. *Br Med J* 291:1671, 1985.
153. Bilheimer DW, Goldstein JL, Grundy SM, Starzle TE, Brown MS: Liver transplantation to provide low density lipoprotein receptors and lower plasma cholesterol in a child with homozygous familial hypercholesterolemia. *N Engl J Med* 311:1658, 1984.
154. Hoeg JM, Starzle TE, Brewer HP Jr: Liver transplantation for treatment of cardiovascular disease: Comparison of medication and plasma exchange in homozygous familial hypercholesterolemia. *Am J Cardiol* 59:705, 1987.
155. Innerarity TL, Weisgraber KH, Arnold KS, Grundy SM, Mahley RW: Familial defective apolipoprotein B-100: Low density lipoproteins with abnormal receptor binding. *Proc Natl Acad Sci USA* 84:6919, 1987.
156. Schuster H, Rauh G, Kormann B, Hepp T, Humphries S, Keller C, Wolfram G, Zollner N: Familial defective apolipoprotein B-100: Comparison with familial hypercholesterolemia in eighteen cases detected in Munich. *Arteriosclerosis* 10:577, 1990.
157. Myant MB, Gallagher JJ, Knight BL, McCarthy SN, Frostegard J, Nilsson J, Hamsten A, Talmud P, Humphries SE: Clinical signs of familial hypercholesterolemia in patients with familial defective apoprotein B-100 and normal low density lipoprotein receptor function. *Arteriosclerosis Thromb* 11:691, 1991.
158. Illingworth DR, Vakar F, Mahley RW, Weisgraber KH: Hypocholesterolemic effects of lovastatin in familial defective apolipoprotein B-100. *Lancet* 339:598, 1992.
159. Innerarity TL, Mahley RW, Weisgraber KH, Bersot TP, Krauss RM, Vega GL, Grundy SM, Friedel W, et al: Familial defective apolipoprotein B-100: A mutation of apolipoprotein B that causes hypercholesterolemia. *J Lipid Res* 31:1337, 1990.
160. Hansen PS, Rudigen N, Tybjærg-Hansen A: Detection of the apo B 3,500 mutation (glutamine arginine) by gene amplification and cleavage with Mspl. *J Lipid Res* 32:1229, 1991.
161. Vega GL, Grundy SM: *In vivo* evidence for reduced binding of low density lipoproteins to receptors as a cause of primary moderate hypercholesterolemia. *J Clin Invest* 78:1410, 1986.
162. Corsini A, Mazzotti M, Fumagalli R, Catapano AL, Romano L, Romano C: Poor response to simvastatin in familial defective apolipoprotein B-100. *Lancet* 337:305, 1991.
163. Maher VMG, Gallagher JJ, Thompson GR, Myant NB: Response to cholesterol-lowering drugs in familial defective apolipoprotein B-100. *Atherosclerosis* 91:73, 1991.
164. Schmidt EB, Illingworth DR, Bacon S, Mahley RW, Weisgraber KH: Hypocholesterolemic effects of nicotinic acid in patients with familial defective apoprotein B-100. *Metabolism* 42:137, 1993.
165. Vega GL, Illingworth DR, Grundy SM, Lindgren FT, Connor WE: Normocholesterolemic tendon xanthomas with overproduction of apolipoprotein B. *Metabolism* 32:118, 1983.
166. Goldstein JL, Schrott HG, Hazzard WR: Hyperlipidemia in coronary heart disease: Genetic analysis of lipid levels in 176 families and delineation of a new inherited disorder, combined hyperlipidemia. *J Clin Invest* 52:1544, 1973.
167. Babirak SP, Inverius P-H, Fujimoto WY, Brunzell JD: Detection and characterization of the heterozygote state for lipoprotein lipase deficiency. *Arteriosclerosis* 9:326, 1989.
168. Wojciechowski AP, Farrall M, Cullen P, Wilson TME, Bayliss JD, Farren B, Griffin BA, Caslake MJ, et al: Familial combined hyperlipidemia linked to the apolipoprotein AI-CIII-AIV gene cluster on chromosome 11q23-q24. *Nature* 349:161, 1991.
169. Sniderman AD, Shapiro S, Marpole D, Skinner B, Tang G, Kwiterovich PO Jr: Association of coronary atherosclerosis with hyperapobetalipoproteinemia. *Proc Natl Acad Sci USA* 77:604, 1980.
170. Sniderman AD, Wolfson C, Tang B, Franklin FA, Bachorik PS, Kwiterovich PO Jr: Association of hyperapobetalipoproteinemia with endogenous hypertriglyceridemia and atherosclerosis. *Ann Intern Med* 97:833, 1982.
171. Janus ED, Nicoll AM, Turner PL, Lewis B: Kinetic basis of

the primary hyperlipoproteinemias: Studies of apolipoprotein B turnover in genetically defined subjects. *Eur J Clin Invest* 10:161, 1980.
172. Deeb SS, Motulsky AG, Albers JJ: A partial cDNA clone for human apolipoprotein B. *Proc Natl Acad Sci USA* 82:4983, 1985.
173. Knott TJ, Rall SC, Innerarity TL, Jacobson SF, Urdea MS, Wilson BL, Powell LM, Pease RJ, et al: Human apolipoprotein B: Structure of carboxyterminal domains, cytogenic expression and chromosomal localization. *Science* 230:37, 1985.
174. Illingworth DR: Fibric acid derivatives, in Rifkind BM (ed): *Drug Treatment of Hyperlipidemia.* New York, Marcel Dekker, 1991, p 103.
175. Goffman JW, Dipalla O, Glazier F, Freeman NK, Linguen FT, Nichols AV, Strisower EH, Tamplan AR: The serum lipoprotein transport system and health, metabolic disorders, atherosclerosis and coronary heart disease. *Plasma* 2:413, 1954.
176. Brewer HB, Zech LA, Gregg RE, et al: Type III hyperlipoproteinemia: Diagnosis, molecular defects, pathology and treatment. *Ann Intern Med* 98:623, 1983.
177. Morganroth J, Levy RI, Fredrickson DS: The biochemical, clinical and genetic features of Type III hyperlipidemia. *Ann Intern Med* 82:158, 1975.
178. Davignon J, Gregg RE, Sing CF: Apoprotein E polymorphism and atherosclerosis. *Arteriosclerosis* 8:1, 1988.
179. Mahley RW, Angelin B: Type III hyperlipoproteinemia: Recent insights into the genetic defects of familial dysbetalipoproteinemia. *Adv Intern Med* 29:395, 1984.
180. Fredrickson DS, Morganroth J, Levy RI: Type III hyperlipidemia: An analysis of two contemporary definitions. *Ann Intern Med* 82:150, 1975.
181. Ghiselli G, Schaffer EJ, Gascon P, Brewer HB Jr: Type III hyperlipoproteinemia associated with apolipoprotein E deficiency. *Science* 214:1239, 1981.
182. Havel RJ: Familial dysbetalipoproteinemia: New aspects of pathogenesis and diagnosis. *Med Clin North Am* 66:441, 1982.
183. Kushwaha RS, Hazzard WR, Gagne C, Chait A, Albers JJ: Type III hyperlipoproteinemia: Paradoxical hypolipidemic response to estrogen. *Ann Intern Med* 87:517, 1977.
184. Zelis R, Mason DT, Braunwald E, Levy RI: Effects of hyperlipoproteinemias and their treatment on the peripheral circulation. *J Clin Invest* 49:1007, 1970.
185. Breckenridge WC, Little JA, Alaupovic P, Wang CS, Kuksis A, Lundgren A, Gardiner G: Lipoprotein abnormalities associated with a familial deficiency of hepatic lipase. *Atherosclerosis* 45:161, 1982.
186. Brunzell JD: Familial lipoprotein lipase deficiency and other causes of the chylomicronemia syndrome, in Scriver CR, Beaudet AL, Sly WS, Valler D (eds): *The Metabolic Basis of Inherited Disease,* 6th ed. New York, McGraw-Hill, 1989, pp 1165–1180.
187. Fredrickson DS, Levy RI: Familial hyperlipoproteinemia, in Stanbury JB, Wyngaarden JB, Fredrickson DS (eds): *The Metabolic Basis of Inherited Disease,* 3d ed. New York, McGraw-Hill, 1972, p 545.
188. Brown WV, Baginsky ML, Ehnholm C: Primary type I and V hyperlipoproteinemia, in Rifkind BM, Levy RI (eds): *Hyperlipidemia: Diagnosis and Therapy.* New York, Grune & Stratton, 1977, p 93.
189. Brunzell JD, Bierman EL: Chylomicronemia syndrome: Interaction of genetic and acquired hypertriglyceridemia. *Med Clin North Am* 66:455, 1982.
190. Kwiterovich PO, Farah JR, Brown WV, Bachorik PS, Baylin SB, Neill CA: The clinical, biochemical, and familial presentation of type V hyperlipoproteinemia in childhood. *Pediatrics* 59:513, 1977.
191. Greenberg BM, Blackwelder WC, Levy RI: Primary type V hyperlipoproteinemia. *Ann Intern Med* 87:526, 1977.
192. Fallat RW, Glueck CJ: Familial and acquired type V hyperlipoproteinemia. *Atherosclerosis* 23:41, 1976.
193. Lesser PB, Warshaw AL: Diagnosis of pancreatitis masked by hyperlipidemia. *Ann Intern Med* 82:795, 1975.
194. Harlan WR, Winesett PS, Wasserman AJ: Tissue lipoprotein lipase in normal individuals and in individuals with exogenous hypertriglyceridemia and the relation of this enzyme to the assimilation of fat. *J Clin Invest* 46:239, 1967.
195. Santamarina-Fojo S, Brewer HB Jr: The familial hyperchylomicronemia syndrome. *JAMA* 265:904–908, 1991.
196. Sigurdson G, Nicoll A, Lewis B: Metabolism of very low density lipoproteins in hyperlipidemia: Studies of apoprotein B kinetics in man. *Eur J Clin Invest* 6:167, 1976.
197. Leaf DA, Connor WE, Illingworth DR, Bacon SP, Sexton G: The hypolipidemic effects of gemfibrozil in type V hyperlipidemia: A double blind crossover study. *JAMA* 262:3154–3160, 1989.
198. McMurry MP, Connor WE, Goplerud CP: Effects of dietary cholesterol upon the hypercholesterolemia of pregnancy. *Metabolism* 30:869–879, 1981.
199. Sanderson SL, Iverius PH, Wilson DE: Successful hyperlipidemic pregnancy. *JAMA* 265:1858–1860, 1991.
200. DenBesten L, Reyna RH, Connor WE, Stegink LD: The different effects on the serum lipids and fecal steroids of high carbohydrate diets given orally or intravenously. *J Clin Invest* 52:1384–1393, 1973.
201. Mishkel MA, Stein EA: Primary type IV hyperlipoproteinemia, in Rifkind BM, Levy RI (eds): *Hyperlipidemia: Diagnosis and Therapy.* New York, Grune & Stratton, 1977, p 177.
202. Goldstein JL, Hazzard WR, Schrott HG, Bierman EL, Motulsky AG, Levinski MJ, Campbell ED: Hyperlipidemia in coronary heart disease: I. Lipid levels in 500 survivors of myocardial infarction. *J Clin Invest* 52:1533, 1973.
203. Brunzell JD, Bierman EL: Plasma triglyceride and insulin levels in familial hypertriglyceridemia. *Ann Intern Med* 87:198, 1977.
204. Kannel WB: Lipids, diabetes, and coronary heart disease: Insights from the Framingham study. *Am Heart J* 110:1100, 1985.
205. Kannel WB, McGee DL: Diabetes and cardiovascular disease—the Framingham study. *JAMA* 241:2035, 1979.
206. Garcia MJ, McNamara PM, Gordon T, Kannel WB: Morbidity and mortality in diabetics in the Framingham population: Sixteen year follow-up study. *Diabetes* 23:105, 1974.
207. Kirkland RT, Keenan BS, Probstfield JL, et al: Decrease in plasma high density lipoprotein cholesterol levels at puberty in boys with delayed adolescence. *JAMA* 257:502, 1987.
208. Mellies MJ, Gartside PS, Galtfelter L, Blueck CJ: Effect of probucol on plasma cholesterol high and low density lipoprotein cholesterol and apolipoprotein AI and AII in adults with primary familial hypercholesterolemia. *Metabolism* 29:956, 1980.
209. Schaefer EJ, Heaton WH, Wetzel MG, Brewer HG Jr: Plasma apolipoprotein AI absence associated with a marked reduction of high density lipoproteins and premature coronary artery disease. *Arteriosclerosis* 2:16, 1982.
210. Norum RA, Lakier JB, Goldstein S, Angel A, Goldberg RB, Block WD, Noffze DK, Dolphin PJ, et al: Familial deficiency of apolipoproteins AI and CIII and precocious coronary artery disease. *N Engl J Med* 306:1513, 1982.
211. Karathanasis SK, Norum RA, Zannis VI, Breslow JL: An inherited polymorphism in the human apolipoprotein AI gene locus related to the development of atherosclerosis. *Nature* 301:718, 1983.
212. Schaefer EJ, Ordovas JM, Law S, et al: Familial lipolipoprotein AI and CIII deficiency, variant II. *J Lipid Res* 26:1089, 1985.
213. Assman G, Schmitz G, Brewer HB Jr: Familial high density lipoprotein deficiency: Tangier disease, in Scriver CR, Beaudet AL, Sly WS, Valle D (eds): *The Metabolic Basis of Inherited Disease,* 6th ed. New York, McGraw-Hill, 1989, p 1267.
214. Frederickson DA: The inheritance of high density lipoprotein deficiency (Tangier disease). *J Clin Invest* 43:228, 1964.

215. Lindeskog GR, Gustafson A, Enerback L: Serum lipoprotein deficiency and diffuse planar xanthoma. *Arch Dermatol* 106:529, 1972.
216. Gustafson A, McCounathy W, Alaupovic P, Curry MD, Persson B: Identification of apoprotein families in a variant of human plasma apolipoprotein A deficiency. *Scand J Clin Lab Invest* 39:377, 1979.
217. Norum KR, Gjone E, Glomset JA: Familial lecithin: Cholesterol acyltransferase deficiency, including fish eye disease, in Scriver CR, Beaudet AL, Sly WS, Valle D (eds): *The Metabolic Basis of Inherited Disease,* 6th ed. New York, McGraw-Hill, 1989, p 1181.
218. Gjone E, Norum KR: Familial serum cholesterol ester deficiency: Clinical study of a patient with a new syndrome. *Acta Med Scand* 183:107, 1968.
219. Carlson LA, Phillipson B: Fish eye disease: A new familial condition associated with massive corneal opacities and dyslipoproteinemia. *Lancet* 2:921, 1979.
220. Carlson LA: Fish eye disease: A new familial condition with massive corneal opacities and dyslipoproteinemia. *Eur J Clin Invest* 12:41, 1982.
221. Weisgraber KH, Rall SC Jr, Bersot TP, et al: Apolipoprotein AI Milano: Detection of normal AI in affected subjects and evidence for a cysteine for arginine substitution in the variant AI. *J Biol Chem* 258:2508, 1983.
222. Rall SC, Menzel HG, Assmann G, et al: Identification of amino acid substitutions in five human apolipoproteins AI variants. *Arteriosclerosis* 3:515a, 1983.
223. Utermann G, Feussner G, Franceschini G, et al: Genetic variants of group A apolipoproteins, lipid methods for screening and characterization without ultracentrifugation. *J Biol Chem* 257:501, 1982.
224. Menzel HJ, Kladetzky RG, Assmann G: One step screening method for the polymorphisms of apolipoprotein AI, AII, and AIV. *J Lipid Res* 23:9156, 1982.
225. Vergani C, Bettale A: Familial hypoalphalipoproteinemia. *Clin Chim Acta* 114:45, 1981.
226. Third JHLC, Montag J, Freidel J, et al: Primary and familial hypoalphalipoproteinemia. *Metabolism* 33:136, 1984.
227. Glueck DJ, Fallet RW, Millet F, Gottside P, Elston RC, Go RCP: Familial hyperalphalipoproteinemia: Studies in 28 kindreds. *Metabolism* 24:1243, 1975.
228. Schaefer EJ: Clinical, biochemical and genetic features in familial disorders of high density lipoprotein deficiency. *Arteriosclerosis* 4:303, 1984.
229. Franceschini G, Sirtori CR, Capurso A, Weisgraber KH, Mahley RW: AI Milano apoprotein: Decreased high density lipoprotein cholesterol levels with significant lipoprotein modifications and with clinical atherosclerosis in an Italian family. *J Clin Invest* 66:892, 1980.
230. Breslow JL: Familial disorders of high density lipoprotein metabolism, in Scriver CR, Beaudet AL, Sly WS, Valle D (eds): *The Metabolic Basis of Inherited Disease,* 6th ed. New York, McGraw-Hill, 1989, p 1251.
231. Daniels SR, Bates S, Lutkin RR, Benton C, Third JLHC, Glueck CJ: Cerebral vascular arteriopathy (arteriosclerosis) and ischemic childhood stroke. *Stroke* 13:360, 1982.
232. Schaefer EJ, Zech LA, Schwartz DS, Brewer HP Jr: Coronary heart disease prevalence and other clinical features in familial high density lipoprotein deficiency (Tangiers disease). *Ann Intern Med* 93:261, 1980.
233. Schmitz G, Assmann G, Rall SE Jr, Mahley RW: Tangier disease: Defective recombination of a specific Tangier apolipoprotein AI isoform (proapo AI) with high density lipoproteins. *Proc Natl Acad Sci USA* 80:6081, 1983.
234. Zannis VI, Lees AM, Lees RS, Breslow JL: Abnormal apo AI isoprotein composition in patients with Tangier disease. *J Biochem* 257:4978, 1982.
235. Kay L, Ronan R, Schaefer EJ, Brewer HG Jr: Tangier disease: A structural defect in apolipoprotein AI. *Proc Natl Acad Sci USA* 79:2485, 1982.
236. Glueck CJ, Kostis PM, Tsang RC, Mellies MJ, Steiner PM: Neonatal familial hyperalphalipoproteinemia. *Metabolism* 26:469, 1977.
237. Koizumi J, Mabuchi H, Yoshimura A, Michishita I, Takeda M, Itoh H, Sakai Y, Sakai T, et al: Deficiency of serum cholesterol-ester transfer activity in patients with familial hyperalphalipoproteinemia. *Atherosclerosis* 58:175, 1985.
238. Kurasawa T, Yokoyama S, Miyake Y, Yamamura T, Yamamoto A: Rate of cholesterol-ester transfer between high and low density lipoproteins in human serum and a case with decreased transfer rate in association with hyperalphalipoproteinemia. *J Biochem* 98:1499, 1985.
239. Kane JP, Havel RJ: Disorders of the biogenesis and secretion of lipoproteins containing the B apoproteins, in Scriver CR, Beaudet AL, Sly WS, Valle D (eds): *The Metabolic Basis of Inherited Disease,* 6th ed. New York, McGraw-Hill, 1989, p 1139.
240. Malloy MJ, Kane JP, Hardman DA, Hamilton RL, Dalal KB: Normotriglyceridemic abetalipoproteinemia: Absence of the B100 apolipoprotein. *J Clin Invest* 67:1441, 1981.
241. Takashimo Y, Kodama T, Lida H, Kawamura M, Aburatani H, Itakura H, Akanuma Y, Takaku F, Kawade M: Normotriglyceridemic abetalipoproteinemia in infancy: An isolated apolipoprotein B100 deficiency. *Pediatrics* 75:541, 1985.
242. Caballero FM, Buchanan GR: Abetalipoproteinemia presenting as severe vitamin K deficiency. *Pediatrics* 65:161, 1980.
243. Muller DPR, Lloyd JK, Bird AC: Long term management of abetalipoproteinemia: Possible role for vitamin E. *Arch Dis Child* 52:209, 1977.
244. Illingworth DR, Connor WE, Miller RG: Abetalipoproteinemia: Report of two cases and review of therapy. *Arch Neurol* 37:659, 1980.
245. Illingworth DR, Kenny TA, Orwolll ES: Adrenal function in heterozygous and homozygous hypobetalipoproteinemia. *J Clin Endocrinol Metab* 54:27, 1982.
246. Illingworth DR, Kenny TA, Connor WE, Orwoll ES: Corticosteroid production in abetalipoproteinemia: Evidence for an impaired response to ACTH. *J Lab Clin Med* 100:115, 1982.
247. Parker CR Jr, Illingworth DR, Bissonnette J, Carr BR: Endocrinology of pregnancy in abetalipoproteinemia: Studies in a patient with heterozygous familial hypobetalipoproteinemia. *N Engl J Med* 314:557, 1986.
248. Muller DPR, Lloyd JK: Effect of large oral doses of vitamin E on the neurological sequelae of patients with abetalipoproteinemia. *Ann NY Acad Sci* 393:133, 1982.
249. Hegele RA, Angel A: Arrest of neuropathy and myopathy in abetalipoproteinemia with high dose vitamin E therapy. *Can Med Assoc J* 132:41, 1985.
250. Runge P, Muller DPR, McCallister J, Calver D, Lloyd JK, Taylor D: Oral vitamin E supplements can prevent the retinopathy of abetalipoproteinemia. *Br J Ophthalmol* 70:166, 1986.
251. Illingworth DR, Connor WE, Buist NRM, Jhaveri DJ, Lin DS, McMurray MP: Sterol balance in abetalipoproteinemia: Studies in a patient with homozygous familial hypobetalipoproteinemia. *Metabolism* 28:1152, 1979.
252. Wang CS, Illingworth DR: Lipid composition and lipolytic activities in milk from a patient with homozygous familial hypobetalipoproteinemia. *Am J Clin Nutr* 45:730, 1987.
253. Lackner KJ, Monge JC, Greg RE, Hoeg JM, Triche TJ, Law SW, Brewer HB Jr: Analysis of the apoprotein B gene and messenger ribonucleic acid in abetalipoproteinemia. *J Clin Invest* 78:1707, 1986.
254. Young SG, Hubi ST, Smith RS, Snyder SM, Terdiman JF: Familial hypobetalipoproteinemia caused by a mutation in the apolipoprotein gene that results in a truncated species of apolipoprotein B (B31). *J Clin Invest* 85:933, 1990.
255. Talmud P, King-Underwood L, Krul E, Schonfeld G, Humphries SE: The molecular basis of truncated forms of apolipoprotein B in a kindred with compound heterozygous hypobetalipoproteinemia. *J Lipid Res* 30:1773, 1989.
256. Hardman DA, Pulinger CR, Hamilton RL, Kane JP, Malloy

MJ: Molecular and metabolic basis for the metabolic disorder normotriglyceridemic abetalipoproteinemia. *J Clin Invest* 88:1722, 1991.

257. Bieri JG, Hoeg JM, Schaefer EJ, Zech LA, Brewer HB Jr: Vitamin A and vitamin E replacement in abetalipoproteinemia. *Ann Intern Med* 100:238, 1984.
258. Kayden HJ, Hatem LJ, Traber MG: The measurement of nanograms of tocopherol from needle aspiration biopsies of adipose tissue: Normal and abetalipoproteinemic subjects. *J Lipid Res* 24:652, 1983.
259. Partin JS, Partin JC, Schubert WK, McAdams AJ: Liver ultrastructure in abetalipoproteinemia: Evolution of micronodular cirrhosis. *Gastroenterology* 67:107, 1974.
260. Noseda G, Riesen W, Schlumph E, Morrell A: Hypobetalipoproteinemia associated with autoantibodies against betalipoproteins. *Eur J Clin Invest* 2:342, 1972.
261. Cottrill C, Glueck CJ, Leuba V, Millett F, Puppinone D, Brown WV: Familial homozygous hypobetalipoproteinemia. *Metabolism* 23:779, 1974.
262. Salt HB, Wolff OH, Lloyd JK, Fosbrooke AS, Cameron AH, Hubble DV: On having no betalipoprotein: A syndrome comprising abetalipoproteinemia, acanthocytosis, and steatorrhea. *Lancet* 2:325, 1960.
263. Andersen GE, Brokhatting NK, Lous P: Familial hypobetalipoproteinemia in nine children diagnosed as the result of cord blood screening for hypolipoproteinemia in 10,000 Danish newborns. *Arch Dis Child* 54:691, 1979.
264. Glueck CJ, Gartside PS, Steiner PM, Miller M, Todd-Hunter T, Haaf J, Puck EM, Terrana M, et al: Hyperalpha and hypobetalipoproteinemia in octogenarian kindreds. *Atherosclerosis* 27:387, 1977.
265. Frohlich J, McLeod R, Pritchard PH, Fesmire J, McConathy W: Plasma lipoprotein abnormalities in heterozygotes for familial lecithin: Cholesterol acyltransferase deficiency. *Metabolism* 37:3, 1988.
266. Rapp JH, Connor WE, Lin DS, Inahara T, Porter JM: The lipids of human atherosclerotic plaques and xanthomas: Clues to the mechanism of plaque progression. *J Lipid Res* 24:1329–1335, 1983.
267. Austin MA: Plasma triglyceride as a risk factor for coronary heart disease: The epidemiologic evidence and beyond. *Am J Epidemiol* 129:249–259, 1989.
268. Gordon T, Castelli WP, Hjortland MC, Kannel WM: High density lipoprotein as a protective factor against coronary heart disease: The Framingham study. *Am J Med* 62:707, 1977.
269. Bhattacharyya AK, Preacher AB, Connor WE: Ectopic xanthomas in familial (Type II) hypercholesterolemia. *Atherosclerosis* 37:319–323, 1980.
270. Bhattacharyya AK, Connor WE, Mausolf FA, Flatt AE: Turnover of xanthoma cholesterol in hyperlipoproteinemic patients. *J Lab Clin Med* 87:503, 1976.
271. Schmidtz G, Assmann G: Acid lipase deficiency, Wolman disease and cholesterol ester storage disease, in Scriver CR, Beaudet AL, Sly WS, Valle D (eds): *The Metabolic Basis of Inherited Disease,* 6th ed. New York, McGraw-Hill, 1989, p 1623.
272. Tarrantino MD, McNamarra DJ, Granstrom P, Ellefson RD, Unger EC, Udall JM Jr: Lovastatin therapy for cholesterol ester storage disease in two sisters. *J Pediatr* 118:131, 1991.
273. Leone L, Ippoliti PF: Use of simvastatin plus Cholestyramine in the treatment of lysosomal acid lipase deficiency. *J Pediatr* 119:1008, 1991.
274. Bisceglie AND, Ishak KG, Rabin L, Hoeg JN: Cholesterol ester storage disease: Hepatopathology and effects of therapy with lovastatin. *Hepatology* 11:764, 1990.
275. Mbewu AD, Durrington PN: Lipoprotein (a): Structure, properties and possible involvement in thrombogenesis and atherogenesis. *Atherosclerosis* 85:1, 1990.
276. Vessby B, Kostner G, Lithell J, Thomas J: Diverging effects of Cholestyramine on apolipoprotein B and lipoprotein Lp(a): A dose response study of the effects of Cholestyramine in hypercholesterolemia. *Atherosclerosis* 44:61, 1982.
277. Berg K, Laren TP: Unchanged serum lipoprotein (a) concentrations with lovastatin. *Lancet* 2:812, 1989.
278. Kostner GM, Gavish O, Leopold B, Bolzano K, Weintraub MS, Breslow JL: HMG CoA reductase inhibitors lower LDL cholesterol without reducing Lp(a) levels. *Circulation* 80:1313, 1989.
279. Carlson LA, Hamsten A, Asplund A: Pronounced lowering of serum levels of lipoprotein Lp(a) in hyperlipidemic subjects treated with nicotinic acid. *J Intern Med* 226:271, 1989.
280. Soma M, Fumagalli R, Paolett R, Meschia M, Maini MC, Crosignani P, Ghanen K, Gaubatz J, Morrisett JD: Plasma Lp(a) concentration after estrogen and progesterone in post menopausal women. *Lancet* 337:612, 1991.
281. Bhattacharyya AK, Connor WE: Familial diseases with storage of sterols other than cholesterol (cerebrotendinous xanthomatosis and β-sitosterolemia and xanthomatosis), in Stanbury JB, Wyngaarden JB, Fredrickson DS (eds): *The Metabolic Basis of Inherited Disease,* 4th ed. New York, McGraw-Hill, 1978, p 656.
282. Bjorkem I, Skrede S: Familial diseases with storage of sterols other than cholesterol: Cerebrotendinous xanthomatosis and phytosterolemia, in Scriver CR, Beaudet AL, Sly WS, Valle D (eds): *The Metabolic Basis of Inherited Disease,* 6th ed. New York, McGraw-Hill, 1989, pp 1283–1304.
283. Salen G, Shefer S, Cheng FW, Dayal B, Batta AK, Tint GS: Cholic acid biosynthesis: The enzymatic defect in cerebrotendinous xanthomatosis. *J Clin Invest* 63:38, 1979.
284. Berginer VN, Salen G, Shefer S: Longterm treatment of cerebrotendinous xanthomatosis with chenodeoxycholic acid. *N Engl J Med* 311:1649, 1984.
285. Bhattacharyya AK, Connor WE: β-Sitosterolemia and xanthomatosis: A newly described lipid storage disease in two sisters. *J Clin Invest* 53:1033–1043, 1974.
286. Salen G, Horak I, Rothkopf M, Cohen JL, Speck J, Tint GS, Shore V, Dayal B, et al: Lethal atherosclerosis associated with abnormal plasma and tissue sterol composition in sitosterolemia with xanthomatosis. *J Lipid Res* 26:1126, 1985.
287. Gregg RA, Connor WE, Lin DS, Brewer H Jr: Abnormal metabolism of shellfish sterols in a patient with sitosterolemia and xanthomatosis. *J Clin Invest* 77:1864–1872, 1986.
288. Connor WE, Connor SL: The key role of nutritional factors in the prevention of coronary heart disease. *Prev Med* 1:49, 1972.
289. Lin DS, Connor WE: The long-term effects of dietary cholesterol upon the plasma lipids, lipoproteins, cholesterol absorption, and the sterol balance in man: The demonstration of feedback inhibition of cholesterol biosynthesis and increased bile acid excretion. *J Lipid Res* 21:1042, 1981.
290. Taylor CB, Patton DE, Cox GE: Atherosclerosis in rhesus monkeys: VI. Fatal myocardial infarction in a monkey fed fat and cholesterol. *Arch Pathol* 76:404, 1963.
291. Armstrong ML, Warner ED, Connor WE: Regression of coronary atheromatosis in rhesus monkeys. *Circ Res* 27:59, 1970.
292. Connor WE, Connor SL: The dietary treatment of hyperlipidemia: Rationale, technique and efficacy, in Havel RJ (ed): Lipid disorders. *Med Clin North Am* 66:485, 1982.
293. Brown MS, Goldstein FL: A receptor-mediated pathway for cholesterol homeostasis. *Science* 232:34, 1986.
294. Spady DK, Dietschy JM: Interaction of dietary cholesterol and triglycerides in the regulation of hepatic low density lipoprotein transport in the hamster. *J Clin Invest* 81:300, 1988.
295. Sorci-Thomas M, Wilson MD, Johnson FL, Williams DL, Rudel LL: Studies on the expression of genes encoding apolipoproteins B100 and B48 and the low density lipoprotein receptor in nonhuman primates. *J Biol Chem* 264:9039, 1989.
296. Fox JC, Mcgill HC Jr, Carey KD, Getz GS: In vivo regulation of hepatic LDL receptor mRNA in the baboon—differential effects of saturated and unsaturated fat. *J Biol Chem* 262:7014, 1987.

297. Hopkins PN: Effects of dietary cholesterol on serum cholesterol: A meta-analysis and review. *Am J Clin Nutr* 55:1060, 1992.
298. Connor WE, Hodges RE, Bleiler RE: The serum lipids in men receiving high cholesterol and cholesterol-free diets. *J Clin Invest* 40:894, 1961.
299. Connor WE, Stone DB, Hodges RE: The interrelated effects of dietary cholesterol and fat upon the human serum lipid levels. *J Clin Invest* 43:1691, 1964.
300. Roberts SL, McMurry M, Connor WE: Does egg feeding (i.e. dietary cholesterol) affect plasma cholesterol levels in humans? The results of a double-blind study. *Am J Clin Nutr* 34:2092, 1981.
301. Gordon T, Fisher M, Ernst M, et al: Relation of diet to LDL cholesterol, VLDL cholesterol and plasma total cholesterol and triglycerides in white adults. *Atherosclerosis* 2:502, 1982.
302. Mensink RP, Katan MB: Effect of dietary trans fatty acids on high-density and low-density lipoprotein cholesterol levels in healthy subjects. *N Engl J Med* 323:439, 1990.
303. Mattson FH, Grundy SM: Comparison of effects of dietary saturated, monounsaturated and polyunsaturated fatty acids on plasma lipids and lipoproteins in men. *J Lipid Res* 26:194, 1985.
304. Neuringer MD, Connor WE: Omega-3 fatty acids in the brain and retina: Evidence for their essentiality. *Nutr Rev* 44:285, 1986.
305. Goodnight SH Jr, Harris WS, Connor WE, Illingworth DR: Polyunsaturated fatty acids, hyperlipidemia and thrombosis. *Arteriosclerosis* 2:87, 1982.
306. Connor WE, Connor SL: Diet, atherosclerosis and fish oil, in Stollerman H, Siperstein MD (eds): *Advances in Internal Medicine*. Chicago, Year Book, 1989, p 139.
307. Harris WS, Connor WE, McMurry MP: The comparative reductions of the plasma lipids and lipoproteins by dietary polyunsaturated fats: Salmon oil versus vegetable oils. *Metabolism* 32:179, 1983.
308. Phillipson BE, Rothrock DW, Connor WE, Harris WS, Illingworth DR: The reduction of plasma lipids, lipoproteins, and apoproteins in hypertriglyceridemic patients by dietary fish oils. *N Engl J Med* 312:1210, 1985.
309. Burr ML, Gilbert JF, Holliday RM, Elwood PC, Fehly AM, Rogers S, Sweetnam PM, Deadman NM: Effects of changes in fat, fish, and fibre intakes on death and myocardial infarction: Diet and reinfarction trial (DART). *Lancet* 2:757, 1989.
310. Harris WS, Connor WE, Alam N, Illingworth DR: The reduction of postprandial triglyceridemia in humans by dietary n-3 fatty acids. *J Lipid Res* 29:1451, 1988.
311. Weintraub MS, Zechner R, Brown A, Eisenberg S, Breslow JL: Dietary polyunsaturated fats of the w-6 and w-3 series reduce postprandial lipoprotein levels: Chronic and acute effects of fat saturation on postprandial lipoprotein metabolism. *J Clin Invest* 82:1884, 1988.
312. Olefsky J, Reaven GM, Farquhar JW: Effects of weight reduction on obesity. *J Clin Invest* 53:64, 1974.
313. Schwartz RS, Brunzell JD: Increase of adipose tissue lipoprotein lipase activity with weight loss. *J Clin Invest* 67:1425, 1981.
314. McMurry MP, Cerqueira MT, Connor SL, Connor WE: Changes in lipid and lipoprotein levels and body weight in Tarahumara Indians after consumption of an affluent diet. *N Engl J Med* 325:1704, 1991.
315. Ullmann D, Connor WE, Hatcher LF, Connor SL, Flavell DP: Will a high carbohydrate, low-fat diet lower plasma lipids and lipoproteins without producing hypertriglyceridemia? *Arteriosclerosis Thromb* 11:1059, 1991.
316. Anderson JW, Story L, Sieling B, Chen WJL, Petro MS, Story J: Hypocholesterolemic effects of oat-bran or bean intake for hypercholesterolemic men. *Am J Clin Nutr* 40:1146, 1984.
317. Malinow MR, Connor WE, McLaughlin P, Stafford C, Lin DS, Livingston AL, Dohler GO, McNulty WP: Sterol balance in Macaca fascicularis: Effects of alfalfa saponins. *J Clin Invest* 67:156, 1981.
318. Witzam JL, Steinbert D: Role of oxidized low density lipoprotein in atherogenesis. *J Lipid Res* 26:194, 1985.
319. Princen HMG, van Poppel G, Vogelezang C, Buytenhek R, Kok FJ: Supplementation with vitamin E but not B-carotene in vivo protects low density lipoprotein from lipid peroxidation in vitro: effect of ciagarette smoking. *Arteriosclerosis Thromb* 12:554, 1992.
320. Marmot M, Brunner E: Alcohol and cardiovascular disease—the status of the U shaped curve. *Br Med J* 303:565, 1991.
321. Hennekens CH, Rosner B, Cole DS: Daily alcohol consumption and coronary heart disease. *Am J Epidemiol* 107:196, 1978.
322. Hegsted DM, Ausman LM: Diet, alcohol and coronary heart disease in men. *J Nutr* 118:1184, 1988.
323. Suh IL, Shaten BJ, Cutler JA, Kuller LH: Alcohol use and mortality from coronary heart disease: The role of high-density lipoprotein cholesterol. *Ann Intern Med* 116:881, 1992.
324. Fry MM, Spector AA, Connor SL, et al: Intensification of hypertriglyceridemia by either alcohol or carbohydrate. *Am J Clin Nutr* 26:798, 1973.
325. Zock PL, Katan MB, Merkus MP, van Dusseldorp M, Harryvan JL: Effect of a lipid-rich fraction from boiled coffee on serum cholesterol. *Lancet* 335:1235, 1990.
326. Fried RE, Levine DM, Kwiterovich PO, Diamond EL, Wilder LB, Moy TF, Pearson TA: The effect of filtered-coffee consumption on plasma lipid levels. *JAMA* 267:811, 1992.
327. Connor WE, Connor SL: The dietary prevention and treatment of coronary heart disease, in Connor WE, Bristow JD (eds): *Coronary Heart Disease: Prevention, Complications, and Treatment*. Philadelphia, Lippincott, 1985, pp 43–64.
328. Connor SL, Connor WE: *The New American Diet*. New York, Simon & Schuster, 1986.
329. Connor SL, Connor WE: *The New American Diet System*. New York, Simon & Schuster, 1991.
330. Connor WE, Connor SL: Dietary treatment of hyperlipidemia: Rationale and benefit. *Endocrinologist* 1:33, 1991.
331. Knuiman JT, Hermus RJJ, Hautvast JGAJ: Serum total and high density lipoprotein (HDL) cholesterol concentrations in rural and urban boys from 16 countries. *Atherosclerosis* 36:529, 1980.
332. Miller GJ, Miller NE: Dietary fat, HDL cholesterol, and coronary disease: One interpretation. *Lancet* 2:1270, 1982.
333. Brinton EA, Eisenberg S, Breslow JL: A low-fat diet decreases high density lipoprotein (HDL) cholesterol levels by decreasing HDL apolipoprotein transport rates. *J Clin Invest* 85:144, 1990.
334. Connor SL, Artand-Wild SM, Classick-Kohn CJ, Gustafson JR, Flavell DP, Hatcher LF, Connor WE: The cholesterol/saturated fat index: An indication of the hypercholesterolemic and atherogenic potential of food. *Lancet* 1:1229, 1986.
335. Connor SL, Gustafson JR, Artand-Wild SM, Classick-Kohn CJ: The cholesterol-saturated fat index for coronary prevention: Background, use, and a comprehensive table of foods. *J Am Diet Assoc* 89:807, 1989.
336. Connor SL, Gustafson JR, Sexton G, Becker N, Artand-Wild SM, Connor WE: The Diet Habit Survey: A new method of dietary assessment that relates to plasma cholesterol changes. *J Am Diet Assoc* 92:41, 1992.
337. Hegsted DM, McGandy RB, Myers ML, Stare FJ: Quantitative effects of dietary fat on serum cholesterol in man. *Am J Clin Nutr* 17:281, 1965.
338. The Lipid Research Clinics Program: The Lipid Research Clinic's Coronary Prevention Trial Results. *JAMA* 251:365, 1984.
339. Frick MH, Elo O, Haapa K, et al: Helsinki Heart Study: Primary Prevention Trial with gemfibrozil in middle-aged men with dyslipidemia: Safety and treatment, changes in risk factors and instance of coronary heart disease. *N Engl J Med* 317:1237, 1987.

340. Kane JP, Malloy MJ, Ports TA, Philips NR, Diehl JC, Havel RJ: Regression of coronary atherosclerosis during treatment of familial hypercholesterolemia with combined drug regimens. *JAMA* 264:3007, 1990.
341. Watts GF, Lewis B, Brunt JNH, Lewis ES, Coltart DJ, Smith LDR, Mann JI, Swan AV: Effects on coronary artery disease of lipid-lowering diet or diet plus Cholestyramine in the St. Thomas' Atherosclerosis Regression Study. *Lancet* 339:563, 1992.
342. Grundy SM: HMG CoA reductase inhibitors for treatment of hypercholesterolemia. *N Engl J Med* 319:24, 1988.
343. Illingworth DR: Treatment of hyperlipidemia. *Br Med Bull* 46:1025, 1990.
344. Shepherd J, Packard CJ, Bicker S, Laurie TDV, Morgan HG: Cholestyramine promotes receptor mediated low density lipoprotein catabolism. *N Engl J Med* 302:1029, 1980.
345. Kovanen PT, Bilheimer DW, Goldstein JL, Jaramillow JJ, Brown MS: Regulatory role for hepatic low density lipoprotein receptors *in vivo* in the dog. *Proc Natl Acad Sci USA* 78:194, 1981.
346. Dujovne CA, Krehbiel P, DeCoursey S, Jackson B, Chernoff SB, Pitteman A, Garty M: Probucol with Colestipol in the treatment of hypercholesterolemia. *Ann Intern Med* 100: 477, 1984.
347. Altschul R, Hoeffer A, Stephen JD: Influence of nicotinic acid on serum cholesterol in man. *Arch Biochem Biophys* 54:558, 1955.
348. Grundy SM, Mok HYI, Zack L, Berman M: The influence of nicotinic acid on metabolism of cholesterol and triglycerides in man. *J Lipid Res* 22:24, 1981.
349. Olsson AG, Carlson LA, Anggard E, Ciabattoni G: Prostacyclin production augmented in the short term by nicotinic acid. *Lancet* 2:565, 1983.
350. Knopp RH, Ginsberg J, Albers JJ, Hoff C, Ogilvie JT, Warnick GR, Burrows E, Retzliff B, Poole M: Contrasting effects of unmodified and time released forms of niacin on lipoproteins in hyperlipidemic subjects: Clues to mechanism of action of niacin. *Metabolism* 34:642, 1985.
351. Mullin GE, Greenson JK, Mitchell MC: Fulminant hepatic failure after ingestion of sustained release nicotinic acid. *Ann Intern Med* 111:253, 1989.
352. Tobert JA: Efficacy and long-term adverse effect pattern of lovastation. *Am J Cardiol* 62:28J, 1988.
353. Tsugita Y, Kuroda M, Shimada Y: CS 514, a competitive inhibitor of 3-hydroxy-3-methylglutaryl-coenzyme reductase: Tissue selective inhibition of sterol synthesis and hypolipidemic effect in various animal species. *Biochim Biophys Acta* 877:50, 1986.
354. Alberts AW: Discovery, biochemistry and biology of lovastatin. *Am J Cardiol* 62:10J, 1988.
355. Koga T, Shimada Y, Kuroda M, Tsujita Y, Hasegawa K, Yamazaki M: Tissue selective inhibition of ch synthesis *in vivo* by pravastatin sodium: A 3-hydroxy-3-methylglutaryl-coenzyme reductase inhibitor. *Biochim Biophys Acta* 1045: 115, 1990.
356. Raasch RH: Pravastatin sodium: A new HMG CoA reductase inhibitor. *DICP* 25:388, 1991.
357. Pappu AS, Illingworth DR, Bacon S: Reduction in plasma low density lipoprotein cholesterol in urine and mevalonic acid by lovastatin in patients with heterozygous familial hypercholesterolemia. *Metabolism* 38:542, 1989.
358. Hagemenas FC, Pappu AS, Illingworth DR: The effects of simvastatin on plasma lipoproteins and cholesterol homeostasis in patients with heterozygous familial hypercholesterolemia. *Eur J Clin Invest* 20:150, 1990.
359. Ginsberg HN, Le NA, Short MP, Ramakrishnan R, Desnick RJ: Suppression of apolipoprotein B production during treatment of cholesterol ester storage disease with lovastatin: Implication for regulation of apolipoprotein synthesis. *J Clin Invest* 80:1692, 1987.
360. Bradford RH, Shear CL, Chremos AN: Expanded clinical evaluation of lovastatin (EXCEL): Study results: I. Efficacy in modifying plasma lipoproteins and adverse event profile in 8,245 patients with moderate hypercholesterolemia. *Arch Intern Med* 151:43, 1991.
361. Stalenhoef AF, Mol MGT, Stuyt PM: Efficacy and tolerability of simvastatin. *Am J Med* 87:39S, 1989.
362. Illingworth DR, Bacon S, Larson KK: Long-term experience with HMG CoA reductase inhibitors in the therapy of hypercholesterolemia. *Atherosclerosis Revs* 18:161, 1988.
363. Maher VM, Pappu AS, Illingworth DR, Thompson GR: Plasma mevalonate response in lovastatin-related myopathy. *Lancet* 2:1098, 1989.
364. Pierce LR, Wysowski DK, Gross TP: Myopathy and rhabdomyolysis associated with lovastatin/gemfibrozil combination therapy. *JAMA* 264:71, 1990.
365. Prihoda JS, Pappu AS, Smith FE, Illingworth DR: The influence of simvastatin on adrenal corticosteroid production and urine mevalonate during adrenal corticotropin stimulation in patients with heterozygous familial hypercholesterolemia. *J Clin Endocrinol Metab* 72:567, 1991.
366. Everett DW, Chando TJ, Didonato GC, Signhvi SM, Pan HY, Weinstein SH: Biotransformation of pravastatin sodium in humans. *Drug Metab Dispos* 19:740, 1991.
367. Malini PL, Ambrosioni E, Rosiello G, Trimarco B: Simvastatin *versus* pravastatin: Efficacy and tolerability in patients with primary hypercholesterolemia. *Clin Ther* 13:500, 1991.
368. McTavish D, Sorkin EM: Pravastatin: A review of its pharmacological properties and therapeutic potential in hypercholesterolemia. *Drugs* 42:65, 1991.
369. Todd PA, Goa KL: Simvastatin: A review of its pharmacological properties and therapeutic potential in hypercholesterolemia. *Drugs* 40:583, 1990.
370. Illingworth DR: Use and abuse of lovastatin. *Endocrinologist* 1:323, 1991.
371. Illingworth DR: New horizons in combination drug therapy for hypercholesterolemia. *Cardiology* 76(Suppl 1):83, 1989.
372. Witztum JR: Intensive drug therapy of hypercholesterolemia. *Am Heart J* 113:603, 1987.
373. Illingworth DR, Bacon S: Influence of lovastatin plus gemfibrozil on plasma lipids and lipoproteins in patients with heterozygous familial hypercholesterolemia. *Circulation* 79:590, 1989.
374. Nestel PJ, Billington T: Effects of probucol on low density lipoprotein removal and high density lipoprotein synthesis. *Atherosclerosis* 38:203, 1981.
375. Miettinen TA, Huttenen LK, Kusi T: Effect of probucol on the activity of post heparin plasma lipoprotein lipase and hepatic lipase. *Clin Chim Acta* 113:59, 1981.
376. Franceschini G, Sirtori M, Vaccarino V, Sirtori C: Mechanisms of LDL reduction after probucol: Changes in HDL subfractions and increased reverse cholesterol ester transfer. *Arteriosclerosis* 9:462, 1989.
377. Coronary Drug Project Research Group: Clofibrate and Niacin in Coronary Artery Disease. *JAMA* 231:360, 1975.
378. Committee of Principal Investigators: A cooperative trial in the primary prevention of eschemic heart disease using clofibrate. *Br Heart J* 40:1069, 1978.
379. Committee of Principal Investigators, WHO: A cooperative trial on primary prevention of eschemic heart disease using clofibrate to lower cholesterol: Final mortality follow-up. *Lancet* 2:600, 1984.
380. Davey Smith G, Pekkanen J: Should there be a moratorium on the use of cholesterol-lowering drugs? *Br Med J* 304:431, 1992.
381. Vega GL, Grundy SM: Gemfibrozil therapy in primary hypertriglyceridemia associated with coronary artery disease: Effects on metabolism of low density lipoproteins. *JAMA* 253:2398, 1985.
382. Samuel P: Treatment of hypercholesterolemia with neomycin: A time for reappraisal. *N Engl J Med* 301:595, 1979.
383. Hoeg JM, Maher MB, Bou E, Zeck LA, Bailey KR, Gregg RE, Sprecher EL, Susser JK, et al: Normalization of plasma lipoprotein concentrations in patients with Type II hyper-

lipoproteinemia by combined use of neomycin and niacin. *Circulation* 70:1004, 1984.

384. Bantle JP, Oppenheimer JH, Schwartz HL, Hunninghake DB, Probstielz JL, Hansom RL: TSH response to TRH in euthyroid hypercholesterolemic patients treated with graded doses of dextrothyroxin. *Metabolism* 30:63, 1981.
385. Glueck CJ: Effects of oxandrolone on plasma triglycerides and post-heparin lipolytic activity in patients with Types III, IV and V familial hyperlipoproteinemia. *Metabolism* 20:691, 1971.
386. Glueck CJ, Levy RI, Fredrickson DS: Norethindrone acetate, post-heparin lipolytic activity and plasma triglycerides in familial Type I, III, IV and V hyperlipoproteinemia: Studies in twenty-six patients and five normal patients. *Ann Intern Med* 75:343, 1971.
387. Coronary Drug Project: Findings leading to discontinuation of the 2.5 mg per day estrogen group. *JAMA* 226:652, 1973.
388. Levy RI, Fredrickson DS, Shulman R: Dietary and drug treatment of primary hyperlipoproteinemia. *Ann Intern Med* 77:267, 1972.
389. Meinertz H: Effects of gemfibrozil on plasma lipoproteins in patients with Type II hyperlipoproteinemia and familial hypercholesterolemia, in *Royal Soc Med Int Congress and Symposium Series: Further Progress with Gemfibrozil*. London, Royal Society of Medicine, 1987, vol 15.
390. Eisenberg S, Gavish D, Oschry Y, Fainaru M, Deckelbaum RJ: Abnormalities in very low, low and high density lipoproteins in hypertriglyceridemia: Reversal toward normal with bezafribrate treatment. *J Clin Invest* 74:470, 1984.
391. Illingworth DR, Olson DG, Cook SF, Wendell H, Connor WE: Ciprofibrate in the therapy of Type II hypercholesterolemia: A double-blind trial. *Atherosclerosis* 44:211, 1982.
392. Rouffy J, Chanu B, Bakir R: Comparative evaluation of the effects of Ciprofibrate and fenofibrate on lipids, lipoproteins and apoproteins A and B. *Atherosclerosis* 54:273, 1985.
393. Weisweiler P, Merck W, Janetschek P, Schwandt P: Effect of fenofibrate on serum lipoproteins in subjects with familial hypercholesterolemia and combined hyperlipidemia. *Atherosclerosis* 53:321, 1984.
394. Fattore PC, Sirtori CR: Nicotinic acid and derivatives. *Curr Opinion Lipidol* 2:43, 1991.
395. Series JJ, Caslake MJ, Kilday C, Crookshank A, Demant T, Packard CJ, Shepherd J: Influence of etofibrate on low density lipoprotein metabolism. *Atherosclerosis* 69:233, 1988.
396. Sirtori CR, Gianfranceschi G, Sirtori M, Bernini F, Descovich GC, Montaguti V, Fuccella L, Musatti M: Reduced triglyceridemia and increased high density lipoprotein cholesterol levels after treatment with acipimox, a new inhibitor of lipolysis. *Atherosclerosis* 38:267, 1981.
397. Angerbauer R, Fey P, Hubsch W, Phillips T, Schmidt D: BAY w 6228, a new generation HMG CoA reductase inhibitor: Synthesis and structure activity relationships. *Proc XIth Int Symp on Drugs Affecting Lipid Metabolism,* Florence, Italy, 69, 1992.
398. Bergstrom JD: The Zaragozic acids: Pontent natural product derived inhibitors of squalene synthesis and cholesterol synthesis. *Proc XIth Int Symp on Drugs Affecting Lipid Metabolism,* Florence, Italy, 120, 1992.
399. McCarthy AD, Fitzgerald BJ, Hutson JL, Motteram JM, Sappora M, Snowden MA, Watson NS, Williams RJ, Wright C: Squalene synthesis inhibition: Effects of a novel natural product on cholesterol metabolism. *Proc XIth Int Symp on Drugs Affecting Lipid Metabolism*, Florence, Italy, 120, 1992.
400. Suckling KE: Drugs working on the intestine. *Curr Opinion Lipidol* 2:31, 1991.
401. Harris WS, Dujovne CA, vonBergman K, Neal J, Akester J, Windsor SL, Greene D, Look Z: Effects of the ACAT inhibitor CL277082 on cholesterol metabolism in humans. *Clin Pharmacol Ther* 48:189, 1990.
402. Koivisto P, Miettinen TA: Long-term effects of ileal bypass on lipoproteins in patients with familial hypercholesterolemia. *Circulation* 70:290, 1984.
403. Madras PN: Portacaval shunt for familial heterozygous hypercholesterolemia. *Surg Gynecol Obstet* 152:187, 1981.
404. Forman MB, Baker SG, Many CJ: Treatment of homozygous familial hypercholesterolemia with portacaval shunt. *Atherosclerosis* 41:349, 1982.
405. Lerner DJ, Kannel WB: Patterns of coronary heart disease morbidity and mortality in the sexes: A 26-year follow-up of the Framingham population. *Am Heart J* 111:383, 1986.
406. Erikson M, Bergman L, Rudling M, Henriksson T, Angelin B: Effect of estrogen on low density lipoprotein metabolism in males: Short-term and long-term studies during hormonal treatment of prostatic carcinoma. *J Clin Invest* 84:802, 1989.
407. Crouse JR III: Gender lipoproteins, diet and cardiovascular risk: Sauce for the goose may not be sauce for the gander. *Lancet* 1:318, 1989.
408. Castelli WP: Cardiovascular disease in women. *Am J Obstet Gynecol* 158:1553, 1988.
409. Castelli WP: The triglycerides issue: A view from Framingham. *Am Heart J* 112:432, 1986.
410. Bush TL, Fried LP, Barrett-Connor E: Cholesterol, lipoproteins and coronary heart disease in women. *Clin Chem* 34:B60, 1988.
411. Denke MA, Grundy SM: Hypercholesterolemia in elderly persons: Resolving the treatment dilema. *Ann Intern Med* 112:780, 1990.
412. Bilheimer DW: Clinical considerations regarding treatment of hypercholesterolemia in the elderly. *Atherosclerosis* 91:S35, 1991.
413. Wysowski DK, Kennedy DL, Gross TT: Prescribed use of cholesterol-lowering drugs in the United States, 1978–1988. *JAMA* 263:2185, 1990.
414. West RJ, Lloyd JK, Leonard JV: Long-term follow-up of children with familial hypercholesterolemia treated with Cholestyramine. *Lancet* 2:873, 1980.
415. Bachorik PS, Wood PDS: Laboratory considerations in diagnosis and management of hyperlipidemia, in Rifkind BM, Levy RI (eds): *Hyperlipidemia: Diagnosis and Therapy*. New York, Grune & Stratton, 1977, p 41.
416. Lipid Research Clinics Program: *Manual of Laboratory Operations:* vol 1: *Lipid and Lipoprotein Analysis*. Bethesda, Md., NIH, DHEW Publication (NIH) 75-628, 1974.
417. Brown MS, Kovanen PT, Goldstein JL, Eeckles R, Vandenberg K, Vandenberg H, Fryns JP, Cassiman JJ: Prenatal diagnosis of homozygous familial hypercholesterolemia. *Lancet* 1:526, 1978.
418. Grundy SM, Vega GL: Causes of high blood cholesterol. *Circulation* 81:412, 1990.
419. Russell DW, Esser V, Hobbs HH: Molecular basis of familial hypercholesterolemia. *Arteriosclerosis* 9:8, 1989.

P A R T VII

Calcium and Bone Metabolism

CHAPTER 23

Mineral Metabolism

Gordon J. Strewler

Michael Rosenblatt

CELLULAR AND EXTRACELLULAR CALCIUM METABOLISM

The divalent calcium cation (Ca^{2+}; ionized calcium) serves an important role in the physiology and metabolism of virtually all living things from unicellular organisms to mammals. Extracellular levels of calcium in humans and other mammals are tightly regulated within a narrow physiologic range to assure appropriate excitation-contraction of the heart, expression of bioactivity for a number of hormones, and normal functioning of muscles, nerves, platelets, neutrophils, and several coagulation factors. The central physiologic role of calcium derives mechanistically from its actions as a cofactor for certain enzymes and as an electrochemical agent involved in membrane activation, permeability, or stabilization and from its ability to serve as an intracellular second messenger. Calcium also plays a role in cell growth and division and in cellular secretion for exocrine function, endocrine function, and neurotransmitter release, when the ion bonds to the membrane of preformed secretory vesicles and promotes fusion with the plasma membrane or stimulates the intracellular microtubule/microfilament system.

Within the cell, calcium concentrations are integrated as a result of a number of complex and interacting component calcium fluxes created by the activity of several plasma membrane "pumps" or "exchangers" (Fig. 23-1).

Furthermore, the activity of these transmembrane macromolecules which transport calcium can be modulated by extracellular calcium levels, membrane electric activity or potential gradient, physical distension ("stretch"), or hormonal activity.

When cells are bathed in extracellular fluid (ECF) containing calcium ion at a concentration of 10^{-3} *M*, the concentration of calcium ions in cytosol is 10^{-6} *M*.[1] Most (90 to 99 percent) of the intracellular calcium is stored within mitochondria or in microsomes, where it is largely complexed to phosphate. From these locales, it leaks into the cytosol. The low intracellular calcium level is preserved by calcium pumps (analogous to those present on the plasma membrane) which return calcium to the intramitochondrial or intramicrosomal space in an energy-dependent fashion or transport calcium out of the cell (Fig. 23-1). However, the levels of intracellular calcium can be self-modulating. Because calcium can serve as an intracellular signal, or "second messenger,"[1] calcium is directly linked to calmodulin function and the inositol polyphosphate–protein kinase C pathway. In many cases, several second messengers interact to produce an integrated intracellular calcium response (see Chap. 5).

It is the ionized or "free" calcium which is metabolically active and critical for normal physiologic function; hence, it is the form of calcium that is regulated. In the ECF, calcium is present in a free form, which accounts for 50 percent of ECF calcium, while 40 percent is bound reversibly to proteins and 10 percent is complexed with citrate and phosphate.[2,3] About 90 percent of the protein-bound calcium is associated with albumin, bound to its carboxyl groups in a pH-dependent manner. Since the amount of calcium present in the blood and ECF represents 1 percent of the total calcium in the body,[4–6] only 0.5 percent of total body calcium is ionized and plays the critical role in physiologic functions described above (Fig. 23-2). The picture is complicated by the fact that calcium normally circulates at a concentration approaching its saturation point—the solubility product constant for calcium phosphate [$K_{sp} = (Ca^{2+})(PO_4^{-})$]—and this accounts for some of the major clinical problems encountered in patients with hypercalcemia, such as soft tissue calcification and kidney stones.

The maintenance of blood calcium levels within the narrow range dictated by normal physiology requires the action of at least two hormones acting on three organs. Parathyroid hormone (PTH, a polypep-

The authors have taken or modified for this chapter portions of the corresponding section of the second edition of this textbook written by Andrew F. Stewart and Arthur E. Broadus. We gratefully acknowledge this contribution to our chapter.

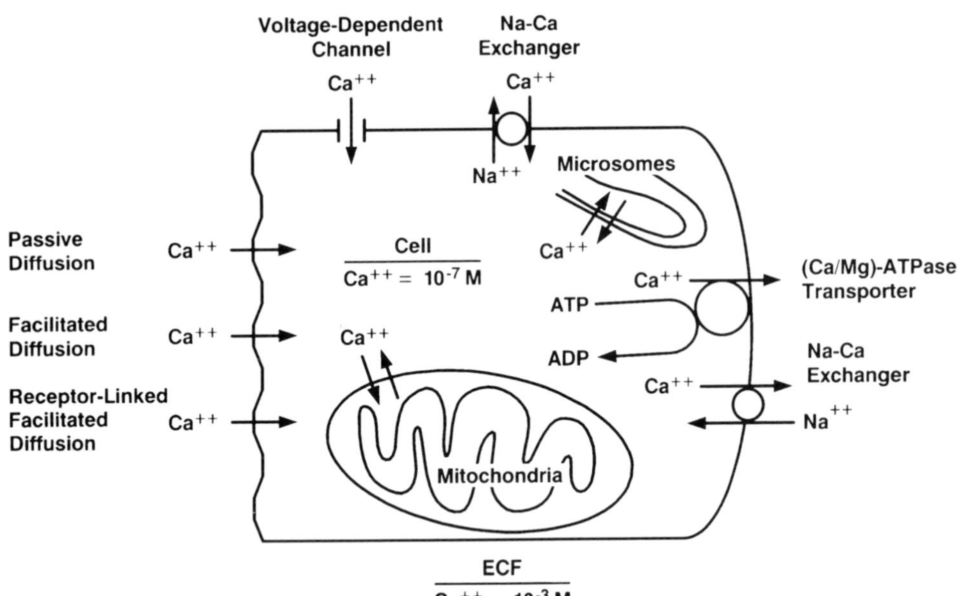

FIGURE 23-1 Schematic representation of calcium flux across the plasma membrane of cells and between the cytoplasm and organelles.

tide hormone) and vitamin D (a steroid hormone) act on bone, kidney, and gut to assure calcium homeostasis and close regulation of extracellular calcium levels. In humans and other mammals, this hormonal system is designed to defend the organism against the major metabolic threat of hypocalcemia. In fish, calcitonin acts to lower blood calcium levels and protects against hypercalcemia. Therefore, it follows logically that this regulatory system did not appear in evolution until the time when animals left the calcium-rich sea.

FIGURE 23-2 Illustration of relative amounts of calcium within the total body calcium pool.

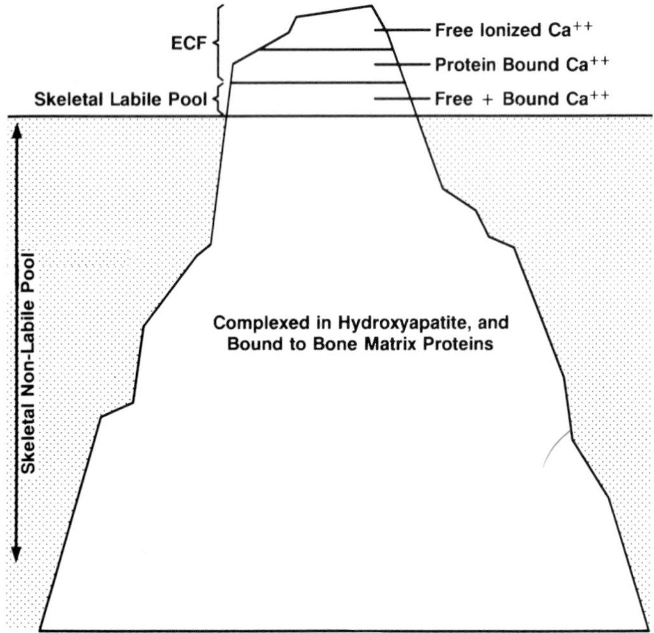

Although the absolute quantity of ionized calcium that is tightly regulated is small, calcium flux at various organs over time is extremely large in comparison (Fig. 23-3). The kidney filters 5 to 7 g of calcium per day, a quantity in large excess over the total amount present at any time in the circulation and ECF. Although the kidney reabsorbs 96 to 98 percent of the calcium it filters, it cannot recover 100 percent of this calcium even when it is maximally stimulated. In addition, there is an obligatory loss of calcium from sweat and from the gut as a result of gastrointestinal secretions and the sloughing of lining cells of the gastrointestinal tract into its lumen.

Bone, which contains 99 percent of the calcium present in the body, not only plays a structural role for the organism but also acts as an internal reservoir for calcium. Calcium stored in the skeleton can be used as a defense against hypocalcemia if the dietary intake of calcium is deficient for a short period or chronically. A substantial amount of calcium can be rapidly mobilized from bone. In fact, quantities of calcium comparable to the total amount present in the ECF can be released within hours. The reservoir is also large enough to sustain normal physiologic function without the development of hypocalcemia for months to years.

Hormonal regulation of calcium by PTH and vitamin D plays two roles: tight regulation of calcium levels in the ECF and maintenance of long-term calcium balance. PTH is responsible for the minute-to-minute regulation of ECF calcium levels. It acts on

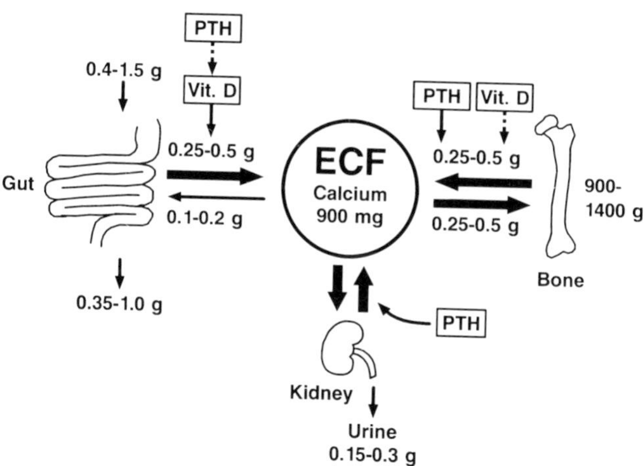

FIGURE 23-3 Schematic representation of calcium flux and balance in a normal human. Arrows indicate direction of movement of calcium between the gut, bone, kidneys, and extracellular fluid (ECF). Modulation of flux by vitamin D (Vit. D) or parathyroid hormone (PTH) is shown. Solid arrows depict a direct effect; dashed arrows depict an indirect effect. The numeric values indicate quantities of elemental calcium stored or transferred in a 24-h period. Thickness of arrows indicates relative magnitude of flux.

the kidney to stimulate calcium reabsorption and on bone to stimulate bone resorption and the release of calcium stores into the ECF. However, reliance of the organism on PTH alone for the maintenance of normocalcemia without adequate calcium intake can lead in the long term only to negative calcium balance (particularly from bone) because of the obligatory calcium losses. This loss of bone mineral ultimately compromises the biomechanical strength of bone.

Therefore, the struggle for calcium homeostasis ultimately is won or lost at the level of the gut, which is the point of entry for calcium to replace the obligatory losses described above. The principal hormone responsible for enhancing the absorption of dietary calcium is vitamin D.[7–9] Its effects on the absorption of dietary calcium from the gut are discussed in the Vitamin D section. Vitamin D levels are determined in part by the circulating levels of PTH, which act on an enzyme in the kidney, 1α-hydroxylase, to convert 25-hydroxyvitamin D_3 into the active form of the hormone, 1α,25-$(OH)D_3$. The average American diet contains 0.4 to 1.5 g of calcium per day (1 quart of milk contains approximately 1 g of calcium). However, the dietary intake of many individuals, particularly the elderly, falls well below this amount (Fig. 23-3). In some countries, such as Japan, the majority of elderly people have diets frankly deficient in calcium. Under these circumstances, even maximally stimulated and efficient calcium absorption cannot offset the cumulative obligatory losses.

PARATHYROID HORMONE

Anatomy and Embryology of the Parathyroid Glands

Anatomy

The four parathyroid glands weigh an average of 40 mg each. Although they are usually found in two symmetric pairs in proximity to the thyroid, their adult location is variable. The two superior glands are usually found near the posterior aspect of the thyroid capsule; the inferior glands are most often located near the inferior thyroid margin. The position of the inferior glands is more variable than that of the superior glands, and they are sometimes found within or near the thymus in the anterior superior mediastinum. Interthyroidal and retroesophageal glands also occur. Five percent of the population has only three parathyroid glands. A supernumerary fifth gland is found in 12 to 15 percent of individuals, and six or more parathyroids are occasionally present. The vagaries of parathyroid number and position are important features of their surgical anatomy.[10]

The parathyroids are composed of epithelial cells and stromal fat. The predominant epithelial element is the chief cell, with clear cytoplasm and a slightly hyperchromatic nucleus. The other epithelial component is the oxyphil cell, which is slightly larger than the chief cell, with eosinophilic granular cytoplasm and a small, extremely hyperchromatic nucleus. Both cell types contain PTH, and it is not known whether they have separate secretory regulation.

Embryology

The two pairs of parathyroid glands arise from the dorsal endoderm of the branchial pouches at the end of the sixth week of gestation. The superior parathyroid glands (parathyroids 4) are derived from the fourth, and the inferior glands (parathyroids 3) from the third branchial pouch. The parathyroids 4 migrate a short distance caudad to assume their superior position; the inferior glands migrate farther caudad with the thymus, ordinarily separating from the thymus at the inferior thyroid margin. If they do not separate, they may be found in association with the thymus or its fat pad in the upper anterior mediastinum.

Biosynthesis, Processing, and Secretion of Parathyroid Hormone

Physiology of Parathyroid Hormone Secretion

Consistent with the function of PTH as an acute regulator of extracellular calcium homeostasis, the secretion of the hormone is under negative feedback regulation by the concentration of ionized calcium in the extracellular fluid. The dynamics of PTH secretion in normal humans are shown in Fig. 23-4.[11] To maintain the serum concentration of calcium within the very narrow normal range, the secretion of PTH must be exquisitely sensitive to the calcium concentration. Thus, the relation of serum ionized calcium to serum PTH levels (Fig. 23-4) is steeply sigmoidal. The steep portion of the curve corresponds precisely to the normal range of ionized calcium, so that the level of PTH is maximal at the lower limit and minimal at the upper limit of the normal range—precisely the desirable relation to maximize the sensitivity of these glands to small changes in ionized calcium and assure maintenance of the normal calcium level by PTH. Small changes in ionized calcium produce large changes in PTH secretion; that is, the system displays "high gain." The macromolecular calcium "sensor" responsible for detecting extracellular levels of calcium and transmitting an intracellular signal to parathyroid cells has recently been cloned.[31] It is a G-protein-coupled seven transmembrane spanning receptor. Its role in the physiology and pathophysiology of PTH secretion is discussed later.

Note that the PTH level is still detectable in the face of markedly elevated ionized calcium concentrations. The nonsuppressible secretion, or "leak," of PTH from suppressed glands may play a role in the development of primary hyperparathyroidism and in secondary hyperparathyroidism in chronic renal failure and after renal transplantation. The regulation of PTH secretion by calcium has also been studied in vitro, using dispersed human parathyroid cells, and similar results have been obtained.[12] As will be discussed below in detail, other factors also influence the secretion of PTH. However, the only physiologically significant regulator of minute-to-minute changes in PTH secretion is the ionized calcium concentration.

FIGURE 23-4 The relation between the serum ionized calcium level and the simultaneous serum concentration of intact PTH in normal humans. The serum calcium concentration was altered by the infusion of calcium (closed circles) or citrate (closed triangles). Parathyroid sensitivity to changes in serum calcium is maximal within the normal range (the shaded area). Low concentrations of PTH persist in the face of hypercalcemia. *(Modified from Conlin PR, Fajtova VT, Mortensen RM, Brown EM,[11] by permission of Journal of Clinical Endocrinology and Metabolism.)*

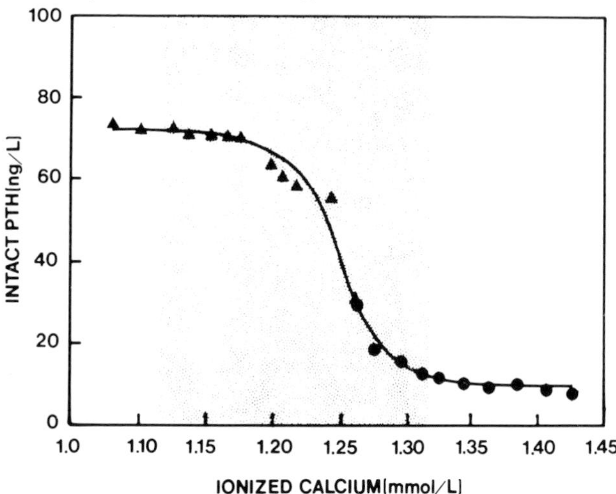

Like many other hormones, PTH is secreted episodically, and PTH levels in blood display both a circadian rhythm, with a peak at midnight, and episodic pulses with a mean interpulse interval of 60 min.[13] The episodic nature of PTH secretion is preserved in primary hyperparathyroidism.

Chemistry, Biosynthesis, and Processing of Parathyroid Hormone

Parathyroid hormone is an 84-amino acid linear peptide with a molecular weight of 9300 (Fig. 23-5). Its sequence is strongly conserved among mammalian species. Structure-function relations for PTH will be discussed extensively in a later section. However, it is noteworthy that all the recognized biological actions of the intact hormone are encoded by the amino-terminal amino acids 1-34.

The human PTH gene is located on the short arm of chromosome 11. It contains three exons: The first encodes a short 5′ untranslated domain, the second a prepro region consisting of a 29-amino acid precursor sequence, and the third the last two amino acids of pro-PTH, the mature 84-amino acid peptide, and the 3′ untranslated domain.[14] After nuclear processing of primary transcripts to remove introns, PTH mRNA is transported into the cytoplasm, where the coding sequence is translated by the ribosomal machinery into the 115-amino acid precursor prepro-PTH.[15] Nascent peptide chains emerging from the ribosome are guided through the membrane of the rough endoplasmic reticulum by a signal recognition particle that recognizes the "signal" sequence in the prepro region of the hormone precursor and guides it to a docking protein on the outer surface of the endoplasmic reticulum (see Chap. 4). As the signal peptide sequence emerges into the lumen of the endoplasmic reticulum, it is cleaved at position -6/-7, leaving the 90-amino acid pro-PTH (Fig. 23-6). The process of binding of nascent chains by the signal recognition particle, docking, insertion, and cleavage of the prepro sequence occurs cotranslationally and so rapidly that nascent chains containing the prepro sequence of PTH are barely detectable unless translation is carried out in vitro in the absence of endoplasmic reticulum.[15,16]

The sequence of prepro-PTH has many of the general features of signal sequences that direct secretory proteins into the lumen of the endoplasmic reticulum[17]: at least one positively charged residue near the amino terminus, an uninterrupted segment of hydrophobic or neutral amino acids, and small

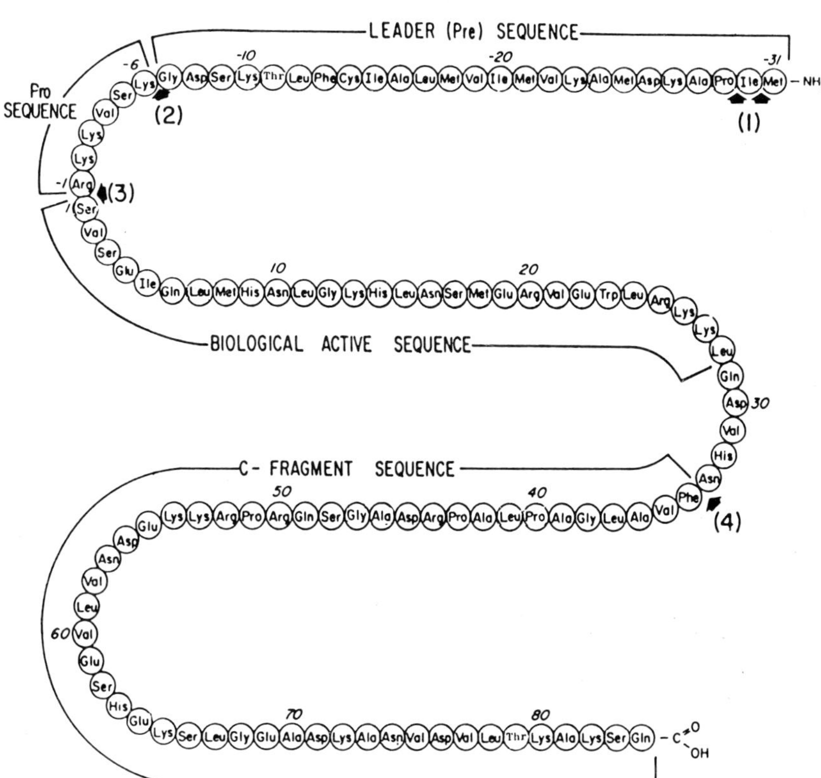

FIGURE 23-5 Primary structure of human preparathyroid hormone. The arrows indicate sites of specific cleavages which occur in the sequence of biosynthesis and peripheral metabolism of the hormone. The biologically active sequence is enclosed in the center of the molecule.

amino acids just proximal to and two residues removed from the cleavage site (i.e., positions -7 and -9). A synthetic fragment of the prepro sequence from PTH can block the processing of PTH and also that of bovine pregrowth hormone and other hormone precursors,[18] illustrating the relative interchangeability of signal sequences and suggesting that many, if not all, secreted proteins utilize the same processing apparatus for intracellular transport. The sequence features of prepro-PTH required for efficient processing have been studied by expressing mutants of the prepro region in cell-free systems or in intact cells. Deletion of the first six amino acids results in translation initiation at met^{-25}, but the truncated peptide is processed normally. In contrast, the deletion of 10 or more residues, including portions of the hydrophobic core, results in peptides that do not enter the secretory pathway and are degraded rapidly.[19,20] Thus, the first six residues of prepro-PTH are relatively dispensable, the hydrophobic core is required for entry into the endoplasmic reticulum, and cleavage of the signal sequence is required for secretion. Along these lines, the signal peptidase—the enzyme that cleaves the signal region from the nascent protein—has an unusually large recognition sequence, requiring 11 amino acids of the PTH signal sequence for recognition as substrate. Another unusual feature of the enzyme is that conformation (secondary structure) appears more critical for recognition than does the primary amino acid sequence per se. A spontaneous mutation that disrupts the hydrophobic core of the signal sequence and blocks translocation is associated with familial hypoparathyroidism,[21] as discussed below.

In contrast to the evanescent existence of prepro-PTH, pro-PTH has a life span of about 15 min in pulse-chase studies and is converted to mature PTH coincidentally with arrival in the Golgi apparatus.[15,22] The Golgi cleavage enzyme presumably recognizes the dibasic sequence lys^{-2}-arg^{-1}; similar dibasic sequences are present at the cleavage sites of other prohormones, e.g., insulin. However, the processing of pro-PTH is more efficient than insulin processing, since pro-PTH, unlike proinsulin, is not secreted.[23] The functional significance of the two-step cleavage of prepro-PTH is not fully understood, but mutational analysis suggests that the hexapeptide pro-PTH sequence is necessary for the correct transport and cleavage of prepro-PTH. Mutants in which the hydrophobic core is intact but the pro sequence is deleted are translocated and cleaved inefficiently. In such mutants, both the correct cleavage site and an incorrect one in the signal sequence are utilized[24]; only the cleaved forms are secreted. Since a normal amino terminus of mature PTH is critical for its biological activity, the pro sequence may have evolved as an "adaptor," first assuring correct cleavage of prepro-PTH and then being cleaved off itself.

After its biogenesis in the Golgi apparatus, mature PTH is packaged in dense secretory granules

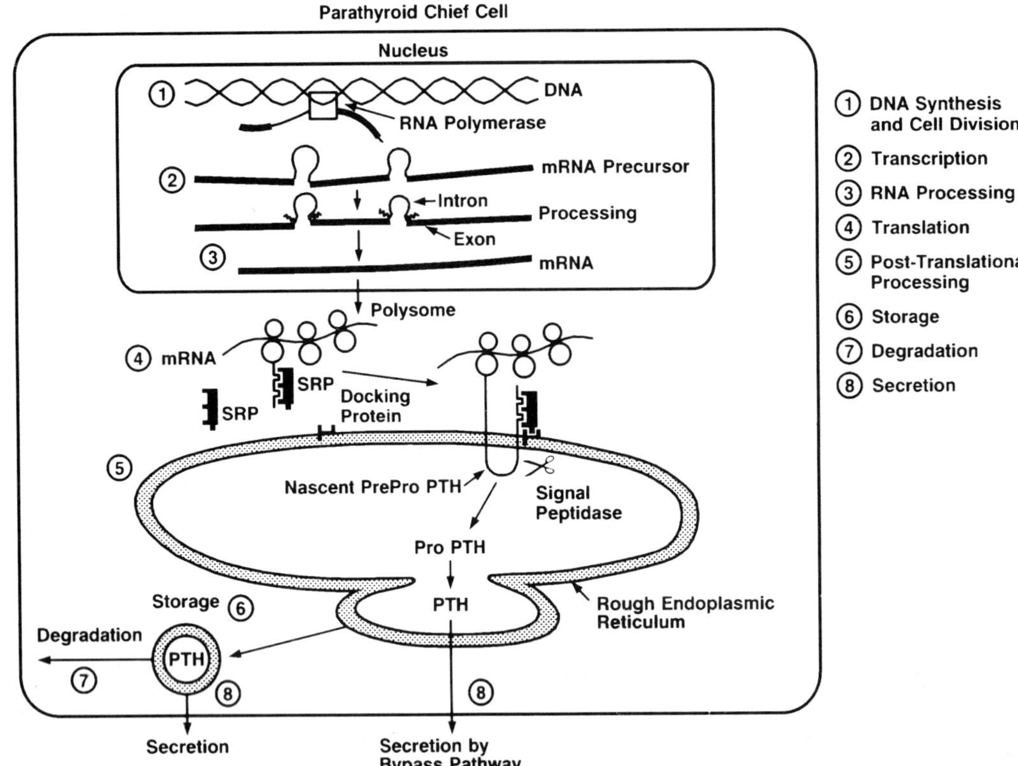

FIGURE 23-6 Schematic representation of major points at which the level of PTH biosynthesis and secretion appears to be regulated. Each point represents a potential site of dysfunction in hyperparathyroid disorders. *(Reprinted with permission from Lynn H. Caporale and Michael Rosenblatt, Parathyroid hormone secretion: Molecular events and regulation, Contributions to Nephrology 50:73–95, 1986.)*

like those of other endocrine cells and stored to await secretion. It has been estimated that glandular stores of PTH are sufficient to maintain maximal rates of secretion for about 1.5 h.[16] PTH is stored and cosecreted with the peptide chromogranin A (parathyroid secretory protein-1).[25] The significance of the presence of chromogranin A as a passenger in secretory granules of parathyroid and other endocrine cells is unknown. It appears that 10 to 20 percent of PTH is postranslationally modified by phosphorylation on serine residues near the amino terminus before secretion[26]; this is also of unknown significance.

Regulation of PTH Synthesis

Acutely, extracellular calcium regulates the secretion of preformed PTH rather than the synthesis of PTH. However, over a period of hours to days, increases in extracellular calcium inhibit the transcription of the PTH gene.[27] The converse is also true: Hypocalcemia also increases the transcription of the PTH gene.[28] The increase in the synthesis of PTH is appropriate in the face of relatively small glandular stores of the hormone, serving to maintain high secretory rates during sustained hypocalcemia.

The synthesis of PTH is also regulated by vitamin D. High levels of 1α,25-dihydroxyvitamin D inhibit transcription of the PTH gene,[29] providing yet another short loop of negative feedback in the remarkably complex interrelations of PTH and vitamin D in the control of calcium homeostasis. This effect occurs within 2 h and involves a vitamin D response element within the first 690 base pairs upstream of the cap site of the PTH gene.[30] The inhibition of PTH gene expression by 1α,25-dihydroxyvitamin D has been observed both in dispersed parathyroid cells in vitro and with the administration of vitamin D analogues in vivo under conditions where the serum calcium does not perceptibly change.[29] Whether or not vitamin D plays a physiologic role in the minute-to-minute regulation of PTH secretion, the effect of 1α,25-dihydroxyvitamin D is relevant therapeutically in the treatment of secondary hyperparathyroidism in chronic renal failure (see Chap. 24).

Cellular Regulation of PTH Secretion by Calcium

The parathyroid cell is unique in its ability to sense and respond to changes in the ambient calcium concentration. For PTH to be secreted in response to hypocalcemia, it must function differently from other secretory cells, which require calcium for stimulus-secretion coupling and are paralyzed by exposure to low calcium concentrations. The regulation of PTH secretion by extracellular calcium has been studied in collagenase-dispersed parathyroid cells from bovine and human glands.[12,31] Like other mammalian cells, the parathyroid cell maintains a large $[Ca^{2+}]$ gradient between the extracellular fluid (free $[Ca^{2+}]$ about 10^{-3} M) and its cytosol (free $[Ca^{2+}]$ about 10^{-7} M). Unlike most other cells, in which the cytosolic calcium concentration is well buffered against changes in extracellular calcium, the parathyroid cell responds to acute increases in extracellular calcium with a transient rise in cytoplasmic free calcium[12,32]; this transient rise is followed by a sustained plateau. Most of the calcium entering the cytosolic compartment in response to increased extracellular calcium appears to originate from intracellular stores. However, the sustained increase in intracellular calcium that follows is dependent on the presence of extracellular calcium. Experiments using the calcium ionophore ionomycin suggest that the regulation of cytoplasmic free calcium is important in the regulation of PTH secretion by extracellular calcium. Intracellular calcium transients induced by ionomycin treatment are associated with inhibition of PTH secretion.[32] It is possible that other potential cellular second messengers (cAMP, protein kinase C) also play a role in the inhibition of PTH secretion by calcium.[12,31,33]

One of the most exciting discoveries in the field of calcium metabolism has been the discovery of an extracellular calcium-sensing receptor on the surface of parathyroid cells.[31] The receptor contains seven transmembrane-spanning domains and belongs to the superfamily of G-protein-coupled receptors (Fig. 23-77, see Addendum). It has a molecular mass of approximately 120 kDa and shares limited homology with metabotropic glutamate receptors. It possesses a large extracellular domain containing clusters of acid amino acids that may be involved in calcium-binding. The receptor appears to be present in kidney, thyroid, brain, as well as parathyroid gland cells. It has a relatively low (millimolar) affinity for calcium, consistent with its role in regulating PTH secretion. It is coupled to the phosphoinositide and cytosolic calcium signal transduction system, presumably through the G-protein, Gq (see Chap. 5 for general description). An acute increase in extracellular calcium stimulates increased synthesis of the intracellular second messenger 1,4,5-inositol trisphosphate (1,4,5-IP_3) and other phosphoinositides.[33,34] In other cells, phospholipase C, the enzyme that generates 1,4,5-IP_3, is coupled to hormone receptors by a guanine nucleotide regulatory or G protein. It has been suggested that the parathyroid calcium sensor may also be G protein–coupled.[31] Besides 1,4,5-IP_3, the action of phospholipase C generates another cellular second messenger, diacylglycerol, which activates protein kinase C. Activation of protein kinase C potentially entrains an additional set of cellular responses to the signal of increased extracellular calcium. In the simplest model, active protein kinase C would cooperate with the intracellular calcium transient to inhibit the secretion of PTH. However, agents that activate protein kinase C tend to reduce the inhibitory effect of high extracellular calcium concentrations on the secretion of PTH.[35] The role of protein kinase C in the regulation of PTH release is obscure.

Other Parathyroid Hormone Secretagogues

Magnesium

Like its sister divalent cation, magnesium inhibits the secretion of PTH at high concentrations and stimulates it at low concentrations.[36] On a molar basis, magnesium is severalfold less potent than calcium as a modulator of PTH secretion, making it unlikely that changes in the physiologic range have an important influence on the gland. However, the high serum magnesium concentrations attained during treatment of premature labor have been shown to inhibit PTH secretion and occasionally to produce hypocalcemia.[37] In contrast to the stimulatory effects of mild hypomagnesemia, profound chronic magnesium deficiency, as seen with chronic gastrointestinal or renal magnesium wasting, can produce a state of functional hypoparathyroidism. This is discussed further in Hypoparathyroidism. However, from the perspective of control of PTH secretion, it is likely that in the parathyroid gland magnesium is required for the release of parathyroid hormone from secretory granules, fulfilling the essential role in stimulus-secretion coupling that calcium subserves in most other secretory tissues, and that depletion of glandular stores of magnesium interferes with the secretory mechanism.

Catecholamines

Acting through beta-adrenergic receptors, catecholamines acutely stimulate the secretion of PTH from parathyroid cells in vitro. This effect is mediated by cAMP. Stimulation of alpha-adrenergic receptors inhibits cAMP accumulation and PTH release. Although early studies showed a small effect of the beta-adrenergic antagonist propranolol in reducing basal levels of PTH,[38] evidence for a tonic role of catecholamines in the parathyroid gland is rather sparse.[39] Hypercalcemia is rarely seen in the state of catecholamine excess produced by a pheochromocytoma, but this phenomenon is probably caused by secretion of the homologous peptide parathyroid hormone–related protein (PTHrP) by some pheochromocytomas (discussed in Malignancy-Associated Hypercalcemia).

Other Secretagogues

Acute administration of phosphate is a powerful stimulus to the secretion of PTH, but this effect is indirect and is entirely attributable to the fall in ionized calcium produced by a phosphate bolus. Exposure of parathyroid cells in vitro to lithium induces a shift to the right in the set point for the secretion of PTH, i.e., decreased sensitivity to suppression by extracellular calcium.[40] The administration of lithium in therapy for bipolar affective disorders is associated with increased PTH secretion and sometimes with hypercalcemia (see Hypercalcemia). Ingestion of alcohol acutely inhibits the secretion of PTH.[41]

Metabolism of Parathyroid Hormone

Heterogeneity of Circulating PTH

In Berson and Yalow's pioneering studies, it was recognized that circulating PTH differs immunochemically from glandular PTH, and it soon became clear that PTH circulates in several distinct forms.[42] These forms have different tissue origins, plasma half-lives, and metabolic fates and are affected differentially by disease states such as chronic renal failure. An understanding of the heterogeneous forms of circulating PTH has been crucial to the interpretation of clinical assay data using region-specific assays, and considerable effort has been expended in this quest.

It is now clear that there are two major forms of circulating PTH. One is the intact, biologically active hormone PTH(1-84); the other is a family of closely related fragments that constitute the midportion and carboxyl terminus of PTH and are biologically inactive in calcium homeostasis, since they do not contain the biologically active 1-34 domain. These will be referred to as carboxyl-terminal fragments.

Clearance of PTH from Plasma

The clearance of intact PTH(1-84) from plasma is very rapid, with a half-life of 2 to 3 min. The principal sites of clearance are the liver and kidney, with the liver accounting for up to two-thirds of the total[43,44] (Fig. 23-7). The major route of clearance is into a degradative pathway. In the liver, this pathway is located primarily in the Kupffer's cells.[45] In the kidney, degradation of PTH(1-84) takes place mainly in tubule cells after uptake either directly from the peritubular circulation or from the tubule lumen after filtration of PTH(1-84) at the glomerulus.[43,44,46]

PTH is also taken up by its target tissues, including osteoblasts in bone, renal tubule cells, and hepatocytes.[15] This is a receptor-mediated process that has a low capacity (probably less than 1 percent of the overall clearance rate) and a high affinity for PTH, in contrast to the high-capacity, nonsaturable uptake of PTH(1-84) by bulk degradative sites in the liver and kidney.[47] Although evidence from experiments in vivo has been interpreted as indicating that PTH(1-34) is preferentially taken up by bone and is more active than PTH(1-84) on adenylyl cyclase in bone,[48] these results are difficult to reconcile with the equivalent binding of the two species to bone cell receptors both in vivo and in vitro. At present, the weight of evidence does not support the view that PTH(1-84) is a prohormone with respect to bone.

Origins of Circulating Fragments of PTH

In vivo, both of the main circulating forms of PTH are probably secreted directly from the gland. Secretion of carboxyl-terminal fragments of PTH is detectable in careful gel filtration studies of parathyroid venous effluent sera.[49] However, parathyroid venous effluents do not appear to contain fragments that possess the amino-terminal domain of PTH or are bioactive. The principal enzyme thought to be responsible for the intraglandular cleavage of PTH is the lysosomal proteinase cathepsin B, which cleaves PTH between residues 36 and 37.[50] Intraglandular degradation of PTH appears to be calcium-dependent[51] and could be a mechanism for diminishing glandular stores of PTH under conditions of chronic suppression of the glands. Pro-PTH, the storage form of PTH, does not appear to be secreted.

At its principal sites of uptake, the liver and kidney, PTH(1-84) is cleaved at the 33-34 and 36-37 positions to produce fragments identical to the major circulating forms.[44,45] The enzymes involved appear to be catheptic proteinases. The primary site of production of circulating fragments is the Kupffer's cell of the liver, and hepatectomy but not nephrectomy eliminates the predominant carboxyl-terminal fragments from the circulation.[44] Cleavage at these sites will also give rise to biologically active amino-terminal fragments. However, release of biologically active fragments has not been detected,[20] although low levels of amino-terminal fragments are present in the liver and kidney. In most circumstances, the only

FIGURE 23-7 Secretion and metabolism of intact PTH and carboxyl-terminal fragments. Secretion is indicated by solid arrows, and major directions of metabolism by open arrows.

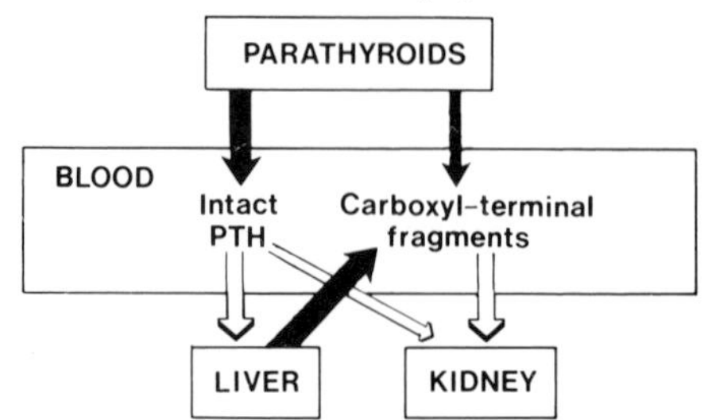

biologically active form of PTH in the circulation is PTH(1-84). Using a highly sensitive cytochemical bioassay for PTH, a smaller fragment was detected in the sera of patients with chronic renal failure.[52] However, in view of the results from a number of other types of experiments, the biological significance of this finding is uncertain.

Carboxyl-terminal fragments of PTH are cleared in the kidney (Fig. 23-7). While intact PTH is cleared by a combination of peritubular uptake from blood and glomerular filtration, carboxyl-terminal fragments are cleared mainly by glomerular filtration.[46] Hormone that is filtered at the glomerulus is efficiently reabsorbed along the nephron, and very little reaches the final urine. The half-life of circulating carboxyl-terminal fragments is much longer than the half-life of intact PTH. Their clearance half-time has been estimated at 20 to 30 min with normal renal function and is greatly prolonged in the presence of renal failure, reflective of the importance of glomerular filtration in this process. Clinically, the accumulation of carboxyl-terminal fragments has complicated the use of PTH radioimmunoassays that are specific for the midregion and carboxyl terminus to quantitate the degree of secondary hyperparathyroidism present in patients with renal insufficiency. Although true secondary hyperparathyroidism is present in most such patients, its effect on circulating levels of PTH is greatly magnified by the reduced clearance of carboxyl-terminal fragments.

Assay of Parathyroid Hormone

Historically, the interpretation of assays for PTH has been complicated greatly by the immunoheterogeneity of the circulating hormone. A variety of different radioimmunoassays have been developed, mostly using antisera to the intact hormone. With the availability of synthetic and natural fragments of the hormone, it became clear that one major class of radioimmunoassays for PTH was directed toward amino-terminal determinants, and another toward determinants in the carboxyl-terminal domain, often to a "midregion" consisting of amino acids 43-68. The predominant species of PTH recognized by "midregion" assays are carboxyl-terminal fragments, which, by virtue of their long half-life, are the major circulating forms of PTH. Surprisingly, antisera to the biologically inactive midregion provided assays that were both sensitive and highly reliable in the diagnosis of primary hyperparathyroidism.[53] For the past 20 years, such assays have been in wide use.

Despite their utility in the diagnosis of hyperparathyroidism, to varying degrees all first- and second-generation radioimmunoassays for PTH shared certain problems. None were sensitive or specific enough to detect the suppression of PTH consistently, for example, in patients with nonparathyroid hypercalcemia. Quantitative comparison of results from different assays was rendered nearly impossible by the immunoheterogeneity of circulating PTH, coupled with limited information about the relevant epitopes for different polyclonal antisera and by the use of different standard PTH preparations in different laboratories. None of the assays clearly measured biologically active hormone, and the potential for excess accumulation of biologically inactive fragments in renal failure complicated the interpretation of assay results in that setting.

The development of two-site assays for PTH in the mid-1980s was a great step forward. Several different assays have been developed and are available commercially.[54,55] They have in common the use of two antibodies, one directed toward an amino-terminal determinant and the other directed toward a carboxyl-terminal determinant. One is immobilized and used as a capture antibody; the other is labeled and used for the detection of bound hormone. The antibody used for detection is labeled either with radioactive iodine (immunoradiometric assays, IRMA) or with a luminescent tag (immunochemiluminescent assays) (Fig. 23-8). Since the only major circulating form of PTH that possesses both amino- and carboxyl-terminal determinants is PTH(1-84), such assays should theoretically be specific for the intact hormone.

The normal range for immunoreactive PTH(1-84) in serum determined using two-site techniques is about 10 to 60 pg/ml (Fig. 23-9). It is likely that this corresponds closely to the concentration of biologically active PTH. The normal range in two-site assays is in good agreement with bioassay results, and

FIGURE 23-8 Two-site immunoradiometric assay for intact PTH. The hormone is captured by anti-carboxyl-terminal antibodies (anti-PTH 39-84) coupled to a bead. Captured PTH is detected by binding of radioactively labeled anti-amino-terminal antibodies (anti-PTH 1-34). *(After SR Nussbaum.)*

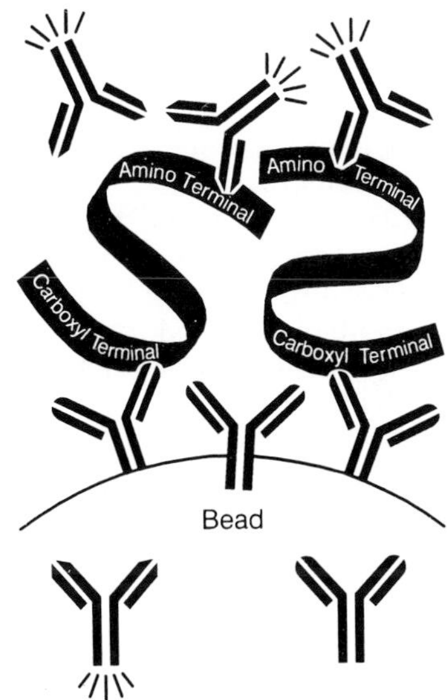

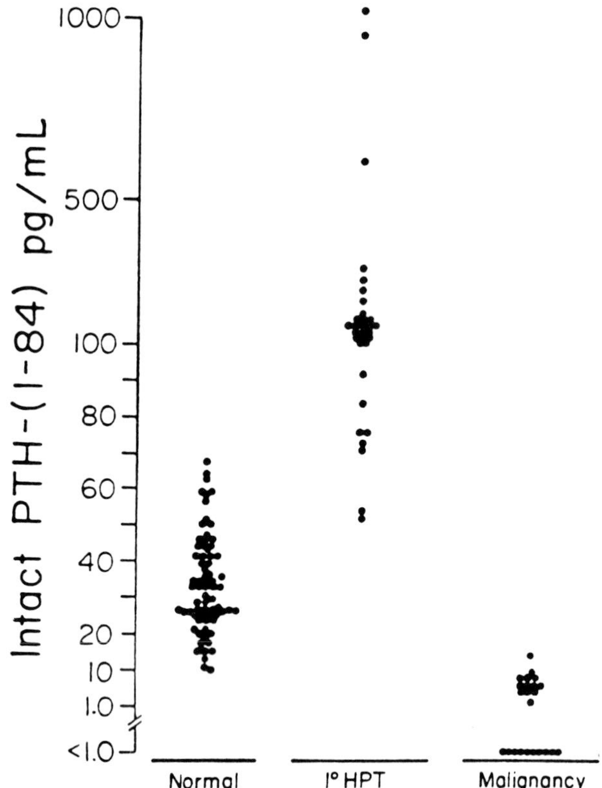

FIGURE 23-9 Levels of intact PTH in primary hyperparathyroidism and malignancy using the two-site technique. The serum level of PTH is typically elevated in hypercalcemic subjects with hyperparathyroidism but is uniformly suppressed in hypercalcemic patients with malignancy. *(From Nussbaum SR, Zahradnik RJ, Lavigne JR, et al[54] by permission of Clinical Chemistry.)*

the ability of such assays to detect dynamic changes in the secretion of PTH suggests that a labile species such as authentic PTH(1-84) is being measured. In practical terms, two-site assays for PTH have two distinct advantages over previous techniques: They are more sensitive, and they are less subject to nonspecific effects of serum. Together, these characteristics provide for the ability to quantitate PTH throughout the normal range and detect the suppression of PTH when present, as illustrated by the results in sera from patients with malignancy-associated hypercalcemia (Fig. 23-9). Wide experience with assays performed in commercial laboratories or using commercially available kits indicates that the level of performance shown in Fig. 23-9 is maintained.

With the advantages of two-site assays for intact PTH, is there a compelling reason to use a region-specific PTH assay in specific clinical circumstances? Midregion assays and amino-terminal assays remain excellent for the detection of primary hyperparathyroidism. They have been widely used for the management of secondary hyperparathyroidism in renal osteodystrophy, and clinicians are accustomed to using results in region-specific PTH assays to adjust treatment. However, aside from familiarity, no clear advantage is gained by the use of region-specific assays. Levels of intact PTH correlate well with midregion PTH levels in chronic renal failure, and while the sensitivity of assays for intact PTH for the detection of primary hyperparathyroidism is no better than that of region-specific assays (and in the authors' experience probably not as good), their enhanced specificity, in particular their ability to detect the suppression of PTH in nonparathyroid hypercalcemia, makes them superior instruments for the differential diagnosis of hypercalcemia.

Bioactive PTH can also be determined using bioassay techniques. A cytochemical technique is based on quantitating the effect of PTH on glucose-6-phosphate dehydrogenase activity measured microspectrophotometrically in distal tubules of guinea pig renal cortex.[52,56] This is a remarkably sensitive assay but is rather cumbersome and not suited to routine use. Glucose-6-phosphate dehydrogenase is not recognized as being directly in the pathway for the primary renal transport effects of PTH, and the assay may respond nonspecifically to otherwise biologically inactive carboxyl-terminal fragments of the hormone. Assays based on the determination of adenylyl cyclase have also been used[57]; these assays require the extraction of PTH from serum for reliable results.

Because the renal PTH receptor is coupled to adenylyl cyclase and a fraction of the cAMP produced in the proximal tubule in response to PTH is secreted into the urine, determination of urinary cAMP can be used as a bioassay for PTH. In research studies, the excretion of the secreted component, called *nephrogenous* cAMP, can be determined specifically by subtracting the filtered load of cAMP [plasma (cAMP) $\times$ glomerular filtration rate (GFR)] from the total urinary excretion. When measured carefully, nephrogenous cAMP is a reliable test of parathyroid function (Fig. 23-10), and determination of total urinary cAMP, which is technically easier, is also useful.[58] Bioassays have the advantage of detecting other molecules that mimic PTH, and determination of urinary cAMP was critical in the detection of a PTH-like peptide in malignancy-associated hypercalcemia. However, this same property makes them nonspecific for true hyperparathyroidism. At present, the principal use of urinary cAMP assays is in the differential diagnosis of hypocalcemic disorders, where the unresponsiveness of urinary cAMP to PTH is the hallmark of pseudohypoparathyroidism.

Biological Effects and Mechanism of Action of Parathyroid Hormone

Parathyroid hormone plays a critical role in the acute regulation of calcium levels in the ECF, while vitamin D plays an important long-term role in overall calcium balance by modulating the efficiency of the absorption of dietary calcium from the gut. PTH

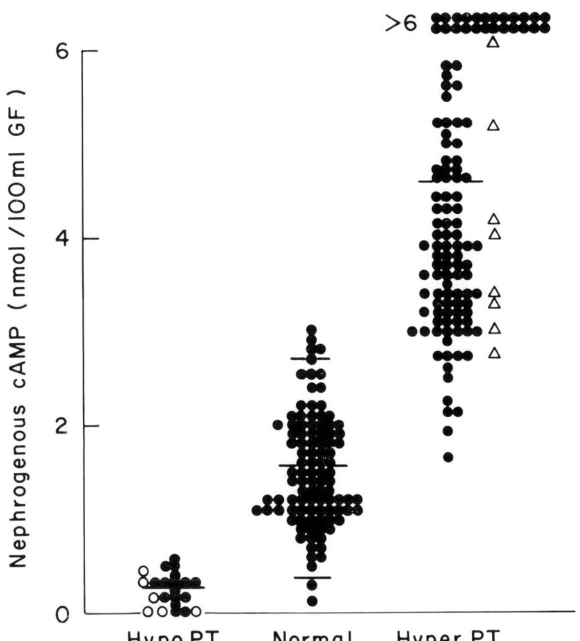

FIGURE 23-10 Values for nephrogenous cAMP in normal subjects and patients with hypoparathyroidism (HypoPT), nonparathyroid hypercalcemia (0), primary hyperparathyroidism (HyperPT), and nonazotemic secondary hyperparathyroidism (△). The marginated bars represent mean ± 2 SD in the normal subjects and mean values in the patients with hypoparathyroidism and hyperparathyroidism. *(By permission of Broadus AE, Nephron 23:136, 1978).*

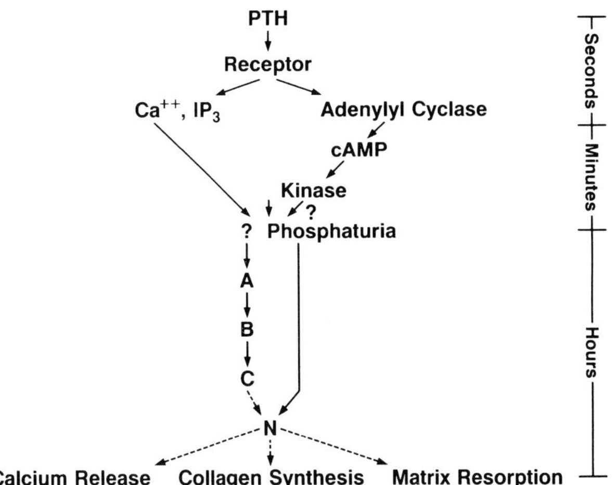

FIGURE 23-11 Sequential events in the expression of PTH biological activity from receptor interaction to cellular metabolic consequences. A time scale is depicted at the right margin. Events in bone occur over a longer time frame than do events in the kidney. A, B, and C indicate the possible requirement for several different steps for PTH actions on bone. N denotes the penultimate biochemical event or a final common pathway leading to the metabolic consequences depicted. The question mark reflects the speculative link, based on currently available data, between activation of kinase activity and phosphaturia.

"fine-tunes" the blood levels of calcium, which otherwise would be subject to peaks and troughs related to intermittent dietary intake. PTH acts directly on bone to stimulate its resorption and the release of calcium salts into the ECF. Similarly, PTH acts directly on the kidney to promote phosphate excretion and increase calcium reabsorption. While the response to PTH at the level of the kidney is rapid, the response in bone typically occurs much more slowly, probably reflecting a more complex cascade of events which must be put in motion to effect bone resorption (Fig. 23-11). The action of PTH in promoting increased dietary absorption of calcium is indirect: The hormone acts at the level of the kidney to stimulate 25-hydroxyvitamin D 1α-hydroxylase. The latter enzyme acts on the weakly active precursor form of vitamin D, 25-hydroxyvitamin D_3, to generate the fully active form, 1α,25-$(OH)D_3$. The active hormone then acts on the gut to stimulate increased activity of calcium-binding protein and facilitated transport of calcium from the gut lumen into the bloodstream (Fig. 23-3). The activity of the 1α-hydroxylase enzyme is in part regulated by PTH, as discussed below.

It is the action of PTH in concert on bone, kidney, and gut which increases the inflow of calcium into the ECF and defends the organism against hypocalcemia[15] (Fig. 23-3). The relative contribution of each of these three principal target organs to calcium homeostasis as a result of PTH action has not been definitively delineated and almost certainly varies with the nature of the stress to homeostasis. However, the contribution of PTH is clear: Surgical removal of the parathyroid glands in animals or humans without replacement of the hormone or other maneuvers designed to increase calcium influx (such as the administration of vitamin D and a high-calcium diet) leads to hypocalcemia, tetany, and even death within hours.

Mechanism of Action and Structure-Activity Relations of Parathyroid Hormone

Parathyroid hormone, like other peptide hormones, produces its biological actions by interacting with a hormone-specific receptor on the cell surface of target tissue cells. This interaction results in the production of intracellular second messengers which initiate a series of metabolic events.

The expression of PTH bioactivity is classically regarded as resulting from its action of increasing the intracellular levels of cAMP.[59,60] cAMP levels increase before a number of intracellular and organ-based events, such as phosphorylation of specific intracellular proteins by PTH-activated kinases, phosphaturia, and bone resorption.[59,61] The role of other potential intracellular second messengers in the expression of PTH action has not been determined. Intracellular calcium levels increase in part as a result of the entry of extracellular calcium or the release of intracellular calcium stores into the cytoplasm.[62–64] Stimulation of the phosphoinositol pathway by PTH is evident in some systems.[65–67] Only recently has it been possible to address these issues experimentally.

The PTH receptor has now been cloned,[68] using an expression screening approach, and its sequence has been elucidated. The successful cloning came after a considerable body of knowledge regarding the physiochemical (molecular weight, glycoprotein character, etc.) properties of the receptor had already been collected using affinity and photoaffinity cross-linking techniques. Studies of the prime initiating event in hormonal action—the biomolecular interaction of the hormone with its receptor—can now be undertaken in a manner not previously possible. Answers to many of the following questions are anticipated in the next months to years: Is there more than one receptor subtype? Are different receptors present on different target tissues, such as bone and kidney? What are the functional domains of the receptor involved in hormone binding and signal transduction? Is a different receptor subtype involved in stimulating the production of each second messenger, or can the same receptor activate more than one second messenger pathway? What is the tissue distribution of the receptor? What is the difference in the nature of the interaction of agonists vs. antagonists vs. partial agonists with the receptor? What complementary groups are involved in the interaction between the hormone molecule and the receptor? What are the defects in receptor or postreceptor signaling events that account for genetic disorders such as pseudohypoparathyroidism and pseudopseudohypoparathyroidism?

Biochemical Events in Parathyroid Hormone Action

The Receptor-Effector Model

In the 1980s, a well-supported model of hormone action emerged which can be applied to the mechanism of action of PTH.[69,70] For peptide hormones which activate adenylyl cyclase and generate increased levels of cAMP intracellularly, a multicomponent complex translates the hormonal signal into biochemical action. In this model, neither the hormone nor the receptor interacts directly with the effector molecule, namely, the enzyme adenylyl cyclase. Rather, the receptor contains specific domains which interact with a membrane protein termed the "guanyl nucleotide-regulatory" (N), or G protein. This G protein interacts directly with adenylyl cyclase, which is the catalytic protein, termed C. When hormone binds to receptor, a complex is formed involving the hormone, the receptor, and the guanyl nucleotide-regulatory protein (Fig. 23-12). Since adenylyl cyclase, the guanyl nucleotide–binding protein, and in many cases the receptors and hormones themselves are composed of multiple subunits, as many as 6 to 12 different protein subunits participate in the transduction of the hormonal signal into the expression of its biological activity.

There are many variations of this model depending on hormone and target tissue, and this topic is reviewed extensively elsewhere[71–73] and in Chap. 5. The interaction of the hormone with the receptor is thought to induce a conformational change in the receptor. Although this change is termed *receptor activation*, the ligand-bound receptor does not actually "activate" another protein. Rather, the ensuing event is one of "disinhibition." The steric change induced in the receptor when hormone binds leads to a dissociation of the receptor and G that "disinhibits" an active subunit of G called α_s (Fig. 23-12). The α_s subunit dissociates from the β-γ heterodimer of the G protein. The GDP present in α_s is released, freeing GTP to enter the α_s binding site, which allows the conformation of α_s and activates it. The α_s subunit then moves to another part of the plasma membrane, where it associates with and then activates adenylyl cyclase.[74–78] GTP is hydrolyzed to GDP in the process, terminating the signal. The α_s then recomplexes with the β-γ subunits to make an intact G protein, which in turn now associates with a ligand-free receptor, thus completing the cycle.

The hormone-bound receptor can activate more than one G_s complex, and the activated α_s in turn can activate more than one adenylyl cyclase molecule, which can generate many molecules of cAMP. Thus, inherent in the cascade is a mechanism for the amplification of hormonal signaling.

Although the β and γ subunits which are tightly associated are functionally interchangeable with many α subunits, approximately 20 different G protein α subunits have been identified. These α subunits provide functional diversity to the G proteins. The PTH receptor appears to be linked to a 52-kDa α_s and perhaps to other α subunits. It is also possible that activated receptor, either through direct linkage to transmembrane ion channels or through linkage to other G proteins (G proteins containing an α subunit other than α_s), can produce other hormonal actions. Similarly, activation of phospholipase C, a critical enzyme in the polyphosphoinositol pathway, is also dependent on a receptor–G protein interaction. The wide array of G protein α subunits can account for multiple hormonal actions. In some cases, a single receptor appears to be able to activate more than one α subunit; in other cases, a different receptor subtype is linked to interaction with each α subunit.

Receptors thus far characterized which are

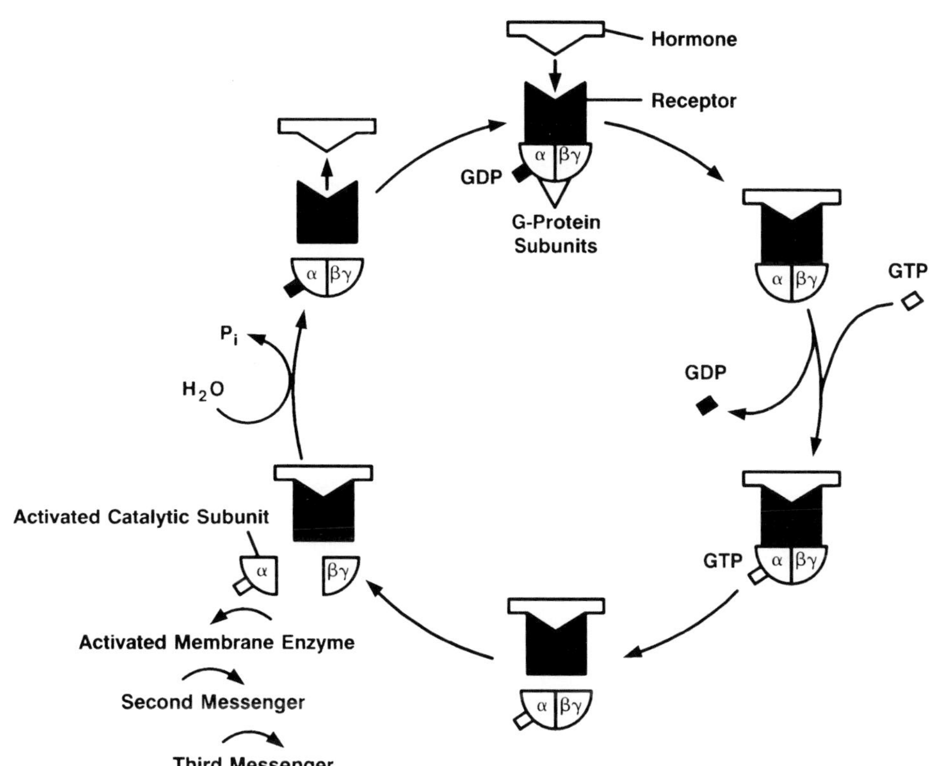

FIGURE 23-12 Cycle of receptor activation and deactivation for a guanyl nucleotide (G) regulatory protein–linked receptor. Description of the events is provided in the text.

linked to adenylyl cyclase activation[79,80] and other G-linked second messenger systems contain a number of common structural features. These include the receptors for rhodopsin,[79] the beta-adrenergic receptor agonists,[81] acetylcholine (muscarinic),[82,83] luteinizing hormone (LH),[84] thyrotropin stimulating hormone,[85] and others.[86] They possess seven membrane-spanning domains, although they may vary in the size of the extracellular N-terminal domain, which in many cases interacts with hormone, and the size of the cytoplasmically oriented C-terminal domain and intracellular loops (which may be involved in signal transduction or regulation of receptor number) varies from receptor to receptor. Interestingly, despite their common interaction with G proteins, the specific transmembrane domains involved in G protein interaction display considerable sequence heterogeneity across receptors.

PTH receptors from rat osteoblast-like bone [ROS 17(2.8)] and opossum kidney (OK) cell lines have recently been cloned;[68] structure-function analysis is still emerging. These receptors encode for 591- and 585-amino acid proteins, respectively, which are 78 percent identical despite differences in species and organ of origin. The receptor, as expected, appears to contain seven membrane-spanning regions (Fig. 23-13). However, the receptor contains little homology to other guanyl nucleotide regulatory protein–linked receptors. There is less than 10 percent conservation of 35 "signatures" present to a level of 80 percent in 120 other G protein–linked receptors, including those which interact with an α_s G protein subunit responsible for activating adenylyl cyclase. However, there is striking homology to the sequence of the recently cloned calcitonin receptor,[87] as well as the receptors for glucagon, secretin, and VIP, indicating that these receptors form a new subgroup in the family of G protein-linked receptors. For example, transmembrane domain number VII is nearly identical (17 of 18 amino acid identity) to the corresponding domain in the calcitonin receptor (see Fig. 23-32). The overall similarity between the PTH and calcitonin receptors is approximately 50 percent; there is 32 percent identity in amino acid sequence.

Because the receptor binds both PTH and the tumor-secreted parathyroid hormone–related protein (PTHrP), it is termed the PTH/PTHrP receptor. The PTH/PTHrP receptor also contains an N-terminal extracellularly oriented domain intermediate in size (approximately 155 amino acids) between that found in the beta-adrenergic receptor (which is stimulated when a small molecule of catecholamine interacts directly with receptor transmembrane domains)[88] and the large extracellular receptor domains present in receptors which interact with glycoprotein hormones such as LH and follicle stimulating hormone (FSH) (where the hormone is thought to interact exclusively with the extracellular

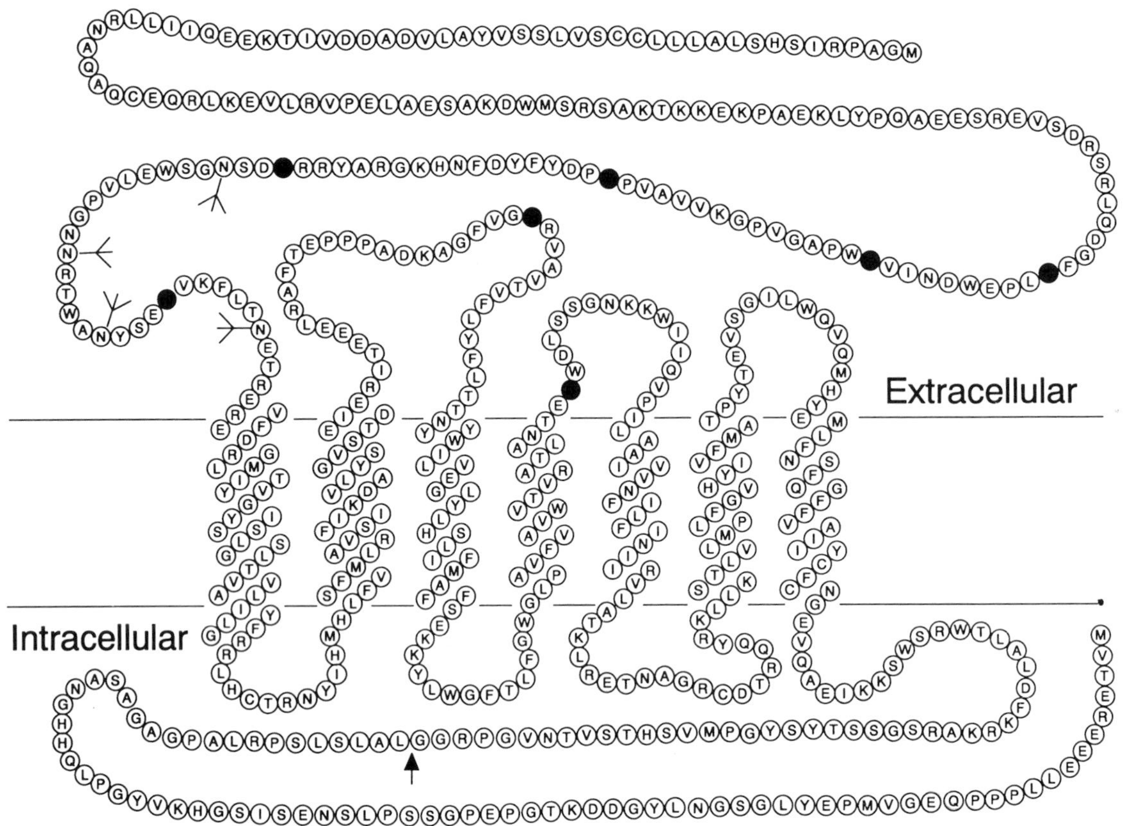

FIGURE 23-13 Schematic representation of the PTH/PTHrP receptor (NH_2 terminus at top) from opossum kidney cells, potential N-glycosylation sites (⅄), and cysteine residues that are conserved in the calcitonin receptor (●). In OK-H, residues 508 to 515 (to the left of the arrow) are WPCSALD. The peptide ends eight residues after the arrow. *(Reprinted with permission from Jüppner et al.[68])*

portion of the receptor by virtue of the hormone's large size, which precludes it from entering the membrane).

The PTH/PTHrP receptor, like the CT receptor and the receptor for large glycoprotein hormones but unlike the beta-adrenergic receptor, contains a signal sequence at the N terminus. In the exoplasmic domain, there are four potential sites for N-linked glycosylation and six cysteines in each of the first two extracellular loops which are thought to be important in maintaining a bioactive conformation for the receptor (two additional cysteines in the signal sequence). The third intracellular loop and the carboxyl-terminal intracellular tail contain potential phosphorylation sites. The gene encoding the receptor contains 4 introns and 4 exons, in contrast to the intronless beta-adrenergic receptor.

In other systems, extensive structural modification of receptor by site-directed mutagenesis has revealed considerable information regarding the functionality of various domains of the receptor.[89–95] Hormone-binding regions can be differentiated from domains which interact with guanyl nucleotide regulatory proteins and subtle structural changes introduced into the receptor can selectively alter interactions with agonists or antagonists.[96,97]

These kinds of insights into hormone-receptor interaction and structure-function relations for the receptor are now becoming available for the PTH/PTHrP receptor. Work in this area should be facilitated by the wide array of hormone analogues available in the PTH system. Already evidence is accumulating that agonists and antagonists may bind to different regions of the receptor.

An important observation already made with the cloned expressed receptor is that both the rat bone and OK receptors stimulate both adenylyl cyclase/cAMP signal transduction and the phospholipase C/IP_3/intracellular Ca^{2+} second messenger pathway. Different domains of the same receptor may be responsible for the activation of these pathways. A mutant form of the OK receptor (in which 69 amino acids are deleted from the C-terminal tail and the 8 terminal residues differ from the native sequence) is still able to bind PTH and PTHrP and stimulate adenylyl cyclase but fails to stimulate the IP_3/intracellular Ca^{2+} second messenger system. These findings indicate that the same PTH/PTHrP receptor can interact with both $G_s\alpha$ and another α subunit involved in phospholipase C/IP_3 signal transduction, similar to the coupling of TSH to these signal pathways. The C terminus of the receptor appears to be particularly important for the activation of the latter pathway.

Extensive structure-activity studies have defined important structural features responsible for hormonal binding to receptor and activation of the receptor subsequent to binding[98,99] (Fig. 23-14). Some analogues can bind to the PTH receptor without causing activation of cAMP or other events in the biochemical cascade of hormonal action[100,101] and can serve as effective antagonists of PTH both in vitro and in vivo.[102,103] These antagonist analogues can be generated by deleting several amino acids from the N terminus of the fully biologically active 1-34 fragment of PTH.[99] Deletion of only two amino acids from the N terminus yields analogues of the 3-34 sequence (Fig. 23-15), which compete with PTH on a one-to-one molar basis for receptor occupancy and display kinetics characteristic of a true competitive antagonist.[100] While these antagonists were highly potent in vitro, they retained weak but definite PTH-like agonist activity in vivo, and this precluded their use as hormone antagonists.[104–106] Nevertheless, the conceptual framework for further design of antagonists was established by these and other studies.[101,107,108] The receptor-binding domain of the hormone lies at the C terminus of the active fragment, principally in the region 28-34, and a domain necessary for activation of receptors once hormone binding occurs lies at the N terminus. Since the receptor "binding" and "activation" domains are largely separable, it appears to be possible to design analogues which could bind to receptors without leading to the activation and expression of hormonal activity.

FIGURE 23-14 A functional map of the parathyroid hormone molecule. All the structural determinants required for full biological activity reside within the N-terminal 1-34 sequence. Contained within this region is a domain critical for activation of the receptor, positions 1-6. The sequence 7-34 forms the core for most PTH antagonists. Within this inhibitory domain lies the principal binding domain of the hormone, positions 25-34. *(Modified and reprinted with permission from Rosenblatt.[99])*

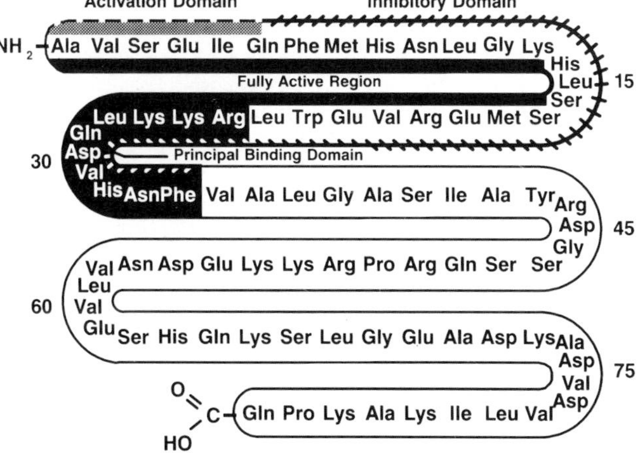

More extensive truncation, to position 7, yielded analogues of 7-34 which were devoid of PTH-like agonist activity yet possessed sufficient receptor avidity to serve as effective PTH agonists both in vitro and in vivo.[102,103,109] These analogues (Fig. 23-16) incorporated other modifications which enhanced receptor binding in order to offset the loss in affinity that accompanies truncation at the N terminus. The combination of these modifications in a single analogue enabled the design of potent in vivo antagonists to be accomplished without restoring partial agonism back into the molecule (Fig. 23-17).[102,103,109]

Just as the analogue design approach has evolved over the last several years, so too has the sensitivity of in vitro bioassays. Until recently, it was possible to detect weak retained PTH agonist-like activity in an analogue only by testing it at high concentration in vivo; the conventional in vitro bioassays failed to detect and predict agonist properties in vivo. However, a bone cell–based bioassay has been modified to enhance sensitivity.[110] When cells are treated with dexamethasone and pertussis toxin, the cAMP signal is amplified. Therefore, this assay can detect retained weak agonist properties and appears to predict the in vivo biological profile of analogues. As such, it will be extremely useful in improving the accuracy and efficiency of selecting compounds for extensive evaluation in vivo.

Other analogues of PTH, such as oxidation stable sulfur-free analogues, have proved suitable for radiolabeling[111] and have served as the foundation for radioligand–membrane receptor binding assays and for photoaffinity or affinity cross-linking of the receptor,[112–117] allowing its physicochemical characterization. The novel PTH agonists, antagonists, and partial agonists which have been designed should facilitate studies of the mechanism of the hormonal[118–120] expression of bioactivity for PTH.

The elucidation of the N-terminal protein structure,[118–120] followed by the cloning[121–123] of PTHrP, has permitted an entirely new avenue for study of the structural determinants important in hormonal binding and activation of PTH receptors.[124–128] More details regarding the PTH-like tumor-secreted factor are provided in Malignancy-Associated Hypercalcemia, but for the purposes of this discussion, some background is provided.

It has been well documented that both PTH and PTHrP are able to bind to what has been conventionally regarded as the PTH receptor.[125–130] Powerful evidence along these lines comes from the observation that each hormone can downregulate receptors for subsequent response to the other hormone, mimicking "homologous desensitization"[128–131] (Fig. 23-18). This occurs despite limited homology between

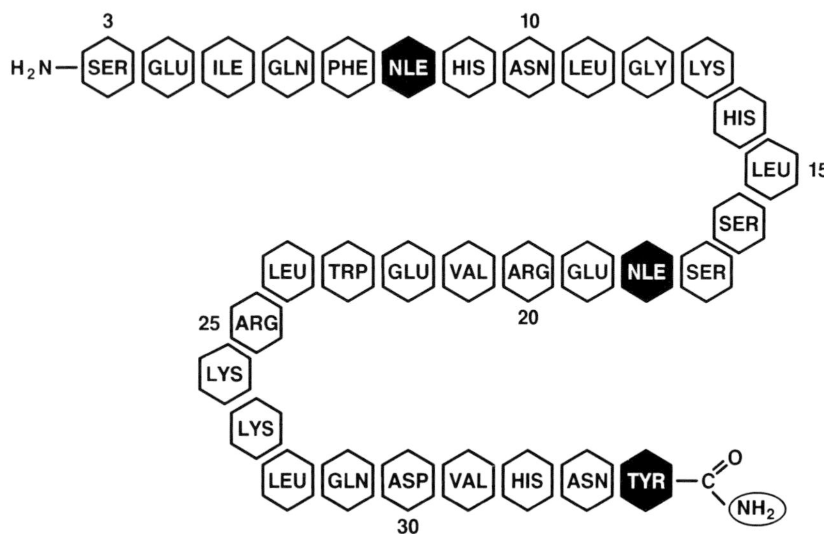

FIGURE 23-15 Structure of [Nle-8,Nle-18,Tyr-34]bPTH-(3-34)amide, a potent antagonist of PTH action in vitro. In vivo, the analogue was found to possess weak but definite PTH agonist-like activity. *(Reprinted with permission from Rosenblatt.[99])*

the two hormones.[118–120] In fact, although the homology is strong at the N terminus of both molecules (a region known to be critically important for PTH bioactivity), beyond position 13 there is a divergence of sequence with very little homology present. Nevertheless, fragments of the hormone from a position distal to residue 13, such as 14-34 of each hormone, are able to bind to PTH receptors.[132] The 7-34 analogue of PTH, described above, is able to block PTHrP action in vitro and in vivo despite deletion of much of the region of homology between the two hormones[133] (Fig. 23-19). Chimeric molecules have been synthesized in which the N-terminal half of the 1-34 sequence of one hormone have been linked contiguously to the C-terminal segment of the other (Fig. 23-20). In both constructs, the chimeric hormones bind and stimulate PTH receptors with nearly identical avidity and efficacy,[132,134] indicating that the PTH/PTHrP receptor accepts and recognizes

FIGURE 23-16 Structure of an in vivo antagonist of parathyroid hormone. The analogue contains a tyrosine amide substitution for phenylalanine at the carboxyl terminus. Shaded residues indicate positions of amino acid identity with PTHrP. Deleted from the truncated analogue are residues 1-6, which contain the major region of homology with PTHrP, yet the PTH antagonist is able to inhibit both PTH and PTHrP actions in vitro and in vivo. *(Reprinted with permission from Horiuchi et al.[133])*

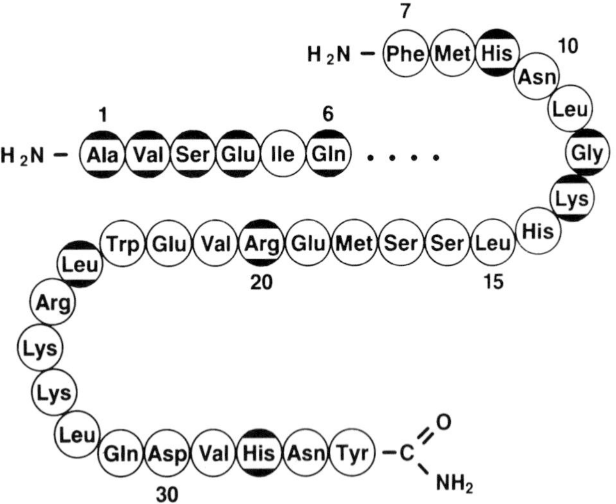

FIGURE 23-17 Evaluation of the effects of [Tyr-34]bPTH-(7-34)NH_2, a PTH antagonist, on urinary phosphate excretion in rats. The data shown were compiled from a total of 40 animals. Fifteen control rats (●) received native bPTH-(1-84) alone intravenously at a rate of 0.27 nmol/h. Twenty-one rats (■) received [Tyr-34]bPTH-(7-34)NH_2 and the native peptide through separate intravenous cannulas at rates of 54 nmol and 0.27 nmol per hour, respectively (a molar ratio of 200 to 1). Infusion of the antagonist was begun 1 h before the beginning of the infusion of native PTH. Four animals (▲) received antagonist alone. *(Reprinted with permission from Roth.[433])*

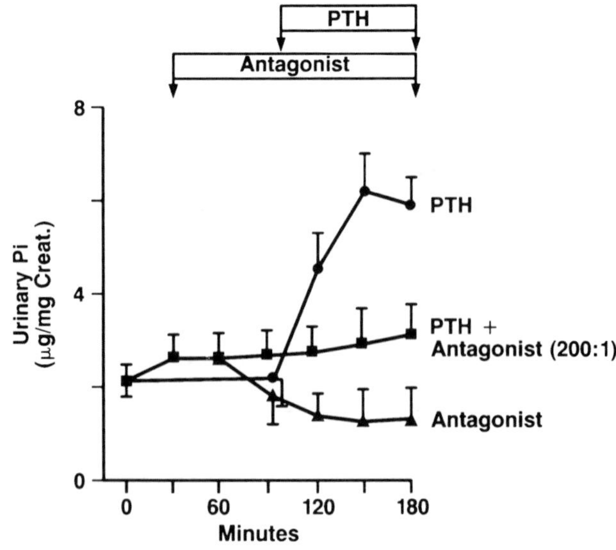

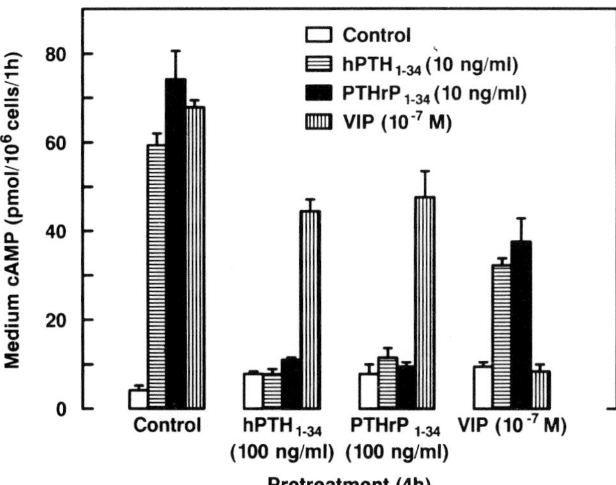

FIGURE 23-18 Preincubation for 4 h with hPTH-(1-34) (100 ng/ml) or PTHrP-(1-34) (100 ng/ml) caused complete loss of response to a second 1-h challenge with 10 ng/ml of either PTH or PTHrP and only modest (to ~70 percent of control value) attenuation of the response to VIP (10^{-7} *M*). Preincubation with VIP (10^{-7} *M*) caused complete homologous desensitization but only partial (to ~50% of control value) loss of response to PTH or PTHrP. Each bar gives the mean value, and the brackets give the SE of three or six dishes per group. *(Reprinted with permission from Fukayama et al.[131])*

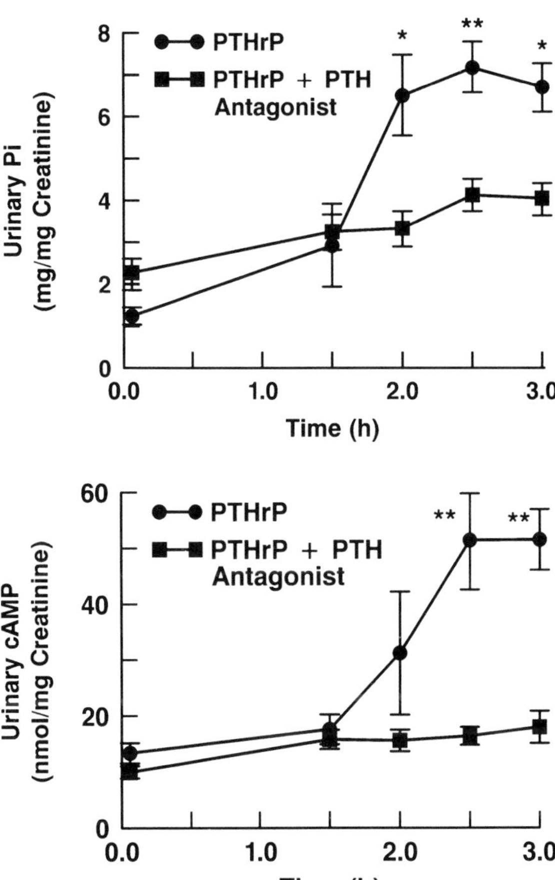

FIGURE 23-19 [Tyr-34]bPTH-(7-34)NH_2 inhibits PTHrP-(1-34)NH_2–stimulated increases in cAMP and phosphate excretion. Coinfusion of PTHrP-(1-34)NH_2 and [Tyr-34]bPTH-(7-34)NH_2 (0.16 and 32 nmol/h, respectively) or PTHrP-(1-34)NH_2 (0.16 nmol/h) administered alone. Values are the mean ± SEM (n = 7–10). Significance was determined using a one-sided Student's *t*-test; $*p < 0.05$; $**p < 0.01$. *(Reprinted with permission from Horiuchi et al.[133])*

domains from two hormones with very different primary amino acid sequences. This observation suggests that despite sequence differences, the two sequences are able to mimic each other in secondary and tertiary conformation, presenting similar topology to the receptor's binding site.

A 7-34 fragment of PTHrP was expected to act as a pure hormone antagonist, analogous to that of the 7-34 fragment of PTH. However, this sequence retained weak but definite residual agonist activity in the newer, more sensitive in vitro bioassays described above[135] and in vivo.[136] This finding suggested that the region 10-13 is potentially important in hormonal action and indicated that the boundary of the "activation" domains of the hormone extend beyond positions 1-6 into the midrange of the active fragments. Substitution of the amino acids present in positions 10 and 11 of PTH into PTHrP generated a hybrid molecule which was a potent antagonist and was completely devoid of agonist-like activity in vitro.[137] Conversely, substitution of two amino acids from the same positions in PTHrP into the PTH molecule generated an analogue which for the first time displayed weak agonist activity on the 7-34 scaffolding of PTH[137] (Fig. 23-21). These observations indicate that the molecular code for hormonal action can be contained in a small number of structural features and that it is possible to insert or delete hormonal activity in "cassette" fashion for these two hormones (Fig. 23-22).

Based on these findings, much of the direction of analogue design for PTH and PTHrP has shifted to region 10-18 of the molecule. Conformational analysis and structure-function studies of the region indicate the presence of an α-helical structure in the neighborhood of the glycine at position 12.[138,139] Substitution with D-tryptophan at position 12 in either the PTH or PTHrP molecule leads to the most potent antagonists yet designed.[140] Other efforts have been made to increase the hydrophobic interactions in the hormone-receptor biomolecular interaction[141] and to chemically "lock" the hormone's conformation into one favored by the receptor. Formation of a lactam "bridge" on one surface of the helix between positions 13 and 17 has been found to increase antagonist potency[142] (Fig. 23-23).

Despite these advances in PTH antagonist design, none of the antagonists prepared to date have

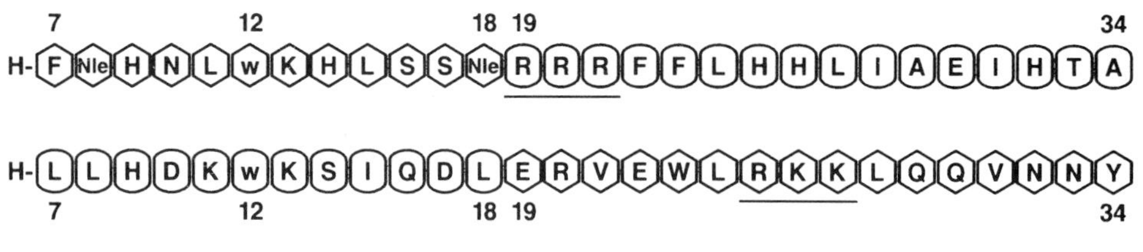

FIGURE 23-20 Hybrid molecules demonstrate the interchangeability of PTH and PTHrP sequences. In the analogue whose sequence is shown in the upper portion, the N-terminal sequence of PTH (diamonds) is contiguous with the C-terminal portion of PTHrP (rounded boxes). In the lower analogue, the converse is true. Both analogues demonstrated comparable binding to PTH/PTHrP receptors and possess affinity comparable to that of both intact native sequences.

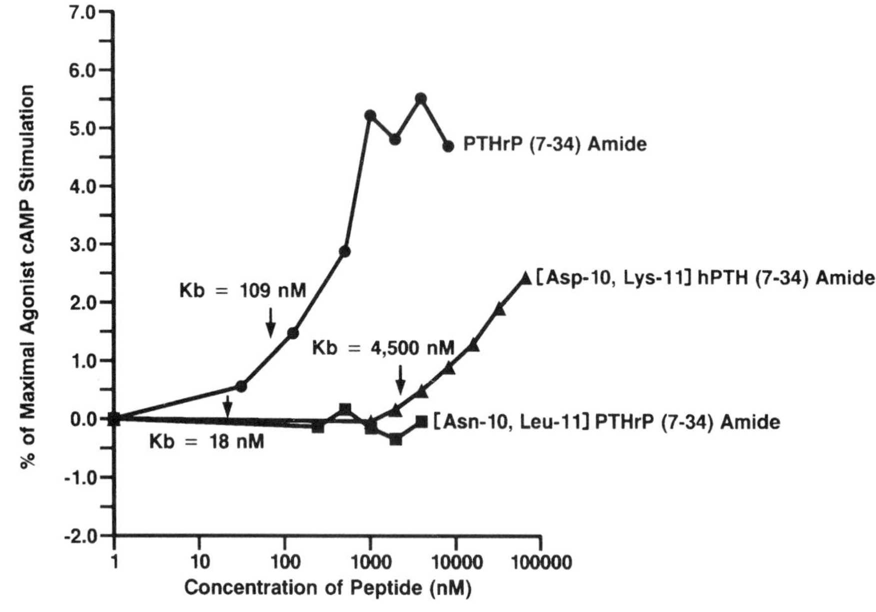

FIGURE 23-21 Role of positions 10 and 11 in agonist activity of PTH and PTHrP antagonists. Peptides were assayed for their ability to stimulate cAMP production in ROS 17/2.8 cells. The PTHrP analogue includes two substitutions from the PTH sequence. The PTH analogue contains two substitutions from the PTHrP sequence. *(Reprinted with permission from Nutt et al.[137])*

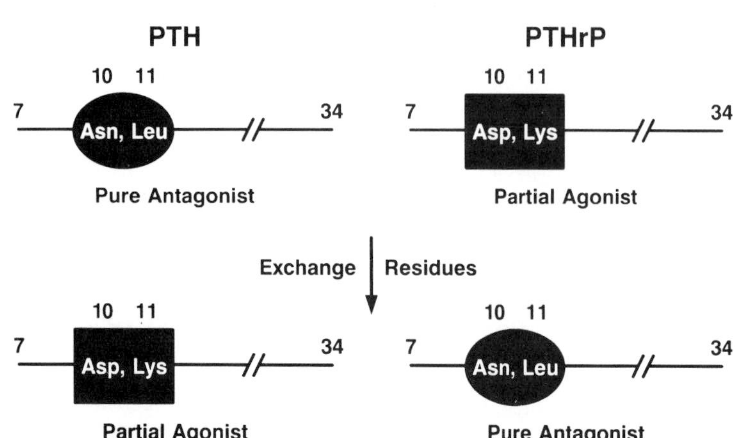

FIGURE 23-22 A structure-function study of the 7-34 sequence of PTH and PTHrP. Two amino acids residues within this region contain structural determinants responsible for the activation of the PTH/PTHrP receptor once binding has occurred. Substituting the asparagine and leucine at positions 10 and 11 (oval), respectively, with the aspartic acid and lysine (rectangle) of PTHrP converts the pure PTH antagonist into a partial agonist. Conversely, substitution of the amino acid residues from PTH into PTHrP at positions 10 and 11 converts the weak partial agonist into a pure antagonist. Therefore, receptor activation can be inserted or removed from one molecular scaffold to the other in "cassette" form. *(Reprinted with permission from Caulfield et al.[132])*

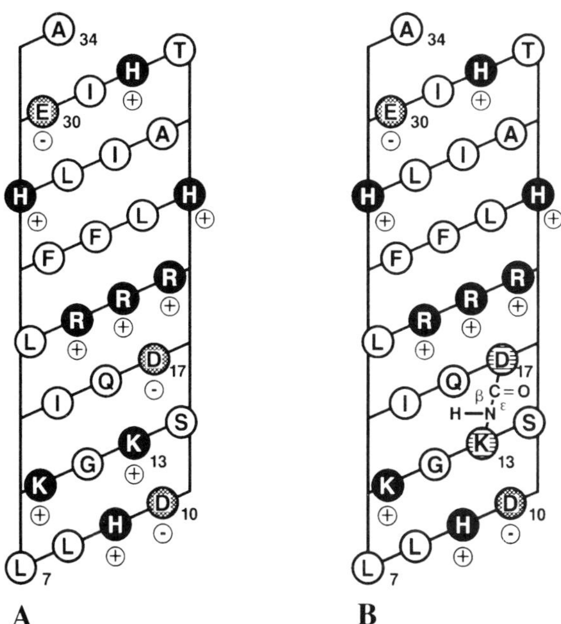

FIGURE 23-23 Linear PTHrP(7-34) schematically presented in an α-helical conformation *(A)*. Cyclic lactam formed between Lys[13] and Asp[17] in an α-helical conformation *(B)* [(Lys[13], Asp[17]) PTHrP (7–34)]. Key amino acids are highlighted: positively charged (●) and negatively charged residues (◎) and residues participating in the cyclization (⊜).

sufficient potency or duration of action to permit their practical use as therapeutic agents in the treatment of hypercalcemic disorders due to excess PTH or PTHrP levels in the circulation (Table 23-1). It is hoped that further insights into hormone-receptor interactions will permit reduction of the size of analogues down to a few critical structural elements, allowing the design of small molecule (and perhaps nonpeptide) mimetics or antagonists for PTH and PTHrP. Another question which we anticipate will soon be answered is, Does this newly discovered hormone interact exclusively with PTH receptors, or does it also interact with a different set of receptors?

TABLE 23-1 Potential Uses of Parathyroid Hormone Antagonists

Short-term treatment of hypercalcemic crisis ("parathyroid storm" due to parathyroid adenoma, hyperplasia, or carcinoma); for preoperative optimization of blood calcium levels
Long-term treatment of hyperparathyroidism
In high-risk surgical candidates
In patients who have undergone unsuccessful surgery
In parathyroid carcinoma (inoperable)
For general medical management of hyperparathyroidism (?)
Adjunct treatment
After renal transplantation, when there is persistent "secondary" hyperparathyroidism

Postreceptor Responses to PTH

Chase and Aurbach,[59,60] following the studies of Rall and Sutherland,[143] documented an association between PTH and cAMP. Since that time, considerable evidence has linked the action of PTH to cAMP. In vivo, perfusion with PTH produces increases in intracellular cAMP in renal cells and a spillover of cAMP extracellularly into urine as nephrogenous cAMP.[59,61,144,145] An analogue of cAMP, dibutyryl cAMP, which is able to penetrate cells and is long-lived, produces PTH-like effects in the kidney.[146,147] PTH-responsive sites for ion transport along the nephron coincide with regions where adenylyl cyclase is stimulated, as documented by micropuncture techniques.[148] Elevated intracellular levels of cAMP presumably activate macromolecules responsible for ion transport, such as the sodium/calcium exchanger in renal cortical tubular cells.[149] Supporting evidence regarding other cAMP-dependent functions is derived from the findings that a series of analogues of PTH display a close correlation between their actions on the kidney in vivo and in vitro and their potency in adenylyl cyclase assays.[52,98,99,149–153]

Intracellular levels of calcium also increase after exposure to PTH.[62–64] Again, the influx of calcium is temporally in advance of "macroscopic" mineral ion flux in blood and urine. This rise in intracellular calcium may result from PTH activation of a calcium channel which permits calcium influx from the extracellular fluid into the cytosol.[1,154,155] However, PTH also stimulates the formation of IP_3[156–158] and both cloned kidney and bone PTH/PTHrP receptors are able to stimulate increases in intracellular cAMP and IP_3 second messengers. The IP_3 second messenger stimulates the release of intracellular stores of calcium from microsomes and may amplify an alternate or overlapping cascade of metabolic events. However, no definitive linkage between IP_3 and any single PTH-mediated metabolic effect has been established.

For bone, the findings are very similar to those observed in kidney. Namely, cAMP appears to be the principal second messenger for hormonal action. Osteoblasts clearly respond to PTH by generating cAMP in a dose-dependent fashion.[159] Skeletal tissue responds to dibutyryl cAMP in a manner parallel to that of PTH.[160,161] In vivo, the administration of dibutyryl cAMP elevates serum calcium as a result of the skeletal release of calcium salts.[162,163]

However, for bone too, cAMP alone may not be responsible for all the metabolic consequences of hormonal bioactivity. PTH-stimulated calcium release from bone (calvaria) organ culture is not affected by substantial blockade of adenylyl cyclase by inhibitors of the enzyme.[164] Furthermore, PTH has been documented to stimulate protein kinase C[165,166] and the formation of IP_3.[65–67]

Whether one or more intracellular second messengers is responsible for PTH action is not known at this time, nor is the potential balance between second messengers and integration of the signals understood. Much of the research leading to our understanding of the cellular cascade involved in PTH action in bone is based on data obtained from stable rat osteosarcoma cell lines, such as ROS 17/2.8 and UMR-106, which possess phenotypic characteristics of osteoblasts.[167,168]

Information about events subsequent to the production of second messengers is limited; the full cascade leading to the expression of hormonal activity and mineral ion fluxes remains to be established. Phosphorylation of certain proteins by PTH-dependent phosphokinases has been documented.[169,170] In addition, dephosphorylation of certain proteins occurs.[169] However, the biological role of these proteins and their full characterization have not been achieved.

Regulation of Receptor Number

Eventual elucidation of the structure of the gene encoding the PTH receptor will undoubtedly identify potential regulatory sites (perhaps for calcium, hormonal second messengers, or steroid hormones) within the promoter region of the gene. Glucocorticoids are known to increase responsiveness to PTH in osteoblast-like cells (osteosarcoma clonal cell lines),[167,171,172] possibly increasing the transcription of the PTH receptor gene.

For many hormones, prior exposure to hormone leads to subsequent diminished responsiveness to the same hormone by many target cells, organs, or even the whole organism (see Chap. 5). Such tachyphylaxis is due partly to down regulation or desensitization of receptors. The existence of the down regulation phenomenon for PTH receptors has been clearly documented: Exposure to hormone in vitro and in vivo can produce a subsequent and dramatic down regulation of receptor number and accompanying tachyphylaxis (Fig. 23-24).[113,173–175] After exposure to PTH, it may take as long as 36 to 48 h for full hormonal responsiveness to be restored. Occupation of receptors alone does not seem to account for the decline in receptor number because antagonists, which act by competitively occupying the receptor, do not produce down regulation.[113,176] Rather, postreceptor events, probably unrelated to the production of cAMP,[177,178] appear to be responsible. Other events, perhaps modeled on those described for phosphorylation of the beta receptor by a specific receptor kinase [the beta-adrenergic receptor kinase (BARK)],[179,180] can account for the marked decline in available receptors after exposure to the hormone. The cloned PTH/PTHrP receptor contains such potential phosphorylation sites in its third intracellular loop and C-terminal intracellular tail. The importance of this phenomenon in physiology or the pathophysiology of hyperparathyroidism is not known. Clearly, down regulation is not complete in

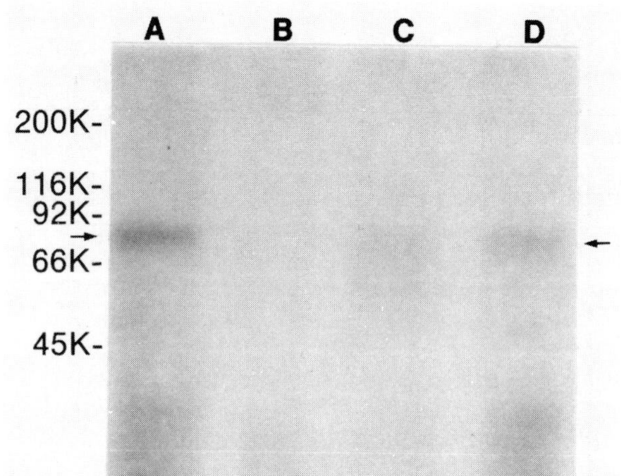

FIGURE 23-24 Desensitization of PTH receptors. Effect of preincubation with PTH or with a PTH inhibitory analogue on labeling of the PTH-binding component in cells cultured from human giant cell tumor of bone. Cells were preincubated without hormone or with PTH (1.0×10^{-7} *M*) or the PTH inhibitor [Nle^8,Nle^{18},Tyr^{34}]b-PTH-(3-34)amide (3.0×10^{-7} *M*). Cells were washed and then reacted with the photolabile PTH radioligand in the presence or absence of excess unlabeled PTH. The PTH-binding components were examined by autoradiography. Lane A represents the labeling pattern in cells preincubated without hormone. The effect of the addition of unlabeled PTH (acutely) before exposure to light is shown in lane B. The effect of preincubation with PTH is shown in lane C, and the effect of preincubation with the PTH inhibitor is shown in lane D.

hyperparathyroidism because these patients are hypercalcemic. However, a relatively diminished response to elevated levels of hormone cannot be ruled out. Some investigators have linked the diminished responsiveness to PTH that accompanies aging to down regulation of receptors.[181]

PTH Effects on the Kidney

At the level of the kidney, the link between cAMP and hormonal action is strongest. Increased cytoplasmic cAMP activates protein kinase A,[182] which phosphorylates specific membrane-bound proteins which are thought to then alter tubular ion transport. Although the analysis is not complete, there appears to be linkage between protein phosphorylation and PTH-mediated inhibition of phosphate reabsorption by tubular cells. Phosphate transport in the proximal tubule is linked to sodium. This transport system is inhibited by PTH and appears to be linked to cAMP and the cAMP-dependent protein kinase system. PTH promotes phosphaturia by directly inhibiting phosphate resorption. The activity of the Na/P_i cotransporter diminishes[183] in association with phosphorylation and subsequent endocytic removal of an apical brush border membrane protein.[170] Similarly, PTH-mediated inhibition of bicarbonate transport is thought to result from the inhibition,[184] perhaps by translocation,[185] of the Na-H antiporter out of the brush border membrane of proximal epithelial tubular cells.

PTH also acts on the tubule to promote the reabsorption of calcium (Fig. 23-25). Since large quantities of calcium (7 to 10 g/day) are filtered, even a small increase in an already efficient process, such as going from 95 to 98 percent efficacy, can have a dramatic salutary effect when calcium homeostasis and balance are stressed. PTH action on the distal tubule stimulates transport against both a calcium concentration and an electric potential gradient.[186–190] Although this observation indicates the presence of an active transport system for calcium, the biochemical linkage of this transporter to postreceptor events is not known. In the distal convoluted tubule, where PTH exerts its greatest effect on renal conservation of calcium,[186–188] a Na^+/Ca^{2+} exchanger is present and its activity is modulated by PTH and cAMP (or its analogues).[64,149] In addition, other calcium transporters may participate in effecting Ca^{2+} flux in the kidney.[149a] The effects of PTH on anion (such as chloride) permeability may produce membrane hyperpolarization, which in turn would drive calcium entry into distal convoluted cells.

PTH also stimulates the formation of the active form of vitamin D, 1α,25-(OH)D, in the nephron. PTH stimulates the activity of the renal 25-hydroxyvitamin D 1-α hydroxylase present in proximal tubular cells.[191] The mechanism of regulation of this enzyme by PTH has not been clearly established but appears to be linked to PTH-dependent production of cAMP; however, low phosphate levels intracellularly, which occur secondarily as a result of PTH action, can also stimulate the enzyme.[192,193]

FIGURE 23-25 Contribution of different portions of the renal nephron to PTH-dependent and PTH-independent calcium absorption. *(Courtesy of Dr. Maurice Attie, University of Pennsylvania School of Medicine.)*

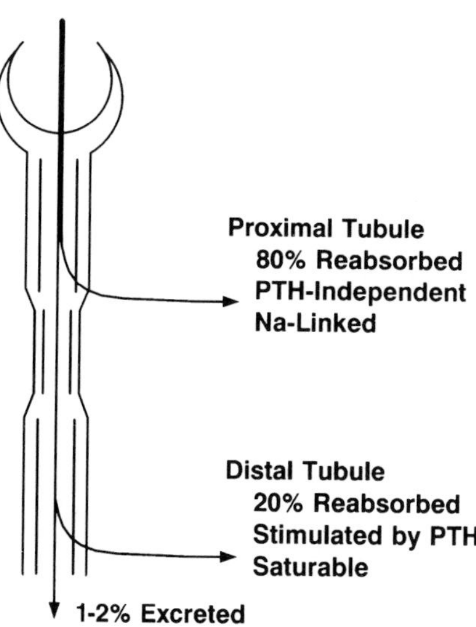

Actions on Bone

To understand the actions of parathyroid hormone on bone and appreciate the contribution of PTH to mineral metabolism, it is necessary to provide some general information regarding bone biology. Bone is a complex organ. It is not metabolically static, but is in dynamic balance. Throughout life, bone is actively involved in remodeling. The continuous resorption of discrete quanta of the skeleton followed by stepwise "programmed" replacement (formation) is termed *bone turnover* (Fig. 23-26). Throughout bone, there are thousands of sites involved in the asynchronous process of first removing and then replacing bone along its surfaces. The discussion that follows is not intended to be comprehensive. Rather, it provides a background oriented toward a discussion of the participation of bone in mineral ion homeostasis.

Bone is composed of cells and extracellular matrix. Cells account for 2 percent of the total volume of bone. The extracellular matrix is rich in collagen and glycosaminoglycans. A unique feature of the extracellular matrix in this connective tissue is that it can be calcified. Bone can be subdivided into cortical (compact) bone and trabecular (cancellous) bone. Approximately 80 to 90 percent of the volume of compact bone is calcified, while 15 to 25 percent of trabecular bone is calcified; the rest is occupied by marrow. Therefore, much of the biomechanical strength of bone is derived from the cortical component, while trabecular bone participates more fully in the metabolic function of mineral ion homeostasis.

FIGURE 23-26 Schematic representation of the cycle of bone resorption by osteoclasts followed by bone formation by osteoblasts. Formation of a Howship lacuna by an osteoclast is depicted in step 2.

1. Osteoclast recruitment and activation

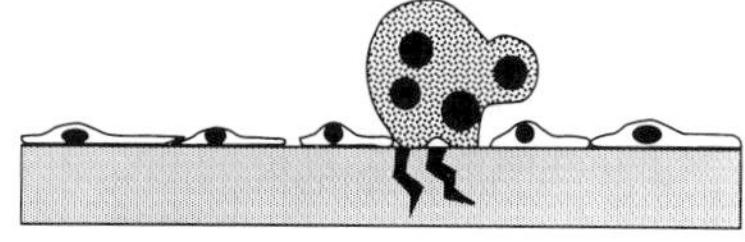

2. Resorption and osteoblast recruitment

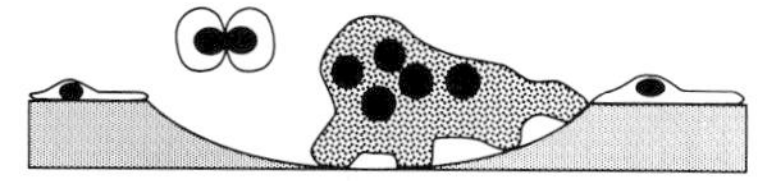

3. Osteoblastic bone formation

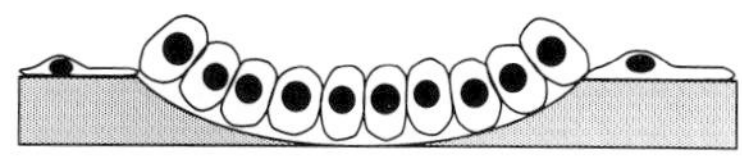

4. Completed remodelling cycle

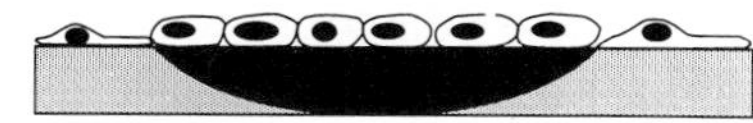

However, it is important to emphasize that both categories of bone participate in structural and metabolic functions. Cortical bone is largely found in the appendicular regions and accounts for 80 percent of the adult skeleton, whereas the vertebrae and axial skeleton are rich in trabecular bone.

In mature bone, collagen fibers are arranged in layers, termed *lamellae*, which are concentrically deposited around a central channel based on a blood vessel (haversian system). These lamellae become calcified. The combination of hydroxyapatite [$Ca_{10}(PO_4)_6(OH)_2$] and matrix proteins (especially collagen) gives bone its strength. Given the correct ionic milieu in ECF, the organic matrix of bone will mineralize spontaneously. In humans, the calcification process is complete within 10 to 20 days after the biosynthesis of organic matrix. If an appropriate ionic environment is not present, mineralization will be delayed. A prolonged lag between matrix formation and mineralization is the hallmark of certain diseases, such as osteomalacia and rickets.

When bone is formed rapidly, the organization of collagen fibers is sacrificed: Fiber bundles are oriented randomly. Such bone is found in healing fractures and in certain metabolic bone diseases; it is termed "woven" bone.

Although there are at least 13 types of collagen, type 1 collagen is the only form found in bone. Several noncollagenous proteins constitute the 10 to 15 percent of bone protein that is not type 1 collagen. The most abundant of these proteins is osteonectin, a phosphorylated glycoprotein. This protein binds ionic calcium and hydroxyapatite. Other proteins synthesized in bone which bind calcium are osteocalcin, bone sialoprotein (BSP), thrombospondin (TSP), and osteopontin (OP). Osteocalcin contains residues of γ-carboxyl glutamic acid (gla), an amino acid which is biosynthesized posttranslationally by a vitamin K–dependent process. Chondroitin sulfate and heparin sulfate are also present.

A separate process for the mineralization of cartilage (endochondral calcification) involves exocytosis of matrix vesicles from the plasma membrane of osteoblasts. Mineralization occurs at specific gap regions in the matrix fibers. These gaps provide space for inorganic ions within the fibril structure.

The *osteoblast* is the principal bone-forming cell. It is responsible for the biosynthesis of the components of the matrix: collagen and ground substance. The enzyme alkaline phosphatase is displayed on the plasma membrane of osteoblasts and plays a critical role in matrix calcification. In fact, genetic alkaline phosphatase deficiency (hypophosphatasia) leads to osteomalacia. Hence, the osteoblast not only synthesizes the organic matrix of bone but also plays a role in its subsequent mineralization. Hence, serum alkaline phosphatase is a marker for bone formation. Osteoblasts arise from stem cells within the bone marrow, different from those which give rise to hematopoietic cells. Under appropriate stimulation, these cells proliferate and differentiate into osteoblast precursors and then mature osteoblasts. The osteoblast is always found adjacent to the lining layer of bone matrix which these cells are synthesizing, the osteoid seam, which is not yet calcified. Osteoblasts possess receptors for parathyroid hormone but not for calcitonin. In addition, they contain intracellular estrogen receptors.

Eventually osteoblasts trap themselves within the calcified matrix they have formed. Now embedded within the bone, they are termed *osteocytes*. They remain bathed in ECF via a network of canaliculi, which are the remnants of a network of thin cellular processes extending from the osteoblast along the bone surface during its formation. Whether an osteocyte is capable of resorbing calcified matrix around its perimeter is a subject of controversy. For the most part, osteocytes are considerably less active metabolically than are osteoblasts and osteoclasts.

The *osteoclast* is the bone cell responsible for resorption of matrix and release of calcium salts from the large reservoir of mineralized matrix into the ECF. Like the osteoblast, the osteoclast lines the calcified bone surface (Fig. 23-27). The osteoclast etches a pit, or Howship lacuna, also termed a resorption bay. The progenitor of the osteoclast appears to be a member of the monocyte/macrophage family. Differentiation occurs from the promonocyte stage; promonocyte precursor cells fuse to generate osteoclasts. The osteoclast is a giant multinucleated

FIGURE 23-27 Photomicrograph of osteitis fibrosa characteristic of severe hyperparathyroidism. Increased osteoclastic activity is evident. In some portions, the osteoclasts have cut through a microspicule of bone. Osteoblasts are depositing new osteoid on the surfaces of bone which has recently undergone osteoclastic resorption.

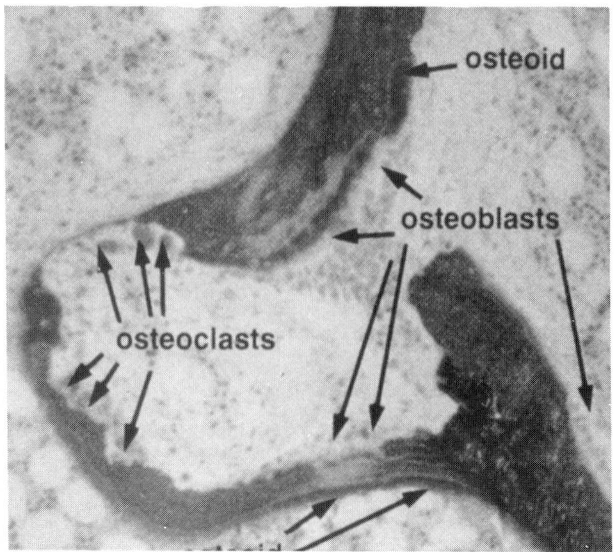

cell which contains 4 to 20 nuclei. It contains receptors for calcitonin but not for parathyroid hormone. The osteoclast adheres to the bony surface through a receptor-mediated attachment process.

When activated, osteoclasts mediate bone resorption by attaching to mineralized matrix of bone that has had surface collagen removed by collagenase, which is latent in bone and is activated by osteoclasts or secreted by the osteoclast itself. It has also been suggested that osteoblasts or bone lining cells may produce collagenase which is activated by the acid and lysosomal enzymes released by osteoclasts. Thus, the osteoblasts "prepare" the bone surface for osteoclastic resorption. Other studies using electron microscopy, however, indicate that osteoclasts can resorb bone without a need for other supporting cells. Heterodimeric plasma membrane receptors on the surface of the osteoclast, termed *integrins*, interact with macromolecules present in the matrix of bone, such as osteocalcin, osteopontin, and other proteins.[194,195] These macromolecules share a common sequence of arginine-glycine-aspartic acid (R-G-D). When enough integrins on the cell surface of an osteoclast bind to bone matrix, the osteoclast is anchored and a microscopic sealed environment is created[196] (Fig. 23-28) which has been termed the *ruffled border*; in reality, this is a series of folds and invaginations of the plasma membrane. Contractile proteins within the cytoplasm of an activated osteoclast help the osteoclast form and maintain this sealed environment as well as move along the surface of bone, resulting in the excavation of a trough.

The space between the ruffled border and the mineralized bone matrix becomes the functional equivalent of an extracellular lysosome. The osteoclast releases numerous enzymes and acid via the hydrogen-potassium-ATPase (proton) pump[197–200] into this sequestered space. The enzyme carbonic anhydrase (type II) also contributes to the creation of an acid microenvironment.[201,202] The coordinated action of these enzymes and acid results in catabolism of bone by breakdown of bone proteins and release of calcium salts into the ECF. Cysteine proteinases such as cathepsin B are also released and/or activated.[203] The importance of each of these individual components to the process of osteolysis is demonstrated by the fact that blockade of the cysteine proteases, carbonic anhydrase, or the proton pump can independently block bone resorption in vitro and in vivo in animal models and in human genetic disorders such as one type of osteopetrosis in which there is a deficiency of carbonic anhydrase type II and vastly diminished bone resorption.[204,205]

These processes of resorption and formation are closely coupled, resulting in the maintenance of bone volume and structural integrity as well as mineral ion homeostasis. The sequence of events is a cycle of activation-resorption-formation (Figs. 23-26 and 23-29). Once osteoclasts have been activated and have formed a pit, they depart. Osteoblasts are then able to move into the resorption bay and fill it with new bone matrix.

The local regulation or coupling of bone resorption and formation is not well understood. There is intensive research under way to identify a coupling factor or factors. It is clear that osteoclastic activity can be influenced by cytokines such as interleukin 1, tumor necrosis factor (TNF), interferons, prostaglan-

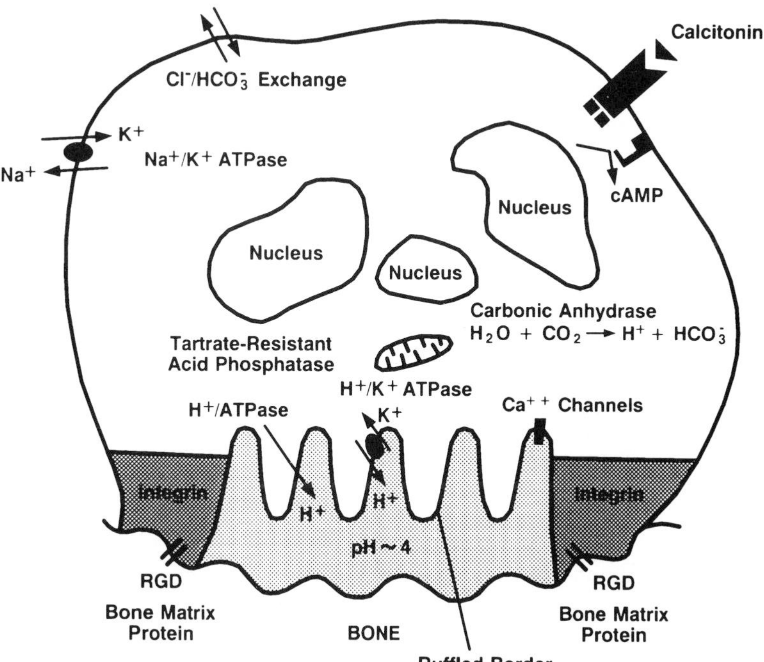

FIGURE 23-28 Osteoclast-mediated bone resorption. The osteoclast attaches to the bone surface via integrin-mediated binding to bone matrix bone proteins. When enough integrin binding has occurred, the osteoclast is anchored and a sealed space is formed. The repeatedly folded plasma membrane creates a "ruffled" border. Secreted into the sealed space are acid and enzymes forming an extracellular "lysosome."

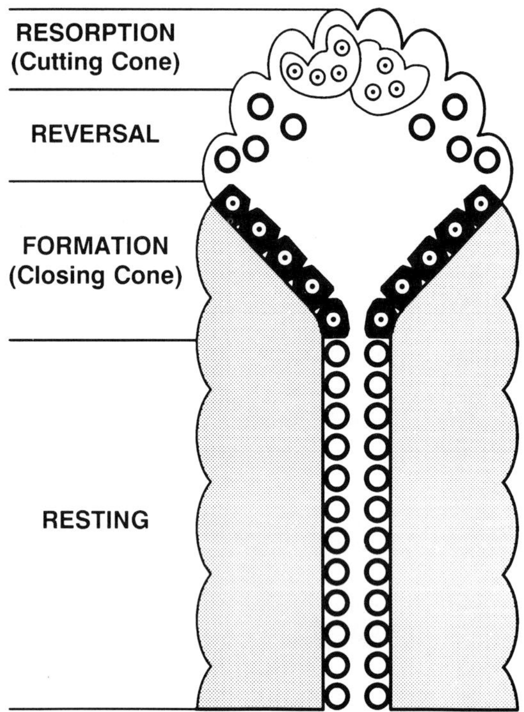

FIGURE 23-29 Schematic representation of the four principal stages involved in the formation of a new basic structural unit in cortical bone. *(Reprinted with permission from Parisien et al.[447])*

dins, and growth factors. These substances may be produced by bone cells and act in an autocrine or paracrine fashion or enter through the circulation. There is speculation that osteoblasts may "seed" their own anabolic activity for bone. It is known that osteoblasts secrete insulin-like growth factor-I (IGF-I), transforming growth factor β (TGF-β), or other growth factors. These proteins may be encased within the bone matrix during formation. Later, during resorption by osteoclasts, they may be released and recruit osteoblasts to the resorption pit and stimulate their biosynthetic activity. TGF-β may also inhibit osteoclastic activity at the same resorption site, setting the stage for osteoblastic activity. Hence, sequestered growth factors within the bone matrix may be the actual coupling factors. Their diffusion locally may result in the proliferation and differentiation of osteoblast precursors.

The actions of PTH on bone are expressed through an unusual cascade. An increase in the number and activity of osteoclasts is the hallmark of PTH action (Fig. 23-27). Yet when examined in vitro, osteoclasts appear to have few if any PTH receptors.[206] Rather, the hormonally responsive cell is the osteoblast, the cell normally associated with bone formation.[207] Presumably, when exposed to PTH, osteoblasts secrete a cytokine(s) which acts locally and directly on osteoclasts to recruit them to sites ready for bone resorption and increase the resorptive activity of osteoclasts.[208,209] Alternatively, PTH-stimulated osteoblasts may secrete factors which act through an intermediate cell, such as a monocyte, which in turn secretes a factor that stimulates or recruits osteoclasts (Fig. 23-30). Candidate molecules which are secreted locally in bone and are known to stimulate bone resorption include interleukin 1 (IL-1), tumor necrosis factor (TNF-α), interleukin 6 (IL-6), prostaglandin E_2 (PGE_2), granulocyte-macrophage colony-stimulating factor (GM-CSF), and leukemia inhibitory factor (LIF or DIF),[210–218] as discussed earlier.

The concept of a "coupling" factor which is secreted by the osteoblast and tightly regulates osteoclast activity has also been put forth. It is not certain whether any of the locally (in bone) secreted molecules cited above are candidates to be this factor or indeed whether the factor actually exists. Nevertheless, at least two groups have attempted to isolate and characterize a putative osteoblast-secreted bone-resorbing or "coupling" factor.[219,220]

Through its action on osteoblasts, PTH can have effects which stimulate bone formation and result in an overall anabolic rather than catabolic effect on the skeleton.[221–227] It seems likely that bone formation mediated by PTH results from an osteoblast autocrine mechanism. Exposure of osteoblasts to PTH leads to increased secretion or activity of certain growth factors, such as insulin-like growth factors I and II, TGF-β, and fibroblast growth factor

FIGURE 23-30 Parathyroid hormone activates osteoclasts indirectly. Receptors for the hormone are present on osteoblasts. Intercellular mediators secreted by the osteoblast act either on the osteoclast directly or on intermediate cells to recruit and activate osteoclasts. Osteoclasts then attach to the bony surface, resorb mineralized matrix, and release calcium salts into the extracellular fluid. *(Modified from Rodan and Martin.[208])*

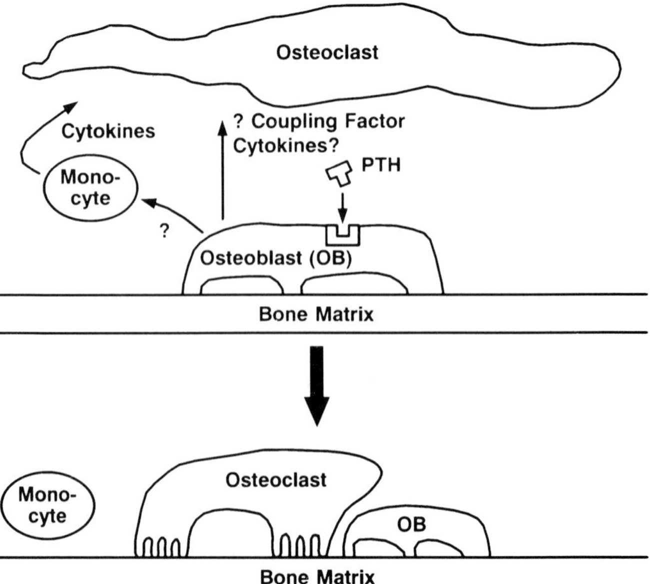

(FGF). These factors may then, in an autocrine manner, stimulate osteoblastic activity and bone formation,[228–230] as discussed above.

Again, the second messengers responsible for expression of PTH bioactivity have not been determined definitively. PTH clearly stimulates adenylyl cyclase activity, and the administration of cAMP analogues such as dibutyryl cAMP is capable of producing PTH-like cellular responses such as increased alkaline phosphatase activity in osteoblasts. In isolated perfused bone organ assays, infusion of PTH results in increased cAMP excretion in the draining vein.[231–234] However, the ultimate outcome of PTH action, such as bone resorption and release of calcium from the mineralized matrix, lags several hours behind the rapid and transitory increase in cAMP levels (Fig. 23-11).

Increases in intracellular calcium serving as a second messenger for PTH action in osteoblasts have also been proposed, but conflicting data have been obtained. While some investigators have been able to show a brisk increase in intracellular calcium after exposure to PTH,[168] the time course of response has been less compelling in many other studies. Furthermore, the quantity of calcium released is small compared to the amounts observed in other hormonal systems where calcium has been more clearly established as a second messenger. The interpretation of the results is also confounded by the observation that only a minority of the osteoblasts present respond to PTH by increasing intracellular calcium levels. Finally, there is no clear linkage between the changes in intracellular calcium and any distal parameter of hormonal action, such as increased alkaline phosphatase activity and activation of osteoclasts.

Although the discussion has focused on osteoblasts as the PTH target cell, it is fair to say that the true target cell has not been definitively identified. Osteoblast progenitor cells may represent the actual target cell, as has been proposed in recent studies.[235–237]

In addition to osteoblasts and their precursors, it is possible (but less likely) that osteocytes respond to PTH. These cells have been particularly difficult to study. The small size of the population and their microenvironment (lining endosteal surfaces) have limited access to these cells. At present, there are no representative cell lines which can be studied in isolation.

Receptor Distribution

The rather surprising finding that the osteoblasts and/or the osteoblast precursor contain many more receptors than do osteoclasts[238,239] and appear to be the target cells for PTH raises important questions regarding tissue distribution for the receptor in cells other than bone and kidney. PTH receptors have been found on other cell types, such as mononuclear leukocytes, fibroblasts, and vascular tissue.[113,240–242] The discovery of PTHrP raises even more intriguing questions regarding the distribution of receptors that interact with PTH. Even though both hormones appear to interact with the same receptors,[125–130] as discussed above, the novel biological properties and tissue distribution of the new hormone (described elsewhere in this chapter) make it likely that new PTH receptor–containing tissues will be identified.[243–252]

CALCITONIN

Introduction and Historical Notes

Although calcitonin has potent effects on mineral ion flux through its actions on kidney and bone, its role in the normal physiology of humans is not known. The hormone was discovered by Copp and coworkers in the early 1960s.[253,254] It is a 32-amino acid peptide whose amino terminus contains a cyclic structure involving seven amino acids bridged by a disulfide bond (Fig. 23-31). The hormone decreases blood calcium levels by inhibiting bone resorption and promoting renal excretion of calcium.[255–257] Phosphaturia is also stimulated by calcitonin.

FIGURE 23-31 The sequence of human calcitonin. The molecule contains a seven-membered ring linked by a disulfide bridge at the N terminus.

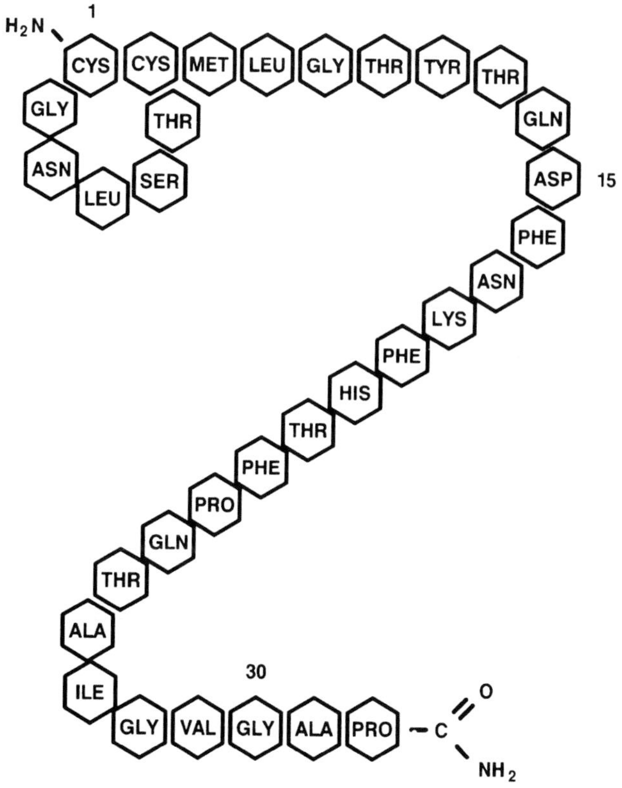

The existence of the hormone was postulated after Copp and colleagues found that perfusion of the parathyroid and thyroid glands with a hypercalcemic perfusate produced a more rapid fall in systemic blood calcium than that produced by surgical removal of the parathyroid glands.[258] Although there was initial confusion regarding the glandular and cellular origin of calcitonin and although for a period of time the parathyroid glands were thought to be the source,[258] the hormone has been documented to be biosynthesized by the parafollicular or C cells of the thyroid gland, which have a different embryologic origin than the rest of the gland, arising from neural crest cells.[259] Calcitonin clearly plays an important role in calcium regulation in lower species such as fish, in which the major homeostatic challenge is maintenance of blood calcium levels when the organism is literally bathed in an external environment (the sea) containing a high concentration of calcium. The evolutionary precursor of the thyroid C cell in fish is the ultimobranchial gland, an older structure (phylogenetically) than the parathyroid gland.

In humans and other terrestrial animals, it is unlikely that calcitonin plays an essential physiological role. Evidence supporting this notion includes the finding that the hormone circulates at very low levels in humans and that surgical removal of the thyroid gland (normally the only source of the hormone) has no appreciable effect on calcium metabolism. Furthermore, the high levels of circulating calcitonin that occur with medullary carcinoma of the thyroid are not accompanied by hypocalcemia. In humans, calcitonin remains "a hormone in search of a function."[257]

Therefore, much of the medical interest in calcitonin arises because this hormone serves as a tumor marker: Calcitonin is secreted by medullary carcinoma of the thyroid (one of the neoplasms which occur as part of the hereditary disorders of multiple endocrine neoplasia type II and type III[257,260]) (see Chap. 11). Removal of the tumor is accompanied by the return of calcitonin to normal or undetectable levels; recurrence of tumor is often heralded by renewed elevation of blood calcitonin levels. Thus, the CT radioimmunoassay can be used to monitor the status of the malignancy and the efficacy of surgical treatment. In addition to basal secretion of calcitonin by such tumors, secretagogues of calcitonin such as calcium and gastrin can be used in stimulatory tests to reveal the presence of early and otherwise undetectable or premalignant lesions[255–257] in subjects with a hereditary predisposition to developing the disease. Protocols for provocative testing of calcitonin are provided in Chap. 28.

Clinical interest in calcitonin also stems from its use as therapeutic agent for the treatment of hypercalcemia, Paget disease of bone, and osteoporosis (discussed below). The hormone is available in several homologues from different species,[255,256] and there is a 10- to 40-fold range in potency between human calcitonin and the highly potent salmon form of the hormone. It was first chemically synthesized in 1968.[261,262]

At the basic level, the biosynthesis and intracellular processing of calcitonin (discussed below) are complex and make a fascinating story, serving as one of the paradigms for hormonal biosynthesis in modern molecular biology.

Biological Effects and Mechanism of Action

When administered intravenously, calcitonin produces a rapid and dramatic decline in levels of serum calcium and phosphorus. These fluxes in mineral ions result from the action of the hormone directly on bone and kidney. At the level of bone, calcitonin directly inhibits bone resorption by inhibiting osteoclast activity. Calcitonin receptors have been documented to be present on mammalian osteoclasts, the principal bone-resorbing cell.[263,264] Calcitonin appears to have no influence on the inhibition of bone formation or mineralization.[265] The magnitude of its action is increased in conditions which increase bone turnover and therefore the number of active osteoclasts recruited to mineralized surfaces of bone, such as skeletal growth in young animals, immobilization, Paget disease, disorders of increased parathyroid hormone levels, or Graves' disease (of the thyroid).

After exposure to calcitonin, the morphology of the active osteoclast changes rapidly.[266] The multinucleated cell shrinks in size, and its ruffled border, which is presumed to be the essential morphologic feature for the conduct of bone resorption, retracts from the resorptive surface.

At the level of the kidney, calcitonin, like PTH, decreases the threshold for urinary reabsorption of phosphorus, thus promoting increased urinary phosphorus excretion.[255,256] In addition, calcitonin promotes an increase in the renal fractional excretion of calcium. These effects are thought to result from the action of the hormone on the proximal tubule. However, these renal actions are unlikely to be of physiologic or even pathophysiologic consequence, as demonstrated by the presence of normal mineral metabolism in patients with medullary carcinoma of the thyroid who exhibit extraordinarily high levels of calcitonin in the blood.

Calcitonin appears to utilize cAMP as the second messenger for expression of bioactivity on bone and on the renal tubule. Although calcitonin works through cAMP, it is not a contributor to nephrogenous cAMP and therefore does not complicate the evaluation of patients with hyperparathyroidism or hypercalcemia of malignancy.

The newest insights into the CT system come

from the recent cloning of the porcine CT receptor.[87] The deduced nucleotide sequence of the receptor cDNA encodes a 482-amino acid protein. Like other receptors which stimulate adenylyl cyclase activity, the CT receptor interacts with a guanyl nucleotide regulatory protein and therefore possesses the characteristic scaffold of seven membrane-spanning domains (Fig. 23-32). In one of the transmembrane domains (domain VII, discussed above), the CT receptor shares great homology (17 of 18 amino acids) with the PTH/PTHrP receptor (Fig. 23-13) and approximately 32 percent homology and 56 percent similarity across four of the seven (IV, V, VI, VII) transmembrane domains. Except for the secretion receptor, the homology of the CT receptor and the PTH/PTHrP receptor with other G protein–linked receptors is low (<12 percent). Therefore, these three receptors, together with the glucagon, VIP, and secretin receptors, may represent a newly identified subgroup of the family of G protein–linked rhodopsin-like receptors. Like the PTH/PTHrP receptor, but unlike the beta-adrenergic receptor, the CT receptor contains a signal sequence at the N terminus. The N-terminal exoplasmic domain contains three potential N-linked glycosylation sites and conserved extracellular cysteine residues (Fig. 23-32). As predicted, the CT receptor has a moderate- to large-sized N-terminal extracellular domain 147 amino acids long, intermediate in size between that of the beta-adrenergic receptor and the luteinizing hormone receptor, which is thought to bind the hormone, and a unique long C-terminal intracellular region which contains several potential phosphorylation sites. Like the PTH receptor,[68] the CT receptor appears to be able to interact not only with $G_s\alpha$ but also with the G protein involved in the activation of protein kinase C.[267] The structural domain(s) within the receptor responsible for this biological property has not been identified. The cloned expressed receptor binds CT with 6 nM affinity and also binds calcitonin gene–related peptide (CGRP) (see below), but less avidly than CT (as predicted), and displays down regulation. It is found in osteoclasts and human giant cell tumors of bone but not in osteoblasts. Preliminary Southern blot analysis indicates the presence of only one gene encoding the CT receptor.

Biochemistry and Molecular Biology

Although many questions remain regarding the role of calcitonin in normal physiology and its contribution to pathophysiology, considerable information

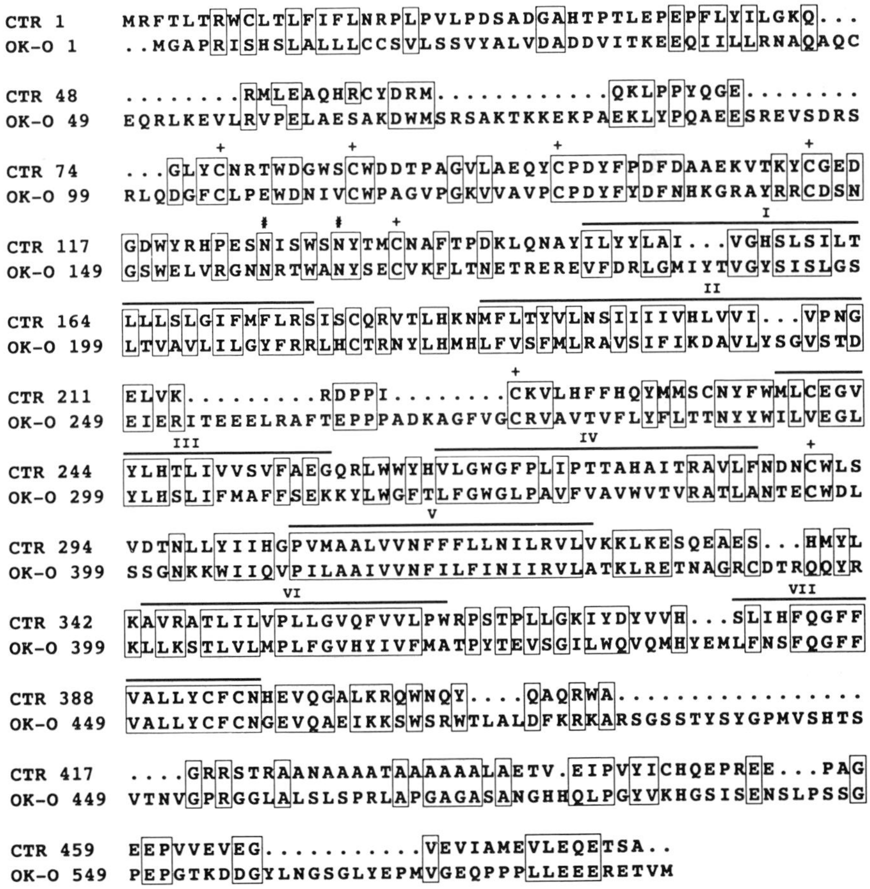

FIGURE 23-32 An alignment of the calcitonin receptor vs. the PTH/PTHrP receptor (OK-O) from opossum kidney cells. Shaded boxes represent identity or similarity. The bars above the sequences represent the transmembrane domains. The symbol # indicates N-linked glycosylation sites, and + indicates conserved cysteins. The GenBank accession number is M74420 for the calcitonin receptor and M74445 for the PTH/PTHrP receptor. *(Reprinted with permission from Lin et al.[87])*

```
CTR 1      MRFTLTRWCLTLFIFLNRPLPVLPDSADGAHTPTLEPEPFLYILGKQ...
OK-O 1     ..MGAPRISHSLALLLCCSVLSSVYALVDADDVITKEEQIILLRNAQAQC

CTR 48     ........RMLEAQHRCYDRM............QKLPPYQGE........
OK-O 49    EQRLKEVLRVPELAESAKDWMSRSAKTKKEKPAEKLYPQAEESREVSDRS

           +  +  +  +
CTR 74     ...GLYCNRTWDGWSCWDDTPAGVLAEQYCPDYFPDFDAAEKVTKYCGED
OK-O 99    RLQDGFCLPEWDNIVCWPAGVPGKVVAVPCPDYFYDFNHKGRAYRRCDSN

           #  #  +  I
CTR 117    GDWYRHPESNISWSNYTMCNAFTPDKLQNAYILYYLAI...VGHSLSILT
OK-O 149   GSWELVRGNNRTWANYSECVKFLTNETREREVFDRLGMIYTVGYSISLGS

           II
CTR 164    LLLSLGIFMFLRSISCQRVTLHKNMFLTYVLNSIIIIVHLVVI...VPNG
OK-O 199   LTVAVLILGYFRRLHCTRNYLHMHLFVSFMLRAVSIFIKDAVLYSGVSTD

           +
CTR 211    ELVK.........RDPPI........CKVLHFFHQYMMSCNYFWMLCEGV
OK-O 249   EIERITEEELRAFTEPPPADKAGFVGCRVAVTVFLYFLTTNYYWILVEGL

           III  IV  +
CTR 244    YLHTLIVVSVFAEGQRLWWYHVLGWGFPLIPTTAHAITRAVLFNDNCWLS
OK-O 299   YLHSLIFMAFFSEKKYLWGFTLFGWGLPAVFVAVWVTVRATLANTECWDL

           V
CTR 294    VDTNLLYIIHGPVMAALVVNFFFLLNILRVLVKKLKESQEAES...HMYL
OK-O 399   SSGNKKWIIQVPILAAIVVNFILFINIIRVLATKLRETNAGRCDTRQQYR

           VI  VII
CTR 342    KAVRATLILVPLLGVQFVVLPWRPSTPLLGKIYDYVVH...SLIHFQGFF
OK-O 399   KLLKSTLVLMPLFGVHYIVFMATPYTEVSGILWQVQMHYEMLFNSFQGFF

CTR 388    VALLYCFCNHEVQGALKRQWNQY....QAQRWA.................
OK-O 449   VALLYCFCNGEVQAEIKKSWSRWTLALDFKRKARSGSSTYSYGPMVSHTS

CTR 417    ....GRRSTRAANAAAATAAAAALAETV.EIPVYICHQEPREE...PAG
OK-O 449   VTNVGPRGGLALSLSPRLAPGAGASANGHHQLPGYVKHGSISENSLPSSG

CTR 459    EEPVVEVEG...........VEVIAMEVLEQETSA..
OK-O 549   PEPGTKDDGYLNGSGLYEPMVGEQPPPLLEEERETVM
```

has emerged from basic investigations regarding its interaction with receptors and its molecular biology.

The 32-amino acid size of the hormone is invariant across species.[255,256] In addition, all the homologues contain a 7-amino acid cyclic structure at the N terminus and a proline amide at the carboxyl terminus. While homology within the ring structure is largely conserved across various species, the central linear portion of the hormone displays great diversity (Fig. 23-33). Only 9 of the 32 amino acid residues across the 10 species which have been structurally elucidated are constant. Interestingly, the nonmammalian calcitonins have higher potency than do mammalian calcitonins even when used in mammalian-based systems or in vivo in humans. Salmon CT, for instance, appears to be approximately 10- to 40-fold more active than human calcitonin in humans.[268] In fact, the interaction of salmon CT with receptors is so avid that almost no dissociation is observed: The interaction with receptor is functionally irreversible.[269–271] This is a very unusual feature of the calcitonin hormone-receptor system.

Beyond the information regarding structure-function relations for the hormone provided by the great sequence diversity present in nature, numerous structure-activity studies have been performed with synthetic analogues of the hormone.[268,272,273]

Shortening of the peptide at either end of the molecule results in nearly complete loss of biological activity,[268,274] although there is at least one exception to this general observation.[275] In the central portion of the molecule, many of the amino acids appear to serve a spacer role and can be substituted without having much of an impact on bioactivity. The 7-amino acid disulfide-linked ring is important for bioactivity but is not essential. The sulfur atoms can be replaced with methylenes,[276] and there is one example of opening of the ring with preservation of bioactivity.[277]

The biosynthesis of calcitonin from its gene occurs by a complex and intriguing process[278,279] (Fig. 23-34). The calcitonin gene is composed of six exons. The gene has the potential to generate at least two different mature mRNAs and the peptides each of them encodes. By one set of splicing routes, the calcitonin precursor of 141 amino acids is generated. Calcitonin is encoded at the C terminus of the precursor molecule and is the major processed peptide. The thyroid C cell follows this pattern of splicing to produce calcitonin. In other tissues, such as neurons, a 128-amino acid precursor is generated which contains a peptide termed calcitonin gene–related peptide (CGRP) but no calcitonin.[279] CGRP is a 37-amino acid peptide with considerable homology to calcitonin. Like calcitonin, it contains a cyclic disulfide bridge region and an amidated C terminus. CGRP biosynthesis has been localized to the dorsal spinal cord and the pituitary.[280] Like calcitonin, it is located at the C terminus of its precursor protein and is encoded by the fourth exon in the series of five which are spliced together to generate the mature mRNA. The calcitonin-coding exon is excised in this splicing arrangement and therefore is not present in the mature mRNA encoding CGRP.

Through interaction with its own receptor, CGRP possesses striking vasodilatory activity: It is one of the most potent vasodilators known.[281] It causes vascular dilatation whether administered intravenously or into the cerebrospinal fluid,[282] leading to the speculation that the hormone may play a role in cerebral vascular regulation. Arterial dilatation stimulated by CGRP appears to involve the activation of K^+ channels,[283] particularly a K^+/ATPase channel. In this regard, CGRP appears to act through a mechanism shared by that of vasoactive intestinal peptide (VIP) and endothelium-derived relaxant factor (EDRF). CGRP probably can also act as a neurotransmitter.[284] It has been shown to have effects on food intake in laboratory rats when administered into the central nervous system, decreasing food intake and spontaneous nocturnal eating[285] and inhibiting gastric acid secretion.[286] CGRP is also able to interact with and activate the calcitonin receptor.[287,288] The calcitonin-like biological properties of CGRP on osteoclasts and elsewhere are therefore directly traceable to the hormone's interaction with calcitonin receptors.[289–291] This ability of both CT and CGRP to interact with the other hormone's receptor has provided the impetus for the synthesis of new "hybrid" analogues which combine structural elements of each hormone in a new molecule.[292]

Interestingly, both calcitonin and CGRP precursor mRNAs also code for additional peptides which are presumed to be translated, termed "cryptic" peptides.[293–296] For the calcitonin precursor, which contains a signal sequence and a pro region, there is also a 16-amino acid carboxyl-terminal adjacent peptide (C-CAP) and an N-terminal adjacent peptide (N-CAP). C-CAP is known to be cosecreted with calcitonin by medullary carcinomas.[297] Such cryptic peptides have now been found in the precursors of many other peptide hormones. Their physiologic role in the CT/CGRP precursor is still uncertain, although some calcium-regulating actions have been reported.[295,298] However, the discovery of new and potentially biologically active peptides within the genes for established hormones indicates that there is a capacity for diversity of biological active peptides not previously envisioned in the endocrine system.

Calcitonin as a Therapeutic Agent

Calcitonin is effective in the acute treatment of hypercalcemia of malignancy.[299–306] Both humoral hypercalcemia of malignancy and hypercalcemia associated with extensive metastases to bone are associated with recruitment by tumor of the normal cellular apparatus for bone resorption: osteoclasts.

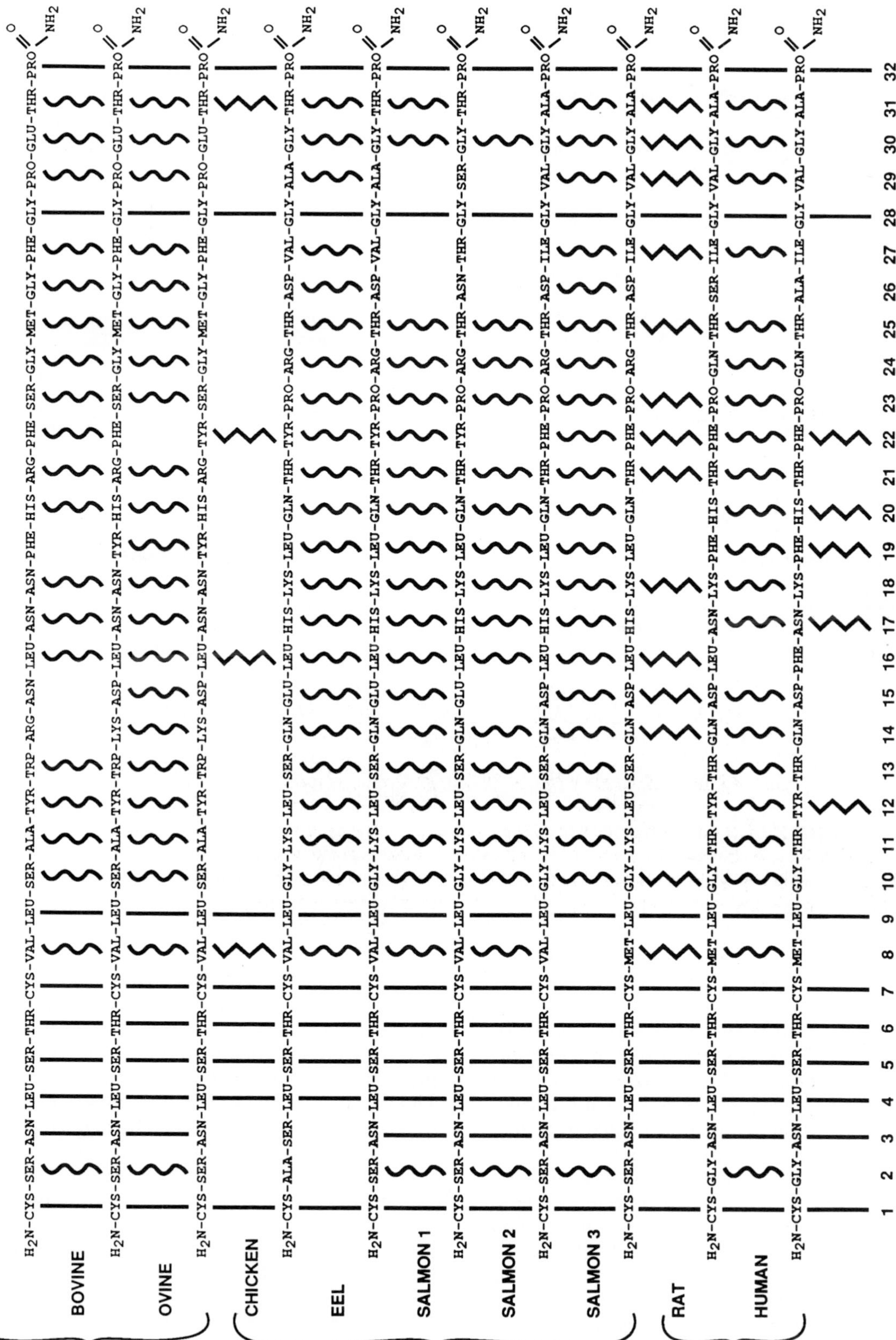

FIGURE 23-33 Comparison of the sequence of homologues of calcitonin from various species. Straight lines indicate conservation across all species. Wavy lines indicate conservation within groups only. *(Modified and reprinted with permission from Leonard J. Deftos, Calcitonin, in Primer on the Metabolic Bone Diseases and Disorders of Mineral Metabolism, Murray J. Favus, ed., Am. Soc. Bone and Mineral Research, Kelseyville, California, p. 53, 1990).*

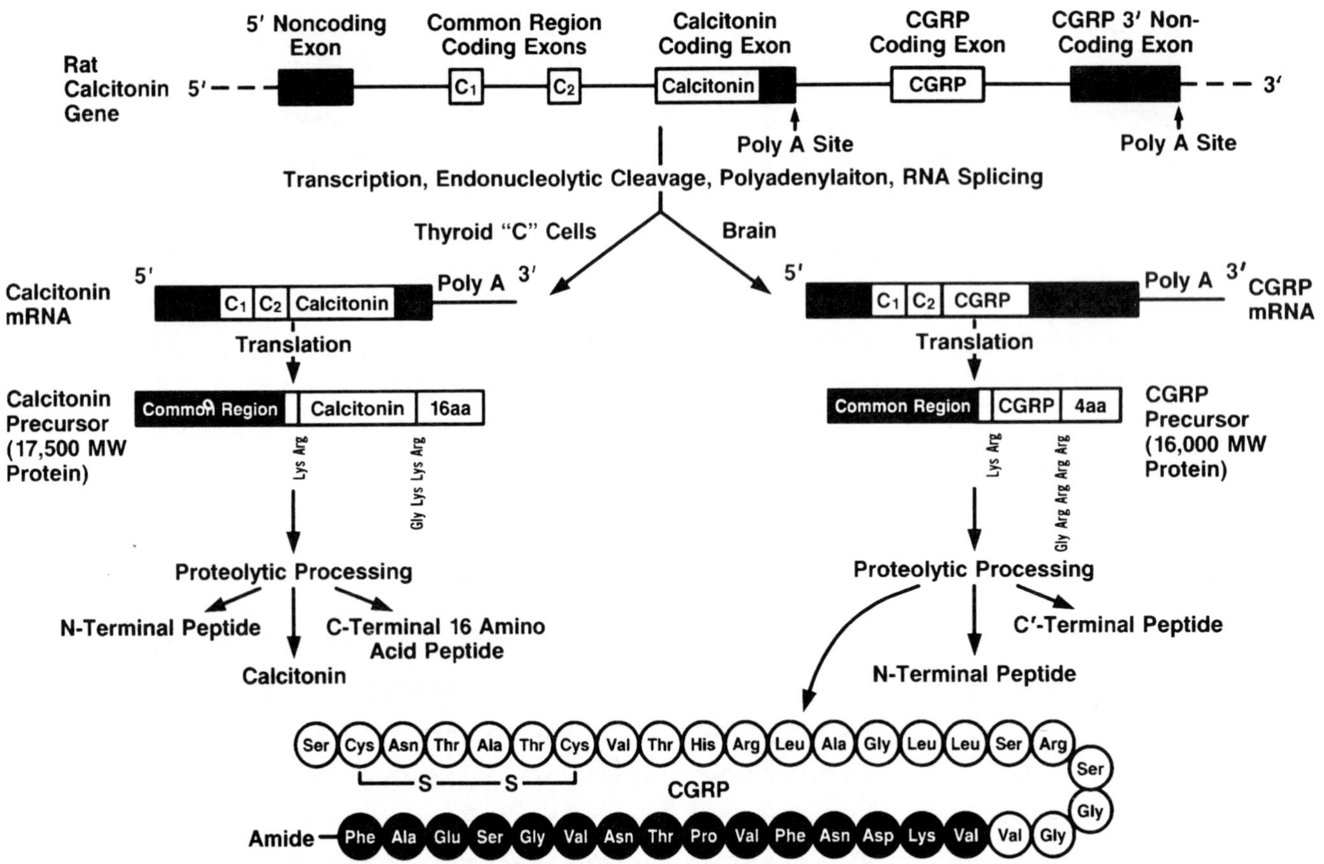

FIGURE 23-34 Alternative RNA processing pathways in the expression of the calcitonin gene. Calcitonin is biosynthesized in thyroid C cells; CGRP mRNA is produced in the brain. In addition to calcitonin and CGRP, N-terminal and C-terminal peptides are encoded in both the precursor of calcitonin and the precursor of CGRP. *(Reprinted with permission from Rosenfeld et al.*[279]*)*

Therefore, calcitonin, which acts on osteoclasts, is effective in blocking further bone resorption and produces a rapid lowering of serum calcium levels. Although the effects of administered calcitonin on mineral ion flux are prompt and large in magnitude, in many instances they are limited to the acute period. Chronic administration of calcitonin leads to a classic picture of tachyphylaxis within days.[299] It seems most likely that this tachyphylaxis is due to down regulation of receptors.[307] In some patients, tachyphylaxis of the response to calcitonin may be delayed for a few days by the coadministration of glucocorticoids.[308] Similarly, although acute hypercalcemia is a documented stimulus for calcitonin secretion, chronic hypercalcemia has not been consistently associated with increased levels of calcitonin.

In Paget disease of bone, there are many localized regions throughout bone where bone turnover (both formation and resorption) is highly accelerated. Although the linkage of formation and resorption in Paget disease is close enough to prevent the development of hypercalcemia, calcitonin is nevertheless able to reduce the metabolic activity and associated pain resulting from increased bone turnover.[306] Symptomatic relief occurs within weeks in approximately two-thirds of patients. Biochemical indexes of improvement such as reduction in serum alkaline phosphatase usually follow within 3 to 6 months. The usual starting dose is 100 units per day subcutaneously. After biochemical efficacy is evident, the dose can be reduced, but usually not below 50 units three times per week. Unfortunately, "escape" from calcitonin's effects occurs commonly, perhaps acutely as a result of down regulation of receptors or long-term via the development of anticalcitonin (salmon) antibodies.[309]

At this time, calcitonin is available in the United States and both parenteral and intranasal formulations are available in Europe. Salmon calcitonin is used more widely in the United States because of its enhanced potency and for historical reasons, while human calcitonin is used more widely in Europe. The clinical use of salmon calcitonin generates antibodies in most patients. However, despite the differences in amino acid sequence between the isoforms (Fig. 23-33), the antibodies generated usually are not neutralizing, and their presence does not seem to correlate with resistance to the hormone.[310,311] In cases where resistance to salmon calcitonin develops after long-term administration and is presumed to be antibody-mediated, switching to the human form is indicated.[306] A more detailed discussion of Paget disease and its treatment can be found in Chap. 24.

The use of calcitonin as a therapeutic agent for the treatment of osteoporosis varies in different regions of the world. In Europe, calcitonin is used to prevent loss of bone mineral and ameliorate the pain associated with osteoporosis-related vertebral fractures and sometimes with metabolic bone disease. How calcitonin produces analgesia is uncertain; this may be due to a central, perhaps endorphin-mediated, effect. Calcitonin treatment may increase bone mineral density for 1 or 2 years. However, the positive effects of calcitonin or bone mineral density in postmenopausal osteoporosis are modest and may begin to plateau or even reverse within 12 to 24 months despite continued treatment.[312] Furthermore, there is no convincing evidence that calcitonin treatment reduces fractures.[313,314] Therefore, in the United States, calcitonin is used less frequently than in Europe for the treatment of osteoporosis, although it does have Food and Drug Administration approval for this indication.

VITAMIN D

Historical Introduction

Rickets became endemic in European cities during their explosive growth in the industrial revolution. By the late nineteenth century epidemiologic investigations in several European countries had found that environmental factors having to do with crowding rather than poor nutrition made city dwellers prone to rickets, which was virtually unheard of among impoverished children in the countryside. As early as 1822, the Polish physician Sniadecki wrote that "if the parents' financial status permits, it is best to take the children [with rickets] out into the country and keep them as much as possible in the dry, open and pure air. If not, at least they should be carried out in the open air, especially in the sun, direct action of which on our bodies must be regarded as one of the most efficient methods for the prevention and cure of the disease."[315] In the British Isles, "systematic use of sunbaths . . . and the education of the public to the appreciation of sunshine as a means of health" was proposed by Palm in 1890. However, this simple notion never caught on. In 1919 Huldschinsky cured rickets with phototherapy[316]; by then, the nutritional and photochemical approaches to rickets were about to merge.

Cod liver oil had been used for treatment of rickets in the nineteenth century. In 1922, McCollum and colleagues identified a specific antirachitic activity in cod liver oil by showing that destruction of vitamin A activity by oxidation did not abolish antirachitic activity.[317] Shortly thereafter, two groups showed that UV irradiation of food substances could also produce the antirachitic activity that by then was called vitamin D.[318,319] By the 1930s milk in the United States was fortified with vitamin D by irradiation, leading to the virtual abolition of rickets. The form of vitamin D produced by the irradiation of yeast extract was shown to be ergocalciferol (vitamin D_2); that produced in skin was cholecalciferol (vitamin D_3). What was referred to as vitamin D_1 turned out to be a mixture of two forms, and the term is now obsolete.

Knowledge of the chemistry of vitamin D did not advance until the late 1960s, when work in the laboratories of DeLuca, Fraser, Norman, and others established that vitamin D is a prohormone which is converted to highly active forms by successive hydroxylation at the 25- and 1-positions.[320] This work emphasized what was clear from their forerunners: Vitamin D is both a vitamin when ingested from nutritional sources and a hormone which they showed is produced in the skin and activated sequentially in the liver and kidney.

Biosynthesis and Chemistry

Cholecalciferol (vitamin D_3) is produced nonenzymatically in the skin from 7-dehydrocholesterol upon exposure to ultraviolet (UV) light of 290 to 310 nm. Upon absorption of photons of this wavelength by the 5,7-diene, the B ring is split and an unstable intermediate (previtamin D_3) is formed. Previtamin D is then slowly converted to cholecalciferol by a temperature-dependent nonenzymatic process.[321] The concentration of 7-dehydrocholesterol in skin is not limiting; the amount of cholecalciferol produced is a function of the dose of UV light and the solar zenith angle. At northern latitudes, where the incident angle of the sun's rays is low, little vitamin D is produced, particularly during the winter months. This probably accounts for the appearance of nutritional rickets in late winter. Ultraviolet light of 290 to 310 nm is efficiently absorbed by sunscreens and by the endogenous pigment melanin, so that for a given exposure blacks produce considerably smaller amounts of vitamin D than do whites.[322]

Cholecalciferol (vitamin D_3) is the form of vitamin D in fish liver oils and other animal sources, whereas the other major calciferol, ergocalciferol (vitamin D_2), is similarly produced from its precursor ergosterol by irradiation in plants and irradiated yeast. Cholecalciferol differs from ergocalciferol only in the side chain (Fig. 23-35), and the two compounds have equivalent biological activity in humans (40,000 IU/mg) and undergo identical metabolic conversion to active forms. Thus, both the endogenous

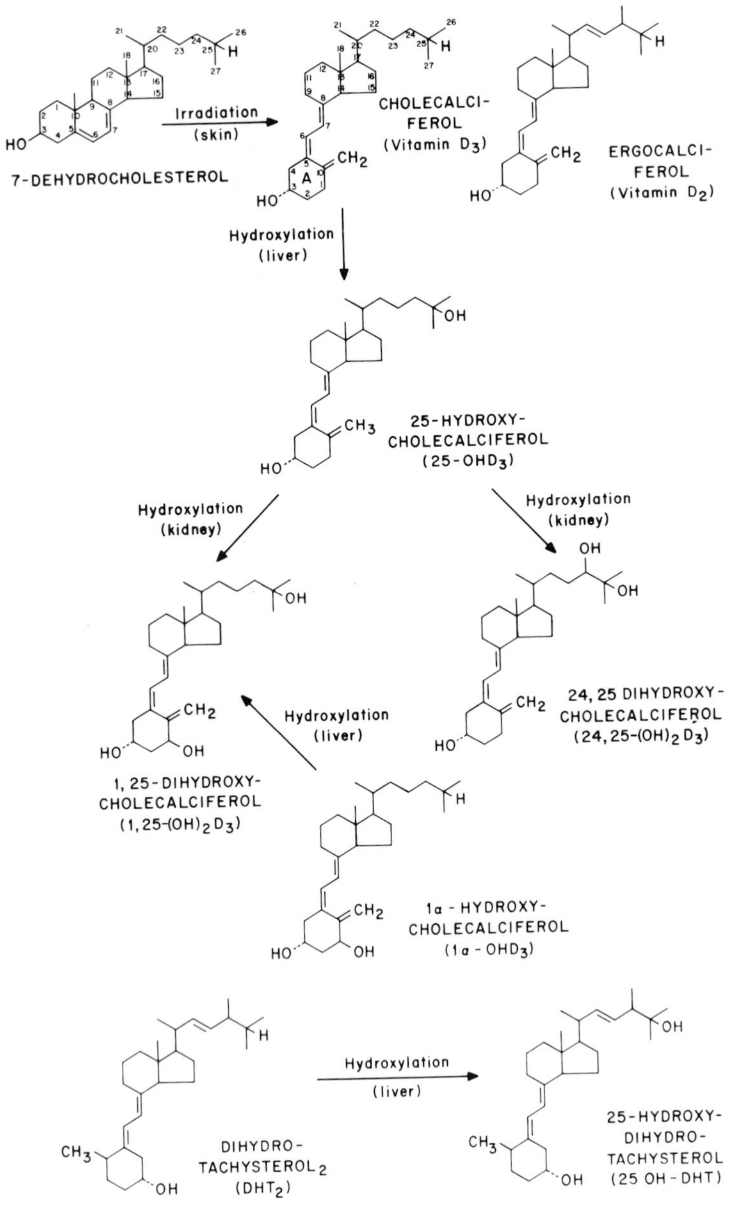

FIGURE 23-35 Chemical structures of the major vitamin D metabolites and analogues. The numbering system is based on that of cholesterol, and the A ring of cholecalciferol is so designated.

form of vitamin D, cholecalciferol, and the plant form, ergocalciferol, can be ingested in foodstuffs. In this chapter, the term *vitamin D* without a subscript will be used generically to apply to both forms.

As will be discussed in detail below, vitamin D is activated by sequential hydroxylations in the 25- and 1α-positions (Fig. 23-35). The structures of two therapeutically useful analogues are also shown there. 1α-Hydroxycholecalciferol can be synthesized from cholesterol and is useful as an analogue of 1α,25-dihydroxycholecalciferol. Dihydrotachysterol (DHT) is a synthetic analogue in which the A ring is rotated 180° so that the position of the 3-hydroxyl sterically resembles that of the 1α-hydroxyl in active vitamin D metabolites. Although its potency is only threefold higher than that of vitamin D, it has a rapid onset of action. Both 1α-hydroxycholecalciferol and DHT appear to require 25-hydroxylation for full activity in vivo. However, because these analogues do not require 1α-hydroxylation in vivo, they are useful in vitamin D–resistant states where 1α-hydroxylation is impaired, such as chronic renal failure and hypoparathyroidism.

Absorption, Activation, and Transport of Vitamin D

Absorption

Vitamin D_3 produced in the skin by exposure to ultraviolet light enters the circulation by a process that is not well understood but may involve a serum binding protein for vitamin D.[321] Vitamin D has a circulating half-life of approximately 48 h and is stored in adipose tissue and muscle. Dietary forms of vitamin D are fat-soluble substances that are primarily absorbed from the proximal small bowel and transported through the lymphatic system bound to chylomicrons. Absorption may fail in individuals with generalized or fat malabsorption disorders (Whipple's disease, celiac disease, pancreatic insufficiency).

Activation

Vitamin D is transported from the skin and body stores to the liver bound to a specific protein, vitamin D–binding protein, whose role is discussed in detail below. In the liver, vitamin D undergoes hydroxylation at the 25-position by enzymes in the microsomes and mitochondria of parenchymal cells (Fig. 23-36). The enzyme system is a mixed-function oxidase that utilizes reduced NADP and molecular oxygen.[323] 25-Hydroxylation of vitamin D is not a closely regulated process. The effect of 1α,25-dihydroxyvitamin D [1α-25-$(OH)_2$D] in reducing circulating levels of 25-hydroxyvitamin D in vivo[324] is attributable primarily to an increase in the metabolic clearance rate of 25-hydroxyvitamin D[325] (see metabolism of vitamin D). Whether 1α,25-$(OH)_2$D affects hepatic synthesis of 25-hydroxyvitamin D directly is controversial.[326]

25-Hydroxyvitamin D is the principal circulating form of the vitamin. Its concentration in serum is 10 to 50 ng/ml (25 to 125 nmol/liter). The circulating pool is presumed to be in equilibrium with body stores in muscle and fat, and the half-life of 25-hydroxyvitamin D has been estimated at 15 to 20 days. As 25-hydroxyvitamin D is produced in a relatively unregulated fashion from either endogenous or exogenous sources of the hormone and enters a large stable circulating pool, the serum concentration of 25-hydroxyvitamin D is the best clinical measure of nutritional vitamin D status, and chronic vitamin D deficiency is reflected in low serum 25-hydroxyvitamin D levels. Note that in vitamin D–replete individuals, acute increases in serum levels of vitamin D induced by brief exposure to sunlight have little impact on the much larger circulating pool of 25-hydroxyvitamin D (Fig. 23-37). Assay of the serum concentration of 25-hydroxyvitamin D is thus a key part of the evaluation of certain disorders of mineral metabolism (see Assay of Vitamin D Metabolites).

FIGURE 23-36 Transport and metabolic sequence of activation of vitamin D in humans.

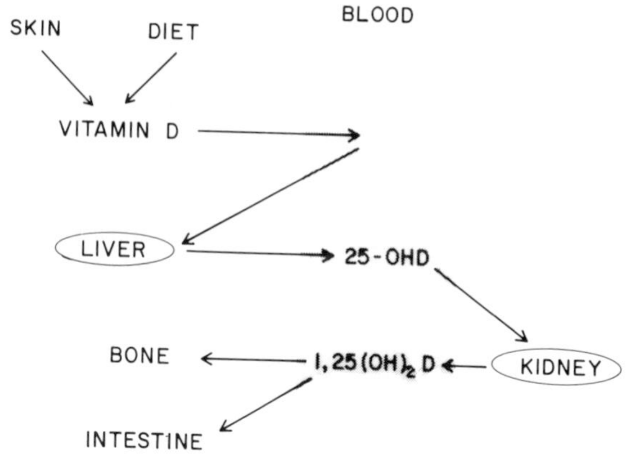

FIGURE 23-37 Changes in serum concentrations of vitamin D and its metabolites after exposure to ultraviolet radiation (UVR). Normal subjects (solid circle, solid square) were exposed to one (solid circle) or three (solid square) minimal erythemal doses of UVR. Vitamin D–deficient subjects (open triangles) were exposed to one minimal erythemal dose of UVR. The transient increase in serum vitamin D levels does not affect the serum level of 25-OH-D or 1α,25-$(OH)_2$D in normal subjects but markedly increases the serum level of both metabolites in patients with vitamin D deficiency. *(From Adams JS, Clemens TL, Parrish JA, Holick MF, N Engl J Med 306:722, 1982, by permission of the New England Journal of Medicine.)*

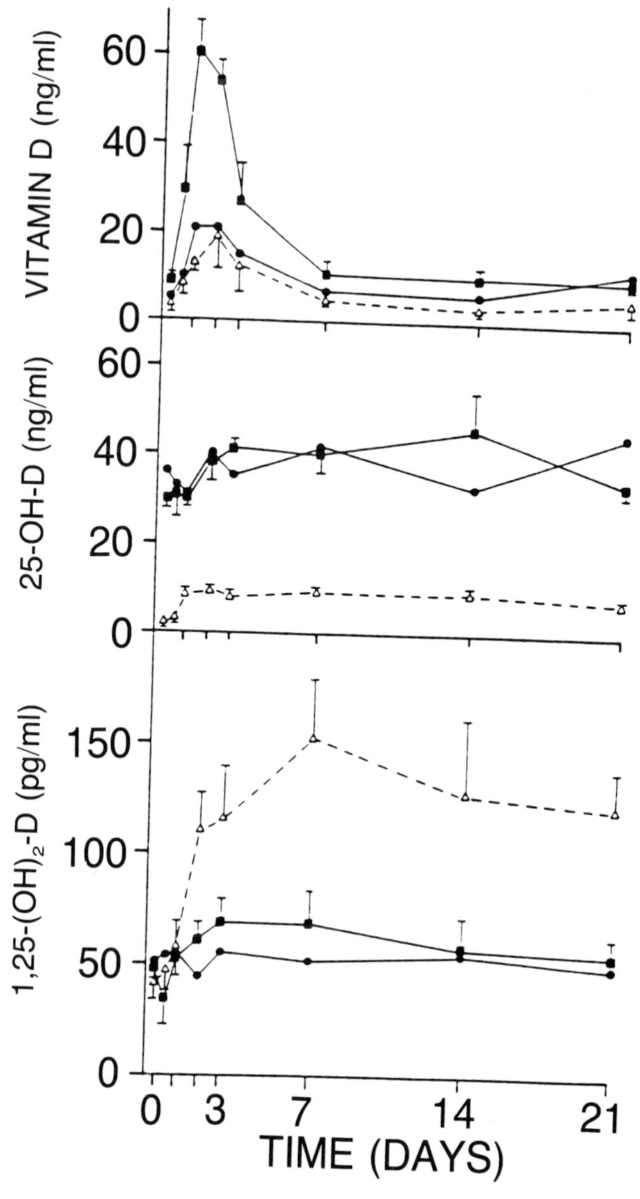

The liver has a large excess capacity to 25-hydroxylate vitamin D, and in the United States chronic liver disease is not generally associated with a clinically significant deficiency of this metabolite. Although circulating levels of 25-hydroxyvitamin D are reduced in liver disease, this is largely a consequence of reduced hepatic synthesis of the carrier protein, vitamin D–binding protein, as discussed in Transport of Vitamin D Metabolites. Treatment with anticonvulsants (phenytoin, phenobarbital) can also reduce 25-hydroxyvitamin D levels, presumably by inducing hepatic microsomal enzymes that inactivate vitamin D and its metabolites. In addition, 25-hydroxyvitamin D undergoes accelerated clearance, together with its binding protein, in the nephrotic syndrome, leading to lower circulating levels of this metabolite. The role of vitamin D therapy in bone disease associated with liver disease, chronic anticonvulsant use, and the nephrotic syndrome is discussed in Chap. 24.

With the discovery of 25-hydroxyvitamin D, it was briefly thought that the most active metabolite of the vitamin had been identified, but within a few years it became clear that a further hydroxylation would produce a thousandfold increase in biological activity. 25-Hydroxyvitamin D is further hydroxylated in the kidney to 1α,25-(OH)D [1α,25-$(OH)_2$D] or 24,25-dihydroxyvitamin D (Fig. 23-36). In contrast to 25-hydroxylation in the liver, 1α-hydroxylation is under exquisite metabolic control (Table 23-2), providing for integration of vitamin D activation into the overall schema for the regulation of mineral homeostasis.[327,328]

The renal 1α-hydroxylase is a mitochondrial cytochrome P450 mixed-function oxidase that requires reduced NADP and molecular oxygen. Although the amino acid sequence of the enzyme is unknown, it appears to function similarly to steroidogenic enzymes of the adrenal cortex. The cytochrome P450 probably participates directly in the hydroxylation of 25-hydroxyvitamin D, transferring electrons from reduced NADP via a reductase and renal renodoxin.[7,329] The enzyme has been localized to the proximal convoluted tubule and the pars recta of the rat nephron. At the former site, it is regulated by parathyroid hormone but not calcitonin; at the latter, it is regulated by calcitonin exclusively.[193] 25-Hydroxyvitamin D 24-hydroxylase is a separate mixed-function oxidase which is also located in the proximal renal tubule and under many circumstances is regulated inversely to the 1α-hydroxylase, as discussed below. The cloned enzyme has less than 30 percent homology to other cytochrome P450s and is thus part of a new family.[330]

TABLE 23-2 Factors That Influence Renal 1α-Hydroxylase Activity

Parathyroid hormone
Phosphate
1,25-$(OH)_2$D
Serum calcium
Growth hormone
Glucocorticoids
Prolactin
pH
Calcitonin
Estrogen

Parathyroid Hormone

Parathyroid hormone stimulates renal 1α-hydroxylase activity and reciprocally decreases the activity of 24-hydroxylase.[327,328,331] Based on the ability of cAMP analogues and the nonhormonal activator of adenylyl cyclase forskolin to mimic the effect of PTH, the second messenger for this effect appears to be cAMP.[332,333] PTH exerts its effects within hours, a time course consistent with the induction of new enzyme protein, but a direct effect of phosphorylating a regulatory component of the complex has not been excluded. The effect of PTH on 24-hydroxylase activity appears to be transcriptional.[333a] It is also conceivable that part of the effect of PTH on the enzyme in vivo could result from PTH action to change intrarenal handling of phosphate and ultimately serum phosphorus levels (see below).

In hyperparathyroidism, the serum level of 1α-25$(OH)_2$D tends to be increased, although many patients have levels in the high-normal range, presumably because of the countervailing influence of hypercalcemia.[334] PTH is the primary mediator of the marked increases in renal 1α-hydroxylase activity in hypocalcemic states. The response to hypocalcemia is blunted in hypoparathyroid states, so that the serum level of 1α,-25-$(OH)_2$D is low or low-normal in hypocalcemic patients with hypoparathyroidism and pseudohypoparathyroidism.[335] However, hypocalcemia per se probably can increase 1α-hydroxylase activity in the absence of PTH[327] (see below).

The plasma level of 1α,25-$(OH)_2$D is regulated by changes in calcium intake within the normal range,[336] and increased 1α,25-$(OH)_2$D levels in response to a low calcium intake play a role in the adaptation of intestinal calcium absorption. Diet-induced changes in 1α,25-$(OH)_2$D are highly correlated with changes in the level of PTH, suggesting that the system is sufficiently sensitive for PTH to play a role in homeostatic adjustments to changing calcium intake within the usual dietary range.

Phosphorus

Although early studies suggested that only extreme changes in phosphate intake might affect the production of 1α,25-$(OH)_2$D, it is now clear that the production of this metabolite can be regulated by alterations in phosphate intake within the range of normal (Fig. 23-38) and that this occurs independently of changes in PTH.[337] It is also clear that

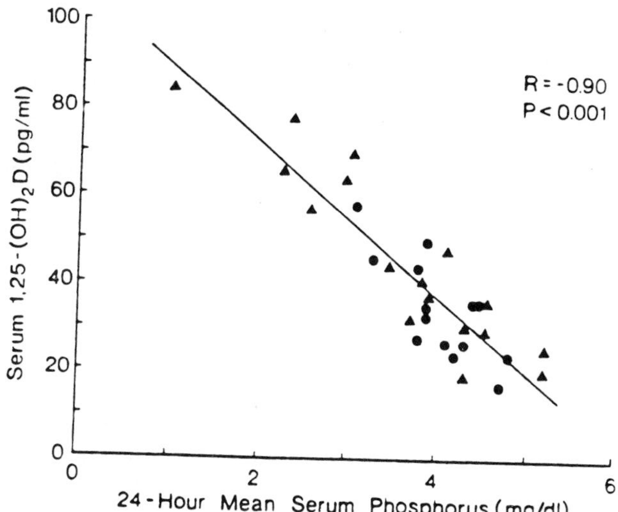

FIGURE 23-38 The relation between serum levels of phosphorus and serum levels of 1α,25-$(OH)_2D$ in normal men in whom serum phosphorus was manipulated by varying phosphate intake. Data are combined from two studies in which dietary phosphorus was maintained at <50, 1500, or >3000 mg/day (closed triangles) or at 625 or 2300 mg/day (closed circles). Changes in dietary phosphorus within the normal range (closed circles) regulate 1α,25-$(OH)_2D$ levels similarly to extreme changes (closed traingles). *(From Portale, Halloran, and Morris[337] by copyright permission of the American Society for Clinical Investigation.)*

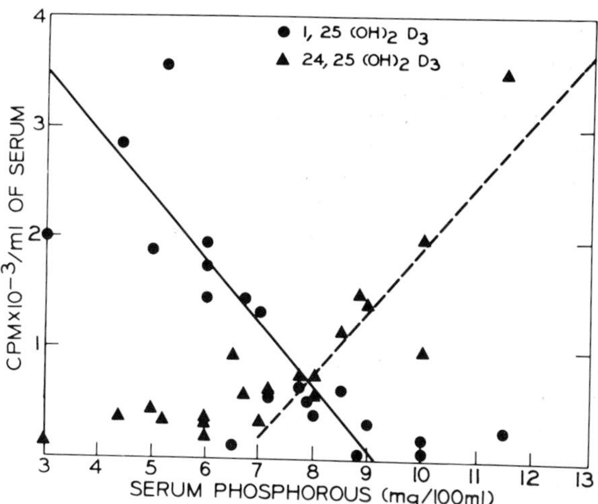

FIGURE 23-39 Relation between serum phosphorus and accumulation of radioactive vitamin D metabolites in the serum of thyroparathyroidectomized rats in which serum phosphorus was manipulated by variations in phosphate intake. The high level of serum phosphorus in these studies reflects both the effects of parathyroidectomy and the fact that serum phosphorus is normally higher in rats than it is in humans. *(By permission of Tanaka Y, DeLuca HF, Arch Biochem Biophys 154:566, 1973.)*

dietary phosphate intake can override the effect of PTH on the production of 1α,25-$(OH)_2D$ in several circumstances. Oral phosphate therapy for primary hyperparathyroidism or idiopathic hypercalciuria decreases the serum 1α,25-$(OH)_2D$ level in the face of a rise in the PTH level[338]; conversely, phosphate restriction in children with moderate chronic renal insufficiency increases the serum concentration of 1α,25-$(OH)_2D$ as PTH levels fall.[339] The changes in the production of 1α,25-$(OH)_2D$ induced by alterations in dietary phosphate are correlated with changes in the serum phosphorus level, but it is not clear how changes in phosphorus intake are sensed and transmitted to the enzymes of vitamin D metabolism. Altered dietary phosphate intake produces adaptive changes in phosphate transport, but the effect of altered phosphate transport on phosphate levels in intracellular compartments relevant to vitamin D metabolism cannot be predicted. This process may also be under hormonal control. The adaptation of 1α-hydroxylase activity to a low phosphate intake requires the presence of growth hormone, acting through IGF-I.[340] There is evidence for humoral factors that simultaneously produce increased renal phosphate clearance and decreased 1α,25-$(OH)_2D$ levels in tumor-induced osteomalacia.[341] Renal 24-hydroxylase activity is regulated inversely to 1α-hydroxylase activity at the extremes of phosphate intake (Fig. 23-39), but it is not known whether the 24-hydroxylase is subject to fine control by smaller changes.

Vitamin D Status

Renal 1α-hydroxylase activity is markedly increased (Fig. 23-37) and 24-hydroxylase activity is negligible in vitamin D deficiency.[328,342] Both are rapidly restored to normal by the administration of 1α,25-$(OH)_2D$. These effects are blocked by inhibitors of RNA and protein synthesis, suggesting that they occur at the transcriptional level. The reduction in 24-hydroxylase activity has been shown directly to involve a reduction in the level of mRNA.[333a] Conversely, vitamin D excess is associated with a reduction in renal 1α-hydroxylase activity, protecting against vitamin D intoxication.

Serum and Intracellular Calcium

Studies in animals and in normal humans indicate that sustained hypercalcemia produces a reduction in the serum concentration of 1α,25-$(OH)_2D$, which can override the stimulatory effect of PTH in experimental hyperparathyroidism.[343] This effect of hypercalcemia may explain the finding of normal serum levels of 1α,25-$(OH)_2D$ in some patients with primary hyperparathyroidism[334] and could contribute to the finding of low serum concentrations of 1α,25-$(OH)_2D$ in malignancy-associated hypercalcemia.

It appears (as discussed above) that the stimulation of 1α-hydroxylase activity in hypocalcemic states is primarily attributable to secondary hyperparathyroidism, with a minor direct effect of hypocalcemia.[7] However, the normal levels sometimes observed in hypoparathyroidism despite the combined effects of PTH deficiency and hyperphosphatemia are compatible with an independent effect of hypocalcemia to stimulate 1α-hydroxylase activity. This has been shown directly in the rat.[344]

In isolated mitochondria, normal metabolism of vitamin D appears to require a fixed range of ionized calcium.[345] However, it is not clear whether acute changes in cytoplasmic [Ca^{2+}] in the intact cell are involved in the physiologic regulation of enzyme activity.

Other Regulators

Estrogen treatment increases serum levels of 1α,25-$(OH)_2D$. This is attributable partly to increased synthesis of the vitamin D–binding protein, but free 1α,25-$(OH)_2D$ concentrations are also elevated.[346,347] The level of 1α,25-$(OH)_2D$ is markedly elevated in the third trimester of pregnancy,[348] a situation to which estrogen-dependent increases in renal synthesis, placental production of 1α,25-$(OH)_2D$ (see below), and other hormones such as prolactin may all contribute. The plasma level of 1α,25-$(OH)_2D$ may be increased in markedly hypercalcitonemic states,[349] but there is no evidence for physiologic regulation of renal production by calcitonin. A number of other factors, including growth hormone, prolactin, glucocorticoids, thyroid hormone, and systemic metabolic acidosis, have been shown to affect the activity of renal 1α-hydroxylase in animal studies, but data supporting significant effects of any of these agents on the activity of the human enzyme are lacking or conflicting.[328]

Integrated Control

The fine control of its synthesis in the kidney serves to integrate 1α,25-$(OH)_2D$ into the regulatory scheme for calcium homeostasis. The most important regulators of vitamin D metabolism in the kidney are PTH and phosphate. The parathyroids can respond to minute-to-minute changes in serum calcium and can sense changes induced by altered calcium intake within the normal dietary range. In pathologic states, the various regulators interact in complex ways. In nutritional vitamin D deficiency hypophosphatemia, secondary hyperparathyroidism and the reduced supply of vitamin D act in concert to increase enzyme activity. Their combined effect may maintain normal serum levels of 1α,25-$(OH)_2D$ in the face of reduced substrate levels (Fig. 23-37). Note that in vitamin D–deficient individuals, exposure to sunlight produces a small increase in 25-(OH)D pool but an exaggerated rise in serum levels of 1α,25-$(OH)_2D$ up to high levels, reflecting the high activity state of 1α-hydroxylase. In vitamin D excess, the combined effects of substrate, product, hypercalcemia, and hyperphosphatemia act to inhibit 1α-hydroxylase activity strongly, maintaining relatively normal levels of 1α,25-$(OH)_2D$. Thus, the integrated control of renal 1α-hydroxylase activity is remarkably successful in protecting the circulating level of the most important vitamin D metabolite against changes in intake or production. In other circumstances, individual factors work in opposition, with a hierarchy of dominance that is not fully predictable. For example, a large increase in phosphate intake suppresses 1α-hydroxylase activity even though it induces secondary hyperparathyroidism. The contrary effects of hypercalcemia, hypophosphatemia, and PTH excess produce variable increases in 1α,25-$(OH)_2D$ in primary hyperparathyroidism.

Circulating and Extrarenal 1α,25-$(OH)_2D$

The circulating concentration of 1α,25-$(OH)_2D$ is 20 to 60 pg/ml (50 to 150 pmol/liter), and its plasma half-life is 12 to 15 h. The relatively rapid turnover of 1α,25-$(OH)_2D$ is a factor in its physiologic role as a day-to-day regulator of calcium homeostasis. The most important extrarenal source of 1α,25-$(OH)_2D$ in humans is the placenta.[350] Production of 1α,25-$(OH)_2D$ at that site probably contributes to high circulating 1α,25-$(OH)_2D$ levels in the third trimester of pregnancy,[348] which in turn probably contribute to physiologic calcium hyperabsorption in pregnancy and lactation.[351] The plasma concentration of 1α,25-$(OH)_2D$ is greatly reduced in anephric individuals, suggesting that in nonpregnant humans there is no major extrarenal source of circulating 1α,25-$(OH)_2D$, although 1α-hydroxylase activity is clearly present at other extrarenal sites. Low levels of 1α-hydroxylase activity are detectable in dermal keratinocytes in vitro[352] in bone[353] and in other target tissues. It is not known whether there is a paracrine tissue role of 1α,25-$(OH)_2D$ produced at extrarenal sites. However, extrarenal production can be pathophysiologically critical. 1α-Hydroxylase is present in activated macrophages,[354] and excessive production of 1α,25-$(OH)_2D$ can lead to hypercalcemia in sarcoidosis and other granulomatous diseases, as discussed below.

Role of 24,25-$(OH)_2D$

24,25-$(OH)_2D$ is the principal circulating metabolite of 25-hydroxyvitamin D. Its serum concentration of 2 to 4 ng/ml (5 to 10 nmol/liter) is 100-fold higher than the concentration of 1α,25-$(OH)_2D$ and, in contrast to 1α,25-$(OH)_2D$, is a function of the 25-hydroxyvitamin D concentration. In most circumstances, the renal production of 1α,25-$(OH)_2D$ and 24,25-$(OH)_2D$ is regulated reciprocally. However, the actual biological role of 24,25-$(OH)_2D$ is obscure. There have been reports that 24,25-$(OH)_2D$ has several biological actions that are not fully mimicked by 1α,25-$(OH)_2D$. These include increased bone formation in vitro in the presence of PTH and 1α,25-$(OH)_2D$, increased proteoglycan synthesis in chondrocytes, and improved mineralization of bone when it is added to 1α,25-$(OH)_2D$ in therapy for vitamin D–deficient osteomalacia.[355] However, studies in intact animals are complicated by renal conversion of 24,25-$(OH)_2D$

to the biologically active trihydroxylated 1α,24,25-trihydroxyvitamin D. Difluoro analogues in which C-24 is incapable of hydroxylation have the same biological activity as 25-hydroxyvitamin D with regard to intestinal calcium transport and healing of rickets in rats. This has been taken as evidence that hydroxylation at the 24-position is not essential for the actions of vitamin D.[355]

Transport of Vitamin D Metabolites

All forms of vitamin D are transported in blood predominantly bound to a specific carrier protein, vitamin D–binding protein (also called Gc-globulin). This is an alpha globulin with a molecular weight of 58,000 which is a member of the same gene family as albumin and α-fetoprotein, and it binds actin in addition to vitamin D.[356] The protein has a single binding site for vitamin D metabolites. Its affinity for 25-hydroxyvitamin D and 24,25-$(OH)_2D$ is equivalent and is higher than its affinity for 1α,25-$(OH)_2D$. In addition to the fraction bound to the specific vitamin D–binding protein, a small fraction of vitamin D metabolites circulates bound to albumin. Vitamin D–binding protein is produced in the liver. Its levels are increased by estrogen therapy[346,347] and reduced in severe liver disease and in the nephrotic syndrome.[356] The latter two states are not generally associated with the development of osteomalacia, and free levels of 25-hydroxyvitamin D are normal.[357]

It is uncertain whether the physiologic actions of vitamin D in vivo occur in conformity with the "free hormone hypothesis," that is, whether only the free fraction is biologically active. However, it is clear that the presence of vitamin D–binding protein limits the availability of 1α,25-$(OH)_2D$ to its receptor and that when levels of vitamin D–binding protein are varied in vitro, the cellular effects of 1α,25-$(OH)_2D$ are tightly correlated with the free concentration of the hormone.[358]

Further Metabolism of 1α,25-$(OH)_2D$

1α,25-$(OH)_2D$ is metabolized by several pathways[328] (Fig. 23-40). A monoglucuronide and sulfates are produced in the liver, and 1α,25-$(OH)_2D$ undergoes enterohepatic recirculation. Side-chain oxidation gives rise to the biologically inert metabolite calcitroic acid (1α-hydroxy-23-carboxy-tetranor vitamin D). 1α,25-$(OH)_2D$ is also hydroxylated in the 24-position to 1α,24,25-$(OH)_3D$, which circulates at 4 to 15 pg/ml in human plasma. In the rat, side-chain oxidation and 24-hydroxylation account for about 40 percent of 1α,25-$(OH)_2D$ metabolism. The quantitative importance of these pathways in humans is less well defined. Other polar metabolites of 1α,25-$(OH)_2D$ include 22-oxo-1α,25-$(OH)_2D$, 1α,25-$(OH)_2D$-26,23-lactone, and 1α,25,26-$(OH)_3D$. All these metabolites have reduced biological activity relative to 1α,25-$(OH)_2D$. In all, some 30 metabolites of vitamin D have been identified to date.

The clearance of vitamin D metabolites is regulated by 1α,25-$(OH)_2D$.[325] In the rat, the administration of 1α,25-$(OH)_2D$ lowers the serum concentrations of 25-(OH)D and 24,25-$(OH)_2D$ by 50 percent and 70 percent, respectively, by increasing their metabolic clearance rate. The administration of 1α,25-$(OH)_2D$ also increases its own metabolic clearance rate. Part of these effects is probably attributable to the sevenfold increase in renal 24-hydroxylase activity induced by 1α,25-$(OH)_2D$ administration. It is likely that a human counterpart to this phenomenon exists, as the administration of 1α,25-$(OH)_2D$ has also been shown to decrease the serum concentration of 25-(OH)D in humans.[324]

Vitamin D Nutrition

In much of the world, the requirement for vitamin D is satisfied by endogenous synthesis. In temperate zones, serum levels of 25-hydroxycholecalciferol reflect seasonal variations in cutaneous exposure to UV light, being lowest in the spring and highest in the period August–October.[359–361] The elderly may manifest this seasonal variation at a lower overall concentration of 25-hydroxyvitamin D because of decreased capacity for cutaneous synthesis of vitamin D[362] or decreased absorption of dietary vitamin D.[363] A substantial fraction of healthy individuals in the northern United States have 25-hydroxyvitamin D levels at the lower limit of normal in the spring.[360]

The recommended daily allowance of vitamin D for adults is 200 IU. In the United States, food is supplemented with vitamin D. Both ergocalciferol and cholecalciferol are used as additives in milk and, in some locales, in cereals. Milk is supplemented with 400 IU per quart. Presumably as a consequence of these practices, Americans have higher 25-hydroxyvitamin D levels than do the residents of European countries in which dietary supplementation is not practiced (for example, Great Britain), and many researchers believe that this accounts for a decreased incidence of vitamin D insufficiency in the United States, particularly in those in whom the system is additionally stressed by illness that compromises the absorption or metabolism of the vitamin (e.g., liver disease, anticonvulsant therapy, nephrotic syndrome).

Some researchers believe that the elderly should receive more than the current recommended daily allowance (RDA), up to 400 to 800 IU of vitamin D. In this regard, it may be significant that among postmenopausal women in New England, seasonal variations in 25-hydroxyvitamin D levels are correlated inversely with the level of PTH.[361] This relation is accounted for by seasonal increases in PTH in women whose intake of vitamin D is <220 IU per day. This suggests that in the late winter and spring, when body stores of vitamin D are at their nadir, secondary hyperparathyroidism may develop to com-

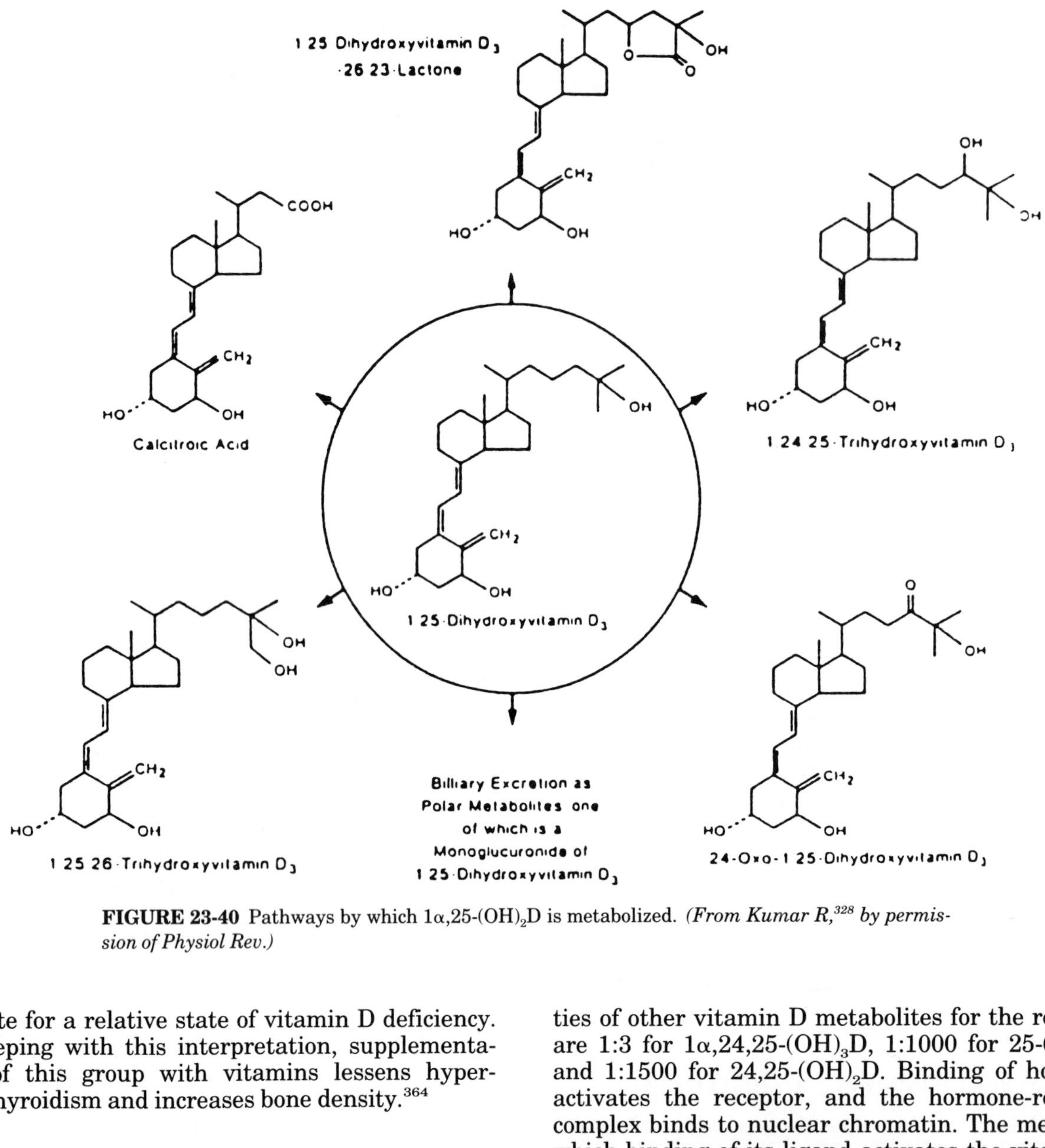

FIGURE 23-40 Pathways by which 1α,25-$(OH)_2D$ is metabolized. *(From Kumar R,[328] by permission of Physiol Rev.)*

pensate for a relative state of vitamin D deficiency. In keeping with this interpretation, supplementation of this group with vitamins lessens hyperparathyroidism and increases bone density.[364]

Cellular Basis of Vitamin D Action

The vitamin D receptor is a member of the steroid hormone receptor supergene family (see Chap. 5). It is a 50,000-molecular-weight protein with a DNA-binding domain whose sequence is 39 to 55 percent homologous to other members of the family.[365] Evidence that the cloned receptor is physiologically relevant comes from studies of patients with hereditary 1α,25-$(OH)_2D$–resistant rickets. These individuals have receptor mutations that interfere with the binding of hormone or association of the occupied receptor with DNA[366] (see Chap. 5). The vitamin D receptor binds 1α,25-$(OH)_2D$ with an affinity of 50 pmol/liter, consistent with the binding of 1α,25-$(OH)_2D$ from a cellular pool that is in diffusion equilibrium with circulating 1α,25-$(OH)_2D$. The relative affinities of other vitamin D metabolites for the receptor are 1:3 for 1α,24,25-$(OH)_3D$, 1:1000 for 25-(OH)D, and 1:1500 for 24,25-$(OH)_2D$. Binding of hormone activates the receptor, and the hormone-receptor complex binds to nuclear chromatin. The means by which binding of its ligand activates the vitamin D receptor are relatively less well understood than for other members of the superfamily[367,368] (see Chap. 5).

The number of receptors is controlled at the transcriptional level, as 1α,25-$(OH)_2D$ is known to induce the synthesis of receptor mRNA and protein in several target tissues, including the intestine, kidney, and parathyroid glands.[369,370] This increase in available receptor is potentially important in the adaptation to states such as a low calcium intake, amplifying the effects of increased 1α,25-$(OH)_2D$ concentrations on intestinal calcium transport. The vitamin D receptor is a phosphoprotein, and phosphorylation may be important for its function.[371]

Direct evidence that the vitamin D receptor is a transcriptional activator has come from studies of the gene for osteocalcin, a bone matrix–specific protein.[368] A vitamin D response element about 500 base pairs upstream of the transcriptional start site of the osteocalcin gene has been shown to confer vitamin D responsivity to this and heterologous promoters. The vitamin D response element in the osteocalcin gene consists of three copies of the half palindrome GGGTGA and an overlapping site for the transcription factor AP-1.[372] It appears that the vitamin D receptor has options of binding to its response elements as a homodimer, or as a heterodimer with a member of the retinoic acid receptor family, RXRβ.[372a,372b] The complex structure of the response element provides for complex regulatory interactions between vitamin A, vitamin D, and AP-1 binding factors such as the products of the proto-oncogenes *jun* and *fos*, which are responsive to serum, to activation of the protein kinase C pathway, or to interleukin 1. Thus, steroid hormones which bind to soluble receptors and hormones and growth factors which activate cell surface receptors may induce coordinated responses at key target genes.

It is likely that not all the effects of vitamin D are genomic. In fibroblasts and liver, exposure to 1α,25-$(OH)_2D$ produces rapid increases in cGMP[373] or in the intracellular calcium concentration.[374] Although these effects are likely to be nongenomic, those in fibroblasts require the presence of the vitamin D receptor. As we shall see, there is also evidence for a nongenomic effect of vitamin D on intestinal calcium transport, and this probably involves the vitamin D receptor as well. Thus, the same receptor may mediate the genomic and nongenomic actions of vitamin D.

Actions of Vitamin D in Intestine, Bone, and Kidney

Intestinal Transport of Calcium

The primary effect of vitamin D on mineral metabolism is the induction of increased calcium absorption across the intestinal epithelium. This conclusion is strongly supported by observations in individuals with hereditary 1α,25-$(OH)_2D$–resistant rickets, in whom active vitamin D receptors are lacking. Their severe bone disease can be healed by supplying calcium in the form of chronic intravenous infusions.[375]

The average diet contains 400 to 1500 mg of calcium. From this dietary load, the net absorption of calcium averages 100 to 250 mg, or about 20 percent of dietary calcium (Fig. 23-3); the remainder is excreted as fecal calcium. Calcium is absorbed throughout the small bowel. In animal studies, the efficiency of absorption per unit length of bowel is duodenum > jejunum ⩾ ileum. In humans, the absolute rates of transport are similar in the jejunum and the ileum. However, because of the prolonged transit through the lengthy ileum, the bulk of calcium is absorbed at this site. Net absorption of calcium varies with the dietary load of calcium, the ambient serum concentration of 1α,25-$(OH)_2D$, and the bioavailability of dietary calcium. In cow's milk, 40 percent of calcium is in solution. Acidification of food in the stomach tends to solubilize calcium, and absorption of calcium may be reduced in achlorhydric states,[376,377] but the fraction that is available for absorption varies with dietary composition. Less calcium may be available in foods, such as leafy vegetables, which are high in oxalate, or in cereals, which may be high in nondigestible organic phosphates such as phytate. Finally, the ability of the intestine to absorb calcium probably decreases with age,[378] an important consideration in the pathogenesis of osteoporosis.

The jejunum and ileum are relatively leaky to calcium, so that there is net diffusion of calcium passively from the intestinal lumen to the plasma through a paracellular pathway when the luminal concentration of calcium is high, but net diffusion is in the opposite direction when the luminal concentration is low. The intestinal calcium transport system that is induced by vitamin D is superimposed on this passive process (Fig. 23-41). The hormonally sensitive transport process is transcellular, unidirectional, and saturable. Thus, at a given calcium intake and a given ambient concentration of vitamin D, the rate of intestinal transport is the sum of an inwardly directed, saturable active component and a linear diffusive component.[379,380]

The vitamin D–sensitive cellular transport of calcium through the intestinal epithelial cell can be

FIGURE 23-41 The active and passive components of intestinal calcium absorption in normal humans. The data were obtained by perfusion of jejunal segments. *(Modified from Ireland P, Fordtran JS, J Clin Invest 52:2672, 1973, by copyright permission of the American Society for Clinical Investigation.)*

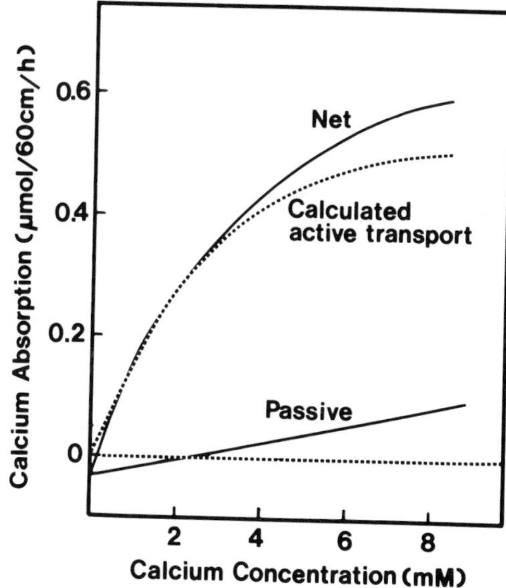

viewed as occurring in three steps (Fig. 23-42). Vitamin D increases the uptake of calcium through the brush border membrane of intestinal microvilli. This is presumably the rate-limiting step in the hormone-sensitive transport of calcium. Subsequently, calcium crosses the cell, probably bound to specific carrier proteins that are induced by vitamin D. Finally, calcium is actively extruded from the cell by an energy-requiring process whose activity is stimulated by vitamin D.

Uptake of calcium across the brush border is a passive process driven by the large electrochemical gradient of calcium (luminal concentration > 1 mM, cytoplasmic concentration ~ 100 nM). Several lines of evidence support the view that the induction of this process is a nongenomic action of vitamin D: Uptake is rapid, occurring within 4 min after exposure to the hormone; it is not blocked by inhibitors of RNA synthesis; and it is also not blocked by inhibitors of de novo protein synthesis.[381,382] However, it presumably requires either the binding of vitamin D to its receptor or cellular components induced by vitamin D–receptor complexes, as intestinal calcium transport is drastically reduced in the absence of a functional receptor in patients with 1α,25-$(OH)_2$D–resistant rickets. Both increased calmodulin binding to a specific brush border membrane–associated protein[383] and increased membrane fluidity[384] have been found after exposure to vitamin D.

Intestinal epithelial cells possess two specific cytosolic calcium-binding proteins called calbindins, with molecular mass of 9 and 28 kDA.[385,386] The calbindins are members of the troponin-C superfamily of calcium-binding proteins. The 9-kDa and 28-kDa forms bind two and four moles of calcium per mole, respectively, to $\sim$29-amino acid domains known as EF hands. With an affinity for calcium of about $1 \times 10^{-6}\,M$, these proteins are suited to buffer intracellular calcium and potentially to shuttle calcium from the lumen of the microvillus to the basolateral surface of the intestinal epithelial cell, from which it can be extruded. The synthesis of both forms of calbindin is induced by vitamin D, with a time course that lags behind the onset of calcium transport but parallels the achievement of maximal rates of transepithelial calcium flux after exposure to 1α,25-$(OH)_2$D. However, the evidence for a direct role in calcium absorption is still circumstantial.

An ATP-driven calcium pump present in the basolateral membrane of the intestinal epithelial cell is capable of active extrusion of calcium into the blood against the existing electrochemical gradient. Calcium transport across the basolateral membrane is stimulated by the exposure of cells to 1α,25-$(OH)_2$D, and it is thought that this could be a third site at which vitamin D acts to stimulate transepithelial transport of calcium.[379,387] Calcium exit could also be driven by a basolateral Na/Ca exchanger driven by the sodium gradient. The overall schema presented in Fig. 23-42—that the transport of calcium across the intestinal epithelium is composed of a passive vitamin D–sensitive entry step, transcellular shuttling of calcium via the vitamin D–inducible calbindins, and active extrusion via a vitamin D–sensitive ATP-driven calcium pump—is attractive and consistent with a mass of data but remains to be proved in detail.

Adaptation to Calcium Intake

The regulation of calcium absorption in response to a changing intake[380] illustrates the way in which metabolism is integrated. Adaptation to a low cal-

FIGURE 23-42 Proposed mechanism of action of 1α,25-$(OH)_2$ D in the intestine. Binding of 1α,25-$(OH)_2$D to the vitamin D receptor (VDR) affects the transcription of genes including calbindin and may also permit calcium entry through channels in the luminal (brush border) membrane by a nongenomic mechanism. Calbindin is proposed to ferry calcium through the cell. The exit step through the basolateral membrane may involve a calcium pump (Ca-ATPase) and/or Na/Ca exchange.

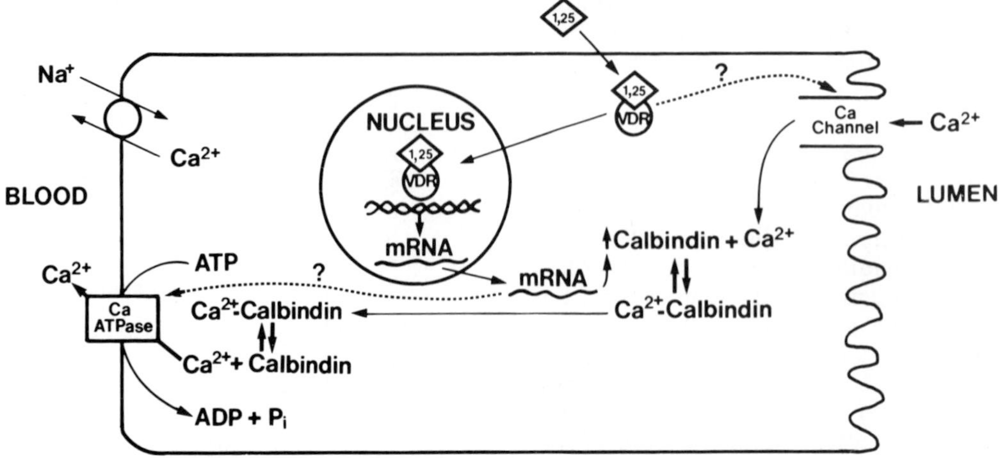

cium intake is thought to begin with an imperceptible fall in the serum calcium concentration, which is a stimulus to secondary hyperparathyroidism. The resultant increment in PTH is the primary driver for accelerated renal synthesis of $1\alpha,25\text{-}(OH)_2D$,[336] and the ensuing increase in serum $1\alpha,25\text{-}(OH)_2D$ concentration has several compensatory actions: Intestinal $1\alpha,25\text{-}(OH)_2D$ receptors are induced,[369] the active component of intestinal calcium absorption is increased by the direct action of $1\alpha,25\text{-}(OH)_2D$ on these receptors, and bone resorption is increased by a direct action of $1\alpha,25\text{-}(OH)_2D$.[338] Of course, PTH participates directly in the response to a low calcium intake, decreasing urinary calcium excretion and increasing bone resorption. Adaptation to a high calcium intake has the opposite effects, with suppression of $1\alpha,25\text{-}(OH)_2D$ and reduced active calcium transport.[380] The total absorption of calcium increases progressively with intake, however, because the passive influx pathway is not saturable (Fig. 23-41). Thus, adequate levels of calcium absorption can be achieved at high levels of intake even in individuals with impaired metabolism of vitamin D (hypoparathyroidism, chronic renal failure). Very high intakes of calcium (greater than 10 g per day) can produce hypercalcemia despite activation of all the compensatory mechanisms discussed above.

Intestinal Absorption of Phosphate

Phosphate is principally absorbed passively, with a smaller component of active transport; the details are discussed under Disorders of Phosphate Metabolism. It is likely that vitamin D stimulates cellular uptake of phosphate by a sodium-coupled phosphate transporter by increasing the V_{max}, most likely by increasing the number of carriers.[389] However, because the vitamin D–dependent component of phosphate absorption is small, the impact of vitamin D deficiency on phosphate absorption is much smaller than it is on calcium absorption. The hypophosphatemia that accompanies osteomalacia results not from this but primarily from resetting of the renal phosphate threshold by associated hyperparathyroidism.

Actions of Vitamin D in Bone

The most prominent clinical effect of vitamin D deficiency is *osteomalacia*, or defective mineralization of bone matrix. Whether this form of bone disease is a direct consequence of defective vitamin D action on bone cells or an indirect effect of impaired absorption of calcium and phosphates, with a reduction in the concentrations of calcium and phosphate available for mineralization of the organic matrix of bone, has been debated for many years. Several lines of evidence support the view that the development of osteomalacia is a secondary result of the systemic effects of vitamin D deficiency. Rachitic cartilage will mineralize in vitro in the presence of adequate concentrations of calcium and phosphate. Experimental vitamin D–deficient osteomalacia will heal after the provision of calcium and phosphorus. Most impressively, the severe form of rickets seen in patients with hereditary resistance to $1\alpha,25\text{-}(OH)_2D$ can be healed by a chronic intravenous infusion of calcium that bypasses the defect in intestinal calcium absorption. Healing of osteomalacia is apparent by both radiologic and histomorphometric examination in individuals who lack functional vitamin D receptors.[375]

Despite the evidence that the clinically most apparent osseous effects of vitamin D deficiency may be indirect, vitamin D has a number of direct effects on bone cells.[390] The primary target cell is the osteoblast. Vitamin D receptors are demonstrable by autoradiographic effects in mature rat osteoblasts and in osteoprogenitor cells. Receptors have also been identified in the direct binding studies of a variety of cultured osteoblast-like cells and osteosarcoma cells from humans and rodents. Most osteoblast functions that have been carefully studied are affected by vitamin D. Transcription of type I collagen genes and collagen synthesis are inhibited by the administration of $1\alpha,25\text{-}(OH)_2D$ in vivo,[391] and collagen synthesis is also inhibited by vitamin D in isolated rat and mouse calvaria in organ culture and cultured bone cells. However, collagen synthesis is stimulated by vitamin D in other bone cell lines.[390] Exposure to vitamin D also has bidirectional effects on the activity of alkaline phosphatase in different bone-derived cell lines. Transcription of the gene encoding the bone matrix protein osteocalcin is stimulated by vitamin D in vivo and in vitro. Exposure to $1\alpha,25\text{-}(OH)_2D$ also affects the synthesis of bone growth factors such as TGF-β.

Vitamin D also stimulates bone resorption in organ culture[390] and in vivo.[388] The hypercalcemia that accompanies vitamin D intoxication is sustained by increased resorption of bone. Mature osteoclasts are reportedly lacking in vitamin D receptors, and coculture experiments suggest that activation of the osteoclast by vitamin D requires the release of a trophic factor from the osteoblast.[392] Besides its effects on the mature osteoclast, $1\alpha,25\text{-}(OH)_2D$ accelerates the maturation of osteoclast precursors in bone organ culture,[393,394] an effect that may be related to its ability to induce the differentiation of circulating mononuclear cells, discussed below.

Administration of pharamacologic doses of $1\alpha,25\text{-}(OH)_2D$ in excess of the replacement dose results in the appearance of large amounts of undermineralized osteoid on bone surfaces.[395] There is a certain irony in these observations, considering the origins of vitamin D as an antirachitic agent. However, it is not clear whether a primary defect in the mineralization of osteoid is indeed present in this circumstance.

It is not possible at present to create a coherent picture of the physiology of vitamin D action in bone.

In individual cells, the hormone can act as a differentiation factor, as a regulator of various differentiated functions, and to modulate cell-cell interactions. This may account for some of the complexity of its effects in various bone-derived systems. In any case, it is difficult to reconcile the remarkably diverse direct effects of vitamin D on bone cells with the view that only its systemic actions (i.e., providing an adequate supply of calcium and phosphate) are required for the health of bone.

Actions of Vitamin D in the Kidney

Because of the complex interrelations among vitamin D, PTH, and phosphate intake, the nature of the direct renal effects of vitamin D has been controversial. However, there is an emerging consensus that 1α,25-$(OH)_2D$ acutely stimulates phosphate reabsorption in the proximal tubule.[396] It is unlikely that vitamin D is a primary regulator of renal phosphate handling under physiologic circumstances. Indeed, in the chronic state, the direct tubular effect of 1α,25-$(OH)_2D$ administration is counterbalanced by a fall in proximal tubule phosphate reabsorption induced by the simultaneous increase in intestinal phosphate absorption that results from the administration of 1α,25-$(OH)_2D$, as discussed under Phosphate Homeostasis. Thus, although the systemic effects of 1α,25-$(OH)_2D$ on phosphate transport can be conceptualized as serving to maintain the availability of phosphate for mineralization of bone by enhancing intestinal absorption and diminishing renal excretion, the superimposed homeostatic effects of increased phosphate absorption by the intestine and of PTH tend to minimize the physiologic importance of the direct renal effects of 1α,25-$(OH)_2D$.

The same complexities that have confused the interpretation of the role of vitamin D in renal phosphate transport apply to the renal handling of calcium. The most convincing interpretation is that vitamin D deficiency impairs renal calcium reabsorption and that the administration of vitamin D restores a normal threshold for renal calcium reabsorption and also sensitizes the tubule to PTH.[397] The tubule site of this action of vitamin D is not known, although calbindins induced by vitamin D are present in the distal tubule segments where PTH-regulated reabsorption of calcium occurs and preliminary data suggest that the effects of vitamin D on calcium transport occur in these cells.[385,386]

Actions of Vitamin D in Other Tissues

Outside the classic target tissues, vitamin D receptors are widely distributed in fibroblasts, skin, brain, pituitary, parotid, stomach, testis, ovary, placenta, breast, and other tissues. In several tissues 1α,25-$(OH)_2D$ has been shown to regulate physiologic functions. The role of vitamin D as a regulator of PTH synthesis in the parathyroids was discussed earlier.

The Immune System

The finding that exposure to 1α,25-$(OH)_2D$ induced the maturation of M-1 and HL-60 myeloblastic leukemia cells to a macrophage phenotype led to demonstrations that 1α,25-$(OH)_2D$ at physiologic concentrations induces the maturation of human peripheral monocytes.[398] Activated T lymphocytes also express vitamin D receptors, and exposure to 1α,25-$(OH)_2D$ inhibits their proliferation and the production of interleukin 2. The physiologic significance of these observations in vitro is unclear.[398] Vitamin D–deficient individuals may have recurrent infections, but rachitic individuals lacking vitamin D receptors do not, even though the receptor deficiency is expressed in their peripheral monocytes. However, the effect of 1α,25-$(OH)_2D$ on monocyte maturation may be related to its ability to influence the maturation of osteoclast precursors in bone.[393,394]

Skin

Keratinocytes can metabolize 25-(OH)D to 1α,25-$(OH)_2D$[352], and 1α,25-$(OH)_2D$ is a potent inducer of the differentiation of keratinocytes.[399] The antiproliferative effects of 1α,25-$(OH)_2D$ have led to its use as an experimental treatment for psoriasis. Although abnormalities of the epidermis are not prominent in vitamin D–deficient individuals, alopecia totalis is present in many kindreds with 1α,25-$(OH)_2D$–resistant rickets. This suggests a possible role of 1α,25-$(OH)_2D$ in the differentiation of the hair follicle.

Tissue-specific analogues

Several vitamin D analogues are reported to have tissue-specific effects.[399a] The best studied is 22-oxa-1α,25-$(OH)_2D$, which is a potent activator of the differentiation of myeloid leukemia cells[400] and inhibits the secretion of PTH but is not a potent bone-resorbing agent in vitro and does not readily produce hypercalcemia in vivo.[400,401] It thus may be of use in treating secondary hyperparathyroidism. Preferential activity in myeloid differentiation over systemic calcemic effects has also been reported for 24-homo-1α,25-$(OH)_2D$ and an analogue with a cyclopropyl group at the end of the side chain.[390,399a,402]

Summary

In cells of the osteoclast lineage, leukocytes, and keratinocytes, 1α,25-$(OH)_2D$ is a differentiation factor with antiproliferative effects. The absence of prominent defects in these systems in vitamin D–deficient or receptor-deficient humans suggests that the effects of the hormone are not essential but modulatory.

Assay of Vitamin D Metabolites

The two metabolites whose assay is clinically vital are 25-(OH)D and 1α,25-$(OH)_2D$. Assay of 25-(OH)D gives the best available measure of body stores of vitamin D and is the assay of choice for the diagnosis of suspected vitamin D deficiency and vitamin D intoxication. The 25-hydroxyvitamin D level can be used to follow therapy in patients treated with vitamin D or 25-hydroxycholecalciferol (calcifediol). In patients with liver disease, the nephrotic syndrome, or hyperestrogenemic states, the results must be interpreted in light of possible changes in levels of the vitamin D–binding protein. Direct assays of the vitamin D–binding protein or free 25-(OH)D are not commercially available.

Assays of 25-(OH)D employ competitive binding to the serum vitamin D–binding protein. Preparative chromatography of serum on LH-20 or silicic acid is necessary to remove other metabolites.[403] For research purposes, 25-$(OH)D_2$ and 25-$(OH)D_3$ can be separated by normal-phase high-performance liquid chromatography (HPLC) and determined independently. As foods may contain either cholecalciferol or ergocalciferol, separate measurement of their metabolites cannot distinguish between dietary and endogenous production of vitamin D.

Despite its central role in calcium homeostasis, there are only a few clinical indications for assay of 1α,25-$(OH)_2D$ in serum. Because the production of 1α,25-$(OH)_2D$ is so closely regulated, assay of this metabolite is not a good measure of body stores of vitamin D in suspected states of deficiency or excess. Specific indications for assay of 1α,25-$(OH)_2D$ involve states in which the activity of 25-(OH)D-1α-hydroxylase is thought to be reduced (heritable defects in vitamin D metabolism, renal failure) or increased (hypercalcemic patients with sarcoidosis, other granulomatous disorders, idiopathic hypercalcemia of infancy, or lymphoma) and suspected intoxication with exogenous 1α-$(OH)D_3$ or 1α,25-$(OH)_2D_3$.

Nearly all methods for determinations of 1α,25-$(OH)_2D$ in clinical use utilize the vitamin D receptor as a binding protein in a competitive binding assay. Many assays now use the receptor present in extracts of calf thymus, which binds 1α,25-$(OH)_2D_2$ and 1α,25-$(OH)_2D_3$ with equivalent affinity.[404] Other vitamin D metabolites that bind to the receptor, of which there are many, must be separated before the assay. This is classically done by HPLC of lipid extracts of serum, but a technique that uses a C-18-OH cartridge to purify 1α,25-$(OH)_2D$ from lipid extracts of small quantities of serum (0.5 to 1.0 ml) has been introduced.[405]

HYPERCALCEMIA

Introduction

Although many diseases are associated with hypercalcemia, they each produce hypercalcemia through only a limited number of mechanisms: (1) increasing gastrointestinal absorption of calcium, (2) decreasing urinary calcium excretion, (3) increasing bone resorption (either generalized or localized, such as at the site of malignant metastases) and release of calcium into the systemic circulation, or combinations of these mechanisms. Furthermore, once established, hypercalcemia can become self-perpetuating or can be aggravated through a "vicious cycle" (Fig. 23-43). Table 23-3 summarizes the differential diagnosis of hypercalcemia. A number of symptoms and signs accompany the hypercalcemic state: central nervous system effects such as lethargy, depression, stupor or coma, ataxia, and psychosis; neuromuscular effects such as weakness, proximal myopathy, and hypertonia; cardiovascular effects such as hypertension, bradycardia and eventually asystole, and a shortened QT interval on electrocardiogram; renal effects such as renal stones, decreased glomerular filtration, polyuria, hyperchloremic acidosis, and nephrocalcinosis; gastrointestinal effects such as nausea, vomiting, constipation, and anorexia; eye findings such as band keratopathy; and systemic metastatic calcification (Table 23-3). This constellation of clinical findings has led to the mnemonic for tallying the signs and symptoms of hypercalcemia: stones, bones, abdominal groans, and psychic moans (Fig. 23-44 and Table 23-4).

The Defense Against Hypercalcemia

The central feature of the adaptive response to an increased calcium load is suppression of the secretion of PTH. This produces a decrease in physiologic calcium release from the skeleton and—along with the direct effects of hypercalcemia—turns off the renal synthesis of 1α,25-$(OH)_2D$, leading to a diminution in intestinal calcium absorption. Most important, the suppression of PTH permits a marked increase in renal calcium excretion. The kidney provides the principal route by which a calcium load can be cleared. Urinary calcium excretion is profoundly

FIGURE 23-43 Once established, hypercalcemia can be maintained or aggravated as depicted. *(Courtesy of Dr. Maurice Attie, University of Pennsylvania School of Medicine.)*

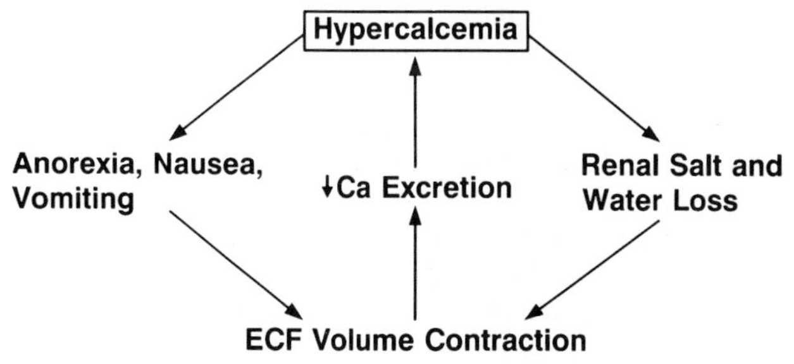

TABLE 23-3 Causes of Hypercalcemia

Hyperparathyroidism
- Idiopathic
- Associated with multiple endocrine neoplasia type 1 or type 2a
- Familial
- After renal transplantation

Malignancies
- Humoral hypercalcemia of malignancy
- Solid tumors with local osteolysis (breast, lung, kidney, etc.)
- Hematologic malignancies (multiple myeloma, lymphoma, leukemia, etc.)

Sarcoidosis or other granulomatous disease

Endocrinopathies
- Thyrotoxicosis
- Adrenal insufficiency
- Pheochromocytoma
- Acromegaly
- VIPoma

Drug-induced
- Vitamin D excess
- Vitamin A excess
- Thiazide diuretics
- Lithium
- Milk-alkali syndrome
- Estrogens, androgens, tamoxifen (in breast carcinoma)

Miscellaneous
- Familial hypocalciuric hypercalcemia (FHH)
- Dehydration
- Immobilization (in growing children or adults with increased bone turnover)
- Acute renal failure
- Idiopathic hypercalcemia of infancy
- ICU hypercalcemia
- Serum protein disorders

enhanced when the filtered load is increased by hypercalcemia and PTH is suppressed; elimination of 1000 mg calcium per day is not uncommon (Fig. 23-45). The only alternative clearance mechanism is deposition in the tissues as a phosphate salt, a physicochemical consequence of the limited solubility product of calcium · phosphate. Calcium phosphate deposition into bone may be adaptive but is usually accompanied by deposition into soft tissues to produce the untoward complications of nephrocalcinosis and calcifications in arterial walls, lungs, skin, and stomach.

Because of the efficiency of the renal response to a calcium load, hypercalciuria is more common than hypercalcemia in most situations where a calcium load is imposed; the exception is primary hyperparathyroidism, where the hypocalciuric effect of PTH persists and the ability of the kidney to respond is thus impaired (Fig. 23-45). However, profoundly hypercalciuric patients are in precarious balance because several factors conspire against the renal adaptation to hypercalcemia (Fig. 23-43). Glomerular filtration is impaired by hypercalcemia. The urinary concentrating ability is diminished, poor mentation may interfere with access to fluids, and nausea or vomiting may occur, so that the patient is subject to dehydration and prerenal azotemia. Renal insufficiency in turn compromises calcium clearance, potentially leading to a downward spiral that can culminate in severe hypercalcemia and renal failure. Thus, a vacation at the beach can set off an episode of hypercalcemia in a patient with sarcoidosis, and a crisis of severe hypercalcemia induced by dehydration may punctuate a long history of mild asymptomatic primary hyperparathyroidism.

Approach to the Hypercalcemic Patient

The approach to the hypercalcemic patient takes account of the demographics and pathophysiology of hypercalcemia. Thus, the causes of hypercalcemia can be divided into three categories: primary hyperparathyroidism, malignancy, and everything else. This division emphasizes that the combined incidence of primary hyperparathyroidism and malignancy is 10-fold higher than that of all other causes of hypercalcemia taken together. To differentiate nonparathyroid hypercalcemia from primary hyperparathyroidism, the clinician relies on shared clinical features of nonparathyroid hypercalcemia, the consequences of suppression of PTH secretion. Once nonparathyroid hypercalcemia has been diagnosed, its cause can usually be found by using other features of its presentation to identify the underlying disorder.

In ambulatory patients with asymptomatic or mildly symptomatic hypercalcemia, primary hyperparathyroidism is the likely diagnosis. The prevalence of primary hyperparathyroidism is much higher than that of all other causes of hypercalcemia combined. A high level of intact PTH in a hypercalcemic patient is virtually diagnostic of primary hyperparathyroidism, since in assays for the intact hormone, the PTH level in nonparathyroid hypercalcemia is suppressed. It is these considerations of the prevalence of primary hyperparathyroidism and the relative ease of diagnosis which led to the recommendation presented below for an abbreviated work-up of hypercalcemia in asymptomatic ambulatory patients. Other laboratory features, such as hypophosphatemia and hyperchloremia, are often present in primary hyperparathyroidism, reflecting the renal actions of excess PTH, but need not be relied on to make the diagnosis.

Although the *incidence* of malignancy-associated hypercalcemia is about half the incidence of primary hyperparathyroidism, the *prevalence* of malignancy-associated hypercalcemia is much lower owing to the short survival in malignancy-associated hypercalcemia (mean life expectancy, 30 days). However, malignancy is the most common etiology of hypercalcemia in hospitalized patients. If the underlying

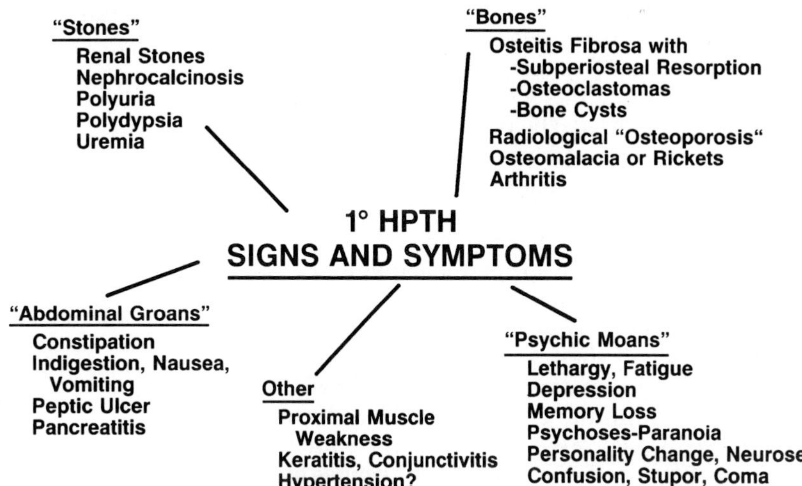

FIGURE 23-44 Mnemonic used for categorizing the signs and symptoms of hyperparathyroidism.

malignancy is not already recognized, it is readily apparent by physical examination or laboratory screening of the hypercalcemic patient. Because PTHrP is the etiologic agent that produces hypercalcemia in most patients with malignant tumors, other features reminiscent of hyperparathyroidism are often present: The serum phosphorus level is often low, and the tubular maximum for phosphate/glomerular filtration rate (TmP/GFR) is correspondingly decreased.

The other causes of hypercalcemia are diverse but have some common features. A key feature is suppression of PTH secretion. The intact PTH level is suppressed below 2 pmol/liter (20 pg/ml). Thus, a determination of the intact PTH level using a two-site assay readily distinguishes all other entities from primary hyperparathyroidism (Fig. 23-9). The suppression of PTH also has several consequences that are useful in making the diagnosis of nonparathyroid, non-PTHrP–related hypercalcemia. The urinary excretion of calcium is significantly increased (Fig. 23-45). The TmP/GFR is generally normal or increased, setting the serum phosphorus concentration in the midnormal range or above (the occasional finding of a low-normal serum phosphorus in nonparathyroid hypercalcemia is probably attributable to a direct effect of hypercalcemia in decreasing renal phosphate reabsorption).

TABLE 23-4 Clinical Characteristics of 51 Patients with Primary Hyperparathyroidism in Rochester, Minnesota

Characteristic	July 1, 1974, to December 31, 1976, %
Urolithiasis	4
Hypercalciuria (>250 mg/dl)	22
Emotional disorder (depression, psychosis, or severe neurosis)	20
Osteoporosis	12
Diminished renal function	15
Hyperparathyroid bone disease	8
Peptic ulcer disease	8
Pancreatitis	0
No problems related to primary hyperparathyroidism	51

Source: Heath et al.[415]

FIGURE 23-45 The effect of hyperparathyroidism and hypoparathyroidism on the relation between serum and urinary calcium. At any level of serum calcium, the urinary calcium is increased in hypoparathyroidism (open and closed triangles) and decreased in hyperparathyroidism (closed circles) compared with normal subjects. Normal subjects were studied in the basal state (shaded area) or during the infusion of calcium, where the response is shown as the mean (—) plus or minus 2 standard deviations (----). *(By permission of BEC Nordin and M Peacock, Lancet 2:1280, 1969.)*

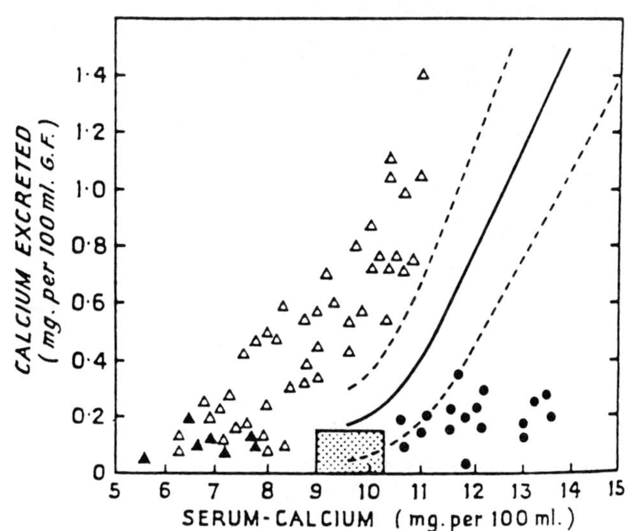

A patient with hypercalcemia in the setting of chronic renal failure presents the physician with a special challenge. Because secondary hyperparathyroidism is common in such patients and phosphorus excretion is impaired, the interpretation of the intact PTH and serum phosphorus levels must be tempered with caution. This special case is discussed further in Chap. 24.

Hypercalcemia is usually caused by increased bone resorption. Bone resorption involves destruction of the collagen-rich bone matrix as well as the release of mineral. This often leads to increased urinary excretion of the metabolites of type I collagen, such as the collagen-specific amino acid hydroxyproline and pyridinium cross-links. Measurement of urinary hydroxyproline is the traditional test for bone resorption, but it is insensitive because hydroxyproline is also released from dietary collagen in meats and gelatin and from collagen-rich tissues other than bone. The pyridinium compounds are the cross-links between collagen chains that remain after extensive hydrolysis, and they are more sensitive and specific than hydroxyproline as measures of bone resorption.[406,407] One (hydroxylysylpyridinoline, or simply pyridinoline) is derived mainly from the degradation of type I collagen in bone and type II collagen in cartilage. The other (lysylpyridinoline or deoxypyridinoline) has been found only in type I collagen of bone. Hence, determination of pyridinolines in urine is coming into use as the preferred clinical assay for bone resorption.

Because bone formation usually remains coupled to bone resorption, most states of increased bone resorption are also characterized by high rates of bone formation. This is sometimes manifested as an increase in serum alkaline phosphatase levels. However, because alkaline phosphatase has multiple sources, determination of serum alkaline phosphatase is lacking in both sensitivity and specificity as a measure of bone formation. Assays for the bone matrix–specific protein osteocalcin (bone gla protein) are now generally available and provide a highly specific measure of bone formation.[406] The osteocalcin level is elevated in many hypercalcemic states.[406,408]

Intestinal absorption of calcium is increased in primary hyperparathyroidism, granulomatous disorders, vitamin D intoxication, and the milk-alkali syndrome. The milk-alkali syndrome may be the only disorder in which increased intestinal absorption of calcium is the primary cause of hypercalcemia, as excessive bone resorption plays a role in all the other states, including vitamin D intoxication. Intestinal absorption of calcium can be estimated from metabolic balance studies or from a variety of tests that measure the unidirectional or bidirectional flux of isotopic calcium. These are all research procedures, and which is best is disputed.[380] However, there is no reliable and readily available clinical measure of intestinal calcium absorption.

Primary Hyperparathyroidism

The most common cause of hypercalcemia is primary hyperparathyroidism. The incidence is approximately 0.2 percent in women over 65 years old and 0.1 percent in men over 65 years old. Approximately 100,000 to 200,000 new causes occur each year in the United States.[197,198] The disease occurs more commonly in women (2:1 ratio) than in men, and the incidence increases markedly with age, particularly over age 60. The majority of these cases occur sporadically; however, hyperparathyroidism also has a hereditary association. It is a component of two of the three multiple endocrine neoplasia syndromes (discussed below). Although any or all of the symptoms and signs described above (Table 23-4) can be produced by primary hyperparathyroidism, the majority of cases arise without symptoms (discussed in the section on Diagnosis and Management of Asymptomatic Primary Hyperparathyroidism).

History

The history of hyperparathyroidism is recounted in a review by Schwartz.[409] The first description of a parathyroid gland was made by Sandstrom in 1880.[410] Although von Recklinghausen described osteitis fibrosis cystica in 1891, the connection between bone disease and parathyroid tumors was not made until more than a decade later by Askanazy.[409] The link between the hormone secreted by the parathyroid gland and calcium mobilization from bone was later established by Erdheim in Vienna. Until that time, the causes of excessive levels of calcium in the blood were not known. In fact, one school of thought held that inadequate parathyroid hormone was the etiology of hypercalcemia and that the parathyroid enlargement observed with hypercalcemia resulted secondarily as a response to elevated blood calcium levels. Therefore, some physicians advocated transplantation with parathyroid glands as a treatment for the disorder.[409] The causal link between the increased activity of one or more parathyroid glands and hyperparathyroidism and hypercalcemia became most clearly established in American medicine by the pioneering efforts of Fuller Albright in his famous studies of the patient (and coinvestigator!) Captain Martell[411] (Fig. 23-46). Linking the abnormal gland to the disease hyperparathyroidism would require an exceptional effort because it was a novel concept: "This gland is so small that few doctors have ever seen one on the dissecting table. . . . This little gland is so powerful, however, that its over- or underfunction can be fatal."[412]

The remarkable story of Captain Martell and the intensive clinical investigation for which he served as the subject is one of the most dramatic accounts of biomedical research in the history of American medicine. Martell's disease was severe; skeletal involvement was dramatic. His habitus was altered remarkably by years of excess secretion of parathyroid hormone. Albright described the situation as follows:

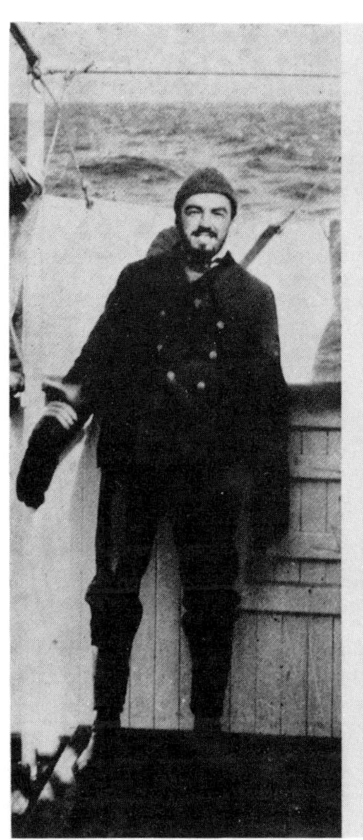
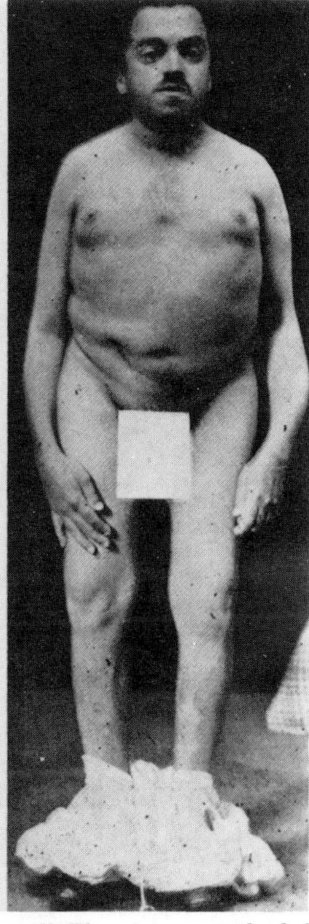

FIGURE 23-46 Captain Charles Martell. The picture on the left shows him a few months before his first symptom. On the right, he is pictured 8 years later at the time of entry to the hospital in 1926. *(Reprinted with permission from W. Bauer and D. D. Federman, Hyperparathyroidism epitomized: The case of Captain Charles Martell, Metabolism 11:22, 1962.)*

"The Captain . . . lay in a ward slowly excreting his skeleton into his urine."[412] Captain Martell's case exemplified the course of others severely incapacitated with the disease, which was fatal at the time because there was no medical or surgical treatment: "The patients [became] more and more skeletonless, more and more plant-like, until finally they were jellyfish incapable of locomotion, in some cases dying of suffocation, unable to move the chest in respiration."[412] Martell underwent six unsuccessful surgical neck explorations in an attempt to identify and remove the abnormally functioning parathyroid gland before an adenoma finally was found ectopically located in the mediastinum.[412]

Albright's efforts to elucidate the pathophysiology of hyperparathyroidism represent a brilliant chapter in endocrine research. While Albright championed the concept that PTH acts principally on kidney to produce its systemic effects on calcium metabolism, the Canadian physician James Bertram Collip argued that the hormone acts principally on bone to mobilize calcium; he thought that the renal effects were secondary. The controversy sparked experimentation for over a decade before the researchers finally realized that both hypotheses were actually correct[409]: The hormone acts directly on both bone and kidney. Using nephrectomized animals, Collip and coworkers showed a direct effect of PTH on bone.[413] The decisive proof that the hormone acts on bone came from later experiments by Barnicot, who transplanted parathyroid glands into a position adjacent to cranial bone, producing local bony resorption.[409,414]

Primary hyperparathyroidism affects women more commonly than men (ratio 2:1) and increases in prevalence progressively after age 30. Postmenopausal women have the highest risk of having not only hyperparathyroidism but also osteoporosis.[415] Hence, a postmenopausal woman who has hyperparathyroidism is at risk for compromise of bone strength because of the combined accelerated bone loss which accompanies both disorders.

The incidence of hyperparathyroidism appears to have increased by an order of magnitude since the advent of multiphasic screening of blood on a routine basis some three decades ago.[415] This vast increase in the detection of the syndrome in the general population has raised controversy regarding the natural history and management of the disease. It now seems likely that many, perhaps most, patients with this disorder have normal life expectancy and do not suffer from the dramatic bone, renal, and other disorders associated with the disease in an earlier era. In fact, it is likely that many patients suffer no symptoms or adverse sequelae from the disorder. Therefore, the important issues regarding the management of "asymptomatic" hyperparathyroidism will be discussed below in a separate section.

Etiology

The "anatomic" etiology of hyperparathyroidism can be divided into several categories. The pathology in 80 to 85 percent of cases of hyperparathyroidism is caused by a single adenoma of one of the four parathyroid glands. These adenomas are monoclonal in origin, as recently documented using recombinant DNA techniques,[416,417] lending strong support to the surgical approach of removing only the single abnormal gland. It is not known why adenomas arise spontaneously, but in at least one (minor) subgroup of patients there was previous exposure to neck irradiation.[410,418,419]

The molecular mechanisms responsible for the development of parathyroid adenomas have only recently begun to be elucidated, and the insights obtained apply thus far to only a minority of cases but may yet prove true for the majority. An apparently common mechanism, possibly accounting for approximately 25 percent of the sporadic adenomas examined thus far,[420] appears to be loss of a tumor suppressor gene, but this has not been established unequivocally. This mechanism is suggested by the finding of deletions in chromosome 11 that have been mapped to 11q12-13. This region of chromosome 11 also is often deleted in parathyroid tumors from patients with multiple endocrine neoplasia syndrome type 1 (discussed later) who have four-gland disease.[421,422] This model for adenoma development may parallel the paradigm described for oncogenesis in retinoblastoma by loss of a tumor suppressor gene product or antioncogene,[423–425] although parathyroid adenomas are benign.

An intriguing mechanism accounting for at least 4 percent of adenomas examined is a DNA rearrangement in the region of the PTH gene.[426–428] This genetic alteration is present in all the cells of the adenoma but not in the same patient's normal tissue. In these cases, one PTH gene has been severed between its coding region and the upstream regulatory domain. The chromosome then inverts and is ligated together, resulting in a new linkage of the PTH gene regulatory domain to an unrelated gene. The alteration is termed a pericentromeric inversion. It brings the PRAD1 gene (for *par*athyroid *ad*enoma) (Fig. 23-47) under the influence of the putative tissue-specific PTH regulatory domain. PRAD1 is markedly overexpressed in this arrangement and appears to be an oncogene. The same oncogene may be involved in lymphoma and breast cancer.[429,430] The PTH produced by the adenoma presumably arises from the unaffected remaining PTH allele, although this does not explain the "set point" error which may be present in some adenomas. PRAD1 is not known to be calcium-regulated.

The role of PRAD1 in normal physiology is not known. The proto-oncogene's product has structural homology to the cyclin families of proteins involved in the cell division cycle,[431] and PRAD1 may regulate the crucial cell cycle checkpoint between the GI and S phases.[431] Whether overexpression of PRAD1 or other cell cycle regulators is involved more generally in parathyroid adenomas without detectable PTH rearrangement is not known.

The pathology of an adenoma may differ only subtly from that of a normal gland. The balance between parenchymal hormone-secreting chief cells or oxyphil cells and fat cells is shifted toward the former group. Since the proportion of fat cells in the gland increases normally with age, an adenomatous gland may simply resemble the "normal" gland of a younger patient. Sometimes the pathologic diagnosis is facilitated by the presence of a rim of normal or "compressed" parathyroid tissue at the edge of the adenoma. The noninvolved glands, which are "suppressed" and hence are synthetically inactive, are not usually distinctive in appearance and appear "normal."

The observed pathology in 10 to 15 percent of patients with primary hyperparathyroidism is four-gland hyperplasia, which typically is polyclonal in origin in the nonfamilial forms but involves a genomic mutation when associated with the multiple endocrine neoplasia (MEN) syndromes (discussed later).[416,432,433] It presents in two pathologic variants. Primary chief cell hyperplasia is the more common form and predominates (or is the only form which occurs) in the hereditarily associated disorders such as the MEN syndromes and familial hyperparathyroidism. Clear cell hyperplasia is much more rare; the cell type of origin is not known. Both kinds of pathology can arise sporadically. Although four-gland hyperplasia can arise spontaneously, its presence should always raise the possibility of a MEN syndrome in the patient and should therefore alert the physician to perform a diagnostic evaluation for the related hereditary disorders as well as the relevant endocrine evaluation of relatives.

The pathology in the remaining small proportion (<1 percent) of patients is a parathyroid carcinoma which secretes parathyroid hormone autonomously. Calcium levels typically are markedly elevated in

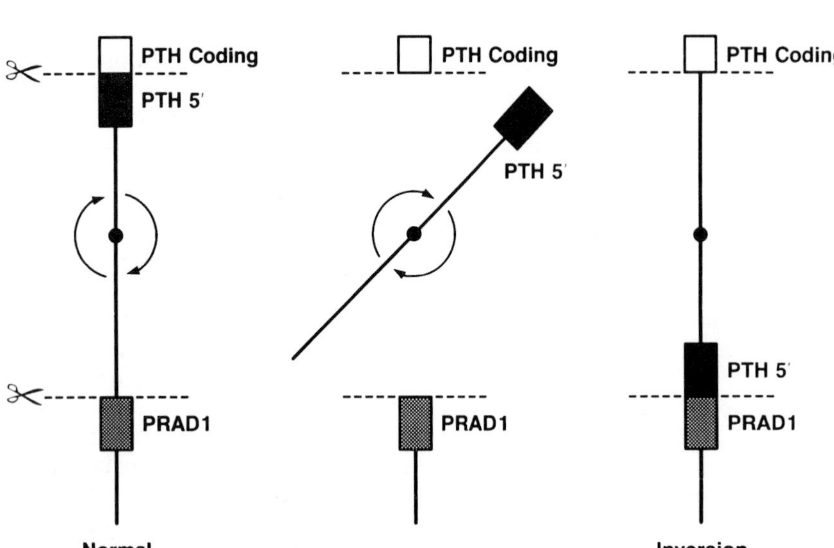

FIGURE 23-47 The genetic abnormality present in a subset of parathyroid adenomas has been structurally elucidated. The abnormality appears to arise from a gene rearrangement (inversion) in which the 5′ regulatory region of PTH is separated from the coding region of the hormone. Instead, the PRAD1 gene occupies the position adjacent to the 5′ regulatory region of PTH. *(Courtesy of Dr. Andrew Arnold, Massachusetts General Hospital.)*

these patients, as are PTH levels; both are considerably higher than usual in typical hyperparathyroidism. The course of the disease usually is rapid, in contrast to the indolent course of primary hyperparathyroidism.

The pathophysiologic mechanism responsible for inappropriately elevated secretion of parathyroid hormone by adenomas and hyperplastic tissue appears to be complex. Much of the increased secretion appears to result from an inappropriate "set point" for hormonal secretion by the abnormal cells.[16,434,435] In other words, the dose-response curve for PTH secretion as regulated by extracellular calcium levels is inappropriately shifted to the right so that higher calcium levels are required to suppress PTH secretion (Fig. 23-48). Once higher levels of calcium are achieved, normal "suppression" of secretion occurs. This "thermostat-like" error appears to be present in both adenomatous and hyperplastic parathyroid tissue. However, for both normal and abnormal parathyroid tissue, total suppression of hormonal secretion cannot be achieved.[16,434] There is always a small but obligatory secretion of hormone which persists even at extremely high levels of extracellular calcium. Therefore, it is reasonable to suppose that when the absolute quantity of parathyroid tissue increases, the obligatory secretion or "nonsuppressible" component of PTH secretion increases and becomes sufficiently high to produce hyperparathyroidism and hypercalcemia (Fig. 23-48). In fact, hyperparathyroidism can be created experimentally in rats by transplanting multiple isologous glands into a single animal.[436] In parathyroid carcinomas, secretion is autonomous and is not affected by extracellular calcium concentrations: Continuously high levels of hormone are released by carcinomatous cells.

The particular step(s) in hormonal biosynthesis and secretion which fails to be appropriately regulated and is therefore responsible for excess secretion of PTH is unknown. All the steps in the biosynthesis, processing, and secretion of the hormone are potential sites of malfunction, including transcription, translation, posttranslational modification, packaging, and release of secretory granules (Fig. 23-6). Thus far, efficiency of transcription and translation, conversion of precursor mRNA to mature mRNA, and the intracellular metabolism of preproparathyroid hormone to proparathyroid hormone and then to native parathyroid hormone appears to be normal. Only the actual regulation of release of hormone into the circulation appears to be defective in primary hyperparathyroidism.[432]

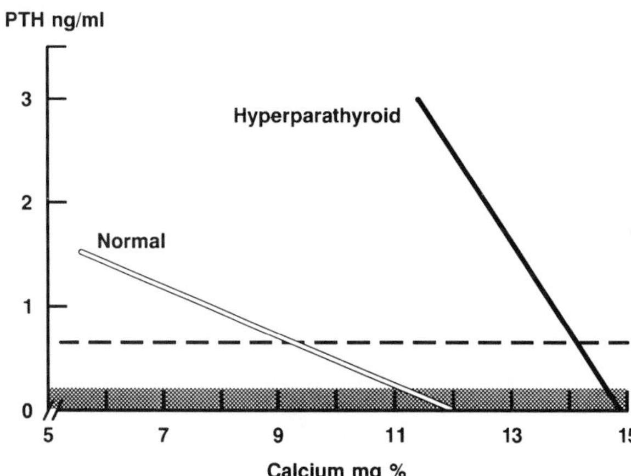

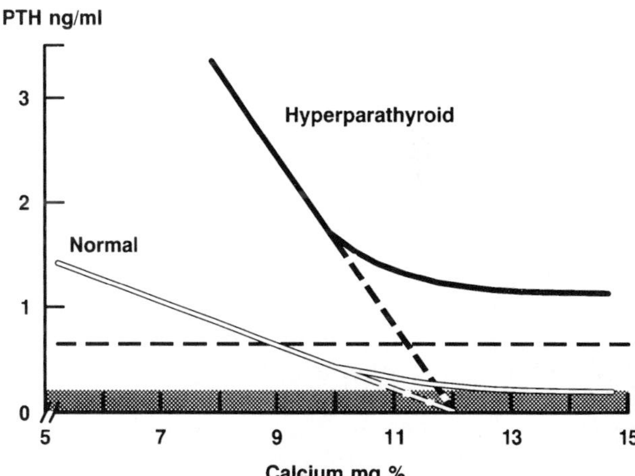

FIGURE 23-48 Possible mechanism for parathyroid hormone oversecretion in various disorders. In instances such as lithium-induced hyperparathyroidism, familial hypercalciuric hypercalcemia, and many parathyroid adenomas, a "set point" error appears to account for the abnormality *(top)*. Glands from such hyperparathyroid individuals show steeper slopes of response than normal, and a higher level of calcium is required to suppress hormone secretion. When the total mass of parathyroid hormone (PTH) is increased, the amount of hormone secreted as a result of the "nonsuppressed" component of PTH secretion is sufficient to produce hypercalcemia without evoking any other abnormality in stimulus-secretion coupling owing to a larger mass of tissue *(bottom)*. The hypothesis requires that a small amount of hormone secretion persists despite elevated calcium. In the normal parathyroid gland, this secretion is small and insignificant. In hyperparathyroidism, greatly increased tissue mass leads to persistent secretion of the hormone above the normal range (dashed line). The slopes of both normal and hyperparathyroid states extrapolate to the same calcium subpoint (12 mg/100 ml). PTH values within the shaded area are below the limits of assay detection. *(Reprinted with permission from Lynn H. Caporale and Michael Rosenblatt, Parathyroid Hormone Secretion: Molecular Events and Regulation, Contributions to Nephrology 50:73–95, 1986.)*

Clinical Presentation and Pathophysiology

The presentation of hyperparathyroidism has evolved considerably since the early days of identification of the syndrome.[415,437] As was mentioned previously, the hallmark of the disease used to be severe bone changes associated with osteitis fibrosa cystica. Over the next several decades, the association with kidney stones was recognized and became the most common presenting sign of hyperparathyroidism, approximately 3 to 10 times more common than bone complications. The routine screening of blood chemistry values in large portions of the population has led to the current clinical profile, in which "asymptomatic" hyperparathyroidism predominates (Fig. 23-49).

It is difficult to specifically attribute signs and symptoms other than renal stones and bone disease to primary hyperparathyroidism for several reasons (Table 23-4 and Fig. 23-44). First, there can be a concurrence of common disorders such as hyperparathyroidism and hypertension or hyperparathyroidism and peptic ulcer disease.[415,437–440] These illnesses previously were thought to be associated with hyperparathyroidism. With the exception of the linkage that occurs between hyperparathyroidism and peptic ulcers caused by the Zollinger-Ellison syndrome as part of multiple endocrine neoplasia syndrome type I (discussed below), there does not appear to be an increased incidence of hypertension or peptide ulcer disease with hyperparathyroidism. Similarly, pancreatitis appears to be associated by chance with primary hyperparathyroidism.[441] Other findings, such as fatigue, weakness, and depression, are common in the general population and therefore are not specific or readily quantified. While physicians who care for patients with primary hyperparathyroidism believe that many of these patients have subtle complaints either originating from the metabolic consequences of hyperparathyroidism or exacerbated by the disease,[442] these disturbances often cannot be reversed by surgical intervention.

A variety of articular manifestations are observed in patients with primary hyperparathyroidism. The most common is chronic chondrocalcinosis, with or without acute attacks of pseudogout. Chondrocalcinosis may affect as many as 5 percent of patients with primary hyperparathyroidism and is seen radiologically as calcification of articular cartilage, most often in the knee. Pseudogout occurs less frequently. It is usually an acute arthritis of the large joints, most commonly the knee, induced by deposition of calcium pyrophosphate crystals. The diagnosis of pseudogout can be made by demonstrating rhomboidal calcium phosphate crystals in joint fluid. Attacks of acute gouty arthritis also occur in a few percent of patients. Both pseudogout and urate gout may occur after parathyroidectomy.

FIGURE 23-49 Clinical presentation of primary hyperparathyroidism in the current era. *(Courtesy of Maurice Attie, University of Pennsylvania School of Medicine.)*

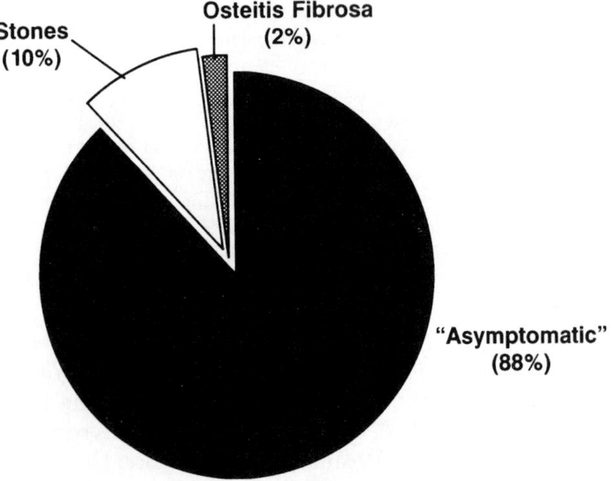

Distinguishing hyperparathyroidism from malignancy (the second most common cause of hypercalcemia) is one of the most challenging diagnostic problems facing the clinician. The chronicity of hypercalcemia strongly favors hyperparathyroidism over malignancy. Typically, the calcium levels are lower in hyperparathyroidism than in hypercalcemia of malignancy. Furthermore, in hypercalcemia of malignancy, the malignant etiology of the hypercalcemia is often obvious at the time of presentation.

Hyperparathyroid Bone Disease

Increased bone turnover is characteristic of primary hyperparathyroidism. However, in most cases, bone formation and bone resorption remain nearly balanced and there are no short-term clinical sequelae of the increased metabolic bone turnover other than hypercalcemia. In severe cases, osteitis fibrosa is present and is associated with bone pain, which can be the presenting complaint. An x-ray is shown in Fig. 23-50. The disorder is characterized by distorted and disorganized remodeling of bone, accelerated bone resorption leading to pathologic fractures, and fibrotic infiltrates. The cortical surfaces of bone are thinned, and much of the bone is demineralized (Fig. 23-51). The fibrotic bulging lesions within bone are histologically termed "brown tumors" (Fig. 23-52). Often, fluid-filled cysts also occur, termed osteitis fibrosa cystica (Fig. 23-53). Present in the hands is a characteristic subperiosteal resorption on the medial aspects of the middle phalanges of the third and fourth fingers (Fig. 23-50); this is also present in the toes and ribs. Subperiosteal resorption in the hand is pathognomonic of hyperparathyroidism. A similar process in the skull leads to a so-called salt and pepper appearance (Fig. 23-54). Disappearance of the lamina dura of the teeth is also seen, but this is a nonspecific finding which occurs commonly in periodontal disease.

During the period 1925–1950, as many as 50 percent of patients presented with skeletal complications. Today, this number has fallen sharply to below 10 percent[415,437] (Table 23-4 and Fig. 23-49). Of greater concern now is osteopenia and its potential aggravation of underlying osteoporosis. Loss of bone mineral density is known to be accompanied by a loss of the biomechanical strength of bone. Such a loss of bone mineral density is clinically silent until the appearance of the first fracture. In most surveys of

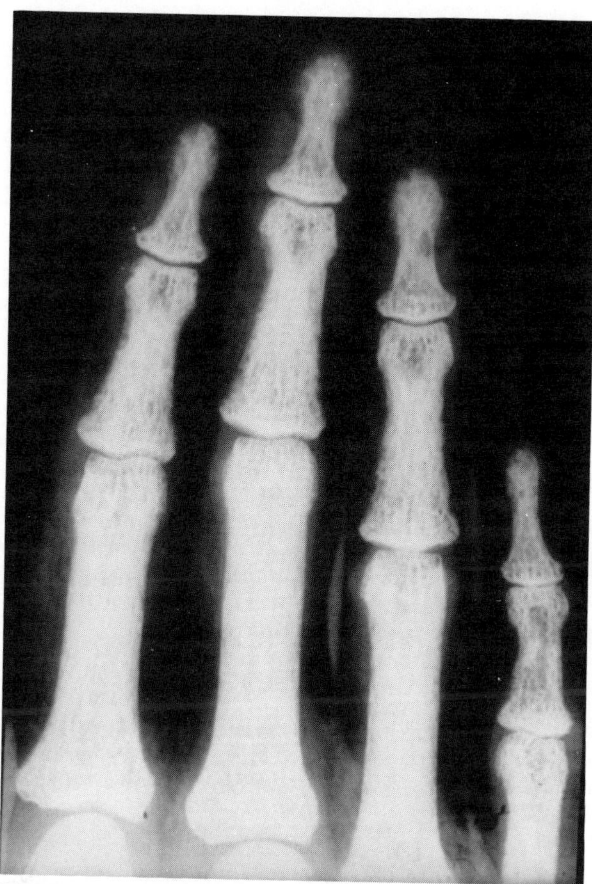

FIGURE 23-50 Radiograph of osteitis fibrosa in primary hyperparathyroidism. Subperiosteal resorption of the medial aspects of the middle phalanges is present. This finding is thought to be pathognomonic for hyperparathyroidism. *(Courtesy of Dr. Maurice Attie, University of Pennsylvania School of Medicine.)*

patients with documented hyperparathyroidism, it is clear that the levels of bone mineral density are below those found in age-, sex-, and race-matched normal cohorts (Figs. 23-55 and 23-56).[443–446] However, there is some controversy regarding the clinical significance of the loss of bone mineral in hyperparathyroid states and the predisposition to fracture. Some evidence suggests an internal shift of bone mineral within the anatomic architecture of bone. Although the cortex of bone is thinned, trabecular bone may be preserved or there may be an increase in the thickness of trabecular bone[447] (Fig. 23-51). Such a local shift of calcium within bone might actually strengthen vertebral bone and prevent crush fractures, although the risk for hip fracture might be increased. Although these observations are provocative, determinations of bone mineral density remain among the most important parameters used in assessing the clinical status of primary hyperparathyroidism and in directing surgical vs. medical management.

Hyperparathyroid Kidney Disease

The occurrence of calcium-containing kidney stones is clearly associated with hyperparathyroidism and can lead to renal compromise[415,437] (see Chap. 25). Hence, nephrolithiasis is generally considered an indication for surgery.[448] However, currently less than 15 percent of these patients have kidney stones at the time of presentation. In addition to the increased calcium clearance, the decreased acid content of the urine may contribute as a risk factor for the development of kidney stones. Although there have been reports indicating an increased incidence of kidney stones in patients whose vitamin D levels are higher than average for hyperparathyroidism,[334] increased vitamin D levels do not predict the future occurrence of kidney stones and certainly should not be used as an indication for surgery.[449] Nephrocalcinosis occurs even less commonly, is mostly associated with more severe disease, and is rare in the modern era. Typically, calcium deposits ectopically in the kidney in an anatomic distribution corresponding to locales where the solute-concentrating function of the kidney is greatest. Nephrocalcinosis can lead to renal failure. However, more subtle renal disturbances occur commonly, such as increased urinary calcium excretion and mild electrolyte disorders. In general, these disturbances are correctable surgically.[446] Renal concentrating ability also may be compromised by long-standing hyperparathyroidism, as occurs with hypercalcemia of other causes but does not necessarily reverse with surgical treatment.

Nonspecific Features of Primary Hyperparathyroidism

Although many symptoms have been commonly ascribed to primary hyperparathyroidism, it has been difficult to establish a true causal relation between primary hyperparathyroidism and many of these symptoms. This is especially true for central nervous system symptoms,[450] for extremes of hypercalcemia, lethargy, stupor, and even coma occur and clearly are attributable to hypercalcemia. However, more subtle or often nonspecific symptoms such as fatigue, difficulty concentrating, and a decline in one's general sense of well-being occur in certain individuals in association with hyperparathyroidism.[442] Along the same lines, constipation, mild nausea, polyuria, polydipsia, and nocturia are difficult to link to hyperparathyroidism. These symptoms can be vague, are difficult to quantify, and are prevalent in the general population. There are undoubtedly many patients with hyperparathyroidism who report an improvement in symptoms as a result of surgery. Some patients report not realizing that they were not feeling well until the contrast they experienced after parathyroidectomy. However, in many cases, surgery does not reverse mild or nonspecific symptoms. Furthermore, surgery is known to

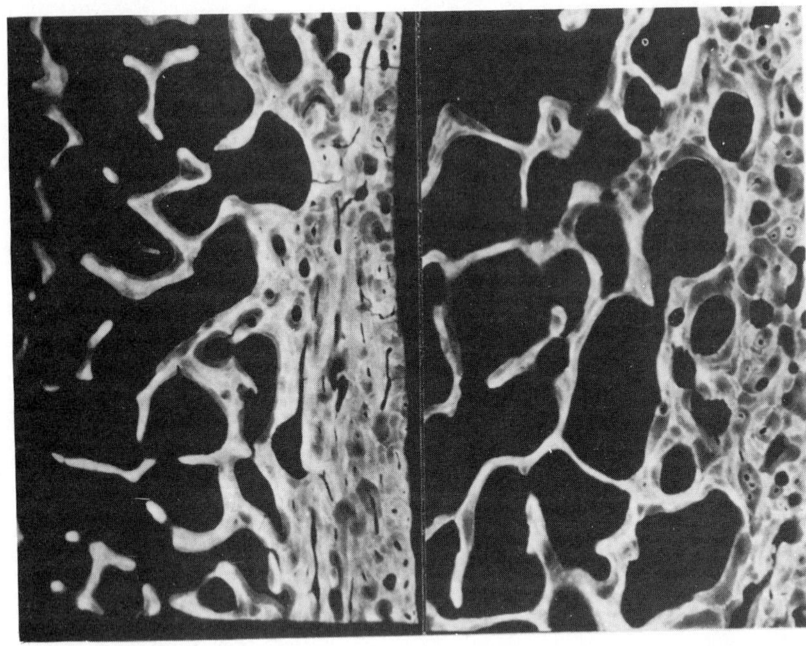

FIGURE 23-51 Normal bone *(left)* vs. bone from a patient with chronic hyperparathyroidism *(right)*. The cortex and the trabecular meshwork are thinned in hyperparathyroidism, compromising biomechanical strength and predisposing to fracture. *(Reprinted with permission from Jenifer Jowsey, Bone histology and hyperparathyroidism, Clinics in Endocrinology and Metabolism, vol. 3, p. 268, 1974.)*

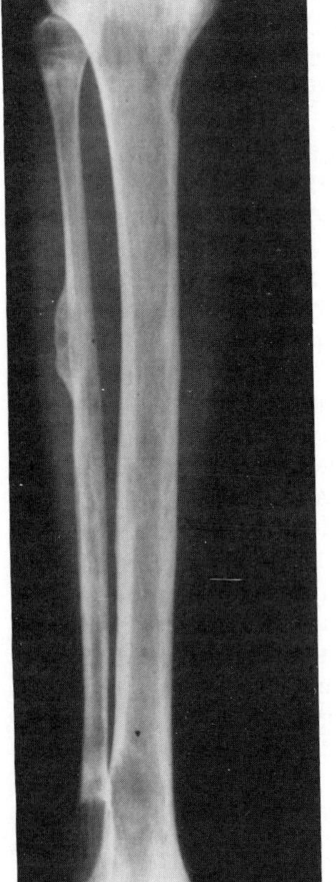

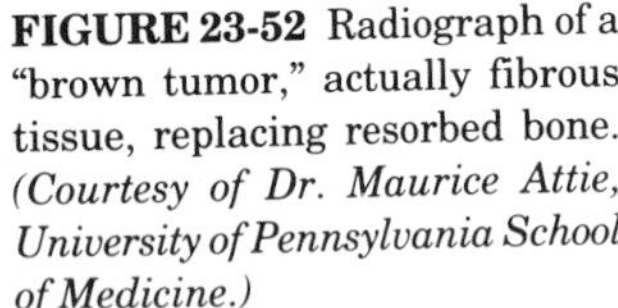

FIGURE 23-52 Radiograph of a "brown tumor," actually fibrous tissue, replacing resorbed bone. *(Courtesy of Dr. Maurice Attie, University of Pennsylvania School of Medicine.)*

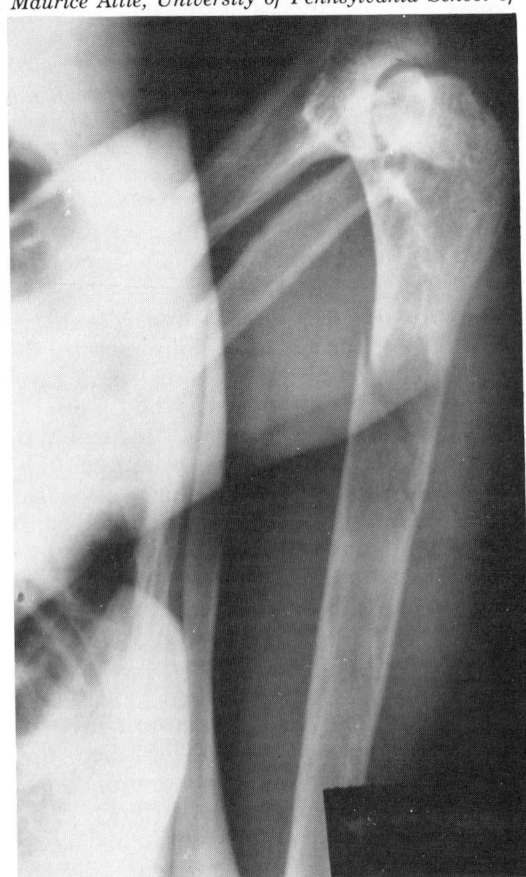

FIGURE 23-53 Osteitis fibrosa cystica. "Brown tumors" can appear "cystic" on a radiograph. The fibrous infiltrate is weaker than normal bone, predisposing to fracture, as seen in this case. *(Courtesy of Dr. Maurice Attie, University of Pennsylvania School of Medicine.)*

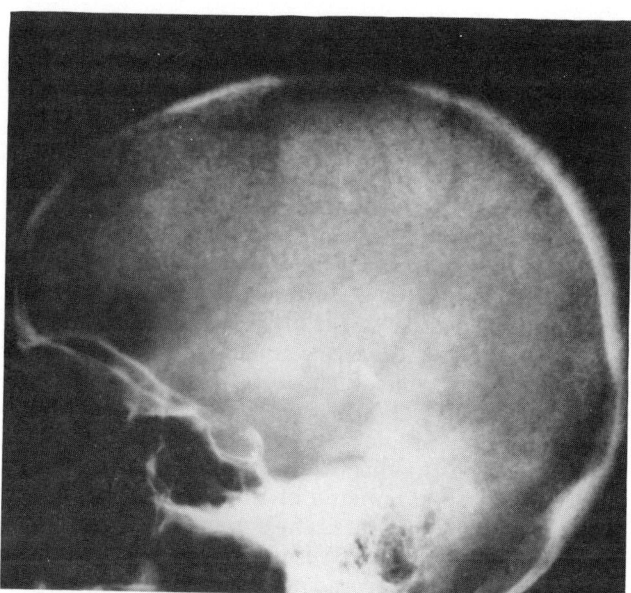

FIGURE 23-54 Radiograph of a "salt and pepper" skull reflecting resorption and demineralization. *(Courtesy of Dr. Maurice Attie, University of Pennsylvania School of Medicine.)*

have a large placebo effect, complicating the evaluation of its benefit in hyperparathyroidism. In any case, it can be said with certainty that it is difficult to predict which patients will respond symptomatically to surgical intervention.

For some disorders, such as the muscle weakness which accompanies hyperparathyroidism, a neuromuscular deficit has been defined which appears to

FIGURE 23-55 The Z-score, an index of bone mineral density in the distal radius in asymptomatic primary hyperparathyroidism (open bars) compared to that in normal subjects (darkened arrow). Diminished bone mineral density is evident for the population with this disorder. *[Reprinted with permission from B.H. Mitlak, et al, Asymptomatic Primary Hyperparathyroidism, J Bone Mineral Res 6(Suppl 2):S103–S110, 1991.]*

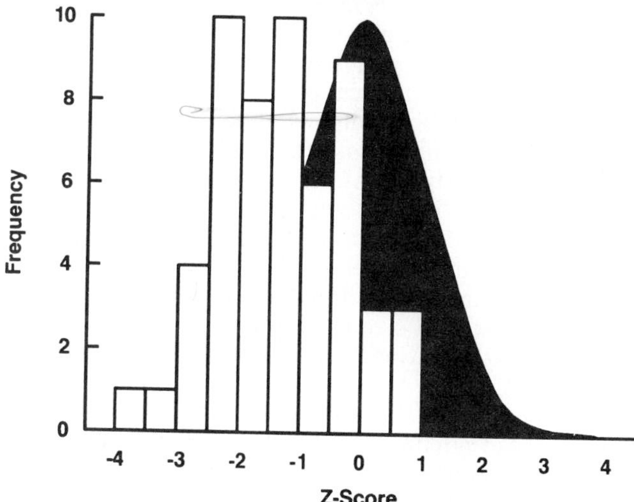

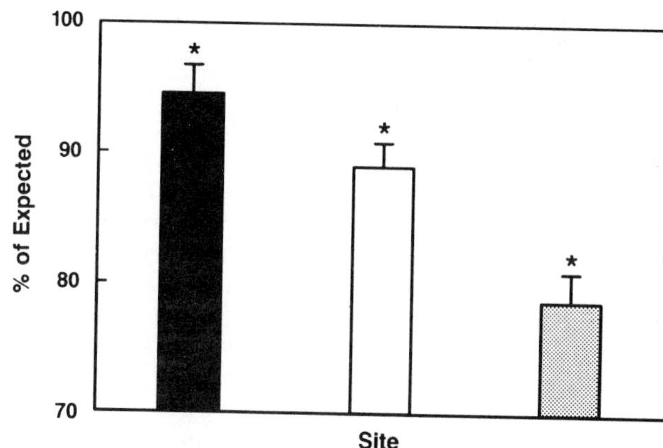

FIGURE 23-56 Decreased bone mineral density in primary hyperparathyroidism at several skeletal sites. ■, Lumbar; □, femoral; ▨, radius. *(Reprinted with permission from Silverberg et al.[449])*

be specific to primary hyperparathyroidism. Characteristic electromyographic (EMG) changes have been observed.[451,452] Some clinicians contend that these abnormalities are neurogenic. Although the muscle weakness and EMG changes seem to be less common now than in earlier times,[452] when present, they may be reversed by parathyroid surgery.[451]

Therefore, in considering a recommendation for surgery in patients with mild elevations of calcium, the physician should be careful to avoid advocating surgery in hopes of reversing nonspecific symptoms. Rather, the recommendation for surgery should be based on biochemical indexes of the disease, evidence of end organ compromise or deterioration, or the presence of fairly clear changes in mental status (such as confusion or altered psyche and mood, which generally occur at moderate to severe elevations of calcium and PTH). A more specific set of guidelines for surgical intervention is provided later, in the section on Diagnosis and Management of Asymptomatic Primary Hyperparathyroidism.

Multiple Endocrine Neoplasia

While hyperparathyroidism occurs most often sporadically, in a minority of cases there is a link to a familial syndrome. Familial hyperparathyroidism without other associated endocrine abnormalities has been reported in a few kindreds.[453] In general, it is inherited as an autosomal dominant pattern, and the pathology is four-gland chief cell hyperplasia. An even more rare form has single-gland parathyroid adenoma as the underlying pathology and is inherited in an autosomal recessive pattern.[454] Clinically, there appear to be no particular features that distinguish these forms of hyperparathyroidism from sporadic primary hyperparathyroidism.

The multiple endocrine neoplasia (MEN) syndromes constitute a well-defined set of hereditary endocrine disorders, some of which include hyperparathyroidism as a component. The MEN syndromes are discussed extensively in Chap. 28. For the purpose of this chapter, some aspects of the MEN syndromes as they relate to hyperparathyroidism are highlighted. Hyperparathyroidism is a prominent component in two of the three MEN syndromes (type 1 and type 2a) and is rare in or absent from the third (type 2b). In these syndromes, hyperparathyroidism occurs as a result of four-gland hyperplasia. Table 23-5 lists the components of MEN type 1 (Wermer's syndrome: the three P's),[455] in which hyperparathyroidism is almost always present (penetrance approaches 100 percent by age 50) and is associated with tumors of the pituitary gland (usually chromophobe prolactin-secreting adenomas) and pancreatic adenomas (which typically secrete gastrin, insulin, or glucagon). The age of onset of hyperparathyroidism tends to be younger (between age 15 and 35) than in primary hyperparathyroidism, and the ratio of afflicted men to women is approximately equal, as opposed to a ratio of 2:1 for women to men in sporadic primary hyperparathyroidism.

The pattern of inheritance is that of an autosomal dominant trait. Using restriction fragment length polymorphism (RFLP) analysis, the genetic defect has been mapped to the long arm of chromosome 11, 11q12-13, in all kindreds with MEN 1 that have been examined.[456] The mutation is thought to result in inactivation of a tumor suppressor gene or antioncogene, as occurs with retinoblastoma, and is thought to be the cause of some parathyroid adenomas. Since both alleles for the tumor suppressor are inactivated or altered, the disease must represent a "two-hit" phenomenon. The germ line may contain a point mutation with no clinical consequences. However, on this background, a second event, such as somatic mutation, will lead to tumorigenesis. Hence, the glandular abnormality is "monoclonal" even though all four glands become hyperplastic (the hyperplasia can be asymmetric across the glands). The markedly increased gland mass per se can account for the excess PTH secretion without a set point abnormality based on the nonsuppressible component of PTH secretion by parathyroid cells.

TABLE 23-5 Multiple Endocrine Neoplasia Syndromes

Type 1
>95% hyperparathyroidism (four-gland hyperplasia)
~50% pancreatic tumors (gastrinoma, insulinoma, glucagonoma, etc.)
15–50% pituitary adenomas (prolactinoma, growth hormone–secreting, etc.)
Type 2 (2a)
100% medullary carcinoma of the thyroid
<50% pheochromocytoma or adrenal medullary hyperplasia
10–50% hyperparathyroidism (four-gland hyperplasia)
Type 3 (2b)
100% medullary carcinoma of the thyroid
<50% pheochromocytoma or adrenal medullary hyperplasia
100% mucosal neuromas

By producing hypercalcemia, the primary hyperparathyroidism of MEN 1 can exacerbate gastrin and acid secretion in patients who also harbor a gastrinoma (Zollinger-Ellison syndrome). Hence, parathyroidectomy is often indicated when the two disorders coexist and some improvement in peptic ulcer disease can be expected after parathyroidectomy.

Primary hyperparathyroidism occurs in approximately 10 percent of cases (although it may be present histologically in 50 percent) of the MEN type 2a syndrome (Sipple's syndrome).[457,458] The other components of the disorder are pheochromocytomas and medullary carcinoma of the thyroid gland, the latter of which dominates the syndrome (Table 23-5). The different endocrine tumors share a common developmental origin from the neuroectoderm. Any of the tumor types can present first, not all the types in each syndrome arise in each individual, and there is no set pattern of appearance. The allelic mutations responsible for both MEN type 2a and MEN type 2b (3) map to a different chromosome than do the abnormalities in MEN type 1; both are found on the same locus of chromosome 10 as opposed to chromosome 11.[459]

It is always important to obtain a family history regarding the presence of any of the other components of the MEN type 1 or 2a syndromes in a patient suspected of having primary hyperparathyroidism. Certainly in patients who are discovered to have four-gland hyperplasia at the time of surgery, it is important to undertake diagnostic evaluation not only of the patient but also of close relatives for the potential relevant endocrine abnormalities.

Familial Hypocalciuric Hypercalcemia

Familial hypocalciuric hypercalcemia (FHH), although rare, has fascinated clinical investigators. It may be an atypical form of primary hyperparathyroidism which could potentially provide insights into the pathophysiology of hyperparathyroidism.[460–462] This disorder is characterized by chronically elevated serum calcium, somewhat depressed phosphorus, and PTH values that are usually detectable and normal or slightly elevated in some cases. Even normal levels of PTH are "inappropriate" in the setting of hypercalcemia and imply that PTH may play an etiologic role in maintenance of the hypercalcemia. Along the same lines, the parathyroid glands are usually normal in size or slightly enlarged. On microscopic examination, they are normal or somewhat hyperplastic.

Patients with this disorder tend to excrete low quantities of calcium in the urine, typically one-third of the value observed in patients with primary hyperparathyroidism and below a value of 0.10 for the ratio of calcium to creatinine clearance. This appears to reflect a renal defect, since the increased tubular reabsorption of calcium persists even after parathyroidectomy. These patients also display somewhat elevated blood magnesium levels. While these biochemical parameters are true of the population with the disorder, they cannot be used to make the diagnosis in any given individual, because the values overlap with those present in classical primary hyperparathyroidism (Fig. 23-57). The disorder is lifelong and is inherited as an autosomal dominant trait with virtually 100 percent penetrance. The age of onset is much earlier than in hyperparathyroidism; hypercalcemia can be demonstrated from birth and is usually detected by age 20. However, since FHH is asymptomatic, the disorder may not be detected until much later in life.

Although the low urine calcium excretion, presentation early in life, and positive family history are findings which strongly suggest the diagnosis of FHH, none of these features alone can distinguish the disorder from primary hyperparathyroidism. Fortunately, however, as far as can be determined at this point, these patients develop no long-term sequelae of the disease other than rare instances of relapsing pancreatitis. If they mistakenly undergo neck exploration, an adenoma is not found. Normal or somewhat hyperplastic-appearing glands may be found. If one or more of these glands are removed, the hypercalcemia remains unchanged; therefore, it is important not to send such patients for unnecessary surgery.

FIGURE 23-57 Biochemical abnormalities in familial hypocalciuric hypercalcemia (FHH). As shown, there is considerable overlap between patients with primary hyperparathyroidism and patients with FHH. ○, FHH; •, 1° PTH. *(Modified from Marx et al.[464])*

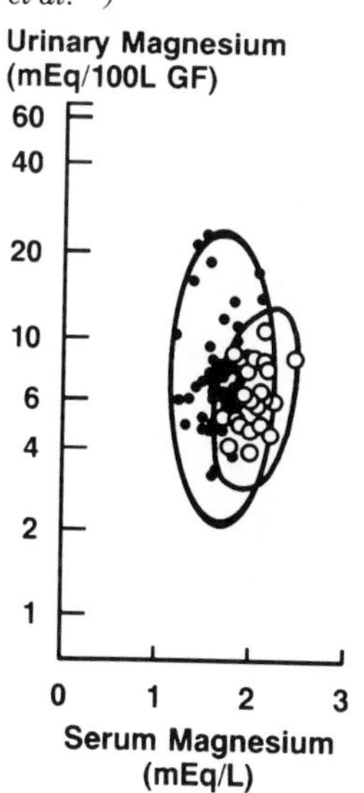

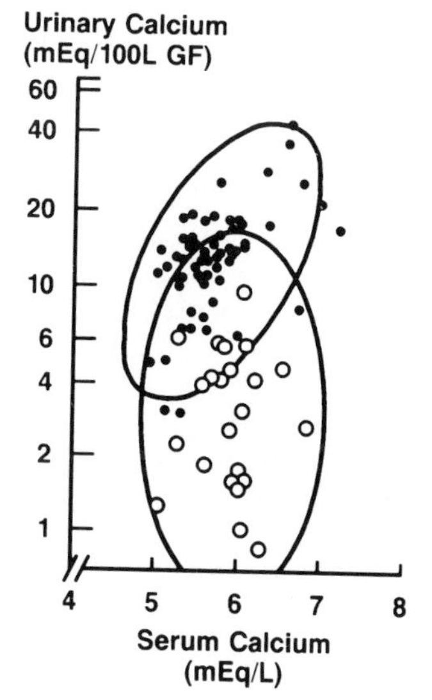

The etiology of FHH has been elucidated recently.[463,464,464a] The pathophysiology seems to derive from a set point error in the response of parathyroid tissue to calcium that is directly related to a mutation in the calcium-sensing receptor[31] (Fig. 23-77, see Addendum). Several distinct mutations have been elucidated which render the calcium sensor's responsiveness markedly diminished. This error accounts for the normal levels of PTH accompanying hypercalcemia. However, the tissues which are exposed to elevated PTH and calcium levels also may respond less than normally; hence, adverse effects do not seem to develop. Since the disorder is inherited as an autosomal dominant trait with high penetrance, it is important to identify family members with the disorder in order to avoid unnecessary surgery.

Although the disease is usually benign, occasionally it presents in the neonate as severe life-threatening hypercalcemia. Individuals with this disorder are homozygous for a defective calcium-sensing receptor gene.[463,464,464a] The double dose cases represent one of the few instances where surgical total parathyroidectomy is recommended.

Physical Findings

There are a limited number of physical findings associated with hyperparathyroidism. Band keratopathy is seen at the outer edge of the cornea at the upper and lower poles (Fig. 23-58). This finding must be distinguished from age-related nonspecific or inflammatory calcification in the limbic girdle by slit-lamp examination. Weakness may be apparent on physical examination, particularly of the proximal muscles of the lower extremities. Confusion or altered mental status may also be present. Only rarely can an abnormal parathyroid gland (sometimes a parathyroid carcinoma) be palpated. In fact, according to "Albright's dictum," if a mass is detected in the neck, it usually is in the thyroid gland or may represent a parathyroid carcinoma. Bone involvement can sometimes be detected by finding tenderness in the region of the distal tibia. Collapse of the terminal phalanges may occur, giving rise to "pseudo clubbing."

Laboratory Findings and Definitive Diagnosis

Consistent elevations in serum calcium above the normal level are the sine qua non of hyperparathyroidism. The measurement of serum calcium is accurate in clinical laboratories nearly universally now that multiphasic automated screening devices are employed. Detection of a calcium level above 10.4 mg/dl (2.6 mmol/liter) should always raise the suspicion of hypercalcemia. This is true regardless of the normal range listed by the laboratory, since some laboratories failed to change the normal range indicated on their lab reports after switching to automated analyzers. While the entity of "normocalcemic

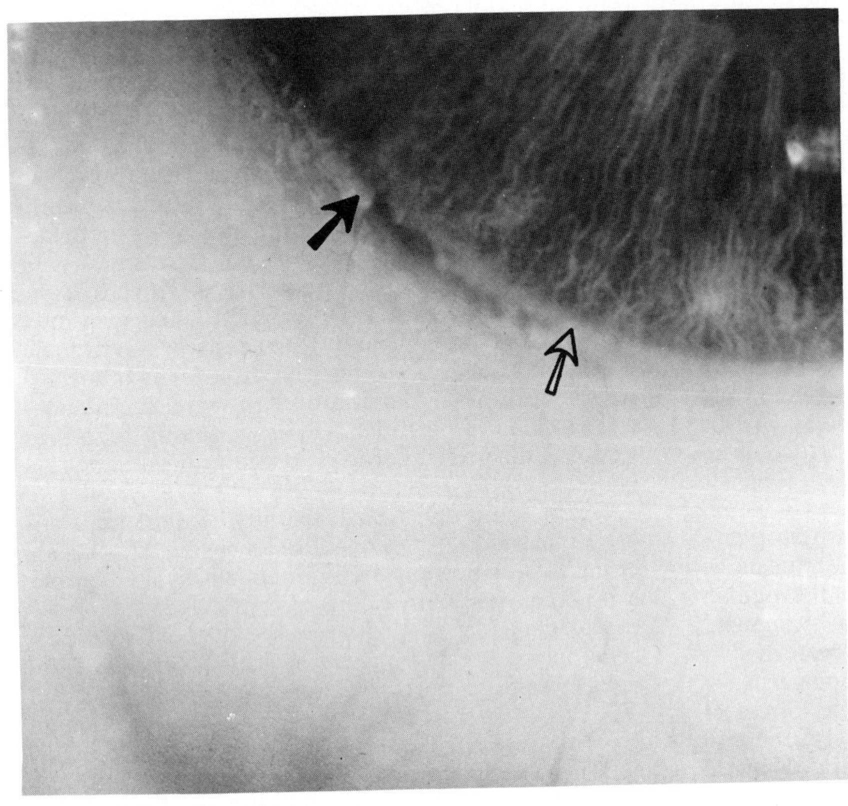

FIGURE 23-58 Band keratopathy. The open arrow identifies the limbic girdle, a region of linear calcium salt deposition associated with aging. Band keratopathy (solid arrow) is a moth-eaten and irregular region of calcium deposition, usually at the medial and lateral limbic margins. These locations are thought to result from diffusion of carbon dioxide from air-exposed regions of the cornea, with local precipitation of calcium phosphate crystals.

hyperparathyroidism" or "intermittent hypercalcemia" has received some attention in the literature,[465] when truly hyperparathyroid patients with borderline or occasional elevations in calcium are monitored and serial calcium determinations are obtained, a clear pattern of repeatedly frank hypercalcemia generally becomes evident. Chronicity of calcium elevation is also a hallmark of hyperparathyroidism. Since the disease is usually asymptomatic in the early stages, it is often possible to look back over a medical record and discover that a patient had documented mild elevations of calcium over a period of years. Hyperparathyroidism and its associated familial disorders are the only clinical disorders which produce hypercalcemia without other signs or symptoms for a period of years. It is also important to avoid misinterpretation of the calcium determination reported by the clinical laboratory. Since calcium circulates bound principally to albumin, abnormalities in the albumin level can alter the total serum calcium value without having a true physiologic consequence. In general, a deviation in serum albumin of 1.0 mg/dl results in a change of 0.8 mg/dl in the same direction for calcium; this shift needs to be taken into account when one is assessing a potential calcium abnormality. If the significance of a total calcium determination is in question, ionized calcium should be measured.

In recent years, definitive establishment of the diagnosis of hyperparathyroidism has been greatly facilitated by the development of reliable, sensitive, and accurate radioimmunoassays for PTH (discussed elsewhere in this chapter). In particular, the two-site IRMA[54] can accurately determine the quantity of biologically active full-length PTH present in the circulation. In almost all cases of hyperparathyroidism, PTH levels are found to be clearly elevated using such assays (Fig. 23-9), obviating the need for provocative testing or calcium-PTH histograms or other devices for assigning a diagnosis based on a combination of laboratory values. For the most part, it is no longer necessary to invoke previously employed diagnostic principles in which an "inappropriately" normal PTH level at the time of hypercalcemia was used to establish the diagnosis of hyperparathyroidism. Using the IRMA, PTH levels are usually elevated in hyperparathyroidism. Furthermore, there is a general correlation between the level of PTH detected, the degree of hypercalcemia, and the mass of abnormal parathyroid tissue. When this assay method is employed in complex clinical situations, many previously confusing diagnostic issues are clarified. Hypercalcemia caused by hyperparathyroidism as opposed to that caused by malignancy can be readily distinguished using the newer assays: PTH levels are depressed or undetectable in patients with hypercalcemia due to malignancy. Even in renal failure, where earlier radioimmunoassay (RIA) systems indicated increased levels of PTH (as a result of accumulation of carboxyl-terminal inactive fragments detected by the RIA system), the IRMA reveals elevated levels of PTH only when biologically active hormone and true secondary hyperparathyroidism are present. While not essential for determining the status of PTH secretion, use of the PTH IRMA can be advantageous compared to previous RIAs for detecting PTH levels in blood.

Other indicators of increased PTH activity such as low fasting serum phosphorus and bicarbonate levels and elevated chloride levels can be helpful in an ancillary manner in supporting the diagnosis. The action of PTH on the proximal tubule inhibits the reabsorption of bicarbonate, resulting in bicarbonate wasting. Consequently, in chronic states of parathyroid excess such as hyperparathyroidism, renal tubular acidosis develops. The resulting retention of hydrogen ions obligates chloride, resulting in a hyperchloremic acidosis. X-ray changes in bone can also corroborate the diagnosis. A determination of bone mineral density, while not helpful in establishing the diagnosis, will provide a useful baseline measurement of bone status by which to later monitor the course of the disease. Once the diagnosis of hyperparathyroidism has been made, an abdominal radiograph should be obtained to assist in the search for calcified renal stones. Elevations in alkaline phosphatase serve as a biochemical indicator of bone involvement before x-ray changes are apparent. The QT interval on the electrocardiogram may be shortened, reflecting hypercalcemia, not hyperparathyroidism specifically. Measurement of 24-h urine calcium should be performed once the diagnosis of hyperparathyroidism has been confirmed to investigate the possibility of FHH syndrome, to evaluate the need for surgery in asymptomatic patients, and as a baseline for future monitoring. However, measurements of vitamin D levels or 24-h urine phosphorus excretion are not necessary. Therefore, it is emphasized that in the current era the diagnosis of hyperparathyroidism can be established definitively and exclusively or disproven by the biochemical determinations of blood calcium and PTH levels.

Preoperative Localization Studies

Several techniques are available for localizing abnormal parathyroid glands before surgery. These include venous catheterization with determination of PTH levels, angiography, ultrasound, and radiothallium/technetium imaging.[466–468] However, each of these methods fails to achieve a high level of detection and can incorrectly suggest the presence of an abnormal parathyroid gland. The combined problem of false negatives and false positives greatly limits their utility. In fact, the skilled surgeon has a much higher rate of identification of the abnormal gland or glands than do any of the preoperative localization techniques.

These techniques also do not help guide the surgeon to the correct side of the neck, reduce operating time, or decrease the morbidity for the patient.[469] Furthermore, techniques such as venous catheterization are expensive and invasive. For some patients, the stress and time required for venous catheterization approximate those of a surgical procedure. Therefore, as Doppman at NIH (an expert in catheterization) has said, "The only localization study needed in a patient with hyperparathyroidism is to locate an experienced parathyroid surgeon."

However, preoperative localization studies can be very useful if they are limited to patients in whom there has been previous surgery and failure to identify the abnormal gland in the neck.[469] In such cases, computed tomography of the mediastinum or angiography should be used to search for the rare abnormal parathyroid gland within the mediastinum (intrathymic or otherwise); CT is noninvasive and less expensive than angiography. If a mediastinal mass is not discovered, selective venous catheterization with measurement of PTH values should be considered to identify secretion from an abnormal gland in the neck. Because the success of invasive techniques depends in part on the skill of the practitioner, patients should be referred to one of the small number of institutions with substantial experience in these procedures. Localization techniques, particularly selective venous catheterization, should also be considered when there has been previous neck surgery which has altered the local anatomy, complicating the anticipated parathyroid surgery, whether or not the previous neck surgery was for hyperparathyroidism. In some cases, localization can be coupled with an ablation technique, such as destructive infusion of angiographic contrast medium, to effectively treat the disease.[470] Ablative methods should be considered when previous surgery has been unsuccessful and the patient is at high risk for complications of neck exploration and no longer amenable to surgery or when the abnormal gland has been localized to the mediastinum and an attempt is being made to avoid sternotomy. Looking back on all the effort undertaken thus far to develop localization techniques for the parathyroids, one is reminded of Albright's quip, "There is no time like the initial operation to find and remove the tumor."

Parathyroid Surgery

Parathyroid surgery can be technically difficult. The adjacent vital structures in the neck require that surgery be performed with considerable skill. Complications from surgery in this area include hypoparathyroidism and vocal cord paralysis from damage to the recurrent laryngeal nerve, causing permanent hoarseness. If the laryngeal nerves are damaged bilaterally, respiratory compromise or death can result. The variation in the anatomic location of abnormal glands in ectopic sites such as the lateral neck, retroesophageal region, intrathyroidal position, and mediastinum may complicate surgery.

Furthermore, the differences in pathology between single-gland adenoma, four-gland hyperplasia, and parathyroid carcinoma dictate different operative treatments. Hence, the need for engaging a surgeon experienced in parathyroid surgery cannot be overemphasized. As was mentioned above, the surgeon can expect to find a single abnormal parathyroid gland in approximately 85 percent of cases. When found, this gland should be removed and at least one other gland should be identified by biopsy as normal.

In the 10 to 15 percent of cases where four-gland hyperplasia is found, the surgeon should remove three glands and a portion of the fourth. Such surgery can be extremely difficult and runs the risk of inadequately treating the condition, thus leaving residual persistent hyperparathyroidism, or removing too much parathyroid tissue, thus producing hypoparathyroidism.[471,472] Even when normocalcemia is achieved postoperatively, within months some patients with hyperplasia develop recurrent hyperparathyroidism, especially those whose hyperplasia results from an MEN syndrome. Within 12 years, 50 percent of MEN patients who underwent successful subtotal parathyroidectomy for hyperplasia developed recurrent hyperparathyroidism.[471] For these reasons, some surgeons have resorted to removing all the abnormal parathyroid glands and then autotransplanting a portion of the abnormal parathyroid tissue into an antecubital position in the brachioradialus muscle in the forearm, where it is more accessible if hyperparathyroidism recurs and the tissue has to be removed.[473–475] Unfortunately, this approach runs the risk of transplanting too much parathyroid tissue or losing all the parathyroid tissue if the transplant fails, producing hypoparathyroidism. Furthermore, although the transplanted tissue is theoretically located in a more accessible site than the neck, it often cannot be found after transplantation. Finally, the autotransplant approach does not preclude possible recurrent disease from remaining and growing parathyroid tissue in the neck or mediastinum. The best surgical approach toward four-gland hyperplasia therefore remains controversial, with most surgeons preferring to remove three glands and a portion of the fourth. Some also cryopreserve the extracted parathyroid tissue for possible future transplantation.

For parathyroid carcinoma, the surgeon must be careful to excise around a margin of the gland. Parathyroid carcinomas are notorious for seeding locally and recurring. Therefore, the capsule of the carcinoma should not be disrupted.[433,476,477] Unusually high calcium or PTH levels should alert the surgeon to the possible presence of a parathyroid carcinoma preoperatively. Metastases occur frequently, however, with parathyroid carcinoma. Since PTH secretion appears to correlate with the size of the tumor, periodic surgical removal of one or a few parathyroid carcinoma metastases should be used to manage the patient. Since the tumors are usually slow-growing and hypercalcemia is often the worst or only complication of the malignancy, such patients can often be maintained in this manner for years. Nevertheless, the level of serum calcium increases progressively and at a rate more rapid than is typical of hyperparathyroidism. The tumors become truly inoperable when the location or number of metastases precludes this surgical approach.

In the immediate postoperative period, some patients become mildly or even severely hypoparathyroid until the remaining suppressed glands, which have been "dormant" for months or years, resume normal function. This situation can last for several days. It is typified by low serum calcium and elevated serum phosphorus. Hence, calcium should be monitored every 12 h until a stable plateau has been reached or the levels have returned to normal. Postoperative transient hypoparathyroidism usually can be managed with dietary calcium supplementation (1 to 2 g/day) alone. Some patients even develop symptoms of hypocalcemia with tingling in the fingertips and around the mouth or even a positive Chvostek's sign on physical examination despite absolute values of calcium level within the normal range. It appears that the rapid relative decline in calcium alone can produce "hypocalcemic" symptoms. Permanent hypoparathyroidism can also develop either in the immediate postoperative period or rarely after a long delay. Treatment with vitamin D analogues and calcium along the lines described elsewhere in this chapter is required in such cases.

Patients with extensive bone disease characterized by changes apparent on x-ray and elevated serum alkaline phosphatase levels are at risk for developing a severe and life-threatening hypocalcemic syndrome postoperatively. It is important to distinguish this syndrome, termed "hungry bones," from transient postoperative hypoparathyroidism.[478] It arises because bone has been under a tremendous resorptive stimulus chronically, which is then abruptly interrupted by removal of the overactive parathyroid tissue. Bone formation is now unopposed and is able to catch up with resorption. As a result, a large calcium influx into bone ensues, depleting the ECF of calcium and sometimes resulting in marked hypocalcemia. This hypocalcemia is distinguished from transient hypoparathyroidism by the serum phosphorus levels, which, instead of being elevated, are below normal because both calcium and phosphate move into bone as part of the remineralization process. This condition usually persists for days to weeks and requires large amounts of calcium supplementation, often administered intravenously, as well as large doses of vitamin D, preferably a relatively short-acting analogue (see Vitamin D, above). Once normocalcemia is established after subtotal parathyroidectomy, calcium should be tested at 1-, 3- to 6-, and 12-month intervals and annually thereafter.

Diagnosis and Management of Asymptomatic Primary Hyperparathyroidism

The diagnosis and management of asymptomatic primary hyperparathyroidism remain one of the most controversial areas in endocrinology and internal medicine. The majority of patients who present with hypercalcemia in an ambulatory setting have primary hyperparathyroidism. The vast majority of these patients are asymptomatic (Fig. 23-49). It appears likely that this management problem will confront internists with increasing frequency as the population ages and more patients are detected by multiphasic screening.

In 1990, the NIH convened a Consensus Development Conference on the diagnosis and management of this disorder.[469] The panel reaffirmed the common practice of recommending surgery as the treatment of choice for primary hyperparathyroidism. However, although control of serum calcium, recurrent kidney stones, and osteitis fibrosa cystica clearly can be managed effectively with surgery, complications and symptoms such as muscle weakness, neuropsychiatric effects, and hypertension do not necessarily respond to surgical treatment, as was discussed earlier.

Although all these patients should be considered candidates for surgery since surgery is relatively safe and is the only proven treatment for primary hyperparathyroidism, some patients are truly asymptomatic and can be considered for medical management under rigorous conditions of selection and monitoring. These patients have neither symptoms nor signs commonly attributable to primary hyperparathyroidism. Because the natural history of the disease is uncertain, there are no signs or absolute laboratory criteria which can be used to predict the future development of long-term complications in any given patient. The current state of understanding of primary hyperparathyroidism and its natural history is analogous to the understanding of hypertension or hypercholesterolemia before large-scale epidemiologic and clinical studies were conducted.

Even if a patient is asymptomatic, the presence of any of the following will make the patient no longer suitable for medical monitoring: markedly elevated serum calcium levels [above 11.4 to 12 mg/dl or 1 to 1.6 mg/dl above normal (above 2.8 to 3 mmol/liter or 2.5 to 2.7 mmol/liter above normal)], a previous episode of life-threatening hypercalcemia, reduced creatinine clearance (30 percent below normal), presence of a kidney stone on radiography, markedly elevated 24-h urine calcium excretion (>400 mg), or substantially reduced bone mass (approximately 2 standard deviations below normal for age, sex, and race). Hence, medical monitoring can be undertaken in selected patients who are defined by not meeting the criteria for surgery listed above.

In addition, medical surveillance is not considered desirable or suitable for patients who (1) requested surgery, (2) are unlikely to be monitored regularly because of issues of patient compliance or because of the physician's circumstances, (3) have a coexisting illness complicating their management, or (4) are young (less than 50 years old, particularly premenopausal women). Finally, physician judgment in consultation with the patient should be applied instead of rigorous adherence to these guidelines.

Not enough is known to predict the occurrence of fractures in primary hyperparathyroidism on the basis of determinations of bone mass or bone mineral density. No subgroup at risk for future fractures can be clearly identified. However, it is assumed that the same paradigm which is operative for osteoporosis—that decreased bone mineral density is associated with increased fractures—is applicable to primary hyperparathyroidism. This would be of special importance when there is a combination of postmenopausal status and primary hyperparathyroidism. At this time, however, there have been no controlled studies with the requisite power (in terms of numbers of patients or duration of follow-up) to resolve the fracture issue for asymptomatic primary hyperparathyroidism. Certainly, in established hyperparathyroidism, bone mineral density is known to be below normal (Figs. 23-55 and 23-56) and fracture rates are increased (Fig. 23-59). Furthermore, surgery only partially restores whatever bone mineral density was lost before the intervention.

A somewhat related issue is the question of hyperparathyroidism contributing to the etiology of

FIGURE 23-59 Increased incidence of fractures at multiple skeletal sites in patients with primary hyperparathyroidism. □, Observed; ■, expected; $P < 0.001$. *(Reprinted with permission from M. Peacock, Osteoporosis 1:463, 1984.)*

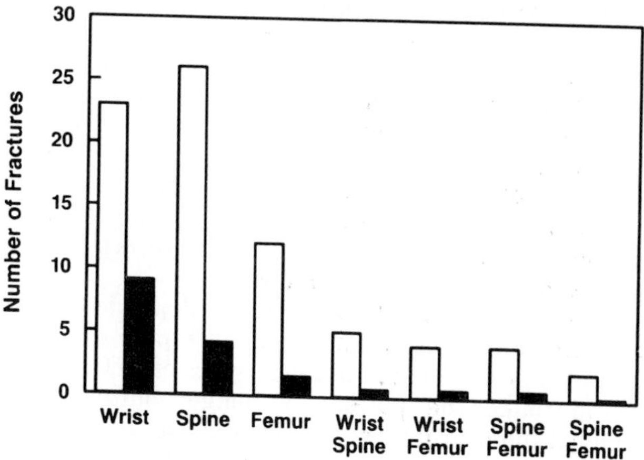

postmenopausal osteoporosis. There has been speculation that subtle hyperparathyroidism or increased sensitivity to normal circulating levels of PTH may cause or exacerbate osteoporosis. This hypothesis has not been proved conclusively even for a subset of osteoporotic patients. Therefore, osteoporosis per se is not an indication for subtotal parathyroidectomy.

Once a decision has been made to follow a patient with medical surveillance, subsequent deterioration in organ status should be considered an indication for surgery. Although definite numbers cannot be recommended and individual physician judgment is paramount, deterioration of renal or bone parameters or elevation of serum calcium to the values previously listed as initial criteria for surgery or the development of kidney stones would seem to warrant surgical intervention. Many physicians will intervene in the presence of a less marked abnormality for any of the parameters cited above.

After an initial determination to ascertain a baseline, monitoring of bone mineral density should be performed on a semiannual basis until lack of progression is confirmed. Thereafter, if a patient is stable, monitoring should be performed at 1- to 3-year intervals, depending on the status of the patient and the particular techniques available for determinations of bone mineral density. It remains unclear whether patients with asymptomatic hyperparathyroidism, once diagnosed, actually continue to lose bone at a more rapid rate than do their peers.

Concerns about the long-term complications of the disease on other organs have not been specifically addressed. For instance, one pathologic survey found that chronic hypercalcemia was associated with accelerated deposition of calcium in cardiac annuli and valvular cusps and in the media and intima of coronary arteries.[479] The coronary intimal calcification might be accelerated in the presence of hypercholesterolemia and thus contribute as a risk factor for atherosclerosis.

Medical Management of Primary Hyperparathyroidism and Asymptomatic Hyperparathyroidism

A limited number of general mechanistic approaches can be used to treat hypercalcemia.[480] Urinary calcium excretion should be increased first by expanding intravascular volume and then by prescribing loop diuretics, if needed and tolerated. Several medical agents inhibit bone resorption: Plicamycin, bisphosphonates, calcitonin, and gallium nitrate all diminish osteoclastic bone resorption by different biochemical mechanisms.

The treatment of hypercalcemia depends on the severity of the abnormality. For "asymptomatic" hyperparathyroidism and in the absence of factors that would make the patient no longer suitable for medical monitoring, as described above, no specific treatment is recommended except avoidance of dehydration, immobilization, and thiazide diuretics. Estrogens provide the theoretical advantage of lowering calcium, perhaps by reducing the action of PTH on bone and simultaneously providing known beneficial effects on the cardiovascular system and bone (osteoporosis) in postmenopausal women.[481–483] Weighing against the use of estrogen, however, is its potential for promoting malignancies of the uterus and breast and the side effects it produces, including uterine bleeding, all of which limit the practical use of estrogens for many patients. Furthermore, estrogen administration results in raised levels of PTH. Although estrogen appears promising, we feel that if a patient requires treatment to control calcium levels, it is more appropriate to recommend surgery. For calcium levels of 12 mg/dl (3 mmol/liter) or less, promotion of urinary excretion of calcium is the best approach. This can usually be accomplished by increasing the oral intake of salt and fluids. Patients with even mild hypercalcemia tend to be relatively dehydrated as a result of the obligatory loss of water that accompanies hypercalciuria. Correction of the fluid derangement alone will usually substantially correct the blood calcium level.

Although diuretics such as furosemide may promote calciuria, they should be used with caution since they can dehydrate the patient further, leading to decreased glomerular filtration and thus exacerbating the hypercalcemia. Thiazide diuretics should be avoided since they may worsen hypercalcemia. Dietary restriction of calcium is controversial: If the pathophysiology of the disease is a set point error in calcium regulation of PTH secretion by the parathyroid gland, dietary restriction will have the adverse effect of raising PTH levels and promoting bone resorption to maintain elevated levels of calcium. Therefore, we favor a moderate calcium intake.

While some clinicians have advocated the use of oral phosphate salts in treating mild cases of hypercalcemia under carefully controlled conditions,[484] it is our feeling that this merely treats the biochemical abnormality of elevated serum calcium. Furthermore, diminishing calcium levels by administering phosphate salts is not without risk. First, such treatment has the undesirable effect of elevating PTH levels.[484] Second, if the solubility product constant for calcium and phosphate is exceeded, ectopic precipitation of calcium phosphate can occur in the soft tissues, including the kidney, where it can lead to renal compromise or failure. Finally, the dose of oral phosphate required to reduce calcium levels into the normal range regularly produces diarrhea.

In the past, several other agents appeared promising for the management of mild hypercalcemia due to primary hyperparathyroidism. Preliminary reports indicated that propranolol[485] or cimetidine[486] might be useful, but ultimately their efficacy was not observed consistently. Another agent, WR-2721, was found to inhibit PTH secretion and diminish serum calcium levels,[487] but the use of WR-2721 remains experimental.

Hypercalcemic Crisis

Patients with calcium levels of 12.5 mg/dl (3.1 mmol/liter) or greater, who are often said to have a "parathyroid storm" or "crisis," require aggressive or emergency treatment since these levels can be life-threatening. Although surgery is definitely required, it should not be undertaken when calcium levels are higher than 12.5 mg/dl because of a substantially increased risk of mortality. Only after reduction of calcium levels to below 12.5 mg/dl should surgery be performed. If it is not known whether the patient's calcium level has been stably but markedly elevated, hospitalization should be considered because of the seriousness of the metabolic disturbance. Again, saline rehydration is the first line of treatment. One to 4 liters of saline should be administered intravenously over a 2- to 6-h period if the patient's cardiovascular status will tolerate such an infusion. Only after complete rehydration should intravenous loop diuretics such as furosemide be administered to promote calcium along with sodium excretion. Calcitonin (100 to 400 units/day) parenterally alone or in conjunction with corticosteroids can effectively decrease calcium levels.[308] Calcium levels will generally fall within 24 to 48 h. However, tachyphylaxis to calcitonin usually occurs within a period of 4 to 6 days, thus limiting its utility to acute treatment.[299,307] Therefore, once calcium has been restored to normal or nearly normal levels by any of the maneuvers described above, parathyroidectomy should be performed before hypercalcemia recurs.

For patients with parathyroid carcinoma who are inoperable (described above), it is necessary to eventually achieve a maintenance regimen. The physican should consider the addition of other therapeutic modalities early in the treatment of acute hypercalcemia described above, especially since these other agents are effective only after a lag period of several days. If orchestrated properly, their beneficial effects can begin just as calcitonin's effectiveness is declining and attempts are being made to discontinue intravenous fluid infusions. These drugs are discussed in more detail in the section on the treatment of hypercalcemia of malignancy, below.

Plicamycin (mithramycin) (25 μg/kg for 3 to 4 days) is quite effective in treating the hypercalcemia of malignancy as well as primary hyperparathyroidism or parathyroid carcinoma since it blocks bone resorption, probably through a toxic effect on the osteoclast.

Bisphosphonates (diphosphonates) have also been shown to be effective. Etidronic acid (etidronate) is effective intravenously, but only in a subset of patients. Because of its gastrointestinal side effects, it is difficult to administer orally in amounts sufficient to effectively treat hypercalcemia. Dichloromethylene diphosphonate, which unlike etidronate does not inhibit bone mineralization or produce osteomalacia, was effective in short-term studies.[488] However, the drug is not available in the United States, although it is used commonly in Europe. In the future, it is possible that newer bisphosphonates with greater oral efficacy and fewer side effects, such as pamidronate and alendronate, will be useful in both acute and maintenance regimens for the treatment of parathyroid carcinoma or hyperparathyroidism in cases where medical control of hypercalcemia is required.[489–491]

Gallium nitrate has recently been approved in the United States for the treatment of hypercalcemia of malignancy.[492] Experience with this agent in treating severe hypercalcemia due to hyperparathyroidism has not been reported, although the agent has been used effectively on a short-term basis in treating parathyroid carcinoma.[493]

Malignancy-Associated Hypercalcemia

Historical Introduction

The association of tumors with hypercalcemia was first made by Zondek and associates in 1924.[38,494] Until 1941 it was generally assumed that hypercalcemia stems directly from local destruction of bone by a metastatic tumor. In that year Albright, in discussing hypercalcemia in a clinicopathological conference, pointed out that in a patient with renal cell carcinoma and a single bone metastasis hypercalcemia had occurred in conjunction with hypophosphatemia and on that basis suggested that the tumor was secreting parathyroid hormone.[495] This brief comment was recounted in his book *The Parathyroid Glands and Metabolic Bone Disease* and is thought to be the first proposal of ectopic production of a hormone by a malignant tumor. In the next two decades there were reports of "humoral hypercalcemia" that was produced by tumors that were not metastatic to bone and was reversed by resection of the tumor,[496] and the combination of hypercalcemia and hypophosphatemia secondary to a malignant tumor without bone metastases was dubbed "pseudohyperparathyroidism."[497] However, the role of PTH was controversial. In some RIAs for PTH cross-reacting substances were detected in such patients; in others, iPTH was undetectable. Thus, the substance in question appeared to differ immunochemically from PTH but was thought by some researchers to be related.[498]

In 1980, Stewart, Broadus, and colleagues[499] reported that not only a decreased renal phosphate threshold but also increased excretion of nephrogenous cAMP was characteristic of patients with malignancy-associated hypercalcemia (Fig. 23-60). None of these patients had high levels of iPTH. Based on the assumption that in these patients, as in hyperparathyroidism, nephrogenous cAMP was pro-

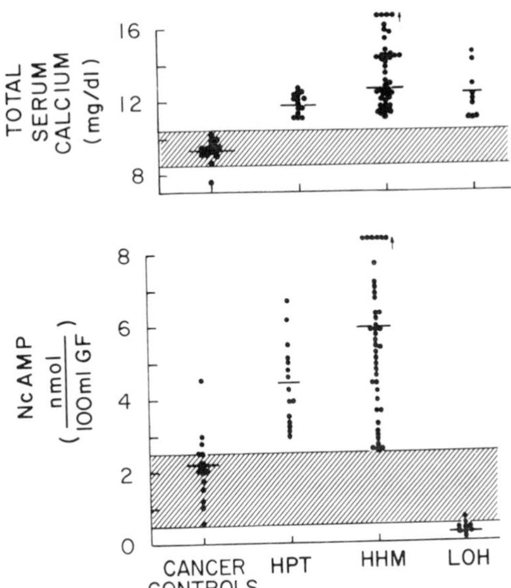

FIGURE 23-60 Serum calcium and excretion of nephrogenous cAMP (NcAMP) in hyperparathyroidism and malignancy. Patient groups are normocalcemic patients with cancer ("cancer controls"), patients with primary hyperparathyroidism (HPT), patients with humoral hypercalcemia of malignancy (HHM), and patients with local osteolytic hypercalcemia (LOH). The HHM group includes patients with squamous carcinomas, renal carcinoma, bladder carcinomas, and miscellaneous tumors; the LOH group includes patients with breast carcinoma, multiple myeloma, lymphoma, and pulmonary adenocarcinoma. *(From Stewart, Horst, Deftos, Cadman, Lang, and Broadus,[499] by permission of the New England Journal of Medicine.)*

duced by activation of the PTH receptor in renal tubule cells, they proposed that a humoral parathyroid hormone–like substance was present not just in unusual patients but in up to 80 percent of patients with the syndrome. This seminal result led over the next decade to the purification and molecular cloning of PTHrP, which is now recognized as the principal cause of the syndrome.[117–123] The discovery of PTHrP thus fits a classic paradigm of biomedical research, with astute observations by clinicians providing the direct impetus for basic investigations.

Clinical Features

Hypercalcemia is the most common symptomatic paraneoplastic complication of malignancy, occurring in 5 to 10 percent of all cancer patients. This makes malignancy the second most common etiology of hypercalcemia, with an estimated incidence about one-half that of primary hyperparathyroidism.[437] Hypercalcemia typically appears late in the course of malignant diseases. It presents with anorexia, nausea, polyuria, confusion, or coma. Evidence of malignancy is seldom subtle at the onset of hypercalcemia: The tumor is already known or readily evident in at least 98 percent of these patients.[500] Often, hypercalcemia ushers in a final phase of the disease. The median survival of hypercalcemic patients is only 30 to 90 days.[501] As discussed below, the pathogenesis and specific clinical features of hypercalcemia differ depending on tumor type. In the following sections, the properties of PTHrP and the general features of the most common form of hypercalcemia are presented first; then the forms of the disorder associated with different tumors are discussed individually.

PTH-Related Peptide

The existence of a PTH-like substance associated with hypercalcemia in malignancy was postulated from clinical studies, most directly from measurements of nephrogenous cAMP as a parathyroid function test (see Historical Introduction, above). The proposal that the humoral mediator of hypercalcemia stimulates the excretion of cAMP led directly to its purification. Assays of adenylyl cyclase activation in bone or kidney cells were subsequently used to identify peptides from squamous lung, breast, and renal carcinomas,[118–120] and molecular cloning of their cDNAs then proved that the peptides produced by these different tumors were identical.[121–123] PTHrP has isoforms of 139, 141, and 173 amino acids, compared with 84 amino acids in PTH. (The isoforms, which arise from alternative RNA splicing at a site corresponding to the carboxyl terminus of the peptide,[123,502–504] have a common sequence through amino acid 139. It is not known whether all are secreted or whether they have distinct functions.) The tumor peptide strongly resembles PTH only at its amino terminus (Fig. 23-61), with 8 amino acid identities among the first 13 residues of the mature peptides. Thereafter, the two peptide sequences have little in common. The PTHrP gene is located on chromosome 12 and is more complex than the PTH gene on chromosome 11,[502,504] yet the two

FIGURE 23-61 The sequence of PTHrP(1-34). Amino acids that are identical to those in PTH are partly shaded.

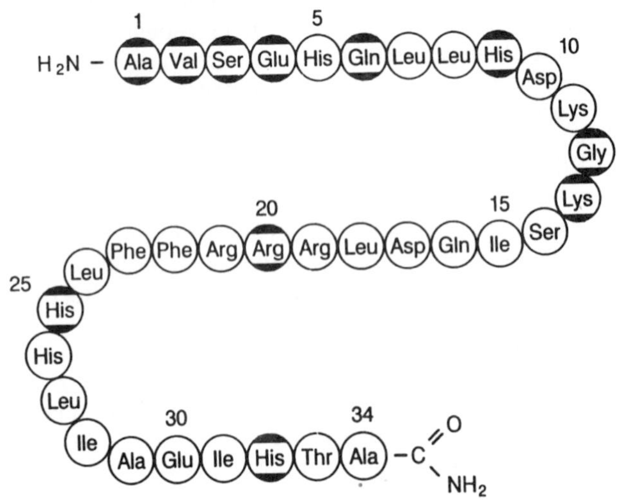

share certain structural features. The homology of their amino acid sequences at the amino terminus, together with these similarities of gene structure, indicates that PTH and PTHrP are the products of a common ancestral gene.

As with PTH, the amino-terminal peptides that constitute the 1-34 sequence of PTHrP are fully active at the PTH receptor.[130,403,505] Surprisingly, PTH and PTHrP are equipotent for receptor binding and for most of their acute effects despite the divergence of their primary sequences in the 14-34 domain that is required for binding. In fact, PTH(14-34) and PTHrP(14-38), fragments with entirely divergent sequences, both compete for PTH receptor binding, albeit weakly.[134] This is an unusual and important example of shared function, presumably owing to shared secondary/tertiary structure, in the face of a remote relation of primary amino acid sequence.

It may be surmised from its binding to the PTH receptor that PTHrP mimicks all the classical acute effects of PTH. In the kidney, PTHrP or amino-terminal peptides of PTHrP indeed produce phosphaturia, hypocalciuria, and activation of 25-hydroxyvitamin D-1α-hydroxylase, stimulating the synthesis of 1α,25-dihydroxyvitamin D.[124,125,506] Moreover, PTHrP is approximately equipotent with PTH in producing bone resorption and hypercalcemia.[506,507] PTH antagonists, which inhibit PTH actions by competitively occupying PTH receptors, are also able to block the actions of PTHrP, demonstrating that both hormones interact with the same receptors in vitro and in vivo.[133]

PTHrP is more highly conserved in evolution than is PTH,[243,506,508] suggesting that it has an important physiologic function. The peptide is expressed at low levels in a variety of normal tissues, including the skin,[247,252] central nervous system,[249] pancreatic islets,[507] uterine smooth muscle at parturition,[250] and lactating mammary tissue.[243] It is secreted into milk at levels 10,000-fold higher than its serum concentration,[244] consistent with the possibility that it subserves some function in the neonate. PTHrP is also expressed in a variety of smooth muscle beds: Besides the uterus, these include the urinary bladder and vascular smooth muscle. In the uterus and urinary bladder its expression is stimulated by stretch. Expressed also in a variety of embryonic tissues, PTHrP modulates the differentiation of embryonic cells in a model system, acting through the PTH/PTHrP receptor.[509] It has been suggested that fetal secretion of PTHrP may regulate placental calcium transport.[245,246] From the presumption that PTHrP probably plays a unique physiologic role, one might infer the existence of specific PTHrP receptors. However, no specific, high-affinity receptor for PTHrP has been identified.[505] With a circulating concentration of less than 1 pmol/liter, compared with a concentration of 1 to 5 pmol/liter for PTH,[510,511] PTHrP has not been shown to function in systemic mineral homeostasis.

Pathogenesis of Humoral Hypercalcemia

PTHrP is probably the mediator of hypercalcemia in most patients with malignant neoplasms. As was discussed above, PTHrP can produce hypercalcemia as well as renal phosphate wasting and is as potent as PTH. Serum levels of PTHrP are increased in most hypercalcemic patients, including 85 percent of patients who develop hypercalcemia in the absence of bone metastases, but levels of PTHrP are normal in most normocalcemic cancer patients and in other hypercalcemic states (Fig. 23-62).[510,511] In addition, hypercalcemia is blocked by affinity-purified neutralizing antibodies to PTHrP in an animal model where hypercalcemia is induced by the growth of human squamous tumors in the nude mouse.[512] Thus, secretion of PTHrP appears to be necessary to produce malignancy-associated hypercalcemia.

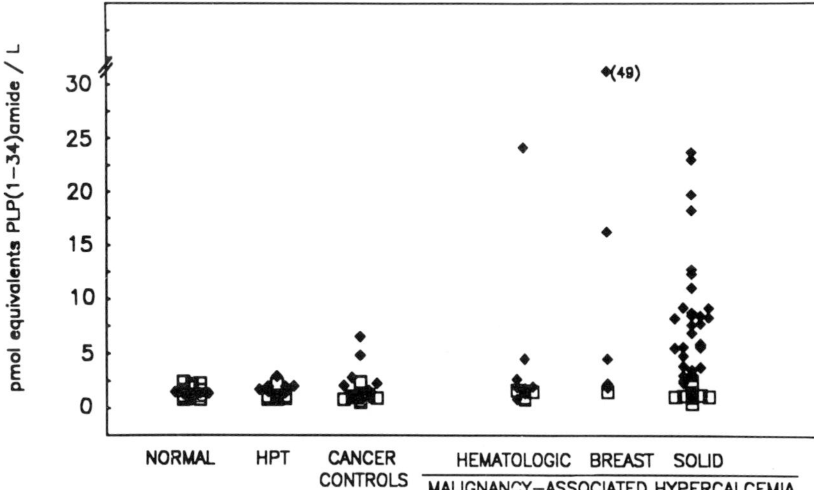

FIGURE 23-62 Serum levels of PTHrP in normal subjects, hyperparathyroidism (HPT), and malignancy. "Cancer controls" are normocalcemic patients with cancer. *(From Budayr, Nissenson, Klein, Pun, Clark, Diep, Arnaud, Strewler,[510] permission of the Annals of Internal Medicine.)*

Nearly all these patients respond to potent inhibitors of bone resorption (e.g., bisphosphonates; see below), indicating that increased bone resorption is the primary pathogenetic mechanism of hypercalcemia produced by PTHrP. However, the ability of PTHrP to decrease renal calcium excretion is probably also important,[513,514] even though it has been difficult to devise conditions to quantitate the relative contributions of bone resorption and hypocalciuria to the pathogenesis of hypercalcemia in humans. Part of the response to saline diuresis in cancer patients probably reflects reversal of the hypocalciuric state induced by PTHrP.

Plasma levels of 1α,25-$(OH)_2D$ tend to be low in malignancy (Fig. 23-63)[499,515] despite the ability of PTHrP to stimulate acutely the synthesis of 1α,25-$(OH)_2D$.[124,506] This contrasts with normal to high levels of 1α,25-$(OH)_2D$ in primary hyperparathyroidism.[334,499] Part of the explanation for this difference may come from the ability of hypercalcemia to suppress the production of 1α,25-$(OH)_2D$, which tends to counteract the acute stimulatory effect of PTH or PTHrP. By this mechanism, a chronic continuous infusion of PTH, in contrast to primary hyperparathyroidism, produces suppression rather than stimulation of 1α,25-$(OH)_2D$ levels.[343] It seems likely that either the pattern of secretion of PTHrP (continuous?) or associated ancillary factors[516] will cause a greater suppressive effect of hypercalcemia on 1α,25-$(OH)_2D$ levels in malignancy than in primary hyperparathyroidism.

Increased bone resorption induced by malignant neoplasms is associated with decreased bone formation which is detected biochemically as a decreased serum osteocalcin level or is detected histologically.[408,517] This uncoupling of resorption and formation contrasts with primary hyperparathyroidism and most other resorptive states, where bone remodeling remains coupled. Under conditions where exogenous PTH is anabolic for bone, PTHrP is variably less so.[506] Yet the in vitro effects of PTHrP on the bone-forming cell, the osteoblast, are similar to those of PTH. It remains to be determined whether the depression of bone formation in malignancy results from a subtle intrinsic difference between PTH and PTHrP, from differences in the secretion of PTH and PTHrP (e.g., intermittent vs. continuous), or from ancillary factors in malignancy such as illness, inanition, the decreased level of 1α,25-$(OH)_2D$, or concomitant secretion of other cytokines. Interleukin 1 is sometimes cosecreted with PTHrP and can diminish bone formation.

FIGURE 23-63 Values for plasma 1α,25-$(OH)_2D$ in the patients described in Fig. 23-60. Plasma 1α,25-$(OH)_2D$ values are elevated in patients with hyperparathyroidism (HPT) but are normal or reduced in patients with humoral hypercalcemia of malignancy (HHM) or local osteolytic hypercalcemia (LOH). *(From Stewart, Horst, Deftos, Cadman, Lang, and Broadus,[499] by permission of the New England Journal of Medicine.)*

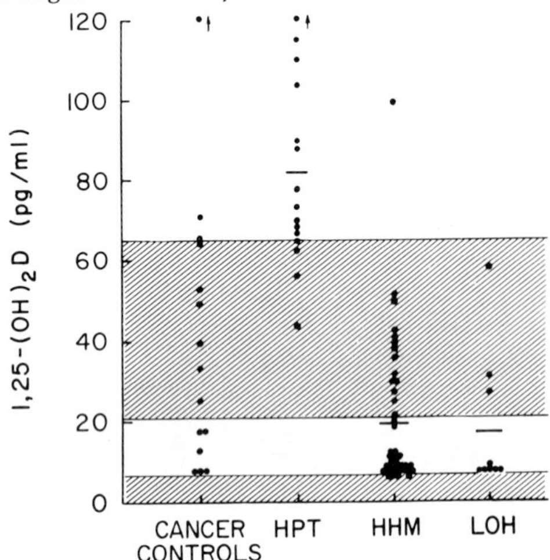

Solid Tumors

The solid tumors most often associated with hypercalcemia are lung carcinoma (25 percent of all cases); breast carcinoma (20 percent); squamous carcinomas of the head, neck, esophagus, or female-genital tract (19 percent); and renal carcinoma (8 percent) (Table 23-6). Among patients with lung carcinoma, 23 percent of those with epidermoid (squamous) carcinoma and smaller fractions of those with large cell or adenocarcinoma will develop hypercalcemia, but hypercalcemia is very rare in small cell lung carcinoma.[518] Overall, about a third of tumors complicated by hypercalcemia have a squamous histology.

Hypophosphatemia and a decreased renal phosphate threshold are seen in 75 percent of hypercalcemic patients.[499] The serum concentration of 1α,25-$(OH)_2D$ is sometimes increased,[515] but most

TABLE 23-6 Malignancy-Associated Hypercalcemia

Primary Site	No. Cases, %	Known Metastic Disease, %
Lung	111 (25.0)	62
Breast	87 (19.6)	92
Multiple myeloma	43 (9.7)	100
Head and neck	36 (8.1)	73
Renal and urinary tract	35 (7.9)	36
Esophagus	25 (5.6)	53
Female genital	24 (5.2)	81
Unknown primary	23 (5.2)	—
Lymphoma	14 (3.2)	91
Colon	8 (1.8)	—
Liver/biliary	7 (1.6)	—
Skin	6 (1.4)	—
Other	25 (5.7)	—
Total	444 (100)	—

Source: Strewler GJ, Nissenson RA, *Adv Intern Med* 32:235, 1987.

often it is at or below the lower limit of normal.[499] The level of PTHrP in serum is increased in 70 to 80 percent of cases, including nearly all pateints with squamous or renal carcinomas.[510,511] The serum concentration of PTHrP is correlated with the level of nephrogenous cAMP and with the serum calcium level.[511] Increased concentrations of PTHrP in malignancy-associated hypercalcemia have been found using assays directed toward the amino terminus of PTHrP [PTHrP(1-34)], toward its carboxyl terminus [PTHrP(109-138)], and toward two sites in the sequence PTHrP(1-74). In chronic renal failure, the carboxyl-terminal assay detects increased PTHrP levels but amino-terminal PTHrP levels are not increased. This immunoheterogeneity of circulating PTHrP presumably means that like PTH, PTHrP is subject to cleavage in the circulation and that carboxyl-terminal PTHrP fragments are probably cleared by the kidney. Given the strong evidence that PTHrP is capable of producing humoral hypercalcemia, these data suggest that hypercalcemia in fact has a humoral basis in most patients. Indeed, a third to a half of squamous and renal carcinomas associated with hypercalcemia do not have demonstrable bone metastases, fitting the classic definition of humoral hypercalcemia. However, the majority of solid tumors causing hypercalcemia have metastasized to bone. Although the role of local osteolysis in these patients cannot be fully defined, the extent of bone metastases correlates poorly with hypercalcemia.[519] For example, among bronchogenic carcinomas, osseous involvement most frequently occurs in small cell carcinoma (66 percent), but these patients rarely manifest hypercalcemia.[518] It seems likely that contrary to the conventional thinking of the past 70 years, local osteolysis is rarely the primary cause of hypercalcemia with solid neoplasms. It may contribute, however.

Numerous substances other than PTHrP have been proposed as mediators of hypercalcemia with solid tumors. Some cases are clearly caused by ectopic secretion of PTH.[520–522] This rare event has been described convincingly only since the advent of two-site assays for PTH, which establish that the hormone is suppressed in typical patients. Ectopic production of PTH has not been shown clearly in small cell carcinomas and in ovarian adenocarcinoma. Hypercalcemia may rarely be caused by the secretion of prostaglandins, as a few patients have responded to inhibition of prostaglandin synthesis.[523] Convincing evidence for a role of cytokines and other tumor cell products is scanty.

Hematologic Neoplasms

Hypercalcemia occurs in a third of patients with multiple myeloma. Occasional patients presenting with asymptomatic hypercalcemia prove to have paraproteins that bind calcium[524] and a normal ionized calcium. However, the great majority of patients who develop hypercalcemia have increased ionized as well as total serum calcium levels. Chronic hypercalciuria heralds episodes of hypercalcemia, frequently induced by failure to clear the increased renal load of calcium because of dehydration or the renal effects of myeloma.[525] Such episodes may respond to treatment with glucocorticoids[526] or to measures aimed at reducing bone resorption and do not invariably usher in a terminal phase of disease. In patients with extensive lytic bone disease, the serum phosphorus level is usually normal and the serum level of 1α,25-$(OH)_2D$ is decreased. Serum levels of PTH and excretion of nephrogenous cAMP are suppressed by hypercalcemia, and the serum concentration of PTHrP is usually normal.[499,510,511] These characteristics define the syndrome of *local osteolytic hypercalcemia*. The systemic manifestations of this disorder differ little from the forms of hypercalcemia seen in other disorders characterized by increased bone resorption, such as immobilization, thyrotoxicosis, and vitamin A intoxication.

The cause of local osteolysis is not fully understood. However, osteolytic metastases are usually surrounded by active osteoclasts, suggesting that it is activation of the osteoclast, not direct resorption of bone by tumor cells, that produces osteolysis.[527] It has been postulated that local release of cytokines with bone-resorbing activity occurs, but this has not been proved. The term *osteoclast activating factor* was formerly used to identify the bone-resorbing activity in supernatants of normal or malignant leukocytes. This term is no longer useful now that individual cytokines with bone-resorbing activity can be identified. These include IL-1α, IL-1β, IL-6, tumor necrosis $factor_\alpha$, tumor necrosis $factor_\beta$ (also called lymphotoxin), leukemia inhibitory factor, and $TGF\alpha$.[528] Given systemically in rodents, these are weak hypercalcemic agents, consistent with a predominantly local role in lymphoma and myeloma. It is unclear which of the cytokines is involved in local osteolytic hypercalcemia. The bone-resorbing substance in normal monocyte supernatants is IL-1β.[529] Myeloma cell supernatants may induce bone resorption in vitro by secretion of tumor necrosis factor-β (lymphotoxin)[530] or IL-1β.[531] Determining which factors actually produce local osteolytic hypercalcemia (as opposed to bone resorption in vitro) will require the use of neutralizing reagents for individual cytokines in a suitable animal model or in human patients. Unfortunately, no animal model of hypercalcemia induced by local osteolysis is currently available.

Hypercalcemia occurs in 1 to 2 percent of lymphomas and leukemias.[532] Bone involvement is often evident in hypercalcemic patients, and lymphoma and leukemia are usually thought of as producing local osteolytic hypercalcemia, with the same etiologic possibilities as multiple myeloma. However, in some lymphomas, 1α,25-$(OH)_2D$ is the mediator of hypercalcemia.[533,534] These patients present with increased serum levels of 1α,25-$(OH)_2D$; with corticosteroid therapy, the serum calcium and serum 1α,25-$(OH)_2D$ levels usually fall in tandem. Although the original studies suggested that this was an uncommon occurrence, in a recent series high levels of 1α,25-$(OH)_2D$ were found in 47 percent of lymphomas.[535] We assume that like activated macrophages in sarcoidosis, lymphoma cells can probably carry out 1α-hydroxylation of vitamin D metabolites, but this has not been shown directly. If this is the case, this is potentially a general property of malignant lymphocytes, since high 1α,25-$(OH)_2D$ levels have been reported across a spectrum of lymphomas, including in Hodgkin's disease and a variety of non-Hodgkin's lymphomas.

A special and remarkable case is the adult T-cell leukemia syndrome, which is caused by the retrovirus HTLV-1. Hypercalcemia develops in fully two-thirds of cases. Hypercalcemic individuals have increased urinary cAMP,[516] and their leukemia cells have been shown to produce a PTH-like substance in vitro[248] and high serum levels of PTHrP (unpublished data, AA Budayr and GJ Strewler). Although these cells also produce IL-1 and rarely 1α,25-(OH) D,[533,536] the secretion of PTHrP probably causes most cases of hypercalcemia in this syndrome.

Breast Cancer

Hypercalcemia occurs in 15 percent of patients with advanced breast carcinoma, and hypercalciuria occurs in an additional 20 percent.[525] In contrast to other solid tumors, hypercalcemia is seen almost exclusively in patients with extensive bone metastasis. Episodic hypercalcemia in these patients can be triggered by hormonal therapy with estrogens, androgens, or the antiestrogen tamoxifen. Hypophosphatemia is commonly present in hypercalcemic patients. In one-third to one-half of these patients, the serum level of PTHrP or the excretion of nephrogenous cAMP is increased.[510,511] It seems likely that this group has a form of humoral hypercalcemia similar to that seen with other solid tumors, even though the strong association of hypercalcemia with bone metastasis suggests a role for local osteolysis. It is reasonable to surmise that the remaining patients, who have extensive bone metastases and normal levels of PTHrP, have a form of local osteolytic hypercalcemia in which PTHrP acts on osteoclasts in the vicinity of osseous tumor deposits. Perhaps many breast cancers secrete PTHrP at levels sufficient to cause local but not systemic effects. However, there are no grounds for excluding the alternative possibility that breast cancer produces hypercalcemia by entirely different mechanisms in patients with and without evidence of humoral hypercalcemia.

Diagnosis

When the diagnosis of malignancy-associated hypercalcemia is entertained, the offending neoplasm is known already or is immediately obvious in 98 percent of cases. Occult malignancy rarely produces hypercalcemia. (The most common exception is multiple myeloma. Determination of serum and urinary immunoglobulins is indicated in hypercalcemia presenting with a suppressed PTH level.) In 80 percent of patients with solid tumors, the diagnosis can be confirmed by determining the serum level of PTHrP, assays for which are commercially available. There is no specific diagnostic test for the 20 percent of solid tumor patients in whom PTHrP levels are normal or for patients with multiple myeloma. Determination of the serum 1α,25-$(OH)_2D$ level should be performed in patients with lymphoma. Intercurrent primary hyperparathyroidism is common in cancer patients and should always be ruled out by assay of intact PTH. A serum PTH level of less than 20 ng/liter excludes primary hyperparathyroidism. The finding of an inappropriately high level of PTH in a patient with a malignant tumor and hypercalcemia is an indication for neck exploration if the clinical circumstances warrant definitive treatment. It is difficult to distinguish intercurrent hyperparathyroidism from the rarer syndrome of true ectopic secretion of PTH. Unsuccessful exploration of the neck led to the recognition of the ectopic disorder in the few instances in which it has been diagnosed.[520–522]

Treatment

Because the kidney is the route by which calcium can be cleared, initial management consisting of rehydration and saline diuresis is generally appropriate. Maintaining a diuresis will correct the dehydration that is commonly present in hypercalcemic patients, will combat the hypocalciuric effect of PTHrP, and in combination with antiresorptive therapy provides a two-pronged attack on the hypercalcemia. Once the patient is rehydrated (urine output > 2 liters/day), a vigorous saline diuresis, supplemented if necessary with intermittent administration of a loop diuretic such as furosemide, will induce substantial calciuresis and further lower the serum calcium level. It is important not to use diuretics until rehydration has been achieved so that urinary calcium clearance is not compromised by further dehydration and to monitor and replace urinary losses of potassium and magnesium. Synthetic salmon calcitonin or plicamycin may be of use as an adjunctive agent at the initiation of treatment. Calcitonin rapidly lowers the serum calcium level, with a nadir at 24 to 48 h. Synthetic salmon calcitonin may be administered at a dose of 4 to 8 IU per kilogram subcutaneously or intramuscularly every 12 h. However, patients generally become refractory to calcitonin within a few days, and it is rarely useful in chronic therapy.[492] The use of plicamycin is discussed below.

Agents suitable for chronic therapy for hypercalcemia should be introduced early in the hospital course so that the patient can be documented to respond before discharge. Some patients benefit from aggressive chemotherapy, radiation, or resection of the underlying neoplasm. Treatment with glucocorticoids is beneficial in multiple myeloma, in lymphoma, and probably in breast carcinoma. Their effect is predominantly on the tumor rather than on bone; glucocorticoids are also used in combination chemotherapy for hematologic neoplasms. Hypercalcemia caused by solid tumors is often unresponsive to glucocorticoids, and bisphosphonates are the preferred first line of defense.

Bisphosphonates (also known as diphosphonates) are analogues of inorganic pyrophosphate which bind tightly to hydroxyapatite crystals in bone and, when resorbed along with mineralized matrix, specifically inhibit osteoclastic bone resorption by a mechanism which is poorly understood.[537] Dichloromethylene diphosphonate has had considerable use in Europe, but is not on the U.S. market. Two bisphosphonates are currently available in the United States. Pamidronate is the bisphosphonate of first choice because of its superior efficacy and the convenience of single-dose therapy. Pamidronate disodium [(3-amino-1-hydroxypropylidene)-1, 1-bisphosphonate (APD)] has recently been approved for use in the United States. Administered intravenously at a dose of 60 mg in a single 24-h infusion, pamidronate normalized serum calcium in 70 percent of patients, compared with 41 percent who were given etidronate in a randomized clinical trial.[538] Over 90 percent responded to an infusion of 90 mg. Similar results were reported in a European study.[539] The nadir of serum calcium does not occur until 4 to 5 days after treatment. Increased serum creatinine ($\geq$0.5 mg/dl) occurs in about 15 percent of patients. Pamidronate and other bisphosphonates should be used cautiously and at reduced doses in patients whose baseline serum creatinine exceeds 2.5 mg/dl. In contrast to etidronate treatment, the use of pamidronate is associated with a fall in the serum phosphorus level. Transient fever and myalgia occur in 20 percent of patients. Etidronate disodium [(1-hydroxyethylidene) diphosphonic acid (EHDP)] is administered intravenously for the treatment of hypercalcemia in a dose of 7.5 mg/kg per day for 3 to 7 days. About 50 to 70 percent of patients will respond with normalization of serum calcium; the duration of the response is from 1 to 6 weeks.[537,538,540] Oral etidronate disodium is not adequate for the treatment of hypercalcemia, probably owing to poor absorption from the gastrointestinal tract, but may provide a more durable remission of hypercalcemia when used as an adjunct to intravenous therapy at a dose of 20 mg/kg per day.[541]

Etidronate disodium is generally well tolerated. The serum phosphorus level typically rises during therapy and may occasionally reach dangerous levels. Increases in serum creatinine may also occur, but renal failure is rare. A third bisphosphonate, alendronate [(3-amino-1-hydroxybutylidene)-1,1-bisphosphonate], is in advanced clinical trials in the United States at this writing and promises superior results compared with etidronate disodium, with about a 90 percent response rate and rather durable responses in large clinical trials employing a shorter duration of treatment (1 to 3 days).[542]

Gallium nitrate has recently been approved in the United States for the treatment of hypercalcemia. It blocks bone resorption through an undefined mechanism, probably a direct action on the osteoclast. The administration of gallium nitrate in a dose of 200 mg/m^2 per day for 5 days results in normalization of serum calcium in 60 to 70 percent of patients.[492] The nadir of the serum calcium level occurs at 5 to 7 days, and the mean duration of the response is about 7 days. During treatment, the serum phosphorus concentration falls by an average of 0.3 mmol/liter.

The cytotoxic antibiotic plicamycin (mithramycin) is also useful in therapy for hypercalcemia. Plicamycin blocks osteoclastic bone resorption. Used in a dose of up to 25 μg/kg per day intravenously, it is a highly effective treatment for hypercalcemia. The nadir of the response to a single dose of plicamycin occurs at 48 to 72 h, and the response may be maintained for a week or more.[543] Treatment with plicamycin may then be repeated as necessary, but the cytotoxic side effects of the agent (renal, bone marrow, and hepatic) may eventually necessitate delaying therapy or reducing the dose. The systemic toxicity of this agent is related to the cumulative dose administered. The incidence of bleeding from thrombocytopenia and/or decreased prothrombin time, renal dysfunction, and liver abnormalities increases markedly after approximately 10 doses are given, and patients must be monitored appropriately after commencing therapy. Because of this potential for major toxic side effects, chronic use of plicamycin should generally be reserved for patients who have failed on therapy with the bisphosphonates or gallium nitrate.

The serum calcium, phosphorus, and creatinine should be monitored closely during treatment of hypercalcemia. The agents that are effective for chronic therapy may produce mild hypocalcemia, although this is rarely symptomatic. All are associated with decreased renal function in some patients and should be used with caution in patients with a baseline serum creatinine $>$ 2 mg/dl. It is important that a high oral salt intake be maintained to assure adequate calciuresis. Calcium supplements should be eliminated. However, maintenance of a low calcium intake is not generally helpful, as $1\alpha,25\text{-}(OH)_2$ D levels are often low and intestinal calcium absorption may be reduced on this basis. With an average survival of as little as 30 days after the onset of hypercalcemia,[501] not all patients will benefit from aggressive medical management, and treatment decisions must be individualized.

Other Hypercalcemic Disorders

Sarcoidosis and Other Granulomatous Disorders

Hypercalcemia occurs in about 10 percent of patients with sarcoidosis, and hypercalciuria is considerably more common, although precise figures are not available. It was originally thought that hypercalcemia reflects direct bone involvement, but in the 1950s it was found that patients with sarcoidosis had findings suggestive of unusual sensitivity to vitamin D[544] and 25 years later the serum concentration of 1α,25-$(OH)_2D$ was found to be increased in hypercalcemic patients.[545] A remarkable case report subsequently documented that 1α,25-$(OH)_2D$ levels were high in an anephric patient with sarcoidosis, establishing unexpectedly that the source of 1α,25-$(OH)_2D$ was extrarenal.[546] More recently, it has been shown that sarcoid tissue and macrophages lavaged from the lungs in pulmonary sarcoidosis are capable of 1α-hydroxylation of 25-(OH)D to produce 1α,25-$(OH)_2D$.[547]

As macrophages from normocalcemic sarcoidosis patients[547] and even normal macrophages[354] metabolize vitamin D to its active form, factors other than intrinsic enzyme activity may be responsible for hypercalciuria and hypercalcemia. Thus, one determinant of hypercalcemia is the mass and activity of sarcoid tissue. A second is the availability of substrate. In contrast to the kidney, macrophages from sarcoid granulomas synthesize 1α,25-$(OH)_2D$ in an unregulated fashion. When challenged with vitamin D, normal individuals regulate the 1α,25-$(OH)_2D$ concentration tightly,[548] but in sarcoidosis patients serum levels of 1α,25-$(OH)_2D$ increase concomitantly with the increase in serum 25-(OH)D levels. This occurs even in normocalcemic patients, suggesting that the development of hypercalcemia may be substrate-limited. Similarly, exposure to UV light increases cutaneous vitamin D synthesis but does not affect the serum concentration of 1α,25-$(OH)_2D$ in normal humans (Fig. 23-37). In sarcoidosis, hypercalcemia has long been recognized as occurring in the summer months, and episodes of hypercalcemia with increased 1α,25-$(OH)_2D$ levels have been reported in English patients after vacations on the Costa del Sol. Most hypercalcemic patients are azotemic, consistent with the notion that impairment of renal function by compromising renal calcium excretion is probably a key element in tipping chronically hypercalciuric patients over into hypercalcemia, although this scenario is not well documented in longitudinal studies.

Hypercalcemia generally presents in patients with active and obvious disease, manifesting high serum levels of angiotensin converting enzyme.[549] The serum 25-(OH)D level is normal, and the serum level of 1α,25-$(OH)_2D$ is increased. Urinary calcium excretion is increased, and calcium-containing renal stones may occur. Serum phosphorus is usually normal. When present, increased levels of alkaline phosphatase most commonly reflect the presence of liver disease. When assayed with immunoradiometric techniques capable of detecting suppression, the serum concentration of intact PTH is in the suppressed range. Hypercalcemia responds over a few days to corticosteroid therapy, and the serum 1α,25-$(OH)_2D$ level falls pari passu with the serum calcium. Doses of 40 mg prednisone daily can be used initially; most patients can be titrated to a lower maintenance dose. Chloroquine has also been used to treat hypercalcemia.[550] The differential diagnosis of hypercalcemia in suspected sarcoidosis has historically been vexing, and short-term suppression tests with hydrocortisone (40 mg tid for 10 days) have been used to rule out hyperparathyroidism, in which hypercalcemia does not respond to corticosteroid therapy. With the advent of assays for 1α,25-$(OH)_2D$ and intact PTH, the hydrocortisone suppression test is often formally unnecessary, but the effect of corticosteroid therapy can be observed during a therapeutic trial of prednisone.

Hypercalcemia is also seen in a variety of other granulomatous disorders. Mild hypercalcemia may be relatively common in untreated pulmonary tuberculosis (up to 28 percent of patients).[551–553] Hypercalcemia also occurs in berylliosis, disseminated candidiasis, disseminated coccidiomycosis, pulmonary eosinophilic granuloma, histoplasmosis, leprosy, and with silicone granulomas. The role of 1α,25-$(OH)_2D$ in these disorders is controversial.[554–558]

Endocrinopathies

Hyperthyroidism

Mild hypercalcemia is observed in about one-fourth of patients with thyrotoxicosis,[559] and the ionized calcium may be high in up to one-half. The serum phosphorus is in the high-normal range or slightly elevated, and the TmP/GFR is correspondingly high. The serum calcium and serum phosphorus levels are correlated with the level of thyroid hormone, and patients with significant hypercalcemia usually have clinically obvious thyrotoxicosis. The serum alkaline phosphatase and urinary hydroxyproline may also be mildly increased. The urinary excretion of calcium is high. Both PTH and 1α,25-$(OH)_2D$ levels are reduced.[559,560] Severe hypercalcemia occurs rarely, usually in patients with high levels of thyroid hormone who have coexisting hyperparathyroidism or are further compromised by immobilization or impaired renal function. Hypercalcemia is best understood as a manifestation of hyperthyroid bone disease. Thyrotoxicosis is a state of increased bone turnover resulting from a direct ability of thyroid hormone to stimulate bone resorption.[561] Despite compensatory increases in bone formation, losses of bone mineral may be substantial, as reflected in persistent hypercalciuria in the face of reduced $1\alpha,25\text{-(OH)}_2D$ levels. Osteopenia is now recognized as common even in mild hyperthyroidism, although symptomatic osteoporosis is found mainly in postmenopausal women. Even hypothyroid patients who are overreplaced with thyroid hormone, as indicated by suppression of thyroid stimulating hormone (TSH), may have significant reductions in bone density. The manifestations of hypercalcemia in hyperthyroid patients thus reflect accelerated bone resorption with suppression of PTH and $1\alpha,25\text{-(OH)}_2D$. Hypercalcemia responds to antithyroid therapy and may respond to beta-adrenergic blocking agents.

Adrenal Insufficiency

Hypercalcemia can be a feature of acute adrenal crisis and responds to corticosteroid replacement therapy. Animal studies suggest that hemoconcentration is a critical factor in elevating total serum calcium; in experimental adrenal insufficiency, plasma ionized calcium is normal.[562] However, the ionized calcium is reported to be elevated in some patients,[563] and the pathogenesis of hypercalcemia is not fully understood.

Pheochromocytoma

Hypercalcemia occurring in a patient with pheochromocytoma is generally due to concomitant hyperparathyroidism, most often as part of MEN type 2A. However, hypercalcemia is also found occasionally in uncomplicated pheochromocytoma. Recent evidence favors production of PTHrP by the pheochromocytoma as the cause of hypercalcemia in such patients.[564,565]

Pheochromocytoma is the only benign neoplasm for which there is evidence that PTHrP is secreted, although the PTHrP gene is also expressed in certain parathyroid adenomas.[566]

VIPoma

Hypercalcemia has been recorded in about 40 percent of patients with the watery diarrhea, hypokalemia, achlorhydria syndrome (WDHA syndrome, Verner-Morrison syndrome). Some patients may have intercurrent primary hyperparathyroidism, but reversal of hypercalcemia has occurred with resection of the VIP-producing tumor. In view of the role of PTHrP in pheochromocytoma and the association of ganglioneuromas and pheochromocytomas with the WDHA syndrome, PTHrP seems to be a good candidate for the etiologic agent.

Drug-Induced Hypercalcemia

Thiazide Diuretics

The administration of thiazides and related diuretics such as chlorthalidone, metolazone, and indapamide can produce an increase in the total serum calcium. This results in part from hemoconcentration, but ionized calcium is also increased.[567] Hypercalcemia is usually transient, lasting for days or weeks, but occasionally persists. Thiazide administration can also exacerbate the effects of mild primary hyperparathyroidism; in fact, a several-week course of thiazides has been employed as a provocative test in patients with borderline hypercalcemia. It appears that most cases of thiazide-associated hypercalcemia involve underlying hyperparathyroidism. In a large cross-sectional screening study in Sweden, the prevalence of hypercalcemia was increased threefold in thiazide users. In one-fourth of patients, hypercalcemia remitted after the thiazide medication was stopped; most thiazide users with persistent hypercalcemia when the drug was stopped proved to have primary hyperparathyroidism.[568]

The mechanism by which thiazide diuretics cause hypercalcemia is controversial. The hypocalciuric effect of thiazides is well known and is used therapeutically in the treatment of renal stone disease and hypoparathyroidism[569] (see Chap. 25). Urinary calcium excretion is reduced by about 40 percent with chronic thiazide use. Thiazides inhibit calcium reabsorption in the early distal convoluted tubule; the cellular basis for this effect is incompletely understood but may be secondary to the effects of the drugs on sodium chloride or sodium entry.[570] In addition, extracellular volume depletion will increase proximal sodium reabsorption and thus reduce delivery to distal sites. Increased sodium intake blunts the hypocalciuric effect of thiazides. However, in the presence of intact calcium homeostasis, a simple reduction in urinary calcium excretion should be compensated. Indeed, thiazide administration has extrarenal effects, increasing the serum calcium concentration in end-stage renal failure.[571] Thus, there may be effects of thiazides on bone either directly or by potentiating the effect of PTH on bone resorption. Theoretically, thiazides could also stimulate the secretion of PTH or intestinal calcium absorption, but there is no compelling evidence for such actions.

Vitamin D

Hypercalcemia occurs in patients taking large doses of vitamin D (usually greater than 50,000 units daily).[571a] It is seen in hypoparathyroid patients treated with vitamin D and in patients who self-administer large amounts as an anodyne. In the latter instance, the history of drug use may not be readily obtainable. The presenting symptoms and signs are those of hypercalcemia. The glomerular filtration rate is reduced, and calcium urolithiasis may also occur. Hypercalcemia persists in fasting patients, indicating a contribution of bone resorption as well as increased intestinal calcium absorption. In patients taking ergocalciferol, cholecalciferol, or calcifediol [25-(OH)D_3], the diagnosis may be established by measurement of the serum 25-(OH)D level, which is often 5 to 10 times normal. The level of 1α,25-$(OH)_2D$ may be normal or slightly raised, a tribute to the tight control of its synthetic rate.[571a,572,573] Thus, much of the toxicity of vitamin D probably results from the action of 25-(OH)D, which has an appreciable affinity for the receptor [one-thousandth that of 1α,25-$(OH)_2D$]. Hypercalcemia in vitamin D intoxication is treated with withdrawal of vitamin D and calcium, increased intake of fluids, and high-dose corticosteroid therapy; it responds to corticosteroids within a few days. In contrast to the effects of corticosteroids on the production of 1α,25-$(OH)_2D$ in sarcoidosis, the effect of steroids seen here appears to be attributable to blockade of vitamin D action. Intoxication with calcitriol [1α,25-$(OH)_2D_3$] can be diagnosed by determining its serum level; the other available short-acting agent, dihydrotachysterol, produces a metabolite that cross-reacts in some assays for 1α,25-$(OH)_2D$ but not in assays that use the calf thymus receptor.

Vitamin A

Large doses of vitamin A (50,000 to 200,000 units daily) produce a syndrome of lassitude, headache, anorexia, cheilitis, glossitis, a scaly pruritic rash, alopecia, hepatomegaly, and bone pain and tenderness. This syndrome is sometimes complicated by hypercalcemia. In hypercalcemic patients, the serum phosphorus is normal and the alkaline phosphase and other hepatic enzymes may be increased. Bone radiographs may show characteristic periosteal calcifications.[574] The vitamin A level in serum is elevated. Food faddism and self-medication with high-dose vitamin preparations are the most common causes of this rare disorder, and a history of excessive vitamin A intake may be difficult to obtain. It appears that dialysis patients are sensitive to smaller doses of vitamin A.[575] Hypercalcemia has also been reported as a complication of treatment with the retinoic acid derivative isotretinoin. The occurrence of hypercalcemia is probably attributable to a direct effect of vitamin A on bone resorption. Hypercalcemia responds to corticosteroids.

Lithium

Hypercalcemia is one of several endocrine complications in lithium-treated patients. As with lithium-induced hypothyroidism and nephrogenic diabetes insipidus, hypercalcemia occurs in patients with therapeutic serum levels of lithium. The serum calcium level is increased in populations of lithium-treated patients, and about 10 percent have frank hypercalcemia.[463,576] PTH levels tend to be increased in hypercalcemic patients, and studies in vitro indicate that lithium increases the set point for calcium suppression of PTH secretion.[40] Lithium therapy also decreases urinary calcium excretion and increases the serum magnesium.[576] Overall, the constellation of hypercalcemia with detectable PTH levels, hypocalciuria, and hypermagnesemia is reminiscent of familial benign hypercalcemia (familial hypocalciuric hypercalcemia), discussed earlier, and it is conceivable that lithium therapy induces abnormalities of calcium sensing that closely resemble those in the familial disorder. Lithium may also increase parathyroid gland growth.[576a,b] It also appears that like other drugs that predispose to hypercalcemia, lithium can exacerbate the hypercalcemia of primary hyperparathyroidism. The diagnosis of "true" primary hyperparathyroidism in the face of lithium therapy may be difficult, particularly since withdrawal of lithium from a well-controlled patient may be unacceptable.[577] Some patients with good evidence for a parathyroid tumor have been operated on, partly in the hope that the psychiatric disturbance would be ameliorated, but in this regard the results of surgery have been disappointing. Expectant management of mild hypercalcemia is often indicated.

The Milk-Alkali Syndrome

The ingestion of large quantities of calcium together with an absorbable alkali can produce hypercalcemia with alkalosis, renal impairment, and often nephrocalcinosis.[578] The serum phosphorus is normal. Hypercalciuria is classically absent despite the high filtered load of calcium. The syndrome was commonplace when the Sippy diet consisting of a milk-cream mixture and either sodium bicarbonate or bismuth subcarbonate was a standard peptic ulcer regimen. It is seen less frequently now that nonabsorbable antacids are in common use but still occurs, as witnessed by a recent epidemic of 65 cases in cardiac transplant patients treated prophylactically for peptic ulcer disease with large doses of calcium carbonate (8 to 12 g daily).[579] The pathophysiology of the syndrome is incompletely known: Clearly, large amounts of calcium can be absorbed passively from the intestine even if 1α,25-$(OH)_2D$ is suppressed; presumably hypercalcemia occurs when renal calcium excretion is impaired.

Miscellaneous Conditions

Immobilization

From the perspective of bone, immobilization is an example of a pure resorptive state. Histomorphometric studies indicate that immobilization produces an uncoupling of bone remodeling, with a decreased rate of bone formation and less pronounced increases in bone resorption.[580] The net effect is a loss of mineral from bone, and the consequences are predictable: osteoporosis, marked hypercalciuria, suppression of PTH, decreased 1α,25-$(OH)_2D$ levels, and an increased renal phosphate threshold.[581]

Hypercalcemia is seen predominantly in immobilized individuals with a preexisting state of high bone turnover: the young, in whom physiologic remodeling is active; the pagetic patient, with extensive osteolysis from a bony neoplasm (e.g., multiple myeloma); and in thyrotoxicosis. After a spinal cord injury, peak levels of hypercalciuria occur between 1 and 4 months, and the incidence of hypercalcemia is also highest during this period. Overall, 24 percent of children under age 16 experience hypercalcemia after a spinal cord injury, usually in conjunction with a decreased GFR.

The treatment of immobilization hypercalcemia consists of early resumption of weight bearing. Passive range-of-motion exercises are not helpful. In situations such as spinal cord injury where weight bearing is not possible, a variety of pharmacologic approaches have been tried. Glucocorticoids, calcitonin, and oral phosphate have been used with minimal success. Several cases have been reported in which bisphosphonate treatment promptly returned serum calcium levels to normal.[582]

Acute Renal Failure

Hypercalcemia is occasionally seen in acute renal failure, usually in the early diuretic phase. It has most commonly been reported in renal failure induced by rhabdomyolysis, which is characterized by severe hyperphosphatemia and hypocalcemia in the oliguric phase. Hypercalcemia appears in the early diuretic phase, at a time when the serum phosphorus level is falling but often still above normal, and resolves over a few weeks.[583] It is not certain what leads to transient hypercalcemia. Substantial amounts of calcium and phosphate are deposited in the injured muscle and are released during recovery. This occurs at a time when levels of PTH and 1α,25-(OH)$_2$D are reported to be high. Treatment consists of low-calcium dialysis, phosphate binders, and hydration.

ICU Hypercalcemia

An apparently new form of hypercalcemia has been reported over the past decade in critically ill patients. The etiology is unclear but may be multifactorial. At lease two of the following factors are commonly present: immobilization, parenteral nutrition, and renal insufficiency.[584] The underlying illnesses are diverse, but the disorder is prevalent in patients with end-stage liver disease.[585] Hypoalbuminemia is often present, serum phosphorus concentrations are normal, and marked hypercalciuria is sometimes observed. The serum level of 25-(OH)D is normal, and intact PTH and 1α,25-(OH)$_2$D are usually suppressed. In a few patients, serum PTHrP levels have been normal. Fluctuating hypercalcemia may persist for weeks but is reversible in patients who survive the ICU. Parenteral nutrition may be a key factor in some patients, as hypercalcemia has also been reported in patients maintained on chronic parenteral nutrition, often in association with low-turnover bone disease. However, hypercalcemia generally does not respond to the removal of calcium or vitamin D from the total parenteral nutrition (TPN) solution. No satisfactory therapy is available.

Idiopathic Hypercalcemia of Infancy

There are at least three forms of hypercalcemia in the newborn. Severe neonatal hypercalcemia is seen in families with familial benign hypercalcemia (familial hypocalciuric hypercalcemia), and some cases may be homozygotes for this autosomal dominant trait.[464] Hypercalcemia responds to subtotal parathyroidectomy. A second form occurs in Williams syndrome, which includes supravalvular aortic stenosis, other cardiac anomalies, mental retardation, and a characteristic elfin facies. High plasma concentrations of 1α,25-(OH)$_2$D have been found in some patients with this disorder,[586] but vitamin D metabolite levels are normal in other patients and the role of 1α,25-(OH)$_2$D is disputed. A third form of neonatal hypercalcemia occurs transiently in patients who lack the somatic features of Williams syndrome.

Serum Protein Disorders

Hemoconcentration leads to hyperalbuminemia and a consequent increase in the total serum calcium; ionized calcium levels are normal. Binding of calcium by myeloma paraproteins has also been reported.[524] These patients present with chronic hypercalcemia and a normal ionized calcium level. Measurement of ionized calcium is unnecessary in patients with symptomatic hypercalcemia but should be performed in asymptomatic myeloma patients.

HYPOCALCEMIA

Classification of Hypocalcemic Disorders

Both PTH and 1α,25-(OH)$_2$D take part in the coordinated defense against hypocalcemia (Fig. 23-64). The increased secretion of PTH that is evoked by hypocalcemia results in increased resorption of calcium from bone, increased reabsorption of calcium by the kidney, and increased renal synthesis of 1α,25-(OH)$_2$D. The active vitamin D metabolite activates intestinal calcium absorption, bone resorption, and probably calcium resorption from the renal tubule. The presence of hypocalcemia provides presumptive evidence of the failure of this homeostatic system (Table 23-7). This can occur because of a failure to secrete PTH (hypoparathyroidism), resistance to the action of PTH (pseudohypoparathyroidism, renal failure, plicamycin therapy), failure to produce 1α,25-(OH)$_2$D normally (vitamin D deficiency, hereditary 1α-hydroxylase deficiency, renal failure), or resistance to the action of vitamin D (heredi-

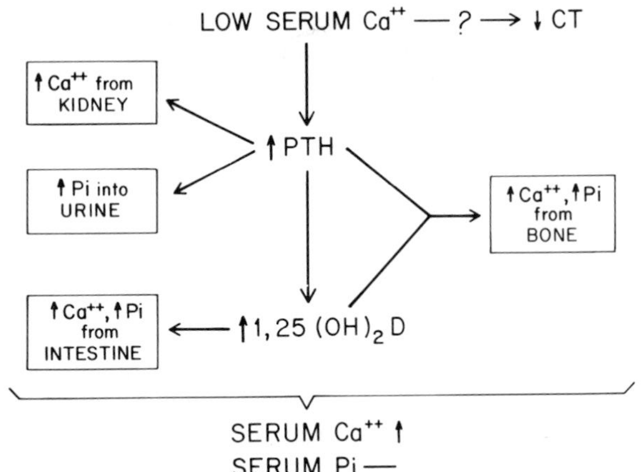

FIGURE 23-64 The sequence of adjustments initiated in response to hypocalcemia.

tary 1α,25-$(OH)_2D$–resistant rickets). Acutely, overwhelming challenges to the calcium homeostatic system that result from rapid complexation or tissue deposition of calcium can outstrip the ability of an intact system to respond. In these conditions (e.g., acute hyperphosphatemia, acute pancreatitis, rapid skeletal mineralization, hungry bones syndrome, massive transfusion of citrated blood), hypocalcemia may persist for hours, days, or weeks but not chronically.

TABLE 23-7 Causes of Hypocalcemia

- Hypoparathyroidism
  - Surgical
  - Idiopathic
  - Neonatal
  - Familial
  - Disposition of metals (iron, copper, aluminum)
  - Postradiation
  - Infiltrative
  - Functional (in hypomagnesemia)
- Resistance to PTH action
  - Pseudohypoparathyroidism
  - Renal insufficiency
  - Medications that block osteoclastic bone resorption
    - Plicamycin (mithramycin)
    - Calcitonin
    - Bisphosphonates
- Failure to produce 1α,25$(OH)_2D$ normally
  - Vitamin D deficiency
  - Hereditary 1α-hydroxylase deficiency
  - Renal insufficiency
- Resistance to 1α,25$(OH)_2D$ action: hereditary 1α,25$(OH)_2D$–resistant rickets
- Acute complexation or deposition of calcium
  - Hyperphosphatemia
    - Crush injury
    - Rapid tumor lysis
    - Parenteral phosphate administration
    - Excessive enteral phosphate
      - Oral
      - Phosphate-containing enemas
  - Acute pancreatitis
  - Citrated blood transfusion
  - Rapid excessive skeletal mineralization
    - Hungry bones syndrome
    - Osteoblastic metastases
    - Vitamin D therapy for vitamin D deficiency

Approach to the Hypocalcemic Patient

Together with knowledge of the clinical circumstances, the serum levels of calcium, magnesium, and phosphorus and a confirmatory determination of the serum PTH level will often suffice for the differential diagnosis of hypocalcemia. Unless there is a history of recent neck surgery, acute development of hypocalcemia suggests that one of the acute antecedent conditions listed above has overwhelmed the homeostatic system. When one is armed with this idea, the cause of hypocalcemia (Table 23-7) is usually obvious. In addition to measuring serum phosphorus, creatinine, and PTH, it is important to exclude hypomagnesemia as a cause of functional hypoparathyroidism.

In a chronically hypocalcemic patient, the presence of *hyper*phosphatemia suggests a failure of secretion of PTH (hypoparathyroidism) or of the response to PTH (pseudohypoparathyroidism) unless renal insufficiency is present. The genesis of hypocalcemia in renal failure is a complex issue that is discussed in Chap. 24, but renal failure rarely causes hypocalcemia unless it is profound (creatinine clearance less than 15 ml/min). Conversely, *hypo*phosphatemia will often be present in a chronically hypocalcemic patient if the parathyroid glands can respond. The combination of hypocalcemia and hypophosphatemia is seen in states of excessive skeletal mineralization (hungry bones syndrome) and in disorders of the vitamin D endocrine system. In both instances, the presence of secondary hyperparathyroidism can be confirmed by direct assay of PTH. Vitamin D disorders are discussed in detail in Chap. 24.

Clinical Manifestations of Hypocalcemia

Most of the symptoms and signs of hypocalcemia result from either increased neuromuscular excitability (tetany, paresthesias, seizures, organic brain syndrome) or calcium deposition (cataract, calcification of basal ganglia).

Tetany

Tetany is a state of spontaneous tonic muscular contraction induced by hypocalcemia or other stimuli.[587] Overt tetany begins with a tingling sensation in the fingers and about the mouth, spreading to become general and sometimes followed by numbness. The muscular component is classically manifested as carpopedal spasm. This begins with adduction of the thumb, followed by flexion of the metacarpophalangeal joints, extension of the interphalangeal joints, and flexion of the wrists and elbows to produce the main d'accoucheur posture (Fig. 23-65). The contractions may be severely painful. Despite the appellation *carpopedal*, the feet are much more rarely involved than are the hands. When severe, tetany can involve spasm of other muscle groups, including life-threatening laryngeal spasm. Electromyographically, tetany is typified by repetitive motor-unit action potentials, usually grouped as doublets. These changes are characteristic of tetany but not of hypocalcemia per se. Extracellular calcium and magnesium are thought to affect the local electric field of the membrane near ion channels in such a fashion that hypocalcemia or hypomagnesemia reduces the amount of depolarization necessary to induce an increase in sodium conductance and depolarize nerve cells.[587]

Lesser degrees of neuromuscular excitability may result in latent tetany, which is elicited by testing for Chvostek's and Trousseau's signs. Chvostek's sign is elicited by tapping the facial nerve about 2 cm anterior to the earlobe just below the zygoma. The reaction can be graded semiquantitatively: grade 1, twitching of the angle of the mouth; grade 2, additional twitching of the alae nasi; grade 3, contraction of the orbicularis oculi; grade 4, hemifacial contractions. A grade 1 Chvostek's sign is present in 25 percent of normal individuals. Trousseau's sign is elicited by inflating a blood pressure cuff to about 20 torr above systolic pressure for 3 min to evoke an attack of carpal spasm. The response depends on the induction of regional ischemia in the ulnar nerve, not generalized ischemia of the forearm. This can be shown by deflating the cuff after placing a second cuff distally. The carpal spasm will recede and then reoccur after several minutes, a response that can be used to outwit the occasional malingerer. Trousseau's sign is more specific than Chvostek's sign, but a positive Trousseau's sign may occur in 1 to 4 percent of normal subjects.

FIGURE 23-65 Carpal spasm in tetany. The wrist is flexed, the thumb is adducted, the metacarpophalangeal joints are flexed, and the interphalangeal joints are extended. *[By permission of Arnaud CD, The calcitropic hormones and metabolic bone disease in FS Greenspan (ed): Basic and Clinical Endocrinology, 3d ed. Norwalk, CT Appleton and Lange, p. 264, 1991.]*

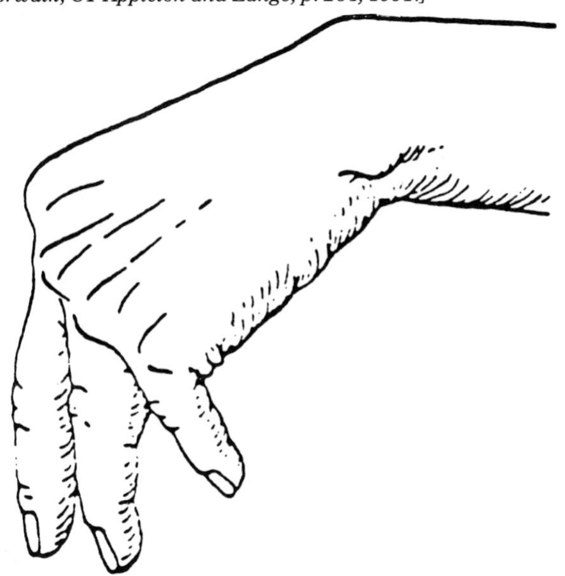

The most important cause of normocalcemic tetany is hyperventilation. Although respiratory alkalosis lowers the ionized calcium by increasing protein binding, alkalosis causes tetany primarily by an independent effect on neuromuscular excitability.[588] However, latent tetany in hypocalcemic persons may become overt during hyperventilation. Other causes of tetany include metabolic alkalosis and hypomagnesemia. Regardless of its cause, tetany worsens during pregnancy and lactation. Tetany in hypocalcemic individuals may be masked by uremia, hypokalemia, or hypermagnesemia.

Other Neuromuscular Effects of Hypocalcemia

Hypocalcemia predisposes to seizures. These may be focal, jacksonian, petit mal, or grand mal. In addition, there may be a distinct hypocalcemic seizure syndrome consisting of tonic spasms after generalized tetany. The most characteristic electroencephalographic finding in hypocalcemia is bursts of high-voltage slow waves (2 to 5 Hz) whose frequency of occurrence is correlated with the serum calcium level. This finding is not pathognomic of hypocalcemia, since it is also seen in other metabolic disturbances.

Other effects of chronic hypocalcemia on the central nervous system include papilledema and pseudotumor cerebri, confusion, lassitude, depression, incontinence, psychosis, and organic brain syndrome. Chronic hypocalcemia is associated with mental retardation in about 20 percent of affected children. Cognitive performance may improve with treatment of the hypocalcemia.

Hypocalcemia in patients with long-standing hypoparathyroidism or pseudohypoparathyroidism is sometimes accompanied by calcification of the basal ganglia. The pathogenesis of basal ganglia calcification is unknown. Calcification is often evident on the plain film, although computed tomography is a more sensitive diagnostic procedure.[589] Calcification of the basal ganglia is usually asymptomatic but may produce a variety of movement disorders, including choreoathetosis and parkinsonian states. Treatment of hypocalcemia can arrest the progression of the extrapyramidal symptoms and may produce some improvement. Calcification of the basal ganglia is also detected rarely in otherwise normal individuals and in a familial form.

Hypocalcemia delays cardiac repolarization, producing prolongation of the QT interval, occasionally accompanied by second-degree heart block. Given the critical role of calcium in excitation-contraction coupling, it is not surprising that refractory congestive heart failure is seen in hypocalcemic patients and responds to the correction of hypocalcemia.[590] Studies in hemodialysis patients suggest that cardiac contractility may vary acutely with smaller changes in the serum calcium level.

Other Manifestations of Hypocalcemia

Cataract is the most common structural complication of hypocalcemia. These are subcapsular lenticular opacities whose severity is correlated with the duration of hypocalcemia. It has been suggested that hypocalcemia interferes with the function of a sodium pump in the lens, leading to swelling and degeneration. *Dental abnormalities* occur in patients in whom hypocalcemia was present during development of the teeth and include hypoplasia of the enamel, delayed eruption, and failure of eruption. The *skin* in hypocalcemic persons may be dry and flaky, with brittle nails and coarse, dry hair. Also associated with hypocalcemia is a particular dermatosis known as impetigo herpetiformis or pustular psoriasis.[591] Part of the autoimmune polyglandular syndrome associated with hypoparathyroidism is chronic mucocutaneous candidiasis, a disorder that is not seen with hypocalcemia of other causes.

Hypoparathyroidism

Clinical Manifestations

The signs and symptoms of hypoparathyroidism are those of hypocalcemia. Biochemically, the serum level of phosphorus is high or high-normal as a result of a high renal phosphate threshold (see Renal Phosphate Handling, below). This results primarily from absence of the phosphaturic effect of PTH. However, hypocalcemia per se may independently increase the renal phosphate threshold, accounting for the variable improvement in hyperphosphatemia when hypoparathyroid patients are treated with vitamin D.[592]

Surgical Hypoparathyroidism

By far the most common form of hypoparathyroidism occurs postoperatively after injury to the parathyroid glands during neck surgery. The frequency of hypoparathyroidism varies with the amount of cervical dissection: It is highest after cancer surgery, it is more common after total than after subtotal thyroidectomy, and with skilled hands it occurs in less than 1 percent of parathyroidectomies.[593] The skill and experience of the surgeon are probably as important a variable as the nature of the procedure. The mechanism of injury to the parathyroid glands is obscure, but ischemia due to excessive use of ligatures in the vicinity of the glands is the most likely cause; rarely are all the parathyroid glands identified in the surgical specimen.

Most patients experience a fall of about 1 mg/dl in the serum calcium during the 24 to 48 h after neck exploration as a nonspecific response to surgery. Patients who develop severe hypocalcemia with overt symptoms of tetany are suspect for the development of postsurgical hypoparathyroidism. Tetany usually appears during the first two postoperative days. About half of patients with postoperative tetany will recover sufficiently to require no chronic therapy, but most of them will have a decreased parathyroid reserve. Some patients with transient tetany and some patients who were asymptomatic in the immediate postoperative period will go on to develop late hypoparathyroidism months or years after neck surgery. Thus, surgical hypoparathyroidism must always be suspected in a hypocalcemic individual with a scar on the neck.[594]

There is a wide spectrum of postsurgical hypoparathyroidism, from decreased parathyroid reserve on testing, through intermittent hypocalcemia, to the requirement for chronic therapy with vitamin D and calcium.[595] Levels of intact PTH may range from inappropriately normal in the face of hypocalcemia to frankly low in patients who require vitamin D and calcium therapy. Older PTH assays were not reliable in making these distinctions. Patients with chronic, poorly treated hypocalcemia are subject to most of the complications of hypocalcemia listed in the previous section.

The usual postoperative fall in serum calcium may be exaggerated in hyperparathyroidism or hyperthyroidism, where the presence of overt bone disease predisposes to the hungry bones syndrome.[478] This represents rapid uptake of calcium into remineralizing bones under conditions where the parathyroid glands may not have recovered fully from suppression. The syndrome may be particularly severe and prolonged after parathyroidectomy for severe secondary hyperparathyroidism in chronic renal failure. The differentiation of the hungry bones syndrome from postoperative hypoparathyroidism often can be made by following the serum phosphorus concentration, which is typically depressed in the hungry bones syndrome but high in hypoparathyroidism. The presence of preexisting hyperparathyroid bone disease may be manifested as radiographic changes or an increased serum alkaline phosphatase level. Patients with hyperthyroidism are also in a preoperative state of high bone turnover, particularly if they are not adequately treated medically, and are at risk for a mild form of the hungry bones syndrome. As many as a third will develop frank hypocalcemia after subtotal thyroidectomy.[596]

Other Causes of Acquired Hypoparathyroidism

Deposition of Metals

Hypoparathyroidism is sometimes seen in congenitally transfusion-dependent patients with thalassemia or pure red cell aplasia who survive until the third decade of life.[597] Pathologically, abundant iron and a fibrous reaction are present in the glands. Hypoparathyroidism is rare in hemochromatosis. Frank hypoparathyroidism and decreased parathyroid reserve can occur in Wilson's disease, presumably because of copper deposition.[598] Aluminum deposition may impair the parathyroid reserve in renal osteodystrophy (see Chap. 24).

Radiation

The parathyroids are quite resistant to radiation damage, but rare cases of hypoparathyroidism have occurred after radioactive iodine therapy for hyperthyroidism.[599]

Other Infiltrative Processes

Metastases to the parathyroids are not uncommon, but only a few cases of hypoparathyroidism have been attributable to neoplastic infiltration, usually from breast cancer.[594] The parathyroid glands can be infiltrated with amyloid and also can be the site of granulomas in sarcoidosis, tuberculosis, and syphilis, but these conditions rarely if ever produce hypoparathyroidism.

Functional Hypoparathyroidism in Hypomagnesemia

Severe magnesium depletion may prevent the secretion of PTH. The clinical settings include chronic gastrointestinal magnesium losses, nutritional deficiency accompanying alcoholism, and renal magnesium wasting. Patients present with the combination of hypocalcemia and hypomagnesemia, and hypocalcemia is rather refractory to therapy until magnesium is repleted. Hypoparathyroidism is rarely seen unless the serum magnesium concentration falls below 0.4 mmol/liter (1 mg/dl). The serum phosphorus level is usually normal. A burst of PTH secretion may occur within minutes of the intravenous administration of magnesium, and sustained therapy reverses the disorder[600] (Fig. 23-66). The basis of the permissive role of magnesium in the secretion of PTH has already been discussed. It appears that relative resistance to the effects of PTH in bone and kidney may also be present in hypomagnesemic patients and could contribute to hypocalcemia.[601,602] In addition, the serum concentration of $1\alpha,25\text{-(OH)}_2D$ may be reduced.[603]

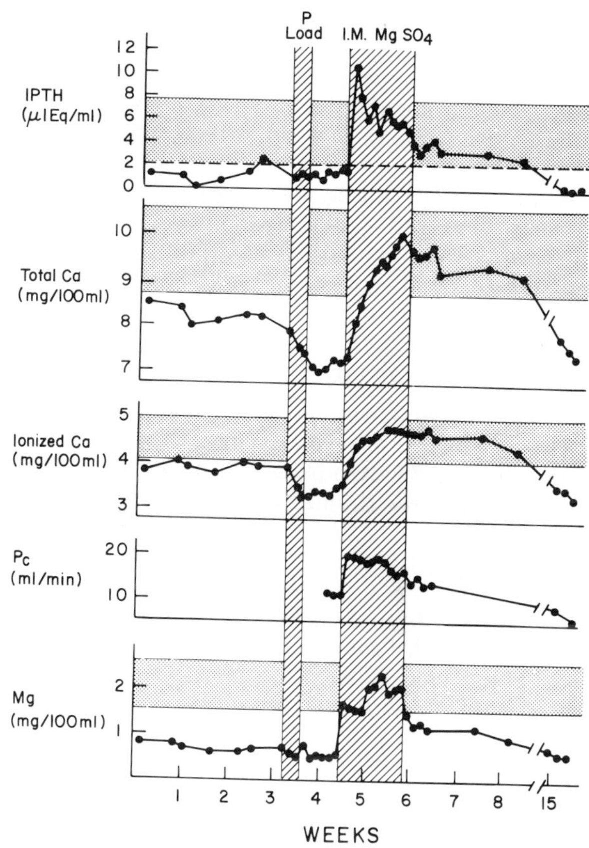

FIGURE 23-66 Response of serum calcium, parathyroid hormone, and phosphorus clearance (P_c) to magnesium replacement in a patient with severe hypomagnesemia. The hypocalcemia produced by an oral phosphate challenge before magnesium replacement did not result in an increase in PTH secretion. The shaded areas represent the normal ranges, and the dotted line represents the detection limit of the PTH assay. *(Adapted from and by permission of Anast CS, Mohs JM, Kaplan SL, Burns TW, Science 177:606, 1972.)*

Idiopathic Hypoparathyroidism

The best defined form of idiopathic hypoparathyroidism occurs as part of a syndrome of pluriglandular endocrine insufficiency (also known as polyglandular autoimmune syndrome; see Chap. 28). Hypoparathyroidism is associated with primary adrenal insufficiency (Addison's disease) and chronic mucocutaneous candidiasis (HAM syndrome, or hypoparathyroidism, Addison's disease, and moniliasis). Candidiasis appears first, in early childhood, followed by idiopathic hypoparathyroidism and finally adrenal insufficiency.[604] The mean age of onset of hypoparathyroidism is 5 to 9 years. Less common associations with the syndrome include premature ovarian failure, alopecia, and vitiligo. The disorder of mineral metabolism may be complicated by intestinal malabsorption or chronic active hepatitis, which are commonly present. Circulating parathyroid antibodies are comparatively common, even in the absence of overt hypoparathyroidism.[605] In rare instances where the parathyroids have been examined, they have shown lymphocytic infiltrates or have not been identifiable. Multiple siblings are often affected, suggesting autosomal recessive inheritance. The management of hypoparathyroidism is confounded by malabsorption, which may improve with restoration of normocalcemia.

Isolated idiopathic hypoparathyroidism also occurs sporadically. The age of onset is 2 to 10 years, and there is a preponderance of female cases. About a third of these patients have parathyroid antibodies.[605]

Neonatal Syndromes

DiGeorge Syndrome

This is a sporadic developmental disorder involving the third and fourth branchial clefts that results in dysgenesis of the thymus and the parathyroids.[606] Hypoparathyroidism presents as tetany in infancy, but defective T-cell function dominates the subsequent course unless thymic tissue is transplanted. Associated cardiac abnormalities and craniofacial anomalies are also common.[606,607] It was recently reported that deletion of both copies of the homeobox gene hox 1.5 in the mouse produces a similar development defect.[608]

Other Neonatal Syndromes

Persistent neonatal hypoparathyroidism is assumed to result from congenital aplasia of the parathyroid glands in most cases, but this has rarely been verified.[609] The disorder may be sporadic or familial; the familial form is described below. *Transient hypoparathyroidism* occurs in the infants of mothers with gestational hyperparathyroidism. Hypocalcemia may persist for several weeks after childbirth and require therapy.[609] Transient hypoparathyroidism probably also plays a role in both forms of *idiopathic hypocalcemia of infancy.* An early form that appears in the first 24 to 48 h after delivery is associated with prematurity, maternal diabetes, and birth asphyxia. A late form occurs after 1 week. It generally occurs in infants who are fed cow's milk and is probably caused by the high phosphate content of cow's milk.[609]

Familial Hypoparathyroidism

This rare disorder can be inherited in autosomal dominant, autosomal recessive, and X-linked patterns. It presents in infancy and can thus be considered a subcategory of persistent neonatal hypoparathyroidism. Linkage analysis of multiple kindreds has excluded a parathyroid gene mutation in about half the families examined; in these families, a developmental syndrome may lead to congenital aplasia.[610] In two kindreds the prepro-PTH gene was abnormal. In a family with autosomal dominant inheritance of hypoparathyroidism, a missense mutation ($Cys^{18} \rightarrow Arg$) disrupts the hydrophobic core of the signal sequence; expression of this trait results in inefficient uptake of prepro-PTH into the endoplasmic reticulum.[21] A family with an autosomal recessive disorder carries a splicing mutation that deletes the prepro sequence in exon 2.[611]

Pseudohypoparathyroidism

Historical Introduction

That end-organ resistance to PTH can produce a syndrome that resembles true hypoparathyroidism was first recognized by Albright. His classic paper in 1942 defining the syndrome reported three hypocalcemic patients with hyperphosphatemia who shared some unusual somatic features (Fig. 23-67). Unlike patients with idiopathic hypoparathyroidism, these individuals had no response to the infusion of parathyroid extract, and one had normal parathyroid glands. Albright proposed that their hypocalcemia had resulted from unresponsiveness to PTH and entitled the paper "Pseudo-hypoparathyrodism—an example of 'Seabright-Bantam syndrome' "[612] after a strain of domestic fowl in which the roosters have female feathering. Albright's report was the first clear description of end-organ resistance to a hormone, since the Seabright bantam syndrome, ironically, has now been shown to be caused by abnormal aromatization of androgen rather than resistance to the tissue effects of androgens.[613] In 1969, shortly after the discovery of cAMP, it was found that the normally brisk increase in urinary cAMP in response to PTH was markedly blunted in pseudohypoparathyroidism (Fig. 23-68), providing a clue that the molecular defect lay in the PTH receptor–adenylyl cyclase complex.[614] The rare opportunity to study renal tissue from a pseudohypoparathyroid patient subsequently led to the discovery of abnormalities in guanosine triphosphate (GTP) stimulation of renal adenylyl cyclase, focusing attention directly on the coupling of the PTH receptor–adenylyl cyclase complex, which is known to be GTP-dependent.[615] Subsequently, it was shown that many patients with pseudohypoparathyroidism display a 50 percent reduction in the content of the stimulatory G-protein subunit of adenylyl cyclase, G_s, as described in detail below, providing a presumptive molecular basis for one form of the disorder.[616,617]

Clinical and Biochemical Features

The symptoms and signs of hypocalcemia develop in childhood. The average age at the onset of symptoms is 8 years, although the diagnosis is not made until adulthood in some relatively asymptomatic persons. As in other hypocalcemic disorders, the presenting symptoms are tetany and seizures.[618] Subsequently, pseudohypoparathyroid patients are prone to the complications of chronic hypocalcemia: calcification of the basal ganglia, which occurs in 50 percent; cognitive defects; cataracts; and dental abnor-

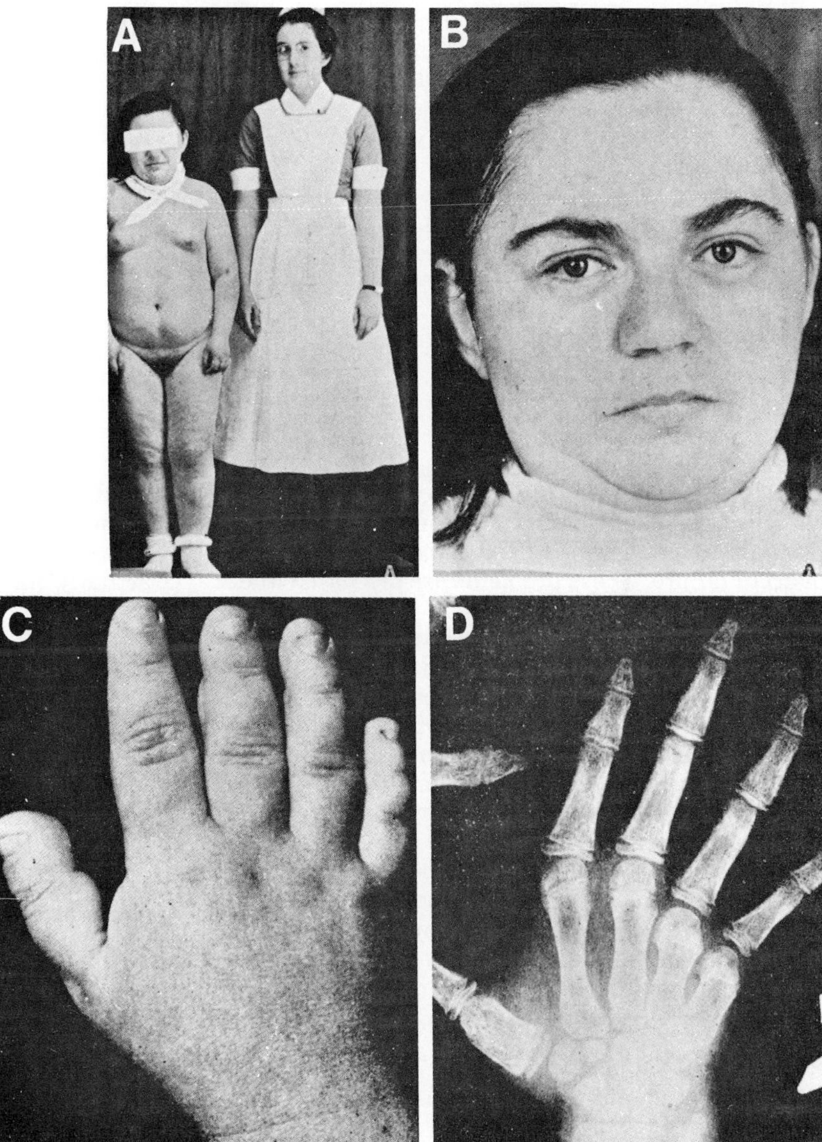

FIGURE 23-67 Phenotypic abnormalities in pseudohypoparathyroidism: *(A)* short, stocky habitus; *(B)* round face; (*C* and *D*) short metacarpals. *(A, B, and C by permission of Albright F, Burnett CH, Smith PH, Parson W, Endocrinology 30:922, 1942. D by permission of Kolb FO, Steinbach HJ, J Clin Endocrinol Metab 22:59, 1962.)*

malities, including hypoplasia of dentin or enamel and delay or absence of eruption (Table 23-8).

Many patients present with the somatic features described in the original report. The combination of short stature, brachydactyly (short digits), and soft tissue calcification is distinctive and is known as Albright's hereditary osteodystrophy (AHO). Patients are short (usually less than 150 cm) and obese and have round faces and short necks (Fig. 23-67). Brachydactyly most commonly affects the fourth and fifth metacarpal bones (brachymetacarpia), but shortened metatarsals (brachymetatarsia) are seen in 43 percent and brachyphalangia in 50 percent of patients (Table 23-8). Brachydactyly may be diagnosed on physical examination or radiographs. On examination of the clenched fists, knuckles that would represent the ends of normal metacarpals are absent; instead, dimples overlie the shortened metacarpals. A straight edge laid over the fourth and fifth metacarpal heads in a clenched fist will normally miss the third metacarpal head but may touch it if the fourth is short. Similarly, on hand films, a line tangential to the fourth and fifth metacarpal heads should not intersect the third. Subcutaneous calcifications which histologically represent ectopic ossification are seen in over half of these patients. These forms of soft tissue calcification are not seen in hypoparathyroidism or other chronic hypocalcemic states. Numerous other syndromes involving brachydactyly are recognized, but the complete picture of AHO is virtually pathognomic of pseudohypoparathyroidism or the related disorder pseudopseudohypoparathyroidism (see below).

In addition to their disorder of mineral metabo-

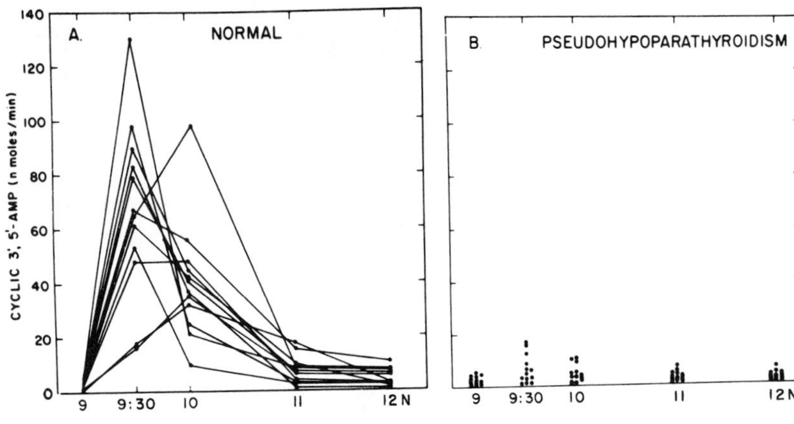

FIGURE 23-68 Urinary cAMP response to parathyroid hormone administration in normal subjects and patients with pseudohypoparathyroidism. *(From Chase, Melson, and Aurbach,[614] by permission of the Journal of Clinical Investigation.)*

lism, patients with AHO may have clinical or biochemical evidence of other hormone resistance syndromes, most prominently hypothyroidism and ovarian failure. These problems are discussed under Pathogenesis.

Pseudohypoparathyroidism presents with hypocalcemia, hyperphosphatemia, and secondary hyperparathyroidism. The urinary excretion of calcium may be lower than in hypoparathyroid patients with a similar serum calcium level, and it is not clear whether the renal defect in responsiveness to PTH extends to the distal site of calcium reabsorption.[619] However, the serum 1α,25-$(OH)_2D$ level is in the low-normal range in the face of hyperparathyroidism and hypocalcemia and does not respond normally to the infusion of PTH.[620] The serum level of alkaline phosphatase is normal. The bones may appear to be dense radiographically. However, in contrast to patients with hypoparathyroidism, pseudohypoparathyroid patients have evidence of increased bone turnover, with increased urinary excretion of hydroxyproline and reduced bone density, and some actually have hyperparathyroid bone disease (see below).[621]

TABLE 23-8 Symptoms and Signs in Pseudohypoparathyroidism

Symptom or Sign	Incidence, %
Somatotype	
Short stature	80
Round face	92
Stocky or obese habitus	50
Mental retardation	75
Dystrophic changes in bone	
Short metacarpals	68
Short metatarsals	43
Calvarial thickening	62
Ectopic ossification	56
Symptoms or signs of hypocalcemia	
Tetany	86
Seizures	59
Cataracts	44
Calcification of the basal ganglia	45
Dental abnormalities	55

Source: Adapted from Nagant de Deuxchaisnes C, Krane SM: Hypoparathyroidism, in Avioli LV, Krane SM (eds): *Metabolic Bone Disease*. New York, Academic Press, 1978, vol. 2, pp 217–445.

Pathogenesis

The finding of Chase, Melson, and Aurbach that the urinary cAMP response to PTH was markedly blunted (but not abolished) in pseudohypoparathyroidism (Fig. 23-68) provides strong evidence that the molecular defect has to do with the synthesis or metabolism of cAMP.[614] In confirmation of this conclusion, infusion of dibutyryl cAMP has a normal effect on urinary phosphorus excretion and serum levels of 1α,25-$(OH)_2D$.[622,623] Theoretical possibilities for the underlying defect include defective function of the PTH receptor, reduced coupling of the occupied receptor to the catalytic subunit of adenylyl cyclase, abnormal synthesis of cAMP by the catalytic subunit, and rapid degradation of cAMP. Subsequent work has shown that the disorder is heterogeneous. Some patients have a reduced level of the coupling protein component of adenylyl cyclase, G_s; this disorder has been termed pseudohypoparathyroidism type IA. The etiology in the remaining patients (pseudohypoparathyroidism type IB) is unknown, but they are thought to have deficient levels of the PTH receptor.

Pseudohypoparathyroidism Type IA

In this disorder, pseudohypoparathyroidism is associated with a deficiency of functional G_s resulting from mutations in the subunit $G_s\alpha$ and the PTH receptor occupied by hormone is coupled inefficiently by G_s to the catalytic subunit of adenylyl cyclase, with defective production of cAMP in response to PTH and a consequent defect in PTH action. The level of the coupling protein G_s in erythrocytes[616,617] or other tissues (fibroblasts, lymphocytes, platelets[624]) was reduced to 50 percent of normal in a group of pseudohypoparathyroid patients (Fig. 23-69), as

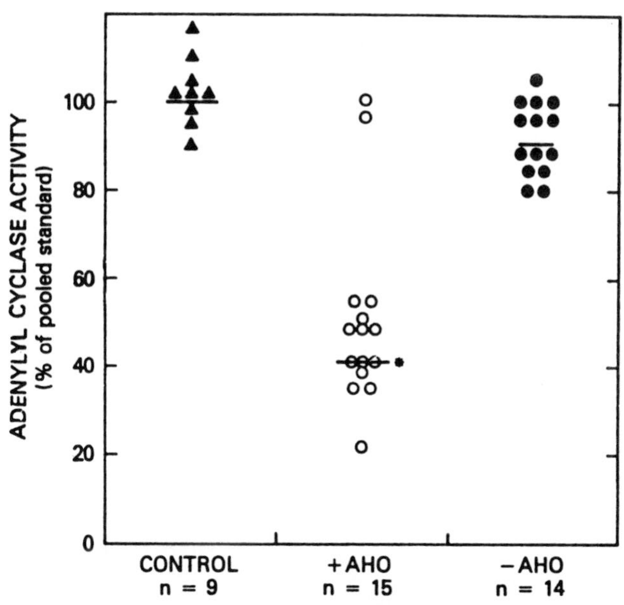

FIGURE 23-69 Activity of G_s in erythrocyte membranes from control subjects and from patients with pseudohypoparathyroidism, with or without Albright's hereditary osteodystrophy (AHO). The activity of G_s was assayed as the ability to reconstitute the adenylyl cyclase activity of turkey erythrocyte membranes containing the catalytic subunit of adenylyl cyclase. *(From Levine, Downs, and Moses,[635] by permission of the American Journal of Medicine.)*

measured either by a functional assay or by labeling its α-subunit with cholera toxin. As discussed under Biochemical Events in Parathyroid Hormone Action, the G proteins are heterotrimeric GTP-binding proteins which couple occupied receptors to effector molecules, including catalytic adenylyl cyclase (Fig. 23-12). The G proteins share common β and γ subunits. The specificity of a G protein for a receptor and for its cognate effector moiety are properties of the GTP-binding α subunit, and $G_s\alpha$ specifically couples stimulatory receptors to catalytic adenylyl cyclase. Thus, a generalized reduction in functional $G_s\alpha$ to one-half of normal levels would be expected to uncouple a fraction of occupied PTH receptors from the catalytic subunit of adenylyl cyclase and also to uncouple from adenylyl cyclase other receptors that normally stimulate the enzyme, engendering a generalized disorder of unresponsiveness of the hormones that utilize this signaling system.

As we shall see, the reduction in $G_s\alpha$ levels is not uniformly associated with unresponsiveness to PTH, as some members of families with pseudohypoparathyroidism have normal mineral metabolism despite a 50 percent reduction in $G_s\alpha$ levels (pseudopseudohypoparathyroidism). However, most patients with reduced levels of $G_s\alpha$ have AHO (Fig. 23-69). Thus, the defect in adenylyl cyclase function, independently of abnormal mineral metabolism, must directly produce the complex developmental abnormalities that eventuate in AHO.

A number of mutations can produce the phenotype of pseudohypoparathyroidism type IA. Most of these patients have an approximately 50 percent reduction in levels of $G_s\alpha$ mRNA,[625] and in the families that have been studied, this is associated with mutations in one allele that affect RNA splicing.[626] These mutations could produce abnormal mRNA species that are presumed to be unstable. Some patients have normal levels of $G_s\alpha$ mRNA, yet plasma membranes of their cells contain reduced quantities of $G_s\alpha$ protein.[627] The nonsense, missense, or frameshift mutations that have been found in such patients are predicted to produce abnormal $G_s\alpha$ proteins that are unstable and do not associate normally with the adenylyl cyclase complex in the plasma membrane.[626,628] In all cases examined, the nucleotide sequence of one allele has been normal, and translation of mRNA transcribed from the normal allele is thought to produce the reduced complement of functional $G_s\alpha$ protein that has uniformly been detected. Thus, the molecular defect displays autosomal dominant inheritance.

The association of peripheral resistance to PTH with an abnormality of the protein that is responsible for coupling the PTH receptor provides a very powerful inference of causality, yet these findings raise as many questions as they answer. What is the basis for hypocalcemia in these individuals? Why do some individuals in families with pseudohypoparathyroidism inherit an abnormal G_s protein and AHO but respond normally to PTH? Since the abnormality in G_s is expressed in many tissues, it would be expected to affect the action of many hormones coupled to adenylyl cyclase. This appears to be the case, but it is not clear why the clinical syndrome is often limited to abnormal PTH action.

Although renal unresponsiveness to PTH, with consequent hyperphosphatemia and possibly increased renal calcium excretion, would predispose a patient to hypocalcemia, it is likely that the genesis of hypocalcemia is multifactorial and involves bone and the gut as well as the kidney. In pseudohypoparathyroid patients, PTH does not mobilize calcium normally from bone, yet there is evidence of increased bone remodeling, with increased urinary hyroxyproline and decreased bone density,[621] and some patients actually manifest the skeletal changes of osteitis fibrosa cystica that occur in other forms of hyperparathyroidism.[624,629] Thus, in patients with pseudohypoparathyroidism, the remodeling function of PTH in bone seems to be dissociated from its function in calcium homeostasis. One theoretical explanation involves the use of multiple cellular second messengers by the PTH receptor (or receptors) in bone cells. Thus, cAMP may be the intracellular second messenger for the regulation of calcium homeostasis by bone cells, which would thus be abnormal in pseudohypoparathyroidism, whereas a different effector for the bone remodeling effects of PTH (e.g., phospholipase C, which is probably coupled to the PTH receptor by a G protein other than G_s) is unaffected in the disorder.

It is also likely that reduced $1\alpha,25\text{-(OH)}_2D$ levels are important in the pathogenesis of hypocalcemia. Evidence from several circumstances suggests that $1\alpha,25\text{-(OH)}_2D$ may be required for PTH to mobilize calcium from bone,[630] and normalization of plasma $1\alpha,25\text{-(OH)}_2D$ concentrations in patients with pseudohypoparathyroidism may normalize plasma calcium.[631] In addition, intestinal calcium absorption is reduced in patients with pseudohypoparathyroidism. Another possible explanation for the syndrome is secretion of PTH with reduced biological activity. Based on bioassay of PTH by a cytochemical method, it was reported that bioactive PTH levels were not increased in pseudohypoparathyroidism.[632,633] However, it is difficult to reconcile this finding with other data on the molecular basis of the syndrome, with the findings of hyperparathyroidism in the bone of many patients, or with the demonstration of increased intact PTH by a variety of two-site assays.

Albright recognized that in families with pseudohypoparathyroidism there are individuals who inherit AHO without a clinical disorder of mineral metabolism and called this state pseudopseudohypoparathyroidism.[634] These individuals have the same inherited abnormality of G_s as do their kin with pseudohypoparathyroidism but have a normal urinary cAMP response to the infusion of PTH.[614] Thus, the inheritance of abnormal G_s is closely linked to the inheritance of AHO. It is not clear why PTH action is normal in these individuals. It is conceivable that they have higher levels of G_s in kidney than do their kin with peripheral resistance to PTH or, more generally, that the action of a nonallelic modifier gene is required to express the mineral disorder. For example, increased phosphodiesterase activity in pseudopseudohypoparathyroid individuals compared with their pseudohypoparathyroid kin could modulate the effect of the mutation in $G_s\alpha$ by increasing the degradation of cAMP.

As expected in view of the defect in $G_s\alpha$, resistance to the action of other hormones whose receptors are coupled to adenylyl cyclase is common in patients with pseudohypoparathyroidism type IA, although this resistance does not usually cause clinically apparent disorders.[635] Most of these patients have compensated primary hypothyroidism, in which thyroid hormone levels are slightly low and TSH is increased, but some present with frank hypothyroidism. Most women patients are oligomenorrheic, and some have increased gonadotropins and an exaggerated LH and FSH response to gonadotropin releasing hormone (GnRH). The cAMP response to glucagon and isoproterenol may be blunted, but resistance to the action of these hormones is not otherwise evident. The spectrum of impaired hormone action observed in pseudohypoparathyroidism type IA parallels the spectrum of impairment in PTH action in individuals with deficient $G_s\alpha$. The modifying factors that account for the differences in hormone responsiveness among tissues and among individuals are unidentified.

Pseudohypoparathyroidism Type IB

This is a syndrome of peripheral resistance to PTH, including a severely blunted urinary cAMP response to the infusion of PTH, without either AHO or a deficiency of G_s. The responsiveness to other hormones is normal.[635] These findings would appear to localize the disorder either to a different part of the PTH receptor–adenylyl cyclase complex or to an abnormality in cAMP metabolism. One attractive possibility is that patients with pseudohypoparathyroidism type IB have an inherited defect in the PTH receptor itself. Consistent with this possibility, these patients do not manifest the generalized impairment in hormone action that is present in patients with the defective G_s associated with pseudohypoparathyroidism type IA.[635] Insight into the molecular defect in this disorder is likely to emerge now that the PTH receptor has been cloned and the presence of normal or abnormal receptor can be detected in tissues.

Pseudohypoparathyroidism Type II

This disorder was originally described as consisting of resistance to the phosphaturic effect of PTH despite a normal increase in urinary cAMP. It is rare and is likely to be heterogeneous.[636,637] Some cases may result from a defect in renal cAMP action leading to impairment of its second messenger function. Others may actually represent forms of vitamin D resistance. Syndromes of vitamin D resistance characterized by hyperphosphatemia have been recognized.[631] In them, osteomalacia may be mild or inapparent. In some cases of vitamin D resistance, the urinary cAMP responses to PTH are normal while the phosphaturic response may be impaired. Finally, the phosphaturic response to PTH is variable in normal subjects, and one must be cautious in ascribing a blunted response to a primary defect in the action of PTH.[638]

Genetics

Clinical evidence supports an autosomal dominant pattern of inheritance of pseudohypoparathyroidism type IA; this is consistent with the biochemical data on $G_s\alpha$ and with molecular genetic studies of some families. However, affected women outnumber men by 2 to 1, suggesting sex modification of inheritance.[639] One example of autosomal recessive inheritance of pseudohypoparathyroidism type IA has been reported.[640] The mode of inheritance of pseudohypoparathyroidism type IB is not precisely known.

Diagnosis

Pseudohypoparathyroidism should be considered in the differential diagnosis of hypocalcemia with hyperphosphatemia and normal renal function regardless of somatic features, as pseudohypoparathyroidism in the absence of AHO is not unusual. The elevated serum concentration of PTH in a patient with chronic hypocalcemia, hyperphosphatemia, and normal renal function excludes hypoparathyroidism and is suggestive of pseudohypoparathyroidism. The diagnosis of pseudohypoparathyroidism type I can be confirmed by a short infusion of PTH (the Ellsworth-Howard test; see Testing for Pseudohypoparathyroidism, below). The primary responses to PTH that are of value in a short infusion protocol are the increase in urinary phosphorus and the increase in urinary cAMP excretion. Although the former is the classic index of renal responsiveness, the phosphaturic effect of PTH is variable, and marked blunting of the robust normal urinary cAMP response to PTH is the most reliable diagnostic maneuver.[614,638] The response of serum $1\alpha,25\text{-(OH)}_2D$ levels and of serum calcium levels to the Ellsworth-Howard protocol is too small to use these as diagnostic criteria; a more prolonged infusion of PTH is necessary for this purpose.

Other Hypocalcemic Disorders

The causes of hypocalcemia are shown in Table 23-7. *Hypoalbuminemia* results in decreased total serum calcium with a normal ionized calcium concentration. *Medications* that predispose to hypocalcemia are those which directly inhibit osteoclastic bone resorption. In general, asymptomatic or mildly symptomatic hypocalcemia is seen with calcitonin or with the doses of the bisphosphonates that are employed in clinical practice. Aggressive plicamycin treatment can produce severe hypocalcemia.

Acute hyperphosphatemia resulting from myonecrosis occurs in compartment syndromes caused by crush injury.[583] Hyperphosphatemia may also occur by lysis of highly responsive tumors (e.g., lymphoma, leukemia) with the induction of aggressive chemotherapy.[641] Renal function is impaired in both settings by concomitant myoglobinuria and acute uric acid nephropathy, respectively. Thus, a massive phosphate load coincides with an impaired ability to excrete phosphate. Hyperphosphatemia can also be produced by oral or parenteral phosphate therapy, especially in the presence of renal failure.

In *acute pancreatitis*, significant hypocalcemia is an ominous prognostic sign. The pathogenesis of hypocalcemia has been debated for decades; factors that have been proposed include relative hypoparathyroidism, hypomagnesemia, and hyperglucagonemia leading to excessive calcitonin secretion. Recent evidence from patients and from an experimental model favors the old proposal that hypocalcemia in acute pancreatitis results from saponification of calcium with fatty acids produced by lipase action in the pancreatic bed, resulting in precipitation of calcium as "soaps."[642,643]

Transfusion

Citrate anticoagulates banked blood by chelating calcium. The excess calcium chelating capacity is approximately 150 mg per unit. Therefore, rapid massive transfusions can result in symptomatic reductions in ionized calcium. This is a special problem in liver transplantation, where metabolism of citrate may also be impaired.[644] However, measurements of total calcium, which include the citrate complexed component, may be increased. It is advisable to monitor ionized calcium and to replace calcium pari passu when large-volume transfusion is indicated.

Skeletal Mineralization

Rapid or excessive *skeletal mineralization* occurs postoperatively in the hungry bones syndrome discussed above,[478] with osteoblastic metastases from prostate or breast carcinoma,[645,646] and in the early phase of vitamin D therapy for severe osteomalacia.

Sepsis and Critical Illness

Hypocalcemia and reduced ionized calcium levels occur acutely in gram-negative sepsis.[647] The underlying cause is unknown, but renal insufficiency may be a contributory factor. The response of calciotropic hormones is variable: Many patients have reduced levels of $1\alpha,25\text{-(OH)}_2D$, and some have inappropriately normal PTH levels. Hypocalcemia is also seen in 20 percent of critically ill patients. Besides sepsis, contributory factors include renal failure, hypomagnesemia, transfusion, and acute pancreatitis.[648]

Treatment of Hypocalcemia

Acute Hypocalcemia

A patient with tetany should be treated intravenously with calcium as calcium chloride (272 mg elemental calcium per 10 ml), calcium gluconate (90 mg calcium per 10 ml), or calcium gluceptate (90 mg calcium per 10 ml). Approximately 200 mg should be given over several minutes, preferably diluted in dextrose in water, because concentrated calcium solutions are irritating. Intravenous calcium should be administered with caution to patients on digitalis therapy, in whom it predisposes to digitalis toxic arrhythmias.[649] The patient can simultaneously be started on oral calcium, and the infusion can be repeated in several hours if symptoms recur. If repeated intravenous administration of calcium is necessary, it is preferable to begin a continuous infusion of approximately 500 to 1000 mg calcium per day and add a rapidly acting form of vitamin D. The objective of therapy is relief of symptoms, which will generally be accomplished if the serum calcium remains above 7.0 mg/dl.

The vitamin D preparations best suited for acute therapy for hypocalcemia are the rapidly acting agents 1α,25-$(OH)_2D$ (calcitriol) and dihydrotachysterol (DHT). DHT can be started with a dose of 4 mg/day for 2 days, then 2 mg/day for 2 days, then 1 mg/day with subsequent adjustments based on serum calcium measurements. Calcitriol can be given similarly with a loading dose of 4 μg/day. Alternatively, either agent can be begun at an estimated maintenance dose (Table 23-9) without loading.

Chronic Therapy

The objective of chronic therapy is to keep the patient asymptomatic and with a serum calcium of approximately 8.5 to 9.2 mg/dl. This should not only control symptoms but prevent the complications of chronic asymptomatic hypocalcemia, such as cataracts. There is debate about how best to accomplish this.[594] In hypoparathyroidism, the ideal therapy would be replacement with the deficient hormone, but this is not practical. Therefore, less optimal treatment with vitamin D must be undertaken. On the one hand, long-acting vitamin D preparations [vitamin D, 25-hydroxycholecalciferol (calcifediol)] provide smooth therapy but may accumulate to toxic levels over time; when this occurs, their effects are slow to reverse (Table 23-9). Vitamin D is converted to 25-(OH)D, and an assay of serum 25-(OH)D levels can be used to aid in dose adjustment for either preparation. The amount of either drug that is converted to active 1α-hydroxylated metabolites is a function of the level of residual parathyroid function and other factors and is difficult to estimate. On the other hand, the short-acting preparations (calcitriol, DHT) may require some adjustment of the dose,[650] but their effects will wane rapidly when they are stopped. Both require 25-hydroxylation to assume an active configuration. The cost of therapy with calcitriol is substantially greater than that of therapy with other preparations. Some experts prefer long-acting, others short-acting calciferols for the treatment of hypoparathyroidism.

Oral calcium therapy should be provided to hypocalcemic individuals treated with vitamin D to assure the availability of calcium for intestinal absorption. The authors prefer to give relatively large doses of oral calcium (1.5 to 3 g elemental calcium per day) to minimize the vitamin D dose and provide a means to lower the serum calcium rapidly in patients who become vitamin D–intoxicated. This is particularly valuable in patients on long-acting vitamin D preparations. Other researchers believe that these considerations do not outweigh the inconvenience to the patient of large calcium doses. Calcium carbonate has the highest calcium content, 40 percent by weight, and is available in several inexpensive formulations containing 200 to 500 mg calcium per tablet. Some studies suggest that calcium carbonate may be absorbed erratically in achlorhydria and is best given with meals.[376,377] Calcium citrate contains 21 percent calcium by weight, is readily soluble, is well absorbed, and is a reasonable alternative to calcium carbonate. Some patients with mild surgical hypoparathyroidism can be managed on oral calcium alone. Thiazide diuretics or chlorthalidone can be added as an adjunct to oral calcium therapy.[569]

Once a satisfactory combination of vitamin D and calcium treatment has been found, it can often be maintained for years. However, hypercalcemia from vitamin D intoxication may occur unexpectedly after months or years of tight control. The serum calcium should be monitored monthly at first and at longer intervals thereafter. The requirement for vitamin D usually goes up during the last trimester of pregnancy and falls after delivery; some patients have been entirely weaned from chronic vitamin D ther-

TABLE 23-9 Pharmacology of Vitamin D and Its Analogues

Characteristic	Calciferol (Ergocalciferol, Vitamin D_2)	Calcifediol (25-OH-D_3)	Dihydrotachysterol (DHT)	Calcitriol [1α,25$(OH)_2D_3$]	1α-Hydroxy-cholecalciferol*
Need for 25-hydroxylation	+	—	+	—	—
Need for l-hydroxylation	+	+	—	—	—
Time for normocalcemia (weeks)†	4–8	2–4	1–2	0.5–1	1–2
Persistence after cessation (weeks)	6–18	4–12	1–3	0.5–1	1–2
Approximate daily dose (μg)	1000–3000 (40,000–120,000 U)‡	75–225	300–1000	0.75–2.25	1–3
Dosage forms	50,000 U‡	20,50 μg	0.125, 0.2, 0.4 mg	0.25, 0.5 μg	*

* Not available in United States.

† Can be decreased by use of loading dose.

‡ 40,000 U = 1 mg.

Source: Parfitt AM, Surgical, idiopathic, and other varieties of parathyroid hormone-deficient hypoparathyroidism, DeGroot (ed): *Endocrinology,* Philadelphia, Saunders, pp 1049–1064, 1989.

apy during the postpartum period, only to resume after lactation.[651] Hypercalcemia has also been reported after the withdrawal of estrogen therapy. Hypoparathyroid patients whose calcium is maintained in the normal range on therapy are often markedly hypercalciuric because the normal ability of PTH to reduce urinary calcium excretion is absent (Fig. 23-45). The principal risk of chronic vitamin D therapy in the hypoparathyroid patient is renal damage from nephrolithiasis or nephrocalcinosis. Therefore, the serum calcium is maintained near the lower limit of normal to minimize hypercalciuria. The introduction of thiazides can acutely reduce urinary calcium excretion and provoke an episode of severe hypercalcemia.[652]

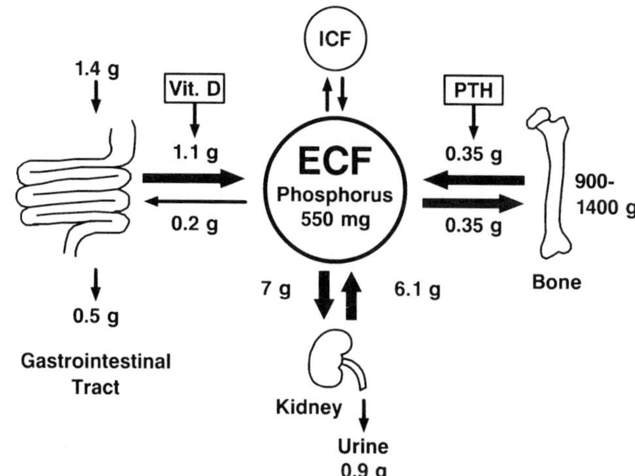

FIGURE 23-70 Schematic representation of phosphorus flux and balance in a normal human. Arrows indicate the direction of movement of phosphorus between the gut, kidneys, and extracellular fluid (ECF). Modulation of flux by vitamin D (Vit. D) or parathyroid hormone (PTH) is shown; the direction of hormonal influence on flux is indicated by the positioning of each hormone directly over the effect which that hormone increases. The numeric values indicate quantities of elemental phosphorus stored or transferred in a 24-h period. The intensities of the arrows indicate relative magnitude of flux.

DISORDERS OF PHOSPHATE METABOLISM

Phosphate Homeostasis

Intracellular and Extracellular Phosphate

The total body content of phosphate is about 1 percent of body weight. About 85 percent is contained in the skeleton, and most extraskeletal phosphate is intracellular. Phosphate is the principal intracellular anion, with a total cellular concentration of 100 mmol/liter, most of which is present as metabolically crucial organic phosphates (ATP, other nucleotides, sugar phosphates, etc). Organic phosphate in cells plays a number of roles: When linked to the purines or pyrimidines of DNA, it has a structural role; in membranes, phosphate-containing phospholipids help create the physicochemical features of membrane bilayers with hydrophobic interiors and hydrophilic (charged) layers to interface with the cytoplasm on one side and ECF on the other side. Phosphate is covalently attached to or removed from ATP and ADP via high-energy bonds for the generation, storage, or utilization of energy. It has been estimated that the intracellular concentration of *free* inorganic phosphate is only about 1 mmol/liter,[653] and because of metabolic demands, this small pool must turn over rapidly. It is not understood how intracellular free phosphate levels are regulated, although they appear to be,[653] but the rapid entry of phosphate into cells that occurs together with the entry and metabolism of carbohydrates can be viewed as a mechanism for maintaining this pool.

Phosphate in plasma and extracellular fluid is in dynamic equilibrium not only with the exterior and with bone (Fig. 23-70) but also with the larger intracellular pool. In adults, the serum concentration of inorganic phosphorus is 0.8 to 1.5 mmol/liter (2.5 to 4.5 mg/dl). In growing children, the serum concentration is higher, averaging 1.5 to 1.6 mmol/liter (4.5 to 5.0 mg/dl) during the first 15 years of life. Because the buffer pair $HPO_4^{-2}/H_2PO_4^-$ has a pK_a of 6.8, both monovalent and divalent phosphate ions are present in blood at a ratio which is dependent on the blood pH. For clinical purposes, the level in serum or urine is expressed as the concentration of phosphorus, because precise conversion to a molar concentration of phosphate would require knowledge of the blood pH. Thus, we refer clinically to measurements of serum phosphorus, recognizing that the ion in question is actually phosphate. About 25 percent of inorganic phosphate in serum is protein-bound, but 90 percent is filterable because of the Gibbs-Donnan equilibrium.

The serum concentration of phosphorus is not as closely regulated as is the concentration of calcium. The fasting concentration is set primarily by the renal phosphate threshold. This contrasts markedly with the complex regulation of the serum calcium concentration, which occurs at the boundaries of the extracellular fluid with bone, the gut, and the kidney. Serum phosphorus levels may fall after meals as phosphate enters cells together with carbohydrates. This postcibal change is superimposed on a marked diurnal variation, with the nadir at 11 A.M. and a peak at about 4 A.M.[654]

Intestinal Absorption of Phosphate

The normal diet contains 800 to 2000 mg of phosphorus per day. Throughout this range, approximately 60 percent of dietary phosphate is absorbed (Fig. 23-70). This is higher than the 20 percent of calcium normally absorbed and is relatively independent of the intake of phosphate. The linearity of phosphate absorption is consistent with absorption primarily by a diffusional process without a large saturable component.

Most foods contain phosphates, but the most important dietary sources are dairy products, grains, and meats. In the American diet, food additives present in baked goods, cheeses, and carbonated beverages can contribute as much as 30 percent of the dietary phosphate intake. Organic phosphate is released during the digestive process. Phosphate is absorbed most efficiently in the duodenum and jejunum, but as with calcium, the greatest net absorption may be from the ileum. Phosphate absorption can be reduced by a high intake of calcium or by aluminum hydroxide–containing compounds, because both calcium and aluminum bind phosphate to form relatively insoluble salts in the intestinal lumen.

Little is understood about the cellular basis of phosphate absorption.[389] With a transepithelial potential difference of 3 mV (lumen negative), the Ussing equation predicts passive phosphate reabsorption of phosphate anion by the paracellular route when the luminal concentration exceeds 1.5 mmol/liter, as probably occurs postprandially. This is probably the quantitatively most significant process. A separate cellular pathway for phosphate uptake involves sodium-coupled phosphate entry by a carrier in the brush border membrane. Energy for this electrochemically uphill process is provided by the sodium gradient, which is maintained by sodium-potassium ATPase. The exit of phosphate across the basolateral membrane into the blood may be passive. It is thought that vitamin D primarily regulates sodium-coupled phosphate entry[389] (see above), but this has little impact on the adaptation to changing dietary intake.

Renal Phosphate Handling

Of the filtered load of phosphate, 80 to 97 percent is normally reabsorbed. The level of renal phosphate reabsorption defines the concentration of phosphate in serum and is thus an important contributor to extracellular mineral homeostasis. Renal phosphate reabsorption can be quantified as the fractional excretion (C_P/C_{creat}) or as tubular resorption of phosphorus ($1 - C_P/C_{creat}$) but is best expressed as the theoretical renal phosphate threshold (TmP/GFR).[655] Because the renal phosphate threshold sets the serum phosphorus concentration, the normal range of TmP/GFR (2.5 to 4.2 mg/dl) closely mirrors the normal range of serum phosphorus. Although the TmP/GFR can be measured by infusion of phosphate (Fig. 23-71), this is impractical clinically, and so it is usually estimated from measurements of serum and urinary phosphorus and creatinine using a nomogram (Fig. 23-72), see also Testing, below). Renal phosphate handling is deranged in renal insufficiency,

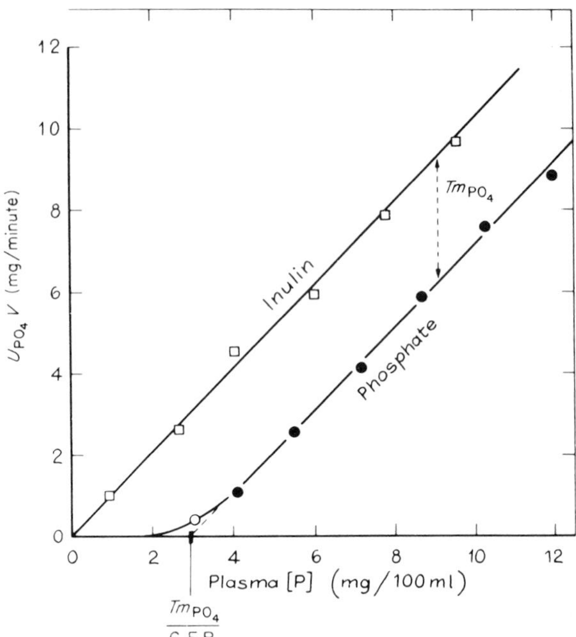

FIGURE 23-71 The relation between the plasma phosphorus concentration (mg/dl) and the urinary excretion rate of phosphate (mg/min) in a normal individual while fasting (○) and during an intravenous infusion of phosphate (●). Also shown is the relation between the urinary excretion rate and the plasma concentration of inulin when inulin was simultaneously infused. The slopes of the lines through the inulin and phosphate data are identical and are numerically equal to the glomerular filtration. The vertical distance between the two lines is the maximum rate of tubular reabsorption of phosphate (TmP/GFR) in mg/dl. *(By permission of Bijvoet OLM, Clin Sci 37:23, 1969.)*

and the TmP/GFR is not readily interpretable with a GFR less than 30 ml/min.

Under normal circumstances, phosphate reabsorption is essentially limited to the proximal tubule.[656,657] The proximal convoluted tubule reabsorbs about 75 percent of filtered phosphate, and most of the remainder is reabsorbed in the proximal straight tubule. Although distal tubule segments may have a limited capacity for reabsorption of phosphate (5 percent of filtered load), this is evident experimentally mainly after acute parathyroidectomy and is probably not of physiologic importance.

The rate-limiting step for phosphate reabsorption in the proximal tubule is sodium-coupled phosphate entry through the apical membrane via a carrier.[657–659] Entry is thus driven by the energy of the sodium gradient, which is maintained by Na-K ATPase. This process is largely electroneutral, involving carriage of divalent phosphate with two equivalents of sodium, but a small component is electrogenic, probably involving the transport of monovalent phosphate together with two equivalents of sodium. Phosphate exit across the basolateral membrane is primarily diffusive and is driven by the elec-

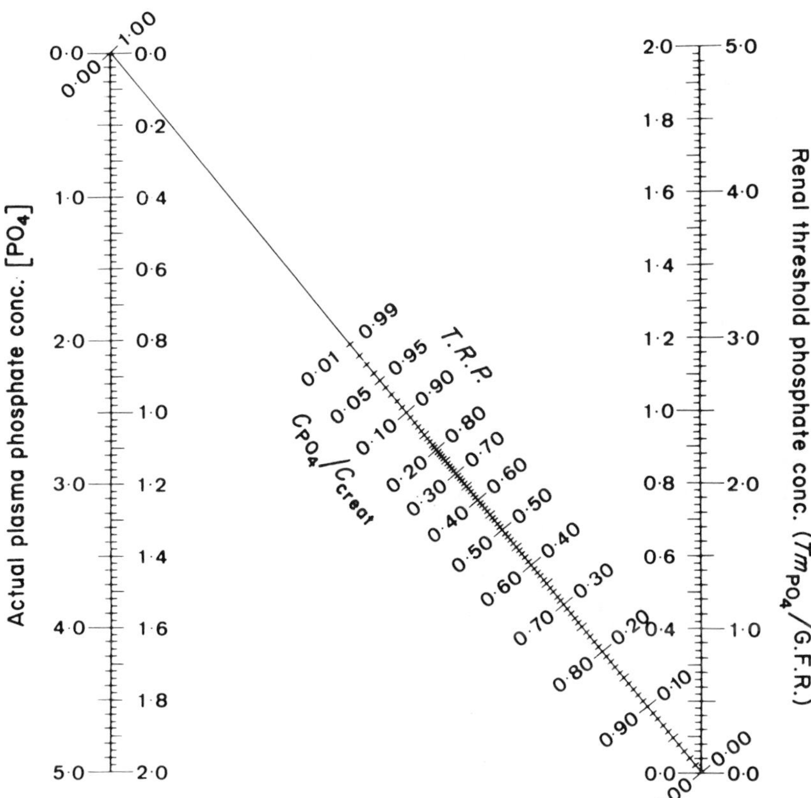

FIGURE 23-72 Nomogram for deriving TmP/GFR from known values for serum phosphorus and the fractional excretion of phosphorus (C_{P_i}/C_{creat}) or TRP. The estimation of (C_{P_i}/C_{creat}) and TRP is described in the section on testing. The outer scale on each ordinate represents units as mg/dl, and the inner scale on each ordinate represents units as mmol/liter. The diagonal connecting the two ordinates has a scale for values for TRP to the right and a scale for values for (C_{P_i}/C_{creat}) to the left. A straight line through the appropriate values for serum phosphorus concentrations and C_{P_i}/C_{creat} (or TRP) intersects the TmP scale at the appropriate value for TmP/GFR. The scale used (mg/dl or mmol/liter) must be the same. All data in the text are presented as mg/dl. For example, at a serum phosphorus concentration of 2.5 mg/dl and a C_{P_i}/C_{creat} of 0.14, the TmP/GFR is 2.3 mg/dl. *(By permission of Walton RJ, Bijvoet OLM, Lancet, i:309, 1975.)*

trochemical potential difference (interior negative) maintained by Na-K ATPase. An anion exchange mechanism also may contribute to the exit of phosphorus, but the counterion has not been identified.[657,658,660]

The most important factors regulating proximal phosphate reabsorption are PTH and the dietary phosphate intake. The cellular basis for the effect of PTH was discussed above. It is dependent on cAMP as an intracellular mediator, requires a cAMP-dependent protein kinase,[661] and probably involves phosphorylation of the apical sodium-phosphate transporter or a regulatory component, although this has not been demonstrated directly. By resetting the renal phosphate threshold, PTH allows the kidney to compensate for changes in bone resorption. Teleologically, the phosphaturic effect of PTH tends to prevent increases in serum phosphate, which would result from release of phosphate from bone together with calcium in hyperparathyroid states, from dampening the homeostatic increase in the serum calcium concentration by complexing calcium. This protective mechanism is inoperative in renal failure, where the hypocalcemic effect of phosphate released from bone in patients with secondary hypoparathyroidism is an important contributor to progressive hyperparathyroidism as part of a positive feedback loop.

The effect of phosphate intake on urinary phosphate handling is independent of PTH. Under conditions of phosphate deprivation, the TmP is increased until phosphate reabsorption is virtually quantitative.[662] The adaptation involves an increase in the V_{max} for phosphate without a change in K_m and probably reflects the insertion of additional transporters into the apical membrane.[656,657,663] This process occurs over days and probably involves both genomic and nongenomic mechanisms. It cannot be overridden by infusion of phosphaturic agents such as PTH. With continual phosphate deprivation, the serum phosphorus concentration eventually falls. In this circumstance, homeostatic mechanisms have been overridden and the renal tubule is no longer able to regulate the serum phosphorus levels.

Other clinically relevant factors that regulate phosphate reabsorption include other hormones, acid-base status, and the level of serum calcium.[656,657] *Growth hormone* increases renal phosphate reabsorption,[664] largely accounting for the finding of hyperphosphatemia in acromegaly. *Insulin* also appears to have a direct ability to increase proximal phosphate reabsorption, independent of its effects on glucose entry. *Glucocorticoids* directly inhibit phosphate reabsorption, and this may be evident clinically as hypophosphatemia in Cushing's syndrome.[665] *Calcitonin* in high concentrations has a phosphaturic effect; it is not clear that this is physiologically significant.[255,256] The ability of *vitamin D* to increase proximal reabsorption of phosphate was discussed above. The bisphosphonate etidronate disodium also increases renal phosphate reabsorption.

Acidosis, both acute and chronic, causes phosphaturia. This is at least partly due to titration of phosphate as tubule fluid is acidified, since monovalent phosphate is transported less well than is the divalent form. Chronically, the number of transporters may also be increased.[666] The increased phosphate excretion provides a urinary buffer for the excretion of acid and also provides for the excretion of phosphate liberated as part of the buffering of metabolic acidosis by bone. In this way, the kidney and bone cooperate in the response to acidosis. Although acute *hypercalcemia* has complex effects on renal phosphate handling, chronic hypercalcemia appears uniformly to decrease renal phosphate reabsorption.[592] This may account for the fall in serum phosphate often observed with treatment of hypoparathyroidism and in some cases for the hypophosphatemia associated with hypercalcemia in malignancy.

Disorders Causing Hypophosphatemia

Hypophosphatemia and phosphate depletion can result from decreased intake or dietary absorption, increased renal losses, or shifts of phosphate into the intracellular space (Table 23-10). The elements of the defense against hypophosphatemia are shown in Fig. 23-73. The primary lines of defense are adaptive increases in the intrinsic phosphate-reabsorbing capacity of the renal tubule, increased renal synthesis of $1\alpha,25\text{-(OH)}_2D$, and probably increases in resorption of bone. The net effect is to protect the serum phosphorus concentration and body phosphate stores, with secondary increases in calcium influx from bone and gut, which, together with suppression of PTH and $1\alpha,25\text{-(OH)}_2D$, may give rise to hypercalciuria. Hypophosphatemia can be a manifestation of depleted body phosphate stores, but the correlation is imperfect. With acute shifts of phosphate induced by glucose and insulin or by respiratory alkalosis, transient severe hypophosphatemia may occur in the face of unchanged stores of total body phosphate. A reduction in the renal phosphate threshold (e.g., in hyperparathyroidism) will also induce mild hypophosphatemia without by itself influencing body stores of phosphate. Conversely, in states of chronically diminished phosphate intake, renal adaptation will essentially eliminate urinary excretion and thus maintain a relatively normal serum phosphorus level in the face of reduced stores until body stores have been markedly depleted.

Hypophosphatemia with levels below 0.3 mmol/liter (1 mg/dl) is thought of as severe.[667,668] As indicated in Table 23-10, profound hypophosphatemia is primarily associated with chronic antacid abuse, alcohol abuse, diabetic ketoacidosis, respiratory alkalosis, hyperalimentation, and the nutritional recovery syndrome. There are many clinical consequences of severe hypophosphatemia with phosphate deficiency. Metabolic encephalopathy may occur. Erythrocyte glycolysis is impeded by dysfunction of glyceraldehyde-3-phosphate dehydrogenase, limiting the formation of ATP and 2,3-DPG.[669] Reduced levels of erythrocyte 2,3-DPG and ATP shift the oxyhemoglo-

TABLE 23-10 Causes of Hypophosphatemia

Disorders of phosphorus intake and absorption
Starvation
Malabsorption, diarrhea
Continuous nasogastric suction
Phosphorus-binding antacids*
Renal phosphorus losses
Diuresis (saline infusion, loop and thiazide diuretics, acetazolamide, osmotic diuresis)
First-, second-, or third-degree hyperparathyroidism
Humoral hypercalcemia of malignancy
Oncogenic osteomalacia
X-linked hypophosphatemia
Chronic metabolic acidosis
Bicarbonate therapy
Hypercalcemia
Calcitonin therapy
Cushing's syndrome
After renal transplant
Extracellular-intracellular shifts
Respiratory alkalosis*
Diabetic ketoacidosis*
Glucose and insulin therapy*
Nutritional recovery*
Shifts into bone
Osteoblastic metastases
Hungry bones syndrome
Miscellaneous conditions
Alcoholism*
Burns
Sepsis
Dialysis against phosphorus-poor dialysate

*Causes severe hypophosphatemia.

FIGURE 23-73 The sequence of adjustments initiated in response to hypophosphatemia.

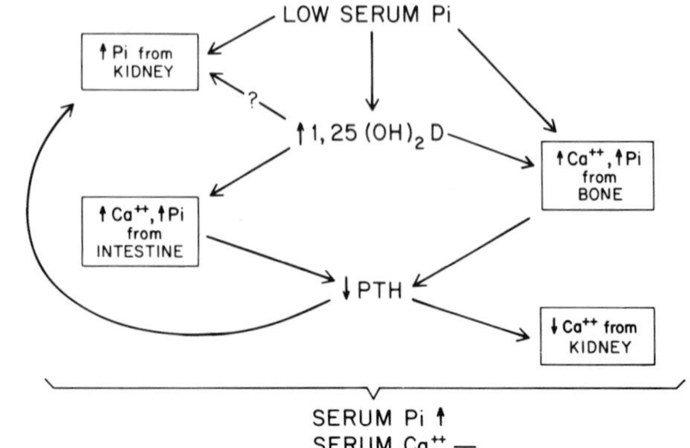

bin dissociation curve to the left, reducing oxygen release in the periphery, and can rarely produce hemolytic anemia, which is generally not life-threatening. Depletion of muscle phosphocreatine can induce clinically significant weakness or even rhabdomyolysis. Rhabdomyolysis occurs in profoundly phosphate-depleted patients with alcoholism or during nutritional recovery.[670] Myocardial dysfunction has been reported.[671] Phosphate is required for the mineralization of bone, and chronic hypophosphatemia can produce osteomalacia.[672,673] Profound hypophosphatemia with phosphate deficiency may also produce metabolic acidosis. It is plausible that many of these complications result from a reduction in tissue ATP stores, but this has rarely been shown directly.

Increased Renal Excretion

A variety of systemic states and renal disorders can result in a fall in the renal phosphate threshold and hypophosphatemia (Table 23-10). In general, these disorders produce only moderate hypophosphatemia that is rarely symptomatic and do not by themselves lead to phosphate depletion. Hyperparathyroidism and malignancy-associated hypercalcemia are among the systemic disorders that give rise to hypophosphatemia. Renal tubule disorders include heritable diseases such as X-linked hypophosphatemic rickets and acquired tubule disorders such as oncogenic osteomalacia,[341] renal tubule disorders, osmotic diuresis, diuretic therapy, bicarbonate administration, and glucocorticoid therapy.

Decreased Absorption

Phosphate is ubiquitous in foodstuffs, and dietary deficiency short of starvation does not by itself produce profound hypophosphatemia. Chronic diarrheal states do not by themselves induce severe phosphate wasting. However, chronic abuse of phosphate-binding antacids can produce osteomalacia with bone pain, increased alkaline phosphatase, marked hypercalciuria, and increased levels of $1\alpha,25\text{-(OH)}_2D$.[672,673]

Respiratory Alkalosis

Acute respiratory alkalosis from hyperventilation may produce transient severe hypophosphatemia.[674] It is thought that the resulting intracellular alkalosis markedly activates glycolysis with a rapid flux of free phosphate into sugar phosphates, leading to a dramatic shift of phosphate into the intracellular space. The finding of severe hypophosphatemia in a patient presenting with tetany sometimes leads to an extensive evaluation of calcium and phosphate metabolism when the only real disorder is hyperventilation. In recent years, it has become evident that moderate hypophosphatemia often results from treatment of respiratory failure.[675,676] The acute shifts with mechanical hyperventilation may be superimposed on previous renal losses of phosphate occasioned by respiratory acidosis or by therapy with glucocorticoids, diuretics, or xanthines. Hypophosphatemia produces reversible respiratory muscle dysfunction[677] and sometimes acute respiratory failure.[678] Respiratory muscle weakness is associated with depleted stores of phosphocreatine in muscle.[679] Treatment of moderate hypophosphatemia may markedly improve respiratory muscle function.[677,678]

Diabetic Ketoacidosis

Both metabolic acidosis and osmotic diuresis produce urinary phosphate wasting, but the resultant phosphate deficit is obscured by shifts of phosphate into the extracellular space because of acidosis and insulin deficiency, and ketoacidotic patients present with normal or elevated serum phosphorus levels. Treatment with insulin and glucose produces rapid shifts into the intracellular space and a fall in the serum phosphorus (Fig. 23-74). The serum phosphorus rarely falls below 0.3 mmol/liter (1 mg/dl) unless there was a long prodrome of polyuria with chronic phosphate wasting. Controlled studies indicate that routine treatment of hypophosphatemia in diabetic ketoacidosis is not beneficial.[680] However, severely hypophosphatemic patients could benefit from phosphate replacement. Precise guidelines for phosphate replacement in diabetic ketoacidosis have not been agreed on.

Nutritional Recovery

Severe hypophosphatemia is precipitated by refeeding after chronic protein-calorie malnutrition. Originally seen as a fatal complication of refeeding survivors of concentration camps after World War II, hypophosphatemia also occurs during the first 2 to 5 days of enteral and parenteral hyperalimentation

FIGURE 23-74 Approximate time course of the development of severe hypophosphatemia in patients with diabetic ketoacidosis, chronic alcoholics, and patients receiving intravenous hyperalimentation without phosphorus supplementation. *(From Knochel,[667] by permission of the Archives of Internal Medicine.)*

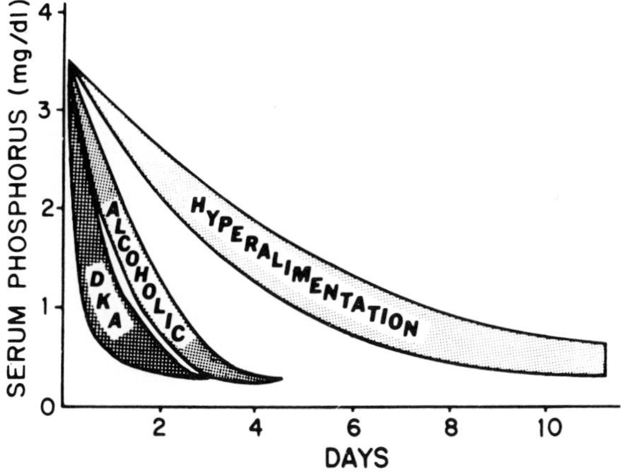

(Fig. 23-74) as large quantities of phosphate enter cells. Central nervous system manifestations, peripheral neuropathy, and respiratory muscle failure dominate the clinical picture when hyperalimentation is instituted.[667,681] It is important that hyperalimentation solutions contain phosphate and that serum phosphorus levels be monitored and phosphate be replaced as necessary.

Alcoholism

The pathogenesis of hypophosphatemia in alcoholism is complex and not fully understood.[667,682] Contributory factors are poor intake, vomiting, antacid use, and urinary wasting due to magnesium depletion. Hospitalization and alcohol withdrawal may precipitate severe hypophosphatemia with rhabdomyolysis, respiratory failure, or CNS manifestations. Respiratory alkalosis occurring with alcohol withdrawal and glucose feeding probably contributes to the rapid appearance of hypophosphatemia.

Miscellaneous

Hypophosphatemia also occurs in thermal burns, where hyperventilation may be the proximate cause; in leukemia during blast crisis; and after renal transplantation in which persistent hyperparathyroidism, glucocorticoid therapy, and poor graft function are probably involved.

Treatment

The decision to treat is based on the evidence for a phosphate depletion state, the level of hypophosphatemia, and the presence of symptoms. Hypophosphatemia does not always require treatment. The syndrome associated with acute respiratory alkalosis or with nutritional recovery may be self-limited and may not require specific therapy. Symptomatic phosphate depletion can usually be treated orally with 1 g per day of elemental phosphorus provided as milk (contains about 1 g per liter) or as a phosphate supplement (Table 23-11). Intravenous therapy should be approached cautiously and only in patients with severe, symptomatic hypophosphatemia [0.3 mmol/liter (1.0 mg/dl)] because of the risk of overshooting and producing hypocalcemia with tetany or soft tissue calcification. Great caution must be exercised in treating renal insufficiency. A dose of 2.5 mg phosphorus/kg body weight as a slow infusion is recommended.[683] This can be administered as sodium phosphate or potassium phosphate (Table 23-11). Close monitoring of serum levels of calcium, phosphorus, and creatinine is necessary.

TABLE 23-11 Oral and Intravenous Preparations of Phosphate

Preparation	Phosphorus, mg	Na, mEq	K, mEq
Oral			
Cow's milk	1000 mg/liter	25	35
Fleet Phospho-Soda	645 mg/5 ml	24	0
K-Phos Neutral	250 mg/capsule	13	1.1
K-Phos Original	114 mg/capsule	0	3.7
Neutra-Phos	250 mg/capsule	7.1	7.1
Neutra-Phos K	250 mg/capsule	14.2	
Parenteral			
K phosphate	93 mg/ml	0	4.4
Na phosphate	93 mg/ml	4	0

Disorders Causing Hyperphosphatemia

Chronic hyperphosphatemia with normal renal function reflects an increased renal phosphate threshold. This occurs in hypoparathyroidism and pseudohypoparathyroidism, in acromegaly, and in some patients treated with the bisphosphonate drug etidronate disodium. Chronic hyperphosphatemia is also part of the tumoral calcinosis syndrome characterized by massive ectopic calcification around large joints. Renal insufficiency is the most common cause of hyperphosphatemia. The ability to excrete phosphate falls off sharply when the GFR is reduced below 30 ml/min, and the TmP/GFR and serum phosphorus levels rise. The hyperphosphatemia of chronic renal failure is a major clinical problem because it leads to soft tissue calcification and contributes significantly to the progression of secondary hyperparathyroidism and renal osteodystrophy. Its treatment with dietary phosphate restriction and phosphate-binding antacids is discussed in Chap. 24.

Acute hyperphosphatemia occurs with rhabdomyolysis in crush and compartment syndromes[583] and in the tumor lysis syndrome[641] and may produce hypocalcemia and tetany. It is also seen because of cellular shifts in acute respiratory acidosis and in metabolic acidosis (both ketoacidosis and lactic acidosis). A decreased GFR probably contributes to all these conditions by decreasing phosphate excretion.

DISORDERS OF MAGNESIUM METABOLISM

Although the intracellular environment is relatively poor in calcium, it is rich in magnesium. The ratio of magnesium to calcium is critically important for maintenance of an electrochemical gradient across the plasma membrane and for transmembrane excitation. Therefore, magnesium is maintained within a tight physiologic concentration range both intracellularly and extracellularly. Magnesium is often handled by the same transporters which act on calcium, and so it may often share the same pattern of flux. Nevertheless, there appears to be no direct hormonal regulation of magnesium levels in blood, in ECF, or within the cell[684–687]; no classical feedback loops for magnesium regulation are known. Rather, maintenance of magnesium levels is achieved by modifying the efficiency of dietary absorption or urinary excretion of the mineral (Figs. 23-75 and 23-76).

Within cells, magnesium is the most abundant divalent cation and is second only to potassium as a cation. The actions of magnesium are similar to those of calcium in some cases, but since magnesium is present in lower concentrations, it has little or no effect unless extremes of magnesium concentration are present. However, magnesium is a cofactor for many enzymes, especially those involved in phosphorylation and dephosphorylation. These include enzymes which catalyze energy production and storage, such as those involved in making and breaking high-energy bonds in ATP, in intracellular metabolism, and in the polymerization reactions involved in the biosynthesis of DNA and RNA.

The normal adult has approximately 25 g (2000 mEq) of magnesium present in total throughout the body.[688] Approximately two-thirds of this magnesium is found in the skeleton; the remaining one-third is present in soft tissues.[688] Within the skeleton, magnesium is not part of the crystalline lattice; rather, it is present on the crystalline surface of mineralized bone, from which location it is not freely exchangeable with magnesium in the ECF.

Although the stores of total body magnesium are large and the role of magnesium is vital, only 1 percent of magnesium is found in the ECF. Furthermore, total body magnesium and the levels present intracellularly or in soft tissue do not necessarily correspond with the ECF level. The normal plasma range for magnesium is 1.5 to 2.2 mEq/liter (1.8 to 2.6 mg/dl). Of the magnesium present in the ECF, 55 percent is ionized. Of the remaining 45 percent, two-thirds is bound to proteins such as albumin and one-third is complexed to counterions. Intracellularly, 60 percent of magnesium is found in the mitochondria (concentration = 1×10^{-3} *M*); the remaining intracellular magnesium is in the cytosol (concentration = 5×10^{-4} *M*). Only 5 to 10 percent of intracellular magnesium is present in a free ionic form.

FIGURE 23-75 Schematic representation of magnesium flux and balance in a normal human. Arrows indicate direction of movement of magnesium between the gut, kidneys, and extracellular fluid (ECF). The numeric values indicate quantities of elemental magnesium stored or transferred in a 24-h period. The thickness of arrows indicates the relative magnitude of flux.

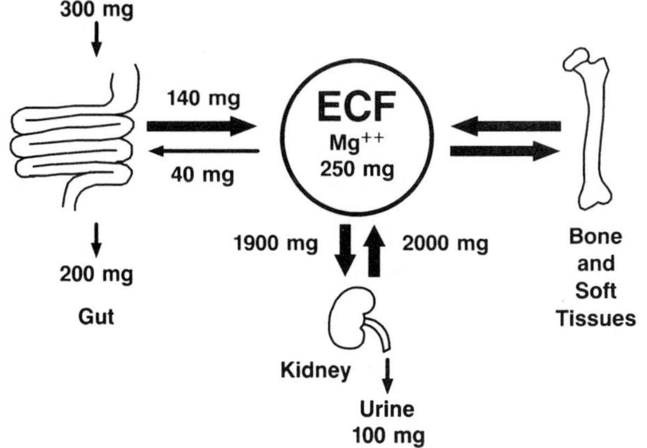

Magnesium Balance

It is possible to construct a diet which is calorically sufficient yet deficient in calcium. However, this is very difficult to do with magnesium. Magnesium is present in all cells; therefore, all normal diets have magnesium present in approximate proportion to caloric intake. The normal adult needs 0.3 to 0.35 mEq/kg of magnesium per day (Fig. 23-75). The average diet exceeds this amount, containing 20 to 40 mEq per day, found principally in green vegetables and meat. The amount of magnesium absorbed from the diet varies linearly with the intake and on average is approximately 30 to 40 percent of the total ingested.[689]

Therefore, the principal homeostatic challenge for the maintenance of normal magnesium levels rests with excretion of the excess magnesium which enters through the diet.[690] This is accomplished by the kidney. The kidney filters an enormous quantity of magnesium. Seventy percent of the magnesium in blood is ultrafilterable, but 95 percent of this filtered magnesium is reabsorbed and only 5 to 10 percent of the filtered load is excreted. Reabsorption within the nephron occurs in the thick limb of the ascending loop of Henle. Hence, renal efficiency of reabsorption is very high and can be most impressive under conditions of dietary deficiency. Under such conditions, magnesium excretion can fall to less than 1 mEq/day in the urine. The excretion of magnesium by the kidney appears to be regulated by the mechanism of a tubular maximum for reabsorption of the ion. Levels in the tubule which exceed a predetermined threshold spill into the urine. The Tm-limited renal process is the principal determinant of ambient serum magnesium. Therefore, in conditions of renal failure, magnesium excretion is inadequate and the mineral accumulates systemically (Fig. 23-76).

Parathyroid hormone, calcitonin, and vitamin D do not play a regulatory role for magnesium but can influence magnesium flux since magnesium tends to be handled similarly to calcium by many cellular transport apparatuses. In fact, the tubular mechanism for the reabsorption of magnesium may be shared with calcium and appears to be sodium-linked. In contrast, vitamin D does not influence magnesium intestinal absorption; the calcium-binding protein responsible for the absorption of dietary calcium does not transport magnesium.

Hypomagnesemia

For hypomagnesemia to develop, increased losses or inadequate intake of magnesium must occur for a

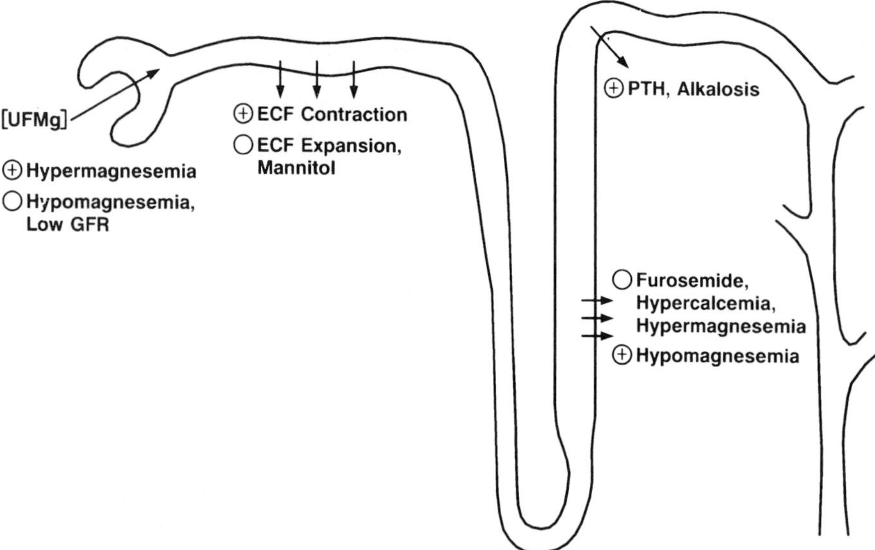

FIGURE 23-76 Handling of magnesium by the nephron. *(Reprinted with permission from Lemann.[689])*

prolonged period.[691] Diffuse intestinal disease can lead to failure to absorb magnesium adequately from the diet. However, inadequate intake is more often the cause. Alcoholism is the leading cause of hypomagnesemia, which occurs in 50 percent of alcoholics because of decreased dietary intake, vomiting or diarrhea, secondary aldosteronism, or a direct effect of alcohol on promoting renal magnesium excretion. Certain drugs, such as loop diuretics, cyclosporin, gentamicin, and cisplatin, can also cause renal magnesium wasting and hypomagnesemia.Magnesium can be depleted in total body stores even in the presence of a normal plasma level (Table 23-12). Treatment of diabetic ketoacidosis with fluid replacement can lead to decreased serum magnesium and unmask the preexisting total body magnesium depletion; therefore, magnesium supplementation is often required along with other components of the treatment regimen. The hungry bones syndrome, in which calcium influx into bone can be extraordinary, is often accompanied by hypomagnesemia. In such instances, calcium replacement alone is not adequate; magnesium needs to be replaced as well in order to relieve tetany. In addition, hypomagnesium per se can produce hypocalcemia and its complications by causing functional hypoparathyroidism.

The symptoms of hypomagnesemia are similar to those of hypocalcemia, but the electrocardiogram changes differ.[691] The ST segments are depressed, and T waves are inverted in the precordial leads in hypomagnesemia. Such findings usually do not occur until magnesium levels are substantially decreased in the blood, usually below 1 mg/dl. Seizures, arrhythmias, coarse tremors, muscle fasciculations, and a positive Trousseau's sign are also part of the syndrome. Once plasma levels of magnesium fall below normal, repletion may take a long time as a result of the large total body deficit which has occurred. Parenteral administration for several days may be required with up to 200 to 400 mEq of magnesium. This can be administered as $MgSO_4 \cdot 7H_2O$ given intravenously during emergent situations, such as seizures. Five hundred mg (40 mEq) can be

TABLE 23-12 Causes of Hypomagnesemia and Magnesium Depletion

Decreased intake or absorption
Dietary deficiency: protein-calorie malnutrition
Vomiting, diarrhea, nasogastric suction
Malabsorption syndromes: pancreatic and intestinal
Parenteral hyperalimentation without adequate magnesium
Primary hypomagnesemia
Renal disorders
Osmotic diuresis: mannitol, glucose, urea
After relief of obstructive uropathy or resolution of acute tubular necrosis
After renal transplantation
Drug-induced: loop diuretics, cisplatin, gentamicin, amphotericin, digoxin, capreomycin, viomycin, tobramycin, amikacin
ECF expansion, hyperaldosteronism, Bartter's syndrome
Congenital, hereditary renal magnesium wasting
Miscellaneous disorders
Alcoholism
Diabetes mellitus/diabetic ketoacidosis
Primary hyperparathyroidism
After parathyroidectomy
Thyrotoxicosis
Syndrome of inappropriate ADH
Chronic hypoparathyroidism
Hypoalbuminemia
Dialysis against a magnesium-deficiency dialysate
Excessive lactation
Pancreatitis
Combinations of the above

given under such circumstances, but the administration rate should not exceed 15 mg/min. Thereafter, 600 mg of magnesium sulfate can be given in the first 3 to 4 h; subsequently, another 900 mg can be given over the next 24 h.[692] Magnesium acetate and other magnesium salts can also be used.

Maintenance dosing can be achieved with oral formulations of magnesium salts such as magnesium oxide or magnesium chloride. A total of 300 mg elemental magnesium in divided doses should be administered. In our experience, magnesium oxide appears to cause less diarrhea than do other forms of magnesium supplementation. When diarrhea limits oral treatment, intramuscular administration may be required.

Caution must be taken to avoid producing hypermagnesemia as a result of treatment in patients with renal impairment.

Hypermagnesemia

Hypermagnesemia most often occurs when there is normal or increased intake of magnesium in the setting of renal failure. Both patients and physicians often fail to recognize that antacids, enemas, and laxatives commonly contain quantities of magnesium sufficient to aggravate hypermagnesemia in the setting of renal compromise (Fig. 23-76). Magnesium-containing enemas and treatment with hemiacidrin can produce hypermagnesia in the absence of renal compromise. $MgSO_4$ administration is the conventional treatment for preeclampsia and eclampsia and can readily produce hypermagnesemia and hypocalcemia. Levels of magnesium above 5 mEq/liter can actually block the action of PTH at its target organs or inhibit its secretion by the gland and can cause hypotension and somnolence. Hence, like hypomagnesemia, hypermagnesemia can produce hypocalcemia. Electrocardiogram changes include a prolonged PR interval and a widened QRS wave. Extremely high magnesium levels—above 15 mEq/liter—lead to muscular flaccidity, respiratory paralysis, and cardiac asystole. Treatment usually is effected simply by stopping the source of magnesium intake. The kidney will usually clear the excess magnesium over time. In emergent situations, dialysis against a low magnesium bath can be performed.

TESTING

Serum Chemistries

1. Calcium, phosphorus, magnesium, intact PTH, 25-hydroxyvitamin D, 1α,25-$(OH)_2D$, alkaline phosphatase, and osteocalcin are measured in fresh serum. Determinations of serum calcium, phosphorus, and PTH should be done in the fasting state. Spurious elevations in serum calcium are produced by venostasis and hemoconcentration. Prolonged standing will spuriously reduce, and hemolysis will spuriously increase, the serum phosphorus level. Osteocalcin levels are increased in renal failure because of decreased renal clearance.
2. Ionized calcium is usually measured on heparinized plasma collected anaerobically. The details of sample collection vary depending on the analytic instrument used and should be specified by the testing laboratory.

Urinary Determinations

1. Twenty-four-hour samples for urinary calcium, phosphorus, magnesium, cAMP, and creatinine are collected in 20 ml of 6 *N* HCl. All are influenced by diet, as discussed in Chap. 25.
2. Fasting urinary calcium excretion, TmP/GFR, total urinary cAMP, and nephrogenous cAMP can be determined on a "spot" or 2-h timed urine sample after a 12- to 15-h overnight fast. Water (200 ml/h) can be given for 2 h before and during the period of sample collection to assure an adequate urinary flow rate.

Fasting calcium excretion is expressed as milligrams of calcium per 100 ml of glomerular filtrate (GF):

$$\text{Fasting calcium excretion (mg/100 ml/GF)} = \frac{U_{Ca}\text{ (mg/dl)}}{U_{creat}\text{ (mg/dl)}} \times S_{creat}\text{ (mg/dl)}$$

TmP/GFR is obtained from simultaneous measurements of serum and urinary phosphorus and creatinine in fasting early morning specimens, calculation of C_P/C_{creat}, and use of the nomogram shown in Fig. 23-72.

$$\frac{C_P}{C_{creat}} = \frac{S_{creat}\text{ (mg/dl)} \times U_p\text{ (mg/dl)}}{S_p\text{ (mg/dl)} \times U_{creat}\text{ (mg/dl)}}$$

Total urinary cAMP can be measured on 24-h or fasting specimens collected as described above. The excretion of cAMP is best expressed as a function of the glomerular filtration rate (nmol per 100 ml GF):

$$\text{Total urinary cAMP (nmol/100 ml GF)} = \frac{U_{cAMP}\text{ (nmol/ml)}}{U_{creat}\text{ (ml/dl)}} \times S_{creat}\text{ (mg/dl)}$$

Nephrogenous cAMP is best measured on fasting morning specimens. The required measurement of plasma cAMP is technically difficult, and determination of nephrogenous cAMP is primarily a research procedure.

3. Total hydroxyproline and urinary pyridinium cross-links are determined on 24-h collections in 20 ml of 6 *N* HCl or on 2-h "spot" urines collected

in 2 ml of 6 N HCl after an overnight fast. Determinations of hydroxyproline excretion should be carried out on a diet with limited quantities of meat and gelatin. Excretion of pyridinium cross-links is not as dependent on diet.

Testing for Pseudohypoparathyroidism

Synthetic human PTH(1-34) (teriparatide acetate) is available for provocative testing of the renal response to parathyroid hormone.[614,693] The stimulation test (Ellsworth-Howard test) should be carried out after an overnight fast. Hydration is achieved with 200 ml/h of water, beginning two h before the study. After three basal 30-min urine collections, hPTH(1-34) (3 U per kg body weight, up to a maximum of 200 U) is administered intravenously over 10 min. Two 30-min collections are then obtained, followed by a 60-min collection. It is important to achieve adequate hydration so that accurate urine collections can be obtained. Samples are assayed for cAMP, phosphorus, and creatinine. The results can be expressed per milligram of creatinine or, preferably, per 100 ml GF using the above formula. The maximal cAMP response occurs in the first 30-min period after the administration of hormone. The response of urinary phosphorus excretion is more variable, and the maximum may occur in the first or second 30-min period.

Acknowledgments

The authors gratefully acknowledge the excellent secretarial assistance of Sandra Camburn, Marcie Gelb, and Jean Jajan.

ADDENDUM

FIGURE 23-77 Proposed structural model for the Ca^{2+}-sensing receptor. The large N-terminal domain is located extracellularly and contains 9 potential N-linked glycosylation sites (shown as branched chains). Potential phosphorylation sites for PKC are shown. Amino acids that were identical or in the following groups in all metabotropic glutamate receptors and the calcium-sensing receptor are shown: acidic, ▲, D, E; nonacidic, ●, {M,I,L,V}, {F,Y,W}, {A,G}, {S,T}, {Q,N}, and {K,R,H}. *(Reprinted with permission from Brown et al.[31])*

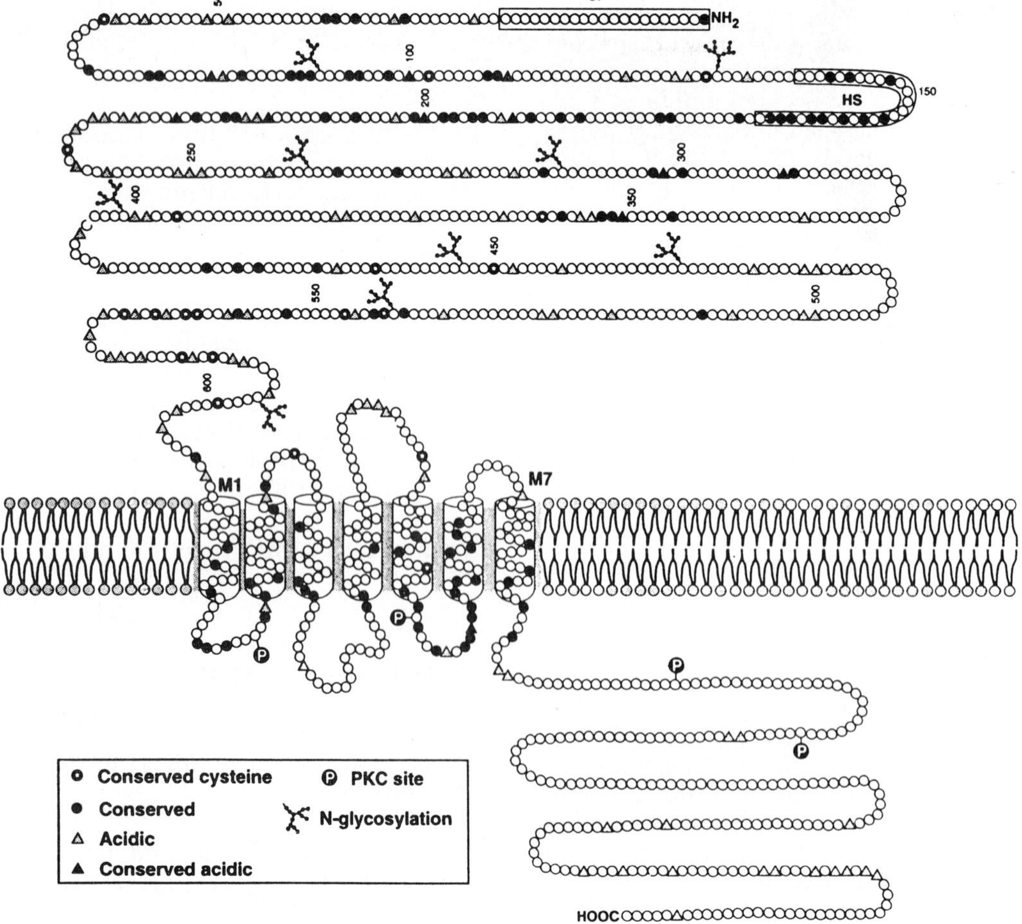

REFERENCES

1. Rasmussen H: The calcium messenger system: Parts 1 and 2. *N Engl J Med* 314:1094, 1986.
2. McLean FC, Hastings AB: A biological method for the estimation of calcium ion concentration. *J Biol Chem* 107:337, 1934.
3. Marshall RW: Plasma fractions, in Nordin BEC (ed): *Calcium, Phosphate and Magnesium Metabolism.* London, Churchill Livingstone, 1976, p 162.
4. Krane SM: Calcium, phosphate and magnesium, in Rasmussen H (ed): *International Encyclopedia of Pharmacology and Therapeutics.* Oxford, Pergamon, 1970, p 19.
5. Bronner F: Dynamics in function of calcium, in Comar LC, Bronner F (eds): *Mineral Metabolism.* New York, Academic Press, 1964, p 342.
6. Neer R, Berman M, Fisher L, Rosenberg LE: Multicompartmental analysis of calcium kinetics in normal adult males. *J Clin Invest* 46:1364, 1967.
7. DeLuca HF, Schnoes HK: Vitamin D: Recent advances. *Annu Rev Biochem* 52:411, 1983.
8. Norman AW, Roth J, Orci L: The vitamin D endocrine system: Steroid metabolism, hormone receptors, and biological response. *Endocr Rev* 3:331, 1982.
9. Haussler MR, McCain TA: Basic and clinical concepts related to vitamin D metabolism and action. *N Engl J Med* 297:974, 1977.
10. Akerström G, Malmaeus J, Bergstrom R: Surgical anatomy of human parathyroid glands. *Surgery* 95:14, 1983.
11. Conlin PR, Fajtova VT, Mortensen RM, LeBoff MS, Brown EM: Hysteresis in the relationship between serum ionized calcium and intact parathyroid hormone during recovery from induced hyper- and hypocalcemia in normal humans. *J Clin Endocrinol Metab* 69:593, 1989.
12. Brown EM, LeBoff MS, Oetting M, Posillico JT, Chen C: Secretory control in normal and abnormal parathyroid tissue, in Clark JH (ed): *Recent Prog Horm Res.* New York, Harcourt Brace Jovanovich, 1987, p 337.
13. Kitamura N, Shigeno C, Shiomi K, Lee K, Ohta S, Sone T, Katsushima S, Tadamura E, et al: Episodic fluctuation in serum intact parathyroid hormone concentration in men. *J Clin Endocrinol Metab* 70:252, 1990.
14. Vasicek TJ, McDevitt BE, Freeman MW, Fennick BJ, Hendy GN, Potts JT Jr, Rich A, Kronenberg HM: Nucleotide sequence of the human parathyroid hormone gene. *Proc Natl Acad Sci USA* 80:2127, 1983.
15. Rosenblatt M, Kronenberg M, Potts JT Jr: Parathyroid hormone: Physiology, chemistry, biosynthesis, secretion, metabolism, and mechanism of action, in DeGroot LJ (ed): *Endocrinology.* Philadelphia, Saunders, 1989, p 848.
16. Habener JF, Rosenblatt M, Potts JT Jr: Parathyroid hormone: Biochemical aspects of biosynthesis, secretion, action, and metabolism. *Physiol Rev* 64:985, 1984.
17. Von Heijne G: Patterns of amino acids near signal-sequence cleavage sites. *Eur J Biochem* 133:17, 1983.
18. Majzoub JA, Rosenblatt M, Fennick B, Maunus R, Kronenberg HM, Potts JT Jr, Habener JF: Synthetic pre-proparathyroid hormone leader sequence inhibits cell-free processing of placental, parathyroid, and pituitary prehormones. *J Biol Chem* 255:11478, 1980.
19. Szczesna-Skorupa E, Mead DA, Kemper B: Mutations of the NH2-terminal domain of the surgical peptide of preproparathyroid hormone inhibit translocation without affecting interaction with signal recognition particle. *J Biol Chem* 262:8896, 1987.
20. Freeman M, Wiren K, Rapoport A, Lazar M, Potts JT Jr, Kronenberg HM: Consequences of amino-terminal deletions of preproparathyroid hormone signal sequence. *Mol Endocrinol* 1:628, 1987.
21. Arnold A, Horst SA, Gardella TJ, Baba H, Levine MA, Kronenberg HM: Mutation of the signal peptide-encoding region of the preproparathyroid hormone gene in familial isolated hypoparathyroidism. *J Clin Invest* 86:1084, 1990.
22. Habener JF, Amherdt M, Ravazzola M, Orci L: Parathyroid hormone biosynthesis: Correlation of conversion biosynthetic precursors with intracellular protein migration as determined by electron microscope autoradiography. *J Cell Biol* 80:715, 1979.
23. Habener JF, Stevens TD, Tregear GW, Potts JT Jr: Radioimmunoassay of human proparathyroid hormone: Analysis of hormone content in tissue extracts and in plasma. *J Clin Endocrinol Metab* 42:520, 1976.
24. Wiren KM, Potts JT Jr, Kronenberg HM: Importance of the propeptide sequence of human preproparathyroid hormone for signal sequence function. *J Biol Chem* 263:19771, 1988.
25. Cohn DV, Zangerle R, Fischer-Colbrie R, Chu LLH, Elting JJ, Hamilton JW, Winkler H: Similarity of secretory protein-I from parathyroid gland to chromogranin-A from adrenal medulla. *Proc Natl Acad Sci USA* 79:6056, 1982.
26. Rabbani SA, Kremer R, Bennett HPJ, Goltzman D: Phosphorylation of parathyroid hormone by human and bovine parathyroid glands. *J Biol Chem* 259:2949, 1984.
27. Russell J, Sherwood LM: The effects of 1,25-dihyroxyvitamin D_3 and high calcium on transcription of the pre-proparathyroid hormone gene are direct. *Trans Assoc Am Physicians* 100:256, 1987.
28. Naveh-Many T, Silver J: Regulation of parathyroid hormone gene expression by hypocalcemia, hypercalcemia, and vitamin D in the rat. *J Clin Invest* 86:1313, 1990.
29. Silver J, Naveh-Many T, Mayer H, Schmeizer HJ, Popovtzer MM: Regulation of vitamin D_3 metabolites of parathyroid hormone gene transcription in vivo in the rat. *J Clin Invest* 78:1296, 1986.
30. Okazaki I, Igarashi T, Kronenberg HM: 5′-Flanking region of the parathyroid hormone gene mediates negative regulation by 1,25-$(OH)_2D_3$. *J Biol Chem* 263:2203, 1988.
31. Brown EM, Gamba G, Riccardi D, Lombardi M, Butters R, Kifor O, Sun A, Hediger MA, Lytton J, Hebert SC: Cloning and characterization of an extracellular Ca^{2+}-sensing receptor from bovine parathyroid. *Nature* 366:575, 1993.
32. Brown EM, Chen CJ, Kifor O, Leboff MS, El-Hajj G, Fajtova V, Rubin LT: Ca^{2+}-sensing, second messengers, and the control of parathyroid hormone secretion. *Cell Calcium* 11:333, 1990.
33. Brown EM, Enyedi P, LeBoff MS, Rotberg J, Preston J, Chen C: High extracellular Ca^{2+} and Mg^{2+} stimulate accumulation of inositol phosphates in bovine parathyroid cells. *FEBS Lett* 218:113, 1987.
34. Shoback DM, Membreño LA, McGhee JG: High calcium and other divalent cations increase inositol triphosphate in bovine parathyroid cells. *Endocrinology* 123:382, 1988.
35. Membreño L, Chen T-H, Woodley S, Gaucas R, Shoback D: The effects of protein kinase C agonists on parathyroid hormone release and intracellular Ca^{2+} in bovine parathyroid cells. *Endocrinology* 124:789, 1989.
36. Brown EM, Thatcher JG, Watson EJ, Leombruno R: Extracellular calcium potentiates the inhibitory effects of magnesium on parathyroid function in dispersed bovine parathyroid cells. *Metabolism* 33:171, 1984.
37. Cholst IN, Steinberg SF, Tropper PJ, Fox HE, Segre GV, Bilezikian JP: The influence of hypermagnesemia on serum calcium and parathyroid hormone levels in human subjects. *N Engl J Med* 310:1221, 1984.
38. Broadus AE, Mangin M, Ikeda K, Insogna KL, Weir EC, Burtis WJ, Stewart AF: Humoral hypercalcemia of cancer: Identification of a novel parathyroid hormone-like peptide. *N Engl J Med* 319:556, 1988.
39. Heath H: Biogenic amines and the secretion of parathyroid hormone and calcitonin. *Endocr Rev* 1:319, 1980.
40. Brown EM: Lithium induces abnormal calcium-regulated PTH release in dispersed bovine parathyroid cells. *J Clin Endocrinol Metab* 52:1046, 1981.
41. Laitinen K, Lamberg-Allardt C, Tunninen R, Karonen S-L, Tähtelä R, Ylikahri R, Välimäki M: Transient hypopar-

athyroidism during acute alcohol intoxication. *N Engl J Med* 324:721, 1991.
42. Berson SA, Yalowe RS: Immunochemical heterogeneity of parathyroid hormone in plasma. *J Clin Endocrinol Metab* 28:1037, 1968.
43. Martin KJ, Hruska KA, Greenwalt A: Selective uptake of intact parathyroid hormone by the liver: Differences between hepatic and renal uptake. *J Clin Invest* 60:808, 1977.
44. Segre GV, D'Amour P, Hultman A, Potts JT Jr: Effects of hepatectomy, nephrectomy, and nephrectomy/uremia on the metabolism of parathyroid hormone in the rat. *J Clin Invest* 67:438, 1981.
45. Segre GV, Perkins AS, Witters LA, Potts JT Jr: Metabolism of parathyroid hormone by isolated rat Kupffer cells and hepatocytes. *J Clin Invest* 67:449, 1981.
46. Martin KJ, Hruska KA, Lewis J, Anderson C, Slatopolsky E: The renal handling of parathyroid hormone: Role of peritubular uptake and glomerular filtration. *J Clin Invest* 60:808, 1977.
47. Rouleau MF, Warshawsky H, Goltzman D: Parathyroid hormone binding in vivo to renal, hepatic, and skeletal tissues of the rat using a radioautographic approach. *Endocrinology* 118:919, 1986.
48. Martin KJ, Freitag JJ, Conrades M, Hruska KA, Klahr S, Slatopolsky E: Selective uptake of the synthetic amino terminal fragment of bovine parathyroid hormone by isolated perfused bone. *J Clin Invest* 62:256, 1978.
49. Flueck JA, Dibella FB, Edis AJ, Kehrwald JM, Arnaud CD: Immunoheterogeneity of parathyroid hormone in venous effluent serum from hyperfunctioning parathyroid glands. *J Clin Invest* 60:1367, 1977.
50. MacGregor RR, Hamilton JW, Shofstall RE, Cohn DV: Isolation and characterization of porcine parathyroid cathepsin B. *J Biol Chem* 254:4423, 1979.
51. Habener JF, Kemper B, Potts JT Jr: Calcium-dependent intracellular degradation of parathyroid hormone: A possible mechanism for the regulation of hormone stores. *Endocrinology* 97:431, 1975.
52. Goltzman D, Henderson B, Loveridge N: Cytochemical bioassay of parathyroid hormone. *J Clin Invest* 65:1309, 1980.
53. Arnaud CD, Tsao HS, Littledike T: Radioimmunoassay of human parathyroid hormone in serum. *J Clin Invest* 50:21, 1971.
54. Nussbaum SR, Zahradnik RJ, Lavigne JR, Brennan GL, Nozawa-Ung K, Kim LY, Keutmann HT, Wang C, et al: Highly sensitive two-site immunoradiometric assay of parathyrin and its clinical utility in evaluating patients with hypercalcemia. *Clin Chem* 33:1364, 1987.
55. Brown RC, Aston JP, Weeks I, Woodhead JS: Circulating intact parathyroid hormone measured by a two-site immunochemiluminometric assay. *J Clin Endocrinol Metab* 6:407, 1987.
56. Chambers DJ, Dunham J, Zanelii JM, Parsons JA, Bitensky L, Chaven J: A sensitive bioassay of parathyroid hormone in plasma. *Clin Endocrinol (Oxf)* 9:375, 1978.
57. Nissenson RA, Abbott SR, Teitelbaum AP, Clark OH, Arnaud CD: Endogenous biologically active human parathyroid hormone: Measured by a guanyl nucleotide-amplified renal adenylate cyclase assay. *J Clin Endocrinol Metab* 52:840, 1981.
58. Broadus AE: Nephrogenous cyclic AMP. *Recent Prog Horm Res* 37:667, 1981.
59. Chase LR, Aurbach GD: Parathyroid function and the renal excretion of 3′,5′-adenylic acid. *Proc Natl Acad Sci USA* 58:518, 1967.
60. Chase LR, Aurbach GD: Renal adenyl cyclase: Anatomically separate sites for parathyroid hormone and vasopressin. *Science* 159:545, 1968.
61. Kaminsky NH, Broadus AE, Hardman JG: Effects of parathyroid hormone on plasma and urinary adenosine 3′,5′-monophosphate in man. *J Clin Invest* 49:2387, 1970.
62. Borle AB: Calcium, parathyroid hormone and cell calcium, in Talmage VT, Munson PL (eds): *Proceedings of the 4th Parathyroid Conference*. Amsterdam, Excerpta Medica, 1972, p 484.
63. Borle AB: Calcium and phosphate metabolism. *Annu Rev Physiol* 36:361, 1974.
64. Bourdeau JE, Eby BK: cAMP-stimulated rise of [Ca^{2+}] in rabbit connecting tubules: Role of peritubular Ca. *Am J Physiol* 27:F751, 1990.
65. Civitelli R, Reid IR, Westbrook S, Avioli LV, Hruska KA: PTH elevates inositol polyphosphates and diacylglycerol in a rat osteoblast-like cell line. *Am J Physiol* 255:E660, 1988.
66. Cosman F, Morrow B, Kopal M, Bilezikian JP: Stimulation of inositol phosphate formation in ROS 17/2.8 cell membranes by guanine nucleotide, calcium, and parathyroid hormone. *J Bone Min Res* 4:413, 1989.
67. Coleman DT, Bilezikian JP: Parathyroid hormone stimulates formation of inositol phosphates in a membrane preparation of canine renal cortical tubular cells. *J Bone Min Res* 5:299, 1990.
68. Jüppner H, Abou-Samra AB, Freeman M, Kong XF, Schipani E, Richards J, Kolakowski LF Jr., Hock J: A G protein-linked receptor for parathyroid hormone and parathyroid hormone-related peptide. *Science* 254:1024, 1991.
69. Ross EM, Gilman AG: Biochemical properties of hormone-sensitive adenlyate cyclase. *Annu Rev Biochem* 49:533, 1980.
70. Spiegel AM, Gierschik P, Levine MA, Downs RW Jr: Clinical implications of guanine nucleotide-binding proteins as receptor-effector couplers. *N Engl J Med* 312:26, 1985.
71. Simon MI, Strathmann MP, Gautam N: Diversity of G proteins in signal transduction. *Science* 252:802, 1991.
72. Casey PJ, Gilman AG: G protein involvement in receptor-effector coupling. *J Biol Chem* 263:2577, 1988.
73. Bourne HR: Who carries what message? *Nature* 337:504, 1989.
74. Cerione RA, Sibley DR, Codina J: Reconstitution of a hormone-sensitive adenylate cyclase system. *J Biol Chem* 259:9979, 1984.
75. Robishaw JD, Russell DW, Harris BA: Deduced primary structure of the alpha subunit of the GTP-binding stimulatory protein of adenylate cyclase. *Biochemistry* 83:1251, 1986.
76. Verkman AS, Skorecki KL, Ausiello DA: Radiation inactivation of multimeric enzymes: Application to subunit interactions of adenylate cyclase. *Am J Physiol* 250:C103, 1986.
77. Skorecki KL, Verkman AS, Jung CY, Ausiello DA: Evidence for vasopressin activation of adenylate cyclase by subunit dissociation. *Am J Physiol* 250:C115, 1986.
78. Dunn WA, Hubbard AL: Receptor-mediated endocytosis of epidermal growth factor by hepatocytes in the perfused rat liver: Ligand and receptor dynamics. *J Cell Biol* 98:2148, 1984.
79. Nathans J, Hogness DS: Isolation and nucleotide sequence of the gene encoding human rhodopsin. *Proc Natl Acad Sci USA* 81:4851, 1984.
80. Lefkowitz RJ: Variations on a theme. *Nature* 351:353, 1991.
81. Dixon RAF, Kobilka BK, Strader DJ, Benovic JL, Dohlman HG, Frielle T, Bolanowski MA, Bennett CD, et al: Cloning of the gene and cDNA for mammalian β-adrenergic receptor and homology with rhodopsin. *Nature* 321:75, 1986.
82. Kubo T, Fukuda K, Mikami A, Maeda A, Takahashi H, Mishina M, Haga T, Haga K, et al: Cloning, sequencing and expression of complementary DNA encoding the muscarinic acetylcholine receptor. *Nature* 323:411, 1986.
83. Colquhoun D: Structure and function of acetylcholine-receptor ion channels. *Nature* 321:382, 1986.
84. McFarland KC, Sprengel R, Phillips HS, Kohler M, Rosemblit N, Nikolics K, Segaloff DL, Seeburg PH: Lutropin-choriogonadotropin receptor: An unusual member of the G protein-coupled receptor family. *Science* 245:494, 1989.

85. Parmentier M, Libert F, Maenhaut C, Lefort A, Gerard C, Perret J, Van Sande J, Dumont JE, et al: Molecular cloning of the thyrotropin receptor. *Science* 246:1620, 1989.
86. Hanley MR, Jackson T: Return of the magnificent seven. *Nature* 329:766, 1987.
87. Lin HY, Harris TL, Flannery MS, Aruffo A, Kaji EH, Gorn A, Kolakowski LF Jr, Lodish HF, et al: Expression cloning of an adenylate cyclase-coupled calcitonin receptor. *Science* 254:1022, 1991.
88. Dixon RAF, Sigal IS, Rands E, Register RB, Candelore MR, Blake AD, Strader CD: Ligand binding to the β-adrenergic receptor involves its rhodopsin-like core. *Nature* 326:73, 1987.
89. Kobilka BK, Kobilka TS, Daniel K, Regan JW, Caron MG, Lefkowitz RJ: Chimeric α_2-,β_2-adrenergic receptors: Delineation of domains involved in effector coupling and ligand binding specificity. *Science* 240:1310, 1988.
90. Hausdorff WP, Hnatowich M, O'Dowd BF, Caron MG, Lefkowitz RJ; A mutation of the β_2-adrenergic receptor impairs agonist activation of adenylyl cyclase without affecting high affinity agonist binding. *J Biol Chem* 265:1388, 1990.
91. Strader CD, Candelore MR, Hill WS, Sigal IS, Dixon RAF: Identification of two serine residues involved in agonist activation of the β-adrenergic receptor. *J Biol Chem* 264:13572, 1989.
92. Fraser CM, Chung F-Z, Wang C-D, Venter JC: Site-directed mutagenesis of human β-adrenergic receptors: Substitution of aspartic acid-130 by asparagine produces a receptor with high-affinity agonist binding that is uncoupled from adenylate cyclase. *Proc Natl Acad Sci USA* 85:5478, 1988.
93. Yoshimura A, Longmore G, Lodish H: Point mutation in the exoplasmic domain of the erythropoietin receptor resulting in hormone-independent activation and tumorigenicity. *Nature* 348:647, 1990.
94. Franke RR, Sakmar TP, Oprian DD, Khorana HG: A single amino acid substitution in rhodopsin (lysine 248—leucine) prevents activation of transducin. *J Biol Chem* 263:2119, 1988.
95. Riedel H, Dull TJ, Schlessinger J, Ullrich A: A chimaeric receptor allows insulin to stimulate tyrosine kinase activity of epidermal growth factor receptor. *Nature* 324:68, 1986.
96. Strader CD, Sigal IS, Candelore MR, Rands E, Hill WS, Dixon RAF: Conserved aspartic acid residues 79 and 113 of the β-adrenergic receptor have different roles in receptor function. *J Biol Chem* 263:10267, 1988.
97. Strader CD, Candelore MR, Hill WS, Dixon RAF, Sigal IS: A single amino acid substitution in the β-adrenergic receptor promotes partial agonist activity from antagonists. *J Biol Chem* 264:16470, 1989.
98. Potts JT Jr, Kronenberg HM, Rosenblatt M: Parathyroid hormone: Chemistry, biosynthesis, and mode of action. *Adv Protein Chem* 35:323, 1982.
99. Rosenblatt M: Peptide hormone antagonists that are effective in vivo: Lessons from parathyroid hormone. *N Engl J Med* 315:1004, 1986.
100. Rosenblatt M, Callahan EN, Mahaffey JE, Pont A, Potts JT Jr: Parathyroid hormone inhibitors: Design, synthesis, and biologic evaluation of hormone analogues. *J Biol Chem* 252:5847, 1977.
101. Nussbaum SR, Rosenblatt M, Potts JT Jr: Parathyroid hormone renal receptor interactions: Demonstration of two receptor-binding domains. *J Biol Chem* 255:10183, 1980.
102. Horiuchi N, Holick MF, Potts JT Jr, Rosenblatt M: A parathyroid hormone inhibitor in vivo: Design and biological evaluation of a hormone analog. *Science* 220:1053, 1983.
103. Doppelt SH, Neer RM, Nussbaum SR, Federico P, Potts JT Jr, Rosenblatt M: Inhibition of the in vivo parathyroid hormone-mediated calcemic response in rats by a synthetic hormone antagonist. *Proc Natl Acad Sci USA* 83:7557, 1986.
104. Segre GV, Rosenblatt M, Tully GL III, Laugharn J, Reit B, Potts JT Jr: Evaluation of an in vitro parathyroid hormone antagonist in vivo in dogs. *Endocrinology* 116:1024, 1985.
105. McGowan JA, Chen TC, Fragola J, Puschett JB, Rosenblatt M: Parathyroid hormone: Effects of the 3-34 fragment in vivo and in vitro. *Science* 219:67, 1983.
106. Gray DA, Parsons JA, Potts JT Jr, Rosenblatt M, Stevenson RW: In vivo studies on an antagonist of parathyroid hormone [Nle-8,Nle-18,Tyr-34]bPTH-(3-34)amide. *Br J Pharmacol* 76:259, 1982.
107. Rosenblatt M, Segre GV, Tyler GA, Shepard GL, Nussbaum SR, Potts JT Jr: Identification of a receptor-binding region in parathyroid hormone. *Endocrinology* 107:545, 1980.
108. Rosenblatt M, Potts JT Jr: Analogues of an in vitro parathyroid hormone inhibitor: Modifications at the amino terminus. *Calcif Tissue Int* 33:153, 1981.
109. Horiuchi N, Rosenblatt M: Evaluation of a parathyroid hormone antagonist in an in vivo multiparameter bioassay. *Am J Physiol* 253:E187, 1987.
110. McKee RL, Caulfield MP, Rosenblatt M: Treatment of bone-derived ROS 17/2.8 cells with dexamethasone and pertussis toxin enables detection of partial agonist activity for parathyroid hormone antagonists. *Endocrinology* 127:76, 1990.
111. Rosenblatt M, Goltzman D, Keutmann HT, Tregear GW, Potts JT Jr: Chemical and biological properties of synthetic, sulfur-free analogues of parathyroid hormone. *J Biol Chem* 251:159, 1976.
112. Coltrera MD, Potts JT Jr, Rosenblatt M: Identification of a renal receptor for parathyroid hormone by photoaffinity radiolabeling using a synthetic analogue. *J Biol Chem* 256:10555, 1981.
113. Goldring SR, Tyler GA, Krane SM, Potts JT Jr, Rosenblatt M: Photoaffinity labeling of parathyroid hormone receptors: Comparison of receptors across species and target tissues and after desensitization to hormone. *Biochemistry* 23:498, 1984.
114. Nissenson RA, Karpf D, Bambino T: Covalent labeling of a high-affinity, guanyl nucleotide sensitive parathyroid hormone receptor in canine renal cortex. *Biochemistry* 26:1874, 1987.
115. Karpf DB, Arnaud CD, King K, Bambino T, Winer J, Nyiredy K, Nissenson RA: The canine renal parathyroid hormone receptor is a glycoprotein: Characterization and partial purification. *Biochemistry* 26:7825, 1987.
116. Shigeno C, Hiraki Y, Westerberg DP, Potts JT Jr, Segre GB: Parathyroid hormone receptors are plasma membrane glycoproteins with asparagine-linked oligosaccharides. *J Biol Chem* 263:3872, 1988.
117. Brennan DP, Levine MA: Characterization of soluble and particulate parathyroid hormone receptors using a biotinylated bioactive hormone analog. *J Biol Chem* 262:14795, 1987.
118. Moseley JM, Kubota M, Diefenbach-Jagger J: Parathyroid hormone-related protein purified from a human lung cancer cell line. *Proc Natl Acad Sci USA* 84:5048, 1987.
119. Stewart AF, Wu T, Goumas D, Burtis WJ, Broadus AE: N-Terminal amino acid sequence of two novel tumor-derived adenylate cyclase-stimulating proteins: Identification of parathyroid hormone-like and parathyroid hormone-unlike domains. *Biochem Biophys Res Commun* 146:672, 1987.
120. Strewler GJ, Stern PH, Jacobs JW, Eveloff J, Klein RF, Leung SC, Rosenblatt M, Nissenson RA: Parathyroid hormone-like protein from human renal carcinoma cells: Structural and functional homology with parathyroid hormone. *J Clin Invest* 80:1803, 1987.
121. Suva LJ, Winslow GA, Wettenhall REH, Hammonds RG, Moseley JM, Diefenbach-Jagger H, Rodda CP, Kemp BE, et al: A parathyroid hormone-related protein implicated in malignant hypercalcemia: Cloning and expression. *Science* 237:893, 1987.

122. Mangin M, Webb AC, Dreyer BE: Identification of a cDNA encoding a parathyroid hormone-like peptide from a human tumor associated with humoral hypercalcemia of malignancy. *Proc Natl Acad Sci* USA 85:597, 1988.
123. Thiede MA, Strewler GJ, Nissenson RA, Rosenblatt M, Rodan GA: Human renal carcinoma expresses two messages encoding a parathyroid hormone-like peptide: Evidence for the alternative splicing of a single-copy gene. *Proc Natl Acad Sci USA* 85:4605, 1988.
124. Kemp BE, Moseley JM, Rodda CP, Ebeling PR, Wetttenhall REH, Stapleton D, Diefenbach-Jagger J, Ure F, et al: Parathyroid hormone-related protein of malignancy: Active synthetic fragments. *Science* 238:1568, 1987.
125. Horiuchi N, Caulfield MP, Fisher JE, Goldman ME, McKee RL, Reagan JE, Levy JJ, Nutt RF, et al: Similarity of synthetic peptide from human tumor to parathyroid hormone in vivo and in vitro. *Science* 238:1566, 1987.
126. Donahue HJ, Fryer MJ, Heath H III: Structure-function relationships for full-length recombinant parathyroid hormone-related peptide and its amino-terminal fragments: Effects on cytosolic calcium ion mobilization and adenylate cyclase activation in rat osteoblast-like cells. *Endocrinology* 126:1471, 1990.
127. Nissenson RA, Diep D, Strewler GJ: Synthetic peptides comprising the amino-terminal sequence of a parathyroid hormone-like protein from human malignancies. *J Biol Chem* 263:12866, 1988.
128. Rabbani SA, Mitchell J, Roy DR, Hendy GN, Goltzman D: Influence of the amino-terminus on in vitro and in vivo biological activity of synthetic parathyroid hormone-like peptides of malignancy. *Endocrinology* 123:2709, 1988.
129. Jüppner H, Abou-Samra A-B, Uneno S, Gu W-X, Potts JT Jr, Segre GV: The parathyroid hormone-like peptide associated with humoral hypercalcemia of malignancy and parathyroid hormone bind to the same receptor on the plasma membrane of ROS 17/2.8 cells. *J Biol Chem* 263:8557, 1988.
130. Shigeno C, Yamamoto I, Kitamura N, Noda T, Lee K, Sone T, Shiomi K, Ohtaka A, et al: Interaction of human parathyroid hormone-related peptide with parathyroid hormone receptors in clonal rat osteosarcoma cells. *J Biol Chem* 263:18369, 1988.
131. Fukayama S, Bosma TJ, Goad DL, Voelkel EF, Tashjian AH Jr: Human parathyroid hormone (PTH)-related protein and human PTH: Comparative biological activities on human bone cells and bone resorption. *Endocrinology* 123:2841, 1988.
132. Caulfield MP, McKee RL, Goldman ME, Duong LT, Fisher JE, Gay CT, DeHaven PA, Levy JJ, et al: The bovine renal parathyroid hormone (PTH) receptor has equal affinity for two different amino acid sequences: The receptor binding domains of PTH and PTH-related protein are located within the 14-34 region. *Endocrinology* 127:83, 1990.
133. Horiuchi N, Hongo T, Clemens TL: The synthetic human tumor hypercalcemia factor is inhibited by a parathyroid hormone antagonist in rats in vivo. *J Bone Min Res* 5:541, 1990.
134. Abou-Samra A-B, Uneno S, Jüppner H, Keutmann H, Potts JT Jr, Segre GV, Nussbaum SR: Non-homologous sequences of parathyroid hormone and the parathyroid hormone related peptide bind to a common receptor on ROS 17/2.8 cells. *Endocrinology* 125:2215, 1989.
135. McKee RL, Goldman ME, Caulfield MP, DeHaven PA, Levy JJ, Nutt RF, Rosenblatt M: The 7-34-fragment of human hypercalcemia factor is a partial agonist/antagonist for parathyroid hormone-stimulated cAMP production. *Endocrinology* 122:3008, 1988.
136. Horiuchi N, Hongo T, Clemens TL: A 7-34 analog of the parathyroid hormone-related protein has potent antagonist and partial agonist activity in vivo. *Bone Mineral* 12:181, 1991.
137. Nutt RF, Caulfield MP, Levy JJ, Gibbons SW, Rosenblatt M, McKee RL: Removal of partial agonism from parathyroid hormone (PTH)-related protein-(7-34)NH_2 by substitution of PTH amino acids at positions 10 and 11. *Endocrinology* 127:491, 1990.
138. Chorev M, Goldman ME, McKee RL, Roubini E, Levy JJ, Gay CT, Reagan JE, Fisher JE, et al: Modifications of position 12 in parathyroid hormone and parathyroid hormone related protein: Toward the design of highly potent antagonists. *Biochemistry* 29:1580, 1990.
139. Caulfield MP, Rosenblatt M: Parathyroid hormone-receptor interactions. Trends Endocrinol Metab 164, 1990.
140. Goldman ME, Chorev M, Reagan JE, Nutt RF, Levy JJ, Rosenblatt M: Evaluation of novel parathyroid hormone analogs using a bovine renal membrane receptor binding assay. *Endocrinology* 123:1468, 1988.
141. Chorev M, Roubini E, McKee RL, Gibbons SW, Reagan JE, Goldman ME, Caulfield MP, Rosenblatt M: Biological activity of parathyroid hormone antagonists substituted at position 13. *Peptides* 12:57, 1991.
142. Chorev M, Roubini E, McKee RL, Gibbons SW, Goldman ME, Caulfield MP, Rosenblatt M: Cyclic parathyroid hormone related protein antagonists: Lysine 13 to aspartic acid 17[i to (i + 4)] side chain to side chain lactamization. *Biochemistry* 30:5968, 1991.
143. Rall TW, Sutherland EW: Formation of a cyclic adenine ribonucleotide by tissue particles. *J Biol Chem* 232:1065, 1958.
144. Michelakis AM: Hormonal effects on cyclic AMP in a renal-cell suspension system. *Proc Soc Exp Biol Med* 135:13, 1970.
145. Steiner AL, Pagliara AS, Chase LR, Kipnis DM: Radioimmunoassay for cyclic nucleotides: II. Adenosine 3′,5′-monophosphate and guanosine 3′,5′-monophosphate in mammalian tissues and body fluids. *J Biol Chem* 347:1114, 1972.
146. Rasmussen H, Pechet N, Fast D: Effect of dibutyryl cyclic adenosine 3′,5′-monophosphate, theophylline, and other nucleotides upon calcium and phosphate metabolism. *J Clin Invest* 47:1843, 1968.
147. Russell RGG, Casey PA, Fleisch H: Stimulation of phosphate excretion by the renal arterial infusion of 3′,5′-AMP (cyclic AMP)—a possible mechanism of action of parathyroid hormone. *Calcif Tissue Res* 2 (suppl):54, 1968.
148. Chabardes D, Imbert M, Clique A: PTH sensitive adenyl cyclase activity in different segments of the rabbit nephron. *Pflugers Arch* 354:229, 1975.
149. Hanai H, Ishida M, Liang CT, Sacktor B: Parathyroid hormone increases sodium/calcium exchange activity in renal cells and the blunting of the response in aging. *J Biol Chem* 261:5419, 1986.
149a. Gesek FA, Friedman PA: On the mechanism of parathyroid hormone stimulation of calcium uptake by mouse distal convoluted tubule cells. *J Clin Invest* 90:749, 1992.
150. Chambers DJ, Shafer H, Laugharn JA Jr: Dose-related activation by PTH of specific enzymes in various regions of the kidney, in Copp DH, Talmage RV (eds): *Endocrinology of Calcium Metabolism.* Amsterdam, Excerpta Medica, 1978, p 216.
151. Sakaguchi K, Fukase M, Kobayashi I, Fujita T: Characteristics of parathyroid hormone-specific cyclic changes of glucose-6-phosphate dehydrogenase activity in the distal convoluted tubule of the guinea pig. *J Bone Min Res* 1:259, 1986.
152. Tregear GW, van Rietschoten J, Greene E: *Principles and Recent Applications in the Solid-Phase Synthesis of Peptide Hormones.* Amsterdam, Excerpta Medica, 1974.
153. Parsons JA, Rafferty B, Gray D: Pharmacology of parathyroid hormone and some of its fragments and analogs, in Talmadge RV, Owens M, Parsons JA (eds): *Calcium-Regulating Hormones: Proceedings of the Fifth Parathyroid Conference, 1974.* Amsterdam Elsevier, Excerpta Medical International Congress Services, 1975, p 33.

154. Bacskai BJ, Friedman PA: Activation of latent Ca^{2+} channels in renal epithelial cells by parathyroid hormone. *Nature* 347:388, 1990.
155. Filburn CR, Harrison S: Parathyroid hormone regulation of cytosolic Ca^{2+} in rat proximal tubules. *Am J Physiol* 258: F545, 1990.
156. Bidot-Lopez P, Farese RV, Sabir MA: Parathyroid hormone and adenosine-3',5'-monophosphate acutely increase phospholipids of the phosphatidate-polyphosphoinositide pathway in rabbit kidney cortex tubules in vitro by a cycloheximide-sensitive process. *Endocrinology* 108:2078, 1981.
157. Meltzer V, Weinreb S, Bellorin-Font E, Hruska KA: Parathyroid hormone stimulation of renal phosphoinositide metabolism is a cyclic nucleotide-independent effect. *Biochim Biophys Acta* 712:258, 1982.
158. Farese RV, Bidot-Lopez P, Sabir MA, Larson RE: Activation by parathyroid hormone and dibutryl-cAMP in rabbit kidney cortex. *Ann NY Acad Sci* 372:539, 1981.
159. Rodan SB, Rodan GA: The effect of parathyroid hormone and thyrocalcitonin on the accumulation of cyclic adenosine 3',5'-monophosphate in freshly isolated bone cells. *J Biol Chem* 249:3068, 1974.
160. Raisz LG, Brand JS, Klein DC, Au WYW: Hormone regulation of bone resorption, in Gaul C, Ebling SG (eds): *Progress in Endocrinology.* Amsterdam, Excerpta Medica, 1969, p 696.
161. Raisz LG: Parathyroid gland: Mechanisms of bone resorption, in Greep R, Astwood EB (eds): *Handbook of Physiology, Section 7: Endocrinology.* Baltimore, Williams & Wilkins, 1976, p 117.
162. Wells H, Lloyd W: Hypercalcemic and hypophosphatemic effects of dibutyryl cyclic AMP in rats after parathyroidectomy. *Endocrinology* 84:861, 1969.
163. Vaes G: Parathyroid hormone-like action of N^6-2'-O-dibutyryladenosine-3',5'-(cyclic)-monophosphate on bone explants in tissue culture. *Nature* 219:939, 1968.
164. Reid IR, Lowe C, Cornish J, Gray DH, Skinner SJM: Adenylate cyclase blockers dissociate PTH-stimulated bone resorption from cAMP production. *Am J Physiol* 258(Endocrinol Metab 21):E708, 1990.
165. Iida-Klein A, Varlotta V, Hahn TJ; Protein kinase C activity in UMR-106-01 cells: Effects of parathyroid hormone and insulin. *J Bone Min Res* 4:767, 1989.
166. Tamura T, Sakamoto H, Filburn CR: Parathyroid hormone 1-34, but not 3-34 or 7-34, transiently translocates protein kinase C in cultured renal (OK) cells. *Biochem Biophys Res Commun* 159:1352, 1989.
167. Rodan GA, Rodan SB: Expression of the osteoblastic phenotype, in Peck WA (ed): *Bone and Mineral Research.* Amsterdam, Elsevier, 1983, p 244.
168. Yamaguchi DT, Hahn TJ, Iida-Klein A, Kleeman CR, Muallem S: Parathyroid hormone-activated calcium channels in an osteoblast-like osteosarcoma cell line: cAMP-dependent and cAMP-independent calcium channels. *J Biol Chem* 262:7711, 1987.
169. Ausiello DA, Rosenblatt M, Dayer J-M: Parathyroid hormone modulates protein kinase in giant cell tumors of human bone. *Am J Physiol* 239:E144, 1980.
170. Reshkin SJ, Wuarin F, Biber J, Murer H: Parathyroid hormone-induced alterations of protein content and phosphorylation in enriched apical membranes of opossum kidney cells. *J Biol Chem* 265:15261, 1990.
171. Rodan SB, Fischer MK, Egan JJ: The effect of dexamethasone on parathyroid hormone stimulation of adenylate cyclase in ROS 17/2.8 cells. *Endocrinology* 115:951, 1984.
172. Yamamoto I, Potts JT Jr, Segre GV: Regulation of parathyroid hormone receptor on clonal rat osteosarcoma cells, in Cohn DV, Fujita T, Potts JT Jr, Talmage RV (eds): *Endocrine Control of Bone and Calcium Metabolism.* Amsterdam, Excerpta Medica, 1984, p 250.
173. Goldring SR, Dayer JM, Russell RGG: Response to hormones of cells cultured from human giant cell tumors of bone. *J Clin Endocrinol Metab* 46:425, 1978.
174. Goldring SR, Mahaffey JE, Rosenblatt M: Parathyroid hormone inhibitors: Comparison of biological activity in bone and skin-derived tissue. *J Clin Endocrinol Metab* 48:655, 1979.
175. Mahoney CA, Nissenson RA: Canine renal receptors for parathyroid hormone: Down-regulation in vivo by exogenous parathyroid hormone. *J Clin Invest* 72:411, 1983.
176. Yamamoto I, Shigeno C, Potts JT Jr, Segre GV: Characterization and agonist-induced down-regulation of parathyroid hormone receptors in clonal rat osteosarcoma cells. *Endocrinology* 122:1208, 1988.
177. Abou-Samra A-B, Jüppner H, Potts JT Jr, Segre GV: Inactivation of pertussis toxin-sensitive guanyl nucleotide-binding proteins increase parathyroid hormone receptors and reverse agonist-induced receptor down-regulation in ROS 17/2.8 cells. *Endocrinology* 125:2594, 1989.
178. Pun K-K, Ho PWM, Nissenson RA, Arnaud CD: Desensitization of parathyroid hormone receptors on cultured bone cells. *J Bone Min Res* 5:1193, 1990.
179. Benovic JL, Staniszewski C, Mayor F Jr, Caron MG, Lefkowitz RJ: β-Adrenergic receptor kinase. *J Biol Chem* 263:3893, 1988.
180. Hausdorff WP, Caron MG, Lefkowitz RJ: Turning off the signal: Desensitization of β-adrenergic receptor function. *FASEB J* 4:2881, 1990.
181. Hanai H, Brennan DP, Cheng L, Goldman ME, Chorev M, Levine MA, Sacktor B, Liang CT: Downregulation of parathyroid hormone receptors in renal membranes from aged rats. *Am J Physiol* 259(Renal Fluid Electrolyte Physiol 28):F444, 1990.
182. Martin KJ, McConkey CL, Garcia JC, Montani D, Betts CR: Protein kinase-A and the effects of parathyroid hormone on phosphate uptake in opossum kidney cells. *Endocrinology* 125:295, 1989.
183. Caverzasio J, Rizzoli R, Bonjour J-P: Sodium-dependent phosphate transport inhibited by parathyroid hormone and cyclic AMP stimulation in an opossum kidney cell line. *J Biol Chem* 261:3233, 1986.
184. Weinman EJ, Shenolikar S, Kahn AM: cAMP-associated inhibition of Na^+-H^+ exchanger in rabbit kidney brush-border membranes. *Am J Physiol* 252(Renal Fluid Electrolyte Physiol 21):F19, 1987.
185. Hensley CB, Bradley ME, Mircheff AK: Parathyroid hormone-induced translocation of Na-H antiporters in rat proximal tubules. *Am J Physiol* 257(Cell Physiol 26):C637, 1989.
186. Pullman TN, Lavender AR, Aho I, Rasmussen H: Direct renal action of a purified parathyroid extract. *Endocrinology* 67:570, 1960.
187. Widrow SH, Levinsky NG: Effect of parathyroid extract on renal tubular calcium reabsorption in the dog. *J Clin Invest* 41:2151, 1962.
188. Agus ZS, Gardner LB, Beck LH, Goldberg M: Effects of parathyroid hormone on renal tubular reabsorption of calcium, sodium, and phosphate. *Am J Physiol* 224:1143, 1973.
189. Scoble JE, Mills S, Hruska KA: Calcium transport in canine renal basolateral membrane vesicles: Effects of parathyroid hormone. *J Clin Invest* 75:1096, 1985.
190. Bouhtiauy D, Lajeunesse D, Brunette MG: The mechanism of parathyroid hormone action on calcium reabsorption by the distal tubule. *Endocrinology* 128:251, 1991.
191. Kurokawa K, Kawashima H, Torikai S: Parathyroid hormone (PTH)-sensitive and calcitonin (CT)-sensitive 25-(OH)-D_3-1-alpha-hydroxylase along the nephron—distinct distribution and mechanisms of action. *Clin Res* 29:541, 1981.
192. Horiuchi N, Suda T, Takahashi H: In vivo evidence for the intermediary role of 3',5'-cyclic AMP in parathyroid hormone-induced stimulation of 1α,25-dihydroxyvitamin D_3 synthesis in rats. *Endocrinology* 101:969, 1977.
193. Kawashima H, Torikai S, Kurokawa K: Localization of 25-

hydroxyvitamin D_3-1α- and -24-dihydroxylase along the rat nephron. *Proc Natl Acad Sci USA* 78:1199, 1981.
194. Sato M, Sardana MK, Grasser WA, Garsky VM, Murray JM, Gould RJ: Echistatin is a potent inhibitor of bone resorption in culture. *J Cell Biol* 111:1713, 1990.
195. Horton MA, Davies J: Perspectives: Adhesion receptors in bone. *J Bone Min Res* 4:803, 1989.
196. Blair HC, Ghandur-Mnaymneh L: Macrophase-mediated bone resorption occurs in an acidic environment. *Calcif Tissue Int* 37:547, 1985.
197. Vaes G: The role of lysosomes and of their enzyme in the development of bone resorption induced by parathyroid hormone, in Talmage RV, Belanger LF, Clerk I (eds): *Proceedings of the 3rd Parathyroid Conference*. Amsterdam, Excerpta Medica, 1968, p 318.
198. Walker DG, Lapier CM, Gross J: A collagenolytic factor in rat bone promoted by parathyroid extract. *Biochem Biophys Res Commun* 15:397, 1964.
199. Tuukkanen J, Vaananen HK: Omeprazole, a specific inhibitor of H^+-K^+ ATPase, inhibits bone resorption in vitro. *Calcif Tissue Int* 38:123, 1986.
200. Blair HC, Teitelbaum SL, Ghiselli R, Gluck S: Osteoclastic bone resorption by a polarized vacuolar proton pump. *Science* 245:855, 1989.
201. Waite LC: Carbonic anhydrase inhibitors, parathyroid hormone and calcium metabolism. *Endocrinology* 91:1160, 1972.
202. Mahgoub A, Stern PH: Carbon dioxide and the effect of parathyroid hormone on bone in vitro. *Am J Physiol* 226:1272, 1974.
203. Delaisse J-M, Eeckhout Y, Vaes G: In vivo and in vitro evidence for the involvement of cysteine proteinases in bone resorption. *Biochem Biophys Res Commun* 125:441, 1984.
204. Sly WS, Whyte MP, Sundaram V: Carbonic anhydrase II deficiency in 12 families with the autosomal recessive syndrome of osteopetrosis with renal tubular acidosis and cerebral calcification. *N Engl J Med* 313:139, 1985.
205. Sly WS, Hewett-Emmett D, Whyte MP: Carbonic anhydrase II deficiency identified as the primary defect in the autosomal recessive syndrome of osteopetrosis with renal tubular acidosis and cerebral calcification. *Proc Natl Acad Sci USA* 80:2752, 1983.
206. Barling PM, Bibby NJ: Study of the localization of [^{3}H] bovine parathyroid hormone in bone by light microscope autoradiography. *Calcif Tissue Int* 37:441, 1985.
207. Silve CM, Hradek GT, Jones AL, Arnaud CD: Parathyroid hormone receptor in intact embryonic chicken bone: Characterization and cellular localization. *J Cell Biol* 94:379, 1982.
208. Rodan GA, Martin TJ: Role of osteoblasts in hormonal control of bone resorption—a hypothesis. *Calcif Tissue Int* 33:349, 1982.
209. McSheehy PMJ, Chambers TJ: Osteoblastic cells mediate osteoclastic responsiveness to parathyroid hormone. *Endocrinology* 118:824, 1986.
210. Raisz LG, Martin TJ: Prostaglandins in bone and mineral metabolism, in Peck WA (ed): *Bone and Mineral Research*. Amsterdam, Excerpta Medica, 1984, p 286.
211. Rodan GA, Heath JK, Yoon K, Noda M, Rodan SB: Diversity of the osteoblastic phenotype, in Evered D, Harnett S (eds): *CIBA Symposium on Cell and Molecular Biology of Vertebrate Hard Tissues*. Chichester, UK, Wiley, 1988, p 79.
212. Ralston SH, Russell RGG, Gowen M: Estrogen inhibits release of tumor necrosis factor from peripheral blood mononuclear cells in postmenopausal women. *J Bone Min Res* 5:983, 1990.
213. Pacifici R, Rifas L, McCracken R, Vered I, McMurtry C, Avioli LV, Peck WA: Ovarian steroid treatment blocks a postmenopausal increase in blood monocyte interleukin 1 release. *Proc Natl Acad Sci USA* 86:2398, 1989.
214. Girasole G, Sakagami Y, Hustmyer FG, Yu XP, Derrigs HG, Boswell S, Peacock M, Boder G, et al: 17β-Estradiol inhibits cytokine induced IL-6 production by bone marrow stromal cells and osteoblasts. *J Bone Min Res* 5(suppl 2):S273, 1990.
215. Tabibzadeh SS, Santhanam U, May L, Sehgal P: Cytokine-induced production of IL-6 by freshly explanted human endometrial stromal cells: Modulation by estradiol-17β. *Ann NY Acad Sci* 557:543, 1989.
216. Ishimi Y, Miyaura C, Jin CH, Akatsu T, Abe E, Nakamura Y, Yamaguchi A, Yoshiki S, et al: IL-6 is produced by osteoblasts and induces bone resorption. *J Immunol* 145:3297, 1990.
217. Gearing DP, Gough NM, King JA, Hilton DJ, Nicola NA, Simpson RJ, Nice EC, Kelso A, et al: Molecular cloning and expression of cDNA encoding a murine myeloid leukemia inhibitory factor (LIF). *EMBO J* 6:3995, 1987.
218. Weir EC, Insogna KL, Horowitz MC: Osteoblast-like cells secrete granulocyte-macrophage colony-stimulating factor in response to parathyroid hormone and lipopolysaccharide. *Endocrinology* 124:899, 1989.
219. Perry HM III, Skogen W, Chappel J, Kahn AJ, Wilner G, Teitelbaum SL: Partial characterization of a parathyroid hormone-stimulated resorption factor(s) from osteoblast-like cells. *Endocrinology* 125:2075, 1989.
220. Morris CA, Mitnick ME, Weir EC, Horowitz M, Kreider BL, Insogna KL: The parathyroid hormone-related protein stimulates human osteoblast-like cells to secrete a 9,000 dalton bone-resorbing protein. *Endocrinology* 126:1783, 1990.
221. Slovik DM, Neer RM, Potts JT Jr: Short term effects of synthetic human parathyroid hormone-(1-34) administration on bone mineral metabolism in osteoporotic patients. *J Clin Invest* 68:1261, 1981.
222. Howard GA, Bottemiller BL, Turner RT, Rader JI, Baylink DJ: Parathyroid hormone stimulates bone formation and resorption in organ culture: Evidence for a coupling mechanism. *Proc Natl Acad Sci USA* 78:3204, 1981.
223. Tam CS, Heersche JNM, Murray TM, Parsons JA: Parathyroid hormone stimulates the bone apposition rate independently of its resorptive action: Differential effects of intermittent and continual administration. *Endocrinology* 110:506, 1982.
224. Reeve J, Davies UM, Hesp R, McNally E, Katz D: Treatment of osteoporosis with human parathyroid peptide and observations on effect of sodium fluoride. *Br Med J* 301:314, 1990.
225. Reeve J, Williams D, Hesp R, Hulme P, Klenerman L, Zanelli JM, Darby AJ, Tregear GW, et al: Anabolic effect of low doses of a fragment of human parathyroid hormone on the skeleton in postmenopausal osteoporosis. *Lancet* 1:1035, 1976.
226. Tada K, Yamamuro T, Okumura H, Kasai R, Takahashi H: Restoration of axial and appendicular bone volumes by h-PTH(1-34) in parathyroidectomized and osteopenic rats. *Bone* 11:163, 1990.
227. Hock JM, Gera I, Fonseca J, Raisz LG: Human parathyroid hormone-(1-34) increases bone mass in ovariectomized and orchidectomized rats. *Endocrinology* 122:2899, 1988.
228. McCarthy TL, Centrella M, Canalis E: Parathyroid hormone enhances the transcript and polypeptide levels of insulin-like growth factor I in osteoblast-enriched cultures from fetal rat bone. *Endocrinology* 124:1247, 1989.
229. Linkhart TA, Keffer MJ: Differential regulation of insulin-like growth factor-I (IGF-I) and IGF-II release from cultured neonatal mouse calvaria by parathyroid hormone, transforming growth factor-β, and 1,25-dihydroxyvitamin D_3. *Endocrinology* 128:1511, 1991.
230. Centrella M, McCarthy TL, Canalis E: Parathyroid hormone modulates transforming growth factor β activity and binding in osteoblast-enriched cell cultures from fetal rat parietal bone. *Proc Natl Acad Sci USA* 85:5889, 1988.

231. Galceran T, Slatopolsky E, Martin KJ: Differences in the reponse to intact b-PTH 1-84 and synthetic b-PTH 1-34 in isolated perfused bones from young and adult dogs. *Calcif Tissue Int* 41:290, 1987.
232. Calvo MS, Fryer MJ, Laakso KJ, Nissenson RA, Price PA, Murray TM, Heath H III: Structural requirements for parathyroid hormone action in mature bone: Effects on release of cyclic adenosine monophosphate and bone gamma-carboxyglutamic acid-containing protein from perfused rat hindquarters. *J Clin Invest* 76:2348, 1985.
233. Sugimoto T, Fukase M, Tsutsumi M, Imai Y, Hiskikawa R, Yoshimoto Y, Fujita T: Additive effects of parathyroid hormone and calcitonin on adenosine 3′,5′-monophosphate release in newly established perfusion system of rat femur. *Endocrinology* 117:1901, 1985.
234. Morrison NE, Ramanathan S, Suh SM: Skeletal contribution of cyclic adenosine monophosphate in response to parathyroid hormone and calcitonin in vivo in the rat. *J Bone Min Res* 3:629, 1988.
235. Rouleau MF, Mitchell J, Goltzman D: In vivo distribution of parathyroid hormone receptors in bone: Evidence that a predominant osseous target cell is not the mature osteoblast. *Endocrinology* 123:187, 1988.
236. Bellows CG, Ishida H, Aubin JE, Heersche JNM: Parathyroid hormone reversibly suppresses the differentiation of osteoprogenitor cells into functional osteoblasts. *Endocrinology* 127:3111, 1990.
237. Rouleau MF, Mitchell J, Goltzman D: Characterization of the major parathyroid hormone target cell in the endosteal metaphysis of rat long bones. *J Bone Min Res* 5:1043, 1990.
238. Duong LT, Grasser W, DeHaven PA, Sato M: Parathyroid hormone receptors identified on avian and rat osteoclasts. *J Bone Min Res* 5(suppl 2):518, 1990.
239. Teti A, Rizzoli R, Zallone AZ: Parathyroid hormone binding to cultured avian osteoclasts. *Biochem Biophys Res Commun* 174:1217, 1991.
240. Yamamoto I, Potts JT Jr, Segre GV: Circulating bovine lymphocytes contain receptors for parathyroid hormone. *J Clin Invest* 71:404, 1983.
241. Perry HM III, Chappel JC, Bellorin-Font E: Parathyroid hormone receptors in circulating human mononuclear leukocytes. *J Biol Chem* 259:5531, 1984.
242. Nickols GA, Nickols MA, Helwig J-J: Binding of parathyroid hormone and parathyroid hormone-related protein to vascular smooth muscle of rabbit renal microvessels. *Endocrinology* 126:721, 1990.
243. Thiede MA, Rodan GA: Expression of a calcium-mobilizing parathyroid hormone-like peptide in lactating mammary tissue. *Science* 242:278, 1988.
244. Budayr AA, Halloran BP, King JC, Diep D, Nissenson RA, Strewler GJ: High levels of a parathyroid hormone-like protein in milk. *Proc Natl Acad Sci USA* 86:7183, 1989.
245. Barlet JP, Davicco M-J, Coxam V: Synthetic parathyroid hormone-related peptide(1-34) fragment stimulates placental calcium transfer in ewes. *J Endocrinol* 127:33, 1990.
246. Rodda CP, Kubota M, Heath JA, Ebeling PR, Moseley JM, Care AD, Caple IW, Martin TJ: Evidence for a novel parathyroid hormone-related protein in fetal lamb parathyroid glands and sheep placenta: Comparisons with a similar protein implicated in humoral hypercalcaemia of malignancy. *J Endocrinol* 117:261, 1988.
247. Hayman JA, Danks JA, Ebeling PR, Moseley JM, Kemp BE, Martin TJ: Expression of parathyroid hormone related protein in normal skin and in tumours of skin and skin appendages. *J Pathol* 158:293, 1989.
248. Motokura T, Fukumoto S, Matsumoto T, Takahashi S, Fujita A, Yamashita T, Igarashi T, Ogata E: Parathyroid hormone-related protein in adult T-cell leukemia-lymphoma. *Ann Intern Med* 111:484, 1989.
249. Weir EC, Brines ML, Ikeda K, Burtis WJ, Broadus AE, Robbins RJ: Parathyroid hormone-related peptide gene is expressed in the mammalian central nervous sytem. *Proc Natl Acad Sci USA* 87:108, 1990.
250. Thiede MA, Daifotis AG, Weir EC, Brines ML, Burtis WJ, Ikeda K, Dreyer BE, Garfield RE, et al: Intrauterine occupancy controls expression of the parathyroid hormone-related peptide gene in preterm rat myometrium. *Proc Natl Acad Sci USA* 87:6969, 1990.
251. Asa SL, Henderson J, Goltzman D, Drucker DJ: Parathyroid hormone-like peptide in normal and neoplastic human endocrine tissues. *J Clin Endocrinol Metab* 71:1112, 1990.
252. Merendino JJ Jr, Insogna KL, Milstone LM, Broadus AE, Stewart AF: A parathyroid hormone-like protein from cultured human keratinocytes. *Science* 231:388, 1986.
253. Copp DH: Parathyroids, calcitonin and control of plasma calcium. *Recent Prog Horm Res* 20:59, 1964.
254. Copp DH, Cameron EC, Cheney BA, Davidson AGF, Henze KG: Evidence for calcitonin—a new hormone from the parathyroid that lowers blood calcium. *Endocrinology* 70:638, 1962.
255. Foster GV, Byfield PGH, Gudmundsson TV: Calcitonin. *Clin Endocrinol Metab* 1:93, 1972.
256. Munson PL: Physiology and pharmacology of thyrocalcitonin, in Aurbach GD (eds): *Handbook of Physiology, Section 7: Endocrinology*. Washington, D.C., American Physiological Society, 1976, p 443.
257. Austin LA, Heath H: Calcitonin physiology and pathophysiology. *N Engl J Med* 304:269, 1981.
258. MacIntyre I: Calcitonin: physiology, biosynthesis, secretion, metabolism, and mode of action, in DeGroot, LJ (ed): *Endocrinology*. Philadelphia, Saunders, 1989, p 892.
259. Pearse AGE, Carvalheira AF: Cytochemical evidence for an ultimobranchial origin of rodent thyroid C cells. *Nature* 214:929, 1967.
260. Goltzman D, Tischler AS: Characterization of the immunochemical forms of calcitonin released by a medullary thyroid carcinoma in tissue culture. *J Clin Invest* 61:449, 1978.
261. Seiber P, Brugger M, Kamber B: Menschliches calcitonin: IV. Die synthese von calcitonin M. *Helv Chir Acta* 51:2057, 1968.
262. Guttmann S, Pless J, Sandrin E: Synthese des thyrocalcitonins. *Helv Chir Acta* 51:1155, 1968.
263. Nicholson GC, Moseley JM, Sexton PM, Mendelsohn FAO, Martin TJ: Abundant calcitonin receptors in isolated rat osteoclasts: Biochemical and autoradiographic characterization. *J Clin Invest* 78:355, 1986.
264. Warshawsky H, Goltzman D, Rouleau MF, Bergeron JM: Direct in vivo demonstration by radioautography of specific binding sites for calcitonin in skeletal and renal tissues of the rat. *J Cell Biol* 85:682, 1980.
265. Raisz LG, Kream BE: Regulation of bone formation. *N Engl J Med* 309:29, 1983.
266. Kallio DM, Garant PR, Minkin C: Ultrastructural effects of calcitonin on osteoclasts in tissue culture. *J Ultrastruct Res* 39:205, 1972.
267. Chakraborty M, Chatterjee D, Kellokumpu S, Rasmussen H, Baron R: Cell cycle-dependent coupling of the calcitonin receptor to different G proteins. *Science* 251:1078, 1991.
268. Potts JT Jr, Niall HD, Keutmann HT, Lequin RM: Chemistry of the calcitonins: Species variation plus structure-activity relations, and pharmacologic implications, in Talmage RV, Munson PL (eds): *Calcium, Parathyroid Hormone, and the Calcitonins: Proceedings of the Fourth Parathyroid Conference*. Amsterdam, Excerpta Medica, 1972, p 121.
269. Tashjian AH, Wright DR, Ivey JL, Pont A: Calcitonin binding sites in bone: Relationships to biological response and "escape." *Recent Prog Horm Res* 34:285, 1977.
270. Lamp SJ, Findlay DM, Moseley JM, Martin TJ: *J Biol Chem* 256:12269, 1981.
271. Michelangeli VP, Findlay DM, Moseley JM, Martin TJ: *J Cyclic Nucleotide Protein Phosphor Res* 9:129, 1983.

272. D'Santos CS, Nicholson GC, Moseley JM, Evans T, Martin TJ, Kemp BE: Biologically active, derivatizable salmon calcitonin analog: Design, synthesis, and applications. *Endocrinology* 123:1483, 1988.
273. Findlay DM, Michelangeli VP, Martin TJ, Orlowski RC, Seyler JK: Conformational requirements for activity of salmon calcitonin. *Endocrinology* 117:801, 1985.
274. Rittel W, Maier R, Brugger M, Kamber B, Riniker B, Siefer P: Structure-activity relationships of human calcitonin III: The biologic activity of systemic analogues with the shortened or terminally modified peptide chains. *Experientia* 32:246, 1976.
275. Schwartz K, Orlowski R, Marcus R: Des-Ser^2 salmon calcitonin: A biologically potent synthetic analog. *Endocrinology* 108:831, 1981.
276. Morikawa T, Munekata E, Sakakibara S, Noda T, Otari MA: Synthesis of ERI calcitonin and (Asu$^{1\text{-}7}$)-eel calcitonin: Contribution of the disulphide bond to hormonal activity. *Experientia* 32:1104, 1979.
277. Yates AJ, Gutierrez GE, Garrett IR, Mencel JJ, Nuss GW, Schriber AB, Mundy GR: A noncyclical analog of salmon calcitonin (N alpha-PropionylDi-Ala^{1,7},des-Leu^{19}sCT) retains full potency without inducing anorexia in rats. *Endocrinology* 126:2845, 1990.
278. Amara SG, Jonas V, Rosenfeld MG, Ong ES, Evans RM: Alternative RNA processing in calcitonin gene expression generates mRNAs encoding different polypeptide products. *Nature* 298:240, 1982.
279. Rosenfeld MG, Mermond J-J, Amara SG, Swanson LW, Sawchenko PE, Rivier J, Vale WW, Evans RM: Production of a novel neuropeptide encoded by the calcitonin gene via tissue-specific RNA processing. *Nature* 304:129, 1983.
280. Petermann JB, Born W, Chang J-Y, Fischer JA: Identification in the human central nervous system, pituitary, and thyroid of a novel calcitonin gene-related peptide, and partial amino acid sequence in the spinal cord. *J Biol Chem* 262:542, 1987.
281. Brain SD, Williams TJ, Tippins JR, Morris HR, MacIntyre I: Calcitonin gene-related peptide is a potent vasodilator. *Nature* 313:54, 1985.
282. McCulloch J, Uddman R, Kingman TA, Edvinsson L: Calcitonin gene-related peptide: Functional role in cerebrovascular regulation. *Proc Natl Acad Sci USA* 83:5731, 1986.
283. Nelson MT, Huang Y, Brayden JE, Hescheler J, Standen NB: Arterial dilations in response to calcitonin gene-related peptide involve activation of K^+ channels. *Nature* 344:770, 1990.
284. Goodman EC, Iversen LL: Calcitonin gene-related peptide: Novel neuropeptide. *Life Sci* 38:2169, 1986.
285. Krahn DD, Gosnell BA, Levine AS, Morley JE: Effects of calcitonin gene-related peptide on food intake. *Peptides* 5:861, 1984.
286. Hughes JJ, Levine AS, Morley JE, Gosnell BA, Silvis SE: Intraventricular calcitonin gene-related peptide inhibits gastric acid secretion. *Peptides* 5:665, 1984.
287. Goltzman D, Mitchell J: Interaction of calcitonin and calcitonin gene-related peptide at receptor sites in target tissues. *Science* 227:1343, 1985.
288. Seitz PK, Thomas ML, Cooper CW: Binding of calcitonin and calcitonin gene-related peptide to calvarial cells and renal cortical membranes. *J Bone Min Res* 1:51, 1986.
289. Zaidi M, Chambers TJ, Gaines Das RE, Morris HR, MacIntyre I: A direct action of human calcitonin gene-related peptide on isolated osteoclasts. *J Endocrinol* 115:511, 1987.
290. D'Souza SM, MacIntyre I, Girgis SI, Mundy GR: Human synthetic calcitonin gene-related peptide inhibits bone resorption in vitro. *Endocrinology* 119:58, 1986.
291. Tannenbaum GS, Goltzman D: Calcitonin gene-related peptide mimics calcitonin actions in brain on growth hormone release and feeding. *Endocrinology* 116:2685, 1985.
292. Zaidi M, Brain SD, Tippins JR, DiMarzo V, Moonga BS, Chambers TJ, Morris HR, MacIntyre I: Structure-activity relationship of human calcitonin-gene-related peptide. *Biochem J* 269:775, 1990.
293. Craig RK, Hall L, Edbrooke MR, Allison J, MacIntyre I: Partial nucleotide sequence of human calcitonin precursor mRNA identifies flanking cryptic peptides. *Nature* 295:345, 1982.
294. Jacobs JW, Goodman RH, Chin WW, Dee PC, Habener JF, Bell NH, Potts JT Jr: Calcitonin messenger RNA encodes multiple polypeptides in a single precursor. *Science* 213:457, 1981.
295. MacIntyre I, Hillyard CJ, Murphy PK, Reynolds JJ, Gaines Das RE, Craig RK: A second plasma calcium-lowering peptide from the human calcitonin precursors. *Nature* 300:460, 1982.
296. Birnbaum RS, Mahoney W, Roos BA: Purification and amino acid sequence of a noncalcitonin secretory peptide derived from preprocalcitonin. *J Biol Chem* 258:5463, 1983.
297. Roos BA, Huber MB, Birnbaum RS, Aron DC, Lindall AW, Lips K, Baylin SB: Medullary thyroid carcinomas secrete a noncalcitonin peptide corresponding to the carboxyl-terminal region of preprocalcitonin. *J Clin Endocrinol Metab* 56:802, 1983.
298. Roos BA, Fischer JA, Pignat W, Alander CB, Raisz LG: Evaluation of the in vivo and in vitro calcium-regulating actions of noncalcitonin peptides produced via calcitonin gene expression. *Endocrinology* 118:46, 1986.
299. Martin TJ: The therapeutic uses of calcitonin. *Scott Med J* 23:161, 1978.
300. Nilsson O, Almqvist S, Karlberg B: Salmon calcitonin in the acute treatment of moderate and severe hypercalcemia in man. *Acta Med Scand* 204:249, 1978.
301. Silva O, Becker K: Salmon calcitonin in the treatment of hypercalcemia. *Arch Intern Med* 132:337, 1973.
302. Sjöberg H, Hjern B: Acute treatment with calcitonin in primary hyperparathyroidism and severe hypercalcemia of other origin. *Acta Chir Scand* 141:90, 1975.
303. Vaughn C, Vitkevicium K: The effects of calcitonin in hypercalcemia in patients with malignancy. *Cancer* 34:1268, 1974.
304. Deftos L, Neer R: Medical management of the hypercalcemia of malignancy. *Annu Rev Med* 23:323, 1974.
305. Wisneski L, Croom W, Silva O, Becker K: Salmon calcitonin in hypercalcemia. *Clin Pharmacol Ther* 24:219, 1978.
306. Deftos LJ, First BP: Calcitonin as a drug. *Ann Intern Med* 95:192, 1981.
307. Deftos LJ: Calcitonin, in Gray CH, James VHT (eds): *Hormones and Blood.* London, Academic Press, 1979, p 97.
308. Au WYW: Calcitonin treatment of hypercalcemia due to parathyroid carcinoma: Synergistic effect of prednisone on long-term treatment of hypercalcemia. *Arch Intern Med* 135:1594, 1975.
309. Singer F, Ginger K: Resistance to calcitonin, in Singer F, Wallach S (eds): *Paget's Disease of Bone: Clinical Assessment, Present and Future Therapy, Procedings of the Symposium on Treatment of Paget's Disease of Bone, 1989.* New York, Elsevier, 1991, p 75.
310. Staehelin A: Possible therapeutic value of calcitonin in disorders of arterial circulation. *Schweiz Med Wochenshcr* 107:1865, 1977.
311. Carman JS, Wyatt RJ: Use of calcitonin in psychotic agitation or mania. *Arch Gen Psychiatry* 35:72, 1979.
312. McDermott MT, Kidd GS: The role of calcitonin in the development and treatment of osteoporosis. *Endocr Rev* 8:377, 1987.
313. Synthetic calcitonin for postmenopausal osteoporosis. *Med Lett Drug Ther* 27:53, 1985.
314. Fatourechi V, Heath H III: Salmon calcitonin in the treatment of postmenopausal osteoporosis. *Ann Intern Med* 107:923, 1987.
315. Mozolowski W: Jedrzej Sniadecki (1768–1838) on the cure of rickets. *Nature* 143:121, 1939.

316. Huldschinsky K: Heilung von rachitis durch kunstlicht hohensonne. *Dtsch Med Wochenschr* 45:712, 1919.
317. McCollum EV, Simmonds N, Becker JE, Shipley PG: Studies on experimental rickets: An experimental demonstration of the existence of a vitamin which promotes calcium deposition. *J Biol Chem* 53:293, 1922.
318. Steenbock H, Black A: The induction of growth promoting and calcifying properties in a ration by exposure to ultraviolet lights. *J Biol Chem* 61:408, 1924.
319. Hess AF, Weinstock M: Antirachitic properties imparted to inert fluids and green vegetables by ultraviolet irradiation. *J Biol Chem* 62:301, 1924.
320. DeLuca HF: Remembrance: Discovery of the vitamin D endocrine system. *Endocrinology* 130:1763, 1992.
321. Holick MF, MacLaughlin JA, Clark MB, Holick SA, Potts TJ Jr, Anderson RR, Blank IH, Parrish JA, et al: Photosynthesis of previtamin D_3 in human skin and the physiologic consequences. *Science* 210:203, 1980.
322. Clemens TL, Adams JS, Henderson SL, Holick MF: Increased skin pigment reduces the capacity of the skin to synthesize vitamin D. *Lancet* 1:74, 1982.
323. Yoon PS, DeLuca HF: Resolution and reconstitution of soluble components of rat liver microsomal vitamin D_3-25 hydroxylase. *Arch Biochem Biophys* 203:529, 1980.
324. Bell NH, Shaw S, Turner RT: Evidence that 1,25-dihydroxyvitamin D_3 inhibits the hepatic production of 25-hydroxyvitamin D in man. *J Clin Invest* 74:1540, 1984.
325. Halloran BP, Bikle DD, Levens MJ, Castro ME, Globus RK, Holton E: Chronic 1,25-dihydroxyvitamin D_3 administration in the rat reduces the serum concentration of 25-hydroxyvitamin D by increasing metabolic clearance rate. *J Clin Invest* 78:622, 1986.
326. Haddad P, Gascon-Barre M, Brault G, Plourde V: Influence of calcium or 1,25-dihydroxyvitamin D_3 supplementation on the hepatic microsomal and in vivo metabolism of vitamin D_3 in vitamin D-depleted rats. *J Clin Invest* 78:1529, 1986.
327. Breslau NA: Normal and abnormal regulation of 1,25-$(OH)_2D$ synthesis. *Am J Med Sci* 296:417, 1988.
328. Kumar R: Metabolism of 1,25-dihydroxyvitamin D_3. *Physiol Rev* 64:478, 1984.
329. Mandel ML, Moorthy B, Ghazarian JG: Reciprocal post-translational regulation of renal 1 alpha- and 24-hydroxylases of 25-hydroxyvitamin D_3 by phosphorylation of ferredoxin: mRNA-directed cell-free synthesis and immunoisolation of ferredoxin. *Biochem J* 266:385, 1990.
330. Ohyama Y, Noshiro M, Okuda K: Cloning and expression of cDNA encoding 25-hydroxyvitamin D_3 24-hydroxylase. *FEBS Lett* 278:195, 1991.
331. Henry HL: Regulation of the hydroxylation of 25-hydroxyvitamin D_3 in vivo and in primary cultures of chick kidney cells. *J Biol Chem* 254:2722, 1979.
332. Henry HL: Parathyroid hormone modulation of 25-hydroxyvitamin D_3 metabolism by cultured chick kidney cells is mimicked and enhanced by forskolin. *Endocrinology* 116:503, 1985.
333. Korkor AB, Gray RW, Henry HL, Kleinman JG, Blumenthal SS, Garancis JC: Evidence that stimulation of $1,25(OH)_2D_3$ production in primary cultures of mouse kidney cells by cyclic AMP requires new protein synthesis. *J Bone Min Res* 2:517, 1987.
333a. Shinki T, Jin CH, Nishimura A, Nagai Y, Ohyama Y, Noshiro M, Okunda M, Sude T: parathyroid hormone inhibits 25-hydroxyvitamin D_3-24-hydroxylase mRNA expression stimulated by 1 α, 25-dihydroxyvitamin D_3 in rate kidney but not in intestine. *JBiol Chem* 267: 13757, 1992.
334. Broadus AE, Horst RL, Lang R, Littledike ET, Rasmussen H: The importance of circulating 1,25-dihydroxyvitamin D in the pathogenesis of hypercalciuria and renal-stone formation in primary hyperparathyroidism. *N Engl J Med* 302:421, 1980.
335. Lund B, Srenson OH, Lund B, Bishop JE, Norman AW: Vitamin D metabolism in hypoparathyroidism. *J Clin Endocrinol Metab* 51:606, 1980.
336. Adams ND, Gray RW, Lemann J: The effects of oral $CaCO_3$ loading and dietary calcium deprivation on plasma 1,25-dihydroxyvitamin D concentrations in healthy adults. *J Clin Endocrinol Metab* 48:1008, 1979.
337. Portale AA, Halloran BP, Morris RC Jr: Physiologic regulation of the serum concentration of 1,25-dihydroxyvitamin D by phosphorus in normal men. *J Clin Invest* 83:1494, 1989.
338. Van den Berg CJ, Kumar R, Wilson DM, Heath H III, Smith LH: Orthophosphate therapy decreases urinary calcium excetion and serum 1,25-dihydroxyvitamin D concentrations in idiopathic hypercalciuria. *J Clin Endocrinol Metab* 51:998, 1980.
339. Portale AA, Booth BE, Halloran BP, Morris RC Jr: Effect of dietary phosphorus on circulating concentrations of 1,25-dihydroxyvitamin D and immunoreactive parathyroid hormone in children with moderate renal insufficiency. *J Clin Invest* 73:1580, 1984.
340. Halloran PB, Spencer EM: Dietary phosphorus and 1,25-dihydroxyvitamin D metabolism: Influence of insulin-like growth factor I. *Endocrinology* 123:1225, 1988.
341. Ryan EA, Reiss E: Oncogenous osteomalacia: Review of the world literature of 42 cases and report of two new cases. *Am J Med* 77:501, 1984.
342. Colston KW, Evans IMA, Spelsberg TC, MacIntyre I: Feedback of regulation of vitamin D metabolism by 1,25-dihydroxycholecalciferol. *Biochem J* 164:83, 1977.
343. Hulter HN, Halloran BP, Toto RD, Peterson JC: Long-term control of plasma calcitriol concentrations in dogs and humans. *J Clin Invest* 76:695, 1985.
344. Trechsel U, Eisman JA, Fischer JA, Bonjour JP, Fleisch H: Calcium-dependent, parathyroid hormone-independent regulation of 1,25-dihydroxyvitamin D. *Am J Physiol* 239:E119, 1980.
345. Bikle DD, Rasmussen H: The ionic control of 1,25-dihydroxyvitamin D_3 production in isolated chick renal tubules. *J Clin Invest* 55:292, 1975.
346. Bikle DD, Gee E, Halloran BP, Haddad JG: Free 1,25-dihydroxyvitamin D levels in serum from normal subjects, pregnant subjects, and subjects with liver disease. *J Clin Invest* 74:1966, 1984.
347. Cheema C, Grant BF, Marcus R: Effects of estrogen on circulating "free" and total 1,25-dihydroxyvitamin D and on the parathyroid-vitamin D axis in postmenopausal women. *J Clin Invest* 83:537, 1989.
348. Kumar R, Cohen WR, Silva P, Epstein FH: Elevated 1,25-dihydroxyvitamin D plasma levels in normal human pregnancy and lactation. *J Clin Invest* 63:342, 1979.
349. Emmersten K, Melsen F, Mosekilde L, Lund BI, Lund BJ, Sorensen OH, Nielsen HE, Solling H, et al: Altered vitamin D metabolism and bone remodelling in patients with medullary thyroid carcinoma and hypercalcitoninemia. *Metab Bone Dis Rel Res* 4:17, 1981.
350. Gray TK, Lester GE, Lorenc RS: Evidence for extrarenal 1α-hydroxylation of 25-dihydroxyvitamin D_3 in pregnancy. *Science* 204:1311, 1979.
351. Gertner JM, Coustan DR, Kliger AS, Mallette LE, Ravin N, Broadus AE: Pregnancy is a state of physiological absorptive hypercalciuria. *Am J Med* 81:451, 1986.
352. Bikle DD, Nemanic MK, Whitney JO, Elias PW: Neonatal human foreskin keratinocytes produce 1,25-dihydroxyvitamin D_3. *Biochemistry* 25:1545, 1986.
353. Howard GA, Turner RT, Sherrard DJ, Baylink DJ: Human bone cells in culture metabolize 25-hydroxyvitamin D_3, and 24,25-dihydroxyvitamin D_3. *J Biol Chem* 256:7738, 1981.
354. Reichel H, Koeffler HP, Bishop JE, Norman AW: 25-Hydroxyvitamin D_3 metabolism by lipopolysaccaride-stimulated normal human macrophages. *J Clin Endocrinol Metab* 64:519, 1987.
355. Brommage R, DeLuca HF: Evidence that 1,25-dihydroxyvitamin D_3 is the physiologically active metabolite of vitamin D_3. *Endocr Rev* 6:491, 1985.

356. Cooke NE, Haddad JG: Vitamin D binding protein (Gc-globulin). *Endocr Rev* 10:294, 1989.
357. Bikle DD, Halloran BP, Gee E, Haddad JG: Free 25-hydroxyvitamin D levels are normal in subjects with liver disease and reduced total 25-hydroxyvitamin D levels. *J Clin Invest* 78:748, 1986.
358. Bikle DD, Gee E: Free, and not total, 1,25-dihydroxyvitamin D regulates 25-hydroxyvitamin D metabolism by keratinocytes. *Endocrinology* 124:649, 1989.
359. McLaughlin M, Raggatt PR, Fairney A, Brown DJ, Lester E, Wills MR: Seasonal variation in serum 25-hydroxycholecalciferol in healthy people. *Lancet* 1:536, 1974.
360. Arnaud SB, Matthusen M, Gilkinson JB, Goldsmith RS: Components of 25-hydroxyvitamin D in serum of young children in upper midwestern United States. *Am J Clin Nutr* 30:1082, 1977.
361. Krall EA, Sahyoun N, Tannenbaum S, Dallal GE, Dawson-Hughes B: Effect of vitamin D intake on seasonal variations in parathyroid hormone secretion in postmenopausal women. *N Engl J Med* 321:1777, 1989.
362. MacLaughlin J, Holick MF: Aging decreases the capacity of human skin to produce vitamin D_3. *J Clin Invest* 76:1536, 1985.
363. Barragry JM, France MW, Corless D, Gupta SP, Switala S, Boucher BJ, Cohen RD: Intestinal cholecalciferol absorption in the elderly and in younger adults. *Clin Sci Mol Med* 55:213, 1978.
364. Dawson-Hughes B, Dallal GE, Krall EA, Harris S, Sokoll LJ, Falconer G: Effect of vitamin D supplementation on wintertime and overall bone loss in healthy postmenopausal women. *Ann Intern Med* 115:505, 1991.
365. Baker AR, McDonnell DP, Jughes M, Crisp TM, Mangelsdorf DJ, Haussler MR, Pike JW, Shine J, et al: Cloning and expression of full-length cDNA encoding human vitamin D receptor. *Proc Natl Acad Sci USA* 85:3294, 1988.
366. Hughes MR, Malloy PJ, Kieback DK, Kesterson RA, Pike JW, Feldman D, O'Malley BW: Point mutation in the human vitamin D receptor gene associated with hypocalcemic rickets. *Science* 242:1702, 1988.
367. Liao J, Ozono K, Sone T, McDonnell DP, Pike JW: Vitamin D receptor interaction with specific DNA requires a nuclear protein and 1,25-dihydroxyvitamin D_3. *Proc Natl Acad Sci USA* 87:9751, 1990.
368. Ozono K, Sone T, Pike JW: The genomic mechanism of action of 1,25-dihydroxyvitamin D_3. *J Bone Min Res* 6:1021, 1991.
369. Strom M, Sandgren ME, Brown TA, DeLuca HF: 1,25-Dihydroxyvitamin D_3 up-regulates the 1,25-dihydroxyvitamin D_3 receptor in vivo. *Proc Natl Acad Sci USA* 86:9770, 1989.
370. Naveh-Many T, Marx R, Keshet E, Pike JW, Silver J: Regulation of 1,25-dihydroxyvitamin D_3 receptor gene expression by 1,25-dihydroxyvitamin D_3 in the parathyroid in vivo. *J Clin Invest* 86:1968, 1990.
371. Hsieh JC, Jurutka PW, Galligan MA, Terpening CM, Haussler CA, Shimizu YK, Shimizu N, Haussler MR: Human vitamin D receptor is selectively phosphorylated by protein kinase C on serine 51, a residue crucial to its trans-activation function. *J Bone Min Res* 6:S118, 1991.
372. Schüle R, Umesono K, Pike JW, Evans RM: Jun-Fos and receptors for vitamins A and D recognize a common response element in the human osteocalcin gene. *Cell* 61:497, 1990.
372a. Yu VC, Delsert C, Andersen B, Holloway JM, Devary OV, Naar AM, Kim SY, Boutin JM, Glass CK, Rosenfeld MG: RXR beta: a coregulator that enhances binding of retinoic acid, thyroid hormone, and vitamin D receptors to their cognate response elements. *Cell* 67:251, 1991.
372b. Carlberg C, Bendik I, Wyss A, Meier E, Sturzenbecker LJ, Grippo JF, Hunziker W: Two nuclear signalling pathways for vitamin D. *Nature* 361:657, 1993.
373. Barsony J, Marx SJ: Receptor-mediated rapid action of 1 alpha, 25-dihydroxycholecalciferol: Increase of intracellular cGMP in human skin fibroblasts. *Proc Natl Acad Sci USA* 85:1223, 1988.
374. Baran DT, Milne ML: 1,25 Dihydroxyvitamin D increases hepatocyte cytosolic calcium levels: A potential regulator of vitamin D-25-hydroxylase. *J Clin Invest* 77:1622, 1986.
375. Balsan S, Garabédian M, Larchet M, Gorski A-M, Cournot G, Tau C, Bourdeau A, Silve C, et al: Long-term nocturnal calcium infusions can cure rickets and promote normal mineralization in hereditary resistance to 1,25-dihydroxyvitamin D. *J Clin Invest* 77:1661, 1986.
376. Recker RR: Calcium absorption and achlorhydria. *N Engl J Med* 313:70, 1985.
377. Sheikh MS, Santa Ana CA, Nicar MJ, Schiller LR, Fordtran JS: Gastrointestinal absorption of calcium from milk and calcium salts. *N Engl J Med* 317:532, 1987.
378. Heaney RP, Gallagher JC, Johnston CC, Neer R, Parfitt AM, Whedon GD: Calcium nutrition and bone health in the elderly. *Am J Clin Nutr* 36:986, 1982.
379. Favus MJ: Factors that influence absorption and secretion of calcium in the small intestine and colon. *Am J Physiol* 248:G147, 1985.
380. Sheikh MS, Schille LR, Fordtran JS: In vivo intestinal absorption of calcium in humans. *Miner Electrolyte Metab* 16:130, 1990.
381. Bikle DD, Zolock DT, Morrissey RL, Herman RH: Independence of 1,25-dihydroxyvitamin D_3-mediated calcium transport from de novo RNA and protein synthesis. *J Biol Chem* 253:484, 1978.
382. Norman AW: Intestinal calcium absorption: A vitamin D-hormone-mediated adaptive response. *Am J Clin Nutr* 51:290, 1990.
383. Bikle DD, Munson S: 1,25-Dihydroxyvitamin D increases calmodulin binding to specific proteins in the chick duodenal brush border membrane. *J Clin Invest* 76:2312, 1985.
384. Rasmussen H, Matsumoto T, Fontaine O, Goodman DBP: Role of changes in membrane lipid structure in the action of 1,25-dihydroxyvitamin D_3. *Fed Proc* 41:72, 1982.
385. Christakos S, Gabrielides C, Rhoten WB: Vitamin D-dependent calcium binding proteins: Chemistry, distribution, functional considerations, and molecular biology. *Endocr Rev* 10:3, 1989.
386. Gross M, Kumar R: Physiology and biochemistry of vitamin D-dependent calcium binding proteins. *Am J Physiol* 259: F195, 1990.
387. Ghijsen WEJM, Van Os CH: 1,25-Dihydroxyvitamin D_3 regulates ATP-dependent calcium transport in basolateral plasma membranes of rat enterocytes. *Biochim Biophys Acta* 689:170, 1982.
388. Maierhofer WJ, Lemann J Jr, Gray RW, Cheung HS: Dietary calcium and serum 1,25-$(OH)_2$-vitamin D concentrations as determinants of calcium balance in healthy men. *Kidney Int* 26:752, 1984.
389. Cross HS, Debiec H, Peterlik M: Mechanism and regulation of intestinal phosphate absorption. *Miner Electrolyte Metab* 16:115, 1990.
390. Stern PH: Vitamin D and bone. *Kidney Int* 38:S17, 1990.
391. Rowe DW, Kream BE: Regulation of collagen synthesis in fetal rat calvaria by 1,25-dihydroxyvitamin D_3. *J Biol Chem* 257:8009, 1982.
392. McSheehy PMJ, Chambers TJ: 1,25-dihydroxyvitamin D_3 stimulates rat osteoblastic cells to release a soluble factor that increases osteoclastic bone resorption. *J Clin Invest* 80:425, 1987.
393. Abe E, Miyaura C, Tanaka H, Shina Y, Kuribayashi T, Suda S, Nishii Y, DeLuca HF, et al: 1α, 25-dihydroxyvitamin D_3 promotes fusion of mouse alevolar macrophages both by a direct mechanism and by a spleen cell-mediated indirect mechanism. *Proc Natl Acad Sci USA* 80:5583, 1983.
394. Udagawa N, Takahashi N, Akatsu T, Tanaka H, Sasaki T, Nishihara T, Koga T, Martin TJ, et al: Origin of osteoclasts: Mature monocytes and macrophages are capable of differentiating into osteoclasts under a suitable microenviron-

ment prepared by bone marrow-derived stromal cells. *Proc Natl Acad Sci USA* 87:7260, 1990.

395. Bikle DD, Halloran BP, McGalliard-Cone C, Morey-Holton E: Different responses of trabecular and cortical bone to $1,25(OH)_2D_3$ infusion. *Am J Physiol* 259:E715, 1990.
396. Hruska KA, Kurnik BRC: Regulation of renal phosphate transport, in Avioli LV, Krane SM (eds): *Metabolic Bone Disease*. Philadelphia, Saunders, 1990, p 222.
397. Yamamoto M, Kawanobe Y, Takahashi H, Shimazawa E, Kimura S, Ogata E: Vitamin D deficiency and renal calcium transport in the rat. *J Clin Invest* 74:507, 1984.
398. Manolages SC, Hystmyer FG, Yu XP: 1,25-Dihydroxyvitamin D_3 and the immune system. *Proc Soc Exp Biol Med* 191:238, 1989.
399. Hosomi J, Hosoi J, Abe E, Suda T, Kuroki T: Regulation of terminal differentiation of cultured mouse epidermal cells by 1α,25-dihydroxyvitamin D_3. *Endocrinology* 113:1950, 1983.
399a. Bikle DD; Clinical counterpoint: *Vitamin D:* new actions, new analogs, new therapeutic potential. *Endocr Rev* 13:765, 1992.
400. Abe J, Takita Y, Nakano T, Miyuara C, Suda T, Nishii Y: A synthetic analog of vitamin D_3, 22-oxa-1α,25-dihydroxyvitamin D_3, is a potent modulator of in vivo immunoregulating activity without inducing hypercalcemia in mice. *Endocrinology* 124:2654, 1989.
401. Brown AJ, Ritter CR, Finch JL, Morrissey J, Martin KJ, Murayama E, Nishii Y, Slatopolsky E: The noncalcemic analogue of vitamin D, 22-oxacalcitriol, suppresses parathyroid hormone synthesis and secretion. *J Clin Invest* 84:728, 1989.
402. Zhou J-Y, Norman AW, Lubbert M, Collins ED, Uskokovic MR, Koeffler HP: Novel vitamin D analogs that modulate leukemic cell growth and differentiation with little effect on either intestinal calcium absorption or bone calcium mobilization. *Blood* 74:82, 1989.
403. Horst RL, Littledike ET, Tiley JL, Napoli JL: Quantitation of vitamin D and its metabolites and their plasma concentrations in five species of animals. *Anal Biochem* 116:189, 1981.
404. Shepard RM, Horst RL, Hamstra AJ, DeLuca HF: Determination of vitamin D and its metabolites in plasma from normal and anephric man. *Biochem J* 182:55, 1979.
405. Horst RL, Reinhardt TA, Hollis BW: Improved methodology for the analysis of plasma vitamin D metabolites. *Kidney Int* 38:S28, 1990.
406. Delmas PD: Biochemical markers of bone turnover for the clinical assessment of metabolic disease. *Endocrinol Metab Clin North Am* 19:1,1990.
407. Eyre D: New biomarkers of bone resorption (editorial). *J Clin Endocrinol Metab* 74:470, 1992.
408. Delmas PD, Demiaux B, Malaval L, Chapuy MC, Edouard C, Meunier PJ: Serum bone gamma carboxyglutamic acid-containing protein in primary hyperparathyroidism and in malignant hypercalcemia. *J Clin Invest* 77:985, 1986.
409. Schwartz TB: Giants with tunnel vision: The Albright-Collip controversy. *Perspec Biol Med* 34:327, 1991.
410. Schachner SH, Hall A: Parathyroid adenoma and previous head-and-neck irradiation. *Ann Intern Med* 88:804, 1978.
411. Albright F: A page out of the history of hyperparathyroidism. *J Clin Endocrinol Metab* 8:637, 1948.
412. Albright F, Ellsworth R: *Unchartered Seas*. Portland, OR, Kalmia Press, 1990.
413. Collip JB, Pugsley LI, Selye H, Thomson DH: Observations concerning the mechanism of action of parathyroid hormone. *Br J Exp Pathol* 15:335, 1934.
414. Barnicot NA: The local action of the parathyroid and other tissues on bone in intracerebral grafts. *J Anat* 82:233, 1948.
415. Heath H, Hodgson SF, Kennedy MA: Primary hyperparathyroidism: Incidence, morbidity and potential economic impact in a community. *N Engl J Med* 302:189, 1980.
416. Arnold A, Staunton CE, Hyung Goo Kim BS, Gaz RD, Kronenberg HM: Monoclonality and abnormal parathyroid hormone genes in parathyroid adenomas. *N Engl J Med* 318:658, 1988.
417. Marx SJ: Genetic defects in primary hyperparathyroidism. *N Engl J Med* 318:699, 1988.
418. Tissell LE, Carlsson S, Lindberg S, Ragnhult I: Autonomous hyperparathyroidism—a possible late complication of neck radiotherapy. *Acta Chir Scand* 142:367, 1976.
419. Paloyan E, Lawrence AM, Prinz RA, Pickleman JR, Braithwaite S, Brooks MH: Radiation-associated hyperparathyroidism (letter). *Lancet* 1:949, 1977.
420. Arnold A, Kim HG: Clonal loss of one chromosome 11 in a parathyroid adenoma. *J Clin Endocrinol Metab* 69:496, 1989.
421. Bystrom C, Larsson C, Blomberg C, Sandelin K, Falkmer U, Skogseid B, Oberg K, Werner S, et al: Localization of the MEN1 gene to a small region within chromosome 11q13 by deletion mapping in tumors. *Proc Natl Acad Sci USA* 87:1968, 1990.
422. Friedman E, Sakaguchi K, Bale AE, Falchetti A, Streeten E, Zimering MB, Weinstein LS, McBridge WO, et al: Clonality of parathyroid tumors in familial multiple endocrine neoplasia type 1. *N Engl J Med* 321:213, 1989.
423. Bishop JM: The molecular genetics of cancer. *Science* 235:305, 1987.
424. Bishop JM: Molecular themes in oncogenesis. *Cell* 64:235, 1991.
425. Friend SH, Horowitz JM, Gerber MR: Deletions of a DNA sequence in retinoblastomas and mesenchymal tumors: Organization of the sequence and its encoded protein. *Proc Natl Acad Sci USA* 84:9059, 1987.
426. Rosenberg CL, Kim HG, Shows TB, Kronenberg HM, Arnold A: Rearrangment and overexpression of D11S287E, a candidate oncogene, on chromosome 11q13 in benign parathyroid tumors. *Oncogene* 6:449, 1991.
427. Friedman E, Bale AE, Marx SJ, Norton JA, Arnold A, Tu T, Aurbach GD, Spiegel AM: Genetic abnormalities in sporadic parathyroid adenomas. *J Clin Endocrinol Metab* 71:293, 1990.
428. Arnold A, Kim HG, Gaz RD, Eddy RL, Fukushima T, Byers MG, Shows TB, Kronenberg HM: Molecular cloning and chromosomal mapping of DNA rearranged with the parathyroid hormone gene in a parathyroid adenoma. *J Clin Invest* 83:2034, 1989.
429. Lammie GA, Fantl V, Smith R, Schuuring E, Brookes S, Michalides R, Dickson C, Arnold A, et al: D11S287, a putative oncogene on chromosome 11q13, is amplified and expressed in squamous cell and mammary carcinomas, and linked to BCL-1. *Oncogene* 6:439, 1991.
430. Rosenberg CL, Wong E, Petty EM, Bale AE, Tsujimoto Y, Harris NL, Arnold A: PRAD1, a candidate BCL1 oncongene: Mapping and expression in centrocytic lymphoma. *Proc Natl Acad Sci USA* 88:9638, 1991.
431. Motokura T, Bloom T, Kim HG, Jüppner H, Ruderman JV, Kronenberg HM, Arnold A: A novel cyclin encoded by a BCL1-linked candidate oncogene. *Nature* 350:512, 1991.
432. Habener JF, Potts JT Jr: Parathyroid physiology and primary hyperparathyroidism, in Avioli LV, Krane SM (eds): *Metabolic Bone Disease*. New York, Academic Press, 1978, p 1.
433. Roth SI: Recent advances in parathyroid gland pathology. *Am J Med* 50:612, 1971.
434. Brown EM: Four-parameter model of the sigmoidal relationship between parathyroid hormone release and extracellular calcium concentration in normal and abnormal parathyroid tissue. *J Clin Endocrinol Metab* 56:572, 1983.
435. Brown EM, Garner DG, Brennan MF, Marx SJ, Spiegel AM, Attie MF, Downs RW Jr, Doppman JL, et al: Calcium-regulated parathyroid hormone release in primary hyperparathyroidism. *Am J Med* 66:923, 1979.
436. Gittes RR, Radde IC: Experimental hyperparathyroidism from multiple isologous parathyroid transplants: Homo-

static effect of simultaneous thyroid transplants. *Endocrinology* 78:1015, 1966.

437. Mundy GR, Cove DH, Fisken R: Primary hyperparathyroidism: Changes in the pattern of clinical presentation. *Lancet* 1:1317, 1980.
438. Barreras RF: Calcium and gastric secretion. *Gastroenterology* 64:1168, 1973.
439. Ostrow JD, Blandshard G, Gray SJ: Peptic ulcer in primary hyperparathyroidism. *Am J Med* 24:769, 1960.
440. Wilson SD, Singh RB, Kalkhoff RK, Go VLW: Does hyperparathyroidism cause hypergastrinemia? *Surgery* 80:231, 1976.
441. Bess MA, Edis AJ, van Heerden JA: Hyperparathyroidism and pancreatitis. *JAMA* 243:246, 1980.
442. Joborn C, Hetta J, Lind L, Rastad J, Akerstrom G, Ljunghall S: Self-rated psychiatric symptoms in patients operated on because of primary hyperparathyroidism and in patients with long-standing mild hypercalcemia. *Surgery* 105:72, 1989.
443. Wishart J, Horowitz M, Need A, Nordin BEC: Relationship between forearm and vertebral mineral density in postmenopausal women with primary hyperparathyroidism. *Arch Intern Med* 150:1329, 1990.
444. Mautalen C, Reyes HR, Ghiringhelli G, Fromm G: Cortical bone mineral content in primary hyperparathyroidism: Changes after parathyroidectomy. *Acta Endocrinol (Copenh)* 111:494, 1986.
445. Christiansen P, Steiniche T, Mosekilde L, Hessov I, Melsen F: Primary hyperparathyroidism: Changes in trabecular bone remodeling following surgical treatment—evaluated by histomorphometric methods. *Bone* 11:75, 1990.
446. Potts JT Jr: Management of asymptomatic hyperparathyroidism. *J Clin Endocrinol Metab* 70:1489, 1990.
447. Parisien M, Silverberg SJ, Shane E, Dempster DW, Bilezikian JP: Bone disease in primary hyperparathyroidism. *Endocrinol Metab Clin N Amer* 19:19, 1990.
448. Bilezikian JP: Surgery or no surgery for primary hyperparathyroidism. *Ann Intern Med* 102:402, 1985.
449. Silverberg SJ, Shane E, Jacobs TP, Siris ES, Gartenberg F, Seldin D, Clemens TL, Bilezikian JP: Nephrolithiasis and bone involvement in primary hyperparathyroidism. *Am J Med* 89:327, 1990.
450. Cogan MG, Covey CM, Arieff AI, Wisniewski A, Clark OH, Lazarowitz V, Leach W: Central nervous system manifestations of hyperparathyroidism. *Am J Med* 65:963, 1978.
451. Patten BM, Bilezikian JP, Mallette LE, Prince A, Engel WK, Aurbach GD: Neuromuscular disease in primary hyperparathyroidism. *Ann Intern Med* 80:182, 1974.
452. Turken SA, Cafferty M, Silverberg SJ, de la Cruz L, Cimino C, Lange DJ, Lovelace RE, Bilezikian JP: Neuromuscular involvement in mild, asymptomatic primary hyperparathyroidism. *Am J Med* 87:553, 1989.
453. Goldsmith RE, Sizemore GW, Chen IW, Zalme E, Altemeier WA: Familial hyperparathyroidism. *Ann Intern Med* 84:36, 1976.
454. Law WM, Hodgson SF, Heath H: Autosomal recessive inheritance of familial hyperparathyroidism. *N Engl J Med* 309:650, 1983.
455. Wermer P: Genetic aspects of adenomatosis of endocrine glands. *Am J Med* 16:363, 1954.
456. Larsson C, Skogseid B, Oberg K, Nakamura Y, Nordenskjold M: Multiple endocrine neoplasia type 1 maps to chromosome 11 and is lost in insulinoma. *Nature* 332:85, 1988.
457. Keiser HR, Beaven MA, Doppman J, Wells S, Buja LM: Sipple's syndrome: Medullary thyroid carcinoma, pheochromocytoma, and parathyroid disease. *Ann Intern Med* 78:1973.
458. Sizemore GW, Heath H, Carney JA: Multiple endocrine neoplasia type 2. *Clin Endocrinol Metab* 9:299, 1980.
459. Norum RA, Lafreniere RG, O'Neal LW: Linkage of the multiple endocrine neoplasia type 2B gene (MEN2B) to chromosome 10 markers linked to MEN2A. *Genomics* 8:313, 1990.
460. Marx SJ, Spiegel AM, Levine MA, Rizzoli RE, Lasker RD, Santora AC, Downs RW, Aurbach GD: Familial hypocalciuric hypercalcemia. *N Engl J Med* 307:416, 1982.
461. Marx SJ, Attie MF, Levine MA, Spiegel AM, Downs RW, Lasker RD: The hypocalciuric or benign variant of familial hypercalcemia: Clinical and biochemical features in fifteen kindreds. *Medicine (Baltimore)* 60:397, 1981.
462. Law WM, Heath H: Familial benign hypercalcemia (hypocalciuric hypercalcemia). *Ann Intern Med* 102:511, 1985.
463. Pollak MR, Brown EM, Chou YHW, Hebert SC, Marx SJ, Steinmann B, Levi T, Seidman CE, Seidman JG: Mutations in the human Ca^{2+}-sensing receptor gene cause familial hypocalciuric hypercalcemia and neonatal severe hyperparathyroidism. *Cell* 75:1297, 1993.
464. Pollak MR, Chou YHW, Marx SJ, Steinmann B, Cole DEC, Brandi ML, Papapoulos SE, Menko FH, Hendy GN, Brown EM, Seidman CE, Seidman JG: Familial hypocalciuric hypercalcemia and neonatal severe hyperparathyroidism: Effects of mutant gene dosage on phenotype. *J Clin Invest* 93:1108, 1994.

464a. Clapham DE: Mutations in G protein-linked receptors: Novel insights on disease. *Cell* 75:1237, 1993.

465. Broadus AE, Horst RL, Littledike ET, Mahaffey JE, Rasmussen H: Primary hyperparathyroidism with intermittent hypercalcemia: Serial observations and simple diagnosis by means of an oral calcium tolerance test. *Clin Endocrinol (Oxf)* 12:225, 1980.
466. Winzelberg GG: Parathyroid imaging. *Ann Intern Med* 107:64, 1989.
467. Mallette LE, Gomez L, Fisher RG: Parathyroid angiography: A review of current knowledge and guidelines for clinical application. *Endocr Rev* 2:124, 1981.
468. Eisenberg H, Pallotta J, Sacks B, Brickman AS: Parathyroid localization, three-dimensional modeling, and percutaneous ablation techniques. *Endocrinol Metab Clin North Am* 18:659, 1989.
469. CDC Panel: Diagnosis and management of asymptomatic primary hyperparathyroidism: Consensus development conference statement. *Ann Intern Med* 114:593, 1991.
470. Pallotta JA, Sacks BA, Moller DE, Eisenberg H: Arteriographic ablation of cervical parathyroid adenomas. *J Clin Endocrinol Metab* 69:1249, 1989.
471. Rizzoli R, Green J III, Marx SJ: Primary hyperparathyroidism in familial multiple endocrine neoplasia type 1: Long term follow-up of serum calcium levels after parathyroidectomy. *Am J Med* 78:467, 1985.
472. Wang C: Parathyroid re-exploration: A clinical and pathological study of 112 cases. *Ann Surg* 186:140, 1977.
473. Niederle B, Roka R, Brennan MF: The transplantation of parathyroid tissue in man: Development, indications, techniques, and results. *Endocr Rev* 3:245, 1982.
474. Wells SA, Ellis GJ, Gunnells JC, Schneider AB, Sherwood LM: Parathyroid autotransplantation in primary parathyroid hyperplasia. *N Engl J Med* 295:57, 1976.
475. Cope O: Hyperparathyroidism—too little, too much surgery? *N Engl J Med* 295:100, 1976.
476. Schantz A, Castleman B: Parathyroid carcinoma. *Cancer* 31:600, 1973.
477. Shane E, Bilezikian JP: Parathyroid carcinoma: A review of 62 patients. *Endocr Rev* 3:218, 1982.
478. Brasier AR, Nussbaum SR: Hungry bone syndrome: Clinical and biochemical predicators of its occurrence after parathyroid surgery. *Am J Med* 84:654, 1988.
479. Roberts WC, Waller BF: Effect of chronic hypercalcemia on the heart: An analysis of 18 necropsy patients. *Am J Med* 71:371, 1981.
480. Bilezikian JP: The medical management of primary hyperparathyroidism. *Ann Intern Med* 96:198, 1982.
481. Selby PL, Peacock M: Ethinyl estradiol and norethindrone in the treatment of primary hyperparathyroidism in postmenopausal women. *N Engl J Med* 314:1481, 1986.

482. Coe FL, Favus MJ, Parks JH: Is estrogen preferable to surgery for postmenopausal women with primary hyperparathyroidism? *N Engl J Med* 314:1508, 1986.
483. Horowitz M, Wishart J, Need AG, Morris H, Philcox J, Nordin BEC: Treatment of postmenopausal hyperparathyroidism with norethindrone. *Arch Intern Med* 147:681, 1987.
484. Broadus AE, Magee JS, Mallette LE, Horst RL, Lang R, Jensen PS, Gertner JM, Baron R: A detailed evaluation of oral phosphate therapy in selected patients with primary hyperparathyroidism. *J Clin Endocrinol Metab* 56:953, 1983.
485. Caro JF, Castro JC, Glennon JA: Effect of long-term propanolol administration on parathyroid hormone and calcium concentration in primary hyperparathyroidism. *Ann Intern Med* 91:740, 1979.
486. Glaser B, Kraiem Z, Rotem M, Gonda M, Bernheim J, Sheinfeld M: Effect of acute cimetidine administration on indices of parathyroid hormone action in healthy subjects and patients with primary and secondary hyperparathyroidism. *J Clin Endocrinol Metab* 59:993, 1984.
487. Glover D, Riley L, Carmichael K, Spar B, Glick J, Kligerman MM, Agus ZS, Slatopolsky E, et al: Hypocalcemia and inhibition of parathyroid hormone secretion after administration of WR-2721 (a radioprotective and chemoprotective agent). *N Engl J Med* 309:1137, 1983.
488. Shane E, Baquiran DC, Bilezikian JP: Effects of dichloromethylene diphosphate on serum and urinary calcium in primary hyperparathyroidism. *Ann Intern Med* 95:23, 1981.
489. Attie MF: Bisphosphonate therapy for osteoporosis. *Hosp Pract* 26:87, 1991.
490. Pedrazzoni M, Palummeri E, Ciotti G, Davoli L, Pioli G, Girasole G, Passeri M: Short-term effects on bone and mineral metabolism of 4-amino-1-hydroxybutylidene-1,1-diphosphonate (ABDP) in Paget's disease of bone. *Bone Min* 7:301, 1989.
491. Thompson DD, Seedor JG, Weinreb M, Rosini S, Rodan GA: Aminohydroxybutane bisphosphonate inhibits bone loss due to immobilization in rats. *J Bone Min Res* 5:279, 1990.
492. Warrell RP Jr, Israel R, Frisone M, Synder T, Gaynor JJ, Bockman RS: Gallium nitrate for acute treatment of cancer-related hypercalcemia: A randomized, double-blind comparison to calcitonin. *Ann Intern Med* 108:669, 1988.
493. Warrell RP Jr, Issacs M, Alcock NW, Bockman RS: Gallium nitrate for treatment of refractory hypercalcemia from parathyroid carcinoma. *Ann Intern Med* 107:683, 1987.
494. Zondek H, Petow H, Siebert W: Die bedeutung der calciumbestimmung im blute für die diagnose der niereninsuffizientz. *Z Klin Med* 99:129, 1924.
495. Case ReportMGH: Case 27461. *N Engl J Med* 225:789, 1941.
496. Plimpton CH, Gellhorn A: Hypercalcemia in malignant disease without evidence of bone destruction. *Am J Med* 21:750, 1956.
497. Lafferty FW: Pseudohyperparathyroidism. *Medicine (Baltimore)* 45:247, 1966.
498. Benson RC, Riggs BL, Pickard BM, Arnaud CD: Radioimmunoassay of parathyroid hormone in hypercalcemic patients with malignant disease. *Am J Med* 56:821, 1974.
499. Stewart AF, Horst R, Deftos LJ, Cadman EC, Lang R, Broadus AE: Biochemical evaluation of patients with cancer-associated hypercalcemia. *N Engl J Med* 303:1377, 1980.
500. Fisken RA, Heath DA, Bold AM: Hypercalcaemia—a hospital survey. *Q J Med* 49:405, 1980.
501. Ralston SH, Gallacher SJ, Patel U, Campbell J, Boyle IT: Cancer-associated hypercalcemia: Morbidity and mortality. *Ann Intern Med* 112:499, 1990.
502. Yasuda T, Banville D, Hendy GN, Goltzman D: Characterization of the human parathyroid hormone-like peptide gene: Functional and evolutionary aspects. *J Biol Chem* 264:7720, 1989.
503. Mangin M, Ikeda K, Dreyer BE, Milstone L, Broadus AE: Two distinct tumor-derived, parathyroid hormone-like peptides result from alternative ribonucleic acid splicing. *Mol Endocrinol* 2:1049, 1988.
504. Mangin M, Ikeda K, Dreyer BE, Broadus AE: Isolation and characterization of the human parathyroid hormone-like peptide gene. *Proc Natl Acad Sci USA* 86:2408, 1989.
505. Orloff JJ, Wu TL, Stewart AF: Parathyroid hormone-like proteins: Biochemical responses and receptor interactions. *Endocr Rev* 10:476, 1989.
506. Strewler GJ, Nissenson RA: Peptide mediators of hypercalcemia in malignancy. *Annu Rev Med* 41:35, 1990.
507. Drucker DJ, Asa SL, Henderson J, Goltzman D: The parathyroid hormone-like peptide gene is expressed in the normal and neoplastic human endocrine pancreas. *Mol Endocrinol* 3:1589, 1989.
508. Schermer DT, Chan SD-H, Bruce R, Nissenson RA, Wood WI, Strewler GJ: Chicken parathyroid hormone-related protein and its expression during embryologic development. *J Bone Min Res* 6:149, 1991.
509. Chan SD-H, Strewler GJ, King KL, Nissenson RA: Expression of a parathyroid hormone-like protein and its receptor during differentiation of embryonal carcinoma cells. *Mol Endocrinol* 4:638, 1990.
510. Budayr AA, Nissenson RA, Klein RF, Pun KK, Clark OH, Diep D, Arnaud CD, Strewler GJ: Increased serum levels of a parathyroid hormone-like protein in malignancy-associated hypercalcemia. *Ann Intern Med* 111:807, 1989.
511. Burtis WJ, Brady TG, Orloff JJ, Ersbak JB, Warrell RP Jr, Olson BR, Wu TL, Mitnick ME, et al: Immunochemical characterization of circulating parathyroid hormone-related protein in patients with humoral hypercalcemia of cancer. *N Engl J Med* 322:1106, 1990.
512. Kukreja SC, Shevrin DH, Wimbiscus SA, Ebeling PR, Danks JA, Rodda CP, Wood WI, Martin TJ: Antibodies to parathyroid hormone-related protein lower serum calcium in athymic mouse models. *J Clin Invest* 82:1798, 1988.
513. Hirschel-Scholz S, Caverzasio J, Rizzoli R, Bonjour J-P: Normalization of hypercalcemia associated with a decrease in renal calcium reabsorption in Leydig cell tumor-bearing rats treated with WR-2721. *J Clin Invest* 78:319, 1986.
514. Harinck HIJ, Bijvot OLM, Plantingh AST, Body J-J, Elte JWF, Sleeboom HP, Wildiers J, Neijt JP: Role of bone and kidney in tumor-induced hypercalcemia and its treatment with bisphosphonate and sodium chloride. *Am J Med* 82:1133, 1987.
515. Yamamoto I, Kitamura N, Aoki J, Kawamura J, Dokoh S, Morita R, Torizuka K: Circulating 1,25-dihydroxyvitamin D concentrations in patients with renal cell carcinoma-associated hypercalcemia are rarely suppressed. *J Clin Endocrinol Metab* 64:175, 1987.
516. Fukumoto S, Matsumoto T, Yamoto H, Kawashima H, Ueyama Y, Taaoki N, Ogata E: Suppression of serum 1,25-dihydroxyvitamin D in humoral hypercalcemia of malignancy is caused by elaboration of a factor that inhibits renal 1,25-dihydroxyvitamin D_3 production. *Endocrinology* 124:2057, 1989.
517. Stewart AF, Vignery A, Silverglate A, Ravin ND, LiVolsi V, Broadus AE, Baron R: Quantitative bone histomorphometry in humoral hypercalcemia of malignancy: Uncoupling of bone cell activity. *J Clin Endocrinol Metab* 55:219, 1982.
518. Bender RA, Hansen H: Hypercalcemia in bronchogenic carcinoma. *Ann Intern Med* 80:205, 1974.
519. Ralston S, Gardner MD, Fogelman I, Boyle IT: Hypercalcemia and metastic bone disease: Is there a causal link? *Lancet* 2:903, 1982.
520. Yoshimoto K, Yamasaki R, Sakai H, Tezuka U, Takahashi M, Iizuka M, Sekiya T, Saito S: Extopic production of parathyroid hormone by small cell lung cancer in a patient with hypercalcemia. *J Clin Endocrinol Metab* 68:976, 1989.
521. Strewler GJ, Budayr AA, Clark OH, Nissenson RA: Production of parathyroid hormone by a malignant nonparathy-

roid tumor in a hypercalcemic patient. *J Endocrinol Metab* 76:1373, 1993.
522. Nussbaum SR, Gaz RD, Arnold A: Hypercalcemia and ectopic secretion of parathyroid hormone by an ovarian carcinoma with rearrangement of the gene for parathyroid hormone. *N Engl J Med* 323:1324, 1990.
523. Brereton HD, Halushka PV, Alexander RW, Mason DM, Keiser HR, DeVita VT Jr: Indomethacin-responsive hypercalcemia in a patient with renal-cell adenocarcinoma. *N Engl J Med* 291:83, 1974.
524. Lingärde F, Zettervall O: Hypercalcemia and normal ionized serum calcium in a case of myelomatosis. *Ann Intern Med* 37:396, 1973.
525. Heyburn PJ, Child JA, Peacock M: Relative importance of renal failure and increased bone resorption in the hypercalcaemia of myelomatosis. *J Clin Pathol* 34:54, 1981.
526. Bentzel CJ, Carbone PP, Rosenberg L, Bean M: The effect of prednisone on calcium metabolism and Ca^{47} kinetics in patients with multiple myeloma and hypercalcemia. *J Clin Invest* 43:2132, 1964.
527. Valentin-Opran A, Charon S, Meunier PJ, Edouard CM, Arlot ME: Quantitative histology of myeloma-induced bone changes. *Br J Haematol* 52:602, 1982.
528. Mundy G: Hypercalcemic factors other than parathyroid hormone-related protein. *Endocrinol Metab Clin North Am* 18:795, 1989.
529. Dewhirst FE, Stashenko PP, Mole JE, Tsurumachi T: Purification and partial sequence of human osteoclast-activating factor: Identity with interleukin 1beta. *J Immunol* 135:2562, 1985.
530. Garrett IR, Durie BGM, Nedwin GE, Gillespie A, Bringman T, Sabatini M, Bertolini DR, Mundy GR: Production of lymphotoxin, a bone-resorbing cytokine, by cultured human myeloma cells. *N Engl J Med* 317:526, 1987.
531. Kawano M, Yamamoto I, Iwato K, Tanaka H, Asaoku H, Tanabe O, Ishikawa H, Nobuyoshi M, et al: Interleukin-1 beta rather than lymphotoxin as the major bone resorbing activity in human multiple myeloma. *Blood* 73:1646, 1989.
532. Canellos GP: Hypercalcemia in malignant lymphoma and leukemia. *Ann NY Acad Sci* 230:240, 1974.
533. Breslau NA, McGuire JL, Zerwekh JE, Frenkel EP, Pak CYC: Hypercalcemia associated with increased serum calcitriol levels in three patients with lymphoma. *Ann Intern Med* 100:1, 1984.
534. Rosenthal N, Insogna KL, Godsall JW, Smaldone L, Waldron JA, Stewart AF: Elevations in circulating 1,25-dihydroxyvitamin D in three patients with lymphoma-associated hypercalcemia. *J Clin Endocrinol Metab* 60:29, 1985.
535. Adams JS, Fernandez M, Gacad MA, Gill PS, Endres DB, Rasheed S, Singer F: Vitamin D metabolite-mediated hypercalcemia and hypercalciura patients with AIDS- and non-AIDS-associated lymphoma. *Blood* 73:235, 1989.
536. Dodd RC, Winkler CF, Williams ME, Bunn PA, Gray TK: Calcitriol levels in hypercalcemic patients with adult T-cell lymphoma. *Arch Intern Med* 146:1971, 1986.
537. Canfield RE: Etidronate disodium: A new therapy for hypercalcemia of malignancy. *Am J Med* 82(2A):1, 1987.
538. Gucalp R, Ritch P, Wiernik PH, Sarma PR, Keller A, Richman SP, Tauer K, Neidhart J, et al: Comparative study of pamidronate disodium and etidronate disodium in the treatment of cancer-related hypercalcemia. *J Clin Oncol* 10:134, 1992.
539. Ralston SH, Patel U, Fraser WD, Gallacher SJ, Dryburgh FJ, Cowan RA, Boyle IT: Comparison of three intravenous bisphosphates in cancer-associated hypercalcemia. *Lancet* 2:1180, 1989.
540. Singer FR, Ritch PS, Lad TE, Ringenberg QS, Schiller JH, Recker RR, Ryzen E: Treatment of hypercalcemia of malignancy with intravenous etidronate. *Arch Intern Med* 151: 471, 1991.
541. Schiller JH, Rasmussen P, Benson AB, Witte RS, Bockman RS, Harvey HA, Siris ES, Citrin DL, et al: Maintenance etidronate in the prevention of malignancy-associated hypercalcemia. *Arch Intern Med* 147:963, 1987.
542. Adami S, Bolzicco GP, Rizzo A, Salvagno G, Bertoldo F, Rossini M, Suppi R, Lo Cascio V: The use of dichloromethylene bisphonate and aminobutane bisphosphonate in hypercalcemia of malignancy. *Bone Min* 2:395, 1987.
543. Ralston SH, Drybaugh FJ, Cowan RA, Gardner MD, Jenkins AS, Boyle IT: Comparison of aminohydroxypropylidene diphosphonate, mithramycin, and corticosteroids/calcitonin in treatment of cancer-associated hypercalcemia. *Lancet* 2:907, 1985.
544. Henneman PH, Dempsey EF, Carroll EL, Albright F: The cause of hypercalciuria in sarcoid and its treatment with cortisone and sodium phytate. *J Clin Invest* 35:1229, 1956.
545. Bell NH, Stern PH, Pantzer E, Sinha TK, DeLuca HF: Evidence that increased circulating 1α,25-dihydroxyvitamin D is the probable cause for abnormal calcium metabolism in sarcoidosis. *J Clin Invest* 64:218, 1979.
546. Barbour GL, Coburn JW, Slatopolsky E, Norman AW, Horts RL: Hypercalcemia in an anephric patient with sarcoidosis: Evidence for extrarenal generation of 1,25-dihydroxyvitamin D. *N Engl J Med* 305:440, 1981.
547. Adams JS, Sharma OP, Gacad MA, Singer FR: Metabolism of 25-hydroxyvitamin D_3 by cultured pulmonary alveolar macrophages in sarcoidosis. *J Clin Invest* 72:1856, 1983.
548. Stern PH, De Olazabal J, Bell NH: Evidence for abnormal regulation of circulating 1α,25-dihydroxyvitamin D in patients with sarcoidosis and normal calcium metabolism. *J Clin Invest* 66:852, 1980.
549. DeRemee RA, Lufkin EG, Rohrbach MS: Serum angiotensin-converting enzyme activity. *Arch Intern Med* 145:677, 1985.
550. Adams JS, Diz MM, Sharma OP: Effective reduction in the serum 1,25-dihydroxyvitamin D and calcium concentration in sarcoidosis-associated hypercalcemia with short-course chloroquine therapy. *Ann Intern Med* 111:437, 1989.
551. Abbasi AA, Chemplavil JK, Farah S, Muller BF, Arnstein AR: Hypercalcemia in active pulmonary tuberculosis. *Ann Intern Med* 90:324, 1979.
552. Gkonos PJ, London R, Hendler ED: Hypercalcemia and elevated 1,25-dihydroxyvitamin D levels in a patient with end-stage renal disease and active tuberculosis. *N Engl J Med* 311:1683, 1984.
553. Epstein S, Stern PH, Bell NH, Dowdeswell I, Turner RT: Evidence for abnormal regulation of circulating 1α,25-dihydroxyvitamin D in patients with pulmonary tuberculosis and normal calcium metabolism. *Calcif Tissue Int* 36:541, 1984.
554. Kantarjian HM, Saad MF, Estey EH, Sellin RV, Samaan NA: Hypercalcemia in disseminated candidiasis. *Am J Med* 74:721, 1983.
555. Parker MS, Dokoh S, Woolfenden JM, Buchsbaum HW: Hypercalcemia in coccidioidomycosis. *Am J Med* 76:341, 1984.
556. Murray JJ, Heim CR: Hypercalcemia in disseminated histoplasmosis. *Am J Med* 78:881, 1985.
557. Ryzen E, Rea TH, Singer FR: Hypercalcemia and abnormal 1,25-dihydroxyvitamin D concentrations in leprosy. *Am J Med* 84:325, 1988.
558. Kozeny GA, Barbato AL, Bansal VK, Vertuno LL, Hano JE: Hypercalcemia associated with silicone-induced granulomas. *N Engl J Med* 311:1103, 1984.
559. Mosekilde L, Christensen MS: Decreased parathyroid function in hyperthyroidism: Interrelationships between serum parathyroid hormone, calcium-phosphorus metabolism and thyroid function. *Acta Endocrinol (Copenh)* 84:566, 1977.
560. Bouillon R, Muls E, DeMoor P: Influence of thyroid function on the serum concentration of 1,25-dihydroxyvitamin D. *J Clin Endocrinol Metab* 51:793, 1980.
561. Mosekilde L, Melsen F, Bagger JP, Myhre-Jensen O, Sorensen NS: Bone changes in hyperthyroidism: Interrela-

tionships between bone morphometry, thyroid function and calcium-phosphorus metabolism. *Acta Endocrinol (Copenh)* 85:515, 1977.
562. Walser M, Robinson BHB, Duckett JW Jr: The hypercalcemia of adrenal insufficiency. *J Clin Invest* 42:456, 1963.
563. Muls E, Bouillon R, Boelaert J, Lamberigts G, Van Imschoot S, Daneels R, De Moor P: Etiology of hypercalcemia in a patient with Addison's disease. *Calcif Tissue Int* 34:523, 1982.
564. Stewart AF, Hoecker JL, Mallette LE, Segre GV, Amatruda TT: Hypercalcemia in pheochromocytoma. *Ann Intern Med* 102:776, 1985.
565. Kimura S, Nishimura Y, Yamaguchi K, Nagasaki K, Shimada K, Uchida H: A case of pheochromocytoma producing parathyroid hormone-related protein and presenting with hypercalcemia. *J Clin Endocrinol Metab* 70:1559, 1990.
566. Ikeda K, Arnold A, Mangin M, Kinder B, Vydelingum NA, Brennan MF, Broadus AE: Expression of transcripts encoding a parathyroid hormone-related peptide in abnormal human parathyroid tissues. *J Clin Endocrinol Metab* 69:1240, 1989.
567. Stote RM, Smith LH, Wilson DM, Dube WJ, Goldsmith RS, Arnaud CD: Hydrochlorothiazide effects on serum calcium and immunoreactive parathyroid hormone concentrations. *Ann Intern Med* 77:587, 1972.
568. Christensson T, Hellström K, Wengle B: Hypercalcemia and primary hyperparathyroidism. *Arch Intern Med* 137:1138, 1977.
569. Porter RH, Cox BG, Heaney D, Hostetter TH, Stinbaugh BJ, Suki WN: Treatment of hypoparathyroid patients with chlorthalidone. *N Engl J Med* 298:577, 1978.
570. Kelepouris E, Agus ZS: Effects of diuretics on calcium and phosphate transport. *Semin Nephrol* 8:273, 1988.
571. Koppel MH, Massry SG, Shinaberger JH, Hartenbower DL, Coburn JW: Thiazide-induced rise in serum calcium and magnesium in patients on maintenance hemodialysis. *Ann Intern Med* 72:895, 1970.
571a. Jacobus CH, Holick MF, Shao Q, Chen TC, Holm IA, Kolodny JM, Fuleihan GE, Seely EW: Hypervitaminosis D associated with drinking milk. *N Engl J Med* 326:1173, 1992.
572. Mawer EB, Hann JT, Berry JL, Davies M: Vitamin D metabolism in patients intoxicated with ergocalciferol. *Clin Sci* 68:135, 1985.
573. Mason RS, Lissner D, Grunstein HS, Posen S: A simplified assay for dihydroxylated vitamin D metabolites in human serum: Application to hyper- and hypovitaminosis D. *Clin Chem* 26:444, 1980.
574. Frame B, Jackson CE, Reynolds WA, Umphrey JE: Hypercalcemia and skeletal effects in chronic hypervitaminosis A. *Ann Intern Med* 80:44, 1974.
575. Farrington K, Miller P, Varghese Z, Baillod RA, Moorhead JF: Vitamin A toxicity and hypercalcaemia in chronic renal failure. *Br Med J* 282:1999, 1981.
576. Christiansen C, Baastrup PC, Lindgreen P, Transbol I: Endocrine effects of lithium: II. "Primary" hyperparathyroidism. *Acta Endocrinol (Copenh)* 88:528, 1978.
576a. Saxe AW, Gibson G: Lithium increases tritated thymidine uptake by abnormal human parathyroid tissue. *Surgery* 110:1067, 1991.
576b. Mellette LE, Khouri K, Zengotita H, Hollis BW, Malini S: Lithium treatment increases intact and midregion parathyroid hormone and parathyroid volume. *J Clin Endocrinol Metab* 68:654, 1989.
577. Mallette LE, Eichhorn E: Effects of lithium carbonate on human calcium metabolism. *Arch Intern Med* 146:770, 1986.
578. Orwoll ES: The milk-alkali syndrome: Current concepts. *Ann Intern Med* 97:242, 1982.
579. Kapsner P, Langsdorf L, Marcus R, Kraemer FB, Hoffman AR: Milk-alkali syndrome in patients treated with calcium carbonate after cardiac transplantation. *Arch Intern Med* 146:1965, 1986.
580. Minaire P, Meunier P, Edouard C, Bernard J, Courpron P, Bourret J: Quantitative histological data on disuse osteoporosis—comparison with biological data. *Calcif Tissue Res* 17:57, 1974.
581. Stewart AF, Adler M, Byers CM, Segre GV, Broadus AE: Calcium homeostasis in immobilization: An example of resorptive hypercalciuria. *N Engl J Med* 306:1136, 1982.
582. Merli GJ, McElwain GE, Adler AG, Martin JH, Roberts JDD, Schnall B, Ditunno JF: Immobilization hypercalcemia in acture spinal cord injury treated with etidronate. *Arch Intern Med* 144:1286, 1984.
583. Llach F, Felsenfeld AJ, Haussler MR: The pathophysiology of altered calcium metabolism in rhabdomyolysis-induced acute renal failure. *N Engl J Med* 305:117, 1981.
584. Forster J, Querusio L, Burchard KW, Gann DS: Hypercalcemia in critically ill surgical patients. *Ann Surg* 202:512, 1985.
585. Gerhardt A, Greenberg A, Reilly JJ Jr, Van Thiel DH: Hypercalcemia: A complication of advanced chronic liver disease. *Arch Intern Med* 147:274, 1987.
586. Garabédian M, Jacqz E, Guillozo H, Grimberg R, Guillot M, Gagnadoux M-F, Broyer M, Lenoir G, et al: Elevated plasma 1,25-dihydroxyvitamin D concentrations in infants with hypercalcemia and an elfin facies. *N Engl J Med* 312:948, 1985.
587. Layzer RB: *Neuromuscular Manifestations of Systemic Disease.* Philadelphia, Davis, 1985.
588. Edmondson JW, Brashear RE, Li T-K: Tetany: Quantitative interrelationships between calcium and alkalosis. *Am J Physiol* 228:1082, 1975.
589. Illum F, Dupont E: Prevalence of CT-detected calcification in the basal ganglia in idiopathic hypoparathyroidism and pseudohypoparathyroidism. *Neuroradiology* 27:32, 1985.
590. Connor TB, Rosen BL, Blaustein MP, Applefeld MM, Doyle LA: Hypocalcemia precipitating congestive heart failure. *N Engl J Med* 307:869, 1982.
591. Stewart AF, Battaglini-Sabetta J, Milstone LM: Hypocalcemia-induced psoriasis of von Zumbusch: New experience with an old syndrome. *Ann Intern Med* 100:677, 1984.
592. Eisenberg E: Effect of serum calcium level and parathyroid extracts on phosphate and calcium excretion in hypoparathyroid patients. *J Clin Invest* 44:942, 1965.
593. Parfitt AM: The incidence of hypoparathyroid tetany after thyroid operations: Relationship to age, extent of resection and surgical experience. *Med J Aust* 1:1103, 1971.
594. Parfitt AM: Surgical, idiopathic, and other varieties of parathyroid hormone-deficient hypoparathyroidism, in DeGroot LJ (ed): *Endocrinology.* Philadelphia, Saunders, 1989, p 1049.
595. Parfitt AM: The spectrum of hypoparathyroidism. *J Clin Endocrinol Metab* 34:152, 1972.
596. Michie W, Duncan T, Hamer-Hodges DW, Brewsher PD, Stowers JM, Pegg CAS, Hems G, Hedley AJ: Mechanism of hypocalcemia after thyroidectomy for thyrotoxicosis. *Lancet* 1:508, 1971.
597. Brezis M, Shalev O, Leibel B, Bernheim J, Ben-Ishay D: Phosphorus retention and hypoparathyroidism associated with transfusional iron overload in thalassaemia. *Min Elect Metab* 4:57, 1980.
598. Carpenter TO, Carnes DL Jr, Anast CS: Hypoparathyroidism in Wilson's disease. *N Engl J Med* 309:873, 1983.
599. Burch WM, Posillico JT: Hypoparathyroidism after ^{131}I therapy with subsequent return of parathyroid function. *J Clin Endocrinol Metab* 57:398, 1983.
600. Anast CS, Winnocker JL, Forte LR, Burns TW: Impaired release of parathyroid hormone in magnesium deficiency. *J Clin Endorinol Metab* 42:707, 1976.
601. Estep H, Shaw WA, Waltington C, Hobe W, Holland SG, Tucker J: Hypocalcemia due to hypomagnesemia and reversible parathyroid hormone unresponsiveness. *J Clin Endocrinol Metab* 29:842, 1969.

602. Rude RK, Oldham SB, Singer FR: Functional hypoparathyroidism and parathyroid hormone end-organ resistance in human magnesium deficiency. *Clin Endocrinol (Oxf)* 5:209, 1976.
603. Rude RK, Adams JS, Ryzen E, Endres DB, Niimi H, Horst RL, Haddad JG, Singer FR: Low serum concentrations of 1,25 dihydroxyvitamin D in human magnesium deficiency. *J Clin Endocrinol Metab* 61:933, 1985.
604. Neufeld M, MacLaren NK, Blizzard RM: Two types of autoimmune Addison's disease associated with different polyglandular autoimmune (PGA) syndromes. *Medicine (Baltimore)* 60:355, 1981.
605. Blizzard RM, Chee D, Davis W: The incidence of parathyroid and other antibodies in the sera of patients with idiopathic hypoparathyroidism. *Clin Exp Immunol* 1:119, 1966.
606. Conley ME, Beckwith JB, Mancer JFK, Tenckhoff L: The spectrum of the DiGeorge syndrome. *J Pediatr* 94:883, 1979.
607. Mallette LE, Cooper JB, Kirkland JL: Transient congenital hypoparathyroidism: Possible association with anomalies of the pulmonary valve. *J Pediatr* 101:928, 1982.
608. Chisaka O, Capecchi MR: Regionally restricted developmental defects resulting from targeted disruption of the mouse homeobox gene hox-1.5. *Nature* 350:473, 1991.
609. Salle BL, Delvin E, Glorieux F, David L: Human neonatal hypocalcemia. *Biol Neonate* 58(Suppl 1):22, 1990.
610. Ahn TG, Antonarakis SE, Kronenberg HM, Igarashi T, Levie MA: Familial isolated hypoparathyroidism: A molecular genetic analysis of 8 families with 23 affected persons. *Medicine (Baltimore)* 65:73, 1986.
611. Parkinson DB, Thakker RV: Hypoparathyroidism due to a donor splice site mutation in the parathyroid hormone gene. *J Bone Min Res* 6(Suppl 1):S300, 1991.
612. Albright F, Burnett CH, Smith PH, Parson W: Pseudo-hypoparathyroidism—an example of "Seabright-Bantam syndrome." *Endocrinology* 30:922, 1942.
613. Wilson JD, George FW, Leshin M: Genetic control of extraglandular aromatase activity in the chicken. *Steroids* 50:235, 1987.
614. Chase LR, Melson GL, Aurbach GD: Pseudohypoparathyroidism: Defective excretion of 3′,5′-AMP in response to parathyroid hormone. *J Clin Invest* 48:1832, 1969.
615. Drezner MK, Burch WM JR: Altered activity of the nucleotide regulatory site in the parathyroid hormone-sensitive adenylate cyclase from the renal cortex of a patient with pseudohypoparathyroidism. *J Clin Invest* 62:1222, 1978.
616. Farfel Z, Brickman AS, Kaslow HR, Brothers VM, Bourne HR: Deficiency of receptor-cyclase coupling protein in pseudohypoparathyroidism. *N Engl J Med* 303:237, 1980.
617. Levine MA, Downs RW, Singer MJ, Marx SJ, Aurbach GD, Spiegel AM: Deficient activity of guanine nucleotide regulatory protein in erythrocytes from patients with pseudohypoparathyroidism. *Biochem Biophys Res Commun* 94:1319, 1980.
618. Nagant de Deuxchaisnes C, Kane SM: Hypoparathyroidism, in Avioli LV, Krane SM (eds): *Metabolic Bone Disease*. New York, Academic Press, 1978, p217.
619. Yamamoto M, Takuwa Y, Masuko S, Ogata E: Effects of endogenous and exogenous parathyroid hormone on tubular reabsorption of calcium in pseudohypoparathyroidism. *J Clin Endocrinol Metab* 66:618, 1988.
620. Drezner MK, Neelon FA, Haussler M, McPherson HT, Lebovitz HE: 1,25-Dihydroxycholecalciferol deficiency: The probable cause of hypocalcemia and metabolic bone disease in pseudohypoparathyroidism. *J Clin Endocrinol Metab* 42:621, 1976.
621. Breslau NA, Moses AM, Pak CYC: Evidence for bone remodeling but lack of calcium mobilization response to parathyroid hormone in pseudohypoparathyroidism. *J Clin Endocrinol Metab* 57:638, 1983.
622. Bell NH, Avery S, Sinha T, Clark CM Jr, Allen DO, Johnston C Jr: Effects of dibutyryl cyclic adenosine 3′,5′-monophosphate and parathyroid extract on calcium and phosphorus metabolism in hypoparathyroidism and pseudohypoparathyroidism. *J Clin Invest* 51:816, 1972.
623. Yamaoka K, Seino Y, Ishida M, Ishii T, Shimotsuji T, Tanaka Y, Kurose H, Matsuda S, et al: Effect of dibutyryl adenosine 3′,3′-monophosphate administration on plasma concentrations of 1,25-dihydroxyvitamin D in pseudohypoparathyroidism type I. *J Clin Endocrinol Metab* 53:1096, 1981.
624. Spiegel AM: Pseudohypoparathyroidism, in Scriver CR, Beaudet AL, Sly WS, Valle D (eds): *The Metabolic Basis of Inherited Disease*. New York, McGraw-Hill, 1989, p 2013.
625. Levine MA, Ahn TG, Klupt SF, Kaufman KD, Smallwood PM, Bourne HR, Sullivan KA, Van Dop C: Genetic deficiency of the alpha subunit of the guanine nucleotide-binding protein G_s as the molecular basis for Albright's hereditary osteodystrophy. *Proc Natl Acad Sci USA* 85:617, 1988.
626. Weinstein LS, Gejman PV, Friedman E, Kadowaki T, Collins RM, Gershon ES, Spiegel AM: Mutations of the G_s alpha-subunit gene in Albright's hereditary osteodystrophy detected by denaturing gradient gel electrophoresis. *Proc Natl Acad Sci USA* 87:8287, 1990.
627. Patten JL, Levine MA: Immunochemical analysis of the alpha-subunit of the stimulatory G-protein of adenyl cyclase in patients with Albright's hereditary osteodystrophy. *J Clin Endocrinol Metab* 71:1208, 1990.
628. Kidd GS, Schaaf M, Adler RA, Lassman MN, Wray HL: Skeletal responsiveness in pseudohypoparathyroidism: A spectrum of clinical disease. *Am J Med* 68:772, 1980.
629. Kolb FO, Steinbach HL: Pseudohypoparathyroidism with secondary hyperparathyroidism and osteitis fibrosa. *J Clin Endocrinol Metab* 22:59, 1962.
630. Stogmann W, Fischer JA: Pseudohypoparathyroidism: Disappearance of the resistance to parathyroid extract during treatment with vitamin D. *Am J Med* 59:140, 1975.
631. Metz SA, Baylink DJ, Hughes MR, Haussler MR, Robertson RP: Selective deficiency of 1,25-dihydroxycholecalciferol: A cause of isolated skeletal resistance to parathyroid hormone. *N Engl J Med* 292:1084, 1977.
632. Nagant de Deuxchaisnes C, Fischer JA, Dambacher MA: Dissociation of parathyroid hormone bioactivity and immunoreactivity in pseudohypoparathyroidism type I. *J Clin Endocrinol Metab* 53:1105, 1981.
633. Mitchell J, Goltzman D: Examination of circulating parathyroid hormone in pseudohypoparathyroidism. *J Clin Endocrinol Metab* 61:328, 1985.
634. Albright F, Forbes AP, Henneman PH: Pseudo-pseudohypoparathyroidism. *Trans Assoc Am Physicians* 65:337, 1952.
635. Levine MA, Downs RW Jr, Moses AM: Resistance to multiple hormones in patients with pseudohypoparathyroidism: Association with deficient activity of the guanine nucleotide regulatory protein. *Am J Med* 74:919, 1983.
636. Drezner M, Neelon FA, Lebovitz HE: Pseudohypoparathyroidism type II: A possible defect in the reception of the cyclic AMP signal. *N Engl J Med* 289:1056, 1973.
637. Rodriguez HJ, Villarreal H Jr, Klahr S, Slatopolsky E: Pseudohypoparathyroidism type II: Restoration of normal renal responsiveness to parathyroid hormone by calcium administration. *J Clin Endocrinol Metab* 39:693, 1974.
638. Aurbach GD, Marcus R, Winickoff RN, Epstein EH Jr, Nigra TP: Urinary excretion of 3′,5′-AMP in syndromes considered refractory to parathyroid hormones. *Metabolism* 19:799, 1970.
639. Fitch N: The identification and inheritance of Albright's hereditary osteodystrophy. *Am J Med Genet* 11:11, 1982.
640. Farfel Z, Brothers VM, Brickman AS, Conte F, Neer R, Bourne HR: Pseudohypoparathyroidism: Inheritance of deficient receptor-cyclase coupling activity. *Proc Natl Acad Sci USA* 78:3098, 1981.
641. Zusman J, Brown DM, Nesbit ME: Hyperphosphatemia,

hyperphosphaturia and hypocalcemia in acute lymphoblastic leukemia. *N Engl J Med* 289:1335, 1973.
642. Stewart AF, Longo W, Kreutter D, Jacob R, Burtis WJ: Hypocalcemia associated with calcium soap formation in a patient with a pancreatic fistula. *N Engl J Med* 315:496, 1986.
643. Dettelbach MA, Deftos LJ, Stewart AF: Intraperitoneal free fatty acids induce severe hypocalcemia in rats: A model for the hypocalcemia of pancreatitis. *J Bone Min Res* 5:1249, 1990.
644. Wu AHB, Bracey A, Bryan-Brown CW, Harper JV, Burritt MF: Ionized calcium monitoring during liver transplantation. *Arch Pathol Lab Med* 111:935, 1987.
645. Raskin P, McClain CJ, Medsger TA Jr: Hypocalcemia associated with metastic bone disease. *Arch Intern Med* 132:539, 1973.
646. Abramson EC, Gajardo H, Kukreja SC: Hypocalcemia in cancer. *Bone Min* 10:161, 1990.
647. Zaloga GP, Chernow B: The multifactorial basis for hypocalcemia during sepsis. *Ann Intern Med* 107:36, 1987.
648. Desai TK, Carlson RW, Geheb MA: Prevalence and clinical implication of hypocalcemia in acutely ill patients in a medical intensive care setting. *Am J Med* 84:209, 1988.
649. Chopra D, Janson P, Sawin CT: Insensitivity to digoxin associated with hypocalcemia. *N Engl J Med* 296:917, 1977.
650. Markowitz ME, Rosen JF, Smith C, DeLuca HF: 1,25- Dihydroxyvitamin D_3-treated hypoparathyroidism: 35 patient years in 10 children. *J Clin Endocrinol Metab* 55:727, 1982.
651. Cundy T, Haining SA, Guilland-Cumming DF, Butler J, Kanis JA: Remission of hypoparathyroidism during lactation: Evidence for a physiological role of prolactin in the regulation of vitamin D metabolism. *Clin Endocrinol (Oxf)* 26:667, 1987.
652. Parfitt AM: Thiazide-induced hypercalcemia in vitamin D-treated hypoparathyroidism. *Ann Intern Med* 77:557, 1972.
653. Freeman D, Bartlett S, Radda G, Ross B: Energetics of sodium transport in the kidney: Saturation transfer 31P-NMR. *Biochem Biophys Acta* 762:325, 1983.
654. Markowitz M, Rotkin L, Rosen JF: Circadian rhythms of blood minerals in humans. *Science* 213:672, 1981.
655. Bijvoet OLM: Relation of plasma phosphate concentration to renal tubular reabsorption of phosphate. *Clin Sci* 37:23, 1969.
656. Suki WN, Rouse D: Renal transport of calcium, magnesium, and phosphorus, in Brenner BM, Rector FC Jr (eds): *The Kidney*. Philadelphia, Saunders, 1991, p 380.
657. Murer H, Werner A, Reshkin S, Wuarin F, Biber J: Cellular mechanisms in proximal tubular reabsorption of inorganic phosphate. *Am J Physiol* 260:C885, 1991.
658. Hammerman MR: Phosphate transport across renal proximal tubular cell membranes. *Am J Physiol* 251:F385, 1986.
659. Cheng L, Sacker B: Sodium gradient-dependent phosphate transport in renal brush border membrane vesicles. *J Biol Chem* 246:1556, 1981.
660. Low I, Friedrich T, Burckhardt G: Properties of an anion exchanger in rat renal basolateral membrane vesicles. *Am J Physiol* 246:F334, 1984.
661. Segal JH, Pollock AS: Transfection-mediated expression of a dominant cAMP-resistant phenotype in the opposum kidney (OK) cell line prevents parathyroid hormone-induced inhibition of Na-phosphate co-transport: A protein kinase-A mediated event. *J Clin Invest* 86:1442, 1990.
662. Trohler V, Bonjour JP, Fleisch J: Inorganic phosphate homeostasis: Renal adaptation to the dietary intake in intact and thyroparathyroidectomized rats. *J Clin Invest* 57:264, 1976.
663. Stoll R, Kinne R, Murer H: Effect of dietary phosphate intake in phosphate transport by isolated rat renal brush border vesicles. *Biochem J* 180:465, 1978.
664. Corvilain J, Abramow M: Effect of growth hormone on tubular transport of phosphate in normal and parathyroidectomized dogs. *J Clin Invest* 43:1608, 1964.
665. Anderson J, Forster JB: Effect of cortisone on urinary phosphate excretion in man. *Clin Sci* 18:437, 1959.
666. Kempson SA: Effect of metabolic acidosis on renal brush border membrane adaptation to low phosphorus diet. *Kidney Int* 22:225, 1982.
667. Knochel JP: The pathophysiology and clinical characteristics of severe hypophosphatemia. *Arch Intern Med* 137:203, 1977.
668. Rubin MF, Narins RG: Hypophosphatemia: Pathophysiological and practical aspects of its therapy. *Semin Nephrol* 10:536, 1990.
669. Travis SF, Sugarman HJ, Ruberg RL: Alterations of red cell glycolytic intermediates and oxygen transport as a consequence of hypophosphatemia in patients receiving intravenous hyperalimentation. *N Engl J Med* 285:763, 1971.
670. Knochel JP, Barcenas C, Cotton JR, Fuller TJ, Haller R, Carter NW: Hypophosphatemia and rhabdomyolysis. *J Clin Invest* 62:1240, 1978.
671. O'Connor LR, Wheeler WS, Bethune JG: Effect of hypophosphatemia on myocardial performance in man. *N Engl J Med* 297:901, 1978.
672. Lotz M, Zisman E, Bartter FC: Evidence for a phosphorus-depletion syndrome in man. *N Engl J Med* 278:409, 1968.
673. Godsall JW, Baron R, Insogna KL: Vitamin D metabolism and bone histomorphometry in a patient with antacid-induced osteomalacia. *Am J Med* 77:747, 1984.
674. Mostellar ME, Tuttle EP: The effects of akalosis on plasma concentrations and urinary excretion of inorganic phosphate in man. *J Clin Invest* 43:138, 1964.
675. Laaban JP, Waked M, Laromiguiere M, Vuong T-K, Rochemaure J: Hypophosphatemia complicating management of acute severe asthma. *Ann Intern Med* 112:68, 1990.
676. Fiaccadori E, Coffrini E, Ronda N, Vezzani A, Cacciani G, Fracchia C, Rampulla C, Borghetti A: Hypophosphatemia in course of chronic obstructive pulmonary disease. *Chest* 97:857, 1990.
677. Aubier M, Murciano D, Lecocguic Y, Viires N, Jacquens Y, Squara P, Patiente R: Effect of hypophosphatemia on diaphragmatic contractility in patients with acute respiratory failure. *N Engl J Med* 313:420, 1985.
678. Newman JH, Neff RA, Ziporin P: Acute respiratory failure associated with hypophosphatemia. *N Engl J Med* 296:1101, 1977.
679. Lewis JF, Hodsman AB, Driedger AA, Thompson RT, McFadden RG: Hypophosphatemia and respiratory failure: Prolonged abnormal energy metabolism demonstrated by nuclear magnetic resonance spectroscopy. *Am J Med* 83: 1139, 1987.
680. Fisher JN, Kitabchi AE: A randomized study of phosphate therapy in the treatment of diabetic ketoacidosis. *J Clin Endocrinol Metab* 57:177, 1983.
681. Hayek ME, Eisenberg PG: Severe hypophosphatemia following the institution of enteral feedings. *Arch Surg* 124:1325, 1989.
682. Angeli P, Gatta A, Caregaro L, Luisetto G, Menon F, Merkel C, Bolognesi M, Ruol A: Hypophosphatemia and renal tubular dysfunction in alcoholics. *Gastroenterology* 100: 502, 1991.
683. Lentz RD, Brown DM, Kjellstrand CM: Treatment of severe hypophosphatemia. *Ann Intern Med* 89:941, 1978.
684. Wacker WEC, Parisi AF: Magnesium metabolism. *N Engl J Med* 278:658, 1968.
685. Agus ZS, Wasserstein A, Goldfarb S: Disorders of calcium and magnesium homeostasis. *Am J Med* 72:473, 1982.
686. Dirks JH: The kidney and magnesium regulation. *Kidney Int* 23:771, 1983.
687. Broadus AE: Physiological functions of calcium, magnesium, and phosphorus, in Favus MJ (ed): *Primer on the Metabolic Bone Diseases and Disorders of Mineral Metabolism*. Richmond, VA, American Society for Bone and Mineral Research, William Byrd Press, 1990, p 29.
688. Silverberg SJ: The distribution and balance of calcium, magnesium and phosphorus, in Favus MJ (ed): *Primer on*

the Metabolic Bone Diseases and Disorders of Mineral Metabolism. Richmond, VA, American Society for Bone and Mineral Research, William Byrd Press, 1990, p 30.

689. Lemann J Jr: Intestinal absorption of calcium, magnesium, and phosphorus, in Favus MJ (ed): *Primer on the Metabolic Bone Diseases and Disorders of Mineral Metabolism.* Richmond, VA, William Byrd Press, 1990, p 32.
690. Lemann J Jr: The urinary excretion of calcium, magnesium, and phosphorus, in Favus MJ (ed): *Primer on the Metabolic Bone Diseases and Disorders of Mineral Metabolism.* Richmond, VA, William Byrd Press, 1990, p 36.
691. Rude RK: Magnesium deficiency and hypermagnesemia, in Favus MJ (ed): *Primer on the Metabolic Bone Diseases and Disorders of Mineral Metabolism.* Richmond, VA, American Society for Bone and Mineral Research, William Byrd Press, 1990, p 141.
692. Flink EF: Therapy of magnesium deficiency. *Ann NY Acad Sci* 162:901, 1969.
693. Mallette L, Kirkland J, Gagel R, Law WJ, Heath H: Synthetic human parathyroid hormone-(1-34) for the study of pseudohypoparathyroidism. *J Clin Endocrinol Metab* 67:964, 1988.

CHAPTER 24

Metabolic Bone Disease

Frederick R. Singer

A *metabolic bone disease* can best be defined as a skeletal disorder which is generalized in extent.[1] This may not always be clinically apparent, as in patients with osteoporosis, in whom the vertebral lesions are often the clinical focus of attention. However, more subtle abnormalities of a generalized nature can be demonstrated in these patients with bone biopsy or bone densitometry.

Metabolic bone diseases, particularly osteoporosis, constitute a growing public health problem which to a great extent is a consequence of the longer life span of the population. These disorders often have a complex pathogenesis which includes abnormal hormone secretion rates, deficiency of vitamin D, impaired metabolic activation of vitamin D or resistance to its actions, other nutritional deficiencies, immobilization, genetic abnormalities of connective tissue matrix and enzyme synthesis, and failure of normal bone stem cell differentiation. In addition, osteoporosis is associated with a number of unrelated primary disorders, such as rheumatoid arthritis, in which the pathogenetic relation between bone loss and the primary disorder is ill defined. Finally, there are instances of "idiopathic" bone disease in which no clues to the pathogenesis are apparent.

CLINICAL EVALUATION OF METABOLIC BONE DISEASE

History and Physical Examination

Patients with a metabolic bone disease may have a prolonged asymptomatic course during which only the appropriate laboratory tests will reveal an abnormality. Such a situation is typical of postmenopausal osteoporosis before bone mass has decreased enough to allow a compression fracture of a vertebral body to occur.

The most common symptoms which occur in adult patients with bone disease are pain and deformity. Pathologic fractures of the vertebral bodies or femoral neck are sometimes the first indication of underlying disease. In children, failure of normal growth is a common feature. Rarely, neurologic deficits may develop as a consequence of abnormal remodeling of bone; for example, optic and auditory nerve compression may complicate osteopetrosis. In patients with hypocalcemia, tetany and seizures may be present. In vitamin D–deficient and phosphate-deficient states, muscle weakness and tenderness may be striking features of the physical examination.

It is particularly important to ascertain the dietary history and the family history and to find out whether there was a period of prolonged immobilization in the past, since these are important determinants of normal skeletal development.

Clinical Chemistry

Important information concerning the type and underlying etiology of metabolic bone disease can be obtained from several routine blood and urine analyses. These are discussed in detail in Chap. 23 and will be only briefly reviewed here.

The fasting serum calcium, phosphorus, and alkaline phosphatase concentrations, usually a part of screening chemistry panels, are simple but valuable parameters in assessing metabolic bone disease.

The serum calcium concentration may be normal, high, or low in patients with bone disease. An elevated concentration suggests that bone resorption is increased, and a low concentration may indicate a failure of adequate release of bone mineral to maintain a normocalcemic state. The presence of a normal serum calcium concentration should not be taken as evidence of normal bone metabolism, since crippling bone disease may be present in normocalcemic patients with osteoporosis, osteomalacia, and renal osteodystrophy.

The serum phosphorus concentration is almost always reduced in osteomalacia and rickets, excluding patients with chronic renal failure. Patients with osteoporosis usually have a normal serum phosphorus concentration. It should be stressed that the serum phosphorus is best measured after an overnight fast to avoid dietary influences and diurnal variation.

The serum alkaline phosphatase activity can be used as an index of osteoblastic activity in the absence of a concomitant disorder which raises extraskeletal enzyme activity. As is stressed in Chap. 23, this parameter is a rather insensitive measure of osteoblastic activity, and mild degrees of bone disease in which increased osteoblasts are found on bone biopsy may be associated with normal circulating alkaline phosphatase activity. More recently a commercially available assay for the measurement of bone-specific alkaline phosphatase activity has become available.[2] This offers the promise of much greater sensitivity in detecting abnormal osteoblast function.

A second index of osteoblast activity—serum osteocalcin (also termed *bone GLA protein*)—has been available for more than a decade. This osteoblast-specific protein is found in increased concentrations in the circulation of individuals with a variety of disorders in which there is increased osteoblastic activity,[3] including primary hyperparathyroidism, acromegaly, hyperthyroidism, and postmenopausal osteoporosis. Low levels of serum osteocalcin have been found in patients with glucocorticoid excess and hypoparathyroidism. Although circulating alkaline phosphatase activity and osteocalcin concentrations may be similarly increased or decreased in most disorders affecting the skeleton, discordant results have been observed in patients with glucocorticoid excess, Paget disease, renal failure, and osteolytic metastases.[3] Factors such as sex, age, renal function, and time of day may influence the levels of osteocalcin in the circulation,[4–6] although all studies have not been in complete agreement. Full understanding of the physiologic and pathologic role of this bone matrix protein has not been achieved, but measurement of serum osteocalcin levels may provide one of the best indexes of skeletal metabolic activity in postmenopausal women.[7]

Acid-base status, renal function, and liver function tests may be useful in the differential diagnosis of bone disease but are secondary tests.

Twenty-four-hour urinary calcium and phosphorus excretion have commonly been measured in the evaluation of patients with disturbed mineral homeostasis. These measurements, particularly phosphorus excretion, are often of little use when obtained under uncontrolled conditions, since urinary excretion of these substances is influenced by a variety of factors. More relevant information can be obtained by spot urine collections after an overnight fast. The fasting calcium excretion (expressed as milligrams Ca per 100 ml glomerular filtrate) provides an indirect index of bone mineral resorption. Occasionally, fasting calcium excretion may be increased as a result of impaired renal tubular reabsorption of calcium. The best index of phosphorus excretion is the maximum tubular reabsorption of phosphate (TmP) expressed as a function of the glomerular filtration rate (GFR), or TmP/GFR (Chap. 23). The TmP/GFR is decreased in hyperparathyroidism; however, a markedly reduced TmP/GFR is typical of various states of primary renal phosphorus wasting unrelated to parathyroid hormone secretion.

Radioimmunoassays for parathyroid hormone provide a more specific test for parathyroid function. Measurements of circulating parathyroid hormone are helpful in determining the pathogenesis of bone disease in patients with primary and secondary hyperparathyroidism. The more recently developed assays for intact parathyroid hormone in the circulation are excellent.[8] Unlike previous assays, the best of the present two-site immunometric assays exhibit little overlap between hormone levels in normal individuals and those in hyperparathyroid patients.

Urinary cAMP or nephrogenous cAMP measurements are sensitive indexes of parathyroid hormone activity. They are particularly useful in patients in whom parathyroid hormone resistance is suspected. These patients fail to exhibit a normal increase in cAMP production after the administration of parathyroid extract.

Hydroxyproline is an amino acid which occurs almost exclusively in the collagen molecule.[9] Hydroxyproline-containing peptides and free hydroxyproline are found in plasma and urine.[10] The peptides in urine are primarily of low molecular weight and represent degradation products of bone matrix. About 10 percent of hydroxyproline-containing peptides are larger than 5 kDa and appear to reflect recently synthesized collagen fragments.[11] Urinary free hydroxyproline excretion is insignificant, since free hydroxyproline is metabolized by the enzyme hydroxyproline oxidase. Because hydroxyproline released from bone matrix is not reutilized for collagen biosynthesis, urinary hydroxyproline excretion has been used clinically as an index of bone matrix resorption.[10] In normal persons, there is a positive correlation between age and urinary total hydroxyproline excretion. In growing children, the upper limit of normal excretion may be as high as 150 mg per 24 h; this high level occurs at the time of the adolescent growth spurt.[10] In adults, the normal range is approximately 20 to 40 mg per 24 h on a low-gelatin diet. A fasting spot urine to determine the ratio of hydroxyproline to creatinine excretion may provide a simpler and more meaningful estimate of bone resorption than is possible with 24-h samples. The use of this test after an overnight fast avoids, for the most part, the influences of dietary collagen and careless urine collection. The upper limit of normal is approximately 0.02 in adults.[12] Hydroxyproline excretion may be increased fivefold to 10-fold in patients with severe metabolic bone disease but may be within the normal range in patients with mild disease. Increased hydroxyproline excretion is also associated with extensive dermatoses and burns.[10]

Measurement of urinary hydroxylysine has also been proposed as an index of bone matrix resorption.[13] Although not widely evaluated, this parameter may be superior to urinary hydroxyproline measurements, since hydroxylysine and its glycosides are less extensively metabolized. Another advantage is that skin and bone collagen contain different ratios of the various glycosides, so that the tissue source of urinary hydroxylysine can be estimated if desired.[13,14]

The most promising new assay for estimating the rate of bone resorption is the measurement of urinary deoxypyridinoline, an amino acid involved in the covalent cross-linking between collagen chains in bone matrix. Preliminary studies utilizing this assay suggest that this parameter of bone resorption may be superior to a hydroxyproline assay in assessing patients with metabolic bone disease.[15]

Calcium balance studies, as devised by Albright and Reifenstein, have been extensively used as a research tool in the investigation of bone disease but can be carried out only in a research ward. Various isotopic studies of intestinal calcium absorption have been devised but also have not been widely applied to patients outside research centers.

Radiology and Nuclear Medicine

Radiologic evaluation of the skeleton is a valuable noninvasive means of determining the extent, severity, and nature of bone disease. The "metabolic bone survey" usually consists of a lateral skull x-ray, hand x-rays, lateral thoracic and lumbar x-rays, and a pelvic x-ray. In most patients with a severe generalized bone disease, an abnormal radiologic finding will be apparent in one or more of these sites. If hyperparathyroidism is in the differential diagnosis, films of the clavicles or lamina dura may prove revealing. If osteomalacia is suspected, a search for pseudofractures in the long bones and scapulae is worthwhile if they are not discovered in other areas.

The types of radiologic abnormality which should be sought are a reduction in bone density, unusual bone texture, widening of the epiphyseal cartilage growth plate, thinning or thickening of the cortex, periosteal new bone formation, endosteal scalloping, fractures, pseudofractures, and abnormalities in the size and shape of a bone. These types of abnormality are illustrated in subsequent sections.

Quantitative assessment of bone mineral is of particular importance in view of the high incidence of osteoporosis. Numerous techniques have been devised to assess this, including visual assessment of lateral radiographs of the spine, radiogrammetry, photodensitometry, single energy photon absorptiometry, dual energy photon absorptiometry, neutron activation analysis, study of Compton scattering, and quantitative computed tomography.[16] Single energy photon absorptiometry of the radius, dual energy photon absorptiometry of the spine, and quantitative computed tomography of the spine have been widely applied in clinical studies.[16–18] A more recently introduced technique for measuring both vertebral and proximal femoral mineral density—dual x-ray absorptiometry or dual energy radiography—utilizes a dual energy source of x-rays and is more accurate and precise than dual photon absorptiometry or quantitative computerized tomography. Further refinement of this technology, in particular the ability to measure accurately vertebral density on a lateral view to avoid sclerosis of the facet joints,[19] has made this technique the preferred method for the foreseeable future.

The development of high-resolution bone scanners and the use of technetium-labeled bisphosphonates have brought about major improvements in the quality of bone scans. The bone scan provides a visual display of the metabolic activity in different regions of the skeleton. Scans are used primarily to detect occult bone metastases in patients with cancer. Approximately 4 h after receiving an intravenous injection of the radiolabeled bone-seeking agent, the patient is scanned in the supine position. An example of the scan of a patient with metastatic breast carcinoma is shown in Fig. 24-1. The asymmetry of radioisotopic activity is thought to reflect both increased osteoblastic activity adjacent to metastatic tumor and an increased blood flow in the involved region. Patients with purely osteolytic lesions, such as those in multiple myeloma, often have normal bone scans unless pathologic fractures are present. It has been suggested that estimation of total isotope uptake by the skeleton would be a valuable parameter of skeletal metabolic activity.[20] Whole body retention of technetium-labeled methylene bisphosphonate has been utilized in categorizing postmenopausal women with osteoporosis into high-bone-turnover and low-bone-turnover groups.[21]

Bone Biopsy

A bone biopsy may provide valuable information which is not supplied by other techniques. This is particularly true in patients with milder forms of metabolic bone disease, in whom the radiologic and biochemical parameters are nearly normal or are not specific for a particular disease entity. Unfortunately, the application of bone biopsies and appropriate histologic techniques to clinical problems in the United States has been quite limited. The lack of a sufficient number of physicians trained in obtaining bone biopsies and the limited number of routine pathology laboratories which have experience in the proper processing of bone specimens account for the underutilization of this important technique.

In the past, bone biopsy material was obtained by resecting part of a rib and required the services of a surgeon. Fortunately, the design of a trocar by Bordier and colleagues[22] has made it possible to obtain an iliac crest biopsy specimen in an outpatient setting. After infiltration of the skin, soft tissues, and

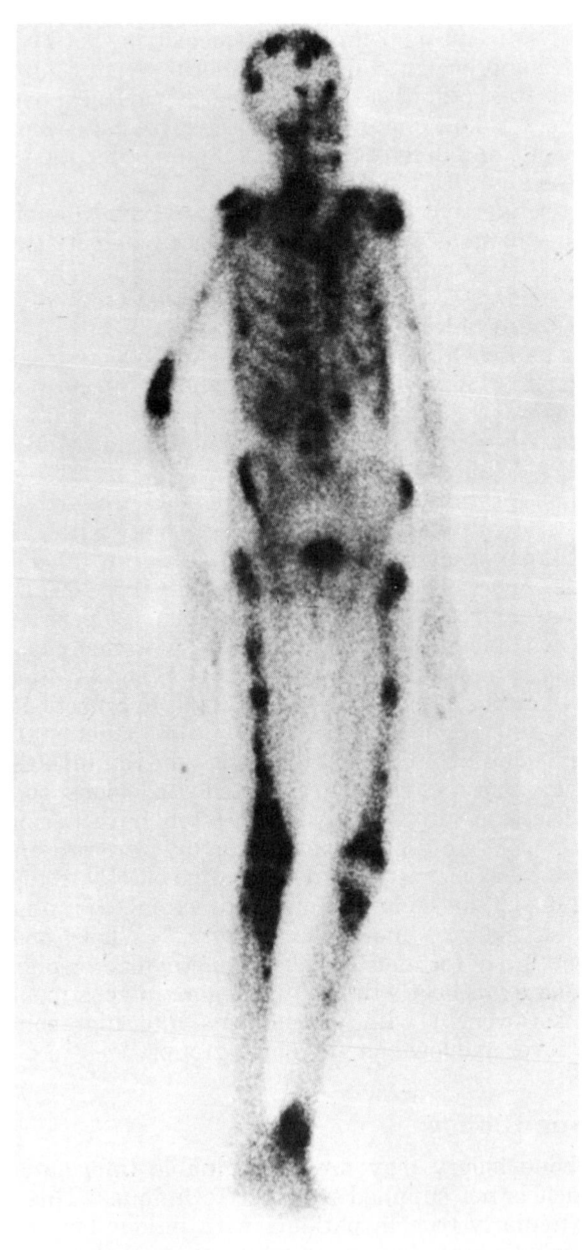

FIGURE 24-1 Technetium-labeled bisphosphonate bone scan of a patient with widespread metastases from a breast carcinoma. Note the numerous foci of increased radioisotope uptake.

marrow cavity with lidocaine (Xylocaine) a biopsy can be obtained from the iliac crest adjacent to the anterior superior spine with minimal discomfort in most cases. A repeat biopsy after therapeutic intervention can be carried out on the opposite iliac crest.

In most pathology departments, the bone biopsy is fixed in formalin, decalcified, and embedded in paraffin prior to staining with hematoxylin and eosin (H&E). Examination of a bone specimen prepared in this manner allows identification of the number and types of bone cells present and of the overall structure of the bone. Unfortunately, the H&E stain of decalcified bone sections does not allow consistent identification of the unmineralized osteoid which may be present in increased amounts in a variety of disorders. This requires the preparation of undecalcified bone sections. The bone specimen is fixed and then embedded in plastic before sectioning with a special microtome. Several stains can be used to delineate the amount of unmineralized osteoid in the sections. In laboratories which do not have the appropriate equipment for preparing undecalcified sections, an alternative technique can be used to demonstrate unmineralized osteoid.[23] After appropriate demineralization of the specimen, an azan stain of the section will produce a blue color at sites of previously unmineralized osteoid and a red color in normally mineralized bone.

Quantitative histomorphometry of bone biopsies is available in a few centers and is the most sophisticated approach to analyzing histologic sections.[24] With a variety of specialized microscopes as well as computerized instrumentation, precise quantitation of many parameters can be achieved, including assessment of the bone volume, the percentage of bone surface covered by osteoid, the average thickness of osteoid, the surface of bone undergoing resorption and formation, and the number of osteoclasts.

The discovery that the antibiotic tetracycline localizes at the sites of mineralization in bone led to the development of a dynamic test of bone metabolic activity.[25] A patient receives 500 mg of tetracycline on 2 consecutive days, nothing for 10 days, and 500 mg daily for 3 days; a bone biopsy is done the next day. The iliac crest bone specimen is processed, and the sections are evaluated by fluorescent microscopy. Two types of tetracycline which fluoresce differently can be used. In a normal subject, two bands of tetracycline fluorescence will be found on the surfaces of bone at which new bone was formed during the period of tetracycline labeling. The inner tetracycline band represents the initial course, and the outer band represents the second course of the antibiotic. The rate of bone formation can then be calculated by measuring the average width between the bands and dividing this by the number of days between tetracycline administration. In normal adults, this approaches 1 μg per day.[26] In patients with osteomalacia, in whom the principal defect is in mineralization, tetracycline uptake by bone is impaired.

The indications for bone biopsy are still evolving, but in general a biopsy is indicated when there is a need to establish a diagnosis in patients in whom noninvasive parameters of bone disease are not definitive. Patients with subclinical osteomalacia particularly require bone biopsies for confirmation of the diagnosis. The bone biopsy may also be used to monitor the results of therapy in patients with disorders such as osteoporosis and renal osteodystrophy. It is likely that as more effective therapies become available for these problems, sequential bone biopsies will be more widely used to confirm the efficacy of therapy.

OSTEOMALACIA AND RICKETS

Osteomalacia is characterized by an excess of unmineralized bone which results from an impairment of bone mineralization. It is a disorder of diverse etiology which can be subdivided into two main categories: disorders associated with a reduction in circulating vitamin D metabolites and those associated with hypophosphatemia.

In children, the term *rickets* is used to indicate a disorder characterized by epiphyseal dysplasia, retardation of longitudinal growth, and a variety of skeletal deformities. Osteomalacia is the predominant histologic lesion. Rickets arises from etiologic factors similar to those which produce osteomalacia in adults.

Clinical Presentation

Symptoms and Signs

The manifestations of rickets depend not only on the severity and duration of the underlying disorder but to a great extent on the patient's age, because rickets affects the areas of bone which are growing most rapidly, and these vary at different ages.[27] Short stature reflects the epiphyseal dysplasia at the ends of the long bones of the lower extremities. The types of skeletal deformity associated with rickets include areas of thinning and softening of the cranium, protuberance of the frontal bone, thickening of the rib ends (rachitic rosary), lateral indentation of the chest wall (Harrison's groove), bowing of long bones, and knock-knee (Fig. 24-2).

In adult-onset disease, skeletal deformities are seldom encountered except in the most severe cases. Abnormal spinal curvature, a bell-shaped thorax, or pelvic deformity may develop.

Bone pain is common in both children and adults. It is often experienced in the pelvis, lower extremities, spine, and ribs. The pain is worsened by activity in weight-bearing regions. In severe cases, bone tenderness is present on palpation. This is best elicited by thumb pressure on the distal tibia.

Muscle weakness and tenderness, particularly of the proximal musculature of the lower extremities, may be the dominant features in some patients. This is much more likely to occur in vitamin D–deficient patients than in hypophosphatemic patients.

In vitamin D–deficient patients, hypocalcemia may be reflected by the presence of paresthesias, tetany, seizures, and impaired mentation.

Radiologic Features

Radiologic examination of the skeleton can provide information of a highly specific nature with regard to the diagnosis of rickets or osteomalacia.[28] The radiologic signs of advanced rickets include widening of the epiphyseal growth plates, a frayed appearance of the metaphyses, and cupping and widening of the metaphyses (Fig. 24-3). These abnormalities are most readily detected at the metaphyseal sites which are growing most rapidly. Up to the age of 1 year, both the upper and lower extremities are likely to exhibit these findings. After 1 year, the lower extremities are more likely to reveal the abnormalities of rickets. Within several weeks of the initiation of appropriate therapy, mineralization of

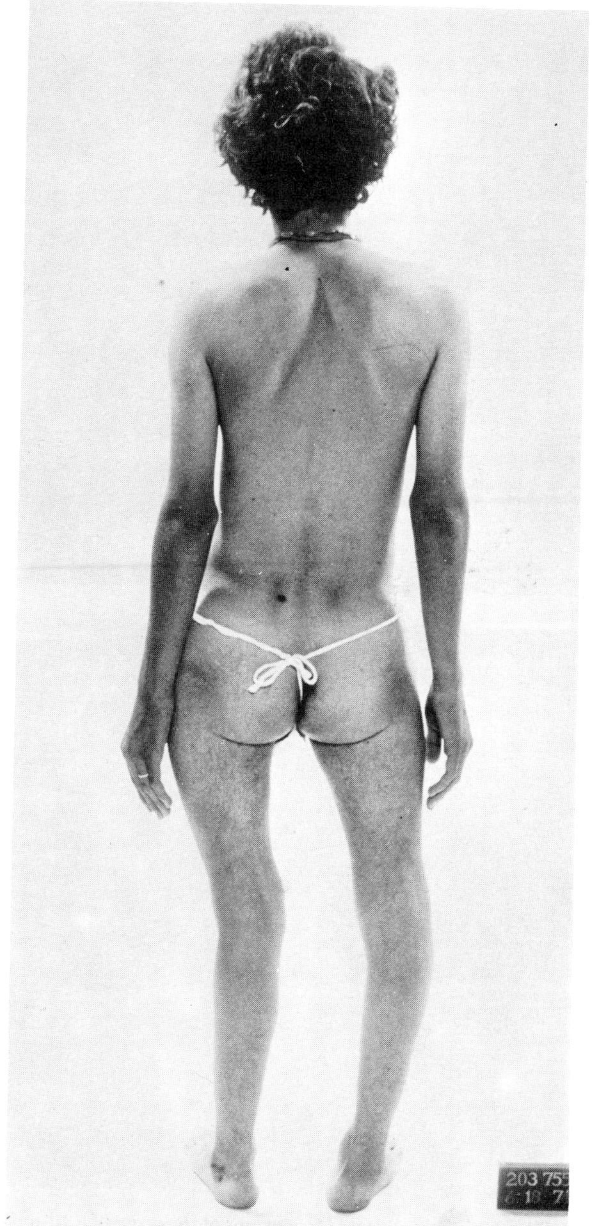

FIGURE 24-2 Bowing and knock-knee deformities in a 19-year-old male with familial X-linked hypophosphatemic rickets.

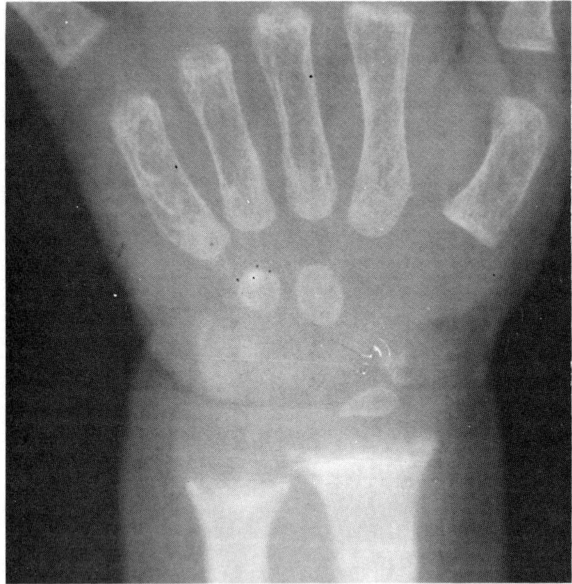

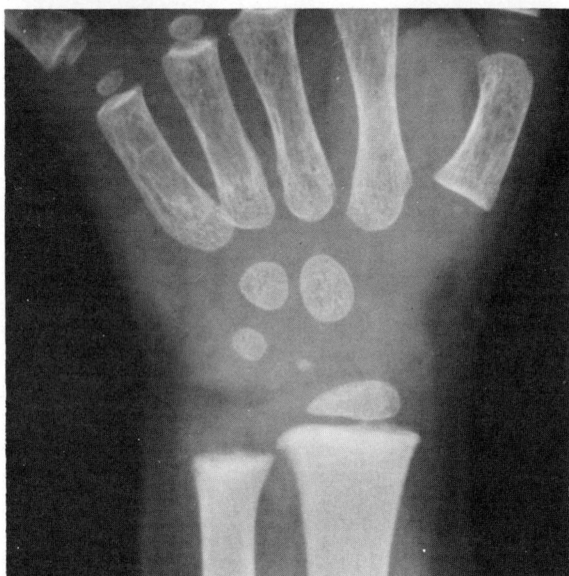

FIGURE 24-3 (*Top*) Roentgenograms of the wrist of a 13-month-old child with rickets due to vitamin D deficiency. Note the frayed appearance associated with widening and cupping of the metaphyses. A pseudofracture is present at the distal radius. (*Bottom*) Nearly total healing of the rickets after 5 months of treatment with vitamin D_2.

the epiphyseal cartilage can be discerned as a radiodense line adjacent to the metaphyses. In subsequent years, Harris lines, which are transverse radiodense lines across the shafts of long bones, may be noted in patients who have had a fluctuating degree of activity of the disease.

Gross deformity of the skeleton is more likely to occur in children than in adults. Kyphoscoliosis, a bell-shaped thorax, a triangular configuration of the pelvic lumen, and bowing of the upper and lower extremities are abnormalities that may be encountered in patients with severe long-standing disease.

In the adult, the radiologic findings in patients with osteomalacia often mimic those found in osteoporosis. A generalized loss of bone density with thinning of the cortex may be impossible to distinguish from that found in patients with osteoporosis. Expansion of intervertebral disk spaces and pathologic compression fractures of the vertebral bodies may be observed. Occasionally the trabecular pattern of bone is thickened, and mottled radiolucencies may be discerned. Osteosclerosis may rarely occur in isolated bones, most often affecting vertebral bodies. This unexpected finding remains unexplained. It is much more likely to be seen in the healing phase of the disease, when the mineralization defect is corrected.

In osteomalacic patients who have vitamin D deficiency, secondary hyperparathyroidism may be reflected by subperiosteal resorption of the phalanges, loss of the lamina dura, widening of the spaces at the symphysis pubis and sacroiliac joints, and the presence of brown tumors or bone cysts. These abnormalities rarely if ever occur in hypophosphatemic patients.

The pathognomonic radiologic feature of osteomalacia is the presence of pseudofractures, also known as Looser zones or Milkman fractures (Fig. 24-4). These narrow zones of rarefaction are often bilateral and symmetric. Common sites at which they may be found include the femoral neck and shaft, ulna and radius, pubic and ischial rami, clavicles, ribs, scapulae, and metacarpals, metatarsals, and phalanges. The origin of these lesions is not known with certainty. There is an underlying excess of unmineralized osteoid which may reflect healing of a microfracture. In severe long-standing cases, the borders of a pseudofracture may appear sclerotic.

Laboratory Findings

Biochemical abnormalities in patients with rickets and osteomalacia can be classified into two categories. In patients whose disorder develops as a consequence of vitamin D lack, abnormal vitamin D metabolism, or vitamin D resistance, the concentrations of serum calcium and phosphorus are usually reduced and the serum alkaline phosphatase activity is elevated.[29–31] Patients who develop bone disease on the basis of chronic hypophosphatemia also have elevated serum alkaline phosphatase activity but have a normal serum calcium concentration.[27] The hypocalcemic state of vitamin D–deficient patients is associated with elevated serum parathyroid hormone levels.[32] The state of secondary hyperparathyroidism is further manifested by a decreased renal phosphate threshold,[29] elevated urinary cAMP excretion,[33] and generalized aminoaciduria,[29] including hydroxyprolinuria.[10] The hypophosphatemic group has seldom been reported to have elevated

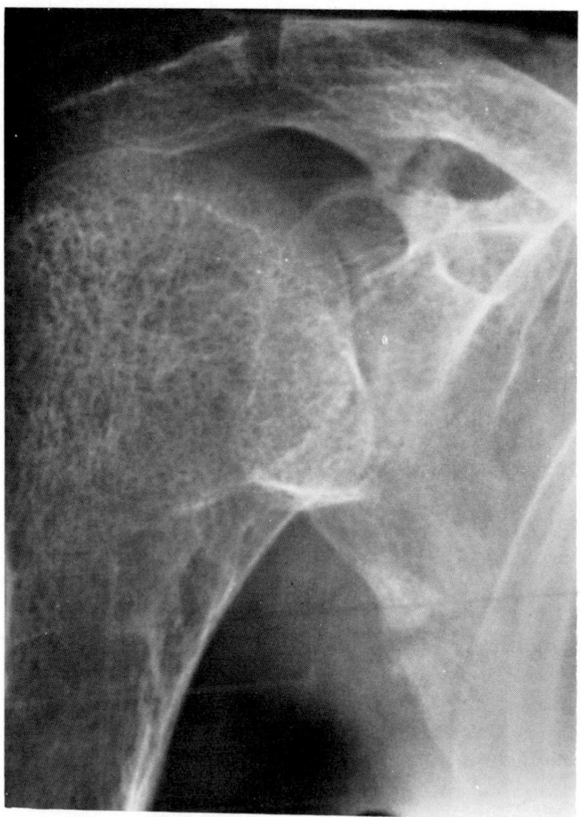

FIGURE 24-4 Pseudofractures of the medial border of the scapula and acromion in a 52-year-old man with malabsorption syndrome.

serum parathyroid hormone levels,[34] but a lowered renal phosphate threshold is usually present, and renal wasting of a single amino acid may be found.[27] Urinary calcium excretion is markedly reduced in hypocalcemic patients but may be less so in hypophosphatemic patients.[27]

Assays of vitamin D metabolites have also been applied to the assessment of patients with rickets and osteomalacia.[35] The best measure of vitamin D status is the serum 25-hydroxyvitamin D concentration, since it is the major vitamin D metabolite in the circulation (Chap. 23). As expected, 25-hydroxyvitamin D and 24,25-dihydroxyvitamin D are found in low concentrations in the circulation of patients with classical vitamin D deficiency. Levels of serum 1α,25-dihydroxyvitamin D may be within the normal range in such patients,[36] but in the context of hypocalcemia these "normal" levels reflect inadequate synthesis of the renal vitamin D metabolite. Other quantitative abnormalities of circulating vitamin D metabolites have been described and are discussed under Classification and Pathogenesis, below.

Bone Pathology

To allow for a better understanding of the pathologic features of rickets, the histology of endochondral ossification at the epiphyseal growth plate is briefly described here.

Longitudinal bone growth occurs at the epiphyseal growth plate, a cartilaginous band separating the epiphysis from the metaphyseal region of the shaft.[28] In the proliferative zone of the growth plate, hypertrophic cartilage cells form orderly columns extending toward the shaft. These cell columns are then penetrated by blood vessels extending from the marrow and subsequently are destroyed by chondroclasts. Simultaneously, calcification of the cartilage matrix occurs, and osteoblasts arise around the blood vessels. They synthesize the bone matrix adjacent to the calcified cartilage, and this is rapidly mineralized.

In rickets, replication of cartilage cells in the proliferative zone proceeds in a normal fashion. However, the proliferating cells fail to form orderly columns advancing toward the shaft.[28] The marrow vessels also fail to penetrate the cartilage, and the cartilage cells are only partially removed. Thus the zone of proliferating cartilage widens. Inadequate mineralization of cartilage and osteoid is noted, along with penetration of this zone by vessels from the perichondrium and adjacent resting cartilage. The weakened structure at the cartilage shaft junction and the proliferation of cartilage account for the deformities which become apparent on radiologic and clinical examination.

Biopsy of the growth plate of a long bone is not recommended, since future bone growth may be impaired. Biopsy of the iliac apophysis can be carried out with less likelihood of skeletal distortion.

The hallmark of osteomalacia is the accumulation of unmineralized osteoid.[37] This occurs as a result of impairment of matrix mineralization and despite a reduction in the rate of bone matrix formation. The increase in osteoid volume is reflected by a greater extent of osteoid seams covering both cortical and trabecular bone surfaces and by an increased width of the osteoid seams. Because excess osteoid may also be a feature of disorders such as thyrotoxicosis, primary hyperparathyroidism, and Paget disease, it may be necessary to label the bone with tetracycline to establish definitively whether an osteomalacic state is present. In osteomalacic patients, the percentage of osteoid seams labeled with tetracycline is reduced; tetracycline uptake, when present, may be diffuse rather than concentrated at the calcification front; bone matrix formation is reduced; and there is an increased mineralization lag time.[37] In states of high bone turnover, tetracycline labels most osteoid seams, and bone matrix formation and mineralization rates are increased. The width of the osteoid seams is usually normal.

Numerous active osteoblasts are usually found lining trabecular bone surfaces in most types of osteomalacia. They are not found in patients with adult hypophosphatasia, in patients with bone disease associated with total parenteral nutrition, and in a small minority of patients with renal osteodystrophy.

Patients with vitamin D deficiency exhibit features of secondary hyperparathyroidism, including increased numbers of osteoclasts and a fibrovascular marrow. Evidence of secondary hyperparathyroidism is generally not found in patients with osteomalacia associated with hypophosphatemic states. The latter patients exhibit increased osteoid volume and a mineralization defect indistinguishable from that found in simple vitamin D deficiency. A partially reversible decrease in mineral surrounding osteocyte lacunae has been reported in hypophosphatemic patients. This may reflect abnormal osteocyte function.[38]

Classification and Pathogenesis

Osteomalacia or rickets may develop as an isolated pathologic state or as a complication of another disorder. Table 24-1 shows a classification of osteomalacia and rickets. In the majority of patients, the pathogenesis can be ascribed to an abnormality of vitamin D supply, metabolic activation or action, or chronic hypophosphatemia. Patients who have an abnormality of vitamin D metabolism are unable to absorb sufficient calcium and phosphorus from their diets to allow normal mineralization of osteoid. A direct effect of vitamin D metabolites on bone mineralization has not been demonstrated convincingly. Patients who develop osteomalacia or rickets as a result of hypophosphatemia probably do so because phosphorus is an essential constituent of hydroxyapatite.

Vitamin D Abnormalities

Vitamin D Deficiency

Classic vitamin D deficiency can develop only in a subject whose skin exposure to ultraviolet light is inadequate *and* whose diet contains insufficient vitamin D.[39] Vitamin D–deficiency rickets has been considered an extremely uncommon disorder since vitamin D supplementation of dairy products and other foods in the United States became a national policy. However, it has been noted that there is an increased susceptibility to rickets in infants of mothers who follow certain dietary practices. Children who are breast-fed but not given vitamin D supplements and those on vegetarian diets without vitamin D supplementation are susceptible to rickets.[40,41] These "outbreaks" of rickets have occurred in northern cities where air pollution may reduce ultraviolet exposure. Dressing in long garments and the use of hoods and veils were contributing factors in one group.[40]

Fraser and Scriver have described three stages in the pathogenesis of human rickets.[34] In stage I, hypocalcemia is the only significant biochemical abnormality. In stage II, the calcium concentration returns to the normal range and hypophosphatemia is apparent, presumably because of secondary hyperparathyroidism. Stage III is associated with severe clinical manifestations of rickets and the return of hypocalcemia.

Vitamin D Malabsorption

Malabsorption of vitamin D may occur in patients with small intestine disease, pancreatic insufficiency, and/or inadequate bile salts.[42] Since osteomalacia may develop in malabsorption states despite adequate ultraviolet light exposure, it is possible that malabsorption of 25-hydroxyvitamin D also occurs after the latter is excreted into the small intestine as a constituent of bile.[43] Evidence for and against this proposal has been obtained.[44] The pathogenesis of bone disease in malabsorption syndromes may be more complex than simply malabsorption of dietary vitamin D and its liver metabolite, since other important nutrients, such as trace elements, may be poorly absorbed. The heterogeneity of bone disease was striking in a study of 21 patients after intestinal bypass surgery for obesity.[45] Only six patients had clear evidence of osteomalacia by rigorous histomorphometric criteria. The majority had evidence of bone loss without osteomalacia.

Abnormal Vitamin D Metabolism

Osteomalacia appears to be a very uncommon complication of severe parenchymal liver disease.[46] In some patients, poor nutrition and lack of exposure to ultraviolet light may produce low levels of circulating vitamin D metabolites and osteomalacia. In others, reduced serum vitamin D–binding protein levels account for low serum total 25-hydroxyvitamin D levels.[47] The latter patients have normal free 25-hydroxyvitamin D levels.

In patients with chronic renal failure, there is a reduction in both 1α,25-dihydroxyvitamin D and 24,25-dihydroxyvitamin D in the circulation.[35,48] The pathogenesis of renal osteodystrophy will be discussed later.

Patients who are treated with anticonvulsant drugs are at risk of developing rickets and/or osteomalacia,[49] although a study of 20 patients revealed only a modest increase in osteoid volume and no impairment of the mineralization rate.[50] The development of bone disease has been attributed to increased liver metabolism of 25-hydroxyvitamin D to more polar metabolites,[51] but not all anticonvulsant-treated patients have low levels of this metabolite,[50] and in some patients inadequate vitamin D intake or ultraviolet light exposure appears to account for reduced levels.[52] While low levels of 24,25-dihydroxyvitamin D have also been found,[53,54] normal, elevated, or low levels of circulating 1α,25-dihydroxyvitamin D have been reported.[54,55] Therefore it is difficult to

TABLE 24-1 Classification of Causes of Osteomalacia and Rickets

I. Reduction of circulating vitamin D metabolites
   A. Inadequate ultraviolet light exposure and inadequate dietary vitamin D
   B. Vitamin D malabsorption
      1. Small intestine disease or surgical bypass
      2. Pancreatic insufficiency
      3. Insufficient bile salts
   C. Abnormal vitamin D metabolism
      1. Liver disease
      2. Chronic renal failure
      3. Drugs (anticonvulsants, glutethimide)
      4. Mesenchymal tumors, prostatic cancer
      5. Vitamin D-dependent rickets type I (25-hydroxyvitamin D-1α-hydroxylase deficiency)
   D. Renal loss
      1. Nephrotic syndrome
II. Peripheral resistance to vitamin D
   A. Vitamin D-dependent rickets, type II
   B. Anticonvulsant drugs
   C. Chronic renal failure
III. Hypophosphatemia
   A. Renal phosphate wasting
      1. Hypophosphatemic rickets
         a. Familial X-linked
         b. Autosomal recessive
         c. Sporadic
      2. Hypophosphatemic osteomalacia
         a. Familial X-linked
         b. Sporadic
      3. Familial renal phosphate leak with hypercalciuria, nephrolithiasis, and osteomalacia and rickets
      4. Fanconi's syndrome
      5. Mesenchymal tumors, fibrous dysplasia, epidermal nevus syndrome, prostatic cancer
      6. Primary hyperparathyroidism
   B. Malnutrition
   C. Malabsorption due to gastrointestinal disease or phosphate-binding antacids
   D. Chronic dialysis
IV. Miscellaneous
   A. Inhibitors of calcification
      1. Sodium fluoride
      2. Etidronate disodium
   B. Calcium deficiency
   C. Hypoparathyroidism
   D. Hypophosphatasia
   E. Fibrogenesis imperfecta ossium
   F. Systemic acidosis
   G. Total parenteral nutrition

be certain that anticonvulsant-induced bone disease is attributable solely to impaired vitamin D metabolism. Anticonvulsant-induced bone disease has been prevented with 3000 units of vitamin D_3 per week, but exposure to sunlight may be more effective.[52] 1α,25-Dihydroxyvitamin D_3 has also been recommended as a safe and effective treatment for reversing this form of bone disease in children.[56]

The association of osteomalacia with a variety of vascular and mesenchymal tumors has been observed in more than 72 patients.[57] An identical syndrome has also been observed in patients with prostatic cancer,[58] oat-cell carcinoma of the lung,[59] and, perhaps, cholangiocarcinoma of the liver.[60] The patients are usually adults and often present with bone pain and generalized muscle weakness. In most patients, a marked reduction in circulating 1α,25-dihydroxyvitamin D levels has been found. The patients were normocalcemic and often markedly hypophosphatemic because of renal phosphate wasting. Complete excision of the neoplasm generally produces resolution of the biochemical abnormalities and osteomalacia, whereas treatment with phosphate and 1α,25-dihydroxyvitamin D_3 has generally been ineffective. No tumor factor has been isolated which could account for the syndrome.

Vitamin D–dependent rickets type I is a rare autosomal recessive disorder which is thought to be due to a deficiency of renal 25-hydroxy-1α-hydroxylase.[30] This has been deduced from the finding of low circulating levels of 1α,25-dihydroxyvitamin D in affected children even when they received high doses of vitamin D[61] and from the demonstration of radiologic healing of the bone lesions with physiologic amounts of 1α,25-dihydroxyvitamin D_3.[30]

Renal Loss

Subtle degrees of osteomalacia and secondary hyperparathyroidism may develop in patients with the nephrotic syndrome, presumably on the basis of renal losses of vitamin D–binding protein and 25-hydroxyvitamin D.[62,63] However, in the absence of renal failure, bone disease may not develop.[64]

Peripheral Resistance to Vitamin D

Since 1978 it has been recognized that a subset of patients with early-onset rickets, termed *vitamin D–dependent rickets type II,* develop this disorder as a consequence of tissue insensitivity to 1α,25-dihydroxyvitamin D.[31] These patients characteristically have hypocalcemia, secondary hyperparathyroidism, elevation of circulating 1α,25-dihydroxyvitamin D_3 and a normal intake of vitamin D as well as adequate exposure to sunshine. In some patients, alopecia is a striking clinical feature.[65] A poor response to high doses of 1α,25-dihydroxyvitamin D_3 has also been reported.[66] The syndrome is often found in siblings whose parents have no detectable biochemical or skeletal abnormalities. Assays of 1α,25-dihydroxyvitamin D_3 binding to receptors and of receptor properties may reveal no detectable abnormality, a decreased binding capacity with normal affinity and decreased nuclear binding of the hormone-receptor complexes, or normal ligand binding with decreased nuclear binding of the complexes.[67–69] In two families in which the receptor gene was examined, an abnormality in the receptor's DNA-binding domain with defective DNA binding of the receptor was found in one family[70] and a mutation that affected the ligand binding was found in the other family[71] (see Chap. 5). Thus, it appears that the vitamin D–resistant state in many patients arises from structural abnormalities in the receptor molecule, not from diminished receptor synthesis. Recently two types of mutations have been described in affected kindreds which explain vitamin D resistance in homozygous individuals. Two different single nucleotide mutations in the DNA-binding domain of the receptor gene account for a decreased affinity of the vitamin D receptor for DNA.[70] In another kindred, a single base substitution resulted in a deletion of a major portion of the steroid hormone–binding domain of the gene and thus prevented binding of 1α,25-dihydroxyvitamin D_3 to its receptor.[71] In addition, defective induction of 25-hydroxyvitamin D_3-24-hydroxylase by 1α,25-dihydroxyvitamin D_3 in cultured skin fibroblasts has been shown to predict the in vivo response to calciferol therapy.[66] In addition, profound resistance to 1α,25-dihydroxyvitamin D appears to be present in alopecic patients.[66]

Since patients with anticonvulsant drug–associated rickets and osteomalacia may have normal or elevated 1α,25-dihydroxyvitamin D levels, it is possible that peripheral resistance to this metabolite is a factor in the pathogenesis of the bone disease in those patients.[50,55] In vitro studies have demonstrated impairment of the action of 25-hydroxyvitamin D_3 on bone and a reduction of calcium transport by the intestine in the presence of diphenylhydantoin.[72,73]

Patients with chronic renal failure require supraphysiologic doses of 1α,25-dihydroxyvitamin D_3 to increase intestinal calcium absorption.[74] This suggests that peripheral resistance to vitamin D is a factor in the impaired calcium absorption found in patients with chronic renal failure.

Hypophosphatemia

It is generally thought that chronic hypophosphatemia produces metabolic bone disease as a consequence of decreased body stores of phosphorus. A chronic hypophosphatemic state may arise from inadequate dietary phosphorus, reduced intestinal absorption of dietary phosphorus, or renal wasting of phosphorus. Renal wasting is the mechanism most commonly encountered clinically.

Renal Phosphate Wasting

The most common cause of rickets in the United States is the dominantly inherited genetic disorder termed *familial X-linked hypophosphatemic* or *vitamin D–resistant rickets.* This entity was first recognized by Albright in 1937.[75] The phenotypic trait of hypophosphatemia is transmitted on the X chromosome. Bone disease and short stature are usually more severe in males who carry the abnormal genotype, whereas heterozygous females exhibit a more variable penetrance of these somatic traits.[76] Spinal stenosis and cord compression are late complications of the disorder which are produced by new bone formation in the ligamentum flavum.[77]

Hypophosphatemia develops as a consequence of a reduction in TmP/GFR. The exact nature of the abnormality in renal transepithelial phosphorus transport is not known. It cannot be attributed to excessive secretion of parathyroid hormone, since hormone levels in blood are usually normal[34] or only modestly elevated.[78] In one study, an increased phosphaturic response to exogenous parathyroid hormone was found and led the investigators to speculate that an increased responsiveness to normal levels of the hormone might be a factor.[79] However, in a careful study of one patient with idiopathic hypoparathyroidism and familial X-linked hypophosphatemic rickets, a marked renal tubular phosphorus leak was present when the serum calcium was restored to normal by calcium and 1α,25-dihydroxyvitamin D_3 therapy.[80] A few patients have been reported to have reduced intestinal phosphorus absorption,[81] but this is not an invariable finding.

Studies of vitamin D metabolites in the circulation of patients with hypophosphatemic rickets have raised questions concerning the pathogenesis of the bone disease in these patients. It would be expected that chronic hypophosphatemia would raise the level of circulating 1α,25-dihydroxyvitamin D. Instead, normal or frankly reduced levels of this metabolite have been reported by several laboratories.[82–84] Low levels of the metabolite are usually found in patients treated with vitamin D.[82,84] Further evidence of an abnormality in renal hydroxylation of vitamin D was provided by a study which demonstrated a subnormal rise in serum 1α,25-dihydroxyvitamin D levels in untreated patients in response to an infusion of parathyroid hormone.[85] Impaired synthesis of 1α,25-dihydroxyvitamin D might explain the diminished rate of intestinal calcium absorption found in some patients,[75] but the normocalcemic state which is typical of the disorder suggests that significant 1α,25-dihydroxyvitamin D deficiency is not present. The low levels of 1α,25-dihydroxyvitamin D do not account for the hypophosphatemic state, since physiologic doses of the metabolite do not correct the abnormality.[86]

At least two inherited forms of hypophosphatemic rickets other than the X-linked type have been described. In two families evaluated with autosomal recessive inheritance patterns,[87,88] an unusual clinical aspect was gross osteosclerosis. A Bedouin tribe with a probable autosomal recessive inheritance pattern has been described in which striking hypercalciuria appeared to develop as a consequence of marked elevation of 1α,25-dihydroxyvitamin D levels.[89] Members of the tribe with milder degrees of hypophosphatemia and slight elevations of 1α,25-dihydroxyvitamin exhibited hypercalciuria only.

Sporadic hypophosphatemic rickets may occur in the absence of hypophosphatemia and/or bone disease in any other family member. This form of rickets is clinically indistinguishable from familial X-linked hypophosphatemic rickets and presumably arises from the same mutation responsible for that disorder.

Hypophosphatemic osteomalacia in adults occurs most commonly as a sporadic condition,[90] but a familial X-linked syndrome has been described in a single large kindred.[91] The biochemical findings in this syndrome are similar to those of familial X-linked hypophosphatemic rickets, but untreated adults have no stigmata of rickets and hypophosphatemic children demonstrate no radiologic evidence of epiphyseal dysplasia.

Osteomalacia and rickets may develop as a complication of a variety of generalized renal tubular disorders.[27] These disorders have been classified under the general term *Fanconi's syndrome.* Not only renal phosphate wasting but excessive renal loss of bicarbonate, glucose, uric acid, and amino acids may be detected in affected patients. The bone disease may then be a manifestation of chronic hypophosphatemia and/or systemic acidosis. Acquired renal tubular disorders of phosphate transport differ in one major respect from X-linked hypophosphatemia. Muscle pain and weakness often are prominent features of the acquired disorders but are seldom a problem in X-linked hypophosphatemia. Distal renal tubular acidosis also may cause bone disease in the absence of hypophosphatemia.[27] Rarely, hypophosphatemic rickets may be associated with reversible renal tubular acidosis.[92]

Patients with a variety of benign or malignant mesenchymal tumors,[57] fibrous dysplasia,[93,94] epidermal nevus syndrome,[95] and prostatic cancer[58] may develop rickets and/or osteomalacia in association with hypophosphatemia. In most of these patients there is renal phosphate wasting, normal or slightly low serum calcium concentrations, normal serum parathyroid hormone concentrations, and reversal of the syndrome after removal of the pathologic lesions. It is likely that the lesions secrete a phosphaturic substance, and in one study an extract of a fibroangioma produced a phosphaturic response in dogs.[95] As discussed previously, the significance of low levels of 1α,25-dihydroxyvitamin D in these patients is uncertain, although therapy with 1α,25-dihydroxyvitamin D_3 is often ineffective.[57]

Primary hyperparathyroidism is associated with hypophosphatemia in approximately 70 percent of cases. It is conceivable that osteomalacia could develop in certain patients with severe hypophosphatemia. In one study, quantitative histomorphometry of bone biopsies revealed a reduction of the calcification rate in some patients, but there was no increase in the width of osteoid seams.[96] At present, it does not appear that uncomplicated primary hyperparathyroidism produces significant osteomalacia. However, a patient with primary hyperparathyroidism may more readily develop osteomalacia in the presence of risk factors such as inadequate exposure to sunshine and anticonvulsant therapy. Also, during the postoperative period after parathyroid surgery, osteomalacia may develop as a consequence of the increased need for phosphorus and calcium in the process of healing of osteitis fibrosa.

Malnutrition and Malabsorption

An isolated deficiency of phosphorus due to malnutrition or malabsorption is distinctly uncommon. It is more likely that a combination of vitamin D deficiency and inadequate supplies of calcium and phosphorus would be responsible for osteomalacia or rickets. Persistent use of phosphate-binding antacids is rarely associated with clinical osteomalacia.[97]

Chronic Dialysis

Hypophosphatemia may occur during the course of chronic dialysis in patients with chronic renal failure.[98] Presumably, this occurs as a consequence of excessive loss of phosphorus from the extracellular fluid into the dialysate. The use of phosphate-binding antacids to control hyperphosphatemia may also contribute. Osteomalacia may be severe in a hypophosphatemic patient on dialysis but is promptly reversible with appropriate therapy. The involvement of aluminum in the production of osteomalacia in certain patients with renal failure is described in a later section.

Miscellaneous

Inhibitors of Calcification

Fluoride is a potent inhibitor of bone mineralization and may cause severe rickets and osteomalacia in areas of endemic fluorosis[99] and in patients treated with pharmacologic doses of sodium fluoride. The latter patients usually receive sodium fluoride, 40 mg or more daily, for the treatment of osteoporosis. Osteomalacia is much less likely to develop if at least 1 g of elemental calcium is also taken orally each day.[100]

Etidronate disodium, a bisphosphonate used to treat Paget disease and prevent heterotopic ossification, is an inhibitor of mineralization at doses of 10 to 20 mg per kilogram per body weight.[101] Fortunately, at a dose of 5 mg/kg, Paget disease can be suppressed without diffuse impairment of mineralization. However, focal osteomalacia has been found in bone biopsies of patients treated with low doses of etidronate disodium.[102] Mineralization defects of uncertain clinical significance have also been reported in patients treated with intravenous pamidronate.[102a]

Calcium Deficiency

Radiologic evidence of rickets has been observed in a child with severe dietary calcium restriction in the presence of normal vitamin D intake and normal circulating 25-hydroxyvitamin D levels.[103] Hypocalcemia, hypophosphatemia, secondary hyperparathyroidism, and elevated alkaline phosphatase were biochemical features in this patient. A group of South African children with poor calcium intake were also found to have a similar ricketslike syndrome, which was corrected by increasing dietary calcium intake.[104] However, these children inexplicably had normal serum calcium and phosphorus levels. Histologic evidence of osteomalacia in three South African children on calcium-deficient diets has been reported.[105] Each of these patients was hypocalcemic. Three Belgian infants who were given soya milk developed severe rickets but had a rapid reversal of bone disease when placed on regular diets.[106] It is not known whether isolated calcium deficiency can produce osteomalacia in adults.

Hypoparathyroidism

Rickets and/or osteomalacia have been reported in a few patients with hypoparathyroidism.[107,108] The pathogenesis is unclear, but successful treatment of the hypocalcemia produced healing of the bone disease. Rickets has also been thought to be present in an infant whose mother had hyperparathyroidism[109] and in two infants whose mothers had received long-term intravenous $MgSO_4$ therapy.[110] At least one patient with pseudohypoparathyroidism has been reported with convincing features of rickets and osteomalacia.[111]

Hypophosphatasia

Hypophosphatasia is a rare cause of rickets and osteomalacia.[112] It is usually inherited as an autosomal recessive trait. A missense mutation in the liver/bone/kidney alkaline phosphatase gene has been reported in an infant with lethal perinatal hypophosphatasia.[113] The milder adult form of the disorder may be inherited as an autosomal dominant trait. The biochemical abnormalities which are characteristic of this disorder are (1) low serum alkaline phosphatase activity, (2) elevated serum and urine inorganic pyrophosphate and phosphorylethanolamine levels, and (3) frequently hypercalcemia in children. Since inorganic pyrophosphate and phosphorylethanolamine are substrates for alkaline phosphatase, it is likely that the high levels of these substances reflect decreased alkaline phosphatase activity in bone and perhaps other organs. Inorganic pyrophosphate may be an important intermediary in the initiation of bone mineralization by extracellular matrix vesicles. It is not known whether phosphorylethanolamine has any function in bone mineralization. The pathogenesis of hypercalcemia in hypophosphatasia is unknown, although one report suggests that parathyroid hormone levels may be elevated in infantile hypophosphatasia.[114]

A study of bone histology in a kindred of patients with adult hypophosphatasia demonstrated a paucity of osteoblasts despite the excess of osteoid.[115] The authors proposed that osteoblast dysfunction might be manifested first by mineralization defects and later by a reduction in the numbers of osteoblasts.

Fibrogenesis Imperfecta Ossium

Fibrogenesis imperfecta ossium is a rare disorder which affects previously healthy males over age 50.[116] Skeletal pain and tenderness may be so severe as to cause total incapacitation. Pseudofractures may be seen on roentgenograms, but, unexpectedly, there is a generalized increase in bone density with a lack of trabeculation and a mottled appearance. Bone histology reveals an increased amount of osteoid, impaired uptake of tetracycline, and absence of a normal lamellar pattern of the collagen fibers. The latter finding suggests an underlying defect in collagen synthesis. Consistent with this hypothesis are the findings of normal plasma calcium and phosphorus concentrations. Plasma alkaline phosphatase activity is increased.

Systemic Acidosis

Systemic acidosis due to isolated renal tubular acidosis, Fanconi's syndrome, or chronic renal failure may be an important factor in the pathogenesis of osteomalacia associated with these disorders.[27] Normal levels of vitamin D metabolites have been found in the circulation of patients with renal tubular acidosis[117] and in volunteers with induced metabolic acidosis.[118] The mineralization defect associated with chronic acidosis probably arises as a direct consequence of acidemia.[119]

Total Parenteral Nutrition

Long-term use of total parenteral nutrition has been associated with bone pain, patchy osteomalacia, low serum levels of parathyroid hormone and 1α,25-dihydroxyvitamin D, hypercalciuria, and intermittent hypercalcemia.[120,121] In patients receiving casein hydrolysate, inadvertent infusion of aluminum has been implicated as the factor responsible for the syndrome. Such patients have been demonstrated to have aluminum localized to the surface of mineralized bone from which tetracycline uptake was absent.[122] However, the syndrome has also been found in patients infused with free amino acids which are relatively devoid of aluminum.[120]

Treatment

The treatment of osteomalacia and rickets is as heterogeneous as are the underlying causes. Knowledge of the pathogenesis of the disease is critical in assuring an optimum result of therapy, particularly in infants.

Classic vitamin D deficiency can be prevented by the ingestion of 400 IU (10 μg) of vitamin D_2 daily by children and 100 IU daily by adults. These amounts of vitamin D_2 may be used to treat patients with established bone disease, but doses as much as two- to tenfold greater have been used to produce a more rapid clinical recovery.[37] Patients also must receive adequate calcium and phosphorus from their diets or, if necessary, from supplementation. In most patients, the recommended normal daily intake is adequate.

The earliest biochemical response to vitamin D therapy is a rise in serum 1α,25-dihydroxyvitamin D levels.[37] Serum phosphorus concentrations usually increase to normal within 4 to 8 days. Initially, serum calcium may actually decline and alkaline phosphatase may rise, but both move toward normal levels within weeks. Vitamin D intoxication can be avoided or minimized by measuring the plasma calcium concentration every 2 to 4 weeks. The dose should be reduced, if pharmacologic, when the biochemical parameters approach the normal range and when radiologic healing of rickets is apparent.

Patients with vitamin D malabsorption require only short-term vitamin D therapy if the underlying disorder can be treated effectively. This is particularly true in patients with celiac disease, in whom a gluten-free diet will produce a complete remission of the malabsorptive state and concomitant vitamin D deficiency. If the disorder is irreversible, pharmacologic doses of vitamin D are required. The dose of vitamin D varies widely, but up to 100,000 IU per day by the oral route may be necessary. In some patients, parenteral administration of smaller doses is required. Greater than usual amounts of calcium and phosphorus also may be needed to overcome the inefficiency of intestinal absorption.

In patients with impaired vitamin D metabolism, vitamin D_2 therapy in pharmacologic amounts is usually effective in preventing or reversing rickets and osteomalacia. Up to 15,000 IU daily has been used to induce healing of established bone disease. Lower doses of 25-hydroxyvitamin D_3 have been effective in these patients.[123] In patients with low circulating levels of 1α,25-dihydroxyvitamin D, near-physiologic doses of this metabolite can produce healing of bone lesions. This has been demonstrated in patients with vitamin D–dependent rickets type I[30] and in some patients with chronic renal failure. In children with vitamin D–dependent rickets type II, pharmacologic doses of vitamin D_2 or its metabolites may be effective. In resistant patients, intravenous or oral calcium (one patient) has been demonstrated to heal rickets.[124,125] The role of 1α,25-dihydroxyvitamin D_3 in the treatment of renal osteodystrophy is discussed further under Renal Osteodystrophy, below.

The main principle in the treatment of hypophosphatemic bone disease is restoration of the serum phosphorus concentration to the normal range. This may prove difficult if administration of vitamin D_2 or a vitamin D analogue is the sole therapy given to patients with renal phosphate wasting. Pharmacologic doses of vitamin D_2 or dihydrotachysterol were the earliest forms of treatment for patients with familial X-linked hypophosphatemic rickets. These drugs often were administered at toxic levels and caused hypercalciuria and hypercalcemia. Despite this high dosage, the rickets was not uniformly healed and there was seldom a significant reversal of short stature.

In 1972, Glorieux and colleagues reported a major improvement in the clinical course of children with X-linked hypophosphatemic rickets who received oral phosphate supplementation.[126] The phosphate was administered every 4 h throughout a 24-h period to maintain the serum phosphorus concentration within the normal range. The children experienced a marked increase in linear growth velocity. Because phosphate therapy alone usually induces hypocalcemia and secondary hyperparathyroidism because of an increased rate of bone mineralization, it has become customary to simultaneously administer vitamin D_2[126,127] or, more recently, 1α,25-dihydroxyvitamin D_3.[128–130] The latter agent is preferable since it has a more rapid onset of action, has a shorter half-life, and has been observed to correct the mineralization defect in trabecular bone more fully than does vitamin D_2.[129,130] Careful observation of the patients is mandatory to avoid hypercalcemia, particularly as bone mineralization nears normalization,[129] and to prevent chronic hypocalcemia, which may result in parathyroid hyperplasia and hypercalcemia after many years of therapy.[131] Urinary calcium excretion should be monitored since a high percentage of patients treated with vitamin D or its renal metabolite have evidence of medullary nephrocalcinosis determined by renal ultrasonography.[132]

If optimum treatment is begun early in the course of hypophosphatemic bone disease in children, dwarfism and rachitic deformities should be reversible or prevented. However, there is some controversy as to whether the achieved adult height is actually increased in treated individuals. After a retrospective analysis of patients at the Mayo Clinic, it was concluded that there was no evidence that any form of treatment had any effect on adult height, symptoms, or alkaline phosphatase levels.[133] Unfortunately, documentation of the serum phosphorus concentrations maintained in these patients was not available. In three studies in which metabolic control was emphasized, combined phosphate and 1α,25-dihydroxyvitamin D_3 or 1α-hydroxyvitamin D_3 did appear to enhance the mature height level.[134–136] The doses of these agents which are needed to achieve maximal benefit are empiric. Phosphate is used in divided doses approximately every 4 h, providing from 1 g of elemental phosphorus daily in infants to 3 to 5 g daily in children or adults, depending on the achievement of normal serum phosphorus concentrations. Diarrhea may limit the dose in some patients. From 0.25 to 1 μg of 1 α,25-dihydroxyvitamin D_3 daily is needed to prevent hypocalcemia and stimulate healing of rickets and osteomalacia. It is uncertain whether treatment should be continued in adults if metabolic parameters are normal and bone pain is absent. Bone biopsies in untreated adults have revealed persistent osteomalacia in a similar degree in asymptomatic and symptomatic individuals,[137] although mineralized bone volume was normal in all specimens. Controlled trials of combined therapy are needed in both children and adults to settle the uncertainties regarding medical management.

Surgical intervention to correct skeletal deformities may be needed in patients who have not received appropriate medical therapy. Procedures such as osteotomy and epiphyseal stapling may increase the mobility of the patient and prevent the long-term complication of degenerative joint disease. Preoperative and postoperative metabolic control have been found to be important in avoiding the recurrence of lower extremity deformity.[138]

Patients with autosomal recessive hypophosphatemic rickets, sporadic hypophosphatemic rickets or osteomalacia, and Fanconi's syndrome with hypophosphatemia all respond well to phosphate–vitamin D regimens.[37]

In patients with hypophosphatemia due to mesenchymal tumors, treatment with 1α,25-dihydroxyvitamin D_3 and phosphate is generally effective if the tumor is not resectable.[57]

No effective treatment program for hypophosphatasia has been developed. The infusion of alkaline phosphatase–rich plasma in several patients failed to produce any clinical benefit despite increasing the circulating alkaline phosphatase activity into the normal range during a 2-month period.[139] Calcitonin, sodium fluoride, and vitamin D have proved to be ineffective therapies, but one patient has been reported to have experienced a dramatic remission after prednisone and melphalan.[140]

Correction of systemic acidosis with oral alkali therapy can fully heal the osteomalacic lesions. Vitamin D therapy is not necessary.

OSTEOPOROSIS

Osteoporosis is the most common metabolic bone disease and is responsible for significant morbidity in elderly men and women and in patients who are treated chronically with glucocorticosteroids in pharmacologic doses.

The disorder is not a single entity but rather a pathologic state which can arise from a variety of disturbances of skeletal homeostasis. It is characterized in all instances by a decreased mass of bone which is normally mineralized.

Clinical Presentation

Symptoms and Signs

In the clinical evolution of osteoporosis, there is a long subclinical phase which occurs in most patients before recognition of the disorder. During this time no symptoms or signs may be detected, but radiologic and histologic abnormalities would be noted if sought. The term *osteopenia* is sometimes used to describe the existence of a reduced bone mass in the absence of symptoms or signs of osteoporosis.[141]

The initial complaint often experienced by these patients is back pain. This may occur suddenly without warning and may be of great intensity. It frequently results from lifting a heavy object. The pain is sharp or burning in quality, is aggravated by movement or weight bearing, and reflects an underlying compression fracture of a vertebral body. The twelfth thoracic and first lumbar vertebrae are most often affected. After healing of the bone, back pain may resolve completely. More commonly, residual pain reflects spasm of the paravertebral muscles.

Spinal deformity may develop after repeated acute episodes of compression fracture or may slowly evolve in the absence of severe back pain. A progressive loss in stature occurs as a result of reduction in the height of multiple vertebral bodies. Dorsal kyphosis is typical of long-standing spinal osteoporosis. In the most severely affected persons the spinal curvature may be so great as to cause the lower ribs to touch the iliac crests.

Osteoporosis does not produce deformities of the extremities unless fractures occur. The common sites of extremity fractures are the femoral neck and the distal radius.

Radiologic Features

The radiologic feature most characteristic of osteoporosis is a decreased density of bone. This is best visualized with routine films of the spine. Cortical thinning and loss of transverse trabeculation are common findings. If the latter feature dominates, a paradoxic accentuation of cortical density and vertical trabeculation may result. The weakened vertebral bodies allow ballooning of the nuclei pulposi into the classical biconcave "codfish" deformities of the intervertebral disk spaces (Fig. 24-5). A localized herniation of a nucleus pulposus into a vertebral body, a *Schmorl's node,* may occasionally occur. Anterior wedging of vertebral bodies is usually a sign of a marked decrease in bone density but may arise at an earlier stage as a complication of trauma.

Radiologic manifestations of osteoporosis at sites other than the spine include a patchy loss of density of the calvarium, decreased cortical density of phalanges and long bones, and vertical striation of long bones. Bowing of the bones of the lower extremity is not typical of osteoporosis but does occur in patients with osteogenesis imperfecta.

Quantitative assessment of bone mineral in the radius, spine, and hip has revolutionized the assessment of patients with osteoporosis. Previously used routine radiographs of the spine could not detect the presence of osteopenia until a 30 to 50 percent deficit of bone mineral was present. The new techniques provide great sensitivity in diagnosis and in follow-up after therapeutic intervention. The possibility of assessing vertebral fracture risk has been suggested by studies utilizing quantitative computed tomography.[142] Vertebral mineral values above 110 mg/cm^3 were generally associated with no vertebral fractures or wedging, whereas below 65 mg/cm^3 almost all patients had fractures (Fig. 24-6). Recently, it has also been suggested that the risk of hip fractures may be predicted by hip mineral estimates using dual energy photon absorptiometry[143] or dual x-ray absorptiometry.[143a]

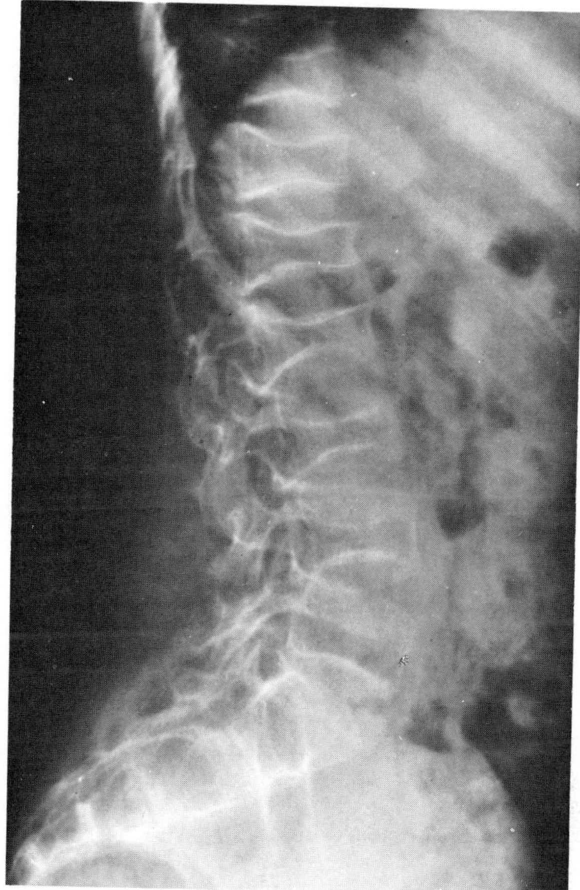

FIGURE 24-5 "Codfish" deformities of the lower thoracic and lumbar spine in a 13-year-old male with juvenile osteoporosis.

Cortical bone density also has been assessed by a variety of techniques. Visual examination of radiographs of the hands and the shafts of long bones is commonly used but is only semiquantitative. Single energy photon absorptiometry of the radius provides a reproducible quantitative means of measuring cortical bone mineral, and dual energy photon absorptiometry or dual energy radiography can give an assessment of cortical bone in the hip.

There has been considerable discussion concerning the use of bone densitometry in clinical practice.[144] Thus far, the cost of the measurements has precluded any widespread use of these technologies for population-based screening for osteoporosis. In

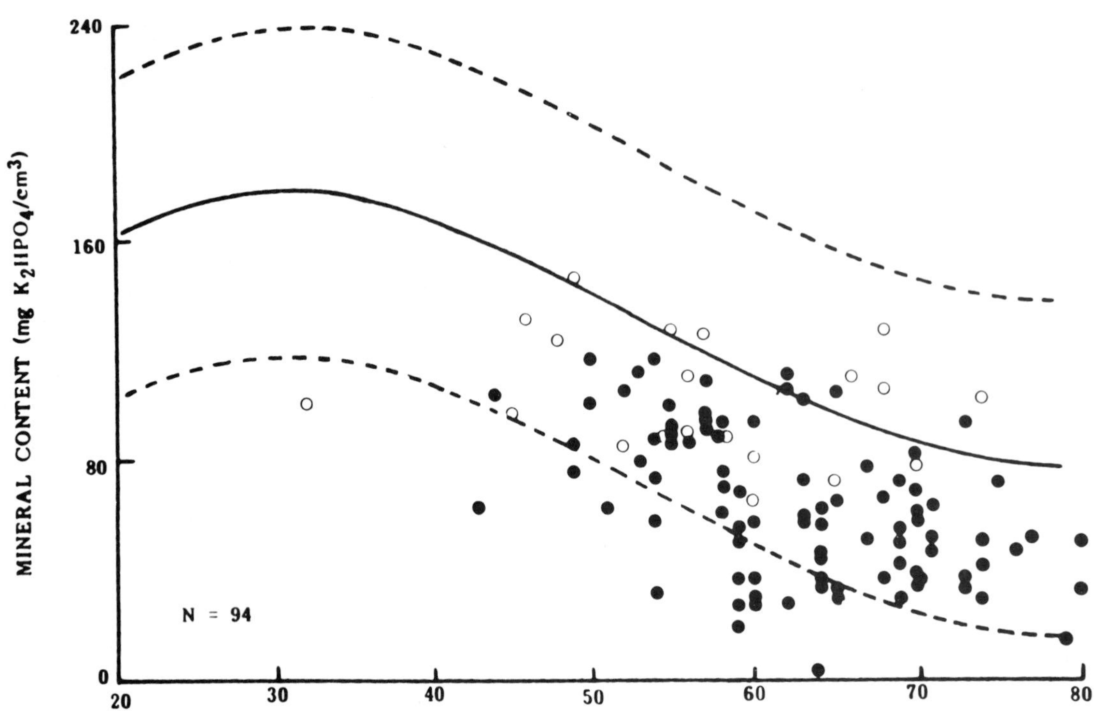

FIGURE 24-6 Vertebral mineral content in osteoporotic (●, with vertebral fractures) and osteopenic (○) females superimposed on mean and 95 percent confidence interval for control women of differing ages (abscissa). None of the osteoporotic women with fractures had values higher than 110 mg/cm^3. Only 1 of 23 women with osteopenia but no fracture had a mineral value below 65 mg/cm^3. *(From Cann CE, Genant HK, Kolb FO, Ettinger B, Bone 6:1, 1985.)*

the future, this may be possible if the cost can be reduced significantly.

Laboratory Findings

In the great majority of patients, there are no significant abnormalities of the calcium, phosphorus, or alkaline phosphatase concentrations in the circulation. A subset of patients who have thyrotoxicosis may have elevated concentrations of all three parameters,[145] and patients with primary hyperparathyroidism may be hypercalcemic, hypophosphatemic, and hyperphosphatasemic (Chap. 23).

The concentration of immunoreactive parathyroid hormone in the circulation of osteoporotic women has been reported to be normal, low, or elevated. In a recent study using an immunochemiluminometric two site assay for parathyroid hormone (Chap. 23), it was reported that the hormone was significantly lower in postmenopausal women with fractures than in age-matched normal women.[146] Bone biopsies in the osteoporotic women indicated a direct correlation between parathyroid hormone levels and bone resorption. It was suggested that in estrogen deficiency, the bone may be more sensitive to parathyroid hormone and that this may account in part for bone loss in estrogen deficiency. In another study, parathyroid hormone secretion was found to be reduced in response to phosphate loads in women with postmenopausal osteoporosis.[147]

Studies of total immunoreactive calcitonin concentrations in the circulation indicate that men have higher levels than women do[148] and that the levels in women decline with age.[149] Comparison of total immunoreactive calcitonin levels in untreated postmenopausal women and those receiving estrogen replacement therapy has produced conflicting results. In two studies, estrogen therapy increased calcitonin levels,[150,151] but in one long-term study, baseline and calcium-stimulated levels were indistinguishable between untreated and treated women.[152] In two other studies, baseline calcitonin levels also failed to increase after estrogen therapy.[153,154] The concept that estrogens stimulate calcitonin secretion has also been challenged by studies of circulating monomeric calcitonin in which levels of this biologically active form of calcitonin have been similar in premenopausal and postmenopausal women.[155] Conflicting results have also been obtained in studies comparing calcitonin levels in osteoporotic and normal postmenopausal women. Decreased and normal baseline total immunoreactive calcitonin levels have been reported in osteoporotic women,[156,157] and in one study total immunoreactive calcitonin levels after calcium infusion failed to increase significantly.[158] In the only study of calcitonin production rates, there was a marked decrease in this index of calcitonin secretory capacity in 11 women with postmenopausal osteoporosis compared to 5 age-matched normal women.[159] However, no difference between osteoporotic and normal women was found in two studies in which calcium infusions were used to stimulate calcitonin secretion. In one study, immunoextraction of calcitonin from plasma was done before the assay,[160] and in the other study, monomeric calcitonin was assayed after column purification of plasma calcitonin.[161] There has been no resolution of the significance of calcitonin in the pathogenesis of postmenopausal osteoporosis.

Intestinal calcium absorption decreases with aging.[162,163] This has been attributed to a reduction of 1α,25-dihydroxyvitamin D in the circulation of the elderly[163,164] because of an impaired ability of the aging kidney to synthesize 1α,25-dihydroxyvitamin D. Indirect evidence for this interpretation has been provided by the observations that the rise in serum 1α,25-dihydroxyvitamin D levels in response to parathyroid hormone infusion is blunted in elderly women[164] and that phosphate loads in osteoporotic postmenopausal women suppress 1α,25-dihydroxyvitamin D levels compared to no change in age-matched women.[147] In countries where there is minimal ultraviolet light exposure and no dietary vitamin D supplementation, calcium malabsorption may also commonly develop as consequence of vitamin D deficiency, as evidenced by low levels of 25-hydroxyvitamin D in the circulation.[165] There is controversy as to whether elderly patients with osteoporosis have lower levels of 1α,25-dihyroxycholecalciferol in the circulation than do subjects of similar age without clinical bone disease, as has been found in some studies[164,165] but not all.[166] It has been suggested that resistance to the action of vitamin D metabolites on the intestine was a factor in the pathogenesis of calcium malabsorption based on the observation that calcium absorption relative to serum 1α,25-dihydroxyvitamin D levels was significantly lower in osteoporotic women than in normal women.[167]

In patients with evolving osteoporosis, urinary calcium excretion may be significantly elevated, a reflection of an increased rate of bone resorption.[168] This is most likely to be found in patients with hyperthyroidism or in a completely immmobilized patient. Urinary hydroxyproline excretion is also elevated in these patients because of increased bone matrix resorption.[168] Urinary pyridinium cross-link measurements provide a more specific index of bone matrix resorption[15] and may replace hydroxyproline measurement as an index of bone resorption in the future (see Chap. 23).

The renal handling of phosphorus has been reported to be abnormal in women with postmenopausal osteoporosis. The TmP/GFR was significantly higher in 24 patients compared with 18 age-matched normal subjects.[169] This may reflect the modest decrease in serum parathyroid hormone levels found in these patients.

Bone Pathology

The histologic features of osteoporosis are quite heterogeneous and, in some respects, still controversial. Two findings are universally agreed on: (1) Bone volume is decreased, and (2) existing bone is normally mineralized.

The rates of bone formation and bone resorption in women with postmenopausal osteoporosis have been estimated by quantitative histomorphometry of iliac crest bone biopsies in several laboratories. Jowsey and colleagues reported that resorptive surfaces were greater than normal and bone-forming surfaces were usually normal in postmenopausal osteoporosis.[170] A similar conclusion was reached in an English study.[171] The former study utilized quantitative microradiography, a technique which measures the density of the mineral phase of bone, and the latter study evaluated the extent of osteoid-covered surfaces and the fraction of surfaces occupied by resorption cavities. The conclusions of these studies have been challenged by investigators who have demonstrated with tetracycline labeling that in many patients bone formation in the iliac crest is reduced.[172,173] A decrease in the mean wall thickness and duration of formation periods of trabecular bone in women with postmenopausal osteoporosis has also been stressed as indicative of impaired osteoblast function.[174] The reason for the discrepancies among these histologic studies is not entirely clear, but the concept has developed that there is considerable heterogeneity of bone histology in postmenopausal osteoporosis.[175–178] Biopsy parameters could be classified as indicative of high, low, or normal turnover. Uncoupling of bone resorption and formation is undoubtedly an important factor in determining bone loss and apparently can occur in either a high-turnover or a low-turnover state. Unfortunately, it has not been possible to consistently correlate biochemical parameters with the histologic indexes. This may relate to the observation that the skeleton does not respond in a homogeneous manner to the influences of hormones[179] and perhaps other influences. Thus, it should not be surprising if local parameters of bone turnover do not correlate with overall skeletal metabolism.

The heterogeneity of the bone pathology of osteoporosis is further reflected by studies of patients with adrenal glucocorticosteroid excess and hyperthyroidism. Cushing's syndrome, spontaneous or iatrogenic, is associated with a marked reduction in bone volume. Studies utilizing either quantitative microradiography or quantitative histomorphometry have demonstrated evidence of increased bone resorption and decreased bone formation in these patients.[180–183] In steroid-induced osteoporosis, a decrease in trabecular width associated with decreased bone formation has been suggested to be a characteristic feature.[183]

The histology of hyperthyroidism is characterized by a marked increase in bone remodeling.[145] Numerous osteoclasts and osteoblasts are present, as well as a fibrous bone marrow. The percentage of trabecular bone covered with osteoid is increased, but there is no widening of the osteoid seams, and the mineralization rate is normal. Decreased cortical and trabecular bone volume must ensue if the rate of bone resorption exceeds that of bone formation. Bone disease induced by hyperthyroidism may be difficult to distinguish from that produced by hyperparathyroidism. It has been reported that the two disorders can be distinguished by measuring the size of the periosteocytic lacunae.[145] There is no increase in this parameter in hyperthyroidism, unlike hyperparathyroidism.

Osteoporosis associated with prolonged immobilization has not been studied extensively. In one study, osteoclastic bone resorption was increased and osteoblastic activity was decreased.[184]

Three studies of bone histology in patients with idiopathic juvenile osteoporosis have been reported.[185–187] In a study utilizing quantitative microradiography, there was an increase in bone resorption surfaces and bone formation surfaces were normal.[185] Quantitative histomorphometry revealed normal osteoclast numbers and a reduced osteoblast surface.[186] In the only study utilizing tetracycline labeling, a single patient was observed to have normal bone formation and resorption.[187]

The histologic findings in patients with osteogenesis imperfecta are unique.[188] There is persistence of primitive woven bone and an absence of well-organized haversian systems. Osteoclasts are not present in excessive numbers, and the osteoblasts which are present are spindle-shaped and flattened, like those of inactive cells.

TABLE 24-2 Classification of Causes of Osteoporosis

1. Aging
2. Endocrine abnormality
   - *a.* Estrogen deficiency
   - *b.* Testosterone deficiency
   - *c.* Cushing's syndrome
   - *d.* Thyrotoxicosis
   - *e.* Primary hyperparathyroidism
   - *f.* Diabetes mellitus
3. Immobilization or weightlessness
4. Genetic
   - *a.* Osteogenesis imperfecta
   - *b.* Ehlers-Danlos syndrome
   - *c.* Homocystinuria
   - *d.* Marfan syndrome
   - *e.* Menkes' syndrome
   - *f.* Lysinuric protein intolerance
5. Juvenile osteoporosis
6. Chronic hypophosphatemia
7. Renal hypercalciuria
8. Chronic alcholism
9. Cigarettes
10. Nutritional abnormality
    - *a.* Calcium deficiency
    - *b.* Vitamin C deficiency
    - *c.* Protein deficiency
11. Systemic mastocytosis
12. Anticonvulsant therapy
13. Heparin therapy
14. Rheumatoid arthritis
15. Chronic liver disease
16. Hematologic malignancy
    - *a.* Multiple myeloma
    - *b.* Leukemia
    - *c.* Lymphoma
17. Idiopathic

Classification and Pathogenesis

Osteoporosis is associated with aging, hormonal deficiencies and excesses, nutritional deficiencies, genetic disorders, hematologic malignancy, immobilization, and a variety of other unrelated disorders (Table 24-2). The pathogenesis of bone disease in many of these states is not completely understood, but modern biochemical and histologic techniques have increased our knowledge to a great extent in the past three decades.

Aging

The incidence of osteoporosis and fractures rises with advancing age in women and men. It has been suggested that two distinct syndromes of osteoporosis may occur in the aging population.[189] Type I osteoporosis is thought to occur in a small group of women age 51 to 65 years and to result in fractures in bones in which trabecular bone is dominant, i.e., vertebral bodies. Type II osteoporosis is believed to affect a high proportion of men and women over 75 years of age and produce fractures involving areas containing large amounts of cortical and trabecular bone. Type I osteoporosis may be accounted for in women in large part by gonadal hypofunction, as discussed below, but epidemiologic studies indicate that a variety of other factors may contribute to the pathogenesis of osteoporosis by preventing the establishment of an individual's peak bone mass or by causing a loss of bone mass before menopause. Cigarette smoking and alcohol intake of moderate degree are reported risk factors for osteoporosis.[190–192] Decreased exercise as a consequence of degenerative arthritis in weight-bearing joints, poor nutrition, impaired intestinal calcium absorption, and reduced renal function are additional factors which may contribute to abnormal skeletal homeostasis in the elderly and to the development of type II osteoporosis. Obesity and black ancestry seem to confer protection against both types of osteoporosis.[191–193]

Although symptomatic osteoporosis in the elderly may arise as a consequence of a slowly progressive pathologic process, there is another viewpoint. Its proponents suggest that a major factor leading to osteoporosis in the elderly is the failure to acquire a normal skeletal mass during intrauterine development, childhood, and adolescence.[194] This may result from poor nutrition,[195] delayed puberty,[196] gonadal dysfunction,[197] and genetic influences.[198] The "physiologic" loss of bone mass which is a universal finding in aging people[141] may lead preferentially to symptomatic disease in those who never achieved a normal bone mass during the critical years of growth and development.

Estrogen and Testosterone Deficiency

The incidence of osteoporosis is highest in postmenopausal females. Evidence has accumulated which implicates estrogen deficiency as a major factor in the pathogenesis of the disorder in these persons, although there is no clear evidence that estrogen levels are lower in postmenopausal individuals who develop osteoporosis than in those who do not.

Estrogens may interact at several areas in the control of calcium homeostasis. Estrogens appear to modulate the action of parathyroid hormone on bone, since physiologic doses of estrogens reduce serum calcium, urinary calcium, and hydroxyproline levels in postmenopausal women with primary hyperparathyroidism.[199] The effect of estrogen on bone appears to be direct since estrogen receptors have been found in human osteoblastlike cells.[200] It is unclear how estrogen's action on osteoblasts translates to inhibition of bone resorption, but it is possible that modulation of cytokine production is an important mechanism. For example, it has been shown that increased osteoclast development in ovariectomized mice is mediated by interleukin 6,[200a] a cytokine produced by osteoblasts as well as by bone marrow cells. Estrogen may also influence vitamin D metabolism and/or action. Postmenopausal women have a mild impairment in intestinal calcium absorption which may be linked to reduced circulating levels of 1α,25-dihydroxyvitamin D.[163] Treatment with estrogen has been reported to reverse both abnormalities.[201] However, in one study, the rise in total plasma 1α,25-dihydroxyvitamin D levels induced by estrogen therapy could be accounted for entirely by an increase in vitamin D–binding protein levels.[153] More recently, measurement of "free" 1α,25-dihydroxyvitamin D has indicated that estrogen does increase this metabolite in postmenopausal women.[202] Although it has been proposed that estrogen stimulation of calcitonin secretion accounts for the estrogen effect on inhibition of bone resorption, studies of monomeric calcitonin in the circulation indicate that calcitonin secretion is similar in normal and osteoporotic postmenopausal women.[161] Therefore, while it may be true that low circulating levels of calcitonin in women account for their lower bone mass compared with men, it is still uncertain whether impaired calcitonin secretion is a major factor in the pathogenesis of osteoporosis in postmenopausal women, as has previously been discussed.

Since the ovary is a source of both estrogens and androgens, several investigators have examined blood androgen levels as a factor in normal and osteoporotic postmenopausal women. Both androstenedione and testosterone blood production rates were reduced in osteoporotic subjects in one study.[203] Serum dehydroepiandrosterone was somewhat reduced in osteoporotic women in another study.[204] In postmenopausal women with Addison's disease, bone mineral density of the wrist is much lower than expected and may have been related to low concentrations of adrenal androgens in the circulation.[205]

The central issue of the mechanism of the bone loss in postmenopausal osteoporosis is still unsettled. Albright proposed that this occurs as a consequence of diminished osteoblastic activity.[206] This view is supported by quantitative histologic analyses of bone biopsies and by dynamic studies utilizing tetracycline labeling but not by measurements of serum osteocalcin, the osteoblast protein which is found to increase in most women with postmenopausal osteoporosis. Consideration of other biochemical characteristics of postmenopausal patients suggests a different or complementary mechanism, i.e., increased bone resorption. Urinary calcium, hydroxyproline, and pyridinium cross-links are increased,[15,168] and radiocalcium kinetic studies are compatible with accelerated bone resorption in these patients.[207] These findings are unlikely to be explained by a combination of reduced osteoblastic function and normal osteoclastic activity. A full understanding of the pathogenesis of postmenopausal osteoporosis awaits future studies.

Reversible estrogen deficiency with associated reduced bone density is now well documented in premenopausal women with athletic oligomenorrhea-amenorrhea,[208] anorexia nervosa,[209,209a] hyperprolactinemia,[210] and endometriosis treated with gonadotropin releasing hormone agonists.[211] It is generally felt that decreased bone density can be attributed to estrogen deficiency in these individuals, although the cortisol excess found in anorexia nervosa may also contribute.[209] The complexity of the reduced bone density in patients with anorexia nervosa is further underscored by the observation that oral contraceptive therapy is only partially effective in preventing bone loss.[209a]

Osteoporosis is less common in elderly men, and there are few studies of its pathogenesis.[212] Bone loss with aging is not found to the same degree in males as in females.[16] Gonadal hypofunction may be a factor in the bone loss found in elderly males, since a positive correlation has been found between the percentage of cortical area of the second phalanx and plasma levels of testosterone, androstenedione, and estrone in a group of 60- to 90-year-old males.[213] There are relatively few studies of bone histomorphometry in hypogonadal males.[214,215] No consistent features have been observed. A recent study in younger males emphasized that a history of constitutionally delayed puberty was associated with decreased bone density in both the radius and the spine.[216] It is likely that these individuals will be at increased risk for osteoporotic fractures in later years. The identification of androgen receptors in normal human osteoblast-like cells suggests, as in the case of estrogen, that androgens have a direct influence on skeletal metabolism.[217]

Cushing's Syndrome

Chronic therapy for disorders such as rheumatoid arthritis, systemic lupus erythematosus, and asthma with glucocorticosteroids often produces a virulent form of osteoporosis. The morbidity resulting from the bone disease may approach or even surpass that of the primary disease being treated. Spontaneous Cushing's syndrome may also cause a severe form of osteoporosis, but spontaneous Cushing's syndrome is a rare finding in the osteoporotic population.

The pathogenesis of glucocorticosteroid-induced osteoporosis is complex and probably involves both direct and indirect effects of glucocorticoids on bone.[218] There is evidence that glucocorticosteroids can inhibit bone formation by existing osteoblasts[219] as well as interfere with mesenchymal cell differentiation into osteoblasts.[220] In children, glucocorticoids produce both osteoporosis and decreased linear bone growth[221] as a consequence of inhibition of cartilage growth.[222] The moderate increase in bone resorption found in bone biopsies has been explained by the presence of secondary hyperparathyroidism,[181] although elevated serum parathyroid hormone levels have not been found in all studies.[223–226] The sequence of events that may lead to parathyroid stimulation is unclear, since frank hypocalcemia has not been observed in these patients. The anti-vitamin D actions of glucocorticosteroids may be involved. Pharmacologic doses of glucocorticoids inhibit intestinal calcium absorption,[227] and it is possible that minimal hypocalcemia is the initial stimulus to parathyroid secretion. Hypercalciuria is a prominent feature of steroid-treated patients which could arise from impaired renal tubular calcium reabsorption, but since it is associated with increased urinary hydroxyproline excretion, it may reflect increased bone resorption.[218] Studies of the interaction of glucocorticosteroids with vitamin D metabolism and action have produced confusing results. In animals, glucocorticoids have been reported to be without effect on the hepatic hydroxylation step[228] and to variably inhibit,[229] stimulate,[230] or be without effect[228] on the renal 1α-hydroxylation step. In humans, both normal and decreased levels of 25-hydroxyvitamin D have been found in the circulation of patients receiving these steroids.[225,231] In two pediatric studies, reduced levels of 1α,25-dihydroxyvitamin D were reported in steroid-treated children with nephritis or systemic lupus erythematosus.[232,233] However, in two studies in adults, normal baseline levels were found.[226,234] It has also been suggested that end organ resistance is a major factor in the impairment of intestinal calcium absorption produced by glucocorticosteroids. Administration of 1α,25-dihydroxyvitamin D_3 failed to completely restore calcium transport to normal in cortisone-treated rats.[235] However, near-physiologic doses of 1α,25-dihydroxyvitamin D_3 significantly increased calcium absorption in five patients receiving high-dose prednisone therapy for rheumatologic disorders.[231] The conflicting results which have been reported may in part be explained by species differences and experimental design. Since glucocorticoids are known to inhibit pituitary gonadotropin secretion and gonadal steroid secretion, it is likely that a deficiency of sex steroids also contributes to the osteoporosis of glucocorticoid excess.[218]

Thyrotoxicosis

Spontaneous thyrotoxicosis is a relatively uncommon cause of osteoporosis, but with the increasing use of bone densitometry, it has become apparent that excessive thyroid hormone replacement therapy in women may have a deleterious impact on bone density.[236] Thyroid hormone has been shown to stimulate bone resorption in vitro.[237] Radioactive calcium turnover studies[238] and bone histology[145] indicate that the rates of both bone resorption and bone formation are increased in thyrotoxicosis. The loss of bone in patients with this "high-turnover" type of osteoporosis must reflect a dominance of bone resorption, but the factors which account for a relative uncoupling of resorption from formation are not known. The role of reduced intestinal calcium absorption, probably due to low levels of 1α,25-dihydroxyvitamin D in the circulation, is uncertain, but this may also contribute to the reduced bone mass found in thyrotoxicosis.[239,240]

Primary Hyperparathyroidism

Severe long-standing primary hyperparathyroidism is known to produce major skeletal abnormalities. More commonly, patients are now discovered in an asymptomatic state, and it is not clear whether mild hyperparathyroidism is a significant risk factor for osteoporosis and fractures.[240a] This problem is discussed in Chap. 23.

Diabetes Mellitus

Decreased bone density has been found in association with diabetes mellitus,[241] particularly in young insulin-dependent patients. Despite this, the incidence of fractures in diabetic subjects does not appear to be high.[242] Since insulin promotes amino acid uptake by bone cells and stimulates bone collagen synthesis, it is possible that insulin deficiency or resistance reduces bone formation directly. Alternatively, the hypercalciuria associated with poor diabetic control or impaired vitamin D metabolism may be an important factor.[241,243,244] In rats, experimental diabetes mellitus produces a reduction in serum 1α,25-dihydroxyvitamin D levels,[244] but this has not been found in humans[245] except in young insulin-dependent diabetic patients[246] and patients with severe diabetic ketoacidosis.[247]

Immobilization and Weightlessness

Osteoporosis is a serious complication in patients confined to bed for prolonged periods as a consequence of spinal trauma or neuromuscular disorders. Bone loss appears to arise from a combination of increased osteoclastic activity and diminished osteoblastic activity.[184] Patients under 30 years of age may become hypercalcemic and hypercalciuric. The absence of weight bearing and of muscular activity, rather than hormonal abnormalities, is responsible for the derangement in skeletal homeostasis. A related loss of bone density occurs during space flight and is not influenced by exercise in the weightless state.

Genetic Disorders

A variety of rare genetic disorders are associated with osteoporosis. Osteogenesis imperfecta, Ehlers-Danlos syndrome, homocystinuria, Menkes' syndrome, and Marfan syndrome all appear to evolve as a consequence of specific gene defects resulting in abnormal bone matrix synthesis.[248,249] A more subtle genetic influence may account for the finding of reduced bone mass in the premenstrual daughters of women with postmenopausal osteoporosis.[250] In one study, serum osteocalcin levels were highly correlated in monozygotic twins,[250a] suggesting that bone formation could be under strong genetic control. More recently it has been proposed that common allelic variants in the gene encoding the vitamin D receptor could account for up to 75 percent of the total genetic effect on bone density in normal individuals.[250b]

Juvenile Osteoporosis

Juvenile osteoporosis is a rare disorder which is characterized by a rapid loss of bone in prepubertal children of both sexes.[251] Multiple fractures of long bones, ribs, and vertebral bodies may occur in the absence of any apparent abnormality of skin, sclera, joints, or endocrine function. With the onset of puberty, most patients go into remission. The reason for the remarkable spontaneous improvement in bone density is not known, but low serum 1α,25-dihydroxyvitamin D levels were found in four children in one study.[252] Three of the four received replacement 1α,25-dihydroxyvitamin D_3 therapy and exhibited major improvement in bone mineral density.

Chronic Hypophosphatemia

Osteoporosis has been demonstrated in the bone biopsies of 19 adults with chronic hypophosphatemia due to renal tubular wasting of phosphate.[253] This was associated with hypercalciuria, increased urinary hydroxyproline excretion, and low levels of serum immunoreactive parathyroid hormone. How this syndrome relates to the more common problems of hypophosphatemic rickets and osteomalacia is unclear.

Renal Hypercalciuria

Relatively few studies have been done to evaluate the status of bone mineral content in hypercalciuric renal stone patients. Conceivably, patients who have a renal leak of calcium and secondary hyperparathyroidism could become osteopenic. This was the case in a group of patients with renal hypercalciuria in whom single energy photon absorptiometry of the radius was done.[254] The mean density in these subjects was about 10 percent below that of age- and sex-matched controlled subjects, whereas the mean density in patients with absorptive hypercalciuria was normal.

Chronic Alcoholism

Bone density and histomorphometric measurements in eight middle-aged males with a history of high alcohol intake for at least 10 years revealed a significant degree of osteoporosis.[255] The patients were otherwise generally in good health and had no evidence of cirrhosis of the liver. Impaired osteoblast function leading to reduced bone formation has been proposed as the mechanism by which osteoporosis emerges in alcoholism.[256]

Miscellaneous

There is an association of osteoporosis with cigarette smoking.[257] The pathogenesis of bone loss in smokers has not been defined but in part may be related to the reduction in weight found in heavy smokers.

Nutritional abnormalities, particularly during growth and development, may produce a reduced skeletal mass. Low calcium intake, which is a common feature of the American diet, seems particularly important in the pathogenesis of osteoporosis.[258] There is some evidence of osteoporosis in patients treated with heparin[259] or anticonvulsants.[260] An association of osteoporosis with rheumatoid arthritis,[261] chronic liver disease,[256] hematologic malignancies,[262] and systemic mastocytosis[263] has been reported, but the pathogenesis in each case is unclear.

Prevention

If the present body of knowledge pertaining to the prevention of osteoporosis were applied to the population, it is likely that in the future the incidence of osteoporosis would be reduced dramatically. This would begin with an attempt to optimize nutrition and exercise in children and deal with the gonadal dysfunction that may arise through anorexia and overexercise. Young adults would be encouraged to maintain an adequate intake of calcium, approximately 1000 mg daily, and avoid harmful habits such as cigarette smoking and excessive alcohol.

At the menopause there are several approaches to retarding the expected bone loss and preventing symptomatic osteoporosis. Estrogen replacement therapy has been conclusively demonstrated to diminish the loss of bone mass in women who undergo either spontaneous or artificial menopause.[264–267] This can be achieved with relatively modest doses of estrogens (0.2 mg ethinyl estradiol or 0.625 mg conjugated equine estrogens orally daily for 25 days each month or 0.05 mg β-estradiol twice weekly by skin patch). Bone resorption is reduced as indicated by a reduction of urinary calcium and hydroxyproline excretion,[206] calcium balance becomes more positive,[206] and intestinal calcium absorption is improved.[201,268] There is now ample evidence that estrogen replacement therapy in postmenopausal women not only inhibits bone loss but reduces the fracture rate compared with that in untreated women,[269] and should be considered the treatment of choice to prevent postmenopausal osteoporosis. Although the greatest benefits of estrogen replacement therapy are believed to occur if the hormone is administered at the onset of the menopause,[265] there is growing evidence that later use can also be beneficial. In a group of postmenopausal women with established osteoporosis who were on average 65 years old, transdermal estrogen slightly increased vertebral and hip density and reduced the incidence of vertebral fractures.[269a]

Estrogen therapy has additional beneficial effects outside the skeleton but may also produce a variety of disturbing complications.[269b] The common menopausal symptoms of hot flashes and increased perspiration are well controlled by estrogen replacement. Estrogen decreases the risk of coronary artery disease by 35 to 45 percent in retrospective studies, but a beneficial effect on stroke prevention is less certain. It has been reported that the hormone prevents the progressive loss of skin collagen in aging women, but this has not been verified in randomized trials. Similarly, improved mood and resolution of urinary symptoms have been observed in uncontrolled studies.

Unopposed estrogen therapy clearly increases the incidence of endometrial carcinoma, although there is no evidence that mortality rates from this tumor have increased as a consequence. Fortunately, progestin therapy prevents endometrial hyperplasia and carcinoma. Cyclic medroxyprogesterone, 10 mg daily for 10 to 14 days a month, and continuous medroxyprogesterone, 2.5 mg daily, are generally effective. However, it is uncertain whether progestins dampen the beneficial effect of estrogen on coronary artery disease. A major controversy continues over the question of an increased risk for breast cancer in estrogen users. Statistical analysis of pooled studies in women who used estrogen for 8 years or more indicated a relative risk of 1.25. As in the case of endometrial carcinoma, it appears that the rate of death from breast cancer is not increased in estrogen users.[270] Whether added progestins have an effect on the incidence of breast cancer is not known. Estrogen usage is associated with a twofold increase in gallbladder disease. Approximately 5 to 10 percent of women experience dose-dependent side effects such as breast tenderness, bloating, edema, and headache, but discontinuation of estrogen is rarely necessary.

Guidelines for the use of estrogen replacement therapy continue to evolve and are particularly difficult to develop for asymptomatic women at the menopause.[270a] As more knowledge about the benefits and risks of hormone replacement develops, the individual patient, with the help of her physician, should have less difficulty deciding whether hormone therapy is appropriate. In postmenopausal women who have had a breast cancer, the synthetic antiestrogen tamoxifen has shown surprising efficacy in preventing vertebral bone loss.[271]

A possible alternative means of inhibiting bone loss in postmenopausal women is manipulation of calcium intake. Correction of negative calcium balance by raising calcium intake to 1500 mg daily has been reported.[268] The data suggest that an absolute increase in net calcium absorption may be achieved in postmenopausal women in whom the efficiency of intestinal calcium absorption is impaired and that this can result in reduced bone turnover and conservation of bone. However, measurement of regional bone mineral content and total body bone mineral in early postmenopausal women who were given 2000 mg of supplemental calcium daily revealed that there was some decrease in the loss of compact bone but that trabecular bone loss in the spine and distal forearm was the same as in a placebo group[272] (Fig. 24-7). Estrogen-treated subjects experienced no decrease in total body bone mineral or regional loss of bone mineral content. An impressive effect of calcium supplementation was subsequently reported in a group of late postmenopausal (at least 65 years)

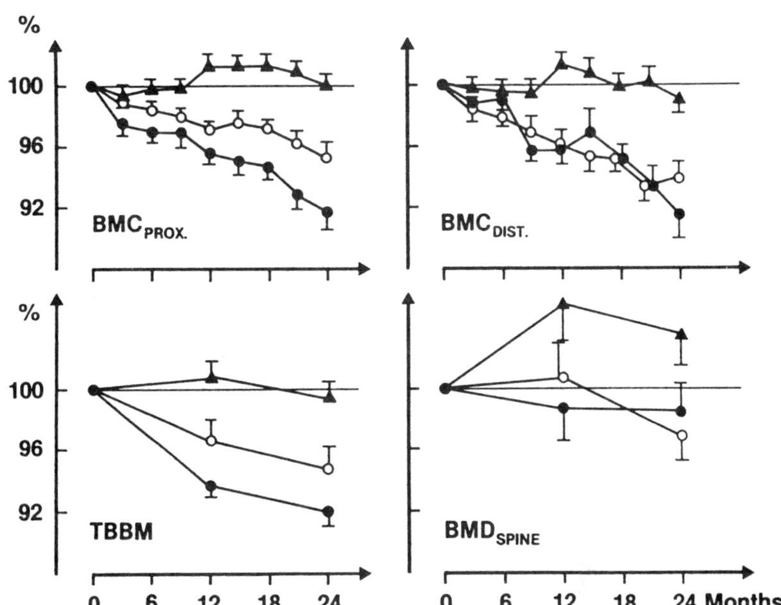

FIGURE 24-7 Bone-mass measurements in groups of early menopausal women treated with percutaneous estrogens (▲), 2000 mg calcium (○), and placebo (●). BMC_{prox} and BMC_{dist} denote bone mineral content in the proximal and distal forearm; TBBM denotes total body bone mineral, and BMD_{spine} denotes bone mineral density in the lumbar spine. *(From Riis B, Thomsen K, Christiansen C, N Engl J Med 316:173, 1987.)*

women who were on a <400 mg daily intake.[273] No decrease was observed in bone mineral density of the spine, femoral neck, and radius over 2 years with supplementation of 500 mg calcium in the form of calcium citrate malate. Calcium carbonate was less effective.

A third means of attempting to prevent bone loss is the administration of physiologic doses of 1α,25-dihydroxyvitamin D_3 to reverse the defect in intestinal calcium absorption commonly present in postmenopausal women. Calcium absorption has been improved with doses of 0.25 to 0.75 μg daily.[274,275] While there have been no trials of 1α,25-dihydroxyvitamin D_3 in healthy postmenopausal women addressing preservation of bone mass, in patients with postmenopausal osteoporosis and vertebral fractures, spinal bone mineral density and total body calcium have been reported to increase slightly[276] and the rate of new vertebral fractures to decrease threefold.[277] However, not all reported studies have documented the efficacy of this therapy.[278] If 1α,25-dihydroxyvitamin D_3 is used to prevent postmenopausal bone loss, careful monitoring of serum and urine calcium levels is necessary to avoid hypercalciuria and hypercalcemia.

Salmon calcitonin administered chronically has been demonstrated to produce a small increase in total body calcium[279] and to stabilize or even increase regional bone density measurements.[280] Most studies have utilized subcutaneous injections of the hormone, but there is evidence that administration by nasal spray can also be effective.[281] There have been no long-term large trials reported which might demonstrate a reduction in fracture rates.

Thiazide diuretics produce a significant lowering of urinary calcium excretion, a property which suggests that they might be beneficial in preventing postmenopausal bone loss. Retrospective analyses of large numbers of patients on these drugs have provided conflicting results. Some studies indicate that there is increased bone mineral content and a reduced prevalence of fractures in treated individuals,[282] but other studies report no reduction in fracture risk.[283]

The bisphosphonates are synthetic analogues of inorganic pyrophosphate which bind to the surface of bone and inhibit bone resorption. Cyclic administration of etidronate sodium (2 weeks on, 13 weeks off) for 2 to 3 years has been reported to increase vertebral density slightly and reduce new vertebral fractures in postmenopausal women with osteoporosis.[284,285] The low dose of etidronate sodium did not produce histologic evidence of osteomalacia in the patients who had bone biopsies. These promising early results may establish bisphosphonates as a major therapy for osteoporosis prevention if the efficacy and safety can be established over a considerably longer period. Newer bisphosphonates such as tiludronate are effective in preventing bone loss[285a] and do not produce osteomalacia at the dose levels used to inhibit bone resorption.

Glucocorticoid-induced osteoporosis is second in clinical importance only to postmenopausal osteoporosis. The management of this problem has proved difficult, particularly when it is not possible to discontinue or reduce the dose of steroid. In one study, changing from daily to alternate-day use of glucocorticosteroids did not seem to reduce the degree of bone loss in arthritic patients.[286]

Because of the known anti-vitamin D effect of glucocorticosteroid therapy, most regimens of therapy for glucocorticoid-induced osteoporosis have included vitamin D and calcium supplementation. Doses of vitamin D_2 ranging from a few thousand to 50,000 IU daily have been administered in combination with 1000 to 1500 mg of dietary and/or supplemental calcium. There is little rigorous documentation of the efficacy of such a therapeutic program. If it is undertaken, serum and urinary calcium levels should be monitored carefully, since hypercalciuria and hypercalcemia are frequent complications of such therapy. If urinary calcium excretion exceeds 300 mg per day, the calcium intake should be reduced to a level which maintains calcium excretion below this amount. In general, doses of vitamin D_2 above 10,000 IU daily should be avoided because of a greater chance of complications. Studies with vitamin D metabolites have suggested a role for these agents in a patient receiving glucocorticosteroid therapy. In one study, nearly physiologic doses of 1α,25-dihydroxyvitamin D_3 (0.4 μg daily) produced a significant increase in intestinal calcium absorption in patients receiving high-dose steroids.[231] In a second study, treatment with 25-hydroxyvitamin D_3 also increased calcium absorption and prevented a decrease in bone density.[287] A third study reported on a double-blind controlled trial of 2 μg of 1α-hydroxyvitamin D_3 in glucocorticosteroid-treated patients.[288] It was concluded that over a 6-month period the drug inhibited bone resorption without suppressing bone formation in iliac crest bone biopsies. No difference in radial bone mineral content was demonstrated between the control and the treated groups. In a large randomized trial 1α,25-dihydroxyvitamin D_3 (mean dose 0.6 μg/day) and calcium supplementation (1000 mg/day), with or without salmon calcitonin, prevented bone loss in the lumbar spine but not in the hip or radius.[288a] Despite these encouraging results the vitamin D metabolites have not been approved for general use in steroid-treated patients. Postmenopausal women receiving chronic glucocorticoid therapy are especially prone to lose bone and ideally should be on estrogen therapy.[289] The role of testosterone therapy in males on glucocorticoid therapy should be explored since serum testosterone levels may be reduced by glucocorticoids. Both salmon calcitonin[290] and the bisphosphonate pamidronate[291] have been reported to prevent steroid-induced osteoporosis.

Treatment

Patients with moderate to severe osteoporosis often have spinal deformities which are associated with intermittent or persistent back pain. The recurrence of back pain may indicate a new compression fracture, perivertebral muscle spasm, or, rarely, spinal cord or nerve root irritation. Chronic back pain may also be related to degenerative arthritis in the area of deformed vertebrae as manifested by osteophyte formation and facet joint sclerosis. Acute compression fractures are usually treated with rest and short-term analgesics. Short-term salmon calcitonin therapy has been reported to reduce pain and improve mobility in patients with recent fractures.[292] In most patients, it is important to arrange a carefully planned long-term program of exercise and physical therapy to attempt to alleviate much of the back pain which may remain after compression fractures are healed.

A long-term goal of treatment of severe osteoporosis is to stimulate bone formation to such a degree that fractures are prevented. The use of agents which primarily inhibit bone resorption can result in mild to even moderate increases in bone mineral content.[267,280,284,285] It has been suggested that this is more likely to occur in patients with high metabolic turnover in the skeleton,[280] but this has not been documented extensively. Moreover, most studies suggest that the gains occur only during the first or second year of treatment. Presumably, bone formation drops as a physiologic response to inhibition of bone resorption. The only agent which has been shown to produce a long-term significant stimulation of bone formation is sodium fluoride.[293] There is general agreement that sodium fluoride therapy given for 4 years or more produces a continuous increase in bone mineral density of the lumbar vertebrae in 65 to 80 percent of patients. However, there is no concensus with respect to the benefits of this therapy in the prevention of vertebral fractures and the potential risk of increasing the number of nonvertebral fractures. Some investigators have found that chronic fluoride administration reduces the frequency of vertebral fractures without increasing the frequency of nonvertebral fractures,[294–297] but none of the studies were double-blind, randomized, and placebo-controlled. The only reported study of this nature found an impressive gain in lumbar spine density, a modest increase in femoral neck and trochanter bone, and a slight decrease in radial cortical bone.[298] Disappointingly, the fluoride-treated patients had no decrease in the vertebral fracture rate. There were more nonvertebral fractures in the fluoride-treated group. Many of these were stress or incomplete fractures, and there was no significant increase in complete hip fractures. Side effects were more frequent with fluoride, mainly gastric irritation and lower extremity pain (58 percent associated with stress fractures). There has been considerable discussion concerning the possibility that the reason for the contrasting outcomes in the fully controlled study versus the other studies is the differences in the dose and the form of fluoride used. In the controlled study, the patients received 30-mg sodium fluoride tablets two or three times daily, and in the other studies, most of the patients received slow-release forms of fluoride. It is thus conceivable that higher fluoride blood levels were achieved in the patients who received plain sodium fluoride tablets and that this produced deleterious effects on bone structure. In a follow-up report of the controlled study, patients were followed for an additional two years.[298a] Lower fluoride doses were administered to more than half the patients because of side effects with the higher dose. Patients who received a lower dose did have an overall reduced vertebral fracture rate. Although these patients were not in a controlled study during the two years, these results support the possibility that fluoride, at appropriate doses, can restore mechanically sound bone in patients with severe osteoporosis.

Growth hormone,[299] human parathyroid hormone (1-34),[300] anabolic steroids,[301] and progestins[302] have been evaluated as agents for the reversal of osteoporosis, but the results have been too fragmentary to allow firm conclusions.

In patients with other endocrine abnormalities which produce osteoporosis, treatment of the underlying abnormality is of greatest value. Resolution of thyrotoxicosis results in an increase in bone mass, although this is less evident in postmenopausal women.[303] Insulin therapy in juvenile-onset diabetes mellitus appears to exert a protective effect on the skeleton.

The osteoporosis of immobilization is best managed by early mobilization of the patient, if this is possible. Although calcitonin is effective in controlling associated hypercalcemia,[304] there is no evidence that osteoporosis can be prevented or corrected by this drug.

The treatment of the osteoporoses associated with genetic disorders has been disappointing. Although several studies suggested a beneficial effect of calcitonin in patients with osteogenesis imperfecta, the most recent study showed no benefits.[305]

A study of a boy with juvenile osteoporosis demonstrated a dramatic effect of the bisphosphonate pamidronate on the clinical course of the disease.[306] A rapid reduction in bone resorption followed by signs of sclerosis near the growth plates of affected metaphyses and at the end plates of the vertebrae was observed over a period of 3 months of treatment with this experimental drug. The improvement of bone density in three children treated with 1α,25-dihydroxyvitamin D_3 has already been discussed.[252]

OSTEOPETROSIS

Osteopetrosis *(Albers-Schönberg disease, marble bone disease, osteosclerosis fragilis generalisata)* is a rare heritable disorder of bone which is characterized by increased skeletal density.[307] The pattern of inheritance is either autosomal recessive or autosomal dominant. Patients with recessive inheritance usually have a more severe form of clinical involvement. Common abnormalities include an enlarged skull, hearing loss, optic atrophy, pathologic fractures, osteomyelitis, retarded growth, leukoerythroblastosis, anemia, thrombocytopenia, lymphadenopathy, and hepatosplenomegaly. Patients often do not survive past age 20 and usually die as a consequence of infection, anemia, or hemorrhage. In approximately 50 percent of patients with an autosomal dominant pattern of inheritance, osteopetrosis is asymptomatic. Fractures, osteomyelitis, and cranial nerve palsies may occur in some patients. Serum calcium, phosphorus, and alkaline phosphatase concentrations are generally normal in both types of osteopetrosis. Serum acid phosphatase is often increased. Occasionally a patient with infantile osteopetrosis will be found to have hypocalcemia, hypophosphatemia, and elevated alkaline phosphatase. A rare recessive syndrome of osteopetrosis, type I renal tubular acidosis, and basal ganglia calcification has been found to be associated with erythrocyte carbonic anhydrate II deficiency.[308,309] Another rare autosomal recessive form of osteopetrosis is associated with a more benign clinical course.[310]

The radiologic features of osteopetrosis are often quite striking. A generalized increase in skeletal density may be associated with a diminution in or absence of marrow cavities, clublike deformities of the long bones, and a "bone within a bone" appearance of the vertebral bodies (Fig. 24-8).

Bone biopsies in patients with osteopetrosis may be difficult to obtain because of increased bone density. Histologic examination of the bone reveals an increased density of bone, often with obliteration of the marrow cavities. The bone may be woven in character in an adult, and remnants of fetal calcified cartilage are a characteristic feature. Numerous osteoclasts may be present, but there is an absence of Howship lacunae, a finding indicative of inactivity of the osteoclasts. This is probably explained by the poorly developed ruffled borders of the osteoclasts observed by electron microscopy.[311] In some patients, few or no osteoclasts may be found in bone specimens. In children, features of rickets may be apparent.[312]

The studies of Walker in osteopetrotic mice have dramatically increased our understanding of the pathogenesis of osteopetrosis.[313] He demonstrated that impaired bone resorption in osteopetrotic mice could be restored by transplanting normal bone marrow or splenic cells and that infusions of splenic cells from osteopetrotic mice to lethally irradiated normal littermates could produce osteopetrosis. These elegant studies have provided strong evidence for the hematopoietic origin of osteoclasts and have stimulated clinical studies of a similar nature. Bone marrow transplantation has been attempted in children with the lethal form of osteopetrosis. Remarkable radiologic and histologic improvement in bone and amelioration of hematologic abnormalities have been reported.[314] In one 5-month-old girl who received a marrow transplant from her normal twin

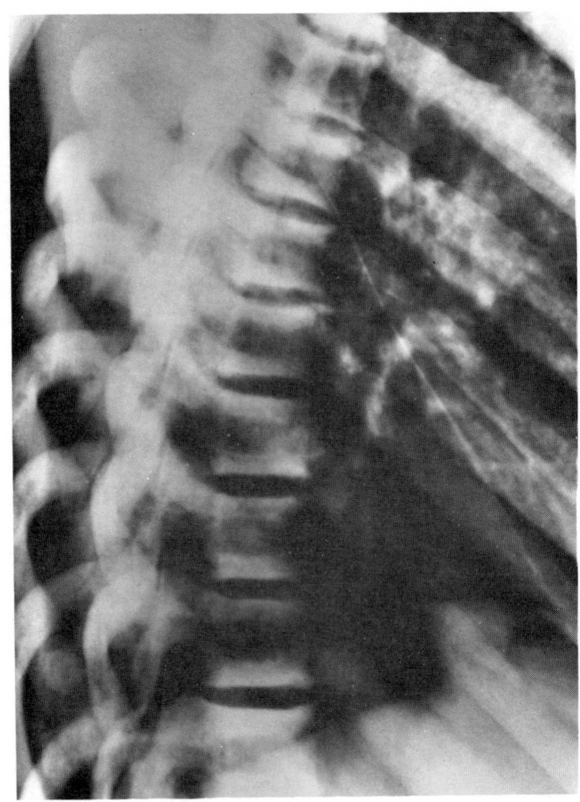

FIGURE 24-8 Roentgenogram of the thoracic spine of a 54-year-old patient with osteopetrosis. Note the marked density of the vertebral end plates, the "bone within a bone" appearance of two vertebral bodies, and the great density of the ribs.

brother, anemia, thrombocytopenia, and leukoerythroblastosis were corrected within 12 weeks.[314] Bone biopsy after transplantation indicated active resorption by osteoclasts, and this was reflected by bony remodeling that was observed radiologically. Normal bone marrow was found in the medullary cavities. Utilizing fluorescent Y-body analysis, it was demonstrated after transplantation that 22 to 67 percent of the osteoclast nuclei were of male origin. None of the osteoclast nuclei had Y bodies before transplantation. Such studies are consistent with the hypothesis that a normal hematopoietic stem cell is not present in some osteopetrotic subjects and that transplantation of normal marrow provides normal osteoclast precursors, which, when fully differentiated, restore normal osteoclast function.

It is likely that new means of treating the various other forms of osteopetrosis will evolve as further knowledge of its pathogenesis emerges. Studies of animal models may again give guidance to therapy in humans. Recently, treatment of *op/op* osteopetrotic mice with macrophage colony stimulating factor has caused a restitution of osteoclasts and resolution of the osteopetrotic state.[315] An analogous syndrome in humans has not been discovered yet.

RENAL OSTEODYSTROPHY

Renal osteodystrophy is the general term used in connection with the variety of skeletal abnormalities which may complicate the clinical course of patients with chronic renal failure. Osteomalacia, secondary hyperparathyroidism, osteoporosis, and osteosclerosis may be encountered in a given patient either as isolated abnormalities or in combination.

Clinical Presentation

Symptoms and Signs

Bone pain, muscle weakness and tenderness, and, rarely, gangrene of the fingers or toes are dramatic complications in patients with renal osteodystrophy.[316] In children, short stature and rachitic deformities are additional features.

Soft tissue calcification often can be detected in the corneas and conjunctivas and gives rise to "red eye." Calcinosis cutis may be associated with generalized pruritus. Calcium deposits may occur around large joints and in muscle. Cardiac and pulmonary calcification may cause congestive heart failure and pulmonary insufficiency.

Radiologic Features

The radiologic findings in patients with renal osteodystrophy are highly variable and reflect the presence of osteomalacia, secondary hyperparathyroidism, osteoporosis, or osteosclerosis in adults and rickets in children. Pseudofractures and rachitic deformities, subperiosteal bone resorption and other lesions of hyperparathyroidism, and, uncommonly, generalized osteopenia may be observed. Osteosclerosis is a common finding, primarily in the spine. A "rugger jersey spine" is characterized by sclerosis of the inferior and superior borders of the vertebral bodies. Sclerosis of the skull and long bones is less common.

Laboratory Findings

Serum calcium concentrations may be low, normal, or even elevated. Serum magnesium is normal or moderately elevated. Serum phosphorus is usually elevated but may fall within the normal range. Alkaline phosphatase activity is often elevated. Serum immunoreactive parathyroid hormone concentrations may be markedly elevated, but this is partly dependent on the type of antiserum used (see Chap. 23). Antisera with carboxy-terminal specificity will measure biologically inactive fragments of parathyroid hormone which are cleared at a reduced rate by diseased kidneys.[317] A small group of dialysis patients will have normal or suppressed levels of immunoreactive parathyroid hormone, even when measured with carboxy-terminal assays.[318] Serum 1α,25-dihydroxyvitamin D and 24,25-dihydroxyvitamin D levels are low,[35,48] but 25-dihydroxyvitamin D is normal if vitamin D intake or sun exposure is adequate.[319] Impaired intestinal calcium absorption is a common finding in severe renal failure.[316] Urinary calcium excretion is low as a consequence of a decreased filtered load of calcium. In patients with elevated serum parathyroid hormone, urinary cAMP excretion is increased and the renal TmP/GFR is reduced. However, the measurement of urinary cAMP and TmP/GFR may not provide a reliable measure of parathyroid function if the GFR is less than 20 to 30 ml/min.

Bone Pathology

The two types of histologic abnormalities in renal osteodystrophy are those of osteomalacia and hyperparathyroidism.[320] Patients who develop osteomalacia as the dominant lesion exhibit all the characteristic features of osteomalacia, including widened osteoid seams which cover an increased percentage of the trabecular bone surface and impaired uptake of tetracycline. There is usually evidence of some degree of secondary hyperparathyroidism as manifested by increased osteoclasts and marrow fibrosis. A small percentage of dialysis patients with aluminum excess have osteomalacic histologic features but no features of secondary hyperparathyroidism in the bone biopsy.[318] Serum parathyroid hormone concentrations are not elevated significantly in these patients.

When hyperparathyroidism is dominant, a marked increase in osteoclastic bone resorption, severe marrow fibrosis, and osteocytic osteolysis are present.[321] The rate of bone formation in these patients may be increased, in contrast to the osteomalacic type of renal osteodystrophy.

Osteosclerosis is characterized by increased bone density. Widened osteoid seams may be seen, but the amount of mineralized bone is greater than normal. Amorphous calcium phosphate rather than hydroxyapatite may be deposited. This may be a consequence of an abundance of woven bone in the osteosclerotic lesions.[316]

Decreased bone volume is rarely found in patients with chronic renal failure. This complication is always accompanied by the histologic features of osteomalacia and/or secondary hyperparathyroidism.

Pathogenesis

The pathogenesis of osteomalacia in patients with renal osteodystrophy is multifactorial. Although circulating levels of 1α,25-dihydroxyvitamin D decrease as the functional renal mass decreases,[322,323] this may not be the critical determinant of osteomalacia, since it is a very common finding, yet only a relatively small proportion of patients with end-stage renal failure develop full-blown osteomalacia. It is likely that factors such as aluminum content of bone, prior parathyroidectomy, metabolic acidosis, and dialysis-induced hypophosphatemia are additional important risk factors in producing clinically relevant defects in bone mineralization.[98,324–326]

The syndrome of aluminum-induced osteomalacia in hemodialysis patients has received considerable attention because of the severity of the symptoms and the potential for reversal of the problem. As was previously discussed, these patients exhibit osteomalacia without evidence of secondary hyperparathyroidism. They may develop hypercalcemia despite modest parathyroid hormone levels,[327] probably as a consequence of the failure of bone to take up calcium from the extracellular fluid. If vitamin D of any type is administered in even small doses to treat the osteomalacic state, severe hypercalcemia may ensue because of increased intestinal calcium absorption,[318] together with the defective mineralization.

Secondary hyperparathyroidism is the most common abnormality in chronic renal failure. A complex series of metabolic interactions leads to the development of parathyroid hyperplasia and high levels of both intact parathyroid hormone and fragments in the circulation.[316] For many years it has been postulated that phosphate retention with resultant transient hypocalcemia is a major factor in producing parathyroid stimulation. A second underlying abnormality is a reduction in circulating 1α,25-dihydroxyvitamin D levels, which may contribute to hypocalcemia through impairing intestinal calcium absorption and may permit greater rates of transcription of the parathyroid hormone gene. The latter could account for an increase in the set point for parathyroid hormone secretion by the ambient calcium. Skeletal resistance to parathyroid hormone may also contribute to secondary hyperparathyroidism. The mechanism which accounts for the dampened calcemic response to exogenous parathyroid hormone in patients with renal failure is not known. Dietary phosphate restriction can prevent the development of secondary hyperparathyroidism in uremic dogs,[328] and the same result has been convincingly confirmed in humans.[329] At the same time, phosphate restriction produces a rise in 1α,25-dihydroxyvitamin D levels in patients with moderate renal failure.[329] The administration of 1α,25-dihydroxyvitamin D_3 can partially restore responsiveness to parathyroid hormone in uremic dogs, and the administration of both 1α,25-dihydroxyvitamin D_3 and 24,25-dihydroxyvitamin D_3 restores full responsiveness to parathyroid hormone.[330] The relevance of this study to human disease has not been established.

The pathogenesis of osteosclerosis in patients with chronic renal failure is unknown. It has been suggested that osteosclerosis is more likely to occur in patients with severe secondary hyperparathyroidism.

Treatment

Successful renal transplantation restores vitamin D metabolism to normal and usually produces healing of osteomalacia within 1 year. Resolution of secondary hyperparathyroidism may take longer because the glomerular filtration rate frequently remains slightly reduced. Persistence of elevated parathyroid hormone levels and long-term posttransplant hypercalcemia are well documented.[316] Other complications of renal transplantation affecting the skeleton include steroid-induced osteoporosis, growth retardation in children, and aseptic necrosis of bone.[316]

Measures which are likely to be helpful in the prevention of renal osteodystrophy are outlined in Table 24-3. Maintenance of normal serum calcium and phosphorus concentrations usually can be achieved by providing an adequate calcium intake, as high as 1500 mg daily, and by restricting dietary phosphorus to 1000 mg daily. Phosphate-binding antacids (Aludrox, Amphojel, Gaviscon, Gelusil, Maalox, and Mylanta) should be used cautiously because of their aluminum content. Calcium carbonate supplements have also been shown to be effective phosphate binders.[331] Dialysis patients should be dialyzed with a dialysate calcium concentration of 6 to 6.5 mg/dl. Careful use of alkali will correct systemic acidosis. Hypocalcemia can be corrected with 1α,25-dihydroxyvitamin D_3 in early renal failure and can reverse resistance to parathyroid hormone and other metabolic abnormalities.[332] The institution of a prophylactic regimen to prevent renal osteodystrophy requires close follow-up to avoid hypophosphatemia, hypercalcemia, and extraskeletal calcification.

TABLE 24-3 Prevention of Renal Osteodystrophy

1. Maintain normal serum phosphorus concentration
2. Calcium intake of 1500 mg daily
3. Maintain normal acid-base status
4. Prophylactic use of 1α,25-dihydroxyvitamin D_3

The treatment of renal osteodystrophy with 25-hydroxyvitamin D_3, 1α,25-dihydroxyvitamin D_3, and 1α-hydroxyvitamin D_3 has received intensive scrutiny because of the greater potency and shorter half-life of these agents. The 1α derivatives of vitamin D have been demonstrated to be particularly effective in hypocalcemic patients with secondary hyperparathyroidism. Chronic therapy with 2 μg or less daily of 1α,25-dihydroxyvitamin D_3 produces normocalcemia, suppression of the parathyroid hormone concentration, and a decrease in alkaline phosphatase activity (Fig. 24-9) as well as reversal of the histologic lesions of secondary hyperparathyroidism.[333] Relief of bone pain and muscle weakness and an increased growth rate in children have been documented in numerous clinical trials. Less consistent results have been reported in respect to improvement of bone mineralization. In some studies, 1α,25-dihydroxyvitamin D_3 has been reported to produce healing of histologic lesions of osteomalacia,[334] but other investigators have reported incomplete healing with this metabolite.[335] It has been claimed that 25-hydroxyvitamin D_3 is a more effective agent in

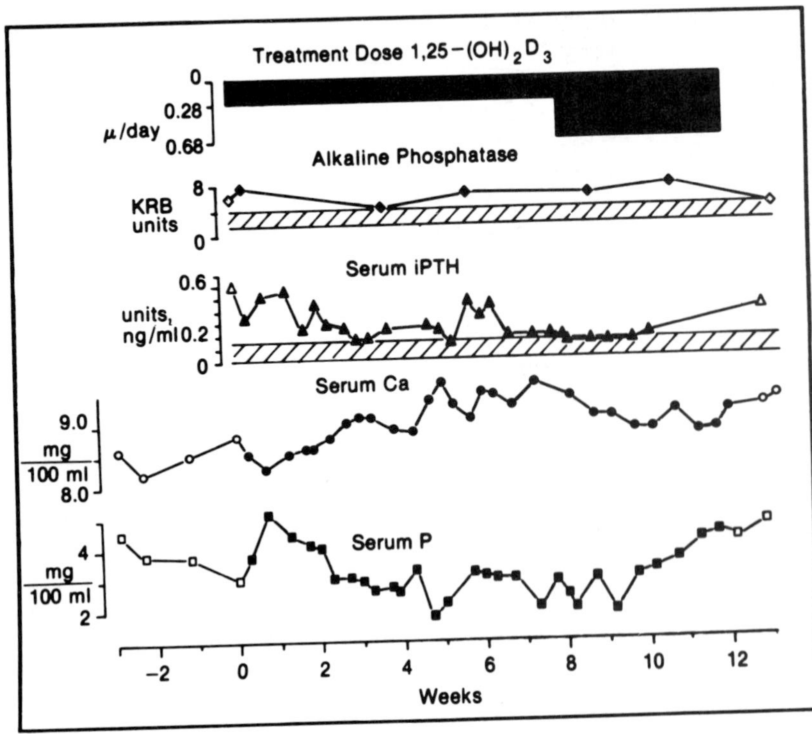

FIGURE 24-9 The effect of 1α,25-dihydroxycholecalciferol therapy in a patient with chronic renal failure. The cross-hatched areas indicate the normal range for serum alkaline phosphatase and immunoreactive parathyroid hormone (iPTH). (*From Brickman AS, Sherrard DJ, Jowsey J, Singer FR, Baylink DJ, Maloney N, Massry SG, Norman AW, Arch Intern Med 134:883, 1974.*)

healing osteomalacia.[336] It is not known at present whether 25-hydroxyvitamin D_3 or the induction of 24,25-dihydroxyvitamin D_3 synthesis is responsible for superior healing or whether inadequate doses of 1α,25-dihydroxyvitamin D_3 in some trials account for the above observations.

If these potent agents are used, the physician must be aware of the danger of hypercalcemia as a complication. A previously normocalcemic patient often becomes hypercalcemic shortly after a significant fall in alkaline phosphatase activity is observed. Hypercalcemia is also likely to occur early in the course of treatment in patients with severe secondary hyperparathyroidism who are normocalcemic or have borderline hypercalcemia before therapy. These patients may require subtotal parathyroidectomy because of massive parathyroid hyperplasia.[316] Symptomatic hypercalcemia, intractable pruritus, bone pain, fractures, extraskeletal calcifications, and cutaneous gangrene are indications for parathyroid surgery. The studies of Wells suggest that total parathyroidectomy with transplantation of parathyroid tissue in a forearm is the surgery of choice.[337]

In hemodialysis patients with secondary hyperparathyroidism, it may prove difficult to control bone disease with oral vitamin D metabolites because small doses may induce hypercalcemia. Another approach is to infuse 1α,25-dihydroxyvitamin D_3 three times weekly (1 to 2.5 μg) in the dialysis tubing. This has been reported to markedly improve osteitis fibrosa in bone biopsies and lower serum parathyroid hormone concentrations in dialysis patients who are refractory to oral 1α,25-dihydroxyvitamin D_3.[338] The efficacy of this form of therapy is probably related to the direct inhibition of parathyroid hormone gene transcription by the vitamin D metabolite.

A particularly difficult group of patients to treat is the subset of dialysis patients with aluminum excess who have severe osteomalacia in the absence of biochemical or histologic evidence of secondary hyperparathyroidism.[318,324] These patients often do not respond adequately to treatment with 1α,25-dihydroxyvitamin D_3. Deferoxamine infusions may remove aluminum from bone and reverse the osteomalacic lesion. Fortunately, aluminum-induced renal osteodystrophy has become much less common because of a reduced aluminum content in the dialysate and reduced use of aluminum hydroxide.

HEREDITARY HYPERPHOSPHATASIA

Hereditary hyperphosphatasia is a rare autosomal recessive disorder which usually presents during infancy.[340] This condition has been described by a variety of eponyms, including chronic idiopathic hyperphosphatasia, hyperostosis corticalis deformans juvenilis, osteochalasia desmalis familiaris, familial osteoectasia, chronic progressive osteopathy with hyperphosphatasia, hereditary bone dysplasia with hyperphosphatasemia, and juvenile Paget disease. Enlargement of the skull and facial bones and bowing of the extremities are common features of the disease. Skin temperature may be increased over affected bones. Bone pain and pathologic features are common.

The radiologic features of hereditary hyperphosphatasia include loss of the normal cortical architecture, disruption of the corticomedullary border, expansion of the diaphysis, and strikingly increased density of the calvarium with a patchy "cotton-wool" pattern. The latter abnormality is quite similar to the radiologic appearance of the skull in patients with advanced Paget disease of bone.

The laboratory characteristics of this disorder are identical to those of polyostotic Paget disease of bone. Serum calcium and phosphorus concentrations are normal. Serum alkaline phosphatase activity and urinary hydroxyproline excretion may be markedly elevated.

The reported histologic findings in patients with hereditary hyperphosphatasia have been heterogeneous, an indication that the classification of patients may be imperfect. There is agreement that the bone is laid down in a chaotic manner indistinguishable from the mosaic pattern of bone characteristic of Paget disease. Numerous osteoblasts and a fibrovascular bone marrow are present. There is disagreement about whether woven or lamellar bone is the dominant type of bone formed. Another point of controversy concerns which bone cells are responsible for the increased rate of bone resorption. In one study of several patients,[340] numerous osteoclasts were present in bone biopsies, but in another study, osteoclasts were rarely observed.[341] Instead, the investigators found a marked degree of osteocytic osteolysis and concluded that the osteocytes were responsible for the accelerated rate of bone resorption. They also described ultrastructural abnormalities in both the osteocytes and the osteoblasts of their patients.[342] Intramitochondrial microcrystalline bodies that were thought to represent calcium deposits were observed. The significance of these intracellular deposits is unknown, but they have been reported to disappear after calcitonin therapy.

The pathogenesis of hereditary hyperphosphatasia is unknown. The disease is clearly not a childhood form of Paget disease, since it is generalized in its distribution and the characteristic nuclear and cytoplasmic inclusions found in the osteoclasts of Paget disease are not present.

Despite the lack of understanding of the pathogenesis of hereditary hyperphosphatasia, remarkable progress has been made in treating this disorder. Chronic treatment with calcitonin is associated with dramatic clinical improvement of both subjective and objective parameters.[341–345] Reduction in bone pain and in the incidence of pathologic fractures has been reported. The rate of bone turnover is decreased, as manifested by a reduction of alkaline phosphatase activity and urinary hydroxyproline excretion. Improvement of radiologic abnormalities has been observed, as well as improvement of the histologic abnormalities in bone biopsies. These improvements in skeletal structure and metabolism appear to be maintained during years of therapy.

FIBROUS DYSPLASIA

Fibrous dysplasia of bone (Albright's syndrome, Albright-McCune-Sternberg syndrome) is a rare disorder of unknown etiology which may be monostotic or polyostotic in distribution. It is clearly not a metabolic bone disease, but because of numerous associated endocrinopathies it seems appropriate to include this entity in a discussion of metabolic bone disease.

The disorder was lucidly described by Albright and colleagues in 1937,[346] but Albright subsequently pointed out that the first cases in the medical literature were reported by von Recklinghausen in 1891.[347] Cases 5 and 6 of von Recklinghausen's monograph were mistakenly believed to be examples of osteitis fibrosa generalisata.[348]

Fibrous dysplasia is usually recognized between the ages of 3 and 10. There is no evidence of genetic transmission. A triad of abnormalities is often present: bone lesions, sexual precocity (primarily in girls), and café-au-lait skin lesions which have serrated edges.[346] The bone lesions most often affect the femur, tibia, pelvis, hand, rib, humerus, and skull.[349] In patients with polyostitic fibrous dysplasia, there is a tendency to unilateral distribution of the disease. Skeletal deformity, pain, and pathologic fractures are the main manifestations of the bone lesions. Sarcomas may rarely arise in a lesion of fibrous dysplasia.[35] Intramuscular myxomas are a rare associated condition.[351] A great variety of endocrinopathies have been described in patients with fibrous dysplasia since the initial reports of sexual precocity. These include acromegaly, gigantism, hyperprolactinemia, hyperthyroidism, hyperparathyroidism, Cushing's syndrome, hypothalamic hypogonadism, and hypophosphatemic rickets.[352–355] The skin pigmentation occurs most frequently over the sacrum, buttocks, and cervical spine.

The characteristic radiologic feature of fibrous dysplasia is a ground-glass appearance of the lesions. Focal cortical thinning, expansion of the diaphysis, and a multilocular configuration of the lesions are also features (Fig. 24-10). Gross deformities of the skeleton are often apparent. Shepherd's-crook deformity of the femur, coxa vara, tibial bowing, protrusio acetabuli, and enlarged facial bones are common abnormalities. Increased radiodensity of the base of the skull and thickening of the occiput may be observed.

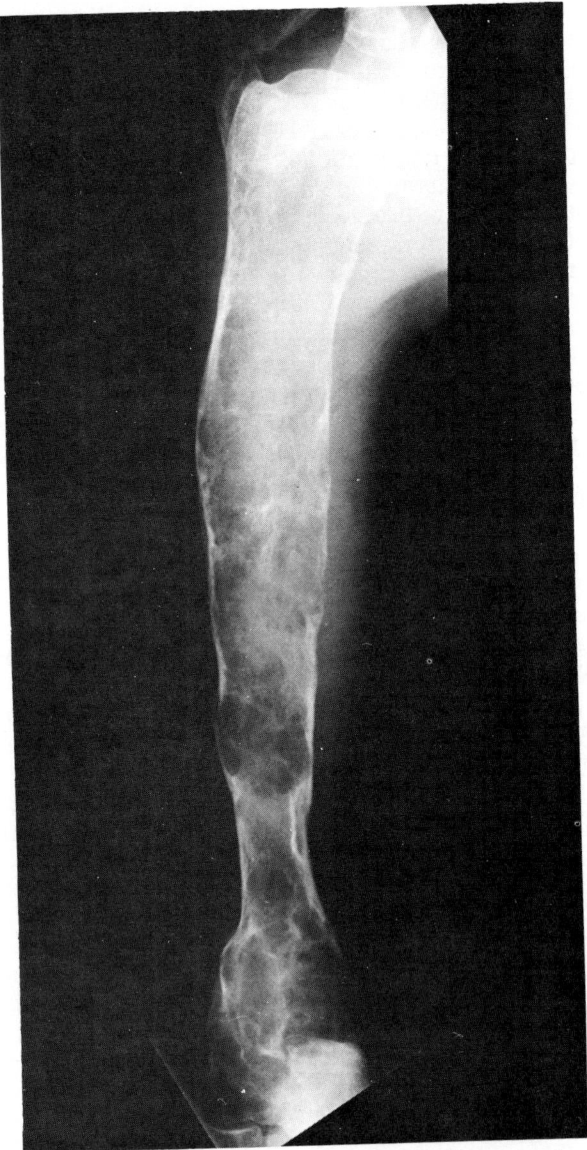

FIGURE 24-10 Roentgenogram of the right humerus of a 32-year-old man with polyostotic fibrous dysplasia. Note the cortical thinning, diaphyseal expansion, and multiloculated appearance of the lesions.

Serum calcium and phosphorus determinations are usually normal, except in the few patients who have associated hyperparathyroidism or hypophosphatemic rickets. Serum alkaline phosphatase activity and urinary hydroxyproline excretion may be increased, a reflection of accelerated bone turnover. The turnover of fibrous connective tissue in bone lesions may also contribute to the level of hydroxyproline excretion.

Pathologically, fibrous dysplasia is dominated by the dense fibrous connective tissue which surrounds the trabeculae[349] (Fig. 24-11). The bone is woven in character, and the randomly oriented collagen fibers appear to extend into the adjacent fibrous tissue. Numerous fibroblasts and osteoblasts may be present in areas of new bone formation. Widened osteoid seams occasionally are noted at sites where there are few osteoblasts. Osteoclasts may be present in areas adjacent to those in which there is increased osteoblastic activity. Islands of cartilage may represent remnants of the epiphysis or abortive callus formation. Callus formation after trauma may be inadequate. Fluid-filled cysts sometimes develop in areas of previous trauma or surgery. Pathologic examination of the endocrine glands in patients with endocrine disease has revealed hyperplasia and adenomas of the pituitary, thyroid, parathyroid, and adrenal glands.[352] The ovaries of girls with sexual precocity have not shown evidence of ovulation in the few such patients who have been studied.

The pathogenesis of fibrous dysplasia may be related to somatic mutations that have been found within exon 8 of the α subunit of the stimulatory guanine nucleotide-binding protein (see Chap. 5) in a variety of tissues.[355a] The resolution of associated hypophosphatemic bone disease after resection of the lesions of fibrous dysplasia in one patient does suggest that a phosphaturic factor may be secreted by the bone lesions.[93]

FIGURE 24-11 A trabecula of bone surrounded by dense fibrous connective tissue from a patient with fibrous dysplasia. Decalcified, H&E.

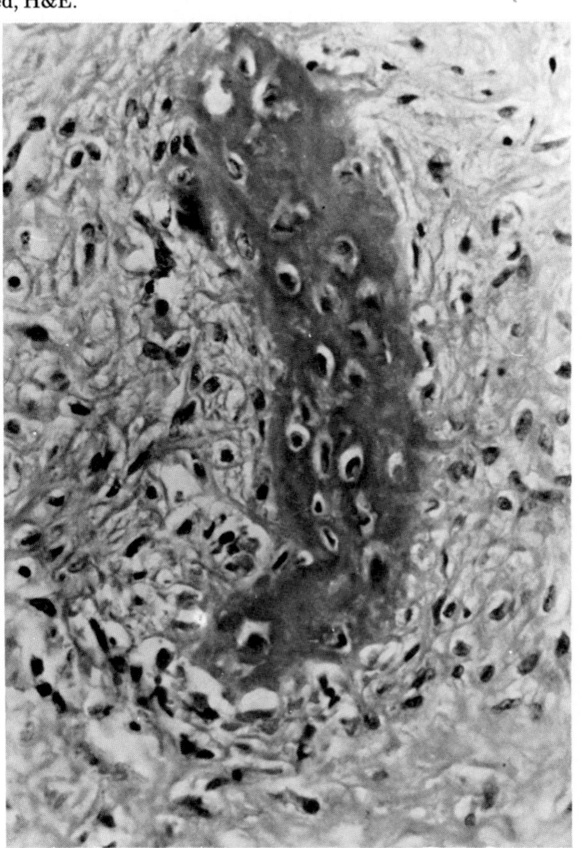

No satisfactory medical treatment of fibrous dysplasia is known. Radiation therapy may lead to sarcomatous degeneration. Because of the finding of osteoclasts in bone biopsies, calcitonin, mithramycin, and etidronate sodium have been administered to several patients[93,356,357]; no significant improvement has been demonstrated. In one patient who had an ovarian cyst, treatment with an analogue of luteinizing hormone releasing hormone failed to suppress cyclical ovarian function.[358] Testolactone, an inhibitor of estrogen synthesis, has been demonstrated to reduce estradiol levels, ovarian volume, and growth rates in young girls with precocious puberty.[359] Standard treatments of the other endocrinopathies are usually successful.

Various orthopedic procedures on the upper extremities, spine, pelvis, and lower extremities are necessary to treat pain, deformity, and fractures.[360]

PAGET'S DISEASE OF BONE

Paget's disease of bone is a common localized disorder of bone which is often included in a consideration of metabolic bone diseases because in its polyostotic form the level of metabolic activity of the skeleton is as great as that in any bone disease.

Sir James Paget provided a brilliant description in 1876 of a crippling bone disorder he termed *osteitis deformans*.[361] Although he thought that it was a rare disorder, the advent of roentgenograms revealed it to be a common albeit often asymptomatic affliction. An incidence of 3 percent in persons over age 40 has been found in regions of the world where there are large concentrations of people of Anglo-Saxon origin.[362] The disease is rare in the Orient, India, and Scandinavia. Males and females are almost equally affected. A positive family history of Paget's disease has been reported in up to 25 percent of patients.

Clinical Presentation

Symptoms and Signs

A significant proportion of patients with Paget's disease do not have symptoms of the disease. In these patients, the disease is discovered because of screening blood chemistry or chance findings on radiologic examinations.

Pain and skeletal deformity are the most common presenting complaints in patients with symptomatic Paget's disease. The pain may arise in bone or joints or from spinal cord or nerve impingement.[363] Bone pain is usually not severe and is only slightly worsened by weight bearing if present in the spine, pelvis, or lower extremities. There is a puzzling lack of correlation between the degree of pain and the severity of skeletal deformity. Patients with polyostotic disease, which is associated with marked deformity, may never experience bone pain, whereas moderate pain may arise in a lesion which is demonstrable only by radiologic examination. Joint pain due to degenerative arthritis is usually more severe than bone pain. The most common sites are the hip and knee joints. Weight bearing typically increases the severity of the joint pain. The most excruciating pain occurs as a consequence of impingement by deformed vertebrae on the spinal cord or nerve roots. This pain is often felt in the back and/or lower extremities. Some patients experience pain as a result of a combination of Paget's involvement, degenerative changes, and nerve impingement, and it may be difficult to judge the relative contributions of each type of pain in these patients.

The deformities which may appear in patients with long-standing Paget's disease are most readily appreciated by examining the skull, clavicles, and long bones. The involved bones are generally both increased in size and of an abnormal contour. An increase in skin temperature over affected long bones is a typical finding and is explained by soft tissue vascularity surrounding the bones.[364]

Loss of auditory acuity occurs in approximately 50 percent of patients with skull involvement. A combined conductive and sensorineural hearing deficit is common.

In about 15 percent of patients, disruptions of Bruch's membrane produce cracks in the retina which are termed *angioid streaks*. They rarely produce visual impairment.

A variety of other complications may occur in patients with Paget's disease. Pathologic fractures of the femur, tibia, and vertebral bodies are not uncommon.[362] Nonunion is usually not a major problem. Bone tumors present with an increase in pain and/or a rapidly growing mass at sites of Paget's disease. Sarcomas are most common but fortunately occur in less than 1 percent of patients.[362] Benign giant-cell tumors may arise in skull and facial lesions. Multiple myeloma and metastatic carcinoma appear to be chance associations. Gout has been reported to affect males with great frequency, but this has not been a uniform finding.[363] An increase in cardiac output may be found in patients whose disease involves 20 percent or more of the skeleton,[365] but intractable high-output cardiac failure is seldom encountered.

Radiologic Features

The earliest lesions of Paget's disease which can be detected radiologically are osteolytic in nature. In the skull, these early lesions have been termed *osteoporosis circumscripta* (Fig. 24-12). Osteolytic lesions in the extremities are usually found at either end of the affected bone and advance as a V-shaped osteolytic front at an average rate of 1 cm per year.

The evolution of osteolytic lesions into an osteoblastic phase may require years or even decades. In the skull, there is thickening of the calvarium with a loss of definition of the inner and outer tables. A "cotton wool" appearance due to a patchy increase in bone density is common (Fig. 24-13). Platybasia or

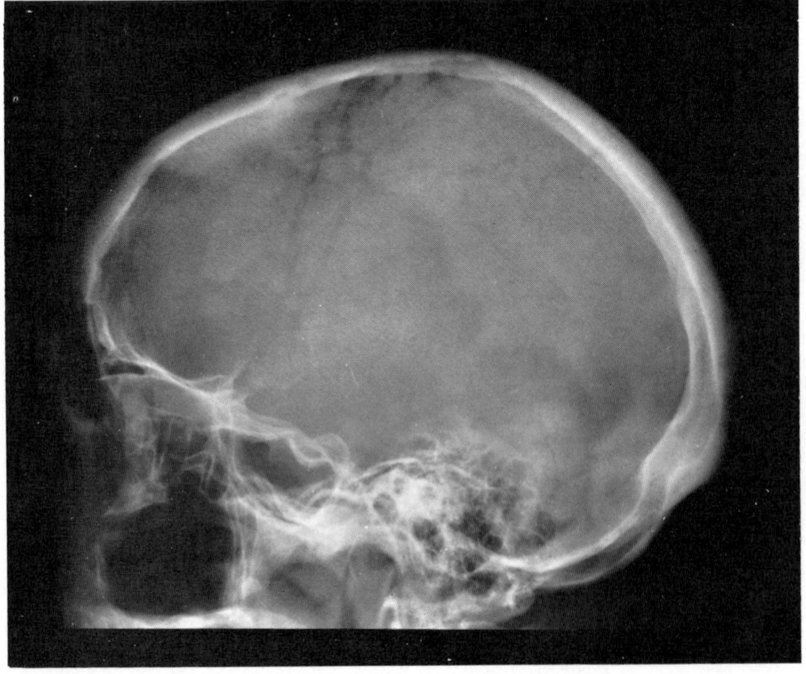

FIGURE 24-12 Roentgenogram of the skull of a 48-year-old patient with osteoporosis circumsripta cranii due to Paget's disease.

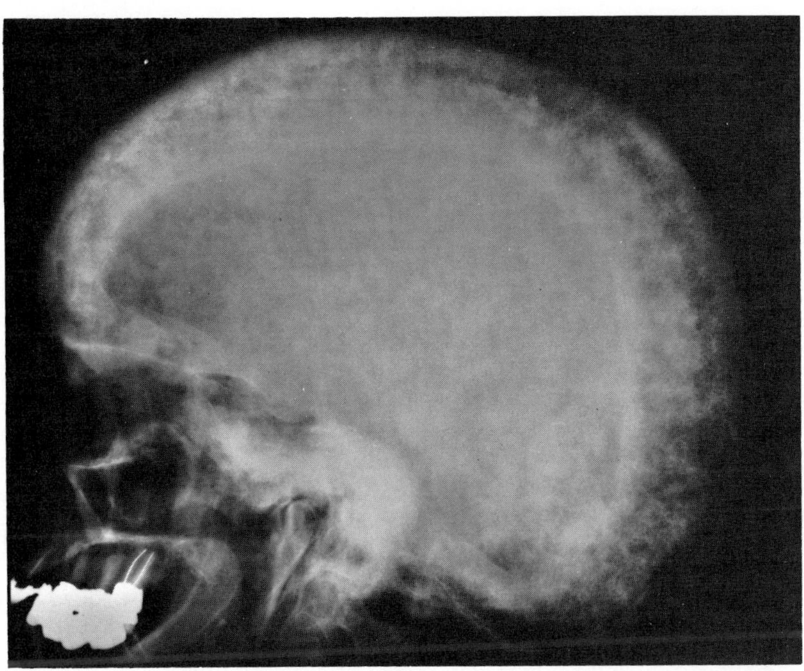

FIGURE 24-13 Roentgenogram of the skull of a 63-year-old patient with the osteoblastic phase of Paget's disease.

basilar invagination may occur in far advanced disease. In the long bones, the osteolytic lesions are replaced by thickened trabeculae which obscure the corticomedullary border. Anterior and lateral bowing of the femur and tibia may develop. Incomplete fissure fractures can be seen on the convex surface of the femur. Pathologic fractures of the lower extremity produce a "chalk stick" rather than a spiral disruption of the bone. Osteoblastic lesions of the vertebrae may produce a "picture frame" appearance because of sclerosis of the vertebral borders, or they may produce a homogeneous increase in density.

Narrowing of the joint spaces of the hip and knee is observed in patients with Paget's disease and degenerative arthritis.[363] Osteophyte formation may be present at these sites and in the spine. Protrusio acetabuli may occur with extensive pagetic involvement of the pelvis.

The radiologic features of a sarcoma include cortical destruction and a soft tissue mass which may exhibit patchy calcification.

Computed tomography of the spine is a valuable technique for demonstrating lesions such as spinal stenosis and is extremely useful in the evaluation of patients with severe back pain.

The metabolic activity of the lesions of Paget's disease is most easily assessed by nuclear medicine techniques (Fig. 24-14). The administration of bone-seeking radioisotopes such as technetium-labeled bisphosphonates to patients with localized disease may be the only noninvasive means of demonstrating disease activity, since biochemical parameters may be normal in monostotic cases.[366] Bone scans also can detect early lesions of Paget's disease before there is a discernible radiologic abnormality.[367] During treatment of Paget's disease with a variety of agents, bone scans can reflect suppression of disease activity. In one study,[368] gallium scans were found to correlate better with suppression of biochemical parameters than did technetium bisphosphonate bone scans. Since gallium is thought to localize within cells, the gallium scan may be a better index of the action of drugs on the abnormal cells of Paget's disease.

Laboratory Findings

The serum calcium and phosphorus concentrations are usually normal in ambulatory patients with Paget's disease. Immobilization because of neurologic complications or after a fracture may cause serious hypercalcemia.[369] Hypercalcemia also may reflect the presence of associated primary hyperparathyroidism, and it has been suggested that there is an increased incidence of hyperparathyroidism in patients with Paget's disease.[370] Control studies of an age-matched population have not been adequate to establish this association convincingly.

Radiocalcium kinetic studies have revealed a markedly increased rate of bone turnover in patients with polyostotic Paget's disease.[369] This is more easily demonstrated by the elevated serum alkaline phosphatase activity and increased urinary hydroxyproline excretion found in these patients. In patients with monostotic disease involving a small bone such as a vertebra, all the above studies may be normal. Serum osteocalcin and urinary pyridinium cross-link levels may be abnormal in Paget's disease but do not clearly provide a better index of bone formation

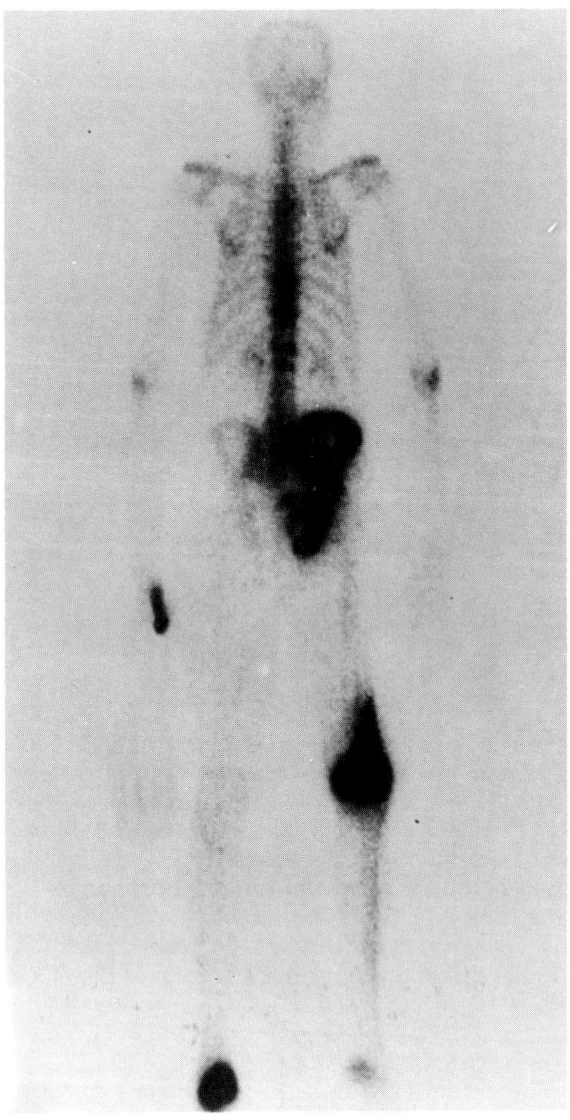

FIGURE 24-14 Bone scan of a 73-year-old patient with Paget's disease involving the left hemipelvis, the distal left femur, the right hand, and the right foot.

and bone resorption in most patients than do alkaline phosphatase and hydroxyproline measurements.

Urinary calcium excretion is usually normal, although hypercalciuria may be present if the rate of bone resorption exceeds that of bone formation.[369] This occurs primarily in immobilized patients. In ambulatory patients, even with extensive active Paget's disease, the resorption and formation rates are usually closely coupled.

Bone Pathology

The earliest lesion of Paget's disease is a localized area of osteolysis which is produced by an increased number of osteoclasts.[371] The osteoclasts of Paget's disease are heterogeneous in size; some may have up to 100 nuclei in a single cross section (Fig. 24-15). Giant osteoclasts of this size are rarely found in metabolic bone disease.

Most bone biopsies or surgical specimens show a combination of intensive osteoclastic bone resorption and large numbers of active osteoblasts which are forming bone at sites of previous osteoclastic resorption (Fig. 24-15). The marrow is also found to contain dense fibrovascular tissue containing numerous fibroblasts and osteoprogenitor cells.

In the quiescent, or "burned-out," phase of Paget's disease, the number of bone cells is markedly reduced and the bone marrow consists mainly of fat cells. A single bone may harbor an advancing osteolytic front, a trailing mixed osteoclastic-osteoblastic pattern, and a burned-out stage of the disease.

The intense cellular activity of Paget's disease produces a characteristic chaotic pattern of bone matrix termed the *mosaic pattern*. The bone is primarily lamellar in character, with woven bone interspersed between incomplete osteons. A high percentage of bone surface is covered by osteoid, but mineraliza-

FIGURE 24-15 Several large multinucleated osteoclasts in Howship lacunae. More than 50 nuclei are present in the osteoclast at the bottom. Note the numerous osteoblasts at the far right of the bone matrix. Decalcified, H&E.

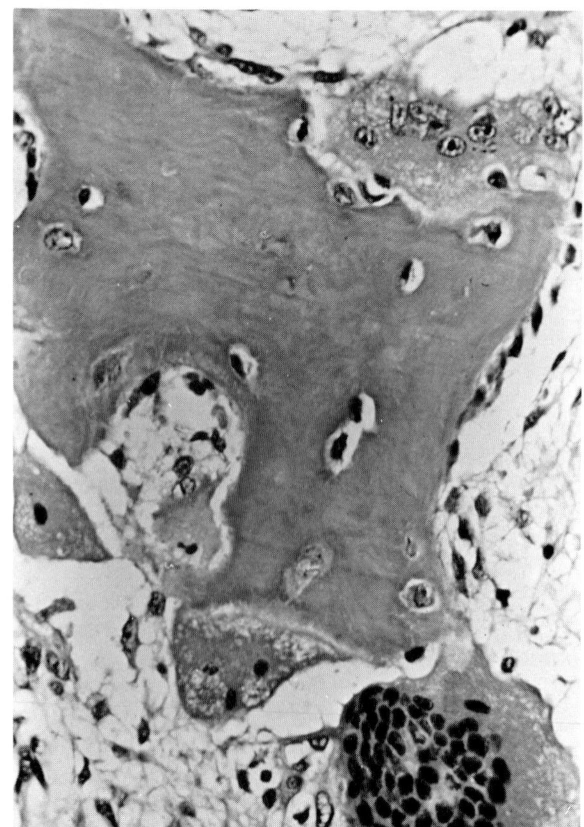

tion is usually normal. The rate of bone formation as determined by double labeling with tetracycline is often increased.

Studies of the ultrastructure of bone cells in Paget's disease have demonstrated characteristic nuclear and cytoplasmic inclusions in the osteoclasts of all patients whose cells have been examined.[372,373] These inclusions consist of numerous microfibrillar structures which are similar in appearance to the viral nucleocapsids of paramyxoviruses and pneumoviruses (Fig. 24-16). The inclusions have not been found in the osteoblasts or osteocytes of Paget's disease or in bone cells from normal subjects. In variable degree, they have been also observed in the osteoclasts of some patients with pycnodysostosis, giant-cell tumor of bone, and osteopetrosis.[374]

Pathogenesis

Sir James Paget believed that Paget's disease is inflammatory in nature—hence the term *osteitis deformans*.[361] Because no infectious agent could be recovered from pathologic specimens, this hypothesis was discarded early in this century. The uniform finding of nuclear and cytoplasmic inclusions in the osteoclasts of Paget's disease has revived the search for an infectious cause of the disorder. It is now appreciated that viruses may produce chronic indolent disorders of the nervous system, termed *slow virus infections,* which share many clinical and pathologic features with Paget's disease.[375] These shared features include involvement of a single organ, a prolonged latent period, absence of fever and an acute inflammatory process, giant cells, and intracellular inclusions. Immunocytologic evidence indicates that measles and/or respiratory syncytial virus antigens are present in the osteoclasts of Paget's disease.[376,377] In a French study, measles virus nucleocapsid mRNA was localized to a variety of pagetic bone and marrow cells by in situ hybridization.[378] This result was not confirmed in a second study in England, where canine distemper virus mRNA was localized to bone and marrow cells by in situ hybridization.[379] A third study from Scotland failed to detect any paramyxovirus sequences in pagetic bone using a polymerase chain reaction.[380] The reasons for the discrepancies among these studies are unclear. Further application of the techniques of molecular biology to the study of pagetic specimens should finally resolve the identity of the nuclear and cytoplasmic inclusions. Then it will have to be determined what the relation of the inclusions is to the pathogenesis of the disease.

A variety of other hypotheses have been proposed to explain the pathogenesis of Paget's disease.[371] It has been suggested that the disease results from an autoimmune process, from an inborn error of connective tissue metabolism, from an abnormality of hormone secretion, from an abnormality of the vascular supply of bone, and from neoplastic transformation of bone cells. Little evidence has been marshaled in support of any of these hypotheses.

FIGURE 24-16 Characteristic microfibrillar nuclear inclusion found in osteoclasts of patients with Paget's disease. ×32,000. (*Courtesy of BG Mills.*)

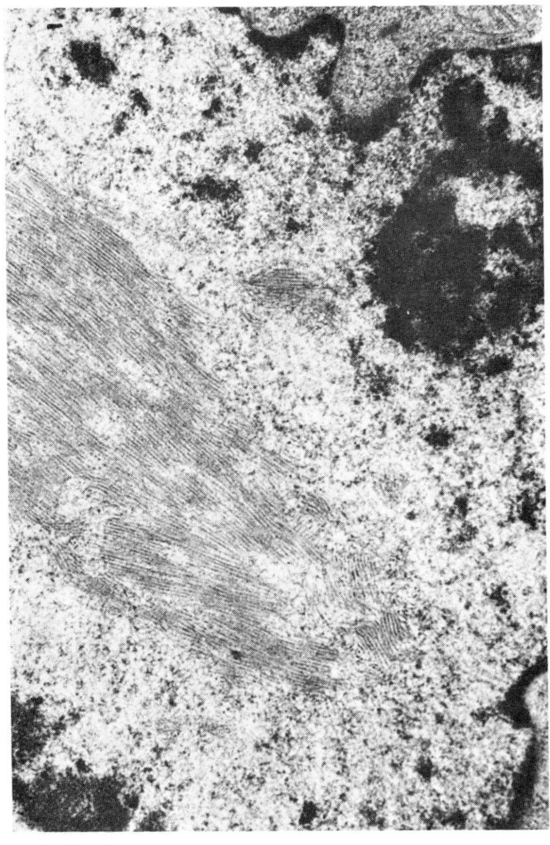

Treatment

A variety of medical and surgical therapies can now be offered to patients with Paget's disease who previously would have had little chance for relief of their symptoms.

Before 1970, no safe and effective drugs were available for the treatment of Paget's disease. Clinical trials with calcitonin began at that time. This agent was chosen because of its known inhibitory effect on osteoclastic bone resorption. Within 30 min after the injection of calcitonin, osteoclasts appear to detach from trabeculae, lose their well-defined ruffled borders, and be reduced in number.[381] Simultaneously, patients with Paget's disease experience a reduction in serum calcium, phosphorus, and serum and urinary hydroxyproline levels, biochemical reflections of an inhibition of bone mineral and matrix resorption. During chronic administration of calcitonin, both histologic and biochemical parameters indicate inhibition of bone formation as well as bone resorption, so that the agent ultimately produces a reduced rate of coupled bone turnover.[371]

Salmon and human calcitonin are currently approved for general use in the United States. Salmon calcitonin is administered by subcutaneous injection at a dose of 50 to 100 MRC units daily until symptoms are improved. Subsequently, the dose usually can be reduced to 50 MRC units three times a week with maintenance of clinical benefit. Occasionally a dose of more than 100 MRC units daily is required to induce maximal radiologic improvement. Relief of bone pain and a reduction in skin temperature over affected extremities are usually observed after 2 to 6 weeks of treatment. Therapy with salmon calcitonin also has been reported to improve neurologic disability, stabilize auditory acuity, decrease cardiac output, decrease the complications of orthopedic surgery, and induce healing of osteolytic bone lesions.[371] Human calcitonin at a dose of 0.5 mg daily produces a similar clinical benefit.

Treatment with calcitonin produces an average reduction of 50 percent in both serum alkaline phosphatase activity and urinary hydroxyproline excretion within 3 to 6 months (Fig. 24-17). Urinary hydroxyproline excretion decreases during the first day of treatment, and serum alkaline phosphatase activity decreases only after 1 or 2 weeks. This suggests that the effect of calcitonin on osteoblastic activity is indirect and is a consequence of inhibition of bone resorption.

Side effects occur in approximately 20 percent of patients treated with salmon calcitonin but seldom require discontinuation of treatment. Side effects are surprisingly more common in patients treated with human calcitonin and are more likely to be intolerable. Nausea, facial flushing, and a metallic taste sensation are most common. Abdominal pain, vomiting, diarrhea, and tetany are rare. Allergic reactions also are rare. The transient hypocalcemia which occurs after each injection in patients with polyostotic disease produces a transient rise in serum parathyroid hormone concentration. There is no evidence that this leads to the development of a persistent state of secondary hyperparathyroidism.[371]

Since salmon calcitonin is a foreign protein, it is not surprising that more than 50 percent of patients who are treated with this agent develop circulating antibodies.[381] In the largest series of patients studied,[381] 22 of 85 patients (26 percent) became resistant to salmon calcitonin treatment after an initial

FIGURE 24-17 The effect of long-term treatment with subcutaneous injections of human calcitonin on the biochemical parameters of a patient with polyostotic Paget's disease. Serum alkaline phosphatase activity (normal, 1 to 3 Bessey-Lowrey-Brock units) and urinary hydroxyproline excretion (normal, < 40 mg per 24 h) both decreased by more than 50 percent of baseline values.

A.S.A.

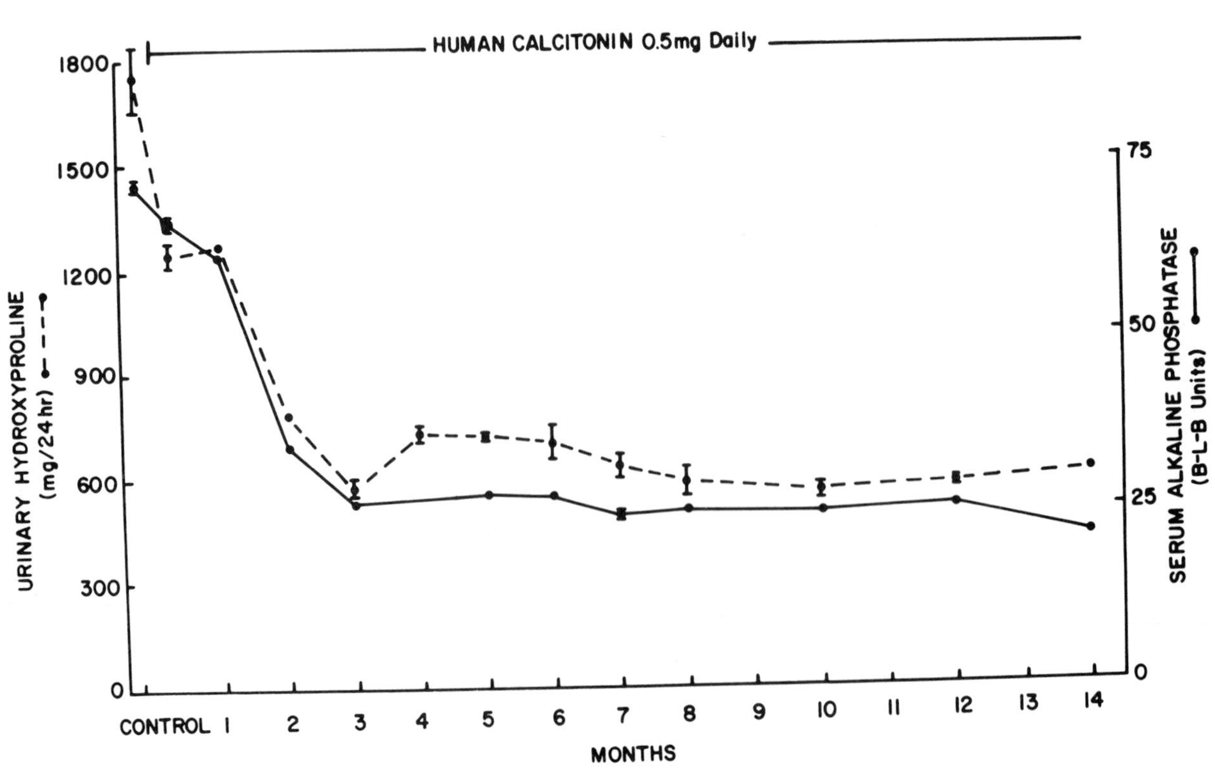

biochemical remission was produced. Nineteen of these patients had high titers of antibodies to salmon calcitonin, and three had no detectable antibodies. The development of neutralizing antibodies appears to be a common cause of resistance to salmon calcitonin. In such patients, therapy with salmon calcitonin should be stopped. Human calcitonin therapy has been uniformly effective in these patients.[382] Bisphosphonates and mithramycin can also be used if warranted (see below). The reason for resistance to salmon calcitonin in patients who have no antibodies is unknown but is apparently not related to the foreign nature of salmon calcitonin, since resistance to human calcitonin can also occur in the absence of antibodies.[382]

The indications for treatment with calcitonin are still evolving. Bone pain, neurologic deficits, and immobilization hypercalcemia are indications for initiating treatment. The use of calcitonin in preparing patients for orthopedic surgery is reviewed in a later section. The prevention of future complications of Paget's disease has not been studied but should be considered in relatively young patients whose disease affects the skull or weight-bearing bones.

The optimum duration of treatment with calcitonin has not been established. In patients treated for an average of 22 months, the biochemical parameters of Paget's disease remained suppressed for at least 1 year after calcitonin was discontinued.[383] However, in patients with a healed osteolytic lesion, reactivation of the osteolytic front occurred within several months of discontinuing therapy.[384] It may be appropriate to continue such patients on treatment indefinitely. Patients whose lesions are predominantly osteoblastic may do well on a regimen of 1 or 2 years, followed by a treatment-free period. If symptoms return, the drug can be reinstituted.

A second group of compounds which have proved useful in the treatment of Paget's disease are the bisphosphonates. These agents are analogues of pyrophosphate (POP), a substance in bone believed to influence calcification and bone cell metabolism.[385] Bisphosphonates have been shown to suppress bone resorption and formation in experimental animals and humans,[385] although the exact mode of action is not known. Etidronate disodium (disodium ethane-1-hydroxyl-1,1-bisphosphonate) has been approved for the treatment of Paget's disease and hypercalcemia and the prevention of heterotopic ossification in the United States.

Etidronate disodium is administered orally, although gastrointestinal absorption of the drug is variable. After absorption, it localizes mainly in the skeleton or is excreted by the kidney. The clinical effects of the drug are similar to those of calcitonin, but there are some differences. In general, greater suppression of biochemical parameters is achieved with the bisphosphonates compared with calcitonin.[386] This is most often achieved at doses of 10 to 20 mg per kilogram of body weight. Unfortunately, high doses of etidronate disodium cause a mineralization defect which may predispose to osteomalacia and pathologic fractures.[387] Since doses of 5 mg per kilogram of body weight usually suppress the disease without producing a mineralization defect, it is best to begin therapy with this lower dose. If the patient does not respond, perhaps because of inadequate intestinal absorption of the drug, a higher dose can be tried, but the patient must be followed carefully to avoid the induction of osteomalacia. Hyperphosphatemia may be a warning of the potential for that complication. Another unusual feature of etidronate disodium therapy is the heterogeneity of the pain response. Most patients are relieved of bone pain, but in about 10 percent of patients there is a paradoxic increase in pain. The severity of pain decreases after the drug is stopped and may not return if treatment is resumed. Another difference between the effects of etidronate disodium and calcitonin is observed in the healing of osteolytic lesions. Roentgenograms of osteolytic lesions seldom have been reported to demonstrate healing after etidronate disodium therapy. In one study, osteolytic lesions progressed despite improvement of biochemical parameters. In patients with osteolytic lesions, calcitonin therapy is preferable.

The incidence of side effects in patients who receive etidronate disodium is low. Loose bowel movements may occur, and asymptomatic hyperphosphatemia may be observed in patients who are given high doses.

A major advantage of etidronate disodium is that a 6-month course of treatment may produce a prolonged biochemical remission of 1 year or more (Fig. 24-18). If symptoms recur, the drug can be readministered for another 6-month period.

A large number of clinical trials have been carried out using second- and third-generation bisphosphonates.[388] Clodronate, pamidronate, alendronate, tiludronate, and risedronate, among others, have been demonstrated to be more potent than etidronate and, importantly, not to induce clinically significant osteomalacia at doses which readily inhibit bone resorption. It can be expected in the future that one or two intravenous infusions or 2 to 3 months of oral therapy with a potent bisphosphonate will produce long-term remissions of Paget disease in most patients.

An alternative therapy for Paget's disease is with the cytotoxic antibiotic mithramycin. This drug is a potent inhibitor of RNA synthesis and acutely inhibits osteoclast activity. It is approved in the United States for the treatment of cancer and severe hypercalcemia but not for Paget's disease. Mithramycin is administered by intravenous injection or infusion. It has been used at a dose of 15 to 50 μg per kilogram of body weight with a variety of treatment schedules. Early studies employed daily infusions of up to 10

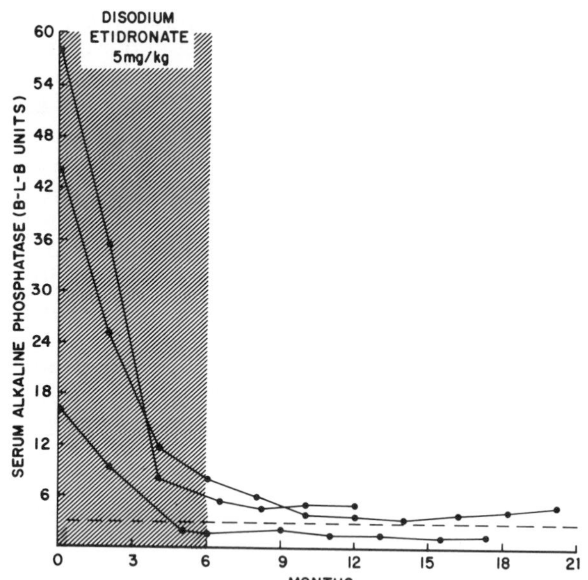

FIGURE 24-18 The effect of 6 months of therapy (hatched lines) with etidronate disodium on serum alkaline phosphatase activity in three patients with Paget's disease. The interrupted line indicates the upper limit of normal. Note the prolonged suppression of the disease after treatment was discontinued.

days.[389] Subsequently, weekly infusions have been used.[390] Relief of bone pain and marked suppression of biochemical parameters have been reported. However, side effects and toxicity are more likely to occur with mithramycin than with other agents. Nausea and malaise may persist for days. Platelet abnormalities leading to hemorrhage, transient elevation of liver enzymes, and impairment of renal function are other toxic effects of mithramycin. Because of this, mithramycin therapy should be reserved for patients who fail to respond to calcitonin and etidronate disodium.

Another proposed therapy is the use of oral calcium supplementation with chlorthalidone.[391] This combination has been given in an attempt to stimulate endogenous calcitonin secretion and thus suppress disease activity. This inexpensive regimen can produce modest decreases in serum alkaline phosphatase activity and urinary hydroxyproline excretion and has been reported to reduce bone pain in most patients. Healing of osteolytic lesions has not been demonstrated.

The most recent new potential therapy for Paget's disease is gallium nitrate.[392] This compound has been shown to inhibit bone turnover in Paget's disease. The drug must be given parenterally at this time, and it remains to be seen whether it will have any advantages over the current standard therapies.

Elective surgery is required in the management of certain patients with Paget's disease and may produce benefits which cannot be achieved by medical means. Occipital decompression may be needed in patients with neurologic deficits secondary to basilar impression. Neurosurgery also may be necessary in patients with vertebral disease. Total hip replacement in patients with severe degenerative arthritis may permit pain-free normal ambulation. Patients with severe bowing of the tibia may have difficulty in ambulation not only because of deformity but also because of painful degenerative arthritis of the knee. Tibial osteotomy can correct the anatomic abnormality as well as reduce the pain resulting from the arthritis, greatly improving ambulation.

In a series of patients undergoing tibial osteotomy, treatment with calcitonin appeared to prevent excessive hemorrhage and postoperative hypercalcemia.[393] It is likely that any patient with Paget's disease requiring orthopedic surgery can benefit from treatment with a drug which suppresses the activity of the disease. Ideally, the treatment should be administered for a minimum of 2 to 3 months before surgery.

REFERENCES

1. Albright FA, Reifenstein EC Jr: *The Parathyroid Glands and Metabolic Bone Disease.* Baltimore, Williams & Wilkins, 1948, p 81.
2. Farley JR, Chestnut CH III, Baylink DJ: Improved method for quantitative determination in serum of alkaline phosphatase of skeletal origin. *Clin Chem* 27:2002, 1981.
3. Duda RJ Jr, O'Brien JF, Katzmann JA, Peterson JM, Mann KG, Riggs BL: Concurrent assays of circulating bone Gla-protein and bone alkaline phosphatase: Effects of sex, age and metabolic bone disease. *J Clin Endocrinol Metab* 66:951, 1988.
4. Epstein S, Poser J, McClintock R, Johnston CC Jr, Bryce G, Hui S: Differences in serum bone GLA protein with age and sex. *Lancet* 1:307, 1984.
5. Delmas PD, Wilson DM, Mann KG, Riggs BL: Effect of renal function on plasma levels of bone GLA-protein. *J Clin Endocrinol Metab* 57:1028, 1983.
6. Grundberg CM, Markowitz ME, Mizruhi M, Rosen JF: Osteocalcin in human serum: A circadian rhythm. *J Clin Endocrinol Metab* 60:736, 1985.
7. Johansen JS, Riss BJ, Delmas PD, Christiansen C: Plasma BGP: An indicator of spontaneous bone loss and of the effect of oestrogen treatment in postmenopausal women. *Eur J Clin Invest* 18:191, 1988.
8. Endres DB, Villanueva R, Sharp CF Jr, Singer FR: Immunochemiluminometric and immunoradiometric determinations of intact and total immunoreactive parathyrin: Performance in the differential diagnosis of hypercalcemia and hypoparathyroidism. *Clin Chem* 37:162, 1991.
9. Adams E: Metabolism of proline and of hydroxyproline. *Int Rev Connect Tissue Res* 5:1, 1970.
10. Kivirikko KI: Urinary excretion of hydroxyproline in health and disease. *Int Rev Connect Tissue Res* 5:93, 1970.
11. Krane SM, Munoz AJ, Harris ED Jr: Urinary polypeptides related to collagen synthesis. *J Clin Invest* 49:716, 1970.
12. Aaron J: Diagnostic procedures, in Nordin BEC (ed): *Calcium, Phosphate and Magnesium Metabolism.* London, Churchill Livingstone, 1976, p 469.
13. Cunningham LW, Ford JD, Segrest JP: The isolation of identical hydroxylysyl glycosides from hydroxylysates of soluble collagen and from human urine. *J Biol Chem* 242:2570, 1967.

14. Pinnell SR, Fox R, Krane SM: Human collagens: Differences in glycosylated hydroxylysines in skin and bone. *Biochim Biophys Acta* 229:119, 1971.
15. Uebelhart D, Gineyts E, Chapuy M-C, Delmas PD: Urinary excretion of pyridinium crosslinks: A new marker of bone resorption in metabolic bone disease. *Bone Mineral* 8:87, 1990.
16. Richardson ML, Genant HK, Cann CE, Ettinger B, Gordan GS, Kolb FO, Reiser UJ: Assessment of metabolic bone diseases by quantitative computed tomography. *Clin Orthop* 195:224, 1985.
17. Cameron JR, Mazess RB, Sorenson JA: Precision and accuracy of bone mineral determination by direct photon absorptiometry. *Invest Radiol* 3:141, 1968.
18. Mazess RB, Peppler WW, Chesney RW, Lange TA, Lindgren U, Smith E Jr: Total body and regional bone mineral by dual-photon absorptiometry in metabolic bone disease. *Calcif Tissue Int* 36:8, 1984.
19. Rupich R, Pacifici R, Griffin M, Vered I, Susman N, Avioli LV: Lateral dual energy radiography: A new method for measuring vertebral bone density: A preliminary study. *J Clin Endocrinol Metab* 70:1768, 1990.
20. Fogelman I, Bessent RG, Turner JG, Citrin DL, Boyle IT, Greig WR: The use of whole-body retention of Tc-99m diphosphonate in the diagnosis of metabolic bone disease. *J Nucl Med* 19:270, 1978.
21. Civitelli R, Gonnelli S, Zacchei F, Bigazzi S, Vattimo A, Avioli LV, Gennari C: Bone turnover in postmenopausal osteoporosis: Effect of calcitonin treatment. *J Clin Invest* 82:1268, 1988.
22. Bordier P, Matrajt H, Miravet L, Hioco D: Mésure histologique de la masse et de la résorption des travées osseuses. *Pathol Biol (Paris)* 12:1238, 1964.
23. Rališ ZA, Rališ HM: A simple method for demonstration of osteoid in paraffin sections. *Med Lab Technol* 32:203, 1975.
24. Parfitt AM, Drezner MK, Glorieux FH, Kanis JA, Malluche H, Meunier PJ, Ott SM, Recker RR: Bone histomorphometry: Standardization of nomenclature, symbols, and units. *J Bone Mineral Res* 2:595, 1987.
25. Harris WH, Jackson RH, Jowsey J: The in vivo distributions of tetracyclines in canine bone. *J Bone Joint Surg [Am]* 44A:1308, 1962.
26. Epker BN, Hattner R, Frost HM: Radial sites of osteon closure. *J Lab Clin Med* 64:643, 1964.
27. Dent CE, Stamp TCB: Vitamin D, rickets and osteomalacia, in Avioli LV, Krane SM (eds): *Metabolic Bone Disease.* New York, Academic, 1977, vol 1, p 237.
28. Mankin H: Rickets, osteomalacia and renal osteodystrophy. *J Bone Joint Surg [Am]* 56A:101, 1974.
29. Fraser D, Kooh SW, Scriver CR: Hyperparathyroidism as the cause of hyperaminoaciduria and phosphaturia in human vitamin D deficiency. *Pediatr Res* 1:425, 1967.
30. Fraser D, Kooh SW, Kind HP, Holick MF, Tanaka Y, DeLuca HF: Pathogenesis of hereditary vitamin D–dependent rickets: An inborn error of vitamin D metabolism involving defective conversion of 25-hydroxyvitamin D to 1α,25-dihydroxyvitamin D. *N Engl J Med* 289:817, 1973.
31. Brooks MH, Bell NH, Love L, Stern PH, Orfei E, Queener SF, Hamstra AJ, DeLuca HF: Vitamin D dependent rickets type II: Resistance of target organs to 1,25-dihydroxyvitamin D. *N Engl J Med* 298:996, 1978.
32. Arnaud CD, Glorieux F, Scriver CR: Serum parathyroid hormone levels in acquired vitamin D deficiency. *Pediatrics* 49:837, 1972.
33. Vainsel M, Manderlier T, Otten J: Urinary excretion of adenosine 3′,5′-monophosphate in vitamin D deficiency. *Eur J Clin Invest* 6:127, 1976.
34. Fraser D, Scriver CR: Disorders associated with hereditary or acquired abnormalities in vitamin D function: Hereditary disorders associated with vitamin D resistance or defective phosphate metabolism, in De Groot LJ (ed): *Endocrinology.* New York: Grune & Stratton, 1979, vol 2, p 797.
35. Haussler MR, McCain TA: Basic and clinical concepts related to vitamin D metabolism and action. *N Engl J Med* 297:1041, 1977.
36. Eastwood JB, DeWardener HE, Gray RW, Lemann JL Jr: Normal plasma 1,25-$(OH)_2$-vitamin D concentrations in nutritional osteomalacia. *Lancet* 1:1377, 1979.
37. Parfitt AM: Osteomalacia and related disorders, in Avioli LV, Krane SM (eds): *Metabolic Bone Disease and Clinically Related Disorders,* 2d ed. Philadelphia, Saunders, 1990, p 329.
38. Marie PJ, Glorieux FH: Relation between hypomineralized periosteocytic lesions and bone mineralization in vitamin D–resistant rickets. *Calcif Tissue Int* 35:443, 1983.
39. Loomis WF: Rickets. *Sci Am* 223:77, 1970.
40. Bachrach S, Fisher J, Parks JS: An outbreak of vitamin D deficiency rickets in a susceptible population. *Pediatrics* 64:871, 1979.
41. Dwyer JT, Dietz WH Jr, Hass G, Suskind R: Risk of nutritional rickets among vegetarian children. *Am J Dis Child* 133:134, 1979.
42. Thompson GR, Lewis B, Booth CC: Absorption of vitamin D_3-^3H in control subjects and patients with intestinal malabsorption. *J Clin Invest* 45:94, 1966.
43. Arnaud SB, Goldsmith RS, Lambert PW, Go VLW: 25-Hydroxyvitamin D_3: Evidence of an enterohepatic circulation in man. *Proc Soc Exp Biol Med* 149:570, 1975.
44. Clements MR, Chalmers TM, Fraser DR: Enterohepatic circulation of vitamin D: A reappraisal of the hypothesis. *Lancet* 1:1376, 1984.
45. Parfitt AM, Podenphant J, Villanueva AR, Frame B: Metabolic bone disease with and without osteomalacia after intestinal bypass surgery: A bone histomorphometric study. *Bone* 6:211, 1985.
46. Stellon AJ, Webb A, Compston J, Williams R: Lack of osteomalacia in chronic cholestatic liver disease. *Bone* 7:181, 1986.
47. Bikle DD, Halloran BP, Gee E, Ryzen E, Haddad JG: Free 25-hydroxyvitamin D levels are normal in subjects with liver disease and reduced total 25-hydroxyvitamin D levels. *J Clin Invest* 78:748, 1986.
48. Horst RL, Jorgensen NA, DeLuca HF: The determination of 24,25-dihydroxyvitamin D and 25,26-dihydroxyvitamin D in plasma from normal and nephrectomized man. *J Lab Clin Med* 93:277, 1979.
49. Richens A, Rowe DJF: Disturbance of calcium metabolism by anticonvulsant drugs. *Br Med J* 4:73, 1970.
50. Weintein RS, Bryce GF, Sappington LJ, King DW, Gallagher BB: Decreased serum ionized calcium and normal vitamin D metabolite levels with anticonvulsant drug treatment. *J Clin Endocrinol Metab* 58:1003, 1984.
51. Hahn TJ: Drug-induced disorders of vitamin D and mineral metabolism. *Clin Endocrionol Metab* 9:107, 1980.
52. Morijiri Y, Sato T: Factors causing rickets in institutionalized handicapped children on anticonvulsant therapy. *Arch Dis Child* 56:446, 1981.
53. Weisman Y, Fattal A, Eisenberg Z, Harel S, Spirer Z, Harell A: Decreased serum 24,25-dihydroxyvitamin D concentrations in children receiving chronic anticonvulsant therapy. *Br Med J* 2:521, 1979.
54. Christensen CK, Lund B, Lund BJ, Sorensen OH, Nielsen HE, Mosekilde L: Reduced 1,25-dihydroxyvitamin D and 24,25-dihydroxyvitamin D in epileptic patients receiving chronic combined anticonvulsant therapy. *Metab Bone Dis Rel Res* 3:17, 1981.
55. Jubiz W, Haussler MR, McCain TA, Tolman KG: Plasma 1,25-dihydroxyvitamin D levels in patients receiving anticonvulsant drugs. *J Clin Endocrinol Metab* 44:617, 1977.
56. Hunt PA, Wu-Chen ML, Handal NJ, Chang CT, Gomez M, Howell TR, Hartenberg MA, Chan JCM: Bone disease induced by anticonvulsant therapy and treatment with calcitriol (1,25-dihydroxyvitamin D_3). *Am J Dis Child* 140:715, 1986.

57. Nuovo MA, Dorfman HD, Sun CJ, Chalew SA: Tumor-induced osteomalacia and rickets. *Am J Surg Pathol* 13:588, 1989.
58. Lyles KW, Berry WR, Haussler M, Harrelson JM, Drezner MK: Hypophosphatemic osteomalacia: Association with prostatic carcinoma. *Ann Intern Med* 93:275, 1980.
59. Taylor HC, Fallon MD, Velasco ME: Oncogenic osteomalacia and inappropriate antidiuretic hormone secretion due to oat-cell carcinoma. *Ann Intern Med* 101:786, 1984.
60. Eulderink F: Adenomatoid changes in Bowman's capsule in primary carcinoma of the liver. *J Pathol* 87:251, 1964.
61. Delvin EE, Glorieux FH, Marie PJ, Pettifor JM: Vitamin D dependency: Replacement therapy with calcitriol. *J Pediatr* 99:26, 1981.
62. Schmidt-Gayk H, Schmitt W, Grawunder C, Ritz E, Tschoepe W, Pietsch V, Andrassy K, Bouillon R: 25-Hydroxy-vitamin D in nephrotic syndrome. *Lancet* 2:105, 1977.
63. Malluche HH, Goldstein DA, Massry SG: Osteomalacia and hyperparathyroid bone disease in patients with nephrotic syndrome. *J Clin Invest* 63:494, 1979.
64. Korkor A, Schwartz A, Bergfeld M, Teitelbaum S, Avioli L, Klahr S, Slatopolsky E: Absence of metabolic bone disease in adult patients with the nephrotic syndrome and normal renal function. *J Clin Endocrinol Metab* 56:496, 1983.
65. Liberman UA, Samuel R, Halabe A, Kauli R, Edelstein S, WeismanY, Papapoulos SE, Clemens TL, et al: End-organ resistance to 1,25-dihydroxycholecalciferol. *Lancet* 1:504, 1980.
66. Marx SJ, Bliziotes MM, Nanes M: Analysis of the relation between alopecia and resistance to 1,25-dihydroxyvitamin D. *Clin Endocrinol (Oxf)* 25:373, 1986.
67. Pike JW, Dokoh S, Haussler MR, Liberman UA, Marx SJ, Eil C: Vitamin D_3-resistant fibroblasts have immunoassayable 1,25-dihydroxyvitamin D_3-resistant receptors. *Science* 224:879, 1984.
68. Liberman UA, Eil C, Marx SJ: Resistance to 1,25-dihydroxyvitamin D: Association with heterogeneous defects in cultured skin fibroblasts. *J Clin Invest* 71:192, 1983.
69. Liberman UA, Eil C, Holst P, Rosen JF, Marx SJ: Hereditary resistance to 1,25-dihydroxyvitamin D: Defective function of receptors for 1,25-dihydroxyvitamin D in cells cultured from bone. *J Clin Endocrinol Metab* 57:958, 1983.
70. Hughes MR, Malloy PJ, Kieback DG, Kesterson RA, Pike JW, Feldman D, O'Malley BW: Point mutations in the human vitamin D receptor gene associated with hypocalcemic resistant rickets. *Science* 242:1702, 1988.
71. Ritchie HH, Hughes MR, Thompson ET, Malloy PJ, Hochberg Z, Feldman D, Pike JW, O'Malley BW: An ochre mutation in the vitamin D receptor gene causes hereditary 1,25-dihydroxyvitamin D_3-resistant rickets in three families. *Proc Natl Acad Sci USA* 86:9783, 1989.
72. Jenkins MV, Harris M, Wills MR: The effect of phenytoin on parathyroid extract and 25-hydroxycholecalciferol–induced bone resorption: Adenosine 3′,5′-cyclic monophosphate production. *Calcif Tissue Res* 16:163, 1974.
73. Corradino RA: Diphenylhydantoin: Direct inhibition of the vitamin D_3-mediated calcium absorptive mechanism in organ cultured duodenum. *Biochem Pharmacol* 25:863, 1976.
74. Brickman AS, Coburn JW, Massry SG: 1,25-Dihydroxyvitamin D_3 in normal man and patients with renal failure. *Ann Intern Med* 80:161, 1974.
75. Albright F, Butler AM, Bloomberg E: Rickets resistant to vitamin D therapy. *Am J Dis Child* 54:529, 1937.
76. Winters RW, Graham JB, Williams TF, McFalls VW, Burnett CH: A genetic study of familial hypophosphatemia and vitamin D resistant rickets with a review of the literature. *Medicine (Baltimore)* 37:97, 1958.
77. Adams JE, Davies M: Intra-spinal new bone formation and spinal cord compression in familial hypophosphatemic vitamin D resistant osteomalacia. *Q J Med* (new series) 61:117, 1986.
78. Reitz R, Weinstein RL: Parathyroid hormone seretion in familial vitamin-D-resistant rickets. *N Engl J Med* 289:941, 1973.
79. Short E, Morris RC Jr, Sebastian A, Spencer M: Exaggerated phosphaturic response to circulating parathyroid hormone in patients with familial X-linked hypophosphatemic rickets. *J Clin Invest* 58:152, 1976.
80. Lyles KW, Burkes EJ Jr, McNamara CR, Harrelson JM, Pickett JP, Drezner MK: The concurrence of hypoparathyroidism provides new insights to the pathophysiology of X-linked hypophosphatemic rickets. *J Clin Endocrinol Metab* 60:711, 1985.
81. Condon JR, Nassim JR, Rutter A: Defective intestinal phosphate absorption in familial and non-familial hypophosphatemia. *Br Med J* 3:138, 1970.
82. Chesney RW, Mazess RB, Rose P, Hamstra AJ, DeLuca HF: Supranormal 25-hydroxyvitamin D and subnormal 1,25-dihydroxyvitamin D: Their role in X-linked hypophosphatemic rickets. *Am J Dis Child* 134:140, 1980.
83. Seino Y, Shimotsuji T, Ishii T, Ishida M, Ikehara C, Yamaoka K, Yabwichi H, Dokoh S: Treatment of hypophosphatemic vitamin D–resistant rickets with massive dose of 1α-hydroxyvitamin D_3 during childhood. *Arch Dis Child* 55:49, 1980.
84. Delvin EE, Glorieux FH: Serum 1,25-dihydroxyvitamin D concentration in hypophosphatemic vitamin D–resistant rickets. *Calif Tissue Int* 33:173, 1981.
85. Lyles KW, Drezner MK: Parathyroid hormone effects on serum 1,25-dihydroxyvitamin D levels in patients with X-linked hypophosphatemic rickets: Evidence for abnormal 25-hydroxyvitamin D–1-hydroxylase activity. *J Clin Endocrinol Metab* 54:638, 1982.
86. Brickman AS, Coburn JW, Kurokawa K, Bethune JE, Harrison HE, Norman AW: Actions of 1,25-dihydroxycholecalciferol in patients with hypophosphatemic, vitamin D–resistant rickets. *N Engl J Med* 289:495, 1973.
87. Stamp TCB, Baker LRI: Recessive hypophosphatemic rickets, and possible etiology of the "vitamin D–resistant" syndrome. *Arch Dis Child* 51:360, 1976.
88. Perry W, Stamp TCB: Hereditary hypophosphatemic rickets with autosomal recessive inheritance and severe osteosclerosis. *J Bone Joint Surg [Br]* 60B:430, 1978.
89. Tieder M, Modai D, Shaked U, Samuel R, Arie R, Halabe A, Maor J, Weissgarten J, et al: "Idiopathic" hypercalciuria and hereditary hypophosphatemic rickets. *N Engl J Med* 316:125, 1987.
90. Nagant de Deuxchaisnes C, Krane SM: The treatment of adult phosphate diabetes and Fanconi syndrome with neutral sodium phosphate. *Am J Med* 43:508, 1967.
91. Frymoyer JW, Hodgkin W; Adult-onset vitamin D–resistant hypophosphatemic osteomalacia: A possible variant of vitamin D–resistant rickets. *J Bone Joint Surg [Am]* 59A:101, 1977.
92. Minari M, Castellani A, Garella S: Renal tubular acidosis associated with vitamin D–resistant rickets: Role of phosphate depletion. *Miner Electrolyte Metab* 10:371, 1984.
93. Dent CE, Gertner JM: Hypophosphatemic osetomalacia in fibrous dysplasia. *Q J Med* 45:411, 1976.
94. McArthur RG, Hayles AB, Lambert PW: Albright's syndrome with rickets. *Mayo Clin Proc* 54:313, 1979.
95. Aschinberg LC, Solomon LM, Zeis PM, Justice P, Rosenthal IM: Vitamin D–resistant rickets associated with epidermal nevus syndrome: Demonstration of a phosphaturic substance in the dermal lesions. *J Pediatr* 91:56, 1977.
96. Bressot C, Courpron P, Edouard C, Meunier P: *Histomorphometrie des ostéopathies endocriniennes.* Lyon, Association Corporative des Étudiants en Médecine de Lyon, 1976, p 117.
97. Dent CE, Winter CE: Osteomalacia due to phosphate depletion from excessive aluminum hydroxide ingestion. *Br Med J* 1:551, 1974.
98. Ahmed KY, Varghese Z, Wills MR, Meinhard E, Skinner

RK, Baillod RA, Moorhead JE: Persistent hypophosphatemia and osteomalacia in dialysis patients not on oral phosphate binders: Response to dihydrotachysterol therapy. *Lancet* 2:439, 1976.

99. Teotia SPS, Teotioa M: Secondary hyperparathyroidism in patients with endemic skeletal fluorosis. *Br Med J* 1:637, 1973.
100. Jowsey J: The long-term treatment of osteoporosis with fluoride, calcium and vitamin D, in Barzel US (ed): *Osteoporosis II*. New York, Grune & Stratton, 1979, p 123.
101. Khairi MRA, Altman RD, DeRosa GP, Zimmerman J, Schenk RK, Johnston CC: Sodium etidronate in the treatment of Paget's disease of bone: A study of long-term results. *Ann Intern Med* 87:656, 1977.
102. Boyce BF, Smith L, Fogelman I, Johnston E, Ralston S, Boyle IT: Focal osteomalacia due to low dose diphosphonate therapy in Paget's disease. *Lancet* 1:821, 1984.
102a. Adamson BB, Gallacher SJ, Byars J, Ralston SH, Boyle IT, Boyce BF: Mineralisation defects with pamidronate therapy for Paget's disease. *Lancet* 342:1459, 1993.
103. Kooh SW, Fraser D, Reilly BJ, Hamilton JR, Gall DG, Bell L: Rickets due to calcium deficiency. *N Engl J Med* 297:1264, 1977.
104. Pettifor JM, Ross FP, Travers R, Glorieux FH, DeLuca HF: Dietary calcium deficiency: A syndrome associated with bone deformities and elevated serum 1,25-dihydroxyvitamin D concentrations. *Metab Bone Dis Rel Res* 2:301, 1981.
105. Marie PJ, Pettifor JM, Ross FP, Glorieux FH: Histological osteomalacia due to dietary calcium deficiency in children. *N Engl J Med* 307:584, 1982.
106. Legius E, Proesmans W, Eggermont E, Vandamme-Lombaerts R, Bouillon R, Smet M: Rickets due to dietary calcium deficiency. Eur J Pediatr 148:784, 1989.
107. Albright F: Hypoparathyroidism as a cause of osteomalacia. *J Clin Endocrinol Metab* 16:419, 1956.
108. Schutt-Aine JC, Young MA, Pescovitz OH, Chrousos GP, Marx SJ: Hypoparathyroidism: A possible cause of rickets. *J Pediatr* 106:255, 1985.
109. Hanukoglu A, Chalew S, Sowarski AA: Late-onset hypocalcemia, rickets, and hypoparathyroidism in an infant of a mother with hyperparathyroidism. *J Pediatr* 112:751, 1988.
110. Lamm CI, Norton KI, Murphy RJC, Wilkins IA, Rabinowitz JG: Congenital rickets associated with magnesium sulfate infusion for tocolysis. *J Pediatr* 113:1078, 1988.
111. Wilson JD, Hadden DR: Pseudohypopariathyroidism presenting with rickets. *J Clin Endocrinol Metab* 51:1184, 1980.
112. Whyte MP: Hypophosphatasia, in Scriver CR, Beaudet AL, Sly WS, Valle D (eds): *The Metabolic Basis of Inherited Disease,* 6th ed. New York, McGraw-Hill, 1989, p 2843.
113. Weiss MJ, Cole DEC, Ray K, Whyte MP, Lafferty MA, Mulivor RA, Harris H: A missense mutation in the human liver/bone/kidney alkaline phosphatase gene causing a form of lethal hypophosphatasia. *Proc Natl Acd Sci USA* 85:7666, 1988.
114. Maesaka H, Niitsu N, Suwa S, Fujita T: Neonatal hypophosphatasia with elevated serum parathyroid hormone. *Eur J Pediatr* 12:71, 1977.
115. Whyte MP, Teitelbaum SL, Murphy WA, Bergfeld MA, Avioli LV: Adult hypophosphatasia: Clinical, laboratory, and genetic investigation of a large kindred with review of the literature. *Medicine (Baltimore)* 58:329, 1979.
116. Frame B, Frost HM, Pak CYC, Reynolds W, Argen RJ: Fibrogenesis imperfecta ossium: A collagen defect causing osteomalacia. *N Engl J Med* 285:769, 1971.
117. Chesney RW, Kaplan BS, Phelps M, DeLuca HF: Renal tubular acidosis does not alter circulating values of calcitriol. *J Pediatr* 104:51, 1984.
118. Kraut JA, Gordon EM, Ransom JC, Horst R, Slatopolsky E, Coburn JW, Kurokawa K: Effect of chronic metabolic acidosis on vitamin D metabolism in humans. *Kidney Int* 24:644, 1983.
119. Phelps KR, Einhorn TA, Vigorita VJ, Lieberman RL, Uribarri J: Acidosis-induced osteomalacia: Metabolic studies and skeletal histomorphometry. *Bone* 79:171, 1986.
120. Shike M, Harrison JE, Sturtridge WC, Tam CS, Bobechko PE, Jones G, Murray TM, Jeejeebhoy KN: Metabolic bone disease in patients receiving long-term total parenteral nutrition. *Ann Intern Med* 92:343, 1980.
121. Klein GL, Targoff CM, Ament ME, Sherrard DJ, Bluestone R, Young JH, Norman AW, Coburn JW: Bone disease associated with total parenteral nutrition. *Lancet* 2:1041, 1980.
122. Ott SM, Maloney NA, Klein GL, Alfrey AC, Ament ME, Coburn JW, Sherrard DJ: Aluminum is associated with low bone formation in patients receiving chronic parenteral nutrition. *Ann Intern Med* 98:910, 1983.
123. Stamp TCB, Round MM, Rowe DJF, Haddad JG: Plasma levels and therapeutic effect of 25-hydroxycholecalciferol in epileptic patients taking anticonvulsant drugs. *Br Med J* 4:9, 1972.
124. Balsan S, Garabedian M, Larchet M, Gorski AM, Cournot G, Tau C, Bourdeau A, Silve C, Ricour C: Long-term nocturnal calcium infusions can cure rickets and promote normal mineralizaton in hereditary resistance to 1,25-dihydroxyvitamin D. *J Clin Invest* 77:1661, 1986.
125. Sakati N, Woodhouse NJY, Niles N, Harfi H, de Grange DA, Marx S: Hereditary resistance to 1,25-dihydroxyvitamin D: Clinical and radiological improvement during high-dose oral calcium therapy. *Hormone Res* 24:280, 1986.
126. Glorieux FH, Scriver CR, Reade TM, Goldman H, Roseborough A: Use of phosphate and vitamin D to prevent dwarfism and rickets in X-linked hypophosphatemia. *N Engl J Med* 287:481, 1972.
127. Lyles KW, Harrelson JM, Drezner MK: The efficacy of vitamin D and oral phosphorus therapy in X-linked hypophosphatemic rickets and osteomalacia. *J Clin Endocrinol Metab* 54:307, 1982.
128. Kirschman GH, DeLuca HF, Chan JCM: Hypophosphatemic vitamin D–resistant rickets: Metabolic balance studies in a child receiving 1,25-dihydroxyvitamin D_3, phosphate, and ascorbic acid. *Pediatrics* 61:451, 1978.
129. Glorieux FH, Marie PJ, Pettifor JM, Delvin EE: Bone response to phosphate salts, ergocalciferol, and calcitriol in hypophosphatemic rickets. *N Engl J Med* 303:1023, 1980.
130. Harrell RM, Lyles KW, Harrelson JM, Friedman NE, Drezner MK: Healing of bone disease in X-linked hypophosphatemic rickets/osteomalacia: Induction and maintenance with phosphorus and calcitriol. *J Clin Invest* 75:1858, 1985.
131. Firth RG, Grant CS, Riggs BL: Development of hypercalcemic hyperparathyroidism after long-term phosphate supplementation in hypophoshatemic osteomalacia. *Am J Med* 78:669, 1985.
132. Goodyer PR, Kronick JB, Jequier S, Reade TM, Scriver CR: Nephrocalcinosis and its relationship to treatment of hereditary rickets. *J Pediatr* 3:700, 1986.
133. Stickler GB, Morgenstern BZ: Hypophosphatemic rickets: Final height and clinical symptoms in adults. *Lancet* 2:902, 1989.
134. Balsan SB, Tieder M: Linear growth in patients with hypophosphatemic vitamin D–resistant rickets: Influence of treatment regimen and parental height. *J Pediatr* 116:365, 1990.
135. Scriver CR, Tenenhouse HS, Glorieux FH: X-linked hypophosphatemia: An appreciation of a classic paper and a survey of progress since 1958. *Medicine (Baltimore)* 70:218, 1991.
136. Verge CF, Lam A, Simpson JM, Cowell CT, Howard NJ, Silink M: Effects of therapy in X-linked hypophosphatemic rickets. *N Engl J Med* 325:1843, 1991.
137. Marie PJ, Glorieux FH: Bone histomorphometry in asymptomatic adults with hereditary hypophosphatemic vitamin D resistant osteomalacia. *Metab Bone Dis Rel Res* 4:249, 1982.
138. Rubinovitch M, Said SE, Glorieux FH, Cruess RL, Rogala

E: Principles and results of corrective lower limb osteotomies for patients with vitamin D–resistant hypophosphatemic rickets. *Clin Orthop* 237:264, 1988.
139. Whyte MP, McAlister WH, Patton LS, Magill HL, Fallon MD, Lorentz WB Jr, Herrod HG: Enzyme replacement therapy for infantile hypophosphatasia attempted by intravenous infusions of alkaline phosphatase–rich Paget plasma: Results in three additional patients. *J Pediatr* 105:926, 1984.
140. Stamp TCB, Byers PD, Ali SY, Jenkins MV, Willoughby JMT: Fibrogenesis imperfecta ossium: Remission with melphalan. *Lancet* 1:582, 1985.
141. Thomson DL, Frame B: Involutional osteopenia: Current concepts. *Ann Intern Med* 85:789, 1976.
142. Cann CE, Genant HK, Kolb FO, Ettinger B: Quantitative computed tomography for prediction of vertebral fracture risk. *Bone* 6:1, 1985.
143. Libanati CR, Schulz E, Shook JE, Bock M, Baylink DJ: Hip mineral density in females with a recent hip fracture. *J Clin Endocrinol Metab* 74:351, 1992.
143a. Cummings SR, Black DM, Nevitt MC, Browner W, Cauley J, Ensrud K, Genant HK, Palermo L, et al: Bone density at various sites for prediction of hip fractures. *Lancet* 34:72, 1993.
144. Johnston CC Jr, Slemenda CW, Melton LJ III: Clinical use of bone densitometry. *N Engl J Med* 324:1105, 1991.
145. Meunier PJ, Bianchi GGS, Edouard CM, Bernard JC, Coupron P, Vignon GE: Bony manifestations of thyrotoxicosis. *Orthop Clin North Am* 3:745, 1975.
146. Kotowicz MA, Klee GG, Kao PC, O'Fallon WM, Hodgson SF, Cedel SL, Eriksen EF, Gonchoroff DG, et al: Relationship between serum intact parathyroid hormone concentrations and bone remodeling in type 1 osteoporosis: Evidence that skeletal sensitivity is increased. *Osteoporosis Int* 1:14, 1990.
147. Silverberg SJ, Shane E, de la Cruz L, Segre GV, Clemens TL, Bilezikian JP: Abnormalities in parathyroid hormone secretion and 1,25-dihydroxyvitamin D_3 formation in women with osteoporosis. *N Engl J Med* 320:277, 1989.
148. Heath H, Sizemore GW: Plasma calcitonin in normal man: Differences between men and women. *J Clin Invest* 60: 1135, 1977.
149. Shamonki IM, Frumar AM, Tataryn IV, Meldrum DR, Davidson BH, Parthemore JG, Judd HL, Deftos LJ: Age-related changes of calcitonin secretion in females. *J Clin Endocrinol Metab* 50:437, 1980.
150. Morimoto S, Tsuji M, Okada Y, Omishi T, Kumahara Y: The effect of oestrogens on human calcitonin secretion after calcium infusion in elderly female subjects. *Clin Endocrinol (Oxf)* 13:135, 1980.
151. Stevenson JC, Abeyasekera G, Hillyard CJ, Phang K-G, McIntyre I, Campbell S, Lane G, Townsend PT, et al: Regulation of calcium-regulating hormones by exogenous sex steroids in early postmenopause. *Eur J Clin Invest* 13:481, 1983.
152. Leggate J, Farish E, Fletcher CD, McIntosh W, Hart DM, Sommerville JM: Calcitonin and postmenopausal osteoporosis. *Clin Endocrinol (Oxf)* 20:85, 1984.
153. Selby PL, Peacock M, Barkworth SA, Brown WB, Taylor GA: Early effects of ethinyloestradiol and norethisterone treatment in post-menopausal women on bone resorption and calcium regulating hormones. *Clin Sci* 69:265, 1985.
154. Lobo RA, Roy S, Shoupe D, Endres DB, Adams JS, Rude RK, Singer FR: Estrogen and progestin effects on urinary calcium and calciotropic hormones in surgically-induced postmenopausal women. *Horm Metab Res* 17:370, 1985.
155. Body JJ, Heath H III: Estimates of circulating monomeric calcitonin: Physiologic studies in normal and thyroidectomized man. *J Clin Endocrinol Metab* 57:897, 1983.
156. Milhaud G, Benezech-Leferre M, Moukhtar MS: Deficiency of calcitonin in age related osteoporosis. *Biomedicine* 29:272, 1978.
157. Chestnut CH III, Baylink DJ, Sisom K, Nelp WB, Roos BA: Basal plasma immunoreactive calcitonin in postmenopausal osteoporosis. *Metabolism* 29:559, 1980.
158. Taggart HM, Chestnut CH III, Ivey JL, Baylink DJ, Sisom K, Huber MB, Roos BA: Deficient calcitonin response to calcium stimulation in postmenopausal osteoporosis. *Lancet* 1:475, 1982.
159. Reginster JY, Deroisy R, Albert A, Denis D, Lecart MP, Collette J, Franchimont P: Relationship between whole plasma calcitonin levels, calcitonin secretory capacity, and plasma levels of estrone in healthy women and postmenopausal osteoporotics. *J Clin Invest* 83:1073, 1989.
160. Sjoberg HE, Torring O, Granberg B, Ehrnsten U, Bucht E: Postmenopausal osteoporosis: Response of immunoextracted calcitonin to a calcium clamp. *Bone* 10:15, 1989.
161. Tiegs RD, Body JJ, Wahner HW, Barta J, Riggs BL, Heath H III: Calcitonin secretion in postmenopausal osteoporosis. *N Engl J Med* 312:1097, 1985.
162. Avioli LV, McDonald JE, Lee SW: The influence of age on the intestinal absorption of ^{47}Ca absorption in postmenopausal osteoporosis. *J Clin Invest* 44:1960, 1965.
163. Gallagher JC, Riggs BL, Eisman J, Hamstra A, Arnaud SB, De Luca HF: Intestinal calcium absorption and serum vitamin D metabolites in normal subjects and osteoporotic patients: Effect of age and dietary calcium. *J Clin Invest* 64:729, 1979.
164. Tsai K-S, Heath H III, Kumar R, Riggs BL: Impaired vitamin D metabolism with aging in women: Possible role in pathogenesis of senile osteoporosis. *J Clin Invest* 73:1668, 1984.
165. Francis RM, Peacock M, Taylor GA, Storer JH, Nordin BEC: Calcium malabsorption in elderly women with vertebral fractures: Evidence for resistance to the action of vitamin D metabolites on the bowel. *Clin Sci* 66:103, 1984.
166. Christiansen C, Rodbro P: Serum vitamin D metabolites in younger and elderly postmenopausal women. *Calcif Tissue Int* 36:19, 1984.
167. Morris HA, Need AG, Horowitz M, O'Loughlin PD, Nordin BEC: Calcium absorption in normal and osteoporotic postmenopausal women. *Calcif Tissue Int* 49:240, 1991.
168. Gallagher JC, Nordin BEC: Oestrogens and calcium metabolism. *Front Horm Res* 2:98, 1973.
169. Gallagher JC, Riggs BL, Jerpbak CM, Arnaud CD: The effect of age on serum immunoreactive parathyroid hormone in normal and osteoporotic women. *J Lab Clin Med* 95:373, 1980.
170. Jowsey J, Kelly PJ, Riggs BL, Bianco AL Jr, Scholz DA, Gershon-Cohen J: Quantitative microradiographic studies of normal and osteoporotic bone. *J Bone Joint Surg [Am]* 47A:785, 1965.
171. Nordin BEC, Aaron J, Speed R, Crilly RB: Bone formation and resorption as the determinants of trabecular bone volume in postmenopausal osteoporosis. *Lancet* 2:77, 1981.
172. Meunier P, Courpron P, Edouard C, Bernard J, Bringuier J, Vignon G: Physiological senile involution and pathological rarefaction of bone. *Clin Endocrinol Metab* 2:239, 1973.
173. Rasmussen H, Bordier P: *The Physiological and Cellular Basis of Metabolic Bone Disease*. Baltimore, Williams & Wilkins, 1974, p 272.
174. Darby AJ, Meunier PJ: Mean wall thickness and formation periods of trabecular bone packets in idiopathic osteoporosis. *Calcif Tissue Int* 33:199, 1981.
175. Arlot M, Edouard C, Meunier PJ, Neer RM, Reeve J: Impaired osteoblast function in osteoporois: Comparison between calcium balance and dynamic histomorphometry. *Br Med J* 289:517, 1984.
176. Johnston CC, Norton J, Khairi MRA, Kernek C, Edouard C, Arlot M, Meunier PJ: Heterogeneity of fracture syndromes in postmenopausal women. *J Clin Endocrinol Metab* 61:551, 1985.
177. Lips P, Netelenbos JC, Jongen MJM, van Ginkel FC, Althuis AL, van Schaik CL, van der Vijgh WJF, Vermeiden

JPW, van der Meer C: Histomorphometric profile and vitamin D status in patients with femoral neck fracture. *Metab Bone Dis Rel Res* 4:85, 1982.
178. Whyte MP, Bergfeld MA, Murphy WA, Avioli LV, Teitelbaum SL: Postmenopausal osteoporosis: A heterogeneous disorder as assessed by histomorphometric analysis of iliac crest bone from untreated patients. *Am J Med* 72:193, 1982.
179. Seeman E, Wahner HW, Offord KP, Kumar R, Johnson WJ, Riggs BL: Differential effects of endocrine dysfunction on the axial and appendicular skeleton. *J Clin Invest* 69:1302, 1982.
180. Riggs BL, Jowsey J, Kelly PJ: Quantitative microradiographic study of bone remodeling in Cushing's syndrome. *Metabolism* 15:773, 1966.
181. Jowsey J, Riggs BL: Bone formation in hypercortisonism. *Acta Endocrinol (Copenh)* 63:21, 1970.
182. Bressot C, Meunier PJ, Chapuy MC, Lejeune E, Edouard C, Darby AJ: Histomorphometric profile, pathophysiology and reversibility of corticosteroid-induced osteoporosis. *Metab Bone Dis Relat Res* 1:303, 1979.
183. Aaron JE, Francis RM, Peacock M, Makins NB: Contrasting microanatomy of idiopathic and corticosteroid-induced osteoporosis. *Clin Orthop* 243:294, 1989.
184. Minaire P, Meunier P, Edouard C, Bernard J, Courpron P, Bouret J: Quantitative histological data on disuse osteoporosis: Comparison with biological data. *Calcif Tissue Res* 17:57, 1974.
185. Jowsey J, Johnson KA: Juvenile osteoporosis: Bone findings in seven patients. *J Pediatr* 81:511, 1972.
186. Smith R: Idiopathic osteoporosis in the young. *J Bone Joint Surg [Br]* 62-B:417, 1980.
187. Evans RA, Dunstan CR, Hills E: Bone metabolism in idiopathic juvenile osteoporosis: A case report. *Calcif Tissue Int* 35:5, 1983.
188. Jaffe HL: *Metabolic, Degenerative, and Inflammatory Diseases of Bones and Joints*. Philadelphia, Lea & Febiger, 1972, p 162.
189. Riggs BL, Melton LJ III: Evidence for two distinct syndromes of involutional osteoporosis. *Am J Med* 75:899, 1983.
190. Daniell HW: Osteoporosis of the slender smoker: Vertebral compression fractures and loss of metacarpal cortex in relation to postmenopausal cigarette smoking and lack of obesity. *Arch Intern Med* 136:298, 1976.
191. Seeman E, Melton LJ III, O'Fallon WA, Riggs BL: Risk factors for spinal osteoporosis in men. *Am J Med* 75:977, 1983.
192. Aloia JF, Cohn SH, Vaswani A, Yeh JK, Yuen K, Ellis K: Risk factors for postmenopausal osteoporosis. *Am J Med* 78:95, 1985.
193. Melton LJ, Riggs BL: Epidemiology of age-related fractures, in Avioli LV (ed): *The Osteoporotic Syndrome: Detection, Prevention and Treatment*. New York, Grune & Stratton, 1983, p 45.
194. Morgan DB: *Osteomalacia, Renal Osteodystrophy, and Osteoporosis*. Springfield, Ill, Charles C Thomas, 1973, p 248.
195. Biller BMK, Saxe V, Herzog DB, Rosenthal DI, Holzman S, Klibanski A: Mechanisms of osteoporosis in adult and adolescent women with anorexia nervosa. *J Clin Endocrinol Metab* 68:548, 1989.
196. Finkelstein JS, Neer RM, Biller BMK, Crawford JD, Klibanski A: Osteopenia in men with a history of delayed puberty. *N Engl J Med* 326:600, 1992.
197. Drinkwater BL, Bruemner B, Chestnut CH III: Menstrual history as a determinant of current bone density in young athletes. *JAMA* 263:545, 1990.
198. Seeman E, Hopper JL, Bach LA, Cooper ME, Parkinson E, McKay J, Jerums G: Reduced bone mass in daughters of women with osteoporosis. *N Engl J Med* 320:554, 1989.
199. Gallagher JC, Wilkinson R: The effect of ethinylestradiol on calcium and phosphorus metabolism of postmenopausal women with primary hyperparathyroidism. *Clin Sci Mol Med* 45:785, 1973.
200. Eriksen EFL, Colvard DS, Berg NJ, Graham ML, Mann KG, Spelsberg TC, Riggs BL: Evidence of estrogen receptors in normal human osteoblast-like cells. *Science* 241:84, 1988.
200a. Jilka RL, Hangoc G, Girasole G, Passeri G, Williams DC, Abrams JS, Boyce B, Broxmeyer H, Manolagos SC: Increased osteoclast development after estrogen loss: Mediation by interleukin-6. *Science* 257:88, 1992.
201. Gallagher JC, Riggs BL, DeLuca HF: Effect of estrogen on calcium absorption and serum vitamin D metabolites in postmenopausal osteoporosis. *J Clin Endocrinol Metab* 51:1359, 1980.
202. Cheema C, Grant BF, Marcus R: Effects of estrogen on circulating "free" and total 1,25-dihydroxyvitamin D and on the parathyroid vitamin D axis in postmenopausal women. *J Clin Invest* 83:537, 1989.
203. Longcope C, Baker RS, Hui SL, Johnston CC Jr: Androgen and estrogen dynamics in women with vertebral crush fractures. *Maturitas* 6:309, 1984.
204. Nordin BEC, Robertson A, Semark RF, Bridges A, Philcox JC, Need AG, Horowitz M, Morris HA, Deam S: The relation between calcium absorption, serum dehydroepiandrosterone, and vertebral mineral density in postmenopausal women. *J Clin Endocrinol Metab* 60:651, 1985.
205. Devogelaer JP, Crabbe J, Nagant de Deuxchaishes C: Bone mineral density in Addison's disease: Evidence for an effect of adrenal androgens on bone mass. *Br Med J* 294:798, 1987.
206. Forbes AP: Fuller Albright: His concept of postmenopausal osteoporosis and what's come of it. *Clin Orthop* 269:128, 1991.
207. Heaney RP, Recker RR, Saville PD: Menopausal changes in bone remodelling. *J Lab Clin Med* 92:964, 1978.
208. Drinkwater BL, Bruemner B, Chestnut CS III: Menstrual history as a determinant of current bone density in young athletes. *JAMA* 263:545, 1990.
209. Biller BMK, Saxe V, Herzog DB, Rosenthal DI, Holzman S, Klibanski A: Mechanisms of osteoporosis in adult and adolescent women with anorexia nervosa. *J Clin Endocrinol Metab* 68:548, 1989.
209a. Seeman E, Szmukler GI, Formica C, Tsalamandris C, Mestrovic R: Osteoporosis in anorexia nervosa: The influence of peak bone density, bone loss, oral contraceptive use, and exercise. *J Bone Mineral Res* 7:1467, 1992.
210. Klibanski A, Biller BMK, Rosenthal DI, Schoenfeld DA, Saxe V: Effects of prolactin and estrogen deficiency in amenorrheic bone loss. *J Clin Endocrinol Metab* 67:124, 1988.
211. Johansen JS, Riis BJ, Hassager C, Moen M, Jacobson J, Christiansen C: The effect of a gonadotropin-releasing hormone agonist analog (Nafarelin) on bone metabolism. *J Clin Endocrinol Metab* 67:701, 1988.
212. Jackson JAL, Kleerekoper M: Osteoporosis in men: Diagnosis, pathophysiology, and prevention. *Medicine (Baltimore)* 69:137, 1990.
213. Foresta C, Ruzza G, Mioni R, Guarnieri G, Gribaldo R, Meneghello A, Mastrogiacomo I: Osteoporosis and decline of gonadal function in the elderly. *Horm Res* 19:18, 1984.
214. Francis RM, Peacock M, Aaron JE, Selby PL, Taylor GA, Thompson J, Marshall DH, HorsmanA: Osteoporosis in hypogonadal men: Role of decreased plasma 1,25-dihydroxyvitamin D, calcium malabsorption, and low bone formation. *Bone* 7:261, 1986.
215. Jackson JA, Kleerekoper M, Parfitt AM, Rao DS, Villanueva AR, Frame B: Bone histomorphometry in hypogonadal and eugonadal men with spinal osteoporosis. *J Clin Endocrinol Metab* 65:53, 1987.
216. Finkelstein JS, Neer RM, Biller BMK, Crawford JD, Klibanski A: Osteopenia in men with a history of delayed puberty. *N Engl J Med* 326:600, 1992.

217. Colvard DS, Eriksen EF, Keeting PE, Wilson EM, Lubahn DB, French FS, Riggs BL, Spelsberg TC: Identification of androgen receptors in normal human osteoblast-like cells. *Proc Natl Acad Sci USA* 86:854, 1989.
218. Lukert BP, Raisz LG: Glucocorticoid-induced osteoporosis: Pathogenesis and management. *Ann Intern Med* 112:352, 1990.
219. Peck WA, Brandt J, Miller I: Hydrocortisone-induced inhibition of protein synthesis and uridine incorporation in isolated bone cells in vitro. *Proc Natl Acad Sci USA* 57:1599, 1967.
220. Jett S, Wu K, Duncan H, Frost HM: Adrenalcorticosteroid and salicylate actions on human and canine haversian bone formation and resorption. *Clin Orthop* 68:301, 1970.
221. Blodgett FM, Burgin L, Jezzoni D, Gribetz D, Talbot NB: Effects of prolonged cortisone therapy on the statural growth, skeletal maturation and metabolic status of children. *N Engl J Med* 254:636, 1956.
222. Barrett AJ, Sledge CB, Dingle JT: Effect of cortisol on the synthesis of chondroitin sulfate by embryonic cartilage. *Nature* 221:83, 1966.
223. Fucik RF, Kukreja SC, Hargis GK, Bowser EN, Henderson WJ, Williams GA: Effects of glucocorticoids on function of the parathyroid glands in man. *J Clin Endocrinol Metab* 49:152, 1975.
224. Lukert BP, Adams JS: Calcium and phosphorus homeostasis in man. *Arch Intern Med* 136:1249, 1976.
225. Slovik DM, Neer RM, Ohman JL, Lowell FC, Clark MB, Segre GV, Potts JT Jr: Parathyroid hormone and 25-hydroxyvitamin D levels in glucocorticoid-treated patients. *Clin Endocrinol (Oxf)* 12:243, 1980.
226. Findling JW, Adams ND, Lemann J Jr, Gray RW, Thomas CJ, Tyrell BJ: Vitamin D metabolites and parathyroid hormone in Cushing's syndrome: Relationship to calcium and phosphorus homeostasis. *J Clin Endocrinol Metab* 54:1039, 1982.
227. Harrison HE, Harrison HC: Transfer of Ca^{45} across intestinal wall in vitro in relation to action of vitamin D and cortisol. *Am J Physiol* 199:265, 1960.
228. Kimberg DV, Baerg RD, Gershon E, Graudusius RT: Effect of cortisone treatment on the active transport of calcium by the small intestine. *J Clin Invest* 50:1309, 1971.
229. Edelstein S, Noff D: The functional metabolism of vitamin D in rats treated with cortisol. *FEBS Lett* 82:115, 1977.
230. Spanos E, Colston KW, MacIntyre I: Effect of glucocorticoids on vitamin D metabolism. *FEBS Lett* 75:73, 1977.
231. Klein RG, Arnaud SB, Gallagher JC, DeLuca HF, Riggs BL: Intestinal calcium absorption in exogenous hypercortisonism. *J Clin Invest* 60:253, 1977.
232. Chesney RW, Mazess RB, Hamstra AJ, DeLuca HF, O'Reagan S: Reduction of serum 1,25-dihydroxyvitamin D_3 in children receiving glucocorticoid. *Lancet* 2:1123, 1978.
233. O'Reagan S, Chesney RW, Hamstra A, Eisman JA, O'Gorman AM, DeLuca HF: Reduced serum 1,25-$(OH)_2$-vitamin D_3 levels in prednisone-treated adolescents with systemic lupus erythematosus. *Acta Paediatr Scand* 68:109, 1979.
234. Rickers H, Deding A, Christiansen C, Rodbro P, Naestoft J: Corticosteroid-induced ostopenia and vitamin D metabolism: Effect of vitamin D_2, calcium phosphate and sodium fluoride administration. *Clin Endocrinol (Oxf)* 16:409, 1982.
235. Favus MJ, Walling MW, Kimberg DV: Effects of 1,25-dihydroxycholecalciferol on intestinal calcium transport in cortisone treated rats. *J Clin Invest* 52:1680, 1973.
236. Stoll GM, Harris S, Sokoll LJ, Dawson-Hughes B: Accelerated bone loss in hypothyroid patients overtreated with L-thyroxine. *Ann Intern Med* 113:265, 1990.
237. Mundy GR, Shapiro JL, Bardelin JG, Canalis EM, Raisz LG: Direct stimulation of bone resorption by thyroid hormones. *J Clin Invest* 58:529, 1976.
238. Krane SM, Brownell GL, Stanbury JB, Corrigan H: The effect of thyroid disease on calcium metabolism in man. *J Clin Invest* 35:874, 1956.
239. Singhelakis P, Alevizaka CC, Ikkos DG: Intestinal calcium absorption in hyperthyroidism. *Metabolism* 23:311, 1974.
240. Bouillon R, Muls E, DeMoor P: Influence of thyroid function on the serum concentration of 1,25-dihydroxyvitamin D_3. *J Clin Endocrinol Metab* 51:793, 190.
240a. Melton LJ III, Atkinson EJ, O'Fallon WM, Heath H III: Risk of age-related fractures in patients with primary hyperparathyroidism. *Arch Intern Med* 152:2269, 1992.
241. McNair P, Madsbad S, Chistensen MS, Christiansen C, Faber OK, Binder C, Transbol I: Bone mineral loss in insulin-treated diabetes mellitus. Studies on pathogenesis. *Acta Endocrinol (Copenh)* 90:463, 1979.
242. Heath H III, Melton LJ III, Chu C-P: Diabetes mellitus and risk of skeletal fracture. *N Engl J Med* 303:567, 1980.
243. Raskin P, Stevenson MRM, Barilla DE, Pak CYC: The hypercalciuria of diabetes mellitus: Its amelioration with insulin. *Clin Endocrinol (Oxf)* 9:329, 1978.
244. Schneider LE, Schedl HP, McCain T, Haussler MR: Experimental diabetes reduces circulating 1,25-dihydroxyvitamin D in the rat. *Science* 196:1452, 1977.
245. Heath H III, Lambert PW, Service FJ, Arnaud SB: Calcium homeostasis in diabetes mellitus. *J Clin Endocrinol Metab* 49:462, 1979.
246. Frazer TE, White NH, Hough S, Santiago JV, McGee BR, Bryce G, Mallon J, Avioli LV: Alterations in circulating vitamin D metabolites in the young insulin-dependent diabetic. *J Clin Endocrinol Metab* 53:1154, 1981.
247. Storm TL, Sorensen OH, Lund B, Lund B, Christiansen JS, Andersen AR, Lumholtz IB, Parving H-H: Vitamin D metabolism in insulin-dependent diabetes mellitus. *Metab Bone Dis Rel Res* 5:107, 1983.
248. Prockop DJ, Kivirikko KK: Heritable diseases of collagen. *N Engl J Med* 311:376, 1984.
249. Rowe DW, Shapiro JR: Osteogenesis imperfecta, in Avioli LV, Krane SM (eds): *Metabolic Bone Disease and Clinically Related Disorders,* 2d ed. Philadelphia, Saunders, 1990, p 659.
250. Seeman E, Hopper JL, Bach LA, Cooper ME, Parkinson E, McKay J, Jerums G: Reduced bone mass in daughters of women with osteoporosis. *N Engl J Med* 320:554, 1989.
250a. Kelly PJ, Hopper JL, Macaskill GT, Pocock NA, Sambrook PN, Eisman JA: Genetic factors in bone turnover. *J Clin Endocrinol Metab* 72:808, 1991.
250b. Morrison NA, ChengQi S, Tokita A, Kelly PJ, Crofts L, Nguyen TV, Sambrook PN, Eisman JA: Prediction of bone density from vitamin D receptor alleles. *Nature* 367:284, 1994.
251. Smith R: Idiopathic juvenile osteoporosis. *Am J Dis Child* 133:889, 1979.
252. Saggese G, Bertelloni S, Baroncelli GI, Perri G, Calderazzi A: Mineral metabolism and calcitriol therapy in idiopathic juvenile osteoporosis. *Am J Dis Child* 145:457, 1991.
253. de Vernejoul MC, Marie P, Kuntz D, Gueris J, Miravet L, Ryckewaert A: Non-osteomalacic osteopathy associated with chronic hypophosphatemia. *Calcif Tissue Int* 34:219, 1982.
254. Lawoyin S, Sismilich S, Browne R, Pak CYC: Bone mineral content in patients with calcium urolithiasis. *Metabolism* 28:1250, 1979.
255. Bikle DD, Genant HK, Cann C, Recker RR, Halloran BP, Strewler GJ: Bone disease in alcohol abuse. *Ann Intern Med* 103:42, 1985.
256. Diamond T, Stiel D, Lunzer M, Wilkinson M, Posen S: Ethanol reduces bone formation and may cause osteoporosis. *Am J Med* 86:282, 1989.
257. Slemenda CW, Hui SL, Longcope C, Johnston CC Jr: Cigarette smoking, obesity, and bone mass. *J Bone Mineral Res* 4:737, 1989.
258. Matkovic V, Fontana D, Tominac C, Goel P, Chesnut CH III: Factors that influence peak bone mass formation: A

study of calcium balance and the inheritance of bone mass in adolescent females. *Am J Clin Nutr* 52:878, 1990.
259. Griffith GC, Nichols G, Asher JD, Flanagan B: Heparin osteoporosis. *JAMA* 193:91, 1965.
260. Weinstein RS, Bryce GF, Sappington LJ, King DW, Gallagher BB: Decreased serum ionized calcium and normal vitamin D metabolite levels with anticonvulsant drug treatment. *J Clin Endocrinol Metab* 58:1003, 1984.
261. Sambrook PN, Reeve J: Bone disease in rheumatoid arthritis. *Clin Sci* 74:225, 1988.
262. Resnick D, Niwayama G: *Diagnosis of Bone and Joint Disorders,* 2d ed. Philadelphia, Saunders, 1988.
263. Chines A, Pacifici R, Avioli LV, Teitelbaum SL, Korenblat PE: Systemic mastocytosis presenting as osteoporosis: A clinical and histomorphometric study. *J Clin Endocrinol Metab* 72:140, 1991.
264. Meema S, Bunker ML, Meema HE: Preventive effect of estrogen on postmenopausal bone loss. *Arch Intern Med* 135:1436, 1975.
265. Aitken JM, Hart DM, Lindsay R: Oestrogen replacement therapy for prevention of osteoporosis after oophorectomy. *Br Med J* 3:515, 1973.
266. Ettinger B, Genant HK, Cann CE: Long-term estrogen replacement therapy prevents bone loss and fractures. *Ann Intern Med* 102:319, 1985.
267. Stevenson JC, Cost MP, Gangor KF, Hillard TC, Lees B, Whitehead MI: Effects of transdermal versus oral hormone replacement therapy on bone density in spine and proximal femur in postmenopausal women. *Lancet* 335:265, 1990.
268. Heaney RP, Recker RR, Saville PD: Menopausal changes in calcium balance performance. *J Lab Clin Med* 92:953, 1978.
269. Weiss NS, Ure CL, Ballard JH, Williams AR, Daling JR: Decreased risk of fractures of the hip and lower forearm with postmenopausal use of estrogen. *N Engl J Med* 303:1195, 1980.
269a. Lufkin EG, Wahner HW, O'Fallon WM, Hodgson SF, Kotowicz MA, Lane AW, Judd HL, Caplan RH, Riggs BL: Treatment of postmenopausal osteoporosis with transdermal estrogen. *Ann Intern Med* 117:1, 1992.
269b. Grady D, Rubin SM, Petiti DB, Fox CS, Black D, Ettinger B, Ernster VL, Cummings SR: Hormone therapy to prevent disease and prolong life in postmenopausal women. *Ann Intern Med* 117:1016, 1992.
270. Henderson BE, Paganini-Hill A, Ross RK: Decreased mortality in users of estrogen replacement therapy. *Arch Intern Med* 151:75, 1991.
270a. American College of Physicians: Guidelines for counseling postmenopausal women about preventive hormone therapy. *Ann Intern Med* 117:1038, 1992.
271. Love RR, Mazess RB, Barden HS, Epstein S, Newcomb PA, Jordan VC, Carbone PP, DeMets DL: Effects of tamoxifen on bone mineral density in postmenopausal women with breast cancer. *N Engl J Med* 326:852, 1992.
272. Riis B, Thomsen K, Christiansen C: Does calcium supplementation prevent postmenopausal bone loss? A double-blind, controlled study. *N Engl J Med* 316:173, 1987.
273. Dawson-Hughes B, Dallal GE, Krall EA, Sadowski L, Sahyoun N, Tannenbaum S: A controlled trial of the effect of calcium supplementation on bone density in postmenopausal women. *N Engl J Med* 323:878, 1990.
274. Need AG, Horowitz M, Philcox JC, Nordin BEC: 1,25-dihydroxycholecalciferol and calcium therapy in osteoporosis with calcium malabsorption. *Mineral Electrolyte Metab* 11:35, 1985.
275. Riggs BL, Nelson KI: Effect of long term treatment with calcitriol on calcium absorption and mineral metabolism in postmenopausal osteoporosis. *J Clin Endocrinol Metab* 61:457, 1985.
276. Gallagher JC, Goldgar D: Treatment of postmenopausal osteoporosis with high doses of synthetic calcitriol: A randomized controlled study. *Ann Intern Med* 113:649, 1990.
277. Tillyard MW, Spears GFS, Thomson J, Dovey S: Treatment of postmenopausal osteoporosis with calcitriol or calcium. *N Engl J Med* 326:357, 1992.
278. Ott SM, Chestnut CH III: Calcitriol treatment is not effective in postmenopausal osteoporosis. *Ann Intern Med* 110:267, 1989.
279. Gruber HE, Ivey JL, Baylink DJ, Matthews M, Nelp WB, Sisom K, Chestnut CH III: Long-term calcitonin therapy in postmenopausal osteoporosis. *Metabolism* 33:295, 1984.
280. Civitelli R, Gonnelli S, Zacchei F, Bigazzi S, Vattimo A, Avioli LV, Gennari C: Bone turnover in postmenopausal osteoporosis: Effect of calcitonin treatment. *J Clin Invest* 82:1268, 1988.
281. Reginster JY, Denis D, Albert A, Deroisy R, Lecart MP, Fontaine MA, Lambelin P, Franchimont P: 1-year controlled randomised trial of prevention of early postmenopausal bone loss by intranasal calcitonin. *Lancet* 2:1481, 1987.
282. Wasnich RD, Ross PD, Heilbrun LK, Vogel JM, Yano K, Benfante RJ: Differential effects of thiazide and estrogen upon bone mineral content and fracture prevalence. *Obstet Gynecol* 67:457, 1986.
283. Heidrich FE, Stergachis A, Gross KM: Diuretic drug use and the risk for hip fracture. *Ann Inter Med* 115:1, 1991.
284. Storm T, Thamsborg G, Steiniche T, Genant HK, Sorensen OH: Effect of intermittent cyclic etidronate therapy on bone mass and fracture rate in women with postmenopausal osteoporosis. *N Engl J Med* 322:1265, 1990.
285. Watts NB, Harris ST, Genant HK, Wasnich RD, Miller PD, Jackson RD, Licata AA, Ross P, et al: Intermittent cyclical etidronate therapy of postmenopausal osteoporosis. *N Engl J Med* 323:73, 1990.
285a. Reginster JY, Lecart MP, Deroisy R, Sarlet MP, Denis D, Ethgen D, Collette J, Franchimont P: Prevention of postmenopausal bone loss by tiludronate. *Lancet* 2:1469, 1989.
286. Gluck OS, Murphy WA, Hahn TJ, Hahn B: Bone loss in adults receiving alternate day glucocorticoid therapy: A comparison with daily therapy. *Arthritis Rheum* 24:892, 1981.
287. Hahn TJ, Halstead LR, Teitelbaum SL, Hahn BH: Altered mineral metabolism in glucocorticoid-induced osteopenia: Effect of 25-hydroxyvitamin D administration. *J Clin Invest* 64:655,1979.
288. Braun JJ, Birkenhager-Frenkel DH, Rietveld AH, Juttmann JR, Visser TJ, Birkenhager JC: Influence of 1α-$(OH)D_3$ administration on bone and bone mineral metabolism in patients on chronic glucocorticoid treatment: A double blind controlled study. *Clin Endocrinol* 18:265, 1983.
288a. Sambrook P, Birmingham J, Kelly P, Kempler S, Nguyen T, Pocock N, Eisman J: Prevention of corticosteroid osteoporosis. A comparison of calcium, calcitriol, and calcitonin. *N Engl J Med* 328:1747, 1993.
289. Nagant de Deuxchaisnes C, Devogelaer JP, Esselinck W, Bouchez B, Depresseux G, Rombouts-Lindemans C, Huaux JP: The effect of low dosage glucocorticoids on bone mass in rheumatoid arthritis: A cross-sectional and a longitudinal study using single photon absorptiometry. *Adv Exp Med Biol* 171:209, 1984.
290. Ringe J-D, Welzel D: Salmon calcitonin in the therapy of corticoid-induced osteoporosis. *Eur J Clin Pharmacol* 33:35, 1987.
291. Reid IR, King AR, Alexander CJ, Ibbertson HK: Prevention of steroid-induced osteoporosis with (3-amino-1-hydroxypropylidene)-1, 1-bis-phosphonate (APD). *Lancet* 1:143, 1988.
292. Gennari C, Agnusdei D, Camporeale A: Use of calcitonin in the treatment of bone pain associated with osteoporosis. *Calcif Tissue Int* 49(Suppl 2):S9, 1991.
293. Murray TM, Singer FR (eds): Proceedings of the International Workshop on Fluoride and Bone. *J Bone Mineral Res* 5(Suppl 1):1990.

294. Namelle N, Meunier PJ, Dusan R, Guillaume M, Martin JL, GaucherA, Prost A, Zeigler G, Netter P: Risk-benefit ratio of sodium fluoride treatment in primary vertebral osteoporosis. *Lancet* 2:361, 1988.
295. Pak CYC, Sakhaee K, Zerwekh JE, Parcel C, Peterson R, Johnson K: Safe and effective treatment of osteoporosis with intermittent slow release sodium fluoride: Augmentation of vertebral bone mass and inhibition of fractures. *J Clin Endocrinol Metab* 68:150, 1989.
296. Nagant de Deuxchaisnes C, Devogelaer J-P, Depresseux G, Malghem J, Maldague B: Treatment of the vertebral crush fracture syndrome with enteric-coated sodium fluoride tablets and calcium supplements. *J Bone Mineral Res* 5(Suppl 1):S5, 1990.
297. Farley SM, Wergedal JE, Farley JR, Javier GN, Schulz EE, Talbot JR, Libanati CR, Lindegren L, et al: Spinal fractures during fluoride therapy for osteoporosis: Relationship to spinal bone density. *Osteoporosis Int* 2:213, 1992.
298. Riggs BL, Hodgson SF, O'Fallon WM, Chao EYS, Wahner HW, Muhs JM, Cedel SL, Melton LJ III: Effect of fluoride treatment on the fracture rate in postmenopausal women with osteoporosis. *N Engl J Med* 322:802, 1990.
298a. Riggs BL, O'Fallon WM, Lane A, Hodgson SF, Wahner HW, Muhs J, Chao E, Melton LJ III: Clinical trial of fluoride therapy in postmenopausal osteoporotic women: Extended observations and additional analysis. *J Bone Mineral Res* 9:265, 1994.
299. Aloia JF, Vaswani A, Kapoor A, Yeh JK, Cohn SH: Treatment of osteoporosis with calcitonin, with and without growth hormone. *Metabolism* 34:124, 1985.
300. Slovik DM, Rosenthal DI, Doppelt SH, Potts JT Jr, Daly MA, Campbell JA, Neer RM: Restoration of spinal bone in osteoporotic men by treatment with human parathyroid hormone (1-34) and 1,25-dihydroxyvitamin D. *J Bone Mineral Res* 1:377, 1986.
301. Chestnut CH III, Ivey JL, Gruber HE, Mathews M, Nelp WB, Sisom K, Baylink DJ: Stanozolol in postmenopausal osteoporosis: Therpeutic efficacy and possible mechanisms of action. *Metabolism* 32:571, 1983.
302. Christiansen C, Riis BJ: 17β-estradiol and continuous norethisterone: A unique treatment for established osteoporosis in the elderly. *J Clin Endocrinol Metab* 71:836, 1990.
303. Mosekilde L, Melsen F: Effect of antithyroid treatment on calcium-phoshorus metabolism in hyperhythyroidism: II. Bone histomorphometry. *Acta Endocrinol (Copenh)* 87:751, 1978.
304. Rosen JF, Wolin DA, Finberg L: Immobilization hypercalcemia after single limb fractures in children and adolescents. *Am J Dis Child* 132:560, 1978.
305. Pedersen V, Charles P, Hansen HH, Elbrond D: Lack of effects of human calcitonin in osteogenesis imperfecta. *Acta Orthop Scand* 56:260, 1985.
306. Hoekman K, Papapoulos SE, Peters ACB, Bijvoet OLM: Characteristics and bisphosphonate treatment of a patient with juvenile osteoporosis. *J Clin Endocrinol Metab* 61:952, 1985.
307. Singer FR, Chang SS: Osteopetrosis. *Semin Nephrol* 12:191, 1992.
308. Whyte MP, Murphy WA, Fallon MD, Sly WS, Teitelbaum SL, McAlister WH, Avioli LV: Osteopetrosis, renal tubular acidosis and basal ganglia calcification in three sisters. *Am J Med* 69:64, 1980.
309. Sly WS, Whyte MP, Sundaram V, Tashian RE, Hewett-Emmett D, Geribaud P, Vainsel M, Baluarte HJ, et al: Carbonic anhydrase II deficiency in 12 families with the autosomal recessive syndrome of osteopetrosis with renal tubular acidosis and cerebral calcification. *N Engl J Med* 313:139, 1985.
310. Kahler SG, Burns JA, Aylsworth AS: A mild autosomal recessive form of osteopetrosis. *Am J Med Genet* 17:451, 1984.
311. Shapiro F, Glimcher MJ, Holtrop ME, Tashjian AH Jr, Brickley-Parsons D, Kenzora JE: Human osteopetrosis: A histological, ultrastructural and biochemical study. *J Bone Joint Surg [Am]* 62-A:384, 1980.
312. Milgram JW, Jasty M: Osteopetrosis: A morphological study of twenty-one cases. *J Bone Joint Surg [Am]* 64-A:912, 1982.
313. Walker DG: Bone resorption restored in osteopetrotic mice by transplants of normal bone marrow and spleen cells. *Science* 190:784, 1975.
314. Coccia PF, Krivit W, Cervenka J, Clawson C, Kersey J, Kim TH, Nesbit ME, Ramsay NKC, et al: Successful bone-marrow transplantation for infantile malignant osteopetrosis. *N Engl J Med* 302:701, 1980.
315. Felix R, Cecchini MG, Fleisch H: Macrophage colony stimulating factor restores in vivo bone resorption in the op/op osteopetrotic mouse. *Endocrinology* 127:2592, 1990.
316. Slatopolsky E, Delmez J: Bone disease in chronic renal failure and after renal transplantation, in Coe FL, Favus MJ (eds): *Disorders of Bone and Mineral Metabolism.* New York, Raven Press, 1991, p 905.
317. Freitag J, Martin KJ, Hruska KA, Anderson C, Conrades M, Ladenson J, Klahr S, Slatopolsky E: Impaired parathyroid hormone metabolism in patients with chronic renal failure. *N Engl J Med* 298:29, 1978.
318. Hodsman AB, Sherrard DJ, Wong EGC, Brickman AS, Lee DBN, Alfrey AC, Singer FR, Norman AW, Coburn JW: Vitamin D–resistant osteomalacia in hemodialysis patients lacking secondary hyperparathyroidism. *Ann Intern Med* 94:629, 1981.
319. Eastwood JB, Harris E, Stamp TCB, DeWardener HE: Vitamin D deficiency in the osteomalacia of chronic renal failure. *Lancet* 2:1209, 1976.
320. Sherrard DJ, Baylink DJ, Wergedahl JE, Maloney N: Quantitative histological studies on the pathogenesis of uremic bone disease. *J Clin Endocrinol Metab* 39:119, 1974.
321. Bressot C, Courpron P, Edouard C, Meunier P: *Histomorphométrie des ostéopathies endocriniennes.* Lyon, Association Corporative des Etudiants en Médecine de Lyon, 1976, p 85.
322. Mason RS, Lissner D, Wilkinson M, Posen S: Vitamin D metabolites and their relationship to azotaemic osteodystrophy. *Clin Endocrinol (Oxf)* 13:375, 1980.
323. Portale AA, Booth BE, Tsai HC, Morris RC Jr: Reduced plasma concentration of 1,25-dihydroxyvitamin D in children with moderate renal insufficiency. *Kidney Int* 21:627, 1982.
324 Hodsman AB, Sherrard DJ, Alfrey AC, Ott S, Brickman AS, Miller NL, Maloney NA, Coburn JW: Bone aluminum and histomorphometric features of renal osteodystrophy. *J Clin Endocrinol Metab* 54:539, 1982.
325. Teitelbaum SL, Bergfeld MA, Freitag J, Hruska KA, Slatopolsky E: Do parathyroid hormone and 1,25-dihydroxyvitamin D modulate bone formation in uremia? *J Clin Endocrinol Metab* 51:247, 1980.
326. Weinstein RS: Decreased mineralization in hemodialysis patients after subtotal parathyroidectomy. *Calcif Tissue Int* 34:16, 1982.
327. Sherrard DJ, Ott SM, Andress DL: Pseudohyperparathyroidism: Syndrome associated with aluminum intoxication in patients with renal failure. *Am J Med* 79:127, 1985.
328. Slatopolsky E, Caglar S, Gradowska L, Canterbury JM, Reiss E, Bricker NS: On the prevention of secondary hyperparathyroidism in experimental chronic renal disease using "proportional reduction" of dietary phosphorus intake. *Kidney Int* 2:147, 1972.
329. Portale AA, Booth BE, Halloran BP, Morris RC Jr: Effect of dietary phosphorus on circulating concentrations of 1,25-dihydroxyvitamin D and immunoreactive parathyroid hormone in children with moderate renal insufficiency. *J Clin Invest* 73:1580, 1984.

330. Massry SG, Tuma S, Dua S, Goldstein DA: Reversal of skeletal resistance to parathyroid hormone in uremia by vitamin D metabolites: Evidence for the requirement of $1,25(OH)_2D_3$ and $24,25(OH)_2D_3$. *J Lab Clin Med* 94:152, 1979.
331. Mak RHK, Turner C, Thompson T, Powell H, Haycock GB, Chantler C: Suppression of secondary hyperparathyroidism in children with chronic renal failure by high dose phosphate binders: Calcium carbonate versus aluminum hydroxide. *Br Med J* 291:623, 1985.
332. Wilson L, Felsenfeld A, Drezner MK, Llach F: Altered divalent ion metabolism in early renal failure: Role of $1,25(OH)_2D$. *Kidney Int* 27:565, 1985.
333. Brickman AS, Sherrard DJ, Jowsey J, Singer FR, Baylink DJ, Maloney N, Massry SG, Norman AW, Coburn JW: 1,25-Dihydroxycholecalciferol: Effect on skeletal lesions and plasma parathyroid hormone levels in uremic osteodystrophy. *Arch Intern Med* 134:883, 1974.
334. Masry SG: Requirements of vitamin D metabolites in patients with renal disease. *Am J Clin Nutr* 33:1530, 1980.
335. Bordier P, Zingraff J, Gueris J, Jungers P, Marie P, Pechet M, Rasmussen H: The effect of $1\alpha(OH)D_3$ and $1\alpha,25(OH)_2D_3$ on the bone in patients with renal osteodystrophy. *Am J Med* 64:101,1978.
336. Eastwood JB, Stamp TCB, DeWardener HE, Bordier PJ, Arnaud CD: The effect of 25-hydroxyvitamin D_3 in the osteomalacia of chronic renal failure. *Clin Sci Mol Med* 52:499, 1977.
337. Wells SA Jr, Ross AJ III, Dale JK, Gray RS: Transplantation of the parathyroid glands: Current status. *Surg Clin North Am* 59:167, 1979.
338. Andress DL, Norris KC, Coburn JW, Slatopolsky EA, Sherrard DJ: Intravenous calcitriol in the treatment of refractory osteitis fibrosa of chronic renal failure. *N Engl J Med* 321:274, 1989.
339. Malluche HH, Smith AJ, Abreo K, Faugere M-C: The use of deferoxamine in the management of aluminum accumulation in bone in patients with renal failure. *N Engl J Med* 311:140, 1984.
340. Thompson RC Jr, Gaull GE, Horwitz SJ, Schenk RK: Hereditary hyperphosphatasia: Studies of three siblings. *Am J Med* 47:209, 1969.
341. Whalen JP, Horwith M, Krook L, McIntyre I, Mena A, Viteri F, Town B, Nunez EA: Calcitonin treatment in hereditary bone dysplasia with hyperphosphatasemia: A radiographic and histologic study of bone. *AJR* 129:29, 1977.
342. Nunez EA, Horwith M, Krook L, Whalen JP: An electron microscopic investigation of human familial bone dysplasia: Inhibition of osteocytic osteolysis and induction of osteocytic formation of elastic fibers following calcitonin treatment. *Am J Pathol* 94:1, 1979.
343. Doyle FH, Woodhouse NJY, Glen CA, Joplin CF, MacIntyre I: Healing of the bones in juvenile Paget's disease treated by human calcitonin. *Br J Radiol* 47:9, 1974.
344. Blanco O, Stivel M, Mautalen C, Schajowicz F: Familial idiopathic hyperphosphatasia. A study of two siblings treated with porcine calcitonin. *J Bone Joint Surg [Br]* 59B:421, 1977.
345. Dunn V, Condon VR, Rallison ML: Familial hyperphosphatasemia: Diagnosis in early infancy and response to human thyrocalcitonin therapy. *AJR* 132:541, 1979.
346. Albright F, Butler AM, Hampton AO, Smith P: Syndrome characterized by osteitis fibrosa disseminata, areas of pigmentation and endocrine dysfunction, with precocious puberty in females: Report of five cases. *N Engl J Med* 216:727, 1937.
347. Albright F: Polyostotic fibrous dysplasia: A defense of the entity. *J Clin Endocrinol* 7:307, 1947.
348. Von Recklinghausen F: Die Fibrose oder deformirende Ostitis, die Osteomalacie und die osteoplastische Carcinose in ihren gegenseitigen Beziehungen, in *Festschrift für Rudolf Virchow*. Berlin, G Reimer, 1891.
349. Harris WH, Dudley HR Jr, Barry RJ: The natural history of fibrous dysplasia: An orthopaedic, pathological and roentgenographic study. *J Bone Joint Surg [Am]* 44A:207, 1962.
350. Schwartz DT, Alpert M: The malignant transformation of fibrous dysplasia. *Am J Med Sci* 247:35, 1964.
351. Gianoutsos MP, Thompson JF, Marsden FW: Mazabraud's syndrome: Intramuscular myxoma associated with fibrous dysplasia of bone. *Aust N J Surg* 60:825, 1960.
352. Benedict PH: Endocrine features in Albright's syndrome (fibrous dysplasia of bone). *Metabolism* 11:30, 1962.
353. McArthur RG, Hayles AB, Lambert PW: Albright's syndrome with rickets. *Mayo Clin Proc* 54:313, 1979.
354. Shires R, Whyte MP, Avioli LV: Idiopathic hypothalamic hypogonadotropic hypogonadism with polyostotic fibrous dysplasia. *Arch Intern Med* 139:1187, 1979.
355. Cuttler L, Jackson JA, Saeed uz-Zafar M, Levitsky LL, Mellinger RC, Frohman LA: Hypersecretion of growth hormone and prolactin in McCune-Albright syndrome. *J Clin Endocrinol Metab* 68:1148, 1989.
355a. Weinstein LS, Shenker A, Gejman PV, Merino MJ, Friedman E, Spiegel AM: Activating mutations of the stimulatory G protein in the McCune-Albright syndrome. *N Engl J Med* 325:1688, 1991.
356. Bell NH, Avery S, Johnston CC: Effects of calcitonin in Paget's disease and polyostotic fibrous dysplasia. *J Clin Endocrinol Metab* 31:283, 1970.
357. Long A, Loughlin T, Towers RP, McKenna TJ: Polyostotic fibrous dysplasia with contrasting responses to calcitonin and mithramycin: Aetiological and therapeutic implications. *Ir J Med Sci* 157:229, 1988.
358. Comite F, Shawker TH, Pescovitz OH, Loriaux DL, Cutler GB Jr: Cyclical ovarian function resistant to treatment with an analogue of luteinizing hormone releasing hormone in McCune-Albright syndrome. *N Engl J Med* 311:1032, 1984.
359. Feuillan PP, Foster CM, Pecovitz OH, Hench KD, Shawker T, Dwyer A, Malley JD, Barnes K, Loriaux DL, Cutler GB Jr: Treatment of precocious puberty in the McCune-Albright syndrome with the aromatase inhibitor testolactone. *N Engl J Med* 315:1115, 1986.
360. Stephenson RB, London MD, Hankin FM, Kaufer H: Fibrous dysplasia: An analysis of options for treatment. *J Bone Joint Surg* 69-A:400, 1987.
361. Paget J: On a form of chronic inflammmation of bones (osteitis deformans). *Med Chir Trans* 60:27, 1877.
362. Barry HC: *Paget's Disease of Bone*. Baltimore, Williams & Wilkins, 1969.
363. Franck WA, Bress NM, Singer FR, Krane SM: Rheumatic manifestations of Paget's disease of bone. *Am J Med* 56:592, 1974.
364. Heistad DD, Abboud FM, Schmid PG, Mark AL, Wilson WR: Regulation of blood flow in Paget's disease of bone. *J Clin Invest* 55:69, 1975.
365. Arnalich F, Plaza I, Sobrino JA, Oliver J, Barbado J, Pena JM, Vazquez JJ: Cardiac size and function in Paget's disease of bone. *Int J Cardiol* 5:491, 1984.
366. Waxman AD, Ducker S, McKee D, Siemsen JK, Singer FR: Evaluation of ^{99m}Tc diphosphonate kinetics and bone scans in patients with Paget's disease before and after calcitonin treatment. *Radiology* 125:761, 1977.
367. Khairi MRA, Wellman HN, Robb JA, Johnston CC Jr: Paget's disease of bone (osteitis deformans): Symptomatic lesions and bone scan. *Ann Intern Med* 79:348, 1973.
368. Waxman AD, McKee D, Siemsen JK, Singer FR: Gallium scanning in Paget's disease of bone: The effects of calcitonin. *AJR* 134:303, 1980.
369. Nagant de Deuxchaisnes C, Krane SM: Paget's disease of bone: Clinical and metabolic observations. *Medicine (Baltimore)* 43:233, 1964.
370. Posen S, Clifton-Bligh P, Wilkinson M: Paget's disease of bone and hyperparathyroidism: Coincidence or causal relationship? *Calcif Tissue Res* 26:107, 1978.

371. Singer FR: *Paget's Disease of Bone*. New York, Plenum, 1977.
372. Rebel A, Malkani K, Baslé M, Bregeon C: Osteoclast ultrastructure in Paget's disease. *Calcif Tissue Res* 20:187, 1976.
373. Mills BG, Singer FR: Nuclear inclusions in Paget's disease of bone. *Science* 194:201, 1976.
374. Mills BG, Yabe H, Singer FR: Osteoclasts in human osteopetrosis contain viral-nucleocapsid-like nuclear inclusions. *J Bone Mineral Res* 3:101, 1988.
375. Singer FR: Paget's disease of bone: A slow virus infection? *Calcif Tissue Int* 31:185, 1980.
376. Rebel A, Baslé M, Pouplard A, Kouyoumdjian S, Filon R, Lepatezour A: Viral antigens in osteoclasts from Paget's disease of bone. *Lancet* 2:344, 1980.
377. Mills BG, Singer FR, Weiner LP, Suffin SC, Stabile E, Holst P: Evidence for both respiratory syncytial virus and measles virus antigens in the osteoclasts of patients with Paget's disease of bone. *Clin Orthop* 183:303, 1984.
378. Baslé MF, Fournier JG, Rozenblatt S, Rebel A, Bouteille M: Measles virus RNA detected in Paget's disease bone tissue by in situ hybridization. *J Gen Virol* 67:907, 1986.
379. Gordon MT, Anderson DC, Sharpe PT: Canine distemper virus localized in bone cells of patients with Paget's disease of bone. *Bone* 12:195, 1991.
380. Ralston SH, di Giovine FS, Gallacher SJ, Boyle IT, Duff GW: Failure to detect paramyxovirus sequences in Paget's disease of bone using polymerase chain reaction. *J Bone Mineral Res* 6:1243, 1991.
381. Singer FR, Melvin KEW, Mills BG: Acute effects of calcitonin on osteoclasts in man. *Clin Endocrnol (Oxf)* 5:333s, 1976.
382. Singer FR, Fredericks RS, Minkin C: Salmon calcitonin therapy for Paget's disease of bone: The problem of acquired clinical resistance. *Arthritis Rheum* 23:1148, 1980.
383. Avramides A, Flores A, DeRose J, Wallach S: Paget's disease of bone: Observations after cessation of long-term synthetic salmon calcitonin treatment. *J Clin Endocrinol Metab* 42:459, 1976.
384. Nagant de Deuxchaisnes C, Rombouts-Lindemans C, Huaux JP, Devogelaer JP, Malghem J, Maldague B: The action of the main therapeutic regimes of Paget's disease of bone, with a note on the effect of vitamin D deficiency. *Arthritis Rheum* 23:1215, 1980.
385. Fleisch H: Bisphosphonates: Mechanisms of action and clinical applications, in Peck WA (ed): *Bone and Mineral Research Annual I*. Amsterdam, Elsevier, 1983, p 319.
386. Khairi MRA, Altman RD, DeRosa GP, Zimmerman J, Schenk RK, Johnston CC: Sodium etidronate in the treatment of Paget's disease of bone: A study of long-term results. *Ann Intern Med* 87:656, 1977.
387. Canfield R, Rosner W, Skinner J, McWhorter J, Resnick L, Feldman F, Kammerman S, Ryan K, et al: Diphosphonate therapy of Paget's disease of bone. *J Clin Endocrinol Metab* 44:96, 1977.
388. Kanis JA, McCloskey EV, O'Doherty D, Hamdy NAT, Bickerstaff D, Beneton M, Thavarajah M: Treatment of Paget's disease with the new bisphosphonates, in Singer R, Wallach S (eds): *Paget's Disease of Bone: Clinical Assessment, Present and Future Therapy*. New York, Elsevier, 1991, p 112.
389. Ryan WG, Schwartz TB, Northrop G: Experiences in the treatment of Paget's disease of bone with mithramycin. *JAMA* 213:1153, 1970.
390. Lebbin D, Ryan WG, Schwartz TB: Outpatient treatment of Paget's disease of bone with mithramycin. *Ann Intern Med* 81:635, 1974.
391. Evans RA, Dunstan CR, Wong SYP, Hills E: Long-term experience with a calcium-thiazide treatment for Paget's disease of bone. *Mineral Electrolyte Metab* 8:325, 1982.
392. Matkovic V, Apseloff G, Shepard DR, Gerber N: Use of gallium to treat Paget's disease of bone: A pilot study. *Lancet* 335:72, 1990.
393. Meyers M, Singer FR: Osteotomy for tibia vara in Paget's disease under cover of calcitonin. *J Bone Joint Surg [Am]* 60A:810, 1978.

CHAPTER 25

Nephrolithiasis

Bruce Ettinger

Karl L. Insogna

INTRODUCTION

Epidemiology

About 10 to 12 percent of men and 3 to 5 percent of women in the United States have *urolithiasis* during their lifetimes.[1] The incidence in men is about 1.3 in 1000 yearly and is apparently increasing.[1] Stones are the cause of 1 in every 1000 hospital admissions in the United States, or about 200,000 admissions yearly. Patients with calcium stone disease or magnesium ammonium phosphate (struvite) stones typically show clinical evidence of disease during midlife, whereas patients with uric acid stones tend to be older and patients with cystine stones tend to be younger (Fig. 25-1).

Classification of Calculi by Clinical Presentation

The term *nephrolithiasis* refers specifically to stones which form in the renal pelvis or calices. Such stones, which represent 90 to 95 percent of the urinary tract calculi encountered in industrialized countries, are responsible for the ureteral colic with which stone disease is associated. Stones in the upper tract that grow or coalesce to mold the collecting system of the kidney are aptly termed *staghorn calculi*. Staghorn stones usually result from infection and are most often composed of struvite, or magnesium ammonium phosphate (MAP), but are occasionally composed of uric acid or cystine. In cases of extreme supersaturation, copious amorphous, semisolid precipitates may be formed by uric acid, cystine, or calcium phosphate crystals; these precipitates produce bilateral intrarenal or extrarenal obstruction, either of which may cause acute renal failure.

Nephrocalcinosis, or calcification within the renal parenchyma, is an uncommon radiologic finding and is usually bilateral, affecting the medullary or corticomedullary areas of the kidneys. *Cortical* nephrocalcinosis (e.g., in acute cortical necrosis of chronic glomerulonephritis) is rare. *Medullary* nephrocalcinosis is often due to dystrophic calcification related to local tissue injury; examples are renal tuberculosis, infarction, mercury poisoning, and tumor. Nephrocalcinosis and nephrolithiasis coexist in only a few conditions, including medullary sponge kidney, renal tubular acidosis (RTA), primary hyperparathyroidism, and other hypercalcemic conditions. Nephrocalcinosis in a patient with nephrolithiasis strongly suggests one of these conditions.

Bladder stones, which account for ≤5 percent of urinary tract stones in the United States, occur principally in elderly men with prostatic obstruction. About 60 percent of bladder stones are composed of calcium salts, 40 percent of struvite, and <10 percent of uric acid. In a few rare cases these patients also have nephrolithiasis. Bladder stones are endemic among children in southern Asia, southern Europe, and the Middle East. These stones are composed predominantly of ammonium acid urate admixed with various proportions of calcium oxalate, a stone composition almost never found in industrialized nations. Although the pathogenesis of endemic bladder stones is unknown, diet apparently plays a major role: Such stones are sometimes referred to as *malnutrition stones*. The same stones were common in young boys in the western world a century ago but became rare after industrialization.[2]

Classification of Calculi by Crystalline Structure

Stones are classified into five major types on the basis of their crystalline components. The term *mixed* is used when the second largest crystalline component contributes >15 percent to stone mass. Based on the results from three large stone analysis centers, the data in Table 25-1 give the relative frequencies of the five stone types.[3–5] Almost all the stones reported in these three series were composed of calcium oxalate; the other principal stone types occur rarely.

Crystallographic analysis of urinary calculi is a key diagnostic step. Classification by crystallographic type (1) provides information about stone

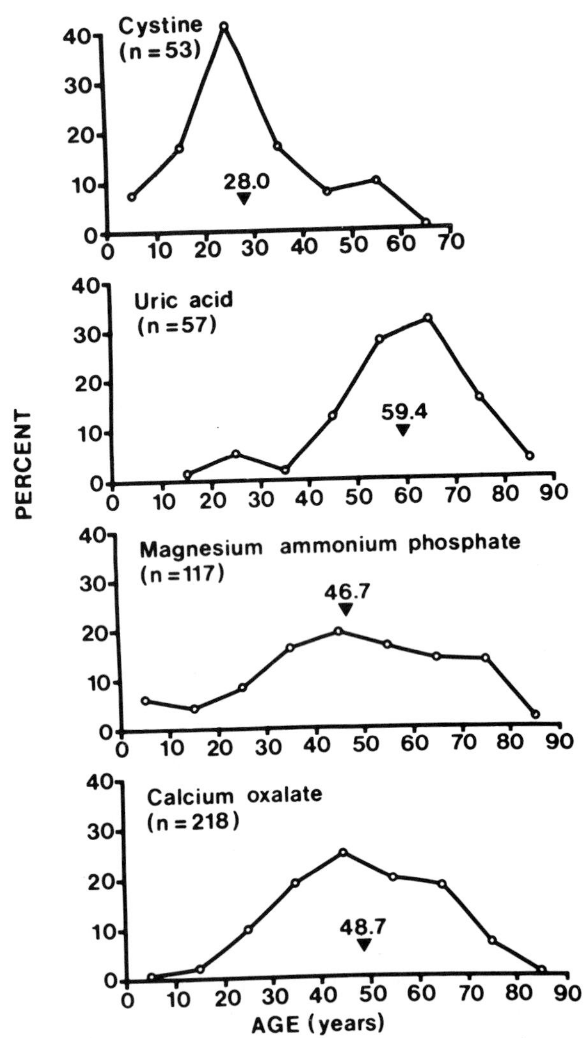

FIGURE 25-1 Age distribution of four major types of renal calculi; mean age of onset shown by arrow. [*Reproduced by permission of the author, editor, and publisher from Hodgkinson A, Nordin BEC: Prevention of urolithiasis, in Coggins CH, Cummings NB (eds): Prevention of Kidney and Urinary Tract Diseases. Washington D.C., U.S. Government Printing Office, 1978, p 198.*]

pathogenesis, (2) provides the diagnosis in some cases, and (3) defines general or specific approaches (or both) to medical or surgical therapy. Stone analysis is diagnostically useful when it reveals one of the less common stone types, in which case analysis either makes the diagnosis obvious (struvite and cystine stones) or limits diagnostic considerations to a few associated conditions (e.g., calcium phosphate and uric acid stones). Stone analysis may directly affect the choice of treatment. For example, a calculus composed of a uric acid nucleus surrounded by calcium oxalate crystals indicates a different mechanism and mandates different therapy than would be the case if the components were reversed. Because calculi of different crystalline structures respond differently to shock-wave lithotripsy, knowledge of stone analysis may facilitate the determination of specific therapy.

Quantitating Clinical Stone Events

Numerous terms and concepts have been introduced in an attempt to clarify and standardize the assessment of the morbidity of stone disease. The Mayo Clinic group[6] uses the term *metabolic activity* to define clinical or radiographic evidence (or both) of new stone formation or stone growth; a patient who shows no such evidence during a 12-month period is considered to have metabolically inactive stone disease. Similarly, the term *surgical activity* describes urologic surgical intervention as a function of time. Coe and associates[2,7] described five interrelated characteristics of stone disease which together define stone morbidity: (1) stone "burden," or the number of stones seen on x-ray films, (2) the rate of formation of new stones, (3) the rate of growth of existing stones, (4) the number and extent of clinical events (infections, surgical procedures, and hospitalizations), and (5) the extent of renal damage caused by stones.

Theories of Stone Pathogenesis

Three theories have been proposed for stone pathogenesis: the matrix theory, the inhibitor theory, and the crystalloid theory. Each has been modified since it was first proposed, and each has current proponents; none of these theories, however, is exclusive of the others.

The *matrix theory* holds that the organic matrix in all stones is critical to stone formation. The process is considered analogous to mineralization of the *osteoid*, the organized organic matrix of bone. Matrix proteins (mostly mucoproteins) in urine and stone material were studied most extensively by Boyce.[8] Critics of this theory note that the matrix substance is similar or identical in stones of all crystalline types as well as in concretions artificially precipitated from urine, suggesting that the material is trapped as an "innocent bystander" instead of causing stone formation. The authors of a recent comprehensive review of urinary stone matrix commented on the paucity of new research in this area.[9]

The *inhibitor theory* maintains that stone formation results from a deficiency of urinary substances which normally inhibit crystallization and crystal growth or aggregation. This theory became attractive more than three decades ago, when Thomas and Howard[10] found that urine from stone patients readily calcified rachitic rat cartilage, whereas urine from normal subjects did not. The authors introduced the terms *good urine* and *evil urine*, attributing their findings to the relative absence of inhibitor substances in evil urine which were first identified

TABLE 25-1 Approximate Prevalence Rates of Five Major Stone Types Reported by Four Large Stone Analysis Centers

	Investigator			
	Prien[3]	Herring[4]	Smith[5]	Mandel*
Total no. stones	24,000	10,000	4,525	28,900
Stone type				
Calcium oxalate	80–84†	72	70	60
Calcium phosphate	1–2	2	9	13
MAP-struvite	6–9	16	9	11
Uric acid	6–10	7	10	13
Cystine	1–2	0.9	0.7	0.6

Note: In cases of mixed composition, the predominant crystal form is reported.

* Personal communication, Gretchen S. Mandel, Ph.D., September 1991.

† Ranges of annual prevalence data during the years 1952–1961.

as low-molecular-weight peptides. The alternative view—that evil urine might be more supersaturated by mineralizing substances—was not critically tested. Other natural inhibitors of crystallization and crystal growth—including pyrophosphate, citrate, magnesium, and other poorly defined substances—have been implicated by various investigators.[2,7,11] Such substances may be more important in preventing crystals from growing and aggregating into clinically significant stone masses than in preventing crystallization. The essential issue, however, is not whether inhibitor substances are present in human urine but whether a deficiency of one or more of these substances contributes to stone pathogenesis.

The *crystalloid* (or precipitation-crystallization) *theory* considers stone formation in strictly physical chemical terms. This theory relates crystallization and the growth of calculi in urine to supersaturation by stone-forming constituents. Of the three classic theories of stone pathogenesis, this theory has the most experimental support and also provides a conceptual framework on which a clinical approach to stone disease can be based.

Physical Chemical Aspects of Stone Formation

Figure 25-2 shows the relative zones and ranges of saturation of the five major stone-forming constituents in normal urine. The three zones of saturation—undersaturated, metastably supersaturated, and oversaturated—are segregated by two limits: the solubility product and the formation product. These terms may be better understood by using several examples. If excess solid material such as calcium oxalate is added to distilled water and left to dissolve for a prolonged period, the solution and the remaining solid phase eventually reach a stable equilibrium. This equilibrium defines the solubility of the material in aqueous solution; to determine the *solubility product*, the concentration of calcium is multi-

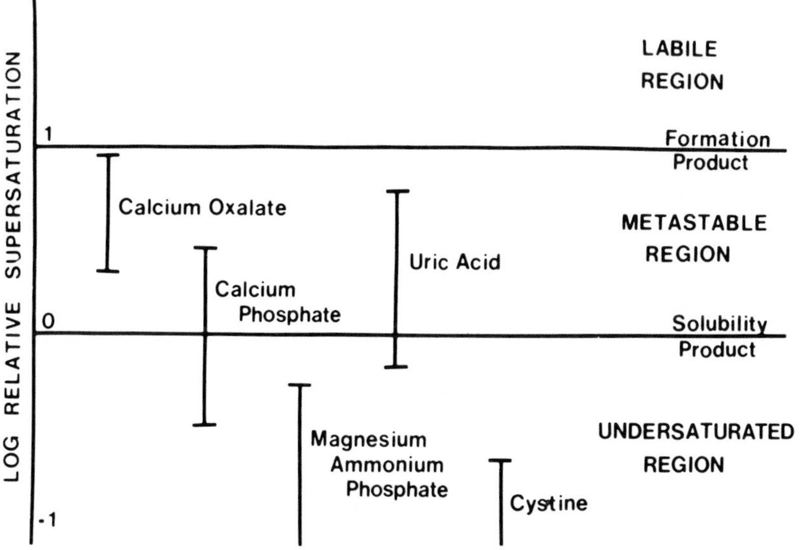

FIGURE 25-2 Three zones of saturation in urine: undersaturation, metastable, saturation, and oversaturation (labile region). Ranges of saturation of five major crystalline stone constituents in normal urine are shown. [*Adapted and reproduced by permission of the author, editor, and publisher from Hodgkinson A, Nordin BEC; Prevention of urolithiasis, in Coggins CH, Cummings NB (eds): Prevention of Kidney and Urinary Tract Diseases. Washington D.C., U.S. Government Printing Office, 1978, p 203.*]

plied by oxalate ions in solution. The solid material is then removed, leaving a saturated solution of calcium oxalate with no solid phase. If a concentrated calcium or oxalate solution is added to the saturated solution, it remains clear and free of solid phase to a critical concentration: the *formation product*. The solution then clouds as solid calcium oxalate crystals form and begin to grow. The zone between the solubility product and the formation product defines a metastable, saturated solution in which spontaneous precipitation does not occur (the metastably supersaturated zone shown in Fig. 25-2). A metastable solution can lead to crystallization and support crystal growth. At and above the formation product, spontaneous nucleation inevitably occurs (the labile, or oversaturated, zone shown in Fig. 25-2). A supersaturated solution produces both spontaneous nucleation and crystal growth.

The term *nucleation* (instead of *precipitation*) is used to define the initiation of a crystalline solid phase in aqueous solution. Crystal nuclei contain only about 100 atoms and are of no clinical consequence; enlargement of these nascent particles into a solid phase of substantial mass produces clinical consequences. Although related, crystal nucleation and crystal growth must be considered separately. Urinary calculi occur through the combined processes of homogeneous crystal growth, epitaxial crystal growth, and crystal aggregation. The first two processes require that crystals be laid on a lattice structure: Homogeneous crystallization occurs when crystals are laid on the surface of an identical crystal lattice; epitaxial crystallization occurs when a crystal lattice provides an acceptable fit for the crystalline and atomic structure of added nonidentical crystals. Aggregation, or agglomeration, depends on crystals adhering to each other to form large clusters. The binding forces that bring about aggregation may be promoted or inhibited by substances which affect neither nucleation nor other processes of crystal growth.

The crystalloid theory can readily explain the four "minor" types of stones: cystine, uric acid, struvite, and pure calcium phosphate. Each stone type can be understood in relatively straightforward terms of supersaturation with respect to the ionic constituents of urine. In contrast, understanding calcium oxalate stone disease in terms of crystalloid theory is complicated by the interaction of numerous other ions that can alter the solubility of calcium oxalate (see Calcium Oxalate and Mixed Calcium Stones, below).

Evaluation and Treatment

The Role of the Internist

The internist is usually expected to identify, interpret, and treat metabolic abnormalities that lead to stone formation. Patients referred for medical management often have had multiple stone events or surgical procedures. The finding of an unusual stone type (e.g., cystine) sometimes prompts a referral. The internist is rarely asked to help make decisions involving urologic surgery. However, anyone providing medical care to patients with nephrolithiasis should be aware of the latest advances in the urologic management of this disease.

Clinical Presentation

The principal clinical consequences of renal stones are pain, hematuria, obstruction, and infection. Impaired renal function is not a natural or predictable outcome of stone disease but results from stone-related complications such as chronic obstruction, infection, postoperative scarring, and surgical removal of renal tissue.

Ureteral colic produces pain of incredible intensity. The term *colic* is a misnomer because the pain typically begins as a vague discomfort and increases gradually, reaching maximum intensity about an hour after onset and rendering the patient incapable of lying down or sitting still. Obstruction of the ureteropelvic junction produces pain in the flank and is often associated with nausea and vomiting. A stone too large to negotiate the ureteropelvic junction may produce intermittent obstruction in a ball-valve fashion. Obstruction lower in the ureter causes pain that radiates from the flank toward the anterior pelvis. Obstruction of the ureterovesical junction produces pain that radiates to the ipsilateral testicle or labium; stones in this region that have passed into the bladder often cause urgency and dysuria, symptoms that mimic cystitis. Staghorn stones or other stones that remain adherent to the renal papillae usually do not produce symptoms, although microscopic or gross hematuria often occurs. Few of these patients experience nagging, chronic flank discomfort.

Surgical Management of Nephrolithiasis

In the past 20 years, considerable improvements have been made in basic kidney surgery; new techniques include anatrophic nephrolithotomy and coagulum pyelolithotomy. However, urologic treatment of stones has been revolutionized by two less invasive techniques: percutaneous nephrolithotomy and lithotripsy. *Lithotripsy*, or stone smashing, is now routinely accomplished through percutaneous nephrostomy or by focusing high-energy waves produced by external devices [extracorporeal shock-wave lithotripsy (ESWL)]. Estimates indicate that percutaneous lithotripsy is associated with one-tenth of the morbidity of surgical nephrolithotomy and that ESWL is associated with one-tenth the morbidity of percutaneous lithotripsy.[12]

Although the urologist chooses the stone removal procedure, the internist should have a basic knowledge of shock-wave principles, the effects of shock waves in tissue and animal studies, and the clinical results obtained with ESWL therapy. Overall, ESWL is 80 percent successful in completely eliminating stones; its effectiveness in eliminating large stones (2.5 to 3.0 cm), however, is <50 percent, particularly for stones in the lower renal calices. In such cases, urologists thus use percutaneous lithotripsy as the initial treatment. For patients in whom stone material is still evident after percutaneous lithotripsy or ESWL, the usual practice now is to give ESWL immediately. Complete elimination of stones is imperative to reduce the likelihood of stone recurrence.

The immediate complications of ESWL include severe pain (sometimes requiring hospitalization), hematuria, perinephric hematoma, obstruction by large stone fragments or by minute stone fragments filling the ureter (*steinstrasse*), and rarely hemorrhage or septicemia. About 5 to 10 percent of patients receiving ESWL must be hospitalized as a result of these complications. ESWL traumatizes the kidney in a way analogous to the pounding it might receive in a boxing match. Subcapsular and intrarenal hematomas as well as less dramatic signs of renal injury occur in most patients who receive ESWL.[13] The long-term effects of such injury are not known, but early reports of elevated blood pressure after ESWL were confirmed in a large series of patients.[14] The incidence of hypertension ranges from <1 to 9 percent, but follow-up has been too short to provide a basis for an estimate of the long-term effects of ESWL on blood pressure or renal function.

Much still must be learned about the biological effects of ESWL. The efficacy and safety of ESWL depend largely on the way in which the shock-wave energy is generated (spark-gap, piezoelectric crystals, lasers, ultrasound), wave power (total number and kilovoltage of shocks delivered), and the amount of energy transferred to the stone and surrounding tissue. ESWL technology in clinical use today is much different from that used 10 years ago because of new devices which have numerous advantages: No anesthesia is required, the patient need not be immersed in a water bath, and improved methods of delivering the energy to the stone reduce renal trauma.[15]

Medical Management of Nephrolithiasis

The medical management of patients with stone disease can be subdivided into several phases. In phase I, risk factors that predispose to stone formation are identified. This evaluation includes careful radiologic identification of the number, location, and size of preexisting stones. In phase II, therapy is begun and elimination or amelioration of the risk factors associated with stone formation is documented. The end result of this phase is the choice of a final regimen for long-term treatment. For some patients, this regimen includes only increased fluid intake and restricted dietary intake; for others, it also includes an agent chosen to reduce excretion or enhance the solubility of a stone-forming constituent. In phase III, the results of long-term treatment are monitored. For patients with preexisting stones, clinical stone events must be differentiated in terms of old vs. new stones; this differentiation requires radiologic assessment either after each symptomatic stone event or, if no symptoms have occurred, yearly. In phase IV, all or part of a therapeutic regimen is discontinued in a patient determined to no longer need it.

Evaluation: Phase I

In working with patients, internists should clarify from the outset that their role in care differs from the role of urologists and that patients should maintain continuity of care with the referring urologist. Patients should be made aware that they are important participants in their own care. Empiric therapy should be discontinued several weeks before analytic screening. Collapsible 24-h urine collection containers and instructions for urine collection may be mailed to patients so that they can bring to the first visit an initial urine specimen collected while they were on a customary (or so-called free or usual) diet. The history and physical examination should be complete; particular care should be given to history of stone events, family history of stones, medications, and diet. The number, composition, and location of stones as well as the outcome of stone events (e.g., stones passed, nephrolithotomy) should be chronologically recorded to serve as the basis for determining stone morbidity. A brief diet history, focusing particularly on the consumption of animal protein, dairy products, and salt, should be obtained; a detailed, quantitative diet history is not essential.

When stones are radiopaque, their number, size, and location should be documented on plain x-ray films. Plain film preceding a previous intravenous pyelogram (IVP) is usually unacceptable; most are not done with the care necessary to delineate clearly the number, size, and location of existing stones and are thus a notorious source of misinformation. Patients should be prepared with diet instruction and laxatives as for an IVP, and a coned-down view of the kidneys should be obtained instead of a kidney, ureter, and bladder (KUB) view. Because it includes the lower pelvis, the KUB view usually does not show the upper poles of the kidneys clearly. We prefer to use the balloon device originally designed to apply ureteral compression during an IVP. Placing the balloon device over the upper abdomen and inflating it (Fig. 25-3) moves intestinal gas as well as gastric and colonic contents away from the kidneys, improving the diagnostic quality of the x-ray films. The IVP should have no role in defining stone burden, response to therapy, or both; serial IVPs are a commonly misused approach to monitoring stone disease

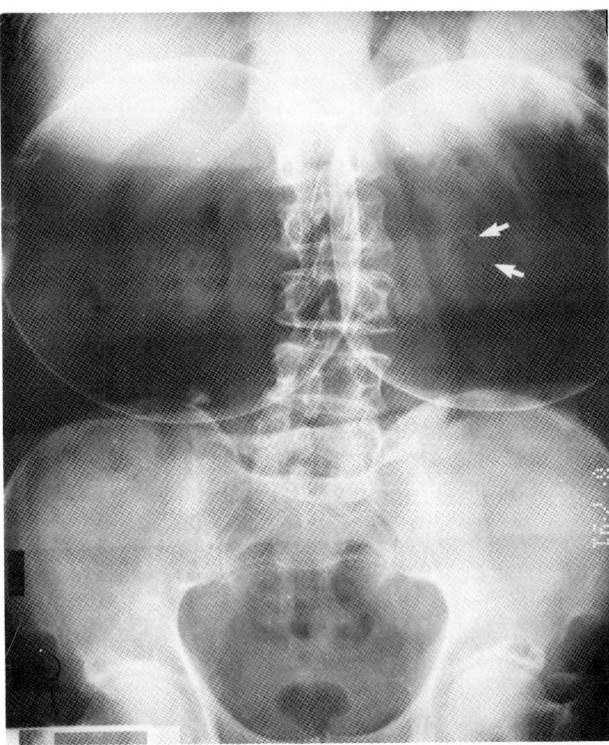

FIGURE 25-3 X-ray film showing coned-down view of kidneys done using a balloon device to enhance imaging of renal calculi.

and expose the patient to an unacceptable dose of radiation.

Ultrasonography should be used to image calculi that are nonopaque. Although ultrasound can also be used for imaging opaque stones, we do not recommend its routine use for this purpose because ultrasound is expensive, is less sensitive, and does not define stone size as well as x-ray films do. All calculi produce a similar ultrasound picture: an echogenic focus with posterior acoustic shadowing. Ultrasound easily distinguishes nonopaque stones, such as those composed of uric acid, from masses such as tumor or blood clot. In a group of 64 patients evaluated after lithotripsy for residual stone fragments, both abdominal x-ray films and sonography showed stones in 53 percent, sonography alone was positive in 16 percent, and x-ray films alone were positive in 31 percent.[16]

Computed tomography (CT) is also an excellent method for imaging nonopaque renal calculi. All calculi appear as bright objects on CT. Some researchers have suggested that the CT number can be used to distinguish stone composition, but technical problems such as partial volume effects make this distinction impractical. The current clinical practice in diagnosing nonopaque calculi is to use ultrasound first and reserve CT for selected patients. CT has the advantage of being more reproducible and less operator-dependent; moreover, if contrast material is used, CT can more accurately define renal collecting structures and obstruction. The disadvantages of CT include higher cost and radiation exposure.

The results of previous stone analyses should be examined, and a recent stone, if available, should be sent to a reference laboratory for crystallographic analysis; simple chemical stone analysis is inadequate. An initial fasting serum autochemistry panel should include calcium, phosphorus, bicarbonate, chloride, creatinine, uric acid, and albumin concentrations. If a stone is unobtainable for analysis, a spot urine sample should be screened for cystine (see Cystinuria, Laboratory Evaluation, below). A 24-h urine specimen collected while the patient is on a free diet should be analyzed for creatinine, sodium, calcium, oxalate, uric acid, and citrate. Urine volume should be noted. Excretion of creatinine serves as an index of completeness of the collection. We recommend that no preservative be added to the 24-h urine container; instead, the aliquot used for measuring calcium, oxalate, and cystine is acidified with 6 *N* hydrochloric acid, and the remainder of the sample is frozen until analyzed.

A clean-voided spot fasting urine sample should be obtained for culture and pH determination by nitrazine paper or pH meter. If cystinuria is suspected or if stone analysis is unavailable, a nitroprusside test for cystine should be done on this specimen; cystine crystals can be seen if the specimen is acidified by adding a few drops of glacial acetic acid and is then cooled.

If the initial urinary pH is extreme (<6.0 or >7.0), serum electrolyte concentrations should be repeated and the patient should be given a roll of nitrazine paper to record variations in urinary pH for several days by making pH measurements upon arising and after meals; such measurements should show normal pH variability. If uric acid stone disease is suspected, serial monitoring of urinary pH is indicated to search for the low, relatively fixed pH seen in many such patients.

When making biochemical determinations for patients with urolithiasis, remember this admonition:

> In stone disease, everything is measurement. What the laboratory cannot tell you, you will not know; what it tells you in error, you will not correct by using your instincts, your medical experience, or your art; what you take from the measurements directs your treatments. When measurements vary, repeat them. If they seem ambiguous, repeat them. If you suspect an error . . . measure again. No expense is as unreasonable as years of misdirected treatment, as great as the cost of treating the urologic consequences of preventable stones.[17]

Evaluation of the Patient with a Single Stone Event
It is universally agreed that patients in whom even one cystine, uric acid, calcium phosphate, or magne-

sium ammonium phosphate stone has formed should be considered as having a chronic disease that requires extensive evaluation and aggressive medical management. For patients who have a single calcium oxalate stone, no clear-cut and accepted rules exist to guide the extent of evaluation or treatment. Some researchers view the first calcium oxalate stone as an indication for extensive evaluation and suggest that treatment for any risk factors identified during the evaluation will be cost-effective. They argue that risk factors are found as frequently in patients with a single stone as in patients with recurrent stone disease and believe that patients with one stone are simply at the beginning of a chronic process.[18,19] In contrast, some researchers quote reports of relatively low recurrence rates, low morbidity, and relatively low success rates for medical treatments[20] and thus advise minimal evaluation. This issue is difficult to resolve because of a lack of both strong epidemiologic data and rigorously designed clinical trials in such patients (see Calcium Oxalate and Mixed Calcium Stones, below).

The authors recommend that minimal evaluation include coned-down x-ray films of the kidneys to detect additional "silent" stones, crystallographic stone analysis, and chemical screening, including a serum autochemistry panel, determination of urinary pH, and collection of a 24-h urine specimen on a free diet. Urinary chemical analysis should include total volume, calcium, uric acid, oxalate, and citrate. When ordered together as a panel, the entire chemistry evaluation costs about $200 at most commercial laboratories.

Extensive Metabolic Evaluations Within the biomedical literature, opinion varies widely about which tests are needed, particularly in evaluating calcium oxalate lithiasis, in which the extremes are a simple serum biochemical panel and a 3-day hospital stay for extensive measurement of serum and urinary response to manipulation of diet and calcium intake.

A tiered approach may be the most appropriate. Almost all experts favor simple, empiric, and nonselective therapy for calcium oxalate lithiasis. Decisions about initial clinical management can be made without an extensive metabolic evaluation. For patients in whom stone disease remains active after treatment, more extensive studies can be done to help guide further management.

Therapy: Phase II

The therapeutic program usually consists of forced hydration, dietary moderation, and drug therapy.

Forced Hydration Water, as a universal solvent, should be the mainstay of therapy for all types of nephrolithiasis. The desirable daily urine output is 2 liters, for which a daily intake of 3 liters of fluid is necessary, provided that fluid loss via the skin or gastrointestinal tract is not accelerated. Most clinical trials of stone disease indicate that patients do not fully comply with high fluid intake; the observed mean daily increase in volume is only 300 to 500 ml.

A definite plan of forced fluids should be designed. Patients should drink a glass of water at bedtime, refill the glass, and keep it near the lavatory. Patients who follow this regimen will invariably awaken early in the morning and can then drink the waiting glass of water; they should drink another glass of water immediately upon arising. When setting a goal for daily urine volume, physicians should emphasize nocturnal hydration.

Restriction of Animal Protein in the Diet All patients with nephrolithiasis should be advised to moderate their intake of animal protein. The average American man consumes 108 g of protein daily, 54 percent more than the Recommended Daily Allowance (RDA); about half this protein intake comes from animal flesh. Reducing the intake of animal protein may help reduce the excretion of cystine, uric acid, calcium, oxalate, and phosphorus. A reduced intake of animal protein can also reduce the load of nonvolatile (fixed) acid, limiting excessive urinary acidity.

Because many patients are unable or unwilling to change their lifelong practice of eating meat, a rigid diet is often impractical and unacceptable. Table 25-2 shows a sample diet which provides 97 g of total protein but limits protein from animal flesh to 35 g; additional protein must come from cereals, vegetables, and legumes. Because severe restriction of dairy products does not prevent recurrence of calculi[21] and because dairy products are a good source of protein, two low-fat dairy portions are allowed. This diet conforms with cholesterol-lowering guidelines which recommend that fat contribute no more than 30 percent to total caloric intake.

Reduced Sodium Intake High sodium intake increases cystine excretion in patients with cystinuria[22] and may cause hypercalciuria or augment the hypercalciuria caused by other mechanisms.[23] High sodium excretion reduces urinary citrate, a substance important in solubilizing calcium and inhibiting calcium oxalate crystal agglomeration.[23] The adverse effects of a high intake of salt and animal protein are apparently additive.[23] Salt intake can be reasonably moderated by avoiding obviously salty foods and by not salting food at the table. Salt may be used lightly in cooking. By following these simple suggestions, patients can conveniently reduce their daily salt intake to the range of 4 to 5 g, reducing daily sodium excretion to $<$100 mEq.

What Can Be Expected from Medical Treatment? Most medical treatments for nephrolithiasis have

TABLE 25-2 Mean U.S. Dietary Protein Intake vs. Reduced Animal Protein Diet Prescribed for Patients with Kidney Stones (grams)

	Sources of Protein					
	Red Meat, Fish, Poultry	Cereal Products	Dairy Products	Egg Products	Other Protein	Total Protein
U.S. diet	52 (7.5 oz)	22	18	4	12	108
Stone diet	35 (5.0 oz)	26	15	4	18	97

Both diets are calculated to provide 2400 kcal/day, sufficient for a moderately active 80-kg man. The following food allocations are offered as an illustration. This diet provides 16 percent of calories in the form of protein and 30 percent in the form of fat.

Meat	5 oz
Cheese	1 slice
Milk	1 cup
Egg	Half
Bread	6 slices
Cereal	1½ cups
Starches	2½ cups
Beans	½ cup
Vegetables	3 servings
Fruit	5 servings
Fat	6 tsp

been accepted without definitive and critical experimental studies. When evaluating a clinical trial, the reader should look for the following design criteria: (1) adequate number of treated subjects and controls (a minimum of 20 receiving active treatment), (2) adequate characterization of subjects, including pretreatment stone rate, stone burden, and metabolic profile, (3) adequate follow-up (a minimum of 2 years and preferably 3 years), and (4) objectively measured and impartially determined end points, including the growth of preexisting stones, the appearance of new stones on x-ray films, and the passage of new stones.

Referral bias may complicate the evaluation of clinical trial results. Many patients seek care and are thus entered into treatment programs soon after one stone event or a cluster of events. Such early treatment, however, creates a substantial bias toward the apparent efficacy of treatment, given that stone events are usually plotted before and after therapy is initiated (i.e., stones per patient-year). This bias, statistically termed *regression to the mean*, is a problem particularly when follow-up is short.

Cointervention may also obscure the meaning of clinical trials. Patients typically begin a program of fluids, dietary control, and a therapeutic agent simultaneously, but the drug is usually credited with reducing stone events and often with reducing biochemical abnormalities.[24]

Careful, regular radiologic assessment of stone burden and the differentiation of new and old stones are critical in determining the efficacy of therapy. Greater credence should be given to reports of clinical trials in which regular radiologic follow-up is part of the outcome assessment.

What criteria can be used to determine the adequacy and scientific validity of such trials? Certainly, a trial showing nearly total stone prevention in 30 patients with recurrent stones during a 3-year period cannot be disputed even if a double-blind randomized design was not employed. In this hypothetical trial, about 11 failures would be predicted if treatment were ineffective. However, few therapies yield such convincing results. In clinical trials of patients with calcium oxalate stones, mean recurrence rates among placebo-treated subjects are often about 10 to 15 percent yearly.[20,25] A convenient guideline is that effective treatment halves the odds of stone recurrence or reduces recurrence to 5 percent yearly.

If a treatment produces salutary changes in the urinary biochemical profile or in vitro tests of crystallization, is its efficacy sufficiently established? For nephrolithiasis caused by cystine or uric acid, urinary biochemical analysis provides reliable indicators of stone risk that may be considered surrogates for stone events. However, this is not true for calcium oxalate stones.[25]

Long-Term Follow-Up: Phase III

After the initial therapeutic period, the patient is seen at 6-month or yearly intervals, depending on preexisting activity of stone disease, presence of stones on x-ray films, and perceived need for supervision, reinforcement of the program, or both. Appropriate analyses and plain x-ray films are obtained at least yearly.

Discontinuation of Treatment: Phase IV

Patients are best advised that the first goal of therapy is to control stone formation for a few years. Assuming that this has been achieved, for which patients should drug treatment be stopped? The following risk factors contribute strongly to recurrence: previous rate of stone events, stone burden, and extreme deviation in the urinary biochemical profile. We recommend discontinuing part or all of the therapeutic program after 3 years of successful treatment if the pretreatment stone event rate was <0.5 stone yearly and if no stones are visible on x-ray films.

CYSTINURIA

Although nephrolithiasis is rarely caused by cystinuria, we describe cystinuria first because we understand its heredity and metabolic basis as well as why calculi develop and how they can be diagnosed, dissolved, and prevented.

History

Cystine stones were recognized as a distinctive stone type in 1810, and their familial occurrence was described shortly afterward.[26,27] The relation between excessive cystine excretion and cystine stones was recognized as early as 1855. However, nearly a century passed before reports of increased orthinine, lysine, and arginine excretion enabled Dent and Rose[28] to synthesize the classic transport hypothesis. They noted that each contributing amino acid had two amino or guanidine groups and suggested that these structurally related amino acids share a common resorptive mechanism, which is located in the renal tubule and is defective in patients with cystinuria.

Genetics

Cystinuria is a classic example of simple autosomal recessive inheritance. In homozygotes, cystinuria increases the excretion rates of cystine and the dibasic amino acids markedly, and the incidence of cystine stones is extremely high. Heterozygotes, however, are at almost no risk for developing cystine stones; such patients can be identified biochemically by their slightly increased excretion of cystine and the dibasic amino acids.[29] Three distinct genetic patterns can be identified by studying both intestinal transport and urinary amino acid excretion in cystinuric pedigrees. These patterns differ according to the presence or degree (or both) of abnormal transport of the four amino acids in the intestine and the presence or absence of abnormal amino acid excretion rates in heterozygotes.[26] Some apparently homozygous patients are "double heterozygotes" in that they have two different allelic mutations instead of a double mutation of a single gene. Double heterozygotes cannot be clinically distinguished from homozygotes. Homozygous cystinuria affects about 1 in 18,000 people, indicating that 1 in 60 or 70 persons is heterozygous.[26]

Pathophysiology of Cystinuria

Five group-specific amino acid transport systems have been recognized. Each system mediates the transport of a group of structurally related amino acids. The mutant genes in cystinuria code for an abnormality in intestinal and kidney transport systems specific for dibasic amino acids: cystine, ornithine, lysine, and arginine (COLA).

Cystine is not an essential amino acid. Cystinuric patients, who cannot absorb cystine, produce it endogenously from methionine. Loss of amino acids into the urine in cystinuria is not nutritionally meaningful. Children with cystinuria have normal intellectual and physical development.

Amino acids in plasma are freely filtered at the glomerulus. Normally, 97 to 99 percent of the filtered amino acid load is resorbed by specific transport systems in the proximal tubule. The system in the luminal brush border is shared by all four dibasic amino acids and is normally responsible for their nearly quantitative resorption. This system is defective in patients with cystinuria.

The entire load of filtered cystine may be spilled by patients with homozygous cystinuria. The daily cystine excretion rate in these patients is more than 400 mg (1664 μmol) and is usually in the range of 600 to 1300 mg (2497 to 5399 μmol). Because maximum cystine solubility at usual urinary pH is 300 mg/L (1248 μmol/L), the predisposition of cystinuric patients to the formation of cystine stones is self-evident.

One or more cystine stones develop in almost all patients with cystinuria; about 10 percent have no stones for unknown reasons. Cystine stones may first occur any time from infancy to the eighth decade,[28] but mean age at onset is about 20 years (Fig. 25-1). Although men and women are affected equally, morbidity is greater in men for unexplained reasons.

Dependence of Cystine Solubility on Urinary pH

Figure 25-4 shows the slope of the curve of cystine ionization and solubility as a function of pH; because the pK_a of cystine is 8.4, variations in urinary pH within the usual physiologic range (pH 5.0 to 7.0) have little influence on cystine solubility, but maximal urine alkalinization (pH 7.8 to 8.0) increases cystine solubility by a factor of 2 to 3.

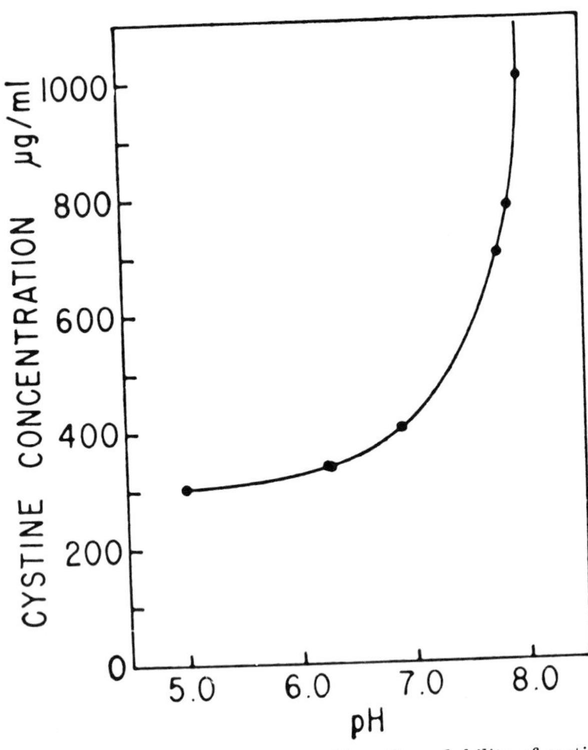

FIGURE 25-4 Effect of urinary pH on the solubility of cystine. *(Adapted and reproduced by permission of the author and publisher from Dent CE, Senior B: Studies on the treatment of cystinuria. Br J Urol 27:317–332, 1955.)*

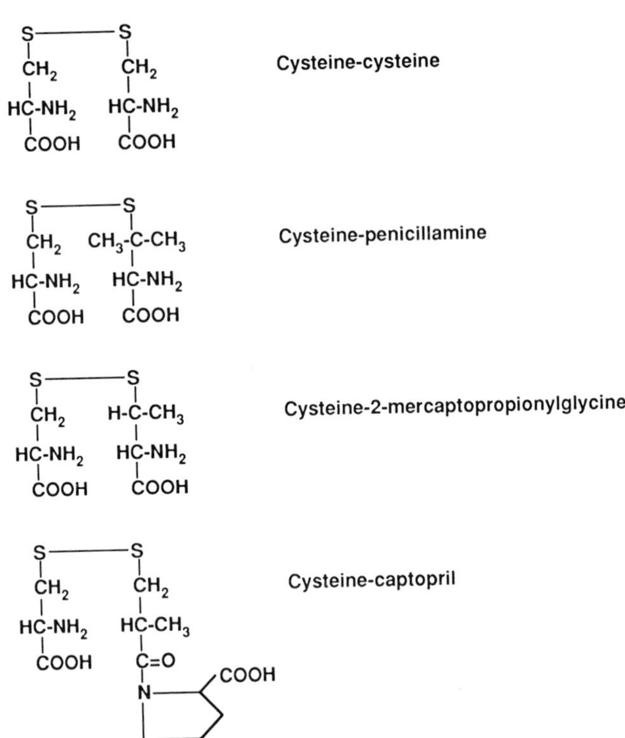

FIGURE 25-5 Chemical structures of cystine and related cysteine disulfides.

Dependence of Cystine Excretion on Salt Intake

The dependence of cystine excretion on sodium intake was recognized during a study of the effect of glutamine on cystine excretion.[30] Glutamine administration was reported to reduce cystine excretion in one patient,[31] but this result was not confirmed in other patients.[32] Jaeger and coworkers found that glutamine reduced cystine excretion only in subjects whose sodium intake was high (150 to 300 mEq/day); these investigators also showed that simply reducing salt intake can lower cystine excretion profoundly.[30] These observations were confirmed by Norman and Manette, who found that reducing the mean daily sodium intake of five cystinuric patients from 184 to 87 mEq reduced urinary cystine excretion by 46 percent.[22]

Effect of Cysteine-Complexing Agents

D-Penicillamine (β,β-dimethylcysteine) is the prototype of a group of sulfhydryl compounds used as cysteine-complexing agents. When these agents are present, cysteine combines with the complexing agent to form a mixed disulfide instead of forming a sulfhydryl linkage with another cysteine (Fig. 25-5). The cysteine-penicillamine disulfide is about 50 times more soluble than cystine. Penicillamine not only prevents cystine stones but can dissolve preexisting stones.[26,27,33]

Clinical Findings

In cystinuric patients, stones are usually multiple and bilateral. A particularly characteristic pattern is a staghorn calculus with multiple small "satellite" stones (Fig. 25-6). A few patients with cystinuria have stones of mixed composition or may alternatively have cystine stones and either calcium oxalate, pure calcium phosphate, or MAP stones.[26,33,34] This observation is explained by the occasional coincidence of cystinuria with other stone risk factors, the adverse influence of alkali treatment on calcium phosphate solubility, and chronic infection resulting from urologic instrumentation.

Extracorporeal shock-wave lithotripsy and other stone-fragmenting techniques are only marginally effective in breaking large cystine stones into particles small enough to be passed spontaneously. Further information about urologic procedures specific to cystine stones is available.[35] Renal transplantation (from a noncystinuric donor) has been successful in patients with cystinuria. This procedure "cures" cystinuria but is used only in patients with end-stage renal failure.

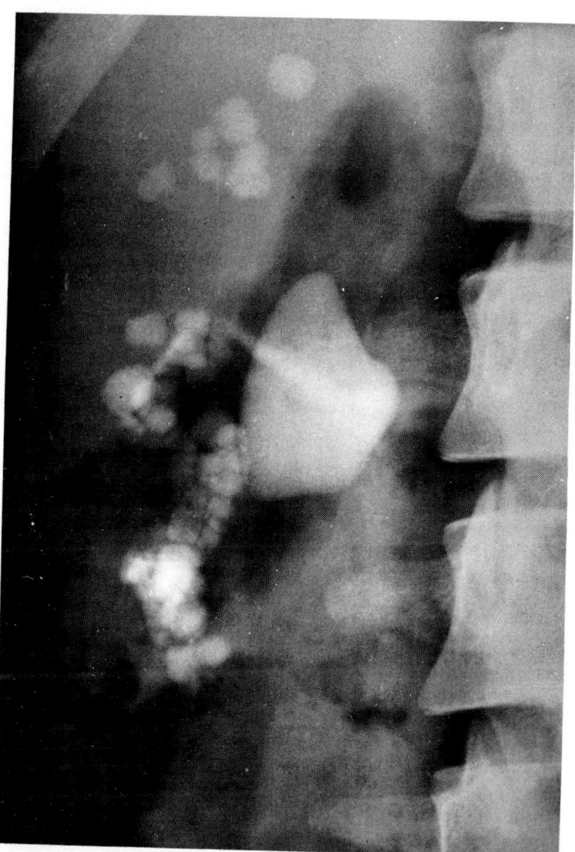

FIGURE 25-6 Multiple cystine stones assuming a characteristic pattern of a staghorn calculus and multiple satellite stones. [*Adapted and reproduced by permission of the author, editor, and publisher from Insogna KL, Broadus AE: Nephrolithiasis, in Felig P, Baxter JD, Broadus AE, Frohman LA (eds): Endocrinology and Metabolism 2d ed. New York, McGraw-Hill, 1987, p 1514.*]

Clinical Evaluation

Clinical Diagnosis

Cystinuria should be considered in any patient with recurrent renal calculi. The diagnosis is suggested by an early onset of stone disease or by a characteristic radiologic stone pattern. Because of their sulfur content, cystine stones are radiopaque, but they are less dense than calcium stones. A family history of stones is common in patients with stone disease and thus is not a useful diagnostic clue. However, cystinuria is improbable if the family history is negative.

Laboratory Evaluation

Cystinuria is diagnosed by stone analysis, demonstrated cystine crystalluria, urinary cystine screening, and (ultimately) quantitative urinary amino acid analysis. Cystine forms unmistakable flat, hexagonal ("benzene ring") crystals in urine which are best observed in cooled, concentrated specimens. The specimen should be acidified to a pH of 4 to 5 by adding a few drops of glacial acetic acid to enhance the formation of cystine crystals. A demonstration of cystine crystals is pathognomonic, but they may not be detected in a dilute, fresh urine specimen.

The cyanide-nitroprusside test is the simplest and most useful chemical screen for cystinuria. The test is based on alkaline reduction of cystine to cysteine and a colorimetric reaction of free sulfhydryl groups with nitroprusside. The test is positive (the solution turns purple) when the cystine concentration reaches 150 mg/dl (6242 μmol/L); a positive result is occasionally seen in heterozygotes and is rarely seen in dehydrated normal persons.[36] A simplified screening test takes advantage of the impregnation of ketone test strips with nitroprusside[37]; after the absence of ketones in the specimen is confirmed, two drops of 1 *M* sodium cyanide are added to six drops of urine. A ketone test strip wetted with this solution turns purple in the presence of elevated levels of urine cystine.

A positive nitroprusside test should be followed by quantitation of 24-h urinary cystine excretion. Amino acid column chromatography can quantitate each of the four related amino acids but is expensive ($250 to $300). Because only cystine excretion is clinically important, simpler and less expensive techniques are preferred. When one is monitoring the effects of penicillamine and other cysteine-complexing agents (see Treatment, below), a quantitative technique that distinguishes cystine from the mixed cysteine-penicillamine disulfide should be used. We prefer the anion-exchange–high-performance liquid chromatography method employing an abbreviated amino acid column analysis optimized for cystine; its upper limit of normal is 31 mg (130 μmol) daily. This analysis is commercially available.

Screening for Other Types of Stones

Stones formed by cystinuric patients may be composed entirely of calcium salts or may be admixtures of cystine and calcium salts. The prevalence of mixed stone diathesis was 15 percent[33] in one series and 30 percent in another.[34] Screening cystinuric patients for calcium stone risk factors (hypercalciuria, hyperuricosuria, and hypocitraturia) yields about the same prevalence of these abnormalities as would be expected in patients with calcium stones.[35]

Treatment

The treatment of cystinuria is guided by urinary cystine concentration and awareness that the maximum solubility of cystine within the physiologic pH range is 300 mg/L (1248 μmol/L). Therapeutic measures include hydration, sodium restriction, alkalinization, and cysteine-complexing drugs.

Hydration

Forced hydration is important in treating all stone disease but is the cornerstone of treatment in cystinuria. Urine volume should be sufficient to ensure a cystine concentration <250 mg/L (1040 μmol/L).

Alkalinization of the Urine

Alkali must be given in a daily dose of 60 to 100 mEq, an amount sufficient to buffer the acid production rate and produce a urinary pH of 7.5 to 8.0. This dose is given as bicarbonate or citrate salts in four divided doses; many physicians prefer citrate because it is metabolized to bicarbonate in the liver, producing alkalinization that is more prolonged and constant. Some physicians advocate a single dose of acetazolamide (350 to 500 mg) at bedtime, but we discourage this approach because the induced RTA may further increase the risk of calcium phosphate stones or cause deposition of calcium phosphate salts on preexisting cystine stones.[33] Table 25-3 lists some commonly used alkali preparations.

Dietary Advice

Daily salt intake should be restricted to <100 mEq. We thus encourage the use of alkali preparations which contain potassium instead of sodium. In addition, patients should be instructed to moderate animal protein intake to reduce the fixed acid load. Diets sufficiently restricted in methionine to substantially reduce cystine excretion are unpalatable and thus are not recommended.

Cysteine-Complexing Drugs

Penicillamine

Given in four divided doses, usually 1000 to 1500 mg daily, penicillamine reduces the excretion of cystine to the range of 300 to 400 mg (1248 to 1664 μmol) daily.[29,33,38] Alkali therapy should be maintained when one is using penicillamine to enhance the formation of the cysteine-penicillamine complex. Stone burden can be diminished or eliminated in about two-thirds of such patients within about 12 months.[33]

Penicillamine causes side effects in about half of patients.[29,33,38] The most common serious toxicity is a hypersensitivity syndrome characterized by fever and rash that typically occurs within the first few weeks of treatment. Lymphadenopathy, arthralgia, thrombocytopenia, and granulocytopenia may accompany these symptoms. In addition, long-term treatment is associated with a risk of loss of skin turgor, especially in the intertriginous areas, resulting in disfiguring cosmetic changes. Penicillamine is also associated with a rare but serious skin disease, elastosis perforans serpiginosa. Other, relatively minor side effects of long-term treatment include minor gastrointestinal distress, malodorous breath and urine, and loss of taste. Potentially serious renal toxicity has been reported in about 10 percent of cases. This toxicity is heralded by proteinuria and may progress to frank nephrotic syndrome; renal biopsy specimens show membranous glomerulonephritis. Because this side effect may occur even after many months with no apparent toxicity, patients should monitor urine protein weekly using urinary test strips. Penicillamine may antagonize the effect of vitamin B_6; pyridoxine in daily doses of 50 mg should thus be prescribed. Penicillamine should be avoided in pregnancy because of reported fetal scalp anomalies.

In some patients, side effects are clearly dose-related, resolve rapidly after penicillamine is discontinued, and may not reappear when the drug is reintroduced at a lower dose. In cases of hypersensitivity reaction, desensitization is readily accomplished; once the reaction has subsided, the drug is started again at a daily dose of 125 mg, which is increased gradually over a few weeks. We give a glucocorticoid when a penicillamine rash first occurs and continue the glucocorticoid, at a low dose, during the period of drug desensitization.

Because of its toxicity and cost, penicillamine should be used selectively in patients with cystinuria. A regimen of vigorous hydration and alkalinization prevents stone recurrence in about 30 to 50

TABLE 25-3 Alkali Therapy: Drug Formulations, Daily Doses, and Costs

				To Provide 60 mEq BASE/D	
Drug	Supplier	Dose Form	Type of Salts(s)	Total Dose	Mean Cost Wholesale, $
Sodium bicarbonate	Lilly	Tablet (648 mg)	Sodium	8 tablets	0.39
Bicitra	Willen	Solution: citrate	Sodium	4 tbsp	0.45
Polycitra	Willen	Solution: citrate	Sodium plus potassium	2 tbsp	0.36
Polycitra K	Willen	Solution: citrate	Potassium	2 tbsp	0.39
Polycitra K	Willen	Crystals: citrate	Potassium	2 packages	0.38
Urocit-K	Mission	Tablet (wax matrix): citrate	Potassium	12 tablets	1.50
Klyte	Bristol	Tablet (effervescent): citrate	Potassium	2 tablets*	1.35
Effer-K	Nomax	Tablet (effervescent): bicarbonate	Potassium	2 tablets*	0.42

* Dose provides only 50 mEq daily.

percent of patients and diminishes rates of stone complications in many others. Indications for penicillamine include (1) inability to control stones with conservative measures (such patients frequently excrete >1000 mg of cystine daily), (2) cystine stones in a single functioning kidney, and (3) a large stone burden. For most patients who have been rendered free of stones, we recommend stopping penicillamine. The rare patient who shows a severe cystine stone diathesis may be maintained on long-term penicillamine at a reduced level; half the usual dose is generally used, an amount sufficient to maintain a 24-h urinary cystine concentration of about 400 mg/L (1664 μmol/L).

Other Cysteine-Complexing Drugs

Because of the frequent side effects of penicillamine, other sulfhydryl compounds have attracted interest (Fig. 25-5). Mercaptopropionylglycine (MPG), which has a higher oxidation-reduction potential than penicillamine and is thus more efficient in binding to cysteine, is usually given at two-thirds the dose of penicillamine.[39,40] Early use suggested that MPG was associated with fewer serious side effects than penicillamine, but more widespread experience has shown that the two drugs have a similar potential for causing serious reactions.[39] In a multicenter trial, 35 percent of patients who had reacted previously to penicillamine developed MPG toxicity. In this study, among 49 patients treated first with penicillamine and subsequently with MPG, fewer instances of rash and gastrointestinal reactions were observed in patients taking MPG. However, clinically significant proteinuria developed in 12.2 percent of patients taking penicillamine and 10.2 percent of patients taking MPG. Renal glomerular damage is apparently an autoimmune reaction, and IgG antinuclear antibodies were found in 22 percent of patients who took MPG for a mean of 6 years.[41] The cost of prescribing 1500 mg daily of penicillamine or 1000 mg daily of MPG is about $2000 per year.

N-acetyl-D-penicillamine has been reported to be effective in reducing cystine concentration in patients with cystinuria and may have fewer side effects than penicillamine. However, experience with this drug is limited,[26] and 1600 mg daily costs about $10,000 a year.

A mixed disulfide also forms between cysteine and the antihypertensive drug captopril. Although initial reports indicated a profound reduction in cystine excretion in patients who were given 75 to 150 mg of captopril daily,[42,43] other studies did not show any benefit.[44,45] The clinical response to captopril has not been entirely satisfactory.[46] Among eight patients, urinary cystine was reduced a mean 44 percent (range, 18 to 89 percent), but after a year stone diathesis was controlled in only two of these patients.

The effect of captopril on cystine excretion is probably mediated by the formation of a cysteine-captopril disulfide (Fig. 25-5), but because small doses occasionally have profound effects on cystine excretion, some researchers have hypothesized that this drug also affects renal tubular amino acid transport.[46] Because the effectiveness of captopril is unproven, we do not recommend that it be used for treating cystinuria unless it is also prescribed for cardiac or hypertensive effects. Perhaps further study of this drug's mechanism of action will lead to the development of safer, better tolerated therapy for cystinuria.

URIC ACID STONES

Epidemiology

The prevalence of uric acid stones in the United States is estimated to be about 1 in 1000.[47–49] Uric acid stones are usually pure, affect predominantly middle-aged and older men (Fig. 25-1), and represent only 5 percent of stone disease in western countries. In some countries, such as Israel, uric acid stones are more common, accounting for 40 percent of all stones.

The pathogenesis of uric acid stones is well understood, and preventive treatment is highly effective.[50,51] The relations among hyperuricosuria, uric acid, and calcium oxalate stone formation are described later in this chapter (see Calcium Oxalate and Mixed Calcium Stones, below).

Purine Metabolism and Uric Acid Excretion

In humans, uric acid is the end product of purine catabolism. Both dietary and endogenous purines contribute to the metabolic pool (Fig. 25-7). About half the nucleic acid purines in the diet can be recovered as urinary uric acid.[47] The rate of metabolism of endogenous purines normally remains constant, and

FIGURE 25-7 Fate of urate in an average 70-kg man. [*Adapted and reproduced by permission of the editor and publisher from Ettinger B: Allopurinol for the treatment of uric acid and calcium calculi, in Pak CYC (ed): Pharmacologic Treatment of Endocrinopathies. Basel, S. Karger, 1991, pp 16–36.*]

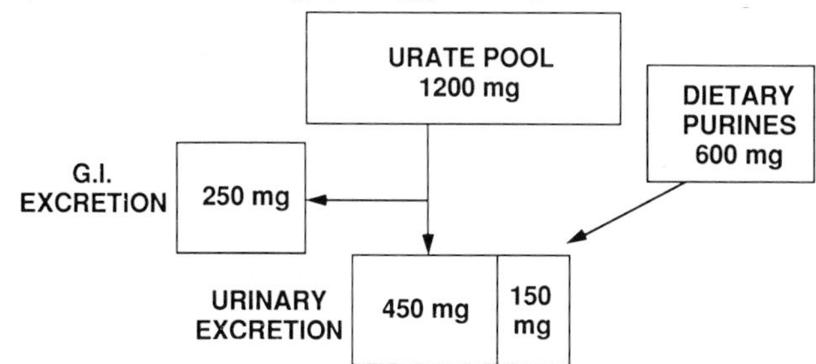

so purine intake accounts for much of the variation in uric acid production rates. Uric acid is eliminated by two routes: About a quarter to a third of the uric acid produced daily enters enteric secretions and is destroyed by intestinal flora (*intestinal uricolysis*); the remaining two-thirds to three-quarters is excreted in urine.

Uric Acid Solubility in Urine

Uric acid stones form when urine is oversaturated by undissociated uric acid; this occurs at a concentration of 100 mg/L (0.6 mmol/L). Urinary pH is a major determinant of uric acid saturation. At pH 5.5 (the pK_a of uric acid), half the total urate is in the form of insoluble undissociated uric acid and half is in the form of soluble urate salt (Fig. 25-8). A small change in pH has a dramatic effect: For example, increasing urinary pH from 5.2 to 5.8 halves the amount of undissociated uric acid; increasing urinary pH from 5.2 to 6.4 reduces the amount of undissociated uric acid by 84 percent.

Risk Factors for Uric Acid Stones

Risk factors for uric acid stones are hyperuricosuria, acidic urine, and low urine volume. Of these, persistently acidic urine is the most important; in some patients with uric acid stones, it may be the only abnormality.

FIGURE 25-8 Effect of urinary pH on free uric acid at two levels of total urate excretion (500 and 1000 mg). Increasing urinary pH from 5.2 to 5.8 (A→C) has the same effect as halving total urate excretion (A→B). [*Adapted and reproduced by permission of the editor and publisher from Ettinger B: Allopurinol for the treatment of uric acid and calcium calculi, in Pak CYC (ed): Pharmacologic Treatment of Endocrinopathies. Basel, S. Karger, 1991, pp 16–36.*]

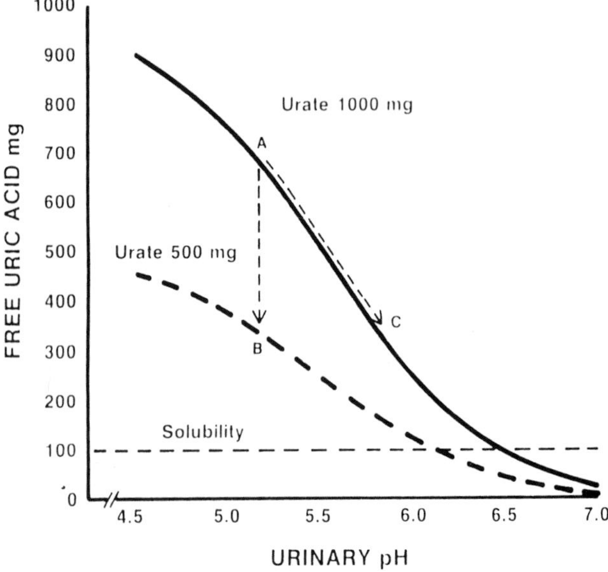

Effect of Diet on Urinary pH and Uric Acid Excretion

Altering the intake of dietary animal protein causes major changes in urinary excretion of uric acid. By consuming 140 g of protein daily (instead of 70 g), a purine glutton may double the body's total uric acid excretion.[52] This additional 70-g protein load contributes fixed acid sufficient to lower urinary pH by 0.5 to 1.0, shifting the equilibrium between urate and undissociated uric acid toward the latter. Dietary excess may thus quadruple the excretion of the insoluble undissociated uric acid moiety.

Gout and Uric Acid Stones

Uric acid stones form in about 20 percent of patients with primary gout, or 1000 times more often than in the general population.[47–49] In half the affected patients, stone disease is recurrent. Stone symptoms precede articular symptoms (occasionally by many years) in 40 percent of these patients.[47]

The gouty population usually has two combined risk factors for uric acid stone formation: hyperuricosuria and excessive urine acidity. A strong correlation exists between the excretion rate of uric acid and the frequency of uric acid stones (Table 25-4); uric acid stones form in almost half of gouty patients excreting >1000 mg (5.9 mmol) daily.[53] About 20 percent of the gouty population in whom uric acid stones form do not have hyperuricosuria; the sole cause of stone diathesis in such patients is excessive urinary acidity. In fasting morning specimens, urinary pH is ≤5.0 in about half these patients compared with 15 percent of normal subjects.[49] The abnormality is also manifested by the absence of the normal postprandial alkaline tide.

In spite of numerous investigations, the reason for excessively acidic urine among patients with uric acid lithiasis is still unknown. Patients with gout excrete relatively more titratable acid and relatively less ammonia than do normal subjects. The defect in

TABLE 25-4 Relation between Rate of Uric Acid Excretion and Frequency of Uric Acid Stones in 1319 Patients with Primary Gout

Urinary Uric Acid	Percentage of Gout Population	Percentage of Patients with Stones
<400	12	24
400–599	36	24
600–799	30	32
800–999	16	31
1000–1600	6	49

Source: Adapted by permission of the author and publisher from Yü T-F: Uric acid nephrolithiasis, in Kelley WN, Weiner IM (eds): *Uric Acid*. New York, Springer-Verlag, 1978, pp 397–422.

ammonia production may be primary or may be secondary to an abnormality in the excretion of titratable acid, or both abnormalities may reflect an unknown fundamental defect in acid-base regulation.

Other Clinical Disorders Associated with Uric Acid Stones

Several rare inborn metabolic defects are associated with a marked overproduction of uric acid and a particularly fulminant diathesis of articular gout and uric acid stone disease. These defects include hypoxanthine-guanine pyrophosphoribosyl transferase (HPRT) deficiency (Lesch-Nyhan syndrome), phosphoribosyl pyrophosphate (PRPP) synthetase overactivity, and glucose-6-phosphatase deficiency (type 1 glycogen storage disease). Affected patients have extreme uric acid overproduction rates and usually have a serum uric acid concentration exceeding 10 mg/dl (6 mmol/L) as well as daily uric acid excretion rates >1000 mg. Uric acid stones form in about three-quarters of such patients, often before age 20 years.[47–49]

Patients with polycythemia vera, myeloid metaplasia, and myelocytic leukemia frequently have hyperuricemia and hyperuricosuria because of increased nucleic acid turnover rates. Gouty arthritis occurs in only 10 percent of patients with myeloproliferative disorders, but uric acid stones form in up to half of such patients. The stones tend to recur and are occasionally the first clinical manifestation leading to a diagnosis of the underlying disorder. Such patients are also at risk for acute uric acid nephropathy.

Numerous drugs (such as probenecid, salicylates, ascorbic acid, and x-ray contrast agents) produce acute uricosuria by inhibiting net uric acid resorption. Continued therapy with these agents, however, results in a new steady state in which uric acid excretion rates should be no greater than pretreatment rates. Nevertheless, probenecid treatment is associated with apparent increased frequency of stone formation in patients with primary gout.[49] Clearly, uricosuric drugs should not be used to treat patients with uric acid overproduction.

The frequency of uric acid stones is increased in patients with inflammatory bowel disease.[47,49] The association is particularly strong in patients who have had an ileostomy, in whom the loss of both bicarbonate and volume as a result of the ileostomy leads to persistently acidic, concentrated urine. Uric acid excretion rates are usually normal in such patients.

Differentiating Uric Acid from Other Purine-Related Stones

Other purine bases or metabolites are sparingly soluble in urine and can form stones in unusual circumstances. Xanthine stones occur in patients with xanthinuria, a rare autosomal recessive disorder caused by a deficiency of xanthine oxidase; xanthinuria is associated with hypouricemia and hypouricosuria. Xanthine stones occasionally develop in patients with rare inborn errors of urate metabolism who are given allopurinol.[6,48,49] Stones composed of 2,8-dihydroxyadenine have been found in a few patients with deficient adenine phosphoribosyl transferase activity.[47] A specific diagnosis of these rare disorders depends on crystallographic analysis of stones.

Mechanisms of the Effect of Allopurinol on Uric Acid

Allopurinol is an analog of hypoxanthine, and both allopurinol and its principal metabolite, oxypurinol, are competitive inhibitors of xanthine oxidase. If this were the only metabolic effect of the drug, xanthine and hypoxanthine would accumulate and might precipitate in urine. However, two metabolic processes prevent this result (Fig. 25-9). First, hypoxanthine is recycled via a "salvage pathway"; this process lets hypoxanthine be reincorporated into nucleic acid production. The enzyme hypoxanthine guanine phosphoribosyltransferase (HGPRtase) directs this salvage process. Second, the adenylic and guanylic acids formed from hypoxanthine salvage inhibit de novo purine synthesis by blocking glutamine phosphoribosylpyrophosphate amidotransferase, the enzyme that directs the first step in purine synthesis.[54]

Absorption of dietary purine is decreased by allopurinol.[55,56] Consequently, its ability to reduce total oxypurine and urate excretion is far greater in subjects whose dietary purine intake is high (Fig. 25-10). This effect has been confirmed by in vitro studies using the rat jejunum.[57]

FIGURE 25-9 Ways in which allopurinol reduces uric acid production. PRPP = phosphoribosyl pyrophosphate; H-Gprtase = hypoxanthine-guanine phosphoribosyl transferase. *(Adapted and reproduced by permission of the publisher and author from Rastegar A, Thier SO: The physiologic approach to hyperuricemia. N Engl J Med 286:470–476, 1972.)*

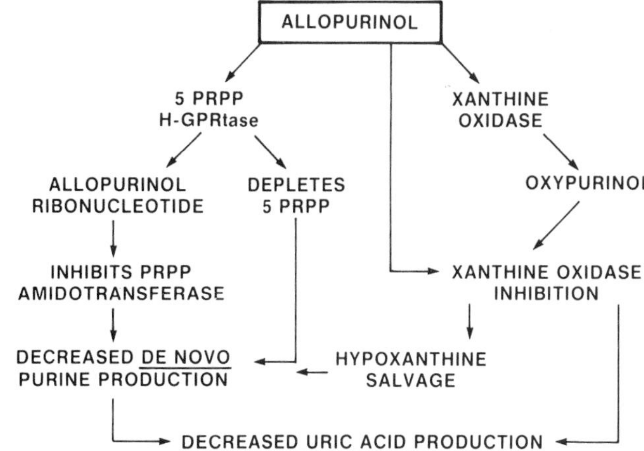

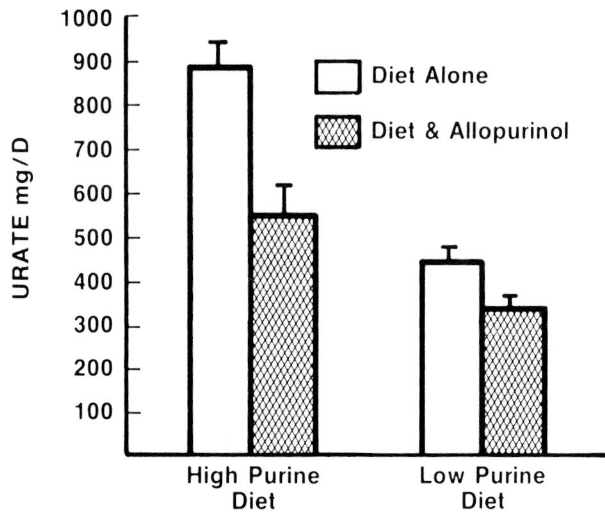

FIGURE 25-10 Reduction of urinary urate excretion with allopurinol is greater in subjects on a high-purine diet. *(Adapted and reproduced by permission of the author and publisher from Pak CYC, Barilla DE, Holt K, Brinkley L, Tolentino R, Zerwekh JC: Effect of oral purine load and allopurinol on the crystallization of calcium salts in urine of patients with hyperuricosuric calcium urolithiasis. Am J Med 65:593–599, 1978.)*

Efficacy of Medical Treatment of Uric Acid Lithiasis

Medical treatment of uric acid lithiasis is highly successful in controlling stone diathesis. Uric acid stones should dissolve within several weeks of treatment. Calculi that are not dissolved after 3 months must be suspected of being admixed or covered with calcium salts or possibly misdiagnosed cystine, triamterene, or some other rare nonopaque calculi.

The efficacy of allopurinol in treating uric acid lithiasis has never been evaluated in a controlled trial and has never been compared with diet or alkali therapy. The results of two recent prospective studies of medical treatment[58,59] have a bearing on this question. Using only potassium citrate (75 mEq/day), Hosking dissolved uric acid calculi in 75 percent of patients.[58] Using potassium citrate (90 mEq/day) combined with allopurinol, Erickson and coworkers dissolved uric acid stones in 71 percent of patients.[59]

Evaluation

Imaging Uric Acid Stones

Uric acid stones are radiolucent and are identified on x-ray films only by the "filling defect" seen after the introduction of a contrast agent. Renal ultrasound and CT are both useful in establishing an accurate diagnosis. Both methods help distinguish uric acid stones from other lesions of the collecting system (e.g., clot, tumor, or rarely sloughed renal papilla).

Urinary Collection

All patients with uric acid stones should be screened for the three risk factors which predispose to uric acid stone formation: low urine volume, excessively acidic urine, and hyperuricosuria. This screening requires that patients collect a 24-h urine specimen while on a free diet.

The collection container should be free of acid. The uricase method is the most reliable for measuring the concentration of uric acid in serum and urine. Recent use of uricosuric agents may invalidate the urine test; the most common of these errors is collecting urine samples shortly after the administration of contrast material, which produces uricosuria.

Researchers do not agree about what constitutes hyperuricosuria. Most consider the upper limit to be 750 mg (4.5 mmol) for women and 800 mg (4.8 mmol) for men. Total urate excretion is not as meaningful as the concentration of undissociated uric acid, which can be estimated from urine volume, total uric acid excretion, and mean urinary pH.

Measuring Urinary Acidity

Nitrazine paper provides an accurate measure of urinary pH within the physiologic range and is convenient for determining urinary pH during outpatient visits and at home. When we screen patients for excessively acidic urine, we instruct them to test the pH of urine voided throughout the day, particularly upon arising and after meals. Normal subjects show peaks and troughs of urinary pH with at least some values >6.0.

Therapy

Correction of Aciduria

Moderation of the intake of animal protein is crucial in a therapeutic program. A diet rigidly restricted in purines and protein is unpalatable, but patients who reduce the total ingestion of meat, poultry, and fish from 8 oz (56 g) to 5 oz (35 g) daily (a realistic goal) derive two benefits: Less total uric acid is excreted, and reduced urine acidity reduces undissociated and insoluble uric acid.[52]

The use of alkali (Table 25-3) is an integral part of therapy, especially for patients whose urine is persistently acidic. Using nitrazine paper, patients can adjust the dose of alkali to maintain a urinary pH between 6.0 and 6.5. Because of the solubility characteristics of uric acid, the goal of alkali therapy is different for patients with uric acid stones than for patients with cystinuria (compare Figs. 25-4 and 25-8). When one is prescribing alkali to patients with uric acid lithiasis, pH must not exceed 7.0. This degree of alkalinization not only is unnecessary but is potentially dangerous because it increases the risk of the formation of calcium phosphate stones. Because of its longer action and possible protection against calcium stone formation, potassium citrate may be preferred to sodium-containing alkali.[60,61]

Treatment with Allopurinol

Indications for the Use of Allopurinol

Because it is effective and easy to use, allopurinol has become a popular agent for treating uric acid stones. However, treatment using only diet modification and alkali is preferred in many cases.

Although the half-life of allopurinol is only a few hours, its metabolite, oxypurinol, has a half-life of 15 to 20 h, extending the biological effects of the drug and enabling effectiveness with a single daily dose, usually 300 mg. This dose reduces uric acid excretion a mean 30 to 40 percent; the hypouricosuric effect may increase slightly during the first few weeks of use. Many physicians do not recognize that the concentration of undissociated uric acid can be reduced much more substantially using diet modification and alkali. Allopurinol is sometimes inappropriately given to patients with uric acid lithiasis who do not excrete excessive uric acid.

Indications for allopurinol therapy include one or all of the following: hyperuricemia, gouty arthritis, recurrent uric acid stone disease, and substantial overproduction [>800 mg/day (>4.8 mmol/day)] of uric acid. Patients with a single uric acid stone in whom overproduction of uric acid is not marked and articular symptoms are not present should be managed conservatively.

Hazards of Allopurinol Therapy

Allopurinol is usually well tolerated and is relatively nontoxic. Gastrointestinal intolerance occurs in about 1 percent of cases, and hypersensitivity reactions occur in about 2 percent. The first sign of a hypersensitivity reaction is pruritus, which nearly always develops during the first few weeks of treatment. If treatment is not stopped, the reaction progresses to a rash, usually maculopapular. Again, prompt discontinuation of the drug prevents the potentially life-threatening hypersensitivity reaction that occurs in about 1 in 1000 patients. This advanced phase of the reaction, which is heralded by fever and chills as well as by an extensive skin rash, may progress to nephritis and hepatitis, resulting in death in 20 percent of cases.[62] When initiating allopurinol therapy, physicians should always advise patients that at the first signs of itching or rash, use of the drug should be discontinued.

CALCIUM PHOSPHATE STONES

Although calcium phosphate in the form of hydroxyapatite may be admixed in typical calcium oxalate stones, pure calcium phosphate stones are rare (Table 25-1). Calcium phosphate stones are given separate status to emphasize the unique aspects of their pathogenesis and because their presence is often an important diagnostic clue to the basis of stone formation.

Crystalline Forms of Calcium Phosphate

Pure calcium phosphate stones form in sterile, alkaline urine. The major crystalline form of calcium phosphate is hydroxyapatite $[Ca_{10}(PO_4)_6(OH)_2]$. Brushite ($CaHPO_4 \cdot 2H_2O$) is not commonly identified in calculi but may form a nidus which later develops into the more mature, hydroxyapatite crystalline form.

Effect of pH on Solubility of Calcium Phosphate

HPO_4^{2-} concentration increases markedly as pH increases; the solubility and formation products for calcium phosphate are both reduced (Fig. 25-11). Pure calcium phosphate stones suggest an underlying disorder of urine acidification manifested by persistently alkaline urine.

Renal Tubular Acidosis

The process of renal acidification normally maintains the pH of extracellular fluids in two ways: by reclaiming filtered bicarbonate and by excreting a quantity of acid equal to the daily systemic production of fixed acid.[2,63] The proximal tubular resorptive mechanism is a high-capacity system which resorbs 90 percent of filtered bicarbonate. The distal tubular mechanism is a low-capacity, high-gradient system which resorbs the remaining bicarbonate and sets the final urinary pH. The gradient of the distal process is sufficient to produce a pH of ≤5.0 and enables the kidney to excrete ammonium and titratable acid in quantities sufficient to balance systemic acid production and regenerate the bicarbonate consumed in buffering the daily production of acid.

Renal tubular acidosis is a rare but important cause of calcium phosphate stones.[2,63,64] Several types of RTA have been identified, but only patients with the distal (classic, or type 1) form are at risk for developing calcium phosphate stones. Patients with complete distal RTA typically have systemic hyperchloremic acidosis and persistently alkaline urine. The exact nature of the defect in distal tubular acidification is unknown, but affected patients are only rarely capable of generating a urinary pH <5.5. Calcium phosphate nephrolithiasis or nephrocalcinosis (or both) has been reported in more than half of such patients[64]; nephrocalcinosis is more common than nephrolithiasis.

The pathogenesis of distal RTA is largely unknown. A familial form associated with an autosomal dominant pattern of inheritance causes growth retardation, rickets, and nephrocalcinosis or nephrolithiasis during childhood. Eighth-nerve deafness and RTA associated with an autosomal recessive pattern of inheritance have also been reported. Sjögren's syndrome and other hyperglobulinemic

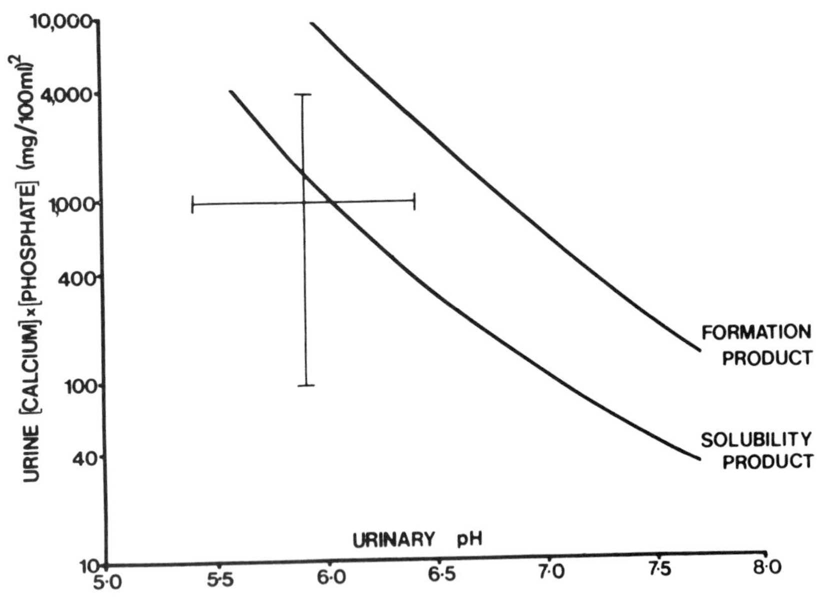

FIGURE 25-11 Relation between urinary pH and calculated solubility and formation products of octocalcium phosphate. Cross represents approximate range of normal urine. [*Adapted and reproduced by permission of the author, editor, and publisher from Robertson WG: Urinary tract calculi, in Nordin BEC (ed): Metabolic Bone and Stone Disease, 2d ed. London, Churchill Livingstone, 1984, pp 271–326.*]

states cause acquired distal RTA in adults. Rare causes of distal RTA include medullary sponge kidney, amphotericin B administration, and obstructive uropathy.[2] No pathogenetic unifying link has been found between these disorders and the distal acidification defect.

Patients with proximal (type 2, or bicarbonate-losing) RTA typically have systemic hyperchloremic acidosis and osteopenia. The distal acidification mechanism is normal in these patients, and stones do not occur. Proximal RTA is also frequently associated with aminoaciduria, glycosuria, and other elements of Fanconi's syndrome; these features are not found in patients with distal RTA.

Pathophysiology of Stone Disease in Renal Tubular Acidosis

Patients with distal RTA usually have multiple risk factors for calcium phosphate stone formation. The most consistent abnormality is alkaline urine, usually fixed at pH $\geqslant$6.5. Acidosis inhibits the production of citrate in the renal cortex, and so citrate excretion is reduced in patients with RTA.[65] Citrate is normally responsible for binding and solubilizing urinary calcium. Most patients also have hypercalciuria; at least two mechanisms contribute to it: Systemic acidosis is buffered to some extent by bone mineral dissolution that releases both calcium and phosphate for eventual renal excretion. In addition, renal calcium resorption is reduced, possibly because of an acidosis-induced defect in calcium resorption in the distal nephron.[2] Intestinal calcium absorption is usually normal or decreased in patients with RTA. The principal risk factors for stone formation in distal RTA are thus alkaline urine, reduced citrate excretion, and hypercalciuria.

Incomplete Renal Tubular Acidosis

RTA is considered complete when systemic acidosis accompanies the acidification defect and incomplete when the process is not severe enough to produce systemic acidosis. Incomplete distal RTA is far more common than complete RTA among stone-forming patients and can be identified by acid-loading studies in about 5 percent of patients with recurrent calcium stones. Among 518 consecutive patients with stone disease, the prevalence of incomplete distal RTA was 7 percent.[66] Several other small series emphasized the association of incomplete distal RTA and the recurrent formation of calcium phosphate stones.[67–69] In some patients, the defect apparently results from tubular damage caused by severe stone disease, medullary sponge kidney, staghorn calculi, or associated pyelonephritis. In other patients, the acidification defect is the apparent primary cause of renal stone formation.[66,70]

The mechanisms by which this partial defect contributes to the formation of kidney stones are apparently similar to, although less severe than, the mechanisms observed in patients who have complete RTA syndrome. Relatively alkaline urine, hypercalciuria, and hypocitraturia are thus all seen in patients with incomplete RTA.[66–71]

Acetazolamide is a noncompetitive carbonic anhydrase inhibitor used primarily in treating glaucoma. Although inhibition of bicarbonate resorption in the proximal tubule is the principal action of this drug, it also inhibits citrate production, decreases the excretion of ammonia as well as titratable acid, and raises urinary pH, in essence producing an iatrogenic RTA.[72] Pure calcium phosphate stones develop in about 5 to 10 percent of patients receiving acetazolamide.

Patients with primary hyperparathyroidism, sarcoidosis, and vitamin D intoxication may also have pure calcium phosphate stones. Although the stones which form in patients with primary hyperparathyroidism as a group appear to have increased calcium phosphate content, calcium oxalate and mixed stones are most commonly found.[73] Parathyroid hormone (PTH) may cause renal bicarbonate wasting and predispose a patient to the formation of calcium phosphate stones (see Chap. 23).

No large series have reported patients with stones composed entirely or predominantly of calcium phosphate. Among 363 consecutive patients seen at the Yale Renal Stone Clinic, 5 percent had pure calcium phosphate stones. As a group, these patients tended to have higher fasting urinary pH values, and the urine tended to have a reduced ability to acidify after ammonium chloride loading. A specific etiology could be established for half the patients: Five had distal RTA, two were ingesting absorbable alkali, one was taking acetazolamide, and one had primary hyperparathyroidism.

Evaluation

Identification

Calcium phosphate stones can be identified only by crystallographic analysis and should be suspected in patients with coincident nephrocalcinosis or specific diseases known to cause RTA. The medication history of patients with stone disease should always include information about acetazolamide or antacid intake.

Renal Acidification Tests

The presence of calcium phosphate stones mandates extensive evaluation of renal acidification. When a urea-splitting infection is present, urinary pH results are uninterpretable. In a spot early-morning check, if urinary pH is ≤ 5.5, complete RTA can be ruled out. Patients with a pH of ≥ 6.0 at initial evaluation may be given a roll of nitrazine paper to record urinary pH at each voiding for a few days. This simple maneuver documents normal acidification capability in almost all patients and precludes acid-loading studies in all but a small percentage of cases. Patients whose urinary pH remains ≥ 6.0 should obtain serum electrolyte measurements.

Equivocal laboratory results indicate acid-loading studies for clarification. In the "acute" acid load study, which is used most commonly, 0.1 g of oral ammonium chloride is given per kilogram of body weight; urinary pH, venous blood pH, and P_{CO_2} are then measured at baseline and hourly for 6 h.[2] Although this study is convenient, the results may be uninterpretable because the medication causes vomiting; a nonabsorbable antacid should be given with the drug to help prevent gastric irritation and vomiting. The normal renal response to the induced acidosis is manifested by urinary pH <5.3. Incomplete RTA is diagnosed on the basis of normal serum electrolyte concentrations and nonmaximal acidification of urine. If test results are equivocal or a patient has gastric intolerance, a "long" acid-loading test lasting 3 consecutive days can be done.[70]

Treatment

Complete Distal RTA

Patients with complete distal RTA are treated with alkali in quantities sufficient to normalize serum bicarbonate concentration. In adults, this is usually 1 mEq per kilogram of body weight daily. In children, acid production rates and dose per kilogram are several times higher.[74] The alkali is given daily in four to six divided doses. Sodium bicarbonate tablets are inexpensive and effective, but many physicians and some patients prefer citrate preparations (Table 25-3).

Alkalinization has a dramatic effect on the skeletal manifestations of RTA and can restore normal growth rates in children.[74] Any hypercalciuria is reduced or eliminated, and excretion of citrate is normalized.

Incomplete Distal RTA

The preferred treatment is potassium citrate because it corrects the hypercalciuria and hypocitraturia which occur in patients with incomplete distal RTA. In an uncontrolled trial of such patients, oral potassium citrate therapy prevented the formation of new stones during a 34-month period.[69]

MAGNESIUM AMMONIUM PHOSPHATE STONES

Terminology

Various synonymous terms, including *struvite stone*, *infection stone*, and *triple phosphate stone*, are used to describe MAP stones. Struvite stones are composed of MAP ($MgNH_4PO_4 \cdot 6H_2O$) admixed with minor amounts of carbonate-apatite [$Ca_{10}(PO_4)_6 \cdot CO_3$]. *Triple phosphate* refers to the three different cations (magnesium, ammonium, and calcium) found together with the phosphate anion. Urologists use the term *infection stone* to distinguish such stones from metabolic stones.

History and Epidemiology

MAP stones are an ancient disease manifestation. Before surgery or antibiotics were available, the outlook for affected patients was bleak. Surgical and medical advances have dramatically altered this outlook, and both the prevalence and the recurrence rates of MAP stones have clearly decreased in the past two decades, perhaps by up to 75 percent.[75,76]

The peak prevalence of MAP stones occurs in three sectors of the population: young boys, middle-aged women, and elderly patients of both sexes. MAP stones represent only a small percentage of total stones (Table 25-1). Nevertheless, because of the high morbidity as well as the difficulty of medical and surgical management, their importance far outweighs their frequency.

Pathophysiology

The formation of MAP stones results from supersaturation of urine with magnesium ammonium phosphate and carbonate-apatite. Such supersaturation occurs only when infection with urea-splitting bacteria is present. MAP stone formation can be reproduced in vitro simply by adding purified urease to normal urine[75]; urease initiates the sequence of reactions shown in Fig. 25-12. Increased concentration of ammonium, carbonate, and alkaline pH that changes PO_{4-1} into PO_{4-2} oversaturates the urine with both MAP and carbonate-apatite.

An in vitro model has been suggested in which urease-producing bacteria, such as *Proteus* species, adhere to renal epithelial cells and form small colonies enclosed in a glycocalix coat secreted by the bacteria.[77] The glycocalix may protect the bacteria from antibiotic action and also traps struvite and apatite crystals. These crystal-encrusted microcolonies then combine with inflammatory cells, debris, and urinary mucoproteins to form a stone matrix. The matrix of MAP stones may have an important role in calculus growth. The large, soft, gel-like matrix may mineralize rapidly and assumes a classic staghorn calculous appearance within weeks.[78]

Bacteriology

About 90 percent of clinical isolates of *Proteus* species, *Staphylococcus aureus*, and *Bacteroides* species produce urease. About 30 percent of *Klebsiella* and *Pseudomonas* isolates are urease-positive. In contrast, *Escherichia coli* rarely if ever produce urease. Although all urea-splitting bacterial strains have been implicated, *Proteus* species are identified in almost 90 percent of these patients.[72] Colony counts are frequently <100,000/ml, a finding important for proper diagnosis and management.

FIGURE 25-12 Biochemical steps leading to the formation of magnesium ammonium phosphate (MAP) stones in urine.

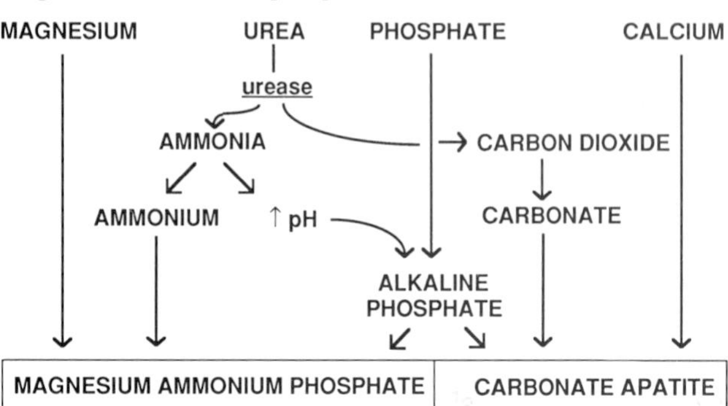

Clinical Risk Factors

Two major categories of patients are at risk for MAP stones: (1) patients with anatomic or functional abnormalities of the urinary tract (or both), which predispose to infection, and (2) patients with antecedent metabolic stones in whom infection introduced by urologic procedures is established at the stone site. The first category includes patients with megaloureter, ureteral reflux or obstruction, ileal conduits, nephrostomy drainage, or bladder outlet obstruction necessitating either intermittent catheterization or an indwelling catheter. The second category includes patients with metabolic stones, particularly patients who need frequent instrumentation for stones. Stone disease in such patients ultimately becomes self-perpetuating: Stones predispose to infection, and infection predisposes to stone formation.

Serious Morbidity from MAP Stones

Untreated staghorn calculi can grow and invade locally in a way similar to a neoplasm. Untreated patients have about a 50 percent chance of losing the affected kidney within 5 years.[75] Renal impairment associated with a unilateral staghorn stone is usually insufficient to greatly alter renal function tests but can be evaluated by visualization of a shrunken or scarred (or both) cortical outline during the nephrogram phase of the IVP. Patients with staghorn calculi in a single functioning kidney or with bilateral staghorn stones may have azotemia. About 25 percent of patients with bilateral staghorn stones die within 5 years.[77]

Evaluation

Identifying MAP stones is usually not difficult. Such stones are diagnosed by the characteristic staghorn configuration of the stone, crystallographic analysis, or both. The apatite content confers radiopacity on MAP stones, which are less dense than oxalate stones but—except for occasional matrix concretions—are readily seen on plain x-ray films.

The bacteriologic aspect of diagnosis is less straightforward. The colony count of urease-producing bacteria is <100,000/ml in half and <10,000/ml in 20 percent of patients.[76] Mixed infections are common, and a tendency exists to neglect the importance of the urea-splitting organisms when they are overshadowed by larger numbers of other organisms (e.g., *E coli*). Thus, for patients suspected of having

MAP stones, obtaining colony counts of all gram-negative organisms in the urine culture is important. Moreover, regardless of the colony count or presence of mixed infection, urease-producing organisms can be cultured from stone material.[76] Surgical specimens should thus be cultured to establish a clear bacteriologic diagnosis.

Other aspects of diagnosis relate to metabolic screening and the search for structural or functional abnormalities of the urinary tract. A careful IVP is essential. Cystoscopy and retrograde pyelography may be indicated. Patients with MAP stones should have a careful and complete urinary biochemical evaluation. Smith reported that more than 60 percent of patients with MAP stones have urinary biochemical abnormalities which predispose to metabolic stone formation.[72] For such patients, it may be possible to document a historical sequence of stones with differing composition.

Treatment

The prognosis for patients with MAP stones has improved considerably as medical and surgical approaches to the disease have become better coordinated and more sophisticated.[79] In a recent series of patients followed for 7 years, a meticulous medical-surgical approach rendered >90 percent of patients free of both stones and infection.[80] This optimistic report is tempered by general experience showing a mean 30 percent stone recurrence rate and a mean 40 percent infection recurrence rate.[75]

For patients in whom metabolic stone diathesis is complicated by MAP stones, fewer specific data are available. In Smith's experience,[76] when all stone material was removed at the time of surgery, the prognosis was good; 81 percent of such patients remained stone-free.

Antibiotic Therapy

The approach to antimicrobial therapy differs at different times in a patient's course. Short-term administration of antibiotics almost never eliminates infection when a MAP stone is present. In preparing for surgery, culture-specific bactericidal drugs are given 24 to 48 h before the procedure and are continued for 10 to 14 days after all urologic devices have been removed. Patients considered free of stones and infection after surgery are usually maintained on either low-dosage bactericidal agents or broad-spectrum drugs for 6 to 12 months, with serial urine cultures every 1 to 3 months during treatment. However, in one series, stopping antibiotics after only 2 weeks in stone-free patients had no adverse consequences.[80]

Patients in whom stones remain after surgery and patients in whom surgery cannot be attempted are treated with long-term antibiotic therapy. Low-dose, culture-specific bactericidal agents are preferred to broad-spectrum agents.[75,78] The goal in these patients is to render the urine sterile during therapy and limit both stone growth and the frequency of infection symptoms; therapy is continued indefinitely. Most reports suggest that if the urine is successfully and permanently sterilized, patients will remain stable.[81,82] Long-term antimicrobial treatment is occasionally associated with reduced stone mass.[75,78]

Complete removal of all stone material is the goal of surgical therapy and represents the only reliable method of cure in patients with MAP stones. The success of this approach depends on meticulous attention to detail during surgery and in the periods immediately before and after surgery. Complete removal of MAP stones is hampered by their friability and tendency to mold to inaccessible areas of the collecting system. These difficulties led to development of various surgical techniques, including coagulum lithotomy, irrigation of the renal pelvis and collecting system, and nephroscopy. Percutaneous and extracorporeal lithotripsy of staghorn calculi may substantially simplify MAP stone surgery. These two procedures combined are likely to become the preferred treatment because they can eliminate all stone material in about three-quarters of these patients. Urologic treatment of MAP stones has been reviewed comprehensively.[79]

Urease Inhibitors

Because the production of urease by the offending organism is the main pathogenic event in MAP stone formation, enzyme-specific inhibitors have been developed. Acetohydroxamic acid, a potent urease inhibitor, has been approved for this use. In a recent review of three randomized, double-blind trials using 341 patients, those who took acetohydroxamic acid up to 2 years had about half the prevalence of stone growth of patients taking placebo.[79] In about 20 percent of patients, the drug caused serious side effects, including rash, headache, phlebitis, thromboembolism, hemolytic anemia, and iron deficiency anemia. The usual dose of acetohydroxamic acid is 10 to 15 mg per kilogram of body weight divided into three or four oral doses; the maximal daily dose is 1.5 g. Patients with moderate renal insufficiency require lower doses; patients with substantial renal failure should not receive this drug. Acetohydroxamic acid should be prescribed by physicians experienced in its use and competent to integrate it into a comprehensive urologic treatment program. Other, less toxic urease inhibitors are being sought.[79]

CALCIUM OXALATE AND MIXED CALCIUM STONES

Epidemiology

Calcium stone disease predominantly affects persons living in industrialized nations and accounts for

75 percent of all cases of nephrolithiasis (Table 25-1). The incidence of calcium stone disease has steadily increased during the last few decades.[1,83] This increase has occurred mostly in men: The man-to-woman ratio increased from 1.8:1.0 in 1954 to 3.8:1.0 in 1970.[1] The incidence of calcium stones peaks for an extended period during the middle four decades of life.[1]

Calcium stone prevalence varies widely, both throughout the world and within countries. The concept of high-prevalence "stone belts" in the United States derives largely from the survey of Boyce and associates of U.S. nationwide hospital admissions for stone disease between 1948 and 1952.[84] The prevalence of stone disease varied as much as fivefold in different geographic regions, with the southeastern United States being the principal stone belt. A similar but more recent study yielded a different distribution of high-prevalence regions,[85] although both studies pinpointed the eastern half of the country as a stone belt. Similar wide geographic variations in stone prevalence exist in Sweden.[86]

About half these stones are composed of pure calcium oxalate, and half are admixtures of calcium oxalate and calcium phosphate. Calcium oxalate crystals may exist as either the monohydrate (whewellite) or dihydrate (weddellite) species; an admixture of the two is most common. We do not know whether the presence of calcium phosphate in mixed stones is important for crystal nucleation or growth, but the calcium phosphate content of these stones apparently reflects urinary pH.[2,87] The percentages of pure calcium phosphate stones and of stones composed of calcium phosphate admixed with calcium oxalate have decreased in recent years[88]; the apparent decreases have been attributed to altered diet, particularly decreased animal protein intake.[83]

Evidence shows that diet plays a major role in the increasing incidence of calcium stones. Surveys in the United Kingdom found that intake of animal protein (meat, poultry, and fish) is the primary dietary variable associated with an increased incidence of calcium oxalate stones; the intake of calcium, oxalate, magnesium, and carbohydrate is relatively unimportant.[83] Increased dietary protein adds to urinary excretion of calcium, uric acid, and oxalate and reduces urinary pH; all these factors predispose to calcium oxalate instead of the other stone types.[23,83]

Physical Chemistry

The concepts of saturation chemistry apply to calcium stone formation, but a single discrete biochemical abnormality, such as that which defines cystine stone disease or cystinuria, is not seen in patients with calcium stone disease.

The solution chemistry of calcium oxalate is complex but can be appreciated by considering the activity of calcium ions in a solution such as urine. At a given pH, calcium may form soluble complexes with citrate, oxalate, sulfate, and four species of phosphate ions. These anions then form soluble complexes with other cations besides calcium, and so anion activity is also variable. Computing calcium ion activity in such a system necessitates solving about a dozen simultaneous equations.

Although techniques and interpretations differ, the implications of findings from several laboratories in regard to saturation and predisposition to crystal formation and growth in stone-forming urine are similar.[89–91] The *activity product ratio* (*APR*) describes the saturation of urine by calcium oxalate. An APR of unity indicates that urine is saturated, a value less than unity indicates undersaturation, and values progressively greater than unity define increasing degrees of supersaturation. Patients with recurrent calcium stones typically have APR values higher than those of normal persons. These results can usually be attributed to increased calcium concentration in the urine of stone patients and a variable tendency toward increased oxalate concentration. Similar observations have been made about brushite, suggesting that the calcium phosphate system may be an important crystal nidus, particularly in alkaline urine.[89]

The *formation product ratio* (*FPR*) is a measurement of the minimum supersaturation needed to cause spontaneous nucleation. The measurement is made by adding calcium to urine and noting the activity product at which cloudiness appears. The FPR is normally 8 to 10 times the APR of calcium oxalate.[89–91] The FPR (or an equivalent parameter) in patients with recurrent calcium stones is often less than normal, indicating an unexplained predisposition to crystallization in stone-forming urine.

This predisposition has been attributed to the process of heterogeneous nucleation (e.g., of crystals of calcium oxalate and either monosodium urate or uric acid), a deficiency of unidentified inhibitors in stone-forming urine, and the presence of "promoters" of crystallization in stone-forming urine. Stone formation apparently results from an imbalance of forces which cause and prevent crystallization and the growth of calcium salts in urine.

Natural History of Calcium Oxalate Lithiasis

In quantitating the risk of stone recurrence, epidemiologists have relied on three methods of data acquisition: retrospective, retrolective, and prospective. A *retrospective*, or population-based, study either asks all subjects to recall previous stone events or reviews health records and other data bases. Although limited by the accuracy of a person's recall and the incompleteness of medical data collection, this method is less biased than a *retrolective* study, which relies on data collection from stone clinic patients. When such patients are asked to recall initial and subsequent stone events, recurrence rates and risk of stone morbidity are exaggerated. Bek-Jensen and Tiselius quantitated the bias introduced in this manner.[92] Among patients seen at a stone clinic, the annual stone passage rate was 0.19 stone per patient-year for 3 years after the first stone event but was 0.66 stone per patient-year during the 3 years just before the stone clinic visit. Others, using the retrolective method, have concluded that the interval between stone events shortens with time.[93] Among six retrospective and retrolective studies recently reviewed,[20] mean cumulative recurrence reached 25 percent after 5 years and 52 percent after 10 years.[1,94–98] Recurrence rates were predictably lower by about half in the population-based studies. For example, Marshall and associates, analyzing stone clinic patients, reported an 8 percent annual recurrence rate in men after the first stone event.[94] In contrast, Johnson and associates, studying the population of Rochester, Minnesota, found a recurrence rate of <4 percent annually for men.[1] Both groups of investigators found relatively low annual recurrence rates for women: 6 percent in the stone clinic study and 2 percent in the population-based study.

Estimates of stone morbidity from stone treatment centers also tend to exaggerate rates of hospitalization and urologic surgery. For example, a history of hospitalization was positive for 90 percent of patients seen at a stone evaluation center after the first stone[18] but for only 23 percent of such patients identified by a population survey.[99] Among patients referred to two centers for stone evaluation, 38 percent (19) and 74 percent (18) had a history of surgical removal. In contrast, a population-based study found that only 5 percent of stone patients needed surgery.[100]

Ideally, *prospective* studies are used to define the natural history of calcium stone disease. To conduct such a study, however, new patients with single stones must be identified soon after the clinical event, patients with additional existing stones must be identified and excluded, and a sufficient number of subjects must be followed long enough to obtain sufficiently robust statistics for recurrence. Ljunghall and Danielson identified 54 such patients who were seen at emergency departments.[101] Figure 25-13 shows that the annual recurrence rate in this study was about 10 percent during the first 4 years of follow-up; recurrence was less frequent thereafter. Recurrence was three times as probable in men as in women. Patients seen at the Mayo Clinic for evaluation of a first stone[102] received fluid and diet advice and were then followed for 5 years; the annual recurrence rate was about 5 percent. In a prospective trial of single-stone patients who were health plan members of the Kaiser Permanente Medical Care Program in northern California (R.A. Hiatt, M.D., unpublished data), the annual recurrence rate was <3 percent during a 3.5-year period among 99 patients who were given general dietary advice.

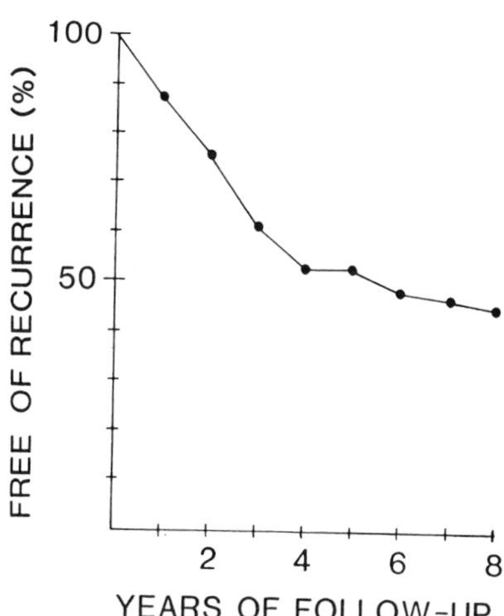

FIGURE 25-13 Percentage of untreated patients free of recurrence after a single renal stone in relation to time of follow-up. *(Adapted and reproduced by permission of the author and publisher from Broadus AE, Thier SO: Metabolic basis of renal-stone disease. N Engl J Med 300:839–845, 1979.)*

The risk of subsequent recurrence is about two to three times greater in patients who have had two or more stone events compared with single-stone patients. Stone patients who have had a relapse may be expected to have stones frequently. These aspects of risk determination are germane to (1) consideration of metabolic screening in patients who have had a single stone event, (2) initiation of treatment in patients who have had one or more stone events, and (3) proposed duration of therapy (see Evaluation and Treatment, below).

Risk Factors

The risk factors which predispose to calcium stone formation can be separated into two categories (Table 25-5): (1) general risk factors (e.g., a family his-

TABLE 25-5 Risk Factors for Calcium Stone Formation

General	Specific
Family history	Low urine volume
Medications	Hypercalciuria
Urinary pH	Hyperoxaluria
Diet	Hyperuricosuria
	Hypocitraturia

Source: Adapted by permission of the author, editor, and publisher from Insogna KL, Broadus AE: Nephrolithiasis, in Felig P, Baxter JD, Broadus AE, Frohman LA (eds): *Endocrinology and Metabolism,* 2d ed. New York, McGraw-Hill, 1987, p 1529.

tory) and (2) specific, treatable metabolic risk factors (e.g., hypercalciuria).

Family History

A family history of renal stones in one or more first-degree relatives is found in 35 to 50 percent of patients with calcium stone disease.[103–105] The most commonly found association is between the patient (male or female) and male first-degree relatives, in whom the risk for stone formation may be 5 to 10 times the risk in the general population. The lifetime risk for brothers of index case patients is nearly 50 percent.[103] The severity of calcium stone disease is not different in these kindreds than in other stone patients.

Coe and associates examined the familial association between hypercalciuria and calcium stone disease.[104] Among 44 first-degree relatives, 43 percent were hypercalciuric, suggesting an autosomal-dominant mode of inheritance. A history of renal stones was also common in these first-degree relatives, but a history of stone disease and the presence of hypercalciuria were unrelated; equal percentages of normocalciuric and hypercalciuric relatives reported a history of stones.

Family history information was evaluated for 206 patients seen at the Yale Renal Stone Clinic for common calcium stones (K.L. Insogna, M.D., unpublished data).* A history of stone disease in one or more first-degree relatives was found for half these patients. Familial patterns of identified risk factors—low urine volume, hyperuricosuria, and hypercalciuria—were analyzed by isolating patients with only one risk factor and excluding patients with combined risk factors. Family history was positive in 71 percent of patients with low urine volume, 62 percent of hyperuricosuric patients, 50 percent of hypercalciuric patients, and 41 percent of patients in whom no risk factor was identified; inherited risks, environmental risks, or a combination were not explained by a simple metabolic pattern.

The marked familial tendency toward calcium stone formation is unexplained. Specific, rare disorders with an autosomal dominant or autosomal recessive inheritance pattern, such as RTA, familial forms of hyperparathyroidism, and primary hyperoxaluria, account for only a small percentage of affected family members.

Medication

Vitamin A and vitamin D intoxication as well as the milk-alkali syndrome are described in detail in Chap. 23. All three conditions are characterized by hypercalcemia, nephrocalcinosis, and azotemia and are only rarely associated with renal stone formation. Large doses of ascorbic acid (≥4 g/day) have been reported to lead to increased urinary oxalate excretion, although considerable disagreement exists about both the reproducibility and the clinical significance of this effect.[106–107] Little evidence shows that vitamin C intake predisposes to the formation of calcium oxalate stones in persons with no history of stone disease, but exacerbation of calcium oxalate stone disease in patients with a history of stones has been reported.

Urinary pH

The solubility of calcium oxalate in aqueous solution is not influenced by an alteration in pH within the limits of the physiologic range. However, the concentration of urinary citrate is dependent on urinary pH, and citrate has an important role in complexing and solubilizing calcium (see Hypocitraturia, below).

Low Urine Volume

When patients with common calcium stones are screened, an initial urine volume of <1 L daily is observed in about 25 percent.[93,108] Pak and associates showed that dilution not only reduces the concentration of calcium and oxalate but enhances the solubility of calcium oxalate.[109] However, the subgroup of patients that habitually avoids fluids tends to resist repeated instructions about hydration. Failure to increase urine volume has been associated with stone recurrence.[103,110]

Hypercalciuria

The term *idiopathic hypercalciuria* was introduced by Albright and colleagues in 1953[111] and was further defined by Henneman and coworkers in 1958[112]; the latter group both defined idiopathic hypercalciuria and broached the question of its pathogenesis, initiating a controversy that still persists. The term idiopathic hypercalciuria encompassed three apparent abnormalities: normocalcemic hypercalciuria, a tendency toward hypophosphatemia, and frequent infection of the urinary tract. The investigators reasoned that the primary abnormality in their patients was a pyelonephritis-induced defect in renal calcium resorption which led to hypercalciuria, secondary hyperparathyroidism, and a consequent tendency toward hypophosphatemia. The finding of bacteriuria was spurious (*Staphylococcus albus* was the organism frequently identified) but was a central feature of their hypothesis. The same investigators presented evidence for increased intestinal calcium absorption in these patients but interpreted this finding as a secondary response to the renal calcium "leak." This study introduced the key elements of the controversy about the diagnosis and pathogenetic importance of "renal" hypercalciuria, "absorptive" hypercalciuria, and subtle ("normocalcemic") primary hyperparathyroidism.

---

* Yale University School of Medicine, New Haven, Connecticut.

Hypercalciuria is a difficult subject; the biomedical literature cannot be summarized easily, reflecting in part the complexity of the putative pathogenetic mechanisms responsible for hypercalciuria and in part the fact that many published series have been flawed in design, methodology, and/or interpretation. Readers should pay particular attention to (1) the limits used in defining hypercalciuria in view of established calcium excretion limits expressed on an absolute basis (milligrams per day), which are not necessarily interchangeable with limits expressed on a weight basis (miligrams per kilogram of body weight daily), (2) the impact of dietary influences on both the detection and the definition of hypercalciuria, particularly calcium and sodium, (3) the shortcomings of certain widely used diagnostic criteria (e.g., classification on the basis of results for fasting calcium excretion), and (4) the importance of study conditions in collecting and interpreting metabolic data. These four points explain much of the controversy.

Investigators find even the simple issues of defining hypercalciuria and estimating its frequency problematic; the many problems and variables include (1) the use of multiple definitions of hypercalciuria, (2) differences in patterns of calcium excretion in different populations, (3) the influence of dietary factors besides calcium on calcium excretion, and (4) the difficulty of assigning a statistical upper limit of calcium excretion in the normal population because of the apparent upward skew of values in this population.[2,6,7,12,88,113–116] Among these issues, dietary influences are by far the most important.

The biomedical literature contains reports of two main types of metabolic studies: those using groups of outpatients, almost all of whom were on a free diet for metabolic screening, and those using groups of inpatients on rigidly defined "metabolic" diets. Each approach reflects a bias. The free-diet approach seems relevant because stone disease develops in patients on habitual diets and because dietary factors may play a role in causing hypercalciuria, stones, or both. Investigators using metabolic diets and conducting predominantly inpatient studies note that only controlled studies are likely to generate consistent data. A clear understanding of hypercalciuria may require that elements of both approaches be used: Patients should be screened both on a free diet and under more defined conditions; moreover, research studies aimed at elucidating the details of pathogenesis must be done in carefully controlled conditions.

At the Yale Renal Stone Clinic (K.L. Insogna, M.D., unpublished data), the results of metabolic screening of outpatients on free diets were systematically compared with the results for patients on a defined metabolic diet (containing 1 g calcium, 1 g protein per kilogram of body weight, and 100 mEq sodium daily). The defined diet (see Evaluation, below) is designed to facilitate the detection of hypercalciuria in patients with a true underlying defect in calcium metabolism and minimize other dietary influences.

As shown in Table 25-6, some patients were hypercalciuric only when on the free diet (group A); some were hypercalciuric on both free and defined diets but showed a moderate to marked reduction in calcium excretion on a defined diet, even though calcium intake had increased on this diet (group B); some had an equal degree of hypercalciuria on both diets (group C); and some were hypercalciuric only on the defined diet (group D). In the first two groups, dietary factors besides calcium must have at least contributed to hypercalciuria in patients on the free diet. Conversely, hypercalciuria in group D patients would have been missed entirely if they had not also been screened on the defined, unrestricted calcium diet.

Hypercalciuria in patients on the defined diet was highly correlated with underlying alterations in calcium metabolism: About 80 percent of these patients clearly had abnormalities.[113,117,118] In contrast, detailed investigation showed that <20 percent of patients found to be hypercalciuric on only the free diet had true abnormalities of mineral metabolism.

TABLE 25-6 Results of Screening 122 Hypercalciuric Patients for Hypercalciuria on a Free or Defined Diet

Diet on Which Hypercalciuria Was Detected	Calcium Excretion on Free Diet, mg/day*	Calciuim Excretion on Defined Diet, mg/day†	No. Patients
A. Free diet only	334	236	27
B. Both free and defined diets: calcium excretion fell >50 mg/day on defined diet	422	331	17
C. Both free and defined diets	354	365	41
D. Defined diet only	224	328	37

* Mean values for daily sodium excretion on the free diet in the four groups were 190, 214, 172, and 121 mEq, respectively.

† Defined diet contained 100 mg calcium, 100 mEq sodium, and 1 g protein per kilogram of body weight daily.

Source: Insogna KL, Broadus AE: Nephrolithiasis, in Felig P, Baxter JD, Broadus AE, Frohman LA (eds): *Endocrinology and Metabolism,* 2d ed. New York, McGraw-Hill 1987, p 1533.

To maximize the detection of hypercalciuria associated with calcium stone disease, patients must be screened on both a free diet and a defined diet with high-normal calcium content. The free intake specimen is critical in assessing numerous risk factors for calcium stone formation, including low urine volume, hyperuricosuria, and hypercalciuria.[113] This specimen allows the detection of dietary hypercalciuria in patients (22 percent in Table 25-6) who are not hypercalciuric on a defined diet. The defined 1000-mg (25-mmol) calcium diet specimen maximizes the detection of true underlying defects in calcium metabolism and minimizes dietary influences besides calcium. Hypercalciuria would not have been detected in 30 percent of the patients listed in Table 25-6 if they had been screened on only a free diet because calcium intake was restricted at screening. When one is screening for hypercalciuria, the circumstances should be such that the abnormality in patients is expressed.

In normal persons, increasing calcium intake from low normal (400 mg/day) to high normal (1000 mg/day) has a moderate impact on calcium excretion, increasing it a mean 6 mg per 100-mg increase in dietary calcium intake. In contrast, in most patients with hypercalciuria and stone disease, the slope of calcium excretion vs. calcium intake is steep (about 20 percent). Evaluating patients whose calcium intake is increased distinguishes them further from normal subjects (Fig. 25-14).[113,115,116,118]

The defined high-normal calcium diet for screening outpatients has been used in inpatient studies and gives equivalent results. Given these findings and the ease with which this diet can be used by outpatients, a sophisticated metabolic ward is unnecessary for identifying hypercalciuric patients.

What Is the Clinical Utility of Diagnosing Hypercalciuria?

Although hypercalciuria is the most common risk factor identified in patients with calcium stone disease, the statistical relation between calcium excretion and calcium stone formation is weak. Many patients with calcium stone disease are not hypercalciuric. Moderate hypercalciuria imparts some risk; however, the risk of developing stone disease increases markedly at daily excretion rates ≥400 mg (≥10 mmol/day).[90]

Calcium Homeostasis and Mechanisms for Hypercalciuria

Readers should review the discussion of calcium and phosphorus homeostasis in Chap. 23, particularly the sections on control of bone mineral exchange, proximal and distal processes of calcium resorption in the renal tubule, sequence of activation and metabolism of vitamin D, mechanisms and control of intestinal calcium absorption, and calcium and phosphorus homeostasis and balance.

Figure 25-15 illustrates calcium homeostasis in a normal person in calcium balance. Hypercalciuria can be produced by three mechanisms individually or in some combination: (1) defective renal tubular calcium resorption, (2) increased net calcium absorption, and (3) increased bone resorption. Regardless of the cause, calcium excreted in the urine must ultimately be derived from dietary calcium, bone mineral, or both. Subtle abnormalities are sufficient to

FIGURE 25-14 Urinary calcium excretion determined on both 400-mg and 1000-mg calcium diets; 30 normal subjects (closed circles), 25 patients with absorptive hypercalciuria (closed triangles), 2 patients with renal hypercalciuria (open triangles), and 8 patients with subtle primary hyperparathyroidism (open circles). Diets were identical except for calcium intake.

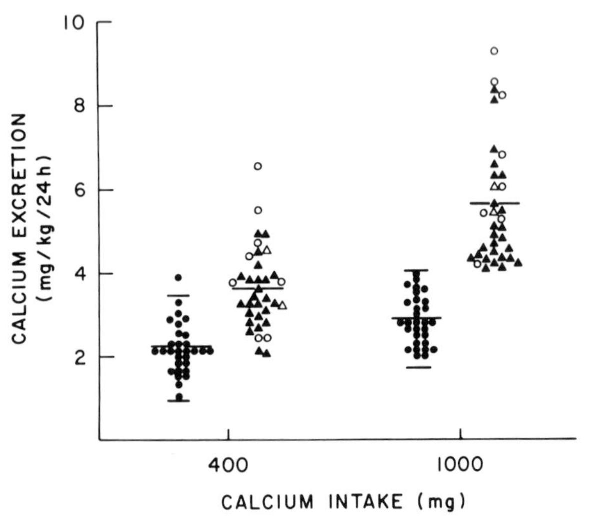

FIGURE 25-15 Schema of calcium metabolism in normal subject in calcium balance. Open arrows denote unidirectional fluxes; solid arrows denote net fluxes. Three mechanisms that can lead to hypercalciuria are denoted A, B, and C (see text). [*Adapted and reproduced by permission of Insogna KL, Broadus AE: Nephrolithiasis, in Felig P, Baxter JD, Broadus AE, Frohman LA (eds): Endocrinology and Metabolism, 2d ed. New York, McGraw-Hill, 1987, p 1536.*]

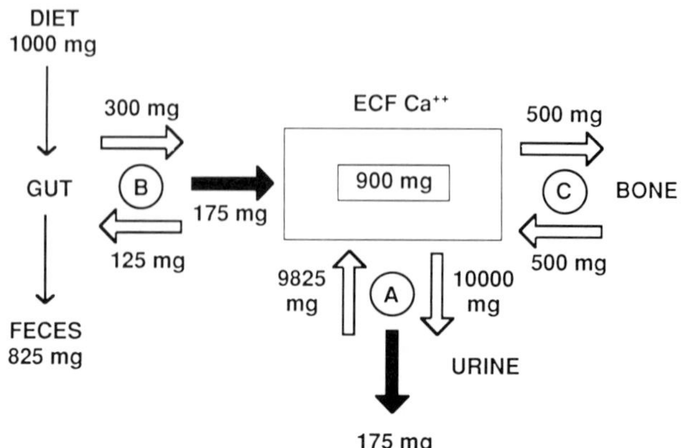

produce hypercalciuria. For example, a 1 to 2 percent error in renal tubular handling of calcium will result in clinically significant hypercalciuria.

Classification of Forms of Hypercalciuria

Secondary Hypercalciuria Among the secondary forms of hypercalciuria listed in Table 25-7, only the first four are encountered with any frequency in an adult population with stone disease. The most important form of secondary hypercalciuria is primary hyperparathyroidism, which was identified in a mean 7.2 percent of 3084 patients with calcium stone disease in eight large series.[73] The "subtle" variety of this disease can easily be overlooked and requires special diagnostic attention (see below). Among patients seen at the Yale Renal Stone Clinic (K.L. Insogna, M.D., unpublished data) for calcium oxalate or calcium phosphate stones, 5 percent had primary hyperparathyroidism, 2 percent had complete RTA, and 5 percent had sarcoidosis.

Constitutional Hypercalciuria The term *constitutional hypercalciuria* refers to patients of large size who appear to be hypercalciuric in absolute terms but are not hypercalciuric relative to weight and who appear to be metabolically normal by detailed evaluation. Expressing calcium excretion on a weight-adjusted basis is the only way to normalize for the wide range of body sizes in the patient population, particularly the size difference between the sexes. In persons whose diets include a 1000-mg daily calcium intake, hypercalciuria exists if daily calcium excretion exceeds 4 mg (0.1 mmol) per kilogram of body weight. When one adjusts calcium excretion for body weight, metabolic evaluation may allow better discrimination. If absolute hyperexcretion of calcium is used as the criterion for metabolic evaluation (groups B, C, and D in Table 25-6), 78 percent of these patients had absorptive hypercalciuria, 14 percent had constituional hypercalciuria, and 8 percent could not be classified. If only patients in whom daily calcium excretion exceeded 4 mg (0.1 mmol) per kilogram of body weight on the defined diet were considered truly hypercalciuric, about 90 percent of these patients would have clear-cut absorptive hypercalciuria.[117,118]

Like any other type of hypercalciuria, constitutional hypercalciuria is a risk factor for calcium stone formation. The volume of urine excreted by patients of large body size is not proportionately larger than that excreted by patients of small size. Thus, like other stone patients, patients with constitutional hypercalciuria should be considered for medical treatment.

TABLE 25-7 Classification of Hypercalciuria

Secondary hypercalciuria due to
- Primary hyperparathyroidism
- Sarcoidosis
- Distal renal tubular acidosis
- Vitamin D excess
- Immobilization, rapidly progressive osteoporosis
- Uncontrolled diabetes mellitus
- Glucocorticoid excess
- Thyrotoxicosis
- Acromegaly
- Furosemide administration

Constitutional hypercalciuria

Dietary hypercalciuria

Idiopathic hypercalciuria
- Resorptive
- Subtle primary hyperparathyroidism
- Renal
- Absorptive

Source: Insogna KL, Broadus AE: Nephrolithiasis, in Felig P, Baxter JD, Broadus AE, Frohman LA (eds): *Endocrinology and Metabolism* 2d ed. New York, McGraw-Hill, 1987, p. 1536.

Dietary Hypercalciuria The 44 patients in groups A and B in Table 25-6 show that hypercalciuria can be profoundly affected by dietary factors besides calcium. Although daily calcium intake was several hundred milligrams higher on the defined diet than on the free diet, mean daily calcium excretion in these 44 patients decreased almost 100 mg on the defined diet.[118] Calcium excretion can be increased by dietary protein, sodium, and carbohydrate and can be decreased by dietary oxalate and phosphate,[2,6,7,11,116,118] although carbohydrate, oxalate, and phosphate appear to be relatively unimportant.

Of the dietary constituents (calcium, protein, sodium) considered to possibly account for dietary hypercalciuria, sodium is the most strongly correlated with calcium excretion. Sodium inhibits the resorption of calcium in the proximal tubule and possibly in more distal segments of the nephron; available evidence suggests that sodium-induced hypercalciuria is renal in origin.[119–121] Hypercalciuric patients studied on a low-calcium, high-sodium diet are in negative calcium balance, and the imposition of a high sodium intake increases fasting calcium excretion.[120] Uncontrolled sodium intake frequently leads to misclassification of patients as having renal hypercalciuria, i.e., as having a primary renal calcium leak.

Increasing sodium intake is commonly believed to increase calcium excretion by only about 25 mg per 100 mEq of sodium in normal subjects, implying that only wide swings in sodium intake have a clinically significant impact on calcium excretion.[120] Considerable disagreement exists about this value; some researchers have reported that the influence of sodium intake on calcium excretion may be as great as 60 to 100 mg (1.5 to 2.5 mmol) of calcium per 100 mEq of sodium in normal persons (those with no stones).[121] Although some disagreement exists about the quantitative influence of sodium intake on calcium excretion, overall sodium intake may have a major effect, and reasonable limits for calcium excretion cannot be defined without close attention to sodium intake, sodium excretion, or both. Furthermore, several investigators have reported that hypercalciuria appeared and disappeared depending on sodium intake.[121,122] In one such study (the results of which are shown in Fig. 25-16), 18 patients previously defined as hypercalciuric on an unrestricted diet were instructed to use a diet containing 500 to 700 mg (12.5 to 17.5 mmol) of calcium and 80 to 200 mEq of sodium.[119] About half the patients were normocalciuric on the 80-mEq-sodium diet. Higher sodium intake caused calcium excretion to increase by a mean of about 100 mg (2.5 mmol) daily.

Some researchers have suggested that idiopathic hypercalciuria results from disordered proximal tubular function. Defects have been shown in proximal tubular resorption of multiple ions, including sodium and calcium.[123,124] Such patients may be more sensitive than normal persons to variations in sodium intake. Whether the slope of calcium excretion vs. sodium intake is steeper in patients who are considered hypercalciuric than in nonhypercalciuric patients with stone disease, normal persons, or both is unclear.

Protein ingestion profoundly influences urinary calcium: Increasing protein ingestion from 0.5 g per kilogram of body weight daily (a restricted intake) to 2 g per kilogram daily (a liberal intake) can double calcium excretion in normal persons.[116] In a study of normal persons, daily dietary protein in the form of red meat was increased from 1 g to 2 g per kilogram of body weight.[19] In addition, the effect of increasing sodium intake from 100 to 310 mEq was measured. Increasing dietary protein or sodium raised urinary calcium by 33 percent; increasing both raised urinary calcium by 73 percent. These dietary manipulations also reduced citrate excretion by 29 percent and increased the tendency for calcium oxalate crystal agglomeration. Breslau and coworkers found that when dietary protein was changed from vegetable sources to animal sources while total dietary protein was kept constant at 75 g/day, urinary calcium increased by half.[125] These investigators postulated that the higher sulfur content of the animal protein diet increased the load of fixed acid and thus caused bone dissolution. This interpretation was supported by reduced urinary cAMP, serum immunoreactive PTH, and 1,25-$(OH)_2D$ and failure to find a compensatory increase in intestinal calcium absorption.

Idiopathic Hypercalciuria As shown in Table 25-7, patients can be subdivided by mechanisms responsible for hypercalciuria. The four subtypes of idiopathic hypercalciuria described here are somewhat unconventional and are outlined to encourage consideration of physiologic mechanisms.

Resorptive Hypercalciuria In resorptive hypercalciuria, a primary disorder associated with increased rates of resorption of bone mineral results in secondary hypercalciuria. Skeletal calcium mobilization increases the ambient concentration of calcium in extracellular fluids, thus suppressing parathyroid function, 1,25-$(OH)_2D$ synthesis, and intestinal calcium absorption as well as increasing the filtered load of calcium; this process is associated with increased fractional calcium excretion resulting from the suppression of PTH (Fig. 25-17). The best-studied example of resorptive hypercalciuria is the immobilization syndrome.[126] Other examples of resorptive hypercalciuria are rapidly progressive osteoporosis, cancer-associated osteolysis, and hyperthyroidism. Hypercalciuria observed in patients with complete distal RTA, primary hyperparathyroidism, glucocorticoid excess, sarcoidosis, and (pos-

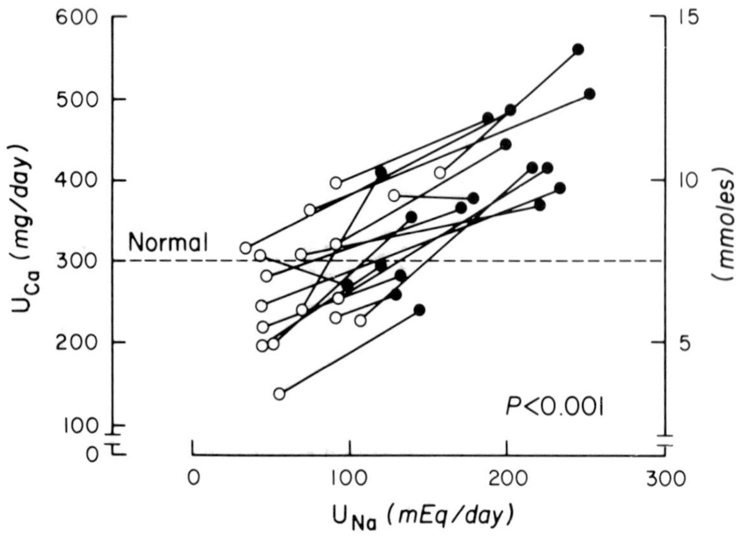

FIGURE 25-16 Twenty-four-hour calcium excretion plotted as a function of sodium excretion in 18 patients first identified as hypercalciuric on a free diet. Patients were allowed 500 to 700 mg of daily calcium; daily sodium intake varied from 80 mEq (open circles) to 200 mEq (closed circles). *(Reproduced by permission of the author and publisher from Muldowney FP, Freaney R, Moloney MF: Importance of dietary sodium in the hypercalciuria syndrome. Kidney Int 22:292–296, 1982.)*

	CALCIUM ABSORPTION	BONE RESORPTION	EXTRACELLULAR CALCIUM	PT FUNCTION	CALCIUM EXCRETION FL	CALCIUM EXCRETION Reab	1,25 (OH)$_2$ D$_3$	SERUM P$_i$
RESORPTIVE HC	↓	[↑]	N, ↑	↓	↑	↓	↓	N, ↑
SUBTLE 1° HPT	↑	↑	N, ↑	[↑]	↑	↑	↑	N, ↓
RENAL HC	↑	N, ↑	N, ↓	↑	↓	[↓]	↑	N, ↓
ABSORPTIVE HC	[↑]	N, ↑	N, ↑	N, ↓	↑	↓	[N, ↑]	N, [↓]

FIGURE 25-17 Pathophysiologic features of four categories or subtypes of hypercalciuria. Features enclosed in rectangle in each subtype denote the known or putative primary pathogenetic defect. Increased intestinal calcium absorption and circulating 1,25-$(OH)_2D$ concentrations as well as a tendency toward hypophosphatemia are common to the three main hypercalciuric subtypes. HC=hypercalciuria; 1°HPT=primary hyperparathyroidism; PT= parathyroid; FL=filtered load; Reab=tubular calcium resorption; P_i=inorganic phosphate. [*Reproduced by permission of the author, editor, and publisher from Insogna KL, Broadus AE: Nephrolithiasis, in Felig P, Baxter JD, Broadus AE, Frohman LA (eds): Endocrinology and Metabolism, 2d ed. New York, McGraw-Hill, 1987, p 1541.*]

sibly) absorptive or renal hypercalciuria (or both) may have a resorptive component (see below).

Subtle Primary Hyperparathyroidism The term *subtle primary hyperparathyroidism* describes the disorder in patients who have a slightly abnormal serum calcium concentration as well as marked hypercalciuria and stone disease. The term *normocalcemic primary hyperparathyroidism* was previously used in describing such patients, but this term should be avoided because these patients usually have a characteristic pattern of intermittent hypercalcemia which deviates 0.5 mg/dl above and below the upper normal limit and a mean fasting serum calcium concentration of about 10.2 to 10.3 mg/dl.[73,127–129] A mean serum calcium concentration in this range should not be considered normal in ambulatory, healthy young adults, especially those with hypercalciuria and stone disease.

Studies have clarified the pathophysiologic features leading to hypercalciuria in patients with primary hyperparathyroidism, particularly those with subtle primary hyperparathyroidism.[127,130] As shown in Table 25-8, the fasting serum calcium concentration in patients A and B was nearly identical, but marked hypercalciuria was present in patient A, who was on an unrestricted-calcium diet and had a history of stones, whereas patient B was normocalciuric and had no stones. The disproportionate hypercalciuria in patient A resulted from the markedly elevated circulating concentration of 1,25-$(OH)_2D$; in contrast, the 1,25-$(OH)_2D$ level was within the normal range in patient B. The disproportionate hypercalciuria in patient A was thus predominantly absorptive in nature and was markedly similar to that observed in patients with absorptive hypercalciuria syndrome, except that the primary pathogenetic abnormality in patient A was parathyroid hyperfunction.

Patient C (Table 25-8) was similar to patient A except that the mean fasting serum calcium concentration was 10.2 mg/dl. Representative measurements of fasting serum calcium concentration during several months were 10.1, 10.3, 10.7, 10.1, and 10.0 mg/dl. Like patient A, patient C had a marked in-

TABLE 25-8 Pathophysiologic Features in Three Patients with Primary Hyperparathyroidism

Feature	Patient A	Patient B	Patient C
Fasting serum calcium concentration (mg/dl)	11.0	11.3	10.2
24-h calcium excretion (mg)	439	275	452
History of renal stones	Yes	No	Yes
Plasma 1,25-$(OH)_2D$ concentration (pg/ml)	90	57	90

Source: Values shown are mean data from Broadus et al.[127,130] Adapted and reproduced by permission of the author and publishers from Broadus AE, Horst RL, Littledike ET, Mahaffey JE, Rasmussen H: Primary hyperparathyroidism with intermittent hypercalcaemia: Serial observations and simple diagnosis by means of an oral calcium tolerance test. *Clin Endocrinol (Oxf)* 12:225–235, 1980; Broadus AE, Horst RL, Lang R, Littledike ET, Rasmussen H: The importance of circulating 1,25-dihydroxyvitamin D in the pathogenesis of hypercalciuria and renal stone formation in primary hyperparathyroidism. *N Engl J Med* 302:421–426, 1980.

crease in circulating 1,25-$(OH)_2D$ concentration, had excessive gastrointestinal tract absorption of calcium, and was hypercalciuric on this basis. Patient C is an extreme case of the disproportionate hypercalciuria which characterizes some patients with primary hyperparathyroidism.[124,130,131]

Subtle primary hyperparathyroidism should be strongly suspected in any hypercalciuric patient with a mean fasting serum calcium concentration >10 mg/dl.

Renal Calcium Leak Patients with a renal leak of calcium (renal hypercalciuria) are considered to have a primary tubular defect in calcium absorption. The increase in fractional calcium excretion in these patients reduces the ambient concentration of ionized calcium, leading to secondary hyperparathyroidism, reduced renal tubular phosphate resorption and serum phosphorus concentration, stimulated 1,25-$(OH)_2D$ synthesis, increased intestinal calcium absorption, and increased mineral resorption from bone (Fig. 25-18). Total hypercalciuria in patients with renal hypercalciuria thus has both renal absorptive and bone resorptive components.

The renal leak hypothesis dates from the 1950s and was the pathogenetic formulation then favored by Henneman and associates.[112] Studies done in the mid-1970s generated considerable evidence to support this hypothesis.[132–134] The most important of these studies historically is that of Coe and associates, who reported increased circulating immunoreactive PTH in two-thirds of hypercalciuric patients and showed that both hypercalciuria and secondary hyperparathyroidism can be reversed by using a thiazide diuretic.[134] The same investigators created a model of renal hypercalciuria in normal subjects by giving them furosemide.[134] Pak and coworkers introduced additional diagnostic criteria for renal hypercalciuria, including increased fasting calcium excretion with abnormal or inappropriate values for serum immunoreactive PTH, total cAMP excretion, or both; these investigators also reported that such abnormalities can be partially reversed using a thiazide diuretic.[133,135,136]

The frequency of renal hypercalciuria and the validity of the criteria for diagnosis remain controversial. What the diagnostic criteria should be is rarely debated. Patients should have both decreased renal calcium absorption and secondary hyperparathyroidism. In practice, this debate focuses mainly on the interpretation of fasting calcium excretion values in hypercalciuric patients.

Most researchers agree that hypercalciuric patients have higher calcium excretion rates than do normal subjects at all levels of calcium intake, including the fasting state.[117,123,124,135] Two laboratories have reported increased fasting fractional calcium excretion in hypercalciuric patients, providing conclusive evidence for a renal calcium leak.[118,137]

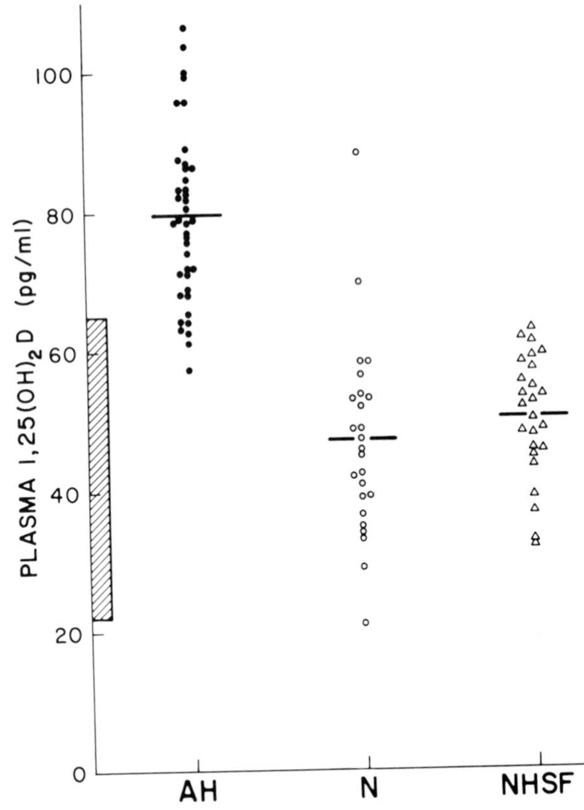

FIGURE 25-18 Plasma 1,25-$(OH)_2D$ concentrations in 50 patients with absorptive hypercalciuria (AH), 25 normal subjects (N), and 25 nonhypercalciuric stone-forming patients (NHSF). All samples were obtained after patients had been on calcium-restricted (400 mg/day), sodium-restricted (about 100 mEq/day) diets for at least 10 days. Horizontal bars represent mean values; hatched bar represents normal range for plasma 1,25-$(OH)_2D$ concentration. *(Reproduced by permission of the author and publisher from Broadus AE, Insogna KL, Lang R, Mallette LE, Oren DA, Gertner JM, Kliger AS, Ellison AF: A consideration of the hormonal basis and phosphate leak hypothesis of absorptive hypercalciuria. J Clin Endocrinol Metab 58:161–169, 1984.)*

However, whether such a "calcium leak" is of primary or secondary pathogenetic importance is unclear.

Several points bear on this controversy. First, a renal calcium leak can be induced in normal subjects by the administration of 1,25-$(OH)_2D$. The sequence of events in this model is 1,25-$(OH)_2D$–induced hyperabsorption of calcium from the intestine, parathyroid suppression, and a resultant increase in fasting fractional calcium excretion.[138,139] Second, identical results were observed in 45 patients with absorptive hypercalciuria.[126] In these patients, a strong correlation was found between the degree of parathyroid suppression in the fasting state and fasting fractional calcium excretion. Third, although fasting calcium excretion was excessive in about half of the hypercalciuric patients studied whose calcium intake was restricted, immunoreactive PTH was normal[118,123,124,140–142] or reduced[137,143–145] in almost all cases. Given the sensitivity of modern parathyroid function tests, it is irrational to regard such patients as having a primary renal calcium leak. Finally, increased sodium intake was reported to increase fasting excretion,[120] yet sodium intake was controlled in only a few published series.[118,136]

Although renal tubular calcium resorption is often reduced in hypercalciuric patients, a renal calcium leak is only rarely of primary pathogenetic importance. The terms *fasting hypercalciuria* and *unclassifiable hypercalciuria* are thus used in describing such patients.[118,136] Using both increased fasting calcium excretion and evidence of secondary hyperparathyroidism as required criteria, one group estimated that renal hypercalciuria accounts for about 10 percent of hypercalciuric patients and that unclassifiable hypercalciuria accounts for about 15 percent.[123,124,146] At the Yale Renal Stone Clinic, patients who fulfill the criteria for primary renal hypercalciuria are exceedingly rare.[118]

Absorptive Hypercalciuria In absorptive hypercalciuria, excessive intestinal absorption of calcium leads to a postprandial increase in extracellular calcium concentration, which both increases the filtered load of calcium and suppresses parathyroid function; the absorbed calcium load is spilled directly into the urine (Fig. 25-18). Suppression of parathyroid function adds a secondary renal component to hypercalciuria in these patients. In patients who have severe absorptive hypercalciuria[118] or are on a rigid calcium-restricted diet,[147] a bone-resorptive component also may exist, but this component is considered neither quantitatively important nor a particular threat to skeletal health.

Postulated mechanisms of absorptive hypercalciuria include (1) hyperabsorption of calcium resulting from a primary intestinal defect, (2) increased circulating 1,25-$(OH)_2D$ concentration resulting from a primary renal phosphate leak, and (3) increased circulating 1,25-$(OH)_2D$ concentration resulting from disordered control of its production. Some patients in whom the production of 1,25-$(OH)_2D$ is disordered may have a fundamental proximal tubular abnormality which results in several presumably related abnormalities, including decreased resorption of phosphate and other ions and increased 1,25-$(OH)_2D$ production. These hypotheses may not be mutually exclusive.

Most of the evidence supporting a primary intestinal abnormality in calcium absorption in patients with absorptive hypercalciuria was found by Pak and coworkers.[133,148–151] Their intestinal perfusion studies revealed selective jejunal hyperabsorption of calcium.[149] In contrast, exogenous 1,25-$(OH)_2D$ increases calcium absorption in both the jejunum and the ileum and stimulates jejunal uptake of magnesium as well as calcium. The intestinal hyperabsorption hypothesis predicts that affected patients should have low circulating 1,25-$(OH)_2D$ values. Although a spectrum of circulating 1,25-$(OH)_2D$ values has been reported in hypercalciuric patients, a subpopulation with low or low-normal values has not been identified.

The frequency with which increased plasma concentration of 1,25-$(OH)_2D$ is observed in patients in whom hypercalciuria has not been classified by metabolic subtype and in patients who are thought to have absorptive hypercalciuria is somewhat controversial.[118,141,142,144,145,151,152] More than 80 percent of patients with absorptive hypercalciuria have frank elevations in circulating 1,25-$(OH)_2D$ concentration; high-normal values are seen in the remaining 20 percent of patients (Fig. 25-19). Issues of patient selection and study conditions generate the most disagreement about the role of 1,25-$(OH)_2D$ in hypercalciuria.

In most studies, patients were both selected and studied while on a free diet. These series reported increased circulating 1,25-$(OH)_2D$ concentrations in about 40 to 50 percent of the patients studied. A study population selected on the basis of calcium excretion while on a free diet would include many patients with dietary and constitutional hypercalciuria; the population of patients with true idiopathic hypercalciuria would thus be considerably diluted. In the series conducted at Yale, the criteria for inclusion were (1) hypercalciuria on a defined high-normal calcium intake, (2) hyperabsorption of calcium as shown by calcium tolerance testing, and (3) normal or low concentration of serum immunoreactive PTH and nephrogenous cAMP.[118] These criteria should substantially increase the number of patients with true "metabolic" idiopathic hypercalciuria in a study population and select for clear-cut instead of borderline cases.

The studies described reveal the importance of dietary calcium as a determinant of circulating 1,25-$(OH)_2D$ concentration (Fig. 25-19). On a low-calcium diet, most hypercalciuric patients had elevated levels of 1,25-$(OH)_2D$, and segregation of plasma 1,25-$(OH)_2D$ values in hypercalciuric and nonhypercalciuric patients was nearly complete. In contrast, the 1,25-$(OH)_2D$ levels of patients on the high-normal 1000-mg (25-mmol) calcium diet were reduced into the normal range in hypercalciuric patients, and overlap of the values between the two groups was nearly complete. Thus, although these short-term studies do not necessarily reflect steady-state conditions,[153] such studies emphasize the need to study patients in defined conditions.

Absorptive hypercalciuria in most cases may be viewed as a 1,25-$(OH)_2D$–mediated syndrome. Increased circulating 1,25-$(OH)_2D$ concentrations in these patients have also been shown to result from increased production of the hormone.[154] What mechanisms lead to increased 1,25-$(OH)_2D$ production?

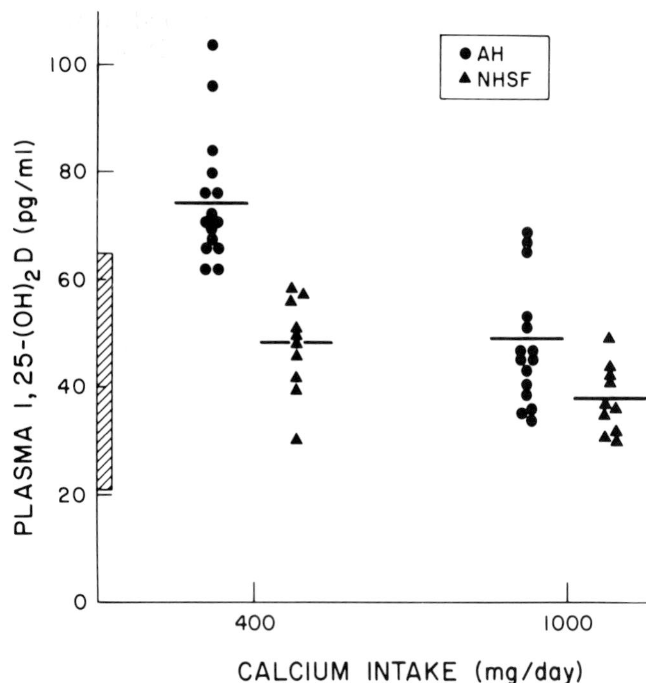

FIGURE 25-19 Values for plasma 1,25-$(OH)_2D$ concentrations in 15 patients with absorptive hypercalciuria (AH) (circles) and 10 nonhypercalciuric stone-forming patients (NHSF) (triangles) studied on a 400-mg daily calcium diet and again 3 days after being placed on a 1000-mg daily calcium diet. Daily sodium intake was controlled at about 100 mEq. Horizontal bars represent mean values, and cross-hatched bar represents normal range for plasma 1,25-$(OH)_2D$ concentration. Note marked suppressibility of plasma 1,25-$(OH)_2D$ concentrations in patients with absorptive hypercalciuria as well as extensive overlap between the values for the two groups on 100-mg daily calcium diet. *(Reproduced by permission of the author and publisher from Broadus AE, Insogna KL, Lang R, Ellison AF, Dreyer BE: Evidence for disordered control of 1,25-dihydroxyvitamin D production in absorptive hypercalciuria. N Engl J Med 311:73–80, 1984.)*

The phosphate leak hypothesis holds that the primary pathogenetic abnormality in patients with absorptive hypercalciuria is a renal tubular leak of phosphate; the resultant hypophosphatemia stimulates 1-hydroxylase activity and thus stimulates 1,25-$(OH)_2D$ synthesis.[155]

Evidence supporting the phosphate leak hypothesis includes (1) a tendency toward hypophosphatemia in some hypercalciuric patients,[112,123,142,152] (2) an increase in circulating 1,25-$(OH)_2D$ concentrations observed in normal subjects in response to a phosphopenic stimulus,[142,156] (3) a statistically significant inverse correlation between plasma concentration of 1,25-$(OH)_2D$ and serum phosphorus concentration in hypercalciuric patients compared with normal subjects,[142,145,152] and (4) partial reversal of elements of the syndrome in patients treated with oral phosphate.[141,145,157] A phosphate leak in such patients is apparently not a fixed abnormality because the serum phosphorus concentration has normal diurnal variation; in the early afternoon, values approach those found in normal subjects.[158]

Evidence against the phosphate leak hypothesis includes (1) the comparative rarity with which hypophosphatemia is observed in hypercalciuric patients,[124,144,157,159] (2) a tendency of stone patients to manifest hypophosphatemia without hypercalciuria,[118,150,158,160] and (3) the hypocalciuric response to phosphate treatment, which is not proportional to pretreatment serum phosphorus concentration.[141,145,160]

The aggregate data can be interpreted in three ways. First, the relation of serum phosphorus concentration to hypercalciuria and specifically to 1,25-$(OH)_2D$ production is a classic example of "guilt by association" in that no direct pathogenic link exists between these abnormalities. Second, absorptive hypercalciuria is pathogenetically heterogeneous; certain patients have hypophosphatemic absorptive hypercalciuria, whereas 1,25-$(OH)_2D$ production is increased in others on some other basis. Third, phosphate loss and disordered control of 1,25-$(OH)_2D$ may be due to a fundamental proximal tubular lesion.

The disordered control hypothesis has received attention only recently and is suggested by the extreme sensitivity of circulating 1,25-$(OH)_2D$ concentration to variations in calcium intake among patients with absorptive hypercalciuria. More direct evidence is provided by the response in these patients when a high-normal calcium diet is continued for several weeks: An apparent "escape" phenomenon is observed, with a rebound increase in circulating 1,25-$(OH)_2D$ level and a pronounced decrease in the tubular maximum for phosphate/glomerular filtration rate (TmP/GFR).[153] Hypercalciuric patients may have numerous abnormalities in proximal tubular function, including defective resorption of calcium, phosphate, sodium, magnesium, and fluid.[123,124,161] However, debate remains as to the specificity of these findings in hypercalciuric vs. nonhypercalciuric patients.

A hypothesis which would explain increased 1,25-$(OH)_2D$ production, the tendency toward hypophosphatemia, and the marked sensitivity to dietary calcium intake in hypercalciuric patients is that such patients are hypersensitive to the proximal tubular effects of PTH.[153] However, no direct evidence supports this hypothesis.

The disordered control hypothesis for absorptive hypercalciuria pathogenesis is suggested by numerous observations and is favored, in various forms, by several current investigators. The evidence is insufficient to substantiate this hypothesis.

Bone Effects in Hypercalciuria

Overt bone disease causing fracture, bone pain, or deformity is rare in hypercalciuric patients. Evidence has been reported of subclinical bone effects in hypercalciuric patients, including abnormal bone histomorphometry,[162,163] an increased bone turnover rate on the basis of calcium kinetic data,[164] and increased hydroxyproline excretion in a small percentage of patients.[118,132] The data in these studies are difficult to summarize because the selection criteria varied. Histomorphometric abnormalities were found in patients thought to have absorptive hypercalciuria[132,165] or renal hypercalciuria.[132] Secondary hyperparathyroidism, hypophosphatemia, an increased circulating 1,25-$(OH)_2D$ concentration, or a combination of these variables would predictably affect the skeleton; however, a history of kidney stones in patients with osteoporosis is rare. Because clinical bone disease is not the predictable consequence of any common form of hypercalciuria, routine radiologic assessment of bone density is not warranted in these patients.

Hyperoxaluria

Although oxalate is the major anionic constituent of calcium stones, patients rarely manifest disorders of oxalate metabolism. However, relatively subtle abnormalities in oxalate metabolism could easily pass undetected because until recently, methods for measuring urinary oxalate were inaccurate. Subtle abnormalities could have a major impact on the tendency for calcium stone formation because of the extreme insolubility of oxalate in aqueous solution. Calcium stone disease could be better controlled if oxalate production could be inhibited in a way analogous to the inhibition of uric acid synthesis by allopurinol or if oxalate could be complexed in a way analogous to the penicillamine-cysteine disulfide (see Treatment of Hyperoxaluria, below).

Oxalate Metabolism

Oxalate is a metabolic end product and serves no known function. Although it forms numerous complexes and salts in urine, oxalate is clinically relevant because of the insolubility of its calcium salt. The metabolic pool of oxalate is derived from intestinal absorption and endogenous production.[166,167] Oxalate is absorbed throughout the small intestine and large intestine by diffusion.[166–169] This process, which was first considered simple, passive diffusion, occurs via a facilitated anion exchange mechanism.[169] When a simple isotopic solution of oxalate is given to a patient in the fasting state, about 15 percent is absorbed. However, only 5 to 10 percent is absorbed from foods. We lack good methods for measuring oxalate in food, and our knowledge of dietary oxalate content is limited. Depending on dietary habits and the particular food table used, estimates of typical adult daily intake of oxalate vary from 100 to 900 mg (1111 to 9999 μmol).[166] Table 25-9 lists foods believed to have a high oxalate content. Even less is known about the bioavailability of oxalate in foods and beverages.

The two main metabolic sources of oxalate are ascorbic acid and glyoxylate (Fig. 25-20).[166,167,170] The metabolism of ascorbic acid accounts for about 30 percent of daily oxalate production and excretion, but the exact metabolic pathway responsible for ascorbic acid oxidation is unknown. Glyoxylate oxidation accounts for most other oxalate production. Lactic dehydrogenase is the most important enzyme in the conversion of glyoxylate to oxalate. Much of the metabolic pool of glyoxylate is also transaminated to glycine by an enzyme that requires pyridoxine (vitamin B_6) as a cofactor. Another important

TABLE 25-9 Some Common Foods Rich in Oxalate

Vegetables	Fruits	Starches	Miscellaneous
Beans, green	Blackberries	Fruit cake	Chocolate
Beans, dried	Blueberries	Grits, corn	Cocoa
Beets	Currants, red	Soy crackers	Peanut butter
Eggplant	Grapes, Concord	Wheat germ	Pecans
Green pepper	Peels, citrus		Tofu (soy curd)
Greens*	Raspberries		
Okra	Rhubarb		
Parsley	Strawberries		
Potato, sweet	Tangerines		
Rutabagas			
Squash, summer			
Watercress			

* Dark green leafy vegetables such as chard, kale, spinach, beet greens and collard greens.

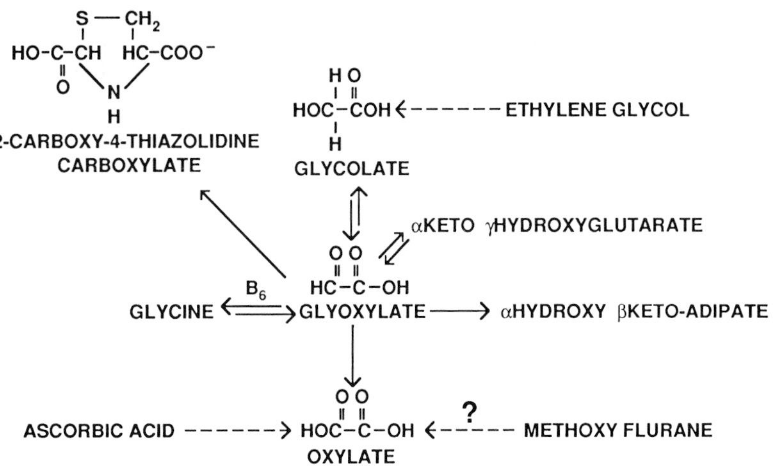

FIGURE 25-20 Pathways of oxalate metabolism. [*Adapted and reproduced by permission of the author and publisher from Dobbins JW, Binder HJ: Derangements of oxalate metabolism in gastrointestinal disease and their mechanisms, in Glass GBJ (ed): Progress in Gastroenterology. New York, Grune & Stratton, 1977, vol 3, pp 505–518.*]

pathway in glyoxylate metabolism is the formation of α-hydroxy-β-ketoadipate from α-ketoglutarate and glyoxylate. A deficiency of the enzyme (2-oxoglutarate:glyoxylate carboligase) responsible for this process occurs in primary hyperoxaluria type 1.[166,167,170]

Although a small amount of oxalate is present in bile and intestinal secretions, the principal route of elimination of oxalate from the extracellular pool is excretion into the urine. Circulating oxalate is filtered freely at the glomerulus. In all species studied, fractional excretion of oxalate exceeds unity, indicating net tubular secretion of oxalate.[166,167,171]

Classification of Hyperoxaluric States

Hyperoxaluria is conventionally classified as a disorder associated with either increased endogenous oxalate production or increased oxalate absorption (Table 25-10).

TABLE 25-10 Classification and Causes of Hyperoxaluria

Increased endogenous oxalate production
Primary hyperoxaluria, types 1 and 2
Administration or increased intake of oxalate precursors
Ethylene glycol
Methoxyflurane
Ascorbic acid
Pyridoxylate
Pyridoxine deficiency
Increased oxalate intake or absorption (or both)
Excessive dietary oxalate
Enteric hyperoxaluria
Low calcium intake
Hyperabsorption of calcium

Source: Modified and reproduced by permission of the author, editor, and publisher from Insogna KL, Broadus AE: Nephrolithiasis, in Felig P, Baxter JD, Broadus AE, Frohman LA (eds): *Endocrinology and Metabolism*, 2d ed. New York, McGraw-Hill, 1987, p. 1557.

All forms of primary hyperoxaluria are rare inborn errors of oxalate metabolism and are the most malignant crystal deposition diseases known.[166,167,170] Type 1 hyperoxaluria (glycolic aciduria), inherited as an autosomal recessive trait, results from deficiency of the soluble carboligase that converts glyoxylate to α-hydroxy-β-ketoadipate (Fig. 25-20). This deficiency results in the accumulation of glyoxylate and increased production and excretion of glyoxylate, oxalate, and glycolate. Heterozygotes are clinically unaffected and cannot be identified by chemical screening. Type 2 hyperoxaluria (glyceric aciduria) results from a deficiency of glyceric dehydrogenase, an enzyme active in the gluconeogenic pathway of serine metabolism.[166,167,170] The mechanism by which a deficiency of this enzyme leads to increased production of oxalate is unknown. Affected patients have increased rates of glyceric acid and oxalate excretion and decreased rates of glyoxylate and glycolate excretion. Few patients with the type 2 syndrome have been described; the mechanism of inheritance is unknown but is presumed to be autosomal recessive.

Patients with type 1 hyperoxaluria typically have calcium oxalate stones in early childhood, usually before age 6 years. In addition to particularly virulent, recurrent stone formation, deposits of oxalate (oxalosis) also usually develop in soft tissue, including the heart, blood vessels, central nervous system, bone marrow, and kidney. Most untreated patients die before age 20 years of renal insufficiency produced by stone complications, infections, and oxalosis-induced interstitial nephritis. Patients with type 2 hyperoxaluria have recurrent calcium oxalate stones at an early age, but soft tissue oxalosis does not occur. Hyperoxaluric patients who are seen for calcium oxalate stones in adulthood are described occasionally; some researchers speculate that such patients may have a mild form of primary hyperoxaluria.

The enzyme alcohol dehydrogenase initiates the conversion of ethylene glycol to oxalate (Fig. 25-20). A common ingredient in antifreeze preparations and industrial solvents, ethylene glycol is a rare cause of poisoning from accidental or intentional ingestion. Poisoning produces massive hyperoxaluria and oxalosis, commonly resulting in acute renal failure and death.

The anesthetic agent methoxyflurane is partially metabolized to oxalate in the liver. Acute renal failure after methoxyflurane anesthesia is occasionally reported and apparently results from hyperoxaluria and renal oxalosis.[166,167]

Oxidation of ascorbic acid normally accounts for much of the endogenous production of oxalate. "Megadoses" of ascorbic acid increase endogenous oxalate production and excretion, although such an increase may have no clinical effect.[106] Ingestion of vitamin C has been reported to possibly exacerbate stone disease, and its use is discouraged in stone patients.[107] Whether taking megadoses of ascorbic acid increases the prevalence of stone disease in the general population is unclear.

Pyridoxine is a cofactor in the transamination of glyoxylate to glycine (Fig. 25-20), and pyridoxine deficiency has been reported to increase oxalate production and excretion in humans and experimental animals.[166,167] Clinical examples of this association, however, are rare. Pharmacologic doses of pyridoxine are used as therapy in patients with calcium stone disease in an attempt to force the transamination reaction toward glycine, thus reducing the conversion of glyoxylate to oxalate. Pyridoxilate, a drug combination containing glyoxylate and pyridoxine, was used in some European countries for treating coronary heart disease until calcium oxalate lithiasis developed in some of the patients receiving this drug.[172] Although 435 mg of pyridoxine was included in the daily dose of the drug, patients excreted twice as much oxalate when taking the drug than they did when it was withdrawn.

Because of poor total intestinal absorption of oxalate from foods, frank hyperoxaluria rarely results solely from excessive oxalate intake. Massive ingestion of one or more of the foods considered high in oxalate content (Table 25-9) occurs only in persons with unusual dietary habits and is usually readily identified by dietary history. Rhubarb gluttony is often cited as causing dietary hyperoxaluria.[166]

Enteric hyperoxaluria, by far the most common and clinically important hyperoxaluric state, is identified in 2 to 5 percent of patients seen for calcium oxalate stones.[2,6,7,165–167] The frequency of stone disease in patients with chronic inflammatory bowel disease is estimated to be about double the frequency in the general population. Enteric hyperoxaluria was described as a distinct entity in the early 1970s.[173] Hyperoxaluria and a predisposition to calcium stone disease were associated with various gastrointestinal conditions, including regional enteritis, nontropical sprue, chronic pancreatic and biliary tract disease, blind loop syndrome, and ileal resection or jejunoileal bypass.[166–168,174] Calcium oxalate stones were particularly common in patients after jejunoileal bypass surgery for obesity, occurring with a reported frequency of 17 to 32 percent. Ulcerative colitis is not associated with enteric hyperoxaluria.

The main abnormality in affected patients is increased intestinal oxalate absorption[174] related directly to fat malabsorption and steatorrhea. The colon is the major site of oxalate absorption[166–168]: Enteric hyperoxaluria is found in jejunoileal bypass patients in whom only a small percentage of the small intestine's absorptive surface is functional.[168] The terms *colonic hyperoxaluria* and *absorptive hyperoxaluria* are thus equally descriptive synonyms for this disorder.

Two hypotheses may explain increased colonic oxalate absorption in patients with enteric hyperoxaluria. The *solubility theory* holds that malabsorbed fatty acids bind calcium and keep it within the intestine, decreasing the quantity of calcium oxalate formed and freeing more oxalate for passive absorption. The *permeability theory* holds that exposure of the colonic mucosa to unabsorbed bile acids and fatty acids produces a nonspecific increase in the diffusion of oxalate across the mucosa. Considerable evidence supports each of these hypotheses, and both mechanisms probably apply.[166–168] In addition, patients with enteric disorders may have other stone risk factors, including intestinal fluid loss and low urine volume, malabsorption of magnesium with hypomagnesuria, reduced pyrophosphate excretion, and hypocitraturia.[166,175]

Moderately increased oxalate excretion is observed in patients with calcium stone disease who show no evidence of primary or enteric hyperoxaluria.[166,176–178] Reported daily excretion rates in these patients are only slightly elevated, in the range of 50 to 80 mg (556 to 889 μmol). Nevertheless, oxalate is believed to have a relatively greater impact than calcium on urine supersaturation; moderate increases in oxalate excretion could thus represent an important risk factor for stone formation. Several mechanisms might explain the observed variable and moderate increases in oxalate excretion. First, patients with recurrent calcium stone disease are almost always instructed to avoid dietary calcium, and reduced calcium in the intestinal lumen may enable more oxalate absorption. Second, patients with increased intestinal calcium absorption and hypercalciuria show a coincident increase in oxalate absorption.[178,179] This mechanism was shown directly in normal subjects in whom absorptive hypercalciuria was created by the administration of 1,25-$(OH)_2D$.[180] Increased oxalate absorption and excretion are particularly evident in hypercalciuric patients who are on a calcium-restricted diet[178–181] or who are treated with calcium-binding agents such as cellulose phosphate.[182,183]

Hyperuricosuria

Identification of Hyperuricosuric Calcium Oxalate Lithiasis Syndrome

An apparent association between calcium stone disease and clinical gout, hyperuricemia, or both was first reported in the late 1960s.[53,184] In 1968, Gutman and Yü reported that subjects with gouty arthritis tended to form calcium-containing calculi; in that series, 8 percent of calculi were composed of calcium oxalate, 4 percent were composed of calcium phosphate, and 4 percent were admixtures of calcium and uric acid.[53] Hyperuricosuria, not hyperuricemia, was subsequently recognized as a risk factor for calcium stone formation; this clinical syndrome was termed *hyperuricosuric calcium oxalate nephrolithiasis*.[2,7,185,186]

Crystallographic identification of mixed calcium-uric stones is unusual; 4 to 8 percent of patients with clinical stone disease have mixed stones or have a history of passing both calcium oxalate and uric acid stones.[187] Patients in whom mixed calculi form resemble patients with uric acid lithiasis but usually are older, are often Asian, and excrete acidic urine.[188]

The strongest evidence for the role of uric acid in calcium oxalate lithiasis is the effectiveness of allopurinol in preventing calcium oxalate stones among the subset of patients with isolated hyperuricosuria.[189–193] Numerous hypotheses, none of them adequate, explaining why hyperuricosuria is a risk factor for calcium oxalate stone lithiasis are reviewed below.

Definition and Prevalence of Hyperuricosuria

About a third of patients with calcium stones are hyperuricosuric.[2,7,186] About half also have hypercalciuria. In most hyperuricosuric patients with calcium stone disease, hyperuricosuria is mild; only about 15 percent of patients excrete more than 1000 mg (5.9 mmol) daily. In addition, mild hyperuricosuria is frequently intermittent, presumably because of dietary variation.

Two mechanisms may account for hyperuricosuria in patients with calcium stone disease: (1) uric acid overproduction and (2) gluttony for a purine-rich diet. Coe emphasized the clinical significance of excessive purine intake by such patients.[2,186] He found by diet survey that purine intake was about 70 percent higher in hyperuricosuric calcium stone patients than in a control population. In addition, restricting purine intake eliminated hyperuricosuria in 70 percent of these patients, suggesting that only 30 percent had true overproduction of uric acid.

Most epidemiologic studies, when comparing normal patients with those who have calcium oxalate nephrolithiasis, did not find an increased prevalence of hyperuricosuria among stone patients.[51,110,194–197] However, by examining urinary uric acid saturation of urine specimens passed in the early morning, Tiselius and Larsson found that 63 percent of patients with calcium oxalate nephrolithiasis had uric acid supersaturation.[198] This highly unstable situation resulted mainly from the transient decrease in urinary pH and partly from more highly concentrated urine in the early morning.

Does hyperuricosuria increase the severity of calcium oxalate nephrolithiasis? Stone recurrence rates of hyperuricosuric patients are not higher than rates observed in stone patients with other metabolic profiles.[188,194,199] Whereas some researchers have found that hyperuricosuria is frequently associated with past calculus surgery,[194,199] others have reported the opposite.[188] Although hyperuricosuric patients may have one or more additional risk factors for calcium stone formation, combined abnormalities do not influence the severity of stone disease.[2,186,188]

Several hypotheses could explain the pathogenetic relation between hyperuricosuria and the formation of calcium stones. Lonsdale first reported similarities in lattice structure among crystals of calcium oxalate monohydrate, calcium oxalate dihydrate, uric acid, and monosodium urate and suggested that epitaxy may occur between any of these crystal pairs.[200] Investigators have induced heterogeneous nucleation and crystal growth of calcium oxalate by both uric acid and monosodium urate.[2,7,186,201–203]

An alternative hypothesis is that crystals of uric acid or monosodium urate may adsorb normally occurring macromolecular inhibitors of calcium oxalate crystallization.[204–207] Microcrystalline or colloidal urates have not been found in urine, and more recent experiments thus refute this hypothesis.[208,209]

The most probable cause of the observed interaction between uric acid and calcium oxalate is a simple "salting-out" effect. Pak and associates reported that oral purine loading is associated with a reduction of the calcium oxalate formation product.[55] In the same study, allopurinol treatment slowed calcium oxalate crystallization and crystal growth. Ryall and coworkers showed that uric acid in solution reduces the calcium oxalate formation product.[208] Increasing urinary urate by 3 to 4 mmol/L doubled calcium oxalate crystal volume and created a marked tendency for these crystals to aggregate into large masses.

Allopurinol is effective in reducing stone recurrence only in calcium oxalate stone patients in whom hyperuricosuria is the only metabolic abnormality. In four of five trials in which allopurinol was given to such patients,[189–193] recurrence rates were low (Table 25-11). In a double-blind, placebo-controlled study, subjects receiving allopurinol 300 mg daily had 51 percent fewer recurrences than subjects treated with

TABLE 25-11 Outcomes of Clinical Trials Using Allopurinol Unselectively or Selectively

Reference	No. Patients Given Allopurinol	Selective Therapy*	Annual Recurrence, %
Ahmad and associates[210]	24	No	Placebo†
Fellström and associates[211]	31	No	28
Marangella and associates[212]	34	No	Advice†
Robertson and associates[213]	12	No	Advice†
Scott and associates[214]	33	No	17
Smith[215]	49	No	20
Sonoda and associates[216]	134	No	30
Tiselius and associates[217]	99	No	15
Ulshöfer and associates[218]	70	No	9
Wilson and associates[219]	17	No	25
Coe[190]	48	Yes	4
Ettinger and associates[189]	29	Yes	11
Oka and associates[192]	44	Yes	20
Okada and associates[191]	15	Yes	12
Pak[193]	21	Yes	8

* Allopurinol was given selectively only to those showing hyperuricosuria without hypercalciuria.

† Data are insufficient for calculations of rate, but no differences were noted between allopurinol treatment and placebo or general advice.

Source: Adapted and reproduced by permission of the publisher from Ettinger B: Does hyperuricosuria play a role in calcium oxalate lithiasis? *J Urol* 141:738–741, 1989.

placebo (Fig. 25-21),[189] and the growth of preexisting calculi was 39 percent less frequent in patients receiving allopurinol. In 10 other clinical trials[210–219] that were reviewed recently,[188] allopurinol was given to patients with calcium oxalate lithiasis regardless of the urinary metabolic profile; 9 of 10 trials showed no benefit (Table 25-11). Allopurinol and its metabolites do not affect calcium oxalate crystallization or solubility in vitro,[220,221] and numerous studies have shown that allopurinol does not alter levels of calcium or oxalate.[54,212,217,222] Both laboratory and clinical trial results provide compelling evidence for a specific metabolic effect that is mediated through uric acid.

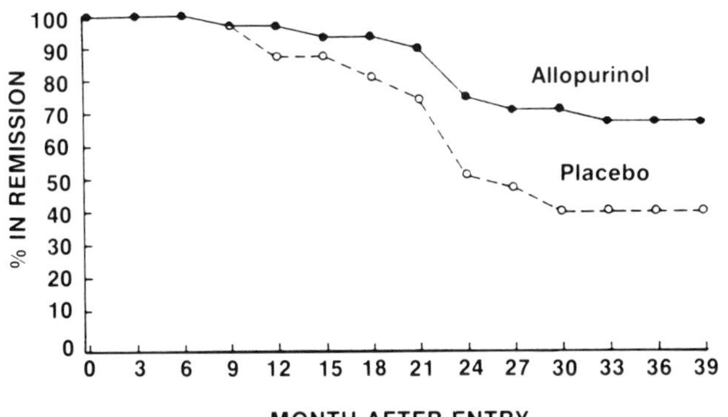

FIGURE 25-21 Life-table plot showing proportion of patients with no calculus events during treatment with allopurinol or placebo. *(Reproduced by permission of the publisher from Ettinger B, Tang A, Citron JT, Livermore B, Williams T: Randomized trial of allopurinol in the prevention of calcium oxalate calculi. N Engl J Med 315:1386–1389, 1986.)*

Hypocitraturia

Various conditions associated with disturbances in acid-base balance are accompanied by hypocitraturia. Among these conditions, distal RTA and enteric hyperoxaluria have received the most attention.

In distal RTA, renal tubular dysfunction leads to systemic acidosis and hypocitraturia.[223] In enteric hyperoxaluria, multiple factors have been implicated in contributing to hypocitraturia. In many patients, metabolic acidosis is caused by bicarbonate losses from the gastrointestinal tract. In other patients, a combination of factors, including hypocitratemia, a reduced renal filtered load, and increased renal citrate resorption due to hypomagnesuria, may contribute to hypocitraturia.[175]

Acetazolamide induces exogenous RTA accompanied by hypocitraturia (see Calcium Phosphate Stones, above).[224] Potassium depletion causes intracellular metabolic acidosis in the renal cortex and is also associated with hypocitraturia.[225]

Many reports describe hypocitraturia in patients with calcium oxalate nephrolithiasis who have normal acid-base status and do not have gastrointestinal disease; prevalence estimates range from 15 to 40 percent.[226–229] In the largest series to date, which studied both men and women, no relation was found between the severity of stone disease and 24-h excretion of citrate, calcium, or both combined.[227] In contrast, Parks and Coe found that compared with normal women, those with stones excreted about 25 percent less citrate.[229] Such differences were not found between normal men and men with calcium stones. Using discriminant analysis, the investigators found that stone risk depended more on the excess of calcium over citrate content than on absolute calcium and citrate concentrations. This "imbalance" theory, though provocative, remains untested.

A major difficulty in assessing the importance of hypocitraturia in calcium stone formation is that most studies do not control for the many dietary factors that may influence citrate excretion. Urinary citrate excretion may vary considerably; in one study, the citrate level was elevated on one occasion but normal on another in about two-thirds of the subjects.[227]

Metabolism of Citrate

Although the average American diet contains about 4 g of citrate, dietary citrate appears to have little influence on final urinary citrate content.

Both filtered at the glomerulus and extracted from peritubular blood, citrate is the most abundant organic acid found in urine. Citrate is metabolized extensively by the kidneys. Metabolic alkalosis induces a prompt, dramatic increase in citrate excretion. Although several processes contribute to this effect, the primary mechanism appears to be inhibition of citrate metabolism in renal tubular cells. Conversely, systemic acidosis is associated with decreased citrate excretion, which results partly from an increased rate of renal citrate metabolism.[230]

Effect of Citrate on Urinary Crystallization

By complexing about half the total urinary calcium, citrate reduces the saturation of urine by calcium oxalate and brushite. Citrate also increases the limits of metastability for these two salts, tending to decrease their tendency to nucleate spontaneously.[231] Citrate may have other salutary effects on one or more steps in crystal growth. Using an artificial crystal growth system, Kok and associates found that citrate therapy doubled both urinary excretion of citrate and the ability of urine to inhibit crystal agglomeration.[232]

Clinical Trials of Citrate Therapy

In one study, treatment with potassium citrate for periods ranging from 1 year to 4 years decreased the stone formation rate in almost all the 89 patients studied.[233] These patients were heterogeneous, and hypocitraturic calcium oxalate stone disease was associated with various metabolic abnormalities; even in patients with no diarrheal syndromes or RTA, the response to treatment was impressive. In another study, 13 patients with hypercalciuria which was apparently refractory to thiazide therapy were found to be hypocitraturic; stone disease in these patients responded clinically to potassium citrate supplementation.[234]

No Metabolic Abnormality: Idiopathic Calcium Oxalate Stones

In the older biomedical literature, the term *idiopathic calcium oxalate stone disease* was used frequently as a synonym for calcium stone disease in general, presumably because stone pathogenesis was viewed as enigmatic in all patients. However, meticulous evaluation should identify one or more risk factors for stone formation in about 80 to 90 percent of patients with recurrent calcium stone disease. The term *idiopathic calcium stone disease* now is used to describe only cases in which no clinical risk factors for stone formation can be identified.

In patients with idiopathic calcium stone disease, the natural history and morbidity of stone formation do not differ from those observed in patients with well-recognized risk factors for stone formation.

Evaluation: Calcium Oxalate Stones

The first section of this chapter gives recommendations for urine collection and biochemical tests.

Evaluating Hypercalciuria

When one is screening for hypercalciuria, samples must be collected both while patients are on a free diet and while they are on a high-normal calcium diet. This approach maximizes the detection of hypercalciuria and also provides some information about its pathogenesis, particularly in dietary hypercalciuria. The high-normal calcium diet is easily adapted for outpatient use by instructing patients to limit their intake of calcium, protein, and sodium and by giving them calcium supplements in tablet form. Patients should be instructed to (1) limit protein intake to about 1 g per kilogram of body weight daily (Table 25-2), (2) limit sodium intake to about 100 mEq daily by avoiding salty foods and adding no salt, (3) eliminate all milk products from the diet (limiting dietary calcium to about 400 to 500 mg daily), and (4) supplement the diet with calcium gluconate tablets 2 g three times daily with meals [adding 540 mg (13.5 mmol) of elemental calcium]. Calcium tablets should be chewed thoroughly before being swallowed. The use of dairy products instead of calcium tablets is not recommended because the protein content of milk may have little effect on calcium excretion and because no normative data are available. One day of equilibration on the diet should precede each urine collection.

Hypercalciuria in patients on a free calcium diet is usually defined as a calcium excretion rate exceeding 300 mg (7.5 mmol) daily in men and 250 mg (6.2 mmol) daily in women.[116,118] By these criteria, hypercalciuria is found in about 40 percent of patients with calcium nephrolithiasis.[2,6,7,93,100,105] Calcium excretion can be expressed on a weight-adjusted basis as well; hypercalciuria is defined as calcium exceeding 4 mg (0.1 mmol) per kilogram of body weight daily in men, women, and children. We recommend using both absolute and weight-adjusted limits and considering a patient hypercalciuric if either limit is exceeded. The most useful definition is calcium exceeding 4 mg (0.1 mmol) per kilogram of body weight daily; in patients in whom this limit is exceeded on a defined high-normal calcium diet, a true disorder of calcium metabolism is highly probable.

Some investigators continue to employ a calcium-restricted diet in screening patients for hypercalciuria, and a daily calcium excretion rate >200 mg in a patient on a 400-mg calcium diet is considered abnormal.[10,132,133,135] We do not recommend that 24-h urine samples be collected for patients on either restricted or unrestricted calcium diets to measure the impact of calcium intake on calcium excretion or to assess the potential benefit of therapeutic restriction of dietary calcium. Such an approach is not optimal in regard to either specificity or sensitivity (Fig. 25-14).

Evaluating Subtle Hyperparathyroidism

An essential goal of diagnosis is to identify patients with subtle primary hyperparathyroidism. This diagnosis (see Chap. 23) should be considered if mean total fasting serum calcium concentration exceeds 10 mg/dl (2.5 mmol/L) on more than one occasion. In most clinical laboratories, serum calcium is determined using an autochemistry method; the usual upper limits are 10.2 to 10.3 mg/dl (2.54 to 2.57 mmol/L). The borderline to elevated serum calcium level should be confirmed by measurement of the serum ionized calcium. The diagnosis of primary hyperparathyroidism in these patients depends on the simultaneous finding of intermittent hypercalcemia and elevated or clearly inappropriate serum PTH levels determined by a sensitive PTH assay. Recently improved immunoreactive PTH assays have eliminated many of the problems encountered with older assays. The calcium tolerance test is rarely necessary, and the thiazide challenge test is unpredictable and nonspecific. Parathyroid ultrasound, venous sampling, and other such techniques are useful for localization but not for diagnosis. The data must be interpreted with great care; needless and inappropriate neck explorations should not be done in patients in whom hyperparathyroidism is suspected and confirmatory biochemical evidence is not found.

Evaluating Dietary Hypercalciuria

Dietary hypercalciuria is most easily detected by having patients collect specimens while on both a free diet and a defined diet. Sodium should be measured in the free intake specimen; excretion >100 mEq daily is considered excessive. Dietary hypercalciuria may account for the wide swings in calcium excretion observed in some "hypercalciuric" patients.

Evaluating Subtypes of Hypercalciuria

After secondary forms of hypercalciuria, dietary hypercalciuria, and subtle primary hyperparathyroidism have been excluded, are further diagnostic measures warranted to distinguish renal from absorptive hypercalciuria? Although the literature reflects disagreement on this point, the pragmatic answer is probably no. Absorptive hypercalciuria is the most common subtype of idiopathic hypercalciuria, primary renal hypercalciuria is rare, and clinical bone disease does not appear to result from either renal or absorptive hypercalciuria. The differential diagnosis is extremely subtle and may necessitate the use of techniques that are not usually available. Empiric therapy with a thiazide is equally effective in each hypercalciuric subtype.

However, a more precise understanding by both patients and physicians of the underlying pathophysiology clarifies the rationale and improves compliance with long-term therapy. For clinicians who intend to conduct such testing, we describe the method.

Appropriate study conditions are crucial to obtaining accurate data. For 10 days before testing, patients should be on a diet restricted in both calcium [about 400 mg/day (10 mmol/day)] and sodium (about 100 mEq/day).[117–119] Compliance should be monitored by 24-h urine collection and determination of calcium and sodium excretion on the day before testing.

The diagnosis of a primary renal calcium leak requires the demonstration of both increased fasting calcium excretion (or fasting fractional calcium excretion) and an elevated serum immunoreactive PTH concentration.

Diagnosing absorptive hypercalciuria requires evidence that a patient absorbs calcium excessively and has normal or depressed parathyroid function. Means of demonstrating excessive gastrointestinal absorption of calcium include a calcium tolerance test and the collection of 24-h urine samples on both a calcium-restricted and unrestricted diet.

Performing the Calcium Tolerance Test

Figure 25-22 shows a flow diagram of the calcium tolerance test and lists data which can be derived from the test. Patients must fast, ingesting only distilled water, for 10 to 12 h before the test. Hourly ingestion of 8 oz of distilled water begins 1 h before the urine is first voided and discarded ($t = 0$) and ends 1 h before the test is completed. An oral dose of about 1000 mg (25 mmol) of elemental calcium (given as 35 ml calcium glubionate syrup plus 8 oz of milk) is given promptly after the first collection period (instead of water). Lactase-treated milk or syn-

I. FLOW DIAGRAM

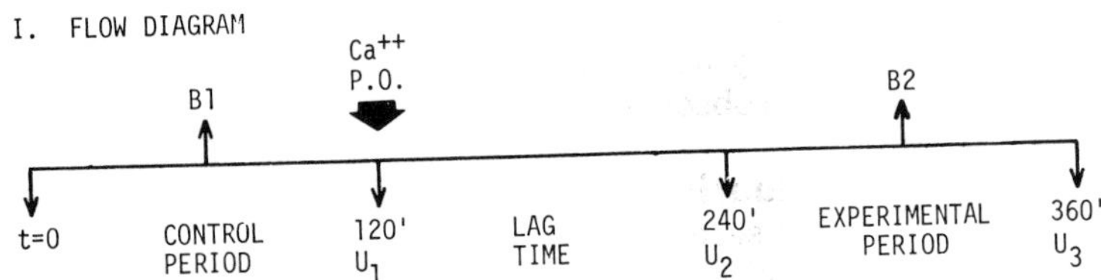

II. DATA BASE

A. STATIC MEASUREMENTS (CONTROL PERIOD)

1. BASAL SERUM CALCIUM & PHOSPHORUS
2. FASTING CALCIUM EXCRETION
3. FASTING TMP/GFR
4. BASAL NEPHROGENOUS OR TOTAL cAMP EXCRETION
5. BASAL VITAMIN D METABOLITES

B. DYNAMIC MEASUREMENTS (EXPERIMENTAL VS CONTROL PERIOD)

1. CALCEMIC RESPONSE AS INDEX OF "CALCIUM TOLERANCE"
2. CALCIURIC RESPONSE (Δ mg CALCIUM/100 ML GF) AS INDEX OF GI ABSORPTION
3. SUPPRESSIBILITY OF NEPHROGENOUS OR TOTAL cAMP EXCRETION

FIGURE 25-22 Flow diagram and data base derived from oral calcium tolerance test. [*Reproduced by permission of the author, editor, and publisher from Insogna KL, Broadus AE: Nephrolithiasis, in Felig P, Baxter JD, Broadus AE, Frohman LA (eds): Endocrinology and Metabolism, 2d ed. New York, McGraw-Hill, 1987, p 1569.*]

thetic liquid meal preparations can be used instead of milk in lactose-intolerant patients. The three collection periods are a fasting control period, a 2-h lag period (necessary for peak calcium absorption), and an experimental period showing the effects of the absorbed calcium. Midpoint blood specimens are drawn during the first and third collection periods.

Measurements are made of calcium, cAMP, and creatinine concentrations in the serum and calcium, creatinine, and cAMP in the urine. Plasma cAMP varies little during the morning, and a single determination of this during the control may be used to calculate nephrogenous cAMP. Plasma 1,25-$(OH)_2D$ and tubular phosphate resorption measurements are not particularly helpful in distinguishing among the subtypes.

From these data, the increase in serum calcium, the induced change in nephrogenous or total cAMP, and the calcemic responses are measured.[117,127] The increase in serum calcium is an index of calcium intolerance. The calcemic response in normal individuals is usually less than 0.4 mg/dl (0.1 mmol/L). The induced change in nephrogenous or total cAMP is an index of parathyroid suppressibility. Nephrogenous cAMP excretion is about twice as sensitive as total cAMP excretion, but the latter is usually adequate for diagnostic purposes. PTH measurements will probably replace cAMP measurements, but firm data on the PTH response are not yet available. The calciuric response is an index of intestinal calcium absorption and is computed by subtracting the control-period rate of calcium excretion from that during the experimental period expressed per 100 ml of glomerular filtrate. In normal persons, the increase in urinary calcium is <0.2 mg/100 ml glomerular filtrate (GF) (0.005 mmol/100 ml GF).

With careful attention to detail, the calcium tolerance test can provide information sufficient to categorize 90 percent of hypercalciuric patients.

Evaluating Hyperoxaluria

The available methods for measuring oxalate concentration include colorimetric, isotope dilution, and enzymatic techniques.[235] The outmoded, inaccurate precipitation method should be avoided. The most difficult and demanding aspect of measurement is sample extraction. The normal range for daily oxalate excretion is usually 15 to 40 mg per day (167 to 144 μmol/day).[173] A difference in oxalate excretion between men and women has not been observed. Daily oxalate excretion among consecutive calcium stone patients exceeded 40 mg (444 μmol) in 21 percent[181] but rarely exceeded 80 mg (888 μmol). Oxalate excretion correlates closely with calcium excretion.[54,181]

Daily excretion of >100 mg (1111 μmol) indicates probable primary hyperoxaluria.[166,167,170] Primary hyperoxaluria should be considered in any child who is seen for calcium stones. The siblings of affected patients should be routinely screened. Type 1 and type 2 syndromes can be distinguished by the different patterns of excretion of glyoxylate, glycolate, and glyceric acid.

Enteric hyperoxaluria should be suspected in stone patients who have a characteristic, chronic enteric disorder and can be confirmed by a demonstrated increase in oxalate excretion. In these patients, daily urinary excretion rates depend greatly on oxalate intake but usually exceed 60 mg (667 μmol).[166–168] In addition to measurement of oxalate excretion, patients should be completely screened for other risk factors for stone formation. Patients with enteric hyperoxaluria are often relatively hypocalciuric, and this may be an important clue to accurate diagnosis if the manifestations of intestinal disease are subtle. If not previously documented and quantified, steatorrhea should be assessed by fecal fat determination.

Evaluating Hyperuricosuria

Hyperuricosuria is best shown in an outpatient setting while patients are on their usual diets. Coincident fasting hyperuricemia and hyperuricosuria suggest overproduction of uric acid, whereas concurrent normouricemia and hyperuricosuria suggest that the patient is a "purine glutton." A thorough diet history can help identify patients whose diet is too rich in purine because of overconsumption of animal protein and may provide a basis for subsequent instructions to moderate purine intake.

Suggested daily upper-normal limits for uric acid excretion are 800 mg (4.8 mmol) for men and 750 mg (4.5 mmol) for women.[52,185,186] By these criteria, 10 percent of normal men and 5 percent of normal women are hyperuricosuric.[186] Pak and coworkers used an upper limit of 600 mg (3.6 mmol) daily for both sexes and considered this limit a "functional definition" of hyperuricosuria on the basis of the quantity of uric acid usually needed to supersaturate urine with monosodium urate.[150] This definition, however, is unusually permissive, classifying 60 percent of normal men as hyperuricosuric; in addition, monosodium is not the uric acid moiety responsible for increasing calcium stone formation.

Evaluating Hypocitraturia

Citrate is measured enzymatically using the citrate lyase method, which is available in commercial laboratories. The excretion of citrate varies widely from day to day, depending on diet. About a third of calcium oxalate stone patients excrete less than the lower limit of normal, which is 320 mg (1666 μmol) daily. Urinary citrate excretion in normal subjects is reported to increase with age, about 70 mg (364 μmol) per decade, but data are scarce, and an age-related increase in citrate excretion was not seen in patients with stone disease.[227] In most studies, citrate excretion is about 20 percent higher in women than in men, regardless of age.[226–229]

Evaluating Combinations of Metabolic Risk Factors

Because stone formation is believed to result when forces promoting crystallization overcome those preventing it, some researchers have suggested the use of a saturation-inhibition index that quantifies these forces.[90] The usefulness of a stone probability index has been challenged on theoretical and practical grounds.[108] Since most of the variables measured are closely correlated with at least two other variables, a multiplicative model is inappropriate. Moreover, Ryall and coworkers showed considerable overlap between stone patients and normal subjects for urinary volume, pH, calcium, oxalate, uric acid, and glycosaminoglycan.[108] Finally, the predictive value of these biochemical tests, alone or in combination, has never been validated.

Treatment of Calcium Oxalate Nephrolithiasis

Is Treatment Needed?

As was previously emphasized, treating patients with any form of stone disease is a program, not simply a pill. This treatment program consists of (1) specific instructions to force fluids,[236,237] (2) guidelines for dietary moderation,[236–238] and, for some patients, (3) an agent to reduce stone recurrence.

When trying to predict the future risk of stone formation in a person who has recurrent stone events, physicians should rely on the adage "history repeats itself." By far the most important predictors of stone events are the number and frequency of past events. Among 155 patients with a history of recurrent calcium oxalate stones who received either placebo or no medication, each increment of 0.5 stone yearly in the previous stone rate was associated with a 36 percent increase in subsequent recurrence rates.[239] Similarly, for each additional stone seen on baseline kidney x-ray films, subsequent annual rates of recurrence doubled. In these patients, none of the usual urinary biochemical tests helped predict recurrence.

Treatment Goals

What constitutes an effective response to treatment? In most clinical trials of calcium oxalate lithiasis, recurrence rates are about 20 to 30 percent in subjects assigned to placebo or "no active treatment."[25] These rates are about half those calculated from reports by these patients describing stone activity before entering the trial. Readers should thus be skeptical of the purported clinical benefits of specific therapy unless treatment reduces yearly stone recurrence rates to between 5 and 10 percent, or about half the rates observed with placebo.

Choosing a Treatment

After deciding to add a medication to the stone prevention program, the physician must choose between directing the medication at correcting one or all metabolic deviations and giving empiric therapy. This issue is controversial, and clinical investigations have not compared these two approaches. Gaining extensive clinical experience with one or two types of therapy may be wiser than using many treatments without fully understanding their risks and benefits. The current therapies are described below. Readers should remember that the success of medical treatment of calcium oxalate lithiasis must be measured by prevention of stone events, not by alterations in urinary biochemistry.

Treatment of Subtle Hyperparathyroidism Associated with Nephrolithiasis

Patients with both subtle primary hyperparathyroidism and nephrolithiasis should have a neck exploration. They should be treated by an experienced surgeon, since about 80 percent of such patients have a single, small parathyroid adenoma, consistent with the view that the disorder is simply a mild form of primary hyperparathyroidism.[240] In a series reported in 1980, before improved PTH assays were available,[241] of 52 patients presumed to have subtle hyperparathyroidism and recurrent calcium lithiasis who had surgery, 17 had normal parathyroid glands, 14 had hyperplasia, and 12 had a single adenoma. After about 5 years, stone disease remission occurred only in the 12 in whom adenomas were removed; stones recurred in 61 percent of the patients with hyperplasia. These poor results dampened enthusiasm about an aggressive approach to subtle hyperparathyroidism. However, improved diagnostic methods, particularly measurements of plasma immunoreactive PTH, justify reevaluation.

Patients who are not considered good candidates for neck exploration or who have persistent hyperparathyroidism after exploration can be managed successfully with oral neutral phosphate sufficient to provide 1500 mg of daily elemental phosphorus. This has been shown in short-term studies to reduce circulating 1,25-$(OH)_2D$, calcium absorption and excretion, and stone formation rates.[242] This therapy is basically antihypercalciuric instead of antihypercalcemic and is not recommended for patients with moderate to severe hypercalcemia.

Treatment of Hypercalciuria

Dietary Hypercalciuria

Patients with dietary hypercalciuria are managed with a program of forced fluids as well as moderation of sodium intake (about 100 mEq/day), calcium intake [about 400 to 600 mg/day (10 to 15 mmol/day)], and animal protein intake (about 35 g of flesh daily) (Table 25-2). The effects of fluid and dietary therapy can be monitored by 24-h urine collection; measurement of sodium excretion monitors compliance.

Renal Hypercalciuria

Given adequate grounds for a diagnosis of primary renal hypercalciuria, the preferred agents are thiazide diuretics.[190,243] Thiazides are also preferred in treating hypercalciuric patients with coincident hypertension. Conventional antihypertensive doses of thiazides are used in treating stone disease. Their hypocalciuric effect results from both volume contraction and direct action to increase calcium resorption in the distal nephron.[244] This effect is shared by all thiazide congeners and related diuretics (e.g., chlorthalidone); no single agent is preferred. Giving single daily doses improves compliance. On average, thiazides halve calcium excretion rates.[190,243] High salt intake can usually overcome the antihypercalciuric effect of the drug. The most common side effect is a feeling of lassitude, which is usually transient and apparently is unrelated to hypokalemia. Triamterene-containing agents are not used in patients with urolithiasis because triamterene and its products have been identified in kidney stones.[245]

Absorptive Hypercalciuria

Patients with absorptive hypercalciuria are instructed to follow a program of forced fluids and dietary moderation (Table 25-2). Additional measures may include the administration of either neutral phosphates or a thiazide diuretic, which appear to have an equivalent antihypercalciuric effect in such patients.[160,190,242–244] Neutral phosphate sufficient to provide 1500 to 2000 mg of daily elemental phosphorus is given in three or four divided doses. This treatment has never been rigorously evaluated in a randomized, double-blind clinical trial. Acidic phosphate preparations are ineffective.[246] Patients tend to prefer phosphate salt tablets to liquid forms. All phosphate salts are cathartic, and this side effect may reduce compliance and often necessitates limiting the dose; beginning with a small dose and slowly increasing to tolerance may help overcome this problem.

Sodium cellulose phosphate is a nonabsorbable cation exchange resin which binds to calcium and prevents its absorption from the intestine.[182,183] It is specifically intended for patients with absorptive hypercalciuria. Magnesium supplements must also be taken, and calcium and oxalate intake must be restricted. Backman and coworkers reported side effects—mainly gastrointestinal discomfort and synovitis—in 9 of 35 patients.[183] In contrast, Pak noted that the drug was "well tolerated" by 18 patients.[182] The question of cellulose phosphate's efficacy is unresolved. Stones recurred in 22 percent of Pak's patients[182] during a mean 2.4-year follow-up and in 47 percent of patients studied by Backman and coworkers[183] in a 2-year trial. The marked difference in efficacy might have resulted because Backman and coworkers neither gave magnesium supplements nor restricted the diets of their subjects. The effects and required dose of sodium cellulose phosphate must be monitored by serial measurement of urinary calcium excretion to avoid creating calcium malabsorption, secondary hyperparathyroidism, or a negative calcium balance. Cellulose phosphate is expensive; 15 g of the drug plus 116 mg of magnesium daily costs more than $1500 a year. The drug is not easy to use: It must be taken three times daily, mixed in water, and taken with or just after each meal; the magnesium supplements (a mandatory part of the regimen) must be taken separately three times daily. We suggest that the drug be used only in rare cases of severe absorptive hypercalciuria which cannot be managed by other means.

Empiric Therapy for Hypercalciuria

By far the most extensive experience with either thiazides or phosphate therapy is in empiric treatment of hypercalciuric patients who are not classified by metabolic subtype. Each form of treatment appears to result in a roughly equivalent decrease in rates of calcium excretion, and each has been reported to reduce stone formation.[2,6,7,190,243,246–250] Given the simplicity, high patient acceptance, low cost, and more extensive documentation of the efficacy of thiazide therapy,[251] we prefer it to phosphate therapy.

Although about 10 percent of patients treated with either thiazides or phosphates do not have the anticipated hypocalciuric response, the dose need not be increased or the treatment altered immediately. Biochemical changes correlate poorly if at all with the success or failure of treatment.[25,236]

Treatment of Hyperoxaluria

Primary Hyperoxaluria

Patients with primary hyperoxaluria are given particularly detailed instructions about hydration, similar to those given to patients with cystinuria. In addition, these patients are usually placed on a low-oxalate diet even though little urinary oxalate excretion is derived from this diet. Large doses of pyridoxine (200 to 400 mg/day) are reported to variably decrease oxalate excretion rates in patients with primary hyperoxaluria, presumably by increasing the conversion of glyoxylate to glycine[252] (Fig. 25-20). In rare cases, much smaller doses of pyridoxine (as little as 2 mg/day) were effective.[253] Pyridoxine in daily doses of 500 to 2000 mg may cause sensory ataxia as a result of neuropathy affecting the peripheral nerves responsible for vibration and position sense.[254,255] Magnesium supplements and phosphate have been reported to reduce stone formation in uncontrolled studies,[166,170] but both agents should be used cautiously, if at all, in patients with moderate or advanced renal insufficiency. Dialysis does not effectively control progressive systemic oxalosis, and primary hyperoxaluria is currently considered a contraindication for renal transplantation.

Enteric Hyperoxaluria

Treatment of patients with enteric hyperoxaluria is multifaceted; general measures include hydration, control of steatorrhea, and the prescription of an oxalate-restricted diet.[166–168,256] Patients with a short bowel have difficulty consuming large quantities of fluid and maintaining adequate urine output. A low-fat diet may improve steatorrhea, but a diet rigidly restricted in fat is unpalatable, and many patients prefer to use medium-chain triglycerides.[257] For many patients, these measures suffice; for others, hyperoxaluria and other risk factors cannot be controlled and other measures are required.

Numerous agents have been used in attempts to bind oxalate in the intestinal contents and limit its bioavailability. These agents include calcium, magnesium, aluminum, cholestyramine, and colestipol.[256] Many such agents also bind bile acids and fatty acids. Calcium 1000 to 2000 mg (25 to 50 mmol) daily is probably the best choice. A considerable margin of safety in calcium dosage exists because many patients absorb calcium poorly and are relatively hypocalciuric before therapy. The antacid Camalox is a useful combination agent because it contains calcium carbonate, aluminum hydroxide, and magnesium hydroxide; a typical daily starting dose of 900 mg (22.5 mmol) is provided by 15 ml (or three tablets) taken three times daily with meals. Long-term trials of such binding agents have not been reported. Major stone complications are considered an indication for restoring intestinal continuity in patients with a jejunoileal bypass.[166]

Oxalate Complexation by Cysteine

Recent reports indicate progress in the search for an oxalate-complexing agent.[257] In rats poisoned with ethylene glycol, excessive urinary oxalate was dramatically reduced by giving cysteine, which apparently binds the oxalate molecule between its sulfhydryl and amino nitrogen groups (Fig. 25-20). Further studies are needed to evaluate long-term safety and efficacy.

Treatment of Hyperuricosuria

Patients with hyperuricosuric calcium oxalate nephrolithiasis are treated with a program of high fluid intake, moderation of purine and animal protein, and often allopurinol. The principle of dietary moderation instead of restriction is emphasized because compliance with a diet low in animal protein is poor. Sodium restriction is also advised for patients who have coincident dietary hypercalciuria.

Allopurinol is effective in preventing stone recurrence in patients with hyperuricosuric calcium oxalate stone disease (Fig. 25-21).[189–193] The mechanism of action, dosage, and toxicity of allopurinol are described in detail in Uric Acid Stones, above. When 300 mg of the drug is given daily, uric acid excretion may be reduced by 40 percent, a reduction which should suffice to reduce daily uric acid excretion to about 500 mg (3 mmol). A single daily dose of allopurinol is adequate and enhances compliance.

Thiazides are effective in patients with hyperuricosuric calcium oxalate nephrolithiasis.[25,258] Using thiazides in such patients, Lærum and Larsen[258] reported an annual stone recurrence rate of 6 percent, and Ettinger and coworkers[25] reported a recurrence rate of 9 percent. Allopurinol has far fewer minor side effects but is associated with a risk of developing rare serious allergic reactions. About half of patients with hyperuricosuria also have hypercalciuria. In patients with such combined overexcretion, allopurinol alone clearly does not stop stone recurrence.[188] In a few patients, combined allopurinol and thiazide therapy was evaluated; stone recurrence was reduced substantially.[186,244] Because the contribution of each therapy and the possible additive benefits of multiple therapies have not been examined rigorously and because the risk of serious allergic reactions increases when thiazides are used with allopurinol,[259] beginning with a thiazide alone is wise.

Whether careful use of alkali would also be beneficial is unknown. As additional therapy, a single dose of 30 mEq at bedtime to offset early-morning urine acidity can be considered; this dose could reduce the saturation of urine by uric acid and inhibit the growth of calcium oxalate crystals.[260] In a preliminary report, the administration of 60 to 80 mmol daily of potassium citrate to hyperuricosuric stone patients was associated with an 8 percent annual stone recurrence rate.[261] Several factors limit the applicability of these results: Hyperuricosuria was liberally defined as exceeding 600 mg (3.6 mmol) daily; two-thirds of subjects had low citrate excretion, about twice the usual prevalence expected; only 14 subjects were followed for $\geq$2 years; and three subjects also received thiazide.

Treatment of Hypocitraturia

Numerous citrate-containing drugs are available (Table 25-3). Potassium citrate embedded in a wax matrix tablet may produce a more sustained increase in citrate excretion than other forms of oral alkali do. Potassium is more useful than sodium citrate in correcting thiazide-induced potassium depletion. Until more carefully controlled studies determine the efficacy of potassium citrate in various clinical settings, its role in treating patients with calcium stone disease will remain uncertain. Citrate has also been given empirically without consideration of the urinary metabolic profile; the preliminary results appear promising. Among 72 patients followed for a mean 3.5 years, a mixture of sodium and potassium citrate in daily doses of 18.5 to 28 mmol was associated with an 8 percent annual recurrence rate.[262] Using 50 mmol of potassium citrate, we found a similar annual recurrence rate after 2 years (B. Ettinger, unpublished data).

Treatment of Patients Free of Metabolic Abnormalities

Idiopathic calcium stone disease is diagnosed by exclusion. The decision to treat such a patient, as for any patient with stone disease, is made by assessing stone-related morbidity. Almost all agents used to treat patients with calcium stones were first introduced on empiric grounds and were reported to be beneficial in patients with no obvious risk factors for stone formation. Although uncontrolled studies have reported the efficacy of oral phosphates[248–252] and thiazides,[24,191,244] more credence should be given to the results of adequate double-blind controlled studies using thiazides (Fig. 25-23).[25,258]

Discontinuing Treatment

The decision to stop medical therapy for calcium oxalate stones is often made by the patient. After a few symptom-free years, patients appear to forget past pain and may come to consider medication an unnecessary nuisance. Joost and Putz reported 5-year follow-up of 26 patients with recurrent stone disease who had been prescribed thiazides, allopurinol, or magnesium hydroxide; 80 percent had stopped treatment after 2 to 3 years.[263] Nevertheless, the annual recurrence rate among these pa-

FIGURE 25-23 Life-table plot showing percentage of patients with no calculus events during treatment with 25 mg chlorthalidone, 50 mg chlorthalidone, or placebo.

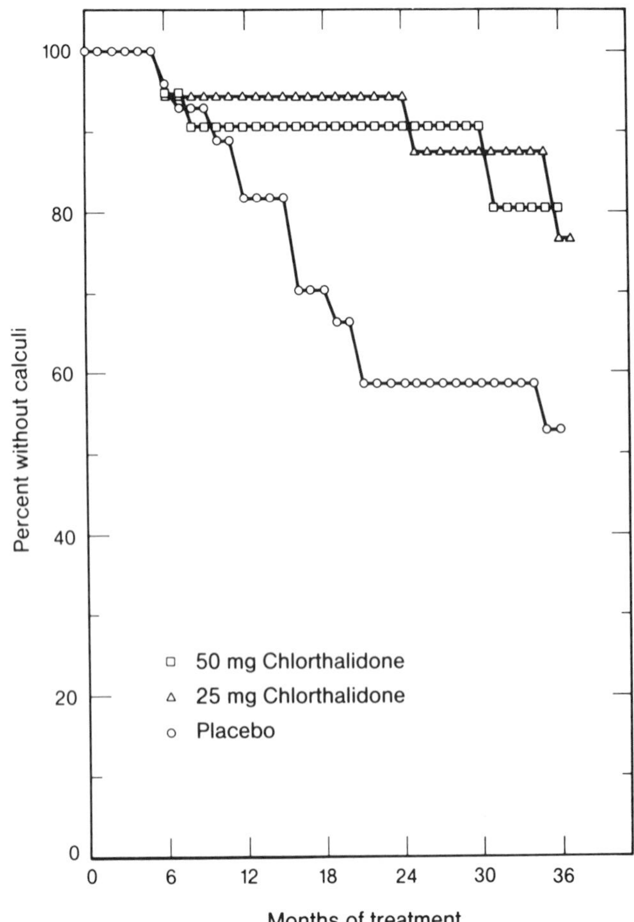

tients was only about 7 percent. Mean urine volume in this cohort was 600 ml higher during follow-up, which may account for the low recurrence rate. Another posttreatment follow-up study also showed a high remission rate.[264] After 3 years of receiving ineffective treatment (potassium acid phosphate), placebo, or diet advice, 71 patients with recurrent stone disease were followed for 3 more years while receiving no treatment (Fig. 25-24). Recurrence was rare, and only one lithotomy was necessary. As in other studies, residual stones were associated with a higher risk of recurrence. On the basis of these studies, for the average calcium oxalate stone patient, we usually recommend stopping medication after 3 years, provided that no residual stones remain in the kidneys. Because residual stones and a history of frequent stone events both portend much higher recurrence rates, we suggest continuing therapy in such cases for 5 years or more. After stopping treatment, patients should be recalled for annual follow-up radiographic evaluation.

CLOSING COMMENTS

We close this chapter with the words of Lynwood H. Smith, who contributed much to our understanding and treatment of nephrolithiasis:

> [W]e have gone through several phases in our studies of idiopathic calcium urolithiasis. In the 1970s it seemed that this was a syndrome made up of precise conditions. With further study it is clear that multiple abnormalities often may be present with significant overlap of risk factors. This situation suggests that we do not as yet understand basic pathophysiology in many patients who are believed to have this syndrome. Fresh approaches with new ideas challenging former concepts clearly are needed.[5]

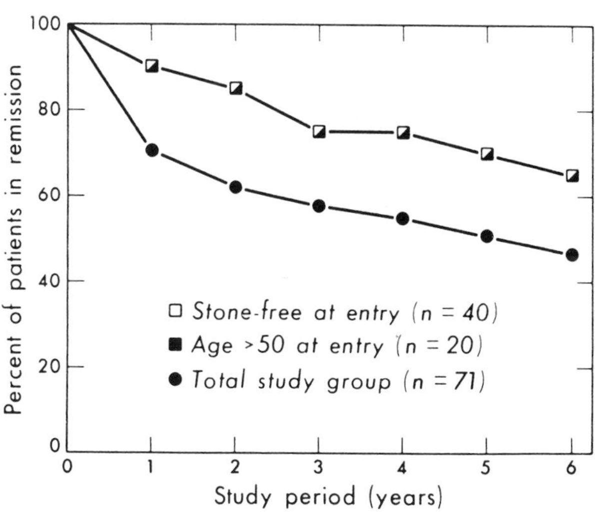

FIGURE 25-24 Life-table plot showing percentage of 71 patients with no calculus events during 3-year treatment with acid phosphate, calcium restriction, or placebo and 3 additional years of follow-up with no treatment. About 45 percent of the entire group remained stone-free after 6 years. Patients older at the start or free of stones at the start were less likely to have recurrences. *(Adapted and reproduced by permission of the publisher from Ettinger B: Recurrence of nephrolithiasis: A six-year prospective study. Am J Med 67:245–248, 1979.)*

Acknowledgments

The medical editing department of Kaiser Foundation Hospitals provided editorial assistance.

REFERENCES

1. Johnson CM, Wilson DM, O'Fallon WM, Malek RS, Kurland LT: Renal stone epidemiology: A 25-year study in Rochester, Minnesota. *Kidney Int* 16:624–631, 1979.
2. Coe FL: *Nephrolithiasis: Pathogenesis and Treatment.* Chicago, Year Book, 1978.
3. Prien EL: Crystallographic analysis of urinary calculi: A 23-year survey study. *J Urol* 89:917–924, 1963.
4. Herring LC: Observations on the analysis of ten thousand urinary calculi. *J Urol* 88:545–562, 1962.
5. Smith LH: The medical aspects of urolithiasis: An overview. *J Urol* 141:707–710, 1989.
6. Smith LH: Urolithiasis, in Schrier RW, Gottschalk CW (eds): *Diseases of the Kidney,* 4th ed. Boston, Little, Brown, 1988, pp 785–813.
7. Coe FL, ed: *Nephrolithiasis.* New York, Churchill Livingstone, 1980.
8. Boyce WH: Organic matrix of human urinary concretions. *Am J Med* 45:673–683, 1968.
9. Morse RM, Resnick MI: Urinary stone matrix. *J Urol* 139:602–606, 1988.
10. Thomas WC Jr, Howard JE: Studies in the mineralizing propensity of urine from patients with and without renal calculi. *Trans Assoc Am Physicians* 72:181–187, 1959.
11. Pak CYC: *Calcium Urolithiasis: Pathogenesis, Diagnosis, and Management.* New York, Plenum, 1978.
12. Drach GW: Surgical overview of urolithiasis. *J Urol* 141:711–713, 1989.
13. Kelley JM: Extracorporeal shock wave lithotripsy of urinary calculi: Theory, efficacy, and adverse effects. *West J Med* 153:165–169, 1990.
14. Lingeman JE, Woods JR, Toth PD: Blood pressure changes following extracorporeal shock wave lithotripsy and other forms of treatment for nephrolithiasis. *JAMA* 263:1789–1794, 1990.
15. Miller HC, Collins LA, Turbow AM, Turbow BA, Beall ME, Berger RM, Lebowitz JM, Young IS, Kahn RI, Karol JB: Initial EDAP LT-01 lithotripsy group experience in the United States. *J Urol* 142:1412–1414, 1989.
16. Coughlin BF, Risius B, Streem SB, Lorig RJ, Siegel SW: Abdominal radiograph and renal ultrasound versus excretory urography in the evaluation of asymptomatic patients after extracorporeal shock wave lithotripsy. *J Urol* 142: 1419–1424, 1989.
17. Coe FL, Parks JH: Pathophysiology of kidney stones and strategies for treatment. *Hosp Pract* 23:185–207, 1988.
18. Strauss AL, Coe FL, Parks JH: Formation of a single calcium stone of renal origin: Clinical and laboratory characteristics of patients. *Arch Intern Med* 142:504–507, 1982.
19. Pak CYC: Should patients with single renal stone occurrence undergo diagnostic evaluation? *J Urol* 127:855–858, 1982.
20. Uribarri J, Oh MS, Carroll HJ: The first kidney stone. *Ann Intern Med* 111:1006–1009, 1989.
21. Nordin BEC, Barry H, Bulusu L, Speed R: Dietary treatment of recurrent calcium stone disease, in Cifuentes De-

latte L, Rapado A, Hodgkinson A: *Urinary Calculi: Recent Advances in Aetiology, Stone Structure, and Treatment.* International Symposium on Renal Stone Research, Madrid, 1972. Basel, Karger, 1973, pp. 170–176.

22. Norman RW, Manette WA: Dietary restriction of sodium as a means of reducing urinary cystine. *J Urol* 143:1193–1195, 1990.
23. Kok DJ, Iestra JA, Doorenbos CJ, Papapoulos SE: The effects of dietary excesses in animal protein and in sodium on the composition and the crystallization kinetics of calcium oxalate monohydrate in urines of healthy men. *J Clin Endocrinol Metab* 71:861–867, 1990.
24. Churchill DN: Medical treatment to prevent recurrent calcium urolithiasis: A guide to critical appraisal. *Miner Electrolyte Metab* 13:294–304, 1987.
25. Ettinger B, Citron JT, Livermore B, Dolman LI: Chlorthalidone reduces calcium oxalate calculus recurrence but magnesium hydroxide does not. *J Urol* 139:679–684, 1988.
26. Rosenberg LE, Scriver CR: Disorders of amino acid metabolism, in Bondy PK, Rosenberg LE (eds): *Metabolic Control and Disease.* Philadelphia, Saunders, 1980, pp 73–102.
27. Segal S, Thier SO: Cystinuria, in Scriver CR, Beaudet AL, Sly WS, Valle D (eds): *The Metabolic Basis of Inherited Disease,* 6th ed. New York, McGraw-Hill, 1989, pp 2479–2496.
28. Dent CE, Rose GA: Amino acid metabolism in cystinuria. *Q J Med* 20:205–219, 1951.
29. Crawhall JC, Purkiss P, Watts RW, Young EP: The excretion of amino acids by cystinuric patients and their relatives. *Ann Hum Genet* 33:149–169, 1969.
30. Jaeger P, Portmann L, Saunders A, Rosenberg LE, Thier SO: Anticystinuric effects of glutamine and of dietary sodium restriction. *N Engl J Med* 315:1120–1123, 1986.
31. Miyagi K, Nakada F, Ohshiro S: Effect of glutamine on cystine excretion in a patient with cystinuria. *N Engl J Med* 301:196–198, 1979.
32. Van Den Berg CJ, Jones JD, Wilson DM, Smith L: Glutamine therapy of cystinuria. *Invest Urol* 18:155–157, 1980.
33. Dahlberg PJ, Van Den Berg CJ, Kurtz SB, Wilson DM, Smith LH: Clinical features and management of cystinuria. *Mayo Clin Proc* 52:533–542, 1977.
34. Sakhaee K, Poindexter JR, Pak CYC: The spectrum of metabolic abnormalities in patients with cystine nephrolithiasis. *J Urol* 141:819–821, 1989.
35. Singer A, Das S: Cystinuria: A review of the pathophysiology and management. *J Urol* 142:669–673, 1989.
36. Smith A: Evaluation of the nitroprusside test for the diagnosis of cystinuria. *Med J Aust* 2:153–155, 1977.
37. David RM, Shihabi ZK, O'Connor ML: Simplified method for cystinuria screening (abstract). *Clin Chem* 32:1417, 1986.
38. Halperin EC, Thier SO, Rosenberg LE: The use of D-penicillamine in cystinuria: Efficacy and untoward reactions. *Yale J Biol Med* 54:439–446, 1981.
39. Denneberg T, Jeppsson J-O, Stenberg P: Alternative treatment of cystinuria with alpha-merkaptopropionylglycine, Thiola. *Proc Eur Dial Transplant Assoc* 20:427–433, 1983.
40. Harbar JA, Cusworth DC, Lawes LC, Wrong OM: Comparison of 2-mercaptopropionylglycine and D-penicillamine in the treatment of cystinuria. *J Urol* 136:146–149, 1986.
41. Lindell Å, Denneberg T, Eneström S, Fich C, Skogh T: Membranous glomerulonephritis induced by 2-mercaptopropionylglycine (2-MPG). *Clin Nephrol* 34:108–115, 1990.
42. Sloand JA, Izzo JL Jr: Captopril reduces urinary cystine excretion in cystinuria. *Arch Intern Med* 147:1409–1412, 1987.
43. Sandroni S, Stevens P, Barraza M, Tolaymat A: Captopril therapy of recurrent nephrolithiasis in a child with cystinuria. *Child Nephrol Urol* 9:347–348, 1988.
44. Aunsholt NA, Ahlbom G: Lack of effect of captopril in cystinuria (letter). *Clin Nephrol* 34:92–93, 1990.
45. Dahlberg PJ, Jones JD: Cystinuria: Failure of captopril to reduce cystine excretion (letter). *Arch Intern Med* 149:713, 1989.
46. Streem SB, Hall P: Effect of captopril on urinary cystine excretion in homozygous cystinuria. *J Urol* 142:1522–1554, 1989.
47. Yü T-F: Uric acid nephrolithiasis, in Kelley WN, Weiner IM (ed): *Uric Acid.* New York, Springer-Verlag, 1978, pp 397–422.
48. Levinson DJ, Sorensen LB: Uric acid stones, in Coe FL (ed): *Nephrolithiasis: Pathogenesis and Treatment.* Chicago, Year Book, 1978, pp 172–202.
49. Holmes EW: Uric acid nephrolithiasis, in Coe FL (ed): *Nephrolithiasis.* New York, Churchill Livingstone, 1980, pp 188–207.
50. Preminger GM: Pharmacologic treatment of uric acid calculi. *Urol Clin North Am* 14:335–338, 1987.
51. Wilson DM: Uric acid lithiasis, in Rous SN (ed): *Stone Disease: Diagnosis and Management.* Orlando, Grune & Stratton, 1987, pp 109–123.
52. Fellström B, Danielson RG, Karlström B, Lithell H, Ljunghall S, Vessby B: The influence of a high dietary intake of purine-rich animal protein on urinary urate excretion and supersaturation in renal stone disease. *Clin Sci* 64:399–405, 1983.
53. Gutman AB, Yü TF: Uric acid nephrolithiasis. *Am J Med* 45:756–779, 1968.
54. Elion GB: Allopurinol and other inhibitors of urate synthesis, in Kelley WN, Weiner IM (eds): *Uric Acid.* Berlin, Springer-Verlag, 1978, vol 51, pp 485–514.
55. Pak CYC, Barilla DE, Holt K, Brinkley L, Tolentino R, Zerwekh JE: Effect of oral purine load and allopurinol on the crystallization of calcium salts in urine of patients with hyperuricosuric calcium urolithiasis. *Am J Med* 65:593–599, 1978.
56. Morris GS, Simmonds HA, Toseland PA, Van Acker KJ, Davies PM, Stuchbury JH: Urinary oxalate levels are not affected by dietary purine intake or allopurinol. *Br J Urol* 60:292–300, 1987.
57. Shaw MI, Parsons DS: Absorption and metabolism of allopurinol and oxypurinol by rat jejunum in vitro: Effects on uric acid transport. *Clin Sci* 66:257–267, 1984.
58. Hosking DH: The use of K-Lyte (potassium citrate) in uric acid lithiasis, in Walker VR, Sutton RAL, Cameron ECB, Pak CYC, Robertson WG (eds): *Urolithiasis.* Proceedings of the 6th International Symposium on Urolithiasis and Related Clinical Research, Vancouver, Canada, July 24–28, 1988. New York, Plenum, 1989, pp 809–812.
59. Erickson SB, Wilson DM, Smith LH: Dissolution of uric acid stones, in Walker VR, Sutton RAL, Cameron ECB, Pak CYC, Robertson WG (eds): *Urolithiasis.* Proceedings of the 6th International Symposium on Urolithiasis and Related Clinical Research, Vancouver, Canada, July 24–28, 1988. New York, Plenum, 1989, pp 821–823.
60. Sakhaee K, Nicar M, Hill K, Pak CYC: Contrasting effects of potassium citrate and sodium citrate therapies on urinary chemistries and crystallization of stone-forming salts. *Kidney Int* 24:348–352, 1983.
61. Pak CYC, Sakhaee K, Fuller C: Successful management of uric acid nephrolithiasis with potassium citrate. *Kidney Int* 30:422–428, 1986.
62. Hande KR, Noone RM, Stone WJ: Severe allopurinol toxicity: Description and guidelines for prevention in patients with renal insufficiency. *Am J Med* 76:47–56, 1984.
63. Cogan MG, Rector FC Jr: Acid-base disorders, in Brenner BM, Rector FC Jr (eds): *The Kidney,* 3d ed. Philadelphia, Saunders, 1986, pp 457–517.
64. Brenner RJ, Spring DB, Sebastian A, McSherry EM, Genant HK, Palubinskas AJ, Morris RC Jr: Incidence of radiographically evident bone disease, nephrocalcinosis, and nephrolithiasis in various types of renal tubular acidosis. *N Engl J Med* 307:217–221, 1982.
65. Simpson DP: Regulation of renal citrate metabolism by bicarbonate ion and pH: Observations in tissue slices and mitochondria. *J Clin Invest* 46:225–238, 1967.

66. Danielson BG, Backman U, Fellström B, Johansson G, Ljunghall S, Wikström B: Experience with the short ammonium chloride test, in Smith LH, Robertson WG, Finlayson B (eds): *Urolithiasis: Clinical and Basic Research.* New York, Plenum, 1981, pp 71–76.
67. Tannen RL, Falls WF Jr, Brackett NC Jr: Incomplete renal tubular acidosis: Some clinical and physiological features. *Nephron* 15:111–123, 1975.
68. Konnak JW, Kogan BA, Lau K: Renal calculi associated with incomplete distal renal tubular acidosis. *J Urol* 128:900–902, 1982.
69. Preminger GM, Sakhaee K, Skurla C, Pak CYC: Prevention of recurrent calcium stone formation with potassium citrate therapy in patients with distal renal tubular acidosis. *J Urol* 134:20–25, 1985.
70. Batlle DC, Kurtzman NA: Distal renal tubular acidosis, in Coe FL (ed): *Hypercalciuric States: Pathogenesis, Consequences, and Treatment.* Orlando, Grune & Stratton, 1984, pp 239–274.
71. Backman U, Danielson BG, Fellström B, Johansson G, Ljunghall S, Wikström B: The clinical importance of renal tubular acidosis in recurrent renal stone formers, in Smith LH, Robertson WG, Finlayson B (eds): *Urolithiasis: Clinical and Basic Research.* New York, Plenum, 1981, pp 67–69.
72. Parfitt AM: Acetazolamide and sodium bicarbonate induced nephrocalcinosis and nephrolithiasis: Relationship to citrate and calcium excretion. *Arch Intern Med* 124:736–740, 1969.
73. Broadus AE: Nephrolithiasis in primary hyperparathyroidism, in Coe FL (ed): *Nephrolithiasis.* New York, Churchill Livingstone, 1980, pp 59–85.
74. McSherry E, Morris RC Jr: Attainment and maintenance of normal stature with alkali therapy in infants and children with classic renal tubular acidosis. *J Clin Invest* 61:509–527, 1978.
75. Griffith DP: Struvite stones. *Kidney Int* 13:372–382, 1978.
76. Smith LH: Renal lithiasis and infection, in Thomas WC Jr (ed): *Renal Calculi: A Guide to Management.* Springfield, IL, Thomas, 1976, pp 77–96.
77. McLean RJ, Nickel JC, Noakes VC, Costerton JW: An in vitro ultrastructural study of infectious kidney stone genesis. *Infect Immun* 49:805–811, 1985.
78. Griffith DP, Bruce RR, Fishbein WN: Infection (urease)-induced stones, in Coe FL (ed): *Nephrolithiasis.* New York, Churchill Livingstone, 1980, pp 231–260.
79. Lerner SP, Gleeson MJ, Griffith DP: Infection stones. *J Urol* 141:753–758, 1989.
80. Silverman DE, Stamey TA: Management of infection stones: The Stanford experience. *Medicine (Baltimore)* 62:44–51, 1983.
81. Chinn RH, Maskell R, Mead JA, Polak A: Renal stones and urinary infection: A study of antibiotic treatment. *Br Med J* 2:1411–1413, 1976.
82. Feit RM, Fair WR: The treatment of infection stones with penicillin. *J Urol* 122:592–594, 1979.
83. Robertson WG, Peacock M: The pattern of urinary stone disease in Leeds and in the United Kingdom in relation to animal protein intake during the period 1960–1980. *Urol Int* 37:394–399, 1982.
84. Boyce WH, Garvey FK, Strawcutter HE: Incidence of urinary calculi among patients in general hospitals, 1948 to 1952. *JAMA* 161:1437–1442, 1956.
85. Sierakowski R, Finlayson B, Landes RR, Finlayson CD, Sierakowski N: The frequency of urolithiasis in hospital discharge diagnoses in the United States. *Invest Urol* 15:438–441, 1978.
86. Ljunghall S: Regional variations in the incidence of urinary stones (letter). *Br Med J* 1:439, 1978.
87. Robertson WG, Peacock M, Heyburn PJ, Marshall DH, Clark PB: Risk factors in calcium stone disease of the urinary tract. *Br J Urol* 50:449–454, 1978.
88. Hodgkinson A, Marshall RW: Changes in the composition of urinary tract stones. *Invest Urol* 13:131–135, 1975.
89. Pak CYC, Holt K: Nucleation and growth of brushite and calcium oxalate in urine of stone-formers. *Metabolism* 25:665–673, 1976.
90. Robertson WG, Peacock M, Marshall RW, Marshall DH, Nordin BEC: Saturation-inhibition index as a measure of the risk of calcium oxalate stone formation in the urinary tract. *N Engl J Med* 294:249–252, 1976.
91. Finlayson B: Physicochemical aspects of urolithiasis. *Kidney Int* 13:344–360, 1978.
92. Bek-Jensen H, Tiselius H-G: Stone formation and urine composition in calcium stone formers without medical treatment. *Eur Urol* 16:144–150, 1989.
93. Coe FL, Keck J, Norton ER: The natural history of calcium urolithiasis. *JAMA* 238:1519–1523, 1977.
94. Marshall V, White RH, Chaput de Saintonge M, Tresidder GC, Blandy JP: The natural history of renal and ureteric calculi. *Br J Urol* 47:117–124, 1975.
95. Blacklock NJ: The pattern of urolithiasis in the Royal Navy, in Hodgkinson A, Nordin BEC (eds): *Renal Stone Research Symposium,* 1968, Leeds, England. London, Churchill, 1969, pp 33–47.
96. Williams RE: Long-term survey of 538 patients with upper urinary tract stone. *Br J Urol* 35:416–437, 1963.
97. Ljunghall S, Christensson T, Wengle B: Prevalence and incidence of renal stone disease in a health-screening programme. *Scand J Urol Nephrol [Suppl]* 41:39–53, 1977.
98. Sutherland JW, Parks JH, Coe FL: Recurrence after a single renal stone in a community practice. *Miner Electrolyte Metab* 11:267–269, 1985.
99. Ljunghall S, Hedstrand H: Epidemiology of renal stones in a middle-aged male population. *Acta Med Scand* 197:439–445, 1975.
100. Ljunghall S: Incidence and natural history of renal stone disease and its relationship to calcium metabolism. *Eur Urol* 4:424–430, 1978.
101. Ljunghall S, Danielson BG: A prospective study of renal stone recurrences. *Br J Urol* 56:122–124, 1984.
102. Wilson DM: Clinical and laboratory approaches for evaluation of nephrolithiasis. *J Urol* 141:770–774, 1989.
103. Resnick M, Pridgen DB, Goodman HO: Genetic predisposition to formation of calcium oxalate renal calculi. *N Engl J Med* 278:1313–1318, 1968.
104. Coe FL, Parks JH, Moore ES: Familial idiopathic hypercalciuria. *N Engl J Med* 300:337–340, 1979.
105. Ljunghall S, Backman U, Danielson BG, Fellström B, Johansson G, Wikström B: Epidemiological aspects of renal stone disease in Scandinavia. *Scand J Urol Nephrol [Suppl]* 53:31–36, 1979.
106. Sestili MA: Possible adverse health effects of vitamin C and ascorbic acid. *Semin Oncol* 10:299–304, 1983.
107. Smith LH: Risk of oxalate stone from large doses of vitamin C. *N Engl J Med* 298:856, 1978.
108. Ryall RL, Darroch JN, Marshall VR: The evaluation of risk factors in male stone-formers attending a general hospital out-patient clinic. *Br J Urol* 56:116–121, 1984.
109. Pak CYC, Sakhaee K, Crowther C, Brinkley L: Evidence justifying a high fluid intake in treatment of nephrolithiasis. *Ann Intern Med* 93:36–39, 1980.
110. Strauss AL, Coe FL, Deutsch L, Parks JH: Factors that predict relapse of calcium nephrolithiasis during treatment: A prospective study. *Am J Med* 72:17–24, 1982.
111. Albright F, Henneman P, Benedict PH, Forbes AP: Idiopathic hypercalciuria: A preliminary report. *Proc R Soc Med* 46:1077–1081, 1953.
112. Henneman PH, Benedict PH, Forbes AP, Dudley HR: Idiopathic hypercalciuria. *N Engl J Med* 259:802–807, 1958.
113. Broadus AE, Thier SO: Metabolic basis of renal-stone disease. *N Engl J Med* 300:839–845, 1979.
114. Nordin BEC, Peacock M, Wilkinson R: Hypercalciuria and calcium stone disease. *Clin Endocrinol Metab* 1:169–183, 1972.
115. Peacock M, Hodgkinson A, Nordin BEC: Importance of di-

etary calcium in the definition of hypercalciuria. *Br Med J* 3:469–471, 1967.

116. Lemann J Jr, Adams ND, Gray RW: Urinary calcium excretion in human beings. *N Engl J Med* 301:535–541, 1979.
117. Broadus AE, Dominguez M, Bartter FC: Pathophysiological studies in idiopathic hypercalciuria: Use of an oral calcium tolerance test to characterize distinctive hypercalciuric subgroups. *J Clin Endocrinol Metab* 47:751–760, 1978.
118. Broadus AE, Insogna KL, Lang R, Mallette LE, Oren DA, Gertner JM, et al: A consideration of the hormonal basis and phosphate leak hypothesis of absorptive hypercalciuria. *J Clin Endocrinol Metab* 58:161–169, 1984.
119. Breslau NA, McGuire JL, Zerwekh JE, Pak CYC: The role of dietary sodium on renal excretion and intestinal absorption of calcium and on vitamin D metabolism. *J Clin Endocrinol Metab* 55:369–373, 1982.
120. Muldowney FP, Freaney R, Moloney MF: Importance of dietary sodium in the hypercalciuria syndrome. *Kidney Int* 22:292–296, 1982.
121. Sabto J, Powell MJ, Breidahl MJ, Gurr FW: Influence of urinary sodium on calcium excretion in normal individuals: A redefinition of calciuria. *Med J Aust* 140:354–356, 1984.
122. Silver J, Rubinger D, Friedlaender MM, Popovtzer MM: Sodium-dependent idiopathic hypercalciuria in renal stone formers. *Lancet* 2:484–486, 1983.
123. Lau YK, Wasserstein A, Westby GR, Bosanac P, Grabie M, Mitnick P, et al: Proximal tubular defects in idiopathic hypercalciuria: Resistance to phosphate administration. *Miner Electrolyte Metab* 7:237–249, 1982.
124. Sutton RAL, Walker VR: Responses to hydrochlorothiazide and acetazolamide in patients with calcium stones. *N Engl J Med* 302:709–713, 1980.
125. Breslau NA, Brinkley L, Hill KD, Pak CYC: Relationship of animal protein-rich diet to kidney stone formation and calcium metabolism. *J Clin Endocrinol Metab* 66:140–146, 1988.
126. Stewart AF, Adler M, Byers CM, Segre GV, Broadus AE: Calcium homeostasis in immobilization: An example of resorptive hypercalciuria. *N Engl J Med* 306:1136–1140, 1982.
127. Broadus AE, Horst RL, Littledike ET, Mahaffey JE, Rasmussen H: Primary hyperparathyroidism with intermittent hypercalcaemia: Serial observations and simple diagnosis by means of an oral calcium tolerance test. *Clin Endocrinol (Oxf)* 12:225–235, 1980.
128. Yendt ER, Gagne RJA: Detection of primary hyperparathyroidism, with special reference to its occurrence in hypercalciuric females with "normal" or borderlin serum calcium. *Can Med Assoc J* 98:331–336, 1968.
129. Muldowney FP, Freaney R, McMullin JP, Towers RP, Spillane A, O'Connor P, et al: Serum ionized calcium and parathyroid hormone in renal stone disease. *Q J Med* 45:75–86, 1976.
130. Broadus AE, Horst RL, Lang R, Littledike ET, Rasmaussen H: The importance of circulating 1,25-dihydroxyvitamin D in the pathogenesis of hypercalciuria and renal stone formation in primary hyperparathyroidism. *N Engl J Med* 302: 421–426, 1980.
131. Parks J, Coe F, Favus M: Hyperparathyroidism in nephrolithiasis. *Arch Intern Med* 140:1479–1481, 1980.
132. Bordier P, Ryckewart A, Gueris J, Rasmussen H: On the pathogenesis of so-called idiopathic hypercalciuria. *Am J Med* 63:398–409, 1977.
133. Pak CYC: Physiological basis for absorptive and renal hypercalciurias. *Am J Physiol* 237:F415–F423, 1979.
134. Coe FL, Canterbury JM, Firpo JJ, Reiss E: Evidence for secondary hyperparathyroidism in idiopathic hypercalciuria. *J Clin Invest* 52:134–142, 1973.
135. Pak CYC, Galosy RA: Fasting urinary calcium and adenosine 3′,5′-monophosphate: A discriminant analysis for the identification of renal and absorptive hypercalciurias. *J Clin Endocrinol Metab* 48:260–265, 1979.
136. Pak CYC, Kaplan R, Bone H, Townsend J, Waters O: A simple test for the diagnosis of absorptive, resorptive and renal hypercalciurias. *N Engl J Med* 292:497–500, 1975.
137. Muldowney FP, Freaney R, Ryan JG: The pathogenesis of idiopathic hypercalciuria: Evidence for renal tubular calcium leak. *Q J Med* 49:87–94, 1980.
138. Broadus AE, Erickson SB, Gertner JM, Cooper K, Dobbins JW: An experimental human model of 1,25-dihydroxyvitamin D-mediated hypercalciuria. *J Clin Endocrinol Metab* 59:202–206, 1984.
139. Adams ND, Gray RW, Lemann J Jr, Cheung HS: Effects of calcitriol administration on calcium metabolism in healthy men. *Kidney Int* 21:90–97, 1982.
140. Von Lilienfeld-Toal H, Bach D, Hesse A, Franck H, Issa S: Parathyroid hormone is normal in renal stone patients with idiopathic hypercalciuria and high fasting urinary calcium. *Urol Res* 10:205–207, 1982.
141. Van Den Berg CJ, Kumar R, Wilson DM, Heath H 3d, Smith LH: Orthophosphate therapy decreases urinary calcium excretion and serum 1,25-dihydroxyvitamin D concentrations in idiopathic hypercalciuria. *J Clin Endocrinol Metab* 51:998–1001, 1980.
142. Gray RW, Wilz DR, Caldas AE, Lemann J Jr: The importance of phosphate in regulating plasma 1,25-$(OH)_2$-vitamin D levels in humans: Studies in healthy subjects, in calcium-stone formers and in patients with primary hyperparathyroidism. *J Clin Endocrinol Metab* 45:299–306, 1977.
143. Burckhardt P, Jaeger P: Secondary hyperparathyroidism in idiopathic hypercalciuria: Fact or theory? *J Clin Endocrinol Metab* 53:550–555, 1981.
144. Coe FL, Favus MJ, Crockett T, Strauss AL, Parks JH, Porat A, et al: Effects of low-calcium diet on urine calcium excretion, parathyroid function and serum $1,25(OH)_2D_3$ levels in patients with idiopathic hypercalciuria and in normal subjects. *Am J Med* 72:25–32, 1982.
145. Shen FH, Ivey JL, Sherrard DJ, Nielsen RL, Haussler MR, Baylink DJ: Further evidence supporting the phosphate leak hypothesis of idiopathic hypercalciuria. *Adv Exp Med Biol* 103:217–223, 1978.
146. Pak CYC: Pathogenesis, consequences, and treatment of the hypercalciuric states. *Semin Nephrol* 1:356–365, 1981.
147. Maierhofer WJ, Gray RW, Cheung HS, Lemann J Jr: Bone resorption stimulated by elevated serum 1,25-(OH)2-vitamin D concentrations in healthy men. *Kidney Int* 24:555–560, 1983.
148. Brannan PG, Morawski S, Pak CYC, Fordtran JS: Selective jejunal hyperabsorption of calcium in absorptive hypercalciuria. *Am J Med* 66:425–428, 1979.
149. Krejs GJ, Nicar MJ, Zerwekh JE, Normann DA, Kane MG, Pak CYC: Effect of 1,25-dihydroxyvitamin D_3 on calcium and magnesium absorption in the healthy human jejunum and ileum. *Am J Med* 75:973–976, 1983.
150. Pak CYC, Britton F, Peterson R, Ward D, Northcutt C, Breslau NA, et al: Ambulatory evaluation of nephrolithiasis: Classification, clinical presentation and diagnostic criteria. *Am J Med* 69:19–30, 1980.
151. Kaplan RA, Haussler MR, Deftos LJ, Bone H, Pak CYC: The role of 1 alpha, 25-dihydroxyvitamin D in the mediation of intestinal hyperabsorption of calcium in primary hyperparathyroidism and absorptive hypercalciuria. *J Clin Invest* 59:756–760, 1977.
152. Shen FH, Baylink DJ, Nielsen RL, Sherrard DJ, Ivey JL, Haussler MJ: Increased serum 1,25-dihydroxyvitamin D in idiopathic hypercalciuria. *J Lab Clin Med* 90:955–962, 1977.
153. Broadus AE, Insogna KL, Lang R, Ellison AF, Dreyer BE: Evidence for disordered control of 1,25-dihydroxyvitamin D production in absorptive hypercalciuria. *N Engl J Med* 311:73–80, 1984.
154. Insogna KL, Broadus AE, Dreyer BE, Ellison AF, Gertner JM: Elevated production rate of 1,25-dihydroxyvitamin D in patients with absorptive hypercalciuria. *J Clin Endocrinol Metab* 61:490–495, 1985.
155. Tanaka Y, Deluca HF: The control of 25-hydroxyvitamin D

metabolism by inorganic phosphorus. *Arch Biochem Biophys* 154:566–574, 1973.
156. Insogna KL, Broadus AE, Gertner JM: Impaired phosphorus conservation and 1,25-dihydroxyvitamin D generation during phosphorus deprivation in familial hypophosphatemic rickets. *J Clin Invest* 71:1562–1569, 1983.
157. Barilla DE, Zerwekh JE, Pak CYC: A critical evaluation of the role of phosphate in the pathogenesis of absorptive hypercalciuria. *Miner Electrolyte Metab* 2:302–309, 1979.
158. Tschöpe W, Ritz E, Schmidt-Gayk H: Is there a renal phosphorus leak in recurrent renal stone formers with absorptive hypercalciuria? *Eur J Clin Invest* 10:381–386, 1980.
159. Edwards NA, Hodgkinson A: Phosphate metabolism in patients with renal calculus. *Clin Sci* 29:93–106, 1965.
160. Insogna KL, Ellison AS, Burtis WJ, Sartori L, Lang RL, Broadus AE: Trichlormethiazide and oral phosphate therapy in patients with absorptive hypercalciuria. *J Urol* 141:269–274, 1989.
161. Lemann J Jr, Gray RW, Wilz DR: Evidence for a renal PO_4 leak in patients with calcium nephrolithiasis. *Adv Exp Med Biol* 103:225–226, 1978.
162. Lawoyin S, Sismilich S, Browne R, Pak CYC: Bone mineral content in patients with calcium urolithiasis. *Metabolism* 28:1250–1254, 1979.
163. Alhava EM, Juuti M, Karjalainen P: Bone mineral density in patients with urolithiasis: A preliminary report. *Scand J Urol Nephrol* 10:154–156, 1976.
164. Liberman UA, Sperling O, Atsmon A, Frank M, Modan M, deVries A: Metabolic and calcium kinetic studies in idiopathic hypercalciuria. *J Clin Invest* 47:2580–2590, 1968.
165. Malluche HH, Tschoepe W, Ritz E, Meyer-Sabellek W, Massry SG: Abnormal bone histology in idiopathic hypercalciuria. *J Clin Endocrinol Metab* 50:654–658, 1980.
166. Smith LH: Enteric hyperoxaluria and other hyperoxaluric states, in Coe JL (ed): *Nephrolithiasis.* New York, Churchill Livingstone, 1980, pp 136–164.
167. Williams HE: Oxalic acid and the hyperoxaluric syndromes. *Kidney Int* 13:410–417, 1978.
168. Dobbins JW, Binder HJ: Derangements of oxalate metabolism in gastrointestinal disease and their mechanisms, in Glass GBJ (ed): *Progress in Gastroenterology.* New York, Grune & Stratton, 1977, vol 3, pp 505–518.
169. Knickelbein RG, Aronson PS, Dobbins JW: Oxalate transport by anion exchange across rabbit ileal brush border. *J Clin Invest* 77:170–175, 1986.
170. Hillman RE: Primary hyperoxaluria, in Scriver CR, Beaudet AL, Sly WS, Valle D (eds): *The Metabolic Basis of Inherited Disease,* 6th ed. New York, McGraw-Hill, 1989, pp 933–944.
171. Weinman EJ, Frankfurt SJ, Ince A, Sansom S: Renal tubular transport of organic acids: Studies with oxalate and para-aminohippurate in the rat. *J Clin Invest* 61:801–806, 1978.
172. Daudon M, Reveillaud R-J, Normand M, Petit C, Jungers P: Piridoxilate-induced calcium oxalate calculi: A new drug-induced metabolic nephrolithiasis. *J Urol* 138:258–261, 1987.
173. Smith LH, Fromm H, Hofmann AF: Acquired hyperoxaluria, nephrolithiasis, and intestinal disease: Description of a syndrome. *N Engl J Med* 286:1371–1375, 1972.
174. Chadwick VS, Modha K, Dowling RH: Mechanism for hyperoxaluria in patients with ileal dysfunction. *N Engl J Med* 289:172–176, 1973.
175. Rudman D, Dedonis JL, Fountain MT, Chandler JB, Gerron GG, Fleming GA, et al: Hypocitraturia in patients with gastrointestinal malabsorption. *N Engl J Med* 303:657–661, 1980.
176. Hodgkinson A: Evidence of increased oxalate absorption in patients with calcium-containing renal stones. *Clin Sci Mol Med* 54:291–294, 1978.
177. Galosy R, Clarke L, Ward DL, Pak CYC: Renal oxalate excretion in calcium urolithiasis. *J Urol* 123:320–323, 1980.
178. Marangella M, Fruttero B, Bruno M, Linari F: Hyperoxaluria in ideopathic calcium stone disease: Further evidence of intestinal hyperabsorption of oxalate. *Clin Sci* 63:381–385, 1982.
179. Jaeger P, Portmann L, Jacquet AF, Burckhardt P: Influence of the calcium content of the diet on the incidence of mild hyperoxaluria in idiopathic renal stone formers. *Am J Nephrol* 5:40–44, 1985.
180. Erickson SB, Cooper K, Broadus AE, Smith LH, Werness PG, Binder HJ, et al: Oxalate absorption and postprandial urine supersaturation in an experimental human model of absorptive hypercalciuria. *Clin Sci* 67:131–138, 1984.
181. Yendt ER: Hyperoxaluria in idiopathic calcium oxalate nephrolithiasis. *Md Med J* 37:857–860, 1988.
182. Pak CYC: A cautious use of sodium cellulose phosphate in the management of calcium nephrolithiasis. *Invest Urol* 19:187–190, 1981.
183. Backman U, Danielson BG, Johansson G, Ljunghall S, Wikström B: Treatment of recurrent calcium stone formation with cellulose phosphate. *J Urol* 123:9–13, 1980.
184. Smith MJV, Hunt LD, King JS Jr, Boyce WH: Uricemia and urolithiasis. *J Urol* 101:637–642, 1969.
185. Coe FL, Raisen L: Allopurinol treatment of uric-acid disorders in calcium-stone formers. *Lancet* 1:129–131, 1973.
186. Coe FL: Hyperuricosuric calcium oxalate nephrolithiasis. *Kidney Int* 13:418–426, 1978.
187. Coe FL: Uric acid and calcium oxalate nephrolithiasis. *Kidney Int* 24:392–403, 1983.
188. Ettinger B: Does hyperuricosuria play a role in calcium oxalate lithiasis? *J Urol* 141:738–741, 1989.
189. Ettinger B, Tang A, Citron JT, Livermore B, Williams T: Randomized trial of allopurinol in the prevention of calcium oxalate calculi. *N Engl J Med* 315:1386–1389, 1986.
190. Coe FL: Treated and untreated recurrent calcium nephrolithiasis in patients with idiopathic hypercalciuria, hyperuricosuria, or no metabolic disorder. *Ann Intern Med* 87:404–410, 1977.
191. Okada Y, Nonomura M, Takeuchi H, Kawamura J, Yoshida O: Experimental and clinical studies on calcium lithiasis: II. Prevention of recurrent calcium stones with thiazides and allopurinol. *Hinyokika Kiyo* 32:1247–1257, 1986.
192. Oka T, Koide T, Sonoda T: A study on the effect of the treatment for idiopathic calcium urolithiasis on the prevention of recurrence: Estimation of stone episodes and clinical effect. *Nippon Hinyokika Gakkai Zasshi* 76:65–73, 1985.
193. Pak CYC: Medical management of nephrolithiasis. *J Urol* 128:1157–1164, 1982.
194. Fellström B, Backman U, Danielson BG, Johansson G, Ljunghall S, Wikström B: Urinary excretion of urate in renal calcium stone disease and in renal tubular acidification disturbances. *J Urol* 127:589–592, 1982.
195. Hodgkinson A: Uric acid disorders in patients with calcium stones. *Br J Urol* 48:1–5, 1976.
196. Schwille P, Samburger N, Wach B: Fasting uric acid and phosphate in urine and plasma of renal calcium-stone formers. *Nephron* 16:116–125, 1976.
197. Pylypchuk G, Ehrig U, Wilson DR: Idiopathic calcium nephrolithiasis: I. Differences in urine crystalloids, urine saturation with brushite and urine inhibitors of calcification between persons with and persons without recurrent kidney stone formation. *Can Med Assoc J* 120:658–665, 1979.
198. Tiselius H-G, Larsson L: Urinary excretion of urate in patients with calcium oxalate stone disease. *Urol Res* 11:279–283, 1983.
199. Coe FL, Kavalach AG: Hypercalciuria and hyperuricosuria in patients with calcium nephrolithiasis. *N Engl J Med* 291:1344–1350, 1974.
200. Lonsdale K: Epitaxy as a growth factor in urinary calculi and gallstones. *Nature* 217:56–58, 1968.
201. Meyer JL, Bergert JH, Smith LH: The epitaxially induced crystal growth of calcium oxalate by crystalline uric acid. *Invest Urol* 14:115–119, 1976.
202. Pak CYC, Arnold LH: Heterogeneous nucleation of calcium

oxalate by seeds of monosodium urate. *Proc Soc Exp Biol Med* 149:930–932, 1975.
203. Coe FL, Lawton RL, Goldstein RB, Tembe V: Sodium urate accelerates precipitation of calcium oxalate in vitro. *Proc Soc Exp Biol Med* 149:926–929, 1975.
204. Robertson WG, Knowles F, Peacock M: Urinary acid mucopolysaccharide inhibitors of calcium oxalate crystallisation, in Fleish H, Robertson WG, Smith LH, Vahlensieck W (eds): *Urolithiasis Research.* New York, Plenum, 1976, pp 331–335.
205. Tiselius H-G: Effects of sodium urate and uric acid crystals on the crystallization of calcium oxalate. *Urol Res* 12:11–15, 1984.
206. Fellström B, Backman U, Danielson BG, Holmgren K, Ljunghall S, Wikström B: Inhibitory activity of human urine on calcium oxalate crystal growth: Effects of sodium urate and uric acid. *Clin Sci* 62:509–514, 1982.
207. Pak CYC, Holt K, Zerwekh JE: Attenuation by monosodium urate of the inhibitory effect of glycosaminoglycans on calcium oxalate nucleation. *Invest Urol* 17:138–140, 1979.
208. Ryall RL, Hibberd CM, Marshall VR: The effect of crystalline monosodium urate on the crystallisation of calcium oxalate in whole human urine. *Urol Res* 14:63–65, 1986.
209. Goldwasser B, Sarig S, Azoury R, Wax Y, Many M: Hyperuricosuria and calcium oxalate stone formation, in Schwille PO, Smith LH, Robertson WG, Vahlensieck W (eds): *Urolithiasis and Related Clinical Research.* New York, Plenum, 1985, pp 859–862.
210. Ahmad R, Goldsmith HJ, Lovatt G: Allopurinol and recurrent renal stone formation, in *Abstracts of the 20th Congress of the European Dialysis and Transplant Association,* 12th Annual Conference of the European Dialysis and Transplant Nurses Association, London, June 19–22, 1983, p. 2.
211. Fellström B, Backman U, Danielson BG, Holmgren K, Johansson G, Lindsjö M, et al: Allopurinol treatment of renal calcium stone disease. *Br J Urol* 57:375–379, 1985.
212. Marangella M, Tricerri A, Ronzani M, Martini C, Petrarulo M, Daniele PG, et al: The relationship between clinical outcome and urine biochemistry during various forms of therapy for idiopathic calcium stone disease, in Schwille PO, Smith LH, Robertson WG, Vahlensieck W (eds): *Urolithiasis and Related Clinical Research.* New York, Plenum, 1985, pp 561–564.
213. Robertson WG, Peacock M, Selby PL, Williams RE, Clark P, Chisholm GD, et al: A multicentre trial to evaluate three treatments for recurrent idiopathic calcium stone disease: A preliminary report, in Schwille PO, Smith LH, Robertson WG, Vahlensieck W (eds): *Urolithiasis and Related Clinical Research.* New York, Plenum, 1985, pp 545–548.
214. Scott R, Mathieson A, McLelland A: The reduction in stone recurrence and oxalate excretion by allopurinol, in Rose GA, Robertson WG, Watts RWE (eds): *Oxalate in Human Biochemistry and Clinical Pathology.* Proceedings of an international meeting in London, October 26–27, 1979. London, Wellcome Foundation, 1979, pp 191–197.
215. Smith MJV: Placebo versus allopurinol for renal calculi. *J Urol* 117:690–692, 1977.
216. Sonoda T, Koide T, Oka T, Sakaguchi H, Itatani H, Ohkawa T, et al: A study of allopurinol in the prevention of recurrent calcium oxalate stones. *Hinyokika Kiyo* 31:2071–2079, 1985.
217. Tiselius H-G, Larsson L, Hellgren E: Clinical results of allopurinol treatment in prevention of calcium oxalate stone formation. *J Urol* 136:50–53, 1986.
218. Ulshöfer B, Zenke J, Achilles W, Rodeck G: The effect of long-term treatment with allopurinol on stone recurrence in calcium urolithiasis, in Schwille PO, Smith LH, Robertson WG, Vahlensieck W (eds): *Urolithiasis and Related Clinical Research.* New York, Plenum 1985, pp 517–519.
219. Wilson DR, Strauss AL, Manuel MA: Comparison of medical treatments for the prevention of recurrent calcium nephrolithiasis. *Urol Res* 12:39–40, 1984.
220. Finlayson B, Reid F: The effect of allopurinol on calcium oxalate (whewellite) precipitation. *Invest Urol* 15:489–492, 1978.
221. Finlayson B, Burns J, Smith A, Du Bois L: Effect of oxipurinol and allopurinol riboside on whewellite crystallization: In vitro and in vivo observations. *Invest Urol* 17:227–229, 1979.
222. Baggio B, Gambaro G, Paleari C, Cicerello E, Marchi A, Bragantini L, et al: Hydrochlorothiazide and allopurinol vs. placebo on urinary excretion of stone promoters and inhibitors. *Curr Ther Res* 34:145–151, 1983.
223. Morrissey JF, Ochoa M Jr, Lotspeich WO, Waterhouse C: Citrate excretion in renal tubular acidosis. *Ann Intern Med* 58:159–166, 1963.
224. Gordon EE, Sheps SG: Effect of acetazolamide on citrate excretion and formation of renal calculi: Report of a case and study of five normal subjects. *N Engl J Med* 256:1215–1219, 1957.
225. Fourman P, Robinson JR: Diminished urinary excretion of citrate during deficiencies of potassium in man: A preliminary communication. *Lancet* 2:656–657, 1953.
226. Menon M, Mahle CJ: Urinary citrate excretion in patients with renal calculi. *J Urol* 129:1158–1160, 1983.
227. Hosking DH, Wilson JWL, Liedtke RR, Smith LH, Wilson DM: Urinary citrate excretion in normal persons and patients with idiopathic calcium nephrolithiasis. *J Lab Clin Med* 106:682–689, 1985.
228. Nicar MJ, Skurla C, Sakhaee K, Pak CYC: Low urinary citrate excretion in nephrolithiasis. *Urology* 21:8–14, 1983.
229. Parks JH, Coe FL: A urinary calcium-citrate index for the evaluation of nephrolithiasis. *Kidney Int* 30:85–90, 1986.
230. Simpson DP: Citrate excretion: A window on renal metabolism. *Am J Physiol* 244:F223–F234, 1983.
231. Nicar MJ, Hill K, Pak CYC: Inhibition by citrate of spontaneous precipitation of calcium oxalate *in vitro. J Bone Miner Res* 2:215–220, 1987.
232. Kok DJ, Papapoulos SE, Bijvoet OLM: Excessive crystal agglomeration with low citrate excretion in recurrent stone formers. *Lancet* 1:1056–1058, 1986.
233. Pak CYC, Fuller C, Sakhaee K, Preminger GM, Britton F: Long-term treatment of calcium nephrolithiasis with potassium citrate. *J Urol* 134:11–19, 1985.
234. Pak CYC, Peterson R, Sakhaee K, Fuller C, Preminger G, Reisch J: Correction of hypocitraturia and prevention of stone formation by combined thiazide and potassium citrate therapy in thiazide-unresponsive hypercalciuric nephrolithiasis. *Am J Med* 79:284–288, 1985.
235. Barlow IM, Harrison SP: Improved urinary oxalate kit (letter). *Clin Chem* 36:1523, 1990.
236. Hosking DH, Erickson SB, Van Den Berg CJ, Wilson DM, Smith LH: The stone clinic effect in patients with idiopathic calcium urolithiasis. *J Urol* 130:1115–1118, 1983.
237. Insogna KL, Broadus AE: Nephrolithiasis, in Krieger DT, Bardin CW (eds): *Current Therapy in Endocrinology and Metabolism, 1985–1986.* St. Louis, Mosby, 1985, pp 353–363.
238. Pak CYC, Smith LH, Resnick MI, Weinerth JL: Dietary management of idiopathic calcium urolithiasis. *J Urol* 131:850–852, 1984.
239. Citron J, Tang A, Ettinger B: A model for predicting stone recurrences (abstract). *Urol Res* 12:97, 1984.
240. Yendt ER, Cohanim M: Clinical and laboratory approaches for evaluation of nephrolithiasis. *J Urol* 141:764–769, 1989.
241. Ljunghall S, Källsen R, Backman U, Danielson BG, Grimelius L, et al: Clinical effects of parathyroid surgery in normocalcaemic patients with recurrent renal stones. *Acta Chir Scand* 146:161–169, 1980.
242. Broadus AE, Magee JS, Mallette LE, Horst RL, Lang R, Jensen PS, et al: A detailed evaluation of oral phosphate therapy in selected patients with primary hyperparathyroidism. *J Clin Endocrinol Metab* 56:953–961, 1983.
243. Yendt ER, Cohanim M: Prevention of calcium stones with thiazides. *Kidney Int* 13:397–409, 1978.
244. Costanzo LS, Windhager EE: Calcium and sodium transport by the distal convoluted tubule of the rat. *Am J Physiol* 235:F492–F506, 1978.

245. Ettinger B, Oldroyd NO, Sörgel F: Triamterene nephrolithiasis. *JAMA* 244:2443–2445, 1980.
246. Ettinger B: Recurrent nephrolithiasis: Natural history and effect of phosphate therapy: A double-blind controlled study. *Am J Med* 61:200–206, 1976.
247. Thomas WC Jr: Use of phosphates in patients with calcareous renal calculi. *Kidney Int* 13:390–396, 1978.
248. Wikström B, Backman U, Danielson BG, Fellström B, Johansson G, Ljunghall S, et al: Phosphate treatment of calcium urolithiasis, in Schwille PO, Smith LH, Robertson WG, Vahlensieck W (eds): *Urolithiasis and Related Clinical Research.* New York, Plenum, 1985, pp 495–498.
249. Heyburn PJ, Robertson WG, Peacock M: Phosphate treatment of recurrent calcium stone disease. *Nephron* 32:314–319, 1982.
250. Smith LH, Thomas WC Jr, Arnaud CD: Orthophosphate therapy in calcium renal lithiasis, in Cifuentes Delatte L, Rapado A, Hodgkinson A (eds): *Urinary Calculi: Recent Advances in Aetiology, Stone Structure, and Treatment.* International Symposium on Renal Stone Research, Madrid, 1972. Basel, Karger, 1973, pp 188–197.
251. Ettinger B: Thiazide treatment of recurrent calcium stones, in Drach GW (ed): *Common Problems in Infections and Stones.* Chicago, Mosby–Year Book, 1991, pp 191–204.
252. Mitwalli A, Ayiomamitis A, Grass L, Oreopoulos DG: Control of hyperoxaluria with large doses of pyridoxine in patients with kidney stones. *Int Urol Nephrol* 20:353–359, 1988.
253. Yendt ER, Cohanim M: Response to a physiologic dose of pyridoxine in type I primary hyperoxaluria. *N Engl J Med* 312:953–957, 1985.
254. Schaumburg H, Kaplan J, Windebank A, Vick N, Rasmus S, Pleasure D, et al: Sensory neuropathy from pyridoxine abuse: A new megavitamin syndrome. *N Engl J Med* 309:445–448, 1983.
255. Berger A, Schaumburg HH: More on neuropathy from pyridoxine abuse (letter). *N Engl J Med* 311:986–987, 1984.
256. Dobbins JW: Nephrolithiasis and intestinal disease. *J Clin Gastroenterol* 7:21–24, 1985.
257. Bais R, Rofe AM, Conyers RAJ: The inhibition of metabolic oxalate production by sulfhydryl compounds. *J Urol* 145: 1302–1305, 1991.
258. Laerum E, Larsen S: Thiazide prophylaxis of urolithiasis: A double blind study in general practice. *Acta Med Scand* 215:383–389, 1984.
259. Young JL Jr, Boswell RB, Nies AS: Severe allopurinol hypersensitivity: Association with thiazides and prior renal compromise. *Arch Intern Med* 134:553–558, 1974.
260. Tiselius H-G: The effect of pH on the urinary inhibition of calcium oxalate crystal growth. *Br J Urol* 53:470–474, 1981.
261. Pak CYC, Peterson R: Successful treatment of hyperuricosuric calcium oxalate nephrolithiasis with potassium citrate. *Arch Intern Med* 146:863–867, 1986.
262. Berg C, Larsson L, Tiselius H-G: The effects of a single evening dose of alkaline citrate on urine composition and calcium stone formation. *J Urol* 148(3 Pt 2):979–985, 1992.
263. Joost J, Putz A: Calcium oxalate stone formers five years later, in Schwille PO, Smith LH, Robertson WG, Vahlensieck W (eds): *Urolithiasis and Related Clinical Research.* New York, Plenum, 1985, pp 557–560.
264. Ettinger B: Recurrence of nephrolithiasis: A six-year prospective study. *Am J Med* 67:245–248, 1979.

PART VIII

Miscellaneous Disorders

CHAPTER 26

Disorders of Growth and Development

Margaret H. MacGillivray

The growth of the human organism from the zygote stage to its culmination in adult stature is a complex phenomenon involving a multitude of regulatory mechanisms which control tissue differentiation, generation, and maturation. In practical terms, growth is the net of mass produced and retained minus that destroyed or lost. Terminal or mature size represents an equilibrium between the incremental and decremental processes, while aging signifies an imbalance in which more tissue is lost than is replaced. Tissue differentiation and maturation, although not explicit in this definition, are essential components of growth.

Throughout childhood and adolescence, gains in height and weight are sensitive and reasonably accurate indexes of the health and well-being of an individual. In general, stature or height is a more accurate basis for evaluating the overall growth process because healthy children show wide variability in weight. However, in chronically malnourished children weight is the more sensitive indicator of disease; linear growth is disturbed to a lesser degree.

This chapter discusses the mechanisms which control the overall growth processes of healthy children as well as the many factors which disturb or enhance growth and provides criteria for differentiating children with pathologic growth from those with short or tall stature at either limit of the normal growth channels. Practical information on diagnostic procedures and therapy is also given.

BIOLOGICAL STAGES OF GROWTH

The growth of all tissues consists of an initial, critical phase of rapid cell division *(hyperplasia)*. During this period, diseases that interfere with DNA replication may have a permanent stunting effect because tissues are denied their full complement of cells. The second phase is attributable to both hyperplasia and increased cell size *(hypertrophy)*. In the final stage, cellular enlargement is responsible for the attainment of full organ size.[1–3] Maturity is a period of equilibrium. It is followed by the process of aging, which is characterized by more tissue degeneration than regeneration (Fig. 26-1). Most studies support the hypothesis that tissues grow first by cellular multiplication and later by cellular size increase; a notable exception is the report by Sands and colleagues,[4] who observed that cell size increased during the early phase of tissue growth and that cellular multiplication continued throughout all the stages.

The phases of cellular hyperplasia, hyperplasia plus hypertrophy, and hypertrophy alone do not occur simultaneously in all organs; also, the length of time spent in each of these stages varies from one tissue to another (Fig. 26-2). Hence, growth in terms of cellular behavior is not the homogeneous process suggested by external body measurements.[2,5] Nevertheless, the adult state is achieved by virtue of smooth integration of these growth phenomena.

A comparison of brain growth with musculoskeletal growth illustrates the individualistic growth characteristics of different tissues. The greatest rates of DNA synthesis in the brain take place before birth. After birth, there is a gradual reduction in mitotic rates; by 6 to 8 months of life, the critical period of brain growth is completed and the infant possesses the total number of brain cells needed for the remainder of its life. In contrast, the critical phase of growth for the musculoskeletal system lasts 15 to 20 years and extends from fetal life to early adulthood.

The long-range impact of disease on the growth process depends on the timing, duration, and severity of the insult. In general, the prognosis for recovery is better if the injury occurs during the stage of hypertrophy rather than that of hyperplasia. The risk of irreparable damage to the growth process is especially high if prolonged injury occurs during both stages, e.g., microcephaly due to fetal alcohol syndrome and viral infections of the central nervous system (CNS).

CONTROL OF GROWTH PROCESSES

Normal growth is controlled by a number of interacting forces, including genetic mechanisms, tissue-

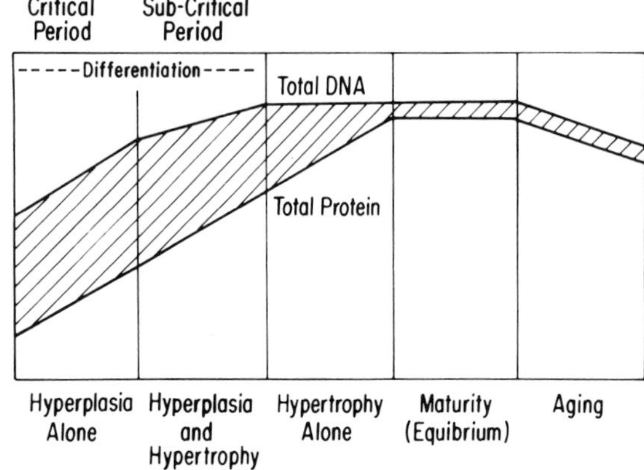

FIGURE 26-1 Representation of the various stages of organ growth and differentiation. During the phase of hyperplasia, growth is due entirely to cellular multiplication, which is represented by the steepness of the DNA slope. In the next phase, the rate of DNA synthesis is less rapid but the rate of protein synthesis is unchanged; consequently, tissue growth is now the result of both cellular multiplication and cellular enlargement. This is followed by a stage of growth due to hypertrophy alone as DNA synthesis plateaus but protein synthesis persists at its previous rate. At maturity, constancy of size is due to equilibrium between tissue gained and tissue lost. During the aging process, tissue loss exceeds replacement. (*From Weiss and Kavanau.*[3])

specific factors, hormone regulators, the responsiveness of tissues, and nutritional influences.

Genetic Factors

Two aspects of growth are influenced by genetic mechanisms which are polygenic in nature: The first is regulation of the rate of cellular multiplication and therefore overall size, and the second is control of the pace of maturation. Studies indicate that birth size does not correlate with midparental height (mean height of parents) or with paternal size or subsequent adult stature but does correlate with maternal size (prepregnancy weight of the mother). On this basis, it has been concluded that genetic factors may not play a dominant role in the growth of the fetus.[6,7] However, during the first 12 to 18 months of postnatal life, genetic influences become increasingly apparent. In this period the linear growth curves of two-thirds of infants shift; the direction of the change correlates best with the mean height of the parents. Approximately one-half drift upward and the remainder downward in growth percentile. From age 2 years to adulthood, genetic mechanisms play a dominant role; thus, a close correlation exists between midparental height and the child's stature.[8,9] Genetic controls also regulate the pace of biological maturation in children, which is best illustrated by familial patterns of delayed or early sexual maturation and age of attainment of adult stature.

Both the X and Y chromosomes contain growth-regulating genes. The special influence of the X chromosome is inferred from growth studies in females. As a rule, girls develop 2 years earlier than boys do, and sisters are more similar in pattern of osseous maturation than are brothers.[10] Also, girls with total or partial loss of the X chromosome are short in stature. A study has revealed a possible influence of Yq heterochromatin on the attainment of body height; i.e., the length of the heterochromatic band Y(q12) was found to correlate with height.[11]

Genetic factors are also known to influence size by race. Although black infants at birth are smaller than white infants, their stature and pace of osseous maturation during the childhood years are equal to or even a little ahead of those of white children from families of comparable income.[12] Japanese children raised in the United States and Chinese children raised in the United Kingdom are taller than are Japanese and Chinese children raised in Japan and Hong Kong, respectively. However, final heights of the Asian emigrés are somewhat lower than those of adult Americans and Europeans.[13,14]

FIGURE 26-2 Critical periods of high mitotic rate with increasing cell number for various tissues. By 6 to 8 months of postnatal life, cellular multiplication in the brain is completed. In contrast, rapid rates of DNA synthesis persist for years in muscle, skeleton, and adipose tissues. (*From Smith and Bierman.*[5])

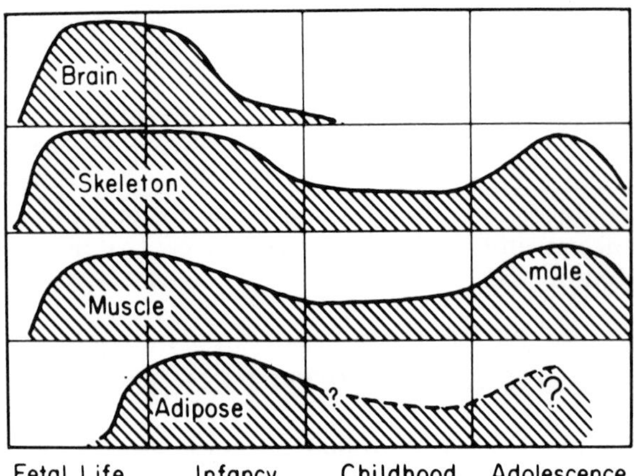

Peptide Growth Factors and Hormonal Influences

The early concept of the endocrine system consisted of an organized network of ductless glands which secreted the classical hormones into the bloodstream; these chemical messengers traveled to distal organs and enhanced their growth and activity. Currently, the endocrine system is viewed in a much broader context which includes the classical network of ductless glands as well as a large number of peptide growth factors which are produced in many tissues. These factors may work locally on the cells from which they originate via *autocrine mechanisms* or may influence adjacent tissues via *paracrine mechanisms*. Alternatively, peptide growth factors may be transported through the bloodstream like classical hormones and work through endocrine mechanisms.

In many instances, the classical hormones regulate the production of specific peptide growth factors which control cell proliferation; as such, these growth factors are the mediators or proximal effectors by which the classical hormones control the growth of tissues. A good example of this type of interaction is the one exhibited by growth hormone (GH) on insulin-like growth factor-I (IGF-I) production and somatic growth. However, other examples include parathyroid hormone (PTH) and estrogen stimulation of IGF-I production in cartilage explants and the uterus, respectively.[15] Table 26-1 summarizes the interrelations between peptide growth factors and the classical hormones.[16]

Insulin-Like Growth Factors

In the late 1950s, Daughaday and Salmon observed that GH administration to hypophysectomized rats resulted in increased incorporation of sulfate and thymidine into cartilage in vivo. In subsequent experiments, GH itself did not produce these effects in vitro, whereas serum from GH-treated hypophysectomized rats did. They concluded that the enhanced uptake of sulfate and thymidine was due to a substance in serum which was GH-dependent and which they called sulfation factor.[17,18] Subsequently, other names were given to this serum factor—i.e.,

TABLE 26-1 Interrelations between Growth Factors and Classic Hormones

Growth Factor*	Sources	Properties	Hormone Regulators
IGFs	Synthesized by liver, fetal lung, kidney, heart, limb, mesenchyme	See text	GH, placental lactogen, prolactin(?), insulin(?)
Epidermal growth factor	First isolated from male mouse submaxillary gland; urogastrone in human urine may be equivalent of mouse EGF	In mice, stimulates early eyelid opening and incisor eruption; role in humans unclear	Androgens, thyroxine
Nerve growth factor	First isolated from male mouse submaxillary gland; shares ~50% homology with brain-derived neurotropic factor	Regulates growth of sensory and sympathetic neurons; stimulates axon outgrowth; regulates levels of peptide neurotransmitters; may play a role in peripheral neurofibromatosis, familial dysautonomia, MEN 2b	Thyroxine
Fibroblast pneumonocyte factor	Secreted by human fetal lung fibroblasts; present in human amniotic fluid	Stimulates surfactant synthesis by type 2 pneumonocytes in vitro	Glucocorticoids
Erythropoietin		Mitogen for proerythrocytes	GH, androgens
Fibroblast growth factor	First isolated from bovine pituitary gland	Mol wt 13,400; mitogen for endodermal, mesodermal, amniotic fluid-derived cells; stimulates angiogenesis	?
Platelet-derived growth factor	Released by human platelets during blood coagulation in vivo	May influence connective tisue response to injury and development of atherosclerotic lesions	?
Thymic hormone		Controls development of mature thymocytes	?
Endothelin	Vascular endothelial cells	Mitogenic for vascular smooth muscle cells, fibroblasts, glomerular mesangial cells, and osteoblasts	?

* See Refs. 16, 196.

EGF = epidermal growth factor; MEN 2b = multiple endocrine neoplasia type 2b.

nonsuppressible insulin-like growth factor (NSILA), somatomedin C (Sm C), and insulin-like growth factor (IGF). The data derived from many pioneering investigations formed the basis for the somatomedin hypothesis of GH action, which proposed that GH regulates the growth of skeletal and extraskeletal tissues through its ability to control the production of IGF-I. This peptide growth factor increases skeletal growth via chondrocyte proliferation and stimulates the growth of many extraskeletal tissues (fibroblasts, muscle, etc.) by increasing cell division and protein synthesis.

Recently, Isaakson and colleagues reported that GH and IGF-I stimulate chondrocytes at different stages of maturation.[19] They observed that isolated epiphyseal chondrocytes suspended in culture contain chondrocyte progenitor cells which form large colonies, while more differentiated chondrocytes form small colonies. GH selectively stimulated the formation of large colonies, whereas IGF-I promoted the formation of small or normal-sized colonies. As a result of these observations with prechondrocytes and somewhat similar effects of GH on preadipocytes, the dual effector theory of GH action was proposed. It states that GH directly stimulates the differentiation of chondrocyte and adipocyte progenitor cells; and also stimulates local production of IGF-I, which enhances the proliferation of the differentiating cells via autocrine/paracrine mechanisms.

Historically, the term *somatomedin* ("mediator of growth") was proposed by investigators whose research focus was somatic growth. By contrast, the name *IGF* was used by researchers working in the field of insulin physiology. By definition, IGFs are peptides which have potent mitogenic and metabolic properties. Although they are biologically and structurally related to proinsulin, in early studies the insulin-like properties of these peptides were not neutralized in the presence of excess anti-insulin antibodies; hence, the origin of the term *NSILA*.

The main IGFs in human serum are IGF-I, a 70 amino acid (molecular weight of 7649) straight-chain, basic peptide (isoelectric point 8.1–8.5) which has greater GH dependency than does IGF-II, a neutral peptide (molecular weight of 7471) containing 67 amino acids. The latter has structural homology with rat multiplication-stimulating activity (MSA) isolated from rat hepatocyte cultures. MSA is now referred to as rIGF-II. IGF-I appears to be the major regulator of somatic growth postnatally, whereas IGF-II plays a predominant role during fetal life. Conclusive evidence about the role of IGF-I in stimulating postnatal growth was provided by studies demonstrating increased somatic growth after IGF-I administration to GH-deficient animals and accelerated postnatal growth of transgenic mice that overexpress the IGF-I gene.[20,21]

In well-nourished subjects, the circulating level of IGF-I reflects the 24-h secretion of GH from the pituitary gland. Theoretically, measurement of IGF-I should give insight into the output of pituitary GH, which is difficult to quantitate because of its pulsatile secretion. In contrast to GH, serum IGF-I has a prolonged half-life because the vast majority of circulating IGF-I is complexed to binding proteins (IGFBP). The measurement of serum IGF-I is complicated because it is contained mainly within the 150kDa IGFBP complex which interferes with interaction between IGF-I and the antisera used in radioimmunoassays (RIAs). Recent assay improvements include the availability of highly specific antisera that do not cross-react with IGF-II, separation of IGF-I from the binding proteins (acid-ethanol extraction, acid-gel chromatography, and Sep-pak chromatography), and the use of biosynthetic IGF-I standards (ng/mL) instead of serum standards (U/mL).

Circulating levels of IGF-I are age-dependent and to some extent sex-dependent. Values are low in newborns and young infants, gradually rise during childhood, and reach a peak during the most rapid growth phase of puberty.[22–27] Pubertal increases occur earlier in females than in males; thereafter they decline to adult levels. Elderly adults have low IGF-I levels because GH production falls. Previous studies showed that IGF-I levels in childhood correlate better with bone age and Tanner stage than with chronologic age. Eighty percent of children with classical GH deficiency have IGF-I levels that are 2 SD or more below the mean for chronologic age. Also, many pathologically short children with normal GH provocative tests have IGF-I levels which are as low as those seen in classical GH deficiency. Whether these children have a subtle defect in GH secretion or action remains to be determined.

In addition to GH, nutrition is the principal regulator of postnatal IGF-I production. During starvation, nutritional factors override the importance of GH.[28–31] Fasting lowers IGF-I levels to approximately 10 percent of basal values, and refeeding restores concentrations toward normal. Studies have shown that food-deprived animals develop a state of GH resistance which leads to low IGF-I levels because the number of GH receptors decreases. Animals experiencing milder forms of nutritional deprivation (i.e., reduced-protein diets) also develop GH resistance and low IGF-I levels, but this occurs before a significant fall in GH receptor numbers; presumably, the mechanism is a post-GH receptor defect.

In addition to GH resistance, diet-restricted rats also exhibit IGF-I resistance because infusions of IGF-I fail to increase weight gain and linear growth. Nevertheless, when IGF-I was administered to diet-restricted human volunteers, it appeared to have some beneficial effects because the protein losses due to nutritional deprivation were reduced.

Low serum IGF-I levels are observed in patients with GH deficiency, GH resistance (Laron syndrome), hypothyroidism, malnutrition, and hepatic failure; in infancy and old age; and in many children with idiopathic growth failure (neurosecretory defect, bioinactive GH, normal-variant short stature [NVSS], idiopathic short stature, etc.).

High serum IGF-I levels are present in acromegaly, pituitary gigantism, and IGF-I resistance syndrome. Transient physiologic elevations also occur during the adolescent growth spurt. The interpretation of IGF-I levels must be based on the normal range for age. For example, a 70-year-old individual with a value which is normal for a 20-year-old may have GH excess.

The IGF-I and IGF-II genes are large and complex; the organization of each is remarkably well conserved among the mammalian species, suggesting that the two growth factors diverged from a common ancestral gene.[32] The human IGF-I gene spans about 95 kilobases (kb) of the genome and is located on the long arm of chromosome 12. It contains 4 coding exons and at least two 5′ UT exons. The human IGF-II gene is about 35 kb and is on the short arm of chromosome 11 immediately downstream from the insulin gene. It contains 8 exons, 3 of which are 5′ UT exons. The promotors and regulatory elements of two 5′ UT exons appear to control the abundant expression of IGF-II in the fetus; however, the factors which stimulate fetal IGF-II gene expression and later cause postnatal suppression have not been defined. Both IGF genes are transcribed and processed into a variety of messenger RNA (mRNA) species which result from the use of different promotors as well as from alternative mRNA splicing mechanisms. The ontogeny of both IGF-I and IGF-II mRNA expression indicates that they are regulated by developmental factors as well as by determinants within the tissues from which the peptide growth factors originate. The functional significance of the various transcripts has not been defined. The main IGF-I transcripts resulting from alternative mRNA splicing generate two precursor species (IGF-IA and IGF-IB mRNAs); these result in translation products containing 153 and 195 amino acid residues, respectively. Within each, the 70 amino acid residue IGF-I molecule occupies positions 49–118. Despite the impressive similarity among IGF-I precursors from different species, very little is known about the biosynthesis and processing of the mature IGF-I peptide. Unlike classical endocrine peptides, the IGF genes are expressed in multiple tissues, and their products—the IGFs—are not stored in secretory granules before secretion.

The IGFs exert their growth-promoting effects postnatally through the type 1 IGF receptor, which has a high degree of structural and functional similarity to the insulin receptor. The insulin and IGF-I receptors are composed of two α subunits and two β subunits which are disulfide-linked into a $\alpha_2\beta_2$ heterotetromeric complex. The α subunits reside on the extracellular side of the plasma membrane and encode the high-affinity ligand-binding domain. The β subunits contain a single membrane-spanning region and an intracellular portion which contains an ATP-binding domain, tyrosine-specific autophosphorylation sites, and intrinsic substrate protein kinase activity (Fig. 26-2). The type 2 IGF receptor is identical to the mannose-6-phosphate receptor and has a binding site for IGF-II. It appears that this receptor is bifunctional only in mammals; i.e., it facilitates the translocation of lysosomal enzymes to lysosomes and also binds IGF-II. Thus it facilitates IGF-II biological effects and enhances degradation of extracellular IGF-II by receptor-mediated internalization. The hypoglycemic properties of the IGFs are due to free IGFs working through the insulin receptor, since this effect can be blocked by the presence of antibody to the insulin receptor but not by antibody to the type 1 IGF receptor.

The bioavailability of IGFs is regulated by the IGF binding proteins (IGFBPs), which carry the IGFs in all extracellular fluid.[33–36] The factors that regulate the synthesis of IGFBPs include tissue-specific factors, developmental factors, hormones (GH, IGFs, insulin, etc.), and metabolic factors (glucose, fasting). Approximately six IGFBPs have been identified. The most important forms are IGFBP-I, IGFBP-II, and IGFBP-III (Table 26-2). Although the liver is the most important source of IGFBPs, a diverse pattern of IGFBP expression exists in many organs and tissues. The IGFBPs serve as a reservoir for IGFs and protect circulating IGFs from enzymatic degradation. They also prolong the half-life of the IGFs and prevent them from crossing the capillary barrier. In serum the amounts of free IGFs are very low because of the abundance of IGFBPs, while in saliva the IGFs are present in free form with low levels of IGFBPs. Approximately 90 percent of the IGFs (IGF-I, IGF-II) circulate in plasma as part of a very large 150-kDa ternary IGFBP complex which is composed of three subunits: the IGF peptide (growth factor or γ subunit), an IGF binding protein (IGFBP-III, β subunit, a 40- to 60-kDa glycosylated derivative of a 29-kDa protein), and a non-IGF-binding glycoprotein which is labile in acid (α subunit, ALS, 85

TABLE 26-2 Terminology of the IGF Binding Proteins

IGFBP-I	GH independent binding protein Amniotic fluid binding protein (AFBP) Placental protein (PP12) Binding protein (BP28)
IGFBP-II	BRLA3A cell-line-derived IGFBP MDBK cell-line-derived IGFBP IBP-2
IGFBP-III	GH-dependent binding protein Acid-stable subunit of the 140-K complex BP53 or BP291

kDa). Little or no interaction occurs between the α and β subunits in the absence of the IGFs (Fig. 26-3). IGFs bound to the ternary complex are unable to exert their insulin-like effects, whereas free IGFs possess 5 to 10 percent of the hypoglycemic potency of insulin. The total circulating IGF concentration is approximately 100 nmol/L compared to the usual insulin concentration of 100 pmol/L. If the circulating IGFs were not complexed, their hypoglycemic potential would be 50- to 100-fold more than that of insulin. Problems with hypoglycemia have been observed when IGF-I infusions are administered in high doses because of the elevated levels of free IGF. Although the ternary complex blocks the passage of IGFs across the capillary barrier, it is possible that the binary β-γ complex becomes dissociated from the 150-kDa ternary complex, after which it traverses the capillary barrier and facilitates IGF actions on tissues.

IGFBP-III has been regarded as a GH-dependent IGF binding protein because concentrations are low in GH-deficient patients and high in patients with acromegaly; however, it is not entirely clear whether GH or IGF-I regulates IGFBP-III production. Since IGF-I administration increases IGFBP-III in cultured chondrocytes and fibroblasts as well as in hypophysectomized rats, it would appear that IGF-I is the main regulator of IGFBP-III production. However, hypophysectomized rats treated with IGF-I produce IGFBP-III, which is not contained in the 150-kDa ternary complex. In contrast, GH treatment of hypophysectomized rats increases IGFBP-III contained within the 150-kDa ternary complex. These observations suggest that GH is the major regulator of the 150-kDa complex, with the α subunit being GH-dependent while the β subunit is IGF-I–dependent. Measurements of IGFBP-III appear to be of diagnostic value in patients with GH deficiency or GH excess.[35] However, interpretations of IGFBP-III levels must take age and nutritional status into account. IGFBP-III concentrations, like IGF-I levels, are low in early childhood, rise with age, and peak during the rapid growth phase of puberty. Thereafter, the levels fall to the adult range (Fig. 26-4). As has already been mentioned, IGFBP-III levels are low in hypopituitarism and high in acromegaly. Not surprisingly, IGFBP-III levels are also low in GH-resistant syndromes (e.g., Laron syndrome) which are characterized by high GH levels and low IGF-I levels. Normal concentrations have been observed in Turner's syndrome and Russell-Silver syndrome. Low levels of IGFBP-III have also been observed in some patients with non-islet-cell tumor hypoglycemia due to overproduction of IGF-II by mesenchymal tumors (Wilms' tumor, neuroblastoma, leiomyomata, leiomyosarcoma, fibrosarcoma). The IGF-II gene is expressed in these tumors, and the product is a high-molecular-weight IGF-II peptide (10 to 15 kDa). Serum levels of IGF-II in hypoglycemic individuals with these tumors range from low to high. The serum IGF-II is present in a 60-kDa complex rather than the normal 150-kDa IGFBP, presumably because of defective binding of the binary IGF-II–IGFBP-III complex to the α subunit. Consequently, IGF-II is able to exert its hypoglycemic effects. The levels of IGFBP-III in late pregnancy have been reported to fall because of protease activity. However, measurements of low IGFBP-III dose by ligand blotting after SDS-PAGE electrophoresis have not been confirmed by analytic methods that do not involve protein denaturation.

Less is known about the physiologic role of human IGFBP-II, which is a nonglycosylated protein with a predicted molecular mass of 34 kDa; it has a preferential affinity for IGF-II. IGFBP-II is found in human cerebrospinal fluid (CSF) and is secreted by the human rhabdomyosarcoma cell line A673. The rat counterpart of human IGFBP-II has been puri-

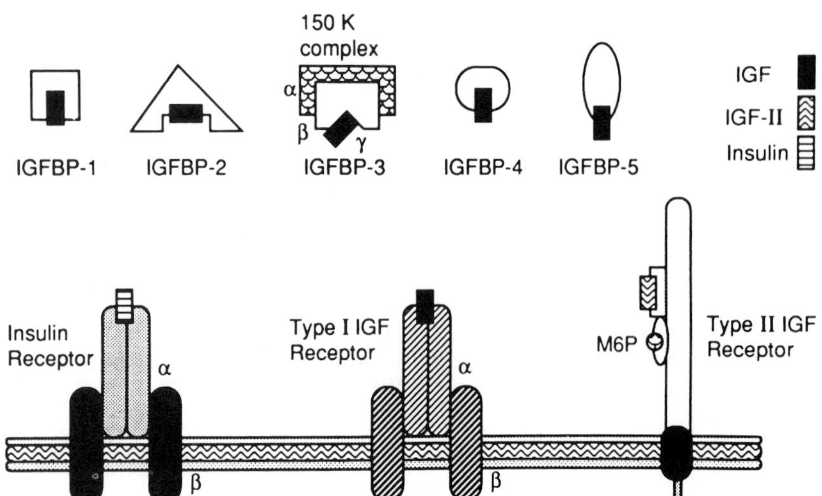

FIGURE 26-3 Schematic representation of IGF binding proteins and IGF receptors on the cell surface. The type I IGF receptor and the insulin receptor share structural and functional properties. The postnatal growth-promoting actions of the IGFs are mediated through the type I IGF receptor, while the hypoglycemic actions of the IGFs are exerted through the insulin receptor. The type II IGF receptor is identical to the mannose-6-phosphate receptor; it has not been linked to the growth-promoting effects of the IGFs. (*From Pinchas et al.*[33])

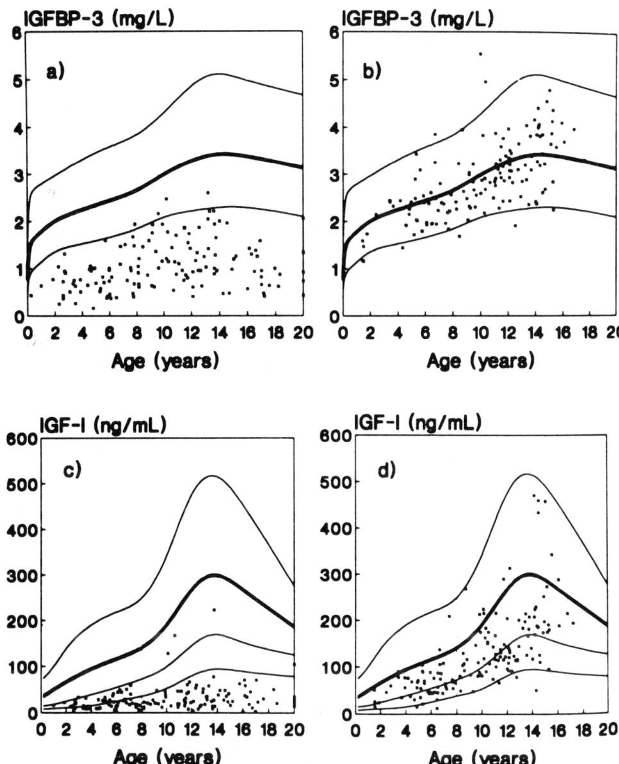

FIGURE 26-4 The normal range (5th to 95th percentiles) for plasma concentrations of IGFBP-III are shown for chronologic age in *A* and *B*. *C* and *D* depict the normal range (1st to 95th percentiles) of IGF-I plasma concentrations. IGFBP-III and IGF-I measurements from growth hormone–deficient children are displayed in *A* and *C*, respectively, while IGFBP-III and IGF-I levels from short children with normal GH secretion are depicted in *B* and *D*, respectively. Note the similarity of IGFBP-III and IGF-I profiles based on chronologic age in normal children. (*From Blum and Ranke.*[35])

fied from the buffalo rat liver cell line, BRL3a. IGFBP-II and IGFBP-I are proteins that are predominantly expressed in fetal tissues; production of IGFBP-II is rapidly turned off after birth except in the choroid plexus of the brain, hence its appearance in CSF.

The second most important IGF binding protein in human plasma is IGFBP-I, which carries about 10 percent of the circulating IGFs in a smaller complex weighing about 40 kDa. Other names which have been given to IGFBP-I include amniotic fluid binding protein (AFBP), placental protein 12 (PP12), and binding protein 28. The molecular mass of IGFBP-I is 28 kDa; it possesses an equal affinity for IGF-I and IGF-II, which is fivefold lower than the affinity of IGFBP-III for these peptides. Unlike IGFBP-III, serum IGFBP-I is independent of GH and has a marked diurnal rhythmicity, with a peak to basal ratio of 13-fold to 20-fold. The diurnal pattern is characterized by a nocturnal rise and high early morning levels followed by a decline. Because glucose suppresses and hypoglycemia, fasting, and exercise increase circulating IGFBP-I levels, a role for IGFBP-I as a regulator of glucose has been proposed. Enhanced hepatic synthesis of IGFBP-I appears to be the mechanism responsible for elevations in the circulating levels of this binding protein, possibly via intracellular cyclic nucleotide accumulation. Serum levels of IGFBP-I have an inverse relation to GH, i.e., elevated levels in GH-deficient states and decreased levels in acromegaly.

IGFBP-I is present in abundance in amniotic fluid and in prenatal and postnatal serum; it is also elevated in patients with chronic renal failure. Amniotic fluid IGFBP is identical to the peptide secreted by the human hepatoma cell line (HEP G2) and to placental protein 12 (PP12), the major protein secreted by the human decidua. HEP G2 secretion of IGFBP-I is suppressed by insulin acting through its own receptor. Other species of IGFBPs include IGFBP-IV, a 25-kDa protein which was identified in human osteosarcoma cells and human prostate tumor cells (PC3); human seminal plasma; and adult rat serum. Additional distinct IGFBP proteins have been identified in serum, in CSF, and in media of various cells in culture; these include IGFBP-V and IGFBP-VI, which await further characterization.

In contrast to the impressive gains made in our understanding of how GH and IGF-I control postnatal somatic growth, knowledge about their contributions to fetal growth is incomplete. It is generally accepted that neither GH nor thyroid hormone has a significant effect on fetal somatic growth because infants with congenital hypopituitarism or hypothyroidism are of normal or nearly normal size at birth.

Recently, the role of IGF-II in fetal growth was conclusively established by DiChiara and colleagues, who noted marked fetal growth retardation in mice bearing a hemizygous deletion of the IGF-II gene which caused a 10-fold reduction in IGF-II expression.[20] Although IGF-I and IGF-II transcripts in the fetus are widely distributed in predominantly mesenchymal cells, IGF-II gene expression dominates over that of IGF-I. Furthermore, the ontogeny of the two transcripts differs in that IGF-II mRNAs have been identified as early as 18 days while IGF-I mRNAs appear at 12 to 14 weeks gestation.[37,38]

Presumably, IGF-II and IGF-I influence fetal growth by stimulating cellular proliferation as well as by inducing differentiation. However, the evidence that IGF-I contributes to fetal growth is less conclusive than that for IGF-II.

The factors regulating tissue-specific expression of the IGF-I and IGF-II genes during fetal life are not fully understood. Placental somatomammotropin (CS, placental lactogen) appears to stimulate IGF-I and IGF-II synthesis, while nutrition affects IGF-I but not IGF-II production. Nutritional influences and GH have fewer effects in fetal life than in postnatal life.[39–41]

The type 1 IGF receptor is widely expressed during fetal organogenesis and is considered to be the receptor through which IGF-I and IGF-II transduce growth-promoting signals. The type 2 IGF receptor mRNA is also widely expressed throughout organogenesis. Both the cellular distribution and the ontogeny of expression of type 2 IGF receptor mRNA are similar to those of IGF-II mRNA, suggesting that the receptor is coupled to the peptide. The type 2 IGF receptor is abundant in the fetus and falls markedly during late gestation and early postnatal life. These observations suggest that IGF-II and its receptor are essential components of the fetal growth process.[42,43]

Of the six IGF binding proteins, IGFBP-I and IGFBP-II are the ones most abundantly expressed during fetal life. The exact role of the IGFBPs is uncertain since evidence exists for an inhibitory influence as well as a stimulatory influence on IGF action. The high levels of IGFBP-I and IGFBP-II present in fetal blood and fluids (e.g., amniotic fluid) suggest that these binding proteins serve in the translocation and/or disposal of the IGFs. IGFBP-III production is initiated in the third trimester, but the level of expression is reduced, presumably as a result of the low levels of IGF-I.[44]

During fetal life, it is evident that all components of the IGF system are present and appear to be developmentally regulated and tissue-specific. The mode of IGF action appears to be either autocrine or paracrine in nature. Evidence for a paracrine mode of action is based on studies which showed that the cells expressing IGF-I differed from the cells expressing type 1 IGF receptor and from cells associated with IGFBP-I. These observations do not, however, exclude an endocrine mechanism of IGF action in fetal life.

Hormonal Regulation

In infancy growth is primarily dependent on nutrition, whereas during childhood GH is the major determinant of growth. Sex hormones and GH control the adolescent growth spurt. Normal thyroid function is essential to each of these stages of growth. Insulin and glucocorticoids influence carbohydrate, fat, and protein metabolism; provide sources of energy needed for growth; and exert a permissive influence on the anabolic actions of GH. Whether insulin acts only permissively or whether it also functions as a growth factor is still unsolved because of the inseparable link between insulin and nutrition. The growth excess of hyperinsulinemic obese children appears to result from increased insulin concentration coupled with increased nutrient intake. Conversely, poor growth in insulin-deficient (type 1) diabetic youngsters is associated with intracellular undernutrition. Skeletal growth and ossification are dependent on PTH, the vitamin D metabolites, and, possibly, calcitonin.

Growth Hormone

The growth hormone molecule secreted by the somatotrophs of the anterior pituitary gland is predominantly a single-chain polypeptide (molecular weight of 22,000) containing 191 amino acid residues with two intrachain disulfide bridges. A form with a molecular weight of 20,000 is produced in lower abundance by means of alternative splicing of GH mRNA. Approximately 4 to 10 percent of the wet weight of the pituitary gland consists of GH (5 to 15 mg per gland). Although GH shares structural homology with prolactin and chorionic somatomammotropin, it is the only member of this family of peptides that exhibits postnatal growth-promoting activity in humans.

Synthesis of GH by the somatotroph is genetically controlled by the GH N gene, one of five genes in the GH gene cluster located on the long arm of chromosome 17.[45,46] The genes in the cluster from 5′ to 3′ are hGH-N, human chorionic somatomammotropin-L (hCS-L), hCS-A, hGH-V, and hCS-B (Fig. 26-5). A closely related gene which codes for prolactin is located on chromosome 6.[47] The hGH-N gene is expressed only in the somatotrophs of the pituitary gland, while the other genes—hCS-A, hCS-B, and hGH-V—are expressed in the syncytiotrophoblastic epithelial cells of the placenta. Little is known about the hCS-L gene. The major product of the GH-V gene is a 22-kDa basic peptide (GH variant, GH-V or placental GH) which differs from GH-N by only 13 amino acids (Fig. 26-6). The second product of the GH-V gene is a membrane-bound 26-kDa peptide (GH-V2) that contains 104 carboxyterminal amino acids. GH-V2 derives from an alternatively spliced GH-V transcript that retains intron 4 of the GH-V gene. The GH-V gene is developmentally regulated, and the ratio of GH-V2 to GH-V is higher in late pregnancy than in early pregnancy. GH-V is a biologically active somatogen and lactogen; it binds more efficiently to somatogenic than to lactogenic receptors and is equal to GH-N in stimulating weight gain in hypophysectomized rats.[48–50] Serum levels of GH-V rise in pregnancy and are presumed to play a role in suppressing maternal pituitary production of GH-N late in gestation. Based on numerous studies, it would appear that GH-V gene serves an important function in pregnancy, but its specific contribution has not been defined.[51,52] The assumption has been made that GH-V regulates placental and fetal growth, but this seems unlikely because deletions of GH-V with or without deletions of the hCS genes do not compromise placental and fetal development. It is possible that redundancy within the robust GH gene family provides backup mechanisms for such gene deletions.[53–55]

GH secretion is regulated primarily by two hypothalamic hormones; *somatostatin* (SRIH), which inhibits, and *growth hormone releasing hormone* (GHRH), which stimulates GH secretion. Each pulse

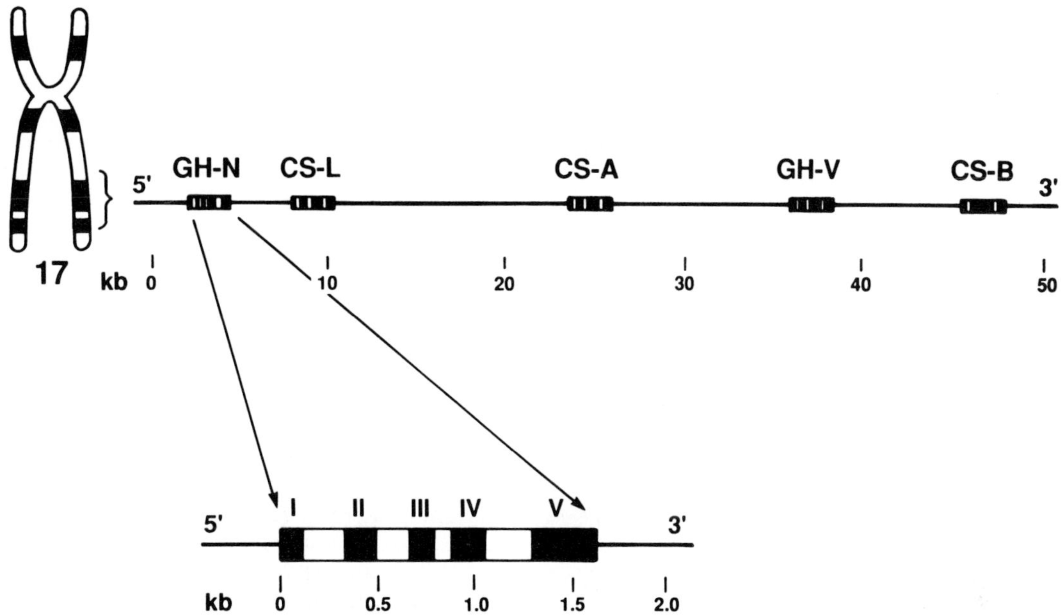

FIGURE 26-5 The five genes in the human GH gene cluster on the long arm of chromosome 17. From 5′ to 3′, the genes in the cluster are GH-N, CS-L, CS-A, GH-V, and CS-B. The GH-N gene is expressed only in the pituitary gland, whereas the remaining genes are active only in the placenta. The five genes have extensive DNA sequence homology, and each is composed of five coding regions or exons (I–V) and four introns. (*From Phillips and Venencak-Jones.*[45])

FIGURE 26-6 The products of the GH-N and GH-V genes. The major products of the GH-N gene, which is expressed in the pituitary gland, are 22-kDa and 20-kDa peptides. The latter are derived from alternative splicing of the GH-N mRNA, which results in omission of the amino acids shown in solid circles (●). The products of the GH-V gene, which is expressed exclusively in the syncytiotrophoblastic cells of the placenta, are a 22-kDa peptide which differs from GH-N by only 13 amino acid substitutions, which are shown as solid circles (●). By alternative splicing of the GH-V mRNA, intron 4 of the GH-V gene is retained and the product is predicted to be a 26-kDa peptide. Unlike GH-V, which is secreted, the GH-V2 product is membrane-bound. (*From Cooke et al.*[47])

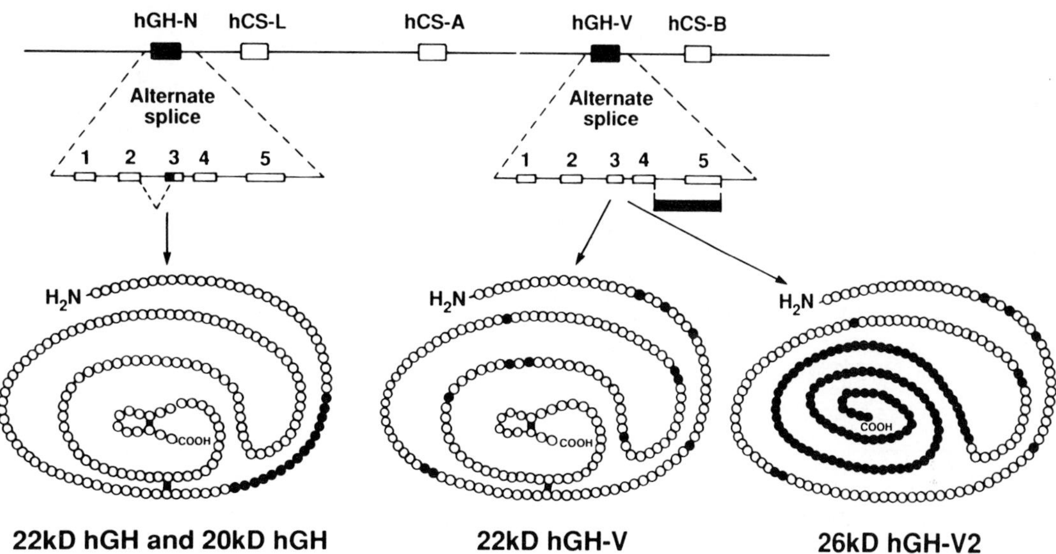

of GH is generated by a combination of a rise in GHRH and a decline in SRIH. Current hypotheses concerning the mechanisms which regulate GH secretion are illustrated in Fig. 26-7. Somatostatin, a tetradecapeptide isolated from ovine hypothalamic tissue in 1973, is present in high concentrations in the preoptic basal area of the hypothalamus, CNS, and GI tract, particularly the pancreas.[56,57] Somatostatin suppresses the GH response to insulin hypoglycemia, arginine infusion, levodopa ingestion, and deep sleep. Somatostatin also blocks thyrotropin releasing hormone (TRH)-induced thyroid stimulating hormone (TSH) release but does not block the prolactin rise following TRH stimulation. The extrapituitary effects of somatostatin include suppression by glucagon and insulin secretion by the pancreas. GH secretion is also inhibited by IGF-I and by GH itself; IGF-I acts directly on the pituitary gland, and both GH and IGF-I act on hypothalamic regulatory centers (i.e., by stimulating somatostatin production and suppressing GHRH release) (Fig. 26-7).

The main areas of the hypothalamus which secrete GHRH are the arcuate nucleus and adjacent ventromedial nucleus (VMN). Final proof of the existence of GHRH was provided when the hormone was isolated from the pancreatic tumors of two patients who had developed acromegaly as a result of tumor-derived GHRH.[58,59] The structure of human hypothalamic GHRH is identical to GHRH isolated from pancreatic tumors.[60,61] Isolation of GHRH from the pancreatic tumors culminated many years of frustrating research. Its existence had been suggested by animal studies carried out over two decades ago and later by clinical and laboratory documentation of acromegaly due to hypersecretion of biologically active GHRH from pancreatic tumors.[62] The two human GHRH peptides which have been recently purified and synthesized contain 40 and 44 amino acid residues; they have similar properties in vivo and in vitro. Synthetic GHRH administration to normal subjects [1 to 10 μg per kilogram of body weight intravenously (IV)] results in rapid and large increments in serum GH concentration; peak GH concentration occurs 30 to 60 min after IV bolus injection. Synthetic GHRH also stimulates modest elevations of serum GH and IGF-I concentrations in many patients with idiopathic hypopituitarism. Accelerated growth rates have been reported in GH-deficient children who received pulses of GHRH by infusion pump.[63]

Synthetic human GHRH appears to be highly specific for the somatotroph: No change has been observed in serum concentrations of glucose, gonadotropins [follicle stimulating hormone (FSH) or

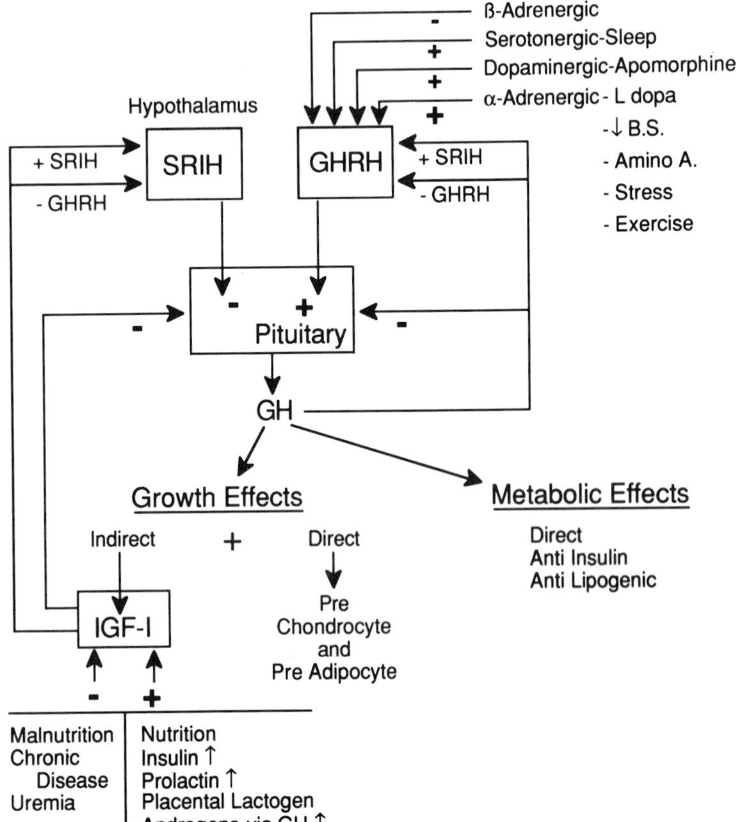

FIGURE 26-7 GH secretion is regulated by hypothalamic hormones: Somatostatin inhibits and growth hormone releasing hormone (GHRH) stimulates GH secretion. GHRH production is enhanced by α-adrenergic, dopaminergic, and serotoninergic neurons and suppressed by β-adrenergic tracts. GH and IGF-I inhibit GHRH secretion and enhance somatostatin production. These phenomena indirectly suppress GH secretion. GH production at the pituitary level is directly suppressed by the negative feedback effects of IGF-I and GH. GH acts directly on carbohydrate and lipid metabolism and directly and indirectly on growth. IGF-I production is enhanced by nutrition, insulin, prolactin, placental lactogen, and androgens. IGF-I production is suppressed by malnutrition, chronic diseases, glucocorticoids (?), and high doses of estrogen.

luteinizing hormone (LH)], TSH, prolactin, or hydrocortisone. The only side effect observed to date has been slight facial flushing.

Release of the hypothalamic hormones GHRH and somatostatin is in turn regulated by biogenic amines derived from neurosecretory neurons in the CNS. Somatostatin secretion is regulated primarily by cholinergic mechanisms (i.e., agonists inhibit and antagonists stimulate SRIH production). In contrast, secretion of GHRH is enhanced by alpha-adrenergic, dopaminergic, and serotoninergic neurons, and suppressed by β-adrenergic tracts. Presumably, β-adrenergic agonists stimulate SRIH and thereby inhibit GH secretion. Alpha-adrenergic pathways (norepinephrine and α-adrenergic receptors) are primary regulators of GHRH release. Drugs which mimic the action of norepinephrine (α-adrenergic agonists, e.g., clonidine) enhance GHRH production; those which block the alpha receptors (e.g., phentolamine) inhibit GHRH release. Dopaminergic receptor stimulation (e.g., by apomorphine) also enhances GHRH release. However, oral administration of levodopa appears to enhance GHRH release via α-adrenergic rather than dopaminergic pathways. Evidence for this was derived from studies which reported that phentolamine prevents levodopa-induced GH release. The normal somatotroph has no demonstrable dopamine receptor. However, GH-secreting pituitary adenomas paradoxically have a dopamine receptor which inhibits GH secretion when stimulated. This accounts for the suppression of plasma GH levels in approximately 80 percent of acromegalic patients treated with either levodopa or the dopaminergic agent bromocriptine. The actual significance of the serotoninergic pathways in the control of GH is less well understood. Administration of 5-hydroxytryptophan, a serotonin precursor, enhances GH release, and cyproheptadine, a serotonin antagonist, decreases GH responses to exercise, hypoglycemia, and 5-hydroxytryptophan. Beta-adrenergic blocking agents (e.g., propranolol) augment GH responses to levodopa, glucagon, and antidiuretic hormone (ADH), and the β-adrenergic agonist isoproterenol inhibits GH release.

In the past 6 years, two additional GH stimuli have been described. A hexapeptide enkephalin analog with GH-releasing activity (GHRP, his-D-trp-ala-trp-D-phe-lys NH_2) has been synthesized. It is not homologous to GHRH, and its activity in humans is not blocked by SRIH. When it is given with submaximal doses of GHRH, the effects of GHRP are additive. The mechanism of action of this peptide and of its native homologue, if it exists, is unknown; however, its therapeutic potential is intriguing.[64]

Galanin, a naturally occurring neuropeptide that is present in the median eminence, has been shown to enhance GH responses to GHRH. The physiologic significance of galanin is poorly understood; it may influence pulsatile GH secretion by lowering the inhibitory effects of SRIH, but it does not appear to be as important as GHRH.[65]

Under physiologic conditions, the pituitary gland secretes approximately eight discrete peaks of GH each day, with very low basal levels between the episodic bursts. In children and young adults, approximately 50 to 75 percent of the daily production of GH occurs during the early nighttime hours that follow the onset of deep sleep; in contrast, prolactin and cortisol concentrations rise progressively during the later hours of sleep. GH secretion is stimulated by exercise, emotional stress, high-protein meals, rapid onset of hypoglycemia, and prolonged fasting; it is suppressed by elevated glucose levels in healthy nondiabetic subjects.

Many investigators have reported that sex steroids increase GH production twofold or threefold during puberty. This increase in GH secretion results from greater pulse amplitude, not from an increased frequency of GH peaks.

Approximately 50 percent of GH in circulation is bound to a high-affinity GH binding protein (GHBP) which is identical to the extracellular domain of the GH receptor[66,67] (Fig. 26-8). Most of the remaining GH in circulation is free except for the 5 percent that is bound to a low-affinity 100-kDa GHBP. The levels of GHBP are low in the fetus and the newborn, rise gradually in childhood, and increase further in puberty. The main GH in circulation has a molecular mass of 22 kDa. Less abundant is the 20-kDa GH, which retains growth-promoting activity. Larger forms of GH (45 kDa) represent aggregations of 22-kDa molecules.

In general terms, GH is an anabolic hormone which stimulates postnatal growth, antagonizes the action of insulin, and possesses lipolytic activity. Direct influences of GH on isolated extraskeletal tissues (e.g., heart muscle, diaphragm, adipocytes, hematopoietic cells, hepatocytes) and on perfused organs (e.g., liver) have been documented. GH also plays an important role in carbohydrate, fat, protein, and mineral metabolism (Table 26-3).

Although the GH receptor is widely expressed in many tissues, the mechanisms by which GH binds to its receptors and initiates cellular responses are not well understood. The GH receptor is a single-chain polypeptide which contains a signal peptide of 12 to 24 amino acids and a mature protein of 614 to 626 amino acids. The mature protein contains an extracellular hormone-binding domain of about 250 amino acids, a single membrane-spanning domain, and an intracellular domain of about 350 amino acids (Fig. 26-8). The extracellular domain of the GH receptor is identical to the soluble GHBP found in circulation. Multiple membrane-associated GH receptors have been identified; at least three have been shown to be immunologically distinct, but their roles have not been defined. Analysis of GH mRNA by

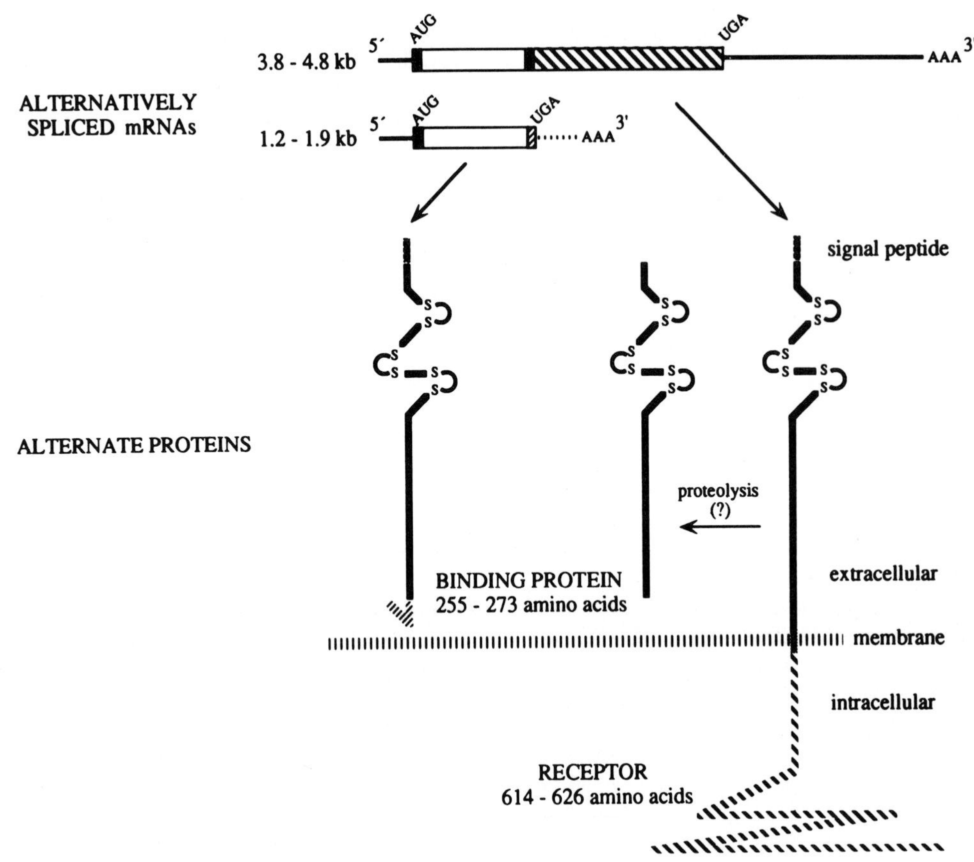

FIGURE 26-8 Schematic representation of GH receptor mRNAs and the GH receptor. Circulating GH binding protein is derived from either alternative splicing of the GH receptor mRNA as shown or from proteolytic cleavage of the extracellular domain of the GH receptor. The GH receptor consists of an extracellular domain, a membrane-spanning domain, and an intracellular domain. (*From Matthews.*[67])

Northern blot hybridization has revealed at least two transcripts which correspond to the smaller soluble and larger membrane-associated GH receptors. This observation suggests that soluble GHBP in circulation is derived from alternative splicing of GH receptor mRNA but does not exclude the possibility that it is also generated by proteolysis of the membrane receptor.[67,68]

The human GH receptor gene spans 87 kb on chromosome 5 and consists of 9 coding exons and several 5′ noncoding exons. Children with GH resistance syndrome (Laron-type) have a deficiency of the GH receptor and lack soluble GHBP in circulation. Some of these patients have extensive deletions of the GH receptor gene, and this eliminates large portions of the GH binding domain; thus cells are unable to bind and respond to GH.[69–74]

The GH receptor, which is primarily somatogenic, has 30 percent sequence identity with the prolactin receptor, which is mainly lactogenic. Both GH and prolactin receptors are members of a newly defined family of hormone receptors in which the extracellular domains are related to a diverse group of proteins, including the receptors for the interleukins, erythropoietin, and granulocyte macrophage colony-stimulating factor.

The intracellular signaling mechanisms which are activated by the GH receptor are poorly under-

TABLE 26-3 Metabolic Effects of Growth Hormone

Increases DNA, RNA, protein synthesis; mitosis; sulfate incorporation
Lowers urinary nitrogen concentration and blood urea nitrogen; raises urinary hydroxyproline concentration
Fat: stimulates lipolysis, liberates free fatty acids
Carbohydrate
Early: insulin-like effect
Late: insulin antagonism
Prolonged GH excess causes carbohydrate intolerance and diabetes mellitus
Mineral: decreases urinary phosphorus excretion, increases urinary calcium excretion
Electrolyte: permits retention of K^+, Na^+, Cl^-, Mg^+

stood. The ligand-binding domain may be directly involved in the regulation of gene expression. This assumption was proposed after GH binding protein was determined by several methods to be localized in the nucleus. Conceivably, the nuclear form of the GH receptor exerts the transcriptional actions of GH and the longer cell surface receptor mediates metabolic changes. Other possible signal transduction mechanisms include induction of c-Fos and c-Jun, nuclear proteins that are involved in the mitogenic responses of many growth factors, and activation of a GH-dependent tyrosine kinase.

Thyroid Hormone

Thyroid hormone by itself does not fulfill the criteria needed to classify it as a true growth-promoting hormone because it is unable to stimulate cellular multiplication directly if GH is absent. Nevertheless, the importance of the synergism between these hormones has been demonstrated in studies which showed that maximal GH stimulation of tissues requires the presence of T_4. Furthermore, primary hypothyroidism causes a reduction in both the number of somatotrophs and the GH content of the anterior pituitary; it also leads to GH unresponsiveness to stimulation by insulin hypoglycemia or L-arginine.[75] The growth spurt which follows thyroid replacement therapy is accompanied by a return of normal pituitary gland GH content and response to stimuli.

It has been suggested that during fetal life, somatic growth is not dependent on T_4 because infants with congenital hypothyroidism due to thyroid dysfunction or pituitary-hypothalamic disorders are of normal body size at birth. This conclusion requires reexamination, since a majority of congenitally hypothyroid infants have lingual or hypoplastic glands and those with anencephaly or other types of hypopituitarism have variable degrees of thyroid function. Evidence that thyroid hormone may influence fetal somatic growth is derived from experiments which documented that growth in three animal species (rat, sheep, and monkey) is impaired after fetal thyroidectomy.[76]

In contrast to the uncertainties about the role of T_4 in fetal somatic growth, it is evident that T_4 is essential for normal brain development, specifically neuronal and neuroglial cell growth in the cerebrum and cerebellum, nerve terminal maturation, axonal and dendritic proliferation, and normal myelinization. Studies suggest that T_4 increases the production of nerve growth factor, which stimulates axon outgrowth and increased neuron cell size and plays a crucial role in the development and survival of sympathetic and sensory neurons. If these data are confirmed, thyroid hormone may have an indirect rather than a direct influence on brain development.[77]

Acquired hypothyroidism in childhood usually delays puberty, but, rarely, a child exhibits precocious sexual development, ovarian cysts, galactorrhea, diabetes insipidus, and a large sella without bony erosion; all these abnormalities regress with thyroid replacement.

Gonadal Steroids: Androgens, Estrogens, and the Pubertal Growth Spurt

The growth spurt of puberty is dependent mainly on gonadal steroids and GH; adrenal steroids are probably not essential. Studies indicate that males experience rapid growth during puberty because of androgen-mediated enhancement of GH secretion; this in turn stimulates increased production of IGF-I and accounts for the elevated levels observed in adolescence.[26] Growth rates in males with isolated GH deficiency do not accelerate sufficiently during puberty, yet osseous maturation progresses and epiphyseal fusion occurs. Consequently, their adult height is compromised. Treatment of these individuals with GH during puberty is essential. Normal thyroid function is a fundamental requirement of the pubertal growth process. Hypothyroid children usually have delayed adolescence; those who experience puberty do not exhibit a growth spurt.

The precise mechanisms which control the onset of puberty have not been fully defined. In human and nonhuman primates, the pituitary gland releases increased quantities of FSH and LH at three periods of life: during fetal life, during the first 6 months of infancy, and during adolescence and adulthood. Suppression of gonadotropin production during the decade of "childhood," between infancy and adolescence, has been attributed to two mechanisms: (1) intrinsic CNS inhibitory influences operating independently of sex steroids (this accounts for the diphasic pattern of gonadotropin secretion seen during childhood in patients with gonadal dysgenesis) and (2) increased sensitivity of the hypothalamic-pituitary regulatory centers (the "gonadostat") to the negative feedback effects of low childhood levels of gonadal steroids.[78] Coincident with the onset of puberty, the arcuate nucleus of the hypothalamus becomes progressively less sensitive to the inhibitory effects of the sex steroids and the intrinsic CNS inhibitory influences gradually are suppressed. Removal of these restraints on gonadotropin releasing hormone (GnRH) secretion allows the pulsatile production of GnRH in increasing amounts, which in turn stimulates augmented secretion of pituitary gonadotropins.[78–83] A model of the mechanisms which control gonadal sex steroid production is shown in Fig. 26-9.

Two separate processes—*gonadarche* and *adrenarche*—account for the increased production of sex steroids in the peripubertal and pubertal periods. Gonadarche, the final activation and maturation of the hypothalamic-pituitary-gonadal axis, is the sine qua non of puberty. It is responsible for the adolescent growth spurt, development of secondary sexual

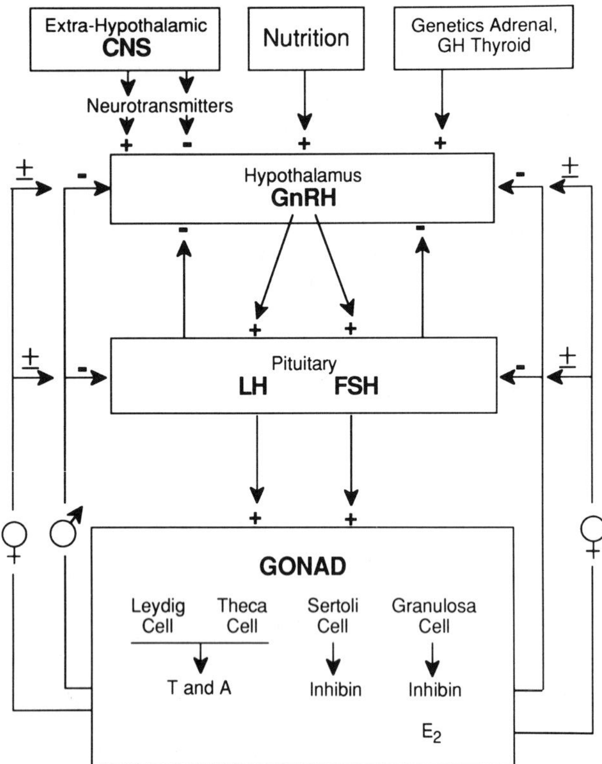

FIGURE 26-9 Schematic representation of the CNS-hypothalamic-pituitary-gonadal axis in males and females. Stimulatory effects are represented by +, and inhibition is shown by −. Gonadotropin releasing hormone (GnRH) stimulates secretion of luteinizing hormone (LH) and follicle stimulating hormone (FSH), which have negative feedback effects on GnRH via a short-loop mechanism. In males, LH stimulates the Leydig cells to produce testosterone (T) and androstenedione (A), which inhibit hypothalamic and pituitary production of GnRH and LH, respectively. In females, LH stimulates the production of testosterone and androstenedione from the theca and interstitial cells. The granulosa cells aromatize these androgens to form E_2 which has a biphasic effect on the mature female pituitary-hypothalamic centers. Testosterone appears to exert a minor influence on female gonadotropin production. FSH stimulation of inhibin production by Sertoli's cells in males and granulosa cells in females results in a suppression of FSH production. In females, FSH stimulates E_2 production by granulosa cells. In the preantral follicle, theca cells with LH receptors encircle granulosa cells with FSH receptors. LH stimulates theca cell development and enhances 17-α-hydroxylase activity and lyase activity, which are necessary for androgen production; the latter becomes the substrate for E_2 production in granulosa cells. The rising E_2 levels in the late follicular phase augment LH responsiveness to (GnRH), which causes further androgen production by the theca cells. Early in the gonadotropin surge, FSH induces LH receptors on the granulosa cells which have been primed by E_2; with luteinization of the granulosa cell, progesterone and E_2 production is enhanced by LH as well as FSH. The increasing progesterone production synergizes with the rising E_2 production to stimulate a further surge in pituitary gonadotropin production, leading to ovulation.

characteristics, and eventual attainment of fertility. Adrenarche signifies increased androgen production from the zona reticularis of the adrenal gland; it occurs about 2 years before gonadarche. Serum concentration of dehydroepiandrosterone (DHEA) usually begins to increase by 8 years of age in boys and girls; this serves as a biochemical marker of adrenal androgenesis. The temporal relation between adrenarche and gonadarche suggested that adrenal androgen may have a regulatory influence on the timing of puberty; it is now evident that adrenarche is not essential for the onset of gonadarche and that the two events are independent processes. The mechanisms responsible for adrenarche have not been fully defined; hypotheses include (1) an intrinsic alteration in the activity of the enzymes involved in adrenal androgen synthesis (*"escalator" theory*), (2) the production of a pituitary androgen stimulating hormone (ASH), although ASH has yet to be isolated (*zonal theory*), and (3) an extrapituitary stimulating factor such as estrogen.[78,84] The role of adrenal androgens in puberty is not clearly understood aside from the stimulation of sexual hair growth in females.

During puberty the Leydig cells of the testes secrete increasing amounts of testosterone, which circulates either bound to protein (i.e., sex hormone–binding globulin, SHBG) or in biologically active free form. Testosterone stimulation of DNA, RNA, and protein synthesis and cell mitosis requires the entrance of free hormone into the cytoplasm of androgen-sensitive cells, where it is metabolized to either 5α- or 5β-dihydrotestosterone (DHT) by 5α- or 5β-reductase. Both testosterone and DHT form complexes with the cytoplasmic receptor which enter the nucleus; there they interact with nuclear acceptor sites and stimulate cellular multiplication. The relative importance of testosterone compared to DHT in stimulating statural growth during puberty is not fully understood. In adult males and females, DHT is not present in skeletal muscle; it thus appears that testosterone may directly promote muscular growth during sexual maturation.[85–87]

During early fetal life in males, conversion of testosterone to DHT via the action of 5α-reductase in the external genital tissues is essential for the complete sexual differentiation of male external genitalia. The wolffian duct system develops normally in XY individuals who lack 5α-reductase. Therefore, it can be concluded that the internal genital duct system is testosterone- rather than DHT-dependent. During adolescence, XY subjects with 5α-reductase deficiency develop muscular, virile physiques even though they were phenotypic females during their prepubertal years.[87] These observations support the hypothesis that testosterone directly contributes to musculoskeletal growth in adolescence.

The characteristic actions of androgens on the skeletal system involve augmentation of bone length and acceleration of bone maturation. Because of the latter, the width of the growth plate is gradually reduced throughout the period of rapid statural growth until epiphyseal fusion occurs and adult height is attained.

There is suggestive evidence that androgens increase GH responses to hypoglycemic stimulation, enhance responsiveness to GnRH stimulation, and promote the onset of puberty.[88,89]

In females, the onset of the adolescent growth spurt coincides with breast development and ovarian production of estrogens. The magnitude of the growth spurt is less than in the male. Estrogens increase the width of the pelvic bones and hips, which are characteristic features of sexually mature women. Increased adiposity and body weight in pubertal girls are estrogen-mediated. Estrogens have less growth-promoting capacity than androgens do yet are capable of accelerating the pace of osseous maturation.

Nutrition

The rate of growth and sexual maturation in children is influenced by their nutritional state.[90] Frisch and McArthur have proposed that the onset of menses in healthy girls occurs at a critical weight which approximates the 10th percentile.[91] Improved nutrition and freedom from chronic infections are factors which have contributed to the taller stature and earlier puberty of European and American children. In countries where malnutrition is prevalent, poor linear growth and delayed adolescence are common. In this country, anorexia nervosa and chronic inflammatory bowel disease are examples of malnutrition interfering with normal growth because of both inadequate availability of substrates for cell replication and suppression of gonadotropin and somatomedin production. Recommended nutrient intakes based on age are given in Table 26-4.

TABLE 26-4 Daily Requirement of Nutrients

	Energy, kcal	Protein, g
Infants		
<6 months	117 × kg	2.2
6–12 months	108 × kg	2.0
Children		
1–3 years	1360	16
4–6 years	1830	20
7–9 years	2190	25
Male adolescents		
10–12 years	2600	30
13–15 years	2900	37
16–19 years	3070	38
Female adolescents		
10–12 years	2350	29
13–15 years	2490	31
16–19 years	2310	30

Source: *WHO Monograph Series*, no. 61, 1974.

PHYSIOLOGY OF SKELETAL GROWTH

Skeletal growth, which is the determinant of stature, is achieved by means of two types of ossification. First, transformation of cartilage into bone, defined as *endochondral ossification*, is responsible for the growth of the long bones, cuboid bones, base of the skull, vertebral bodies, and parts of the pelvis. Second, bone formation directly from fibrous membrane, or *membranous ossification*, occurs in the calvaria, clavicles, body of the mandible, vertebral spinous processes, and parts of the pelvis.

Elongation of long bones is responsible for statural growth. In the growth plate, chondrocytes produce the cartilaginous matrix consisting of type 2 collagen, mucopolysaccharides, and core proteins. The matrix undergoes an initial period of calcification followed by a stage of breakdown and chondrocyte degeneration. Finally, there is a phase of inward osteoblast migration via vascular channels from the metaphyses; bone is deposited on the remaining calcified cartilage, which is gradually resorbed and replaced by true bone. Disturbances in chondrocyte proliferation, matrix formation, calcification, and ossification cause short stature.

Endochondrial ossification is hormonally controlled. An excess of glucocorticoids disturbs the protein matrix and causes osteoporosis. Vitamin D deficiency or PTH excess leads to abnormalities in mineralization and osteomalacia.

Bone width is determined by the thickness of the diaphyseal cortex, which is formed by membranous ossification directly from the periosteum.

The fetus develops primary centers of ossification in the cartilaginous anlage of long bones at 7 weeks. By the third fetal month, the process of ossification extends to the metaphyses and the growth plate begins to contain chondrocytes. In early fetal life, the epiphyseal ends of long bones exist mainly as cartilage; later in gestation, secondary centers of ossification convert the cartilaginous epiphyses to bone. Bone age or biological age is defined by the size and appearance of these secondary centers of epiphyseal ossification.

Osteocalcin (bone Gla protein), which is secreted by osteoblasts, is an important noncollagenous protein which is contained in the bone matrix and also circulates in blood. The serum concentration is believed to reflect the rate of bone formation and osteoblast activity. In healthy children, osteocalcin levels vary with age and sex and parallel the growth velocity curve. A sharp increase in serum osteocalcin concentrations occurs during the growth spurt of normal as well as precocious puberty. Growth hormone–deficient children have low serum levels of osteocalcin which rise after GH therapy. Presumably, GH therapy stimulates IGF-I production in bone, increasing the number of functional osteoblasts as well as bone mineralization. Osteocalcin levels are reliable biochemical markers of altered bone metabolism; levels are low in patients with type I diabetes mellitus and in children receiving glucocorticoid therapy. The rise in serum osteocalcin after GH therapy correlates with the linear growth response and may predict which children are likely to benefit from GH administration.

DEVELOPMENTAL STAGES

Intrauterine Life

The initial growth period of the fetus is one of rapid cellular generation, differentiation, and organogenesis. During this embryonic period, the fetus grows primarily by a process of cellular multiplication. Extraordinary linear growth rates are observed during fetal life. Peak velocities of 10 to 11 cm/month occur at 4 to 5 months gestation; the growth rate gradually declines during the last trimester as uterine constraints become a limiting force. However, even this growth rate is spectacular: 2 cm/month (Fig. 26-10).

FIGURE 26-10 Linear growth by lunar months during fetal life and in the first postnatal year. The slowing of the late fetal growth rate is compatible with the concept of constraints to growth by the uterus and is followed postnatally by a brief period of accelerated "catch-up" growth. (*From Smith.*[93])

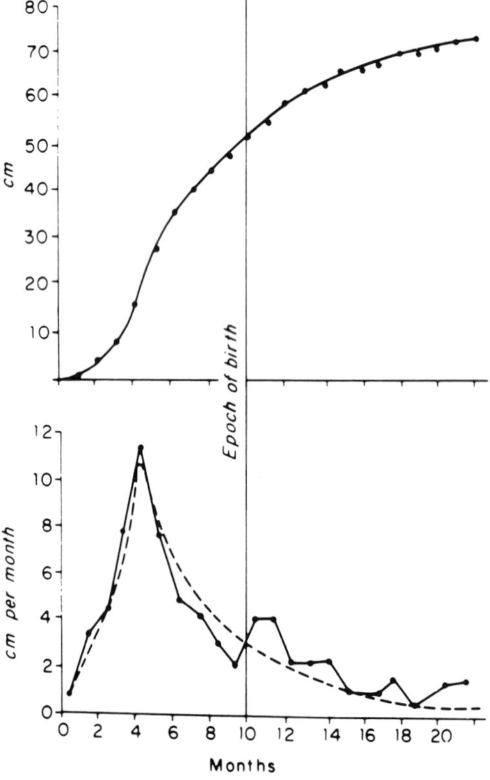

In the last trimester, adipose tissue is formed at an increasing rate; fetal weight doubles during the last 2 months of pregnancy.

The size of a full-term newborn is mainly dependent on the size of the mother, not the father. In controlled animal studies, the offspring of large mothers and small fathers are larger than the products of matings between small mothers and large fathers.[92] This observation indicates that lifelong adequate nutrition is essential for girls in order to enhance their adult height and the size of their offspring.

An additional factor which influences fetal growth is uterine size in the late gestational period. In women with twins or triplets, uterine constraints may limit fetal size.

The placenta is yet another determinant of fetal growth and well-being since it is the portal for the delivery of nutrients and the removal of metabolic wastes. The placenta is a fetal organ which grows by cellular multiplication until the 35th week of gestation; thereafter, it enlarges by cellular hypertrophy until full size is achieved at the 38th to 40th week. Any disturbance of early placental growth due to embryologic abnormalities, infections, or vascular insults may cause permanent growth retardation.[1]

Gender plays a minor role in determining fetal growth rate. Males grow faster after 32 weeks gestation and at birth are more muscular and have less adipose tissue than females. Newborn boys have a slightly larger head circumference and are, on average, 0.9 cm longer and 150 g heavier than girls.[93] However, osseous maturation is more rapid in girls than in boys after 30 weeks gestation. At birth, bone age in females is 2 weeks ahead of that in males; by 1 year, this difference has increased to 8 weeks.

Infancy: Birth to 2 Years of Age

In the first year of life, linear growth and weight gain continue at a rate which is still remarkable although less spectacular than during fetal life. The fastest gains in length occur in the first months after birth, when uterine constraints are no longer present. By 1 year, the infant has accumulated generous stores of adipose tissue, has tripled its birth weight, and has grown 25 additional cm (an increase of 50 percent of birth length). Male infants continue to grow slightly faster in length, weight, and head circumference during the first 3 to 6 months after birth. These phenomena have been attributed to increased testosterone production in males, which gradually diminishes by 6 months of postnatal age.[94] In the second year, there is continued deceleration of linear growth rates; by the age of 2 years, linear growth has stabilized at a rate which is characteristic of the childhood years (Fig. 26-11).

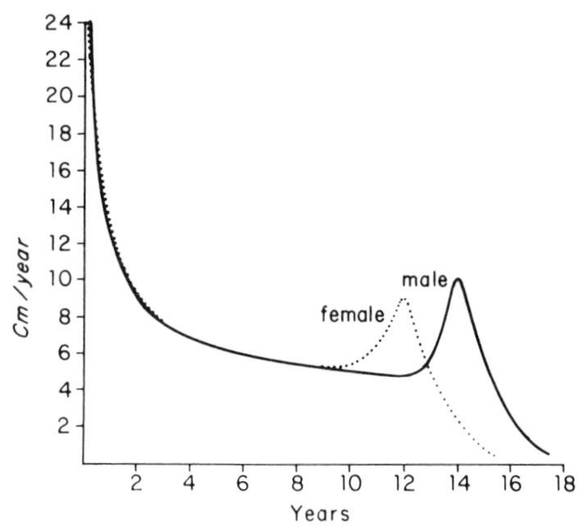

FIGURE 26-11 Velocity curves for length (<2 years) and height (2 to 28 years) for females and males show deceleration of the growth rate from infancy until the onset of adolescence. (*From Smith*[93] *and Tanner et al.*[99,194])

Childhood

The period of childhood, which extends from age 2 years to the onset of puberty, is characterized by relatively stable rates of gain in height (5 to 7.5 cm/year) and weight (2 to 2.5 kg/year). Throughout these years, there is a slight deceleration in the linear growth rate (Fig. 26-11) and an acceleration in weight gain (Fig. 26-12). The major period of brain growth has already been completed, and cellular multiplication in the musculoskeletal and adipose systems continues at a slower pace than is evident during infancy or adolescence. In the years before puberty, there is an increased gain in adipose tissue. During this period, lymphoid tissue reaches its maximum size relative to body size.

Adolescence

Adolescence is the last period of major growth; during this period, there is attainment of adult stature, sexual maturation, and reproductive function.

FIGURE 26-12 Growth velocity curves for females and males show gradual increases in rates of weight gain from 2 years until adolescence. (*From Smith*[93] *and Tanner et al.*[99,194])

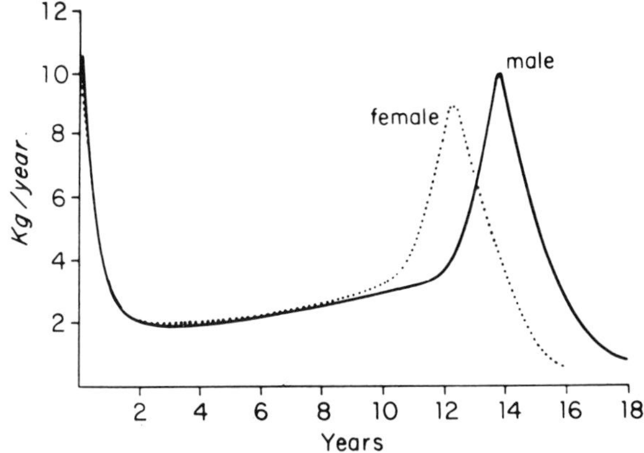

Among healthy children, chronologic age at the onset of puberty and the rate of sexual maturation are highly variable. These differences are largely dependent on genetic factors. The individual's sex also plays a role; the average girl enters and completes pubertal development 1 to 2 years ahead of the average boy. The most accurate criterion for the assessment of adolescence is not chronologic age but the individual's biological age (bone age) and physical stage of sexual maturation, based on Tanner's criteria.[95]

The sequence of physiologic and hormonal events during adolescence in girls is shown in Fig. 26-13. The first signs of puberty in females are the appearance of breast buds and the beginning of the adolescent growth spurt; for the average girl, these events occur at 11 years of age. They are followed by the appearance of pubic hair at 11.5 years, peak growth rates (approximately 9 cm/year) at 12 years, the appearance of axillary hair at 12.5 to 13 years, and menarche at 12.5 years. Almost invariably, menarche occurs after the attainment of peak growth velocity. Slower rates of linear growth continue after menarche until age 16 to 17 years, when epiphyseal fusion occurs; this information has relevance to the management of girls who are concerned about genetic tall stature. Adolescence in females is also associated with widening hips due to fat deposition and a general increase in body adipose tissue. The normal ranges in chronologic age for each pubertal event in girls are listed in Table 26-5.

In boys, the first signs of adolescence are axillary sweat, body odor, testicular enlargement, and thinning of the scrotal skin. The average boy gains 25 cm and 20 kg during adolescence.[95] The mechanisms of gonadotropin action on testicular growth and function have not been fully clarified. FSH is primarily responsible for growth of the seminiferous tubules and thus for increments in testes size in addition to sperm development. LH is the regulator of androgen, primarily testosterone, production by the Leydig cells. Evidence suggests that optimal sexual maturation depends on the interaction of FSH and LH in the testes.[96]

The sequence of physiologic events and their relation to the hormonal changes in adolescent boys are depicted in Fig. 26-14. Unlike girls, who simultaneously exhibit increased growth velocity and breast buds at the outset of puberty, boys begin their growth spurt approximately 1 year after the first signs of testicular enlargement and achieve greater peak rates of linear growth (mean 10.3 cm/year) at age 14, compared to age 12 in girls. The male adolescent growth spurt is largely due to the increased secretion of testosterone, which enhances the production of GH; deficiencies of either of these hormones or a lack of T_4 will impair the adolescent growth spurt. Males achieve greater growth velocities, muscular development, and statural height

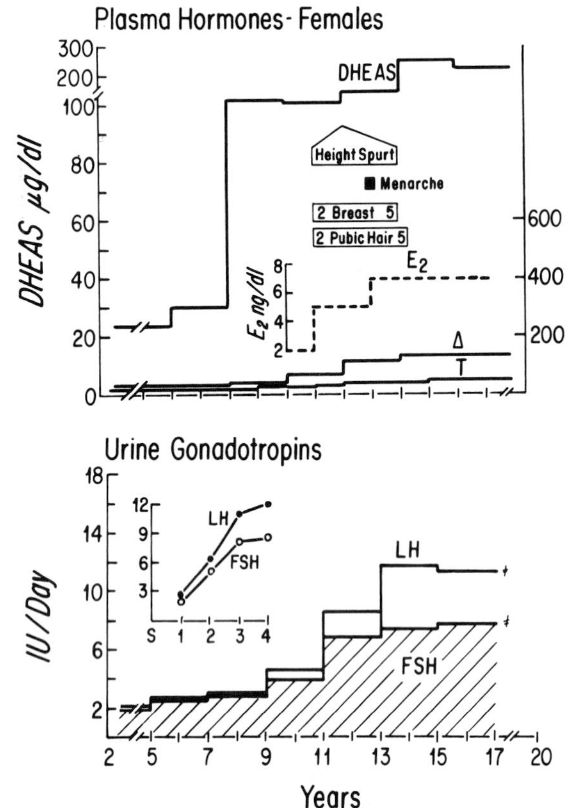

	FSH Excretion, IU/day	LH Excretion, IU/day
S1 (completely prepubertal, t1)	1–5	1–5
S2 (only breast tissue, t2 or t3)	4–9	4–9
S3 (breasts and sexual hair, t3 to t4)	5–11	6–16
S4 adult breasts and hair, t4 to t5)	5–12	7–28
Midcycle peak	39–49	108–122

Not shown in the diagram is the sleep-associated increase in LH secretion during early and midpuberty. (*Tanner criteria from Tanner*[95]; *hormonal events of puberty from Grumbach et al,*[81] *Kelch et al,*[86] *Penny et al.*[196])

FIGURE 26-13 Relation between the stages of pubertal development in girls based on Tanner (t) criteria and the hormonal events of puberty. Increased plasma levels of DHEA sulfate from the adrenal gland (adrenarche) are detected before increased secretion of gonadotropins or gonadal steroids (gonadarche). E_2 = estradiol, = androstenedione, T = testosterone. Based on chronologic age, urinary gonadotropin levels appear to increase before the average age of breast development. However, when urinary gonadotropin excretion is based on stage of sexual maturation (S), a positive correlation exists with stages 2 and 3.

than do females because of augmented androgen production.

In the average male, testicular size increases at age 12 years. This is followed 1 year later by the onset of penis enlargement. The first ejaculation of seminal fluid and nocturnal emissions occur at approximately 14 years of age. Pubic hair growth begins at approximately 12.5 to 13 years; the first signs of axillary and facial hair occur 2 years later (i.e., 14.5 to 15 years). Acne and apocrine sweat are characteristic features of adolescence. The male physique undergoes striking changes as a result of androgen action: Shoulder width increases, facial bone structure enlarges, vocal cords expand to deepen the voice, muscle cell number doubles, and muscle mass and strength show striking gains. Early developers are athletically superior with regard to strength and coordination to late developers. However, the later onset of adolescence may contribute to the tall stature seen in some adult males.[95]

TABLE 26-5 Range of Chronologic Ages for Pubertal Events in Healthy Girls

	Age, years	
Event	Onset	Completion
Height spurt	9½–14½	12–17½
Breast bud*	8–13	10½–16
Pubic hair	8–14	11–17½
Menarche	10–16†	

* Asymmetry when breast = Tanner 5; will not resolve spontaneously.

† Nine to 16 years in other series.

Source: Based on Tanner.[95]

Approximately one-half of boys develop a small amount of breast tissue (2 to 3 cm in diameter) midway through adolescence. Usually this lasts for 12 to 18 months and resolves completely. Progressive breast enlargement over a period of 1 to 2 years is not likely to resolve spontaneously, and mastectomy via a periareolar incision should be considered before excessive stretching of breast skin occurs. In most instances, these boys have idiopathic gynecomastia; however, the possibility of Klinefelter's syndrome, true hermaphroditism, choriocarcinoma, or estrogen-producing lesions must be considered.

Adult height in males is usually attained by age 18; growth cessation occurs first in the hands and feet, followed by the legs, trunk, and shoulder girdle. The ranges in age for the events of male adolescence are shown in Table 26-6.

SHORT STATURE

Clinical Approach to Short Stature

It is important to emphasize that many healthy children who are growing along a normal lower growth channel (3d to 10th percentile) and whose size is compatible with genetic endowment have innocent short stature that requires psychological support but no medical treatment.

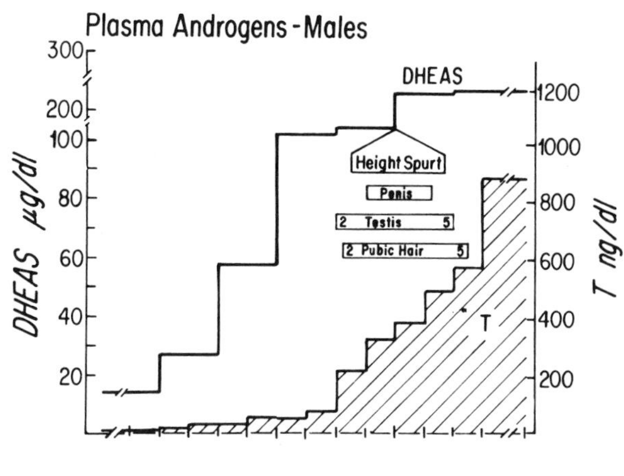

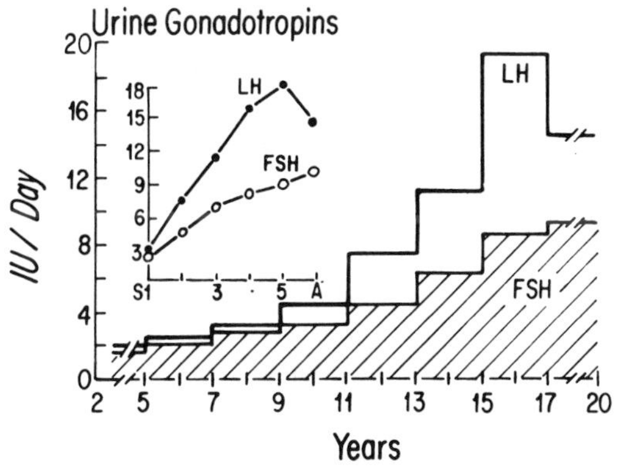

	FSH Excretion, IU/day	LH Excretion, IU/day
S1 (prepubertal)	0.5–5	0.5–6
S2 (testes ⩾ 2 cm, scrotal changes)	2–9	2–13
S3 (penis > 7 cm)	3–12	5–23
S4 (further penis and testes growth)	3–14	9–29
S5 (prostate palpable, sexual hair)	5–16	9–39
SA [adult testes (> 4cm) and penis (> 13 cm stretched)]	5–16	8–24

Sleep-associated increases in LH secretion have been documented in early and midpuberty. After adolescence, daytime and nighttime excretion of LH are equal. (*From Grumbach et al,*[81] *Tanner,*[95] *Reiter et al*[95] *Penny et al.*[197])

FIGURE 26-14 Relation between the stages of pubertal development in boys and the hormonal events during adolescence. As noted in girls, DHEA sulfate levels are increased before any evidence of sexual maturation. Based on chronologic age, increased gonadotropin excretion appears to precede the onset of testicular enlargement. However, when gonadotropin excretion is related to stages of sexual maturation (S), there is a positive correlation between increased gonadotropin output and stages 2, 3, and 4. Positive correlations also exist for increases in LH excretion, testes enlargement, and testosterone concentration (T).

TABLE 26-6 Range of Chronologic Ages for Pubertal Events in Healthy Boys

Event	Age, years: Onset	Age, years: Completion
Testis enlargement	10–13½	14½–18
Height spurt	10½–16	2½–3*
Penis enlargement	11–14½	13½–17
Pubic hair	10–15	14–18

* Years after onset.

Source: Based on Tanner.[95]

The care of children with short stature has become controversial because questions have been raised about the validity of the traditional GH provocative tests and because more physicians are willing to prescribe GH treatment for "short children" because they believe that such therapy has long-term benefits. Also, some of the current disagreement is due to confusion about the precise meaning of the term *short stature* when it is applied to heterogeneous populations of children receiving empiric GH treatment.

The problem with nomenclature arose when the term *short stature* was used increasingly to describe children with pathologic heights or growth rates when in fact they could be described more accurately as having growth failure. Examples of the innocent-sounding terminology which was used to describe these children include NVSS, idiopathic short stature (ISS), and constitutional short stature (CSS).

Most physicians try to avoid using stigmatizing names for children with growth problems; therefore, terms such as *dwarf* and *midget* are seldom used now. However, there is a clear need for language which conveys whether a child has innocent short stature in contrast to growth failure due to an idiopathic cause or other causes.

The following is a practical approach to the management of children with a growth disorder. There is general agreement that an abnormally low growth rate for chronologic age with abnormal or normal height is a warning sign of growth failure which requires investigation. When first seen, children whose heights are 2 to 3 SD below the mean should be remeasured at 6-month intervals to determine the growth velocity; if it is pathologic for chronologic age, the child should be thoroughly evaluated. Children with more severe growth failure (i.e., height more than 3 SD below the mean and abnormal or normal growth velocity) require prompt and thorough investigation. The causes of short stature and growth failure are shown in Table 26-7.

Before the first examination, it is advisable to ask parents to send in previous heights and weights obtained from school health records, personal physicians, or clinics. Annual school photographs are particularly valuable in growth problems which are

TABLE 26-7 Differential Diagnosis of Short Stature

- **Causes of normal short stature**
  - Genetic or familial short stature
  - Constitutional growth delay with or without delayed adolescence
  - Genetic short stature and constitutional growth delay
- **Pathologic growth**
  - Intrauterine disturbances
    - Placental dysfunction
    - Maternal factors
      - Malnutrition
      - Diseases
      - Drug use
    - Fetal disease
      - Infections
      - Congenital abnormalities
      - Chromosomal abnormalities
    - Premature delivery
    - Genetic syndromes: Bloom, Hallermann-Streiff-François, Russell-Silver, Seckel's, Donahue's, Dubowitz', progeria, de Lange's, Williams
  - Postnatal malnutrition
    - Poverty, ignorance, neglect
    - Mechanical gastrointestinal disorders
      - Esophageal stenosis, web, reflux
      - Pyloric stenosis
      - Duodenal atresia, stenosis, bands, annular pancreas
      - Malrotation, volvulus
      - Foreign body
      - Aganglionosis (Hirschsprung's)
      - Short-bowel syndrome
    - Digestive diseases
      - Enzyme deficiencies
        - Proteolytic enzymes: trypsin, cystic fibrosis
        - Disaccharidases: sucrase, isomaltase, lactase
        - α_1-Antitrypsin: liver cirrhosis
      - Intolerance: milk-protein allergy
      - Chronic infection: *Escherichia coli,* salmonella, giardiasis, shigella, staphylococcus, etc.
      - Inflammatory bowel disease: ulcerative colitis, granulomatous ileocolitis
      - Tumor: neural crest tumors
      - Miscellaneous: celiac disease, gluten sensitivity, immunologic disorders, acrodermatitis enteropathica, abetalipoproteinemia
  - Endocrine causes
    - Hypothyroidism: congenital or aquired; primary, secondary (TSH), or tertiary (TRH)
    - GH deficiency (also assess anterior pituitary function: TSH, ACTH, prolactin, FSH-LH) (see Table 26-8)
    - Cushing's syndrome: glucocorticoid excess
    - Short adult stature due to precocious sexual maturation
  - Metabolic disorders
    - Glycogen storage disease
    - Cystinosis
    - Fructose intolerance
    - Galactosemia
    - Mucopolysaccharidoses
    - Diabetes insipidus: vasopressin-resistant, vasopressin-sensitive
  - Bone disorders (skeletal dysplasias)
    - Chondrodystrophies: achondroplasia, hypochondroplasia
    - Rickets: hypophosphatemia, vitamin D deficiency or resistance
    - Epiphyseal dysplasia
    - Metaphyseal dysplasia
    - Spondyloepiphyseal dysplasia, metaphyseal dysplasia
    - Osteogenesis imperfecta
    - Multiple exostoses syndrome
  - Chromosomal abnormalities
    - X chromosome abnormalities: gonadal dysgenesis, Turner's syndrome
    - Trisomy syndromes
  - Environmental deprivation syndrome: emotional(?), parental(?), nutritional(?)
  - Anoxemia
    - Pulmonary disease: cystic fibrosis, hypoplastic lung, fibrous dysplasia(?)
    - Hemoglobinopathies
    - Cardiovascular disease
  - Chronic disease in a major organ
    - Kidney: renal insufficiency, acidosis
    - Neurologic system: microcephaly, hydrocephalus, diencephalic syndrome, degenerative disease, neurofibromatosis
    - Hepatic cirrhosis
    - Malignancy
  - Primordial dwarfism
  - Drugs: daily cortisone therapy for asthma, collagen disease, nephrotic syndrome, rheumatoid arthritis, aplastic anemia, malignancy (leukemia, Hodgkin's, etc.)

associated with changing facial appearance, e.g., hypothyroidism and Cushing's syndrome. The initial medical evaluation involves taking the patient's history and performing a physical examination and laboratory and radiographic studies.

History

A complete history includes details of the child's health from conception to the time of examination; specifics of maternal health, including drug use and diseases before and during the pregnancy; information on height, weight, rate of maturation, and health of family members; and assessment of emotional stresses within the family. Questions should focus on the presence and location of headaches, visual problems, frequency of respiratory or other infections, presence of chronic disease, use of medications, character of stools, frequency of urination, and details of nutritional intake.

Physical Examination

A thorough examination either indicates excellent health or provides clues to an endocrinopathy or an underlying chronic disease in a major organ (GI tract, kidney, heart, lungs, CNS) or stigmata of one of the many growth-deficiency syndromes.[97] Malnutrition due to inadequate food intake, malabsorption, or underlying chronic disease tends to disturb weight gain more severely than it affects linear growth.

Measurements

Carefully maintained growth records (accurate measurements displayed on standard growth charts) are essential for the early detection of growth problems due to nutritional inadequacies, endocrine disorders, or the onset of an underlying chronic disease.[98] The presence of disproportionate short stature points to problems in bone growth (e.g., chondrodystrophies or other skeletal dysplasias), while normal body proportions are characteristic of most of the remaining growth disorders (Table 26-7).

1. Length: From birth to 1½ to 2 years, measure infant on a flat, horizontal board which has one vertical, immovable end to brace the head; the other vertical end slides along a track until it touches the soles of the feet. Place the infant supine and hold the knees flat.[93]
2. Height: For children > age 2, stand child with buttocks and heels (remove shoes and socks) against a vertical rule which has a movable device at right angles to the rule that can be lowered until it touches the top of the cranium.
3. Weight: Measure with a minimum of clothing.
4. Head circumference: Place nonstretchable tape over maximal occipital prominence and just above eyebrows.
5. Body proportions:
   a. Lower segment length (L) is the distance from the upper level of the pubic bone to the point where the medial aspect of the heel touches the floor.
   b. Derive upper segment length (U) by subtracting L from height (H); i.e., $U = H - L$.
   c. Calculate the U/L ratio. At birth, $U/L = 1.7$; it decreases as leg length increases until it equals 1.0 at 7 to 10 years of age. The U/L ratio for adult white males (0.95) is greater than that for adult black males (0.85), who tend to have longer leg length. The current standards for U/L ratio have many deficiencies.
6. Span: Stand patient flat against wall with arms outstretched at shoulder height. With nonstretchable tape held against wall (i.e., behind patient), measure the widest distance between extended fingers. Usually, span and height measurements are similar. Marked discrepancies point to disproportionate growth of limb versus trunk.
7. Other measurements include: *sitting height* measures trunk length; *triceps skin fold thickness* estimates subcutaneous adipose tissue (use calipers and measure at midpoint between shoulder and elbow posteriorly); *testis length* and *width* or *volume* (latter measured with Prader orchidometer); and *penis* stretched *length, width,* and *circumference.*

Plotting Growth Data on Standard Growth Curves

The most recently developed growth curves for American children are based on cross-sectional measurements of a nationally representative sample; they do not make allowances for genetic and ethnic influences on height or for the variability of age of onset of adolescence in normal children. The Tanner-Whitehouse growth charts,[99] based on data collected in English children, are the ones most widely used internationally. The disadvantages of the available charts are not serious if the physician is aware that children whose growth follows the 3d percentile and whose parents are short are growing normally based on midparental height. Growth curves which are adjusted to correct for parental height have been developed by Tanner et al.[99] Standardized growth charts for specific growth disorders such as Turner's syndrome, Noonan's syndrome, achondroplasia, Marfan syndrome, and Down syndrome have also become available.[98]

The physical measurements (height, weight, etc.) of an individual can be expressed either in terms of percentiles for chronologic age, with the range of normal being the 3d to 97th percentiles, or in terms of standard deviations (SD) above or below the mean. One SD extends from the 16th to the 84th percentile; 2 SD extends from the 2½th to the 97½ percentile, approximating the 3d and 97th percentiles on the growth curve. Data have been collected which give the SD in centimeters for each age and sex. Thus, a child's height can be given an SD score or a Z score by performing the following calculations. Subtract the child's height (cm) from the mean height (cm) for chronologic age and divide the difference by the SD (in cm) for chronologic age. A child with a Z score of −3 has a height 3 SD below the mean for chronologic age. This approach provides a method for comparing heights of children with diverse ages and a means of assessing the effects of a particular therapy on the growth process.

The growth curves also allow for the expression of an individual's size in terms of height age (HA) and weight age (WA). HA is defined as the chronologic age at which the patient's height would fall at the 50th percentile. This is calculated by drawing a horizontal line from the patient's position on the growth curve to the 50th percentile and dropping a vertical line to age in years. It does not take into account genetic influences on stature and pace of maturation. Nevertheless, it is extremely valuable when used to compare an individual's stature with his or her biological age (i.e., bone age). For example, a healthy 15-year-old male with delayed adolescence and a height age of 11 and bone age of 11 has a much better prognosis for adult height than does a 15-year-old sexually maturing young man with genetic short stature whose height age is 13 and whose bone age is 15.

The method for calculating WA is similar to that for HA but is more subject to error. The relation among chronologic age, HA, WA, and bone age in a patient helps delineate the etiology of the growth disorder; e.g., a 2-year-old with HA = 18 months and WA = 6 months is likely to have a nutritional problem which impairs weight gain more seriously than it impairs linear growth. Conversely, a 6-year-old child with HA = 3, WA = 4, and a bone age of 3 may have GH or thyroid deficiency.

Radiographic Studies

Skeletal maturation (bone age) is based on the size, shape, and number of the secondary centers of ossification in the epiphyses. To minimize x-ray exposure, the left hand and wrist, and occasionally the knee, are most commonly used for radiographic study. The carpal, metacarpal, and phalangeal epiphyses are compared with standards obtained on healthy children at different ages. When there is variation in the maturation of these epiphyses more weight is given to the metacarpal and phalangeal centers than to the carpal epiphyses. The standard in the Greulich and Pyle *Radiographic Atlas* which most closely approximates that of the child indicates his or her bone age.[100] Bone age is of great value in children with significant growth disorders due to endocrine disturbances. In situations where a problem in mineralization exists or bone growth is disordered (skeletal dysplasia), cautious interpretation of bone age is advisable.

Prediction of estimated adult height based on present height and bone age can be made from the Bayley and Pinneau predictive tables[101] in the Greulich and Pyle atlas. This requires consideration of midparental height. Height prediction cannot be made accurately in children with pathologic growth but is useful in healthy children with normal types of short stature. However, patients must be advised that these estimations do not make allowances for rapid progress in sexual maturation, which may accelerate bone age disproportionately to height gain and result in stature which is lower than predicted.

Laboratory Studies

Additional laboratory tests may be ordered on the basis of evidence obtained during the history, physical, growth-curve, and radiographic evaluations. Further information concerning hormone determinations, hematologic tests, chromosome analyses, blood chemistry determinations, and elaborate radiologic procedures (e.g., CT scan and MRI) is discussed in the sections below dealing with specific growth disorders.

Causes of Short Stature

Introduction

Two examples of normal short stature discussed below are genetic short stature and constitutional growth delay. In both entities, growth rate is normal, height is within 2 SD of the mean, body proportions are normal, and general health is good. These children are different from the subgroups of pathologically short patients who have been classified as having NVSS or simple "short stature."[102–104] The characteristics of the children in the latter subgroups are heights greater than 2 SD from the mean and abnormally low growth rates. GH responses to provocative stimuli are normal and IGF-I levels are low or normal in many. GH treatment was beneficial for a majority. There is disagreement over whether these children have atypical forms of GH deficiency or insufficiency. They represent a heterogeneous group of children who have growth failure of unknown etiology.[105,106]

Causes of Normal Short Stature

Genetic or Familial Short Stature

Throughout childhood and adolescence, growth in children with genetic short stature remains consistently at lower percentiles, with rates equal to or greater than 5 cm/year. These children's heights are in the normal range based on midparental stature, and they are healthy, well-proportioned young individuals. Bone age based on radiologic examination of the left wrist is usually within 2 SD of chronologic age. Occasionally, a child inherits both short stature and constitutional growth delay (Table 26-7). This combination increases the severity of the growth problem. The greatest burden to these families is the emotional stress which results from teasing, feelings of inadequacy, and parental guilt. Diagnostic studies can usually be kept to a minimum (bone age determination, T_4 assay) if the history and physical and growth data implicate genetic short stature.

The ultimate height of these children can be estimated directly from midparental height or calculated using either predictive data which include allowances for midparental height or the unadjusted predictive tables of Bayley and Pinneau.[101] A simple way of determining whether a short child with short parents is growing normally is to calculate midparental height by averaging the parents' heights and adding 6.5 cm if the child is a boy and subtracting 6.5 cm if the child is a girl. Then the percentile on which the midparental height falls is determined. The child's growth curve followed to adult height should fall within ±5 cm of midparental height after skeletal age has been taken into account. There is no effective treatment for genetic short stature. Androgen therapy is contraindicated because of the risk of acceleration in bone maturation, which further compromises adult height. Oxandrolone, a synthetic androgen, when given during adolescence, has not enhanced the ultimate heights of genetically short boys. There is considerable interest in determining whether pharmacologic doses of GH might increase the adult height of these children; at present such evidence is lacking. The potential adverse effects of such treatment (eliciting antibodies to GH, generating glucose intolerance, etc.) and the enormous costs are the reasons why most endocrinologists advise against this therapy. At present, the management of genetic short stature consists mainly of supportive counseling, career planning, and encouraging the child to engage in appropriate physical activities which build self-confidence.

Constitutional Growth Delay with or without Delayed Adolescence

Children with constitutional growth delay have a more gradual rate of biological aging. The slow growth pattern starts at about 2 years of age. By kindergarten, the child is shorter and younger-appearing than the majority of his or her schoolmates, although health is good and body proportions are normal. Bone age is lower than chronologic age and is equal or close to height age. Growth rates are 5 cm or more per year; linear growth, with height at a lower percentile, is a characteristic feature. A dip in the growth rate before the start of puberty is usually seen. The family has a history of slow maturation and delayed onset of adolescence. Parental heights are average to tall, although an occasional family with genetic short stature has the added burden of familial slow maturation. Males are affected more often than females; most such boys are also delayed in sexual maturation, although an occasional patient enters puberty at age 12 years. Those with delayed adolescence continue to grow at approximately 5 cm/year and do not have a growth spurt until age 15 to 16; in contrast, the average boy's growth velocity accelerates at 13 years. This is the chronologic age when all growth charts show a steeper slope, representative of the mean increase in growth velocity during puberty. Consequently, the growth curve of the delayed developer often falls below the 5th percentile around age 13 and steepens later as puberty begins. As long as the prepubertal linear growth rate is over 5 cm/year, there is usually no need for concern. These young men reach their adult height at 20 to 21 years of age instead of the usual 18 years; they may not begin shaving regularly until age 20 years or more.

The criteria for diagnosing delayed adolescence include absence of testicular enlargement and other signs of secondary sexual maturation in a boy who is 14 years of age.[95]

The management of delayed adolescence in a boy depends on his chronologic age when first seen and his history and physical characteristics. If a young man of 14 to 15 is healthy but has no evidence of testicular enlargement or sexual hair, the management can be limited to determining his bone age, plotting his growth curve, and giving him reassurance. Alternatively, the assessment may be extended to include a complete blood count (CBC) and sedimentation rate, biochemical profile, T_4 assay, and urinalysis. These tests exclude the possibility that chronic diseases such as renal insufficiency, hypothyroidism, and chronic inflammatory bowel disease are present. If the data support the clinical diagnosis of delayed adolescence, the patient is reassured and examined every 6 months. Most boys enter puberty within the following 12 to 18 months and agree to allow sexual maturation to proceed without androgen supplementation. If, however, the patient is very emotionally distressed, modest doses of androgens may be used for 3 to 6 months in conjunction with psychological counseling.

A patient who presents at age 16 years without any evidence of puberty may still have an innocent delay of adolescence; however, a search for organic disease is indicated before this diagnosis is made. Boys who grow less than 5.0 cm/year or who have an abnormal physical sign or symptom (small penis, hypoplastic testes, pallor, dry skin, cushingoid features, headaches, visual disturbances, or anosmia) require thorough investigation. The differential diagnoses of delayed adolescence include (1) gonadotropin deficiency (either idiopathic or due to organic disease in the hypothalamus or pituitary, i.e., GnRH or FSH-LH deficiency, respectively), (2) primary testicular disease (hypoplastic testes, Leydig cell deficiency or dysfunction), (3) sex chromosome defects (Klinefelter's syndrome), (4) hypothyroidism (primary hypothyroidism or TSH or TRH deficiency), (5) Cushing's syndrome or disease (glucocorticoid treatment of asthma, rheumatoid arthritis, etc., or lesions in the hypothalamus, pituitary, or adrenal gland), and (6) chronic disease (chronic inflammatory bowel disease, cystic fibrosis, cardiac disease, CNS lesions, renal insufficiency, etc.).

The extent of the diagnostic evaluation must be individualized for each patient. The following are diagnostic procedures which aid in confirming or excluding diseases listed in the differential diagnoses:

1. CBC, sedimentation rate, biochemical profile
2. Assays for TSH, T_4 (RIA), T_3 (RIA), free T_4; TRH stimulation test (optional)
3. Assays of urine and/or plasma FSH and LH concentrations
4. GnRH testing (optional; may not differentiate hy-

pothalamic from pituitary dysfunction with a single injection or infusion)
5. Measurement of plasma GH and cortisol responses to insulin hypoglycemia and L-arginine infusion
6. Plasma testosterone and DHEA sulfate assays
7. Determinations of diurnal patterns of plasma cortisol and 24-h urinary 17-ketosteroid, 17-hydroxycorticosteroid, and cortisol output before and after low- and high-dose dexamethasone administration for suspected Cushing's syndrome
8. Chromosome analysis for Klinefelter's syndrome
9. hCG stimulation to test Leydig cell function
10. Radiologic studies: bone age, skull x-rays (optional: CT scan or MRI of head, skeletal survey for bone disease, GI series, chest x-ray for heart or lung disease, kidney studies)
11. Visual acuity, fields, and funduscopic examinations and visual evoked response for suspected organic lesions in the hypothalamic-pituitary axis

One of the following treatment programs may be used in healthy boys with delayed adolescence who need treatment for psychological reasons. If chronic disease (e.g., Crohn's disease) is discovered to be the cause of delayed adolescence, these treatment programs are not applicable because they may advance bone age without promoting linear growth or sexual maturation.

1. Testosterone enanthate 75 to 100 mg every 3 to 4 weeks for 3 to 6 months. This treatment may trigger the onset of puberty. If a permanent lack of androgens exists and satisfactory height has been achieved, the full virilizing dose is 200 mg intramuscularly (IM) every 2 to 3 weeks. Bone age is measured at the beginning and every 6 months if the effect of therapy on osseous maturation is an important factor.
2. Oxandrolone 0.05 to 0.1 mg per kilogram of body weight per day for 3 to 6 months (oxandrolone is an oral synthetic androgen with potent anabolic and weak androgenic properties). Oxandrolone is used in situations in which the priority is linear growth and sexual maturation can be postponed.
3. Human chorionic gonadotropin (hCG) 500 to 1000 units (U) IM three times weekly for 1 to 2 months; plasma testosterone concentration is monitored, and the dose is adjusted accordingly. hCG is useful only if Leydig cell function is intact.

Delayed adolescence in girls is present when breast tissue and/or sexual hair have not appeared by 14 years of age. Usually, menarche occurs 2.3 years after the onset of breast development, but it can occur as late as 4.5 years after breast budding.[95]

The differential diagnoses of delayed menarche in girls include (1) emotional disorders (e.g., anorexia nervosa), (2) gonadotropin deficiency, (3) primary ovarian disease (embryologic defects or acquired disease, e.g., agenesis, polycystic ovarian disease, or torsion of the ovary), (4) chronic disease, (5) absence of the uterus, (6) X chromosome abnormalities (Turner's syndrome), and (7) XY male pseudohermaphrodism (androgen insensitivity, 17α-hydroxylase deficiency, embryologic defects in the testes, e.g., agenesis or absence of Leydig cells).

On the initial evaluation, the history and physical examination guide the extent to which the patient is investigated. A healthy-appearing girl who presents at age 15 years without breast tissue and with a normal height and growth rate probably will begin puberty in the following 6 to 12 months and needs only reexamination and reassurance. However, if she is short or if her growth rate is 4.5 cm or less per year, a search must be initiated for chromosomal abnormalities, pituitary-hypothalamic disorders, and chronic diseases. On rare occasions, girls have presented with excellent breast growth, normal sexual hair, and primary amenorrhea due to congenital absence of the uterus; the vaginal examination shows an absence of the cervix. Pelvic sonography and peritoneoscopic examination are indicated if a normal female karyotype and elevated gonadotropin concentrations are discovered or if absence of the uterus is suspected. Gonadectomy must be performed in females who possess a Y chromosome because of the increased risk of gonadal malignancy.

Estrogen therapy for simple delayed adolescence in girls is unnecessary except for psychological reasons.

Pathologic Short Stature (Table 26-7)

Intrauterine Growth Disturbances

Abnormal intrauterine growth must be considered in any newborn whose birth weight is inappropriately low for gestational age. These babies are usually referred to as small-for-date infants; the prognosis for their recovery depends on the timing, severity, and duration of the intrauterine insult. As a rule, small-for-date infants whose growth accelerates and achieves a normal channel by 6 months postnatal age grow normally thereafter. If they show persistence of an abnormal growth rate at 2 years of age, they are likely to be short throughout childhood and adulthood.

A careful evaluation of the health of the mother, the placenta, and the fetus is needed to determine the likely cause of the fetal growth abnormality.

Placenta Abnormal embryologic development of the placenta or injuries from infection or vascular accidents interrupt the supply of essential nutrients to the fetus. The size and gross appearance as well as the histologic characteristics of the placenta should be documented in all cases of intrauterine growth failure.

Mother Many factors related to maternal health and well-being influence fetal growth. Chronic malnutrition throughout the childhood and early adult years of prospective mothers places their infants in jeopardy physically and intellectually. Maternal diseases such as toxemia, hypertension, compromised cardiac status, and renal insufficiency may impair fetal growth because of placental dysfunction.

Drugs ingested by pregnant women are a potential hazard to fetal growth and well-being. The teratogenic effects to the fetus of excessive alcohol ingestion *(fetal alcohol syndrome)*[107] include (1) intrauterine growth failure, (2) microcephaly (and possibly hydrocephalus), (3) mental retardation, which may be mild or severe (IQ range 15 to 105; in 16 of 20 infants the IQ was < 80), (4) facial abnormalities, including small midface, strabismus, ptosis, short palpebral fissures, epicanthal folds, thin upper lip, short nose, micrognathia, and maxillary hypoplasia, (5) minor joint and limb abnormalities, including limited range of movement and altered palm creases, and (6) behavioral problems, mainly hyperactivity, short attention span, and learning difficulties, but not rebelliousness, negativism, or psychosis.[107] Narcotic (heroin and morphine) addiction during pregnancy causes intrauterine growth failure in half the offspring and also increases the risk of prematurity and intrauterine infection. Anticoagulants (e.g., warfarin) used in mothers with prosthetic mitral valves have resulted in infants with mental retardation, hypotonia, seizures, optic atrophy, flat facies, hypoplastic nose, and stippled epiphyses. Anticonvulsants (e.g., phenytoin) have caused intrauterine growth failure, mental retardation, hypertelorism, cleft lip and palate, and hypoplastic distal phalanges with small nails. Aminopterin used for abortion in the first trimester causes poor fetal growth, microcephaly, craniofacial abnormalities, and shortness of limbs. Heavy cigarette smoking is associated with an increased incidence of prematurity as well as smaller-sized offspring.

Fetus The fetal diseases which interfere most frequently with growth are intrauterine infections which are maternally transmitted, congenital abnormalities of major organ systems, chromosomal defects, and a variety of growth-deficiency syndromes of genetic or unknown origin.

Maternally transmitted infections include (1) rubella, which causes microcephaly, mental retardation, deafness, cataracts, chorioretinitis, microphthalmus, congenital heart disease (patent ductus arteriosus, pulmonary stenosis, septal defects, etc.), (2) toxoplasmosis, caused by a protozoan agent, which causes fetal growth retardation, hepatosplenomegaly, microcephaly or hydrocephalus, retinal pigmentation, mental retardation, and intracranial calcification, (3) cytomegalovirus, which causes poor fetal growth, hepatosplenomegaly, jaundice, retinopathy, mental retardation, and intracranial calcification, and (4) syphilis, which is associated with small fetal size, brain and bone abnormalities, and nasal mucous membrane lesions.

Congenital malformations of the brain, lung, etc., may interfere with fetal growth. Many chromosomal defects cause intrauterine growth failure: trisomy 18, trisomy 13, Down syndrome (trisomy 21), etc. The phenotypic characteristics of these and many other syndromes of unknown etiology are fully described by Smith.[97]

Postnatal Malnutrition

Malnutrition due to inadequate food supplies is the major cause worldwide of poor growth in infancy and childhood. In this country, poverty and parental neglect or ignorance are the usual reasons for growth failure due to malnutrition. Poor weight gain and sometimes actual weight loss are the main findings. A careful history with particular emphasis on caloric intake and a thorough physical examination are essential. Characteristically, these infants are hungry and have very little subcutaneous fat and muscle mass. They are prone to develop gastroenteritis and dehydration, which further compromise their nutritional state. The cachexia, dehydration, and electrolyte abnormalities in these infants may mimic salt loss due to Addison's disease or adrenogenital syndrome but can be easily differentiated from those disorders by documenting stress elevations of plasma cortisol and aldosterone concentrations.

Management consists of hospitalizing the child in a clean area, avoiding unnecessary diagnostic tests, and providing optimal nutrition. Weight gain on this simple regimen provides adequate proof of the diagnosis. The need for cultures, blood chemistry studies, and hormone determinations (plasma cortisol and 17-hydroxyprogesterone and urinary 17-ketosteroid, allopregnanetriol, aldosterone, etc., concentrations) must be individualized. Dietary counseling and psychological support for the mother, plus home supervision after discharge by a visiting nurse, suffice if the mother-child relation is a healthy one. The prognosis for catch-up growth and subsequent normal stature is good if the duration and severity of the period of malnutrition are not excessive. If parental neglect has placed the infant in jeopardy, removal to a good foster home is advisable.

Gastrointestinal diseases which compromise growth in infants and young children include esophageal reflux, obstructive lesions of the bowel, and deficiencies of the digestive enzymes. Cystic fibrosis of the pancreas produces malabsorption due to insufficiency of pancreatic enzymes (trypsin, lipase, amylase). It also causes chronic pulmonary disease because of airway obstruction from abnormally thick mucus, combined with bacterial superinfection. Persistent elevation of sweat sodium concentration above 70 mEq/L is diagnostic for this disorder; concentrations above 50 mEq/L should elicit suspicion. Children with disaccharidase enzyme abnormalities need the expertise of a pediatric gastroenterologist who is skilled in performing endoscopic biopsies of the proximal small bowel for histology and quantitative enzyme determinations. Diarrheal stools which are acidic (pH < 6) and contain reducing substance by Clinitest Reagent tablet (> 0.25 percent) strongly suggest this disorder.

Chronic inflammatory bowel disease (Crohn's disease) occurs most frequently (78 percent of cases) between the ages of 10 and 29 years. Growth failure and delayed sexual maturation result from decreased caloric intake and increased fetal losses of nutrients. Hypoalbuminemia occurs in 50 percent of patients; anemia (iron and folate deficiencies) is also a frequent complication. Improved growth has occurred in prepubertal children treated with nutritional support or by surgical resection of the diseased bowel. If bone age is greater than 13 years, surgery may not result in catch-up growth. Androgens should be used with extreme caution because they do not enhance growth in the absence of adequate protein and caloric intake and may compromise adult height.

Endocrine Causes of Short Stature

Hypothyroidism *Congenital Hypothyroidism* Congenital hypothyroidism occurs in approximately 1 of 4000 newborns; the female/male ratio is 4:1. Data from screening programs indicate that 84 percent of congenitally hypothyroid infants have thyroid dysgenesis or agenesis, 8 percent have enzymatic defects in hormonogenesis, and 8 percent have either TSH or TRH deficiency. Early recognition and treatment afford the best hope of ameliorating or reversing the harmful effects of hypothyroidism on the brain. The placenta is relatively impermeable to maternal thyroid hormones; thus, the factors which influence the infant's prognosis for intelligence are the severity of intrauterine hypothyroidism, postnatal age at diagnosis, and adequacy of treatment.

After birth, linear growth is poor in hypothyroid infants. The diagnosis of congenital primary hypothyroidism is confirmed by low serum T_4, low free T_4, and high TSH concentrations. Additional criteria include absence or dysgenesis of the tibial epiphysis on knee x-ray and absence, hypoplasia, or maldescent of the thyroid gland by technetium scan. Breast-fed infants were once believed to be partially protected by breast milk because of its thyroid hormone content. This concept is no longer considered valid because breast milk contains insignificant amounts of thyroid hormone.

Early signs of congenital hypothyroidism include a large posterior fontanel, suture separation, feeding difficulties, prolonged unconjugated hyperbilirubinemia, and hypothermia. These subtle features usually go unnoticed by most physicians; therefore, the advantage of screening is detection of these infants before the development of obvious signs such as cretinous facies, myxedematous protruding tongue, hypotonia, umbilical hernia, mottling, lethargy, and constipation. The benefits of early detection and treatment justify the approximate cost of $5000 per case identified: Approximately 80 percent of congenitally hypothyroid infants treated before 3 months of age have IQs > 90, whereas only 45 percent of infants treated before 6 months have IQs > 90.[108–110] Recent studies indicate that the mean IQ of congenitally hypothyroid children identified by neonatal screening programs is similar to that of the general population; however, about 15 percent of these children have IQ scores below the normal range.

Management consists of administering L-thyroxine 6 to 10 μg per kilogram of body weight per day for the first year.[111,112] The thyroxine tablet is crushed and mixed in a teaspoon of formula or cereal. The criteria for judging response to treatment include improvements in the infant's behavior and appearance, increased growth rate, assessment of developmental milestones, and serum T_4 and TSH concentrations. In a few infants, TSH elevations have persisted even though the clinical response was excellent and the serum T_4 concentration was normal for age; therefore, TSH concentrations have not been relied on exclusively.[113] Initially, these infants must be seen every 4 to 6 weeks to monitor growth and T_4 levels and adjust the thyroid hormone dose. From age 6 months to 1 year, they are examined at 2- to 3-month intervals and then every 6 months until the age of 4 to 5 years. Thereafter, yearly examinations are sufficient to monitor progress and adjust the dose. Assessment of developmental progress and intelligence must be made before the child's entry into kindergarten to determine whether there is a need for special educational support.

Acquired Hypothyroidism The onset of acquired hypothyroidism in childhood can be readily diagnosed from the linear growth curve. Deceleration or complete cessation of growth is the earliest sign. The myxedematous physical findings seen in adults are usually absent. Features of acquired hypothyroidism include pallor, stocky physique, coarseness of facial features and puffiness about the eyes, delayed dental development, cool hands and feet, constipation, and sluggish behavior; occasionally, muscle hypertrophy is present. Scalp hair may be normal or sparse and dry. Rarely, children with hypothyroidism exhibit precocious sexual development, ovarian cysts, hyperprolactinemia, and diabetes insipidus which regress after thyroid replacement is begun. A goiter, usually due to thyroiditis, may be present, or there may be no palpable thyroid tissue. These children tend to socialize with inappropriately young playmates and by nature are quiet and studious. School performance is usually satisfactory until thyroid hormone is prescribed, after which there is frequently an adjustment period characterized by deterioration in school performance, rebelliousness, and "acting-out" behavior. Gradual increments in thyroid dosage have been tried but have not significantly altered this difficult transition period. Family members and school authorities should be informed of the changes in personality which follow the patient's discovery of new energies and interests. With time, there is a return to behavior patterns which are appropriate for chronologic age. The intelligence of these children is not adversely affected by the period of hypothyroidism.

The possible etiologies of acquired hypothyroidism include embryologic defects (thyroid hypoplasia), maldescent (lingual thyroid), chronic lymphocytic thyroiditis (Hashimoto's disease), acute and subacute thyroiditis, and pituitary hypothalamic disease. Lingual thyroid, when present, may be seen as a mass in the midline posterior portion of the extended tongue. Hypothyroidism develops in 40 to 50 percent of children who clinically have a goiter due to chronic lymphocytic thyroiditis. Primary hypothyroidism is characterized by elevated serum concentrations of TSH and low serum T_4, free T_4, and T_3 levels. In secondary hypothyroidism, the TSH concentration is low or normal and fails to increase after TRH stimulation. In tertiary hypothyroidism, the disease is in the hypothalamus; TRH stimulation elevates serum TSH levels.

The thoroughness of the diagnostic evaluation depends on the suspected etiology. It should include construction of a growth curve; measurement of serum T_4, free T_4, T_3, and TSH concentrations; determinations of thyroid antibody titers against thyroglobulin and microsomal antigens; and a ^{99m}Tc or ^{123}I thyroid scan. Measurement of bone age gives valuable data concerning the patient's biological age, the estimated age of onset of disease, and remaining growth potential. Skull x-rays (anteroposterior and lateral views) are useful for evaluating sella size and detecting bony erosion. Long-standing primary hypothryoidism may result in pituitary hypertrophy and sella enlargement; the sella is free of erosion and returns to normal size with thyroid replacement. Electrocardiograms show low voltage; they are not essential. Anemia is a common finding which disappears with thyroid medication. Pituitary function tests (e.g., TRH stimulation, GH responses) and special radiologic (CT or MRI of the pituitary and hypothalamus), neurologic, and ophthalmologic studies must be considered in children with hypothyroidism and low serum TSH concentrations.

Treatment consists of oral L-thyroxine, 0.1 mg per square meter of body surface (3 to 4 μg per kilogram of body weight) per day, given as a single dose. The dose must be individualized since absorption and metabolism vary among patients.

The clinical response to treatment in primary hypothyroidism consists of a catch-up growth spurt, disappearance of the abnormal physical stigmata, and improvement in facial features, including a loss of puffiness and pallor. The most valuable laboratory data are serum T_4, TSH, and hemoglobin concentrations and hematocrit; these indexes should be monitored every 2 months for the first 6 months. Bone age x-rays (at 6 to 12 months) are optional during the growth spurt and are not needed after the patient resumes growth at a normal percentile. After the patient is stabilized, the growth response and serum T_4 and TSH concentrations can be evaluated every 6 to 12 months to be certain of compliance. The prognosis for adult height is excellent if the patient is compliant and if the bone age is young. In cases where noncompliance is persistent, the entire weekly dose can be administered by a visiting nurse or school nurse once a week.[114] This therapy cannot safely be used in adults or in children with compromised cardiac or adrenal function. Excessive daily doses of thyroid should be avoided because it causes disproportionate acceleration of bone maturation and aggravates behavioral problems.

The thyroid treatment doses for patients with secondary or tertiary hypothyroidism are slightly lower than those for primary hypothyroidism. Usually, two-thirds or even one-half of the normal dose provides satisfactory serum thyroxine concentrations. It is especially important to avoid overtreatment in these children because undue acceleration of osseous maturation shortens the period of responsiveness if GH therapy is also needed. The prognosis for normal intelligence is excellent in children who acquire hypothyroidism after 1 to 2 years of age.

GH Deficiency The clinical features of patients with GH deficiency vary with the etiology, age at onset, and severity of the disorder. Those with congenital GH deficiency have characteristic growth patterns which distinguish them from children with acquired disease. In general, the idiopathic form is more common than the organic variety (disease due to tumor, trauma, embryologic defect, etc.).

The prevalence of GH deficiency was estimated to be as low as 1 in 30,000 births and as high as 1 in 4018 in two studies carried out in Great Britain.[115,116] It is possible that identification of the milder forms of GH deficiency will result in a disease frequency greater than 1 in 4000.

A classification of the causes of GH deficiency and GH resistance is outlined in Table 26-8. No attempt is made to distinguish whether the defect in GH secretion is due to disease in the hypothalamus or the pituitary gland.

Congenital GH Deficiency Infants with congenital GH deficiency usually have normal birth length and weight. They grow normally for 3 to 6 months, but

TABLE 26-8 Causes of GH Deficiency or Defective GH Action

Congenital GH Deficiency	
Decreased GH secretion	
Idiopathic	
Hereditary: autosomal recessive, autosomal dominant	
Embryologic defects	
Aplasia, hypoplasia, ectopia	
Anencephaly, arhinencephalia	
Septo-optic dysplasia	
Midline facial dysplasia	
Empty sella syndrome	
Miscellaneous syndromes	
Biologically inactive GH	
Neurosecretory defects	
GH resistance	
Laron dwarfism	
Pygmy	
Acquired GH Deficiency	
Idiopathic	
Neurosecretory defects	
CNS tumors	
Craniopharyngioma	Dysgerminoma
Optic glioma	Hamartoma
Trauma	
Perinatal insult: breech deliveries, hypoxemia, asphyxia, difficult forceps delivery, intracranial hemorrhage, precipitate or prolonged delivery, twin pregnancy	
Child abuse	
Accidental trauma	
Inflammatory diseases	
Viral encephalitis	
Bacteria, group B streptococcal meningitis, etc.	
Fungal	
Granulomatous: tuberculosis, syphilis, sarcoidosis, unknown etiology	
Autoimmunity: lymphocytic hypophysitis	
Irridiation: CNS radiation for brain tumors, leukemia	
Vascular lesions	
Aneurysms, pituitary vessels	
Infarction	
Hematologic disorders	
Hemochromatosis	
Sickle cell disease	
Thalassemia	
Histiocytosis	
Transient defects in GH secretion or action	
Peripuberty (secretion)	
Primary hypothyroidism (secretion, action)	
Psychosocial stress (secretion, action)	
Malnutrition (action)	
Glucocorticoid excess (?)	
Drug use	

linear growth rates decelerate thereafter. Their linear growth curves deviate progressively from the mean. The severity of the growth disorder is not usually appreciated until the child is 2 to 5 years of age, at which time it is obvious that a marked height discrepancy exists between the patient and his or her peers. After 3 years of age, growth rates in affected children are almost always less than 5 cm/year. Characteristically, these patients have normal body proportions for chronologic age. Most but not all children with GH deficiency are overweight for height; some are frankly obese. Excessive accumulation of fat occurs predominantly in the chest and abdominal areas, and the overlying skin has a grossly ripply or bosselated appearance. The general appearance of the child is always younger than is appropriate for chronologic age. In early childhood, the facies are frequently cherubic, infantile, or doll-like and the voice may be high-pitched. Frontal bossing, a common feature, is due to undergrowth of facial bones. Eruption and shedding of primary teeth usually are delayed. The permanent teeth also may appear late and are often crowded and irregularly positioned. Muscle mass is diminished. The hair is thin, and nail growth is poor. Skeletal age in a prepubertal hypopituitary patient is always delayed, and the degree of retardation of bone maturation is proportional to that of height age. Head circumference is within the normal range for age, but the sella turcica is often small. Closure of the anterior fontanel is usually very much delayed.

During early infancy and childhood, patients with GH deficiency may experience recurring episodes of fasting hypoglycemia and convulsions which, if untreated, may result in mental retardation, a seizure disorder, and even death. Therapy with GH is highly effective. Some of these infants have a concomitant deficiency of ACTH; their treatment includes maintenance doses of hydrocortisone (10 to 15 mg per square meter of surface per day in two or three divided doses PO) in addition to GH (0.18 to 0.3 mg per kilogram of body weight per week divided and given daily SC). During illnesses, stress doses of hydrocortisone given orally (60 mg/m^2 per day in three divided doses) or parenterally (60 mg/m^2 IM or IV given in two or three divided doses) are required. Glucose-containing electrolyte solutions must frequently be used IV when oral intake is curtailed in these children. The tendency to fasting hypoglycemia usually disappears by 5 years of age but may reappear if severe illnesses prevent oral intake for prolonged periods. Apart from the problems of hypoglycemia and seizures during the early childhood years, children with idiopathic GH deficiency are generally healthy and have normal intelligence. Emotional problems are more frequent, however, in this population, because patients are perceived to be much younger than their chronologic age and are treated accordingly. Excessive teasing and social isolation are common complaints in older untreated patients.

GH-deficient boys with microphallus and hypoplastic testes are likely to also have gonadotropin deficiency, which may be partial or complete. Usually, the gonadotropin status cannot be accurately assessed until their adolescent years. Small doses of androgen should be prescribed during infancy and early childhood to bring the penis size into the normal range for age. During the adolescent and adult years, testicular growth and enhanced virilization can be facilitated in gonadotropin-deficient hypopituitary males through the use of hCG in combination with human menopausal gonadotropin (hMG).[117] In children with isolated idiopathic GH deficiency who are treated with GH from an early age, pubertal maturation is likely to begin normally, whereas puberty is often delayed in those who begin treatment late in childhood. Hypopituitarism of organic origin (birth trauma, embryologic brain defects, etc.) carries a high risk of multiple pituitary hormone deficiencies.

There are several causes of congenital GH deficiency (Table 26-8). *Idiopathic hypopituitarism* is the most common type of hypopituitarism. By definition, no organic lesion or etiologic factor can be identified. Males are affected more frequently than are females. The disorder may involve only GH *(isolated GH deficiency)* or may be associated with deficiencies of TSH and/or gonadotropins and/or ACTH *(idiopathic multiple primary deficiencies)*. Prepubertal children with GH plus TSH or ACTH deficiency are likely to exhibit gonadotropin deficiency (partial or complete) in their adolescent years.

Magnetic resonance imaging (MRI) studies of the hypothalamus and pituitary gland in patients with idiopathic GH deficiency have shown that the sella volume tends to be small and that stalk abnormalities are most frequent in children with multiple pituitary hormone deficiencies. Those with diabetes insipidus frequently had an absent or ectopic posterior pituitary gland, and the bright spot indicating the neurohypophyses was absent. It is not certain that imaging studies are necessary in all children with isolated idiopathic GH deficiency, but they should be performed when multiple hormone deficiencies are present.

Genetic transmission of GH deficiency has been documented in six types of single-gene disorders. The modes of inheritance are autosomal recessive, autosomal dominant, and X-linked. Genetic types of GH deficiency have been caused by two mechanisms: (1) Mutations within or close to the GH gene cluster on the long arm of chromosome 17, or (2) mutations within the regulatory gene loci which are distant from the GH gene cluster, causing underproduction of biologically normal GH.[118]

A unique genetic disorder with GH deficiency, *isolated GH deficiency type 1A*, was described by Illig and colleagues. This entity is characterized by familial occurrence of early, extremely severe dwarfism. Patients have a typical appearance; they respond well initially to GH therapy but then may develop anti-GH antibodies and resistance to GH therapy. These patients are believed to have a total absence of GH during prenatal life, which causes them to lack immune tolerance to exogenous GH. The mechanism of inheritance is autosomal recessive.[119]

Patients with other forms of inherited GH deficiency continue to respond to exogenous GH therapy and present with variable degrees of growth failure. Those with X-linked recessive forms of GH deficiency have two distinct clinical phenotypes; this suggests that at least two loci on the X chromosome influence GH production.

Embryologic defects include aplasia, hypoplasia, and ectopic location of the pituitary. They may occur as isolated, congenital defects or in association with anencephaly or arhinencephalia. The latter comprises a spectrum of embryologic abnormalities which interfere with midline cleavage of the forebrain and cause midline dysplasia of the face.

The syndrome of septo-optic dysplasia (De Morsier's syndrome) consists of optic nerve and optic disk hypoplasia with or without abnormalities of the septum pellucidum and corpus callosum. Growth failure and hypopituitarism occur in 60 percent of cases. Other features include median facial cleft, hyperprolactinemia, and diabetes insipidus. Septo-optic dysplasia may represent a mild form of arhinencephalia.[120–122]

An increased incidence of hypopituitarism has been documented in patients with cleft lip and palate.[123]

Extension of the subarachnoid space into the sella turcica is responsible for the *empty sella syndrome*. It is presumed to result from an incompetent sella diaphragm and an increase in CSF pressure.[124–126] In the absence of surgery or radiation, the condition is called *primary* empty sella syndrome. Familial cases are rare. In most patients, pituitary function is normal and the sella turcica is diffusely enlarged. Empty sella syndrome is seen most frequently in obese middle-aged women; it is rarely recognized during childhood. The disorder can be readily distinguished from pituitary tumor by CT or MRI studies of the hypothalamus and pituitary gland. Most of the reported cases have associated cranial defects. One kindred has been described in which empty sella syndrome was transmitted as an autosomal dominant trait in association with Rieger's anomaly of the anterior chamber of the eye.[127]

Children with *biologically inactive GH* present with growth failure and have the following characteristics: height that is below the mean by > 3 SD, abnormal growth rate (< 4 cm/year), apparent good health, normal body proportions, normal plasma GH responses by RIA but abnormally low ratios of radioreceptor-measured/RIA-measured GH concentrations, low serum IGF-I concentrations which improve after 3 to 10 daily injections of GH, and improvement of linear growth when given GH therapy.[105] The assumption is made that the endogenous GH in these children has reduced biological activity but is immunologically reactive. Biologically inactive GH is thought to be one of the etiologic factors in NVSS.[102]

GH neurosecretory dysfunction was first described in children who had received prior cranial radiation and in very short children with unexplained poor growth (i.e., growth velocity < 4 cm/year, peak GH concentration > 10 ng/mL after provocative testing, low serum IGF-I levels, and abnormally low diurnal frequency and amplitude of GH pulses).[106] Spontaneous GH secretion in these children was found to be lower than in controls but higher than in patients with classical GH deficiency. The data suggested that these children have a subtle deficiency of GH as a result of defective neuroregulation of GH secretion. Treatment with exogenous GH enhanced linear growth velocity in the majority. Assessment of spontaneous GH secretion is labor-intensive because serum samples for GH measurement must be obtained at 15- to 20-min intervals, or alternatively, a plasma sample can be collected by means of a constant withdrawal portable pump for an integrated GH concentration. These studies cannot be carried out safely in small children.

Recently, the validity of spontaneous GH secretion studies has been questioned because additional investigations have shown that mean GH levels in very short children are not significantly different from those of control subjects matched for age and pubertal stage. The use of both GH and IGF-I measurements in these children may better distinguish them from normally growing subjects.

GH Resistance Syndrome (Laron Syndrome) Children with Laron syndrome resemble GH-deficient subjects except that they are small at birth and have high resting levels of serum GH and exaggerated GH responses to provocative testing. They lack circulating GHBP and have a deficiency of cell surface GH receptors. Deletions of the GH receptor gene have been documented in some patients.[68–72] Serum concentrations of IGFBP-III and IGF-I are low in these patients and do not rise after GH administration. The endogenous GH produced by these children is biologically active and binds normally in standard GH receptor assays. Adults with GH resistance syndrome rarely exceed 130 cm in height and appear to be fertile. This syndrome is seen most commonly in the offspring of consanguineous marriages involving Jewish parents of Middle Eastern extraction. Transmission is by an autosomal recessive mode of inheritance. Recently a large population of patients with growth hormone resistance syndrome was identified in southern Equador; they differed from the Israeli patients by exhibiting a distorted sex distribution (19 females: 1 male). Affected children are responsive to human biosynthetic IGF-I therapy, which is available through clinical research protocols.[128,129]

Pygmies represent another example of individuals with GH resistance in whom IGF-I levels are low and IGF-II levels are normal. Treatment with exogenous GH fails to correct the IGF-I deficiency. Merimee and colleagues postulated that pygmies have isolated deficiencies of IGF-I due to a defect in GH receptor.[130,131] Malnutrition is an alternative explanation for the low IGF-I in pygmies.[132]

Acquired GH Deficiency Children with acquired GH deficiency by definition grow normally during early childhood and then fail to grow because they develop GH deficiency. It is essential that organic disease be excluded. The causes of acquired GH deficiency are discussed briefly here.

Craniopharyngioma is the most common *CNS tumor* that causes GH deficiency in childhood. The tumor is believed to rise from embryonic squamous cell rests located at the junction of the adenohypophysis and neurohypophysis. Because of its location, expansion may cause permanent injury to the hypothalamus, optic nerves, and pituitary gland. The only complaint may be growth failure. Other clinical features include visual field defects, signs and symptoms of increased intracranial pressure, and multiple pituitary endocrine deficiencies. After surgical extirpation of the tumor, a majority of children have panhypopituitarism. Destruction of the satiety center may result in uncontrolled hyperphagia and obesity. Normal or excessive growth has been observed after surgery in some hyperphagic patients who have abnormally low GH responses and normal somatomedin levels.[133] Recent studies suggest that hyperprolactinemia or hyperinsulinism may account for the normal IGF-I levels and sustained growth in these children.[134–136] Other CNS tumors which cause hypopituitarism in childhood are optic gliomas, germinomas, ependymomas, meningiomas, colloid cysts of the third ventricle, and, rarely, chromophobe adenomas.

Trauma may also produce GH deficiency. Perinatal injury to the pituitary and/or hypothalamus may account for a significant number of childhood cases of presumed congenital idiopathic GH deficiency. A careful review of the birth histories of these children has shown that 50 to 65 percent of patients had one or more significant perinatal insults. Birth size is generally normal. The male/female ratio is 4:1. Perinatal risk factors include intrapartum hypoxemia or asphyxia, breech deliveries, difficult forceps deliveries, intracranial hemorrhage, precipitate or prolonged labor, twin pregnancies, and postnatal seizures. Other risk factors include bleeding during pregnancy and toxemia.[137,138] Throughout childhood, accidental head trauma or child abuse may result in hypopituitarism.

Inflammatory diseases, including bacterial meningitis, viral encephalitis, and fungal infections of the CNS, may cause permanent injury to the pituitary and hypothalamus. Giant cell granuloma of the pituitary gland is a rare cause of hypopituitarism. Its presentation may be indistinguishable from that of pituitary adenoma[139]; the diagnosis is usually made at autopsy or by obtaining pituitary tissue for histologic examination. The disease is usually of unknown etiology but has been seen in association with tuberculosis, syphilis, and sarcoidosis.

Lymphocytic hypophysitis is considered an *autoimmune disorder,* the clinical characteristics of which resemble those of pituitary tumors; hypopituitarism is frequently present. The disease has been described most frequently in women who are pregnant or were recently pregnant.[140–142]

Irradiation for tumors of the head and neck carries a high risk for impaired hypothalamic-pituitary function.[143–145] The doses of radiation usually exceed 4000 rads. GH deficiency is the most common abnormality; TSH and ACTH secretion usually are preserved. Less is known about the gonadotropin status of these children. Primary thyroid dysfunction due to radiation injury of the thyroid gland is not uncommon. Usually, the patient appears euthyroid and has an elevated TSH level with normal T_4 and T_3 concentrations. Clinical hypothyroidism with low T_4 and T_3 levels has also been observed in these children. In the early stages after cranial radiation, GH responses to pharmacologic stimulation may be normal, but spontaneous GH secretion is low.

Aneurysms of the pituitary vessels and infarction of the pituitary gland due to vascular malformations are extremely rare causes of hypopituitarism in childhood.[146]

Impaired hypothalamic-pituitary function may be observed in patients with *thalassemia major* who have iron overload. Normal GH responses and low somatomedin levels have been documented.[147–149]

Permanent vasopressin deficiency and diabetes insipidus are the most common CNS complications of *disseminated histiocytosis.* Most affected children have inadequate GH responses to provocative tests but grow satisfactorily and do not require treatment. Those with growth failure and abnormal GH responses benefit from GH therapy. Usually TSH, ACTH, FSH, and LH secretion remain normal.[150]

Transient Defects in GH Secretion or Action Transient or functional hypopituitarism has been documented in prepubertal males; it has been called "lazy pituitary syndrome."[151] Therapy with GH or androgens accelerates growth velocity. Normal GH responses to provocative stimuli have been observed after the onset of puberty.[152,153]

Hypopituitarism has been documented in young children with growth failure who come from hostile home environments. Psychological stress and nutritional factors are the probable causes of the entity known as *psychosocial dwarfism.* These patients have delayed onset of speech, are withdrawn, and have abnormal sleep patterns and bizarre eating habits. After these children are placed in foster homes or after the home stresses are resolved, pituitary function returns to normal, growth accelerates, and they exhibit improved behavior and normal dietary habits.[154–157]

Transient GH deficiency due to depletion of pituitary GH has been documented in primary hypothyroidism. Treatment with thyroid hormone is associated with catch-up growth and normal GH responses to provocative stimuli.

Diagnosis of GH Deficiency The diagnostic evaluation and treatment of GH deficiency depends on the age of the child and the presence or absence of hypoglycemia. Small infants with hypoglycemia require immediate evaluation and treatment but are able to undergo only limited diagnostic studies. The most practical test involves measurement of glucose, plasma cortisol, GH, and insulin concentrations during a documented episode of spontaneous hypoglycemia. Serum T_4 and TSH concentrations should be determined. Insulin-induced hypoglycemia is a hazardous diagnostic test in small infants. L-Arginine stimulation is safe but requires an infusion and six or more blood samples. The diagnosis of GH and ACTH deficiency in the neonatal period is based on a plasma GH level < 10 ng/ml and a plasma cortisol concentration < 5 μg/dL during fasting hypoglycemia or L-arginine challenge. Frequent feedings at 3- to 4-h intervals coupled with GH and hydrocortisone treatment usually restore carbohydrate homeostasis. With advancing age, the tendency to hypoglycemia lessens. During illness, therapy with stress doses of hydrocortisone (see above) may be needed to protect the patient from hypoglycemia and seizures. Parents can also be taught to give rectal glucose (25 mL of 50% glucose diluted in equal parts with tap water and dispensed from a pediatric Fleet's enema container which has been emptied of enema solution).

Opinions differ concerning the appropriate age for conducting pituitary function tests beyond infancy. If growth failure is the child's only problem, it may be preferable to wait until 3 or 4 years of age; however, diagnostic evaluation can be performed at an earlier age depending on the circumstances. No child should undergo GH testing while hypothyroid, because the results are unreliable. Treatment with T_4 for 1 or 2 months prior to assessment of GH responsiveness is recommended.

The usual indications for the evaluation of GH deficiency include (1) pathologic short stature in a child with normal body proportions (height > 2 SD below the mean, (2) abnormal growth rate for chronologic age (< 7 cm/year prior to age 3, < 5 cm/year from age 3 to onset of puberty, and < 6 cm/year during the pubertal years), (3) delayed skeletal maturation (bone age > 2 SD below the mean for chronologic age), and (4) special clinical considerations (e.g., microgenitalia, prior hypoglycemia, history of head trauma, CNS tumor, hypoxemia, or intracranial hemorrhage). In addition, tests of pituitary function are necessary when linear growth in children with suspected acquired hypopituitarism decelerates or ceases, even if height is within the normal range.

Valuable information is obtained from the following: construction of growth curves, serum T_4 and TSH assays (T_3 and TRH stimulation tests are optional), insulin hypoglycemia challenge for GH and cortisol secretion (if GH deficiency is suspected, use only 0.05 U regular insulin per kilogram of body weight as an IV bolus and take the precautions noted in Table 26-13), L-arginine stimulation test for GH, prolactin determination, urine specific gravity and/or osmolality (on the second voided urine after an overnight water-deprivation test to assess vasopressin secretion), CBC, urinalysis, biochemical profile, bone age determination, anteroposterior and lateral skull x-rays for sella size and shape, examinations of visual fields and acuity, funduscopic examination, and CT scan or MRI of hypothalamus and pituitary (in selected cases only). GHRH stimulation tests are not routinely performed in pathologically short children because a majority of these patients have excellent reserves of pituitary GH; only children with severe classical GH deficiency show poor GH responses to GHRH.

The diagnosis of classical GH deficiency is based on a peak GH of <8 to 10 ng/mL after two provocative stimuli. Severe GH deficiency is present when the peak GH level is <4 ng/mL. Since monoclonal IRMA GH assays give lower concentrations than do standard polyclonal GH RIAs, the diagnostic criteria must be adjusted in accordance with the GH assay used. Many studies have suggested that GH treatment should not be confined exclusively to children with classical GH deficiency since a majority of subjects with severe idiopathic growth failure will benefit from GH treatment. Characteristically, this group has normal GH responses to provocative tests, low IGF-I and GHBP-III levels, and pathologic height, growth rate, and bone age for chronologic age.

Treatment At present, hypopituitary children are being treated exclusively with recombinant DNA–derived human GH. The dose is 0.18 to 0.3 mg/kg per week divided and given subcutaneously daily or 5 to 6 days a week. Pulsatile infusions of GH are not widely used.

Two recombinant GH preparations have been approved for treatment. Somatrem, or met-GH, is a 192 amino acid product with an extra methionine residue. Somatropin has 191 amino acids and is identical to pituitary GH. Both products have been given orphan drug status by the FDA. The efficacy and safety of the two GH preparations are similar. Neither product stimulates significant titers of antibodies which interfere with the response to GH treatment. The potential adverse effects of GH include glucose intolerance and salt and water retention. Neither has caused significant problems. Healthy children receiving GH treatment do not appear to have a significantly increased risk of developing leukemia. However, a higher incidence of leukemia has been observed in GH-treated subjects who have had prior brain tumors, radiation treatment, or chemotherapy. During the era of human pituitary GH therapy, which ended in 1985, no one anticipated the development of spongiform encephalopathy (Creutzfeldt-Jakob disease). Consequently, the risks of unknown potential adverse effects due to recombinant GH therapy must always be kept in mind.

Until 1985, the standard GH used for treatment was purified GH extracted from human pituitary glands. This preparation was withdrawn from human use in 1985 because four young adults who had received GH in the late 1960s and early 1970s died of Creutzfeldt-Jakob disease (CJD).[158–160] CJD is a slow degenerative disease of the central nervous system caused by a transmissible unconventional prion. It has been classified as one of the subacute spongiform encephalopathies. Clinically, the disease is characterized by progressive truncal ataxia, tremors of the head and extremities, speech disturbances, involuntary movements, dementia, and death. Seldom is CJD seen in patients before age 30 years.

During the first treatment periods, the growth response is 9 to 12 cm/year; subsequently, it is 7 to 8 cm/year. Within a few months of starting therapy, there is a loss of subcutaneous fat and the children lose their cherubic, babyish facial appearance and look more mature.

Small doses of androgens given simultaneously with GH during the prepubertal years enhance linear growth responses.[161,162] A regimen of oxandrolone, 0.05 to 0.1 mg per kilogram of body weight per day PO, plus GH increases growth rates without significant enlargement of the phallus. When microphallus is present, GH treatment can be combined with a small dose of depot testosterone (25 mg IM monthly for 2 or 3 months). Androgen therapy should never be used without concurrent GH administration, because bone maturation usually accelerates without compensatory increases in height and ultimate stature may be compromised. Bone age must be evaluated at both the start and the completion of each treatment period to assess the effects of therapy on bone maturation relative to height gain. Lastly, androgens should not be combined with GH if bone age has moved significantly ahead of height age during the previous treatment period. In these circumstances, it is safer to use only GH treatment. Thyroid hormone determination should be performed at 6- to 12-month intervals because hypopituitary children with previously normal serum T_4 levels have been known to develop hypothyroidism during GH treatment. This may be due to a stimulation of somatostatin release by GH which in turn suppresses TSH secretion. In this situation, thyroid replacement must be administered concurrently to ensure an optimal growth response to administered GH. At present, GH therapy should be continued until the epiphyses close or the patient ceases to respond to therapy.

Assessment of gonadotropin secretion is usually postponed until the adolescent years. In a male who has reached age 14 years and has no increase in testicular size, 24-h urinary FSH and LH excretion (by RIA) and plasma testosterone concentration should be determined. Stimulation of pituitary FSH and LH by GnRH is now being standardized. Unfortunately, a single GnRH injection may not indicate whether dysfunction exists in the pituitary or the hypothalamus. Absence of a rise in plasma and/or urinary FSH and LH concentration is indicative of either pituitary disease or prolonged endogenous lack of GnRH. Repeated GnRH stimulation has been used to differentiate pituitary from hypothalamic dysfunction.

The treatment of gonadotropin deficiency depends on the height and bone age of the patient. If the patient is 14 years old, bone age is $<$ 14 years, and height is approximately 5 ft, GH or testosterone 17β-cypionate or testosterone enanthate (50 to 100 mg every 3 to 4 weeks) results in increased growth velocity as well as penis and sexual hair growth. After the patient has achieved a height of 5 ft 4 in. or has begun epiphyseal fusion (bone age = 16 years), larger doses of testosterone (200 mg every 2 to 3 weeks IM) are needed to promote sexual maturation. For reasons which are poorly understood, many gonadotropin-deficient hypopituitary males do not achieve satisfactory beard growth or muscular development. An alternative treatment program for gonadotropin-deficient males involves simultaneous administration of hMG and hCG to promote testicular maturation, virilization, and fertility. The treatment of pituitary hormone deficits is summarized in Table 26-9.

Cushing's Syndrome Obesity, linear growth failure, and delayed adolescence may be the only signs of Cushing's syndrome in childhood. In contrast to obese normal children who grow rapidly, those with Cushing's syndrome exhibit linear growth deceleration and subtle or obvious cushingoid facial features. Annual school photographs often document the onset of a cushingoid facial appearance. The diagnostic protocol includes measurement of diurnal plasma cortisol concentrations: plasma ACTH concentration; 24-h excretion of 17-hydroxycorticosteroids, 17-ketosteroids, and cortisol; low-dose dexamethasone suppression test (20 μg per kilogram of body weight per day divided into four doses and given at 6-h intervals); high-dose dexamethasone suppression test (80 μg/kg per day given in four doses); ACTH stimulation test; skeletal x-rays for osteoporosis and bone age; and CT scans of the head and abdomen. Abdominal ultrasonography may also aid in the detection of an adrenal lesion. These less invasive diagnostic tests have almost entirely replaced adrenal arteriography and/or angiography, which were once the only means for localizing an adrenal tumor.

The treatment of Cushing's syndrome due to ade-

TABLE 26-9 Treatment of Hormone Deficits and Monitoring Schedule for Hypopituitary Patients

Hormone Deficit	Treatment	Monitoring System
TRH-TSH	1. L-Thyroxine 2 μg/kg^2 per day PO	Growth rate, serum T_4 concentration
GH	2. rhGH 0.04 mg/kg/day SC (range = 0.18–0.3 mg/kg per week)	Linear growth rate, bone age, clinical appearance, T_4, IGF-I
ACTH	1. Oral hydrocortisone or cortisone acetate, 10–15 mg/m^2 per day divided into 2 or 3 doses, *or* 2. IM cortisone acetate maintenance dose, 10–15 mg/m^2 per day; stress dose, 60–75 mg/m^2 per day	Fasting blood sugar, plasma cortisol concentrations
FSH-LH	1. Testosterone, 100–200 IM every 2–4 weeks after completion of GH therapy, *or* 2. hCG, 1000–2000 U in 0.2–0.4 mL diluent, IM, three times weekly; Pergonal menotropins, one vial in 1 mL diluent, IM, three times weekly; hCG and Pergonal menotropins may be combined in single syringe	1. Plasma testosterone concentration, penis size, sexual hair growth 2. Plasma testosterone concentration, penis and testis size, sexual hair and beard growth, sperm analysis
Vasopressin	1. DDAVP,* 50 μL at bedtime, 25–50 μL every morning 2. Pitressin in oil, 0.5–1.0 mL IM every 1–3 days is used on rare occasions	Clinical response (thirst, etc.), specific gravity , volume of urine , serum Na, Cl, and osmolality in normal range

* DDAVP-desmopressin (1-desamino-8-D-arginine vasopressin).

noma or carcinoma is unilateral adrenalectomy and supportive glucocorticoid therapy during and after surgery until function is restored in the contralateral adrenal gland. Bilateral adrenalectomy is necessary for Cushing's syndrome due to micronodular adrenal disease, a non-ACTH-dependent form of glucocorticoid excess. The choices of therapy for bilateral adrenal hyperplasia (Cushing's disease) include (1) transsphenoidal pituitary microadenectomy, (2) pituitary irradiation, and (3) bilateral adrenalectomy. A study documented the presence of pituitary microadenoma in 14 of 15 children with Cushing's disease.[163] Only three displayed radiographic evidence of an abnormal sella turcica. In the hands of an experienced neurosurgeon, pituitary microadenectomy has been reported to cause rapid amelioration of glucocorticoid excess, resumption of growth, and progression through puberty; other pituitary functions generally improve or remain unchanged. Jennings and coworkers reported favorable results after cranial irradiation for childhood Cushing's disease.[164] However, the long-range impact of cranial irradiation on pituitary function and behavior is unknown. Bilateral adrenalectomy has been widely used as therapy in children with Cushing's disease. Unfortunately, 25 to 45 percent of patients develop hyperpigmentation and enlargement of the sella turcica due to Nelson's syndrome. Glucocorticoid (hydrocortisone, 12 to 15 mg per square meter of body surface per day PO, or cortisone acetate, 30 mg/m^2 per day PO) and mineralocorticoid replacement (9α-fluorocortisone, 0.1 mg/day PO) also are needed after a bilateral adrenalectomy. These patients also require stress doses of hydrocortisone (60 to 75 mg per square meter of body surface per day) with febrile illness, trauma, anesthesia, etc. Careful periodic evaluation for Nelson's syndrome is mandatory. Cyproheptadine, bromocriptine, metyrapone, and mitotane are agents which are seldom used in childhood Cushing's disease.

Short Adult Stature due to Precocious Sexual Maturation

During the early childhood years, children who have had precocious puberty or who secrete excessive amounts of androgens, as in non-salt-losing congenital virilizing adrenal hyperplasia (CVAH), are at risk for short stature in their adult years. Before epiphyseal fusion, these children are tall, but their markedly accelerated pace of bone maturation without compensatory increases in height results in epiphyseal fusion and growth cessation at an inappropriately young age.

Bone Disorders (Chondrodystrophies or Skeletal Dysplasias)

Disproportionate short stature is the distinguishing characteristic of the chondrodystrophies, a heterogeneous group of bone diseases which disturb, to varying degrees, the length and shape of long bones, trunk, and skull. The 50 or more chondrodystrophies have been classified by clinical, radiographic, and pathophysiologic criteria.

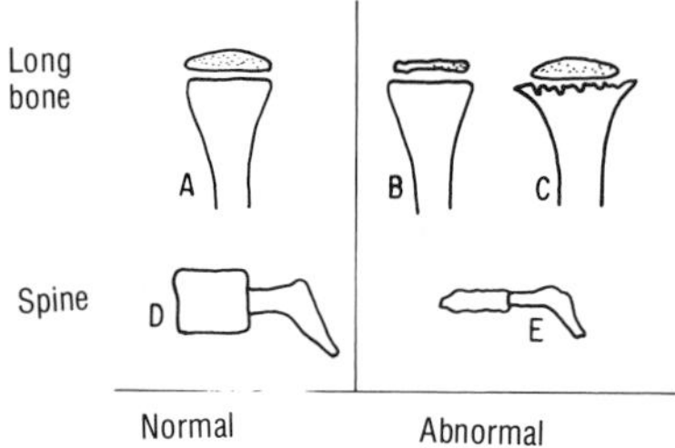

Involvement	Classification
A + D	Normal
B + D	Epiphyseal dysplasia
C + D	Metaphyseal dysplasia
B + E	Spondyloepiphyseal dysplasia
C + E	Spondylometaphyseal dysplasia

FIGURE 26-15 Classification of the chondrodystrophies based on radiographic abnormalities in the long bones. (*From Rimoin DL: The Chondrodystrophies. Adv Hum Genet 5:1, 1975.*)

One clinical classification divides the chondrodystrophies into those with predominantly short limbs (e.g., achondroplasia) and those with predominantly short trunk (e.g., spondyloepiphyseal dysplasia). Other clinical features used to classify these patients include age of onset; location of the defect, i.e., in proximal, medial, or distal segments of limbs; and presence of associated physical abnormalities, e.g., polydactylism in Ellis–van Creveld syndrome (chondroectodermal dysplasia) or fine hair in cartilage-hair hypoplasia.

The radiographic classifications are based on the location of the abnormality in the long bones, e.g., epiphyses (epiphyseal dysplasia), metaphyses (metaphyseal dysplasia), or diaphysis (Fig. 26-15). When both the spine and the long bones have disordered growth, the terms *spondyloepiphyseal* and *spondylometaphyseal* dysplasia have been used. Further subdivision of these groups has been based on other distinguishing abnormalities. The clinical and radiographic classifications are descriptive and do not provide information on the cellular abnormalities responsible for abnormal bone growth.

The pathophysiologic classification is based on the histochemical and ultrastructural characteristics of cartilage and bone; it thus gives more detailed information on the possible pathogenesis of many of these disorders. Examples include abnormal chondrocyte metabolism (mucopolysaccharidoses), chondrocyte proliferation (achondroplasia), chondrocyte maturation and degeneration (metaphyseal dysplasia), and epiphyseal ossification (epiphyseal dysplasia).[165]

None of the present methods of grouping the chondrodystrophies is perfect because the precise biochemical defect in many of these disorders is unknown, and there is much overlap in their clinical and radiographic features. Nevertheless, more order now exists because of the progress made in classifying the skeletal dysplasias.

This group of disorders is characterized by poor linear growth from early life, abnormal body proportions, distinguishing physical and radiographic data, bone age close to chronologic age (and ahead of height age), normal sexual maturation, and appropriate age of epiphyseal fusion. Detailed endocrine evaluation is seldom needed. The genetic implications must be shared with patients as adulthood approaches.

Chondrodystrophies Two treatments for achondroplasia have become available. The first involves the use of GH administration, which improves growth velocity mainly in the first year, with fewer effects in the second and third years of treatment. It appears that modest gains in final height can be achieved with GH therapy, but the evidence is inconclusive. The second approach involves limb-lengthening operations using small percutaneous incisions through which the long bones of the extremities are broken.[166] The method developed by Villarubias in Barcelona involves the use of one externally fixated bar which controls the gradual distraction of the callus. This device allows for limb stretching at a rate of 1.2 mm/day. Bilateral tibial lengthening is done first. Subsequently, the femurs are lengthened, along with percutaneous tenotomies of the adductors and the internal rectorus. The Villarubias technique does not permit weight bearing, so that after a brief hospitalization of 3 to 5 days the patient must spend many months in a wheelchair. This approach is said to be associated with less pain and discomfort than alternative approaches. Prophylactic tenotomies prevent the contractures encountered with other techniques. Care must be taken to preserve the blood supply, which is essential for good callus healing. Complications include muscle contractions, stretching of nerves, joint stiffness, vascular complications, problems at the pin site, and various psychological difficulties. This procedure has yielded as much as 12 in of height and has corrected the lordosis which is a constant feature of achondroplasia. Expert care by skilled orthopedists, geneticists, psychologists, and physical therapists is required for a successful outcome. Most important, the patient should be the individual who makes the decision. Emotional maturity and stability are prerequisites. It has been recommended that surgery be postponed until children reach the age of 14 to 20 years. Finally, it is important to inform patients and their families that experience with these procedures is very limited and that the risks are significant (Fig. 26-16).

Chromosome Abnormalities: Turner's Syndrome

Turner's syndrome occurs in approximately 1 in 2500 to 5000 female live births. The frequency in female fetuses is as high as 3 percent, but most are lost through spontaneous abortion.[167] Monosomy X (45,X) accounts for 90 percent of affected fetuses, whereas liveborn girls with Turner's syndrome have a wide variety of karyotypes (50 percent are 45,X, and the remainder may have isochromosomes of the long arm of X, ring X, deletions of the short arm of X, or various mosaicisms).

The phenotype of Turner's syndrome is diverse; most girls have easily recognizable physical characteristics, while in some the fetuses may consist only of short stature and absence of sexual maturation in adolescence. For this reason, it is advisable to perform a karyotype in all girls with unexplained growth failure. In infancy, the usual clues are loose skin folds in the posterior neck region (Bonnevie-Ullrich syndrome), which later form the pterygium colli (webbed neck); lymphedema of the dorsum of the feet and hands; increased carrying angles and various nail abnormalities, such as rudimentary, dysplastic, or hyperconvex nails surrounded by abundant soft tissue. In childhood and adolescence, the most constant feature is short stature, which may be accompanied by some of the well-recognized features of Turner's syndrome. Characteristically, the facial appearance is triangular in shape with midfacial hypoplasia, micrognathia, epicanthal folds, ptosis, prominent low set, rotated or malformed ears, and a short, broad webbed neck with a low posterior hairline. The webbed neck is a residual of intrauterine edema, which is presumed to result from failure to open lymphatic channels. Other features include a broad or shieldlike chest with widely set nipples, increased carrying angles, numerous pigmented nevi, bicuspid aortic valve, wide aortic root diameter, and coarctation of the aorta. The renal anomalies are malrotation, horseshoe-shaped kidney, duplication of renal pelvis and ureter, and hydronephrosis from ureteropelvic obstruction. Numerous skeletal abnormalities have been described, including bone rarefaction of the hands, elbows, and feet; vertebral hypoplasia; osteochondrosis-like changes in the spine; angular configuration of proximal carpal bones described by Kosowicz; short fourth metacarpals and metatarsals; bayonet or Madelung's deformity of the radius; and deformities of medial tibial and femoral condyles. The main health problems result from recurrent otitis media and conductive hearing loss, hypertension (coarctation of the aorta or renal arteries or idiopathic), autoimmune diseases (type 1 diabetes mellitus and Hashimoto's thyroiditis), and rarely GI hemorrhage from intestinal telangiectasia. Intelligence is normal in girls with Turner's syndrome; however, mean performance IQ is lower than that of the general popula-

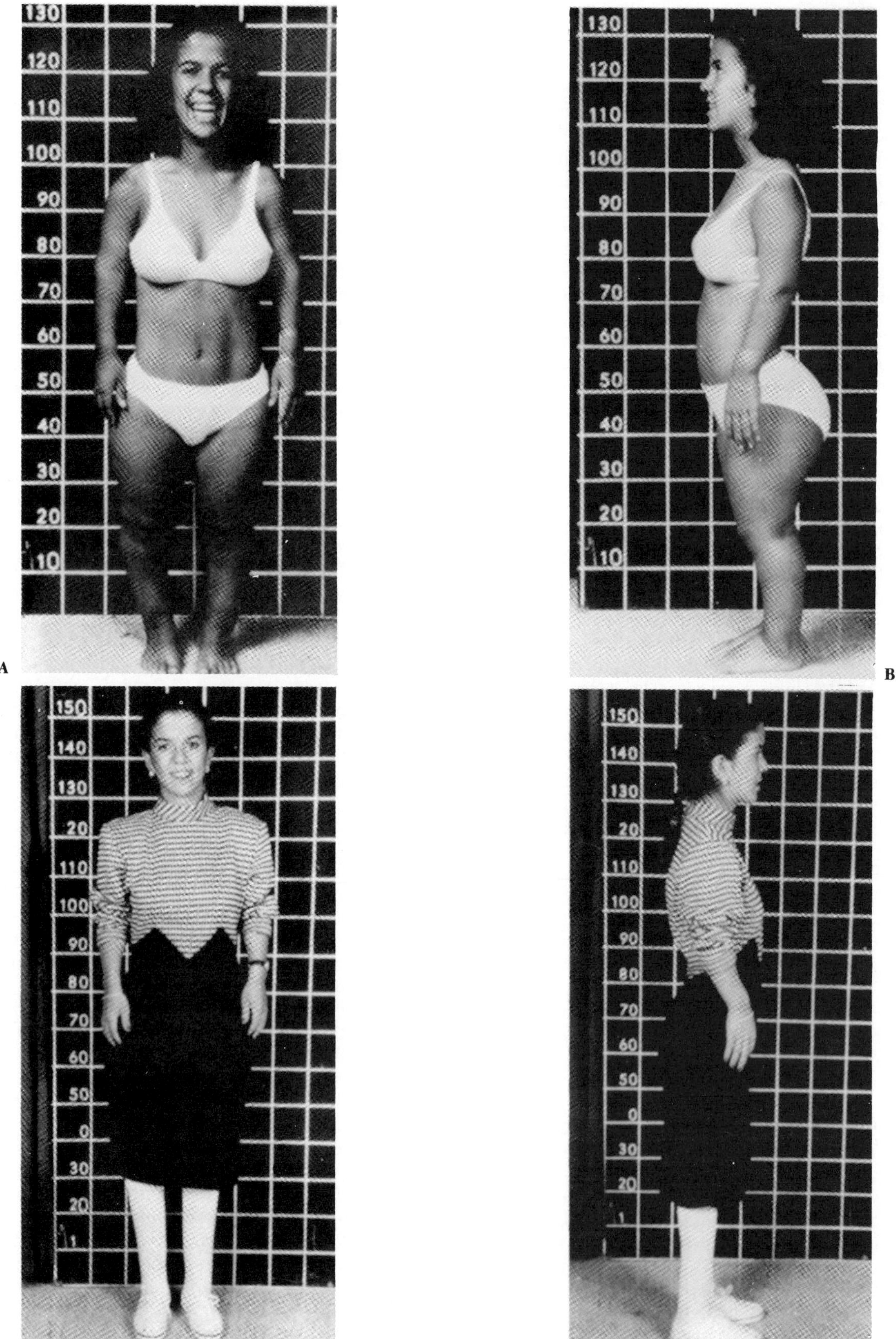

FIGURE 26-16 A young woman with achondroplasia is shown before (*A* and *B*) and after (*C* and *D*) leg lengthening. Final height (61.5 inches) was increased by approximately 12 in. (*From Rimoin.*[166])

tion because space-form perception is deficient while verbal IQ abilities are normal. Poor performance in mathematics is a common complaint. Difficulty in socializing is common, but the incidence of psychopathology is not greater in girls with Turner's syndrome.

In a fetus with X chromosomal abnormalities, ovarian differentiation and function appear to be normal until 14 to 18 weeks gestation. Thereafter, oocytes are lost at a rapid rate and the streak gonad develops through a process of accelerated stromal fibrosis. Oocyte loss and stromal fibrosis are not absolute in all girls with Turner's syndrome. It has been estimated that 5 percent of these girls will have spontaneous puberty, but the actual incidence of transient ovarian function may be higher. Maintenance of ovarian function is more frequent in patients with mosaic karyotypes but also is seen in 45,X individuals. In most instances, ovarian function will fail over time; however, a few women with Turner's syndrome have experienced persistence of ovulatory menses and successful pregnancies.

The diagnosis of Turner's syndrome is confirmed by chromosome analysis of peripheral leukocytes. The presence of Y chromosome material is likely if clitoromegaly or posterior labial fusion is seen in a girl with Turner's syndrome. The risk of gonadoblastoma is as high as 25 percent in Y-bearing dysgenetic gonads. Examination of the patient's DNA with Y-specific probes is necessary. In girls with a Y fragment, ultrasound examination of the pelvis can be used to monitor gonadal size, but early prophylactic gonadectomy is strongly recommended by most endocrinologists. Selection of other laboratory tests is individualized on the basis of age and therapeutic goals. Plasma gonadotropins, especially FSH, are high in the first years of life, return to normal values until about 10 years of age, and then become elevated again. This pattern of FSH secretion has been described as diphasic. Other diagnostic studies include thyroid function tests, GH responsiveness to provocative stimuli, echocardiography, renal ultrasound, and bone age determination.

Short stature is the most constant feature of Turner's syndrome. Moderate intrauterine growth retardation is usually the rule, with birth length and weight falling below the 10th percentile for full-term infants. Birth length is reduced 2.8 cm below the mean. In the first 3 years growth rates are normal, but thereafter gradual deceleration in growth velocity occurs. Without treatment, there is no pubertal growth spurt and the epiphyses remain open, permitting a prolonged period of slow growth (Fig. 26-17). Greater retardation of leg growth is responsible for the disproportionate ratio of upper limbs to lower limbs. Skeletal maturation remains normal or slightly delayed during childhood but falls increasingly behind in adolescence unless sex steroids are administered. The cause of the growth disorder in

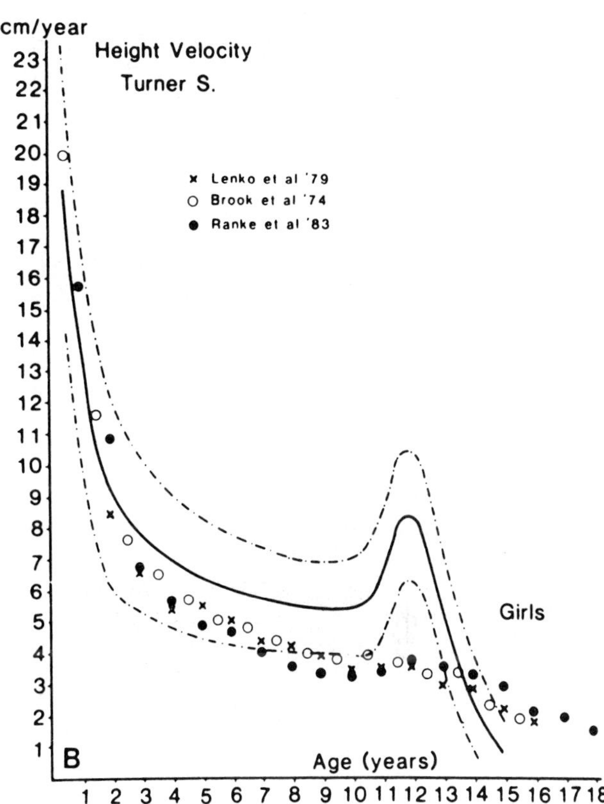

FIGURE 26-17 Depicted on the normal female height velocity curve are the mean growth velocities of untreated girls with Turner's syndrome. The data were obtained from three growth studies of patients with Turner's syndrome. Note the normal growth velocity in Turner's syndrome during the first 3 years of life, followed by declining growth rates in childhood and absence of a pubertal growth spurt in adolescence. (*From Neely and Rosenfeld*[168] *and Ranke et al.*[169])

Turner's syndrome remains unexplained. Spontaneous GH secretion and GH responses to provocative stimuli are normal in childhood, but during the pubertal years they appear to be lower than in sexually maturing adolescents who increase their GH production. Serum IGF-I levels follow a similar pattern. Deficiencies of gonadal or adrenal steroids are also not the explanation, since linear growth is preserved in children who lack these hormones and have normal chromosomes. It is possible that tissue responses to trophic stimuli are suboptimal in Turner's syndrome since decreased cell turnover has been observed in patients with aneuploidy. Also, the long-range adverse effects of intrauterine edema on growing fetal tissues are unknown.

The mean adult height of 366 girls with Turner's syndrome was 143 cm, with a range of 136 to 147 cm.[168] In 1983, Ranke and colleagues described the growth patterns of 150 untreated German girls with Turner's syndrome.[169] This information and data from three other growth studies were used by Lyon and associates to construct normative growth velocity curves for untreated girls with Turner's syndrome[170] (Fig. 26-18). They determined that a strong correlation (0.95) existed between the height centile of a girl in childhood and her final height centile on the Turner curves and that the accuracy of the prediction was not influenced by prior estrogen treatment or initial bone age. They concluded that it is possible to predict or project the adult height of a girl with Turner's syndrome and to use that information to evaluate the efficacy of current hormonal treatments.

Growth-promoting therapies for girls with Turner's syndrome currently include biosynthetic growth hormone administered alone or in combination with oxandrolone, oxandrolone alone, and low-dose estrogen therapy.[171] In a 5-year study involving 70 girls with Turner's syndrome, growth hormone treatment (0.375 mg/kg per week divided into seven doses and given daily SC) significantly increased growth velocity to means of 5 to 6 cm/year. Based on the observation that the mean height of 22 older girls was approximately 150 cm after 5 years of treatment, the authors believe that GH treatment will lead to adult heights in the range of 150 cm in most girls with Turner's syndrome. Oxandrolone administered concurrently with GH yielded even faster growth rates (7 to 10 cm/year) over a 3-year period; however, the long-range outcome is uncertain since bone maturation tended to advance more rapidly with combination therapy. Also, greater weight gains and hyperinsulinemia in the presence of euglycemia were observed in the combination treatment group. The dose of oxandrolone was initially 0.125 mg/kg per day, whereas subsequently it was lowered to 0.0625 mg/kg per day. Based on current data, the long-term impact of oxandrolone therapy when used concomitantly with GH remains uncertain in Turner's syndrome; however, it would appear that lower doses (0.05 mg/kg per day) may be efficacious and have fewer adverse effects.

The use of oxandrolone treatment *alone* for patients with Turner's syndrome has also improved growth velocity during the first 1 or 2 years of therapy. However, declining responsiveness with continued treatment has been reported in almost all studies, and final heights do not appear to exceed predicted untreated adult heights based on the Turner growth curve. Usually oxandrolone treatment is reserved for older girls (>9 to 10 years), preferably with delayed bone ages (2 years or more), because of the risk of more rapid bone maturation in young children and the declining growth responses over time.

The use of low-dose estrogen treatment to promote growth acceleration in patients with Turner's syndrome is controversial. Ethinyl estradiol has been administered in doses ranging from 25 to 125 ng/kg per day. When given alone, ethinyl estradiol treatment (100 ng/kg per day) has yielded short-term modest improvements in growth velocity followed by declining responsiveness. Potentially adverse effects on bone maturation and final height have been observed. Lower doses (25 to 50 ng/kg per day) do not improve growth velocity. When it is given in combination with GH, the growth response is not greater than the response to GH alone. When used for growth promotion, ethinyl estradiol should be reserved for girls who are older than 11 years since breast budding has been observed in young girls who were given doses as low as 25 ng/kg per day.

Replacement therapy with estrogen and progesterone for breast development and menstruation is usually started between ages 12 and 14 years. It is usual practice to start with a low dose of daily estrogen (Premarin 0.3 to 0.6 mg) for 6 to 9 months, after which cyclic treatment is begun with a combination of estrogen and progesterone. A frequently prescribed regimen consists of Premarin 0.6 to 1.25 mg per day PO for 24 days each month and medroxyprogesterone 5 to 10 mg/day PO on the last 10 days of estrogen treatment. Usually the dose of estrogen is low at the beginning and is increased gradually to promote breast growth. On rare occasions, breast development is poor because of possible injury to the

FIGURE 26-18 The mean heights of untreated girls with Turner's syndrome are placed on the normal female growth curve. The data were derived from four European studies.[169] Note the progressive decline in growth velocity during childhood and the absence of a pubertal growth spurt. (*From Lyon et al.*[170]) Growth curves based on these studies are used to project adult height of girls with Turner's syndrome and to estimate the effect of various therapies on final height.

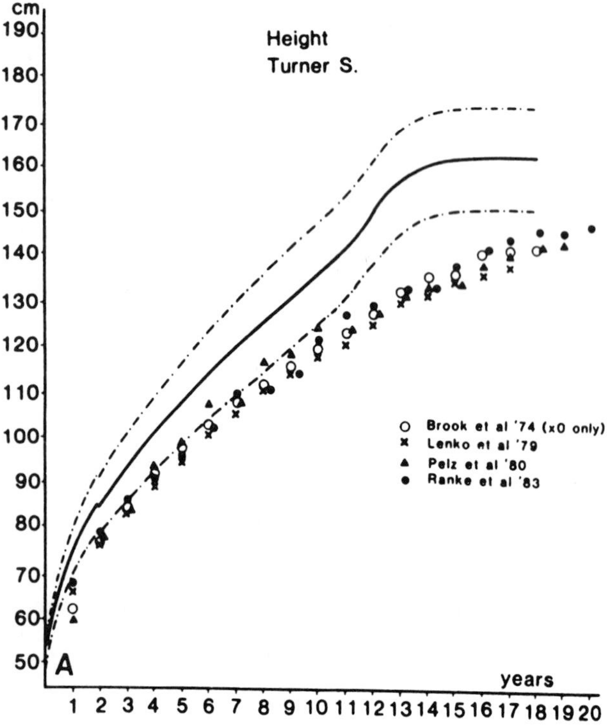

breast primordium in utero. In such patients, the option of undergoing breast augmentation in late adolescence can be reviewed.

Sex education should be started at age 8 years. These girls need to be told that a majority of individuals with Turner's syndrome have underdeveloped ovaries and that they will need hormone therapy for breast development and menstruation. Also, information about adoption and in vitro fertilization procedures with a donor egg should be provided. In the rare patient with functioning ovaries, genetic transmission is possible and genetic counseling is advisable.

Many of the phenotypic abnormalities which characterize Turner's syndrome are present also in Noonan's syndrome, a familial growth disorder with an autosomal dominant mode of inheritance.[172] Approximately 70 percent of males with Noonan's syndrome have cryptorchism and hypogonadism, whereas gonadal function tends to be normal in affected females; hence, transmission usually occurs through the affected female. The cardiovascular defects include pulmonary stenosis, peripheral branch stenosis, and asymmetric septal hypertrophy. In contrast, the cardiovascular lesions of Turner's syndrome are extracardiac, mainly coarctation of the aorta or renal arteries. The main features of Noonan's syndrome are short stature; triangular facies with micrognathia; prominent, low-set ears; hypertelorism; ptosis; epicanthal folds; antimongoloid slant of eyes; low posterior hairline; pterygium colli; shield-shaped chest with hypoplastic, widely spaced nipples; cubitus valgus; lymphedema of the dorsum of hands and feet; clinodactylism; scoliosis; kyphosis; pectus excavatum (funnel chest); pigmented nevi; dystrophic nails; and a tendency to keloid formation. The karyotype is normal in affected individuals. Varied incidences of mental retardation have been reported. Genetic counseling is essential because this is a heritable growth disorder.

Environmental Deprivation Syndrome (Psychosocial Dwarfism and Emotional, Maternal, and Parental Deprivation Syndromes)

Environmental deprivation syndrome is a growth disorder which occurs in young infants and children from infancy to early childhood whose family life is filled with turmoil. Usually, one child exhibits "psychosocial dwarfism" and the others are not affected. Previous studies implicated disturbed mother-child interaction, but the problem may result from conflict between the child and either or both parents or be due to entire family pathology. The importance of emotional stress vs. malnutrition in a particular child with deprivation syndrome is not readily evident from the history. These children are said to have large appetites, and their eating behavior is abnormal; e.g., they may have pica, eat from garbage cans or the toilet bowl, or eat animal food. Foul, bulky stools may occur. Restless sleep patterns have been described. These children are developmentally delayed and frequently display temper tantrums. The physical features resemble those seen in hypopituitarism; a fraction of these patients actually have laboratory evidence of GH, TSH, and ACTH deficiencies. In addition, they exhibit abdominal protuberance, body hypertrichosis, and sparse scalp hair, all signs of long-standing malnutrition.[154–157]

The management of these children consists of placing them in a happy environment and providing optimal nutrition; improvement in growth and behavior may then be observed. Usually, this can be achieved with hospitalization, but the child should be protected from infection, and diagnostic studies should be avoided or postponed in order to minimize stress during this recuperative period. Blood count, serum T_4 determination, biochemical profile, and urinalysis are usually adequate at the start. The behavioral changes in the child should be recorded along with the daily caloric intake and changes in stool character. At the outset, a psychologist or health worker should follow the child and work with the parents. If the child is sent home, home visits should be regularly carried out and the growth progress of the child should be monitored every 1 to 2 months. If weight loss or lack of progress in growth is observed, attempts should be made to move the child to a secure and supportive foster home.

Anoxemia

Optimal cellular growth requires an adequate supply of oxygen. Poor linear growth, weight gain, and delayed adolescence are frequently seen in patients who have severe anoxemia due to chronic pulmonary disorders (cystic fibrosis of pancreas), cardiovascular deficits (right-to-left shunts), or red blood cell diseases (hemoglobinopathies, sickle cell or Cooley's anemia, aplastic anemia, etc.). Marked improvement in growth has resulted from prolonged transfusion programs aimed at correcting anemia in children with sickle cell disease or Cooley's anemia. Unfortunately, the risk of hemosiderosis due to iron overload limits the length of time during which transfusion programs can be used at present.

GROWTH EXCESS

The normal and abnormal causes of excessive growth during childhood and adolescence are listed in Table 26-10.

Normal Variants

Familial, Genetic, or Constitutional Tall Stature

Healthy girls and boys with extremely tall predicted adult height may seek medical help to slow or

TABLE 26-10 Causes of Growth Excess in Childhood and Adolescence

Normal variants
- Familial, genetic, or constitutional tall stature
- Familial early maturation
- Abnormal overgrowth
- Endocrine causes
  - Congenital virilizing hyperplasia
  - Precocious sexual maturation (puberty, etc.)
  - Acromegaly
  - Hyperthyroidism
- Chromosome abnormalities
  - XYY
  - XXY Klinefelter's syndrome
- Tumor: granulosa cell tumor of ovary, interstitial cell tumor of testis
- Miscellaneous
  - Marfan syndrome
  - Homocystinuria
  - Cerebral gigantism (Sotos' syndrome)
  - Obesity
  - Beckwith-Wiedemann syndrome
  - Infant of diabetic mother
  - Gigantism and lipodystrophy

arrest linear growth. The only treatment available at present is sex steroids. This presents a dilemma for the physician, who must decide whether the risks of treatment with high-dose estrogens or androgens are greater or lesser than the psychosocial trauma of very tall stature. These hormones can suppress the hypothalamic-pituitary-gonadal axis and have carcinogenic potential. In addition, there is always the possibility of error in height prediction. Some children show extremely rapid rates of sexual maturation and may have adult heights which are shorter than predicted. Despite these shortcomings, useful information can be obtained from the patient's growth curve and from estimations of bone age and adult height.

The indications for treating genetic tall stature in healthy girls [predicted height > 183 cm (6 ft)] are psychosocial only. Treatment is nonphysiologic and should be undertaken only after careful estimation of predicted final height and evaluation of the physical and mental health of the patient. Girls exposed to stilbestrol during fetal life must not be placed at risk with pharmacologic doses of sex steroids. Mean height reduction is 6 cm if treatment is begun when the chronologic and bone ages are less than 13 years; the earlier treatment is begun, the greater is the curtailment of predicted adult stature. Treatment schedules vary considerably; ethinyl estradiol, 0.15 to 0.3 mg/day continuously, and 10 mg of medroxyprogesterone or 5 mg of norethindrone on the first 7 to 10 days of each calendar month are examples. Curtailment of adult height is due to estrogen-mediated reduction of somatomedin concentration and growth velocity coupled with acceleration of bone maturation. Hormone therapy is usually prescribed for 18 months to 2 years and is discontinued after linear growth has ceased for three consecutive monthly measurements. Careful follow-up of these patients includes menstrual history and determination of reproductive capacity and changes in vaginal cytology. If a young woman is postmenarchal and has a bone age of 14 years, estrogen treatment provides negligible benefits and should not be used.[173]

Similarly, in tall boys whose predicted adult height is 195 to 200 cm (approximately 6 ft 6 in.), testosterone treatment (500 mg per square meter of body surface of long-acting testosterone per month IM given at 2- to 3-week intervals) reduces estimated adult stature by about 8 cm if the starting bone age is 12 to 14 years. At a later bone age, the benefits of treatment are insufficient to justify the risks. Normal testicular function has been reported in a series of 29 boys after cessation of treatment.[174]

In summary, reduction in adult height can be accomplished only if pharmacologic doses of sex hormones are used to promote early adolescence and rapid maturation of bone age. Physicians who prescribe these steroids must advise parents that the long-term effects on patients and their offspring are unknown.

Familial Early Maturation

Children with familial early maturation are different from patients with genetic tall stature because they grow physically and biologically at a rapid pace during childhood and achieve adolescence and adult height at the earliest limits of normal. During childhood, they are tall and look more mature than their chronologic age; unfortunately, they are expected to behave accordingly. Their bone age and height age are proportionately advanced ahead of their chronologic age. Usually their parents are of average height, and there is a family history of early development. The predicted adult height is compatible with parental height, and medical therapy is not needed. Psychological support and sex education should be offered to these children and their families to help them understand and accept the psychosocial stresses which accompany early development.

Pathologic Overgrowth

Congenital Virilizing Adrenal Hyperplasia

CAH is an inherited disorder of adrenal steroidogenesis. The most common form of the disease is due to a deficiency of the enzyme 21-hydroxylase with or without salt loss. Molecular genetic studies have identified two structural genes that code for the microsomal P_{450} enzyme involved in 21-hydroxylation (P_{450}-C_{21}). Less common defects are deficiencies of 11β-hydroxylase or 3β-hydroxysteroid dehydrogenase. In patients with deficient cortisol synthesis there is overproduction of ACTH, adrenal cortical hyperplasia, and excessive production of intermediary steroid metabolites with androgenic activity. In the rare patients with 17α-hydroxylase deficiency, gonadal and adrenal sex steroids cannot be synthesized; thus, genetic males have a female phenotype and genetic females do not become sexually mature. The disease follows an autosomal recessive pattern of inheritance[175] (see Chap. 12).

Exposure of the female fetus to excessive amounts of adrenal androgens results in varying degrees of masculinization of the external genitalia, manifested by labioscrotal fusion, a urogenital sinus, and clitoral hypertrophy. The vaginal orifice and urinary meatus frequently are located within the perineal opening of the urogenital sinus. Since müllerian duct development is not suppressed by excesses of adrenal androgen, the fallopian tubes, uterus, and upper vagina are normal, as are the ovaries.

The external genitalia of the male fetus are not affected significantly by the overproduction of adrenal androgens and are structurally normal, but scrotal hyperpigmentation may be present. There are exceptions: In boys born with 3β-hydroxysteroid dehydrogenase deficiency, synthesis of fetal testicular hormones is defective; they cannot achieve full virilization of the external genitalia. XY male pseudohermaphrodites with a 17α-hydroxylase deficiency totally lack sex steroid production and are hypertensive, phenotypic females with no müllerian structures.

Females with non-salt-losing CAH usually are diagnosed and treated in the newborn period because of their genital abnormalities. Failure to make an early diagnosis and provide cortisone therapy results in excessive androgen production, which causes heterosexual precocious development with masculinization and clitoromegaly. The problem is often not suspected in boys with the non-salt-losing form of the disease until several years have passed because their genitalia are normal at birth. By then, the continued overproduction of androgens has caused acceleration in the rate of somatic growth, accompanied by even more rapid osseous maturation, virilization with acne, deepening of the voice, increased musculature, growth of sexual hair, and enlargement of the penis. The testes usually remain prepubertal in size, however, because of the absence of gonadotropin stimulation.

Both males and females with the salt-losing variety of CAH have a normal early neonatal course but after 7 days of age are at risk for developing vomiting, diarrhea, severe dehydration, and shock, with the clinical and biochemical features of classic addisonian crisis. Patients with the 11β-hydroxylase defect develop hypertension as a result of overproduction of deoxycorticosterone.

A nonclassical or late-onset form of adrenal hyperplasia due to 21-hydroxylase deficiency has been identified. It is inherited by an autosomal recessive mode of transmission. The clinical manifestations include virilization in late childhood or adolescence and even postpubertally. Initially, the presentation in childhood resembles premature pubarche, while in adolescent or adult females the picture resembles that of polycystic ovarian disease. At birth, affected females have normal external genitalia. During the adolescent years, affected girls are likely to develop hirsutism, severe acne, menstrual irregularities, and later infertility. The diagnosis is confirmed by elevated 17-hydroxyprogesterone (17-OHP) levels before and after ACTH stimulation. Low-dose glucocorticoid therapy is necessary to correct the hyperandrogenic state and restore normal menstrual cycles.

Diagnosis

The biochemical abnormalities in CAH are determined by the position of the deficient enzyme in the biosynthetic pathways involving cortisol, aldosterone, and androgen production. In the newborn period, elevated serum 17-OHP and Δ^4-androstenedione in the presence of reduced serum cortisol levels are diagnostic of classic CAH due to a deficiency of 21-hydroxylase enzyme. Increased serum testosterone is present in genetic females, but the level may not reach diagnostic significance in genetic males. Urine 17-ketosteroid and pregnanetriol measurements are used less frequently now because serum assays are more practical. Hyponatremia, hyperkalemia, metabolic acidosis, and high plasma renin levels are indicators of mineralocorticoid deficiency. Plasma renin measurements are helpful in screening for hypovolemia due to subtle defects in aldosterone biosynthesis. In different forms of CAH, the hormone profiles needed for diagnosis vary with the enzyme abnormality.

Newborn screening for 21-hydroxylase deficiency has been carried out in selected geographic areas using RIA measurement of 17-OHP concentrations in a drop of blood deposited on microfilter paper.[176] When the diagnosis of classic CAH is made by means of neonatal screening, the incidence of affected males is equal to that of females; a majority (75 percent) are salt wasters. When the diagnosis is made by case detection, females outnumber males; this observation indicates that many males die undiagnosed in infancy. The incidence worldwide varies from 1 in 5000 to 1 in 15,000. The Yupik Eskimos in Alaska have the highest frequency, approximately 1 in 500.

Prenatal diagnosis of CAH can be made as early as 8 to 11 weeks gestation using chorionic villus tissue for HLA typing by standard means or molecular genetics techniques. Later in gestation, prenatal diagnosis is made by HLA genotyping of amniocytes and measurement of amniotic fluid 17-OHP and Δ^4-androstenedione levels.

Prenatal treatment with dexamethasone, 0.5 mg tid, should be initiated as soon as pregnancy is diagnosed in a woman at risk of transmitting CAH to her offspring. After the diagnostic studies are completed, treatment can be discontinued if the fetus is a male or an unaffected female. This treatment has prevented or lessened the masculinization of the external genitalia in affected female infants. The maximum daily dose of dexamethasone should not exceed 20 μg/kg of maternal prepregnancy weight per day. To date, no fetus exposed to dexamethasone has died or has developed cleft palate or placental degeneration; however, the sample size is very small, and further assessment is essential.[177]

Treatment

The treatment of CAH involves the replacement of deficient hormones. Children with 21-OH deficiency and salt wasting require hydrocortisone and mineralocorticoid therapy. Although aldosterone deficiency is not obvious in the simple form of 21-OH deficiency, many of these children have elevated plasma renin levels which respond favorably to 9α-fludrocortisone treatment. Combined hormone treatment frequently makes it possible to reduce the glucocorticoid dose which improves linear growth; androgen levels also fall on this regimen. The daily dose of oral hydrocortisone now used (12 to 15 mg/m^2 in two or three divided doses) is lower than the one previously administered. During stress, the glucocorticoid dose must be increased. Mineralocorticoid therapy consists of 9α-fludrocortisone 0.15 to 0.2 mg/day in infancy and 0.05 to 0.1 mg/day in childhood. Blood pressure is monitored at each visit. Longer-acting glucocorticoid preparations are avoided because they slow linear growth.

Measurement of serum 17-OHP, Δ^4-androstenedione, testosterone, and plasma renin are performed at approximately 3- to 4-month intervals to monitor biochemical control and compliance. Linear growth, bone maturation, and pubertal development are also regularly assessed, since this clinical information and the biochemical monitors form the basis for decisions concerning adjustments in medication.

A sodium supplement (2 to 4 g/day of sodium chloride) is frequently provided to salt wasters in the first 6 to 12 months of life. In early childhood, the risk of hypoglycemia is significant during periods of severe illness and curtailed food intake. Intravenous therapy with glucose containing electrolyte solution (5 to 10% in half-normal saline) will protect these children from developing hypoglycemia. Within the first 6 months of life, the clitoris is usually recessed and the vaginal orifice is exteriorized. Additional reconstructive surgery may be needed in adolescence if the size of the vaginal orifice cannot be adequately enlarged by means of dilators.

Psychological support, sex education, and personalized medical care in an atmosphere of privacy are essential to the emotional well-being of young women with CAH.

Precocious Sexual Maturation

A classification of the causes of sexual precocity is given in Table 26-11. True or pituitary gonadotropin–dependent precocious puberty is defined as activation of the hypothalamic-pituitary-gonadal axis at an abnormally early age. In girls, breast enlargement, sexual hair, accelerated rates of linear growth, and menstruation before age 8 years are seen. Boys with precocious puberty exhibit progessive enlargement of the testes and penis, development of sexual hair, and growth spurt before age 10 years. Early onset of acne is common. Precocious puberty occurs more frequently in girls than in boys. Seventy-five percent of these females have no identifiable organic lesion; they are classified as having idiopathic or constitutional precocious puberty. The long-range

TABLE 26-11 Classification of Precocious Sexual Maturation

- True precocious puberty (pituitary gonadotropin–dependent)
  - Complete
    - Idiopathic
      - Sporadic (more common in females)
      - Familial
        - Autosomal recessive
        - Autosomal dominant (males)
    - Organic lesions of the hypothalamic-pituitary region
      - Congenital: hydrocephalus, cysts
      - Acquired
        - Tumors: pinealoma, glioma, hamartoma, teratoma, ependymoma, chorioepithelioma
        - Trauma
        - Inflammation: meningitis, encephalitis
        - Hydrocephalus
      - Associated with other conditions
        - Neurofibromatosis
        - McCune-Albright syndrome
        - Primary hypothyroidism
  - Incomplete
    - Premature thelarche
    - Premature adrenarche (pubarche)
    - Premature menarche
- Precocious pseudopuberty (pituitary gonadotropin–independent)
  - Isosexual
    - Ectopic gonadotropin production: hepatoblastoma, choriocarcinoma, dysgerminoma
    - Ovarian tumors, testicular tumors
    - Boys with non-salt-losing congenital adrenal hyperplasia or virilizing tumors
    - McCune-Albright syndrome
    - Iatrogenic
    - Primary Leydig cell hyperplasia (testitoxicosis)
  - Heterosexual
    - Girls with congenital adrenal hyperplasia, adrenal virilizing tumors, ovarian virilizing tumors
    - Boys with feminizing tumors (adrenal or testicular), gynecomastia
    - Iatrogenic

prognosis for health is good; fertility and age of menopause are normal. The major physical abnormality is eventual short stature. The prognosis for adult height is especially poor if precocious puberty begins in the first years of life and if bone age advances rapidly without compensatory gains in height.

In contrast to girls, boys are at greater risk of having a space-occupying lesion (over 50 percent of boys in some series are thus affected). Careful neuroradiologic and endocrine evaluation is required to rule out CNS tumors, especially in boys. The most common CNS tumors are hamartomas, teratomas, ependymomas, and, less frequently, optic gliomas, astrocytomas, chorioepitheliomas, and neurofibromas. These tumors tend to be located in the posterior hypothalamus, pineal gland, median eminence, or floor of the third ventricle. Conditions which may be associated with true precocious puberty include prenatal anoxia, microcephaly, hydrocephalus, head trauma, CNS infections, severe primary hypothyroidism, poorly controlled CAH, and, rarely, McCune-Albright syndrome. Precocious puberty also may be transmitted by either autosomal recessive or autosomal dominant inheritance; the latter occurs only in males and may be transmitted by an affected father or an unaffected mother.[79]

Incomplete or partial precocious puberty is the early appearance of one of the characteristics of complete puberty, e.g., isolated breast development (premature thelarche), isolated sexual hair growth (premature pubarche or adrenarche), or isolated premature menarche.

Premature thelarche is seen only in girls, usually is bilateral, and is not accompanied by estrogenization of the vaginal mucosa, growth of pubic or axillary hair, or acceleration of linear growth or bone maturation. Most commonly, it presents in the second year of life, persists for a variable period, and regresses within 2 years. Subsequently, puberty occurs at the appropriate age in a majority of cases. These children and their families need reassurance and psychological support; medications should be avoided. Careful follow-up every 6 months by a single observer is advisable because early breast development may be the first sign of complete puberty. When this occurs, the child will exhibit progressive changes, including appearance of sexual hair and rapid linear growth. Premature thelarche is presumed to result from a transient elevation of gonadotropin concentrations; however, its precise etiology is unknown.

Premature adrenarche (or pubarche) is the isolated early appearance of sexual hair. Pubic hair alone may appear (pubarche), or hair in both the pubic and axillary areas may appear. It occurs more frequently in healthy girls than in boys and also is seen with severe CNS dysfunction. Increased production of adrenal androgens (e.g., DHEA, DHEA sulfate) from the zona reticularis has been reported in these children. Linear growth and bone maturation may accelerate slightly in some children; however, these patients never exhibit the features of intense androgen stimulation. In affected children, height age and hormone levels (plasma DHEA sulfate, testosterone, 17-hydroxyprogesterone, urinary 17-ketosteroids) are appropriate for bone age. Management consists of reassurance and psychological support. Careful follow-up examinations every 4 to 6 months are advisable because premature pubarche may be the first sign of precocious puberty, androgen-producing tumors, or adrenal dysfunction (late-onset congenital adrenal hyperplasia).

Isolated premature menarche presents as vaginal spotting or frank menstruation without other signs of sexual maturation. The phenomenon is poorly understood. It is more frequently seen in children with McCune-Albright syndrome and may precede the appearance of the bony lesions. An ultrasound examination of the pelvis may document the presence of an ovarian cyst.

Precocious pseudopuberty, or pituitary gonadotropin–independent precocity, is characterized by sexual maturation due to autonomous production of sex steroids (ovarian, testicular, or adrenal hormones) or to ectopic gonadotropin-like hormones (e.g., hCG). The hypothalamic-pituitary axis is suppressed; LH and FSH measured by RIA are in the prepubertal range and have a negligible response to GnRH stimulation. In patients who have ectopic production of hCG, care must be taken to use specific antisera which distinguish hCG from LH; the antisera used in routine RIAs cross-react with hCG and give falsely elevated levels of LH.

In girls, the ovarian lesions include granulosa cell tumors, thecal lipoid tumors, and functional ovarian cysts. The mass is frequently palpable by abdominal and rectal examination and is readily confirmed by pelvic ultrasound or CT. In boys with autonomously functioning testicular tumors (embryonal testicular carcinomas) or ectopic tumors that secrete androgens or hCG (dysgerminomas, hepatoblastomas), the clinical picture mimics true puberty. Testicular tumors usually cause unilateral testicular enlargement. Boys with untreated or poorly managed CAH exhibit sexual precocity; their testes remain prepubertal in size, in contrast to the generous testicular volumes observed in boys with true puberty.

Precocious pseudopuberty is also observed in a majority of girls who have McCune-Albright syndrome, a poorly understood disease which is characterized by many large areas of skin hyperpigmentation (café au lait spots), bony lesions (polyostotic fibrous dysplasia), and sexual precocity.[178] The disease is sporadic and occurs predominantly in females. Gonadotropin production is suppressed in a majority of these patients, who usually have autonomously functioning ovarian follicular cysts. Rarely, a child with McCune-Albright syndrome may present with isolated menses before the appearance of skin or bone lesions. Abnormalities involving the thyroid gland (autonomous multinodular goiter), pituitary (acromegaly, hyperprolactinemia), and adrenal gland (non-ACTH-dependent Cushing's syndrome) are part of the syndrome. The variable presentation of patients with McCune-Albright syndrome requires that this diagnosis be considered in all children with atypical sexual precocity and that careful physical examinations, cranial and skeletal x-rays, and endocrine diagnostic tests be repeated at regular intervals. A unique syndrome of precocious pseudopuberty has been described in males with gonadotropin-independent familial primary Leydig cell hyperplasia (testitoxicosis). It appears to be inherited by an autosomal dominant mode of transmission. GnRH analog therapy fails to suppress testosterone hypersecretion in these boys; greater androgen suppression and clinical improvement were noted with ketoconazole therapy.[178] However, prolonged treatment with ketoconazole has been associated with an escape phenomenon characterized by increased LH and FSH levels and pubertal LH responses to exogenous GnRH. When this occurred, combined treatment with GnRH analog and ketoconazole was effective in suppressing gonadotropin and testosterone production. Testolactone and spironolactone have also been efficacious in treating this disorder.[179]

Children who exhibit precocious sexual maturation which is not compatible with their phenotype are said to have *heterosexual precocity*. Examples include girls who are masculinized because of CAH (noncompliance or untreated non-salt losers) or androgen-producing tumors; feminizing tumors may similarly cause heterosexual precocity in boys. Heterosexual precocity is pathologic and requires immediate investigation and treatment.

The diagnostic approach to precocious puberty should be individualized. In general, a personal and family history should be obtained for each patient, with previous and current growth data; each child should undergo ophthalmologic examination, complete physical examination, bone age determination, and (in females) vaginal cytology for maturation index. The diagnosis of central precocious puberty is confirmed by documentation of exaggerated gonadotropin responses to exogenous GnRH stimulation and increased frequency and amplitude of spontaneous secretory gonadotropin pulses. In select patients it is necessary to obtain a 24-h urine collection for FSH, LH, hCG, 17-ketosteroids, and pregnanetriol determinations and measure the serum concentrations of FSH, LH, hCG, alpha-fetoprotein, prolactin, testosterone, estradiol, and 17-hydroxyprogesterone. MRI or CT scans of the head, abdomen, and pelvis are indicated if a tumor in one of these areas is suspected. Pelvic and/or abdominal ultrasound examination aids in the detection of cysts or tumors in abdominal or pelvic organs. The extent of the diagnostic evaluation depends on the nature of the clinical problem. For example, a 3-year-old girl with a 1-year history of isolated, nonprogressive breast enlargement probably needs minimal testing, e.g., bone age determination and vaginal cytology for maturation index. The same holds true for an 8-year-old girl with a 6-month history of breast enlargement, growth of sexual hair, and accelerated linear growth. However, patients with rapid appearance of complete puberty in the first years of life should have a thorough endocrine and radiologic evaluation, especially boys. The diagnosis of idiopathic constitutional precocious puberty can be made only after a thorough evaluation has excluded the presence of organic disease.

The treatment of precocious sexual maturation depends on the etiology of the disorder. Surgery with or without radiation and chemotherapy may be required if a tumor is found. Precocious thelarche or adrenarche does not require treatment. The aims of treatment for idiopathic precocious puberty are suppression of sexual maturation (in girls: regression of breast size, cessation of menses, return to normal rate of linear growth and bone maturation; in boys: cessation of erections, curtailment of phallic growth, reduction of testicular volume, return to normal rate of linear growth and bone maturation).

Currently, the GnRH agonists are the agents most widely used to suppress gonadotropin production.[180,181] The increased potency and duration of action of the GnRH agonists have resulted from chemical alteration of the sequence of amino acids in the native decapeptide, GnRH. Prolonged exposure to the agonists down regulates the GnRH receptors on pituitary gonadotrophs, leading to decreased LH and FSH secretion. Permission to use these agents in patients with precocious puberty is awaiting FDA approval. Thus, agonist therapy is currently available through informed consent protocols or the off-label use of agents such as leuprolide which have become available in pharmacies for the treatment of prostatic cancer. A depot preparation, leuprolide acetate, at a dose of 0.3 mg/kg per dose to a maximum of 7.5 mg injected intramuscularly every 4 weeks, is being used by many endocrinologists who formerly used daily subcutaneously administered GnRH agonists. The efficiency of the GnRH agonist depends on the use of a treatment dose which fully suppresses gonadotropin production. Serum gonadotropin and sex steroid levels as well as LH responses to GnRH stimulation should return to the prepubertal range within 1 month of the initial depot injection. Clinically, the treatments lead to regression of breast size in girls and of testis volume of boys along with reduction of the growth rate and bone maturation. Final heights are still not available for a large number of children; however, it would appear that predicted adult height in many has been increased over the pretreatment height estimate. Approximately one-quarter of patients receiving GnRH agonist therapy grow at a pathologically slow rate, prompting concern that the predicted height gains may not be attained in some subjects. Apart from an occasional skin reaction and a single report of an anaphylactic reaction, the GnRH agonists appear to provide a relatively safe means of achieving reversible suppression of gonadotropin production. However, the long-range safety of these agents has not been proved conclusively.

Prior to the availability of GnRH analogues, the most widely used treatment for precocious puberty was medroxyprogesterone acetate; 100 to 300 mg is given IM every 2 weeks. Medroxyprogesterone acetate administration usually suppresses menstruation and curtails breast growth. However, its effects on linear growth, bone maturation, and adult height are variable and controversial.

Outside of the United States, cyproterone acetate (70 to 150 mg per square meter of body surface per day PO) has been widely used as treatment for precocious puberty. In children whose bone age was less than 11 years, the drug reduced both growth velocity and the rate of osseous maturation. Among the potential side effects of medroxyprogesterone and cyproterone acetate is mild adrenal suppression. The long-term effects of these agents have also not been carefully evaluated.

Children with precocious puberty need supportive counseling and sex education in order to adjust to the extra demands encountered because of their mature appearance. The emotional and social development of these children has been reported to be between the chronologic age and the physical age, depending on the patient's range of experience. Their emotional adjustment is generally satisfactory, and their verbal IQs are higher than their performance IQs, which tend to be average.[182]

Acromegaly and Gigantism

Gigantism in childhood is a rare disease which is characterized by rapid linear growth in the presence of normal rates of osseous maturation. Therefore, the patient is at risk for extraordinarily tall stature in adulthood (7 ft or more).[183] Acromegalic features usually accompany the excessive growth velocity. Extremely large hands and feet, overgrowth of the mandible and supraorbital ridges, coarse facies, splanchnomegaly, joint discomfort, and weakness are common features. Radiologic examination of the skull may reveal thick calvaria, enlargement of the sella with erosion, and increased size of the sinuses. Cortical thickening of bones with tufting of the terminal phalanges and overgrowth of soft tissues are additional characteristic radiologic findings. Longstanding active acromegaly may cause diabetes mellitus and cardiac decompensation. In most patients, excessive GH secretion can be demonstrated. Fasting GH levels may be elevated and nonsuppressible, or GH concentration may paradoxically increase during a glucose tolerance test. However, deficiencies of other pituitary hormones may result from intrasellar pressure from the tumor. In rare cases, all the clinical features of acromegaly are present and the GH concentration is normal or low. The IGF-I concentration is elevated in active acromegaly. The usual lesion is a GH-secreting pituitary adenoma or, less commonly, somatotroph hyperplasia. Rare causes include pancreatic malignancies which produce ectopic GHRH or ectopic GH.[184] Treatment consists mainly of surgical removal of the tumor; radiation and/or chemotherapy may also be necessary. Pharmacologic doses of estrogen are palliative; newer agents, such as the somatostatin analog octreotide, have proved useful.[185]

Hyperthyroidism

Hyperthyroidism during fetal life and in early childhood causes acceleration in linear growth and osseous maturation. Early closure of the fontanels and craniosynostosis have been reported in young infants. However, hyperthyroidism in late childhood is not likely to compromise adult stature because there is proportional advancement of height and osseous maturation, which return to normal after therapy has been initiated.[186]

Chromosome Abnormalities

XYY Genotype

The distinguishing feature of adult males with XYY syndrome is their tendency to have tall stature which is not caused by overproduction of androgens. Chromosome analysis confirms the diagnosis; endocrine testing and therapy usually are not needed. Surprisingly, during childhood, boys with XYY genotype are not taller than their XY peers.[187] A large-scale prospective study of growth in XYY males is needed to clarify the true incidence of excessive height and the growth characteristics of asymptomatic patients. A recent evaluation of XYY males in a general population has shown that they are not more aggressive than height-matched XY males although, as a group, they have significantly lower mean intelligence scores; the increased crime rate previously reported for the XYY population was mainly accounted for by property offenses rather than acts of violence. Criminal behavior by this group correlates only with low intelligence and not with height or an inherent tendency toward overaggressiveness. A similar explanation has been offered for the increased frequency of XYY individuals in penal mental institutions. Psychological support and career counseling should be offered to these patients.

Klinefelter's Syndrome

The XXY genotype is associated with tall stature, eunuchoid appearance, and arm span greater than height. Gynecomastia during the adolescent and adult years often is present. If Leydig cell function is intact, phallic size is normal. However, in patients with a deficiency of testosterone, penile growth is inadequate. The testes are small because of tubular dysgenesis, and facial and body hair are sparse. Infertility is almost always present. Confirmation of the diagnosis depends on chromosome analysis. Elevated plasma and urinary concentrations of the gonadotropins and low to normal levels of plasma testosterone are characteristic. During adolescence, especially after age 14, boys with high gonadotropin and low plasma testosterone levels should receive long-acting testosterone preparations (testosterone enanthate or testosterone 17β-cypionate, 200 to 400 mg/month, given at 2- or 4-week intervals) to increase penis size, sexual hair growth, and muscle mass and to enhance psychosocial well-being. Androgen treatment for emotionally disturbed patients with personality disorders should be undertaken only if approved by the patient's psychotherapist and under close supervision.

In the general population, young men with the XXY genotype have mean intelligence scores which are substantially lower than those of height-matched XY controls. The increased frequency of XXY males in penal mental institutions is attributable to psychosocial pathology which correlates with low intelligence in specific patients, not to a genotypic or height-determined tendency toward criminality or overaggressiveness in the group as a whole.[188]

Miscellaneous Syndromes

Marfan Syndrome and Homocystinuria

The tall, slender stature which characterizes both Marfan syndrome and the homocystinuria syndrome is associated with a generalized disease of connective tissue which involves the eye, cardiovascular system, and skeletal system. The etiology of Marfan syndrome is unknown, but a defect in mucopolysaccharide metabolism is suspected. The genetic defect has been mapped to the long arm of chromosome 15, but the specific gene has not been identified. A deficiency of fibrillin in skin sections from Marfan patients was recently demonstrated. In homocystinuria, the enzyme activity of cystathionine synthetase is decreased, causing an accumulation of homocystine and methionine and a deficiency of cystathionine and cystine. Mental retardation is present in more than 50 percent of patients with homocystinuria, whereas normal intelligence is characteristic of patients with Marfan syndrome. The similarities and differences of these two phenotypically similar diseases are listed in Table 26-12.

Skovby and McKusick[189] have reported impressive benefits from the use of conjugated estrogens (Premarin 10 mg/day) or ethinyl estradiol 0.15 mg/day in young girls with Marfan syndrome age 4½ to 9½ years. The final height ranged from 156 to 165 cm, a reduction of 12.5 to 17 cm of predicted height. Treatment lasted from 33 to 78 months and was not discontinued until bone age was 16 and growth had ceased for 12 months. There was no benefit of estrogen treatment in girls with Marfan syndrome after spontaneous menarche had occurred. The authors concluded that estrogen treatment must be started before or early in the growth spurt, preferably when the bone age is less than 10 years.

Cerebral Gigantism (Sotos' Syndrome)

Children with Sotos's syndrome are large from birth and have accelerated osseous maturation. The most common findings are gigantism, prominent

TABLE 26-12 Comparison of Marfan Syndrome with Homocystinuria

	Marfan Syndrome	Homocystinuria
Intelligence	Normal	60% of patients retarded
Skeletal	Tall, slender stature	Tall, slender stature
	Long limbs, arachnodactyly	Osteoporosis, collapsed vertebrae
	Span > height	Scoliosis (variably present)
	Scoliosis, kyphosis	Pectus excavatum or carinatum
	Pectus excavatum or carinatum	Increased fractures
	Hypotonic muscles	
Joints	Hyperextensible	Asymmetric spasticity (variable)
Eye	Lens subluxation—upward	Lens subluxation—downward
	Myopia, blue sclerae	Myopia, occasional cataracts
		Retinal detachment (variable)
Cardiovascular	Dilation of ascending aorta with or without dissecting aneurysm	Medial degeneration of aorta
	Aortic regurgitation	Irregular inner surface of vessels due to fibrosis and hyperplasia
		Frequent thromboses
Other	Hernias	Hernias
Inheritance	Autosomal dominant	Autosomal recessive
Biochemical defect	Unknown disease of connective tissue, abnormal mucopolysaccharide metabolism(?)	Connective tissue disease due to cystathionine synthetase deficiency

forehead, hypertelorism, dolichocephalus, large hands and feet, pointed chin, poor coordination, delayed development early in infancy, and mental retardation (IQ range 18 to 119, mean 72). No chromosomal abnormalities have been found, and numerous investigations have failed to show any endocrine abnormalities (GH and somatomedin levels are normal). Compared with healthy children, glucose intolerance is more frequently found; 14 percent of affected children are glucose-intolerant. At birth, these children are large (mean weight 3400 g, 75th percentile) and long (55.2 cm, 97th percentile). Growth is most rapid in the first 3 to 4 years, followed by normal rates during childhood; stature in adulthood is variably tall. The major handicaps are intellectual retardation and emotional disorders. Genetic mechanisms, an autosomal recessive or dominant mode of inheritance, are presumed to be the cause of this syndrome.[190]

Obesity

Obese boys and girls are taller by 6 cm or more than normal-weight children of comparable age and have a larger bony frame.[191] Bone age, height age, and dental maturation are advanced during childhood. Usually, obese children reach adolescence early and are of average height as adults. Occasionally, the diagnosis of Cushing's syndrome is considered, but it can be readily disproved because these children are tall and have normal growth rates and pubertal development, features which are not seen in states of glucocorticoid excess. Psychological stress, especially in late childhood and adolescence, is the main problem of obese children; as a rule, they are otherwise healthy. Metabolic and endocrine testing may cause unnecessary concern. Glucose intolerance with elevated insulin levels may be a result of the obesity; they usually return to normal with weight reduction. Increased urinary 17-hydroxycorticosteroid excretion and poor GH responses to stimulation tests have been reported in obese subjects. Treatment consists of restricted caloric intake and vigorous physical activities. Only highly motivated patients have long-term success in controlling their weight.

Beckwith-Wiedemann Syndrome

This syndrome (omphalocele, macroglossia, and gigantism) was first recognized in 1963. Splanchnomegaly, hemihypertrophy, earlobe malformation, and port-wine nevus (nevus flammeus) may occur. Hypoglycemia has been observed in the majority of patients.[192]

Infant of a Diabetic Mother

Gigantism is a common finding in infants born of mothers with poorly controlled diabetes and in some infants born many years before a diagnosis of maternal diabetes. The excess tissue is mostly fat resulting from increased fetal adipogenesis. Hypoglycemia due to hyperinsulinism and respiratory disease are commonly found in the newborn period.

Gigantism and Lipodystrophy

Total and partial lipodystrophy have been reported in children. In addition to partial or generalized fat loss, affected individuals may have increased height, advanced bone age, hirsutism, muscle hypertrophy, abdominal protuberance, penile or clitoral enlargement, liver and renal disease, hyperglycemia, hyperlipemia, and hypermetabolism. No specific treatment is available.[193]

APPENDIX: DETAILS OF TESTING PROCEDURES IN CHILDREN

Pituitary-Hypothalamic Evaluation

Growth Hormone

Preparation of Patient

Do not evaluate GH responses to stimuli while patient is hypothyroid. Administer L-thyroxine, 3 to 4 μg per kilogram of body weight per day PO, 1 to 2 months before performing GH stimulation tests if patient is hypothyroid.
Nothing by mouth after 10 P.M.
Keep patient at rest and fasting except for water throughout test.
Insert a no. 21 butterfly needle which is kept patent by flushing with dilute heparinized saline (0.1 mL heparin added to 30 mL saline) after each sample is obtained, or use a slow saline infusion to prevent the needle from clogging.

Diagnostic Tests for GH

See Table 26-13.

Interpretation of GH Tests

Severe GH deficiency: peak GH concentration < 4 ng/mL on two of the above tests
Normal response: peak GH concentration > 10 ng/mL on any test at any time (polyclonal RIA)

Factors which Modify GH Stimulation Tests

Food (suppresses)
Obesity (suppresses)
Hypothyroidism (suppresses)
Glucocorticoids (suppress)
Puberty (enhances)
Estrogens (enhance)
Androgens (enhance)

TABLE 26-13 Diagnostic Tests for Growth Hormone

Test	Method	Comment
Insulin hypoglycemia	Give regular insulin, 0.05–0.1 U/kg IV; glucose nadir <40 mg/dL at 20–30 min; take samples at −15,0,+15,30, 45,60,90,120 min	Peak GH concentration at 45–75 min; peak cortisol >15 μg/dL; required constant supervision
Arginine	L-Arginine monohydrochloride (10%), 0.5 g/kg IV over 30 min Same sampling times as for insulin	No discomfort; may cause hypoglycemia in hypopituitary children
Arginine-insulin	Same doses as in above two tests; give arginine from 0 to +30 min; give insulin at +60 min	Same precautions as insulin hypoglycemia test
Clonidine	0.075–0.15 mg/m² PO; take samples at 0, +30,45,60,90,120 min (25 μg PO also used)	Peak GH concentration at 60–90 min; somnolence and fall in blood pressure result; dose-related side effects
Levodopa	10 mg/kg PO; maximum dose = 500 mg; take samples at 0,+30,60,90,120 min; crush tablet or open capsule	Keep patient recumbent; nausea, vomiting result; peak GH concentration at 45–120 min
Propranolol	Give 0.75 mg/kg PO 30–60 min before glucagon, insulin, or arginine (20 mg for patients who weigh <20 kg; 40 mg for all others)	Do not use in asthmatic or cardiac patients; weakness, pallor, sweating, confusion result
Glucagon	Give 0.03 mg/kg IM or subcutaneously; sample times same as for insulin, plus 150 and 180 min	Nausea, vomiting result; peak GH at 45–120 min
Sleep	Take samples at 60 and 90 min after onset of deep sleep	Questionable reliability
Exercise	Have patient exercise strenuously for 20 min; take samples at 0,+20,40,60 min	Questionable reliability
Diurnal GH profile	Take samples at 20-min intervals over 24 h	Requires special staff and diagnostic unit; interpretation based on number and amplitude of GH pulses; questionable reliability

ACTH Reserve

See Table 26-14.

TSH Reserve

See Table 26-15.

FSH and LH Concentrations

The reported plasma FSH and LH concentrations in normal children and adolescents vary greatly depending on the source of the standards [Second International Reference Preparation/Human Menopausal Gonadotropin (IRP/HMG) or pituitary FSH-LH] and the definition of international unit (IU). The normal range for the laboratory performing the assay must be the basis for interpreting basal gonadotropin values in plasma or urine and for evaluating FSH and LH responses to GnRH (Figs. 26-13 and 26-14).

LH and FSH Levels: Responses to GnRH Stimulation

Mean 24-h plasma FSH and LH levels rise with increasing pubertal stage in boys and girls. Also, the output of FSH and LH in 24-h urine collections increases progressively throughout puberty (Figs. 26-13 and 26-14).

Spontaneous LH pulse amplitude also increases progressively throughout puberty, whereas FSH

TABLE 26-14 Test for ACTH Reserve

Test	Dose and Sampling Times	Comments and Results
Insulin hypoglycemia	Give insulin dose (see Table 26-13) Measure plasma cortisol concentration at 0, 30, 60, 90, and 120 min	Normal response Basal cortisol concentration = 10–25 μg/dL Peak concentration > 15 μg/dL

TABLE 26-15 Test for TSH Reserve

Test	Dose and Sampling Times	Comments and Results
TRH	Give 10 μg/kg IV or 200 μg/1.7 m^2 IV; measure plasma TSH concentration at 0, +30, and 60 min	Normal response Basal = 4.5 ± 3.6 μU/mL (varies with assay) Peak TSH = 20–40 μU/mL (increment in TSH exceeds 10 μU/mL) Peak at 15–30 min

pulse amplitude does not change significantly. Nocturnal increases in mean plasma LH levels and LH pulse amplitude and frequency are characteristic of pubertal stages 1 through 4. In stage 5 of puberty, gonadotropin pulses are similar throughout the day and night.

The pubertal gonadotropin response to GnRH stimulation (100 μg IV) is defined as a peak LH level which is at least twice the baseline concentration, which is 5 mIU/mL or more. The ratio of the peak LH to FSH expressed in mIU/mL is considered diagnostic of puberty if it exceeds 1 (i.e., an LH-predominant response). During childhood, the peak LH to FSH ratio is characteristically below 1. The ratio of peak LH to peak FSH increases progressively during puberty in both boys and girls.

Prolactin Concentration

Basal prolactin concentration < 20 ng/mL
Peak prolactin concentration after TRH administration = 10 to 150 ng/mL in prepubertal child

Vasopressin

See Table 26-16.

Adrenal Function Tests

Basal Hormone Levels

Urinary 17-Hydroxycorticosteroid Excretion

Age 6 months to 15 years: 3.1 ± 1.0 mg per square meter of body surface per 24 h
Adult males: 3 to 9 mg/24 h
Adult females: 2 to 8 mg/24 h

Urinary 17-Ketosteroid Excretion

Age 0 to 1 month: < 2.5 mg/24 h
1 month to 5 years: < 0.5 mg/24 h
6 to 9 years: 1 to 2 mg/24 h
Puberty: progressive increase to adult values
Adult males: 7 to 17 mg/24 h
Adult females: 5 to 15 mg/24 h

TABLE 26-16 Vasopressin Tests

Test	Dose and Sampling Times	Comments and Results
Water deprivation, overnight test, 8 P.M.–8 A.M.	Void and discard 7 A.M. urine; void and record 8 A.M. specific gravity	Use if no history of polydipsia or polyuria Normal response: specific gravity > 1.020
Daytime	At 0 time, record body weight; serum Na^+, Cl^-, and osmolality; and urine specific gravity and volume Recheck these indexes every 2 h	Use when polydipsia or polyuria present; criteria for vasopressin-sensitive diabetes insipidus Weight loss > 5% of body weight Serum osmolality > 290 mOsm Serum [Na^+] > 150 mEq/L Urine specific gravity < 1.005 Plasma vasopressin < 2 pg/mL Positive response to vasopressin Constant supervision necessary, especially for infants and small children Stop test if weight loss exceeds 5%

Plasma Cortisol Concentration

8 A.M.: 10 to 25 μg/dL
8 P.M.: 1 to 8 μg/dL

ACTH Suppression Tests

1. Days 1 and 2: obtain control 24-h urine collections.
2. Days 3 and 4 (and possibly day 5): give low-dose dexamethasone, 20 μg per kilogram of body weight per day (in four doses per day, every 6 h).
3. Days 6 and 7 (and possibly day 8): give high-dose dexamethasone, 80 μg/kg per day (in four doses per day, every 6 h).
4. Obtain 24-h urine collection on days 1, 2, 4 (possibly day 5), 6, 7 (and possibly day 8) for 17-hydroxycorticosteroids and creatinine determinations (17-ketosteroids and free cortisol determinations optional).
5. Measure plasma cortisol concentration every 12 to 24 h on days 1, 4, and 7.

Normal response: by day 4, urinary 17-hydroxycorticosteroid excretion is less than 2 mg/24 h or less than 1 mg per gram of creatinine, and plasma cortisol concentration is less than 5 μg/dL.

Abnormal values: Cushing's syndrome is diagnosed if 17-hydroxycorticosteroid excretion is greater than 2 mg/24 h on days 4 and 5. If Cushing's syndrome is due to bilateral adrenal hyperplasia, urinary 17-hydroxycorticosteroid excretion is less than 2 mg/24 h by days 7 and 8, except if hyperplasia is due to an autonomous ACTH-producing tumor or to adrenal carcinoma; then urinary 17-hydroxycorticosteroid excretion exceeds 2 mg/24 h on days 7 and 8. Rarely, a hypothalamic tumor is not suppressed.

ACTH Stimulation Tests

Intravenous Synthetic ACTH (Cosyntropin) Bolus

Use a dose of 0.25 mg IV.
Measure plasma cortisol concentration at 0, 30, 60, and 90 min. A normal response is a peak plasma cortisol concentration exceeding 20 μg/dL.

IV Infusion of ACTH

Administer 0.25 mg cosyntropin in 250 mL saline over 6 h. Measure plasma cortisol concentration at 0 and 6 h. A normal response is a plasma cortisol concentration exceeding 30 μg/dL at 6 h.

Unresponsiveness occurs in patients with Addison's disease or Cushing's syndrome due to adrenal carcinoma. The test is unreliable in patients with prolonged adrenal suppression.

IM Injection of ACTH Gel (Corticotropin)

Collect two control 24-h urine samples for 17-hydroxycorticosteroid (with or without 17-ketosteroid) determination. Administer 20 mg of corticotropin per square meter of body surface every 12 h for 3 to 6 days (40 mg/m^2 per day). Measure plasma cortisol concentration at 0 and 48 h and then every 24 h. Collect a 24-h urine sample for 17-hydroxycorticosteroid (with or without 17-kerosteroid) determination on days 3 to 6.

A normal response is an increase in urinary 17-hydroxycorticosteroid excretion to 5 to 10 times the normal basal value.

Use 4 to 6 days of stimulation in states associated with long-standing ACTH deficiency and adrenal suppression. An inadequate response is seen in some patients with Cushing's syndrome.

REFERENCES

1. Winick M: Fetal malnutrition and growth processes. *Hosp Pract* 34:33, 1970.
2. Winick M: Nutrition, growth and development, in Freinkel N (ed): *The Year in Metabolism*. New York, Plenum, 1977, p 379.
3. Weiss P, Kavanau JL: A model of growth and growth control in mathematical terms. *J Gen Physiol* 41:1, 1957.
4. Sands J, Dobbing J, Gratrix C: Cell number and cell size: Organ growth and development and the control of catch-up growth in rats. *Lancet* 2:503, 1979.
5. Smith DW, Bierman EL: *The Biologic Ages of Man*. Philadelphia, Saunders, 1973.
6. Tanner JM, Healy MJR, Lockhart RD, MacKenzie JD, Whitehouse RH: The prediction of adult body measurements from measurements taken every year from birth to 5 years. *Arch Dis Child* 31:372, 1956.
7. Garn SM, Pesick SD: Relationship between various maternal body mass measures and size of the newborn. *Am J Clin Nutr* 36:664, 1982.
8. Smith DW, Truog W, Rogers JE, Greitzer LJ, Skinner AL, McCann JJ, Harvey MS: Shifting linear growth during infancy: Illustration of genetic factors in growth from fetal life through infancy. *J Pediatr* 89:225, 1976.
9. Tanner JM: Regulation of growth in size of mammals. *Nature* 199:845, 1963.
10. Garn SM, Rohmann CG: X-linked inheritance of developmental timing in men. *Nature* 196:695, 1962.
11. Yamada K, Ohta M, Yoshimura K, Hasekura H: A possible association of Y chromosome heterochromatin with stature. *Hum Genet* 58:268, 1981.
12. Wingerd J, Solomon IL, Schoen EJ: Parent-specific height standards for preadolescent children of three racial groups. *Pediatrics* 52:555, 1973.
13. Wheeler E, Tan SP: Trends in the growth of ethnic Chinese children living in London. *Ann Hum Biol* 10:441, 1983.
14. Barr GD, Allen CM, Shinefield HR: Height and weight of 7500 children of three skin colors: Pediatric multiphasic program: Report 3. *Am J Dis Child* 124:866, 1972.
15. Spencer EM: *Modern Concepts of Insulin-Like Growth Factors*. New York, Elsevier, 1991.
16. Sara VR, Hall K, Low H: *Growth Factors: From Genes to Clinical Application*. New York, Raven, 1990.
17. Daughaday WH, Herington AC, Phillips LS: The regulation of growth by endocrines. *Annu Rev Physiol* 37:211, 1975.
18. Daughaday WH: Growth hormone and the somatomedins, in Daughaday WN (ed): *Endocrine Control of Growth*. New York, Elsevier, 1981, p 1.
19. Isaksson OGP, Lindahl A, Isgaard J, Nilsson JT, Carlsson B: Dual regulation of cartilage growth, in Spencer EM (ed): *Modern Concepts of Insulin-Like Growth Factors*. New York, Elsevier, 1991, p 121.

20. DeChiara TM, Efstratiadis A, Robertson EJ: A growth-deficiency phenotype in heterozygous mice carrying an insulin-like growth factor II gene disrupted by targeting. *Nature* 345:78, 1990.
21. Matthews LS, Hammer RE, Behringer RR, D'Ercole AJ, Bell GI, Brinster RL, Palmeter RD: Growth enhancement of transgenic mice expressing human insulin-like growth factor I. *Endocrinology* 123:2827, 1988.
22. Clemmons DR, Van Wyk JJ: Factors controlling blood concentrations of somatomedin-C. *Clin Endocrinol Metab* 13: 113, 1984.
23. Clemmons DR, Underwood LE, Van Wyk JJ: Hormonal control of immunoreactive somatomedin production by cultured human fibroblasts. *J Clin Invest* 67:10, 1981.
24. Underwood LE, D'Ercole AJ, Van Wyk JJ: Somatomedin-C and the assessment of growth. *Pediatr Clin North Am* 27:771, 1980.
25. Chernausek SD, Underwood LE, Utiger RD, Van Wyk JJ: Growth hormone secretion and plasma somatomedin-C in primary hypothyroidism. *Clin Endocrinol (Oxf)* 19:337, 1983.
26. Parker MW, Johanson AJ, Rogol AD, Kaiser DL, Blizzard RM: Effect of testosterone on somatomedin-C concentrations in pre-pubertal boys. *J Clin Endocrinol Metab* 58:87, 1984.
27. Rosenfeld RG, Wilson DM, Lee PD, Hintz RL: Insulin-like growth factors I and II in evaluation of growth retardation. *J Pediatr* 109:428, 1986.
28. Underwood LE, Clemmons DR, Maes M, D'Ercole AJ, Ketelslegers JM: Regulation of somatomedin-C/insulin-like growth factor I by nutrients. *Horm Res* 24:166, 1986.
29. Clemmons DR, Klibanski A, Underwood LE, McArthur JW, Ridgway EC, Beitins IZ, Van Wyk JJ: Reduction of plasma somatomedin-C during fasting in humans. *J Clin Endocrinol Metab* 53:1247, 1981.
30. Hintz RL, Suskind R, Amatayakul K, Thanagkul O, Olson R: Plasma somatomedin and growth hormone values in children with protein calorie malnutrition. *J Pediatr* 92:153, 1978.
31. Underwood LE, Thissen JP, Moats-Staats BM, Bruton E, Maes M, Ketelslegers JM: Nutritional regulation of IGF-I and post-natal growth, in Spencer EM (ed): *Modern Concepts of Insulin-Like Growth Factors.* New York, Elsevier, 1991, p 37.
32. Daughaday WH, Rotwein P: Insulin-like growth factors I and II, peptide, messenger ribonucleic acid and gene structures, serum and tissue concentrations. *Endocr Rev* 10:68, 1989.
33. Pinchas C, Fielder PJ, Yukihuro H, Frisch H, Giudiec LC, Rosenfeld RG: Clinical aspects of insulin-like growth factor binding proteins. *Acta Endocrinol (Copenh)* 124:72, 1991.
34. Drop SLS, Brinkman A, Kortleve DJ, Groffen CAH, Schuller A, Swarthoff EC: The evolution of the insulin-like growth factor binding protein family, in Spencer EM (ed): *Modern Concepts of Insulin-Like Growth Factors.* New York, Elsevier, 1991, p 311.
35. Blum WF, Ranke MB: Plasma $IGFBP_3$ levels as clinical indicators, in Spencer EM (ed): *Modern Concepts of Insulin-Like Growth Factors.* New York, Elsevier, 1991, p 381.
36. Baxter RC: Physiological roles of the IGF binding proteins, in Spencer EM (ed): *Modern Concepts of Insulin-Like Growth Factors.* New York, Elsevier, 1991, p 371.
37. D'Ercole AJ: The insulin-growth factors and fetal growth, in Spencer EM (ed): *Modern Concepts of Insulin-Like Growth Factors.* New York, Elsevier, 1991, p 9.
38. Han VK, D'Ercole AJ, Lund PK: Cellular localization of somatomedin insulin-like growth factor messenger RNA in the human fetus. *Science* 236:193, 1987.
39. Hurley TW, D'Ercole AJ, Handwerger S, Underwood LE, Furlanetto RW, Fellows RE: Ovine placental lactogen induces somatomedin: A possible role in fetal growth. *Endocrinology* 101:1635, 1977.
40. Davenport ML, D'Ercole AJ, Underwood LE: Effect of maternal fasting on fetal serum insulin-like growth factors (IGFs) and tissue IGF messenger ribonucleic acids. *Endocrinology* 126:2062, 1990.
41. Hill DJ, Davidson P, Milner RDG: Retention of plasma somatomedin activity in the fetal rabbit following decapitation in utero. *J Endocrinol* 81:93, 1979.
42. Rechler MM, Nissley SP: Insulin-like growth factor (IGF)/ somatomedin receptor subtypes: Structure, function and relationships to insulin receptors and IGF carrier proteins. *Horm Res* 24:152, 1986.
43. Bondy CA, Werner H, Roberts CT Jr, LeRoith D: Cellular pattern of insulin-like growth factor-I (IGF-I) and type I IGF receptor gene expression in early organogenesis; comparison with IGF-II gene expression. *Mol Endocrinol* 4:1386, 1990.
44. Baxter RC, Martin JL: Binding proteins for the insulin-like growth factors: Structure, regulation and function. *Prog Growth Factor Res* 1:49, 1989.
45. Phillips JA, Venencak-Jones CL: Genetics of growth hormone and its disorders. *Adv Hum Genet* 18:305, 1989.
46. Chen EY, Liao YC, Smith DH, Barrera-Saldana HA, Gelinas RE, Seeburg PH: The human growth hormone locus: Nucleotide sequence biology and evolution. *Genomics* 4:479, 1989.
47. Cooke NE, Emery JG, Ray J, Urbanek M, Estes PA, Liebhaber SA: Placental expression of the human growth hormone-variant gene. *Trophoblast Res* 5:61, 1991.
48. Liebhaber SA, Urbanek M, Ray J, Tuan R, Cooke NE: Characterization and histologic localization of Human Growth Hormone-variant gene expression in the placenta. *J Clin Invest* 83:1985, 1989.
49. Cooke NE, Ray J, Watson MA, Kuo BA, Liebhaber SA: The human growth hormone gene and the highly homologous growth hormone variant gene display different splicing patterns. *J Clin Invest* 82:270, 1988.
50. Cooke NE, Ray J, Emery JG, Liebhaber SA: Two distinct species of human growth hormone-variant mRNA in the human placenta predict the expression of novel growth hormone proteins. *J Biol Chem* 263:9001, 1988.
51. Frankenne F, Closset J, Gomez F, Scippo ML, Smal J, Hennen G: The physiology of growth hormones (GH) in pregnant women and partial characterization of the placental GH variant. *J Clin Endocrinol Metab* 66:1171, 1988.
52. Selden RF, Wagner TE, Blethen S, Yun JS, Rowe ME, Goodman HM: Expression of the human growth hormone variant gene in cultured fibroblasts and transgenic mice. *Proc Natl Acad Sci USA* 85:8241, 1988.
53. Goossens M, Brauner R, Czernichow Duquesnoy P, Rappaport R: Isolated growth hormone (GH) deficiency type 1A associated with a double deletion in the human GH gene cluster. *J Clin Endocrinol Metab* 62:712, 1986.
54. Parks JS, Nielsen PV, Sexton LA, Jorgensen EH: An effect of gene dosage on production of human chorionic somatomammotropin. *J Clin Endocrinol Metab* 60:994, 1985.
55. Simon P, Decoster C, Brocas H, Schwers J, Vassart G: Absence of human chorionic somatomammotropin during pregnancy associated with two types of gene deletion. *Hum Genet* 74:235, 1986.
56. Guillemin R, Gerich JE: Somatostalin: Physiological and clinical significance. *Annu Rev Med* 27:379, 1976.
57. Brazeau P, Vale W, Burgus R, Ling N, Butcher M, Rivier J, Guillemin R: Hypothalamic peptide that inhibits the secretion of immunoreactive pituitary growth hormone. *Science* 179:77, 1973.
58. Rivier J, Spress J, Thorner M, Vale W: Characterization of a growth hormone releasing factor from a human pancreatic islet tumour. *Nature* 300:276, 1982.
59. Guillemin R, Brazeau P, Bohlen P, Esch F, Ling N, Wehrenberg W: Growth hormone releasing factor from a human pancreatic tumor that caused acromegaly. *Science* 218:585, 1982.
60. Bloch B, Brazeau P, Ling N, Bohlen P, Esch F, Wehrenberg

WB, Benoit R, Bloom F, Guillemin R: Immunochemical detection of growth hormone releasing factor in brain. *Nature* 301:607, 1983.
61. Bohlen P, Brazeau P, Bloch B, Ling N, Gaillard R, Guillemin R: Human hypothalamic growth hormone releasing factor (GRF): Evidence for two forms identical to tumor derived GRF-44-NHz and GRF 40. *Biochem Biophys Res Commun* 114:930, 1983.
62. Frohman LA, Szabo M, Berelowitz M, Stachura ME: Partial purification and characterization of a peptide with growth hormone releasing activity from extrapituitary tumors in patients with acromegaly. *J Clin Invest* 65:43, 1980.
63. Thorner MO, Reschke J, Chitwood J, Rogol AD, Furlanetto RW, Rivier J, Vale J, Blizzard RM: Acceleration of growth in two children treated with human growth hormone releasing factor. *N Engl J Med* 312:4, 1985.
64. Bowers CY, Reynolds GA, Durham D, Barrera CM, Pezzole SS, Thorner MO: Growth hormone releasing peptide stimulates GH release in normal men and acts synergistically with GH releasing hormone. *J Clin Endocrinol Metab* 70:975, 1990.
65. Ottlecz A, Snyder GD, McCann SM: Regulatory role of galanin in control of hypothalamic anterior pituitary function. *Proc Natl Acad Sci USA* 85:9861, 1988.
66. Baumann G, Amburn K, Shaw MA: The circulatory growth hormone (GH) binding protein complex a major constituent of plasma GH in man. *Endocrinology* 122:976, 1988.
67. Matthews LS: Molecular biology of growth hormone receptors. *Trends Endocrinol Metab* 2:176, 1991.
68. Leung DW, Spencer SA, Cachianes G, Hammonds RG, Collins C, Henzel WJ, Barnard R, Waters MJ, Wood WI: Growth hormone receptor and serum binding protein: Purification, cloning, expression. *Nature* 330:537, 1987.
69. Godowski P, Leung DW, Meachaem LR, Galgani JP, Hellmiss R, Keret R, Rotwein PS, Parks JS, et al: Characterization of human growth hormone receptor gene and demonstration of a partial gene deletion in two patients with Laron-type dwarfism. *Proc Natl Acad Sci USA* 86:8083, 1989.
70. Amselem S, Duquesnoy P, Attree O, Novelli G, Bousnina S, Postal-Vinay MC, Goossens M: Laron dwarfism and mutations of the growth hormone receptor gene. *N Engl J Med* 321:989, 1989.
71. Baumann G, Shaw MA, Winter RJ: Absence of the plasma growth hormone-binding protein in Laron type dwarfism. *J Clin Endocrinol Metab* 65:814, 1987.
72. Daughaday WH, Trivedi B: Absence of serum growth hormone binding protein in patients with growth hormone receptor deficiency (Laron dwarfism). *Proc Natl Acad Sci USA* 84:4636, 1987.
73. Rosenbloom AL, Guevara-Aguirre J, Vaccarello M, Rosenfeld RG, Fielder PJ, Diamond FB: Growth hormone receptor deficiency (Laron syndrome), in Spencer EM (ed): *Modern Concepts of Insulin-Like Growth Factors.* New York, Elsevier, 1991, p 49.
74. Rosenbloom AL, Guevara-Aguirre J, Rosenfeld RG, Fielder PJ: The little women of Loja—Growth hormone receptor deficiency in an inbred population of Southern Equador. *N Engl J Med* 323:1367, 1990.
75. MacGillivray MH, Aceto T, Frohman LA: Plasma growth hormone response and growth retardation of hypothyroidism. *Am J Dis Child* 115:273, 1979.
76. Kerr GK, Tyson IB, Allen JR, Wallace JH, Scheffler G: Deficiency of thyroid hormone and development of the fetal rhesus monkey. *Biol Neonate* 21:282, 1972.
77. Walker P, Weichsel ME, Fisher DA, Guo SM: Thyroxine increases nerve growth factor concentration in adult mouse brain. *Science* 204:427, 1979.
78. Reiter EO, Grumbach MM: Neuroendocrine control mechanisms and the onset of puberty. *Annu Rev Physiol* 44:595, 1982.
79. Ducharme JR, Collu R: Pubertal development: Normal, precocious and delayed. *Clin Endocrinol Metab* 11:57, 1982.
80. Ducharme JR, Forest MG, De Peretti E, Sempe M, Collu R, Bertrand J: Plasma adrenal and gonadal sex steroids in human pubertal development. *J Clin Endocrinol Metab* 42:468, 1976.
81. Grumbach MM, Roth JC, Kaplan SL, Kelch RP: Hypothalamic pituitary regulation of puberty: Evidence and concepts derived from clinical research, in Grumbach MM et al (eds): *The Control of the Onset of Puberty.* New York: Wiley, 1974, p 115.
82. Lee PA, Jaffe RB, Midgley AR Jr: Serum gonadotropin, testosterone and prolactin concentrations throughout puberty in boys: A longitudinal study. *J Clin Endocrinol Metab* 39:664, 1974.
83. Lee PA, Xenakis T, Winer J, Matsenbaugh S: Puberty in girls; correlation of serum levels of gonadotropins, prolactin, androgens, estrogens and progestins with physical changes. *J Clin Endocrinol Metab* 43:775, 1976.
84. Anderson DC: The adrenal androgen-stimulating hormone does not exist. *Lancet* 2:454, 1980.
85. Mainwaring WIP: The mechanism of action of androgens, in *Monographs on Endocrinology.* New York, Springer-Verlag, 1977, vol 10.
86. Kelch RP, Lindolm UB, Jaffe RB: Testosterone metabolism in target tissues: II. Human fetal and adult reproductive tissues, perineal skin and skeletal muscle. *J Clin Endocrinol Metab* 32:449, 1971.
87. Peterson RE, Imperato-McGinley J, Gautier T, Sturla E: Male pseudohermaphroditism due to steroid 5α-reductase deficiency. *Am J Med* 62:170, 1977.
88. Martin LG, Clark JW, Conner TB: Growth hormone secretion enhanced by androgens. *J Clin Endocrinol Metab* 28:425, 1968.
89. Rosenfeld RG, Northcraft GB, Hintz RL: A prospective, randomized study of testosterone treatment of constitutional delay of growth and development in male adolescents. *Pediatrics* 69:681, 1982.
90. Marshall WA, Tanner JM: Puberty, in David JA, Dobbing J (eds): *Scientific Foundations of Paediatrics.* Philadelphia, Saunders, 1974.
91. Frisch RE, McArthur JW: Menstrual cycles: Fatness as a determinant of minimum weight for height necessary for their maintenance or onset. *Science* 185:949, 1974.
92. Walton A, Hammond J: The maternal effects of growth and conformation in shire-horse-Shetland pony crosses. *Proc R Soc London [Biol]* 125:311, 1938.
93. Smith DW: Growth and its disorders, in *Major Problems in Clinical Pediatrics.* Philadelphia, Saunders, 1977, vol 15.
94. Forest MG: Plasma androgens in normal and premature newborns and infants: Evidence for maturation of the gonadostat's regulation. *Proceedings of the Fourteenth International Congress of Pediatrics.* Buenos Aires, 1974.
95. Tanner JM: *Growth at Adolescence,* 2d ed. Oxford, Blackwell, 1955.
96. Odell WD, Swerdloff RS: Etiologies of sexual maturation. A model system based on the sexually maturing rat. *Recent Prog Horm Res* 32:245, 1976.
97. Jones KL: *Smiths' Recognizable Patterns of Human Malformations,* 4th ed. Philadelphia, Saunders, 1988.
98. Brunner KM, Recker B: Reference charts used frequently by endocrinologists in assessing the growth and development of children, in Lifshitz F (ed): *Pediatric Endocrinology,* 2d ed. New York, Marcel Dekker, 1990, p 983.
99. Tanner JM, Whitehouse RH, Marshall WA, Carter BS: Prediction of adult height, from height, bone age, and occurrence of menarche at ages 4 to 16 with allowance for mid parent height. *Arch Dis Child* 50:14, 1975.
100. Greulich WW, Pyle SE: *Radiographic Atlas of Skeletal Development of the Hand and Wrist,* 2d ed. Stanford, Stanford University Press, 1959.

101. Bayley N, Pinneau S: Tables for predicting adult height from skeletal age. *J Pediatr* 40:432, 1952.
102. Rudman D, Kutner MH, Blackston RD, Cushman RA, Bain RP, Patterson JH: Children with normal-variant short stature: Treatment with human growth hormone for six months. *N Engl J Med* 305:123, 1981.
103. Van Vliet G, Styne DM, Kaplan SL, Grumbach MM: Growth hormone treatment for short stature. *N Engl J Med* 309:1016, 1983.
104. Gertner JM, Genel M, Granfredi SP, Hintz RL, Rosenfeld RG, Tamborlane WV, Wilson DM: Prospective clinical trial of human growth hormone in short children without growth hormone deficiency. *J Pediatr* 104:172, 1984.
105. Kowarski AA, Schneider J, Ben-Galim E, Weldon VV, Daughaday WH: Growth failure with normal serum RIA-GH and low somatomedin activity: Somatomedin restoration and growth acceleration after exogenous GH. *J Clin Endocrinol Metab* 47:461, 1978.
106. Spiliotis BE, August GP, Hung W, Sonis W, Mendelson W, Bercu BB: Growth hormone neurosecretory dysfunction. *JAMA* 251:2223, 1984.
107. Clarren SK, Smith DW: The fetal alcohol syndrome. *N Engl J Med* 298:1063, 1978.
108. Klein AH, Melner S, Kenny FM: Improved prognosis in congenital hypothyroidism treated before three months. *J Pediatr* 81:912, 1972.
109. Glorieux J, Dussault JH, Letarte J, Guyda H, Morissette J: Preliminary results on the mental development of hypothyroid infants detected by the Quebec Screening Program. *J Pediatr* 102:19, 1983.
109a. New England Congenital Hypothyroidism Collaborative: Characteristics of infantile hypothyroidism discovered on neonatal screening. *J Pediatr* 104:539, 1984.
110. Smith DW, Blizzard RM, Wilkins L: The mental prognosis in hypothyroidism of infancy and childhood. *Pediatrics* 19:1011, 1957.
111. Abbassi V, Aldige C: Evaluation of sodium L-thyroxine (T4) requirement in replacement therapy of hypothyroidism. *J Pediatr* 90:298, 1977.
112. Rezvani I, DiGeorge AM: Reassessment of the daily dose of oral thyroxine for replacement therapy in hypothyroid children. *J Pediatr* 90:291, 1977.
113. Schultz RM, Glassman MS, MacGillivray MH: Elevated threshold for thyrotropin suppression in congenital hypothyroidism. *Am J Dis Child* 134:19, 1980.
114. Sekadde CB, Slaunwhite WR Jr, Aceto T Jr, Murray KA: Administration of thyroxine once a week. *J Clin Endocrinol Metab* 39:759, 1974.
115. Vimpani GV, Vimpani AF, Lidgard GP, Cameron EHD, Farquhar JW: Prevalence of severe growth hormone deficiency. *Br Med J* 2:427, 1977.
116. Parkin JM: Incidence of growth hormone deficiency. *Arch Dis Child* 49:905, 1974.
117. Clopper RR, Mazur T, MacGillivray MH, Peterson RE, Voorhess MJ: Data on virilization and erotosexual behavior in male hypopituitarism during gonadotropin and androgen treatment. *J Androl* 4:303, 1983.
118. Phillips JA III: The growth hormone (hGH) gene and human disease, in *Banbury Report 14: Recombinant DNA Applications to Human Disease*. Cold Spring Harbor, N.Y., Cold Spring Laboratory, 1983.
119. Illig R, Prader A, Ferrandez A: Hereditary prenatal growth hormone deficiency with increased tendency to growth hormone antibody formation ("A-type" of isolated growth hormone deficiency). *Acta Paediatr Scand* 60:607, 1971.
120. Kaplan SL, Grumbach MM, Hoyt WF: A syndrome of hypopituitary dwarfism, hypoplasia of optic nerves and malformation of the prosencephalon. *Pediatr Res* 4:480, 1970.
121. Patel H, Tze WJ, Crichton JU, McCormick AQ, Robinson GC, Dolman CL: Optic nerve hypoplasia with hypopituitarism. *Am J Dis Child* 129:175, 1975.
122. Stewart C, Castro-Magana M, Sherman J, Angulo M, Collipp PJ: Septo-optic dysplasia and median cleft face syndrome in a patient with isolated growth hormone deficiency and hyperprolactinemia. *Am J Dis Child* 137:484, 1983.
123. Rudman D, Davis GT, Priest JH, Patterson JH, Kutner MH, Heymsfield SB, Bethel RA: Prevalence of growth hormone deficiency in children with cleft lip or palate. *J Pediatr* 93:378, 1978.
124. Berke JP, Buxton LF, Kokmen E: The empty sella. *Neurology* 25:1137, 1975.
125. Jordan RM, Kendall JW, Kerber CW: The primary empty sella syndrome: Analysis of the clinical characteristics, radiographic features, pituitary function and cerebrospinal fluid adenohypophysial hormone concentrations. *Am J Med* 62:569, 1977.
126. Onur K, Lala V, Zimmer J, Juan CS, AvRuskin TW: The primary empty sella syndrome in a child. *J Pediatr* 90:425, 1977.
127. Kleinmann RE, Kazarian EL, Raptopoulos V, Braverman LE: Primary empty sella and Rieger's anomaly of the anterior chamber of the eye. *N Engl J Med* 304:90, 1981.
128. Walker JL, Ginalska-Malinowska M, Romer TE, Pucilowska J, Young S, Clemmons DR, Underwood LE: Infusion of recombinant IGF-I is anabolic in growth hormone insensitivity syndrome. *2nd Intl Symposium on Insulin-Like Growth Factors/Somatomedins,* San Francisco, 1991, p. 283 (abstract).
129. Froesch ER, Guler HP, Schmid C, Binz K, Zapf J: Therapeutic potential of insulin-like growth factor I. *Trends Endocrinol Metab* 1:254, 1990.
130. Merimee TJ, Zapf J, Hewlett B, Gavilli-Sforza LL: Insulin-like growth factors in pygmies. *N Engl J Med* 316:906, 1987.
131. Merimee TJ, Baumann G, Daughaday W: Growth hormone binding protein: Studies in pygmies and normal statured subjects. *J Clin Endocrinol Metab* 71:1183, 1990.
132. Bode H, Bailey RC, Underwood LE: Somatomedin C in EFE pygmy of the Ituri forest. *Pediatr Res* 20:211a, 1986.
133. Thomsett MJ, Conte FA, Kaplan SL, Grumbach MM: Endocrine and neurologic outcome in childhood craniopharyngioma: Review of effect of treatment in 42 patients. *J Pediatr* 97:728, 1980.
134. Clemmons DR, Underwood LE, Ridgway EC, Kliman B, Van Wyk JJ: Hyperprolactinemia is associated with increased immunoreactive somatomedin C in hypopituitarism. *J Clin Endocrinol Metab* 52:731, 1981.
135. Blethen SL, White NH, Santiago JV, Daughaday WH: Plasma somatomedins in children with hyperinsulinism. *J Clin Endocrinol Metab* 52:748, 1981.
136. Bucher J, Zapf J, Torresani T, Prader A, Froesch ER, Illig R: Insulin-like growth factors I and II, prolactin, and insulin in 19 growth hormone-deficient children with excessive, normal, or decreased longitudinal growth after operation for craniopharyngioma. *N Engl J Med* 309:1142, 1983.
137. Rona RJ, Tanner JM: Aetiology of idiopathic growth hormone deficiency in England and Wales. *Arch Dis Child* 52:197, 1977.
138. Craft WH, Underwood LE, Van Wyk JJ: High incidence of perinatal insult in children with idiopathic hypopituitarism. *J Pediatr* 96:397, 1980.
139. Del Pozo JM, Roda JE, Montoya JG, Iglesias JR, Hurtado A: Intrasellar granuloma. *J Neurosurg* 53:717, 1980.
140. Bottazzo GF, McIntosh C, Stanford W, Preece M: Growth hormone cell antibodies and partial growth hormone deficiency in a girl with Turner's syndrome. *Clin Endocrinol (Oxf)* 12:1, 1980.
141. Portocarrero CJ, Robinson AG, Taylor AL, Klein I: Lymphoid hypophysitis. *JAMA* 246:1811, 1981.
142. Asa SL, Bilbao JM, Kovacs K, Josse RG, Kreines K: Lymphocytic hypophysitis of pregnancy resulting in hypopitu-

itarism: A distinct clinicopathologic entity. *Ann Intern Med* 95:166, 1981.
143. Richard GE, Wara WM, Grumbach MM, Kaplan SL, Sheline GE, Conte FA: Delayed onset of hypopituitarism: Sequelae of therapeutic irradiation of central nervous system, eye and middle ear tumors. *J Pediatr* 89:553, 1976.
144. Samaan NA, Bakdash MM, Caderao JB, Cangir A, Jesse RH, Ballantyne AJ: Hypopituitarism after external irradiation: Evidence for both hypothalamic and pituitary origin. *Ann Intern Med* 83:771, 1975.
145. Duffner PK, Cohen ME, Anderson SW, Voorhess ML, MacGillivray MH, Panahon A, Brecher ML: Long-term effects of treatment on endocrine function in children with brain tumors. *Ann Neurol* 14:528, 1983.
146. Russell JD, Wise PH, Rischbieth HG: Vascular malformation of the hypothalamus: A cause of isolated growth hormone deficiency. *Pediatrics* 66:306, 1980.
147. Saenger P, Schwartz E, Markenson AL, Graziano JH, Levine LS, New MI, Hilgartner MW: Depressed serum somatomedin activity in beta-thalassemia. *J Pediatr* 96:214, 1980.
148. Costin G, Kogut MD, Hyman CB, Ortega JA: Endocrine abnormalities in thalassemia major. *Am J Dis Child* 133:497, 1979.
149. McIntosh N: Endocrinopathy in thalassaemia major. *Arch Dis Child* 51:195, 1976.
150. Braunstein GD, Kohler PO: Pituitary function in Hand-Schuller-Christian disease: Evidence for deficient growth hormone release in patients with short stature. *N Engl J Med* 286:1225, 1972.
151. Underwood LE, Van Wyk JJ: Hormones in normal and aberrant growth, in Williams RH (ed): *Textbook of Endocrinology*. Philadelphia, Saunders, 1981, p 1177.
152. Penny R, Blizzard RM: The possible influence of puberty on the release of growth hormone in 3 males with apparent growth hormone deficiency. *J Clin Endocrinol Metab* 34:82, 1972.
153. Gourmelen M, Pham-Huu-Trung MT, Girard F: Transient partial hGH deficiency in prepubertal children with delay of growth. *Pediatr Res* 13:221, 1979.
154. Patton RG, Gardner LI: Influence of family environment on growth: The syndrome of "maternal deprivation." *Pediatrics* 30:957, 1962.
155. Powell GF, Brasel JA, Blizzard RM: Emotional deprivation and growth retardation simulating idiopathic hypopituitarism: I. Clinical evaluation of the syndrome. *N Engl J Med* 276:1271, 1967.
156. Powell GF, Brasel JA, Raiti S, Blizzard RM: Emotional deprivation and growth retardation simulating idiopathic hypopituitarism: II. Endocrinologic evaluation of the syndrome. *N Engl J Med* 276:1279, 1967.
157. Krieger I, Mellinger RC: Pituitary function in the deprivation syndrome. *J Pediatr* 79:216, 1971.
158. Gibbs CJ Jr, Joy A, Heffner R, Franko M, Miyazaki M, Asher DM, Parisi JE, Brown PW, Gajdusek DC: Clinical and pathological features and laboratory confirmation of Creutzfeldt-Jakob disease in a recipient of pituitary-derived human growth hormone. *N Engl J Med* 313:734, 1985.
159. Koch TK, Berg BO, De Armond SJ, Gravina RF: Creutzfeldt-Jakob disease in a young adult with idiopathic hypopituitarism: Possible relation to the administration of cadaveric human growth hormone. *N Engl J Med* 313:731, 1985.
160. Powell-Jackson J, Kennedy P, Whitcombe EM, Weller RO, Preece MA, Newsom-Davis J: Creutzfeldt-Jakob disease after administration of human growth hormone. *Lancet* 3:244, 1985.
161. Raiti S, Trias E, Levitsky L, Grossman MS: Oxandrolone and human growth hormone: Comparison of growth stimulating effects in short children. *Am J Dis Child* 126:597, 1973.
162. MacGillivray MH, Kolotkin M, Munschauer RW: Enhanced linear growth responses in hypopituitary dwarfs treated with growth hormone plus androgen versus growth hormone alone. *Pediatr Res* 8:103, 1974.
163. Styne DM, Grumbach MM, Kaplan SL, Wilson CB, Conte FA: Treatment of Cushing's disease in childhood and adolescence by transsphenoidal microadenomectomy. *N Engl J Med* 310:899, 1984.
164. Jennings AS, Liddle GW, Orth DN: Results of treating childhood Cushing's disease with pituitary irradiation. *N Engl J Med* 297:957, 1977.
165. Shohat M, Remoin DL: The skeletal dysplasias, in Lifshitz F (ed): *Pediatric Endocrinology,* 2d ed. New York, Marcel Dekker, 1990, p 147.
166. Rimoin DL: Limb lengthening: Past, present, future. *Growth Genet Horm* 7:1, 1991.
167. Lippe B: Turner syndrome. *Endocrinol Metab Clin North Am* 20:121, 1991.
168. Neely EK, Rosenfeld RG: Growth in Turner syndrome. *Endocrinologist* 1:313, 1991.
169. Ranke MB, Pflüger H, Rosendahl W, Stubbe P, Enders H, Bierich JR, Majewski F: Turner syndrome: Spontaneous growth in 150 cases and review of the literature. *Eur J Pediatr* 141:81, 1983.
170. Lyon AJ, Preece MA, Grant DB: Growth curve for girls with Turner syndrome. *Arch Dis Child* 60:932, 1985.
171. Rosenfeld RG: Non-conventional growth hormone therapy in Turner syndrome: The United States experience. *Horm Res* 33:131, 1990.
172. Collins E, Turner G: The Noonan syndrome—a review of the clinical and genetic features of 27 cases. *J Pediatr* 83:941, 1973.
173. Frasier SD: Tall stature and excessive growth syndrome, in Lifshitz F (ed): *Pediatric Endocrinology,* 2d ed. New York, Marcel Dekker, 1990, p 197.
174. Zachman M, Ferrandez A, Murset G, Guehn HG, Prader A: Testosterone treatment of excessively tall boys. *J Pediatr* 88:116, 1976.
175. Speiser PW, New MI: An update on congenital adrenal hyperplasia, in Lifshitz F (ed): *Pediatric Endocrinology,* 2d ed. New York, Marcel Dekker, 1990, p 307.
176. Pang S, Wallace MA, Hofman L, Thuline HC, Dorche C, Lyon ICT, Dobbins RH, Kling S, et al: Worldwide experience in newborn screening for classical congenital adrenal hyperplasia due to 21 hydroxylase deficiency. *Pediatrics* 81:866, 1988.
177. Speiser PW, Laforgia N, Kato K, Pareira J, Khan R, Yang SY, Whorwood C, White PC, et al: First trimester prenatal treatment and molecular genetic diagnosis of congenital adrenal hyperplasia (21 hydroxylase deficiency). *J Clin Endocrinol Metab* 70:838, 1990.
178. Holland FJ: Gonadotropin—independent precocious puberty. *Endocrinol Metab Clin North Am* 20:191, 1991.
179. Laue L, Kenigsberg D, Pescovitz OH, Hench KD, Barnes KM, Loriaux DL, Cutler GB: Treatment of familial male precocious puberty with spironolactone and testolactone. *N Engl J Med* 320:496, 1989.
180. Wheeler MD, Styne DM: The treatment of precocious puberty. *Endocrinol Metab Clin North Am* 20:183, 1991.
181. Manasco PK, Pescovitz OH, Hill SC, Jones JM, Barnes KM, Hench KD, Loriaux DL, Cutler GB: Six-year results of luteinizing hormone releasing hormone (LHRH) agonist treatment in children with LHRH-dependent precocious puberty. *J Pediatr* 115:105, 1989.
182. Solyom AE, Austad CC, Sherick I, Bacon GG: Precocious sexual development in girls: The emotional impact on the child and her parents. *J Pediatr Psychol* 5:385, 1980.
183. Spence HJ, Trias EP, Racti S: Acromegaly in a 9½ year old boy. *Am J Dis Child* 123:504, 1972.
184. Melmed S: Acromegaly. *N Engl J Med* 322:966, 1990.
185. Barkan AL, Kelch RP, Hopwood NJ, Beitins IZ: Treatment of acromegaly with the long-acting somatostatin analogue SMS 201-999. *J Clin Endocrinol Metab* 66:16, 1988.

186. Schlesinger S, MacGillivray MH, Munschauer RW: Acceleration of growth and bone maturation in childhood thyrotoxicoses. *J Pediatr* 83:233, 1973.
187. Higurashi M, Iijima K, Ikeda Y, Egi S, Ohzeki T: Anthropometric study of cases with Turner's syndrome and XYY, in *Birth Defects: Original Article Series*. New York, Alan R. Liss, 1982, vol 18, p 155.
188. Watkin HA, Mednick LSA, Schulsinger F, Bakkestrom E, Christensen KO: Criminality in XYY and XXY men. *Science* 193:547, 1976.
189. Skovby F, McKusick VA: Estrogen treatment of tall stature in girls with Marfan's syndrome, in *Birth Defects: Original Article Series*. New York, Alan R. Liss, 1977, vol 13, p 155.
190. Sotos JF: Cerebral gigantism. *Am J Dis Child* 131:625, 1977.
191. Garn SM, Clark DC: Nutrition, growth, development and maturation. Findings from the ten state nutrition survey of 1968–70. *Pediatrics* 56:306, 1975.
192. Filippi G, McKusick VA: The Beckwith-Wiedemann syndrome. *Medicine (Baltimore)* 49:279, 1970.
193. Senior B, Gellis SS: The syndrome of total lipodystrophy and of partial lipodystrophy. *Pediatrics* 33:593, 1964.
194. Tanner JM, Whitehouse RH, Takaishi M: Standards from birth to maturity for height, weight, height velocity and weight velocity: British children. *Arch Dis Child* 41:613, 1966.
195. Reiter EO, Fuldauer VG, Root AW: Secretion of adrenal androgen, dehydroepiandrosterone during normal infancy, childhood and adolescence in sick infants and in children with endocrinologic abnormalities. *J Pediatr* 90:766, 1977.
196. Penny R, Goldstein IP, Frasier SD: Overnight gonadotropin excretion in normal females. *J Clin Endocrinol* 44:780, 1977.
197. Penny R, Goldstein IP, Frasier SD: Overnight follicle stimulating hormone (FSH) and luteinizing hormone (LH) excretion in normal males. *J Clin Endocrinol* 43:1394, 1976.

CHAPTER 27

Gastrointestinal Hormones and Carcinoid Syndrome

Jan Redfern
Thomas M. O'Dorisio

Bayliss and Starling discovered the first gastrointestinal peptide hormone—*secretin*—in extracts of intestinal mucosa 90 years ago.[1] Since that time the number of putative gastrointestinal regulatory substances has increased rapidly, especially over the past 10 to 15 years; more than 30 peptides have been identified.

Our understanding of the biochemistry, physiology, and clinical significance of gut hormones continues to grow at an astounding rate: Over the period 1986–1991, there have been nearly 14,000 journal publications on gastrointestinal peptides. It is clear from the voluminous literature that these peptides have a wide variety of absorptive, secretory, digestive, motor, and trophic actions not only on the gastrointestinal (GI) tract but also on other endocrine and nonendocrine organ systems.[2–4] Collectively these peptide substances play a pivotal role in coordinating the physiologic activities of the gut, and some are indispensable for the maintenance of life.

In light of their wide-ranging biological effects, it is not surprising that several GI peptides have found applications in clinical diagnostic settings. Gastrointestinal peptides have been utilized in the evaluation of the secretory functions of the stomach and pancreas, as aids in radiologic and endoscopic evaluations of the GI tract, and as diagnostic probes for the presence of endocrine tumors.[2] Although useful in diagnostic evaluations, GI peptides have not been extensively used as therapeutic agents. Only somatostatin and its clinically approved synthetic analog, octreotide, have clearly shown potential in the treatment of a variety of clinical abnormalities, including endocrine tumors and secretory diarrhea.[5]

The hyposecretion and hypersecretion of several GI peptides are associated with a variety of disease states. Several clinical syndromes have been described in which tumors of neuroendocrine cell origin elaborate specific tumor products which give rise to distinctive clinical features.[2,6] For example, carcinoid tumors, one of the most frequently occurring and well-known primary endocrine tumors of the small intestine, can secrete several peptide substances (substance P, motilin, and growth hormone releasing factor) and amines (5-hydroxytryptamine and histamine).[7–12] These secretory products collectively give rise to the *carcinoid syndrome*, which is characterized clinically by diarrhea, flushing, and metastases to the liver[7–9] (see below).

This chapter reviews the overall cellular localization and distribution of GI peptides and, in selected cases, summarizes their biological effects, clinical significance, and potential diagnostic and therapeutic uses in disease states. The final section focuses on the clinical presentation, diagnosis, pathophysiology, and treatment of carcinoid tumors, the most common adult neuroendocrine tumors of the gastroenteropancreatic system.

LOCALIZATION AND DISTRIBUTION OF GI PEPTIDES

Identifying the cellular location of GI peptides is important in understanding their physiologic and pathophysiologic roles in regulating gastrointestinal functions.[13,14] A variety of immunohistochemical and radioimmunologic methodologies have permitted a detailed analysis of the cellular and subcellular localization of GI peptides and regional differences in the distribution of peptides in the GI tract and other tissues.[15,16] Using these techniques, several peptides, such as vasoactive intestinal polypeptide (VIP) and substance P, have been colocalized in nerve fibers and ganglion cells that originate in the submucosal (Meissner's) plexus and the myenteric (Auerbach's) plexus, both of which constitute the intrinsic nervous system (Table 27-1).[13] Indeed, most enteric nerve cells appear to contain one or more peptides, which may coexist with nonpeptide neurotransmitters such as acetylcholine and norepinephrine.[3]

Other GI peptides have been localized in endocrine cells in the mucosal layer of the GI tract [e.g., glucose-dependent insulinotropic polypeptide (GIP)], in pancreatic islet cells (e.g., insulin and somatostatin), or in both sites (e.g., glucagon) (Table 27-1).[15–17]

TABLE 27-1 Predominant Cellular Distribution of Gastrointestinal Peptides

Nerve Fibers and Ganglion Cells	Endocrine Cells in the GI Tract	Pancreatic Islets
Somatostatin	Somatostatin	Somatostatin
Vasoactive intestinal polypeptide	Gastrin	Insulin
Peptide histidine isoleucine (PHI)	Secretin	Glucagon
Substance P	Cholecystokinin	Pancreatic polypeptide
Met-enkephalin	Glucose-dependent insulinotropic peptide	
Neuropeptide Y (NPY)	Motilin	
Galanin	Neurotensin	
Bombesin-like immunoreactive peptides	Enteroglucagon	
Calcitonin gene-related peptide	Peptide YY	

Source: From Go and Koch with permission.[13]

In the human small and large intestines, it has been estimated that 3 billion endocrine cells are present, with the greatest density occurring in the proximal duodenum and the lowest density occurring in the distal colon.[18]

Ultrastructural and immunohistochemical studies of endocrine cells in the GI tract and pancreas [collectively called the gastroenteropancreatic (GEP) system] have revealed the existence of at least 15 different types.[17] According to the APUD (amine precursor uptake and decarboxylation) concept proposed by Pearse, the endocrine cells of the gut and pancreas belong to a larger group of cells which have a similar neuroectodermal origin (neural crest tissue) and share a number of cytochemical (cholinesterase positivity), ultrastructural (amine storage), and functional characteristics.[19,20] However, the neuroectodermal origin of gut and pancreatic endocrine cells is controversial, and a number of investigators have presented evidence refuting this hypothesis.[21–23] Pancreatic endocrine cells are now believed to have an endodermal rather than neuroectodermal origin.

Many of the individual endocrine cell types are confined to a specific region of the GI tract or pancreas (Fig. 27-1).[2] For example, G endocrine cells containing gastrin occur principally in the stomach, whereas S, CCK, M, and GIP endocrine cells (containing secretin, cholecystokinin, motilin, and GIP) occur only in the duodenum and jejunum.[17] Somatostatin is unusual in that this key regulatory peptide and the cells that produce it occur in the stomach, pancreas, upper and lower intestine, and colon.[24–26] Its wide distribution in the GEP system implies a pivotal regulatory role for this peptide.

Based on the cellular location of GI peptides (nerve fibers/ganglion cells or endocrine cells) and the manner in which peptides are delivered from

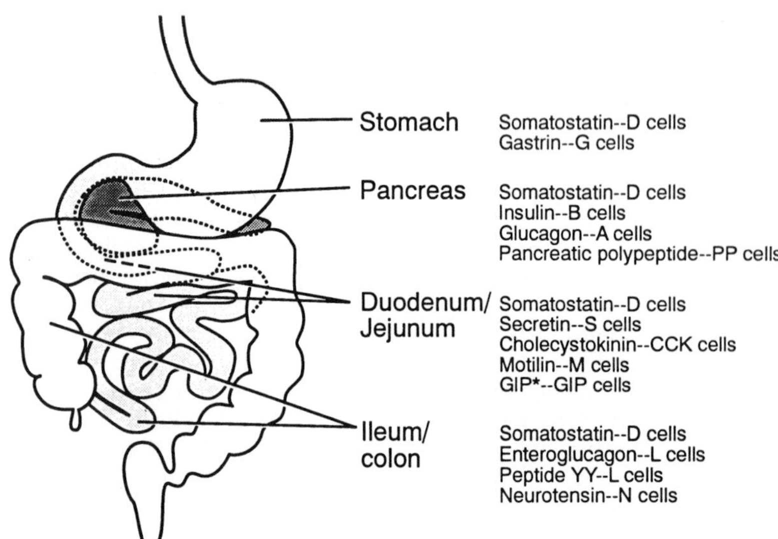

FIGURE 27-1 Distribution of gastrointestinal peptides and corresponding endocrine cells. GIP = gasric inhibitory peptide or glucose-dependent insulinotropic peptide. (*Adapted from Walsh with permission.*[2])

their storage sites to their target cells, GI peptides can be broadly classified into several functional (or regulating) groups: endocrine, paracrine, neurocrine, and autocrine (Table 27-2).[14] *Endocrine* peptides such as gastrin, cholecystokinin (CCK), secretin, GIP, and possibly motilin achieve their biological effects on target tissues through the general circulation.

In contrast, other peptides, such as somatostatin and probably motilin, may function in a local (*paracrine*) manner and achieve their regulatory effects on target cells after release into the interstitial space rather than into the general circulation. *Neurocrine* peptides such as VIP, neuropeptide Y, and substance P influence the postsynaptic membranes on their target cells after release into the synaptic cleft. Finally, some peptides may inhibit their own release through an ultrashort feedback loop. For example, somatostatin congeners [(D-Trp^8-D-Cys^{14})-somatostatin and des-Asn^5-(D-Try^8)-somatostatin] block CCK- and arginine-induced release of somatostatin from pancreatic D cells, suggesting that somatostatin is able to regulate its own secretion (*autocrine* effect).[27]

To date, somatostatin is the only GI peptide known to function as a neurotransmitter, paracrine, and autocrine substance depending on the tissue in which it is located.[5] In addition, somatostatin occurs in numerous hypothalamic nuclei, especially the anterior periventricular region, and may also be classified as a neuroendocrine substance.[28] The cell bodies of neurons in this hypothalamic region synthesize somatostatin, which then passes down the axons as far as the median eminence. Depolarization of axonal terminal swellings in the median eminence releases somatostatin into the capillary plexus of the superior hypophyseal artery. Somatostatin ultimately reaches the anterior pituitary through the long portal veins.

BIOLOGICAL ACTIONS AND CLINICAL APPLICATIONS

Somatostatin

Somatostatin exists in two biologically active forms: somatostatin-14 (SS-14) and somatostatin-28 (SS-28 or prosomatostatin).[5] SS-14 is a 14-amino acid peptide with a cyclic molecular structure.[29] SS-28 is identical to SS-14 from the carboxy terminus but has 14 additional amino acids attached to the amino-terminal end.[30] Recombinant DNA technology has revealed another, much larger somatostatin peptide (preprosomatostatin).[31] Both SS-14 and SS-28 appear in the human circulation, but in dogs the principal circulating molecular species of somatostatin is SS-14.[32–34]

Biological Actions

The biological effects of somatostatin are extremely diverse (Table 27-3).[5] In the anterior pituitary, somatostatin plays an integral physiologic role in regulating the release of growth hormone and possibly thyroid stimulating hormone.[35–39] Both native somatostatin and its congener (see below) appear to exert their regulatory action by first binding to somatostatin receptors.[5]

TABLE 27-2 Functional Classification of GI Regulatory Peptides

Peptide	Endocrine	Paracrine	Neurocrine	Autocrine
Somatostatin	+	+	+	+
Gastrin	+			
CCK*	+		+	
Secretin, GIP enteroglucagon	+			
Motilin	+			
Neurotensin	+		+	
PP, PYY	+			
NPY			+	
VIP/PHI			+	
Tachykinins (SP, SK, NK)			+	
Bombesins (GRP, NB)			+	
Opioids (dynorphin, met-enk)			+	
Galanin			+	
CGRP			+	

* CCK = cholecystokinin; CGRP = calcitonin gene-related peptide; GIP = glucose-dependent insulinotropic peptide; GRP = gastrin-releasing peptide; met-enk = methionine-enkephalin-Arg-Gly-Leu; NB = neuromedin B; NK = neuromedin K; NPY = neuropeptide Y; PHI = peptide histidine isoleucine; PP = pancreatic polypeptide; PYY = peptide YY; SK = substance K; SP = substance P; VIP = vasoactive intestinal polypeptide.

Source: From Makhlouf et al. with permission.[14]

TABLE 27-3 Summary of the Effects of Somatostatin

System	Effect Product/Function	Affected
Anterior pituitary		
Endocrine	Inhibition of secretion	Growth hormone Thyrotropin
Gastrointestinal tract		
Endocrine	Inhibition of gut hormone secretion	Gastrin Vasoactive intestinal polypeptide Motilin Neurotensin Gastric inhibitory peptide
Exocrine	Inhibition of secretion	Acid Pepsin Fluid/electrolytes
Absorption	Inhibition of absorption	Calcium Glucose Amino acids Triglycerides
Motility	Inhibition	Gastric emptying Small bowel transit time
Mucosal protection	Cytoprotection	Stomach Duodenum
Hemodynamics	Decrease in blood flow	Mesenteric and celiac arteries
Pancreas		
Endocrine	Inhibition of secretion	Insulin Glucagon Pancreatic polypeptide
Exocrine	Inhibition of secretion	Digestive enzymes Bicarbonate
Liver		
Hemodynamics	Decrease in blood flow	Portal vein
Exocrine	Inhibition of secretion	Bile acid–independent bile flow
Kidney		
Homeostasis	Fluid/electrolyte balance	Diuresis

Source: From O'Dorisio and Redfern with permission.[5]

In the stomach, somatostatin inhibits basal acid secretion and acid secretion stimulated by pentagastrin or a meal.[40,41] In addition, somatostatin may protect the gastroduodenal mucosa against injury (cytoprotective action) independently of the inhibition of acid secretion.[42,43] In the small intestine, somatostatin inhibits absorption (glucose, amino acids, triglycerides, and calcium) and suppresses fluid and electrolyte secretion induced by secretagogues (e.g., VIP and prostaglandins).[44–48] Intravenous administration of exogenous somatostatin in humans induces splanchnic arterial vasoconstriction, leading to a rapid and marked decrease in portal venous pressure and blood flow.[49]

Somatostatin inhibits both the exocrine and endocrine secretory functions of the pancreas. SS-14 and SS-28 inhibit the secretion of electrolytes and enzymes stimulated by a meal or by the administration of exogenous secretin, CCK, or a combination of the two.[50,51] Somatostatin strongly inhibits insulin, glucagon, and pancreatic polypeptide release and may also block its own release from pancreatic D cells.[27,50,52–54]

Clinical Relevance and Applications

Excess secretion of somatostatin resulting from somatostatinoma has been described.[55–57] Primary somatostatinomas usually occur in the pancreas but may also occur in the small intestine.[58] The major clinical manifestations of somatostatin hypersecretion include diabetes mellitus, steatorrhea, cholelithiasis, and achlorhydria.[59,60]

Hyposomatostatinemic states are not easily detectable, and no disease has been attributed to a deficiency of somatostatin secretion. However, patients with duodenal ulcer disease have been shown to have lower levels of somatostatin in the antral mucosa.[61,62] It is intriguing to speculate that diseases such as diabetic retinopathy, with its attendant neovascularization, may be related in part to a loss of somatostatin nerve fibers that are known to innervate the retina.[5]

Many of the inhibitory actions of somatostatin have important clinical applications in the treatment of acromegaly, endocrine tumors of the GEP system, the dumping syndrome, and secretory diarrhea.[5] However, the short half-lives of SS-14 and SS-28 (1.0 min and 2.3 min, respectively) limit their clinical usefulness.[63–65] Chemical synthesis of somatostatin-like peptides with considerably longer half-lives (e.g., octreotide with a half-life of 1.5 h) obviates this problem.[66,67]

The ability of somatostatin and octreotide to inhibit growth hormone and thyrotropin secretion has been successfully applied in the treatment of acromegaly and some forms of hyperthyroidism.[66,68] Both conditions can result from peptide-secreting tumors. Excess production of growth hormone results in the stimulation of hepatic somatomedin-C (also termed insulin-like growth factor-I or IGF-I) generation, which in turn acts at the tissue level to produce the characteristic clinical features of acromegaly.[69] Long-term treatment of patients with severe acromegaly resistant to surgery and/or radiation results in marked reduction in growth hormone and somatomedin-C levels (many patients return to normal levels) and a dramatic improvement in symptoms and physical findings (Fig. 27-2).[70]

Somatostatin or octreotide administration has been shown to reduce both the early and late symptoms of the dumping syndrome.[71–73] *Dumping syndrome*, a collective term for the symptoms associated with rapid gastric emptying, typically occurs in patients who have undergone gastric sugery (e.g., vagotomy and pyloroplasty, subtotal gastectomy, or gastroenterostomy). The mechanism by which somatostatin reduces the symptoms of the dumping syndrome has not been clearly established, but it may involve decreases in gastric emptying, intestinal motility, and gut hormone secretion (e.g., VIP, peptide YY, neurotensin, serotonin, insulin, glucagon, motilin, and bradykinin).[74–76]

The intestinal antisecretory effect of somatostatin and octreotide has clinical implications in the control of secretory diarrhea (Table 27-4). Somatostatin effectively inhibits diarrhea in patients with endocrine tumors that produce a neurohumoral agent that is capable of stimulating intestinal secretion [e.g., carcinoid syndrome, VIPomas/watery diarrhea syndrome (WDS)] and in some patients with AIDS (cryptosporidial diarrhea) in whom the secretagogue is an endotoxin.[77–82] In addition, there have

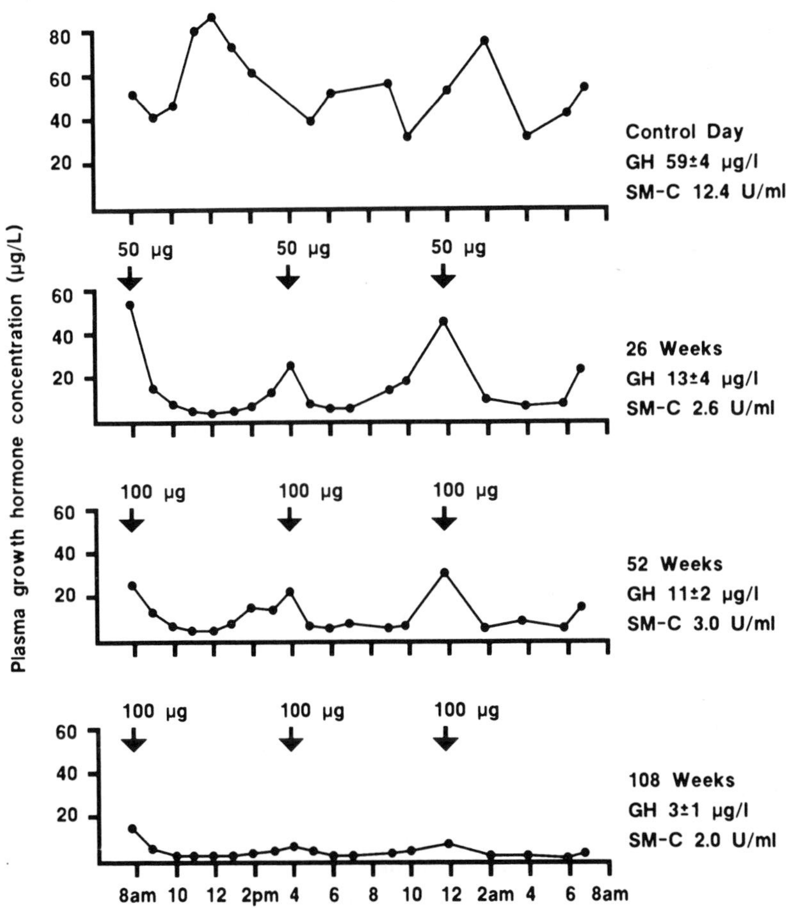

FIGURE 27-2 Plasma growth hormone levels measured over 24 h in an acromegalic patient at baseline and after 26, 52, and 108 weeks of octreotide therapy. Margin: mean 24-h plasma growth hormone and somatomedin-C levels. (*From Lamberts et al. with permission.*[70])

TABLE 27-4 Use of Octreotide in Controlling Secretory Diarrhea

Condition	Dose/Route	Comments	Reference
Carcinoid syndrome	50–150 μg SC bid	25 patients; 72% had decreased 5-HIAA in urine and 88% had symptomatic improvement	85
	100 μg SC bid, increased to 1000 μg/day	Diarrhea reduced in 83% of 12 patients; treatment up to 4 years slowed tumor growth in 67% of cases	86
VIPoma (pancreatic cholera syndrome)	100 μg SC bid	65-year-old female; reduced K^+, HCO_3^-, water loss; also lowered plasma levels of neurotensin, motilin, VIP, PP, GIP, glucagon	87
	100 μg SC bid	72-year-old female; decreased stool weight and plasma VIP	88
	50 μg SC bid	43-year-old male; possible shrinkage of tumor; diarrhea controlled for 14 months	89
	50 μg SC bid	2 patients; decreased hormone release with symptomatic improvement	90
	50 μg SC bid	5 patients; 4 patients had decreased VIP concentrations, and all showed symptomatic improvement	91
	50 μg/h IV	1 patient; male, 5 months; ganglioneuroblastoma; NPY also present; administration of up to 300 μg SC ineffective	92
	50 μg SC bid increased to tid	44-year-old female; reduction in jejunal and ileal secretion of fluid in perfusion study; decrease in stool output	93
	100–600 μg SC daily	4 patients; suppressed release of peptides with symptomatic improvements	94
	50–1000 μg daily	86% of patients improved or completely resolved diarrhea in 3 months	82
Gastrinoma	220–675 μg SC daily	25 patients; 60% improved, 30% unchanged, 10% worse	82
	1500 μg daily	9 patients with metastatic disease, 6 had reduction in symptoms; in 2, dose of H_2 blockers could be reduced	95
AIDS	100–300 μg SC, tid	1 patient; maintained 8 months 300 μg/kg tid without diarrhea; eats normal diet	77
	50 μg SC bid, increased to 200 μg SC, tid	1 patient; no demonstrable cryptosporidial infection; stopped diarrhea, and patient gained weight	78
	10–100 μg/hr IV	1 patient, cryptosporidiosis-positive; maintained on 75 μg/h for 9 months with a reduced severity of diarrhea	79
	100 μg SC bid	2 patients with cryptosporidiosis responded with reduced diarrhea; 2 patients with concomitant CMV infection did not respond well	96
Idiopathic diarrhea of infancy	1.9 μg/kg SC bid	1 patient; 60% decrease in stool output; possible tolerance at 26 weeks	84

SC = subcutaneous; bid = 2 times daily; tid = 3 times daily; 5-HIAA = 5-hydroxyindoleacetic acid; VIP = vasoactive intestinal peptide; IV = intravenous; GIP = gastric inhibitory peptide; PP = pancreatic polypeptide; NPY = neuropeptide Y; AIDS = acquired immunodeficiency syndrome; CMV = cytomegalovirus.

Source: Modified from Redfern et al. with permission.[97]

been reports of octreotide being used successfully in the treatment of infants with idiopathic secretory diarrhea.[83,84]

Somatostatin and octreotide are effective in inhibiting the release not only of regulatory peptides from neuroendocrine APUD cells but also of the target cells of specific tumor peptides. Therefore, octreotide has applications in the treatment of several types of neuroendocrine tumors of the GI tract, including carcinoid tumors, VIPomas, gastrinomas, glucagonomas, and insulinomas (Table 27-5), and their target organ manifestations (e.g., secretory diarrhea, gastric acid hypersecretion, skin rash).

Because of the excellent safety profile and virtual lack of significant dose-limiting side effects of octreotide, it will undoubtedly continue to be useful for many clinically expressed GEP endocrine tumors. Further, octreotide represents a prototype of future long-acting gut peptide congeners.

Gastrin

Gastrin belongs to the gastrin/cholecystokinin peptide family, which is characterized by the presence of a common amino acid sequence at the carboxy-terminal end: Gly-Trp-Met-Asp-Phe amide.[98] The biological activity of all peptides in this family is believed to reside in this carboxy-terminal sequence.[2] This similarity in sequence results in some degree of overlap in the biological actions of these peptides and the ability of CCK to antagonize gastrin's interaction with its receptor.[99]

Gastrin exists in several biologically active molecular forms: G17 ("little" gastrin), G34 ("big" gastrin), and G14 (minigastrin).[100] The amino acid sequence of G14 is identical to the first 14 amino acids of G17 from the C-terminal end; the amino acid sequence of G17 is identical to G34 for the first 16 amino acids from the C-terminal end. G34 and G17 are the most abundant circulating gastrin species, followed by smaller amounts of G14.[101] A larger precursor called preprogastrin (101 amino acids) also exists and gives rise to smaller gastrin peptides after posttranslational enzymatic cleavage.[102] All gastrin species may exist in both nonsulfated (gastrin I) and sulfated (gastrin II) forms.[101] However, sulfation is not necessary for biological activity, and both forms appear in approximately equal amounts in blood and tissues.[101]

TABLE 27–5 Efficacy of Octreotide (Sandostatin) on GEP Peptide-Producing Tumors

Tumor	Sign/Symptom	Dose	Clinical Response (1–10)*	Comment
Gastrinoma[82,103,104]	Zollinger-Ellison syndrome	220–675 μg daily	6	Diarrhea, abdominal pain improved; very high dose may be needed
Carcinoid syndrome[66,80,85,86]	Carcinoid syndrome Flushing/diarrhea	150–450 μg tid	9.5	Flushing and wheezing most responsive; tumor shrinkage (>50%) at very high doses noted in 17% of patients
VIPomas[66,82,103]	Watery diarrhea syndrome	250 μg daily	8	Excellent direct correlation between somatostatin receptors and clinical response to octreotide
Glucagonoma[82,94,103]	Glucagonoma syndrome	200–300 μg daily	8, rash 10, diarrhea	Rash responds over time Diarrhea responds Diabetes mellitus improves in 50% of patients
Insulinoma[66,82]	Hypoglycemia	200–675 μg daily	4.5	Must watch for worsening of hypoglycemia
PPoma[66,82]	Asymptomatic or diarrhea (rare)	250–320 μg daily	10	Diarrhea, when present, resolves

* 1 = poor response; 10 = best response.

PP = pancreatic polypeptide.

Source: Modified from O'Dorisio and Redfern with permission.[5]

Biological Actions

Gastrin has a wide range of biological effects on the epithelium and smooth muscle of the GI tract, although many of these actions are probably pharmacologic rather than physiologic (Table 27-6).[100,101,105] The most notable physiologic action of gastrin is its potent ability to stimulate gastric acid secretion.[106,107] Gastrin released into the circulation in response to a protein meal can completely account for the meal-induced increase in gastric acid secretion.[108] This observation substantiates the physiologic role of gastrin in the regulation of acid secretion.[108] Gastrin plays a major role in mediating the acid secretory response to gastric distension but only a minor role in mediating the cephalic phase of gastric acid secretion.[2]

Gastrin exhibits a trophic effect on the GI tract (especially the pyloric mucosa) and pancreas, an action clearly demonstrated by its ability to stimulate mucosal cell proliferation and the synthesis of DNA, RNA, and protein.[100,109] Hypertrophy of the pyloric (but not antral) gastric mucosa is a notable feature of the Zollinger-Ellison syndrome, a disease characterized by hypergastrinemia (see Gastrinoma below).[110]

Clinical Relevance and Applications

Excess secretion of gastrin is associated with a number of disease states, the best known of which is the Zollinger-Ellison syndrome.[111] This syndrome, which is characterized by excess secretion of gastric acid, severe peptic ulcer disease, and profuse diarrhea, occurs as a consequence of a gastrin-producing, non-beta-islet cell tumor (gastrinoma).[58] Hypergastrinemia is also associated with antral G-cell hyperfunction,[112,113] isolated retained antrum (after a Billroth II gastrectomy),[114] atrophic gastritis,[115] pernicious anemia,[116] vagotomy,[117] uremia,[2] and antisecretory drugs.[118,119] No disease states are known to be associated with hyposecretion of gastrin.

Gastrin has no clinical therapeutic applications, but pentagastrin, a synthetic short-acting analogue of the carboxy-terminal pentapeptide, is used diagnostically to identify patients with achlorhydria and to evaluate gastric acid secretion in patients with peptic ulcer disease who are undergoing vagotomy.[2] Pentagastrin is also useful in the diagnosis of medullary carcinoma of the thyroid. A circulating calcitonin concentration of >400 pg/mL after intravenous infusion of pentagastrin (0.5 μg/kg body weight) is highly suggestive of medullary thyroid carcinoma. It should be noted that the pentagastrin/gastrin-induced calcitonin response is not paradoxic but consists of accentuation of the normal response. Pentagastrin is also used clinically to assess the severity of symptoms (especially flushing attacks induced by eating) associated with carcinoid tumor or medullary carcinoma of the thyroid.[120] Measurement of basal and secretin-stimulated circulating gastrin concentrations by radioimmunoassay is commonly used to detect patients with gastrinomas.[121,122]

TABLE 27-6 Actions of Gastrin

Water and electrolyte secretion Stomach Pancreas Liver Small intestine Brunner's glands	Stimulation of smooth muscle Lower esophageal sphincter Stomach Small intestine Colon Gallbladder
Enzyme secretion Stomach Pancreas Small intestine	Release of hormones Insulin Calcitonin
Inhibition of water/salt/glucose absorption Small intestine	Increase in blood flow Stomach Small intestine Pancreas
Inhibition of smooth muscle Pyloric sphincter Ileocecal sphincter	Trophic action Gastric mucosa Small intestinal mucosa Pancreas

Source: From Dockray and Gregory with permission.[100]

Cholecystokinin

CCK, like gastrin, exists in a variety of biologically active molecular forms, each of which is derived from prepro-CCK (114-amino acid peptide): CCK-58, CCK-39, CCK-33, CCK-22, CCK-8, CCK-5, and CCK-4.[123] However, whether all these molecular forms function as true circulating hormones or whether some simply represent degradation products remains to be elucidated. Hydrolytic products of luminal fat and protein digestion are potent stimulators of CCK release into the circulation. In humans, the principal circulating molecular species after the ingestion of a meal are CCK-8, CCK-22, and CCK-33.[124]

In contrast to gastrin, which naturally exists in both sulfated and nonsulfated forms, all circulating molecular forms of CCK are sulfated.[99] Indeed, sulfation of the tyrosine residue at position 7 (from the C-terminal end) is critical for full biological potency.[101]

Biological Actions

One of the principal effects of CCK is stimulation of gallbladder contraction and pancreatic enzyme secretion.[123] These effects are the key physiologic actions of CCK after the ingestion of a meal.[2,125] CCK also has a wide range of biological actions, including secretory, absorptive, and motor actions on the GI tract (Table 27-7). In addition, this peptide exhibits a trophic effect on the pancreas and may mediate the satiety response after eating.[123]

TABLE 27-7 Biological Effects of CCK

Gastrointestinal secretion
Stimulates pancreatic enzyme secretion
Induces hypertrophy and hyperplasia of pancreas
Stimulates gastric acid secretion (weak agonist)
Increases intestinal lymph flow
Releases intestinal peptidases
Gastrointestinal motility
Causes gallbladder contraction
Relaxes Oddi's sphincter
Decreases gastric emptying rate
Decreases LES* pressure
Increases small intestinal motility and decreases transit time
Increases colonic motility
Hormone release
Enhances insulin release
Increases secretion of
Somatostatin (pancreas)
Pancreatic polypeptide
Gastric inhibitory polypeptide
Calcitonin
Food intake
Decreases after intraventricular administration

* LES = lower esophageal sphincter.

Source: From Walsh with permission.[101]

Clinical Relevance and Applications

No recognized disease states are associated with hypersecretion or hyposecretion of CCK. Because of its extensive biological actions, however, CCK has a number of potential clinical applications.[2] For example, the ability of exogenous CCK to stimulate gallbladder contraction is used in radiographic and ultrasonic evaluation of gallbladder emptying.[126] CCK may also have potential clinical use in the treatment of obesity (by suppressing appetite) and the treatment of exocrine pancreatic deficiency (by increasing the size of the pancreas).[2]

Secretin

The secretin family of peptides is the largest group of GI hormones and includes vasoactive intestinal polypeptide and gastric inhibitory peptide.[4] This group also includes pancreatic glucagon, peptide histidine isoleucine [or peptide histidine methionine (PHM)], growth hormone releasing factor (GHRF), oxyntomodulin, and glicentin [glucagon-like peptide (GLP)]. GIP and VIP are discussed below.

Secretin, a linear 27-amino acid peptide, was discovered in 1902 by Bayliss and Starling and represents the first gastrointestinal hormone described.[1] The principal stimulus for the release of secretin into the circulation is acidification of the duodenum ($pH < 4.5$), although fatty acids and amino acids are also capable of inducing secretin release.[127]

Biological Actions

The primary physiologic action of circulating secretin is stimulation of pancreatic secretion of water and bicarbonate.[128,129] Secretin potentiates the actions of CCK in stimulating pancreatic water and bicarbonate secretion and inhibits gastrin release and gastric acid secretion.[127,101] Secretin also has a wide range of effects, such as delaying gastric emptying; relaxing the lower esophageal sphincter; stimulating secretion of hepatic bile, pepsinogen, and gastric mucus; inducing adipose tissue lipolysis; and releasing insulin (Table 27-8).[127] However, it is not established whether these effects are physiologic or pharmacologic phenomena.

Clinical Relevance and Applications

Hypersecretinemia has been reported to be associated with the Zollinger-Ellison syndrome, duodenal ulcer disease (in combination with gastric acid

TABLE 27-8 Biological Effects of Secretin

System Affected	Response
Water-electrolyte secretion	
Stomach acid	↓
Pancreas	↑
Liver	↑
Brunner's glands	↑
Enzyme secretion	
Stomach	↑
Pancreas	↑↓
Intestine	↑
Endocrine secretion	
Gastrin	↓
Insulin	↑
Glucagon	↑↓
Somatostatin	↑
Smooth muscle	
Lower esophageal sphincter	↓
Stomach	↓
Small and large intestine	↓
Gallbladder	↑
Oddi's sphincter	↓
Growth	
Gastric mucosa	↓
Pancreas	↑↓
Metabolic	
Lipolysis	↑
Cardiovascular system	
Heart rate	↑
Stroke volume	↑
Blood flow	
Superior mesenteric artery	↑
Hepatic artery	↓
Gastric mucosal artery	↓
Pancreatic artery	↑
Small intestinal artery	↑

↓ = inhibition; ↑ = stimulation; ↑↓ = inconclusive.

Source: From Chey and Chang with permission.[127]

hypersecretion), and chronic renal failure.[130] The underlying cause of increased circulating levels of secretin in these disease states is unclear, although decreased renal clearance of secretin may contribute to hypersecretinemia in renal failure.[131] This supposition is strengthened by the prolonged $t_{1/2}$ of secretin in azotemic patients compared to normal subjects (6 min vs. 2.4 min).[130] Further, elevation of circulating secretin levels (in addition to gastrin) in gastrinoma patients may produce mild antagonism of endogenous gastrin, since secretin is known to inhibit gastric acid secretion.

Hyposecretinemia occurs in some patients with celiac disease and achlorhydria.[132,133] Malabsorption in patients with celiac disease may be a consequence of a diminished pancreatic secretory response to the ingestion of a meal as well as the marked loss of intestinal absorptive area associated with denudation of the villi.[2] Patients with celiac sprue exhibit a markedly attenuated secretin response to acidification of the duodenum, an observation which may explain the poor meal-stimulated pancreatic secretory output.[132]

Secretin has two principal diagnostic uses in gastroenterology: evaluation of the secretory function of the exocrine pancreas and identification of patients with gastrin-secreting tumors (gastrinomas).[2] Typically, pancreatic secretory testing is performed in duodenally intubated patients by means of intravenous secretin administration in a dose of 2 U/kg, alone or in combination with CCK.[134] The volume, electrolyte composition, and amylase output of pancreatic juices secreted into the duodenum are subsequently determined. This approach is useful in evaluating the involvement of the pancreas in patients who exhibit intestinal malabsorption and identifying patients with pancreatic cancer or chronic pancreatitis.

In the majority of patients with gastrinoma, the condition may be diagnosed by the prompt increase in circulating gastrin concentrations after the intravenous administration of secretin (Fig. 27-3).[135,136] The mechanism for this increase is unknown, but is considered paradoxic. In normal subjects, secretin produces a minimal effect on basal gastrin concentrations and actually inhibits gastrin release induced by the ingestion of a meal. An absolute gastrin rise of 200 pg/mL following 2 U/kg secretin bolus is considered diagnostic of gastrinoma.[137]

By increasing pancreatic blood flow, secretin may also be helpful in localizing vascular or endocrine tumors by angiography.[138]

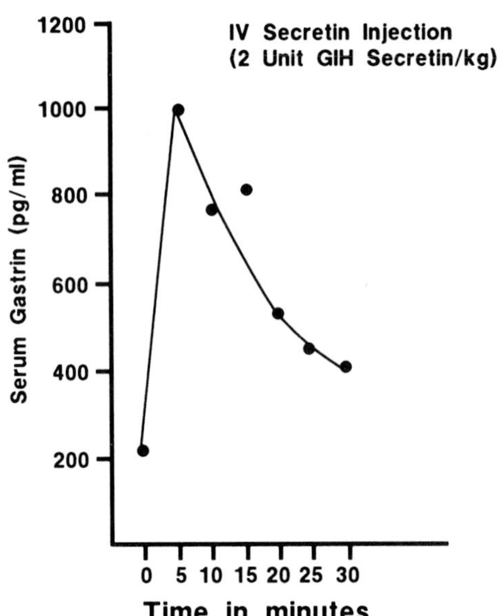

FIGURE 27-3 Rapid increase in serum gastrin concentrations in response to secretin in patients with gastrinoma. Note that an absolute increase of 200 pg/ml over basal values is very suggestive of gastrinoma. (*From McGuigan with permission.*[137])

Vasoactive Intestinal Polypeptide

Vasoactive intestinal polypeptide, which was first isolated from hog intestine by Said and Mutt, is a 28-amino acid single-chain linear peptide.[139–142] VIP is released from the peripheral nervous system, specifically after stimulation of preganglionic parasympathetic nerves or stimulation by a local electrical field.[143] Release of VIP into the circulation occurs after the introduction of hydrochloric acid, fat, or ethanol into the duodenum.[144] Amino acids, glucose, and a mixed meal do not affect VIP release.[144] It has been suggested that the appearance of VIP in the circulation represents a spillover phenomenon resulting from the release of neural VIP.[4,143] Indeed, the primary regulatory role of VIP is one of neurocrine rather than endocrine function.[58]

Biological Actions

The physiologic function of VIP has not been unequivocally established. However, neural release of VIP has been implicated in several physiologic events in animals, including gastric relaxation produced by vagal stimulation or lower esophageal distension, intestinal vasodilation after mechanical stimulation of the mucosa, colonic vasodilation induced by stimulation of pelvic nerves, and atropine-resistant vagal stimulation of pancreatic bicarbonate secretion.[101]

While VIP has a limited known physiologic role, its pharmacologic effects are diverse (Table 27-9). VIP administered in vivo or in vitro influences gastrointestinal and respiratory smooth muscle, gastrointestinal secretion, hormone release, hepatic and adipocyte metabolism, and the central nervous system.[143]

Clinical Relevance and Applications

No clinical abnormality of the GI tract has been attributed to a deficiency of VIP. However, VIP may

TABLE 27-9 Pharmacologic Actions of VIP

Cardiovascular system	Digestive system
Vasodilation	Esophagus
Chronotropic effect	Relaxation of lower esophageal sphincter
Inotropic effect	Contraction in body
Endocrine system	Stomach
Pancreas	Relaxation of antral/fundic smooth muscle
Release of insulin, glucagon, somatostatin, pancreatic polypeptide	Relaxation of muscularis mucosa
Thyroid	Inhibition of acid/pepsin secretion
Hormone secretion	Small intestine
Adrenal	Relaxation/contraction of circular smooth muscle
Steroidogenesis	Contraction of longitudinal smooth muscle
Kidney	Stimulation of water and ion secretion
Stimulation of renin secretion	Stimulation of Brunner's gland secretion
Pituitary-hypothalamus	Large intestine
Stimulation of prolactin release	Relaxation of smooth muscle
Inhibition of somatostatin release	Water and chloride secretion
Urogenital system	Gallbladder
Inhibition of myoelectrical and smooth muscle activity	Relaxation of smooth muscle
Potentiation of electrically induced and pilocarpine-induced prostatic secretion	Inhibition of fluid and NaCl absorption
Respiratory system	Liver
Bronchodilation	Stimulation of biliary secretion
Stimulation of submucosal gland secretion	Pancreas
Metabolism	Stimulation of water and bicarbonate secretion
Lipolysis	
Glycogenolysis	

Source: From Fahrenkrug with permission.[143]

be deficient in the pulmonary nerve fibers of patients with asthma.[145] Decreased VIP levels in asthmatic patients may contribute to the bronchial smooth muscle hyperreactivity that is characteristic of this disease.[146,147]

Excess secretion of VIP occurs as a result of non-beta-cell pancreatic tumors (VIPomas).[58] Prolonged hypersecretion of VIP produces severe watery diarrhea, profound hypokalemia, flushing, hypochlorhydria, and hypercalcemia.[148–152] This syndrome, which has been described by two independent groups,[150,151] was initially called watery diarrhea syndrome (WDS) but is now commonly referred to as VIPoma/WDS.[150,151] The efficacy of octreotide in the treatment of VIPoma was discussed above (Table 27-4). Other tumors associated with increased levels of circulating VIP include ganglioneuroblastoma, pheochromocytoma, and medullary carcinoma of the thyroid[58]; the latter rarely has high circulating VIP levels.

Currently, VIP has no therapeutic applications, and its clinical usefulness is limited to serving as a marker for VIP-producing tumors.

Gastric Inhibitory Polypeptide (Glucose-Dependent Insulinotropic Peptide)

GIP, which originally was isolated as a contaminant of partially purified CCK by Brown in 1970, is a 42-amino acid peptide and one of the largest members of the secretin family.[153,154] The peptide was named gastric acid inhibitory polypeptide because of its potent ability to inhibit gastric acid secretion. Indeed, GIP was identified and isolated on the basis of its gastric acid inhibitory actions.[155]

GIP circulates in at least two molecular forms: One species corresponds to GIP_{1-42} with a molecular mass of 5 kDa, and the other species probably corresponds to a prohormone with a higher molecular mass of 8 kDa.[155] GIP is released into the circulation in response to the ingestion of a mixed meal or specific meal components, such as carbohydrates (glucose), triglycerides (long-chain fatty acid triglycerides), and amino acids (arginine, histidine, isoleucine, lysine, and threonine).[156–160] Typically, circulating GIP remains elevated for approximately 6 h postprandially, and peak levels may be up to six times the basal values.

Biological Actions

GIP has diverse actions on the GI tract, pancreas, and other organ systems (Table 27-10).[155] The major biological actions of GIP include enhancement of insulin release; inhibition of gastric acid, pepsin, and gastrin secretion; and inhibition of intestinal electrolyte and water absorption, leading to a net secretory state. The principal physiologic role of GIP appears to be augmentation of insulin release in response to

TABLE 27-10 Biological Effects of GIP

Reduction in gastric secretion
 Acid
 Pepsin
 Gastrin
Augmentation of insulin secretion in the presence of glucose or amino acids
Inhibition of gastrointestinal motility
 Lower esophageal sphincter
 Stomach
 Small intestine
Increase in small intestinal secretion
Increase in mesenteric blood flow
Stimulation of exocrine pancreatic secretion (in vitro)
Release of anterior pituitary hormones

orally or intraduodenally administered glucose or amino acids.[4,101,155] In studies conducted by Duprè on humans, GIP administered intravenously with glucose augmented insulin secretion and improved glucose tolerance.[161–163] This insulinotropic effect was also achieved with intravenous amino acid combined with GIP.[164] GIP may also participate in the physiologic regulation of gastric acid secretion, although this role has not been fully established.[4,101,155]

Clinical Relevance and Applications

Clearly defined clinical syndromes associated with an excess or deficiency of GIP have not been described. However, in patients with diabetes mellitus, chronic pancreatitis, duodenal ulcer, dumping syndrome, or obesity, an exaggerated GIP response to glucose or fat has been noted (Fig. 27-4).[165–170] The clinical significance of these observations remains to be established.

FIGURE 27-4 Enhanced release of GIP into the circulation in response to oral glucose (50 g) in patients with adult-onset diabetes mellitus. Mean integrated increment in GIP from 0 to 2 h was significantly different between normals and diabetics ($p < 0.01$). *(From Brown et al. with permission.*[165]*)*

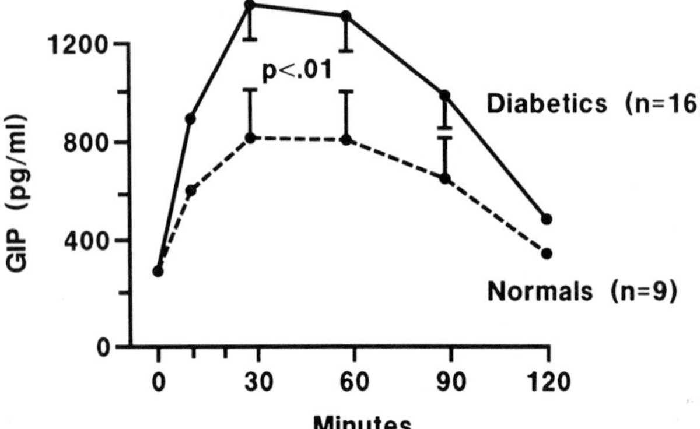

Motilin

Motilin, a 22-amino acid peptide, was originally isolated and purified from the canine small intestine by Brown and colleagues in 1971.[171,172] Based on the ability of the purified material to stimulate gastric motor activity, Brown named the peptide motilin. As with members of the secretin family, the biological activity of motilin is attributed to the amino-terminal sequence rather than the carboxy-terminal sequence.[173]

In humans, circulating levels of motilin are increased after acidification of the duodenum and decreased or unaltered after alkalinization.[174–177] Small increases in plasma motilin occur in response to fat, although a mixed meal produces a sustained decrease in circulating motilin levels.[177–179] The primary action of motilin is probably that of a paracrine versus endocrine regulatory substance.

Biological Actions

Motilin primarily affects the GI tract.[173] In humans and dogs, motilin induces the appearance of activity fronts corresponding to phase III of migrating motor complexes in the antroduodenal region (similar to those seen during fasting).[180–182] These complexes subsequently migrate along the small intestine from their gastric point of origin. The induction of activity fronts can also be achieved by alkalinization or acidification of the duodenum.[178] In this experimental situation, fluctuations in migrating motor complexes correlate closely with increases in circulating motilin concentrations, suggesting that motilin is intimately involved in the regulation of interdigestive motility.[178]

Motilin also increases lower esophageal pressure, delays gastric emptying of a liquid meal (but accelerates gastric emptying of a solid meal), and stimulates gastric pepsin secretion.[173]

Clinical Relevance and Applications

Several disease states have been associated with hyper- or hypomotilinemia, but the clinical significance of this association has not been elucidated. Although specific endocrine tumors that secrete motilin have not been identified, elevated circulating (fasting) motilin concentrations have been reported in patients with diabetes and patients with diarrhea associated with carcinoid syndrome, inflammatory bowel disease, infectious diarrhea, tropical malabsorption, and small bowel resection.[183–186] Reduced circulating motilin levels are associated with hyperthyroidism and pregnancy.[187,188] Motilin may have therapeutic potential in restoring normal intestinal motility patterns after abdominal surgery, although the preliminary results have been disappointing.[189] Recent work suggests that the antibiotic erythromycin and its derivatives stimulate GI motor activity by interacting with motilin receptors.[190–193] Erythromycin has been demonstrated to enhance motility in patients with gastroparesis, possibly through the motilin receptor on smooth muscle.[194]

Pancreatic Polypeptide Family

Members of this group of peptides include pancreatic polypeptide (PP), peptide tyrosine tyrosine (PYY), and neuropeptide Y (NPY). Each member consists of a 36-amino acid linear peptide with a carboxy-terminal tyrosine amide.[4] PP is the most extensively studied peptide in this family and is predominantly located in the islets of the pancreas and to a lesser extent in the exocrine parenchyma.[195] PYY, which originally was isolated and characterized by Tatemoto in the duodenum, is primarily localized in the hindgut (terminal ileum, colon, and rectum).[196,197] The neurotransmitter NPY, which was identified initially in extracts of porcine brain, is widely distributed in the central nervous system (e.g., frontal, parietal, and temporal lobes; hypothalamus; caudate; median eminence; and pineal gland) and the peripheral nervous system, notably in the GI tract, respiratory tract, heart, peripheral blood vessels, kidney, and spleen.[195,198]

The release of PP into the circulation occurs in a biphasic manner after a meal.[195] This pattern of meal-induced PP secretion may represent the overall effects of three phases of PP release: cephalic-vagal, gastric, and intestinal. In the *cephalic-vagal phase*, the release of PP occurs as a result of the sight, smell, and taste of food.[199] In the *gastric phase*, PP release is induced by gastric distension (possibly involving vagovagal or gastropancreatic reflexes) and by direct interaction of food components (e.g., amino acids) with receptors within the gastric mucosa.[195] In the *intestinal phase*, PP release results from the presence of fat, amino acids, and glucose in the proximal small intestine.[200] It remains unclear whether the intestinal phase of PP release is an indirect result of the release of other GI peptides (e.g., CCK) which subsequently induce the release of PP from the pancreas, or a direct result of absorbed nutritients stimulating the pancreas to release PP.[195]

Biological Actions

The biological actions of PP are varied and include alterations in gastric, intestinal, and pancreatic secretion; GI and gallbladder motility; and hormone release (Table 27-11). The actions of PP vary considerably among species, and whether they are inhibitory or stimulatory often depends on the experimental conditions. For example, in humans PP produced no effect on basal or pentagastrin-stimulated gastric acid and pepsin secretion, whereas in dogs PP stimulated basal gastric acid secretion but inhibited pentagastrin-stimulated gastric acid secretion.[201,202] The physiologic significance of PP secretion in humans remains to be clarified.

TABLE 27-11 Biological Actions of Pancreatic Polypeptide

Gastric secretion
Increases basal secretion
Inhibits pentagastrin-stimulated secretion
Intestinal secretion
Induces fluid and electrolyte secretion (small/large intestine)
Pancreatic secretion
Inhibits fluid, bicarbonate, and protein secretions
Motility
Esophagus: increases lower esophageal sphincter
Stomach: stimulates gastric emptying
Intestine: increases transit time
Gallbladder: relaxes gallbladder smooth muscle
Hormone secretion
Decreases plasma motilin and somatostatin levels

Clinical Relevance and Applications

Several endocrine tumors may be associated with excess secretion of PP, including carcinoid tumors, VIPomas, glucagonomas, gastrinomas, insulinomas, and multiple endocrine adenomatosis type I (MEAI).[203–205] Elevated circulating levels of PP are frequently observed in patients with VIPomas, and PP is thought to contribute to the clinical diarrheal symptoms of the VIPoma syndrome.[195,206] Elevated circulating concentrations of PP have also been reported in patients with juvenile and maturity-onset diabetes mellitus and renal disease.[207,208]

Clinical conditions associated with decreased secretion of PP include cystic fibrosis, obesity, and acute pancreatitis, especially in patients who exhibit steatorrhea and pancreatic calcification.[209–211] Indeed, several animal studies have indicated that PP may have potential in the treatment of acute pancreatitis.[212] However, clinical studies of the therapeutic potential of PP in treating pancreatitis have not been reported.

Neurotensin

Neurotensin was initially discovered in extracts of bovine hypothalami in 1973 by Carraway and Leeman.[213] These investigators sequenced and synthesized this 13-amino acid peptide several years later.[214,215] In several species, including humans, neurotensin appears to be preferentially localized in the small intestinal mucosa and is particularly concentrated in the ileum.[216] The functional properties of neurotensin reside in the carboxy-terminal region, as indicated by full intrinsic biological activity of the peptide NT_{8-13}.[217]

Neurotensin is released into the circulation after the ingestion of a mixed meal or fat but not in response to isocaloric amino acid and glucose solutions.[218,219] Several neuropeptides, notably bombesin and its relative, gastrin-releasing peptide, induce neurotensin release in humans, but the significance of this effect is unknown.[220,221]

Biological Actions

Neurotensin produces a myriad of effects on the GI system, including inhibition of gastric acid secretion, motility, and emptying; alterations in intestinal blood flow and motility; and modulation of endocrine and exocrine pancreatic function (Table 27-12).[216] Many of the biological effects of exogenously administered neurotensin are similar to the alterations in GI function observed after the ingestion of lipid, suggesting that neurotensin may play a pivotal role in postprandial lipid digestion.[216] However, the physiologic role of neurotensin in regulating GI function has not been fully delineated.

Clinical Relevance and Applications

Disease states correlated with a deficiency of neurotensin have not been described. However, elevated circulating levels of neurotensin may occur in some patients with pancreatic endocrine tumors and carcinoid tumors.[222] Specific symptoms attributed to hypersecretion of neurotensin have not been defined. Currently, neurotensin has no clinical therapeutic applications.

Substance P

Substance P, an 11-amino acid peptide, was discovered in 1931 in extracts of equine intestine by von Euler and Gaddum.[223] The letter P, an abbreviation for "preparation," was used by those authors to mark a perturbation on a kymograph tracing produced by the substance contained in intestinal extracts. Substance P belongs to the tachykinin peptide family, of which bombesin, substance K, neuromedin K, neuromedin B, and gastrin-releasing peptide are members.[224] Eleven nonmammalian tachykinins have also been identified, including eledoisin, physalaemin, and phyllomedusin.[224]

Substance P is distributed widely in the GI tract, but the highest concentrations are found in the proximal small intestine.[225,226] Most of the substance P in the GI tract is located in the myenteric and submucosal plexuses, but small amounts are also present in endocrine cells.[4,227] Substance P is also found outside the gut in the spinal cord, the spinal ganglia, the vagus, and most peripheral nerves.[101]

Although functioning primarily as a neurotransmitter or neuromodulator in the central and peripheral nervous systems, substance P appears in the vasculature of the small intestine during peristalsis, suggesting a physiologic role.[228,229] However, the factors that influence the release of substance P have not been fully elucidated.

TABLE 27-12 Gastrointestinal Actions of Neurotensin

Stomach
Decrease in gastric acid and pepsin secretion, motility, emptying, blood flow
Alteration in antroduodenal motor activity
Small intestine
Inhibition of motility, intestinal absorption of water and electrolytes
Increase in intestinal fluid secretion and blood flow
Increase in intestinal capillary permeability
Pancreas
Stimulation of pancreatic exocrine secretion
Release of glucagon, insulin, pancreatic polypeptide

Biological Actions

Substance P markedly decreases systemic blood pressure, stimulates smooth muscle contractions and salivary flow, and induces small intestinal secretion.[224] The most striking effect of substance P is its potent spasmogenic effect on GI smooth muscle.[224] Whether this spasmogenic response represents a direct action on smooth muscle or an indirect effect via myenteric neurons is unclear. It remains to be determined whether substance P functions as a physiologic modulator of GI function.

Clinical Relevance and Applications

Clinical conditions associated with decreased tissue content of substance P include Hirschsprung's disease and Huntington's chorea.[230] Hirschsprung's disease (congenital megacolon) is characterized by a narrowing of the rectosigmoid colon caused by the congenital absence of ganglion cells from the myenteric and submucosal plexuses (aganglionosis). Decreased content of substance P has been observed in aganglionic segments of the large intestine, suggesting the involvement of substance P in the pathophysiology of this disease.[231]

Elevated tissue content and significantly increased circulating concentrations of substance P have been noted in patients with carcinoid tumors, suggesting that substance P contributes to the clinical features of the carcinoid syndrome.[8] The involvement of substance P and other peptide hormones in the carcinoid syndrome is discussed in detail in the following section.

CARCINOID SYNDROME

Carcinoid syndrome represents a spectrum of symptoms and physical findings resulting from the release of potent biologically active products from primary carcinoid tumors and their associated metastases. Carcinoid tumors are slow-growing neoplasms that originate from the ubiquitous Kulchitsky's or enterochromaffin cells, which in turn form part of the APUD system.[19,232] These tumors constitute a relentlessly progressive type of cancer and represent well the indolent, episodic clinically expressed behavior of endocrine cancers of the GEP system.

Carcinoid tumors are the most frequently occurring primary APUD tumors of the small intestine and, for that matter, of the whole GEP endocrine system. Approximately 25 percent of all small bowel tumors and 46 percent of all malignant tumors of the small bowel are attributable to carcinoid tumors.[10–12] Although the incidence of carcinoid tumors is relatively low (estimated incidence of 1.5 cases per 100,000 population per year), these neoplasms are among the best-known tumors of the GI tract, partly because of their dramatic symptoms when they metastasize to the liver.[10]

The first description of a tumor with the morphological characteristics of carcinoid tumors appeared in 1838,[233] but it was not until 1907 that the name *Karzinoide* ("carcinoid") was used.[234] The collection of symptoms and physical findings now termed the carcinoid syndrome was first described in 1954 by Thorson and associates, who observed right-sided valvular disease, asthma, cyanosis, and peripheral vascular disease in a series of patients with small intestinal primary carcinoids and liver metastases.[235]

Although once exclusively attributed to secretion of biogenic amines, notably 5-hydroxytryptamine (5-HT), the symptoms that often accompany carcinoid tumors are now believed to result from secretion of additional substances such as motilin, neuropeptide K, kinins, and prostaglandins.[7–9]

Pathology

Typically, primary carcinoid tumors develop in the GI tract, especially in the appendix, terminal ileum, and rectum.[7] Other GI sites include the colon, stomach, duodenum, and Meckel's diverticulum. In rare instances, primary carcinoid tumors may also occur in the biliary tract, pancreatic duct, bronchus, esophagus, thymus, and ovary.[9,58]

Carcinoid tumors in the GI tract may be classified as foregut, midgut, or hindgut, based on their anatomic location.[236] *Foregut* carcinoid tumors are located in the stomach and proximal duodenum; *midgut* tumors are located in the distal duodenum, small intestine, ascending colon, and proximal transverse colon; and *hindgut* tumors are located in the distal transverse colon, descending colon, and rectum. Midgut tumors, which are associated most frequently with carcinoid syndrome, are described as classical carcinoids, whereas foregut and hindgut tumors are described as atypical carcinoids.[7]

Primary tumors are usually small (<1 cm in diameter) and consequently are rarely identified during routine radiologic procedures. Furthermore, primary tumors are usually asymptomatic; for example, in a review of 3718 carcinoid tumor cases by Wilson and associates, only 3.7 percent of patients with carcinoid tumors exhibited signs and symptoms of the carcinoid syndrome.[237] Carcinoid syndrome is frequently associated with primary tumors of the ileum and jejunum but not usually with tumors of the stomach, duodenum, and ovary. Bronchial carcinoid tumors give rise to the most severe clinical features of carcinoid syndrome, including prolonged flushing attacks, disorientation, anxiety, rhinorrhea, bronchospasm, and fever.[9]

Large primary tumors (>2 cm in diameter), especially of the midgut, almost inevitably metastasize, whereas smaller tumors (<1 cm) metastasize in only 2 percent of patients.[10,11,237] Mesenteric lymph nodes, liver, and peritoneum represent the principal metastatic sites, but the tumor may also spread to the lung, bone, skin, ovary, brain, mediastinum, and spleen.[7] Mesenteric lymphatic metastases may induce abnormal bowel distension, fixation, or filling patterns that may become visible with barium contrast radiography.[9]

Histologically, carcinoid tumor cells from the midgut, appendix, and colon are monomorphous with small, dark oval nuclei; they display few mitotic figures. Tumors in the small intestine take the form of insular-like tumor buds that occasionally anastomose.[7] Tumor cells from these locations show an argentaffin reaction with silver stains, whereas tumor cells from bronchial, gastric, and pancreatic carcinoids exhibit an argyrophilic reaction.[7]

Immunohistochemical studies of carcinoid tumor tissue from the stomach, small and large intestines, liver, lung, ovary, prostate, and thymus reveal the presence of chromogranin A and synaptophysin.[238–241] Chromogranin A belongs to a family of proteins (the chromatogranins/secretogranins) that are stored with peptide hormones and neuropeptides in secretory granules of endocrine cells and neurons.[238–241] The presence of chromogranin A in carcinoid tumors (together with neuronal-specific enolase) suggests that these tumors are derived from neuroendocrine tissue. Interestingly, chromogranin A may be the precursor for pancreastatin, a 49-amino acid peptide that is capable of inhibiting glucose-stimulated insulin release and acid secretion in rats.[241] Synaptophysin, which originally was isolated from neuronal presynaptic vesicles, is an integral membrane protein of small vesicular organelles in both endocrine cells and neurons.[238]

Although their precise biological function is unclear, chromogranin A, pancreastatin, and synaptophysin may serve as useful markers for both normal and neoplastic neuroendocrine cells and tissues.[238] Indeed, immunohistochemical localization of chromatogranin A is becoming an established technique to help identify a variety of endocrine and neuroendocrine tumors, including carcinoid tumors.[240] Further, chromogranin A levels are elevated in the plasma of patients with endocrine tumors such as carcinoid (most likely a consequence of increased secretion of peptides costored with chromogranin A).[241] Thus, measurement of plasma chromogranin A levels may be of clinical benefit in the early diagnosis of some endocrine tumors (see below).[241,242]

Symptoms

In the early stages of growth (typically for the first 6 to 12 years), primary carcinoid tumors are often accompanied by vague abdominal symptoms and consequently are frequently not recognized.[86] Overt, sustained clinical symptoms such as flushing and diarrhea do not usually develop until the primary tumor metastasizes to the liver, mesenteric lymph nodes, or other regions (Fig. 27-5).

The principal symptoms of carcinoid syndrome include flushing (precipitated by stress, alcohol, and/or food), diarrhea (secretory, malabsorptive, colicky, and hypermotile in nature), cramping, abdominal pain (colicky and often partially obstructive), cardiac fibrosis, peptic ulcer disease (possibly resulting from the production of gastrin by some tumors and local release of histamine or another undetermined acid-producing substance), and pellagra (Table 27-13).[12,232,243] The chronologic sequence of clinical manifestations of carcinoid tumors shows considerable heterogeneity. Flushing may develop with or without diarrhea; this suggests that a combination of secretagogues is required for the expression of the complete syndrome.[5]

The symptoms of carcinoid syndrome vary according to the regional location of the carcinoid tumor.[7] For example, the carcinoid syndrome associated with bronchial carcinoid tumors exhibits the most severe clinical features. Flushing attacks are usually severe and protracted (lasting up to 4 days) and often are accompanied by facial edema, anxiety, tremulousness, agitation, lacrimation, sweating, salivation, nausea, vomiting, fever, and explosive diarrhea.[9]

The carcinoid syndrome associated with gastric carcinoid tumors is unique in that the flushes start as bright red erythematous patches that eventually coalesce.[9] The flushes may be triggered by spicy foods, cheese, and low doses of pentagastrin.[9]

FIGURE 27-5 Natural history of carcinoid tumor growth and associated symptom complex. (*From Vinik and Moattari with permission.*[86])

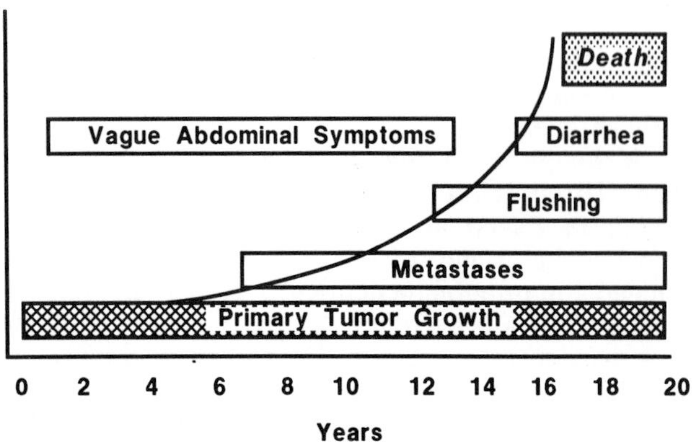

Pathophysiology

The full spectrum of clinical features associated with carcinoid syndrome results from the secretion of a wide variety of biologically active peptides, amines, and prostaglandins (Table 27-14). However, the rarity of carcinoid tumors that produce the recognized syndrome, combined with incomplete information regarding peptide tumor secretagogues, precludes full identification of carcinoid tumor pathophysiology.

Carcinoid tumors originating from the midgut (ileum and jejunum) synthesize the amine 5-hydroxytryptamine (serotonin) from dietary tryptophan.[7] Tryptophan is initially hydroxylated to form 5-hydroxytryptophan (5-HTP) (the rate-limiting step) and then decarboxylated by the enzyme aromatic L-amino acid decarboxylase (or dopa decarboxylase) in the tumor to form 5-HT (Fig. 27-6). Once synthesized, 5-HT is released into the circulation, where it is taken up by platelets and stored in secretory granules or catabolized to 5-hydroxyindoleacetic acid (5-HIAA) and subsequently excreted in the urine.

Excessive secretion of 5-HT from carcinoid tumors leads to elevated urinary concentrations of 5-HIAA in the majority of carcinoid patients.[7,8,232] Urinary 5-HT secretion may be within the normal range or only slightly increased because of extensive renal catabolism of 5-HT to 5-HIAA. However, in a small number of carcinoid patients, typically those with foregut tumors (e.g., bronchus, pancreas, and stomach), urinary levels of 5-HT and 5-HTP may be markedly elevated whereas levels of 5-HIAA may be only modestly increased.[7,8,232] One explanation for this change in 5-HT excretory products is that some carcinoid tumors lack dopa decarboxylase and thus are unable to synthesize 5-HT from 5-HTP. In these patients, the 5-HTP enters the circulation and is excreted by the kidney. Some 5-HTP is converted to 5-HT by the kidney, leading to elevated urinary 5-HT excretion.

5-HT has a wide variety of physiologic effects which can give rise to the flushing, diarrhea, malabsorption, intestinal hypermotility, abdominal cramps, nausea, and vomiting associated with carcinoid syndrome.[245] 5-HT is also believed to be involved in the etiology of the cardiac fibrosis (primarily of the tricuspid heart valve) commonly seen in carcinoid syndrome.[12]

Flushing in carcinoid syndrome may result not

TABLE 27-13 Principal Clinical Signs and Symptoms of the Carcinoid Syndrome

Clinical Signs/Symptom	Frequency, %	Comments
Flushing	80	Episodic; precipitated by stress, associated with hypotension
Diarrhea	76	Secretory, malabsorptive, obstructive, hypermotile
Pain	70	Dull or aching, midepigastric location, partial obstruction
Wheezing	10–20	May be asthmatic; bronchospasm
Cardiac fibrosis	50	Serotonin implicated in pathogenesis
Peptic ulcers	Rare	Thought to be due to gastrin-producing tumors
Pellagra	Rare	Thought to be due to niacin deficiency caused by diarrhea

Source: From O'Dorisio and O'Dorisio with permission.[58] Data incorporated from refs. 12, 86, 243.

only from serotonin release but also from the actions of a plethora of other vasoactive agents, including histamine, bradykinin, substance P, neurotensin, motilin, somatostatin, prostaglandins, neuropeptide K, gastrin-releasing peptide, and VIP (unusual).[8] However, the involvement of many of these peptides has not been completely delineated. For example, Feldman and O'Dorisio measured substance P and neurotensin levels in patients with carcinoid syndrome before and after a flushing attack induced by alcohol (30 mL of dry sherry).[246] The development of facial flushing 1.5 to 5.0 min after the ingestion of alcohol was not preceded by an elevation in the plasma concentration of substance P or neurotensin.

Diagnosis

The diagnosis of a carcinoid tumor and its syndrome may not be made unequivocally for several years. Early primary carcinoid tumors are especially difficult to diagnose because the associated symptoms are vague and mimic other GI complaints (e.g., irritable bowel syndrome and spastic colon).[8] An accurate diagnosis usually hinges on the results of specific diagnostic tests for tumor markers and the results of imaging techniques such as CT, endoscopy, and radiology (Table 27-15).

Laboratory Diagnostic Tests

The presence of a variety of tumor markers in urine, plasma, or serum may be indicative of carcinoid tumor, although the diagnostic usefulness of each tumor marker varies with the location of the carcinoid tumor (Table 27-16).[7] No single marker is capable of identifying all patients with carcinoid tumors. However, the most widely used, inexpensive, and effective screening procedure is measurement of urinary 5-HIAA.[247] Urinary excretion of 5-HIAA and plasma serotonin should be measured in *all* patients suspected of having carcinoid tumor or syndrome. Urinary excretion of ⩾30 mg 5-HIAA over a 24-h period is considered a positive result (normal range, 2 to 8 mg/24 h); some patients may excrete as much as 1000 mg/24 h.[9] However, these values may vary according to the analytic procedure used (e.g., radioenzymatic assay or high-pressure liquid chromatography). In a study of 75 patients with carcinoid syndrome, urinary and platelet 5-HIAA concentrations were elevated in 64.[248] Similarly, Wilander and colleagues found that 88 percent of patients with carcinoid tumors (most of whom had carcinoid syndrome) had increased levels of 5-HIAA; the degree of increase was associated with the size of the tumor mass in midgut carcinoid tumors.[7]

TABLE 27-14 Secretory Products of Carcinoid Tumors

Peptides	Amines	Other
Bradykinin, lysyl-bradykinin	Serotonin	$PGE_{2\alpha}$, PGE_2
Substance P	Dopamine	
Neurotensin	Histamine	
Motilin	5-Hydroxyindoleacetic acid	
VIP		
Neuropeptide K		
GRP		
Calcitonin		
Somatostatin		

VIP = vasoactive intestinal polypeptide; GRP = gastrin-releasing peptide; PG = prostaglandin.

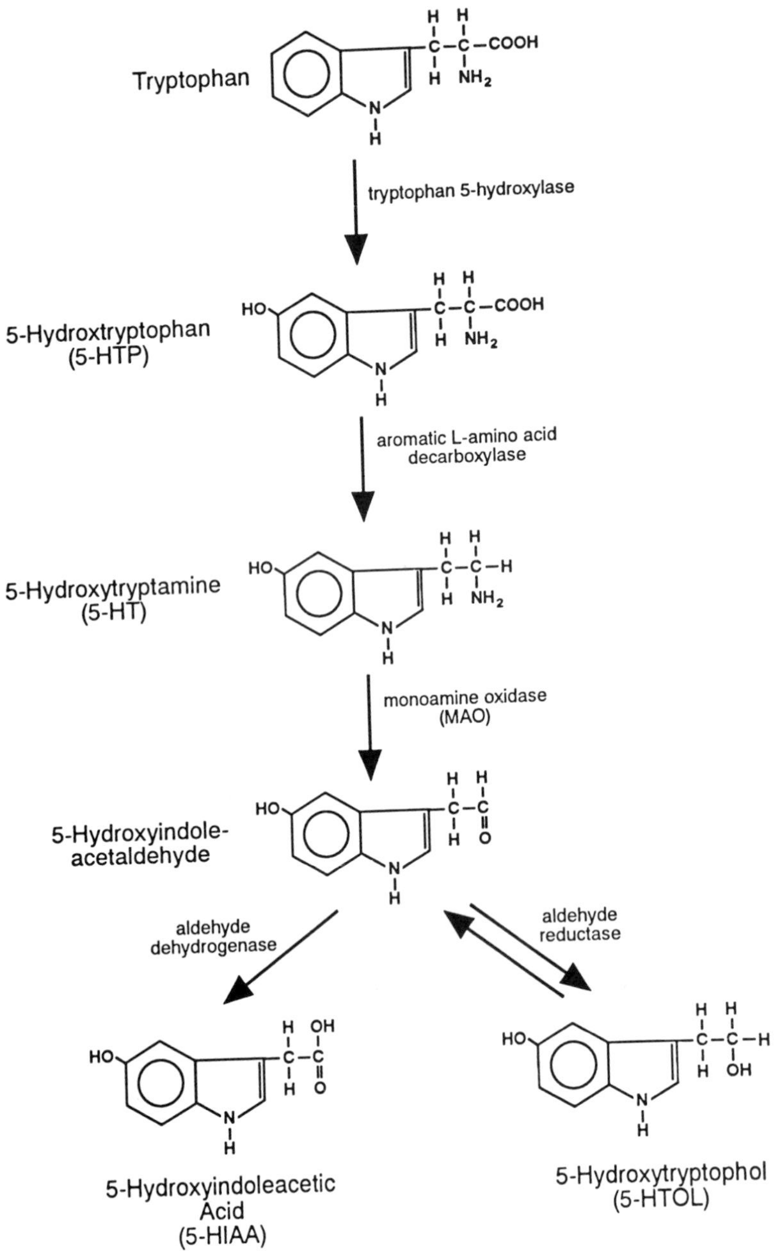

Tryptophan

tryptophan 5-hydroxylase

5-Hydroxtryptophan (5-HTP)

aromatic L-amino acid decarboxylase

5-Hydroxytryptamine (5-HT)

monoamine oxidase (MAO)

5-Hydroxyindole-acetaldehyde

aldehyde dehydrogenase

aldehyde reductase

5-Hydroxyindoleacetic Acid (5-HIAA)

5-Hydroxytryptophol (5-HTOL)

FIGURE 27-6 Synthesis and catabolism of 5-hydroxytryptamine. (*From Douglas with permission.*[244])

In addition to 5-HIAA, some investigators measure fasting, whole-blood concentration of 5-HT in patients with suspected carcinoid tumors.[9] Measurement of 5-HT is especially valuable because the consumption of foods containing large amounts of this amine does not influence the results (in contrast to 5-HIAA levels, which increase after consumption of 5-HT-rich foods as a result of catabolism during intestinal absorption) and because this method rarely detects anything but carcinoid tumors.[232] 5-HT concentrations in whole blood (or plasma prepared from blood collected in ascorbic acid tubes) from carcinoid patients range from 790 to 4500 ng/dL (normal range, 71 to 310 ng/dL).[9] However, as in the case of urinary 5-HIAA measurements, 5-HT values in blood may vary according to the method used (HPLC or enzymatic).

A high percentage of patients with carcinoid tumors also have elevated plasma or serum concentrations of neuropeptide (66 percent), pancreatic polypeptide (60 percent), human chorionic gonadotropin-α (69 percent), a novel anterior pituitary gland protein called APPG or IR-7B2 (64 percent), chromogranin A, and motilin (52 percent).[250–256] Plasma levels of pancreatic polypeptide are especially elevated in patients with bronchial and midgut carcinoids.[252] Plasma concentrations of other GI peptides, such as substance P and neurotensin, are also ele-

TABLE 27-15 Diagnostic Approaches in Suspected Carcinoid Syndrome

Determine 5-HIAA and 5-HT levels
Measure fasting peptide profile, including substance P, neurotensin, and pancreastatin
Localize tumor with venous catheterization—measure arterial-venous gradients of peptides (e.g., substance P)
Examine patient for curable ovarian, testicular, or bronchial primary carcinoid tumors if 5-HIAA/5-HT levels are elevated
Consider surgical exploration in any symptomatic patient if metastases are detected by CT, scintillation scanning, arteriography, or ultrasonography
Consider surgical resection of hepatic metastases after
  Evaluation of hepatic/cardiac function
  Identification of possible extrahepatic metastases (e.g., bone)
Evaluate possible nutrient malabsorption in patients with severe diarrhea
All patients suspected of carcinoid syndrome should have ^{111}In-octreotide scan (when available in the United States)

5-HIAA = 5-hydroxyindoleacetic acid; 5-HT = 5-hydroxytryptamine; CT = computed tomography.
Source: Adapted from Oates and Roberts with permission.[249]

vated in carcinoid patients.[246] However, these peptides are of limited diagnostic value in confirming the presence of carcinoid tumors.[246]

Diagnostic Imaging Techniques

A variety of diagnostic imaging techniques are available to identify primary and secondary carcinoid tumor sites and determine the extent of disease.[8] These techniques include CT, ultrasound, magnetic resonance imaging, radiography, hepatic and mesenteric artery angiography, endoscopy, barium contrast studies, and ^{131}I-metaiodobenzylguanidine (^{131}I-MIBG) or ^{99m}Tc scintigraphy.[12,232,257–259] Recently, a new technique, somatostatin receptor imaging, has been used to localize carcinoid tumors and other endocrine tumors. This approach exploits the propensity of most endocrine tumors to express high-affinity receptors for somatostatin; surgically excised carcinoid tumor tissue has been shown to bind somatostatin analogs in vitro.[260] The method involves the intravenous administration of ^{123}I-labeled Tyr$_3$-octreotide followed by gamma camera scintigraphy of the abdomen and thorax.[261] Somatostatin receptor–positive tumors in the abdomen as small as 1 cm in diameter can be visualized safely and quickly (within 30 min after isotope administration) using this technique. Nevertheless, because ^{123}I-labeled Tyr$_3$-octreotide has a short half-life and is difficult to prepare, this isotope will probably be replaced with ^{111}Indium-coupled octreotide, an isotope that is already available in Europe.[262]

Many of these imaging techniques are particularly applicable to tumor identification in specific locations. For example, bronchial carcinoid tumors are readily detectable by CT scan, while small intestinal tumors are too small to be detected with this technique and are best evaluated using other methods, such as mesenteric angiography.[8] Small bowel

TABLE 27-16 Usefulness of Tumor Markers in Diagnosing Carcinoid Syndrome

Tumor Marker	Specimen	Foregut	Midgut	Hindgut
5-HIAA	Urine	+	+++	−
Chromogranin A (pancreastatin)	Plasma	+++	+++	+++
APGP (IR-7B2)	Plasma	++	+++	++
NPK	Plasma	−	++	−
PP	Serum	++	+	+
hCG_α	Serum	++	+	+
hCG_β	Serum	+	+	+
Gastrin	Serum	++	−	−
Neurotensin	Plasma	+	−	−

Foregut = stomach and proximal duodenum; midgut = distal duodenum, small intestine, ascending colon, and proximal transverse colon; hindgut = distal transverse colon, descending colon, and rectum; 5-HIAA = 5-hydroxyindoleacetic acid; APGP (IR-7B2) = immunoreactive pituitary protein 7B2; NPK = neuropeptide K; PP = pancreatic polypeptide; $hCG_{\alpha/\beta}$ = human chorionic gonadotropin; +++ = very useful; ++ = useful; + = may be useful; − = not useful.

Source: From Wilander et al. with permission.[7]

tumors may be identified by a barium contrast series, a method that may reveal abnormal bowel distension, fixation, or filling defects associated with mesenteric lymph node metastastic tumors.[257] Liver metastases (>2 cm) may be identified using hepatic angiography but can also be evaluated using ^{99m}Tc liver-spleen scintiscan or CT scan of the abdomen.[8] When routine procedures are not successful, tumor localization with venous catheterization and measurement of blood levels and arterial-venous gradients of peptides (e.g., substance P) may be a useful alternative diagnostic approach.

Differential Diagnosis

Patients with systemic mastocytosis may also develop attacks of flushing, hepatomegaly, and diarrhea, symptoms very similar to those of carcinoid syndrome. Panic attacks, menopause, medullary carcinoma of the thyroid, and the rare VIPoma syndrome may also be accompanied by flushing attacks (Table 27-17). Occasionally, patients with pheochromocytoma (a catecholamine-secreting tumor) may also exhibit flushing attacks, although this is a rare occurrence. These diseases can be differentiated from carcinoid tumors by the absence of elevated levels of 5-HIAA or 5-HT and the lack of a flushing response to the intravenous administration of epinephrine.[8] However, the flushing response to epinephrine is not always a reliable diagnostic test.

Treatment

In patients with carcinoid tumor who develop carcinoid syndrome, the principal clinical manifestations requiring therapy include flushing, diarrhea, cardiac disease (e.g., congestive heart failure, fibrotic valvular lesions, or carcinoid tumor involvement of myocardium or pericardium), bronchospasm, and painful enlargement of the liver.[263] In a small percentage of patients, development of peptic ulcer disease, severe hypoalbuminemia, pellagra, muscle wasting, myopathy, arthropathy, retroperitoneal fibrosis, edema, hypertension, and hyperglycemia may also necessitate therapeutic intervention.

The therapeutic options for treating carcinoid tumors include surgical removal of the tumor, antineoplastic chemotherapy to decrease tumor size, and pharmacologic therapy to block the actions of secretagogues (e.g., somatostatin analogues and antagonists of alpha-adrenergic, 5-HT, and H_1 and H_2 histamine receptors).[86,264–268]

Surgery

Surgical extirpation may be appropriate in any patient in whom the primary carcinoid tumor can be localized. If the primary carcinoid tumor is detected in an early stage, surgical removal is usually curative. However, surgical removal of carcinoid tumors in patients who exhibit the carcinoid syndrome is associated with a high risk of complications. These complications, which are due to inherent properties of the carcinoid tumor rather than the surgical procedure, may include adhesion formation, development of short bowel syndrome, and precipitation of a carcinoid crisis resulting from anesthesia or tumor manipulation during surgery (see below).[9]

Antitumor Chemotherapy

Chemotherapy using combinations of a number of cytotoxic agents (such as 5-fluorouracil and streptozotocin, 5-fluorouracil and lomustine, and carmustine and etoposide) is frequently used in the treatment of carcinoid tumor patients.[269] However, some patients who exhibit severe carcinoid symptoms may experience a paradoxic aggravation of their symptoms in response to chemotherapy. The potential for an adverse response to chemotherapy in some patients necessitates a reduction in the usual chemotherapeutic dose and pretreatment with agents such as octreotide to lessen the severity of carcinoid symptoms.[263] Antineoplastic chemotherapy is generally not recommended unless the patient's daily activities are impaired, the tumor is growing rapidly, or the tumor becomes life-threatening.[232] Further, the risks of chemotherapy-induced renal toxicity preclude the chronic use of agents such as streptozotocin.

TABLE 27-17 Differential Diagnosis of Flushing Syndromes

Flushing Syndrome	Features	Hormone Assay
Carcinoid	Diarrhea, wheezing, myopathy	Urinary 5-HIAA, substance P, NKA
Medullary carcinoma, thyroid	Mass in neck, familial	TCT (pentagastrin provocative test)
Pheochromocytoma	Paroxysmal hypertension, tachycardia	Urine VMA
Menopause	—	FSH
Panic attacks	Phobias, anxiety	—
Mastocytosis	Dyspepsia, ulcer disease, dermatographia	Histamine
Idiopathic	—	—

5-HIAA = 5-hydroxyindoleacetic acid; NKA = neuropeptide K; TCT = thyrocalcitonin; VMA = vanillylmandelic acid; FSH = follicle stimulating hormone.

Source: Adapted from Vinik et al. with permission.[8]

TABLE 27-18 Clinical and Biochemical Effects of Octreotide in 14 Patients with Carcinoid Syndrome

Response to Octreotide	Diarrhea, %	Flushing, %	Wheezing, %	Urinary 5-HIAA, %	Blood 5-HT, %
Positive responders*	58	89	67	63	10
Partial responders†	17	11	33	12	10
Negative responders‡	0	0	0	0	10

* Positive responders: 75% drop in intensity or frequency of symptom or level of biochemical marker.

† Partial responders: 25 to 75% improvement.

‡ Negative responders: clinical and/or biochemical values increased by more than 25% of initial values.

5-HIAA = 5-hydroxyindoleacetic acid; 5-HT = 5-hydroxytryptamine.

Source: From Vinik et al. with permission.[247]

Pharmacologic Therapy

A wide variety of pharmacologic agents have been proposed to alleviate the symptoms of carcinoid syndrome, including somatostatin and octreotide, 5-HT receptor antagonists, H_1 and H_2 receptor antagonists, synthetic antiestrogen (tamoxifen), steroids, methyldopa, human leukocyte interferon, and cholestyramine.[9,267,268,270] H_1 and H_2 receptor antagonists are especially effective in preventing the patchy, bright red flushing attacks that occur postprandially in patients with gastric carcinoids.[271] 5-HT receptor antagonists such as methysergide maleate and cyproheptadine ameliorate the flushing associated with carcinoid tumors but are rarely effective in lessening the often severe diarrhea.[9] However, more recently developed antagonists of the 5-HT-M receptor (ketanserin A) decrease the volume of diarrhea induced by carcinoid tumors.[272]

Octreotide, a long-acting synthetic analogue of naturally occurring somatostatin, provides the most dramatic and effective control of the symptoms of carcinoid syndrome.[86,264,265,273] Octreotide administration markedly inhibits diarrhea, flushing, wheezing, myopathy, and secretion of gut hormones associated with carcinoid tumors.[86,265]

Vinik and colleagues investigated the clinical and biochemical effects of octreotide in 14 patients with histologically proven carcinoid tumors.[247] Patients initially received octreotide at a dose of 100 μg subcutaneously every 12 h; this was later increased to a maximum of 375 μg every 6 h. Octreotide treatment abolished or significantly improved diarrhea (75 percent of patients), flushing (100 percent of patients), and wheezing (100 percent of patients) (Table 27-18).

In a similar study involving 53 malignant carcinoid patients, Kvols reported that octreotide (450 μg/day subcutaneously) resolved both flushing and diarrhea (89 percent of patients) and urinary output of 5-HIAA (≥50 percent) (72 percent of patients).[267] Hepatic pain, impairment of liver function, and tumor mass also decreased during octreotide therapy.

Kvols also reported that octreotide was dramatically effective in reducing the symptoms of carcinoid crisis. Carcinoid crisis, which usually occurs in carcinoid patients during the induction of anesthesia before surgery, is characterized by abrupt severe hypotension, prolonged cutaneous flushing, confusion, and sometimes death. Octreotide is now routinely used and kept available during surgery involving carcinoid patients.

Prognosis

The prognosis of carcinoid tumor patients is good, with an overall survival of 82 percent.[86,268] However, the 5-year survival is directly related to the size and location of the tumor at the time of surgery. Five-year survival is greater than 95 percent if the tumor that is found is less than 2 cm in size but drops to 64 percent if an ileal or jejunal tumor greater than 2 cm is found at time of surgery and is accompanied by regional lymph node involvement. The 5-year survival is only 18 percent if a distant metastasis (especially to the liver) is found at the time of surgery. A sharp increase in the appearance of the carcinoid syndrome symptom complex occurs over the 7-year period from the first appearance of symptoms (diarrhea and flushing) to death (Figure 27-5). Mean survival time from the occurrence of the initial flushing episode has been estimated to be 38 months, with approximately 25 percent of patients living longer than 6 years.[274]

Acknowledgment

The authors wish to recognize Stephanie Phillips, Ph.D., for both her creative and constructive contributions toward this manuscript.

REFERENCES

1. Bayliss WM, Starling EH: The mechanism of pancreatic secretion. *J Physiol (Lond)* 28:325–353, 1902.
2. Walsh JH: Gastrointestinal peptide hormones, in Sleisenger MH, Fordtran JS (eds): *Gastrointestinal Disease: Pathophysiology, Diagnosis, Management,* 4th ed. Philadelphia, Saunders and Harcourt Brace Jovanovich, 1989, pp 78–107.
3. Sundler F, Böttcher E, Ekblad E, Håkanson R: The neuroendocrine system of the gut. *Acta Oncol* 28:303–314, 1989.
4. Green DW, Gomez G, Greeley GH Jr: Gastrointestinal peptides. *Gastroenterol Clin North Am* 18:695–733, 1989.
5. O'Dorisio TM, Redfern JS: Somatostatin and somatostatin-

like peptides: Clinical research and clinical applications, in Mazzaferri EL (ed): *Advances in Endocrinology and Metabolism,* vol 1. Chicago, Mosby Year Book, 1990, pp 175–230.
6. Bloom SR: Clinical syndromes of gut hormones, in Thompson JC, Cooper CW, Rayford PL, Greeley GH Jr, Singh P, Townsend CM Jr (eds): *Gastrointestinal Endocrinology: Receptors and Post-Receptor Mechanisms.* San Diego, Academic Press, 1990, pp 479–490.
7. Wilander E, Lundqvist M, Öberg K: Gastrointestinal carcinoid tumors: Histogenetic, histochemical, immunohistochemical, clinical and therapeutic aspects. *Prog Histochem Cytochem* 19:S1–S88, 1989.
8. Vinik AI, McLeod MK, Fig LM, Shapiro B, Lloyd RV, Cho K: Clinical features, diagnosis, and localization of carcinoid tumors and their management. *Gastroenterol Clin North Am* 18:865–896, 1989.
9. Kowlessar OD: The carcinoid syndrome, in Sleisenger MH, Fordtran JS (eds): *Gastrointestinal Disease. Pathophysiology, Diagnosis, Management,* 4th ed. Philadelphia, Saunders, 1989, pp 1560–1570.
10. Godwin JD II: Carcinoid tumors: An analysis of 2837 cases. *Cancer* 36:560–569, 1975.
11. Beaton HL: Carcinoid tumors of the alimentary tract. *CA* 32:92–99, 1982.
12. Strodel WE, Vinik AI, Thompson NW, Eckhauser FE, Talpos GB: Small bowel carcinoid tumors and the carcinoid syndrome, in Thompson NW, Vinik AI (eds): *Endocrine Surgery Update.* New York, Grune & Stratton, 1983, pp 277–291.
13. Go VLW, Koch TR: Distribution of gut peptides, in Schultz SG, Makhlouf GM (eds): *Handbook of Physiology: The Gastrointestinal System II.* Bethesda, MD, American Physiological Society, 1989, pp 111–122.
14. Makhlouf GM, Grider JR, Schubert ML: Identification of physiological function of gut peptides, in Schultz SG, Makhlouf GM (eds): *Handbook of Physiology: The Gastrointestinal System II.* Bethesda, MD, American Physiological Society, 1989, pp 123–131.
15. Polak JM: Endocrine cells of the gut, in Schultz SG, Makhlouf GM (eds): *Handbook of Physiology: The Gastrointestinal System II.* Bethesda, MD, American Physiological Society, 1989, pp 79–96.
16. Solcia E, Capella C, Buffa R, Usellini L, Fiocca R, Sessa F: Endocrine cells of the digestive system, in Johnson LR (ed): *Physiology of the Gastrointestinal Tract.* New York, Raven Press, 1981, pp 39–58.
17. Solcia E, Capella C, Fiocca R, Cornaggia M, Bosi F: The gastroenteropancreatic endocrine system and related tumors. *Gastroenterol Clin North Am* 18:671–693, 1989.
18. Sjölund K, Sandén G, Håkanson R, Sundler F: Endocrine cells in human intestine: An immunocytochemical study. *Gastroenterology* 85:1120–1130, 1983.
19. Pearse AGE: The APUD concept and hormone production. *Clin Endocrinol Metab* 9:211–222, 1980.
20. Pearse AGE: Common cytochemical properties of cells producing polypeptide hormones, with particular reference to calcitonin and the thyroid C-cells. *Vet Rec* 79:587–590, 1966.
21. Le Douarin N: A biological cell labeling technique and its use in experimental embryology. *Dev Biol* 30:217–222, 1973.
22. Andrew A: Further evidence that enterochromaffin cells are not derived from the neural crest. *J Embryol Exp Morphol* 31:589–598, 1974.
23. Like AA, Orci L: Embryogenesis of the human pancreatic islets: A light and electron microscopic study. *Diabetes* 21(Suppl 2):511–534, 1972.
24. Baldissera FG, Holst JJ, Jensen SL, Krarup T: Distribution and molecular forms of peptides containing somatostatin immunodeterminants in extracts from the entire gastrointestinal tract of man and pig. *Biochim Biophys Acta* 838:132–143, 1985.
25. Polak JM, Pearse AGE, Grimelius L, Bloom SR, Arimura A: Growth-hormone release-inhibiting hormone in gastrointestinal and pancreatic D cells. *Lancet* 1:1220–1222, 1975.
26. Yamada T, Chiba T: Somatostatin, in Schultz SG, Makhlouf G (eds): *Handbook of Physiology: The Gastrointestinal System II.* Bethesda, MD, American Physiology Association, 1989, pp 431–453.
27. Ipp E, Rivier J, Dobbs RE, Brown M, Vale W, Unger RH: Somatostatin analogs inhibit somatostatin release. *Endocrinology* 104:1270–1273, 1979.
28. Sagar SM, Martin JB: Hypothalamohypophysiotropic peptide system, in Bloom FE (ed): *Handbook of Physiology: The Nervous System IV.* Bethesda, MD, American Physiological Society, 1986, pp 413–462.
29. Brazeau P, Vale W, Burgus R, Ling N, Butcher M, Rivier J, Guillemin R: Hypothalamic polypeptide that inhibits the secretion of immunoreactive pituitary growth hormone. *Science* 179:77–79, 1973.
30. Pradayrol L, Jörnvall H, Mutt V, Ribet A: N-terminally extended somatostatin: The primary structure of somatostatin-28. *FEBS Lett* 109:55–58, 1980.
31. Shen LU, Pictet RL, Rutter WJ: Human somatostatin: I. Sequence of the cDNA. *Proc Natl Acad Sci USA* 79:4575–4579, 1982.
32. Kronheim S, Berelowitz M, Pimstone BL: The characterization of somatostatin-like immunoreactivity in human serum. *Diabetes* 27:523–529, 1978.
33. Baldissera FG, Munoz-Perez MA, Holst JJ: Somatostatin 1-28 circulates in human plasma. *Regul Pept* 6:63–69, 1983.
34. Conlon JM, Srikant CB, Ipp E, Schusdziarra V, Vale W, Unger RH: Properties of endogenous somatostatin-like immunoreactivity and synthetic somatostatin in dog plasma. *J Clin Invest* 62:1187–1193, 1978.
35. Patel YC, Srikant CB: Somatostatin mediation of adenohypophysial secretion. *Annu Rev Physiol* 48:551–567, 1986.
36. Arimura A, Fishback JB: Somatostatin: Regulation of secretion. *Neuroendocrinology* 33:246–256, 1981.
37. Delitala G, Tomasi P, Virdis R: Neuroendocrine regulation of human growth hormone secretion: Diagnostic and clinical applications. *J Endocrinol Invest* 11:441–462, 1988.
38. Reichlin S: Somatostatin: I. *N Engl J Med* 309:1495–1501, 1983.
39. Reichlin S: Somatostatin: II. *N Engl J Med* 309:1556–1563, 1983.
40. Colturi TJ, Unger RH, Feldman M: Role of circulating somatostatin in regulation of gastric acid secretion, gastrin release, and islet cell function: Studies in healthy subjects and duodenal ulcer patients. *J Clin Invest* 74:417–423, 1984.
41. Konturek SJ, Tasler J, Cieszkowski M, Coy DH, Schally AV: Effect of growth hormone release-inhibiting hormone on gastric secretion, mucosal blood flow, and serum gastrin. *Gastroenterology* 70:737–741, 1976.
42. Szabo S, Usadel KH: Cytoprotection-organoprotection by somatostatin: Gastric and hepatic lesions. *Experientia* 38:254–256, 1982.
43. Palitzsch KD, Schuler H, Schwedes U, Usadel KH: Protection against duodenal ulceration by somatostatins. *Klin Wochenschr* 64(Suppl 7):93–96, 1986.
44. Lucey MR: Endogenous somatostatin and the gut. *Gut* 27:457–467, 1986.
45. Dueno MI, Bai JC, Santangelo WC, Krejs GJ: Effect of somatostatin analog on water and electrolyte transport and transit time in human small bowel. *Dig Dis Sci* 32:1092–1096, 1987.
46. Carter RF, Bitar KN, Zfass AM, Makhlouf GM: Inhibition of VIP-stimulated intestinal secretion and cyclic AMP production by somatostatin in the rat. *Gastroenterology* 74:726–730, 1978.
47. Krejs GJ: Effect of somatostatin infusion on VIP-induced transport changes in the human jejunum. *Peptides* 5:271–276, 1984.
48. Dharmsathaphorn K, Sherwin RS, Dobbins JW: Somatostatin inhibits fluid secretion in the rat jejunum. *Gastroenterology* 78:1554–1558, 1980.
49. Morgan JS, Groszmann RJ: Somatostatin in portal hypertension. *Dig Dis Sci* 34:40S–47S, 1989.

50. Walsh JH: Gastrointestinal hormones, in Johnson LR (ed): *Physiology of the Gastrointestinal Tract,* 2d ed. New York, Raven Press, 1987, pp 181–253.
51. Solomon TE: Control of exocrine pancreatic secretion, in Johnson LR (ed): *Physiology of the Gastrointestinal Tract,* 2d ed. New York, Raven Press, 1987, pp 1173–1207.
52. Moreau JP, DeFeudis FV: Pharmacological studies of somatostatin and somatostatin-analogues: Therapeutic advances and perspectives. *Life Sci* 40:419–437, 1987.
53. Koerker DJ, Ruch W, Chideckel E, Palmer J, Goodner CJ, Ensinck J, Gale CC: Somatostatin: Hypothalamic inhibitor of the endocrine pancreas. *Science* 184:482–484, 1974.
54. Unger RH, Dobbs RE, Orci L: Insulin, glucagon, and somatostatin secretion in the regulation of metabolism. *Annu Rev Physiol* 40:307–343, 1978.
55. Larsson LI, Hirsch MA, Holst JJ, Ingemansson S, Kühl C, Lindkaer Jensen S, Lundqvist G, Rehfield JF, Schwartz TW: Pancreatic somatostatinoma: Clinical features and physiological implications. *Lancet* 1:666–668, 1977.
56. Ganda OP, Weir GC, Soeldner JS, Legg MA, Chick WL, Patel YC, Ebeid AM, Gabbay KH, Reichlin S: "Somatostatinoma": A somatostatin-containing tumor of the endocrine pancreas. *N Engl J Med* 296:963–967, 1977.
57. Krejs GJ, Orci L, Conlon JM, Ravazzola M, Davis GR, Raskin P, Collins SM, McCarthy DM, Baetens D, Rubenstein A, Aldor TAM, Unger RH: Somatostatinoma syndrome: Biochemical, morphologic and clinical features. *N Engl J Med* 301:285–292, 1979.
58. O'Dorisio TM, O'Dorisio MS: Endocrine tumors of the gastroenteropancreatic (GEP) axis, in Mazzaferri EL (ed): *Textbook of Endocrinology*, 3d ed. New York, Elsevier, 1986, pp 764–817.
59. O'Dorisio TM, Vinik AI: Pancreatic polypeptide and mixed hormone producing tumors of the gastrointestinal tract, in Cohen S, Soloway RD (eds): *Contemporary Issues in Gastroenterology.* Edinburgh, Churchill-Livingstone, 1984, pp 117–128.
60. Kelly TR: Pancreatic somatostatinoma. *Am J Surg* 146:671–673, 1983.
61. Chayvialle JAP, Descos F, Bernard C, Martin A, Barbe C, Partensky C: Somatostatin in mucosa of stomach and duodenum in gastroduodenal disease. *Gastroenterology* 75:13–19, 1978.
62. Sumii K, Fukushima T, Hirata K, Matsumoto Y, Sanuki E, Tsumaru S, Sumioka M, Miyoshi A, Miyachi Y: Antral gastrin and somatostatin concentrations in peptic ulcer patients. *Peptides* 2(Suppl 2):281–283, 1981.
63. Patel YC, Wheatley T: In vivo and in vitro plasma disappearance and metabolism of somatostatin-28 and somatostatin-14 in the rat. *Endocrinology* 112:220–225, 1983.
64. Polonsky K, Jaspan J, Berelowitz M, Pugh W, Moossa A, Ling N: The in vivo metabolism of somatostatin-28: Possible relationship between diminished metabolism and enhanced biological action. *Endocrinology* 111:1698–1703, 1982.
65. Seal A, Yamada T, Debas HT, Debas H, Hollinshead J, Osadchey B, Aponte G, Walsh J: Somatostatin-14 and -28: Clearance and potency on gastric function in dogs. *Am J Physiol* 243:G97–G102, 1982.
66. Battershill PE, Clissold SP: Octreotide: A review of its pharmacodynamic and pharmacokinetic properties, and therapeutic potential in conditions associated with excessive peptide secretion. *Drugs* 38:658–702, 1989.
67. Pless J, Bauer W, Briner U, Doepfner W, Marbach P, Maurer R, Petcher TJ, Reubi JC, Vonderscher J: Chemistry and pharmacology of SMS 201-995, a long-acting octapeptide analogue of somatostatin. *Scand J Gastroenterol* 21(Suppl 119):54–64, 1986.
68. Katz MD, Erstad BL: Octreotide, a new somatostatin analogue. *Clin Pharm* 8:255–273, 1989.
69. Daughaday WH: The anterior pituitary, in Wilson JD, Foster DW (eds): *Williams Textbook of Endocrinology.* Philadelphia, Saunders, 1985, pp. 568–613.
70. Lamberts SWJ, Uitterlinden P, Del Pozo E: SMS 201-995 induces a continuous decline in circulating growth hormone and somatomedin-C levels during therapy of acromegalic patients for over two years. *J Clin Endocrinol Metab* 65:703–710, 1987.
71. Hopman WPM, Wolberink RGJ, Lamers CBHW, Van Tongeren JHM: Treatment of the dumping syndrome with the somatostatin analogue SMS 201–995. *Ann Surg* 207:155–159, 1982.
72. Primrose JN, Johnston D: Somatostatin analogue SMS 201-995 (octreotide) as a possible solution to the dumping syndrome after gastrectomy or vagotomy. *Br J Surg* 76:140–144, 1989.
73. Woltering E, O'Dorisio T, Williams ST, Lebrado L, Fletcher WS: Treatment of nonendocrine gastrointestinal disorders with octreotide acetate. *Metabolism* 39:176–179, 1990.
74. Thirlby RC: Somatostatin and postgastrectomy dumping. *Gastroenterology* 97:1344, 1989.
75. Richards WO, Geer R, O'Dorisio TM, Robarts T, Parish KL, Rice D, Woltering G, Abumrad NN: Octreotide acetate induces fasting small bowel motility in patients with dumping syndrome. *J Surg Res* 49:483–487, 1990.
76. Geer RJ, Richards WO, O'Dorisio TM, Woltering EO, Williams S, Rice D, Abumrad NN: Efficacy of octreotide acetate in treatment of severe postgastrectomy dumping syndrome. *Ann Surg* 212:678–687, 1990.
77. Cook DJ, Kelton JG, Stanisz AM, Collins SM: Somatostatin treatment for cryptosporidial diarrhea in a patient with the acquired immunodeficiency syndrome (AIDS). *Ann Intern Med* 108:708–709, 1988.
78. Robinson EN Jr, Fogel R: SMS 201-995, a somatostatin analogue, and diarrhea in the acquired immunodeficiency syndrome (AIDS). *Ann Intern Med* 109:680–681, 1988.
79. Katz MD, Erstad BL, Rose C: Treatment of severe cryptosporidium-related diarrhea with octreotide in a patient with AIDS. *Drug Intell Clin Pharm* 22:134–136, 1988.
80. Kvols LK: Therapy of the malignant carcinoid syndrome and metastatic islet cell carcinoma, in O'Dorisio TM (ed): *Sandostatin in the Treatment of Gastroenteropancreatic Endocrine Tumors.* New York, Springer-Verlag, 1989, pp 65–82.
81. Maton PN, O'Dorisio TM, O'Dorisio MS, Malarkey WB, Gower WR Jr, Gardner JD, Jensen RT: Successful therapy of pancreatic cholera with the long-acting somatostatin analogue SMS 201-995: Relation between plasma concentrations of drug and clinical and biochemical responses. *Scand J Gastroenterol* 21(Suppl 119):181–186, 1986.
82. Dunne MJ, Elton R, Fletcher T, Hofker P, Shui J: Sandostatin and gastroenteropancreatic endocrine tumors: Therapeutic characteristics, in O'Dorisio TM (ed): *Sandostatin in the Treatment of Gastroenteropancreatic Endocrine Tumors.* New York, Springer-Verlag, 1987, pp 93–114.
83. Smith SS, Shulman DI, O'Dorisio TM, McClenathan DT, Borger JA, Bercu BB, Root AW: Watery diarrhea, hypokalemia, achlorhydria syndrome in an infant: Effect of the long-acting somatostatin analogue SMS 201-995 on the disease and linear growth. *J Pediatr Gastroenterol Nutr* 6:710–716, 1987.
84. Jaros W, Biller J, Greer S, O'Dorisio TM, Grand R: Successful treatment of idiopathic secretory diarrhea of infancy with the somatostatin analogue SMS 201-995. *Gastroenterology* 94:189–193, 1988.
85. Kvols LK, Moertel CG, O'Connell MJ, Schutt AJ, Rubin J, Hahn RG: Treatment of the malignant carcinoid syndrome: Evaluation of a long-acting somatostatin analogue. *N Engl J Med* 315:663–666, 1986.
86. Vinik A, Moattari AR: Use of somatostatin analog in management of carcinoid syndrome. *Dig Dis Sci* 34:14S–27S, 1989.
87. Maton PN, O'Dorisio TM, Howe BA, McArthur KE, Howard JM, Cherner JA, Malarkey TB, Collen MJ, Gardner JD, Jensen RT: Effect of a long-acting somatostatin analogue (SMS 201-995) in a patient with pancreatic cholera. *N Engl J Med* 312:17–21, 1985.

88. Santangelo WC, O'Dorisio TM, Kim JG, Severino G, Krejs GJ: Pancreatic cholera syndrome: Effect of a synthetic somatostatin analog on intestinal water and ion transport. *Ann Intern Med* 103:363–367, 1985.
89. Kraenzlin ME, Ch'ng JLC, Wood SM, Carr DH, Bloom SR: Long-term treatment of a VIPoma with somatostatin analogue resulting in remission of symptoms and possible shrinkage of metastases. *Gastroenterology* 88:185–187, 1985.
90. Wood SM, Kraenzlin ME, Adrian TE, Bloom SR: Treatment of patients with pancreatic endocrine tumours using a new long-acting somatostatin analogue: Symptomatic and peptide responses. *Gut* 26:438–444, 1985.
91. Ch'ng JLC, Anderson JV, Williams SJ, Carr DH, Bloom SR: Remission of symptoms during long term treatment of metastatic pancreatic endocrine tumours with long acting somatostatin analogue. *Br Med J* 292:981–982, 1986.
92. Öberg K, Jakobsson A, Gustafsson G, Willander E, Lundqvist G, Stridsberg M: WDHA syndrome caused by a ganglioneuroblastoma producing vasoactive intestinal polypeptide and neuropeptide Y: Treatment with SMS 201-995, a somatostatin analogue. *Scand J Gastroenterol* 21(Suppl 119):228–229, 1986.
93. Edwards CA, Cann PA, Read NW, Holdsworth CD: The effect of somatostatin analogue SMS 201-995 on fluid and electrolyte transport in a patient with secretory diarrhoea. *Scand J Gastroenterol* 21(Suppl 119): 259–261, 1986.
94. Anderson JV, Bloom SR: Neuroendocrine tumours of the gut: Long-term therapy with the somatostatin analogue SMS 201-995. *Scand J Gastroenterol* 21(Suppl 119):115–128, 1986.
95. Kvols LK, Buck M, Moertel CG, Schutt AJ, Rubin J, O'Connell MJ, Hahn RG: Treatment of metastatic islet cell carcinoma with a somatostatin analogue (SMS 201-995). *Ann Intern Med* 107:162–168, 1987.
96. Rene E, Regnier B, Laine MJ, Bonfils S: Somatostatin and cryptosporidial diarrhea during AIDS. *Can J Physiol Pharmacol* 64:70, 1986.
97. Redfern JS, Mekhjian HS, O'Dorisio TM: Use of somatostatin-like peptides in the treatment of diarrhea, in Lebenthal E, Duffey M (eds): *Textbook of Secretory Diarrhea*. New York, Raven Press, 1990, pp 421–428.
98. Gregory RA: A review of some recent developments in the chemistry of the gastrins. *Bioorg Chem* 8:497, 1979.
99. O'Dorisio TM: Gastrointestinal hormones, in Mazzaferri EL (ed): *Endocrinology: A Clinical Review of Endocrinology*, 2d ed. Flushing, N.Y., Medical Examination Publishing Co, 1980, pp 772–807.
100. Dockray GJ, Gregory RA: Gastrin, in Schultz SG, Makhlouf GM (eds): *Handbook of Physiology: The Gastrointestinal System II*. Bethesda, MD, American Physiological Society, 1989, pp 311–336.
101. Walsh JH: Gastrointestinal hormones and peptides, in Johnson LR (ed): *Physiology of the Gastrointestinal Tract*. New York, Raven Press, 1981, pp 59–144.
102. Boel E, Vuust J, Norris F, Norris K, Wind A, Rehfield JF, Marcker KA: Molecular cloning of human gastrin cDNA: Evidence for evolution of gastrin by gene duplication. *Proc Natl Acad Sci USA* 80:2866–2869, 1983.
103. Maton PN, Gardner JD, Jensen RT: Use of long-acting somatostatin analog SMS 201-995 in patients with pancreatic islet cell tumors. *Dig Dis Sci* 34:28S–39S, 1989.
104. Ruszniewski P, Elouaer-Blanc L, Mignon M, Bonfils S: Long term treatment of Zollinger-Ellison syndrome (ZES) with long acting somatostatin: Efficacy on gastric acid and gastrin secretions. *Gastroenterology* 92:1606, 1987.
105. Mulholland MW, Debas HT: Physiology and pathophysiology of gastrin: Review. *Surgery* 103:135–147, 1988.
106. Makhlouf GM, McManus JPA, Card WI: A comparative study of the effects of gastrin, histamine, histalog and mechothane on the secretory capacity of the human stomach in two normal subjects over 20 months. *Gut* 6:525–534, 1965.
107. Grossman MI: Gastrin: II. Physiology: Hormonal effects, in Berson SA, Yalow RS (eds): *Investigative and Diagnostic Endocrinology: Peptide Hormones*. Amsterdam, North-Holland, 1973, pp 1034–1037.
108. Feldman M, Walsh JH, Wong HC, Richardson CT: Role of gastrin heptadecapeptide in the acid secretory response to amino acids in man. *J Clin Invest* 61:308–313, 1978.
109. Johnson LR: Regulation of gastrointestinal growth, in Johnson LR (ed): *Physiology of the Gastrointestinal Tract*. New York, Raven Press, 1981, pp 169–196.
110. Ellison EH, Wilson SD: Further observations on factors influencing the symptomatology manifest by patients with Zollinger-Ellison syndrome, in Shnitka TK, Gilbert JAL, Harrison RC (eds): *Gastric Secretion*. New York, Pergamon, 1967, pp 363–369.
111. Zollinger RM, Ellison EH: Primary peptide ulcerations of the jejunum associated with islet cell tumors of the pancreas. *Ann Surg* 142:709–723, 1955.
112. Lewin KJ, Yang K, Ulrich T, Elashoff JD, Walsh JH: Primary gastrin cell hyperplasia: Report of five cases and a review of the literature. *Am J Surg Pathol* 8:821–832, 1984.
113. Keuppens F, Willems G, De Graef J, Woussen-Colle MC: Antral gastrin cell hyperplasia in patients with peptic ulcer. *Ann Surg* 191:276–281, 1980.
114. Webster MW, Barnes EL, Stremple JF: Serum gastrin levels in the differential diagnosis of recurrent peptic ulceration due to retained gastric antrum. *Am J Surg* 135:248–252, 1978.
115. Strickland RG, Bhathal PS, Korman MG, Hansky J: Serum gastrin and the antral mucosa in atrophic gastritis. *Br Med J* 4:451, 1971.
116. McGuigan JE, Trudeau WL: Serum gastrin concentrations in pernicious anemia. *N Engl J Med* 282:358–361, 1970.
117. Becker HD, Reeder DD, Thompson JC: Effect of truncal vagotomy with pyloroplasty or with antrectomy on food-stimulated gastrin values in patients with duodenal ulcer. *Surgery* 74:580–586, 1973.
118. Gehling N, Lawson MJ, Alp MH, Rofe SB, Butler RN: Antral gastrin concentrations in duodenal ulcer patients after cimetidine and highly selective vagotomy. *Aust N Z J Surg* 56:793–796, 1986.
119. Festen HPM, Thijs JC, Lamers CBHW, Jansen JMBJ, Pals G, Frants RR, Defize J, Meuwissen SGM: Effect of oral omeprazole on serum gastrin and serum pepsinogen I levels. *Gastroenterology* 87:1030–1034, 1984.
120. Ahlman H, Dahlström A, Grönstad K, Tisell LE, Oberg K, Zinner MJ, Jaffe BM: The pentagastrin test in the diagnosis of the carcinoid syndrome: Blockade of gastrointestinal symptoms by ketanserin. *Ann Surg* 201:81–86, 1985.
121. Regan PT, Malagelada JR: A reappraisal of clinical, roentgenographic, and endoscopic features of the Zollinger-Ellison syndrome. *Mayo Clin Proc* 53:19–23, 1978.
122. Jensen RT, Gardner JD, Raufman JP, Pandol SJ, Doppman JL, Collen MJ: Zollinger-Ellison syndrome: Current concepts and management. *Ann Intern Med* 98:59–75, 1983.
123. Rehfeld JF: Cholecystokinin, in Schultz SG, Makhlouf GM (eds): *Handbook of Physiology: The Gastrointestinal System II*. Bethesda, MD, American Physiological Society, 1989, pp 337–358.
124. Liddle RA, Goldfine ID, Rosen MS, Taplitz RA, Williams JA: Cholecystokinin bioactivity in human plasma: Molecular forms, responses to feeding, and relationship to gallbladder contraction. *J Clin Invest* 75:1144–1152, 1985.
125. Loewe CJ, Grider JR, Gardiner J, Vlahcevic ZR: Selective inhibition of pentagastrin- and cholecystokinin-stimulated exocrine secretion by proglumide. *Gastroenterology* 89:746–751, 1985.
126. Hopman WPM, Rosenbusch G, Jansen JBMJ, de Jong AJL, Lamers CBHW: Gallbladder contraction: Effects of fatty meals and cholecystokinin. *Radiology* 157:37–39, 1985.
127. Chey WY, Chang T-M: Secretin, in Schultz SG, Makhlouf GM (eds): *Handbook of Physiology: The Gastrointestinal*

System II. Bethesda, MD, American Physiological Society, 1989, pp 359–402.
128. Hubel KA: Secretin: A long progress note. *Gastroenterology* 62:318–341, 1972.
129. Chey WY, Kim MS, Lee KY, Chang TM: Effect of rabbit antisecretin serum on postprandial pancreatic secretion in dogs. *Gastroenterology* 77:1268–1275, 1979.
130. Chey WY, Rhodes RA, Tai HH: Role of secretin in man, in Bloom SR (ed): *Gut Hormones*. Edinburgh, Churchill-Livingstone, 1978, pp 183–196.
131. Thompson JC, Llanos OL, Schafmayer A, Teichmann RK, Rayford PL: Mechanism of release and catabolism of secretin, in Bloom SR (ed): *Gut Hormones*. Edinburgh, Churchill-Livingstone, 1978, pp 176–181.
132. Rhodes RA, Tai HH, Chey WY: Impairment of secretin release in celiac sprue. *Dig Dis Sci* 23:833–839, 1978.
133. Rominger JM, Chey WY, Chang TM: Plasma secretin concentrations and gastric pH in healthy subjects and patients with digestive diseases. *Dig Dis Sci* 26:591–597, 1981.
134. Meyer JH: Pancreatic physiology, in Sleisenger MH, Fordtran JS (eds): *Gastrointestinal Disease: Pathophysiology, Diagnosis, Management,* 4th ed. Philadelphia, Saunders, 1989, pp 1777–1788.
135. Mignon M, Rigaud D, Cambray S, Chayvialle JA, Accary JP, René E, Vatier J, Bonfils S: A comparative evaluation of secretin bolus and secretin infusion as secretin provocation tests in the Zollinger-Ellison syndrome. *Scand J Gastroenterol* 20:791–797, 1985.
136. Lamers CBH, Van Tongeren JHM: Comparative study of the value of the calcium, secretin, and meal stimulated increase in serum gastrin to the diagnosis of the Zollinger-Ellison syndrome. *Gut* 18:128–134, 1977.
137. McGuigan JE: The Zollinger-Ellison syndrome, in Sleisenger MH, Fordtran JS (eds): *Gastrointestinal Disease: Pathophysiology, Diagnosis, Management,* 4th ed. Philadelphia, Saunders, 1989, pp 909–925.
138. Debas HT, Soon-Shiong P, McKenzie AD, Bogoch A, Greig JH, Dunn WL, Magill AB: Use of secretin in the roentgenologic and biochemical diagnosis of duodenal gastrinoma. *Am J Surg* 145:408–411, 1983.
139. Said SI, Mutt V: Long-acting vasodilator peptide from lung tissue. *Nature* 224:699–700, 1969.
140. Said SI, Mutt V: Polypeptide with broad biological activity: Isolation from small intestine. *Science* 169:1217–1218, 1970.
141. Said SI, Mutt V: A peptide fraction from lung tissue with prolonged peripheral vasodilator activity. *Scand J Clin Lab Invest* 24(Suppl 107): 51–57, 1969.
142. Mutt V, Said SI: Structure of the procine vasoactive intestinal octacosapeptide: The amino-acid sequence: Use of kallikrein in its determination. *Eur J Biochem* 42:581–589, 1974.
143. Fahrenkrug J: Vasoactive intestinal peptide, in Schultz SG, Makhlouf GM (eds): *Handbook of Physiology: The Gastrointestinal System II*. Bethesda, MD, American Physiological Society, 1989, pp 611–629.
144. Schaffalitzky de Muckadell OB, Fahrenkrug J, Holst JJ, Lauritsen KB: Release of vasoactive intestinal polypeptide (VIP) by intraduodenal stimuli. *Scand J Gastroenterol* 12:793–799, 1977.
145. Ollerenshaw S, Jarvis D, Woolcock A, Sullivan C, Scheibner T: Absence of immunoreactive vasoactive intestinal polypeptide in tissue from the lungs of patients with asthma. *N Engl J Med* 320:1244–1248, 1989.
146. Said S: Vasoactive intestinal polypeptide (VIP) in asthma. *Ann NY Acad Sci* 629:305–3418, 1991.
147. Said SI: Vasoactive intestinal polypeptide and asthma. *N Engl J Med* 320:1271–1273, 1989.
148. O'Dorisio TM, Mekhjian HS: VIPoma syndrome, in Cohen S, Soloway RD (eds): *Contemporary Issues in Gastroenterology*. Edinburgh, Churchill Livingstone, 1984, pp 101–116.
149. Marks N, Bank S, Louw JH: Islet cell tumor of the pancreas with reversible watery diarrhea and achlorhydria. *Gastroenterology* 52:695–708, 1967.
150. Verner JV, Morrison AB: Islet cell tumor and a syndrome of refractory watery diarrhea and hypokalemia. *Am J Med* 29:529, 1958.
151. Priest WM, Alexander MK: Islet-cell tumor of the pancreas with peptic ulceration, diarrhea and hypokalemia. *Lancet* 2:1145–1147, 1957.
152. Bloom SR, Polak JM: VIPomas, in Said SI (ed): *Vasoactive Intestinal Peptide*. New York, Raven Press, 1982, p 457.
153. Brown JC, Pederson RA: A multiparameter study on the action of preparations containing cholecystokinin-pancreozymin. *Scand J Gastroenterol* 5:537–541, 1970.
154. Brown JC, Mutt V, Pederson RA: Further purification of a polypeptide demonstrating enterogastrone activity. *J Physiol (Lond)* 209:57–64, 1970.
155. Brown JC, Buchan AMJ, McIntosh CHS, Pederson RA: Gastric inhibitory polypeptide, in Schultz SG, Makhlouf GM (eds): *Handbook of Physiology: The Gastrointestinal System II*. Bethesda, MD, American Physiological Society, 1989, pp 403–430.
156. Jorde R, Burhol PG, Waldum HL, Schulz TB, Lygren I, Florholmen J: Diurnal variation of plasma gastric inhibitory polypeptide in man. *Scand J Gastroenterol* 15:617–619, 1980.
157. Kuzio M, Dryburgh JR, Malloy KM, Brown JC: Radioimmunoassay for gastric inhibitory polypeptide. *Gastroenterology* 66:357–364, 1974.
158. Cataland S, Crockett SE, Brown JC, Mazzaferri EL: Gastric inhibitory polypeptide (GIP) stimulation by oral glucose in man. *J Clin Endocrinol Metab* 39:223–228, 1974.
159. Falko JM, Crockett SE, Cataland S, Mazzaferri EL: Gastric inhibitory polypeptide (GIP) stimulated by fat ingestion in man. *J Clin Endocrinol Metab* 41:260–265, 1975.
160. Thomas FB, Sinar D, Mazzaferri EL, Cataland S, Mekhjian HS, Caldwell JH, Fromkes JJ: Selective release of gastric inhibitory polypeptide by intraduodenal amino acid perfusion in man. *Gastroenterology* 74:1261–1265, 1978.
161. Duprè J, Ross SA, Watson D, Brown JC: Stimulation of insulin secretion by gastric inhibitory polypeptide in man. *J Clin Endocrinol Metab* 37:826–828, 1973.
162. Duprè J: An intestinal hormone affecting glucose disposal in man. *Lancet* 2:672–673, 1964.
163. Duprè J, Beck JC: Stimulation of release of insulin by an extract of intestinal mucosa. *Diabetes* 15:555–559, 1966.
164. Yovos JG, O'Dorisio TM, Pappas TN, Cataland S, Thomas FB, Mekhjian H, Carey LC: Effects of amino acids and gastric inhibitory polypeptide on insulin release in dogs. *Am J Physiol* 242:E53–E58, 1982.
165. Brown JC, Dryburgh JR, Ross SA, Duprè J: Identification and actions of gastric inhibitory polypeptide. *Recent Prog Horm Res* 31:487–532, 1975.
166. Crockett SE, Cataland S, Falko J, Mazzaferri EL: Gastric inhibitory polypeptide: Responses to variable doses of glucose in normal subjects and abnormal responses to oral glucose in patients with adult-onset diabetes mellitus. *Diabetes* 24:413, 1975.
167. Creutzfeldt W, Ebert R: GIP in obesity, diabetes and hyperlipoproteinemia, in Hessel LW, Krans HMJ (eds): *Lipoprotein Metabolism and Endocrine Regulation*. New York, Elsevier North Holland, 1979, pp 65–73.
168. Creutzfeldt W, Ebert R, Willms B, Frerichs H, Brown JC: Gastric inhibitory polypeptide (GIP) and insulin in obesity: Increased response to stimulation and defective feedback control of serum levels. *Diabetologia* 14:15–24, 1978.
169. Ebert R, Creutzfeldt W, Brown JC, Frerichs H, Arnold R: Response of gastric inhibitory polypeptide (GIP) to test meal in chronic pancreatitis—relationship to endocrine and exocrine insufficiency. *Diabetologia* 12:609–612, 1976.
170. Arnold R, Creutzfeldt W, Ebert R, Becker HD, Börger HW, Schafmayer A: Serum gastric inhibitory polypeptide (GIP) in duodenal ulcer disease: Relationship to glucose tolerance, insulin, and gastrin release. *Scand J Gastroenterol* 13:41–47, 1978.

171. Brown JC, Mutt V, Dryburgh JR: The further purification of motilin, a gastric motor activity stimulating polypeptide from the mucosa of the small intestine of hogs. *Can J Physiol Pharmacol* 49:399–405, 1971.
172. Brown JC, Cook MA, Dryburgh JR: Motilin, a gastric motor activity stimulating polypeptide: The complete amino acid sequence. *Can J Biochem* 51:533–537, 1973.
173. Vantrappen G, Peeters TL: Motilin, in Schultz SG, Makhlouf GM (eds): *Handbook of Physiology: The Gastrointestinal System II*. Bethesda, MD, American Physiological Society, 1989, pp 545–558.
174. Bloom SR, Mitchell SJ, Greenberg GR, Christofides N, Domschke W, Domschke S, Mitznegg P, Demling L: Release of VIP, secretin and motilin after duodenal acidification in man. *Acta Hepatogastroenterol*. 25:365–368, 1978.
175. Mitznegg P, Bloom SR, Domschke W, Domschke S, Wünsch E, Demling L: Release of motilin after duodenal acidification. *Lancet* 1:888–889, 1976.
176. Mitznegg P, Bloom SR, Christofides N, Besterman H, Domschke W, Domschke S, Wünsch E, Demling L: Release of motilin in man. *Scand J Gastroenterol* 11(Suppl 39):53–56, 1976.
177. Collins SM, Lewis TD, Fox JET, Track NS, Meghji MM, Daniel EE: Changes in plasma motilin concentration in response to manipulation of intragastric and intraduodenal contents in man. *Can J Physiol Pharmacol* 59:188–194, 1981.
178. Fox JET, Track NS, Daniel EE: Relationship of plasma motilin concentration to fat ingestion, duodenal acidification and alkalinization and migrating motor complexes in dogs. *Can J Physiol Pharmacol* 59:180–187, 1981.
179. Imura H, Seino Y, Mori K, Itoh Z, Yanaihara N: Plasma motilin levels in normal subjects and patients with diabetes mellitus and certain other diseases: Fasting levels and responses to food and glucose. *Endocrinol Jpn* 27(Suppl 1):151–155, 1980.
180. Wingate DL, Ruppin H, Green WER, Thompson HH, Domschke W, Wünsch E, Demling L, Ritchie HD: Motilin-induced electrical activity in the canine gastrointestinal tract. *Scand J Gastroenterol* 11(Suppl 39):111–118, 1976.
181. Vantrappen G, Janssens J, Peeters TL, Bloom SR, Christofides ND, Hellemans J: Motilin and the interdigestive migrating motor complex in man. *Dig Dis Sci* 24:497–500, 1979.
182. Vantrappen GR, Peeters TL, Janssens J: The secretory component of the interdigestive migrating motor complex in man. *Scand J Gastroenterol* 14:663–667, 1979.
183. Besterman HS, Bloom SR, Christofides ND, Mallinson CN, Pera A, Modigliani R: Gut hormone profile in inflammatory bowel disease. *Gut* 19:A988–A989, 1978.
184. Besterman HS, Christofides ND, Welsby PD, Adrian TE, Sarson DL, Bloom SR: Gut hormones in acute diarrhoea. *Gut* 24:665–671, 1983.
185. Besterman HS, Cook GC, Sarson DL, Christofides ND, Bryant MG, Gregor M, Bloom SR: Gut hormones in tropical malabsorption. *Br Med J* 2:1252–1255, 1979.
186. Besterman HS, Adrian TE, Mallinson CN, Christofides ND, Sarson DL, Pera A, Lombardo L, Modigliani R, Bloom SR: Gut hormone release after intestinal resection. *Gut* 23:854–861, 1982.
187. Aoyagi K, Mishima Y, Murakami S, Ito K: Serum gastrin and motilin in treated and untreated hyperthyroidism. *Bull Tokyo Med Dent Univ* 29:153–159, 1982.
188. Christofides ND, Ghatei MA, Bloom SR, Borberg C, Gillmer MDG: Decreased plasma motilin concentrations in pregnancy. *Br Med J* 285:1453–1454, 1982.
189. Ruppin H, Kirndörfer D, Domschke S, Domschke W, Schwemmle K, Wünsch E, Demling L: Effect of 13-Nle-motilin in postoperative ileus patients: A double-blind trial. *Scand J Gastroenterol* [Suppl]39:89–92, 1976.
190. Sarna SK, Soergel KH, Koch TR, Stone JE, Wood CM, Ryan RP, Arndorfer RC, Cavanaugh JH, Nellans HN, Lee MB: Gastrointestinal motor effects of erythromycin in humans. *Gastroenterology* 101:1488–1496, 1991.
191. Tomomasa T, Kuroume T, Arai H, Wakabayashi K, Itoh Z: Erythromycin induces migrating motor complex in human gastrointestinal tract. *Dig Dis Sci* 31:157–161, 1986.
192. Depoortere I, Peeters TL, Vantrappen G: The erythromycin derivative EM-523 is a potent motilin agonist in man and in rabbit. *Peptides* 11:515–519, 1990.
193. Inatomi N, Satoh H, Maki Y, Hashimoto N, Itoh Z, Omura S: An erythromycin derivative, EM-523, induces motilin-like gastrointestinal motility in dogs. *J Pharmacol Exp Ther* 251:707–712, 1989.
194. Janssens J, Peeters TL, Vantrappen G, Tack J, Urbain JL, De Roo M, Muls E, Bouillon R: Improvement of gastric emptying in diabetic gastroparesis by erythromycin. *N Engl J Med* 322:1028–1031, 1990.
195. Taylor IL: Pancreatic polypeptide family: Pancreatic polypeptide, neuropeptide Y, and peptide YY, in Schultz SG, Makhlouf GM (eds): *Handbook of Physiology: The Gastrointestinal System II*. Bethesda, MD, American Physiological Society, 1989, pp 475–543.
196. Tatemoto K: Isolation and characterization of peptide YY (PYY), a candidate gut hormone that inhibits pancreatic exocrine secretion. *Proc Natl Acad Sci USA* 79:2514–2518, 1982.
197. Jeng Y-J, Hill FLC, Lluis F, Gomez G, Izukura M, Kern K, Chuo S, Ferrar S, Greeley GH Jr: Peptide YY release and actions, in Thompson JC, Cooper CW, Rayford PL, Greeley GH Jr, Singh P, Townsend CM Jr (eds): *Gastrointestinal Endocrinology: Receptors and Post-Receptor Mechanisms*. San Diego, Academic Press, 1990, pp 371–386.
198. Tatemoto K, Mutt V: Isolation of two novel candidate hormones using a chemical method for finding natural occurring polypeptides. *Nature* 285:417–418, 1980.
199. Taylor IL, Feldman M, Richardson CT, Walsh JH: Gastric and cephalic stimulation of pancreatic polypeptide release. *Gastroenterology* 75:432–437, 1978.
200. Scarpello JH, Vinik AI, Owyang C: The intestinal phase of pancreatic polypeptide release. *Gastroenterology* 82:406–412, 1982.
201. Greenberg GR, McCloy RF, Adrian TE, Boron JH, Bloom SR: Effect of bovine pancreatic polypeptide on gastric acid and pepsin output in man. *Acta Hepatogastroenterol* 25:384–387, 1978.
202. Lin TM, Evans DC, Chance RE, Spray GF: Bovine pancreatic peptide: Action on gastric and pancreatic secretion in dogs. *Am J Physiol* 232:E311–E315, 1977.
203. Friesen SR, Tomita T, Kimmel JR: Pancreatic polypeptide update: Its roles in detection of the trait for multiple endocrine adenopathy syndrome, type I and pancreatic polypeptide-secreting tumors. *Surgery* 94:1028–1037, 1983.
204. Lamers CBH, Diemel J, Roeffen W: Serum levels of pancreatic polypeptide in Zollinger-Ellison syndrome, and hyperparathyroidism from families with multiple endocrine adenomatosis type I. *Digestion* 18:297–302, 1978.
205. Polak JM, Bloom SR, Adrian TE, Heitz P, Bryant MG, Pearse AGE: Pancreatic polypeptide in insulinomas, gastrinomas, VIPomas and glucagonomas. *Lancet* 1:328–330, 1976.
206. Schwartz TW: Pancreatic-polypeptide (PP) and endocrine tumours of the pancreas. *Scand J Gastroenterol* 14(Suppl 53):93–100, 1979.
207. Floyd JC, Fajans SS, Pek S, Chance RE: Regulations in healthy subjects of the secretion of human pancreatic polypeptide, a newly recognized pancreatic islet polypeptide. *Trans Assoc Am Physicians* 89:146–158, 1976.
208. Hållgren R, Lundqvist G, Chance RE: Serum levels of human pancreatic polypeptide in renal disease. *Scand J Gastroenterol* 12:923–927, 1977.
209. Adrian TE, McKiernan J, Johnstone DI, Hiller EJ, Vyas H, Sarson DL, Bloom SR: Hormonal abnormalities of the pancreas and gut in cystic fibrosis. *Gastroenterology* 79:460–465, 1980.

210. Lassmann V, Vague P, Vialettes B, Simon MC: Low plasma levels of pancreatic polypeptide in obesity. *Diabetes* 29:428–430, 1980.
211. Lassmann V, Cabrerizzo Garcia L, Vialettes B, Vague P: Impaired pancreatic polypeptide response to insulin hypoglycemia in obese subjects. *Horm Metab Res* 17:663–666, 1985.
212. Coelle EF, Taylor IL, Lewin K, Adham N: Beneficial effect of pancreatic polypeptide in experimental pancreatitis. *Dig Dis Sci* 28:1083–1088, 1983.
213. Carraway R, Leeman SE: The isolation of a new hypotensive peptide, neurotensin, from bovine hypothalami. *J Biol Chem* 248:6854–6861, 1973.
214. Carraway R, Leeman SE: The amino acid sequence of a hypothalamic peptide, neurotensin. *J Biol Chem* 250:1907–1911, 1975.
215. Carraway R, Kitabgi P, Leeman SE: The amino acid sequence of radioimmunoassayable neurotensin from bovine intestine. *J Biol Chem* 253:7996–7998, 1978.
216. Ferris CF: Neurotensin, in Schultz SG, Makhlouf GM (eds): *Handbook of Physiology: The Gastrointestinal System II*. Bethesda, MD, American Physiological Society, 1989, pp 559–586.
217. Granier C, Van Rietschoten J, Kitabgi P, Poustis C, Freychet P: Synthesis and characterization of neurotensin analogues for structure/activity relationship studies: Acetyl-neurotensin-(8-13) is the shortest analogue with full binding and pharmacological activities. *Eur J Biochem* 124:117–125, 1982.
218. Go VLW, Demol P: Role of nutrients in the gastrointestinal release of immunoreactive neurotensin. *Peptides* 2(Suppl 2):267–269, 1981.
219. Rosell S, Rökaeus A: The effect of ingestion of amino acids, glucose and fat on circulating neurotensin-like immunoreactivity (NTLI) in man. *Acta Physiol Scand* 107:263–267, 1979.
220. Fletcher DR, Shulkes A, Bladin PH, Hardy KJ: The effect of atropine on bombesin and gastrin releasing peptide stimulated gastrin, pancreatic polypeptide and neurotensin release in man. *Regul Pept* 7:31–40, 1983.
221. Yanaihara N, Sato H, Inoue A, Sakura N, Sakagami M, Mochizuki T, Nakamura H, Yanaihara C: Comparative study on distribution of bombesin-, neurotensin-, and α-endorphin-like immunoreactivities in canine tissues. *Adv Exp Med Biol* 120A:29–37, 1979.
222. Theodorsson-Norheim E, Öberg K, Rosell S, Boström H: Neurotensinlike immunoreactivity in plasma and tumor tissue from patients with endocrine tumors of the pancreas and gut. *Gastroenterology* 85:881–889, 1983.
223. Von Euler US, Gaddum JH: An unidentified depressor substance in certain tissue extracts. *J Physiol (Lond)* 72:74–87, 1931.
224. Maggio JE, Mantyh PW: Gut tachykinins, in Schultz SG, Makhlouf GM (eds): *Handbook of Physiology: The Gastrointestinal System II*. Bethesda, MD, American Physiological Society, 1989, pp 661–690.
225. Pearse AGE, Polak JM: Immunocytochemical localization of substance P in mammalian intestine. *Histochemistry* 41:373–375, 1975.
226. Holzer P, Bucsics A, Saria A, Lembeck F: A study of the concentrations of substance P and neurotensin in the gastrointestinal tract of various mammals. *Neuroscience* 7:2919–2924, 1982.
227. Wattchow DA, Furness JB, Costa M: Distribution and coexistence of peptides in nerve fibers of the external muscle of the human gastrointestinal tract. *Gastroenterology* 95:32–41, 1988.
228. Hökfelt T, Johansson O, Ljungdahl A, Lundberg JM, Schultzberg M: Peptidergic neurons. *Nature* 284:515–521, 1980.
229. Donnerer J, Barthó L, Holzer P, Lembeck F: Intestinal peristalsis associated with release of immunoreactive substance P. *Neuroscience* 11:913–918, 1984.
230. Powell D, Cannon P, Skrabanek P, Kirrane J: The pathophysiology of substance P in man, in Bloom SR (ed): *Gut Hormones*. Edinburgh, Churchill Livingstone, 1978, pp 524–529.
231. Phillips SF: Megacolon: Congenital and acquired, in Sleisenger MH, Fordtran JS (eds): *Gastrointestinal Disease: Pathophysiology, Diagnosis, Management,* 4th ed. Philadelphia, Saunders, 1989, pp 1389–1402.
232. Feldman JM: Carcinoid tumors and the carcinoid syndrome. *Curr Probl Surg* 26:829–885, 1989.
233. Rosenberg JM, Welch JP: Ileal tumor causing carcinoid syndrome without hepatic metastases. *Arch Surg* 119:485, 1984.
234. Oberndorfer S: Karzinoide tumoren des dünndarms. *Frankfurt Z Path* 1:426–432, 1907.
235. Thorson A, Biorck G, Björkman G, Waldenström J: Malignant carcinoid of the small intestine with metasteses to the liver, valvular disease of the right side of the heart (pulmonary stenosis and tricuspid regurgitation with septal defects), peripheral vasomotor symptoms, bronchoconstrictions and an unusual type of cyanosis: A clinical and pathological syndrome. *Am Heart J* 47:795–817, 1954.
236. Williams ED, Sandler M: The classification of carcinoid tumours. *Lancet* 1:238–239, 1963.
237. Cheek RC, Wilson H: Carcinoid tumors. Curr Probl Surg Nov:4–31, 1970.
238. Wiedenmann B, Huttner WB: Synaptophysin and chromogranins/secretogranins—widespread constituents of distinct types of neuroendocrine vesicles and new tools in tumor diagnosis. *Virchows Arch [B]* 58:95–121, 1989.
239. Huttner WB, Gerdes HH, Rosa P: The granin (chromogranin/secretogranin) family. *Trends Biochem Sci* 16:27–30, 1991.
240. Deftos LJ: Chromogranin A: Its role in endocrine function and as an endocrine and neuroendocrine tumor marker. *Endocr Rev* 12:181–187, 1991.
241. Simon J-P, Aunis D: Biochemistry of the chromogranin A protein family. *Biochem J* 262:1–13, 1989.
242. O'Connor DT, Takiyyuddin MA, Cervenka JH, Parmer RJ, Barbosa JA, Chang YM, Hsiao RJ: Circulating chromogranin A as a diagnostic tool in clinical chemistry. *Acta Histochem* 38:27–33, 1990.
243. Woods HF, Bax HDS, Thorpe JAC, Smith JAR: Carcinoid tumors and the carcinoid syndrome, in O'Dorisio TM (ed): *Sandostatin in the Treatment of GEP Endocrine Tumors.* Berlin, Springer-Verlag, 1989, pp 15–22.
244. Douglas WW: Histamine and 5-hydroxytryptamine (serotonin) and their antagonists, in Gilman AG, Goodman LS, Gilman A (eds): *The Pharmacological Basis of Therapeutics,* 6th ed. New York, Macmillan, 1980, pp 609–646.
245. Sjoerdsma A, Weissbach H, Terry LL, Udenfriend S: Further observations on patients with malignant carcinoid. *Am J Med* 23:5, 1957.
246. Feldman JM, O'Dorisio TM: Role of neuropeptides and serotonin in the diagnosis of carcinoid tumors. *Am J Med* 81(Suppl 6B):41–48, 1986.
247. Vinik AI, Thompson N, Eckhauser F, Moattari AR: Clinical features of carcinoid syndrome and the use of somatostatin analogue in its management. *Acta Oncol* 28:389–402, 1989.
248. Feldman JM: Urinary serotonin in the diagnosis of carcinoid tumors. *Clin Chem* 32:840–844, 1986.
249. Oates JA, Roberts LJ II: Carcinoid syndrome, in Braunwald E, Isselbacher KJ, Petersdorf RJ, Wilson JD, Martin JB, Fauci AS (eds): *Harrison's Principles of Internal Medicine,* 11th ed. New York, McGraw-Hill, 1987, pp 1585–1588.
250. Norheim I, Theodorsson-Norheim E, Brodin E, Öberg K: Tachykinins in carcinoid tumors: Their use as a tumor marker and possible role in the carcinoid flush. *J Clin Endocrinol Metab* 63:605–612, 1986.
251. Norheim I, Theodorsson-Norheim E, Brodin E, Öberg K, Lundqvist G, Rosell SJ: Antisera raised against eledoisin and kassinin detect elevated levels of immunoreactive mate-

rial in plasma and tumor tissue from patients with carcinoid tumors. *Regul Pept* 9:245–257, 1984.
252. Öberg K, Grimelius L, Lundqvist G, Lörelius LE: Update on pancreatic polypeptide as a specific marker for endocrine tumours of the pancreas and gut. *Acta Med Scand* 210:145–152, 1981.
253. Öberg K, Wide L: hCG and hCG subunits as tumor markers in patients with endocrine pancreatic tumours and carcinoids. *Acta Endocrinol (Copenh)* 98:256–260, 1981.
254. Suzuki H, Ghatei MA, Williams SJ, Uttenthal LO, Facer P, Bishop AE, Polak JM, Bloom SR: Production of pituitary protein 7B2 immunoreactivity by endocrine tumors and its possible diagnostic value. *J Clin Endocrinol Metab* 63:758–765, 1986.
255. O'Connor DT, Deftos LJ: Secretion of chromogranin A by peptide-producing endocrine neoplasms. *N Engl J Med* 314: 1145–1151, 1986.
256. Öberg K, Theodorsson-Norheim E, Norheim I: Motilin in plasma and tumor tissues from patients with carcinoid syndrome. *Scand J Gastroenterol* 22:1041–1048, 1987.
257. Bancks NH, Goldstein HM, Dodd GD: The roentgenologic spectrum of small intestinal carcinoid tumors. *AJR* 123:274–280, 1975.
258. Hulnick DH: Small intestine, in Megibow AJ, Balthazar EJ (eds): *Computed Tomography of the Gastrointestinal Tract.* St. Louis, Mosby, 1986, pp 257–259.
259. Kressel HY: Strategies for magnetic resonance imaging of focal liver disease. *Radiol Clin North Am* 26:607–615, 1988.
260. Reubi JC, Maurer R, von Werder K, Torhorst J, Klijn JGM, Lamberts SWJ: Somatostatin receptors in human endocrine tumors. *Cancer Res* 47:551–558, 1987.
261. Lamberts SWJ, Bakker WH, Reubi JC, Krenning EP: Somatostatin-receptor imaging in the localization of endocrine tumors. *N Engl J Med* 323:1246–1249, 1990.
262. Patel YC: Somatostatin-receptor imaging for the detection of tumors. *N Engl J Med* 323:1274–1276, 1990.
263. Warner RRP: Carcinoid, in Bardin CW (ed): *Current Therapy in Endocrinology and Metabolism,* 4th ed. Philadelphia, Decker, 1991, pp 491–496.
264. Arnold R: Therapeutic strategies in the management of endocrine GEP tumours. *Eur J Clin Invest* 20(Suppl 1):S82–S90, 1990.
265. Gorden P: NIH Conference: Somatostatin and somatostatin analogue (SMS 201-995) in treatment of hormone-secreting tumors of the pituitary and gastrointestinal tract and non-neoplastic diseases of the gut. *Ann Intern Med* 110:35–50, 1989.
266. Ahlman H, Scherstén T, Tisell LE: Surgical treatment of patients with the carcinoid syndrome. *Acta Oncol* 28:403–407, 1989.
267. Kvols LK: Therapeutic considerations for the malignant carcinoid syndrome. *Acta Oncol* 28:433–438, 1989.
268. Moertel CG: Treatment of the carcinoid tumor and the malignant carcinoid syndrome. *J Clin Oncol* 1:727–740, 1983.
269. Kvols LK: Metastatic carcinoid tumors and the carcinoid syndrome: A selective review of chemotherapy and hormonal therapy. *Am J Med* 81(Suppl 6B):49–55, 1986.
270. Nobin A, Lindblom B, Månsson B, Sundberg M: Interferon treatment in patients with malignant carcinoids. *Acta Oncol* 28:445–449, 1989.
271. Roberts LJ II, Marney SR Jr, Oates JA: Blockade of the flush associated with metastatic gastric carcinoid by combined histamine H_1 and H_2 receptor antagonists: Evidence for an important role of H_2 receptors in human vasculature. *N Engl J Med* 300:236–238, 1979.
272. Antonsen S, Hansen MGJ, Bukhave K, Rask-Madsen J: Influence of a new selective 5-HT_2 receptor antagonist (ketanserin) on jejunal PGE_2 release and ion secretion due to malignant carcinoid syndrome. *Gut* 23:A887, 1982.
273. Oates JA: The carcinoid syndrome. *N Engl J Med* 315:702–704, 1986.
274. Davis Z, Moertel CG, McIlrath DC: The malignant carcinoid syndrome. *Surg Gynecol Obstet* 137:637–644, 1973.

CHAPTER 28

Multiglandular Endocrine Disorders

Leonard J. Deftos
Bayard D. Catherwood
Henry G. Bone III

MULTIPLE ENDOCRINE NEOPLASIA TYPE 1 (MEN 1)

Definition and History

Since early in this century, individuals have been reported to have tumors affecting multiple glands in various combinations. Over time, consistent patterns of such tumors were found to occur in several members of affected families. From these observations, certain widely recognized hereditary syndromes of multiglandular endocrine neoplasia have emerged. These include multiple endocrine neoplasia type 1 (MEN 1), also known as the *multiple endocrine adenomatosis* (MEA)–*peptic ulcer syndrome,* or *Wermer's syndrome,* and the two variants of multiple endocrine neoplasia type 2 (MEN 2) which are described below. It should be understood that not every example of polyglandular endocrine neoplasia fits one of these well-defined hereditary syndromes. As knowledge advances, it may be possible to delineate additional distinct genetic disorders manifested by various combinations of tumors of endocrine glands beyond the classic syndromes described in this chapter.

MEN 1 is an autosomal dominant disorder with a high degree of penetrance and some variability of expression. Affected individuals typically have tumors of the parathyroid and pituitary glands and the endocrine pancreas; they may have other tumors as well. The early reports which led to the recognition of this syndrome were based on autopsy studies. Erdheim appears to have been the first to describe the appearance of more than one endocrine tumor in a single individual in his report of autopsy studies published in 1903.[1] In a subsequent autopsy study, Cushing and Davidoff reported thyroid, parathyroid, and adrenal hyperplasia in four acromegalic patients.[2] Lloyd described a case of "hypophyseo-parathyreo-insular syndrome" in 1929.[3] An early premortem description of patients with what would probably now be recognized as MEN 1 was published by Rossier and Dressler in 1939.[4] They reported sisters with multiple endocrine disorders whose brothers had peptic ulcer disease. These authors were apparently the first to recognize the familial nature of multiple endocrine neoplasia. The specific association among adenomas of the parathyroid glands, the pituitary, and the pancreatic islets was recognized by Underdahl et al.[5] in 1953 and by Moldawer et al.[6] in 1954. Current understanding of the syndrome is largely attributable to Wermer,[7] who in 1954 described the familial aggregation of multiple adenomas of these glands and proposed that they constituted a distinct syndrome inherited as an autosomal dominant disorder. He noted the association with peptic ulcer disease in these patients and suggested the possibility of a genetic relationship between the ulcer disease and the endocrine adenomatosis. In 1955, an independent investigation led Zollinger and Ellison to the recognition of the syndrome that bears their names.[8] They described the association of severe peptic ulcer disease and gastric hypersecretion with non-insulin-producing islet-cell tumors of the pancreas. It was subsequently recognized that the same syndrome may also be manifested by malabsorption or watery diarrhea.[9,10] It was gradually appreciated that the Zollinger-Ellison syndrome is produced by gastrin-secreting pancreatic neoplasms and can occur as a component of MEA syndrome along with insulinomas and parathyroid and pituitary tumors.[11–13] Recent studies (see Pathogenesis) have brought us much closer to an understanding of the cause of this disorder.

Components of the Syndrome

The approximate relative frequencies of the various glandular tumors constituting the MEN 1 syndrome are indicated in Table 28-1. This table is based on a large number of reports and reviews; it should be understood that generally uncommon associations may occur quite frequently within particular pedigrees. As shown in the table, primary hyperparathyroidism is the most common manifestation of the syndrome, occurring in as many as 100 percent of affected individuals in some series.[14–16] The next most common among the site of involvement is the pancreas. The two kinds of pancreatic lesions generally recognized in this syndrome are insulinomas arising from the beta cells of the islets of Langerhans and gastrinomas of delta cell origin, which produce the Zollinger-Ellison syndrome. Both types of pancreatic tumor are often multifocal; either may appear as areas of hyperplasia rather than well-localized nodular adenomas, and either may be malignant. Pituitary adenomas may be slightly less common. In the past, they were thought to be nonfunctional in the majority of cases, although functional tumors were recognized, especially those causing acromegaly. More recently, it has been recognized that some pituitary adenomas are prolactin-producing.[17–20] As Table 28–1 indicates, adenomas of the other endocrine glands are much less common. Their etiologic relation to the genetic disorder is uncertain. Lipomas occur regularly in the affected members of certain pedigrees.[21]

TABLE 28-1 Approximate Relative Frequencies of Elements of the MEN 1 Syndrome

	Frequency, % of patients
Hyperparathyroidism	>80
Pancreatic tumors	
Gastrinomas	
Benign	20
Malignant	30
Insulinomas	
Benign	20
Malignant	5
Nonfunctioning	
Benign	<5
Malignant	<5
Pituitary tumors	
Chromophobe or nonfunctioning	
Benign	40
Malignant	<5
Eosinophilic or acromegalic (benign)	15
Cushing's disease, basophilic	5
Mixed and other types (benign)	<5
Prolactic-secreting	15(?)
Other tumors	
Carcinoid and bronchial adenoma	<5
Lipoma/liposarcoma	5
Adrenal cortical adenoma	10
Thyroid adenomas	5

Note: These figures are based on the reviews cited in the text but are adjusted to reflect moderate diagnostic criteria and to reduce ascertainment bias.

Primary Hyperparathyroidism

Primary hyperparathyroidism is the single most common feature of MEN 1, occurring in 80 to 90 percent of cases. It has become clear that although one or more of the parathyroid glands may appear at surgery to be normal, all these glands have the potential for neoplastic enlargement. If only one or two enlarged glands are removed at the time of the original operation, the likelihood of persistent or recurrent hyperparathyroidism is great. This has led to the recommendation of subtotal parathyroidectomy.[22,23]

There has been considerable difference of opinion about the proper description of the pathologic process in these parathyroid glands. Although the contemporaneous enlargement of multiple glands has prompted some authors to use the term *hyperplasia,* others have preferred to use the term *multiple adenomas.* The latter term carries the implication that the neoplastic changes are primary processes which may arise concurrently but independently in the different glands; it is more in keeping with current theories of pathogenesis. From a pragmatic standpoint, the use of the term *multiglandular primary hyperparathyroidism* has considerable appeal.[22] Histologically, these glands are usually dominated by chief cells, but clear-cell dominance may be seen, as well as a mixed picture. Parathyroid carcinoma is not a feature of typical MEN 1, although a case has been reported in association with familial primary hyperparathyroidism and a suspect family history.[24] Patients with primary multiglandular hyperparathyroidism are fairly often found to have relatives with either familial primary hyperparathyroidism or MEN 1, but sporadic instances of isolated primary multiglandular parathyroid disease occur as well.[25–27]

Evidence has recently been reported of a circulating factor in the plasma of MEN 1 patients which acts as a mitogen on parathyroid cells.[28,29] This factor resembles basic fibroblast growth factor (bFGF).[30] There is also new evidence for a clonal origin of neoplastic parathyroid cells.[31]

Pancreatic Tumors

Malignant Potential

The pancreatic tumors differ markedly from the other elements of the MEN 1 syndrome in that both insulin- and gastrin-producing tumors may take a malignant course, with invasion and metastasis in as many as half of affected individuals in some series.[12,13,32]

Insulinoma

Insulinoma is a fairly common and often clinically striking feature of the MEN 1 syndrome. This tumor arises from the beta cells of the islets of Langerhans; it secretes excessive amounts of insulin. The clinical presentation is similar to that seen with sporadic insulinomas; the principal features are hypoglycemia and its associated symptoms. These symptoms may include seizures, loss of consciousness, and symptoms associated with the counterregulatory response. Typically, patients have a constant sensation of hunger, and the hypoglycemia may be masked by a constant carbohydrate intake. These patients often have nightmares or other nocturnal symptoms when their carbohydrate intake is interrupted by sleep. They are frequently affected by marked weight gain and may have hypoglycemic symptoms when they attempt to restrict their caloric intake in order to lose weight. Insulinomas may be single or multiple and may be poorly demarcated. The common occurrence of multiple insulinomas or nodular hyperplasia of the beta cells makes selective resection extremely difficult, and so a subtotal pancreatectomy is frequently required. Of all the components of the MEN 1 syndrome, insulinoma probably constitutes the most severe hazard to the patient because of the neurologic effects of hypoglycemia.

Gastrinoma

Gastrin-producing tumors, which are derived from the delta cells of the islets of Langerhans, may occur in patients with insulin-producing tumors; more often, though, patients are afflicted with only one or the other type of pancreatic tumor. Although for some time the Zollinger-Ellison syndrome was treated as a completely separate entity, it is now recognized that individual patients may have the gastrinoma syndrome alone or as a feature of MEA. The Zollinger-Ellison syndrome is quite likely to be diagnosed because of the severe symptoms of the ulcer diathesis, with gastric hypersecretion and/or secretory diarrhea and malabsorption. For this reason, it is often the presenting complaint of the index case in an affected family. It should be borne in mind that hyperparathyroidism may mimic or unmask the Zollinger-Ellison syndrome.[33,34]

Glucagonoma and Somatostatinoma

There have been several reports of pancreatic alpha cell tumors which secrete glucagon, usually in association with a distinctive rash.[35–37] A kindred has been reported with glucagonoma and MEN 1.[38] There have also been reports of pancreatic tumors which secrete somatostatin.[38–40] While these somatostatinomas have not yet been described in association with typical MEN 1, with further investigation such an association may be noted. The relatively mild and nonspecific symptoms that might be associated with subtle excesses of glucagon or somatostatin could cause underrecognition of cases of glucagonoma and somatostatinoma. As the clinical features of glucagonoma and somatostatinoma are more completely described and radioimmunoassays (RIAs) for glucagon and somatostatin are made more widely available, a better understanding of these disorders and their possible relationship to MEN 1 may be achieved.

Vipoma

Pancreatic tumors secreting vasoactive intestinal peptide, also called vipomas, have been reported with MEN 1. Such tumors produce a clinical picture of pancreatic cholera.[41] (See Chap. 23.)

Pituitary Tumors

Chromophobe Adenomas

A variety of functional and histologic types of pituitary tumors have been described in association with multiple endocrine neoplasia. Historically, the most commonly described tumor type appears to be the nonfunctioning chromophobe adenoma.[12,13,42] While these tumors do not produce hormones, they may cause significant endocrine effects when their mass impinges on normal pituitary cells and interferes with the hypothalamic-pituitary axis. It now appears that a number of the reported "nonfunctional" tumors may well have been prolactinomas.[43–46] Patients from the family originally studied by Wermer were reevaluated and were found to have evidence of prolactinomas.[47]

Functioning Adenomas

In addition to reports of chromophobe adenomas, there have been a substantial number of reports of acromegaly, which is associated with eosinophilic pituitary adenomas.[13] There have also been reports of Cushing's syndrome in MEN 1, perhaps caused by pituitary disease, although pancreatic tumor cells also may secrete adrenocorticotropic hormone (ACTH).[48] Although precocious puberty has been described in endocrine polyneoplasia,[49,50] gonadotropin-secreting pituitary adenomas have not been demonstrated in the MEN 1 syndrome.

Recent reports indicate that prolactinomas occur fairly commonly in the MEN 1 syndrome.[43–46] The possibility that hyperprolactinemia was caused by the tumor mass interfering with the transfer of hypothalamic prolactin inhibitory factor to the appropriate pituitary cells has not been rigorously excluded in every case. In several cases, however, it has been demonstrated by immunohistology and electron microscopy that the pituitary tumor cells contain prolactin.[19,20]

For the most part, the pituitary adenomas recognized in multiple endocrine neoplasia have been associated with enlargement of the sella turcica; the frequency and clinical significance of microadenomas have not been established. Presumably, early detection of pituitary adenomas while they are still small would permit surgical removal with improved preservation of pituitary function. Whether additional adenomas might form subsequently is unknown.

Other Associations

Lipomas

In certain kindreds[13,42] lipomas are closely associated with the more typical features of parathyroid, pituitary, and pancreatic tumors. The lipomas may be small and few in number or may be large and quite prominent.[21] In kindreds in which lipomas occur, they are often a useful sign, indicating which members will be affected by the other features of the syndrome.[50]

Bronchial Adenomas and Carcinoid Tumors

Rarely, bronchial adenomas and intestinal carcinoid tumors have been reported in association with the fully expressed MEN 1 syndrome.[50–52] In a few other cases, these tumors have been associated with individual components of the MEN 1 syndrome.[52] These patients may have the typical carcinoid syndrome or may be found to have carcinoid tumors incidentally.

Adrenal Cortical Adenomas

Although there have been case reports of steroid-producing adrenocortical adenomas and hyperplasia in association with the MEN 1 syndrome,[13,51,52] they are extraordinarily rare. Somewhat more commonly, small adrenocortical nodules are discovered at autopsy.[2,13,52] Such nodules may be found in as many as half of autopsied adults[53]; thus, they may be only incidental findings in patients with MEN 1. Generally, they do not appear to have caused any clinical symptoms and are thought to have been nonfunctional.

Thyroid Adenomas

Some patients with MEN 1 have been noted to have thyroid hyperplasia or follicular adenomas.[2,12,13] These are nonfunctioning lesions which may occur in as many as 50 percent of carefully examined autopsy specimens from unselected subjects.[54] Therefore, the significance of these findings in MEN 1 is questionable. Hyperthyroidism has only rarely been associated with cases of MEA, and its etiologic relationship to MEN 1 is uncertain.

Other Associated Tumors

Renal adenomas and leiomyomas[13,55] have been reported as incidental findings in patients with other endocrine tumors. It is particularly important to interpret the older reports with care because of the uncertain relationship of many of those cases to what is now recognized as the MEN 1 syndrome.

Clinical Evaluation

Patient Evaluation

There are two principal settings in which diagnostic studies are likely to be undertaken. A patient may appear with the clinical features of one or more of the component disorders and therefore be evaluated for other features of the syndrome, or asymptomatic subjects may be investigated because of their familial relationship to a patient with the disorder. Patients may present with such common problems as nephrolithiasis or other features of hyperparathyroidism, peptic ulcer disease, or symptoms of hypoglycemia. They may have such manifestations of pituitary tumors as headaches, visual field disturbances, amenorrhea, impotence, secondary hypothyroidism, or evidence of pituitary hyperfunction as in acromegaly. In the absence of suggestive clinical signs or symptoms or a suspicious family history, patients with typical primary hyperparathyroidism have a very low risk of developing MEN 1.[56] In patients with positive family histories, multiglandular parathyroid involvement, or symptoms or signs of other glandular tumors, the risk is greater. In such cases, the diagnostic yield is great enough to justify investigation of such patients to determine whether other components of the MEN 1 syndrome are present. Fortunately, such an assessment is fairly easily carried out.

Determination of the serum calcium level should be made in order to detect hyperparathyroidism. An x-ray examination of the sella turcica is generally a satisfactory method of ascertaining whether pituitary enlargement has occurred. Newer imaging procedures to detect microadenomas are probably necessary only if there is other evidence of pituitary dysfunction or if the patient or a relative is known to have MEN. Prolactin levels should be checked in both men and women.

Hypergastrinemia is usually symptomatic, and determination of the serum gastrin level or gastric acid secretion, perhaps employing a secretin test, helps exclude or confirm the diagnosis of Zollinger-Ellison syndrome. The diagnosis of Zollinger-Ellison syndrome may be problematic in occasional patients with hyperparathyroidism because hypercalcemia may cause hypergastrinemia and increased gastric acid secretion, mimicking gastrinoma (see Chap. 23). For this reason, it has been recommended that definitive evaluation for gastrinoma be carried out *after* parathyroidectomy in such cases.[33] Some investigators have found that a secretin test generally provides adequate discrimination between gastrinoma and the effects of hyperparathyroidism,[57] although others have disagreed.[31,58] Most reports indicate that extremely high gastrin levels can usually be attributed to gastrinoma, although hypercalcemia causes amplification of gastrin secretion. The use of a standard test meal, with hormone levels determined before and during the meal, has reportedly been useful in diagnosing pancreatic tumors in patients with MEN 1.[59]

Evaluation of the adrenal glands is called for only in rare cases in which there appears to be abnormal adrenal function. Thyroid nodules may be detected by means of palpation of the gland. The benign nature of the thyroid lesions reported with MEN 1 should not distract the physician from proper evaluation of any thyroid nodule for possible malignancy. It is generally not necessary to screen patients or relatives for disorders only rarely associated with this syndrome unless there is a specific reason for suspecting such abnormalities.

Family Evaluation

Initial Evaluation

Once it has been ascertained that the proband has two or more of the typical components of the MEA syndrome, family studies should be carried out; such studies may also be indicated in patients with multiglandular parathyroid disease alone[25,26] or multifocal insulinoma.[60] It should be realized that thorough family evaluation is a detailed and often difficult process. Although genetic testing may greatly simplify the work-up in the foreseeable future, at present repeated evaluation is required because individuals may appear to be normal when first studied but develop abnormalities some years later. The siblings, parents, and children of the index patients should be evaluated.

The first step is a meticulous review of the family members' medical histories, searching for manifestations that the family may be able to recall, such as kidney stones, peptic ulcers, low blood sugar, and premature menopause. Considerations of compliance, time, and cost require that screening be performed simply, quickly, and cheaply: Physical examination, determinations of serum calcium and prolactin concentrations and fasting blood sugar level, and x-ray examination of the sella turcica, together with the review of the medical history, should generally constitute an adequate screening examination. In some reported kindreds, primary hyperparathyroidism has consistently been a feature of MEN 1 in virtually all the affected members.[14–16] Further studies should be undertaken if there are specific indications for them. Although many affected individuals do not manifest the complete syndrome, the degree of penetrance in this disorder is high. Therefore, it is generally sufficient to study first-degree relatives of affected individuals. More distant relatives require investigation if there are historical or clinical findings suggestive of the disorder or if findings indicating MEN 1 are present in intermediate relatives.

Further Evaluation

Once the diagnosis of MEN 1 has been established in a family, the occurrence of any one feature of this disorder in an individual family member provides presumptive evidence of the genetic disease. It is important that relatives of the propositus understand that negative tests at the initial evaluation do not exclude the possibility of future development of features of the disease. Furthermore, members of such families should understand that often the adenomas do not develop concurrently and that another organ may be affected years after the treatment of the initial tumor.

Epidemiology

All studies of MEN 1 have indicated that the inheritance follows an autosomal dominant pattern; thus, approximately equal numbers of males and females are affected. The degree of penetrance is quite high, although the expression is variable; the pattern, or combination, of adenomas may differ between family members. Therefore, the family history is usually strongly positive and screening of the relatives of affected individuals is highly productive. This disorder has been found in both white and black families in North America and in families from Europe and Central America as well.[61]

The prevalence of MEN 1 in the general population is not known. Its apparent prevalence has been steadily increasing owing to the increased awareness of this syndrome and the improvement in diagnostic methods. The frequency of MEN 1 appears to be sufficient to warrant a screening investigation in patients who present with any of the typical features.

MEN in Other Species

Endocrine polyneoplasia with a pattern similar to that of MEN 1 in humans has been observed in a variety of species, but spontaneously occurring examples are extremely rare.[62] Quite a high incidence has been observed in irradiated rats,[63,64] suggesting that multiple somatic mutations are present in irradiated animals.

Pathogenesis

In his landmark paper in 1954, Wermer[7] demonstrated the autosomal dominant inheritance of this syndrome. He postulated that the heritable abnormality is in a gene responsible for regulation of the growth of the affected glands. The generalized character of the defect was inferred from the multiple parathyroid adenomas and multiple islet-cell tumors found in his patients.

The gene for MEN 1 has been localized to chromosome 11.[65–69] It appears that mutations are required at both alleles at locus 11q13, where the MEN 1 gene is closely linked to the gene for bFGF.[67] Apparently, the inherited characteristic is a mutation at one allele. When a somatic mutation at the corresponding site occurs in an endocrine cell, neoplastic daughter cells are produced. This is consistent with the two-hit mutation model for tumor formation[68,69] and with recent evidence for clonal origin of neoplastic cells.[31] It is not clear how this information relates to the older evidence against the clonal origin of parathyroid tumors or to the reported bFGF-like parathyroid mitogen which would presumably promote glandular hyperplasia. Possibly, a single clone could become dominant under the influence of such a mitogen.

The nature of the MEN 1 gene has not been well characterized. It is suspected to be an "antioncogene" whose loss permits neoplastic cell proliferation. When the nature of the gene is better characterized, it may be possible to test specifically for the gene or its product, permitting early identification of affected members of MEN 1 kindreds.

Relation to Other Syndromes

A small number of cases have been reported in which patients had elements associated with MEN 1 and other elements associated with MEN 2.[70,71] In some of these cases, the findings reported were not definite diagnostic features of the syndrome to which they were ascribed. In other cases, certain major features of both categories of MEN were present. However, these reports do not describe concurrence of two or more of the *distinguishing* diagnostic features of each syndrome (e.g., a patient with medullary thyroid carcinoma and pheochromocytoma as well as an islet-cell tumor and a pituitary adenoma). The lack of evidence for inheritance of these atypical combinations is consistent with sporadic occurrence.

Management

The management of the component disorders of MEN is presented in detail in other chapters. There are, however, some special considerations when these disorders occur in cases of MEN 1. In general, surgical treatment is the basis of management.

Parathyroid

When parathyroidectomy is undertaken, it must be borne in mind that the patient has (or will have) multiglandular involvement.[72] In general, a subtotal parathyroidectomy is the preferred procedure, even though gross enlargement may not be obvious in all parathyroid glands. If a less extensive procedure is performed, the likelihood of persistence or recurrence of hyperparathyroidism is great. If a patient with a small remnant of one gland again develops hyperparathyroidism, completion of a total parathyroidectomy and medical management of hypocalcemia are generally satisfactory. Autografting of parathyroid tissue (e.g., to the forearm) may prove useful,[73] but concern exists because of the neoplastic nature of the tissue and the potential risk of recurrent hyperparathyroidism as observed in an autografted adenoma.[74]

Pituitary

The rebirth of transsphenoidal hypophysectomy[75,76] has inaugurated a new era in the management of pituitary neoplasms and has made surgery of the pituitary gland by an experienced neurosurgeon much safer and more reliable than was previously the case. Suprasellar extension of the pituitary gland, even to the extent of affecting visual fields, does not necessarily preclude a satisfactory result from transsphenoidal surgery. Such a surgical approach permits the resection of small tumors that are entirely within the sella turcica and allows more complete removal of an intrasellar tumor than is possible with the transcranial approach. The early detection of pituitary adenomas by advanced radiologic techniques combined with microsurgery of the hypophysis may permit early resection of adenomas in patients in whom their occurrence can be anticipated because of a positive family history or the presence of other features of MEN 1. This may permit preservation of pituitary function that might otherwise be lost. Only experience will determine whether such tumors will recur.

Gastrinoma

Current surgical management of the Zollinger-Ellison syndrome is largely based on total gastrectomy by such improved methods as the Hunt-Lawrence[77] and modified Roux-19[78] gastrectomies. The gastrinoma may be resected if it is apparent; however, as gastrinomas are often multiple or obscure, resection is generally an adjunctive part of the management. It has been reported that duodenal gastrinomas may occur with some frequency in MEN 1.[79] Histamine-2 antagonists are of considerable value in the preoperative management of Zollinger-Ellison syndrome and in the long-term management of selected cases.[80] Streptozotocin has also been useful.[81] For further discussion of the management of the Zollinger-Ellison syndrome, see Chap. 27.

Insulinoma

Insulinomas are often multiple in the MEN 1 syndrome, usually requiring a subtotal or nearly total pancreatectomy for adequate resection. In cases of metastatic insulinomas and other instances in which adequate resection is not possible, or for interim management, diazoxide may be useful,[82] as may streptozotocin[83] in the case of unresectable tumors.

In both gastrinoma and insulinoma, resection of the tumor is important, if it can be accomplished, because of the malignant potential of the pancreatic tumors as well as their endocrine effects.

The most important general considerations in the management of MEN 1 are recognition of other elements of the syndrome in patients who present with one of its components and awareness of the implications for the families of patients with this heritable disease.

MULTIPLE ENDOCRINE NEOPLASIA TYPE 2 (MEN 2)

A second clinical syndrome involving tumors of multiple endocrine glands has been defined.[84] This syndrome can be clearly distinguished from MEN 1; it has been designated MEN 2. The signal tumor of MEN 2 is *medullary thyroid carcinoma* (MTC), a neoplasm of the calcitonin-secreting cells (C cells) of the thyroid gland.[85] In the early reports of MTC as part of a multiple endocrine disorder, the associated lesions were pheochromocytomas, hyperparathyroidism, and a syndrome consisting of multiple mucosal neuromas (MMN) and a marfanoid habitus.[84] More experience with MEN 2 has led to the appreciation that two distinct clinical syndromes of associated endocrinopathies can be defined: MEN 2a and MEN 2b. Both involve MTC; this tumor thus remains the signal neoplasm of both syndromes.

MEN 2a consists of MTC, pheochromocytoma, and hyperparathyroidism (Sipple's syndrome); MEN 2b consists of MTC and pheochromocytoma with MMN and a marfanoid habitus. The component tumors of MEN 2a and MEN 2b vary in their incidence and prevalence. In MEN 2a, the frequency of pheochromocytoma is less than 50 percent and the frequency of hyperparathyroidism ranges from 10 to 60 percent. In MEN 2b, the prevalence of pheochromocytoma exceeds 50 percent and hyperparathyroidism is rare or nonexistent; MMN syndrome is part of MEN 2b only.[85,86] In addition to these clinical differences, there are other features that distinguish these two syndromes. MEN 2a seems to be transmitted as an autosomal dominant characteristic. MEN 2b also exhibits this genetic pattern, but a number of sporadic cases have also been described.[87]

With one exception, the clinical behavior of the component tumors in both syndromes seems to be similar; the exception is the clinical behavior of the MTC. In patients with MEN 2a the MTC may run an indolent course, whereas in MEN 2b patients it is likely to be more aggressive.[88] There are, however, dramatic exceptions to these generalities, and patient management must be individualized.

There is an embryologic as well as a genetic basis for the association of MTC with these other tumors. The cells of MTCs, pheochromocytomas, and the neurogangliomas are all of neural crest origin.[89] The associated hyperparathyroidism does not fit into this unitary concept of embryogenesis, since parathyroid cells are not classically considered to be of neural crest origin. However, some authorities have suggested that the parathyroid gland is of neural crest origin.[90] An alternative explanation for the hyperparathyroidism is a functional relation between it and MTC. According to this hypothesis, the abnormal concentrations of calcitonin produce hyperparathyroidism that is a consequence of the hypocalcemic actions of the calcitonin.[91] Although this type of functional relation between the neoplasias may exist, the most convincing evidence supports a genetic relation between MTC and hyperparathyroidism.[92]

There are important clinical consequences of the association of MTC with other tumors. When they occur, mucosal neurogangliomas may be the first manifestation of the MEN syndrome. These lesions thus may provide an early warning of the presence of two potentially lethal tumors: MTC and pheochromocytoma. Additionally, the existence of either pheochromocytoma or MTC should suggest that the other entity may coexist. Hyperparathyroidism can be similarly regarded. It is therefore important for physicians to recognize that the presence of MTC in their patients should stimulate a search for other tumors in the patients' families. If diagnosed early, all the serious features of MEN 2 are treatable and even curable.

The gene responsible for the MEN 2a and MEN 2b forms of this syndrome has been localized to chromosome 10.[93–95] Genetic deletions have also been reported in some of the tumors of MEN 2a, but their significance is unclear.[96] Clarification of the genetic abnormalities underlying this disorder should make genetic counseling an important component in managing patients with MEN 2a and MEN 2b.[97] A negative family history is not reliable in excluding familial disease.

Medullary Thyroid Carcinoma

In contrast to the follicular cells of the thyroid, the presence of C cells within the human thyroid gland has been established only recently. This population of cells had attracted little attention until the discovery of (thyro)calcitonin in the early 1960s. Williams[98] suggested in 1966 that C cells may be the cells of origin of MTC. This tumor had been recognized by Hazard and his colleagues[99] as a distinct pathologic entity that could be distinguished from other thyroid tumors. Williams's hypothesis was proved correct when several investigators demonstrated by bioassay the presence of calcitonin in MTC.[100–103] These findings were later confirmed by specific RIAs of human calcitonin in tumor and blood[104] and by histochemical studies.[105] Subsequently, the tumor was also shown to produce a wide variety of other bioactive substances.[106] The unique histologic and biochemical features of MTC were soon embellished by its unique clinical associations with other endocrine and nonendocrine neoplasms (Table 28-2), most of which share with MTC a common embryologic origin, the neural crest.[90,107]

Embryology

Thyroidal C cells, which become neoplastic in MTC, are now generally accepted to be of neural crest origin.[107] These cells migrate to the ultimobranchial bodies from the neural crest. In nonmammalian species, the cells form a distinct organ, the ultimobranchial organ, which becomes the residence of the C cells and their secretory product, calcitonin. In mammals, the C cells become incorporated into the thyroid gland and perhaps other sites. The neural crest origin of C cells offers an explanation for the association of MTC with other tumors of neural crest origin; it also appears to explain the production by these tumors of a wide variety of bioactive substances.[90] Since these cells do not participate in iodine metabolism, they do not usually produce thyroglobulin.[108]

Pathology

An MTC is usually a firm, rounded tumor located in the middle or upper lobes of the thyroid gland.[98] It is commonly bilateral and multifocal, especially in familial cases. The histologic features of the tumor vary and in general cannot be used for prognosis. However, immunohistochemical studies suggest that cellular heterogeneity of calcitonin production may indicate a grave prognosis.[109] The cells usually are polyhedral or polygonal in shape and are arranged in a variety of patterns.[110] The arrangement of the cells can be influenced by the distribution of stromal elements, which can be scanty or predominant. Calcification is commonly found in the tumor; the calcifications are more dense and irregular than the homogeneous psammoma bodies which occur in other thyroid cancers. Dense calcifications may be visible on x-ray. A common feature of MTC is the presence of amyloid. The amyloid has the histochemical characteristics of the immune amyloids, but immunochemical and immunohistologic studies suggest that it is also secreted by the C cells and is structurally related to calcitonin. Although the presence of amyloid has long been considered to be important in the diagnosis of medullary thyroid carcinoma, the diagnosis is best established through the use of specific immunohistochemical procedures for calcitonin which demonstrate the abnormal C cells.[111,112] Specimens collected by needle biopsy are usually not adequate for diagnosis, even with immunohistology.[84] However, immunohistologic evaluation of sputum may demonstrate pulmonary metastases.[113] Mixed tumors containing malignant elements of thyroid follicles are rare.[114]

C Cell Hyperplasia

C cell hyperplasia has emerged as a distinct pathologic entity.[115] This had been preceded by the description of increased C cell populations in animals[98] and humans[110] with MTC. Wolfe and colleagues[115] were studying three patients at risk for MTC because of their family history. These patients had small but progressive increases in plasma calcitonin concentration during calcium infusion; they consequently underwent thyroidectomy. The extirpated thyroid glands did not display the presence of MTC but did show clusters of hyperplastic parafollicular cells which were calcitonin-positive on immunohistologic studies. The presence of increased calcitonin levels in these cells was confirmed by means of bioassay and immunoassay. These hyperplastic parafollicular cells were found to be localized to the areas where C cells are usually most prominent: the upper and middle portions of the lateral thyroid lobes. These cells exhibited no nuclear atypia or invasive tendencies. These observations suggest that, at least in familial cases of MTC, the frank malignancy is preceded by progressive hyperplasia of C cells.

This predecessor of MTC can become manifest in early childhood or as late as the second decade.[115–117] These early stages of MTC are of fundamental importance to cancer pathogenesis; detection of them is of considerable clinical significance. The early stages of MTC, when the neoplastic process is confined to the thyroid gland, are the most amenable to surgery; C cell hyperplasia and even more subtle histologic

TABLE 28-2 Approximate Frequency of Endocrine and Nonendocrine Neoplasms Associated with MEN 2a and 2b

MEN 2a	Frequency, %	MEN 2b	Frequency, %
Medullary thyroid carcinoma	97	Medullary thyroid carcinoma	90
Pheochromocytoma	50	Pheochromocytoma	45
Hyperparathyroidism	30	Multiple mucosa neuromas	100
		Marfanoid habitus	65

changes are below the threshold of clinical detection but may be identifiable with a calcitonin assay. Such early identification offers the best hope for effective therapy and even cure. Provocative testing is especially valuable in such patients, who may have normal basal levels of plasma calcitonin.[118]

Although oncogene abnormalities have been reported in MTC, a cascade of oncogene expression has not been defined for the progression of MTC through its hyperplastic stage.[119,120] Such a cascade, which apparently is present for colon cancer and its premalignant precursors, is consistent with the well-documented progression of C cells through a hyperplastic stage to frank malignancy.

C Cell Adenoma

Several instances of C cell adenoma have been reported.[121,122] These results must be considered as providing only preliminary evidence for the existence of such an adenoma. Definitive evidence will have to be provided by specific immunohistochemic studies which demonstrate the presence of calcitonin in tumor and perhaps in peripheral blood.

Occurrence

MTC has been reported to account for 4 to 12 percent of all thyroid cancer; it is a relatively uncommon tumor.[123] The ratio of affected females to males is closer to unity than in other thyroid tumors. Although the majority of cases reported in the earlier literature appeared to occur sporadically, an appreciation of the familial incidence of the tumor is resulting in an increasing identification of inherited cases,[106] especially in patients with MEN 2a. Approximately 25 percent of new cases of MTC are familial.[124] Despite its rarity, the tumor has acquired a clinical importance that far outweighs its prevalence. This has occurred because the tumor commonly exists in a familial distribution with an autosomal dominant pattern, because its presence can be established by measuring the concentration of calcitonin, and because it is associated with an intriguing constellation of clinical features (Table 28-2). Since the tumor is often inherited as an autosomal dominant characteristic, screening the family of an affected individual is often fruitful. In fact, with biochemical testing, the tumor can be diagnosed even when there has been no clinical evidence of its presence.[125]

Natural History

The natural history of MTC can vary greatly; this may make decisions regarding therapy difficult. The tumor is generally regarded as intermediate between the aggressive behavior of anaplastic thyroid carcinoma and the more indolent behavior of papillary and follicular thyroid carcinoma. However, it can be rapidly progressive and widely metastatic and can lead to death within weeks of diagnosis. By contrast, it can be indolent and compatible with decades of life.[123] Chromosomal abnormalities in the tumor may be predictive of a poorer prognosis.[126] In patients with MEN 2b, MTC develops at an earlier age, metastasizes earlier, and has a higher mortality rate.[88] MTC commonly spreads via regional lymphatics; local metastases have been present in the majority of tumors reported. Distant metastases can involve any organ; the lung, liver, bone, and adrenal gland are relatively common sites.[127] The most common presentation is a thyroid nodule, and the most common symptom is diarrhea.[84]

Secretory Products and Screening for the Tumor

The neoplastic cells in MTC produce a wide variety of secretory products. While all these products are of biological interest, some of them can also account for certain manifestations of the syndrome. A few of these secretory products can be used as markers for the tumor. This tumor has recently been demonstrated to concentrate ^{131}I-metaiodobenzylguanidine. (^{131}I-MIBG). This agent might thus be useful for scintigraphic examination of MTC, as it is for pheochromocytoma.[128]

Calcitonin and Related Peptides and Proteins

Since MTC is a neoplastic disorder of the C cells of the thyroid gland, the tumor produces abnormally high amounts of calcitonin. The calcitonin content of the tumor can exceed that of the normal thyroid by orders of magnitude. As a result, patients with this tumor have elevated concentrations of calcitonin in peripheral blood and urine. In most patients, basal concentrations of the hormone are sufficiently elevated to be diagnostic of the presence of the tumor. Therefore, the RIA for calcitonin can be used to diagnose the presence of MTC with an exceptional degree of accuracy and specificity when applied to measurements in random plasma samples. However, in a small but increasing percentage of patients with this tumor, basal levels of the hormone are indistinguishable from normal.[129] Many of these cases represent early stages of C cell neoplasia or perhaps even hyperplasia; these early stages are the most amenable to surgical cure. Thus, provocative tests have been developed for the diagnosis of MTC and its histologic antecedents.[92] These tests have led to the identification of the tumor in patients in whom the diagnosis could have been missed by basal calcitonin determinations.[84]

It has been shown that the calcitonin gene encodes other peptides (Fig. 28-1).[130–132] Although the function of these peptides is unknown, they are secreted by MTC and may thus serve as tumor markers. C cells also secrete chromogranin A (CgA), a high-molecular-weight protein originally discovered in the secretory granules of pheochromocytomas and

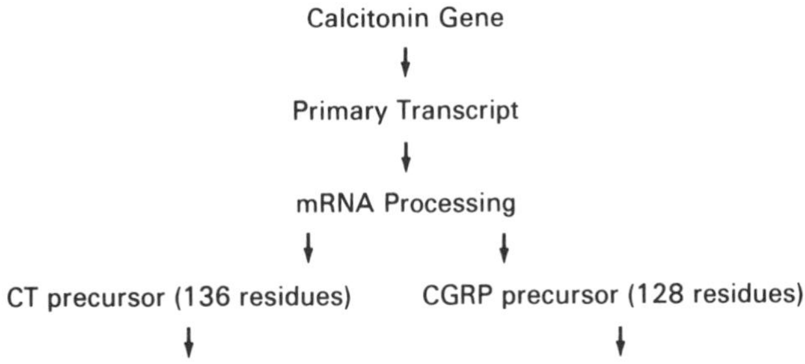

FIGURE 28-1 Summary of human calcitonin (CT) gene expression. The CT pathway occurs primarily in endocrine tissue (e.g., C cells), and the calcitonin gene–related peptide (CGRP) pathway primarily in neural tissue. The gene has six exons whose primary RNA transcript is differentially spliced into an mRNA for the CT precursor and for the CGRP precursor. A common 25-residue leader sequences is removed, and these two polypeptide precursors are each processed into their three respective peptide products. (Alternative designations for some of these peptides are as follows: for N-pro CT, PAS-57; for C-pro CT, PDN-21 and katacalcin; for N-pro CGRP, PAS-55.) The function of the other one of these peptides is not firmly established.

now known to be present in other endocrine tissues, among them the parathyroid, pancreas, and pituitary.[133] This protein could thus be a marker for each of the endocrine neoplasias of both MEN 1 and MEN 2.[134] CgA has also been reported to be produced by CT-negative MTC.[135]

Provocative Testing *Calcium* The intravenous (IV) infusion of calcium has been the most widely used technique for stimulating calcitonin secretion in MTC. In early studies, calcium was infused at doses ranging from 3 to 5 mg per kilogram of body weight per hour for periods varying from 2 to 4 h. The increase in serum calcium concentration produced by such infusions, usually several milligrams per deciliter, consistently produced an abnormal increase in plasma calcitonin concentration in patients with MTC.[125] The abnormal increase in plasma calcitonin concentration occurred even in patients who had basal concentrations of the hormone that were indistinguishable from normal.[129]

Prolonged calcium infusions have several disadvantages. The length of the procedure is inconvenient, and the dose of calcium used often produces untoward effects such as hypertension, nausea, and even vomiting. This necessitates hospitalization in research wards under constant professional supervision. For these reasons, shorter infusions of calcium have been developed which are more convenient and safer than the longer procedures and yet seem to be reliable in stimulating calcitonin secretion.[136] In these procedures, the increase in plasma calcium concentration usually is less than 1 mg/dl, but calcitonin secretion is reliably stimulated. The procedure can be completed in several minutes and is generally well tolerated.[136]

Pentagastrin Pentagastrin is another widely used provocative agent for calcitonin secretion in patients with MTC.[136] When administered IV at a dose of 0.5 μg per kilogram of body weight, pentagastrin produces a rapid increase in plasma calcitonin concentration. This pattern of calcitonin response, however, probably is a function of the dose and rapidity of administration of pentagastrin rather than of any innate properties of this secretagogue. When calcium is given in a similar IV manner over a few seconds, a calcitonin response similar to that seen with pentagastrin infusion is observed; when pentagastrin is infused over several minutes, a response similar to that produced by calcium infusion is seen.[106]

Although the rapidity of the pentagastrin infusion is advantageous, this provocative test does have drawbacks. The administration of pentagastrin produces an unpleasant (but poorly described) sensation in the recipient which is commonly called "burning" or "flushing." Also, the use of pentagastrin as a diagnostic test for suspected MTC has not been approved by the U.S. Food and Drug Administration; therefore, an institutionally approved protocol may be required for its administration.[137]

Wells and colleagues[138] have described interesting modifications of the pentagastrin test. They administered the peptide to patients with MTC while an indwelling catheter was located in the inferior thyroid veins to permit plasma sampling for calcitonin assay. During this procedure they were able to demonstrate a dramatic increase in thyroidal vein as well as peripheral calcitonin concentration. In some patients, however, there was a diagnostic increase in thyroid vein calcitonin concentration, while the increase in peripheral calcitonin concentration was not diagnostic. However, such procedures cannot be considered routine, and they require considerable competence. Not only is the normal concentration of thyroidal venous calcitonin not well established, it can be influenced by a small change in the position of the indwelling catheter used to collect the sample for assay. The improved diagnostic potential of these catheterization procedures is certainly diminished by their technical difficulty and may be obviated by the increased sensitivity of newer calcitonin RIAs. These newer assays have better defined normal and abnormal ranges of both basal and stimulated calcitonin concentrations in peripheral human plasma.[139] Accordingly, patients in whom provocative testing was previously necessary for establishing the diagnosis of MTC can now often be identified by basal calcitonin measurements with assays of improved sensitivity.

A more practical use of selective venous catheterization is in the evaluation of the location and extent of an MTC or an ectopic calcitonin-producing tumor.[138] This procedure may be able to localize a recurrence of MTC precisely and thus may result in more effective treatment.[140] However, considerable skill is necessary for these procedures; even when they are technically successful, a calcitonin gradient from the tumor may be obscured by high basal circulating concentrations of hormone.

Pentagastrin vs. Calcium Differences of opinion have appeared in the literature regarding the relative clinical value of pentagastrin and calcium infusion in the diagnosis of MTC.[138] The most important point to keep in mind is that most tumors respond to either agent and that both infusion procedures have a small incidence of false-negative results; i.e., some tumors (or hyperplasia) respond to calcium but not to pentagastrin and vice versa.[84] Therefore, if one procedure gives negative results in a patient suspected of having MTC, the alternative procedure should be considered before the diagnosis is excluded.[106] There is, however, some preliminary evidence that calcium infusion may be more valuable in diagnosing early forms of the tumor.[118] In general, both the sensitivity and the specificity of the calcitonin assay are probably just as important as the choice between calcium and pentagastrin in provocative testing of suspected MTC. With a sensitive assay (of the appropriate specificity), either pentagastrin or calcium will identify a patient with this tumor in most instances. Preliminary results of combined calcium-pentagastrin infusions have not been consistent.[118,138]

Other Provocative Agents Several other agents have been reported to be useful in the diagnosis of MTC. They include the oral administration of whiskey and the infusion of magnesium and glucagon. These agents have not been widely used, and their clinical value has not been established.[84,137,141,142]

Venous Catheterization Procedures The presence as well as the location of MTC can be established by means of a calcitonin assay in conjunction with selective venous catheterization. A gradient of hormone concentration in a specific vein may localize the tumor to the site draining that vein. This procedure requires accurate catheter placement and confirmation of location with appropriate venography studies. Several factors limit the usefulness of catheterization procedures. The high incidence of bilaterality in familial MTC mandates bilateral neck surgery, so that the procedure has limited use in primary diagnosis and preoperative localization. If recurrence or persistence after surgical treatment is being evaluated, catheterization must be done in an area in which the venous anatomy has been distorted by prior surgery.[143] Therefore, accurate correlation between venous samples and anatomic sites necessitates preliminary arteriography studies to establish blood flow patterns. Such studies add considerable risk, time, and expense to venous catheterization. Therefore, the greatest potential value of catheterization studies is probably in the location of tumor metastases (or ectopic calcitonin production). Prior knowledge of the presence of metastatic (or ectopic) disease can greatly influence therapy.[139] The value of newer radiologic and radionuclear imaging procedures in detecting MTC continues to be explored.[128]

Calcitonin Measurements in the Evaluation of Therapy The effectiveness of therapy in patients with calcitonin-producing tumors can be monitored by means of serial measurements of plasma calcitonin concentration.[84] This application of the calcitonin assay pertains to surgical as well as chemotherapeutic treatment. In addition to determining the relatively immediate effects of a given treatment regimen, periodic surveillance with appropriate provocative testing can be conducted for recurrence of the tumor.[144]

Immunochemical Heterogeneity There are multiple immunochemical forms of calcitonin in tumor tissue and in plasma.[145,146] When plasma or tumor extracts from a patient with MTC are immunoassayed after gel filtration chromatography, multiple peaks of immunoreactive calcitonin are observed. The number of peaks can be influenced by the size of the column, the nature of the matrix gel, and the elution conditions. Under such influences, calcitonin auto- or homoaggregation (dimerization or polymerization) or heteroaggregation (with other proteins) may influence the elution profile. Thus, only some of the peaks may actually reflect the biosynthesis, secretion, and metabolism of calcitonin. The complex pathway for CT gene expression (Fig. 28–1) may also account for the multiple calcitonin forms found in blood.[132,147] And, since calcitonin is metabolized after secretion and perhaps also inside cells, such metabolic derivatives may also be represented in plasma. Therefore, the multiple forms of immunoassayable plasma calcitonin represent a complex mixture of actual as well as operatively created species of calcitonin, its biosynthetic precursors, and its metabolites.

Certain characteristics of the immunochemical heterogeneity of plasma calcitonin are also conferred by the immunochemical specificity of the antiserum used to make hormone measurements.[148] Antibodies of a given specificity for the calcitonin molecule react with (and therefore detect) preferentially species of the hormone which have that specificity. For example, if calcitonin is metabolized to a fragment which contains a carboxy-terminal peptide, an antiserum with specificity for the carboxy-terminal region of calcitonin will detect that fragment, whereas an antiserum with specificity for another region of the molecule may not. Therefore, immunochemical heterogeneity is a function of the hormone species being measured as well as the assay procedure employed.

Assessment of the immunochemical heterogeneity of plasma calcitonin can provide fundamental information about C cell function as well as information of clinical importance. Perhaps the most important clinical implication of calcitonin heterogeneity will be in screening patients for early diagnosis of MTC or other calcitonin-producing tumors. Some assay procedures may identify better than other assay systems the slightly increased basal concentrations of calcitonin which occur in early MTC. Furthermore, different provocative agents may stimulate the secretion (or release) of different species of calcitonin.[147] Thus, the optimal diagnostic combination may depend on choosing the correct provocative test for a given assay system and the correct assay system for a given provocative test. Clearly, optimum results are provided by sensitive assay systems which have been well characterized and extensively applied.

Serial Calcitonin Measurements Patients at risk for MTC should be evaluated periodically for the manifestations of the tumor. Sensitive and specific assays for calcitonin should be applied at frequent intervals.[149] In general, screening should begin no later than age 5 and continue until at least age 35 at intervals of approximately 6 to 9 months; more aggressive screening may be indicated in some patients.[134] The initial 50 percent risk of developing this tumor declines to approximately 10 percent if the stimulated calcitonin response remains normal until age 25.[150] Since other endocrine tumors occur later, screening procedures for them should be conducted indefinitely.[84]

Other Secretory Products

In addition to calcitonin and the other products of its gene (Fig. 28-1), MTC produces other substances, nonpeptides as well as peptides (Table 28-3). This unusual biosynthetic capacity of MTC may be related to the neural crest origin of C cells.[151,152]

Prostaglandins Abnormal concentrations of prostaglandins (PGs) are present in the tumor and blood of some patients with MTC. These excess PGs have been implicated in the pathogenesis of the diarrhea commonly seen in patients with this tumor. It is known that PGs can stimulate intestinal smooth muscle, and diarrhea seems to be a more prominent symptom in patients with an extensive tumor burden. Furthermore, diarrhea may be decreased by surgical removal of the tumor and treatment with PG inhibitors. However, patients with diarrhea and MTC may have normal PG levels, and patients with elevated PG levels may not have diarrhea. Furthermore, excess PG production occurs in a variety of other tumors which are not associated with diarrhea.[132]

TABLE 28-3 Products of Medullary Thyroid Carcinoma

Calcitonin (CT)	Substance P
Calcitonin gene-related peptide	Neurotension
PDN21 (katacalcin)	Vasoactive intestinal polypeptide
N-pro CT	Corticotropin releasing hormone
L-Dopa decarboxylase	Gastrin releasing peptide
Histaminase	Prolactin releasing factor
Serotonin	Nerve growth factor
Prostaglandins	Amyloid
Kallikrein and kinins	Carcinoembryonic antigen
Adenocorticotropin	Melanin
Melanocyte stimulating hormone	Neuron-specific enolase
Somatostatin	Synaptophysin
β-Endorphin	Chromogranin A

Serotonin MTC can be associated with abnormal serotonin production and the carcinoid syndrome. In some patients, the carcinoid syndrome is uncovered by procedures, such as calcium infusion, which stimulate the secretory activity of MTC. The tumor can also produce peptides such as bradykinin and kallikrein, which are integral to the carcinoid syndrome. As with prostaglandins, serotonin and its metabolites may contribute to the diarrhea commonly seen in patients with MTC.[132]

Histaminase Elevated levels of histaminase, an enzyme which catalyzes the deamination of histamine, are commonly found in the tumor and serum of patients with MTC. This may play a role in the abnormal result of a histaminase test observed in some patients with this tumor, although alternative explanations are possible. Unlike PGs and serotonin and like calcitonin, abnormal histaminase production seems to be somewhat specific for MTC as opposed to other tumors. Thus, the measurement of histaminase level may have some clinical value in the diagnosis and management of a patient with MTC. Although histaminase is generally not as sensitive a marker for MTC as is calcitonin, it may be useful in identifying patients with metastatic MTC.[153]

Peptide Hormones In addition to calcitonin and the other products of the CT gene, MTC can produce a variety of other peptide hormones, including ACTH, melanocyte stimulating hormone (MSH), somatostatin, and β-endorphin.[153] This group of peptides, including calcitonin, is also commonly represented in other tumors of neural crest origin, notably oat-cell carcinoma of the lung. It has also been reported that pituitary cells produce calcitonin or a substance immunochemically related to calcitonin. The concurrent production of this variety of peptide hormones may represent an independent expression of the malignant state. However, it has been postulated that the production of some of these peptide hormones may be regulated by closely related genes and that there may even be a precursor molecule common to some of them.[132]

Pheochromocytoma

In 1961 Sipple presented evidence for an association between pheochromocytoma and thyroid tumor.[154] He reported the case of a 33-year-old male with bilateral pheochromocytomas and a poorly differentiated invasive thyroid tumor thought to be a follicular adenocarcinoma. Sipple reviewed the literature and presented five other patients with pheochromocytoma and thyroid tumor. The pheochromocytomas were bilateral in four of the patients. The thyroid tumors were variously described as follicular adenocarcinoma, papillary adenocarcinoma, adenocarcinoma, and anaplastic carcinoma.

In the early 1960s there were additional case reports of the simultaneous occurrence of pheochromocytomas and thyroid carcinomas (reviewed in ref. 84). In 1967 Williams reported 2 cases of pheochromocytomas and thyroid cancer; he reviewed 15 others.[155] He was able to establish that at least 11 of the total of 17 cases of thyroid tumor actually were MTC. In the same year Schimke and Hartmann[156] also reviewed the previous reports of the simultaneous occurrence of pheochromocytoma and MTC and added studies of their own of two families in which these two tumors occurred simultaneously in each of five patients.[156] Thus, the association between pheochromocytomas and MTC has become well established only in the past 25 years.[106]

The classical tests of catecholamine metabolism may not be adequate for pheochromocytoma diagnosis in MEN 2. Therefore, the diagnosis should be vigorously pursued if appropriate even when urinary and serum metabolites are normal. Serum chromogram A measurements may be useful since they are not affected by the drugs used in the medical management of these patients.[84,153]

Occurrence

Since different reports have emphasized different aspects of the MEN syndrome, it is difficult to determine how commonly pheochromocytomas occur in association with MTC. It has become apparent that the frequency of pheochromocytomas is much higher than previously appreciated. In MEN 2b the prevalence of pheochromocytomas usually approaches 50 percent,[157] whereas in MEN 2a it usually is less than 20 percent.[122] However, it is likely that these represent underestimates, especially in MEN 2b, since most recent studies suggest a much higher frequency.[106]

There are several distinct features of pheochromocytomas occurring in association with MTC. In this circumstance, bilateral and multifocal pheochromocytomas are very common and have a prevalence greater than 70 percent; this contrasts with a prevalence of bilateral pheochromocytoma of usually less than 10 percent for sporadic MTC. Pheochromocytomas are much more likely to occur in patients with familial rather than sporadic MTC.[157,158] When pheochromocytomas and MTC occur together in the same patient, the MTC is likely to be diagnosed first.[123,157,158] The thyroid tumor may antedate the pheochromocytomas by as much as 21 years. Furthermore, a second pheochromocytoma may become manifest after removal of the first.[123] This sequence of events results in a greater incidence of pheochromocytomas in older patients with MTC. Less often, the thyroid and adrenal tumors may be discovered contemporaneously; in some cases, pheochromocytomas may be diagnosed before MTC. If hyperparathyroidism also exists, it, too, is likely to be diagnosed before the pheochromocytoma.[123,157,158] Computerized abdominal tomography and other imaging procedures are helpful in identifying these tumors.

Adrenal Medullary Hyperplasia

Adrenal medullary hyperplasia may be a predecessor of the pheochromocytomas seen with MTC, just as C cell hyperplasia may be a predecessor of MTC.[110,159] Although cases of adrenal medullary hyperplasia had been reported previously in the literature, none of them occurred in patients with MTC.[84] DeLellis and colleagues described the adrenal glands of 10 patients from a large kindred with familial MTC.[160] There was an increase in the medullary volume of adrenal glands compared with controls. The increase in medullary mass resulted from diffuse and/or multifocal proliferation of adrenal medullary cells, primarily those found within the head and body of the glands. Multifocal proliferation can produce an adenomatous appearance.[101] There is hypertrophy as well as hyperplasia of the cells, and they show increased mitotic activity and increased total catecholamine content.[159] In addition, the ratio of epinephrine to norepinephrine was increased in the tumor.[160] These findings suggest that a sequence of events similar to that postulated for MTC and hyperparathyroidism takes place in the development of pheochromocytomas: Hypertrophy develops into hyperplasia; multifocal hyperplasia develops into nodularity; nodularity undergoes neoplastic transformation to pheochromocytomas. This transformation is the final stage of the sequence in most tumors, but malignant transformation can also be seen.

Hyperparathyroidism

Cushman described the simultaneous occurrence of a parathyroid adenoma in a patient with MTC who also had a pheochromocytoma.[161] Additional reports of the association of hyperparathyroidism and MTC subsequently appeared, and the two additional cases of Steiner et al. in 1968 brought the literature total to 13 at that time.[158] In the ensuing years other reports have clearly established the association between MTC and hyperparathyroidism.

Occurrence

It is difficult to establish the exact prevalence of hyperparathyroidism in patients with MTC. Melvin and colleagues made the diagnosis of hyperparathyroidism in 10 of 12 patients of a kindred with MTC,[92] whereas Hill et al. could establish the diagnosis of hyperparathyroidism in only 2 of 73 patients with MTC.[123] The most recent literature suggests that hyperplasia is more common than adenoma.[106] There are several possible explanations for this disparity. For one, there is disagreement regarding the criteria necessary to distinguish between a normal and an abnormal parathyroid gland as well as the criteria used to classify parathyroid abnormalities.[84] Another possible explanation involves the developing appreciation that hyperparathyroidism is considerably more common in MEN 2a than in MEN 2b. Despite these differences, the concurrence of hyperparathyroidism and MTC is well established; although the frequency with which they occur together cannot be specified, the presence of one tumor should always arouse suspicion of the presence of the other.

Pathology

Steiner and colleagues reviewed the literature on MEN 2a in 1968 and recorded 10 cases with parathyroid adenoma and 3 cases with parathyroid hyperplasia.[158] In later reports the prevalence of parathyroid hyperplasia in patients with MTC has increased and has even approached 100 percent.[117,162] The controversy regarding parathyroid pathology in patients with MTC is reflective of the general difficulties in this area of histologic diagnosis.[117,163]

Relation to MTC

Two hypotheses prevail regarding the link between hyperparathyroidism and MTC. One possibility is that the hyperparathyroidism is a functional disorder representing a compensatory response of the parathyroid glands to a hypocalcemic effect of calcitonin. This view does have some clinical and experimental support.[91] There are, however, more convincing data indicating that the hyperparathyroidism is an inherited rather than a functional component of the syndrome.[106] The genetic view would be more attractive if the embryologic origin of the parathyroid gland were the neural crest, in keeping with the embryologic origin of the other prominent features of the syndrome, i.e., pheochromocytoma, MTC, and mucosal neuromas. Most evidence suggests that the parathyroid glands are of entodermal origin, arising from the third and fourth branchial pouches. However, if the data which suggest that the parathyroid glands are of neural crest origin[90] are confirmed, a more unifying genetic basis for MEN 2a and MEN 2b would be provided.

Multiple Mucosal Neuromas (MMN)

In 1966 Williams and Pollock described two patients with MTC and pheochromocytomas who had neuromas involving the mucous membranes of the lips, tongue, and eyes.[164] In 1968 Schimke and colleagues described three additional patients with this syndrome; they recorded the presence of megacolon in each patient.[165] In one patient rectal biopsy was consistent with ganglioneuromatosis of the submucous and myenteric plexuses. In the same year Gorlin and coworkers reemphasized the association between MMNs, pheochromocytomas, and MTC by reviewing 17 published cases.[166] In several patients the neuromas were congenital or were noticed within the first few years of life, thus becoming manifest before the other features of the syndrome. These authors also commented on the presence of a marfanoid habitus, intestinal ganglioneuromatosis, and medullated corneal nerve fibers in this group of patients and thus articulated the features of this syndrome as it is currently appreciated: MTC, pheochromocytomas, diffuse neurogangliomatosis involving the mucosa of the gastrointestinal tract, and a marfanoid habitus.[157]

Mucosal Neuromas

The presence of neuromas with a centrofacial distribution is the most consistent component of the MMN syndrome. The most prominent microscopic feature of the neuromas is an increase in the size and number of nerves. The nerves are tortuous and highly branched and are often surrounded by a thickened perineurium; both medullated and unmedullated fibers are involved. Ganglion cells and connective tissue may be present, but the connective tissue often is not prominent. This latter feature usually distinguishes these neuromas from the neurofibromas of von Recklinghausen's neurofibromatosis.[132]

The most common location of neuromas is in the oral cavity. The lips, tongue, and buccal mucosa are the most common sites for oral MMN. The oral lesions usually are the first components of the syndrome to appear. They are almost invariably present by the first decade and can even be present at birth.[157] The mucosal neuromas, along with the ocular findings described below, give the affected patients a very characteristic facial appearance. Because of this, there is a striking similarity in the appearance of different subjects with the syndrome, even though they may be unrelated and of the opposite sex.

Mucosal neuromas can be present in the eyelids, conjunctiva, and cornea. The tarsal neuromas result in thickened eyelids and retracted eyelashes, which give the eye a hooded, sleepy look. In addition to the neuromas, a variety of other ocular abnormalities have been reported. The medullated corneal nerves are thickened; they traverse the cornea and anastomose in the pupillary area. These hypertrophied nerve fibers are seen readily with the slit lamp but occasionally may be evident on direct funduscopic examination.[157]

Gastrointestinal Abnormalities

One of the most prominent features of MEN 2a and 2b is the presence of gastrointestinal (GI) abnormalities.[116,123] Diarrhea is a common symptom in affected patients.[123] Its etiology is multifactoral. The diarrhea seen in these patients often can be ascribed to one of the many humors produced by MTC.[106] Most of these agents have been variably described as increasing GI motility either directly or indirectly. Some of the GI symptoms of diarrhea and constipation additionally can be ascribed to GI abnormalities that are part of the mucosal neuroma syndrome. The most common of these is gastrointestinal ganglioneuromatosis. The lesions of GI ganglioneuromatosis are reminiscent of those which occur in the facial mucosal neuromas. In fact, all cases of diffuse GI ganglioneuromatosis occur in association with mucosal neuromas; isolated intestinal ganglioneuromatosis is not associated with MTC. The ganglioneuromatosis is best observed in the small intestine and large intestine but has also been noted in the esophagus and stomach.[116] There is a proliferation of the neural elements of the myenteric and submucosal plexuses. The anatomic lesions can be associated with functional difficulties in swallowing, megacolon, diarrhea, and constipation.[157] Another common GI finding which may contribute to the diarrhea is the presence of diverticulosis.

Marfanoid Habitus

A marfanoid habitus is seen commonly in the MMN syndrome.[157] The marfanoid habitus refers to a tall, slender body with an abnormal upper- to lower-body-segment size ratio and poor muscle development. The extremities are thin and long; there may be lax joints and hypotonic muscles. Associated with the marfanoid habitus may be dorsal kyphosis, pectus excavatum (funnel chest), pectus carinatum (pigeon breast), pes cavus, and a high-arched palate. In contrast to patients with true Marfan syndrome, no patients with MMN have been reported to have aortic abnormalities, ectopia lentis, homocystinuria, or mucopolysaccharide abnormalities.

Treatment

The treatment of patients with MEN 2 is guided by the same general principles that are used for the treatment of the individual tumor components.[132] Thus, surgery is the treatment of choice for the three neoplasias of this disorder.[167–169] Since all of the tumors are potentially lethal, aggressive surgical treatment is warranted.[84] Early treatment before tumor spread can be curative, emphasizing the importance of early diagnosis.[169] It is important to consider the multifocal nature of the tumors when planning surgery.[84] For the thyroid tumor, this means bilateral and total thyroidectomy.[167,170] For the pheochromocytoma, both adrenals and ancillary tissues should be thoroughly explored,[149] and for the parathyroid tumor, the possibility of hyperplasia or multiple tumor sites should be kept in mind.[132,171] Although a variety of antineoplastic drugs and radiotherapeutic approaches have been tried, none seems to be effective.[172–176]

PLURIGLANDULAR ENDOCRINE INSUFFICIENCY SYNDROMES

Physicians have noted the coincidence of diabetes mellitus and Addison's disease in the same patient since the nineteenth century.[177] In 1926 Schmidt described a "biglandular illness" in two patients with nontuberculous Addison's disease and lymphocytic thyroiditis. In 1964 Carpenter et al.[178] reviewed Schmidt's syndrome and found coexisting diabetes mellitus in 10 of 15 patients with Addison's disease and thyroiditis. They expanded the definition of the syndrome to nontuberculous Addison's disease associated with either of these other endocrinopathies. It has since become apparent that there are multiple associations among presumed autoimmune diseases of endocrine organs, including the adrenals, endocrine pancreas, thyroid, parathyroids, ovaries, and, probably, testes and adenohypophysis. Schmidt's syndrome, as defined by Carpenter et al.[178] (and as used in this chapter), is characteristic of only one subset of patients with pluriglandular endocrine failure. In addition, these endocrine disorders are frequently associated with other disorders of tissue-specific autoimmunity, notably pernicious anemia and vitiligo. The clinical and immunologic relationships among the autoimmune endocrinopathies are reviewed here.

Immunologic tissue injury can result from six mechanisms (Table 28-4). The primary agents in autoimmune reactions are immunoglobulins, effector T cells (thymus-dependent lymphocytes which become sensitized to specific antigens and release soluble nonimmunoglobulin mediators), and monocytes (which possess receptors for the Fc region of immunoglobulins and cytotoxic capabilities in the pres-

TABLE 28-4 Types of Immunologic Tissue Injury

1. IgE-mediated immediate hypersensitivity
2. Complement-dependent direct humoral cytotoxicity
3. Antigen-antibody complex deposition
4. T-cell-mediated immunity
5. Antireceptor antibody binding (blocking or stimulating)
6. Antibody-dependent cell-mediated cytotoxicity

ence of tissue-specific antibody). Table 28-5 shows some of the methods which have been used to detect tissue-specific immunity and the mechanism of injury implied. The indirect immunofluorescence technique for autoantibodies to cytoplasmic microsomal antigens has been especially versatile; a pathogenetic role for these antibodies is suggested by observations that they also react with the cell-surface antigens of living cells.[179] Antibodies to thyroid stimulating hormone (TSH), ACTH, and possibly other receptors are also involved.[180,181]

The pathogenesis of autoimmune endocrine disease has been most extensively studied in Hashimoto's thyroiditis and Graves' disease and has been the subject of several recent reviews.[182] T-cell-mediated immunity and antibody-dependent cell-mediated cytotoxicity (ADCC) have received the greatest attention as mechanisms of target organ destruction in Hashimoto's thyroiditis.[183] In addition, in vitro evidence for T cells specifically sensitized against other endocrine tissues exists.[179,184–186] Although immune complexes are present in the sera of some patients with Hashimoto's thyroiditis (and Graves' disease), the pathologic significance of this finding is unclear.[187] Volpe[182] has proposed a unifying theory of pathogenesis of autoimmune thyroid disease based on a defect in immunoregulation by suppressor T cells (thymus-dependent lymphocytes which suppress immune responses, possibly including recognition of autoantigens).

Evidence to support this hypothesis is building.[188,189] Experiments assessing the function of normal suppressor T cells in vitro have demonstrated that these cells can depress the production of migration-inhibiting lymphokines by cultured leukocytes and repress the differentiation of antithyroid B cells from patients with Hashimoto's thyroiditis. A defect in these functions is confined to patients with autoimmune thyroid disease.[190] However, the precise events that initiate immune recognition of antigens in the endocrine system remain unclear. Class II histocompatibility molecules (see below), which are crucial to antigen recognition, are normally expressed only on the surface of monocytic and other antigen-presenting cells. These glycoproteins appear on the surface of endocrine cells in the course of the autoimmune disorder.[191–193] It has therefore been suggested that an environmental event (e.g., viral infection) may initiate the process by causing internal cellular proteins to be displayed on the endocrine cell surface along with class II HLA glycoproteins bearing required structural features. However, since endocrine cell HLA-DR expression has also been found in areas of lymphocyte accumulation in diseases such as multinodular goiter, carcinoma of the thyroid, and tuberculous Addison's disease, HLA molecules are not generally sufficient for progression to an outright autoimmune state. It has not been determined whether the combination of three factors (display of cell-specific proteins, expression of antigen-presenting molecules, and coexistence of an antigen-specific suppressor cell defect) is sufficient for the development of autoimmunity.

Pluriglandular Autoimmunity with Addison's Disease

For several reasons, Addison's disease has provided a good focus for investigation of the pluriglandular endocrine insufficiency syndromes. First, the clinical impact of this disease is such that few of these patients should escape medical attention. This is confirmed by the low prevalence of subclinical antiadrenal autoimmunity as detected serologically. Second, tuberculous destruction of the adrenal glands provides a natural control group for clinical and immunologic comparison.

Some variation in the criteria for making a diagnosis of idiopathic Addison's disease exists in the

TABLE 28-5 Tests of Tissue-Specific Immunity

Antibody determinations	Tests for cell-mediated immunity (type 4)
Immunoprecipitation (gel counterdiffusion)	Direct lymphocytotoxicity
Complement fixation	Lymphocyte blast transformation
Indirect immunofluorescence	Leukocyte migration inhibition
Demonstration of direct serum cytotoxicity (type 2)	Intradermal skin testing
Inhibition of trophic hormone binding and/or action (type 5)	Lymphocyte Ia antigen (HLA-DR)
Facilitation of cell-mediated cytotoxicity (type 6)	

literature. Pulmonary tuberculosis and radiographic evidence of adrenal calcification allow a presumptive diagnosis of tuberculous Addison's disease to be made; idiopathic Addison's disease is diagnosed when there is no evidence of tuberculosis or another reasonable etiology. In patients with tuberculous disease on x-ray film of the chest but without adrenal calcification, no definitive assignment of etiology can be made (i.e., the etiology is indeterminate). Age of onset does not permit a distinction between idiopathic and tuberculous Addison's disease except that tuberculous Addison's disease is uncommon under age 10. However, there is an approximate 2:1 female predominance in idiopathic Addison's disease, whereas the sex ratio in tuberculous Addison's disease is approximately unity. Table 28-6 shows the high frequency of one or more second diseases in patients with idiopathic Addison's disease and notes the much lower prevalence of associated disorders in patients with tuberculous Addison's disease. Cumulation of five series shows that 39 percent of 419 patients with idiopathic Addison's disease had an associated tissue-specific autoimmune disease, compared with only 8 percent of patients with tuberculous Addison's disease. The diseases found with tuberculous Addison's disease have generally been diabetes and thyroid disease.[177] Additionally, among 90 patients with tuberculous Addison's disease (as defined above), none had adrenal antibodies, whereas the prevalence of adrenal antibodies in idiopathic Addison's disease ranges from 48 to 74 percent.[177] In vitro evidence of cell-mediated immunity to adrenal antigens is present in many patients with idiopathic Addison's disease but not in patients with tuberculous Addison's disease.[186] These findings reinforce the conclusion that idiopathic Addison's disease is part of an autoimmune endocrine syndrome and that the in vitro immunologic abnormalities found in idiopathic Addison's disease (and by inference in the other disorders) are not simply a result of tissue destruction.

Nerup[194] has studied the frequency of associated endocrine disorders and antibodies in the group of patients with Addison's disease of indeterminate etiology. He detected adrenal antibodies in 39 percent of patients in this group by means of indirect immunofluorescence, compared with 74 percent in idiopathic Addison's disease and none in tuberculous Addison's disease patients. Five percent of these patients had an associated endocrinopathy, compared with 5 percent of tuberculous Addison's disease patients and 39 percent of idiopathic Addison's disease patients. These results suggest that this group is mixed with respect to etiology. Some studies of idiopathic Addison's disease have included these patients, and other studies have excluded them. If found, mineralocorticoid deficiency with partial if not complete preservation of glucocorticoid secretory reserve may suggest idiopathic Addison's disease.[195] Testing of adrenal medullary function[196] also discriminates between tuberculous and idiopathic Addison's disease, but this has not become a generally accepted procedure.

Adrenal antibodies in blood, which are detected most commonly by indirect immunofluorescence and precipitation, correlate with the presence of clinical Addison's disease and associated diseases. Table 28-7 shows the frequency of adrenal antibody by immunofluorescence according to sex of the patient or the age of onset of adrenal insufficiency in patients with and without associated disease. Adrenal antibodies may disappear in patients studied later than 1 to 5 years after the onset of Addison's disease.[194,197] The higher prevalence of antibodies in Addison's disease associated with other disorders is particularly striking; conversely, the association of a second autoimmune disease is 2.5 to 2.7 times greater in antibody-positive compared with antibody-negative patients.[186,198] Most investigators[186,198] have found adrenal antibodies to be more frequent in women, although this has not been uniformly reported.[194] Patients with Addison's disease alone who are male or whose adrenal insufficiency began prior to age 20 have adrenal antibodies much less frequently. Adrenal antibodies have been found in 12 of a total of 95 patients with idiopathic hypoparathyroidism in three separate studies.[177,194,199] Such antibodies are found rarely in patients with Cushing's disease,

TABLE 28-6 Frequencies of Other Disorders in Idiopathic Addison's Disease

Ref.	No. patients	Diabetes*	Hyper-thyroidism*	Hashimoto's myxedema*	Pernicious anemia*	Hypo-gonadism*	Hypopara-thyroidism*	One or more*
235	23	3 (13)	1 (4)	4 (17)	1 (4)	7 (30)	0	9 (40)
236	46	4 (10)	5 (10)	4 (10)	1 (3)	2 (5)	0	18 (45)
237	18	1 (6)	1 (6)	2 (12)	0	3 (18)	3 (18)	8 (44)
194	71	13 (18)	7 (10)	4 (5)	2 (2)	8 (11)	0	28 (39)
177	261	21 (8)	19 (7)	23 (9)	12 (5)	47 (18)	16 (6)	101 (39)
Total	419	42 (10)	33 (8)	37 (9)	16 (4)	67 (16)	19 (5)	164 (39)

* Percentages are denoted by numbers in parentheses.
Note: Among 114 patients with tuberculous Addison's disease in the five series, 9 (8 percent) had one or more other disorders.
Source: Modified from Irvine and Barnes.[177]

TABLE 28-7 Frequency* of Antiadrenal Antibodies in Patients with Idiopathic Addison's Disease Alone and with Other Disorders Classified by Sex and Age at Onset of Addison's Disease

	Sex			Age at onset†		
	Female‡	Male‡	Total‡	<17‡	≥17‡	Total‡
Addison's alone	14/27 (52)	7/40 (18)	21/67 (31)	4/26 (15)	16/36 (44)	20/62 (32)
Addison's + other disease	23/30 (77)	13/21 (62)	36/51 (71)	15/21 (71)	20/28 (71)	35/49 (71)
		Total	57/118 (48)			55/111 (50)

* Fraction of patients of sex or age category with antiadrenal antibodies; percentages in parentheses.
† Of patients whose age at onset of Addison's disease was known.
‡ Percentages are denoted by numbers in parentheses.
Source: Modified from Blizzard et al.[198]

Hashimoto's thyroiditis, or diabetes alone or in first-degree relatives of patients with idiopathic Addison's disease.[177,194] The prevalence of adrenal antibodies in the general population is <1 in 1000.[194]

Many investigators have also found an increased frequency of other tissue-specific antibodies in patients with antibody-positive Addison's disease, including antibodies to parathyroid, islet-cell, and thyroid tissue, in the absence of clinical disease of these tissues.[177,194,198,199] Nerup[194] found a sixfold increase in the prevalence of thyroid antibodies and a tenfold increase in the frequency of parietal cell antibodies in patients with adrenal antibody-positive Addison's disease compared with age- and sex-matched controls, but no difference was observed between Addison's disease patients without adrenal antibodies and controls. A group of 118 patients with idiopathic Addison's disease was studied by Blizzard et al.[198] for associated autoimmune diseases and the presence of three extraadrenal antibodies; the prevalence of one of these abnormalities was 84 percent in patients who were adrenal antibody-positive compared with 44 percent of patients who were adrenal antibody-negative. The prevalence of at least one additional autoimmune disease or extraadrenal antibody was 82 percent in females with Addison's disease and 46 percent in males.

These findings suggest that (1) idiopathic Addison's disease is not a homogeneous disorder with a random coincidence of other autoimmune endocrine disease and (2) patients with pluriglandular endocrine insufficiency may also be heterogeneous. Figure 28-2 supports this thesis, showing the distribution of age of onset or diagnosis for each sex for isolated Addison's disease and Addison's disease with other endocrine disorders. Differences in the percentage of childhood-onset patients between the two series shown are probably attributable to the pediatric orientation of one set of investigators. It is clear that the Addison's disease associated with hypoparathyroidism has a much younger age of onset than do the other two major groups; in all three groups a trend toward earlier onset of disease in males may be noted. Spinner et al.[199,200] analyzed 140 families containing 182 patients with idiopathic Addison's disease, idiopathic hypoparathyroidism, or both disorders. They found evidence for genetic as well as clinical heterogeneity among these patients. They divided their patients into four groups: Addison's disease with hypoparathyroidism, isolated hypoparathyroidism, isolated Addison's disease, and Schmidt's syndrome. Immunologic findings in the patients with isolated Addison's disease or isolated hypoparathyroidism suggest that the abnormality in some of these patients may represent a forme fruste

FIGURE 28-2 Clinical heterogeneity of Addison's disease. Distribution of age of onset (*top*) and age of diagnosis (*bottom*) of Addison's disease alone and Addison's disease with hypoparathyroidism or Schmidt's syndrome. The open area represents females; the closed area represents males. (*Data from Spinner et al.*[200] *and Irvine and Barnes.*)[177]

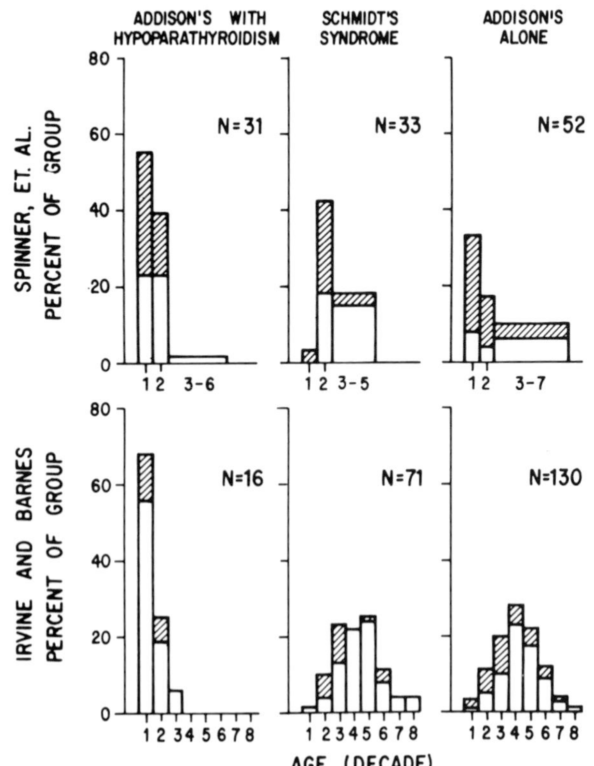

of pluriglandular endocrine insufficiency. Furthermore, evidence discussed below indicates that diabetes and autoimmune thyroid disease frequently coexist in the absence of adrenal autoimmunity. Thus, pluriglandular endocrine autoimmunity can be divided into the major types and variations shown in Fig. 28-3.

Addison's Disease with Hypoparathyroidism

As shown in Fig. 28-2, the group of patients with Addison's disease plus hypoparathyroidism is distinguished by a much earlier onset of Addison's disease in both sexes. Taken together, the two series shown in Fig. 28-2 demonstrate only a slight excess of female patients in this category. Chronic mucocutaneous candidiasis occurs frequently in this group; in 84 percent of patients with this infection and an associated endocrinopathy, the endocrine disorder is hypoparathyroidism.[201] The onset of candidiasis and hypoparathyroidism (usually in that order) is even earlier than that of Addison's disease: hypoparathyroidism occurs before age 10 in 88 percent of patients[200] (Fig. 28-4). Addison's disease follows within 2 years in half the patients, and within 9 years in three-fourths. These patients are occasionally afflicted by a third endocrine disorder, including thyroid disease, diabetes, pernicious anemia, or ovarian failure.

Addison's disease with hypoparathyroidism is frequently familial; the probability is estimated to be 0.35 that the sibling of an affected person will have Addison's disease, hypoparathyroidism, or any one of the above-mentioned secondary disorders.[200] It is relatively uncommon, however, for the sib to have both Addison's disease and hypoparathyroidism. Spinner et al.[200] found 10 siblings with either Addison's disease or hypoparathyroidism but only 2 with both disorders among the families of probands with both endocrinopathies. It is, of course, likely that some siblings with only one of the two disorders will eventually develop the second.

Antibodies to parathyroid tissue, as demonstrated by indirect immunofluorescence, occur in 38 percent of patients with idiopathic hypoparathyroidism[202]; in addition, they are found in 26 percent of patients with idiopathic Addison's disease without hypoparathyroidism (see below). Among patients with Addison's disease and hypoparathyroidism there is also an increased frequency of thyroid and parietal cell antibodies.[199]

A variety of immunologic defects have been reported in patients with chronic mucocutaneous candidiasis with or without endocrinopathies, including impaired blast transformation, impaired macrophage migration inhibition, and impaired lymphocytotoxicity.[203] The pathogenetic relation between these defects and those responsible for immune sensitization to endocrine tissue is unclear.

FIGURE 28-3 The three major clinical categories of pluriglandular autoimmune endocrinopathy (center column), with forme fruste variants (dashed boxes) and less frequently associated endocrine disorders and nonendocrine disorders. Graves' disease may substitute for thyroiditis. Gonadal failure is associated with a pansteroid cell antibody in Addison's disease; candidiasis is strongly associated with hypoparathyroidism.

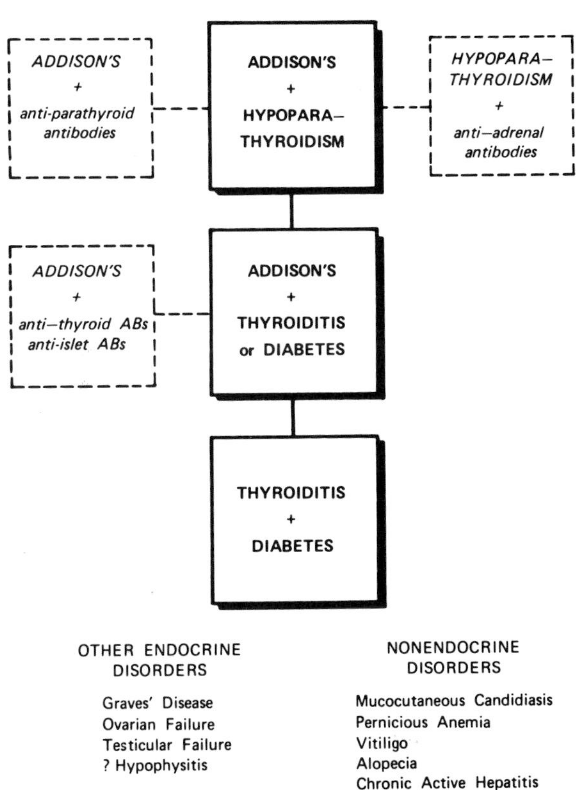

Hypoparathyroidism without Addison's Disease

Patients with hypoparathyroidism but no Addison's disease have an early onset of hypoparathyroidism (73 percent prior to age 10) and chronic candidiasis, similar to those with Addison's disease. In the group of patients reported by Spinner et al.,[200] the time elapsed after the onset of hypoparathyroidism was sufficient to make it unlikely that many of these patients would later develop Addison's disease. Familial aggregation is infrequent, although a few patients or their sibs have developed thyroid disease or pernicious anemia. The prevalence of parathyroid antibodies in this group is similar to that of the group with Addison's disease and hypoparathyroidism.[202] In hypoparathyroid patients there is a 7 percent rate of immunofluorescent adrenal antibody detection,[199] but in hypoparathyroidism with candidiasis subclinical antiadrenal autoimmunity may occur in more than half.[204] The occurrence of

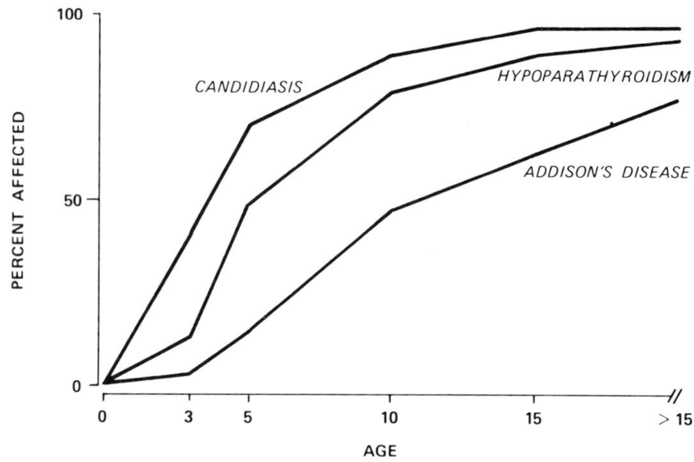

FIGURE 28-4 Typical sequence of childhood onset of chronic mucocutaneous candidiasis, autoimmune hypoparathyroidism, and Addison's disease. Patients with hypoparathyroidism may not develop Addison's disease, but frequent adrenal antibodies suggest that the polyendocrine diathesis is still present. (*Data from Neufeld et al, Medicine 60:355, 1981.*)

adrenal antibodies and candidiasis in this group suggests that this subset may represent a forme fruste of pluriglandular endocrine insufficiency. Thyroid and parietal cell antibodies do not appear to be significantly more prevalent than they are in control subjects. Nonimmunologic forms of familial isolated hypoparathyroidism also exist.[205]

Isolated Addison's Disease

As noted above, isolated idiopathic Addison's disease is associated with a lower prevalence of adrenal antibodies than is the case in patients who have other endocrinopathies associated with Addison's disease. However, this group still has an increased frequency of thyroid, parathyroid, and islet-cell antibodies compared with control populations.[198,199] Although these patients do not have clinically evident involvement of any other endocrine glands, the immunologic findings suggest that they should not be excluded from the spectrum of pluriglandular endocrine disease, and some may ultimately develop an associated endocrinopathy. Patients with isolated Addison's disease may have one or more affected siblings, especially if the onset occurred before 20 years of age.[200]

Schmidt's Syndrome

Schmidt's syndrome (Addison's disease with diabetes mellitus and/or chronic thyroiditis) has a predominantly adult age of onset and a 2:1 female predominance[200] (Fig. 28-2). In half the cases there is familial aggregation; the probability that a given sibling will also be affected is estimated to be 0.25. Table 28-6 shows that the overall frequency of diabetes mellitus in idiopathic Addison's disease is 10 percent, while that of Hashimoto's thyroiditis and primary myxedema is 9 percent. Diabetes mellitus in these patients may begin in either childhood or adulthood, but most of the patients have been treated with insulin.[177] The onset of Hashimoto's thyroiditis and diabetes is not closely linked to Addison's disease; they start an average of 7 years later. Schmidt's syndrome is frequently associated with additional disorders, including ovarian failure and pernicious anemia. As mentioned above, some patients with idiopathic Addison's disease without associated endocrinopathies may be at risk for the later development of Schmidt's syndrome. In the absence of a sibling with established Schmidt's syndrome, these individuals cannot be clinically identified.

As might be expected, patients with Schmidt's syndrome have a higher prevalence of thyroid antibodies than does any other group of patients with Addison's disease. Assays for antibodies against thyroglobulin and thyroid cytoplasmic antigens are widely available. The latter antibody is more prevalent in Hashimoto's thyroiditis and appears to be more discriminative; thyroperoxidase is one of the major cytoplasmic antigens detected in this procedure.[206] The presence of thyroid antibodies in Addison's disease indicates an increased risk for thyroid failure. McCarthy-Young et al.[207] found elevated serum TSH concentrations in 10 of 13 patients with idiopathic Addison's disease and thyroid antibodies compared with 3 of 14 patients without thyroid antibodies. Parents and siblings of patients with Schmidt's syndrome have a significantly greater prevalence of thyroid antibodies (50 and 18 percent, respectively) compared with age- and sex-matched controls.[199]

Islet-cell antibodies may also be a feature of Schmidt's syndrome. Bottazzo et al.[208] and MacCuish et al.[209] originally detected islet-cell antibodies by immunofluorescence in a group of 18 patients with diabetes and other tissue-specific autoantibodies: one-half had Addison's disease. Subsequent studies have shown such antibodies to be present in 60 percent of patients with insulin-dependent diabetes when they were tested within 1 year of diagnosis, irrespective of the presence of autoimmune disease.[210] Islet-cell antibodies disappear with time in patients with isolated diabetes; however, among patients in whom islet-cell antibodies persist for 3 to 5 years after the diagnosis of diabetes, another autoimmune disease occurs in 29 percent[210] and 67 percent have thyroid or parietal cell antibodies.[211] Islet-cell antibodies were present in 16 percent of nondiabetic patients with Addison's disease plus another autoimmune disease.[210]

Addison's Disease with Other Endocrinopathies

There is a striking incidence of ovarian failure in women with idiopathic Addison's disease. In the large series of Irvine and Barnes,[177] 24 percent of women whose menstrual history was known had amenorrhea and an additional 6 percent had oligomenorrhea. Abnormal menstrual function is not related to a deficiency of adrenal corticosteroids, since it usually persists after replacement therapy and is uncommon in tuberculous Addison's disease. Figure 28-5 shows the age of diagnosis of amenorrhea compared with the age of diagnosis of idiopathic Addison's disease in a group of these patients. Many patients with childhood onset of Addison's disease developed primary amenorrhea; in the patients with secondary amenorrhea, the ages of diagnosis of the two disorders were close, with ovarian failure usually preceding Addison's disease by a few years.

Ovarian failure in Addison's disease is associated with a special type of antibody against multiple steroid-producing cells, including Leydig cells and cells of the theca interna, corpus luteum, placenta, and adrenal cortex.[212,213] Absorption studies with these tissues distinguish between those antibodies to common antigens and others which react only with adrenal cortex. Sera containing steroid cell antibodies have direct cytotoxicity for granulosa cells in monolayer cell culture. These steroid cell antibodies are found in 20 percent of women with Addison's disease but in only 4 percent of men.[177] The frequency of amenorrhea or other menstrual disorders in women with Addison's disease is significantly greater than in those without steroid cell antibodies (Table 28-8). In a small number of patients with idiopathic Addison's disease, steroid cell antibodies, and gonadal failure, ovarian biopsy has shown lymphocytic infiltration or, in some cases, streak gonads. This type of antibody also indicates more active autoimmune disease, as shown by a higher frequency of other components of the pluriglandular endocrine insufficiency syndrome (Table 28-8). Steroid cell antibodies occur only rarely in other autoimmune diseases and have not been demonstrated in nonaddisonian patients with menstrual disorders. Although steroid cell antibodies are uncommon in men with Addison's disease, two cases of testicular failure associated with Addison's disease have been reported.[177,214]

Although most autoimmune disorders of the endocrine glands cause decreased function or failure, Graves' disease is intimately associated with these disorders. Thyrotoxicosis occurs in about 8 percent of patients with Addison's disease. In patients with idiopathic Addison's disease, pernicious anemia may occur with or without diabetes, thyroid disease, hypoparathyroidism, or ovarian failure. The prevalence of pernicious anemia in Addison's disease is

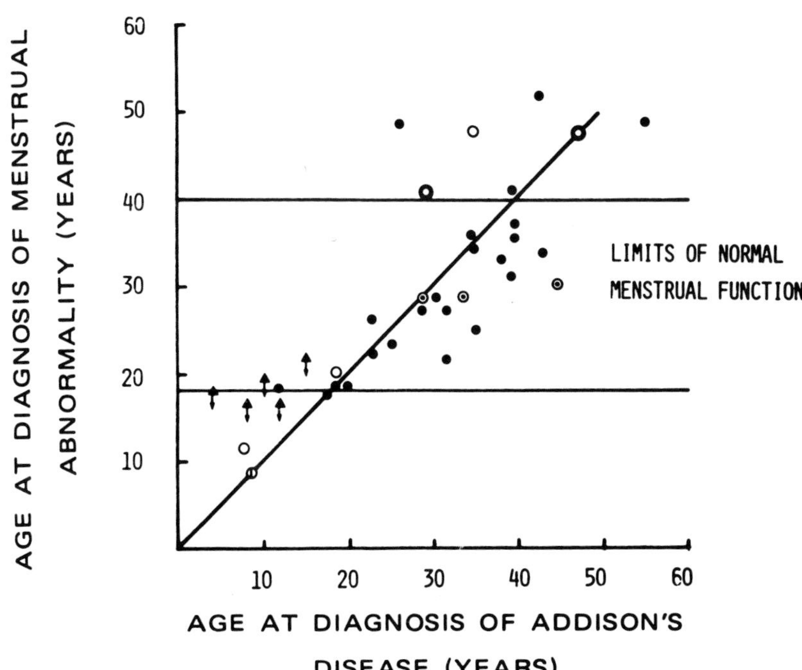

FIGURE 28-5 Correlation between age at diagnosis of menstrual abnormality and age at diagnosis of Addison's disease in patients with steroid cell antibodies (△ = primary amenorrhea, ● = secondary amenorrhea or normal menopause, = oligomenorrhea, **O** = menorrhagia, ○ = normal menses, ⦶ = prepubertal). (*From Irvine and Barnes.*[177])

TABLE 28-8 Occurrence of Associated Disorders in Idiopathic Addison's Disease Patients with and without Steroid Cell Antibodies

	Amenorrhea or oligomenorrhea*	Other associated disorders	No associated disorder
Steroid cell antibody-positive ($n = 40$)	27†	9‡	4
Steroid cell antibody-negative ($n = 221$)	20	45	156

* In women with known menstrual histories (36 antibody-positive, 121 antibody-negative).
† Statistically significant difference between seropositive and seronegative groups, $p < 0.00025$.
‡ $p < 0.0005$; independent risk of associated autoimmune disorder, excluding oligomenorrhea and Addison's disease.
Source: Modified from Irvine and Barnes.[177]

approximately 4 percent (Table 28-6). (The association of thyroid disease, diabetes, and pernicious anemia is discussed below.)

Thyroid Disease and Diabetes Mellitus without Addison's Disease

The greater prevalence of diabetes and thyroid disease in the general population makes the quantitative study of an association between these disorders difficult. Nevertheless, many authors have cited an increased frequency of autoimmune thyroid disease in diabetics; pernicious anemia is also associated. This has been confirmed by studies of tissue-specific autoantibodies in diabetics compared with age- and sex-matched controls (Fig. 28-6). Table 28-9 summarizes representative studies of the interrelationships of autoimmune sensitivities to these three tissues.

Other Disorders

Vitiligo may occur with any of the above-mentioned pluriglandular endocrine insufficiency syndromes. The suspicion that this disorder represents another tissue-specific autoimmune disease is supported by the identification of antibodies to melanin-producing cells.[219]

A dozen cases of lymphocytic infiltration of the adenohypophysis have been reported. All these cases have been temporally related to pregnancy and have presented as sellar masses or sudden collapse; half were associated with autoimmune diseases, particularly lymphocytic thyroiditis and atrophic gastritis. In several cases, the adrenals were atrophic and the patient appeared to have died in adrenal crisis; however, hypopituitarism was diagnosed during life in at least one of these patients.[220] This entity may represent "autoimmune hypophysitis." One case of diabetes insipidus associated with Addison's disease and hypoparathyroidism has been reported, but the pathogenesis of the diabetes insipidus is unclear.[221]

Diagnosis, Complications, and Surveillance

The signs, symptoms, diagnostic testing, and therapy of the individual endocrinopathies discussed in this section are generally the same as they are when these disorders occur individually (see Chaps. 10, 12, 19, and 23). Some observed or theoretically possible pitfalls in diagnosis caused by hormonal interactions are discussed in this section.

The most serious possible error in the diagnosis of multiple endocrine failure would be to attribute adrenal, thyroid, and ovarian failure solely to hypo-

FIGURE 28-6 Frequency of antibodies to thyroglobulin, thyroid cytoplasm, and parietal cell cytoplasm in diabetics over 10 years of age and in age- and sex-matched controls. (*From Irvine et al.*[215])

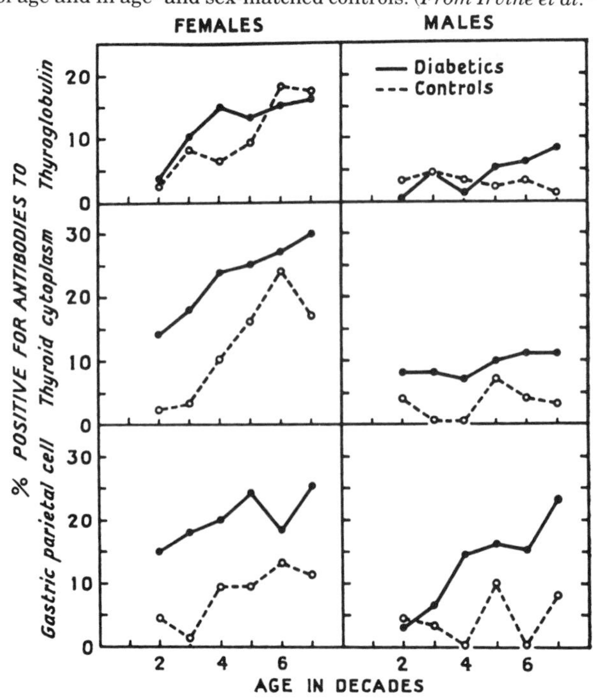

TABLE 28-9 Interrelationship of Thyroid, Gastric, and Islet-Cell Autoimmunity

Index disease	Associated finding	Frequency (%)	Ref.
Diabetes	Thyroid antibodies	16	215
	↑ TSH (males)	6	216
	↑ TSH (females)	17	216
	Parietal cell antibodies	17	215
Thyroiditis	Islet-cell antibodies	9	199
	Intrinsic factor antibodies	2	217
	Pernicious anemia	9	217
Hyperthyroidism	Islet-cell antibodies	3	199
	Intrinsic factor antibodies	3	217
	Pernicious anemia	3	217
Pernicious anemia	Islet-cell antibodies	11	199
	Thyroid antibodies	38	218
	Hypothyroidism	12	218
	Hyperthyroidism	9	218

pituitarism. This is easily avoided, as the diagnosis of autoimmune primary end organ failures should be considered in every case, and the integrity of pituitary function should be proved by detecting elevated blood levels of TSH, luteinizing hormone (LH), or ACTH. The coexistence of hypoparathyroidism or diabetes is an obvious indicator of autoimmune endocrinopathy. Conversely, the entity of lymphocytic hypophysitis should be kept in mind in the setting of pregnancy.

Failure to effect normal regulation because of glucocorticosteroid deficiency in Addison's disease patients may alter the secretion and action of other hormones. Lack of the suppressive effect of glucocorticosteroids on TSH release can result in elevated TSH levels in the absence of intrinsic thyroid disease.[222] TSH levels are therefore unreliable indicators of thyroid failure in untreated Addison's disease and should be reevaluated after adrenal steroid replacement. Adrenal insufficiency could theoretically also mask the development of glucose intolerance during early insulitis, but this has not been documented clinically. Calcium is an important controller of stimulus-secretion coupling in many endocrine cell types, but clinically important effects of hypocalcemia on the secretion of other hormones have not been observed.

A number of interactions with thyroid hormone status must be kept in mind in the diagnostic evaluation of untreated patients with pluriglandular failure. Hypothyroidism can cause macrocytic anemia, especially in children[223] but also in adults. This should be differentiated from pernicious anemia by clinical assessment of other effects of B_{12} deficiency, response to thyroid hormone replacement, and Schilling test, as indicated. Hypothyroidism can also cause a blunted adrenal response to ACTH and abnormal menses. Conversely, low serum T_4 and T_3 concentrations can be caused by a variety of acute and chronic nonthyroid illnesses ("euthyroid sick syndrome"). This phenomenon could lead to the suspicion of associated hypothyroidism in patients with poorly controlled diabetes.

In surveillance for the development of new endocrine gland involvement, emphasis should be placed on patients with Addison's disease, as these individuals are at greater risk. Hypothyroidism and pernicious anemia may have a prolonged, insidious onset; the physician should be highly suspicious that these problems are present, especially in patients with Addison's disease. Hypothyroidism should be considered in children with sudden deceleration of growth, but poorly controlled diabetes may be a more frequent cause.[224] Determination of serum TSH concentration, antithyroid antibody assay, complete blood count, and serum B_{12} assay are useful laboratory screens. Elevated serum TSH concentration alone is not a good predictor of future clinical hypothyroidism, but in patients in whom an elevated TSH level is combined with a positive test for antithyroid antibodies, the incidence of clinical hypothyroidism is 4 percent per year. When antibody titers are markedly elevated, the incidence may be as high as 26 percent per year.[225] Healthy relatives of patients with Addison's disease should also receive careful explanation of their susceptibility and close observation; an ACTH stimulation test is indicated if they develop any autoimmune disorder or nonspecific symptoms compatible with adrenal insufficiency. The appearance of complement-fixing adrenal antibodies may predict the development of Addison's disease,[226] but this is not a readily available diagnostic test.

Therapeutic implications of pluriglandular endocrine failure are less well characterized. It is known that cortisol antagonizes the intestinal calcium transport effects of vitamin D and its metabolites, which are used to treat hypoparathyroidism. The subsequent development of adrenal insufficiency can result in sudden vitamin D intoxication in these patients.[227] Secondary amenorrhea has remitted after the treatment of associated Addison's disease.[228] However, the combination of Addison's disease and loss of ovarian function, even physiologic menopause, may result in more severe postmenopausal osteoporosis if sex steroid replacement therapy is not given.[229] The loss of a protective effect of adrenal androgens has been postulated.

Genetics of Pluriglandular Endocrine Insufficiency Syndromes

Early genetic analyses of the pluriglandular endocrine insufficiency syndromes attempted to estimate the probability that the sib of a proband would be affected. With the assumption of complete ascertainment (no affected sibs unknown owing to mild disease), one study[200] gave probabilities of 0.25 to 0.35 for Schmidt's syndrome and Addison's disease with hypoparathyroidism. More recently, the application of human histocompatibility (HLA) typing has provided new information. Histocompatibility antigens are expressions of a gene complex located on chromosome 6 and are detectable with panels of test sera. The presumed defect in immune regulation resulting in sensitization to autoantigens in these disorders may reside in a gene of the HLA region. An increased incidence of some HLA antigens has been noted in patients with diabetes (antigens HLA-B8, B15, DR3, and DR4) and Addison's disease (antigens HLA-B8, DR3, and DR4).

Among the three major classes of HLA glycoproteins, autoimmune endocrine disease is most closely linked to the class II HLA genes (DR, DQ, and DP). Further HLA-D polymorphism can be detected by means of functional assays on lymphocytes and analysis of restriction endonuclease-digested genomic DNA as well as probes for specific DNA sequences within the HLA-DR and HLA-DQ genes. The presence or absence of specific amino acid residues at positions within the antigen-binding domains of the class II molecule subunits may indicate a substantial portion of the genetic risk for developing autoimmune disease.[230,231] HLA typing has been performed on a number of kindreds with pluriglandular endocrine insufficiency. In most families, this type of analysis has suggested dominant inheritance linked to either HLA-DR3 or HLA-DR4.[232,233] In a few kindreds, the predictive value of HLA typing appeared questionable, and no HLA association has yet been reported for Addison's disease with hypoparathyroidism.[233]

Nonautoimmune Pluriglandular Dysfunction

Bardwick et al.[234] reviewed a syndrome which had previously been reported mostly in Japan. Seventy-five percent of these patients are male; they have plasma cell dyscrasias occurring in the fourth or fifth decade, usually sclerotic plasmacytomas. This has been given the acronym POEMS syndrome (polyneuropathy, organomegaly, endocrinopathy, M protein, and skin changes). Hypogonadism, gynecomastia, and diabetes mellitus are frequent endocrine disorders, while adrenal failure is uncommon. In one of the cases of Bardwick et al., fasting hyperglycemia requiring insulin resolved with radiotherapy of the patient's plasmacytoma, recurred 3 years later with the appearance of a new bone lesion, and resolved again with radiation treatment. Neither the polyneuropathy nor the endocrinopathy appears to be explainable on the basis of infiltration by amyloid protein, nor were the investigators able to demonstrate tissue-specific endocrine antibodies, as are present in many patients with the autoimmune endocrinopathies. The mechanism of this interesting syndrome remains obscure.

REFERENCES

1. Erdheim J: Zur normalen und pathologischen histologie der glandula thyreodea, parathyreoidea, und hypophysis. *Beitr Pathol Anat* 33:158, 1903.
2. Cushing H, Davidoff LM: The pathological findings in four autopsied cases of acromegaly with a discussion of their significance. The Rockefeller Institute for Medical Research Monograph 22, 1927.
3. Lloyd PC: Hypophyseo-parathyreo-insular syndrome. *Bull Johns Hopkins Hosp* 45:1, 1929.
4. Rossier PH, Dressler M: Familare Erkrankunginnersekretorischer Drusen kombiniert mit Ulcuskrankheit. *Schweiz Med Wochenschr* 20:985, 1939.
5. Underdahl LO, Woolner LB, Black BM: Multiple endocrine adenomas: Report of eight cases in which parathyroids, pituitary, and pancreatic islets were involved. *J Clin Endocrinol* 13:20, 1953.
6. Moldawer MP, Nordi GL, Raker W: Concomitance of multiple adenomas of the parathyroids and pancreatic islets with tumor of the pituitary: A syndrome with familial incidence. *Am J Med Sci* 228:190, 1954.
7. Wermer P: Genetic aspects of adenomatosis of endocrine glands. *Am J Med* 16:363, 1954.
8. Zollinger RM, Ellison EH: Primary peptic ulceration of the jejunum associated with islet cell tumors of the pancreas. *Ann Surg* 142:709, 1955.
9. Verner JF, Morrison AB: Islet cell tumor and a syndrome of refractory watery diarrhea and hypokalemia. *Am J Med* 25:374, 1958.
10. Spencer SS, Summerskill WHJ: Malabsorption induced by gastrin hypersecretion due to ectopic islet cell adenoma. *Am J Gastroenterol* 39:26, 1963.
11. Schmid JR, Labhart A, Rossier PH: Relationship of multiple endocrine adenomas to syndrome of ulcerogenic islet cell adenomas (Zollinger-Ellison): Occurrence of both syndromes in one family. *Am J Med* 31:343, 1961.
12. Huizenga KA, Goodrick WIM, Summerskill WHJ: Peptic ulcer with islet cell tumor. *Am J Med* 37:564, 1964.
13. Ballard HS, Frame B, Harstock RJ: Familial multiple endocrine adenoma–peptic ulcer complex. *Medicine (Baltimore)* 43:481, 1964.
14. Benson L, Ljunghall S, Akerstrom G, Oberg K: Hyperparathyroidism presenting as the first lesion in multiple endocrine neoplasia type 1. *Am J Med* 82(4):731–737, 1987.
15. Marx SJ, Vinik AI, Santen RJ, Floyd JC Jr, Mills JL, Green J III: Multiple endocrine neoplasia type I: Assessment of labo-

ratory tests to screen for the gene in a large kindred. *Medicine (Baltimore)* 65:226, 1986.
16. Lamers CBHW, Froeling PGAM: Clinical significance of hyperparathyroidism in familial multiple endocrine adenomatosis type I (MEA 1). *Am J Med* 66:422, 1979.
17. Vanderweghe M, Schutyser J, Braxer K, Vermeulen A: A case of multiple endocrine adenomatosis with primary amenorrhea. *Postgrad Med J* 54:618, 1978.
18. Carlson HE, Levine JA, Goldberg NJ, Hershman JM: Hyperprolactinemia in multiple endocrine adenomatosis, type 1. *Arch Intern Med* 138:1807, 1978.
19. Tourniaire J, Trouillas J, Maillet P, David L, Pallo D, Tran Minh V, Pressot C: Polyadénomatose endocrinienne associant un adénome hypophysaire à prolactine et un adénome parathyroïdien intrathyroïdien. *Ann Endocrinol* 38:1, 1977.
20. Levine JH, Sagel J, Rosebrock GL Jr, Gonzalez J: Hyperprolactinemia in the multiple endocrine adenomatosis type 1 (MEA-1) syndrome. *Arch Intern Med* 38:1777, 1977.
21. Wermer P: Endocrine adenomatosis and peptic ulcer in a large kindred. Inherited multiple tumors and mosaic pleotropism in man. *Am J Med* 35:205, 1963.
22. Paloyan E, Lawrence AM: Laboratory diagnosis of parathyroid tumors. *Ann Clin Lab Sci* 4:241, 1974.
23. Block MA, Frame B: The extent of operation for primary hyperparathyroidism. *Arch Surg* 109:798, 1974.
24. Mallete LE, Bilezikian JP, Ketcham AS, Aurbach GD: Parathyroid carcinoma in familial hyperparathyroidism. *Am J Med* 7:642, 1974.
25. Marx SJ, Spiegel AM, Brown EM, Aurbach GD: Family studies in patients with primary parathyroid hyperplasia. *Am J Med* 2:698, 1977.
26. Jung RT, Davie M, Grant AM, Jenkins D, Chalmers TM: Multiple endocrine adenomatosis (type I) and familial hyperparathyroidism. *Postgrad Med J* 54:92, 1978.
27. Scholz DA, Purnell DC, Edis AJ, van Heerden JA, Woolner LB: Primary hyperparathyroidism with multiple parathyroid gland enlargement: Review of 53 cases. *Mayo Clin Proc* 53:792, 1978.
28. Brandi ML, Aurbach GD, Fitzpatrick LA, Quarto R, Spiegel AM, Bliziotes MM, Norton JA, Doppman JL, Marx SJ: Parathyroid mitogenic activity in plasma from patients with familial multiple endocrine neoplasia type I. *N Engl J Med* 314:1287, 1986.
29. Marx SJ, Sakagucki K, Green J III, Aurbach GD, Brandi ML: Mitogenic activity on parathyroid cells in plasma from members of a large kindred with multiple endocrine neoplasia type 1. *J Clin Endocrinol Metab* 67(1):149–153, 1988.
30. Zimering MB, Brandi ML, DeGrange DA, Marx SJ, Streeten E, Katsumata N, Murphy PR, Sato Y, et al: Circulating fibroblast growth factor-like substance in familial multiple endocrine neoplasia type 1. *J Clin Endocrinol Metab* 70:149–154, 1990.
31. Friedman E, Sakaguchi K, Bale AE, Falchetti A, Streeten E, Zimering MB, Weinstein LS, McBride WO, et al: Clonality of parathyroid tumors in familial multiple endocrine neoplasia type 1. *N Engl J Med* 321(4): 213–218, 1989.
32. Isenberg JI, Walsch JH, Grossman MI: Zollinger-Ellison syndrome. *Gastroenterology* 65:140, 1973.
33. McGuigan JE, Colwell JA, Franklin J: Effect of parathyroidectomy on hypercalcemic hypersecretory peptic ulcer disease. *Gastroenterology* 66:269, 1974.
34. Gogel HK, Buckman MT, Cadieux D, McCarthy DM: Gastric secretion and hormonal interactions in multiple endocrine neoplasia type I. *Arch Intern Med* 145:855, 1985.
35. McGavaran MH, Unger RH, Recant L, Polk HC, Kilo C, Levin ME: A glucagon-secreting alpha-cell carcinoma of the pancreas. *N Engl J Med* 274:1408, 1966.
36. Mallinson CN, Bloom SR, Warin AP, Salmon PR, Cox B: A glucagonoma syndrome. *Lancet* 2:1, 1974.
37. Stacpoole PW, Jaspan J, Kasselberg AG, Halter SA, Polonsky K, Gluck FW, Liljenquist JE, Rabin D: A familial glucagonoma syndrome. *Am J Med* 70:1017, 1981.
38. Krejs GJ, Orci L, Conlon JM, Ravazzola M, Davis GR, Raskin P. Collins SM, McCarthy DM, et al: Somatostatinoma syndrome. *N Engl J Med* 301:285, 1979.
39. Ganda OP, Weir GC, Soeldner JS, Legg ML, Chick WL, Patel YC, Ebeid AM, Gabbay KH, Reichlin S: "Somatostatinoma": A somatostatin-containing tumor of the endocrine pancreas. *N Engl J Med* 296:963, 1977.
40. Larsson L-I, Hirsch MA, Holst JJ, Ingemansson S, Kuhl C, Jensen SL, Lundqvist G, Rehfeld JF, Schwartz TW: Pancreatic somatostatinoma: Clinical features and physiological implications. *Lancet* 1:666, 1977.
41. Namihira Y, Achord JL, Subramony C: Multiple endocrine neoplasia type 1 with pancreatic cholera. *Am J Gastroenterol* 82(8):794–797, 1987.
42. Rimoin DL, Schimke RN: *Genetic Disorders of the Endocrine Glands:* St. Louis, Mosby, 1971.
43. Prosser PR, Karam JH, Townsend JJ, Forsham P: Prolactin-secreting pituitary adenomas in multiple endocrine adenomatosis, type-1. *Ann Intern Med* 91:41, 1979.
44. Stabile BE, Passaro E, Carlson HE: Elevated serum prolactin level in the Zollinger-Ellison syndrome. *Arch Surg* 116:449, 1981.
45. Farid NR, Buehler S, Russell NA, Maroun FB, Allerdice P: Prolactinomas in familial multiple endocrine neoplasia syndrome type I. *Am J Med* 69:874, 1980.
46. Veldhuis JD, Green JE, Kovacs E, Worgul TJ, Murray FT, Hammond JM: Prolactin-secreting pituitary adenomas. *Am J Med* 67:830, 1979.
47. Goldman M, Holub D: Prolactinomas and the multiple endocrine adenomatosis type-I complex. *Ann Intern Med* 91:791, 1979.
48. O'Neal LW, Kipnis DM, Luse SA, Lacy PE, Jarrett L: Secretion of various endocrine substances by ACTH-secreting tumors—gastrin, melanotropin, norepinephrine, serotonin, parathormone, vasopressin, glucagon. *Cancer* 21:1219, 1968.
49. Vance JE, Stoll RW, Kitabachi AE, Williams RH, Wood FC Jr: Nesidioblastosis in familial endocrine adenomatosis, *JAMA* 207:1679, 1969.
50. Snyder N III, Scurry MT, Deiss WP: Five families with multiple endocrine adenomatosis. *Ann Intern Med* 76:53, 1972.
51. Williams ED, Celestin LR: The association of bronchial carcinoid and pluriglandular adenomatosis. *Thorax* 17:120, 1962.
52. Amano S, Hazama F, Haebara H, Tsurusawa M, Kaito H: Ectopic ACTH-MSH producing carcinoid with multiple endocrine hyperplasia in a child. *Acta Pathol Jpn* 28:721, 1978.
53. Sommers SC: Adrenal glands, in Anderson WAD (ed): *Pathology*. St. Louis, Mosby, 1971, pp 1464–1487.
54. Mortensen JD, Woolner LB, Bennett WA: Gross and microscopic findings in clinically normal thyroid glands. *J Clin Endocrinol Metab* 15:1270, 1955.
55. Friedman NB: Chronic hypoglycemia: Report of two cases with islet adenoma and changes in the hypophysis. *Arch Pathol* 27:994, 1939.
56. Muhr C, Ljunghall S, Akerstrom G, Palmer M, Bergstrom K, Enoksson P, Lundquist G, Wide L: Screening for multiple endocrine neoplasia syndrome (type 1) in patients with primary hyperparathyroidism. *Clin Endocrinol (Oxf)* 20(2): 153–162, 1984.
57. Lamers CB, Buis JT, van Tongeren J: Secretin-stimulated serum gastrin levels in hyperparathyroid patients from families with multiple endocrine adenomatosis. *Ann Intern Med* 86:719, 1977.
58. Selking O, Johansson H, Lundqvist G: Serum gastrin and its response to secretin in hyperparathyroid patients. *Acta Chir Scand* 147:649, 1981.
59. Skogseid B, Oberg K, Benson L, Lindgren PG, Lorelius LE, Lundquist G, Wide L, Wilander E: A standardized meal stimulation test of the endocrine pancreas for early detection of pancreatic endocrine tumors in multiple endocrine neoplasia type 1 syndrome: Five years experience. *J Clin Endocrinol Metab* 64(6): 1233–1240,1987.

60. Service FJ, Dale AJD, Elveback LR, Jiang N-S: Insulinoma: Clinical and diagnostic features of 60 consecutive cases. *Mayo Clin Proc* 51:417, 1976.
61. Goldstein JL: Multiple endocrine adenoma–peptic ulcer syndrome, in *Medical Grand Rounds, Parkland Memorial Hospital*. Jan. 30, 1975, p 1.
62. Effron M, Griner L, Benirschke K: Nature and rate of neoplasia found in captive wild mammals, birds, and reptiles at necropsy. *JNCI* 59:185, 1977.
63. Berdjis CC: Pluriglandular syndrome: I. Multiple endocrine adenomas in irradiated rats. *Oncologia* 13:441, 1960.
64. Rosen VJ Jr, Castanera TJ, Jones DC, Kimeldorf DJ: Islet-cell tumors of the pancreas in the irradiated and non-irradiated rat. *Lab Invest* 10:608, 1961.
65. Nakamura Y, Larsson C, Julier C, Bystrom C, Skogseid B, Wells S, Oberg K, Carlson M, et al: Localization of the genetic defect in multiple endocrine neoplasia type 1 within a small region of chromosome 11. *Am J Hum Genet* 44(5):751–755, 1989.
66. Yoshimoto K, Iizuka M, Iwahana H, Yamasaki R, Saito H, Saito S, Sekiya T: Loss of the same alleles of HRAS1 and D11S151 in two independent pancreatic cancers from a patient with multiple endocrine neoplasia type 1. *Cancer Res* 49(10):2716–2721, 1989.
67. Bale SJ, Bale AE, Stewart K, Dachowski L, McBride OW, Glaser T, Green JE III, Mulvihill JJ, et al: Linkage analysis of multiple endocrine neoplasia type 1 with INT2 and other markers on chromosome 11. *Genomics* 4(3):320–322, 1989.
68. Larsson C, Skogseid B, Oberg K, Nakamura Y, Nordenskjold M: Multiple endocrine neoplasia type 1 gene maps to chromosome 11 and is lost in insulinoma. *Nature* 332(6159):85–87, 1988.
69. Thakker RV, Bouloux P, Wooding C, Chotai K, Broad PM, Spurr NK, Besser GM, O'Riordan JL: Association of parathyroid tumors in multiple endocrine neoplasia type 1 with loss of alleles on chromosome 11. *N Engl J Med* 321(4):218–224, 1989.
70. Hansen OP, Hansen M, Hansen HH, Rose B: Multiple endocrine adenomatosis of mixed type. *Acta Med Scand* 200:327, 1976.
71. Berg B, Biorklund A, Grimelius L, Ingemansson S, Larsson L-I, Stenram U, Akerman M: A new pattern of multiple endocrine adenomatosis. *Acta Med Scand* 200:321, 1976.
72. Wells SA Jr, Ellis GJ, Gunnells JC, Schneider AB, Sherwood LM: Parathyroid autotransplantation in primary parathyroid hyperplasia. *N Engl J Med* 295:57, 1976.
73. Van Heerden JE, Kent RB, Sizemore GW, Grant CS, Remine WH: Primary hyperparathyroidism in patients with multiple endocrine neoplasia syndromes. *Arch Surg* 118:533, 1983.
74. Brennan MF, Brown EM, Marx SJ, Spiegel AM, Broadus AE, Doppman JL, Webber B, Aurbach GD: Recurrent hyperparathyroidism from an autotransplanted parathyroid adenoma. *N Engl J Med* 299:1057, 1978.
75. Guiot G: Transsphenoidal approach in surgical treatment of pituitary adenomas: General principles and indications in nonfunctioning adenomas, in Kohler PO, Ross GT (eds): *Diagnosis and Treatment of Pituitary Tumors*. New York, American Elsevier, 1973, pp 159–178.
76. Hardy J: Transsphenoidal surgery of hyper-secreting pituitary tumors, in Kohler PO, Ross GT (eds): *Diagnosis and Treatment of Pituitary Tumors,* New York, American Elsevier, 1973, pp 179–194.
77. Scott HW Jr, Gobbel WG Jr, Law DH IV: Clinical experience with a jejunal pouch (Hunt-Lawrence) as a substitute stomach after gastrectomy. *Surg Gynecol Obstet* 121:1231, 1965.
78. Turner WW, McLelland RN, Fry WJ: Roux-19 esophagojejunostomy following total gastrectomy. *Curr Surg* 35:64, 1978.
79. Pipeleers-Marichal M, Somers G, Willems G, Foulis A, Imrie C, Bishop AE, Polak JM, Path FRC, et al: Gastrinomas in the duodenums of patients with multiple endocrine neoplasia type 1 and the Zollinger-Ellison syndrome. *N Engl J Med* 322(11):723–727, 1990.
80. McCarthy DM: Report on the United States experience with cimetidine in Zollinger-Ellison syndrome and other hypersecretory states. *Gastroenterology* 74:453, 1978.
81. Cryer PE, Hill GJ: Pancreatic islet cell carcinoma with hypercalcemia and hypergastrinemia. Response to streptozotocin. *Cancer* 38:2217, 1976.
82. Graber AL, Porte D Jr, Williams RH: Clinical use of diatoxide and mechanism for its hyperglycemic effects. *Diabetes* 15:143, 1966.
83. Schein PS: Chemotherapeutic management of the hormone-secreting malignancies. *Cancer* 30:1616, 1972
84. Deftos LJ: *Medullary Thyroid Carcinoma*. Basel, Karger, 1983.
85. Sizemore GW, Carney JA, Heath H: Epidemiology of medullary carcinoma of the thyroid gland. *Surg Clin North Am* 57:633, 1977.
86. Chang GC, Beahrs O, Sizemore GW, Woolner CH: Medullary carcinoma of the thyroid gland. *Cancer* 35:695, 1975.
87. Carney JA, Sizemore GW, Hayles AB: C-cell disease of the thyroid gland in multiple endocrine neoplasia, type 2b. *Cancer* 44:2173, 1979.
88. Norton JA, Froome LC, Farrell RE, Wells SA: Multiple endocrine neoplasia type IIb: The most aggressive form of medullary thyroid carcinoma. *Surg Clin North Am* 59:109, 1979.
89. Pearse AGE: Common cytochemical and ultrastructural characteristics of cells producing polypeptide hormones (the APUD series) and their relevance to thyroid and ultimobranchial C-cells and calcitonin. *Proc R Soc Lond* 170:71, 1968.
90. Pearse AGE, Takor TT: Neuroendocrine embryology and the APUD concept. *Clin Endocrinol* 5:299, 1976.
91. Deftos LJ, Parthemore JG: Secretion of parathyroid hormone in patients with medullary thyroid carcinoma. *J Clin Invest* 54:416, 1974.
92. Melvin KEW, Tashjian AH Jr, Miller HH: Studies in familial thyroid cancer. *Trans Assoc Am Physicians* 84:144, 1971.
93. Simpson NE, Kidd KK, Goodfellow PJ, McDermid H, Myers S, Kidd JR, Jackson CE, Duncan AMV, et al: Assignment of multiple endocrine neoplasia type 2A to chromosome 10 by linkage. *Nature* 328:528–530, 1987.
94. Mathew CGP, Smith BA, Thorpe K, Wong Z, Royle NJ, Jeffreys AJ, Ponder BAJ: Deletions of genes on chromosome 1 in endocrine neoplasia. *Nature* 328:524–526, 1987.
95. Lairmore TC, Howe JR, Korte JA, Dilley WG, Aine L, Aine E, Wells SA Jr, Donis-Keller H: Familial medullary thyroid carcinoma and multiple endocrine neoplasia type 2B map to the same region of chromosome 10 as multiple endocrine neoplasia type 2A. *Genomics* 9:181–192, 1991.
96. Landsvater RM, Mathew CGP, Smith BA, Marcus EM, Te-Meerman GJ, Lips CJM, Geerdink RA, Nakamura K, et al: Development of multiple endocrine neoplasia type 2A does not involve substantial deletions of chromosome 10. *Genomics* 4:246–250, 1989.
97. Ponder BAJ, Coffey R, Gagel RF, Semple P, Ponder MA, Pembrey ME, Telenius-Berg M, Easton DF: Risk estimation and screening in families of patients with medullary thyroid carcinoma. *Lancet* 1:397, 1988.
98. Williams ED: Medullary carcinoma of the thyroid. *J Clin Pathol* 19:114, 1966.
99. Hazard JB, Hawk WA, Crile G: Medullary (solid) carcinoma of the thyroid—a clinicopathologic entity. *J Clin Endocrinol Metab* 19:152, 1959.
100. Cunliffe WJ, Black MM, Hall R, Johnston IDA, Hudgson P, Shuster S, Gudmundsson TV, Joplin GF, et al: A calcitonin-secreting thyroid carcinoma. *Lancet* 2:63, 1968.
101. Melvin KEW, Tashjian AH Jr: The syndrome of excessive thyrocalcitonin produced by medullary carcinoma of the thyroid. *Proc Natl Acad Sci USA* 59:1216, 1968.
102. Meyer JS, Abdel-Bari W: Granules and thyroidcalcitonin-like activity in medullary carcinoma of the thyroid. *N Engl J Med* 278:523, 1968.

103. Milhaud G, Tubiana M, Parmentier C, Coutris G: Epithelioma de la thyroide secretant de la thyrocalcitonine. *C R Seances Acad Sci [III]* 266:608, 1968.
104. Clark MB, Byfield PGH, Boyd GW, Foster GV: A radioimmunoassay for human calcitonin M. *Lancet* 2:74, 1969.
105. Kalina M, Foster GV, Clark MB, Pearse AGE: C-cells in man, in Taylor S, Foster G (eds): *Calcitonin, 1969*. New York, Heinemann, 1970, pp 268–273.
106. Deftos LJ: Calcitonin in clinical medicine, in Stollerman GH (ed): *Advances in Internal Medicine*. New York, Year Book, 1978, pp 159–193.
107. LeDourain N, LeLievre C: Demonstration de l'origine neural des cellules à calcitonine du corps ultimobranchial chez l'embryon de poulet. *C R Seances Acad Sci [III]* 270:2857, 1970.
108. Holm R, Sobrinho-Simoes M, Nesland JM, Sambade C, Johannessen JV: Medullary thyroid carcinoma with thyroglobulin immunoreactivity—a special entity? *Lab Invest* 57:258, 1987.
109. Lippman SM, Mendelsohn G, Trump DL, Wells SA, Baylin SB: The prognostic and biological significance of cellular heterogeneity in medullary thyroid carcinoma: A study of calcitonin, L-dopa decarboxylase, and histaminase. *J Clin Endocrinol Metab* 54:233, 1982.
110. Ljungberg O: On medullary carcinoma of the thyroid: A clinicopathologic entity. *Acta Pathol Microbiol Scand* 231:1, 1972.
111. Livolsi VA, Feind CR, LoGerfo P. Tashjian AH Jr: Demonstration by immunoperoxidase staining of hyperplasia of parafollicular cells in the thyroid gland in hyperparathyroidism. *J Clin Endocrinol Metab* 37:550, 1973.
112. McMillan PJ, Hooker WM, Deftos LJ: Distribution of calcitonin-containing cells in human thyroid. *Am J Anat* 140:73, 1974.
113. Hamilton CW, Bigner SH, Wells SA, Johnston WW: Metastatic medullary thyroid carcinoma in sputum. *Acta Cytol (Baltimore)* 27:49, 1983.
114. Lamberg BA, Reissel P, Stenman S, Koivuniemi A, Ekblom M, Makinen J, Franssila K: Concurrent medullary and papillary thyroid carcinoma in the same lobe and in siblings. *Acta Med Scand* 209:421, 1981.
115. Wolfe HJ, Melvin KEW, Cervi-Skinner SJ, Al Saadi AA, Juliar JF, Jackson CE, Tashjian AH Jr: C-cell hyperplasia preceding medullary thyroid carcinoma. *N Engl J Med* 289:437, 1973.
116. Carney AJ, Sizemore GW, Lovestedt SA: Mucosal ganglioneuromatosis, medullary thyroid carcinoma, and pheochromocytoma: MEN, type 2B. *Oral Surg* 41:739, 1976.
117. Keiser JR, Beaven MA, Doppman J, Wells S, Buja LM: Medullary thyroid carcinoma, pheochromocytoma, and parathyroid disease. *Ann Intern Med* 78:561, 1973.
118. McKenna TJ, McLean D, Lorber DL, Bone HG, Parthemore JG, Deftos LJ: Comparison of calcitonin stimulation tests used in screening for medullary carcinoma of the thyroid, *Proceedings of the 60th Annual Meeting of the Endocrine Society,* 1978, p 370.
119. Santoro M, Rosati R, Grieco M, Berlingieri MT, D'Amato L-C, de Franciscis V, Fusco A: The ret proto-oncogene is consistently expressed in human pheochromocytomas and thyroid medullary carcinomas. *Oncogene* 5:1595–1598, 1990.
120. Yang K-P, Castillo SG, Nguyen CV, Hickey RC, Samaan NA: C-myc, N-myc, N-ras, and c-erb-B: Lack of amplification or rearrangement in human medullary thyroid carcinoma in a derivative cell line. *Anticancer Res* 10:189–192, 1990.
121. Beskid M: Thyroid C-cells in normal and goitrous gland: A histochemical study. *Acta Histochem* 54:313, 1975.
122. Milhaud G, Calmettes C, Jullienne A, Tharaud D, Bloch-Michel H, Cavaillon JP, Colin R, Moukhtar MS: A new chapter in human pathology: Calcitonin disorders and therapeutic use, in Talmage RV, Munson PL (eds): *Calcium, Parathyroid Hormone, and the Calcitonins*. Amsterdam, Excerpta Medica, 1972, pp 56–70.
123. Hill CS Jr, Ibanez ML, Samaan NA, Ahearn MJ, Clark RL: Medullary (solid) carcinoma of the thyroid gland: An analysis of the M.D. Anderson Hospital experience with patients with the tumor, its special features, and its histogenesis. *Medicine (Baltimore)* 52:141, 1973.
124. Block MA: Clinical characteristics distinguishing hereditary from sporadic medullary thyroid carcinoma. *Arch Surg* 115:142, 1980.
125. Tashjian AH Jr, Howland BG, Kenneth BA, Melvin KEW, Hill CS Jr: Immunoassay of human calcitonin. (Clinical measurement, relation to serum calcium and studies in patients with medullary thyroid carcinoma.) *N Engl J Med* 283:890, 1970.
126. Galera-Davidson H, González-Cámpora R, Mora-Marín JA, Matilla-Vicente A, Hytch HE, Bartels PH, Lerma-Puertas E, Andrada-Becerra E, Bibbo M: Cytophotometric DNA measurements in medullary thyroid carcinoma. *Cancer* 65:2255–2260, 1990.
127. Ibanez ML, Cole VW, Russell WO, Clark RI: Solid carcinoma of the thyroid gland. *Cancer* 20:706, 1967.
128. Zanin DEA, van Dongen A, Hoefnagel CA, Bruning PF: Radioimmunoscintigraphy using iodine-131-anti-CEA monoclonal antibodies and thallium-201 scintigraphy in medullary thyroid carcinoma: A case report. *J Nucl Med* 31:1854–1855, 1990.
129. Deftos LJ: Radioimmunoassay for calcitonin in medullary thyroid carcinoma. *JAMA* 227:403, 1974.
130. MacIntyre I, Hillyard CJ, Murphy PK, Reynolds JJ, Gaines RE, Craig RK: A second plasma calcium-lowering peptide from the human calcitonin precursor. *Nature* 300:460, 1982.
131. Roos BA, O'Niel JA, Muszynski M, Birnbaum RS: Noncalcitonin secretory products of calcitonin gene expression. Proceedings of the International Conference on Calcium Regulating Hormones, Japan, 1983, in Cohn PV, Fujita T, Potts JT Jr, Talmage RV (eds): *Endocrine Control of Bone and Calcium Metabolism*. Amsterdam, Elsevier, 1984, pp 169–175.
132. Deftos LJ, Roos B: Medullary thyroid carcinoma and calcitonin gene expression, in Peck WA (ed): *Bone and Mineral Research*. New York, Elsevier, pp 267–316.
133. O'Connor DT, Burton D, Deftos LJ: Immunoreactive human chromagranin A in diverse polypeptide hormone producing human tumors and normal endocrine tissues. *J Clin Endocrinol Metab* 57:1084, 1983.
134. O'Connor DT, Burton D, Deftos LJ: Chromagranin A: Immunohistology reveals its universal occurrence in normal polypeptide hormone producing endocrine glands. *Life Sci* 33:1657, 1983.
135. Sobol RE, Memoli V, Deftos LJ: Hormone-negative, chromogranin A-positive endocrine tumors. *N Engl J Med* 320:444–447, 1989.
136. Parthemore JG, Bronzert D, Roberts G, Deftos LJ: A short calcium infusion in the diagnosis of medullary thyroid carcinoma. *J Clin Endocrinol Metab* 39:108, 1974.
137. Hennessey JF, Wells SA, Ontjes DA, Cooper CW: A comparison of pentagastrin injection and calcium infusion as provocative agents for the detection of medullary thyroid carcinoma. *J Clin Endocrinol Metab* 39:487, 1974.
138. Wells SA Jr, Ontjes DA, Cooper CW, Hennessey JF, Ellis GJ, MacPherson HT, Sabiston DC Jr: The early diagnosis of medullary carcinoma of the thyroid gland in patients with multiple endocrine neoplasia, type II. *Ann Surg* 182:362, 1975.
139. Parthemore JG, Deftos LJ: Calcitonin secretion in normal human subjects. *J Clin Endocrinol Metab* 47:184, 1978.
140. Wells SA Jr, Baylin SB, Leight GS, Dale JK, Dilley WG, Farndon JR: The importance of early diagnosis in patients with hereditary medullary thyroid carcinoma. *Ann Surg* 195:595, 1982.
141. Cohen SL, MacIntyre I, Grahame-Smith D, Walker JG: Alcohol-stimulated calcitonin release in medullary carcinoma of the thyroid. *Lancet* 2:1172, 1973.

142. Anast C, David L, Winnacker J, Glass R, Baskin W, Brubaker L, Burns T: Serum calcitonin-lowering effect of magnesium in patients with medullary thyroid carcinoma. *J Clin Invest* 56:1615, 1975.
143. Norton JA, Doppman JL, Brennan MF: Localization and resection of clinically inapparent medullary carcinoma of the thyroid. *Surgery* 87:616, 1980.
144. Silva OL, Becker KL, Primack A, Doppman JL, Snider RH: Hypercalcitoninemia in bronchogenic cancer. *JAMA* 234: 183, 1975.
145. Deftos LJ, Roos BA, Bronzert D, Parthemore JG: Immunochemical heterogeneity of calcitonin in plasma. *J Clin Endocrinol Metab* 40:407, 1975.
146. Sizemore GW, Heath H: Immunochemical heterogeneity of calcitonin in plasma of patients with medullary thyroid carcinoma. *J Clin Invest* 55:111, 1975.
147. Amara SG, Jones V, Rosenfeld MG: Alternative RNA processing in calcitonin gene expression. *Nature* 298:240, 1982.
148. Lee JC, Parthemore JG, Deftos LJ: Calcitonin secretion in renal disease. *Calcif Tissue Res* 22S:154, 1977.
149. Bigner SH, Mendelsohn G, Wells SA, Cox EB, Baylin SB, Eggleston JC: Medullary carcinoma of the thyroid in the multiple endocrine neoplasia IIA syndrome. *Am J Surg Pathol* 5:459, 1981.
150. Gagel RF, Tashjian AH, Cummings T, Papathanasopoulas N, Kaplan MM, DeLellis RA, Wolfe H, Reichlin S: The clinical outcome of prospective screening for multiple endocrine neoplasia type 2a: An 18-year experience. *Medicine (Baltimore)* 318:478, 1988.
151. Lloyd RV, Sisson JC, Marangos PL: Calcitonin, carcinoembryonic antigen and neuron-specific enolase in medullary thyroid carcinoma. *Cancer* 51:2234, 1982.
152. Marcus JN, Dise CA, Livolsi VA: Melanin production in a medullary thyroid carcinoma. *Cancer* 49:2518, 1982.
153. Deftos LJ: Calcitonin and medullary thyroid carcinoma, in Wyngaarden JB, Smith LH, Bennett JC, Plum F (eds): *Cecil Textbook of Medicine,* 19th ed. Philadelphia, Saunders, 1991, pp 1420–1423.
154. Sipple JH: The association of pheochromocytoma with carcinoma of the thyroid gland. *Am J Med* 31:163, 1961.
155. Williams ED: Medullary carcinoma of the thyroid. *J Clin Pathol* 20:395, 1967.
156. Schimke RN, Hartmann WH: Familial amyloid-producing medullary thyroid carcinoma and pheochromocytoma. A distinct genetic entity. *Ann Intern Med* 63:1027, 1965.
157. Khairi MRA, Dexter RN, Burzynski NJ, Johnston CC Jr: Mucosal neuroma, pheochromocytoma, and medullary thyroid carcinoma: MEN, type III. *Medicine (Baltimore)* 54:89, 1975.
158. Steiner AL, Goodman AD, Powers SR: Study of kindred with pheochromocytoma, medullary thyroid carcinoma, hyperparathyroidism, and Cushing's disease: MEN, type II. *Medicine (Baltimore)* 47:371, 1968.
159. Carney AJ, Sizemore GW, Tyce GM: Bilateral adrenal medullary hyperplasia in MEN, type 2. *Mayo Clin Proc* 50:3, 1975.
160. DeLellis RA, Wolfe HJ, Gagel RF, Feldman ZT, Miller HH, Gang DL, Reichlin S: Adrenal medullary hyperplasia. *Am J Pathol* 83:177, 1976.
161. Cushman P Jr: Familial endocrine tumors: Report of two unrelated kindred affected with pheochromocytomas, one also with multiple thyroid carcinomas. *Am J Med* 32:352, 1962.
162. Melvin KEW, Miller HH, Tashjian AH Jr: Early diagnosis of medullary thyroid carcinoma of the thyroid gland by means of calcitonin assay. *N Engl J Med* 285:1115, 1971.
163. Potts JT Jr, Deftos LJ: Parathyroid hormone, thyrocalcitonin, vitamin D, and diseases of bone and bone mineral metabolism, in Bondy PK, Rosenberg LE (eds): *Duncan's Diseases of Metabolism,* 6th ed. Philadelphia, Saunders, 1969, pp 904–1082.
164. Williams ED, Pollock DJ: Multiple mucosal neuromata with endocrine tumors: A syndrome allied to von Recklinghausen's disease. *J Pathol Bacteriol* 91:71, 1966.
165. Schimke RN, Hartmann WH, Prout TE, Rimoin DL: Syndrome of bilateral pheochromocytoma, medullary thyroid carcinoma, and multiple neuromas. *N Engl J Med* 279:1, 1968.
166. Gorlin RJ, Sedano HO, Vicker RA, Cervenka J: Multiple mucosal neuromas, pheochromocytomas, and medullary carcinoma of the thyroid—a syndrome. *Cancer* 22:293, 1968.
167. Russell CF, van Heerden JA, Sizemore GW, Edis J, Taylor WF, Remine WH, Carney JA: The surgical management of medullary thyroid carcinoma. *Ann Surg* 197:42, 1982.
168. Block MA: Management of carcinoma of the thyroid. *Ann Surg* 185:133, 1977.
169. Jones BA, Sisson JC: Early diagnosis and thyroidectomy in multiple endocrine neoplasia, type 2b. *J Pediatr* 102:219, 1983.
170. Block MA, Horn RC Jr, Miller JM, Barrett JL, Brush BE: Familial medullary carcinoma of the thyroid. *Ann Surg* 166:403, 1967.
171. Block MA, Xavier A, Brush BE: Management of primary hyperparathyroidism in the elderly. *J Am Geriatr Soc* 23:385, 1975.
172. Nusynowitz ML, Pollard E, Benedetto AR, Leckitner ML, Ware RW: Treatment of medullary carcinoma of the thyroid with I-131. *J Nucl Med* 23:143, 1981.
173. Saad M, Guido JJ, Samman NA: Radioactive iodine in the treatment of medullary carcinoma of the thyroid. *J Clin Endocrinol Metab* 57:124, 1983.
174. Gottlieb JA, Hill CS Jr: Adriamycin (NSC-123127) therapy in thyroid carcinoma. *Cancer Chemother Rep* 6:283, 1975.
175. Deftos LJ, Catherwood BD: Syndrome involving multiple endocrine glands, in Greenspan FS (ed): *Basic and Clinical Endocrinology,* 3d ed. 1991, pp 725–740.
176. Mahler C, Verhelst J, De Longueville M, Harris A: Long-term treatment of metastatic medullary thyroid carcinoma with the somatostatin analogue octreotide. *Clin Endocrinol (Oxf)* 33:261–269, 1990.
177. Irvine WJ, Barnes EW: Addison's disease, ovarian failure and hypoparathyroidism. *Clin Endocrinol Metab* 4:379, 1975.
178. Carpenter CCJ, Solomon N, Silverberg SG, Bledsoe T, Northcutt RC, Klinenberg JR, Bennett IL Jr, Harvey AM: Schmidt's syndrome (thyroid and adrenal insufficiency): A review of the literature and a report of fifteen new cases including ten instances of coexistent diabetes mellitus. *Medicine (Baltimore)* 43:153, 1964.
179. Khoury EL, Hammond L, Bottazzo GF, Doniach D: Surface reactive antibodies to human adrenal cells in Addison's disease. *Clin Exp Immunol* 45:48, 1981.
180. Chiovato L, Vitti P, Santini F, Lopez G, Mammoll C, Bassi P, Giusti L, Tonacchera M, et al: Incidence of antibodies blocking thyrotropin effect in vitro in patients with euthyroid or hypothyroid autoimmune thyroiditis. *J Clin Endocrinol Metab* 71:40, 1990.
181. Wulffraat NM, Drexhage HA, Bottazzo GF, Wiersinga WM, Jeucken P, Van der Gaag R: Immunoglobulins of patients with idiopathic Addison's disease block the in vitro action of adrenocorticotropin. *J Clin Endocrinol Metab* 69:231, 1989.
182. Volpe R: Autoimmune thyroid disease—a perspective. *Mol Biol Med* 3:25, 1986.
183. Chan JY, Walfish PG: Activated (Ia+) T-lymphocytes and their subsets in autoimmune thyroid diseases: Analysis by microfluorocytometry. *J Clin Endocrinol Metab* 62:403, 1986.
184. Drell DW, Notkins AL: Multiple immunological abnormalities in patients with type 1 (insulin-dependent) diabetes mellitus. *Diabetologia* 30:132, 1987.
185. Rabinowe SL, Jackson RA, Dluhy RG, Williams GH: Ia-positive T lymphocytes in recently diagnosed idiopathic Addison's disease. *Am J Med* 77:597, 1984.
186. Nerup J, Bendixen G: Anti-adrenal cellular hypersensitivity

in Addison's disease: II. Correlation with clinical and serological findings. *Clin Exp Immunol* 5:341, 1969.

187. Calder EA, Penhale WJ, Barnes EW, Irvine WJ: Evidence for circulating immune complexes in thyroid disease. *Br Med J* 2:30, 1974.
188. Okita N, Row VV, Volpe R: Suppressor T-lymphocyte deficiency in Graves' disease and Hashimoto's thyroiditis. *J Clin Endocrinol Metab* 52:528, 1981.
189. Sridama V, Pacini F, DeGroot L: Decreased suppressor T-lymphocytes in autoimmune thyroid diseases detected by monoclonal antibodies. *J Clin Endocrinol Metab* 54:316, 1982.
190. Iitaka M, Aguayo JF, Iwatani Y, Row VV, Volpe R: Studies of the effect of suppressor T lymphocytes on the induction of antithyroid microsomal antibody-secreting cells in autoimmune thyroid disease. *J Clin Endocrinol Metab* 66:708, 1988.
191. Pujol-Borrell R, Todd I, Londei M, Foulis A, Feldmann M, Bottazzo GF: Inappropriate major histocompatibility complex class II expression by thyroid follicular cells in thyroid autoimmune disease and by pancreatic beta cells in type I diabetes. *Mol Biol Med* 3:159, 1986.
192. Piccinini LA, Goldsmith NK, Schachter BS, Davies TF: Localization of HLA-DR alpha-chain messenger ribonucleic acid in normal and autoimmune human thyroid using in situ hybridization. *J Clin Endocrinol Metab* 66:1307, 1988.
193. Jackson R, McNicol AM, Farquharson M, Foulis AK: Class II MHC expression in normal adrenal cortex and cortical cells in autoimmune Addison's disease. *J Pathol* 155:113, 1988.
194. Nerup J: Addison's disease. *Acta Endocrinol (Copenh)* 76:127, 1974.
195. Marieb NJ, Melby JC, Lyall SS: Isolated hypoaldosteronism associated with idiopathic hypoparathyroidism. *Arch Intern Med* 134:424, 1974.
196. Wegienka LC, Grasso SG, Forsham PH: Estimation of adrenomedullary reserve by infusion of 2-deoxy-D-glucose. *J Clin Endocrinol* 26:37, 1966.
197. Wuepper KD, Wegienka LC, Fudenberg HH: Immunologic aspects of adrenocortical insufficiency. *Am J Med* 45:206, 1969.
198. Blizzard RM, Chee D, Davis W: The incidence of adrenal and other antibodies in the sera of patients with idiopathic adrenal insufficiency (Addison's disease). *Clin Exp Immunol* 2:19, 1967.
199. Spinner MW, Blizzard RM, Gibbs J, Abeey H, Childs B: Familial distribution of organ specific antibodies in the blood of patients with Addison's disease and hypoparathyroidism and their relatives. *Clin Exp Immunol* 5:461, 1969.
200. Spinner MW, Blizzard RM, Childs B: Clinical and genetic heterogeneity in idiopathic Addison's disease and hypoparathyroidism. *J Clin Endocrinol* 28:795, 1968.
201. Blizzard RM, Gibbs JH: Candidiasis: Studies pertaining to its association with endocrinopathies and pernicious anemia. *Pediatrics* 42:231, 1968.
202. Blizzard RM, Chee D, Davis W: The incidence of parathyroid and other antibodies in the sera of patients with idiopathic hypoparathyroidism. *Clin Exp Immunol* 1:119, 1966.
203. Dwyer JM: Chronic mucocutaneous candidiasis. *Annu Rev Med* 32:491, 1981.
204. Krohn K, Perheentupa J, Heinonen E: Precipitating anti-adrenal antibodies in Addison's disease. *Clin Immunol Immunopathol* 3:59, 1974.
205. Ahn TG, Antonarakis SE, Kronenberg HM, Igarashi T, Levine MA: Familial isolated hypoparathyroidism: A molecular genetic analysis of 8 families with 23 affected persons. *Medicine (Baltimore)* 65:73, 1986.
206. Phillips D, McLachlan S, Stephenson A, Roberts D, Moffitt S, McDonald D, AdHiah A, Stratton A, et al: Autosomal dominant transmission of autoantibodies to thyroglobulin and thyroid peroxidase. *J Clin Endocrinol Metab* 70:742, 1990.
207. McCarthy-Young S, Lessof MH, Maisey MN: Serum TSH and thyroid antibody studies in Addison's disease. *Clin Endocrinol (Oxf)* 1:45, 1972.
208. Bottazzo GF, Florin-Christensen A, Doniach D: Islet-cell antibodies in diabetes mellitus with autoimmune polyendocrine deficiencies. *Lancet* 2:1279, 1974.
209. MacCuish AC, Jordan J, Campbell CJ, Duncan LJP, Irvine WJ: Cell-mediated immunity to human pancreas in diabetes mellitus. *Diabetes* 23:693, 1974.
210. Irvine WJ, McCallu CJ, Gray RS, Campbell CJ, Duncan LJP, Farquhar JW, Vaughn H, Morris PJ: Pancreatic islet-cell antibodies in diabetes mellitus correlated with the duration and type of diabetes, coexistent autoimmune disease, and HLA type. *Diabetes* 26:138, 1977.
211. Bottazzo GF, Mann JI, Thorogood M, Baum JD, Doniach D: Autoimmunity in juvenile diabetics and their families. *Br Med J* 2:165, 1978.
212. De Moraes Ruehsen M, Blizzard RM, Garcia-Bunuel R, Seegar Jones G: Autoimmunity and ovarian failure. *Am J Obstet Gynecol* 112:693, 1972.
213. Irvine WJ, Chan MMW, Scarth L, Kolb FO, Hartog M, Bayliss RIS, Drury MI: Immunological aspects of premature ovarian failure associated with idiopathic Addison's disease. *Lancet* 2:883, 1968.
214. Weinberg U, Kraemer FB, Kammerman S: Coexistence of primary endocrine deficiencies: A unique case of male hypergonadism [*sic*] associated with hypoparathyroidism, hypoadrenocorticism, and hypothyroidism. *Am J Med Sci* 272:215, 1976.
215. Irvine WJ, Scarth L, Clarke BF, Cullen DR, Duncan LJP: Thyroid and gastric autoimmunity in patients with diabetes mellitus. *Lancet* 2:164, 1970.
216. Gray RS, Borsey DQ, Seth J, Herd R, Brown NS, Clarke BF: Prevalence of subclinical thyroid failure in insulin-dependent diabetes. *J Clin Endocrinol Metab* 50:1034, 1980.
217. Ardeman S, Chanarin I, Krafchik B, Singer W: Addisonian pernicious anemia and intrinsic factor antibodies in thyroid disorders. *Q J Med* 35:421, 1965.
218. Carmel R, Spencer CA: Clinical and subclinical thyroid disorders associated with pernicious anemia. *Arch Intern Med* 142:1465, 1982.
219. Hertz KC, Gazze LA, Kirkpatrick CH, Katz SI: Autoimmune vitiligo: Detection of antibodies to melanin-producing cells. *N Engl J Med* 297:634, 1971.
220. Asa SL, Bilbao JM, Kovacs K, Josse RG, Kreines K: Lymphocytic hypophysitis of pregnancy resulting in hypopituitarism: A distinct clinicopathologic entity. *Ann Intern Med* 95:166, 1981.
221. Clifton-Bligh P, Lee C, Smith H, Posen S: The association of diabetes insipidus with hypoparathyroidism, Addison's disease and mucocutaneous candidiasis. *Aust NZ J Med* 10:548, 1980.
222. Topliss DJ, White EL, Stockigt JR: Significance of thyrotropin excess in untreated primary adrenal insufficiency. *J Clin Endocrinol Metab* 50:52, 1980.
223. Chu J-Y, Monteleone JA, Peden VH, Graviss ER, Vernava AM: Anemia in children and adolescents with hypothyroidism. *Clin Pediatr* 20:696, 1981.
224. Court S, Parkin JM: Hypothyroidism and growth failure in diabetes mellitus. *Arch Dis Child* 57:622, 1982.
225. Gordin A, Lamberg B-A: Spontaneous hypothyroidism in symptomless autoimmune thyroiditis. A long-term follow-up study. *Clin Endocrinol (Oxf)* 15:537, 1981.
226. Betterle C, Zanette F, Zanchetta R, Pedini B, Trevisan A, Mantero F, Rigon F: Complement-fixing adrenal autoantibodies as a marker for predicting onset of idiopathic Addison's disease. *Lancet* 1:1238, 1983.
227. Walker DA, Davies M: Addison's disease presenting as a hypercalcemic crisis in a patient with idiopathic hypoparathyroidism. *Clin Endocrinol (Oxf)* 14:419, 1981.
228. Rabinowe SL, Berger MJ, Welch WR, Dluhy RG: Lymphocyte dysfunction in autoimmune oophoritis: Resumption of menses with corticosteroids. *Am J Med* 81:347, 1986.

229. Devogelaer JP, Crabbe J, Nagant de Deuxchaisnes C: Bone mineral density in Addison's disease: Evidence for an effect of adrenal androgens on bone mass. *Br Med J* 294:798, 1987.
230. Todd JA, Bell JI, McDevitt HO: A molecular basis for genetic susceptibility to insulin-dependent diabetes mellitus. *Trends Genet* 4:129, 1988.
231. Khalil I, d'Auriol L, Gobet M, Morin L, Lepage V, Deschamps I, Park MS, Degos L, et al: A combination of HLA-DQ beta Asp57-negative and HLA DQ alpha Arg52 confers susceptibility to insulin-dependent diabetes mellitus. *J Clin Invest* 85:1315, 1990.
232. Allen DB, MacDonald MJ, Gottschall JL, Hunter JB: Autoimmune thyroid phenomena are not evidence for human lymphocyte antigen-genetic heterogeneity in insulin-dependent diabetes. *Am J Med Genet* 33:405, 1989.
233. Maclaren NK, Riley WJ: Inherited susceptibility to autoimmune Addison's disease is linked to human leukocyte antigens-DR3 and/or DR4, except when associated with type I autoimmune polyglandular syndrome. *J Clin Endocrinol Metab* 62:455, 1986.
234. Bardwick PA, Zvaifler NJ, Gill GN, Newman D, Greenway GD, Resnick DL: Plasma cell dyscrasia with polyneuropathy, organomegaly, endocrinopathy, M protein, and skin changes: The POEMS syndrome. *Medicine (Baltimore)* 59:311, 1980.
235. Turkington RW, Lebovitz HE: Extra-adrenal endocrine deficiencies in Addison's disease. *Am J Med* 43:449, 1967.
236. Maisey MN, Lessof MH: Addison's disease: A clinical study. *Guy's Hosp Rep* 118:363, 1969.
237. Males JL, Spitler AL, Townsend JL: Addison's disease: A review of 32 cases. *Okla Med J* 64:298, 1971.

CHAPTER 29

Ectopic Hormone Production

Glenn D. Braunstein

GENERAL PRINCIPLES

Paraneoplastic Syndromes

Most clinical abnormalities found in patients with cancer are directly related to the growth of the primary tumor and to metastases, infections, or therapy. In addition, these patients may exhibit one or more remote effects of cancer. Such remote effects, or *paraneoplastic syndromes,* include the signs, symptoms, and biochemical abnormalities that occur in patients as a result of cancer which are not due to the mass effects of the primary neoplasm or its metastases. The spectrum of paraneoplastic syndromes is large and covers every organ system (Table 29-1). Paraneoplastic syndromes are relatively common in patients with cancer, being found in approximately 20 percent at any time period and in up to 75 percent at some time during the course of disease.[1,2] The most common paraneoplastic syndromes involve ectopic hormone production, neurologic dysfunction, and hematologic abnormalities.

Many of the nonendocrine paraneoplastic syndromes result from immunologic abnormalities. Some syndromes are associated with the production of site-specific antibodies. Examples include subacute cerebellar degeneration, which is associated with anti-Purkinje cells cytoplasmic antibodies, the peripheral motor neuropathy found with lymphomas and plasma cell dyscrasias in which antibodies against the GM_1 and GD_{1b} gangliosides are present, the antiacetylcholine receptor antibodies found in patients with myasthenia gravis associated with thymomas, and autoantibodies to desmoplakin I and other skin antigens in paraneoplastic pemphigus.[3,4] Circulating antibodies may also cause a paraneoplastic syndrome through the formation of immune complexes. The deposition of an immune complex composed of carcinoembryonic antigen and anticarcinoembryonic antigen has been described in patients with nephrotic syndrome associated with cancer.[5] Similarly, glomerular membrane deposition of IgG and IgM in patients with the nephrotic syndrome and lung carcinoma has been noted.[6,7] Cell-mediated immune dysfunction in patients with cancer is well known and accounts for the anergy found in patients with late-stage disease. Lymphocytes that are cytotoxic for muscle cells have been found in patients with cancer-associated dermatomyositis.[8] The alterations in normal immunity found in cancer patients also account for some of the unusual infections that occur. For many years the syndrome of progressive multifocal leukoencephalopathy was thought to be a paraneoplastic syndrome primarily found in lymphoproliferative and myoproliferative neoplasms. However, it is now known that this syndrome is the consequence of central nervous system (CNS) infection with a papovavirus (JC virus or SV40-PML virus).[9]

Another mechanism by which tumors may give rise to a paraneoplastic syndrome is through the depletion of substrates. Examples include a pellagra-like dermatitis secondary to the niacin deficiency found in some patients with carcinoid tumors and the necrolytic migratory erythema from amino acid depletion in the hypercatabolic state induced by glucagon-secreting tumors. Also, the hypoglycemia found in markedly cachectic patients may result from a lack of sufficient quantities of gluconeogenic amino acids to allow the liver to synthesize adequate quantities of glucose during a fasting state.[10]

Tumors also may secrete excessive quantities of normally occurring proteins. A number of growth factors that have generally been considered to be local or paracrine regulators of cell function may be secreted in sufficient quantities to act systemically. Eosinophilopoietin production in lymphoproliferative disorders may be responsible for the eosinophilia associated with these tumors.[11] Disseminated intravascular coagulation has been associated with mucin-producing adenocarcinomas in which the mucin appears to activate factor X.[12] These examples illustrate the wide range of pathophysiologic mechanisms that may give rise to nonendocrine paraneoplastic syndromes.

Eutopic versus Ectopic Hormone Production

Until recently, the definition of eutopic and ectopic hormone production was relatively straightforward.

TABLE 29-1 Spectrum of Paraneoplastic Syndromes

Ectopic hormone syndromes (see Table 29-2)	Dermatologic syndromes
Neurologic syndromes	Acanthosis nigricans
Dementia	Leser-Trelat Sign
Limbic encephalitis	Bowen's disease
Subacute cerebellar degeneration	Melanosis
Necrotizing myelopathy	Bazex's syndrome
Subacute sensory neuropathy	Erythema gryatum repens
Peripheral neuropathies	Erythema annulare centrifugum
Paraneoplastic retinopathy	Exfoliate dermatitis
Myesthesia gravis	Pemphigoid
Eaton-Lambert syndrome	Dermatitis herpetiformis
Myopathies	Hypertrichosis lanuginosa
Dermatomyositis-polymyositis	Acquired icthyosis
Carcinomatous neuromyopathy	Pachydermoperiostosis
Acute necrotizing myopathy	Pruritis
Hemotologic syndromes	Gastrointestinal syndromes
Erythrocytosis	Protein losing enteropathy
Red cell aplasia	Anorexia-cachexia
Megaloblastic anemia	Dysgeusia/hypogeusia
Autoimmune hemolytic anemia	Rheumatologic syndromes
Microangiopathic hemolytic anemia	Hypertrophic pulmonary osteoarthropathy
Granulocytosis	Rheumatoid arthritis-like arthropathy
Granulocytopenia	Polyarteritis
Eosinophilia	Secondary gout
Thrombocytosis	Vascular syndromes
Disseminated intravascular coagulation	Venous thrombosis
Cryoglobulinemia	Nonbacterial thrombotic endocarditis
Cold hemagglutinin disease	Miscellaneous syndromes
Circulating anticoagulant	Fever
Hyperviscosity syndrome	Lactic acidosis
Hypogammaglobulinemia	Hyperlipidemia
T- and B-cell dysfunction	Porphyria cutanea tarda
Renal syndromes	
Glomerulonephritis	
Nephrotic syndrome	
Renal tubular acidosis	
Secondary amyloidosis	

Eutopic hormone production referred to the secretion of a hormone by a neoplasm derived from a tissue or organ which normally produces the hormone, while *ectopic hormone production* was defined as the secretion of a hormone by a neoplasm derived from a tissue or organ which does not normally produce that hormone. Using these definitions, excessive production of adrenocorticotropin (ACTH) by a corticotroph cell adenoma of the pituitary represents eutopic production of ACTH, while Cushing's syndrome resulting from production of ACTH by a small cell carcinoma of the lung represents ectopic production. However, many normal tissues, including lung, contain small amounts of immunoreactive ACTH or proopiomelanocortin (POMC).[13] This finding has resulted in the hypothesis that the elevated serum and tumor levels of immunoreactive ACTH or POMC are due to a quantitative difference in the amounts of ACTH/POMC synthesized by tumor cells in contrast to normal cells. In addition, if cancer cells contain the enzymes that process the biologically inactive POMC to the biologically active ACTH molecule, Cushing's syndrome may result.[13] Growth hormone, insulin, corticotropin releasing factor (CRF), human chorionic gonadotropin (hCG), somatostatin, calcitonin, vasoactive intestinal peptide (VIP), and parathyroid hormone–related protein (PTH-rp) have also been demonstrated in normal nonendocrine tissues.[14–23] In an effort to maintain the concept of ectopic hormone production while recognizing the possibility that all normal tissues may secrete small quantities of at least immunoreactive forms of peptide hormones, ectopic hormone production may be redefined as the excessive secretion of a hormone by a neoplasm derived from a tissue or organ which is not the known *physiologic* source of that hormone. This definition is not wholly satisfactory since the small quantities of peptide hormones that are secreted by normal tissues may have a physiologic autocrine or paracrine function. Nevertheless, this is a satisfactory working definition which encompasses the current state of knowledge.

A large number of hormones are produced ectopically, although not all are associated with clinical syndromes (Table 29-2). It is of interest that neither the thyronines nor the steroid hormones are on this list. Presumably, the synthesis of these classes of hormones requires orderly enzymatic steps which are absent in tumors that are not derived from the thyroid, adrenals, or steroid-secreting gonadal cells. Although nonendocrine tumors do not synthesize steroid hormones from cholesterol, they may have enzyme systems that convert one steroid hormone to another. Indeed, the gynecomastia found in some males with lung, gastric, and hepatic carcinomas is caused by the conversion of dehydroepiandosterone to estrone and estradiol by the tumors.[24,25]

Importance of Ectopic Hormone Production

There are several reasons why consideration of ectopic hormone production is important. First, the recognition of the syndrome may lead to the diagnosis of the tumor. Although most patients are known to harbor a tumor when the ectopic hormone syndrome is diagnosed, there are many examples of ectopic hormone syndromes occurring months to years before the diagnosis of a tumor. This is most commonly seen in patients who have slowly growing neoplasms such as bronchial carcinoids, malignant thymomas, or islet-cell carcinomas. With these tumors, Cushing's syndrome from ectopic production of ACTH or CRF or acromegaly from secretion of growth hormone releasing factor (GHRF) commonly antedates the other manifestations of the underlying malignancy, and it is during the evaluation of these patients for this syndrome that the underlying tumor is discovered. In some patients, the tumor may be discovered at such an early stage that the patient can be cured through surgical resection.

A second reason why ectopic hormone production

TABLE 29-2 Hormones Produced Ectopically and Their Associated Clinical Syndromes

Eutopic Source of Hormone	Hormone	Syndrome
Hypothalamus	Corticotropin releasing factor	Cushing's syndrome
	Growth hormone releasing hormone	Acromegaly
	Somatostatin	None
	Gonadotropin releasing hormone	None
	Thyrotropin releasing hormone	None
	Antidiuretic hormone	SIAD
	Oxytocin	None
Pituitary	Pro-opiomelanocortin/ACTH	Cushing's syndrome
	Growth hormone	Acromegaly
	Prolactin	Galactorrhea
Placenta	Human chorionic gonadotropin	Precocious puberty (childhood) Gynecomastia (adults)
	Placental lactogen	None
Gastrointestinal tract	Gastrin	Zollinger-Ellison syndrome
	Glucagon	Glucagonoma syndrome
	Vasoactive intestinal peptide	Diarrhea hypokalemia
	Cholecystokinin	None
	Bombesin/gastrin-releasing peptide	Cushing's syndrome
	Secretin	None
Kidney	Erythropoietin	Polycythemia
	Prorenin/renin	Hypertension, hypokalemia
Parafollicular cells	Calcitonin	None
Liver	Insulin-like growth factors	Hypoglycemia
Multiple sites	Parathyroid hormone–related peptide	Hypercalcemia
	Transforming growth factor	?Hypercalcemia
	Epidermal growth factor	?Hypercalcemia
	Platelet-derived growth factor	?Hypercalcemia
Unknown	Hypophosphatemia-producing factor	Oncogenic osteomalacia

is important is that the patient may succumb to the metabolic effects of the hormone rather than to the direct effects of the neoplasm. The intense catabolic state induced by the full-blown ectopic ACTH syndrome, the severe hyponatremia that may occur with the syndrome of inappropriate secretion of antidiuretic hormone (SIADH), and the hypercalcemic crisis that occurs with excessive production of PTH-rp are examples. Prompt treatment of these metabolic abnormalities can be expected to prolong survival, assuming that the patient is not preterminal from the other effects of the neoplasm.

An understanding of ectopic hormone syndromes is also important because failure to recognize the presence of a syndrome may lead to erroneous diagnosis in a patient with known cancer. The hypercortisolemia found with ectopic ACTH production, the hyponatremia found with SIADH, and humoral hypercalcemia are each associated with neurologic abnormalities, including behavioral disorders and alterations of consciousness. These conditions may be mistaken for the presence of CNS metastases or infections which in turn may result in inappropriate therapy.

Furthermore, the hormone itself may serve as a tumor marker for localizing the neoplasm, monitoring the effects of therapy, and detecting a recurrence. For instance, approximately 70 percent of tumors associated with the clinical ectopic ACTH syndrome are located between the jaw and the diaphragm. The finding of an elevated, nonsuppressible ACTH level in such a patient should lead to a careful search for a lung, thymic, or thyroid tumor. Once a tumor is identified, serial measurements of the ectopic hormone may provide objective evidence of the effects of therapy. In many instances, the changes in the serum or plasma concentrations of a hormone accurately reflect changes in the mass of the tumor. Although a persistently elevated hormone level is indicative of a persistent tumor, the reverse is not always true, as the ectopically produced hormone may decrease at a time when the tumor mass is increasing. Immunohistologic staining for hormone-secreting cells in tumor tissues has demonstrated that most tumors are quite heterogeneous, with much variability in the proportion of cells that synthesize the hormone.[26] Either selective loss of the hormone-producing cells from overgrowth by more rapidly dividing cells that do not secrete the hormone or selective destruction of hormone-producing cells from chemotherapy or radiotherapy may account for the discordance between changes in the marker levels and tumor growth.[27] This phenomenon is also illustrated by studies in which multiple tumor markers were measured.[28,29] Indeed, it is the exception rather than the rule that all tumor markers and tumor growth remain concordant throughout the course of disease. Nevertheless, a rising level of the ectopically produced hormone is almost always indicative of recurrence or progression of the disease. The only exception occurs immediately after surgical manipulation of the tumor or shortly after radiation therapy or induction chemotherapy. In these situations, necrosis of tumor tissue may lead to the release of preformed hormone into the circulation, which may result in a transient increase in the hormone level.

Finally, ectopic hormone syndromes are important because their study may lead to the discovery of new hormones. The discovery, purification, and structural characterization of GHRF and PTH-rp are recent examples of hormones that were initially isolated from cancers causing acromegaly and hypercalcemia, respectively.

Criteria for Ectopic Hormone Production

Multiple criteria have been developed to establish ectopic hormone production (Table 29-3). Most of the clinical criteria are sufficient to lead to a presumptive diagnosis of ectopic hormone production but are not sufficient for an unequivocal diagnosis. Both the presence of an endocrine syndrome associated with a nonendocrine neoplasm and the finding of increased quantities of a circulating hormone associated with a neoplasm derived from the tissue that is not the physiologic source of the hormone are not definitive because of the possibility of coexistence of an endocrine neoplasm with a nonendocrine cancer. For example, several studies have shown that hyperparathyroidism due to parathyroid adenomas or hyperplasia occurs with a greater than expected frequency in patients with cancer.[30–32] A patient with an ectopic CRF-producing neoplasm will present with Cushing's syndrome associated with elevated plasma ACTH. In this situation, it may be erroneously concluded that the tumor was secreting ACTH when in fact the source of the ACTH was actually the anterior pituitary corticotroph cells responding to the ectopic CRF. A third example of how an erroneous conclusion may be reached utilizing clinical criteria alone is seen in the case of the SIADH in association with some neoplasms. Chemotherapeutic drugs such as cyclophosphamide and vincristine may cause hyponatremia which could be mistakenly attributed to the secretion of antidiuretic hormone (ADH) by the tumor. A lung tumor associated with SIADH may actually not be secreting ADH but may have so altered intrathoracic pressure that the stretch receptors present in the great pulmonary veins and left atrium may be inappropriately stimulated, which in turn may lead to the release of ADH from the hypothalamus and posterior pituitary. Removal of the lung tumor may reestablish normal intrathoracic pressure, and the excessive ADH release will cease. Recurrence of the tumor may again alter intrathoracic pressure in such a manner that ADH release from the hypothalamus and posterior pitu-

TABLE 29-3 Criteria for Ectopic Hormone Production

1. Presence of an endocrine syndrome associated with a neoplasm derived from a tissue that is not the physiologic source of the hormone known to cause the syndrome
2. Disappearance of the endocrine syndrome after removal or effective treatment of the tumor recurrence of syndrome with relapse of tumor
3. Excessive quantities of circulating hormone associated with a neoplasm derived from a tissue that is not the physiologic source of the hormone
4. Return of circulating hormone to normal or subnormal levels after removal or effective treatment of the tumor; recurrence of elevated hormone levels with relapse of tumor
5. Persistence of syndrome or excessive hormone production after removal or suppression of the normal physiologic endocrine source of the hormone
6. Extraction of the hormone from the tumor tissue in quantities greater than expected from blood contamination
7. Greater concentration of the hormone in the tumor than in the surrounding nonneoplastic tissue
8. Immunochemical or histochemical localization of the hormone in the tumor cells, especially in secretory granules
9. Arteriovenous hormone concentration difference across the tumor, with higher levels in the venous effluent
10. Detection of messenger RNA for the hormone in the tumor tissue by Northern analysis, in situ hybridization, or in vitro cell-free translation systems
11. In vitro synthesis and secretion of the hormone by the tumor, especially with incorporation of radiolabeled precursors into the hormone
12. Demonstration of in vivo hormone production after tumor transplantation into an animal model

itary is again stimulated. Thus, recurrence of the syndrome or an elevation of ADH levels cannot be used as evidence that the tumor is secreting the hormone directly.

Although in most instances persistence of a syndrome or excessive hormone production after the removal or suppression of the normal physiologic endocrine source of that hormone is indicative of ectopic production of the hormone, there are exceptions. The most frequent exceptions are seen in some patients with Cushing's disease in whom ACTH is not suppressed after the administration of even very high doses of dexamethasone. Another example is the presence of hyperparathyroidism due to a parathyroid adenoma in an accessory parathyroid gland in a patient who also harbors a cancer. A neck exploration may reveal four suppressed parathyroid glands, and it may be erroneously concluded that the cancer is responsible for elaborating the parathyroid hormone.

If the tumor contains a greater concentration of the hormone than does the surrounding normal tissue or than can be accounted for by the amount of contaminating blood, a stronger case can be made for ectopic production of the hormone by the tumor. However, there are potential exceptions. Several tumors have been shown to possess receptors for hormones, and it is conceivable that some concentrate hormones from the circulation.[33,34] A much stronger criterion is the specific localization of the hormone in secretory granules within the tumor tissue. Although the presence of a hormone in such secretory granules does not necessarily indicate that the hormone is secreted, a reasonable cause-and-effect relation may be assumed if the tumor contains the hormone in the secretory granules and the patient exhibits the appropriate clinical syndrome with an elevation of the same hormone in the blood. The last four criteria for ectopic hormone production in Table 29-3 unequivocally establish the production of the hormone by the tumor. Of course, each criterion assumes that the methods used for detecting the hormone or its messenger RNA are specific.

An example of how these various criteria may be used to establish the presence of an ectopic hormone syndrome is provided in the report of Melmed and colleagues, who described a 60-year-old male with acromegaly and elevated serum growth hormone and insulin-like growth factor-I (IGF-I) concentrations.[35] The finding of a normal pituitary on high-resolution CT scan prompted a search for a possible GHRF-producing neoplasm. A CT scan of the abdomen (Fig. 29-1) revealed a large mass in the region of the head of the pancreas, which at surgery was found to be a partially cystic vascular mass consistent with an intramesenteric pancreatic islet-cell tumor. At the time of surgery, an arteriovenous gradient of growth hormone was present across the tumor; the growth hormone concentration in a peripheral artery was 34 ng/ml, and that in a tumor vein was 368 ng/ml. Postoperatively, the serum growth hormone levels rapidly fell from 34 to 2 ng/ml over the expected rate of disappearance based on the half-life of growth hormone (Fig. 29-2). GHRF was not detected in the peripheral blood or in a tumor vein. Six months postoperatively, the patient's acromegaly had remitted, the serum growth hormone was 1.4 ng/ml, and the serum IGF-I was normal. Elevated levels of immunoreactive growth hormone were found in the tumor tissue, and immunoreactive growth hormone was localized in juxtanuclear granules in the tumor cells by both immunohistochemistry and immunoelectron microscopy (Fig. 29-3). The tumor growth hormone comigrated with pituitary growth hormone on Sephadex column chromatography. In addition, dispersed tumor cells secreted im-

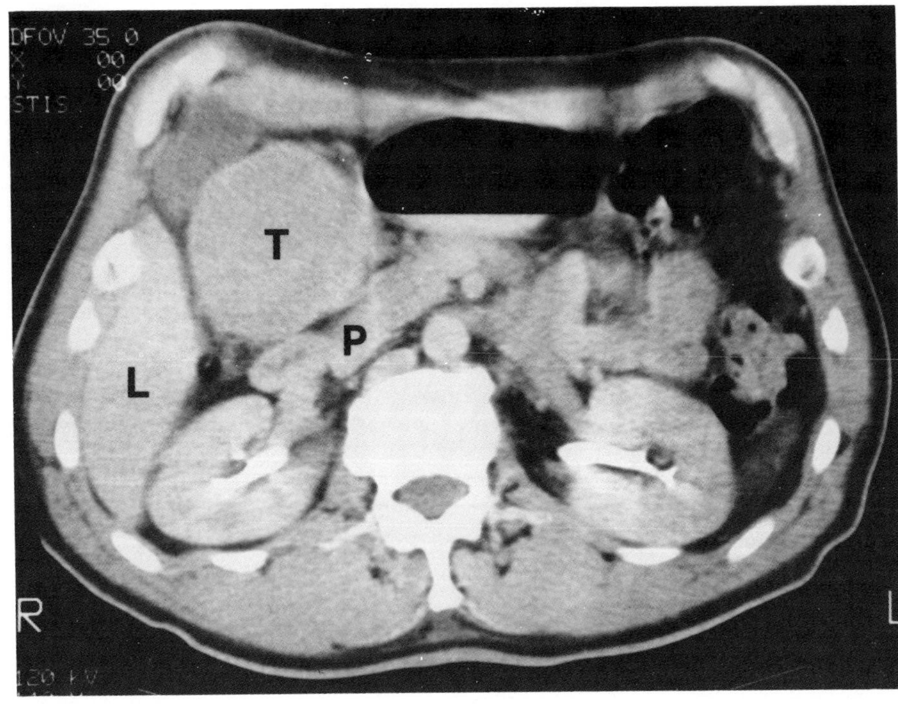

FIGURE 29-1 Abdominal CT scan of the acromegalic male described in the text showing an 8.1 × 6.6-cm mass adjacent to the liver. T = tumor mass; L = liver; P = pancreas. (*Reprinted from Melmed and coworkers,*[35] *with permission.*)

munoreactive growth hormone into tissue culture medium for several weeks, and the tumor cells were able to synthesize growth hormone. Finally, messenger RNA extracted from the tumor cells hybridized with a cDNA probe for human growth hormone in a dose-dependent fashion (Fig. 29-4). Subsequent to the published report, the patient was found to have a return of the clinical features of acromegaly associated with a rising growth hormone level, and evaluation revealed the presence of liver metastases from the original tumor (Melmed, personal communication). Thus, virtually all the criteria for ectopic hormone production outlined in Table 29-3 were satisfied in this case study.

Frequency of Ectopic Hormone Production

The frequency of ectopic hormone production varies considerably, depending to a great extent on the population of patients studied and whether clinical or biochemical criteria are utilized for making the diagnosis. Table 29-4 summarizes a number of studies that have examined the frequency of the most common paraneoplastic endocrine syndromes.[36–58] Hypercalcemia is the most frequently recognized syndrome, being found in 10 to 14 percent of patients with cancer. However, the frequency among the different types of cancers varies considerably. Thus, patients with multiple myeloma and breast carcinoma tend to have a higher incidence of hypercalcemia than do patients with lung carcinoma. Even among patients with lung carcinoma, there is substantial variability in the frequency of hypercalcemia; patients harboring squamous cell carcinomas have a much higher frequency than do patients with small cell carcinoma. If the incidence of hypercalcemia in carcinoma patients is assessed in a population in which breast carcinoma is overrepresented, the incidence of hypercalcemia will be higher than that in a population in which breast carcinoma is underrepresented. Thus, the incidence figures are heavily prone to ascertainment bias. In addition, the various reported frequencies are dependent on the criteria used to diagnose ectopic hormone production. Incidence figures based on clinical criteria are uniformly lower than are those based on biochemical criteria. For example, less than 5 percent of patients with small cell carcinoma of the lung have clinically recognizable Cushing's syndrome.[39,47,51,52] In contrast, between 24 and 78 percent of patients with small cell carcinoma of the lung have elevated ACTH levels, and between one-quarter and one-half of these patients have elevated serum cortisol concentrations which do not suppress appropriately after dexamethasone administration.[39,47,48,59–63] The same phenomenon is also true in regard to SIADH in patients with small cell carcinoma of the lung. Approximately 10 to 15 percent of patients with this tumor have symptomatic or asymptomatic hyponatremia.[44,49,51,53] However, 40 to 68 percent fail to excrete a standardized water load appropriately,[49,58,63] and close to half of these patients have elevated plasma or urinary ADH or neurophysin lev-

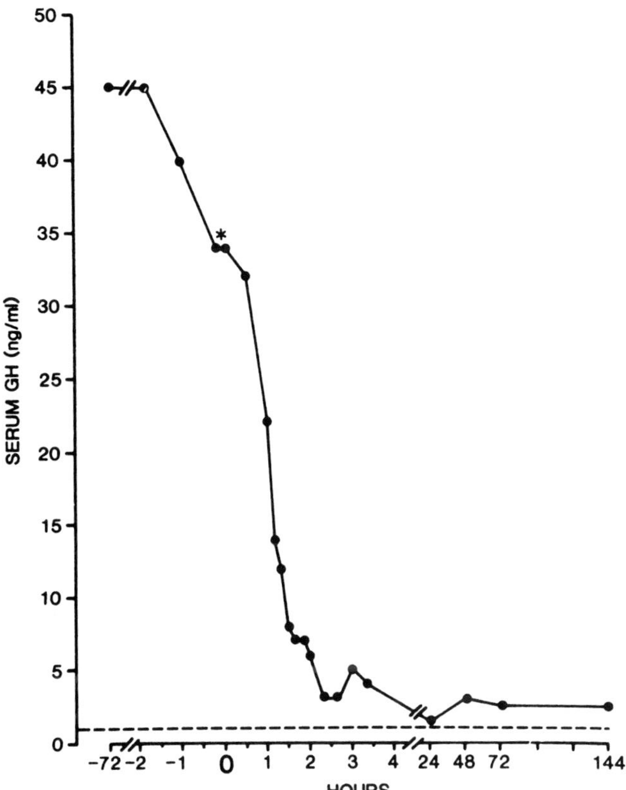

FIGURE 29-2 Serum growth hormone levels in the patient with a growth hormone–secreting islet-cell tumor described in the text. Preoperative growth hormone levels varied between 25 and 60 ng/ml. Abdominal surgery was begun at −2 h and just before tumor removal at 0 h (*), blood was drawn from a tumor vein and peripheral artery for growth hormone measurements. The simultaneous arteriovenous gradient of GH levels across the tumor: peripheral artery, 34 ng/ml; tumor vein, 368 ng/ml. (*Reprinted from Melmed and coworkers,*[35] *with permission.*)

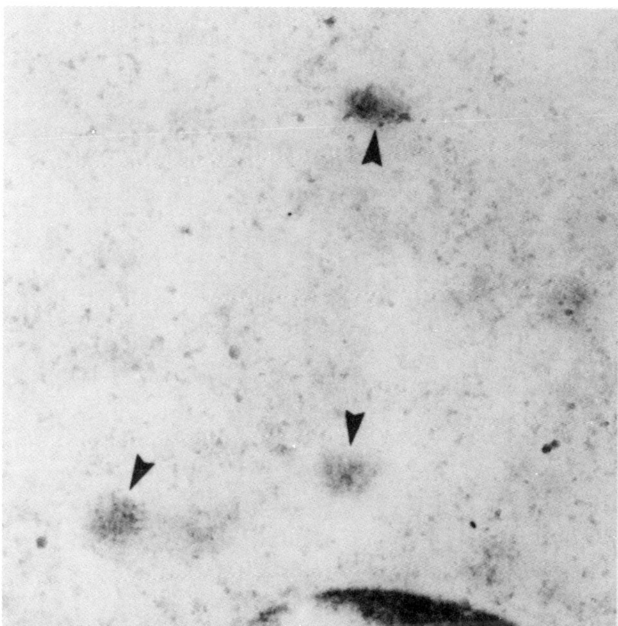

FIGURE 29-3 Immunoelectron micrographs of a growth hormone–secreting islet-cell tumor demonstrating the presence of cytoplasmic growth hormone in secretory granules (arrow) (×40,800). (*Reprinted from Melmed and coworkers,*[35] *with permission.*)

els.[46–48,52,58–64] Thus, relying only on the presence or absence of a clinical syndrome will give a spuriously low frequency of ectopic hormone production.

Several other factors are responsible for the low frequency of diagnosis of ectopic hormone production (Table 29-5).[65–68] The physician caring for the patient may have a low index of clinical suspicion that an ectopic hormone syndrome is present. Patients with the ectopic ACTH syndrome, SIADH, or hypercalcemia may complain of weakness and anorexia which may be attributable to other effects of cancer or therapy rather than to the hypokalemic alkalosis and catabolic effects of large amounts of circulating cortisol seen with the ectopic ACTH syndrome, the hyponatremia seen with excessive ADH, or the direct effects of an increase in serum calcium. Early in the course of ectopic hormone production, the ectopic hormone may actually replace the eutopic hormone, and therefore a hormone excess syndrome may not be clinically apparent. Low levels of ACTH from a tumor may stimulate cortisol production from the adrenals, and the cortisol will suppress pituitary ACTH production. The patient will not exhibit the signs or symptoms of Cushing's syndrome until the cortisol production rate rises above normal for several weeks or months. In addition, the clinical features of an ectopic hormone syndrome may actually be obscured by other manifestations of the neoplasm. One reason why patients with the ectopic ACTH syndrome associated with small cell carcinoma of the lung generally do not have cushingoid features with centripetal redistribution of fat may be the coexistence of cancer cachexia. Also, some paraneoplastic endocrine syndromes occur as a late manifestation of the neoplasm and therefore may not be apparent to the clinician unless the patient is followed over a long period. The phenomenon of periodic hormonogenesis may account for an underdiagnosis of ectopic hormone production. Bailey originally described this phenomenon in which some neoplasms secrete excessive quantities of their hormones intermittently and in an autonomous fashion.[69] This has been well described for the ectopic ACTH syndrome. Biochemical testing during the intervals between excessive hormone production may give normal results.

There are many situations in which hormones are produced ectopically without clinical expression, and a diagnosis of ectopic hormone production will thus be missed unless a battery of hormone determinations are made in blood or urine samples from such patients. In some instances, the hormone ex-

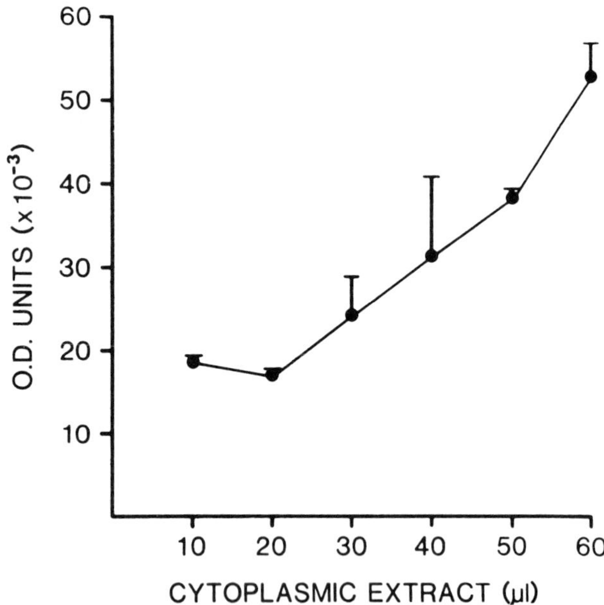

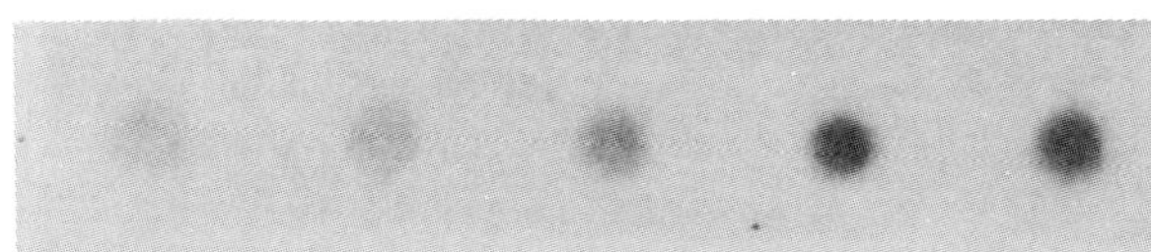

FIGURE 29-4 Nitrocellulose dot hybridization of ^{32}P-labeled growth hormone cDNA with dilutions of islet-cell tumor cytoplasmic mRNA. Each point represents the mean optical density (O.D.) of two or three separate immobilized dots visualized by autoradiography. *(Reprinted from Melmed and coworkers,[35] with permission.)*

TABLE 29-4 Frequency of Paraneoplastic Endocrine Syndromes

Syndrome	Tumor	Frequency %
Cushing's syndrome	Small cell lung carcinoma	1.3–4.8
	Squamous cell lung carcinoma	0
	Adenocarcinoma of lung	0
SIADH	Small cell lung carcinoma	9.5–14
	Lung carcinoma (all)	1.6
Hypercalcemia	Carcinomas in general	10–14
	Breast carcinoma	7.2–22.8
	Multiple myeloma	21.2–28.1
	Renal cell carcinoma	5–12.7
	Lung cancer (all)	6.8–12.5
	Squamous cell carcinoma	24
	Small cell carcinoma	1
	Adenocarcinoma	3
	Large cell carcinoma	8
	Lymphoma	9.8
	Leukemia	11.5
Polycythemia	Renal cell carcinoma	0.9–3.5
	Cerebellar hemangioblastoma	9–20

Source: From references 36–58.

cess may not be associated with a clinical syndrome. Mild hypercalcemia is usually asymptomatic and is detected as part of a multiphasic panel of tests run on a blood sample. In addition, there may be situations in which the body's homeostatic mechanisms are able to compensate for the excessive concentration of the ectopic hormone. For instance, prolonged elevation of human chorionic gonadotropin (hCG) may lead to down regulation of testicular Leydig cell receptors, which in turn may lead to a decrease in the Leydig cells' responsiveness to the effects of hormones.[70] There are numerous examples of tumors which secrete hormone precursors that do not undergo processing to the active hormone. One of the best studied examples concerns the ectopic ACTH syndrome, in which the major form of the hormone circulating in the blood and present in the tumor tissue is a large molecular form ("big" ACTH; pro-ACTH, POMC) which is immunologically active but biologically inactive. This precursor of ACTH may be converted into biologically active ACTH by trypsin exposure. Indeed, a high frequency (17 to 88 percent) of elevated concentrations of immunoreactive ACTH has been found in the circulation of patients with all types of lung cancer.[48,60,62,71–74] This is in contrast to the low (less than 5 percent) prevalence of clinical Cushing's syndrome in such patients. It has been proposed that this difference is due to the inability of

TABLE 29-5 Factors Responsible for the Low Frequency of Diagnosis of Ectopic Hormone Production

- Low index of clinical suspicion
  - Minimal clinical expression
  - Ectopic hormone replaces eutopic hormone
  - Syndrome obscured by other effects of cancer
- Inadequate long-term follow-up of patient
- Periodic hormonogenesis
- Hormone production without clinical expression
  - Hormone excess not associated with clinical syndromes
  - Secretion of hormone precursor without processing to active hormone
  - Secretion of hormone subunits
  - Secretion of hormone fragments
- Ectopic secretion of unidentified hormones
- Hormone assay factors
  - Insensitive assay
  - Presence of interfering substances

Source: Adapted from references 66–68.

the majority of lung cancers to convert the POMC molecule to ACTH. In addition to hormone precursor molecules, some tumors secrete biologically inactive hormone subunits, such as the α and β subunits of hCG, or biologically inactive fragments of hormones.

Ectopic hormone production may be undiagnosed if the tumor secretes an unidentified hormone. Most recently, this has been demonstrated with PTH-rp. Before the discovery of PTH-rp, ectopic production of the PTH-like hormone was diagnosed only when the patient developed hypercalcemia. Since the advent of radioimmunoassays (RIAs) for measuring PTH-rp, it has been found that some patients with cancer but without hypercalcemia also have elevated levels of this hormone.[21] Alternatively, the patient may exhibit a full-blown syndrome from the ectopic production of an unidentified hormone. In this situation, the fact that the syndrome is actually a paraneoplastic syndrome may not be appreciated. This was the case with the description of the first patient with a hypoglycemia-inducing mesenchymal tumor who had an intrathoracic fibrosarcoma associated with neuroglucopenic symptoms that responded to a rectal glucose drip.[75] The symptoms were attributed to the mechanical displacement of the heart and blood vessels by the tumor, which resulted in "lack of nourishment to the brain and accumulation of toxemia in the brain [which] could induce mental disturbance."[75] Another theory stated that such tumors, being quite large, consume more glucose than the body's homeostatic mechanisms can cope with.[76] It is now recognized that the hypoglycemia occurring with these non-islet-cell tumors is due to excessive production of insulin-like growth factors, especially insulin-like growth factor-II.[77]

Hormone assay factors may also be responsible for the low frequency of diagnosis of ectopic hormone production. Some assays may be too insensitive to detect ectopic hormone production, especially when the hormone levels are too low to elicit a clinical syndrome. Thus, before the advent of a sensitive and relatively specific RIA for hCG based on antibodies generated against the β subunit of the hormone, hCG RIAs exhibited substantial cross-reaction with human luteinizing hormone. Therefore, hCG could not be measured with confidence until the quantities measured exceeded the normal physiologic levels of luteinizing hormone. This resulted in the development of pregnancy tests that required that 500 mIU of hCG/ml of urine or serum be reached or exceeded before the test would become positive. The beta-hCG RIA allowed the detection of 5 mIU/ml of hCG in the presence of physiologic concentrations of luteinizing hormone, a 100-fold increase in sensitivity over the earlier pregnancy tests.[78] Since most patients with ectopic hCG production have levels under 15 mIU/ml of blood, the earlier urinary pregnancy tests would not have been sufficiently sensitive to detect the ectopic production of this hormone.[79] Another problem with immunomimetric assays is their susceptibility to interference by many different substances, including proteases, circulating binding proteins for the ligand, heterophilic antibodies, hyperlipidemia, contaminant radioactivity in serum, and other nonspecific serum factors.

Etiology of Ectopic Hormone Production

Any etiologic theory of the mechanisms of ectopic hormone production must provide an adequate explanation for two observations. First, the ectopically produced hormones closely resemble the eutopic hormone, at least in their amino acid sequences. Some tumors produce prohormones, hormone subunits, or fragments of hormones. When analyzed, these proteins are structurally identical to the analogous sequence in the native hormone or prohormone. Alterations in the carbohydrate composition of several ectopically produced glycoproteins have been noted.[80–82] These findings indicate that the translation of the RNA sequence into the protein proceeds normally and that the differences between ectopically and eutopically produced hormones relate to posttranslational modifications such as glycosylation and enzymatic modification of prohormones or of the hormone itself.

Second, ectopic hormone production is not random. Certain tumor types are associated with specific clinical syndromes and hormone production. Even within the same organ system, different histologic varieties of a tumor give rise to different syndromes. Thus, hypercalcemia is found with squamous cell carcinoma of the lung, while Cushing's syndrome is associated primarily with small cell carcinoma of the lung (Table 29-4). In a thorough analysis of the literature, Levine and Metz concluded that the majority of the ectopic hormone–producing tumors could be segregated into two main groups (Table 29-6).[67] The tumors in each group share embryologic, morphologic, and hormone-producing capabilities. Each of the group I tumors is capable of secreting any of the hormones characteristic of that group, and several have been shown to secrete multiple hormones.[43] The group I tumors are derived from neuroectoderm cells, which constitute the APUD system of Pearse (see below). The group II tumors are derived from endoderm and mesoderm and primarily secrete glycoprotein hormones, peptides, and growth factors. A small group of tumors of neural crest origin which embryologically and histologically resemble group I tumors are associated with the secretion of hormones of groups I and II and therefore constitute a transitional group. Although the Levine-Metz classification is reasonably accurate for the association between tumor types and clinical syndromes, it is not as useful when ectopic hormone production per se is considered. Thus, hCG is produced by a wide variety of neoplasms, not just

TABLE 29-6 Levine-Metz Classification of Tumors Producing Ectopic Hormones

	Group I (APUD)	Group II	Transitional
Tumors	Foregut carcinoid Small cell carcinoma Pancreatic islet-cell tumors Some tumors of pancreatic and biliary ducts Thyroid medullary carcinoma Malignant epithelial thymomas	Hepatoma Cholangioma Wilms' tumor Hypernephroma Adrenocortical carcinoma Nongerminal gonadal tumors Vascular tumors Connective tissue and mesodermal tumors Reticuloendothelial tumors Non-small-cell lung carcinoma GI tumors (except APUD) Melanoma	Pheochromocytoma Melanoma
Hormones	Insulin Calcitonin ACTH/POMC ADH Gastrin Glucagon Secretin Biogenic amines	PTH-rp Erythropoietin hCG hPL PRL GH IGF Renin	Biogenic amines ACTH Calcitonin Glucagon Secretin hPL PTH-rp Erythropoietin

Source: Adapted from Levine and Metz.[67]

those associated with group II, even though the clinical syndromes of gynecomastia in adults and precocious puberty in children are seen only with group II tumors. Similarly, elevated concentrations of pro-ACTH are found in patients with squamous cell carcinoma of the lung (a group II tumor) as well as small cell carcinoma of the lung (a group I tumor), although clinical Cushing's syndrome is seen primarily in association with group I tumors.

De Novo Synthesis from Gene Mutation

According to this theory, the process of oncogenesis involves a variety of gene mutations. The resulting alterations in the DNA may then lead to the synthesis of new proteins, some of which may possess biological activity resembling that found with hormones. Since hormone production is not entirely random and the tumor hormones, prohormones, fragments, and subunits that are produced ectopically are identical to the eutopic hormones, at least in regard to the translated protein, this theory cannot explain ectopic hormone production.

Sponge Theory

In 1964, Unger and colleagues suggested that some tumors concentrate hormones from the circulation and release them at the time of cell death.[33] Support for this hypothesis includes the observation that some adrenocortical carcinomas apparently develop "ectopic" receptors for gonadotropins and beta-adrenergic hormones.[34,83] Since virtually all the ectopically produced hormones described to date have been shown to be synthesized and secreted by tumor cells in culture, this hypothesis cannot account for ectopic hormone production.

Endocrine Cell Hypothesis

In a series of studies, Pearse and colleagues showed the wide distribution of cells of neuroectodermal origin which have the properties of concentrating amine precursors such as dopa and 5-hydroxytryptophan, decarboxylating them, and converting them into biogenic amines.[84,85] These APUD (*a*mine *p*recursor *u*ptake and *d*ecarboxylation) cells contain multiple decarboxylating enzymes and chromogranin A.[84–86] Histologically, these cells exhibit secretory granules, a prominent rough endoplasmic reticulum, and a Golgi apparatus indicating active peptide synthesis. As was noted above, these cells are widely distributed throughout the body (Table 29-7), and neoplasms of these cells all can produce a variety of polypeptides, primarily those associated with group I tumors of the Levine-Metz classification (Table 29-6), as well as biogenic amines. A substantial

TABLE 29-7 APUD Cell Distribution

APUD Cell Type	Tumor
Thyroid parafollicular cells	Medullary carcinoma of the thyroid
Adrenal medullary cells	Pheochromocytoma
Gastrointestinal neuroendocrine cells	Gastrointestinal carcinoids
Pancreatic neuroendocrine cells	Islet-cell tumors
Respiratory tract Kultschitsky's cells	Small cell carcinoma; bronchial carcinoid
Argyrophil cells of the thymus	Thymomas
Anterior pituitary cells	Pituitary adenomas
Carotid body and sympathetic ganglia cells	Paragangliomas; neuroblastoma
Melanocytes	Melanomas
Urogenital neuroendocrine cells	Prostate carcinoma
?Parathyroid chief cell	Parathyroid adenoma

amount of experimental evidence indicates that APUD cells are derived from the neural crest.[87] However, some studies suggest that the gastrointestinal (GI) tract and pancreatic APUD cells, and possibly those found in the respiratory tract, may be of endodermal origin.[88,89] In addition, the finding that thyroid C cells contain immunoreactive thyroglobulin[90] and that both islet-cell β granules and zymogen granules may coexist in the same pancreatic cell[91,92] raises the possibility that cells may develop APUD characteristics through cellular differentiation of totipotential local tissue progenitor cells rather than through migration of cells from the neural crest.

It has been hypothesized that ectopic hormone production is a result of secretion of the hormones by APUD cells in tumors.[87] Certainly this is a viable hypothesis for the group I tumors of the Levine-Metz classification (Table 29-6) and the tumors listed in Table 29-7. However, this theory cannot account for the production of the hormones by the Levine-Metz group II tumors, which do not have APUD cell characteristics, or explain the ectopic production of APUD (group I) hormones by group II tumors. The APUD cells contain convertases and other processing enzymes that allow the secretion of biologically active hormones. This may explain why clinical syndromes due to the ectopic secretion of group I hormones are seen more frequently with tumors that have APUD characteristics than with group II tumors, which may not be capable of appropriately processing group I prohormones.

A variation of the APUD hypothesis of ectopic hormone production is the cell hybridization hypothesis of Warner.[93] It has been proposed that ectopic hormone production represents the fusion of a malignant cell with an APUD-type "bystander" cell which results in the malignant cell secreting the polypeptide that APUD-type cells can secrete. Warner further suggested that the production of the hormones by these fused cells may give the clone of hormone-producing cells a survival advantage. Support for this theory is circumstantial and based on histologic and histochemical findings such as the demonstration of mucin-secreting carcinoid tumors, the presence of argentophil cells in some adenocarcinomas of the GI tract, and the existence of carcinosarcomas and adenocanthomas. There is no direct evidence that such cell hybridization takes place in vivo; even if it did, the same criticisms that have been used to discount the APUD theory as a unifying hypothesis for ectopic hormone production would apply to the cell hybridization theory.

Gene Derepression

All nucleated diploid cells in any individual contain the same genetic information that was initially present in the zygote. During the process of cellular differentiation and specialization, portions of the genome become repressed and are no longer expressed. It has been estimated that the average cell expresses less than 10 percent of its genetic information.[94] According to the depression hypothesis, during the process of neoplastic transformation, portions of the tumor cell's DNA become derepressed and the gene is then allowed to be expressed. If the derepressed portion of the genome normally codes for a hormone, that tumor may express the hormone ectopically. The possibility of derepression has clearly been shown in the frog experiments of Gurdon, who transplanted the nucleus from a differentiated adult frog cell into an enucleated frog egg which subsequently developed into an adult frog.[95] Similarly, when the nucleus from a frog kidney carcinoma is placed into an enucleated frog ovum, differentiation to the tadpole stage occurs.[96] Derepression is an attractive concept because it could account for the production of hormones by nonendocrine tumors that are structurally identical to the hormone secreted by the normal endocrine gland and could also account for the production of prohormones, fragments, and subunits. The production of prohormones could reflect the lack of derepression of the genes responsible for directing the synthesis of the cytoplasmic hormone-processing enzymes. However, this hypothesis does not account for the nonrandom association of certain tumors with specific hormones or explain why polypeptide hormones such as calcitonin, ACTH, and hCG are more frequently produced than are hormones such as growth hormone and placental lactogen.

Cellular Dedifferentiation

The cellular dedifferentiation hypothesis is an extension of the gene derepression hypothesis. This theory suggests that tumor tissues regress from a differentiated state to an undifferentiated state.[97,98] At each step in this process, the dedifferentiated cell resembles a stage in normal cell development during the process of differentiation. The dedifferentiated cell will have the ability to make all the products normal for that particular stage of differentiation. The nonrandom nature of ectopic hormone production provides strong evidence against this hypothesis.

Dysdifferentiation or Blocked Ontogenesis

According to this theory, every tissue in the body contains stem or renewal cells that are either totipotential or relatively undifferentiated. These cells are normally responsible for replenishing cells that are lost through disease or injury. The genome of these cells is either unrepressed or not fully repressed. During the process of differentiation, the genome of the stem cells undergoes progressive repression until the adult, specialized state is reached. At each stage, the differentiating cell may express a variety of proteins specific for that stage. Thus, a stem cell in the skin may be capable of secreting fetal and placental proteins, while in the adult state these cells are not able to produce these proteins. According to this theory, neoplasia takes place in these progenitor cells and the morphologic and functional characteristics of the tumor depend on the stage of the differentiation process in which oncogenesis occurs.[99,100] This theory differs from the dedifferentiation theory in that the neoplasm is derived from cells that have not fully differentiated rather than from cells that have gone from a differentiated state to a less differentiated state.

This theory is attractive because it accounts for several phenomena that are observed with cancer. It is well established that tumor populations are heterogeneous, and immunohistochemical studies have shown that different tumors contain variable numbers of hormone-secreting cells.[26] This theory also accounts for the phenomenon of hormone production by granulomas and inflammatory lesions.[101,102] It also provides a possible explanation for the nonrandom association of certain hormones with specific tumors. Local factors such as cell surface contact and the presence of growth factors or other paracrine substances may modulate the proliferation and differentiation of the stem cells in a particular organ. The experimental work with small cell carcinoma carried out by Baylin and colleagues has shown how the dysdifferentiation theory can account for the APUD characteristics of tumor cells. This does not necessarily indicate that the tumor originated from a neuroectodermal cell but rather that APUD characteristics may be a feature of the degree of cell maturation.[103]

Excessive Expression of Normal Genes

As was previously noted, many immunoreactive polypeptide hormones have been detected in normal nonendocrine tissues using sensitive immunoassay techniques. The low levels of these hormones may represent incomplete repression of the portion of the genome that is responsible for the hormone production (gene leakage) or may reflect the production of the hormones from the stem cells present in the tissues. If the process of repression is incomplete, ectopic hormone production may merely represent excessive expression of normal genes and may be directly related to proliferation of the neoplastic cells and tumor mass. If this is correct, ectopic peptide synthesis may be a "universal concomitant of neoplasia," as suggested by Odell and colleagues.[65] Clinical syndromes occur only when tumors elaborate bioactive forms of hormones.

Therapy

Specific therapies have been devised for the treatment of each of the ectopic hormone syndromes and will be discussed later under the specific syndromes. In general, several therapeutic approaches may be used for the treatment of ectopic hormone syndromes. The first approach is to remove the tumor, if possible. If the primary neoplasm is unresectable or if metastases are present, hormone production may be inhibited through the use of chemotherapy or radiation therapy. If these approaches are unsuccessful and the metabolic derangements from the ectopic hormone syndrome substantially contribute to morbidity, therapy directed at the target organ or target organ products may be instituted. Using the ectopic ACTH syndrome as an example, Cushing's syndrome may be reversed through bilateral adrenalectomy and the administration of physiologic doses of glucocorticoids and mineralocorticoids. In some patients, a medical adrenalectomy may be accomplished through the use of mitotane (o,p′-DDD). Alternatively, the function of the target organ, in this case the adrenal, may be blocked. The block may take place at the target organ receptor or at an intracellular step in target organ activity. In some tissues, it is possible to block the cell membrane receptors for hormones through hormone antagonists or agonists, with the agonists causing down regulation of the receptor. In the case of the ectopic ACTH syndrome, there are no clinically effective ACTH agonists or antagonists that are useful for the treatment of Cushing's syndrome. Instead, target organ activity is blocked through the use of inhibitors of the enzymatic pathways required for steroid hormone production. Such inhibitors include aminoglutethimide, ketoconazole, and metyrapone. Finally, if the metabolic derangements are due to overproduction of a target organ product, this product may be antagonized. For the ectopic ACTH syndrome, mifepristone (RU-486) is an effective glucocorticoid antagonist and has been useful in the treatment of some patients with Cushing's syndrome.[104] As we gain further insight into the biochemical mediators of hormone action, it is likely that additional approaches to therapy will be forthcoming.

Hormones as Tumor Markers

The experience gained from the use of hCG as a tumor marker in patients with gestational and nongestational trophoblastic disease served as a major impetus for the search for hormones, enzymes, oncofetal proteins, and other cellular components that could be used as markers of neoplasms. In fact, in patients with gestational trophoblastic disease, hCG measurements fulfill virtually all the criteria for an ideal tumor marker (Table 29-8). hCG may be measured in the blood or urine through rapidly performed, technically simple, and inexpensive immunomimetric assays. If one uses a cutoff level of 50 mIU/ml of serum, only pregnancy and an occasional nontrophoblastic neoplasm will be positive and virtually all patients with trophoblastic disease will have measurable quantities of hCG (no false negatives). The levels of hCG in the serum and urine accurately reflect tumor burden and fluctuate concordantly with changes in tumor growth. In addition, the approximately 24-h half-life of hCG allows for an assessment of the efficacy of therapy within a few days of the initiation of treatment. After the initial disappearance of the hormone, an early recurrence of the trophoblast disease may be detected through serial measurements of hCG levels.[105]

Unfortunately, the excellent experience with the use of hCG as a marker of gestational trophoblastic disease has not been duplicated for most other tumor markers, including carcinoembryonic antigen, alpha-fetoprotein, CA-125, and prostate-specific antigen. The major limitations to the use of tumor markers involve *sensitivity* and *specificity*. To detect as many cancers as possible, the method of measuring the tumor marker should be highly sensitive. However, as the sensitivity of the test increases, the number of patients without cancer who are either normal or have benign disease processes and test positive increases. Therefore, the test loses its specificity, or the ability to rule out disease when none is present. In fact, the sensitivity and specificity of a test, along with the prevalence of the disease in the population being studied, determine the utility of that test as a screen for cancer.

TABLE 29-8 The Ideal Tumor Marker

1. Present in blood or urine
2. No false positives (specific)
3. No false negatives (sensitive)
4. Levels fluctuate appropriately with changes in tumor growth
5. Rapid half-life in blood
6. Rapidly performed
7. Technically simple
8. Inexpensive

The interaction of test sensitivity and specificity and cancer prevalence can be illustrated by examining the experience with the use of measurements of immunoreactive hCG in the sera of patients with nontrophoblastic neoplasms. The combined data from 66 published studies are shown in Tables 29-9 and 29-10 for patients with cancer and those without cancer, respectively.[105] Overall, approximately 18 percent of patients with cancer are found to have immunoreactive hCG in their circulation, while 2.4 percent of control patients without cancer have circulating immunoreactive hCG by assays that have a sensitivity of 5 mIU/ml. Thus, the sensitivity of hCG measurements as a tumor marker is 18 percent, while the specificity is 97.6 percent (100 percent − 2.4 percent). Table 29-11 illustrates the effect of cancer prevalence on the diagnostic accuracy of hCG measurements. If we assume that the prevalence of cancer in the population being examined is 1 percent (Table 29-11, top), we find that for every 100,000 patients screened, 1000 will have cancer. Of this 1000, 18 percent (180) will have immunoreactive hCG present in the circulation (true positives), while 820 patients with cancer will not have immu-

TABLE 29-9 Immunoreactive hCG in Sera of Patients with Cancer

Tumor or Site	N		% Positive	
Islet cell	104		39.4	
Gynecologic	2,010		28.9	
Ovary		633		28.6
Endometrium		348		16.7
Cervix		976		33.8
Vulva/vagina		37		27.0
Carcinoid	41		26.8	
Gastrointestinal	2,165		18.0	
Oropharynx		298		14.8
Esophagus		124		17.7
Gastric		232		20.7
Small intestine		24		16.7
Colon/rectum		693		9.8
Hepatic		281		22.1
Biliary		26		30.7
Pancreatic		200		20.0
Lung	1,365		17.4	
Breast	3,031		16.8	
Melanoma	244		13.9	
Genitourinary	658		11.8	
Renal		119		6.7
Bladder		176		23.3
Prostate		363		8.0
Sarcoma	136		11.8	
Hemopoietic	544		6.1	
Lymphoma	339		5.3	
Miscellaneous	576		10.4	
Total	11,213		18.0	

Source: From Braunstein,[105] with permission.

TABLE 29-10 Immunoreactive hCG in Sera of Control Patients without Cancer

Type of Control	*N*		% Positive	
Premenopausal females	430		0.7	
Postmenopausal females	242		0	
Normal males	438		0.2	
Castrate males	4		0	
Blood donors	165		2.4	
Benign disease	1,963		3.6	
Gynecologic		528		6.6
Gastrointestinal		318		6.0
Breast		254		4.3
Lung		174		2.9
Genitourinary		84		0
Neurologic		10		0
Hypothyroid		10		0
Unspecified		650		0
Other normal	172		0	
Miscellaneous	691		2.7	
Total	4,105		2.4	

Source: From Braunstein,[105] with permission.

TABLE 29-11 Predictive Value of hCG Measurements for Cancer Screening

Sensitivity of test: 18% (105
Specificity of test: 97.6% (105)

Example 1
Assumed prevalence of cancer: *1%*

	Test Result		
	Positive	*Negative*	*Total*
Cancer	180 (TP)	820 (FN)	1000
Benign disorders	2376 (FP)	96,624 (TN)	99,000
Total	2556	97,444	100,000

Predictive value of a positive test ($\frac{TP}{TP+FP} \times 100$): 7%
False positives: 93%
Predictive value of a negative test ($\frac{TN}{TN+FN} \times 100$): 99%
False negatives: 1%

Example 2
Assumed prevalence of cancer: *10%*

	Test Result		
	Positive	*Negative*	*Total*
Cancer	1800	8200	10,000
Benign disorders	2160	87,840	90,000
Total	3960	96,040	100,000

Predictive value of a positive test: 45%
False positives: 55%
Predictive value of a negative test: 91%
False negatives: 9%

TP = true positives; FP = false positives; FN = false negatives; TN = true negatives.

noreactive hCG detected by these tests (false negatives). Of the 99,000 patients without cancer, 96,624 (99,000 × 97.6 percent) will not have hCG detected in their circulation (true negatives), while 2376 patients without cancer (99,000 × 2.4 percent) will have hCG detected (false positives). In this situation, the predictive value of a positive test—that is, the percentage of patients who have immunoreactive hCG in the circulation who actually have cancer—is 7 percent, while the false-positive rate (100 percent − 7 percent) is 93 percent. The predictive value of a negative test (the percentage of noncancerous patients with negative hCG results) is 99 percent with only 1 percent false negatives. Thus, in this population, the number of false positives markedly exceeds the number of true positives; therefore, approximately 9 of every 10 patients with detectable immunoreactive hCG in the circulation will undergo unnecessary further diagnostic evaluation.

If the prevalence of cancer in the population being evaluated is 10-fold higher (10 percent) (Table 29-11, bottom), the predictive value of a positive test rises to 45 percent and the number of false positives decreases to 55 percent. However, the number of false negatives rises dramatically to 9 percent. In this population, a patient with a positive test result is more likely to harbor a neoplasm than is the case in a population with a 1 percent prevalence of cancer, but almost 10 percent of patients with cancer will be missed.

These calculations suggest that hCG measurements are not particularly useful as a screening test for nontrophoblastic cancer. In actuality, hCG and other potential tumor markers generally perform worse in a screening situation than is suggested in much of the medical literature. This occurs because of biases in the ascertainment of many of the patient populations which have been the subject of reports. To establish the value of a tumor marker, investigators usually measure the marker in the blood or urine of patients with well-established neoplasms. Most markers are more likely to be positive in patients with advanced disease than in patients with minimal disease. Therefore, the sensitivity of the test established in research laboratories with well-defined populations often overestimates the actual sensitivity of the test in terms of detection of early cancer, a stage when the disease is potentially curable and not diagnosable with other screening tests. Some investigators have tried to increase the sensitivity of tumor marker tests by measuring multiple markers in the blood and evaluating patients further if any of the markers are positive. This strategy (parallel testing) increases the sensitivity of the test but markedly decreases the specificity because each test will give false-positive results. Another strategy is to measure a tumor marker and subject all samples that give positive test results to measurements of a different tumor marker and to consider a combined test positive only if both are positive (serial testing).

This increases the specificity of tumor marker testing but reduces the sensitivity. Indeed, for any test that is less than 100 percent sensitive or 100 percent specific, an increase in sensitivity of the testing strategy will lead to a decrease in specificity and vice versa.[106]

SPECIFIC SYNDROMES

Hypercalcemia of Malignancy

Hypercalcemia is the most frequently encountered paraneoplastic endocrine abnormality, being found in 10 to 14 percent of patients with cancer (Table 29-4). A wide spectrum of neoplasms are associated with hypercalcemia (Table 29-12).[107–114] Metastatic adenocarcinoma of the breast and squamous cell carcinoma of the lung and head and neck region account for over half the patients with tumor-associated hypercalcemia. If patients with documented bony metastases are excluded, approximately half of patients with hypercalcemia have a squamous cell carcinoma of the lung or clear cell carcinoma of the kidney.[115–117]

Pathophysiology of Hypercalcemia (Table 29-13)

Bony Metastases

The idea that osseous metastases are directly associated with calcium abnormalities was first suggested by Virchow, who in 1855 described three patients with bone metastases who had ectopic calcification in various tissues.[117] The association of hypercalcemia with tumor types such as breast carcinoma and multiple myeloma, almost exclusively when the tumors involve the bone, led to the hypothesis that direct tumor-induced osteolysis can account for the hypercalcemia.[118] Indeed, various tumor cells have been shown to release prostaglandins, epidermal growth factor, lymphotoxins, PTH-rp, and other substances that are capable of stimulating osteoclastic bone resorption.[21,109,119] Thus, some tumor cells may directly stimulate osteoclastic bone resorption and lead to an uncoupling of bone resorption and formation characteristic of the hypercalcemia of malignancy.[120] In addition, monocytes and lymphocytes in close proximity to the tumor cells may be responsible for the release of bone-resorbing cytokines.

It is clear that the presence of tumor cells in bone alone is not sufficient to cause hypercalcemia. Some tumors, such as small cell carcinoma of the lung, adenocarcinoma of the colon, and adenocarcinoma of the prostate, metastasize to the bone and are only rarely associated with hypercalcemia[117] (Table 29-4), indicating that the tumor cell type is an important factor determining whether the patient will develop hypercalcemia with bone metastases. Ralston and coworkers demonstrated that there was no association between the presence or extent of osseous metastases and the frequency or severity of hypercalcemia in a large group of cancer patients assessed by bone scan.[118] In fact, patients with a light bone tumor load had a higher mean serum calcium level than did those with a heavy bone tumor load. When analysis was restricted to patients who had hypercalcemia, the highest mean serum calcium levels were found in patients without evidence of metastatic bone disease. These data indicate that although 60 to 80 percent of patients with hypercalcemia and cancer have skeletal metastases,[109,118] the cause of the hypercalcemia is probably multifactorial and includes both direct and indirect local production of stimulators of osteoclastic bone resorption, including prostaglandins and cytokines, as well as the secretion of PTH-rp, the substance responsible for the majority of cases of humoral hypercalcemia in patients with nonmetastatic solid tumors (see below).

TABLE 29-12 Tumor Types Associated with Hypercalcemia

Tumor Type	Percent
Breast	36
Lung	15
Head and neck	8
Lymphoma	7
Multiple myeloma	7
Kidney	6
Gastrointestinal tract	4
Leukemia	2
Ovary	1
Miscellaneous*	15

*Carcinomas of the endometrium, cervix, vagina, vulva, penis, testis, adrenal, and prostate; pheochromocytoma; neuroblastoma; melanoma; thymoma; osteogenic sarcoma; lymphosarcoma; reticulum cell sarcoma; hemangiosarcoma; fibrosarcoma; rhabdomyosarcoma; leiomyosarcoma.

Source: Based on data on 1055 patients from eight series of patients.[107-114]

TABLE 29-13 Pathophysiologic Mechanisms of Hypercalcemia in Cancer

Bony metastasis
Elaboration of humoral substances
Parathyroid hormone
Parathyroid hormone–related protein
Prostaglandins
Cytokines
Conversion of 25(OH)-vitamin D to 1,25$(OH)_2$-vitamin D
Coexistence of cancer and another disease
Primary hyperparathyroidism
Other causes of hypercalcemia

Systemic Elaboration of Humoral Substances

Historical Perspective The development of our understanding of the humoral hypercalcemia of cancer and the mediators involved parallels the history of endocrinology. The early studies were observational. In 1924, Zondek and coworkers described a patient with hypercalcemia who at autopsy was found to have normal parathyroid glands and carcinoma of the gallbladder.[121] In 1936, Gutman and associates described a patient with symptomatic hypercalcemia and bronchogenic carcinoma who had normal parathyroid glands, no skeletal metastases, and a small focus of monostotic Paget disease.[122] The next major step was conceptual and was provided by Fuller Albright in his discussion of a 51-year-old man with a renal cell carcinoma that was metastatic to the ilium.[123] Because of the presence of hypophosphatemia associated with the hypercalcemia, this patient underwent a parathyroid exploration with a finding of three normal parathyroid glands. Subsequently, the patient's tumor and iliac metastases were treated with radiation therapy, which led to a concomitant decrease in the serum calcium concentration and a rise in the serum phosphate concentration. A normal fourth parathyroid gland was found at necropsy. Albright hypothesized that the tumor was secreting a parathormone (PTH)-like substance, since hypercalcemia resulting from osteolysis alone would be expected to be associated with hyperphosphatemia. However, bioassay of the tumor tissue for the presence of PTH was negative. In 1956, two groups reported on several patients with malignancies, normal bone x-rays, hypercalcemia, and hypophosphatemia whose biochemical abnormalities normalized after surgical resection of the tumors. With tumor recurrence, there was a temporally associated increase in serum calcium.[124,125] No parathyroid bone or renal abnormalities were found at surgery or autopsy in the patients studied. These observations supported Albright's contention that the tumors were producing a PTH-like substance that was responsible for the hypercalcemia. As additional patients with the syndrome were reported, the term *pseudohyperparathyroidism* was applied to this condition.[126] After the purification of PTH, immunoassays were developed, and in 1964 the presence of a material immunologically similar to bovine PTH was extracted from several tumor tissues.[115,127,128]

With the advent of RIAs, there was initial support for the concept that the PTH-like substance is actually PTH. One study found that 95 percent of paients with hypercalcemia associated with cancer had inappropriately high PTH levels as measured by an RIA directed against the carboxy-terminal portion of the molecule.[129] Sherwood and colleagues demonstrated immunoreactive PTH in several tumor extracts, and other investigators showed arteriovenous differences in PTH concentrations across tumors.[130–132] However, several investigators found that there were differences between the immunoreactive PTH-like substances in the sera of patients with cancer and hypercalcemia and in the sera of patients with hypercalcemia from primary hyperparathyroidism.[133,134] Since both amino- and carboxy-terminal fragments of PTH were known to be present in circulation, it was conceivable that the differences between pseudohyperparathyroidism and hyperparathyroidism reflected differences in the processing of the hormone at the time of or after secretion. The difficulties in interpreting RIA data were highlighted by the study of Raisz and colleagues, who had the same serum samples from patients with primary hyperparathyroidism and humoral hypercalcemia of cancer measured for immunoreactive PTH by four different laboratories.[135] There were marked differences in the results. However, it was generally found that PTH assays that used antisera generated against amino-terminal portions of the molecule gave lower serum concentrations of PTH than did RIAs that used antisera against the carboxy-terminal portion of the molecule. Since the carboxy-terminal fragment of PTH is elevated in patients with renal insufficiency and also appears to be released continuously even when the amino-terminal fragment of PTH release is suppressed, it is understandable how some of these immunoassay discrepancies could occur.

An important study was reported in 1973 by Powell and coworkers who described 11 patients with nonparathyroid neoplasms associated with hypercalcemia and hypophosphatemia in the absence of bony metastases.[136] Remission of biochemical abnormalities occurred in nine patients after antitumor therapy. These investigators were unable to demonstrate PTH in the patients' blood or the tumor tissue despite using three different RIAs that covered virtually all regions of the PTH molecule. However, the tumor extracts did cause bone resorption by bioassay, leading to the conclusion that the humoral hypercalcemia factor was not PTH. During the 1970s a variety of other substances were found to stimulate osteoclastic bone resorption in vitro, and this fueled the effort to determine whether one or more of these substances could be the humoral hypercalcemic factor produced by cancers. The two substances which received the most attention were prostaglandins of the E series and "osteoclastic activating factor."[137–139]

Major strides in unraveling the pathogenesis of humoral hypercalcemia of malignancy were made during the last decade through the use of molecular biological tools. Early studies showed the absence of PTH messenger RNA by in situ hybridization in tumors associated with nonmetastatic hypercalcemia.[140] Subsequently, several tumor cell lines derived from patients with this syndrome were established and secreted a biologically active bone-resorbing factor.[141,142] This led to purification and sequencing of the PTH-rp protein and the cloning of the gene.[143] Synthetic peptides based on the structure of the PTH-rp protein were used as immunogens for the development of immunoassays to measure the concentrations of the protein in body fluids and tissues. The use of these assays has established the fact that the majority of patients with humoral hypercalcemia of malignancy have elevated levels of PTH-rp, establishing this factor as Albright's predicted PTH-like substance that is responsible for the syndrome.

Parathyroid Hormone As was noted above, the majority of patients who had been diagnosed as having "pseudohyperparathyroidism" due to the ectopic production of PTH most likely had the syndrome on the basis of excessive production of PTH-rp. The close homology between the PTH and PTH-rp molecules in their first 13 amino acids might have accounted for some of the positive results reported in early PTH immunoassays. In addition, the presence of renal insufficiency in some patients and the inability to completely shut off the release of the carboxy-terminal fragments of PTH even in the face of hypercalcemia might have been important factors in accounting for the spurious diagnosis of ectopic PTH production by tumors.[109] Finally, the coexistence of hyperparathyroidism and cancer may have accounted for some of the examples of "pseudohyperparathyroidism."

Although the bona fide ectopic production of PTH appears to be exceedingly rare, it does occur. For instance, Yoshimoto and associates recently described a 70-year-old man with a small cell carcinoma of the lung, multiple metastases, and normal parathyroid glands at autopsy. He had markedly elevated serum PTH levels by three separate assays as well as high concentrations of PTH in a tumor extract that cochromatographed with human PTH on gel filtration chromatography. Northern blot analysis also showed the presence of PTH mRNA in the tumor.[144] Similarly, authentic ectopic PTH secretion was reported recently in a patient with an ovarian carcinoma and a patient with a primitive neuroectodermal tumor.[145,146]

Parathyroid Hormone–Related Protein After the 1973 report of Powell and colleagues[136] which demonstrated that the syndrome of humoral hypercalcemia of malignancy is not due to the production of immunoreactive PTH, several groups of investigators sought the putative PTH-like factor. In 1980, Stewart and associates examined 50 consecutive patients with humoral hypercalcemia of malignancy and found that they segregated into two groups that were distinguishable primarily on the basis of nephrogenous cyclic AMP excretion.[110] Over 80 percent of these patients had elevated nephrogenous cyclic AMP and harbored squamous cell carcinomas of the head and neck, lung, esophagus, and vulva; squamous metaplasia; renal cell carcinomas; or transitional cell carcinomas. The patients with low cyclic AMP excretion had hematologic malignancies including myeloma and lymphoma as well as breast carcinoma. The patients with elevated nephrogenous cyclic AMP excretion exhibited hypercalcemia, hypophosphatemia, decreased tubular reabsorption of phosphate, increased fasting calcium excretion for a given level of serum calcium and low $1,25(OH)_2D_3$ serum concentrations compared with patients with primary hyperparathyroidism, and undetectable serum immunoreactive PTH levels.[110,147] The sera from patients in this group were active in a kidney cortex cytochemical bioassay for PTH, and the biological activity could not be completely inhibited by preincubation with antiserum against PTH.[148] Several tumor cell lines elaborating the PTH-like substance were established.[141,142] One such line, when transplanted into nude mice, led to the development of hypercalcemia, hypophosphatemia, and elevation of $1,25(OH)_3D_3$ serum concentrations.[149] The biochemical abnormalities were inhibited by analogues to PTH that also inhibited PTH activity in vitro and in vivo. The biologically active components of these cell lines were purified and found to reside in a protein with a molecular mass of 17 to 18 kDa. Amino-terminal sequence analysis demonstrated significant homology with the first 13 amino acids of PTH and also allowed the preparation of synthetic oligonucleotides which were used to isolate the cDNA for PTH-rp.[143] The full-length DNA coding for the protein was isolated, and the amino acid structure was predicted.[142]

PTH-rp has been found to exist in three isoforms of 139, 141, and 173 amino acids resulting from alternate splicing of exons. There is a 36-amino acid prepropeptide. Eight of the first 13 amino-terminal amino acids are homologous with those found in PTH, and this accounts for the PTH-like biological activity both in vivo and in vitro. The amino acid sequence of PTH and PTH-rp diverges completely after the first 13 amino acids. It is likely that the genes for both PTH and PTH-rp are derived from a common ancestral gene. Synthetic amino-terminal peptides containing the first 34 amino acids retain full biological activity, while no biological activity has been demonstrated for the carboxy-terminal fragments.[21,142,150]

PTH-rp fulfills the criteria for the humoral hypercalcemic factor for the majority of nonmetastatic solid tumors. First, serum immunoreactive PTH-rp is elevated in 53 to 83 percent of patients with nonmetastatic hypercalcemia,[111–113,151] and serum concentrations of PTH-rp have been correlated with total serum calcium concentrations.[111] Second, therapy for tumors associated with hypercalcemia has led to a decrease in serum calcium and a parallel reduction in PTH-rp levels.[113,151] Third, serum PTH-rp concentrations have been correlated with nephrogenous cyclic AMP excretion in patients with this syndrome.[151] Fourth, PTH-rp has been isolated from tumors associated with this syndrome, and the tumors contain PTH-rp mRNA.[152,153] Fifth, the infusion of PTH-rp into animals leads to the development of hypercalcemia, and the administration of anti-PTH-rp antibodies reverses the hypercalcemia in animal models.[154–156]

PTH-rp production by tumors is not limited to nonmetastatic solid neoplasms, and elevated levels have been found in patients with metastases to the bone as well as in one-third to one-half of patients with hematologic malignancies.[111–113]

Depending on the assay utilized, between 5 and 90 percent of normal individuals have detectable concentrations of immunoreactive PTH-rp in their blood.[157] Normal concentrations are generally below 2.5 pmol/L with assays based on antisera to the 1-34 fragment of PTH-rp, and below 2.1 pmol/L for carboxy-terminal assays (amino acids 109–138).[111–113,151] PTH-rp is widely distributed throughout the body as assessed by immunoassay, immunohistochemistry, and mRNA determinations. Thus, it is present in keratinocytes of the epidermis, pancreatic islet cells, stomach, adrenal cortex and medulla, hypothalamus, pituitary, brain, thyroid, bone marrow, myometrium, placenta, and lactating mammary glands.[158–161] In fact, the highest concentrations of the protein are found in milk.[151,160] Although the physiologic functions of PTH-rp are unknown, it has been speculated that it may play a role in calcium transport in the breast, where the production of PTH-rp is under the control of prolactin, and in transplacental calcium transport.[161–163] PTH-rp may also have an important autocrine function. The protein has been shown to be produced by lectin-stimulated T lymphocytes. When it was incubated with synthetic PTH-rp (1–34), suppression of the lymphocyte DNA synthesis was found.[164] The widespread distribution of PTH-rp raises the possibility that production of the hormone by neoplasms is not strictly ectopic but may represent excessive eutopic production.

Prostaglandins In 1970 prostaglandins of the E series (PGEs) were found to stimulate osteoclastic bone resorption and increase cyclic AMP in vitro.[165,166] A few years later, Tashjian and associates studied mouse $HSDM_1$ fibrosarcoma and rabbit VX_2 carcinoma tumors, which are associated with nonmetastatic hypercalcemia.[167,168] The tumor tissues from these animals contain high quantities of PGE_2, and the tumor cells secrete the prostaglandin in vitro and stimulate osteoclastic bone resorption. Arteriovenous concentration differences of PGE_2 across the tumor confirm the in vivo production, and the administration of an inhibitor of prostaglandin synthesis—indomethacin—to tumor-bearing animals lowers the elevated serum calcium and plasma PGE_2 levels in a parallel fashion.[169] Indomethacin also inhibits PGE_2 and bone resorption–stimulating activity produced by tumor cells grown in vitro. Finally, infusion of PGE_2 into rats was found to produce hypercalcemia.[170] These studies provided strong support for the concept that some tumors may cause hypercalcemia through osteoclastic bone resorption stimulated by the excessive production by prostaglandins.

The first study in humans appeared in 1974 with the description of a hypercalcemic patient with a renal cell carcinoma associated with a high concentration of E-type prostaglandin in liver metastases and a low plasma prostaglandin level.[171] The administration of indomethacin was associated with a decline in serum calcium, which again rose after the cessation of the medication. Additional cases of patients with renal cell carcinoma and hypercalcemia who were responsive to indomethacin were reported[138,172] In 1975, Seyberth and colleagues studied 29 patients with solid tumors, including 14 with hypercalcemia.[137] They evaluated prostaglandin production in these patients by measuring the urinary excretion of the major urinary metabolite of PGE_1 and PGE_2, 7 alpha-hydroxy-5,11-diketotetranorprostane-1, 16-dioic acid (PGE-M). They found that 12 of the 14 patients with humoral hypercalcemia associated with solid tumors had elevations of urinary PGE-M, as did 2 patients who were normocalcemic at the time of study but subsequently developed hypercalcemia. Patients who were hypercalcemic as a result of hyperparathyroidism or hematologic malignancies had normal urine concentrations of PGE-M. Five of 13 normocalcemic patients who had solid tumors also had elevations of this urinary metabolite. Six hypercalcemic patients with solid tumors received inhibitors of prostaglandin synthesis and had a concomitant decrease in serum calcium and urinary PGE-M levels. These investigators subsequently found that urinary cyclic AMP excretion was normal in patients with elevated PGE-M levels, in contrast to patients who had nonmetastatic hypercalcemia with normal PGE-M levels, who demonstrated elevated urinary cyclic AMP concentrations.[173]

Despite this initial positive report, relatively few hypercalcemic patients with neoplasms have been found to have a reduction in serum calcium with the use of inhibitors of prostaglandin synthesis.[174,175] In addition, it has been noted that there is no correlation between PGE levels and the degree of hypercalcemia or the presence or absence of metastases.[117,176] It is of interest that indomethacin may lower the urinary excretion of PGE without consistently altering plasma PGE levels or serum calcium.[176] Since PGE is extensively metabolized during the first pass through the lungs and liver, it has been calculated that the venous blood concentration of PGE_2 would need to be greater than 10 times the upper limit of normal to result in an arterial PGE_2 blood concentration that is the minimal effective concentration required to increase bone resorption in vitro.[176] Concentrations of that magnitude have not been found in patients with hypercalcemia associated with nonmetastatic solid tumors.

As noted above, prostaglandin production by tumor cells is probably most important in inducing osteolysis in the region surrounding osseous tumor deposits. It is clear that tumors do synthesize and secrete prostaglandins, as do monocytes and macrophages, which are also found in the area of bone metastases.[109] In this regard, it has long been known that after the initial administration of estrogens or antiestrogens, patients with breast cancer metastatic to the bone may develop acute, severe hypercalcemia. Breast cancer cells have been shown to release E-series prostaglandins after exposure to estrogens in vitro, and there is a concomitant increase in bone resorbing activity, which can be inhibited by indomethacin and flufenamic acid.[177] Unfortunately, the administration of prostaglandin synthesis inhibitors has not been shown to be effective in lowering serum calcium in hypercalcemic patients with metastatic breast cancer. Although the reasons for this are unclear, concentrations of the prostaglandin synthesis inhibitors in the area of the bone metastases that can be achieved after oral administration may be insufficient to inhibit prostaglandin synthesis in vivo. Alternatively, since elevated concentrations of PTH-rp have been found in some patients with metastatic breast cancer, the hypercalcemia associated with such tumors may be multifactorial.

Cytokines Interest in cytokines as potential mediators of hypercalcemia in patients with cancer began in 1974, when Mundy and associates described the production of an osteoclast-activating factor produced in vitro by multiple myeloma cells.[139] This substance was similar to a material produced by phytohemagglutinin-transformed normal lymphocytes. Similar osteoclast-activating-factor activity was found in cells derived from hypercalcemic patients with Burkitt's lymphoma, T-cell lymphoma, and some leukemias. Subsequent work has indicated that the osteoclast-activating-factor activity can be accounted for by a group of cytokines and growth factors including interleukin-Iα, interleukin-Iβ, transforming growth factor-α, transforming growth factor-β, tumor necrosis factor-β (lymphotoxin), colony-stimulating factors, and epidermal growth factor.[21,119] These cytokines may be produced by the tumor cells or by transformed lymphocytes, monocytes, or macrophages in the vicinity of the tumor cells. Several different mechanisms for stimulation of bone reabsorption by the cytokines have been described, including the activation of preexisting osteoclasts, stimulation of the proliferation of osteoclast progenitor cells without activation of preexisting osteoclasts, and stimulation of PGE_2 synthesis in the bone.[178] Thus, as is the case with prostaglandins, cytokines appear to be local mediators of bone resorption in patients with metastatic solid tumors associated with hypercalcemia as well as patients with hematologic and lymphoproliferative disorders involving the bone.

Conversion of 25(OH)-vitamin D to 1,25(OH)$_2$-vitamin D

In addition to renal tubular cells, the vitamin-D-1α-hydroxylase enzyme is present in keratinocytes, fibroblasts, trophoblasts, alveolar macrophages, and lymphocytes. Several tumors, including HIV-I–associated and unassociated lymphomas, HTLV-I–mediated adult T-cell leukemia/lymphoma, small cell carcinoma of the lung, and melanoma, have been found to be associated with elevated 1,25(OH)$_2$-vitamin D levels with dysregulated 25(OH)-1α-vitamin D hydroxylase activity.[179–184] High levels of 1,25(OH)$_2$-vitamin D have been found in close to half of patients with lymphomas.[184] In patients with lymphomas associated with elevated 1,25-dihydroxy vitamin D levels and hypercalcemia, therapy with glucocorticoids reduces both the serum calcium and 1,25-dihydroxy vitamin D concentrations in a parallel fashion.[179]

Coexistence of Cancer and Primary Hyperparathyroidism

The association of hyperparathyroidism and nonparathyroid malignancies is well established in patients with both type I and type II multiple endocrine neoplasia syndromes. Additionally, numerous investigators have reported an increased incidence of malignant breast, thyroid, GI, genitourinary, and pulmonary neoplasms in patients with hyperparathyroidism.[30–32,185–188] These studies have suggested that between 34 and 42 percent of patients with parathyroid adenomas or hyperplasia have an associated neoplasm, raising the possibility that hypercalcemia or hyperparathyroidism predisposes a patient to neoplasia. Alternatively, neoplasms may produce a parathyrotropic substance that leads to the development of parathyroid hyperplasia or adenoma(s).

However, caution should be exercised in interpreting the literature because of three considerations. First, both hyperparathyroidism and neoplasms are relatively common, and the frequency of both increases with age.[189] This, coupled with the increased scrutiny that a patient undergoes during an evaluation for one of the conditions which incidentally could uncover the other, may account for the apparent association. Second, some of these studies utilized histologic criteria for the diagnosis of parathyroid hyperplasia or adenoma in patients with cancer. One of the major criteria for parathyroid chief cell hyperplasia is a reduction in stromal fat. In a study of hypercalcemic patients with nonmetastatic tumors and undetectable parathyroid hormone who exhibited the clinical features of the humoral hypercalcemia of cancer syndrome, 70 percent had markedly reduced amounts of parathyroid stromal fat, giving a histologic appearance that was indistinguishable from that of chief cell hyperplasia. Similar data were found in 20 percent of normocalcemic cancer patients.[120] These histologic findings undoubtedly represent the effects of weight loss and cachexia on the parathyroid glands rather than functional parathyroid abnormalities. Third, the association between well-differentiated thyroid cancer and hyperparathyroidism in some of these series may have been due to the inclusion of patients who received head and neck irradiation for benign disorders during childhood and adolescence, a known risk factor for both problems.[190,191]

Clinical Manifestations of Diagnosis

Hypercalcemia is generally a late and often preterminal manifestation of malignancy, with death usually occurring within 3 months of the diagnosis.[114,192–194]

The signs and symptoms of hypercalcemia fall into four groups. Nonspecific general complaints of fatigue, weakness, headaches, behavioral abnormalities, and malaise are present in over half the patients and are an especially prominent complaint in individuals with calcium concentrations below 14 mg/dl.[114] Gastrointestinal manifestations include anorexia, nausea, vomiting, constipation, and abdominal discomfort and are present in one-half to three-quarters of patients at the time of presentation.[108,114] Neurologic abnormalities are also prominent, especially in patients with serum calcium above 14 mg/dl.[108,114] Patients often complain of drowsiness, visual abnormalities, confusion, and memory impairment and are frequently found to be lethargic, confused, stuporous, or comatose. There are usually no localizing signs. Finally, the hypercalcemia may lead to a nephrogenic diabetes insipidus resulting in polyuria, thirst, and polydipsia. If fluid intake is insufficient, findings of dehydration may be present.

Patients who have humoral hypercalcemia of malignancy share many of the clinical and biochemical findings of primary hyperparathyroidism, although there are clinical and biochemical differences between these diseases (Table 29-14).[115,195–197] Considering the close biochemical similarity in the actions of PTH and PTH-rp, it is of interest that three laboratory abnormalities cannot be explained on the

TABLE 29-14 Comparison of Primary Hyperparathyroidism and Humoral Hypercalcemia of Malignancy

Feature	Primary Hyperparathyroidism	Humoral Hypercalcemia of Malignancy
History	Long, indolent course (1–25 years)	Short, rapidly progressive course (weeks to months)
Sex	60% female	75% male
Major symptoms	None; renal stones, peptic ulcer, pancreatitis, bone pain, memory impairment	Weight loss, lethargy, obtundation, polyuria, nocturia, nausea, vomiting
Serum calcium	Rarely >14 mg/dl	Often >14 mg/dl
Urine calcium/serum calcium	Lower	Higher
Serum phosphate	Normal or decreased	Normal or decreased
Serum chloride	Often >102 mEq/L	Often ≤102 mEq/L
Serum HCO_3	Normal or low	Elevated
Serum Cl/PO_4	Usually >35	Usually <35
Alkaline phosphatase	Usually normal	Often elevated
Nephrogenous cAMP	Elevated	Elevated
$1,25(OH)_2D_3$	Normal to elevated	Normal to low
Hematocrit	>38% in 90%	<38% in 75%
Serum PTH	Normal to elevated	Low
Serum PTH-rp	Low	High
Bone biopsy	Elevation of osteoclastic bone resorption and osteoblastic bone formation (coupled resorption formation)	Elevated osteoclastic bone resorption, depressed bone formation (uncoupled resorption formation)

Source: From references 115 and 195–197.

basis of the direct biochemical effects of these two hormones. Patients with hyperparathyroidism generally have hyperchloremic acidosis, while individuals with humoral hypercalcemia of malignancy have hypochloremic alkalosis and do not exhibit the renal bicarbonate wasting found with primary hyperparathyroidism. Although in vitro both PTH and PTH-rp stimulate renal 25(OH)-vitamin D1α-hydroxylase activity, clinically patients with primary hyperparathyroidism have elevated levels of $1,25(OH)_2D_3$ while patients with the humoral hypercalcemia of malignancy generally have normal or low levels of this vitamin D metabolite. Finally, patients with malignancy-associated hypercalcemia exhibit uncoupling of bone resorption and bone formation as assessed through histomorphometric evaluation, while patients with primary hyperparathyroidism usually demonstrate coupling of the resorption and formation activity. Thus, some of the clinical manifestations of humoral hypercalcemia of malignancy may not be explained by simply implicating excessive production of PTH-rp. Instead, it is likely that other humoral factors, nutritional deficiencies, and metabolic abnormalities contribute to the observed differences between the two diseases.

Figure 29-5 provides an algorithm for evaluating patients with hypercalcemia and cancer. A bone scan is the most sensitive screening test for detecting osteolytic metastases. If lytic lesions are found, the hypercalcemia may be due to local prostaglandin or cytokine production or may represent osteoclastic reabsorption from secretion of PTH-rp. If the bone scan is normal, a determination of serum concentrations of PTH and PTH-rp should be performed. Elevated levels of PTH are almost always due to the coexistence of primary hyperparathyroidism, while elevations of PTH-rp point to the neoplastic production of PTH-rp as the etiology of the hypercalcemia. If the PTH and PTH-rp concentrations are normal or low, a measurement of 1,25-dihydroxyvitamin D should be performed; if it is elevated, this suggests the presence of lymphoma or leukemia or the possibility of an associated granulomatous disease or vitamin D intoxication. If the 1,25-dihydroxyvitamin D levels are normal, a therapeutic trial of indomethacin or another prostaglandin synthesis inhibitor may be given. A decrease in calcium provides presumptive evidence of prostaglandin-mediated hypercalcemia. An absence of change in the calcium concentration suggests the presence of bony micrometastases which are too small to be seen by bone scan or the coexistence of another cause of hypercalcemia.

Therapy

The mainstays of therapy for humoral hypercalcemia include the treatment of the underlying tumor and therapies directed toward directly reducing serum calcium. Hydration with normal saline not only expands intravascular fluid volume, which decreases the serum calcium, but also promotes urinary calcium excretion. The rate of urine flow may be enhanced with diuretics such as furosemide or ethacrynic acid with careful attention to and replacement of the potassium lost in urine. Concurrently, medications may be administered to inhibit bone resorption. Glucocorticoids are effective in patients with prostaglandin-mediated hypercalcemia and patients with hematologic and lymphoproliferative neoplasms with cytokine production or enhanced conversion of 25(OH)-vitamin D to $1,25(OH)_2$ vitamin D. Calcitonin, mithramycin, bisphosphonates, and gallium nitrate are medications that inhibit osteoclas-

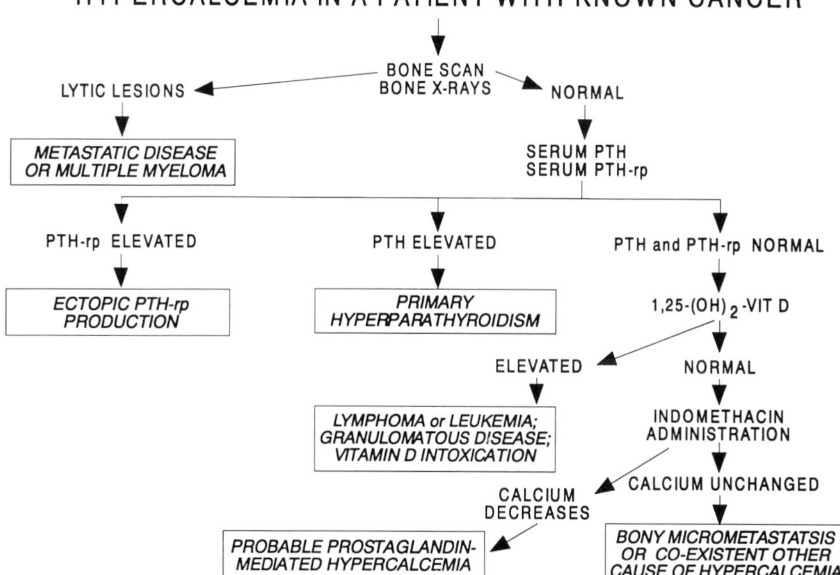

FIGURE 29-5 Algorithm for evaluating patients with cancer and hypercalcemia. See text for details.

tic bone resorption. Finally, if these measures are not effective, a dangerously elevated serum calcium may be reduced through peritoneal dialysis or hemodialysis using a calcium-free dialysis solution.[198–202]

Once the acute hypercalcemia has been effectively treated, further exacerbations of hypercalcemia may be prevented through the maintenance of adequate hydration, ambulation, and exercise and the administration of oral bisphosphonates or phosphates. In the rare patient with prostaglandin-mediated hypercalcemia due to systemic overproduction of prostaglandin, indomethacin or another prostaglandin synthesis inhibitor may be effective.

Ectopic POMC/ACTH Syndrome

The first recorded example of the ectopic POMC/ACTH syndrome was reported in 1928 by Brown, 4 years before Cushing's classic paper describing the syndrome which bears his name.[203] Brown's patient was a 45-year-old obese female with hyperpigmentation, glucose intolerance, hypertension, hirsutism, weakness, and plethora who was found to have bilateral adrenal hyperplasia associated with a small cell carcinoma of the lung. In 1961, Christy demonstrated the presence of an adrenal weight-maintaining factor in the plasma of two patients with neoplasms and this syndrome.[204] This was followed shortly by the demonstration of immunoreactive ACTH in tumor tissue and plasma.[205,206] Subsequent studies by Liddle and colleagues showed that the ACTH present in tumors from patients with Cushing's syndrome closely resembled the biologically active moiety present in the pituitary.[207]

Prevalence and Tumor Types

Cushing's syndrome is a relatively uncommon paraneoplastic syndrome associated with cancer. The ectopic production of POMC/ACTH accounts for 15 to 20 percent of patients with Cushing's syndrome.[117,208] Close to half the patients with this syndrome have a small cell carcinoma of the lung, while an additional 11 percent harbor a bronchial carcinoid and 13 percent have an epithelial thymic neoplasm or thymic carcinoid (Table 29-15).[209–212] Thus, close to 70 percent of patients presenting with this syndrome have a tumor between the clavicles and the diaphragm. Islet-cell tumors of the pancreas, carcinoid tumors arising from sites other than the lung, pheochromocytomas and other tumors of chromaffin tissue, ovarian neoplasms, and medullary carcinoma of the thyroid account for the majority of the remaining 30 percent of tumor types associated with this syndrome.[209–212] Altogether, 84 percent of the tumor types associated with this syndrome have APUD characteristics, while the remaining 16 percent are squamous cell tumors, adenocarcinomas, or hepatomas.[210]

Between 1.3 and 4.8 percent of patients with small cell carcinoma of the lung have clinically recognizable ectopic POMC/ACTH syndrome (Table 29-4).[39,47,48,51,52] In contrast, 19 percent of patients with small cell carcinoma of the lung examined at autopsy have unequivocal pathologic evidence of ACTH excess as reflected by bilateral adrenal hyperplasia and the presence of Crooke's hyaline changes in the pituitary.[213] Using biochemical criteria, between one-fourth and one-half of patients with small cell carcinoma of the lung have elevations of plasma or urine cortisol and do not show appropriate suppression of plasma cortisol after an overnight dexamethasone suppression test.[39,47,63,214] In addition, between 24 and 78 percent of patients with small cell carcinoma have elevated concentrations of immunoreactive POMC/ACTH in the serum or plasma.[48,59,60,62,65,71,81,215] The dichotomy between the high prevalence of elevated blood immunoreactive ACTH concentrations and the low frequency of the clinical ectopic POMC/ACTH syndrome is due to the secretion by these tumors of immunologically active forms of POMC/ACTH with little or no biological activity (see below).

TABLE 29-15 Tumors Associated with the Ectopic POMC/ACTH Syndrome ($N = 220$)

Tumor	Percent
Small cell carcinoma of lung	45
Thymic carcinoma/carcinoid	13
Bronchial carcinoid	11
Islet-cell tumor	10
Other carcinoid	4
Pheochromocytoma	2
Ovarian carcinoma	2
Other*	13

* Esophageal, gastric, ileal, appendicular, colonic, cervical, breast, prostate, and laryngeal carcinomas; medullary carcinoma of the thyroid; acute myelogenous leukemia.

Source: From references 209-212.

POMC Products Produced by Tumors

In the anterior pituitary, the 1200-base POMC mRNA encodes for the pre-POMC protein which contains a 26-amino acid signal peptide along with the 241-amino acid POMC protein (Fig. 29-6). POMC is glycosylated and has a molecular mass of approximately 31 kDa. In the anterior pituitary it undergoes posttranslational processing through convertases, with the generation of ACTH, N-terminal fragment, joining peptide, and β-lipotropin (β-LPH). β-LPH is further processed to γ-LPH and β-endorphin.[81,208] A small quantity of pro-ACTH, a 22 kDa glycosylated form of ACTH, has also been detected in pituitary extracts.[81,216] In the human fetal pituitary intermediate lobe, the amino-terminal peptide is further processed to generate gamma melanocyte stimulating hormone (γ-MSH), and ACTH is cleaved to form α-MSH [N-α-acetyl-($ACTH^{1-13}$)-NH_2] and corticotro-

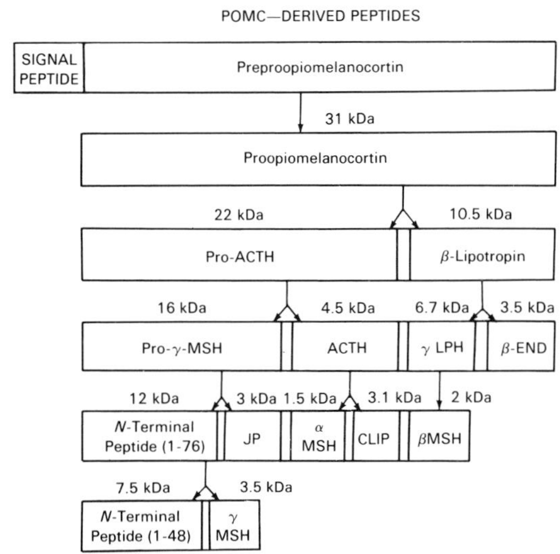

FIGURE 29-6 Proopiomelanocortin–derived peptides. JP = joint-ing peptide; CLIP = corticotropin-like intermediate peptide; MSH = melanocyte stimulating hormone; β-END = β-endorphin.

pin-like intermediate peptide (CLIP). γ-LPH is also cleaved to form the 18-residue β-MSH (Fig. 29-6).

Each of the POMC-derived peptides produced by the normal anterior pituitary and the fetal intermediate lobe has been found in extracts of tumors removed from patients with the ectopic PMOC/ACTH syndrome.[82,208,217–223] Met-enkephalin has also been found in tumor extracts.[224,225] Although this molecule was originally thought to be derived from β-lipotropin molecules since it shares a common amino acid sequence with the C-terminal portion of β-LPH, met-enkephalin is actually derived from a separate precursor, pro-enkephalin.

In patients with the clinical syndrome, the biologically active nonglycosylated 39-amino acid ACTH moiety is the predominant immunoreactive form of the hormone present in the tumor and circulation. As has been noted previously, a number of investigations have found that the majority of patients with lung cancer of any histologic type have elevations of immunoreactive ACTH in the circulation but do not exhibit any clinical syndrome. In addition, the majority of extracts derived from lung cancers of all histologic types, including squamous cell carcinoma, adenocarcinoma, small cell carcinoma, and poorly differentiated carcinoma, have been found to contain immunoreactive ACTH, and over one-third also contain immunoreactive β-LPH.[61] The immunoreactive ACTH in the tumors and blood of patients without the clinical syndrome lacks biological activity, as reflected by absent or reduced binding in a radioreceptor assay.[60] This form of ACTH represents the glycosylated 22,000-dalton pro-ACTH molecule initially described by Yalow as "big ACTH."[81,215] Digestion of this intermediate form of ACTH with trypsin generates biologically active ACTH.

It is of interest that POMC mRNA has been found to be widely distributed in normal tissues, including the stomach, pancreas, brain, placenta, adrenal medulla, and testis.[226] In addition, POMC peptides have been found in many normal tissues.[61,65,227,228] In this regard, Odell and colleagues hypothesized that all normal tissues produce small amounts of the ACTH precursor and carcinomas produce increased quantities of this material. Selected carcinomas are capable of converting this ACTH precursor into biologically active ACTH, thereby producing the ectopic POMC/ACTH syndrome.[65,229] However, recent studies suggest an alternative mechanism. The POMC mRNA in nonpituitary tissues and tumors that is not associated with the ectopic POMC/ACTH syndrome is smaller (approximately 800 bases) than the 1200-base POMC mRNA present in the pituitary.[226,230–232] In contrast, the 1200-base POMC mRNA has been found in tumors associated with the clinical syndrome.[233] This, together with the observation that the ratio of POMC mRNA to POMC peptides present in nonpituitary tissues is much greater than that in the pituitary, suggests that POMC gene expression in normal tissues and tumors not associated with the clinical syndrome is inefficient or defective.[208]

Clinical Manifestations

There are two major modes of presentation of patients with the ectopic PMOC/ACTH syndrome. The first is found in individuals with clinically apparent neoplasms, especially small cell carcinoma of the lung, in which there is rapid onset of clinical and biochemical aberrations. The usual patient is a male 45 to 60 years old, often with a cigarette smoking history of multiple packs over many years, who has the acute onset of profound proximal muscle weakness; pitting edema of the lower extremities; neuropsychiatric symptoms such as mood change, mania, depression, and obtundation; and hypertension. Either weight loss from the underlying neoplasm or weight gain may be present. Polyuria and polydipsia may also be present as a result of glucose intolerance. Women may note the onset of acne and hirsutism. Biochemically, these patients generally exhibit a profound hypokalemic ($K < 3$ mEq/L) alkalosis ($HCO_3 > 28$ mEq/L) and usually have either overt diabetes mellitus or glucose intolerance. Although some patients may appear to be cushingoid, most presenting in this manner do not presumably because they have not had enough time to develop the centripetal fat redistribution and moon facies characteristic of Cushing's disease. Alternatively, the highly malignant nature of the underlying neoplasm in these patients, along with the attendant weight loss and cachexia, may obscure the more typical cushingoid features. The average survival of patients presenting in this manner is 4 months or less.[211–213,234]

The second major mode of presentation is seen

primarily in patients with occult tumors, especially pulmonary and thymic carcinoids.[212] These patients usually harbor small neoplasms, some of which may be benign, and generally present with signs and symptoms closely mimicking Cushing's disease. Thus, typical cushingoid features are common, with centripetal obesity, moon facies, buffalo hump, increased supraclavicular fat pads, thinning of the skin with purplish stria, easy bruising, plethora, hirsutism, acne, psychiatric symptoms, polydipsia, polyuria, and hypertension. Virtually all these patients have significant proximal muscle weakness, and approximately one-third exhibit hyperpigmentation. Hypokalemic alkalosis may also be present, but it is generally of a milder degree than in patients with more overt neoplasms.[211,212] This group of patients is most difficult to differentiate clinically and biochemically from patients with Cushing's disease.

The Ectopic Corticotropin Releasing Hormone Syndrome

In 1971, Upton and Amatruda described two patients, one with a pancreatic tumor and the other with a small cell carcinoma of the lung, who exhibited the clinical ectopic POMC/ACTH syndrome but whose tumors contained bioactive corticotropin releasing hormone (CRH).[235] Subsequently, several additional patients have been reported with the spectrum of tumors including bronchial carcinoid, prostatic carcinoma, medullary carcinoma of the thyroid, and intrasellar gangliocytoma.[236–242] Both the rapid-onset and slow-onset types of presentation described above have been noted in these patients. Some but not all of these tumors also contain POMC and related peptides, including biologically active ACTH. The pituitary in these patients demonstrates corticotroph hyperplasia, indicating that the CRH is biologically active.[236,237,243] It appears that the clinical features of Cushing's syndrome result from CRH stimulation of pituitary ACTH secretion with or without concomitant secretion of biologically active ACTH from the tumor. It is also of interest that materials closely related immunologically to CRH have been found in normal stomach, pancreas, and adrenal glands, along with various tumors, including those not associated with Cushing's syndrome.[244]

Diagnosis

In patients with overt neoplasms and a rapid onset of the ectopic POMC/ACTH syndrome, the biochemical diagnosis does not present difficulties (Fig. 29-7). The 24-h urine free cortisol concentration is generally four or more times above the upper limit of normal, and these patients fail to demonstrate a 50 percent or greater suppression of serum or urine cortisol concentrations after the administration of either low-dose (1 mg overnight; 0.5 mg orally every 6 h for eight doses) or high-dose (2 mg orally every 6 h for eight doses) dexamethasone because of the autonomous secretion of ACTH from the tumor. Measurement of serum or plasma ACTH can differentiate between the ectopic POMC/ACTH syndrome and the presence of an adrenal adenoma or carcinoma that autonomously secretes excessive quantities of cortisol. In the latter group of patients, blood ACTH levels are suppressed, while in patients with the ectopic POMC/ACTH syndrome, the levels are usually over 200 pg/ml.[117,211]

Unfortunately, not all patients with the ectopic POMC/ACTH syndrome follow this classical scheme. Close to 80 percent of patients with pituitary-dependent Cushing's disease have over 50 percent suppression of plasma or 24-h urine cortisol levels after 2 days of ingesting 8 mg of dexamethasone each day, while 11 percent of patients with the ectopic POMC/ACTH syndrome also show such suppression.[212] Similarly, close to 90 percent of patients with Cushing's disease and 63 percent of patients with ectopic POMC/ACTH syndrome demonstrate a 100 percent or greater rise in either plasma ACTH or urinary 17-hydroxysteroids after metyrapone administration.[212] This overlap in biochemical responses between patients who have Cushing's disease and those with the ectopic POMC/ACTH syndrome is seen primarily in individuals who have occult neoplasms as well as patients with the ectopic CRH syndrome. Indeed, in the group of patients with occult tumors and Cushing's syndrome, an incorrect diagnosis is initially made in approximately 70 percent.[245]

In 1982, CRH became available for clinical use on an investigational basis. When it is administered as an intravenous bolus over 30 s at a dose of 1 μg/kg, normal individuals show a prompt rise in ACTH followed by an increase in plasma cortisol (Fig. 29-8).[246] As expected, patients with ACTH-independent Cushing's syndrome resulting from primary adrenocortical disease demonstrate little or no rise in either ACTH or cortisol. In contrast, individuals with pituitary ACTH-dependent Cushing's disease have elevations of the basal ACTH and cortisol concentrations and exhibit an exuberant rise in both hormones after CRH administration. Patients with ectopic POMC/ACTH Cushing's syndrome also have elevated plasma ACTH and cortisol concentrations and demonstrate no further increase after receiving CRH. Unfortunately, only 90 percent of patients with pituitary ACTH-dependent Cushing's disease show a rise in ACTH, while 8 percent of patients with the ectopic POMC/ACTH syndrome show a similar rise. Because of the four-fold greater prevalence of pituitary ACTH-dependent Cushing's disease, the predictive value of a positive CRH test in identifying Cushing's disease is 99 percent, but the predictive value of a negative test with an insufficient rise in ACTH is only 63 percent.[247] Thus, this test is not as useful in differentiating between the two diseases as the initial reports suggested. It is of interest that

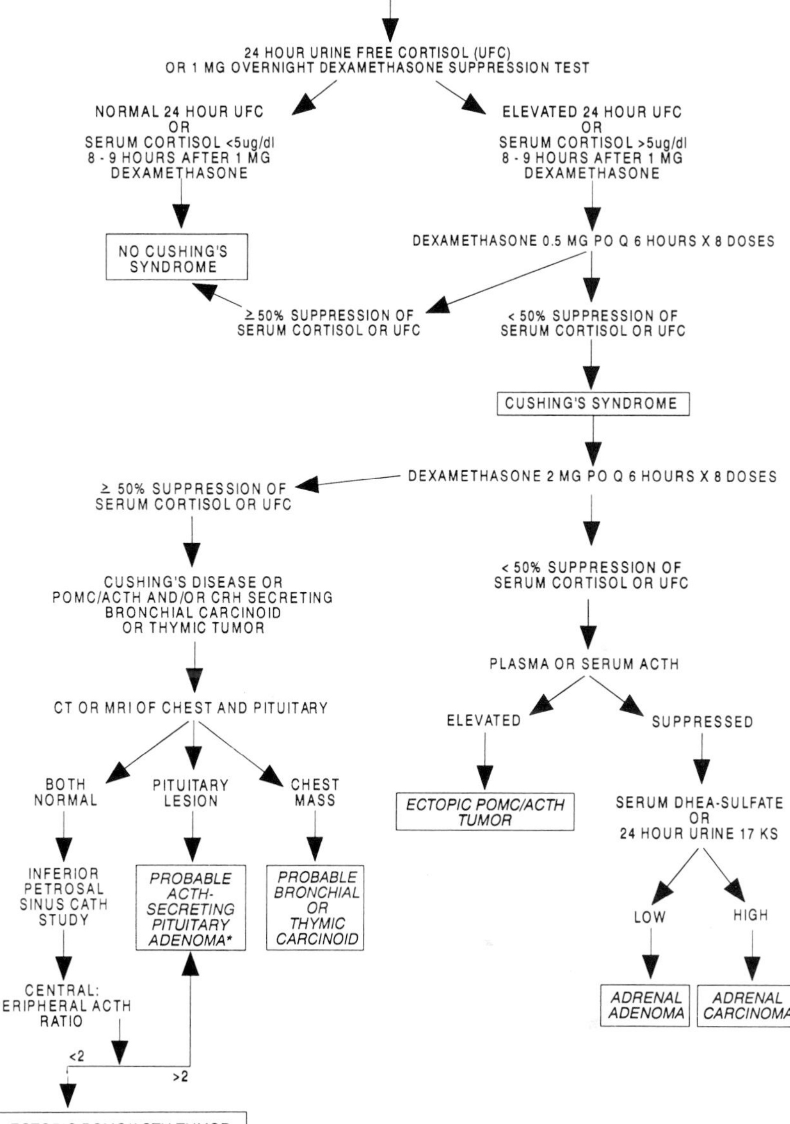

FIGURE 29-7 Algorithm for the evaluation of a patient with suspected Cushing's syndrome. See text for details. (*The rare pure CRH-secreting tumor potentially may give similar results. Plasma CRH levels should help differentiate these entities.)

CRH has been found in tumors from patients with the ectopic POMC/ACTH syndrome who have an increase in ACTH after a CRH test, suggesting that the false-positive responses in this syndrome are due to the ectopic production of CRH by the tumor, which leads to hyperplasia of the pituitary corticotrophs which are responsive to exogenous CRH.[240]

Another technique developed to differentiate eutopic pituitary ACTH-dependent Cushing's syndrome from ectopic POMC/ACTH Cushing's syndrome is selective venous blood sampling from multiple sites with measurement of ACTH. Because the pituitary venous effluent drains into the inferior petrosal sinuses, catheterization of the sinuses with simultaneous blood sampling of both sinuses and a peripheral vein will show a gradient of 2 or greater in the unstimulated state or 3 or greater during a simultaneous infusion of CRH in patients with an ACTH-secreting pituitary adenoma.[247–249] In contrast, patients with the ectopic POMC/ACTH syndrome have a gradient below 2 in the basal state or during CRH infusion. The localization of the tumor producing the syndrome may be accomplished through sampling of blood from a variety of other sites throughout the venous vascular tree. Because of the potential for microsecretory bursts of ACTH secretion, it is important to carry out the procedure as rapidly as possible.[248,250]

Serum serotonin or urine 5-hydroxyindolacetic acid measurements are occasionally useful in patients with the ectopic POMC/ACTH syndrome due to carcinoid tumors or small cell carcinoma of the

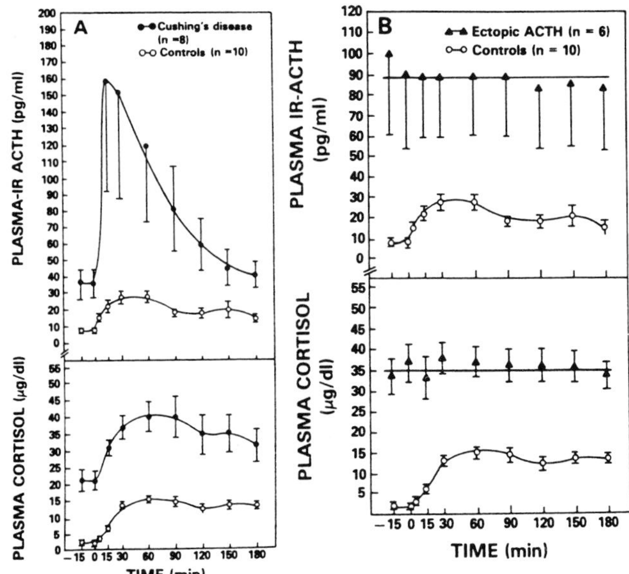

FIGURE 29-8 Plasma ACTH and cortisol responses to the administration of CRH in 8 patients with untreated Cushing's disease, 6 patients with ectopic POMC/ACTH secretion, and 10 control patients. (*Reprinted from Chrousos and colleagues,*[246] *with permission.*)

lung.[251] Since the majority of patients with this syndrome harbor a neoplasm within the chest, a CT or MRI scan of the chest and mediastinum should be performed on all patients who do not have an overt tumor but fulfill the biochemical criteria for the ectopic POMC/ACTH syndrome. Similarly, patients who appear to have classical Cushing's disease should also have a CT or MRI scan of the chest unless radiographic procedures or inferior petrosal sinus studies have clearly demonstrated the presence of an ACTH-secreting pituitary adenoma.

Treatment

Slow-growing, well-localized bronchial or thymic carcinoids may be successfully removed surgically. Bilateral adrenalectomy is certainly effective in reversing the metabolic abnormalities but may be inappropriate in a patient with a highly malignant neoplasm such as small cell carcinoma of the lung. Inhibitors of glucocorticoid synthesis including aminoglutethimide, metyrapone, and ketoconazole have been successfully used in treating this syndrome.[208,252,253] Combinations of inhibitors and the adrenalytic agent o,p′-DDD have also been used.[254] Similarly, glucocorticoid receptor blockade with the glucocorticoid antagonist RU-486 has been effective in a limited number of patients.[104] Finally, octreotide, a long-acting somatostatin analogue, was used in two patients with pancreatic neoplasms and the ectopic POMC/ACTH syndrome and led to the rapid correction of the hypercortisolemia.[255,256]

Syndrome of Inappropriate Antidiuresis in Cancer

The first description of the syndrome of inappropriate antidiuresis (SIAD) in patients with cancer appeared in 1938.[257] In 1957, Schwartz and coworkers published the classic description of two patients with bronchogenic carcinoma who exhibited hyponatremia, continual loss of sodium in urine, and an impaired ability to dilute their urine.[258] Recognizing the similarity between the biochemical features in the two patients with lung cancer and normal subjects given injections of pitressin tannate-in-oil and free access to fluid, Schwartz et al proposed that the syndrome is due to the inappropriate secretion of antidiuretic hormone [arginine vasopressin (AVP)].[259] In 1963, an increased concentration of antidiuretic hormone was found to be present in the urine of a patient with a lung tumor and this syndrome[260] and in tumor tissue by bioassay.[261] That a tumor could be the source of AVP was suggested by the finding in 1964 of increased concentrations of AVP in the plasma and tumor tissue of a patient with a bronchogenic carcinoma who also exhibited destruction of the posterior pituitary from a metastatic lesion.[262] More direct evidence of tumor production was provided by the studies of George et al, who demonstrated the incorporation of radiolabeled amino acids into AVP by lung tumor cells in vitro.[263] The similarity of the biosynthetic pathway for tumor and hypothalamic production of AVP was shown by Yamaji and colleagues in 1981 with the in vitro production of provasopressin by a small cell carcinoma of the lung maintained in vitro.[264] In the same year, a nude mouse bearing a small cell carcinoma of the lung derived from a patient with SIAD exhibited increased blood and tumor levels of AVP, excessive sodium loss in the urine, and decreased free water clearance, mimicking the human syndrome.[265]

Prevalence and Tumor Types

Between one-half and two-thirds of patients in reported series of SIAD have an underlying malignancy as the etiology.[266,267] This undoubtedly represents a reporting bias, since transient SIAD is frequently seen in patients with conditions such as meningitis and head trauma. The vast majority of patients with SIAD associated with cancer have a bronchogenic carcinoma, especially small cell carcinoma, which accounts for three-quarters of the patients with cancer-associated SIAD (Table 29-16).[210,266–269] Other histologic types of lung tumors, lymphomas, and an array of different types of tumors account for the remaining cases.

The prevalence of SIAD depends on how the condition is defined. The clinical syndrome associated with small cell carcinoma of the lung occurs in 7 to 14 percent of patients.[44,47–49,51,53,58,270,271] Even within this group, the patients may be asymptomatic and merely demonstrate hyponatremia and a urinary

TABLE 29-16 Tumor Types Associated with SIAD

	Cases, %	
Bronchogenic carcinoma	83	
Small cell carcinoma		59
Non-small-cell carcinoma		24
Lymphoma	3	
Pancreatic carcinoma	2	
Laryngeal carcinoma	1	
Duodenal carcinoma	1	
Miscellaneous tumors*	10	

* Prostate (small cell), cervical (small cell), bladder, colon, thymoma, mesothelioma, olfactory neuroblastoma, sarcoma, lymphosarcoma, reticulum cell sarcoma, Ewing's sarcoma, malignant histiocytosis.

Source: From references 210 and 266–269.

concentrating defect. On the basis of an abnormal water load test, between 35 and 66 percent of patients with small cell carcinoma of the lung are classified as having SIAD.[49,58,63,266] However, close to 70 percent of patients with other malignancies also exhibit abnormalities in the ability to excrete a water load, raising the possibility that this test gives nonspecific results in all patients.[63] Increased concentrations of plasma or urinary AVP levels are found in 33 to 71 percent of these patients.[46–49,52,58,65] Elevated AVP levels have also been noted in 43 percent of patients with colon carcinoma who do not exhibit clinical SIAD.[65] Using immunoassays for neurophysins, North and colleagues found that approximately 65 percent of patients with small cell carcinoma of the lung have elevated concentrations of neurophysins in the circulation.[64,272] Close to one-third have increased quantities of vasopressin-associated neurophysin alone, 12 percent have elevations of oxytocin-associated neurophysin alone, and 22 percent have elevations of both neurophysins.[64] Approximately 20 percent of patients with non-small-cell carcinoma of the lung also have elevations of neurophysins in the serum. Since AVP and AVP-associated neurophysin are synthesized together, along with a glycopeptide as provasopressin, and are normally secreted in equimolar amounts, it is not surprising that both are elevated in about half the patients with small cell carcinoma of the lung. Immunohistologic staining for AVP-associated neurophysin in small cell carcinoma of the lung has shown the presence of the antigen in 72 percent of the tissue specimens examined.[273] Thus, it appears that many patients with small cell carcinoma of the lung have a propensity for developing SIAD, although only a minority exhibit the clinical syndrome.

Tumor Peptides and Pathophysiology

Early studies demonstrated that the substance with antidiuretic activity extracted from tumors closely resembles that extracted from the posterior pituitary in terms of the dose-response effect in bioassay and inactivation by thioglycolate, vasopressinase, and vasopressin antibodies.[269,274,275] In addition, these materials appear to be identical to AVP immunologically and physiochemically. Direct evidence of in vitro synthesis was provided through immunoassay measurements of AVP production in vitro and through the incorporation of tritiated phenylalanine into a peptide resembling AVP.[263,276–278] Finally, in carefully performed pulse-chase experiments using labeled cysteine and glucosamine, Yamaji and associates found a small cell carcinoma of the lung that synthesized and secreted a 20,000-dalton glycosylated provasopressin which could be cleaved by trypsin to yield neurophysin, AVP, and a glycopeptide.[264,279] The mRNA for preprovasopressin also has been demonstrated in small cell carcinoma of the lung.[280]

Although it is clear that some lung tumors are capable of synthesizing and secreting AVP, it is safe to conclude that many cases of SIAD cannot be accounted for by ectopic production of AVP by these tumors, since only three-fourths of patients with SIAD associated with lung cancer have been found to have inappropriately elevated concentrations of AVP.[281] Also, some patients with typical SIAD actually have resetting of the hypothalamic osmostat, as manifested by a lowered osmotic threshold for the release of AVP from the hypothalamus.[282] In the latter situation, the rise of AVP with increasing plasma osmolality during a hypertonic saline infusion has a normal slope but the entire curve is shifted to the left.

Since the normal physiologic regulation of AVP secretion from the hypothalamus and posterior pituitary is mediated through baroreceptors as well as osmoreceptors, there are multiple situations in which neoplasms may lead to a release of hypothalamic-pituitary AVP as opposed to ectopic production of the hormone by the tumor. Such mechanisms include obstruction of the vena cava, infiltration of the vagus nerve leading to baroreceptor denervation, hypothalamic metastases, carcinomatous neuropathy, CNS or pulmonary infections, pain, and alterations of intrathoracic pressure sufficient to stimulate the baroreceptors in the left atrium and great veins.[117,282,283] Similarly, a number of medications used in patients with cancer may be associated with hyponatremia. These drugs include cyclophosphamide, vincristine, cisplatin, doxorubicin, vinblastine, and bleomycin.[284,285]

It has also been proposed that some tumors may synthesize an AVP-releasing factor.[282] In patients who have SIAD without measurable levels of AVP, another antidiuretic substance may be produced by the tumor. One candidate substance is arginine vasotocin, a fetal peptide related to AVP, which may be produced by some tumors.[65] The natriuresis found in this syndrome may be due in part to the secretion of atrial natriuretic peptide (ANP), since plasma levels of this hormone are elevated in some patients with SIAD[286–288] and the mRNA for ANP has been isolated from small cell carcinomas associated with hyponatremia.[289]

Criteria for SIAD and Clinical Features

Vasopressin acts on the renal collecting tubule by binding with the V_2 AVP receptor, an interaction which stimulates adenyl cyclase activity and ultimately allows the collecting ducts to become permeable to water. This results in the reabsorption of water from the hypotonic urine entering the collecting ducts which pass through the hypertonic renal medullary region. The net effect is the excretion of more concentrated urine and the delivery of the reabsorbed water to the intravascular and extravascular spaces. Normally, the secretion of AVP by the hypothalamus and posterior pituitary is tightly regulated through osmolar and volume mechanisms. With inappropriate secretion of AVP, inappropriate water retention and a reduction of body tonicity occur. The cardinal features of SIAD include the following:

1. Dilutional hyponatremia ($Na^+ < 130$ mEq/L), hypoosmolality (<280 mOsmol/kg), and low serum blood urea nitrogen (BUN), creatinine, uric acid, and albumin.
2. The presence of a urine osmolality that is inappropriately high for the serum hypoosmolality. This does not imply that urine osmolality must always be greater than serum osmolality in patients with SIAD, although it usually is; it implies only that the urine is not maximally dilute (50 to 60 mOsmol/kg), which it should be when AVP is suppressed. This criterion is reflected in the inability of patients with SIAD to excrete a water load normally.
3 The presence of continued natriuresis with a urine sodium concentration greater than 20 mEq/L despite the hyponatremia. The urine sodium excretion reflects sodium intake so that the administration of increasing quantities of sodium results in an equivalent loss of sodium in the urine. The natriuresis may be absent if the patient's sodium intake is severely restricted. The cause of the natriuresis is multifactorial and includes an increase in the glomerular filtration rate from the expanded extracellular fluid space, which in turn results in an increased filtered load of sodium. Additionally, serum aldosterone levels are either normal or low but are inappropriately low relative to the hyponatremia, which is a stimulus for aldosterone secretion. In the face of extracellular volume expansion, there is a decrease in the proximal tubular sodium reabsorption because of factors that are incompletely understood. Finally, atrial natriuretic factor levels are increased in these patients, and this may also enhance the natriuresis.[283]
4. Little or no edema despite the approximately 4 to 5 liters of water retention in this syndrome. There is an escape from the effects of the ADH which ultimately occurs in these patients. The reasons include a decrease in the tonicity of the normally hypertonic renal medullary interstitial space as a result of the dilutional effects, an increase in the water delivered to the distal nephron from the elevated glomerular filtration rate, and the hypokalemia that is present in approximately half these patients, which antagonizes the effect of AVP at the renal tubular level.[269]
5. The absence of a condition which results in a reduced effective vascular volume, including dehydration, congestive heart failure, and liver disease associated with ascites. These conditions are associated with an appropriate increase in hypothalamic and posterior pituitary secretion of AVP.
6. Normal renal, adrenal, thyroid, and anterior pituitary function.

The clinical manifestations of SIAD depend on the rate of development of hyponatremia and hypoosmolality as well as the actual level of serum sodium. Only a quarter of patients with SIAD exhibit clinical symptoms.[270] Symptoms may be precipitated through the ingestion of a thiazide diuretic, the administration of excessive oral or intravenous fluids during chemotherapy, or acutely as a result of tumor lysis with release of stored AVP. Also, water intoxication in predisposed patients may theoretically be precipitated by the ingestion of nonsteroidal analgesics which potentiate the antidiuretic effect of AVP by blocking PGE_2, an inhibitor of AVP action.[283]

It is uncommon for symptoms other than nonspecific malaise to occur above a serum sodium of 120 mEq/L. Between 115 and 120 mEq/L, the signs and symptoms of water intoxication include anorexia, nausea, vomiting, abdominal cramps, bloating, ileus, myoclonus, muscle weakness, restlessness, irritability, hostility, withdrawal, confusion, and headache. Serum sodium levels below 110 mEq/L are associated with severe muscle weakness, hyporeflexia, ataxia, extrapyramidal signs such as rigidity, bulbar or pseudobulbar palsies, positive Babinski signs, hemiparesis, stupor, coma, and seizures.

The diagnosis of SIAD is rarely difficult in patients with symptoms that fulfill the classical criteria. Secondary causes of ADH secretion from volume depletion due to adrenal insufficiency, diuretic use, diarrhea, or hemorrhage are associated with typical signs and symptoms, including orthostatic hypotension and tachycardia, dry mucous membranes, and decreased skin turgor. In addition, dehydration leads to a low urinary sodium concentration, as do the conditions associated with volume overload and decreased effective vascular volume, such as congestive heart failure, cirrhosis of the liver, and the nephrotic syndrome. Pseudohyponatremia from elevations of serum glucose, lipids, or proteins is excluded through the measurement of plasma osmolality, which is normal rather than decreased, or correction of the serum sodium concentration for the level of glucose, triglycerides, or protein. Patients with primary polydipsia may have a low plasma osmolality but uniformly have a low urine osmolality and thus may be easily differentiated from patients with SIAD.

Plasma AVP measurements are of interest but add little to the management of these patients. The presence of an inappropriately elevated plasma AVP concentration in a patient with a neoplasm does not in itself indicate that the neoplasm is secreting the hormone ectopically. Tumors may be associated with SIAD through multiple mechanisms, as outlined above.

In small cell carcinoma of the lung, there is a tendency for patients with more extensive disease to have a higher prevalence of an inability to excrete a water load than is seen in patients with limited disease.[49] However, taking into account the stage of the disease, there is no difference in the survival of patients who have SIAD vs. those who do not.[49,63,270,271] The abnormalities in water load tests as well as the concentrations of AVP and neurophysins reasonably parallel the clinical course of patients with small cell carcinoma of the lung and therefore may be used as markers of the disease.[49,272,283]

Therapy

Mild water intoxication is treated with fluid restriction to 800 ml per day or less. This reduces intravascular volume, resulting in a lowering of the glomerular filtration rate and a decrease in renal sodium loss.

For severe water intoxication, especially in patients with serum sodium levels below 110 mEq/L, a combination of 3% hypertonic sodium chloride with a loop diuretic such as furosemide or ethacrynic acid with replacement of urine sodium and potassium losses usually increases the serum sodium effectively. Because individuals with SIAD are fluid overloaded to begin with, the administration of hypertonic saline alone may result in congestive heart failure and hypertension. Also, since these patients excrete an amount of sodium in their urine equivalent to their sodium intake, hypertonic saline alone rarely leads to a sustained increase in serum sodium. The loop diuretics increase free water clearance and, together with the hypertonic saline, result in a rise in the sodium concentration.[283,284,290]

When one is using hypertonic saline and a loop diuretic, it is important to monitor the rate of rise of serum sodium. Overzealous correction of hyponatremia in severely debilitated patients has been associated with central pontine myelinosis. This problem can be avoided if the rate of rise of serum sodium is kept at less than 2 mEq/L per h until a level of serum sodium of 120 mEq/L is achieved, at which time the rate should be reduced. This therapy should be discontinued before the sodium reaches 130 mEq/L in order to avoid hypernatremia and hyperchloremia.[291]

For patients who are mildly symptomatic or exhibit chronic SIAD, three drugs are currently available. The first is demeclocycline, a tetracycline antibiotic which induces a nephrogenic diabetes insipidus by inhibiting the formation and action of cyclic AMP in the collecting ducts of the renal tubules. This drug may be initiated at a dose of 1200 mg a day in divided doses. Urine osmolality decreases in 3 to 6 days, at which time the dose may be gradually decreased to a maintenance level of 300 to 900 mg/day. The goal is to maintain serum sodium within the normal range while the patient has free access to fluid. The side effects of this medication include nausea, vomiting, diarrhea, photosensitivity dermatitis, a dose-related rise in BUN without renal dysfunction, and nephrotoxicity, especially in patients with hepatic insufficiency.

Another drug which induces a nephrogenic diabetes insipidus is lithium carbonate in doses of 900 to 2100 mg/day. The CNS, renal, and cardiac toxicities of this drug render it inferior to demeclocycline as a treatment for SIAD.[292]

Oral urea acts as an osmotic diuretic and enhances water clearance. Thirty grams of urea is dissolved in 100 ml of water or juice and is administered with 15 g of magnesium and aluminum hydroxide once a day.[284] The only adverse reaction to this medication is the potential for hypernatremic dehydration if the patient does not drink enough fluid. This therapy is reasonable to use if demeclocycline is not tolerated.

Finally, with small cell carcinoma of the lung, chemotherapy is effective in resolving SIAD in the majority of patients at the time of initial presentation.[53] Indeed, Hainsworth and colleagues found that 16 of 17 patients with small cell carcinoma had resolution of their SIAD between 8 and 26 days after the institution of chemotherapy.[53] Unfortunately, the majority have a return of SIAD at the time of progression, and one of the other therapies must be administered.

Hypoglycemia Associated with Malignancy

The first report of hypoglycemia associated with a neoplasm was published in 1929 when Nadler and Wolfer[293] and Elliot[294] described a patient with a hepatoma who had neuroglucopenic symptoms and a blood sugar as low as 13 mg/dl. The following year,

Doege and Potter independently described a patient with low-grade fibrosarcoma and hypoglycemia whose hypoglycemia remitted after removal of the tumor, only to return with the recurrence of the malignancy.[75,295]

In the same year, Anderson described the association of hypoglycemia and adrenocortical carcinoma.[296] Since that time, hundreds of patients with the association have been reported and extensively reviewed.[297,298] Several eponyms have been used to describe specific associations, including Doege-Potter syndrome (mesenchymal tumors), Nadler-Wolfer-Elliot syndrome (hepatoma), Anderson's syndrome (adrenocortical tumors), and Rosenfeldt's syndrome (pseudomyxoma).[297]

Incidence and Tumor Types

Paraneoplastic hypoglycemia is rare. Hypoglycemia was found to occur in 1.2 percent of hospitalized patients, most often as a result of complications of diabetes mellitus, renal insufficiency, malnutrition, liver disease, infection, and shock.[299] In the few patients who had an underlying malignancy, hypoglycemia was associated with insulin therapy, extensive liver metastases, and malnutrition.[299] Despite its low prevalence, hypoglycemia is associated relatively frequently with some tumor types.

Approximately half the patients with tumor-associated hypoglycemia harbor neoplasms of mesenchymal origin, which include fibrosarcomas, mesotheliomas, leiomyosarcomas, rhabdomyosarcomas, and hemangiopericytomas, as well as a variety of other histologic types (Table 29-17).[297,300–302] Approximately 10 percent are benign tumors or of very low grade malignancy.[297,300] Many of these tumors have a spindle cell morphology.[297] They tend to be large neoplasms, ranging from 310 g to 20 kg.[298,301] A third of these tumors are located within the thorax, one-half in the retroperitoneal area, 11 percent intraabdominally, and approximately 6 percent in unique sites.[303] Both sexes are effected equally.[297]

TABLE 29-17 Tumor Types Associated with Hypoglycemia ($N = 246$)

	Patients, %	
Sarcoma	46	
Fibrosarcoma		24
Mesothelioma		9
Leiomyosarcoma/rhabdomyosarcoma		6
Hemangiopericytoma		4
Other		3
Hepatoma	19	
Adrenocortical carcinoma	10	
Lymphoma	6	
Neuroectodermal tumors	2	
Gastric carcinoma	2	
Colon carcinoma	1	
Other*	14	

* Cholangiocarcinoma, teratomas, pseudomyxoma, Wilms' tumor, lung carcinoma, melanoma.

Source: From references 297 and 300-302.

Hepatocellular carcinoma is the second most common tumor associated with hypoglycemia. Approximately 1 to 2 percent of hepatocellular carcinomas have been found to be associated with hypoglycemia, although the incidence is as high as 26 percent in hepatocellular carcinomas found in Asian patients.[304–307] Males are affected approximately four times more frequently than females are. McFadzean and Yueng divided these patients into two groups.[307] The first group consisted of 87 percent of the patients, who had rapidly growing, poorly differentiated hepatomas with marked replacement of the liver parenchyma. These patients experienced muscle weakness and wasting, and hypoglycemia was found in the terminal or preterminal state and could easily be controlled with glucose infusions. In contrast, the second group, composed of 13 percent of the patients, had slow-growing, well-differentiated neoplasms without evidence of substantial cachexia or muscle weakness when the hypoglycemia appeared. In this group, death occurred 2 to 10 months after the onset of hypoglycemia, whereas in the other group, death generally occurred within 2 weeks.[307]

Adrenocortical carcinoma accounts for approximately 10 percent of patients with tumor-associated hypoglycemia. The tumors generally are highly malignant and are associated with metastases at the time of diagnosis. Both sexes are affected equally, and survival is generally less than 6 months from diagnosis. The tumors may be functional or nonfunctional; when they are functional, about half are associated with Cushing's syndrome and half with virilization.[297]

Pathophysiology

Abnormalities of glucose metabolism have been noted in patients with malignancy-associated hypoglycemia. Tumor cells exhibit a high rate of glycolysis, and it was proposed that large mesenchymally derived tumors weighing multiple kilograms may consume enough glucose to overwhelm the body's conterregulatory mechanisms.[297,308] However, calculations based on an arterial-venous glucose difference across a tumor and in vitro glucose uptake studies suggest that even tumors in the range of 1.4 to 6.0 kg consume less than 400 g of glucose per day, while the liver is capable of producing more than 800 g of glucose per day.[308,309] Thus, overutilization of glucose by the tumor is insufficient to account for the hypoglycemia. These patients also exhibit an increase in glucose utilization by peripheral tissues, as shown by the large amount of glucose that must be infused to keep the blood glucose within the normal range.[308] Of interest in this regard, Stuart and coworkers demonstrated insulin receptor proliferation in the liver and muscle of a patient with a hypoglycemia-producing colon carcinoma that metastasized to the liver.[309] The threefold to fivefold increase in insulin receptors associated with elevations of IGF-II, which can act through insulin receptors, may account for the high total body glucose utilization.

In addition to overutilization of glucose by tumor and peripheral tissues, there is evidence of deficient hepatic glucose production in these patients.[300,308,310,311] With the exception of patients with slowly growing hepatomas that extensively replace the normal liver parenchyma, most patients with tumor-associated hypoglycemia do not exhibit sufficient destruction of the normal liver to account for the deficient hepatic glucose production, since experimental studies have shown that over 75 percent of the liver must be destroyed before hypoglycemia ensues.[312] A problem in glycogenolysis is present, as histologic studies have shown that glycogen is present in the livers of these patients and the administration of glucagon and epinephrine to some patients results in an increase in hepatic glucose output.[312,313] Also, there is an inadequate amount of gluconeogenesis, as reflected in increased blood lactate levels and possible reductions in gluconeogenic amino acids.[300,308,314] Part of the reduction in hepatic glucose production may reflect an absent or sluggish response to the hypoglycemia of the insulin counterregulatory hormones. Indeed, growth hormone, ACTH, cortisol, and glucagon may be inappropriately low considering the level of the blood sugar in these patients, a response that may be due to a slow decrease in blood sugar which does not activate the sympathetic nervous system and stress-induced release of the counterregulatory hormones.[312] Also, the low levels of growth hormone noted in the basal state in these patients as well as after arginine infusion may reflect suppression of growth hormone secretion directly by IGF-II.[314–316]

Several different humoral factors secreted by these tumors have been implicated in the pathogenesis of the disorder. In 1962, after the development of the insulin immunoassay, Olefesky and associates reported elevated serum insulin levels in a patient with a fibrosarcoma.[317] During the next two decades, more than 100 patients were described as having elevated concentrations of bioactive or immunoactive insulin or insulin-like activity in blood or tumor tissue. An in-depth analysis of the data by Skrabanek and Powell suggested that insulin production by non-islet-cell tumors is rarely if ever responsible for the hypoglycemia.[298] Occasional carcinoid tumors that resemble islet-cell tumors have been associated with excessive insulin secretion.[318] More recently, a neuroectodermal pelvic tumor was shown to contain insulin, proinsulin, and secretory granules and to be responsible for elevated insulin levels and hypoglycemia in a patient.[319] Nevertheless, ectopic insulin production is exceedingly rare, and in most series immunoreactive insulin levels are low and insulin mRNA is absent from tumor tissue.[316] Although there have been occasional suggestions that tumors may release a pancreatic beta-cytotrophic substance that stimulates insulin secretion, no such substance has been identified in these tumors, and pancreatic hyperplasia has not been found at autopsy.[297,298,320]

Before the development of insulin RIAs, insulin biological activity was divided into that which could be suppressed with insulin antibodies, which represented the true insulin activity, and that which could not be suppressed by these antibodies, designated nonsuppressible insulin-like activity (NSILA). Subsequently, NSILA was fractionated by acid-ethanol, which separated the activity into high-molecular-weight proteins, NSILA-p or NSILAP, and a soluble fraction containing low-molecular-weight proteins, NSILA-s.[312,321] NSILA-s was found to consist of several peptides, including IGF-I and IGF-II, with molecular masses of approximately 7650 and 7500 dalton, respectively.[312] In 1974, Megyesi and coworkers used a radioreceptor assay for NSILA-s that was primarily responsive to IGF-II and noted that three of seven patients with non-islet-cell tumors associated with hypoglycemia had elevated serum concentrations of IGF-II.[322] Further studies by this group indicated that nearly 40 percent of patients with the syndrome had elevated serum IGF-II-like activity.[304,312] Daughaday and coworkers, using a different radioreceptor assay, found that over 90 percent of patients had elevated IGF-II concentrations in their serum.[77] However, Zapf and colleagues were unable to demonstrate elevated IGF-II concentrations using a different radioreceptor assay or an RIA.[302,323] These discrepancies were partially explained by Merimee, who noted elevated serum IGF-II concentrations in two patients with non-islet-cell tumors as measured by a radioreceptor assay; however, 2 to 4 months later, when the sera were remeasured in the same assay, the activity was lost, indicating that the IGF-II molecule produced by these tumors was unstable during storage.[315]

Chromatography of serum and tumor extracts from these patients has revealed that 60 percent exhibit an increased proportion of a high-molecular-weight precursor of IGF-II compared to that in normal serum, and in some patients virtually all the IGF-II is in the "big" 10- to 15-kDa fraction.[314,324,325] Finally, several investigators have shown that tumors contain IGF-II mRNA.[314,316,324,325] Although it has been suggested that NSILP may be responsible for the hypoglycemia found in some patients, levels of this protein have been inconsistently elevated and have been noted to increase in some patients after the removal of hypoglycemia-producing tumors at a time when the blood sugar levels have returned to normal.[321,324]

From the available data, it would appear that the pathogenesis of non-islet-cell-tumor-associated hypoglycemia is multifactorial. These tumors produce an increased quantity of a high-molecular-weight form of IGF-II, probably as a result of incomplete processing of the protein.[314,325] This 10- to 15-kDa IGF-II binds poorly to the circulating IGF-binding proteins.[325,326] In contrast, approximately 99 percent of normal 7.5-kDa IGF-II binds avidly to IGF-binding proteins.[325] With less protein binding, the high-molecular-weight IGF-II is free to interact with IGF receptors or insulin receptors present throughout the body, leading to an increase in glucose uptake by both the tumor and peripheral tissues. In contrast to proACTH (POMC), the high-molecular-weight form of IGF-II retains receptor-binding activity.[324] The elevated IGF-II probably inhibits pituitary growth hormone secretion in a manner analogous to the inhibition observed with IGF-I and insulin, probably mediated through IGF-I receptors.[327] This would account for the observed reduction in serum growth hormone levels during periods of hypoglycemia or after arginine infusion and would also account for the lowered concentrations of IGF-I observed in patients with this syndrome.[328] The decreased growth hormone also lowers some of the species of IGF-binding proteins, and this would further account for an increase in free IGF-II in the circulation. Finally, the elevated IGF-II concentrations may lead to an inhibition of the release of gluconeogenic amino acids from muscle tissue, accounting for some of the decrease in hepatic glucose output observed with this syndrome.[314]

Clinical Manifestations and Diagnosis

In general, hypoglycemic symptoms may be divided into the sympathomimetic types of symptoms, such as tachycardia, diaphoresis, piloerection, and tremulousness, which reflect a relatively rapid rate of fall of blood sugar, and the CNS symptoms, which reflect the actual level of blood sugar. In patients with non-islet-cell-tumor hypoglycemia, the neuroglucopenic symptoms predominate because the rate of fall of blood sugar is generally slow.[77,297,300,312] Thus, episodes of behavioral abnormalities, obtundation, seizures, or coma, especially in the early morning or after fasting, are commonly observed. The symptoms are usually insidious and may be intermittently present for weeks, months, or years before the diagnosis of the underlying neoplasm.

Other symptoms are related to the location and size of the neoplasm. Mesenchymal tumors are usually located in the retroperitoneal, intraabdominal, or thoracic regions and are associated with pain, abdominal fullness, cough, dyspnea, or peripheral neurologic symptoms. When they are located within the abdomen or retroperitoneal space, a mass is often palpable. Hepatomegaly, jaundice, fever, abdominal pain, and nonspecific symptoms including malaise, weakness, anorexia, and weight loss are commonly seen in patients with hepatocellular carcinoma. The other large group of non-islet-cell tumors associated with hypoglycemia—adrenocortical carcinomas—may have associated clinical findings of excessive glucocorticoids, mineralocorticoids, or adrenal androgens.

The diagnosis of this syndrome requires the demonstration of fasting hypoglycemia with suppressed serum insulin concentrations in association with the presence of a non-islet-cell neoplasm. It is important to keep in mind that during a 72-h fast, normal men generally maintain a plasma glucose above 55 mg/dl, while normal women may have plasma glucose levels of 30 mg/dl or less.[329] The other causes of fasting hypoglycemia with suppressed insulin levels must be ruled out. These include fulminant liver failure, chronic renal failure, severe malnutrition, adrenal insufficiency, alcohol use, and the ingestion of drugs that interfere with gluconeogenesis. Measurements of IGF-II may be helpful if the levels are elevated but are not useful in the differential diagnosis if they are normal, since some patients with this syndrome have normal total levels of IGF-II with an elevated proportion of high-molecular-weight IGF-II, which binds poorly to the IGF-binding proteins.

Therapy

The only therapy that is uniformly effective in this syndrome is that directed at the primary tumor. Surgical extirpation, radiation therapy, or chemotherapy may be effective in reducing the tumor bulk to the extent that the hypoglycemia disappears. If such therapy is ineffective, frequent carbohydrate feedings and the administration of glucocorticoids, growth hormone, or glucagon may ameliorate the symptoms. Diazoxide, phenytoin, and somatostatin are rarely effective.[312]

The prognosis depends to a great extent on the underlying disease. In a review of mesenchymal tumors associated with hypoglycemia, Anderson and Lokich noted that approximately 20 percent of the tumors are inoperable and that those which are operable generally recur locally rather than with distant metastases.[303] Most recurrences occur within 2 years of the primary surgery. A little more than a third of patients with resected thoracic tumors exhibit a recurrence, while close to two-thirds of abdominal lesions recur locally after the initial surgery. Approximately 25 percent of patients with thoracic tumors die of the disease, while almost half with abdominal tumors die as a direct result of the neoplasm. The prognosis for patients with primary hepatocellular carcinomas and malignant adrenocortical carcinomas associated with hypoglycemia is poor, with the majority of patients succumbing within 1 year of diagnosis.

Oncogenic Osteomalacia

In 1947, McCance described a teenage female with an osteoid tumor of the femur associated with osteomalacia which improved after removal of the tumor.[330] However, it was Prader and coworkers who suggested a cause-and-effect relation while describing an 11-year-old girl with osteomalacia associated with a giant cell reparative granuloma of a rib.[331] The osteomalacia improved after removal of the granuloma.[331] Subsequently, approximately 75 cases of oncogenic osteomalacia have been reported in the literature.[332]

Incidence and Tumor Types

Oncogenic osteomalacia appears to be rare, although it is likely that the association is underreported because these tumors are often small, usually measuring 1 to 4 cm in diameter, and are often located in unusual areas.[332] Since these tumors may be quite indolent, it is likely that many patients with mild "idiopathic hypophosphatemic osteomalacia" may actually have this syndrome. Indeed, this syndrome may occur relatively frequently with tumors such as prostatic carcinoma. Lyles and associates studied in detail two hypophosphatemic patients with prostatic carcinoma who had the typical clinical and biochemical findings of oncogenic osteomalacia.[333] They noted that 21 percent of the patients they studied with prostatic carcinoma had hypophosphatemia, raising the possibility that they also suffered from a milder form of oncogenic osteomalacia.[333]

The vast majority of tumors associated with this syndrome are mesenchymal-derived neoplasms that contain multinucleated giant cells, extensive vascularity, fibrous tissue, and often osteoid formation. The spectrum of tumors includes giant cell granulomas and tumors, hemangiomas, fibromas, hemangiopericytomas, fibroangiomas, osteoblastomas, chondromas or chondroblastomas, and fibrous xanthanomas.[334,335] Weidner and Santa Cruz classified the majority of these tumors into four groups: mixed connective tissue tumors in soft tissue with prominent vascularity and osteoclast-like giant cells, osteoblastoma-like tumors in the bone, nonossifying fibroma-like tumors in the bone, and ossifying fibroma-like tumors in the bone.[336] Although most tumors fall into this classification, not all do: Tumors such as prostatic carcinoma are of endodermal origin, and oat cell carcinoma, which has also been associated with this syndrome, is of neuroectodermal origin.[337] Other tumors associated with this syndrome include sarcoma, multiple myeloma, fibrous malignant histocytoma, neurofibromatosis, and neurinomas.[338–341] Electron microscopic studies of these tumors have not shown the presence of secretory granules.[332,340]

Approximately 10 percent of these tumors are malignant, and 5 percent are multiple.[334] Fifty-five percent are located in bone, approximately half of which are found in the long bones, including the femur and tibia.[332,342] Another common site of involvement is the head, with lesions being noted in the mandible, maxilla, skull, and ethmoid regions. Approximately 45 percent of these tumors are found in soft tissues including skin, with two-thirds of the soft tissue tumors being located in the legs.[332] The nasopharyngeal region is another site of soft tissue involvement.

Clinical Features and Biochemical Abnormalities

Over 90 percent of these patients present with generalized bone pain, especially involving the weight-bearing bones of the legs, ankles, hips, and lower back. Profound muscle weakness is present in two-thirds, with approximately 40 percent exhibiting abnormal gait or being bedridden. Fatigue, myalgias, and multiple fractures are also common complaints.[332,334,335,342] The average age at the time of diagnosis is 40 years, with a range of 7 to 73 years, and symptoms are present for an average of 5 years, with a range of 3 months to 17 years.[334,335,342] Both sexes are affected equally.

Hypophosphatemia is uniformly present, with a mean phosphate level of approximately 1.5 mg/dl.[332,334,335] Serum calcium concentrations are generally normal, and alkaline phosphatase levels are elevated. Virtually all these patients have a marked decrease in the renal tubular reabsorption of phosphate with phosphaturia. Calcium and phosphorus balance studies have also demonstrated a decrease in GI tract absorption of both minerals.[343] Parathyroid hormone and calcitonin levels are normal,[334,344] as are serum 25(OH)-vitamin D and 24,25$(OH)_2$-vitamin D levels.[334] 1,25$(OH)_2$-vitamin D levels are undetectable or low in over 80 percent of the patients in whom this metabolite has been measured.[332,334,343] One-third of these patients have aminoaciduria, and nearly half have glycosuria.[334,335,343,345]

Pathophysiology

These patients exhibit an acquired Fanconi-like proximal renal tubular reabsorption dysfunction manifested by phosphaturia, glycosuria, and aminoaciduria. In addition, they have a defect in the conversion of 25(OH)-vitamin D levels to 1,25$(OH)_2$-vitamin D in the proximal tubules, suggesting an inhibition of the 25(OH)-vitamin D-1α-hydroxylase enzyme present in the proximal tubule.

The etiology of the proximal tubular defect in these patients is unknown but is clearly humoral in nature and is associated with an underlying neoplasm. The evidence includes the association of the syndrome with the neoplasms, most of which are very similar pathologically; the disappearance of the syndrome after removal of the tumor; and the recurrence of the syndrome with recurrence of the neoplasm. The most convincing data come from experimental studies with tumor extracts and heterotransplantation. Saline extracts of tumors have been shown to induce phosphaturia and decrease tubular reabsorption of phosphate in puppies, rats, and mice.[346–350] Tumors propagated in nude mice have resulted in hypophosphatemia, hyperphosphaturia, and a defect in the conversion of 25(OH)-vitamin D to 1,25(OH)-vitamin D.[351–353] There are conflicting data concerning whether the material stimulates renal adenylate cyclase, with the most convincing data suggesting that it does not.[249,354] The nature of the material is unknown. It is destroyed by heat but not by trypsin treatment.[353] Fukumoto and coworkers pointed out the similarity between this syndrome and the features of maleic acid–induced proximal tubular dysfunction but were unable to demonstrate the presence of maleic acid in the serum or urine of the patient they studied.[345]

The clinical features clearly reflect the profound hypophosphatemia and reduced $1,25(OH)_2$-vitamin D levels. Bone biopsies demonstrate osteomalacia with increased osteoclastic bone resorption, which probably accounts for the maintenance of the normal serum calcium and normal parathyroid hormone level.[355] The decrease or inhibition of the 25(OH)-vitamin D-1α-hydroxylase enzyme is all the more striking considering the profound degree of hypophosphatemia, which should be a potent stimulus for the conversion of 25(OH)-vitamin D to $1,25(OH)_2$-vitamin D.

Differential Diagnosis

A number of conditions that result in osteomalacia and hypophosphatemia must be considered. These include nutritional deficiency in elderly housebound individuals, adult-onset hypophosphatasia, intestinal malabsorption, renal tubular acidosis, vitamin D–resistant rickets, chronic renal failure, phosphate-binding antacids, familial or acquired defects of renal tubular phosphate transport seen with X-linked hypophosphatemic rickets, Fanconi's syndrome, heavy metal poisoning, and cystinosis.[332,334,356]

These conditions can usually be eliminated from consideration through a careful family history, occupational and drug history, consideration of the age at onset, and performance of tests for urinary phosphoethanolamine and serum alkaline phosphatase to rule out adult-onset hypophosphatasia; fecal fat and D-xylose excretion for the evaluation of steatorrhea; ability of the urine to be acidified after ammonium chloride administration; and a screen for heavy metal poisoning with cadmium, lead, or copper.[343,356]

Therapy

Over 80 percent of patients are cured with removal of the tumor.[332] If one considers only symptomatic patients, over 90 percent have a complete disappearance of symptoms between 1 day and 1 year after total removal of the tumor. Within 1 to 2 days, the serum phosphate usually increases, the tubular reabsorption of phosphate returns to normal, and the phosphaturia ceases.[335] If the tumor recurs, the syndrome generally also recurs.[332]

Massive doses of vitamin D, 1-α-(OH)-D_3, and dihydrotachysterol have rarely been effective. Similarly, the administration of phosphate alone has not induced symptomatic remissions, although 15 to 30 percent of patients show some degree of improvement with the combination of phosphate and vitamin D administration.[332,334] The most effective medical therapy is the supplementation with $1,25(OH)_2$-vitamin D, which has led to improvement in up to 70 percent of the patients in whom it has been tried.[334,343] However, $1,25(OH)_2$-vitamin D alone rarely completely corrects the syndrome.

The prognosis for these patients is excellent, reflecting the generally benign nature of the majority of the underlying neoplasms.

Ectopic Growth Hormone and Growth Hormone Releasing Hormone Production

Ectopic Growth Hormone Production

In 1968, Steiner and associates described a patient with hypertrophic osteoarthropathy, adenocarcinoma of the lung, and elevated serum levels of growth hormone, which reverted to normal after removal of the tumor.[357] The following year, Cameron and coworkers described a similar patient with normal serum concentrations of growth hormone (GH) but elevated concentrations in the lung tumor in comparison to the surrounding normal lung tissue.[358] Subsequently, Greenberg and coworkers demonstrated the synthesis and release of GH from a poorly differentiated lung carcinoma associated with hypertrophic osteoarthropathy maintained in tissue culture for 4 months.[359] The tumor incorporated [^{14}C]leucine into growth hormone that comigrated with monomeric pituitary GH on both paper and Sephadex chromatography.

Immunoreactive GH has been found in 39 percent of bronchogenic carcinomas, including adenocarcinoma, large cell carcinomas, and small cell carcinoma, although no arterial-venous difference in GH concentrations across the tumors were found.[360] Close to two-thirds of gastric carcinomas have also been found to contain immunoreactive GH,[360] and all 12 breast carcinomas studied through immunohistochemistry by Ghosh and colleagues showed the presence of growth hormone–containing tumor cells.[361] The significance of these findings is open to question in view of the presence of both immunoreactive GH and receptor-assayable GH-like material that is present in a number of normal tissues including the liver, kidney, lung, muscle, colon, stomach, and brain.[18] In addition, the possibility that proteolytic enzymes present in tissues may degrade the radiolabeled GH used in the RIAs must be kept in mind. This possibility was illustrated by Caplan and associates, who described a young woman with acromegaly associated with a cystic beta cell adenoma of the pancreas.[362] The tumor tissue extract contained immunoreactive GH, which comigrated with GH extracted from normal human pituitary, and serial dilutions of the tumor extract also demonstrated parallelism to the reference GH. However, further investigation showed that the GH activity was spurious and was due to proteolytic enzyme damage of the tracer used in the RIA. The acromegaly in that patient was subsequently shown to be due to the secretion of growth hormone releasing hormone (GHRH) rather than GH.[363]

The clinical significance of the presence of GH in tumors is unclear. Many patients with lung cancer, carcinoids, and endometrial carcinoma either fail to suppress serum GH after a glucose load or show a paradoxic increase.[364–366] For a time, GH was considered a prime candidate for the humoral mediator of hypertrophic pulmonary osteoarthropathy. However, growth hormone is not uniformly elevated in patients with osteoarthropathy.[357,365] Full-blown acromegaly would be anticipated to be the consequence of the ectopic secretion of growth hormone. However, to date, only the patient described by Melmed and colleagues with acromegaly and an intramesenteric pancreatic islet-cell tumor fulfills the criteria for ectopic growth hormone production, attesting to its rarity.[35] Also, some of the abnormalities in GH secretion in patients with tumors may be due to the secretion of GHRH, somatostatin, or other substances.

Ectopic Production of Growth Hormone Releasing Hormone

In 1959, Altmann and Schutz described a patient who had acromegaly that did not respond to pituitary radiotherapy but remitted after the removal of a pulmonary carcinoid tumor.[367] In 1976, Sonksen and coworkers reported a patient with acromegaly whose hormonal abnormalities remitted after the removal of a bronchial carcinoid tumor that did not contain immunoreactive GH.[368] Subsequently, Shalet and colleagues described a similar patient and showed that the tumor cells grown in culture released a substance that stimulated GH secretion from rat pituitary cells.[369] Partial purification and characterization of GHRH was described by Frohman and associates in 1980, and in 1982 both Rivier and coworkers and Guillemin and colleagues independently isolated and clinically characterized GHRH from patients with GHRH-secreting pancreatic islet-cell tumors associated with acromegaly.[363,370–372]

Tumor Types

To date, there have been 33 well-described patients with ectopic GHRH production associated with clinical acromegaly (Table 29-18).[373–376] Most of these patients harbor a carcinoid, especially a bronchial carcinoid, or a pancreatic islet-cell tumor. Immunoreactive GHRH is present in a large proportion of carcinoids, islet-cell tumors, small cell carcinomas of the lung, pheochromocytomas, endometrial carcinomas, and medullary carcinomas of the thyroid tumor tissue extracts.[374–376] GHRH has been localized immunohistochemically in islet-cell tumors; carcinoid tumors of the lung, thymus, appendix, and cecum; medullary carcinoma of the thyroid; small cell carcinoma of the lung; and pheochromocytoma.[377–380]

Many of these tumors contain other hormones as assessed by immunohistochemical means. Thus, somatostatin, gastrin, gastrin-releasing peptide, calci-

TABLE 29-18 Tumors Associated with Ectopic GHRH Production

	Clinical Acromegaly	Immunochemical Studies			
		Immunohistochemical presence of GHRH in tumor		Immunoreactive GHRH in tumors	
Tumor Type	Total (malignant)	N	Positive, %	N	Positive, %
Carcinoid	19 (7)	92	17	15	87
Bronchial	16 (5)	10	10		
Intestinal	3 (2)	82	18		
Pancreatic islet-cell	9 (3)	81	17	49	37
Small cell carcinoma of lung	2 (2)			13	69
Sympathetic neural tumors	2 (0)	13	15	38	53
Adrenal adenoma	1 (0)	—	—	—	—
Medullary carcinoma of thyroid		—	—	8	50

Source: From references 373–376.

tonin, insulin, glucagon, vasoactive intestinal peptide, pancreatic polypeptide, and ACTH have been described in association with GHRH-secreting tumors.[374,375]

There is molecular heterogeneity of the GHRH produced by tumors. The predominant forms are GHRH (1-40)OH and GHRH (1-44)NH_2, with lesser amounts of GHRH (1-37)OH.[374,375] Additionally, a single patient was found to have the biologically inactive GHRH (3-40)OH in his serum.[374] These findings suggest that variable posttranslation proteolysis occurs to modify the forms of GHRH produced by the tumors.

Clinical Features

Patients with GHRH-secreting tumors associated with acromegaly present at an average age of approximately 40 years with typical acromegalic features. The diagnosis is made approximately 8 years after the onset of the disease and is somewhat shorter in patients with pancreatic islet-cell tumors and longer in patients with pulmonary carcinoid neoplasms. There is a female predominance, with a female to male ratio of 2.7:1. In addition to the acromegalic features, other endocrine abnormalities may coexist. These include the Zollinger-Ellison syndrome, insulin-induced hypoglycemia, galactorrhea, and hyperparathyroidism with pancreatic islet-cell tumors; galactorrhea, Cushing's syndrome, and carcinoid syndrome with carcinoid tumors; and catecholamine excess with pheochromocytomas.[375] GHRH-secreting tumors may also be present as part of the multiple endocrine neoplasia 1 (MEN 1) syndrome. Symptoms from the mass effects of the underlying neoplasm also may be present and are especially apparent with the bronchial carcinoids, which may produce cough, hemoptysis, atelectasis, and recurrent pneumonias that follow obstructive pulmonary infections. Slightly over one-third of these tumors are malignant, although most are slow-growing.

Diagnosis

The diagnosis of GHRH-secreting tumors is often made serendipitously after an attempt at neurosurgical removal of a suspected growth hormone-secreting pituitary adenoma, at which time somatotroph hyperplasia is found rather than a pituitary adenoma (with one exception in a patient with MEN).[381,382] Since somatotroph hyperplasia and the excessive secretion of GH from the hyperplastic somatotrophs are direct results of excessive GHRH stimulation, a search for a source of GHRH may then uncover the neoplasm. In addition to peripheral sources of ectopic GHRH secretion, the possibility that the GHRH excess is due to eutopic secretion from a hypothalamic hamartoma, choristoma, glioma, or gangliocytoma must be considered.[383]

The standard diagnostic tests for acromegaly do not differentiate GH-secreting pituitary adenomas from GHRH-secreting tumors. In both conditions, the sella turcica may be enlarged and there may appear to be an intrasellar tumor. Similarly, with both conditions, GH does not suppress appropriately after the administration of glucose, immunoreactive GH in the serum may rise after a bolus injection of thyrotropin releasing hormone (TRH) of after insulin-induced hypoglycemia, and either no response or a rise in serum GH may occur after the administration of exogenous GHRH.[375,376,383] The only test that clearly differentiates the two conditions is measurement of peripheral levels of GHRH. Normal individuals generally have GHRH levels of 10 pg/ml or less, while patients with GHRH-secreting tumors have levels that range between 300 pg/ml and 50 ng/ml.[375]

Therapy

The most effective therapy for these patients is removal of the neoplasm. When this is accomplished, the acromegaly in virtually all patients remits and the GH secretory dynamics return to normal. Even after partial debulking of tumors in the presence of metastatic disease, there may be improvement in the acromegaly.[375] In patients with persistent disease, the somatostatin analogue octreotide has led to clinical and biochemical improvement in the acromegaly as well as reduction in GH and GHRH levels, indicating that the drug has a peripheral effect on the tumor as well as its known effect on the pituitary somatotrophs.[383] Dopamine agonists are not useful. The long-term prognosis of these patients is unclear, although only approximately 10 to 15 percent have died directly from the disease.[375]

Ectopic Production of Placental Proteins

Human Chorionic Gonadotropin

Human chorionic gonadotropin is a eutopic product of gestational and nongestational trophoblastic disease. Before the development of the β-hCG RIA, several case reports described patients with the ectopic production of hCG. The associated tumors were bronchogenic carcinoma, hepatoma or hepatoblastoma, adrenocortical carcinoma, melanoma, an undifferentiated retroperitoneal carcinoma, breast carcinoma, and renal cell carcinoma.[384] Two clinical syndromes were present in most of the patients reported. Adult males exhibited gynecomastia and occasionally other signs of feminization, and isosexual precocious puberty was present in young boys with hCG-secreting hepatoblastomas.[384,385] After the development of sensitive and specific hCG RIAs, immunoreactive hCG was found to be present in approximately 18 percent of patients with a wide variety of nontrophoblastic neoplasms (Table 29-9).[105] Most of these patients do not have clinical symptoms attributable to the hCG primarily because the quantities of hCG are quite low in all but a fraction of them. Since an hCG-like substance is present in the blood of normal individuals and patients with a variety of benign diseases (Table 29-10), hCG measurements are not useful as a screening test for nontrophoblastic neoplasms. In addition, the presence or absence of hCG and the quantitative levels generally show poor correlation with the stage of disease, may not show concordant changes with disease progression or regression, and have little or no prognostic value.[105] Recently, there has been interest in the measurement of a fragment of the β subunit of hCG, the β-core fragment, which is present in the urine of one-half to three-quarters of patients with cancer and 6 percent of nonpregnant healthy individuals.[386,387] Whether this will be a useful tumor marker for patients with nontrophic neoplasms is unknown.

Human Placental Lactogen

Human placental lactogen (hPL), which, like hCG, is normally secreted by the syncytiotrophoblast of the placenta during pregnancy, is also found in patients with gestational and nongestational trophoblastic disease. However, unlike hCG, serial measurements of hPL in those conditions are not useful for monitoring the effects of therapy because the concentrations of this hormone are generally low. hPL has also been noted to be produced ectopically by nontrophoblastic neoplasms, especially those of gynecologic or GI tract origin (Table 29-19).[105] Although overall approximately 14 percent of patients with cancers may have small quantities of immunoreactive hPL in their sera, close to half the tumor specimens that have been examined immunohistochemically for the presence of hPL have been found to contain cells that stain positively for this hormone.[388–391] However, hPL has also been detected by immunohistochemical techniques in approximately 13 percent of benign breast disease, and the specificity of hPL as a tumor marker thus is questionable.[390,391] As with hCG, hPL measurements do not consistently correlate with disease stage or changes in tumor mass or provide prognostic information.[28,382–394]

TABLE 29-19 Immunoreactive hPL in Sera of Patients with Cancer and Control Patients

Tumor or Site	*N*		Positive, %	
Patients with cancer				
Gynecologic	344		30.8	
Ovary		219		38.4
Cervix		125		17.6
Gastrointestinal	274		13.5	
Esophagus		16		0
Gastric		46		26.1
Colon/rectum		174		9.2
Hepatic		24		29.2
Biliary		13		15.4
Leukemia	13		7.7	
Lung	64		4.7	
Prostate	57		0	
Miscellaneous	60		15	
Total	812		14.3	
Controls	*N*		Positive, %	
Normal volunteers	455		0	
Benign disease	180		0	
Breast		57		0
Gastrointestinal		54		0
Genitourinary		19		0
Other		50		0
Total	630		0	

Source: From Braunstein[105] with permission.

Paraneoplastic Erythrocytosis

Polycythemia is associated with benign and malignant lesions of the kidney as well as neoplasms of the liver, cerebellum, uterus, and adrenal (Table 29-20).[395–399] In the majority of the patients studied, elevations of the serum or tissue levels of erythropoietin have been noted (Table 29-21).[395,400–405] Approximately 3 to 4 percent of patients with hypernephroma, 3 to 12 percent of patients with hepatocellular carcinoma, and 9 to 20 percent of patients with cerebellar hemangioblastoma exhibit erythrocytosis.[45,396,406,407]

Since erythropoietin is normally produced by the kidney and liver, the production of excessive quantities of this hormone in benign and malignant renal and hepatic disorders probably represents eutopic production. Most of the data concerning erythropoietin production by tumors have come from studies of renal cell carcinoma. Several investigators have

TABLE 29-20 Paraneoplastic Erythrocytosis Associated with Neoplasms and Other Pathologic Conditions in 340 Patients

Site of Pathology	% of Total	
Kidney	52.6	
Hypernephroma		35.3
Cystic kidney		10.3
Hydronephrosis		4.1
Wilms' tumor		0.9
Hemangioma		0.9
Adenoma		0.6
Sarcoma		0.6
Liver (primarily hepatoma)	18.8	
Central nervous system (cerebellar hemangioblastoma)	14.7	
Uterus (fibromyoma)	7.4	
Adrenal (adrenocortical adenoma, carcinoma; pheochromocytoma)	3.2	
Ovary	2.1	
Lung	0.9	
Thymus	0.3	

Source: From Hammond and Winnick,[395] with permission. Also noted with leiomyoma of esophagus and skin,[396] fibrous histiocytoma of parotid,[397] hepatic hemangioma,[398] and breast cancer.[399]

TABLE 29-21 Proportion of Patients with Paraneoplastic Erythrocytosis Who Exhibit Elevations of Serum and Tissue Erythropoietin Concentrations

	Increased Serum Erythropoietin		Increased Tissue Erythropoietin	
Condition	*N* total	*N* elevated (%)	*N* total	*N* elevated (%)
Cystic kidney	11	5 (45)	12	10 (83)
Hypernephroma	10	9 (90)	13	11 (85)
Hepatoma	9	6 (67)	8	2 (25)
Cerebellar hemangio-blastoma	10	6 (60)	6	6 (100)
Uterine fibromyoma	6	0 (0)	6	2 (33)
Hydronephrosis	5	4 (80)	2	0 (0)
Pheochromocytoma	2	2	1	1
Wilms' tumor	2	2	2	2

Source: From references 395 and 400–405.

demonstrated the secretion of erythropoietin by tumor cells in vitro[408–410] as well as the presence of erythropoietin mRNA by in situ hybridization in several hypernephromas with an absence of the mRNA in adjacent normal kidney cells.[405] The erythropoietin from a cerebellar cyst was physiochemically similar to erythropoietin derived from anemic patients.[411] In addition to the eutopic or ectopic production of erythropoietin, other mechanisms may be responsible for erythrocytosis. Thus, virilizing ovarian or adrenal tumors which secrete androgens may lead to the stimulation of erythropoiesis. Glucocorticoid-producing adrenal tumors may result in "stress polycythemia," and excessive production of prostaglandin A or E may stimulate erythropoiesis through enhancement of erythropoietin action on the erythrocyte progenitor cells in the marrow.[395]

The diagnosis of polycythemia is generally made fortuitously when a serum hematocrit is found to be elevated above 55 percent in a male and 50 percent in a female, reflecting the increase in total red cell mass. In most instances, the erythrocytosis is asymptomatic, although venous thrombosis may occur as an unusual complication.[402] Paraneoplastic erythrocytosis may be differentiated from dehydration with hemoconcentration and stress polycythemia through the absence of clinical findings of dehydration and the presence of an increase in the total red cell mass, which is elevated in paraneoplastic erythrocytosis but normal in stress polycythemia. Measurements of the partial pressure of oxygen in arterial blood and hemoglobin electrophoresis allow differentiation from secondary polycythemia due to hypoxia or the presence of a hemoglobinopathy. Erythrocytosis is a prominent feature of polycythemia vera, but these patients also exhibit pancytosis with elevations of the white cell and platelet counts as well as splenomegaly. Erythropoietin RIAs are available commercially, and elevated serum erythropoietin concentrations are found in patients with paraneoplastic erythrocytosis as well as other secondary causes of polycythemia, while the levels tend to be normal or low in patients with polycythemia vera.[401]

Successful removal of the erythropoietin-producing tumor is associated with a decrease in erythropoietin levels and a decrease in the erythrocytosis.[395] If tumor removal is not possible and the patient develops the symptomatic form of polycythemia, phlebotomy may relieve the symptoms.[402]

Ectopic Production of Calcitonin

Serum calcitonin measurements are useful for the diagnosis and monitoring of therapy in patients with medullary carcinoma of the thyroid or C cell hyperplasia. In 1970, Milhaud and coworkers described a patient with hypercalcitonemia associated with a bronchial carcinoid tumor.[412] Since then, several investigators have measured calcitonin in the serum of patients with neoplasms and overall have found elevations in approximately half the patients studied and 6.7 percent of patients with benign disorder (Table 29-22).[413–424] Many of the tumors associated with hypercalcitonemia have APUD characteristics and include small cell carcinoma of the lung, carcinoid tumors, pheochromocytomas, melanoma, and islet-cell tumors. Elevated tissue calcitonin concentrations have been found in 95 percent of APUD-type tumors and close to 40 percent of tumors without APUD characteristics.[425] Although some investigators have been unable to detect calcitonin in normal tissues,[419,425] others have been able to extract calcitonin from a variety of normal tissues or demonstrate calcitonin by immunohistochemical techniques in normal tissues.[426,427] Between 16 and 38 percent of the patients studied have had a rise in serum calcitonin levels after pentagastrin administration, although the increase is proportionally less than that found in patients with medullary carcinoma of the thyroid.[417,418,424]

The source of the calcitonin excess in patients

TABLE 29-22 Serum Immunoreactive Calcitonin Levels in Patients with Malignancies and Benign Diseases

Tumor	Number Positive/ Total Number		Positive, %	
Lung	127/257		49.4	
Small cell		91/147		61.9
Squamous		15/55		27.3
Adenocarcinoma		16/38		42.1
Anaplastic/ large cell		4/13		30.8
Alveolar		1/4		25.0
Carcinoid	5/11		45.5	
Breast	36/73		49.3	
Colon	8/30		26.7	
Stomach	4/11		36.4	
Esophagus	0/2		0	
Pancreatic	6/15		40	
Melanoma	4/10		40	
Leukemia	48/57		84.2	
CGL		32/33		97
AML		8/8		100
Other myeloproliferative		8/11		72.7
CLL		0/10		0
ALL		0/2		0
Miscellaneous	3/10		30	
Total	289/540		52.0	
Benign				
Normal and miscellaneous controls	2/100		2	
Benign breast	0/75		0	
GI	13/59		22	
Benign pulmonary	5/65		7.7	
Total	20/299		6.7	

Source: From references 413-424.

with nonmedullary cancers is unclear, since a catheterization study in such patients demonstrated that four of six patients had elevated calcitonin levels emanating from the thyroid rather than from the tumor.[416,428] The apparent high frequency of hypercalcitonemia in patients with neoplasms may actually be an artifact in some assays. Roos and colleagues showed that heating of serum from patients with squamous cell carcinoma and hypercalcitonemia abolished the elevated immunoreactive calcitonin but did not alter the immunoreactive calcitonin present in patients with small cell carcinoma of the lung or adenocarcinoma of the lung.[429] Nevertheless, it is clear that some tumors are capable of synthesizing and secreting calcitonin. Tumor cells derived from squamous cell carcinoma of the lung, small cell carcinoma of the lung, and breast carcinoma have been shown to produce immunoreactive calcitonin in vitro.[415,430–432] A calcitonin-producing breast carcinoma was propagated in nude mice and continued to proliferate and secrete calcitonin.[415]

In culture, several of these tumors produce high-molecular-mass species of calcitonin including 40-, 13-, and 10-kDa proteins.[415,432,433] In the BEN squamous cell carcinoma of the lung cell line, both high-molecular-mass species and biologically active 3500-dalton calcitonin are secreted.[431] A greater proportion of the immunoreactive calcitonin present in the circulation of patients with nonthyroid tumors exists in large-molecular-weight forms than is found in the plasma of patients with medullary carcinoma of the thyroid.[429] The calcitonin mRNA from the BEN cell line closely resembles the calcitonin mRNA from medullary carcinoma of the thyroid, as do the translation products produced in a wheat germ system. However, other human lung tumor cell lines which contain mRNA for both calcitonin and calcitonin gene–related product have calcitonin mRNA that is larger than that found in medullary thyroid carcinoma.[434] Thus, as is the case with ectopic ACTH-secreting tumors, some calcitonin-secreting neoplasms may exhibit abnormalities in transcription of the calcitonin mRNA or posttranslational processing of the synthesized preprocalcitonin or procalcitonin.

There are no clinical manifestations of calcitonin excess in patients with nonthyroid neoplasms. The differential diagnosis of hypercalcitonemia in these patients includes the presence of chronic renal failure, acute pancreatitis, sepsis, hypercalcemia, and pernicious anemia.[103,435]

Other Hormones Produced by Tumors

Prolactin

In 1971, Turkington described a 53-year-old male with an undifferentiated bronchogenic carcinoma who exhibited hyperprolactinemia, which decreased after a course of radiation therapy to the tumor.[436] He also described a 49-year-old woman with hypernephroma, hyperprolactinemia, and galactorrhea who exhibited a return of prolactin to the normal range after surgical resection of the tumor. The hypernephroma was grown in culture and continued to release prolactin over a 2-week period.[436] Turkington noted that only 1 of 21 patients with lung cancer had hyperprolactinemia. In contrast, one-third of 21 patients with lung cancer studied by Davis and colleagues had hyperprolactinemia, although none exhibited gynecomastia, galactorrhea, or hypogonadism.[437] In patients who were tested, there was a normal prolactin response to L-dopa and TRH. There was no correlation with the presence or absence of hyperprolactinemia or the quantitative level of the prolactin elevation and the histology or tumor burden in these patients.[437] In a larger study, Molitch and coworkers examined 215 patients with cancer and found that 15 (7 percent) had hyperprolactinemia.[438] However, 12 of these 15 patients were receiving phenothiazines or opiates or had undergone prior radiation therapy to the chest wall or brain, which could account for the prolactin elevation. In fact, only two patients (1 percent) had hyperprolactinemia without another known cause being present. Immunoreactive prolactin has been found in a variety of tumor tissues and cell lines.[439,440] Nevertheless, true ectopic secretion of prolactin by tumors in vivo appears to be quite limited.

Vasoactive Intestinal Peptide

The syndrome of "pancreatic cholera," also referred to as the WDHA syndrome (*w*atery *d*iarrhea, *h*ypokalemia, and *a*chlorhydria) or Verner-Morrison syndrome, is associated with excessive production of VIP and is usually associated with a non-β-cell tumor of the pancreatic islets. Using a sensitive RIA, Said and Faloona found elevated VIP concentrations in five of six patients with lung carcinoma and in a patient with a ganglioneuroblastoma of the adrenal and another patient with a pheochromocytoma.[441] Elevated levels of VIP were also present in the tumor tissue.[441] Subsequent studies demonstrated an arterial-venous difference in VIP concentration across a malignant renal APUDoma associated with this syndrome[442] and the presence of VIP by immunoperoxidase staining in ganglioneuromas, ganglioneuroblastomas, and neuroblastomas.[443,444] Removal of the tumor is effective in lowering plasma VIP concentrations and reversing the syndrome. For tumors that are nonmetastatic or nonoperable, the long-acting somatostatin analogue octreotide may be effective in suppressing VIP production by these tumors, as has been shown in patients with VIP-secreting non-β-islet-cell tumors of the pancreas.[445]

Somatostatin

Elevated concentrations of plasma immunoreactive somatostatin have been identified in patients with small cell carcinoma of the lung and carcinoid tumors, often in association with the ectopic production of ACTH.[425,446] Elevated concentrations of somatostatin have also been identified in tumor extracts from carcinoids and small cell cancer of the lung as well as in small cell cancer of the lung cell lines.[425,446,447] There is a substantial amount of heterogeneity in the somatostatin molecules that have been extracted from tumor tissues, with species measuring 13, 3 to 4, and 1.6 kDas being noted.[446] No clinical manifestations have been described from the excessive production of somatostatin by these tumors, probably because the actual concentrations of somatostatin in the plasma are rather low in comparison to the concentrations in patients with pancreatic somatostatinomas.[446]

Other Gastrointestinal Hormones

Ectopic gastrin production associated with the Zollinger-Ellison syndrome has been noted with an ovarian cystadenoma and a pancreatic cystadenocarcinoma.[448,449]

Glucagon has been described in a patient with a renal endocrine tumor who exhibited edema, rash, malabsorption, villous hypertrophy of the small intestine, and decreased motility of the jejunum and colon, which reversed after removal of the tumor.[450] Hunstein and coworkers reported a 76-year-old male with a glucagon-secreting large cell carcinoma of the lung who exhibited a typical glucagonoma syndrome with necrolytic migratory erythema, glucose intolerance, and weight loss.[451] Elevated glucagon levels were present in the patient's plasma, and immunoreactive glucagon was found in the carcinoma cells, with no abnormalities noted in the pancreas.[451] Immunoreactive glucagon also has been found in lung carcinoma and ovarian carcinoid tumors.[451,452]

Immunoreactive bombesin-like peptide, which probably represents its mammalian counterpart, gastrin-releasing peptide, has been found in a variety of tumors, including lung cancers associated with ectopic ACTH, carcinoid tumors, medullary carcinoma of the thyroid, and pheochromocytoma. Increased levels have also been found in the peripheral circulation of two patients with bronchial carcinoids and one with medullary carcinoma of the thyroid.[453] No clinical symptoms have been attributed to excessive quantities of this peptide.

Renin

Renin production has been associated with several tumors, including Wilms' tumor (nephroblastoma), juxtaglomerular cell tumors (hemangiopericytomas), and hypernephroma, which may be considered to be eutopic sources of the hormone.[454–459] Ectopic production has been found in ovarian carcinomas, pancreatic adenocarcinomas, and lung tumors.[460–463] Some of the renin-producing tumors are associated with hypokalemic alkalosis and hypertension, while other are not. In addition to renin, prorenin may be secreted by these tumors.[460,463] Removal of the tumors cures the hypertension and hypokalemia. Unresectable lesions may be treated with inhibitors of angiotensin-converting enzyme.[462]

REFERENCES

1. Hall TC: Ectopic synthesis and paraneoplastic syndromes. *Cancer Res* 34:2088, 1974.
2. Naschitz JE, Abrahamson J, Yeshurun D: Clinical significance of paraneoplastic syndrome. *Oncology* 46:40, 1989.
3. Antel JP, Moumdjian R: Paraneoplastic syndromes: A role for the immune system. *J Neurol* 236:1, 1989.
4. Anhalt GJ, Kim SC, Stanley JR, et al: Paraneoplastic pemphigus. An autoimmune mucocutaneous disease associated with neoplasia. *N Engl J Med* 323:1729, 1990.
5. Costanza ME, Perin V, Schwartz RS, Nathansen L: Carcinoembryonic antigen-antibody complexes in a patient with colonic carcinoma and nephrotic syndrome. *N Engl J Med* 289:520, 1973.

6. Richard-Mendes da Costa C, Dupont E, Hamers R, Hooghe R, Dupuis F, Potuliege R: Nephrotic syndrome in bronchogenic carcinoma: Report of two cases with immunochemical studies. *Clin Nephrol* 2:245, 1974.
7. Fichman M, Bethune J: Effects of neoplasms on renal electrolyte function. *Ann NY Acad Sci* 230:448, 1974.
8. Friou GJ: Current knowledge and concepts of the relationship of malignancy, autoimmunity, and immunologic disease. *Ann NY Acad Sci* 230:23, 1974.
9. Richardson EP Jr: Our evolving understanding of progressive multifocal leukoencephalopathy. *Ann NY Acad Sci* 230:358, 1974.
10. Marks LJ, Steinke J, Podolsky S, Egdahl RH: Hypoglycemia associated with neoplasia. *Ann NY Acad Sci* 230:147, 1974.
11. Miller AM, McGarry MP: A diffusible stimulator of eosinophilopoiesis produced by lymphoid cells as demonstrated with diffusion chambers. *Blood* 48:293, 1976.
12. Pineo GF, Brain MC, Gallus AS, Hirsch J, Hatton MWC, Regoeczi E: Tumors, mucus production, and hypercoagulability. *Ann NY Acad Sci* 230:262, 1984.
13. Odell WD: Paraendocrine syndromes of cancer. *Adv Intern Med* 34:325, 1989.
14. Braunstein GD, Rasor JL, Wade ME: Presence in normal human testes of a chorionic-gonadotropin-like substance distinct from human luteinizing hormone. *N Engl J Med* 293:1339, 1975.
15. Braunstein GD: Production of human chorionic gonadotropin by nontrophoblastic tumors and tissues, in Tomoda Y, Mitzutani S, Narita O, Klopper A (eds): *Placental and Endometrial Proteins: Basic and Clinical Aspects*. Utrecht, The Netherlands, VNU Science Press, 1988, pp 493–502.
16. Yoshimoto Y, Wolfsen AR, Odell WD: Human chorionic gonadotropin-like substance in nonendocrine tissues of normal subjects. *Science* 197:575, 1977.
17. Rosenzweig JL, Havrankova J, Lesniak MA, Brownstein M, Roth J: Insulin is ubiquitous in extra pancreatic tissues of rats and humans. *Proc Natl Acad Sci* USA 77:572, 1980.
18. Kyle CV, Evans MC, Odell WD: Growth hormone-like material in normal human tissues. *J Clin Endocrinol Metab* 53:1138, 1981.
19. Saito E, Iwasa S, Odell WD: Widespread presence of large molecular weight adrenocorticotropin-like substances in normal rat extrapituitary tissues. *Endocrinology* 113:1010, 1983.
20. Suda T, Tomori N, Tozawa F, Demura H, Shizume K, Mouri T, Miura Y, Sasano N: Immunoreactive corticotropin and corticotropin-releasing factor in human hypothalamus, adrenal, lung cancer and pheochromocytoma. *J Clin Endocrinol Metab* 58:919, 1984.
21. Strewler GJ, Nissenson RA: Hypercalcemia in malignancy. *West J Med* 153:635, 1990.
22. Said SI, Rosenberg RN: Vasoactive intestinal polypeptide: Abundant immunoreactivity in neural cell lines and normal nervous tissue. *Science* 192:907, 1976.
23. Fischer JA, Tobler PH, Kaufmann M, Born W, Henke H, Copper PE, Sagar SM, Martin JB: Calcitonin: Regional distribution of the hormone and its binding sites in the human brain pituitary. *Proc Natl Acad Sci USA* 78:7801, 1981.
24. Kew MC, Kirschner MA, Abrahams GE, Katz M: Mechanism of feminization in primary liver cancer. *N Engl J Med* 296:1084, 1977.
25. Kirschner MA, Lippman A, Berkowitz R, Mayrer E, Drejka M: Estrogen production as a tumor marker in patients with gonadotropin-producing neoplasms. *Cancer Res* 41:1447, 1981.
26. Kuida CA, Braunstein GD, Shintaku P, Said JW: Human chorionic gonadotropin expression in lung, breast, and renal carcinoma. *Arch Pathol Lab Med* 112:282, 1987.
27. Braunstein GD, McIntire KR, Waldmann TA: Discordance of human chorionic gonadotropin and alpha-fetoprotein in testicular teratocarcinomas. *Cancer* 31:1065, 1973.
28. Samaan NA, Smith JP, Rutledge FN, Schultz PN: The significance of measurement of human placental lactogen, human chorionic gonadotropin, and carcinoembryonic antigen in patients with ovarian carcinoma. *Am J Obstet Gynecol* 126:186, 1976.
29. Sussman HH, Weintraub BD, Rosen SW: Relationship of ectopic placental alkaline phosphatase to ectopic chorionic gonadotropin and placental lactogen: Discordance of three "markers" for cancer. *Cancer* 33:820, 1974.
30. Samaan NA, Hickey RC, Hill CS Jr, Medellin H, Gates RB: Parathyroid tumors: Preoperative localization and association with other tumors. *Cancer* 33:933, 1974.
31. Farr HW, Fahey TJ Jr, Nash AG, Farr CM: Primary hyperparathyroidism and cancer. *Am J Surg* 126:539, 1973.
32. Drezner MK, Lebovitz HE: Primary hyperparathyroidism in paraneoplastic hypercalcemia. *Lancet* 1:1004, 1977.
33. Unger RH, Lochner J de V, Eisentraut AM: Identification of insulin and glucagon in a bronchogenic metastasis. *J Clin Endocrinol Metab* 24:823, 1964.
34. Schorr I, Rathnam P, Saxena BB, Ney RL: Multiple specific hormone receptors in the adenylate cyclase of an adrenocortical carcinoma. *J Biol Chem* 246:5806, 1971.
35. Melmed S, Ezrin C, Kovacs K, Goodman RS, Frohman LA: Acromegaly due to secretion of growth hormone by an ectopic pancreatic islet-cell tumor. *N Engl J Med* 312:9, 1985.
36. Woodard HQ: Changes in blood chemistry associated with carcinoma metastatic to bone. *Cancer* 6:1219, 1953.
37. Jessiman AG, Emerson K Jr, Shah RC, Moore FD: Hypercalcemia in carcinoma of the breast. *Ann Surg* 157:377, 1963.
38. Galasko CSB, Burn JI: Hypercalcemia in patients with advanced mammary cancer. *Br Med J* 2:573, 1971.
39. Kato Y, Ferguson TB, Bennett DE, Burford TH: Oat cell carcinoma of the lung: A review of 138 cases. *Cancer* 23:517, 1969.
40. Warren MM, Utz DG, Kelalis PP: Concurrence of hypernephroma and hypercalcemia. *Ann Surg* 174:863, 1971.
41. Davis HL Jr, Wiseley AN, Ramirez G, Ansfield FJ: Hypercalcemia complicating breast cancer: Clinical features and management. *Oncology* 28:126, 1973.
42. Bender RA, Hansen H: Hypercalcemia in bronchogenic carcinoma: A prospective study of 200 patients. *Ann Intern Med* 80:205, 1974.
43. Rees LH, Ratcliffe JG: Ectopic hormone production by nonendocrine tumours. *Clin Endocrinol (Oxf)* 2:263, 1974.
44. Eagan RT, Maurer LH, Forcier RJ, Tulloh M: Small cell carcinoma of the lung: Staging, paraneoplastic syndromes, treatment and survival. *Cancer* 33:527, 1974.
45. Chisholm GD: Nephrogenic ridge tumors and their syndromes. *Ann NY Acad Sci* 230:403, 1974.
46. Richardson RL, Greco FA, Oldham RK, Liddle GW: Tumor products and potential markers in small cell lung cancer. *Semin Oncol* 5:253, 1978.
47. Hansen M, Hammer M, Hummer L: Diagnostic and therapeutic implications of ectopic hormone production in small cell carcinoma of the lung. *Thorax* 35:101, 1980.
48. Hansen M, Hansen HH, Hirsch FR, Arends J, Christensen JD, Christensen JM, Hummer L, Kuhl C: Hormonal polypeptides and amine metabolites in small cell carcinoma of the lung, with special reference to stage and subtypes. *Cancer* 45:1432, 1980.
49. Comis RL, Miller M, Ginsberg SJ: Abnormalities in water homeostasis in small cell anaplastic lung cancer. *Cancer* 45:2414, 1980.
50. Burt ME, Brennan MF: Incidence of hypercalcemia and malignant neoplasm. *Arch Surg* 115:704, 1980.
51. Lokich J: The frequency and clinical biology of the ectopic hormone syndromes of small cell carcinoma. *Cancer* 50:2111, 1982.
52. Merrill WW, Bondy PK: Production of biochemical marker substances by bronchogenic carcinomas. *Clin Chest Med* 3:307, 1982.
53. Hainsworth JD, Workman R, Greco FA: Management of the syndrome of inappropriate antidiuretic hormone secretion in small cell lung cancer. *Cancer* 51:161, 1983.

54. De la Monte SM, Hutchins GM, Moore GW: Paraneoplastic syndromes and constitutional symptoms in prediction of metastatic behavior of small cell carcinoma of the lung. *Am J Med* 77:851, 1984.
55. Laski ME, Vugrin D: Paraneoplastic syndromes in hypernephroma. *Semin Nephrol* 7:123, 1987.
56. Amatruda TT Jr, Upton GV: Hyperadrenocorticism and ACTH-releasing factor. *Ann NY Acad Sci* 230:168, 1974.
57. Canellos GP: Hypercalcemia in malignant lymphoma and leukemia. *Ann NY Acad Sci* 230:240, 1974.
58. Gilbey ED, Bondy PK, Fosling M: Impaired water excretion in oat cell lung cancer. *Br J Cancer* 34:323, 1976.
59. Gewirtz G, Yalow RS: Ectopic ACTH production in carcinoma of the lung. *J Clin Invest* 53:1022, 1974.
60. Wolfsen AR, Odell WD: ProACTH: Use for early detection of lung cancer. *Am J Med* 66:765, 1979.
61. Odell WD, Wolfsen AR, Bachelot I, Hirose F: Ectopic production of lipotropin by cancer. *Am J Med* 66:631, 1979.
62. Ratcliffe JG, Podmore J, Stack BHR, et al: Circulating ACTH and related peptides in lung cancer. *Br J Cancer* 45:230, 1982.
63. Trump DL, Abeloff MD, Hsu TH: Frequency of abnormalities of cortisol secretion and water metabolism in patients with small cell carcinoma of the lung and other malignancies. *Chest* 81:576, 1982.
64. Maurer LH, O'Donnell JF, Kennedy S, Faulkner CS, Rist K, North WG: Human neurophysins in carcinoma of the lung: Relation to histology, disease stage, response rate, survival, and syndrome of inappropriate antidiuretic hormone secretion. *Cancer Treat Rep* 67:971, 1983.
65. Odell WD, Wolfsen AR, Yoshimoto Y, Weitzman R, Fisher D, Hirose FM: Ectopic peptide synthesis: A universal concomitant of neoplasia. *Trans Assoc Am Physicians* 90:204, 1977.
66. Rees LH: Concepts in ectopic hormone production. *Clin Endocrinol (Oxf)* 5:363s, 1976.
67. Levine RJ, Metz SA: A classification of ectopic hormone-producing tumors. *Ann NY Acad Sci* 230:533, 1974.
68. Orth DN: Ectopic hormone production, in Felig P, Baxter JD, Broadus AE, Frohman LA (eds): *Endocrinology and Metabolism,* 2d ed. New York, McGraw-Hill, 1987, pp 1692–1735.
69. Bailey RE: Periodic hormonogenesis—a new phenomenon: Periodicity in function of a hormone-producing tumour in man. *J Clin Endocrinol Metab* 32:317, 1971.
70. Kirschner MA, Wider JA, Ross GT: Leydig cell function in men with gonadotrophin producing testicular tumors. *J Clin Endocrinol Metab* 30:504, 1970.
71. Gropp C, Havemann K, Scheuer A: Ectopic hormones in lung cancer patients at diagnosis and during therapy. *Cancer* 46:347, 1980.
72. Yalow RS, Eastridge CE, Higgins G, Wolf J: Plasma and tumour ACTH in carcinoma of the lung. *Cancer* 44:1789, 1979.
73. Ayvazian LF, Schneider B, Gewirtz G, Yalow RS: Ectopic production of big ACTH in carcinoma of the lung. *Am Rev Respir Dis* 111:279, 1975.
74. Torstensson S, Thoren M, Hall K: Plasma ACTH in patients with bronchogenic carcinoma. *Acta Med Scand* 207:353, 1980.
75. Doege DW: Fibrosarcoma of the mediastinum. *Ann Surg* 92:955, 1930.
76. Landau BR, Wills N, Craig JW, Leonards JR, Moriwaki T: The mechanism of hepatoma-induced hypoglycemia. *Cancer* 15:1188, 1962.
77. Daughaday WH: Hypoglycemia in patients with non-islet cell tumors. *Endocrinol Metab Clin North Am* 18:91, 1989.
78. Vaitukaitis JL, Braunstein GD, Ross GT: A radioimmunoassay which specifically measures human chorionic gonadotropin in the presence of human luteinizing hormone. *Am J Obstet Gynecol* 113:751, 1972.
79. Braunstein GD, Rasor J, Thompson R, Van Scoy-Mosher M, Wade ME: Prospective evaluation of serum chorionic gonadotropin measurements for the immunodiagnosis of cancer. *Clin Res* 29:98A, 1981.
80. Fein HG, Rosen SW, Weinstraub DB: Increased glycosylation of serum human chorionic gonadotropin and subunits from eutopic and ectopic sources: Comparison with placental and urinary forms. *J Clin Endocrinol Metab* 50:1111, 1980.
81. Orth DN, Nicholson WE: Different molecular forms of ACTH. *Ann NY Acad Sci* 297:27, 1977.
82. Tanaka I, Nakai Y, Nakao K, Oki S, Fukata J, Imura H: γ-melanotrophin-like immunoreactivities in human pituitaries, ACTH-producing pituitary adenomas, and ectopic ACTH-producing tumours: Evidence for an abnormality in glycosylation in ectopic ACTH-producing tumours. *Clin Endocrinol (Oxf)* 15:353, 1981.
83. Katz MS, Kelley TM, Dax EM, Pineyro MA, Partilla JS, Gregerman RI: Ectopic β-adrenergic receptors coupled to adenylate cyclase in human adrenocortical carcinomas. *J Clin Endocrinol Metab* 60:900, 1985.
84. Pearse AGE: The cytochemistry and ultrastructure of polypeptide hormone-producing cells of the APUD series and the embryologic, physiologic and pathologic implications of the concept. *J Histochem Cytochem* 17:303, 1969.
85. Smith LH: The APUD cell concept. *J Surg Oncol* 8:137, 1976.
86. O'Connor DT, Deftos LJ: Secretion of chromogranin A by peptide-producing endocrine neoplasms. *N Engl J Med* 314:1145, 1986.
87. Weichert AF III: The neural ectodermal origin of the peptide-secreting endocrine glands: Unifying concept for the etiology of multiple endocrine adenomatosis and the inappropriate secretion of peptide hormones by nonendocrine tumors. *Am J Med* 49:232, 1970.
88. Sidhu GS: The endodermal origin of digestive and respiratory tract APUD cells: Histopathologic evidence and a review of the literature. *Am J Pathol* 96:5, 1979.
89. Baylin SB: "APUD" cells: Fact and fiction. *Trends Endocrinol Metab* 1:198, 1990.
90. Kameda Y, Ikeda A: Immunochemical and immunohistochemical studies on the 27S iodoprotein of dog thyroid with reference to thyroglobulin-like reaction of the parafollicular cells. *Biochim Biophys Acta* 577:241, 1979.
91. Melmed RN, Turner RC, Holt SJ: Intermediate cells of the pancreas: II. The effects of dietary soybean trypsin inhibitor on acinar-β cell structure and function in the rat. *J Cell Sci* 13:279, 1973.
92. Melmed RN, Benitez CJ, Holt SJ: Intermediate cells of the pancreas: III. Selective autophagy and destruction of β-granules in intermediate cells of the rat pancreas induced by alloxan and streptozotocin. *J Cell Sci* 13:297, 1973.
93. Warner TFCS: Cell hybridisation in the genesis of ectopic hormone-secreting tumours. *Lancet* 1:1259, 1974.
94. Tagnon HJ, Hildebrand J: Paraneoplastic syndromes. *Eur J Cancer Clin Oncol* 17:969, 1981.
95. Gurdon JB: Adult frogs derived from the nuclei of single somatic cells. *Dev Biol* 4:256, 1962.
96. King TJ, DiBerardino MA: Transplantation of nuclei from the frog renal adenocarcinoma: I. Development of tumor nuclear-transplant embryos. *Ann NY Acad Sci* 126:115, 1965.
97. Uriel J: Cancer, retrodifferentiation, and the myth of Faust. *Cancer Res* 36:4269, 1976.
98. Shields R: Gene derepression in tumours. *Nature* 269:752, 1977.
99. Pierce GB: Neoplasms, differentiations and mutations. *Am J Pathol* 77:103, 1974.
100. Anderson NG, Coggin JH Jr: Molecular mechanisms in blocked ontogeny and retrogenesis. *Ann NY Acad Sci* 230:508, 1974.
101. Vorherr H, Massry SG, Fallet R, Kaplan L, Kleeman CR: Antidiuretic principle in tuberculous lung tissue of a patient with pulmonary tuberculosis and hyponatremia. *Ann Intern Med* 72:383, 1970.
102. Dupont AG, Somers G, Van Steirteghem AC, Warson F, Vanhaelst L: Ectopic andrenocorticotropin productions: Disappearance after removal of inflammatory tissue. *J Clin Endocrinol Metab* 58:654, 1984.

103. De Bustros A, Baylin SB: Hormone production by tumours: Biological and clinical aspects. *Clin Endocrinol Metab* 14: 221, 1985.
104. Nieman LK, Chrousos GP, Kellner C, et al: Successful treatment of Cushing's syndrome with the glucocorticoid antagonist RU 486. *J Clin Endocrinol Metab* 61:536, 1985.
105. Braunstein GD: Placental proteins as tumor markers, in Herberman RB, Mercer DW (eds): *Immunodiagnosis of Cancer,* 2d ed. New York, Marcel Dekker, 1991, pp 673–701.
106. Galen RS: Predictive value of immunodiagnostic cancer tests, in Herberman RB, Mercer DW (eds): *Immunodiagnosis of Cancer,* 2d ed. New York, Marcel Dekker, 1991, pp 3–11.
107. Myers WPL: Hypercalcemia in neoplastic disease. *AMA Arch Surg* 80:140, 1960.
108. Warwick OH, Yendt ER, Olin JS: The clinical features of hypercalcemia associated with malignant disease. *Can Med Assoc J* 85:719, 1961.
109. Singer FR, Sharp CF Jr, Rude RK: Pathogenesis of hypercalcemia in malignancy. *Miner Electrolyte Metab* 2:161, 1979.
110. Stewart AF, Horst R, Deftos LJ, Cadman EC, Lang R, Broadus AE: Biochemical evaluation of patients with cancer-associated hypercalcemia: Evidence for humoral and nonhumoral groups. *N Engl J Med* 303:1377, 1980.
111. Budayr AA, Nissenson RA, Klein RF, Pun KK, Clark OH, Diep D, Arnaud CD, Strewler GJ: Increased serum levels of a parathyroid hormone-like protein in malignancy-associated hypercalcemia. *Ann Intern Med* 111:807, 1989.
112. Kao PC, Klee GG, Taylor RL, Heath H III: Parathyroid hormone-related peptide in plasma of patients with hypercalcemia and malignant lesions. *Mayo Clin Proc* 65:1399, 1990.
113. Henderson JE, Shustik C, Kremer R, Rabbani SA, Hendy GN, Goltzman D: Circulating concentrations of parathyroid hormone-like peptide in malignancy and in hyperparathyroidism. *J Bone Min Res* 5:105, 1990.
114. Ralston SH, Gallacher SJ, Patel U, Campbell J, Boyle IT: Cancer-associated hypercalcemia: Morbidity and mortality: Clinical experience in 126 treated patients. *Ann Intern Med* 112:499, 1990.
115. Lafferty FW: Pseudohyperparathyroidism. *Medicine (Baltimore)* 45:247, 1966.
116. Skrabanek P, McPartlin J, Powell D: Tumor hypercalcemia and "ectopic hyperparathyroidism." *Medicine (Baltimore)* 59:262, 1980.
117. Howlett TA, Rees LH. Ectopic hormones: *Spec Topics Endocrinol Metab* 7:1, 1985.
118. Ralston S, Fogelman I, Gardner MD, Boyle IT: Hypercalcaemia and metastatic bone disease: Is there a causal link? *Lancet* 2:903, 1982.
119. Mundy GR: Ectopic production of calciotropic peptides. *Endocrinol Metab Clin North Am* 20:473, 1991.
120. Sharp CF Jr, Rude RJ, Terry R, Singer FR: Abnormal bone and parathyroid histology in carcinoma patients with pseudohyperparathyroidism. *Cancer* 49:1449, 1982.
121. Zondek H, Petow H, Siebert W: Bie Bedeutung der Kalzium Bestimmung im Blut fur diagnose der Niereninsuffizienz. *Z Klin Med* 99:129, 1924.
122. Gutman AB, Tyson TL, Gutman EB: Serum calcium, inorganic phosphorous and phosphatase activity in hyperparathyroidism, Paget's disease, multiple myeloma, and neoplastic disease of the bones. *Arch Intern Med* 57:379, 1936.
123. Case records of the Massachusetts General Hospital. *N Engl J Med* 225:789, 1941.
124. Connor TB, Thomas WC Jr, Howard JE: Etiology of hypercalcemia associated with lung carcinoma. *J Clin Invest* 35:697, 1956.
125. Plimpton CH, Gellhorn A: Hypercalcemia in malignant disease without evidence of bone destruction. *Am J Med* 21:750, 1956.
126. Fry L: Pseudohyperparathyroidism with carcinoma of bronchus. *Br Med J* 1:301, 1962.
127. Tashjian AH Jr, Levine L, Munson PL: Immunochemical identification of parathyroid hormone in non-parathyroid neoplasms associated with hypercalcemia. *J Exp Med* 119:467, 1964.
128. Goldberg MF, Tashjian AH Jr, Order SE, Dammin GJ: Renal adenocarcinoma containing a parathyroid hormone-like substance and associated with marked hypercalcemia. *Am J Med* 36:805:1964.
129. Benson RC Jr, Riggs BL, Pickard BM, Arnaud CD: Radioimmunoassay of parathyroid hormone in hypercalcemic patients with malignant disease. *Am J Med* 56:821, 1974.
130. Sherwood LM, O'Riordan JLH, Aurbach GD, Potts JT Jr: Production of parathyroid hormone by nonparathyroid tumors. *J Clin Endocrinol Metab* 27:140, 1967.
131. Knill-Jones RP, Buckle RM, Parson V, Calne RY, Williams R: Hypercalcemia and increased parathyroid-hormone activity in a primary hepatoma: Studies before and after hepatic transplantation. *N Engl J Med* 282:704, 1970.
132. Buckle RM, McMillan M, Mallinson C: Ectopic secretion of parathyroid hormone by a renal adenocarcinoma in a patient with hypercalcaemia. *Br Med J* 4:724, 1970.
133. Roof BS, Carpenter B, Fink DJ, Gordan GS: Some thoughts on the nature of ectopic parathyroid hormones. *Am J Med* 50:686, 1971.
134. Riggs BL, Arnaud CD, Reynolds JC, Smith LH: Immunologic differentiation of primary hyperparathyroidism from hyperparathyroidism due to nonparathyroid cancer. *J Clin Invest* 50:2079, 1971.
135. Raisz LG, Yajnik CH, Bockman RS, Bower BF: Comparison of commercially available parathyroid hormone immunoassays in the differential diagnosis of hypercalcemia due to hyperparathyroidism or malignancy. *Ann Intern Med* 91: 739, 1979.
136. Powell D, Singer FR, Murray TM, Minkin C, Potts JT Jr: Nonparathyroid humoral hypercalcemia in patients with neoplastic diseases. *N Engl J Med* 289:176, 1973.
137. Seyberth HW, Segre GV, Morgan JL, Sweetman BJ, Potts JT Jr, Oates JA: Prostaglandins as mediators of hypercalcemia associated with certain types of cancer. *N Engl J Med* 293:1278, 1975.
138. Robertson RP, Baylink DJ, Marini JJ, Adkison HW: Elevated prostaglandins and suppressed parathyroid hormone associated with hypercalcemia and renal cell carcinoma. *J Clin Endocrinol Metab* 41:164, 1975.
139. Mundy GR, Raisz LG, Cooper RA, Schechter GP, Salmon SE: Evidence for the secretion of an osteoclast stimulating factor in myeloma. *N Engl J Med* 291:1041, 1974.
140. Simpson EL, Mundy GR, D'Souza SM, Ibbotson KJ, Bockman R, Jacobs JW: Absence of parathyroid hormone messenger RNA in nonparathyroid tumors associated with hypercalcemia. *N Engl J Med* 309:325, 1983.
141. Strewler GJ, Williams RD, Nissenson RA: Human renal carcinoma cells produce hypercalcemia in the nude mouse and a novel protein recognized by parathyroid hormone receptors. *J Clin Invest* 71:769, 1983.
142. Martin TJ, Ebeling PR, Rodda CP, Kemp BE: Humoral hypercalcemia of malignancy: Involvement of a novel hormone. *Aust N Z J Med* 18:287, 1988.
143. Suva LJ, Winslow GA, Wettenhall REH, et al: A parathyroid hormone-related protein implicated in malignant hypercalcemia: Cloning and expression. *Science* 237:893, 1987.
144. Yoshimoto K, Yamasaki R, Sakai H, Tezuka U, Takahashi M, Iizuka M, Sekiya T, Saito S: Ectopic production of parathyroid hormone by small cell lung cancer in a patient with hypercalcemia. *J Clin Endocrinol Metab* 68:976, 1989.
145. Nussbaum S, Gaz R, Arnold A: Ectopic secretion of parathyroid hormone from an ovarian cancer with DNA rearrangement of the 5′ regulatory region of the PTH gene. *Clin Res* 38:462A, 1990.
146. Strewler GJ, Budayr AA, Bruce RJ, Clark OH, Nissenson RA: Secretion of authentic parathyroid hormone by a malignant tumor. *Clin Res* 38:462A, 1990.
147. Rude RK, Sharp CF Jr, Fredericks RS, Oldham SB, Elbaum

N, Link J, Irwin L, Singer FR: Urinary and nephrogenous adenosine 3′,5′-monophosphate in the hypercalcemia of malignancy. *J Clin Endocrinol Metab* 52:765, 1981.
148. Goltzman D, Stewart AF, Broadus AE: Malignancy-associated hypercalcemia: Evaluation with a cytochemical bioassay for parathyroid hormone. *J Clin Endocrinol Metab* 53:899, 1981.
149. Strewler GJ, Wronski TJ, Halloran BP, Miller SC, Leung SC, Williams RD, Nissenson RA: Pathogenesis of hypercalcemia in nude mice bearing a human renal carcinoma. *Endocrinology* 119:303, 1986.
150. Goltzman D, Hendy GN, Banville D: Parathyroid hormone-like peptide: Molecular characterization and biological properties. *Trends Endocrinol Metab* 1:39, 1989.
151. Burtis WJ, Brady TG, Orloff JJ, et al: Immunochemical characterization of circulating parathyroid hormone-related protein in patients with humoral hypercalcemia of cancer. *N Engl J Med* 322:1106, 1990.
152. Honda S, Yamaguchi K, Suzuki M, Sato Y, Adachi I, Kimura S, Abe K: Expression of parathyroid hormone-related protein mRNA in tumors obtained from patients with humoral hypercalcemia of malignancy. *Jpn J Cancer Res* 79:677, 1988.
153. Ikeda K, Mangin M, Dreyer BE, et al: Identification of transcripts encoding a parathyroid hormone-like peptide in messenger RNAs from a variety of human and animal tumors associated with humoral hypercalcemia of malignancy. *J Clin Invest* 81:2010, 1988.
154. Stewart AF, Mangin M, Wu T, Goumas D, Insogna KL, Burtis WJ, Broadus AE: Synthetic human parathyroid hormone-like protein stimulates bone resorption and causes hypercalcemia in rats. *J Clin Invest* 81:596, 1988.
155. Rabbani SA, Mitchell J, Roy DR, Hendy GN, Goltzman D: Influence of the amino-terminus on in vitro and in vivo biological activity of synthetic parathyroid hormone-like peptides of malignancy. *Endocrinology* 123:2709, 1988.
156. Kukreja SC, Shevrin DH, Wimbiscus SA, Ebeling PR, Danks JA, Rodda CP, Wood WI, Martin TJ: Antibodies to parathyroid hormone-related protein lower serum calcium in athymic mouse models of malignancy-associated hypercalcemia due to human tumors. *J Clin Invest* 82:1798, 1988.
157. Bilezikian JP: Measurement of parathyroid hormone-related peptide in the circulation. *Trends Endocrinol Metab* 2:1, 1991.
158. Ikeda K, Weir EC, Mangin M, Dannies PS, Kinder B, Deftos LJ, Brown EM, Broadus AE: Expression of messenger ribonucleic acids encoding a parathyroid hormone-like peptide in normal human and animal tissues with abnormal expression in human parathyroid adenomas. *Mol Endocrinol* 2:1230, 1988.
159. Thiede MA, Rodan GA: Expression of a calcium-mobilizing parathyroid hormone-like peptide in lactating mammary tissue. *Science* 242:278, 1988.
160. Budayr AA, Halloran BP, King JC, Diep D, Nissenson RA, Strewler GJ: High levels of a parathyroid hormone-like protein in milk. *Proc Natl Acad Sci USA* 86:7183, 1989.
161. Thiede MA: The mRNA encoding a parathyroid hormone-like peptide is produced in mammary tissue in response to elevations in serum prolactin. *Mol Endocrinol* 3:1443, 1989.
162. Rodda CP, Kubota M, Heath JA, Ebeling, PR, Moseley JM, Care AD, Caple IW, Martin TJ: Evidence for a novel parathyroid hormone-related protein in fetal lamb parathyroid glands and sheep placenta: Comparisons with a similar protein implicated in humoral hypercalcaemia of malignancy. *J Endocrinol* 117:261, 1988.
163. Abbas SK, Pickard DW, Rodda CP, Heath JA, Hammonds RG, Wood WI, Caple IW, Martin TJ, Care AD: Stimulation of ovine placental calcium transport by purified natural and recombinant parathyroid hormone-related protein (PTHrP) preparations. *Q J Exp Physiol* 74:549, 1989.
164. Adachi N, Yamaguchi K, Miyake Y, Honda S, Nagasaki K, Akiyama Y, Adachi I, Abe K: Parathyroid hormone-related protein is a possible autocrine growth inhibitor for lymphocytes. *Biochem Biophys Res Commun* 166:1088, 1990.
165. Klein DC, Raisz LG: Prostaglandins: Stimulation of bone resorption in tissue culture. *Endocrinology* 86:1436, 1970.
166. Chase LR, Aurbach GD: The effect of parathyroid hormone on the concentration of adenosine 3′,5′-monophosphate in skeletal tissue in vitro. *J Biol Chem* 245:1520, 1970.
167. Tashjian AH Jr, Voelkel EF, Levine L, Goldhaber P: Evidence that the bone resorption-stimulating factor produced by mouse fibrosarcoma cells is prostaglandin E_2: A new model for the hypercalcemia of cancer. *J Exp Med* 136:1329, 1972.
168. Voelkel EF, Tashjian AH Jr, Franklin R, Wasserman E, Levine L: Hypercalcemia and tumor-prostaglandins: The VX_2 carcinoma model in the rabbit. *Metabolism* 24:973, 1975.
169. Flower RJ: Drugs which inhibit prostaglandin biosynthesis. *Pharmacol Rev* 26:33, 1974.
170. Franklin RB, Tashjian AH Jr: Intravenous infusion of prostaglandin E_2 raises plasma calcium concentration in the rat. *Endocrinology* 97:240, 1975.
171. Brereton HD, Halushka PV, Alexander RW, Mason DM, Keiser HR, DeVita VT: Indomethacin-responsive hypercalcemia in a patient with renal-cell adenocarcinoma. *N Engl J Med* 291:83, 1974.
172. Ito H, Sanada T, Katayama T, Shimazaki J: Indomethacin-responsive hypercalcemia. *N Engl J Med* 293:558, 1975.
173. Seyberth HW, Segre GV, Hamet P, Sweetman BJ, Potts JT Jr, Oates JA: Characterization of the group of patients with the hypercalcemia of cancer who respond to treatment with prostaglandin synthesis inhibitors. *Trans Assoc Am Physicians* 89:92, 1976.
174. Tashjian AH Jr: Prostaglandin, hypercalcemia and cancer. *N Engl J Med* 293:1317, 1975.
175. Coombes RC, Neville AM, Bondy PK, Powles TJ: Failure of indomethacin to reduce hydroxyproline excretion of hypercalcemia in patients with breast cancer. *Prostaglandins* 12:1027, 1976.
176. Caro JF, Besarab A, Flynn JT: Prostaglandin E and hypercalcemia in breast carcinoma: Only a tumor marker? *Am J Med* 66:337, 1979.
177. Valentin-Opran A, Eilon G, Saez S, Mundy GR: Estrogens and antiestrogens stimulate release of bone resorbing activity by cultured human breast cancer cells. *J Clin Invest* 75:726, 1985.
178. Tashjian AH Jr, Voelkel EF, Lazzaro M, Singer FR, Roberts AB, Derynck R, Winkler ME, Levine L: Alpha and β human transforming growth factors stimulate prostaglandin production and bone resorption in cultured mouse calvaria. *Proc Natl Acad Sci USA* 82:4535, 1985.
179. Breslau NA, McGuire JL, Zerwekh JE, Frenkel EP, Pak CYC: Hypercalcemia associated with increased serum calcitriol levels in three patients with lymphoma. *Ann Intern Med* 100:1, 1984.
180. Rosenthal LN, Insogna KL, Godsall JW, Smaldone L, Waldron JA, Stewart AF: Elevations in circulating 1,25-dihydroxyvitamin D in three patients with lymphoma-associated hypercalcemia. *J Clin Endocrinol Metab* 60:29, 1985.
181. Zaloga GPL, Eil C, Medbery CA: Humoral hypercalcemia in Hodgkin's disease. *Arch Intern Med* 145:155, 1985.
182. Davies M, Hayes ME, Mawer EB, Lumb GA: Abnormal vitamin D metabolism in Hodgkin's lymphoma. *Lancet* 1:1186, 1985.
183. Schaefer K, Saupe J, Pauls A, von Herrath D: Hypercalcemia and elevated serum 1,25-$(OH)_2$-D_3 in a patient with Hodgkin's lymphoma. *Klin Wochenschr* 64:89, 1986.
184. Adams JS, Fernandez M, Gacad MA, Gill PS, Endres DB, Rasheed S, Singer FR: Vitamin D metabolite-mediated hypercalcemia and hypercalciuria patients with AIDS- and non-AIDS-associated lymphoma. *Blood* 73:235, 1989.
185. Katz A, Kaplan L, Massry SG, Heller R, Plotkin D, Knight I: Primary hyperparathyroidism in patients with breast carcinoma. *Arch Surg* 101:582, 1970.

186. Kaplan L, Katz AD, Ben-Isaac C, Massry SG: Malignant neoplasms and parathyroid adenoma. *Cancer* 28:401, 1971.
187. Petro AB, Hardy JD: The association of parathyroid adenoma and non-medullary carcinoma of the thyroid. *Ann Surg* 181:118, 1975.
188. Newman HK, Plucinski TE: Unsuspected nonmedullary carcinoma of the thyroid in patients with hyperparathyroidism. *Am J Surg* 134:799, 1977.
189. Heath H, Hodgson SF, Kennedy MA: Primary hyperparathyroidism: Incidence, morbidity and potential economic impact in a community. *N Engl J Med* 302:189, 1980.
190. Rao SD, Frame B, Miller MJ, Kleerekoper M, Block MA, Parfitt AM: Hyperparathyroidism following head and neck irradiation. *Arch Intern Med* 140:205, 1980.
191. Katz A, Braunstein GD: Clinical biochemical and pathologic features of patients with radiation-associated hyperparathyroidism. *Arch Intern Med* 143:79, 1983.
192. Fisken RA, Heath DA, Bold AM: Hypercalcaemia—a hospital survey. *Q J Med* 49:405, 1980.
193. Blomqvist CP: Malignant hypercalcaemia—a hospital survey. *Acta Med Scand* 220:455, 1986.
194. Warrell RP Jr, Israel R, Frisone M, Snyder T, Gaynor JJ, Bockman RS: Gallium nitrate for acute treatment of cancer-related hypercalcemia: A randomized, double-blind comparison to calcitonin. *Ann Intern Med* 108:669, 1988.
195. Buckle RM: Ectopic PTH syndrome, pseudohyperparathyroidism; hypercalcemia of malignancy. *Clin Endocrinol Metab* 3:237, 1974.
196. Burtis WJ, Wu TL, Insogna KL, Stewart AF: Humoral hypercalcemia of malignancy. *Ann Intern Med* 108:454, 1988.
197. Boyd JC, Ladenson JH: Value of laboratory tests in the differential diagnosis of hypercalcemia. *Am J Med* 77:863, 1984.
198. Ebie N, Ryan W, Harris J: Metabolic emergencies in cancer medicine. *Med Clin North Am* 70:1151, 1986.
199. Singer FR, Fernandez M: Therapy of hypercalcemia of malignancy. *Am J Med* 82(suppl 2A):34, 1987.
200. Schaiff RA, Hall TG, Bar RS: Medical treatment of hypercalcemia. *Clin Pharm* 8:108, 1989.
201. Siris ES, Hyman GA, Canfield RE: Effects of dichloromethylene diphosphonate in women with breast carcinoma metastatic to the skeleton. *Am J Med* 74:401, 1983.
202. Elomaa I, Blomqvist C, Grohn P, Porkka L, Kairento A-L, Selander K, Lamberg-Allardt C, Holmstrom T: Long-term controlled trial with diphosphonate in patients with osteolytic bone metastases. *Lancet* 1:146, 1983.
203. Brown WH: A case of pluriglandular syndrome: "Diabetes of bearded woman." *Lancet* 2:1022, 1928.
204. Christy NP: Adrenocorticotrophic activity in the plasma of patients with Cushing's syndrome associated with pulmonary neoplasms. *Lancet* 1:85, 1961.
205. Holub DA, Katz FH: A possible etiological link between Cushing's syndrome and visceral malignancy. *Clin Res* 9:194, 1961.
206. Meador CK, Liddle GW, Island DP, Nicholson WE, Lucas CP, Nockton JG, Luetscher JA: Cause of Cushing's syndrome in patients with tumors arising from nonendocrine tissue. *J Clin Endocrinol Metab* 22:693, 1962.
207. Liddle GW, Nicholson WE, Island DP, Orth DN, Abe K, Lowder SC: Clinical and laboratory studies of ectopic humoral syndromes. *Recent Prog Horm Res* 25:283, 1969.
208. Schteingart DE: Ectopic secretion of peptides of the proopiomelanocortin family. *Endocrinol Metab Clin North Am* 20:453, 1991.
209. Azzopardi JG, Williams ED: Pathology of 'nonendocrine' tumors associated with Cushing's syndrome. *Cancer* 22:274, 1968.
210. Imura H, Matsukura S, Yamamoto H, Hirata Y, Nakai Y, Eno J, Tanaka A, Nakamura M: Studies on ectopic ACTH-producing tumors: II. Clinical and biochemical features of 30 cases. *Cancer* 35:1430, 1975.
211. Jex RK, van Heerden JA, Carpenter PC, Grant CS: Ectopic ACTH syndrome: Diagnostic and therapeutic aspects. *Am J Surg* 149:276, 1985.
212. Howlett TA, Drury PL, Perry L, Doniach I, Rees LH, Besser GM: Diagnosis and management of ACTH-dependent Cushing's syndrome: Comparison of the features in ectopic and pituitary ACTH production. *Clin Endocrinol (Oxf)* 24:699, 1986.
213. Singer W, Kovacs K, Ryan N, Horvath E: Ectopic ACTH syndrome: Clinicopathological correlations. *J Clin Pathol* 31:591, 1978.
214. Kohler PC, Trump DL: Ectopic hormone syndromes. *Cancer Invest* 4:543, 1986.
215. Yalow RS: Big ACTH and bronchogenic carcinoma. *Annu Rev Med* 30:241, 1979.
216. Ratter SJ, Gillies G, Hope J, et al: Pro-opiocortin related peptides in human pituitary and ectopic ACTH secreting tumours. *Clin Endocrinol (Oxf)* 18:211, 1983.
217. Jeffcoate WJ, Rees LH, Lowry PJ, Besser GM: A specific radioimmunoassay for human β-lipotropin. *J Clin Endocrinol Metab* 47:160, 1978.
218. Ueda M, Takeuchi T, Abe K, Miyakawa S, Ohnami S, Yanaihara N: β-melanocyte-stimulating hormone immunoreactivity in human pituitaries and ectopic adrenocorticotropin-producing tumors. *J Clin Endocrinol Metab* 50:550, 1980.
219. Kleber G, Hollt V, Oelkers W, Quabbe HJ: Elevated plasma and tissue concentrations of β-endorphin and β-lipotropin associated with an ectopic ACTH-producing lung tumor. *Horm Metab Res* 12:385, 1980.
220. Pullan PT, Clement-Jones V, Corder R, Lowry PJ, Besser GM, Rees LH: ACTH, LPH and related peptides in the ectopic ACTH syndrome. *Clin Endocrinol (Oxf)* 13:437, 1980.
221. Baker J, Holdaway IM, Jagusch M, Kerr AR, Donald RA, Pullan PT: Ectopic secretion of ACTH and met-enkephalin from a thymic carcinoid. *J Endocrinol Invest* 5:33, 1982.
222. Sheng SL, Seurin D, Bertagna X, Girard F: Molecular forms of beta-endorphin in ACTH/LPH hypersecretion syndromes in man. *Horm Res* 20:95, 1984.
223. Hale AC, Besser GM, Rees LH: Characterization of pro-opiomelanocortin-derived peptides in pituitary and ectopic adrenocorticotrophin-secreting tumours. *J Endocrinol* 108: 49, 1986.
224. Pullan PT, Clement-Jones V, Corder R, Lowry PJ, Rees GM, Rees LH, Besser GM, Macedo MM, Galvao-Teles A: Ectopic production of methionine enkephalin and beta-endorphin. *Br Med J* 1:758, 1980.
225. Lundberg JM, Hamberger B, Schultzberg M, et al: Enkephalin- and somatostatin-like immunoreactivities in human adrenal medulla and pheochromocytoma. *Proc Natl Acad Sci USA* 76:4079, 1979.
226. DeBold CR, Menefee JK, Nicholson WE, Orth DN: Proopiomelanocortin gene is expressed in many normal tissues and in tumors not associated with ectopic adrenocorticotropin syndrome. *Mol Endocrinol* 2:862, 1988.
227. Odell WD, Saito E: Protein hormone-like materials from normal and cancer cells: "Ectopic" hormone production. *Proceedings of the 13th International Cancer Congress,* Part E: *Cancer Management.* New York, Liss, 1983, p 247.
228. Orwoll ES, Kendall JW: β-endorphin and adrenocorticotropin in extrapituitary sites: Gastrointestinal tract. *Endocrinology* 107:438, 1980.
229. Odell WD: Ectopic ACTH secretion. *Endocrinol Metab Clin North Am* 20:371, 1991.
230. Bardin CW, Shaha C, Mather J, Salomon Y, Margioris AN, Liotta AS, Gerendai I, Chen CL, Krieger DT: Identification and possible function of proopiomelanocortin derived peptides in the testis. *Ann NY Acad Sci* 438:346, 1984.
231. Chen CLC, Chang CC, Krieger DT, Bardin WC: Expression and regulation of proopiomelanocortin-like gene in the ovary and placenta: Comparison with the testis. *Endocrinology* 118:2382, 1986.
232. Jingami H, Nakanishi S, Imura I, Numa S: Tissue distribu-

tion of messenger RNAs coding for opioid peptide precursors and related RNA. *Eur J Biochem* 142:441, 1984.
233. DeKeyzer Y, Rousseau-Merck MF, Luton J-P, Girard F, Kahn A, Bertagna X: Pro-opiomelanocortin gene expression in human phaeochromocytomas. *J Mol Endocrinol* 2:175, 1989.
234. Abeloff MD, Trump DL, Baylin SB: Ectopic adrenocorticotrophic (ACTH) syndrome and small cell carcinoma of the lung—assessement of clinical implications in patients on combination chemotherapy. *Cancer* 48:1082, 1981.
235. Upton GV, Amatruda TT Jr: Evidence for the presence of tumor peptides with corticotropin-releasing-factor-like activity in the ectopic ACTH syndrome. *N Engl J Med* 285:419, 1971.
236. Carey RM, Varma SK, Drake CR Jr, Thorner MO, Kovacs K, Rivier J, Vale W: Ectopic secretion of corticotropin-releasing factor as a cause of Cushing's syndrome: A clinical, morphologic, and biochemical study. *N Engl J Med* 311:12, 1984.
237. Asa S, Kovacs K, Tindal GT, Barrow DL, Horvath E, Vecsei P: Cushing's disease associated with an intraseller gangliocytoma producing corticotrophin-releasing factor. *Ann Intern Med* 101:789, 1984.
238. Belsky JL, Cuello B, Swanson LW, Simmons DM, Jarrett RM, Braza F: Cushing's syndrome due to ectopic production of corticotropin-releasing factor. *J Clin Endocrinol Metab* 60:496, 1985.
239. Schteingart DE, Lloyd RV, Akil H, Chandler WF, Ibarra-Perez G, Rosen SG, Olgetree R: Cushing's syndrome secondary to ectopic CRH-ACTH secretion. *J Clin Endocrinol Metab* 63:770, 1986.
240. Suda T, Kondo M, Totani R, et al: Ectopic adrenocorticotropin syndrome caused by lung cancer that responded to corticotropin-releasing hormone. *J Clin Endocrinol Metab* 63:1047, 1986.
241. Fjellestad-Paulsen A, Abrahamsson P-A, Bjartell A, Grino M, Grimelius L, Hedeland H, Falkmer S: Carcinoma of the prostate with Cushing's syndrome. *Acta Endocrinol (Copenh)* 119:506, 1988.
242. Tourniaire J, Rebattu B, Conte-Devolk B, Trouillas J, Grino M, Berger-Dutrieux N, Peix JL, Pugeat M: Syndrome de Cushing secondaire à la production ectopique de CRF par un carcinome medullaire du corps thyroide. *Ann d'Endocrinol (Paris)* 4:61, 1988.
243. Adams EF, Skrabal F, Carroll D, Loizou M, White MC, Biggins JA, Mashiter K: Ectopic corticotrophin-releasing-factor and growth hormone releasing factor secretion: Diagnosis using human pituitary cell culture. *Horm Res* 25:80, 1987.
244. Wakabayashi I, Ihara T, Hattori M, Tonegawa Y, Shibasaki T, Hashimoto K: Presence of corticotropin-releasing factor-like immunoreactivity in human tumors. *Cancer* 55:995, 1985.
245. Findling JW, Tyrrell JB: Occult ectopic secretion of corticotropin. *Arch Intern Med* 146:929, 1986.
246. Chrousos GP, Schulte HM, Oldfield EH, Gold PW, Cutler GB Jr, Loriaux DL: The corticotropin-releasing factor stimulation test: An aid in the evaluation of patients with Cushing's syndrome. *N Engl J Med* 310:622, 1984.
247. Loriaux DL, Nieman L: Corticotropin-releasing hormone testing in pituitary disease. *Endocrinol Metab Clin North Am* 20:363, 1991.
248. Findling JW, Aron DC, Tyrrell JB, Shinsako JH, Fitzgerald PA, Norman D, Wilson CB, Forsham PH: Selective venous sampling for ACTH in Cushing's syndrome: Differentiation between Cushing's disease and the ectopic ACTH syndrome. *Ann Intern Med* 94:647, 1981.
249. Oldfield EH, Doppman JL, Nieman LK, Chrousos GP, Miller DL, Katz DA, Cutler GB Jr, Loriaux DL: Petrosal sinus sampling with and without corticotropin-releasing hormone for the differential diagnosis of Cushing's syndrome. *N Engl J Med*.325:897, 1991.
250. Drury PL, Ratter S, Tomlin S, Williams J, Dacie JE, Rees LH, Besser GM: Experience with selective venous sampling in diagnosis of ACTH-dependent Cushing's syndrome. *Br Med J* 284:9, 1982.
251. Horai T, Nishihara H, Tateishi R, Matsuda M, Hattori S: Oat-cell carcinoma of the lung simultaneously producing ACTH and serotonin. *J Clin Endocrinol Metab* 37:212, 1973.
252. Sonino N, Boscaro M, Merola G, Mantero F: Prolonged treatment of Cushing's disease by ketoconazole. *J Clin Endocrinol Metab* 61:718, 1985.
253. Jeffcoate WJ, Rees LH, Tomlin S, Jones AE, Edwards CRW, Besser GM: Metyrapone in long-term management of Cushing's disease. *Br Med J* 2:215, 1977.
254. Carey RM, Orth DN, Hartmann WH: Malignant melanoma with ectopic production of adrenocorticotropic hormone: Palliative treatment with inhibitors of adrenal steroid biosynthesis. *J Clin Endocrinol Metab* 36:482, 1973.
255. Bertagna X, Favrod-Coune C, Escourolle H, Beuzeboc P, Christoforov B, Girard F, Luton J-P: Suppression of ectopic adrenocorticotropin secretion by the long-acting somatostatin analog octreotide. *J Clin Endocrinol Metab* 68:988, 1989.
256. Lamberts SWJ, Tilanus HW, Klooswijk AIJ, Bruining HA, VanDerLely AJ, DeJong FH: Successful treatment with SMS 201-995 of Cushing's syndrome caused by ectopic adrenocorticotropin secretion from a metastatic gastrin-secreting pancreatic islet cell carcinoma. *J Clin Endocrinol Metab* 67:1080, 1988.
257. Winkler AW, Cranshaw OS: Chloride depletion conditions other than Addison's disease. *J Clin Invest* 17:1, 1938.
258. Schwartz WB, Bennett W, Curelop S, Bartter FC: A syndrome of renal sodium loss and hyponatremia probably resulting from inappropriate secretion of antidiuretic hormone. *Am J Med* 23:529, 1957.
259. Leaf A, Bartter FC, Santos RF, Wrong O: Evidence in man that urinary electrolyte loss induced by pitressin is a function of water retention. *J Clin Invest* 32:868, 1953.
260. Thorn NA, Transbol I: Hyponatremia and bronchogenic carcinoma associated with renal excretion of large amounts of antidiuretic material. *Am J Med* 35:257, 1963.
261. Amatruda TT, Mulrow PJ, Gallagher JC, Sawyer WH: Carcinoma of the lung with inappropriate antidiuresis: Demonstration of antidiuretic-hormone-like activity in tumor extract. *N Engl J Med* 269:544, 1963.
262. Bower BF, Mason DM, Forsham PH: Bronchogenic carcinoma with inappropriate antidiuretic activity in plasma and tumor. *N Engl J Med* 271:934, 1964.
263. George JM, Capen CC, Phillips AS: Biosynthesis of vasopressin in vitro and ultrastructure of a bronchogenic carcinoma. *J Clin Invest* 51:141, 1972.
264. Yamaji T, Ishibashi M, Katayama S, Itabashi A, Ohsawa N, Kondo Y, Mizumoto Y, Kosaka K: Neurophysin biosynthesis in vitro in oat cell carcinoma of the lung with ectopic vasopressin production. *J Clin Invest* 69:1441, 1981.
265. Kondo Y, Mizumoto Y, Katayama S, Murase T, Yamaji T, Ohsawa N, Kosaka K: Inappropriate secretion of antidiuretic hormone in nude mice bearing a human bronchogenic oat cell carcinoma. *Cancer Res* 41:1545, 1981.
266. Moses AM, Miller M, Streeten DHP: Pathophysiologic and pharmacologic alterations in the release and action of ADH. *Metabolism* 25:697, 1976.
267. DeTroyer A, Demanet JC: Clinical, biological and pathogenic features of the syndrome of inappropriate secretion of antidiuretic hormone: A review of 26 cases with marked hyponatraemia: *Q J Med* 45:521, 1976.
268. Bartter FC, Schwartz WB: The syndrome of inappropriate secretion of antidiuretic hormone. *Am J Med* 42:790, 1967.
269. Vorherr H: Para-endocrine tumor activity with emphasis on ectopic ADH secretion: Genetic, diagnostic, prognostic and therapeutic aspects. *Oncology* 29:382, 1974.
270. List AF, Hainsworth JD, Davis BW, Hande KR, Greco FA, Johnson DH: The syndrome of inappropriate secretion of antidiuretic hormone (SIADH) in small-cell lung cancer. *J Clin Oncol* 4:1191, 1986.
271. Lockton JA, Thatcher N: A retrospective study of thirty-two

patients with small-cell bronchogenic carcinoma and inappropriate secretion of antidiuretic hormone. *Clin Radiol* 37:47, 1986.

272. North WG, Maurer LH, Valtin H, O'Donnell JF: Human neurophysins as potential tumor markers for small cell carcinoma of the lung: Application of specific radioimmunoassays. *J Clin Endocrinol Metab* 51:892, 1980.
273. Memoli VA, North WG: A monoclonal antibody to human neurophysin recognizes pulmonary neuroendocrine carcinomas. *Lab Invest* 56:50a, 1987.
274. Edwards CRW: Vasopressin and oxytocin in health and disease. *Clin Endocrinol Metab* 6:223, 1977.
275. Baumann G, Lopez-Amor E, Dingman JF: Plasma arginine vasopressin in the syndrome of inappropriate antidiuretic hormone secretion. *Am J Med* 52:19, 1972.
276. Rees LH, Bloomfield GA, Rees GM, Corrin B, Franks LM, Ratcliffe JB: Mutiple hormones in a bronchial tumour. *J Clin Endocrinol Metab* 38:1090, 1974.
277. Pettengill OS, Faulkner CS, Wurster-Hill DH, Maurer LH, Sorenson GD, Robinson AG, Zimmerman EA: Isolation and characterization of a hormone-producing cell line from human small cell anaplastic carcinoma of the lung. *JNCI* 58:511, 1977.
278. Martin TJ, Greenberg PB, Beck C, Johnston CI: Synthesis of peptide hormones by human tumours in cell culture, in Scow RO (ed): *Endocrinology*. Amsterdam, Excerpta Medica, 1973, p 1198.
279. Yamaji T, Ishibashi M, Katayama S: Nature of the immunoreactive neurophysins in ectopic vasopressin-producing oat cell carcinomas of the lung: Demonstration of a putative common precursor to vasopressin and neurophysin. *J Clin Invest* 68:388, 1981.
280. Sausville E, Carney D, Battey J: The human vasopressin gene is linked to the oxytocin gene and is selectively expressed in a cultured lung cancer cell line. *J Biol Chem* 260:10236, 1985.
281. Padfield PL, Morton JJ, Brown JJ, Lever AF, Robertson JIS, Wood M, Fox R: Plasma arginine vasopressin in the syndrome of antidiuretic hormone excess associated with bronchogenic carcinoma. *Am J Med* 61:825, 1976.
282. Zerbe R, Stropes L, Robertson G: Vasopressin function in the syndrome of inappropriate antidiuresis. *Annu Rev Med* 31:315, 1980.
283. Moses AM, Scheinman SJ: Ectopic secretion of neurohypophyseal peptides in patients with malignancy. *Endocrinol Metab Clin North Am* 20:489, 1991.
284. Kinzie BJ: Management of the syndrome of inappropriate secretion of antidiuretic hormone. *Clin Pharm* 6:625, 1987.
285. Sorensen JB, Kristjansen PEG, Osterlind K, Hammer M, Hansen M: Syndrome of inappropriate antidiuresis in small-cell lung cancer: Classification and effect of tumor regression. *Acta Med Scand* 222:155, 1987.
286. Cogan E, DeBieve M-F, Pepersack T, Abramow M: Natriuresis and atrial natriuretic factor secretion during inappropriate antidiuresis. *Am J Med* 84:409, 1988.
287. Kothe MJC, Prins JM, DeWit R, Velden KVD, Schellekens PTA: Small-cell carcinoma of the cervix with inappropriate antidiuretic-hormone secretion: Case report. *Br J Obstet Gynaecol* 97:647, 1990.
288. Manoogian C, Pandian M, Ehrlich L, Fisher D, Horton R: Plasma atrial natriuretic hormone levels in patients with the syndrome of inappropriate antidiuretic hormone secretion. *J Clin Endocrinol Metab* 67:571, 1988.
289. Bliss DP Jr, Battey JF, Linnoila RI, Birrer MJ, Gazdar AF, Johnson BE: Expression of the atrial natriuretic factor gene in small cell lung cancer tumors and tumor cell lines. *JNCI* 82:305, 1990.
290. Hantman D, Rossier B, Zohlman R, Schrier R: Rapid correction of hyponatremia in the syndrome of inappropriate secretion of antidiuretic hormone: An alternative treatment to hypertonic saline. *Ann Intern Med* 78:870, 1973.
291. Ayus JC, Krothapalli RK, Arieff AI: Changing concepts in treatment of severe symptomatic hyponatremia. *Am J Med* 78:897, 1985.
292. Forrest JN Jr, Cox M, Hong C, Morrison G, Bia M, Singer I: Superiority of demeclocycline over lithium in the treatment of chronic syndrome of inappropriate secretion of antidiuretic hormone. *N Engl J Med* 298:173, 1978.
293. Nadler WH, Wolfer JA: Hepatogenic hypoglycemia associated with primary liver cell carcinoma. *Arch Intern Med* 44:700, 1929.
294. Elliott CA: Hepatic hypoglycemia associated with primary liver cell carcinoma. *Trans Assoc Am Physicians* 44:121, 1929.
295. Potter RP: Intrathoracic tumors. *Radiology* 14:60, 1930.
296. Anderson HB: Tumor of adrenal gland with fatal hypoglycemia. *Am J Med Sci* 180:71, 1930.
297. Laurent J, Debry G, Floquet J: *Hypoglycemia Tumors*. Amsterdam, Excerpta Medica, 1971.
298. Skrabanek P, Powell D: Ectopic insulin and Occam's razor: Reappraisal of the riddle of tumour hypoglycaemia. *Clin Endocrinol (Oxf)* 9:141, 1978.
299. Fischer KF, Lees JA, Newman JH: Hypoglycemia in hospitalized patients: Causes and outcomes. *N Engl J Med* 315:1245, 1986.
300. Marks V: Hypoglycaemia: II. Other causes. *Clin Endocrinol Metab* 5:769, 1976.
301. Gorden P, Hendricks CM, Kahn CR, Megyesi K, Roth J: Hypoglycemia associated with non-islet-cell tumor and insulin-like growth factors: A study of the tumor types. *N Engl J Med* 305:1452, 1981.
302. Widmer U, Zapf J, Froesch ER: Is extrapancreatic tumor hypoglycemia associated with elevated levels of insulin-like growth factor II? *J Clin Endocrinol Metab* 55:833, 1982.
303. Anderson N, Lokich JJ: Mesenchymal tumors associated with hypoglycemia: Case report and review of the literature. *Cancer* 44:785, 1979.
304. Edmondson HA, Steiner PE: Primary carcinoma of the liver. *Cancer* 7:462, 1954.
305. McDonald RA. Primary carcinoma of liver: *Arch Intern Med* 99:266, 1957.
306. Anderson IF, Webster AL, Wypkema W: Primary malignant hepatoma associated with hypoglycaemia. *S Afr Med J* 41:505, 1967.
307. McFadzean AJS, Yeung RTT: Further observations on hypoglycemia in hepatocellular carcinoma. *Am J Med* 47:220, 1969.
308. Unger RH: The riddle of tumor hypoglycemia. *Am J Med* 40:325, 1966.
309. Stuart CA, Prince MJ, Peters EJ, Smith FE, Townsend CM III, Poffenbarger PL: Insulin receptor proliferation: A mechanism for tumor-associated hypoglycemia. *J Clin Endocrinol Metab* 63:879, 1986.
310. Butterfield WJH, Kinder CH, Mahler RF: Hypoglycemia associated with sarcoma. *Lancet* 1:703, 1960.
311. Landau BR, Wills N, Craig JW, Leonards JR, Moriwakis A: The mechanism of hepatoma-induced hypoglycemia. *Cancer* 15:1188, 1962.
312. Kahn CR: The riddle of tumour hypoglycaemia revisited. *Clin Endocrinol Metab* 9:335, 1980.
313. Volpe R, Evans J, Clarke DW, Forbath N, Ehrlich R: Evidence favoring the sarcomatous origin of an insulin-like substance in a case of fibrosarcoma with hypoglycemia. *Am J Med* 38:540, 1965.
314. Daughaday WH, Deuel TF: Tumor secretion of growth factors. *Endocrinol Clin North Am* 20:539, 1991.
315. Merimee TJ: Insulin-like growth factors in patients with nonislet cell tumors and hypoglycemia. *Metabolism* 35:360, 1986.
316. Ron D, Powers AC, Pandian MR, Godine JE, Axelrod L: Increased insulin-like growth factor II production and consequent suppression of growth hormone secretion: A dual mechanism for tumor-induced hypoglycemia. *J Clin Endocrinol Metab* 68:701, 1989.

317. Olefesky S, Bailey I, Samols E, Bilkus D: A fibrosarcoma with hypoglycaemia and a high serum-insulin level. *Lancet* 2:378, 1962.
318. Shames JM, Dhurandhar NR, Blackard WG: Insulin-secreting bronchial carcinoid tumor with widespread metastases. *Am J Med* 44:632, 1968.
319. Shetty MR, Boghossian HM, Duffell D, Freel R, Gonzales JC: Tumor-induced hypoglycemia: A result of ectopic insulin production. *Cancer* 49:1920, 1982.
320. Lyall SS, Marieb NJ, Wise JK, Cornog JL, Neville EC, Felig P: Hyperinsulinemic hypoglycemia associated with a neurofibrosarcoma. *Arch Intern Med* 135:865, 1975.
321. Plovnick H, Ruderman NB, Aoki T, Chideckel EW, Poffenbarger PL: Non-β-cell tumor hypoglycemia associated with increased nonsuppressible insulin-like protein (NSILP). *Am J Med* 66:154, 1979.
322. Megyesi K, Kahn CR, Roth J, Gorden P: Hypoglycemia in association with extrapancreatic tumors: Demonstration of elevated plasma NSILA-s by a new radioreceptor assay. *J Clin Endocrinol Metab* 38:931, 1974.
323. Zapf J, Rinderknecht E, Humbel RE, Froesch ER: Nonsuppressible insulin-like activity (NSILA) from human serum: Recent accomplishments and their physiologic implications. *Metabolism* 27:1803, 1978.
324. Daughaday WH, Emanuele MA, Brooks MH, Barbato AL, Kapadia M, Rotwein P: Synthesis and secretion of insulin-like growth factor II by a leiomyosarcoma and associated hypoglycemia. *N Engl J Med* 319:1434, 1988.
325. Shapiro ET, Bell GI, Polonsky KS, Rubenstein AH, Kew MC, Tager HS: Tumor hypoglycemia: Relationship to high molecular weight insulin-like growth factor II. *J Clin Invest* 85:1672, 1990.
326. Daughaday WH, Kapadia M: Significance of abnormal serum binding of insulin-like growth factor II in the development of hypoglycemia in patients with non-islet-cell tumors. *Proc Natl Acad Sci USA* 86:6778, 1989.
327. Weber MM, Melmed S, Rosenbloom J, Yamasaki H, Prager D: Insulin-like growth factor 2 action in rat somatotrophs is mediated by the insulin-like growth factor I receptor. *Clin Res* 40:24A, 1992.
328. Teale JD, Marks V: Inappropriately elevated plasma insulin-like growth factor II in relation to suppressed insulin-like growth factor I in the diagnosis of non-islet cell tumour hypoglycemia. *Clin Endocrinol (Oxf)* 33:87, 1990.
329. Merimee TJ, Tyson JE: Stabilization of plasma glucose during fasting: Normal variations in two separate studies. *N Engl J Med* 291:1275, 1974.
330. McCance RA: Osteomalacia with Losser's nodes (Milkman's syndrome) due to a raise resistance to vitamin D acquired about the age of 15 years. *Q J Med* 16:33, 1947.
331. Prader VA, Illig R, Vehlinger E, Stalder G: Rachitis infolge Knochentumors. *Helv Paediatr Acta* 14:554, 1959.
332. Nuovo MA, Dorfman HD, Sun C-CJ, Chalew SA: Tumor-induced osteomalacia and rickets. *Am J Surg Pathol* 13:588, 1989.
333. Lyles KW, Berry WR, Haussler M, Harrelson JM, Drezner MK: Hypophosphatemic osteomalacia: Association with prostatic carcinoma. *Ann Intern Med* 93:275, 1980.
334. Ryan EA, Reiss E: Oncogenous osteomalacia: Review of the world literature of 42 cases and report to two new cases. *Am J Med* 77:501, 1984.
335. Cotton GE, Van Puffelen P: Hypophosphatemic osteomalacia secondary to neoplasia. *J Bone Joint Surg* 68A:129, 1986.
336. Weidner N, Santa Cruz D: Phosphaturic mesenchymal tumors: A polymorphous group causing osteomalacia or rickets. *Cancer* 59:1442, 1987.
337. Taylor HC, Fallon MD, Velasco ME: Oncogenic osteomalacia and inappropriate antidiuretic hormone secretion due to oat-cell carcinoma. *Ann Intern Med* 101:786, 1984.
338. Stanbury SW: Tumour-associated hypophosphataemic osteomalacia and rickets. *Clin Endocrinol (Oxf)* 1:256, 1972.
339. Sirota JH, Hamerman D: Renal function studies in an adult subject with Fanconi syndrome. *Am J Med* 16:138, 1954.
340. Rico H, Fernandez-Miranda E, Sanz J, Gomez-Castresana F, Escriba A, Hernandez ER, Krsnik I: Oncogenous osteomalacia: A new case secondary to a malignant tumor. *Bone* 7:325, 1986.
341. Hauge BN: Vitamin D resistant osteomalacia. *Acta Med Scand* 153:271, 1956.
342. Weidner N, Bar RS, Weiss D, Strottmann MP: Neoplastic pathology of oncogenic osteomalacia/rickets. *Cancer* 55:1691, 1985.
343. Drezner MK, Feinglos MN: Osteomalacia due to 1α,25-dihydroxycholecalciferol deficiency: Association with a giant cell tumor of bone. *J Clin Invest* 60:1046, 1977.
344. Parker MS, Klein I, Haussler MR, Mintz DH: Tumor-induced osteomalacia: Evidence of a surgically correctable alteration in vitamin D metabolism. *JAMA* 245:492, 1981.
345. Fukumoto Y, Tarui S, Tsukiyama K, et al: Tumor-induced vitamin D-resistant hypophosphatemic osteomalacia associated with proximal renal tubular dysfunction and 1,25-dihydroxyvitamin D deficiency. *J Clin Endocrinol Metab* 49:873, 1979.
346. Aschinberg LC, Solomon LM, Zeis PM, Justice P, Rosenthal IM: Vitamin D-resistant rickets associated with epidermal nevus syndrome: Demonstration of a phosphaturic substance in the dermal lesions. *J Pediatr* 91:56, 1977.
347. Jefferis AF, Taylor PCA, Walsh-Waring GP: Tumour-associated hypophosphataemic osteomalacia occurring in a patient with an odontogenic tumour of the maxilla. *J Laryngol Otol* 99:1011, 1985.
348. Yoshikawa S, Nakamura T, Takagi M, Imamura T, Okano K, Sasaki S: Benign osteoblastoma as a cause of osteomalacia. *J Bone Joint Surg* 59:279, 1977.
349. Lau K, Stom MC, Goldberg M, Goldfarb S, Gray RW, Lemann J Jr, Agus ZS: Evidence for a humoral phosphaturic factor in oncogenic hypophosphatemic osteomalacia. *Clin Res* 27:421A, 1979.
350. Popovtzer MM: Tumor-induced hypophosphatemic osteomalacia (TUO): Evidence for a phosphaturic cyclic AMP-independent action of tumor extract. *Clin Res* 29:418A, 1981.
351. Lyles KW, Lobaugh B, Paulson DF, Drezner MK: Heterotransplantation of prostatic cancer from an affected patient creates an animal model for tumor-induced osteomalacia (TIO) in the athymic nude mouse. *Calcif Tissue Int* 34:533, 1982.
352. Gitelis S, Ryan WG, Rosenberg AG, Templeton AC: Adult-onset hypophosphatemic osteomalacia secondary to neoplasm: A case report and review of the pathophysiology. *J Bone Joint Surg* 68A:134, 1986.
353. Miyauchi A, Fukase M, Tsutsumi M, Fujita T: Hemangiopericytoma-induced osteomalacia: Tumor transplantation in nude mice causes hypophosphatemia and tumor extracts inhibit renal 25-hydroxyvitamin D-1-hydroxylase activity. *J Clin Endocrinol Metab* 67:46, 1988.
354. Papotti M, Foschini MP, Isaia G, Rizzi G, Betts CM, Eusebi V: Hypophosphatemic oncogenic osteomalacia: Report of three new cases. *Tumori* 74:599, 1988.
355. Siris ES, Clemens TL, Dempster DW, Shane E, Segre GV, Lindsay R, Bilezikian JP: Tumor-induced osteomalacia: Kinetics of calcium, phosphorus, and vitamin D metabolism and characteristics of bone histomorphometry. *Am J Med* 82:307, 1987.
356. Case records of the Massachusetts General Hospital: Case 52–1989. *N Engl J Med* 321:1812, 1989.
357. Steiner H, Dahlback O, Waldenstrom J: Ectopic growth hormone production and osteoarthropathy in carcinoma of the bronchus. *Lancet* 1:783, 1968.
358. Cameron DP, Burger HD, DeKretzer DM, Catt KJ, Best JB: On the presence of immunoreactive growth hormone in a bronchogenic carcinoma. *Aust Ann Med* 18:143, 1969.
359. Greenberg PB, Beck C, Martin TJ, Burger HG: Synthesis and release of human growth hormone from lung carcinoma in cell culture. *Lancet* 1:350, 1972.

360. Beck C, Burger HG: Evidence for the presence of immunoreactive growth hormone in cancers of the lung and stomach. *Cancer* 30:75, 1972.
361. Ghosh L, Ghosh BC, Gupta TKD: Intracellular demonstration of growth hormone in human mammary carcinoma cells. *Am J Surg* 135:215, 1978.
362. Caplan RH, Koob L, Abellera RM, Pagliara AS, Kovacs K, Randall RV: Cure of acromegaly by operative removal of an islet cell tumor of the pancreas. *Am J Med* 64:874, 1978.
363. Frohman LA, Szabo M, Berelowitz M, Stachura ME: Partial purification and characterization of a peptide with growth hormone-releasing activity from extrapituitary tumors in patients with acromegaly. *J Clin Invest* 65:43, 1980.
364. Benjamin F, Casper DJ, Sherman L, Kolodny HD: Growth-hormone secretion in patients with endometrial carcinoma. *N Engl J Med* 281:1448, 1969.
365. Sparagana M, Phillips G, Hoffman C, Kucera L: Ectopic growth hormone syndrome associated with lung cancer. *Metabolism* 20:730, 1971.
366. Oberg K, Norheim I, Wide L: Serum growth hormone in patients with carcinoid tumours: Basal levels and response to glucose and thyrotrophin releasing hormone. *Acta Endocrinol (Copenh)* 109:13, 1985.
367. Altmann HW, Schutz W: Uber ein Knochenhaltiges Bronchuscarcinoid. *Beitr Pathol Anat* 120:455, 1959.
368. Sonksen PH, Ayres AB, Braimbridge M, et al: Acromegaly caused by pulmonary carcinoid tumours. *Clin Endocrinol (Oxf)* 5:503, 1976.
369. Shalet SM, Beardwell CG, MacFarlane IA, Ellison ML, Norman CM, Rees LH, Hughes M: Acromegaly due to production of a growth hormone releasing factor by a bronchial carcinoid tumour. *Clin Endocrinol (Oxf)* 10:61, 1979.
370. Cronin MJ, Rogol AD, Dabney LG, Thorner MO: Selective growth hormone and cyclic AMP stimulating activity is present in a human pancreatic islet cell tumor. *J Clin Endocrinol Metab* 55:381, 1982.
371. Rivier J, Spiess J, Thorner MO, Vale W: Characterization of a growth hormone-releasing factor from a human pancreatic islet tumor. *Nature* 300:276, 1982.
372. Guillemin R, Brazeau P, Bohlen P, Esch F, Ling N, Wehrenberg WB: Growth hormone-releasing factor from a human pancreatic tumor that caused acromegaly. *Science* 218:585, 1982.
373. Scheithauer BW, Carpenter PC, Bloch B, Brazeau P: Ectopic secretion of a growth hormone-releasing factor: Report of a case of acromegaly with bronchial carcinoid tumor. *Am J Med* 76:605, 1984.
374. Frohman LA, Downs TR: Ectopic GRH syndromes, in Robbins RJ, Melmed S (eds): *Acromegaly: A Century of Scientific and Clinical Progress*. New York, Plenum, 1987, pp 115–125.
375. Sano T, Asa SL, Kovacs K: Growth hormone-releasing hormone-producing tumors: Clinical, biochemical, and morphological manifestations. *Endocr Rev* 9:357, 1988.
376. Frohman LA, Thominet JL, Szabo M: Ectopic growth hormone-releasing factor syndromes, in Raiti S, Tolman RA (eds): *Human Growth Hormone*. New York, Plenum, 1986, pp 347–360.
377. Asa Sl, Kovacs K, Thorner MO, Leong DA, Rivier J, Vale W: Immunohistochemical localization of growth hormone-releasing hormone in human tumors. *J Clin Endocrinol Metab* 60:423, 1985.
378. Bostwick DG, Quan R, Hoffman AR, Webber RJ, Chang J-K, Bensch KG: Growth hormone-releasing factor immunoreactivity in human endocrine tumors. *Am J Pathol* 117:167, 1984.
379. Christofides ND, Stephanou A, Suzuki H, Yiangou Y, Bloom SR: Distribution of immunoreactive growth hormone-releasing hormone in the human brain and intestine and its production by tumors. *J Clin Endocrinol Metab* 59:747, 1984.
380. Dayal L, Lin HD, Tallberg K, Reichlin S, DeLellis RA, Wolfe HJ: Immunocytochemical demonstration of growth hormone-releasing factor in gastrointestinal and pancreatic endocrine tumors. *Am J Clin Pathol* 85:13, 1986.
381. Thorner MO, Perryman RL, Cronin MJ, et al: Somatotroph hyperplasia: Successful treatment of acromegaly by removal of a pancreatic islet tumor secreting a growth hormone-releasing factor. *J Clin Invest* 70:965, 1982.
382. Aida M, Furukawa Y, Hanyu K, et al: Familial multiple endocrine neoplasia with a pancreatic carcinoid tumor. *J Clin Exp Med* 101:152, 1977.
383. Melmed S: Extrapituitary acromegaly. *Endocrinol Metab Clin North Am* 20:507, 1991.
384. Braunstein GD, Vaitukaitis JL, Carbone PP, Ross GT: Ectopic production of human chorionic gonadotropin by neoplasms. *Ann Intern Med* 78:39, 1973.
385. Braunstein GD, Bridson WE, Glass A, Hull EW, McIntire WR: *In vivo* and *in vitro* production of human chorionic gonadotropin and alpha-fetoprotein by a virilizing hepatoblastoma. *J Clin Endocrinol Metab* 35:857, 1972.
386. Kato Y, Kelley L, Braunstein GD: Beta-core fragment of human chorionic gonadotropin, in Tomoda Y, Mizutani S, Narita O, Klopper A (eds): *Placental and Endometrial Proteins: Basic and Clinical Aspects*. Utrecht, The Netherlands, VNU Science Press, 1988, pp 87–90.
387. Blithe DL, Wehmann RE, Nisula BC: β-Core: Chemical and clinical properties. *Trends Endocrinol Metab* 1:394, 1990.
388. Horne CHW, Reid IN, Milne GD: Prognostic significance of inappropriate production of pregnancy proteins by breast cancers. *Lancet* 2:279, 1976.
389. Harach HR, Skinner M, Gibbs AR: Biological markers in human lung carcinoma: An immunopathological study of six antigens. *Thorax* 38:937, 1983.
390. Eiermann W, Brutting G, Prechtel K: Detection of pregnancy specific proteins β_1-(SP1) glycoprotein and human placental lactogen in benign breast disease, in Lehmann FG (ed): *Carcino-Embryonic Proteins,* vol II. Amsterdam, Elsevier/North Holland, 1979, pp 477–480.
391. Prechtel K, Eiermann W, Groh M, Brutting G, Hogel B: Ein Beitrag zur Bewertung des Nachweises von schwangerschaftsspezifischen Hormonen (Human placental lactogen and beta-1-glycoprotein) in Brustdrusenexzidaten bei Mastopathie und mammacarcinom. *Pathologe* 4:12, 1983.
392. Muggia FM, Rosen SW, Weintraub BD, Hansen HH: Ectopic placental proteins in nontrophoblastic tumors. *Cancer* 36: 1327, 1975.
393. Stanhope CR, Smith JP, Britton JC, Crosley PK: Serial determination of marker substances in ovarian cancer. *Gynecol Oncol* 8:284, 1979.
394. Szymendera JJ, Kaminska JA, Nowacki MP, Szawlowski A, Gadek A: The serum levels of human α-fetoprotein, AFP, choriogonadotropin, hCG, placental lactogen, hPL, and pregnancy-specific β_1-glycoprotein, SP_1, are of no clinical significance in colorectal carcinoma. *Eur J Cancer Clin Oncol* 17:1047, 1981.
395. Hammond D, Winnick S: Paraneoplastic erythrocytosis and ectopic erythropoietins. *Ann NY Acad Sci* 230:219, 1974.
396. Doll DC, Weiss RB: Neoplasia and the erythron. *J Clin Oncol* 3:429, 1985.
397. VanWingerden JJ, VanRensburg PG, Coetzee BP: Malignant fibrous histiocytoma of the parotid gland associated with polycythemia. *Head Neck Surg* 8:218, 1986.
398. Taillan B, Sanderson F, Fuzibet JG, Vinti H, Pesce A, Dujardin P: Polycythemia secondary to hepatic hemangioma with abnormal secretion of erythropoietin. *Am J Med* 87:700, 1989.
399. Bohnen RF, Banisadre M, Gulbrandson RN, Zanjani ED: Erythrocytosis caused by an erythropoietin-producing breast adenocarcinoma. *West J Med* 152:417, 1990.
400. Anagnostou A, Chawla MS, Pololi L, Fried W: Determination of plasma erythropoietin levels: An early marker of tumor activity. *Cancer* 44:1014, 1979.
401. Koeffler HP, Goldwasser E: Erythropoietin radioimmunoassay in evaluating patients with polycythemia. *Ann Intern Med* 94:44, 1981.

402. Shulkin BL, Shapiro B, Sisson JC: Pheochromocytoma, polycythemia, and venous thrombosis. *Am J Med* 83:773, 1987.
403. Nielsen OJ, Jespersen FF, Hilden M: Erythropoietin-induced secondary polycythemia in a patient with a renal cell carcinoma: A case report. *APMIS (Copenh)* 96:688, 1988.
404. Rigatti P, Montorsi F, Guazzoni G, Viale G, Bulfamante G, Coggi G: Adult nephroblastoma induced erythrocytosis: Report of a case and review of the literature. *Scand J Urol Nephrol* 24:159, 1990.
405. DaSilva J-L, Lacombe C, Bruneval P, et al: Tumor cells are the site of erythropoietin synthesis in human renal cancers associated with polycythemia. *Blood* 75:577, 1990.
406. Thorling EB: Paraneoplastic erythrocytosis and inappropriate erythropoietin production. *Scand J Hematol [Suppl]* 17:1, 1972.
407. Jacobson RJ, Lowenthal MN, Kew MC: Erythrocytosis in hepatocellular carcinoma. *S Afr Med J* 53:658, 1978.
408. Sherwood JB, Goldwasser E: Erythropoietin production by human renal carcinoma cells in culture. *Endocrinology* 99:504, 1976.
409. Sytkowski AJ, Richie WR, Bicknell KA: New human renal carcinoma cell line established from a patient with erythrocytosis. *Cancer Res* 43:1415, 1983.
410. Sytkowski AJ, Bicknell KA, Smith GM, Garcia JF: Secretion of erythropoietin-like activity by clones of human renal carcinoma cell line GKA. *Cancer Res* 44:51, 1984.
411. Waldmann TA, Rosse WF: Tumors producing erythropoiesis-stimulating factors, in Sundermann FW, Sundermann FW Jr (eds): *Hemoglobin: Its Precursors and Metabolism.* Philadelphia, Lippincott, 1964, pp 276–280.
412. Milhaud G, Calmette C, Raymond JP, Bignon J, Moukhtar MS: Carcinoid secretant de la thyrocalcitonin. *Compte Rendu Hebdomadaire des Séances de l'Academie des Sciences,* Series D, 270:2192, 1970.
413. Milhaud G, Calmette C, Taboulet J, Julienne A, Moukhtar MS: Hypersecretion of calcitonin in neoplastic conditions. *Lancet* 1:462, 1974.
414. Coombes RC, Hillyard C, Greenberg PB, MacIntyre I: Plasma-immunoreactive-calcitonin in patients with non-thyroid tumours. *Lancet* 1:1080, 1974.
415. Coombes RC, Ellison ML, Easty GC, Hillyard CJ, James R, Galante L, Girgis S, Heywood L, et al: The ectopic secretion of calcitonin by lung and breast carcinomas. *Clin Endocrinol (Oxf)* 5:387s, 1976.
416. Silva OL, Becker KL, Primack A, Doppman JL, Snider RH: Increased serum calcitonin levels in bronchogenic cancer. *Chest* 69:495, 1976.
417. Hansen M, Hansen HH, Tryding N: Small cell carcinoma of the lung: Serum calcitonin and serum histaminase (diamine oxidase) at basal levels and stimulated by pentagastrin. *Acta Med Scand* 204:257, 1978.
418. Mulder H, Hackeng WHL: Ectopic secretion of calcitonin. *Acta Med Scand* 204:253, 1978.
419. Schwartz KE, Wolfsen AR, Forster B, Odell WD: Calcitonin in nonthyroidal cancer. *J Clin Endocrinol Metab* 49:438, 1979.
420. Silva OL, Broder LE, Doppman JL, Snider RH, Moore CF, Cohen MH, Becker KL: Calcitonin as a marker for bronchogenic cancer: A prospective study. *Cancer* 44:680, 1979.
421. Hillyard CJ, Oscier DG, Foa R, Catovsky D, Goldman JM: Immunoreactive calcitonin in leukaemia. *Br Med J* 2:1392, 1979.
422. Becker KL, Nash DR, Silva OL, Snider RH, Moore CF: Urine calcitonin levels in patients with bronchogenic carcinoma. *JAMA* 243:670, 1980.
423. Mulder H, Silberbusch J, Hackeng WHL, VanDerMeer C, DenOttolander GJH: Hypercalcitoninaemia in patients with chronic inflammatory disease. *Neth J Med* 23:129, 1980.
424. Samaan NA, Castillo S, Schultz PN, Khalil KG, Johnston DA: Serum calcitonin after pentagastrin stimulation in patients with bronchogenic and breast cancer compared to that in patients with medullary thyroid carcinoma. *J Clin Endocrinol Metab* 51:237, 1980.
425. Abe K, Adachi I, Miyakawa S, Tanaka M, Yamaguchi K, Tanaka N, Kameya T, Shimosato Y: Production of calcitonin, adrenocorticotropic hormone, and β-melanocyte-stimulating hormone in tumors derived from amine precursor uptake and decarboxylation cells. *Cancer Res* 37:4190, 1977.
426. Becker KL, Snider RH, Moore CF, Monaghan KG, Silva OL: Calcitonin in extrathyroidal tissues of man. *Acta Endocrinol (Copenh)* 92:746, 1979.
427. Becker KL, Monaghan KG, Silva OL: Immunocytochemical localization of calcitonin in Kulchitsky cells of human lung. *Arch Pathol Lab Med* 104:196, 1980.
428. Silva OL, Becker KL, Primack A, Doppman JL, Snider RH: Hypercalcitonemia in bronchogenic cancer: Evidence for thyroid origin of the hormone. *JAMA* 234:183, 1975.
429. Roos BA, Lindall AW, Baylin SB, O'Neil JA, Frelinger AL, Birnbaum RS, Lambert PW: Plasma immunoreactive calcitonin in lung cancer. *J Clin Endocrinol Metab* 50:659, 1980.
430. Ellison M, Woodhouse D, Hillyard C, Dowsett M, Coombes RC, Gilby ED, Greenberg PB, Neville AM: Immunoreactive calcitonin production by human lung carcinoma cells in culture. *Br J Cancer* 32:3731, 1975.
431. Zajac JD, Martin TJ, Hudson P, Niall H, Jacobs JW: Biosynthesis of calcitonin by human lung cancer cells. *Endocrinology* 116:749, 1985.
432. Lumsden J, Ham J, Ellison ML: Purification and partial characterization of high-molecular-weight forms of ectopic calcitonin from a human bronchial carcinoma cell line. *Biochem J* 191:239, 1980.
433. Bertagna XY, Nicholson WE, Pettengill OS, Sorenson GD, Mount CD, Orth DN: Ectopic production of high molecular weight calcitonin and corticotropin by human small cell carcinoma cells in tissue culture: Evidence for separate precursors. *J Clin Endocrinol Metab* 47:1390, 1978.
434. Nelkin BD, Rosenfeld KI, deBustros A, Leong SS, Roos BA, Baylin SB: Structure and expression of a gene encoding human calcitonin and calcitonin gene related peptide. *Biochem Biophys Res Commun* 123:648, 1984.
435. Mulder H: Ectopic secretion of calcitonin as a tumor marker. *Anticancer Res* 3:247, 1983.
436. Turkington RW: Ectopic production of prolactin. *N Engl J Med* 285:1455, 1971.
437. Davis S, Proper S, May PB, Ertel NH: Elevated prolactin levels in bronchogenic carcinoma. *Cancer* 44:676, 1979.
438. Molitch ME, Schwartz S, Mukherji B: Is prolactin secreted ectopically? *Am J Med* 70:803, 1981.
439. Podmore J, Wilson B, Cowden EA, Beastall GH, Ratcliffe JG: Multiple hormones in human tumors, in Lehman GF (ed.): *Carcino-Embryonic Proteins,* vol 1. New York, Elsevier/North Holland, 1979, pp 457–463.
440. Rosen SW, Weintraub BD, Aaronson SA: Non random ectopic protein production by malignant cells: Direct evidence in vitro. *J Clin Endocrinol Metab* 50:834, 1980.
441. Said SI, Faloona GR: Elevated plasma and tissue levels of vasoactive intestinal polypeptide in the watery-diarrhea syndrome due to pancreatic bronchogenic and other tumors. *N Engl J Med* 293:155, 1975.
442. Hamilton I, Reis L, Bilimoria S, Long RG: A renal vipoma. *Br Med J* 281:1323, 1980.
443. Mendelsohn G, Eggleston JC, Olson JL, Said SI, Baylin SB: Vasoactive intestinal peptide and its relationship to ganglion cell differentiation in neuroblastic tumors. *Lab Invest* 41:144, 1979.
444. Cooney DR, Voorhess ML, Fisher JE, Brecher M, Karp MP, Jewett TC: Vasoactive intestinal peptide producing neuroblastoma. *J Pediatr Surg* 17:821, 1982.
445. Maton PN, O'Dorisio TM, Howe BA, et al: Effect of a long-acting somatostatin analogue (SMS 201-995) in a patient with pancreatic cholera. *N Engl J Med* 312:17, 1985.
446. Penman E, Wass JAH, Besser GM, Rees LH: Somatostatin secretion by lung and thymic tumours. *Clin Endocrinol (Oxf)* 13:613, 1980.
447. Szabo M, Berelowitz M, Pettengill OS, Sorenson GD, Froh-

man LA: Ectopic production of somatostatin-like immuno- and bioactivity by cultured human pulmonary small cell carcinoma. *J Clin Endocrinol Metab* 51:978, 1980.
448. Long TT III, Barton TK, Draffin R, Reeves WJ, McCarty KS Jr: Conservative management of Zollinger-Ellison syndrome: Ectopic gastrin production by an ovarian cystadenoma. *JAMA* 243:1837, 1980.
449. Margolis RM, Jang N: Zollinger-Ellison syndrome associated with pancreatic cystadenocarcinoma. *N Engl J Med* 311:1380, 1984.
450. Gleeson MH, Bloom SR, Polak JM, Henry K, Dowling RH: Endocrine tumour in kidney affecting small bowel structure, motility, and absorptive function. *Gut* 12:773, 1971.
451. Hunstein W, Trumper LH, Dummer R, Schwechheimer K: Glucagonoma syndrome and bronchial carcinoma. *Ann Intern Med* 109:920, 1988.
452. Sakura H, Hamada Y, Tsuruta S, Okamoto K, Nakamura S: Large glucagon-like immunoreactivity in a primary ovarian carcinoid. *Cancer* 55:1001, 1985.
453. Price J, Nieuwenhuijzen-Kruseman AC, Doniach I, Howlett TA, Besser GM, Rees LH: Bombesin-like peptides in human endocrine tumors: Quantitation, biochemical characterization, and secretion. *J Clin Endocrinol Metab* 60:1097, 1985.
454. Ganguly A, Gribble J, Tune B, Kempson RL, Luetscher JA: Renin-secreting Wilms' tumor with severe hypertension: Report of a case and brief review of renin-secreting tumors. *Ann Intern Med* 79:835, 1973.
455. Mitchell JD, Baxter TJ, Blair-West JR, McCredie DA: Renin levels in nephroblastoma (Wilms' tumour): Report of a renin secreting tumour. *Arch Dis Child* 45:376, 1970.
456. Sheth KJ, Tang TT, Blaedel ME, Good TA: Polydipsia, polyuria, and hypertension associated with renin-secreting Wilms' tumor. *J Pediatr* 92:921, 1978.
457. Spahr J, Demers LM, Shochat SJ: Renin producing Wilms' tumor. *J Pediatr Surg* 16:32, 1981.
458. Kihara I, Kitamura S, Hashimo T, Seida H, Watanabe T: A hitherto unreported vascular tumor of the kidney: A proposal of juxtaglomerular cell tumor. *Acta Pathol Jpn* 18:197, 1968.
459. Hollifield JW, Page DL, Smith C, Michelakis AM, Staab E, Rhamy R: Renin-secreting clear cell carcinoma of the kidney. *Arch Intern Med* 135:859, 1975.
460. Ruddy MC, Atlas SA, Salerno FG: Hypertension associated with a renin-secreting adenocarcinoma of the pancreas. *N Engl J Med* 307:993, 1982.
461. Hauger-Klevene JH: High plasma renin activity in an oat cell carcinoma: A renin-secreting carcinoma? *Cancer* 26:1112, 1970.
462. Aurell M, Rudin A, Tisell L-E, Kindblom LG, Sandberg G: Captopril effect on hypertension in patient with renin-producing tumour. *Lancet* 2:149, 1979.
463. Atlas SA, Hesson TE, Sealey JE, Dharmgrongartama B, Laragh JH, Ruddy MC, Aurell M: Characterization of inactive renin ("Prorenin") from renin-secreting tumors of nonrenal origin: Similarity to inactive renin from kidney and normal plasma. *J Clin Invest* 73:437, 1984.

CHAPTER 30

Hormone-Responsive Tumors

Christopher C. Benz

Tumorigenesis can be defined as a form of uncontrolled tissue growth and can be thought of as a potential dysfunction in the multiplicity of hormonal, autocrine, and paracrine mechanisms that govern normal tissue proliferation and maturation. Tumors are typically composed of proliferating cells of larger size and lesser histologic differentiation than those found in normal mature tissue, mimicking the hyperplastic and hypertrophic states these tissues assume during their normal prenatal and postnatal growth periods. Thus, it may be logical to suppose that the hormones and factors that support somatic growth also contribute to tumorigenesis. As discussed in Chap. 26, however, most hormones do not directly stimulate tissue or organ growth. Recent evidence indicates that cell growth is controlled and coordinated by growth factors whose local production is hormonally mediated; this evidence is consistent with our current understanding of tumorigenesis.

Among the growth-permissive hormones (growth hormone, thyroid hormone, insulin, glucocorticoids, and sex steroids), only sex steroids are known to stimulate cell growth directly, and some of these steroids have proved to have mutagenic and carcinogenic properties. In contrast, many of the known growth factors and their receptors can be readily shown to have transforming or tumorigenic properties under appropriate circumstances; in fact, they are structurally homologous to known oncogenes (Table 30-1; see Chap. 5 for a review of oncogene-regulated cell growth). The notion that autonomous tumor growth is driven by the dysregulated expression of locally produced and locally acting growth factors is now generally accepted, and humoral models of growth stimulation at the cellular level illustrate the functional relation that exists between growth factors and oncogenes in addition to their known structural relations (Table 30-1). When the cellular mechanisms underlying autonomous tissue growth are linked to the growth-promoting effects of sex steroids, the clinical result is a hormone-responsive tumor.

There are many *in vitro* and *in vivo* models showing localized production of growth factors by tumors that have receptors for these autostimulating factors *(autocrine loop)*. Autocrine factors produced by certain activated oncogenes (e.g., c-*sis*) may not even be secreted extracellularly; rather, they may simply be factors that, alone or bound to internally sequestered receptors, result in malignant transformation. Perhaps as important as the autocrine loop in tumorigenesis is another, more insidious humoral process in which the transformed cells recruit local normal cells of stromal or epithelial origin to secrete growth factors required by the receptor-bearing malignant cells *(paracrine loop)*. This paracrine interdependence between adjacent normal tissues and malignant tissues has been used to explain a variety of neoplastic phenomena, including site-specific metastases, fibroblast and endothelial chemotaxis and proliferation (leading to stromal reactivity and tumor neovascularity), local bone resorption and malignant hypercalcemia, and the suppression of normal immune reactions, that are commonly observed features of advancing malignancy. In hormonally responsive tumors, all these neoplastic and paraneoplastic phenomena can be controlled with endocrine intervention, indicating that the interruption of autocrine and paracrine loops represents a successful therapeutic strategy.

Hormonally responsive human tumors may be few in type, but they are prevalent in number. They account for 20 percent of all newly diagnosed male cancers and 40 percent of all newly diagnosed female cancers and are best represented by breast, endometrial, and prostate adenocarcinomas. These three particular forms of cancer arise in the target organs most responsive to the growth regulatory influences of estrogens, progestins, and androgens. The early observations of Bittner, Huggins, Furth, and others first established the association between sex steroids and these target gland tumors.[1–6] The early theory that hormones influence the growth of some human cancers has been extended by Henderson and colleagues, who have suggested that sex steroids play a pathogenic role in about 30 percent of all human cancers in the United States.[7]

In a general sense, it is probably true that endocrine dependency can develop as an associated trait

TABLE 30-1 Common Growth Factors and Receptors Probably Involved in the Autocrine and Paracrine Stimulation of Hormone-Responsive Human Tumors

Extracellular Growth Factors [Homologous Oncogenes]	Growth Factor Receptors [Homologous Oncogenes]
Epidermal growth factor (EGF)	170-kDa tyrosine kinase [c-*erb* B-1] on epithelial and mesenchymal cell membranes
Transforming growth factor α (TGF-α)	Cross-reacts with EGF receptor on same cells
Transforming growth factor β (TGF-β)	Family of tyrosine kinase and proteoglycan membrane receptors on epithelial and mesenchymal cells as well as an extracellular matrix proteoglycan receptor
Platelet-derived growth factor (PDGF) [c-*sis* with beta chain]	185-kDa tyrosine kinase on smooth muscle and mesenchymal cell membranes
Insulin-like growth factor-I (IGF-I/somatomedin C)	450-kDa tyrosine kinase [c-*ros* and c-*src* with beta chain] on epithelial and mesenchymal cell membranes
Insulin-like growth factor-II (IGF-II/somatomedin A)	250-kDa glycoprotein on epithelial and mesenchymal cell membranes
Fibroblast growth factors (FGFs) [*int*-2 with basic form]	Family of membrane tyrosine kinases on endothelial and mesenchymal cells whose binding is dependent on glycosaminoglycans or proteoglycans present in membrane and extracellular matrix

Source: Adapted from references 97–103.

of any malignancy arising in a tissue whose normal growth is controlled by sex hormones. Studies have demonstrated links between estrogens and vaginal, ovarian, laryngeal, pancreatic, and other gastrointestinal carcinomas as well as melanomas and meningiomas.[6–8] Epidemiologic data indicate that 10 years of oral contraceptive use can reduce the risk of developing ovarian cancer by about 50 percent,[9] yet mechanisms directly linking sex steroids with the growth control of ovarian cancer have not been discovered. With further epidemiologic and basic study, it is likely that other tumors will be added to the list of proven and putative hormone-responsive human tumors shown in Table 30-2. Interesting clinical leads include the fact that the incidence of osteosarcoma closely parallels the age-specific growth patterns of men and women, implicating pubertal hormonal changes in the etiology of this tumor; also, meningiomas and thyroid and renal cell carcinomas all show a marked discrepancy in male-female incidence and prognosis, and these tumors occasionally possess steroid receptors, suggesting that sex steroids also regulate their growth[8] (see Receptor Mechanisms Mediating Hormone Response).

In contrast to the growth-promoting effects of sex steroids, glucocorticoids are normally capable of inducing cytolytic responses in some human lymphocytes mediated by steroid-induced intracellular enzymes. With this realization, glucocorticoids have been employed extensively in the treatment of leukemia and lymphoma[10,11]; thus, some clinicians consider these hematologic malignancies to be hormonally responsive. With regard to nonsteroidal hormones, thyroid, testicular, and ovarian tumors,

TABLE 30-2 Classification of Hormone-Responsive Tumors

	Hormone Dependency		
	Sex Steroids	Glucocorticoids	Polypeptides
Primary therapy based on hormones			
Breast cancer	X		
Uterine (endometrial) cancer	X		
Prostate cancer	X		
Antitumor therapy that may include hormones			
Leukemia/lymphomas		X	
Ovarian cancer	X		
Renal cell carcinoma	X		
Melanoma	X		X
Pancreatic carcinoma	X		
Thyroid carcinoma			X
Pituitary adenoma			X
Carcinoid and other APUDomas			X

as well as melanoma and APUDomas (tumors from cells capable of amine precursor uptake and decarboxylation), all occur in tissues that are under the tropic influences of various polypeptide hormones. Many of these tumors retain their endocrine dependencies and, like papillary thyroid carcinomas responsive to thyroid stimulating hormone (TSH)–suppressing doses of thyroid hormone, they are appropriately considered hormone-responsive. In this chapter, however, we will focus on hormonal issues related to sex steroid–responsive breast, endometrial, and prostate cancers. Among these, breast cancer will be discussed in the greatest detail because it is the most common and life-threatening of these epithelial malignancies. Breast cancer has also received greater attention by basic scientists; thus, it provides a rich source of examples to illustrate concepts that probably are applicable to all hormone-responsive tumors.

GENERAL ASPECTS CONCERNING THE DEVELOPMENT OF HORMONE-RESPONSIVE TUMORS

A consideration of some general aspects of cancer development is relevant for hormone-responsive tumors, and the reader is advised to consult more general texts on cancer for a broader overview.[12] Central to modern precepts is the notion that cancers are caricatures of normal tissue development and renewal processes, driven by DNA mutations and the abnormal expression of genes otherwise critical for normal cellular ontogeny.

Substantial evidence over the past decade indicates that human cancers do not result from a single mutagenic event. Like most solid epithelial tumors, hormonally responsive cancers appear to arise from stepwise genetic changes that produce clonal chromosomal abnormalities. From epidemiologic studies and animal models, the essential carcinogenic events can be grouped into three basic steps: tumor *initiation*, tumor *promotion* (early and late), and tumor *progression*. In the common human epithelial cancers, these steps typically appear to require 1 to 2 days (initiation), 10 to 20 years (promotion), and 1 to 5 years (progression). The experimentally observed in vivo events associated with tumor latency, preneoplasia, and the clinical outgrowth of a hormonally responsive tumor are illustrated in Fig. 30-1. Carcinogen-induced initiation may involve not only subcellular and intercellular mechanisms that stimulate cell growth but also other genetic events that relieve the cell of influences that keep it from dividing, such as the inactivation of so-called antioncogenes or tumor suppressor genes.[13] Promotion and progression involve influences that allow the tumor to proliferate and spread, such as suppression of a host's immunologic responses and the diverse effects of activated oncogenes as discussed below (see The Role of Oncogenes and Tumor Suppressor Genes in Hormone-Responsive Tumors).

While carcinogens may be encountered in either inactive (precarcinogen) or active forms, most precarcinogens are first activated in the large intestine or liver and then are distributed to specific host tissues where the activated carcinogen damages cellular constituents. The ultimate subcellular site of action of a carcinogen is DNA. However, the genetic damage is achieved either directly by the activated compound or indirectly by host molecules, such as membrane-bound lipids, and the subsequent generation of toxic intermediates that damage DNA structure. In the case of radiation and chemically alkylating aromatic hydrocarbons, DNA damage can occur either directly or indirectly through intracellular free radicals.

Steroids as Carcinogens and Tumor Promoters

Among the wide variety of catalogued carcinogens, natural and synthetic steroids or steroidlike compounds represent some of the most prevalent endogenously or exogenously contacted carcinogens. These compounds act as tumor initiators or promoters, often in cooperation with host effects from lipids and other nutritionally derived chemicals that are capable of altering tissue metabolism.

Hormonally induced tumors have been observed for over 50 years in experimental animals. In particular, many mammalian species, including primates, are known to be susceptible to the tumorigenic properties of estrogens.[14] Steroidal estrogens are mild carcinogens that are structurally related to the more toxic cholanthrene carcinogens. A variety of naturally occurring phytoestrogens and synthetic xenobiotic stilbene estrogens [e.g., diethylstilbesterol (DES)] are known to be metabolically activated by organs such as the liver and kidney into catechols, whose conversion into more reactive intermediates (inhibitable by antioxidants) generates free radicals and mutagenic DNA adducts and strand breaks.[15–19]

These steroid-induced events in animals appear to be remarkably similar to clinical events observed in patients with breast and prostate cancers, except that the human time scale of tumorigenesis involves years rather than months. Of note, the antiestrogen tamoxifen can dramatically inhibit estrogen-induced tumor development in these animals. In such cases, however, tamoxifen does not appear to affect the level of estrogen-induced DNA damage, suggesting that at least part of the steroid's tumorigenic role is nonreversible tumor initiation that is not mediated by a classical steroid receptor mechanism.[20] However, in typical animal models of estrogen-induced renal and hepatic cancers (Fig. 30-1), both steroid receptor–mediated mechanisms and the microsomal

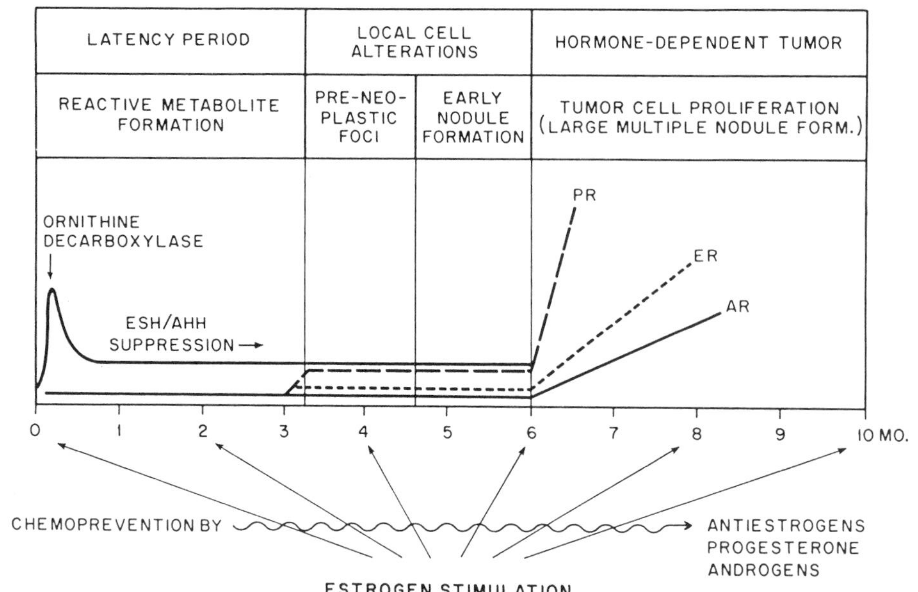

FIGURE 30-1 Experimentally observed progression of events associated with the formation of estrogen-induced hormone-dependent tumors. In typical animal models of renal and hepatic tumor initiation and promotion following repeated estrogen stimulation, steroid receptor levels [progesterone receptor (PR), estrogen receptor (ER), androgen receptor (AR)] increase well above normal levels many months after the tumor-initiating DNA damage. The mutagenic and irreversible DNA damage is produced by excess free radicals and unrepaired DNA adducts and strand breaks that occur with the estrogen induction of microsomally activated catechols by aryl hydrocarbon hydroxylase (AHH) and estrogen 2-/4-hydroxylase (ESH). Throughout the entire interval of tumor promotion, which typically requires 10 to 20 years in humans, antiestrogens and various other compounds may act as chemoprevention agents and inhibit tumor formation; however, there is no evidence that these chemoprevention agents can reverse the tumor-initiating DNA damage. (*Modified from Li and Li.*[19])

activation by estrogen of aryl hydrocarbon hydroxylase (AHH) and estrogen 2-/4-hydroxylase (ESH) are necessary for tumor formation. In such models, nontoxic dietary supplements have been shown to be critically important in modulating the microsomal oxidative activation of catechols,[19] providing experimental support for the epidemiologic role of diet in human tumorigenesis. The observed inability of tamoxifen to prevent steroid-induced DNA damage and tumor initiation in animals is clinically relevant as tamoxifen tumor prevention trials begin in humans.[21]

In mammalian models of carcinogen-induced breast cancer, tumors usually develop only after females become sexually mature, supporting the tumor-promoting role of endogenous sex hormones.[22] Also, carcinogens are rarely effective in rodent breast tumor models if given before puberty, suggesting that the tumor-initiating DNA damage occurs in genes transcriptionally activated by endogenous sex steroids.[23] These observations are consistent with epidemiologic data in humans. Higher incidences of breast cancers are observed in women who have been exposed to ionizing radiation at puberty (age 10 to 12) and before first pregnancy and lactation,[24] and early and prolonged exposure to exogenous estrogens is associated with an increased risk for the later development of vaginal, uterine, and breast carcinomas.[25] Detailed studies of rodent mammary tumorigenesis have pointed out the critical status of undifferentiated breast ductal tissue and its susceptibility to tumor initiation. Comparative histomorphologic analyses indicate that mammary cancers in both rats and humans appear to arise from the steroid-responsive terminal end buds and pubertal type I lobular units (composed of ducts and ductules) abundant in developing mammary tissue.[22] Not only are these immature breast structures the most actively proliferating and hormonally responsive mammary elements throughout life, they remain the breast elements most vulnerable to oncogenic transformation.[22]

In contrast to the well-established tumor-initiating and tumor-promoting influences of estrogenic steroids, the tumorigenic role of nonaromatic steroids such as androgens is less well documented. Androgenizing testis tumors are known to produce rodent prostate cancers. Testosterone and its 5α-reduced metabolite, dihydrotestosterone, can induce prostatic adenocarcinomas in experimental animals in which it is particularly difficult to induce tumors by any other means.[26] The embryologic origins of the human prostate from both endodermal and mesodermal tissues appears to provide the most important discriminant for the development of androgen-dependent benign and malignant prostate growth later in life. Although both prostate tissue components are sensitive to androgens, benign prostatic hypertrophy (BPH) develops only in the mesodermally derived periurethral tissue component, while prostate cancer usually develops in the peripheral glandular cells and long-branched ducts of the endodermally derived tissue component. This may explain why BPH is not in itself a premalignant condition, but it provides no rationale for the tumorigenic propensity of the endodermally derived epithelium unless the hypertrophic tissues release paracrine factors that stimulate the growth of the endodermally derived cells, as has been suggested with respect to the tumorigenic role of prostatic mesenchyme. Perhaps recent experimental models of prostate cancer development by transfection of *ras* and *myc* oncogenes into murine fetal cloacal tissue will assist in the study of this question.[27]

The abundant mesenchyme present in the endodermal zone of the prostate may play an important tumorigenic role, since recent studies have shown that it is critical in conferring androgenic differentiation on both normal and neoplastic prostate epithelium. Using androgen receptor–containing rat urogenital mesenchyme and the serially transplantable R3327 Dunning prostate tumor, investigators have shown that androgenic influences on prostatic epithelium can be either tumor growth–promoting or tumor growth–inhibiting, depending on the absence or presence of functioning prostatic mesenchyme, respectively.[28–31] The nature of these hormone-mediated paracrine influences within the prostate gland must still be defined, since this experimental model suggests that prostate tumors lack an androgen-induced paracrine mechanism of growth control and differentiation. The hypothesis that an aberrant stromal-epithelial interaction leads to hormone-responsive tumorigenesis may similarly apply to breast and endometrial cancers, but it has been proposed only for prostate cancer because of the novel mesenchyme-tumor animal model recently developed from the older R3327 prostate cancer model. The serially transplantable Dunning prostate tumor was developed 30 years ago from a spontaneous prostate cancer arising in an aged Copenhagen rat; it requires androgen for growth in vivo, behaves much as human prostate cancer does, and remains one of the few good animal models for studying hormone-responsive prostate cancer.[32]

The Role of Oncogenes and Tumor Suppressor Genes in Hormone-Responsive Tumors

Oncogenes activated by DNA amplification, gene rearrangement, mutation, or deletion have been identified in isolated cases of virtually every type of human malignancy. With few exceptions, however, there is only preliminary evidence to implicate specific oncogenes in the etiology or progression of hormonally responsive human tumors.[33] Chemical carcinogens and the genomic integration of viral DNA can each induce hormone-dependent tumor growth through tissue-specific activation of transforming (dominant acting) proto-oncogenes. Mouse mammary cancers are commonly induced by the murine mammary tumor virus (MMTV), which is a weakly oncogenic type B retrovirus.[34,35] A less well studied pathogen is the rat C-type retrovirus, R-35 (possibly the same as the endogenous RaLV retrovirus sequence), which may be an important cause of spontaneous rat mammary cancers.[35] The regional insertion of MMTV DNA activates the genomic c-*int* family of proto-oncogenes, any number of which are then constitutively expressed in mammary epithelium, leading first to premalignant hyperplastic lesions and finally to infiltrating adenocarcinomas.[36] Since there is a closely linked steroid receptor–binding sequence (hormone response element; see Chap. 5) within the integrated MMTV long terminal repeat (LTR) segment of this retrovirus, this transforming process is promoted in vivo by endogenous exposure to steroids. Although the MMTV retrovirus does not infect humans and although there are no proven viral etiologies for hormonally responsive human cancer, there have been provocative observations implicating similar viruses in human breast cancer. In particular, morphologic, immunologic, enzyme, and nucleic acid evidence exists for MMTV-like viral involvement in breast cancer patients, including the temporal association of seroconversion with the clinical onset of human breast cancer.[37–40] Malignant transformation through the activation of c-*int* proto-oncogenes independent of viral integration may be important in human tumorigenesis, moreover, as judged by the ability of c-*int*-1 to partially transform normal mammary epithelial cells[41] and the recent finding of amplified c-*int*-2 sequences in at least 15 percent of human breast cancer specimens.[42]

The transfection of activated oncogenes into mammalian cells has been useful in shedding light on the molecular mechanisms operative in hormone-responsive tumors such as breast cancer. Kasid and colleagues transfected an activated Ha-*ras* oncogene into human MCF-7 breast cancer cells and found that in contrast to normal MCF-7 cells, the transfected breast cancer cells were no longer dependent on exogenous estrogen for tumorigenic growth in nude mice.[43] As will be discussed later, breast, endometrial, and prostate cancers that are normally responsive to hormones in their early clinical stages invariably evolve to become hormonally independent during tumor progression, at which time the diseases behave more aggressively and the tumors are no longer responsive to endocrine therapy. Although *ras* mutations are not commonly found in human breast tumors,[33] the *ras* transfection study with MCF-7 cells demonstrated that activated oncogene products may assist in the conversion of cancers to a hormonally unresponsive and clinically more aggressive state. In another revealing set of oncogene transfer studies, Leder and colleagues produced transgenic mice carrying the c-*erbB*-2 (HER2/*neu*) oncogene, activated by a point mutation and fused to a MMTV-LTR sequence which acted as the steroid-inducible promoter/enhancer.[44] This oncogene encodes a transmembrane tyrosine kinase growth factor receptor with extensive homology to the epidermal growth factor (EGF) receptor (Table 30-1). All female founders possessed the MMTV-LTR/*erbB*-2 transgene in all the tissues analyzed and passed it on to progeny mice of both sexes in a Mendelian fashion. Among the few murine tissues found to express this transgene in subsequent progeny, the breast glands preferentially developed infiltrating and metastasizing adenocarcinomas. Unlike the stochastic occurrence of solitary breast tumors found in similar transgenic animals carrying either MMTV-LTR/*myc* or MMTV-LTR/Ha-*ras* fusion genes, mice expressing MMTV-LTR/*erbB*-2 showed rapid growth of polyclonal cancers throughout the epithelial tissue of every mammary gland. Thus, unlike the effect of constitutively overexpressed c-*myc* or activated Ha-*ras* genes in mammalian breast tissue, activated c-*erbB*-2 under a steroid-inducible promoter appears to be sufficient to induce a single-step malignant transformation of mammary tissue into hormonally responsive breast cancer. The mammary tissue tropism of the transforming oncogene is probably specified by the transgene's promoter since a milk fat whey acidic protein (Wap) gene promoter can also be used in such transgenic constructs to produce breast-specific hormone-dependent breast cancers in vivo.[45]

Oncogene and tumor suppressor gene studies have provided important clues to the molecular mechanisms underlying hormone-dependent tumorigenesis in humans. A recent review of activated oncogenes putatively implicated in human mammary cancer indicated that the amplification of c-*erbB*-2 represents the most clinically important dominant transforming gene found in breast cancer specimens to date, present in 17 to 35 percent of all invasive breast tumors and predicting less favorable patient survival.[46] More recently, recessive genetic changes associated with the inactivation of tumor-suppressing gene products such as RB (retinoblastoma protein) and p53 have also been identified as important and common contributing events in human tumorigenesis. As can be seen in surveys of breast tumor samples, genetic or transcriptional abnormalities relating to RB and p53 may occur in 13 to 50 percent of cases, although molecular links between inactivated tumor suppressor genes and the tissue specificity or hormone dependency of given tumors have not been described.[46] Fewer studies have addressed the importance of oncogenes and tumor suppressor genes in prostate and endometrial cancers.[33] Preliminary evidence indicates that c-*myc* may be overexpressed in prostate cancer,[47] but there is perhaps more convincing evidence for the clinical importance of c-*ras*, as suggested by the studies of Viola and colleagues[48] in which overexpression of this oncogene product appeared to correlate with more aggressive (poor nuclear grade and histologic differentiation) and presumably hormonally independent prostate cancers. A mechanistic association between oncogene activation or tumor suppressor gene inactivation and the hormone sensitivity of either prostate or endometrial cancers has not been uncovered.

Epidemiologic Features of Hormone-Responsive Tumors

Age, geography, diet, and genetics result in common epidemiologic associations supporting a tumorigenic role for sex steroids in the development of breast, endometrial, and prostate cancers. These associations are summarized in Table 30-3.

Age and Hormones

Age is the predominant determinant of overall cancer risk in the general population, with most life-threatening cancers occurring in people over age 65.[49] The explanation for this age-related increase in incidence is believed to be multifactorial, including a natural decline in immune and mesenchymal tissue function, impaired subcellular repair mechanisms, and accumulated damage from oxidation and environmental carcinogens combined with the prolonged

TABLE 30-3 Common Clinical Associations between Breast, Endometrial, and Prostate Cancers

Latent increase in incidence with age beyond puberty
Congenital risk increased with hypergonadal function (e.g., Klinefelter's syndrome, polycystic ovaries) and reduced with hypogonadal function (e.g., Turner's syndrome, eunuchoidism)
Geographic profile of excess risk correlates with population's nutritional profile (dietary fat, obesity)
Multiple risk factors related to endogenous and/or exogenous imbalance in estrogen/androgen exposure
Prognosis and therapy related to tumor steroid receptor levels (ER, PR, AR) and hormonal intervention

effects of endogenous risk factors such as obesity and exposure to sex steroids. Figure 30-2 compares the age-specific incidence rates of breast, endometrial, and prostate cancers relative to cancers of all sites in men and women. For breast and endometrial cancers, the incidence curves begin to plateau or decline by age 65, presumably as a delayed response to the changes in ovarian sex steroid levels that occur with menopause (about age 50) that result in a 60 percent decline in circulating progesterone and estrogen (estrone, estradiol) levels and a 50 percent decline in androgenic precursors such as dehydroepiandrosterone (DHEA) and androstenedione. The incidence of endometrial cancer reportedly rose during the years 1960–1973 in parallel with the increased use of exogenous estrogens as postmenopausal replacement therapy. Studies showing increased cancer risks from exogenous estrogens also indicate that it takes larger amounts and longer exposures to estrogen to affect breast cancer risk rates than is the case for endometrial cancer which arises in a more estrogen-sensitive target organ. This presents an interesting paradox, since breast cancers occur with greater overall frequency while endometrial cancers occur later in life (80 percent are diagnosed after menopause). To reconcile these disparate facts, it has been suggested that endometrial tissue is protected early on by progestins from the carcinogenic influence of estrogens, while additional nonhormonal factors contribute to the risk of developing early breast cancer.

FIGURE 30-2 Age-specific incidence rates of individual hormone-responsive cancers (breast, uterine/endometrial, prostate) in comparison to the combined incidence of cancers from all sites in men and women. (*Incidence curves reproduced from Fraumeni et al,[49] originally derived from N.C.I./S.E.E.R. program data on U.S. white population, 1981–1985.*)

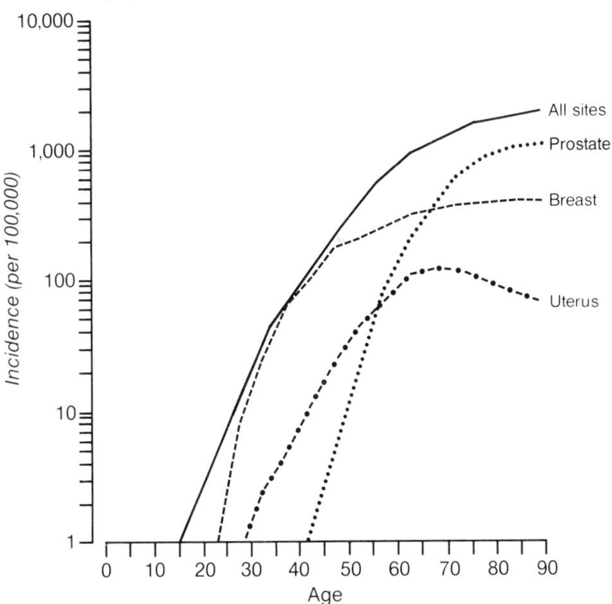

Despite reports to the contrary and after more than 30 years of investigation into the relations between breast and endometrial cancers and sex steroids, there is no clear-cut pattern of abnormal hormone production or excretion involving estrogens, androgens, progesterone, or prolactin in women who (after weight and diet are accounted for) are at increased risk for these malignancies. The details of these studies have been reviewed, and the lack of a conclusion does not refute the basic hypothesis that one or more abnormalities in endogenous steroid metabolism contribute to the eventual development of breast or endometrial cancer.[50,51] Henderson, Pike, and colleagues have measured higher serum and urinary estradiol levels in postmenopausal breast cancer patients compared to healthy individually matched control women; these groups had no significant differences with regard to prolactin or androgen levels.[52] These investigators also found significantly higher serum estrone and estradiol levels in healthy postmenopausal American women compared to a cohort of postmenopausal Japanese women at low risk for breast cancer.[53] From these studies they concluded that the risk for developing postmenopausal (but not premenopausal) breast cancer is related to serum estrogen levels. While they were controlled for women's weight, these studies were not controlled for diet or fat intake, factors which could certainly affect serum estrogen levels. Pike has suggested that high American rates of breast, endometrial, and ovarian cancers are completely explained by an increased total number of menstrual cycles associated with earlier menarche, low parity, less intensive breast-feeding, a high-fat diet, and obesity.[54]

In contrast to breast and endometrial cancers, prostate cancer shows an even more marked and steadily rising incidence associated with age, as shown in Fig. 30-2.[49,55,56] Men at age 80 have a 40-fold higher risk than those at age 50, and over 80 percent of all prostate cancers arise in men over age 65. This age-related difference in incidence from that seen with breast and endometrial cancers is consistent with the relative lack of change in circulating sex steroid levels in men over age 50, perhaps allowing the tumor-promoting effect of androgens to accumulate after age 65. Alternatively, the presence of estrogen receptor in prostatic tissue and tumors and the well-documented accelerated aromatization of androgens to estrogens that occurs with advancing age also argue that androgenic precursors or estrogen conversion is important in determining the age-related increase in prostate cancer incidence.[49] Of interest, black American males have the highest rates of prostate cancer in the world, with an incidence that peaks between 80 and 84 years of age, unlike white American males, in whom a continuously increasing incidence rate is observed beyond age 85. This ethnic and geographic difference in the incidence of prostate cancer appears to be independent of socioeconomic factors and may be related to dietary influences and/or the higher mean serum testosterone levels measured in American blacks compared to American white males.[57] Nonetheless, the hypothesis that sex steroids account for the age-related increase in human prostate cancer is somewhat more speculative than that for breast and endometrial cancers, in which the tumorigenic potential of estrogens is better understood.

Geography, Diet, and Genetics

The human diet has changed profoundly over a short period of recent evolutionary time. Hunter-gatherer societies today subsist as they did 10,000 years ago, on fewer calories, 50 percent less fat, and 300 percent more fiber compared with the present-day U.S. diet. We are essentially trying to alter the dietary habits of our 10,000-year-old physiology with western-style diets acquired within the past 250 years. A compelling body of evidence indicates that these dietary changes, along with a more sedentary and stress-filled lifestyle, account for the increased obesity, earlier maturity, and greater amount of cardiovascular disease and cancer, which were uncommon even in the eighteenth and nineteenth centuries.[58] In particular, it is now accepted that the worldwide geographic variations in organ-specific and age-specific cancer rates are attributable less to genetic and ethnic differences than to environmental influences, of which diet must be considered the most prominent. This is certainly true for our most common epithelial malignancies, including breast, prostate, and endometrial cancers.

The observed shifts in ethnic incidences of breast, prostate, and gastrointestinal cancers occurring within two generations of immigrants from low-incidence areas (Japan, Poland) living in high-incidence regions (Hawaii, California) are generally attributable to changes in dietary habits.[49,58] Figure 30-3 shows the strong linear correlation that exists between per capita dietary fat consumption and breast cancer mortality in many different nations.[58,59] As economic advances affect low-cancer-incidence countries such as Japan, Iceland, Italy, and Greece, dietary shifts toward more fat and higher total caloric

FIGURE 30-3 Correlation between per capita dietary fat consumption and reported breast cancer mortality in different nations. *(Reproduced from Cohen,[58] previously published in Carroll KK, Cancer Res 35:3374–3383, 1975.)*

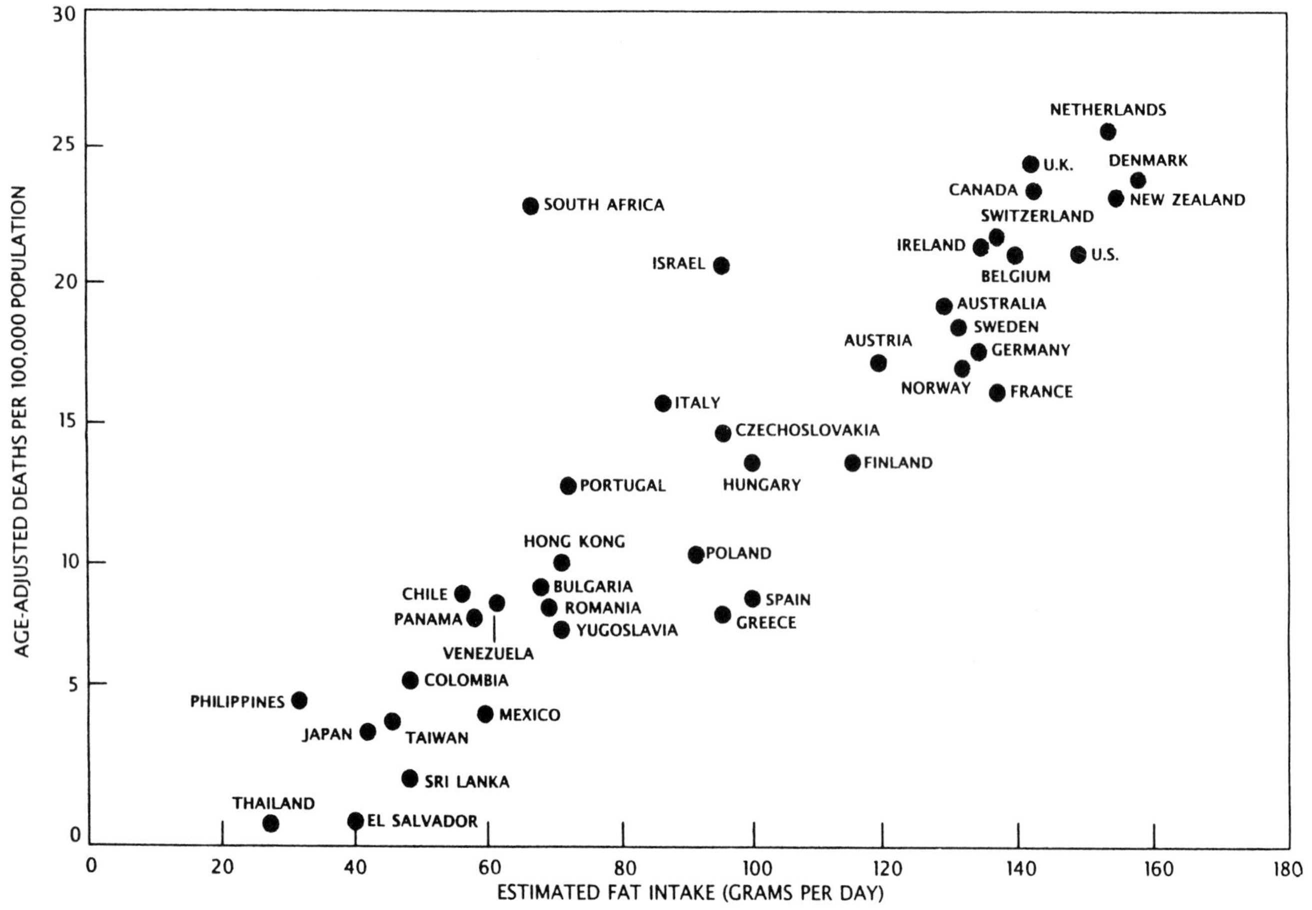

consumption (with a lower intake of fiber and complex carbohydrates) occur in parallel with rising breast, prostate, and colon cancer rates.

The majority of animal experiments and human population data studies indicate strong positive correlations between breast and prostate cancer incidences and total dietary fat intake[60–66]; however, some studies do not directly support the fat hypothesis but indicate that specific types of fat, total caloric intake, and/or obesity are more important links to cancer.[49] An important hormonal connection is found in the close association between obesity and breast and endometrial cancer incidences, generally attributable to the increased conversion of circulating androestenedione to estrogen within excess adipose tissue.[49] Putative associations between the incidence of hormone-responsive cancers, dietary fiber, and other dietary components including vitamins, micronutrients (selenium, calcium), and naturally occurring phytochemicals (carotenoids, flavonoids, isoflavones, polyacetylenes, saponins, lignans, and triterpenoids) are provocative but unproven.[59] In particular the potential tumor-promoting role of phytoestrogens, which are found in over 300 different plants, must be carefully evaluated against their possible antiestrogenic constituents, as shown for isoflavones, or the anticarcinogenic properties of carotenoids, saponins, and triterpenoids. Soy products, rich in isoflavones, protease inhibitors, phytosterols, and saponins as well as metal-chelating inositol hexaphosphate are of special interest since they have been linked to altered fertility rates in some mammals and lower incidence rates of breast cancer in Asian women.[67] This decade will see an unprecedented effort to initiate clinical trials with dietary intervention and antihormonal therapies to reduce the increasing incidence of hormonally responsive cancers.[21,68] It is hoped that these efforts will be associated with an improved understanding of the tumorigenic mechanisms by which dietary factors and hormones interact.

Only a small fraction of all cancers appear to be inherited in a Mendelian fashion despite the fact that over 200 single-gene disorders have been linked to malignancy.[49] Familial aggregations of prostate cancer cases have been described, but there are no data suggesting a role for genetic determinants; the same can be said of endometrial cancer. However, this absence of genetic data for prostate and endometrial cancers partially reflects a lack of study in these areas, since molecular defects in families with increased risk for breast cancer have been discovered.[69] In each of three uncommon familial breast cancer syndromes (breast cancer with Li-Fraumeni syndrome, early-onset familial breast cancer, and familial predisposition to breast and ovarian cancer), kindreds have been linked by chromosome 17 markers located on either the short or long arms.[69–71] The genes involved or encoded by these chromosome markers must be identified to confirm their specific roles in breast carcinogenesis. Despite these encouraging first steps, breast, prostate, and endometrial cancers should be considered largely nonfamilial disorders whose increasing sporadic incidence in industrialized countries is most likely related to endogenous hormonal factors and exogenous dietary factors.[49]

Primary Modalities of Endocrine Intervention

The specific applications of endocrine therapy to breast, endometrial, and prostate cancers and the prognostic utility of tumor steroid receptors in predicting therapeutic outcome will be discussed later in this chapter. For each of the different hormone-responsive tumors, however, different strategies and combinations of endocrine therapies are optimal, with all endocrine modalities based on the same hypothalamic-pituitary-gonadal axis of endocrine control that is illustrated in Fig. 30-4. Therapeutic options are commonly categorized as ablative (removal of endogenous hormone production), additive (administration of superphysiologic hormone doses), antagonistic (competition for receptor binding by antagonists such as antiestrogens or antiandrogens), or inhibitory (blocking of steroid-metabolizing enzymes). Excellent current reviews are available that detail the principles and practice of these endocrine options for breast,[72–76] endometrial,[77,78] and prostate cancers.[79–82]

When Beatson and associates first observed the regression of breast cancer after bilateral oophorectomy in the 1890s,[83] this marked the beginning of ablative endocrine therapy and the awareness of endocrine-dependent tumors. Likewise, Huggins and coworkers first ushered in the era of hormonal management of advanced prostate cancer by demonstrating the beneficial clinical effect of orchiectomy in 1941.[84] Surgical castration, resulting in over 95 percent reduction of circulating testosterone in males and a 60 percent reduction in estrogen levels in females (relative to follicular phase levels in normal premenopausal women), produces the gold standard response rates for both prostate and premenopausal breast cancers to which all other forms of hormonal therapy are compared. Sixty to 80 percent of men with metastatic prostate cancer respond to bilateral orchiectomy.[79–82] Approximately 30 percent of unselected premenopausal women and 60 to 80 percent of patients with estrogen receptor (ER) and progesterone receptor (PR)–positive breast tumors respond to bilateral oophorectomy.[72–76] As expected, oophorectomy is not beneficial for postmenopausal patients (<10 percent response rates) or perimenopausal patients (<20 percent response rates). Ovarian irradiation (450 to 1000 cGy) as a substitute for surgery can effectively ablate ovarian function but requires sev-

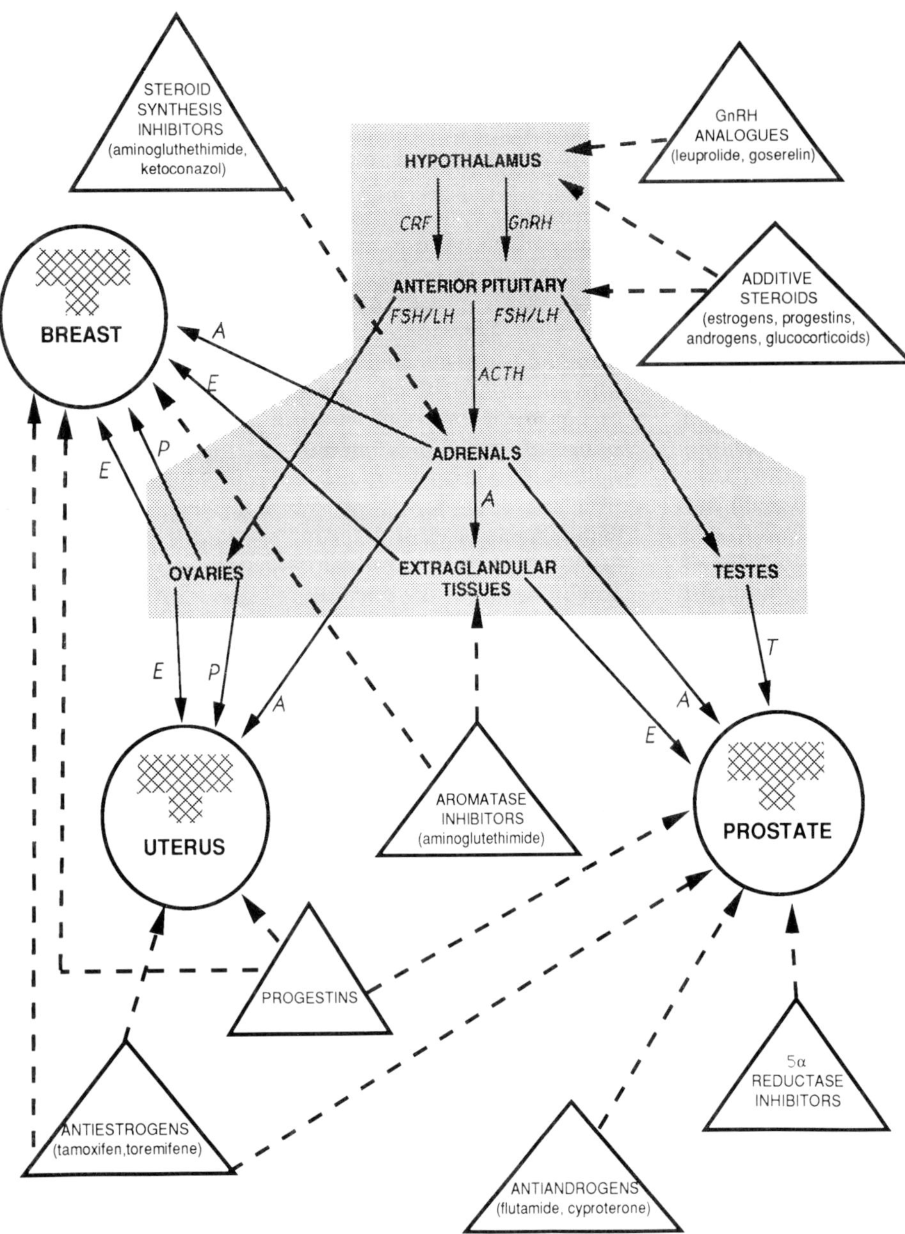

FIGURE 30-4 The hypothalamic-pituitary-gonadal axis of endocrine control which forms the basis for endocrine therapy for hormone-responsive tumors. Tumors within breast, uterus, and prostate end organs (hatched circles) are stimulated by estrogenic (E), progestational (P), and androgenic (A) steroids produced by the gonads, adrenals, and certain extraglandular tissues (e.g., fat). Therapeutic options (triangles) target the tumors directly or deprive them of their stimulatory steroids by inhibiting their production in other organs within the axis of endocrine control. The specific uses of these therapies are discussed in the text.

eral weeks to achieve a full effect. The response rates with ablative therapy are consistent with the concept that breast and prostate cancers are induced or stimulated by circulating sex steroids and that tumor regression occurs as a direct result of the removal of these hormonal stimuli. Ablative therapy is not clinically relevant for endometrial cancer because 80 percent of these estrogen-sensitive tumors arise in postmenopausal patients.

Residual estrogen levels in castrated or postmenopausal women persist because of adrenally secreted androgenic precursors (DHEA and androstenedione) which are converted to estrogen (estrone) by aromatization in extraglandular tissues.[85,86] Furthermore, the remaining 5 percent of androgens circulating in castrated males consists of testosterone and adrenally synthesized androstenedione or its precursor, DHEA[87]; the influence of these residual androgens on prostate cancer growth may be disproportionate to their circulating levels.[88,89] Because of this residual androgen production, adrenalectomy and hypophysectomy have been tried with some success in prostate cancer patients who have relapsed after orchiectomy,[90–92] although these procedures are much more successful in breast cancer patients relapsing after oophorectomy, in whom second responses are commonly seen in about 40 to 50 percent of cases, some lasting for 2 or more years.[93,94]

The advent of receptor antagonists and steroid synthesis inhibitors over the past 20 years has reduced the need for all ablative surgical procedures, particularly adrenalectomy and hypophysectomy, which have been replaced by aminoglutethimide and blockers of gonadotropin releasing hormone (GnRH), respectively. The additive hormonal agents, diethylstilbestrol (DES) and progestins, have proved to be effective first-line endocrine therapies for prostate, endometrial, and postmenopausal breast cancers. The number of hormonal agents and endocrine treatment modalities is increasing rapidly, while the number of clinical indications for endocrine treatment is increasing more gradually.[95] The relatively low toxicity of most endocrine agents and our improved understanding of the cellular and molecular mechanisms that mediate hormone-dependent tumor regression have fueled the development of newer endocrine modalities. Some of the more promising endocrine agents currently in clinical trials and/or recently approved for use are listed in Table 30-4. Additional discussion of the basic mechanisms of action of ablative therapies and receptor antagonists (especially antiestrogens) will be given in the next two sections, while the therapeutic use of many of these modalities, including GnRH analogs and aromatase inhibitors, will be covered in the clinical sections.

Cellular Mechanisms Mediating Hormone Response

The subcellular mechanisms underlying steroid-induced and receptor-mediated gene transcription are detailed in Chaps. 3 and 5. In vitro and in vivo studies of hormone-dependent human breast and endometrial cancers using cultured cell lines and nude mouse animal models have begun to clarify the mechanistic interactions between sex steroids and autocrine and paracrine growth factors. Estrogen receptor–rich MCF-7 human breast cancer cells are a widely studied transformed cell line first established from a malignant pleural effusion nearly two decades ago.[96] After exposure to physiologic concentrations of estradiol, these cells show a variably increased rate of proliferation in culture; more dramatic, however, is their absolute dependence on estrogen for tumorigenic growth in castrated nude mice. In culture, estrogen regulates the transcription rate of various MCF-7 gene products, including the progesterone receptor, secreted pS2 protein, proteases such as cathepsin D and uroplasminogen activator (urokinase), and autocrine growth factors such as EGF, transforming growth factor alpha (TGF-α), IGF-I, IGF-II, as well as paracrine acting factors such as PDGF and FGF(s).[97–99] While there is much evidence to support autocrine mediation of estrogenic growth,[100,101] other data indicate that estrogen-induced tumor growth is not entirely explained by autocrine growth factor production.[102] The ability of estrogen to induce paracrine-mediated growth and the secretion of proteases whose function may be to facilitate tumor invasion and metastasis has received recent attention.

Estradiol depresses the synthesis of the bifunctional autocrine and paracrine growth factor, TGF-β, that inhibits the proliferation of breast cancer epithelial cells while paradoxically stimulating the growth of local mesenchymal cells.[103] The net paracrine effect after estrogen induction of PDGF, IGF-II, and TGF-β includes a rapid increase in the expression in fibroblasts of several oncogenes (c-*myc*, c-*fos*, c-*jun*) and release into the interstitial space of additional growth factors and growth-promoting proteoglycans that enable breast cancer cells to proliferate and invade the local tissue and extracellular matrix.[104] Thus, paracrine induction recruits otherwise normal fibroblasts and stromal elements to remodel the basement membrane and extracellular matrix into constituents digestible by tumor-secreted proteases, facilitating local invasion and metastasis by a tumor. Recent surveys of resected breast tumor specimens indicate that the tumor content of secreted proteases such as cathepsin D and urokinase is independently correlated with clinically aggres-

TABLE 30-4 Antitumor Endocrine Agents Currently in Clinical Trials and/or Recently Approved

Endocrine Agent	Mechanism	Tumor Targets
ICI-164384	Pure antiestrogen	Breast
RU-486, onapristone	Antiprogestins	Breast, endometrial
Anandron, casodex	Antiandrogens	Prostate
Goserelin, buserelin, others	GnRH analogs	Prostate, breast, endometrial, ovarian
CGS-16949A, 4-hydroxyandrostenedione (4-OHA)	Aromatase inhibitors	Breast, endometrial, ovarian
Finasteride, 4-OHA	5α-reductase inhibitors	Prostate
Suramin	Polyanionic growth factor (bFGF) inhibitor	Prostate, breast
Sandostatin, others	Somatostatin receptor antagonists	Breast, ovarian, prostate

Source: Adapted from reference 95.

sive tumor behavior and poor patient survival.[105,106] These findings suggest that the role of normal breast stroma in maintaining breast epithelial differentiation and response to estrogen is at least as important as the paracrine interaction between prostatic epithelium and its mesenchyme that was discussed earlier.

The study of hormone-dependent breast and endometrial cancer cell lines has provided key molecular and cellular explanations for clinically observed remissions after endocrine therapy using receptor-binding agents such as antiestrogens and progestins. The primary antitumor action of an antiestrogen results from the binding of the parent compound or an in vivo generated metabolite to ER.[107–110] In general, antiestrogens are classified either as pure estrogen antagonists (e.g., ICI-164384) or, more commonly, as antagonists with partial agonist activity (e.g., tamoxifen). Mechanistically, antiestrogens may be antagonistic by preventing ER dissociation from its oligomeric complex with the heat-shock protein, hsp-90, by inhibiting ER dimerization and binding to DNA or by inhibiting its two transcriptional activating functions (TAF-1 and TAF-2; see Chap. 5).

ICI-164384, by interfering with ER dimerization and receptor binding to DNA, effectively inhibits both transcriptional activating functions of ER. Tamoxifen, by contrast, promotes DNA binding by ER and is thought to inhibit only the estrogen-induced activity of TAF-2 without affecting the constitutive activity of TAF-1. Thus, the partial antagonistic activity of tamoxifen depends on the particular ER target gene response being examined and the normal contribution of TAF-1 and TAF-2 activities in promoting or inhibiting that gene's expression.[111–113] By promoting DNA binding by ER and permitting the constitutive activity of TAF-1, tamoxifen can exert partial agonist activity on certain genes in some tissues or cells. ER-positive (ER^+) breast cancer cells treated with tamoxifen are arrested in G_0/G_1 stages of the cell cycle; thus, the breast cancer growth inhibitory properties of tamoxifen are considered to be cytostatic rather than cytocidal. One postulated set of tamoxifen effects on estrogen-induced autocrine growth regulation is illustrated in Fig. 30-5. As a result of its ER antagonistic properties, tamoxifen causes an increase in TGF-β production and a decrease in tumor secretion of estrogen-induced proteases and autocrine growth factors. Because of its partial agonistic ER properties on other tissues, tamoxifen also appears to have estrogenic effects on cholesterol and bone metabolism as well as on uterine and vaginal epithelium. In particular, tamoxifen stimulates the synthesis of PR in endometrial cells and sex hormone–binding globulin (SHBG) in hepatocytes. Normally synthesized by the liver, SHBG is the major blood transport protein for estro-

FIGURE 30-5 Opposing effects of tamoxifen on estrogen-stimulated autocrine regulation of breast cancer cell growth. Estrogen growth stimulation of an estrogen receptor (ER)–positive tumor cell is thought to occur through increased expression of autocrine growth factors such as TGF-α and IGF-I (see definitions in Table 30-1) that interact with their respective membrane receptors (EGFR, IGFR), decreased expression of the bifunctional growth factor TGF-β, and enhanced secretion of proteases and other proteins that facilitate local tissue invasion and tumor cell metastasis. Tamoxifen's ability to cause a G_1 block in the cell cycle of ER-positive tumor cells may result from both its antagonistic effect on ER-mediated mechanisms (see text for explanation of its agonistic-like effect on SHBG production) and its ability to influence non-ER-mediated mechanisms such as antiestrogen binding sites (AEBS), protein kinase C and calmodulin inhibition, and induction of natural killer (NK) immune cell function. Moreover, tamoxifen's induction of TGF-β activity may be mediated by either an ER-dependent autocrine mechanism or an ER-independent paracrine mechanism, as discussed in the text. *(Modified from Jordan VC, Cancer Invest 6:589–595, 1988.)*

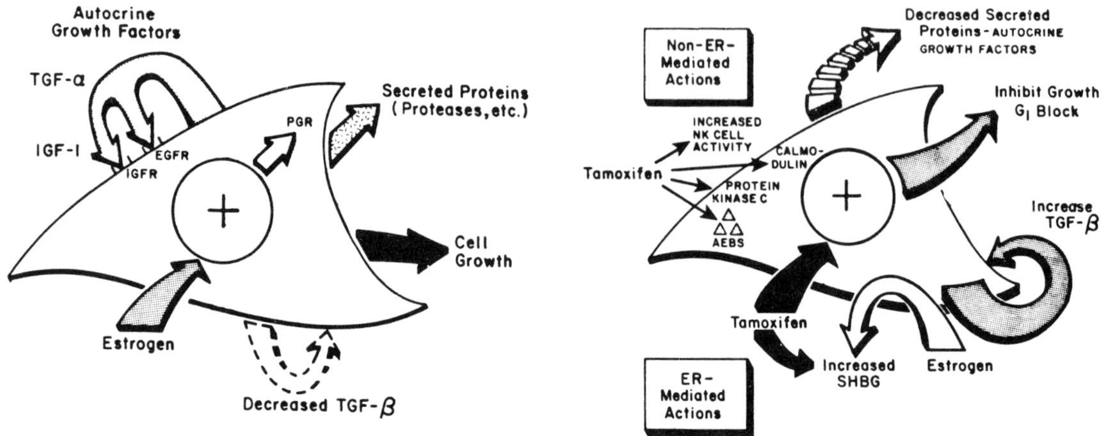

genic steroids. Thus, in premenopausal women taking tamoxifen, a reactive increase in ovarian steroidogenesis combines with enhanced liver production of SHBG to result in an elevation in both total and free plasma steroid levels.[108–110] In postmenopausal women, the partial agonist properties of tamoxifen probably account for beneficial clinical side effects such as improved blood lipid profiles and increased bone density.[109,110,114] However, the same agonist properties also enhance the risk that a woman on long-term tamoxifen therapy may develop a liver neoplasm or endometrial cancer.[115] Finally, micromolar concentrations of tamoxifen can produce ER-independent and estrogen-irreversible effects, such as the induction of TGF-β in ER-negative stromal cells, possibly mediated by lower-affinity antiestrogen-binding proteins.[116] At such concentrations, tamoxifen is known to be a potent inhibitor of calmodulin, protein kinase C, and other important regulators of cell viability and function; it also has the curious ability to increase natural killer cell activity.[107]

When MCF-7 cells are used to produce tumors in nude mice, the antitumor effects of tamoxifen are observed to be very similar to those of ovarian ablation or estrogen withdrawal, since estrogen is an absolute requirement for MCF-7 tumorigenic growth.[117] In contrast, when various estrogen-dependent human endometrial cancer cell lines are implanted into nude mice, tamoxifen has no growth inhibitory effects and actually can be used to support their in vivo tumorigenic growth in the absence of estrogens.[118] These implanted ER^+/PR^+ endometrial tumors can be growth-inhibited by progestins, however, and are even more profoundly inhibited by a tamoxifen and progestin combination.[118]

When estrogen-dependent MCF-7 tumor growth has been arrested for months by either estrogen withdrawal or tamoxifen therapy, in vivo tumor growth can be fully restored by resuming estrogen treatment, indicating that endocrine intervention results in dormant tumor cells that can remain viable and potentially tumorigenic for long periods. Tumor dormancy is now recognized as a commonplace clinical occurrence produced by the loss of essential tumor growth factors or hormones.[119] The release of tumor cells from dormancy occurs when access to the essential growth-promoting hormone or factor is restored or when an intracellular event occurs that allows the tumor cell to circumvent the essential requirement. Long-term tamoxifen treatment of implanted MCF-7 tumors inevitably leads to the emergence of tamoxifen-resistant breast tumors that still contain abundant ER[117]; similarly, in vivo endocrine resistance develops in human endometrial tumors that initially respond to progestin or the tamoxifen-progestin combination.[118] These models of acquired endocrine resistance, along with the recent development of variant ER-positive human breast cancer cell lines resistant to tamoxifen,[120] are helping investigators understand the perplexing clinical problems of de novo and acquired endocrine resistance.

The eventual and inevitable loss of endocrine responsiveness observed in the clinical management of advanced breast, endometrial, and prostate cancers is commonly ascribed to the selective outgrowth of hormone-resistant tumor clones. In 30 to 50 percent of breast cancers and in a smaller percentage of endometrial and prostate cancers, these resistant tumors contain steroid receptors and retain some degree of endocrine sensitivity, as demonstrated by their subsequent response to another form of hormone therapy.[121] An alternative explanation is that hormonal responsiveness is lost when a tumor autonomously synthesizes an autocrine growth factor, perhaps by newly activating an oncogene.[43] Clinical observations such as the nude mouse models substantiate the fact that endocrine therapies do not all work through the same steroid receptor pathways. Apart from the varying number of different steroid receptors [ER, PR, and androgen receptor (AR)] that may be present in a given tumor and may offer alternative mechanisms for endocrine attack, many steroids are also capable of exerting pharmacologic action on target organs through receptors other than their own, such as progestins acting through AR, glucocorticoid receptor (GR), or PR and androgens acting through either ER or AR.[121] Feedback mechanisms and interactions between various hormones and receptors may be important in explaining secondary responses after acquired endocrine resistance in breast cancer or the induction of PR synthesis in endometrial cancer by tamoxifen, which leads to an enhanced response by progestin.

The altered cellular distribution and metabolism of specific endocrine agents may also lead to hormone resistance patterns that are independent of steroid receptor mechanisms. In ER^+ breast cancers, tamoxifen in its *trans* isomer form (the clinically administered formulation) is a receptor antagonist, while its *cis* isomer acts as a weak agonist. Furthermore, in both humans and mice, approximately 10 percent of *trans*-tamoxifen is metabolized to *trans*-4-hydroxytamoxifen, and this metabolite is a far more potent antiestrogen since it binds to the estrogen receptor 50-fold more tightly. *Trans*-4-hydroxytamoxifen can then isomerize to the much less potent metabolite, *cis*-4-hydroxytamoxifen. In tamoxifen-resistant breast tumors compared to sensitive tumors, there is an overall reduction in intracellular tamoxifen levels along with a relative increase in the ratio of *cis*- to *trans*-tamoxifen metabolites and an excess production of estrogenic metabolites.[122,123] These recent studies indicate that one way in which breast cancers acquire tamoxifen resistance is by developing mechanisms to both extrude the parent drug and metabolize it into less antiestrogenic compounds. Unlike acquired hormonal resistance, de novo resistance invariably includes all forms of endocrine therapy and probably results from a failure of steroid receptor function.

Receptor Mechanisms Mediating Hormone Response

The measurement of steroid receptors by either ligand binding or specific monoclonal antibody techniques is discussed in Chap. 6. Steroid receptor binding by ligand was the earliest and simplest assay for receptor function and was proved to be of clinical value when Jensen and colleagues first demonstrated a direct correlation between the ER content of a tumor and the likelihood of that tumor responding to endocrine therapy.[124] Since then, ER has been demonstrated in a variety of human tumors, including breast, uterine, ovarian, prostate, colon, and pancreatic cancers; hepatomas and sarcomas; meningiomas; melanomas; and renal cell carcinomas.[6,125] Except for breast and endometrial tumors, however, these tumor types have such low ER content and reduced frequencies of ER positivity that their routine assay is of little prognostic value.

ER, PR, and occasionally AR are used clinically to select hormonally sensitive tumor subsets and to predict therapeutic responses.[126] Immmunohistochemical assays for ER, PR, and AR have provided important new clinical methods for assessing tumor receptor heterogeneity and determining tumor receptor status amid a tissue background normally abundant in receptor, like that of the uterus and prostate.[127–131] An immunohistochemical receptor assay also allows the identification of hormonally responsive tumor cells in small cytologic samples such as fine-needle aspirates. Table 30-5 relates the incidence of ER positivity (assayed by monoclonal antibody) in newly diagnosed breast, endometrial, and ovarian cancer samples with clinical response rates observed after unselected patients were treated with endocrine therapy. These relations confirm what has been known for some time about the response rate of breast cancers that are ER^{+} [132,133]; that is, only a selected fraction of ER^{+} tumors respond de novo to any form of endocrine therapy. Explanations for this lack of complete endocrine responsiveness include false-positive receptor assays, nonfunctional steroid receptors, and tumor heterogeneity with respect to other components of estrogen responsiveness. A tumor may have a sufficient number of ER^{+}/PR^{+} cells to give a positive assay result yet be composed of enough ER^{+}/PR^{-} or ER^{-}/PR^{-} cells that the clinical response to endocrine therapy is minimal or not detectable. The quantitative relation between the amount of breast tumor ER and the likelihood of an endocrine response supports this possibility.[132] Tumors with trace or no detectable ER content (fmol receptor/mg tumor protein) have little chance (≤15 percent) of responding to any form of endocrine therapy. Increasing breast cancer ER content correlates with an increasing chance (30 to 80 percent) that the tumor will respond to endocrine therapy by showing a cessation in tumor growth or an actual reduction in tumor size. Likewise, intratumor variations in PR content probably explain the lower than expected response rates of endometrial cancer to progestins.[118] While receptor heterogeneity is well documented in immunohistochemical assays[118,127] and may account for changing patterns of hormonal sensitivity during tumor progression,[126] it probably does not provide the full explanation for de novo endocrine resistance. In fact, given the fact that sex steroids act by regulating the levels of other gene products that in turn have profound growth-altering effects on the cell, it would be expected that variations in postreceptor elements of the cellular response will commonly result in the hormone resistance of tumors.

The likelihood that a breast tumor will respond to an endocrine agent such as tamoxifen is correlated not only with the tumor level of ER but also with tumor PR content. PR is determined because it provides some indication that the tumor ER is functional through its ability to induce PR synthesis,[134] even though examples of breast cancers that express PR independent of ER are well known.[135,136] Why 20 to 30 percent of ER^{+}/PR^{+} tumors and up to 60 to 70 percent of ER^{+}/PR^{-} breast tumors fail to respond to endocrine therapy is unknown.[133] Some studies suggest that these endocrine-resistant tumors contain dysfunctional ER, and researchers have been trying to develop assays to detect such abnormal ER.[137–141] To date, however, these assays have been difficult to implement and have not identified specific enzymatic or structural defects that account for the clinical prevalence of endocrine-resistant ER^{+} breast cancers. There are, however, emerging data suggesting that transcriptional and posttranscriptional ER defects are associated with human breast tumors and that these defects may account for some forms of de novo hormone resistance. These receptor abnormalities have been detected using newer and more specific molecular assays, with the recognition that current immunochemical and radioligand binding assays for receptor content recognize only limited portions of the ER protein and ignore important re-

TABLE 30-5 Response to Endocrine Therapy of Tumors Known to Contain Estrogen Receptors

Tumor Type	Positive for ER, %	Rate of Response to Endocrine Therapy,% *
Breast carcinoma	50–60	30
Endometrial carcinoma	40–50	30
Ovarian carcinoma	30–40	<20

* Objective clinical response after antiestrogen or progestin therapy in advanced cases not selected with regard to ER status.

Source: Adapted from references 72–78, 132, 133, 161, 176, 177.

ceptor domains such as the amino(n)-terminal TAF-1 region and the highly conserved zinc-finger DNA-binding domains.[142–148] As with all members of the nuclear receptor superfamily, ER-regulated gene expression occurs through the binding of a ligand-occupied receptor dimer to a defined hormone-responsive DNA sequence, such as the estrogen-responsive element (ERE), usually located within the promoter region of a given target gene[146–148] (see Chap. 5). Rare and heritable clinical disorders involving defective steroid receptors have been linked to genetic mutations in specific receptor domains[149] (see Chap. 5). In fact, mutations resulting in altered amino acids in the ER ligand-binding domain as well as transcriptional splicing errors yielding deletions of entire ER domains have recently been found in some human breast tumors and cell lines.[150–152] To date, Fuqua and McGuire have identified nearly 20 different ER sequence variants occurring throughout encoded mRNA extracted from a number of receptor-positive human breast tumors; a list of these variants and their resulting mutations or expected receptor protein truncations are shown in Table 30-6.

In addition to transcriptional or splicing errors, it is possible that posttranslational receptor modifications occur in some breast tumors, potentially leading to functionally disabled ER with intact ligand-binding domains.[153,154] The differential susceptibility of specific ER domains to endoproteolytic cleavage has long been recognized and accounts for the ligand-binding meroreceptors (3S) that are commonly isolated along with intact (4-8S) ER from estrogen-responsive tissues.[153] In fact, a steroid-inducible protease activity has been found in normal rodent uterine tissue that produces n-terminally truncated nuclear-localizing ER, suggesting that there may be a physiologic role for this form of posttranslational ER modification.[155–157] Endogenous truncation of ER may occur with tumor progression to hormone independence in some murine breast cancer models, and this has led investigators to suggest that truncated DNA-binding ER can compete for available target gene response elements, interfering with normal receptor-regulated gene transcription.[158] Alternatively, altered ER could interfere with normal ER function by competing with normal ER or other regulatory proteins for binding to critical transcription factors (so-called squelching; see Chap. 5). Benz and colleagues have found evidence for truncated DNA-binding ER in a significant proportion of ER^+/PR^- human breast tumors, implicating posttranslational receptor modifications that underlie some forms of de novo endocrine-resistant breast cancers.[159]

TABLE 30-6 Sequence Variants Identified within the Human Estrogen Receptor

Domain	Sequence (Amino Acid No.)	Nucleotide Change	Amino Acid Change
A/B	30	T→C	—
C	584	A→G	Tyr→Cys
	644–760	Exon 3 Δ	Deletion
	644	+GTAATA	+Asn Arg
D	874	T→C	Trp→Arg
	887	T→C	Leu→Pro
	896	A→G	Lys→Arg
	911	A→G	Asn→Ser
	932	C→T	Thr→Met
E	975	C→G	—
	1008	C→T	—
	1139	A→G	Glu→Gly
	1265	T→C	Val→Ala
	1272	C→T	—
	1097–1235	Exon 5 Δ	Truncation
	1576	T→C	Tyr→His
	1370–1553	Exon 7 Δ	Truncation
	1674	A→G	—

Source: S. Fuqua and W. McGuire, 1991.

CLINICAL CHARACTERISTICS OF HORMONE-RESPONSIVE CANCERS

Breast Cancer

Breast cancer is a major worldwide health problem. In the United States in 1992, approximately 175,000 new cases were diagnosed, with 45 percent occurring in women over age 65. Breast cancer is the most common of all life-threatening malignancies in western countries and represents about a third of all female cancers. Approximately 45,000 American women die yearly from this malignancy, second only to lung cancer deaths; for women age 15 to 54, breast cancer is the leading cause of cancer death. The clinical characteristics and management of female breast cancer have been extensively reviewed recently.[160–162] By contrast, breast cancer in men is a relatively uncommon disease, with an incidence rate less than 1 percent that of females. Despite its rarity, nearly a third of men diagnosed with breast cancer die of the disease, probably because their tumors present in a more locally advanced form, partially as a result of delayed medical attention. Unlike female breast cancer, 80 percent of male breast tumors contain hormone receptors (ER, PR) and respond to hormonal therapy (tamoxifen or orchiectomy); in most other respects, the management of male breast cancer is similar to that for postmenopausal women.[163,164]

Risk Factors

The major risk factors for breast cancer are listed in Table 30-7. As was discussed earlier, exposure of the breast ductal epithelium to estrogen constitutes the major known risk factor for breast cancer, with

TABLE 30-7 Risk Factors for Breast Cancer

Family history (genetics)
Number of ovulatory cycles (early menarche, late menopause)
Parity and age of first full-term pregnancy
Geographic and ethnic differences
Endogenous hormone levels
Exogenous hormone use
Benign breast disease (hyperplasia with cellular atypia)
Obesity
Diet (caloric intake, alcohol intake)
Exposure to ionizing radiation in youth
Prior history of breast, endometrial, or ovarian cancer

the total duration of a woman's menstrual history correlating positively with the risk of developing breast cancer. Most of this risk can be attributed to the length of time between menarche and first pregnancy, suggesting that pregnancy has a protective effect against breast cancer. A delay in first pregnancy beyond age 30 provides a fourfold to fivefold increase in risk for the subsequent development of breast cancer. Age at menarche and menopause correlates less well with breast cancer risk. A woman who experiences menopause after age 55 has twice the risk of developing breast cancer that a woman who undergoes menopause before age 45 has. Likewise, an artificial and/or premature menopause resulting from surgery, radiation, or drugs confers some protection against breast cancer.

The relation of oral contraceptive use to breast cancer risk remains controversial. Unlike ovarian and endometrial cancers as well as some forms of benign breast disease, oral contraceptives certainly do not reduce the risk of developing breast cancer; in fact, oral contraceptive use may slightly increase the risk of breast cancer in young women.[9,54,165,166] The risk potential of estrogen replacement therapy (ERT) is also somewhat controversial, but most investigators believe that ERT increases the risk of breast cancer; on a population basis, however, ERT actually reduces overall mortality in this age group of women.[9,54,114,167–170] It has been estimated that for every eight heart attack deaths prevented by ERT, one breast cancer death may result.[54,170]

Radiation exposure is an environmental risk factor for breast cancer. Extrapolating from the atomic bomb survivors in Hiroshima and Nagasaki and from women who received radiotherapy for mastitis or Hodgkin's disease or repeated diagnostic radiography for scoliosis or tuberculosis during youth, a latency of 10 to 15 years is expected before the clinical appearance of radiation-induced breast cancer. Of note, radiation exposure beyond age 40 does not seem to pose additional risk, and present-day diagnostic chest radiographs and mammography screening constitute no significant risk for developing radiation-induced breast cancer.

Benign breast disease used to be considered a controversial risk factor because there are so many different forms of so-called fibrocystic breast disease. Now the excess risk for developing breast cancer is known to exist only for women whose fibrocystic breast disease contains elements of hyperplasia with cellular atypia.[171]

Diagnosis

A palpable breast mass is still the most common clinical presentation of breast cancer; however, nonpalpable mammographic abnormalities are increasingly more common presentations now that screening mammography is recommended for all women age 40 years or older. A mammographically detectable mass or clustering of microcalcifications that leads to a suspicion of carcinoma frequently occurs in the absence of any palpable breast abnormality. Conversely, up to 10 to 15 percent of palpable breast lesions may not be detectable by mammography. A palpable mass, an ill-defined thickening of the breast, and a bloody nipple discharge are worrisome clinical signs which should prompt further medical evaluation. The palpable mass or mammographic area of suspicion can be biopsied by fine-needle aspiration (FNA) or surgical excision. FNA is a quick, simple, and accurate office procedure without significant complications. When cancer is discovered by means of FNA or surgical biopsy, a staging evaluation is undertaken before the start of definitive treatment.

Breast cancer presenting during pregnancy or lactation is a relatively rare problem that poses difficult medical and psychosocial problems, as discussed in a recent review.[172] The diagnosis is frequently and unintentionally delayed because of the normal breast changes resulting from pregnancy that obscure detection, leading to more locally advanced tumors on diagnosis. When such tumors are matched for patient age and stage, however, patients diagnosed during pregnancy have the same prognosis that other breast cancer patients have. Since the termination of pregnancy does not improve survival in these cases, a decision to terminate pregnancy should be based only on patient desires and the urgency for radiation or chemotherapy that could potentially harm the fetus. In addition, subsequent pregnancy after a diagnosis of breast cancer does not have any proven detrimental effect on tumor recurrence rates or patient survival.[172]

Pathology and Prognosis

After surgical excision, the primary breast tumor specimen is measured, the margins of the resection are characterized, and a piece of tumor is cryopreserved for determination of ER and PR as well as other tumor markers (e.g., S phase and ploidy, HER2/*neu* and cathepsin D expression) which may have prognostic utility in identifying more aggressive tumors and patients at greatest risk of relapsing after definitive therapy. The tumor is histologically typed and graded, with the most common type of breast cancer being infiltrating ductal (70 percent). Lobular (5 to 10 percent), medullary (5 percent), colloid (3 percent), and tubular (1 percent) types are much less prevalent. Paget's disease of the breast accounts for 3 percent of all breast cancers; it presents as an erythematous, scaling, weeping lesion of the nipple that is associated with an underlying cancer in at least 60 percent of cases. Inflammatory breast carcinoma is an uncommon but particularly lethal form of breast cancer that presents with skin inflammation (often mistaken for infection), edema, warmth, erythema, and induration. The characteristic pathologic finding underlying inflammatory breast cancer is tumor cells infiltrating throughout the dermal lymphatic vessels.

Ductal carcinoma in situ (DCIS) is an increasingly prevalent premalignant disorder with malignant-like cells proliferating within ductal lumens and lobular units. Since the proliferating cells have not yet invaded the basement membrane of the ductal-lobular unit, DCIS is considered to be a premalignant tumor stage that will eventually invade and become fully malignant if it is not surgically excised. DCIS tumors can range in size from microscopic lesions to palpable lumps 5 cm or more in diameter. Lobular carcinoma in situ (LCIS), by contrast, is a poorly understood neoplastic disorder. Unlike DCIS, LCIS is not likely to become invasive and is considered to be a high-risk marker for the subsequent development of invasive breast cancer somewhere else in the breast. Up to 15 to 20 percent of women with LCIS eventually develop invasive cancer in the same or opposite breast, even after the original LCIS lesion has been completely excised.

The upper outer breast quadrant contains the greatest volume of breast tissue, and thus most (nearly 50 percent) breast tumors arise there; however, a patient's clinical outcome is not determined by breast tumor location. Axillary lymph node involvement on the same side in a primary breast tumor is the first sign of regional tumor spread (metastasis), and this is the most powerful prognostic factor determining the clinical outcome. Approximately 50 percent of primary breast tumors have already spread to the axillary lymph nodes at diagnosis, and the likelihood of this having occurred increases with tumor size. Recurrence rates and the subsequent mortality from metastatic breast cancer vary inversely with the number of lymph nodes involved at the time of breast tumor diagnosis. Patients whose tumors contain ER and/or PR have a better short-term prognosis than do those with receptor-poor tumors, which have higher S-phase fractions and growth rates and thus recur earlier. ER is abundant in about half of all breast cancers, and this finding is even more common in older patients. As was discussed earlier, ER and PR levels are determinants for endocrine therapy. Breast cancers containing both ER and PR (ER^+/PR^+) have a 70 percent response rate to various types of hormonal therapy, ER^-/PR^+ tumors have about a 50 percent response rate, ER^+/PR^- tumors have only a 30 percent response rate, and ER^-/PR^- tumors have less than a 15 percent response rate to endocrine therapy.[132,133]

Treatment

Surgical treatment of breast cancer has evolved from the Halstedian approach of radical surgery that removes all breast, chest wall muscle, and supporting tissue to the present multimodality approach requiring either a modified radical mastectomy or more conservative surgery (lumpectomy, segmental resection, or quadrantectomy) followed by local radiation therapy and systemic adjuvant therapy (hormonal or chemotherapy). Axillary lymph nodes usually are removed in a sampling manner that is designed not for therapeutic but for prognostic purposes. A recent controversial issue is the importance of timing primary breast surgery with the patient's menstrual cycle. At least two studies have suggested that when breast cancer resection is performed 3 to 12 days after the last menstrual cycle (during the follicular phase with unopposed estrogen synthesis), survival rates appear to be worse than those for patients whose tumors are excised during the luteal phase (with lower estrogen and high progesterone synthesis) of the menstrual cycle.[173,174]

Large ulcerating or inflammatory breast cancers are difficult if not impossible to resect completely and are best treated with preoperative chemotherapy before a mastectomy. Radiation therapy may be used preoperatively or postoperatively to establish local control of these regionally advanced breast tumors. Surgery also plays an important role in the palliative control of recurrent or metastatic disease. Among the unfortunate 10 percent of women who present with metastatic breast cancer, some may still desire breast surgery for cosmetic rather than curative reasons.

The use of radiation therapy after breast-conserving surgery is an integral part of primary therapy designed to prevent local tumor recurrence. Nearly a third of patients treated only with breast-conserving surgery will develop local tumor relapse, compared to less than 10 percent of patients who are given postoperative radiation therapy. Radiation therapy is also used for local control of advanced breast cancer and is an effective palliative modality for patients with metastatic disease. Painful bone metastases respond quickly to local radiotherapy, which is often more effective and more rapid in achieving symptomatic control than is systemic chemotherapy or endocrine therapy.

Chemotherapy and hormonal therapy are now commonly used adjuvant therapies for eradicating

TABLE 30-8 Breast Cancer Recurrence Rates and Relapse Reductions with Adjuvant Tamoxifen or Chemotherapy, Including Comparisons for Lymph Node, Age, and Receptor Status

	Control (C) vs. Tamoxifen (TAM)			Control (C) vs. Chemotherapy (CTX)		
	10-year Recurrence-Free Survival Rates, %		Annual Reduction in Relapse with TAM, %	10-year Recurrence-Free Survival Rates, %		Annual Reduction in Relapse with CTX, %
Patient Group	C	TAM		C	CTX	
Lymph node status						
Node-negative	63.1	68.1	26	54.5	61.5	26
Node-positive	33.1	41.9	28	29.8	38.5	30
All patients	44.7	51.2	25	36.6	44.0	28
Age						
<50 years			12			36
50–59 years			33			27
60–69 years			29			20
Receptor status						
ER-poor*			13			—
ER-pos*			32			—

(All C vs. TAM and CTX comparisons significant, $p < 0.001$).

* ER-poor = <10 fmol/mg; ER-pos = ≥10 fmol/mg.

Source: Data abstracted and summarized from reference 175.

micrometastases after primary surgical removal of a tumor. Over 15 years of clinical experience and 133 randomized clinical trials involving about 75,000 women worldwide have confirmed the value of adjuvant therapy in reducing the incidence of subsequent tumor recurrence in patients with node-positive (stage II) and node-negative (stage I) breast cancer.[175] Premenopausal patients and those with receptor-negative tumors are treated with adjuvant chemotherapy. Postmenopausal patients and those whose tumors contain abundant ER or PR are treated with adjuvant tamoxifen therapy for at least 2 years. Despite the fact that tamoxifen is believed to be a cytostatic rather than cytocidal agent, the fractional improvement in the survival curve of patients following only 2 years of tamoxifen therapy persists undiminished more than 10 years after the cessation of treatment, suggesting that tamoxifen is not simply a cytostatic form of therapy capable of inducing dormancy in micrometastatic tumor deposits only for as long as it is administered.[175] The relative reduction in recurrence rates after either chemotherapy or tamoxifen adjuvant therapy is shown in Table 30-8.

Tamoxifen (10 to 20 mg administered orally twice daily) is the standard first-line agent for both hormonal adjuvant therapy and the hormonal management of patients with metastatic breast cancer because tamoxifen is effective, orally administered, and very well tolerated. Patients with metastatic breast cancer are treated in accordance with the strategy shown in Fig. 30-6. Patients who are given tamoxifen as a first-line agent have a 30 to 60 percent objective response rate (remission or tumor reduction of 50 percent or more) that lasts an average of 12 to 15 months. Patients who first respond to endocrine therapy and then relapse have a good likelihood of responding to a second endocrine modality.[121] Breast cancer recurrences in the skin, lymph nodes, soft tissue, or bone have the highest likelihood of responding to hormonal therapy. When tumor

FIGURE 30-6 Clinical algorithm for the treatment of advanced breast cancer. Tumor content of estrogen and progesterone receptors (ER, PR) is determined at the time of histologic diagnosis, and endocrine therapy or chemotherapy is offered as first-line therapy for patients with metastatic disease according to tumor receptor positivity (+) and negativity (−), as shown. This algorithm applies to both premenopausal and postmenopausal patients, although oophorectomy is reserved for premenopausal patients only. Adrenalectomy and hypophysectomy are now accomplished medically rather than surgically, as discussed in the text. →, Initial therapy; – → response, then progression; - - →, no response.

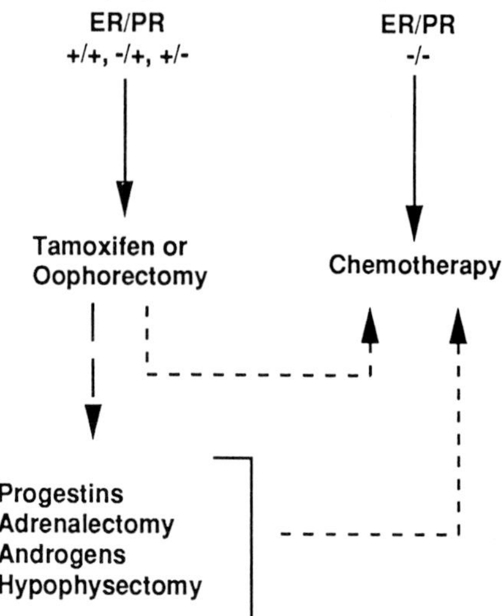

growth resumes during tamoxifen therapy (tumor relapse), the administration of progestins (e.g., megestrol acetate 40 mg orally four times daily) or treatment with medical adrenalectomy (aminoglutethimide) is usually tried and produces a 15 to 40 percent chance of a second remission. Subsequent endocrine therapies include the administration of androgen [e.g., fluoxymesterone (halotestin) 10 mg orally three times daily], high-dose estrogen (e.g., DES), or GnRH analogues. When hormonal therapy fails to produce a clinical response and for patients with receptor-negative tumors, chemotherapy is recommended. Breast cancer is sensitive to a large number of chemotherapy agents; however, the standard combination chemotherapy regimens usually recommended include cyclophosphamide, methotrexate, and 5-fluorouracil (CMF), and 5-fluorouracil, adriamycin, and cyclophosphimide (FAC). These combinations are preferred since they produce higher (about 60 percent) objective clinical response rates. Empirically derived combinations of endocrine agents with chemotherapy are also used for the treatment of metastatic breast cancer [e.g., vinblastine, adriamycin, thio-TEPA (triethylenethiophosphamide), halotestin (VATH)], usually for tumor relapses occurring after CMF or FAC therapy. The administration of tamoxifen along with adriamycin and cyclophosphamide (AC) appears promising and is under clinical evaluation as adjuvant therapy for patients with ER^+ breast cancers.

Endometrial Cancer

The most common pelvic malignancy in women is endometrial cancer, which causes 9 percent of all female cancers, amounting to over 30,000 American cases diagnosed yearly. While this represents nearly half of all gynecologic malignancies, endometrial cancer accounts for only 13 percent of gynecologic cancer deaths and 4 percent of total female cancer deaths. Despite the relative prevalence of this form of uterine cancer, there has been a steady decline in deaths from endometrial cancer over the past 50 years. The median age at diagnosis is 61 years, with 75 to 80 percent of patients diagnosed after menopause. The clinical presentation and management of endometrial cancer have been reviewed recently.[77,176]

Risk Factors

The risk factors for endometrial cancer have been clearly delineated (Table 30-9). More so than for breast cancer, the use of exogenous estrogens (ERT) is associated with a significantly (twofold to fivefold) increased risk of developing endometrial cancer, and this is dependent on both the dose and duration of ERT.[9] Unlike the case of breast cancer, the concomitant use of progestin with ERT reduces this risk for developing endometrial cancer.[9] Of interest, endometrial cancer associated with established metabolic and endocrine risk factors appears to have a more favorable prognosis as a result of its better-differentiated histologic grade, its more superficial extent of myometrial invasion, the presence of steroid receptors, and an increased sensitivity to endocrine therapy.[177]

TABLE 30-9 Risk Factors for Endometrial Cancer

Obesity
Nulliparity
Late menopause
Polycystic ovarian disease
Exogenous estrogens
Estrogen-secreting tumors
Hypertension
Diabetes mellitus

Diagnosis

Endometrial cancer usually presents with postmenopausal bleeding. Fortunately, only 20 percent of such patients with spotting or bleeding actually have cancer; with increasing age, however, this association becomes more likely. Pap smears are generally not helpful, but endometrial biopsies have become a safe and reliable office procedure that is performed routinely in response to a patient's report of postmenopausal bleeding. A tissue biopsy made with evaluation under anesthesia, dilation and curettage (D&C), serves to confirm the diagnosis, since additional tissue is often necessary for a full histologic analysis if the diagnosis is first made by means of outpatient endometrial biopsy. With the diagnosis of endometrial cancer, a full staging evaluation is performed to rule out metastatic disease and determine the extent of pelvic invasion by the tumor.

Pathology and Prognosis

The histologic types of noncervical uterine carcinoma include adenocarcinoma (60 to 65 percent), adenoacanthoma (19 to 22 percent), adenosquamous (7 to 14 percent), clear cell (1 to 6 percent), and papillary serous (5 percent) types.[77] Adenoacanthomas behave like adenocarcinomas, which are the most common type of endometrial carcinoma. The remaining histologic types of uterine cancer have a worse prognosis because of their more aggressive clinical behavior. The recognized prognostic factors for endometrial cancer include histologic type, tumor grade (differentiation) and size, depth of myometrial invasion, DNA content, lymph node involvement, patient age, and hormone receptor content. High-grade or poorly differentiated tumors, large tumors, deep myometrial invasion, lymph node involvement, positive peritoneal cytology, low or absent hormone receptors, and age of patient greater than 59 years are poor prognostic factors.

Treatment

Almost 90 percent of endometrial cancers present as early-stage cancers that can be treated with surgical resection of all tumor-bearing tissue. This usually involves a total abdominal hysterectomy and bilateral salpingoöphorectomy (TAH/BSO). Radiation therapy is given preoperatively and/or postoperatively for deep myometrial invasion and cervical or adnexal tumor involvement. Alternatively, radical hysterectomy with pelvic and paraaortic lymph node sampling or resection is indicated for more locally advanced disease. There is no evidence that hormone therapy enhances the outcome in patients with early-stage cancers or more locally advanced disease. Patients with regionally advanced primary tumors or metastatic disease are usually not candidates for surgery. For these patients, radiation therapy, hormonal agents, and chemotherapy are used for cytoreduction or palliation.

Treatment of metastatic or recurrent endometrial cancer rests on the location and extent of the recurrence. A single focus of recurrent disease may be treated with surgery or radiotherapy ablation; if there is no further evidence of remaining disease after these modalities, systemic therapy can be used to try to sustain the remission. Hormonal therapy with progestins or antiestrogens is effective and produces 20 to 40 percent response rates in patients with metastatic disease. The response to either of these hormonal agents depends on tumor cell expression of ER and PR.

Progestins were first reported to cause regression of endometrial cancer 30 years ago; since then, a number of different agents with progestational activity have been evaluated, with most recent interest focused on oral preparations such as megestrol acetate and medroxyprogesterone acetate. Whether clinical response rates vary according to the choice of progestational agent, dose, or route of administration is still controversial; however, clinical response is clearly dependent on the tumor's histologic grade and receptor (ER/PR) status, as shown in Table 30-10.[78] In particular, the presence of PR within the tumor tissue is essential for eliciting a clinical response to progestin. While there is generally a good (>80 percent) concordance between biochemical and immunohistochemical determination of PR in endometrial tumors, immunohistochemical determination has provided important data regarding tumor heterogeneity, PR expression, and endocrine response. Tumors with abundant PR content (800 to 2000 fmol/mg of protein) can show intratumor proportions of PR^+ immunostaining cells that range from 20 to 90 percent.[118] Immunohistochemical studies also indicate that the failure of some PR^+ endometrial cancers to respond to progestin therapy is due to PR^- tumors that were falsely designated as PR^+ by biochemical assays, contamination with receptor-positive nonneoplastic endometrium and myometrium, or tumors with endocrine-unresponsive PR^- tumor cell subpopulations admixed with PR^+ tumor cells.

TABLE 30-10 Endometrial Cancer: Characteristics and Response to Progestins

Tumor Characteristic	Clinical Response Rate, %
Tumor Grade	
Well differentiated	52
Poorly differentiated	16
Tumor Receptor Status	
ER^+/PR^+	77
ER^-/PR^-	9

Source: Adapted from references 77, 78, 126, 176, 177.

The antiestrogen tamoxifen is the only other form of hormonal manipulation which has been evaluated and found to be effective in treating endometrial cancer. Of interest, tamoxifen has been shown in multiple studies to produce an average 25 percent response rate in patients with endometrial cancer that has become resistant to progestins.[78] These clinical responses to tamoxifen are interesting because in studies with nude mice implanted with human endometrial cancer cell lines, tamoxifen not only appeared to be ineffective as an antitumor agent but produced estrogen-like acceleration of tumor growth.[118] Further investigations are necessary to resolve this paradox and define the mechanism that accounts for the efficacy of tamoxifen in patients with advanced endometrial cancer. Patients who respond to hormonal therapy have a more prolonged survival than do those who do not respond, and the side effects of hormonal therapy are generally mild.[78] Chemotherapy is reserved for patients who do not respond to hormonal therapy.

Single-agent chemotherapy produces response rates no greater than 20 to 35 percent, and the commonly used combination chemotherapy regimen of cyclophosphamide, doxorubicin, and cisplatin produces objective clinical responses in 40 to 60 percent of patients. Combinations of hormonal and chemotherapeutic agents have not yet been shown to improve these response rates. Patient survival after a diagnosis of endometrial cancer ranges from ≥75 percent (at 5 years) for the earliest stage tumors (confined to endometrium with or without myometrial invasion) to 10 percent for endometrial cancers presenting with bladder, bowel, or abdominal invasion or more distant metastatic lesions. Current clinical trials are assessing the potential value of adjuvant chemotherapy or hormonal therapy for patients with high-risk, surgically resected endometrial cancer. Preliminary studies using high-dose progestin adjuvant therapy suggest that reduced tumor recurrence rates may be achievable, but at the expense of excess progestin-induced cardiovascular deaths.[78]

Further clinical studies with other hormonal agents are needed.

Prostate Cancer

There are large geographic and racial differences in the incidence of clinically diagnosed prostate cancer; these differences range over 100-fold when one compares low-incidence populations such as that in Shanghai, China, with high-incidence populations such as black Americans in Alameda, California. Cancer of the prostate is now the most common cancer in American males, having overtaken lung and colorectal cancer incidences during the 1980s. Estimates indicate that over 100,000 American men were diagnosed with this malignancy in 1991 and that about 29,000 died from it, making it the third leading cause of male cancer deaths. Pathologists find microscopic foci of well-differentiated adenocarcinomas in clinically normal autopsied prostate glands with an incidence ranging from 10 percent (in 50-year-old men) to 70 percent (in men over 80 years of age). Since there is less than an 8 percent average lifetime chance of being diagnosed with prostate cancer, it is possible that 90 percent of all prostate cancers are "latent" or incidental, remaining undetected and clinically unimportant for decades. Despite this apparent indolent growth rate, less than half of all clinically diagnosed prostate cancers are detected early enough to achieve complete tumor resection before there has been tumor spread beyond the prostate gland. Problems associated with prostate cancer can be expected to increase. As the average life expectancy is prolonged, the proportion of elderly people in the population will increase (the population over age 60 will increase more than 60 percent over the next 30 years), as will the incidence rate of this age-related malignancy. Uncontrolled carcinoma of the prostate has a major impact on the quality and duration of life, although many men with prostate cancer die from other comorbid illnesses rather than from prostate cancer. The management and treatment of prostate cancer have been extensively reviewed recently.[178–180]

Risk Factors

While prostatic cancer and BPH are often found concurrently in older men and have the same risk factors of age, geography, and hormone factors, BPH is not a proven risk factor for the development of prostate cancer.[178,179] As was discussed earlier, age, diet, and hormones all appear to play a significant role in the etiology of prostate cancer. An etiological association between hormones and prostate cancer is supported by the clinical observations that prostatic cancer does not develop in eunuchs and that latent prostatic cancer is lower than expected in cirrhotic males who have elevated blood levels of endogenously produced estrogens.[178,179] Some studies confirm a higher frequency of previous venereal disease in patients with prostate cancer, but there is no proven risk association with coital frequency or circumcision.[178] Thus, there is little to support the possibility of a viral-venereal relation with prostate cancer. Of interest, smoking and alcohol appear not to be associated with prostate cancer, and past exposure to radiation, as in Hiroshima and Nagasaki survivors, does not increase the incidence of prostate cancer.

Diagnosis

About 65 percent of prostate cancers are clinically localized at the time of diagnosis, and only about half of these prove to be confined to the prostate at the time of surgery. Thus, nearly two-thirds of these cancers have spread beyond the prostate gland when first identified, and this has led to a search for more sensitive screening and detection methods. Until recently, the digital rectal exam with FNA of any clinically palpable prostate irregularity was the two-step process commonly used to detect most prostate cancers. A more recent approach employs a simple blood test for prostate-specific antigen (PSA), formerly used only to track therapeutic response in advanced disease, and transrectal ultrasonography that can locate hypoechoic tumors as small as 5 mm in diameter confined within the prostate gland. Ultrasound-guided biopsy is performed in any area of specific sonographic abnormality. This new combined screening approach is capable of detecting 30 to 40 percent more cases than can either digital exam or ultrasonography used alone.[181] PSA is a serine protease secreted exclusively by prostatic epithelial cells. From 30 to 50 percent of patients with BPH also have elevated PSA serum levels, and serum PSA levels are increased in 25 to 92 percent of prostate cancer patients. In practice, all men older than 50 years with serum PSA levels over 10 μg/liter who have an abnormal or suspicious finding on rectal exam, ultrasonography, or both should be biopsied, since about two-thirds will be found to have prostate cancer.[181]

The symptoms of locally advanced prostate cancer are difficult to discern from those of BPH and include painful or frequent urination, a sudden decrease in the size and force of the urinary stream, or blood in the urine. Symptoms commonly related to metastatic prostate cancer include bone pain (in the back, hips, thighs, and shoulders), weight loss, and generalized fatigue. After the initial diagnosis is made from a cytology or biopsy specimen, a full staging evaluation is performed to determine the extent of local tumor invasion or metastatic spread.

Pathology and Prognosis

The most common tumor arising in the prostate is adenocarcinoma originating from the peripheral acinar glands. These tumors are classified according to degree of cellular differentiation and histologic grade or Gleason rating, a scale from 1 to 10 with the highest rating associated with the poorest clinical outcome.[178,179] Tumor stage based on tumor size, degree of local tissue invasion, spread to pelvic or periaortic lymph nodes, and metastatic involvement by hematogenous spread to distant organs are the most encompassing and important prognostic variables. There is a striking correlation among clinical stage, tumor histology and grade; response to therapy; and patient survival 5 and 10 years after diagnosis. For patients without lymph node involvement, disease-free survival exceeds 85 percent; for those with a tumor involving the periaortic nodes, it is only about 30 percent. Androgen receptors as well as ER and PR are found in prostate tumor tissue and appear to correlate with the response to hormonal therapy, indicating that about 80 percent of receptor-positive tumors respond to hormonal therapy while only 20 percent of receptor-negative tumors respond.[182] Until recently, however, the following technical problems have precluded the clinical use of ligand-binding receptor measurements in human prostate cancers: (1) intermixed epithelial and stromal cells all possessing receptor, with normal, benign hyperplastic, and malignant cells all appearing in the same small surgical specimen, (2) tissue contamination with sex hormone–binding globulin, (3) high concentrations of competing androgens present in the prostate tissue, (4) high prostate content of receptor-degrading proteases, (5) competition between PR and AR for ligand, and (6) lack of suitable monoclonal antibodies to detect AR by immunohistochemical assay. In the past 2 years, however, antibodies and immunohistochemical assays for AR have been developed; these show promise in identifying receptor-negative cancers for which endocrine therapy would not be indicated.[131,183] Another prostate tumor marker of prognostic importance is DNA ploidy.[180] The serum markers, PSA and prostatic acid phosphatase (PAP), which are elevated in proportion to tumor load, are useful for monitoring regression and relapse during systemic therapy.[178]

Treatment

Prostate cancer treatment depends on tumor grade and size and the degree of local or distant spread. If a cancer is detected when confined to the prostate gland, it is curable. Curative treatment choices include surgery and radiation therapy, and there continues to be controversy about the issue of optimal management of local tumors by one or another of these modalities.[178,179]

Endocrine therapy for prostate cancer, first employed by Huggins 50 years ago,[84] has remained the mainstay of systemic therapy and clearly benefits 60 to 80 percent of patients with metastatic prostate cancer.[79–82] Ablative therapy based on the withdrawal of growth-stimulating androgens has focused on two pathways of endogenous androgen production: (1) gonadal production of testosterone that can bind receptor or become converted in androgen target tissues (including normal and malignant prostate cells) to the more potent receptor-binding androgen dihydrotestosterone by the microsomal enzyme 5α-reductase and (2) adrenal cortex production of androstenedione and DHEA, less potent androgens which constitute about 5 percent of the total androgenic stimulation available to the prostate gland.[79–82,184] As schematically shown in Fig. 30-4, the current choices of endocrine treatment modalities for prostate cancer are antitestosterone interventions and antiadrenal androgen interventions. Together, these modalities can be employed in a complementary fashion known as total androgen blockade.

There continues to be vigorous debate about the relative benefit of total androgen blockade versus single-modality endocrine treatment with either orchiectomy or medical castration using agents such as DES, megestrol acetate, and GnRH analogues to treat patients with locally advanced or metastatic prostate cancer.[81] The surgical and medical options appear to be equally effective in reducing circulating testosterone levels and producing subjective and objective clinical responses.[79–82] The median durations of tumor response are in the range of 12 to 18 months with these treatments, and patient survival is about 30 months beyond the initiation of therapy for metastatic disease.[79–82] Thus, the medical advances made over the past 50 years should not be measured by response rates and survival duration (which remain about the same) but rather by the availability of medical alternatives (DES, GnRH) to orchiectomy, which many patients prefer, and the recent option of avoiding DES-induced painful gynecomastia and cardiovascular complications by using GnRH. With monthly administered depot formulations of a GnRH agonist such as leuprolide, medical therapy is now much more convenient, and also more expensive. The excess thrombotic and cardiovascular risks of DES (even at a 1.0-mg daily dose) and other estrogen formulations will probably make this form of additive endocrine therapy obsolete.

The importance of the role of adrenal androgen production was first assessed in patients relapsing from primary endocrine therapy after either orchiectomy or DES. Adrenalectomy became a safe procedure 40 years ago with the advent of glucocorticoids and replacement therapy. Short-lived responses were reported in 20 to 40 percent of relapsing patients treated with adrenalectomy.[184] DES, megestrol acetate, ketoconazole, and aminoglutethimide all block adrenal androgen production to varying degrees yet produce no more than 20 percent objective response rates in patients relapsing from initial endocrine therapy. Such variable second response rates might be expected depending on the percentage of androgen-independent tumor cells present after initial androgen deprivation therapy. Labrie and associates first championed the hypothesis that combined androgen blockade should be therapeutically attempted earlier in the disease process, when a higher fraction of prostate tumor cells are androgen-dependent.[185] Their encouraging results in uncontrolled trials using medical castration combined with the antiandrogen flutamide have since been reevaluated in randomized studies comparing castration with or without antiandrogen (flutamide or anandron) therapy. For the most part, these studies have revealed small but statistically significant improvements in patient outcome for those treated with complete androgen blockade, especially patients with minimal metastatic disease.[186–189] Some studies have failed to show any statistically significant advantage in favor of total androgen blockade.[179] It is generally agreed that the use of nonsteroidal antiandrogens such as flutamide and anandron has consistently eliminated the painful clinical flare-up of tumor lesions that typically occurs within 72 h of starting GnRH agonist therapy, which has been attributed to the transient rise in luteinizing hormone (LH) and testosterone. Additional studies indicate that antiandrogens have significant activity as first-line endocrine agents when given alone.

At present, the marginal advantage of total androgen blockade must be weighed against its side effects, especially diarrhea, and its much higher cost.[179] If the improved results seen in patients with minimal metastatic disease are borne out after further study, however, early aggressive therapy with total androgen blockage will become the standard of care.[82] Since chemotherapy is of little value in treating prostate cancer patients because of the lack of effective single agents and combination regimens, more attention is being paid to the development of new endocrine therapies for prostate cancer, as shown in Table 30-4. Inhibitors of 5α-reductase, such as finasteride, appear to have significant potential for treating BPH but only limited activity against prostatic cancer. Agents such as suramin, in contrast, by blocking paracrine-mediated tumor cell mechanisms, are showing early clinical promise and may usher in a new treatment era for prostate cancer.[95,190]

References

1. Bittner JJ: The causes of mammary cancer in mice. *Harvey Lect* 42:221, 1947.
2. Huggins C: Endocrine-induced regression of cancers. *Science* 156:1050, 1967.
3. Furth J: Hormones as etiological agents in neoplasia, in Becker FF (ed): *Cancer: A Comprehensive Treatise,* vol 1, New York, Plenum, 1975, pp 75–120.
4. Miller AB: An overview of hormone-associate cancer. *Cancer Res* 38:3985–3990, 1978.
5. Thomas DB: Do hormones cause breast cancer? *Cancer* 53:595–604, 1984.
6. Hawkins RA, Miller WR: What is the role of sex hormones in cancer development? *Rev Endocr Related Cancer* 30:13–18, 1988.
7. Henderson BE, Ross RK, Pike MC, Casagrande JT: Endogenous hormones as a major factor in human cancer. *Cancer Res* 42:3232–3269, 1982.
8. Benz CC, Lewis BJ: Hormones and cancer, in Greenspan FJ, Baxter JD (eds): *Basic and Clinical Endocrinology,* 4th ed. San Mateo, Calif., Appleton and Lange, 1993.
9. Bernstein L, Ross RK, Henderson BE: Relationship of hormone use to cancer risk. *J Natl Cancer Inst Monogr* 12:137–147, 1992.
10. Claman HN: Corticoids and lymphoid cells. *N Engl J Med* 287:388–397, 1972.
11. Baxter JD, Forsham PH: Tissue effects of glucocorticoids. *Am J Med* 53:573–589, 1972.
12. DeVita VT Jr, Hellman S, Rosenberg SA (eds): *Cancer: Principles and Practice of Oncology,* 3d ed. Philadelphia, Lippincott, 1989, Chaps. 5–10.
13. Hollingsworth RE, Lee W-H: Tumor suppressor genes: New prospects for cancer research. *JNCI* 83:91–96, 1991.
14. Li JJ, Nandi S: Hormones and carcinogenesis: Laboratory studies, in Becker KL (ed): *Principles and Practice of Endocrinology and Metabolism.* Philadelphia, Lippincott, 1987.
15. Buenaventura SK, Jacobson-Kram D, Dearfield KL, Williams JR: *Cancer Res* 44:3851, 1984.
16. Purdy RH, Marshall MV: Enhancement of the mutagenicity of carcinogenic arylamines by ethinyl estradiol. *Carcinogenesis* 5:1709–1715, 1984.
17. Liehr JG, Avitts TA, Randerath E, Randerath K: Estrogen-induced endogenous DNA adduction: Possible mechanism of hormonal cancer. *Proc Natl Acad Sci USA* 803:5301–5305, 1986.
18. Metzler M: Metabolic activation of xenobiotic stilbene estrogens. *Fed Proc* 46:1855–1857, 1987.
19. Li JJ, Li SA: Estrogen carcinogenesis in Syrian hamster tissues: Role of metabolism. *Fed Proc* 46:1858–1863, 1987.
20. Liehr JG, Sirbasku DA, Jurka E, Randerath K, Randerath E: Inhibition of estrogen-induced renal carcinogenesis in male Syrian hamsters by tamoxifen without decrease in DNA adduct levels. *Cancer Res* 48:779–783, 1988.
21. Kiang DT: Chemoprevention for breast cancer: Are we ready? *JNCI* 7:462–463, 1991.
22. Russo J, Gusterson BA, Rogers AE, Russo IH, Wellings SR, VanZwietein MJ: Biology of disease: Comparative study of human and rat mammary tumorigenesis. *Lab Invest* 62: 244–278, 1990.
23. Ethier SP, Heppner GH: Biology of breast cancer in vivo and in vitro, in Harris JR, Hellman S, Henderson IC, Kinne DW, (eds): *Breast Disease,* Philadelphia, Lippincott, 135–146, 1987.
24. McGregor DH, Land CE, Choi K, Tokuoka S, Liu PI, Wakabayaski I, Beebe GW: Breast cancer incidence among atomic bomb survivors, Hiroshima and Nagasaki, 1950–1969. *JNCI* 59:799, 1977.
25. Thomas DB: Role of exogenous female hormones in altering the risk of benign and malignant neoplasms in humans. *Cancer Res* 38:3991–4000, 1978.
26. Noble RL: The development of prostatic adenocarcinoma in N6 rats following prolonged sex hormone administration. *Cancer Res* 37:1929, 1977.
27. Thompson TC, Southgate J, Kitchener G, Land H: Multistage carcinogenesis induced by *ras* and *myc* oncogenes in a reconstituted organ. *Cell* 56:917–930, 1989.
28. Mawhinney MG: Etiological considerations for the growth of stroma in benign prostatic hyperplasia. *Fed Proc* 45:2615–2617, 1986.
29. Neubauer BL, Best KL, Hoover DM, Slisz ML, VanFrank RM, Goode RL: Mesenchymal-epithelial interactions as factors influencing male accessory sex organ growth in the rat. *Fed Proc* 45:2618–2626, 1986.

30. Hayashi N, Cunha GR, Wong YC: Influence of male genital tract mesenchymes on differentiation of Dunning prostatic adenocarcinoma. *Cancer Res* 50:4747–4754, 1990.
31. Chung LWK, Zhau HE, Ro JY: Morphologic and biochemical alterations in rat prostatic tumors induced by fetal urogenital sinus mesenchyme. *Prostate* 17:165–174, 1990.
32. Murphy GP (ed): Models for prostate cancer, in *Progress in Clinical and Biological Research,* vol 37. New York, Alan R. Liss, 1980.
33. Rochlitz CF, Benz CC: Oncogenes in human solid tumors, in Benz C, Liu E (eds): *Oncogenes*. Boston, Kluwer, pp 199–240, 1989.
34. Cardiff R: Protoneoplasia: The molecular biology of murine mammary hyperplasia. *Adv Cancer Res* 42:107–190, 1984.
35. Teich N: Taxonomy of retroviruses, in Weiss R, Teich N, Varmus H, Coffin J (eds): *RNA Tumor Viruses: Molecular Biology of Tumor Viruses*. Cold Spring Harbor Laboratory, Cold Spring Harbor, NY, pp 25–207, 1984.
36. Dickson C, Smith R, Brookes S, Peters G: Tumorigenesis by mouse mammary virus: Proviral activation of a cellular gene in the common integration region *int*-2. *Cell* 37:529–536, 1984.
37. May FEB, Westley BR, Rochefort H: Mouse mammary tumour virus related sequences are present in human DNA. *Nucleic Acids Res* 11:4127–4139, 1983.
38. Poon M-C, Tomana M, Niedermeier W: Serum antibodies against mouse mammary tumor virus-associated antigen detected nine months before appearance of a breast carcinoma. *Ann Intern Med* 98:937–938, 1983.
39. Holder WD Jr, Wells SA Jr: Antibody reacting with the murine mammary tumor virus in the serum of patients with breast carcinoma: A possible serological detection method for breast carcinoma. *Cancer Res* 43:239–244, 1983.
40. Dion AS, Girardi AJ, Williams CC, Pomenti AA, Redfield ES: Responses of serum from breast cancer patients to murine mammary tumor virus: Fact or artifact? *JNCI* 79:207–211, 1987.
41. Brown AMC, Wilding RS, Prendergast TJ, Varmus HE: A retrovirus vector expressing the putative mammary oncogene *int*-1 causes partial transformation of a mammary epithelial cell line. *Cell* 46:1001–1009, 1986.
42. Leidereau R, Callahan R, et al: Amplification of the *int*-2 gene in primary human breast tumors. *Oncogene Res* 2:285–291, 1988.
43. Kasid A, Lippman M, et al: Transfection of v-*ras*H DNA into MCF-7 human breast cancer cells bypasses dependence on estrogen for tumorigenicity. *Science* 228:725–728, 1985.
44. Muller W, Sinn E, Puttengale P, Wallace R, Leder P: Single-step induction of mammary adenocarcinomas in transgenic mice bearing the activated c-*neu* oncogene. *Cell* 54:105–115, 1988.
45. Schoenenberger CA, Andres A-C, Groner B, Van der Valk M, LeMeur M, Gerlinger P: Targeted *c-myc* gene expression in mammary glands of transgenic mice induces mammary tumours with constitutive milk protein gene transcription. *EMBO J* 7:169–176, 1988.
46. Benz CC, Tripathy D: Activated oncogenes and putative tumor suppressor genes involved in human breast cancers, in Benz C, Liu E (eds): *Oncogenes and Tumor Suppressor Genes in Human Malignancies*. Boston, Kluwer, 1993.
47. Fleming W, Hamel A, et al: Expression of the c-*myc* protooncogene in human prostatic carcinoma and benign prostatic hyperplasia. *Cancer Res* 46:1535–1538, 1986.
48. Viola M, Formowitz F, et al: Expression of *ras* oncogene p21 in prostate cancer. *N Engl J Med* 314:133–137, 1986.
49. Fraumeni JF Jr, Hoover RN, Devesa SS, Kinlen LJ: Epidemiology of cancer, in DeVita VT Jr, Hellman S, Rosenberg SA (eds): *Cancer: Principles and Practice of Oncology*. Philadelphia, Lippincott, 1989, pp 196–235.
50. Lippman ME: Endocrine responsive cancers of man, in Wilson JB, Foster DW (eds): *Williams Textbook of Endocrinology,* 8th ed. Philadelphia, Saunders, 1990, pp 1577–1598.
51. Fishman J: Endocrine participation in the etiology of breast cancer, in Harris JR, Hellman S, Henderson IC, Kinne DW (eds): *Breast Diseases*. Philadelphia, Lippincott, 1987, pp 103–109.
52. Bernstein L, Rose RK, Pike MC, Brown JB, Henderson BE: Hormone levels in older women: A study of post-menopausal breast cancer patients and healthy population controls. *Br J Cancer* 61:298–302, 1990.
53. Shimizu H, Ross RK, Bernstein L, Pike MC, Henderson BE: Serum estrogen levels in postmenopausal women: Comparison of American whites and Japanese in Japan. *Br J Cancer* 61:451–453, 1990.
54. Pike M: Commentary. *Oncology* 5:14–22, 1991.
55. Ross RK, Paganini-Hill A, Henderson BE: Epidemiology of prostatic cancer, in Skinner DG, Lieskovsky G (eds): *Diagnosis and Management of Genitourinary Cancer*. Philadelphia, Saunders, 1988, pp 40–45.
56. Scott R Jr, Mutchnik DL, Laskowski TZ, Schmalhorst WR: Carcinoma of the prostate in elderly men: Incidence, growth characteristics, and clinical significance. *J Urol* 101:602–607, 1969.
57. Ross RK, Bernstein L, Judd H, Hanisch R, Pike M, Henderson B: Serum testosterone levels in healthy young black and white men. *JNCI* 76:45–48, 1986.
58. Cohen LA: Diet and cancer. *Sci Am* 257:42–48, 1987.
59. Willet W, London S: Dietary factors and the etiology of breast cancer, in Harris JR, Hellman S, Henderson IC, Kinne DW (eds): *Breast Diseases,* 2d ed. Philadelphia, Lippincott, 1991, pp 136–142.
60. Freedman LS, Clifford C, Messina M: Analysis of dietary fat, calories, body weight, and the development of mammary tumors in rats and mice: A review. *Cancer Res* 50:5710–5719, 1990.
61. National Academy of Sciences, National Research Council, Committee on Diet, Nutrition and Cancer: *Diet, Nutrition and Cancer*. Assembly of Life Sciences. National Academy Press, Washington, D.C., 1982.
62. National Academy of Sciences, National Research Council, Food and Nutrition Board: *Diet and Health: Implications for Reducing Chronic Disease Risk*. Council on Life Sciences. National Academy Press, Washington, D.C., 1989.
63. U.S. Department of Health and Human Services, Public Health Service: *The Surgeon General's Report on Nutrition and Health*. DHHS (PHS) publication no. 88-50211, U.S. Government Printing Office, Washington, D.C., 1988.
64. Schatzkin A, Greenwald P, Byar DP, Clifford CK: The dietary fat-breast cancer hypothesis is alive. *JAMA* 261:3284–3287, 1989.
65. Prentice RL, Kakar F, Hursting S, et al: Aspects of the rationale for the Women's Health Trial. *JNCI* 80:802–814, 1988.
66. Boyd NF, Cousins M, Beaton M, et al: Clinical trial of low-fat, high carbohydrate diet in subjects with mammographic dysplasia: Report of early outcomes. *JNCI* 80:1244–1248, 1988.
67. Messina M, Barnes S: The role of soy products in reducing risk of cancer. *JNCI* 83:541–546, 1991.
68. Byar DP, Freedman LS: Clinical trials in diet and cancer. *Prev Med* 18:203–219, 1989.
69. Malkin D, Li FP, Strong LC, et al: Germ-line p53 mutations in a familial syndrome of breast cancer, sarcomas and other neoplasms. *Science* 250:1233–1250, 1990.
70. Hall JM, Lee MK, Newman B, et al: Linkage of early-onset familial breast cancer to chromosome 17q21. *Science* 250:1604–1689, 1990.
71. Breast cancer genetics: some clues, more questions (editorial). *Lancet* 337:329–331, 1991.
72. Henderson IC: Endocrine therapy of metastatic breast cancer, in Harris JR, Hellman S, Henderson IC, Kinne DW (eds): *Breast Diseases,* 2d ed. Philadelphia, Lippincott, 1991, pp 559–603.
73. Harmsen HA Jr, Prosins AJ: Endocrine therapy of breast cancer. *Eur J Clin Oncol* 24:1099–1116, 1988.

74. Rose C, Morridsen HT: Endocrine therapy of advanced breast cancer. *Acta Oncol* 27:721–728, 1988.
75. Manni A: Endocrine therapy of metastatic breast cancer. *J Endocrinol Invest* 12:357–372, 1989.
76. Schacter LP, Rozencweig M, Canetta R, Kelley S, Nicaise C, Smaldone L: Overview of hormonal therapy in advanced breast cancer. *Semin Oncol* 17:38–46, 1990.
77. DiSaia PJ, Cressman WT: Adenocarcinoma of the uterus, in *Clinical Gynecologic Oncology*. St. Louis, Mosby, 1989, pp 161–197.
78. Thigpen T: Systemic therapy with single agents for advanced or recurrent endometrial carcinoma, in Surwit EA, Alberts DS (eds): *Endometrial Cancer*. Boston, Kluwer, 1989, pp 93–106.
79. Grayhack JT, Keeler TC, Koslowski JM: Carcinoma of the prostate—hormonal therapy. *Cancer* 60:589–601, 1987.
80. Wollin M, Diamond DA, Menon M: Hormonal therapy for advanced carcinoma of the prostate, in Williams R (ed): *Advances in Urologic Oncology,* vol I, New York, Macmillan, 1987, pp 131–162.
81. Venner PM: Therapeutic options in treatment of advanced carcinoma of the prostate. *Semin Oncol* 17:73–77, 1990.
82. Crawford ED, Nabors W: Hormone therapy of advanced prostate cancer: Where we stand today. *Oncology* 5:21–30, 1991.
83. Beatson GT: On the treatment of inoperable cases of carcinoma of the mamma: Suggestions for a new method of treatment with illustrative cases. *Lancet* 2:104–107, 1896.
84. Huggins C, Stevens RE, Hodges CL: Studies on prostatic cancer: II. The effect of castration on clinical patients with carcinoma of the prostate. *Arch Surg* 43:209, 1941.
85. Longcope C: Metabolic clearance and blood production rates of estrogens in post-menopausal women. *Am J Obstet Gynecol* 111:778–781, 1971.
86. Grodin JM, Siiteri PK, MacDonald PC: Source of estrogen production in postmenopausal women. *J Clin Endocrinol* 36:207–214, 1973.
87. Sciaria F, Sarcini G, DiSilverio F, Gagliardi V: Plasma testosterone and androstenedione after orchiectomy in prostatic adenocarcinoma. *Clin Endocrinol (Oxf)* 2:101–109, 1973.
88. Geller J: Rationale for blockade of adrenal as well as testicular androgens in the treatment of advanced prostate cancer. *Semin Oncol* 12:28–35, 1985.
89. Labrie F, Dupont A, Giguere M, et al: Advantages of combination therapy in previously treated and untreated patients with advanced prostate cancer. *J Steroid Biochem* 25:877–883, 1986.
90. Murphy P, Reynoso G, Schoonees R, et al: Hypophysectomy and adrenalectomy for disseminated prostatic carcinoma. *J Urol* 105:817–825, 1971.
91. Maddy JA, Winteroritz WW, Norrell H: Cryohypophysectomy in the management of advanced prostatic cancer. *Cancer* 28:322–328, 1971.
92. Silverberg GD: Hypophysectomy in the treatment of disseminated prostatic carcinoma. *Cancer* 39:1727–1731, 1977.
93. Legha SS, Davis HL, Muggia FM: Hormonal therapy of breast cancer: New approaches and concepts. *Ann Intern Med* 88:69–77, 1978.
94. MacDonald I: Endocrine ablation in disseminated mammary carcinoma. *Surg Gynecol Obstet* 115:215–222, 1962.
95. Klijn JGM: Second international symposium on hormonal manipulation of cancer: Peptides, growth factors and new (anti)steroidal agents. *Ann Oncol* 2:183–189, 1991.
96. Soule HD, Vazquez J, Lucy A, Albert S, Brennan M: A human breast cancer line from a pleural effusion derived from a breast carcinoma. *JNCI* 51:1409–1413, 1973.
97. Bronzert DA, Pantazis P, Antoniades HN, Kasid A, Davidson N, Dickson RB, Lippman ME: Synthesis and secretion of platelet-derived growth factor by human breast cancer cell lines. *Proc Natl Acad Sci USA* 84:5763–5767, 1987.
98. Huff KK, Knabbe C, Lindsey R, Kaufman D, Bronzert D, Lippman ME, Dickson RB: Multihormonal regulation of insulin-like growth factor-I-related protein in MCF-7 human breast cancer cells. *Mol Endocrinol* 2:200–208, 1988.
99. Bates SE, Davidson NE, Valverius EM, Freter CE, Dickson RB, Tam JP, Kudlow JE, Lippman ME, Salomon DS: Expression of transforming growth factor α and its messenger ribonucleic acid in human breast cancer: Its regulation by estrogen and its possible functional significance. *Mol Endocrinol* 2:543–555, 1988.
100. Harris AL, Sainsbury JRC: Local growth factors and tumor stimulation, in Stoll BA (ed): *Breast Cancer Treatment and Prognosis*. Oxford, Blackwell, 1986, pp 312–327.
101. Dickson RB, Lippman ME: Estrogenic regulation of growth and polypeptide growth factor secretion in human breast carcinoma. *Endocr Rev* 8:29–43, 1987.
102. Arteaga CL, Coronado E, Osborne CK: Blockade of the epidermal growth factor receptor inhibits transforming growth factor α induced but not estrogen induced growth of hormone-dependent human breast cancer. *Mol Endocrinol* 2:1064–1069, 1988.
103. Knabbe C, Lippman ME, Wakefield LM, Flanders KC, Kasid A, Derynck R, Dickson RB: Evidence that transforming growth factor-β is a hormonally regulated negative growth factor in human breast cancer cells. *Cell* 48:417–428, 1987.
104. Ruoslahti E, Yamaguchi Y: Proteoglycans as modulators of growth factor activities. *Cell* 64:867–869, 1991.
105. Duffy MJ, Reilly D, O'Sullivan C, O'Higgins N, Fennelly JJ, Andreasen P: Urokinase-plasminogen activator, a new and independent prognostic marker in breast cancer. *Cancer Res* 50:6827–6829, 1990.
106. Tandon TK, Clark GM, Chamness GC, Chirgwin JM, McGuire ML: Cathepsin D and prognosis in breast cancer. *N Engl J Med* 322:297–302, 1990.
107. Wakeling AE: Cellular mechanisms in tamoxifen action on tumours: *Rev Endocr Related Cancer* 30:27–33, 1988.
108. Jordan VC: Chemosuppression of breast cancer with tamoxifen—laboratory evidence and future clinical investigation. *Cancer Invest* 6:589–595, 1988.
109. Love RR: Tamoxifen therapy in primary breast cancer: Biology, efficacy, and side effects. *J Clin Oncol* 7:803–815, 1989.
110. Lerner LJ, Jordan VC: Development of antiestrogens and their use in breast cancer: Eighth Cain memorial award lecture. *Cancer Res* 50:4177–4189, 1990.
111. Lees JA, Fawell WE, Parker MG: Identification of two transactivation domains in the mouse oestrogen receptor. *Nucleic Acids Res* 17:5477–5488, 1989.
112. Tora L, White J, Brou C, Tasset D, Webster N, Scheer E, Chambon P: The human estrogen receptor has two independent nonacidic transcriptional activation functions. *Cell* 59:477–487, 1989.
113. Pham TA, Elliston JF, Nawaz Z, McDonnell DP, Tsai M-J, O'Malley BW: Antiestrogen can establish nonproductive receptor complexes and alter chromatin structure at target sites. *Proc Natl Acad Sci USA* 88:3125–3129, 1991.
114. Spicer D, Pike MC, Henderson BE: The question of estrogen replacement therapy in patients with a prior diagnosis of breast cancer. *Oncology* 4:49–62, 1990.
115. Fornander T, Cedermark B, Mattsson A, et al: Adjuvant tamoxifen in early breast cancer: Occurrence of new primary cancers. *Lancet* 2:117–120, 1989.
116. Colletta AA, Wakefield LM, Howell FV, vanRoozendaal KEP, Danielpour D, Ebbs SR, et al: Anti-oestrogens induce the secretion of active transforming growth factor beta from fetal fibroblasts. *Br J Cancer* 62:405, 1990.
117. Osborne CK, Coronado EB, Robinson JP: Human breast cancer in the athymic nude mouse: Cytostatic effects of long-term antiestrogen therapy. *Eur J Cancer Clin Oncol* 23:1189–1196, 1987.
118. Satyaswaroop PG, Zaino RJ, Mortel R: Carcinoma of the endometrium and hormonal receptors, in Surwit EA, Alberts DS (eds): *Endometrial Cancer*. Boston, Kluwer, 1989.
119. Brown GE: New concepts in tumour cell dormancy. *Rev Endocr Related Cancer* 32:23–28, 1989.

120. Mullick A, Chambon P: Characterization of the estrogen receptor in two antiestrogen-resistant cell lines, LY2 and T47D. *Cancer Res* 50:333–338, 1990.
121. Stoll BA: Second endocrine response in breast, prostate and endometrial cancers. *Rev Endocr Related Cancer* 30:19–25, 1988.
122. Osborne CK, Wiebe VJ, McGuire WL, Ciocca DR, DeGregorio MW: Tamoxifen and the isomers of 4-hydroxytamoxifen in tamoxifen-resistant tumors from breast cancer patients. *J Clin Oncol* 10:304–310, 1992.
123. Wiebe VJ, Osborne CK, McGuire WL, DeGregorio MW: Identification of estrogenic tamoxifen metabolite(s) in tamoxifen-resistant human breast tumors. *J Clin Oncol* 10:990–994, 1992.
124. Jensen EV, DeSombre ER, Jungblut PP: Estrogen receptors in hormone responsive tissues and tumors, in Wissler RV, Dao TL, Wood S (eds): *Endogenous Factors Influencing Host Tumor Balance*. Chicago, University of Chicago Press, 1967.
125. Stedman K, Moore G, Morgan R: Estrogen receptor proteins in diverse human tumors. *Arch Surg* 115:244–248, 1980.
126. Merkel DE, Osborne CK: Use of steroid receptor assay in cancer management. *Rev Endocr Related Cancer*. 30:5–12, 1988.
127. Green GL, Sobel NB, King WJ, Jerson EV: Immunochemical studies of estrogen receptors. *J Steroid Biochem* 20:51–56, 1984.
128. Marchetti E, Querzoli P, Moncharmont B, et al: Immunocytochemical demonstration of estrogen receptors by monoclonal antibodies in human breast cancer: Correlation with estrogen receptor assay by dextran-coated charcoal method. *Cancer Res* 47:2508–2513, 1987.
129. Pertschuk LP, Feldman JG, Eisenberg KD, et al: Immunocytochemical detection of progesterone receptor in breast cancer with monoclonal antibody: Relation to biochemical assay, disease-free survival, and clinical endocrine response. *Cancer* 62:342–349, 1988.
130. Elashry-Stowers D, Zava DT, Speers WC, Edwards DP: Immunocytochemical localization of progesterone receptors in breast cancer with anti-human receptor monoclonal antibodies. *Cancer Res* 48:6462–6474, 1988.
131. Demura T, Kuzumaki N, Oda A, Fujita H, Ishibashi T, Koyanagi T: Establishment and characterization of monoclonal antibody against androgen receptor. *J Steroid Biochem* 33:845–851, 1989.
132. McGuire WL: Steroid receptors in human breast cancer. *Cancer Res* 38:4289–4291, 1978.
133. McGuire WL: Steroid receptors in human breast cancer treatment strategy. *Recent Prog Horm Res* 36:135–156, 1980.
134. McGuire WL, Clark GM: The prognostic role of progesterone receptors in human breast cancer. *Semin Oncol* 10:2–6, 1983.
135. Horwitz KB, Mockus MB, Lessey BA: Variant T47D human breast cancer cells with high progesterone-receptor levels despite estrogen and antiestrogen resistance. *Cell* 28:633–642, 1982.
136. Reiner GCA, Katzenellenbogen BS: Characterization of estrogen and progesterone receptors and the dissociated regulation of growth and progesterone receptor stimulation by estrogen in MDA-MB-134 human breast cancer cells. *Cancer Res* 46:1124–1131, 1986.
137. Horwitz KB, McGuire WL, Pearson OH, Segaloff A: Predicting response to endocrine therapy in human breast cancer: A hypothesis. *Science* 189:726–727, 1975.
138. Raam S, Robert N, Pappas CA, Tamura H: Defective estrogen receptors in human mammary cancers: Their significance in defining hormone dependence. *JNCI* 80:756–761, 1988.
139. Berkenstam A, Glaumann H, Martin M, Gustafsson J, Norstedt G: Hormonal regulation of estrogen receptor messenger ribonucleic acid in $T47D_{co}$ and MCF-7 breast cancer cells. *Mol Endocrinol* 3:22–28, 1989.
140. May E, Mouriesse H, May-Levin F, Contesso G, Delarue J-C: A new approach allowing an early prognosis in breast cancer: The ratio of estrogen receptor (ER) ligand binding activity to the ER-specific mRNA level. *Oncogene* 4:1037–1042, 1989.
141. Sklarew RJ, Bodmer SC, Pertschuk LP: Quantitative imaging of immunocytochemical (PAP) estrogen receptor staining patterns in breast cancer sections. *Cytometry* 11:359–378, 1990.
142. Greene GL, Gilna P, Kushner P: Estrogen and progesterone receptor analysis and action in breast cancer, in Ceriani RL (ed): *Breast Cancer: Immunodiagnosis and Immunotherapy*. New York, Plenum, 1989, pp 119–129.
143. Kumar V, Green S, Stack G, Berry M, Jin J-R, Chambon P: Functional domains of the human estrogen receptor. *Cell* 51:941–951, 1987.
144. Green S, Kumar V, Theulaz I, Wahli W, Chambon P: The N-terminal DNA-binding zinc-finger of the oestrogen and glucocorticoid receptors determines target gene specificity. *EMBO J* 7:3037–3044, 1988.
145. Klein-Hitpass L, Ryffel GU, Heitlinger E, Cato ACB: A 13 bp palindrome is a functional estrogen responsive element and interacts specifically with estrogen receptor. *Nucleic Acids Res* 16:647–663, 1988.
146. Evans R: The steroid and thyroid hormone receptor superfamily. *Science* 240:889–895, 1988.
147. Green S, Chambon P: Nuclear receptors enhance our understanding of transcriptional regulation. *Trends Genet* 4:309–314, 1988.
148. Beato M: Gene regulation by steroid hormones. *Cell* 56:335–344, 1989.
149. Hughes MR, Malloy PJ, Kieback DG, Kesterson RA, Pike JW, Feldman D, O'Malley BW: Point mutations in the human vitamin D receptor gene associated with hypocalcemic rickets. *Science* 242:1702–1705, 1988.
150. Tora L, Mullick A, Metzger D, Ponglikitmongkol M, Park I, Chambon P: The cloned human oestrogen receptor contains a mutation which alters its hormone binding properties. *EMBO J* 8:1981–1986, 1989.
151. Fuqua SAW, Fitzgerald SD, Chamness GC, Tandon AK, McDonnell DP, Nawaz Z, O'Malley BW, McGuire WL: Variant human breast tumor estrogen receptor with constitutive transcriptional activity. *Cancer Res* 51:105–109, 1991.
152. Horwitz KB, Graham ML II, Miller LA: Hormone resistant breast cancer: Genetic instability and mutant estrogen receptors (abstract). *Proc Am Assoc Cancer Res* 31:1269, 1990.
153. Vedeckis WV: Steroid hormone receptor structure in normal and neoplastic cells, in Hollander VP (ed): *Hormonally Responsive Tumors*. Orlando, Academic, 1985, pp 3–61.
154. Migliaccio A, Di Domenico M, Green S, de Falco A, Kajtaniak EL, Blasi F, Chambon P, Auricchio F: Phosphorylation on tyrosine of *in vitro* synthesized human estrogen receptor activates its hormone binding. *Mol Endocrinol* 3:1061–1069, 1989.
155. Danzo BJ: A protease acting on the estrogen receptor may modify its action in the adult rabbit epididymis. *J Steroid Biochem* 25:511–519, 1986.
156. Faye JC, Fargin A, Bayard F: Dissimilarities between the uterine estrogen receptor in cytosol of castrated and estradiol-treated rats. *Endocrinology* 118:2276–2283, 1986.
157. Horigome T, Ogata F, Golding TS, Korach KS: Estradiol-stimulated proteolytic cleavage of the estrogen receptor. *Endocrinology* 123:2540–2548, 1988.
158. Sluyser M: Steroid/thyroid receptor-like proteins with oncogenic potential: A review. *Cancer Res* 50:451–458, 1990.
159. Scott GK, Kushner P, Vigne J-L, Benz CC: Truncated forms of DNA binding estrogen receptors in human breast cancer. *J Clin Invest* 88: 700–706, 1991.
160. Harris JR, Hellman S, Henderson IE, Kinne DW (eds): in *Breast Diseases*. Philadelphia, Lippincott, 1991, pp 347–486.
161. Henderson IC, Harris JR, Kinne DW, Hellman S: Cancer of the breast, in DeVita VT Jr, Hellman S, Rosenberg SA (eds):

Cancer: Principles and Practice of Oncology. Philadelphia, Lippincott, 1989, pp 1197–1268.

162. Bonadonna G: Conceptual and practical advances in the management of breast cancer. *J Clin Oncol* 7:1380–1397, 1989.
163. Griffith H, Muggia FM: Male breast cancer: Update on systemic therapy. *Rev Endocr Related Cancer* 31:5–11, 1989.
164. Kinne DW: Management of male breast cancer. *Oncology* 5:45–47, 1991.
165. Thomas DB: Role of exogenous female hormones in altering the risk of benign and malignant neoplasms in humans. *Cancer Res* 38:3991–4000, 1978.
166. Olsson H, Moller TR, Ranstam J: Early oral contraceptive use and breast cancer among premenopausal women: Final report from a study in southern Sweden. *JNCI* 81:1000–1004, 1989.
167. Judd HL: Estrogen replacement therapy: Indications and complications. *Ann Intern Med* 98:195–205, 1983.
168. Haber RJ: Should postmenopausal women be given estrogen? *West J Med* 142:672–677, 1985.
169. Bergkvist L, Adami H-O, Persson I, Hoover R, Schairer C: The risk of breast cancer after estrogen and estrogen-progestin replacement. *N Engl J Med* 321:293–297, 1989.
170. Henderson BE, Paganini-Hil A, Ross RF: Decreased mortality in users of estrogen replacement therapy. *Arch Intern Med* 151:75–78, 1991.
171. Dupont WD, Page DL: Risk factors for breast cancer in women with proliferative breast disease. *N Engl J Med* 312:146–151, 1985.
172. Gallenberg MM, Loprinzi CL: Breast cancer and pregnancy. *Semin Oncol* 16:369–376, 1989.
173. Hrushesky WJM, Bluming AZ, Gruber SA, Sothern RB: Menstrual influence on surgical cure of breast cancer. *Lancet* 2:949–952, 1989.
174. Badwe RA, Gregory WM, Chaudary MA, Richards MA, Bentley AE, Rubens RD, Fentiman IS: Timing of surgery during menstrual cycle and survival of premenopausal women with operable breast cancer. *Lancet* 337:1261–1264, 1991.
175. Early Breast Cancer Trialists' Collaborative Group: Systemic treatment of early breast cancer by hormonal, cytotoxic, or immune therapy. *Lancet* 339:1–15, 71–85, 1992.
176. Surwit EA, Alberts DS (eds): *Endometrial Cancer*. Boston, Kluwer, 1989, pp 1–116.
177. Barrett RJ, Geisinger KR, McCarty K-S Jr: Endometrial carcinoma: Prognostic factors. *Rev Endocr Related Cancer* 32:11–16, 1990.
178. Perez CA, Fair WR, Ihde DC: Carcinoma of the prostate, in DeVita VT Jr, Hellman S, Rosenberg SA (eds): *Cancer: Principles and Practice of Oncology*. Philadelphia, Lippincott, 1989, pp 1023–1058.
179. Gittes RF: Carcinoma of the prostate. *N Engl J Med* 324:236–245, 1991.
180. Zincke H: The role of pathologic variables and hormonal treatment after radical prostatectomy for stage D1 disease. *Oncology* 5:129–139, 1991.
181. Catalona WJ, Smith DS, Ratliff TL, Dodds KM, Coplen DE, Yuan JJ, Petros JA, Andriole GL: Measurement of prostate-specific antigen in serum as a screening test for prostate cancer. *N Engl J Med* 324:1156–1161, 1991.
182. Ekman P, Snochowski M, Zetterberg A, et al: Steroid receptor content in human prostate carcinoma and response to endocrine therapy. *Cancer* 44:1173–1181, 1979.
183. Liao S, Kokontis J, Sai T, Hiipakka RA: Androgen receptors: Structures, mutations, antibodies and cellular dynamics. *J Steroid Biochem* 34:41–51, 1989.
184. Bhanalaph T, Varkarakis MJ, Murphy GP: Current status of bilateral adrenalectomy for advanced prostatic carcinoma. *Ann Surg* 179:17–23, 1974.
185. Labrie F, Dupont A, Cusan L, et al: Combination therapy with flutamide and castration (LHRH agonist or orchiectomy) in previously untreated patients with clinical stage D2 prostate cancer: Today's therapy of choice. *J Steroid Biochem* 30:107–117, 1988.
186. Crawford ED, Eisenberger MA, McLeod DG, et al: A controlled trial of leuprolide with and without flutamide in prostatic carcinoma. *N Engl J Med* 321:419–424, 1989.
187. Beland G, Elhilali M, Fradel Y, et al: Total androgen blockade for metastatic cancer of the prostate. *Am J Clin Oncol* 11:187–190, 1988.
188. Namer M, Amiel J, Toubol J: Anadron (RU-23908) associated with orchiectomy in stage D prostate cancer. *Am J Clin Oncol* 11:191–196, 1988.
189. Crawford ED, Kasimis BS, Gandara D, et al: A randomized controlled clinical trial of leuprolide and anandron versus leuprolide and placebo for advanced prostate cancer. *Proc Am Soc Clin Oncol* 9:135, 1990.
190. Myers C, Cooper M, Stein C, LaRocca R, Walther MM, et al: Suramin: A novel growth factor antagonist with activity in hormone-refractory metastatic prostate cancer. *J Clin Oncol* 10:881–889, 1992.

CHAPTER 31

Hormones, Aging, and Endocrine Disorders in the Elderly

John E. Morley

The human population is growing progressively older (Fig. 31-1). In ancient Rome the average human being could expect to live 22 years. In the Middle Ages life expectancy was 33 years, and at the turn of this century it had risen to 40 years. At the end of World War II life expectancy for whites in the United States was 66.7 years, and by 1990 it was 72.1 years for males and 78.9 years for females. At present the Japanese are the most long-lived population, with an average life expectancy at birth of 75.9 years for males and 81.8 years for females. In contrast, life expectancy in Ethiopia today is 39.4 years for males and 42.6 years for females. Increasing life expectancy has led to an increase in the percentage of the population over 65 years old such that in 1900, 4 percent of the U.S. population was over 65 years old, while by 1990, this proportion was 12.7 percent; it is projected to rise to 21.2 percent by 2030. While the largest proportion of persons over 60 years of age live in the developed nations, by the year 2000 almost two-thirds of the world's 600 million older persons will be living in developing countries, making aging a truly international issue. Finally, it should be recognized that a female who reaches 65 years still has 19.2 years on average to live, and a male has 14.5 years. This extended longevity of those who reach old age is particularly important in light of the potential for the development of microvascular complications in older persons with diabetes mellitus.

The demographic aging imperative has resulted in an increasing awareness of the importance of the interaction of aging and a variety of disease processes. With advancing age there is often a blurring of the distinctions between health and disease, with the two existing as extremes on a continuum rather than as static, distinct entities. This is particularly true in regard to endocrine disorders, where the age-related decline in glandular function often results in an older person having hormonal values which would be considered borderline abnormal in a young person. This often leads to diagnostic dilemmas and results in an increasing frequency of endocrine deficiency diseases such as hypothyroidism, diabetes mellitus, and hypogonadism. Table 31-1 lists the putative effects of aging on endocrine disorders.

In addition to the decreased functional reserve, aging is also associated with decreased T-suppressor lymphocytes and increased circulating autoantibodies; this increases the propensity to develop an autoimmune disease and further increases the prevalence of hypoendocrine disease with advancing age. It also increases the likelihood of more than one endocrine disorder occurring in the same person (polyglandular failure syndromes).[1] Altered receptor and postreceptor responsiveness leads to an increased prevalence of diabetes mellitus and can also result in atypical presentations, e.g., apathetic thyrotoxicosis. The atypical presentation of excessive thyroid hormone secretion in older persons results in part from the decrease in adrenergic β-receptor and postreceptor responsiveness.[2] Table 31-2 compares the differences in the presentation of hyperthyroidism in young and old persons.

Older persons often have nonspecific presenting symptoms of disease, e.g., weight loss, delirium, dementia, depression, and fatigue. This often leads to delays in seeing a physician or missed diagnoses. Table 31-3 lists the endocrine and metabolic causes of dementia, delirium, and depression in older persons.

Most normal laboratory test values have been established using young, healthy persons, and abnormal results may reflect the aging process, e.g., low IGF-I or a diminished thyroid stimulating hormone (TSH) response to thyrotropin releasing hormone (TRH). This can be further complicated by the presence of an intercurrent disease, such as euthyroid sick syndrome, which can also alter basal and stimulated hormone levels.

Malignant neoplasias are more prevalent with advancing age, and ectopic hormone production from neoplasms can mimic endocrine diseases. Consideration of ectopic hormone production in older persons can result in the early diagnosis of an occult cancer or the solution of a clinical problem. It can help prevent an inadequate or incorrect treatment of an en-

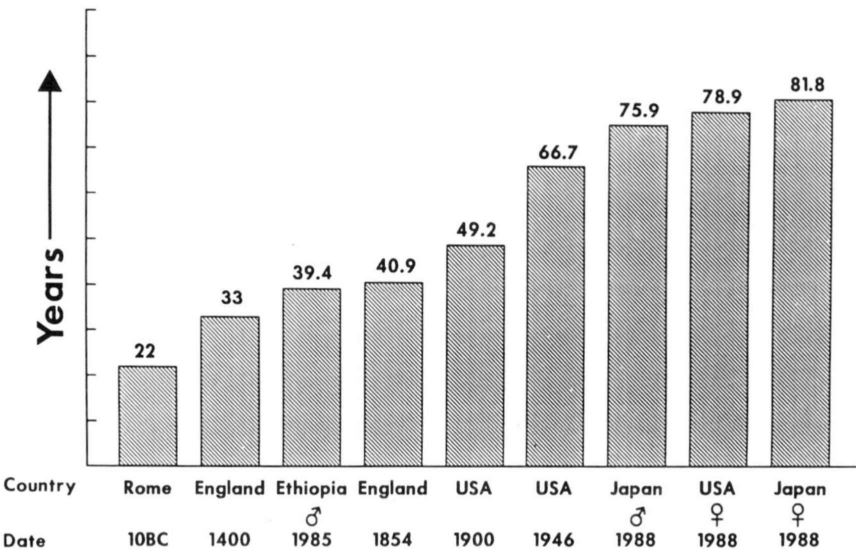

FIGURE 31-1 The aging of the human population.

docrinopathy. The effectiveness of therapy or the demonstration of a recurrence of a cancer may be facilitated by the monitoring of ectopic hormone production. Cancer anorexia may be due to the production of ectopic hormones such as bombesin and calcitonin.[3] The presence of hyperendocrine disease in older persons, especially when the biochemical parameters are out of proportion to the clinical presentation, should suggest the possibility of ectopic hormone secretion.

Changes due to aging may mimic endocrine disease. In 1886 Victor Horsley suggested that older persons resembled myxedematous monkeys and that thyroid deficiency could result in "mere senility." Table 31-4 summarizes the similarities between hypothyroidism and the aging process. Despite these similarities, there is little evidence that the aging process is related to thyroid deficiency, and an excess of thyroid hormone may in fact aggravate the aging process, for example, by producing accelerated osteoporosis. However, recently Mooradian et al. found an age-related decrease in the responsiveness to thyroid hormone of both mRNA levels and the enzyme activities of hepatic cytosolic malate dehydrogenase.[4] The major defect appears to occur at the pretranslational level. There is also an in vivo decrease in plasma membrane T_3 transport with advancing age.[5]

Older persons often have a decreased functional reserve of endocrine target organs as a result of aging per se or secondary to an intercurrent disease. This can lead to a need for lower than normal replacement doses of hormones in older persons.

If an older person has chronic obstructive pulmonary disease or angina, keeping the replacement dose of thyroid hormone at a level that just restores the circulating hormonal values to normal may ameliorate the symptoms of the disease and improve the functional quality of life. Similarly, an older person

TABLE 31-1 Effects of Aging and Related Diseases on Endocrine Disorders

Effect	Consequence
Decreased functional reserve of endocrine organs	Increased prevalence of endocrine deficiency diseases
Decreased T-suppressor lymphocytes/increased circulating autoantibodies	Increased autoimmune endocrine diseases
Decreased receptor and postreceptor responsiveness	Atypical presentations; delayed diagnosis, increased prevalence of diabetes mellitus
Nonspecific response to hormonal imbalance, e.g., weight loss, fatigue, delirium, depression, dementia	Delayed or missed diagnosis
Altered normal ranges	Inappropriate diagnosis
Intercurrent disease	Diagnostic dilemma
Increased prevalence of neoplasia	Ectopic hormone production
Aging changes mimicking endocrine deficiency disease	Delayed or missed diagnosis or inappropriate diagnosis
Decreased functional reserve of target organs	Decreased replacement dose of hormones Increased propensity to develop untoward effects from hormone replacement
Polypharmacy	Interference with hormonal measurement Altered circulating hormones Decreased hormonal responsiveness Increased or decreased replacement dose Poor compliance Adverse drug reactions

TABLE 31-2 Differences in the Presentation of Hyperthyroidism between Young and Old Persons

	Signs and Symptoms, %					
	Nordyke et al.*				Tibaldi et al.†	Davis et al.‡
Age Range	20–40	60	70	80	75–95	60–82
Appetite increased	50–61	31	10	36	—	11
Appetite decreased	5–9	14	21	27	—	36
Weight loss	29–52	76	78	82	44	69
Palpitations	58–67	58	52	45	36	63
Tachycardia	83–84	79	76	70	28§	11¶
Nervousness	59–73	64	69	55	20	55
Dizziness/syncope	—	—	—	—	20	—
Memory loss	—	—	—	—	8	—
Tremor	69	62	67	73	36	89
Atrial fibrillation	0–1	1	8	17	32	39
Eyelid lag	19	18	17	0	12	35
Thyroid enlargement	97–99	84	83	73	32	63

* Nordyke RA, Gilbert FI, Harada ASM: Influence of age on clinical findings. *Arch Intern Med* 148:626, 1988.

† Tibaldi JM, Barzel US, Albin J, Surks M: Thyrotoxicosis in the very old. *Am J Med* 81:619, 1986.

‡ Davis PJ, Davis FB: Hyperthyroidism in patients over the age of 60 years. *Medicine* 53:161, 1974.

§ >90/min.

¶ >120/min.

with osteopenia may develop worsening bone disease if the thyroid replacement dose results in hormonal levels in the upper half of the normal range. Calcitonin therapy for Paget disease may result in severe anorexia and weight loss in older persons.[6]

Persons over 65 years take, on the average, four to six prescription drugs and three to four nonprescription drugs a day.[7] This can result in altered circulating hormone levels (e.g., phenytoin and thyroid hormone levels) and decreased hormone responsiveness (e.g., cimetidine and testosterone). Drugs such as rifampin and phenytoin increase thyroid hormone turnover and thus may result in a requirement for a relatively higher replacement dose. Patients on β blockers may have elevated thyroid hormone levels, resulting in inappropriate treatment for hyperthyroidism.[8] Nonprescription cough mixtures containing iodine may precipitate thyroid disorders or interfere with the uptake of radioactive iodine. Vitamin ingestion in a megadosage may mimic endocrine disease; for example, vitamin A may produce hypercalcemia by activating cathepsin D in the parathyroid gland, resulting in increased circulating parathyroid hormone (PTH). Megadoses of vitamin C interfere with the ability to measure glucose in the blood. Ginseng tea used as a health food may produce hypertension secondary to its ability to increase the hypothalamic-pituitary-adrenal

TABLE 31-3 Metabolic Causes of Psychiatric Disturbances in Older Persons

Delirium	Dementia
Hypoxemia	Hypoxemia
Electrolyte disturbances	Electrolyte disturbances
Acid-base abnormalities	Hyperlipidemia
Uremia	Hypothyroidism
Hepatic failure	Hypoglycemia
Thyroid disorders	Diabetes mellitus
Hypoglycemia	Hypoparathyroidism
Hypoparathyroidism	Hyperparathyroidism
Hyperparathyroidism	Hypoadrenalism
Hypoadrenalism	Malnutrition
Hypopituitarism	Pernicious anemia
Isolated ACTH deficiency	Folate deficiency
Exogenous corticosteroids	Dehydration
Thiamine deficiency	
Pellagra	
Porphyria	
Depression	
Hypokalemia	
Apathetic thyrotoxicosis	
Hypothyroidism	
Diabetes mellitus	
Hyperparathyroidism	
Cushing disease	
Addison disease	
Malnutrition	
Pernicious anemia	
Folate deficiency	
Impotence	

TABLE 31-4 Similarities between Hypothyroidism and the Aging Process

Bradycardia	Muscular weakness
Hypertension	Lethargy
Hypercholesterolemia	Cognitive dysfunction
Weight gain	Impotence
Cold intolerance	Dry skin
Constipation	

axis.[9] Theophylline may interact with thyroid hormones to produce tachycardia and weight loss. Multiple drugs may interact with oral hypoglycemic agents to precipitate hypoglycemia.

Noncompliance with prescription medications is common in older persons and increases with the number of medications. Special care needs to be paid to improving compliance to hormone replacement therapy in older persons with memory problems and dementia, e.g., through the use of calendar pill boxes and by writing down medication instructions.

Certain endocrine disorders are peculiar to older persons or are most common in older persons; examples include type II (age-related) osteopenia and Paget's disease.

THEORIES OF AGING

The major theories of aging are summarized in Table 31-5. No single theory adequately describes all the features of aging. A major group of theories (stochastic theories) suggest that aging results from environmental insults. One stochastic theory suggests that random background radiation damage produces genetic mutations that shorten the life span.[10] The finding that the maximal life span of different species correlates with DNA excision-repair capacity suggests that this theory may be viable. Although hymenopteran wasp haploids are more sensitive to radiation than are diploids, when they were not exposed to radiation, both had the same life span.[11] The error catastrophe theory of Orgel suggests that the formation of error-containing proteins that are involved in the regulation of genetic material or protein synthesis results in an amplification of the original error, eventually leading to an "error crisis."[12] There is little experimental evidence for an increase in the frequency of errors with cellular aging.[13]

Increasing levels of glucose with advancing age can lead to an increase in protein cross-linking.[14] This has been best studied in collagen cross-linking, but other molecules, such as DNA, can also cross-link. The DNA unwinding rate is slowed with aging. In addition, glycosylation of lipoproteins can result in their cross-linking with protein molecules in the arterial wall, resulting in atherosclerosis, an almost universal pathologic concomitant of aging.[14]

System-based theories of aging suggest that alteration of the endocrine system or immune system with advancing age leads to deterioration of the organism and the aging process. Neuroendocrine theories of aging suggest that a central pacemaker results in endocrine organ failure which leads to the aging process. The finding by Snowdon that the age of menopause predicts the age of death provides support for this theory.[15] Denckla found that hypophysectomy and hormone replacement lead to life extension. This prompted him to suggest the presence of a "death hormone" that decreases oxygen consumption and accelerates the aging process.[16] The failure of Denckla to ascertain the adequacy of hypophysectomy and the possibility that hypophysectomy had merely removed pituitary tumors have cast doubt on this possibility. The role of a multiple hormone lack in the aging process remains to be determined.

It has been suggested that multiple age-related alterations in the immune system accelerate the aging process. Some of these alterations in immunity may in fact lead to autoimmune endocrine gland failure. Walford has suggested that these immune changes with aging are related to genes of the major histocompatibility complex.[17] Congenic animals differing only at the major histocompatibility locus have different life spans. This locus also regulates the superoxide dismutase enzyme, linking the immune theory of aging to the free radical theory of aging. In addition, the production of interleukin-1 α accelerates senescence in cellular systems.[18]

The life span of most species is inversely related to their metabolic rates. Cellular metabolism results in free radical formation. The activity of superoxidase dismutase correlates with life span,[13] and dietary restriction which reduces free radical production results in life extension.[19] Deprenyl, which reduces free radical formation from dopamine, has been demonstrated to prolong life in rats.[20]

When RNA from senescent cells is injected into young cells, it causes an inhibition of growth.[21] Proto-oncogenes drive cellular proliferation, and one proto-oncogene, c-fos, is decreased with aging.[22] In addition, the retinoblastoma gene product ($p110^{Rb}$) which inhibits cell proliferation shows increased activity with aging.[23] Finally, it has been shown that mitochondrial DNA may play an important role in aging in some species.[24]

Overall, it appears that the regulation of aging is a complex process that involves both genetic and environmental components. It seems likely that different aspects of aging are regulated by different processes. Alterations in the endocrine system with

TABLE 31-5 Theories of Aging

Environmental theories
Background radiation produces genetic mutations
Error catastrophe theory
Large molecule cross-linking theory (glucose-driven)
System-based theories
Endocrine failure
Neuroendocrine pacemaker
"Death" hormone
Immune theory
Cellular theories
Free radical theory
Oncogene theory
Mitochondrial DNA theory
DNA and RNA-based theories

aging may play an important role in coordinating the aging process in different organs.

HORMONAL CHANGES

Table 31-6 summarizes the major hormonal changes associated with the aging process.

Growth Hormone and IGF-I

There is an age-related decline in growth hormone pulses in older persons.[25] This is associated with an age-related decrease in the number and size of somatotrophs.[26] The growth hormone response to growth hormone releasing hormone is attenuated with advancing age.[27,28] The major decrease in the growth hormone response in males occurs at about 40 years of age,[27] explaining the failure of Pavlov et al., who utilized controls up to 49 years of age, to find a significant decrease in the growth hormone response to growth hormone releasing hormone.[29] The decrease in the growth hormone response in the female appears to occur approximately a decade later.[30] In postmenopausal females estrogen administration can restore the growth hormone response to growth hormone releasing hormone.[31] Repeated administration of growth hormone releasing hormone results in an increased response to the releasing hormone after a number of days of administration. The growth hormone response to insulin hypoglycemia is diminished with the decreased responsiveness, again starting at middle age.[32,33] There is also a decrease in the response to apomorphine with advancing age.[34]

Animal studies have strongly supported the concept that increased somatostatin secretion is responsible for the diminished secretion of growth hormone seen with advancing age.[25] Somatostatin produces this effect both by inhibiting the effect of growth hormone releasing hormone on the pituitary and by decreasing the secretion of growth hormone releasing hormone. In humans, arginine increases growth hormone secretion by inhibiting hypothalamic somatostatin release.[35] Arginine administration in older humans results in a growth hormone response equivalent to that seen in younger persons.[36,37]

IGF-I levels are reduced in older males and females, and this reduction is correlated with 24-h growth hormone release.[38–41] In institutionalized malnourished older persons IGF-I levels are even further reduced compared with age-matched controls.[42]

The alterations in the hypothalamic-pituitary-liver growth hormone axis with aging are summarized in Fig. 31-2.

Prolactin

There appears to be a mild but significant increase in prolactin levels with advancing age.[43] This parallels

TABLE 31-6 Major Changes Associated with the Aging Process

Hormone	Effect of Aging
Pituitary hormones	
Growth hormone	
24-h secretion	Decreased
Response to GHRH	Decreased
Response to repetitive GHRH	Restored
Response to arginine	Unchanged
Prolactin	Mild increase
TSH	
Basal	Normal
Response to TRH	Decreased (males)
ACTH	
Basal	Normal
Response to CRF	Mild increase
β-endorphin	Blunting of circadian rhythm
Gonadotropins	
Males	Inappropriately low (LH) and increased (FSH)
Females	Increased
Thyroid hormones	
Thyroxine	Normal
Triiodothyronine	Mild decrease
Adrenal hormones	
Cortisol, basal	Normal
Dexamethasone suppression	Less efficient
Aldosterone	Decreased
Dehydroepiandrosterone sulfate	Decreased
Epinephrine	Unchanged
Calcitropic hormones	
PTH	Increased
Calcitonin	Decreased
25(OH) Vitamin D	Decreased
1,25(OH)$_2$ Vitamin D	Normal or decreased
Pancreatic hormones	
Insulin	Increased
Amylin	Increased
Glucagon	Unchanged
Pancreatic polypeptide	Increased
Sex hormones:	
Males Testosterone	Normal or decreased
Bioavailable testosterone	Decreased
Dehydrotestosterone	Decreased
Sex hormone-binding globulin	Normal or increased
Estradiol	Normal
Females Estradiol	Decreased
Estrone	Decreased
Androstenedione	Decreased
Testosterone	Decreased
Miscellaneous	
Norepinephrine	Increased
Renin	Decreased
Gastric inhibitory polypeptide	Unchanged
Cholecystokinin	Increased
Vasoactive intestinal peptide	Increased; loss of circadian rhythm
Atrial natriuretic factor	Increased
Arginine vasopressin	Increased

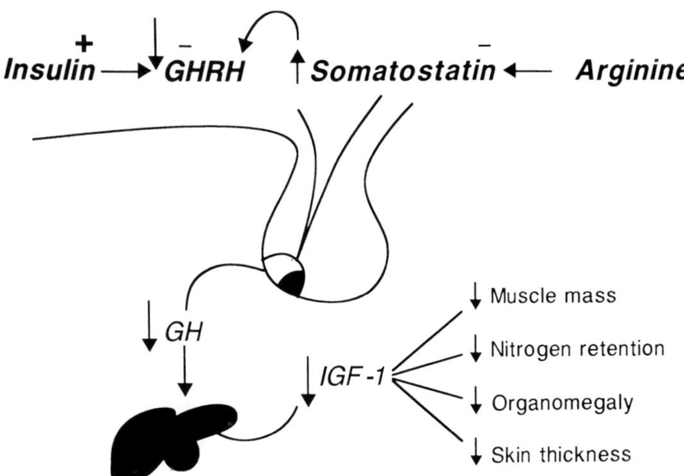

FIGURE 31-2 Alterations in the hypothalamic-pituitary-liver growth hormone axis with aging.

the decrease in dopaminergic activity seen with aging. Older persons with diabetes mellitus have been reported to have even greater increases in prolactin levels.[44]

Hypothalamic-Pituitary-Thyroid Axis

Overall there are no major age-related changes in basal TSH levels with aging, though 2.7 to 3.5 percent of older men and 7.1 to 17.4 percent of older women may have elevated serum TSH levels, representing incipient hypothyroidism in many older persons.[45–47] The TSH response to TRH is suppressed in elderly men but not in older women.[48]

With advancing age there is a decrease in the thyroxine production rate from 80 μg to 60 μg per day.[49] This is balanced by a decrease in the metabolic clearance rate of thyroxine with aging.[50] Free thyroxine levels are not altered with aging. Triiodothyronine levels decrease with advancing age as a result of the decreased production rate and no change in the metabolic clearance rate.[51,52] There is a progressive decline in radioactive iodine uptake in the thyroid gland from middle age to 90 years of age.[53]

It should also be remembered that many older persons may have marked changes in thyroid hormone levels because of an intercurrent illness that results in the development of the euthyroid sick syndrome (Table 31-7).

Hypothalamic-Pituitary-Adrenal Axis

With advancing age there is a reduction in the secretion rate of cortisol and a decrease in the metabolic clearance rate, resulting in plasma levels of cortisol that remain unchanged with aging.[54–56] The cortisol acrophase tends to occur earlier with aging.[57] The adrenal maintains its ability to produce cortisol in response to exogenous ACTH administration throughout life, though in view of the decreased plasma clearance of cortisol, this is suggestive of a decreased adrenal responsiveness.[58] There is a tendency for ACTH levels to be greater in response to corticotropin releasing factor (CRF), insulin, hypoglycemia, metyrapone, and surgical stress.[59] Older persons often fail to appropriately suppress the hypothalamic-pituitary-adrenal axis after the administration of dexamethasone, though this may result from dementia, depression, or an intercurrent illness.[9]

TABLE 31-7 Comparison between the Changes in Aging and Changes due to the Euthyroid Sick Syndrome

	Aging	Euthyroid Sick Syndrome
Thyroxine (T_4) level	Normal	Normal or decreased
Thyroxine production rate	Decreased	Decreased
Thyroxine clearance rate	Decreased	Decreased
T_4 binding to TBG	Unchanged	Decreased
Triiodothyronine (T_3) level	Decreased	Markedly decreased
Triiodothyronine production rate	Decreased	Decreased
Triiodothyronine clearance rate	Unchanged	Decreased
Reverse T_3 levels	Unchanged	Increased
TSH	Unchanged or increased*	Normal, decreased, or increased
TSH response to TRH (males)	Decreased	Decreased
TSH response to TRH (females)	Unchanged	Decreased

* Increase is due to incipient hypothyroidism, which occurs with increasing frequency in old age.

Older persons have a blunting of the circadian rhythm of β-endorphin secretion compared with younger persons.[60] β-Endorphin levels in the cerebrospinal fluid (CSF) are reduced in older persons compared with younger persons.[61] Age-related differences in β-endorphin to exercise[62] and the cold pressor test[63] have not been demonstrated.

Basal aldosterone levels, 24-h urinary aldosterone excretion, and the aldosterone plasma clearance rate decrease with aging.[9] Aldosterone and plasma resin activity levels show diminished responses with advancing age.[64] These changes tend to increase the propensity of older persons to develop hyporeninemic hypoaldosteronism.

The secretion of dehydroepiandrosterone (DHEA) declines linearly from 20 to 96 years of age.[65,66] DHEA sulfate has been associated inversely with future mortality, especially from coronary heart disease.[67] Both DHEA and DHEA sulfate are also inversely correlated with hypocholesterolemia and hypertension.[68] DHEA can cause weight loss without decreasing food intake.[69] In experimental animals, DHEA exerts a protective effect against tumorigenesis, immune disorders, and diabetes mellitus.[70]

Norepinephrine levels increase with advancing age, while circulating epinephrine levels are unchanged.[9] The increase in norepinephrine levels parallels the increase in systolic blood pressure seen in older persons.[71] There is both an increase in norepinephrine appearance in plasma and a decrease in the norepinephrine clearance rate.[72,73] Stepwise multiple linear regression analysis suggests that norepinephrine appearance rates play a more important role in increasing norepinephrine levels than does the decrease in clearance rates,[74] and compartment analysis has suggested that the increased appearance rate occurs mainly in the extravascular space, suggesting an increased tone of the sympathetic nervous system.[74] Both age and percentage of body fat play an important role in producing the increased norepinephrine appearance rate. Older persons have increased norepinephrine responsiveness to both upright posture and oral glucose ingestion.[9]

Isoproterenol produces less of an increase in the heart rate in older persons, suggesting a decrease in adrenergic responsiveness with advancing age.[9] There is a small decrease in the proportion of β-adrenergic receptors in the high-affinity state, a reduction in receptor affinity, and a reduced activity of the catalytic unit of adenylate cyclase.[75] α-Adrenergic receptor function is altered less with advancing age, with only a mild decrease in the affinity for agonist binding[76] and a reduction in epinephrine-mediated inhibition of NaF-stimulated platelet membrane adenylate cyclase activity in elderly persons.[77] These findings are compatible with an uncoupling of the platelet α_2-adrenergic receptor adenylate cyclase complex with advancing age.

Sex Hormones

Male

While the effects of aging on testosterone levels in males once were controversial, it is now clear that testosterone levels decrease with age.[78] This is seen even more dramatically in the decrease in bioavailable testosterone that occurs with advancing age (Fig. 31-3).[79] The circadian rhythm of testosterone is also lost with advancing age.[80]

Dihydrostestosterone is decreased in older persons unless there is significant prostatic hypertrophy, in which case it may be increased.[81] The testosterone production rate is decreased in subjects over 70 years of age (mean 4.0 mg/24 h) compared to subjects under 50 years of age (mean 6.6 mg/24 h).[82] The decreased production rate is partially balanced by a decrease in the plasma clearance rate of testosterone in older adults (530 ± 35 mg/liter per 24 h). The plasma clearance rate of testosterone is directly proportional to the free testosterone levels. There is a decrease in testicular weight and the total number of Leydig cells with advancing age.[78] There is an impaired testosterone response to exogenous human chorionic gonadotropin (hCG) with advancing age, though whether this is secondary to the decrease in basal testosterone production or is due to refractoriness to gonadotropin stimulation is uncertain.[83]

Estradiol levels are unchanged with age, resulting in an increase in the ratio of estradiol to testosterone.[78] Estradiol production rates are unchanged with age, but there is a decrease in the clearance rates.[84] Peripheral conversion of testosterone to estradiol and androstenedione to estrone increases with aging.[84] This increased aromatization is presumably secondary to the increased obesity seen in old males. Sex hormone–binding globulin (SHBG) levels are unchanged or slightly increased with aging.[85,86] As testosterone is bound with greater avidity to SHBG than is estradiol, the ratio of free estradiol to bioavailable testosterone is greatly increased.

While it has been stated that luteinizing hormone (LH) levels increase with age,[87,88] recent studies have reevaluated this issue. As can be seen in Fig. 31-3, older persons with markedly depressed bioavailable testosterone levels fail to show the expected increase in LH levels.[79] There is a decrease in LH amplitude with aging without a change in the pulse frequency, suggesting a hypothalamic defect.[89,90] There is also a decreased response to naloxone, suggesting increased opioid tone in older males.[91] Furthermore, there is a blunted response to gonadotropin releasing hormone (GnRH) in older compared with younger men[92] and a mild age-related decline in the ratio of LH bioactivity to immunoreactivity,[85] suggesting a pituitary defect. Testosterone is less effective at inhibiting LH in older

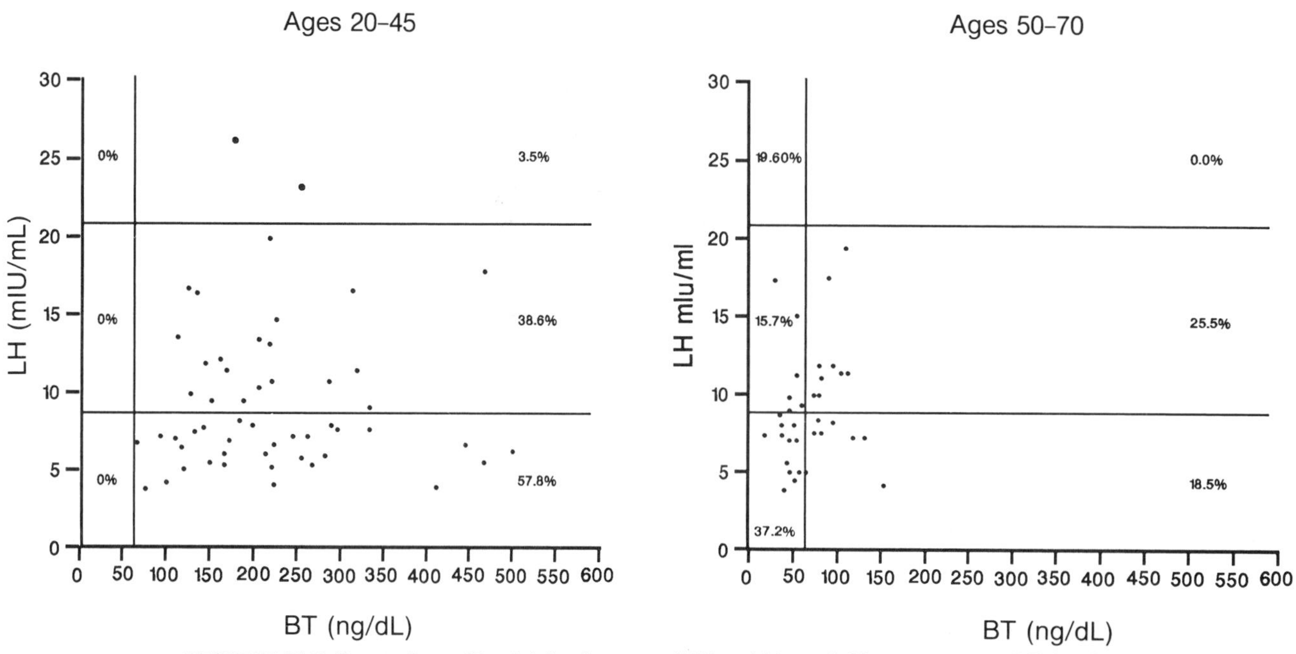

FIGURE 31-3 Comparison of luteinizing hormone (LH) and bioavailable testosterone (BT) levels with aging. Demonstrates the failure of LH to rise appropriately in response to the falling BT levels seen with aging. (*Data from Korenman et al.*[79])

males than in younger males.[93] Thus, it appears that with advancing age there is a defect in the testicular secretion of testosterone (primary hypogonadism) coupled with a failure of the hypothalamic-pituitary axis to sense the falling testosterone level (secondary hypogonadism). This central failure results in only a minority of older men having elevated LH levels, while the majority have inappropriately normal LH levels for the decreased levels of circulating testosterone (Fig. 31-4).

Testes from older men histologically show thickening of the basement membrane, peritabular fibrosis, and impaired spermatogenic maturation. The areas of testicular degeneration are patchy in distribution, allowing normal spermatogenesis to occur in over half of males over 70 years of age.[94] Sperm

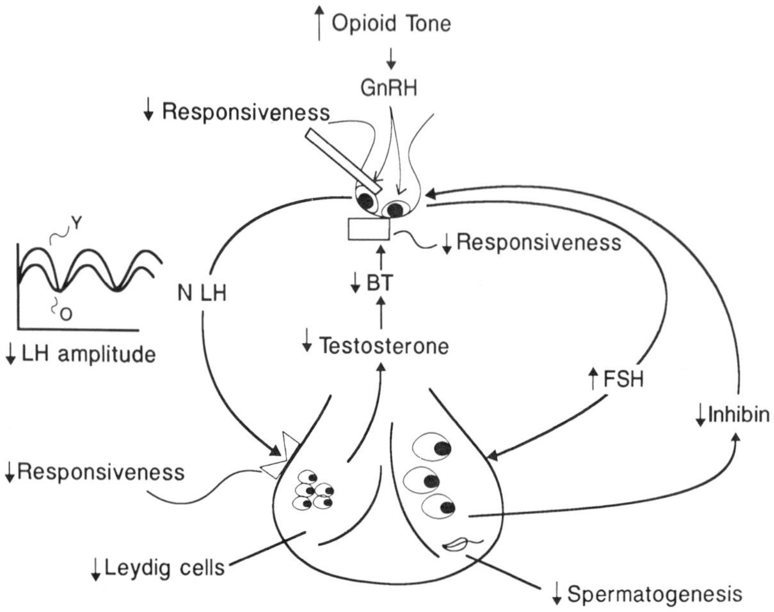

FIGURE 31-4 Major changes in the hypothalamic-pituitary-gonadal axis that occur with aging. BT = bioavailable testosterone; LH = luteinizing hormone; FSH = follicle stimulating hormone; GnRH = gonadotropin releasing hormone.

counts tend to decrease with advancing age, and there is diminished sperm motility and altered morphology in older men.[95] Increased follicle stimulating hormone (FSH) levels with advancing age are inversely correlated with daily sperm production.[84] Inhibin levels appear to decrease with advancing age.[85]

Female

The average age at menopause in the United States is 51 years, with the majority of women experiencing menopause between 45 and 55 years. Cigarette smoking results in menopause occurring 1 to 2 years earlier than might be predicted. With the onset of menopause, estrone replaces estradiol as the major circulating estrogen.[96] After menopause, estradiol levels decrease by 35-fold, estrone levels by 20-fold, testosterone levels by 1.5-fold, and androstenedione levels by 1.5-fold. Progesterone levels are not altered with advancing age. After menopause, the estradiol production rate is 12 μg/24 h and the plasma clearance rate is reduced by 30 percent.[97] Estrone production rates are 55 μg/24 h, and there is a 20 percent reduction in the clearance rate. Postmenopausally, the major source of estrogens is the adrenal gland, with most estrone being produced by peripheral aromatization of androstenedione.[97] The rate of peripheral conversion in postmenopausal women is double that in premenopausal women.

The changes in the hypothalamic-pituitary-ovarian axis with aging are delineated in Fig. 31-5. Postmenopausally, both LH and FSH levels are increased, with FSH levels increasing to a greater extent.[96] These increases represent alterations in production rates, as gonadotropin clearance rates are not altered postmenopausally.[97] The relatively higher FSH levels may be secondary to the slower clearance rate of FSH. After menopause, there appears to be no alteration in LH and FSH levels.[98]

The lack of estrogen postmenopausally results in a decrease in the opioid inhibitory tone of GnRH secretion.[99] This effect of estrogen appears to be mediated through a decrease in central nervous system (CNS) dopaminergic activity.[100]

Hormones Associated with Water Metabolism

Older persons with loss of the activities of daily living are at major risk of developing either dehydration or hyponatremia. Older persons also have an impaired thirst response to dehydration.[101] Both animal[102] and human[103] studies have suggested that this is due to a failure of the opioid drinking drive. There is also evidence that the impaired release of peripheral angiotensin II, a potent dipsogen in animals, may play a role in the development of dehydration in older persons.[104]

Basal arginine vasopressin (AVP) levels tend to be increased in older subjects at any level of osmolality.[105] Older persons fail to show the normal nocturnal increase in vasopressin, and this may explain the nocturnal diuresis seen in older persons.[106] Older subjects fail to show prolonged inhibition of AVP after an ethanol infusion.[107] By contrast, the volume-pressure (baroreceptor)–mediated release of AVP is impaired in older humans.[105] The borderline vasopressin excess provides a partial explanation for the fact that 53 percent of patients over 60 years of age in a nursing home develop hyponatremia at least once a year.[9] The majority of these older persons who

FIGURE 31-5 Alterations in the hypothalamic-pituitary-ovarian axis with aging.

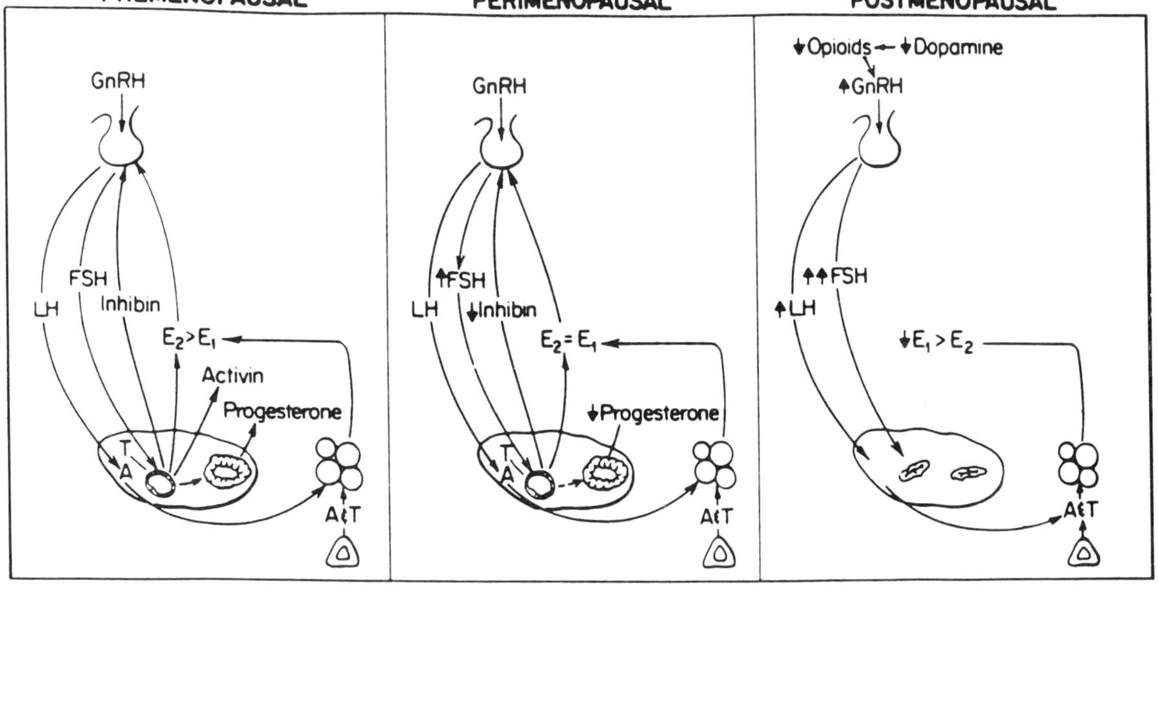

develop hyponatremia have evidence of the syndrome of inappropriate antidiuretic hormone (ADH). Other causes of hyponatremia in institutionalized patients include tube feeding with insufficient salt in the supplements and malnutrition.[108]

Atrial natriuretic hormone (ANH) levels are increased in older persons.[109] The increased levels are much lower than are those seen in patients with cardiac failure.[113] There is an attenuation of the cAMP response to ANH with advancing age, suggesting a reduction in the ability of ANH to activate its receptors with advancing age.[109]

FRAILTY, HORMONES, AND AGING

With advancing age there is an increase in functional dependence as well as an increased propensity to fall and suffer injuries. Four major factors appear to be involved in the development of frailty syndromes in older persons: (1) a decrease in muscle mass, (2) a decrease in bone mass, (3) a decrease in the ability to maintain balance coupled with an increased reliance on visual cues, and (4) a decrease in cognitive processing. Four hormonal systems whose function is often decreased with aging play an important role in maintaining the integrity of muscle and bone mass: the growth hormone–IGF-I system, testosterone, estradiol, and vitamin D. The physiologic changes seen with aging and the effects of those hormones on these systems are described in Table 31-8. In addition, low levels of DHEA in older institutional subjects have been correlated with a loss in the ability of these persons to carry out the activities of daily living,[110] and DHEA has been shown to improve cognitive function in old animals.[111] Alterations in balance in older persons and animals appear to be related predominantly to a decreased input of beta-adrenergic tone from the locus ceruleus to the cerebellum as a result of a decrease in β receptor and postreceptor function.[112] This loss of β-adrenergic tone results in an inability to appropriately regulate the flow of neuronal messages in the cerebellum.

Growth Hormone

Marcus et al. studied the effects of growth hormone treatment for 7 days in humans over 60 years of age.[114] They found an increase in IGF-I and nitrogen retention, phosphate, parathormone, osteocalcin, $1,25(OH)_2$ vitamin D, and urinary calcium. There was a decrease in cholesterol and sodium excretion and a mild impairment of glucose tolerance with hyperinsulinemia.

Rudman et al. examined the effect of growth hormone treatment for 6 months in healthy males over 60 years of age with low IGF-I plasma levels.[115] This growth hormone replacement dose resulted in a return of IGF-I levels to values seen in normal young men. This resulted in a significant increase in lean body mass (14.4 percent) and a decrease in adipose tissue mass (8.8 percent) which was not significant. There was a tendency for skin thickness to increase. A minimal increase in bone mass (1.6 percent) was also reported. It should be noted that another study found no benefit in adding growth hormone to calcitonin for the treatment of osteoporosis.[116]

Two studies have evaluated the utility of growth

TABLE 31-8 A Comparison of the Effects of Aging and Growth Hormone, Testosterone in Males, Estrogen in Females, and Vitamin D

	Aging	Growth Hormone	Testosterone	Estrogen	Vitamin D
Nitrogen balance	↓*	↑	↑	—	—
Muscle mass/strength	↓	↑	↑	↑	↑
Body fat content	↑	↓	↑	↑	—
Bone mass	↓	±	↑	↑	↑
Body water content	↓	↑	—	—	—
Hematocrit	↓ (m)	—	↑	—	—
Renal blood flow	↓	↑	—	—	—
Glomerular filtration	↓	↑	—	—	—
Libido	↓	—	↑	↑ (?)	—
Facial hair	↓	—	↑	—	—
Cognition	↓	—	↑	—	—
Immune system					
Autoimmune complexes	↑	—	—	—	—
T-cell helper function	↓	—	—	—	—
Macrophage inhibition of tuberculosis	↓	↑	—	—	↑
Atherosclerosis	↑	↑	↑	↓	—
Neoplasia	↑	↑	—	↑	—

* ↑ = increase; ↓ = decrease; — = no effect or unknown; m = males.

hormone treatment in older persons with protein-energy malnutrition. In a short-term study, growth hormone produced weight gain and increased nitrogen retention.[117] Kaiser et al. treated five older patients with protein-energy malnutrition with growth hormone and compared the results to those seen in five patients who received normal supportive treatment.[118] There was one death in the control group. Growth hormone increased IGF-I in these malnourished individuals. The growth hormone–treated group showed an increase in weight and midarm circumference compared with the loss seen in the group which did not receive growth hormone. Growth hormone also enhanced nitrogen retention in these malnourished patients. The growth hormone–treated group showed no evidence of impaired glucose metabolism.

Overall, these studies suggest a possible place for growth hormone replacement in the frail elderly, particularly those with protein-energy malnutrition. There is a need for trials examining the effect of growth hormone on muscle strength and a need to establish the cost-effectiveness and risk/benefit ratio of long-term therapy.

Testosterone

Hypogonadism occurs in up to half of healthy males over 50 years of age.[119] Testosterone produces important effects on muscle strength.[120] In addition, the fall in hematocrit which is present in males but not in females with advancing age may be related to testosterone deficiency. Testosterone also plays a role in cognitive function and the maintenance of bone mass. Many of the changes seen with aging are similar to those associated with hypogonadism.[119] There are few data on the nonsexual effects of testosterone replacement in older males.

Hartnell et al. reported that testosterone therapy in older males with low bioavailable testosterone levels resulted in increased energy, better sleep, less depression, and an increased hemotocrit.[121] This form of therapy did not increase myocardial infarction or hospitalizations. One male with an elevated hematocrit did have a stroke. Griggs et al. found that testosterone can enhance muscle strength in normal males.[122] Tenover et al. (unpublished data) reported salutary effects of testosterone on calcium metabolism in older persons.

Two studies have demonstrated a correlation between testosterone and bone density in older males.[123,124] Testosterone therapy increased 1,25$(OH)_2$ vitamin D and intestinal calcium absorption.[123] Baran et al. found an increase in bone formation and mineralization in a patient who received 6 months of testosterone therapy.[124] Hypogonadal males have an increase in osteoclastic activity similar to that seen in postmenopausal females.[125]

Overall, these studies suggest that low testosterone levels may play an important role in the pathogenesis of frailty syndromes. The lack of well-designed interventional trials in older hypogonadal males makes it difficult to draw firm conclusions regarding the efficacy of testosterone replacement in elderly males.

Estrogens

The utility of estrogen therapy in white females in the 10 years after menopause has been clearly established. Estrogen decreases overall mortality and the death rate from cardiovascular disease.[126] Estrogens decrease the levels of high-density lipoprotein$_2$ (HDL_2) and apoprotein AI and AII.[127] It should be noted that the addition of progesterone to estrogen negates the beneficial effects of estrogen on HDL and HDL_2 levels.[128] Numerous studies have demonstrated that estrogens slow the rate of bone loss in postmenopausal women for at least the first 10 years after menopause and reduce the future risk of fracture by at least 50 percent.[129] Estrogen therapy may also increase muscle strength and enhance cognitive function even in older females.[130]

Vitamin D, Type II (Age-Related) Osteopenia, and Hip Fracture

Hip fracture represents a major cause of morbidity and mortality in older persons.[131] There is a 20 percent excess mortality in the first year after a hip fracture. One-half of older whites and one-third of older blacks suffering from a hip fracture will be discharged to a nursing home.[131] Approximately one-half of persons who suffer a hip fracture require significant assistance with the activities of daily living for a short period, and one-quarter require long-term assistance. The incidence of hip fractures in the United States in persons over 65 years of age is 6.63 fractures per 1000 per year, with the peak incidence of 35.4 per 1000 per year occurring in 95-year-old white females. Two-thirds of all hip fractures occur in those over the age of 75 years. While hip fractures occur most commonly in older white women (80.7 per 1000 per year), appreciable numbers of hip fractures occur in white men (4.28 per 1000), black women (3.06 per 1000), and black men (2.38 per 1000).

The major factors in hip fracture are osteopenia, falls, and the mechanics of landing. In three-quarters of women with hip fractures, the bone density is 3 or more SD below the young normal mean.[132] However, bone mass does not decrease as rapidly as hip fractures increase, and the rate of Colles' fracture remains relatively stable with advancing age. This suggests the importance of other factors in the pathogenesis of hip fractures. With advancing age, a number of factors make people more vulnerable to falling when they encounter simple environmental hazards such as a throw rug. These factors include drugs (especially barbiturates and psychotropics[133,134] and polypharmacy),[135] visual disturbances, poor balance (related to altered neuronal input to the cerebellum, such as decreased β-adrenergic activity), cognitive dysfunction, muscle weakness, and postural and meal-associated hypotension. Another important factor in the pathogenesis of hip fracture is the mechanics of the fall. Older persons often react more slowly than do younger persons and fail to protect themselves with their hands. Older persons also often fall sideways rather than forward or backward, increasing the mechanical stress on the femur. Decreased muscle strength also leads to a decrease in protection of the femur and an increase in hip fractures.[136]

Vitamin D deficiency may play a crucial role in the pathogenesis of many hip fractures and of frailty in general. A number of studies have suggested that vitamin D deficiency plays a role in up to 40 percent of hip fractures.[132] However, these studies did not utilize tetracyline labeling techniques, making the diagnosis suspect. Vitamin D deficiency not only predisposes to osteomalacia but also may result in decreased muscle strength. Numerous studies have suggested that a number of older persons have decreased 25(OH) vitamin D levels and, in a lower number of cases, a decrease in its active metabolite 1,25(OH)$_2$ vitamin D (Table 31-6).[132] This appears to be particularly true of the institutionalized elderly, who are at greater risk of suffering a hip fracture. Nagraj et al. reported that bone density in males in nursing homes ranged from 71 to 92 percent of that of age-matched normal males.[137] The major factor correlating with decreased bone density was low body weight, suggesting a role for malnutrition in the development of decreased bone density in this population. Factors associated with hip fracture in this population include IGF-I, 25(OH) vitamin D, and 1,25(OH)$_2$ vitamin D levels.[138]

The reasons for declining vitamin D levels with aging are multifactorial (Fig. 31-6). The major source of vitamin D is synthesis in the skin of cholecalciferol after exposure to ultraviolet light. Some older persons are housebound and do not go out into the sun,

FIGURE 31-6 The major factors responsible for the decline in vitamin D levels with age.

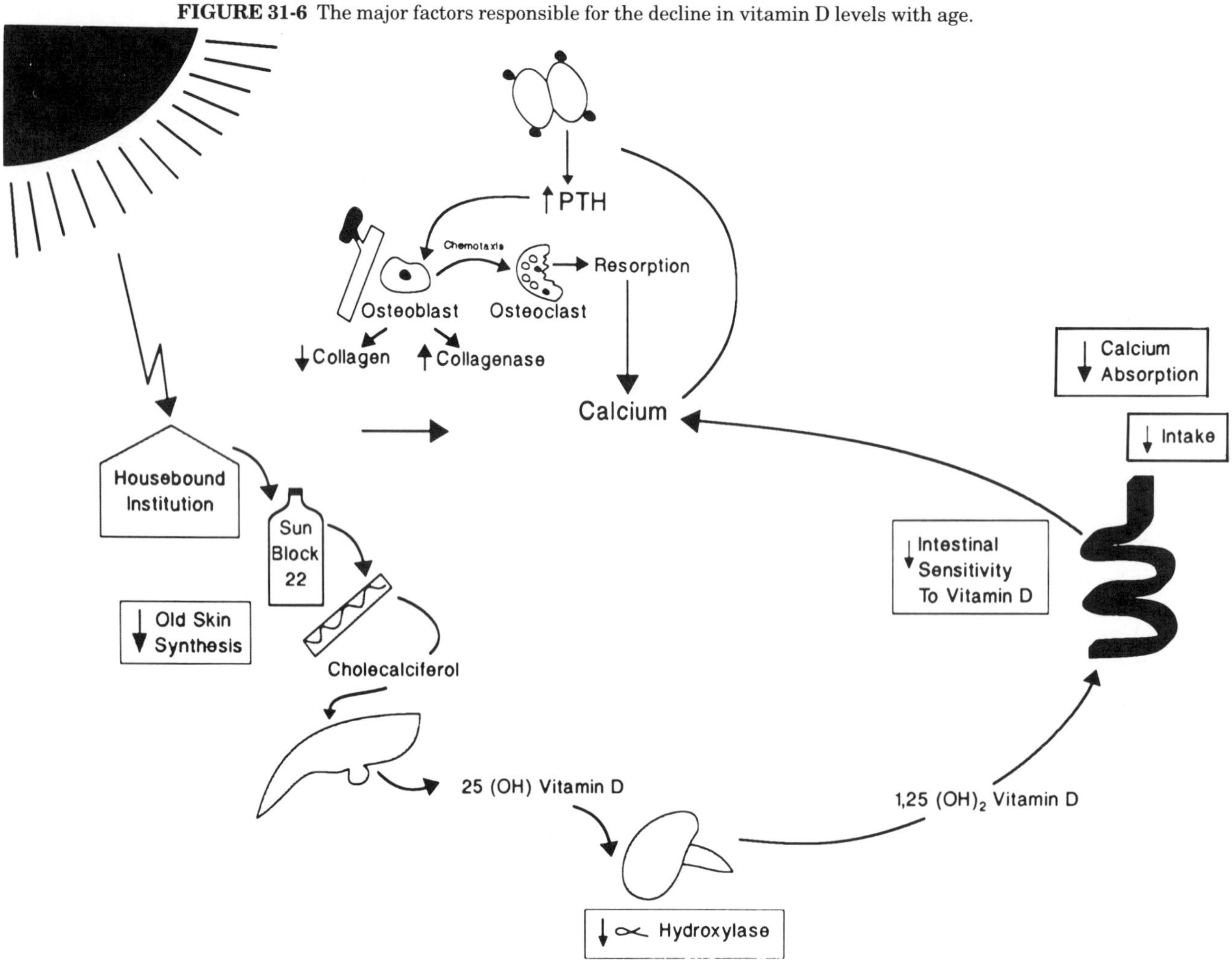

and others who do often bundle themselves to such an extent that they receive no sun exposure. Other older persons with skin cancer apply sun block to prevent further cancers, leading to a decrease in vitamin D levels.[139] Older skin has been demonstrated to be less capable of synthesizing cholecalciferol on exposure to ultraviolet light compared with young skin.[140] Armbrecht et al. have shown that older kidneys fail to synthesize 1,25$(OH)_2$ vitamin D as well as younger kidneys do because of a defect in 1α-hydroxylase activity with advancing age.[141] Finally, older persons with a poor nutritional intake may further compromise their vitamin D status by decreasing their intake of vitamin D. In addition, Horst et al.[210] found a reduction in calcitriol receptors in both bone and intestine. For these reasons, it is recommended that the majority of older persons take a 400 IU vitamin D supplement daily.[142] Clinically, vitamin D deficiency can be suspected when an older person has a low or low normal calcium level and a raised alkaline phosphatase level.

SEXUALITY AND AGING

The full expression of sexuality involves a delicate balance of social, cultural, psychological, hormonal, and physical factors. For many people, sexuality is considered a proclamation of life while aging is a herald of approaching death.[78] For this reason, sexuality plays an important role in the quality of life of many older persons. A number of studies have documented a decrease in sexual activity with advancing age. These changes are due to a variety of factors, including the development of disease and frailty, a decrease in available partners, social and cultural beliefs, psychological factors, hormonal changes, and the development of impotence.

Males

Dionko et al. found that 73.8 percent of married men in the United States over 60 years of age are sexually active.[143] In contrast, only 10 percent of males of a similar age in Japan are still sexually active.[144] In apparently healthy males between the ages of 50 to 70 years, 20 percent were unable to obtain or sustain an erection adequate for intercourse. Slag et al. found that one in three persons over 50 years of age who had at least one illness also had erectile dysfunction.[145] In contrast, a survey of healthy 80-year-old Californians found that 63 percent were still having intercourse "at least several times a year."[146]

Sexual activity in males consists of both libido and potency. *Libido* refers to the sexual desire and drive, thoughts and fantasies, and satisfaction and pleasure associated with sexual activity. Libido is predominantly driven by sex hormones, as was first noted in the fourteenth century B.C. in Assyria when castration was used as a treatment for sexual offenders. *Potency* consists of the ability to obtain and maintain an erection and to ejaculate. Potency and libido are to some extent interdependent.

The major causes of impotence are listed in Table 31-9. Nearly half of older males are impotent as a result of atherosclerotic vascular disease impeding blood flow in the penile artery.[147] In some of these males, blockage of the penile artery is only partial and the person needs to exercise his buttocks to demonstrate the fall in penile blood flow, i.e., the "pelvic steal" syndrome. A rare cause of obstructed arterial blood flow is penile Raynaud's phenomenon, which is seen in some persons with vasculitides.[148] The diagnosis of penile arterial disease is made by measuring the penile blood pressure and comparing it with the brachial blood pressure (penile-brachial pressure index) or by utilizing duplex ultrasonography, which can demonstrate penile blood flow and more accurately delineates the state of the deep penile vessels. Older persons with vascular impotence have a 23 percent greater chance of developing a myocardial infarction or a stroke over the subsequent 2 to 3 years than do impotent persons with normal penile blood pressure.[149] Impotent males with low penile brachial pressure indexes are more likely to have abnormal electrocardiographic stress or dipyridamole thallium testing than are those with normal pressures.[150] These findings strongly suggest that

TABLE 31-9 Causes of Impotence in Older Males

Vascular	Endocrine disorders
Arterial	Increased prolactin
Penile Raynaud's phenomenon	Thyroid disease
Venous leakage	Hypogonadism
Medications	Cushing disease
Diuretics	Neuropathy
Antihypertensive medications	Autonomic
Tranquilizers	Sensory
Antidepressants	Nutritional
H_2 receptor antagonists	Zinc deficiency
Cytotoxic agents	Protein-energy malnutrition
Nonsteroidal anti-inflammatory agents	Peyronie's disease
Estrogens	Psychiatric disorders
Digoxin	Depresion
Anticonvulsants	Widower's syndrome
Carbonic anhydrase inhibitors	Performance anxiety
Metoclopramide	Spinal cord damage
Baclofen	Tumor
Disopyramide	Trauma
Street drugs	Central nervous system
Tobacco	Multiple sclerosis
Alcohol	Temporal lobe epilepsy
Opiates	Stroke
Diabetes mellitus	

arterial vascular impotence is closely correlated with atherosclerotic disease in other parts of the body.

Venous leakage from the corpora cavernosa causes from 14 to 54 percent of all cases of impotence and is increasingly common with advancing age because of age-related alterations in the tunica albuginea.[151,152] These patients cannot maintain an erection after obtaining an adequate response to intracorporeal papaverine injection.[153] The diagnosis is confirmed by cavernosography.[154]

Elevated prolactin levels have been clearly associated with impotence, but hyperprolactinemia in unselected series of impotent male occurs in less than 5 percent.[156] Most of these prolactin elevations are drug-related, and only 0.5 to 1 percent of impotent males have prolactinomas.

Depression results in decreased nocturnal penile tumescence, decreased testosterone levels, and impotence.[78] These changes may be due to increased levels of CRF in many depressed patients, resulting in suppression of LH release and altered autonomic nervous system tone.[155]

Approximately 10 percent of all older impotent males have a psychological problem as the primary cause of their impotence, and nearly half of these men have some degree of performance anxiety (i.e., inability to obtain an adequate erection related to anxiety because of a previous failure) associated with their organic impotence.[156] Widower's syndrome occurs in older males who develop impotence to protect them from amorous advances while still grieving for the former spouse.[157]

Medications play a role in 25 percent of all cases of impotence in older persons.[156] Impotence in older persons is often multifactorial, with two-thirds of impotent patients having more than one contributory factor.[156]

The major treatment modalities available for the management of impotence are outlined in Table 31-10. After excluding treatable causes of impotence such as depression and endocrine disorders, the majority of older persons have three options for the treatment of impotence: a penile prosthesis, a vacuum tumescence device, and intracavernosal injection therapy. The decision about which therapy to use is based on the patient's needs, e.g., daily versus weekly intercourse, his preference, and the stability of his relationship.

Penile prostheses are the gold standard for the treatment of impotence. The satisfaction rate with penile prostheses is around 80 percent provided that adequate counseling is carried out before the operation. There are two types of prostheses: semirigid (or malleable) and inflatable. The inflatable penile prosthesis may be self-contained within the penis or may have parts in the abdomen and scrotum as well. Inflatable prostheses have a 5-year half-life, are much more expensive than the semirigid form, and require manual dexterity, limiting their use in persons with arthritis or frailty syndromes. Overall, semirigid prostheses are usually the best choice for older persons.

TABLE 31-10 Modalities Available for the Treatment of Impotence in Older Men

1. Vacuum tumescence devices (external suction devices)
2. Penile prosthesis
3. Intracavernosal injections
   - Papaverine
   - Phentolamine
   - Prostaglandin E_1
4. Surgery
   - Arterial revascularization*
   - Venous leakage ligation
5. Psychological treatments
   - Treatment of depression
   - Psychotherapy
6. Hormonal treatments
   - Testosterone
   - Bromocriptine
   - Treatment of thyroid disease
7. Medications*
   - Yohimbine
   - Pentoxifylline
   - Oral phentolamine
   - Isoxsuprine
   - Zinc
   - Transdermal nitroglycerine
   - Opioid antagonists
8. Adjust medications to those less likely to cause impotence or, when possible, discontinue medication

* Experimental.

Direct injections of either papaverine (with or without phentolamine) or prostaglandin E_1 into the corpora cavernosa produce good-quality erections in most persons.[157] Patients can self-inject at home with good success. Side effects include bruising pain on injection, induration, urethral bleeding, and priapism, and long-term use may result in scarring or fibrosis.

Vacuum tumescence devices are clear cylinders that can be placed over the penis. Through a connection with a hand-operated suction pump, they produce external negative pressure around the penis, resulting in an erection. The erection is maintained by slipping a rubber band or ring over the base of the penis. These devices have a high satisfaction rate and can produce erections in some patients who have had penile prostheses removed.[158] Side effects include premature loss of penile rigidity, failure to ejaculate, pain or discomfort, inconvenience, and occasional bruising. They are particularly useful in older persons who are in a well-bonded relationship and wish to have intercourse no more frequently than once or twice a week.

Testosterone therapy has been clearly demonstrated to enhance normal sexual drive, ejaculation, and spontaneous erections in young hypogonadal males.[159] In eugonadal males, testosterone has been shown to produce an increase in sexual interest.[160] In a single-blind crossover study, testosterone therapy increased sexual activity and nocturnal penile tumescence in eugonadal men.[161] However, in older persons this improvement is often short-lived. Transscrotal testosterone patches produce physiologic concentrations of testosterone[162] and have been shown to restore potency.[163] Cost, however, may be a limiting factor in the use of transscrotal patches.

In the last decade there has been dramatic improvement in the understanding of the pathophysiology of impotence. This has been accompanied by major advances in the ability to treat impotence. Impotence has clearly become a major medical disease whose diagnostic work-up and treatment can be undertaken by an endocrinologist. Appropriate management of sexual dysfunction in older males is an important quality of life issue.

Females

Females have been shown in survey studies to have an increased prevalence of sexual dysfunction at the time of menopause.[78] Coital frequency and sexual thoughts decline significantly after menopause.[164] This decline in sexuality is more closely related to the decrease in testosterone than to estradiol levels. Libido and sexual response after bilateral salpingo-oophorectomy was substantially enhanced by ethinyl estradiol treatment.[165] Estrogen replacement therapy in postmenopausal women enhances vaginal expansion and lubrication after sexual arousal. Estrogens also enhance vaginal blood flow and vaginal electropotential difference.[166]

Testosterone was first shown to enhance libido in females in 1943.[167] The antiandrogen cyproterone acetate, which is used to treat hirsutism, decreases libido in 60 percent of females.[168] Two studies have suggested that a combination of testosterone and estradiol is superior to estradiol alone in enhancing libido.[169,170]

In women over age 80, the following were the major sexual problems reported: anorgasmia (30 percent), partner's impotence (30 percent), poor vaginal lubrication (30 percent), and decreased libido (23 percent).[147] The Sarr-Weiner report found that 23 percent of women over 60 had anorgasmia and that 17.6 percent had dyspareunia.[171] Treatment with estrogen or estrogen cream and treatment of depression are important therapeutic modalities for the management of sexual difficulties in older women.

DIABETES MELLITUS

Diabetes mellitus is present in nearly 18 percent of persons between 65 and 74 years of age.[172] Diabetes mellitus is particularly prevalent in African-Americans, occurring in 25.9 percent between 65 and 74 years of age.[173] Older African-Americans with diabetes mellitus have retinopathy twice as often as do whites, have renal disease three times as often, and are two and a half times more likely to have an amputation. Of the 65 million type II diabetics in the United States, 3.1 million are over the age of 65 years.[174] Older diabetics are more likely to be institutionalized, have a greater risk of suffering a disability, and have a greater risk of premature death.[175]

Hyperglycemia of Aging

Blood glucose levels tend to increase with advancing age.[176] The reasons for this are multifactorial. Older persons tend to have a defect in both insulin receptors and postreceptor responsiveness.[177,178] In addition, the second phase of insulin secretion is somewhat attenuated in older persons.[179] Approximately 80 percent of the hyperglycemia of aging can be attributed to environmental factors such as obesity and physical inactivity, with less than 20 percent being due to age per se.[180,181] The possible role of amylopectin in the hyperglycemia of aging remains to be determined.[182]

Should Blood Glucose Be Controlled in Older Individuals?

There are numerous reasons for regulating blood glucose in older persons (Table 31-11).[183] Blood glucose control will prevent the development of diabetic hyperglycemia comas, which are often fatal in older persons.[176] There is evidence that age interacts with

TABLE 31-11 Reasons for Glucose Control in Older Individuals with Diabetes Mellitus

Prevention of hyperglycemic coma	Management of glucose toxicity
Hyperosmolar coma	Pain
Ketoacidosis	Incontinence
Lactic acidosis	Dehydration
Prevention of long-term complications	Increased platelet adhesiveness
Nephropathy	Myocardial infarction
Neuropathy	Stroke
Visual disturbances	Infection
Retinopathy	Poor red cell deformability
Cataracts	Peripheral vascular disease
	Poor recovery from stroke
	Accelerated atherosclerosis
	Trace minimal deficiency
	Accelerated aging

hyperglycemia to accelerate the development of retinopathy, nephropathy, and neuropathy.[184]

The increased urination produced by the osmolar effect of hyperglycemia is a major reason for controlling glucose levels in older persons.[183] Increased urination results in nocturia, with the need to get up more frequently at night and therefore poor sleep and an increased risk of falling. This osmotic diuresis can also result in incontinence in older persons. Finally, older persons fail to have a normal recognition of thirst, resulting in the osmotic diuresis that leads to mild dehydration associated with fatigue.

Hyperglycemia is associated with an increased perception of pain caused by a decreased responsiveness to endogenous opioids.[185] This results in older diabetics complaining of pain more often than do age- and disease-matched controls.[186]

Older diabetic patients with hyperglycemia have been demonstrated to have problems of memory retention to a greater extent than do matched controls.[187] These memory problems appear to play a role in reducing compliance in this population.[188] Animal studies have demonstrated that normalization of glucose can reverse the effects of hyperglycemia on memory dysfunction.[189]

Retrospective studies have suggested that hyperglycemia is associated with a poor outcome after a stroke.[183] Older diabetics who have had a stroke are more likely to have a second stroke than are nondiabetics who have had a stroke, and older diabetics also die sooner.[190]

Diabetes mellitus can be considered a form of accelerated aging, with persons who have diabetes tending to be 5 to 10 years older than are those who do not have diabetes.[176] Hyperglycemia has been suggested to play a role in producing this premature aging. Table 31-12 lists a number of similarities between diabetes mellitus and the aging process.

Special Features in the Management of Older Diabetics

There are a number of special problems seen typically in older persons. These problems may modulate the approach to older diabetics (Table 31-13).

TABLE 31-12 Some Similarities between Diabetes Mellitus and the Aging Process

Decreased DNA unwinding rate
Increased basement membrane thickness
Increased tissue glycolation
Memory problems
Osteopenia
Accelerated atherosclerosis
Decreased renal function
Increased cataracts
Increased propensity to develop incontinence
Increased propensity to develop unusual infection

Of particular concern is the development of depression, which may be more common in older persons with diabetes mellitus.[184] Depression is highly correlated with increased hospital admissions and mortality in older diabetics (unpublished observations). All older diabetics should be screened for depression, utilizing the Yesavage Geriatric Depression Scale.[191] When this scale suggests depression, intervention with low-dose antidepressants is appropriate.[192]

Diet in Older Diabetics

Generally, major dietary changes are not recommended for diabetics over 70 years of age. The majority of diabetics over 70 years of age are not overweight; they are usually underweight. Thus, care should be taken to prescribe weight-reducing diets only when such diets are appropriate. Because of their increased propensity to develop hypoglycemia, all older diabetics on oral hypoglycemic agents or insulin should eat a bedtime snack. Some older diabetics have large variations of glucose immediately after a meal, and this may be associated with symptoms. Under these circumstances, the addition of fiber to the diet may greatly improve a diabetic's quality of life. Glucose is also responsible for meal-associated hypotension in older persons.[193] This drop in blood pressure may be associated with falls after the meal in older individuals.[193] Symptoms 2 or 3 h after a meal often mean that an older diabetic has gastroparesis. Metoclopramide, while improving the gastroparesis, crosses the blood-brain barrier and can result in CNS symptoms such as delirium and parkinsonism. Erythromycin, which activates the motilin receptor, may be an alternative in some older diabetics. Cisparide has fewer CNS effects and is as effective as metoclopromide in the treatment of gastroparesis.

Oral Hypoglycemia Agents

A number of age-associated changes may modulate the action of oral sulfonylureas in older persons. These changes include decreases in hepatic blood flow, hepatic oxidative metabolism, serum albumin, and renal function.[183] Finally, hypoglycemic counter-regulatory hormones, specifically growth hormone and cortisol responses, are reduced in older persons.[194] The end result of these changes is to increase the propensity of older persons to develop hypoglycemia when they take sulfonylureas. The increased occurrence of hypoglycemia in older compared with younger subjects has been clearly demonstrated by the Swedish Spontaneous Adverse Drug Reporting System.[195] Chlorpropramide should be used with caution in older diabetics because of the prolonged hypoglycemia and hyponatremia it produces.[183] The second-generation oral agents glipizide and gly-

TABLE 31-13 Special Problems That Commonly Interfere with the Management of Older Persons with Diabetes Mellitus

Problem	Outcome	Management
Hypodipsia	Dehydration: hyperosmolar coma	Drink 4–8 glasses of water daily
Anorexia	Hypoglycemia	Early detection of weight loss; adjust hypoglycemic agents, diagnose cause, and manage appropriately
Visual disturbance	Inadequate insulin dosing; hyper- or hypoglycemia	Predraw insulin syringes; insulin syringe magnifier
Decreased activities of daily living	Decreased food intake; hypoglycemia	Adaptive devices; Meals on Wheels
Decreased physical activity	Obesity; hyperglycemia	Exercise program
Altered renal and hepatic function	Hypoglycemia	Decreased dose of hypoglycemics
Cognitive impairment	Poor compliance	Memory aids
Depression	Poor compliance; death; suicide	Early detection and management of depression
Impaired baroreceptor response	Orthostatic hypotension made worse by diabetic autonomic neuropathy and dehydration	Detection; adequate fluid intake; nonpharmacologic and pharmacologic management
Multiple medications	Drug interactions; hypoglycemia	Be aware of potential interactions; limit drugs where possible
Multiple disease processes	Multiple medications; anorexia; dehydration; amputations; infection	Treat where appropriate; create priority list for management decisions
Poverty	Poor dietary intake; cannot afford specialized diets	Recognize; advise social worker; realistic management plan

buride (glibenclamide) are generally preferred in older persons because their nonionic binding to albumin reduces their propensity to produce drug-drug interactions in a population which is likely to be on multiple medications.[183] However, in some diabetics over 80 years of age, tolbutamide in a single daily dose may be an excellent therapeutic modality.[183]

Metformin, a biguanide, has been shown to produce lactic acidosis in less than 1 in 10,000 patients per year.[195] A number of the patients in this study were over 75 years of age. Other side effects of metformin which can be worrisome in older persons include gastrointestinal discomfort and weight loss and interference with the absorption of vitamin B_{12} and folate.[183]

Insulin

Older diabetics, especially those with visual disturbances, have been shown to make errors between 10 and 20 percent when drawing up insulin.[183] All older diabetics should have their ability to draw up insulin in the correct amount checked at each visit. If the patient is shown to be incapable of doing this, it is usually best to have the pharmacist supply the patient with predrawn insulin syringes, one week at a time. A syringe magnifier may help some older diabetics. Older diabetics with tremors, arthritis, or muscle weakness may benefit from utilizing needle guides and vial holders, which allow them to place the insulin syringe directly into the vial, eliminating the risk of jabbing themselves during the process.

Monitoring Treatment

Older diabetics adapt well to self-monitoring of blood glucose without negatively altering their perception of the quality of life.[196] Glycosylated hemoglobin levels may be falsely elevated in some older diabetics.[197] Fructosamine has been demonstrated to be a highly effective, cost-effective means of monitoring intermediate diabetic control in older diabetics.[198]

Diabetes in Nursing Home Residents

There are 190,000 diabetics in nursing homes, with 75 percent being over 75 years of age. Among diabetics in nursing homes, 9 percent are overweight and 21 percent are underweight.[199] Diabetics in nursing homes are more likely to have retinopathy, neuropathy, renal failure, amputations, atherosclerotic cardiovascular disease, peripheral vascular disease, and infections than are nondiabetics in nursing homes (Table 31-14). Thus, overall, diabetics in nursing homes are sicker than nondiabetic residents.

Mooradian et al. demonstrated that acceptable glucose control can be obtained in most nursing home residents, with minimal episodes of hypoglycemia.[199] All nursing home residents with diabetes

TABLE 31-14 Comparison of Diabetics and Nondiabetics in the Nursing Home

	Diabetics	Nondiabetics
Age (years)	80	80.1
Overweight (%)	21	25
Underweight (%)	9	0
Cataracts (%)	51	51
Retinopathy (%)	7	2
Renal failure (%)	30	10
Proteinuria (%)	32	0
Nephropathy (%)	28	10
Urinary tract infection (%)	55	30
Skin infections (%)	34	18
Amputations (%)	13	6
Stroke (%)	32	34
Angina/myocardial infarction (%)	60	48
Peripheral vascular disease	26	12

Source: Adapted from Mooradian et al.[199]

mellitus who are receiving either oral sulfonylureas or insulin should have a prescription for 1 mg glucagon intramuscularly when hypoglycemia occurs and oral glucose cannot be given. When a diabetic nursing home resident misses a meal, the insulin dose should be halved and chemstrips should be checked every 6 h until the resident begins to eat again.

Summary

Diabetes mellitus is commonly not diagnosed in older persons; over half the persons over 65 years of age with this disorder may not have the diagnosis made.[172] Older diabetics have a number of unique features to which endocrinologists need to pay careful attention in order to optimize diabetic management. Much evidence supports the use of blood glucose control in older diabetics.

NUTRITIONAL DISORDERS

In older persons, the major nutritional problem is protein-energy malnutrition, which is present in 9 percent of older outpatients, 17 to 65 percent of older hospitalized patients, and between 26 and 59 percent of nursing home residents.[200] An underweight state is much more highly correlated with mortality in older persons than is being overweight.[201] Most older persons with protein-energy malnutrition ingest sufficient calories to maintain their serum albumin at the cost of muscle protein. This results in older persons presenting with a picture where weight loss predominates, i.e., a marasmic picture. When an older person has an infection, cytokines are released and albumin levels fall, resulting in a kwashiorkor-type picture.

Weight loss in older persons has multiple causes, many of which are treatable (Table 31-15).[202] In addition, there is an anorexia of aging which appears to occur in response to the decrease in metabolic rate and the reduced physical activity that occur with advancing age.[201] The decrease in food intake in older persons is in part due to a decrease in the ability to appreciate the hedonic qualities of food because of the alterations in taste and smell that occur with advancing age.[202] In addition, animal studies have demonstrated that with advancing age there is a decrease in the endogenous opioid (dynorphin) feeding drive and an increased satiety effect of the gastrointestinal hormone cholecystokinin.[202] Medroxyprogesterone acetate has been demonstrated to increase food intake in older persons with cancer.[203] Recombinant growth hormone, with its anabolic effects, has been utilized to treat severe protein-energy malnutrition in older persons.[117,118]

Obesity is associated with only a minimal increase in mortality in older persons, and with advancing age it appears to be a problem only when it interferes with carrying out the activities of daily living (e.g., in persons with osteoarthritis) or when it is associated with a specific obesity-associated disease such as diabetes mellitus or hypertension.[203] Older persons are at increased risk for developing

TABLE 31-15 Causes of Weight Loss in Older Persons

I. Social
  A. Poverty
  B. Problems with shopping
  C. Problems with food preparation
II. Psychosocial
  A. Depression
  B. Dementia
  C. Late-life paranoia
  D. Anorexia nervosa (tardive)
  E. Manipulative behaviors
  F. Excessive burden of life
III. Medical
  A. Hypermetabolism/hyperthyroidism
    1. Pheochromocytoma
    2. Parkinson's disease
  B. Anorexia
    1. Hyperparathyroidism
    2. Candidal esophagitis
    3. Abdominal ischemia
    4. Medications, e.g., digoxin, theophylline
    5. Cancer
    6. Unpalatable diets, e.g., low cholesterol, low-salt
    7. Infections (interleukins, cachectin)
  C. Mixed
    1. Chronic obstructive pulmonary disease
      a. Cardiac cachexia
IV. Malabsorption
  A. Gluten enteropathy
  B. Lactose deficiency

obesity because of a decrease in the resting metabolic rate, a decrease in the thermic effect of feeding, and a decrease in habitual physical activity. Despite this, most obesity is seen in middle age in males rather than in old age; 30.5 percent aged 45 to 54 are obese, while only 25.8 percent aged 65 to 74 years are obese.[203] Obesity in females shows a continuous increase to the age of 74, after which the prevalence tends to decrease. Changes in body adipose tissue follow a similar pattern, with a marked increase in the early forties and a decline after age 75 years.[203] Fat distribution changes with age, with the waist/hip ratio increasing in both sexes over the ages of 17 to 96 years.[203]

The decreased risks associated with obesity in advancing age suggest that management intervention should be limited to those who are over 130 percent of average body weight unless they have a specific obesity-associated disease. The utility of different weight-loss methods in older persons is described in Table 31-16.

Cholesterol levels tend to rise with age, plateauing by 55 years in males and 60 years in females.[204] Total cholesterol levels are less predictive of new-onset coronary heart disease in older adults.[205] HDL cholesterol appears to be a better predictor than total cholesterol for coronary heart disease in young-old subjects but not in old-old subjects.[206]

A number of studies have suggested that low cholesterol levels predict total mortality in older persons, particularly those residing in institutions.[207] This appears to be related to the fact that low cholesterol levels are a marker for protein-energy malnutrition[208] and possibly for cytokine activity which results from underlying infections or neoplasms.[209] Major dietary alterations in older persons can be hazardous.[210] For these reasons, it would appear that it is inappropriate to recommend cholesterol-lowering diets in persons over 70 years of age.

TABLE 31-16 Utility of Weight-Loss Methods in Older Persons

Method	Utility in older persons
Exercise	Mall walking programs, swimming, tai chi; chair exercises are primary modality
Diet	Only if over 130% of average weight, associated with diabetes mellitus, or interferes with activities of daily living
Behavior modification	Yes
Low-calorie and very low calorie diets	Should be avoided
Drugs	
Anorectic agents	Rarely indicated
Thermogenic agents	Potentially dangerous
Gastric balloon	Not useful
Surgery	
Gastric restriction	Only when massive obesity is associated with sleep apnea
Jejunoileal bypass	Never used

CONCLUSION

As the individual ages, a panoply of hormonal changes occur. Many of these changes are first evident in the early forties. The role of these hormonal changes in the expression of the phenotypic changes seen with aging is uncertain. However, it appears that hormones may play a role in preventing or treating the frailty syndromes seen in older persons. Atypical presentations of endocrine disorders in older persons often create a diagnostic challenge for the endocrinologist.

REFERENCES

1. Trence DL, Morley JE, Handwerger BS: Polyglandular autoimmune syndromes. *Am J Med* 77:107–116, 1984.
2. Mooradian AD, Scarpace PJ: The response of isoproterenol-stimulated adenylate cyclase activity after administration of L-triiodothyronine is reduced in aged rats. *Horm Metab Res* 21:638–639, 1989.
3. Morley JE, Levine AS: Pharmacology of eating behavior. *Annu Rev Pharmacol Toxicol* 25:127–146, 1985.
4. Mooradian AD, Deebaj L, Wong NCW: Age-related alterations in the response of hepatic lipogenic enzymes to altered thyroid states in the rat. *J Endocrinol* 128:79–84, 1991.
5. Mooradian AD: The hepatic transcellular transport of 3-5-3′ triiodothyronine is reduced in aged rats. *Biochim Biophys Acta* 1054:1–7, 1990.
6. Morley JE, Krahn DD, Gosnell BA, Billington CJ, Levine AS: Interrelationships between calcitonin and other modulators of feeding behavior. *Psychopharmacol Bull* 20:463–465, 1984.
7. Solomon DM, Judd HL, Sur MC, Rubenstein LZ, Morley JE: New issues in geriatric care. *Ann Intern Med* 108:718–732, 1988.
8. Morley JE, Shafer RB: Thyroid function screening in new psychiatric admissions. *Arch Intern Med* 42:591–593, 1982.
9. Mooradian AD, Morley JE, Korenman SG: Endocrinology in aging. *Dis Mon* 34:398–461, 1988.
10. Curtis HF, Miller K: Chromosome aberrations in lower cells of guinea pigs. *J Gerontol* 26:292–293, 1971.
11. Clark AM, Rubin MA: The modification by x-irradiation of the life span of haploid and diploid. *Habrobracon Radiat Res* 15:244–249, 1961.
12. Orgel LE: The maintenance of the accuracy of protein synthesis and its relevance to aging. *Proc Natl Acad Sci USA* 49:517–521, 1963.
13. Cristofalo VJ: Biological mechanisms of aging: An overview, in Hazzard WR, Andres R, Bierman EL, Blass JP (eds): *Principles of Geriatric Medicine and Gerontology,* 2d ed. New York, McGraw-Hill, 1990, pp 3–14.
14. Brownlee M, Cerami A, Vlassarci M: Advanced glycosylation end products in tissue and the biochemical bases of diabetic complications. *New Engl J Med* 318:1315–1321, 1988.
15. Snowdon DA: Early natural menopause and the duration of post menopausal life: Findings from a mathematical model of life expectancy. *J Am Geriatr Soc* 38:402–410, 1990.

16. Denckla WD: Role of the pituitary and thyroid glands in the decline of minimal O_2 consumption with age. *J Clin Invest* 53:572–581, 1974.
17. Walford RL: Multigene families, histocompatibility system, transformation meiosis, stem cells and DNA repair. *Mech Ageing Dev* 9:19–24, 1979.
18. Maier JAM, Voculalas P, Roeder D, Maciaq T: Extension of the lifespan of human endothelial cells by an interleukin-1a antisense oligomer. *Science* 249:1570–1574, 1990.
19. Habib MP, Dickerson F, Mooradian AD: Ethane production rate in vivo is reduced with dietary restriction. *J Appl Physiol* 68:2588–2590, 1990.
20. Knoll J, Dallo J, Yen TT: Striatal dopamine sexual activity and lifespan: Longevity of rats treated with (−) deprenyl. *Life Sci* 45:525–531, 1989.
21. Pereira-Smith OM, Smith JR: Genetic analysis of indefinite division in human cells: Identification of four complementation groups. *Proc Natl Acad Sci USA* 85:6042–6046, 1988.
22. Seshadri T, Campizi J: Repression of c-fos transcription and an altered genetic program in senescent human fibroblasts. *Science* 247:205–209, 1990.
23. Steen GM, Beeson M, Gordon L: Failure to phosphorylate the retinoblastoma gene product in senescent human fibroblasts. *Science* 249:666–669, 1990.
24. Osiewarcz HD: Molecular analysis of aging processes in fungi. *Mutat Res* 237:1–8, 1990.
25. Kelijman M: Age-related alterations of the growth hormone/insulin-like-growth factor I axis. *J Am Geriatr Soc* 39:295–307, 1991.
26. Sun Y-K, Xi X-P, Fenoglio CM, et al: The effect of age on the number of pituitary cells immunoreactive to growth hormone and prolactin. *Hum Pathol* 15:169–180, 1984.
27. Shilaski T, Shizume K, Nakahara M, et al: Age-related changes in plasma growth hormone response to growth hormone-releasing factor in man. *J Clin Endocrinol Metab* 58:212–214, 1984.
28. Giusti M, Lomeo A, Marini G, et al: Role of aging on growth hormone and prolactin release after growth hormone releasing hormone and domperidone in man. *Horm Res* 27:134–140, 1987.
29. Pavlov EP, Harmon SM, Merriam GR, et al: Responses of growth hormone (GH) and somatomedin C to GH-releasing hormone in healthy aging men. *J Clin Endocrinol Metab* 62:595–600, 1986.
30. Lang I, Schernthaner G, Pietschmann P, et al: Effects of sex and age on growth hormone response to growth hormone-releasing hormone in healthy individuals. *J Clin Endocrinol Metab* 65:535–540, 1987.
31. Dawson-Hughes B, Stern D, Goldman J, et al: Regulation of growth hormone and somatomedin C secretion in postmenopausal women: Effect of physiological estrogen replacement. *J Clin Endocrinol Metab* 63:424–432, 1986.
32. Kalk WJ, Vinik AI, Pimstone BL, et al: Growth hormone response to insulin hypoglycemia in the elderly. *J Gerontol* 28:431–433, 1973.
33. Muggeo M, Fedele D, Tiengo A, et al: Human growth hormone and cortisol response to insulin stimulation in aging. *J Gerontol* 39:546–551, 1991.
34. Lal S, Nair NPV, Thavundagil JX, et al: Growth hormone response to apomorphine, a dopamine receptor agonist, in normal aging and in dementia of the Alzheimer type. *Neurobiol Aging* 10:227–231, 1989.
35. Alba-Roth J, Muller OA, Schopohl J, et al: Arginine stimulates growth hormone secretion by suppressing endogenous somatostatin secretion. *J Clin Endocrinol Metab* 67:1186–1189, 1988.
36. Dudl RJ, Ensinek JW, Palmer HE, et al: Effect of age on growth hormone secretion in man. *J Clin Endocrinol Metab* 67:11–16, 1973.
37. Blichert-Toft M: Stimulation of the release of corticotrophen and sommatotrophin by metyrapone and arginine. *Acta Endocrinol [Suppl] (Copenh)* 195:65–85, 1975.
38. Rudman D, Kutner MH, Rogers CM, et al: Impaired growth hormone secretion in the adult population: Relation to age and adiposity. *J Clin Invest* 67:1361–1369, 1981.
39. Vermeulen A: Nyctohemeral growth hormone profiles in young and aged men: Correlation with somatomedin C levels. *J Clin Endocrinol Metab* 64:884–888, 1987.
40. Tan K, Baxter RC: Serum insulin-like growth factor I levels in adult diabetic patients: The effect of age. *J Clin Endocrinol Metab* 63:651–655, 1986.
41. Bennett AE, Wahner MW, Riggs BL, et al: Insulin-like growth factors I and II: Aging and bone density in women. *J Clin Endocrinol Metab* 59:7012–7014, 1984.
42. Rudman D, Nagraj HS, Mattson DE, et al: Hyposommatomedinemia in the nursing home patient. *J Am Geriatr Soc* 34:427–430, 1986.
43. Sawin CT, Carlson HE, Geller A, Castelli WP, Bacharach P: Serum prolactin and aging: Basal values and changes with estrogen use and hypothyroidism. *J Gerontol* 44:131–135, 1989.
44. Mooradian AD, Morley JE, Billington CJ, Slag MF, Elson MK, Shafer RB: Hyperprotactinemia in male diabetics. *Postgrad Med J* 61:11–14, 1985.
45. Sawin CT, Chopra D, Azizi F, Mannix JE, Bacharach P: The aging thyroid: Increased prevalence of elevated serum thyrotropin in the elderly. *JAMA* 242:247–250, 1979.
46. Jeffreys PM, Farran MEA, Hoffenberg R, Fraser PM, Hodkinson HM: Thyroid function tests in the elderly. *Lancet* i:924–927, 1972.
47. Rosenthal MJ, Hun WC, Garry PJ, Goodwin JS: Thyroid function in the elderly: Microsomal antibodies as a discriminant for therapy. *JAMA* 258:209–213, 1987.
48. Kaiser FE: Variability of responses to TRH in normal elderly. *Age Ageing* 16:345–354, 1987.
49. Spaulding SW: Age and the thyroid. *Endocrinol Clin North Am* 16:1013–1025, 1987.
50. Gregerman RI, Gaffney GW, Shock NW: Thyroxine turnover in euthyroid man with special reference to changes in age. *J Clin Invest* 41:2065–2074, 1962.
51. Herrmann J, Heinen E, Kroll MJ, Rodoff KM, Kruskemper ML: Thyroid function and thyroid hormone metabolism in elderly people: Low T3-syndrome in old age. *Klin Wochenschr* 59:315–323, 1981.
52. Burrows AE, Shakespear RA, Mesch RD, Cooper E, Aickin EM, Burke CW: Thyroid hormones in the elderly sick: T_4 euthyroidism. *Br Med J* 4:437–439, 1975.
53. Gaffney GW, Gregerman RI, Shock NW: Relationship of age to the thyroidal accumulation, renal excretion and distribution of radioiodide in euthyroid man. *J Clin Endocrinol Metab* 22:786–794, 1962.
54. Samuels LT: Factors affecting the metabolism and distribution of cortisol as measured by levels of 17-hydroxycorticosteroids in blood. *Cancer* 10:746–751, 1957.
55. West CD, Brown H, Simmons EL, Carter DB, Kumage LF, Engelbert EL: Adrenocortical function and cortisol metabolism in old age. *J Clin Endocrinol Metab* 21:1197–1207, 1961.
56. Romanoff LP, Morris CW, Welch P, Rodriguez RM, Pincus G: The metabolism of cortisol [4]C-14 in young and elderly men: I. Secretion rate of cortisol and daily excretion of tetrahydrocortisone and cortalone (20 alpha and 20 beta). *J Clin Endocrinol Metab* 21:1413–1425, 1961.
57. Touitou Y, Salon J, Bogdan A, Touitou C, Reinberg A, Beck M, Sodiyez JC, Demey-Ponsort E, Van Couwenberge M: Adrenal circadian system in young and elderly human subjects: A comparative study. *J Endocrinol* 93:201–208, 1982.
58. Friedman M, Green MF, Shrland DG: Assessment of hypothalamic-pituitary-adrenal function in the geriatric age group. *J Gerontol* 24:292–297, 1969.
59. Pavlov EP, Hrman SM, Chrousos GP, Lourizux DL, Blackman MR: Responses of plasma adrenocorticotrophin, cortisol, and dehydroepiandrosterone to avine corticotrophin-releasing hormone in healthy aging men. *J Clin Endocrinol Metab* 62:767–772, 1986.

60. Rolandi E, Franceschini R, Marabini A, et al: Twenty-four hour beta-endorphin secretory pattern in the elderly. *Acta Endocrinol (Copenh)* 115:441–446, 1987.
61. Facchinetti G, Petraglia F, Nappi G, et al: Different patterns of central and peripheral beta-endorphin, beta lipoprotein and ACTM throughout life. *Peptides* 4:469–474, 1983.
62. Hatfield BD, Goldfarb AM, Sforzo GA, et al: Serum beta-endorphin and affective responses to graded exercise in young and elderly men. *J Gerontol* 42:429–431, 1987.
63. Casale G, Pecorini M, Cuzzoni G, de Nicola P: Beta endorphin and cold pressor test in the aged. *Gerontology* 31:101–105, 1985.
64. Tsunoda K, Abe K, Goto T, Yasujima M, Sato M, Omata K, Seino M, Yoshinaga K: Effect of age on the renin-angiotensin aldosterone system in normal subjects: Simultaneous measurement of active and inactive renin, renin substrate and aldosterone in plasma. *J Clin Endocrinol Metab* 62:384–389, 1986.
65. Yamaji T, Ibayashi H: Plasma dehydroepiandrosterone sulfate in normal and pathological conditions. *J Clin Endocrinol Metab* 29:273–277, 1969.
66. Oventreich N, Brind JC, Rizer RL, Vogelman JM: Age changes in sex differences in serum dehydroepiandrosterone sulfate concentrations throughout adulthood. *J Clin Endocrinol Metab* 59:531–539, 1984.
67. Barrett-Connor E, Khaw KT, Yen SCC: A prospective study of dehydroepiandrosterone sulfate, mortality and cardiovascular disease. *N Engl J Med* 315:1519–1524, 1986.
68. Sonka J, Fassati M, Fassati P, et al: Serum lipids and dehydroepiandrosterone excretion in normal subjects. *J Lipid Res* 9:769–772, 1968.
69. Coleman DL, Leites EM, Applezweig N: Therapeutic doses of dehydroepiandrosterone metabolites in diabetic mutant mice. *Endocrinology* 115:239–243, 1984.
70. Pashko LL, Schwartz AG: Effect of food restriction, dehydroepiandrosterone or obesity on the binding of 3H-7,12 dimethylbenz(a) anthracene to mouse skin DNA. *J Gerontol* 38:8–12, 1983.
71. Tuck ML, Griffiths RF, Johnson L, Stern N, Morley JE: Hypertension in the elderly. *J Am Geriatr Soc* 36:630–643, 1988.
72. Linares OA, Halter JB: Sympathochromaffin system activity in the elderly. *J Am Geriatr Soc* 35:448–453, 1987.
73. Hoeldtke RD, Cilmi KM: Effects of aging on catecholamine metabolism. *J Clin Endocrinol Metab* 60:479–484, 1985.
74. Linares OA, Supiano MA, Morrow LA, Halter JB: Norepinephrine release and metabolism in the elderly by compartmental analysis: Relationship to dietary salt. *Clin Res* 34:950A, 1986.
75. Scarpace PJ: Decreased beta-adrenergic responsiveness during senescence. *Fed Proc* 45:51–54, 1986.
76. Hyland L, Docherty JR: An investigation of age-related change in pre- and post-functional alpha-adrenoreceptors in human saphenous vein. *Eur J Pharmacol* 114:361–363, 1985.
77. Supiano MA, Linares OA, Halter JB, Reno KM, Rosen SG: Functional uncoupling of the platelet alpha$_2$-adrenergic receptor-adenylate cyclase complex in the elderly. *J Clin Endocrinol Metab* 64:1160–1164, 1987.
78. Morley JE: Endocrine factors in geriatric sexuality clinics. *Geriatr Med* 7:85–94, 1991.
79. Korenman SG, Morley JE, Mooradian AD, Davis SS, Kaiser FE, Silver AJ, Viosca SP, Garza D: Secondary hypogonadism in older men: Its relationship to impotence. *J Clin Endocrinol Metab* 71:963–969, 1990.
80. Zumoff B, Strain GW, Kream J, et al: Age variation of the 24-hour plasma concentrations of androgens, estrogens and gonadotropins in normal adult men. *J Clin Endocrinol Metab* 54:534–538, 1982.
81. Pirke KM, Doerr P: Age-related changes in free plasma testosterone, dihydrotestosterone and estradiol. *Acta Endocrinol (Copenh)* 80:171–178, 1975.
82. Vermeulen A, Reubens R, Verdonck L: Testosterone secretion and metabolism in male senescence. *J Clin Endocrinol Metab* 34:730–735, 1972.
83. Harman SM, Tsitouras PD: Reproductive hormones in aging men, in Measurement of sex steroids, basal luteinizing hormone and Leydig cell response to human chorionic gonadotropin. *J Clin Endocrinol Metab* 51:35–41, 1980.
84. Morley JE, Kaiser FE. Testicular function in the aging male, in Armbrecht HJ, Coe RM, Wongsurawat N (eds): *Endocrine Function and Aging.* New York, Springer-Verlag, 1990, pp 94–114.
85. Tenover JS, Matsumoto AM, Plymate SR, et al; The effects of aging in normal men on bioavailable testosterone and luteinizing hormone secretion: Response to clomiphene citrate. *J Clin Endocrinol Metab* 65:1118–1125, 1987.
86. Vermeulen A, Verdonck L: Some studies on the biological significance of free testosterone. *J Steroid Biochem* 3:421–426, 1972.
87. Deslypere JP, Vermeulen A: Leydig cell function in normal men: Effect of age, lifestyle, residence, diet and activity. *J Clin Endocrinol Metab* 59:955–962, 1984.
88. Baker HWG, Burges HG, DeKretser DM, et al: Changes in the pituitary-testicular system with age. *Clin Endocrinol (Oxf)* 5:349–372, 1976.
89. Tenover JS, Matsumoto AM, Clifton DK, Bremner WJ: Age-related alterations in the circadian rhythms of pulsatile luteinizing hormone and testosterone secretion in healthy men. *J Gerontol* 43:163–169, 1988.
90. Kaiser FE, Viosca SP, Mooradian AD, Morley JE, Korenman SG: Impotence and aging: Alterations in hormonal secretory patterns. *Endo Soc Abstr* 70:778A, 1988.
91. Vermeulen A, Deslypere JP, Kaufman JM: Influence of antiopioids on luteinizing hormone pulsatility in aging men. *J Clin Endocrinol Metab* 68:68–72, 1989.
92. Harman SM, Tsitouras PD, Costa PT, et al: Reproductive hormones in aging men: II. Basal pituitary gonadotropins and gonadotropin responses to luteinizing hormone-releasing hormone. *J Clin Endocrinol Metab* 54:547–551, 1982.
93. Winters SJ, Sherins RJ, Troen P: The gonadotropin-suppressive activity of androgen is increased in elderly men. *Metabolism* 33:1052–1059, 1984.
94. Engle ET: The male reproductive system, in Lansing AI (ed): *Cowdry's Problems of Aging,* 3d ed. Baltimore, Williams & Wilkins, 1952, pp 708–729.
95. Natoli A, Riondino G, Brancati A: Studio delta funizone gonadale ammonia e spermatogenetica nel corso della senescenza muschille. *G Gerontol* 20:1103–1119, 1972.
96. Kaiser FE, Morley JE: The menopause and beyond, in Cassel CR, Reisenberg D (eds): *Geriatric Medicine.* New York, Springer-Verlag, 1990, pp 279–290.
97. Judd HL, Korenman SG: Effects of aging on reproductive function in women, in Korenman SG (ed): *Endocrine Aspects of Aging.* New York, Elsevier, 1982, pp 163–197.
98. Scalgia H, Medina M, Pinto-Ferreira AI, et al: Pituitary LH and FSH secretion and responsiveness in women of old age. *Acta Endocrinol (Copenh)* 81:673–679, 1976.
99. Petraglia A, Porro C, Facchinetti R, et al: Opioid control of LH secretion in humans: Menstrual cycle, menopause and aging reduce effect of naloxone but not of morphine. *Life Sci* 38:2103–2110, 1986.
100. Melis GB, Cagnacci A, Gambacciani M, et al: Chronic bromocriptine administration restores luteinizing hormone response to naloxone in post-menopausal women. *Neuroendocrinology* 47:159–163, 1988.
101. Phillips PA, Rollo BJ, Ledingham JCG, et al: Reduced thirst after water deprivation in healthy elderly men. *N Engl J Med* 311:753–759, 1984.
102. Silver AJ, Flood JF, Morley JE: Effect of aging on fluid ingestion in mice. *J Gerontol* 46:B117–121, 1991.
103. Silver AJ, Morley JE: The role of the opioid system in the hypodysia associated with aging. *J Am Geriatr Soc* (in press).
104. Yanamoto T, Harada H, Fukuyama J, et al: Impaired argi-

nine-vasopressin secretion associated with hypoangiotensinemia in hypernatremic dehydrated elderly patients. *JAMA* 259:1039–1042, 1988.
105. Helderman JH: The impact of normal aging on the hypothalamic-neurohypophyseal-renal axis, in Korenman SG (ed): *Endocrine Aspects of Aging*. New York, Elsevier, 1982, pp 9–32.
106. Asplund R, Aberg H: Diumal variation in the levels of antidiuretic hormone in the elderly. *J Intern Med* 229:131–134, 1991.
107. Helderman JH, Vestal RE, Rowe JW, et al: The response of arginine vasopressin to intravenous ethanol and hypertonic saline in man: The impact of aging. *J Gerontol* 33:39–47, 1978.
108. Rudman D, Rachette D, Rudman IW, Mattson DE, Erve PR: Hyponatremia in tube-fed elderly men. *J Chronic Dis* 39:73–80, 1986.
109. Ohashi M, Fujia N, Nawata M, et al: High plasma concentrations of human atrial natriuretic polypeptide in aged men. *J Clin Endocrinol Metab* 64:81–85, 1987.
110. Rudman D, Shetty KR, Mattson DE: Plasma dehydroepiandrosterone sulfate in nursing home men. *J Am Geriatr Soc* 38:421–427, 1990.
111. Flood JF, Roberts E: Dehydroepiandrosterone sulfate improves memory in aging mice. *Brain Res* 448:178–181, 1988.
112. Rosenthal MJ, Morley JE, Flood JF, Scarpace PJ: Relationship between behavioral and motor responses of mature and old mice and cerebellar adrenergic receptor density. *Mech Ageing Dev* 45:231–237, 1988.
113. Saito Y, Nakao K, Nishimura K, et al: Clinical application of atrial naturetic polypeptide in patients with congestive heart failure: Beneficial effects on left ventricular function. *Circulation* 76:115–124, 1987.
114. Marcus R, Butterfield G, Holloway L, et al: Effects of short term administration of recombinant human growth hormone to elderly people. *J Clin Endocrinol Metab* 70:519–527, 1990.
115. Rudman D, Feller AG, Nagraj HS, et al: Effects of human growth hormone in men over 60 years old. *N Engl J Med* 323:1–6, 1990.
116. Aloia JF, Zanzi I, Vaswani A, et al: Combination therapy for osteoporosis. *Metabolism* 26:787–792, 1977.
117. Binnerts A, Wilson JH, Lamberts SW: The effects of human growth hormone administration in elderly men with recent weight loss. *J Clin Endocrinol Metab* 67:1312–1316, 1988.
118. Kaiser FE, Silver AJ, Morley JE: The effect of recombinant human growth hormone on malnourished older individuals. *J Am Geriatr Soc* 39:235–240, 1991.
119. Morley JE, Kaiser FE: Sexual function with advancing age. *Med Clin North Am* 73:1483–1495, 1989.
120. Mooradian AD, Morley JE, Korenman SG: Biological action of androgens. *Endocr Rev* 8:1–28, 1987.
121. Hartnell J, Korenman SG, Ciosca SP: Results of testosterone enanthate therapy for hypogonadism in older men. *Endocrine Soc Abstr*, No 428, Atlanta, 1990.
122. Griggs RC, Kingston W, Jozefowicz RF: Effect of testosterone on muscle mass protein synthesis. *J Appl Physiol* 66:498–503, 1989.
123. Francis RM, Peacock M, Aaron JE, et al: Osteoporosis in hypogonadal men: Role of decreased plasma, 1,25 dihydroxy vitamin D, calcium malabsorption and low bone formation. *Bone* 7:261–268, 1986.
124. Baran DT, Bergfeld MA, Teitelbaum SL, Avioli V: Effect of testosterone therapy on bone formation in an osteoporotic hypogonadal male. *Calcif Tissue Res* 26:103–106, 1978.
125. Jackson JA, Kleerekoper M, Parfitt AM, et al: Bone histomorphometry in hypogonadal and eugonadal men with spinal osteoporosis. *J Clin Endocrinol Metab* 63:53–58, 1987.
126. Bush TL, Cowan LD, Barrett-Connor E, et al: Estrogen use and all-cause mortality. *JAMA* 249:903–906, 1983.
127. Chetkowski RJ, Meldrum DR, Steingold KA, et al: Biologic effects of transdermal estradiol. *N Engl J Med* 314:1615–1620, 1986.
128. Hirvonen E, Malkonen M, Manninen V: Effects of different progestogens on lipoproteins during postmenopausal replacement therapy. *N Engl J Med* 304:560–563, 1981.
129. Pierron RL, Perry HM II, Grossberg G, et al: The aging hip. *J Am Geriatr Soc* 38:1339–1352, 1990.
130. Birge S, Price S, McGee S, et al: The role of estrogen in the prevention of hip fracture in women over age 69, in Chirstensen C, Overguard K (eds): *3rd International Symposium on Osteoporsis*. Copenhagen, Abstracts, 1990, pp 1196–1197.
131. Kellie SE, Brody JA: Sex-specific and race-specific hip fracture rates. *Am J Public Health* 80:326–328, 1990.
132. Morley JE, Gorbien MJ, Mooradian AD, et al: UCLA Geriatric Grand Rounds: Osteoporosis. *J Am Geriatr Soc* 36:845–859, 1988.
133. MacDonald JB, MacDonald ET: Nocturnal femoral fracture and continued widespread use of barbiturate hypnotics. *Br Med J* 2:483–486, 1977.
134. Ray WA, Griffen MR, Schaffner W, et al: Psychotropic drug use and risk of hip fracture. *N Engl J Med* 316:363–367, 1987.
135. Taggart H, McA: Do drugs affect the risk of hip fracture? *J Am Geriatr Soc* 36:1006–1009, 1988.
136. Frontera WR, Meredith CN, O'Reilly KP, Knuttgen MG, Evans WJ: Strength conditioning in older men: Skeletal muscle hypertrophy and improved function. *J Appl Physiol* 64:1038–1042, 1988.
137. Nagraj MS, Gregans GA, Mattson DE, Rudman IW, Rudman D: Osteopenia in the men of a veterans administration nursing home. *Am J Clin Nutr* 51:100–106, 1990.
138. Rudman D, Rudman IW, Mattson DE, et al: Fractures in the men of a veterans administration nursing home: Relation to 1,25 dihydroxyvitamin D. *J Am Coll Nutr* 8:324–334, 1989.
139. Matsuoka LY, Wortsman J, Hanifan N, Holick MF: Chronic sunscreen use decreases circulating concentrations of 25 hydroxyvitamin D. *Arch Dermatol* 124:1802–1803, 1988.
140. McLaughlin J, Holick MF: Aging decreases the capacity of human skin to produce vitamin D_3. *J Clin Invest* 76:1536–1538, 1985.
141. Armbrecht HJ, Zenser TV, Davis BB: Effect of age on the conversion of 25-hydroxyvitamin D_3 to 1,25 dihydroxyvitamin D_3 by kidney of rat. *J Clin Invest* 66:1118–1123, 1980.
142. Morley JE: A place in the sun does not guarantee adequate vitamin D. *J Am Geriatr Soc* 37:663–664, 1989.
143. Dionko AC, Brown MB, Herzog AR: Sexual function in the elderly. *Arch Intern Med* 150:197–200, 1990.
144. Aoki M, Kumcemoto Y, Mori K: Studies on sexual activity in Japanese males based on inquiry about sexual behavior. *Hinyokika Kiyo* 33:1623–1631, 1987.
145. Slag MF, Morley JE, Elson MK, et al: Impotence in medical clinic outpatients. *JAMA* 249:1736–1740, 1983.
146. Bretschneider JG, McCoy NL: Sexual interest and behavior in healthy 80 to 102-year olds. *Arch Sex Behav* 17:109–129, 1988.
147. Kaiser FE, Viosca SP, Morley JE, et al: Impotence and aging: Clinical and hormonal factors. *J Am Geriatr Soc* 36:511–519, 1988.
148. Mooradian AD, Viosca SP, Kaiser FE, Morley JE, Korenman SG: Penile Raynaud's phenomenon: A possible cause of erectile failure. *Am J Med* 85:748–750, 1988.
149. Morley JE, Korenman SG, Kaiser FE, et al: Relationship of penile brachial pressure index to myocardial infarction and cerebrovascular accidents in older males. *Am J Med* 84:445–448, 1988.
150. Kaiser FE, Udhoji V, Ciosca SP, et al: Cardiovascular stress tests in patients with vascular impotence. *Clin Res* 37:89A, 1989.
151. Shabsighi R, Fishman IJ, Quesada ET, et al: Evaluation of vasculogenic erectile impotence using penile duplex ultrasonography. *J Urol* 142:1469–1474, 1989.
152. Tudoriu T: My views about the applied anatomy on the penis and the physiopathology of erection. *Arch Intern Urol* 61:249–273, 1989.

153. Williams G, Mulachy J, Harnell G, Keely E: Diagnosis and treatment of venous leakage: A curable cause of impotence. *Br J Urol* 61:151–155, 1988.
154. Stig CG, Welterauer U, Sommerkamp H: Intra-individual comparative study of dynamic and pharmacocavernography. *Br J Urol* 64:93–97, 1989.
155. Ono N, Lumpkin MD, Samson WK, et al: Intrahypothalamic action of corticotropin-releasing factor to inhibit growth hormone and LH release in the rat. *Life Sci* 35:1117–1123, 1984.
156. Morley JE: Impotence. *Am J Med* 80:L897–905, 1986.
157. Morley JE, Kaiser FE: Impotence in elderly men. *Drugs Aging* (in press).
158. Korenman SG, Viosca SP, Kaiser FE, Mooradian AD, Morley JE: Use of a vacuum tumescence device in the management of impotence. *J Am Geriatr Soc* 38:217–220, 1990.
159. Davidson JM, Camargo CA, Smith ER: Effects of androgen on sexual behavior in hypogonadal men. *J Clin Endocrinol Metab* 48:955–958, 1979.
160. O'Carrol R, Bancroft J: Testosterone therapy for low sexual interest and erectile dysfunction in men: A controlled study. *Br J Psychiatry* 145:146–151, 1986.
161. Billington CJ, Mooradian AD, Duffy L, et al: Testosterone therapy in impotent patients with normal testosterone. *Clin Res* 31:718A, 1983.
162. Korenman SG, Viosca S, et al: Androgen therapy of hypogonadal men with transscrotal testosterone systems. *Am J Med* 83:471–478, 1987.
163. McClure RD, Oses R, Ernest NL: Hypogonadal impotence treated by transdermal testosterone. *Urology* 37:224–228, 1991.
164. McCoy NC, Davidson JM: A longitudinal study of the effects of menopause on sexuality. *Maturitas* 7:203–210, 1985.
165. Dennerstein L, Burrows GD, Wood C, et al: Hormones and sexuality: Effect of estrogen and progestogen. *Obstet Gynecol* 56:316–322, 1980.
166. Stemmens JP, Tsai CL, Semmens EC, et al: The effects of estrogen therapy on vaginal physiology during menopause. *Obstet Gynecol* 66:15–18, 1985.
167. Salmon TJ, Gast SH: Effect of androgens in libido in women. *J Clin Endocrinol Metab* 3:235–238, 1943.
168. Mazenod B, Pugeat M, Forest MG: Hormones, sexual function and erotic behavior in women, in Sitsen JMA (ed): *Handbook of Sexology,* vol 6. Amsterdam, Elsevier, 1988, pp 316–351.
169. Burger H, Hailes J, Nelson J, et al: Effect of combined implants of estradiol and testosterone on libido in post menopausal women, in Campbell S (ed): *Management of Menopause and Postmenopause Years.* Lancaster Time Press, Lancaster, UK, 1976, p 149.
170. Sherwin BB, Gelfand MM: The role of androgen in maintenance of sexual functioning in oophorectomized women. *Psychosom Med* 49:397–409, 1987.
171. Starr B, Weiner M: *The Starr-Weiner Report on Sex and Sexuality in the Mature Years.* New York, McGraw-Hill, 1981.
172. Harris MI, Hadden WC, Knowlen WC, et al. Prevalence of diabetes and impaired glucose tolerance and plasma glucose levels in US population ages 20–74 years. *Diabetes* 136:523–534, 1987.
173. Lieberman LS: Diabetes and obesity in elderly black Americans, in Jackson JS (ed): *The Black American Elderly.* New York, Springer, 1988, pp 130–189.
174. Huse DM, Oster G, Kellen AR, et al: The economic costs of non-insulin dependent diabetes mellitus. *JAMA* 262:2708–2713, 1989.
175. Waugh NR, Dallas JM, Jung RT, Newton RW: Mortality in a cohort of diabetic patients. *Diabetologia* 32:103–104, 1989.
176. Morley JE, Mooradian AD, Rosenthal MJ, Kaiser FK: Diabetes in elderly persons: Is it different? *Am J Med* 83:533–544, 1987.
177. Bolinder J, Ostman J, Arner P: Influence of aging on insulin receptor binding and metabolic effects of insulin on human adipose tissue. *Diabetes* 32:959–964, 1983.
178. Pogano G, Cassander M, Diana A, et al: Insulin resistance in the aged: The role of peripheral insulin receptors. *Metabolism* 30:46–49, 1981.
179. Chen M, Bergman RN, Pauni G, Porte D Jr: Pathogenesis of age-related glucose intolerance in man: Insulin resistance and decreased B-cell function. *J Clin Endocrinol Metab* 60:13–20, 1985.
180. Zavaroni I, Dall'Aglio E, Bruschi F, et al: Effect of age and environmental factors on glucose tolerance and insulin secretion in a worker population. *J Am Geriatr Soc* 34:271–275, 1986.
181. Shimokata H, Muller DC, Fleg JL, et al: Age as independent determinant of glucose tolerance. *Diabetes* 40:44–51, 1991.
182. Cooper GJS, Willis AC, Clark A, et al: Purification and characterization of a peptide from amyloid-rich pancreases of type 2 diabetic patients. *Proc Natl Acad Sci USA* 84:8628–8632, 1987.
183. Morley JE, Perry HM III: The management of diabetes mellitus in older individuals. *Drugs* 41:548–565, 1991.
184. Naliboff BD, Rosenthal M: Effects of age on complications in adult onset diabetes. *J Am Geriatr Soc* 37:838–843, 1989.
185. Morley GK, Mooradian AD, Levine AS, Morley JE: Why is diabetic peripheral neuropathy painful? The effect of glucose on pain perception in humans. *Am J Med* 77:79–83, 1984.
186. Damsguard EM: Why do elderly diabetics burden the health care system more than non-diabetics? *Dan Med Bull* 36:89–92, 1989.
187. Mooradian AD, Perryman K, Fitten LJ, et al: Cortical function in elderly non-insulin dependent diabetic patients. *Arch Intern Med* 148:2369–2372, 1988.
188. Rost K, Rotes D, Quill T, et al: Recall of prescription medication changes. *Diabetes* 38(Suppl 2): 40A, 1989.
189. Flood JF, Mooradian AD, Morley JE: Characteristics of learning and memory in streptozocin-induced diabetic mice. *Diabetes* 39:1391–1398, 1990.
190. Olson T, Vutanen M, Asplund K, et al: Prognosis after stroke in diabetic patients: A controlled prospective study. *Diabetologia* 33:244–249, 1990.
191. Yesavage JA, Brink TL, Rose TL, et al: Development and validation of a geriatric depression screening scale: A preliminary report. *J Psychiatr Res* 17:37–49, 1983.
192. Fitten LJ, Morley JE, Gross PL, et al: UCLA geriatric grand rounds: Depression. *J Am Geriatr Soc* 37:459–472, 1989.
193. Jansen RWMM, Peeters TL: The effect of oral glucose, protein, fat and water loading on blood pressure and the gastrointestinal peptides VIP and somatostatin in hypertensive elderly subjects. *Eur J Clin Invest* 20:192–198, 1990.
194. Rosenthal MJ, Hartnell JM, Morley JE, et al: Diabetes in the elderly. *J Am Geriatr Soc* 35:435–447, 1987.
195. Wilholm B-E, Westerholm B: Drug utilization and morbidity statistics for the evaluation of drug safety in Sweden. *Acta Med Scand [Suppl]* 683:107–117, 1984.
196. Gilden JL, Casia C, Hendryx M, et al: Effects of self-monitoring of blood glucose on quality of life in elderly diabetic patients. *J Am Geriatr Soc* 38:511–515, 1990.
197. Arnetz BB, Kallner A, Theorell T: The influence of aging on hemoglobin A_{ic}. *J Gerontol* 37:648–650, 1982.
198. Negro H, Morley JE, Rosenthal MJ: Utility of serum fructosamine as a measure of glycemia in young and old diabetic and non-diabetic subjects. *Am J Med* 85:360–364, 1988.
199. Mooradian AD, Osterweil D, Petrasek D, Morley JE: Diabetes mellitus in elderly nursing home patients: A survey of clinical characteristics and management. *J Am Geriatr Soc* 36:391–396, 1988.
200. Morley JE: Nutrition and aging, in Hazzard WR, Andres R, Bierman EL, Blass JP (eds); *Principles of Geriatic Medicine and Gerontology,* 2d ed. New York, McGraw-Hill, 1990 pp, 48–59.
201. Morley JE: Nutritional status of the elderly. *Am J Med* 81:679–695, 1986.
202. Morley JE, Silver AJ: Anorexia of aging. *Neurobiol Aging* 9:9–16, 1988.

203. Morley JE, Glick Z. Obesity. In Morley JE, Glick Z, Rubenstein LZ (eds): *Geriatric Nutrition.* New York, Raven Press, 1990, pp 293–306.
204. Miller NE: Aging and plasma lipoproteins, in Hazzard WR, Andres R, Bierman EL, Blass JP (eds): *Principles of Geriatric Medicine and Gerontology,* 2d ed. New York, McGraw-Hill, 1990, pp 767–776.
205. Anderson KM, Castelli WP, Levy D: Cholesterol and mortality: 30 years of follow-up from the Framingham study. *JAMA* 257:2176–2180, 1987.
206. Castelli WP, Garrison RJ, Wilson PWF, et al: Incidence of coronary heart disease and lipoprotein cholesterol levels: The Framingham study. *JAMA* 256:2835–2838, 1986.
207. Foretta B, Tortsat D, Wolmark Y: Cholesterol as a risk factor for mortality in elderly women. *Lancet* 1:868–870, 1989.
208. Kaiser FE, Morley JE: Cholesterol can be lowered in older persons: Should we care? *J Am Geriatr Soc* 38:84–85, 1990.
209. Noel MA, Smith TK, Ettinger WH: Characteristics and outcomes of hospitalized older patients who develop hypocholesterolemia. *J Am Geriatr Soc* 39:455–461, 1991.
210. Horst RL, Goff JP, Reinhardt TA: Advancing age results in a reduction of intestinal and bone 1,25 dihydroxyvitamin D receptor. *Endocrinology* 126:1053–1057, 1990.

CHAPTER 32

Hormones and Athletic Performance

David C. Cumming

ENERGY SUPPLY AND PHYSICAL WORK

The endocrine system at rest is characterized by endogenous rhythmic fluctuations in hormone levels. Superimposed on these internal rhythms is the capacity to respond to changes in the external environment. Thus, stress, feeding, trauma, and other stimuli are followed by adjustments of hormonal control. Physical activity, both short-term, acute activity and repeated exertion over a longer interval, may induce changes in the circulating levels of a number of hormones. Although much information about endocrine responses to physical exertion has come from investigations of exercise, such research also has important applications in industrial, military, and other forms of work as well as in recreational and competitive sports.

For optimal physical work to be carried out, nervous, cardiac, vascular, pulmonary, and metabolic functions must be coordinated and adjusted. The detailed mechanisms of control of this coordination are unclear, but the central role of the endocrine system in the regulation of energy metabolism, salt and water balance, and cardiac and vascular function, together with neuroendocrine influences on other systems, indicates the importance of the endocrine system in exercise and the capacity for physical work.

Muscular work is dependent on the supply of energy and oxygen. The basic fuel for muscular work is adenosine triphosphate (ATP). Enough ATP is stored for direct use in muscle for less than 1 s of activity. Creatine phosphate can supply ATP for a further 15 to 30 s; after that, stored carbohydrates and fats must be metabolized to supply continuing energy needs.

Oxygen consumption increases dramatically during the first few minutes of exercise until the demands of active tissues are met and a steady state is reached in which oxygen uptake and demand are balanced. In light exercise (10 to 40 percent of maximal oxygen consumption), the demand for oxygen from energy output during the initial 2 to 4 min can be met aerobically by both stored myoglobin and the blood perfusing the muscle. During severe exercise (70 to 90 percent of maximal oxygen consumption), the energy demands cannot be totally accounted for by the aerobic process even in early exercise; therefore, anaerobic sources must contribute so that lactic acid is produced. The point at which this begins is the *anaerobic threshold*. Maximal aerobic capacity or maximal oxygen consumption ($V_{O_{2max}}$) can be defined as the point at which no further increase in oxygen uptake occurs with an increase in energy demand, i.e., the exercise workload. $V_{O_{2max}}$ is used as a measure of fitness by which comparisons of workload are made among individuals of differing fitness.

$V_{O_{2max}}$ can be determined by means of various tests, such as continuous versus discontinuous exercise, bicycle versus treadmill or other form of exercise, and arm versus leg exercise. The duration of the test may also vary. The criteria used to determine $V_{O_{2max}}$ include (1) no further increase in oxygen consumption despite increasing workload (plateau phenomenon), (2) blood lactate levels greater than 80 mg/ml of blood, (3) heart rate greater than 190 beats per minute, and (4) respiratory quotient greater than unity. Determination of $V_{O_{2max}}$ therefore does not provide a specific measure but varies in accordance with the kind of test used. Nevertheless, it is the best single measure of fitness.

Exercise cannot be described as a single entity, as the characteristics of different activities place different demands on the body. The way in which energy is handled varies with exercise load, type, and duration and the fitness of the individual. Energy consumption at strenuous workloads can be 120 times basal levels; at less intense but sustained activity such as distance running, energy utilization is about 23 to 30 times basal levels. The ability to sustain a maximal load is limited, while less strenuous loads can be sustained for longer periods.

EVALUATING HORMONAL RESPONSE TO EXERCISE AND TRAINING

There are many experimental protocols and subjects involved in research on physical activity. Comparisons among investigations are therefore difficult, if not impossible, even when the comparisons are based on V_{O2max}. A comparison of the effects of a weight-lifting experiment with the responses to an endurance activity may produce different results, and a comparison of exhaustive exercise for 15 min with 4 hr of submaximal exercise or a 1000-km race over several days is clearly meaningless.

Nevertheless, exercise in many forms can produce changes in a range of hormonal systems. The variables which determine the response include fitness of the individual, aptitude for the exercise, type of exercise, duration, percentage of maximal aerobic capacity, and workload. The hormonal influences on physical activity are complex, and measurement of responses can be influenced by a large number of variables (Table 32-1). This chapter will review current knowledge about the effects of exercise and training on the endocrine system and will examine the role of endogenous and exogenous hormones in modifying an athlete's ability to perform.

TABLE 32-1 Hormonal Responses to Exercise and Training: Modifying Factors

1. Characteristics of the exercise activity
   a. Intensity of the exercise
   b. Duration of the activity
   c. Type of exercise, e.g., running, cycling, swimming
      (1) Hemoconcentration
      (2) Muscle groups involved
      (3) Posture during exercise
   d. Special effects, e.g., immersion
2. Fitness of the individual
   a. Cardiopulmonary fitness
   b. Strength and flexibility
   c. Familiarity of the subject with specific activity
   d. Training over previous 24 h
3. Baseline endocrine function
   a. Age-related differences
   b. Sex-related differences
   c. Effects of biological rhythms: circadian, menstrual, lifetime, maturational, circhoral
   d. Stress: physical and psychological
   e. Metabolic: glucose, salt, and fluid loads
   f. Endocrine disorders
4. Methods of sampling the hormones
   a. Blood vs. urine
   b. Indwelling cannula versus repeated stabs
   c. Length of presampling baseline
   d. Sampling frequency
   e. Fluids maintaining IV patency
5. Biochemistry of the hormones
   a. Blood production rates, direct and indirect
   b. Protein binding, specific and nonspecific
   c. Clearance rates and systems: target tissues/metabolism and excretion in liver and/or kidney
6. Ambient conditions
   a. Temperature, humidity, altitude, P_{O_2}
   b. Laboratory vs. free range
   c. Competitive vs. noncompetitive

EFFECTS OF PHYSICAL ACTIVITY AND TRAINING ON ENDOCRINE FUNCTION

Growth Hormone in Exercise

The Effect of Exercise and Training

The release of growth hormone (GH) is controlled by the interplay of GH releasing factor[1] and somatostatin,[2] which inhibits the effect of GH releasing factor. Many other hormones and substances influence GH release (Table 32-2) and also can modulate the effect of physical activity on GH levels. Basal release of GH is ultradian and pulsatile, with low levels of GH occurring as a result of an increased influence of somatostatin.[3,4] Training tends to reduce basal GH levels,[5,6] although the added stress of training at altitude produces no further change in trained runners.[7] The influence of training on physiologic rhythms has not been studied, but it may influence responses to pharmacologic stimulation and exercise at the same relative workload.[5,8–10] Increasing age, but not gender differences, influences the GH response to exercise.[10,11]

The observation that GH increases during strenuous exercise in most individuals was among the earliest identified endocrine responses to exercise.[12,13] This effect has been used clinically to examine GH release, particularly in children.[9,14–17] GH response to strenuous exercise is low in GH-deficient children, but even well-controlled strenuous exercise fails to release GH in one-third of children who have a response to other stimuli. The test is simple but relatively imprecise. Estrogen replacement therapy in postmenopausal women increases the GH response to exercise, but priming children with sex steroids fails to increase sensitivity.[18,19] A range of physical activities increase GH levels.[9,20–30] Release is not consistent until at least 30 to 40 percent of maximal oxygen consumption, although prolonged exercise even at 10 percent of maximal oxygen consumption may release GH.[31] Serum GH levels increase progressively with an increasing load until the maximal load is reached, at which time the response may decrease.[9,22,23,25,28,29,32] Responses to the same absolute exercise load and perhaps the same relative load are reduced by training.[9,22] This was not confirmed in a prospective study, and other studies have reported an enhanced response in trained individuals.[23,33]

TABLE 32-2 A Partial List of Factors Which Influence Growth Hormone Secretion

Increase GH Levels	Decrease GH Levels
Stress	
Stage III and IV sleep	REM sleep
α-Adrenergic agonists	α-Adrenergic antagonists
β-Adrenergic antagonists	β-Adrenergic agonists
Hypoglycemia	Hyperglycemia
Low free fatty acids	High free fatty acids
Some forms of diabetes mellitus	Obesity
Glucagon	High glucocorticoid levels
Androgens	Hypothyroidism
Estrogens	IGF-I
Opiates	Substance P
Vasoactive intestinal peptide	Neurotensin
Bombesin	
Motilin	

The Effect of Metabolic and Pharmacologic Manipulations

The control of GH release during exercise has been further examined by means of metabolic and pharmacologic manipulations. The GH response is augmented in accordance with submaximal oxygen debt and hypoxia.[34–38] Although the GH response is proportional to exercise intensity relative to an individual maximum,[9,39,40] lactic acid does not directly mediate the increase in GH levels during exercise in normoxia[40–42] or hypoxia.[36]

Moderately decreased blood glucose induced by fasting[43] or a chronic fat-rich diet[44] enhances the GH increment during exercise, although lowered blood glucose does not appear to be a physiologic stimulus during exercise. Hypoinsulinemia associated with fasting or lowered blood glucose may be a further stimulus to exaggerated GH secretion with exercise in normal humans,[43] as suggested by responses in poorly controlled diabetics.[45] Hyperglycemia induced in normal subjects preceding exercise decreases the normal GH increment during intense exercise[46] and eliminates the normal GH response to mild exercise.[47] This blunted GH response to exercise may be due to hyperinsulinemia, as diabetic subjects do not show the same reduction in GH response.[46–48] Obese women with higher insulin levels also have a substantially reduced GH response to exercise.[49] Free fatty acids (FFA) elevated above 3 mEq/liter induced by an infusion of soybean oil emulsion and heparin can completely block the GH increase seen during exercise.[50] The effects of nonphysiologic levels of FFA, glucose, and possibly insulin are probably mediated at the hypothalamic level.[51,52]

Neuroendocrine Control of GH Release with Exercise

There is considerable and conflicting evidence regarding the neuroendocrine pathways that regulate GH secretion during exercise. Mechanisms involving cholinergic, serotoninergic, α-adrenergic, dopaminergic, and opioidergic pathways have been proposed.[53–57] There may be interactions among the pathways, and they may operate at different exercise intensities.

Relatively light exercise and insulin-induced hypoglycemia increased GH levels in one study, but not through GH releasing hormone; it was postulated that the mechanism involves the inhibition of somatostatin.[58] Exercise also elevated GH even when levels were increased during the infusion of GH releasing hormone, again suggesting that exercise influences GH levels through the inhibition of somatostatin.[57]

Atropine reduced the normal GH response to cycle ergometer work at moderate intensity, suggesting involvement of cholinergic pathways, but failed to affect GH increments during high-intensity work.[53] Specific muscarinic receptor blockade also inhibits the exercise-induced GH response.[59] The γ-aminobutyric acid (GABA) receptor agonist sodium valproate also inhibits exercise-associated GH responses.[60,61]

Pharmacologic agents that affect central serotoninergic pathways have been shown to modify GH secretion in many circumstances.[62,63] Cyproheptadine blunts GH responses by approximately 50 percent during exercise at a moderate work rate (600 kpm/min), but its effects at higher intensities have not been tested.[54] This suppression of the normal GH increment could be due to the anticholinergic properties of cyproheptadine,[53] but this is unlikely since cyproheptadine reduces the increment induced by the serotonin precursor 5-hydroxytryptophan and suppresses GH in a manner similar to that of other serotonin antagonists, such as methysergide and melatonin, during insulin-induced hypoglycemia (IIH).[54,64] GH levels are increased by α-adrenergic[65,66] and decreased by β-adrenergic[67] stimulation. Dopaminergic agents, L-dopa,[68] apomorphine,[69] and bromocriptine[70] can also increase GH levels. As the dopamine-induced GH response can be inhibited by phentolamine,[71] this action may be mediated through an α-adrenergic receptor or a neuronal intermediary with α-adrenergic activity. The involvement of dopaminergic and adrenergic mechanisms in exercise-induced GH increments is shown by the potentiation of GH responses to exercise with L-dopa,[72] bromocriptine,[73] pyridoxine hydrochloride,[74] and propranolol,[75,76] and suppression of exercise-induced GH increases after pimozide and clonidine.[53,77] In contrast, α_2-adrenergic blockade by idazoxan augments the GH response to exercise.[78]

The release of GH and prolactin (PRL) after the

administration of a met-enkephalin analogue can be blocked by naloxone,[79] suggesting that opioid peptides modulate the secretion of these hormones. Naloxone is ineffective in reducing GH responses to moderate exercise,[80–82] but high doses of naloxone and naltrexone obliterate GH and PRL increases even with high-intensity exercise.[57,83] Opiate receptors may therefore mediate GH and PRL increments during intense exercise, inducing peripheral elevations in peripheral levels of β-endorphin.[84–86]

The mechanisms of GH release at different exercise rates are unclear, as is the relation of these mechanisms to the mechanisms that cause GH secretion in other circumstances. A model for GH control in exercise can be postulated as follows: During moderate exercise, increases in GH levels can be modified by drugs affecting dopaminergic, α-adrenergic, β-adrenergic, cholinergic, and serotoninergic pathways.[53,71–74] Stress-induced GH release due to IIH is mediated by a serotoninergic pathway.[64] This increment is accompanied by a synchronous cortisol elevation[87] which could also be mediated by serotoninergic neurons. Although GH increases with exercise up to the anaerobic threshold may occur in the absence of a cortisol increment,[53,88] these increases are still inhibited by serotonin antagonism.

Simultaneous increases in GH, PRL, and cortisol during intense exercise[89] may be due to the concomitant increase of ACTH and β-endorphin,[85,86] since naloxone suppresses exercise-induced GH and PRL increases.[57] Pyridoxine, a coenzyme involved in the conversion of L-dopa to dopamine, enhances the GH increase that occurs with intense exercise.[74] The dopaminergic influence on GH release in this situation may involve a final serotoninergic mechanism, since cyproheptadine reduces the GH response to L-dopa without altering PRL suppression and since serotonin depletion follows the administration of dopamine or L-dopa.[90–92]

The GH increase at high work rates represents a stress similar to IIH as synchronous GH and cortisol increases occur.[87] Both conditions may be similarly mediated by serotonin neurons since serotonin antagonists reduce GH responses to both in exercise and IIH. However, the basic peripheral stimulus is different. Hypoglycemia stimulates GH by means of a direct action at the hypothalamus,[52] whereas the exercise stimulus remains to be elucidated but seems to interact to some degree only with the altered blood glucose mechanism. Opioid peptides do not mediate GH release due to IIH but seem to play a role in the exercise-induced GH rise.[93]

Effects of Increased GH with Exercise

The role for increased GH during exercise has been suggested to be that of mobilizing FFA for fuel.[94] This seems exaggerated, since the FFA response to infused or injected GH is slower than lipolysis during short-term exercise[95,96] and since FFA and glucose levels are not reduced when GH increments are pharmacologically blocked.[53] Norepinephrine is probably more important in this role.[97] The specific functions of GH increments with exercise remain unknown but probably represent a generalized stress response. The anabolic properties of GH may also be important during the recovery phase that follows stress.

ACTH-CORTISOL AXIS

Exercise and the ACTH-Cortisol Axis

The ACTH-cortisol response to acute physical activity depends on the relative intensity of the workload. Levels of cortisol may increase in anticipation of exercise.[22,98] During low-intensity exercise (less than 50 percent of maximal oxygen consumption), cortisol levels usually decrease, probably as a result of increased removal from the circulation.[25,99–103] With prolonged or more intense exercise, circulating cortisol levels increase in proportion to the workload in laboratory settings[25,28,29,104–108] and in free exercise studies.[26,109–116] This increase occurs despite a decrease in the half-life of cortisol and increased tissue uptake.[102,117] Although tissue uptake is generally assumed in vivo,[118] this has not been shown to occur in muscle tissue in vitro.[119] The cortisol increase is ACTH-mediated.[84–86,120–123] The critical value which results in an increase in circulating cortisol levels is 60 to 70 percent of maximal oxygen consumption, and the response increases with greater exercise intensity.[31,124] In contrast, exercise for 30 min at 80 percent of maximal heart rate produces no change in either cortisol or ACTH,[125] emphasizing the need for optimal respiratory measures of exercise load. Hypoxia increases the cortisol response to any workload.[35,101,123] Although the cortisol response parallels lactic acid production,[108] glucose loading and glycogen store depletion have no effect.[43,46,126] Single leg working produces a greater increase than exercise with two legs, probably because of a greater metabolic response from harder-working muscles.[127] Cortisol levels may decline with exhaustive exercise. The increase to exhaustion is not linear, perhaps because of negative feedback of high cortisol levels, depletion or near depletion of the adrenals, or a defense mechanism to avoid total cortisol depletion.[99,128]

The Effect of Physical Training

The response of basal cortisol levels to training seems to depend on the training load. Some but not all reports suggest that highly trained male athletes have high basal cortisol and ACTH levels, perhaps as a result of increased rates of production.[129–132] A sudden increase in the intensity of training produces a further increase in cortisol levels over several days.[133] "Overtraining" may result in chronically elevated cortisol levels and an impaired response to ACTH.[134] Cortisol levels are elevated in eumenorrheic athletes,[135,136] an elevation which persists during the off season.[137] Training programs have been reported to decrease basal ACTH levels, while arguably more accurate but cross-sectional 24-h frequent sampling pulse studies have shown no difference between athletes and nonathletes.[138,139]

Serum ACTH and cortisol levels appear to be elevated in women with exercise-associated amenorrhea and psychogenic hypothalamic amenorrhea.[135,138,140–142] Serum cortisol levels are also elevated in women with psychogenic amenorrhea and anorexia nervosa, but the reported mechanisms appear to be different.[143,144] Cortisol production rates are increased in runners, while in patients with hypothalamic amenorrhea and anorexia hypercortisolism is due to decreased clearance and increased binding. A somewhat unexpected finding is that while ACTH is elevated in amenorrheic athletes, corticotropin releasing hormone (CRH) is not similarly increased.[145] This raises several questions, particularly about the specificity and sensitivity of the assay, the origins of CRH in circulation, and the possibility that the effect of CRH on ACTH release is modulated by another factor at the pituitary level. ACTH and cortisol responses to CRF are blunted in both male and female athletes.[130,131,135] The relative cortisol response (increase from the baseline of cortisol versus increase from the baseline of ACTH) is enhanced in runners, yet the cortisol response to ACTH does not appear to be enhanced.[135]

Cortisol and ACTH responses to the same absolute workload fall with training.[146–149] However, in response to the same relative intensity, well-controlled studies have shown clear potentiation of the cortisol response[25,33] or no change.[22,23] The response to marathon running appears to be proportional to individual fitness,[26,109,111] while other field and laboratory studies have shown no cortisol response to intense exercise in endurance-trained athletes.[21,147,150] ACTH response to short-term supramaximal exercise may be enhanced by training.[121] Many of these investigations have used endurance training as the investigative regime. The response to a maximal treadmill test may differ depending on the training regime which was used; sprint interval training but not endurance training was shown to induce an increased cortisol response to a maximal load.[151] There was no increase in basal cortisol levels over the course of this study.

Influence of Circadian and Other Rhythms

Circadian variation influences the cortisol response to exercise and is substantially lower when cortisol levels are basal.[152,153] Such changes have to be considered in the design of studies to examine the response to cortisol in exercise. Exercise immediately before eating induces increments of cortisol and enhances the response, while exercise during the subsequent decline of cortisol results in a lower response.[152] Psychological stress may also influence the response to a particular exercise load since in one study cortisol levels in rowers were higher on competition days than they were on practice days, when the workload was similar but the psychological stress was different.[98,103]

Physiologic Significance

The physiologic significance of the cortisol response to activity is unclear; possible explanations include defense of fluid volume and blood pressure, catabolic effect of labile protein stores to generate amino acids and energy for the healing of damaged tissues *after* exercise, and psychogenic effects. Exercise in experimental animals has produced an increase in adrenal size which may provide a better response to life-threatening stress.[154,155] More immediate physiologic requirements could be metabolic, but this remains unclear.[156] Glucocorticoid deficiency and short-term administration may, respectively, inhibit and enhance physical activity in animals.[101,157,158] Although athletes may have high-normal or supraphysiologic basal cortisol levels, they are not cushingoid in appearance. The significance of high glucocorticoid levels in loss of muscle in overtrained athletes is unknown. Regular physical activity protects against the muscle atrophy usually induced by glucocorticoids in rats, but changes in the testosterone/cortisol ratio are regarded as significant in muscle loss in overtrained athletes.[159,160] It is important to recognize the influence of activity on cortisol levels when one is evaluating the results of a hormonal investigation. There has been a paucity of studies of the effects of different occupations on hormonal variables; such studies might be revealing.

PROLACTIN AND EXERCISE

Prolactin has received much attention in regard to exercise since increased levels of PRL are associated with menstrual dysfunction in women and impaired spermatogenesis and decreased libido in men. No teleologically satisfactory explanation for the exercise-associated changes in PRL has been suggested. The transient effects of exercise are comparable to other physiologic stimuli on PRL except in extreme situations.[115] Levels increase with exercise in sedentary controls[24,28,43,81,83,93,107,139,161–163] and in recreational and competitive runners.[30,57,114,122,138,164–166] Levels rapidly normalize even after very strenuous activity.[167] The effects of training appear minimal, since equivalent exercise loads produce generally similar serum PRL increases in trained and untrained individuals.[130,168–170] Some researchers have suggested that the PRL response occurs only in trained individuals[33,171] and differs according to the degree of training.[172] Serum PRL may not increase after a typical daily training session[173] or even during intensive exercise in amenorrheic runners.[30,106] This is not solely because of the hypoestrinism, since PRL levels increase in agonadal women in response to exercise.[30] Dopamine agonists are capable of suppressing the prolactin-induced increase associated with exercise;[174] the lack of response in amenorrheic athletes suggests that an increased tonic dopaminergic tone may be present. This could contribute to exercise-associated dysfunction. Levels are elevated after participation in competitive team sports and normalize within 3 to 4 h after the competition.[175,176]

Effects of Training on Prolactin

Basal PRL levels have been described as being reduced in trained male runners and in women runners with an increased training load[129,177,178] but not in swimmers, in whom PRL levels increase with heavier training.[179] It is unclear whether the increase persists when training loads are kept constant for a long period. Relatively light training in previously sedentary individuals and weight training are not sufficient to suppress PRL levels.[7,180] Nocturnal secretion is augmented on days when endurance training takes place.[181] The response to stimulation with metoclopramide is reduced,[170] and domperidone increases the prolactin response to exercise.[182] Clonidine, an α_2 adrenergic agonist, has no effect on exercise-associated changes in prolactin.[77]

Mechanisms

The mechanisms of PRL increase with exercise are unclear. Prolactin levels may increase when the anaerobic threshold is reached, perhaps synchronously with a GH increase.[183] Even prolonged (90-min) exercise below this threshold fails to elicit any response.[184] Other researchers have suggested that the PRL increase may be related to changes in body temperature and dehydration but not to acute changes in fluid balance,[185–189] is reduced by facial cooling,[186,190] is exaggerated by stress, is reduced with habituation[42,191] and hypoxia,[168,192,193] and is unresponsive to metabolic events.

Prolactin increments with exercise appear to be correlated with pro-opiomelanocortin derivatives, ACTH, and beta-endorphins.[194] The increase may be suppressed by naloxone infusion, suggesting that endogenous opiates are involved in the release.[195] Unfortunately, several studies found no effect of a bolus or infusion of naloxone.[83,196,197] One study found an enhanced PRL response.[198] The response to thyrotropin releasing hormone (TRH) may be decreased in trained female subjects[170] and augmented in male subjects.[199] Serotonin may also be a controlling factor.[200] The control of and effects of exercise-associated PRL responses remain enigmatic. Changes clearly do occur, but the inadequacy of many of the studies suggests that a more carefully controlled investigation might provide more definitive answers. The effects of physical activity and other physiologic stimuli on PRL raise concerns that mildly elevated values obtained in clinical circumstances should be reviewed to exclude physiologic elevations.

TSH-THYROID AXIS

The role of thyroxine (T_4), triiodothyronine (T_3), and reverse triodothyronine (rT_3) in modulating the rate of metabolic processes suggests that the thyroid axis may be responsive to physical work. The axis is, however, buffered against sudden change, and responses to acute exercise seem unlikely to be of significance.

Acute Responses

Most studies have found no change in thyroid stimulating hormone (TSH) levels with acute exercise.[28,111,201–205] Some authors have reported a slight fall.[199,206] Increased TSH levels were reported with acute exercise in untrained subjects[202] and after prolonged and strenuous exercise,[207–209] but the increment is minute compared with the response to TRH stimulation. Acute exercise-induced changes varied with exercise load in one study, although all three loads used could be considered fairly light.[163]

Levels of total T_4, total T_3, and their free moieties generally increase slightly with acute exercise, but the increase is usually small.[201,203,206,209–211] Since less than 0.05 percent of circulating T_4 is unbound, it is not surprising that changes in total hormone do not exceed the exercise-induced hemoconcentration. Individual studies have observed a decrease in T_4[212] or T_3.[213] The latter may result from alterations in peripheral conversion to favor the production of rT_3.[209] The different individual responses with acute exercise have been related to fitness and workload by means of measurement of the "double product" (heart rate in beats per minute multiplied by systolic blood pressure in mmHg); fitter individuals have an increase, while the less fit have a decrease.[213] Other researchers have suggested a biphasic response based on the fitness of athletes running marathons and ultramarathons.[214]

Effect of Training

Alterations in thyroid function may occur with repeated exercise.[215] Thyroxine degradation has been estimated to be 75 percent higher in athletes than in nonathletes and approaches levels found in hyperthyroidism. In one study, inactivity for a relatively short time rapidly reduced the rate of degradation, while only 6 days of exercise in a normally sedentary population was sufficient to increase T_4 turnover. T_3 degradation was also found to be enhanced.[216] The findings initially reported during an endurance training study are compatible with this observation. When training load was increased by 30 mi a week, decreased levels of T_3 and rT_3 were observed with an enhanced TSH response to a TRH bolus.[217] The authors suggested that the changes supported a diagnosis of mild hypothyroidism developing in women runners at high mileage. The effect was no longer seen when the training load was increased by 50 mi per week.[218] Similar changes have been described in endurance and resistance training in men and endurance training in women.[219–221] In the latter case the slight change was ascribed to lowered thyroxin-binding globulin (TBG) levels. Short-term training in women has been reported to have no effect.[222] It is unclear how increased turnover might happen since radioiodine uptake has been reported as being lower with training despite an increase in 24-h urinary iodine.[223]

There is a small increase in the resting metabolic rate in endurance-trained athletes when this rate is determined per kilogram of fat-free weight.[224] Basal thyroid hormones were not related to fitness (as assessed by maximal oxygen consumption) or percentage of body fat.

There is little information about physical activity in athletes with hypothyroidism treated with hormone replacement. A case report suggests that TSH and PRL responses to TRH may be increased by training even in non-endurance-trained hypothyroid athletes despite apparently normal thyroid function.[225] Careful monitoring may be advisable in hypothyroid athletes, although the changes are unlikely to be sufficient to produce clinical symptoms.[156]

ENDOGENOUS OPIATES IN EXERCISE AND TRAINING

The wide range of possible effects of endogenous opiates (EO) has encouraged research into their role in exercise performance, their psychological and behavioral effects (including mood, appetite changes, exercise addiction, and pain perception), and their role in a variety of hormonal changes, including exercise-associated reproductive dysfunction.

Response to Acute Physical Activity

Older studies often measured circulating β-endorphin (β-END), using an antibody with cross-reactivity with β-LPH; the problem can be avoided by chromatographic separation of β-LPH and β-END and, more recently, by specific assays which do not cross-react with β-LPH. Unfortunately, many exercise studies do not use chromatography and measure a combined β-END/β-LPH rather than β-END. Sometimes it is unclear exactly what has been measured.

In most physiologic situations, β-END and ACTH are released concurrently from the pituitary and have a common precursor, pro-opiomelanocortin (POMC).[226] There are synchronous increases in β-END and ACTH in response to a treadmill run to exhaustion at 15 km/h in male athletes; this finding suggested that physical exercise stimulates POMC synthesis in a manner similar to that of other stressors.[85,227–230] Maximal treadmill and resistance exercise produced an increase in cortisol, while EO increased only with treadmill running.[231] This suggested that the control mechanisms may not be identical. However, like cortisol, the response of β-END to exercise shows a circadian variation.[232]

Strenuous physical activity is consistently accompanied by an increase in EO, but lesser activity produces an inconsistent response. β-END/β-LPH increase was observed after a strenuous run described as near maximum, but changes with low-intensity running exercise were inconsistent.[233–235] Increases over baseline were lower at the end of a 100-mi supermarathon than at 60 mi, suggesting that, like glucocorticoids, EO tend to be depleted with extremely strenuous exercise.[128,234] Several investigations have suggested that the trigger for β-END release is anaerobiosis.[228,236–238] Below the anaerobic threshold, responses are individual and varied.[239,240] Duration and intensity may both play significant roles.[194,241–244] The return to baseline values after exercise is quite rapid.[166]

The increased physical stress of a hot ambient temperature and dehydration progressively enhance the exercise-associated opiate response.[245] Running at cool temperatures has a varied effect depending on the subject; responses are unchanged in men, partially suppressed in eumenorrheic women, and absent in amenorrheic women. An early suggestion that opiates are involved in the control of core temperature has been disputed.[246–248]

Effects of Training

An early report suggested that the plasma β-END/β-LPH response to acute exercise increases in women with training.[84] If exercise were addictive, an increasing response to exercise might stimulate exercisers into progressively increasing their activity. The conclusion was criticized because the relative load was kept constant, but power output increased with increasing fitness.[249] Since several investigations have suggested that the opiate response varies with workload, the increased opiate response to exercise may not be due to an increase in the endogenous capacity to secrete β-endorphin. An attempt to reproduce the findings was not successful, but in contrast, the exercise-induced increase in plasma met-enkephalin levels decreased with training in women.[250] Met-enkephalin levels were reported to be unchanged with maximal exertion in men,[198] a finding which suggests that there may be a sex difference in the met-enkephalin response. A sex difference in β-END/β-LPH responses to exercise was also reported,[86] but this has not been confirmed. No change was observed in plasma leu-enkephalin levels in men after a 10-mi road race.[251] Several investigations have provided varied views of the effects of fitness, training, and gender on basal and exercise-induced opiate responses.[116,125,151,252–256] Other determining variables have included afferent muscle signals but not psychological status.[257,258]

Physiologic Significance of the Exercise-Associated Opiate Increase

The function of peripheral opiates and their relation to changes of EO within the central nervous system (CNS) and the neuroendocrine regulatory system are in need of investigation. The presence of β-endorphin in cerebrospinal fluid (CSF) at concentrations different from those in the peripheral blood, differential effects of exercise, and the poor penetration of β-END through the blood-brain barrier imply separately regulated CNS manufacture.[258–261] Most studies of the functional importance of EO in exercise have employed the opiate antagonist naloxone. Evidence suggests that opiates may be involved in the regulation of immunity and in insulin regulation, although hyperglycemia has little effect on opiate response to exercise.[262–264]

The Influence of Endogenous Opiates on Exercise Performance

Several investigations of the effect of opioids on cardiopulmonary function in exercise in physiologic and pathologic states have been carried out with entirely negative or physiologically insignificant results.[82,198,265–278] The time to exhaustion in both graded, maximal-intensity exercise and prolonged submaximal exercise depends on a number of physiologic factors, e.g., cardiopulmonary fitness and muscle glycogen stores, as well as determination and pain perception. Opiate receptor blockade does not have a significant effect on the time of exhaustion or other variables of performance.[198,265,269,270,277,278]

Endogenous Opiates, Analgesia, and Exercise

Exercise-associated analgesia[279–281] has been described and is generally regarded as similar to other forms of stress-induced analgesia.[122] Reduced perception of pain associated with ischemic heart disease,[268,282,283] dysmenorrhea,[284] and muscular pain[285] are examples of exercise-associated analgesic effects with clinical significance. "Negative addiction" was described in runners who continued to exercise against medical advice after being injured.[286] Tolerance of pain may be as great a factor in these circumstances as is a psychological dependency on running. The increasing frequency of running-associated injuries may also reflect analgesic effects as runners try to push themselves beyond their physiologic capacity.

Endogenous Opiates, Food Intake, and Exercise

Several lines of research have supported the idea that exercise and training may influence appetite and caloric intake.[287–294] Suppression of 24-h caloric intake in rats may be associated more with high-intensity, short-duration exercise than with low-intensity endurance exercise and may be more common in male than in female rats.[290,295–297] Accurate human studies are much more difficult because measurements of caloric intake and energy expenditure are relatively imprecise. In one study, caloric intake corresponded with physical activity only within the normal activity range, and sedentary individuals did not decrease intake to suit their relatively low energy expenditure.[298] When studies have examined caloric intake in response to an exercise program, the energy intake has in some cases decreased, or, where an increase was found, the change did not correspond to the energy requirements of the increased physical activity.[299–301] Acute exercise may also influence appetite in humans.[302]

Opiate peptides, particularly dynorphin, have been implicated in the regulation of the feeding behavior of animals.[303] Acute administration of opiate agonists induces food and water intake in satiated and nonhungry animals,[304–306] while antagonists inhibit food intake in severely food deprived animals.[307–312] The opiate effect on feeding may be mediated in part by dopaminergic neurons since dopamine blockade inhibits dynorphin-induced feeding and naloxone inhibits dopamine agonist–induced feeding.[303,313]

Rats exposed to a 50-min bout of swimming exercise demonstrate a biphasic response.[314] In this study, an initial hyperphagia lasting 2 h was followed by a time of decreased appetite. The initial hyperphagia was accompanied by elevated peripheral opiate levels and was reduced by high doses of naltrexone. The secondary hypophagia was not accompanied by elevated plasma β-END levels, and there was a tendency for high-dose naltrexone to reduce further food intake during the 2 to 8 h after swimming. During this time, the 2-deoxyglucose-induced increase in appetite was attenuated by exercise. After treadmill running, rats were reported to have decreased appetite without an initial hyperphagia.[297] The discrepancy may reflect differences in the effects of swimming and running on core temperature elevation, which in itself can modulate appetite.[315] A naloxone-reversible increase in water intake was observed in rats for 4 h after exercise but not in the basal state.[311,312] EO may therefore be involved in mediating the rapid replacement of fluid loss but not in basal regulation.

Training (forced swimming for 60 min per day, 5 days per week, for 12 weeks) significantly reduced overnight (12 h) food intake at 4 weeks but not at 10 weeks.[316] The 2-deoxyglucose (2-DG)-induced increase in food intake was attenuated at 4 to 5 weeks but not at 10 weeks. The authors considered that the findings at 4 to 5 weeks of training represented an opiate deficiency. This is inconsistent with the findings at 10 to 11 weeks, when food intake and response to 2-DG were similar in trained and untrained rats and nocturnal β-END/β-LPH levels were substantially higher in trained rats. However, as reported elsewhere, training does not necessarily produce similar changes in central and peripheral opioid levels.[317]

A major weakness of these studies is that it is difficult to differentiate between the metabolic stress of physical activity and stress from forced exercise. Further studies with animals trained to exercise spontaneously would be useful. It is unclear how the animal findings can be applied to the human situation, where research is also lacking.

Opiates, Exercise, and Appetite Suppression in Humans

Excessive physical activity, often described as purposeless, is a common feature of anorexia nervosa.[318] Running is a socially acceptable way of expressing a drive to burn calories, so that at least some patients who present with exercise-associated amenorrhea may in fact have anorexia nervosa. Several authors consider the recent simultaneous increases in the prevalence of anorexia nervosa, "cosmetic emaciation," and habitual exercise to be more than coincidental. Anorectic tendencies have been described anecdotally in athletes.[319–321] One-third of 182 women athletes practiced "pathogenic weight control behavior."[322] Similarities in personalities and behaviors have been described in habitual male athletes and teenage patients with anorexia nervosa.[323,324] The substantial similarities originally described have not been validated, but subtle changes in body image and eating attitudes do occur.[325,326] A particularly important observation was that animals that were allowed free access to a treadmill but were kept on a food schedule tended to increase their activity, self-starve, and die.[327,328] The parallels with strict dieting and intense exercise in humans are obvious.

CSF total opioid activity is elevated in patients with anorexia nervosa, although β-END levels may be normal.[329] Naloxone administration stimulates weight gain in patients with anorexia nervosa, suggesting that EO may have an appetite-inhibitory effect in anorectic patients, in contrast to the findings in animal studies.[330] The chronic elevation of peripheral β-END found in many women exercisers[179] may be related to the pathologic eating behavior common in women athletes. This important area should be studied further, perhaps with a more critical diagnostic appraisal.

Exercise and Mood

Psychologic advantages associated with running and other forms of exercise include reduced anxiety, better stress management, reduction of depression, improved self-esteem, an improved feeling of well-being, and a heightened sense of personal control.[331–336] Acute exercise, particularly running, is associated with a transient elevation in mood,[337–339] so that the "runners' high" has become an accepted part of the folklore of running and is popularly associated with altered EO levels induced by running. The evidence is almost entirely anecdotal, e.g., the account of Mandell,[340] with little objective psychometric data.

In human research, at least four variables have to be considered in the investigation of mood changes with acute exercise: the fitness of the subjects, the exercise activity, the dose of antagonist, and the means of measuring affect. The methodology of the studies has varied and therefore there is some discrepancy among the results. Most investigators have discounted EO involvement in exercise-associated mood changes.[280,281,341–344] Studies do support the concept that exercise has an acute effect on mood, but the changes do not measure up to the powerful images created by Mandell.

Exercise Addiction and Opiates

The "positive addiction" of running has gained credibility despite a lack of systematic evidence.[340,345,346] For running or another activity to be considered addictive, three criteria must be established: pleasurable reward of the activity, tolerance requiring increasing activity to maintain the reward, and withdrawal symptoms if the activity is stopped.[347] Runners who voluntarily discontinued their activity experienced changes in sleep patterns, increased sexual tension, and other effects.[348] Runners forced to rest because of injury also report feelings of restlessness and increased tension. Animal experimentation has also provided evidence suggesting that endorphins may be involved in exercise addiction. Withdrawal symptoms similar to those from withdrawal of morphine were observed when swimming exercise was discontinued in rats, suggesting an opiate-mediated physical dependency.[349] Naloxone reduced voluntary running in hamsters, implying that exercise produced an opiate-mediated reward which could lead to addiction.[350] Fatiguing exercising changed β-END levels in the nucleus accumbens septi, which functions as an interface between locomotor activity and motivated behaviors.[351] The lack of change in β-END levels in other areas of the brain adds emphasis to the possibility that exercise addiction is mediated through endogenous opiates.

Reproductive Dysfunction and Endogenous Opiates

The role of endogenous opiates in exercise-associated reproductive dysfunction has been intensively investigated. This will be dealt with in the sections on the reproductive effects of exercise.

Endogenous Opiates in Acute Exercise-Induced Hormonal Change

The involvement of EO in controlling peripheral hormone levels led to investigations of their importance in exercise-induced hormonal changes, generally looking at acute change and using naloxone as the investigative probe. Unfortunately, the results have been inconsistent. Differences in subjects, fitness, exercise load, and dosage of naloxone make comparison among the studies very difficult. Growth hormone and PRL responses to exercise have been reported to be reduced[57,80] or unchanged[81,198] by naloxone in doses varying from 0.4 to 15 mg. Plasma catecholamines, norepinephrine, and epinephrine have been reported to be enhanced by high-dose naloxone (12.2 mg)[198] and unchanged with a 10-fold lower dose.[197] Similarly, exercise-induced increases in plasma renin activity and aldosterone were increased with high-dose naloxone and were not changed with lower doses of this opiate antagonist. These various findings suggest that EO are involved in the hormonal response to stressful exercise but that their physiologic importance remains to be clarified.

Summary

Physical exercise involves a complex interrelation of cardiac, pulmonary, vascular, metabolic, hormonal, psychological, neurologic, and biochemical functions. It is perhaps the most physiologic stimulus that can be used to "stress" the organism. The involvement of endorphins and other opiates in many of these areas has justifiably stimulated research interest. Such work has clearly shown that endorphins are involved in exercise-associated analgesia and are clearly not involved to a significant degree in determining exercise performance. Involvement in mood alteration and at least some hormonal changes seem likely, but further work is required to demonstrate EO involvement in reproductive dysfunction and exercise addiction. We can only guess at the importance of EO in other areas, such as metabolism and even bowel function, where "runners' trots" are an interesting but poorly explained phenomenon.

It is important that approaches to the problems be multidisciplinary and that subjects' fitness and training, the exercise methodology, and the method of administering antagonists used in acute studies be given careful consideration in designing studies. The emotional responses to impending exercise may vary depending on the familiarity of the subject with physical activity.

The psychological and physiologic responses to exercise are different between habitual exercisers and untrained individuals. Investigations should control for fitness and attempt to diminish stress as a component in the response to exercise. This is also important in animal experiments, where investigators take little account of the stress in animals forced to exercise. It is possible to train animals to run spontaneously and to quantitate such activity.[352] However, it is naive to believe that opiates work in isolation without interaction with other hormones and neuromodulators. Before full understanding can be achieved, the role of many other similarly active substances must be clarified.

ENDOCRINE REGULATION OF FLUID BALANCE DURING PHYSICAL WORK

During strenuous or prolonged physical work there is a considerable loss of water and electrolytes in sweat, since evaporation is the main means for dissipating heat generated from the inefficient muscular use of chemical energy. Substantial changes occur in serum electrolytes with increased levels of K^+ and Na^+.[353] Blood flow is diverted to working muscle and away from the kidneys. To minimize the loss through normal endocrine mechanisms, increases in aldosterone and arginine vasopressin (AVP) would be anticipated. The decreased plasma volume, increased serum sodium and potassium levels, and fluid loss during exercise, together with the activation of the ACTH-adrenal axis, could increase aldosterone and AVP levels through their individual mechanisms. One might expect that as part of training for endurance activity fluid balance is more carefully controlled as part of a physiologic adaptation to fitness. This appears to be the case.

Arginine Vasopressin, Exercise, and Training

It was recognized many years ago that exercise inhibits the diuresis induced by water loading.[354–356] Bioassay evidence of the presence of a humoral factor found in the blood was assumed to explain the exercise-associated antidiuresis.[357] Antidiuretic hormone or arginine vasopressin was found to be increased when specific assay systems became available.[111,358,359] Subsequent studies have generally but not universally concluded that AVP increases with physical exertion.[360,361] This increase is progressive with increasing workload and duration.[362–365] The response is not modified by gender[365] or training,[366,367] although as may be anticipated with increased fitness, the response to the same absolute workload is diminished.[368] The return to basal levels after exercise is quite rapid, occurring within 1 h of ending the activity.[362] This occurs despite continuing hemoconcentration.[369] AVP has also been implicated in the increase in plasma volume which occurs with training.[366]

Various factors have been implicated in the increase in AVP with exercise, including high plasma osmolality, extracellular fluid volume contraction, hydration, body temperature, angiotensin II, psychological factors, altered metabolism, and peripheral nerve stimulation.[362,369,370] The change in response to exercise is greater than would be anticipated from a comparable change if hypertonic fluids were given and from a comparable heat stress.[362] The involvement of angiotensin is unclear since converting enzyme inhibition has been reported to diminish or have no effect on the vasopressin response.[83,371] Dehydration and fluid loading both diminish the response.[372–375] Predictability of exercise reduces the response while unpredictability enhances it, suggesting a significant psychological component.[376] The response is not changed by posture, hypoxia, or opiate inhibitors.[83,376,377] A direct afferent arc from the muscle may induce the release of AVP from neurosecretory cells in the supraoptic nucleus.[378]

Aldosterone, Exercise, and Training

A sixfold increase in aldosterone levels was observed after a marathon run.[112] Small increments have been described with lesser degrees of exertion.[198,358,362,363,369,379–382] The onset is rapid, but the levels return to normal more slowly, depending on the initial exercise load. The increment is workload-related and is mediated at least in part by sodium levels. Training at altitude has little effect.[383] Swimming for 60 min has no effect on either AVP or aldosterone.[384] Plasma renin activity increases two- to fivefold as a result of exercise, and the changes appear to be in direct proportion to the workload. Angiotensinogen levels decrease with exercise, presumably as a result of conversion to angiotensin II. The level of angiotensin II increases with exercise and appears to be at least partly responsible for the increased aldosterone levels. The increase in angiotensin II but not aldosterone can be blocked by the β-blocker propranolol.[385] Other factors are involved in the activation of aldosterone production, including the ACTH-adrenal axis.[367] Energy deprivation has no effect, but manipulation of physiologic saline to minimize fluid loss modulates the changes.[386] A psychological component is present since hypnotic suggestion of running activates the axis.[387] Basal levels of active hormones in the axis and responses are reduced for maximal workloads in trained individuals.[378,379,386,387] Prolonged, repeated competitive exercise does not result in continued activation of the axis, and basal values are regained each day within 12 hr of competition during a 20-day race despite continuing fluid loss.[388] Trained athletes also have a greater tolerance to a fluid load without suppressing their hormonal response.[389] These changes might be expected to improve endurance performance.

INSULIN AND GLUCAGON IN EXERCISE

The supply of fuel to exercising and nonexercising tissues during physical activity is one of the crucial factors which determine performance of a task. Glucagon stimulates both glycogenolysis and gluconeogenesis, resulting in elevated glucose levels. Insulin facilitates glucose transport through cell membranes and increases glycogen synthetase activity, promoting glycogen storage. Since the supply of glucose to working muscle is one of the prime limiting factors in physical activity and since even mild exercise increases glucose uptake from the circulation,[390] it can be expected that both insulin and glucagon are responsive to an increased metabolic load and are likely to be changed with physical activity and training.

Insulin and Exercise

During moderate exercise, insulin levels remain unchanged over the first 40 to 60 min of exercise. More prolonged or strenuous exercise induces a decline in insulin levels.[22,23,25,48,391–400] The insulin decline may not be essential to maintain glucose homeostasis.[401] Counterregulatory hormones, catecholamines, glucagon, GH, and cortisol tend to increase, inducing hepatic glycogenolysis, gluconeogenesis, and lipolysis to provide increased FFA for use as a metabolic fuel. During short-term strenuous exercise, when the counterregulatory hormones increase rapidly, glucose levels may transiently increase.[402] After exercise, insulin levels rapidly return to baseline.

Prior carbohydrate intake may increase preexercise insulin levels and prevent insulin decline, maintaining circulating glucose as the substrate used in exercise until supplies decline.[403–406] Other researchers have not confirmed this finding.[46,407] Fasting induces a reduced insulin response.[408–410] Hypoxia has no effect on either insulin or glucagon.[411]

The remarkable increase in glucose uptake by exercising muscles (30-fold) can result from increased insulin action on the muscles through increased receptor content[412] as well as non-insulin-mediated uptake by muscle.[413] It appears that the muscle glucose uptake which is not directly mediated by insulin still requires at least basal insulin levels to occur.[414–416] Increased insulin availability above basal levels has little effect on glucose transport, and the supply of glucose to the muscle is maintained during exercise despite decreased insulin levels, theoretically reducing insulin to the muscle.[417] The decline in insulin with exercise can be prevented by α-adrenergic blockade but not β-blockade.[394,418] Insulin also plays a role in controlling the sensitivity of hepatic glucose production.[419] Insulin and glucose changes are needed for optimal activity to occur.[420]

Glucagon and Exercise

Glucagon levels increase during strenuous exercise, but the response is variable at lesser intensities.[25,38,394,395,397,417,421,422] However, the rise in glucagon is not necessarily linear with duration or intensity of exercise. Decreasing blood glucose levels stimulate glucagon,[395] and the glucagon response is generally blunted by preloading with glucose.[403,406,407,423,424] Fasting and hypoglycemia have been reported to produce a variable effect on glucagon response, depending on the blood glucose level attained.[408–410]

The increase in glucagon can occur without a prior fall in glucose levels.[156] In general, levels of glucagon correspond significantly with epinephrine and norepinephrine levels,[425] although β-blockade with propranolol has little if any inhibitory effect on the glucagon response to moderate exercise.[394,418] Some researchers have suggested that the sympathoadrenal system is more important in maintaining euglycemia and enhanced hepatic production of glucose.[426]

The response of glucagon and other counterregulatory hormones is usually adequate to maintain glucose levels during exercise, although asymptomatic and symptomatic hypoglycemia can occur with prolonged and strenuous exercise in nondiabetic individuals.[427–430] This emphasizes the importance of maintaining glucose intake during prolonged exercise such as marathon running.

Effects of Training

Training induces a reduction in basal insulin levels and in the exercise-associated changes in both glucagon and insulin.[22,23,394,397,421,431–433] The decline in glucose with exercise may decrease or even be reversed.[25,415,434] There are gender differences in the relative importance of sources of nutrient; women use lipids to a greater degree than do men, who use more carbohydrate and protein.[435] Neither gender nor menstrual cycle has an important effect on glucoregulatory hormones during exercise.[10,436]

Training also increases sensitivity to insulin at rest and in response to a glucose load.[437–443] The increase in insulin sensitivity changes by 20 to 30 percent when maximal oxygen consumption is increased by 15 to 20 percent. These changes could be related to increased tissue binding of insulin or decreased secretion or to a change in somatotype to less adipose tissue and increased muscle mass.[412,437,444,445] Insulin decline with activity is also reduced during acute exercise in trained individuals. This can also be observed in older individuals, although there is some impairment of glucose handling even in well-trained older persons.[11,446–451] The long-term significance of enhanced insulin sensitivity has been questioned.[452] It appears to be very rapidly reversed on refraining from exercise even for a few days, although it is not modified by acute exercise.[441,453–458] The benefits may not be seen in obese hypertryglyceridemic men with impaired carbohydrate tolerance.[459]

CATECHOLAMINES IN EXERCISE

During exercise both epinephrine and norepinephrine levels increase in circulation. This is to be expected, since these hormones are involved in inotropic and chronotropic effects on the heart, redistribution of blood flow, and substrate mobilization through the promotion of glycogenolysis and lipolysis. The differential responses of epinephrine and norepinephrine suggest that there is also some difference in function. Norepinephrine is related to hemodynamic changes, while epinephrine is more clearly related to sympathetic activity and blood glucose levels.[460]

Epinephrine and Norepinephrine

The responses of epinephrine and norepinephrine to physical activity are not necessarily the same for a given exercise intensity. Mild exercise produces little or no response in either hormone, but at moderate exercise levels significant norepinephrine release occurs with minimal change in circulating epinephrine.[156,396,461] The increase in norepinephrine is probably a consequence of release from sympathetic postganglionic neurons. At intense or prolonged exercise levels both hormones increase significantly.[156,396,462,463] Graded exercise produces a lower response than continuous prolonged exercise.[425] The responses are directly related to workload and oxygen uptake and are greater with small muscle groups than with large muscle groups.[23,396,464,465] The increase in epinephrine is abrupt in onset at strenuous workloads, while prolonged work to the point of exhaustion induces a progressive increase in epinephrine.[22,25,396] These increases in catecholamines involve both conjugated and free hormone and may be higher in capillary blood than in venous blood.[466–468] The changes persist for 24 h after prolonged exercise.[469]

Control of Catecholamine Release

The factors responsible for hormone release are not clear. In one study, the response during exercise occurred approximately at the time of reaching the anaerobic threshold, suggesting that the production of lactate may influence the initiation of catecholamine response to exercise.[470] Fasting enhances the catecholamine response to activity, but glucose loading seems to have little effect.[407,410,471,472] Hypoxia enhances the response in trained subjects but not in untrained subjects.[473] The exercise load is much more of a determining factor than is the psychological state, negating the concept of "getting the adrenaline pumping" before exercise.[42] Gender does not influence catecholamine response.[10]

Endogenous opiate inhibition was reported to have no influence on catecholamine release, but β blockade with timolol augmented basal and maximal exercise-stimulated epinephrine levels.[267,474] Other researchers disagree, suggesting that opioid inhibition may influence catecholamine response during exercise.[82,198] The basal levels of norepinephrine were increased, while the response to maximal exercise was blunted. While the immediate effect of β-blockade during exercise is contradictory,[475–477] propranolol and other β-blockers may enhance exercise-induced catecholamine increase after exercise.[478]

Effects of Catecholamine Release

The effects of catecholamine release include increased glycogenolysis and increased FFA concentrations.[469] Although similar glucagon and epinephrine changes are observed, catecholamines are unlikely to be entirely responsible for the increase in glucagon, as decreased glucose availability enhances glucagon and epinephrine secretion during prolonged exercise.[415,495] Cardiovascular but not respiratory adaptations to exercise are mediated at least in part by catecholamines.[479,480] Redistribution of circulation to working muscles and to the skin for heat loss and sweating is mediated through changes in catecholamines directly or indirectly via other intermediate hormones. Evidence has also suggested that mental performance may be improved through exercise; this improvement may be mediated through catecholamines.[481]

Effects of Training

Training results in a diminished catecholamine response to the same absolute level of physical activity but paradoxically may actually increase the ability to secrete epinephrine in response to other stimuli.[23,25,421,482–486] The response is probably unchanged at the same relative workload,[23,484] although some researchers have reported a lower response.[25] The lipase response to circulating epinephrine levels may increase with training.[487–489] Platelet assays of catecholamines, considered as a measure of long-term catecholamine concentration in the circulation, respond little to acute exercise, but basal levels are substantially elevated in athletes.[490] Very prolonged exercise leads to substantial elevations of free catecholamines; levels may also be chronically elevated in highly trained athletes.[256,469]

Dopamine Responses to Exercise

The relationship of dopamine to modulation of hypothalamic-pituitary function is well established; the involvement of dopamine in exercise-associated changes in reproductive hormones has been questioned but involves hypothalamic rather than peripheral dopamine involvement.

Dopamine increases during exercise in a manner similar to that of epinephrine and norepinephrine, although the elevation may persist longer after exercise than that of the other catecholamines.[465,467,469,490–492] There is no dopamine response to exercise that involves small muscle groups; this is in contrast to the responses of other catecholamines.[493] Dopamine levels may also be chronically elevated in highly trained athletes.[274] The significance of elevations of dopamine with exercise remain unclear. Elevations in dopamine β-hydroxylase suggest that dopamine may act as a precursor for other catecholamines.[494] In one study, no differences were found in the dopamine responses to physical activity in eumenorrheic, oligomenorrheic, and amenorrheic runners.[495] Some evidence suggests that dopamine elevation may be involved in exercise-induced asthma and in other aspects of respiratory control.[496,497] Clear roles for epinephrine and norepinephrine have been established, while the significance of dopamine in exercise and fitness is much less clear.

EXERCISE, TRAINING, AND THE HYPOTHALAMIC-PITUITARY-GONADAL AXIS

One area which has long been considered an exception to the rule that exercise is good for you involves the reproductive response to training, particularly in young women. The effects of strenuous physical activity on the reproductive system in women have gained widespread recognition: Delayed menarche, oligoamenorrhea, inadequate luteal phase, and anovulatory cycles occur, although probably not with the frequency that was originally suggested. Research on the effects of exercise on the hypothalamic-pituitary-gonadal (HPG) axis in men has been performed for a considerably longer time, but without the publicity given to studies in women. Attention was focused on the effects of physical activity on men when it became apparent that parallels exist between the sexes in terms of the chronic reproductive effects of exercise. This section will review the acute and chronic effects of strenuous physical activity on the HPG axis in men and women and examine mechanisms which may be involved in those changes.

Acute Exercise and the HPG Axis in Men

Serum testosterone levels at any particular time depend on a number of factors (Table 32-3), some of which can be altered by acute exercise or training. It is important to note that luteinizing hormone (LH) pulses or acute LH increments do not produce a testosterone increment in less than 20 to 30 min.[498] An exercise-associated increase in serum testosterone levels occurring with exercise before this time cannot be the result of an LH effect. Testosterone is bound in circulation to a specific high-affinity plasma protein, sex hormone–binding globulin (SHBG), and to albumin, which has a large capacity but low affinity. Substantial changes in albumin can occur without significant effects on the levels of total testosterone. A small amount (less than 2 percent) of testosterone circulates as the free steroid. The binding of testosterone to SHGB reduces its clearance. It seems likely that the biologically active portion of the hormone is bound to albumin and the small unbound fraction,[499,500] which together amount to approximately 35 percent of the total levels. The majority (>95 percent) of testosterone (4 to 10 mg daily) is secreted directly from the testes. In males, approximately half the testosterone produced is cleared through the liver and the remainder is cleared through extrahepatic metabolism.[501] The androgen target organs, including muscle, are responsible for extrahepatic clearance. It is apparent that along with changes in synthesis and secretion, modifications of binding or clearance could play significant roles in changes in circulating testosterone in response to physical activity. As with other hormonal systems, acute exercise-associated responses of the male HPG axis depend on the intensity and duration of the activity and the fitness of the individual.

TABLE 32-3 Factors Determining Exercise-Associated Changes in Serum Testosterone Levels

Synthesis/secretion	Gonadotropin-mediated (LH and FSH)
	Other (prolactin, catecholamines)
Testicular blood flow	
Protein binding	Specific, high affinity (SHBG, CBG)
	Nonspecific, low affinity (albumin)
Clearance	Target tissue uptake and metabolism
	Hepatic metabolism

Short-Term Exercise and the HPG Axis

The first paper on the effects of short-term strenuous physical activity on testicular androgens, which was published in 1973, summarized most of the questions and problems which still remain to be explained.[21] Increases in circulating testosterone levels have been reported during free and treadmill running, weight training, and ergometer cycling and have ranged from 13 percent to 185 percent.[21,26,28,107,208,502–512] High altitude does not seem to affect the testosterone response.[513] Although a 120-min swim terminating in a maximal effort induced a clear increase in circulating testosterone,[21] a consistent decrease in serum testosterone levels was seen in elite swimmers undertaking a tethered swim graded to maximum over approximately 14 min.[514] There is no clear reason for this unexpected finding. Increases in androstenedione and estrogens have also been reported.[26,107] Conflicting evidence exists with regard to gonadotropin response: LH and FSH levels have been reported as unchanged,[208,503,506] increased,[26,107,504] and decreased.[507]

Mechanism of Exercise-Associated Testosterone Increase

Problems arise in trying to explain the exercise-associated increase in serum testosterone levels because of the inconsistent LH response to short-term intense exercise and because serum testosterone levels increase more quickly than would be anticipated from an increase in serum LH. A variety of mechanisms have been proposed. Nonspecific mechanisms associated with short-term exercise-induced serum testosterone elevations include a decreased metabolic clearance rate (MCR) and decreased plasma volume. Testosterone is cleared via hepatic and extrahepatic mechanisms. Hepatic blood flow approximates 1250 liters/m^2 per day; the MCR of testosterone through the liver is approximately half this value. This implies that the 50 percent reduction in hepatic blood flow which is observed during strenuous exercise[515,516] should have little effect on the MCR of testosterone. However, clearance through the liver depends on protein binding and hepatic blood flow. Binding to a specific protein such as SHBG inhibits hepatic metabolism, whereas albumin binding does not. Thus the splanchnic extraction of testosterone approximates 50 percent. The real hepatic reserve may therefore be smaller than would be anticipated from blood flow and clearance rate figures. The metabolic clearance rate of testosterone has been described as being reduced during physical activity.[517,518] Exercise rates in both studies were moderate, and the time course of clearance changes seems to follow the testosterone increments reported elsewhere.[107,505]

Changes in hemoconcentration were considered important in some[195,505,508,514] but by no means all studies.[26,107,504,507,509,510,517,519,520] The assumptions are that measured components such as hematocrit and hemoglobin accurately reflect the degree of fluid loss, that changes are not influenced by the differential binding of the steroid, and that physiologic changes such as increased temperature do not affect binding. The association constants of testosterone with SHBG (1.6 to 1.9 $\times$ 10^9 liters/mol) and albumin (4 $\times$ 10^4 liters/mol) are very different.[521] Because of the characteristics of testosterone binding, even substantial changes in albumin have little influence on circulating testosterone levels. Based on the association constants, it can be calculated that if the serum albumin doubled without a change in SHBG, the increase in total testosterone would approximate 6 percent. Although variable hemoconcentration has been reported with different forms of exercise, circulating SHBG changes little with short-term or longer-term running, and increases in the testosterone/SHBG ratio suggest that hemoconcentration does not play a significant role.[504]

For nonspecific mechanisms to be responsible for the acute exercise-induced rise in serum testosterone, we would expect all circulating steroids to be affected in the same manner given that MCR and hemoconcentration do not differentiate between hormones. The temporal patterns of change among the various steroid hormones does not provide this picture.[107] In one study, the testosterone increase was distinct from those of androstenedione and dehydroepiandrosterone (DHEA), adrenal androgens whose increments were simultaneous with that of cortisol.[107] The clear difference in responses among the hormones suggests that specific mechanisms are involved.

What mechanism could exist independent of gonadotropin stimulation of testosterone? Overnight dexamethasone did not influence the exercise-induced testosterone response, an expected finding which indicated little adrenal contribution to the increment.[522] The involvement of the sympathetic system in testicular testosterone production has suggested that a direct neural pathway may stimulate testosterone production during exercise in some species.[523,524] As discussed earlier, circulating catecholamine levels also increase substantially during exercise. β-Blockade inhibits testosterone responses to exercise, whereas L-dopa, phentolamine, and clonidine have no effect.[506,525] It remains unclear exactly what mechanisms may be operative in increasing circulating testosterone levels in any exercise protocol, and it is possible that the mechanisms responsible early in exercise differ from those observed subsequently. As a consistent increase in testosterone was observed prior to cycle ergometry[107] and testosterone levels were proportional to anticipated workload,[505] there is an anticipatory rise which is presumably independent of hepatic perfusion or hemoconcentration.

The Effects of Prolonged Exercise on the HPG Axis in Men

Prolonged acute submaximal exercise bouts (exceeding 2 h) may be associated with complex changes in circulating androgen. Responses have been examined under laboratory conditions and during free activity such as marathon and ultramarathon races as well as in cross-country skiing. Several studies have reported an initial testosterone increase with exercise, followed by a decline to or below baseline values.[109,153,167,175,204,507,526–534] The decrease appears to be proportional to the preceding workload.[534] Lowered testosterone levels may follow even relatively short term but strenuous physical activity.[208,519] Stresses such as surgery, myocardial infarction, and simulated warfare training also result in decreased testosterone levels.[534–536] Several mechanisms may be important in decreasing circulating testosterone levels during and after prolonged exercise, including suppressed gonadotropin release and a more direct effect by elevated prolactin, cortisol, or catecholamine levels. Alterations in β-endorphin have been popularly blamed for acute exercise-associated suppression of the HPG axis in both men and women, although this has been difficult to prove since opiate antagonism does not prevent[109] the exercise-induced decrease in LH that has been observed by some but by no means all investigators.[166,167,507,526,530,537,538] Response to gonadotropin releasing hormone (GnRH) has been reduced[539] and increased[167] after prolonged, exhaustive exercise. Pulsatile LH release does not decrease after 60 and 120 min of treadmill running in men, although the area under the multiple sample curve is decreased after exercise.[526,538] The response of testosterone levels to stimulation with HCG has also been described as being reduced.[539]

We are again faced with the difficulty of explaining a change in serum testosterone levels which does not appear to be mediated by alterations in central control. Prolactin responses to intense or prolonged exertion are transient and unlikely to influence postexercise testosterone levels. In one study, decreases in serum testosterone followed increments in cortisol levels induced by insulin hypoglycemia or injection of hydrocortisone hemisuccinate.[540] Increases in serum cortisol accompany prolonged or intense exercise; therefore, a similar mechanism may be operative.[107,109] A decline in serum testosterone levels was observed accompanying an exercise-induced cortisol increment.[107] A persistent increase in catecholamines accompanies and follows physical activity; this may be related to testicular resistance to endogenous gonadotropins.[167] The exercise-associated decline in serum testosterone levels remains unclear. It is possible that the decline results from subtle interference at either the hypothalamic or the gonadal level or because of increased androgen consumption after strenuous exercise to repair structural and metabolic injury to the tissues.

Effect of Endurance Training on the HPG Axis in Men

The consistent testosterone decline that follows prolonged submaximal exercise suggests that there may be a continuing suppression of circulating testosterone associated with chronic involvement in endurance training. Several cross-sectional and prospective studies have supported this idea. A fall in plasma testosterone has been repeatedly observed in trained athletes.[129,153,177,529,541–549] In contrast, military training including a heavy physical exercise component resulted in an increase in mean plasma testosterone, androstenedione, and LH, with no significant change in SHBG.[550] Prospective studies using two relatively light training regimes also found increased levels of testosterone.[551,552] Some cross-sectional studies have reported no change in serum testosterone even with heavy training.[553]

Symptomatic Impairment of the HPG Axis in Men

In contrast to cyclic endocrine control of reproduction in women, endocrine control of the male reproductive system is steady state with a typical endocrine servomechanism. Symptomatic changes in testicular androgenesis and spermatogenesis are slower and less clearly definable. There is some evidence that males with a high level of physical activity may have some impairment of fertility.[542,554] In an artificial insemination program, donors with a high physical activity profile and low semen volume had significantly lower pregnancy rates than those with "normal" activity and low semen volume.[554] When semen volume was normal, there was no reduction in fertility. Normal sperm counts are generally found in runners even with very strenuous training regimes.[553–555]

Anecdotal data have also suggested that libido may be impaired in some runners during periods of intense endurance training.[542] Reduced testosterone levels may play a role in this, but chronic fatigue could also be significant. Only one large-scale study of sexuality in runners has been published.[556] While the scientific validity may be questioned, it is surprising that almost one-quarter of the male respondents to the questionnaire were prepared to give up sex before running and almost half admitted that they sometimes felt too tired from running to engage in sex. The positive replies to this question increased with increasing mileage. So little is known about short- or long-term problems with exercise-induced symptomatic reproductive change in men that it is impossible to provide advice on the management of problems other than to review with an athlete the possibility of decreasing the exercise load.

Androgen-dependent skeletal muscle hypertrophy and synergism with GH are well accepted. The decline in testosterone in rats undergoing endurance training is accompanied by increased excretion of the products of muscle catabolism.[557] Increased utilization of testosterone may be needed to maintain muscle in chronic exercisers, and so basal testosterone or testosterone/cortisol ratios may be important.[558] One consequence of severe training regimes could be to reduce the repair of muscle damage because of lowered circulating testosterone levels. The catabolic effects of high cortisol levels in "overtraining syndrome"[134] and the inability of testosterone to prevent muscle catabolism could be contributory in this regard. Testosterone and GH also interact in stimulating cardiac muscle hypertrophy.[559] It is possible that significant lowering of testosterone levels influences the repair of cardiac muscle.

The number of lower limb injuries, particularly shin splints and stress fractures, has increased dramatically in high-mileage runners.[560] Shin splints represent the effects of chronic mechanical stress on the bone with possible associated impairment of bone repair mechanisms. Maintenance of bone mass is steroid-dependent: The interaction of testosterone and bone mass and testosterone levels has been demonstrated in normal aging men.[561] The declining testosterone levels associated with high-mileage runners, particularly in the fourth and fifth decades of their lives, raises the question of the implications of the early development of osteoporosis in these men. Exercise may indeed prevent age-related decreases in bone mineral content in male runners, but a case report has described osteoporotic fractures in a hypogonadal marathoner with anorexia nervosa.[562,563] Clearly the anorexia is more significant, but the report raised the question of how much exercise-associated hypogonadism could produce a similar, if less dramatic, effect.[564]

The aerobic capacity of runners is dependent on central and peripheral factors. There is a correlation between fitness as judged by maximal oxygen consumption and exercise-associated decreases in testosterone.[550] Testosterone increases the synthesis of erythropoietin, which stimulates erythropoiesis; lowered testosterone levels could be related to exercise-associated anemia, which has been described in endurance-trained athletes. It is, however, difficult to believe that the reductions in serum testosterone levels generally observed in endurance-trained athletes could affect erythropoiesis.

Physical inactivity, male gender, and elevated blood lipids are among the well-recognized risk factors for atherosclerotic heart disease. Androgens are important in regulating blood lipid levels: The levels of high-density lipoprotein cholesterol (HDLC) in the blood of men are significantly lower than values in women. Since HDLC has a cardioprotective effect, the risk of atherosclerosis is increased in men. In contrast, endurance training has been associated with lower overall cholesterol, lower low-density lipoprotein cholesterol (LDLC), and higher HDLC.[565–568] This change in pattern may contribute to the beneficial effects of exercise on atherosclerotic heart disease. It is unclear whether the physiologic reductions in androgens could play a significant role in these changes. Androgens may also be important in hepatic and renal function; in the brain, including effects on aggression; and in the immune system. While there has been concern over the normal functioning of the immune system in endurance-trained athletes, any effect of lowered but still physiologic serum testosterone levels on the immune system and on hepatic and renal function remains speculative. Social and other pressures influence aggression, so that any short-term increases or longer-term reductions in testosterone would be likely to have little influence.

Mechanisms of Long-Term Activity-Associated Suppression of Circulating Testosterone Levels

The fall in serum testosterone levels must result from decreased production rates, decreased binding, or increased clearance. There is scant evidence of decreased binding.[129] No studies have shown long-term increases in hepatic or extrahepatic clearance of testosterone in endurance-trained or other athletes, although basal estradiol clearance is increased in women athletes, presumably through increased hepatic metabolism.[569] Evidence of an altered LH pulsatile release in male runners[526,538] has been disputed.[547,570] LH pulse frequency is not significantly altered in runners with acute exercise.[526,538] The GnRH-induced LH response appears to be impaired.[526] No evidence has supported increased opioidergic tone as being important in the generation of GnRH-LH suppression in athletes, and the effects of catecholamines have received little attention.[166,570] Chronic elevation of serum cortisol levels has been associated with overtraining or a shift in cortisol/testosterone ratios associated with strenuous exercise.[160] It is possible but unlikely that such a change could exert a direct effect on testicular testosterone production. Serum PRL levels are chronically depressed rather than elevated and are therefore not likely to be involved in the fall in testosterone in highly trained male runners.[547]

Suppression of the HPG axis in men is associated with starvation, a vegetarian diet, and a low-fat, high-fiber diet.[571–573] An anorectic subgroup with reduced total and free testosterone and a preoccupation with caloric intake and lean body mass was described among a group of 20 high-mileage runners.[542] Significant reductions in total and free testosterone in wrestlers were associated with their practices in trying to "make weight."[541] The possibility of an association between exercise and anorexia nervosa has been raised,[324,326,574] but the reliability of human data has been criticized.[325] While there were significant correlations among total and free testosterone and body weight and body fat in young male wrestlers, no correlation was observed between physiologic reductions in serum testosterone levels and body fat in cross-sectional studies of runners and controls.[129,326,541]

In summary, it seems likely that the chronic suppressive effects of endurance training on the HPG axis in men result from a mechanism of inhibition that is central and is analogous to that described in women, perhaps involving a nutritional-metabolic influence. The possibility of peripheral effects of increased utilization of steroids is worthy of further investigation. It is unlikely that clinical manifestations of reproductive suppression with training are common in men. Further investigation is essential to provide continuing reassurance that "exercise is good for you" and to define the physiologic boundaries and the effects of overstepping them.

EXERCISE AND THE REPRODUCTIVE SYSTEM IN WOMEN

Acute Exercise-Associated Changes in Reproductive Hormones

There have been few studies of hormonal responses to acute exercise in women.[30,106,108,114,115,164,513,527,575,576] In general, these studies reflect the problems in explaining the responses of male reproductive hormones to acute exercise. Variable responses of LH, follicle stimulating hormone (FSH), estradiol, progesterone, and testosterone have been described. Some studies[106,513] have also addressed the question of how acute responses to exercise might be involved in the genesis of exercise-associated amenorrhea by examining differences in the responses to exercise in normally menstruating and amenorrheic runners. Such differences as there are tend to reflect the suppressed state of the HPG axis rather than provide a reason for the amenorrhea; there is scant evidence that acute exercise-induced hormonal responses play a significant role in the genesis of reproductive dysfunction.[513]

Reproductive Effects of Exercise in Women

A popular picture has emerged in which thin high-mileage runners commonly have reproductive problems. Endurance training, particularly distance running, has become associated with an increased frequency of reproductive dysfunction in women; delayed menarche, an inadequate luteal phase, anovulatory cycles, and oligoamenorrhea have all been reported as being more common in women athletes. The significance of physical activity alone in generating exercise-associated reproductive dysfunction has been increasingly questioned.[577] It seems likely that "runner's amenorrhea" or any other overt reproductive dysfunction usually blamed on endurance training occurs only in individuals in whom another factor is compromising the normal functioning of the HPG-axis. In this section we will examine the accuracy of the runner's amenorrhea stereotype and consider mechanisms which might be responsible for reproductive dysfunction and subclinical changes.

Pubertal development and menarche are delayed in competitive athletes and ballet dancers.[578–584] This delay appears to reflect the level of competition but not the individual sports activity.[578,579] There was no difference in age of menarche among groups of athletes from various sports disciplines[579] or between swimmers and runners,[582] although both groups differed from unathletic girls. Menarche is delayed in ballet dancers to a much greater degree than it is in Olympic athletes.[581] Some authors have offered explanations for the delay in menarche that are unrelated to physical activity. Relatively low body fat gives prepubertal individuals a greater strength/weight ratio, a benefit in sports such as gymnastics. A somatotype with increased height, longer legs, narrower hips, and better neuromuscular coordination occurs more frequently with delayed puberty; this may result in better athletic performance. Early maturers may socialize away from sports activity. Factors related to physical activity and nutritional status are, however, more likely to be involved.

Some aspect of physical activity appears important as only premenarcheally trained athletes have a significant delay in the onset of menses, proportional to the time in training.[582] Advancement of pubertal stages and/or resumption of menses occurred in ballet dancers during inactivity.[583] However, a genetic component may also be present, so that the resolution of the question is very difficult even with studies designed to control for all these factors. In dancers, leanness is the best predictor of menarche and is superior in this regard to activity level and maternal age of menarche.[585]

Subclinical luteal-phase abnormalities and anovulatory cycles are relatively common. Reduced luteal phase length and midluteal progesterone levels in runners and teenage swimmers, abnormalities of basal body temperature graphs, delayed endometrial maturation in runners, and decreased salivary progesterone levels in recreational runners have all been reported.[586–590] The frequency of secondary amenorrhea/oligomenorrhea in runners was examined in a study based on replies received from 128 women not taking birth control pills out of 400 members of U.S. collegiate track and field and cross-country teams.[591] The frequency of amenorrhea (defined as three periods or less in the previous year) varied from 6 to 43 percent depending on weekly mileage. The prevalence of menstrual dysfunction has been considerably lower in subsequent investigations.[592–596] Such surveys are not based on true epidemiologic principles and may be biased because runners with problems are more likely to respond; some researchers have suggested that there is not a significant increase in exercise-associated amenorrhea.[594]

Reproductive dysfunction has been associated mostly with runners, with little investigation of other forms of activity. Swimmers and cyclists have a lower frequency of reproductive dysfunction than do runners.[597] The relatively greater frequency in the runners correlated with body build. Similarly, there is a lower prevalence of oligoamenorrhea in racquet players and sprinters than there is in middle-distance runners (800 to 5000 m).[598] This also correlated with a more linear physique. Surprisingly, ball players were not very different from distance runners despite being clearly different in physique.

Factors Involved in the Genesis of Exercise-Associated Menstrual Dysfunction

It has been suggested that the reproductive changes, clinical and subclinical, may represent hypothalamic adaptations, analogous to physical (cardiopulmonary) conditioning from training.[599] However, little evidence has been presented that amenorrheic runners possess a particular physiologic advantage. Functional abnormalities of the HPG axis have been associated with the extremes of reproductive life, abnormal dietary practices, extremes of body fat content, psychological stress, and pathologic conditions including androgen excess, hyperprolactinemia, hypothyroidism, and ovarian failure. While acute exercise-induced elevations in serum testosterone and prolactin levels occur, they have generally been considered insignificant. Investigation has focused on factors that may be related to hypothalamic amenorrhea (Table 32-4).

The Psychological Stress of Training and Competing

Amenorrheic runners associated significantly more stress with training than normally menstruating

TABLE 32-4 Pathophysiologic Factors in Exercise-Induced Changes in Reproductive Function

Stress of training and/or competing
Physical stresses
Emotional stresses
Nutritional and metabolic
Abnormalities of nutrition and energy drain
Altered lean/fat ratio
Loss of weight
Predisposition
Immature hypothalamus, young gynecologic age
History of menstrual irregularity
Hormonal changes with exertion
Repeated acute changes
Chronic changes

women,[140] but there is little evidence that this produces problems. Studies of psychological well-being found no significant difference between amenorrheic and normally menstruating runners.[140,600] There is no evidence that the menstrual irregularity associated with activity is caused by psychological or psychiatric problems, as no runners in either study approached clinically significant scores on psychological testing.

The Physical Stress of Training and/or Competition

There have been conflicting results from cross-sectional studies to determine whether the frequency of oligoamenorrhea increases with greater training load. Some studies show a clear increase in the frequency of amenorrhea as mileage increases,[591,593,595] but other studies have not related the prevalence of reproductive dysfunction to increased training volume.[140,584,585,594,601] Intensity of exercise (e.g., speed of running) has received little attention. Prospective training studies have suggested that most women who have regular menses continue to do so after increased training.[178,594,597,602,603] In contrast, two studies have shown a clear effect of increasing exercise on reproductive function; 2 months of training (beginning at 4 mi per day and reaching 10 mi per day after 5 weeks) altered the normal menstrual cycles of a group of sedentary women and 5 of 13 regularly menstruating swimmers became oligoamenorrheic when their weekly training volume was increased from 60 to 100 km per week.[179,604,605]

Training intensity and/or mileage in the genesis of reproductive dysfunction seems to be a commonsense finding, but the evidence is far from conclusive. It also remains unclear what mechanism might mediate an exercise effect. The possibilities include alterations in neurotransmitter levels as part of a generalized stress response to the activity and, more indirectly, alteration of the nutritional balance, which seems somewhat precarious in runners.[606,607]

Body Composition and Nutrition

Although the role of nutrition and body composition in determining the onset and maintenance of normal reproductive function has been explored extensively in animals,[608] ethical constraints have resulted in human data that are indirect and observational but consistent in implicating a nutritional component in determining menstrual function.

Over the last century the mean menarcheal age has declined as more young women enter puberty at an early age except in geographic areas where nutrition has not changed.[609,610] Famine and starvation from warfare have provided short-term nutritional stresses, and reproductive consequences (amenorrhea or infertility) were first seen in women with marginally adequate nutrition.[611] The effects of nutrition and/or body composition on age at menarche have been confirmed in different populations.[612–616] Dieting, self-induced weight loss, and low body weight are also associated with delayed menarche.[617]

Body fat has been suggested as a trigger for the onset of menarche and the maintenance of normal cycles.[618] Low body weight, dieting, weight loss, and reduced body fat are associated with primary and secondary amenorrhea.[617,619] Malnutrition reduces gonadotropin levels before puberty[620,621] and in adults.[622,623] Attempts to define the specific nutrient deficiency associated with reduced gonadotropin levels have been inconclusive.[624]

Some studies have supported an association of low body fat with amenorrhea in women who exercise. Amenorrheic athletes were lighter and leaner and had lost more weight after the onset of running than were their normally menstruating counterparts.[140,582,592,593] However, several large-scale studies have failed to find an association between lower body fat and amenorrhea.[584,594,600,625] Some authors suggested that the linear physique of runners is more likely to be associated with amenorrhea but failed to find a correlation within this group.[597,626] The variability of findings suggests that methodologic considerations may influence the conclusions. There are method-specific differences in body fat estimates, and differing conclusions can be drawn from the same population depending on the means of calculation.[627]

One study utilizing the hydrostatic method, the "gold standard," suggested that menstrual irregularity in exercise is more frequent in runners with a low percentage of body fat.[628] However, low body fat is not invariably associated with menstrual irregularity, and menstrual irregularity is not invariably associated with reduced body fat.

Injuries preventing exercise in amenorrheic young ballet dancers precipitated menarche or were followed by the resumption of menses with no weight change.[583] It was postulated that an "energy drain" of exercise may delay menarche or result in amenorrhea without alteration of body composition. A relatively small change in weight of 1 to 2 kg around the critical level can regulate menstruation in some athletes.[140,582] It is unclear how such a small alteration in the lean to fat ratio could directly influence menstrual function, but it is possible that even short-term relative nutritional stresses can influence reproductive function, particularly when nutrition may have been marginal prior to the further insult.

Cross-sectional studies of diet have provided conflicting evidence of macronutrient deficiencies in amenorrheic athletes,[140,626,629–635] although the most consistent finding has been that amenorrheic runners have a caloric deficit compared with their normally menstruating peers. Dietary intake even in normally menstruating runners does not seem to match the increase in energy output which their activity requires.[636] The long-held belief that if dietary intake is constant and energy output is increased, weight will be progressively lost is open to question. Malnutrition is capable of altering the metabolic cost of exercise,[637] and it is possible that the "relative malnutrition" of physical activity can have the same effect. Runners have a consistently superior food efficiency compared with nonrunners.[606] As the requirements for the body to remain efficient become more stringent, reproductive function may be initially compromised and later sacrificed to minimize energy loss. It has been popularly assumed that the mechanism involves a decrease in body fat as a marker with the teleologic goal of preventing pregnancy in the presence of inadequate fat stores, but the low percentage of body fat per se may not be the metabolic signal. Possibly, cumulative changes in several endocrine systems and in neurotransmitters consequent to crossing the fine line of nutritional adequacy prompt the reproductive abnormalities.

The thermal readjustment with luteal levels of progesterone requires an increase of a mean 500 calories per cycle.[638] Suppression of luteal progesterone levels may be the first in a series of energy-saving measures which culminate in total reproductive shutdown. Reproductive shutdown to save the energy cost of the menstrual cycle is a more immediate goal than preventing pregnancy, although the long-term effects are the same. Amenorrheic runners have been shown to have a decrease in the metabolic rate, supporting the concept that energy balance is critical in the development of reproductive dysfunction.[639]

Predisposition to Menstrual Irregularity

Investigations have consistently suggested that amenorrheic athletes may have either immaturity of the HPG axis or a predisposition to menstrual irregularity. College-age women tend to have irregular menses. Studies in which a high prevalence of amenorrhea has been reported have tended to use college-age athletes. Women with reproductive dysfunction induced by exercise tend to be younger than those reporting regular menses, are less likely to have had a previous pregnancy, and are more likely to have a past history of menstrual irregularity.[140,593,595,601] The interaction of nutritional inadequacy or other factors clearly would be more likely to induce problems in such women than in women with a mature gynecologic age (e.g., 10 to 12 years since menarche).

The Endocrinology of Exercise-Associated Reproductive Dysfunction

"Athletic amenorrhea" has generally been considered as hypothalamic with low or normal gonadotropins and estradiol; occasional patients have a more clearly pathologic cause for their amenorrhea.[577]

The abnormalities are apparent in the GnRH-gonadotropin axis, while adrenal androgenesis appears normal.[614] This contrasts with findings in women with primary hypothalamic amenorrhea.[577] As was indicated earlier, serum cortisol levels are elevated in women with exercise-associated amenorrhea and psychogenic hypothalamic amenorrhea.[135,140–143]

Boyden and colleagues tested the functioning of the HPG axis in normally menstruating recreational runners preparing for a marathon on days 8 to 11 in the late follicular phase at baseline (mean of 15 miles per week) and when weekly mileage was 30 and 50 miles above baseline.[178,602,603] Basal prolactin and estradiol levels decreased, but serum LH, FSH, estrone, and testosterone levels were unchanged by the increasing workload.

Gonadotropin responses to GnRH decreased with increasing training volume. Cross-sectional and longitudinal investigations found decreased basal estradiol and progesterone levels as well as lower serum gonadotropin responses to GnRH with increased training.[170,640] This suggests a suppressive effect of physical activity on the HPG axis but does not differentiate between the hypothalamus and the pituitary. Chronically altered frequency and amplitude of LH pulsatile release have been observed in the early follicular phase in normally menstruating and frequently in amenorrheic runners.[641–643] These three studies suggested that the mechanism for exercise-associated reproductive dysfunction involves hypothalamic inhibition.

Neurotransmitter control of the cycle is complex and involves catecholamines, catechol estrogens, EO, and probably other neuromodulators. For normal GnRH pulses to occur, two events are necessary: First, the individual GnRH neurons must release their product in a cyclic fashion; second, that cyclic release must be made synchronous. It is likely that these two events require different stimulatory neurotransmitters. Norepinephrine and GABA may be involved in stimulation. Evidence strongly suggests that dopamine and EO inhibit the GnRH-LH axis physiologically through the menstrual cycle and inappropriately in women with hypothalamic amenorrhea.[644]

As was indicated above, acute exercise releases EO from the pituitary, and peripheral β-endorphin/β-LPH levels were chronically elevated during intensive training when reproductive dysfunction was occurring.[179] Basal plasma β-endorphin/β-LPH levels may be higher in amenorrheic than in eumenorrheic runners,[180,645] but the administration of opiate antagonists to amenorrheic runners has not confirmed the popular view that EO suppress the GnRH-LH axis[89,646,647]; however, increases in pulse amplitude were reported in some subjects.[648] The role of exercise- and-training-associated changes in dopamine and other catecholamines has similarly not been substantiated.[577] It is tempting to believe that neurotransmitters are involved in the hypothalamic-pituitary alterations of exercise, but their involvement is conjectural and the concept of a single neurotransmitter being responsible for menstrual dysfunction in exercise is probably simplistic.

Summary

Prospective studies make it clear that oligoamenorrhea does not occur in healthy, normally menstruating women runners when their exercise load is increased. Nonetheless, there are changes in the function of the hypothalamic-pituitary axis. The changes which occur with training would progressively reduce the luteal phase and its accompanying caloric "waste" resulting from preparations for pregnancy. When nutrition is in question or when another factor is present, the need to conserve calories may be sufficient to stop menstruation altogether. Amenorrheic runners have a greater need to preserve calories through progressive reduction in the resting metabolic rate, but other messengers may be important. Possible signals could include deficiencies of neurotransmitter precursors, alteration in thyroid function, activation of "stress" hormones, alterations in glucoregulatory and other metabolic hormones, changes in steroid metabolism in fat tissue, changes in hepatic metabolism of binding proteins, and an exaggerated peripheral response to exercise in a nutritionally stressed subject.

USE OF PERFORMANCE-ENHANCING ENDOCRINE DRUGS (DOPING) IN COMPETITIVE AND RECREATIONAL SPORTS ACTIVITY

The use of drugs and practices to enhance athletic performance is as old as organized competition. It is, however, now more scientific and widespread at all levels of sport. A universally acceptable definition of *doping* in sport remains elusive, although in a general sense it refers to using an artificial method to gain an unfair advantage in competition. The International Olympic Committee chose not to define doping per se but has banned specific substances or groups of substances and certain physical methods.[649] Groups of drugs which they have banned include stimulants, narcotics, anabolic steroids (Table 32-5), β-blockers, diuretics, and peptide hormones and their analogues. Physical methods also banned include blood doping (autotransfusion) and any chemical, pharmacologic, or physical manipulation such as urine substitution. Drugs such as alcohol, marijuana, local anesthetics, and corticosteroids are subject to restrictions. Sixty-two athletes have been penalized for the use of banned substances at Olympic games since 1968.[650] This compares with estimates of use in the United States, where it is thought that over 1 million individuals, including a quarter of a million adolescents, use or have used anabolic steroids in an industry whose annual receipts exceed $100 million.[651]

Since 1976 two-thirds of the infractions at the Olympic Games have been for the use of anabolic steroids.[650] These drugs are used frequently without detection provided that they are discontinued early enough to allow elimination from the body and are perhaps masked by other substances. They are, therefore, particularly important in sport. Other drug usage relevant to endocrinology includes the use of human growth hormone and, more recently, erythropoietin to enhance muscle size and red blood cell mass, respectively.

Mens Sana in Corpore Sano: Ethical Aspects of Doping in Sports

Sport has meaning, purpose, and values that surpass the physical experience, including self-discipline, dedication, perseverence, and endurance. The sporting ideal is that individuals compete against each other based on their talent and training. Sport

TABLE 32-5 Anabolic Steroids Banned by the International Olympic Committee

Bolasterone	Nandrolone
Boldenone	Norethandrolone
Clostebol	Oxandrolone
Dihydrochlormethyl-testosterone	Oxymesterone
Fluoxymesterone	Oxymetholone
Mesterolone	Stanozolol
Metandienone	Testosterone and related compounds
Methyltestosterone	

is also a focus for local, regional, and national pride. Governments recognize the nation-building role of sport and provide facilities and funding so that individuals can compete optimally in international competitions.

The Canadian Task Force on National Sport Policy established a long-term goal in the area of high-performance sport, attempting to "develop a Canadian Sport system which will provide opportunities to enable athletes with talent and dedication to *win* [emphasis added] at the highest levels of international competition."[652] It tied funding to international success. The task force report was published in 1988, the year in which a Canadian sprinter was deprived of the Olympic 100-m gold medal because his urine was found to contain traces of stanozolol. While there is no direct link between sport policy and the use of anabolic steroids, the atmosphere fostered makes governments that fail to enforce the regulations of the International Olympic Committee at least as culpable as the athletes involved.

Winning at all costs becomes acceptable because of national and personal pride, media pressure to win, and the large financial rewards in some sports for the few who are very successful. When factors other than talent and training, such as the use of banned drugs and practices, enter into the results of competition, this is considered unfair and constitutes cheating. The use of doping—more euphemistic terms include *ergogenic aids* and *performance-enhancing drugs*—is considered to be cheating. There is in sport a moral climate in which such practices are acceptable if the risk of detection is low. Athletes no longer regard striving to win as important; winning even by risking the life or health of the athletes is the only acceptable outcome. Some may argue that the rules should be changed to permit individuals who wish to use anabolic steroids and other drugs to do so.[653] These drugs could be viewed as just another aid, like complex machinery and good training. Permitting the use of drugs may endanger the health of the athletes involved, but sport itself may be dangerous. We do not ban hang gliding or motorcycle racing; therefore, it may be argued, we have no right to interfere with an individual's choice. A physiologic rationale can be used which suggests that strenuous sports activity invariably places the participants in a catabolic state. Providing anabolic steroids merely returns the athlete to physiologic norms.

This question goes beyond the danger of steroids. Pressure to compete on an even basis demands that athletes who wish to compete must take performance-enhancing drugs or remain second class, a situation many people would regard as unfair. Winning should remain a triumph of talent, training, dedication, and character, not a triumph of chemistry. As Thomas Murray says, "If I said that I could put the shot 90 ft with the aid of a sling or 2 mi with a cannon, you would rightly tell me that I had missed the point of the sport."[653]

Physicians must also answer the specific ethical questions which apply to them. Should physicians refuse to provide anabolic steroids to athletes, or should they consider circumstances under which these drugs can be provided? Should doctors consider anabolic steroids as forbidden drugs in the sense of narcotic drugs? Since athletes seem to obtain adequate supplies of drugs from unofficial sources, should physicians refuse to monitor the health of individuals who are self-prescribing anabolic steroids? It is clearly unethical and unacceptable to provide a drug solely for the purpose of enhancing sports performance, but refusal to monitor a patient is less clear from an ethical point of view. Refusing to monitor patients may be a greater evil. Physicians should warn individuals in a nonjudgmental way about the known and possible dangers of steroids but should consider monitoring these patients for several reasons, including the health of the individual, the need for even anecdotal information about people taking these drugs, and because refusal by physicians to become involved, overestimating the benefits and understating the side effects, has probably increased the utilization of anabolic steroids. As care givers, physicians must ask themselves whether individuals taking these drugs are better off unsupervised. Would we abandon those who abuse narcotics or alcohol or prescription drugs?

Anabolic Steroids

Anabolic steroids are the most widely abused performance-enhancing drugs. The recognition that humoral factors, notably testosterone, are responsible for many of the visible differences in secondary sex characteristics and for gender differences in muscle mass and strength led to the attempted development of compounds which could differentially influence the androgenic and anabolic effects of testosterone. Such a disassociation has not been convincingly achieved, and particularly in high doses these drugs have strong androgenic effects. It is unlikely that complete separation will be achieved since the receptors for each effect are common.[654] The medical indications for the use of anabolic steroids are relatively few. Use of anabolic steroids to enhance sport performance is not recognized; therefore, for physicians to prescribe them is at best unethical and at worst illegal.

Medical Indications for Anabolic Steroids

Generally accepted uses for anabolic-androgenic steroids include testosterone deficiency such as that resulting from bilateral orchidectomy, cryptorchidism, bilateral torsion, orchitis, vanishing testis syndrome, gonadotropin deficiency, GnRH deficiency resulting from congenital absence or injury secondary to tumors, trauma, or irradiation.[655] Drugs can also be used with well-characterized pubertal delay. Indications for use in women include metastatic breast cancer and, for some anabolic steroids in low doses, as part of a hormone replacement program for postmenopausal women. Anabolic steroids have also been used in other conditions, including aplastic and hypoplastic anemias, debilitating disease (e.g., burns), and hereditary angioneurotic edema. These drugs have also been used for the promotion of growth and for osteoporosis. Their use in debilitating conditions, promotion of growth, and osteoporosis remains controversial. Some researchers have suggested that these drugs may be effective in speeding the healing of injured tissues,[656] but this is of doubtful validity. There is no other medical reason for their use in sports medicine, where they are being used not to treat illness but to enhance performance in healthy young men and women.

Extent of the Use of Anabolic Steroids in Various Populations

Evidence on the extent of anabolic steroid use is elusive and consists largely of rumor and speculation. Medical authorities associated with the U.S. Olympic squad have identified a relatively small number of athletes but believe that the usage is widespread, particularly among athletes involved in weight lifting and track and field.[657] Other sources of information include the results of drug testing during training and at the time of competition and necessarily incomplete voluntary surveys of athletes at various levels admitting to steroid use. It is, however, apparent that the use of the drugs is frequent and extensive, especially at national and international levels of competition and in sports where a premium is placed on large body size and strength.

Judicial and other official inquiries have been held in Canada, the United States, Australia, and the United Kingdom.[650,658–660] These inquiries generally focused on steroid use in athletes at the highest levels of national and international competition. Testimony was heard that suggested that up to 80 percent of male athletes at international levels use steroids at some time during their training. An Australian senate standing committee heard evidence that 70 percent of Australian athletes competing internationally had used performance-enhancing drugs.[659]

Robert Kerr of San Gabriel, California, testified before the Dubin Commission in Canada that he prescribed anabolic steroids to approximately 20 medalists in the 1984 Olympic Games and had also prescribed steroids to several thousand athletes in various sports, including track and field, baseball, ice hockey, roller hockey, cycling, and swimming.[650] Other steroid-prescribing physicians gave similar testimony. The Australian committee heard testimony that children as young as 10 years of age were given steroids to enhance performance.[659] Forty-nine athletes have been banned for testing positive for anabolic steroids at the Olympic Games, predominantly in weight lifting,[650] but this must substantially underestimate the number of individuals involved. In a survey of athletes participating in track and field at the 1972 Olympic Games (before the drugs were banned), 68 percent admitted to anabolic steroid use.[661] It is doubtful if such an open confession could be obtained from recent Olympic athletes. A 1983 study of 220 international-level Canadian athletes found 11 (5 percent) who admitted using steroids,[662] a finding which is probably an underestimate. In contrast, 79 athletes in four sports admitted to having used anabolic steroids, including 18 of 19 power lifters, 26 of 28 body builders, 14 of 18 football players, and 10 of 14 track and field athletes.[663] Anecdotal evidence suggests that use by weight lifters[664–668] and body builders[669] is particularly high.

Use by Women Athletes

Pat Connolly estimated that 30 percent and 40 percent of the U.S. womens' track and field teams at the 1984 and 1988 Olympic Games, respectively, had used anabolic steroids.[658] Other evidence suggests that substantial numbers of women body builders also abuse anabolic steroids.[670]

Use in College Populations

At collegiate levels of sport, 17 to 20 percent of collegiate athletes from seven universities in the United States who responded to a survey reported that they used anabolic steroids.[671,672]

Use in High School

Ninety-five of 853 responding male high school junior athletes and nonathletes (11 percent) and 5 of 914 female juniors had used or were using anabolic steroids.[673] Other estimates suggest that 5 to 11 percent of male high school athletes use or have used anabolic steroids,[674–677] although others[678] suggest a lower frequency of use. These drugs may be used more frequently in affluent areas than in poorer areas (10.2 percent vs. 2.8 percent).[674] It is likely that usage begins in teenagers and preadolescents.[667] High school women athletes use anabolic steroids much less frequently than their male counterparts (1.4 to 2.5 percent).[673–677]

Use by Nonathletes

A small proportion of nonathletes (1 to 2 percent), both men and women, admit to using anabolic steroids merely to enhance appearance or to improve physique for occupations where this is important (e.g., police, security guards, and fire fighters).[671,672,679]

Sources of Illicit Anabolic Steroids

These drugs are provided in high school predominantly by illicit sources (95 percent), although 15 to

21 percent of individuals indicated a physician as the primary source.[674,676,679] Many athletes began their use with a prescription provided by a physician before they were 16 years of age. Forty-one percent of present or past steroid-using body builders cited physicians as the source of their drugs.[680] Other sources of illicit anabolic steroids may include veterinarians, other countries, mail order, and drugs manufactured in the third world and smuggled in.[651,681] There is little doubt that black market drugs are readily available through gymnasiums.[680] It has been estimated that over 1 million individuals in the United States have taken or currently take anabolic steroids.[651] The annual market for illicit anabolic steroids in the United States probably exceeds $100 million.

Pharmacology of Anabolic Steroids

Testosterone is inactive when given orally since, like other sex steroids, it is substantially metabolized in the gut and what is absorbed intact is degraded in the liver.[655] Alkylation at the 17-alpha position produced orally active derivatives resistant to hepatic degradation, and esterification of the 17 beta-hydroxy group with a range of carboxylic acids produced a range of lipid-soluble, slow-release injectable derivatives[655] (Table 32-5).

The Use of Anabolic Steroids by Athletes

Testosterone is produced in adult males at the rate of 4 to 10 mg daily. Oral replacement dosage using methandrostenolone is 35 to 70 mg per week.[655] The mean daily doses of steroids taken by athletes are substantially larger (10- to 100-fold higher) than the replacement dose, and the pattern of use is characteristically cyclic, with "stacking" and "pyramiding" to minimize the health risk and chance of detection and to maximize the anabolic effects.[680,682–694] The cycles are characteristically 6 to 12 weeks in length and involve a progressive increase (pyramiding) of several oral and injectable steroids (stacking) to a peak followed by a reduction prior to competition. The dose of each drug is severalfold higher than that recommended by the manufacturers and may involve different drugs for different parts of the cycle. This is done to avoid the effects of receptor down regulation by using just one drug and to obtain a balance of anabolic and androgenic effects.[692] Strauss and colleagues observed mean weekly oral and injectable doses of 173 ± 45 mg and 202 ± 34 mg in 20 body builders.[680] A steroid-dependent athlete was using 75 mg of methandrostenolone and 150 mg of methenolone on alternate days and 20 mg of oxandrolone and 100 mg of oxymetholone daily.[695] The average length of a cycle was 8.3 ± 1.2 weeks, with a range of 4 to 22 weeks. Other researchers have reported doses up to 100-fold higher than manufacturers' suggested doses.[688]

There is no scientific evidence that stacking is more effective than single drug regimens and certainly no evidence that it is safer. It is possible that unknown interactions among the various drugs have a greater potential for more adverse effects than does the use of a single preparation. Because anabolic steroids are obtained by athletes from black market sources, the nature and quantity of the drugs are open to question. The lack of monitoring by physicians also means that little scientific data are available on the potential side effects of these drugs.

Human chorionic gonadotropin (hCG) is sometimes combined with anabolic steroid regimens to prevent the testicular atrophy, reduction of spermatogenesis, and decline in endogenous testosterone production which accompany anabolic steroid use.[680]

Anabolic Steroids and Athletic Performance

Mode of Action of Anabolic Steroids

Testosterone at physiologic levels produces its effects by binding to androgen receptors and initiating ribosomal protein synthesis via hormone receptor–initiated messenger RNA transcription.[696–698] In most target tissues, testosterone is converted to dihydrotestosterone (DHT) by 5α-reductase, and it is DHT which binds to the receptor and is the principal intracellular mediator of hormone action. This may not be true of skeletal muscle, where 5α-reductase activity is low and testosterone is the more usual ligand for the androgen receptor.[699] The concentration of androgen receptors is high in skeletal muscle;[699] the direct action of endogenous androgenic steroids is limited by the number and availability of such receptors.[700] Anabolic steroids also bind to androgen receptors.[701,702] At physiologic androgen levels in normal men, the receptors are saturated.[696] Additional androgenic steroids reduce the receptor number,[696] and a receptor-mediated effect of medication therefore should not occur in normal men. In women and hypogonadal men, the low levels of circulating testosterone are not sufficient to fully occupy androgen receptors so that masculizing and anabolic effects could be readily mediated via the receptor.[703]

Potential mechanisms of action for supraphysiologic doses of testosterone and other anabolic steroids include action via the receptor with or without an increase in receptor number, an anabolic effect on cellular activity independent of the receptor, and an antagonistic effect on catabolic hormones, particularly glucocorticoids. It has also been suggested that the response of muscles to anabolic steroids may be genetically different in elite athletes.[697] In a rat model, training alone increased RNA polymerase activity by 50 percent and specific cytoplasmic binding by 90 percent.[704] The additional use of nandrolone decanoate (Retabolil) (0.1 mg/100 g) induced a further increase in RNA polymerase activity but reduced androgen receptor activity by 21 percent.[704]

This supports the concept both of increased receptor effects and of an effect which is independent of the number of available receptors.

It is accepted that anabolic steroids have an anticatabolic effect mediated through antagonistic effects on glucocorticoids, but the exact mechanism through which this occurs is unclear. Binding to the glucocorticoid receptor is low, and androgens have little direct effect on receptor number.[705,706] Androgens do, however, block the glucocorticoid-induced induction of glutamine synthetase.[707] Some evidence does, however, support a direct anticatabolic effect of anabolic steroids via the glucocorticoid receptor.[708]

The relation between testosterone levels and aggression and the supposed role of testosterone in determining social rank in nonhuman primates has led to suggestions that the psychological effects of testosterone may be important.[709–712] The relation in these situations is by association, which does not prove causality. Athletes feel that steroids give them the ability to train with greater intensity and for longer periods.[666,668,697,713,714] The importance of psychological effects remains questionable.[715,716]

Effectiveness of Anabolic Steroids as Ergogenic Aids

Athletes and coaches with personal experience of anabolic steroids are convinced of the effectiveness of these drugs in improving performance.[650,668,689,717] Several possible benefits are claimed (Table 32-6). Physicians and scientists have generally taken the conservative view that there is no consistent scientific proof that anabolic steroids enhance performance. The differences between the medical and scientific views of the effectiveness of the drugs and the coaches' and athletes' views support the view that physicians do not understand the use of steroids. The Council on Scientific Affairs of the American Medical Association agreed in 1988 that improvement in muscular strength may occur with anabolic steroids used in conjunction with strenuous training and a high-protein diet.[715]

Anabolic steroids have been used by athletes in two ways. First, they have been used to increase muscle bulk, strength, and power when combined with increased dietary protein intake. Strenuous exercise induces a catabolic state, and this can be reversed by using anabolic steroids. The steroids permit training at levels which would otherwise induce catabolism.[718] They have also been used in lower doses to enhance athletic performance yet do not have a significant effect on aerobic metabolism or maximal oxygen consumption.[661,703,719–728] There is also speculation that the androgenic action may have psychological benefits by making athletes more aggressive and competitive in both training and competition.[680,729–731] Other researchers have suggested that this contributes to an imagined effect of steroids.[685]

TABLE 32-6 Possible Benefits of Anabolic Steroids

Possible Benefits
Increased muscle bulk and strength
More aggressive approach to competition
Muscle damage repair facilitated (?)
Change in reaction times (?)
Better tolerance to training

Because of the inconsistency in results, several metaanalytic papers have tried to reconcile differences in steroid dose, training, fitness, and dietary intake among athletes. Although some investigators disagree,[685] the evidence suggests that a combination of anabolic steroids, intensive strength training, and a protein-rich diet leads to gain in strength, body weight, and lean body mass.[715,721,732,733]

Forbes's analysis of the literature suggested that progressively larger doses of steroids induce progressively larger increases in lean body mass.[734] Lamb reassessed the literature, finding 18 studies with at least five subjects which employed a placebo group in a crossover design.[693] Of these studies, 12 showed significantly greater gains with steroid therapy.[661,720,722,723,727,732,735–740] The remaining six studies showed no effect of steroid therapy.[702,718,726,741–743] The mean weight gain over this length of time was 2.2 kg, although this may underestimate the increase in lean body mass, since fat may be lost with the training and the use of anabolic steroids.[734] When lean body mass alone was estimated by underwater weighing (the hydrostatic method), gains of 2 to 3 kg were also found where the dose was controlled.[721,733,737] However, with self-administered drugs (presumably in higher doses) a mean gain of 7.8 kg was obtained.[744] Other controlled dosage studies, generally with relatively low doses of anabolic steroid, have revealed no significant change in lean body mass.[685,703,741,742] In general, the studies showing no effect were those in which a low dose of anabolic steroids was used.

Haupt and Rovere, in perhaps the best metaanalysis of the literature,[721] examined 20 variables in 24 studies published prior to 1984 and found 14 that suggested an increase in strength[668,720,723–725,727,733,735,737,739,745–748] and 10 in which no improvement was found.[661,685,703,719,722,726,738,741,742,749] They concluded that anabolic steroids will consistently result in significant strength increases when given to athletes who have been intensively trained in weight lifting immediately before the start of the steroid regimen and who continue intensive weight training during the steroid regimen, when the athletes maintain a high-protein diet, and when the changes in athletes' strength are measured by the single repetition–maximal weight technique for those exercises with which the athlete trains.[721]

A subsequent prospective nonrandomized study of the effects of self-administered drugs has shown greater gains in strength in those using anabolic steroids compared with controls going through a similar training program.[745] The mean doses used in this study were 31 ± 14.4 mg per day of anabolic steroids (methandienone, stanozolol, nandrolone) and 1788.4 ± 82.7 mg per week of testosterone by injection. It seems likely that anabolic steroids alone are ineffective and that concomitant with heavy training in a previously well-trained individual and taken for at least 3 to 4 months, they may play a significant role in enhancing certain types of athletic performance.[750]

Anabolic Steroid Abuse in Women

There is little information on the effects of the drugs in women. Strauss and colleagues described 10 women athletes who reported a significant increase in muscle size, muscle strength, and performance.[680]

Anabolic Steroids, Motor Coordination, and Reaction Time

Some evidence has suggested that latent time for reflex responses is reduced by anabolic steroids.[751]

Animal Data

It is difficult to construct a good animal model for the motivated human athlete. Data from animal investigations have suggested that anabolic steroids, exercise, and adequate protein intake may stimulate skeletal muscle protein synthesis[752] but do not augment the muscle strength in the rat functional overload which results from surgical removal of a synergistic leg muscle.[753]

Problems with Assessing Benefits to Athletes

The published studies are confusing because the dosage, type, and duration of steroid use; the status of training before beginning steroids; and the method of evaluation of strength and body composition differ among studies. The scientific investigations may not be relevant to the issue because they do not encompass the variety of agents, patterns of self-medication, or dosage levels commonly used. The difference between winning and losing at a high-performance sport is relatively small, measured in the 100 m dash, for example, in hundredths of a second. Even minor improvement may substantially improve the performance of an athlete. Windsor and Dimitru suggest that the anabolic effect is not consistent and that nitrogen balance will eventually become negative unless there is a progressive increase in the dosage.[692] It is questionable whether appropriate studies to resolve the issue can even be completed. Certainly they cannot be performed in the normal manner of investigative studies. Regardless of any ability of the medical and scientific world to demonstrate an effect of steroids, their value is accepted within the sports world. They are believed to augment and facilitate but not replace training. The testimony from athletes at the Dubin Enquiry is compelling.[650]

Adverse Effects of Anabolic Steroids in Athletes

Most of the adverse effects of anabolic steroids (Table 32-7) are based on studies at doses substantially below those used to enhance athletic performance. There is little evidence of long-term harmful effects of steroids in the athletic population,[693] but physicians continue to caution against interpreting the lack of evidence as indicating that these drugs are safe to use. Neither the medical community nor the pharmaceutical industry has good reason to study the effects of supraphysiologic doses of anabolic steroids. The effects of duration of treatment, patterns of administration, and drug-drug interactions have never been systematically explored. The descriptions of life-threatening side effects tend to be anecdotal. Accounts of liver cancer,[748,754,755] stroke,[756,757] myocardial infarction and cardiomyopathy,[758] suicide,[759] and homicidal and nearly homocidal rage[760] have been published. The frequency of these problems in relation to that in the general population is not known. The side effects are frequently disregarded by athletes to some degree because of the "immortality of the young," the need to win regardless of health risks, and to some degree because

TABLE 32-7 Side Effects of Anabolic Steroids

- Stunting of growth in children and adolescents
- Changes in blood lipids to an atherogenic pattern (low serum HDL)
- Adverse psychological effects including aggressive behavior and acute psychosis
- Effects on HPG axis in women (changes are generally reversible when the drugs are discontinued)
  - Increased facial and body hair, acne
  - Deepening of the voice
  - Male pattern baldness
  - Clitoromegaly
  - Decreased breast size
  - Alterations in libido
  - Male musculature
  - Amenorrhea, oligomenorrhea, anovulation, infertility
- Effects on HPG axis in men
  - Acne
  - Gynecomastia
  - Changes in libido
  - Testicular atrophy
  - Infertility
- Impaired liver function and biochemical changes
- Benign and malignant tumors of the liver, hepatoma, peliosis hepatis
- Fluid retention with occasional hypertension

of the credibility gap which has emerged on the efficacy of anabolic steroids. The lack of trust in physicians has been recognized for many years.[761] If physicians and scientists cannot accept the fact that these drugs are effective, can athletes trust their judgment about side effects?

Stunting of Growth in Children and Adolescents

Premature epiphyseal closure with consequent failure to attain potential height is perhaps the most significant side effect in children and adolescents.[762,763]

Changes in Blood Lipids to an Atherogenic Pattern

Steroid use produces a rapid and profound lowering of HDLC in healthy trained individuals.[680,682–684,764–772] The lower HDLC levels are accompanied by lower HDLC subfractions 2 and 3, apolipoprotein A-I and A-II levels, and increased LDLC.[770,771,773,774] Strength training, in contrast to endurance training, confers no cardioprotective benefits as lipid patterns are similar to those in nonactive individuals.[565,765,768,775–777] Suppression of HDLC levels continues for up to 7 months after the steroids are discontinued.[565,768,778] It is likely that prolonged use of anabolic steroid increases the risk of infarction in athletes, but there is little evidence that the hearts of steroid takers are different from those of nonsteroid takers.[689,779,780] Diet is of minimal importance in determining the lipid response to steroids.[781] Sudden death in athletes is not rare,[782] but the importance of the atherogenic effects of anabolic steroids is unclear.

Adverse Psychological Effects

Anabolic steroid use is associated with several behavioral effects and psychological symptoms. Early anecdotal reports associated anabolic steroid use and an acute schizophrenic episode in a 17-year-old male athlete, a hypomanic episode in a 27-year-old male body builder, paranoid episodes in five depressed men taking imipramine with an anabolic steroid, and psychotic reactions in two body builders.[759,783–785] Other reported effects have included increased irritability and aggressiveness,[680] dependence compatible with standard (DSM-III) criteria,[786] severe depression and suicide,[787,788] and homicide and nearly homicidal attacks.[789] Other reported effects include euphoria and diminished fatigue, change in libido, and mood swings.

Structured interviews suggested manic or depressive episodes in 9 of 41 steroid users and psychotic episodes in 5 others.[688] Objective evidence of addiction by DSM-III-R criteria was found in eight weight lifters.[789] The authors also observed particularly depressive symptoms in dependent users. A rapid adverse response to a low dose of naloxone in one individual suggested that endogenous opiates may play a role in the dependence.[695]

Anabolic steroids were used with the goal of increasing aggressiveness in soldiers during combat.[759] Anecdotal, self-report, and objective evaluations have suggested a greater degree and frequency of episodes of aggression in steroid-using athletes.[680] The ability to train aggressively with euphoria and diminished fatigue may be potentially beneficial to athletes,[680,731,776,790,791] but the degree to which this contributes to overall performance is not known.[715] Violence away from the sports field is also associated with anabolic steroid use. A number of anecdotal reports have supported this association.[760] Legal defenses based on impaired capacity have also been used in U.S. courts.[760,792] Current steroid users scored higher on anger arousal and hostile outlook scales in answering the Multidimensional Anger Inventory.[793] Former steroid users also scored higher on a steroid symptom Likert-type scale when asked about their psychological symptoms during steroid use.[794]

Reports of possible addiction to anabolic steroids have appeared in the literature.[695,786,789] One questionnaire assessment has provided objective evidence that anabolic steroid users fulfill DSM-III-R criteria for addiction.[789] This should not come as a surprise to those who deal with postmenopausal patients since women receiving androgens as part of a hormone replacement program are notoriouly reluctant to discontinue therapy despite the side effects.

Effects on the HPG Axis in Women

Reported side effects of anabolic steroids in women include increased facial and body hair, acne, deepening of the voice, male pattern baldness, clitoromegaly, decreased breast size, alterations in libido, male musculature, amenorrhea, oligomenorrhea, anovulation, and infertility.[713] Some changes (e.g., facial hair growth, clitoromegaly, laryngeal enlargement, and deepening of the voice) are not reversible when the drugs are discontinued.

Few specific studies have been performed in women athletes. A study of 10 weight-trained women athletes taking doses of anabolic steroids approximately ninefold higher than recommended confirmed these effects.[670] The drugs were taken in 9-week cycles, and the users averaged about three cycles per year. The majority of these women had facial hair growth, clitoromegaly, increased libido, decreased or absent menstruation, acne, and decreased body fat. The side effects described by some of these women included loss of scalp hair, increased body hair, decreased breast size, and aggressiveness.

Effects on the HPG Axis in Men

A long list of reproductive side effects occur in men, including acne,[668,795] changes in libido,[680] testicular atrophy,[680,686] and a dose-dependent effect on sperm production.[683,796] Serum testosterone levels are suppressed during steroid use[669,682,685,690,693,726,728,797–799] and remain suppressed to half their initial values for 3 to 4 months after high-dose anabolic steroid administration.[682,800,801] Rebound after a lower dose is quicker, so that values were higher than baseline at 6 weeks after discontinuation of the medication.[799] The suppression is probably mediated through effects on gonadotropin production and release,[669,686,800,801] although some researchers have found no evidence of this.[703,722,726] Testicular responsiveness to exogenous hCG appears to be intact.[802] Stromme and colleagues reported a normal free testosterone level with decreased SHBG levels.[726] Acne is accompanied by an increase in the size of the sebaceous glands and the quantity of sebum secreted, the cholesterol and FFA content, and the population of *Propionibacterium acnes* on the skin.[803,804]

Gynecomastia has been seen in children using steroids for medical reasons[805] as well as in mature individuals.[680,790] It is ironic that those seeking to sculpt a perfect physique suffer a side effect that is so clearly inappropriate.[719,806] The development of breast tissue is probably a result of peripheral conversion of androgens to estrogens as estradiol levels increase substantially.[682] Attempts to self-treat with tamoxifen, an antiestrogen, have been unsuccessful.[679]

Other Endocrine Changes

The levels of TSH, total and free thyroxine, triiodothyronine, and TBG are all decreased.[800] Growth hormone increases fivefold- to 60-fold,[800] compatible with changes at puberty.[807] Although there is probably little effect on the ACTH-cortisol axis and no effect on cortisol-binding globulin,[682,750] adrenal androgens are suppressed with reduced levels of DHEA and its sulfate.[801] Insulin resistance and diminished glucose tolerance have also been observed.[808]

Impaired Liver Function Tests

Changes in hepatic function are mostly found with the orally active 17-α alkylated testosterone derivatives.[713] Liver damage can result from intrahepatic cholestasis but is rarely fatal.[713] Evidence of liver damage from injectable anabolic steroids is rare.[713,809] Single sample studies of athletes generally show normal[680,728,736,738,810] or minimally elevated liver enzymes.[665,668,669,686,690,732,778,810,811] Some biochemical changes (e.g., elevated AST and ALT levels) probably reflect muscle damage rather than hepatic dysfunction.[680] It is suggested that liver-specific enzymes (e.g., LDH and alkaline phosphatase) should be used to monitor hepatic function.[680,721,812] When this was done, fewer than 10 percent of athletes appeared to have abnormal liver function tests.[721] Tests generally return to normal when the steroid is discontinued.

Benign and Malignant Tumors of the Liver

Peliosis hepatis, the occurrence of blood-filled cysts in the liver, has been reported in patients receiving anabolic steroids[694,721,809,813–815] but not in athletes to date. Liver cancer has also been reported in patients[713,721,809,814–822] and in a small number of athletes[748,754,755] who used anabolic steroids.

Elevation of Muscle Enzymes

As was indicated above, muscle enzymes are substantially higher in athletes using steroids than in nonusers. Creatinine kinase is also elevated.[823–825] This could reflect an effect of these drugs on the muscles or, more likely, the consequences of pushing muscles harder than would be normally possible. It is not clear what effect the presumed muscle damage might have in the long term. Massive rhabdomyolysis has been described in a weight lifter taking anabolic steroids,[826] but this effect is far more common in marathoners and ultramarathoners.[827]

Miscellaneous Tumors

Wilms' tumor has been reported in association with anabolic steroid use,[693,828] and adenocarcinoma of the prostate has been described in a 40-year-old body builder using anabolic steroid drugs.[829]

Fluid Retention with Occasional Hypertension

Fluid retention is not uncommon with steroid use.[668] The occasional occurrence of hypertension is probably idiosyncratic, as with other sex steroids, although some researchers have observed an elevation of mean systolic blood pressure.[772]

Increased Hematocrit

The use of anabolic steroids to stimulate red blood cell production has been recognized and used clinically for many years.[830] It is not surprising that substantial evidence shows that athletes using anabolic steroids also increase their hematocrit.[680,811]

Changes in Immunity

Some evidence suggests that humoral immunity may be impaired by anabolic steroid use. IgG, IgM, and IgA are significantly lower in anabolic steroid users than in controls.[831,832] The number and relative distribution of T cells was unchanged, but the response to a β-cell mitogen, *Staphylococcus aureus* Cowan Strain I, was enhanced. Natural killer cell activity was also significantly greater in anabolic steroid users.[832] Four of 13 steroid-using body builders and 3 of 8 non-steroid-using body builders had positive antinuclear antibodies.[832]

Risks for Injections by Unqualified Individuals

Since steroids are often given by injection and without medical supervision, it is not surprising that complications from the injections occur. Hematomas and abscesses[833] are reported, and HIV transmission has probably occurred through sharing needles.[834]

Detection of Anabolic Steroids

The focus in detecting banned drugs is on the major games. Widespread press coverage was devoted to disqualifications (and desertions) from the 1983 Panamerican Games and the 1984 and 1988 Olympic Games. It is possible to detect anabolic steroids at picomolar levels using gas chromatography/mass spectrophotometry.[835,836]

The methodologies of the laboratories associated with each of the recent Olympic Games has been published.[835,836] Metabolites of all banned anabolic steroids are readily detected in the urine of tested athletes with less than 30 min of testing using gas chromatography/mass spectrophotometry. Particularly important is the security used in the collection, labeling, and handling of the samples.

The problem, however, does not lie in detecting the drugs at major competitions. The value of anabolic steroids is almost entirely during the training period. Clearance times for water-soluble and fat-soluble drugs are recognized, and it should be impossible to detect the drugs in urine when the drugs are stopped at an appropriate time before the likely time of testing. This is likely to be a problem only when the elimination time is prolonged, as in the oil-based depot preparations. Nandrolone, for example, may take up to 9 months to be eliminated from the urine.

Breakdowns in regimes for avoiding detection should occur only on isolated occasions, but the problem of black market drugs which are often unlabeled or mislabeled means that athletes may not know what they are taking. The individual variation in clearance times means that some way of defining the clearance for each individual athlete would be useful. The very high number of positive tests found in athletes during training[837] suggests that testing facilities have been used by athletes with this purpose in mind. The problem of controlling steroid abuse, therefore, does not lie in the laboratory at the major games.

Controlling the Steroid Epidemic

Approaches to controlling the "steroid epidemic" have included identification of users by testing at competition and during training, control of the manufacture and distribution of steroids, banning possession of these drugs, and education of users and potential users.[837] Mandatory random drug testing has been suggested as the only method to control steroid use, but its acceptability remains limited by law courts and in the case of professional sports by player-management agreements.[657,681] Getting caught at the games remains only a slight deterrent.

Warnings of harmful side effects tend to be unheeded.[717,838,839] Knowledge and acceptance of the benefits is quite high among athletes, while knowledge and acceptance of significant side effects is low.[757] Educational interventions at the high school level have had little effect on intent to take steroids,[840] and some researchers have suggested that education would need to occur in the preteen or early teen years. Practical recommendations for teaching have been made but seem inadequate in view of failures.[841]

The use of the drugs may be proscribed and control of the anabolic steroids may be transferred from the U.S. Food and Drug Administration to the Drug Enforcement Agency.[842] This may not have the desired effect if the policing of anabolic steroids has to compete with the problem of policing hard and soft ilicit recreational drugs as well as alcohol and tobacco.[681,842,843] Many would consider that the use of alcohol by 45 percent of teenagers and the use of amphetamines by 8.5 percent are significantly greater social problems.[715] Controlling prescribing by the few physicians involved is not worthwhile since most of these drugs come from the black market.[837]

It is unlikely in the absence of an international will to control anabolic steroids and other ergogenic aids that attempts to reduce anabolic steroid use will be effective. Winning remains too important.

OTHER ERGOGENIC AIDS

Growth Hormone

The extent of use of GH is not known. Until the advent of synthetic GH, its use was retricted by the availability of the drug. Interest has, however, increased in its use.[844] There are animal data which suggest that it may produce some muscle hypertrophy.[845,846] The adverse effect of persistent high GH levels in patients with acromegaly suggests that supraphysiologic doses may be counterproductive. To date, there are few human data. Decrease in fat mass and an increase in lean body mass were observed with 6 weeks of GH administration in supraphysiologic doses during training in highly trained athletes.[847] It remains unclear how this might translate into enhanced performance. Although there are some obvious concerns related to health, nothing is known about complications of its use in athletes.

Erythropoietin

Blood doping has been banned by the International Olympic Committee but is difficult to detect other than by suppression of erythropoietin levels in the circulation.[848] The availability of recombinant erythropoietin has had a profound effect on some patients with chronic renal failure.[849] Problems with hypertension and coagulation of vascular access were complications. There have been few studies of the effects of erythropoietin in athletes. Endurance runners with low-normal hematologic parameters were unchanged by erythropoietin, but exercise performance does not appear to increase perhaps because of an effect on erythrocyte turnover.[850,851] These drugs are being used,[852] but the extent of use is unknown. This use has been associated with deaths.[853] Since, like growth hormone, there are no urine tests for this drug, athletes may be able to continue its use for the present without detection. The use of this drug does, however, seem rather more dangerous than that of GH or anabolic steroids. The combination of an elevated hematocrit in the resting state with the hemoconcentration associated with prolonged exercise may result in a dangerous increase in blood viscosity in athletes taking erythropoietin.

REFERENCES

1. Rivier J, Spiess J, Thorner M, Vale W: Characterization of a growth hormone releasing factor from a human pancreatic islet cell tumor. *Nature* 300:276–278, 1982.
2. Brazeau P, Vale W, Burgus R, Ling N, Butcher M, Rivier J, Guillemin R: Hypothalamic peptide that inhibits the secretion of immunoreactive growth hormone. *Science* 179:77–79, 1973.
3. Tannenbaum GS, Ling N: The interrelationship of growth hormone (GH)–releasing factor and somatostatin in the generation of the ultradian rhythm of GH secretion. *Endocrinology* 115:1952–1957, 1984.
4. Vance ML, Kaiser DL, Evans WS, Furlanetto R, Vale W, Rivier J, Thorner MO: Pulsatile growth hormone secretion in normal man during a continuous 24 hour infusion of human growth hormone releasing factor (1-40): Evidence for intermittent somatostatin excretion. *J Clin Invest* 75:1584–1590, 1985.
5. Tremblay A, Pinsard D, Coveney S, Catellier C, Laferriere G, Richard D, Nadeau A: Counterregulatory response to insulin-induced hypoglycemia in trained and nontrained humans. *Metabolism* 39:1138–1143, 1990.
6. Hackney AC, Ness RJ, Schrieber A: Effects of endurance exercise on nocturnal hormone concentrations in males. *Chronobiol Int* 6:341–346, 1989.
7. Hurley RS, Bossetti BM, O'Dorisio TM, Welch MA, Rice RR, Tenison EB, Wasson CJ, Malarkey WB: The response of serum growth hormone and prolactin to training in weight-maintaining healthy males. *J Sports Med Phys Fitness* 30:45–48, 1990.
8. Dela F, Mikines KJ, Tronier B, Galbo H: Diminished arginine-stimulated insulin secretion in trained men. *J Appl Physiol* 69:261–267, 1990.
9. Sutton JR, Lazarus L: Growth hormone in exercise: Comparison of physiological and pharmacological stimuli. *J Appl Physiol* 41:523–527, 1976.
10. Friedmann B, Kindermann W: Energy metabolism and regulatory hormones in women and men during endurance exercise. *Eur J Appl Physiol* 59:1–9, 1989.
11. Hagberg JM, Seals DR, Yerg JE, Gavin J, Gingerich R, Premachandra B, Holloszy JO: Metabolic responses to exercise in young and older athletes and sedentary men. *J Appl Physiol* 65:900–908, 1988.
12. Hunter WM, Greenwood FC: Studies on the secretion of pituitary growth hormone. *Br Med J* i:804–807, 1964.
13. Glick SM, Roth J, Yalow RS, Berson SA: The regulation of growth hormone secretion. *Recent Prog Horm Res* 21:241–283, 1965.
14. Okada Y, Hirata T, Ishitobi K, Wada M, Santo Y, Harada Y: Human growth hormone secretion after exercise and oral glucose administration in patients with short stature. *J Clin Endocrinol Metab* 34:1055–1058, 1972.
15. Lacey KA, Hewison A, Parkin JM: Exercise as a screening test for growth hormone deficiency in children. *Arch Dis Child* 48:508–512, 1973.
16. Lin T, Tucci JR: Provocative tests of growth hormone release: A comparison of results with seven stimuli. *Ann Intern Med* 80:464–469, 1974.
17. Seip RL, Weltman A, Goodman D, Rogol AD: Clinical utility of cycle exercise for the physiologic assessment of growth hormone release in children. *Am J Dis Child* 144:998–1000, 1990.
18. Lanes R, Lifshitz F, Sekaran C, Fort P, Recker B: Premarin priming does not alter growth hormone release following exercise. *J Endocrinol Invest* 9:443–446, 1986.
19. Dawson-Hughes B, Stern D, Goldman J, Reichlin S: Regulation of growth hormone and somatomedin-C secretion in postmenopausal women: Effect of physiological estrogen replacement. *J Clin Endocrinol Metab* 63:424–432, 1986.
20. Sutton J, Young JD, Lazarus L, Hickie JB, Maksuytis J: Hormonal changes during exercise. *Lancet* 2:1304–1305, 1968.
21. Sutton JR, Coleman MJ, Casey J, Lazarus L: Androgen responses during physical exercise. *Br Med J* i:520–522, 1973.
22. Hartley LH, Mason JW, Hogan RP, Jones LG, Kotchen TA, Mougey EH, Wherry FE, Pennington LL, Ricketts PT: Multiple hormonal responses to prolonged exercise in relation to physical training. *J Appl Physiol* 33:602–606, 1972.
23. Hartley LH, Mason JW, Hogan RP, Jones LG, Kotchen TA, Mougey EH, Wherry FE, Pennington LL, Ricketts PT: Multiple hormonal responses to graded exercise in relation to physical training. *J Appl Physiol* 33:607–610, 1972.
24. Noel GL, Suh HK, Stone JG, Frantz AG: Human prolactin and growth hormone measurement during surgery and other conditions of stress. *J Clin Endocrinol Metab* 35:840–851, 1972.
25. Bloom SR, Johnson RH, Park DM, Rennie MJ, Sulaimen WR: Differences in the metabolic and hormonal responses to exercise between racing cyclists and untrained individuals. *J Physiol* 258:1–18, 1976.
26. Kuoppasalmi K, Naveri H, Rehunen S, Harkonen M, Adlercreutz H: Effect of strenuous anaerobic running on plasma growth hormone, cortisol luteinizing hormone, testosterone, androstenedione and estrone and estradiol. *J Steroid Biochem* 7:823–829, 1976.
27. Fahey TD, Del Valle-Zuris A, Oehlson G, Trieb M, Seymour J: Pubertal stage differences in hormonal and hematological responses to maximal exercise in males. *J Appl Physiol* 46:823–827, 1979.
28. Gawel MJ, Park DM, Alaghband-Zadeh J, Rose FC: Exercise and hormonal secretion. *Postgrad Med J* 55:373–376, 1979.
29. Farrel PA, Garthwaite TL, Gustafson AB: Plasma adrenocorticotropin and cortisol responses to submaximal and exhaustive exercise. *J Appl Physiol* 55:1441–1444, 1983.
30. Cumming DC, Rebar RW, Stern B, Brunsting LA III, Strich G, Greenberg L, Bremer B, Liu J, et al: The effects of acute exercise on endocrine homeostasis, in Laron Z, Rogol AD (eds): *Hormones and Sport.* Proceedings of Serono Symposium, vol. 55. New York, Raven Press, 1989, pp 73–87.
31. Galbo H: Endocrinology and metabolism in exercise. *Int J Sports Med* 2:203–211, 1981.
32. Karagiorgios A, Garcia JF, Brooks GA: Growth hormone response to continuous and intermittent exercise. *Med Sci Sports* 11:302–307, 1979.
33. Bullen BA, Skrinar GS, Beitins IZ, Carr DB, Reppert SM, Dotson CO, Fencl MM, Gervino EV, McArthur JW: Endurance training effects on plasma hormonal responsiveness and sex hormone secretion. *J Appl Physiol* 56:1453–1463, 1984.
34. Lassarre CF, Girard F, Durard J, Raynaud J: Kinetics of

human growth hormone during submaximal exercise. *J Appl Physiol* 37:826–830, 1974.
35. Sutton JR: Effect of acute hypoxia on the hormonal response to exercise. *J Appl Physiol* 42:587–592, 1977.
36. Raynaud J, Drouet L, Martineaud JP, Bordacher J, Coudert J, Durand J: Time course of plasma growth hormone during exercise in humans at altitude. *J Appl Physiol* 50:229–233, 1981.
37. Naveri H: Blood hormone and metabolite levels during graded cycle ergometer exercise. *Scand J Clin Lab Invest* 45:599–603, 1985.
38. Naveri H, Kuoppasalmi K, Harkonen M: Metabolic and hormonal changes in moderate and intense long-term running exercises. *Int J Sports Med* 6:276–281, 1985.
39. Buckler JMH: Exercise as a screening test for growth hormone. *Arch Dis Child* 69:219–229, 1972.
40. Sutton JR, Jones NL, Toews CJ: Growth hormone secretion in acid base alterations at rest and during exercise. *Clin Sci Mol Med* 50:241–247, 1976.
41. Klimes I, Vigas M, Jurcovicova J, Nemeth S: Lack of effect of acid base alterations on growth hormone secretion in man. *Endocrinol Exp (Bratisl)* 11:155–162, 1977.
42. Hyyppa MT, Aunola S, Kuusela V: Psychoendocrine responses to bicycle exercise in healthy men in good physical condition. *Int J Sports Med* 7:89–93, 1986.
43. Galbo H, Christansen NJ, Mikines KJ, Sonne B, Hilsted J, Fahrenkrug J: The effect of fasting on the hormonal response to graded exercise. *J Clin Endocrinol Metab* 52:1106–1112, 1981.
44. Johanesson A, Hagen C, Galbo H: Prolactin, growth hormone, thyrotropin, 3,5,3′-triiodothyronine and thyroxine responses to exercise after fat and carbohydrate enriched diet. *J Clin Endocrinol Metab* 52:56–61, 1981.
45. Tamborlane WV, Sherwin RS, Koivisto V, Handler R, Gawel M, Felig P: Normalization of the growth hormone and catecholamine response to exercise in juvenile onset diabetics treated with a portable insulin infusion pump. *Diabetes* 28:785–788, 1979.
46. Bonen A, Belcastro AN, MacIntyre K, Gardner I: Hormonal responses during intense exercise preceded by glucose ingestion. *Can J Appl Sport Sci* 5:85–90, 1980.
47. Hansen P: The effect of intravenous glucose infusion on the exercise induced serum growth hormone rise in normals and juvenile diabetics. *Scand J Clin Lab Invest* 28:195–205, 1971.
48. Rennie MJ, Johnson RH: Effect of an exercise diet program on metabolic changes in runners. *J Appl Physiol* 231:967–973, 1974.
49. Gustafson AB, Farrell PA, Kalkhoff RK: Impaired plasma catecholamine response to submaximal treadmill exercise in obese women. *Metabolism* 39:410–417, 1990.
50. Casanueva F, Villanueva L, Penalva A, Vila T, Cabezas-Cerato J: Free fatty acid inhibition of exercise induced growth hormone. *Horm Metab Res* 13:348–350, 1981.
51. Taylor LM, Blockard WG: Effects of lipids on growth hormone synthesis by isolated pituitaries. *Proc Soc Exp Biol Med* 137:1026–1028, 1971.
52. Aizawa T, Yasuda N, Greer MA: Hypoglycemia stimulates ACTH secretion through a direct effect on the basal hypothalamus. *Metabolism* 30:996–1000, 1981.
53. Few JD, Davies CTM: The inhibiting effect of atropine on growth hormone release during exercise. *Eur J Appl Physiol* 43:221–228, 1980.
54. Smythe GA, Lazarus L: Suppression of human growth hormone secretion by melatonin and cyproheptadine. *J Clin Invest* 54:116–121, 1974.
55. Hansen AP: The effect of adrenergic receptor blockade on the exercise induced growth hormone rise in normals and juvenile diabetics. *J Clin Endocrinol Metab* 33:807–812, 1971.
56. Schwinn G, Schwarck H, McIntosh C, Milstrey HR, Willms B, Kobberlin J: Effect of dopamine receptor blocking agent, pimozide, on the growth hormone response to arginine and exercise and on the spontaneous growth hormone fluctuations. *J Clin Endocrinol Metab* 43:1183–1189, 1976.
57. Moretti C, Fabbri A, Gnessi L, Cappa M, Calzolari A, Fraioli F, Grossman A, Besser GM: Naloxone inhibits exercise induced release of prolactin and GH in athletes. *Clin Endocrinol* 18:135–138, 1983.
58. Gil-Ad I, Leibowitch N, Josefsberg Z, Wasserman M, Laron Z: Effect of oral clonidine, insulin-induced hypoglycemia and exercise on plasma GHRH levels in short-stature children. *Acta Endocrinol (Copenh)* 122:89–95, 1990.
59. Arends J, Wagner ML, Willms BL: Cholinergic muscarinic receptor blockade suppresses arginine- and exercise-induced growth hormone secretion in type I diabetic subjects. *J Clin Endocrinol Metab* 66:389–394, 1988.
60. Steardo L, Iovino M, Monteleone P, Agrusta M, Orio F: Pharmacological evidence for a dual GABAergic regulation of growth hormone release in humans. *Life Sci* 39:979–985, 1986.
61. Steardo L, Iovino M, Monteleone P, Agrusta M, Orio F: Evidence for a GABAergic control of the exercise-induced rise in GH in man. *Eur J Clin Pharmacol* 28:607–609, 1985.
62. Smythe GA: The role of serotonin and dopamine in hypothalamic-pituitary function. *Clin Endocrinol (Oxf)* 7:325–341, 1977.
63. Smythe GA, Duncan MW, Bradshaw JE, Cai WY: Serotoninergic control of growth hormone secretion: Hypothalamic dopamine, norepinephrine and serotonin levels and metabolism in three hyposomatotropic rat models and normal rats. *Endocrinology* 110:376–383, 1982.
64. Bivens CH, Lebovitz HE, Feldman JM: Inhibition of hypoglycemia induced growth hormone secretion by the serotonin antagonists cyproheptadine and methysergide. *N Engl J Med* 289:236–239, 1973.
65. Blockard WG, Heidnigsfelder SA: Adrenergic receptor control mechanism for growth hormone secretion. *J Clin Invest* 47:1407–1414, 1968.
66. Lal S, Tolis G, Martin JB, Brown GM, Guyda H: Effect of clonidine on growth hormone, prolactin, luteinizing hormone, follicle stimulating hormone and thyroid stimulating hormone in the serum of normal men. *J Clin Endocrinol Metab* 41:827–832, 1975.
67. Parra A, Schultz RB, Foley TP Jr, Blizard RM: Influence of epinephrine-propranolol infusion on growth hormone release in normal and hypopituitary patients. *J Clin Endocrinol Metab* 30:134–137, 1970.
68. Boyd AE, Lebovitz HE, Pfeiffer JB: Stimulation of human growth hormone secretion by I-dopa. *N Engl J Med* 283:1425–1429, 1970.
69. Maany I, Fraser A, Mandels J: Apomorphine: Effect on GH. *J Clin Endocrinol Metab* 40:162–163, 1975.
70. Camanni F, Massara F, Belforte L, Molinatti GM: Changes in plasma growth hormone levels in normal and acromegalic subjects following administration of an infusion of 2-bromo-alpha-ergocryptine. *J Clin Endocrinol Metab* 40:363–366, 1975.
71. Massara F, Camanni F: Effects of various adrenergic receptor stimulating and blocking agents on HGH secretion. *J Endocrinol* 54:195–200, 1972.
72. Liberman B, Cesar FP, Wajchenberg BL: Human growth hormone (hGH) stimulation tests: The sequential exercise and I-dopa procedure. *Clin Endocrinol (Oxf)* 10:649–654, 1979.
73. Mayer G, Schwinn G: Human growth hormone release: Suppression by TRH and augmentation by bromocryptine (abstract). *Acta Endocrinol (Copenh)* 87:10, 1978.
74. Moretti C, Fabbri A, Gnessi L, Bonifacio V, Fraioli F: Pyridoxine (B6) suppresses the rise in prolactin and increases the rise in growth hormone induced by exercise. *N Engl J Med* 307:444–445, 1982.
75. McClaren NK, Taylor GE, Raiti S: Propranolol augmented, exercise induced human growth hormone release. *Pediatrics* 56:804–807, 1975.

76. Shanis BS, Moshang T: Propranolol and exercise as a screening test for growth hormone deficiency. *Paediatrics* 57:712–714, 1976.
77. Joffe BI, Haitas B, Edelstein D, Panz V, Lamprey JM, Baker SG, Seftel HC: Clonidine and the hormonal responses to graded exercise in healthy subjects. *Horm Res* 23:136–141, 1986.
78. Struthers AD, Burrin JM, Brown MJ: Exercise-induced increases in plasma catecholamines and growth hormone are augmented by selective alpha-2-adrenoceptor blockade in man. *Neuroendocrinology* 44:22–28, 1986.
79. Stubbs WA, Delitala G, Jones A, Jeffcoate WL, Edwards CRW, Ratter SJ, Besser GM: Hormonal and metabolic responses to an enkephalin analogue in normal man. *Lancet* 2:1225–1227, 1978.
80. Spiler IJ, Molitch ME: Lack of modulation of pituitary hormone stress response by neural pathways involving opiate receptors. *J Clin Endocrinol Metab* 50:516–520, 1980.
81. Mayer G, Wessel J, Kobberling J: Failure of naloxone to alter exercise-induced growth hormone and prolactin release in normal men. *Clin Endocrinol (Oxf)* 13:413–416, 1980.
82. Staessen J, Fiocchi R, Bouillon R, Fagard R, Hespel P, Lijnen P, Moerman E, Amery A: Effects of opioid antagonism on the haemodynamic and hormonal responses to exercise. *Clin Sci* 75:293–300, 1988.
83. Farrell PA, Gustafson AB, Garthwaite TL, Kalkhoff RK, Cowley AW Jr, Morgan WP: Influence of endogenous opioids on the response of selected hormones to exercise in humans. *J Appl Physiol* 61:1051–1057, 1986.
84. Carr DB, Bullen BA, Skrinar GS, Arnold MA, Rosenblatt M, Beitins IZ, Martin JB, McArthur JW: Physical conditioning facilitates the exercise-induced secretion of beta-endorphin and beta-lipotropin. *N Engl J Med* 305:560–563, 1981.
85. Fraioli F, Moretti C, Paolucci D, Aliciccio E, Crescenzi F, Fortunio G: Physical exercise stimulates marked concomitant release of beta-endorphin and adrenocorticotropic hormone (ACTH) in peripheral blood in man. *Experientia* 36:987–989, 1981.
86. Gambert SR, Garthwaite TL, Pontzer CH, Cook EE, Tristani FE, Duthie EH, Martinson DR, Hagen TC, McCarty DT: Running elevates plasma beta-endorphin immunoreactivity and ACTH in untrained human subjects. *Proc Soc Exp Biol Med* 168:1–4, 1981.
87. Rosak C, Vogel D, Althoff PH, Neubauer M, Brecht HM, Schoffling K: Hormonal and metabolic parameters following insulin-induced hypoglycemia. *Endokrinologie* 79:337–44, 1982.
88. Schnabel A, Kinderman W, Schmitt WM, Biro G, Stegman H: Hormonal and metabolic consequences of prolonged running at the individual anaerobic threshold. *Int J Sports Med* 3:163–168, 1982.
89. Cumming DC, Rebar RW: Effects of exertion on reproductive function. *Am J Ind Med* 5:113–125, 1983.
90. Koenig J, Mayfield MA, McCann SM, Krulich L: Stimulation of prolactin secretion by morphine: Role of the central serotoninergic system. *Life Sci* 25:853–864, 1979.
91. Karebath M, Doaz JL, Huttunen M: Serotonin synthesis by brain synaptosomes, effect of L-dopa, 1-3-methoxytyrosine, and catecholamines. *Biochem Pharmacol* 21:1245–1251, 1972.
92. Goodwin FK, Dunner DL, Gershon ES: Effect of L-dopa treatment on brain serotonin metabolism in depressed patients. *Life Sci* 10:751–759, 1971.
93. Grossman A, Stubbs WA, Gaillard RC, Delitala G, Rees LH, Besser GM: Studies of the opiate control of prolactin, GH and TSH. *Clin Endocrinol (Oxf)* 14:381–386, 1981.
94. Hunter WM, Fonseke CC, Passmore R: The role of growth hormone in the mobilization of fuel for muscular exercise. *Q J Physiol Cogn Med Sci* 50:406–415, 1965.
95. Raben MS, Hollenberg CH: Effect of growth hormone on plasma fatty acids. *J Clin Invest* 59:484–488, 1965.
96. Daughaday WH, Kipnis DM: The growth promoting actions of somatotropin. *Recent Prog Horm Res* 22:49–99, 1966.
97. Galbo H: *Hormonal and Metabolic Adaptations to Exercise.* New York, Springer-Verlag, 1983.
98. Sutton JR, Case JH: The adrenocortical response to competitive athletics in veteran athletes. *J Clin Endocrinol Metab* 40:135–138, 1975.
99. Tharp GD: The role of glucocorticoids in exercise. *Med Sci Sports* 7:6–11, 1975.
100. Shephard RJ, Sydney KH: Effects of physical exercise on plasma growth hormone and cortisol levels in human subjects. *Exerc Sports Sci Rev* 3:1–30, 1975.
101. Davies CTM, Few JD: Effects of exercise on adrenocortical function. *J Appl Physiol* 35:887–891, 1973.
102. Few JD: Effect of exercise on the secretion and metabolism of cortisol in man. *J Endocrinol* 62:341–353, 1974.
103. Hill SR, Goetz FC, Fox HM, Murawski BJ, Krakauer LJ, Reifenstein RW, Gray SJ, Reddy WJ, et al: Studies on the adrenocortical and psychological responses to stress in man. *Arch Intern Med* 97:269–298, 1955.
104. Cornil A, De Coster A, Copinschi G, Franckson JRM: Effects of muscular exercise on the plasma level of cortisol in man. *Acta Endocrinol (Copenh)* 148:163–168, 1965.
105. Staehelin D, Labhart A, Froesch R, Kagi HR: The effect of muscular exercise and hypoglycemia on the plasma levels of 17-hydroxysteroids in normal adults and in patients with the adrenogenital syndrome. *Acta Endocrinol (Copenh)* 18:521–529, 1955.
106. Loucks AB, Horvath SM: Exercise induced stress responses of amenorrheic and eumenorrheic runners. *J Clin Endocrinol Metab* 59:1109–1120, 1984.
107. Cumming DC, Brunsting LA III, Strich G, Greenberg L, Ries AL, Rebar RW: Reproductive hormone increases in response to acute exercise in men. *Med Sci Sports Exerc* 18:369–373, 1986.
108. Cumming DC, Wall SR, Galbraith MA, Belcastro AN: Reproductive hormone responses to resistance exercise. *Med Sci Sports Exerc* 9:234–238, 1987.
109. Dessypris A, Adlercreutz H: Plasma cortisol, testosterone, androstenedione and luteinizing hormone (LH) in a noncompetitive marathon run. *J Steroid Biochem* 7:33–37, 1976.
110. Adlercreutz H, Dessypris A: Effects of exertion on hormone secretion. *Br Med J* ii:726, 1974.
111. Dessypris A, Wagar G, Fyhrquist F, Makinen T, Welin WG, Lamberg BA: Marathon run: Effects on blood cortisol-ACTH, iodothyronine-TSH, and vasopressin. *Acta Endocrinol (Copenh)* 95:151–157, 1980.
112. Newmark SR, Himathongkam T, Martin RP, Cooper KH, Rose LI: Adrenocortical response to marathon running. *J Clin Endocrinol Metab* 42:393–394, 1976.
113. Galbo H, Houston ME, Christensen NJ, Holst JJ, Nielson B, Nygaard E, Suzuki J: The effect of water temperature on the hormonal response to prolonged swimming. *Acta Physiol Scand* 105:326–337, 1979.
114. Baker ER, Mathur RS, Kirk RF, Landgrebe SC, Moody LO, Williamson HO: Plasma gonadotropins, prolactin, and steroid hormone concentrations immediately after a long-distance run. *Fertil Steril* 38:38–41, 1982.
115. Hale RW, Kosasa TW, Krieger J, Pepper S: A marathon: The immediate effect on female runners' luteinizing hormone, follicle stimulating hormone, prolactin, testosterone and cortisol levels. *Am J Obstet Gynecol* 146:550–556, 1983.
116. Mougin C, Baulay A, Henriet MT, Haton D, Jacquier MC, Turnill D, Berthelay S, Gaillard RC: Assessment of plasma opioid peptides, beta-endorphin and met-enkephalin, at the end of an international nordic ski race. *Eur J Appl Physiol* 56:281–286, 1987.
117. Cashmore GC, Davies CTM, Few JD: Relationship between increases in plasma cortisol concentration and rate of cortisol secretion during exercise in man. *J Endocrinol* 72:109–110, 1977.
118. Rennie MJ, Park DM, Sukaimen WR: Uptake and release of hormones and metabolites by the tissues of exercising leg in man. *Am J Physiol* 231:967–973, 1976.

119. Bohesen E, Egense J: Elimination of endogenous corticosteroids in vivo. *Acta Endocrinol (Copenh)* 33:347–369, 1973.
120. Carr DB, Reppert SM, Bullen B, Skrinar G, Beitins I, Arnold MA, Rosenblatt M, Martins JB, McArthur JW: Plasma melatonin increases during exercise in women. *J Clin Endocrinol Metab* 3:224–225, 1981.
121. Farrell PA, Garthwaite TL, Gustafson AB: Plasma adrenocortical and cortisol responses to submaximal and exhaustive exercise. *J Appl Physiol* 55:1441–1444, 1983.
122. Janal MN, Colt EWD, Clarke WC, Glusman M: Pain sensitivity, mood and plasma endocrine levels in man following long distance running: Effects of naloxone. *Pain* 19:13–25, 1984.
123. Davies CTM, Few JD: Effect of hypoxia on adrenocortical response to exercise in man. *J Endocrinol* 71:175–188, 1976.
124. Howlett TA: Hormonal responses to exercise and training: A short review. *Clin Endocrinol (Oxf)* 26:723–742, 1987.
125. Kraemer RR, Blair S, Kraemer GR, Castracane VD: Effects of treadmill running on plasma beta-endorphin, corticotropin, and cortisol levels in male and female 10K runners. *Eur J Appl Physiol* 58:845–851, 1989.
126. Brandenberger G, Follenius M: Influence of timing and intensity of muscular exercise on temporal patterns of plasma cortisol levels. *J Clin Endocrinol Metab* 4:845–849, 1975.
127. Few CTM, Cashmore GC, Turton G: Adrenocortical response to one leg and two leg exercise on a bicycle ergometer. *Eur J Appl Physiol* 44:167–174, 1980.
128. Viru A, Akke H: Effects of muscular work on cortisol and corticosterone content in the blood and adrenals of guinea pigs. *Acta Endocrinol (Copenh)* 59:61–68, 1969.
129. Wheeler GD, Wall SR, Belcastro AN, Cumming DC: Reduced serum testosterone and prolactin levels in male distance runners. *JAMA* 252:514–516, 1984.
130. Luger A, Deuster PA, Gold PW, Loriaux DL, Chrousos GP: Hormonal responses to the stress of exercise. *Adv Exp Med Biol* 245:273–280, 1988.
131. Luger A, Deuster PA, Kyle SB, Gallucci WT, Montgomery LC, Gold PW, Loriaux DL, Chrousos GP: Acute hypothalamic-pituitary-adrenal responses to the stress of treadmill exercise: Physiologic adaptations to physical training. *N Engl J Med* 316:1309–1315, 1987.
132. Bonen A: Effects of exercise on the excretion rates of urinary free cortisol. *J Appl Physiol* 40:155–158, 1976.
133. Kirwan JP, Costill DL, Flynn MG, Mitchell JB, Fink WJ, Neufer PD, Houmard JA: Physiological responses to successive days of intense training in competitive swimmers. *Med Sci Sports Exerc* 20:255–259, 1988.
134. Barron JL, Noakes TD, Levy W, Smith C, Millar RP: Hypothalamic dysfunction in overtrained athletes. *J Clin Endocrinol Metab* 60:803–806, 1985.
135. Villaneuva AL, Schlosser C, Hopper B, Liu JH, Hoffman DI, Rebar RW: Increased cortisol production in women runners. *J Clin Endocrinol Metab* 63:133–136, 1986.
136. Ronkainen HR, Pakarinen AJ, Kauppila AJ: Adrenocortical function of female endurance runners and joggers. *Med Sci Sports Exerc* 18:385–389, 1986.
137. Tegelman R, Johansson C, Hemmingsson P, Eklof R, Carlstrom K, Pousette A: Endogenous anabolic and catabolic steroid hormones in male and female athletes during off season. *Int J Sports Med* 11:103–106, 1990.
138. Loucks AB, Mortola JF, Girton L, Yen SS: Alterations in the hypothalamic-pituitary-ovarian and the hypothalamic-pituitary-adrenal axes in athletic women. *J Clin Endocrinol Metab* 68:402–411, 1989.
139. Keizer HA, Kuipers H, de Haan J, Janssen GM, Beckers E, Habets L, van Kranenburg G, Geurten P: Effect of a 3-month endurance training program on metabolic and multiple hormonal responses to exercise. *Int J Sports Med* 8(Suppl 3):154–160, 1987.
140. Schwartz B, Cumming DC, Riordan E, Selye M, Yen SSC, Rebar RW: Exercise associated amenorrhea: A distinct entity? *AmJ Obstet Gynecol* 1141:662–670, 1982.
141. Laatikainen T, Virtanen T, Apter D: Plasma immunoreactive β-endorphin in exercise associated amenorrhea. *Am J Obstet Gynecol* 154:94–97, 1986.
142. Ding JH, Sheckter CB, Drinkwater BL, Soules MR, Bremner WJ: High serum cortisol levels in exercise-associated amenorrhea. *Ann Intern Med* 108:530–534, 1988.
143. Suh BY, Liu JH, Bergas SL, Quigley ME, Laughlin GA, Yen SSC: Hypercortisolism in patients with functional amenorrhea. *J Clin Endocrinol Metab* 66:733–739, 1988.
144. Boyar RM, Hellman LD, Roffwarg H, Katz J, Zumoff B, O'Connor J, Bradlow L, Fukushima DK: Cortisol secretion and metabolism in anorexia nervosa. *N Engl J Med* 296:190–193, 1977.
145. Hohtari H, Elovainio R, Salminen K, Laatikainen T: Plasma corticotropin-releasing hormone, corticotropin, and endorphins at rest and during exercise in eumenorrheic and amenorrheic athletes. *Fertil Steril* 50:233–238, 1988.
146. Leistl S, Finnila M-J, Kiuru E: Effects of physical training on hormonal responses to exercise in asthmatic children. *Arch Dis Child* 54:524–528, 1979.
147. Sutton JR: Hormonal and metabolic responses to exercise in subjects of high and low work capacities. *Med Sci Sports* 10:1–6, 1978.
148. White JA, Ismail AH, Bottoms GD: Effect of physical fitness on the adrenocortical response to exercise stress. *Med Sci Sports* 8:113–118, 1976.
149. Buono MJ, Yeager JE, Sucec AA: Effect of aerobic training on the plasma ACTH response to exercise. *J Appl Physiol* 63:2499–2501, 1987.
150. Rose LI, Freidman HW, Bering SC, Cooper KH: Plasma cortisol following a mile run in conditioned subjects. *J Clin Endocrinol Metab* 31:339–341, 1970.
151. Kraemer WJ, Fleck SJ, Callister R, Shealy M, Dudley GA, Maresh CM, Marchitelli L, Cruthirds C, et al: Training responses of plasma beta-endorphin, adrenocorticotropin, and cortisol. *Med Sci Sports Exerc* 21:146–153, 1989.
152. Brandenberger G, Follenius M, Hietter B, Reinhardt B, Simeoni M: Feedback from meal related peaks determines diurnal changes in cortisol response to exercise. *J Clin Endocrinol Metab* 54:592–596, 1982.
153. Hakkinen K, Pakarinen A, Alen M, Kauhanen H, Komi PV: Neuromuscular and hormonal responses in elite athletes to two successive strength training sessions in one day. *Eur J Appl Physiol* 57:133–139, 1988.
154. Severson JA, Fell RD, Griffith DR: Adrenocortical function in response to myocardial necrosis in exercise-trained rats. *J Appl Physiol* 44:104–108, 1978.
155. Song MK, Ianuzzo, Saubert CW, Gollnick PD: The mode of adrenal gland enlargement in the rat. *Pflugers Arch* 339:59–68, 1973.
156. Terjung R: Endocrine response to exercise. *Exerc Sport Sci Rev* 7:153–180, 1979.
157. Huston RL, Askew EW, Tsue JM, Oermann BE: Effect of physical training, exhaustion and cortisol treatment on gluconeogenesis, glycogen stores and endurance in the rat (abstract). *Fed Proc* 32:889, 1973.
158. Issekutz B, Allen M: Effects of methylprednisolone on carbohydrate metabolism of exercise dogs. *J Appl Physiol* 31:813–818, 1871.
159. Czerwinski SM, Kurowski TG, O'Neill TM, Hickson RC: Initiating regular exercise protects against muscle atrophy from glucocorticoids. *J Appl Physiol* 63:1504–1510, 1987.
160. Adlercreutz H, Harkonen M, Kuopposalmi, Naveri H, Huhtaniemi H, Tikkanen H, Remes K, Dessypris A, Karvonen J: Effect of training on plasma anabolic and catabolic steroid hormones and their responses during physical exercise. *Int J Sports Med* 7(suppl):27–28, 1986.
161. Zaworonok ME, Hudson RW, Orban WA: The prolactin response of males to a standard MVO2 treadmill test. *J Androl* 8:378–382, 1987.
162. Keizer HA, Kuipers H, de Haan J, Beckers E, Habets L: Multiple hormonal responses to physical exercise in eumen-

orrheic trained and untrained women. *Int J Sports Med* 8(Suppl 3):139–150, 1987.
163. Hashimoto T, Migita S, Matsubara F: Response of thyrotropin, prolactin and free thyroid hormones to graded exercise in normal male subjects. *Endocrinol Jpn* 33:735–741, 1986.
164. Shangold MM, Gatz JM, Thysen B: Acute effects of exercise on plasma concentrations of prolactin and testosterone in recreational women runners: *Fertil Steril* 35:699–702, 1981.
165. Chang FE, Dodds WG, Sullivan M, Kim MH, Malarkey WB: The acute effects of exercise on prolactin and growth hormone secretion: Comparison between sedentary women and women runners with normal and abnormal cycles. *J Clin Endocrinol Metab* 62:551–556, 1986.
166. Elias AN, Fairshter R, Pandian MR, Domurat E, Kayaleh R: Beta-endorphin/beta-lipotropin release and gonadotropin secretion after acute exercise in physically conditioned males. *Eur J Appl Physiol* 58:522–527, 1989.
167. Tanaka H, Cleroux J, de Champlain J, Ducharme JR, Collu RJ: Persistent effects of a marathon run on the pituitary-testicular axis. *Endocrinol Invest* 9:97–101, 1986.
168. Bouissou P, Brisson GR, Peronnet F, Helie R, Ledoux M: Inhibition of exercise-induced blood prolactin response by acute hypoxia. *Can J Sport Sci* 12:49–50, 1987.
169. Odink J, Van der Beek EJ, Van den Berg H, Bogaards JJ, Thissen JT: Effect of work load on free and sulfate-conjugated plasma catecholamines, prolactin, and cortisol. *Int J Sports Med* 7:352–357, 1986.
170. Ronkainen H: Depressed follicle-stimulating hormone, luteinizing hormone, and prolactin responses to the luteinizing hormone-releasing hormone, thyrotropin-releasing hormone, and metoclopramide test in endurance runners in the hard-training season. *Fertil Steril* 44:755–759, 1985.
171. Brisson GR, Volle MA, De Carufel D, Desharnais M, Tanaka M: Exercise induced dissassociation of the blood prolactin response in young women according to their sports habits. *Horm Metab Res* 12:201–205, 1980.
172. Mougin C, Henriet MT, Baulay A, Haton D, Berthelay S, Gaillard RC: Plasma levels of beta-endorphin, prolactin and gonadrotropins in male athletes after an international nordic ski race. *Eur J Appl Physiol* 57:425–429, 1988.
173. Chang FE, Richards SR, Kim MH, Malarkey WB: Twenty-four hour prolactin profiles and prolactin responses to dopamine in long distance running women. *J Clin Endocrinol Metab* 59:631–635, 1984.
174. De Meirleir K, Baeyens L, L'Hermite M, L'Hermite-Baleriaux M, Olbrecht J, Holmann W: Pergolide mesylate inhibits exercise-induced prolactin release in man. *Fertil Steril* 43:628–631, 1985.
175. Tegelman R, Carlstrom K, Pousette A: Hormone levels in male ice hockey players during the night after a 26-hour cup tournament. *Andrologia* 22:261–268, 1990.
176. Carli G, Bonifazi M, Lodi L, Lupo C, Martelli G, Viti A: Hormonal and metabolic effects following a football match. *Int J Sports Med* 7:36–38, 1986.
177. Hackney AC, Sinning WE, Bruot BC: Hypothalamic-pituitary-testicular axis function in endurance-trained males. *Int J Sports Med* 11:98–103, 1990.
178. Boyden TW, Pamenter RW, Grosso D, Stanforth P, Rotkis T, Wilmore JH: Prolactin responses, menstrual cycles and body composition of women runners. *J Clin Endocrinol Metab.* 54:711–714, 1982.
179. Russell JB, Mitchell D, Musey PI, Collins DC: The role of β-endorphins and catechol-estrogens on the hypothalamic-pituitary axis in female athletes. *Fertil Steril* 42:690–695, 1984.
180. Hakkinen K, Pakarinen A, Alen M, Komi PV: Serum hormones during prolonged training of neuromuscular performance. *Eur J Appl Physiol* 53:287–293, 1985.
181. Hackney AC, Ness RJ, Schrieber A: Effects of endurance exercise on nocturnal hormone concentrations in males. *Chronobiol Int* 6:341–346, 1989.
182. Mannelli M, Pupilli C, Fabbri G, Musante R, De Feo ML, Franchi F, Giusti G: Endogenous dopamine (DA) and DA2 receptors: A mechanism limiting excessive sympathetic-adrenal discharge in humans. *J Clin Endocrinol Metab* 66: 626–631, 1988.
183. De Meirleir KL, Baeyens L, L'Hermite-Baleriaux M, L'Hermite M, Hollmann W: Exercise-induced prolactin release is related to anaerobiosis. *J Clin Endocrinol Metab* 60:1250–1252, 1985.
184. Mastrogiacomo I, Toderini D, Bonanni G, Bordin D: Gonadotropin decrease induced by prolonged exercise at about 55% of the $V_{O_{2max}}$ in different phases of the menstrual cycle. *Int J Sports Med* 11:198–203, 1990.
185. Melin B, Cure M, Pequignot JM, Bittel J: Body temperature and plasma prolactin and norepinephrine relationships during exercise in a warm environment: Effect of dehydration. *Eur J Appl Physiol* 58:146–151, 1988.
186. Brisson GR, Bouchard J, Peronnet F, Boisvert P, Garceau F: Evidence for an interference of selective face ventilation on hyperprolactinemia induced by hyperthermic treadmill running. *Int J Sports Med* 8:387–391, 1987.
187. Brisson GR, Peronnet F, Ledoux M, Pellerin-Massicotte J, Matton P, Garceau F, Boisvert P Jr: Temperature-induced hyperprolactinemia during exercise. *Horm Metab Res* 18: 283–284, 1986.
188. Brisson GR, Audet A, Ledoux M, Matton P, Pellerin-Massicotte J, Peronnet F: Exercise-induced blood prolactin variations in trained adult males: A thermic stress more than an osmotic stress. *Horm Res* 23:200–206, 1985.
189. Christensen SE, Jorgensen O, Moller J, Moller N, Orskov H: Body temperature elevation, exercise and serum prolactin concentrations. *Acta Endocrinol (Copenh)* 109:458–462, 1985.
190. Brisson GR, Boisvert P, Peronnet F, Quirion A, Senecal L: Face cooling-induced reduction of plasma prolactin response to exercise as part of an integrated response to thermal stress. *Eur J Appl Physiol* 58:816–820, 1989.
191. Voigt K, Ziegler M, Grunert-Fuchs M, Bickel U, Fehm-Wolfsdorf G: Hormonal responses to exhausting physical exercise: The role of predictability and controllability of the situation. *Psychoneuroendocrinology* 15:173–184, 1990.
192. Knudtzon J, Bogsnes A, Norman N: Changes in prolactin and growth hormone levels during hypoxia and exercise. *Horm Metab Res* 21:453–454, 1989.
193. Utsunomiya T, Kadota T, Yanaga T: Pituitary hormone responses to exercise at high altitudes. *Nippon Naibunpi Gakkai Zasshi* 60:1214–1226, 1984.
194. Oleshansky MA, Zoltick JM, Herman RH, Mougey EH, Meyerhoff JL: The influence of fitness on neuroendocrine responses to exhaustive treadmill exercise. *Eur J Appl Physiol* 59:405–410, 1990.
195. Mesaki N, Sasaki J, Motobu M, Nabeshima Y, Shoji M, Iwasaki H, Asano K, Eda M: Effect of naloxone on hormonal changes during exercise. *Nippon Sanka Fujinka Gakkai Zasshi* 41:1991–1998, 1989.
196. Coiro V, Passeri M, Davoli C, Bacchi-Modena A, Bianconi L, Volpi R, Chiodera P: Oxytocin reduces exercise-induced ACTH and cortisol rise in man. *Acta Endocrinol (Copenh)* 119:405–412, 1988.
197. Bramnert M, Hokfelt B: The influence of naloxone on exercise-induced increase in plasma pituitary hormones and the subjectively experienced level of exhaustion in healthy males. *Acta Endocrinol (Copenh)* 115:125–130, 1987.
198. Grossman A, Bouloux P, Price P, Drury PL, Lam KS, Turner T, Thomas J, Besser GM, Sutton J: The role of opioid peptides in the hormonal responses to acute exercise in man. *Clin Sci* 67:483–491, 1984.
199. Smallridge RC, Whorton NE, Burman KD, Ferguson EW: Effects of exercise and physical fitness on the pituitary-thyroid axis and on prolactin secretion in male runners. *Metabolism* 34:949–954, 1985.
200. De Meirleir K, L'Hermite-Baleriaux M, L'Hermite M, Rost R, Hollmann W: Evidence for serotoninergic control of exercise-

induced prolactin secretion. *Horm Metab Res* 17:380–381, 1985.

201. Terjung RL, Tipton CM: Plasma thyroxine and thyroid stimulating hormone levels during submaximal exercise in humans. *Am J Physiol* 220:1840–1845, 1971.
202. Mason JW, Hartley LH, Kotchen TA, Wherry FE, Pennington LL, Jones LG: Plasma thyroid stimulating hormone response in anticipation of muscular exercise in the human. *J Clin Endocrinol Metab* 37:403–406, 1973.
203. Stock MJ, Chapman C, Stirling JL, Campbell IT: Effects of exercise, altitude and food on blood hormone and metabolite levels. *J Appl Physiol* 45:350–354, 1978.
204. Berchtold P, Berger M, Cuppers HJ, Herrmann J, Nieschlag E, Rudorff K, Zimmerman H, Kruskemper HL: Non-glucoregulatory hormones (T4, T3, rT3, TSH, testosterone) during physical exercise in juvenile-type diabetics. *Horm Metab Res* 10:269–273, 1978.
205. Federspil G, Franchimont P, Hazee-Hagelstein MT: Serum TSH and prolactin levels during prolonged muscular exercise in man. *Horm Metab Res* 8:323–324, 1977.
206. Opstad PK, Falch D, Oktedalen O, Fonnum F, Wergeland R: The thyroid function in young men during prolonged exercise and the effect of energy and sleep deprivation. *Clin Endocrinol (Oxf)* 20:657–669, 1984.
207. Refsum HE, Stromme SB: Serum thyroxine, tri-iodothyronine and thyroid stimulating hormone after prolonged heavy exercise. *Scand J Clin Lab Invest* 39:455–459, 1979.
208. Galbo H, Hummer L, Petersen IB, Christensen NJ, Bie N: Thyroid and testicular hormone responses to graded and prolonged exercise in man. *Eur J Appl Physiol* 36:101–106, 1977.
209. Sander M, Rocker L: Influence of marathon running on thyroid hormones. *Int J Sports Med* 9:123–126, 1988.
210. Kirkeby K, Stromme SB, Bjerkedahl I, Hertzenberg L, Refsum HE: Effects of prolonged, strenuous exercise on lipids and thyroxine in serum. *Acta Med Scand* 202:463–467, 1977.
211. DeNayer P, Malvaux P, Ostyn M, Vand Den Schreick HG, Beckers C, DeVisscher M: Serum free thyroxine and binding proteins after muscular exercise. *J Clin Endocrinol Metab* 28:714–716, 1968.
212. O'Connell M, Robbins DC, Horton ES, Sims EAH, Danforth E Jr: Changes in serum concentration of 3,5,3′-triiodothyronine during prolonged moderate exercise. *J Clin Endocrinol Metab* 49:242–246, 1979.
213. Caralis DG, Edwards L, David PJ: Serum total and free thyroxine and triiodothyronine during dynamic muscular exercise in man. *Am J Physiol* 233:E115–E118, 1977.
214. Hesse V, Vilser C, Scheibe J, Jahreis G, Foley T: Thyroid hormone metabolism under extreme body exercises. *Exp Clin Endocrinol* 94:82–88, 1989.
215. Irvine CHG: Effect of exercise on thyroxine degradation in athletes and non-athletes. *J Clin Endocrinol Metab* 28:942–948, 1968.
216. Balsam A, Leppo E: Effect of physical training on the metabolism of thyroid hormones in man. *J Appl Physiol* 38:212–215, 1975.
217. Boyden TW, Parmenter RW, Stanforth P, Rotkin T, Wilmore JH: Evidence for mild thyroidal impairment in women undergoing endurance training. *J Clin Endocrinol Metab* 53:53–56, 1982.
218. Boyden TW, Parmenter RW, Rotkis TC, Stanforth P, Wilmore JH: Thyroidal changes associated with endurance training. *Med Sci Sports Exerc* 16:243–248, 1984.
219. Pakarinen A, Alen M, Hakkinen K, Komi P: Serum thyroid hormones, thyrotropin and thyroxine binding globulin during prolonged strength training. *Eur J Appl Physiol* 57:394–398, 1988.
220. Poehlman ET, Tremblay A, Nadeau A, Dussault J, Theriault G, Bouchard C: Heredity and changes in hormones and metabolic rates with short-term training. *Am J Physiol* 250:E711–E717, 1986.
221. Hohtari H, Pakarinen A, Kauppila A: Serum concentrations of thyrotropic, thyroxine, triiodothyronine and thyroxine binding globulin in female endurance runners and joggers. *Acta Endocrinol (Copenh)* 114:41–46, 1987.
222. Caron PJ, Sopko G, Stolk JM, Jacobs DR, Nisula BC: Effect of physical conditioning on measures of thyroid hormone action. *Horm Metab Res* 18:206–208, 1986.
223. Hooper PL, Rhodes BA, Conway MJ: Exercise lowers thyroid radioiodine uptake: Concise communication. *J Nucl Med* 21:835–837, 1980.
224. Poehlman ET, McAuliffe TL, Van Houten DR, Danforth E Jr: Influence of age and endurance training on metabolic rate and hormones in healthy men. *Am J Physiol* 259:E66–E72, 1990.
225. Cumming DC, Grainger JA, Campbell LG, Wall SR: TSH and prolactin responses to TRH in a treated hypothyroid athlete: Effect of activity and rest. *J Sports Med Phys Fitness* 25:243–245, 1985.
226. Eipper BA, Mains RE: Structure and biosynthesis of pro-adrenocorticotropin/endorphin and related peptides. *Endocr Rev* 1:1–27, 1980.
227. Kjaer M, Secher NH, Bach FW, Sheikh S, Galbo H: Hormonal and metabolic responses to exercise in humans: Effect of sensory nervous blockade. *Am J Physiol* 257:E95–E101, 1989.
228. De Meirleir K, Naaktgeboren N, Van Steirteghem A, Gorus F, Olbrecht J, Block P: Beta-endorphin and ACTH levels in peripheral blood during and after aerobic and anaerobic exercise. *Eur J Appl Physiol* 55:5–8, 1986.
229. Oltras CM, Mora F, Vives F: Beta-endorphin and ACTH in plasma: Effects of physical and psychological stress. *Life Sci* 40:1683–1686, 1987.
230. Kraemer WJ, Patton JF, Knuttgen HG, Marchitelli LJ, Cruthirds C, Damokosh A, Harman E, Frykman P, Dziados JE: Hypothalamic-pituitary-adrenal responses to short-duration high-intensity cycle exercise. *J Appl Physiol* 66:161–166, 1986.
231. Elliot DL, Goldberg L, Watts WJ, Orwoll E: Resistance exercise and plasma beta-endorphin/beta-lipotrophin immunoreactivity. *Life Sci* 34:515–518, 1984.
232. McMurray RG, Hill D, Field KM: Diurnal variations of beta-endorphin at rest and after moderate intensity exercise. *Chronobiol Int* 7:135–142, 1990.
233. Colt EWD, Wardlaw SL, Franz AG: The effect of running on plasma beta-endorphin. *Life Sci* 28:1637–1640, 1981.
234. Bortz WM II, Angwin P, Mefford IN, Boarder MR, Noyce N, Barachas JD: Catecholamines, dopamine and endorphin levels during extreme exercise (letter). *N Engl J Med* 305:466–467, 1981.
235. Dearman J, Francis KT: Plasma levels of catecholamines, cortisol, and β-endorphins in male athletes after running 26.2, 6, and 2 miles. *J Sports Med* 23:30–38, 1983.
236. Goldfarb AH, Hatfield BD, Armstrong D, Potts J: Plasma beta-endorphin concentration: Response to intensity and duration of exercise. *Med Sci Sports Exerc* 22:241–244, 1990.
237. Rahkila P, Hakala E, Alen M, Salminen K, Laatikainen T: Beta-endorphin and corticotropin release is dependent on a threshold intensity of running exercise in male endurance athletes. *Life Sci* 43:551–558, 1988.
238. McMurray RG, Forsythe WA, Mar MH, Hardy CJ: Exercise intensity-related responses of beta-endorphin and catecholamines. *Med Sci Sports Exerc* 19:570–574, 1987.
239. Farrell PA, Gates WK, Maksud MG, Morgan WP: Increases in plasma beta-endorphin/beta-lipotropin activity after treadmill running in humans. *J Appl Physiol* 52:1245–1259, 1982.
240. Langenfeld ME, Hart LS, Kao PC: Plasma beta-endorphin responses to one-hour bicycling and running at 60% $V_{O_{2max}}$. *Med Sci Sports Exerc* 19:83–86, 1987.
241. Petraglia F, Bacchi Modena A, Comitini G, Scazzina D, Facchinetti F, Fiaschetti D, Genazzani AD, Barletta D, et al: Plasma beta-endorphin and beta-lipotropin levels increase in well trained athletes after competition and non competitive exercise. *J Endocrinol Invest* 13:19–23, 1990.

242. Brooks S, Burrin J, Cheetham ME, Hall GM, Yeo T, Williams C: The responses of the catecholamines and beta-endorphin to brief maximal exercise in man. *Eur J Appl Physiol* 57:230–234, 1988.
243. Petraglia F, Barletta C, Facchinetti F, Spinazzola F, Monzani A, Scavo D, Genazzani AR: Response of circulating adrenocorticotropin, beta-endorphin, beta-lipotropin and cortisol to athletic competition. *Acta Endocrinol (Copenh)* 118:332–336, 1988.
244. Lartigue M, Louisy F, Habrioux G, Guezennec CY, Galen FX: La réponse du peptide natriuretique auriculaire à l'exercise physique, est inhibée par un antagoniste des récepteurs opiaces. *Pathol Biol (Paris)* 37:831–835, 1989.
245. Kelso TB, Herbert WG, Gwazdauskas FC, Goss FL, Hess JL: Exercise, thermoregulatory stress and increased plasma β-endorphin/β-lipotropin in humans. *J Appl Physiol* 57:444–449, 1984.
246. De Meirleir K, Arentz T, Hollmann W, Vanhaelst L: The role of endogenous opiates in thermal regulation of the body during exercise. *Br Med J* 290:739–740, 1985.
247. Schwellnus MP, Gordon NF: The role of endogenous opioids in thermoregulation during submaximal exercise. *Med Sci Sports Exerc* 19:575–578, 1987.
248. Schwellnus MP, Gordon NF: Effect of opioid antagonism on esophageal temperature during exercise. *Med Sci Sports Exerc* 20:381–384, 1988.
249. Farrel PA: Exercise and the endogenous opioids. *N Engl J Med* 305:1591–1592, 1981.
250. Howlett TA, Tomlin S, Ngahfong L, Rees LH, Bullen BA, Skrinar GS, McArthur JW: Release of β-endorphin and met-enkephalin during exercise in normal women: Response to training. *Br Med J* 288:1950–1952, 1984.
251. Farrell PA: Exercise and endorphins—male responses. *Med Sci Sports Exerc* 17:89–93, 1985.
252. Donevan RH, Andrew GM: Plasma beta-endorphin immunoreactivity during graded cycle ergometry. *Med Sci Sports Exerc* 19:229–233, 1987.
253. Farrell PA, Kjaer M, Bach FW, Galbo H: Beta-endorphin and adrenocorticotropin response to supramaximal treadmill exercise in trained and untrained males. *Acta Physiol Scand* 130:619–625, 1987.
254. Rahkila P, Hakala E, Salminen K, Laatikainen T: Response of plasma endorphins to running exercises in male and female endurance athletes. *Med Sci Sports Exerc* 19:451–455, 1987.
255. Lobstein DD, Ismail AH: Decreases in resting plasma beta-endorphin/-lipotropin after endurance training. *Med Sci Sports Exerc* 21:161–166, 1989.
256. Pestell RG, Hurley DM, Vandongen R: Biochemical and hormonal changes during a 1000 km ultramarathon. *Clin Exp Pharmacol Physiol* 16:353–361, 1989.
257. Thoren P, Floras JS, Hoffmann P, Seals DR: Endorphins and exercise: Physiological mechanisms and clinical implications. *Med Sci Sports Exerc* 22:417–428, 1990.
258. McMurray RG, Hardy CJ, Roberts S, Forsythe WA, Mar MH: Neuroendocrine responses of type A individuals to exercise. *Behav Med* 15:84–92, 1989.
259. Nakao K, Nakai Y, Oki S, Matsubara S, Konishi T, Nishitani H, Imura H: Immunoreactive β-endorphin in human cerebrospinal fluid. *J Clin Endocrinol Metab* 50:230–233, 1980.
260. Rapoport SI, Klee WA, Pettigrew KD, Ohno K: Entry of opioid peptides into the central nervous system. *Science* 207:84–86, 1980.
261. Radosevich PM, Nash JA, Lacy DB, O'Donovan C, Williams PE, Abumrad NN: Effects of low- and high-intensity exercise on plasma and cerebrospinal fluid levels of ir-beta-endorphin, ACTH, cortisol, norepinephrine and glucose in the conscious dog. *Brain Res* 498:89–98, 1989.
262. Fiatarone MA, Morley JE, Bloom ET, Benton D, Makinodan T, Solomon GF: Endogenous opioids and the exercise-induced augmentation of natural killer cell activity. *J Lab Clin Med* 112:544–552, 1988.
263. Farrell PA, Sonne B, Mikines K, Galbo H: Stimulatory role for endogenous opioid peptides on postexercise insulin secretion in rats. *J Appl Physiol* 65:744–749, 1988.
264. Farrell PA, Mikines KJ, Bach FW, Sonne B, Galbo H: Plasma beta endorphin immunoreactivity: Effects of sustained hyperglycemia with and without prior exercise. *Life Sci* 39:965–971, 1986.
265. Surbey GS, Andrew GM, Cervenko FW, Hamilton PP: Effects of naloxone on exercise performance. *J Appl Physiol* 57:674–679, 1984.
266. Tal A, Pasterkamp H, Chernick V: Endogenous opiates and response to exercise in asthmatic children and adolescents. *Pediatr Pulmonol* 1:46–51, 1985.
267. Bramnert M, Hokfelt B: Lack of effect of naloxone in a moderate dosage on the exercise induced increase in blood pressure, heart rate, plasma catecholamines, plasma renin activity and plasma aldosterone in healthy males. *Clin Sci* 68:185–191, 1984.
268. Ellestad MH, Kuan P: Naloxone and asymptomatic ischemia: Failure to induce angina during exercise testing. *Am J Cardiol* 54:982–984, 1984.
269. McMurray RG, Sheps DS, Guinan DM: Effects of naloxone on maximal stress testing in females. *J Appl Physiol* 56:436–440, 1984.
270. Leslie RGD, Bellamy D, Pyke DA: Asthma induced by enkephalin. *Br Med J* 1:18–19, 1980.
271. Staessen J, Fiocchi R, Fagard R, Hespel P, Amery A: Carotid baroreflex sensitivity at rest and during exercise is not influenced by opioid receptor antagonism. *Eur J Appl Physiol* 59:131–137, 1989.
272. Kirsch JL, Muro JR, Stansbury DW, Fischer CE, Monfore R, Light RW: Effect of naloxone on maximal exercise performance and control of ventilation in COPD. *Chest* 96:761–766, 1989.
273. Mahler DA, Cunningham LN, Skrinar GS, Kraemer WJ, Colice GL: Beta-endorphin activity and hypercapnic ventilatory responsiveness after marathon running. *J Appl Physiol* 66:2431–2436, 1989.
274. Imai N, Stone CK, Woolf PD, Liang CS: Effects of naloxone on systemic and regional hemodynamic responses to exercise in dogs. *J Appl Physiol* 64:1493–1499, 1988.
275. Griffis C, Kaufman RD, Ward SA: Naloxone and the ventilatory response to exercise in man. *Eur J Appl Physiol* 55:624–629, 1986.
276. Gaillard RC, Bachman M, Rochat T, Egger D, de Haller R, Junod AF: Exercise induced asthma and endogenous opioids. *Thorax* 41:350–354, 1986.
277. Gordon NF, Duncan JJ, Kohl HW: Effect of opioid antagonism on the ability to tolerate maximal anaerobic exercise. *S Afr Med J* 76:268–269, 1989.
278. Strassman RJ, Appenzeller O, Lewy AJ, Qualls CR, Peake GT: Increase in plasma melatonin, beta-endorphin, and cortisol after a 28.5-mile mountain race: Relationship to performance and lack of effect of naltrexone. *J Clin Endocrinol Metab* 69:540–545, 1989.
279. Black J, Chesher JB, Starmer GA, Egger G: The painlessness of the long distance runners. *Med J Aust* 1:522–523, 1979.
280. Haier RJ, Quaid K, Mills JSC: Naloxone alters pain perception after jogging. *Psychiatry Res* 5:231–232, 1981.
281. Shyu B-C, Andersson SA, Thoren P: Endorphin mediated increase in pain threshold induced by long-lasting exercise in rats. *Life Sci* 30:833–840, 1982.
282. Colt EWD: Coronary artery disease in marathon runners (letter). *N Engl J Med* 302:57, 1980.
283. Droste C, Meyer-Blankenburg H, Greenlee MW, Roskamm H: Effect of physical exercise on pain thresholds and plasma beta-endorphins in patients with silent and symptomatic myocardial ischaemia. *Eur Heart J* 9(Suppl N):25–33, 1988.
284. Timonen S, Procope B-J: Premenstrual syndrome and physical exercise. *Acta Obstet Gynecol Scand* 50:331–337, 1971.
285. Paulev PE, Thorboll JE, Nielsen U, Kruse P, Jordal R, Bach

FW, Fenger M, Pokorski M: Opioid involvement in the perception of pain due to endurance exercise in trained man. *Jpn J Physiol* 39:67–74, 1989.
286. Morgan WP: Negative addiction in runners. *Med Sci Sports Exerc* 7:52–67, 1979.
287. Mayer J, Marshall NB, Vitale JJ, Christensen JH, Mashanlkhi MB, Stone FJ: Exercise, food intake and body weight in normal rats and genetically obese adult mice. *Am J Physiol* 177:544–548, 1954.
288. Thomas BM, Miller AT: Adaptation to forced exercise in the rat. *Am J Physiol* 193:350–354, 1958.
289. Stevenson JAF, Fox BM, Feleki V, Beaton JR, Bouts of exercise and food intake in the rat. *J Appl Physiol* 21:118–122, 1966.
290. Oscai LB, Holloszy JO: Effects of weight changes produced by exercise, food restriction or overeating on body composition. *J Clin Invest* 48:2124–2128, 1969.
291. Pitts GC, Bull LS: Exercise, dietary obesity and growth in the rat. *Am J Physiol* 232:R38–R44, 1977.
292. Nickoletseas MM: Food intake in the exercising rat: A brief review. *Neurosci Biobehav Rev* 4:265–267, 1980.
293. Tsuji K, Katayama Y, Oishi N: Effects of dietary protein level on energy metabolism of rats during exercise. *J Nutr Sci Vitaminol (Tokyo)* 21:437–449, 1975.
294. Brownell KD, Stunkard AJ: Physical activity in the development and control of obesity, in Stunkard AJ (ed): *Obesity*. Philadelphia, Saunders, 1980, pp 300–324.
295. Nance DM, Bromley B, Barnard RJ, Gorski RA: Sexually dimorphic effects of forced exercise on food intake and body weight in the rat. *Physiol Behav* 19:155–158, 1977.
296. Crews J, Aldinger EA: Effect of chronic exercise on myocardial function. *Am Heart J* 74:536–547, 1967.
297. Katch VL, Martin R, Martin J: Effects of exercise intensity on food consumption in the male rat. *Am J Clin Nutr* 32:1401–1407, 1979.
298. Mayer J, Roy P, Mitra KP: Relation between caloric intake, body weight and physical work: Studies in an industrial population in West Bengal. *Am J Clin Nutr* 4:169–175, 1956.
299. Watt EW, Wiley J, Fletcher G: Effect of dietary control and exercise training on daily food intake and serum lipids in postmyocardial infarction patients. *Am J Clin Nutr* 29:900–904, 1976.
300. Katch FI, Michael ED, Jones EM: Effect of physical training on the body composition and diet of females. *Res Quart* 40:99–103, 1969.
301. Johnson RE, Mastropoulos JA, Wharton MA: Exercise dietary intake and body composition. *J Am Diet Assoc* 61:399–403, 1972.
302. Edholm OG, Fletcher JG, Widdowson EM, McCance RA: Energy expenditure and food intake of individual men. *Br J Nutr* 9:286–300, 1955.
303. Morley JE, Levine AS: The central control of appetite. *Lancet* 2:398–401, 1983.
304. Grandison L, Guidotti A: Stimulation of food intake by muscimol and beta-endorphin. *Neuropharmacology* 16:533–536, 1977.
305. Leibowitz SF, Hor L: Endorphinergic and alpha-adrenergic systems in the paraventricular nucleus: Effects on eating behaviour. *Peptides* 3:421–428, 1982.
306. Mckay LD, Kenney NJ, Edens NK, Williams RH, Woods SC: Intracerebroventricular beta-endorphin increases food intake in rats. *Life Sci* 29:1429–1434, 1981.
307. Holtzman SG: Effects of narcotic antagonists on fluid intake in the rat. *Life Sci* 16:1465–1470, 1975.
308. Holtzman SG: Suppression of appetite behaviour in the rat by naloxone: Lack of effect of prior morphine dependance. *Life Sci* 24:219–226, 1979.
309. Margules DL, Moisset B, Lewis MJ, Shibuya H, Pert CB: β-endorphin is associated with overeating in genetically obese mice (ob/ob) amd rats (fa/fa). *Science* 202:988–991, 1978.
310. Maikel RP, Brauch MC, Zabik JE: The effects of various narcotic agonists and antagonists on deprivation induced fluid consumption. *Neuropharmacology* 16:863–866, 1977.
311. Kirkham TC, Blundell JE: Dual action of naloxone on feeding revealed by behavioural analysis: Separate effects on initiation and termination of eating. *Appetite* 5:47–54, 1984.
312. Fishman SM, Carr DB: Naloxone blocks exercise stimulated water intake in the rat. *Life Sci* 32:2523–2527, 1983.
313. Morley JE, Levine AS, Grace M, Kneip J: Dynorphin (1-13), dopamine and feeding in rats. *Pharmacol Biochem Behav* 16:701–705, 1982.
314. Davis JM, Lamb DR, Lowy MT, Yim GKW, Malven PV: Opioid modulation of feeding behaviour following forced swimming exercise in male rats. *Pharmacol Biochem Behav* 23:701–707, 1985.
315. Brobeck JR: Food intake as a mechanism of temperature. *Yale J Biol Med* 20:545–555, 1948.
316. Davis JM, Lamb DR, Yim GKW, Malven PV: Opioid modulation of feeding behaviour following repeated exposure to forced swimming exercise in male rats. *Pharmacol Biochem Behav* 23:709–714, 1985.
317. Rossier J, French ED, Rivier C, Ling N, Guillemin R, Bloom FE: Footshock induced stress increases β-endorphin levels in blood but not brain. *Nature* 270:618–620, 1977.
318. Feighner JP, Robins E, Guze SB, Woodruff RA, Winokur G, Munoz R: Diagnostic criteria for use in psychiatric research. *Arch Gen Psychiatry* 26:57–63, 1972.
319. Smith ND: Excessive weight loss and food aversion in athletes simulating anorexia nervosa. *Pediatrics* 66:139–142, 1980.
320. Norval JD: Running anorexia. *S Afr Med J* 58:1024, 1980.
321. Henry SJP: The price of perfection. *The Runner* 4(6):35–39, 1982.
322. Rosen LW, McKeag DB, Hough DO, Curley V: Pathogenic weight control behaviour in female athletes. *Phys Sports Med* 14(1):79–86, 1986.
323. Sours JA: Running: Anorexia nervosa and perfection, in Sachs MH, Sachs ML (eds): *Psychology of Running*. Champaign, IL, Human Kinetic, 1981, pp 80–91.
324. Yates A, Leehay K, Shisslak CM: Running an analogue of anorexia nervosa. *N Engl J Med* 308:251–255, 1983.
325. Blumenthal JA, O'Toole LC, Chang JL: Is running an analogue of anorexia nervosa? *JAMA* 252:520–523, 1984.
326. Wheeler GD, Wall SR, Belcastro AN, Conger P, Cumming DC: Are anorexic tendencies prevalent in the habitual runner? *Br J Sports Med* 20:77–81, 1986.
327. Routtenberg A, Kuznesof AW: Self-starvation of rats living in activity wheels on a restricted feeding schedule. *J Comp Physiol Psychol* 64:414–421, 1976.
328. Epling WF, Pierce WD, Stefan L: Schedule induced self starvation: Possible implications for anorexia nervosa, in Bradshaw CM, Szabadi E, Lowe CF (eds): *Quantification of Steady State Operant Behaviour*. Amsterdam, Elsevier, 1981, pp 393–397.
329. Kaye WH, Pickar D, Naber D, Ebert MH: Cerebrospinal fluid opioid activity in anorexia nervosa. *Am J Psychiatry* 139:643–645, 1982.
330. Moore R, Mills IH, Forster A: Naloxone in the treatment of anorexia nervosa: Effect on weight gain and lipolysis. *J R Soc Med* 74:129–131, 1981.
331. Folkins CH, Lynch S: Psychological fitness as a function of physical fitness. *Arch Phys Med Rehabil* 53:503–508, 1972.
332. Greist JH, Klein MH, Eischens RR, Faris JT: Running out of depression. *Phys Sports Med* 6(12):49–51, 1978.
333. Jorgensen CB, Jorgensen DE: The effect of running on perception of self and others. *Percept Mot Skills* 48:242–246, 1979.
334. Leonardson GR: Relationship between self-concept and perceived physical fitness. *Percept Mot Skills* 47:1215–1218, 1978.
335. McCann IL, Holmes DS:Influence of aerobic exercise on depression. *J Pers Soc Psychol* 46:1142–1147, 1984.
336. Morgan WP, Roberts JA, Brand FR, Feinerman AD: Psycho-

logical effect of chronic physical activity. *Med Sci Sports Exerc* 2:213–217, 1970.
337. Bahrke MS, Morgan WP; Anxiety reduction following exercise and meditation. *Cogn Ther Res* 2:323–333, 1978.
338. DeVries HA, Wiswell RA, Bulbulian R, Moritani T: Tranquilizer effect of exercise. *Am J Phys Med* 60:57–66, 1981.
339. Morgan WP: Anxiety reduction following acute physical activity. *Psychiatr Ann* 9:36–45, 1979.
340. Mandell AJ: The second second wind. *Psychiatr Ann* 9:57–69, 1979.
341. Markoff RA, Ryan P, Young T: Endorphins and mood changes in long distance running. *Med Sci Sports Exerc* 14:11–15, 1982.
342. Williams JM, Getty D: Effect of levels of exercise on psychological mood states, physical fitness, and plasma beta-endorphin. *Percept Mot Skills* 63:1099–1105, 1986.
343. Goldfarb AH, Hatfield BD, Sforzo GA, Flynn MG: Serum beta-endorphin levels during a graded exercise test to exhaustion. *Med Sci Sports Exerc* 19:78–82, 1987.
344. Kraemer RR, Dzewaltowski DA, Blair MS, Rinehardt KF, Castracane VD: Mood alteration from treadmill running and its relationship to beta-endorphin, corticotropin, and growth hormone. *J Sports Med Phys Fitness* 30:241–246, 1990.
345. Glasser W: *Positive Addiction.* New York, Harper & Row, 1976.
346. Sachs ML: Running addiction, in Sachs MH, Sachs ML (eds): *The Psychology of Running.* Champaign, IL, Human Kinetics, 1981, pp 116–126.
347. Steinberg H, Sykes EA: Introduction to symposium on endorphins and behavioural processes: Review of literature on endorphins and exercise. *Pharmacol Biochem Behav* 23: 857–862, 1985.
348. Baekland F: Exercise deprivation: Sleep and psychological reactions. *Arch Gen Psychiatry* 22:365–369, 1970.
349. Christie MJ, Chesher GB: Physical dependence on physiologically released endogenous opiates. *Life Sci* 30:1173–1177, 1982.
350. Potter CD, Borer KT: Opiate receptor blockade reduces voluntary running but not self-stimulation in hamsters. *Pharmacol Biochem Behav* 18:217–223, 1983.
351. Blake MJ, Stein EA, Vomachka AJ: Effects of exercise on brain opioid peptides and serum LH in rats. *Peptides* 5:953–958, 1981.
352. Shyu BC, Andersson SA, Thoren P: Spontaneous running in wheels: A microprocessor assisted method for measuring physiological parameters in rodents. *Acta Physiol Scand* 121:103–109, 1984.
353. Rose LI, Carroll DR, Lowe SL, Peterson EW, Cooper KH: Serum electrolyte changes after marathon running. *J Appl Physiol* 29:449–451, 1970.
354. Raizy L, Au W, Scheer R: Studies on the renal concentrating mechanism: III. The effect of heavy exercise. *J Clin Invest* 39:8–13, 1959.
355. Castenfors J: Renal function during prolonged exercise. *Ann NY Acad Sci* 301:151–159, 1978.
356. Kachadorian WA, Johnson RE: Renal responses to various rates of exercise. *J Appl Physiol* 28:743–752, 1970.
357. Vera R, Croxatto H: Muscular work and antidiuretic substance in the blood. *J Appl Physiol* 7:172–175, 1954.
358. Beardwell CG, Geleen G, Palmer HM, Roberts D, Salamonson L: Radioimmunoassay of plasma vasopressin in physiological and pathological states in man. *J Endocrinol* 67:189–202, 1975.
359. Baylis PH, Heath DA: The development of a radioimmunoassay for the measurement of human arginine vasopressin. *Clin Endocrinol (Oxf)* 7:91–102, 1977.
360. Viti A, Lupo C, Lodi L, Bonifazi M, Martelli G: Hormonal changes after supine posture, immersion, and swimming. *Int J Sports Med* 10:402–405, 1989.
361. Lenz T, Weiss M, Werle E, Walz U, Kohler U, Pinther J, Weicker H: Influence of exercise in water on hormonal, metabolic and adrenergic receptor changes in man. *Int J Sports Med* 9(suppl 2):S125–131, 1988.
362. Wade CE, Claybaugh J: Plasma renin activity, vasopressin concentration and urinary excretory responses to exercise in man. *J Appl Physiol* 49:930–936, 1980.
363. Convertino VA, Keil LC, Bernauer EM: Plasma volume, osmolality, vasopressin, and renin activity during exercise in man. *J Appl Physiol* 50:123–128, 1981.
364. Nazar K, Jezova D, Kowalik-Borowka E: Plasma vasopressin, growth hormone and ACTH responses to static handgrip in healthy subjects. *Eur J Appl Physiol* 58:400–404, 1989.
365. Maresh CM, Wang BC, Goetz KL: Plasma vasopressin, renin activity, and aldosterone responses to maximal exercise in active college females. *Eur J Appl Physiol* 54:398–403, 1985.
366. Convertino VA, Brock PJ, Keil LC, Bernauer EM, Greenleaf JE: Exercise induced hypervolemia: Role of plasma albumin, renin and vasopressin. *J Appl Physiol* 48:665–669, 1980.
367. Melin B, Eclache JP, Geelen G, Annat G, Allevard AM, Jarsaillon E, Zebidi A, Legros JJ, Gharib CI: Plasma AVP, neurophysin, renin activity, and aldosterone during submaximal exercise performed to exhaustion in trained and untrained men. *Eur J Appl Physiol* 44:141–151, 1980.
368. Convertino VA, Keil LC, Greenleaf JE: Plasma volume, renin, and vasopressin responses to graded exercise after training. *J Appl Physiol* 54:508–514, 1983.
369. Rocker L, Kirsch KA, Heyduck B, Altenkirch HU: Influence of prolonged physical exercise on plasma volume, plasma proteins, electrolytes, and fluid-regulating hormones. *Int J Sports Med* 10:270–274, 1989.
370. Landgraf R, Hacker R, Buhl H: Plasma vasopressin and oxytocin in response to exercise and during a day-night cycle in man. *Endocrinologie* 79:281–291, 1982.
371. Khokhar AM, De Silva P, Harvard CWH, Bird R, Forsling ML, Slater JDH: The mechanism of exercise mediated vasopressin release in man (abstract). *Eur J Clin Invest* 9:111, 1979.
372. Viinamaki O: The effect of hydration status on plasma vasopressin release during physical exercise in man. *Acta Physiol Scand* 139:133–137, 1990.
373. Viinamaki O, Heinonen OJ, Kujala UM, Alen M: Glucose polymer syrup attenuates prolonged endurance exercise-induced vasopressin release. *Acta Physiol Scand* 136:69–73, 1989.
374. Brandenberger G, Candas V, Follenius M, Kahn JM: The influence of the initial state of hydration on endocrine responses to exercise in the heat. *Eur J Appl Physiol* 58:674–679, 1989.
375. Brandenberger G, Candas V, Follenius M, Libert JP, Kahn JM: Vascular fluid shifts and endocrine responses to exercise in the heat: Effect of rehydration. *Eur J Appl Physiol* 55:123–129, 1986.
376. Perrault H, Cantin M, Thibault G, Brisson GR, Brisson G, Beland M: Plasma and atrial natriuretic peptide during brief upright and supine exercise in humans. *J Appl Physiol* 66:2159–2167, 1989.
377. Meehan RT: Renin, aldosterone, and vasopressin responses to hypoxia during 6 hours of mild exercise. *Aviat Space Environ Med* 57:960–965, 1986.
378. Koizumi K, Ishikawa T, McBrooks C: Control of activity neurons in the supraoptic nucleus. *Neurophysiology* 27:878–892, 1964.
379. Luger A, Deuster PA, Debolt JE, Loriaux DL, Chrousos GP: Acute exercise stimulates the renin-angiotensin-aldosterone axis: Adaptive changes in runners. *Horm Res* 30:5–9, 1988.
380. Lijnen P, Hespel P, Vanden Eynde E, Amery A: Urinary excretion of electrolytes during prolonged physical activity in normal man. *Eur J Appl Physiol* 53:317–321, 1985.
381. Freund BJ, Claybaugh JR, Dice MS, Hashiro GM: Hormonal and vascular fluid responses to maximal exercise in trained and untrained males. *J Appl Physiol* 63:669–675, 1987.

382. Hespel P, Lijnen P, Van Hoof R, Fagard R, Goossens W, Lissens W, Moerman E, Amery A: Effects of physical endurance training on the plasma renin-angiotensin-aldosterone system in normal man. *J Endocrinol* 116:443–449, 1988.
383. Maher JT, Jones LG, Hartley H, Williams GH, Rose LI: Aldosterone dynamics during graded exercise at sea level and at altitude. *J Appl Physiol* 26:18–22, 1975.
384. Boning D, Mrugalla M, Maassen N, Busse M, Wagner TO: Exercise versus immersion: Antagonistic effects on water and electrolyte metabolism during swimming. *Eur J Appl Physiol* 57:248–253, 1988.
385. Bonelli J, Waldhausl W, Magometschnigg D, SchwarzMeier J, Korn A, Hitzenberger G: Effect of exercise and prolonged oral administration of propranolol on haemodynamic variables, plasma renin concentration, plasma aldosterone and c-AMP. *Eur J Clin Invest* 7:337–343, 1977.
386. Opstad PK, Oktedalen O, Aakvaag A, Fonnum F, Lund PK: Plasma renin activity and serum aldosterone during prolonged physical strain: The significance of sleep and energy deprivation. *Eur J Appl Physiol* 54:1–6, 1985.
387. Kosunen KJ, Kuopposalmi K, Naveri H, Rehunen S, Narvanen S, Adlercreutz H: Plasma renin activity, angiotensin II, and aldosterone during hypnotic suggestion of running. *Scand J Clin Lab Invest* 37:99–103, 1988.
388. Wade CE, Dressendorfer RH, O'Brien JC, Claybaugh JR: Renal function, aldosterone, and vasopressin secretion following repeated long distance running. *J Appl Physiol* 50:709–712, 1981.
389. Freund BJ, Claybaugh JR, Hashiro GM, Dice MS: Hormonal and renal responses to water drinking in moderately trained and untrained humans. *Am J Physiol* 254:R417–R423, 1988.
390. Wahren J, Ahlborn G, Felig P, Jorfeldt L: Glucose metabolism during exercise in man, in Pernow B, Saltin B (eds): *Muscle Metabolism during Exercise.* New York: Plenum, 1971, pp 189–203.
391. Felig P, Wahren J: Fuel homeostasis in exercise. *N Engl J Med* 293:1078–1084, 1975.
392. Cochran B, Marbach EP, Poucher R, Steinberg T, Gwinup G: The effect of acute muscular exercise on serum immunoreactive concentration. *Diabetes* 15:838–841, 1966.
393. Benadé AJS, Wyndham CH, Jansen CR, Rogers GG, de Bruin EJP: Plasma insulin and carbohydrate metabolism after rest and during prolonged aerobic exercise. *Pflugers Arch* 342:207–218, 1973.
394. Galbo H, Christensen NJ, Holst JJ: Catecholamines and pancreatic hormones during autonomic blockade in exercising man. *Acta Physiol Scand* 101:428–437, 1977.
395. Galbo H, Christensen NJ, Holst JJ: Glucose induced decrease in glucagon and epinephrine responses to exercise in man. *J Appl Physiol* 42:525–530, 1977.
396. Galbo H, Holst JJ, Christensen NJ, Hilsted J: Glucagon and plasma catecholamines during beta-receptor blockade in exercising man. *J Appl Physiol* 42:855–863, 1976.
397. Gyntelberg F, Rennie MJ, Hickson RC, Holloszy JO: Effect of training on the response of plasma glucagon to exercise. *J Appl Physiol* 43:302–305, 1976.
398. Wirth A, Diehm C, Mayer H, Morl H, Vogel I, Bjorntorp P, Schlierf G: Plasma C-peptide and insulin in trained and untrained subjects. *J Appl Physiol* 50:71–77, 1981.
399. Chisholm DJ, Jenkins AB, James DE, Kraegen EW: The effect of hyperinsulinemia on glucose homeostasis during moderate exercise in man. *Diabetes* 31:603–608, 1982.
400. Bjorntorp P, Krotkiewski M: Exercise treatment in diabetes mellitus. *Acta Med Scand* 217:3–7, 1985.
401. Tuttle KR, Marker JC, Dalsky GP, Schwartz NS, Shah SD, Clutter WE, Holloszy JO, Cryer PE: Glucagon, not insulin, may play a secondary role in defense against hypoglycemia during exercise. *Am J Physiol* 254:E713–E719, 1988.
402. Mitchell TH, Abraham G, Schiffrin A, Leiter LA, Marliss E: Hyperglycemia after intense exercise in IDDM during continuous insulin infusion. *Diabetes Care* 11:311–317, 1988.
403. Koivisto VA, Karonen S-L, Nikkila EA: Carbohydrate ingestion before exercise: Comparison of glucose, fructose and sweet placebo. *J Appl Physiol* 51:783–787, 1981.
404. Brouns F, Saris WH, Beckers E, Adlercreutz H, van der Vusse GJ, Keizer HA, Kuipers H, Menheere P, et al: Metabolic changes induced by sustained exhaustive cycling and diet manipulation. *Int J Sports Med* 10(Suppl 1):S49–S62, 1989.
405. Mikines KJ, Farrell PA, Sonne B, Tronier B, Galbo H: Postexercise dose-response relationship between plasma glucose and insulin secretion. *J Appl Physiol* 64:988–999, 1988.
406. Jenkins AB, Chisholm DJ, James DE, Ho KY, Kraegen EW: Exercise-induced hepatic glucose output is precisely sensitive to the rate of systemic glucose supply. *Metabolism* 34:431–436, 1985.
407. Mitchell JB, Costill DL, Houmard JA, Flynn MG, Fink WJ, Beltz JD: Influence of carbohydrate ingestion on counterregulatory hormones during prolonged exercise. *Int J Sports Med* 11:33–36, 1990.
408. Minuk HL, Hanna AK, Marlis EB, Vranic M, Zinman B: Metabolic responses to moderate exercise in obese man during prolonged fasting. *Am J Physiol* 238:E322–E329, 1980.
409. Sotsky MJ, Shilo S, Shamoon H: Regulation of counterregulatory hormone secretion in man during exercise and hypoglycemia. *J Clin Endocrinol Metab* 68:9–16, 1989.
410. Nieman DC, Carlson KA, Brandstater ME, Naegele RT, Blankenship JW: Running endurance in 27-h-fasted humans. *J Appl Physiol* 63:2502–2509, 1987.
411. Bouissou P, Peronnet F, Brisson G, Helie R, Ledoux M: Metabolic and endocrine responses to graded exercise under acute hypoxia. *Eur J Appl Physiol* 55:290–294, 1986.
412. Okuno Y, Fuji S, Okada K, Tabata T, Tanaka S, Wada M: Effects of acute exercise on insulin binding to erythrocytes in normal men. *Horm Metab Res* 15:366–369, 1983.
413. Bonen A, Tan MH, Clune P, Kirby RL: Effects of exercise on insulin binding to human muscle. *Am J Physiol* 248:E403–E408, 1985.
414. Berger M, Hagg S, Ruderman NB: Glucose metabolism in perfused skeletal muscle. *Biochem J* 146:231–238, 1975.
415. Dorchy H, Ego F, Baran D, Loeb H: Effect of exercise on glucose uptake in diabetic adolescents. *Acta Paediatr Belg* 29:83–85, 1976.
416. DeFronzo RA, Ferrannini E, Sato Y, Felig P: Synergistic interaction between exercise and insulin on peripheral glucose uptake. *J Clin Invest* 68:1468–1474, 1981.
417. Felig P, Wahren J, Hendler R, Ahlborg G: Plasma glucagon levels in exercising man. *N Engl J Med* 287:184–185, 1972.
418. Adams JH, Irving G, Koeslag JH, Lochner JD, Sandell RC, Wilkinson C: Beta-adrenergic blockade restores glucose's antiketogenic activity after exercise in carbohydrate-depleted athletes. *J Physiol* 386:439–454, 1987.
419. Jenkins AB, Furler SM, Chisholm DJ, Kraegen EW: Regulation of hepatic glucose output during exercise by circulating glucose and insulin in humans. *Am J Physiol* 250:R411–R417, 1986.
420. Wolfe RR, Nadel ER, Shaw JH, Stephenson LA, Wolfe MH: Role of changes in insulin and glucagon in glucose homeostasis in exercise. *J Clin Invest* 77:900–907, 1986.
421. Winder WW, Hickson RC, Hagberg JM, Ehsani AA, McLane JA: Training induced changes in hormonal and metabolic responses to submaximal exercise. *J Appl Physiol* 46:766–771, 1979.
422. Vanhelder WP, Radomski MW, Goode RC, Casey K: Hormonal and metabolic response to three types of exercise of equal duration and external work output. *Eur J Appl Physiol* 54:337–342, 1985.
423. Felig P, Wahren J: Role of insulin and glucose in the regulation of hepatic glucose production during exercise. *Diabetes* 28(Suppl 1):71–75, 1979.
424. Ahlberg G, Felig P: Influence of glucose ingestion on fuel hormone response during prolonged exercise. *J Appl Physiol* 41:683–688, 1976.

425. Galbo H, Holst JJ, Christensen NJ: Glucagon and plasma catecholamine responses to graded and prolonged exercise in man. *J Appl Physiol* 38:70–76, 1975.
426. Naveri H, Kuoppasalmi K, Harkonen M: Plasma glucagon and catecholamines during exhaustive short-term exercise. *Eur J Appl Physiol* 53:308–311, 1985.
427. Pruett EDR: Glucose and insulin during prolonged work stress in men living on different diets. *J Appl Physiol* 28:199–208, 1970.
428. Felig P, Cherif A, Minagawa A, Wahren J: Hypoglycemia during prolonged exercise in normal men. *N Engl J Med* 306:895–900, 1982.
429. Levine SA, Gordon B, Derick CL: Some changes in the constituents of the blood following a marathon race: With special reference to the development of hypoglycemia. *JAMA* 82:1778–1779, 1924.
430. Sutton J, Coleman MJ, Millar AP, Lazarus L, Russo P: The medical problems of mass participation in athletic competition: The "City-to-Surf" Race. *Med J Aus* 2:127–133, 1972.
431. Brockman RP: Glucagon responses to exercise in sheep. *Aust J Biol Sci* 32:215–220, 1979.
432. Hartung GH, Myhre LG, Tucker DM, Burns JW: Hormone and energy substrate changes during prolonged exercise in the heat. *Aviat Space Environ Med* 58:24–28, 1987.
433. Naveri H: Blood hormone and metabolite levels during graded cycle ergometer exercise. *Scand J Clin Lab Invest* 45:599–603, 1985.
434. Koivisto V, Hendler R, Nadel E, Felig P: Influence of physical training on the fuel-hormone response to prolonged low intensity exercise. *Metabolism* 31:192–197, 1982.
435. Tarnopolsky LJ, MacDougall JD, Atkinson SA, Tarnopolsky MA, Sutton JR: Gender differences in substrate for endurance exercise. *J Appl Physiol* 68:302–308, 1990.
436. Lavoie JM, Dionne N, Helie R, Brisson GR: Menstrual cycle phase dissociation of blood glucose homeostasis during exercise. *J Appl Physiol* 62:1084–1089, 1987.
437. LeBlanc J, Nadeau A, Boulay M, Rousseau-Migneron S: Effects of physical training and adiposity on glucose metabolism and ^{125}I-insulin binding. *J Appl Physiol* 46:235–239, 1979.
438. Lohmann D, Liebold F, Heilmann W, Senger H, Pohl A: Diminished insulin response of highly trained athletes. *Metabolism* 27:521–524, 1978.
439. Dela F, Mikines KJ, Von Linstow M, Galbo H: Effect of training on response to a glucose load adjusted for daily carbohydrate intake. *Am J Physiol* 260:E14–E20, 1991.
440. Oshida Y, Yamanouchi K, Hayamizu S, Sato Y: Long-term mild jogging increases insulin action despite no influence on body mass index or $V_{O_{2max}}$. *J Appl Physiol* 66:2206–2210, 1989.
441. Sato Y, Hayamizu S, Yamamoto C, Ohkuwa Y, Yamanouchi K, Sakamoto N: Improved insulin sensitivity in carbohydrate and lipid metabolism after physical training. *Int J Sports Med* 7:307–310, 1986.
442. Tremblay A, Nadeau A, Despres JP, St-Jean L, Theriault G, Bouchard C: Long-term exercise training with constant energy intake: II. Effect on glucose metabolism and resting energy expenditures. *Int J Obes* 14:75–84, 1990.
443. O'Rahilly SO, Hosker JP, Rudenski AS, Matthews DR, Burnett MA, Turner RC: The glucose stimulus-response curve of the beta-cell in physically trained humans, assessed by hyperglycemia clamps. *Metabolism* 37:919–923, 1988.
444. Hommell HH, Labitzke H: Insulinsekretion nack Langzeitausdauerbelastungen. *Med Sport* 27:204–207, 1987.
445. King DS, Staten MA, Kohrt WM, Dalsky GP, Elahi D, Holloszy JO: Insulin secretory capacity in endurance-trained and untrained young men. *Am J Physiol* 259:E155–E161, 1990.
446. Kahn SE, Larson VG, Beard JC, Cain KC, Fellingham GW, Schwartz RS, Veith RC, Stratton JR, et al: Effect of exercise on insulin action, glucose tolerance, and insulin secretion in aging. *Am J Physiol* 258:E937–E943, 1990.
447. Coon PJ, Bleecker ER, Drinkwater DT, Meyers DA, Goldberg AP: Effects of body composition and exercise capacity on glucose tolerance, insulin, and lipoprotein lipids in healthy older men: a cross-sectional and longitudinal intervention study. *Metabolism* 38:1201–1209, 1989.
448. Tonino RP: Effect of physical training on the insulin resistance of aging. *Am J Physiol* 256:E352–E356, 1989.
449. Van Dam S, Gillespy M, Notelovitz M, Martin AD: Effect of exercise on glucose metabolism in postmenopausal women. *Am J Obstet Gynecol* 159:82–86, 1988.
450. Mikines KJ, Sonne B, Farrell PA, Tronier B, Galbo H: Effect of training on the dose-response relationship for insulin action in men. *J Appl Physiol* 66:695–703, 1989.
451. Craig BW, Everhart J, Brown R: The influence of high-resistance training on glucose tolerance in young and elderly subjects. *Mech Ageing Dev* 49:147–157, 1989.
452. Lavoie JM, Helie R, Peronnet F, Cousineau D, Provencher PJ: Effects of muscle CHO-loading manipulations on hormonal responses during prolonged exercise. *Int J Sports Med* 6:95–99, 1985.
453. Young JC, Enslin J, Kuca B: Exercise intensity and glucose tolerance in trained and nontrained subjects. *J Appl Physiol* 67:39–43, 1989.
454. Tremblay A, Nadeau A, Fournier G, Bouchard C: Effect of a three-day interruption of exercise-training on resting metabolic rats and glucose-induced thermogenesis in training individuals. *Int J Obes* 12:163–168, 1988.
455. King DS, Dalsky GP, Clutter WE, Young DA, Staten MA, Cryer PE, Holloszy JO: Effects of lack of exercise on insulin secretion and action in trained subjects. *Am J Physiol* 254:E537–E542, 1988.
456. Burstein R, Polychronakos C, Toews CJ, MacDougall JD, Guyda HJ, Posner BI: Acute reversal of the enhanced insulin action in trained athletes: Association with insulin receptor changes. *Diabetes* 34:756–760, 1985.
457. Evans WJ, Hughes VA: Dietary carbohydrates and endurance exercise. *Am J Clin Nutr* 41(Suppl 5):1146–1154, 1985.
458. Mikines KJ, Sonne B, Tronier B, Galbo H: Effects of acute exercise and detraining on insulin action in trained men. *J Appl Physiol* 66:704–711, 1989.
459. Lampman RM, Schteingart DE, Santinga JT, Savage PJ, Hydrick CR, Bassett DR, Block WD: The influence of physical training on glucose tolerance, insulin sensitivity, and lipid and lipoprotein concentrations in middle-aged hypertriglyceridaemic, carbohydrate intolerant men. *Diabetologia* 30:380–385, 1987.
460. Christensen NJ, Galbo H, Hansen JF, Hesse B, Richter EA, Trap-Jensen J: Catecholamines and exercise. *Diabetes* 28(Suppl 1):58–62, 1979.
461. Sothmann MS, Gustafson AB, Chandler M: Plasma free and sulfoconjugated catecholamine responses to varying exercise intensity. *J Appl Physiol* 63:654–658, 1987.
462. Holmqvist N, Secher NH, Sander-Jensen K, Knigge U, Warberg J, Schwartz TW: Sympathoadrenal and parasympathetic responses to exercise. *J Sports Sci* 4:123–128, 1986.
463. Schwarz L, Kindermann W: Beta-endorphin, catecholamines, and cortisol during exhaustive endurance exercise. *Int J Sports Med* 10:324–328, 1989.
464. Lewis SF, Taylor FW, Graham RM, Pettinger WA, Schutte JE, Blomquist CG: Cardiovascular responses to exercise as functions of absolute and relative workload. *J Appl Physiol* 54:1314–1323, 1983.
465. Meyer R, Mayer U, Weiss M, Weicker H: Sympathoadrenergic regulation of metabolism and cardiocirculation during and following running exercises of different intensity and duration. *Int J Sports Med* 9(Suppl 2):S132–S140, 1988.
466. Sagnol M, Claustre J, Cottet-Emard JM, Pequignot JM, Fellmann N, Coudert J, Peyrin L: Plasma free and sulphated catecholamines after ultra-long exercise and recovery. *Eur J Appl Physiol* 60:91–97, 1990.
467. Sothmann MS, Blaney J, Woulfe T, Donahue-Fuhrman S, Lefever K, Gustafson AB, Murthy VS: Plasma free and sulfo-

conjugated catecholamines during sustained exercise. *J Appl Physiol* 68:452–456, 1990.
468. Lehmann M, Keul J: Capillary-venous differences of free plasma catecholamines at rest and during graded exercise. *Eur J Appl Physiol* 54:502–505, 1985.
469. Sagnol M, Claustre J, Pequignot JM, Fellmann N, Coudert J, Peyrin L: Catecholamines and fuels after an ultralong run: Persistent changes after 24-h recovery. *Int J Sports Med* 10:202–206, 1989.
470. Lehmann M, Keul J, Wybitul K: Einfluss einer stufenweisen Laufband- und Fahrradergometrie auf die Plasmacatecholamine, energiereichen Substrate, aerobe und anaerobe Kapazitat. *Klin Wochenschr* 59:553–559, 1981.
471. Pequignot JM, Peyrin L, Peres G: Catecholamine-fuel interrelationship during exercise in fasting men. *J Appl Physiol* 48:109–113, 1980.
472. Lavoie JM, Bonneau MC, Roy JY, Brisson GR, Helie R: Effects of dietary manipulations on blood glucose and hormonal responses following supramaximal exercise. *Eur J Appl Physiol* 56:109–114, 1987.
473. Kjaer M Bangsbo J, Lortie G, Galbo H: Hormonal response to exercise in humans: Influence of hypoxia and physical training. *Am J Physiol* 254:R197–R203, 1988.
474. Gullestad L, Dolva LO, Kjeldsen SE, Eide I, Kjekshus J: The effects of naloxone and timolol on plasma catecholamine levels during short-term dynamic exercise. *Scand J Clin Lab Invest* 47:847–851, 1987.
475. Schnabel A, Kindermann W, Salas-Fraire O, Cassens J, Steinkraus V: Effect of beta-adrenergic blockade on supramaximal exercise capacity. *Int J Sports Med* 4:278–281, 1983.
476. Erisksen J, Thaulow E, Mundal R, Opstad P: Comparison of beta-adrenergic receptor blockers under maximal exercise. *Br J Clin Pharmacol* 13:209S–210S, 1982.
477. Irving MH, Britton BJ, Wood WG, Padgham C, Caruthers M: Effects of beta adrenergic blockade on plasma catecholamines in exercise. *Nature* 248:531–533, 1974.
478. Planz G, Planz R: Influence of propranolol on catecholamine concentration in blood of normotensive man during physical exercise and depending of the drug effect on dosage intervals. *Arch Int Pharmacodyn Ther* 1(suppl):58–66, 1980.
479. Christensen NJ, Galbo H: Sympathetic nervous activity during exercise. *Annu Rev Physiol* 45:139–153, 1983.
480. Folgering H Th M, Borm JFE, van Haaren RHLM: Metabolic aspects of maximal exercise performance after slow release metoprolol and after atenolol. *Eur J Clin Pharmacol* 23:283–288, 1982.
481. Peyrin L, Pequignot JM, Lacour JR, Fourcade J: Relationships between catecholamine or 3-methoxy 4-hydroxy phenylglycol changes and the mental performance under submaximal exercise in man. *Psychopharmacology* 93:188–192, 1987.
482. Cousineau D, Ferguson RJ, de Champlain J, Gauthier P, Cote P, Baourassa M: Catecholamines in coronary sinus during exercise in man before and after training. *J Appl Physiol* 43:801–806, 1977.
483. Hickson RC, Hagberg JM, Coulee RK, Jones DA, Ehsairi AA, Winder WW: Effects of training on hormonal response to exercise in competitive swimmers. *Eur J Appl Physiol* 41:211–219, 1979.
484. Peronnet F, Cléroux J, Perrault H, Cousineau D, de Champlain J, Nadeau R: Plasma norepinephrine response to exercise before and after training in humans. *J Appl Physiol* 51:812–815, 1981.
485. Korge P, Masso R, Roosson S: The effect of physical conditioning on cardiac response to acute exertion. *Can J Pharmacol Physiol* 42:745–752, 1974.
486. Kjaer M, Galbo H: Effect of physical training on the capacity to secrete epinephrine. *J Appl Physiol* 64:11–16, 1988.
487. Askew EH, Huston RL, Plopper CG, Hecker AL: Adipose tissue cellularity and lipolysis: Response to exercise and cortisol treatment. *J Clin Invest* 56:521–529, 1975.
488. Crampes F, Beauville M, Riviere D, Garrigues M: Effect of physical training in humans on the response of isolated fat cells to epinephrine. *J Appl Physiol* 61:25–29, 1986.
489. Riviere D, Crampes F, Beauville M, Garrigues M: Lipolytic response of fat cells to catecholamines in sedentary and exercise-trained women. *J Appl Physiol* 66:330–335, 1989.
490. Chamberlain KG, Pestell RG, Best JD: Platelet catecholamine contents are cumulative indexes of sympathoadrenal activity. *Am J Physiol* 259:E141–E147, 1990.
491. Van Loon GR, Schwartz L, Sole MJ: Plasma dopamine responses to standing and exercise in man. *Life Sci* 24:2273–2278, 1979.
492. Musso NR, Gianrossi R, Pende A, Vergassola C, Lotti G: Plasma dopamine response to sympathetic activation in man: A biphasic pattern. *Life Sci* 47:619–626, 1990.
493. Hartling OJ, Kelbaek H, Gjorup T, Nielsen MD, Trap-Jensen J: Plasma concentrations of adrenaline, noradrenaline and dopamine during forearm dynamic exercise. *Clin Physiol* 9:399–404, 1989.
494. Peronnet F, Cleroux J, Perrault H, Thibault G, Cousineau D, de Champlain J, Guilland JC, Klepping J: Plasma norepinephrine, epinephrine, and dopamine beta-hydroxylase activity during exercise in man. *Med Sci Sports Exerc* 17:683–688, 1985.
495. Chin NW, Chang FE, Dodds WG, Kim MH, Malarkey WB: Acute effects of exercise on plasma catecholamines in sedentary and athletic women with normal and abnormal menses. *Am J Obstet Gynecol* 157:938–944, 1987.
496. Dosani R, Van Loon GR, Burki NK: The relationship between exercise-induced asthma and plasma catecholamines. *Am Rev Respir Dis* 136:973–978, 1987.
497. Boetger CL, Ward DS: Effect of dopamine of transient ventilatory response to exercise. *J Appl Physiol* 61:2102–2107, 1986.
498. Baker HWG, Santen RJ, Berger HG, de Kretser DM, Hudson B, Peperell RJ, Bardin GW: Rhythms in the secretion of gonadotropins and gonadal steroids. *J Steroid Biochem* 6:793–801, 1975.
499. Pardridge WM: Transport of protein bound hormones into tissues in vivo. *Endocr Rev* 2:103–123, 1981.
500. Vermeulen A, Verdonck L, Van Der Straeten M, Orie N: Capacity of testosterone binding globulin in human plasma and its influence on specific binding of testosterone and its clearance rate. *J Clin Endocrinol Metab* 29:1470–1480, 1969.
501. Baird DT, Horton R, Longcope C, Tait JF: Steroid dynamics under steady state conditions. *Recent Prog Horm Res* 25: 611–625, 1969.
502. Fahey TD, Rolph R, Moongee P, Nagel J, Mortara S: Serum testosterone, body composition, and strength of young adults. *Med Sci Sports Exerc* 1:31–34, 1976.
503. Brisson GR, Volle MA, Desharnais M, Dion M, Tanaka M: Pituitary-gonadal axis in exercising man (abstract). *Med Sci Sports Exerc* 9:47, 1977.
504. Kuopposalmi K: Plasma testosterone and sex-hormone-binding capacity in physical exercise. *Scand J Clin Lab Invest* 40:411–418, 1980.
505. Wilkerson JE, Horvath SM, Gutin B: Plasma testosterone during treadmill exercise. *J Appl Physiol* 49:249–253, 1980.
506. Jezova D, Vigas M: Testosterone response to exercise during blockade and stimulation of adrenergic receptors in man. *Horm Res* 15:141–147, 1981.
507. Schmid P, Pusch PP, Wolf WW, Pilger E, Pessenhofer H, Schwaberger G, Pristautz H, Purstner P: Serum FSH, LH and testosterone in humans after physical exercise. *Int J Sports Med* 3:84–89, 1982.
508. Kindermann W, Schnabel A, Schmitt WM, Biro G, Cassens J, Weber F: Catecholamines, growth hormone, cortisol, insulin and sex hormones in aerobic and anaerobic exercise. *Eur J Appl Physiol* 49:389–399, 1982.
509. Mathur DN, Toriola AL, Dada OA: Serum cortisol and testosterone levels in conditioned male distance runners and

non-athletes after maximal exercise. *J Sports Med Phys Fitness* 26:245–250, 1986.
510. Vogel RB, Books CA, Ketchum C, Zauner CW, Murray FT: Increase of free and total testosterone during submaximal exercise in normal males. *Med Sci Sports Exerc* 17:119–123, 1984.
511. Kraemer WJ, Marchitelli L, Gordon SE, Harman E, Dziados JE, Mello R, Frykman P, McCurry D, Fleck SJ: Hormonal and growth factor responses to heavy resistance exercise protocols. *J Appl Physiol* 69:1442–1450, 1990.
512. Metivier G, Gauthier R, de la Chevotriere J, Grymala D: The effect of acute exercise on the serum levels of testosterone and luteinizing (LH) hormone in human male athletes. *J Sports Med Phys Fitness* 20:235–237, 1980.
513. Karvonen J, Peltola E, Saarela J, Nieminen MM: Changes in running speed, blood lactic acid concentration and hormone balance during sprint training performed at an altitude of 1860 metres. *J Sports Med Phys Fitness* 30:122–126, 1990.
514. Cumming DC, Wall SR, Quinney HA, Belcastro AN: Decrease in serum testosterone levels with maximal intensity swimming exercise in trained male and female swimmers. *Endocr Res* 13:31–41, 1987.
515. Rowell LB: Human cardiovascular adjustments to exercise and thermal stress. *Physiol Rev* 53:75–159, 1974.
516. Wahren J, Felig P, Ahlborg G, Jorfeldt I: Glucose metabolism during leg exercise in man. *J Clin Invest* 50:2715–2725, 1971.
517. Sutton JR, Coleman MJ, Casey JH: Testosterone production rate during exercise, in Landry F, Orban WAR (eds): *3rd International Symposium on Biochemistry of Exercise.* Miami, Symposium Specialists. 1978, pp 227–234.
518. Cadoux-Hudson TA, Few JD, Imms FJ: The effect of exercise on the production and clearance of testosterone in well trained young men. *Eur J Appl Physiol* 54:321–325, 1985.
519. Kuopposalmi K, Naveri H, Harkonen N, Adlerkreutz H: Plasma cortisol, a'dione, testosterone and luteinizing hormone in running exercise of various intensities. *Scand J Clin Invest* 40:403–409, 1980.
520. McConnell TR, Sinning WE: Exercise and temperature effects on human sperm production and testosterone levels. *Med Sci Sports Exerc* 16:51–55, 1984.
521. Burke CW, Anderson DC: Sex hormone binding globulin is an estrogen amplifier. *Nature* 240:38–40, 1972.
522. Sutton JR, Coleman MJ, Casey JH: Adrenocortical contribution to serum androgens during physical exercise (abstract). *Med Sci Sports Exerc* 6:72, 1974.
523. Eik-Nes KB: On the relationship between testicular blood flow and secretion of testosterone in anesthetized dogs stimulated with human chorionic gonadotropin. *Can J Physiol Pharmacol* 42:671–677, 1964.
524. Levin J, Lloyd CW, Lobotsky J, Friedrich EH: The effect of epinephrine on testosterone production. *Acta Endocrinol (Copenh)* 55:184–192, 1967.
525. Kindermann W, Schnabel A, Schmitt A, Biro G, Hippchen M: Catechlamine, STH, cortisol, glucagon, insulin und sexualhormone bei korperlicher belastung und beta1-blockade. *Klin Wohenschr* 60:505–512, 1982.
526. MacConnie SE, Barkan A, Lampman RM, Schork MA, Beitins IZ: Decreased hypothalamic gonadotropin releasing hormone secretion in male marathon runners. *N Engl J Med* 315:411–417, 1986.
527. Webb ML, Wallace JP, Hamill C, Hodgson JL, Mashaly MM: Serum testosterone concentration during two hours of moderate intensity treadmill running in trained men and women *Endocr Res* 10:27–38, 1984.
528. de Lignieres B, Plas J-N, Commandre F, Morville R, Viani J-L, Plas F: Secretion testiculaire d'androgenes après effort physique prolongué chex l'homme. *Nouv Presse Med* 5:2060–2064, 1976.
529. Morville R, Pesquies PC, Guezzenec CY, Serrurier BD, Guignard M: Plasma variations in testicular and adrenal androgens during prolonged physical exercise in man. *Ann Endocrinol* 40:501–510, 1979.
530. Schurmeyer T, Jung K, Nieschlag E: The effects of an 1100 kilometer run on testicular adrenal and thyroid hormones. *Int J Androl* 7:276–282, 1984.
531. Urhausen A, Kinderman W: Behaviour of testosterone, sex hormone binding globulin (SHBG) and cortisol before and after a triathlon. *Int J Sports Med* 8:305–308, 1987.
532. Johansson C, Tsai L, Hultman E, Tegelman R, Pousette A: Restoration of anabolic deficit and muscle glycogen consumption in competitive orienteering. *Int J Sports* 11:204–207, 1990.
533. Mateev G, Djarova T, Ilkov A, Sachanska T, Klissurov L: Hormonal and cardiorespiratory changes following simulated saturation dives to 4 and 11 ATA. *Undersea Biomed Res* 17:1–11, 1990.
534. Keizer H, Janssen GM, Menheere P, Kranenburg G: Changes in basal plasma testosterone, cortisol, and dehydroepiandrosterone sulfate in previously untrained males and females preparing for a marathon. *Int J Sports Med* 10(Suppl 3):S139–S145, 1989.
535. Wang C, Chan V, Tse TF, Yeung RTT: Effect of acute myocardial infarction on pituitary-testicular function. *Clin Endocrinol (Oxf)* 9:249–253, 1978.
536. Wang C, Chan V, Yeung RTT: Effect of surgical stress on pituitary-testicular function. *Clin Endocrinol (Oxf)* 9:255–256, 1978.
537. Aakvaag A, Sand T, Opstad PK, Fonnum F: Hormonal changes in young men during prolonged physical strain. *Eur J Appl Physiol* 39:283–291, 1978.
538. McColl EM, Wheeler GD, Gomes P, Bhambhani Y, Cumming DC: The effects of acute exercise on LH pulsatile release in high mileage male runners. *Clin Endocrinol (Oxf)* 31:617–629, 1989.
539. Kujala UM, Alen M, Huhtaniemi IT: Gonadotrophin-releasing hormone and human chorionic gonadotrophin tests reveal that both hypothalamic and testicular endocrine functions are suppressed during acute prolonged physical exercise. *Clin Endocrinol (Oxf)* 33:219–225, 1990.
540. Cumming DC, Quigley ME, Yen SSC: Acute suppression of circulating testosterone levels by cortisol in man. *J Clin Endocrinol Metab* 57:671–673, 1983.
541. Strauss RH, Lanese RR, Malarkey WB: Weight loss in amateur wrestlers and its effect on testosterone levels. *JAMA* 254:3337–3338, 1985.
542. Ayers JWT, Komesu Y, Romain T, Ansbacher RA: Anthropometric, hormonal and psychologic correlates of semen quality in endurance trained male athletes. *Fertil Steril* 43:917–921, 1985.
543. Hackney AC, Sinning WE, Bruot BC: Reproductive hormonal profiles of endurance-trained and untrained males. *Med Sci Sports Exerc* 2:60–65, 1988.
544. Hakkinen K, Keskinen KL, Alen M, Komi PV, Kauhanen H: Serum hormone concentrations during prolonged training in elite endurance-trained and strength-trained athletes. *Eur J Appl Physiol* 59:233–238, 1989.
545. Craig BW, Brown R, Everhart J: Effects of progressive resistance training on growth hormone and testosterone levels in young and elderly subjects. *Mech Ageing Dev* 49:159–169, 1989.
546. Urhausen A, Kullmer T, Kindermann W: A 7-week follow-up study of the behaviour of testosterone and cortisol during the competition period in rowers. *Eur J Appl Physiol* 56:528–533, 1987.
547. Wheeler GD, Singh M, Pierce WD, Epling WF, Cumming DC: Endurance training decreases serum testosterone levels in men without change in LH pulsatile release. *J Clin Endocrinol Metab* 72:422–425, 1991.
548. Frey MAB, Doerr BM, Srivastava LM, Glueck CJ: Exercise training, sex hormones and lipoprotein relationships in men. *J Appl Physiol* 54:757–762, 1983.

549. Hakkinen K, Pakarinen A, Alen M, Kauhanen H, Komi PV: Relationships between training volume, physical performance capacity and serum hormone concentrations during prolonged weight training in elite weight lifters. *Int J Sports Med* 8(suppl):61–65, 1987.
550. Remes K, Kuopposalmi K, Adlercreutz H: Effects of long-term physical training on plasma testosterone, androstenedione, luteinizing hormone, sex hormone binding globulin capacity. *Scand J Lab Invest* 39:743–749, 1979.
551. Johnson CC, Stone MH, Byrd RJ, Lopez SA: The response of serum lipids and plasma androgens to weight training exercise in sedentary males. *J Sports Med Phys Fitness* 23:39–44, 1983.
552. Peltonen P, Marniemi J, Hietanen E, Vuori I, Enholm C: Changes in serum lipids, lipoproteins and heparin releasable lipolytic enzymes during moderate physical training in man: A longitudinal study. *Metabolism* 30:518–526, 1981.
553. Bagatell CJ, Bremner WJ: Sperm counts and reproductive hormones in male marathoners and lean controls. *Fertil Steril* 53:688–692, 1990.
554. Baker ER, Leuker R, Stumpf PG: Relationships of exercise to semen parameters and fertility success of artificial insemination donors (abstract). *Fertil Steril* 41:107S, 1984.
555. Cumming DC, Wheeler GD, McColl EM: The effects of exercise on reproductive function in men. *Sports Med* 7:1–17, 1989.
556. Editorial. Special survey: Running and sex (abstract). *The Runner* May 1982, pp 26–35.
557. Dohm GL, Louis TM: Changes in androstenedione, testosterone and protein metabolism as a result of exercise. *Proc Soc Exp Biol Med* 158:622–625, 1978.
558. Hakkinen K: Neuromuscular and hormonal adaptations during strength and power training: A review. *J Sports Med Phys Fitness* 29:9–26, 1989.
559. Mooradian AD, Morley JE, Korenman SG: Biological actions of androgens. *Endocr Rev* 8:1–28, 1987.
560. Stanish W: Overuse injuries in athletes: A perspective. *Med Sci Sports Exerc* 16:1–7, 1984.
561. Foresta C, Ruzza G, Mioni R, Guarneri G, Gribaldo R, Meneghello A, Mastrogiacomo I: Osteoporosis and decline of gonadal function in the elderly man. *Horm Res* 19:18–22, 1984.
562. Aloia JF, Cohn SH, Babu T, Abesamic C, Kalici N, Ellis K: Skeletal mass and body composition in marathon runners. *Metabolism* 27:1793–1796, 1978.
563. Rigotti NA, Neer RM, Jameson L: Osteopenia and bone fractures in a man with anorexia nervosa and hypogonadism. *JAMA* 256:385–388, 1986.
564. Riggs BL: Exercise, hypogonadism and osteopenia. JAMA 256:392–393, 1986.
565. Enger S, Herbjornsen K, Erikssen K, Fretland A: High density lipoproteins and physical activity: The influence of physical exercise, age and smoking on HDL-cholesterol and the HDL/total cholesterol ratio. *Scand J Clin Lab Invest* 37:251–255, 1977.
566. Hartung GH, Foreyt JP, Mitchell RE, Vlasek I, Gotto AM: Relation of diet to high-density-lipoprotein cholesterol in middle aged marathon runners, joggers and inactive men. *N Engl J Med* 302:357–361, 1980.
567. Kantor MA, Cullinane EM, Herbert PN, Thompson PD: Acute increase in lipoprotein lipase following prolonged exercise. *Metabolism* 33:454–457, 1984.
568. Schriewer H, Jung K, Gunnewiig V, Assmann G: Serum lipids and lipoproteins during a twenty day run of 1,100 kilometers. *Ann Sports Med* 1:71–74, 1983.
569. Keizer HA, Doorfman J, Bunnik GSJ: Influence of physical exercise on sex hormone metabolism. *Med Sci Sports Exerc* 48:765–769, 1980.
570. Rogol AD, Veldhuis JD, Williams FA, Johnson ML: Pulsatile secretion of gonadotropins and prolactin in male marathon runners: Relation to the endogenous opiate system. *J Androl* 5:21–27, 1984.
571. Hamalainen EK, Adlercreutz H, Puska P, Pietinen P: Decrease of serum total and free testosterone during a low-fat high fibre diet. *J Steroid Biochem* 18:369–370, 1983.
572. Zubiran S, Gomez-Mont F: Endocrine disturbance in chronic human malnutrition. *Vitam Horm* 11:97–102, 1952.
573. Hill P, Wynder E, Garbacrewski L, Garnes H, Walker ARP, Hellman P: Plasma hormones and lipids in men at different risk for coronary heart disease. *Am J Clin Nutr* 33:1010–1018, 1980.
574. Epling WF, Pierce WD, Stefan L: A theory of activity-based anorexia. *Int J Eat Dis* 3:27–46, 1983.
575. Bonen A, Ling WY, MacIntyre KP, Neil R, McGrail JC, Belcastro AN: Effects of exercise on the serum concentrations of FSH, LH, progesterone and estradiol. *Eur J Appl Physiol* 42:15–23, 1979.
576. Jurkowski JE, Jones NL, Walker WC, Younglai EV, Sutton JR: Ovarian hormone response to exercise. *J Appl Physiol* 44:109–114, 1978.
577. Cumming DC: Physical activity and control of the hypothalamic-pituitary gonadal axis. *Semin Reprod Endocrinol* 8:15–24, 1990.
578. Malina RM, Bouchard C, Shoup RF, Demirjian A, Lariviere G: Age at menarche, family size and birth order in athletes at the Olympic Games, 1976. *Med Sci Sports Exerc* 11:354–358, 1979.
579. Malina RM, Spirduso WW, Tate C, Baylor AM: Age at menarche and selected menstrual characteristics in athletes at different competitive levels and in different sports. *Med Sci Sports Exerc* 10:218–222, 1978.
580. Malina RM, Harper AB, Avent HH, Campbell DE: Age at menarche in athletes and non-athletes. *Med Sci Sports Exerc* 5:11–13, 1973.
581. Frisch RE, Wishak G, Vincent L: Delayed menarche and amenorrhea in ballet dancers. *N Engl J Med* 303:17–19, 1980.
582. Frisch RE, Gotz-Welbergen AV, McArthur JV, Albright T, Witschi J, Bullen B, Birnholtz J, Reed RB, Hermann H: Delayed menarche and amenorrhea of college athletes in relation to age of onset of training. *JAMA* 246:1559–1563, 1981.
583. Warren MP: The effects of exercise on pubertal progression and reproductive function in girls. *J Clin Endocrinol Metab* 51:1150–1157, 1980.
584. Wakat DK, Sweeney KA, Rogol AD: Reproductive system function in women cross country runners. *Med Sci Sports Exerc* 14:263–269, 1982.
585. Brooks-Gunn J, Warren MP: Mother-daughter differences in menarcheal age in adolescent girls attending national dance company schools and non-dancers. *Ann Hum Biol* 15:35–44, 1988.
586. Shangold MM, Freeman R, Thysen B, Gatz M: The relationship between long-distance running, plasma progesterone and luteal phase length. *Fertil Steril* 31:130–133, 1981.
587. Bonen A, Belcastro AN, Ling WY, Simpson AA: Profiles of selected hormones during the menstrual cycles of teenage athletes. *J Appl Physiol* 50:545–551, 1981.
588. Prior JC: Menstrual cycle changes with training: Anovulation and short luteal phase. *Can J Appl Sports Sci* 7:173–177, 1982.
589. Prior JC, Ho Yuen B, Clement P, Thomas J: Reversible luteal phase changes associated with marathon training. *Lancet* 1:269–270, 1982.
590. Ellison PT, Lager C: Exercise-induced menstrual disorders. *N Engl J Med* 313:825–826, 1985.
591. Feicht CB, Johnson TS, Martin BJ, Sparkes KE, Wagner WW Jr: Secondary amenorrhoea in athletes. *Lancet* 2:1145–1146, 1978.
592. Speroff L, Redwine DB: Exercise and menstrual dysfunction. *Phys Sports Med* 8(5):42–52, 1979.
593. Dale E, Gerlach DH, Wilhite AL: Menstrual dysfunction in distance runners. *Obstet Gynecol* 54:47–53, 1979.

594. Shangold MM, Levine HS: The effect of marathon training on menstrual function. *Am J Obstet Gynecol* 143:862–869, 1982.
595. Lutter JM, Cushman S: Menstrual patterns in female runners. *Phys Sports Med* 10(9):60–72, 1983.
596. Glass AR, Yahiro JA, Deuster PA, Ferguson EW, Vigersky RA: Amenorrhea in Olympic marathon runners. *Fertil Steril* 48:740–745, 1987.
597. Sanborn CF, Martin BJ, Wagner WW: Is athletic amenorrhea specific to runners? *Am J Obstet Gynecol* 143:859–861, 1982.
598. Toriola AL: Survey of menstrual function in young Nigerian athletes. *Int J Sports Med* 9:29–34, 1988.
599. Prior JC: Endocrine "conditioning" with endurance training. *Can J Appl Sports Sci* 7:148–157, 1982.
600. Galle PC, Freeman EW, Galle MG, Huggins GR, Sondheimer SJ: Physiologic and psychologic profiles in a survey of women runners. *Fertil Steril* 39:633–639, 1983.
601. Baker ER, Mathur RS, Kirk RF, Landgrebe SE: Female runners and secondary amenorrhea: Correlation with age, parity, mileage and plasma hormones and sex-hormone-binding globulin. *Fertil Steril* 36:183–187, 1981.
602. Boyden TW, Pamenter RW, Stanforth P, Rotkis T, Wilmore JH: Sex steroids and endurance running in women runners. *Fertil Steril* 39:629–632, 1983.
603. Boyden TW, Pamenter RW, Stanforth P, Rotkis T, Wilmore JH: Impaired gonadotropin responses to gonadotropin stimulating hormone in endurance trained women. *Fertil Steril* 41:359–363, 1984.
604. Bullen BA, Skrinar GS, Beitins IZ, von Mering G, Turnbull BA, McArthur JW: Induction of menstrual disorders by strenuous exercise in untrained women. *N Engl J Med* 312:1349–1353, 1985.
605. Russell JB, Mitchell D, Musey PI, Collins DC: The relationship of exercise to anovulatory cycles in female athletes: Hormonal and physical characteristics. *Obstet Gynecol* 63:452–456, 1984.
606. Brownell KD, Steen SN, Wilmore JH: Weight regulation practices in athletes: Analysis of metabolic and health effects. *Med Sci Sports Exerc* 19:546–556, 1987.
607. Barr SI: Women, nutrition and exercise: A review of athletes' intakes and a discussion of energy balance in active women. *Prog Food Nutr Sci* 11:307–361, 1987.
608. Kirkwood RF, Cumming DC, Aherne FX: Nutrition and puberty in the female. *Proc Soc Nutr* 46:177–192, 1987.
609. Brown PE: The age at menarche. *Br J Soc Prev Med* 20:9–14, 1966.
610. Bojilen K, Bentzoin M: Influence of climate and nutrition on age at menarche: A historical review and a modern hypothesis. *Hum Biol* 40:69–85, 1968.
611. Stein Z, Susser M: Fertility, fecundity, famine: Food rations in the Dutch famine 1944/5 have a causal relationship to fertility and probably to fecundity. *Hum Biol* 47:131–154, 1975.
612. Weir J, Dunn JE Jr, Jones EG: Race and age at menarche. *Am J Obstet Gynecol* 111:594–596, 1971.
613. Baanders-Van Halewin EA, de Ward F: Menstrual cycles shortly after menarche in European and Bantu girls. *Hum Biol* 40:314–322, 1968.
614. Wolanski N: Environmental modification of human form and function. *Ann NY Acad Sci* 134:826–840, 1968.
615. Kantero R-L, Widholm O: The age of menarche in Finnish girls in 1969. *Acta Obstet Gynecol Scand* 14(suppl):7–18, 1971.
616. Dreizen S, Spirakis CN, Stone RE: A comparison of skeletal growth and maturation in undernourished and well nourished girls before and after menarche. *J Pediatr* 70:256–263, 1967.
617. Kennedy GC: Interactions between feeding behaviour and hormones during growth. *Ann NY Acad Sci* 157:1049–1061, 1969.
618. Frisch RE: Body fat, menarche and reproductive ability. *Semin Reprod Endocrinol* 3:45–54, 1985.
619. Fries H, Nillius SJ, Petterson F: Epidemiology of secondary amenorrhea. *Am J Obstet Gynecol* 118:473–479, 1974.
620. Chakravarty I, Sreedhar R, Ghosh KK, Bulusu S: Circulating gonadotropin profile in severe cases of protein calorie malnutrition. *Fertil Steril* 37:650–654, 1982.
621. Kulin HE, Bwibo N, Mutie D, Santner SJ: Gonadotropin excretion during puberty in malnourished children. *J Pediatr* 105:325–328, 1984.
622. Vigersky RA, Andersen AE, Thompson RH, Loriaux DL: Hypothalamic dysfunction in secondary amenorrhea associated with simple weight loss. *N Engl J Med* 297:1141–1145, 1977.
623. Beumont PJV, George GCW, Pimstone BL, Vinik AI: Body weight and the pituitary response to hypothalamic releasing hormones. *J Clin Endocrinol Metab* 43:487–496, 1976.
624. Steiner RA: Nutritional and metabolic factors in the regulation of reproductive hormone secretion in the primate. *Proc Nutr Soc* 46:159–175, 1987.
625. Deuster PA, Kylem SB, Moser PB, Vigersky RA, Singh A, Schoomaker EB: Nutritional intakes and status of highly trained amenorrheic and eumenorrheic women runners. *Fertil Steril* 46:636–643, 1986.
626. Sanborn CF, Albrecht BH, Wagner WW: Athletic amenorrhea: Lack of association with body fat. *Med Sci Sports Exerc* 19:207–212, 1987.
627. Cumming DC, Rebar RW: Lack of consistency in the indirect methods of estimating body fat. *Fertil Steril* 41:739–742, 1984.
628. Carlberg KA, Buckman MT, Peake GT, Riedesel ML: Body composition of oligo/amenorrheic athletes. *Med Sci Sports Exerc* 15:215–217, 1983.
629. Dale E, Goldberg E: Implications of nutrition in athletes' menstrual cycle irregularity. *Can J Appl Sport Sci* 7:74–78, 1982.
630. Brooks SM, Sanborn CF, Albrecht BH, Wagner WW: Diet in athletic amenorrhea (letters). *Lancet* 1:559–560, 1984.
631. Drinkwater BL, Nilson K, Chesnut CH III, Bremner WJ, Shainoltz S, Southworth M: Bone mineral content of amenorrheic and eumenorrheic athletes. *N Engl J Med* 311:277–281, 1984.
632. Marcus R, Cann C, Madvig P, Minkoff J, Goddard M, Bayer M, Martin M, Guadiani L, et al: Menstrual function and bone mass in elite women distance runners. *Ann Intern Med* 102:158–163, 1985.
633. Nelson ME, Fisher EC, Catsos PD, Meredith CN, Turksoy RN, Evans WJ: Diet and bone status in amenorrheic runners. *Am J Clin Nutr* 43:910–916, 1986.
634. Lloyd T, Buchanan JR, Bitzer S, Waldman CJ, Myers C, Ford BG: Interrelationships of diet, athletic activity, menstrual status and bone density among collegiate women. *Am J Clin Nutr* 46:681–684, 1987.
635. Schweiger UF, Herman R, Laessle W, Riedel M, Schweiger R, Pirke KM: Caloric intake, stress and menstrual function in athletes. *Fertil Steril* 49:447–450, 1988.
636. Cumming DC: Exercise and reproductive dysfunction in women. *J Soc Obstet Gynaecol Can* 13(2):9–17, 1991.
637. Bruce V, Crosby LO, Reicheck N, Pertschuk M, Lusk E, Mullen JL: Energy expenditure in primary malnutrition during standardized exercise. *Am J Phys Med* 63:165–174, 1984.
638. Dalvit SP: The effect of the menstrual cycle on patterns of food intake. *Am J Clin Nutr* 34:1811–1815, 1981.
639. Myerson M, Gutin B, Warren MP, May MT, Contento I, Lee M, Pi-Sunyer FX, Pierson RN Jr, Brooks-Gunn J: Resting metabolic rate and energy balance in amenorrheic and eumenorrheic runners. *Med Sci Sports Exerc* 23:15–22, 1990.
640. Ronkainen H, Pakarinen A, Kirkinen P, Kaupila AJ: Physical exercise-induced changes and season-associated differences in the pituitary-ovarian function of runners and joggers. *J Clin Endocrinol Metab* 60:416–422, 1985.
641. Cumming DC, Vickovic MM, Wall SR, Fluker MR: Defects in pulsatile LH release in normally menstruating runners. *J Clin Endocrinol Metab* 60:810–812, 1985.

642. Cumming DC, Vickovic MM, Wall SR, Fluker MR, Belcastro AN: The effects of acute exercise on pulsatile release of luteinizing hormone in women runners. *Am J Obstet Gynecol* 153:482–485, 1985.
643. Veldhuis JD, Evans WS, Demers LM, Thorner MO, Wakat D, Rogol AD: Altered neuroendocrine regulation of gonadotropin secretion in women distance runners. *J Clin Endocrinol Metab* 61:557–563, 1985.
644. Quigley ME, Sheehan KL, Casper RF, Yen SSC: Evidence for increased dopaminergic and opioid activity in patients with hypothalamic hypogonadotropic amenorrhea. *J Clin Endocrinol Metab* 50:949–952, 1980.
645. Viswanathan M, Van Dijk JP, Graham TE, Bonen A, George JC: Exercise- and cold-induced changes in plasma β-endorphin and β-lipotropin in men and women. *J Appl Physiol* 62:622–627, 1987.
646. Dixon G, Eurman P, Stern B, Schwartz B, Rebar RW: Hypothalamic function in amenorrheic runners. *Fertil Steril* 42:377–383, 1984.
647. Samuels MH, Sanborn CF, Hofeldt F, Robbins R: The role of endogenous opiates in athletic amenorrhea. *Fertil Steril* 55:507–512, 1991.
648. McArthur JW, Bullen BH, Beitins IZ, Pagano M, Badger TM, Klibanski A: Hypothalamic amenorrhea in runners of normal body composition. *Endocr Res Commun* 7:13–25, 1980.
649. International Olympic Committee: *IOC Medical Handbook,* Geneva, Switzerland, 1989.
650. Dubin CL: *Commission of Inquiry into the Use of Drugs and Banned Practices Intended to Increase Athletic Performance.* Ottawa, Supply and Services Canada, 1990.
651. Marshall E: The drug of champions. *Science* 242:183, 1988.
652. Canada: *Report of the Task Force on National Sport Policy Building Canada's Sport System.* Ottawa, Fitness and Amateur Sport, 1988.
653. Berger A, Murray TH, Fost N: Comments from the lay press: Excerpts from three newspaper editorials and commentaries. *Phys Sports Med* 12(3):187–188, 1984.
654. Saartok T, Dahlbey E, Gustaffson JA: Relative binding affinity of anabolic-androgenic steroids: Comparison of the binding to the androgen receptors in skeletal muscle and in prostate, as well as to sex hormone-binding globulin. *Endocrinology* 114:2100–2106, 1984.
655. Wilson JD: Androgens, in Gilman AG, Rall TW, Nies AS, Taylor P (eds): *The Pharmacological Basis of Therapeutics,* 8th ed. New York, Pergamon, 1990, pp 1413–1430.
656. Eriksson E: Comprehensive knee rehabilitation. *Bull Hosp Jt Dis Orthop Inst* 48:117–129, 1988.
657. Cowart VS: Issues of drugs and sports gain attention as Olympic Games open in South Korea. *JAMA* 260:1513–1518, 1988.
658. United States Congress, Senate Judiciary Committee: Hearing on Steroid Abuse in America, April 3, 1989, testimony of Pat Connolly.
659. Australia, Parliament: *Drugs in Sport: An Interim Report of the Senate Standing Committee on Environment, Recreation and the Arts.* Commonwealth of Australia, 1989, p 75.
660. Amateur Athletic Association, Great Britain: *Report of the A.A.A: Drug Abuse Inquiry,* London, 1989.
661. Loughton SJ, Ruling RO: Human strength and endurance responses to anabolic steroid training. *J Sportsmed Phys Fitness* 17:285–296, 1977.
662. Clement DB: Drug use survey: Results and conclusions. *Phys Sports Med* 11(9):64–67, 1983.
663. Barnes L: Steroid use pandemic, strength coaches told. *Phys Sports Med* 11(9):25–29, 1983.
664. Cooper DL: Drugs and the athlete. *JAMA* 221:1007–1011, 1972.
665. Ljungqvist A: Use of anabolic steroids in top Swedish athletes. *Br J Sports Med* 9:82, 1975.
666. Lucking MT: Steroid hormones in sports: Special reference: Sex hormones and their derivatives. *Int J Sports Med* 3(suppl):65–67, 1982.
667. Frankle MA, Cicero GJ, Payne J: Use of androgenic steroids by athletes (letter) *JAMA* 252:482, 1984.
668. Freed DJL, Banks AJ, Longson D, Burley I: Anabolic steroids in athletes: Crossover double blind trial on weightlifters. *Br Med J* ii:471–473, 1975.
669. Shephard RJ, Killinger D, Fried T: Responses to sustained use of anabolic steroids. *Br J Sports Med* 11:170–173, 1977.
670. Strauss RH, Liggett MT, Lanese RR: Anabolic steroid use and perceived effects in ten weight-trained women athletes. *JAMA* 253:2871–2873, 1985.
671. Dezelsky TL, Toohey JV, Shaw RS: Non-medical drug use behavior at five United States universities: A 15-year study. *Bull Narc* 37:49–53, 1985.
672. Pope HG, Katz DL, Champoux R: Anabolic steroid use among 1010 college men. *Phys Sports Med* 16(7):75–83, 1988.
673. Duda M: Gauging steroid use in high school kids. *Phys Sports Med* 16(8):16–17, 1988.
674. Windsor R, Dumitru D: Prevalence of anabolic steroid use by male and female adolescents. *Med Sci Sports Exerc* 21:494–497, 1989.
675. Terney R, McLain LG: The use of anabolic steroids in high school students. *Am J Dis Child* 144:99–103, 1990.
676. Buckley WE, Yesalis CE III, Friedl KE, Anderson WA, Streit AL, Wright JE: Estimated prevalence of anabolic steroid use among male high school seniors. *JAMA* 260:3441–3445, 1988.
677. Johnson MD, Jay MS, Shoup B, Rickert VI: Anabolic steroid use by male adolescents. *Pediatrics* 83:921–924, 1989.
678. Krowchuk DP, Anglin TM, Goodfellow DB, Stancin T, Williams P, Zimet GD: High school athletes and the use of ergogenic aid. *Am J Dis Child* 143:486–489, 1989.
679. Friedl KE, Yesalis CE: Self-treatment of gynecomastia in bodybuilders who use anabolic steroids. *Phys Sports Med* 17(3):67–79, 1989.
680. Strauss RH, Wright JE, Finerman GAM, Catlin DH: Side effects of anabolic steroids in weight trained men. *Phys Sports Med* 11:87–98, 1983.
681. Cowart VS: Some predict increased steroid use despite drug testing, crackdown on suppliers. *JAMA* 257:3025–1987.
682. Alen M, Reinila M, Vihko R: Responses of serum hormones to androgen administration in power athletes. *Med Sci Sports Exerc* 17:354–359, 1985.
683. Alen M, Suominen J: Effect of androgenic and anabolic steroids on spermatogenesis in power athletes. *Int J Sports Med* 5(suppl):189–192, 1984.
684. Cohen JC, Noakes TD, Benade AJS: Hypercholesterolemia in male power lifters using anabolic-androgenic steroids. *Phys Sports Med* 16(8):49–56, 1988.
685. Crist DM, Stackpole PJ, Peake GT: Effects of androgenic substances on neuromuscular power and body composition. *J Appl Physiol* 54:366–370, 1983.
686. Hakkinen K, Alen M: Physiological performance, serum hormones, enzymes, and lipids of an elite power athlete during training with and without androgens and during prolonged detraining. *J Sportsmed Phys Fitness* 26:92–100, 1986.
687. Morey SW, Passariello K: *Steroids—A Comprehensive and Factual Report.* Tampa, SW Morey and K Passariello, 1982.
688. Pope HG Jr, Katz DL: Affective and psychotic symptoms associated with anabolic steroid use. *Am J Psychiatry* 145:487–490, 1988.
689. Salke RC, Roland TW, Burke EJ: Left ventricular size and function in body builders using anabolic steroids. *Med Sci Sports Exerc* 17:701–704, 1985.
690. Thomson DP, Pearson DR, Costill DL: Use of anabolic steroids by national levels athletes (abstract). *Med Sci Sports Exerc* 13:111, 1981.
691. Burkett LN, Falduto MT: Steroid use by athletes in a metropolitan area. *Phys Sports Med* 12(8):69–74, 1984.
692. Windsor RE, Dumitru D: Anabolic steroid use by athletes: How serious are the health hazards? *Postgrad Med* 84:37–49, 1988.

693. Lamb DR: Anabolic steroids and athletic performance, in Laron Z, Rogol AD (eds): *Hormones and Sport*. New York, Serono Symposia Publications, vol. 55. New York, Raven Press 1989, pp 257–273.
694. Wright JE: Anabolic steroids and athletics. *Exerc Sport Sci Rev* 8:149–202, 1980.
695. Tennant F, Black DL, Voy RO: Anabolic steroid dependence with opioid-type features (letter). *N Engl J Med* 219:578, 1988.
696. Rance NE, Max SR: Modulation of the cytosolic androgen receptor in striated muscle by sex steroids. *Endocrinology* 115:862–866, 1984.
697. Wilson JD: Androgen abuse by athletes. *Endocr Rev* 9:181–199, 1988.
698. Rogozkin V: Metabolic effects of anabolic steroid on skeletal muscle. *Med Sci Sports Exerc* 11:160–163, 1979.
699. Sholl SA, Goy RW, Kim KL: 5 alpha-reductase, aromatase, and androgen receptor levels in the monkey brain during fetal development. *Endocrinology* 124:627–634, 1989.
700. Viru A, Korge P: Role of anabolic steroids in the hormonal regulation of skeletal muscle adaptation. *J Steroid Biochem* 11:932, 1979.
701. Hickson RC, Galassi TM, Kurowski TT, Daniels DG, Chatterton RT Jr: Skeletal muscle cytosol [3H]methyltrienolone receptor binding and serum androgens: Effects of hypertrophy and hormonal state. *J Steroid Biochem* 19:1705–1712, 1983.
702. Hickson RC, Kurowski TG: Anabolic steroids and training. *Clin Sports Med* 5:461–469, 1986.
703. Fahey TD, Brown CH: The effects of anabolic steroids on the strength, body composition and endurance of college males when accompanied by a weight training program. *Med Sci Sports Exerc* 5:272–276, 1973.
704. Rogozkin VA: Anabolic steroid metabolism in skeletal muscle. *J Steroid Biochem* 11:923–926, 1979.
705. Hickson RC, Czerwinski SM, Falduto MT, Young AP: Glucocorticoid antagonism by exercise and androgenic-anabolic steroid. *Med Sci Sports Exerc* 22:331–340, 1990.
706. Tanaka H, Gibb W, Ducharme JR, Collu R: Influence of compensatory overload on glucocorticoid receptors in rat skeletal muscle. *Steroids* 51:115–122, 1988.
707. Max SR: Glucocorticoid-mediated induction of glutamine synthetase in skeletal muscle. *Med Sci Sports Exerc* 22:325–330, 1990.
708. Danhaive PA, Rousseau GG: Evidence for sex-dependent anabolic response to androgenic steroids mediated by muscle glucocorticoid receptors in the rat. *J Steroid Biochem* 1988:575–581, 1988.
709. Schiavi RV, Thielgard A, Owen DR, White D: Sex chromosome anomalies, hormones and aggressivity. *Arch Gen Psychiatry* 41:93–99, 1984.
710. Mattson A, Schalling D, Olweus D, Low H, Svensson J: Plasma testosterone, aggressive behavior and personality dimensions in young male delinquents. *J Am Acad Child Adolesc Psychiatry* 19:476–490, 1980.
711. Olweus D, Mattson A, Schalling D, Low H: Testosterone, aggression, physical, and personality dimensions in normal adolescent males. *Psychosom Med* 42:253–269, 1980.
712. Rose RM, Holaday JW, Bernstein IS: Plasma testosterone, dominance rank and aggressive behaviour in male Rhesus monkeys. *Nature* 231:366–368, 1971.
713. Wilson JD, Griffin JE: The use and misuse of androgens. *Metabolism* 29:1278–1295, 1980.
714. Hervey GR: Are athletes wrong about anabolic steroids? *Br J Sports Med* 9:74–77, 1975.
715. Council on Scientific Affairs: Drug abuse in athletes: Anabolic steroids and human growth hormone. *JAMA* 259: 1703–1705, 1988.
716. Ariel G, Saville W: Anabolic steroids: the physiological effect of placebos. *Med Sci Sports Exerc* 4:124–126, 1972.
717. Wade NA: Doctors denounce them but athletes aren't listening. *Science* 176:1399–1403, 1972.
718. Kibble MW, Ross MB: Adverse effects of anabolic steroids in athletes. *Clin Pharmacol* 6:686–692, 1987.
719. Johnson LC, Roundy ES, Allsen PE, Fisher AG, Silvester LJ: Effect of anabolic steroid treatment on endurance. *Med Sci Sports Exerc* 7:287–289, 1975.
720. Johnson LC, Fisher G, Silvester LJ, Hofheins CC: Anabolic steroids: Effect upon strength, body weight, oxygen uptake, and spermatogenesis upon mature males. *Med Sci Sports Exerc* 4:43–45, 1972.
721. Haupt HA, Rovere GD: Anabolic steroids: A review of the literature. *Am J Sports Med* 12:469–484, 1984.
722. Hervey GR, Hutchinson I, Knibbs AV, Burkinshaw L, Jones PRM, Norgan MG, Levell MJ: "Anabolic" effects of methandienone in men undergoing athletic training. *Lancet* 2:699–702, 1976.
723. Bowers RW, Reardon JP: Effects of methandostenolone (Dianabol) on strength development and aerobic capacity (abstract). *Med Sci Sports Exerc* 4:54, 1972.
724. O'Shea JP: A biochemical evaluation of the effects of stanozolol on adrenal, liver, and muscle function in humans. *Nutr Rep Int* 10:381–388, 1974.
725. O'Shea JP, Winkler W: Biochemical and physical effects of an anabolic steroid in competitive swimmers and weightlifters. *Nutr Rep Int* 2:351–362, 1970.
726. Stromme SB, Meen HD, Aakvaag A: Effects of an androgenic-anabolic steroid on strength development and plasma testosterone levels in normal males. *Med Sci Sports Exerc* 6:203–208, 1974.
727. Win-May M, Mya-Tu M: The effects of anabolic steroids on physical fitness. *J Sportsmed Phys Fitness* 15:266–271, 1975.
728. Ballarin E, Guglielmini C, Martinelli S, Casoni I, Borsetto C, Ziglio PG, Conconi F: Unmodified performance in runners following anabolic steroid administration. *Int J Sports Med* 7:302–306, 1986.
729. Chandler JV, Blair SN: The effect of amphetamines on selected physiological components related to athletic success. *Med Sci Sports Exerc* 12:65–69, 1985.
730. Brooks RV: Anabolic steroids and athletes. *Phys Sports Med* 8(3):161–163, 1980.
731. MacDougall D: Anabolic steroids. *Phys Sports Med* 11(9):95–100, 1983.
732. Lamb DR: Androgens and exercise. *Med Sci Sports Exerc* 7:1–5, 1975.
733. Hervey GR, Knibbs AV, Burkinshaw L, Morgan DB, Jones PRM, Chettle DR, Vartsky D: Effects of methandienone on the performance and body composition of men undergoing athletic training. *Clin Sci* 60:457–461, 1981.
734. Forbes GB: The effect of anabolic steroids on lean body mass: The dose response curve. *Metabolism* 34:571–573, 1985.
735. Stamford B, Moffat R: Anabolic steroids: Effectiveness as an ergogenic aid to experienced weight trainers. *J Sports Med Exerc* 14:191–197, 1974.
736. O'Shea JP: The effects of anabolic steroid on dynamic strength levels of weightlifters. *Nutr Rep Int* 10:363–370, 1974.
737. Ward P: The effect of an anabolic steroid on strength and lean body mass. *Med Sci Sports Exerc* 5:277–282, 1973.
738. Casner S, Early R, Carlson BR: Anabolic steroid effects on body composition in normal young men. *J Sports Med Phys Fitness* 11:98–103, 1971.
739. Johnson LC, O'Shea JP: Anabolic steroid: Effects on strength development. *Science* 164:957–959, 1969.
740. Steinbach M: Uber den Einfluss anaboler Wirkstoffe auf Korpergewicht, Muskelkraft und Muskeltraining. *Sportarzt Sportmed* 11:485–492, 1968.
741. Fowler WM Jr, Gardner GW, Egstrom GH: Effect of anabolic steroids on physical performance in young men. *J Appl Physiol* 20:1038–1040, 1965.
742. Golding LA, Freydinger JE, Fishel SS: Weight, size and strength—unchanged with steroids. *Phys Sports Med* 2:39–45, 1974.

743. Weiss V, Muller H: Aur Frage der Beeninflussungdes Krafttrainings durch anabole Hormone. *Schweiz Z Sportsmed* 16:78–89, 1968.
744. Alen M, Hakkinen K, Komi PV: Changes in neuromuscular performance and muscle fibre characteristics of elite power athletes self-administering androgenic and anabolic steroids. *Acta Physiol Scand* 122:535–544, 1984.
745. Ariel G: The effect of anabolic steroid (methandrostenelone) on selected physiological parameters. *Ath Training* 7:190–200, 1972.
746. Ariel G: Residual effect of an anabolic steroid upon isotonic muscular force. *J Sportsmed Phys Fitness* 14:103–111, 1974.
747. Tahmindjis AJ: The use of anabolic steroids by athletes to increase body weight and strength. *Med J Aust* 1:991–993, 1976.
748. Overly WL, Dankoff JA, Wang BK, Singh UD: Androgens and hepatocellular carcinoma in an athlete (letter). *Ann Intern Med* 100:158–159, 1984.
749. Samuels LT, Henschel AF, Keys A: Influence of methyltestosterone on muscular work and creatine metabolism in normal young men. *J Clin Endocrinol Metab* 2:649–654, 1942.
750. Alen M, Hakkinen K: Androgenic steroid effects of serum hormones and on maximal force development in strength athletes. *J Sports Med Phys Fitness* 27:38–46, 1987.
751. Ariel G, Saville W: The effects of anabolic steroids on reflex arc components. *Med Sci Sports Exerc* 4:120–123, 1972.
752. Rogozkin V: Metabolic effects of anabolic steroids on skeletal muscle. *Med Sci Sports Exerc* 11:160–163, 1979.
753. Max SR, Nance RE: No effect of sex steroids on compensatory muscle hypertrophy. *J Appl Physiol* 56:1589–1593, 1984.
754. Creagh TM, Rubin A, Evans DJ: Hepatic tumours induced by anabolic steroids in an athlete. *J Clin Pathol* 41:441–443, 1988.
755. Goldman B: Liver carcinoma in an athlete taking anabolic steroids (letter). *J Am Osteopath Assoc* 85:56, 1985.
756. Frankle MA, Eichberg R, Zachariah SB: Anabolic androgenic steroids and a stroke in an athlete: Case report. *Arch Phys Med Rehabil* 69:632–633, 1988.
757. Mochizuki RM, Richter KJ: Cardiomyopathy and cerebrovascular accident associated with anabolic androgenic steroid use. *Phys Sports Med* 16(11):108–114, 1988.
758. McNutt RA, Ferenchick GS, Kirlin PC, Hamlin NJ: Acute myocardial infarction in a 22-year-old world class weight lifter using anabolic steroids. *Am J Cardiol* 62:164, 1988.
759. Annitto WJ, Layman WA: Anabolic steroids and acute schizophrenic episode. *J Clin Psychiatry* 41:143–144, 1980.
760. Pope HG Jr, Katz DL: Homicide and near-homicide by anabolic steroid users. *J Clin Psychiatry* 51:28–31, 1990.
761. Hearing before the Senate Subcommittee to Investigate Juvenile Delinquency of the Committee on the Judiciary: *Proper and Improper Use of Drugs by Athletes*. United States Senate, 93rd Congress. Washington, DC, U.S. Government Printing Office, 1973.
762. Frasier D: Androgens and athletes. *Am J Dis Child* 125:479–480, 1973.
763. Rogol AD: Drugs to enhance performance in the adolescent. *Semin Adolesc Med* 1:317–324, 1985.
764. Costill DL, Pearson DR, Fink WJ: Anabolic steroid use among athletes: Changes in HDL-C levels. *Phys Sports Med* 12(6):112–117, 1984.
765. Hurley BF, Seals DR, Hagberg JM, Goldberg AC, Ostrove SM, Holloszy JO, Wiest WG, Goldberg AP: High-density-lipoprotein cholesterol in bodybuilders v powerlifters: Negative effects of androgen use. *JAMA* 252:507–513, 1984.
766. Kantor MA, Bianchini A, Bernier D, Sady SP, Thompson PD: Androgens reduce HDL_2-cholesterol and increase hepatic triglyceride lipase activity. *Med Sci Sports Exerc* 17:462–465, 1985.
767. Peterson GE, Fahey TD: HDL-C in five elite athletes using anabolic-androgenic steroids. *Phys Sports Med* 12(6):120–130, 1984.
768. Webb OL, Laskarzewski PM, Glueck CJ: Severe depression of high density lipoprotein cholesterol levels in weight lifters and body builders by self-administered exogenous testosterone and anabolic-androgenic steroids. *Metabolism* 33:971–975, 1984.
769. Alen M, Rahkila P: Reduced high-density lipoprotein-cholesterol in power athletes: Use of male sex hormone derivates, an atherogenic factor. *Int J Sports Med* 5:341–342, 1984.
770. Mueller R, Hollmann W: Akute Lipoproteinbeeinflussung durch ein anaboles Steroid bei Kraftsportlern. *Deutsche Z Sportmed* 39:35–40, 1988.
771. Crist DM, Peake GT, Stackpole PJ: Alphalipoproteinemic effects of androgenic-anabolic steroids in athletes. *Ann Sports Med* 2:125–128, 1985.
772. Lenders JWM, Demacker PNM, Vos JA, Lansen PLM, Hoitsma AJ, van't Laar A, Thien T: Deleterious effects of anabolic steroid on serum lipoproteins, blood pressure, and liver function in amateur body builders. *Int J Sports Med* 9:19–23, 1988.
773. Frohlich J, Kullmer T, Urhausen A, Bergmann R, Kindermann W: Lipid profile of body builders with and without self-administration of anabolic steroids. *Eur J Appl Physiol* 59:98–103, 1989.
774. McKillop G, Ballantyne D: Lipoprotein analysis in bodybuilders. *Int J Cardiol* 17:281–288, 1987.
775. Alen M, Rahkila P, Marniemi J: Serum lipids in power athletes self-administering testosterone and anabolic steroids. *Int J Sports Med* 6:139–144, 1985.
776. Haffner SM, Kushwaha Foster DM, Applebaum-Bowden D, Hazzard WR: Studies of the metabolic mechanism of reduced high density lipoproteins during anabolic steroid therapy. *Metabolism* 32:413–420, 1983.
777. Kiraly CL: Androgenic-anabolic steroid effects on serum and skin surface lipids, on red cells and on liver enzymes. *Int J Sports Med* 9:249–252, 1988.
778. O'Connor JS, Baldini FD, Skinner JS, Einstein M: Blood chemistry of current and previous anabolic steroid users. *Milit Med* 155:72–75, 1990.
779. Urhausen A, Holpes R, Kindermann W: One- and two-dimensional echocardiography in bodybuilders using anabolic steroids. *Eur J Appl Physiol* 58:633–640, 1989.
780. McKillop G, Todd IC, Ballantyne D: Increased left ventricular mass in a bodybuilder using anabolic steroids. *Br J Sports Med* 20:151–152, 1986.
781. Kleiner SM, Calabrese LH, Fiedler KM, Naito HK, Skibinski CI, Fiedler KM: Dietary influences on cardiovascular disease risk in anabolic steroid-using and nonusing bodybuilders. *J Am Coll Nutr* 8:109–119, 1989.
782. Maron BJ, Roberts WC, McAllister HA, Rosing DR, Epstein SE: Sudden death in young athletes. *Circulation* 62:218–229, 1980.
783. Freinhar JP, Alvarez W: Androgen induced hypomania (letter). *J Clin Psychiatry* 46:354–355, 1985.
784. Wilson IC, Prange AJ Jr, Lara PP: Methyltestosterone and imipramine in men: Conversion of depression to a paranoid reaction in men. *Am J Psychiatry* 131:21–24, 1974.
785. Pope HG Jr, Katz DL: Bodybuilders psychosis (letter). *Lancet* 1:863, 1987.
786. Brower KJ, Blow FC, Beresford TP, Fuelling C: Anabolic-androgenic steroid dependence. *J Clin Psychiatry* 50:31–33, 1989.
787. Elofson G, Elofson S: Steroids claimed our son's life. *Phys Sports Med* 18(8):15–16, 1990.
788. Brower KJ, Blow FC, Eliopoulos GA, Beresford TP: Anabolic androgens and suicide (letter). *Am J Psychiatry* 146:1075, 1989.
789. Brower KJ, Eliopoulos GA, Blow FC, Catlin DH, Beresford TP: Evidence for physical and psychological dependence on anabolic androgenic steroids in eight weight lifters. *Am J Psychiatry* 147:510–512, 1990.
790. Limbird TJ: Anabolic steroids in the training and treatment of athletes. *Compr Ther* 11:25–30, 1985.

791. Strauss RH, Wright JE, Finerman GA: Anabolic steroid use and health status among 42 weight trained male athletes (abstract). *Med Sci Sports Exerc* 14:119, 1982.
792. Lubell A: Does steroid abuse cause—or excuse—violence? *Phys Sports Med* 17(2):176–180, 1989.
793. Lefavi RG, Reeve TG, Newland MC: Relationship between anabolic steroid use and selected psychological parameters in male bodybuilders. *J Sport Behav* 13:157–166, 1990.
794. Yesalis CE, Streit AL, Vicary JR, Friedl KE, Brannon D, Buckley W: Anabolic steroid use: Indications of habituation among adolescents. *J Drug Educ* 19:103–116, 1989.
795. Mayerhausen W, Riebel B: Acne fulminans nach Anabolikaeinnahme. *Z Hautkr* 64:875–880, 1989.
796. Holma PK: Effect of an anabolic steroid (metandienone) on spermatogenesis. *Contraception* 15:151–162, 1977.
797. Clerico A, Leoncini R, Ferdeghini M, Sardano G, Palombo C: Effect of anabolic treatment on the serum levels of gonadotropins, testosterone, prolactin, thyroid hormones, and myoglobin of male athletes under physical training. *J Nucl Med Allied Sci* 25:79–88, 1981.
798. Kilshaw BH, Harkness RA, Hobson BM, Smith AWM: The effects of large doses of the anabolic steroid, methandrostenolone, on an athlete. *Clin Endocrinol (Oxf)* 4:537–541, 1975.
799. Remes K, Vuopio P, Jarvinen M, Adlercreutz H: Effect of short term treatment with an anabolic steroid (methandienone) and dehydroepiandrosterone sulphate on plasma hormones, red cell volume and 2,3-diphosphoglycerate in athletes. *Scand J Clin Lab Invest* 37:577–586, 1977.
800. Alen M, Rahkila P, Reinila M, Vihko R: Androgenic-anabolic steroid effects on serum thyroid, pituitary and steroid hormones in athletes. *Am J Sports Med* 15:357–361, 1987.
801. Ruokonen A, Alen M, Bolton N, Vihko R: Response of serum testosterone and its precursor steroids, SHBG and CBG, to anabolic steroid and testosterone self administration in man. *J Steroid Biochem* 23:33–38, 1985.
802. Martikainen H, Alen M, Rahkila P, Vihko R: Testicular responsiveness to human chorionic gonadotrophin during transient hypogonadotrophic hypogonadism induced by androgenic/anabolic steroids in power athletes. *J Steroid Biochem* 25:109–112, 1986.
803. Kiraly CL, Collan Y, Alen M: Effect of testosterone and anabolic steroids on the size of sebaceous glands in power athletes. *Am J Dermatopathol* 9:515–519, 1987.
804. Kiraly CL, Alen M, Korvola J, Horsmanheimo M: The effect of testosterone and anabolic steroids on the skin surface lipids and the population of Propionibacteria acnes in young postpubertal men. *Acta Derm Venereol (Stockh)* 68:21–26, 1988.
805. Laron Z: Breast development induced by methandrostenolone (Dianabol) (letter). *J Clin Endocrinol Metab* 22:450–452, 1962.
806. Taylor WN, Black AB: Pervasive anabolic steroid use among health club athletes. *Ann Sports Med* 3:155–159, 1987.
807. Wall SR, Cumming DC: The effects of physical activity on reproductive function and development in males. *Semin Reprod Endocrinol* 3:65–80, 1985.
808. Cohen JC, Hickman RJ: Insulin resistance and diminished glucose tolerance in powerlifters ingesting anabolic steroids. *J Clin Endocrinol Metab* 64:960–963, 1987.
809. Ishak KG, Zimmerman JH: Hepatologic effects of the anabolic androgenic steroids. *Semin Liver Dis* 7:230–236, 1987.
810. Keul J, Deus H, Kindermann W: Anabole hormone: Schadigung, leistungsfahigkeit und stoffweschel. *Med Klin* 71:497–503, 1976.
811. Alen M: Androgenic steroid effects on liver and red cells. *Br J Sports Med* 19:15–20, 1985.
812. Hough DO: Anabolic steroids and ergogenic aids. *Am Fam Physician* 41:1157–1164, 1990.
813. Bagheri SA, Boyer JL: Peliosis heptis associated with androgenic-anabolic steroid therapy. *Ann Intern Med* 81:610–618, 1974.
814. Johnson FL: Association of androgenic-anabolic steroids and life threatening disease. *Med Sci Sports Exerc* 7:284–286, 1976.
815. Westaby D, Ogle SJ, Paradinas FJ: Liver damage from long term methyltestosterone. *Lancet* 2:261–263, 1977.
816. Farrell GC, Uren RF, Perkins KW, Joshua DE, Baird PJ, Kronenburg H: Androgen induced hepatoma. *Lancet* 1:430–431, 1975.
817. Meadows AT, Naiman JL, Valdes-Dapena M: Hepatoma associated with androgen therapy for aplastic anemia. *J Pediatr* 84:109–110, 1974.
818. Committee on Neoplastic Disease: Is liver cancer induced by treating aplastic anemia with androgenic agents. *Pediatrics* 53:764, 1974.
819. Editorial: Liver tumours and steroid hormones. *Lancet* 2:1481, 1973.
820. Antunes MF, Stolley PD: Cancer induction by exogenous hormones. *Cancer* 39:1896–1898, 1977.
821. Bernstein MS, Hunter RL, Yachnin S: Hepatoma and peliosis hepatis developing in a patient with Fanconi's anemia. *N Engl J Med* 284:1135–1136, 1971.
822. Goldfarb S: Sex hormones and hepatic neoplasia. *Cancer Res* 36:2584–2588, 1976.
823. Hakkinen K, Alen M: Training volume, androgen use and serum creatine kinase activity. *Br J Sports Med* 23:188–189, 1989.
824. McKillop G, Ballantyne FC, Borland W, Ballantyne D: Acute metabolic effects of exercise in bodybuilders using anabolic steroids. *Br J Sports Med* 23:186–187, 1989.
825. Boone JB, Lambert CP, Flynn MG, Michaud TJ, Rodriguez-Zayas JA, Andres FF: Resistance exercise effects on plasma cortisol, testosterone and creatine kinase activity in anabolic-androgenic steroid users. *Int J Sports Med* 4:293–297, 1990.
826. Hageloch W, Appell HJ, Weicker H: Rhabdomyolyse bei Bodybuilder unter Anabolika-Einnahme. *Sportverletz Sportschaden* 2:122–125, 1988.
827. Milne CJ: Rhabdomyolysis, myoglobinuria and exercise. *Sports Med* 6:93–106, 1988.
828. Prat J, Gray GF, Stolley PD, Coleman JW: Wilms tumor in an adult associated with androgen abuse. *JAMA* 237:2322–2323, 1977.
829. Roberts JT, Essenhigh DM: Adenocarcinoma of prostate in a forty-year old body builder. *Lancet* 2:742, 1986.
830. Shahidi NT: Androgens and erythropoiesis. *N Engl J Med* 289:72–80, 1973.
831. Duda M: Steroids lower immunity, lipids. *Phys Sports Med* 16(2):56–60, 1988.
832. Calabrese LH, Kleiner SM, Barna BP, Skibinski CI, Kirkendall DT, Lahita RG, Lombardo JA: The effects of anabolic steroids and strength training on the human immune response. *Med Sci Sports Exerc* 21:386–392, 1989.
833. Rastad J, Joborn H, Ljunghall S, Akerstrom G: Gluteal infektion hos styrkelyftare efter injektion av anabola steroider. *Lakartidningen* 82:3407, 1985.
834. Sklarek HM, Mantovani RP, Erens E, Heisler D, Niederman MS, Fein AM: AIDS in a body builder using anabolic steroid drugs (letter). *N Engl J Med* 311:1701, 1984.
835. Chung BC, Choo HY, Kim TW, Eom KD, Kwon OS, Suh J, Yang J, Park J: Analysis of anabolic steroids using GC/MS with selected ion monitoring. *J Anal Toxicol* 14:91–95, 1990.
836. Hatton CK, Catlin DH: Detection of androgenic anabolic steroids in urine. *Clin Lab Med* 7:655–668, 1987.
837. Hallagan JB, Hallagan LF, Snyder MB: Anabolic-androgenic steroid use by athletes. *N Engl J Med* 321:1042–1045, 1989.
838. Lamb DR: Anabolic steroids in athletics: How well do they work and how dangerous are they? *Am J Sports Med* 12:31–38, 1984.
839. Ryan AJ: Anabolic steroids are fools gold. *Fed Proc* 40:2682–2688, 1981.
840. Goldberg L, Bosworth EE, Bents RT, Trevisan L: Effect of an

anabolic steroid education program on knowledge and attitudes of high school football players. *J Adolesc Health Care* 11:210–214, 1990.
841. Isetts BJ: Preparing community educational presentations on ergogenic drug use. *Am J Hosp Pharm* 46:2028–2030, 1989.
842. Cowart V: Classifying steroids as controlled substances suggested to decrease athletes' supply, but enforcement could be a major problem (news). *JAMA* 257:3029, 1987.
843. Shroyer JA: Getting tough on steroids: Can we win the battle? *Phys Sports Med* 18(2):106–118, 1990.
844. Cowart VJ: Human growth hormone: The latest ergogenic aid? *Phys Sports Med* 16(3):175–192, 1988.
845. Bigland B, Jehring B: Muscle performance in rats normal and treated with growth hormone. *J Physiol* 116:129–136, 1952.
846. Goldberg AL, Goodman HM: Relationship between growth hormone and muscle work in determining muscle size. *J Physiol* 200:655–666, 1952.
847. Crist DM, Peake GT, Egan PA, Walters DL: Body composition response to exogenous GH during training in highly conditioned adults. *J Appl Physiol* 65:579–584, 1988.
848. Berglund B: Development of techniques for detection of blood doping in sport. *Sports Med* 5:27–135, 1988.
849. Canadian Erythropoietin Study Group: Association between recombinant human erythropoietin and quality of life and exercise capacity of patients receiving haemodialysis. *Br Med J* i:573–578, 1990.
850. Ricci G, Masotti M, De Paoli Vitali E, Vedovato M, Zanotti G: Effects of exercise on haematologic parameters, serum iron, serum ferritin, red cell 2,3-diphosphoglycerate and creatine contents, and serum erythropoietin in long-distance runners during basal training. *Acta Haematol (Basel)* 80:95–98, 1988.
851. Schmidt W, Maassen N, Trost F, Boning D: Training induced effects on blood volume, erythrocyte turnover and haemoglobin oxygen binding properties. *Eur J Appl Physiol* 57:490–498, 1988.
852. Albert K: A bad boost (erythropoietin, genetically engineered hormone being abused by athletes). *Sports Illustrated* 73:29–33, 1990.
853. Ramotar JE: Cyclists' deaths linked to erythropoietin? *Phys Sports Med* 18(8):48–50, 1990.

Index

Index

Note: Pages in italics indicate figures; pages followed by t indicate tables.

Abdominal pain, 26–27
Abetalipoproteinemia, 561–562, 1357–1359
 clinical characteristics of, 1357–1358
 definition of, 1357
 genetics of, 1358
 laboratory findings in, 1358
 pathophysiology of, 1358–1359
 treatment of, 1359
Absorptive hypercalciuria, 1595–1597, *1596*
 treatment of, 1606–1607
Absorptive hyperoxaluria, 1599
Acanthosis nigricans, 25
 insulin resistance and, 1144, 1169
Acetohydroxamic acid, for magnesium ammonium phosphate stones, 1585
Acetyl CoA carboxylase, 1120
Acetylcholine, anatomic pathway of, 250
Acetylcholine receptor, nicotinic, 100, *100*
Acid cholesteryl ester hydrolase deficiency, 1362–1363
Acidosis:
 lactic, diabetes mellitus and, 1224–1225
 osteomalacia and, 1529
 renal phosphate handling and, 1492
Aciduria, correction of, 1580
Acne, 26
 Cushing's syndrome and, 666
Acquired immunodeficiency syndrome (AIDS). *See also* Human immunodeficiency virus (HIV) infection
 adrenocortical insufficiency and, 645–646
 hypogonadotropic hypogonadism and, 926
 hypopituitarism and, 315
 treatment of, pharmacologic, 1680t
Acromegaly, 265, 341–349, 1663
 diabetes mellitus and, 1170, *1170,* 1234
 differential diagnosis of, 344–345
 gangliocytomas and, 262
 laboratory studies in, 344
 pathogenesis of, 345–347, *346*
 signs and symptoms of, *342,* 342–344
 treatment of, 347–349
  pharmacologic, 348–349, *349*
  radiation therapy in, 347–348
  surgical, 347
Actin, 1129
Activation, 172
Activity. *See* Exercise
Activity product ratio (APR), 1586
Acute renal failure (ARF), hypercalcemia and, 1477
Acyl CoA cholesterol acyltransferase, inhibitors of, 1389–1390
Addisonian crisis:
 clinical features of, 648, 650, 650t
 treatment of, 654t, 654–655
Addison's disease. *See also* Adrenocortical insufficiency
 acquired immunodeficiency syndrome and, 645–646
 acute, clinical features of, 648, 650, 650t
 adrenal hemorrhage and, 646
  clinical features of, 650, 650t
 adrenal hyperplasia and, 646–647
 adrenoleukodystrophy and, 646
 autoimmune, 643–645
  disorders associated with, 644, 644t
  etiology, pathogenesis, and genetic aspects of, 643–644
  pathology of, 644–645
 bone and calcium metabolism in, 605
 central nervous system function in, 606
 chronic, clinical features of, 647–648, 648t, *649*
 clinical features of, 647–650
  of acute adrenocortical insufficiency, 648, 650, 650t
  adrenal hemorrhage and, 650, 650t
  of chronic pituitary adrenocortical insufficiency, 647–648, 648t, *649*
 familial glucocorticoid deficiency and, 647
 invasive disorders and, 645
 isolated, 1722
 laboratory features of, 650t, 650–651
 pathophysiology of, 647
 pluriglandular autoimmunity with, 1718–1724, 1719t, *1720,* 1720t, *1721, 1723,* 1724t
  hypoparathyroidism and, 1721–1722, *1722*
  isolated Addison's disease and, 1722
  Schmidt's syndrome and, 1722–1723
 tuberculosis and, 642–643, 643t, 645
Adenohypophysis, 230, 290
 acromegaly and, 345–347, *346*
 adenomas of. *See* Pituitary adenomas
 amenorrhea-galactorrhea syndrome and, 352, *353,* 354
 anatomy of, 886
 cell types in, 291–293
 Cushing's disease and, 359, *360,* 873
 Cushing's syndrome and, 660–661, *661*
 disorders of. *See specific disorders*
 gland, anatomy of, 289, *290*
 hormones of, 293–313, 294t. *See also specific hormones*
 lymphocyte infiltration of, 1724
 tumors of. *See* Pituitary adenomas; Pituitary tumors; *specific tumors*
Adenomas:
 adrenal. *See* Adrenal adenomas
 C cell, 1711
 pituitary. *See* Pituitary adenomas
 thyroid:
  thyrotoxicosis and, 474, 485
  toxic. *See* Goiter, toxic
Adenomatosis, endocrine, multiple. *See* Multiple endocrine neoplasia (MEN), type 1
Adenomectomy, for Cushing's disease, 361
Adenosine, 36
Adenosine diphosphate ribosylation factor proteins, 119
Adenosine monophosphate (AMP), cyclic. *See* Cyclic adenosine monophosphate (cAMP)
Adenosine triphosphate (ATP)-citrate lyase, 1119, *1119*
Adenyl cyclase, 1111
Adenylic acid, 36
Adenylyl cyclase, structure and regulation of, 132–133, *133*
Adolescents. *See also* Puberty
 development of, 1635–1636, *1636,* 1636t, *1637,* 1637t
 virilization of, clinical approach to, *1098,* 1099
Adrenal adenomas:
 adrenocortical, 1706
 clinical features of, 668
 Cushing's syndrome and, 662
 deoxycorticosterone-producing, 833
 primary hyperaldosteronism and, 815–817
  treatment of, 830t, 830–832
 treatment of, 676
Adrenal carcinoma:
 clinical features of, 668
 Cushing's syndrome and, 662
 treatment of, 676–677
Adrenal cortex, 555–680

Adrenal cortex (*Cont.*)
- anatomy of, *557,* 557–559, *558*
- Cushing's syndrome and, 661–662
  - hyperplasia and, 661–662
  - tumors and, 662
- embryology and development of, 556–557
- fetal, 556–557
- historical background of, 555–556
- hormones of. *See* Glucocorticoids; Mineralocorticoids; Steroid hormones; *specific hormones*
- hyperfunction of, 659–660. *See also* Cushing's syndrome; Hyperaldosteronism

Adrenal crisis:
- clinical features of, 648, 650, 650t
- treatment of, 654t, 654–655

Adrenal glands. *See also* Adrenal cortex; Adrenal medulla
- accessory, 558–559
- disorders of. *See specific disorders*
- hormones of. *See specific hormones*
- hypothyroidism and, 502
- thyrotoxicosis and, 477

Adrenal hyperplasia:
- adrenocortical insufficiency and, 646–647
- idiopathic, treatment of, 832
- primary, treatment of, 832

Adrenal insufficiency:
- anemia in, 27
- hypercalcemia and, 1475
- hypothyroidism and, 502
- hypovolemic hyponatremia and, 415–416
- primary:
  - diagnosis of, 321
  - hypopituitarism versus, 319–320

Adrenal medulla:
- glucocorticoids and, 607
- hyperplasia of, multiple endocrine neoplasia, type 2 and, 1715

Adrenal stimulation testing, in children, 626, 626t

Adrenal tumors. *See also specific tumors*
- Cushing's syndrome and, 663–664, 665
- treatment of, 676–677

Adrenal vein catheterization, in primary hyperaldosteronism, 827–828

Adrenalectomy:
- for adrenal adenomas, 676
- for Cushing's disease, 361–362, 676
- for primary hyperaldosteronism, idiopathic, 832

Adrenalitis, lymphocytic, diffuse, 645

Adrenarche, 583–584, 1631

Adrenergic receptors, 105–106
- alpha-adrenergic, 105–106
- beta-adrenergic, 106, *107*
  - agonists of, for diabetes mellitus, 1212–1213
- catecholamines and, 718–720, 719t
- desensitization of, 719–720
- hypersensitization of, 720

Adrenocortical adenomas, in multiple endocrine neoplasia, type 1, 1706

Adrenocortical hyperplasia. *See also* Cushing's disease
- Cushing's syndrome and, 661–662

Adrenocortical insufficiency, *642,* 642–659
- hypoaldosteronism and, 657–659
  - hyporeninemic, 657–658
  - normoreninemic or hyperreninemic, 658–659
- hypopituitarism and, 315–316
- primary. *See* Addison's disease
- prognosis and survival and, 657
- pseudohypoaldosteronism and, 659
- secondary, 651–652
  - clinical features of, 652
  - diagnosis of, 652–654, *653*
  - etiology of, 651
  - isolated adrenocorticotropic hormone deficiency and, 651
  - laboratory features of, 652
  - pathophysiology of, 651–652
  - treatment of, 654–657
- treatment of, 654–657
  - for acute Addisonian crisis, 654t, 654–655
  - for chronic adrenocortical insufficiency, 655t, 655–656
  - steroid coverage for illness, surgery, or trauma and, 656t, 656–657

Adrenocorticotropic hormone (ACTH):
- action of, 295, 575–577
  - acute, 575–576
  - on adrenal cortex, 558
  - chronic, 577
  - receptors and, 576–577
- adrenal response to, 557
- assays for, 295, 363–365
  - basal measurements, 363–364
  - hypopituitarism and, 320–322, *321*
  - stimulation tests, 364–365
  - suppression tests, 365
- chemistry of, 293–295, *294*
- coordinate action of growth factors with, 84–85
- Cushing's syndrome and, 659t, 659–660
- deficiency of:
  - hypothalamic, 268
  - isolated, 651
- ectopic. *See* Ectopic ACTH syndrome
- excess of, ectopic ACTH syndrome and, 664–665
- exercise and. *See* Exercise, adrenocorticotropic hormone-cortisol axis and
- extraadrenal effects of, 295, 295t
- extrapituitary, 297
- feedback loops and, 225
- glucocorticoid feedback on release of, 580, *581*
- glucocorticoid suppression of, 876
- hereditary unresponsiveness to, 647
- hypertension and, 771–772
- hypopituitarism and, 318, 324–325
- hypothyroidism and, 502
- metabolism of, 296
- neurotransmitter function of, 576
- pituitary cells secreting, 292–293
- pituitary level of, 296
- pituitary tumors secreting. *See* Cushing's disease
- plasma level of, 296
  - in adrenocortical insufficiency, 653, *653*
  - assays for, 616–617
  - in children, 626
  - in Cushing's disease, 358
- precursor of, 73–74
- receptors for, 576–577
- regulation of, 243–244, *244,* 296, *296*
  - hypothalamic, 573–574
  - pituitary, 574–580, *575, 576*
- rhythm of, 258
- stress and, 272
- synthesis of, rhythms and, 577–579
- therapeutic uses of, 868
- vasopressin and, 398
- venous sampling of, in Cushing's syndrome, 673

Adrenocorticotropic hormone (ACTH) stimulation tests, 320–321, 1668
- rapid, 620–622, *621,* 878
- three-day, 622

Adrenocorticotropic hormone (ACTH) suppression tests, 1668

Adrenodoxin, *566,* 566–567

Adrenodoxin reductase, *566,* 566–567

Adrenogenital syndrome. *See* 21β-Hydroxylase deficiency

Adrenoleukodystrophy, 646

Adsorption, solid-phase, 210

Adult respiratory distress syndrome (ARDS), cerebral, 1224

Adult T-cell leukemia syndrome, malignancy-associated hypercalcemia and, 1471, 1472

Advanced glycosylation end products (AGEs), 1119

Age. *See also* Adolescents; Children; Elderly persons; Infants; Neonates
- hormone-responsive tumors and, 1790–1792, *1791*
- osteoporosis and, 1534–1535
- ovarian activity and, 1004–1009
  - during fetal period, 1004
  - menarche and, 1004–1006, *1005*
  - menopause and, 1008–1009
  - postmenarche, 1006–1008, *1006–1008*
  - premenarche, 1004, *1005*
- solitary thyroid nodules and, 533
- sporadic goiter and, 527
- steroid hormone metabolism and, 593
- thyroid function and, 456

Aging, theories of, 1816t, 1816–1817

Ahumada-del Castillo syndrome. *See* Amenorrhea-galactorrhea syndrome

Alanine aminotransferase, 1115
Alanine cycle, *1115,* 1115–1116
Albers-Schönberg disease, 1541–1542, *1542*
Albright-McCune-Sternberg syndrome, *1546,* 1546–1547, *1547*
Albright's syndrome, *1546,* 1546–1547, *1547*
Albumin:
glucocorticoid binding to, 587
thyroid hormone binding to, 88, 441, 442
Alcohol use:
Cushing's syndrome and, 670
effect on plasma lipids and lipoproteins, 1373
hyperlipidemia and, 1334
hypoglycemia induced by, 1266
hypophosphatemia and, 1494
osteoporosis and, 1537
Aldose reductase, 1117
Aldosterone. *See also* Hyperaldosteronism; Plasma aldosterone/renin ratio
Bartter's syndrome and, 680
binding of, 589
for congenital adrenal hyperplasia, 638t
Cushing's disease and, 664, *664*
edema and, 680
exercise and training and, 1847
hypertension and, 768
menstrual cycle and, 678–679
metabolism of, 591–592
plasma, in primary hyperaldosteronism, 125, 126
plasma level of, 585t
during pregnancy, 678–679
primary hyperaldosteronism and, subtype differentiation and, 828
regulation of, 580–583
secretion rate of, 585t
structure of, *171*
unresponsiveness to, 659
urinary, in primary hyperaldosteronism, 825
Aldosteronism. *See* Hyperaldosteronism
Alendronate, for hypercalcemia, 1473
Alimentary hypoglycemia, 1264–1265
Alkaline phosphatase:
as index of osteoblastic activity, 1517–1518
serum, assays for, 1497
Alkalosis, respiratory, hypophosphatemia and, 1493
Allergy, to insulin, 1205
Allopurinol:
hazards of, 1581
for hyperuricosuria, 1600–1601, 1601t
uric acid and, 1579, *1579, 1580*
for uric acid stones, 1581
Allstrom-Hallgren syndrome, 270t
Alopecia, 25
totalis, 25
$Alpha_1$ antitrypsin deficiency, hyperlipidemia and, 1334
Alpha-adrenergic blocking drugs, for pheochromocytoma, 731
Alpha-adrenergic receptors, 105–106
Aluminum, osteomalacia induced by, 1543
Amenorrhea, 29. *See also* Amenorrhea-galactorrhea syndrome
in Addison's disease, 648
clinical approach to, 1099, *1099*
gonadotropin-releasing hormone deficiency and, 266
thyrotoxicosis and, 477
Amenorrhea-galactorrhea syndrome, 349–357
differential diagnosis of, 351t, 351–352
laboratory studies in, 350–351
in men, 350
pathogenesis of, 352–354, *353*
signs and symptoms of, 349–350
treatment of, 354–357
for macroadenomas, 354–355
for microadenomas, 354, *355*
pharmacologic, 354, 355–357, *356*
radiotherapeutic, 357
surgical, 354–355, 357
in women, 349–350
Amiloride, for adrenal adenomas, 831
Amine precursor uptake and decarboxylation (APUD) series, 1107
Aminergic system, 885
Amino acids:
analogues of, 5–6
insulin secretion and, 1134
metabolism of, 1125–1128, *1127*
diabetes mellitus and, 1171–1172
glucose-alanine cycle and, 1126–1127
insulin and, 1139
protein repletion and feeding and, *1127,* 1127–1128
as neurotransmitters, 251
neutral, large, obesity and, 1287
steroid-binding residues of, 174, *176*
Aminoglutethimide:
for Cushing's disease, 362, 676
for ectopic ACTH syndrome, 676
steroid synthesis inhibition by, 586
Amiodarone, thyroid function and, 465
Amitriptyline, for diabetic neuropathy, 1189
Amniotic fluid, thyroid hormones in, 456
Amphophils, of adenohypophysis, 293
Amplitude-modulated enzyme immunoassays, 210–211, *211*
Amylin, 1179
Amyotrophy, diabetic, 32, 1190
Anabolic steroids:
control of, 1865
detection of, 1865
for hyperlipoproteinemia, 1388
in sports, 1857–1865
adverse effects of, 1862t, 1862–1865
athletic performance and, 1860–1862, 1861t
ethics of, 1857–1858
extent of use of, 1859
illicit, sources of, 1859–1860
medical indications for, 1858–1859
mode of action of, 1860–1861
pharmacology of, 1860
in women, 1859, 1862
Analgesia, endogenous opiates and exercise, 1844
Analog assays, 205
Androgen(s), 555. *See also specific androgens*
action of, 614
assays for, 623–624
binding of, 589–590
cirrhosis and, 273
erythropoietic effect of, 27
feedback and, negative, 904–905
growth and, 1631–1633, *1632*
hypertension and, 772
hypothalamic-pituitary-germ cell axis and. *See* Hypothalamic-pituitary-germ cell axis
hypothalamic-pituitary-Leydig cell axis and. *See* Hypothalamic-pituitary-Leydig cell axis
insensitivity to, 182, 1084–1085
hypogonadotropic hypogonadism and, *934,* 934–935
metabolism of, 592, *592*
defective, 1083–1084
negative feedback and, 904–905
ovarian, synthesis of, 993
plasma level of, assays for, 623–624
regulation of, 583–584
adrenal versus ovarian sex steroids and, 584
adrenarche and, 583–584
structure of, *171*
synthesis of, 81–83
target tissues of, defects in, 1083–1085
therapeutic uses of, for hypogonadism, 936–937
tumors dependent on, 952–955, *953*
complete androgen blockade for, 954–955
secondary endocrine treatments for, 953–954
urinary, assays for, 624
Androgen blockade, for androgen-dependent neoplasia, 954–955
Androstanes, 559
Androstenedione, 558, 899
binding of, 589
Cushing's disease and, 664, *664*
metabolism of, 86
plasma level of, 585t
secretion rate of, 585t
Anemia, 27
normocytic normochromic, 27
adrenocortical insufficiency and, 650–651

Anemia (*Cont.*)
pernicious, 27
adrenocortical insufficiency and, 651
Aneuploidy, 1054
Aneurysms:
growth hormone deficiency and, short stature and, 1649
hypothalamic, 263
of internal carotid artery, pituitary adenoma versus, 336t, 338
microaneurysms, diabetes mellitus and, 1181
Angina pectoris, hypothyroidism and, 500
Angiography, digital subtraction, intravenous, in renovascular hypertension, 808
Angioid streaks, 1548
Angiotensin:
action of, 760
mechanisms of, 761–762
angiotensin receptor antagonists and, 762
Bartter's syndrome and, 680
circulation of, 761
metabolism of, 761
mineralocorticoid regulation by, 581–582
responsiveness to, regulation of, 762
synthesis of, 760
glucocorticoids and, 604
Angiotensin-converting enzyme (ACE), 252, 759–760
expression and action of, 759–760
glucocorticoids and, 604
inhibitors of, 760
for diabetic nephropathy, 1187–1188
for renovascular hypertension, 809
Angiotensinogen. *See* Angiotensin-converting enzyme (ACE)
Anorchia, hypogonadotropic hypogonadism and, 931
Anorexia, 26
hypothalamic, 270
nervosa, Cushing's syndrome and, 670
Anosmia, 26
Anoxemia, short stature and, 1657
Antagonists, administration or abnormal production of, 16
Anterior clinoid processes, 289
Antibiotics, for magnesium ammonium phosphate stones, 1585
Antibodies:
antigen interaction with, 206
heterophilic, interference in assays caused by, 213–214
for immunoassays, 206–207
monoclonal, 207
nature and structure of, 206, 206f
polyclonal, 206–207
production of, 206–207
ligand interaction with, 206
monoclonal. *See* Monoclonal antibodies
Anticancer drugs. *See* Chemotherapeutic agents; Chemotherapy
Anticodon loop, 41
Anticonvulsant drugs, Cushing's syndrome and, 670
Antidiuretic hormone. *See* Vasopressin (ADH; antidiuretic hormone)
Antiestrogens, 182
Antigens:
interaction with antibodies, 206
labeled, for immunoassays, 203–204
Antihypertensive drugs, for diabetic nephropathy, *1187,* 1187–1188
Antineoplastic agents. *See* Chemotherapeutic agents; Chemotherapy Antiresorptive agents, for osteoporosis, in iatrogenic Cushing's syndrome, 861
Antioxidants, dietary, effect on plasma lipids and lipoproteins, 1372–1373
Antithyroglobulin antibodies, 453–454
Antithyroid drugs:
for Graves' disease, 490
hypothyroidism and, 497
for thyrotoxicosis, 480–483
Graves' disease causing, 479–480, 480t
inorganic iodide, 482
during pregnancy, 487
thionamide drugs, 480–482, *481*
Antithyroid peroxidase antibodies, 453–454
Antral follicles, 979, 981–982
Apathy, 31
Apolipoprotein A-I deficiency, familial, 1354
with apolipoprotein C-III and A-IV deficiency, 1355
variants of, 1355
Apolipoprotein A-1 regulatory protein (ARP-1), 186
Apolipoprotein A-VI deficiency, familial, with apolipoprotein A-I and C-III deficiency, 1354
Apolipoprotein B-100, defective. *See* Hypercholesterolemia, familial defective apolipoprotein B-100
Apolipoprotein C-III deficiency, familial, 1354
with apolipoprotein A-I and A-IV deficiency, 1354
Apoproteins, 1318–1320
function of, 1319t, 1319–1320
structure of, 1318–1319
Appetite, 26. *See also* Anorexia; Satiety
endogenous opiates and exercise and, 1845–1846
APUD system, 1688–1689
Arachidonic acid, 601
release and metabolism of, stimulation of, 147–148, *148*
Arcuate nuclei neurons, 227, 229t
Arginine insulin test, for growth hormone, 1666t
Arginine test, for growth hormone, 367–368, 1666t
Arginine vasopressin (AVP). *See* Vasopressin (ADH; antidiuretic hormone)
Aromatase, 83, 86
Arteriography, renal, in renovascular hypertension, 807
Arteriosclerosis, diabetes mellitus and, 1179–1180
Arthritis:
degenerative, 31
gouty, 31
Ascites:
hyperaldosteronism and, 679–680
hypervolemic hyponatremia and, 415
Assays, 18–20, 201–215. *See also specific assays and under specific hormones*
analog, 205
biological. *See* Bioassays
chemiluminescence, 209
chromatographic, 211–212
chromatography and, 211
detection and, 211–212
commercial, for thyroid hormone, 205–206, 206t
competitive binding, 205
cytochemical, 202–203
equilibrium dialysis, 205
fluorescence, 208–209
polarization, 210
future trends for, 215
homogeneous systems for, 210–211
amplitude-modulated, 210–211, *211*
fluorescence polarization, 210
immunoassays. *See* Immunoassays; Radioimmunoassays
interference and, 213–214
complement and rheumatoid factors and, 214
drugs and, 214
enzyme contaminants and, 214
hemodynamic effects and, 214
heterophilic antibodies and, 213–214
sample matrix effects and, 213
latex particle agglutination, 209
multianalyte, 209
nomenclature for, 203
quality control for, 214–215
of receptors, 211
sandwich, 204, 616
separation systems for, 209–210
vesicle, 209
Asthma, glucocorticoid therapy for, 857, *857,* 863, 868
Astrocytomas, 274
Atherosclerosis, 1360–1361
anabolic steroids and, 1863
complications of, renin-angiotensin system and, 767
Cushing's syndrome and, iatrogenic, 862
lipoprotein particle atherogenicity and, 1325t, 1325–1326
renovascular hypertension and, 798–799

Athletic performance. *See* Exercise
Atresia, ovarian follicle development and, 999
Atretic follicles, *981,* 981–982
Atrial fibrillation, thyrotoxicosis and, 475
Atrial natriuretic peptide (ANP), 254, *776,* 776–779, *777*
action of, 778
molecular mechanisms of, 778
hypertension and heart failure and, 778–779
mineralocorticoids and, 583, 612–613
production and forms of, 776–777
regulation of, 777–778
therapeutic uses of, 779
Atrial pacing, for postural hypotension, 735
Autocrine regulation, 5, 93, *93,* 1620–1621, 1785
Autoimmune disorders:
adrenocortical insufficiency. *See* Addison's disease, autoimmune
diabetes mellitus and, 1163–1164
excess syndromes caused by, 17
growth hormone deficiency and, short stature and, 1649
insulin hypoglycemia, 1263–1264
male infertility and, 942
polyglandular autoimmune syndrome, types I and II, 644
thyroiditis. *See* Thyroiditis, autoimmune
Autonomic failure:
generalized, *732,* 732–736
postural hypotension and. *See* Hypotension, postural
hypoglycemia-associated:
classical diabetic autonomic neuropathy versus, 738
pathogenesis of, 738, *738*
progressive, 734
with parkinsonism or multiple system atrophy, 734
Autonomic function, indirect tests of, 742t, 743
Autonomic nervous system, 713. *See also* Sympathochromaffin system
hypertension and, 779–780
insulin secretion and, 1135
obesity and, 1289–1290
Autonomic neuropathy, 31–32
diabetic, 1190–1191
hypoglycemia-associated autonomic failure versus, 738
Autophosphorylation, ligand-induced, 120
Avascular necrosis of bone, Cushing's syndrome and, iatrogenic, 860
Avidin/biotin system, for immunoassays, 207–208
Axons, adrenergic, physiology of, 715–720
Azoospermia. *See specific disorders*

B lymphocytes, glucocorticoids and, 602
Babinski-Froelich syndrome, 270t
Back pain, osteoporosis and, 1531
Bacteriophages, cloning cDNA onto, 49
Bacteroides infection, magnesium ammonium phosphate stones and, 1584
Band keratopathy, 33
primary hyperparathyroidism and, 1461, *1462*
Bardet-Biedl syndrome, 270t, 924–925
Baroregulation, of vasopressin, *390,* 390–391, 391t, *392*
Bartter's syndrome, 680
sympathochromaffin function and, 740
Basal ganglia, calcification of, hypocalcemia and, 1479
Basal lamina, of primordial follicles, 975, *977*
Base(s), in DNA, 35–36
Base change mutations. *See* Point mutations
Basic fibroblast growth factor (bFGF), granulosa cell cytodifferentiation and, 992
Beckwith-Wiedemann syndrome, 1665
Behavioral modification, for weight loss, 1294
Benign intracranial hypertension, 274–275
β oxidation, 1121, *1122, 1123*
Beta-adrenergic agonists, for weight loss, 1300
Beta-adrenergic antagonists:
for renovascular hypertension, 810
thyroid function and, 464
Beta-adrenergic receptors, 106, *107*
Betamethasone, for congenital adrenal hyperplasia, 638t
Bicarbonate, for diabetic ketoacidosis, 1222–1223
Big plasma glucagon (BPG), 1147
Biguanides, for diabetes mellitus, 1211–1212
Bile acid sequestrants:
for hyperlipoproteinemia, 1381–1382
mechanism of action of, 1381
indications and dosage for, 1381–1382, *1382*
side effects of, 1381
Bile duct obstruction, hyperlipidemia and, 1333–1334
Binding, 6–7, 69. *See also* Hormone receptors; *under specific hormones*
Binding proteins. *See also specific proteins and under specific hormones*
functions of, 6–7
for immunoassays, 206–208
antibodies, 206–208
avidin/biotin, 207–208
Bioassays, 201–203
for adrenocorticotropic hormone, 617
cytochemical, 202–203
for follicle-stimulating hormone, 301
of growth hormone, 306
international standards for, 201
for luteinizing hormone, 300–301
of prolactin, 310
reference preparations for, 201
in vitro, 202, *202*
complementarity of in vivo assays and, 203
in vivo, 201, *202*
complementarity of in vitro assays and, 203
Biosynthesis. *See under specific hormones*
Biphosphonates (diphosphonates):
for hypercalcemia, 1473
hypercalcemic crisis, 1467
for osteoporosis:
prophylactic, 1539
in iatrogenic Cushing's syndrome, 861
for Paget's disease of bone, 1553
Bisexual gonadal development, 1071–1072
Bleeding. *See* Hemorrhage
Blood pressure. *See also* Hypertension; Hypotension
maintenance of, renin-angiotensin system and, 762–763
regulation of, 753
thirst and, 399
vasopressin and, *390,* 390–391, 391t, *392,* 398, 399
Blood volume:
thirst and, 399
vasopressin and, *390,* 390–391, 391t, *392*
Blotting, 47
Blunt ends, 45
Body composition:
exercise and reproductive function in women and, 1855–1856
fuel homeostasis and, 1152–1153, 1153t
Body temperature, 25
hypoglycemia and, 1252–1253
regulation of, hypothalamic disorders and, 271
Body weight. *See* Obesity; Weight gain; Weight loss
Bone(s). *See also* Metabolic bone disease; Musculoskeletal disorders; *specific disorders*
avascular necrosis of, Cushing's syndrome and, iatrogenic, 860
biopsy of, in metabolic bone disease, 1519–1521
disorders of, short stature and, *1652,* 1652–1653
glucocorticoids and, 605–606, *606*
growth of, 1633–1634
hypercalciuria and, 1597
hypothyroidism and, 503
mineralization of. *See* Calcification
parathyroid hormone and, *1427–1430,* 1427–1431
primary hyperparathyroidism and, 1456–1457, *1457–1459*

Bone(s) (*Cont.*)
  skeletal mineralization and,
    hypocalcemia and, 1487
  thyrotoxicosis and, 477
  turnover of, 1427, *1427*
  vitamin D and, 1447–1448
Bone GIA protein:
  growth and, 1633–1634
  serum, as index of osteoblastic activity, 1518
Bradykinin, synthesis of, glucocorticoids and, 601
Brain, 221–226. *See also* Central nervous system; Central nervous system disorders
  development of, glucocorticoids and, 606–607
  as endocrine gland, 3–4
  injury of. *See* Head trauma
  neuron-neuron interactions in, 221–223, *223*
Brain natriuretic peptide (BNP), 254
Breast. *See also* Lactation; Nursing
  male. *See* Gynecomastia
  oxytocin and, 398
  prolactin and, 309–310
Breast cancer, 1799–1803
  diagnosis of, 1800
  estrogen and, 182
  malignancy-associated hypercalcemia and, 1471, 1472
  pathology and prognosis of, 1800–1801
  risk factors for, 1799–1800, 1800t
  treatment of, 1801–1803, *1802,* 1802t
BRL 26830A, for weight loss, 1300
Bromocriptine:
  for acromegaly, 348
  for amenorrhea-galactorrhea syndrome, 355–357, *356*
  for Cushing's disease, 676
Bronchial adenomas, in multiple endocrine neoplasia, type 1, 1706
Brownian motion, 210
Bullae, diabetic, 1192
Burns, hypophosphatemia and, 1494
Bypass surgery, for renovascular hypertension, 811

C cell adenomas, 1711
C cell hyperplasia, 1710–1711
C4 genes, 21-hydroxylase deficiency and, 632
C kinase, 9
C peptide, 1129
  in hypoglycemia, 1253–1254
Cachexia, 313
  neuropathic, diabetic, 1191
Calcification. *See* Ossification
Calcitonin, *1431,* 1431–1437
  action of, 1432–1433, *1433*
  assays for, 1712–1714
    serial, 1714
  biochemistry and molecular biology of, 1433–1434, *1435, 1436*
  biological effects of, 1432
  calcitonin gene-related peptide and, 1434
  hypothyroidism and, 503
  medullary thyroid carcinoma and, 1711–1714, *1712*
    calcitonin measurements in evaluation of therapy and, 1713
    immunohistochemical heterogeneity of, 1713–1714
    provocative testing for, 1712–1713
    serial calcitonin measurements and, 1714
    venous catheterization procedures and, 1713
  osteoporosis and, 1532–1533
    in iatrogenic Cushing's syndrome, 861
  paraneoplastic, 1770–1771, 1771t
  renal phosphate handling and, 1491–1492
  serum level of, in medullary carcinoma of the thyroid, 547–548
  therapeutic uses of, 1434, 1436–1437
    for hypercalcemia, 1471, 1472
    for hypercalcemic crisis, 1467
    for osteoporosis prophylaxis, 1539
    for Paget's disease of bone, 1551–1553, *1552*
Calcitonin gene-related peptide (CGRP):
  calcitonin and, 1434
  hypertension and, 773
  mRNA encoding, 41
Calcitonin stimulation test, in medullary carcinoma of the thyroid, 547, 548
Calcitrol, for hypocalcemia, 1488
Calcium. *See also* Hypercalcemia; Hypocalcemia
  action of, 784
  assays for, in metabolic bone disease, 1518
  deficiency of, rickets and, 1528
  dietary, regulation of absorption on response to variations in intake and, 1446–1447
  extracellular calcium-sensing receptor on parathyroid cells and, 1410, 1413, 1461, *1498*
  hypercalciuria and, *1590,* 1590–1591
  hypertension and, 784–785, 785t
  inositol(1,4,5)-triphosphate-induced, 152–153
  intestinal transport of, vitamin D and, *1445,* 1445–1446, *1446*
  intracellular concentration of, regulation of, 140–141
  metabolism of, 1407–1409, *1408, 1409*
    glucocorticoids and, 605
  mineralocorticoids and, 613
  oscillation in agonist-stimulated cells, 153
  osteoporosis and, 1533
  in iatrogenic Cushing's syndrome, 861
  parathyroid hormone secretion and, 1413
  peptide hormone action and, 139–147
    calcium as second messenger and, 141t, 141–147
    regulation of intracellular calcium concentration and, 140–141
  primary hyperparathyroidism and, 1461–1462
  regulation of, 784
  as second messenger, 141t, 141–147
    calcium-calmodulin and enzyme activation and, 141–143, *142*
    protein kinase C and, *143,* 143–147
  serum:
    assays for, 1497
    in rickets and osteomalacia, 1522–1523
  urinary, assays for, 1497–1498
  vitamin D and, 1441–1442
Calcium carbonate, for hypocalcemia, 1488
Calcium channel blockers:
  for adrenal adenomas, 831
  for diabetic nephropathy, 1188
Calcium chloride, for tetany, 1487
Calcium citrate, for hypocalcemia, 1488
Calcium citrate malate, for osteoporosis prophylaxis, 1538–1539, *1539*
Calcium gluceptate, for tetany, 1487
Calcium gluconate, for tetany, 1487
Calcium leak, renal, hypercalciuria and, *1594,* 1594–1595
Calcium phosphate:
  crystalline forms of, 1581
  effect of pH insolubility of, 1581, *1582*
Calcium phosphate stones, 1581–1583
  crystalline forms of calcium phosphate and, 1581
  effect of pH on solubility of calcium phosphate and, 1581, *1582*
  evaluation of, 1574
  renal tubular acidosis and, 1581–1583
    incomplete, 1582–1583
    pathophysiology of stone disease in, 1582
  treatment of, 1574
Calcium provocative test, for calcitonin, 1712, 1713
Calcium stones, 1585–1609
  calcium oxalate, natural history of, 1586–1587, *1587*
  calcium phosphate. *See* Calcium phosphate stones
  epidemiology of, 1585–1586
  evaluation of, 1602–1605
  hypercalciuria and. *See* Hypercalciuria
  hyperoxaluria and. *See* Hyperoxaluria
  hyperuricosuria and, 1600–1601
  hypocitraturia and, 1601–1602
  idiopathic, 1602
  physical chemistry of, 1586
  risk factors for, 1587t, 1587–1588
  treatment of, 1605–1609
    choosing, 1605–1606
    discontinuation of treatment and, 1608–1609, *1609*
    goals of, 1605

with hypercalciuria, 1606–1607
with hyperoxaluria, 1607
with hyperuricosuria, 1607–1608
with hypocitraturia, 1608
need for, 1605
with subtle hyperparathyroidism, 1606
without metabolic abnormalities, 1608, *1608*
Calcium tolerance test, 1603–1604, *1604*
Calcium-regulating hormones, hypertension and, 773
Calculi. *See* Nephrolithiasis
Call-Exner bodies, 978, *979*
Calmodulin, calcium as second messenger and, 141–143, *142*
Calories:
dietary, in diet therapy for hyperlipidemia, 1376, 1378
obesity and, 1372
restriction of, thyroid function and, 463
Cancer. *See also* Hormone(s), ectopic production of; Tumor; *specific cancers and sites*
hypercalcemia associated with. *See* Hypercalcemia, malignancy-associated
obesity and, 1279
research of, molecular biology in, *60,* 60–61
steroid carcinogens and, 1787–1789, *1788*
steroid hormone receptors and, 182–183
Capacitation, 891, 909
Capping, 70
Capsaicin (Zostrix), for diabetic neuropathy, 1189
Captopril:
for cystinuria, 1577
for diabetic nephropathy, 1187–1188
Captopril test:
in primary hyperaldosteronism, 826
in renovascular hypertension, *804,* 804–805
Carbamazepine, thyroid function and, 465
Carbenoxolone, hypertension and, 834
Carbohydrate(s):
dietary:
in diet therapy for hyperlipidemia, 662
effect on plasma lipids and lipoproteins, 1372
interactions with proteins, diabetes mellitus and, 1172
Carbohydrate metabolism, 1108–1119
diabetes mellitus and, *1171,* 1181
during exercise. *See* Exercise
glucocorticoids and, 596–598, *598*
gluconeogenesis and, 1113–1115, *1114*
glucose transport and glucose phosphorylation and, 1109t, 1109–1110, *1110*
glycogenesis and glycogenolysis and, 1110–1111, *1111, 1112*
glycolysis and, 1111–1113, *1112*
insulin and, 1137–1139
interaction with fat metabolism, 1123–1125, 1126t
lactate and alanine cycles and, *1115,* 1115–1116
pentose shunt and, 1117
polyol pathway and, 1117–1118, *1118*
protein glycation and, 1118–1119
protein glycosylation and, 1119
thyroid hormone effects on, 445
thyrotoxicosis and, 476
tricarboxylic acid cycle and, 1116, *1117*
Carbon dioxide. *See* Hypercapnia
Carcinogens, steroids and, 1787–1789, *1788*
Carcinoid syndrome, 1688–1695
diagnosis of, 1691–1694, 1693t
imaging in, 1693–1694
laboratory studies in, 1691–1693, 1693t
differential diagnosis of, 1694, 1694t
pathology of, 1689–1690
pathophysiology of, 1690–1691, 1691t, *1692*
prognosis of, 1695
symptoms of, 1690, *1690,* 1691t
treatment of, 1694–1695
chemotherapy in, 1694
pharmacologic, 1680t, 1695, 1695t
surgical, 1694
Carcinoid tumors, in multiple endocrine neoplasia, type 1, 1706
Carcinoma. *See also specific sites*
primary hyperaldosteronism and, 821
treatment of, 832
Cardiac failure, 28
atrial natriuretic peptide and, 778–779
thyrotoxicosis and, 475
Cardiomyopathy, diabetic, 1191
Cardiovascular disorders, 28. *See also specific disorders*
acromegaly and, 343
adrenocortical insufficiency and, 651
diabetes mellitus and, 1179–1180, *1180,* 1191–1192
hypertension and, 753–754
hypocalcemia and, 1480
hypothyroidism and, 500
obesity and, 1274–1277, *1276, 1277*
pheochromocytomas and, 727–728
thyrotoxicosis and, 475
Cardiovascular system:
glucocorticoids and, *603,* 603–604, *604*
in iatrogenic Cushing's syndromes, 859
regulation of, 14
Carnitine palmitoyl transferase 1 (CPT-1), 1121, *1122, 1123*
Carotid artery aneurysms, internal, pituitary adenoma versus, 336t, 338
Carpal tunnel syndrome, 32
Cataracts, 32
diabetes mellitus and, 5879
glucocorticoids and, 607
in iatrogenic Cushing's syndrome, 859
hypocalcemia and, 1480
Catecholamines, 713. *See also specific catecholamines*
action of, 1150
mechanisms of, 608, 719t
assays for, 722–724, 723t, 740–742, 741t
biological effects of, 720–722, *721,* 722t
chemistry of, *714,* 714–715
degradation of, 715, *716*
exercise and, 1848–1849
control of release during, 1849
effects of release during, 1849
hypertension and, 779–780
inactivation of, 717–718
insulin secretion and, 1134–1135, 1150
kinetics of, 722–724, 723t
parathyroid hormone secretion and, 1413
physiologic adaptation and, 724, *725, 726*
release of, 717
storage of, 717
synthesis of, *714,* 714–715, *715,* 717
thyroid hormone interactions with, 445
Catechol-*O*-methyl transferase (COMT), catecholamine synthesis and, 715
Cavitation, 978–979, *980*
cDNA libraries, screening of, 49–50
Cell growth, glucocorticoid effects on, 856
Cellular differentiation, ectopic hormone production and, 1743–1744
Cellular retinol-binding protein type II (CRBPII), 190
Cellular theories of aging, 1816
Central nervous system:
adrenergic receptors and, 718–720, 719t
anatomy of, 885–886, *886*
peptidergic and aminergic systems and, 885
steroid receptor neurons and, 885
glucocorticoids and, 606–607
hypocalcemia and, 1479
insulin secretion and, 1135
rhythms of, 257–258, *258*
vasopressin and. *See* Diabetes insipidus, neurogenic
Central nervous system disorders, 31. *See also specific disorders*
amenorrhea-galactorrhea syndrome and, 352
diabetes insipidus and, 402, 403t
hypopituitarism and, 316–317
hypopituitarism versus, 320
primary, prolactin secretion and, 351–352
thyrotoxicosis and, 474
Cerebral edema, diabetic ketoacidosis and, 1223–1224
Cerebral gigantism, 275, 1664–1665
Cerebrospinal fluid (CSF):
oxytocin in, 396

Cerebrospinal fluid (CSF) (*Cont.*)
  vasopressin in, 396, 399
Cerebrospinal fluid (CSF) studies, in pituitary adenomas, 336
Cerebrotendinous xanthomatosis, 1363–1364
  clinical manifestations of, 1364
  laboratory and pathologic findings in, 1364
  pathophysiology of, 1364
  treatment of, 1364
Charcot's joints, 1188
  diabetes mellitus and, 1193
Chemical goitrogens, sporadic goiter and, 529, 529t
Chemiluminescence assays, 209
Chemotherapeutic agents:
  hypogonadotropic hypogonadism and, 932–933
  hypopituitarism and, 317
Chemotherapy:
  for breast cancer, 1801–1802, 1803
  for carcinoid tumors, 1694
  for endometrial cancer, 1804
  for thyroid carcinoma, anaplastic, 545
Chiari-Frommel syndrome. *See* Amenorrhea-galactorrhea syndrome
Chicken ovalbumin upstream promoter transcription factor (COUP-TF), 186
Children. *See also* Growth deficiency; Growth excess; Infants; Neonates
  adrenocortical function in, laboratory assessment of, 624–626, 625t
  Cushing's syndrome in, 660, 665
  development of, 1635, *1635*
  glucocorticoid therapy in, 874
  hyperlipidemia and, diet therapy for, 1379–1380
  hyperlipoproteinemia in, surgical treatment of, 1391–1392
  hypothyroidism in, 506–507
  obesity in, 1283
  osteoporosis in, 1537
  thyroid function in, 456
  virilization of, clinical approach to, *1098,* 1099
Chimeric transgenic animals, 54
Chimerism, 1054
Chloride:
  hypertension and, 783
  intracellular pH regulation and, Na^+-independent Cl^--HCO_3^- anion exchanger and, 787
Chlorpropamide (Diabinese):
  for diabetes insipidus:
    gestational, 414
    neurogenic, 412, *413*
  for diabetes mellitus, 1209, 1209t
Chlorthalidone, for Paget's disease of bone, 1554
Cholecalciferol. *See* Vitamin D_3
Cholecystokinin (CCK), 252, 1682–1683
  action of, 1682, 1683t
  clinical relevance and applications of, 1683
Cholestanes, 559
Cholesterol, 560–567. *See also* Hypercholesterolemia
  ceiling amount of, 1368
  conversion to pregnenolone, 565–566
  dietary:
    effect on plasma lipids and lipoproteins, 1367–1368, *1368*
    in single-diet treatment for hyperlipidemia, calories and, 1374–1375, 1375t
  free, binding of, 563
  metabolism of, 1321
    hypothyroidism and, 502
    thyrotoxicosis and, 476
  steroid hormone derivation from. *See* Steroid hormones, synthesis of
  storage of, 563
  synthesis of, 560–561, 1320t, 1320–1321
    inhibitors of, 1389
    thyrotoxicosis and, 476
  threshold amount of, 1368
  transport of, 562–563
  uptake of, 561–562, *562*
Cholesterol gallstones, obesity and, 1279
Cholesterol-saturated fat index (CSI), 1376, 1377t, 1378
Cholesteryl ester storage disease, 1363
Cholesteryl ester transfer protein (CETP), 1322
Cholestyramine (Questran):
  for familial hypercholesterolemia, 1340
  for hyperlipoproteinemia, 1381–1382
  mechanism of action of, 1381
    indications and dosage for, 1381–1382, *1382*
    side effects of, 1381
Chondrodystrophies, short stature and, *1652,* 1652–1653, *1654*
Choriocarcinomas, 274
Chromaffin cells, physiology of, 715–720
Chromatin, *37,* 37–38, 178
  gene transactivation by glucocorticoid receptor and, 180–181
Chromatographic assays, 211
  chromatography and, 211
  detection and, 211–212
Chromosomal walking, 184
Chromosomes:
  cloning of genes of, 50–51
  isochromosomes, 1058
  in oogonia, 995
  ring, 1054
  sex. *See* Sex chromosomes
Chronic renal failure (CRF):
  amenorrhea-galactorrhea syndrome and, 352
  hypopituitarism and, 316
  prolactin secretion and, 313
Chvostek's sign, 1479
Chylomicron(s), 203, 1317t. *See also* Hyperchylomicronemia
  metabolism of, 1322–1323
Chylomicron retention disease, 1359
Cigarette smoking, osteoporosis and, 1537
Cilium, of sperm, 891
Circadian rhythms, 257
  cortisol response to exercise and, 1841
  factors influencing, 257–259, *258*
  feedback loops and, 225
  glucocorticoid therapy and, 871
  of thyroid function, 455, *455*
Circulation, hypertension and, 753–754
Circumventricular organs, 254
Cirrhosis:
  amenorrhea-galactorrhea syndrome and, 352
  glucose intolerance and, 1235
  hypervolemic hyponatremia and, 415
  hypothalamic disorders and, 273
  portal, thyroid function and, 463
Citrate. *See also* Hypocitraturia
  hypocalcemia and, 1487
Citrate synthase, 1116
Classical cloning, 183
Cleft lip/palate, hypothalamus and, 260, 261
Climacteric, male, hypogonadotropic hypogonadism and, 933–934
Clinoid processes:
  anterior, 289
  posterior, 289
Clofibrate (Atromid):
  for diabetes insipidus:
    gestational, 414
    neurogenic, 412–413
  for familial hypercholesterolemia, 1340
  for hyperlipoproteinemia, 1386–1387
  indications and dosage for, 1386–1387
  mechanism of action of, 1386
  for primary type III hyperlipoproteinemia, 1348, *1348*
  side effects of, 1386
Clomiphene citrate, for hypopituitarism, 326
Clomiphene stimulation test:
  for follicle-stimulating hormone, 366, 912–913, *913, 914,* 914t
  for luteinizing hormone, 366, 912–913, *913, 914,* 914t
Clonidine, for postural hypotension, 735
Clonidine stimulation test, for growth hormone, 368, 1666t
Cloning. *See* Recombinant DNA technology
C17,20-lyase, steroid hormone synthesis and, 82–83
Codons, 41
Coffee, effect on plasma lipids and lipoproteins, 1374
Colestipol (Colestid):
  for familial hypercholesterolemia, 1340
  for hyperlipoproteinemia, 1381–1382
  mechanism of action of, 1381
    indications and dosage for, 1381–1382, *1382*

side effects of, 1381
Collagen, in bone, 1428
Colloid, 436
endocytosis of, 439, *439*
Colloid droplets, 439
Colonic hyperoxaluria, 1599
Coma:
hepatic, thyroid function and, 463
myxedema, 507
nonketotic, hyperosmolar, 1224
Competitive binding assays, 205
Competitive protein-binding radioassay, for cortisol, 615
Complement, interference in assays caused by, 214
Compound tumors, testicular, 952
Computed tomography (CT):
in adrenocortical insufficiency, 654
in Cushing's syndrome, 673, *674*
in nephrolithiasis, 1570
in pheochromocytomas, 730
in pituitary adenomas, 332–333
in primary hyperaldosteronism, 827
in renovascular hypertension, 808
in solitary thyroid nodules, 536
in uric acid stones, 1580
Confusion, 31
Congenital adrenal hyperplasia (CAH), 569–570, 626–627
female pseudohermaphroditism and. *See* Female pseudohermaphroditism, congenital adrenal hyperplasia and
21-hydroxylase deficiency and. *See* 21-Hydroxylase deficiency
3β-hydroxysteroid dehydrogenase deficiency and, 628t, 638–639
infertility and, in males, 941
lipoid, 628t, 641–642
nonclassic, 630–631
P450c11 deficiency and, 628t, 640–641
P450c17 deficiency and, 628t, 639–640
P450c21 deficiency and, 628t
prenatal, 635–638
diagnosis of, 636–637
treatment of, 637–638, 638t
salt-wasting, 630
virilizing, 630
diagnosis of, 1659–1660
missense mutations causing, 634
tall stature and, 1658–1660
treatment of, 1660
Congenital anomalies. *See also specific anomalies*
diabetes mellitus in pregnancy and, 1229
short stature and, 1647
Congestive heart failure:
hypervolemic hyponatremia and, 415
steroid hormone metabolism and, 593
Connexin, 979
Consensus hormone response elements, 178–179, *179*
Constipation, 27
Constitutional hypercalciuria, 1591
Constitutional tall stature, 1657–1658
Convulsions, 31
hypocalcemia and, 1479
Cori cycle, *1115,* 1115–1116
Coronary artery disease (CAD), diabetes mellitus and, 1191
Corpus albicans, 973, 987
Corpus luteum, 973, 985–987, *987–989*
cytodifferentiation of, 993–995
luteinization and, 994
luteolysis and, 994–995
Cortex, ovarian, 973
Cortexolone, structure of, *171*
Cortical androgen stimulating hormone (CASH), 584
Corticosteroid(s), urinary, assays for, 617–618
Corticosteroid myopathy, 32
Corticosteroid-binding globulin (CBG), 85
competitive binding assays and, 205
glucocorticoid distribution and, 863
plasma, physical state of, 586–587, 588t
Corticosterone:
metabolism of, 591
plasma level of, 585t
secretion rate of, 585t
Corticosterone methyl oxidase (CMO), 81
deficiency of, 640
Corticotrop(s), of adenohypophysis, 292–293
Corticotropin. *See* Adrenocorticotropic hormone (ACTH)
Corticotropin releasing hormone (CRH), 242–245, *243, 244,* 296
action of, 243–244, *244*
alternate-day steroid therapy and, 871
areas containing, 242–243
assays for, 622–623
glucocorticoid regulation by, 573–574
hyperresponsiveness to, in Cushing's disease, 359
hypothyroidism and, 502
interaction with vasopressin, 243, *244*
receptors for, 243
rhythm of, 578–579
structure of, 242, *243*
therapeutic uses of, 244–245
Corticotropin releasing hormone (CRH) stimulation test, for adrenocorticotropic hormone, 320–321, 364
Corticotropin test, 1668
Cortisol, 558. *See also* Hydrocortisone; Hypercortisolism
assays for, 615–616
in Cushing's syndrome, 668
for free cortisol, 617
binding of, 85, 586–587, 588t
bioavailability of, 862, 863
for congenital adrenal hyperplasia, 638t
distribution of, 63
exercise and. *See* Exercise, adrenocorticotropic hormone-cortisol axis and
free fraction of, metabolism of, 85–86
glucose counterregulation and, 736
glucocorticoid suppression of, 874–875, *875*, 876
hypertension and, 768–769
metabolism of, 590–591
plasma, physical state of, 586, *587*
plasma level of, 585t, 1668
interpretation of, 615–616
renal failure and, 273
rhythm of, 258
secretion rate of, 585t
stress and, 272
structure of, *171*
synthesis of:
rate of, 618
rhythms and, 577–579
therapeutic use of, for adrenocortical insufficiency, 654t, 655, 656, 656t
thyroid-stimulating hormone regulation by, 299
Cortisone:
for hypopituitarism, 324–325
metabolism of, 863–864
Cortisone acetate:
for adrenocortical insufficiency, 655
for congenital adrenal hyperplasia, 638t
for hypopituitarism, 1651t
Cosyntropin. *See* Adrenocorticotropic hormone (ACTH)
Cosyntropin bolus test, 1668
Counterregulatory hormones, 1152, 1153t
Craniopharyngiomas, 328, *329*
hypothalamus and, 261–262
short stature and, 1648
Creatinine, urinary, assays for, 1497–1498
Cremasteric muscle, 886–887
Cretinism:
endemic goiter and, 525
etiology of, 525
nongoitrous, sporadic, hypothyroidism and, 495
Critical illness:
hypercalcemia and, 1477
hypocalcemia and, 1487
Crooke's hyaline degeneration, 293
Cryptorchidism, 944–947, 1086
pathophysiology of, 944–946, *945*
treatment of, 947
rationale for, 946
Crystalloid theory, of stone pathogenesis, 1567
Crystalloids of Reinke, 985
CSII insulin delivery system, 1202–1203
Cultural factors, obesity and, 1283
Cushing's disease, 357–362, 659
clinical features of, 667
differential diagnosis of, 359
etiology of, 359–361, *360,* 662t, 662–663

Cushing's disease (*Cont.*)
hypothalamic disorders and, 268
laboratory studies in, 358–359
pathogenesis of, 662t, 662–663
pathophysiology of, 664, *664*
signs and symptoms of, 358
treatment of, 361–362, 673–676
pharmacologic, 362
radiotherapeutic, 362
surgical, 361–362
Cushing's syndrome, 659–678
in children, 660, 665
classification, occurrence, and age and sex distributions of, 659t, 659–660
clinical features of, 665t, 665–667, *666*
etiology and, 667–668
determination of etiology of, 670–673, *671*
with elevated adrenocorticotropic hormone level, 672
with low normal adrenocorticotropic hormone level, 672
problems in, 672–673
with suppressed plasma adrenocorticotropic hormone, 671–672
diabetes mellitus and, 1170, *1170,* 1234
diagnosis of, 668–673, *669, 670*
etiology and tumor localization in, 670–673, *671*
etiology and pathogenesis of, 662–664
adrenal tumors and, 663–664
clinical features suggesting etiolgy and, 667–668
Cushing's disease and, 662t, 662–663
ectopic ACTH syndrome and, 663, 663t
glucocorticoid therapy for, reproductive function and, 608
hypertension and, 835
iatrogenic, 857–858, 859–862
atherosclerosis and, 862
avascular necrosis of bone and, 860
comparisons with spontaneous Cushing's syndrome, 859
diagnosis of, 862
glucocorticoid dose and time dependency and reversibility and, 862
infections and, 861
myopathy and, 861–862
ocular changes in, 859–860
osteoporosis and, *860,* 860–861, *861*
laboratory features of, 667
osteoporosis and, 1536
pathology of, 660–662
adrenal cortex and, 661–662
anterior pituitary and, 660–661, *661*
pathophysiology of, 664–665
of adrenal tumors, 665
of Cushing's disease, 664, *664*
of ectopic ACTH syndrome, 664–665
plasma adrenocorticotropic hormone level in, 616
prognosis of, 678
short stature and, 1651–1652
treatment of, 673–678
for adrenal tumors, 676–679
for Cushing's disease, 673–676
for ectopic ACTH syndrome, 676
for Nelson's syndrome, 677–678
tumor localization in, 670, 673, *674*
Cutaneous disorders, 25–26. *See also specific disorders*
acromegaly and, 342
in Addison's disease, 648, *649*
Cushing's syndrome and, 665–666
diabetes mellitus and, 1192, *1192*
hypocalcemia and, 1480
hypothyroidism and, 499, *499*
pigmentation of. *See* Hyperpigmentation; Pigmentation
Cyanide-nitroprusside test, in cystinuria, 1575
Cyanoketone, steroid synthesis inhibition by, 586
Cyclic adenosine monophosphate (cAMP):
cAMP regulatory element binding protein and, 43
cAMP-dependent protein kinase and, 95, 134–137, *135*, 135t, 136t
glucocorticoids and, 609
insulin secretion and, 1132
nephrogenous, 1426, *1427*
second messenger system of, biosynthetic enzyme regulation by, 71
signaling system and, *131,* 131–132, *132*
somatostatin gene transcription and, 242
urinary, assays for, 1497–1498
Cyclic guanosine monophosphate (cGMP):
peptide hormone action and, 137
protein kinases dependent on, peptide hormone action and, 138
Cyclic nucleotide phosphodiesterases, 134
Cyclopentanophenanthrene ring, 560, *561*
Cyproheptadine, for Cushing's disease, 676
Cyproterone acetate, structure of, *171*
Cystic fibrosis, male infertility and, 941, 942t
Cystinuria, 1573–1577
clinical diagnosis of, 1575
clinical findings in, 1574, *1575*
cysteine-complexing agents and, 1574, *1574*
dependence of cystine excretion on salt intake and, 1574
dependence of cystine solubility on urinary pH and, 1573, *1574*
genetics of, 1573
history in, 1573
laboratory evaluation in, 1575
pathophysiology of, 1573
screening for other types of stones in, laboratory evaluation in, 1575
treatment of, 1575–1577
alkalinization of urine in, 1576, 1576t
dietary advice in, 1576
hydration in, 1575–1576
pharmacologic, 1576–1577
Cytochemical assays, 202–203
Cytochrome P450:
cholesterol synthesis and, 563–567, *564*
adrenodoxin reductase and adrenodoxin and, *566,* 566–567
cholesterol conversion to pregnenolone and, 565–566
steroid hormone synthesis and, 80–81, *81*
of zona glomerulosa cells, 81
Cytochrome P450 reductase, cholesterol synthesis and, 569, *569*
Cytokines:
hypercalcemia of malignancy and, 1751
malignancy-associated hypercalcemia and, 1471
receptor for, 111
signaling by, 158

Dawn phenomenon, 1205
Decompressive surgery, to orbits, for Graves' disease, 491
Deficiency syndromes, 5, 14–16. *See also specific disorders and under specific hormones*
administration of or abnormal production of antagonists causing, 16
endocrine gland hypofunction causing, 14–15
extraglandular disorders causing, 15
fasting hypoglycemia and, 1262
hyporesponsiveness to hormones causing, 16
Dehydroepiandrosterone (DHEA), 82, 83, 558
adrenarche and, 583–584
binding of, 589–590
Cushing's disease and, 664, *664*
plasma level of, 585t
secretion rate of, 585t
synthesis of, fetal, 573
Dehydroepiandrosterone sulfate (DHEA-S), 558
adrenarche and, 583–584
binding of, 589–590
Cushing's disease and, 664, *664*
plasma level of, 585t
secretion rate of, 585t
Dehydrogenases, steroid hormone synthesis and, 80
5′-Deiodinase, type II, 88–89
Deletions, 45, 1054
Delivery. *See* Parturition
Demeclocycline (Declomycin), for syndrome of inappropriate antidiuretic hormone, 421

Dental disorders, hypocalcemia and, 1480
Deoxycorticosterone (DOC):
binding of, 589
hypertension and, 769
plasma level of, 585t
regulation of, 580–581
secretion rate of, 585t
11-Deoxycorticosterone, metabolism of, 591
Deoxycorticosterone acetate (DOCA):
for congenital adrenal hyperplasia, 638t
diagnostic, in primary hyperaldosteronism, 827
Deoxycorticosterone-excess hypertension, 832–833
adrenocortical adenomas and, 833
congenital adrenal hyperplasia and, 832–833
11-Deoxycortisol:
metabolism of, 591
plasma level of, 585t
secretion rate of, 585t
Deoxypyridiboline, urinary, in metabolic bone disease, 1519
Depression, 24, 31
Cushing's syndrome and, 670
glucocorticoids and, 606
thyroid function and, 464
Dermopathy, diabetic, 1192
Desensitization:
of adrenergic receptors, 719–720
heterologous, 122
homologous, 122–123
of target cell responses, *122,* 122–123
17,20-Desmolase deficiency, testosterone synthesis and, 1082
20,22-Desmolase deficiency, 1079
Desmopressin (DDAVP), 386
for diabetes insipidus:
dipsogenic, 414
gestational, 414
nephrogenic, 414
neurogenic, 412, *413,* 413–414
following pituitary surgery, 340
for nocturnal enuresis, 414
therapeutic trial of, to differentiate between primary polydipsia and neurogenic diabetes insipidus, 422
therapeutic uses of, for hypopituitarism, 1651t
Development:
of brain, glucocorticoids and, 606–607
glucocorticoids and, 607–608
regulation of, 14
stages of, 1634–1636
Dexamethasone:
bioavailability of, 863
for congenital adrenal hyperplasia, 637, 638t
distribution of, 863
for primary hyperaldosteronism, glucocorticoid-remediable, 832
structure of, *171*
for typhoid fever, 871
Dexamethasone sodium phosphate, for septic shock, 871
for primary hyperaldosteronism, glucocorticoid-remediable, 832
Dexamethasone suppression tests, 618–620
in children, 624–626
high-dose, 619–620
overnight 8-mg test, 619, *620*
two-day, 619–620
low-dose, 618–619
in Cushing's syndrome, 668
overnight, 618
two-day, 618–619
overnight:
for adrenocorticotropic hormone, 365
high-dose, for adrenocorticotropic hormone, 365
standard, for adrenocorticotropic hormone, 365
Dexfenfluramine, for weight loss, 1300
Dextrothyroxine, for hyperlipoproteinemia, 1388
Diabetes insipidus, 402–414
dipsogenic, treatment of, 414
etiology of, 402–404, 403t, *404*
gestational:
etiology of, 405
pathophysiology of, 409
treatment of, 414
nephrogenic:
etiology of, 404–405
pathophysiology of, 409
treatment of, 414
neurogenic:
in comatose and postoperative patients, management of, 413–414
desmopressin trial as test for, 422
diagnosis of, 409–411, 410t
familial, 403, *404*
hypertonic saline infusion test for, 422
pathophysiology of, 406, *406, 407*
treatment of, *404,* 412–414
pathophysiology of, 405–406, *405–407,* 409
Diabetes mellitus, 1156–1235. *See also* Insulin
acromegaly and, 343–344, 1234
aging and. *See* Elderly persons, diabetes mellitus in
amyotrophy in, 32
clinical manifestations of, 1181–1193
coronary artery disease, 1191
cutaneous, 1192, *1192*
diabetic foot, 1191–1192
hyperglycemic symptoms, 1181–1182
infectious, 1192–1193
joint disease, 1193
nephropathy, 1185–1188, *1187*
neuropathy, 1188–1191
retinopathy, 1182–1185, *1183, 1184*
Cushing's syndrome and, 1234
definition and classification of, 1156–1159, 1157t, 1158t
diabetic foot and, 1188, 1191–1192
diagnosis of, 1174–1179
fasting plasma glucose concentration in, 1175
glycohemoglobin in, 1178
insulin determination in, 1177
intravenous glucose tolerance test in, 1177
oral glucose tolerance testing in, 1175–1177
urinary glucose determination in, 1177–1178
etiology of, 1159–1164, *1165*
autoimmunity in, 1163–1164
environmental factors in, 1161–1163, *1162*
genetic factors in, *1159,* 1159–1161, 1160t
obesity and nutrition in, 1164
glucagonomas and, 1234–1235
glucocorticoid therapy in, 873
historical background of, 1156
hyperlipidemia and, 1330–1332
diet therapy for, 1379–1380
diet-induced, 1332
genetic, 1332
hyperosmolar nonketotic coma in, 1224
hypoglycemia and, reactive, 1265
hypogonadotropic hypogonadism and, 933
hypothalamic disorders and, 273
insulin-dependent, 1158, 1158t
hypoglycemia in, 736–738
with ketoacidosis, hyperlipidemia and, 1331–1332
ketoacidosis and. *See* Diabetic ketoacidosis (DKA)
lactic acidosis in, 1224–1225
lipoatrophic, 1232–1233
maturity-onset diabetes of young people. *See* Maturity-onset diabetes of young people (MODY)
mortality due to, 1197
multiple endocrine deficiency and, 1235
non-insulin-dependent, 1158, 1158t
obesity and, 1277–1278
osteoporosis and, 1537
pathogenesis of, 1165–1170
glucagon secretion and, 1170, *1170*
glucocorticoids and, 1170
growth hormone and, 1170
insulin resistance and, 1167–1169, *1168*
insulin secretion and, 1165–1167, *1166*
pathogenesis of complications of, 1193–1197
biopsy studies and, 1194
effect of treatment and, 1196–1197
metabolic studies and, 1194–1196
pathology of, 1179–1181
blood vessels and, 1179–1180, *1180*
eye and, 1181

Diabetes mellitus (*Cont.*)
islets and, 1179
kidney and, 1180, *1181*
nervous system and, 1181
pathophysiology of, 1170–1174, *1174*
carbohydrate metabolism and, 1171, *1171*
fat metabolism and diabetic hyperlipidemia and, 1172–1174, *1173*
protein and amino acid metabolism and, 1171–1172
protein-carbohydrate interactions and, 1172
pheochromocytomas and, 1234
polyneuropathy in, 31
poorly controlled, hyperlipidemia and, 1332
prediction and prevention of, 1164–1165, *1165*
pregnancy and:
classification of, 1227–1228
course of diabetes mellitus and, *1228,* 1228–1229
diabetic complications and, 1232
diagnosis of, 1227, 1227t
gestational, 1159, 1179, 1227–1228
maternal and fetal fuel metabolism and, 1225–1227
outcome of pregnancy and, 1229–1232, 1230t
prevalence of, 1179
Schmidt's syndrome and, 1722–1723
secondary, 1158, 1233–1235
endocrine-associated, 1234–1235
pancreoprival, 1233–1234
sympathochromaffin function and, 738–739
tall stature and, 1665
treatment of, 1197–1218
dietary, 1206–1208
exercise in, 1213–1216
future of, 1216–1218
insulin therapy in. *See* Insulin therapy
oral hypoglycemic agents in. *See* Oral hypoglycemic agents
urinary manifestations of, 28
well-controlled, hyperlipidemia and, 1332
without Addison's disease, 1724, *1724,* 1725t
Diabetic amyotrophy, 1190
Diabetic bullae, 1192
Diabetic cardiomyopathy, 1191
Diabetic dermopathy, 1192
Diabetic ketoacidosis (DKA), 1219–1224
clinical manifestations of, 1220–1221
complications of, 1223–1224
diagnosis of, 1221
hyperlipidemia and, 1331–1332
hypophosphatemia and, 1493, *1493*
pathogenesis of, 1219–1220
treatment of, 1221–1223
bicarbonate in, 1222–1223
fluids in, 1222
insulin therapy in, 1221–1222
potassium in, 1223
Diabetic neuropathic cachexia, 1191
Dialysis:
aluminum-induced osteomalacia and, 1543
chronic, hypophosphatemia and, 1528
for diabetic nephropathy, 1188
renal osteodystrophy and, 1544, 1545
Diaphragma sellae, 289
Diarrhea, 27
treatment of, pharmacologic, 1679, 1680t, 1681
Dichloromethylene diphosphonate, for hypercalcemia, 1473
Dictyotene, 996
DIDMOAD syndrome, 403
Diencephalic syndrome, hypothalamic disorders and, 270–271
Diet:
as cholesterol source, 561–562
cystinuria and, 1576
diabetes mellitus and, 1332, 1162–1163
endemic goiter and, 524
hormone-responsive tumors and, *1792,* 1792–1793
hyperlipidemia caused by, 1330, 1330t, *1331*
diabetes mellitus and, 1332
low-fat, high-complex-carbohydrate:
chemical composition of, 1379
in diabetic patients, pregnant patients, children, and hypertensive patients, 1379–1380
predicted plasma cholesterol lowering from, 1379
obesity and, 1283, 1283t
sporadic goiter and, 529
urinary pH and uric acid excretion and, 1578
Diet therapy:
for diabetes mellitus, 1206–1208
in older patients, 1828
during pregnancy, 1231–1232
for familial hypercholesterolemia, 1339
for hyperlipidemia. *See* Hyperlipidemia, dietary treatment of
for weight loss, 1294–1299
Dietary hypercalciuria, 1591–1592, *1592*
treatment of, 1606
Diethylstilbestrol (DES), therapeutic uses of, for prostatic cancer, 1806
Diffuse lymphocytic adrenalitis, 645
Diffuse neuroendocrine system (DNES), 1107
DiGeorge syndrome, 1482
Digital subtraction angiography, intravenous, in renovascular hypertension, 808
Dihydrotachysterol (DHT), 1438
growth and, 1632
therapeutic uses of, for hypocalcemia, 1488
Dihydrotestosterone, aging and, in males, 1819
5α-Dihydrotestosterone, structure of, *171*
Dihydroxyacetone phosphate, 1120
1,25-Dihydroxyvitamin D, 169
circulating and extrarenal, 1442
glucocorticoids and, 605–606, *606*
hypercalcemia of malignancy and, 1751
hyperparathyroidism and, 1543
hypothyroidism and, 503
metabolism of, 1443, *1444*
regulation of, 1440
for renal osteodystrophy, *1544,* 1544–1545
serum, assays for, 1497
synthesis of, 83, *84*
therapeutic uses of, for osteoporosis prophylaxis, 1539
24,25-Dihydroxyvitamin D, 1442–1443
Diphosphonates. *See* Bisphosphonates
Disorientation, 31
Diuresis:
solute, vasopressin and, 396–397
water, vasopressin and, 396, *397*
Diuretics:
for adrenal adenomas, 831
for hypercalcemia, 1471, 1472
for primary hyperparathyroidism, 1466
thiazide:
for diabetes insipidus, nephrogenic, 414
hypercalcemia induced by, 1475
hypovolemic hyponatremia and, 415
for osteoporosis prophylaxis, 1539
Diurnal growth hormone profile, 1666t
Diurnal rhythms:
of corticotropin releasing hormone, 578–579
of cortisol, 577–580
changes in, 579–580, *580*
DNA, 35. *See also* Recombinant DNA technology
degradation of, glucocorticoids and, 600
3′-flanking, 39
5′-flanking, 39
gene expression and, 42
hormone action and, *42,* 42–43
hybridization of, 46–47
movement into existing genes, 40–41
replication of, 36, *37*
retinoic acid receptor binding to, 172
sequencing of, *47,* 47–48
chain termination method for, 47–48
chemical degradation for, 47, *47*
Southern blotting of, 47
steroid receptor binding to, 170, 172
synergistic transactivation by nuclear receptors and, 181
structure of, 35–37, *36*
double helix, 37
synthesis of:
glucocorticoids and, 600
as source of DNA for molecular cloning, 48
thyroid hormone receptor binding to, 172

transcription of, *38,* 38–39, *39*
DNA-binding domain (DBD):
of steroid hormone receptors, 173, *174,* 176, 177
orphan, 184t, 184–185
structure of, 179, 187
Docosahexanoic acid (DHA), 1370
L-Dopa:
for acromegaly, 348
prolactin response to, in amenorrhea-galactorrhea syndrome, 351
L-Dopa suppression test:
for growth hormone, 367
for prolactin, 369
Dopamine:
action of, 235
anatomic pathway of, 248–250
exercise and, 1849
insulin secretion and, 1135
progesterone receptor activation by, 178
prolactin inhibiting factor and, 247
prolactin secretion and, 311, 312
thyroid function and, 464
thyroid-stimulating hormone regulation by, 300, 447–448
Dopamine agonists, prolactin secretion and, 312
Dopamine receptor blockers, prolactin response to, in amenorrhea-galactorrhea syndrome, 350–351
Dopaminergic receptor antagonists, prolactin secretion and, 312
Doppler ultrasonography, duplex, in renovascular hypertension, 807–808
Dorsum sellae, 289
Down regulation, 9
Down's syndrome, hypogonadotropic hypogonadism and, 931
Doxorubicin (Adriamycin), for thyroid carcinoma, anaplastic, 545
Drosophila, orphan receptors in embryonal development, 186
Drug(s). *See also specific drugs and drug types and under specific disorders*
calcium stones and, 1588
glucocorticoid clearance and, 864
growth hormone secretion and, 309
hypercalcemia induced by. *See* Hypercalcemia, drug-induced
hyperlipoproteinemia induced by, hyperlipidemia and, 1334t, 1334–1335
hypocalcemia induced by, 1487
hypogonadotropic hypogonadism and, 927
impotence and, 951
interference in assays caused by, 214
metabolism of:
hypothyroidism and, 501
thyrotoxicosis and, 476
prolactin secretion and, 312, 351
steroid hormone metabolism and, 593
syndrome of inappropriate antidiuretic hormone and, 416
thyroid function and, 464–465
uric acid stones and, 1579
vasopressin and, 394t, 394–395
for weight loss, 1299–1301
Drug delivery systems:
based on recombinant DNA techniques, 57
implantable insulin pumps, 1203, 1218
Drug therapy. *See specific drugs and drug types and under specific disorders*
Dumping syndrome, 1679
Duplications, 1054
Dwarfism:
Laron-type, 309, 1648
psychosocial, 1657
Dynamic testing, 19–20
in amenorrhea-galactorrhea syndrome, 350
of vasopressin, in syndrome of inappropriate antidiuretic hormone, 416–418, *418*
Dynein, 891
Dynorphin, 253–254
Dysdifferentiation, ectopic hormone production and, 1743–1744
Dysgenetic male pseudohermaphroditism, 1077
Dysgerminomas, suprasellar, 262
Dyslipidemia, 1331
Dysphagia, oropharyngeal, 26

E75 gene, 186
Early response genes, hormonal regulation of, 159, 159–161
*Eco*RI, 45, *45*
Ectopic ACTH syndrome:
clinical features of, 667–668
etiology and pathogenesis of, 663, 663t
pathophysiology of, 664–665
treatment of, 676
Ectopic corticotropin releasing hormone syndrome, 1756
Ectopic pro-opiomelanocortin/adreno-corticotropic hormone syndrome, 1754–1758
clinical manifestations of, 1755–1756
diagnosis of, 1756–1758, *1757, 1758*
prevalence and tumor types in, 1754, 1754t
pro-opiomelanocortin products produced by tumors in, 1754–1755, *1755*
treatment of, 1758
Edema, 24
aldosterone and, 680
cerebral, diabetic ketoacidosis and, 1223–1224
hypervolemic hyponatremia and, 415
idiopathic, sympathochromaffin function and, 739
insulin-induced, 1206
periorbital, 33
Edwards syndrome, 270t
egon gene, 186
Eicosanoids, hypertension and, 780
Eicosapentaenoic acid (EPA), 1370
Elderly persons, 1813–1831, *1814,* 1814t, 1815t
diabetes mellitus in, 1827–1830
blood glucose control and, 1827t, 1827–1828, 1828t
diet and, 1828
hyperglycemia of aging and, 1827
insulin and, 1829
management of, 1828, 1829t
among nursing home residents, 1829–1830, 1830t
oral hypoglycemia agents and, 1828–1829
treatment monitoring and, 1829
frailty, hormones, and aging and, 1822t, 1822–1825
estrogens and, 1823
growth hormone and, 1822–1823
testosterone, 1823
vitamin D, type II osteopenia, and hip fracture and, 1823–1825, *1824*
growth hormone in, 1817, *1818*
hormones associated with water metabolism in, 1821–1822
hyperlipoproteinemia in, surgical treatment of, 1391
hypothalamic-pituitary-adrenal axis in, 1818–1819
hypothalamic-pituitary-thyroid axis in, 1818, 1818t
insulin-like growth factor in, 1817, *1818*
nutritional disorders in, 1830t, 1830–1831, 1831t
prolactin in, 1817–1818
sex hormones in, 1819–1821
female, 1821, *1821*
male, 1819–1821, *1820*
sexuality and, 1825–1827
in females, 1827
in males, 1825t, 1825–1827, 1826t
solitary thyroid nodules in, management of, 538
theories of aging and, 1816t, 1816–1817
Ellsworth-Howard test, 1498
Embden-Meyerhof pathway, 1111–1113, *1112*
Emotional deprivation syndrome, short stature and, 1657
Empty sella syndrome, 274–275
hypopituitarism and, 316
pituitary adenoma versus, 336t, *337,* 337–338, 338t
primary, 337
short stature and, 1647
Encephalocele, basal, hypothalamus and, 261
Endarterectomy, for renovascular hypertension, 810

Endemic goiter. *See* Goiter, endemic
Endochondral ossification, 1633
Endocrine cell hypothesis, of ectopic hormone production, 1742–1743, 1743t
Endocrine disorders, 14–18, *15*. *See also specific disorders*
  assessment of, 18–20
  clinical manifestations of, 23–33
    cardiovascular, 28
    central nervous system, 31
    cutaneous, 25–26
    gastrointestinal, 26–27
    generalized symptoms, 23–25
    hematopoietic, 27–28
    musculoskeletal, 30–31
    neuromuscular, 31–32
    olfactory, 26
    ophthalmic, 32–33
    of reproductive system, 29–30
    tongue and, 26
    urinary, 28–29
    voice and, 26
  deficiency syndromes, 14–16
  excess syndromes, 16–17
  multiple endocrine syndromes, 17–18
  not associated with hormonal imbalance, 18
  treatment of, 20–21
Endocrine glands. *See also specific glands*
  disorders of, not associated with hormone imbalance, 18
  evolution of, 11–12
  hyperfunction of, 16
  hypofunction of, 14–15
  serving multiple functions, 4
  specialized, 4
Endocrine peptides, 1677
Endocrine system. *See also* Hormone(s); *specific hormones*
  disorders of. *See* Endocrine disorders; *specific disorders*
  evolution of, 9–12
    diversification of families of hormones and, 11
    origin of hormones and other regulatory ligands and, *10*, 10–11
    glands and, 11–12
    origins of receptors and other mediators and, 11
    simple and complex regulation and, 9–10
  glands of. *See* Endocrine glands; *specific glands*
  hypothyroidism and, 502
  integration of, 12–13
    attenuation and terminating mechanisms and, 13
    of classes of hormones, 12
    hormone antagonisms and, 13
    hormone synergisms and, 12–13
  obesity and, 1289–1290
  response limb of, 5
Endocrinology, definitions and scope of, 3–5, *4*
Endometrial cancer, 1803–1805
  diagnosis of, 1803
  pathology and prognosis of, 1803
  risk factors for, 1803, 1803t
  treatment of, 1804t, 1804–1805
Endonucleases, restriction. *See* Restriction enzymes
Endorphins, 297
  β-endorphin, 252–253, *253*, 297
    chemistry of, 295
    extrapituitary, 297
  prolactin regulation by, 313
Endothelins, 254
  hypertension and, 774
Endothelium-derived hyperpolarizing factor (EDHF), hypertension and, 776
Endothelium-derived releasing factor (EDRF). *See* Nitric oxide
Endozepine, 563
Endurance training. *See* Exercise
Energy expenditure, obesity and, 1283–1286, *1284*
Enhanced dissociation hypothesis, 205
Enkephalins, 297
  growth hormone regulation by, 309
  pentapeptide, 253
Enteric hyperoxaluria, treatment of, 1607
Enuresis, nocturnal:
  diagnosis of, 411–412
  etiology of, 404
  pathophysiology of, 409
  treatment of, 414
Environmental deprivation syndrome, short stature and, 1657
Environmental factors:
  diabetes mellitus and, 1161–1163, *1162*
  hormones, prenatal virilization by, 1096
  hypertension and, 752–753
  obesity and, 1283, 1283t
  sporadic goiter and, 529–530
  temperature:
    male infertility and, 941
    thyroid function and, 456–457
    vasopressin and, 393
  toxins, hypogonadotropic hypogonadism and, 933
Environmental theories of aging, 1816
Enzyme(s):
  calcium-dependent systems of. *See* Calcium
  defects of, hypogonadotropic hypogonadism and, 933
  interference in assays caused by, 214
  lipoprotein metabolism and, 1321–1322
  restriction, 45, *45*
  steroidogenic, 563–573
Enzyme immunoassay (EIA), 208
  amplitude-modulated, 210–211, *211*
Eosinophilia, 28
Eosinophilic granulomas. *See* Histiocytosis X
Ependymal cells, 229
Ependymomas, 274
Epidermal growth factor (EGF):
  granulosa cell cytodifferentiation and, 992
  granulosa cell heterogeneity and, granulosa cell cytodifferentiation and, 992–993
  receptor for, 108–109, *109*
Epinephrine. *See also* Catecholamines
  action of, 1150
  anatomic pathway of, 250
  biological roles of, 724–726, *726*
  corticotropin releasing hormone and, 244
  exercise and, 1848–1849
  glucose counterregulation and, 737
  insulin secretion and, 1134–1135
  metabolic effects of, 722, 722t
  physiologic adaptation and, 724, *725*, 726
Epiphyseal plate, endochondral ossification at, 1523
Epithelial tissue, glucocorticoids and, 603
Equilibrium dialysis (ED) assays, 205
Ergocalciferol. *See* Vitamin D_2
Ergogenic aids, 1857t, 1857–1865. *See also* Anabolic steroids
  erythropoietin as, 1865–1866
  ethical aspects of, 1857–1858
  growth hormone as, 1865
Ergotamines, for postural hypotension, 735
Eruptive xanthomas, diabetes mellitus and, 1192
Erythrocytosis, paraneoplastic, 1769t, 1769–1770, 1770t
Erythroid cells, glucocorticoids and, 603
Erythropoietin:
  as ergogenic aid, 1865
  hypertension and, 772–773
Escalator theory, of adrenarche, 1632
Escherichia coli infection:
  magnesium ammonium phosphate stones and, 1584
  male infertility and, 941
Essential hypertension:
  mineralocorticoids and, 770
  renin-angiotensin system and, 764–767, *765*
    blockade of, 764–765
    low-renin essential hypertension and, 766–767
    normal and high-renin essential hypertension and, 765–766, *766*
Estradiol. *See also* Ethinyl estradiol
  aging and, in males, 1819
  binding of, 85
  metabolism of, 86
  structure of, 171
  transdermal patch (Estraderm), for hypopituitarism, 325
Estranse, 559
Estrogen(s). *See also specific estrogens*
  action of, 237–238, 614
  aging and:

in females, 1821
frailty and, 1823
binding of, 590
cirrhosis and, 273
conjugated (Premarin):
for hypopituitarism, 325
for osteoporosis prophylaxis, 1538
serum thyroid-binding globulin level and, 457
Cushing's syndrome and, 670
deficiency, osteoporosis and, 1535
DNA-binding domain of, 176, *177*
feedback and:
negative, 905–906
positive, 906–907
follicle-stimulating hormone regulation by, 302
growth and, 1631–1633, *1632*
growth hormone regulation by, 309
for hyperlipoproteinemia, 1388
hypertension and, 772
luteinizing hormone regulation by, 302
metabolism of, 592, *592*
prolactin regulation by, 311–312
receptors for:
breast cancer and, 182
dimerization and, 175–176, *177*
genes homologous to, 185
phosphorylation of, 176
serum thyroid-binding globulin level and, 457–458
structure of, *171*
synthesis of, 81–83
therapeutic uses of:
for androgen-dependent neoplasia, 953
for primary hyperparathyroidism, 1466
thyroid-stimulating hormone regulation by, 299–300
vitamin D and, 1442
Estrogen response element (ERE), consensus, 179
Estrone, synthesis of, 83
Ethanol. *See* Alcohol use
Ethinyl estradiol:
for familial tall stature, 1658
for hypopituitarism, 325
for osteoporosis prophylaxis, 1538
serum thyroid-binding globulin level and, 457, 458
for Turner's syndrome, 1075, 1076
Etidronate, for hypercalcemia, 1473
Etidronate disodium, inhibition of bone mineralization by, 1528
Etidronate sodium, for Paget's disease of bone, 1553, *1554*
Etidronic acid, for hypercalcemic crisis, 1467
Etiocholanolone glucuronide:
plasma level of, 585t
secretion rate of, 585t
Etiocholanolone sulfate:
plasma level of, 585t
secretion rate of, 585t
Etomidate, steroid synthesis inhibition by, 586
Eukaryotes:
DNA sequences in, 69, *70*
screening of cDNA library for, 49–50
Eunuchoidal proportions, 929
Eunuchoidism, hypogonadotropic. *See* Kallman's syndrome
Euthyroid sick syndrome, 459–462, *460*, 460t
serum thyroxine concentrations and, 461–462
serum triiodothyronine concentrations and, 461
Excess syndromes, 5, 16–17. *See also specific disorders and under specific hormones*
autoimmune disease causing, 17
biosynthetic or metabolic defects causing, 17
ectopic hormone production causing, 16–17
hormone administration causing, 17
hyperfunction causing, 16
secondary hormone hypersecretion causing, 17
tissue hypersensitivity causing, 17
Exercise, 1837–1866
addiction to, endogenous opiates and, 1845–1846
adrenocorticotropic hormone-cortisol axis and, 1840–1841
circadian and other rhythms and, 1841
physical training and, 1840–1841
physiologic significance of, 1841
carbohydrate metabolism during, in normal humans, 1213–1214
blood glucose concentration and, 1213–1214
glucoregulatory hormones and, 1214, *1215*
glucose production and, 1214
glucose utilization and, 1213
catecholamines and, 1848–1849
control of release and, 1849
effects of release and, 1849
in diabetes mellitus, 1214–1216
alterations in insulin action induced by, 1215–1216
hyperglycemia induced by, 1215
hyperketonemia induced by, 1215
hypoglycemia induced by, 1214–1215
dopamine and, 1849
doping in sports activity and. *See* Anabolic steroids; Ergogenic aids
endogenous opiates and, 1843–1846
acute physical activity and, 1843
appetite suppression and, 1845–1846
physiologic significance of opiate increase and, 1844–1845
reproductive dysfunction and, 1846
training and, 1843–1844
energy supply and physical work and, 1837
evaluation of hormonal response to, 1837–1838, 1838t
fuel requirements and, 1155, *1156*
glucagon and, 1848
glucose homeostasis during, fasting hypoglycemia and, 1255–1256, *1256*
growth hormone and, 1838–1840
exercise and training effects on, 1838, 1839t
increases in, 1840
metabolic and pharmacologic manipulations and, 1839
neuroendocrine control of release of, 1839–1840
hypogonadotropic hypogonadism and, 928
insulin and, 1847–1848
prolactin and, 1841–1842
mechanisms and, 1842
secretion of, 311
training and, 1842
thyroid-stimulating hormone-thyroid axis and, 1842–1843
acute responses of, 1842
training and, 1842–1843
for weight loss, 1291–1294, 1292t, *1293*
Exercise test, for growth hormone, 1666t
Exocytosis, 717
Exons, 39, 41, 69
External plexus, of pituitary, 289
Extracorporeal shock wave lithotripsy (ESWL), 1568–1569
for cystinuria, 1574
Extraglandular disorders. *See* Systemic illness
Eyebrow, loss of lateral third of, 33

Fad diets, 1299
Familial apolipoprotein A-I deficiency, 1354
Familial apolipoprotein C-II deficiency, 1348–1351
Familial apolipoprotein C-III deficiency, 1354
Familial combined hyperlipidemia, 1344–1345
clinical characteristics of, 1344
definition of, 1344
diagnostic laboratory features of, 1345
genetics of, 1344
pathophysiology of, 1345
treatment of, 1345
Familial dysalbuminemic hyperthyroxinemia (FDH), 458
Familial early maturation, tall stature and, 1658
Familial glucocorticoid deficiency, 647
Familial hyperalphalipoproteinemia, 1357
Familial hypercholesterolemia. *See* Hypercholesterolemia, familial
Familial hyperproinsulinemia, 1131
Familial hypoalphalipoproteinemia, 1354
Familial hypocalciuric hypercalcemia (FHH), 1460–1461, *1461*

Familial hypocalciuric hypercalcemia (FHH) (*Cont.*)
extracellular calcium-sensing receptor and, 1461
Familial hypoparathyroidism, 1482
Familial lecithin cholesterol acyltransferase. *See* Lecithin cholesterol acyltransferase deficiency, familial
Familial neurogenic diabetes insipidus (FNDI), 403, *404*
Familial short stature, 1640–1641
Familial tall stature, 1657–1658
Familial thyroid hormone resistance (FTHR), 188–189
Fanconi's syndrome, 1527
Fasting. *See also* Food intake; Malnutrition; Starvation
hypothalamic disorders and, 272
prolonged, supervised, in hypoglycemia, 1254
protein repletion and, *1127,* 1127–1128
thyroid function and, 463
Fasting hypercalciuria, 1595
Fasting hypoglycemia. *See* Hypoglycemia, fasting
Fasting plasma glucose concentration, in diabetes mellitus, 1175
Fat. *See also specific types of fats*
dietary:
effect on plasma lipids and lipoproteins, 1368–1371, *1370, 1371*
obesity and, 1287–1288
saturation of, 1369–1371, *1370, 1371*
in single-diet treatment for hyperlipidemia, 1375–1376, *1376*
Fat-derived substrates, insulin secretion and, 1134
Fatigue, 24
Fatty acid(s):
free. *See* Free fatty acids (FFA); Lipid metabolism
inhibitors of oxidation of, for diabetes mellitus, 1212
mobilization of, 1120–1121
omega-3, *1370,* 1370–1371, *1371*
dietary, in single-diet treatment for hyperlipidemia, 1375
omega-6, *1370,* 1370–1371, *1371*
oxidation of, 1121, *1122, 1123*
synthesis of, *1119,* 1119–1120, *1120*
Fatty acid esters, cholesterol transport and, 562–563
Fed state, fuel homeostasis and, *1154,* 1154–1155, 1155t
Feedback, hypothalamic-pituitary-Leydig cell axis and. *See* Hypothalamic-pituitary-Leydig cell axis, feedback interaction and
Feedback inhibition, 1320–1321
Feedback loops, *224,* 224–226, 225t
perturbation of, 225–226
Feeding cycles, diurnal patterns of adrenocorticotropic hormone and cortisol and, *578,* 578–579
Female pseudohermaphroditism, 1086–1096
congenital adrenal hyperplasia and, 1086–1096
11-hydroxylase deficiency and, 1095
21-hydroxylase deficiency and, 1087–1093, *1088–1090,* 1091t, *1092, 1094,* 1095
3β-hydroxysteroid dehydrogenase deficiency and, 1095–1096
Feminization:
of external genitalia, 1062, *1062*
testicular, 182, 1084–1085
Fenfluramine, for weight loss, 1300
Fetal alcohol syndrome, 1643
α Fetoprotein, pineal region tumors and, 274
Fetus. *See also* Intrauterine growth disturbances; Placenta; Pregnancy
adrenal cortex of, 556–557
adrenal steroid synthesis in, 573
congenital adrenal hyperplasia in. *See* Congenital adrenal hyperplasia (CAH), prenatal
development of, 1634, *1634*
fuel metabolism of, diabetes mellitus and, 1225–1227
intrauterine death of, diabetes mellitus and, 1230
ovarian activity in, 1004
regulation of gonadal function in, 1064–1066
chorionic gonadotropin and, 1064
pituitary gonadotropin and, 1064–1066, *1065, 1066*
sex steroids in circulation of, 1063
teratologic malformations of external genitalia of, 1096
thyroid function in, 455–456
thyrotoxicosis and, 486
virilization of, by environmental hormones, 1096
Fever, hypothalamic disorders and, 271
Fiber, dietary, effect on plasma lipids and lipoproteins, 1372–1373
Fibric acid derivatives, for hyperlipoproteinemia, 1388, 1389t
Fibrillation, atrial, thyrotoxicosis and, 475
Fibroblastic tissue, glucocorticoids and, 603
Fibrogenesis imperfecta ossium, 1528–1529
Fibromuscular dysplasia:
intimal fibroplasia, 799
medial, 799–800
medial dissection, 800
medial fibroplasia, 799–800
medial hyperplasia, 800
perimedial fibroplasia, 800
periarterial hyperplasia, 800
renovascular hypertension and, 788–800
Fibrous dysplasia, of bone, *1546,* 1546–1547, *1547*
Fine-needle aspiratory biopsy. *See* Needle biopsy
Fish, in diet, 1370–1371, *1371*
Fish eye disease, 1354
3′-Flanking DNA, 39
5′-Flanking DNA, 39
Fludrocortisone (Florinef; 9α-fluorocortisol):
for adrenocortical insufficiency, 655–656
for congenital adrenal hyperplasia, 637–638, 638t
virilizing, 1660
diagnostic, in primary hyperaldosteronism, 827
for postural hypotension, 735
Fluid(s):
balance of, regulation during physical work, 1846–1847
aldosterone, exercise, and training and, 1847
vasopressin, exercise, and training and, 1846–1847
for cystinuria, 1575–1576
for diabetic ketoacidosis, 1222
for hypercalcemic crisis, 1467
for nephrolithiasis, 1571
Fluid and electrolyte balance. *See also specific imbalances*
anabolic steroids and, 1864
glucocorticoids and, *603,* 603–604, *604*
in iatrogenic Cushing's syndrome, 859
syndrome of inappropriate antidiuretic hormone and, 418–419
Fluid and electrolyte metabolism:
hypothyroidism and, 501
thyrotoxicosis and, 475
Fluid restriction test, for polyuria, 421–422
Fluorescence assays, 208–209
polarization, 210
Fluoride:
for iatrogenic Cushing's syndrome, 859
inhibition of bone mineralization by, 1528
9α-Fluorocortisol, structure of, 171
Fluoxetine, for weight loss, 1301
Fluoxymesterone (halotestin):
for breast cancer, 1803
for Turner's syndrome, 1075
Fluphenazine, for diabetic neuropathy, 1189
Flutamide, for androgen-dependent neoplasia, 954–955
Follicles, ovarian. *See* Ovarian follicles
Follicle-stimulating hormone (FSH):
action of, 300
aging and, in males, 1821
assays for, 300–301, 366, 911–912, *912,* 1666–1667
basal measurements, 366
hypopituitarism and, 322–323, *323*
stimulation tests, 366
cirrhosis and, 273
disorders of. *See specific disorders*

exercise and, 1853
fasting and malnutrition and, 272
glucocorticoids and, 608–609
granulosa cell cytodifferentiation and, 992
hypopituitarism and, 318, 325–326
in men, 326
in women, 325–326
hypothalamic-pituitary-germ cell axis and. *See* Hypothalamic-pituitary-germ cell axis
hypothalamic-pituitary-Leydig cell axis and. *See* Hypothalamic-pituitary-Leydig cell axis
hypothyroidism and, 502, 503
luteinization and, 994
luteolysis and, 994–995
menarche and, 1004–1005
menstrual cycle and, 1007–1008
metabolism of, 302
ovarian steroid synthesis and, 991
pituitary cells secreting, 292
pituitary level of, 301
pituitary tumors secreting, 363
plasma level of, 301, *301*
regulation of, 235, 236–237, *237, 238,* 302t, 302–303
feedback control and, 909–910
secretion rate of, 302
thyrotoxicosis and, 477
urine level of, 301
Follistatin, negative feedback effects of, 239
Food intake. *See also* Fasting; Malnutrition; Nutrition; Starvation
endogenous opiates and and exercise and, 1844–1845
hypothalamic disorders and, 268–271
obesity and, 1286–1289
Foot, diabetic, 1188, 1191–1192
Forbes-Albright syndrome. *See* Amenorrhea-galactorrhea syndrome
Formation product, stone formation and, 1568
Formation product ratio (FPR), 1586
Fornix, hypothalamic, 226, *228*
Fractures:
of hip, aging and hormones and, 1823–1825, *1824*
in iatrogenic Cushing's syndrome, 860
osteomalacia and, 1522, *1523*
in osteoporosis, treatment of, 1540
Frailty, hormones and aging and. *See* Elderly persons
Free fatty acids (FFA). *See also* Lipid metabolism
metabolism of, 1325
mobilization of, in starvation and diabetes mellitus, 1114
release of, glucocorticoids and, 599
Free hormone assays, 205
Free hormone levels, 18–19
Free thyroxine index, 451–453, *452*
Fructokinase, 1113
FT2-F1 gene, 186
Functional prepubertal castrate syndrome, hypogonadotropic hypogonadism and, 931
Fushi tarazu gene, 186
Fusion proteins. *See* Hybrid proteins

G proteins:
G protein-couple receptors and, 102t, 102–108, *103, 104. See also* Adrenergic receptors
abnormalities of receptor function and, 107–108, *108*
hormone receptors coupled to, 102t, 102–108, *103, 714*
abnormalities of function of, 107–108, *108*
adrenergic. *See* Adrenergic receptors
receptor kinases coupled to, 123–124
signal transduction and. *See* Transmembrane signal transduction, G proteins and
Galactorrhea, 30. *See also* Amenorrhea-galactorrhea syndrome
hypothalamic disorders and, 267–268
normoprolactinemic, 352
Galanin, 254
Gallium nitrate:
for hypercalcemia, 1473
for hypercalcemic crisis, 1467
for Paget's disease of bone, 1554
Gallstones, cholesterol, obesity and, 1279
Gamma-aminobutyric acid (GABA):
anatomic pathway of, 250
as prolactin inhibiting factor, 247
receptors for, 101–102
Gangliocytomas, 262
growth hormone excess and, 265
GAP:
action of, 239
as prolactin inhibiting factor, 247
Gastric bypass, Roux-en-Y, for obesity, 1302–1303
Gastric inhibitory polypeptide (GIP), 1685–1686
action of, 1685–1686, 1686t
clinical relevance and applications of, 1686, *1686*
insulin secretion and, 1133–1134
Gastrin, 1681–1682
action of, 1682, 1682t
clinical relevance and applications of, 1682
paraneoplastic, 1772
Gastrinomas:
in multiple endocrine neoplasia, type 1, 1705
management of, 1708
treatment of, pharmacologic, 1680t, 1681t
Gastrointestinal disorders. *See also specific disorders*
diabetes mellitus and, 1190–1191
hypothyroidism and, 501
multiple mucosal neuromas and, 1717
thyrotoxicosis and, 475–476
Gastrointestinal system, 26–27
glucocorticoids and, 607
hormones of, 1675–1695. *See also* Carcinoid syndrome; *specific hormones*
insulin secretion and, 1133–1134, *1134*
localization and distribution of, 1675–1677, *1676,* 1676t, 1677t
tumors of, treatment of, 1681, 1681t
Gastroplasty:
horizontal, for obesity, 1302, 1303
vertical banded, for obesity, 1302
Gemfibrozil:
for familial hypercholesterolemia, 1340
for hyperchylomicronemia, 1351
for hyperlipoproteinemia, 1387
indications and dosage for, 1387
mechanism of action of, 1387
for primary type III hyperlipoproteinemia, 1348
side effects of, 1387
for type IV hyperlipoproteinemia, 1352
Gender role, 1067–1068
Gene(s), 35–45
chromatin and, *37,* 37–38
chromosomal, as source of DNA for molecular cloning, 50–51
cloning of. *See* Recombinant DNA technology
DNA structure and replication and, 35–37, *36*
early response, hormonal regulation of, *159,* 159–161
evolution of, 44, *44*
expression of, 39–44
excessive, ectopic hormone production and, 1743–1744
hormonal control of, 52, *52*
regulation of, *42,* 42–44
RNA processing and, 40–41, 43–44
mechanisms of genetic disease and, 44–45
mutations of. *See* Missense mutations; Mutations
orphan receptors and. *See* Steroid hormones, orphan receptors for
peptide hormone encoding on, 72, *73*
regulation by nuclear receptors, 178–182
classification of nuclear receptors and, 179
DNA binding and, 178–179, *179*
negative regulation and, 181–182
synergistic transactivation and, 181
transcriptional transactivation and, *180,* 180–181
RNA structure and function and, *38,* 38–39, *39*
tumor suppressor:
hormone-responsive tumors and, 1787–1790, *1788*

Gene(s) (*Cont.*)
identification of, 61
Gene conversions, 633, *634*
Gene depression, ectopic hormone production and, 1743
Gene families, 44, *44*
Gene therapy, 58–60, *59*
Gene transfer, into mammalian cells, 52–53, *53*
Genetic disorders:
DNA probes for diagnosis of, 57–58, *58*
hypergonadotropic hypogonadism and. *See* Hypogonadism, hypergonadotropic
male infertility and, 941–942
mechanisms of, 44–45
obesity and, 1290
osteoporosis and, 1537
Genetic factors:
abetalipoproteinemia and, 1358
autoimmune adrenocortical insufficiency and, 643–644
cystinuria and, 1573
diabetes mellitus and, *1159,* 1159–1161, 1160t
endemic goiter and, 526
familial combined hyperlipidemia and, 1344
familial defective apolipoprotein B-100 and, 1342
familial hypercholesterolemia and, 1338
familial lecithin cholesterol acyltransferase deficiency and, 1360
growth and, 1620
hormone-responsive tumors and, *1792,* 1792–1793
in 21-hydroxylase deficiency. *See* 21-Hydroxylase deficiency, genetics of
hyperchylomicronemia and, 1350
hypertension and, 752–753
obesity and, *1282,* 1282–1283, *1283*
pluriglandular endocrine insufficiency syndromes and, 1726
pseudohypoparathyroidism and, 1486
receptor function defects and, 182
short stature and, 1640–1641, 1647
in sporadic goiter, 527
tall statue and, 1657–1658
Tangier disease and, 1356
type IV hyperlipoproteinemia and, 1352
Genetic sex. *See* Sex chromosomes
Genetic tests, of testicular function, 913–914
Genital ducts, differentiation of, 1060–1061, *1061*
female, 1060
male, 1060–1061
Genitalia. *See also* Sexual differentiation
external, differentiation of, 1061–1062
sex steroid actions on, *1063,* 1063–1064
teratologic malformations of, 1096
Geriatric population. *See* Elderly persons
Germ cells, primordial, 995
Germinal cells, 887
failure of. *See* Infertility, male
Germinal epithelium
testicular, 888–889, 891, *892–896*
ovarian, 973
Germinomas, 274
suprasellar, 274
Gestational diabetes insipidus. *See* Diabetes insipidus, gestational
Gestational diabetes mellitus, 1159, 1179, 1227–1228
Gigantism, 1663, 1665. *See also* Acromegaly
cerebral, 275, 1664–1665
growth hormone excess and, 265
Glands. *See* Endocrine glands; *specific glands*
Glaucoma, 33
diabetes mellitus and, 5879
glucocorticoids and, 607
Glicentin, 1146
Gliomas, 274
Glipizide, for diabetes mellitus, 1209, 1209t
Glomerular filtration rate (GFR), glucocorticoids and, 604–605
Glucagon, 1146–1150
action of, 1147–1149, *1148, 1149*
big plasma, 1147
chemistry of, 1146
circulating, 1147
degradation of, 1150
exercise and, 1848
glucose counterregulation and, 737
paraneoplastic, 1772
secretion of, 1147
diabetes mellitus and, 1170, *1170*
synthesis of, 1146
Glucagon test, for growth hormone, 1666t
Glucagon-like immunoreactivity (GLI), 1146
Glucagonomas:
diabetes mellitus and, 1234–1235
in multiple endocrine neoplasia, type 1, 1705
treatment of, pharmacologic, 1681t
Glucocorticoid(s). *See also specific glucocorticoids*
action of, 593–610, 1150–1151
on adrenal medulla, 607
anti-inflammatory, 855–856
bone and calcium metabolism and, 605–606, *606*
cardiovascular system and fluid and electrolyte balance and, *603,* 603–605, *604*
on central nervous system, 606–607
DNA-binding domain of, 176, *177*
on eye, 607
on gastrointestinal tract, 607
growth and development and, 607–608
immunologic and inflammatory, 600–603, 601t, 602t
kinetics of, 859
mediation through mineralocorticoid receptors, 858, 858t
metabolic, 596–600, *597–599*
mineralocorticoid receptors and, 594
molecular mechanisms of, 593–595
production and clearance of other hormones and, 608
receptors for:
dimerization and, 175–176, 177
heat shock protein and, 175
nuclear localization signals within, 177
phosphorylation of, 176
transactivation of gene activity by, 180–181
reproductive, 608–609
reversibility of, 696
stress and, 609–610
structure of, *171*
synergistic and antagonistic interrelations with other hormones and, 609
therapeutic. *See* Glucocorticoid(s), therapeutic uses of
agonists and antagonists of, 595
binding of, 586–590
to albumin, 587
of aldosterone, 589
of androgens and estrogens, 589–590
to corticosteroid-binding globulin, 586–587, 588t
of deoxycorticosterone, 589
physiologic role of, 587–589
bone loss due to, *860*, 860–861, *861*
deficiency of, 605
familial, 647
definition of, 593
diabetes mellitus and, 1170, *1170*
feedback in adrenocorticotropic hormone release, 580, *581*
for hypercalcemia, 1473
hypertension and, 770–771
hypogonadotropic hypogonadism and, 928
osteoporosis induced by, prevention of, 1539–1540
potency of, 862–865
bioavailability and, 862–863
concentration at sites of action and, 864–865
distribution and, 863
metabolism and clearance and, 863–864, *864*
preparations of, 866–868
of adrenocorticotropic hormone, 868
aerosol, 863, 868
intraarticular, 866–867
orally and parenterally active, 862–863, 866, 867t
steroids with glucocorticoid activity available for therapy and, 866
topical, 863, 867, 867t

prolactin regulation by, 312
receptors for, 594–595, 858, 858t
renal phosphate handling and, 1491
resistance to, primary and secondary, 835
therapeutic uses of, 855–878, 856t, *857*
adjunctive therapy with, 870
adverse effects of, 857–858
reduction of, 871
alternate-day therapy and, 871–872, 872t
bioavailability and, 862–863
in children, 874
circadian rhythm and, 871
clinical applications of, 856t
concentration at sites of action and, 864–865
for congenital adrenal hyperplasia, 637
in diabetes mellitus, 873
distribution and, 863
dose adjustment and, 871
dose-response considerations with, 869–870
drug effectiveness and, 869
evaluating response to, 870
for Graves' disease, 490–491
iatrogenic Cushing's syndrome and. *See* Cushing's syndrome, iatrogenic
Kaposi's sarcoma and, 874
kinetics and, 859
for leukemia, 856, 869
metabolism and clearance and, 863–864, *864,*
molecular mechanisms for therapeutic influences and, 858, 858t
for myxedema coma, 507
objective criteria for, 870
patient selection for, 868–869
peptic ulcer and, 873–874
during pregnancy, 873
preparations for, 866–868
psychological effects of, 873
reduction of side effects and, 871
sensitivity testing for, 869
short- versus long-term, 869
surgery and, 873
therapeutic actions and, 855–857, *857*
molecular mechanisms for, 858, 858t
for thyroid storm, 486
for thyrotoxicosis, thyroiditis causing, 485
withdrawal of glucocorticoids and, 874–879
thyroid function and, 464
thyroid-stimulating hormone regulation by, 448
withdrawal of, suppression of hypothalamic-pituitary-adrenal axis and, 874–879
evaluation of axis function and, 878
kinetics and dosage required for suppression and, *874,* 874–875, *875*
kinetics of return to normal axis function and, *875,* 875–877, *876*
steroid withdrawal syndromes and, 877–878
withdrawal protocols and indications for steroid coverage for, 878–879
Glucocorticoid regulatory element (GRE), *42,* 42–43
negative, 181
Glucokinase, 1109–1110
Gluconeogenesis, 1113–1115, *1114*
glucocorticoids and, 597–598
inhibitors of, for diabetes mellitus, 1212
integration with glycolysis, *1115,* 1115–1116
Glucose. *See also* Carbohydrate metabolism; Hyperglycemia; Hypoglycemia
blood:
concentration of, during exercise, 1213–1214
levels, control in older diabetics, 1827t, 1827–1828, 1828t
self-monitoring of, 1200–1202, 1201t
counterregulation of:
fasting hypoglycemia and, *1257,* 1257–1258
pathophysiology in insulin-dependent diabetes mellitus, 737–738, *738*
physiology of, 736, *737*
homeostasis during fasting and exercise, 1255–1256, *1256*
insulin secretion and, 1131–1133, *1132, 1133*
plasma, fasting concentration of, 1175
regulation of, during exercise, 1214, *1215*
synthesis of, during exercise, 1214
toxicity of, diabetes mellitus and, 1165, 1167
urinary, determination of, 1177–1178
utilization during exercise, 1213
Glucose suppression testing, for growth hormone, 368
Glucose tolerance, impaired, 1158–1159
nonendocrine disease and, 1235
Glucose tolerance testing:
intravenous, 1177
oral, 1175–1177
diagnostic criteria and, 1176, 1176t
factors affecting, 1175t, 1175–1176
flat curve and, 1176–1177
in hypoglycemia, 1254
indications for, 1177
Glucose transporters, 1143
Glucose-alanine cycle, 1126–1127
Glucose-dependent insulinotropic peptide (GIP), 1685–1686
action of, 1685–1686, 1686t
clinical relevance and applications of, 1686, *1686*
Glucose-6-phosphatase (G6Pase), 1113
Glucose-6-phosphate dehydrogenase, 1117
Glutamate, receptors for, 100–101
Glutathione-insulin transhydrogenase, 1145
Glyburide, for diabetes mellitus, 1209, 1209t
Glycation:
diabetes mellitus and, 1195–1196
of protein, 1118–1119
Glycerol, 1119
Glycerol kinase, 1120
Glycerol 3-phosphate, 1120
Glycine, receptors for, 102
Glycogen, 1110, *1111*
metabolism of, glucocorticoids and, 598–599, *599*
synthesis of, indirect, 1116
Glycogen synthase, 1110, *1111*
Glycogenesis, 1110–1111, *1111, 1112*
Glycogenolysis, 1110–1111, *1111, 1112*
Glycohemoglobin, assays for, 1178
Glycolysis, 1111–1113, *1112*
integration with gluconeogenesis, *1115,* 1115–1116
Glycoproteins:
metabolism of, 78
pituitary. *See also* Follicle-stimulating hormone (FSH); Human chorionic gonadotropic (hCG); Luteinizing hormone (LH); Placental chorionic gonadotropin; Thyroid-stimulating hormone (TSH)
chemistry of, 297–298
pituitary tumors secreting α-subunit of, 363
synthesis of, 298
α-Glycosidase inhibitors, intestinal, for diabetes mellitus, 1212
Glycosylation:
of peptide hormones, 76–77
of protein, 1118, 1119
Goiter, 521–532
classification of, 521, 522t
endemic, 524–526
clinical features of, 525
cretinism and, 525–526
development of, 524
genetic factors and, 526
geography, diet, and iodine and, 524, 524t
hyperfunction and, 525
prophylaxis of, 526, *526*
protein-calorie malnutrition and, 526
relation to thyroid cancer, 525
etiology of, 522–524
thyroid-stimulating hormone and, 522–524, *523*
historical background of, 521
nontoxic, 530–532
incidence of, 530
laboratory evaluation of, 531
presentation and complications of, 530
risk of carcinoma in multinodular goiter and, 530–531
treatment of, 531–532, 532t

Goiter (*Cont.*)
sporadic, 526–530
chemical goitrogens and, 529, 529t
dietary goitrogens and, 529
environmental goitrogens and, 529–530
genetic influences on formation of, 527
inherited defects in thyroid hormone synthesis and, *528*, 528–529
during pregnancy, 527
sex and age in relation to, 527
thyrotoxicosis and, 474
toxic:
multinodular, thyrotoxicosis and, 472, 485
uninodular, thyrotoxicosis and, 472
Gonadal dysfunction, Cushing's syndrome and, 666
Gonadal function:
hypothyroidism and, 502–503
thyrotoxicosis and, 477
Gonadal sex. *See* Sexual differentiation, gonadal sex and
Gonadarche, 1631–1632
Gonadotrophs, 886
of adenohypophysis, 292
Gonadotropin(s). *See also specific gonadotropins*
aging and, 1819–1821
in females, 1821, *1821*
in males, 1819–1821, *1820*
chorionic. *See also* Human chorionic gonadotropin (hCG)
fetal, 1064
deficiency of, hypogonadotropic hypogonadism and, 920–925
exogenous, defective virilization due to, 1085–1086
in fetal circulation, 1063
hypothalamic disorders and, 265–267
pituitary, fetal, 1064–1066, *1065, 1066*
synthesis of, 1062–1063
regulation of, 991
tumors producing, 943
Gonadotropin-releasing hormone (GnRH), 235–239, *236–238*
action of, 236–237, *237, 238*
amenorrhea-galactorrhea syndrome and, 350
areas containing, 235–236
follicle-stimulating hormone regulation by, 302–303
hypothalamic-pituitary-germ cell axis and. *See* Hypothalamic-pituitary-germ cell axis
hypothalamic-pituitary-Leydig cell axis and. *See* Hypothalamic-pituitary-Leydig cell axis
luteinizing hormone regulation by, 302–303
puberty and, 584
structure of, 235, *236*
superagonist analogues of, for androgen-dependent neoplasia, 953
therapeutic uses of, 239
for hypogonadism, 938
for hypopituitarism, 326
Gonadotropin-releasing hormone (GnRH) stimulation test:
for follicle-stimulating hormone, 366
for luteinizing hormone, 366
Gonadotropin-releasing hormone (GnRH) test:
for follicle-stimulating hormone, 913, 914t
for luteinizing hormone, 913, 914t
Gout, 31
uric acid stones and, 1578t, 1578–1579
Graafian follicles, 979, 981, *981*
Granulomas, eosinophilic. *See* Histiocytosis X
Granulomatous disorders:
hypercalcemia and, 1474
pituitary adenoma versus, 336t, 338
Granulosa cells:
cytodifferentiation of, 991–992
heterogeneity of, 992–993
mucification of, 1003
progesterone synthesis by, 83
Granulosa-lutein cells, 986, *988*
Graves' disease, 467–470, 474, 488–492
euthyroid, infiltrative ophthalmopathy in, 489–490
infiltrative ophthalmopathy in, 488–491
clinical manifestations of, 488t, 488–489, *489, 490*
course and management of, 490–491
in euthyroid Graves' disease, 489–490
pathogenesis of, 470
localized myxedema in, *491*, 491–492
pathogenesis of, 470
natural history of, *469*, 469–470
pathogenesis of, 468–469, *469*
thyroid acropachy in, *491*, 491–492
thyroid-stimulating antibodies in, 467–468
thyrotoxicosis caused by, treatment of, 479–480, 480t
Growth:
abnormalities of, 30–31. *See also specific abnormalities*
anabolic steroids and, 1863
biological stages of, 1619, *1620*
constitutional delay of, short stature and, 1641
control of, 1619–1633
genetic factors in, 1620
gonadal steroids and, 1631–1633, *1632*
growth hormone and, 1626, *1627, 1628*, 1628–1631, *1630*, 1630t
insulin-like growth factors and, 1621–1626, 1623t, *1624, 1625*
nutrition and, 1633, 1633t
peptide growth factors and hormonal influences in, 1620–1621, 1621t
thyroid hormones and, 1631
glucocorticoids and, 607–608
of oocytes, *996*, 996–998
regulation of, 13
skeletal, 1633–1635
Growth deficiency, 1636–1657
causes of, 1640–1657
anoxemia, 1657
bone disorders, *1652*, 1652–1653
chondrodystrophies, 1653, *1654*
constitutional growth delay with or without delayed puberty, 1641–1642
Cushing's syndrome, 1651–1652
environmental deprivation syndrome, 1657
genetic or familial short stature, 1640–1641
growth hormone deficiency, 1645–1651, 1646t
hypothyroidism, 1644–1645
intrauterine growth disturbances, 1642–1643
normal short status, 1640–1642
postnatal malnutrition, 1643–1644
precocious sexual maturation, 1652
Turner's syndrome, 1653, *1655*, 1655–1657, *1656*
clinical approach to, 1636–1640, 1638t
history and, 1638
laboratory studies in, 1640
physical examination and, 1639–1640
radiographic studies in, 1640
testing procedures for, 1665–1668
Growth excess, 1657–1665, 1658t
acromegaly and. *See* Acromegaly
Beckwith-Wiedemann syndrome and, 1665
congenital adrenal hyperplasia, virilizing, 1658–1660
gigantism and. *See* Acromegaly; Gigantism
homocystinuria and, 1664, 1664t
hyperthyroidism and, 1663
infants of diabetic mothers and, 1665
Klinefelter's syndrome and, 1663–1664
lipodystrophy and, 1665
Marfan syndrome and, 1664, 1664t
normal variants and, 1657–1658
familial, genetic, or constitutional tall stature and, 1657–1658
familial early maturation and, 1658
obesity and, 1665
precocious puberty and, 1660t, 1660–1663
Sotos' syndrome and, 1664–1665
testing procedures for, 1665–1668
XYY genotype and, 1663
Growth factors:
coordinate action of, 84–85
growth and, 1620–1621, 1621t
orphan receptors induced by, 186
ovarian, 1009

phosphoinositide hydrolysis and, 155–156
receptors for. *See* Hormone receptors, growth factor
Growth hormone (GH), 303–313
action of, 304–305, 1151
aging and, 1817, *1818*
frailty and, 1822–1823
assays for, 306, 366–368, 1665, 1666t
basal measurements, 366–367
hypopituitarism and, 323–324
stimulation tests, 367–368
suppression tests, 368
biologically inactive, short stature and, 1647–1648
chemistry of, 303–304
cirrhosis and, 273
deficiency of:
acquired, 1648–1649
congenital, 1645–1648
diagnosis of, 1649–1650
hypothalamus and, 260, *261*, 264–265
isolated, 1647
short stature and, 1645–1651, 1646t
transient defects in secretion or action and, 1649
treatment of, 1650–1651, 1651t
diabetes mellitus and, 1170, *1170*
diurnal profile of, 1666t
ectopic production of, 1766–1767
as ergogenic aid, 1865
evolution of, 44, *44*
excess of, hypothalamic disease and, 265
exercise and. *See* Exercise, growth hormone and
fasting and malnutrition and, 272
feedback loops and, 225
glucose counterregulation and, 736
growth and, 1626, *1627, 1628*, 1628–1631, *1630*, 1630t
hypertension and, 773
hypopituitarism and, 318, 326–327
metabolism of, 306
neurosecretory dysfunction and, short stature and, 1648
pituitary cells secreting, 292
pituitary level of, 306
pituitary tumors secreting. *See* Acromegaly
plasma level of, 306
in acromegaly, 344
receptor for, 110–111
regulation of, 235, 241, 245–246, 306–309, *307*, 308t
hormonal, 309
metabolic, 307–309
neural, 307, *308*
neuropharmacologic agents and, 309
neurotransmitters and, 309
renal failure and, 273
renal phosphate handling and, 1491
resistance to, short stature and, 1648
rhythms of, 257, 258–259
stress and, 272
therapeutic uses of:
for hypopituitarism, 1651t
for Turner's syndrome, 1075
for weight loss, 1300–1301
Growth hormone gene, regulatory elements of, 42
Growth hormone releasing hormone (GRH), 245–246, *246*, 306, *307*
action of, 245–246
areas containing, 245
clinical uses of, 246
ectopic production of, 1767–1768
clinical features of, 1768
diagnosis of, 1768
treatment of, 1768
tumor types and, 1767t, 1767–1768
interaction with somatostatin, 241
structure of, 245
Growth hormone releasing hormone (GRH) stimulation test, for growth hormone, 367
Growth retardation:
hypopituitarism and, 326–327
glucocorticoid therapy and, 874
Guanosine triphosphate (GTP)-binding proteins. *See* Transmembrane signal transduction, guanosine triphosphate-binding proteins and
Guanylyl cyclase, peptide hormone action and, 137–138
Gynecomastia, 30, *947*, 947–951
pathologic, 948–949, 949t, *950*
patient evaluation in, 949–950
physiologic, 948
adult, 948
pubertal, 948
treatment of, 950–951

Hamartomas, hypothalamic, 262
Head injury:
diabetes insipidus and, 402, 403t
hypopituitarism and, 316, 317
hypothalamus and, 263–264
Headache, 31
Heart. *See also* Cardiac *entries;* Cardiovascular *entries*
hypertension and, 753
size of, 28
Heat shock proteins (hsp), 170, 174–175
dissociation from receptor after steroid binding, 172
interaction with receptor at steroid-binding domain, 174–175
steroid receptor binding to DNA and, 170, 172
Hematopoietic system, 27–28. *See also* Anemia
anabolic steroids and, 1864
hypothyroidism and, 501
thyrotoxicosis and, 476
Hemochromatosis:
hypogonadotropic hypogonadism and, 928
hypopituitarism and, 315
Hemodialysis. *See* Dialysis
Hemodynamics:
catecholamines and, 720–721
interference in assays caused by, 214
vasopressin and, *390*, 390–391, 391t, *392*
Hemorrhage:
adrenal, adrenocortical insufficiency and, 646, 650, 650t
pituitary, 330
hypopituitarism secondary to, 315, *315*
in thyroid nodule, 508
Heparin, steroid synthesis inhibition by, 586
Hepatic disorders, 27. *See also specific disorders*
anabolic steroids and, 1864
diabetes mellitus and, 1181
fasting hypoglycemia and, 1262–1263
hypogonadotropic hypogonadism and, 927
serum thyroid-binding globulin level and, 458
steroid hormone metabolism and, 593
thyroid function and, 463
Hepatic lipase, 1322
deficiency of, 1348
Hepatitis:
in iatrogenic Cushing's syndrome, 861
serum thyroid-binding globulin level and, 458
thyroid function and, 463
Hermaphroditism, true, 1071–1072
Hernia uteri inguinalis, 1078
Heterodimerization:
of retinoic acid receptors, 172
of retinoid X receptors, 190–191
of thyroid hormone receptors, 172, 188
Heterologous desensitization, 122
Heterophilic antibodies, interference in assays caused by, 213–214
Hexokinases, 1109–1110
High-density lipoproteins (HDL), 561–562, 1317–1318
disorders of, 1353t, 1353–1357, 1354t. *See also specific disorders*
metabolism of, *1324*, 1324–1325
High-pressure liquid chromatography (HPLC), 211–212
for cortisol, 615
detection methods for, 211–212
Hilus cells, ovarian, 985, *986*
Hirsutism, 25
Cushing's syndrome and, 666
Histaminase:
medullary thyroid carcinoma and, 1714
serum level of, in medullary carcinoma of the thyroid, 547–548
Histamine:
anatomic pathway of, 250
prolactin secretion and, 312–313
Histiocytosis, disseminated, growth hormone deficiency and, short stature and, 1649

Histiocytosis X, 263, *263*
History taking, 18
  in hypertension, 794, 794t
  in metabolic bone disease, 1517
  in primary hyperaldosteronism, 822
  in short stature, 1638
HNF-4, 186
Homocystinuria, tall stature and, 1664, 1664t
Homologous desensitization, 122–123
Homovanillic acid (HVA), in neuroblastomas, 732
Honeymoon phase, in diabetes mellitus, 1165, *1166*
Hormonal sex. *See* Hypothalamic-pituitary-gonadal axis, differentiation of
Hormone(s). *See also specific hormones*
  actions of, 4–5, 13–14, 791–793. *See also under specific hormones*
    cardiovascular regulation as, 14
    classes of, 9, 91–93, *92*
    developmental regulation as, 14
    DNA and, *42,* 42–43
    integration of, 12
    intermediary metabolism and growth regulation as, 13
    local regulation and, 93, *93*
    mechanisms of, 8–9
    mineral and water metabolism regulation as, 14
    molecular mechanisms of steroid hormones. *See* Steroid hormone supergene family, regulation of target cell function by
    receptor phosphorylation and, 119–120
    reproductive regulation as, 14
    tropic, 13–14
  amino acid analogues. *See* Amino acid analogues; *specific hormones*
  antagonisms among, 13
  assays for. *See* Assays; *specific assays and under specific hormones*
  attenuation and termination of response to, 13
  binding of. *See* Binding; *under specific hormones*
  circulation of, 6–7
  counterregulatory, 1152, 1153t
  definition of, 3
  diversification of, 11
  domains of control of, 91–93, *92*
  ectopic production of, 1733–1772
    of calcitonin, 1770–1771, 1771t
    criteria for, 1736–1738, 1737t, *1738–1740*
    ectopic pro-opiomelanocortin/adrenocorticotropic hormone syndrome and, 1754–1758
    etiology of, 1741–1744, 1742t
    eutopic production versus, 1733–1735, 1734t
    frequency of, 1738–1741, 1740t
    of gastrin, 1772
    of glucagon, 1772
    of growth hormone, 1766–1767
    of growth hormone releasing hormone, 1767–1768
    hormones as tumor markers and, 1745t, 1745–1747, 1746t
    hypercalcemia of malignancy and, 1747t, 1747–1754
    hypoglycemia associated with malignancy and, 1761–1764
    of immunoreactive bombesin-like peptide, 1772
    importance of, 1735–1736
    oncogenic osteomalacia and, 1764–1766
    paraneoplastic erythrocytosis and, 1769t, 1769–1770, 1770t
    paraneoplastic syndromes and, 1733, 1734t
    of placental proteins, 1768–1769
    of prolactin, 1771–1772
    of renin, 1772
    of somatostatin, 1772
    syndrome of inappropriate antidiuretic hormone in cancer and, 1758–1761
    treatment of, 1744–1745
    of vasoactive intestinal polypeptide, 1772
  free, 6
  hypophysiotropic, 223–224, 231–248, *233. See also specific hormones*
  interactions with receptors, 196–197
  internalization of, 8
  metabolism of, 7. *See also under specific hormones*
    defects in, 17
  peptide. *See* Peptide hormones; *specific hormones*
  receptors for. *See* Hormone receptors; *under specific hormones*
  regulation by:
    of growth, 1626–1633
    paracrine, autocrine, and intracrine, 5, 93, *93,* 1620–1621, 1785
  regulation of. *See* Regulation; *specific hormones*
  as second messengers, 8
  somatomammotropic. *See* Growth hormone (GH); Placental lactogen; Prolactin (PRL)
  steroid. *See* Steroid hormones; *specific hormones*
  synergisms among, 12–13
  synthesis of. *See under specific hormones*
    defects in, 17
    ectopic, 16–17
  as tumor markers, 1745t, 1745–1747, 1746t
  types of, 5–6
Hormone agonist therapy, 20–21
Hormone antagonist therapy, 20–21
Hormone receptors, 9, *99,* 99–111. *See also under specific hormones*
  assays for, 211
  definition of, 3
  G protein-coupled, *714,* 102t, 102–108, *103*
    abnormalities of function of, 107–108, *108*
    adrenergic. *See* Adrenergic receptors
  for growth factors, 108–111
    cytokine receptors, 111
    epidermal growth factor receptor, 108–109, *109*
    growth hormone receptor, 110–111
    insulin receptor, 109–110, *110*
    prolactin receptor, 110
  ligand-gated ion channels and, 99–102
    gamma-aminobutyric acid receptors, 101–102
    glutamate receptors, 100–101
    glycine receptors, 102
    nicotinic acetylcholine receptor, 100, *100*
  nuclear, gene regulation by. *See* Gene(s), regulation by nuclear receptors
  origin of mediators of, 11
  osmoreceptors, 387–388
  for peptide hormones, *77,* 77–78. *See* Peptide hormones, receptors for
  phosphorylation of, hormone action and, 119–120
  serotonin receptor, 102
  for thyroid hormones, *443,* 443–444
  transmembrane signal transduction and. *See* Transmembrane signal transduction
Hormone response elements (HREs), 43
  binding of nuclear receptors to, 178
  consensus, 178–179, *179*
  glucocorticoids and, 594
  mineralocorticoids and, 610
Hormone-responsive tumors, 1785–1807, 1786t
  breast cancer, 1799–1803
  endocrine therapy and, 1793–1795, *1794,* 1795t
  endometrial cancer, 1803–1805
  epidemiology of, 1790t, 1790–1793
    age and hormones and, 1790–1792, *1791*
    geography, diet, and genetics and, *1792,* 1792–1793
  hormone response and:
    cellular mechanisms mediating, 1795–1798, *1796*
    receptor mechanisms mediating, 1798t, 1798–1799, 1799t
  oncogene and tumor suppressor genes and, 1789–1790
  prostate cancer, 1805–1807
  steroids as carcinogens and tumor promoters and, 1787–1789, *1788*
Hormone-sensitive lipase, 1121
Human chorionic gonadotropin (hCG):
  chemistry of, 297–298
  ectopic production of, 1768–1769

for hypopituitarism, 326
luteinization and, 994
luteolysis and, 994–995
therapeutic uses of:
for cryptorchidism, 947
for hypogonadism, 937, *938*
for hypopituitarism, 1651t
thyroid-stimulating hormone excess and, 473
Human chorionic gonadotropin (hCG) test:
for follicle-stimulating hormone, 913, 914t
for luteinizing hormone, 913, 914t
Human immunodeficiency virus (HIV) infection. *See also* Acquired immunodeficiency syndrome (AIDS)
serum thyroid-binding globulin level and, 458
thyroid function and, 463–464
Human leukocyte antigen (HLA):
class II molecules, Graves' disease and, 468–469, *469*
diabetes mellitus and, *1159,* 1159–1160, 1160t
21-hydroxylase deficiency and, 632
Human menopausal gonadotropin (hMG), therapeutic uses of, for hypogonadism, 937
Human menopausal gonadotropin (hMG) CoA reductase inhibitors:
for hyperlipoproteinemia, 1383–1385
indications and dosage for, 1384–1385, *1385,* 1385t
mechanism of action of, 1383, *1384*
side effects of, 1383–1384
Human placental lactogen (hPL), ectopic production of, 1769, 1770t
Hungry bones syndrome, 1464
Hung-up reflexes, 32
Hybrid arrest, 50
Hybrid proteins, 48
synthesis of, by recombinant DNA techniques, 55, *56*
Hybridization, 46–47, *47*
Hybridization screening, 49
Hybrid-selected translation, 50
Hydrochlorothiazide, for thyroid carcinoma, follicular, 545
Hydrocortisone:
for congenital adrenal hyperplasia, 637
virilizing, 1660
for Cushing's disease, 675
for hypopituitarism, 324–325, 1651t
for myxedema coma, 507
Hydrocortisone butyrate, bioavailability of, 863
Hydropic degeneration, 1179
17-Hydroxycorticosteroids, assays for, 617–618, 1667
18-Hydroxycortisol, diagnostic, in primary hyperaldosteronism, 829–830, 830t
5-Hydroxyindoleacetic acid (5-HIAA),
carcinoid tumors and, 1690, 1691–1692
11-Hydroxylase, deficiency of, female pseudohermaphroditism and, 1095
11β-Hydroxylase, 570–571
17α-Hydroxylase, deficiency of, 639–640
testosterone synthesis and, *1081,* 1081–1082
18-Hydroxylase, 571
21-Hydroxylase, 569–570
extraadrenal, 570
genes for, 570
21-Hydroxylase deficiency, 627–638, 628t. *See also* Congenital adrenal hyperplasia (CAH)
female pseudohermaphroditism and, 1087–1093, *1088–1090,* 1091t, *1092, 1094,* 1095
genetics of, 631–635
21-hydroxylase genes and, *631,* 631–632
P450c21 gene lesions and, 632–635
incidence of, 631
nonclassic congenital adrenal hyperplasia and, 630–631
pathophysiology of, 627–629, *629*
salt-wasting congenital adrenal hyperplasia and, 630
simple virilizing congenital adrenal hyperplasia and, 630
Hydroxylysine, urinary, in metabolic bone disease, 1518–1519
3-Hydroxy-3-methylglutaryl coenzyme A reductase (HMGCoA reductase), cholesterol synthesis and, 560–562, 562
17α-Hydroxyprogesterone (17-OHP), 568
plasma level of, 585t
secretion rate of, 585t
Hydroxyproline, urinary, in metabolic bone disease, 1518
3β-Hydroxysteroid dehydrogenase (3β-HSD):
cholesterol synthesis and, 567–568
deficiency of, 628t, 638–639
female pseudohermaphroditism and, 1095–1096
testosterone synthesis and, 1079–1081
11β-Hydroxysteroid dehydrogenase, 572–573
17β-Hydroxysteroid dehydrogenase (3β-HSD), deficiency of, testosterone synthesis and, 1082–1083
25-Hydroxyvitamin D, *1439,* 1439–1442, 1440t
Hyperalbuminemia, hypercalcemia and, 1477
Hyperaldosteronism, 678–680
primary, 678, 812–832, *813,* 814t
adenomas and, 815–817
autonomous versus nonautonomous, 815, 816t, *817, 818*
biochemical determination of
subtypes and, 828–830
carcinoma and, 821, 832
glucocorticoid-remediable, 819–821, *820,* 820t, 832
history and physical findings in, 822
hyperplasia and, 817–821
hypertension and, 822
idiopathic, 818, *819*
idiopathic hyperplasia and, 832
initial studies in, 822–827, *823*
localization procedures in, 827–828
occurrence and classification of, 812, 814t, 814–821, *815*
pathophysiology of, *821,* 821–822
primary adrenal hyperplasia and, 819, 832
treatment of, 830–832
secondary, 678–680, 679t
Bartter's syndrome and, 680
classification of, 679t
extrarenal sodium loss and sodium restriction in, 678
menstrual cycle and pregnancy and, 678–679
renal electrolyte loss in, 680
sodium excess distribution in, 679–680
Hyperalphalipoproteinemia, familial, 1357
Hypercalcemia, *1449,* 1449–1477, *1451,* 1451t
acute renal failure and, 1477
adrenal insufficiency and, 1475
adrenocortical insufficiency and, 651
approach to patient and, 1450–1452, *1451*
calcitonin for, 1434, 1436
defense against, 1449–1450
drug-induced, 1475–1476
lithium and, 1476
milk-alkali syndrome and, 1476
thiazide diuretics and, 1475
vitamin A and, 1476
vitamin D and, 1475–1476
granulomatous disorders and, 1474
hyperthyroidism and, 1474–1475
hypocalciuric, familial, 1460–1461, *1461*
extracellular calcium-sensing receptor and, 1461
idiopathic, of infancy, 1477
immobilization and, 1476–1477
in infants, idiopathic, 1477
intensive care unit and, 1477
malignancy-associated, 1467–1474, 1747t, 1747–1754
bony metastases and, 1747
breast cancer and, 1472
cancer and primary hyperparathyroidism and, 1751–1752
clinical features of, 1468
clinical manifestations of, 1752t, 1752–1753, *1753*
diagnosis of, 1472

Hypercalcemia (*Cont.*)
1,25-dihydroxyvitamin D and, 1751
hematologic neoplasms and, 1471–1472
historical background of, 1467–1468, *1468*
humoral, pathogenesis of, *1469,* 1469–1470, *1470*
parathyroid hormone-related peptide and, *1468,* 1468–1469
solid tumors and, 1470t, 1470–1471
systemic elaboration of humoral substances and, 1748–1751
treatment of, 1472–1474, 1753–1754
osteolytic, local, 1471
pheochromocytomas and, 1475
primary hyperparathyroidism and. *See* Hyperparathyroidism, primary
renal phosphate handling and, 1492
serum protein disorders and, 1477
VIPomas and, 1475
Hypercalcemic crisis, treatment of, 1467
Hypercalciuria, 1588–1597, 1589t, *1590*
absorptive, treatment of, 1606–1607
bone effects in, 1597
calcium homeostasis and, *1590,* 1590–1591
classification of, 1591–1597
constitutional, 1591
dietary, 1591–1592, *1592*
evaluation of, 1603
treatment of, 1606
evaluation of, 1602–1603, 1603
fasting, 1595
idiopathic, 1588, 1592–1597
absorptive, 1595–1597, *1596*
renal calcium leak and, *1594,* 1594–1595
resorptive, 1592–1593, *1593*
subtle primary hyperparathyroidism, 1593t, 1593–1594
renal:
osteoporosis and, 1537
treatment of, 1606
secondary, 1591, 1591t
treatment of, empiric therapy for, 1607
unclassifiable, 1595
usefulness of diagnosing, 1590
Hypercapnia, vasopressin and, 393–394
Hypercholesterolemia, 1335–1353
familial, 1335–1341
clinical characteristics of, 1335–1337, *1336,* 1337t
definition of, 1335
diagnostic laboratory features of, 1337
genetics of, 1338
homozygous, surgical treatment of, 1390
pathophysiology of, 1337–1338, *1338, 1339*
treatment of, 1339–1341, 1341t
familial defective apolipoprotein B-100, 1342–1343
clinical characteristics of, 1342, *1342*
definition of, 1342
diagnostic laboratory features of, 1343
genetics of, 1342
pathophysiology of, 1343
treatment of, 1343
hypertriglyceridemia and. *See* Hypertriglyceridemia, hypercholesterolemia and
Hyperchylomicronemia, 1348–1351
clinical features of, *1349,* 1349–1350, 1350t
definition of, 1348–1349
diagnostic laboratory features of, 1350–1351
genetics of, 1350
pathophysiology of, 1351
treatment of, 1351
Hypercortisolism:
in Cushing's disease. *See* Cushing's disease
ectopic ACTH syndrome and, 664
Hyperglycemia:
catecholamines and, *721,* 721–722
exercise-induced, 1215
hypothalamic disorders and, 271
postprandial, diabetes mellitus in pregnancy and, 1226–1227
stress-induced, 1156, *1157,* 1235
symptoms of, 1181–1182
Hypergonadism, hypothalamic, 266–267
Hypergonadotropic hypogonadism. *See* Hypogonadism, hypergonadotropic
Hypergonadotropic syndromes, infertility and, 938–940, *939*
Hyperinsulinemia, 1135–1136
hypertension, insulin resistance, and obesity correlated with, 788–789
Hyperkalemia:
adrenocortical insufficiency and, 650
diabetic nephropathy and, 1186
drug-induced, diabetic nephropathy and, 1186
Hyperketonemia, exercise-induced, 1215
Hyperlipidemia, 1326–1335
classification of, 1326t, 1326–1327, *1327*
diabetic, 1172–1174, *1173*
diagnostic criteria for, 1327–1330, *1328,* 1328t, 1329t
dietary treatment of, 1366–1380
effects of specific nutrients on plasma lipids and lipoproteins and, 1367t, 1367–1374
pharmacologic therapy compared with, 1380
phased approach to, 1378t, 1378–1380
single-diet concept and, 1374–1378, 1375t, *1376*
laboratory diagnosis of of, 1392–1394
lipid determinations, 1392
lipoprotein separations, 1392–1393
sample collection and handling for, 1392
lipoprotein(a), 1363
secondary, 1330–1335
alcohol use and, 1334
$alpha_1$ antitrypsin deficiency and, 1334
bile duct obstruction and, 1324–1334
diabetes mellitus and, 1330–1332
dietary, 1330, 1330t, *1331*
drug-induced, 1334t, 1334–1335
hypothyroidism and, 1332–1333
renal disease and, 1333
Hyperlipoproteinemia:
drug-induced, hyperlipidemia and, 1334t, 1334–1335
pharmacologic treatment of, 1380–1390
acyl CoA cholesterol acyltransferase inhibitors in, 1389–1390
anabolic steroids in, 1388
bile acid sequestrants in, 1381–1382
cholesterol synthesis inhibitors in, 1389
clofibrate in, 1386–1387
dextrothyroxine in, 1388
estrogens in, 1388
fibric acid derivatives in, 1388, 1389t
gemfibrozil in, 1387
human menopausal gonadotropin CoA reductase inhibitors in, 1383–1385
neomycin in, 1387–1388
nicotinic acid derivatives in, 1388–1389
nicotinic acid in, 1382–1383
probucol in, 1385–1386
progestational agents in, 1388
primary type III, 1345–1348
clinical characteristics of, 1345–1346, *1346*
definition of, 1345
diagnostic laboratory features of, 1346–1347
pathophysiology of, 1347, *1347*
treatment of, 1347–1348, *1348*
surgical treatment of, 1390–1392
in children, 1391–1392
in homozygous familial hypercholesterolemia, 1390
in older patients, 1391
in women, 1390–1391
type IV, 1351–1353
clinical characteristics of, 1352
definition of, 1351–1352
diagnostic laboratory features of, 1352
genetics of, 1352
pathophysiology of, 1352
treatment of, 1352–1353
types I and V, 1348–1351
Hypermagnesemia, 1497
Hypernatremia:
adipsic:
pathophysiology of, 408
treatment of, 414
essential, pathophysiology of, 408, *408*
hypodipsic, pathophysiology of, 408
Hyperosmolar nonketotic coma, 1224

Hyperoxaluria, 1597–1600
  absorptive, 1599
  classification of, 1598t, 1598–1600
  colonic, 1599
  enteric, treatment of, 1607
  evaluation of, 1604–1605
  oxalate metabolism and, 1597t, 1597–1598, *1598*
  primary, treatment of, 1607
Hyperparathyroidism:
  multiple endocrine neoplasia, type 2 and, 1716
  occurrence of, 1716
  pathology of, 1716
  primary, 1452–1467
    anemia in, 27
    asymptomatic, diagnosis and management of, *1465,* 1465–1466
    bone and, 1456–1457, *1457–1459*
    cancer and, 1751–1752
    clinical presentation of, 1455–1456, *1456*
    etiology of, 1453–1455, *1454, 1455*
    familial hypocalciuric hypercalcemia and, 1460–1461, *1461*
    historical background of, 1452–1453, *1453*
    laboratory findings and definitive diagnosis of, 1461–1463
    medical management of, 1466–1467
    multiple endocrine neoplasia and, 1459–1460, 1460t, 1704
    nonspecific features of, 1457, 1459
    osteoporosis and, 1536
    parathyroid surgery for, 1463–1465
    pathophysiology of, 1456
    physical findings in, 1461, *1462*
    preoperative localization studies in, 1463
    subtle, 1593t, 1593–1594
      evaluation of, 1603
  relation to medullary thyroid carcinoma, 1716
  secondary, renal osteodystrophy and, 1543
  vitamin D and, 1440
Hyperphosphatasia, hereditary, 1545–1546
Hyperphosphatemia, 1494
  acute, hypocalcemia and, 1487
  adrenocortical insufficiency and, 651
Hyperpigmentation, 25
  in Addison's disease, 648, *649*
  Cushing's syndrome and, 666
Hyperplasia, 1619, *1620*
  primary hyperaldosteronism and, 817–821
    glucocorticoid-remediable hyperaldosteronism and, 819–821, *820,* 820t
    idiopathic, 818, *819*
    primary adrenal hyperplasia and, 819
Hyperproinsulinemia, familial, 1131
Hyperprolactinemia. *See also* Amenorrhea-galactorrhea syndrome
  chronic renal failure and, 313
  gonadotropin-releasing hormone deficiency of and, 266
  hypogonadotropic hypogonadism and, 918–920
  hypothalamus and, 261, 267
  idiopathic, 267–268
  renal failure and, 273–274
Hypersecretion. *See also specific hormones and disorders*
  secondary, 17
Hypersensitization, of adrenergic receptors, 720
Hypertension, 749–835
  accelerated, renin-angiotensin system and, 763–764
  adrenocorticotropic hormone and, 771–772
  anabolic steroids and, 1864
  androgens and, 772
  atrial natriuretic peptide and, 778–779
  autonomic nervous system and, 779–780
  blood pressure regulation and, 753
  calcitonin gene-related peptide and, 773
  calcium ion and calcium regulatory hormones and, 784–785
  calcium-regulating hormones and, 773
  carbenoxolone ingestion and, 834
  catecholamines and, 779–780
  chloride and, 783
  classification of blood pressure levels in, 749, 750t
  complications of, 753–754
  Cushing's syndrome and, 666, 835
  iatrogenic, 859
  deoxycorticosterone-excess, 832–833
    adrenocortical adenomas and, 833
    congenital adrenal hyperplasia and, 832–833
  endothelin and, 774
  endothlium-derived hyperpolarizing factor and, 776
  epidemiology of, 750, 752, *752*
  erythropoietin and, 772–773
  essential. *See* Essential hypertension
  estrogens and, 772
  experimental, renin-angiotensin system and, 763
  genetic and environmental influences on, 752–753
  glucocorticoids and, 770–771
    excess of, 603–604
    resistance to, 835
  growth hormone and, 773
  hyperlipidemia and, diet therapy for, 1379–1380
  hypothyroidism and, 500
  intracellular pH regulation and, 786–787
  intracranial, benign, 274–275
  kallikreins and kinins and, 780–781
  licorice ingestion and, 833–834
  low-renin, 832–835
  magnesium and, 785
  mineralocorticoids and, *767,* 767–770
    aldosterone, 768
    cortisol and other mineralocorticoids with glucocorticoid activity and, 768–769
    deoxycorticosterone, 769
    essential hypertension and, 770
    excess syndromes and, 834
    mechanisms of blood pressure elevation and, 769–770
    19-Nor-deoxycorticosterone and, 769
  Na^+,K^+-ATPase and, 785
  Na^+-K^+-Cl^+ cotransport and, 786
  Na^+-Na^+ countertransport and, 786
  nitric oxide and, 774–776, *775*
  obesity, insulin, and insulin resistance and, 788–794, 1278–1279. *See also* Diabetes mellitus; Insulin; Insulin resistance
    correlations between, 788–789
    diabetes mellitus and, 789–790
  ouabain-like factors and, *787,* 787–788
  parathyroid gland hypertensinogenic factor and, 773
  parathyroid hormone and parathyroid hormone-related peptide and, 773
  patient evaluation in, 794–797
    clinical history in, 794, 794t
    laboratory tests in, 795–797, 796t, 798t
    physical examination in, 794–795, 795t
    plasma renin activity and, 796–797, 798t
  pheochromocytomas and, 728
  potassium and, 783–784
  primary hyperaldosteronism and. *See* Hyperaldosteronism, primary
  progestins and, 772
  prostaglandins and other eicosanoids and, 780
  renin-angiotensin system and, 763–767. *See also* Renin-angiotensin system
    accelerated hypertension and, 764
    atherosclerotic complications and, 767
    essential hypertension and, 764–767, *765*
    experimental hypertension and, 763
    genetic linkages and, 764
    renin-secreting tumors and, 763, *764*
    renovascular hypertension and, 763
  renovascular. *See* Renovascular hypertension
  secondary, renin-angiotensin system and, 763–764
  sodium chloride and, 781–783, *782, 783*
  steroid ingestion and, 834
  thyroid hormones and, 772
  types of, 749, 751t

Hypertension (*Cont.*)
  vasopressin and, 772
  vitamin D and, 773
Hyperthermia, paroxysmal, hypothalamic disorders and, 271
Hyperthyroidism. *See also* Thyrotoxicosis
  anemia in, 27
  differentiated from thyrotoxicosis, 466
  endemic goiter and, 525
  hypercalcemia and, 1474–1475
  steroid hormone metabolism and, 593
Hyperthyroxinemia, 451
  dysalbuminemic, familial, 458
Hypertriglyceridemia, 1348–1353
  diabetes mellitus and, 1173
  hypercholesterolemia and, 1343–1348
    familial combined hyperlipidemia, 1344–1345
    hepatic lipase deficiency, 1348
    hyperchylomicronemia, 1348–1351
    primary type III hyperlipoproteinemia, 1345–1348
  hyperchylomicronemia, 1348–1351
  hyperlipoproteinemia and, type IV, 1351–1353
  obesity and, 1278
  pregnancy and, 1351
  type IV hyperlipoproteinemia, 1351–1353
Hypertrophy, 1619
Hyperuricosuria, 1600–1601
  definition and prevalence of, 1600–1601, *1601*, 1601t
  evaluation of, 1605
  identification of, 1600
Hyperventilation, tetany and, 1479
Hypoalbuminemia:
  hyperaldosteronism and, 679
  hypocalcemia and, 1487
Hypoaldosteronism, 657–659
  hyporeninemic, 657–658
  normoreninemic and hyperreninemic, 658–659
  pseudohypoaldosteronism, 659
Hypoalphalipoproteinemia, familial, 1354
Hypobetalipoproteinemia, 1359
Hypocalcemia:
  adrenocortical insufficiency and, 651
  approach to patient and, 1478
  classification of, 1477–1478, *1478*, 1478t
  clinical manifestations of, 1478–1480
    tetany, 1478–1479, *1479*
  critical illness and, 1487
  drug-induced, 1487
  hyperphosphatemia and, 1487
  hypoalbuminemia and, 1487
  hypoparathyroidism and. *See* Hypoparathyroidism
  pancreatitis and, 1487
  pseudohypoparathyroidism and. *See* Pseudohypoparathyroidism
  sepsis and, 1487
  skeletal mineralization and, 1487
  transfusions and, 1487
  treatment of, 1487–1489
    for acute hypocalcemia, 1487–1488
    for chronic hypocalcemia, 1488t, 1488–1489
Hypocitraturia, 1601–1602
  citrate metabolism and, 1602
  effect of citrate on urinary crystallization and, 1602
  evaluation of, 1605
  treatment of, 1602
Hypoglycemia, 736–738, 1251–1267
  in Addison's disease, 648
  of aging, 1827
  awareness of, 737–738
  classification of, 1255, 1255t
  definition of, 1251
  exercise-induced, 1214–1215
  fasting, 1255–1264
    diagnostic and therapeutic approach to, 1266–1267, *1267*
    in endocrine deficiency states, 1262
    glucose counterregulation and, *1257*, 1257–1258
    glucose homeostasis during fasting and exercise and, 1255–1256, *1256*
    hepatic disorders and, 1262–1263
    insulin autoimmune hypoglycemia, 1263–1264
    insulin-producing islet-cell tumors and, 1258–1261
    non-islet-cell tumor hypoglycemia, 1261–1262
    substrate deficiency and, 1263
  fuel requirements and, 1155–1156
  glucose counterregulation and:
    pathophysiology in insulin-dependent diabetes mellitus, 737–738, *738*
    physiology of, 736, *737*
  induced, 1265t, 1265–1266
    ethanol and, 1266
    pentamidine isethionate and, 1265–1266
    sulfonylureas and, 1265
  insulin therapy and, 1203–1204
  malignancy and, 1761–1764
    clinical manifestations and diagnosis of, 1764
    incidence and tumor types and, 1762, 1762t
    pathophysiology of, 1762–1764
    treatment of, 1764
  reactive, 1264–1265
    alimentary, 1264–1265
    definition of, 1264
    diabetes mellitus and, 1265
    symptoms of, 1264, *1264*
    treatment of, 1265
  signs and symptoms of, 1251–1253
    neuroglycopenia, 1252
    sympathoadrenal, 1252
  tests for, 1253–1255
    C peptide, 1253–1254
    oral glucose tolerance test, 1254
    plasma insulin, 1253
    proinsulin, 1254
    supervised prolonged fasting, 1254
  unawareness of, 1200
  vasopressin and, 393
Hypoglycemia-associated autonomic failure (HAAF):
  classical diabetic autonomic neuropathy versus, 738
  pathogenesis of, 738, *738*
Hypogonadism:
  hypergonadotropic, 928–935, *929*, 929t
    androgen insensitivity and, *934*, 934–935
    diabetes mellitus and, 933
    enzyme defects and, 933
    functional prepubertal castrate syndrome and, 932
    genetic disorders and, 929–932
    gonadal toxins and, 932–933
    luteinizing hormone resistance and, 935
    male climacteric and, 933–934
    mumps orchitis and, 933
  hypothalamic, 265–266
    postpubertal, 266
    prepubertal, 265–266
  primary, pituitary adenoma versus, 336t, 338
  treatment of, 935–938, 936t
    delayed puberty and, 935–936
    hypergonadotropic hypogonadism and, *936*, 936–937, *937*
Hypogonadotropic eunuchoidism. *See* Kallman's syndrome
Hypogonadotropic syndromes, 917–928, *919*, 919t
  chronic illnesses and, 926–928
  hyperprolactinemia and, 918–920
  isolated gonadotropin deficiency and, 920–925
  multiple trophic hormone deficiency and, 918
  physiologic delayed puberty and, 928
Hypokalemia:
  primary hyperaldosteronism and, 823–824, *824*
  weakness and, 24
Hypomagnesemia, 1495–1497, 1496t
  hypoparathyroidism and, 1481
Hyponatremia:
  adrenocortical insufficiency and, 650
  euvolemic. *See* Syndrome of inappropriate antidiuretic hormone (SIADH)
  hypervolemic:
    diagnosis of, 419, 420t
    etiology and pathophysiology of, 415
    treatment of, 420
  hypovolemic:
    diagnosis of, 419, 420t
    etiology and pathophysiology of, 415–416
    treatment of, 420–421
Hypoparathyroidism, 1480–1482
  Addison's disease and, 1721–1722, *1722*

clinical manifestations of, 1480
familial, 1482
hypomagnesemia and, 1481, *1481*
idiopathic, 1481–1482
infiltrative diseases and, 1481
metal deposition and, 1481
in neonates, 1482
radiation and, 1481
rickets and osteomalacia and, 1528
surgical, 1480
Hypophosphatasia, rickets and osteomalacia and, 1528
Hypophosphatemia, *1492,* 1492t, 1492–1494, 1526–1528
alcoholism and, 1494
chronic, osteoporosis and, 1537
chronic dialysis and, 1528
decreased absorption causing, 1493
diabetic ketoacidosis and, 1493, *1493*
increase renal excretion causing, 1493
malnutrition and malabsorption and, 1527–1528
nutritional recovery and, 1493–1494
renal phosphate wasting and, 1526–1527
respiratory alkalosis and, 1493
treatment of, 1494, 1494t
Hypophysectomy:
diabetes insipidus and, 402
for diabetic retinopathy, 5879
transsphenoidal, for multiple endocrine neoplasia, type 1, 1708
Hypophysiotropic hormones, 223–224, 231–248, *233. See also specific hormones*
Hypophysiotropic neurons, 221, 227, *230*
Hypophysitis, hypogonadotropic hypogonadism and, 928
Hypopigmentation, 25
Hypopituitarism, 313–327
clinical features of, 317–319
adrenocorticotropic hormone and, 318
follicle-stimulating hormone and, 318
growth hormone and, 318
isolated hormonal deficiencies and, 319
luteinizing hormone and, 318
oxytocin and, 319
prolactin and, 318
thyroid-stimulating hormone and, 318
vasopressin and, 318–319
diagnostic procedures for, 320–324
adrenocorticotropic hormone and, 320–322, *321*
combined pituitary hormone testing and, 324
follicle-stimulating hormone and, 322–323, *323*
growth hormone and, 323–324
luteinizing hormone and, 322–323, *323*
prolactin and, 324
thyroid-stimulating hormone and, 322, *322*
differential diagnosis of, 319–320
neuroendocrine disorders and, 320
target organ and hypothalamic hypofunction and, 319–320
etiology of, 313–316, 314t
of primary hypopituitarism, 313–316, *315*
of secondary hypopituitarism, 326–327
familial, 316
pituitary adenoma versus, 336t, 338–339
hypogonadotropic hypogonadism and, 918
hypothalamus and, 261
idiopathic, short stature and, 1647
primary, 313
etiology of, 313–316, *315*
secondary, 313
etiology of, 326–327
treatment of, 324–327, 1651t
adrenocorticotropic hormone in, 324–325
follicle-stimulating hormone in, 325–326
growth hormone in, 326–327
luteinizing hormone in, 325–326
in men, 326
prolactin in, 327
thyroid-stimulating hormone in, 325
in women, 325–326
Hyporesponsiveness syndromes, 16
Hypospadias:
isolated, 1086
perineoscrotal, pseudovaginal, 1083–1084
Hypotension:
in Addison's disease, 648
glucocorticoid deficiency and, 603, *603, 604*
postural, 732–736
diabetes mellitus and, 1190
mechanisms of, 733–734, 733–735t
treatment of, 735–736
Hypothalamic disorders, 259–271, 260t. *See also specific disorders*
embryopathic, congenital, 260–261, *261*
food intake and, 268–271
hamartomas, 262
hyperglycemia and, 271
inflammatory, 262–264
pituitary function and, 264–268
adrenocorticotropic hormone and, 268
gonadotropins and, 265–267
growth hormone and, 264–265
prolactin and, 267–268
thyroid-stimulating hormone and, 268
polyostotic fibrous dysplasia, 264
radiation-induced, 264
temperature regulation and, 271
traumatic, 263–264
tumors, 261–262
vascular, 263
vasopressin and, 268
Hypothalamic-pituitary axis, anatomy of, 885–886, *886*
Hypothalamic-pituitary portal system, 227, 229–230, *231, 232*
Hypothalamic-pituitary-adrenal axis, 573
aging and, 1818–1819
alternate-day steroid therapy and, 871
corticosteroid withdrawal and. *See* Glucocorticoids, withdrawal of, suppression of hypothalamic-pituitary-adrenal axis and
negative feedback control of, in Cushing's disease, 358–359
Hypothalamic-pituitary-germ cell axis, *907,* 907–910
feedback control of follicle-stimulating hormone release and, 909–910
hypothalamus and, 907
interactions with hypothalamic-pituitary-Leydig cell axis, 910–911
pituitary and, 907–908
testis and, 908–909
Hypothalamic-pituitary-gonadal axis:
abnormal, 1068t, 1068–1096, 1069t
clinical approach to, 1096–1099
errors of primary sex determination, 1068–1078
errors of sexual differentiation, 1078–1096
anabolic steroids and:
in men, 1863–1864
in women, 1863
differentiation of, 1062–1068
control of fetal gonadal function and, 1064–1066
gender role and psychosexual differentiation and, 1067–1068
gonadal steroid synthesis and, 1062–1063
perinatal adaptations of reproductive endocrine system and, 1066–1067
sex steroid actions on genitalia and, *1063,* 1063–1064
sex steroids in fetal circulation and, 1063
exercise and training and, 1849–1853
acute exercise in men and, 1850, 1850t
endurance training in men and, 1852
exercise-associated testosterone release and, 1850–1851
long-term-activity-associated testosterone suppression and, 1853
prolonged exercise in men and, 1851–1852
short-term exercise and, 1850, 1850t
symptomatic impairment of axis in men and, 1852–1853
regulation of, 237–239
Hypothalamic-pituitary-Leydig cell axis, 891–907
feedback interaction and, 903–907, *905, 906*

Hypothalamic-pituitary-Leydig (*Cont.*)
androgen negative feedback, 904–905
estrogen negative feedback, 905–906
estrogen positive feedback, 906–907
hypothalamus and, 892–895
afferent neural input and, 892
behavioral centers of, 894–895
hypothalamic pulse generator and, 892–894, *897*
interactions with hypothalamic-pituitary-germ cell axis, 910–911
Leydig cells and, 898–903, *899–901, 903, 904,* 905t
pituitary and, 895–898
Hypothalamic-pituitary-testicular axis, 911–916
assessment of hormonal status of, 911–913
basal levels and, 911–912, *912*
biological effects of sex steroids on target organs and, 913
dynamic tests and, 912–913, *913, 914,* 914t
genetic tests and, 913–914
pituitary and hypothalamus and, 914
testes and surrounding structures and, 914–916, 915t
Hypothalamic-pituitary-thyroid axis, aging and, 1818, 1818t
Hypothalamus. *See also specific hypothalamic axes*
acromegaly and, 345, *346,* 346–347
amenorrhea-galactorrhea syndrome and, 352–354, *353*
anatomy of, 226–227, *226–228,* 229t, *230*
behavioral centers of, 894–895
activational effects of, 895
organizational effects of, 894–895
Cushing's disease and, *360,* 5273
disorders of. *See* Hypothalamic disorders; *specific disorders*
glucocorticoid regulation by, 573–574
hormones of, 223–224, 231–248, *233.* *See also specific hormones*
hypothyroidism and, 497
interactions between luteinizing hormone-Leydig cell and follicle-stimulating hormone-germ cell axes and, 910, *910*
medial basal, 885
obesity and, 1290
structural and functional assessment of, 914
Hypothyroidism, 492–507
acquired, short stature and, 1644–1645
adaptive, 492
amenorrhea-galactorrhea syndrome and, 352
anemia and, 27
central, 492, 497–498
hypothalamic, 497
pituitary, 497
thyroid-stimulating hormone secretion in, 497–498
clinical manifestations of, 498t, 498–503
cardiovascular, 500
endocrine, 502–503
energy, nutrient, and drug metabolism and, 501–502
fluid and electrolyte metabolism and, 501
gastrointestinal, 501
general appearance and, 499
hematopoietic, 501
illness and surgery and, 503
musculoskeletal, 500
neurologic, 499–500
pulmonary, 500–501
renal function and, 501
skin and appendages and, 499, *499*
thyroid gland and, 499
congenital, short stature and, 1644
etiology of, 492–498, 493t
central hypothyroidism and, 497–498
chronic autoimmune thyroiditis and, 493t, 493–494, *494*
infiltrative disease of thyroid and, 495–496
radiation therapy and, 495
resistance therapy thyroid hormones and, 498
surgery and, 495
thyroid dysgenesis and, 495
thyroid hormone synthetic defects and, 496–497
transient hypothyroidism in autoimmune thyroiditis and, 494–495
hyperlipidemia and, 1332–1333
hypothalamic, 268
laboratory diagnosis of, 503–504, *504*
serum thyroid hormone concentrations and, 503–504
serum thyroid-stimulating hormone concentrations and, 503
myxedema coma and, 507
in neonates and children, 506–507
pathophysiology of, 492, *492*
pituitary (secondary), 318
primary, 492
pituitary adenoma versus, 336t, 338
steroid hormone metabolism and, 593
subclinical, 492, 506
tall stature and, 1663
thyroid hormone withdrawal and, 506
treatment of, 504–506, 505t
Hypothyroxinemia, 451
Hypoventilation, obesity and, 1281
Hypoxia, vasopressin and, 393–394
Hysterectomy, for endometrial cancer, 1804

Idiopathic growth hormone deficiency (IGHD), hypothalamic disease and, 265
Idiopathic hypocalcemia of infancy, 1482
Idiopathic hypoparathyroidism, 1481–1482
Ileal bypass, distal, for familial hypercholesterolemia, 1341
Illness. *See* Critical illness; Systemic illness; *specific disorders*
Imaging. *See specific modalities and disorders*
Immediate early response genes, hormonal regulation of, *159,* 159–161
Immobilization:
hypercalcemia and, 1476–1477
osteoporosis and, 1537
Immotile cilia syndrome, 941, 942t
Immune system:
anabolic steroids and, 1864
glucocorticoids and, 600–603
primary and secondary phases of immune response and, 206
vitamin D and, 1448
Immunization, for production of monoclonal antibodies, 207
Immunoassays, 203–209. *See also specific assays and specific hormones*
binding proteins for, 206–208
antibodies, 206–207
avidin/biotin, 207–208
enzyme, 208, 210–211, *211*
free and total hormone measurements using, 205–206, 206t
labeled analyte and reagent limiting for, 203–204, *204*
labels for, 208–209
nonlabels for, 208–209
radioactive, 208
optimization and validation of, 212–213
detection limits and, 212, *212*
general considerations in, 212
specificity and, 212–213, *213*
reagent excess and labeled antibody for, 204
of thyroid-stimulating hormone, 296
Immunoglobulin G (IgG), structure of, 206, *206*
Immunoreactive bombesin-like peptide, paraneoplastic, 1772
Immunosuppression, for diabetes mellitus, 1216–1217
Implantable devices, for drug delivery, 57
insulin pumps, 1203, 1218
Impotence, 29, 951
contraception, male, 951–952
drug-related, 951
endocrine-related, 951
neuropathic, 951
psychogenic, 951
of vascular insufficiency, 951
Infants. *See also* Lactation; Neonates; Nursing
development of, 1634, *1635*
diabetes mellitus during pregnancy and, 1230–1231
hypercalcemia in, idiopathic, 1477
thyroid function in, 456
Infection(s):

adrenocortical insufficiency and, 645
Cushing's syndrome and, iatrogenic, 861
diabetes mellitus and, 1161–1162, 1192–1193
hypocalcemia and, 1487
male infertility and, 941
Paget's disease of bone and, 1551
Infection stones. *See* Magnesium ammonium phosphate stones
Inferior petrosal sinus sampling, for pituitary hormones, in Cushing's disease, 359
Infertility, 29
clinical approach to, 1099, *1099*
female:
hypopituitarism and, 326
hypothyroidism and, 503
male, 182, 938–943, 939t
autoimmune, 942
diagnosis of, 942–943
eugonadotropic, 940–941
genetic syndromes, 941–942
hypergonadotropic syndromes and, 938–940, *939*
hypopituitarism and, 326
sinopulmonary-infertility syndrome, 941, 942t
Infiltrative disease:
hypoparathyroidism and, 1481
of thyroid, hypothyroidism and, 495–496
Inflammatory disorders. *See also specific disorders*
growth hormone deficiency and, short stature and, 1648–1649
hypothalamic, 262–264
Inflammatory response, glucocorticoids and, 600, 601, 855–856
Infradian rhythms, 257
factors influencing, 257–259, *258*
Infundibular process, of neurohypophysis, 385
Infundibulum:
hypothalamic, 226
neurohypophyseal, 385
pituitary, 289
Infusion pumps, for insulin therapy, 1202–1203
Inhibin:
follicle-stimulating hormone and, 303, 907
negative feedback effects of, 238
Inhibitor theory, of stone pathogenesis, 1566–1567
Inositol:
calcium release induced by, 152–153
inositol-phosphate metabolism and, 150–151, *152*
inositol(1,4,5)-triphosphate receptor and, 153–154, *155*
Insertions, 45
Insulin, 3, 1128–1146. *See also* Diabetes mellitus
action of, 1136–1140, 1137t
amino acid metabolism and, 1139
blood pressure and, *790,* 790–792
on blood vessels, 791
carbohydrate metabolism and, 1137–1139
exercise-induced alterations in, 1215–1216
fat metabolism and, 1139–1140
on ions, 791–792
potassium metabolism and, 1140
protein metabolism and, 1139
renal, 791
sodium metabolism and, 1140
sympathetic, 791
on vascular structure, 791
allergy to, 1205
assays for, 1177
catecholamines and, 721, *721*
chemistry of, 1128–1129
degradation of, 1145–1146
exercise and, 1847–1848
food intake and, 1288
glucose counterregulation and, 736–738, *737, 738*
growth hormone and, 305
historical background of, 1128, *1128*
human, synthesis of, by recombinant DNA techniques, 56
hypertension and, 788–794
diabetes mellitus and, 790–791
insulin actions influencing blood pressure and, *790,* 790–792
insulin resistance and, 788–789, 792–794
insulin resistance and hyperinsulinemia correlated with, 788–789
plasma, in hypoglycemia, 1253
postreceptor events and, 1143–1144
diabetes mellitus and, 1169
potentiators of, for diabetes mellitus, 1213
precursor of, connecting peptide in, 74–75, *75*
receptors for, 109–110, *110,* 1140–1143
in diabetes mellitus, 1168–1169
interaction and structure of, 1140–1142, *1141*
phosphorylation of, 1142–1143
turnover of, 1142, *1142*
renal phosphate handling and, 1491
resistance to. *See* Insulin resistance
responsiveness to. *See also* Insulin resistance
decreased, 1144, *1144*
secretion of, 1130–1136, 1150
amino acids and fat-derived substances and, 1134
basal concentrations and, 1130–1131
carbohydrate and, 1131–1133, *1132, 1133*
diabetes mellitus and, 1165–1167, *1166*
gastrointestinal hormones and, 1133–1134, *1134*
hyperinsulinemia and, 1135–1136
neural and neurohormonal regulation of, 1134–1135
obesity and, 1136
somatostatin and, 1135, *1136*
synthesis of, 1129–1130, *1130, 1131*
Insulin autoimmune hypoglycemia, 1263–1264
Insulin hypoglycemia stimulation test:
for adrenocorticotropic hormone, 364, 623
for growth hormone, 1666t
for prolactin, 369
Insulin lipodystrophy, 1205
Insulin pumps, implantable, 1203, 1218
Insulin resistance, 1144–1145, *1144–1146,* 1145t
diabetes mellitus and, 1166, 1167–1169, *1168*
acanthosis nigricans and, 1169
insulin receptors and, 1168–1169
postreceptor defects and, 1169
syndrome X and, 1169
tissue sites of resistance and, 1168
hypertension and, 788–789, 792–794
essential, 792–793
hyperinsulinemia and obesity correlated with, 788–789
ion transport abnormalities in, 793
therapeutic implications of, 793–794
insulin therapy and, 1205–1206
obesity and, 1278
Insulin secretagogues, for diabetes mellitus, 1212
Insulin therapy, 1198–1206
complications of, 1203–1206
dawn phenomenon, 1205
hypoglycemia, 1203–1204
insulin allergy, 1205
insulin lipodystrophy, 1205
insulin resistance, 1205–1206
insulin-induced edema, 1206
Somogyi phenomenon, 1204–1205
in diabetes mellitus, in older patients, 1828–1829
for diabetic ketoacidosis, 1221–1222
goals of, 1206
insulin delivery devices for, 1202–1203, 1218
insulin preparations and, 1198t, 1198–1199
during pregnancy, 1231
types of diabetic control and, 1199–1202
initiating therapy and, 1199–1200
intensive treatment and, 1200–1202, 1201t
Insulin tolerance test:
for growth hormone, 367
in hypopituitarism, 320, 321, *321*
Insulin-dependent diabetes mellitus (IDDM). *See* Diabetes mellitus, insulin-dependent
Insulin-like growth factors (IGFs):
action of, 1151t, 1151–1152

Insulin-like growth factors (*Cont.*)
aging and, 1817, *1818*
fasting and malnutrition and, 272
growth and, 1621–1626, 1623t, *1624, 1625*
growth hormone and, 305, 309
menarche and, 1005–1006
as ovarian growth factor, 1009
plasma level of, in acromegaly, 344
regulation of, 245–246
Insulinomas:
in multiple endocrine neoplasia, type 1, 1704–1705
management of, 1708–1709
treatment of, pharmacologic, 1681t
Insulitis, 1161
Integrins, 1429
Interleukin-1 (IL-1), corticotropin releasing hormone and, 244
Intermediary metabolism:
glucocorticoids and, 596, *597*
regulation of, 13
Internal carotid artery aneurysms, pituitary adenoma versus, 336t, 338
Internal plexus, of pituitary, 289
Internalization mechanism, 8
International standards, for bioassays, 201
Interstitial cells. *See* Corpus luteum; Leydig cells; Oocytes; Ovaries, interstitial cells of
Intestine:
calcium transport in, vitamin D and, *1445,* 1445–1446, *1446*
phosphate absorption in, 1489–1490, 1493
vitamin D and, 1447
Intracellular signaling. *See* Transmembrane signal transduction
Intracrine regulation, 93
Intranasal drugs, 57
Intraocular pressure, glucocorticoids and, 607
Intrauterine growth disturbances, short stature and, 1642–1643
fetus and, 1643
mother and, 1643
placenta and, 1642
Intravenous pyelography (IVP), in nephrolithiasis, 1569
Introns, 39–40, 69
functions of, 40, 41
Invasive disorders, adrenocortical insufficiency and, 645
Iodinated radiographic contrast agents, thyroid function and, 465
Iodine (iodide). *See also* Radioiodine scanning; Radioiodine therapy
concentration defect of, hypothyroidism and, 496
deficiency of, hypothyroidism and, 496–497
economy of, 437–438
endemic goiter and, 524, 524t
prophylaxis of, 526, *526*
excess of, hypothyroidism and, 497
inorganic, for thyrotoxicosis, 482
metabolism of, *86,* 86–87, *87*
thyroid-stimulating hormone stimulation of, 448
organification defects of, hypothyroidism and, 496
thyroid function and, 465
thyroid hormone secretion and, 448–449
thyroid hormone synthesis and, 437–438
for thyrotoxicosis, in neonates, 487
thyrotoxicosis induced by, 471–472
transport of, 438
Iodocholesterol scanning, in primary hyperaldosteronism, 828
Iodotyrosine deiodinase defect, hypothyroidism and, 496
Ion transport, blood pressure and, 785–787
Na^+,K^+-ATPase and, 785
Na^+-K^+-Cl^+ cotransport and, 786
Na^+-Na^+ countertransport and, 786
Iopanoic acid, for thyrotoxicosis, 483
Ipodate, for thyrotoxicosis, 483
Islet(s), diabetes mellitus and, 1179
Islet amyloid-associated protein (IAAP), 1179
Islet cells, 1107, *1108,* 1108t
alpha, 1107
beta, 1107
delta, 1107
glucagon synthesis in, 1146
insulin-producing tumors of:
clinical characteristics of, 1258–1259
diagnosis of, 1259–1260, *1260*
fasting hypoglycemia and, 1258–1261
treatment of, 1260–1261
transplantation of, for diabetes mellitus, 1217–1218
Isocaproic acid, 989
Isochromosomes, 1058
Isocitrate dehydrogenase, 1116
Isomerase, cholesterol synthesis and, 567–568

Jejunoileal bypass, for obesity, 1302

Kallikreins
hypertension and, 780–781
mineralocorticoids and, 613
Kallman's syndrome, 266, 920–923, *920–925,* 925
hypothalamus and, 261
Kaposi's sarcoma, glucocorticoid therapy and, 874
Karyotype, 1054
Keratitis, glucocorticoids and, 607
Ketoacidosis, diabetic. *See* Diabetic ketoacidosis (DKA)
Ketoconazole (Nizoral):
for Cushing's disease, 362, 676
for ectopic ACTH syndrome, 676
steroid synthesis inhibition by, 586
Ketogenesis, 1121–1123, *1124, 1125*
Ketone(s), utilization of, 1121–1123, *1124, 1125*
17-Ketosteroid(s), assays for, 617–618, 1667t
17-Ketosteroid reductase (17-KSR), 571
estrogenic, 571
Kidneys. *See also* Renal *entries*
diabetes mellitus and, 1180, *1181*
parathyroid hormone and, 1426–1427, *1427*
phosphate excretion by, 1493
phosphate handling in, *1490,* 1490–1492, *1491*
primary hyperparathyroidism and, 1457
renin in, regulation of, 756–758, *759*
vasopressin and. *See* Diabetes insipidus, nephrogenic
vitamin D and, 1448
Kinetics, of glucocorticoid action, 859
glucocorticoid withdrawal and, *874* 874–875, *875*
Kinins, hypertension and, 780–781
Kleine-Levin syndrome, 270t
Klinefelter's syndrome, 929–931, 930t, 1068–1070, *1070*
tall stature and, 1663–1664
variants of, 930
kni gene, 186
knrl gene, 186
Kyphoscoliosis, in osteomalacia, 1522

Laboratory tests, 18–20. *See also* Assays; *specific tests*
assays. *See* Assays
dynamic testing, 19–20
interpretation of, 19
providing direct information, 20
of sensitivity of target cells to hormones, 20
Lactate dehydrogenase, 1113
Lactation:
nonpuerperal. *See* Galactorrhea
oxytocin and, 398
prolactin and, 309–310
thyroid hormones in milk and, 487
Lactic acidosis, diabetes mellitus and, 1224–1225
Lactogen, placental. *See* Placental lactogen
Lactotrophs, of adenohypophysis, 292
Lagophthalmia, 33
Lamellae, in bone, 1428
Large neutral amino acids (LNAAs), obesity and, 1287
Laron-type dwarfism, 309, 1648
Laryngeal hypertrophy, 26
Latex particle agglutination assays, 209
Laurence-Moon syndrome, 270t, 924–925
Lecithin, dietary, effect on plasma lipids and lipoproteins, 1374

Lecithin cholesterol acyltransferase, 1321–1322, *1322*
deficiency of, familial, 1359–1360
clinical features of, 1359–1360
diagnostic laboratory features of, 1360
genetics of, 1360
pathophysiology of, 1360
treatment of, 1360
Lenticular opacities, 32, 33
Lesch-Nyhan syndrome, uric acid stones and, 1579
Lethargy, 31
Leukemia:
acute lymphoblastic, hormone therapy for, 182–183
acute promyelocytic, 182–183
avian erythroblast, 182–183
glucocorticoid therapy for, 856–869
malignancy-associated hypercalcemia and, 1471, 1472
Leukocytes:
function of, glucocorticoids and, 602t, 602–603
movement of, glucocorticoids and, 601t, 601–602
Leukopenia, 27–28
Leuprolide, for androgen-dependent neoplasia, 954–955
Levodopa test, for growth hormone, 1666t
Leydig cell(s), 887–888, *890*. *See also* Hypothalamic-pituitary-Leydig cell axis
hypoplasia of, 1078–1079
Leydig cell tumors, 952
Libido, 29
hypopituitarism and, 326
Licorice, hypertension and, 833–834
Lid lag, thyrotoxicosis and, 474
Lid retraction, thyrotoxicosis and, 474
Liddle's syndrome, 834–835
Ligands, 4. *See also* Binding; Hormones; Receptors; Second messengers; *specific ligands*
autophosphorylation induced by, 120
interaction with antibodies, 206
origin of, *10*, 10–11
origin of mediators of, 11
steroid-hormone antagonists, 177–180
Ligand-gated ion channels. *See* Hormone receptors, ligand-gated ion channels
Light exposure, pineal and biological rhythms and, 256–257
Light-dark cycles, diurnal patterns of adrenocorticotropic hormone and cortisol and, 578
Limited joint mobility (LJM), diabetes mellitus and, 1193
Linkers, 48
Lipemia retinalis, diabetes mellitus and, 1192
Lipid(s). *See also specific types of lipids and specific lipid disorders*
anabolic steroids and, 1863
determinations of, 1392
plasma, effect of nutrients on, 1367t, 1367–1374
protein kinase C activation by, 146–147
Lipid metabolism, 1119–1123, 1315–1394. *See also specific types of lipids*
diabetes mellitus and, 1172–1174, *1173*
disorders of. *See specific disorders*
fatty acid and triglyceride synthesis and, *1119*, 1119–1120, *1120*
fatty acid mobilization and, 1120–1121
fatty acid oxidation and, 1121, *1122*, *1123*
glucocorticoids and, 599
insulin and, 1139–1140
interaction with carbohydrate metabolism, 1123–1125, 1126t
ketogenesis and ketone utilization and, 1121–1123, *1124*, *1125*
thyrotoxicosis and, 476
Lipoatrophic diabetes, 1232–1233
Lipoatrophy, partial, 1233
Lipodystrophy:
insulin, 1205
tall stature and, 1665
Lipogenesis, 1109
thyroid hormone stimulation of, 445
Lipolysis, 1121
glucocorticoids and, 599
inhibitors of, for diabetes mellitus, 1212
thyroid hormone stimulation of, 445
Lipomas, in multiple endocrine neoplasia, type 1, 1706
Lipoprotein(s) (LPH), 296–297, 1315–1320. *See also* Cholesterol
abnormal, 1318
atherogenicity of particles of, 1325t, 1325–1326
chemistry of, 295
classification of, 1316, *1316*, 1317t
composition of, 1316–1318
enzymes and transfer proteins active in, 1321–1322
high-density. *See* High-density lipoproteins (HDL)
hypothyroidism and, 502
low-density. *See* Low-density lipoprotein(s) (LDL)
metabolism of, 1322–1325
plasma, effect of nutrients on, 1367t, 1367–1374
separations of, 1392–1393
available methods for, 1393
indications for, 1392–1393
structure of, 1320, *1320*
thyroid hormone binding to, 441, 442
very low density. *See* Very low density lipoproteins (VLDL)
Lipoprotein(a), 1318
hyperlipidemia and, 1363
Lipoprotein lipase (LPL), 1120, 1322
obesity and, 1288
Lipoprotein X, 1334
β-Lipotropin, chemistry of, 295
Liquid-phase precipitation, 210
Lithium:
hypercalcemia induced by, 1476
hypothyroidism and, 497
parathyroid hormone secretion and, 1413–1414
thyroid function and, 465
for thyrotoxicosis, 483
Lithotripsy, 1568–1569
Liver. *See also* Hepatic disorders; *specific disorders*
glucose and protein metabolism in, glucocorticoids and, 600
Local osteolytic hypercalcemia, 1471
Looser zones, osteomalacia and, 1522, *1523*
Lovastatin:
for familial hypercholesterolemia, 1339–1340
for hyperlipoproteinemia, 1383–1385
indications and dosage for, 1384–1385, *1385*, 1385t
mechanism of action of, 1383, *1384*
for primary type III hyperlipoproteinemia, 1348
side effects of, 1383–1384
Low-density lipoprotein(s) (LDL), 561, 562, *562*, 1317
metabolism of, 1323–1324, *1324*
Low-density lipoprotein (LDL) receptors, steroid hormone synthesis and, 79
Low stringency screening, 183
Lungs. *See* Pulmonary disorders; Respiratory disorders
Luteinization, of ovarian interstitial cells, 994
Luteinizing hormone (LH). *See also specific testicular disorders*
action of, 300
aging and, in males, 1819–1820, *1821*
androgen synthesis and, 993
assays for, 300–301, 366, 911–912, *912*, 1666–1667
basal measurements, 366
hypopituitarism and, 322–323, *323*
stimulation tests, 366
chemistry of, 298
cirrhosis and, 273
exercise and, in women, 1853
fasting and malnutrition and, 272
glucocorticoids and, 608–609
hypopituitarism and, 318, 325–326
in men, 326
in women, 325–326
hypothalamic-pituitary-germ cell axis and. *See* Hypothalamic-pituitary-germ cell axis
hypothalamic-pituitary-Leydig cell axis and. *See* Hypothalamic-pituitary-Leydig cell axis

Luteinizing hormone (LH) (*Cont.*)
hypothyroidism and, 502, 503
luteinization and, 994
luteolysis and, 994–995
menarche and, 1004–1005
menstrual cycle and, 1008
metabolism of, 302
ovarian steroid synthesis and, 991
pituitary cells secreting, 292
pituitary level of, 301
pituitary tumors secreting, 363
plasma level of, 301, *301*
regulation of, 236–237, *237, 238,* 302t, 302–303
resistance to, hypogonadotropic hypogonadism and, 935
secretion rate of, 302
thyrotoxicosis and, 477
urine level of, 301
Luteolysis, 986, 994–995
17,20-Lyase deficiency, 639–640
Lymphocytic adrenalitis, diffuse, 645
Lymphocytosis, 28
Lymphomas. *See specific site*
malignancy-associated hypercalcemia and, 1471–1472
Lypressin (Diapid), for diabetes insipidus:
dipsogenic, 414
neurogenic, 412

McCune-Albright syndrome, 346–347
hypothalamus and, 264
McKenzie mouse bioassay, 201, *202,* 296
Macroadenomas, Cushing's disease and, 675
Macromastia, pubertal, persistent, 948
Macrophages, glucocorticoids and, 602–603
Magnesium:
hypertension and, 785
mineralocorticoids and, 613
parathyroid hormone secretion and, 1413
serum, assays for, 1497
urinary, assays for, 1497–1498
Magnesium ammonium phosphate stones, 1583–1585
bacteriology of, 1584
clinical risk factors for, 1584
evaluation of, 1584–1585
history and epidemiology of, 1583–1584
morbidity from, 1584
pathophysiology of, 1584, *1584*
terminology for, 1583
treatment of, 1585
Magnesium balance, 1494–1497, *1495, 1496*
disorders of. *See* Hypermagnesemia; Hypomagnesemia
Magnetic resonance imaging (MRI):
in Cushing's disease, 359, 673
in pituitary adenomas, *334,* 334–335
in primary hyperaldosteronism, 827
in renovascular hypertension, 808
in solitary thyroid nodules, 536
Malabsorption:
osteomalacia and, 1527–1528
rickets and, 1527–1528
Male climacteric, hypogonadotropic hypogonadism and, 933–934
Male pseudohermaphroditism:
dysgenetic, 1077
of unknown etiology, 1086
cryptorchidism and, 1086
isolated hypospadias and, 1086
multiple malformation syndromes, 1086
Malignancy. *See* Cancer; Ectopic hormone production; Tumor(s); *specific tumors and tumor types*
Malnutrition. *See also* Fasting; Protein-calorie malnutrition (PCM)
hypothalamic disorders and, 272
osteomalacia and, 1527–1528
rickets and, 1527–1528
short stature and, 1643–1644
Malnutrition stones, 1565
Malonyl CoA, 1120
Mammalian cells:
protein synthesis in, by recombinant DNA techniques, 56
ras proteins of, 118, *119*
transfer of cloned genes into, 52–53, *53*
Mammillary bodies, 226
Mammoplasty, for gynecomastia, 950
Marble bone disease, 1541–1542, *1542*
Marfan syndrome, tall stature and, 1664, 1664t
Marfanoid habitus, multiple mucosal neuromas and, 1717
Masculinization. *See* Virilization
Masses. *See* Hormone(s), ectopic production of; Tumor(s); *specific tumors and tumor types*
Mastectomy, 1801
Maternal deprivation syndrome, short stature and, 1657
Matrix effects, interference in assays caused by, 213
Matrix theory, of stone pathogenesis, 1566
Maturity-onset diabetes of young people (MODY), 1158
etiology of, 1161
insulin-dependent, etiology of, 1159–1160, *1160,* 1160t, 1161–1164, *1162*
non-insulin-dependent, etiology of, 1164
Median eminence:
hypothalamic, anatomy of, 227, 229–230, *231, 232*
neurohypophyseal, 385
Medroxyprogesterone:
for familial tall stature, 1658
for osteoporosis prophylaxis, 1538
Medroxyprogesterone acetate, for hypopituitarism, 325
Medulla, ovarian, 973
Medullary carcinoma of the thyroid (MCT). *See* Thyroid carcinoma, medullary
Mefipristone (RU-486), for Cushing's disease, 362
Megestrol acetate, for breast cancer, 1803
Meiosis, in oocyte growth, *997,* 997–998, *998*
Melanocyte stimulating hormone (MSH):
chemistry of, 295
extrapituitary, 297
neurotransmitter function of, 576
Melatonin, 255–256
binding sites for, 255–256
pineal and biological rhythms and, 256–257
substance P and, 255, *256*
Membranous ossification, 1633
Menarche:
obesity and, 272
ovarian activity and, 1004–1006, *1005*
Menopause, 1008–1009
osteoporosis following. *See* Osteoporosis
Menotropins (Pergonal), for hypopituitarism, 326
Menstrual cycle:
aldosterone during, 678–679
disorders of. *See also specific disorders*
obesity and, 1279
exercise and, 1854, 1855t, 1856
onset of, 272, 1004–1006, *1005*
ovarian activity and, 1006–1008, *1006–1008*
thyrotoxicosis and, 477
Mercaptopropionylglycine (MPG), for cystinuria, 1577
Messenger RNA. *See* mRNA
Mestranol, for Turner's syndrome, 1076
Metabolic activity, stone growth and, 1566
Metabolic bone disease, 1517–1554. *See also specific disorders*
clinical evaluation of, 1517–1521
bone biopsy in, 1519–1521
clinical chemistry in, 1517–1519
history and physical examination in, 1517
radiology and nuclear medicine in, 1519, *1520*
Metabolic factors, growth hormone secretion and, 307–309
Metabolic studies, in diabetes mellitus, 1194–1196
Metabolism. *See also* Fuel-hormone interactions; Glucagon; Insulin
of amino acids. *See* Amino acid metabolism
of arachidonic acid, 147–148, *148*
of carbohydrates. *See* Carbohydrate metabolism
catecholamines and, *721,* 721–722, 722t, 1150
disorders of:

hypothalamic disorders and, 272–274
obesity and, 1277–1279
of fats. *See* Lipid metabolism
fuel-hormone interactions and, 1152–1156
basal state and, 1153–1154
body composition and, 1152–1153, 1153t
exercise and, 1155, *1156*
fed state and, *1154,* 1154–1155, 1155t
hypoglycemia and, 1155–1156
starvation and, 1155
stress hyperglycemia and, 1156, *1157*
glucocorticoids and, 1150–1151
of glycogen, glucocorticoids and, 598–599, *599*
growth hormone and, 1151
of hormones. *See under specific hormones*
hypothyroidism and, 501–502
of inositol-phosphate, 150–151, *152*
insulin-like growth factors and, 1151t, 1151–1152
intermediary:
glucocorticoids and, 596, *597*
regulation of, 13
of lipids. *See* Lipid metabolism
of minerals, regulation of, 14
of nucleic acids, glucocorticoids and, 599–600
pancreatic polypeptide and, 1152
pheochromocytomas and, 728
of phospholipids. *See* Phospholipids, metabolism of
during pregnancy, diabetes mellitus and, 1225–1227
of protein. *See* Protein(s), metabolism of
regulatory and counterregulatory hormones and, 1152, 1153t
thyrotoxicosis and, 476
of water, regulation of, 14
Metabotropic receptor, 101
Metal deposition, hypoparathyroidism and, 1481
Metastases:
to adrenal gland, adrenocortical insufficiency and, 645
bony, hypercalcemia of malignancy and, 1747
Metformin, for diabetes mellitus, 1211–1212
Methimazole (MMI):
in breast milk, 487
for Graves' disease, 490
hypothyroidism and, 497
thyroid function and, 464–465
for thyroid storm, 486
for thyrotoxicosis, 480–482, *481*
in neonates, 487
during pregnancy, 487
Methionine-GH, for hypopituitarism, 327
3-Methoxy-4-hydroxyphenylglycol (MHPG), catecholamine synthesis and, 715
Methylprednisolone:
bioavailability of, 863
for congenital adrenal hyperplasia, 638t
Methylprednisolone sodium succinate, for septic shock, 871
α-Methyl-l-tyrosine (Demser), for pheochromocytoma, 731
Metoclopramide stimulation test, for prolactin, 369
Metopirone. *See* Metyrapone (Metopirone) stimulation test; Metyrapone (Metopirone)
Metrorrhagia, 29
Metyrapone (Metopirone):
for Cushing's disease, 362, 676
for ectopic ACTH syndrome, 676
steroid synthesis inhibition by, 586
Metyrapone (Metopirone) stimulation test, 622
for adrenocorticotropic hormone, 321, 364–365
in children, 626
in Cushing's disease, 359
overnight, 622
three-day intravenous test, 622
Microadenomas, Cushing's disease and, 675
Microalbuminuria, diabetes mellitus and, 1186
Microaneurysms, diabetes mellitus and, 1181
Microangiopathy, 1157
diabetes mellitus and, 1180, *1180*
Microdensitometer, 202
Microemulsions, 57
Microsurgery, for renovascular hypertension, 811
Midline cleft syndromes, hypothalamus and, 260, 261, 265
Midodrine, for postural hypotension, 735
Milk-alkali syndrome, 1476
Milkman fractures, osteomalacia and, 1522, *1523*
Mineral(s). *See also specific minerals*
effect on plasma lipids and lipoproteins, 1374
metabolism of, regulation of, 14
Mineralization. *See* Ossification
Mineralocorticoids, 555, 610–614
action of, 612–614
extrarenal, 613–614
molecular mechanisms of, *610,* 610–611
renal, 612–613
agonists and antagonists of, 611–612, *612*
assays for, 623
definition of, 610
excess of, hypertension and, 834
hypertension and. *See* Hypertension, mineralocorticoids and
receptors for, 610
glucocorticoid actions mediated through, 858, 858t
regulation of, 580–583
atrial natriuretic peptide and, 583
potassium ion and, 582–583
pro-opiomelanocortin peptides and, 583
renin-angiotensin system and, 581–582, *582*
sodium ion and, 583
spironolactone-unresponsive, 834–835
structure of, *171*
therapeutic uses of, for congenital adrenal hyperplasia, 637–638
Missense mutations, 44
congenital adrenal hyperplasia and:
nonclassic, 634–635
simple virilizing, 634
familial neurogenic diabetes insipidus and, 403, *404*
Mithramycin, for Paget's disease of bone, 1553–1554
Mitotane:
for adrenal carcinoma, 677
for Cushing's disease, 676
for ectopic ACTH syndrome, 676
steroid synthesis inhibition by, 586
Mixed gonadal dysgenesis, 1072–1073
Mixed-function oxidases, 987, *989*
Monoclonal antibodies:
heterophilic, interference in assays caused by, 213–214
production of, 207
Monokines, corticotropin releasing hormone and, 244
Mononeuritis multiplex, 31, 1190
Mononeuropathy, 32
Monosomy, 1054
Mood:
endogenous opiates and and exercise and, 1845
glucocorticoids and, 606
Moon facies, Cushing's syndrome and, 665
Mosaic pattern, in Paget's disease of bone, 1550
Motolin, 1686–1687
action of, 1686
clinical relevance and applications of, 1686–1687
mRNA, 38, 39
of calcitonin gene, 41
gene expression and, 43–44
gene transcription to produce, *180,* 180–181
glucocorticoid action and, 859
hormone synthesis and, of peptide hormones, 72, *74*
modification of, 40
reverse transcription of, as source of DNA for molecular cloning, 48–50
synthesis of, 69–72, *70, 73*
translation of, 41
Mucification, of granulosa cells, 1003
Müllerian ducts, persistent, 1078

Müllerian inhibiting substance, 1060–1061
Multianalyte assays, 209
Multiple endocrine adenomatosis (MEA). *See* Multiple endocrine neoplasia (MEN), type 1
Multiple endocrine deficiency, diabetes mellitus and, 1235
Multiple endocrine neoplasia (MEN), 17–18. *See also* Pheochromocytomas
  acromegaly and, 343
  primary hyperparathyroidism and, 1454, 1459–1460, 1460t
  type 1, 1703–1709
    clinical evaluation of, 1706–1707
    components of, 1703–1706, 1704t
    definition and historical background of, 1703
    epidemiology of, 1707
    management of, 1708–1709
    in other species, 1707
    pathogenesis of 1707–1708
  type 2, 1709–1717
    adrenal medullary hyperplasia and, 1715
    hyperparathyroidism and, 1716
    medullary thyroid carcinoma and. *See* Thyroid carcinoma, medullary
    multiple mucosal neuromas and, 1716–1717
    pathogenesis of, 1707–1708
    pheochromocytomas and, 1715
    treatment of, 1717
  type 2A, 546, 1709
  type 2B, 546, *547,* 1709
Multiple endocrine syndromes, 17–18
Multiple mucosal neuromas (MMN), 1716–1717
  gastrointestinal abnormalities and, 1717
  marfanoid habitus and, 1717
  treatment of, 1717
Multiple myeloma, malignancy-associated hypercalcemia and, 1471
Mumps orchitis, hypogonadotropic hypogonadism and, 933
Muscle. *See also* Musculoskeletal disorders; *specific disorders*
  glucose and protein metabolism in, glucocorticoids and, 600
Muscle biopsy, in diabetes mellitus, 1194
Musculoskeletal disorders, 30–31. *See also* Metabolic bone disease; *specific disorders*
  acromegaly and, 342
  diabetes mellitus and, 1193
  hypothyroidism and, 500
  obesity and, 1280
Mutations:
  abnormalities resulting from, 45
  ectopic hormone production and, 1742
  hypopituitarism and, 316
  missense. *See* Missense mutations
  nonsense, 44
  point, 44
Myocardial infarction, 28
Myoinositol, 1118
Myopathy, 32
  Cushing's syndrome and, iatrogenic, 861–862
  thyrotoxicosis and, 474–475
Myotonic dystrophy, hypergonadotropic hypogonadism and, 931
Myxedema:
  localized, 491, *491*
    in Graves' disease, pathogenesis of, 470
  syndrome of inappropriate antidiuretic hormone and, 416
Myxedema coma, 507

NAK1, 186
Nausea, vasopressin and, 391–393, *392*
Necrobiosis lipoidica diabeticorum, 1192, *1192*
Needle biopsy:
  of muscle, in diabetes mellitus, 1194
  of thyroid gland, 455
    in solitary thyroid nodules, *536,* 536–537, *537,* 537t
Nelson's syndrome, treatment of, 677–678
Neomycin, for hyperlipoproteinemia, 1387–1388
Neonates. *See also* Lactation; Nursing
  with abnormal genitalia, clinical approach to, 1096–1099, *1097*
  Graves' disease in, 487–488
  hypoparathyroidism in, 1482
  hypothyroidism in, 506–507
  morbidity in, diabetes mellitus during pregnancy and, 1230
Neoplastic disorders. *See* Hormone(s), ectopic production of; Tumor(s); *specific tumors and tumor types*
Neovascularization, ocular, diabetes mellitus and, 1181
Nephrectomy, for renovascular hypertension, 811
Nephrocalcinosis, 28–29, 1565
  cortical and medullary, 1565
Nephrolithiasis, 28–29, 1565–1609
  calcium phosphate stones and. *See* Calcium phosphate stones
  calcium stones and. *See* Calcium stones; Hypercalciuria; Hyperoxaluria
  classification of calculi and:
    by clinical presentation, 1565
    by crystalline structure, 1565–1566, 1567t
  clinical presentation of, 1568
  cystinuria and. *See* Cystinuria
  epidemiology of, 1565
  internist's role in evaluation and treatment of, 1568
  magnesium ammonium phosphate stones and. *See* Magnesium ammonium phosphate stones
  medical management of, 1569–1573
    discontinuation of therapy and, 1573
    evaluation phase of, 1569–1571, *1570*
    follow-up phase of, 1572
    therapy phase of, 1571–1572
  quantitation of clinical stone events in, 1566
  stone formation in, physical chemical aspects of, *1567,* 1567–1568
  surgical management of, 1568–1569
  theories of stone pathogenesis in, 1566–1567
  uric acid stones. *See* Uric acid stones
Nephrons, vasopressin and, 396, *397*
Nephropathy, diabetic, 1185–1188, *1187*
  incipient, 1186
Nephrotic syndrome:
  hypervolemic hyponatremia and, 415
  thyroid function and, 463
Neural factors:
  growth hormone secretion and, 307, *308*
  insulin secretion and, 1134–1135
Neuroblastomas, 731–732
Neurocrine peptides, 1677
Neuroendocrine disorders. *See also specific disorders*
Neuroendocrinology, 3–4, *4,* 221–275, *222*
Neuroglycopenia, 1252
Neurohypophyseal system, 221
Neurohypophysis, 230, 290, 385–423. *See also* Hypopituitarism
  anatomy of, 385, *386*
  hormones of. *See* Vasopressin (ADH; antidiuretic hormone); Oxytocin
Neurologic disorders. *See also specific disorders*
  diabetes mellitus and, 1181
  hypothyroidism and, 499–500
Neuromas, mucosal. *See* Multiple mucosal neuromas (MMN)
Neuromodulation, 222
Neuromuscular disorders, 31–32. *See also specific disorders*
  thyrotoxicosis and, 474–475
Neuron-neuron interactions, in brain, 221–223, *223*
Neuroopthalmologic studies. *See specific studies and disorders*
Neuropathy, 31–32
  diabetic, 1188–1191
    autonomic, 1190–1191
    mononeuropathy, 1190
    symmetric peripheral polyneuropathy, 1188–1190, *1189*
Neuropeptide(s). *See also specific neuropeptides*
  as neurotransmitters, 251–254
Neuropeptide Y (NPY), 254, 1687
Neurophysins, 386
Neurosecretory cells, 221
Neurotensin, 252, 1687–1688
  action of, 1688, 1688t

clinical relevance and applications of, 1688
Neurotransmitters, 3, 221, 248–254. *See also specific neurotransmitters*
amino acid, 251
anatomic pathways of, 248–250
binding of, 221–222
catecholamines as, 724–726, *726*
growth hormone secretion and, 309
metabolism of, 248, *249*
neuropeptide, 251–254
neuropharmacology of, 250–251, *251,* 251t
synthesis of, 221, 248
thyroid-stimulating hormone secretion and, 300
thyrotropin releasing hormone as, 235
Neutrophils, glucocorticoids and, 603
Niacin. *See* Nicotinic acid
NGFI-B, 186
Nicotinic acetylcholine receptor, 100, *100*
Nicotinic acid (niacin):
for familial hypercholesterolemia, 1340
for hyperlipoproteinemia, 1382–1383
indications and dosage for, 1382–1383
mechanism of action of, 1382
for primary type III hyperlipoproteinemia, 1348
side effects of, 1382
Nicotinic acid derivatives, for hyperlipoproteinemia, 1388–1389
Nifedipine, for adrenal adenomas, 831
Nitrazine paper, 1580
Nitric oxide (EDRF; endothelium-derived releasing factor):
hypertension and, 774
peptide hormone action and, *138,* 138–139
Nocturia, 28
Non-insulin-dependent diabetes mellitus (NIDDM). *See* Diabetes mellitus, non-insulin-dependent
Nonsense mutations, 44
Nonsteroidal anti-inflammatory drugs (NSAIDs):
for diabetic neuropathy, 1189
with glucocorticoid therapy, peptic ulcers and 873–874
Nontoxic goiter. *See* Goiter, nontoxic
Noonan's syndrome, 931
19-Nor-deoxycorticosterone, hypertension and, 769
Norepinephrine. *See also* Catecholamines
anatomic pathway of, 250
biological roles of, 724–726, *726*
corticotropin releasing hormone and, 244
exercise and, 1848–1849
metabolic effects of, 722, 722t
physiologic adaptation and, 724, *725,* 726
thyroid-stimulating hormone regulation by, 300
Norethindrone, for familial tall stature, 1658
Normoprolactinemic galactorrhea, 352
Northern blotting, 47
Nortriptyline, for diabetic neuropathy, 1189
Nuclear localization signal, steroid-dependent, 177
Nuclear matrix, 38
Nuclear receptors, gene regulation by. *See* Gene(s), regulation by nuclear receptors
Nucleation, stone formation and, 1568
Nucleic acids, 36
metabolism of, glucocorticoids and, 599–600
Nucleosides, 36
Nucleosomes, 37, *37,* 178
Nucleotides, 36
Nursing. *See also* Lactation
oxytocin and, 398
prolactin secretion and, 311
Nutrition. *See also* Caloric restriction; Diet; Fasting; Food intake; Malnutrition; Starvation
diabetes mellitus and, 1164
exercise and reproductive function in women and, 1855–1856
feedback loops and, 226
growth and, 1633, 1633t
in older patients, 1830t, 1830–1831, 1831t
osteoporosis and, 1537
vitamin D in, 1443–1444

Oat-cell carcinoma, of lung, ectopic ACTH syndrome and, 663
Obesity, 24–25, 1271–1303
calories and, 1372
in children, 1283
complications of, 1273–1281, 1274t, *1275*
cardiovascular, 1274–1277, *1276, 1277*
endocrine, 1279–1280
malignancy, 1279
metabolic, 1277–1279
pulmonary, 1281
skeletal, 1280
Cushing's syndrome and, 665, 669–670
definition of, 1271
diabetes mellitus and, 1164
diagnosis of, 1271–1273, 1272t, 1273t
etiology of, 1281–1290
endocrine systems and autonomic nervous system and, 1289–1290
energy expenditure and, 1283–1286, *1284*
environmental factors in, 1283, 1283t
food intake and, 1286–1289
genetic factors in, *1282,* 1282–1283, *1283*
hypertension and, insulin resistance and hyperinsulinemia correlated with, 788–789
hypogonadotropic hypogonadism and, 927
hypothalamic, *269,* 269–270, 270t
hypothalamic disorders and, 272
insulin secretion and, 1136
menarche and, 272
in older patients, 1830–1831
prevention of, 1290–1291
sympathochromaffin function and, 739
tall stature and, 1665
treatment of, 1290, 1291–1303. *See* Weight loss
Obesity hypoventilation syndrome, 1281
Obstructive sleep apnea, obesity and, 1281
Octreotide:
for acromegaly, 348–349, *349*
action of, 1679, 1680t, 1681, 1681t
for carcinoid tumors, 1695, 1695t
side effects of, 349
Ocular disorders, 32–33. *See also specific disorders*
Cushing's syndrome and, iatrogenic, *860,* 860–861, *861*
diabetes mellitus and, 1181
glucocorticoids and, 607
hypocalcemia and, 1480
primary hyperparathyroidism and, 1461, *1462*
thyrotoxicosis and, 474
Ocular pain, 32–33
Okazaki fragments, 37
Older adults. *See* Elderly persons
Olfaction, loss of, 26
Oligomenorrhea, 29
thyrotoxicosis and, 477
Oligosaccharides, peptide hormone glycosylation and, 76–77
Oligospermia. *See specific disorders*
Omega-3 fatty acids, *1370,* 1370–1371, *1371*
dietary, in single-diet treatment for hyperlipidemia, 1375
Omega-6 fatty acids, *1370,* 1370–1371, *1371*
Oncogenes, *60,* 60–61
hormone-responsive tumors and, promoters of, 1789–1790
recessive. *See* Tumor suppressor genes
Oncogenic osteomalacia. *See* Osteomalacia, oncogenic
Ontogenesis:
blocked, ectopic hormone production and, 1743–1744
steroid hormones and, 182–183
Oocyte meiotic inhibitor (OMI), 998
Oocytes, 995–998
growth of, *996,* 996–998
meiotic maturation and, *997,* 997–998, *998*
oogonia, 995–996
primordial germ cells, 995
Oogonia, 995–996
Operative vasography, 915
Ophthalmic disorders. *See* Ocular disorders; *specific disorders*

Ophthalmopathy, in Graves' disease. *See* Graves' disease, infiltrative ophthalmopathy in
Ophthalmoplegia, 33
Opiates:
  endogenous, exercise and. *See* Exercise, endogenous opiates and
  prolactin secretion and, 313
Opioid peptides:
  endogenous, 252–254, *253*
  food intake and, 1288
  functions of, 254
  receptors for, functions of, 254
Optic atrophy, pigmented, 32
Oral contraceptives, serum thyroid-binding globulin level and, 458
Oral hypoglycemic agents, 1208–1213
  biguanides, 1211–1212
  in diabetes mellitus, in older patients, 1828–1829
  investigational, 1212–1213
  sulfonylureas, 1208–1211
Orchidometer, 914
Orchiectomy, for androgen-dependent neoplasia, 953
Orchiopexy, for cryptorchidism, 947
Orchitis, mumps, hypogonadotropic hypogonadism and, 933
Oropharyngeal dysphagia, 26
Orphan receptors. *See* Steroid hormones, orphan receptors for
Orthostatic hypotension. *See* Hypotension, postural
Osmoreceptors, 387–388
  dysfunction of:
    diagnosis of, 411, 411t
    etiology of, 404, 404t
    treatment of, 414
  set point of, 401–402
Osmoregulation, vasopressin and, *388, 389,* 401–402, 420
Osmotic threshold, for thirst, 399
Ossification:
  endochondral, 1523, 1633
  hypocalcemia and, 1487
  inhibitors of, rickets and osteomalacia and, 1528
  membranous, 1633
Osteitis deformans. *See* Paget's disease of bone
Osteoarthritis, obesity and, 1280
Osteoblasts, 1428
  indexes of activity of, 1517–1518
  in osteomalacia, 1523–1524
Osteocalcin, 1633–1634
  serum:
    assays for, 1497
    as index of osteoblastic activity, 1518
Osteoclast(s), *1428,* 1428–1429
Osteoclast activating factor, 1471
Osteocytes, 1428
Osteodystrophy, renal. *See* Renal osteodystrophy
Osteoid, 1566
  accumulation in osteomalacia, 1523
Osteolysis, glucocorticoids and, 605
Osteomalacia, 30–31, 1521–1530
  bone pathology in, 1523–1524
  calcium deficiency and, 1528
  classification and pathogenesis of, 1524, 1525t
  clinical presentation of, 1521–1523
    laboratory findings, 1522–1523
    radiologic features, 1521–1522, *1522, 1523*
    signs and symptoms, 1521, *1521*
  fibrogenesis imperfecta ossium and, 1528–1529
  hypoparathyroidism and, 1528
  hypophosphatasia and, 1528
  hypophosphatemia and. *See* Hypophosphatemia
  inhibitors of calcification and, 1528
  oncogenic, 1764–1766
    clinical features and biochemical abnormalities in, 1765
    differential diagnosis of, 1766
    incidence and tumor types and, 1765
    pathophysiology of, 1765–1766
    treatment of, 1766
  systemic acidosis and, 1529
  total parenteral nutrition and, 1529
  treatment of, 1529–1530
  vitamin D abnormalities in, 1524–1526
    deficiency, 1524
    malabsorption, 1524
    metabolic, 1524–1526
    peripheral resistance to vitamin D, 1526
    renal loss, 1526
  vitamin D and, 1447
Osteopenia, 30–31, 1530–1531
  diabetes mellitus and, 1181
  in iatrogenic Cushing's syndrome, in children, 860
Osteopetrosis, 1541–1542, *1542*
Osteoporosis, 30–31, 1530–1541
  bone pathology in, 1533–1534
  calcitonin for, 1437
  classification and pathogenesis of, 1534t, 1534–1538
    aging and, 1534–1535
    alcoholism and, 1537
    chronic hypophosphatemia and, 1537
    cigarette smoking and, 1537
    Cushing's syndrome and, 1536
    diabetes mellitus and, 1537
    estrogen and testosterone deficiency and, 1535–1536
    genetic disorders and, 1537
    immobilization and, 1537
    juvenile osteoporosis and, 1537
    nutritional abnormalities and, 1537
    primary hyperparathyroidism and, 1536
    renal hypercalciuria and, 1537
    thyrotoxicosis and, 1536
    weightlessness and, 1537
  clinical presentation of, 1530–1533
    laboratory findings, 1532–1533
    radiologic features, *1531,* 1531–1532, *1532*
    signs and symptoms, 1530–1531
  Cushing's syndrome and, 667
    iatrogenic, *860,* 860–861, *861*
  obesity and, 1280
  prevention of, 1538–1540, *1539*
  treatment of, 1540–1541
Osteoporosis circumscripta, 1548, *1548*
Osteosclerosis fargilis generalista, 1541–1542, *1542*
Ouabain, hypertension and, *787,* 787–788
Ovarian arteries, 973
  spiraling of, 973–975
Ovarian failure, Addison's disease and, 1723, *1723,* 1724t
Ovarian follicles, 975–982, *976*
  atretic, *981,* 981–982
  development of, 998–1004
    atresia and, 999
    ovulation and, *1002,* 1002–1004, *1003*
    recruitment and, 998–999
    selection and, 999–1002, *1000,* 1000t, *1001*
  graafian, 979, 981, *981*
  primary, 976
  primordial, 975–976, *977, 978*
  secondary, 976–978, *978, 979*
  tertiary, 978–979, *980*
Ovaries, 973–1048
  anatomy of, 973–975
    blood vessels and, 973–975, *974*
    innervation and, 975
    morphology, 973, *974*
  cytodifferentiation of, 991–998
    of granulosa cell, 991–993
    of interstitial cells, *993,* 993–998
  defective formation of, 1076–1077
  differentiation of, 1059–1060
  follicles of. *See* Ovarian follicles
  granulosa cells of. *See* Granulosa cells
  growth factors and, 1009
  histology of, 975–987
    of antral follicles, 979, 981–982
    of corpus lutea, 985–987, *987–989*
    of interstitial cells, 982–985
    of ovarian follicles, 975, *976*
    of preantral follicles, 975–979
  hormones of. *See also specific hormones*
    adrenal hormones versus, 584
    synthesis of, 987–991
  interstitial cells of, 973, 982–985. *See also* Corpus luteum; Oocytes
    cytodifferentiation of, *993,* 993–998
    hilus cells, 985, *986*
    primary, 982, *983*
    secondary, 983, 985, *985*
    theca, 979, 982–983, *984*
  polycystic, 1004
    obesity and, 1279–1280
Overweight. *See also* Obesity
  definition of, 1271
Ovulation, follicle development and, *1002,* 1002–1004, *1003*

Oxalate, metabolism of, 1597t, 1597–1598, *1598*
Oxandrolone, for Turner's syndrome, 1075
18-Oxidase, 571
Oxygen. *See also* Hypoxia
consumption of, thyrotoxicosis and, 476
Oxytocin:
action of, 398
chemistry of, 385–386, *387*
hypopituitarism and, 319
metabolism of, 396
plasma level of, 395
regulation of, 395
extrahypophyseal pathways and, 396
synthesis of, 386–387, *388*

Pacemakers, for postural hypotension, 735
Paget's disease of bone, 1547–1554
bone pathology in, *1550,* 1550–1551, *1551*
calcitonin for, 1436
clinical presentation of, 1547–1550
laboratory findings, 1549–1550
radiologic features, 1548–1549, *1548–1550*
signs and symptoms, 1547–1548
pathogenesis of, 1551
treatment of, 1551–1554, *1552, 1554*
Pain:
abdominal, 26–27
ocular, 32–33
of thyroid gland. *See* Thyroid gland, painful
Pamidronate, for hypercalcemia, 1473
Pancreas. *See also* Diabetes mellitus
islet cells of. *See* Islet cells
tumors of, in multiple endocrine neoplasia, type 1, 1704–1705
Pancreatectomy, for insulinomas, 1708–1709
Pancreatic polypeptides (PPs), 1152, 1687
action of, 1687, 1687t
clinical relevance and applications of, 1687
Pancreatic transplantation, for diabetes mellitus, 1217–1218
Pancreatitis, acute, hypocalcemia and, 1487
Pancreoprival diabetes, 1233–1234
Panhypopituitarism, 317
hypopigmentation in, 25
Papilledema, 33
Paracrine regulation, 5, 93, *93,* 1620–1621, 1785
Paraneoplastic syndromes, 1733, 1734t. *See also* Hormone(s), ectopic production of
erythrocytosis, 1769t, 1769–1770, 1770t
Parasellar tumors, pituitary adenoma versus, 336t, 338
Parathyroid gland(s):
anatomy of, 1409
carcinoma of, surgical treatment of, 1464
embryology of, 1409–1410
extracellular calcium-sensing receptor on cells of, 1410, 1413, 1461, *1498*
hyperplasia of, acromegaly and, 343
hypothyroidism and, 503
preoperative localization of, 1463
thyrotoxicosis and, 477
Parathyroid gland hypertensinogenic factor, hypertension and, 773
Parathyroid hormone (PTH), 3, 1410–1431. *See also* Hyperparathyroidism
action of:
mechanism of, 1417–1418
postreceptor responses and, 1425–1426
receptor-effector model of, 1418–1423, *1419–1425,* 1425, 1425t
regulation of receptor number and, 1426, *1426*
structure-activity relations and, 1417–1418
assays for, 1415–1416, *1415–1417,* 1462–1463
in metabolic bone disease, 1518
biological effects of, 1416–1417
on bone, *1427–1430,* 1427–1431
renal, 1426–1427, *1427*
calcium and, 1413
catecholamines and, 1413
chemistry of, 1410, *1411*
glucocorticoids and, 605
hypercalcemia of malignancy and, 1748–1749
hypertension and, 773
magnesium and, 1413
metabolism of, 1411–1412, 1414–1415
clearance from plasma and, 1414, *1414*
heterogeneity of circulating parathyroid hormone and, 1414
origins of circulating fragments and, 1414–1415
osteoporosis and, 1532
receptors for:
distribution of, 1431
receptor-effector model and, 1418–1423, *1419–1425,* 1425, 1425t
regulation of number of, 1426, *1426*
renal phosphate handling and, 1491
secretion of, 1410, *1410*
regulation of, 1413
serum, assays for, 1497
synthesis of, 1410–1411, *1412*
regulation of, 1412
vitamin D and, 1440
Parathyroid hormone (PTH) gene, primary hyperparathyroidism and, 1454, *1454*
Parathyroid hormone (PTH)-related peptide:
hypertension and, 773
malignancy-associated hypercalcemia and, *1468,* 1468–1469, 1749–1750
Parathyroid storm, treatment of, 1467
Parathyroid surgery, 1463–1465
Parathyroidectomy, for multiple endocrine neoplasia, type 1, 1708
Parental deprivation syndrome, short stature and, 1657
P450aro, 571–572
Paroxysmal hyperthermia, hypothalamic disorders and, 271
Pars anterior, 290
Pars distalis, 290
Pars intermedia, 290
Pars nervosa, 385
Pars tuberalis, 290
Parturition:
diabetes mellitus and, 1232
oxytocin and, 398
Paternal deprivation syndrome, short stature and, 1657
P450c11, 570–571
deficiency of, 628t, 640–641
P450c17:
cholesterol synthesis and, 568–569
deficiency of, 628t, 639–640
electron transport to, 569, *569*
P450c21, 569–570
deficiency of, 628t
P450c21 gene, 21-hydroxylase deficiency and, 632–635
gene conversions and, 633, *634*
mapping in normals and congenital adrenal hyperplasia, 633
missense mutations and, 634–635
point mutations and, 633–634, 635t
structure-function inference from mutations of, 635
Pendred's syndrome, 496
Pengastrin stimulation test, in medullary carcinoma of the thyroid, 547
d-Penicillamine, for cystinuria, 1574, *1574,* 1576–1577
Pentagastrin provocative test, for calcitonin, 1712–1713
Pentamidine isethionate, hypoglycemia induced by, 1265–1266
Pentose shunt, 1117
Peptic ulcers. *See also* Multiple endocrine neoplasia (MEN), type 1
glucocorticoid therapy and, 873–874
Peptide histidine methionine (PHM), 248
Peptide hormones, 5, 69–78. *See also specific hormones*
action of, 130–157
calcium and calcium-dependent enzyme systems and, 139–147
cyclic guanosine monophosphate and, 137
guanylyl cyclase and, 137–138
nitric oxide and, *138,* 138–139
phospholipid metabolism and, *147,* 147–157
second messenger hypothesis of, 130–137

Peptide hormones (*Cont.*)
endocrine and nuerocrine, 1677
gastrointestinal. *See* Gastrointestinal hormones; *specific hormones*
medullary thyroid carcinoma and, 1714–1715
metabolism of, 78, *78*
mRNA synthesis and, 69–72, *70, 73*
receptors for, *94,* 94–99, *95,* 96t, 124–130
binding properties of, 95–96
chemical and physical properties of, 98–99
fate of hormone-receptor complex and, *126,* 127–130, *129*
hormonal activation of, 97
hormone-receptor interactions and, 96–97
receptor occupancy and activation of target cell responses and, *97,* 97–98
receptor regulation effects on cell responses and, 127
regulation in endocrine target cells, 125–126
synthesis and expression of plasma membrane receptors, 124–125
secretion of, 77, *77*
synthesis of, 72–77, *74–76*
transport of, *77,* 77–78
Peptidergic system, 885
Percutaneous transluminal angioplasty (PTA), for renovascular hypertension, 810, 811–812
Performance-enhancing drugs. *See* Anabolic steroids; Ergogenic aids
Pergonal, for hypopituitarism, 1651t
Perikarya, hypothalamic, 226
Periorbital edema, 33
Peripheral neuropathy, acromegaly and, 343
Periventricular nuclei neurons, 227, 229t
Permeability theory, of stone formation, 1599
Peroxisome proliferator-activated receptor (PPAR), 185
Pernicious anemia, 27
Persistent müllerian duct syndrome, 1078
Persistent neonatal hypoparathyroidism, 1482
Persistent pubertal macromastia, 948
Peutz-Jeghers syndrome, 952
pH:
calcium phosphate solubility and, 1581, *1582*
intracellular, regulation of, 786–787
Na^+-H^+ exchanger and, 786–787
Na^+-independent Cl^--HCO_3^- anion exchanger and, 787
urinary:
calcium stones and, 1588
dependence of cystine solubility on, 1573, *1574*
in nephrolithiasis, 1570
Phallus, 1061
Pharyngeal pituitary, 290
Phenformin, for diabetes mellitus, 1211
Phenoxybenzamine (Dibenzyline), for pheochromocytoma, 731
Phentermine, for weight loss, 1300
Phentolamine (Regitine), for pheochromocytoma, 731
Phenylethanolamine *N*-methyl transferase (PNMT), glucocorticoids and, 607
Phenytoin, thyroid function and, 465
Pheochromocytomas, 726–731
clinical manifestations of, 727–728
diabetes mellitus and, 1234
diagnosis of, 728–730, *729*
hemoglobin values in, 27
hypercalcemia and, 1475
multiple endocrine neoplasia, type 2 and, 1715
occurrence of, 1715
origin and distribution of, 727
screening for, 730
treatment of, 731
Phosphate:
intestinal absorption of, vitamin D and, 1447
metabolism of, glucocorticoids and, 605
parathyroid hormone secretion and, 1413
for primary hyperparathyroidism, 1466
Phosphate balance, 1489–1492. *See also* Hyperphosphatemia; Hypophosphatemia
intestinal absorption of phosphate and, 1489–1490
intracellular and extracellular phosphate and, 1489, *1489*
renal phosphate handling and, *1490,* 1490–1492, *1491*
Phosphoenolpyruvate carboxykinase (PEPCK), 1113, 1114–1115
Phosphoglucomutase, 1111
Phosphoinositide:
hydrolysis of, growth factors and, 155–156
phospholipase C specific for, 152, *153*
turnover of, stimulation of, 149–150, *150, 151*
Phospholipase A_2, phospholipid metabolism and, 148–149
Phospholipase C, phosphoinositide-specific, 152, *153*
Phospholipids:
metabolism of, *147,* 147–157, 1321
calcium oscillation in agonist-stimulated cells and, 153
growth factors and phosphoinositide hydrolysis and, 155–156
inositol-phosphate metabolism and, 150–151, *152*
inositol(1,4,5)-triphosphate receptor and, 153–154, *155*
inositol(1,4,5)-triphosphate-induced calcium release and, 152–153
phosphoinositide-specific phospholipase C and, 152, *153*
phospholipase A_2 and, 148–149
ryanodine receptors and, 154–155
stimulation of, 156–157
stimulation of arachidonic acid release and metabolism and, 147–148, *148*
stimulation of phosphoinositide turnover and, 149–150, *150, 151*
synthesis of, 1321
Phosphorus:
assays for, in metabolic bone disease, 1518
osteoporosis and, 1533
serum:
assays for, 1497
in rickets and osteomalacia, 1522–1523
urinary, assays for, 1497–1498
vitamin D and, 1440–1441, *1441*
Phosphorylase, 1110–1111, *1112*
Phosphorylase kinase, 1111, *1112*
Phosphorylation, of steroid hormone receptors, 176
Photocoagulation, for diabetic retinopathy, 1184, *1184*
Physical activity. *See* Exercise
Physical examination, 18
in hypertension, 794–795, 795t
in metabolic bone disease, 1517
in primary hyperaldosteronism, 822
in short stature, 1639–1640
growth curves and, 1639–1640
laboratory studies in, 1640
measurements in, 1639
radiographic studies in, 1640
of thyroid gland, 435–436, 436t
Pineal gland, 254–257
anatomy of, 244–245, *245*
hormones and neurotransmitters of, 255–256, *256*
rhythms of, 256–257
Pineal region tumors, 274
Pinealomas, hypopituitarism and, 317
Pineoblastomas, 274
Pineocytomas, 274
Pitressin, for hypopituitarism, 1651t
Pitressin tannate, for diabetes insipidus:
gestational, 414
neurogenic, 412, 413
Pituitary adenomas, 328
adrenocorticotropic hormone-secreting. *See* Cushing's disease
basophilic, 357–358
chromophobe, in multiple endocrine neoplasia, type 1, 1705
Cushing's disease and, 662–663, 664, *664,* 675
Cushing's syndrome and, 660–661, *661*
functioning, in multiple endocrine neoplasia, type 1, 1705–1706
growth hormone-secreting. *See* Acromegaly
hypothalamus and, 261

prolactin-secreting. *See* Amenorrhea-galactorrhea syndrome
Pituitary apoplexy, 330
hypopituitarism secondary to, 315, *315*
Pituitary gland, 289–293. *See also specific hypothalamic-pituitary axes*
anatomy of, 230–231
anterior. *See* Adenohypophysis
blood and nerve supply of, 289–290, *290*
disorders of. *See specific disorders*
embryology of, 290–291
glucocorticoid regulation by, 574–580, *575, 576*
adrenocorticotropic hormone actions and, 575–577
adrenocorticotropic hormone and cortisol synthesis and release and, 577–579
diurnal rhythm of cortisol and, 579–580, *580*
glucocorticoid feedback on adrenocorticotropic hormone release and, 580, *581*
gonadotropin-producing tumors of, 943
hormones of. *See also specific hormones*
feedback loops and, *224,* 224–226, 225t
regulation by hypophysiotropic hormones, 231–248, *233*
hypothalamic disease and. *See* Hypothalamic disorders, pituitary function and
hypothyroidism and, 497, 502
interactions between luteinizing hormone-Leydig cell and follicle-stimulating hormone-germ cell axes and, 910, *910*
pharyngeal, 290
posterior. *See* Neurohypophysis
rhythms of, 257, 258
structural and functional assessment of, 914
surgery of. *See* Pituitary surgery
thyroid-stimulating hormone hypersecretion by, 472–473
thyrotoxicosis and, 477
tumors of. *See* Pituitary tumors; *specific tumors*
Pituitary necrosis, hypopituitarism and, 313–315
Pituitary surgery:
diabetes insipidus and, 406
for hypopituitarism, 316
for tumors, 339–340
Pituitary tumors, 327–363. *See also specific tumors*
adrenocorticotropic hormone-secreting. *See* Cushing's disease
cerebrospinal fluid studies in, 336
classification of, 327–328
differential diagnosis of, 336t, 336–339
empty sella syndrome and, 336t, *337,* 337–338, 338t
parasellar diseases and, 336t, 338
pituitary enlargement associated with other endocrine disease and, 338–339, *339*
functioning, 327
gonadotropin-secreting, 363
growth hormone-secreting. *See* Acromegaly
hypopituitarism due to, 315
imaging of, 331–335
computed tomography, 332–333
initial studies, 331–332, *331–333*
magnetic resonance imaging, *334,* 334–335
in multiple endocrine neoplasia, type 1, 1705–1706
in Nelson's syndrome, 677
neuroophthalmologic diagnostic procedures for, *335,* 335–336
visual evoked response, 335–336
visual fields, 335, *335*
nonfunctioning, 327, 363
prolactin-secreting. *See* Amenorrhea-galactorrhea syndrome
signs and symptoms of, 328–330
endocrinologic manifestations, 329
neuroanatomic manifestations, 329–330
neuroradiologic presentation, 330, 331t
α-subunit-secreting, 363
thyroid-stimulating hormone-secreting, 363
treatment of, 339–341
choice of therapy for, 340–341
radiation therapy in, 340
surgical, 339–340
Pituitary-adrenal reserve, tests of, 620–622
rapid adrenocorticotropic hormone stimulation test, 620–622, *621*
three-day adrenocorticotropic hormone stimulation tests, 622
Placenta:
gonadotropin-releasing hormone and, 239
intrauterine growth disturbances and, 1642
thyroid hormone crossing of, 456
Placental lactogen, 303–313
chemistry of, 303
ectopic production of, 1769, 1770t
synthesis of, 304
Plasma aldosterone/renin ratio, in primary hyperaldosteronism, 825–826, *826*
Plasma binding proteins. *See also specific proteins*
functions of, 6–7
Plasma renin activity (PRA):
in hypertension, 796–797, 798t
in primary hyperaldosteronism, 824–825
in renovascular hypertension, 803–805, *804*
Plasmids:
cloning cDNA onto, 49
gene cloning and, 45–46, *46*
Plasminogen, 1003
Plicamycin (mithramycin):
for hypercalcemia, 1471, 1472, 1473
for hypercalcemic crisis, 1467
Pluriglandular endocrine insufficiency syndromes, 1717–1726, 1718t
Addison's disease and. *See* Addison's disease, pluriglandular autoimmunity with
diagnosis, complications, and surveillance for, 1724–1726
genetics of, 1726
nonautoimmune, 1726
thyroid disease and diabetes mellitus without Addison's disease and, 1724, *1724,* 1725t
Pneumocystis carinii infection:
thyroid function and, 464
thyroiditis and, 509
Poikilothermia, hypothalamic disorders and, 271
Point mutations, 44
of P450c21 gene, 633–634, 635t
Poly A tail, 40
Polyclonal antibodies, production of, 206–207
Polycystic ovary syndrome (PCO), 1004
obesity and, 1279–1280
Polydipsia:
primary:
desmopressin trial as test for, 422
etiology of, 404
hypertonic saline infusion test for, 422
pathophysiology of, 408–409
syndrome of inappropriate antidiuretic hormone and, 416
Polyglandular autoimmune syndrome (PGA), types I and II, 644
Polymerase chain reaction (PCR), *51,* 51–52
Polymorphisms, 57
Polymorphonuclear leukocytes, glucocorticoids and, 601–602
Polyneuropathy, 32
in diabetes mellitus, 31
diabetic, 31
Polyol pathway, 1117–1118, *1118*
Polyostotic fibrous dysplasia. *See* McCune-Albright syndrome
Polysomy, 1054
Polyuria, 28
fluid restriction test for, 421–422
Portal venous system, anatomy of, 885–886, *887*
Porter-Silber reaction, 617–618
Postabsorptive state, fuel homeostasis and, 1153–1154
Posterior clinoid processes, 289
Postpartum thyroiditis, 494–495
Postpartum thyrotoxicosis, 488
Postural hypotension. *See* Hypotension, postural

Postural test, in primary hyperaldosteronism, subtype differentiation and, 828–829
Potassium
  blood pressure and:
    Na^+,K^+-ATPase and, 785
    Na^+-K^+-Cl^+ cotransport and, 786
  for diabetic ketoacidosis, 1223
  hypertension and, 783–784
  metabolism of, insulin and, 1140
  mineralocorticoid regulation by, 582–583
Potassium balance. *See also* Hyperkalemia; Hypokalemia
  glucocorticoids and, 605
  mineralocorticoids and, 613
Potassium perchlorate, for thyrotoxicosis, 483
PPomas, treatment of, pharmacologic, 1681t
Prader orchidometer, 914
Prader-Labhart-Willi syndrome, 923–924
Prader-Willi syndrome, 269–270, 270t
  obesity and, 1290
Pravastatin:
  for hyperlipoproteinemia, 1383–1385
  indications and dosage for, 1384–1385, *1385,* 1385t
  mechanism of action of, 1383, *1384*
  side effects of, 1383–1384
Prazosin (Minipress), for pheochromocytoma, 731
Precipitation:
  liquid-phase, 210
  solid-phase, 210
Precocious pseudopuberty, 1661–1662
Precocious puberty. *See* Puberty, precocious
Prednisolone:
  bioavailability of, 862
  for congenital adrenal hyperplasia, 638t
  metabolism of, 863–864, *864*
Prednisone:
  alternate-day therapy using, 871
  for congenital adrenal hyperplasia, 638t
  discontinuation of, 874–875, *875*
  for hypopituitarism, 325
  for osteoporosis, in iatrogenic Cushing's syndrome, 860
  for subacute thyroiditis, 508
Pregnancy. *See also* Fetus; Intrauterine growth disturbances; Parturition; Placenta
  aldosterone during, 678–679
  diabetes insipidus during. *See* Diabetes insipidus, gestational
  diabetes mellitus and. *See* Diabetes mellitus, pregnancy and
  glucocorticoid therapy during, 873
  hyperlipidemia and, diet therapy for, 1379–1380
  hypertriglyceridemia and, 1351
  hypopituitarism and, 316
  hypothyroidism and, 503
  macroadenomas during, 355
  microadenomas during, 354
  pituitary necrosis and, 313–315
  prolactin secretion and, 311
  sporadic goiter during, 527
  thyroid function and, 455
  thyrotoxicosis during, 486–487
Pregnane, 559
Pregnenolone:
  cholesterol conversion to, 565–566
  metabolism of, 82–83
  structure of, 559, *559, 560*
  synthesis of, 80–81, *81*
Preoptic nucleus, hypothalamic, 227
Preproinsulin, 1129
Previtamin D, 84
  binding of, 85
Primary follicles, ovarian, 976
Primary pigmented nodular adrenocortical disease (PPNAD), 671–672
Primordial follicles, ovarian, 975–976, *977, 978*
Primordial germ cells (PGCs), 995
Probucol:
  for familial hypercholesterolemia, 1340
  for hyperlipoproteinemia, 1385–1386
  indications and dosage for, 1386
  mechanism of action of, 1385–1386
  side effects of, 1386
Progestational agents, for hyperlipoproteinemia, 1388
Progesterone:
  action of, 238–239
  binding of, 85
  follicle-stimulating hormone regulation by, 302
  growth hormone regulation by, 309
  luteinizing hormone regulation by, 302
  as mineralocorticoid antagonist, 612
  plasma level of, 585t
  receptors for:
    activation by dopamine, 178
    dimerization and, 176
  secretion rate of, 585t
  structure of *171*
  synthesis of, 83
Progestins:
  for endometrial cancer, 1804, 1804t
  hypertension and, 772
  receptors for, phosphorylation of, 176
  structure of, *171*
Proinsulin, 1129
  excess of, 1131
  in hypoglycemia, 1254
Prolactin (PRL), 309–313. *See also* Amenorrhea-galactorrhea syndrome; Hyperprolactinemia
  action of, 309–310
  aging and, 1817–1818
  assays for, 310, 368–369
    in amenorrhea-galactorrhea syndrome, 350–351
    basal measurements, 368
    hypopituitarism and, 324
    stimulation tests, 368–369
    suppression tests, 369
  chemistry of, 303
  exercise and, 1841–1842
    mechanisms of, 1842
    training and, 1842
  feedback loops and, 225
  follicle-stimulating hormone regulation by, 303
  hypopituitarism and, 318, 327
  hypothalamic disorders and, 267–268
  luteinizing hormone regulation by, 303
  male reproduction and, 911
  metabolism of, 311
  paraneoplastic, 1771–1772
  pituitary cells secreting, 292
  pituitary level of, 310
  pituitary tumors secreting. *See* Amenorrhea-galactorrhea syndrome
  plasma level of, 311
    in amenorrhea-galactorrhea syndrome, 350
  receptor for, 110
  regulation of, 234–235, 311–313, 312t
  rhythms of, 259
  stress and, 272
  synthesis of, 304
Prolactin (PRL) concentration test, 1667
Prolactin inhibiting factors (PIFs), 247, 311
Prolactin releasing factor (PRF), 248
Promoter, 39, 42
  synergistic transactivation by nuclear receptors and, 181
Pro-opiomelanocortin (POMC), 252–253, *253*
  glucocorticoid regulation by, 574–575, *575*
  mineralocorticoid regulation by, 583
Propranolol (Inderal):
  for pheochromocytoma, 731
  thyroid function and, 464
  for thyroid storm, 486
  for thyrotoxicosis, 483
    in neonates, 487
    thyroiditis causing, 485
Propranolol test, for growth hormone, 1666t
Proptosis, in Graves' disease, 488
Propylthiouracil (PTU):
  in breast milk, 487
  hypothyroidism and, 497
  thyroid function and, 464–465
  for thyroid storm, 486
  for thyrotoxicosis, 480–482, *481*
    in neonates, 487–488
    during pregnancy, 487
Prorenin, 754
Prostaglandins (PG):
  hypercalcemia of malignancy and, 1750–1751
  hypertension and, 780
  medullary thyroid carcinoma and, 1714

synthesis of, glucocorticoids and, 601, 604
Prostate cancer, 1805–1807
  diagnosis of, 1805
  pathology and prognosis of, 1805–1806
  risk factors for, 1805
  treatment of, 1806–1807
Protein(s):
  chaperone. *See* Heat shock proteins (hsp)
  dietary:
    in diet therapy for hyperlipidemia, 662
    effect on plasma lipids and lipoproteins, 1373–1374
    restriction of, in nephrolithiasis, 1571
  interactions with carbohydrates, diabetes mellitus and, 1172
  glycation of, 1118–1119
  glycosylation of, 1118, 1119
  metabolism of:
    diabetes mellitus and, 1171–1172
    glucocorticoids and, 599–600
    insulin and, 1139
    thyrotoxicosis and, 476
  repletion of, *1127*, 1127–1128
  synthesis of, 41
    by recombinant DNA techniques, 55–56, *56*
    thyroid hormone effects on, 445
    thyrotoxicosis and, 476
Protein kinase(s):
  cyclic adenosine monophosphate-dependent, 94, 134–137, *135*, 135t, 136t
  cyclic guanosine monophosphate-dependent, peptide hormone action and, 138
Protein kinase C (PKC):
  activation of, 146–147
  calcium as second messenger and, *143*, 143–147
  lipid activators of, 146–147
  structure and properties of, 144
  superfamily of, 144
Protein tyrosine phosphatases, 121
Protein-calorie malnutrition (PCM):
  endemic goiter and, 526
  hypothalamic disorders and, 272
  refeeding after, hypophosphatemia and, 1493–1494
Proteus infection:
  diabetes mellitus and, 1193
  magnesium ammonium phosphate stones and, 1584
P450scc, 565–566
  action of, 565
  electron transport to, *566*, 566–567
  enzymology of, 565
  genetics of, 566
  interactions with adrenodoxin and adrenodoxin reductase, 567
Pseudocryptorchidism, 944
Pseudofractures, osteomalacia and, 1522, *1523*
Pseudohermaphroditism. *See* Female pseudohermaphroditism; Male pseudohermaphroditism
Pseudohypoaldosteronism, 659
Pseudohypoparathyroidism, 1482–1487
  clinical and biochemical features of, 1482–1484, 1484t
  diagnosis of, 1487
  genetics of, 1486
  historical background of, 1482, *1483*, *1484*
  pathogenesis of, 1484–1486
    type IA, 1484–1486, *1485*
    type IB, 1486
    type IIB, 1486
  sympathochromaffin function and, 740
  test for, 1498
Pseudomonas infection:
  diabetes mellitus and, 1193
  magnesium ammonium phosphate stones and, 1584
Pseudoprolactinomas, 352
Pseudopuberty, precocious, 1661–1662
Pseudotumor cerebri, 274–275
Pseudovaginal perineoscrotal hypospadias, 1083–1084
Psychological disturbances:
  anabolic steroids and, 1863
  Cushing's syndrome and, 666–667
    iatrogenic, 859
  hypogonadotropic hypogonadism and, 926
  thyroid function and, 464
Psychosexual differentiation, 1067–1068
Psychosocial dwarfism, 1657
PTHrP. *See* Parathyroid hormone (PTH)-related peptide
Puberty. *See also* Adolescence
  adrenarche and, 584
  delayed:
    clinical approach to, 1099, *1099*
    hypogonadotropic hypogonadism and, 928
    short stature and, 1641
    treatment of, 935–936
  gonadotropin rhythms and, 258
  growth spurt of, 1631–1633, *1632*
  precocious, 29–30, 943–944, 944t
    central, 266–267
    hamartomas and, 262
    heterosexual, 1662
    pineal region tumors and, 274
    short stature and, 1652
    tall stature and, 1660t, 1660–1663
  testicular function and, 916–917, *917*, *918*
Pulmonary disorders. *See also* Respiratory disorders; *specific disorders*
  hypothyroidism and, 500–501
  obesity and, 1281
Pupillary reflexes, loss of, 33
Purine metabolism, uric acid excretion and, *1577*, 1577–1578
Pyruvate carboxylase (PC), 1113
Pyruvate dehydrogenase (PDH), 1114

Quality control, for assays, 214–215

R1881, structure of, *171*
R2956, structure of, *171*
Rab proteins, 118–119
Rac protein, 119
Radiation, thyroiditis induced by, thyrotoxicosis and, 471
Radiation therapy. *See also* Radioiodine therapy
  for breast cancer, 1801
  for Cushing's disease, 675–676
  for Graves' disease, 491
  growth hormone deficiency and, short stature and, 1649
  of head and neck, solitary thyroid nodules and, 533–534
  hypogonadotropic hypogonadism and, 932
  hypoparathyroidism following, 1481
  hypopituitarism and, 316
  hypothyroidism following, 495
  for Nelson's syndrome, 677
  for pituitary tumors, 340
  for thyroid carcinoma, anaplastic, 545
  thyroid carcinoma following, *540*, 540–541
Radioactive tracers, for immunoassays, 208
  [³H] labeling and, 208
  iodination of, 208
Radioassays, competitive protein-binding, for cortisol, 615
Radiographic contrast agents. *See also* Radioiodine scanning
  iodinated, thyroid function and, 465
Radioimmunoassays:
  for adrenocorticotropic hormone, 295, 363–364, 616–617, 617
  for cortisol, 615
  for follicle-stimulating hormone, 300
  for growth hormone, 306
  for luteinizing hormone, 300
  for prolactin, 310
  sandwich, 204
    for adrenocorticotropic hormone, 616
    for thyroid-stimulating hormone, 296
Radioiodine scanning, 454t, 454–455
  in solitary thyroid nodules, *534*, 534–535
  in thyrotoxicosis, 478
Radioiodine therapy:
  hypothyroidism following, 495
  for nontoxic goiter, 531, 532
  for thyroid carcinoma, 543
    follicular, 544–545
    papillary, 544
  thyroid carcinoma following, *540*, 540–541
  thyroiditis induced by, 508
    thyrotoxicosis and, 471
  for thyrotoxicosis, 483–484

Radioiodine therapy (*Cont.*)
Graves' disease causing, 479, 480, 480t thyroid adenoma causing, 485
toxic multinodular goiter causing, 485
Radioiodine uptake test, 454t, 454–455
in thyrotoxicosis, 478
Radioligand assays:
for follicle-stimulating hormone, 301
for luteinizing hormone, 301
Radiology, in metabolic bone disease, 1519
Radionuclide scanning:
in carcinoid tumors, 1693
in metabolic bone disease, 1519, *1520*
iodocholesterol, in primary hyperaldosteronism, 828
in pheochromocytomas, 730
renographic, in renovascular hypertension, *805,* 805–807, *806*
Radioreceptor assays:
of growth hormone, 306
of prolactin, 310
Ramus ovaricus artery, 973
Rapid adrenocorticotropic hormone stimulation test, in adrenocortical insufficiency, 653–654
ras proteins, 118, *119*
Rathke's pouch, 230, 290
Reactive hypoglycemia. *See* Hypoglycemia, reactive
Reagent(s), for immunoassays. *See* Immunoassays
Reagent excess, immunoassays and, 204
Reagent limiting, immunoassays and, 204, *204*
Receptor(s). *See also* Hormone receptors; *under specific hormones*
for extracellular calcium, on parathyroid cells, 1410, 1413, 1461, *1498*
for neurotransmitters, 221
Receptor activation, 1418
Receptor assays, 211
Receptor-effector model, parathyroid hormone and, 1418–1423, *1419–1425,* 1425, 1425t
Recombinant DNA technology, *45,* 45–61, *46*
in diagnosis of genetic disease, 57–58, *58*
DNA sequencing and, *47,* 47–48
DNA sources for molecular cloning and, 48–51
chromosomal genes as, 50–51
DNA synthesis as, 48
reverse transcription of mRNA as, 48–50
drug delivery systems based on, 57
gene therapy and, 58–60, *59*
hybridization and, 46–47, *47*
medical applications of, *60,* 60–61
medically important protein production by, 55–56, *56*
orphan receptor cloning and, 183t, 183–184
polymerase chain reaction and, *51,* 51–52
products of, 56–57
transfer of cloned genes into mammalian cells and, 52–53, *53*
transgenic animals and, 53–55, *54*
Recruitment, ovarian follicle development and, 998–999
5α-Reductase, 572
deficiency of, 1083–1084
Reference preparations, for bioassays, 201
Reflexes:
prolongation of relaxation time of, 32
pupillary, loss of, 33
Refractoriness. *See* Desensitization
Regulation, 6, *6*. *See also under specific hormones*
of cardiovascular function, 14
of development, 14
of growth, 13
of hormone levels, 7–8, *8*. *See also under specific hormones*
of hormone responsiveness, 9
hypophysiotropic hormones and, 223–224. *See also specific hormones*
of intermediary metabolism, 13
of iodine uptake, 87
of mineral metabolism, 14
regulatory networks and, 7–8, *8*
of reproductive function, 14
simple and complex, 9–10
of target cell function, by steroid hormones. *See* Steroid hormones, regulation of target cell function by
of transcription, 42–43
tropic, of hormone synthesis, 84–85
of water metabolism, 14
Reifenstein syndrome, 1085
Renal acidification tests, for uric acid stones, 1583
Renal arteriography, in renovascular hypertension, 807
Renal artery thrombosis, renovascular hypertension and, 800–801
Renal disorders. *See also specific disorders*
chronic renal failure. *See* Chronic renal failure (CRF)
Cushing's syndrome and, 667
hyperlipidemia and, 1333
hypertrophy, acromegaly and, 343
hypogonadotropic hypogonadism and, 927–928
hypothalamic disorders and, 273–274
steroid hormone metabolism and, 593
thyroid function and, 463
Renal function:
glucocorticoids and, 605
hyperaldosteronism and, 680
hypothyroidism and, 501
mineralocorticoids and, 612–613
thyrotoxicosis and, 475
Renal hypercalciuria:
osteoporosis and, 1537
treatment of, 1606
Renal osteodystrophy, 1542–1545
bond pathology in, 1543
clinical presentation of, 1542–1543
laboratory findings, 1542–1543
radiologic features, 1542
signs and symptoms, 1542
pathogenesis of, 1543
treatment of, *1544,* 1544t, 1544–1545
Renal transplantation:
for cystinuria, 1574
for diabetic nephropathy, 1188
glucocorticoids for, 870–871
hypophosphatemia and, 1494
for renal osteodystrophy, 1544
Renal tubular acidosis (RTA), uric acid stones and, 1581–1583
incomplete acidosis and, 1582–1583
pathophysiology of, 1582
treatment of, 1583
Renin, 5, 754–759. *See also* Plasma aldosterone/renin ratio; Plasma renin activity (PRA); Renin-angiotensin system
angiotensinogen and, 759
Bartter's syndrome and, 680
deficiency of, hypoaldosteronism and, 657–658
differential renal vein determinations of, in renovascular hypertension, 805
excess of, hypoaldosteronism and, 658–659
inhibitors of, 759
low-renin hypertension and, 832–835
mineralocorticoid regulation by, 581, *582*
nonrenin reninlike enzymes and, 755–756
paraneoplastic, 1772
renal, regulation of, 756–758, *759*
sources of, 754–755, *757, 758*
tumors secreting, 763, *764*
renovascular hypertension and, 801
Renin-angiotensin system, 252, 754–767, *755, 756*. *See also* Angiotensin-converting enzyme (ACE); Angiotensin
blockade of, in renovascular hypertension, *804,* 804–805
blood pressure maintenance and, 762–763
components of, 754–759. *See also* Angiotensin; Prorenin; Renin
hypertension and. *See* Hypertension, renin-angiotensin system and
mineralocorticoid regulation by, 571–582
angiotensin and, 581–582
renin and, 581, *582*
renal versus extrarenal, 762

vasopressin and, 393
Renin-angiotensin-aldosterone system, sodium excess distribution and, 679–680
Renography, radioisotope, in renovascular hypertension, *805*, 805–807, *806*
Renovascular hypertension:
diagnostic studies for, 803–808
computed tomography, 808
duplex Doppler ultrasonography, 807–808
intravenous digital subtraction angiography, 808
magnetic resonance imaging, 808
plasma renin activity determination, 803–805, *804*
radioisotope renography, *805*, 805–807, *806*
renal arteriography, 807
selection and sequencing of, 808, *809*
pathology of, 798–801, *799*, *800*, 800t
atherosclerosis and, 798–799
fibromuscular dysplasia and, 799–800
renal artery thrombosis and, 800–801
renin-secreting tumors and, 801
Takayasu's arteritis and, 800
patient evaluation for, initiation of, 802–803
renal artery lesions and, 801–802
clinical characteristics and, 801–802, 802t
renin-angiotensin system and, 763
treatment of, 808–812
medical therapy in, 808–810
revascularization in, 810, 812
surgical, 810–812
Replicons, 37–38
Reproduction:
glucocorticoids and, 608–609
regulation of, 14
Reproductive system. *See also* Follicle-stimulating hormone (FSH); Gonadotropin(s); Human chorionic gonadotropin (hCG); Luteinizing hormone (LH); Ovaries; Testes
exercise and, endogenous opiates and, 1846
exercise by women and:
body composition and nutrition and, 1855–1856
endocrinology of exercise-related reproductive dysfunction and, 1856–1857
hormone changes related to, 1853
menstrual irregularity and, 1854, 1855t, 1856
physical stress of competing and, 1855
psychological stress of competing and, 1854–1855
reproductive effects of, 1854
perinatal adaptations of reproductive endocrine system, 1066–1067
Resection, for thyroid carcinoma, 543
Reserpine, prolactin secretion and, 312
Resorptive hypercalciuria, 1592–1593, *1593*
Respiratory alkalosis, hypophosphatemia and, 1493
Respiratory disorders. *See also* Pulmonary disorders; *specific disorders*
acromegaly and, 343
thyrotoxicosis and, 475
Respiratory distress syndrome (RDS). *See also* Adult respiratory distress syndrome (ARDS)
diabetes mellitus in pregnancy and, 1229–1230
Restriction enzymes, 45, *45*
cleaving of chromosomal DNA by, 50
Restriction fragment length polymorphisms (RFLPs), in diagnosis of of genetic disease, 57–58, *58*
Retinal, biology of, 189, *189*
Retinal disorders, 33
Retinoic acid (RA), biology of, 189, *189*
Retinoic acid receptors (RARs), 189–191
binding to DNA, 172
functional significance of, 189–190
heterodimerization of, 172, 188
retinoid biology and, 189, *189*
RXR mediation of retinoid transduction and, 190–191
structure of, 190
Retinoid X receptors (RXRs), 185, 190
heterodimerization of thyroid receptors with, 188
in retinoic acid receptor and other nuclear receptor functions, 190–191
structure of, 190
Retinol. *See* Vitamin A
Retinopathy:
diabetic, 1182–1185, *1183*, *1184*
background, 1182
proliferative, 1181, 1182–1184, *1183*
transitional, 1184
Retractile testis, 944
Retroviral vectors, for gene therapy, 59, *59*
Revascularization, for renovascular hypertension, 810
results with, 812
Reverse transcription, as source of DNA for molecular cloning, 48–50
Rheumatoid factors, interference in assays caused by, 214
Rho protein, 119
Ribosomal RNA, 38–39
Ribosomes, 38–39
Ribozymes, 40
Rickets, 1521
abnormal vitamin D metabolism and, 1524–1525, 1526
bone pathology in, 1523–1524
calcium deficiency and, 1528
classification and pathogenesis of, 1524, 1525t
clinical presentation of, 1521–1523
laboratory findings, 1522–1523
radiologic features, 1521–1522, *1522*
signs and symptoms, 1521, *1521*
hypoparathyroidism and, 1528
hypophosphatasia and, 1528
hypophosphatemic:
familial X-linked, 1526–1527
sporadic, 1527
inhibition of calcification and, 1528
malnutrition and malabsorption and, 1527–1528
treatment of, 1529–1530
vitamin D deficiency, 1524
vitamin D-dependent, type II, 1526
vitamin D-resistant, 182, 1526–1527
Rifampin, thyroid function and, 465
Ring chromosomes, 1054
RNA. *See also* mRNA; rRNA; tRNA
complexation with snRNPs, 71–72
degradation of, glucocorticoids and, 599–600
function of, 38–39
hybridization of, 46–47, *47*
Northern blotting of, 47
processing of, in lower life forms, 40
structure of, 38, *38*, *39*
synthesis of, glucocorticoids and, 599–600
RNA polymerases, 39
Roux-en-Y gastric bypass, for obesity, 1302–1303
rRNA, 38–39
RU 486, structure of, *171*
Ruffled border, 1429
Rugger jersey spine, renal osteodystrophy and, 1542
Ryanodine, receptors for, 154–155

Salicylates, for subacute thyroiditis, 508
Saline infusions:
hypertonic, to differentiate between primary polydipsia and neurogenic diabetes insipidus, 422
for hypovolemic hyponatremia, 421
for syndrome of inappropriate antidiuretic hormone, 421
Saline infusion test, in primary hyperaldosteronism, subtype differentiation and, 829
Salivary cortisol measurement, 615
Salivary gland enlargement, acromegaly and, 343
Salpingoöphorectomy, for endometrial cancer, 1804
Salt balance. *See also specific electrolytes and imbalances*
vasopressin and, 399–402, *400*, *401*

Sandwich immunoradiometric assays (IRMA), 204
  for adrenocorticotropic hormone, 616
Saponins, dietary, effect on plasma lipids and lipoproteins, 1372–1373
Sarcoidosis:
  hypercalcemia and, 1474
  hypothalamic, 262–263
  pituitary adenoma versus, 336t, 338
Satiety, 1288
  hypothalamus and, 268–269
Schmidt's syndrome, 1722–1723
  diabetes mellitus and, 1235
Schmorl's nodes, osteoporosis and, 1531
Scintigraphy. *See* Radionuclide scanning
Second messenger hypothesis, 8, 130–137
  adenylyl cyclase and, structure and regulation of, 132–134, *133*
  calcium as second messenger and, 141t, 141–147
    calcium-calmodulin and enzyme activation and, 141–143, *142*
    protein kinase C and, *143,* 143–147
  cyclic adenosine monophosphate signaling system and, *131,* 131–132, *132*
  cyclic adenosine monophosphate-dependent protein kinase and, 134–137, *135,* 135t, 136t
  cyclic guanosine monophosphate-dependent protein kinase and, 138
  cyclic nucleotide phosphodiesterases and, 134
Secondary follicles, ovarian, 976–978, *978, 979*
Secretin, 1683–1684
  action of, 1683, 1683t
  clinical relevance and applications of, 1683–1684, *1684*
Seizures, 31
  hypocalcemia and, 1479
Selective sampling, 19
Self-priming effect, 895
Sella turcica, 289
  empty. *See* Empty sella syndrome
Semiconservative replication, 37
Seminal fluid analysis, 915t, 915–916
Seminiferous tubules, 888, *891*
  idiopathic failure with hyalinization, 940
Separation systems, for assays, 209–210
Sepsis, hypocalcemia and, 1487
Septic shock, glucocorticoid therapy for, 871
Serine protease inhibitor (SERPIN) family, 586
Serotonin:
  anatomic pathway of, 250
  carcinoid tumors and, 1690, *1692*
  insulin secretion and, 1135
  medullary thyroid carcinoma and, 1714
  receptors for, 102
  thyroid-stimulating hormone secretion and, 300
Serotonin receptor blockers, prolactin secretion and, 313
Serous epithelium, ovarian, 973
Sertoli cell(s), 887, 888
Sertoli-cell-only syndrome, 939–940
Sertoli cell tumors, 952
Sex:
  solitary thyroid nodules and, 533
  sporadic goiter and, 527
  thyroid function differences and, 456
Sex chromosomes, 1054–1058, *1055*
  anomalies and, 1054–1056
    aneuploidy, 1054
    with bisexual gonadal development, 1071–1072
    with dysgenic gonads, 1072–1076
    with functional testes and male phenotype, 1068–1071
    with ovaries and female phenotype, 1071
    structural anomalies, 1054, 1056
  in oogonia, 995
  properties and functions of, 1056–1058
    X chromosome, 1057–1058
    Y chromosome, *1056,* 1056–1057, *1057*
  Y chromosome, structural anomalies of, 1072
Sex hormone-binding globulin (SHBG), 85
  competitive binding assays and, 205
  hypothyroidism and, 502, 503
Sexual differentiation, 1053–1099
  genetic sex and. *See* Sex chromosomes
  genital ducts and, 1060–1061, *1061*
    female, 1060
    male, 1060–1061
  gonadal sex and, 1058–1060, *1059*
    ovarian differentiation and, 1059–1060
    testicular differentiation and, 1059
  hormonal sex and. *See* Hypothalamic-pituitary-gonadal axis, differentiation of
  urogenital sinus and external genitalia and, 1061–1062
    feminization of genitalia and, 1062, *1062*
    masculinization of genitalis and, 1062
Sexual function, 29–30
Sexuality, aging and, 1825–1827
  in females, 1827
  in males, 1825t, 1825–1827, 1826t
Shock:
  diabetic ketoacidosis and, 1223
  septic, glucocorticoid therapy for, 871
Short stature. *See* Growth deficiency
Signal recognition particle, 38
Signal recognition particle receptor, 72
Signaling, intracellular. *See* Transmembrane signal transduction
Simvastatin:
  for hyperlipoproteinemia, 1383–1385
  indications and dosage for, 1384–1385, *1385,* 1385t
  mechanism of action of, 1383, *1384*
  side effects of, 1383–1384
Sinopulmonary-infertility syndrome, 941, 942t
Sitosterolemia, 1364–1366
  chemistry, absorption, and metabolism of plant sterols and, 1365
  clinical features of, 1365
  diagnosis of, 1366
  laboratory abnormalities in, 1365–1366
  pathophysiology of, 1366
  treatment of, 1366
Skeletal dysplasias, short stature and, *1652,* 1652–1653
Skin. *See also* Cutaneous disorders
  vitamin D and, 1448
Sleep, prolactin secretion and, 311
Sleep apnea, obesity and, 1281
Sleep test, for growth hormone, 1666t
Sleep-wake cycle, 257–259, *258*
Sliding microtubule process, 891
Small nuclear ribonucleoproteins (snRNPs), RNA complexation with, 71–72
Smoking, osteoporosis and, 1537
Sodium:
  blood pressure and:
    Na^+,K^+-ATPase and, 785
    Na^+-K^+-Cl^+ cotransport and, 786
    Na^+-Na^+ countertransport and, 786
  dependence of cystine excretion on, 1574
  hyperaldosteronism and. *See* Hyperaldosteronism
  intracellular pH regulation and:
    Na^+-H^+ exchanger and, 786–787
    Na^+-independent Cl^--HCO_3^- anion exchanger and, 787
  metabolism of, insulin and, 1140
  mineralocorticoid regulation by, 583
  steroids with sodium-retaining actions and, mediation through mineralocorticoid receptors, 858, 858t
Sodium balance. *See also* Hypernatremia; Hyponatremia
  mineralocorticoids and, 612–613
  in syndrome of inappropriate antidiuretic hormone, 418
  vasopressin and, 400, 401–402
Sodium chloride, hypertension and, 781–783, *782, 783*
Sodium fluoride:
  inhibition of bone mineralization by, 1528
  for osteoporosis, 1540–1541
Sodium restriction:
  for diabetes insipidus:
    nephrogenic, 414
    neurogenic, 413
  in nephrolithiasis, 1571
Solid-phase adsorption, 210
Solid-phase precipitation, 210

Solubility product, stone formation and, 1567–1568
Solubility theory, of stone formation, 1599
Solute diuresis, vasopressin and, 396–397
Somatomammotrophs, of adenohypophysis, 293
Somatomammotropic hormones. *See* Growth hormone (GH); Placental lactogen; Prolactin (PRL)
Somatomedin, 305
Somatostatin (somatotroph release inhibiting factor; SRIF), 239–242, *240, 241,* 306, 1677–1681
  for acromegaly, 348
  action of, 235, 1677–1678, 1678t
  areas containing, 240
  clinical relevance and applications of, 1678–1679, *1679,* 1680t, 1681, 1681t
  insulin secretion and, 1135
  interaction with growth hormone releasing hormone, 241
  paraneoplastic, 1772
  receptors for, distribution of, 240–241
  regulation of, 242
  structure of, 239–240, *240*
  therapeutic uses of, 242
  thyroid-stimulating hormone regulation by, 300, 447
Somatostatinomas, in multiple endocrine neoplasia, type 1, 1705
Somatotroph(s):
  of adenohypophysis, 292
  hyperplasia of, acromegaly and, 346–347
Somatotroph release inhibiting factor. *See* Somatostatin (somatotroph release inhibiting factor; SRIF)
Somogyi phenomenon, 1204–1205
Sorbitol, 1117–1118
Sorbitol dehydrogenase, 1117
Sotos' syndrome, 1664–1665
Southern blotting, 47
Southwestern cloning, 183
Specificity, of immunoassays, 212–213, *213*
Sperm, capacitation of, 891, 909
Spermatocytes, primary and secondary, 891
Spermiogenesis, 891
Spinal cord injury, hypogonadotropic hypogonadism and, 928
Spironolactone:
  for adrenal adenomas, 831–832
  diagnostic, in primary hyperaldosteronism, 829
  hypertension unresponsive to, 834–835
  as mineralocorticoid antagonist, 612
  steroid synthesis inhibition by, 586
  stucture of, *171*
Spliceosomes, 39
Splicing mechanism, 39–40, *40*
Spondyloepiphysial dysplasia, short stature and, 1652
Spondylometaphyseal dysplasia, short stature and, 1652
Sponge theory, of ectopic hormone production, 1742
Sporadic goiter. *See* Goiter, sporadic
Squelching, 180
Staghorn calculi, 1565
Staphylococcus aureus infection:
  diabetes mellitus and, 1193
  magnesium ammonium phosphate stones and, 1584
Starvation:
  accelerated, diabetes mellitus in pregnancy and, *1225,* 1225–1226
  fuel requirements and, 1155
Stature. *See* Growth deficiency; Growth excess
Steroid hormone(s), 5, 78–86, 559–573. *See also* Androgens; Estrogens; Glucocorticoids; Mineralocorticoids; *specific hormones*
  action of, 559–560
    mechanism of, 170, 172, *172*
  antagonists of, 177–178
  binding of, 173–174, *175, 176*
  chemistry of, 559–560, *559–561,* 561t
  classes of, 169, 170t
  competitive binding assays for, 205
  free fraction of, metabolism of, 85–86
  gonadal. *See* Follicle-stimulating hormone (FSH); Gonadotropin(s); Human chorionic gonadotropin (hCG); Luteinizing hormone (LH)
    actions on genitalia, *1063,* 1063–1064
  growth hormone regulation by, 309
  hypertension and, 834
  inhibitors of, for Cushing's disease, 362
  metabolism of, 85–86, 590–593, *591*
    variations in, 592–593
  nuclear localization signal and, 177
  orphan receptors for, 183–186
    characteristics of, 183t, 183–185
    grouping of, 183t, 183–184
    homology to classical steroid receptors, 184, *184*
    physiologic roles of, 186
    physiologic roles of, 186
    properties of, 185–186
    zinc finger DNA-binding domain of, 184t, 184–185
  ovarian:
    metabolism of, 989–991
    regulation of, 991
    synthesis of, 987–989, *989,* 991
  plasma, 584–593
    binding of, 173
    inhibitors of synthesis and, 585–586
    metabolism of, 590–593, *591, 592*
    physical state and, 586–590, *587,* 588t
    quantities produced and, 584–585, 585t
  receptors for, 885. *See also* Steroid hormone supergene family
    activation by nonsteroidal entities, 178
    chaperone proteins and. *See* Heat shock proteins (hsp)
    dimerization and, 175–176, *177*
    intracellular localization of, 176–177
    oncogenesis and, 182–183
    orphan. *See* Steroid hormones, orphan receptors for
    phosphorylation of, 176
    regulation of levels and responsiveness of, 178
    structure of, 173, *174*
    synergistic transactivation by nuclear receptors and, 181
    transactivation of gene activity by, *180,* 180–181
  regulation of, 573–584, *574*
    of adrenal androgens, 583–584
    of glucocorticoids, 573–580, *575, 576, 578, 581*
    of mineralocorticoids, 580–583, *582*
  structure of, 169–170, *171,* 559, 561t
  synthesis of, 79–85, 560–584
    cholesterol and, 560–567, *562, 564, 566,* 987–988, *990*
    cholesterol side-chain cleavage and, 989, *990*
    cholesterol substrate for, *79,* 79–80
    cytochrome P450 and, 563–567, *564, 566*
    cytochrome P450 aro and, 571–572
    cytochrome P450c11 and, 570–571
    cytochrome P450c17 and, 568–570, *569*
    fetal, 573
    of gonadal hormones, 1062–1063
    3β-hydroxysteroid dehydrogenase and, 567–568
    11β-hydroxysteroid dehydrogenase and, 572–573
    intracellular cholesterol transport and, 988
    isomerase and, 568
    17-ketosteroid reductase and 17β-hydroxysteroid oxidoreductase and, 571
    pathway of, 81–84, *82–84*
    rate-controlling step in, *80,* 80–81, *81*
    5α-reductase and, 572
    regulation of, 573–580, *574–576, 578, 580–582*
    steroid sulfotransferase and sulfatase and, 572
    synthesis of, 987–991, *989*
    tropic regulation of, 84–85
  transport of, 85
Steroid hormone receptor supergene family, 169

Steroid hormone receptor supergene family (*Cont.*)
regulation of target cell function by, 169–187
genetic defects in receptor function and, 182
mechanism of gene regulation of nuclear receptors and, 178–182
mechanism of hormone action and, 169–179, 170t, *171*, *172*, 172–178
oncogenesis and, 182–183
orphan receptors and, 183–186
receptors for retinoids and, 189–191
Steroid sulfatase, 572
Steroid sulfotransferase, 572
Steroid withdrawal syndromes, 877–878
Steroidogenesis activator peptide (SAP), 563
Sterol carrier protein (SCP), 563
Sterol storage diseases, 1360–1363. *See also* Atherosclerosis
acid cholesteryl ester hydrolase deficiency, 1362–1363
xanthomas, 1362
Sticky ends, 45
Stigma, 1002, *1002*
Stilbestrol, structure of, *171*
Stimulus-secretion hypothesis, 140
Stokes shift, 209
Stress:
of athletic competition by women:
physical, 1855
psychological, 1854–1855
feedback loops and, 226
glucocorticoids and, 609–610
hyperglycemia and, 1156, *1157*, 1235
hypothalamic disorders and, 271–272
physical, cortisol rhythm and, 579
surgical:
cortisol rhythm and, 579, *580*
glucocorticoid therapy and, 873
prolactin secretion and, 313
vasopressin and, 393
Stroke, 28
Struma ovarii, thyrotoxicosis and, 472
Struvite stones. *See* Magnesium ammonium phosphate stones
Substance P (SP), 251–252, 1688
action of, 1688
clinical relevance and applications of, 1688
Substrate deficiency, fasting hypoglycemia die to, 1263
Subtle primary hyperparathyroidism, 1593t, 1593–1594
Subtraction screening, 50
Sulfate storage shunt, 899
Sulfonylureas:
clinical effects of, 1209–1210
for diabetes mellitus, 1208–1211
hypoglycemia induced by, 1265
indications for, 1211
preparations of, 1209, 1209t
toxicity of, 1210–1211
Suprachiasmatic nucleus:
hypothalamic, 227
rhythms and, 257
Supraoptic nucleus, hypothalamic, 227
Surgery. *See also* Stress, surgical; *specific operations and disorders*
hypoparathyroidism following, 1480
for hypothyroidism, 503
hypothyroidism following, 495
for obesity, 1301t, 1301–1303
pituitary. *See* Pituitary surgery
Surgical activity, stone growth and, 1566
Surgical stress:
cortisol rhythm and, 579, *580*
prolactin secretion and, 313
svp gene, 186
Sweating, excessive, 25
Swyer syndrome, 1076–1077
Sympathoadrenal symptoms, hypoglycemia and, 1252
Sympathochromaffin system, 713–743
diagnostic testing and, 740–743
catecholamine measurement and, 740–742, 741t
indirect tests of autonomic function and, 742t, 743
hormones of. *See* Catecholamines; *specific catecholamines*
organization of, 715–717
pathophysiology of, 726–740. *See also* Hypoglycemia; Hypotension, postural; Pheochromocytomas
Bartter's syndrome and, 740
diabetes mellitus and, 738–739
idiopathic edema and, 739
neuroblastomas and, 731–732
obesity and, 739
pseudohypoparathyroidism and, 740
thyroid disorders and, 739
physiology of, 714–726
Synapse, 221
Syndrome of inappropriate antidiuretic hormone (SIADH), 415
aging and, 1822
cancer and, 1758–1761
criteria and clinical features of, 1760–1761
prevalence and tumor types and, 1758–1759, 1759t
treatment of, 1761
tumor peptides and pathophysiology of of, 1759–1760
diagnosis of, 419, 420t
etiology and pathophysiology of, 416–419, *417*, 417t, *418*
treatment of, 421
Syndrome X, 1169
Synthesis. *See* Hormone(s), synthesis of; *under specific hormones*
System-based theories of aging, 1816
Systemic illness. *See also specific disorders*
cortisol rhythm and, 579–580
critical. *See* Critical illness
deficiency syndromes caused by, 15
feedback loops and, 226
glucocorticoid clearance and, 873
hypogonadotropic hypogonadism and, 926–928
hypothalamic disorders and, 272
in hypothyroidism, 503

T lymphocytes, glucocorticoids and, 602
T suppressor cells, in Graves' disease, 469
Tachycardia, 28
Tachyphylaxis, 822
Takayasu's arteritis, renovascular hypertension and, 800
Tall stature. *See* Growth excess
Tamoxifen, 182
for breast cancer, *1802*, 1802–1803
for endometrial cancer, 1804
structure of, *171*
Tangier disease, 1355–1356
clinical features of, 1356
definition of, 1355–1356
diagnostic laboratory features of, 1356
genetics of, 1356
pathophysiology of, 1356
treatment of, 1356
Target cells:
activation of responses of, *97*, 97–98
of androgens, defects in, 1083–1085
desensitization of responses of, *122*, 122–123
peptide receptors and, regulation of, 135–136
regulation by steroid hormones. *See* Steroid hormone supergene family
Target tissues, hypersensitivity of, 17
Tea, effect on plasma lipids and lipoproteins, 1374
Temperature. *See* Body temperature; Environmental factors, temperature
Teratologic malformations, of external genitalia, 1096
Teratomas, 274
Teriparatide acetate provocative test, 1498
Tertiary follicles, ovarian, 978–979, *980*
Testes, 885–955
age-dependent changes in function of, 916–917
prepuberty, 916, *916*
puberty, 916–917, *917*, *918*
anatomy of, 886–891, *888–889*
germinal epithelia and, 888–889, 891, *892–896*
interstitial cell compartment and, 887–888, *890*
seminiferous tubular compartment and, 888, *891*
Sertoli cells and, 888
biopsy of, 915, 915t
central nervous system and hypothalamic-pituitary axis and, 885–886, *886*
defective formation of, 1077–1078
differentiation of, 1059

disorders of. *See specific disorders*
hormones of. *See* Androgens; *specific hormones*
hypothalamic-pituitary-germ cell axis and. *See* Hypothalamic-pituitary-germ cell axis
hypothalamic-pituitary-Leydig cell axis and. *See* Hypothalamic-pituitary-Leydig cell axis
interactions between luteinizing hormone-Leydig cell and follicle-stimulating hormone-germ cell axes and, *910,* 910–911
retractile, 944
structural and functional assessment of, 914–916, 915t
tumors of, 952
Testicular carcinoma, 952
Testicular feminization, 1084–1085
Testicular regression syndrome, 1077–1078, 1078t
Testis toxicosis syndrome, 944
Testosterone, 585t
aging and, frailty and, 1823
amenorrhea-galactorrhea syndrome and, 350
binding of, 85
cirrhosis and, 273
deficiency, osteoporosis and, 1535–1536
exercise-associated testosterone release and, 1850–1851
for familial tall stature, 1658
follicle-stimulating hormone regulation by, 303
genital duct differentiation in male and, 1061
glucocorticoids and, 608
for hypopituitarism, 326
hypothalamic-pituitary-germ cell axis and. *See* Hypothalamic-pituitary-germ cell axis
hypothalamic-pituitary-Leydig cell axis and. *See* Hypothalamic-pituitary-Leydig cell axis
long-term-activity-associated suppression of, 1853
luteinizing hormone regulation by, 303
metabolism of, 86
plasma level of, 585t
structure of, *171*
synthesis of, 83, 614
inborn errors of, 1079–1083, *1080*
therapeutic uses of:
for hypogonadism, 935, 936, 937, *937*
for hypopituitarism, 1651t
Testosterone-estradiol-binding globulin (TeBG), 589–590
Tetany:
hypocalcemia and, 1478–1479, *1479*
treatment of, 1487
Thalassemia major, growth hormone deficiency and, short stature and, 1649
Theca interstitial cells, 979
Theca lutein cells, 986, *989*
Thermogenesis:
hypoglycemia and, 1252–1253
thyroid hormone stimulation of, 444
Thiazide diuretics. *See* Diuretics, thiazide
Thirst. *See also* Polydipsia
osmotic threshold for, 399
vasopressin and, 398–399
Thrombocytes, glucocorticoids and, 603
Thromboxane A_2, hypertension and, 780
Thyroglobulin, 87
assays for, in thyroid carcinoma follow-up, 546
metabolism of, thyroid-stimulating hormone stimulation of, 448
secretion of, thyroid-stimulating hormone stimulation of, 448
serum concentration of, 453
synthesis of, 438–439, *439*
defects of, 496
Thyroid acropachy, 491–492
Graves' disease and, pathogenesis of, 470
Thyroid adenomas:
in multiple endocrine neoplasia, type 1, 1706
thyrotoxicosis and, 474
treatment of, 485
toxic. *See* Goiter, toxic uninodular
Thyroid carcinoma, 539–549
anaplastic, 542, *543*
treatment of, 545
classification of, 539, 539t, 540t
effects of radiation on development of, *540,* 540–541
endemic goiter and, 525
evaluation of, 543
factors predisposing to, 533–534
age as, 533
gender as, 533
previous irradiation of head and neck as, 533–534
follicular, 539, 542, *542*
treatment of, 544–545
follow-up for, 545–546
general, 545–546
thyroglobulin determinations in, 546
incidence of, 539–540
medullary, 546–549, 1709–1715, 1710t
clinical course of, 547, *548*
diagnosis of, 547–548, *548*
embryology of, 1710
natural history of, 546–547, *547,* 1711
occurrence of, 1711
pathology of, 1710–1711
secretory products of, 1711–1715
treatment of, 549
in multinodular goiter, risk of, 530–531
natural history of, 541–542
papillary, 539, *541,* 541–542
treatment of, 543t, 543–544, *544*
thyrotoxicosis and, 472
treatment of, 543–545
for anaplastic carcinoma, 545
for follicular carcinoma, 544–545
for medullary carcinoma, 549
for papillary carcinoma, 543t, 543–544, *544*
undifferentiated, 539
Thyroid function tests, 450t, 450–455
antithyroglobulin antibodies, 454
antithyroid peroxidase antibodies, 453–454
free thyroxine index, 451–453, *452*
needle biopsy, 455
radionuclide tests, 454–455, 463t
serum free thyroxine concentrations, 453
serum reverse triiodothyronine concentrations, 453
serum thyroglobulin concentrations, 453
serum thyroid-stimulating hormone concentrations, 450–451, *451*
serum thyroxine concentrations, 451, 452t
serum triiodothyronine concentrations, 453
of thyroid hormone action in tissue, 455
thyroid hormone-binding capacity, 451–453, *452*
thyrotropin releasing hormone stimulation tests, 454
ultrasonography, 455
Thyroid gland, 435–509
adenoma of. *See* Thyroid adenomas
anatomy of, 435–436, *436*
physical examination and, 435–436, 436t
biopsy of, in solitary thyroid nodules, *536,* 536–537, *537,* 537t
caloric restriction and, 463
carcinoma of. *See* Thyroid carcinoma
disorders of. *See also specific disorders*
sympathochromaffin function and, 739
drug effects on, 464–465
dysgenesis of, hypothyroidism and, 495
fasting and, 463
histology of, 436
hormones of. *See* Thyroid hormones; Thyroxine (T_4); Triiodothyronine (T_3)
human immunodeficiency virus infection and, 463–464
hypothyroidism and, 499
liver disease and, 463
nodules of. *See* Thyroid nodules
nonthyroidal illness and, 459–463, *460,* 460t
decreased extrathyroidal triiodothyronine production in, 461

Thyroid gland (*Cont.*)
decreased serum thyroxine concentrations and, 461–462
increased serum thyroxine concentrations and, 462–463
painful, 507–509
hemorrhage in thyroid nodule and, 508
radiation thyroiditis and, 508
in subacute thyroiditis, 508
suppurative thyroiditis and, 508–509
physiologic variables affecting function of, 455–457
aging, 456
daily variations, 455, *455*
environmental, 456–457
fetal, 455–456
in infants and children, 456
pregnancy, 455
sex, 456
psychiatric disease and, 464
renal disease and, 463
testing of. *See* Thyroid function tests; *specific tests*
thyroid-stimulating hormone stimulation of, 522–524, *523*
thyrotoxicosis and, 474
Thyroid hormone(s), 86–89. *See also* Thyroxine (T_4); L-Thyroxine; Triiodothyronine (T_3); *specific thyroid diseases*
action of, 443–445
on carbohydrate metabolism, 445
interactions with catecholamines and, 445
on lipolysis and lipogenesis, 445
peripheral, drugs ameliorating, 483
on protein synthesis, 445
thermogenic, 444
tissue responses and, 444
triiodothyronine nuclear receptors and, *443,* 443–444
binding of, 442–443, *443,* 457t, 457–459
decreased, 458–459
increased, 457–458
cellular hormone entry and, 442–443, *443*
chemistry of, 436, *437*
exercise and, 1842–1843
acute responses to, 1842
training and, 1842–1843
free, commercial assays for, 205–206, 206t
glucocorticoids and, 608
growth and, 1631
hypertension and, 772
metabolism of, 88–89, *440,* 440t, 440–441, *441*
prolactin regulation by, 312
receptors for, 187–189, *443,* 443–444
binding to DNA, 172
as dominant repressors, 188
functional significance of forms and subtypes of, 188
heterodimers with, 188
mechanism of action of, 187
resistance to thyroid hormone and, 188–189
structure of, 187–188
regulation of, *445,* 445–450
of extrathyroidal triiodothyronine production, *449,* 449t, 449–450
iodide regulation of secretion and, 448–449
thyroid hormone regulation of thyroid-stimulating hormone secretion and, *446,* 446–447
by thyroid-stimulating hormone, 445–446
thyrotropin releasing hormone and, 447, 448
resistance to, 498
serum binding proteins and, *441,* 441–442
albumin, 442
lipoproteins, 442
thyroid-binding globulin, 442
transthyretin, 442, 442t
serum concentration of, in hypothyroidism, 503–504
suppression of, in solitary thyroid nodules, 538
synthesis of, 86–88, 436–441, *438, 440,* 440t, *441*
antithyroid agents and, 497
colloid endocytosis and hormone release and, 439, *439*
congenital defects in, 496
defects in, *528,* 528–529
extrathyroid, 439–440
iodine deficiency and, 496–497
iodine economy and, 437–438
iodine excess and, 497
iodine metabolism and, *86,* 86–87, *87*
iodine transport and, 438
pathway of, 87–88, *88*
thyroglobulin synthesis and, 438–439, *439*
tyrosyl iodination and coupling and, 438
therapeutic use of. *See also* L-Thyroxine
for nontoxic goiter, 531–532, 532t
for solitary thyroid nodules, 538
for thyroid carcinoma, papillary, 544, *544*
thyrotoxicosis induced by, 471
transport of, 88
Thyroid hormone-binding ratio (THBR), 451–453, *452*
Thyroid hormone response elements (TREs), negative, 181
Thyroid lobectomy:
for solitary thyroid nodules, 538–539
for thyroid carcinoma, papillary, 543t, 543–544
Thyroid lymphoma, 545
Thyroid nodules:
hemorrhage in, 508
solitary, 533–539
factors predisposing to carcinoma and, 533–534
laboratory diagnosis of, 534–537
management of, *537,* 537–539
physical characteristics of, 534
Thyroid storm, 485–486
Thyroid-binding globulin (TBG), 88
increased serum level of, 457–458
thyroid hormone binding to, 441, 442
Thyroid-binding prealbumin (TBPA), 88
Thyroidectomy:
for Graves' disease, 490
subtotal:
hypothyroidism following, 495
during pregnancy, 487
for thyroid carcinoma, 543–544
for thyrotoxicosis, 484–485, 487
total, for thyroid carcinoma, 544, 545
Thyroiditis:
autoimmune:
hypothyroidism and, 493t, 493–495, *494*
natural history of, 494
risk factors for, 494
painless (silent), thyrotoxicosis and, 471
primary thyroid failure due to, 224
radiation-induced, thyrotoxicosis and, 471
Schmidt's syndrome and, 1722–1723
subacute, 508
thyrotoxicosis and, 471
thyrotoxicosis and, 470–471, 474
treatment of, 485
without Addison's disease, 1724, *1724,* 1725t
Thyroid-stimulating antibodies (TSab):
in Graves' disease, 467–468, 469, 470
thyroid-stimulating antibodies crossing of, 487
thyrotoxicosis and, 478
transplacental passage of, 487
Thyroid-stimulating hormone (TSH), 298–303
action of, 298
mechanism of, 448
assays for, 296, 298, 322, *322,* 365–366
basal measurements, 365
biological, 201, 202, *202,* 203
hypopituitarism and, 322, *322*
stimulation tests, 365–366
chemistry of, 298
excess of, 472–473
pituitary hypersecretion and, 472–473
trophoblastic tumors and, 473
exercise and, 1842–1843
acute responses to, 1842
training and, 1842–1843
feedback loops and, 224
goiter and, 522–524, *523*
hypopituitarism and, 318, 325

hypothalamic disorders and, 268
iodine uptake and, 87
metabolism of, 299
pituitary cells secreting, 292
pituitary level of, 298
pituitary tumors secreting, 363
plasma level of, 298–299
prolactin regulation by, 311
receptors for, Graves' disease and, 468–469, *469*
regulation of, 88–89, 234–235, 241–242, 299–300, 447–448
by thyrotropin releasing hormone, 447
renal failure and, 274
rhythm of, 258
secretion of, in central hypothyroidism, 497–498
serum concentration of, 450–451, *451*
in hypothyroidism, 503
in thyrotoxicosis, 477, 478
test for reserve of, 1667t
thyroid hormone regulation by, 445–446
thyroid hormone regulation of secretion of, *446,* 446–447
thyroid insensitivity to, hypothyroidism and, 496
Thyromegaly, acromegaly and, 343
Thyrotoxicosis, 465–492. *See also* Graves' disease
apathetic, 473
clinical manifestations of, 473t, 473–477
cardiovascular, 475
endocrine, 477
energy, nutrient, and drug metabolism and, 476
gastrointestinal, 475–476
general appearance and, 473, *474*
hematopoietic, 476
muscular, 474–475
neurologic, 474
ocular, 474
renal, 475
respiratory, 475
skin and appendages and, 473–474
thyroid, 474
differentiated from hyperthyroidism, 466
etiology of, 467t, 467–473
ectopic thyrotoxicosis and, 472
exogenous thyrotoxicosis and, 471–472
Graves' disease and, 467–470
thyroid carcinoma and, 472
thyroiditis and, 470–471
thyroid-stimulating hormone excess and, 472–473
toxic multinodular goiter and, 472
toxic uninodular goiter and, 472
laboratory diagnosis of, 477–479, *478*
radioiodine uptake and scanning and, 478
serum thyroid-stimulating hormone concentrations and, 477
serum thyroxine concentrations and, 477–478
serum triiodothyronine concentrations and, 478
thyroid-stimulating antibodies and, 478
thyrotropin releasing hormone stimulation test and, 478
masked, 473
neonatal, 487–488
osteoporosis and, 1536
pathophysiology of, *466,* 466–467
postpartum, 488
during pregnancy, 486–487
subclinical, 485
thyroid storm and, 485–486
treatment of, 479t, 479–485
antithyroid drugs in, 480–483
Graves' disease and, 479–480, 480t
radioiodine therapy in, 483–484
surgical, 484–485
thyroid adenoma and, 485
thyroiditis and, 485
toxic multinodular goiter and, 485
Thyrotrophs, of adenohypophysis, 292
Thyrotropin releasing hormone (TRH):
action of, 234–235
areas containing, 234
growth hormone and, 344
metabolism of, 234
as neurotransmitter, 235
prolactin regulation by, 311
as prolactin releasing factor, 248
regulation of, 235
structure of, 232, *233,* 234
thyroid hormone regulation by, 447
thyroid-stimulating hormone plasma level and, 298–299
Thyrotropin releasing hormone (TRH) stimulation test, 454
for prolactin, 368–369
for thyroid-stimulating hormone, 365–366
Thyroxine (T_4). *See also* Hyperthyroxinemia; Thyroid hormones; L-Thyroxine; *specific thyroid diseases*
binding of, 88
in breast milk, 487
chemistry of, 436, *437*
growth hormone regulation by, 309
secretion of, 87–88
serum concentration of, 451, 451t
free, 453
in thyrotoxicosis, 477–478
serum level of:
decreased, 461–462
increased, 462–463
structure of, 86, *86*
L-Thyroxine:
for hypopituitarism, 325, 1651t
for hypothyroidism, 504–505, 505t
in infants and children, 506–507
for nontoxic goiter, 532
for thyroid carcinoma, follicular, 545
Thyroxine-binding prealbumin (TBPA). *See* Transthyretin (TTR)
Tolazamide, for diabetes mellitus, 1209, 1209t
Tolbutamine, for diabetes mellitus, 1209, 1209t
Tongue, 26
Total hormone assays, 205–206, 206t
Total parenteral nutrition (TPN), osteomalacia and, 1529
Toxic goiter. *See* Goiter, toxic
Toxins, gonadal, hypogonadotropic hypogonadism and, 932–943
TPA response element (TRE), 43
Tracheostomy, for thyroid carcinoma, anaplastic, 545
Training. *See* Exercise
Transactivation, by nuclear receptors:
mechanism of, *180,* 180–181
synergistic, 181
Transactivation domains, 180
Transcription, *38,* 38–39, *39*
capping and, 70
glucocorticoid action and, 859
hormonal regulation of, 42–43
inhibition by nuclear receptors, 181–182
of P450scc gene, 566
rate of initiation of, regulation of, 70–71
termination of, 72
transactivation by nuclear receptors and, *180,* 180–181
Transfections, 52–53
Transfer RNA, 38, 39
Transformation, 172
Transfusions, hypocalcemia and, 1487
Transgenic animals, 53–55, *54*
chimeric, 54
Transient neonatal hypoparathyroidism, 1482
Translation, hybrid-selected, 50
Translocations, 1054
Transmembrane signal transduction, 94, 111–124
cytokine receptor signaling, 158
desensitization of target cell responses and, *122,* 122–123
G protein-coupled receptor kinases and, 123–124
G proteins and, 111–116, *112,* 113t
abnormalities of, 115–116
beta and gamma subunits and, 114–115, 115t
molecular structure of G proteins and, 114
properties of G proteins and, 113–114
guanosine triphosphate-binding proteins and, 116t, 116–119
Rab and ARF proteins, 118–119
rho and rac proteins, 119
small, *117,* 117–118
yeast and mammalian ras proteins, 118, *119*

Transmembrane signal transduction (*Cont.*)
  hormonal regulation of early response genes and, *159*, 159–161
  intrinsic receptor signaling domains and, 120–121
    ligand-induced autophosphorylation and, 120
    SH2 and SH3 domains and, 120–121
  mediators of peptide hormone action and. *See* Peptide hormones, action of to nucleus, 157–161, *158*
  protein tyrosine phosphatases and, 121
  receptor phosphorylation and hormone action and, 119–120
Transport proteins:
  definition of, 3
  steroid hormone binding to, 85
Transsphenoidal hypophysectomy, for multiple endocrine neoplasia, type 1, 1708
Transsphenoidal microsurgery:
  for Cushing's disease, 674–675
  for pituitary adenoma, 339
Transthyretin (TTR), thyroid hormone binding to, 441, 442, 458, 459
Trauma:
  amenorrhea-galactorrhea syndrome and, 352
  diabetes insipidus and, 406
  growth hormone deficiency and, short stature and, 1648
  to head. *See* Head trauma
  prolactin secretion and, 313
Tremor, thyrotoxicosis and, 474
Triamcinolone:
  bioavailability of, 863
  for congenital adrenal hyperplasia, 638t
Triamcinolone acetonide, bioavailability of, 863
Triamterene, for adrenal adenomas, 831
Tricarboxylic acid (TCA) cycle, 1116, *1117*
Triglycerides, 1119
  hypothyroidism and, 502
  metabolism of, 1321
  synthesis of, *1119*, 1119–1120, *1120*, 1321
Triiodothyronine (T_3). *See also* Thyroid hormones; *specific thyroid diseases*
  in breast milk, 487
  chemistry of, 436, *437*
  secretion of, 87–88
  serum concentration of, 453
    decreased, 461
    in thyrotoxicosis, 478
  serum reverse concentrations of, 453
  structure of, 86, *86*
  synthesis of, 187
    drugs inhibiting, 483
    extrathyroidal, regulation of, *449*, 449t, 449–450
Triiodothyronine (T_3)-resin uptake, 451–453, *452*
Trilostane (Modrastane)
  for Cushing's disease, 362
  steroid synthesis inhibition by, 586
Triple phosphate stones. *See* Magnesium ammonium phosphate stones
Trisomy, 1054
Trisomy X, 1071
tRNA, 38, 39
Trophoblastic tumors, thyroid-stimulating hormone excess and, 473
Tropic hormones, 13–14
Trousseau's sign, 1479
Tuber cinereum, 226, *227*
Tuberculosis:
  Addison's disease and, 642–643, 643t
  adrenocortical insufficiency and, 645
  in iatrogenic Cushing's syndrome, 861
Tuberculum sellae, 289
Tuberoinfundibular dopamine (TIDA) pathway, 247
Tuberoinfundibular tract, 227
Tubulin, 1129
Tumor(s). *See also* Hormone(s), ectopic production of; *specific tumors and tumor types*
  anabolic steroids and, 1864
  androgen-dependent, 952–955, *953*
    complete androgen blockade for, 954–955
    secondary endocrine treatments for, 953–954
  gonadotropin-producing, 943
  hormone-responsive. *See* Hormone-responsive tumors
  insulin-producing:
    islet-cell. *See* Islet cells, insulin-producing tumors of
    non-islet-cell, fasting hypoglycemia and, 1261–1262
  obesity and, 1279
  renin-secreting, 763, *764*
    renovascular hypertension and, 801
Tumor markers, hormones as, 1745t, 1745–1747, 1746t
Tumor suppressor genes:
  hormone-responsive tumors and, 1789–1790
  identification of, 61
Tumorigenesis, 1785
Tunica albuginea:
  ovarian, 973
  testicular, 887
Tunica vaginalis, 887
Turner's syndrome, *1073*, 1073–1076
  diagnosis and treatment of, 1075–1076, *1076*
  male. *See* Noonan's syndrome
  phenotype-karyotype correlations in, 1074–1075
  short stature and, 1653, *1655*, 1655–1657, *1656*
Thyphoid fever, glucocorticoid therapy for, 871
Tyrosyl iodination, 438
Ulcers:
  neuropathic, diabetes mellitus and, 1188, 1191–1192
  peptic. *See also* Multiple endocrine neoplasia (MEN), type 1
    glucocorticoid therapy and, 873–874
Ultradian rhythms, 257
Ultrasonography:
  in solitary thyroid nodules, 535, *535*
  of thyroid gland, 455
  in uric acid stones, 1580
3′-Untranslated region, 41
5′-Untranslated region, 41
Uptake, 8
Ureaplasma urealyticum infection, male infertility and, 941
Urease inhibitors, for magnesium ammonium phosphate stones, 1585
Uremia, glucose intolerance and, 1235
Uric acid stones, 1577–1581
  allopurinol effects on uric acid and, 1579, *1579*, *1580*
  differentiating from other purine-related stones, 1579
  disorders associated with, 1579
  effect of diet on urinary pH and uric acid excretion and, 1578
  epidemiology of, 1577
  evaluation of, 1580
  gout and, 1578t, 1578–1579
  medical treatment of, efficacy of, 1580
  purine metabolism and uric acid excretion and, *1577*, 1577–1578
  risk factors for, 1578
  treatment of, 1580–1581
    allopurinol in, 1581
    correction of aciduria and, 1580
  uric acid solubility in urine and, 1578, *1578*
Urinary frequency, 28
Urinary tract, 28–29
  diabetes mellitus and, 1190
Urine:
  alkalinization of, for cystinuria, 1576, 1576t
  collection of sample for testing, 1580
  concentration of, vasopressin and, 396–397
  crystallization of, citrate and, 1602
  flow of, vasopressin and, 396–397
  low volume of, calcium stones and, 1588
  measuring acidity of, 1580
  output of, vasopressin and, 401, *401*
  uric acid solubility in, 1578, *1578*
Urogenital sinus, differentiation of, 1061–1062
Urolithiasis. *See* Nephrolithiasis
usp gene, 186
Uterus, oxytocin and, 396–397

Vaccines, production by recombinant DNA techniques, 56
Vanillylmandelic acid (VMA):
  assays for, 728

catecholamine synthesis and, 715
in neuroblastomas, 732
in pheochromocytomas, 728
Varicocele, 914, 940–941
Vasoactive agents, glucocorticoids and, 601
Vasoactive intestinal polypeptide (VIP), 251, 1684–1685
action of, 1684, 1685t
clinical relevance and applications of, 1684–1685
paraneoplastic, 1772
prolactin secretion and, 311
Vasography, operative, 915
Vasopressin (ADH; antidiuretic hormone):
action of, 396–398, *397*
aging and, 1821–1822
assays for:
in hyperfunction, 422
in hypofunction, 422
in syndrome of inappropriate antidiuretic hormone, 416–418, *418*
chemistry of, 385–386, *387*
deficiency of, 402–414. *See also* Diabetes insipidus; Enuresis, nocturnal; Osmoreceptors, dysfunction of; Polydipsia, primary
diagnosis of, 409–412
etiology of, 402–405
idiopathic, 403
pathophysiology of, 405–409
tests for, 421–422
treatment of, 412–414
exercise and training and, 1846–1847
following pituitary surgery, 340
glucocorticoid regulation by, 573–574
hypersecretion of, 415–421. *See also* Syndrome of inappropriate antidiuretic hormone (SIADH); Hyponatremia
diagnosis of, 419, 420t
etiology of, 415–419
pathophysiology of, 415–419
tests for, 422–423
treatment of, 420–421
hypertension and, 772
hypopituitarism and, 318–319
hypothalamic disorders and, 268
interaction with corticotropin releasing hormone, 243, *244*
metabolism of, 395–396
plasma level of, 395
regulation of, 387–395
emetic factors in, 391–393, *392*
extrahypophyseal pathways and, 396
glucopenic factors in, 393
hemodynamic factors in, *390,* 390–391, 391t, *392*
hypercapnia and, 393–394
hypoxia and, 393–394
oropharyngeal factors in, 390
osmotic factors in, 387–390, *388, 389*
pharmacologic factors in, 394t, 394–395
renin-angiotensin system and, 393
stress and, 393
temperature and, 393
salt and water balance and, 399–402, *400, 401*
synthesis of, 386–387, *388*
thirst and, 398–399
Vasopressin (ADH; antidiuretic hormone) tests, 1667t
Vasotocin, 256
Venous catheterization, calcitonin measurement and, 1713
Ventromedial nucleus (VMN), food intake and, 268–269
v-*erbA* gene, 182–183
genes homologous to, 185
thyroid hormone receptorα homology with, 187
Very low density lipoproteins (VLDL), 1317
metabolism of, 1323, *1323*
Vesicle assays, 209
VIPomas, 1685, 1687
hypercalcemia and, 1475
in multiple endocrine neoplasia, type 1, 1705
treatment of, pharmacologic, 1680t, 1681t
Virilization, 29
during childhood or adolescence, clinical approach to, *1098,* 1099
congenital adrenal hyperplasia and. *See* Congenital adrenal hyperplasia (CAH)
Cushing's syndrome and, 666
genital, 1062, *1062*
defective, 1078–1086
exogenous sex steroids causing defects in, 1085–1086
of genetic female. *See* Female pseudohermaphroditism
prenatal, by environmental hormones, 1096
Virilizing adrenal hyperplasia. *See* 21β-Hydroxylase deficiency
Visual evoked response, in pituitary adenomas, 335–336
Visual fields, in pituitary adenomas, 335, *335*
Visual impairment, 32
Vitamin(s), effect on plasma lipids and lipoproteins, 1374
Vitamin A:
biology of, 189, *189*
hypercalcemia induced by, 1476
Vitamin D, 1437–1449. *See also* 1,25-Dihydroxyvitamin D
absorption of, 1438–1439
action of:
adaptation to calcium intake and, 1446–1447
on bone, 1447–1448
cellular basis of, 1444–1445
cutaneous, 1448
on immune system, 1448
intestinal absorption of phosphate and, 1447
on intestine, *1445,* 1445–1446, *1446*
renal, 1448
tissue-specific analogues and, 1448
activation of, *1439,* 1439–1442, 1440t
aging and, frailty and, 1823–1825, *1824*
assays for, 1448–1449
chemistry of, 1437–1438, *1438*
circulating and extrarenal, 1442
deficiency of, 1441
dietary, 1443–1444
excess of, 1441
hypercalcemia induced by, 1475–1476
hypertension and, 773
hypothyroidism and, 503
metabolism of, 1443, *1444*
osteomalacia and. *See* Osteomalacia
for osteoporosis, in iatrogenic Cushing's syndrome, 861
parathyroid hormone and, 1440
phosphorus and, 1440–1441, *1441*
regulation of:
calcium and, 1441–1442
estrogens and, 1442
integrated control and, 1442
renal phosphate handling and, 1492
resistance to, 182
rickets and. *See* Rickets
serum, in rickets and osteomalacia, 1523
synthesis of, 1437
therapeutic uses of, for hypocalcemia, 1488–1489
thyrotoxicosis and, 477
transport of, 1443
Vitamin D_2
binding of, 85
synthesis of, 83, *84*
therapeutic uses of, for rickets and osteomalacia, 1529–1530
transport of, 83
Vitamin D_3 (cholecalciferol):
metabolism of, 83–84
synthesis of, 83, *84*
transport of, 83
Vitamin D binding-globulin (DBG), 85
Vitiligo, 1724
in Addison's disease, 648
Vitrectomy, for diabetic retinopathy, 5879
Voice, 26

Water:
excretion of, glucocorticoids and, 604–605
extrarenal loss of, vasopressin and, 398, 401, *401*
intake of, vasopressin and, 390
metabolism of, regulation of, 14
retention of, mineralocorticoids and, 613

Water balance, vasopressin and, 399–402, *400, 401*
Water diuresis, vasopressin and, 396–397, *397*
Water load test, for vasopressin deficiency, 422–423, *423*
Weakness, 24, 32
  Cushing's syndrome and, 667
  of eye muscles, 33
  thyrotoxicosis and, 474, 475
Weight gain, 24–25
  acromegaly and, 343
  hypopituitarism and, 317
Weight loss, 24
  behavioral modification and, 1294
  diet and, 1294–1299
  drugs and, 1299–1301
  exercise and, 1291–1294, 1292t, *1293*
  fad diets and, 1299
  hypopituitarism and, 317
  in older patients, 1830, 1830t, 1831t
  surgery for, 1301t, 1301–1303
Weightlessness, osteoporosis and, 1537
Wermer's syndrome. *See* Multiple endocrine neoplasia (MEN), type 1
Whole-brain irradiation, hypothalamic dysfunction and, 264
Withdrawal, of corticosteroids. *See* Glucocorticoids, withdrawal of, suppression of hypothalamic-pituitary-adrenal axis and
Wolff-Chaikoff effect, 87
Wolfram syndrome, 403
Wolman disease, 1362–1363
Women. *See also* Menstrual cycle; Pregnancy; Sexual differentiation
  hyperlipoproteinemia in, surgical treatment of, 1390–1391
Work. *See* Exercise
WR-2721, for primary hyperparathyroidism, 1466–1467

XR2C gene, 186
X chromosomes
  in oogonia, 995
  properties and functions of, 1057–1058
Xanthomas, 1362
  eruptive, diabetes mellitus and, 1192
  planar, high-density lipoproteins deficiency with, 1354
Xanthomatosis, 1364–1366
  cerebrotendinous, 1363–1364
  chemistry, absorption, and metabolism of plant sterols and, 1365
  clinical features of, 1365
  diagnosis of, 1366
  laboratory abnormalities in, 1365–1366
  pathophysiology of, 1366
  treatment of, 1366
XX gonadal dysgenesis, 1071, 1076–1077
XXY syndrome. *See* Klinefelter's syndrome
XYY syndrome, 931, 1070–1071
  tall stature and, 1663

Y chromosome, properties and functions of, *1056,* 1056–1057, *1057*
Yeasts:
  cloning of genes into, 50–51
  protein synthesis in, by recombinant DNA techniques, 55–56
  ras proteins of, 118, *119*
Yellow exudates, diabetes mellitus and, 1181
Yersinia enterocolitica, Graves' disease and, 468
Young's syndrome, 941, 942t

Zeitgeiber, 257
Zimmerman reaction, 618
Zinc finger structure, of DNA-binding domain:
  of steroid hormone receptors, 179
  of thyroid hormone receptors, 187
Zollinger-Ellison syndrome, 1682, 1683. *See also* Gastrinomas; Multiple endocrine neoplasia (MEN), type 1
Zona fasciculata, 557–558, *558*
Zona glomerulosa, 557, 558
  cytochrome P450 of, 81
Zona reticularis, 557, 558
Zonal theory, of adrenarche, 1632

ISBN 0-07-020448-9